W9-BWF-570

Contents in Brief

UNIT 1 Basic Concepts in Nursing   2

1 Health Care Delivery and Evidence-Based Nursing Practice   4
2 Community-Based Nursing Practice   18
3 Critical Thinking, Ethical Decision Making, and the Nursing Process   27
4 Health Education and Health Promotion   48
5 Adult Health and Nutritional Assessment   62

UNIT 2 Biophysical and Psychosocial Concepts in Nursing Practice   82

6 Individual and Family Homeostasis, Stress, and Adaptation   84
7 Overview of Transcultural Nursing   102
8 Overview of Genetics and Genomics in Nursing   114
9 Chronic Illness and Disability   139
10 Principles and Practices of Rehabilitation   164
11 Health Care of the Older Adult   193

UNIT 3 Concepts and Challenges in Patient Management   222

12 Pain Management   224
13 Fluid and Electrolytes: Balance and Disturbance   251
14 Shock and Multiple Organ Dysfunction Syndrome   296
15 Management of Patients With Oncologic Disorders   324
16 End-of-Life Care   387

UNIT 4 Perioperative Concepts and Nursing Management   416

17 Preoperative Nursing Management   418
18 Intraoperative Nursing Management   436
19 Postoperative Nursing Management   456

UNIT 5 Gas Exchange and Respiratory Function   478

20 Assessment of Respiratory Function   480
21 Respiratory Care Modalities   510
22 Management of Patients With Upper Respiratory Tract Disorders   552
23 Management of Patients With Chest and Lower Respiratory Tract Disorders   583

24 Management of Patients With Chronic Pulmonary Disease   634

UNIT 6 Cardiovascular and Circulatory Function   670

25 Assessment of Cardiovascular Function   672
26 Management of Patients With Dysrhythmias and Conduction Problems   712
27 Management of Patients With Coronary Vascular Disorders   750
28 Management of Patients With Structural, Infectious, and Inflammatory Cardiac Disorders   791
29 Management of Patients With Complications From Heart Disease   818
30 Assessment and Management of Patients With Vascular Disorders and Problems of Peripheral Circulation   841
31 Assessment and Management of Patients With Hypertension   884

UNIT 7 Hematologic Function   900

32 Assessment of Hematologic Function and Treatment Modalities   902
33 Management of Patients With Nonmalignant Hematologic Disorders   925
34 Management of Patients With Hematologic Neoplasms   970

UNIT 8 Immunologic Function   1002

35 Assessment of Immune Function   1004
36 Management of Patients With Immune Deficiency Disorders   1022
37 Assessment and Management of Patients With Allergic Disorders   1057
38 Assessment and Management of Patients With Rheumatic Disorders   1082

UNIT 9 Musculoskeletal Function   1112

39 Assessment of Musculoskeletal Function   1114
40 Musculoskeletal Care Modalities   1131
41 Management of Patients With Musculoskeletal Disorders   1160
42 Management of Patients With Musculoskeletal Trauma   1185

Digestive and Gastrointestinal Function 1222

43 Assessment of Digestive and Gastrointestinal Function 1224
44 Digestive and Gastrointestinal Treatment Modalities 1243
45 Management of Patients With Oral and Esophageal Disorders 1264
46 Management of Patients With Gastric and Duodenal Disorders 1292
47 Management of Patients With Intestinal and Rectal Disorders 1311

 Metabolic and Endocrine Function 1356

48 Assessment and Management of Patients With Obesity 1358
49 Assessment and Management of Patients With Hepatic Disorders 1377
50 Assessment and Management of Patients With Biliary Disorders 1428
51 Assessment and Management of Patients With Diabetes 1456
52 Assessment and Management of Patients With Endocrine Disorders 1502

 Kidney and Urinary Tract Function 1546

53 Assessment of Kidney and Urinary Function 1548
54 Management of Patients With Kidney Disorders 1567
55 Management of Patients With Urinary Disorders 1615

 Reproductive Function 1648

56 Assessment and Management of Patients With Female Physiologic Processes 1650
57 Management of Patients With Female Reproductive Disorders 1686
58 Assessment and Management of Patients With Breast Disorders 1719

59 Assessment and Management of Patients With Male Reproductive Disorders 1752

 Integumentary Function 1788

60 Assessment of Integumentary Function 1790
61 Management of Patients With Dermatologic Disorders 1806
62 Management of Patients With Burn Injury 1845

 Sensory Function 1874

63 Assessment and Management of Patients With Eye and Vision Disorders 1876
64 Assessment and Management of Patients With Hearing and Balance Disorders 1915

 Neurologic Function 1944

65 Assessment of Neurologic Function 1946
66 Management of Patients With Neurologic Dysfunction 1972
67 Management of Patients With Cerebrovascular Disorders 2009
68 Management of Patients With Neurologic Trauma 2033
69 Management of Patients With Neurologic Infections, Autoimmune Disorders, and Neuropathies 2065
70 Management of Patients With Oncologic or Degenerative Neurologic Disorders 2091

 Acute Community Based Challenges 2122

71 Management of Patients With Infectious Diseases 2124
72 Emergency Nursing 2156
73 Terrorism, Mass Casualty, and Disaster Nursing 2193

Appendix A: Diagnostic Studies and Interpretation
Available on thePoint

Index I-1

BRUNNER & SUDDARTH'S

TEXTBOOK OF
Medical-Surgical Nursing

14TH EDITION

BRUNNER & SUDDARTH'S

TEXTBOOK OF
Medical-Surgical
Nursing

14TH EDITION

Janice L. Hinkle, PhD, RN, CNRN
Fellow
Villanova University College of Nursing
Villanova, Pennsylvania

Kerry H. Cheever, PhD, RN
Professor and Chairperson
Helen S. Breidegam School of Nursing
Moravian College
Bethlehem, Pennsylvania

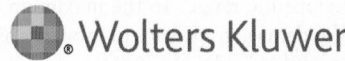

Philadelphia • Baltimore • New York • London
Buenos Aires • Hong Kong • Sydney • Tokyo

Publisher: Julie K. Stegman
Executive Editor: Kelley Squazzo
Director of Product Development: Jennifer K. Forestieri
Senior Development Editor: Meredith L. Brittain
Freelance Development Editor: Rose G. Foltz
Marketing Manager: Katie Schlesinger
Editorial Assistant: Leo Gray
Design Coordinator: Joan Wendt
Art Director, Illustration: Jennifer Clements
Production Project Manager: Marian Bellus
Manufacturing Coordinator: Karin Duffield
Prepress Vendor: Aptara, Inc.

14th Edition

9 8 7 6 5 4 3 2 1

Printed in China.

Library of Congress Cataloging-in-Publication Data

Names: Hinkle, Janice L., author. | Cheever, Kerry H., author.
Title: Brunner & Suddarth's textbook of medical-surgical nursing / Janice L.
   Hinkle, Kerry H. Cheever.
Other titles: Brunner and Suddarth's textbook of medical-surgical nursing |
   Textbook of medical-surgical nursing
Description: 14th edition. | Philadelphia : Wolters Kluwer, [2018] | Includes
   bibliographical references and index.
Identifiers: LCCN 2017026661 | ISBN 9781496347992 (1-volume American edition : hardback : alk. paper)
ISBN 9781496355157 (2-volume American edition : hardback : alk. paper)
Subjects: | MESH: Nursing Care | Medical-Surgical Nursing | Perioperative
   Nursing
Classification: LCC RT41 | NLM WY 150 | DDC 617/.0231—dc23
LC record available at https://lccn.loc.gov/2017026661

Contributors*

Contributors to the 14th Edition

Marianne Adam, PhD, RN, CRNP
Assistant Professor of Nursing
RN to BSN Program Coordinator
Pennsylvania State University
Schuykill Haven, Pennsylvania

Chapter 43: Assessment of Digestive and Gastrointestinal Function

Julie Adkins, DNP, APN, FNP-BC, FAANP
Family Nurse Practitioner
West Frankfort, Illinois

Chapter 63: Assessment and Management of Patients With Eye and Vision Disorders

Jennifer L. Bartlett, PhD, RN-BC, CNE, CHSE
Assistant Professor
Georgia Baptist College of Nursing of Mercer University
Atlanta, Georgia

Chapter 45: Management of Patients With Oral and Esophageal Disorders

Susan Bonini, MSN, RN
Senior Instructor
Integrated Nursing Pathway Program Coordinator
University of Colorado College of Nursing
Anschutz Medical Campus
Aurora, Colorado

Chapter 31: Assessment and Management of Patients With Hypertension

Lisa Bowman, RN, MSN, CRNP, CNRN
Nurse Practitioner
Jefferson Hospital for Neuroscience
Thomas Jefferson University Hospital
Philadelphia, Pennsylvania

Chapter 67: Management of Patients With Cerebrovascular Disorders

Jo Ann Brooks, PhD, RN, FAAN, FCCP
System Vice President, Quality and Safety
Indiana University Health
Indianapolis, Indiana

Chapter 23: Management of Patients With Chest and Lower Respiratory Tract Disorders
Chapter 24: Management of Patients With Chronic Pulmonary Disease

Sherry Burrell, PhD, RN, CNE
Assistant Professor
Villanova University College of Nursing
Villanova, Pennsylvania

Chapter 46: Management of Patients With Gastric and Duodenal Disorders

Wendy Cantrell, DNP, CRNP
Assistant Professor
Manager of Clinical Research
University of Alabama Birmingham Department of Dermatology
Birmingham, Alabama

Chapter 61: Management of Patients With Dermatologic Disorders

Lauren Cantwell, RN, MS, ACNP-BC, ACNPC, CNS, CCNS, CCRN, CHFN
Advanced Heart Failure/Transplant Nurse Practitioner
Inova Heart and Vascular Institute
Falls Church, Virginia

Chapter 28: Management of Patients With Structural, Infectious, and Inflammatory Cardiac Disorders

Kim Cantwell-Gab, MN, ACNP-BC, ANP-BC, CVN, RVT, RDMS
Nurse Practitioner, Cardiology
Providence Medical Group Cardiology
Medford, Oregon

Chapter 30: Assessment and Management of Patients With Vascular Disorders and Problems of Peripheral Circulation

Patricia E. Casey, MSN, RN, CPHQ, AACC
Associate Director, NCDR Training and Orientation
American College of Cardiology
Washington, DC

Chapter 26: Management of Patients With Dysrhythmias and Conduction Problems

Jill Cash, RN, MSN, APRN-BC
Vanderbilt University Medical Center
Westhaven Family Practice
Franklin, Tennessee

Chapter 38: Assessment and Management of Patients With Rheumatic Disorders
Chapter 64: Assessment and Management of Patients With Hearing and Balance Disorders

Kerry H. Cheever, PhD, RN
Professor and Chairperson
Helen S. Breidegam School of Nursing
Moravian College
Bethlehem, Pennsylvania

Chapter 1: Health Care Delivery and Evidence-Based Nursing Practice
Chapter 47: Management of Patients with Intestinal and Rectal Disorders
Chapter 48: Assessment and Management of Patients With Obesity

v

Elise Colancecco, MSN, RN
Instructor
Helen S. Breidegam School of Nursing
Moravian College
Bethlehem, Pennsylvania

Chapter 42: Management of Patients With Musculokeletal Trauma

Moya Cook RN, MSN, APN
Family Nurse Practitioner
Marion, Illinois

Chapter 13: Fluid and Electrolytes: Balance and Disturbance

Linda Carman Copel, PhD, RN, PMHCNS, BC, CNE,
   ANEF, NCC, FAPA
Professor
Villanova University College of Nursing
Villanova, Pennsylvania

Chapter 4: Health Education and Health Promotion
Chapter 6: Individual and Family Homeostasis, Stress, and Adaptation
*Chapter 59: Assessment and Management of Problems Related to
   Male Reproductive Processes*

Tara Bilofsky, ACNP-BC, MS
Acute Care Nurse Practitioner
St. Luke's University Health Network-Allentown
Allentown, Pennsylvania

Chapter 21: Respiratory Care Modalities

Elizabeth Petit deMange, PhD, RN
Assistant Professor
Villanova University College of Nursing
Villanova, Pennsylvania

*Chapter 52: Assessment and Management of Patients With Endocrine
   Disorders*

Nancy Donegan, MPH, RN
Independent Consultant
Washington, DC

Chapter 71: Management of Patients With Infectious Diseases

Paulette Dorney, PhD, RN, CCRN
Assistant Professor
Helen S. Breidegam School of Nursing
Moravian College
Bethlehem, Pennsylvania

Chapter 21: Respiratory Care Modalities

Diane Dressler, MSN, RN, CCRN-R
Clinical Assistant Professor Emerita
Marquette University College of Nursing
Milwaukee, Wisconsin

Chapter 27: Management of Patients With Coronary Vascular Disorders
*Chapter 29: Management of Patients With Complications from Heart
   Disease*

Debra Drew, MS, RN-BC (retired), ACNS-BC (retired),
   AP-PMN
Clinical Nurse Specialist, Pain Management
Minneapolis, Minnesota

Chapter 12: Pain Management

Phyllis Dubendorf, MSN, RN, CCNS, CNRN, CRNP-BC
Clinical Nurse Specialist
Hospital of the University of Pennsylvania
Philadelphia, Pennsylvania

Chapter 66: Management of Patients With Neurologic Dysfunction

Susan M. Fallone, MS, RN, CNN
Retired Clinical Nurse Specialist Adult and Pediatric
   Dialysis
Albany Medical Center Hospital
Albany, New York

Chapter 53: Assessment of Kidney and Urinary Function

Janice Farber, PhD, RN, CNOR
Assistant Professor
Helen S. Breidegam School of Nursing
Moravian College
Bethlehem Pennsylvania

Chapter 7: Overview of Transcultural Nursing

Eleanor Fitzpatrick, RN, MSN, CCRN, AGCNS-BC,
   ACNP-BC
Clinical Nurse Specialist
Thomas Jefferson University Hospital
Philadelphia, Pennsylvania

*Chapter 49: Assessment and Management of Patients With Hepatic
   Disorders*
*Chapter 50: Assessment and Management of Patients With Biliary
   Disorders*

Trudy Gaillard, PhD, RN, CDE
Assistant Professor
University of Cincinnati College of Nursing
Cincinnati, Ohio

Chapter 51: Assessment and Management of Patients With Diabetes

Dawn Goodolf, PhD, RN
Assistant Professor
Director of RN to BSN and Accelerated Postbaccalaureate
   Programs
Helen S. Breidegam School of Nursing
Moravian College
Bethlehem, Pennsylvania

Chapter 39: Assessment of Musculoskeletal Function

Beth Gotwals, PhD, RN
Associate Professor
Helen S. Breidegam School of Nursing
Moravian College
Bethlehem Pennsylvania

Chapter 2: Community-Based Nursing Practice
Home Care Checklists

Theresa Lynn Green, PhD, MScHRM, BScN, RN
Professor
School of Nursing, Queensland University of Technology
Queensland, Australia

Chapter 10: Principles and Practices of Rehabilitation

Debbie Gunter, MSN, APRN, ACHPN
Palliative Care and Family Nurse Practitioner
Emory Healthcare
Atlanta, Georgia

Chapter 22: Management of Patients With Upper Respiratory Tract Disorders

Jamie Heffernan MSN, RN, CCRN-K, NE-BC
Patient Care Director
New York-Presbyterian Weill Cornell
New York, New York

Chapter 62: Management of Patients With Burn Injury

Janice L. Hinkle, PhD, RN, CNRN
Fellow
Villanova University College of Nursing
Villanova, Pennsylvania

Chapter 55: Management of Patients With Urinary Disorders

Lisa J. Jesaitis, RN, MS, CHFN, ACNP
Acute Care Nurse Practitioner
MedStar Georgetown University Hospital Arrhythmia
    Service
Washington, DC

Chapter 28: Management of Patients With Structural, Infectious, and Inflammatory Cardiac Disorders

Tamara Kear, PhD, RN, CNS, CNN
Assistant Professor
Villanova University College of Nursing
Villanova, Pennsylvania

Chapter 54: Management of Patients With Kidney Disorders

Elizabeth Keech, RN, PhD
Adjunct Clinical Assistant Professor
Villanova University College of Nursing
Villanova, Pennsylvania

Chapter 11: Health Care of the Older Adult

Kathleen Kelleher, DMH, WHNP-BC, CBCN, DVS
Coordinator, Women's Health Nurse Practitioner
Breast Surgery Atlantic Health System
 Pompton Plains, New Jersey

Chapter 58: Assessment and Management of Patients With Breast Disorders

Lynne Kennedy, PhD, MSN, RN, RNFA, CHPN, CNOR, CLNC, CHTP, Alumnus CCRN
Program Coordinator
Women's Services, Minimally Invasive Gynecology and
    Palliative Care
Inova Fair Oaks Hospital
Fairfax, Virginia

Chapter 17: Preoperative Nursing Management
Chapter 18: Intraoperative Nursing
Chapter 19: Postoperative Nursing Management

Mary Beth Flynn Makic, PhD, CNS, CCNS, CCRN-K, FAAN, FNAP
Professor
University of Colorado College of Nursing
Denver, Colorado

Chapter 14: Shock and Multiple Organ Dysfunction Syndrome

Katrina Nice Masterson, RN, DNP, FNP-BC, DCNP
Educational Coordinator
Randall Dermatology
West Lafayette, Indiana

Chapter 60: Assessment of Integumentary Function

Jennifer McCaughey, MSN, BS, RNC-MNN, CCE
Clinical Educator
Women and Children's Services
Inova Fair Oaks Hospital
Fairfax, Virginia

Chapter 57: Management of Patients With Female Reproductive Disorders

Melissa V. Moreda, BSN, RN, CCRN, CNRN, SCRN
Clinical Nurse IV
Duke Raleigh Hospital
Raleigh, North Carolina

Chapter 70: Management of Patients With Oncologic or Degenerative Neurologic Disorders

Donna Nayduch, MSN, RN, ACNP, TCRN
Assistant Vice President of Trauma
North Florida Division HCA
Ocala, Florida

Chapter 72: Emergency Nursing
Chapter 73: Terrorism, Mass Casualty, and Disaster Nursing

Kathleen Nokes, PhD, RN, FAAN
Professor Emerita
Hunter College and Graduate Center, CUNY
New York, New York

Chapter 36: Management of Patients With Immunodeficiency Disorders

Kristen Overbaugh, PhD, RN, ACNS-BC, CHPN
Clinical Assistant Professor
School of Nursing
University of Texas Health Science Center San Antonio
San Antonio, Texas

Chapter 20: Assessment of Respiratory Function

Janet Parkosewich, DNSc, RN, FAHA
Nurse Researcher
Yale-New Haven Hospital
New Haven, Connecticut

Chapter 25: Assessment of Cardiovascular Function

Mae Ann Pasquale, PhD, RN
Assistant Professor of Nursing
Cedar Crest College
Allentown, Pennsylvania

Chapter 40: Musculoskeletal Care Modalities

Beth A. Bednarz Pruski, RN, MSN, CCRN
Program Manager, National Cardiovascular Data Registries
(NCDR)
American College of Cardiology
Washington, DC

*Chapter 26: Management of Patients With Dysrhythmias and
Conduction Problems*

Sue Pugh, MSN, RN, CNRN, CRRN, CNS-BC, FAHA
Patient Care Manager
Neuroscience Unit (NSU) & Neuroscience Critical Care
Unit (NSCCU)
Johns Hopkins Bayview Medical Center
Baltimore, Maryland

*Chapter 69: Management of Patients With Neurologic Infections,
Autoimmune Disorders, and Neuropathies*

JoAnne Reifsnyder, PhD, RN, FAAN
Executive Vice President and Chief Nursing Officer
Genesis Health Care
Kennett Square, Pennsylvania

Chapter 16: End-of-Life Care

Rebecca Wildman Repetti, RN, ANP-BC
Nurse Practitioner, Thoracic Oncology Service
Memorial Sloan Kettering Cancer Center
New York, New York

Chapter 35: Assessment of Immune Function

Marylou V. Robinson, PhD, FNP
Associate Professor of Nursing
Pacific Lutheran University
Tacoma, Washington

Chapter 41: Management of Patients With Musculoskeletal Disorders

Erin Sarsfield, MSN, RN, CCRN-K
Clinical Nurse Specialist, Medical and Heart and Vascular
Critical Care
Penn State Health Hershey Medical Center
Hershey, Pennsylvania

Chapter 44: Digestive and Gastrointestinal Treatment Modalities

Susan Scholtz, PhD, RN
Associate Professor
Helen S. Breidegam School of Nursing
Moravian College
Bethlehem, Pennsylvania

*Chapter 3: Critical Thinking, Ethical Decision Making, and the
Nursing Process*
Ethical Dilemma charts

Lindsey R. Siewert, RN, MSN, APRN, CCNS, CCRN-K
Clinical Nurse Specialist Neuroscience/Stroke Coordinator
Norton Healthcare
Louisville, Kentucky

Chapter 65: Assessment of Neurologic Function

Suzanne C. Smeltzer, RN, EdD, ANEF, FAAN
Professor and Director, Center for Nursing Research
Villanova University College of Nursing
Villanova, Pennsylvania

Chapter 9: Chronic Illness and Disability

Jennifer Specht, PhD, RN
Assistant Professor
Widener University
Chester, Pennsylvania

Chapter 5: Adult Health and Nutritional Assessment
Chapter 48: Assessment and Management of Patients With Obesity

Cindy Stern, RN, MSN, CCRP
Senior Administrator, Penn Cancer Network
Abramson Cancer Center of the University of Pennsylvania
Philadelphia, Pennsylvania

Chapter 15: Management of Patients With Oncologic Disorders

Julie G. Stover, RN, MSN, CRNP
Women's Health Nurse Practitioner
Lancaster, Pennsylvania

*Chapter 56: Assessment and Management of Female Physiologic
Processes*

Kimberly A. Subasic, PhD, MS, RN
Associate Professor
University of Scranton
Scranton, Pennsylvania

Chapter 8: Overview of Genetics and Genomics in Nursing
Genetics in Nursing Practice charts

Carole Sullivan, DNP, RN
Director
Deaconess VNA Home Care and Hospice
Eldorado, Illinois

*Chapter 37: Assessment and Management of Patients
With Allergic Disorders*
Unit-opening case studies, Units 1-9

Mary Laudon Thomas, MS, CNS, AOCN
Hematology Clinical Nurse Specialist
VA Palo Alto Health Care System
Palo Alto, California

*Chapter 32: Assessment of Hematologic Function and Treatment
Modalities*
*Chapter 33: Management of Patients With Nonmalignant
Hematologic Disorders*
Chapter 34: Management of Patients With Hematologic Neoplasms

Kristin Weitmann, RN, MSN, ACNP
Acute Care Nurse Practitioner
Optum
Wauwatosa, Wisconsin

*Chapter 27: Management of Patients With Coronary Vascular
Disorders*
*Chapter 29: Management of Patients With Complications
from Heart Disease*

Marie Wilson, RN, MSN, CCRN, CNRN, CRNP
Nurse Manager
Neuroscience Intensive Care Unit
Thomas Jefferson University Hospital
Philadelphia, Pennsylvania

Chapter 68: Management of Patients With Neurologic Trauma

Contributors to the 13th Edition

Christina M. Amidei, PhD, RN, CNRN, CCRN, FAAN
Chicago, Illinois

Chapter 65: Assessment of Neurologic Function
Chapter 70: Management of Patients With Oncologic or Degenerative Neurologic Disorders

Janice M. Beitz, PhD, RN, CS, CNOR, CWOCN, CRNP
Camden, New Jersey

Chapter 48: Management of Patients With Intestinal and Rectal Disorders

Elizabeth Blunt, PhD, RN, FNP-BC
Villanova, Pennsylvania

Chapter 38: Assessment and Management of Patients With Allergic Disorders

Lisa Bowman, MSN, RN, CRNP, CNRN
Philadelphia, Pennsylvania

Chapter 67: Management of Patients With Cerebrovascular Disorders

Jo Ann Brooks, PhD, RN, FAAN, FCCP
Indianapolis, Indiana

Chapter 23: Management of Patients With Chest and Lower Respiratory Tract Disorders
Chapter 24: Management of Patients With Chronic Pulmonary Disease

Kim Cantwell-Gab, MN, ARNP, CVN, RVT, RDMS
Vancouver, Washington

Chapter 30: Assessment and Management of Patients With Vascular Disorders and Problems of Peripheral Circulation

Patricia E. Casey, MSN, RN, CPHQ
Washington, DC

Chapter 26: Management of Patients With Dysrhythmias and Conduction Problems

Jill Cash, MSN, RN, APN
Herrin, Illinois

Chapter 64: Assessment and Management of Patients With Hearing and Balance Disorders

Kerry H. Cheever, PhD, RN
Bethlehem, Pennsylvania

Chapter 43: Management of Patients With Musculoskeletal Trauma

Odette Y. Comeau, MS, RN
Galveston, Texas

Chapter 62: Management of Patients With Burn Injury

Linda Carman Copel, PhD, RN, PMHCNS, BC, CNE, NCC, FAPA
Villanova, Pennsylvania

Chapter 4: Health Education and Promotion
Chapter 6: Individual and Family Homeostasis, Stress, and Adaptation
Chapter 59: Assessment and Management of Problems Related to Male Reproductive Processes

Carolyn Cosentino, RN, ANP-BC
New York, New York

Chapter 58: Assessment and Management of Patients With Breast Disorders

Susanna Garner Cunningham, PhD, BSN, MA, FAAN
Seattle, Washington

Chapter 31: Assessment and Management of Patients With Hypertension

Nancy Donegan, MPH, RN
Washington, DC

Chapter 71: Management of Patients With Infectious Diseases

Diane K. Dressler, MSN, RN, CNRN, CCNS
Milwaukee, Wisconsin

Chapter 27: Management of Patients With Coronary Vascular Disorders
Chapter 29: Management of Patients With Complications From Heart Disease

Phyllis Dubendorf, MSN, RN, CNRN, CCNS
Philadelphia, Pennsylvania

Chapter 66: Management of Patients With Neurologic Dysfunction

Susan M. Fallone, MS, RN, CNN
Albany, New York

Chapter 53: Assessment of Kidney and Urinary Function

Eleanor Fitzpatrick, MSN, RN, CCRN
Philadelphia, Pennsylvania

Chapter 49: Assessment and Management of Patients With Hepatic Disorders
Chapter 50: Assessment and Management of Patients With Biliary Disorders

Kathleen Kelleher Furniss, APN-C, DMH, CBCM, DVS
Pompton Plains, New Jersey

Chapter 57: Management of Patients With Female Reproductive Disorders

Catherine Glynn-Milley, RN, CPHQ, CRNO
Palo Alto, California

Chapter 63: Assessment and Management of Patients With Eye and Vision Disorders

Dawn M. Goodolf, PhD, RN
Bethlehem, Pennsylvania

Chapter 40: Assessment of Musculoskeletal Function

Theresa Green, PhD, RN
Calgary, Alberta, Canada

Chapter 10: Principles and Practices of Rehabilitation

Jamie Moore Heffernan, BSN, RN, CCRN
Galveston, Texas

Chapter 62: Management of Patients With Burn Injury

Melissa Hladek, MSN, RN, FNP-BC
Washington, DC

Chapter 39: Assessment and Management of Patients With Rheumatic Disorders

Joyce Young Johnson, PhD, MSN, RN
Albany, Georgia

Chapter 1: Health Care Delivery and Evidence-Based Nursing Practice
Chapter 2: Community-Based Nursing Practice
Chapter 3: Critical Thinking, Ethical Decision Making, and the Nursing Process
Chapter 7: Overview of Transcultural Nursing

Tamara M. Kear, PhD, RN, CNN
Villanova, Pennsylvania

Chapter 54: Management of Patients With Kidney Disorders
Chapter 55: Management of Patients With Urinary Disorders

Elizabeth K. Keech, PhD, RN
Villanova, Pennsylvania

Chapter 11: Health Care of the Older Adult

Lynne Kennedy, PhD, MSN, RN, CNOR, CHPN
Fairfax, Virginia

Chapter 17: Preoperative Nursing Management
Chapter 18: Intraoperative Nursing Management
Chapter 19: Postoperative Nursing Management

Mary Theresa Lau, MS, APN, CNSN, CRNI
Hines, Illinois

Chapter 45: Digestive and Gastrointestinal Treatment Modalities

Dale Halsey Lea, MPH, RN, CGC, FAAN
Cumberland Foreside, Maine

Chapter 8: Overview of Genetics and Genomics in Nursing Genetics in Nursing Practice Charts

Linda M. Lord, MS, RN, CNSC, NP
Rochester, New York

Chapter 45: Digestive and Gastrointestinal Treatment Modalities

Mary Beth Flynn Makic, PhD, RN, CNS
Aurora, Colorado

Chapter 14: Shock and Multiple Organ Dysfunction Syndrome

Elizabeth Petit de Mange, PhD, MSN, RN
Villanova, Pennsylvania

Chapter 52: Assessment and Management of Patients With Endocrine Disorders

Barbara J. Maschak-Carey, MSN, RN, CDE
Philadelphia, Pennsylvania

Chapter 51: Assessment and Management of Patients With Diabetes

Agnes Masny, BS, MPH, MSN, RN, ANP-BC
Philadelphia, Pennsylvania

Chapter 8: Overview of Genetics and Genomics in Nursing

Phyllis J. Mason, MS, RN, ANP
Baltimore, Maryland

Chapter 44: Assessment of Digestive and Gastrointestinal Function
Chapter 47: Management of Patients With Gastric and Duodenal Disorders

Jennifer D. McPherson, DNP, CRNA
Bethesda, Maryland

Chapter 21: Respiratory Care Modalities

Donna M. Molyneaux, PhD, RN
Gwynedd Valley, Pennsylvania

Chapter 22: Management of Patients With Upper Respiratory Tract Disorders

Barbara Moran, PhD, CNM, RNC, FACCE
Washington, DC

Chapter 56: Assessment and Management of Female Physiologic Processes

Susan Snight Moreland, DNP, CRNP
Bethesda, Maryland

Chapter 35: Assessment of Immune Function
Chapter 36: Management of Patients With Immunodeficiency Disorders

Martha A. Mulvey, MSN, ANP-BC
Newark, New Jersey

Chapter 13: Fluid and Electrolytes: Balance and Disturbance

Donna A. Nayduch, MSN, RN, ACNP, CAIS
Evans, Colorado

Chapter 72: Emergency Nursing
Chapter 73: Terrorism, Mass Casualty, and Disaster Nursing

Kathleen M. Nokes, PhD, RN, FAAN
New York, New York

Chapter 37: Management of Patients With HIV Infection and AIDS

Kristen J. Overbaugh, MSN, RN, ACNS-BC
San Antonio, Texas

Chapter 20: Assessment of Respiratory Function

Janet A. Parkosewich, DNSc, RN, FAHA
New Haven, Connecticut

Chapter 25: Assessment of Cardiovascular Function

Chris Pasero, MS, RN-BC, FAAN
El Dorado Hills, California

Chapter 12: Pain Management

Mae Ann Pasquale, PhD, RN
Allentown, Pennsylvania

Chapter 41: Musculoskeletal Care Modalities

Sue Baron Pugh, MSN, RN, CNS-BC, CRRN, CNRN, CBIS, FAHA
Baltimore, Maryland

Chapter 69: Management of Patients With Neurologic Infections, Autoimmune Disorders, and Neuropathies

Kimberly L. Quinn, BSN, MSN, RN, CRNP, ANP, ACNP, CCRN
Baltimore, Maryland

Chapter 46: Management of Patients With Oral and Esophageal Disorders

JoAnne Reifsnyder, PhD, APRN, BC-PCM
Philadelphia, Pennsylvania

Chapter 16: End-of-Life Care

Marylou V. Robinson, PhD, FNP-C
Aurora, Colorado

Chapter 42: Management of Patients With Musculoskeletal Disorders

Linda Schakenbach, MSN, RN, CNS, CCRN, CWCN, ACNS-BC
Falls Church, Virginia

Chapter 28: Management of Patients With Structural, Infectious, and Inflammatory Cardiac Disorders

Suzanne C. Smeltzer, EdD, RN, FAAN
Villanova, Pennsylvania

Chapter 9: Chronic Illness and Disability

Anthelyn Jean Smith-Temple, DNS, MSN, BSN
Valdosta, Georgia

Chapter 1: Health Care Delivery and Evidence-Based Nursing Practice
Chapter 2: Community-Based Nursing Practice
Chapter 3: Critical Thinking, Ethical Decision Making, and the Nursing Process
Chapter 7: Overview of Transcultural Nursing

Jennifer A. Specht, PhD, RN
Bethlehem, Pennsylvania

Chapter 5: Adult Health and Nutritional Assessment

Karen A. Steffen-Albert, MSN, RN
Philadelphia, Pennsylvania

Chapter 68: Management of Patients With Neurologic Trauma

Cindy L. Stern, MSN, RN, CCRP
Philadelphia, Pennsylvania

Chapter 15: Oncology: Nursing Management in Cancer Care

Candice Jean Sullivan, MSN, RNC, LCCE
Falls Church, Virginia

Chapter 56: Assessment and Management of Female Physiologic Processes

Mary Laudon Thomas, MS, RN
San Francisco, California

Chapter 32: Assessment of Hematologic Function and Treatment Modalities
Chapter 33: Management of Patients With Nonmalignant Hematologic Disorders
Chapter 34: Management of Patients With Hematologic Neoplasms

Lauren M. Weaver, MS, RN, CNS, ACNP, CCRN, CCNS
Washington, DC

Chapter 28: Management of Patients With Structural, Infectious, and Inflammatory Cardiac Disorders

Kristin Weitmann, MSN, RN, ACNP
Milwaukee, Wisconsin

Chapter 27: Management of Patients With Coronary Vascular Disorders
Chapter 29: Management of Patients With Complications From Heart Disease

Iris Woodard, BSN, RN-CS, ANP
Rockville, Maryland

Chapter 60: Assessment of Integumentary Function
Chapter 61: Management of Patients With Dermatologic Problems

Reviewers

Mike Aldridge, CNE
Concordia University Texas
Austin, Texas

Lori Bell, DrPH, MSN, RN
Cecil College
North East, Maryland

Deborah Beyer, MSN, RN
Miami University—Hamilton Campus
Hamilton, Ohio

Charemon Brooks, RN, MSN
Piedmont Virginia Community College
Charlottesville, Virginia

Schvon Bussey, MSN, FNP
Albany Technical College
Albany, Georgia

Michelle Edmonds, RN, MSN, DNP
Southside Virginia Community College
Alberta, Virginia

Janice Eilerman, MSN, RN
Rhodes State College
Lima, Ohio

Jennifer Ellis, DNP, MSN, RN
UC Blue Ash College
University of Cincinnati
Blue Ash, Ohio

Tiffany Losekamp-Roberts, RN, MSN
University of Cincinnati
Cincinnati, Ohio

Larry Maturin, MSN, APN, ACNS-BC, CEN, CCRN
DePaul University
Chicago, Illinois

Anna Moore, MS, RN
J. Sargeant Reynolds Community College
Richmond, Virginia

Darcy Nelson, MSN, RN, ABD
Crown College
St. Bonifacius, Minnesota

Maureen O'Shea, DNP, AGPCNP-BC
Curry College
Milton, Massachusetts

Vicki Plagenz, PhD candidate
Montana State University—Northern
Havre, Montana

Sigrid Sexton, RN, MSN
Long Beach City College
Long Beach, California

Ellis Siegel, RN, BSN, MSN
Norfolk State University
Norfolk, Virginia

Rebecca Sutter, RN, MSN, BC-FNP, DNP
George Mason University
Fairfax, Virginia

Megan Talbot, DNP, MSN, BSN, RN, CNE
Merritt College
Sacramento, California

Virginia Tufano, EdD, MSN, RN
College of Saint Mary
Omaha, Nebraska

Preface

The 1st edition of *Brunner & Suddarth's Textbook of Medical-Surgical Nursing* was published in 1964 under the leadership of Lillian Sholtis Brunner and Doris Smith Suddarth. Lillian and Doris pioneered a medical-surgical nursing textbook that has become a trusted learning resource. Lillian and Doris chose Suzanne Smeltzer and Brenda Bare as their successors. For several decades, Suzanne and Brenda continued the legacy of medical-surgical nursing excellence established by Lillian and Doris, meticulously supervising all updates and revisions for subsequent editions of this textbook. Suzanne and Brenda, in turn, served as our mentors for several editions of this textbook and have passed that legacy of excellence on to us. The result of the seamless and meticulous succession planning for editorship of this textbook is this new 14th edition.

Medical-surgical nursing has significantly advanced since 1964 but continues to be strongly influenced by the expansion of a host of other disciplines and new developments in technology, as well as myriad social, cultural, economic, and environmental changes throughout the world. In today's environment, nurses must be particularly skilled in critical thinking and clinical decision making, as well as in consulting and collaborating with other members of the multidisciplinary health care team.

Along with the challenges that today's nurses confront, there are many opportunities to provide skilled, compassionate nursing care in a variety of health care settings, for patients in the various stages of illness, and for patients across the age continuum. At the same time, there are significant opportunities for fostering health promotion activities for individuals and groups; this is an integral part of providing nursing care.

Continuing the tradition of the first 13 editions, this 14th edition of *Brunner & Suddarth's Textbook of Medical-Surgical Nursing* has evolved to prepare nurses to think critically and practice collaboratively within today's challenging and complex health care delivery system. The textbook focuses on physiologic, pathophysiologic, and psychosocial concepts as they relate to nursing care, and emphasis is placed on integrating a variety of concepts from other disciplines such as nutrition, pharmacology, and gerontology. Content relative to health care needs of nursing research findings, ethical considerations, evidence-based practice, bariatrics, prioritization, and people with disabilities has been expanded to provide opportunities for the nurse to refine clinical decision-making skills.

Organization

Brunner & Suddarth's Textbook of Medical-Surgical Nursing, 14th Edition, is organized into 17 units. These units mirror those found in previous editions with the incorporation of some changes. Content was updated throughout all units, with cross-references to specific chapters included as appropriate. Units 1 through 4 cover core concepts related to medical-surgical nursing practice. Units 5 through 16 discuss adult health conditions that are treated medically or surgically. Each of these units is structured in the following way to better facilitate comprehension:

- The first chapter in the unit covers assessment and includes a review of normal anatomy and physiology of the body system being discussed.
- Subsequent chapters in the unit cover management of specific disorders. Pathophysiology, clinical manifestations, assessment and diagnostic findings, medical management, and nursing management are presented. Nursing Process sections, provided for selected conditions, clarify and expand on the nurse's role in caring for patients with these conditions.

Special Features

When caring for patients, nurses assume many different roles, including practitioner, educator, advocate, and researcher. Many of the features in this textbook have been developed to help nurses fulfill these varied roles. Key updates to practice-oriented features in the 14th edition include new unit-opening Case Studies with QSEN Competency Focus—a feature that highlights a competency from the Quality and Safety Education for Nurses (QSEN) Institute that is applicable to the case study and poses questions for students to consider about relevant knowledge, skills, and attitudes (KSAs). Quality and Safety Nursing Alerts, Genetics in Nursing Practice charts, Ethical Dilemma charts, and Home Care Checklist charts offer updated formats and information.

The textbook also provides pedagogical features developed to help readers engage and learn critical content. Concept Mastery Alerts continue to clarify fundamental nursing concepts to improve the reader's understanding of potentially confusing topics, as identified by Misconception Alerts in Lippincott's Adaptive Learning Powered by prepU. Data from hundreds of actual students using this program in medical-surgical courses across the United States identified common misconceptions for the authors to clarify in this feature. An enhanced suite of online, interactive multimedia resources is also highlighted with icons placed in text near relevant topics. New to this suite of resources in this edition are Unfolding Patient Stories (case study vignettes) based on vSim for Nursing patients.

Read the User's Guide that follows the Preface for a full explanation and visual representation of all special features. See also the "Special Charts in This Book" and "Case Studies in This Book" sections of this front matter for the location of these items in the text.

A Comprehensive Package for Teaching and Learning

To further facilitate teaching and learning, a carefully designed ancillary package has been developed to assist faculty and students.

Instructor Resources

Tools to assist you with teaching your course are available upon adoption of this text on thePoint at http://thepoint. lww.com/Brunner14e.

- A thoroughly revised and augmented **Test Generator** contains more than 2900 NCLEX-style questions mapped to chapter learning objectives.
- An extensive collection of materials is provided for each book chapter:
  - **Lesson Plans** outline learning objectives and identify relevant resources from the robust instructor and student resource packages to help you prepare for your class.
  - **Pre-Lecture Quizzes** (and answers) allow you to check students' reading.
  - **PowerPoint Presentations** provide an easy way to integrate the textbook with your students' classroom experience; multiple-choice and true/false questions are included to promote class participation.
  - **Guided Lecture Notes** are organized by objective and provide corresponding PowerPoint slide numbers to simplify preparation for lecture.
  - **Discussion Topics** (and suggested answers) can be used in the classroom or in online discussion boards to facilitate interaction with your students.
  - **Assignments** (and suggested answers) include group, written, clinical, and Web assignments to engage students in varied activities and assess their learning.
  - **Case Studies** with related questions (and suggested answers) give students an opportunity to apply their knowledge to a client case similar to one they might encounter in practice.
- Sample **Syllabi** are provided for one- and two-semester courses.
- A **QSEN Competency Map** identifies content and special features in the book related to competencies identified by the QSEN Institute.
- An **Image Bank** lets you use the photographs and illustrations from this textbook in your course materials.
- **Strategies for Effective Teaching** provides general tips for instructors related to preparing course materials and meeting student needs.
- Access to all **Student Resources** is provided so that you can understand the student experience and use these resources in your course as well.

Student Resources

An exciting set of free learning resources is available on thePoint to help students review and apply vital concepts in medical-surgical nursing. Multimedia engines have been optimized so that students can access many of these resources on mobile devices. Students can access all these resources at http://thepoint.lww.com/Brunner14e using the codes printed in the front of their textbooks.

- **NCLEX-Style Review Questions** for each chapter, totaling more than 1800 questions, help students review important concepts and practice for NCLEX.
- Interactive learning resources appeal to a variety of learning styles. Icons in the text direct readers to relevant resources:

- **Concepts in Action Animations** bring physiologic and pathophysiologic concepts to life.
- **Interactive Tutorials** review key information for common or complex medical-surgical conditions. Tutorials include graphics and animations and provide interactive review exercises as well as case-based questions.
- **Practice & Learn Case Studies** present case scenarios and offer interactive exercises and questions to help students apply what they have learned.
- **Watch & Learn Video Clips** reinforce skills from the textbook and appeal to visual and auditory learners.
- **Procedural Guidelines charts** review key nursing interventions and rationales for specific patient care situations.
- **Appendix A, Diagnostic Studies and Interpretation**, provides reference ranges and lab values for common laboratory tests.
- A **Spanish–English Audio Glossary** provides helpful terms and phrases for communicating with patients who speak Spanish.
- **Journal Articles** offer access to current articles relevant to each chapter and available in Wolters Kluwer journals to familiarize students with nursing literature.

Study Guide

A comprehensive study aid for reviewing key concepts, *Study Guide for Brunner & Suddarth's Textbook of Medical-Surgical Nursing*, 14th Edition, has been thoroughly revised and presents a variety of exercises, including case studies and practice NCLEX-style questions, to reinforce textbook content and enhance learning.

Quick Reference Tools

Clinical Handbook for Brunner & Suddarth's Textbook of Medical-Surgical Nursing, 14th Edition, presents need-to-know information on nearly 200 commonly encountered disorders in an easy-to-use, alphabetized outline format that is perfect for quick access to vital information in the clinical setting. *Brunner & Suddarth's Handbook of Laboratory and Diagnostic Tests*, 3rd Edition, includes a review of specimen collection procedures followed by a concise, alphabetical presentation of tests and their implications. Information for each test includes reference values or normal findings, abnormal findings and related nursing implications, critical values, purpose, description, interfering factors, precautions, and nursing considerations. Both quick references are available in print or e-book format.

Adaptive Learning Powered by prepU

Updated to accompany the 14th edition, Lippincott's Adaptive Learning Powered by prepU helps every student learn more, while giving instructors the data they need to monitor each student's progress, strengths, and weaknesses. The adaptive learning system allows instructors to assign quizzes or students to take quizzes on their own that adapt to each student's individual mastery level. Visit http://thepoint.lww. com/prepU to learn more.

vSim for Nursing

vSim for Nursing, jointly developed by Laerdal Medical and Wolters Kluwer, offers innovative scenario-based learning modules consisting of Web-based virtual simulations, course learning materials, and curriculum tools designed to develop critical thinking skills and promote clinical confidence and competence. vSim for Nursing | Medical-Surgical includes 10 virtual simulations based on the National League for Nursing Volume I Complex patient scenarios. Students can progress through suggested readings, pre- and postsimulation assessments, documentation assignments, and guided reflection questions, and will receive an individualized feedback log immediately upon completion of the simulation. Throughout the student learning experience, the product offers remediation back to trusted Lippincott resources, including *Brunner & Suddarth's Textbook of Medical-Surgical Nursing*, as well as Lippincott Nursing Advisor and Lippincott Nursing Procedures—two online, evidence-based, clinical information solutions used in health care facilities throughout the United States. This innovative product provides a comprehensive patient-focused solution for learning and integrating simulation into the classroom.

Contact your Wolters Kluwer sales representative or visit http://thepoint.lww.com/vsim for options to enhance your medical-surgical nursing course with vSim for Nursing.

Lippincott DocuCare

Lippincott DocuCare combines web-based academic EHR simulation software with clinical case scenarios, allowing students to learn how to use an EHR in a safe, true-to-life setting, while enabling instructors to measure their progress. Lippincott DocuCare's nonlinear solution works well in the classroom, simulation lab, and clinical practice.

Contact your Wolters Kluwer sales representative or visit http://thepoint.lww.com/DocuCare for options to enhance your medical-surgical nursing course with DocuCare.

A Comprehensive, Digital, Integrated Course Solution

Lippincott CoursePoint+ is an integrated digital learning solution designed for the way students learn. It is the only nursing education solution that integrates:

- **Leading content in context:** Content provided in the context of the student learning path engages students and encourages interaction and learning on a deeper level.
- **Powerful tools to maximize class performance:** Course-specific tools, such as adaptive learning powered by prepU, provide a personalized learning experience for every student.
- **Real-time data to measure students' progress:** Student performance data provided in an intuitive display lets you quickly spot which students are having difficulty or which concepts the class as a whole is struggling to grasp.
- **Preparation for practice:** Integrated virtual simulation and evidence-based resources improve student competence, confidence, and success in transitioning to practice.
  - **vSim for Nursing:** Co-developed by Laerdal Medical and Wolters Kluwer, vSim for Nursing simulates real nursing scenarios and allows students to interact with virtual patients in a safe, online environment.
  - *Lippincott Advisor for Education:* With over 8500 entries covering the latest evidence-based content and drug information, Lippincott Advisor for Education provides students with the most up-to-date information possible, while giving them valuable experience with the same point-of-care content they will encounter in practice.
- **Training services and personalized support:** To ensure your success, our dedicated educational consultants and training coaches will provide expert guidance every step of the way.

Janice L. Hinkle, PhD, RN, CNRN
Kerry H. Cheever, PhD, RN

User's Guide

Brunner & Suddarth's Textbook of Medical-Surgical Nursing, 14th Edition, has been revised and updated to reflect the complex nature of nursing practice today. This textbook includes many features to help you gain and apply the knowledge that you need to pass NCLEX and successfully meet the challenges and opportunities of clinical practice. In addition, features have been developed specifically to help you fulfill the varied roles that nurses assume in practice.

Opening Features That Start With the End in Mind

Unit opening features put the patient first and highlight competent nursing as well as application of the nursing process.

- **All new! A Case Study with QSEN Competency Focus** opens each unit and provides discussion points focusing on one competency from the QSEN Institute: patient-centered care, interdisciplinary teamwork and collaboration, evidence-based practice, quality improvement, safety, and informatics. This feature helps you consider the KSAs required for the delivery of safe, quality patient care. For your convenience, a list of these case studies, along with their location in the book, appears in the "Case Studies in This Book" section later in this front matter.

UNIT 17

Acute Community Based Challenges

Case Study
ENSURING EQUITABLE PATIENT ASSIGNMENTS IN AN EMERGENCY DEPARTMENT

A new charge nurse has just started a 12-hour night shift in a community emergency department (ED). The first order of business is to make patient assignments for the 32-bed unit. Staffing for this shift includes 3 RNs (1 new and 2 seasoned), 1 LPN and 1 unlicensed assistant. What would be a fair assignment and what can be delegated to each of these staff members? How can the nurse foster open communication, mutual respect, and shared decision-making with the team to achieve quality patient care?

QSEN Competency Focus: Teamwork and Collaboration

The complexities inherent in today's health care system challenges nurses to demonstrate integration of specific interdisciplinary core competencies. These competencies are aimed at ensuring the delivery of safe, quality patient care (Institute of Medicine, 2003). The Quality and Safety Education for Nurses project (QSEN, 2017; Cronenwett, Sherwood, Barnsteiner, et al., 2007) provides a framework for the knowledge, skills, and attitudes (KSA) required for nurses to demonstrate competency in these key areas, which include *patient-centered care, interdisciplinary teamwork and collaboration, evidence-based practice, quality improvement, safety,* and *informatics.*

Teamwork and Collaboration Definition: Function effectively within nursing and interprofessional teams, fostering open communication, mutual respect, and shared decision making to achieve quality patient care.

SELECTED PRE-LICENSURE KSAs	APPLICATION AND REFLECTION
Knowledge	
Describe own strengths, limitations, and values in functioning as a member of the team.	Describe the charge nurse's priorities in making a fair assignment for this night shift. How would these intersect with those of other members of the team? Describe roles of each of the team members and how these roles interplay with each other.
Skills	
Function competently within own scope of practice as a member of the healthcare team.	As a novice charge nurse in the ED setting, whom would you rely on to help you develop your skillset? Identify your professional development growth goals so that you would be an effective member of the emergency health care team.
Attitudes	
Contribute to resolution of conflict and disagreement	Reflect upon your preferred communication style and approach to conflict. How might you react if a seasoned nurse challenges the assignment? What skills might you wish to develop to be most effective in this setting with seasoned nurses and other members of the team?

Cronenwett, L., Sherwood, G., Barnsteiner, J., et al. (2007). Quality and safety education for nurses. *Nursing Outlook, 55*(3), 122–131.
Institute of Medicine. (2003). *Health professions education: A bridge to quality.* Washington, DC: National Academies Press.
QSEN Institute. (2017). *QSEN competencies: Definitions and pre-licensure KSAs.* Retrieved on 3/1/2017 at: www.qsen.org/competencies/pre-licensure-ksas

- **Learning Objectives** give an overview of each chapter and identify learning goals to help focus reading and studying.

- A **Glossary** provides a list of key terms and definitions at the beginning of each chapter, providing a review of vocabulary words before reading the material and a useful reference and study tool.

32 Assessment of Hematologic Function and Treatment Modalities

LEARNING OBJECTIVES

On completion of this chapter, the learner will be able to:

1 Describe hematopoiesis and the processes involved in maintaining hemostasis.
2 Discuss the significance of the health history to the assessment of hematologic health.

3 Specify the proper techniques utilized to perform a comprehensive physical assessment of hematologic function.
4 Explain the diagnostic tests and related nursing implications used to evaluate hematologic function.
5 Identify therapies for blood disorders, including nursing implications for the administration of blood components.

GLOSSARY

anemia: decreased red blood cell (RBC) count
band cell: slightly immature neutrophil
blast cell: primitive white blood cell (WBC)
cytokines: proteins produced by leukocytes that are vital to regulation of hematopoiesis, apoptosis, and immune responses
differentiation: development of functions and characteristics that are different from those of the parent stem cell
erythrocyte: a cellular component of blood involved in the transport of oxygen and carbon dioxide (*synonym:* red blood cell)
erythropoiesis: process of the formation of RBCs
erythropoietin: hormone produced primarily by the kidney; necessary for erythropoiesis
fibrin: filamentous protein; basis of thrombus and blood clot
fibrinogen: protein converted into fibrin to form thrombus and clot
fibrinolysis: process of breakdown of fibrin clot
granulocyte: granulated WBC (i.e., neutrophil, eosinophil, basophil); sometimes used synonymously with neutrophil
hematocrit: percentage of total blood volume consisting of RBCs
hematopoiesis: complex process of the formation and maturation of blood cells
hemoglobin: iron-containing protein of RBCs; delivers oxygen to tissues
hemostasis: intricate balance between clot formation and

myeloid: pertaining to nonlymphoid blood cells that differentiate into RBCs, platelets, macrophages, mast cells, and various WBCs
myelopoiesis: formation and maturation of cells derived from myeloid stem cell
natural killer (NK) cells: immune cells that accumulate in lymphoid tissue that are potent killers of virus-infected and cancer cells
neutrophil: fully mature WBC capable of phagocytosis; primary defense against bacterial infection
nucleated RBC: immature form of RBC; portion of nucleus remains within the RBC
oxyhemoglobin: combined form of oxygen and hemoglobin; found in arterial blood
phagocytosis: process of cellular ingestion and digestion of foreign bodies
plasma: liquid portion of blood
plasminogen: protein converted to plasmin to dissolve thrombi and clots
platelet: a cellular component of blood involved in blood coagulation (*synonym:* thrombocyte)
red blood cell (RBC): a cellular component of blood involved in the transport of oxygen and carbon dioxide (*synonym:* erythrocyte)
reticulocytes: slightly immature RBCs, usually only 1% of total circulating RBCs

Features to Develop the Nurse as Practitioner

One of the central roles of the nurse is to provide holistic care to patients and their families, both independently and through collaboration with other health care professionals. Special features throughout chapters are designed to assist readers with clinical practice.

- **Nursing Process sections** are organized according to the nursing process framework—the basis for all nursing practice—and help clarify the nurse's responsibilities in caring for patients with selected disorders.

NURSING PROCESS

The Patient With Anemia

Assessment

The health history and physical examination provide important data about the type of anemia involved, the extent and type of symptoms it produces, and the impact of those symptoms on the patient's life. Weakness, fatigue, and general malaise are common, as are pallor of the skin and mucous membranes (conjunctivae, oral mucosa) (see Fig. 33-1).

Jaundice; angular cheilosis (ulcerated corners of the mouth); and brittle, ridged, concave nails may be present in patients with **megaloblastic anemia** (characterized by the presence of abnormally large, nucleated RBCs) or hemolytic anemia. The tongue may be beefy red and sore in megaloblastic anemia, or smooth and red in iron deficiency anemia. Patients with iron deficiency anemia may infrequently crave ice, starch, or dirt; this craving is known as pica (Broadway-Duren & Klaassen, 2013). Restless leg syndrome is common in as many as 24% of

- **Plans of Nursing Care**, provided for selected disorders, illustrate how the nursing process is applied to meet the patient's health care and nursing needs.

Chart 50-4

PLAN OF NURSING CARE
Care of the Patient With Acute Pancreatitis

NURSING DIAGNOSIS: Acute pain and discomfort related to edema, distention of the pancreas, peritoneal irritation, and excess stimulation of pancreatic secretions
GOAL: Relief of pain and discomfort

Nursing Interventions	Rationale	Expected Outcomes
1. Using a pain scale, assess pain level at baseline, before and after administration of analgesic medications.	1. Baseline assessment and control of pain are important because restlessness increases the body's metabolism, which stimulates the secretion of pancreatic and gastric enzymes.	• Patient rates pain using pain scale • Reports relief of pain, discomfort, and abdominal cramping • Moves and turns without increasing pain and discomfort • Rests comfortably and sleeps for increasing periods • Reports increased feelings of well-being and security with the health care team
2. Administer morphine, fentanyl, or hydromorphone frequently, as prescribed, to achieve level of pain acceptable to patient.	2. Morphine, fentanyl, and hydromorphone act by depressing the central nervous system and thereby increasing the patient's pain threshold. Meperidine (Demerol) is avoided because it has failed acute pain studies and possesses toxic metabolites.	
3. Maintain the patient NPO (nothing by mouth) as prescribed.	3. Pancreatic secretion is increased by food and fluid intake.	
4. Maintain the patient on bed rest.	4. Bed rest decreases body metabolism and thus reduces pancreatic and gastric secretions.	
5. Maintain continuous nasogastric drainage if paralytic ileus or nausea and vomiting, abdominal distention are present. a. Measure gastric secretions at specified intervals.	5. Nasogastric suction relieves nausea, vomiting, and abdominal distention. Decompression of the intestines (if intestinal intubation is used) also assists in relieving respiratory distress.	

- **Assessment charts** focus on data that should be collected as part of the assessment step of the nursing process.

Chart 39-2

ASSESSMENT
Assessing for Peripheral Nerve Function

Assessment of peripheral nerve function has two key elements: evaluation of sensation and evaluation of motion. The nurse may perform one or all of the following during a musculoskeletal assessment.

Nerve	Test of Sensation	Test of Movement
Peroneal	Prick the skin midway between the great and second toe.	Ask the patient to dorsiflex the foot and extend the toes.

- **Risk Factors charts** outline factors that can impair health.

Chart 55-2

RISK FACTORS:
Urinary Tract Infection

- Contributing conditions such as:
  - Female gender
  - Diabetes
  - Pregnancy
  - Neurologic disorders
  - Gout
  - Altered states caused by incomplete emptying of the bladder and urinary stasis
- Decreased natural host defenses or immunosuppression
- Inability or failure to empty the bladder completely
- Inflammation or abrasion of the urethral mucosa
- Instrumentation of the urinary tract (e.g., catheterization, cystoscopic procedures)
- Obstructed urinary flow caused by:
  - Congenital abnormalities
  - Urethral strictures
  - Contracture of the bladder neck
  - Bladder tumors
  - Calculi (stones) in the ureters or kidneys
  - Compression of the ureters

- **Pharmacology charts and tables** display important considerations related to administering medications and monitoring drug therapy.

TABLE 48-2 Medications Prescribed to Treat Obesity

Medication	Adverse Effects	Nursing Considerations[a]
Gastrointestinal Lipase Inhibitor		
Mechanism of Action: Diminishes intestinal absorption and metabolism of fats, particularly triglycerides		
Orlistat (Xenical) *Note: Also available in lower dosages over-the-counter under the trade name of Alli*	Diarrhea Flatus Oily stools Fecal incontinence	Patients may have associated problems with malabsorption of nutrients; advise them to take a concomitant daily multivitamin. Caution in patients with known history of renal insufficiency, liver disease, or gallbladder disease as concomitant use is associated with renal calculi, liver failure, and cholelithiasis. Do not administer with cyclosporine (Neoral).
Selective Serotonergic 5-HT2C Receptor Agonist		
Mechanism of Action: Stimulates central 5-HT2C receptors, causing appetite suppression		
Lorcaserin (Belviq)	Fatigue Dizziness Nausea Headaches Cough Dry mouth Constipation	Can be associated with deficits in attention or memory; administer with caution in patients who drive or work with hazardous equipment when first prescribed until effects are realized. Can cause hypoglycemia in patients with diabetes Patients concomitantly taking antidepressants or migraine medications can have synergistic effects. Discontinue in patients who express suicidal ideation. Rarely, serotonin syndrome may develop—be alert for high fevers, brisk reflexes, agitation, and diarrhea; notify primary provider immediately and hold medication if these occur.

- **Updated! Quality and Safety Nursing Alerts** offer tips for best clinical practice and red-flag safety warnings to help avoid common mistakes.

> **Quality and Safety Nursing Alert**
>
> *Inadvertent removal of an endotracheal tube can cause laryngeal swelling, hypoxemia, bradycardia, hypotension, and even death. Measures must be taken to prevent premature or inadvertent removal.*

- **Critical Care icons** identify nursing considerations for the critically ill patient.

Emergency Management of Upper Airway Obstruction

Upper airway obstruction has a variety of causes. Acute upper airway obstruction may be caused by food particles, vomitus, blood clots, or anything that obstructs the larynx or trachea. It also may occur from enlargement of tissue in the wall of the airway, as in epiglottitis, obstructive sleep apnea, laryngeal edema, laryngeal carcinoma, or peritonsillar abscess, or from thick secretions. Pressure on the walls of the airway, as occurs in retrosternal goiter, enlarged mediastinal lymph nodes, hematoma around the upper airway, and thoracic aneurysm, also may result in upper airway obstruction.

The patient with an altered level of consciousness from any cause is at risk for upper airway obstruction because of loss of the protective reflexes (cough and swallowing) and loss of the tone of the pharyngeal muscles, which causes the tongue to fall back and block the airway.

- **Extensively revised! Genetics in Nursing Practice charts** summarize and highlight nursing assessments and management issues related to the role of genetics in selected disorders.

Chart 49-2 — **GENETICS IN NURSING PRACTICE**
Hepatic Disorders

A number of hepatic disorders have an underlying genetic cause. However, other genetic disorders associated with metabolic, gastrointestinal, or bleeding disorders will also impact the function of the liver. Some examples of hepatic disorders caused by genetic abnormalities include:

Autosomal Dominant:
- Alagille syndrome
- Hereditary coproporphyria
- Polycystic liver disease

Autosomal Recessive:
- Crigler–Najjar syndrome
- Dublin–Johnson syndrome
- Hemochromatosis
- Progressive familial intrahepatic cholestasis
- Thalassemia
- Wilson disease

Inheritance Pattern is not distinct; however, there is a genetic predisposition for the disorder:
- Biliary atresia
- Gilbert syndrome

Other genetic disorders that impact the hepatic system:
- Alpha-1 antitrypsin deficiency
- Cystic fibrosis
- Glycogen storage disease
- Lysosomal storage disease
- Polycystic kidney disease
- Zellweger syndrome

Obesity contributes to back strain by overtaxing the relatively weak back muscles in the absence of abdominal muscle support. Exercises are less effective and more difficult to perform when the patient is overweight. Weight reduction through diet modification is imperative to prevent recurrence of back pain. A sound nutritional plan that includes a change in eating habits and low-impact activities is vital. Noting achievement of weight reduction and providing positive reinforcement facilitate adherence. Back problems may or may not resolve as optimal weight is achieved (MQCI, 2016a).

- **Gerontologic Considerations**, identified with an icon applied to headings, charts, and tables, highlight information that pertains specifically to the care of the older adult patient. In the United States, older adults comprise the fastest-growing segment of the population.

- In addition to a new chapter on obesity, **Obesity Considerations icons** identify content related to obesity or to the nursing care of patients with obesity.

Chart 60-1 Benign Changes in the Skin of the Older Adult

- Cherry angiomas (bright red "moles")
- Diminished hair, especially on scalp and pubic area
- Dyschromias (color variations)
  - Solar lentigo (liver spots)
  - Melasma (dark discoloration of the skin)
  - Lentigines (freckles)
- Neurodermatitis (itchy spots)
- Seborrheic keratoses (crusty brown "stuck-on" patches)
- Spider angiomas (see Fig. 49-3)
- Telangiectasias (red marks on skin caused by stretching of the superficial blood vessels)
- Wrinkles
- Xerosis (dryness)
- Xanthelasma (yellowish waxy deposits on upper and lower eyelids)

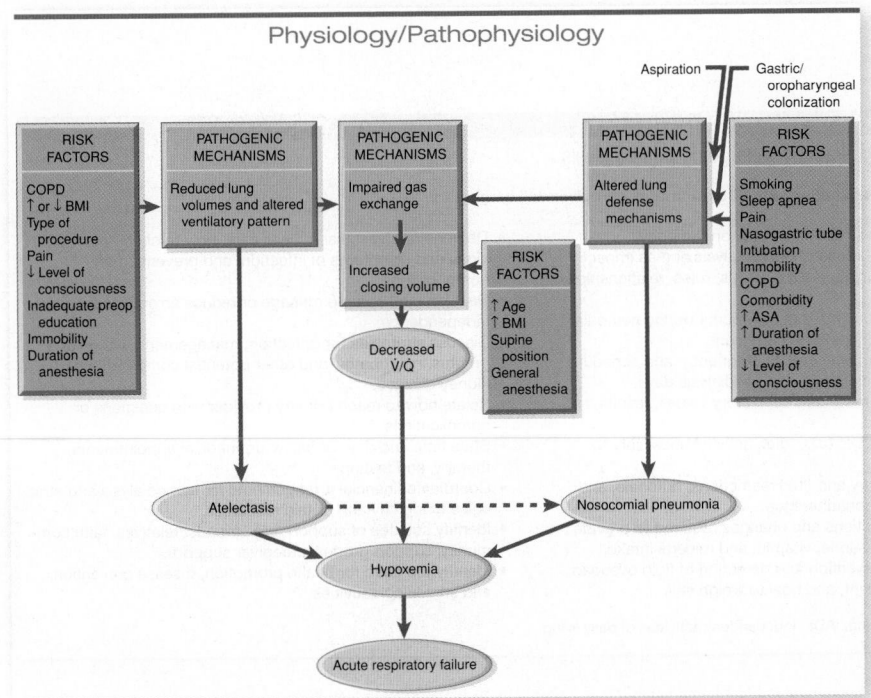

- **Physiology/Pathophysiology figures** include illustrations and algorithms describing normal physiologic and pathophysiologic processes.

Features to Develop the Nurse as Educator

Health education is a primary responsibility of the nursing profession. Nursing care is directed toward promoting, maintaining, and restoring health; preventing illness; and helping patients and families adapt to the residual effects of illness. Patient education and health promotion are central to all of these nursing activities.

- **Patient Education charts and icons** help the nurse prepare the patient and family for procedures, assist them in understanding the patient's condition, and explain to them how to provide self-care.

Chart 24-4   PATIENT EDUCATION

Use of Pressurized Metered-Dose Inhaler (pMDI)

The nurse instructs the patient to:
- Remove the cap and hold the inhaler upright.
- Shake the inhaler.
- Sit upright or stand upright. Breathe out slowly and all the way.
- Use one of two techniques: open-mouth technique or closed-mouth technique.
  - *Open-mouth technique*
    - Place the pMDI 2 finger widths away from lips.
    - With mouth open and tongue flat, tilt outlet of the pMDI so that it is pointed toward the upper back of the mouth.
    - Actuate the pMDI and begin to breathe in slowly. Breathe slowly and deeply through the mouth and try to hold

Chart 70-3   HEALTH PROMOTION

Strategies For the Patient With PD

To promote optimal health, the nurse works closely with the patient and family to ensure that they understand:
- How PD and its treatment impact physiologic functioning, ADLs, IADLs, roles, relationships, and spirituality
- The importance of adhering to the prescribed medication regimen; including knowing the purpose, dose, route, schedule, side effects, and precautions for all medications
- How and when to contact all members of the treatment team (e.g., health care providers, home care professionals, and durable medical equipment and supply vendors)
- Specific types of environmental and safety changes or support that will allow optimum functioning in the home
- The risk of falls/injury and how to implement fall prevention and adaptive measures in the home

In addition, the nurse advises the patient and family about lifestyle changes that are necessary to maintain

- **Health Promotion charts** review important points that the nurse should discuss with the patient to prevent common health problems from developing.

- **Extensively revised! Home Care Checklists** review points that should be covered as part of home care education prior to discharge from the health care facility.

Chart 54-9   HOME CARE CHECKLIST

The Patient Undergoing Hemodialysis

At the completion of education, the patient and/or caregiver will be able to:

- Discuss kidney disease and its effects on the body.
- State the goal and purpose of hemodialysis and its impact on physiologic functioning, ADLs, IADLs, roles, relationships, and spirituality.
- Discuss common problems that may occur during hemodialysis and their prevention and management.
- State the name, dose, side effects, frequency, and schedule for all medications on dialysis and nondialysis days.
- Describe commonly measured laboratory values, results, and implications.
- State changes in lifestyle (e.g., diet, activity) necessary to maintain health.
  - Acknowledge dietary and fluid restrictions, rationale, and consequences of nonadherence.
  - State dietary restrictions and changes required to provide adequate protein, calorie, vitamin, and mineral intake.
- List guidelines for prevention and detection of fluid overload, meaning of "dry" weight, and how to weigh self.
- Demonstrate vascular access care, how to check patency, signs and symptoms of infection, and prevention of complications.
- Develop strategies to manage or reduce anxiety and maintain independence.
- Discuss strategies for detection, management, and relief of pruritus, neuropathy, and other potential complications of kidney disease.
- Relate how to reach primary provider with questions or complications.
- State time and date of follow-up medical appointments, therapy, and testing.
- Coordinate financial arrangements for hemodialysis and strategies to identify and obtain resources.
- Identify sources of support (e.g., friends, relatives, faith community, support groups, caregiver support).
- Identify the need for health promotion, disease prevention, and screening activities.

ADL, activities of daily living; IADL, independent activities of daily living.

Features to Develop the Nurse as Patient Advocate

Nurses advocate for patients by protecting their rights (including the right to health care) and assisting patients and their families in making informed decisions about health care.

- **Extensively revised! Ethical Dilemma charts** provide a clinical scenario, discussion points, and questions to help analyze fundamental ethical principles related to the dilemma.

Chart 36-13 ETHICAL DILEMMA
Under What Circumstances May a Nurse Refuse to Care for a Patient?

Case Scenario

You are the charge nurse in the Intensive Care Unit (ICU). A 52-year-old male patient, who is married but is bisexual, is admitted with pneumocystic pneumonia. His bisexual status is unknown to his spouse. He appears malnourished and emaciated. His laboratory findings indicate he has HIV. His wife has been at his bedside daily but is unaware that he has HIV. The nurse assigned to care for him tells you, "I cannot believe what he has done to his wife! She is at his bedside and has no idea about his double lifestyle. I am a Christian and I want nothing to do with a man with no morals. I think someone needs to tell her the truth but it won't be me! I'm not going to take care of him—give me another assignment."

Discussion

Some health care providers may display a judgmental manner when providing care for patients with HIV/AIDS. The negative attitude often leads to a significant decrease in patient satisfaction regarding their health care. The American Nurses Association (ANA) clearly stipulates that nurses have an obligation to "provide fair and equal treatment to all patients" (ANA, 2016, p. 3) and also stipulates in its *Code of Ethics* that nurses must provide fair and equitable treatment to all individuals regardless of gender, socioeconomic status, religious, culture, or sexual orientation (ANA, 2015).

Analysis

- Does a nurse have the right to refuse treating a patient? What if a nurse refuses to care for a patient because he or she believes that by doing so the nurse may suffer harm or it may conflict with tenets of his or her religious beliefs?
- There are several statements that the staff nurse in this case makes with regard to this patient assignment. Analyze each of these in turn. Does the staff nurse demonstrate respect for the patient's autonomy? Is he or she adhering to the ethical principles of beneficence and nonmaleficence? Is the nurse's actions and statements in conflict with the ANA Code of Ethics? (see Chart 3-3)
- What might be the legal implications of the staff nurse refusing this assignment? As the charge nurse, how would you act to ensure that applicable hospital policies are adhered to, that you do not permit any type of negligent or other potentially criminal act to occur, and that the patient and his partner receive just and equitable health care?
- What responsibility does the health care team have to the patient's wife? Since her health may be at risk due to her husband's disease, does the health care provider have an obligation to disclose the patient's diagnosis? Does the health care team have any responsibility to inform the patient's sexual partners of his HIV status? What health agencies must be notified of this patient's newly diagnosed HIV status?

References

American Nurses Association. (2015). *Code of ethics for nurses with interpretive statements*. Washington, DC: American Nurses Publishing, American Nurses Foundation/American Nurses Association.

American Nurses Association. (2016). Position statement on the nurse's role in ethics and human rights: Protecting and promoting individual worth, dignity, and human rights in practice settings. Retrieved on 8/28/2016 at: www.nursingworld.org/MainMenuCategories/EthicsStandards/Ethics-Position-Statements/NursesRole-EthicsHumanRights-PositionStatement.pdf

Li, L., Comulada, W.S., Wu, Z., et al. (2011). Providers HIV avoidance and attitude and patient satisfaction. *Health Connection, 16*, 105–112.

Resource

See Chapter 3, Chart 3-6 for ethics resources.

Chart 51-6 NURSING RESEARCH PROFILE
Impact of Community Diabetes Education

Gaillard, T., Amponsah, G., & Osei K. (2015). Patient-centered community diabetes education program improves glycemic control in African American patients with poorly controlled type 2 diabetes: Importance of point of care metabolic measurements. *Journal of the National Black Nurses Association, 26*(1), 51–58.

Purpose

The purpose of this study was to evaluate the benefits of a 6-month patient-centered, intensive lifestyle and diabetes self-management education support (DSMES) program on improving glycemic control as assessed by point-of-care (POC) A1C testing, body weight, blood pressure, and lipids and lipoprotein levels in African Americans with poorly controlled type 2 diabetes compared to standard diabetes cares.

Design

This was a single center randomized clinical trial of participants with poorly controlled type 2 diabetes (A1C > 7.0%) residing in the inner city. Participants were randomized to DSMES (n = 58) or to standard diabetes care (n = 38). Participants in the DSMES group received intensive lifestyle and behavioral program that included didactic lectures provided by the Diabetes Care Team at 1 to 2 week intervals for 6 months. A community health worker, trained in diabetes self-management, provided support in the form of weekly phone calls and information about community resources. At the end of each didactic session, goals from the prior week, barriers, and challenges were discussed. The group then discussed alternate strategies for goal attainment. Participants were provided with quarterly POC testing (A1C, blood pressure, cholesterol, weight) and were reminded of targets. Emphasis was placed on how lifestyle changes could assist in meeting targets/goals. Participants in the standard care group attended the initial orientation, but did not attend the didactic nor intensive self-management lectures. General diabetes topics were discussed to increase group participation. POC testing was done in both groups at baseline, 3 and 6 months.

Findings

At 6 months, the DSMES group had significant reduction in A1C (8.2 ± 1.4% vs. 7.5 ± 1.5%, p = 0.02) and random glucose (190.4 ± 77.6 vs. 160.6 ± 59.8 mg/dl, p = 0.03) when compared with the standard care group. However, there were no changes in body weight, blood pressure, or lipids/lipoprotein levels. In addition, participants in the DSMES verbalized enjoying meeting with the group to discuss strategies and challenges faced with controlling type 2 diabetes.

Nursing Implications

Nurses need to encourage patients with diabetes and prediabetes to attend diabetes self-management, education, and support groups. In addition, these programs should be culturally sensitive, located in the community, and offered at times that are convenient to participants. Finally, the addition of POC testing allows individuals to reconcile their results with goals of therapy and provides immediate feedback and suggestions for change.

Features to Develop the Nurse as Researcher

Nurses identify potential research problems and questions to increase nursing knowledge and improve patient care. The use and evaluation of research findings in nursing practice are essential to further the science of nursing.

- **All new and in most chapters! Nursing Research Profiles** identify the implications and applications of nursing research findings for evidence-based nursing practice.

Features to Facilitate Learning

In addition to practice-oriented features, special features have been developed to help readers learn key information.

- **Concept Mastery Alerts** highlight and clarify fundamental nursing concepts to improve understanding of difficult topics, as identified by Misconception Alerts in Lippincott's Adaptive Learning Powered by prepU, an adaptive quizzing platform. Data from hundreds of actual students using this program in medical-surgical courses across the United States continue to be used to identify common misconceptions for the authors to clarify in this feature.

 Concept Mastery Alert

One major difference between cardioversion and defibrillation is the timing of the delivery of electrical current. In **cardioversion**, the delivery of the electrical current is synchronized with the patient's electrical events; in **defibrillation**, the delivery of the current is immediate and unsynchronized.

- **New! Unfolding Patient Stories**, written by the National League for Nursing, are an engaging way to begin meaningful conversations in the classroom. These vignettes, which appear throughout the text near related content, feature patients from Wolters Kluwer's vSim for Nursing | Medical-Surgical (co-developed by Laerdal Medical) and DocuCare products; however, each Unfolding Patient Story in the book stands alone, not requiring purchase of these products. For your convenience, a list of these case studies, along with their location in the book, appears in the "Case Studies in This Book" section later in this front matter.

- Interactive learning tools available online enrich learning and are identified with icons in the text:

  - **Concepts in Action Animations** bring physiologic and pathophysiologic concepts to life.

  - **Interactive Tutorials** review key information for common or complex medical-surgical conditions. Tutorials include graphics and animations and provide interactive review exercises as well as case-based questions.

  - **Practice & Learn Case Studies** present case scenarios and offer interactive exercises and questions to help students apply what they have learned.

  - **Watch & Learn Video Clips** reinforce skills from the textbook and appeal to visual and auditory learners.

- **All new! Critical Thinking Exercises** foster critical thinking and challenge you to apply textbook knowledge to clinical scenarios. Evidence-Based Practice (EBP) questions encourage you to apply best evidence from research findings to nursing interventions. Prioritization (PQ) questions ask you to consider the priorities for nursing care for specific patients and conditions.

- **References** cited are listed at the end of each chapter and include updated, current sources.

- **Resources** lists at the end of each chapter include sources of additional information, Web sites, agencies, and patient education materials.

Unfolding Patient Stories: Doris Bowman • Part 1

Doris Bowman, a 39-year-old diagnosed with uterine fibroids, dysmenorrhea, and menorrhagia, is scheduled for a total abdominal hysterectomy with bilateral salpingoopherectomy. She has a family history of uterine and ovarian cancer. She asks the nurse what she can do to further reduce her risk for cancer and is also concerned for her family members. What patient and family education should the nurse present on risk reduction strategies, health promotion, and cancer screening? (Doris Bowman's story continues in Chapter 57.)

Care for Doris and other patients in a realistic virtual environment: **vSim** *for Nursing* (**thepoint.lww.com/vSimMedicalSurgical**). Practice documenting these patients' care in DocuCare (**thepoint.lww.com/DocuCareEHR**).

CRITICAL THINKING EXERCISES

1 **pq** A 19-year-old patient is admitted with suspected meningitis. Describe the pathophysiology of meningitis. What are the signs of meningeal irritation the nurse should watch for and how are they tested? What is the priority nursing diagnosis in the patient with meningitis? What history and physical findings are common in the patient with meningitis?

2 **pq** Identify the priorities, approach, and techniques you would use to provide care to the patients in your assignment on an intermediate neuroscience unit. Two of the patients have a diagnosis of myasthenia gravis, one is intubated and on a ventilator, one patient has a diagnosis of GBS and the other has meningitis. What tasks can you delegate and to whom?

3 **ebp** A 35-year-old woman is newly diagnosed with Bell palsy. Identify her treatment options. Describe the evidence base for the options that you have identified and the criteria used to evaluate the strength of the evidence for her various treatment options.

REFERENCES

*Asterisk indicates nursing research.

Books

Emergency Nurses Association (ENA). (2013). *Sheehy's manual of emergency care*. St. Louis, MO: Mosby.

Moore, K. L., Agur, A. M. R., Dalley, A. F. II (2015). *Essential clinical anatomy* (5th ed.). Philadelphia, PA: Lippincott Williams & Wilkins

National Association of Orthopedic Nurses (NAON). (2013). *Core curriculum for orthopaedic nursing* (7th ed.). Boston, MA: Pearson.

Porth, C. M. (2015). *Essentials of pathophysiology: Concepts of altered health states.* (4th ed.). Philadelphia, PA: Lippincott Williams & Wilkins

Strickland, J. W., & Graham, T. J. (2005). *Master techniques in orthopaedic surgery: The hand* (2nd ed.). Philadelphia, PA: Lippincott Williams & Wilkins.

Resources

American Cancer Society, www.cancer.org
American College of Surgeons, Ostomy Home Skills Program, www.facs.org/education/patient-education/skills-programs/ostomy-program
American Society of Colon and Rectal Surgeons (ASCRS), www.fascrs.org
Beyond Celiac Disease, www.beyondceliac.org
Celiac Support Association, www.csaceliacs.org
Colon Cancer Alliance, www.ccalliance.org
Crohn's and Colitis Foundation of America (CCFA), www.ccfa.org
Gluten Free Drugs, www.glutenfreedrugs.com
International Foundation for Functional Gastrointestinal Disorders (IFFGD), www.iffgd.org
J-Pouch Group (source for J-Pouch surgery support), www.j-pouch.org
Meet an OstoMate, www.meetanostomate.org
National Association for Continence, www.nafc.org
National Cancer Institute, National Institutes of Health, www.cancer.gov

Contents

UNIT 1 Basic Concepts in Nursing 2

1 Health Care Delivery and Evidence-Based Nursing Practice 4
Nursing 5
The Patient: Consumer of Nursing and Health Care 5
The Patient's Basic Needs: Maslow Hierarchy of Needs 5
Health 5
Wellness 6
Health Promotion 6
Influences on Health Care Delivery 6
Population Demographics 6
Changing Patterns of Disease and Wellness 7
Advances in Technology and Genetics 7
Quality, Safety, and Evidence-Based Practice 7
The Patient Protection and Affordable Care Act 8
Pay for Performance 8
The Joint Commission Best-Practice Initiatives 8
Patient Satisfaction: A Quality Metric 9
The Triple Aim of Effective Health Care Systems 9
TeamSTEPPS 9
Quality and Safety Education for Nurses 11
The Practice of Nursing in Today's Health Care Delivery System 11
Medical-Surgical Nursing 12
Advanced Nursing Roles 12
The Nurse as Coordinator of Care Transitions 12
The Future of Nursing 13
Interprofessional Collaborative Practice 15

2 Community-Based Nursing Practice 18
Key Components of Community-Based Care 19
Discharge Planning for Transition to the Community or Home Care Setting 19
Continuing the Transition Through Community Resources and Referrals 19
Home Health Care 20
Services Provided 20
The Home Setting 21
Home Health Visits 21
Additional Care Settings in the Community 24
Hospice Care 24
Ambulatory Settings 24
Occupational Health Programs 24
School Health Programs 25
Community Nurse–Managed Centers 25
Care for Those Who Are Homeless 25

3 Critical Thinking, Ethical Decision Making, and the Nursing Process 27
Critical Thinking 27
Rationality and Insight 28
Components of Critical Thinking 29
Critical Thinking and Clinical Reasoning in Nursing Practice 29
Ethical Nursing Care 29
Ethics Versus Morals 30
Ethics Theories 30
Approaches to Ethics 31
Moral Situations 31
Types of Ethical Problems in Nursing 32
Preventive Ethics 34
Ethical Decision Making 35
The Nursing Process 35
Definition 35
Using the Nursing Process 37

4 Health Education and Health Promotion 48
Purpose of Health Education 48
Meeting Nursing Standards 48
Supporting Informed Decision Making and Self-Care 49
Promoting Adherence to the Therapeutic Regimen 49
The Nature of Teaching and Learning 51
Learning Readiness 51
The Learning Environment 52
Teaching Techniques and Resources 52
The Nursing Process in Patient Education 52
Assessment 52
Nursing Diagnosis 52
Planning 53
Implementation 54
Evaluation 54
Health Promotion 55
Definition 55
Health Promotion Models 55
Components of Health Promotion 57
Health Promotion Strategies Throughout the Lifespan 58
Adolescents 59
Young and Middle-Aged Adults 59
Gerontologic Considerations 59
Nursing Implications of Health Promotion 60

5 Adult Health and Nutritional Assessment 62
Considerations for Conducting a Health Assessment 62
The Role of the Nurse 62
Effective Communication 63

Ethical Use of Health Assessment Data 63
The Role of Technology 63
Assessment in the Home or Community 63
Health History 63
The Informant 64
Components of the Health History 64
Physical Assessment 71
Examination Considerations 71
Components of the Physical Examination 72
Nutritional Assessment 74
Lifespan Considerations 74
Components of Nutritional Assessment 76
Factors Influencing Nutritional Status in Various
Situations 79
Analysis of Nutritional Status 79

UNIT 2 Biophysical and Psychosocial Concepts in Nursing Practice 82

6 Individual and Family Homeostasis, Stress, and Adaptation 84
Fundamental Concepts 85
Constancy and Homeostasis 85
Stress and Adaptation 85
Overview of Stress 85
Types of Stressors 85
Stress as a Stimulus for Disease 86
Psychological Responses to Stress 86
Physiologic Response to Stress 87
Maladaptive Responses to Stress 90
Indicators of Stress 90
Stress at the Cellular Level 91
Control of the Steady State 91
Cellular Adaptation 92
Cellular Injury 92
Cellular Response to Injury:
Inflammation 94
Cellular Healing 95
Nursing Management 95
Promoting a Healthy Lifestyle 96
Enhancing Coping Strategies 97
Relaxation Techniques 97
Educating About Stress Management 98
Promoting Family Health 98
Enhancing Social Support 99
Recommending Support and Therapy
Groups 99
The Role of Stress in Health Patterns 99

7 Overview of Transcultural Nursing 102
Cultural Concepts 102
Subcultures 103
Minorities 103
Transcultural Nursing 104
Culturally Competent Nursing Care 104
Cross-Cultural Communication 105
Culturally Mediated Characteristics 106

Information Disclosure 106
Space and Distance 107
Eye Contact 107
Time 107
Touch 107
Observance of Holidays 107
Diet 108
Biologic Variations 108
Complementary, Alternative, and Integrative
Health Therapies 108
Causes of Illness 109
Biomedical or Scientific View 109
Naturalistic or Holistic Perspective 109
Magico-Religious View 109
Folk Healers 110
Cultural Nursing Assessment 111
**Additional Cultural Considerations:
Know Thyself 111**
The Future of Transcultural Nursing Care 111

8 Overview of Genetics and Genomics in Nursing 114
Genomic Framework for Nursing Practice 115
Integrating Genetic and Genomic Knowledge 116
Genes and Their Role in Human Variation 116
Inheritance Patterns 119
Chromosomal Differences and
Genetic Conditions 122
Genetic and Genomic Technologies in Practice 122
Genetic Testing 122
Genetic Screening 123
**Testing and Screening for Adult-Onset
Conditions 124**
Single Gene Conditions 124
Genomic Conditions 127
Population Screening 127
The Nursing Role in Testing and Screening for
Adult-Onset Conditions 127
Personalized Genomic Treatments 128
Pharmacogenomics 128
**Ethical, Legal, and Social Issues Surrounding
Genetics 129**
Ethical Concerns 129
Legal Aspects of Personalized Health Care 130
Ancestry, Cultural, Social, and Spiritual
Concerns Related to Genetic and Genomic
Practice 130
**Applications of Genetics and Genomics in Nursing
Practice 131**
Genetics and Genomics in Health
Assessment 131
Genetic Counseling and Evaluation
Services 133
Genetics and Genomics Tomorrow 136

9 Chronic Illness and Disability 139
Overview of Chronicity 139
Multiple Chronic Conditions 140
Health Disparities and Chronic Disease 140

Definition of Chronic Diseases or
Conditions 141
Prevalence and Causes of Chronic
Conditions 142
Prevention of Chronic Disease 143
Characteristics of Chronic Conditions 143
Implications of Managing Chronic
Conditions 145
Phases of Chronic Conditions 145
Gerontologic Considerations 146
**Nursing Care of Patients With Chronic
Conditions 147**
Applying the Nursing Process Using the Phases
of the Chronic Illness System 147
Home, Community-Based and Transitional
Care 148
Nursing Care for Special Populations With
Chronic Illness 149
Overview of Disability 149
Definitions of Disability 149
Prevalence of Disability 150
Characteristics of Disability 150
Federal Legislation 152
Right of Access to Health Care 154
Barriers to Health Care 154
Federal Assistance Programs 157
Nursing Care of Patients With Disabilities 158
Nursing Considerations During
Hospitalization 158
Health Promotion and Prevention 158
Significance of "People-First" Language 159
Gerontologic Considerations 159
Disability in Medical–Surgical Nursing
Practice 159
Home, Community-Based and
Transitional Care 160

10 Principles and Practices of Rehabilitation 164
The Rehabilitation Team 165
Areas of Specialty Rehabilitation 166
Substance Abuse Issues in Rehabilitation 167
Assessment of Functional Ability 167
• *Nursing Process:* The Patient With Self-Care Deficits
in Activities of Daily Living 168
• *Nursing Process:* The Patient With Impaired
Physical Mobility 170
• *Nursing Process:* The Patient With Impaired Skin
Integrity 178
• *Nursing Process:* The Patient With Altered
Elimination Patterns 186
**Promoting Home, Community-Based, and
Transitional Care 188**
Educating Patients About Self-Care 188
Continuing and Transitional Care 190

11 Health Care of the Older Adult 193
Overview of Aging 193
Demographics of Aging 193
Health Status of the Older Adult 194
Nursing Care of the Older Adult 194
Theories of Aging 195
Age-Related Changes 195
Physical Aspects of Aging 195
Psychosocial Aspects of Aging 202
Cognitive Aspects of Aging 204
Pharmacologic Aspects of Aging 205
Mental Health Problems in the Older Adult 207
Depression 207
Substance Abuse 208
Delirium 208
Dementia 209
**Additional Aspects of Health Care of the
Older Adult 215**
Pseudobulbar Affect 215
Geriatric Syndromes 215
Elder Neglect and Abuse 217
Social Services 218
Health Care Costs of Aging 218
Home Health Care 218
Hospice Services 218
Aging With a Disability 219
Ethical and Legal Issues Affecting the
Older Adult 219

UNIT 3 Concepts and Challenges in Patient Management 222

12 Pain Management 224
Fundamental Concepts 225
Definition of Pain 225
Effects of Pain 225
Types and Categories of Pain 225
Pain Assessment 230
Performing the Comprehensive Pain Assessment:
Patient Interview 230
Reassessing Pain 233
Pain Management 233
Pharmacologic Management of Pain:
Multimodal Analgesia 233
Nonpharmacologic Methods of Pain
Management 245
Nursing Implications of Pain Management 247

**13 Fluid and Electrolytes: Balance and
Disturbance 251**
Fundamental Concepts 252
Amount and Composition of Body Fluids 252
Regulation of Body Fluid Compartments 253
Systemic Routes of Gains and Losses 254
Laboratory Tests for Evaluating Fluid
Status 255
Homeostatic Mechanisms 256
Gerontologic Considerations 258
FLUID VOLUME DISTURBANCES 259
Hypovolemia 259
Pathophysiology 259
Clinical Manifestations 259

Assessment and Diagnostic Findings 259
Gerontologic Considerations 260
Medical Management 260
Nursing Management 260
Hypervolemia 262
Pathophysiology 262
Clinical Manifestations 263
Assessment and Diagnostic Findings 263
Medical Management 263
Nursing Management 263
ELECTROLYTE IMBALANCES 264
Sodium Imbalances 264
Sodium Deficit (Hyponatremia) 265
Pathophysiology 265
Clinical Manifestations 265
Assessment and Diagnostic Findings 266
Medical Management 266
Nursing Management 267
Sodium Excess (Hypernatremia) 267
Pathophysiology 267
Clinical Manifestations 267
Assessment and Diagnostic Findings 268
Medical Management 268
Nursing Management 268
Potassium Imbalances 268
Potassium Deficit (Hypokalemia) 268
Pathophysiology 269
Clinical Manifestations 269
Assessment and Diagnostic Findings 269
Medical Management 269
Nursing Management 270
Potassium Excess (Hyperkalemia) 271
Pathophysiology 271
Clinical Manifestations 271
Assessment and Diagnostic Findings 271
Medical Management 272
Nursing Management 272
Calcium Imbalances 272
Calcium Deficit (Hypocalcemia) 273
Pathophysiology 273
Clinical Manifestations 273
Assessment and Diagnostic Findings 274
Medical Management 274
Nursing Management 275
Calcium Excess (Hypercalcemia) 275
Pathophysiology 275
Clinical Manifestations 275
Assessment and Diagnostic Findings 276
Medical Management 276
Nursing Management 276
Magnesium Imbalances 276
Magnesium Deficit (Hypomagnesemia) 277
Pathophysiology 277
Clinical Manifestations 277
Assessment and Diagnostic Findings 278
Medical Management 278
Nursing Management 278
Magnesium Excess (Hypermagnesemia) 278
Pathophysiology 278
Clinical Manifestations 278
Assessment and Diagnostic Findings 278

Medical Management 278
Nursing Management 279
Phosphorus Imbalances 279
Phosphorus Deficit (Hypophosphatemia) 279
Pathophysiology 279
Clinical Manifestations 280
Assessment and Diagnostic Findings 280
Medical Management 280
Nursing Management 280
Phosphorus Excess (Hyperphosphatemia) 280
Pathophysiology 280
Clinical Manifestations 280
Assessment and Diagnostic Findings 280
Medical Management 281
Nursing Management 281
Chloride Imbalances 281
Chloride Deficit (Hypochloremia) 281
Pathophysiology 282
Clinical Manifestations 282
Assessment and Diagnostic Findings 282
Medical Management 282
Nursing Management 282
Chloride Excess (Hyperchloremia) 282
Pathophysiology 282
Clinical Manifestations 282
Assessment and Diagnostic Findings 282
Medical Management 282
Nursing Management 282
ACID–BASE DISTURBANCES 283
Acute and Chronic Metabolic Acidosis (Base Bicarbonate Deficit) 284
Pathophysiology 284
Clinical Manifestations 285
Assessment and Diagnostic Findings 285
Medical Management 285
Acute and Chronic Metabolic Alkalosis (Base Bicarbonate Excess) 285
Pathophysiology 285
Clinical Manifestations 285
Assessment and Diagnostic Findings 285
Medical Management 286
Acute and Chronic Respiratory Acidosis (Carbonic Acid Excess) 286
Pathophysiology 286
Clinical Manifestations 286
Assessment and Diagnostic Findings 286
Medical Management 286
Acute and Chronic Respiratory Alkalosis (Carbonic Acid Deficit) 287
Pathophysiology 287
Clinical Manifestations 287
Assessment and Diagnostic Findings 287
Medical Management 287
Mixed Acid–Base Disorders 287
Compensation 287
Blood Gas Analysis 287
PARENTERAL FLUID THERAPY 288
Purpose 288
Types of Intravenous Solutions 288
Isotonic Fluids 288
Hypotonic Fluids 290

Hypertonic Fluids 290
Other Intravenous Therapies 290
Nursing Management of the Patient Receiving Intravenous Therapy 290
Managing Systemic Complications 290
Managing Local Complications 291
Promoting Home, Community-Based, and Transitional Care 293

14 Shock and Multiple Organ Dysfunction Syndrome 296
Overview of Shock 296
Normal Cellular Function 297
Pathophysiology 297
Stages of Shock 298
Compensatory Stage 299
Clinical Manifestations 299
Medical Management 299
Nursing Management 299
Progressive Stage 301
Pathophysiology 301
Clinical Manifestations 301
Medical Management 302
Nursing Management 302
Irreversible Stage 303
Medical Management 304
Nursing Management 304
General Management Strategies in Shock 304
Fluid Replacement 304
Vasoactive Medication Therapy 306
Nutritional Support 307
Hypovolemic Shock 308
Pathophysiology 308
Medical Management 308
Nursing Management 309
Cardiogenic Shock 310
Pathophysiology 310
Clinical Manifestations 310
Medical Management 310
Nursing Management 312
Distributive Shock 313
Sepsis and Septic Shock 313
Pathophysiology 314
Medical Management 315
Nursing Management 316
Neurogenic Shock 318
Medical Management 318
Nursing Management 318
Anaphylactic Shock 318
Medical Management 319
Nursing Management 319
Multiple Organ Dysfunction Syndrome 319
Pathophysiology 319
Clinical Manifestations 320
Medical Management 320
Nursing Management 320
Promoting Home, Community-Based, and Transitional Care 320
Educating Patients About Self-Care 320
Continuing and Transitional Care 320

15 Management of Patients With Oncologic Disorders 324
Epidemiology 325
Pathophysiology of the Malignant Process 326
Characteristics of Malignant Cells 326
Carcinogenesis 326
Proliferative Patterns 327
Role of the Immune System 330
Detection and Prevention of Cancer 330
Primary Prevention 331
Secondary Prevention 331
Tertiary Prevention 331
Diagnosis of Cancer 333
Tumor Staging and Grading 333
Anatomic Stage Group 334
Management of Cancer 334
Surgery 335
Diagnostic Surgery 335
Surgery as Primary Treatment 336
Prophylactic Surgery 337
Palliative Surgery 337
Reconstructive Surgery 337
Nursing Management 337
Radiation Therapy 338
Radiation Dosage 339
Administration of Radiation 339
Toxicity 340
Nursing Management 341
Protecting Caregivers 341
Chemotherapy 341
Cell Kill and the Cell Cycle 341
Classification of Chemotherapeutic Agents 342
Adjunct Chemotherapeutic Agents 342
Administration of Chemotherapeutic Agents 342
Nursing Management 347
Protecting Caregivers 348
Hematopoietic Stem Cell Transplantation 348
Types of Hematopoietic Stem Cell Transplantation 349
Nursing Management 350
Hyperthermia 352
Nursing Management 352
Targeted Therapies 352
Biologic Response Modifiers 352
Gene Therapy 354
Nursing Management 354
Complementary, Alternative, and Integrative Health Therapies 355
Nursing Care of Patients With Cancer 355
Maintaining Tissue Integrity 355
Promoting Nutrition 371
Relieving Pain 372
Decreasing Fatigue 373
Improving Body Image and Self-Esteem 375
Addressing Sexuality 375
Assisting in the Grieving Process 375
Management of Psychosocial Distress 375
Monitoring and Managing Potential Complications 376

Promoting Home, Community-Based, and
Transitional Care 378
Gerontologic Considerations 379
Cancer Survivorship 379
Providing Care to the Patient
With Advanced Cancer 380

16 End-of-Life Care 387
Nursing and End-of-Life Care 388
Death and Dying in America 388
Technology and End-of-Life Care 388
Sociocultural Context 388
Settings for End-of-Life Care 390
Palliative Care 390
Hospice Care 393
Nursing Care of Terminally Ill Patients 395
Psychosocial and Regulatory Issues 395
Communication 395
Providing Culturally Sensitive Care at the
End of Life 399
Goal Setting in Palliative Care at the End of
Life 400
Spiritual Care 402
Hope 402
Managing Physiologic Responses to Terminal
Illness 402
Palliative Sedation at the End of Life 407
**Nursing Care of Patients
Who Are Close to Death 407**
Expected Physiologic Changes 407
The Death Vigil 409
After-Death Care 409
Grief, Mourning, and Bereavement 410
**Coping With Death and Dying: Professional
Caregiver Issues 412**

UNIT 4
**Perioperative Concepts and
Nursing Management 416**

17 Preoperative Nursing Management 418
Perioperative Nursing 418
Technology and Anesthesia 419
Surgical Classifications 419
Preadmission Testing 419
**Special Considerations During the Perioperative
Period 419**
Gerontologic Considerations 419
Bariatric Patients 421
Patients With Disabilities 421
Patients Undergoing Ambulatory Surgery 422
Patients Undergoing Emergency Surgery 422
Informed Consent 422
Preoperative Assessment 423
Nutritional and Fluid Status 424
Dentition 424
Drug or Alcohol Use 424
Respiratory Status 425
Cardiovascular Status 426

Hepatic and Renal Function 426
Endocrine Function 426
Immune Function 426
Previous Medication Use 426
Psychosocial Factors 427
Spiritual and Cultural Beliefs 427
Preoperative Nursing Interventions 428
Providing Patient Education 428
Providing Psychosocial Interventions 431
Maintaining Patient Safety 432
Managing Nutrition and Fluids 432
Preparing the Bowel 432
Preparing the Skin 432
**Immediate Preoperative Nursing
Interventions 432**
Administering Preanesthetic Medication 432
Maintaining the Preoperative Record 433
Transporting the Patient to the
Presurgical Area 433
Attending to Family Needs 434
Expected Patient Outcomes 434

18 Intraoperative Nursing Management 436
The Surgical Team 436
The Patient 437
The Circulating Nurse 438
The Scrub Role 438
The Surgeon 438
The Registered Nurse First Assistant 439
The Anesthesiologist and CRNA 439
The Surgical Environment 440
Principles of Surgical Asepsis 441
Robotics 442
Health Hazards Associated With the Surgical
Environment 442
The Surgical Experience 443
Types of Anesthesia and Sedation 443
Potential Intraoperative Complications 449
Anesthesia Awareness 449
Nausea and Vomiting 450
Anaphylaxis 450
Hypoxia and Other Respiratory Complications 450
Hypothermia 450
Malignant Hyperthermia 450
Pathophysiology 451
Clinical Manifestations 451
Medical Management 451
Nursing Management 451
• *Nursing Process:* The Patient During Surgery 451

19 Postoperative Nursing Management 456
**Care of the Patient in the Postanesthesia
Care Unit 456**
Phases of Postanesthesia Care 456
Admitting the Patient to the Postanesthesia
Care Unit 457
Nursing Management in the Postanesthesia
Care Unit 457
Preparing the Postoperative Patient for
Direct Discharge 461

Care of the Hospitalized Postoperative
Patient 463
    Receiving the Patient in the Clinical
        Unit 463
    Nursing Management After Surgery 463

• *Nursing Process:* The Hospitalized Patient Recovering
    From Surgery 464

Gas Exchange and Respiratory Function 478

20 Assessment of Respiratory Function 480
Anatomic and Physiologic Overview 480
    Anatomy of the Respiratory System 481
    Function of the Respiratory System 483
    Gerontologic Considerations 488
Assessment 488
    Health History 488
    Physical Assessment of the Respiratory
        System 492
    Assessment of Respiratory Function in the
        Acutely or Critically Ill Patient 500
Diagnostic Evaluation 502
    Pulmonary Function Tests 502
    Arterial Blood Gas Studies 502
    Venous Blood Gas Studies 502
    Pulse Oximetry 503
    Cultures 503
    Sputum Studies 503
    Imaging Studies 504
    Endoscopic Procedures 505
    Biopsy 507

21 Respiratory Care Modalities 510
NONINVASIVE RESPIRATORY THERAPIES 511
Oxygen Therapy 511
    Indications 511
    Complications 512
    Methods of Oxygen Administration 512
    Gerontologic Considerations 515
    Nursing Management 515
**Incentive Spirometry (Sustained Maximal
    Inspiration) 516**
    Indications 516
    Nursing Management 516
**Small-Volume Nebulizer (Mini-Nebulizer)
    Therapy 517**
    Indications 517
    Nursing Management 517
Chest Physiotherapy 517
    Postural Drainage (Segmented Bronchial
        Drainage) 517
    Nursing Management 519
    Chest Percussion and Vibration 519
    Nursing Management 520
    Breathing Retraining 521
    Nursing Management 521

AIRWAY MANAGEMENT 521
**Emergency Management of Upper Airway
    Obstruction 521**
Endotracheal Intubation 521
Tracheostomy 523
    Procedure 523
    Complications 524
    Nursing Management 524
Mechanical Ventilation 525
    Indications 525
    Classification of Ventilators 525
    Ventilator Modes 527
    Adjusting the Ventilator 528
    Monitoring the Equipment 529

• *Nursing Process:* The Patient Receiving
    Mechanical Ventilation 529

    Weaning the Patient from the Ventilator 535
THE PATIENT UNDERGOING THORACIC SURGERY 537
Preoperative Management 537
    Assessment and Diagnostic Findings 537
    Preoperative Nursing Management 537
Postoperative Management 539
    Mechanical Ventilation 540
    Chest Drainage 540
    Postoperative Nursing Management 542

22 Management of Patients With Upper Respiratory
Tract Disorders 552
UPPER AIRWAY INFECTIONS 552
Rhinitis 553
    Pathophysiology 553
    Clinical Manifestations 554
    Medical Management 554
    Nursing Management 555
Viral Rhinitis (Common Cold) 555
    Clinical Manifestations 555
    Medical Management 555
    Nursing Management 556
Rhinosinusitis 556
    Acute Rhinosinusitis 556
    Pathophysiology 556
    Clinical Manifestations 557
    Assessment and Diagnostic Findings 557
    Complications 557
    Medical Management 557
    Nursing Management 558
    Chronic Rhinosinusitis and Recurrent Acute Rhinosinusitis 559
    Pathophysiology 559
    Clinical Manifestations 559
    Assessment and Diagnostic Findings 559
    Complications 559
    Medical Management 560
    Nursing Management 560
Pharyngitis 560
    Acute Pharyngitis 560
    Pathophysiology 561
    Clinical Manifestations 561
    Assessment and Diagnostic Findings 561
    Medical Management 561
    Nursing Management 562

Chronic Pharyngitis 562
  Clinical Manifestations 562
  Medical Management 562
  Nursing Management 562
Tonsillitis and Adenoiditis 562
  Clinical Manifestations 563
  Assessment and Diagnostic Findings 563
  Medical Management 563
  Nursing Management 563
Peritonsillar Abscess 564
  Clinical Manifestations 564
  Assessment and Diagnostic Findings 564
  Medical Management 564
  Nursing Management 564
Laryngitis 565
  Clinical Manifestations 565
  Medical Management 565
  Nursing Management 565

  • *Nursing Process:* The Patient With Upper Airway
  Infection 565

**OBSTRUCTION AND TRAUMA OF THE UPPER
RESPIRATORY AIRWAY 567**
Obstructive Sleep Apnea 567
  Pathophysiology 567
  Clinical Manifestations 568
  Assessment and Diagnostic Findings 568
  Medical Management 568
  Nursing Management 569
Epistaxis (Nosebleed) 569
  Medical Management 569
  Nursing Management 569
Nasal Obstruction 570
  Medical Management 570
  Nursing Management 570
Fractures of the Nose 570
  Clinical Manifestations 570
  Assessment and Diagnostic Findings 571
  Medical Management 571
  Nursing Management 571
Laryngeal Obstruction 571
  Clinical Manifestations 572
  Assessment and Diagnostic Findings 572
  Medical Management 572
Cancer of the Larynx 572
  Clinical Manifestations 572
  Assessment and Diagnostic Findings 572
  Medical Management 573

  • *Nursing Process:* The Patient Undergoing
  Laryngectomy 575

23 Management of Patients With
  Chest and Lower Respiratory
  Tract Disorders 583
ATELECTASIS 584
  Pathophysiology 584
  Clinical Manifestations 584
  Assessment and Diagnostic Findings 584
  Prevention 584
  Management 585

RESPIRATORY INFECTIONS 586
Acute Tracheobronchitis 586
  Pathophysiology 586
  Clinical Manifestations 586
  Medical Management 586
  Nursing Management 587
Pneumonia 587
  Classification 587
  Pathophysiology 589
  Risk Factors 590
  Clinical Manifestations 590
  Assessment and Diagnostic Findings 590
  Prevention 592
  Medical Management 592
  Gerontologic Considerations 596
  Complications 596

  • *Nursing Process:* The Patient With Pneumonia 596

Aspiration 599
  Pathophysiology 599
  Prevention 599
Pulmonary Tuberculosis 600
  Transmission and Risk Factors 600
  Pathophysiology 600
  Clinical Manifestations 601
  Assessment and Diagnostic Findings 601
  Gerontologic Considerations 602
  Medical Management 602
  Nursing Management 604
Lung Abscess 605
  Pathophysiology 605
  Clinical Manifestations 605
  Assessment and Diagnostic Findings 605
  Prevention 606
  Medical Management 606
  Nursing Management 606

PLEURAL CONDITIONS 606
Pleurisy 606
  Pathophysiology 606
  Clinical Manifestations 607
  Assessment and Diagnostic Findings 607
  Medical Management 607
  Nursing Management 607
Pleural Effusion 607
  Pathophysiology 607
  Clinical Manifestations 607
  Assessment and Diagnostic Findings 607
  Medical Management 608
  Nursing Management 608
Empyema 608
  Pathophysiology 608
  Clinical Manifestations 608
  Assessment and Diagnostic Findings 608
  Medical Management 608
  Nursing Management 609
Pulmonary Edema (Noncardiogenic) 609
Acute Respiratory Failure 609
  Pathophysiology 609
  Clinical Manifestations 609
  Medical Management 610
  Nursing Management 610

Acute Respiratory Distress Syndrome 610
  Pathophysiology 610
  Clinical Manifestations 611
  Assessment and Diagnostic Findings 611
  Medical Management 611
  Nursing Management 611
Pulmonary Hypertension 613
  Pathophysiology 613
  Clinical Manifestations 613
  Assessment and Diagnostic Findings 613
  Medical Management 614
  Nursing Management 614
  Pulmonary Heart Disease
    (Cor Pulmonale) 614
Pulmonary Embolism 614
  Pathophysiology 615
  Clinical Manifestations 615
  Assessment and Diagnostic Findings 615
  Prevention 616
  Medical Management 616
  Nursing Management 617
Sarcoidosis 618
  Pathophysiology 618
  Clinical Manifestations 618
  Assessment and Diagnostic Findings 619
  Medical Management 619
OCCUPATIONAL LUNG DISEASES: PNEUMOCONIOSES 619
CHEST TUMORS 620
Lung Cancer (Bronchogenic Carcinoma) 620
  Pathophysiology 621
  Classification and Staging 621
  Risk Factors 621
  Clinical Manifestations 622
  Assessment and Diagnostic Findings 622
  Medical Management 623
  Treatment-Related Complications 624
  Nursing Management 624
  Gerontologic Considerations 624
Tumors of the Mediastinum 624
  Clinical Manifestations 624
  Assessment and Diagnostic Findings 625
  Medical Management 625
CHEST TRAUMA 625
Blunt Trauma 626
  Pathophysiology 626
  Assessment and Diagnostic Findings 626
  Medical Management 626
Sternal and Rib Fractures 626
  Clinical Manifestations 627
  Assessment and Diagnostic Findings 627
  Medical Management 627
Flail Chest 627
  Pathophysiology 627
  Medical Management 627
Pulmonary Contusion 628
  Pathophysiology 628
  Clinical Manifestations 628
  Assessment and Diagnostic Findings 628
  Medical Management 628
Penetrating Trauma 629
  Medical Management 629

Pneumothorax 629
  Types of Pneumothorax 629
  Clinical Manifestations 630
  Medical Management 630
Cardiac Tamponade 631
Subcutaneous Emphysema 631

24 Management of Patients With Chronic
Pulmonary Disease 634
Chronic Obstructive Pulmonary Disease 634
  Pathophysiology 635
  Risk Factors 636
  Clinical Manifestations 637
  Assessment and Diagnostic Findings 637
  Complications 638
  Medical Management 638
  Nursing Management 645
Bronchiectasis 648
  Pathophysiology 648
  Clinical Manifestations 648
  Assessment and Diagnostic Findings 648
  Medical Management 648
  Nursing Management 654
Asthma 654
  Pathophysiology 655
  Clinical Manifestations 655
  Assessment and Diagnostic Findings 655
  Prevention 656
  Complications 656
  Medical Management 656
  Nursing Management 663
Status Asthmaticus 664
  Pathophysiology 664
  Clinical Manifestations 664
  Assessment and Diagnostic Findings 664
  Medical Management 664
  Nursing Management 665
Cystic Fibrosis 665
  Pathophysiology 665
  Clinical Manifestations 666
  Assessment and Diagnostic Findings 666
  Medical Management 666
  Nursing Management 667

UNIT 6 Cardiovascular and Circulatory
Function 670

25 Assessment of Cardiovascular
Function 672
Anatomic and Physiologic Overview 673
  Anatomy of the Heart 673
  Function of the Heart 675
  Gerontologic Considerations 678
  Gender Considerations 678
Assessment of the Cardiovascular System 678
  Health History 679
  Physical Assessment 685

Diagnostic Evaluation 693
 Laboratory Tests 693
 Chest X-Ray and Fluoroscopy 695
 Electrocardiography 695
 Cardiac Stress Testing 699
 Radionuclide Imaging 700
 Additional Imaging 701
 Echocardiography 702
 Cardiac Catheterization 703
 Electrophysiologic Testing 705
 Hemodynamic Monitoring 705

26 Management of Patients With Dysrhythmias and Conduction Problems 712
DYSRHYTHMIAS 713
Normal Electrical Conduction 713
Influences on Heart Rate and Contractility 713
The Electrocardiogram 713
 Obtaining an Electrocardiogram 713
 Components of the Electrocardiogram 715
Analyzing the Electrocardiogram Rhythm Strip 716
 Determining Heart Rate from the Electrocardiogram 717
 Determining Heart Rhythm from the Electrocardiogram 717
Normal Sinus Rhythm 718
Types of Dysrhythmias 718
 Sinus Node Dysrhythmias 718
 Atrial Dysrhythmias 720
 Junctional Dysrhythmias 727
 Ventricular Dysrhythmias 729
 Conduction Abnormalities 732

 • *Nursing Process:* The Patient With a Dysrhythmia 734

ADJUNCTIVE MODALITIES AND MANAGEMENT 736
Cardioversion and Defibrillation 737
 Electrical Cardioversion 737
 Defibrillation 738
Electrophysiology Studies 738
Pacemaker Therapy 739
 Pacemaker Design and Types 739
 Pacemaker Generator Functions 741
 Complications of Pacemaker Use 742
 Pacemaker Surveillance 744
Implantable Cardioverter Defibrillator 744
 Nursing Management 746

27 Management of Patients With Coronary Vascular Disorders 750
Coronary Artery Disease 750
Coronary Atherosclerosis 751
 Pathophysiology 751
 Clinical Manifestations 751
 Risk Factors 752
 Prevention 753
 Gender 757
Angina Pectoris 757
 Pathophysiology 757

Clinical Manifestations 758
 Assessment and Diagnostic Findings 758
 Medical Management 758
 • *Nursing Process:* The Patient With Angina Pectoris 760
Acute Coronary Syndrome and Myocardial Infarction 762
 Pathophysiology 762
 Clinical Manifestations 763
 Assessment and Diagnostic Findings 763
 Medical Management 765
 Cardiac Rehabilitation 766
 • *Nursing Process:* The Patient With Acute Coronary Syndrome 767
INVASIVE CORONARY ARTERY PROCEDURES 771
Percutaneous Coronary Interventions 771
 Types of Procedures 771
 Complications 772
 Postprocedure Care 772
Surgical Procedures: Coronary Artery Revascularization 773
 Traditional Coronary Artery Bypass Graft 773
 Alternative Coronary Artery Bypass Graft Techniques 775
 Complications of Coronary Artery Bypass Graft 775
 Nursing Management 775

28 Management of Patients With Structural, Infectious, and Inflammatory Cardiac Disorders 791
VALVULAR DISORDERS 791
Mitral Valve Prolapse 792
 Pathophysiology 792
 Clinical Manifestations 792
 Assessment and Diagnostic Findings 793
 Medical Management 793
 Nursing Management 793
Mitral Regurgitation 793
 Pathophysiology 793
 Clinical Manifestations 793
 Assessment and Diagnostic Findings 793
 Medical Management 794
Mitral Stenosis 794
 Pathophysiology 794
 Clinical Manifestations 794
 Assessment and Diagnostic Findings 794
 Prevention 794
 Medical Management 794
Aortic Regurgitation 794
 Pathophysiology 794
 Clinical Manifestations 795
 Assessment and Diagnostic Findings 795
 Prevention 795
 Medical Management 795
Aortic Stenosis 795
 Pathophysiology 795
 Clinical Manifestations 795
 Assessment and Diagnostic Findings 796

Prevention 796
Medical Management 796
**Nursing Management: Valvular Heart
Disorders 796**
**SURGICAL MANAGEMENT: VALVE REPAIR AND REPLACEMENT
PROCEDURES 796**
Valvuloplasty 796
Commissurotomy 797
Annuloplasty 798
Leaflet Repair 798
Chordoplasty 798
Valve Replacement 799
Mechanical Valves 800
Tissue Valves 800
**Nursing Management: Valvuloplasty and Valve
Replacement 800**
Cardiomyopathy 801
Pathophysiology 801
Clinical Manifestations 803
Assessment and Diagnostic Findings 803
Medical Management 803
Surgical Management 804

• *Nursing Process:* The Patient With Cardiomyopathy 807

INFECTIOUS DISEASES OF THE HEART 809
Rheumatic Endocarditis 809
Infective Endocarditis 810
Pathophysiology 810
Clinical Manifestations 810
Assessment and Diagnostic Findings 811
Prevention 811
Medical Management 811
Surgical Management 812
Nursing Management 812
Myocarditis 812
Pathophysiology 812
Clinical Manifestations 813
Assessment and Diagnostic Findings 813
Prevention 813
Medical Management 813
Nursing Management 813
Pericarditis 813
Pathophysiology 814
Clinical Manifestations 814
Assessment and Diagnostic Findings 814
Medical Management 814
Nursing Management 814

• *Nursing Process:* The Patient With Pericarditis 815

**29 Management of Patients With Complications
From Heart Disease 818**
HEART FAILURE 818
Chronic Heart Failure 819
Etiology 819
Pathophysiology 820
Clinical Manifestations 821
Assessment and Diagnostic Findings 823
Medical Management 823
Gerontologic Considerations 828

• *Nursing Process:* The Patient With Heart Failure 828

Pulmonary Edema 833
Pathophysiology 833
Clinical Manifestations 834
Assessment and Diagnostic Findings 834
Prevention 834
Medical Management 834
Nursing Management 834
OTHER COMPLICATIONS 835
Cardiogenic Shock 835
Medical Management 835
Nursing Management 835
Thromboembolism 835
Pulmonary Embolism 835
**Pericardial Effusion and Cardiac
Tamponade 836**
Pathophysiology 836
Clinical Manifestations 836
Assessment and Diagnostic Findings 836
Medical Management 836
Cardiac Arrest 837
Clinical Manifestations 837
Emergency Assessment and Management:
Cardiopulmonary Resuscitation 837

**30 Assessment and Management of Patients With
Vascular Disorders and Problems of Peripheral
Circulation 841**
Anatomic and Physiologic Overview 841
Anatomy of the Vascular System 842
Function of the Vascular System 843
Pathophysiology of the Vascular System 844
Gerontologic Considerations 845
Assessment of the Vascular System 845
Health History 845
Physical Assessment 846
Diagnostic Evaluation 847
Doppler Ultrasound Flow Studies 847
Exercise Testing 848
Duplex Ultrasonography 848
Computed Tomography Scanning 849
Angiography 849
Magnetic Resonance Angiography 849
Contrast Phlebography (Venography) 849
Lymphoscintigraphy 849
ARTERIAL DISORDERS 850
Arteriosclerosis and Atherosclerosis 850
Pathophysiology 850
Risk Factors 851
Prevention 852
Clinical Manifestations 852
Medical Management 852
Nursing Management 852
Peripheral Arterial Occlusive Disease 857
Clinical Manifestations 857
Assessment and Diagnostic Findings 858
Medical Management 858
Nursing Management 860
Upper Extremity Arterial Occlusive Disease 860
Clinical Manifestations 860
Assessment and Diagnostic Findings 861

Medical Management 861
Nursing Management 861
Aortoiliac Disease 861
Medical Management 861
Nursing Management 861
Aneurysms 862
Thoracic Aortic Aneurysm 862
Clinical Manifestations 862
Assessment and Diagnostic Findings 862
Medical Management 862
Abdominal Aortic Aneurysm 863
Pathophysiology 863
Clinical Manifestations 863
Assessment and Diagnostic Findings 863
Gerontologic Considerations 863
Medical Management 864
Nursing Management 864
Other Aneurysms 864
Dissecting Aorta 865
Pathophysiology 865
Clinical Manifestations 865
Assessment and Diagnostic Findings 865
Medical Management 865
Nursing Management 865
Arterial Embolism and Arterial Thrombosis 865
Pathophysiology 865
Clinical Manifestations 865
Assessment and Diagnostic Findings 866
Medical Management 866
Nursing Management 867
**Raynaud Phenomenon and Other
Acrosyndromes 867**
Clinical Manifestations 867
Medical Management 867
Nursing Management 867
VENOUS DISORDERS 868
Venous Thromboembolism 868
Pathophysiology 868
Clinical Manifestations 869
Assessment and Diagnostic Findings 869
Prevention 870
Medical Management 870
Nursing Management 871
**Chronic Venous Insufficiency/Postthrombotic
Syndrome 873**
Clinical Manifestations 874
Complications 874
Medical and Nursing Management 874
Leg Ulcers 874
Pathophysiology 874
Clinical Manifestations 874
Assessment and Diagnostic Findings 875
Medical Management 875
• *Nursing Process:* The Patient With Leg Ulcers 877
Varicose Veins 878
Pathophysiology 878
Clinical Manifestations 878
Assessment and Diagnostic Findings 878
Prevention and Medical Management 878
Nursing Management 879

LYMPHATIC DISORDERS 880
Lymphangitis and Lymphadenitis 880
Lymphedema and Elephantiasis 880
Medical Management 880
Nursing Management 881
CELLULITIS 881
Pathophysiology 881
Clinical Manifestations 881
Medical Management 881
Nursing Management 881

**31 Assessment and Management of Patients
With Hypertension 884**
Hypertension 884
Pathophysiology 885
Clinical Manifestations 887
Assessment and Diagnostic Findings 887
Medical Management 887
• *Nursing Process:* The Patient With Hypertension 894
Hypertensive Crises 897

UNIT 7 **Hematologic Function** 900

**32 Assessment of Hematologic Function and
Treatment Modalities 902**
Anatomic and Physiologic Overview 903
Structure and Function of the Hematologic System 903
Bone Marrow 903
Blood Cells 905
Plasma and Plasma Proteins 908
Reticuloendothelial System (RES) 908
Hemostasis 908
Gerontologic Considerations 909
Assessment 909
Health History 909
Physical Assessment 909
Diagnostic Evaluation 909
Hematologic Studies 909
Bone Marrow Aspiration and Biopsy 910
**Therapeutic Approaches to Hematologic
Disorders 913**
Splenectomy 913
Therapeutic Apheresis 913
Hematopoietic Stem Cell Transplantation 914
Therapeutic Phlebotomy 914
Blood Component Therapy 914
Special Preparations 914
Procuring Blood and Blood Products 914
Blood Donation 914
Complications of Blood Donation 916
Blood Processing 916
Transfusion 917
Setting 918
Pretransfusion Assessment 918
Patient Education 919
Complications 919

Nursing Management for Transfusion
Reactions 921
Pharmacologic Alternatives to Blood
Transfusions 922

33 Management of Patients With Nonmalignant
Hematologic Disorders 925
ANEMIA 925
Classification of Anemias 925
Clinical Manifestations 926
Assessment and Diagnostic Findings 927
Complications 927
Medical Management 927
Gerontologic Considerations 927

• *Nursing Process:* The Patient With Anemia 928

Hypoproliferative Anemias 930
Iron Deficiency Anemia 930
Clinical Manifestations 930
Assessment and Diagnostic Findings 930
Medical Management 930
Nursing Management 931
Anemias in Renal Disease 931
Anemia of Inflammation 932
Aplastic Anemia 932
Pathophysiology 932
Clinical Manifestations 932
Assessment and Diagnostic
Findings 932
Medical Management 932
Nursing Management 933
Megaloblastic Anemias 933
Pathophysiology 933
Clinical Manifestations 933
Assessment and Diagnostic Findings 934
Medical Management 934
Nursing Management 934
Hemolytic Anemias 934
Sickle Cell Disease 935
Clinical Manifestations 935
Assessment and Diagnostic Findings 937
Prognosis 937
Medical Management 937

• *Nursing Process:* The Patient With Sickle
Cell Crisis 939

Thalassemias 941
Glucose-6-Phosphate Dehydrogenase
Deficiency 942
Clinical Manifestations 942
Assessment and Diagnostic Findings 942
Medical Management 942
Nursing Management 942
Immune Hemolytic Anemias 943
Clinical Manifestations 943
Assessment and Diagnostic Findings 943
Medical Management 943
Nursing Management 943
Hereditary Hemochromatosis 944
Clinical Manifestations 944
Assessment and Diagnostic Findings 944

Medical Management 944
Nursing Management 944
POLYCYTHEMIA 944
Secondary Polycythemia 945
Medical Management 945
NEUTROPENIA 945
Clinical Manifestations 945
Medical Management 945
Nursing Management 945
LYMPHOPENIA 946
BLEEDING DISORDERS 947
Clinical Manifestations 947
Medical Management 947
Nursing Management 947
Secondary Thrombocytosis 948
Thrombocytopenia 948
Clinical Manifestations 948
Assessment and Diagnostic
Findings 949
Medical Management 949
Nursing Management 949
Immune Thrombocytopenic Purpura 949
Pathophysiology 949
Clinical Manifestations 949
Assessment and Diagnostic Findings 949
Medical Management 950
Nursing Management 950
Platelet Defects 951
Clinical Manifestations 951
Medical Management 951
Nursing Management 951
Hemophilia 951
Clinical Manifestations 951
Medical Management 953
Nursing Management 953
Gerontologic Considerations 954
Von Willebrand Disease (vWD) 954
Clinical Manifestations 954
Assessment and Diagnostic Findings 955
Medical Management 955
ACQUIRED COAGULATION DISORDERS 956
Liver Disease 956
Vitamin K Deficiency 956
Disseminated Intravascular Coagulation 956
Pathophysiology 956
Clinical Manifestations 956
Assessment and Diagnostic Findings 956
Medical Management 958
Nursing Management 959
Thrombotic Disorders 959
Hyperhomocysteinemia 959
Antithrombin Deficiency 959
Protein C Deficiency 961
Protein S Deficiency 962
Activated Protein C Resistance and Factor V
Leiden Mutation 962
Acquired Thrombophilias 962
Etiology 962
Medical Management 963
Nursing Management 965

34 Management of Patients With Hematologic Neoplasms 970

CLONAL STEM CELL DISORDERS 971

LEUKEMIA 971

Acute Myeloid Leukemia 971
Clinical Manifestations 972
Assessment and Diagnostic Findings 972
Medical Management 972
Complications 973
Nursing Management 974

Chronic Myeloid Leukemia 974
Clinical Manifestations 974
Medical Management 974
Nursing Management 974

Acute Lymphocytic Leukemia 975
Clinical Manifestations 975
Medical Management 976
Nursing Management 976

Chronic Lymphocytic Leukemia 976
Pathophysiology 976
Clinical Manifestations 977
Medical Management 977

• Nursing Process: The Patient With Acute Leukemia 978

MYELODYSPLASTIC SYNDROMES (MDS) 981
Clinical Manifestations 982
Assessment and Diagnostic Findings 982
Medical Management 982
Nursing Management 983

MYELOPROLIFERATIVE NEOPLASMS 984
Polycythemia Vera 984
Clinical Manifestations 984
Assessment and Diagnostic Findings 984
Complications 984
Medical Management 984
Nursing Management 985

Essential Thrombocythemia 985
Clinical Manifestations 986
Assessment and Diagnostic Findings 986
Complications 986
Medical Management 986
Nursing Management 987

Primary Myelofibrosis 987
Medical Management 988
Nursing Management 988

LYMPHOMA 988
Hodgkin Lymphoma 988
Pathophysiology 989
Clinical Manifestations 989
Assessment and Diagnostic Findings 989
Medical Management 990
Nursing Management 991

Non-Hodgkin Lymphomas 991
Clinical Manifestations 991
Assessment and Diagnostic Findings 991
Medical Management 992
Nursing Management 992

MULTIPLE MYELOMA 993
Pathophysiology 993
Clinical Manifestations 994

Assessment and Diagnostic Findings 995
Medical Management 995
Gerontologic Considerations 997
Nursing Management 997

UNIT 8 Immunologic Function 1002

35 Assessment of Immune Function 1004

Anatomic and Physiologic Overview 1005
Anatomy of the Immune System 1005
Function of the Immune System 1006

Advances in Immunology 1013
Genetic Engineering 1013
Stem Cells 1013
Cancer and Immunotherapy 1013

Assessment of the Immune System 1014
Health History 1014
Physical Assessment 1018

Diagnostic Evaluation 1019
Nursing Management 1019

36 Management of Patients With Immune Deficiency Disorders 1022

PRIMARY IMMUNE DEFICIENCIES 1022
Pathophysiology 1023
Clinical Manifestations 1023
Assessment and Diagnostic Findings 1023
Prevention 1023
Medical Management 1023
Nursing Management 1023

ACQUIRED IMMUNE DEFICIENCY 1025
HIV Infection and AIDS 1025
Epidemiology 1025
HIV Transmission 1026
Gerontologic Considerations 1027
Prevention of HIV Infection 1027
Reducing the Risk of Transmission to Health Care Providers 1029
Pathophysiology 1030
Stages of HIV Infection 1031
Assessment and Diagnostic Findings in HIV Infection 1031
Treatment of HIV Infection 1033
Clinical Manifestations 1037
Medical Management 1041
Complementary, Alternative, and Integrative Health Therapies 1042
Supportive Care 1043

• Nursing Process: The Patient With HIV/AIDS 1043

Emotional and Ethical Concerns 1053

37 Assessment and Management of Patients With Allergic Disorders 1057

ALLERGIC ASSESSMENT 1058
Physiologic Overview 1058
Function of Immunoglobulins 1058
Function of Antigens 1058

Function of Chemical Mediators 1058
Hypersensitivity 1060
Assessment 1061
Diagnostic Evaluation 1061
Complete Blood Count With Differential 1061
Eosinophil Count 1061
Total Serum Immunoglobulin E Levels 1061
Skin Tests 1061
Provocative Testing 1064
Serum-Specific IgE Test 1064
ALLERGIC DISORDERS 1064
Anaphylaxis 1064
Pathophysiology 1064
Clinical Manifestations 1065
Prevention 1065
Medical Management 1066
Nursing Management 1066
Allergic Rhinitis 1066
Pathophysiology 1067
Clinical Manifestations 1067
Assessment and Diagnostic Findings 1067
Medical Management 1067

• *Nursing Process:* The Patient With Allergic Rhinitis 1071

Contact Dermatitis 1074
Clinical Manifestations 1074
Assessment and Diagnostic Findings 1074
Atopic Dermatitis 1074
Medical Management 1075
Nursing Management 1075
Dermatitis Medicamentosa (Drug Reactions) 1075
Urticaria and Angioneurotic Edema 1075
Hereditary Angioedema 1076
Clinical Manifestations 1076
Medical Management 1076
Cold Urticaria 1076
Clinical Manifestations 1076
Medical Management 1076
Food Allergy 1077
Clinical Manifestations 1077
Assessment and Diagnostic Findings 1077
Medical Management 1077
Nursing Management 1077
Latex Allergy 1078
Clinical Manifestations 1079
Assessment and Diagnostic Findings 1079
Medical Management 1079
Nursing Management 1079

38 Assessment and Management of Patients With Rheumatic Disorders 1082
Rheumatic Diseases 1082
Pathophysiology 1083
Clinical Manifestations 1084
Assessment and Diagnostic Findings 1084
Medical Management 1084
Nursing Management 1087
Gerontologic Considerations 1087
Diffuse Connective Tissue Diseases 1090
Rheumatoid Arthritis 1093
Pathophysiology 1093

Clinical Manifestations 1094
Assessment and Diagnostic Findings 1094
Medical Management 1095
Nursing Management 1096
Systemic Lupus Erythematosus 1098
Pathophysiology 1098
Clinical Manifestations 1098
Assessment and Diagnostic Findings 1099
Medical Management 1100
Nursing Management 1100
Sjögren's Syndrome 1101
Pathophysiology 1101
Clinical Manifestations 1101
Assessment and Diagnostic Findings 1101
Medical Management 1101
Nursing Management 1101
Scleroderma 1101
Pathophysiology 1102
Clinical Manifestations 1102
Assessment and Diagnostic Findings 1102
Medical Management 1102
Nursing Management 1102
Polymyositis 1102
Pathophysiology 1103
Clinical Manifestations 1103
Assessment and Diagnostic Findings 1103
Medical Management 1103
Nursing Management 1103
Polymyalgia Rheumatica and Giant Cell Arteritis 1103
Pathophysiology 1103
Clinical Manifestations 1103
Assessment and Diagnostic Findings 1103
Medical Management 1104
Nursing Management 1104
Osteoarthritis (Degenerative Joint Disease) 1104
Pathophysiology 1104
Clinical Manifestations 1105
Assessment and Diagnostic Findings 1105
Medical Management 1105
Nursing Management 1106
Spondyloarthropathies 1106
Ankylosing Spondylitis 1106
Reactive Arthritis (Reiter's Syndrome) 1106
Psoriatic Arthritis 1106
Medical Management 1107
Nursing Management 1107
Metabolic and Endocrine Diseases Associated With Rheumatic Disorders 1107
Gout 1107
Pathophysiology 1107
Clinical Manifestations 1108
Medical Management 1108
Nursing Management 1108
Fibromyalgia 1109
Pathophysiology 1109
Assessment and Diagnostic Findings 1109
Medical Management 1109
Nursing Management 1109
Miscellaneous Disorders 1109

UNIT 9 Musculoskeletal Function 1112

39 Assessment of Musculoskeletal Function 1114
Anatomic and Physiologic Overview 1115
Structure and Function of the Skeletal
System 1115
Structure and Function of the Articular
System 1117
Structure and Function of the Skeletal Muscle
System 1118
Gerontologic Considerations 1119
Assessment 1119
Health History 1119
Physical Assessment 1122
Diagnostic Evaluation 1126
X-Ray Studies 1126
Computed Tomography 1127
Magnetic Resonance Imaging 1127
Arthrography 1127
Bone Densitometry 1127
Bone Scan 1127
Arthroscopy 1128
Arthrocentesis 1128
Electromyography 1128
Biopsy 1129
Laboratory Studies 1129

40 Musculoskeletal Care Modalities 1131
The Patient in a Cast, Splint, or Brace 1131
Casts 1131
Splints and Braces 1133
Nursing Management of a Patient in a Cast,
Splint, or Brace 1133
Nursing Management of the Patient
With an Immobilized Upper Extremity 1136
Nursing Management of the Patient With an
Immobilized Lower Extremity 1136
Nursing Management of the Patient With a
Body or Spica Cast 1137
The Patient With an External Fixator 1137
Nursing Management 1138
The Patient in Traction 1139
Principles of Effective Traction 1139
Types of Traction 1140
Skin Traction 1140
Skeletal Traction 1141
Nursing Management 1143
The Patient Undergoing Orthopedic Surgery 1144
Joint Replacement 1144
Nursing Interventions 1145
Total Hip Arthroplasty 1147
Total Knee Arthroplasty 1154

• *Nursing Process:* Postoperative Care of the Patient
Undergoing Orthopedic Surgery 1155

41 Management of Patients With Musculoskeletal Disorders 1160
Low Back Pain 1160
Pathophysiology 1160

Clinical Manifestations 1161
Assessment and Diagnostic Findings 1161
Medical Management 1161
Nursing Assessment 1162
Nursing Management 1162
Common Upper Extremity Disorders 1164
Bursitis and Tendonitis 1164
Loose Bodies 1164
Impingement Syndrome 1164
Carpal Tunnel Syndrome 1164
Ganglion 1165
Dupuytren Disease 1165
Nursing Management of the Patient Undergoing Surgery of
the Hand or Wrist 1165
Common Foot Problems 1166
Callus 1166
Corn 1167
Hallux Valgus 1167
Hammer Toe 1167
Ingrown Toenail 1167
Morton Neuroma 1168
Pes Cavus 1168
Pes Planus 1168
Plantar Fasciitis 1168
Nursing Management of the Patient Undergoing
Foot Surgery 1168
Metabolic Bone Disorders 1169
Osteoporosis 1169
Prevention 1169
Gerontologic Considerations 1169
Pathophysiology 1170
Risk Factors 1170
Assessment and Diagnostic Findings 1171
Medical Management 1172

• *Nursing Process:* The Patient With a Spontaneous Vertebral
Fracture Related to Osteoporosis 1172
Osteomalacia 1174
Pathophysiology 1174
Gerontologic Considerations 1174
Assessment and Diagnostic Findings 1174
Medical Management 1175
Paget Disease of the Bone 1175
Pathophysiology 1175
Clinical Manifestations 1175
Assessment and Diagnostic Findings 1175
Medical Management 1175
Gerontologic Considerations 1176
Musculoskeletal Infections 1176
Osteomyelitis 1176
Pathophysiology 1176
Clinical Manifestations 1176
Assessment and Diagnostic Findings 1176
Prevention 1177
Medical Management 1177

• *Nursing Process:* The Patient With Osteomyelitis 1177

Septic (Infectious) Arthritis 1178
Clinical Manifestations 1178
Assessment and Diagnostic Findings 1178
Medical Management 1179
Nursing Management 1179

Bone Tumors 1179
   Types 1179
   Pathophysiology 1180
   Clinical Manifestations 1180
   Assessment and Diagnostic Findings 1180
   Medical Management 1181
   Nursing Management 1181

42 Management of Patients With Musculoskeletal
Trauma 1185
   Contusions, Strains, and Sprains 1185
      Nursing Management 1186
   Joint Dislocations 1186
      Medical Management 1186
      Nursing Management 1187
   Injuries to the Tendons, Ligaments, and
      Menisci 1187
      Rotator Cuff Tears 1187
      Lateral and Medial Epicondylitis 1187
      Lateral and Medial Collateral Ligament Injury 1187
      Medical Management 1188
      Nursing Management 1188
      Cruciate Ligament Injury 1188
      Meniscal Injuries 1188
      Rupture of the Achilles Tendon 1189
   Fractures 1189
      Types of Fractures 1189
      Clinical Manifestations 1189
      Emergency Management 1191
      Medical Management 1191
      Nursing Management 1192
      Fracture Healing and Complications 1193
   Fractures of Specific Sites 1198
      Clavicle 1198
      Humeral Neck 1198
      Humeral Shaft 1199
      Elbow 1199
      Radial Head 1200
      Radial and Ulnar Shafts 1200
      Wrist 1200
      Hand 1200
      Pelvis 1201
      Stable Pelvic Fractures 1201
      Unstable Pelvic Fractures 1202
      Acetabulum 1202
      Hip 1202
      Clinical Manifestations 1203
      Gerontologic Considerations 1203
      Medical Management 1203
      Nursing Management 1203
      Femoral Shaft 1210
      Assessment and Diagnostic Findings 1210
      Medical Management 1210
      Tibia and Fibula 1211
      Assessment and Diagnostic
         Findings 1211
      Medical Management 1211
      Rib 1211
      Gerontologic Considerations 1212
      Thoracolumbar Spine 1212

   Sports-Related Musculoskeletal
      Injuries 1212
      Management 1212
      Prevention 1212
   Occupation-Related Musculoskeletal
      Disorders 1212
      Prevention of Occupation-Related
         Musculoskeletal Disorders in Nursing
         Personnel 1214
   Amputation 1214
      Levels of Amputation 1214
      Complications 1215
      Medical Management 1215
      Rehabilitation 1215

   • *Nursing Process:* The Patient Undergoing an
      Amputation 1216

UNIT 10 Digestive and Gastrointestinal Function 1222

43 Assessment of Digestive and Gastrointestinal
Function 1224
   Anatomic and Physiologic Overview 1224
      Anatomy of the Gastrointestinal System 1224
      Function of the Digestive System 1226
      Gerontologic Considerations 1228
   Assessment of the Gastrointestinal
      System 1229
      Health History 1229
      Physical Assessment 1231
   Diagnostic Evaluation 1232
      Serum Laboratory Studies 1232
      Stool Tests 1233
      Breath Tests 1233
      Abdominal Ultrasonography 1233
      Genetic Testing 1234
      Imaging Studies 1234
      Endoscopic Procedures 1237
      Manometry and Electrophysiologic
         Studies 1240
      Gastric Analysis, Gastric Acid Stimulation Test,
         and pH Monitoring 1240
      Laparoscopy (Peritoneoscopy) 1241

44 Digestive and Gastrointestinal Treatment
Modalities 1243
   Gastrointestinal Intubation 1244
      Tube Types 1244
   Gastrostomy and Jejunostomy 1252

   • *Nursing Process:* The Patient With a Gastrostomy or
      Jejunostomy 1253

   Parenteral Nutrition 1256
      Establishing Positive Nitrogen Balance 1256
      Clinical Indications 1256
      Formulas 1257
      Initiating Therapy 1257

Administration Methods 1257
Discontinuing Parenteral Nutrition 1259

• *Nursing Process:* The Patient Receiving Parenteral
Nutrition 1259

45 Management of Patients With Oral and Esophageal Disorders 1264

DISORDERS OF THE ORAL CAVITY 1264
Dental Plaque and Caries 1265
Prevention 1265
Dental Health and Disease 1268
Periapical Abscess 1268
Clinical Manifestations 1268
Medical Management 1268
Nursing Management 1268
DISORDERS OF THE JAW 1269
Temporomandibular Disorders 1269
Clinical Manifestations 1269
Assessment and Diagnostic Findings 1269
Medical Management 1269
Jaw Disorders Requiring Surgical
Management 1269
Nursing Management 1269
DISORDERS OF THE SALIVARY GLANDS 1269
Parotitis 1270
Sialadenitis 1270
Salivary Calculus (Sialolithiasis) 1270
Neoplasms 1270
CANCER OF THE ORAL CAVITY AND PHARYNX 1270
Pathophysiology 1271
Clinical Manifestations 1271
Assessment and Diagnostic Findings 1271
Human Papillomavirus Prevention 1271
Medical Management 1271
Nursing Management 1271
**NURSING MANAGEMENT OF THE PATIENT WITH DISORDERS
OF THE ORAL CAVITY 1272**
Promoting Mouth Care 1272
Ensuring Adequate Food and Fluid Intake 1272
Minimizing Pain and Discomfort 1272
Preventing Infection 1272
Promoting Home, Community-Based, and
Transitional Care 1273
NECK DISSECTION 1274

• *Nursing Process:* The Patient Undergoing a Neck
Dissection 1274

DISORDERS OF THE ESOPHAGUS 1279
Achalasia 1279
Clinical Manifestations 1279
Assessment and Diagnostic Findings 1279
Management 1279
Esophageal Spasm 1279
Clinical Manifestations 1280
Assessment and Diagnostic Findings 1280
Management 1280
Hiatal Hernia 1280
Clinical Manifestations 1280
Assessment and Diagnostic Findings 1280
Management 1281

Diverticulum 1281
Clinical Manifestations 1281
Assessment and Diagnostic Findings 1281
Management 1282
Perforation 1282
Clinical Manifestations 1282
Assessment and Diagnostic Findings 1282
Management 1282
Foreign Bodies 1282
Chemical Burns 1283
Gastroesophageal Reflux Disease 1283
Clinical Manifestations 1283
Assessment and Diagnostic Findings 1283
Management 1283
Barrett Esophagus 1283
Clinical Manifestations 1283
Assessment and Diagnostic Findings 1283
Management 1284
Benign Tumors of the Esophagus 1284

• *Nursing Process:* The Patient With a Noncancerous
Condition of the Esophagus 1284

Cancer of the Esophagus 1286
Pathophysiology 1286
Clinical Manifestations 1287
Assessment and Diagnostic Findings 1287
Medical Management 1287
Nursing Management 1288

46 Management of Patients With Gastric and Duodenal Disorders 1292

Gastritis 1292
Pathophysiology 1293
Clinical Manifestations 1293
Assessment and Diagnostic Findings 1294
Medical Management 1294
Nursing Management 1294
Peptic Ulcer Disease 1296
Pathophysiology 1297
Clinical Manifestations 1298
Assessment and Diagnostic Findings 1298
Medical Management 1298

• *Nursing Process:* The Patient With Peptic Ulcer Disease 1301

Gastric Cancer 1303
Pathophysiology 1304
Clinical Manifestations 1304
Assessment and Diagnostic Findings 1304
Medical Management 1304
Gerontologic Considerations 1306

• *Nursing Process:* The Patient With Gastric Cancer 1306

Tumors of the Small Intestine 1308
Clinical Manifestations 1308
Assessment and Diagnostic Findings 1309
Management 1309

47 Management of Patients With Intestinal and Rectal Disorders 1311

ABNORMALITIES OF FECAL ELIMINATION 1312
Constipation 1312
Pathophysiology 1312

Clinical Manifestations 1312
Assessment and Diagnostic Findings 1313
Complications 1313
Gerontologic Considerations 1313
Medical Management 1313
Nursing Management 1313
Diarrhea 1314
Pathophysiology 1315
Clinical Manifestations 1315
Assessment and Diagnostic Findings 1315
Complications 1315
Gerontologic Considerations 1315
Medical Management 1316
Nursing Management 1316
Fecal Incontinence 1316
Pathophysiology 1316
Clinical Manifestations 1316
Assessment and Diagnostic Findings 1316
Medical Management 1316
Nursing Management 1317
Irritable Bowel Syndrome (IBS) 1317
Pathophysiology 1318
Clinical Manifestations 1318
Assessment and Diagnostic Findings 1318
Medical Management 1318
Nursing Management 1318
DISORDERS OF MALABSORPTION 1318
Celiac Disease 1319
Pathophysiology 1320
Clinical Manifestations 1320
Assessment and Diagnostic Findings 1321
Medical Management 1321
Nursing Management 1322
ACUTE ABDOMEN 1322
Peritonitis 1322
Pathophysiology 1322
Clinical Manifestations 1322
Assessment and Diagnostic Findings 1323
Medical Management 1323
Nursing Management 1323
Appendicitis 1323
Pathophysiology 1323
Clinical Manifestations 1323
Assessment and Diagnostic Findings 1324
Complications 1324
Gerontologic Considerations 1324
Medical Management 1324
Nursing Management 1324
Diverticular Disease 1325
Pathophysiology 1325
Clinical Manifestations 1325
Assessment and Diagnostic Findings 1326
Gerontologic Considerations 1326
Medical Management 1326
Nursing Management 1327
Intestinal Obstruction 1327
Small Bowel Obstruction 1327
Pathophysiology 1327
Clinical Manifestations 1328
Assessment and Diagnostic Findings 1328

Medical Management 1328
Nursing Management 1328
Large Bowel Obstruction 1329
Pathophysiology 1329
Clinical Manifestations 1329
Assessment and Diagnostic Findings 1329
Medical Management 1329
Nursing Management 1329
INFLAMMATORY BOWEL DISEASE 1329
Crohn's Disease (Regional Enteritis) 1330
Pathophysiology 1330
Clinical Manifestations 1331
Assessment and Diagnostic Findings 1331
Complications 1331
Ulcerative Colitis 1331
Pathophysiology 1331
Clinical Manifestations 1331
Assessment and Diagnostic Findings 1331
Complications 1332
Medical Management of Chronic Inflammatory
Bowel Disease 1332

• *Nursing Process:* Management of the Patient With Chronic
Inflammatory Bowel Disease 1334

**NURSING MANAGEMENT OF THE PATIENT REQUIRING AN
OSTOMY 1336**
COLORECTAL NEOPLASMS 1342
Colorectal Cancer 1343
Pathophysiology 1344
Clinical Manifestations 1344
Assessment and Diagnostic Findings 1344
Complications 1344
Gerontologic Considerations 1344
Prevention 1345
Medical Management 1345

• *Nursing Process:* The Patient With Colorectal Cancer 1347

Polyps of the Colon and Rectum 1349
DISORDERS OF THE ANORECTUM 1350
Proctitis 1350
Anorectal Abscess 1351
Anal Fistula 1351
Anal Fissure 1351
Hemorrhoids 1351
Pilonidal Sinus or Cyst 1352
Nursing Management of Patients
With Anorectal Disorders 1352

UNIT 11 Metabolic and Endocrine Function 1356

48 Assessment and Management of Patients
With Obesity 1358
Obesity 1358
Epidemiology of Obesity 1358
Obesity Risks 1359
Pathophysiology 1360

Assessment and Diagnostic Findings 1361
Medical Management 1362
Gerontologic Considerations 1366
Nursing Management 1367
Surgical Management 1368

- *Nursing Process:* The Patient Undergoing Bariatric
  Surgery 1369

49 Assessment and Management of Patients With
Hepatic Disorders 1377
ASSESSMENT OF THE LIVER 1377
Anatomic and Physiologic Overview 1377
Anatomy of the Liver 1378
Functions of the Liver 1379
Gerontologic Considerations 1380
Assessment 1380
Health History 1380
Physical Assessment 1380
Diagnostic Evaluation 1382
Liver Function Tests 1382
Liver Biopsy 1382
Other Diagnostic Tests 1382
MANIFESTATIONS OF HEPATIC DYSFUNCTION 1382
Jaundice 1384
Hemolytic Jaundice 1384
Hepatocellular Jaundice 1384
Obstructive Jaundice 1384
Hereditary Hyperbilirubinemia 1385
Portal Hypertension 1385
Ascites 1385
Pathophysiology 1385
Clinical Manifestations 1386
Assessment and Diagnostic Findings 1386
Medical Management 1386
Nursing Management 1388
Esophageal Varices 1388
Pathophysiology 1389
Clinical Manifestations 1389
Assessment and Diagnostic Findings 1389
Medical Management 1390
Surgical Management 1392
Nursing Management 1393
Hepatic Encephalopathy and Coma 1393
Pathophysiology 1394
Clinical Manifestations 1394
Assessment and Diagnostic Findings 1395
Medical Management 1395
Nursing Management 1396
Other Manifestations of Hepatic Dysfunction 1397
Edema and Bleeding 1397
Vitamin Deficiency 1397
Metabolic Abnormalities 1397
Pruritus and Other Skin Changes 1397
VIRAL HEPATITIS 1397
Hepatitis A Virus 1398
Clinical Manifestations 1399
Assessment and Diagnostic Findings 1399
Prevention 1399
Medical Management 1399
Nursing Management 1399

Hepatitis B Virus 1400
Gerontologic Considerations 1401
Clinical Manifestations 1401
Assessment and Diagnostic Findings 1401
Prevention 1401
Medical Management 1402
Nursing Management 1403
Hepatitis C Virus 1403
Hepatitis D Virus 1404
Hepatitis E Virus 1404
Hepatitis G Virus and GB Virus-C 1404
NONVIRAL HEPATITIS 1404
Toxic Hepatitis 1404
Drug-Induced Hepatitis 1405
FULMINANT HEPATIC FAILURE 1405
HEPATIC CIRRHOSIS 1406
Pathophysiology 1406
Clinical Manifestations 1406
Assessment and Diagnostic
Findings 1407
Medical Management 1408
Nursing Management 1408
CANCER OF THE LIVER 1417
Primary Liver Tumors 1417
Liver Metastases 1417
Clinical Manifestations 1417
Assessment and Diagnostic Findings 1417
Medical Management 1418
Surgical Management 1418
Nursing Management 1419
LIVER TRANSPLANTATION 1420
Surgical Procedure 1421
Complications 1422
Nursing Management 1423
LIVER ABSCESSES 1425
Pathophysiology 1425
Clinical Manifestations 1425
Assessment and Diagnostic Findings 1425
Medical Management 1425
Nursing Management 1425

50 Assessment and Management of Patients With
Biliary Disorders 1428
ANATOMIC AND PHYSIOLOGIC OVERVIEW 1428
The Gallbladder 1428
The Pancreas 1429
The Exocrine Pancreas 1429
The Endocrine Pancreas 1429
Endocrine Control of Carbohydrate
Metabolism 1430
Gerontologic Considerations 1430
DISORDERS OF THE GALLBLADDER 1430
Cholecystitis 1430
Cholelithiasis 1430
Pathophysiology 1430
Clinical Manifestations 1431
Assessment and Diagnostic Findings 1432
Medical Management 1434

- *Nursing Process:* The Patient Undergoing Surgery for
  Gallbladder Disease 1438

DISORDERS OF THE PANCREAS 1440

Acute Pancreatitis 1440
  Gerontologic Considerations 1441
  Pathophysiology 1441
  Clinical Manifestations 1441
  Assessment and Diagnostic Findings 1442
  Medical Management 1442
  Nursing Management 1443
Chronic Pancreatitis 1445
  Clinical Manifestations 1445
  Assessment and Diagnostic Findings 1445
  Medical Management 1445
Pancreatic Cysts 1449
Cancer of the Pancreas 1450
  Clinical Manifestations 1450
  Assessment and Diagnostic Findings 1450
  Medical Management 1450
  Nursing Management 1451
Tumors of the Head of the Pancreas 1451
  Clinical Manifestations 1452
  Assessment and Diagnostic Findings 1452
  Medical Management 1452
  Nursing Management 1452
Pancreatic Islet Tumors 1453
  Surgical Management 1453
  Nursing Management 1453
Hyperinsulinism 1453
Ulcerogenic Tumors 1453

51 Assessment and Management of Patients With Diabetes 1456
DIABETES 1457
  Epidemiology 1457
  Classification 1457
  Pathophysiology 1457
  Prevention 1460
  Clinical Manifestations 1460
  Assessment and Diagnostic Findings 1460
  Medical Management 1461
  Nursing Management 1473
ACUTE COMPLICATIONS OF DIABETES 1481
Hypoglycemia (Insulin Reactions) 1482
  Gerontologic Considerations 1482
  Clinical Manifestations 1482
  Assessment and Diagnostic Findings 1482
  Management 1482
Diabetic Ketoacidosis 1483
  Pathophysiology 1483
  Prevention 1484
  Clinical Manifestations 1484
  Assessment and Diagnostic Findings 1484
  Management 1485
Hyperglycemic Hyperosmolar Syndrome 1485
  Clinical Manifestations 1486
  Assessment and Diagnostic Findings 1486
  Management 1486
  • *Nursing Process:* The Patient With Diabetic Ketoacidosis or Hyperglycemic Hyperosmolar Syndrome 1487
LONG-TERM COMPLICATIONS OF DIABETES 1488
Macrovascular Complications 1488

  Role of Diabetes in Macrovascular Diseases 1489
  Management 1489
Microvascular Complications 1489
  Diabetic Retinopathy 1489
    Clinical Manifestations 1490
    Assessment and Diagnostic Findings 1490
    Medical Management 1490
    Nursing Management 1491
  Nephropathy 1491
    Clinical Manifestations 1492
    Assessment and Diagnostic Findings 1492
    Management 1492
Diabetic Neuropathies 1493
  Peripheral Neuropathy 1493
    Clinical Manifestations 1493
    Management 1493
  Autonomic Neuropathies 1493
    Clinical Manifestations 1493
    Management 1494
Foot and Leg Problems 1494
  Management 1495
SPECIAL ISSUES IN DIABETES CARE 1496
Patients With Diabetes Who Are Undergoing Surgery 1496
Management of Hospitalized Patients With Diabetes 1496
  Self-Care Issues 1496
  Hyperglycemia During Hospitalization 1497
  Hypoglycemia During Hospitalization 1497
  Common Alterations in Diet 1498
  Hygiene 1499
  Stress 1499
  Gerontologic Considerations 1499
  Nursing Management 1499

52 Assessment and Management of Patients With Endocrine Disorders 1502
ASSESSMENT OF THE ENDOCRINE SYSTEM 1503
Anatomic and Physiologic Overview 1503
  Glands of the Endocrine System 1503
  Function and Regulation of Hormones 1503
  Classification and Action of Hormones 1503
Assessment 1504
  Health History 1504
  Physical Assessment 1504
Diagnostic Evaluation 1505
  Blood Tests 1505
  Urine Tests 1506
  Additional Diagnostic Studies 1506
THE PITUITARY GLAND 1506
Anatomic and Physiologic Overview 1506
  Anterior Pituitary 1507
  Posterior Pituitary 1508
Pathophysiology 1508
  Anterior Pituitary 1508
  Posterior Pituitary 1508
Pituitary Tumors 1508
  Clinical Manifestations 1508
  Assessment and Diagnostic Findings 1509
  Medical Management 1509

Diabetes Insipidus 1509
  Clinical Manifestations 1509
  Assessment and Diagnostic Findings 1509
  Medical Management 1509
  Nursing Management 1510
Syndrome of Inappropriate Antidiuretic Hormone
  Secretion 1510
  Medical Management 1510
  Nursing Management 1510
THE THYROID GLAND 1510
Anatomic and Physiologic Overview 1510
  Thyroid Hormone 1510
  Calcitonin 1511
Pathophysiology 1511
Assessment 1511
  Physical Examination 1511
  Diagnostic Evaluation 1512
Hypothyroidism 1513
  Clinical Manifestations 1514
  Medical Management 1515
  Nursing Management 1515
  Gerontologic Considerations 1518
Hyperthyroidism 1519
  Clinical Manifestations 1519
  Assessment and Diagnostic Findings 1519
  Medical Management 1519
  Gerontologic Considerations 1522

  • *Nursing Process:* The Patient With Hyperthyroidism 1522

Thyroid Tumors 1524
  Endemic (Iodine-Deficient) Goiter 1525
  Nodular Goiter 1525
Thyroid Cancer 1525
  Assessment and Diagnostic Findings 1525
  Medical Management 1525
  Nursing Management 1526
THE PARATHYROID GLANDS 1527
Anatomic and Physiologic Overview 1527
Pathophysiology 1527
Hyperparathyroidism 1527
  Clinical Manifestations 1527
  Assessment and Diagnostic Findings 1528
  Medical Management 1528
  Nursing Management 1528
  Complications: Hypercalcemic Crisis 1529
Hypoparathyroidism 1529
  Clinical Manifestations 1529
  Assessment and Diagnostic Findings 1530
  Medical Management 1530
  Nursing Management 1530
THE ADRENAL GLANDS 1531
  Anatomic and Physiologic Overview 1531
  Adrenal Medulla 1531
  Adrenal Cortex 1531
Pheochromocytoma 1532
  Clinical Manifestations 1532
  Assessment and Diagnostic Findings 1532
  Medical Management 1533
  Nursing Management 1534
Adrenocortical Insufficiency
  (Addison Disease) 1534

Clinical Manifestations 1534
Assessment and Diagnostic Findings 1535
Medical Management 1535
Nursing Management 1535
Cushing Syndrome 1536
  Clinical Manifestations 1536
  Assessment and Diagnostic Findings 1537
  Medical Management 1537

  • *Nursing Process:* The Patient With Cushing
    Syndrome 1538

Primary Aldosteronism 1540
  Clinical Manifestations 1540
  Assessment and Diagnostic Findings 1540
  Medical Management 1540
  Nursing Management 1541
Corticosteroid Therapy 1541
  Side Effects 1541
  Therapeutic Uses of Corticosteroids 1541
  Dosage 1542
  Tapering 1543
  Nursing Management 1543

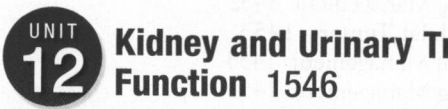

UNIT 12 Kidney and Urinary Tract Function 1546

**53 Assessment of Kidney and Urinary
Function 1548**
Anatomic and Physiologic Overview 1548
  Anatomy of the Kidney and Urinary
    Systems 1548
  Function of the Kidney and Urinary
    Systems 1551
  Gerontologic Considerations 1554
Assessment of the Kidney and Urinary
  Systems 1555
  Health History 1555
  Physical Assessment 1557
Diagnostic Evaluation 1559
  Urinalysis and Urine Culture 1559
  Specific Gravity 1561
  Osmolality 1561
  Renal Function Tests 1562
  Diagnostic Imaging 1562
  Urologic Endoscopic Procedures 1564
  Biopsy 1565

**54 Management of Patients With Kidney
Disorders 1567**
**FLUID AND ELECTROLYTE IMBALANCES IN KIDNEY
DISORDERS 1568**
  Clinical Manifestations 1568
  Gerontologic Considerations 1569
KIDNEY DISORDERS 1569
Chronic Kidney Disease 1569
  Pathophysiology 1569
  Stages of Chronic Kidney Disease 1569
  Clinical Manifestations 1569
  Assessment and Diagnostic Findings 1569

Medical Management 1569
Gerontologic Considerations 1570
Nephrosclerosis 1570
Pathophysiology 1570
Assessment and Diagnostic Findings 1570
Medical Management 1570
Primary Glomerular Diseases 1570
Acute Nephritic Syndrome 1570
Pathophysiology 1570
Clinical Manifestations 1570
Assessment and Diagnostic Findings 1571
Complications 1571
Medical Management 1571
Nursing Management 1571
Chronic Glomerulonephritis 1572
Pathophysiology 1572
Clinical Manifestations 1572
Assessment and Diagnostic Findings 1572
Medical Management 1572
Nursing Management 1573
Nephrotic Syndrome 1573
Pathophysiology 1573
Clinical Manifestations 1573
Assessment and Diagnostic Findings 1574
Complications 1574
Medical Management 1574
Nursing Management 1574
Polycystic Kidney Disease 1574
Pathophysiology 1574
Clinical Manifestations 1574
Assessment and Diagnostic Findings 1574
Medical Management 1574
RENAL CANCER 1574
Clinical Manifestations 1575
Assessment and Diagnostic Findings 1575
Medical Management 1575
Nursing Management 1575
KIDNEY DISEASE 1576
Acute Kidney Injury 1576
Pathophysiology 1576
Classifications of Acute Kidney Injury 1576
Categories of Acute Kidney Injury 1577
Phases of Acute Kidney Injury 1577
Clinical Manifestations 1578
Assessment and Diagnostic Findings 1578
Prevention 1579
Gerontologic Considerations 1579
Medical Management 1579
Nursing Management 1580
End-Stage Kidney Disease or Chronic Kidney Disease 1581
Pathophysiology 1581
Clinical Manifestations 1581
Assessment and Diagnostic Findings 1581
Complications 1583
Medical Management 1583
Nursing Management 1584
Gerontologic Considerations 1584
RENAL REPLACEMENT THERAPIES 1589
Dialysis 1589
Hemodialysis 1589

Dialyzers 1589
Vascular Access 1590
Complications 1591
Nursing Management 1592
Continuous Renal Replacement Therapies 1594
Continuous Venovenous Hemofiltration 1594
Continuous Venovenous Hemodialysis 1595
Peritoneal Dialysis 1595
Procedure 1596
Complications 1597
Approaches 1598
Nursing Management 1599
Special Considerations: Nursing Management of the Patient on Dialysis Who Is Hospitalized 1601
KIDNEY SURGERY 1602
Management of Patients Undergoing Kidney Surgery 1602
Preoperative Considerations 1602
Perioperative Concerns 1602
Postoperative Management 1602
Nursing Management 1603
Kidney Transplantation 1607
Preoperative Management 1608
Medical Management 1608
Nursing Management 1608
Postoperative Management 1609
Medical Management 1609
Nursing Management 1610
RENAL TRAUMA 1612
Medical Management 1613
Nursing Management 1613

55 Management of Patients With Urinary Disorders 1615
INFECTIONS OF THE URINARY TRACT 1615
Lower Urinary Tract Infections 1616
Pathophysiology 1616
Clinical Manifestations 1617
Gerontologic Considerations 1617
Assessment and Diagnostic Findings 1618
Medical Management 1618

• *Nursing Process:* The Patient With a Lower Urinary Tract Infection 1619

Upper Urinary Tract Infections 1621
Acute Pyelonephritis 1622
Assessment and Diagnostic Findings 1622
Medical Management 1622
Chronic Pyelonephritis 1622
Clinical Manifestations 1622
Assessment and Diagnostic Findings 1622
Complications 1622
Medical Management 1622
Nursing Management 1622
ADULT VOIDING DYSFUNCTION 1622
Urinary Incontinence 1623
Types of Urinary Incontinence 1623
Gerontologic Considerations 1624
Assessment and Diagnostic Findings 1624
Medical Management 1624
Nursing Management 1626

Urinary Retention 1627
   Pathophysiology 1627
   Assessment and Diagnostic Findings 1627
   Complications 1627
   Nursing Management 1627
Neurogenic Bladder 1628
   Pathophysiology 1628
   Assessment and Diagnostic Findings 1628
   Complications 1628
   Medical Management 1628
Catheterization 1628
   Indwelling Catheters 1629
   Suprapubic Catheters 1629
   Nursing Management 1629
UROLITHIASIS AND NEPHROLITHIASIS 1632
   Pathophysiology 1632
   Clinical Manifestations 1632
   Assessment and Diagnostic Findings 1633
   Medical Management 1633

   • Nursing Process: The Patient With Kidney Stones 1634

GENITOURINARY TRAUMA 1637
   Specific Injuries 1637
   Medical Management 1637
   Nursing Management 1637
URINARY TRACT CANCERS 1637
Cancer of the Bladder 1637
   Clinical Manifestations 1638
   Assessment and Diagnostic Findings 1638
   Medical Management 1638
URINARY DIVERSIONS 1639
Cutaneous Urinary Diversions 1639
   Ileal Conduit 1639
      Complications 1639
      Nursing Management 1639
   Cutaneous Ureterostomy 1642
Continent Urinary Diversions 1642
   Continent Ileal Urinary Reservoir (Indiana Pouch) 1642
   Ureterosigmoidostomy 1643
   Nursing Management 1643
Other Urinary Diversion Procedures 1643

   • Nursing Process: The Patient Undergoing Urinary
     Diversion Surgery 1643

UNIT 13 Reproductive Function 1648

56 Assessment and Management of Patients With
   Female Physiologic Processes 1650
   ROLE OF NURSES IN WOMEN'S HEALTH 1650
   ASSESSMENT OF THE FEMALE REPRODUCTIVE SYSTEM 1651
   Anatomic and Physiologic Overview 1651
      Anatomy of the Female Reproductive
         System 1651
      Function of the Female Reproductive
         System 1653
   Assessment 1654
      Health History 1654
      Physical Assessment 1660

Diagnostic Evaluation 1663
   Cytologic Test for Cancer (Pap Smear) 1663
   Colposcopy and Cervical Biopsy 1663
   Cryotherapy and Laser Therapy 1663
   Cone Biopsy and Loop Electrosurgical Excision
      Procedure 1663
   Endometrial (Aspiration) Biopsy 1663
   Dilation and Curettage 1664
   Endoscopic Examinations 1664
   Other Diagnostic Procedures 1665
MANAGEMENT OF FEMALE PHYSIOLOGIC PROCESSES 1665
Menstruation 1666
   Psychosocial Considerations 1666
   Cultural Considerations 1666
Menstrual Disorders 1666
   Premenstrual Syndrome 1666
      Clinical Manifestations 1666
      Medical Management 1666
      Nursing Management 1667
   Dysmenorrhea 1667
      Assessment and Diagnostic Findings 1667
      Management 1667
   Amenorrhea 1668
   Abnormal Uterine Bleeding 1668
      Menorrhagia 1668
      Metrorrhagia 1668
Dyspareunia 1668
Contraception 1669
   Contraindications 1669
   Abstinence 1669
   Long-Acting Reversible Contraceptive (LARC) Methods 1669
   Sterilization 1671
   Hormonal Contraception 1671
      Hormonal Contraception 1671
   Mechanical Barriers 1672
      Diaphragm 1672
      Cervical Cap 1672
      Female Condom 1673
      Spermicides 1673
      Male Condom 1673
   Coitus Interruptus or Withdrawal 1674
   Fertility Awareness-Based Methods 1674
   Emergency Contraception 1674
      Methods of Emergency Contraception 1674
      Nursing Management 1674
Abortion 1674
   Spontaneous Abortion 1674
      Habitual Abortion 1675
      Medical Management 1675
      Nursing Management 1675
   Induced Abortion 1675
      Medical Management 1675
      Nursing Management 1676
Infertility 1676
   Diagnostic Findings 1677
   Medical Management 1677
   Nursing Management 1678
Preconception/Periconception
   Health Care 1678
Ectopic Pregnancy 1679
   Clinical Manifestations 1679

Assessment and Diagnostic Findings 1679
Medical Management 1680

- *Nursing Process:* The Patient With an Ectopic Pregnancy 1680

Perimenopause 1681
Nursing Management 1681
Menopause 1681
Postmenopausal Bleeding 1681
Clinical Manifestations 1681
Psychological Considerations 1682
Medical Management 1682
Nursing Management 1683

57 Management of Patients With Female Reproductive Disorders 1686
VULVOVAGINAL INFECTIONS 1687
Candidiasis 1687
Clinical Manifestations 1687
Medical Management 1688
Bacterial Vaginosis 1688
Clinical Manifestations 1689
Medical Management 1689
Trichomoniasis 1689
Clinical Manifestations 1689
Medical Management 1689
Gerontologic Considerations 1689

- *Nursing Process:* The Patient With a Vulvovaginal Infection 1689

Human Papillomavirus 1691
Pathophysiology 1691
Medical Management 1691
Prevention 1692
Herpes Virus Type 2 Infection (Herpes Genitalis, Herpes Simplex Virus) 1692
Pathophysiology 1692
Clinical Manifestations 1692
Medical Management 1692

- *Nursing Process:* The Patient With a Genital Herpes Infection 1693

Endocervicitis and Cervicitis 1694
Chlamydia and Gonorrhea 1694
Medical Management 1694
Nursing Management 1694
Pelvic Inflammatory Disease 1695
Pathophysiology 1695
Clinical Manifestations 1695
Complications 1695
Medical Management 1696
Nursing Management 1696
Human Immune Deficiency Virus Infection and Acquired Immune Deficiency Syndrome 1696
STRUCTURAL DISORDERS 1697
Fistulas of the Vagina 1697
Clinical Manifestations 1697
Assessment and Diagnostic Findings 1698
Medical Management 1698
Pelvic Organ Prolapse: Cystocele, Rectocele, Enterocele 1698

Clinical Manifestations 1699
Medical Management 1699
Uterine Prolapse 1700
Medical Management 1701
Nursing Management 1701
BENIGN DISORDERS 1701
Vulvitis and Vulvodynia 1701
Medical Management 1702
Vulvar Cysts 1702
Medical Management 1702
Vulvar Dystrophy 1702
Medical Management 1702
Nursing Management 1702
Ovarian Cysts 1702
Medical Management 1703
Benign Tumors of the Uterus: Fibroids (Leiomyomas, Myomas) 1703
Clinical Manifestations 1703
Medical Management 1703
Endometriosis 1704
Pathophysiology 1704
Clinical Manifestations 1704
Assessment and Diagnostic Findings 1704
Medical Management 1704
Nursing Management 1705
Chronic Pelvic Pain 1705
Adenomyosis 1705
Endometrial Hyperplasia 1705
MALIGNANT CONDITIONS 1706
Cancer of the Cervix 1706
Clinical Manifestations 1706
Assessment and Diagnostic Findings 1707
Medical Management 1707
Cancer of the Uterus (Endometrium) 1708
Pathophysiology 1709
Assessment and Diagnostic Findings 1709
Medical Management 1709
Cancer of the Vulva 1709
Clinical Manifestations 1709
Medical Management 1709
Nursing Management 1710
Cancer of the Vagina 1711
Medical Management 1711
Cancer of the Fallopian Tubes 1712
Cancer of the Ovary 1712
Epidemiology 1712
Pathophysiology 1712
Clinical Manifestations 1712
Assessment and Diagnostic Findings 1712
Medical Management 1712
Nursing Management 1713
Hysterectomy 1714
Preoperative Management 1714
Postoperative Management 1714

- *Nursing Process:* The Patient Undergoing a Hysterectomy 1714

Radiation Therapy 1716
Methods of Radiation Therapy 1716
Nursing Considerations for Radiation Safety 1717

58 Assessment and Management of Patients With Breast Disorders 1719

BREAST ASSESSMENT 1720
Anatomic and Physiologic Overview 1720
  Assessment 1720
Diagnostic Evaluation 1721
  Breast Self-Examination 1721
  Mammography 1723
  Contrast Mammography 1725
  Ultrasonography 1725
  Magnetic Resonance Imaging 1725
  Procedures for Tissue Analysis 1726
CONDITIONS AFFECTING THE NIPPLE 1728
Nipple Discharge 1728
  Fissure 1728
BREAST INFECTIONS 1728
Mastitis 1728
  Lactational Abscess 1728
BENIGN CONDITIONS OF THE BREAST 1728
Breast Pain 1728
Cysts 1728
Fibroadenomas 1728
Benign Proliferative Breast Disease 1729
Other Benign Conditions 1729
MALIGNANT CONDITIONS OF THE BREAST 1730
Types of Breast Cancer 1730
Risk Factors 1731
Protective Factors 1732
Breast Cancer Prevention Strategies in the
  Patient Who Is at High Risk 1732
Clinical Manifestations 1732
Assessment and Diagnostic Findings 1732
Staging 1732
Prognosis 1733
Surgical Management 1733

• *Nursing Process:* The Patient Undergoing Surgery
  for Breast Cancer 1734

Radiation Therapy 1740
Systemic Treatments 1741
Treatment of Recurrent and Metastatic Breast
  Cancer 1744
Reconstructive Procedures After
  Mastectomy 1745
Prosthetics 1747
Special Issues in Breast Cancer Management 1747
RECONSTRUCTIVE BREAST SURGERY 1748
Reduction Mammoplasty 1749
Augmentation Mammoplasty 1749
Mastopexy 1749
DISEASES OF THE MALE BREAST 1749
Gynecomastia 1749
Male Breast Cancer 1749

59 Assessment and Management of Patients With Male Reproductive Disorders 1752
ASSESSMENT OF THE MALE REPRODUCTIVE SYSTEM 1753
Anatomic and Physiologic Overview 1753
  Gerontologic Considerations 1754
Assessment 1754
  Health History 1754

Physical Assessment 1755
Diagnostic Evaluation 1755
  Prostate-Specific Antigen Test 1756
  Ultrasonography 1756
  Prostate Fluid or Tissue Analysis 1756
  Tests of Male Sexual Function 1756
DISORDERS OF MALE SEXUAL FUNCTION 1756
Erectile Dysfunction 1756
  Assessment and Diagnostic Findings 1756
  Medical Management 1756
  Nursing Management 1760
Disorders of Ejaculation 1760
INFECTIONS OF THE MALE GENITOURINARY TRACT 1761
PROSTATIC DISORDERS 1761
Prostatitis 1761
  Clinical Manifestations 1762
  Medical Management 1762
  Nursing Management 1762
Benign Prostatic Hyperplasia (Enlarged
  Prostate) 1762
  Pathophysiology 1762
  Clinical Manifestations 1763
  Assessment and Diagnostic Findings 1763
  Medical Management 1763
Cancer of the Prostate 1764
  Clinical Manifestations 1764
  Assessment and Diagnostic Findings 1764
  Medical Management 1765
The Patient Undergoing Prostate Surgery 1771
  Surgical Procedures 1771
  Complications 1771

• *Nursing Process:* Patient Undergoing Prostatectomy 1774

DISORDERS AFFECTING THE TESTES AND ADJACENT STRUCTURES 1778
Orchitis 1778
  Epididymitis 1779
  Pathophysiology 1779
  Clinical Manifestations 1779
  Assessment and Diagnostic Findings 1779
  Medical Management 1779
  Nursing Management 1779
Testicular Torsion 1779
Testicular Cancer 1779
  Classification of Testicular Tumors 1780
  Risk Factors 1780
  Clinical Manifestations 1780
  Assessment and Diagnostic Findings 1780
  Medical Management 1780
  Nursing Management 1782
Hydrocele 1782
Varicocele 1783
Vasectomy 1783
  Nursing Management 1783
  Vasovasostomy (Sterilization Reversal) 1784
  Semen Cryopreservation (Sperm Banking) 1784
DISORDERS AFFECTING THE PENIS 1784
Phimosis 1784
Cancer of the Penis 1784
  Clinical Manifestations 1784
  Assessment and Diagnostic Findings 1784

Prevention 1785
Medical Management 1785
Priapism 1785
Peyronie's Disease 1785
Urethral Stricture 1785
Circumcision 1786

UNIT 14 Integumentary Function 1788

60 Assessment of Integumentary Function 1790
Anatomic and Physiologic Overview 1790
Anatomy of the Skin, Hair, Nails, and Glands of the Skin 1790
Functions of the Skin 1793
Gerontologic Considerations 1794
Assessment 1794
Health History 1795
Physical Assessment 1795
Skin Consequences of Selected Systemic Diseases 1803
Diagnostic Evaluation 1803
Skin Biopsy 1803
Patch Testing 1804
Skin Scrapings 1804
Tzanck Smear 1804
Wood Light Examination 1804
Clinical Photographs 1804
Nursing Implications 1804

61 Management of Patients With Dermatologic Disorders 1806
PATIENTS WITH SKIN DISORDERS 1806
Protecting the Skin 1806
Preventing Secondary Infection 1807
Reversing the Inflammatory Process 1807
Wound Dressing Care for Skin Disorders 1807
Autolytic Débridement 1807
Categories of Dressings 1807
Medical Management 1809
Nursing Management 1810
PRURITUS 1811
General Pruritus 1811
Gerontologic Considerations 1812
Pathophysiology 1812
Medical Management 1812
Nursing Management 1812
Perineal and Perianal Pruritus 1812
Nursing Management 1812
SECRETORY DISORDERS 1813
Hidradenitis Suppurativa 1813
Pathophysiology 1813
Clinical Manifestations 1813
Medical Management 1813
Seborrheic Dermatoses 1813
Clinical Manifestations 1813
Medical Management 1814
Nursing Management 1814
Acne Vulgaris 1814

Pathophysiology 1814
Clinical Manifestations 1814
Assessment and Diagnostic Findings 1814
Medical Management 1814
Nursing Management 1816
INFECTIOUS DERMATOSES 1816
Bacterial Skin Infections 1816
Impetigo 1817
Clinical Manifestations 1817
Medical Management 1817
Nursing Management 1818
Folliculitis, Furuncles, and Carbuncles 1818
Medical Management 1818
Nursing Management 1818
Viral Skin Infections 1819
Herpes Zoster 1819
Clinical Manifestations 1819
Medical Management 1819
Nursing Management 1820
Herpes Simplex 1820
Fungal (Mycotic) Skin Infections 1820
Parasitic Skin Infestations 1820
Pediculosis: Lice Infestation 1820
Clinical Manifestations 1820
Medical Management 1821
Nursing Management 1822
Scabies 1822
Clinical Manifestations 1822
Gerontologic Considerations 1822
Assessment and Diagnostic Findings 1822
Medical Management 1822
Nursing Management 1823
NONINFECTIOUS INFLAMMATORY DERMATOSES 1823
Irritant Contact Dermatitis 1823
Clinical Manifestations 1823
Medical Management 1823
Psoriasis 1823
Pathophysiology 1824
Clinical Manifestations 1824
Complications 1824
Assessment and Diagnostic Findings 1824
Medical Management 1824
Nursing Management 1826
Generalized Exfoliative Dermatitis 1826
Clinical Manifestations 1827
Assessment and Diagnostic Findings 1827
Medical Management 1827
Nursing Management 1827
BLISTERING DISEASES 1827
Pemphigus Vulgaris 1827
Assessment and Diagnostic Findings 1828
Medical Management 1828
Bullous Pemphigoid 1828
Assessment and Diagnostic Findings 1828
Medical Management 1828
Dermatitis Herpetiformis 1828
Assessment and Diagnostic Findings 1828
Medical Management 1828
• *Nursing Process:* Care of the Patient With Blistering Diseases 1829

Toxic Epidermal Necrolysis and Stevens–Johnson
Syndrome 1830
 Clinical Manifestations 1830
 Complications 1830
 Assessment and Diagnostic Findings 1830
 Medical Management 1830

• *Nursing Process:* Care of the Patient With Toxic Epidermal
Necrolysis or Stevens–Johnson Syndrome 1831

SKIN TUMORS 1833
Benign Skin Tumors 1833
 Cysts 1833
 Seborrheic and Actinic Keratoses 1833
 Verrucae: Warts 1833
 Angiomas 1833
 Pigmented Nevi: Moles 1833
 Keloids 1833
 Dermatofibroma 1833
 Neurofibromatosis: Von Recklinghausen
  Disease 1833
Malignant Skin Tumors 1834
 Basal Cell Carcinoma and Squamous Cell Carcinoma   1834
 Clinical Manifestations 1834
 Medical Management 1835
 Nursing Management 1835
 Melanoma 1836
 Clinical Manifestations 1836
 Assessment and Diagnostic Findings 1836
 Medical Management 1837

• *Nursing Process:* Care of the Patient With
Melanoma 1837

Metastatic Skin Tumors 1839
Kaposi Sarcoma 1839
PLASTIC, RECONSTRUCTIVE, AND COSMETIC PROCEDURES 1839
Wound Coverage: Grafts and Flaps 1839
 Skin Grafts 1839
 Nursing Management 1840
 Flaps 1840
Cosmetic Procedures 1841
 Chemical Face Peeling 1841
 Dermabrasion 1841
 Facial Reconstructive Surgery 1841
 Face-Lift 1841
Laser Treatment of Cutaneous Lesions 1841
 Nursing Management 1841

62 Management of Patients With
Burn Injury 1845
Overview of Burn Injury 1845
 Incidence 1845
 Gerontologic Considerations 1846
 Prevention 1846
 Outlook for Survival and Recovery 1847
 Severity 1847
 Pathophysiology 1849
Management of Burn Injury 1853
 Emergent/Resuscitative Phase 1853
 On-the-Scene Care 1853
 Medical Management 1853
 Nursing Management 1856
 Acute/Intermediate Phase 1856

 Medical Management 1856
 Nursing Management 1865
Rehabilitation Phase 1868
 Psychological Support 1868
 Abnormal Wound Healing 1869

• *Nursing Process:* Care of the Patient During the
Rehabilitation Phase 1869

Outpatient Burn Care 1872

UNIT 15 Sensory Function 1874

63 Assessment and Management of Patients With
Eye and Vision Disorders 1876
ASSESSMENT OF THE EYE 1877
Anatomic and Physiologic Overview 1877
Assessment 1879
 Ocular History 1879
 Visual Acuity 1879
 External Eye Examination 1880
Diagnostic Evaluation 1881
 Direct Ophthalmoscopy 1881
 Indirect Ophthalmoscopy 1881
 Slit-Lamp Examination 1881
 Tonometry 1881
 Color Vision Testing 1881
 Amsler Grid 1882
 Ultrasonography 1882
 Optical Coherence Tomography 1882
 Fundus Photography 1882
 Laser Scanning 1882
 Angiography 1882
 Perimetry Testing 1883
IMPAIRED VISION 1883
Refractive Errors 1883
Vision Impairment and Blindness 1883
 Assessment and Diagnostic Testing 1883
 Gerontologic Considerations 1884
 Medical Management 1884
 Nursing Management 1884
OCULAR MEDICATION ADMINISTRATION 1886
 Common Ocular Medications 1887
 Nursing Management 1888
GLAUCOMA 1890
 Physiology 1890
 Pathophysiology 1891
 Classification of Glaucoma 1891
 Clinical Manifestation 1891
 Assessment and Diagnostic Findings 1891
 Medical Management 1892
 Nursing Management 1893
CATARACTS 1894
 Pathophysiology 1894
 Clinical Manifestations 1895
 Assessment and Diagnostic Findings 1895
 Medical Management 1895
 Nursing Management 1896
CORNEAL DISORDERS 1897

Corneal Dystrophies 1897
    Keratoconus 1897
    Fuchs Endothelial Dystrophy 1898
Corneal Surgeries 1898
    Phototherapeutic Keratectomy 1898
    Penetrating Keratoplasty 1898
    Additional Keratoplasty Surgeries 1898
    Keratoprosthesis 1898
    Nursing Management 1899
Refractive Surgeries 1899
    Laser Vision Correction Photorefractive
        Keratectomy 1899
    Phakic Intraocular Lenses 1899
    Conductive Keratoplasty 1900
RETINAL DISORDERS 1900
Retinal Detachment 1900
    Clinical Manifestations 1900
    Assessment and Diagnostic Findings 1900
    Surgical Management 1900
    Nursing Management 1901
Retinal Vascular Disorders 1901
    Central Retinal Vein Occlusion 1901
    Branch Retinal Vein Occlusion 1901
    Central Retinal Artery Occlusion 1901
Age-Related Macular Degeneration 1901
    Medical Management 1902
    Nursing Management 1902
Orbital and Ocular Trauma 1902
    Orbital Trauma 1902
    Soft Tissue Injury and Hemorrhage 1902
    Orbital Fractures 1903
    Foreign Bodies 1903
Ocular Trauma 1904
    Assessment and Diagnostic Findings 1904
    Medical Management 1904
INFECTIOUS AND INFLAMMATORY CONDITIONS 1905
Dry Eyes 1905
    Clinical Manifestations 1905
    Assessment and Diagnostic Findings 1905
    Management 1905
Conjunctivitis 1906
    Clinical Manifestations 1906
    Assessment and Diagnostic Findings 1906
    Types of Conjunctivitis 1906
    Medical Management 1907
Uveitis 1908
    Medical Management 1908
Orbital Cellulitis 1909
    Medical Management 1909
ORBITAL AND OCULAR TUMORS 1909
Benign Tumors of the Orbit 1909
Benign Tumors of the Eyelids 1909
Benign Tumors of the Conjunctiva 1909
Malignant Tumors of the Orbit 1909
Malignant Tumors of the Eyelid 1910
Malignant Tumors of the Conjunctiva 1910
Malignant Tumors of the Globe 1910
SURGICAL PROCEDURES AND ENUCLEATION 1910
Orbital Surgeries 1910
Enucleation 1910
    Ocular Prostheses 1911

Medical Management 1911
Nursing Management 1911
OCULAR CONSEQUENCES OF SYSTEMIC DISEASE 1912
Diabetic Retinopathy 1912
Cytomegalovirus Retinitis 1912
    Medical Management 1912
Hypertension-Related Eye Changes 1913

64 Assessment and Management of
Patients With Hearing and Balance
Disorders 1915
ASSESSMENT OF THE EAR 1915
Anatomic and Physiologic Overview 1915
    Anatomy of the External Ear 1916
    Anatomy of the Middle Ear 1916
    Anatomy of the Inner Ear 1917
    Function of the Ears 1918
Assessment 1918
    Inspection of the External Ear 1918
    Otoscopic Examination 1918
    Evaluation of Gross Auditory Acuity 1919
Diagnostic Evaluation 1921
    Audiometry 1921
    Tympanogram 1921
    Auditory Brain Stem Response 1921
    Electronystagmography 1921
    Platform Posturography 1922
    Sinusoidal Harmonic Acceleration 1922
    Middle Ear Endoscopy 1922
HEARING LOSS 1922
    Clinical Manifestations 1923
    Prevention 1923
    Gerontologic Considerations 1924
    Medical Management 1925
    Nursing Management 1925
CONDITIONS OF THE EXTERNAL EAR 1926
Cerumen Impaction 1926
    Management 1926
Foreign Bodies 1926
    Management 1926
External Otitis (Otitis Externa) 1926
    Clinical Manifestations 1926
    Medical Management 1926
    Nursing Management 1926
Malignant External Otitis 1927
Masses of the External Ear 1927
CONDITIONS OF THE MIDDLE EAR 1927
Tympanic Membrane Perforation 1927
    Medical Management 1927
Acute Otitis Media 1927
    Clinical Manifestations 1927
    Medical Management 1928
Serous Otitis Media 1928
    Clinical Manifestations 1928
    Management 1928
Chronic Otitis Media 1928
    Clinical Manifestations 1928
    Medical Management 1929

• *Nursing Process:* The Patient Undergoing Mastoid
    Surgery 1929

Otosclerosis 1931
  Clinical Manifestations 1931
  Medical Management 1931
Middle Ear Masses 1931
CONDITIONS OF THE INNER EAR 1932
Motion Sickness 1932
  Clinical Manifestations 1932
  Management 1932
Ménière Disease 1933
  Clinical Manifestations 1933
  Assessment and Diagnostic Findings 1933
  Medical Management 1933
Benign Paroxysmal Positional Vertigo 1934
Tinnitus 1934
Labyrinthitis 1934
  Clinical Manifestations 1934
  Management 1934
Ototoxicity 1937
Acoustic Neuroma 1938
  Assessment and Diagnostic Findings 1938
  Management 1938
AURAL REHABILITATION 1938
Hearing Aids 1938
Implanted Hearing Devices 1940
Hearing Guide Dogs 1941

UNIT 16   Neurologic Function 1944

65 Assessment of Neurologic Function 1946
Anatomic and Physiologic Overview 1946
  Cells of the Nervous System 1947
  Neurotransmitters 1947
  The Central Nervous System 1947
  The Peripheral Nervous System 1951
  Motor and Sensory Pathways of the
    Nervous System 1954
Assessment of the Nervous System 1957
  Health History 1957
  Physical Assessment 1958
  Gerontologic Considerations 1964
Diagnostic Evaluation 1965
  Computed Tomography Scanning 1965
  Magnetic Resonance Imaging 1966
  Positron Emission Tomography 1967
  Single-Photon Emission Computed
    Tomography 1967
  Cerebral Angiography 1967
  Myelography 1968
  Noninvasive Carotid Flow Studies 1968
  Transcranial Doppler 1968
  Electroencephalography 1968
  Electromyography 1969
  Nerve Conduction Studies 1969
  Evoked Potential Studies 1969
  Lumbar Puncture and Examination of
    Cerebrospinal Fluid 1969
  Promoting Home, Community-Based, and
    Transitional Care 1971

66 Management of Patients With Neurologic Dysfunction 1972
ALTERED LEVEL OF CONSCIOUSNESS 1973
  Pathophysiology 1973
  Clinical Manifestations 1973
  Assessment and Diagnostic Findings 1973
  Medical Management 1974
• *Nursing Process:* The Patient With an Altered Level
of Consciousness 1974
INCREASED INTRACRANIAL PRESSURE 1979
  Pathophysiology 1979
  Clinical Manifestations 1980
  Assessment and Diagnostic Findings 1981
  Complications 1981
  Medical Management 1981
• *Nursing Process:* The Patient With Increased
Intracranial Pressure 1984
INTRACRANIAL SURGERY 1989
Supratentorial and Infratentorial Approaches 1989
  Preoperative Management 1989
  Postoperative Management 1991
    Reducing Cerebral Edema 1991
    Relieving Pain and Preventing Seizures 1991
    Monitoring Intracranial Pressure 1991
• *Nursing Process:* The Patient Who Has Undergone
Intracranial Surgery 1991
Transsphenoidal Approach 1995
  Complications 1995
  Preoperative Management 1995
  Postoperative Management 1995
SEIZURE DISORDERS 1996
  Pathophysiology 1996
  Clinical Manifestations 1996
  Assessment and Diagnostic Findings 1997
  Nursing Management 1997
The Epilepsies 1997
  Pathophysiology 1998
  Epilepsy in Women 1999
  Gerontologic Considerations 1999
  Prevention 2000
  Medical Management 2000
• *Nursing Process:* The Patient With Epilepsy 2001
Status Epilepticus 2003
  Medical Management 2003
  Nursing Management 2003
HEADACHE 2004
  Pathophysiology 2004
  Clinical Manifestations 2004
  Assessment and Diagnostic Findings 2005
  Prevention 2006
  Medical Management 2006
  Nursing Management 2007

67 Management of Patients With Cerebrovascular Disorders 2009
Ischemic Stroke 2009
  Pathophysiology 2010
  Clinical Manifestations 2011

Assessment and Diagnostic Findings 2011
Prevention 2013
Medical Management 2013

- *Nursing Process:* The Patient Recovering From an Ischemic Stroke 2018

Hemorrhagic Stroke 2025
Pathophysiology 2025
Clinical Manifestations 2026
Assessment and Diagnostic Findings 2026
Prevention 2027
Complications 2027
Medical Management 2028

- *Nursing Process:* The Patient With a Hemorrhagic Stroke 2028

68 Management of Patients With Neurologic Trauma 2033
Head Injuries 2033
Pathophysiology 2034
Clinical Manifestations 2035
Assessment and Diagnostic Findings 2035
Gerontologic Considerations 2035
Medical Management 2035
Brain Injury 2035
Types of Brain Injury 2036
Medical Management 2038

- *Nursing Process:* The Patient With a Traumatic Brain Injury 2038

Spinal Cord Injury 2048
Pathophysiology 2048
Clinical Manifestations 2048
Assessment and Diagnostic Findings 2048
Emergency Management 2050
Medical Management (Acute Phase) 2051
Management of Acute Complications
   of Spinal Cord Injury 2053

- *Nursing Process:* The Patient With Acute Spinal Cord Injury 2054

Medical Management of Long-Term
   Complications of Spinal Cord Injury 2058

- *Nursing Process:* The Patient With Tetraplegia or Paraplegia 2059

69 Management of Patients With Neurologic Infections, Autoimmune Disorders, and Neuropathies 2065
INFECTIOUS NEUROLOGIC DISORDERS 2065
Meningitis 2065
Pathophysiology 2065
Clinical Manifestations 2066
Assessment and Diagnostic Findings 2067
Prevention 2067
Medical Management 2067
Nursing Management 2068
Brain Abscess 2068
Pathophysiology 2068
Clinical Manifestations 2068
Assessment and Diagnostic Findings 2068

Medical Management 2069
Nursing Management 2069
Herpes Simplex Encephalitis 2069
Pathophysiology 2069
Clinical Manifestations 2069
Assessment and Diagnostic Findings 2069
Medical Management 2069
Nursing Management 2070
Arthropod-Borne Virus Encephalitis 2070
Pathophysiology 2070
Clinical Manifestations 2070
Assessment and Diagnostic Findings 2070
Medical Management 2070
Nursing Management 2070
Fungal Encephalitis 2070
Pathophysiology 2071
Clinical Manifestations 2071
Assessment and Diagnostic Findings 2071
Medical Management 2071
Nursing Management 2071
Creutzfeldt–Jakob and Variant Creutzfeldt–Jakob Diseases 2071
Pathophysiology 2071
Clinical Manifestations 2072
Assessment and Diagnostic Findings 2072
Medical Management 2072
Nursing Management 2072
AUTOIMMUNE PROCESSES 2072
Multiple Sclerosis 2072
Pathophysiology 2073
Clinical Manifestations 2073
Gerontologic Considerations 2074
Assessment and Diagnostic Findings 2074
Medical Management 2074

- *Nursing Process:* The Patient With MS 2075

Myasthenia Gravis 2079
Pathophysiology 2079
Clinical Manifestations 2079
Assessment and Diagnostic Findings 2079
Medical Management 2080
Complications 2081
Nursing Management 2081
Guillain–Barré Syndrome (GBS) 2082
Pathophysiology 2082
Clinical Manifestations 2082
Assessment and Diagnostic Findings 2083
Medical Management 2083

- *Nursing Process:* The Patient With GBS 2083

CRANIAL NERVE DISORDERS 2085
Trigeminal Neuralgia (Tic Douloureux) 2085
Medical Management 2087
Nursing Management 2088
Bell Palsy 2088
Medical Management 2088
Nursing Management 2089
DISORDERS OF THE PERIPHERAL NERVOUS SYSTEM 2089
Peripheral Neuropathies 2089
Mononeuropathy 2089

70 Management of Patients With Oncologic or Degenerative Neurologic Disorders 2091

ONCOLOGIC DISORDERS OF THE BRAIN AND SPINAL CORD 2091

Brain Tumors 2091
Types of Primary Brain Tumors 2092
Gerontologic Considerations 2093
Clinical Manifestations 2093
Assessment and Diagnostic Findings 2095
Medical Management 2096
Nursing Management 2096

Cerebral Metastases 2097
Medical Management 2097

• *Nursing Process:* The Patient With Nervous System Metastases or Primary Brain Tumor 2097

Spinal Cord Tumors 2100
Assessment and Diagnostic Findings 2100
Medical Management 2100
Nursing Management 2100

DEGENERATIVE DISORDERS 2101

Parkinson Disease 2101
Pathophysiology 2101
Clinical Manifestations 2102
Assessment and Diagnostic Findings 2103
Medical Management 2103

• *Nursing Process:* The Patient With Parkinson Disease 2105

Huntington Disease 2108
Pathophysiology 2108
Clinical Manifestations 2108
Assessment and Diagnostic Findings 2109
Medical Management 2109

Amyotrophic Lateral Sclerosis 2109
Clinical Manifestations 2110
Assessment and Diagnostic Findings 2111
Management 2111

Muscular Dystrophies 2111
Medical Management 2111
Nursing Management 2112

Degenerative Disc Disease 2113
Pathophysiology 2113
Clinical Manifestations 2113
Assessment and Diagnostic Findings 2113
Medical Management 2114

Herniation of a Cervical Intervertebral Disc 2114
Clinical Manifestations 2114
Medical Management 2114

• *Nursing Process:* The Patient Undergoing a Cervical Discectomy 2115

Herniation of a Lumbar Disc 2117
Clinical Manifestations 2117
Assessment and Diagnostic Findings 2117
Medical Management 2117
Nursing Management 2118

Post-Polio Syndrome 2119
Pathophysiology 2119
Assessment and Diagnostic Findings 2119
Management 2119

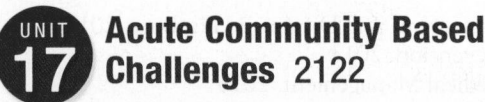

UNIT 17 Acute Community Based Challenges 2122

71 Management of Patients With Infectious Diseases 2124

The Infectious Process 2125
The Chain of Infection 2125
Colonization, Infection, and Infectious Disease 2125

Infection Control and Prevention 2128
Preventing Infection in the Hospital 2129
Preventing Infection in the Community 2133

Home-Based Care of the Patient With an Infectious Disease 2136
Reducing Risk to the Patient 2136
Reducing Risk to Household Members 2137
Nursing Management 2137

Diarrheal Diseases 2138
Transmission 2138
Causes 2138

• *Nursing Process:* The Patient With Infectious Diarrhea 2145

Sexually Transmitted Infections 2146
Syphilis 2147
Stages of Syphilis 2147
Assessment and Diagnostic Findings 2147
Medical Management 2147
Nursing Management 2147
Chlamydia trachomatis and Neisseria gonorrhoeae Infections 2147
Clinical Manifestations 2148
Complications 2148
Assessment and Diagnostic Findings 2148
Medical Management 2148
Nursing Management 2148

• *Nursing Process:* The Patient With a Sexually Transmitted Infection 2148

Emerging Infectious Diseases 2150
Zika Virus 2150
West Nile Virus 2150
Ebola Virus Disease 2151
Pathophysiology 2151
Clinical Manifestations 2151
Medical Management 2151
Nursing Management 2151
Legionnaires Disease 2151
Pathophysiology 2151
Risk Factors 2151
Clinical Manifestations 2152
Assessment and Diagnostic Findings 2152
Medical Management 2152
Nursing Management 2152
Pertussis 2152
Pathophysiology 2152
Clinical Manifestations 2152
Assessment and Diagnostic Findings 2152
Medical Management 2152
Nursing Management 2152

Travel and Immigration 2153
  Immigration and Acquired Immune
    Deficiency Syndrome 2153
  Immigration and Tuberculosis 2153
  Immigration and Vector-Borne Diseases 2153

72 Emergency Nursing 2156
ISSUES IN EMERGENCY NURSING CARE 2157
  Documentation of Consent and Privacy 2157
  Limiting Exposure to Health Risks 2157
  Violence in the Emergency Department 2157
  Providing Holistic Care 2158
EMERGENCY NURSING AND THE CONTINUUM OF CARE 2160
  Discharge Planning 2160
  Community and Transitional Services 2160
  Gerontologic Considerations 2160
  Obesity Considerations 2160
PRINCIPLES OF EMERGENCY CARE 2161
  Triage 2161
  Assess and Intervene 2162
AIRWAY OBSTRUCTION 2163
  Pathophysiology 2163
  Clinical Manifestations 2163
  Assessment and Diagnostic Findings 2163
  Management 2163
HEMORRHAGE 2165
  Management 2165
HYPOVOLEMIC SHOCK 2167
WOUNDS 2167
  Management 2167
TRAUMA 2167
  Collection of Forensic Evidence 2168
  Injury Prevention 2168
  Multiple Trauma 2168
    Assessment and Diagnostic Findings 2169
    Management 2169
  Intra-Abdominal Injuries 2169
    Assessment and Diagnostic Findings 2169
    Management 2170
  Crush Injuries 2170
    Assessment and Diagnostic Findings 2171
    Management 2171
  Fractures 2171
    Management 2171
ENVIRONMENTAL EMERGENCIES 2171
  Heat-Induced Illnesses 2171
    Gerontologic Considerations 2172
    Assessment and Diagnostic Findings 2172
    Management 2172
  Frostbite 2173
    Assessment and Diagnostic Findings 2173
    Management 2173
  Hypothermia 2173
    Assessment and Diagnostic Findings 2174
    Management 2174
  Nonfatal Drowning 2174
    Management 2175
  Decompression Sickness 2175
    Assessment and Diagnostic Findings 2175
    Management 2175
  Animal and Human Bites 2175

Snakebites 2176
  Clinical Manifestations 2176
  Management 2176
Spider Bites 2177
Tick Bites 2177
POISONING 2178
  Ingested (Swallowed) Poisons 2178
  Carbon Monoxide Poisoning 2179
    Clinical Manifestations 2179
    Management 2179
  Skin Contamination Poisoning (Chemical
    Burns) 2179
  Food Poisoning 2180
SUBSTANCE ABUSE 2180
  Acute Alcohol Intoxication 2185
  Alcohol Withdrawal Syndrome/Delirium
    Tremens 2185
VIOLENCE, ABUSE, AND NEGLECT 2186
  Family Violence, Abuse, and Neglect 2186
    Clinical Manifestations 2186
    Assessment and Diagnostic Findings 2186
    Management 2187
  Sexual Assault 2188
    Assessment and Diagnostic Findings 2188
    Management 2188
  Human Trafficking 2189
PSYCHIATRIC EMERGENCIES 2190
  Patients Who Are Overactive 2190
  Posttraumatic Stress Disorder 2190
    Patients Who Are Underactive or
      Depressed 2190
  Patients Who Are Suicidal 2190

73 Terrorism, Mass Casualty, and Disaster
Nursing 2193
  Federal, State, and Local Responses
    to Emergencies 2194
    Federal Agencies 2194
    State and Local Agencies 2195
    The Incident Command System 2195
  Hospital Emergency Preparedness Plans 2195
    Components of the Emergency
      Operations Plan 2196
    Initiating the Emergency Operations Plan 2196
  Preparedness and Response 2200
    Recognition and Awareness 2200
    Personal Protective Equipment 2201
    Decontamination 2201
  Natural Disasters 2201
  Weapons of Terror 2202
    Blast Injury 2202
    Biologic Weapons 2203
    Chemical Weapons 2206
    Nuclear Radiation Exposure 2208

Appendix A: Diagnostic Studies and Interpretation
  Available on thePoint

Index I-1

Case Studies in This Book

QSEN Cases That Open Each Unit

UNIT 1 **Basic Concepts in Nursing**
Using Technology to Improve Care in Community Nursing   2

UNIT 2 **Biophysical and Psychosocial Concepts in Nursing Practice**
Providing Care for a Patient With a Communication Barrier   82

UNIT 3 **Concepts and Challenges in Patient Management**
Managing Pain in End of Life Care   222

UNIT 4 **Perioperative Concepts and Nursing Management**
Empowering Through Informed Consent   416

UNIT 5 **Gas Exchange and Respiratory Function**
Preventing Readmissions in Patients With COPD   478

UNIT 6 **Cardiovascular and Circulatory Function**
Avoiding a Near Miss With Anticoagualtion Therapy   670

UNIT 7 **Hematologic Function**
Preventing Infection in The Patient With Leukemia   900

UNIT 8 **Immunologic Function**
Supporting the Patient With Systemic Lupus Erythematous   1002

UNIT 9 **Musculoskeletal Function**
Developing a Team Approach to Care in the Home Setting   1112

UNIT 10 **Digestive and Gastrointestinal Function**
Promoting Self-Care in the Patient With a New Ostomy   1222

UNIT 11 **Metabolic and Endocrine Function**
Ensuring Open Communication and Appropriate Delegation   1356

UNIT 12 **Kidney and Urinary Tract Function**
Decreasing Central Line–Associated Bloodstream Infections (CLABSI)   1546

UNIT 13 **Reproductive Function**
Incorporating Technology in Managing a Patient With Newly Diagnosed Prostate Cancer   1648

UNIT 14 **Integumentary Function**
Managing a Patient With a Pressure Ulcer   1788

UNIT 15 **Sensory Function**
Supporting a Patient Who Values Independence   1874

UNIT 16 **Neurologic Function**
Evaluating Increased Hypertension in a Neurology Clinic   1944

UNIT 17 **Acute Community Based Challenges**
Ensuring Equitable Patient Assignments in an Emergency Department   2122

Unfolding Cases That Appear Within Chapters

Chapter 4 **Health Education and Health Promotion**
Unfolding Patient Stories: Vincent Brody, Part 1   58

Chapter 6 **Individual and Family Homeostasis, Stress, and Adaptation**
Unfolding Patient Stories: Skyler Hansen, Part 1   97

Chapter 12 **Pain Management**
Unfolding Patient Stories: Stan Checketts, Part 1   245

Chapter 15 **Management of Patients With Oncologic Disorders**
Unfolding Patient Stories: Doris Bowman, Part 1   331

Chapter 17 **Preoperative Nursing Management**
Unfolding Patient Stories: Vernon Watkins, Part 1   429

Chapter 23 **Management of Patients With Chest and Lower Respiratory Tract Disorders**
Unfolding Patient Stories: Kenneth Bronson, Part 1   591

Chapter 24 **Management of Patients With Chronic Pulmonary Disease**
Unfolding Patient Stories: Jennifer Hoffman, Part 1   664

Chapter 26 **Management of Patients With Dysrhythmias and Conduction Problems**
Unfolding Patient Stories: Kenneth Bronson, Part 2   729

Chapter 27 **Management of Patients With Coronary Vascular Disorders**
Unfolding Patient Stories: Carl Shapiro, Part 1   757

Chapter 32 **Assessment of Hematologic Function and Treatment Modalities**
Unfolding Patient Stories: Lloyd Bennett, Part 1   913

Chapter 37 **Assessment and Management of Patients With Allergic Disorders**
Unfolding Patient Stories: Jennifer Hoffman, Part 2   1064

Chapter 42 **Management of Patients With Musculoskeletal Trauma**
Unfolding Patient Stories: Marilyn Hughes, Part 1   1193

Chapter 47 **Management of Patients With Intestinal and Rectal Disorders**
Unfolding Patient Stories: Stan Checketts, Part 2   1329

Chapter 51 **Assessment and Management of Patients With Diabetes**
Unfolding Patient Stories: Skyler Hansen, Part 2   1476

Chapter 53 **Assessment of Kidney and Urinary Function**
Unfolding Patient Stories: Lloyd Bennett, Part 2   1559

Chapter 57 **Management of Patients With Female Reproductive Disorders**
Unfolding Patient Stories: Doris Bowman, Part 2   1716

Chapter 60 **Assessment of Integumentary Function**
Unfolding Patient Stories: Vincent Brody, Part 2   1795

Chapter 63 **Assessment and Management of Patients With Eye and Vision Disorders**
Unfolding Patient Stories: Vernon Watkins, Part 2   1886

Chapter 65 **Assessment of Neurologic Function**
Unfolding Patient Stories: Marilyn Hughes, Part 2   1960

Chapter 72 **Emergency Nursing**
Unfolding Patient Stories: Carl Shapiro, Part 2   2191

Special Charts in This Book*

Assessment

Assessing the Home Environment   23
Assessing the Need for Home Visits   23
Patient Profile   68
Assessing the Health of People With Disabilities   70
Assessing for Stress   90
Assessing for Patients' Cultural Beliefs   111
Assessing Psychosocial Genetic Health   133
Assessing Potential Struggles in Function or
    Movement   168
Assessing Mental Status: Mini-Mental State Examination
    Sample Items   205
Confusion Assessment Method   211
Assessing for Arterial Blood Gases   289
Assessing for Infiltration   292
Assessing for Phlebitis   293
Assessing End-of-Life Care Beliefs, Preferences, and
    Practices   400
Assessing the Patient and Family Perspective: Goal Setting
    in Palliative Care   401
Assessing Symptoms Associated With Terminal
    Illness   403
Assessing for Anticipatory Mourning in the Family Facing
    Life-Threatening Illness   411
Assessing Psychosocial Factors Related to Respiratory
    Function and Disease   491
Assessing for Obstructive Sleep Apnea   568
Assessing Patients With Chronic Obstructive Pulmonary
    Disease   639
Assessing Patients for Postural Hypotension   687
Assessing Angina   760
Assessing for Acute Coronary Syndrome or Acute
    Myocardial Infarction   763
Heart Failure   822
Assessing for Thrombosis and Bleeding in Disseminated
    Intravascular Coagulation   957
Assessing for Immune Dysfunction   1014
Allergy Assessment Form   1062
Assessing for Rheumatic Disorders   1085
Assessing for Peripheral Nerve Function   1126
Assessing Patients Receiving Tube Feedings   1250
Assessing for Home Nutrition Support   1261
Rome IV Diagnostic Criteria for Functional
    Constipation   1312
Assessing for Cirrhosis   1407
Assessing the Patient With Diabetes   1461
Assessing for End-Stage Kidney Disease   1582
Assessing a Woman With a Disability   1659

Abnormal Assessment Findings During Inspection of the
    Breasts   1722
Assessing for Skin Disorders   1795
Assessing the ABCDEs of Moles   1837
Taking a History of Patients With Eye and Vision
    Disorders   1880
Hearing Loss   1923
Glasgow Coma Scale   2039
Assessing for Brain Abscesses   2069
Assessing for Infectious Disease   2137
Food Poisoning   2180
Assessing for Abuse, Maltreatment, and Neglect   2187

Ethical Dilemma

Common Ethical Principles   31
Steps of an Ethical Analysis   35
When May Folk Remedies be Considered Harmful or
    Complementary?   110
Can Predictive Genetic Testing Threaten Patient
    Autonomy?   123
What If a Patient Asks You to Help Her End Her
    Life?   391
Who Makes Difficult Health Care Decisions for Patients
    Who Lack Capacity?   625
Should an Older Adult Be Allowed to Refuse
    Treatment When That Treatment Is Likely to Extend
    Life?   807
What If the Patient Does Not Consent to Blood
    Transfusions?   919
Can Comfort Care at End of Life Equate to Assisted
    Suicide or Active Euthanasia?   981
Under What Circumstances May a Nurse Refuse to Care
    for a Patient?   1054
Should a Health Care Agent Be Allowed to Refuse
    Treatment When That Treatment Is Likely to Extend
    Life?   1214
Is it Ethical to Withhold or Withdraw Nutrition and
    Hydration?   1254
What Ethical Principles Apply When a Candidate
    for a Second Liver Transplantation Abuses
    Alcohol?   1421
The Gift of Life for Whom? Whose Life Is It?   1609
What If the Patient Refuses to Autonomously Make
    Decisions?   1708
How Much Is Enough and What Is Comfort Care?   1885
When Might Someone's Commitment to an Independent
    Lifestyle Put Himself or Others at Risk?   1924
When is it Appropriate to Use Restraints?   2043
Who Receives Care First During a Mass Casualty?   2194

Genetics in Nursing Practice

Genetic Aspects of Health Assessment   67
Genetics Concepts and the Older Adult   196

*Please note that updated versions of the Procedural Guidelines charts that
  appeared in the 13th edition book are now found in the student resources
  on thePoint at http://thepoint.lww.com/Brunner14e.

Genetics Concepts and Oncologic Disorders   327
Genetics Concepts and Perioperative Nursing   424
Respiratory Disorders   491
Cardiovascular Disorders   683
Hematologic Disorders   910
Immunologic Disorders   1017
Musculoskeletal Disorders   1122
Digestive and Gastrointestinal Disorders   1234
Hepatic Disorders   1381
Metabolic and Endocrine Disorders   1506
Kidney and Urinary Disorders   1557
Female Reproductive Processes   1656
Male Reproductive Disorders   1760
Integumentary Conditions   1796
Eye and Vision Disorders   1880
Hearing Disorders   1922
Neurologic Disorders   1958

Health Promotion

Nursing Strategies for Promoting Cognitive Function   205
American Cancer Society Guidelines on Nutrition and
    Physical Activity for Cancer Prevention   331
Promoting Health After Myocardial Infarction and Other
    Acute Coronary Syndromes   770
An Exercise Program for Patients With Heart Failure   829
Facts About Dietary Sodium   830
Protecting Against HIV Infection   1028
Strategies for Preventing Acute Low Back Pain
    Prevention   1162
Strategies for Preventing Osteoporosis   1169
Denture Care   1230
Prevention of Hepatitis   1400
Interventions for Urinary Incontinence   1625
Strategies for Women Approaching Menopause   1682
Strategies for The Patient With Genital Herpes   1693
Preventing Skin Cancer   1836
Burn Prevention   1846
Strategies for the Patient With Epilepsy   2003
Preventing Head and Spinal Cord Injuries   2034
Strategies For the Patient With PD   2107
Preventing Heat-Induced Illnesses   2172

Home Care Checklist

Managing Chronic Illness and Disability at Home   160
Managing the Therapeutic Regimen at Home   189
Managing the Therapeutic Regimen at Home   190
The Patient Receiving Care for an Oncologic
    Disorder   378
Discharge After Surgery   463
Oxygen Therapy   516
Ventilator Care   534
The Patient With a Thoracotomy   549
The Patient With a Laryngectomy   580
Prevention of Recurrent Pulmonary Embolism   619
Use of Peak Flow Meter in Asthma Management   663
Educating the Patient With an Implantable Cardiac
    Device   747
Managing Angina Pectoris   762
Discharge After Cardiac Surgery   782
The Patient With Heart Failure   832
Foot and Leg Care in Peripheral Vascular Disease   857

The Patient at Risk for Infection   946
The Patient at Risk for Bleeding   947
Home Administration of Ig Replacement Therapy   1025
Infection Prevention for the Patient With Immune
    Deficiency   1052
Allergy Management   1073
Managing Food Allergies   1077
The Patient With Rheumatoid Arthritis   1097
The Patient With a Cast, Splint, or Brace   1136
The Patient With an External Fixator   1139
The Patient Who Has Had Orthopedic Surgery   1154
Hand or Foot Surgery   1166
The Patient With Osteomyelitis   1179
The Patient With a Bone Tumor   1182
The Patient With a Closed Fracture   1192
The Patient With an Amputation   1219
The Patient Receiving Tube Feeding   1256
The Patient Receiving Parenteral Nutrition   1261
The Patient With an Oral Disorder   1273
The Patient Recovering From Neck Surgery   1278
The Patient With an Esophageal Disorder   1286
The Patient With Gastritis   1296
The Patient With Peptic Ulcer Disease   1303
The Patient With Gastric Cancer   1308
The Patient with Inflammatory Bowel Disease   1336
Managing Ostomy Care   1343
Management of Ascites   1388
The Patient With Hypothyroidism (Myxedema)   1518
The Patient With Hyperthyroidism   1524
The Patient With Hyperparathyroidism   1529
The Patient With Hypoparathyroidism   1530
The Patient With Adrenal Insufficiency (Addison
    Disease)   1536
The Patient With Cushing Syndrome   1539
The Patient Undergoing Hemodialysis   1594
Peritoneal Dialysis, Continuous Ambulatory Peritoneal
    Dialysis, or Continuous Cycling Peritoneal
    Dialysis   1600
The Patient With Pelvic Inflammatory Disease   1696
Patient With a Drainage Device Following Breast
    Surgery   1738
Self-Administration of Hematopoietic Growth
    Factors   1743
Postprostatectomy Care   1778
The Patient With a Burn Injury   1871
Intraocular Lens Implant   1897
Discharge After Intracranial Surgery   1994
The Patient Recovering From a Stroke   2030
The Patient With a TBI   2047
The Patient With a Halo Vest   2056
The Patient With MS   2078
The Patient With GBS   2085
The Patient With Nervous System Metastases   2099
The Patient With Cervical Discectomy and Cervical
    Collar   2116
Prevention of Infection in the Home Care Setting   2136

Nursing Research Profile

Home Health Services and Telehealth   8
Predicting Rehospitalization in Home Health Care   20

Critical Thinking Skills in Nursing Students   28
Perception and Attitudes Toward Dementia and Dementia
    Risk Reduction   56
Food Patterns Among Hispanic Women   79
Perceived Sources of Stress Among Nursing Students   96
Self-Assessed Cultural Competency of Nurses   112
Family Health History, Genetic Testing and Feasibility of
    Pedigree Development   131
Secondary Health Conditions in Individuals With
    Multiple Sclerosis   151
Understanding Interdisciplinary Teams in Rehabilitation
    Practice   165
Care Transitions for Older Adults Discharged Home from
    the Emergency Department   203
Effects of Patient-Directed Music   246
Monitoring Intake and Output in Patients in the ICU   262
Family Presence During Life-Threatening Events   313
Do Neutropenic Diets Prevent Infection?   351
Perceptions of Helpful Interventions During End-of-Life
    Care   399
The Relationship Between Certification of Nurses and
    Surgical Outcomes   434
Comparing Methods of Intraoperative Temperature
    Monitoring   440
The Effectiveness of Aromatherapy for Relief of
    Postoperative Nausea and Vomiting   460
The Patient Receiving Mechanical Ventilation   532
Patterns of Symptom Severity of Patients With Cancer of
    the Head and Neck   581
Nurses' Knowledge About Neuromuscular Blocking
    Agents   612
Sleep and Quality of Life in Chronic Obstructive
    Pulmonary Disease   647
Electrode Placement, Skin Preparation, and Alarm
    Fatigue   698
Uncertainty Among Couples With Atrial
    Fibrillation   736
Glycemic Control in Patients Post-Cardiac Surgery   785
Quality of Life After Heart Transplant   806
Helping Patients With Heart Failure Adhere to a
    Low-Sodium Diet   827
The Effects of Smoking on Walking and Quality-of-Life in
    Patients With Peripheral Arterial Disease   856
Perceptions of Hypertension and Health Behaviors Among
    African American Women   895
Attitudes Toward Patients With Sickle Cell Disease
    in a Multicenter Sample of Emergency Department
    Providers   941
Sleep Disturbances Among Patients Post-HSCT   980
Peripheral Immune Response Trajectories   1016
Symptom Self-Management Using Technology   1038
Addressing Unmet Needs of Patients With Rheumatoid
    Arthritis   1096
Guided Imagery for Pain Relief after Total Knee
    Replacement   1146
Osteoporosis Risks in Men   1171
Venous Thromboembolism Knowledge of Older Adults
    After Hip Fracture   1205
Experiences of Patients with Acute Abdominal Pain   1229
Enteral Feedings During Repositioning and the Incidence
    of Aspiration   1248

Family Caregivers of Patients with Head and Neck
    Cancers   1276
The Effects of a Dietary Intervention on Patients With
    Gastrectomy   1307
The Efficacy of a Self-Care Program on Symptoms and
    Quality of Life of Patients With Irritable Bowel
    Syndrome   1320
Pressure Ulcers Among Critically Ill Patients With
    Extreme Obesity   1368
Detecting Chronic Liver Diseases in a Primary Care Nurse
    Consultancy   1384
Patients With Advanced Pancreatic Cancer and the
    Psychological Health of Their Family Caregivers   1451
Impact of Community Diabetes Education   1478
Quality of life in Patients Receiving Dialysis   1593
Risk Factors for Catheter-Associated Urinary Tract
    Infections   1621
Isolation in LGBT Youth   1660
Life With HIV Infection   1697
Nurse Navigators and Breast Biopsy   1737
Surviving Testicular Cancer   1782
Quality of Life Among Women With Acne   1817
Family Presence During Dressing Changes in the
    Burn Unit   1861
Does Interferon Beta-1a Contribute to Hearing Loss in
    Patients with Multiple Sclerosis (MS)?   1937
BIS Monitoring for Pain Assessment   1961
Experiences With a New Diagnosis of Epilepsy in Older
    Adults   1999
Awareness of Stroke Risk in Young African
    Americans   2014
Validating the Electronic Medical Record for Measuring
    Increased Intracranial Pressure   2039
Predictors of Fatigue in Patients With MS   2076
When a Partner Has Parkinson Disease   2108
Does Washing the Hands of Patients Decrease
    HAIs?   2133
Barriers to Nurses Screening for Intimate Partner
    Violence   2187
Preparedness for Loss of Electricity after a Natural
    Disaster   2200

Patient Education*

Educating Patients About Activities of Daily Living   169
Educating Patients and Their Families How to Use a Pain
    Rating Scale   231
Preoperative Instructions to Prevent Postoperative
    Complications   430
Wound Care Instructions   471
Performing Incentive Spirometry   516
Breathing Exercises   517
Effective Coughing Technique   519
Performing Arm and Shoulder Exercises   548
Use of Pressurized Metered-Dose Inhaler (pMDI)   647
Self-Management After Cardiac Catheterization   705
Taking Anticoagulant Medications   873
Taking Oral Iron Supplements   931
The Correct Way to Use a Male Condom   1028

**Please note that in addition to the book's Gerontologic Considerations
and Patient Education charts, substantial information on these topics is
indicated elsewhere in the text using the same icons.*

Self-Administration of Epinephrine   1067
Muscle Setting Exercises   1135
Avoiding Hip Dislocation After Arthroplasty With
    Posterior or Posterolateral Approach   1151
Measures to Promote Shoulder Healing of Impingement
    Syndrome   1164
Encouraging Exercise after Treatment for Wrist
    Fracture   1200
Preventing Constipation   1315
Managing Lactose Intolerance   1320
Foods that Contain Gluten   1322
Healthy Eating Strategies   1364
Dietary Guidelines for the Patient Who Has Had Bariatric
    Surgery   1372
Managing Self-Care After Laparoscopic
    Cholecystectomy   1440
General Considerations for Exercise in People With
    Diabetes   1465
Basic Skills for People With Diabetes   1476
Self-Injection of Insulin   1480
Guidelines to Follow During Periods of Illness
    ("Sick Day Rules")   1484
Foot Care Tips   1495
Before and After Urodynamic Testing   1559
Preventing Recurrent Urinary Tract Infections   1621
Strategies for Promoting Urinary Continence   1626
Preventing Kidney Stones   1633
Using Urinary Diversion Collection Appliances   1642
The Pelvic Examination   1660
Using Contraceptives   1669
Performing Kegel (Pelvic Muscle) Exercises   1699
Breast Self-Examination   1724
Hand and Arm Care After Axillary Lymph Node
    Dissection   1737
Exercise After Breast Surgery   1739
Managing Side Effects of Adjuvant Hormonal Therapy in
    Breast Cancer   1744
Testicular Self-Examination   1781
Strategies for Avoiding Contact Dermatitis   1823
Instilling Eye Medications   1889
Managing Glaucoma   1894
Education for Patients About Preventing Eye
    Injuries   1903
Education for Patients With Viral Conjunctivitis   1908
Prevention of Otitis Externa   1927
Self-Care After Middle Ear or Mastoid Surgery   1931
Dietary Guidelines for Patients with Ménière Disease   1933
Tips for Hearing Aid Care   1939
Migraine Headaches   2006
Preventing the Spread of Syphilis   2148

Pharmacology

Self-Administration of Nitroglycerin   759
Administration of Thrombolytic (Fibrinolytic)
    Therapy   766
Administering and Monitoring Diuretic Therapy   826
Contraindications to Anticoagulant Therapy   871
Pharmacologic Alternatives to Blood Transfusions   923
Medications and Substances That Impair Platelet
    Function   952

Agents That Interact With Warfarin (Coumadin)   964
Selected Medications That Affect Body Weight   1363
Selected Medications That May Alter Thyroid Test
    Results   1514
Benefits and Risks of Hormonal Contraceptives   1671
Medications That Induce Ovulation   1677
Medications Associated With Erectile Dysfunction   1757

Plan of Nursing Care

Example of a Plan of Nursing Care for a Patient Post
    Laparoscopic Appendectomy   42
Care of the Patient With Acute Pain   247
The Patient With Cancer   358
Care of the Patient After Thoracotomy   544
Care of the Patient With Chronic Obstructive Pulmonary
    Disease   649
Care of the Patient With an Uncomplicated Myocardial
    Infarction   768
Care of the Patient After Cardiac Surgery   780
The Patient With Peripheral Vascular Problems   854
The Patient With Disseminated Intravascular
    Coagulation   960
Care of the Patient With AIDS   1044
Care of the Patient With a Rheumatic Disorder   1091
The Patient With a Total Hip Arthroplasty   1148
Care of the Older Adult Patient With a Fractured
    Hip   1206
The Patient Undergoing Ostomy Surgery   1337
The Patient With Impaired Liver Function   1409
Care of the Patient With Acute Pancreatitis   1446
Care of the Patient With Hypothyroidism   1516
Care of the Patient Undergoing Diagnostic Testing of the
    Renal–Urologic System   1560
The Patient With End-Stage Kidney Disease   1585
Care of the Patient Undergoing Kidney Surgery   1603
Care of the Patient Undergoing Kidney Surgery   1604
The Patient With Prostate Cancer   1766
Care of the Patient During the Emergent/Resuscitative
    Phase of Burn Injury   1857
Care of the Patient With Vertigo   1935
Care of the Patient With an Infectious Disease   2139

Risk Factors

Pressure Ulcers   178
Hypovolemic Shock   308
Distributive Shock   314
Surgical Complications   423
Respiratory Disease   491
Hypoventilation   501
Surgery-Related Atelectasis and Pneumonia   539
Epistaxis   569
Laryngeal Cancer   572
Pneumonia Based Upon Pathogen Type   587
Aspiration   599
Tuberculosis   600
Acute Respiratory Distress Syndrome   610
Chronic Obstructive Pulmonary Disease   636
Atrial Fibrillation   723
Coronary Artery Disease   752
Infective Endocarditis   810
Atherosclerosis and Peripheral Arterial Disease   851

Deep Vein Thrombosis and Pulmonary Embolism   868
Hypertension   887
Development of Infection and Bleeding in Patients With
     Hematologic Disorders   946
Risks Associated With HIV Infection   1027
Osteoporosis   1171
Colorectal Cancer   1343
Hepatitis B   1400
Hepatitis C   1403
Cholelithiasis   1431
Diabetes   1457

Renal Cancer   1575
Urinary Tract Infection   1616
Urinary Incontinence   1624
Bladder Cancer   1638
Vulvovaginal Infections   1687
Cervical Cancer   1706
Uterine Cancer   1709
Skin Cancer   1834
Glaucoma   1890
Cataract Formation   1894
Hearing Loss   1924
Ischemic Stroke   2014

BRUNNER & SUDDARTH'S

TEXTBOOK OF
Medical-Surgical
Nursing

14TH EDITION

UNIT
1

Basic Concepts in Nursing

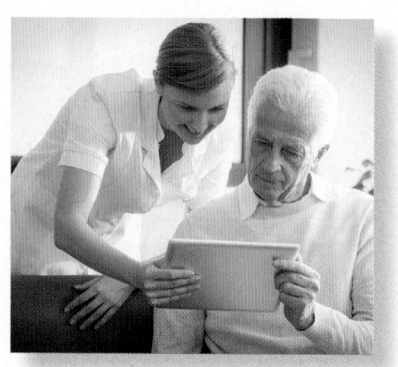

Case Study

USING TECHNOLOGY TO IMPROVE CARE IN COMMUNITY NURSING

The nurse is working in a home health agency that cares for older adults, many with comorbid conditions that require monitoring. The agency has received a grant to implement a home tele-health program for patients in the community. The nurse knows that telehealth is an emerging new technology with potential to increase adherence to prescribed therapy for patients with chronic diseases such as diabetes, heart failure, and chronic obstructive pulmonary disease. In addition, if the nurse identifies early warning signs and intervenes appropriately, hospitalizations for these patients may be prevented. In order for this program to be successful, the nurse must become familiar with the technology and how it works, become an expert in home monitoring, and be able to educate patients about the technology and how it can improve their quality of life.

QSEN Competency Focus: Informatics

The complexities inherent in today's health care system challenge nurses to demonstrate integration of specific interdisciplinary core competencies. These competencies are aimed at ensuring the delivery of safe, quality patient care (Institute of Medicine, 2003). The Quality and Safety Education for Nurses project (QSEN, 2017; Cronenwett, Sherwood, Barnsteiner, et al., 2007) provides a framework for the knowledge, skills, and attitudes (KSA) required for nurses to demonstrate competency in these key areas, which include **patient-centered care, interdisciplinary teamwork and collaboration, evidence-based practice, quality improvement, safety,** and **informatics.**

Informatics Definition: Use information and technology to communicate, manage knowledge, mitigate error, and support decision making.

SELECTED PRE-LICENSURE KSAs	APPLICATION AND REFLECTION
Knowledge	
Identify essential information that must be available in a common database to support patient care.	Describe what type of information the nurse will need to include in reporting results to the project manager for the grant. Describe ways in which the use of telehealth can potentially decrease hospitalization rates for patients monitored in the home for chronic conditions.
Skills	
Seek education about how information is managed in care settings before providing care.	Describe the type of training the nurse would need in order to use tele-health competently. Identify how the nurse can ensure quality outcomes for these older adult patients.
Attitudes	
Value nurse's involvement in design, selection, implementation, and evaluation of information technologies to support patient care.	The role of the nurse is vital in choosing which patients to monitor. How might the nurse determine which patients should be selected for the telehealth program? What barriers can the nurse anticipate with using technology at home?

Cronenwett, L., Sherwood, G., Barnsteiner, J., et al. (2007). Quality and safety education for nurses. *Nursing Outlook*, *55*(3), 122–131.
Institute of Medicine. (2003). *Health professions education: A bridge to quality*. Washington, DC: National Academies Press.
QSEN Institute. (2017). *QSEN competencies: Definitions and pre-licensure KSAs*. Retrieved on 3/1/2017 at: www.qsen.org/competencies/pre-licensure-ksas

1

Health Care Delivery and Evidence-Based Nursing Practice

LEARNING OBJECTIVES

On completion of this chapter, the learner will be able to:

1 Define nursing, health, wellness, and health promotion.
2 Describe how changes in population demographics, changes in patterns of disease and wellness, and advances in technology and genetics have influenced the health care delivery system.
3 Discuss recent laws, provisions, and practices that improve quality and safety and ensure the use of evidence-based practices within the health care system.
4 Discuss behavioral competencies and characteristics of professional nursing practice.
5 Describe models that foster interdisciplinary collaborative practice and promote safety and quality outcomes in the practice of health care.

GLOSSARY

advanced practice registered nurse (APRN): a title that encompasses certified nurse practitioners (CNPs), clinical nurse specialists (CNSs), certified nurse-midwives (CNMs), and certified registered nurse anesthetists (CRNAs)

bundle: a set of three to five evidence-based practices that, when implemented appropriately, can measurably improve patient outcomes

core measures: benchmark standards of best practices used to gauge how well a hospital gives care to its patients who are admitted to seek treatment for a specific disease (e.g., heart failure) or who need a specific treatment (e.g., an immunization)

evidence-based practice (EBP): a best practice derived from valid and reliable research studies that also considers the health care setting, patient preferences and values, and clinical judgment

health: according to the World Health Organization (2006), a "state of complete physical, mental, and social well-being and not merely the absence of disease and infirmity" (p. 1); often viewed as equivalent to wellness

health informatics: the use of health information technology to improve the quality, efficiency, or delivery of health care

health promotion: focuses on the potential for wellness and targets appropriate alterations in personal habits, lifestyle, and environment in ways that reduce risks and enhance health and well-being

interprofessional collaborative practice: employing multiple health professionals to work together with patients, families, and communities to deliver best practices, thus ensuring best patient outcomes

Joint Commission: a nonprofit organization that accredits hospitals and health care organizations

medical-surgical nursing: a specialty area of practice that provides nursing services to patients from adolescence through the end-of-life in hospital medical-surgical units, clinics, ambulatory care units, urgent care centers, home health care agencies, and long-term care facilities

National Patient Safety Goals (NPSGs): areas of patient safety concern identified annually by the Joint Commission that, if rectified, may have the most positive impact on improving patient care and outcomes

nursing: according to the American Nurses Association (2015b), "the protection, promotion, and optimization of health and abilities, prevention of illness and injury, facilitation of healing, alleviation of suffering through the diagnosis and treatment of human response, and advocacy in the care of individuals, families, groups, communities, and populations" (p. 1)

patient: a traditional term used to identify someone who is a recipient of health care

pay for performance: a health insurance model that reimburses health care provider groups, hospitals, and health care agencies for either meeting or exceeding metrics that demonstrate that the care and treatments rendered are both cost-efficient and of best quality; also known as *value-based purchasing*

precision medicine: using advances in research, technology, and policies to develop individualized plans of care to prevent and treat disease

Quality and Safety Education for Nurses (QSEN): a project whose aim is to develop curricula that prepare future nurses with the knowledge, skills, and attitudes (KSAs) required to continuously improve the quality and safety of the health care system through demonstrating competency in patient-centered care, teamwork and collaboration, evidence-based practice, quality improvement, safety, and informatics

telehealth: the use of technology to deliver health care, health information, or health education at a distance

wellness: the ability to perform well, adjust and adapt to varying situations, and report feeling well and harmonious

As American society has undergone changes, so has the nation's health care system. Nursing, as the health care profession with the greatest number of employees and a major contributor to the health care delivery system, has been significantly affected by these changes. Nursing has played an important role in the health care system and will continue to do so. This chapter provides an overview of the practice of nursing in the United States today.

Nursing

Since the time of Florence Nightingale, who wrote in 1858 that the goal of nursing was "to put the patient in the best condition for nature to act upon him," nursing scholars and leaders have described nursing as both an art and a science. However, the definition of nursing has evolved over time. In the American Nurses Association (ANA) Scope and Standards of Practice (ANA, 2015b, p. 1), **nursing** is defined as "the protection, promotion, and optimization of health and abilities, prevention of illness and injury, facilitation of healing, alleviation of suffering through the diagnosis and treatment of human response, and advocacy in the care of individuals, families, groups, communities, and populations." Nurses have a responsibility to carry out their role as described in Nursing's Social Policy Statement (ANA, 2010; Fowler, 2015), to comply with the nurse practice act of the state in which they practice, and to comply with the Code of Ethics for Nurses as spelled out by the ANA (2015a) and the International Council of Nurses (ICN, 2012).

The Patient: Consumer of Nursing and Health Care

The term **patient**, derived from a Latin verb meaning "to suffer," has traditionally been used to describe a person who is a recipient of care. The connotation commonly attached to the word is one of dependence. For this reason, many nurses prefer to use the term *client*, which is derived from a Latin verb meaning "to lean," connoting alliance and interdependence. The term *patient* is used purposely throughout this book; it is most commonly used by clinicians, as evidenced by its usage by the Interprofessional Education Collaborative (IPEC) (2016), whose members include 15 national associations of schools of the health professions, including nursing, allopathic medicine, osteopathic medicine, pharmacy, dentistry, and public health, to name a few (see later discussion of IPEC).

The patient who seeks care for a health problem or problems (increasing numbers of people have multiple health problems) is also an individual person, a member of a family, a member of various social groups, and a citizen of the community. Patients' needs vary depending on problems, associated circumstances, and past experiences. Many patients, who as consumers of health care have become more knowledgeable about health care options, expect a collaborative approach with the nurse in the quest for optimal health (van den Hooff & Goossensen, 2015). Among the nurse's important functions in health care delivery are identifying the patient's immediate, ongoing, and long-term needs and working in concert with the patient to address them.

The Patient's Basic Needs: Maslow Hierarchy of Needs

Certain needs are basic to all people. Some of these needs are more important than others. Once an essential need is met, people often experience a need on a higher level of priority. Addressing needs by priority reflects Maslow hierarchy of needs (see Fig. 1-1).

Maslow ranked human needs to include physiologic needs, safety and security, sense of belonging and affection, esteem and self-respect, and self-actualization. Self-actualization includes self-fulfillment, desire to know and understand, and aesthetic needs. Lower-level needs always remain; however, a person's ability to pursue higher-level needs indicates movement toward psychological health and well-being (Maslow, 1954). Such a hierarchy of needs is a useful framework that can be applied to many nursing models for assessment of a patient's strengths, limitations, and need for nursing interventions.

Health

How health is perceived depends on how health is defined. The World Health Organization (WHO, 2006) defines **health** in the preamble to its constitution as a "state of complete physical, mental, and social well-being and not merely the absence of disease and infirmity" (p. 1). This definition implies that health and illness are not polar opposites. Theoretically, therefore, it is possible for a patient to have a physical illness and yet strive for and perhaps attain health in another domain (e.g., mental, social). Although commonly cited worldwide, this definition has been criticized for being too utopian—after all, it is not possible for anyone to achieve *complete* physical, mental, and social well-being (Pender, Murdaugh, & Parsons, 2015)

Figure 1-1 • This scheme of Maslow hierarchy of needs shows how a person moves from fulfillment of basic needs to higher levels of needs, with the ultimate goal being integrated human functioning and health.

Wellness

Wellness has been defined as being equivalent to health. Wellness involves being proactive and being involved in self-care activities aimed toward a state of physical, psychological, and spiritual well-being. Wellness is conceptualized as having four components: (1) the capacity to perform to the best of one's ability, (2) the ability to adjust and adapt to varying situations, (3) a reported feeling of well-being, and (4) a feeling that "everything is together" and harmonious (Hood, 2013). With this in mind, nurses must aim to promote positive changes that are directed toward health and well-being. The sense of wellness has a subjective aspect that addresses the importance of recognizing and responding to patient individuality and diversity in health care and nursing.

Health Promotion

Today, increasing emphasis is placed on health, wellness, health promotion, and self-care. Health is seen as resulting from a lifestyle oriented toward wellness. **Health promotion** focuses on the potential for wellness and targets appropriate alterations in personal habits, lifestyle, and environment in ways that reduce risks and enhance health and well-being (see Chapter 4).

People are increasingly knowledgeable about health and take more interest in and responsibility for health and well-being. Organized self-care education programs emphasize health promotion, disease prevention, management of illness, self-care, and collaborative use of the professional health care system. Web sites, chat groups, and social media applications promote sharing of experiences and information about self-care with others who have similar conditions, chronic diseases, or disabling conditions. The advent of mobile wireless computer technologies (e.g., Fitbit™) and novel informatics tools (e.g., Step counts) have had the effect of tailoring health promotion activities to meet individual preferences (Pender et al., 2015). Researchers have begun to take advantage of these popular technological advancements by developing population-based registries. For instance, in 2015, more than 41,000 people consented that specific smartphone application data could be used to study the effects of activity on cardiac health (Keller, 2015; Stanford University Medicine, 2016).

Influences on Health Care Delivery

The health care delivery system is constantly adapting to changes in health care needs and expectations. Shifting population demographics; changing patterns of disease and wellness; advances in technology and genetics; and greater emphasis on health care quality, costs, and reform efforts have impacted health care delivery and nursing.

Population Demographics

Changes in the population in general are affecting the need for and the delivery of health care. The US Bureau of the Census estimated that nearly 309 million people reside in the country (Mackun & Wilson, 2011). Not only is the population increasing, but its composition is also changing. The decline in birth rate and the increase in lifespan have resulted in proportionately fewer school-age children and more senior citizens, many of whom are women. Much of the population resides in highly congested urban areas, with a steady migration of members of ethnic minorities to urban settings. Poverty is a greater concern; it is estimated that on any given night, more than 400,000 Americans are homeless, with more than 1.5 million experiencing homelessness annually. Of these, 37.2% of homeless persons come from homeless families, which are mostly headed by women with two children, and tend to be of ethnic minority status (Substance Abuse and Mental Health Services Administration [SAMHSA], 2011).

 Gerontologic Considerations

Both the number and proportion of Americans 65 years of age and older have grown substantially in the past century. In 2013, an estimated 44.7 million older adults resided in the United States; this number is expected to grow to 79.7 million by 2040. The rate of growth among all older adults will continue to climb, with the greatest growth in the Hispanic population (Administration on Aging [AoA], 2014).

The health care needs of older adults are complex and demand significant investments, both professional and financial. Many older adults suffer from multiple chronic conditions that are exacerbated by acute episodes. In particular, older women are frequently underdiagnosed and undertreated. Although older women continue to outnumber older men, the overall number of older men has also increased over the past decade (Howden & Meyer, 2011) (see Chapter 11).

Cultural Diversity

An appreciation for the diverse characteristics and needs of people from varied ethnic and cultural backgrounds is important in health care and nursing. Some projections indicate that by 2030, racial and ethnic minority populations in the United States will triple. The 2010 census classified five distinct races (White, Black, Asian, Native American, and Native Hawaiian/Pacific Islander). The Asian race had the largest growth rate among these five racial groups. The Hispanic population, classified primarily under the White race, was noted to account for more than half of the increased population growth. With increased immigration, this figure could approach 50% by the year 2030 (Humes, Jones, & Ramerez, 2011). By the middle of the 21st century, it is projected that the *majority-minority* crossover will occur, meaning that the non-Hispanic Caucasian population will proportionally decrease so that it will no longer comprise the *majority* population, and other ethnic and racial *minority* populations will collectively comprise the majority of all Americans (Ortman & Guarneri, 2011). As the cultural composition of the population changes, it is increasingly important to address cultural considerations in the delivery of health care. Patients from diverse sociocultural groups not only bring various health care beliefs, values, and practices to the health care setting but also have unique risk factors for some disease conditions and unique reactions to treatment. These factors significantly affect a person's responses to health care problems or illnesses, to caregivers, and to the care itself. Unless these factors are assessed, understood, and respected by nurses, the care delivered may be ineffective, and health care outcomes may be negatively affected (see Chapter 7).

Changing Patterns of Disease and Wellness

During the past several decades, the health problems of the American people have changed significantly. Chronic diseases, including cardiovascular disease, cancers, diabetes, and chronic lung diseases, account for 7 out of 10 leading causes of death (Centers for Disease Control and Prevention [CDC], 2015). Nearly half of all adults live with one diagnosed chronic condition; 60 million live with two or more (Mereya, Raval, & Sambamoorthi, 2015). Tobacco use, substance abuse (e.g., alcohol, illicit drugs), poor physical activity and nutrition habits, and obesity have become major health concerns, and are associated with multiple chronic conditions such as hypertension, coronary artery disease, diabetes, and cancer (CDC, 2015).

As the prevalence of chronic conditions increases, health care broadens from a focus on cure and eradication of disease to include health promotion and the prevention or rapid treatment of exacerbations of chronic conditions. Nursing, which has always encouraged patients to take control of health and wellness, has a prominent role in the current focus on management of chronic illness and disability (see Chapter 9).

Healthy People 2020

The *Healthy People* initiatives identify important periodic goals that, if reached, could have major impacts on improving the nation's health (U.S. Department of Health and Human Services [HHS], 2014). *Healthy People 2020* (HHS, 2014), the most recent of these initiatives, set several goals that are aimed at reducing or eliminating illness, disability, and premature death among individuals and communities. The Leading Health Care Indicators (LHIs) include 26 important goals or indicators that are organized around topics that are aimed at improving access to health services, improving environmental quality, diminishing rates of injury and violence, addressing social determinants of health, improving use of clinical preventive services, improving patterns of nutrition and physical activity while decreasing rates of obesity, decreasing rates of tobacco use, and decreasing rates of substance abuse, among others (HHS, 2014). Enacting the goals set by the LHIs and other health care reforms have contributed to continuous change in health care organization and delivery in the United States.

Advances in Technology and Genetics

Advances in technology and genetics have occurred rapidly during the past several decades. Sophisticated techniques and devices, such as robot assisted technology, have revolutionized treatments making it possible to perform many procedures and tests on an outpatient basis. Increased knowledge and understanding of genetics and genomics have resulted in expanded screening, diagnostic testing, and treatments for a variety of conditions (see Chapter 8).

In January 2015, President Obama announced the launching of the *Precision Medicine Initiative (PMI)*, which has the ambitious aim to leverage advances in research, technology, and policies to develop individualized plans of care to prevent and treat disease (White House, 2015). **Precision medicine** is possible because of the recent development of biologic databases (e.g., human genome sequencing), technological advances that can identify unique characteristics of individual persons (e.g., genomics, cellular assay tests), and computer-driven systems that can mine and analyze datasets. The immediate goal of the PMI is to focus on preventing and curing cancers; however, there are long-term implications that hold promise for preventing and treating many other conditions and diseases (Collins & Varmus, 2015).

Health Informatics

The sophisticated communication systems that connect most parts of the world, with the capability of rapid storage, retrieval, and dissemination of information, have stimulated advances in health information technology (HIT). Using HIT to improve the quality, efficiency, or delivery of health care is an interdisciplinary field of study called **health informatics**. Key examples of recent advances in HIT include the ICD-10 coding system, the electronic health record, and the use of telehealth. Nurses must not only be cognizant of advances in HIT, but also become adept in its use as their practice setting and patient population require. The *Technology Informatics Guiding Education Reform (TIGER)* initiative, now a subsidiary of the Healthcare Information Management Systems Society (HIMSS), provides expert panel reports and guidelines for incorporating HIT into nursing practice (The TIGER Initiative Foundation, 2014).

The *International Classification of Diseases (ICD)* (WHO, 2016) launched its 10th iteration for use in the United States in 2015. The ICD-10 classifies diseases and conditions into nearly 70,000 codes. The Centers for Medicare and Medicaid Services (CMS) (2015) and most other major health insurance programs require utilization of ICD-10 codes when treatment is rendered in order for providers to claim reimbursement. This system provides for common nomenclature and tracking of the incidence and prevalence of various diseases and conditions globally. CMS (2016) also requires that clinicians and health care systems use electronic health records; its final rule for stage 3 of the *Electronic Health Record (EHR) Incentive Program* requires that providers use EHRs by 2018 or face reductions in reimbursement.

In addition to these HIT advancements, **telehealth**, which uses technology to deliver health care, health information, or health education at a distance, is being utilized by both individual clinicians and health care systems more and more frequently. In particular, home health services use telehealth to develop more individualized care plans for patients (see Chart 1-1: Nursing Research Profile). One type of telehealth application uses *real-time communication*, characterized by an exchange of information between people at one point in time. For instance, a nurse practitioner in a rural clinic may consult with a specialist on a webcam about a patient's condition. Another type of telehealth application uses *store-and-forward*, characterized by transmission of digital images that may be retrieved and reviewed at later points in time (HHS, 2016b).

Quality, Safety, and Evidence-Based Practice

At the turn of the millennium, the Institute of Medicine (IOM) (2000) reported an alarming breakdown in quality control in the American health care system. The IOM report *To Err Is Human: Building a Safer Health System* (2000)

Chart 1-1   NURSING RESEARCH PROFILE
Home Health Services and Telehealth

Radhakrishnan, K., Jacelon, C. S., Bigelow, C., et al. (2013). Association of comorbidities with home care service utilization of patients with heart failure while receiving telehealth. *Journal of Cardiovascular Nursing, 28*(3), 216–227.

Purpose

Patients with heart failure frequently have comorbid disorders and diseases. Telehealth is being used more frequently by home health nurses to provide services for patients with heart failure, as it can reduce the number of "live" home nursing visits without decreasing the quality of care delivered. The aims of this study were to identify the most common comorbidities reported by patients with heart failure who were recipients of telehealth services, and to identify the characteristics of those patients with heart failure most likely to withdraw from telehealth services.

Design

A descriptive correlational design that analyzed data obtained from retrospective chart reviews was utilized. The charts of patients with heart failure who used a telehealth program associated with a home care agency in New England between the years of 2008 and 2010 were eligible, as long as the patients had a primary diagnosis of heart failure; were recipients of Medicare; and did not have concomitant Alzheimer disease, extensive wounds, or concomitant fractures or recent surgery ($N = 403$).

Findings

The sample yielded was mostly White (94%), older than 75 years of age (70%), female (55%), urban (79%), and lived with others (69%). The mean nursing contacts was nearly 10 telehealth visits. Logistic regression analysis identified that those patients with heart failure who were more likely to use telehealth more frequently had anxiety, musculoskeletal complaints (e.g., osteoarthritis), depression, acute cardiac events (e.g., dysrhythmias), or anemia ($p <0.05$). The comorbid variables significantly associated with telehealth program withdrawal included renal disorder, cancer, and depression ($p <0.05$).

Nursing Implications

Results from this study suggest that patients with heart failure who require more frequent telehealth follow-up include those with anxiety, musculoskeletal disorders, depression, recent acute cardiac events, and anemia; whereas, those at risk for withdrawing from a telehealth program include those with a concomitant renal disorder, cancer, and depression. Recognizing comorbid complications that require more frequent telehealth interventions or risk for withdrawal from a telehealth program can aid the home health nurse to design care plans that better fit the needs of patients with heart failure receiving telehealth services.

---

noted that nearly 100,000 Americans died annually from preventable errors in hospitals, and many more suffered nonfatal injuries from errors. A subsequent IOM report, *Crossing the Quality Chasm: A New Health System for the 21st Century* (2001), described an inefficient, fragmented, health care system fraught with inequities and inaccessibility. It envisioned a reformed health care system that is evidence-based and systems-oriented. Its proposed six aims for improvement included ensuring that patient care is safe, effective, patient centered, timely, efficient, and equitable (IOM, 2001). The following sections describe a series of recent laws, provisions, and practices that are aimed at improving quality and safety and ensuring use of evidence-based practices (EBPs) within the US health care system.

The Patient Protection and Affordable Care Act

The Patient Protection and Affordable Care Act (ACA), signed into law in 2010, aims to reform the health care system so that all Americans have access to quality, affordable health care. The ACA aims to improve access to innovative and preventive health care programs and therapies and to expand insurance coverage. Key provisions under the ACA include expansion of insurance coverage for young adults up to the age of 26 under their parent's health insurance plan, elimination of lifetime limits on benefit coverage, elimination of arbitrary withdrawals of insurance coverage, and removal of barriers to use of emergency services. The ACA seeks to establish a more integrated and equitable health care system (HHS, 2016a).

Pay for Performance

As a result of the landmark IOM reports (IOM, 2000; IOM, 2001) previously cited, and because of provisions within the ACA (HHS, 2016a), the landscape of health care is rapidly changing to ensure that quality benchmarks are established. Whether or not providers and health care systems meet these benchmarks may then be publicly reported to health care consumers. Many health insurance companies are adopting pay for performance measures, also known as *value-based purchasing*. **Pay for performance** is a health insurance model that reimburses health care provider groups, hospitals, and health care agencies for either meeting or exceeding metrics that demonstrate that the care and treatments rendered are both cost-efficient and of best quality. By the same token, these same insurance companies may disallow reimbursement for care or treatment that either does not meet a predetermined quality metric or for care that is necessary because of provider error (i.e., iatrogenic).

The Joint Commission Best-Practice Initiatives

The **Joint Commission** is a nonprofit organization that accredits hospitals and health care organizations. Over the past decade, it has annually updated and published its **National Patient Safety Goals (NPSGs)**—selected NPSGs include areas of patient safety concern that, if rectified, may have the most positive impact on improving patient care and outcomes. Recently adopted NPSGs revolve around identifying patients correctly, improving staff communication, using medications safely, using alarms safely, preventing infections, identifying patient safety risks, and preventing surgery-related mistakes (Joint Commission, 2016a). Each NPSG has implications for scrutinizing and perhaps changing and improving nursing practices. In addition, the Joint Commission provides EBP solutions for these NPSGs. An **evidence-based practice (EBP)** is a best practice derived from valid and reliable research studies that also considers the health care setting, patient preferences and values, and clinical judgment. The facilitation of EBP involves identifying and evaluating current literature and research findings, and then incorporating these findings into patient care as a means of ensuring quality care (Melnyk & Fineout-Overholt, 2014).

In addition to the NPSGs, the Joint Commission, in cooperation with CMS, has developed sets of performance measures for hospitals called **core measures.** The core measures are used to gauge how well a hospital gives care to patients admitted to seek treatment for a specific disease (e.g., heart failure) or who need a specific treatment (e.g., an immunization) as compared to evidence-based guidelines and standards of care. Benchmark standards of quality are used to compare the care or treatment that patients receive as compared to the best practice standards (Joint Commission, 2016b). The percentage of the patients who receive the best care or treatment as specified at a given hospital is then calculated and reported so that hospitals can use those results to continue to improve processes and performance until they consistently meet the best practice standards 100% of the time.

Patient Satisfaction: A Quality Metric

Patients' satisfaction with the care they receive when hospitalized is an important quality metric. CMS partnered with the Agency for Healthcare Research and Quality (AHRQ) to launch the Hospital Consumer Assessment of Healthcare Providers and Systems (HCAHPS) survey. HCAHPS is a survey that is given to a random sample of recently hospitalized patients within 6 weeks of discharge. Most items on the HCAHPS survey measure patients' satisfaction with the quality of the nursing care they receive, including their satisfaction with communication with the nurses, the responsiveness of the hospital staff, the quietness of the environment, pain management, communication about medications, and discharge information. Discharged patients are also asked to provide an overall rating of the hospital and whether or not they would recommend the hospital. Hospitals' HCAHPS scores are calculated and publicly reported on the HCAHPS Web site (CAHPS Hospital Survey, 2015).

The Triple Aim of Effective Health Care Systems

The Institute for Healthcare Improvement (IHI) is a non-profit organization that advocates that effective health care systems must effect the *Triple Aim*, meaning that effective health care systems must do the following (Stiefel & Nolan, 2012):

- Improve population health
- Improve the patient care experience
- Reduce per capita costs

Under this model, in order for patients to feel that they have experienced excellent care, they must believe that their care is safe, effective, patient-centered, timely, efficient, and equitable, aims for care that are mirrored in the IOM's *Crossing the Quality Chasm* report (IOM, 2001).

Rapid Cycle Testing: A Model for Improving Quality

The credibility of IHI's quality improvement methods has encouraged hospitals to change quality improvement processes and nursing practices. For instance, many hospitals have adopted the IHI's change model (sometimes called the *rapid cycle testing* model) to more rapidly integrate proven performance improvement processes. The principles and steps that guide the Model for Improvement are shown in Chart 1-2 (IHI, 2016a). This model is commonly used by nurses and other health care professionals to monitor quality and performance improvement processes in US hospitals.

Evidence-Based Practice Bundles

The IHI has developed numerous sets of readily implemented EBP sets for use by hospitals. These **bundle**s include a set of three to five EBPs that, when implemented appropriately, can measurably improve patients' outcomes. Many of these practices are within the scope of independent nursing practice. For instance, the IHI Ventilator Bundle advocates that the head of the bed should be elevated and that oral care should be provided using chlorhexidine for all patients on ventilators (IHI, 2016b) (see Chapter 23).

EBP tools used for planning patient care may include not only bundles but also clinical guidelines, algorithms, care mapping, multidisciplinary action plans (MAPs), and clinical pathways. These tools are used to move patients toward predetermined outcomes. Algorithms are used more often in acute situations to determine a particular treatment based on patient information or response. Care maps, clinical guidelines, and MAPs (the most detailed of these tools) help to facilitate coordination of care and education throughout hospitalization and after discharge. Nurses who provide direct care have an important role in the development and use of these tools through participation in researching the literature and then developing, piloting, implementing, and revising the tools as needed.

TeamSTEPPS

Team Strategies and Tools to Enhance Performance and Patient Safety (TeamSTEPPS) is an evidence-based curriculum that trains health care professionals to achieve improved teamwork skills and communication, based upon the assumption that if teamwork improves, quality and safety will also improve (AHRQ, 2015). The premise that undergirds the development of TeamSTEPPS is that teams that train together make fewer mistakes. Hence, TeamSTEPPS developed teamwork competencies based upon four teachable-learnable team skills, including communication, leadership, situation monitoring, and mutual support. Teams that achieve competency demonstrate the knowledge of a shared mental model, the attitudes of mutual trust and team orientation; and demonstrate adaptable, accurate, productive, efficient, and safe performance (AHRQ, 2013). The TeamSTEPPS curriculum features tools that may be used by team members to enhance a given competency; a commonly used example of such a tool is the SBAR format for communicating critical information. SBAR is an acronym, which includes the following components:

- S—Situation—What is going on with the patient?
- B—Background—What is the clinical background or context?
- A—Assessment—What do I think the problem is?
- R—Recommendation or Request—What would I do to correct it?

The TeamSTEPPS 2.0 Framework and Competencies Model is displayed in Figure 1-2.

Chart 1-2   Model for Improvement (Known as Rapid Cycle Testing)

Forming the Team

Including the right people on a process improvement team is critical to a successful improvement effort. Teams vary in size and composition. Each organization builds teams to suit its own needs.

Setting Aims

Improvement requires setting aims. The aim should be time-specific and measurable; it should also define the specific population of patients or other system that will be affected.

Establishing Measures

Teams use quantitative measures to determine if a specific change actually leads to an improvement.

Selecting Changes

Ideas for change may come from the insights of those who work in the system, from change concepts or other creative thinking techniques, or by borrowing from the experience of others who have successfully improved.

Testing Changes

The Plan-Do-Study-Act (PDSA) cycle is shorthand for testing a change in the real work setting—by planning it, trying it, observing the results, and acting on what is learned. This is the scientific method adapted for action-oriented learning (see figure on right side).

Implementing Changes

After testing a change on a small scale, learning from each test, and refining the change through several PDSA cycles, the team may implement the change on a broader scale—for example, for an entire pilot population or on an entire unit.

Spreading Changes

After successful implementation of a change or package of changes for a pilot population or an entire unit, the team can spread the changes to other parts of the organization or in other organizations.

What are we trying to accomplish?

How will we know that a change is an improvement?

What changes can we make that will result in an improvement?

Act | Plan
Study | Do

Reprinted with permission from Institute for Healthcare Improvement. (2016a). *Science of improvement: How to improve.* Retrieved on 3/5/2016 at: www.ihi.org/resources/Pages/HowtoImprove/ScienceofImprovementHowtoImprove.aspx

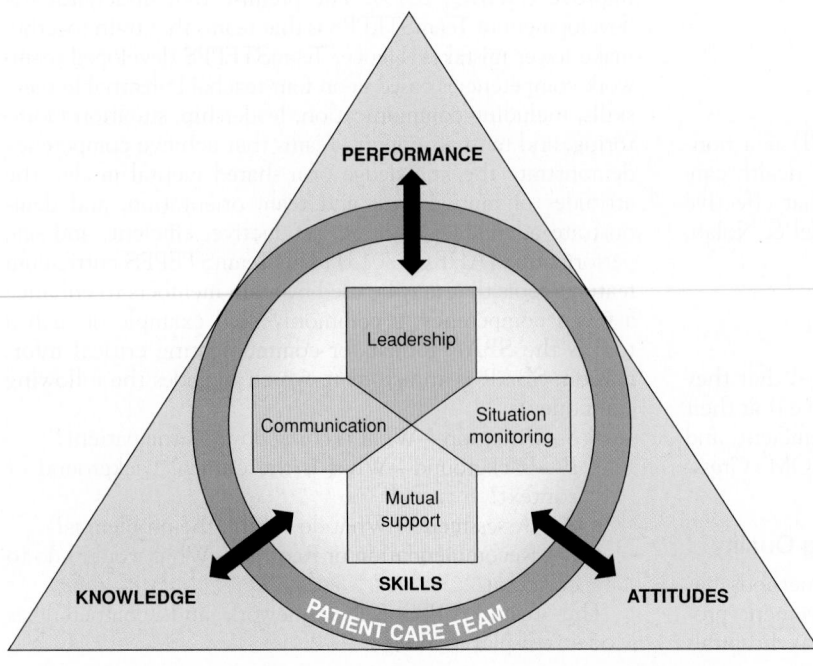

PERFORMANCE

Leadership

Communication | Situation monitoring

Mutual support

KNOWLEDGE   SKILLS   ATTITUDES

PATIENT CARE TEAM

Figure 1-2 • TeamSTEPPS 2.0 Framework and Competencies. TeamSTEPPS has five key principles. It is based on team structure and four teachable–learnable skills: Communication, Leadership, Situation Monitoring, and Mutual Support. The *arrows* depict a two-way dynamic interplay between the four skills and the team-related outcomes. Interaction between the outcomes and skills is the basis of a team striving to deliver safe, quality care and support quality improvement. Encircling the four skills is the team structure of the patient care team, which represents not only the patient and direct caregivers, but also those who play a supportive role within the health care delivery system. From Agency for Healthcare Research and Quality (AHRQ). (2013). *Pocket guide: TeamSTEPPS 2.0: Team strategies & tools to enhance performance and patient safety.* Rockville, MD: Author, AHRQ Pub. No. 14-0001-2. Reproduced with permission.

Quality and Safety Education for Nurses

The **Quality and Safety Education for Nurses (QSEN)** project was initially funded by the nonprofit Robert Wood Johnson Foundation (RWJF) to develop curricula that prepare future nurses with the knowledge, skills, and attitudes (KSAs) required to continuously improve the quality and safety of the health care system. In particular, nurses educated under QSEN concepts demonstrate the KSAs consonant with competency in patient-centered care, teamwork and collaboration, EBP, quality improvement, safety, and informatics (QSEN, 2014). Table 1-1 highlights the QSEN definition of safety and its associated KSAs.

The Practice of Nursing in Today's Health Care Delivery System

Novice, entry-level registered nurses, as well as those with advanced degrees who work in highly specialized settings, all engage in the practice of nursing. The ANA (2015b) notes that the profession of nursing's scope of practice encompasses the full range of nursing practice, pertinent to general and specialty practice. "The depth and breadth in which individual registered nurses and advanced practice registered nurses engage in the total scope of nursing practice is dependent on education, experience, role, and the population served" (p. 2). The ANA (2015b, pp. 7–9) also identifies the following tenets characteristic of all nursing practice:

- Caring and health are central to the practice of the registered nurse.
- Nursing practice is individualized.

- Registered nurses use the nursing process to plan and provide individualized care for health care consumers (see Chapter 2).
- Nurses coordinate care by establishing partnerships.
- A strong link exists between the professional work environment and the registered nurse's ability to provide quality health care and achieve optimal outcomes.

The profession of nursing has a distinct disciplinary body of knowledge, education, and specialty standards of practice (ANA, 2015b); social contract (ANA, 2010; Fowler, 2015); and code of ethics (ANA, 2015a). Nursing's Standards of Practice describe basic competencies in delivering nursing care using the nursing process (see Chapter 2), whereas the Standards of Professional Performance describe expectations for behavioral competencies (ANA, 2015b, pp. 5–6), which include that the registered nurse:

- Practices ethically
- Practices in a manner that is congruent with cultural diversity and inclusion principles
- Communicates effectively in all areas of practice
- Collaborates with the health care consumer and other key stakeholders in the conduct of nursing practice
- Leads within the professional practice setting and the profession
- Seeks knowledge and competence that reflect current nursing practice and promote futuristic thinking
- Integrates evidence and research findings into practice
- Contributes to quality nursing practice
- Evaluates one's own and others' nursing practice

TABLE 1-1 Quality and Safety Education for Nurses (QSEN) Definition of Safety and Knowledge, Skills, and Attitudes (KSAs) for Pre-Licensure Nursing Students

Safety
Definition: Minimizes risk of harm to patients and providers through both system effectiveness and individual performance.

Knowledge	Skills	Attitudes
Examine human factors and other basic safety design principles as well as commonly used unsafe practices (e.g., work-arounds and dangerous abbreviations) Describe the benefits and limitations of selected safety-enhancing technologies (e.g., barcodes, Computer Provider Order Entry, medication pumps, and automatic alerts/alarms) Discuss effective strategies to reduce reliance on memory	Demonstrate effective use of technology and standardized practices that support safety and quality Demonstrate effective use of strategies to reduce risk of harm to self or others Use appropriate strategies to reduce reliance on memory (e.g., forcing functions, checklists)	Value the contributions of standardization/reliability to safety Appreciate the cognitive and physical limits of human performance
Delineate general categories of errors and hazards in care Describe factors that create a culture of safety (e.g., open communication strategies and organizational error reporting systems)	Communicate observations or concerns related to hazards and errors to patients, families, and the health care team Use organizational error reporting systems for near miss and error reporting	Value own role in preventing errors
Describe processes used in understanding causes of error and allocation of responsibility and accountability (e.g., root cause analysis and failure mode effects analysis)	Participate appropriately in analyzing errors and designing system improvements Engage in root cause analysis rather than blaming when errors or near misses occur	Value vigilance and monitoring (even of own performance of care activities) by patients, families, and other members of the health care team
Discuss potential and actual impact of national patient safety resources, initiatives, and regulation	Use national patient safety resources for own professional development and to focus attention on safety in care settings	Value relationship between national safety campaigns and implementation in local practices and practice settings

Reprinted with permission from Cronenwett, L., Sherwood, G., Barnsteiner, J., et al. (2007). Quality and safety education for nurses. *Nursing Outlook, 55*(3), 122–131; QSEN Institute & Frances Payne Bolton School of Nursing, Case Western Reserve University (2014). Competencies: Prelicensure KSAs. Retrieved on 3/5/2016 at: qsen.org/competencies/pre-licensure-ksas/#safety

- Utilizes appropriate resources to plan, provide, and sustain evidence-based nursing services that are safe, effective, and fiscally responsible
- Practices in an environmentally safe and healthy manner

Medical-Surgical Nursing

Medical-surgical nursing is a specialty area of practice that provides nursing services to patients from adolescence through the end-of-life in a variety of inpatient and outpatient clinical settings. These settings may include traditional hospital medical-surgical units, clinics, ambulatory care units, urgent care centers, home health care agencies, and long-term care facilities (Academy of Medical-Surgical Nurses [AMSN], 2012, 2016). The *Scope and Standards of Medical-Surgical Nursing Practice* (AMSN, 2012) mirror the scope of practice and standards for practice set by the ANA (2015b) for professional nursing practice; the AMSN (2012) further delineates specific role expectations for the medical-surgical nurse. Medical-surgical nurses can demonstrate proficiency in their role by completing certification requirements. They may also enhance practice by completing graduate degree programs in nursing (AMSN, 2012).

Advanced Nursing Roles

Nurses may enroll in specialized graduate nursing education programs and pursue role preparation in a myriad of specialties, including as nurse researchers, nurse administrators, nurse informatics specialists, and nurse educators, to name a few. They may also enroll in either master's programs in nursing or doctor of nursing practice (DNP) programs (American Association of Colleges of Nursing [AACN], 2015) and pursue role preparation as certified nurse practitioners (CNPs), clinical nurse specialists (CNSs), certified nurse-midwives (CNMs), and certified registered nurse anesthetists (CRNAs), all of whom are collectively identified as **advanced practice registered nurses (APRNs)** (APRN Consensus Work Group & the National Council of State Boards of Nursing [NCSBN] APRN Advisory Committee, 2008). Each of these programs prepares APRNs to demonstrate competence with a focused population that is the recipient of care. The population foci include family, adult-gerontology, neonatal, pediatrics, women's health, and psychiatric-mental health (APRN Consensus Work Group & the NCSBN APRN Advisory Committee, 2008). The APRN roles that are most relevant to medical-surgical nursing are the CNP and CNS roles, and the most relevant population focus is adult-gerontology.

CNPs who are educationally prepared with a population focus in adult-gerontology or pediatrics receive additional focused training in primary care or acute care. CNPs may practice autonomously, diagnosing and treating individual patients with undifferentiated clinical manifestations as well as those with confirmed diagnoses. The scope of CNP practice includes health promotion and education, disease prevention, and the diagnosis and management of acute and chronic diseases for individual recipients of care (APRN Consensus Work Group & the NCSBN APRN Advisory Committee, 2008).

The primary role of CNSs, on the other hand, is to integrate care across the health care continuum through three spheres of influence—the patient, the nurse, and the health care system. In each of these spheres of influence, the goal of CNS practice is to monitor and improve aggregate patient outcomes and nursing care. CNSs identify their role to include core competency in direct care; consultation; systems leadership; collaboration; coaching; research; evaluation of clinical practice; and ethical decision making, moral agency, and advocacy (National CNS Competency Task Force, 2010).

The Nurse as Coordinator of Care Transitions

Nearly one-third of the $2 trillion spent on health care in the United States is spent on hospitalizations. Of these, approximately 20% are rehospitalizations within 30 days of discharge; and, of these, an estimated 76% are avoidable (Rutherford, Nielsen, Taylor, et al., 2013). These rehospitalizations are not only costly; patients rehospitalized are sicker and tend to become skeptical that the health care system can meet their needs. Health insurance plans are increasingly holding hospitals accountable for readmissions within 30 days of hospital discharge; many times, the plans will not reimburse hospitals for costs associated with these readmissions (Laderman, Loehrer, & McCarthy, 2013). Rehospitalizations can result from problems in discharge planning processes, patients' inability to manage their own care, and poor communication between the hospital and the next level of care (e.g., home health agency, primary care office) regarding patient needs and resources. All of these problems are collectively referenced as breakdowns in care transitions (Rutherford et al., 2013).

Patient care must be coordinated seamlessly from the inpatient hospital environment through transitions into the community setting. Various nursing roles have evolved to provide improved care coordination and care transitions, including the nurse navigator, case manager, and the clinical nurse leader (CNL). Nurse navigators are registered nurses employed by hospitals and health networks who work with a given population of patients with a common diagnosis or disease (e.g., cancer). Their role involves helping the patient and the patient's family transition through different levels of care (e.g., from hospital to a skilled nursing facility, from home care to assisted care). One example of an essential role function for the nurse navigator is patient medication reconciliation, which ensures that the patient adheres to the prescribed medication regimen, including taking medications that are newly prescribed, as well as ceasing to take those that must be discontinued.

Case management is a system of coordinating health care services to ensure cost-effectiveness, accountability, and quality care. Case managers may be nurses or may have backgrounds in other health professions, such as social work. The case manager coordinates the care of a caseload of patients through facilitating communication between nurses, other health care personnel who provide care, and insurance companies. In some settings, particularly the community setting, the case manager focuses on managing the treatment plan of the patient with complex conditions. The case manager may follow the patient throughout hospitalization and at home after discharge in an effort to coordinate health care services that will avert or delay rehospitalization. The caseload is usually limited in scope to patients with similar diagnoses, needs, and therapies (Case Management Society of America, 2016).

A CNL is a certified nurse generalist with a master's degree in nursing educated to help patients navigate the complex health care system (AACN, 2016). The CNL coordinates care for a distinct group of patients, may provide direct care as the situation warrants, and assumes a leadership role among members of the health care team. The CNL integrates evidence-based practices with advocacy, care coordination, outcomes measurement, risk assessment, quality improvement, and interprofessional communication skills (AACN, 2016). Currently, CNLs are being utilized in hospital-based environments as well as in community settings.

The Future of Nursing

The now classic report *The Future of Nursing: Leading Change, Advancing Health* (IOM, 2010) identified that the future of the profession of nursing was inextricably tied into the future of health care in the nation. This report recommended that nurses practice, "to the full extent of their education and training" (p. 1), to meet the growing primary care needs of health care consumers. This recommendation and other IOM recommendations and key messages are included in Chart 1-3. The RWJF partnered with the AARP to introduce the *Future of Nursing: Campaign for Action* to begin implementing recommendations in the report by fostering the development of national and state Action Coalitions (RWJF & AARP, 2015). In 2014, the RWJF requested that the IOM (which became the Health and Medicine Division [HMD] in 2016) reassess progress made on implementing *Future of Nursing* recommendations. The summary recommendations from this follow-up report are included in Chart 1-4 (National Academies of Sciences, Engineering, and Medicine, 2016).

Chart 1-3	The Institute of Medicine's Key Messages and Recommendations for the Future of Nursing
Key Message I	Nurses should practice to the full extent of education and training.
Key Message II	Nurses should achieve higher levels of education and training through an improved education system that promotes seamless academic progression.
Key Message III	Nurses should be full partners, with physicians and other health professionals, in redesigning health care in the United States.
Key Message IV	Effective workforce planning and policy making require better data collection and an improved information infrastructure.
Recommendation 1: Remove scope-of-practice barriers.	Advanced practice registered nurses should be able to practice to the full extent of education and training.
Recommendation 2: Expand opportunities for nurses to lead and diffuse collaborative improvement efforts.	Private and public funders, health care organizations, nursing education programs, and nursing associations should expand opportunities for nurses to lead and manage collaborative efforts with physicians and other members of the health care team to conduct research and to redesign and improve practice environments and health systems. These entities should also provide opportunities to diffuse successful practices.
Recommendation 3: Implement nurse residency programs.	State boards of nursing, accrediting bodies, the federal government, and health care organizations should take actions to support nurses' completion of a transition-to-practice program (nurse residency) after they have completed a prelicensure or advance practice degree program or when they are transitioning into new clinical practice areas.
Recommendation 4: Increase the proportion of nurses with a baccalaureate degree to 80% by 2020.	Academic nurse leaders across all schools of nursing should work together to increase the proportion of nurses with a baccalaureate degree from 50% to 80% by 2020. These leaders should partner with education accrediting bodies, private and public funders, and employers to ensure funding, monitor progress, and increase the diversity of students to create a workforce prepared to meet the demands of diverse populations across the lifespan.
Recommendation 5: Double the number of nurses with a doctorate by 2020.	Schools of nursing, with support from private and public funders, academic administrators and university trustees, and accrediting bodies, should double the number of nurses with a doctorate by 2020 to add to the cadre of nurse faculty and researchers, with attention to increasing diversity.
Recommendation 6: Ensure that nurses engage in lifelong learning.	Accrediting bodies, schools of nursing, health care organizations, and continuing competency educators from multiple health professions should collaborate to ensure that nurses and nursing students and faculty continue education and engage in lifelong learning to gain the competencies needed to provide care for diverse populations across the lifespan.
Recommendation 7: Prepare and enable nurses to lead change to advance health.	Nurses, nursing education programs, and nursing associations should prepare the nursing workforce to assume leadership positions across all levels, while public, private, and governmental health care decision makers should ensure that leadership positions are available to and filled by nurses.
Recommendation 8: Build an infrastructure for the collection and analysis of interprofessional health care workforce data.	The National Health Care Workforce Commission[a], with oversight from the Government Accountability Office and the Health Resources and Services Administration, should lead a collaborative effort to improve research and the collection and analysis of data on health care workforce requirements. The Workforce Commission and the Health Resources and Services Administration should collaborate with state licensing boards, state nursing workforce centers, and the Department of Labor in this effort to ensure that the data are timely and publicly accessible.

[a]The National Health Care Workforce Commission did not receive congressional appropriations to fulfill its mission.
Reprinted with permission from the Institute of Medicine. (2010). *The future of nursing: Leading change, advancing health.* Washington, DC: National Academies Press.

Chart 1-4 Summary of the Committee for Progress on Implementing the Recommendations of the Institute of Medicine Report *The Future of Nursing: Leading Change, Advancing Health*

In the Committee's view, the work of the Campaign and others would best be advanced if it were driven by the following three themes:

- The need to build a broader coalition to increase awareness of nurses' ability to play a full role in health professions practice, education, collaboration, and leadership;
- The need to continue to make promoting diversity in the nursing workforce a priority; and
- The need for better data with which to assess and drive progress.

The Committee hopes that, taken together, the 10 recommendations presented in this report provide a blueprint for advancing implementation of the recommendations of *The Future of Nursing*.

Recommendation 1:
Build common ground around the scope of practice and other issues in policy and practice

The Campaign should broaden its coalition to include more diverse stakeholders. The Campaign should build on its successes and work with other health professions groups, policy makers, and the community to build common ground around removing scope-of-practice restrictions, increasing interprofessional collaboration, and addressing other issues to improve health care practice in the interest of patients.

Recommendation 2:
Continue pathways toward increasing the percentage of nurses with a baccalaureate degree.

The Campaign, the nursing education community, and state systems of higher education should continue efforts aimed at strengthening academic pathways for nurses toward the baccalaureate degree—both entry-level baccalaureate and baccalaureate completion programs.

Recommendation 3:
Create and fund transition-to-practice residency programs.

The Campaign, in coordination with health care providers, health care delivery organizations, and payers, should lead efforts to explore ways of creating and funding transition-to-practice residency programs at both the registered nurse and advanced practice registered nurse levels. Such programs are needed in all practice settings, including community-based practices and long-term care. These efforts should include determining the most appropriate program models; setting standards for programs; exploring funding and business case models; and creating an overarching structure with which to track and evaluate the quality, effectiveness, and impact of transition-to-practice programs.

Recommendation 4:
Promote nurses' pursuit of doctoral degrees.

The Campaign should make efforts, through incentives and expansion of programs, to promote nurses' pursuit of both the doctor of nursing practice (DNP) and PhD degrees so as to have an adequate supply of nurses for clinical care, research, faculty, and leadership positions. More emphasis should be placed on increasing the number of PhD nurses in particular. To maximize the potential value of additional education, nurses should be encouraged to pursue these degrees early in their careers. DNP and PhD programs should offer coursework that prepares students to serve as faculty, including preparing to teach in an evolving health care system that is less focused on acute care than has previously been the case.

Recommendation 5:
Promote nurses' interprofessional and lifelong learning.

The Campaign should encourage nursing organizations, education programs, and professional societies, as well as individual nurses, to make lifelong learning a priority so that nurses are prepared to work in evolving health care environments. Lifelong learning should include continuing education that will enable nurses to gain, preserve, and measure the skills needed in the variety of environments and settings in which health care will be provided going forward, particularly community-based, outpatient, long-term care, primary care, and ambulatory settings. Nurses should work with other health care professionals to create opportunities for interprofessional collaboration and education. The Campaign could serve as a convener to bring together stakeholders from multiple areas of health care to discuss opportunities and strategies for interdisciplinary collaboration in this area.

Recommendation 6:
Make diversity in the nursing workforce a priority.

The Campaign should continue to emphasize recruitment and retention of a diverse nursing workforce as a major priority for both its national efforts and the state Action Coalitions. In broadening its coalition to include more diverse stakeholders (see Recommendation 1), the Campaign should work with others to assess progress and exchange information about strategies that are effective in increasing the diversity of the health workforce.

Recommendation 7:
Expand efforts and opportunities for interprofessional collaboration and leadership development for nurses.

As the Campaign broadens its coalition (see Recommendation 1), it should expand its focus on supporting and promoting (1) interprofessional collaboration and opportunities for nurses to design, implement, and diffuse collaborative programs in care and delivery; and (2) interdisciplinary development programs that focus on leadership. Health care professionals from all disciplines should work together in the planning and implementation of strategies for improving health care, particularly in an interprofessional and collaborative environment.

Recommendation 8:
Promote the involvement of nurses in the redesign of care delivery and payment systems.

The Campaign should work with payers, health care organizations, providers, employers, and regulators to involve nurses in the redesign of care delivery and payment systems. To this end, the Campaign should encourage nurses to serve in executive and leadership positions in government, for-profit and nonprofit organizations, health care delivery systems (e.g., as hospital chief executive officers or chief operations officers), and advisory committees. The Campaign should expand its metrics to measure the progress of nurses in these areas.

Chart 1-4	Summary of the Committee for Progress on Implementing the Recommendations of the Institute of Medicine Report *The Future of Nursing: Leading Change, Advancing Health* (continued)
Recommendation 9: Communicate with a wider and more diverse audience to gain broad support for Campaign objectives.	The Campaign should expand the scope of its communication strategies to connect with a broader, more diverse, consumer-oriented audience and galvanize support at the grassroots level. The Campaign, including its state Action Coalitions, should bolster communication efforts geared toward the general public and consumers using messages that go beyond nursing and focus on improving health and health care for consumers and their families. The Campaign should recruit more allies in the health care community (such as physicians, pharmacists, and other professionals, as well as those outside of health care, such as business leaders, employers, and policy makers) as health care stakeholders to further demonstrate a collaborative approach in advancing the recommendations of *The Future of Nursing*.
Recommendation 10: Improve workforce data collection.	The Campaign should promote collaboration among organizations that collect workforce-related data. Given the absence of the National Health Care Workforce Commission, the Campaign can use its strong brand and partnerships to help improve the collection of data on the nursing workforce.

"Committee" refers to the Committee for Progress on Implementing the Recommendations of the Institute of Medicine Report *The Future of Nursing*. "Campaign" refers to the Campaign for Action launched by the RWJF and AARP to implement the recommendations in the *Future of Nursing* report. Reprinted with permission from the National Academies of Sciences, Engineering, and Medicine. (2016). *Assessing progress on the Institute of Medicine report "The Future of Nursing."* Washington, DC: National Academies Press.

Interprofessional Collaborative Practice

It is worth noting that the IOM has not only made recommendations about the future of the profession of nursing (IOM, 2010), but also about health professions education. Another IOM report, *Health Professions Education: A Bridge to Quality* (IOM, 2003), challenged health professions education programs to integrate interdisciplinary core competencies into respective curricula to include patient-centered care, interdisciplinary teamwork and collaboration, EBP, quality improvement, safety, and informatics.

In response to this report, the Interprofessional Education Collaborative Expert Panel (IPEC) published *Core Competencies for Interprofessional Collaborative Practice* (IPEC, 2011) with the goal to "prepare all health professions students for deliberately working together with the common goal of building a safer and better patient-centered and community/population oriented US health care system" (p. 3). **Interprofessional collaborative practice** involves employing multiple health professionals to work together with patients, families, and communities to deliver best

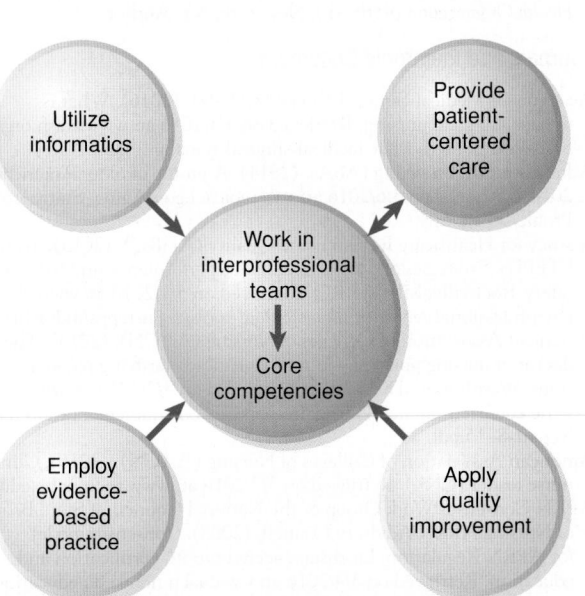

Figure 1-3 • Interprofessional teamwork and Institute of Medicine core competencies. From Interprofessional Education Collaborative Expert Panel. (2011). Core competencies for interprofessional collaborative practice: Report of an expert panel. Washington, DC: Author, p. 14. © 2011 Association of American Medical Colleges. All rights reserved. Reproduced with permission.

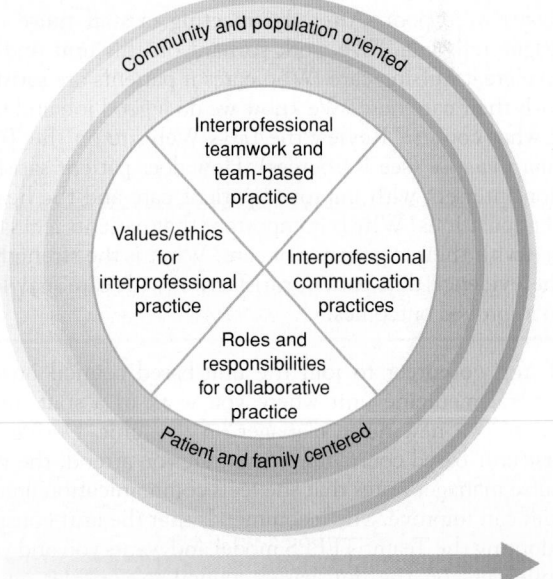

The learning continuum pre-licensure through practice trajectory

Figure 1-4 • Interprofessional collaborative practice domains. From Interprofessional Education Collaborative Expert Panel. (2011). Core competencies for interprofessional collaborative practice: Report of an expert panel. Washington, DC: Author, p. 15. © 2011 Association of American Medical Colleges. All rights reserved. Reproduced with permission.

practices, thus assuring best patient outcomes. Interprofessional teamwork is viewed as central to this model, which incorporates the interdisciplinary core competencies identified in the 2003 IOM report as displayed in Figure 1-3. The IPEC devised four collaborative practice competency domains, which include values/ethics for interprofessional practice, roles and responsibilities for collaborative practice, interprofessional communication practices, and interprofessional teamwork and team-based practice. The interplay between these competency domains, practice settings, and professional learning trajectories is displayed in Figure 1-4. Implementation of the IPEC model should not only result in improved collaborative practice between nurses, physicians, and other health professions, but it should also promote safe, quality care, and best practices.

CRITICAL THINKING EXERCISES

1 `pq` You work on a cardiac unit and are planning the discharge of an older adult patient who has been newly diagnosed with heart failure. The patient lives alone; his nearest relative, an adult daughter, lives 50 miles from his home. He has been prescribed new medications to take home with him. He also must be instructed to make a follow-up visit with his primary provider in 2 weeks. What are your priorities when you devise your discharge education plan for this patient? What referrals will you consider so that he may achieve an ideal transition from hospital to home?

2 `ebp` You work on a general surgery unit as a staff nurse. You attend a staff meeting and hear from the unit nurse manager that the unit's latest HCAHPS survey scores were poor. After the meeting, a staff nurse colleague tells you, "We work so hard on this unit and we give great nursing care. Who cares if patients are satisfied with their care here? We know we do a good job and that is what counts." Review the IHI's Web site on the *Triple Aim Initiative* (see Resources). How does patient satisfaction intersect with improved patient care and the health of populations? Why is it important that patients feel satisfied with their experience of care? What is the strength of the evidence that patient satisfaction with care may lead to improved outcomes?

3 You volunteer to join the unit-based council on the general medicine unit where you work as a staff nurse. There is a new nurse manager on this unit. During the first unit-based council meeting that you attend, the new nurse manager notes that she feels communication among staff can improve. She recommends that the unit consider adopting the TeamSTEPPS model and wants you and your colleagues on the unit-based council to consider implementing its tools (see Resources). Describe some of the TeamSTEPPS tools that could be used to improve communication among staff on your unit. How would you propose implementing them on the unit? How will you evaluate the effectiveness of implementing these tools?

REFERENCES

*Asterisk indicates nursing research article.
**Double asterisk indicates classic reference.

Books

Academy of Medical-Surgical Nurses (AMSN). (2012). *Scope and standards of medical-surgical nursing practice* (5th ed.). Pittman, NJ: Author.
Agency for Healthcare Research and Quality (AHRQ). (2013). *Pocket guide: TeamSTEPPS 2.0: Team strategies & tools to enhance performance and patient safety.* Rockville, MD: Author, AHRQ Pub. No. 14–0001–2.
American Nurses Association. (ANA). (2015a). *Code of ethics for nurses with interpretive statements.* Washington, DC: Nursesbooks.org.
American Nurses Association. (ANA). (2015b). *Nursing: Scope and standards of practice* (3rd ed.). Silver Springs, MD: Nursesbooks.org.
American Nurses Association. (ANA).(2010). *Nursing's social policy statement* (3rd ed.). Silver Springs, MD: Nursesbooks.org.
Fowler, M. D. (2015). *Guide to nursing's social policy statement: Understanding the profession from social contract to social covenant.* Silver Springs, MD: Author.
Hood, L. (2013). *Leddy & Pepper's conceptual bases of professional nursing* (8th ed.). Philadelphia, PA: Lippincott Williams & Wilkins.
**Institute of Medicine. (2000). *To err is human: Building a safer health system.* Washington, DC: National Academies Press.
**Institute of Medicine. (2001). *Crossing the quality chasm: A new health system for the 21st century.* Washington, DC: National Academies Press.
**Institute of Medicine. (2003). *Health professions education: A bridge to quality.* Washington, DC: National Academies Press.
**Institute of Medicine. (2010). *The future of nursing: Leading change, advancing health.* Washington, DC: National Academies Press.
**Interprofessional Education Collaborative Expert Panel (IPEC). (2011). *Core competencies for interprofessional collaborative practice: report of an expert panel.* Washington, DC: Author.
**Maslow, A. (1954). *Motivation and personality.* New York, NY: Harper.
Melnyk, B. M., & Fineout-Overholt, E. (2014). *Evidence-based practice in nursing and healthcare: a guide to best practice* (3rd ed.). Philadelphia, PA: LWW.
National Academies of Sciences, Engineering, and Medicine. (2016). *Assessing progress on the Institute of Medicine report "The Future of Nursing."* Washington, DC: National Academies Press.
Pender, N. J., Murdaugh, C. L., & Parsons, M. A. (2015). *Health promotion in nursing practice* (7th ed.). Upper Saddle River, NJ: Pearson Education.
**World Health Organization (WHO). (2006). *Constitution of the World Health Organization* (45th ed.). New York, NY: Author.

Journals and Electronic Documents

Academy of Medical-Surgical Nurses (AMSN). (2016). What is medical-surgical nursing? Retrieved on 3/5/2016 at: www.amsn.org/practice-resources/what-medical-surgical-nursing
Administration on Aging (AoA). (2014). A profile of older Americans: 2014. Retrieved on 3/6/2016 at: www.aoa.acl.gov/Aging_Statistics/Profile/Index.aspx
Agency for Healthcare Research and Quality (AHRQ). (2015). TeamSTEPPS: Strategies and tools to enhance performance and patient safety. Rockville, MD: AHRQ. Retrieved on 3/7/2016 at: www.ahrq.gov/professionals/education/curriculum-tools/teamstepps/index.html
American Association of Colleges of Nursing (AACN). (2015). The doctor of nursing practice: Current issues and clarifying recommendations. Washington, DC: Author. Retrieved on 3/7/2016 at: www.aacn.nche.edu/aacn-publications/white-papers/DNP-Implementation-TF-Report-8–15.pdf
American Association of Colleges of Nursing (AACN). (2016). Clinical nurse leader (CNL). Retrieved on 3/7/2016 at: www.aacn.nche.edu/cnl
APRN Consensus Work Group & the National Council of State Boards of Nursing APRN Advisory Council. (2008). Consensus model for APRN Regulation: Licensure, accreditation, certification and education. Retrieved on 3/4/2016 at: www.aacn.nche.edu/education-resources/APRNReport.pdf
CAHPS Hospital Survey. (2015). HCAHPS fact sheet. Retrieved on 3/4/2016 at: www.hcahpsonline.org/Files/HCAHPS_Fact_Sheet_June_2015.pdf
Case Management Society of America. (2016). What is a case manager? Retrieved on 3/4/2016 at: www.cmsa.org/Consumer/FindaCaseManager/WhatisaCaseManager/tabid/276/Default.aspx

Centers for Disease Control and Prevention (CDC). (2015). The four domains of chronic disease prevention. Working toward healthy people in healthy communities. Retrieved on 3/6/2016 at: www.cdc.gov/chronicdisease/pdf/four-domains-factsheet-2015.pdf

Centers for Medicare and Medicaid Services (CMS). (2015). ICD-10 next steps for providers: Assessment and maintenance toolkit. Retrieved on 3/6/2016 at: www.cms.gov/Medicare/Coding/ICD10/Downloads/ICD-10NextStepsToolkit20160226.pdf

Centers for Medicare and Medicaid Services (CMS). (2016). Electronic health records (EHR) incentive programs. Retrieved on 3/6/2016 at: www.cms.gov/Regulations-and-Guidance/Legislation/EHRIncentivePrograms/index.html

Collins, F. S., & Varmus, H. (2015). A new initiative on precision medicine. *New England Journal of Medicine, 372*(9), 793–795.

Cronenwett, L., Sherwood, G., Barnsteiner, J., et al. (2007). Quality and safety education for nurses. *Nursing Outlook, 55*(3), 122–131.

Howden, L. A., & Meyer, J. A. (2011). Age and sex composition. 2010 Census Briefs. Washington, DC: U.S. Bureau of the Census.

Humes, K. R., Jones, N. A., & Ramerez, R. R. (2011). Overview of race and Hispanic origin: 2010. 2010 Census Briefs. Washington, DC: U.S. Bureau of the Census.

Institute for Healthcare Improvement (IHI). (2016a). Science of improvement: How to improve. Retrieved on 3/4/2016 at: www.ihi.org/knowledge/Pages/HowtoImprove/ScienceofImprovementHowtoImprove.aspx

Institute for Healthcare Improvement (IHI). (2016b). Ventilator bundle compliance. Retrieved on 3/4/2016 at: www.ihi.org/resources/Pages/Measures/VentilatorBundleCompliance.aspx

International Council of Nurses. (2012). The ICN code of ethics for nurses: Revised 2012. Retrieved on 3/4/2016 at: www.icn.ch/images/stories/documents/about/icncode_english.pdf

Interprofessional Education Collaborative (IPEC). (2016). Interprofessional Education Collaborative announces expansion: Nine new members join organization dedicated to improving patient care. Press release: February 22, 2016, Washington, DC. Retrieved on 3/5/2016 at: ipecollaborative.org/uploads/2016.02.22_IPEC-Press-Release.pdf

Joint Commission. (2016a). 2016 National Patient Safety Goals. Retrieved on 3/4/2016 at: www.jointcommission.org/standards_information/npsgs.aspx

Joint Commission. (2016b). Core measure sets. Retrieved on 3/4/2016 at: www.jointcommission.org/core_measure_sets.aspx

Keller, J. (2015). The MyHeart Counts study leads research kit's international expansion, iMore, August 6, 2015. Retrieved on 3/5/2016 at: www.imore.com/myheart-counts-leads-researchkits-international-expansion

Laderman, M., Loehrer, A., & McCarthy, D. (2013). STAAR issue brief: The effect of Medicare readmissions penalties on hospitals' efforts to reduce readmissions: Perspectives from the field. Cambridge, MA: IHI. Retrieved on 3/7/2016 at: www.ihi.org/resources/Pages/Publications/STAARIssueBriefEffectofMedicareReadmissionsPenalties.aspx

Mackun, P., & Wilson, S. (2011). Population distribution and change: 2000 to 2010. 2010 Census Briefs. Washington, DC: U.S. Bureau of the Census.

Mereya, A. M., Raval, A. D., & Sambamoorthi, U. (2015). Chronic condition combinations and health care expenditures and out-of-pocket spending burden among adults, Medical Expenditure Panel Survey, 2009 and 2011. *Preventing Chronic Disease: Public Health Research, Practices, and Policy, 12*(E12), 1–13.

National CNS Competency Task Force. (2010). *Clinical nurse specialist core competencies*. Philadelphia, PA: NACNS. Retrieved on 3/7/2016 at: www.nacns.org/docs/CNSCoreCompetenciesBroch.pdf

Ortman, J. M., & Guarneri, C. E. (2011). United States population projections: 2000 to 2050. Retrieved on 3/6/2017 at: www.census.gov/population/projections/files/analytical-document09.pdf

QSEN Institute & Frances Payne Bolton School of Nursing, Case Western Reserve University. (2014). Competencies: Prelicensure KSAs. Retrieved on 3/4/2016 at: qsen.org/competencies/pre-licensure-ksas

*Radhakrishnan, K., Jacelon, C. S., Bigelow, C., et al. (2013). Association of comorbidities with home care service utilization of patients with heart failure while receiving telehealth. *Journal of Cardiovascular Nursing, 28*(3), 216–227.

Robert Wood Johnson Foundation (RWJF) & AARP. (2015). Future of Nursing: Campaign for Action. Retrieved on 3/4/2016 at:

campaignforaction.org/sites/default/files/Campaign%20Overview%20Updated%205-13-15.pdf

Rutherford, P., Nielsen, G. A., Taylor, J., et al. (2013). How-to guide: Improving transitions from the hospital to community settings to reduce avoidable rehospitalizations. Cambridge, MA: IHI. Retrieved on 3/7/2016 at: www.ihi.org/resources/Pages/Tools/HowtoGuideImprovingTransitionstoReduceAvoidableRehospitalizations.aspx

Stanford University Medicine. (2016). MyHeart Counts iPhone application: Frequently asked questions. Retrieved on 3/5/2016 at: med.stanford.edu/myheartcounts/faq.html

Stiefel, M., & Nolan, K. (2012). A guide to measuring the Triple Aim: Population health, experience of care, and per capita cost. IHI Innovation Series white paper. Cambridge, MA: Author. Retrieved on 3/6/2016 at: www.ihi.org/resources/Pages/IHIWhitePapers/AGuidetoMeasuringTripleAim.aspx

Substance Abuse and Mental Health Services Administration (SAMHSA). (2011). Current statistics on the prevalence and characteristics of people experiencing homelessness in the United States. Retrieved on 3/6/2016 at: homeless.samhsa.gov/ResourceFiles/hrc_factsheet.pdf

The TIGER Initiative Foundation. (2014). The leadership imperative: TIGER's recommendation for integrating technology to transform practice and education. Retrieved on 3/7/2016 at: www.himss.org/ResourceLibrary/genResourceDetailPDF.aspx?ItemNumber=46421

U.S. Department of Health and Human Services (HHS), Office of Disease Prevention and Health Promotion. (2014). Healthy People 2020 Leading Health Indicators: Progress update, March 2014. Retrieved on 3/5/2016 at: www.healthypeople.gov/sites/default/files/LHI-ProgressReport-ExecSum_0.pdf

U.S. Department of Health and Human Services (HHS). (2016a). About the law: The Affordable Care Act. Retrieved on 3/6/2016 at: www.hhs.gov/healthcare/about-the-law/index.html

U.S. Department of Health and Human Services (HHS) HRSA: Health Information Technology. (2016b). What is telehealth? Retrieved on 3/6/2016 at: www.hrsa.gov/healthit/toolbox/RuralHealthITtoolbox/Telehealth/whatistelehealth.html

*van den Hooff, S. L., & Goossensen, A. (2015). Ethical considerations on the value of patient knowledge in long-term care: A qualitative study of patients suffering from Korsakoff's syndrome. *Nursing Ethics, 22*(3), 377–388.

White House. (2015). The Precision Medicine Initiative. Retrieved on 3/6/2016 at: www.whitehouse.gov/precision-medicine

World Health Organization (WHO). (2016). International classification of diseases. Retrieved on 3/6/2016 at: www.who.int/classifications/icd/en/

Resources

Academy of Medical-Surgical Nurses, www.amsn.org

Agency for Healthcare Research and Quality (AHRQ) TeamSTEPPS, www.ahrq.gov/professionals/education/curriculum-tools/teamstepps/index.html

American Association of Colleges of Nursing (AACN), www.aacn.nche.edu

American Nurses Association (ANA), www.nursingworld.org

Campaign for Action: Future of Nursing, campaignforaction.org

Centers for Medicare and Medicaid Services (CMS), www.cms.gov

Healthy People 2020, www.healthypeople.gov

Institute for Healthcare Improvement (IHI), www.ihi.org

Institute for Healthcare Improvement (IHI) *Triple Aim Initiative*, www.ihi.org/engage/initiatives/TripleAim/Pages/default.aspx

International Council of Nurses (ICN), www.icn.ch

Interprofessional Education Collaborative (IPEC), ipecollaborative.org

Joint Commission, www.jointcommission.org

National Academy of Medicine (formerly the Institute of Medicine [IOM]), iom.nationalacademies.org

National Council of State Boards of Nursing (NCSBN), www.ncsbn.org/index.htm

National League for Nursing, nln.org

QSEN Institute: Quality and Safety Education for Nurses, qsen.org

The TIGER Initiative, www.himss.org/professional-development/tiger-initiative

World Health Organization (WHO), who.int/en

2

Community-Based Nursing Practice

LEARNING OBJECTIVES

On completion of this chapter, the learner will be able to:

1 Discuss the multiple roles and various settings of community health nursing.
2 Compare the differences and similarities between community-based and community-oriented/public health nursing.

3 Describe the discharge planning process.
4 Explain the methods for identifying community resources and making referrals.
5 Discuss how to prepare for a home health care visit and how to conduct the visit.

GLOSSARY

community: an interacting population of individuals living together within a larger society

community-based nursing: nursing care of individuals and families as they transition through the health care system to manage acute and chronic conditions in the community setting

community-oriented nursing: nursing interventions that prevent or reduce illness and promote wellness for groups or communities

community hub: centralized networks with infrastructure focused on coordinating health care and social services to reduce health risks in a given community

primary prevention: health care delivery focused on health promotion and prevention of illness or disease

public health nursing: a specialty practice of nursing that combines the discipline of public health with nursing; it is considered a specialty practice within community-oriented nursing that focuses on population health

secondary prevention: health care delivery centered on health maintenance and aimed at early detection of disease, with prompt intervention to prevent or minimize loss of function and independence

telehealth: the use of technology to provide health care services

tertiary prevention: health care delivery focused on minimizing deterioration associated with disease and improving quality of life through rehabilitation measures

third-party payer: an organization or insurance company that provides reimbursement for services covered by a health plan

The role of nurses in community settings is ever expanding. In the past, the term *community health nursing* was used to define any nurse who practiced out in the community. With changes in health care delivery and accountability, new terms have arisen to better define the types of nursing care and interventions in the community. The shift in health care delivery from inpatient to outpatient is a result of multiple factors, including new population trends (the growing number of older adults), changes in federal legislation, tighter insurance regulations, and decreasing hospital revenues. Transitions in the health care industry, the nursing profession, and changing patterns of disease and wellness have also affected the community setting (see Chapter 1).

On an increasing basis, hospitals and other health care organizations and providers are held accountable for providing health care using best practices, as evidenced by meeting performance benchmarks for quality and efficiency, known as pay for performance or value-based purchasing (see Chapter 1 for further discussion). Under this system, hospitals and other health care organizations and providers can reduce costs and earn additional income by carefully monitoring the types of services they provide, discharging patients as soon as possible, and keeping patients who are discharged from the hospital from being readmitted. Consequently, patients are

discharged from acute care facilities to homes or to residential or long-term care facilities in the early stages of recovery.

Community-based nursing occurs in a variety of settings and is directed toward people and families with needs related to illness, injury, or disability. A **community** is an interacting population of individuals living together within a larger social structure. While community-based nurses may care for patients recovering from an acute illness, many times the interventions needed result from chronic illness (Stanhope & Lancaster, 2014). Home health care is a major aspect of community-based care.

Another group of nurses practicing in the community have a **community-oriented nursing** approach targeted at improving the health status of groups of patients or the community at large (Stanhope & Lancaster, 2014). This community-oriented approach promotes health and wellness, reduces the spread of disease or illness, and improves health status for the whole community. **Public health nursing** combines the discipline of public health with nursing and is considered a specialty practice within community-oriented nursing that focuses on population health.

Together, community-based and community-oriented nurses work in a variety of settings in the community including public health departments, ambulatory health clinics, long-term care

Figure 2-1 • Community-based nursing takes many forms and focuses. Here, the school nurse performs screening for scoliosis. This is an example of secondary prevention.

facilities, schools, faith communities, hospice centers, industrial environments (as occupational nurses), homeless shelters and clinics, nursing centers, home health agencies, urgent care centers, same-day surgical centers, short-stay facilities, and patients' homes (Stanhope & Lancaster, 2014).

Nurses in the community organize interventions based upon primary, secondary, and tertiary levels of preventative care. **Primary prevention** focuses on health promotion and prevention of illness or disease, including interventions such as teaching about healthy lifestyles. **Secondary prevention** centers on health maintenance and is aimed at early detection, with prompt intervention to prevent or minimize loss of function and independence, including interventions such as health screening (see Fig. 2-1) and health risk appraisal. **Tertiary prevention** focuses on minimizing deterioration and improving quality of life, including rehabilitation to assist patients in achieving maximum potential by working through physical or psychological challenges. Depending on the setting and roles, one type of prevention intervention may predominate. For example, home care nurses most often focus on tertiary preventative nursing care, although they may address primary and secondary prevention.

Nurses practicing in the community need to be self-directed, flexible, adaptable, and accepting of various lifestyles and living conditions. To function effectively, nurses in these settings must have expertise in independent decision making, critical thinking, assessment, health education, community resources, and competence in basic nursing care (Allender, Rector, & Warner, 2014).

In addition, nurses in community settings must be culturally competent, as culture plays a role in the delivery of care in all settings. Cultural competence is particularly important in a setting in which most community members share a cultural heritage that is unfamiliar to the nurse. Cultural

competence is not static in the community setting; new population groups may move into a community. Furthermore, established groups' ways of expressing culture grow and change over time. Developing cultural competence involves awareness and self-reflection, willingness to explore cultural expressions in health and illness, and delivery of interventions that are congruent with the patient's culture (Dreachslin, Gilbert, & Malone, 2013) (see Chapter 7).

Key Components of Community-Based Care

As described previously, community-based nursing is a philosophy of care provision for patients and their families as they move among various service providers outside of hospitals, typically after an episode of acute illness or exacerbation of chronic illness. It focuses on promoting and maintaining the health of individuals and families, preventing and minimizing the progression of disease, and improving quality of life (Stanhope & Lancaster, 2014).

Discharge Planning for Transition to the Community or Home Care Setting

Discharge planning is an essential component of facilitating the transition of the patient from the acute care to the community or home care setting, or for facilitating the transfer of the patient from one health care setting to another. A documented discharge plan is mandatory for patients who receive Medicare or Medicaid health insurance benefits. Discharge planning begins with the patient's admission to the hospital or health care setting and must consider the potential for necessary follow-up care in the home or another community setting. Several different personnel (e.g., social workers, home care nurses, case managers) or agencies may be involved in the planning process.

The development of a comprehensive discharge plan requires collaboration between professionals at the referring agency and the home care agency, as well as other community agencies that provide specific resources upon discharge. The process involves identifying the patient's needs and developing a thorough plan to meet them. It is essential to have open lines of communication with family members to ensure understanding and cooperation.

Continuing the Transition Through Community Resources and Referrals

As case managers and discharge planners, community-based nurses often make referrals to other team members, such as home health aides and social workers. These nurses work collaboratively with the health care team and the referring agency or person. Continuous coordinated care among all health care providers involved in a patient's care is essential to avoid duplication of effort by the various personnel caring for the patient.

A community-based nurse must be knowledgeable about community resources available to patients, as well as services provided by local agencies, eligibility requirements for those services, and any possible charges for the services. Most communities have directories or resource booklets that list local health and social service agencies and their offerings. The telephone book and the Internet are often useful in helping patients identify the location and accessibility of grocery and drug stores, banks, health care facilities, ambulances, physicians, dentists, pharmacists, social service agencies, and senior citizens' programs. In addition, a patient's place of worship or faith community may be an important resource for services. The community-based nurse is responsible for informing the patient and family about the community resources available to meet their needs. When appropriate, nurses may make the initial contact.

Home Health Care

Home health care is a unique component of community-based nursing and a major player in posthospital care for patients who return home to complete recuperation following an acute illness episode or exacerbation of chronic illness. Home health agencies can also provide advanced technologies in the home setting. All together, these services provided in the home setting work to maximize the patient's ability to function at his highest level of wellness (Allender et al., 2014).

Holistic care is provided in the home through the collaboration of an interdisciplinary team that includes professional nurses; home health aides; social workers; physical, speech, and occupational therapists; and physicians. This approach provides health and social services with oversight of the total health care plan by a case manager, clinical nurse specialist, or nurse practitioner. Interdisciplinary collaboration is required if a home health agency is to receive Medicare certification (Stanhope & Lancaster, 2014).

Most home health agencies are reimbursed by various sources, including Medicare and Medicaid programs, private insurance, and direct patient payment. Older adults are the most frequent users of home care expenditures financed by Medicare, which allows nurses to manage and evaluate care of seriously ill patients who have complex, labile conditions and are at high risk for rehospitalization. Each funding source has its own requirements for services rendered, number of visits allowed, and amount of reimbursement the agency receives. The Omaha System's care documentation referred to as the Outcome and Assessment Information Set (OASIS) has been required for more than a decade to ensure that outcome-based care is provided for all care reimbursed by Medicare. This system uses sociodemographic, environment, support system, health status, and functional status domains to assess and plan care for adult patients. OASIS is also used to collect data and report on agency case mix and improve performance or quality outcomes (Centers for Medicare and Medicaid Services [CMS], 2015a). Shang, Larson, Liu, et al. (2015) utilized the OASIS to identify factors that led to rehospitalization in patients using home health care services. Chart 2-1 summarizes nursing research findings that suggest that selected direct and indirect patient data collected by the OASIS may predict those at risk for rehospitalization.

Services Provided

Many home care patients are acutely ill or have chronic health problems or disabilities requiring that nurses provide more education and monitoring to patients and families. Home care or visiting nurses make home visits to provide skilled nursing care, follow-up care, and teaching to promote health and prevent complications. Home health care visits may be intermittent or periodic, and case management via

---

Chart 2-1 **NURSING RESEARCH PROFILE**
Predicting Rehospitalization in Home Health Care

Tao, H., & Ellenbecker, C. H. (2013). Is OASIS effective in predicting rehospitalization for home health care elderly patients? *Home Health Care Management and Practice, 25*(6), 250–255.

Purpose

Readmission to the hospital is a costly aspect of our health care system. Not only are there direct economic costs, but also indirect costs to the patient in terms of personal upheaval with each hospitalization. The Affordable Care Act stipulates financial penalties for rehospitalization. Home health care may be able to impact this issue through early recognition and intervention of patients at risk for readmission. The purpose of this study was to find factors that predict rehospitalization using information collected on the OASIS dataset during home health services.

Design

This study used the start of care OASIS data from a population of 1,268 home care patients and the 212 patients who were readmitted to the hospital within 30 days of their discharge date. Through a review of the literature, 10 possible predictors were chosen—2 of the predictors were a synthesis of the patients' clinical status and abilities related to activities of daily living (ADLs) and 8 of the predictors were single items such as age, cognitive status, and living situation. The first part of the statistical analysis used independent *t*-test and chi-square to identify differences between those who were and were not rehospitalized.

OASIS, Outcome and Assessment Information Set.

Regression analyses were conducted to find any association between the predictors and rehospitalization.

Findings

Factors that directly predicted rehospitalization were: male gender; mid-level cognitive impairment; lower ability to perform ADLs; and a variety of support deficits, such as psychosocial, environmental, financial, and assistance with medical care. Decreased functional ability was also found to predict rehospitalization indirectly when associated with advanced age, obesity, poor clinical status, need for assistance with ADLs and instrumental ADLs (IADLs), and infrequent use of informal caregivers.

Nursing Implications

Home health care agencies serving the Medicare population collect OASIS data that can be used to recognize those at risk for readmission to the hospital. Furthermore, the results of this study suggest that successful transition from hospital to home may involve a shift of resources to the community. In particular, the community-based nurse can identify those older adult patients who are especially at risk (e.g., those who are male, or who have mid-level cognitive impairment or functional impairments) so that their care may be specifically managed to avoid rehospitalization. Successful transitions home will prevent health care systems from incurring penalties associated with rehospitalization.

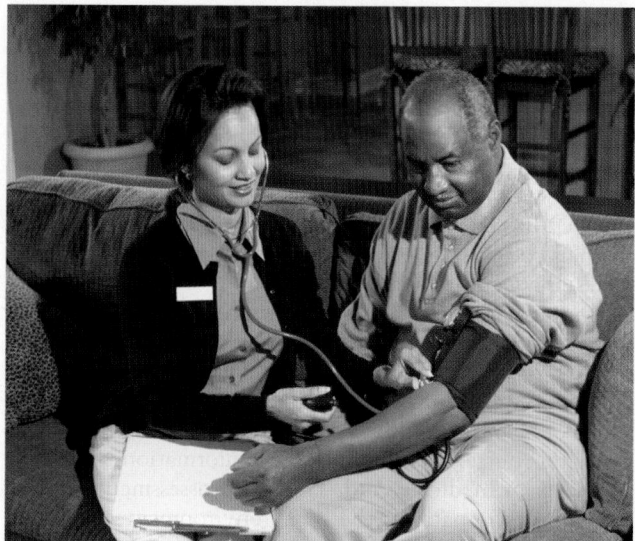

Figure 2-2 • Assessment is an important part of any home health visit.

telephone or Internet may be used to promote communication with home care consumers. The nurse instructs the patient and family about skills, self-care strategies, and health maintenance and promotion activities (e.g., nutritional counseling, exercise programs, stress management). Nursing care includes skilled assessment of the patient's physical, psychological, social, and environmental status (see Fig. 2-2). Nursing interventions may include intravenous (IV) therapy and injections, parenteral nutrition, venipuncture, catheter insertion, pressure ulcer treatment, wound care, ostomy care, and patient and family teaching. Complex technical equipment such as mechanical ventilation and procedures such as peritoneal dialysis may be involved in home health care (Allender et al., 2014; Stanhope & Lancaster, 2014). Nurses have a role in evaluating the safety and effectiveness of technology in the home setting. In addition, **telehealth** is useful in home health care in facilitating exchange of information via telephone or computers between patients and nurses regarding health information such as blood glucose readings, vital signs, and cardiac parameters (Stanhope & Lancaster, 2014). The use of a broad spectrum of computer and Internet resources, such as webcams, also facilitates exchange of information.

The Home Setting

The home care nurse is a guest in the patient's home and must have permission to visit and give care. The nurse has minimal control over the lifestyle, living situation, and health practices of the visited patients. This lack of full decision-making authority can create a conflict for the nurse and lead to problems in the nurse–patient relationship. To work successfully with patients in any setting, the nurse must be nonjudgmental and convey respect for patients' beliefs, even if they differ sharply from those of the nurse. This can be difficult when a patient's lifestyle involves activities that a nurse considers harmful or unacceptable, such as smoking, the use of alcohol, drug abuse, or overeating.

The cleanliness of a patient's home may not meet the standards of a hospital. Although the nurse can provide teaching points about maintaining clean surroundings, the patient and

family decide if they will implement the nurse's suggestions. The nurse must accept their decisions and deliver the care required regardless of the conditions of the setting (Lundy & Janes, 2016). The kind of equipment and the supplies or resources that usually are available in acute care settings are often unavailable in the patient's home. The nurse has to learn to improvise when providing care, such as when changing a dressing or catheterizing a patient in a regular bed that is not adjustable and lacks a bedside table (Allender et al., 2014).

Infection control is as important in the home as it is in the hospital; however, it can be more challenging in the home and requires creative approaches. As in any situation, it is important to perform hand hygiene before and after giving direct patient care, even in a home that does not have running water. If aseptic technique is required, the nurse must have a plan for implementing this technique before going to the home. This applies to universal precautions, transmission-based precautions, and disposal of bodily secretions and excretions. If injections are given, the nurse must use a closed container to dispose of syringes. Injectable and other medications must be kept out of the reach of children during visits and stored in a safe place if the medications remain in the home.

> ### ▷ Quality and Safety Nursing Alert
>
> *Friends, neighbors, or family members may ask the nurse about the patient's condition. The patient has a right to confidentiality, and information should be shared only with the patient's permission. The nurse should be mindful of any sensitive information (e.g., electronic health records [EHRs]) taken into the home and prevent it from being misplaced or picked up by others.*

Home Health Visits

Most agencies have a policy manual that identifies the agency's philosophy and procedures and defines the services provided. The eligibility of a patient and provision of services may be prescribed by the type of insurance the patient carries. For example, Medicare beneficiaries must meet certain eligibility requirements such as homebound criteria and may be permitted only intermittent skilled services of a registered nurse or licensed therapist (CMS, 2015b). Becoming familiar with these policies is essential before initiating a home visit. It is also important to know the state laws regarding what actions to take if the nurse finds a patient dead, suspects abuse, determines that a patient cannot safely remain at home, or observes a situation that possibly indicates malicious harm to the community at large.

Preparing for a Home Visit

Before making a home visit, the nurse should review pertinent data about the patient that is typically provided on a referral form. It may be necessary to contact the referring agency if the purpose for the referral is unclear or important information is missing. The nurse calls the patient to obtain permission to visit, schedules a time for the visit, and verifies the address. This initial phone conversation provides an opportunity to introduce oneself, identify the agency, and explain the reason for the visit. If the patient does not have a telephone, the nurse should see if the person who made the referral is able to contact the patient regarding the visit. If an unannounced visit to a patient's home must be made, the nurse should ask permission to come in before entering the house. Explaining the purpose of the referral at the outset and setting up the times for future visits before leaving are also recommended.

Conducting a Home Visit

Personal Safety Precautions

Community nurses must pay attention to personal safety, because they often practice in unknown environments. Based on the principle of due diligence, agencies should investigate at-risk working environments prior to making the assignment and must inform employees accordingly. Agencies have policies and procedures concerning the promotion of safety for clinical staff, and training is provided to facilitate personal safety. The individual nurse and agency must proactively assess environments for safety. Suggested precautions to take when making a home visit are presented in Chart 2-2.

Initial Home Visit

The first visit sets the tone for subsequent visits and is crucial in establishing the nurse–patient relationship. The situations

---

Chart 2-2	**Safety Precautions in Home Health Care**

- Learn, or preprogram a phone with, the telephone numbers of the agency, police, and emergency services. Most agencies provide phones for nurses so that the agency can contact the nurse and the nurse can easily contact the agency.
- Carry agency identification and a charged phone to make telephone calls if you become lost or have problems; a mobile phone charger provides additional backup.
- Let the agency know your daily schedule and the telephone numbers of your patients (if available) so that you can be located if you do not return when expected.
- Know where the patient lives before leaving to make the visit, and either carry a map or use the navigation system in your car or the GPS software on your smartphone for quick referral.
- Keep your car in good working order, and have sufficient gas in the tank.
- Park the car near the patient's home, and lock the car during the visit.
- Do not drive an expensive car or wear expensive jewelry when making visits.
- Know the regular bus schedule, and know the routes when using public transportation or walking to the patient's house.
- When making visits in high-crime areas, visit with another person rather than alone (if possible).
- Try to schedule visits during daylight hours (when possible).
- Never walk into a patient's home uninvited; be vigilant for unrestrained pets.
- If you do not feel safe entering a patient's home, leave the area.
- Become familiar with the layout of the house, including exits from the house.
- If a patient or family member is intoxicated or hostile, leave and reschedule the visit.
- If a family is having a serious argument or abusing the patient or anyone else in the household, leave, reschedule the visit, contact your supervisor, and report the abuse to the appropriate authorities.

GPS, Global Positioning System.

---

encountered depend on numerous factors. Patients may be in pain and have additional factors that make them unable to care for themselves. Family members may be overwhelmed and doubt their ability to care for loved ones. They may not understand why the patient was sent home from the hospital before being totally rehabilitated. They may not comprehend what home care is or why they cannot have 24-hour nursing services. It is critical that the nurse conveys an understanding of what patients and families are experiencing and how the illness is affecting their lives.

During the initial home visit, which may take 1 hour or more, the patient is evaluated and a plan of care is established that may be modified on subsequent visits. The nurse informs the patient of the agency's practices, policies, and hours of operation. If the agency is to be reimbursed for the visit, the nurse asks for insurance information, such as a Medicare or Medicaid card. The initial assessment includes evaluating the patient, the home environment (see Chart 2-3), the patient's self-care abilities or the family's ability to provide care, and the patient's need for additional resources. After the assessment, necessary skilled interventions are accomplished. Most agencies provide nurses with bags that contain standard supplies and equipment needed during home visits. It is important to keep the bag properly supplied and to bring any additional items that might be needed for the visit. Depending on insurance coverage, supplies may be delivered to the home or may need to be purchased by the patient. Home health nurses need to be prepared for the inevitability that a patient may not have the medical supplies needed for treatment, and work to procure all needed items.

One important aspect of the transition from hospital to home is self-management of the medication regimen. Older adults may have multiple prescribers, or may use alternative therapies such as herbal remedies as well as vitamins and other over-the-counter medications. While under the care of the home health agency, the home health nurse may promote medication management by assisting with discrepancies such as wrong dosages, duplicate medications, omissions, or use of a medication for something other than the prescribed reason (Lancaster, Marek, Bub, et al., 2014). Some home health agencies mandate medication reconciliation at each visit, and the nurse as case manager works to develop a plan for future discharge from home health services.

Determining the Need for Future Visits

While conducting an assessment of a patient's situation, the home care nurse evaluates and clearly documents the need for future visits and the frequency with which those visits may need to be made. To make these judgments, the nurse should consider the questions listed in Chart 2-4. With each subsequent visit, these same factors are evaluated to determine the continuing health needs of the patient. As progress is made and the patient—with or without the help of significant others—becomes more capable of self-care and more independent, the need for home visits may decline.

Ending the Visit

As the visit comes to a close, the nurse summarizes the main points of the visit for the patient and family and identifies expectations for future visits or patient achievements.

Chart 2-3 ASSESSMENT
Assessing the Home Environment

Physical Facilities (check all that apply)

Exterior

❏ Steps
❏ Unsafe steps
❏ Porch
❏ Litter
❏ Noise
❏ Adequate lighting
❏ Other

Interior

❏ Accessible bathroom
❏ Level, safe floor surface
❏ Number of rooms
❏ Privacy
❏ Sleeping arrangements
❏ Refrigeration
❏ Trash management
❏ Animals
❏ Adequate lighting
❏ Steps/stairs
❏ Other

Safety Hazards (check all that apply)

❏ None
❏ Inadequate floor, roof, or windows
❏ Inadequate lighting
❏ Unsafe gas/electric appliances
❏ Inadequate heating
❏ Inadequate cooling
❏ Lack of fire safety devices
❏ Unsafe floor coverings
❏ Inadequate stair rails
❏ Lead-based paint (particularly for homes built prior to 1978) or lead in drinking water (particularly in homes built prior to 1986)
❏ Improperly stored hazardous material
❏ Improper wiring/electrical cords
❏ Other

Safety Factors (check all that apply)

❏ Fire/smoke detectors
❏ Working telephone
❏ Placement of electrical cords
❏ Emergency plan
❏ Emergency phone numbers displayed
❏ Safe portable heaters
❏ Oxygen in use
❏ Obstacle-free paths
❏ Other

The following points should be considered at the end of each visit:

- What are the main points the patient or family should remember from the visit?
- What positive attributes have been noted about the patient and the family that will give a sense of accomplishment?
- What were the main points of the teaching plan or the treatments needed to ensure that the patient and family understand what they must do? A written set of instructions should be left with the patient or family, provided they can read and see (alternative formats include video or audio recordings). Printed material must be in the patient's primary language and in large print when indicated.
- Whom should the patient or family call if someone needs to be contacted immediately? Are current emergency telephone numbers readily available? Is telephone service available, or can an emergency phone service be provided?
- What signs of complications should be reported immediately?
- How frequently will visits be made? How long will they last (approximately)?
- What is the day and time of the next visit? Will a different nurse make the visit?

Chart 2-4 ASSESSMENT
Assessing the Need for Home Visits

Current Health Status

- How well is the patient progressing?
- How serious are the present signs and symptoms?
- Has the patient shown signs of progressing as expected, or does it seem that recovery will be delayed?

Home Environment

- Are safety concerns apparent?
- Are family or friends available to provide care, or is the patient alone?

Level of Self-Care Ability

- Is the patient capable of self-care?
- What is the patient's level of independence?
- Is the patient ambulatory or bedridden?
- Does the patient have sufficient energy, or is he or she frail and easily fatigued?
- Does the patient need and use assistive devices?

Level of Nursing Care Needed

- What level of nursing care does the patient require?
- Does the care require basic skills or more complex interventions?

Prognosis

- What is the expectation for recovery in this particular instance?
- What are the chances that complications may develop if nursing care is not provided?

Educational Needs

- How well has the patient or family grasped the teaching points made?
- Is there a need for further follow-up and retraining?
- What level of proficiency does the patient or family show in carrying out the necessary care?

Mental Status

- How alert is the patient?
- Are there signs of confusion or thinking difficulties?
- Does the patient tend to be forgetful or have a limited attention span?

Level of Adherence

- Is the patient following the instructions provided?
- Does the patient seem capable of following the instructions?
- Are the family members helpful, or are they unwilling or unable to assist in caring for the patient as expected?

Documenting the Visit

Documentation considerations for home visits follow fairly specific regulations. The patient's needs and the nursing care provided must be documented to ensure that the agency qualifies for payment for the visit. Medicare, Medicaid, and other **third-party payers** (i.e., organizations that provide reimbursement for services covered under a health care insurance plan) require documentation of the patient's homebound status and the need for skilled professional nursing care. The medical diagnosis and specific detailed information on the functional limitations of the patient are usually part of the documentation. The goals and the actions appropriate for attaining those goals must be identified. Expected outcomes of the nursing interventions must be stated in terms of patient behaviors and must be realistic and measurable. In addition, the goals must reflect the nursing diagnosis or the patient's problems and must specify those actions that address the patient's problems. Inadequate documentation may result in nonpayment for the visit and care services.

Additional Care Settings in the Community

Hospice Care

Community-based nurses may serve a population that is not moving toward restoration of health but instead toward death. Hospice nursing is a specialty area of nursing practice in which nurses provide palliative care that promotes comfort, peace, and dignity for patients who are dying. During this terminal stage, hospice nurses provide education and support and also coordinate care between various health care and social service agencies. Hospice care can be provided in the home or in specialized facilities designed to assist the patient and family through the death experience (National Hospice and Palliative Care Organization [NHPCO], 2014). Patients are eligible for hospice care services if they are determined to be within the final 6 months of life. Third-party payers cover many hospice services for terminal patients and their families during the final stages of an illness and after death with bereavement support for family members. Beneficiaries must be re-certified by the hospice medical director as terminally ill at the beginning of each benefit period (NHPCO, 2015). Chart 2-5 displays the services that may be covered by hospice care.

Ambulatory Settings

Ambulatory health care is provided for patients in community- or hospital-based settings. The types of agencies that provide such care are medical clinics, ambulatory care units, urgent care centers, cardiac rehabilitation programs, mental health centers, student health centers, community outreach programs, and nursing centers. Some ambulatory centers provide care to a specific population, such as migrant workers or Native Americans. Neighborhood community health centers provide services to patients who live in a geographically defined area. These centers collectively provide affordable, accessible health care services to more than 20 million people in the United States, most of whom are impoverished (Centers for Disease Control and Prevention, 2015). The centers may operate in freestanding buildings, storefronts, or mobile

---

Chart 2-5   Hospice Services

- Nursing care
- Medical social worker services
- Physician services
- Counseling (including dietary, pastoral, and other)
- Inpatient care (including respite care and short-term inpatient care for procedures necessary for pain control and acute and chronic symptom management)
- Hospice aide and homemaker services
- Medical appliances and supplies (including drugs and biologics)
- Physical and occupational therapies
- Speech–language pathology services
- Volunteers
- Bereavement services for families (up to 13 months following a patient's death)

Adapted from National Hospice and Palliative Care Organization. (2014). *Facts and figures: Hospice care in America*. Retrieved on 6/4/2015 at: www.nhpco.org/sites/default/files/public/Statistics_Research/2014_Facts_Figures.pdf

---

units. Agencies may provide ambulatory health care in addition to other services, such as an adult day care or health program. The kinds of services offered and the patients served depend on the agency's mission.

Nursing responsibilities in ambulatory health care settings include providing direct patient care, conducting patient intake screenings, treating patients with acute or chronic illnesses or emergency conditions, referring patients to other agencies for additional services, teaching patients self-care activities, and offering health education programs that promote health maintenance.

Nurses may work as clinic managers, direct the operation of clinics, and supervise other health team members. Nurses can play an important part in facilitating the function of the varied types of ambulatory care facilities. For instance, primary care nurse practitioners often practice in ambulatory care settings that focus on gerontology, pediatrics, family or adult health, or women's health. Some nurse practitioner faculty provide care in nurse-managed clinics as a part of faculty practice appointments. Support for the full utilization of nurse practitioners is addressed in the *Future of Nursing* report produced by the Institute of Medicine (IOM) and the Robert Wood Johnson Foundation (RWJF) (IOM, 2010; see Chapter 1 for full discussion).

Occupational Health Programs

Federal legislation, especially the Occupational Safety and Health Act (OSHA), has been enacted to ensure safe and healthy work conditions. A safe working environment results in decreased employee absenteeism, hospitalization, and disability, as well as reduced costs. Occupational nurses may work in solo units in industrial settings, or they may serve as consultants on a limited or part-time basis. They may be members of an interdisciplinary team composed of various personnel, such as nurses, physicians, exercise physiologists, health educators, counselors, nutritionists, safety engineers, and industrial hygienists.

Occupational health nurses may provide direct care to employees who become ill or injured; conduct health education programs for company staff members; set up programs aimed at establishing specific health outcomes, such as healthy eating and regular exercise; monitor employees' hearing, vision, blood pressure, or blood glucose; and track and report exposure to infectious diseases and agents such as toxic substances.

Occupational health nurses must be knowledgeable about federal regulations pertaining to occupational health and familiar with other pertinent legislation, such as the Americans With Disabilities Act (Stanhope & Lancaster, 2014).

School Health Programs

School health programs provide services to students and may also serve the school's community. Ideally, school health programs have an interdisciplinary health team consisting of physicians, nurses, dentists, social workers, counselors, school administrators, parents, and students. The school may serve as the site for a family health clinic that offers primary health and mental health services to all family members in the community. Advanced practice nurses perform physical examinations and diagnose and treat students and families for acute and chronic illnesses within the scope of their practice. These clinics are cost-effective and benefit students from low-income families who lack access to traditional health care or have no health insurance. The Affordable Care Act has provided funding for expansion and improvement of school-based health center services. This expansion will increase access beyond the approximately 2000 school-based health centers operating in the nation (Health Resources and Services Administration, 2015).

School nurses play several roles, including care provider, health educator, consultant, and counselor. They collaborate with students, parents, administrators, teachers, and other health and social service professionals regarding student health problems. In addition to providing information on health practices, teaching health classes, and participating in the development of the health education curriculum, school nurses educate teachers and classes when a student has a special problem, a disability, or a disease such as hemophilia, asthma, or human immune deficiency virus (HIV) infection.

School nurses perform health screenings, provide basic care for minor injuries and complaints, administer medications, monitor the immunization status of students and families, identify children with health problems, provide teaching related to health maintenance and safety, and monitor the weight of children to facilitate prevention and treatment of obesity. They need to be knowledgeable about state and local regulations affecting school-age children, such as ordinances for excluding students from school because of communicable diseases or parasites such as lice or scabies (Stanhope & Lancaster, 2014).

Community Nurse–Managed Centers

Community nurse–managed centers are another context for care in the community. Frequently initiated or sponsored by academic institutions, these centers typically are designed for the delivery of primary health care and serve people who are vulnerable, underinsured or uninsured, and without access to health services. These centers may have a physical location within an academic institution that patients must travel to in order to be seen, or may be located in a mobile setting (e.g., a van) that travels to the patient. Community nurse–managed

centers, which are usually run by advanced practice nurses, serve numerous patients who are poor, members of minority groups, women, older adults, or homeless. Advanced practice nurses working in these settings report positive perceptions related to their role and the autonomy it provides in this setting (Pron, 2013). The nurses provide health teaching, wellness and illness care, case management services, and psychosocial counseling. In some areas, various community partnership models facilitate care for the growing number of migrant workers (Allender et al., 2014). The concept of **community hubs** to address vulnerable populations is gaining acceptance. These hubs contain the infrastructure to identify those at risk, treat using evidence-based practice, and evaluate benchmarks and outcomes to determine the effectiveness of care (Agency for Healthcare Research and Quality, 2015).

Care for Those Who Are Homeless

Being homeless is defined by the federal government as lacking a regular residence for sleeping at night. Approximately 580,000 people in the United States are homeless on any given night (National Alliance to End Homelessness, 2015). The homeless population is diverse; it includes members of both dysfunctional and intact families, women who have experienced abuse, veterans, older adults, the unemployed, and those who cannot find affordable housing. Adults and children can be experiencing a brief episode of homelessness such as after a natural disaster, or temporary homelessness following loss of a job, or persistent or chronic homelessness where homelessness has become a way of life (Lundy & Janes, 2016).

Those who are homeless are often underinsured or uninsured and have limited or no access to health care. Because of numerous barriers, they often seek health care late in the course of a disease and deteriorate more quickly than patients who are not homeless. Many of their health problems are related in large part to living situation. Street life exposes people to the extremes of hot and cold environments, and it compounds health risks. This population has a lower life expectancy and high rates of trauma, tuberculosis, upper respiratory tract infections, poor nutrition and anemia, lice, scabies, peripheral vascular disorders, sexually transmitted infections (STIs), dental problems, arthritis, hypothermia, skin disorders, and foot problems. Common chronic health problems also include diabetes, hypertension, heart disease, acquired immune deficiency syndrome (AIDS), mental illness, and abuse of alcohol or other drugs (Lundy & Janes, 2016; National Alliance to End Homelessness, 2015). These problems are made more difficult by living on the streets or by being discharged to a transitory homeless situation in which follow-up care is unlikely. Shelters frequently are overcrowded and unventilated, promoting the spread of communicable diseases such as tuberculosis.

Community-based nurses who work with the homeless population must be nonjudgmental, patient, and understanding. They must be skilled in dealing with people who have various health problems and needs and must recognize that individualized treatment strategies are required in highly unpredictable environments. Nursing interventions are aimed at evaluating the health care needs of people who live in shelters and attempting to obtain health care services for those who are homeless. Nurses serve in many capacities in the community setting. As varied as the service settings and roles might be, the common thread lies in the nurse's provision and coordination of evidence-based and outcome-driven care. The focus of nursing care in any community setting is to support the patient, family, and community to live the healthiest life possible (Stanhope & Lancaster, 2014).

CRITICAL THINKING EXERCISES

1 `pq` You are a nurse employed at a school-based health center in an impoverished urban area. In meeting with the school nurse, a problem of increased numbers of students with asthma is recognized. These students have many school absences due to asthma. Together, you decide to form a community hub to impact this illness through support and education. What are your priorities as you begin to organize this hub, and what support would you request from the administration? How might health fairs fit into the hub you are developing? Name the top five areas of concern that you will address.

2 `ebp` An 82-year-old man diagnosed with emphysema is being referred for home care after discharge from the hospital, and he needs regular monitoring and teaching. He has several family members at home; however, they all work. You are concerned about his ability to manage his activities of daily living (ADLs) because of severe decreased activity tolerance and his need for assistance with self-care activities. What resources could you use to assist him to remain in his home for as long as possible? How would you go about obtaining this information? What is needed to ensure appropriate home care follow-up and facilitate maximum independent self-care measures within the limits of activity intolerance owing to decreased cardiac function? What is the strength of the evidence?

3 A 58-year-old woman who is an accountant has just experienced a mild stroke due to undiagnosed hypertension. Assessment reveals complete return of function and ability to perform ADLs. The woman impatiently states that "it's over and done, thank goodness, it's tax season and they need me back at work." Further discussion reveals she has not seen a health care provider since the birth of her children 30 years ago. Develop a teaching plan for this patient with rationale for including specific content and plans to use specific teaching approaches.

REFERENCES

*Asterisk indicates nursing research.

Books

Allender, J. A., Rector, C., & Warner, K. D. (2014). *Community & public health nursing: Promoting the public's health* (8th ed.). Philadelphia, PA: Lippincott Williams & Wilkins.

Dreachslin, J. L., Gilbert, M. J., & Malone, B. (2013). *Cultural competence in health care: A systems approach*. San Fransisco,CA: Jossey-Bass.

Institute of Medicine. (2010). *The future of nursing: Leading change, advancing health*. Washington, DC: Author.

Lundy, K. S., & Janes, S. (2016). *Community health nursing: Caring for the public's health*. (3rd ed.). Burlington, MA: Jones & Bartlett.

Stanhope, M., & Lancaster, J. (2014). *Foundations of nursing in the community: Community-oriented practice* (4th ed.). St. Louis, MO: Mosby.

Journals and Electronic Documents

Agency for Healthcare Research and Quality, U.S. Department of Health and Human Services. (2015). Why create a community hub and pathways? Retrieved on 6/4/2015 at: innovations.ahrq.gov/guide/QuickstartGuide/why_create

Centers for Disease Control and Prevention. (2015). Community health center strengthening: What are community health centers? Retrieved on 6/4/2015 at: www.cdc.gov/nchhstp/PreventionThroughHealthCare/HealthDepartments/CommHealthCenters.html

Centers for Medicare and Medicaid Services. (2015a). Outcome and assessment information set (OASIS) background. Retrieved on 6/4/2015 at: www.cms.gov/Medicare/Quality-Initiatives-Patient-Assessment-Instruments/OASIS/Background.html

Centers for Medicare and Medicaid Services. (2015b). Medicare benefit policy manual Chapter 7—home health services. Retrieved on 6/4/2015 at: www.cms.gov/Regulations-and-Guidance/Guidance/Manuals/downloads/bp102c07.pdf

Health Resources and Services Administration. (2015). School-based health centers. Retrieved on 6/4/2015 at: www.hrsa.gov/ourstories/schoolhealthcenters/

*Lancaster, R., Marek, K. D., Bub, L. D., et al. (2014). Medication regimens of frail older adults after discharge from home health care. *Home Health Nurse, 32*(9), 536–542.

National Alliance to End Homelessness. (2015). The state of homelessness in America. Retrieved on 6/4/2015 at: endhomelessness.org/library/entry/the-state-of-homelessness-in-america-2015

National Hospice and Palliative Care Organization. (2014). Facts and figures: Hospice care in America. Retrieved on 6/4/2015 at: www.nhpco.org/sites/default/files/public/Statistics_Research/2014_Facts_Figures.pdf

National Hospice and Palliative Care Organization. (2015). The Medicare hospice benefit. Retrieved on 6/4/2015 at: www.nhpco.org/sites/default/files/public/communications/Outreach/The_Medicare_Hospice_Benefit.pdf

*Pron, A. L. (2013). Job satisfaction and perceived autonomy for nurse practitioners working in nurse-managed health centers. *Journal of the American Association of Nurse Practitioners, 25*(4), 213–221.

*Shang, J., Larson, E., Liu, J., et al. (2015). Infection in home health care: Results from a national outcome and assessment information data set. *American Journal of Infection Control, 43*, 454–459.

*Tao, H., & Ellenbecker, C.H. (2013). Is OASIS effective in predicting rehospitalization for home health care elderly patients? *Home Health Care Management and Practice, 25*(6), 250–255.

Resources

Case Management Society of America (CMSA), www.cmsa.org
Centers for Disease Control and Prevention (CDC), www.cdc.gov
Centers for Medicare and Medicaid Services (CMS), www.cms.gov
Faith Community Nursing resource: Church Health Center, www.churchhealthcenter.org
Health Resources and Services Administration (HRSA), www.hrsa.gov
Literacy Information and Communication System (LINCS), lincs.ed.gov
National Association for Home Care and Hospice (NAHC), www.nahc.org
National Association of School Nurses (NASN), www.nasn.org
National Guideline Clearinghouse (NGC), www.guideline.gov
National Hospice and Palliative Care Organization, www.nhpco.org
National Nursing Centers Consortium (NNCC), www.nncc.us
U.S. Department of Health and Human Services, Office of Disease Prevention and Health Promotion, *Healthy People 2020*, http://healthypeople.gov
Urban Institute, www.urban.org

3

Critical Thinking, Ethical Decision Making, and the Nursing Process

LEARNING OBJECTIVES

On completion of this chapter, the learner will be able to:

1 Define the characteristics of critical thinking, critical thinkers, and the critical thinking process.
2 Define ethics, nursing ethics, and morals.
3 Identify several ethical dilemmas common to the medical-surgical area of nursing practice.

4 Specify strategies that can aid nurses in ethical decision making.
5 Describe the components of the nursing process.
6 Develop a plan of nursing care for a patient using strategies of critical thinking.

GLOSSARY

assessment: the systematic collection of data, through interview, observation, and examination, to determine the patient's health status and any actual or potential problems

collaborative problems: the physiologic manifestations, which are monitored to detect a new onset of changes in patient status and are managed by nursing, medicine, and allied health professionals

critical thinking: a cognitive process that utilizes thinking that is purposeful, insightful, reflective, and goal directed to develop conclusions, solutions, and alternatives that are appropriate for the given situation

deontologic or formalist theory: an ethical theory that states rational beings are ethically bound to act from a "sense of duty" independent of the ends or consequences

ethics: the formal, systematic approach used to understand, analyze, and evaluate matters of right and wrong as they relate to well-being

evaluation: determination of the patient's responses to the nursing interventions and the extent to which the outcomes have been achieved

implementation: actualization or carrying out of the plan of care through nursing interventions

morals: specific beliefs or actions whose outcomes are often examined through a systematic ethical analysis

moral dilemma: circumstances in which a clear conflict exists between two or more moral principles or competing moral claims that are incompatible

moral distress: conflict that arises within oneself when a person is aware of the correct course of action but institutional constraints stand in the way of pursuing the correct action

moral integrity: virtue composed of honesty, truthfulness, benevolence, wisdom, and moral courage

moral problem: competing moral claim or principle; one claim or principle is clearly dominant

moral uncertainty: conflict that arises within a person when the individual cannot accurately define what the moral situation is or what moral principles apply but has a strong feeling that something is not right

morality: the adherence to informal personal values

nursing diagnoses: a clinical judgment concerning an individual's, family's, group's, or community's actual or potential health problems, state of health promotion, or potential risk that can be managed by independent nursing interventions

nursing process: a systematic, problem-solving approach for meeting people's health care and nursing needs; components include assessment, diagnosis, planning, implementation, and evaluation

planning: development of measurable goals and outcomes, as well as a plan of care designed to assist the patient in resolving the diagnosed problems and achieving the identified goals and desired outcomes

teleologic theory or consequentialism: the theoretical basis of ethics, which focuses on the ends or consequences of actions, such as utilitarianism

utilitarianism: a teleologic theory of ethics based on the concept of promotion of the greatest good for the greatest number of people who may be affected by an action

As scientific advances in healthcare technology continue to proceed, nurses face increasingly complex issues and situations. Greater acuity of patients in both hospital and community settings, an aging population, complex disease processes and end-of-life concerns, as well as ethical issues and cultural factors must be considered. The decision-making part of nurses' problem-solving activities has become increasingly multifaceted and requires critical thinking based upon sound ethical principles.

Critical Thinking

Critical thinking is a cognitive process that utilizes thinking that is purposeful, insightful, reflective, and goal directed in order to develop conclusions, solutions, and alternatives that are appropriate for the given situation. Critical thinking, which includes reasoning and judgment, is based upon a body of knowledge and includes analysis of all information and ideas. Thoughts must not be taken at "face value"; rather, they must be analyzed and assessed for its clarity, accuracy, relevance, depth, breadth, and logicalness (Critical Thinking Community, 2013). Critical thinking leads to the formulation of conclusions and alternatives that are the most appropriate for the situation and is used to plan patient-centered care. Critical thinking has been identified as an essential core competency for nurses by the National League for Nursing and the American Association of Colleges of Nursing (Brudvig, Dirkes, Dutta, et al., 2013). This cognitive process is critical to effective use of the nursing process (Perez-Rivas, Martin-Inglesias, Pacheco del Cerro, et al., 2015).

Critical thinking includes metacognition—the examination of one's own reasoning or thought processes—to help refine thinking skills. Independent nursing judgments and decisions evolve from a sound knowledge base and the ability to synthesize information within the context in which it is presented. Nursing practice in today's society requires the use of high-level critical thinking skills. Critical thinking enhances clinical decision making, helping to identify patient needs and the best nursing actions that will assist patients in meeting those needs. Because critical thinking is a deliberate, outcome-oriented activity, it is logical, organized, and iterative. Critical thinking occurs through inquiry and the "process of intentional higher level thinking to define a client's problem, examine the evidence-based practice in caring for the client, and make choices in the delivery of care"

(Alfaro-LeFevre, 2013, p. 144). It is grounded in a comprehensive knowledge base (Brudvig et al., 2013). Critical thinkers are inquisitive truth seekers who are open to the alternative solutions that might surface. Alfaro-LeFevre (2013) identified critical thinkers as people who ideally are active thinkers, fair minded, open minded, persistent, empathic, independent in thought, good communicators, honest, organized and systematic, proactive, flexible, realistic, humble, cognizant of the rules of logic, curious and insightful, and creative and committed to excellence. The skills involved in critical thinking are developed over time through effort, practice, and experience (see Chart 3-1). Critical thinking is used for clinical reasoning, which is the process used to "gather and analyze client information, evaluate the relevance of the information, and decide on possible nursing actions to improve the client's physiological and psychosocial outcomes" (Alfaro-LeFevre, 2013, p. 144).

Rationality and Insight

Skills needed in critical thinking include interpretation, analysis, inference, explanation, evaluation, self-reflection, and self-regulation. Critical thinking requires strong background knowledge and knowledge of key concepts as well as logical thinking. Nurses use this disciplined process to validate the accuracy of data and the reliability of any assumptions they have made, and they then carefully evaluate the effectiveness of what they have identified as the necessary actions to take. Nurses also evaluate the reliability of sources, being mindful of and questioning inconsistencies. Nurses use interpretation to determine the significance of data that are gathered, analysis to identify patient problems suggested by the data,

---

Chart 3-1 **NURSING RESEARCH PROFILE**
Critical Thinking Skills in Nursing Students

Newton, S. E., & Moore, G. (2013). Critical thinking skills in basic baccalaureate and accelerated second degree nursing students. *Nursing Education Perspectives*, 34(3), 154–158.

Purpose

Many nursing researchers believe that critical thinking is a developmental process that evolves over time. Student experiences, as well as the context in which they learn, all contribute to the development of critical thinking. There is an assumption that accelerated second-degree nursing students (ASDs) have better critical thinking skills than basic baccalaureate nursing students (Basic BSNs) because they have had more time and experiences to develop these skills. The purpose of this study was to examine the critical thinking skills of Basic BSNs and ASDs and identify the educational implications of any differences between the two groups.

Design

The study design was exploratory descriptive. The sample consisted of 2 cohorts of ASDs and 2 cohorts of Basic BSNs. All participants were enrolled as full-time students. The instrument used was the Critical Thinking Entrance Assessment Examination (CTAE). Competencies measured in this test included interpretation, evaluation, analysis, inference, explanation, and self-regulation. The survey was given to all participants (*N* = 283) during the first month of the nursing curriculum, after Institutional Review Board (IRB) approval was obtained.

Findings

Findings indicated that both the ASDs and the Basic BSNs began the nursing curriculum with high CTAE scores; however, the ASDs had higher CTAE scores in the categories of analysis, inference, interpretation, and self-regulation. Although not statistically significant, the ASDs scored higher than Basic BSNs in evaluation and explanation. If critical thinking is a developmental process that requires time and experience, the findings of this study are congruent with the literature. Since the ASDs enter the nursing curriculum with 4 years of previous undergraduate experiences, it can be assumed they have had the opportunity to engage in more critical thinking than the newly admitted Basic BSNs.

Nursing Implications

Findings from this research suggest both Basic BSNs and ASDs have high critical thinking scores. Nurse educators are challenged to create experiences that facilitate further development of the six components of critical thinking. Although the CTAE is a validated instrument, it is not nursing discipline-specific; a nursing-specific instrument that measures how well a student applies knowledge to clinical practice would be most useful. These researchers suggest that nurse educators may want to use a qualitative approach to examine nursing students' ability to critically think. Findings from these studies may be helpful to design pedagogies to foster critical thinking among nursing students in all programs.

and inference to draw conclusions. Explanation is the justification of actions or interventions used to address patient problems and to help patients move toward desired outcomes. Evaluation is the process of determining whether outcomes have been or are being met. Self-regulation is the process of examining the care provided and adjusting the interventions as needed. All processes are iterative.

Critical thinking is also reflective, involving metacognition, active evaluation, and refinement of the thinking process. Metacognition involves reflective thinking as well as awareness of the nursing skills needed for patient-centered care (Alfaro-LeFevre, 2013). Nurses engaged in critical thinking consider the possibility of cultural differences and personal bias when interpreting data and determining appropriate actions (see Chapter 7). Critical thinkers must be insightful and have a sense of fairness and integrity; the courage to question personal ethics; and the perseverance to strive continuously to minimize the effects of egocentricity, ethnocentricity, and other biases on the decision-making process (Alfaro-LeFevre, 2013).

Components of Critical Thinking

Certain cognitive or mental activities are key components of critical thinking as it relates to nurses. Critical thinkers:

- Identify the priorities that will determine the nurse's plan of patient-centered care.
- Gather pertinent data from the patient's chart and assessments to determine why certain developments have occurred and to determine if additional data are needed to address the situation accurately.
- Validate the information presented to make sure that it is accurate and compare it with any pre-existing data. Information should be evidence based.
- Analyze the information to determine its significance and to identify the formation of clusters or patterns that point to certain conclusions.
- Utilize logical thinking, past clinical experiences, theoretical knowledge, and intuitive thinking to assess the status of the patient's condition. Anticipate the patient's needs and outcomes while acknowledging personal bias and cultural influences.
- Maintain a flexible attitude that facilitates thinking and inquiry and consider all possibilities.
- Utilize inductive and deductive reasoning to identify available options and analyze each in terms of its advantages and disadvantages.
- Formulate decisions that reflect creativity and independent decision making.
- Demonstrate personal humility in terms of one's knowledge deficits and willingly seek additional information to assist with decision making.
- Exhibit the courage to seek new, innovative approaches to patient-centered care. Detach their personal viewpoints from situations and look at things objectively, a process called *bracketing*.

Critical thinking requires going beyond basic problem solving into a realm of inquisitive exploration, looking for all relevant factors that affect the issue, and being an "out-of-the-box" thinker. Nurses' ongoing quest for "best practice" clearly demonstrates intellectual integrity, a component of critical thinking.

Critical Thinking and Clinical Reasoning in Nursing Practice

Critical thinking and decision making are thought to be associated with improved clinical expertise. Critical thinking is the foundation of the process of clinical reasoning and clinical judgment (Alfaro-LeFevre, 2013). Using critical thinking to develop a plan of nursing care requires considering the human factors that might influence the plan. Nurses interact with patients, families, and other health care providers in the process of providing appropriate, individualized nursing care.

Nurses must use critical thinking skills in all practice settings—acute care, ambulatory care, extended care, and the home and community—and must view each patient situation as unique and dynamic. The unique factors that patients and nurses bring to the health care situation are considered, studied, analyzed, and interpreted. Interpretation of the information then allows nurses to focus on those factors that are most relevant and most significant to the clinical situation. Decisions about a nursing plan, priority of actions, and measurable outcomes are developed into an action plan.

In decision making related to the nursing process, nurses use cognitive and metacognitive skills as well as logical reasoning to set priorities. These skills include systematic and comprehensive assessment, recognition of assumptions and inconsistencies, verification of reliability and accuracy, identification of missing information, distinguishing relevant from irrelevant information, support of the evidence with facts and conclusions, priority setting with timely decision making, determination of patient-specific outcomes, and reassessment of responses and outcomes (Alfaro-LeFevre, 2013). All of these data are examined within the context of a solid knowledge base. For example, nurses use critical thinking, clinical reasoning, and decision-making skills in providing genetics-related nursing care when they:

- Assess and analyze family history data for genetic risk factors.
- Identify those individuals and families in need of referral for genetic testing or counseling.
- Ensure the privacy and confidentiality of genetic information.
- Maintain a knowledge base that is current and based on evidence-based research.

Because developing the skill of critical thinking involves experiential learning and practice, critical thinking exercises are offered at the end of each chapter as a means of honing the reader's ability to think critically. Some exercises include questions that stimulate the reader to seek information about evidence-based practice relative to the clinical situation described, whereas others challenge the reader to identify priority assessments and interventions. Additional exercises may be found in the study guide that accompanies the text. The questions listed in Chart 3-2 can serve as a guide in working through the exercises. It is important to remember that each clinical situation is unique and calls for an individualized approach that fits its unique set of circumstances. As critical thinking may require consideration of ethical principles and cultural contexts, these concepts are discussed in this chapter and in Chapter 7.

Ethical Nursing Care

In the complex healthcare world, nurses are faced with ethical issues across the lifespan. Consequently, there has been a

Chart 3-2 The Inquiring Mind: Critical Thinking in Action

Throughout the critical thinking process, a continuous flow of questions evolves in the thinker's mind. It is not sufficient to rely solely on the acquisition of knowledge or a set of problem-solving skills; rather, it is the combination of one's application of knowledge, analysis of the situation, synthesis, and evaluation that promotes effective critical thinking inquiry. Although posing questions will vary according to the particular clinical situation, certain general inquiries can serve as a basis for reaching conclusions and determining a course of action.

When faced with a patient situation, seeking answers to some or all of the following questions may help to determine those actions that are most appropriate:

- What relevant assessment information do I need, and how do I interpret this information? What is the most effective way to gather this information? What does this information tell me? What contextual factors must be considered when gathering this information? What are the priority assessments?
- Have I identified the most important assessments and findings? Does the information I have gathered point to any other problems that I should consider?
- Have I gathered all of the necessary information (signs and symptoms, laboratory values, medication history, emotional factors, mental status)? Is anything missing?
- Is there anything that needs to be reported immediately? Do I need to seek additional assistance?
- What risks factors are specific to this patient? Which risk factors are of the highest priority? What must I do to minimize these risks?
- What possible complications must I anticipate?
- What are the most important problems in this situation? Do the patient and the patient's family recognize the same problems?
- What are the desired outcomes for this patient? Which have the highest priority? Do the patient and I agree on these points?
- What is going to be my first action in this situation? Why is this action a priority?
- How can I construct a plan of care to achieve the goals?
- Are there any age-related factors involved, and will they require some special approach? Will I need to make some change in the plan of care to take these factors into account?
- How do the family dynamics affect this situation, and will they affect my actions or the plan of care?
- Are there cultural factors that I must address and consider?
- Am I dealing with an ethical issue here? If so, how am I going to resolve it?
- Has any nursing research been conducted on this subject? What are the nursing implications of this research for care of this patient? What is the strength of the evidence found from research?

Adapted from Brudvig, T. J., Dirkes, A., Dutta, P., et al. (2013). Critical thinking in health care professional students: A systematic review. *Journal of Physical Therapy Education, 27*(3), 12–25.

heightened interest in the field of ethics in an attempt to gain a better understanding of how these issues can be addressed. Specifically, the focus on ethics in healthcare has intensified in response to controversial developments, including advanced technology, genomics, medical futility, scarcity of resources, and end-of-life issues.

Today, sophisticated technology can prolong life well beyond the time when death would have occurred in the past. Expensive experimental procedures, clinical trials, equipment, and treatments are available to prolong life, even when such attempts may not provide quality of life.

The development of technologic support has influenced the quality and delivery of nursing care at all stages of life and also has contributed to an increase in average life expectancy. For example, the prenatal period has been influenced by genetic screening, in vitro fertilization, the harvesting and freezing of embryos, and prenatal surgery. Premature neonates, who once would have died due to a gestational age less than 24 weeks, now may survive because of advances in technology. Patients who would have died of organ failure are living longer because of organ transplantation and stem cell transplant.

These advances in technology have been a mixed blessing. Questions have been raised about whether it is appropriate to use such technology and, if so, under what circumstances. Although many patients do achieve a good quality of life, others face extended suffering as a result of efforts to prolong life, usually at great expense both emotionally and financially. Ethical issues also surround those practices or policies that seem to allocate health care resources unjustly on the basis of age, race, gender, disability, or social mores. Older adults may be at risk for being denied healthcare because of their advanced age and the bias known as ageism. See Chapter 11 for a further discussion of ageism.

Ethical dilemmas that nurses may encounter in the medical-surgical nursing arena are numerous, diverse, and occur in all settings. An awareness of underlying concepts helps nurses use reason to work through these dilemmas. Basic concepts related to moral philosophy, such as ethics and its principles, theories, and approaches, are included in this chapter. Understanding the role of the professional nurse in ethical decision making not only helps nurses articulate their ethical positions and develop the skills needed to make ethical decisions, but also helps them use the nursing process to develop plans of care from an ethical perspective.

Ethics Versus Morals

The terms *ethics* and *morality* are used to describe beliefs about right and wrong and to suggest appropriate guidelines for action. In essence, **ethics** is the formal, systematic study of moral beliefs to understand, analyze, and evaluate matters of right and wrong; whereas, **morality** includes specific values, characters, or actions whose outcomes are often examined through systematic ethical analysis. Because the distinction between ethics and morality is slight, the terms are often used interchangeably.

Ethics Theories

One classic theory in ethics is **teleologic theory or consequentialism**, which focuses on the ends or consequences of actions. The best-known form of this theory, **utilitarianism**, is based on the concept of "the greatest good for the greatest number." The choice of action is clear under this theory, because the action that maximizes good over bad is the correct one. The theory poses difficulty when one must judge intrinsic values and determine whose good is the greatest. In addition, it is important to ask whether good consequences can justify any amoral actions that might be used to achieve them.

Another theory in ethics is the **deontologic or formalist theory**, which argues that ethical standards or principles exist independently of the ends or consequences. In a given situation, nurses have a "sense of duty" to act based on the one relevant principle, or the most relevant of several ethical principles. Their actions must be independent of the ends or consequences. Problems arise with this theory when personal and cultural biases influence the choice of the most primary ethical principle.

Approaches to Ethics

Two approaches to ethics are meta-ethics and applied ethics. An example of meta-ethics (understanding the concepts and linguistic terminology used in ethics) in the health care environment is analysis of the concept of informed consent. Nurses are aware that patients must give consent before surgery; however, sometimes a question arises as to whether a patient is truly informed. Delving more deeply into the concept of informed consent would be a meta-ethical inquiry. See Chapter 17 for more information about informed consent before surgery.

Applied ethics refers to identification of ethical problems relevant to a specific discipline and that discipline's practice. It addresses the implications of actions or practices in terms of their moral permissibility. Various disciplines use the frameworks of general ethical theories and principles and apply them to specific problems within their domain. Nursing ethics may be considered a form of applied ethics because it addresses moral situations that are specific to the nursing profession and patient care. Common ethical principles that can be used to validate moral claims in clinical practice include autonomy, beneficence and nonmaleficence, double effect, and distributive justice. Brief definitions of these important principles can be found in Chart 3-3.

Moral Situations

Many situations exist in which ethical analysis is needed. Some are **moral dilemmas**, or situations in which a clear conflict exists between two or more moral principles or competing moral claims, and nurses must choose the lesser of two evils. Other situations represent **moral problems**, in which there may be competing moral claims or principles, although one claim or principle is clearly dominant. Some situations result in **moral uncertainty**, when one cannot accurately define what the moral situation is or what moral principles apply but has a strong feeling that something is not right. Still other situations may result in **moral distress**, in which one is aware of the correct course of action but institutional constraints stand in the way of pursuing the correct action.

For example, an older adult patient, with a history of Stage 4 adenocarcinoma of the lung, is admitted to the hospital with difficulty breathing. Although she has been advised by the radiation oncologist to begin a course of radiation to her lung, she tells the nurse that she has had radiation before and just wants to go home. She is mentally competent and says, "I have had a good life and I am tired of treatments that don't work. I just want to go home." The radiation oncologist and the patient's adult daughter feel differently and do not support the patient's wishes to go home and not receive the radiation treatment. The nurse believes that since the patient is mentally competent, she has the right to make autonomous decisions about her treatment options. However, the radiation oncologist and the patient's daughter are concerned that if she is discharged home with difficulty breathing and a growing mass of the lung, the patient will likely become even sicker and could die. Thus, the ethical principles of autonomy and nonmaleficence are at odds with each other—a moral problem exists because of the competing moral claims of the patient's daughter and physician, who wish to pursue what is ordinarily considered the best treatment option, and the patient, whose autonomy is advocated by the nurse. If the patient's competency was questionable, a moral dilemma would exist because no dominant principle would be evident. The physician states,

---

Chart 3-3 ETHICAL DILEMMA
Common Ethical Principles

The following common ethical principles may be used to validate moral claims.

Autonomy

This word *autonomy* is derived from the Greek words *autos* ("self") and *nomos* ("rule" or "law") and therefore refers to self-determination. In contemporary discourse, it has broad meanings, including "obtaining informed consent for treatment, facilitating and supporting patients' choices regarding treatment options, allowing patients to refuse treatments, maintaining privacy and confidentiality (Butts & Rich, 2016, pp. 36–37)." The principle of autonomy entails the right of patients to receive adequate and accurate information so that they have the ability to make a choice free from external constraints.

Beneficence and Nonmaleficence

Beneficence is the duty to "perform deeds of mercy, kindness, friendship, charity, and the like (Beauchamp & Childress, 2013, p. 202)" to benefit others. It also entails taking positive action to prevent patients from harming themselves or others, including society as a whole. There is also an implied commitment to help individuals with disabilities.

Nonmaleficence is the duty to not inflict harm. The only time when it is considered morally permissible to exercise power over a competent person against their will is when by doing so, harm to others is prevented.

Double Effect

The double effect is a principle that may morally justify some actions that produce both good and evil effects.

All four of the following criteria must be fulfilled:

1. The action itself is good or morally neutral.
2. The agent sincerely intends the good and not the evil effect (the evil effect may be foreseen but is not intended).
3. The good effect is not achieved by means of the evil effect.
4. There is proportionate or favorable balance of good over evil.

Distributive Justice

From a broad perspective, justice states that like cases should be treated alike. More specifically, distributive justice is an ethical principle commonly applicable to clinical situations. This principle is upheld when benefits and burdens are distributed equitably and fairly without consideration of age, gender, socioeconomic status, religion, ethnicity, or sexual orientation. Simply stated, there is an ethical obligation to distribute or allocate resources fairly.

Adapted from Beauchamp, T. L., & Childress, J. F. (2013). *Principles of biomedical ethics*. New York, NY: Oxford University Press; Butts, J. B., & Rich, K. L. (2016). *Nursing ethics across the curriculum and into practice* (4th ed.). Burlington, MA: Jones and Bartlett Learning.

"If this was my mother, I would insist that she has the radiation." Although the physician is acting under the intent of beneficence, there is a clear violation of patient autonomy, which is called paternalism or "Father Knows Best."

It is essential that nurses freely engage in dialogue concerning moral situations, even though such dialogue is difficult for everyone involved. Improved interdisciplinary collaboration is supported when all members of the health care team can voice their concerns and come to an understanding of the moral situation. Consultation with an ethics committee could be helpful to assist the health care team, patient, and family to identify the moral dilemma and possible approaches to the dilemma (see the Ethics Committees section). Nurses should be familiar with agency policy supporting patient self-determination and resolution of ethical issues.

Types of Ethical Problems in Nursing

As a profession, nursing is accountable to society. Nursing has identified its standards of accountability through formal codes of ethics that explicitly state the profession's values and goals. The International Council of Nurses (ICN) has endorsed a globally applicable *Code of Ethics for Nurses* (ICN, 2012). Likewise, the American Nurses Association (ANA) established a *Code of Ethics for Nurses* that includes ethical standards, each with its own interpretive statements (ANA, 2015b) (see Chart 3-4). The

---

Chart 3-4 | American Nurses Association Code of Ethics for Nurses

1. The nurse practices with compassion and respect for the inherent dignity, worth, and unique attributes of every person.
2. The nurse's primary commitment is to the patient, whether an individual, family, group, community, or population.
3. The nurse promotes, advocates for, and strives to protect the rights, health, and safety of the patient.
4. The nurse has authority, accountability, and responsibility for nursing practice; makes decisions; and takes action consistent with the obligation to promote health and to provide optimal care.
5. The nurse owes the same duties to self as to others, including the responsibility to preserve health and safety, preserve wholeness of character and integrity, maintain competence, and continue personal and professional growth.
6. The nurse, through individual and collective effort, establishes, maintains, and improves the ethical environment of the work setting and conditions of employment that are conducive to safe, quality health care.
7. The nurse, in all roles and settings, advances the profession through research and scholarly inquiry, professional standards development, and the generation of both nursing and health policy.
8. The nurse collaborates with other health professionals and the public to promote human rights, promote health diplomacy, and reduce health disparities.
9. The profession of nursing, collectively through its professional organizations, must articulate nursing values, maintain the integrity of the profession, and integrate principles of social justice into nursing and health policy.

Reprinted with permission from the American Nurses Association, *Code of ethics for nurses with interpretive statements*, © 2015, American Nurses Publishing, American Nurses Foundation/American Nurses Association, Washington, DC.

Chart 3-5 | Position Statements from the American Nurses Association Center for Ethics and Human Rights

Position Statement	Latest Approval/Revision Date
Euthanasia, Assisted Suicide, and Aid in Dying	Revised 4/24/13
Nursing Care and Do Not Resuscitate (DNR) and Allow Natural Death (AND)	Approved 3/12/12
Foregoing Nutrition and Hydration	Revised 3/11/11
Reduction of Patient Restraint and Seclusion in Health Care Settings	Approved 3/11/11
The Nurses' Role in Ethics and Human Rights: Protecting and Promoting Individual Worth, Dignity, and Human Rights in Practice Setting	Approved 6/14/10
Nurses' Role in Capital Punishment	Approved 1/28/10
In Support of Patients' Safe Access to Therapeutic Marijuana	Approved 12/12/08
Stem Cell Research	Approved 1/10/07
Privacy and Confidentiality	Approved 12/8/06
Assuring Patient Safety: The Employers' Role in Promoting Healthy Nursing Work Hours for Registered Nurses in All Roles and Settings to Guard Against Working When Fatigued	Approved 12/8/06
Risk and Responsibility in Providing Nursing Care	Approved 6/21/06
Registered Nurses' Role and Responsibilities in Providing Expert Care and Counseling at End-of-Life	Approved 6/14/10

---

interpretive statements provide guidance to address and resolve ethical dilemmas by incorporating universal moral principles. In addition, the ANA sponsors a Center for Ethics and Human Rights that contains a repository of position statements that can be used to guide nursing practice (see Chart 3-5).

Ethical issues have always affected the role of professional nurses. The accepted definition of professional nursing supports the advocacy role for nurses. The ANA, in *Nursing's Social Policy Statement* (2010), defines *nursing* as "the protection, promotion, and optimization of health and abilities, prevention of illness and injury, alleviation of suffering through the diagnosis and treatment of human response, and advocacy in the care of individuals, families, communities, and populations" (p. 9). This definition supports the claim that nurses must be actively involved in the decision-making process regarding ethical concerns surrounding health care and human responses. Nurses are morally obligated to present ethical conflicts within a logical, systematic framework. Health care settings in which nurses are valued members of the team promote interdisciplinary communication and may enhance patient care. To practice effectively in these settings, nurses must be aware of ethical issues and serve as patient advocates to assist patients in asserting their autonomy in decision making.

Nursing theories that incorporate the biopsychosocial–spiritual dimensions emphasize a holistic viewpoint, with humanism or caring at the core. Caring and compassion are often cited as virtues inherent within the moral foundation for professional nursing practice. For nurses to embrace this professional ethos, they must be aware not only of major ethical dilemmas but also of those daily interactions with health care consumers that frequently give rise to less easily identifiable ethical challenges. Although technologic advances and diminished resources have been instrumental in raising numerous ethical questions and controversies, including life-and-death issues, nurses should not ignore the many routine situations that involve ethical considerations. Some of the most common issues faced by nurses today include confidentiality, the use of restraints, truth-telling, refusing to provide care, and end-of-life decisions and palliative care.

Confidentiality

All nurses should be aware of the confidential nature of information obtained in daily practice. Confidentiality acknowledges and respects each individual's privacy. If information is not pertinent, nurses should question whether it is prudent to document it in a patient's record. In the practice setting, discussion of patients with other members of the health care team is often necessary. However, these discussions should occur in a private area where it is unlikely that the conversation will be overheard. Nurses should also be aware that the use of family members or hospital ancillary personnel as interpreters for patients who are not fluent in English language or who are deaf violates patients' rights of confidentiality. Translation services should be provided for non–English-speaking patients, and interpreters should be provided for those who use sign language by the hospital or institution.

Another threat to confidentiality is the widespread use of computer-based technologies, specifically electronic health records (EHR) and people's easy access to them. The growing demand for telehealth innovations and the increasing use of this method can result in unchecked access to health information. In addition, personal and health information is often made available to numerous individuals and corporate stakeholders, which may increase the potential for misuse of health care information. Because of these possibilities of maleficence, sensitivity to the principle of confidentiality is essential. The ANA (1999) published a position statement that addresses patients' rights to privacy and confidentiality of their health information.

Federal legislation has been developed to protect the right of confidentiality. According to the Health Insurance Portability and Accountability Act (HIPAA) (U.S. Department of Health and Human Services [HHS], 2003), efforts must be made to protect each patient's private health information (PHI), whether it is transmitted by verbal, written, or electronic means of communication. Communication should be confined to the appropriate settings and with appropriate individuals and should occur for the appropriate purposes of facilitating patient care. Violations of protection of any patient's privacy could result in criminal or civil litigation (HHS, 2003).

Restraints

The use of restraints (including physical and pharmacologic measures) and patient seclusion are additional issues with ethical overtones because of the limits on a person's autonomy and human dignity when these measures are used. Nurses must weigh carefully the risks of limiting autonomy and increasing the risks of injury by using restraints against the risks of injury if not using restraints, which have been documented as

resulting in physical harm and death. The ANA (2012) advocates that in situations where restraints and seclusion must be used, all staff must be educated on safety measures. In addition, there must be adequate staff who are vigilant in monitoring their use. These interventions may be utilized only when there is no other viable option available. The Joint Commission and the Centers for Medicare and Medicaid Services (CMS) have designated standards for the use of restraints. See the Joint Commission and CMS Web sites listed in the Resources section.

Trust Issues

Truth-telling or veracity is one of the basic principles in the nurse–patient relationship. Truth-telling is based upon the principle of autonomy and the patient's "rational capacity for self-determination" (Vaughn, 2013, p. 133). For example, failure to disclose a diagnosis to a patient deprives the individual of the right to make informed decisions. Three ethical dilemmas in clinical practice that can directly conflict with this principle are the use of placebos (nonactive substances used for treatment), not revealing a diagnosis to a patient, and revealing a diagnosis to people other than the patient with the diagnosis. All involve the issue of trust, which is an essential element in the nurse–patient relationship.

Placebos may be used in experimental research, in which a patient is involved in the decision-making process and is aware that placebos are being used in the treatment regimen. However, the use of a placebo as a substitute for an active drug to show that a patient does not have actual symptoms of a disease is deceptive, has both ethical and legal implications, and severely undermines the nurse–patient relationship.

Informing a patient of their diagnosis when the family and physician have chosen to delay full disclosure of pertinent information is an ethical dilemma that can occur in nursing practice. The nurse may experience moral distress when asked by the patient for a truthful diagnosis. The nurse may use evasive comments with the patient in these situations. This area is indeed complex, because it challenges a nurse's **moral integrity**. Nurses could consider the following strategies:
- Avoid lying to the patient.
- Provide all information related to nursing procedures and diagnoses.
- Act as a patient advocate and communicate the patient's requests for information to the family and physician. The family is often unaware of the patient's repeated questions to the nurse. With a better understanding of the situation, the family members may change their perspective.
- Make a referral to the institution's ethics committee.

Although providing the information may be the morally appropriate behavior, the manner in which the patient is told is important. Nurses must be compassionate and caring when informing patients; disclosure of information merely for the sake of patient autonomy does not convey respect for others and in some circumstances may result in emotional distress. Family support or the support of a spiritual advisor (e.g., chaplain) may be needed to reduce the impact of distressing information or a poor prognosis.

Disclosing the patient's diagnosis to others without the patient's consent is a HIPAA violation and therefore is not only unethical but also illegal. Failure to protect the patient's right to privacy and a breach of confidentiality is unethical (Vaughn, 2013).

Refusing to Provide Care

Any nurse who feels morally obliged to refuse to provide care for a particular type of patient faces an ethical dilemma. Reasons for refusal range from a conflict of personal values to a fear that the nurse would place either the patient or self in jeopardy. Feelings related to care of people of different ethnicities or sexual orientation also surface as societal changes emerge. The ethical obligation to care for all patients is clearly identified in the *Code of Ethics for Nurses* (ANA, 2015b). Accordingly, the nurse must give patient-centered care to all patients, regardless of their socioeconomic status, sexual orientation, gender expression, ethnicity, or proximity to death. In particular, patients facing end-of-life decisions must receive supportive care, which must be extended to their family and surrogate decision makers (ANA, 2015b).

End-of-Life Issues

Dilemmas that center on death and dying are prevalent in medical-surgical nursing practice. With the availability of increasingly sophisticated and advanced technology, it may be difficult to accept that nothing more can be done to prolong life or that technology may prolong life but at the expense of the patient's comfort and quality of life. When providing end-of-life care, nurses serve as the patient's advocate and manage pain and suffering. Nurses have the moral obligation to facilitate a patient's right to self-determination (Butts & Rich, 2016). Furthermore, nurses should facilitate end-of-life discussions between the patient and the family in order to prevent suffering and preserve the patient's dignity (ANA, 2015b).

Many people who are terminally ill seek legal options for a peaceful and dignified death. Nurses who deliver palliative care must understand that their actions are targeted at relieving pain and suffering and not hastening death. According to Provision 1.4 of the *Code of Ethics for Nurses*, "The nurse should provide interventions to relieve pain and other symptoms in the dying patient consistent with palliative care practice standards and may not act with the sole intent to end life (2015b, p. 3)," even if the intent to end life is motivated by compassion or respect for patient autonomy.

End-of-life issues shift the focus from curative care to palliative and end-of-life care. Focusing on the caring as well as the curing role may help nurses deal with these difficult moral situations. Needs of patients and families require holistic and interdisciplinary approaches. End-of-life issues that often involve ethical dilemmas include pain control, "do not resuscitate" orders, life support measures, and administration of food and fluids. These issues are discussed in detail in Chapter 16.

Preventive Ethics

When a nurse is faced with two conflicting alternatives, it is their moral responsibility to choose the lesser of the two evils. These situations often result in feelings of moral distress in the nurse who is obliged to make a choice.

Patient Self-Determination

Frequently, dilemmas occur when health care practitioners are unsure of the patient's wishes because the patient is unconscious or mentally incompetent and cannot communicate. The Patient Self-Determination Act, enacted in December 1991, encourages people to prepare advance directives in which they indicate their wishes concerning the degree of supportive care they wish if they become incapacitated. This legislation requires that patients be informed about advance directives by the staff of the health care facility.

Advance directives are legal documents that specify a person's wishes before hospitalization and provide valuable information that may assist health care providers in decision making. A living will is one type of advance directive. Typically, living wills are limited to situations in which the patient's medical condition is deemed terminal. Because it is difficult to define *terminal* accurately, living wills are not always honored. Another potential drawback is that living wills are frequently written while people are in good health. It is not unusual for people to change their minds as an illness progresses; therefore, patients retain the option to nullify these documents.

Identifying a health care representative, in which one person identifies another person to make health care decisions on their behalf, is another type of advance directive. It is the responsibility of the health care representative to act as the patient stated in the advance directive. For example, patients may have clarified their wishes concerning various medical situations. If there is no advance directive, the health care representative must act in good faith and make decisions that he or she believes the patient would make if mentally competent. Laws concerning advance directives vary among state jurisdictions. However, even in states where these documents are not legally binding, they provide helpful information to determine the patient's prior expressed wishes in situations in which this information can no longer be obtained.

Advance directives are limited in scope to hospital and long-term care facility environments. Emergency medical system (EMS) personnel (e.g., paramedics) therefore cannot legally follow advance directives. Yet, there are many patients with debilitating long-term chronic and eventually fatal illnesses who reside at home. Some of these patients may not wish to have invasive, life-sustaining emergency interventions should their status rapidly deteriorate. To protect the wishes of these patients to forego life-sustaining treatments, a document titled Physician Orders for Life-Sustaining Treatment (POLST) has been legally endorsed by many states. POLST gives EMS personnel the ability to rapidly determine whether a patient wishes to have cardiopulmonary resuscitation (CPR) or receive any type of emergency interventions that may sustain life in the event when the patient suddenly becomes incapacitated (POLST, 2015).

Ethics Committees

Institutional ethics committees exist in many hospitals to assist clinicians with ethical dilemmas. The purpose of these multidisciplinary committees varies among institutions. In some hospitals, the committees exist solely for the purpose of developing policies; whereas in others, they may have a strong educational or consultation focus. These committees usually are composed of people with some advanced training in ethics and are important resources for the health care team, patient, and family. Nurses with a particular interest or expertise in the area of ethics can serve as members of these committees, which are valuable resources for staff nurses. In addition, physicians, social workers, and hospital chaplains are often members of the team.

Ethical Decision Making

Ethical dilemmas are common and diverse in nursing practice. Situations vary, and experience indicates that there are no clear solutions to these dilemmas, which may be referred to as a slippery slope (Pozgar, 2016). However, the fundamental philosophical principles are the same, and the process of moral reflection helps nurses justify their actions. The systematic approach to ethical decision making can follow the steps of the nursing process. Ethics charts contained in all units within this text present case scenarios that challenge the reader to identify the ethical principles involved that may or may not be in conflict (see Chart 3-2). Chart 3-6 outlines the steps of an ethical analysis that may be used to resolve the moral dilemmas presented in these charts.

The Nursing Process

Definition

The **nursing process** is a deliberate problem-solving approach for meeting people's health care and nursing needs. Although the steps of the nursing process have been stated in various ways by different writers, the common components cited are assessment, diagnosis, planning, implementation, and evaluation (Carpenito, 2017). The ANA's *Scope and Standards of Practice* (ANA, 2015a) includes an additional component entitled outcome identification, defined as identification of expected outcomes for a plan that is tailored to the patient's needs. The sequence of steps in this process is assessment, diagnosis, outcome identification, planning, implementation, and evaluation. For the purposes of this text, the nursing process is based on the traditional five steps and delineates two components in the diagnosis step: nursing diagnoses and collaborative problems. After the diagnoses or problems have been determined, the desired outcomes are often evident. The traditional steps are defined as follows:

1. *Assessment*: The systematic collection of data through interview, observation, and examination to determine the patient's health status as well as any actual or potential health problems (Analysis of data is included as part of the assessment. Analysis may also be identified as a separate step of the nursing process).
2. *Diagnosis*: Identification of the following two types of patient problems:

Chart 3-6 · ETHICAL DILEMMA

Steps of an Ethical Analysis

The following guidelines reflect an active process in decision making, similar to the nursing process detailed in this chapter. Nurses can use these guidelines to engage in ethical decision making. Key resources that may assist in ethical decision making are also included.

Assessment

1. Once the ethical issue has been identified, assess the ethical/moral situations of the problem. This step entails recognition of the ethical, legal, and professional dimensions involved.
   a. Does the situation entail substantive moral problems (conflicts among ethical principles or professional obligations)? Examine the ethical issue using the principles of autonomy, beneficence, justice, and nonmaleficence.
   b. Are there procedural conflicts? (e.g., Who should make the decisions? Any conflicts among the patient, health care providers, family, and guardians?)
   c. Identify the significant people involved and those affected by the decision.
   d. Identify agency or hospital policy or protocol to use when a conflict exists. Is there an ethics committee or council? How is an ethics consult made, and who may request this consultation? What other resources are available to help resolve this conflict?

Planning

2. Collect information.
   a. Include the following information: the medical facts, treatment options, nursing diagnoses, legal data, and the values, beliefs, cultures, and religious components.
   b. Make a distinction between the factual information and the values/beliefs.
   c. Validate the patient's capacity, or lack of capacity, to make decisions.
   d. Identify any other relevant information that should be elicited.
   e. Identify the ethical/moral issues and the competing claims.

f. If it is an end-of-life issue, determine whether an advance directive exists and whether a medical power of attorney or a heath care representative has been identified.

Implementation

3. List the alternatives. Compare alternatives with applicable ethical principles and the 2015 ANA *Code of Ethics for Nurses*. Choose either of the frameworks that follow, or other frameworks, and compare outcomes.
   a. *Utilitarian approach:* Predict the consequences of the alternatives; assign a positive or negative value to each consequence; choose the consequence that predicts the highest positive value or "the greatest good for the greatest number."
   b. *Deontological approach:* Identify the relevant moral principles; compare alternatives with moral principles; appeal to the "higher-level" moral principle if there is a conflict.

Evaluation

4. Decide and evaluate the decision.
   a. What is the best or morally correct action?
   b. Give the ethical reasons for your decision.
   c. What are the ethical reasons against your decision or your biases?
   d. How do you respond to the reasons against your decision?

Resources

American Nurses Association, Center for Ethics and Human Rights: An online resource that contains a repository of positions papers, codes, and other materials aimed at improving the ethical competence of nurses, www.nursingworld.org/ethics

The Hastings Center: A nonprofit, nonpartisan research institute dedicated to interdisciplinary bioethics, www.thehasting scenter.org

National Center for Ethics in Health Care: Provides key analysis of topics in health care ethics, publishes ethics-related news, and posts seminal national reports in ethics, www.ethics.va.gov

- *Nursing diagnoses*: According to Carpenito (2017), "Are clinical judgments about individual, family, or community responses to actual or potential health problems/life processes" that can be managed by independent nursing interventions (p. 9).
- *Collaborative problems*: According to Carpentino (2017), "Certain physiologic complications that nurses monitor to detect onset or changes in status. Nurses manage collaborative problems using physician-prescribed and nurse-prescribed interventions to minimize the complications of the events" (p. 9).

3. *Planning*: Development of measurable goals and outcomes as well as a plan of care designed to assist the patient in resolving the diagnosed problems and achieving the identified goals and desired outcomes
4. *Implementation*: Actualization or carrying out of the plan of care through nursing interventions
5. *Evaluation*: Determination of the patient's responses to the nursing interventions and the extent to which the outcomes have been achieved

Dividing the nursing process into distinct steps serves to emphasize the essential nursing actions that must be taken to address the patient's nursing diagnoses and manage any collaborative problems or complications. However, dividing the process into separate steps is artificial: The process functions as an integrated whole, with the steps being interrelated, interdependent, and recurrent (see Fig. 3-1). Chart 3-7 presents

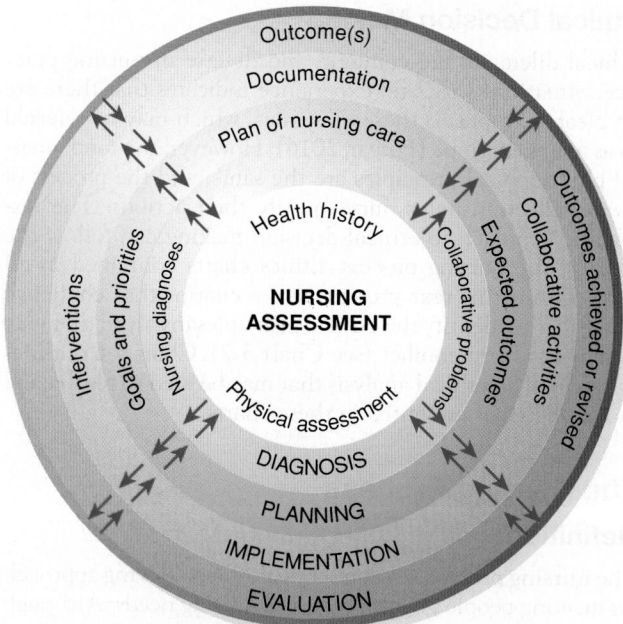

Figure 3-1 • The nursing process is depicted schematically in this circle. Starting from the innermost circle, nursing assessment, the process moves outward through the formulation of nursing diagnoses and collaborative problems; planning, with setting of goals and priorities in the nursing plan of care; implementation and documentation; and, finally, the ongoing process of evaluation and outcomes.

Chart 3-7 — Steps of the Nursing Process

Assessment

1. Conduct the health history.
2. Perform the physical assessment.
3. Interview the patient's family or significant others.
4. Study the health record.
5. Organize, analyze, synthesize, and summarize the collected data.

Diagnosis

Nursing Diagnoses

1. Identify the patient's nursing problems or potential problems.
2. Identify the defining characteristics of the nursing problems.
3. Identify the etiology of the nursing problems.
4. State nursing diagnoses concisely and precisely.

Collaborative Problems

1. Identify potential problems or complications that require collaborative interventions.
2. Identify health care members with whom collaboration is essential.

Planning

1. Assign priority to the nursing diagnoses.
2. Specify the goals.
   a. Develop immediate, intermediate, and long-term goals.
   b. State the goals in realistic and measurable terms.
3. Identify nursing interventions appropriate for goal attainment.
4. Establish expected outcomes.
   a. Make sure that the outcomes are realistic and measurable.
   b. Identify critical times for the attainment of outcomes.

5. Develop the written plan of nursing care.
   a. Include nursing diagnoses, goals, nursing interventions, expected outcomes, and critical times.
   b. Write all entries precisely, concisely, and systematically.
   c. Keep the plan current and flexible to meet the patient's changing problems and needs.
6. Involve the patient, family or significant others, nursing team members, and other health care team members in all aspects of planning.

Implementation

Put the plan of nursing care into action.

1. Coordinate the activities of the patient, family or significant others, nursing team members, and other health care team members.
2. Record the patient's responses to the nursing actions.

Evaluation

1. Collect data.
2. Compare the patient's actual outcomes with the expected outcomes. Determine the extent to which the expected outcomes were achieved.
3. Include the patient, family or significant others, nursing team members, and other health care team members in the evaluation.
4. Identify alterations that need to be made in the nursing diagnoses, collaborative problems, goals, nursing interventions, and expected outcomes.
5. Continue all steps of the nursing process: assessment, diagnosis, planning, implementation, and evaluation.

an overview of the nursing activities involved in applying the nursing process. Note that the use of the nursing process requires critical thinking and consideration of common ethical principles to ensure that a truly comprehensive plan of care is developed.

Using the Nursing Process

Assessment

According to Carpenito (2017), the initial or baseline assessment is a systematic process of collecting predetermined data during the first contact with the patient. Data are gathered through the health history and the physical assessment. In addition, ongoing assessment and monitoring are crucial to remain aware of changing patient needs and the effectiveness of nursing care.

Health History

The health history is conducted to determine a person's state of wellness or illness and is best accomplished as part of a planned interview. The interview is a personal dialogue between a patient and a nurse that is conducted to obtain information. The nurse's approach to the patient largely determines the amount and quality of the information received. To achieve a relationship of mutual trust and respect, the nurse must communicate a sincere interest in the patient. Examples of therapeutic communication techniques are found in Table 3-1.

A health history guide may help in obtaining pertinent information and directing the course of the interview. Various health history formats designed to guide the interview are available; however, they must be adapted to the responses, health problems, and needs of the person. See Chapter 5 for more information about the health history.

Physical Assessment

A physical assessment may be carried out before, during, or after the health history, depending on a patient's physical and emotional status and the immediate priorities of the situation. The purpose of the physical assessment is to identify those aspects of a patient's physical, psychological, and emotional state that indicate a need for nursing care. It requires the use of sight, hearing, touch, and smell as well as

TABLE 3-1 Therapeutic Communication Techniques

Technique	Definition	Therapeutic Value
Listening	Active process of receiving information and examining one's reactions to the messages received	Nonverbally communicates nurse's interest in the patient
Silence	Periods of no verbal communication among participants for therapeutic reasons	Gives patient time to think and gain insights, slows the pace of the interaction, and encourages the patient to initiate conversation while conveying the nurse's support, understanding, and acceptance
Restating	Repeating to the patient what the nurse believes is the main thought or idea expressed	Demonstrates that the nurse is listening and validates, reinforces, or calls attention to something important that has been said
Reflection	Directing back to the patient their feelings, ideas, questions, or content	Validates the nurse's understanding of what the patient is saying and signifies empathy, interest, and respect for the patient
Clarification	Asking the patient to explain what he or she means or attempting to verbalize vague ideas or unclear thoughts of the patient to enhance the nurse's understanding	Helps to clarify the patient's feelings, ideas, and perceptions and to provide an explicit correlation between them and the patient's actions
Focusing	Questions or statements to help the patient develop, explore, or expand an idea or verbalize feelings	Allows the patient to discuss central issues and keeps communication goal directed
Broad openings	Encouraging the patient to select topics for discussion	Indicates acceptance by the nurse and the value of the patient's initiative
Humor	Discharge of energy through the comic enjoyment of the imperfect	Promotes insight by bringing repressed material to consciousness, resolving paradoxes, tempering aggression, and revealing new options; a socially acceptable form of sublimation
Informing	Providing information	Helpful in health teaching or patient education about relevant aspects of the patient's well-being and self-care
Sharing perceptions	Asking the patient to verify the nurse's understanding of what the patient is thinking or feeling	Conveys the nurse's understanding to the patient and has the potential to clarify confusing communication; may promote additional reflection
Theme identification	Underlying issues or problems experienced by the patient that emerge repeatedly during the course of the nurse–patient relationship	Allows the nurse to best promote the patient's exploration and understanding of important problems
Suggesting	Presentation of alternative ideas for the patient's consideration relative to problem solving	Increases the patient's perceived options or choices

Adapted from Stuart, G. W. (2012). *Principles and practice of psychiatric nursing* (10th ed.). St. Louis, MO: CV Mosby.

appropriate interview skills and techniques. Physical examination techniques, as well as techniques and strategies for assessing behaviors and role changes, are presented in Chapter 5 and in the first chapter of each unit of this book, beginning with Unit 5 and continuing through Unit 16.

Other Components of the Assessment

Additional relevant information should be obtained from the patient's family or significant others, from other members of the health care team, and from the patient's health record or chart. Depending on the patient's immediate needs, this information may have been completed before the health history and the physical assessment were obtained. A review of a past medical history or records from previous admissions may provide important information for consideration. Whatever the sequence of events, the nurse should use all available sources of pertinent data to complete the nursing assessment.

Recording the Data

After the health history and physical assessment are completed, the information obtained is recorded in the patient's permanent record. These records are more commonly becoming electronic (i.e., electronic health records [EHRs]). The ANA (2009) advocates that when EHRs are used, "patients should receive written, easily understood notification of how their health records are used and when their individually identifiable health information is disclosed to third parties" (p. 1). It is imperative that the patient's right to privacy and confidentiality are not violated through the use of EHRs. Regardless of whether the record is in a traditional paper format or an EHR, it must provide a means of communication among members of the health care team and facilitate coordinated planning and continuity of care (Perez-Rivas et al., 2015). The record fulfills other functions as well:

- It serves as the legal and business record for a health care agency and for the professional staff members who are responsible for the patient's care. Various systems are used for documenting patient care, and each health care agency selects the system that best meets its needs.
- It serves as a basis for evaluating the quality and appropriateness of care and for reviewing the effective use of patient care services.
- It provides data that are useful in research, education, and short- and long-range planning.

Diagnosis

The assessment component of the nursing process serves as the basis for identifying nursing diagnoses and collaborative problems. Soon after the completion of the health history and the physical assessment, nurses organize, analyze, synthesize, and summarize the data collected and determine the patient's need for nursing care.

Nursing Diagnoses

Nursing diagnoses, the first taxonomy created in nursing, have fostered autonomy and accountability in nursing and have helped to delineate the scope of practice. Many state nurse practice acts include nursing diagnosis as a nursing function, and nursing diagnosis is included in the ANA's *Scope and Standards of Practice* (2015a) and the standards of nursing specialty organizations.

NANDA International (NANDA-I; formerly known as the North American Nursing Diagnosis Association) is the official organization responsible for developing the taxonomy of nursing diagnoses and formulating nursing diagnoses that are acceptable for study. Approved nursing diagnoses, designed by nurses, are compiled and categorized by NANDA-I in a taxonomy that is updated to maintain currency. The revised diagnostic labels identified by NANDA-I (Herdman & Kamitsuru, 2014) have been generally accepted; however, ongoing validation, refinement, and expansion based on clinical use and research are encouraged. Currently, NANDA-I has identified 235 accepted nursing diagnoses, which include defining characteristics as well as risk factors for potential problems.

Choosing a Nursing Diagnosis

When identifying a nursing diagnosis for a particular patient, nurses must first identify the commonalities among the assessment data collected. These common features lead to the categorization of related data that reveal the existence of a problem and the need for nursing intervention. The identified problems are then defined as specific nursing diagnoses. Nursing diagnoses represent actual or potential health problems, state of health promotion, or potential risks that can be managed by independent nursing actions.

It is important to remember that nursing diagnoses are not medical diagnoses; they are not medical treatments prescribed by the physician, and they are not diagnostic studies. Rather, they are succinct statements of specific patient problems that guide nurses in the development of the plan of nursing care.

To give additional meaning to the nursing diagnosis, the characteristics and etiology of the problem are identified and included as part of the diagnosis. For example, the nursing diagnoses and their defining characteristics and etiology for a patient who has anemia may include the following:

- Activity intolerance related to weakness and fatigue
- Ineffective peripheral tissue perfusion related to decreased hemoglobin
- Imbalanced nutrition: less than body requirements related to fatigue and inadequate intake of essential nutrients

Collaborative Problems

In addition to nursing diagnoses and their related nursing interventions, nursing practice involves certain situations and interventions that do not fall within the definition of nursing diagnoses. These activities pertain to potential problems or complications that are medical in origin and require collaborative interventions with the physician and other members of the health care team. The term *collaborative problem* is used to identify these situations.

Collaborative problems are certain physiologic complications that nurses monitor to detect changes in the status or onset of complications. Nurses manage collaborative problems using physician-prescribed and nurse-prescribed interventions to minimize complications (Carpenito, 2017). When treating collaborative problems, the primary nursing focus is monitoring patients for the onset of complications or changes in the status of existing complications. The complications are usually related to the disease process, treatments, medications, or diagnostic studies. The nurse recommends nursing interventions that are appropriate for managing the complications and implements the treatments prescribed by the physician. According to Carpenito (2017), collaborative problems do not have patient goals; therefore, the approach to evaluation is different from a nursing diagnosis. The algorithm in Figure 3-2 depicts the differences between nursing diagnoses and collaborative problems. After the nursing diagnoses and collaborative problems have been identified, they are recorded on the plan of nursing care.

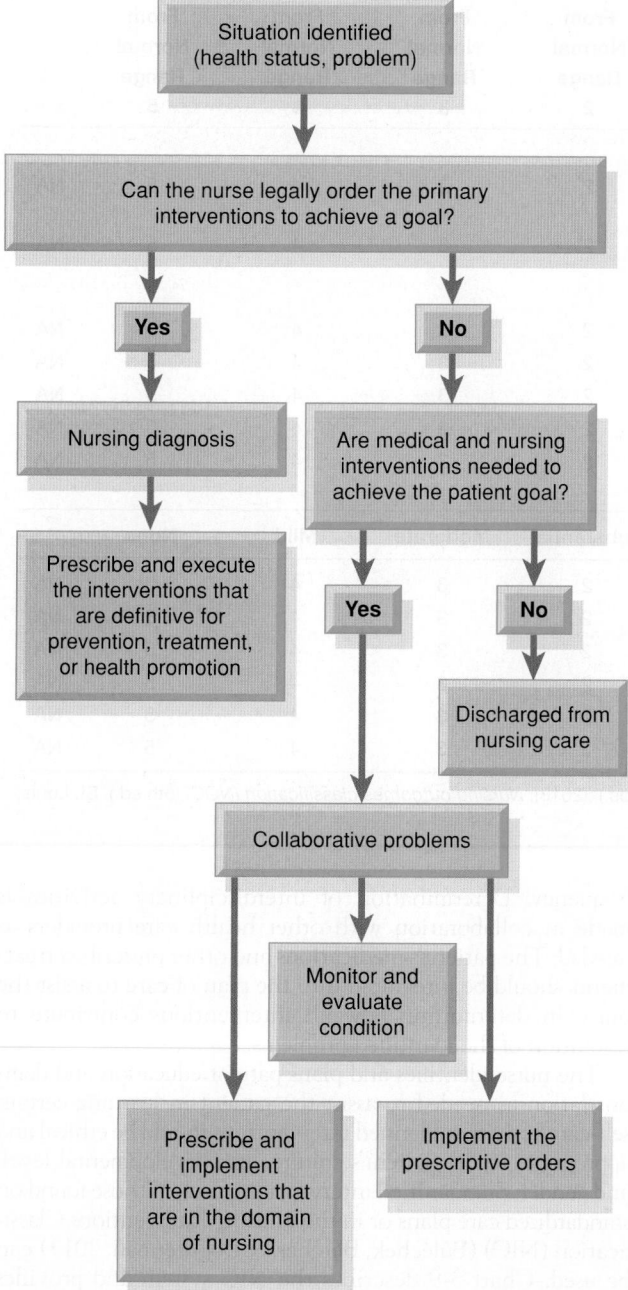

Figure 3-2 • Differentiating nursing diagnoses and collaborative problems. Redrawn from Carpenito, L. J. (2017). *Nursing diagnosis: Application to clinical practice* (15th ed., p. 25). Philadelphia, PA: Lippincott Williams & Wilkins.

Planning

Once the nursing diagnoses have been identified, the planning component of the nursing process begins. This phase involves the following steps:

1. Assigning priorities to the nursing diagnoses and collaborative problems
2. Specifying expected outcomes
3. Specifying the immediate, intermediate, and long-term goals of nursing action
4. Identifying specific nursing interventions appropriate for attaining the outcomes
5. Identifying interdependent interventions
6. Documenting the nursing diagnoses, collaborative problems, expected outcomes, nursing goals, and nursing interventions on the plan of nursing care
7. Communicating to appropriate personnel any assessment data that point to health care needs that can best be met by other members of the health care team

Setting Priorities

Assigning priorities to the nursing diagnoses and collaborative problems is a joint effort by the nurse and the patient or family members. Any disagreement about priorities is resolved in a way that is mutually acceptable. Consideration must be given to the urgency of the problems, with the most critical problems receiving the highest priority. Maslow hierarchy of needs provides one framework for prioritizing problems, with importance being given first to physical needs; once those basic needs are met, higher-level needs can be addressed. See Chapter 1 for a discussion of Maslow hierarchy of needs.

Establishing Expected Outcomes

Expected outcomes of the nursing interventions, identified either as long term or short term, are written in terms of the patient's behaviors and the time period in which the outcomes are to be met. The outcomes must be attainable and quantifiable (Carpenito, 2017). Resources for identifying appropriate expected outcomes include the Nursing Outcomes Classification (NOC) (see Chart 3-8) and standard outcome criteria established by health care agencies for people with specific health problems. These outcomes can be associated with nursing diagnoses and interventions and can be used when appropriate. However, the NOC may need to be adapted to establish realistic criteria for the specific patient involved.

The expected outcomes that define the patient's desired behavior are used to measure the progress made toward resolving the problem. The expected outcomes also serve as the basis for evaluating the effectiveness of the nursing interventions and for deciding whether additional nursing care is needed or whether the plan of care needs to be revised.

Establishing Goals

After the priorities of the nursing diagnoses and expected outcomes have been established, goals (immediate, intermediate, and long-term) and the nursing actions appropriate for attaining the goals are identified. The patient and family are included in establishing goals for the nursing actions. Immediate goals are those that can be attained within a short time frame. Intermediate and long-term goals require a longer time frame to be achieved and usually involve preventing complications and other health problems and promoting

Chart 3-8 Nursing Outcomes Classification

The Nursing Outcomes Classification (NOC) is a classification of patient outcomes that is sensitive to nursing interventions. Each outcome is a neutral statement about a variable patient condition, behavior, or perception, coupled with a rating scale. The outcome statement and scale can be used to identify baseline functioning, expected outcomes, and actual outcomes for individual patients. The following table is an example of a nursing-sensitive outcome.

Respiratory Status: Gas Exchange (0402)

Definition: Alveolar exchange of carbon dioxide and oxygen to maintain arterial blood gas concentrations.

Outcome Target Rating   *Maintain at* _____   *Increase to* _____

Respiratory Status: Gas Exchange Overall Rating		Severe Deviation From Normal Range 1	Substantial Deviation From Normal Range 2	Moderate Deviation From Normal Range 3	Mild Deviation From Normal Range 4	No Deviation From Normal Range 5	
Indicators							
040208	Partial pressure of oxygen in arterial blood (PaO_2)	1	2	3	4	5	NA
040209	Partial pressure of carbon dioxide in arterial blood ($PaCO_2$)	1	2	3	4	5	NA
040210	Arterial pH	1	2	3	4	5	NA
040211	Oxygen saturation	1	2	3	4	5	NA
040212	End-tidal carbon dioxide	1	2	3	4	5	NA
040213	Chest x-ray findings	1	2	3	4	5	NA
040214	Ventilation–perfusion balance	1	2	3	4	5	NA
		Severe	**Substantial**	**Moderate**	**Mild**	**None**	
040203	Dyspnea at rest	1	2	3	4	5	NA
040204	Dyspnea with mild exertion	1	2	3	4	5	NA
040205	Restlessness	1	2	3	4	5	NA
040206	Cyanosis	1	2	3	4	5	NA
040207	Somnolence	1	2	3	4	5	NA
040216	Impaired cognition	1	2	3	4	5	NA

Used with permission from Moorhead, S., Johnson, M., Maas, M. L., et al. (Eds.). (2013). *Nursing outcomes classification (NOC)* (5th ed.). St. Louis, MO: Mosby-Elsevier.

self-care and rehabilitation. For example, goals for a patient with a nursing diagnosis of impaired physical mobility related to pain and edema following total knee replacement may be stated as follows:

- Immediate goal: Stands at bedside for 5 minutes 6 to 12 hours after surgery
- Intermediate goal: Ambulates 15 to 20 minutes with walker or crutches in hospital and home
- Long-term goal: Ambulates independently 1 to 2 miles each day

Determining Nursing Actions

In planning appropriate nursing actions to achieve the desired goals and outcomes, the nurse, with input from the patient and significant others, identifies individualized interventions based on the patient's circumstances and preferences that address each outcome. Interventions should identify the activities needed, who will implement them, as well as the frequency. Determination of interdisciplinary activities is made in collaboration with other health care providers as needed. The patient's medications and other prescribed treatments should be integrated into the plan of care to assist the nurse in determining how all interventions contribute to resolution of the identified problems.

The nurse identifies and plans patient education and demonstration as needed to assist the patient in learning certain self-care activities. Planned interventions should be ethical and appropriate to the patient's culture, age, developmental level, and gender. Standardized interventions, such as those found on standardized care plans or in the Nursing Interventions Classification (NIC) (Bulechek, Butcher, & Dochterman, 2013) can be used. Chart 3-9 describes the NIC system and provides an example of an NIC system intervention. It is important to individualize prewritten interventions to promote optimal effectiveness for each patient. Actions of nurses should be based on established standards.

> ### Chart 3-9 Nursing Interventions Classification

The Nursing Interventions Classification (NIC) is an in-depth, evidence-based taxonomy of interventions that includes independent and collaborative interventions. These interventions are performed in a variety of health care settings. Intervention labels are terms such as *hemorrhage control, medication administration,* or *pain management.* Listed under each intervention are multiple discrete nursing actions that together constitute a comprehensive approach to the treatment of a particular condition. Not all actions are applicable to every patient; nursing judgment and critical thinking will determine which actions to implement. The following is an example of a nursing intervention:

Ventilation Assistance

Definition

Promotion of an optimal spontaneous breathing pattern that maximizes oxygen and carbon dioxide exchange in the lungs

Activities

Maintain a patent airway.
Position to alleviate dyspnea.
Position to facilitate ventilation–perfusion matching ("good lung down"), as appropriate.

Assist with frequent position changes, as appropriate.
Position to minimize respiratory efforts (e.g., elevate head of bed and provide overbed table for patient to lean on).
Monitor the effects of position change on oxygenation (e.g., arterial blood gases, SaO_2, $S\bar{v}\text{-}O_2$).
Encourage slow deep breathing, turning, and coughing.
Assist with incentive spirometer, as appropriate.
Auscultate breath sounds, noting areas of decreased or absent ventilation and presence of adventitious sounds.
Monitor for respiratory muscle fatigue.
Initiate and maintain supplemental oxygen, as prescribed.
Administer appropriate pain medication to prevent hypoventilation.
Ambulate three to four times per day, as appropriate.
Monitor respiratory and oxygenation status.
Administer medications (e.g., bronchodilators and inhalers) that promote airway patency and gas exchange.
Teach pursed lips breathing techniques, as appropriate.
Teach breathing techniques, as appropriate.
Initiate a program of respiratory muscle strength and/or endurance training, as appropriate.
Initiate resuscitation efforts, as appropriate.

Used with permission from Bulechek, G. H., Butcher, H. K., & Dochterman, J. M. (Eds.). (2013). *Nursing interventions classification (NIC)* (6th ed.). St. Louis, MO: Mosby-Elsevier.

Implementation

The implementation phase of the nursing process involves carrying out the proposed plan of nursing care. The nurse assumes responsibility for the implementation and coordinates the activities of all those involved in implementation, including the patient and family, and other members of the health care team so that the schedule of activities facilitates the patient's recovery. The plan of nursing care serves as the basis for implementation as such:

- The immediate, intermediate, and long-term goals are used as a focus for the implementation of the designated nursing interventions.
- While implementing nursing care, the nurse continually assesses the patient and the patient's individual response to the nursing care.
- Revisions are made in the plan of care as the patient's condition, problems, and responses change and when reordering of priorities is required.

Implementation includes direct or indirect execution of the planned interventions. It is focused on resolving the patient's nursing diagnoses and collaborative problems and achieving expected outcomes, thus meeting the patient's health needs. The following are examples of nursing interventions:

- Reposition the patient every 2 hours around the clock
- Teach and reinforce the use of guided imagery to reduce pain prior to invasive procedures
- Monitor oral and intravenous fluid intake to ensure that 2000 mL of fluids has been received
- Position the client in an upright position in a chair for 15 minutes before meals
- Apply lanolin to the patient's lips every 2 hours and as needed (i.e., *pro re nata* [prn])

- Teach the patient and family the correct way to apply a wedge splint prior to sleep
- Promote a therapeutic relationship

Clinical judgment, critical thinking, and good decision-making skills are essential in the selection of appropriate evidence-based and ethical nursing interventions. All nursing interventions are patient focused and outcome directed and are implemented with compassion, skill, confidence, and a willingness to accept and understand the patient's responses.

 Concept Mastery Alert

Implementation is nursing action. Therefore, statements involving implementation always start with a verb.

Although many nursing actions are independent, others are interdependent, such as carrying out prescribed treatments, administering medications and therapies, and collaborating with other health care team members to accomplish specific expected outcomes and to monitor and manage potential complications. Such interdependent functioning is just that—interdependent. Requests or prescriptions from other health care team members should not be followed blindly but must be assessed critically and questioned when necessary. The implementation phase of the nursing process ends when the nursing interventions have been completed.

Evaluation

Evaluation, the final step of the nursing process, allows the nurse to determine the patient's response to the nursing interventions and the extent to which the objectives have been achieved. The plan of nursing care is the basis for evaluation. The nursing diagnoses, collaborative problems, priorities, nursing interventions, and expected outcomes provide the specific guidelines that dictate the focus of the evaluation. Through evaluation, the nurse can answer the following questions:

- Were the nursing diagnoses and collaborative problems accurate?
- Did the patient achieve the expected outcomes within the critical time periods?
- Have the patient's nursing diagnoses been resolved?
- Have the collaborative problems been resolved?
- Do priorities need to be reordered?
- Have the patient's nursing needs been met?
- Should the nursing interventions be continued, revised, or discontinued?
- Have new problems evolved for which nursing interventions have not been planned or implemented?
- What factors influenced the achievement or lack of achievement of the objectives?
- Should changes be made to the expected outcomes and outcome criteria?

Objective data that provide answers to these questions are collected from all available sources (e.g., patients, families, significant others, health care team members). These data are included in patients' records and must be substantiated by direct patient observation before the outcomes are documented.

Documentation of Outcomes and Revision of the Plan

Outcomes are documented concisely and objectively. Documentation should relate outcomes to the nursing diagnoses and collaborative problems, describe the patient's responses to the interventions, indicate whether the outcomes were met, and include any additional pertinent data. As noted previously, the nurse individualizes a plan of care for each patient's

particular circumstances. Chart 3-10 gives an example of a plan of nursing care that has been developed for a 22-year-old woman admitted to a postoperative surgical unit after having an emergent laparoscopic appendectomy.

The plan of care is subject to change as a patient's needs change, as the priorities of needs shift, as needs are resolved, and as additional information about a patient's state of health is collected. As the nursing interventions are implemented, the patient's responses are evaluated and documented, and the plan of care is revised accordingly. A well-developed, continuously updated plan of care is the greatest assurance that the patient's nursing diagnoses and collaborative problems are addressed and their basic needs are met.

Framework for a Common Nursing Language: Combining NANDA-I, NIC, and NOC

Various frameworks or taxonomies can be used for determining nursing diagnoses (e.g., NANDA-I), establishing outcomes (e.g., NOC), and designing interventions (e.g., NIC). Ultimately, a framework that uses a language common to all aspects of nursing, regardless of the classification system, is desirable. In 2001, a taxonomy of nursing practice was developed for the harmonization of NANDA-I, NIC, and NOC. This three-part combination links nursing diagnoses, accompanying interventions, and outcomes, organizing them in the same way. Such organization of concepts in a common language or taxonomy may facilitate the process of clinical judgment and critical thinking, because interventions and outcomes are more accurately matched with appropriately developed nursing diagnoses (Carpenito, 2017). The final taxonomic scheme identifies 13 clinical domains that contain numerous classes of diagnoses, outcomes, and interventions. Chart 3-11 presents the taxonomy of nursing practice.

Chart 3-10 **PLAN OF NURSING CARE**

Example of a Plan of Nursing Care for a Patient Post Laparoscopic Appendectomy

NURSING DIAGNOSIS: Acute pain
GOAL: Relief of pain and discomfort

Nursing Interventions	Rationale	Expected Outcomes
1. When taking vital signs, use pain scale to assess pain and discomfort characteristics: location, quality, frequency, durations, etc., at baseline and on an ongoing basis	1. Provides baseline data	• Reports decreased level of pain and discomfort on pain scale • Reports less disruption in activity and quality of life from pain and discomfort • Reports decrease in other symptoms and psychosocial distress
2. Assure the patient that you know that pain is real and will assist in reducing it	2. Fear that pain will not be considered real increases anxiety and reduces pain tolerance	• Adheres to analgesic regimen as prescribed • Barriers to adequately addressing pain do not interfere with strategies for managing pain
3. Assess other factors contributing to patient's pain: fear; fatigue; other symptoms; psychosocial and/or spiritual distress, etc.	3. Provides data about factors that decrease patient's ability to tolerate pain and increase pain level	• Takes an active role in administration of analgesia • Identifies additional effective pain relief strategies
4. Administer prescribed analgesic regimen, and provide education to patient and family regarding regimen.	4. Analgesics tend to be more effective when given early in pain cycle, around the clock at regular intervals, or when given in long-acting forms; breaks the pain cycle; premedication with analgesics is used for activities that cause increased pain or breakthrough pain.	• Uses previously employed successful pain relief strategies appropriately • Reports effective use of nonpharmacologic pain relief strategies and a decrease in pain • Reports that decreased level of pain permits early ambulation postoperatively

Chart 3-10 **PLAN OF NURSING CARE** (Continued)

Example of a Plan of Nursing Care for a Patient Post Laparoscopic Appendectomy

Nursing Interventions	Rationale	Expected Outcomes
5. Address myths or misconceptions and lack of knowledge about use of opioid analgesics	5. Barriers to adequate pain management involve patients' fear of side effects, fatalism about the possibility of achieving pain control, fear of distracting providers from treating the postoperative pain, belief that pain is indicative of progressive disease, and fears about addiction. Professional health providers also have demonstrated limited knowledge about pain management, potential analgesic side effects, and management and risk of addiction.	
6. Collaborate with patient, primary provider/surgeon, and other health care team members when changes in pain management are necessary	6. New methods of administering analgesia must be acceptable to the patient, primary provider/surgeon, and health care team to be effective; patient's participation decreases sense of powerlessness.	
7. Encourage strategies of pain relief that patient has used successfully in previous pain experience	7. Encourages success of pain relief strategies accepted by patient and family	
8. Offer nonpharmacologic strategies to relieve pain and discomfort: distraction, guided imagery, relaxation, cutaneous stimulation, therapeutic touch, Reiki, etc.	8. Increases options and strategies available to patient that serve as adjuncts to pharmacologic interventions	

NURSING DIAGNOSIS: Risk for infection (i.e., wound infection, pneumonia, urinary tract infection [UTI])
GOAL: No evidence of infection

Nursing Interventions	Rationale	Expected Outcomes
1. Assess wound site for signs of infection or increased inflammation:	1. Some manifestations of inflammation are to be expected (e.g., wound tenderness, slight erythema, and edema); however, this should decrease over time and there should be no evidence of an infection at the wound site.	• No drainage or increased erythema or edema at the laparoscopic wound site • Temperature within normal limits (i.e., between 36.1°C [97°F] and 38.0°C [100.4°F]) • Lung sounds clear to auscultation; no cough • Voids clear yellow urine without complaints of burning on micturition or feelings of bladder fullness • Laboratory results, if assessed, are within normal limits
a. If there is a dressing or bandage present, verify whether and when it will be changed by the primary provider/surgeon	a. The primary provider/surgeon may wish to remove the first dressing or bandage, to assess the status of the wound and presence of drainage first-hand.	
b. Note the color, consistency, and amount of drainage, if present; if so, also note if any odor is present; notify the primary provider/surgeon as indicated	b. Drainage may indicate an infectious process, particularly if it is malodorous.	
c. Note any changes in appearance of wound over time, particularly if it becomes increasingly edematous or erythematous	c. Increased wound edema or erythema may indicate an infection	

(continued on page 44)

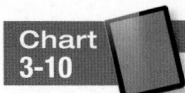

Chart 3-10

PLAN OF NURSING CARE (Continued)

Example of a Plan of Nursing Care for a Patient Post Laparoscopic Appendectomy

Nursing Interventions	Rationale	Expected Outcomes
2. Monitor vital signs, temperature, and laboratory results (if available) for signs of infection	**2.** Changes in vital signs, particularly temperature, may suggest an infection; if these changes are marked, they may suggest sepsis (see Chapter 14 for further discussion of the clinical manifestations of sepsis); laboratory results particularly the presence of leukocytosis with a shift to the left on the differential of the white blood cell count (WBC) on the complete blood count (CBC) may suggest an infection is present. Postoperatively, most patients will have a slightly elevated temperature (up to 38.0°C [100.4°F]), which is consistent with the inflammatory process. A temperature higher than this in a previously healthy adult suggests some type of underlying infectious process	
3. Monitor for manifestations of atelectasis or pneumonia	**3.** Atelectasis and pneumonia are prevalent postoperative pulmonary complications (see Table 19-4)	
a. Assess for adventitious lung sounds (e.g., rales, wheezes) or for decreased air movement	**a.** Lung sounds should be clear to auscultation bilaterally; the presence of adventitious sounds may suggest the development of atelectasis or pneumonia; diminished lung sounds may suggest poor air movement from splinting respirations, which can lead to respiratory compromise	
b. Encourage early movement (e.g., demonstrate and encourage use of incentive spirometer, encourage early ambulation)	**b.** Movement mobilizes respiratory secretions and respiratory effort	
c. Preemptively treat postoperative pain, as described above.	**c.** Pain interferes with the ability to move; pain results in splinting of respiratory effort	
4. Monitor micturition status; note when patient first voids, the amount, and if there are any complaints of burning or bladder fullness; notify the primary provider/surgeon as indicated; monitor laboratory results, including the CBC and urinalysis as indicated	**4.** Urinary retention and urinary tract infections are prevalent postoperative complications (see Chapter 19, Table 19-4); CBC results may reveal leukocytosis with a shift to the left on the WBC differential; urinalysis results may reveal the presence of blood cells (e.g., red blood cells [RBCs], WBCs) that may suggest a urinary tract infection	

NURSING DIAGNOSIS: Imbalanced nutrition: less than body requirements related to perioperative *nil per os* (NPO) status
GOAL: Will consume typical diet by discharge

Nursing Interventions	Rationale	Expected Outcomes

1. Assess for return of gastrointestinal function postoperatively
   a. Auscultate for the presence of bowel sounds
   b. Ask the patient if he/she has passed flatus
   c. Encourage early ambulation as this will assist with return of gastrointestinal function
	1. Gastrointestinal motility is diminished post-surgery; peristalsis should return within hours and is evidenced by return of bowel sounds and passing of flatus	• Will advance diet, as tolerated
		• No complaints of nausea

2. Advance diet as tolerated and prescribed by primary provider/surgeon	**2.** Patient will need to demonstrate ability to tolerate fluids and food prior to discharge	
a. Assess for complaints of nausea. If present, may give antiemetic medications as prescribed (e.g., ondansetron [Zofran]) and delay advancement of diet	**a.** Complaints of nausea are prevalent post laparoscopic surgery; if patient vomits, that may delay recovery (e.g., disrupt wound, delay intake of nutrients); administering antiemetic medications may preempt complications	

Chart 3-10	**PLAN OF NURSING CARE** (Continued)

Example of a Plan of Nursing Care for a Patient Post Laparoscopic Appendectomy

NURSING DIAGNOSIS: Activity intolerance related to fatigue post-surgery
GOAL: Participation in activities of daily living within tolerance

Nursing Interventions	Rationale	Expected Outcomes

1. Assess factors contributing to activity intolerance and fatigue
2. Promote atmosphere conducive to physical and mental rest:
  a. Encourage alternation of rest and activity
  b. Encourage limitation of visitors and stress-producing interactions
	1. Indicates factors contributing to severity of fatigue
	2. Promotes rest, activity tolerance, and decreased overall stress
		• Identifies factors contributing to fatigue
		• Alternates periods of rest and activity
		• Limits visitors to ensure adequate rest periods

NURSING DIAGNOSIS: Deficient knowledge regarding methods to ensure postoperative recovery
GOAL: Increased knowledge about expected postoperative recovery and transition back to preoperative baseline functional status

Nursing Interventions	Rationale	Expected Outcomes

1. Educate patient on expectations for recovery, discharge, and transition to home
  a. Demonstrate wound care to patient, as prescribed by primary provider/surgeon; ask patient to return demonstrate wound care
  b. Educate patient on use of prescribed analgesic medications (e.g., oxycodone), including actions, indications, side effects, and when to take them (e.g., prior to ambulation)
  c. Educate patient on activity restrictions (e.g., bathing, lifting, return to work or school) as prescribed by primary provider/surgeon
  d. Educate patient on when to follow up with primary provider/surgeon postoperatively, for scheduled postoperative appointment and as needed.
	1. Inpatient recovery time after a laparoscopic appendectomy is short (e.g., 1 day, assuming there are no complications [see Chapter 19, Table 19-4]); therefore, preparing patient for discharge must commence expeditiously	• Demonstrates appropriate care of wound
		• Verbalizes understanding of continued analgesic regimen, including when to take prescriptive analgesic medications (e.g., oxycodone [Percocet]), and whether there are any activity restrictions associated with their use (e.g., no driving)
		• Verbalizes understanding of activity restrictions, including bathing, lifting, return to work/school, as prescribed by primary provider/surgeon
		• Verbalizes adherence to scheduled postoperative appointment

Chart 3-11	Domains and Classes in the NANDA-I Taxonomy II

All NANDA-I-approved nursing diagnoses fall under one of these domains and classes. Note that there are some domains and classes that at the present time do not yet feature an articulated nursing diagnosis.

Domain 1. Health Promotion

The awareness of well-being or normality of function and the strategies used to maintain control of and enhance that well-being or normality of function

Class 1. Health Awareness—Recognition of normal function and well-being
Class 2. Health Management—Identifying, controlling, performing, and integrating activities to maintain health and well-being

Domain 2. Nutrition

The activities of taking in, assimilating, and using nutrients for the purposes of tissue maintenance, tissue repair, and the production of energy

Class 1. Ingestion—Taking food or nutrients into the body

Class 2. Digestion—The physical and chemical activities that convert foodstuffs into substances suitable for absorption and assimilation
Class 3. Absorption—The act of taking up nutrients through body tissues
Class 4. Metabolism—The chemical and physical processes occurring in living organisms and cells for the development and use of protoplasm, the production of waste and energy, with the release of energy for all vital processes
Class 5. Hydration—The taking in and absorption of fluids and electrolytes

Domain 3. Elimination and Exchange

Secretion and excretion of waste products from the body

Class 1. Urinary function—The process of secretion, reabsorption, and excretion of urine
Class 2. Gastrointestinal function—The process of absorption and excretion of the end products of digestion
Class 3. Integumentary function—The process of secretion and excretion through the skin

(continued on page 46)

| **Chart 3-11** | Domains and Classes in the NANDA-I Taxonomy II (continued) |

Class 4. Respiratory function—The process of exchange of gases and removal of the end products of metabolism

Domain 4. Activity/Rest

The production, conservation, expenditure, or balance of energy resources

Class 1. Sleep/Rest—Slumber, repose, ease, relaxation, or inactivity

Class 2. Activity/Exercise—Moving parts of the body (mobility), doing work, or performing actions often (but not always) against resistance

Class 3. Energy balance—A dynamic state of harmony between intake and expenditure of resources

Class 4. Cardiovascular/pulmonary responses—Cardiopulmonary mechanisms that support activity/rest

Class 5. Self-care—Ability to perform activities to care for one's body and bodily functions

Domain 5. Perception/Cognition

The human information processing system, including attention, orientation, sensation, perception, cognition, and communication

Class 1. Attention—Mental readiness to notice or observe

Class 2. Orientation—Awareness of time, place, and person

Class 3. Sensation/perception—Receiving information through the senses of touch, taste, smell, vision, hearing, and kinesthesia, and the comprehension of sensory data resulting in naming, associating, and/or pattern recognition

Class 4. Cognition—Use of memory, learning, thinking, problem-solving, abstraction, judgment, insight, intellectual capacity, calculation, and language

Class 5. Communication—Sending and receiving verbal and nonverbal information

Domain 6. Self-Perception

Awareness about the self

Class 1. Self-concept—The perception(s) about the total self

Class 2. Self-esteem—Assessment of one's worth, capability, significance, and success

Class 3. Body image—A mental image of one's own body

Domain 7. Role Relationships

The positive and negative connections or associations between people or groups of people and the means by which those connections are demonstrated

Class 1. Caregiving roles—Socially expected behavior patterns by people providing care who are not healthcare professionals

Class 2. Family relationships—Associations of people who are biologically related or related by choice

Class 3. Role performance—Quality of functioning in socially expected behavior patterns

Domain 8. Sexuality

Sexual identity, sexual function, and reproduction

Class 1. Sexual identity—The state of being a specific person in regard to sexuality, gender, or both

Class 2. Sexual function—The capacity or ability to participate in sexual activities

Class 3. Reproduction—Any process by which human beings are produced

Domain 9. Coping/Stress Tolerance

Contending with life events/life processes

Class 1. Posttrauma responses—Reactions occurring after physical or psychological trauma

Class 2. Coping responses—The process of managing environmental stress

Class 3. Neurobehavioral stress—Behavioral responses reflecting nerve and brain function

Domain 10. Life Principles

Principles underlying conduct, thought, and behavior about acts, customs, or institutions viewed as being true or having intrinsic worth

Class 1. Values—The identification and ranking or preferred modes of conduct or end states

Class 2. Beliefs—Opinions, expectations, or judgments about acts, customs, or institutions viewed as being true or having intrinsic worth

Class 3. Value/belief/action congruence—The correspondence or balance achieved among values, beliefs, and actions

Domain 11. Safety/Protection

Freedom from danger, physical injury, or immune system damage; preservation from loss; and protection of safety and security

Class 1. Infection—Host responses following pathogenic invasion

Class 2. Physical injury—Bodily harm or hurt

Class 3. Violence—The exertion of excessive force or power so as to cause injury or abuse

Class 4. Environmental Hazards—Sources of danger in the surroundings

Class 5. Defensive processes—The processes by which the self protects itself from the nonself

Class 6. Thermoregulation—The physiological process of regulating heat and energy within the body for purposes of protecting the organism

Domain 12. Comfort

Sense of mental, physical, or social well-being or ease

Class 1. Physical comfort—Sense of well-being or ease and/or freedom from pain

Class 2. Environmental comfort—Sense of well-being or ease in/with one's environment

Class 3. Social comfort—Sense of well-being or ease with one's social situation

Domain 13. Growth/Development

Age-appropriate increases in physical dimension, maturation of organ systems, and/or progression through the developmental milestones

Class 1. Growth—Increases in physical dimensions or maturity of organ systems

Class 2. Development—Progress or regression through a sequence of recognized milestones in life

Herdman, T. H., & Kamitsuru, S. (Eds.). (2014). *Nursing diagnoses: Definitions & classification 2015–2017.* Oxford: Wiley-Blackwell. Used with permission.

CRITICAL THINKING EXERCISES

1 `pcg` A 50-year-old man is admitted to the emergency department with complaints of a "vise-like" headache that is accompanied by nausea. His past medical history shows that he has a 20-year history of migraine headaches; however, his headache has not responded to his typical self-administered dose of sumatriptan (Imitrex). What are your priorities for assessing this patient's current condition? Two hours after his admission, you noted he has garbled speech and his level of consciousness has changed. How would your priorities change based on these changes? What nursing diagnosis would be most appropriate for these changes in neurological status?

2 You are assigned to care for a 40-year-old man with terminal metastatic melanoma. Three days ago, he became unresponsive and was admitted to the intensive care unit (ICU). The palliative care physician shares with you that he is going to strongly recommend using terminal sedation for this patient and asks you for your support with the family. The patient's girlfriend, the designated health care representative, is in favor of the palliative care plan; however, the patient's mother vehemently opposes this option and protests that this is "murder." The patient's 16-year-old daughter wants "everything done" for him. You realize the difficulty the family is experiencing and request an ethics committee consult. What ethical principles should be examined when exploring this dilemma? What legal considerations should be taken into consideration? Who has the decision-making authority in this case?

3 `ebp` You are assigned to care for a patient who was admitted to the ICU with diabetic ketoacidosis. The patient has an intravenous (IV) insulin drip and is also prescribed an IV antibiotic. You find the empty IV bag of the last dose of antibiotic piggybacked through the same IV line as the insulin drip. You question the nurse from the previous shift about this finding, but she denies that this route was used. When you return to the patient's room, his level of consciousness is diminished and his blood glucose level is now 40 mg/dL. What actions should be taken? Should this information be communicated to your supervisor? What is the care priority for the patient? What evidence supports or does not support disclosure of medication administration errors to patients? What steps would you take and in what order?

American Nurses Association (ANA). (2010). *Nursing's social policy statement* (3rd ed.). Silver Springs, MD: Nursesbooks.org.

American Nurses Association (ANA). (2015a). *Nursing: Scope and standards of practice* (3rd ed.). Silver Springs, MD: Nursesbooks.org.

American Nurses Association (ANA). (2015b). *Code of ethics for nurses with interpretive statements*. Washington, DC: Nursesbooks.org.

Beauchamp, T. L., & Childress, J. F. (2013). *Principles of biomedical ethics*. New York, NY: Oxford University Press.

Bulechek, G. H., Butcher, H. K., & Dochterman, J. M. (Eds.). (2013). *Nursing interventions classification (NIC)* (6th ed.). St. Louis, MO: Mosby-Elsevier.

Butts, J. B., & Rich, K. L. (2016). *Nursing ethics across the curriculum and into practice* (4th ed.). Burlington, MA: Jones and Bartlett Learning.

Carpenito, L. J. (2017). *Nursing diagnosis: Application to clinical practice* (15th ed.). Philadelphia, PA: Lippincott Williams & Wilkins.

Herdman, T. H., & Kamitsuru, S. (Eds.) (2014). *Nursing diagnoses: Definitions & classification 2015–2017*. Oxford: Wiley-Blackwell.

**International Council of Nurses. (2012). *Code of ethics for nurses* Geneva: Author.

Moorhead, S., Johnson, M., Maas, M. L., et al. (Eds.). (2013). *Nursing outcomes classification (NOC)* (5th ed.). St. Louis, MO: Mosby-Elsevier.

Pozgar, G. D. (2016). *Legal and ethical issues for healthcare professionals*. Burlington, MA: Jones and Bartlett.

Stuart, G. W. (2012). *Principles and practice of psychiatric nursing* (10th ed.). St. Louis, MO: CV Mosby.

Vaughn, L. (2013). *Bioethics: Principles, issues, and cases* New York, NY: Oxford University Press.

Journals and Electronic Documents

**American Nurses Association. (1999). Position statement on privacy and confidentiality. Retrieved on 12/28/2015 at: www.nursingworld.org/MainMenuCategories/Policy-Advocacy/Positions-and-Resolutions/ANAPositionStatements/Position-Statements-Alphabetically/PrivacyandConfidentiality.html

**American Nurses Association. (2009). Position statement on electronic health record. Retrieved on 12/28/2015 at: nursingworld.org/MainMenuCategories/Policy-Advocacy/Positions-and-Resolutions/ANAPositionStatements/Position-Statements-Alphabetically/Electronic-Health-Record.html

**American Nurses Association. (2012). Position statement on reduction of patient restraint and seclusion in health care settings. Retrieved on 12/28/2015 at: nursingworld.org/restraintposition

Brudvig, T. J., Dirkes, A., Dutta, P., et al. (2013). Critical thinking in health care professional students: A systematic review. *Journal of Physical Therapy Education, 27*(3), 12–25.

Critical thinking community. (2013). Critical thinkers. Retrieved on 6/14/2015 at: www.criticialthinking.org.

*Newton, S. E., & Moore, G. (2013). Critical thinking skills in basic baccalaureate and accelerated second degree nursing students. *Nursing Education Perspectives, 34*(3), 154–158.

*Perez-Rivas, F. J., Martin-Inglesias, S., Pacheco del Cerro, J. L., et al. (2015). Effectiveness of nursing process use in primary care. *International Journal of Nursing Knowledge, 27*(1), 43–48. Retrieved on 12/27/2015 at: www.researchgate.net/publication/271449068_Effectiveness_of_Nursing_Process_Use_in_Primary_Care

POLST: Physician's orders for life sustaining orders paradigm (2015). Retrieved on 6/14/2015 at: www.polst.org.

**U.S. Department of Health and Human Services. (2003). Summary of the HIPAA privacy rule. Retrieved on 6/14/2015 at: www.hhs.gov/ocr/privacy/hipaa/understanding/summary/privacysummary.pdf

REFERENCES

*Asterisk indicates nursing research.
**Double asterisk indicates classic reference.

Books

Alfaro-LeFevre, R. (2013). *Critical thinking and clinical judgment: A practical approach to outcome focused thinking* (5th ed.). Philadelphia, PA: Saunders.

Resources

American Nurses Association Center for Ethics and Human Rights, www.nursingworld.org/ethics

Centers for Medicare and Medicaid Services (CMS), www.cms.hhs.gov

The Hastings Center, www.thehastingscenter.org

The Joint Commission, www.jointcommission.org

NANDA International, www.nanda.org

National Center for Ethics in Health Care (NCEHC), www.ethics.va.gov

4 Health Education and Health Promotion

Effective **health education** lays a solid foundation for individual and **community** wellness. All nurses use teaching as a tool to assist patients and families in developing effective health behaviors and altering lifestyle patterns that predispose people to health risks. Health education is an influential factor directly related to positive health outcomes.

Purpose of Health Education

Today's health care environment mandates the use of an organized approach to health education so that patients can meet their specific health care needs. There are many reasons for providing health education.

Meeting Nursing Standards

Teaching, as a function of nursing, is included in all state nurse practice acts and in the American Nurses Association's (ANA) *Scope and Standards of Practice* (ANA, 2015). Health teaching and health promotion are independent functions of nursing practice and essential nursing responsibilities. All nursing care is directed toward promoting, maintaining, and restoring health; preventing illness; and helping people adapt to the residual effects of illness. Many of these nursing activities are accomplished through patient education. Nurses in their role as teachers are challenged to focus on the educational needs of communities and to provide specific patient and family education. Health education is important to nursing care because it affects the abilities of people and families to perform important self-care activities.

Every contact a nurse has with a health care consumer, whether or not that person is ill or has a disability, should be considered an opportunity for health education. Although people have a right to decide whether or not to learn, nurses have the responsibility to present information that motivates people to recognize the need to learn. Therefore, nurses must use opportunities in all health care settings to promote wellness. There are many educational environments. Some examples include homes, hospitals, community health centers, schools, places of business, service agencies, shelters, and consumer action or support groups (deChesnay & Anderson, 2016).

Supporting Informed Decision Making and Self-Care

The emphasis on health education stems in part from the public's right to comprehensive health care, which includes up-to-date health information. It also reflects the emergence of an informed public that is asking more significant questions about health and health care. Because of the importance that American society places on health and the responsibility that each person has to maintain and promote their own health, members of the health care team, specifically nurses, are obligated to make health education available. Significant factors to consider when planning patient education include the availability of health care, the use of diverse health care providers to accomplish care management goals, and the increased use of complementary and alternative strategies rather than traditional approaches to care. Without adequate knowledge and training in self-care skills, consumers cannot make informed decisions about their health. Guidance from nurses may assist consumers to obtain health information from trustworthy, credible, and timely Internet resources (Blanch-Hartigan, Blake, & Viswanath, 2014). People with chronic illnesses and disabilities are among those most in need of health education. As the lifespan of the population increases, the number of people with such illnesses also increases. Health information targeted at identifying and managing the exacerbations or issues commonly associated with having a chronic illness or disability is a major focus of health education. People with chronic illness need health care information to participate actively in and assume responsibility for self-care. Health education can help those with chronic illness adapt to their illness, prevent complications, carry out prescribed therapy, and solve problems when confronted with new situations. It can also help to prevent crisis situations and reduce the potential for rehospitalization resulting from inadequate information about self-care. The goal of health education is to teach people to live life to its healthiest—that is, to strive toward achieving their maximum health potential.

In addition to the public's right to and desire for health education, patient education is also a strategy for promoting self-care at home and in the community, reducing health care costs by preventing illness, effectively managing necessary therapies, avoiding expensive medical interventions, decreasing lengths of hospital stay, and facilitating earlier discharge. For health care agencies, offering community wellness programs is a public relations tool for increasing patient satisfaction and for developing a positive image of the institution. Patient education is also a cost-avoidance strategy in that positive staff–patient relationships may avert malpractice suits. Some insurance companies support health education through reimbursement for programs, such as diabetes management classes and fitness and weight management programs.

Promoting Adherence to the Therapeutic Regimen

One of the goals of patient education is to encourage people to adhere to their **therapeutic regimen**. **Adherence** to treatment usually requires that a person make one or more lifestyle changes to carry out specific activities that promote and maintain health. Common examples of behaviors facilitating health include taking prescribed medications, maintaining a healthy diet, increasing daily activities and exercise, self-monitoring for signs and symptoms of illness and changes in baseline health status, practicing specific hygiene measures, seeking recommended health evaluations and screening, and performing other therapeutic and preventive measures. When using nursing diagnosis language, the term *compliance* is used to discuss patient adherence.

Factors Affecting Adherence

Many people do not adhere to their prescribed regimens; rates of adherence are generally low, especially when the regimens are complex or of long duration (e.g., therapy for tuberculosis, multiple sclerosis, and human immune deficiency virus [HIV] infection and hemodialysis). Nonadherence to prescribed therapy has been the subject of many studies (Bender, Gentry, Brufsky, et al., 2014; Claborn, 2015; Hooper & Huffman, 2014; Martins, de Souza, & da Silva, 2015; Mitchell, Khoukaz, McNeal, et al., 2014). For the most part, findings have been inconclusive, and no one predominant causative factor has been identified. Instead, a wide range of variables influences the degree of adherence, including the following:

- Demographic variables, such as age, gender, race, socioeconomic status, and level of education
- Illness variables, such as the severity of the illness and the relief of symptoms afforded by the therapy
- Therapeutic regimen variables, such as the complexity of the regimen, treatment fatigue, and uncomfortable side effects
- Psychosocial variables, such as intelligence, motivation, availability of significant and supportive people (especially family members), competing or conflicting demands, attitudes toward health professionals, acceptance or denial of illness, substance abuse, and religious or cultural beliefs
- Financial variables, especially the direct and indirect costs associated with a prescribed regimen

Another factor to consider when the nurse is developing strategies to promote patient adherence is the concept of health literacy. A challenge for all health care providers is to improve the health literacy of patients. In establishing suitable health education materials, technological innovations and services, providers must communicate health information in plain language and work with patients to promote accurate processing and understanding of the health information. Nurses must consider their knowledge of the myriad factors that affect health literacy in any given population. The primary factors influencing health literacy are the effective use of communication and cultural skills, along with the presentation of health care information, and a basic background of mathematical skills. Without such skills, patients are at risk for being unable to share personal health information, perform self-care management for both acute and chronic health conditions, navigate through health systems and complete health forms, and calculate information such as nutritional information on food labels (Harris, Thomas, & Fox, 2015; Roundtable on Health Literacy & Institute of Medicine Board on Population Health and Public Health, 2014).

Health literacy skills are basic to understanding the body and how it functions, assessing lifestyle choices along with the variables that cause and perpetuate disease, as well as making health care decisions. If people have low health literacy, the consequence is poor overall health. Deconstructing this cycle of low health literacy leading to poor health status and higher risk of health problems is essential. To increase health literacy, providers must design and distribute accurate health information and must ensure that these health materials are culturally appropriate for various populations. It is imperative to build community partnerships to support education and public health activities. Nurses can be instrumental in performing evaluation research on the educational undertakings that support individuals, groups, or communities. Furthermore, nurses must be directly involved in facilitating change through the development of health care policies that address the promotion of a health literate society (Parnell, 2015).

Nurses' success with health education is determined by both the development of strong health literacy and the ongoing assessment of the variables that affect patients' ability to adopt specific behaviors to obtain resources, and maintain a healthy social environment (Edelman, Kudzma, & Mandle, 2014). Teaching programs are more likely to succeed if patients have improved health literacy and providers pay careful attention to the variables affecting patient adherence. Both health literacy and the concept of adherence must be considered in the patient's teaching plan. Teaching strategies are discussed later in the chapter.

Motivation

The problem of nonadherence to therapeutic regimens is substantial and must be addressed before patients can achieve their maximum health potential. Patients' need for knowledge has not been found to be a sufficient stimulus for acquiring knowledge and thereby enabling complete adherence to a health regimen. Teaching directed toward stimulating patient motivation results in varying degrees of adherence. Research suggests that factors such as medication costs, perceived control, and type of health problem must also be considered (Adam & Folds, 2014; Ryan, Fedders, Jennings, et al., 2014; Theofilou, 2013; Wu & Moser, 2014). The variables of choice, establishment of mutual goals, and quality of the patient–provider relationship also influence the behavioral changes that can result from patient education. Many factors are linked to motivation for learning.

Using a learning contract or agreement can also be a motivator for learning. Such a contract is based on assessment of patient needs; health care data; and specific, measurable goals (Miller & Stoeckel, 2016). The learning contract is recorded in writing and contains methods for ongoing evaluation. A well-designed learning contract is realistic and positive. In a typical learning contract, a series of measurable goals is established, beginning with small, easily attainable objectives and progressing to more advanced goals. Frequent, positive reinforcement is provided as the person moves from one goal to the next. For example, incremental goals such as weight loss of 1 to 2 pounds per week are more appropriate in a weight reduction program than a general goal such as a 30-pound weight loss.

 Gerontologic Considerations

Nonadherence to therapeutic regimens is a significant problem for older adults, leading to increased morbidity, mortality, and cost of treatment (Fang, Robinson, Lauffenburger, et al., 2014; Harold, Briesacher, Peterson, et al., 2013). Many admissions to nursing homes and hospitals are associated with nonadherence.

Older adults frequently have one or more chronic illnesses that are managed with numerous medications, and their disease course may be complicated by periodic acute episodes (Miller, 2015). Older adults may have additional problems that affect adherence to therapeutic regimens, such as increased sensitivity to medications and their side effects, difficulty in adjusting to change and stress, financial constraints, forgetfulness, inadequate support systems, lifetime habits of self-treatment with over-the-counter medications, visual and hearing impairments, and mobility limitations. To promote adherence among older adults, all variables that may affect health behavior should be assessed (see Fig. 4-1). Nurses must also consider that cognitive impairment may be manifested by the older adult's inability to draw inferences, apply information, or understand the major teaching points (Mauk, 2013; Tabloski, 2013; Touhy & Jett, 2013). The person's strengths and limitations must be assessed to encourage the use of existing strengths to compensate for limitations. Above all, health care professionals must work together to provide continuous, coordinated care; otherwise, the efforts of one health care professional may be negated by those of another.

Figure 4-1 • Taking time to teach patients about their medication and treatment program promotes interest and cooperation. Older adults who are actively involved in learning about their medication and treatment program and the expected effects may be more likely to adhere to the therapeutic regimen.

The Nature of Teaching and Learning

Learning can be defined as acquiring knowledge, attitudes, or skills. **Teaching** is defined as helping another person learn. These definitions indicate that the teaching–learning process is an active one, requiring the involvement of both the teacher and the learner in the effort to reach the desired outcome—a change in behavior. The teacher does not simply give knowledge to the learner but instead serves as a facilitator of learning. Although learning can take place without teachers, most people who are attempting to learn new or altered health behaviors benefit from contact with a nurse. The interpersonal interaction between the person and the nurse who is attempting to meet the person's learning needs may be formal or informal, depending on the method and techniques of teaching.

There is no definitive theory about how learning occurs and how it is affected by teaching. However, learning can be affected by factors, such as readiness to learn, the learning environment, and the teaching techniques used (Miller & Stoeckel, 2016).

Learning Readiness

One of the most significant factors influencing learning is a person's **learning readiness**. For adults, readiness is based on culture, personal values, physical and emotional status, and past experiences in learning (Tam, 2014). The "teachable moment" occurs when the content and skills being taught are congruent with the task to be accomplished (Miller & Stoeckel, 2016).

Culture encompasses values, ideals, and behaviors, and the traditions within each culture provide the framework for solving the issues and concerns of daily living. Because people with different cultural backgrounds have different values and lifestyles, choices about health care vary. Culture is a major variable influencing readiness to learn because it affects how people learn and what information can be learned. Sometimes people do not accept health teaching because it conflicts with culturally mediated values. Before beginning health teaching, nurses must conduct an individual cultural assessment instead of relying only on generalized assumptions about a particular culture. A patient's social and cultural patterns must be appropriately incorporated into the teaching–learning interaction. (See Chapter 7, Chart 7-4, which describes cultural assessment components to consider when formulating a teaching plan.)

A person's values include beliefs about behaviors that are desirable and undesirable. The nurse must know what value the patient places on health and health care. In clinical situations, patients express their values through their actions and the level of knowledge pursued (deChesnay & Anderson, 2016). When the nurse is unaware of the patient's values (cultural and personal), misunderstanding, lack of cooperation, and negative health outcomes may occur (McFarland & Wehbe-Alamah, 2015). A person's values and behaviors can be either an asset or a deterrent to readiness to learn. Therefore, patients are unlikely to accept health education unless their values and beliefs about health and illness are respected (Dayer-Berenson, 2013).

Physical readiness is of vital importance, because until the person is physically capable of learning, attempts at teaching and learning may be both futile and frustrating. For example, a person in acute pain is unable to focus attention away from the pain long enough to concentrate on learning. Likewise, a person who is short of breath concentrates on breathing rather than on learning.

Emotional readiness also affects the motivation to learn. A person who has not accepted an existing illness or the threat of illness is not motivated to learn. A person who does not accept a therapeutic regimen, or who views it as conflicting with their present lifestyle, may consciously avoid learning about it. Until the person recognizes the need to learn and demonstrates an ability to learn, teaching efforts may be thwarted. However, it is not always wise to wait for the person to become emotionally ready to learn, because that time may never come unless the nurse makes an effort to stimulate the person's motivation. For example, a person with colon cancer who has a fasting blood sugar twice the expected normal value may focus only on the cancer diagnosis and exclude or deny the health consequences of an abnormal blood sugar.

Illness and the threat of illness are usually accompanied by anxiety and stress. Nurses who recognize such reactions can use simple explanations and instructions to alleviate these anxieties and provide further motivation to learn. Because learning involves behavior change, it often produces mild anxiety, which can be a useful motivating factor.

Emotional readiness can be promoted by creating a warm, accepting, positive atmosphere and by establishing realistic learning goals. When learners achieve success and a feeling of accomplishment, they are often motivated to participate in additional learning opportunities. One example of a strategy that facilitates learner success is the teach-back technique. This technique is used to evaluate the recall and understanding of the learner after health teaching has occurred. It is a useful, in-the-moment feedback and evaluation method because it allows the educator to discover if the learner can effectively verbalize information or demonstrate a particular health behavior (Miller & Stoeckel, 2016). In addition, the teach-back strategy can be used with family members and caregivers to ascertain if they have retained and understood the health content. Having a strategy to actively involve the adult learner in making health care decisions and performing self-management skills promotes learner receptivity and motivation to integrate health principles into one's daily life. Furthermore, **feedback** about progress also motivates learning. Such feedback should be presented in the form of positive reinforcement when the learner is successful, and in the form of constructive suggestions for improvement when the learner is unsuccessful.

Experiential readiness refers to past experiences that influence a person's ability to learn. Previous educational experiences and life experiences in general are significant determinants of a person's approach to learning. People with little or no formal education may not be able to understand the instructional materials presented. People who have had difficulty learning in the past may be hesitant to try again. Many behaviors required for reaching maximum health potential require knowledge, physical skills, and positive attitudes. In their absence, learning may be very difficult and very slow. For example, a person who does not understand the basics of normal nutrition may not be able to understand the restrictions of a specific diet. A person who does not view the desired learning as personally meaningful may reject teaching efforts. A person who is not future oriented may be unable to appreciate many aspects of preventive health teaching. Experiential readiness is closely related to emotional readiness, because motivation tends to be stimulated by an appreciation for the need to learn and by those learning tasks that are familiar, interesting, and meaningful.

The Learning Environment

Learning may be optimized by minimizing factors that interfere with the learning process. For example, the room temperature, lighting, noise levels, and other environmental conditions should be appropriate to the learning situation. In addition, the time selected for teaching should be suited to the needs of the individual person. Scheduling a teaching session at a time of day when a patient is fatigued, uncomfortable, or anxious about a pending diagnostic or therapeutic procedure, or when visitors are present, is not conducive to learning. However, if the family is to participate in providing care, the sessions should be scheduled when family members are present so that they can learn any necessary skills or techniques.

Teaching Techniques and Resources

Teaching techniques and methods enhance learning if they are appropriate to the patient's needs. Numerous techniques are available, including the following:

- *Lectures:* Lectures are explanation methods of teaching and should be accompanied by discussion, because discussion affords learners opportunities to express their feelings and concerns, ask questions, and receive clarification.
- *Group teaching:* Group teaching allows people not only to receive needed information but also to feel secure as members of a group (promoting moral support). Assessment and follow-up are imperative to ensure that each person has gained sufficient knowledge and skills. Not all patients relate or learn well in groups.
- *Demonstration and practice:* Demonstration and practice are especially important when teaching skills. The nurse should demonstrate the skill and then give the learner ample opportunity for practice. When special equipment is involved, such as syringes or colostomy bags, it is important to teach with the same equipment that will be used in the home setting to avoid confusion, frustration, and mistakes.
- *Reinforcement and follow-up:* Nurses must allow ample time for patients to learn and provide reinforcement. Follow-up sessions are imperative to promote the learner's confidence in their abilities and to plan for additional teaching sessions.
- *Motivational interviewing:* Pilot research suggests that using motivational interviewing as an enhanced educational method in an acute inpatient setting can increase both patient and caregiver knowledge as well as patient satisfaction following discharge from the acute care setting (Mehta, Cameron, & Battistella, 2014).
- *Electronic, online, or Internet information:* Electronic technologies are used to provide health information. Examples are interactive or noninteractive Internet learning, an online self-paced program, or a structured online course. There are also DVD, CD-ROM, pod-casts, and recorded programs available over a television channel.
- *Teaching aids:* Teaching aids include books, pamphlets, pictures, films, slides, audiotapes, models, programmed instruction, other visual aids (e.g., charts), and computer-assisted learning modules. They are invaluable when used appropriately and can save a significant amount of personnel time and related cost. However, all such aids should be reviewed before use to ensure that they meet the patient's learning needs and are free of advertisements that may confuse the patient. (See Resources section at the end of the chapter for additional information.)

The chance of success is maximized when nurses, families, and other health care professionals work collaboratively to facilitate learning. Successful learning should result in improved self-care management skills, enhanced self-esteem, confidence, and a willingness to learn in the future. There are specific considerations for teaching special populations. Table 4-1 outlines some of the teaching strategies to use when teaching people with disabilities. (See Chapters 9 and 11 for additional teaching strategies for people with disabilities and older adults.)

 ## The Nursing Process in Patient Education

The nurse relies on the steps of the nursing process when constructing an individualized teaching plan to meet the patient's teaching and learning needs (see Chart 4-1).

Assessment

Assessment in the teaching–learning process is directed toward the systematic collection of data about the patient's and family's learning needs and readiness to learn. The nurse identifies all internal and external variables that affect the patient's readiness to learn. Many learning assessment guides are available. Some guides are directed toward the collection of general health information (e.g., healthy eating), whereas others are specific to medication regimens or disease processes (e.g., stroke risk assessments). Such guides facilitate assessment but must be adapted to the responses, problems, and needs of each person. The nurse organizes, analyzes, synthesizes, and summarizes the assessment data collected and determines the patient's need for teaching.

Nursing Diagnosis

The process of formulating nursing diagnoses makes educational goals and evaluations of progress more specific and meaningful. Teaching is an integral intervention implied by all nursing diagnoses, and for some diagnoses, education is the primary intervention. Examples of nursing diagnoses that help in planning for educational needs are ineffective health maintenance, ineffective self-health management, and decisional conflict. The diagnosis "Deficient knowledge" should be used cautiously, because knowledge deficit is not a human response but a factor relating to or causing the diagnosis. For example, "Ineffective health maintenance related to a lack of information about wound care" is a more appropriate nursing diagnosis than "Deficient knowledge"

TABLE 4-1 Educating People With Disabilities

Type of Disability	Educational Strategy
Physical, Emotional, or Cognitive Disability	Adapt information to accommodate the person's cognitive, perceptual, and behavioral disabilities. Give clear written and oral information. Highlight significant information for easy reference. Avoid medical terminology or "jargon."
Hearing Impairment	Use slow, directed, deliberate speech. Use sign language or interpreter services if appropriate. Position yourself so that the person can see your mouth if speech reading. Use telecommunication devices (TTY or TDD) for the person with hearing impairment. Use written materials and visual aids, such as models and diagrams. Use captioned videos, films, and computer-generated materials. Speak on the side of the "good ear" if unilateral deafness is present.
Visual Impairment	Use optical devices such as a magnifying lens. Use proper lighting and proper contrast of colors on materials and equipment. Use or convert information to auditory and tactile formats if appropriate (e.g., Braille or large-print materials). Obtain audiotapes, CDs, digital audio available on smart phones or tablets, and talking books. Explain noises associated with procedures, equipment, and treatments. Arrange materials in clockwise pattern.
Learning Disabilities Input disability	If visual perceptual disorder: • Explain information verbally; repeat and reinforce frequently. • Use audiotapes, CDs, and digital audio. • Encourage learner to verbalize information received. If auditory perceptual disorder: • Speak slowly with as few words as possible; repeat and reinforce frequently. • Use direct eye contact (as appropriate for the person's culture) to help focus on the task. • Use demonstration and return demonstration, such as modeling, role-playing, and hands-on experiences. • Use visual tools; written materials; and computers, tablets, and smartphones.
Output disability	Use all senses as appropriate. Use written, audiotape, and computerized or other electronic information. Review information, and give time verbally to interact and ask questions. Use hand gestures and motions.
Developmental disability	Base information and teaching on developmental stage, not chronologic age. Use nonverbal cues, gestures, signing, and symbols as needed. Use simple explanations and concrete examples with repetition. Encourage active participation. Demonstrate information, and have person perform return demonstrations.

(Carpenito-Moyet, 2017). A nursing diagnosis that relates specifically to a patient's and family's learning needs serves as a guide in the development of the teaching plan.

Planning

Once the nursing diagnoses have been identified, the planning component of the teaching–learning process is established in accordance with the steps of the nursing process:

1. Assigning priorities to the diagnoses
2. Specifying the immediate, intermediate, and long-term goals of learning
3. Identifying specific teaching strategies appropriate for attaining goals
4. Specifying the expected outcomes
5. Documenting the diagnoses, goals, teaching strategies, and expected outcomes of the teaching plan

The assignment of priorities to the diagnoses should be a collaborative effort by the nurse and the patient or family members. Consideration must be given to the urgency of the patient's learning needs; the most critical needs should receive the highest priority.

 Concept Mastery Alert

The nurse needs to keep in mind that before the teaching strategy can be determined, the goals of learning must be developed.

After the diagnostic priorities have been mutually established, it is important to identify the immediate and long-term goals and the teaching strategies appropriate for attaining the goals. Teaching is most effective when the objectives of both the patient and the nurse are in agreement (Bastable, 2014). Learning begins with the establishment of goals that are appropriate to the situation and realistic in terms of the patient's ability and desire to achieve them. Involving the patient and family in establishing goals and in planning teaching strategies promotes their cooperation in the implementation of the teaching plan.

Outcomes of teaching strategies can be stated in terms of expected behaviors of patients, families, or both. Outcomes should be realistic and measurable, and the critical time periods for attaining them should be identified. The desired outcomes and the critical time periods serve as a basis for evaluating the effectiveness of the teaching strategies.

Chart 4-1 Summary of the Nursing Process for Individualized Patient Education

Assessment

1. Assess the person's readiness for health education.
   a. What are the person's health beliefs and behaviors?
   b. What physical and psychosocial adaptations does the person need to make?
   c. Is the learner ready to learn?
   d. Is the person able to learn these behaviors?
   e. What additional information about the person is needed?
   f. Are there any variables (e.g., hearing or visual impairment, cognitive issues, literacy issues) that will affect the choice of teaching strategy or approach?
   g. What are the person's expectations?
   h. What does the person want to learn?
2. Organize, analyze, synthesize, and summarize the collected data.

Nursing Diagnosis

1. Formulate the nursing diagnoses that relate to the person's learning needs.
2. Identify the learning needs, their characteristics, and their etiology.

Planning

1. Assign priority to the nursing diagnoses that relate to the individual's learning needs.
2. Specify the immediate, intermediate, and long-term learning goals established by teacher and learner together.
3. Identify teaching strategies appropriate for goal attainment.
4. Establish expected outcomes.
5. Develop the written teaching plan.
   a. Include diagnoses, goals, teaching strategies, and expected outcomes.
   b. Put the information to be taught in logical sequence.
   c. Write down the key points.
   d. Select appropriate teaching aids.
   e. Keep the plan current and flexible to meet the person's changing learning needs.

6. Involve the learner, family or significant others, nursing team members, and other health care team members in all aspects of planning.

Implementation

1. Put the teaching plan into action.
2. Use language that the person can understand.
3. Use appropriate teaching aids and provide Internet resources if appropriate.
4. Use the same equipment that the person will use after discharge.
5. Encourage the person to participate actively in learning.
6. Record the learner's responses to the teaching actions.
7. Provide feedback.

Evaluation

1. Collect objective data.
   a. Observe the person.
   b. Ask questions to determine whether the person understands.
   c. Use rating scales, checklists, anecdotal notes, and written tests when appropriate.
2. Compare the person's behavioral responses with the expected outcomes. Determine the extent to which the goals were achieved.
3. Include the person, family or significant others, nursing team members, and other health care team members in the evaluation.
4. Identify alterations that need to be made in the teaching plan.
5. Make referrals to appropriate sources or agencies for reinforcement of learning after discharge.
6. Continue all steps of the teaching process: assessment, diagnosis, planning, implementation, and evaluation.

During the planning phase, the nurse must consider the sequence in which the subject matter is presented. Critical information (e.g., survival skills for a patient with diabetes) and material that the person or family identifies to be of particular importance must receive high priority. An outline is often helpful for arranging the subject matter and for ensuring that all necessary information is included. In addition, appropriate teaching aids to be used in implementing teaching strategies are prepared or selected at this time. Patient Education charts throughout this textbook guide teaching about self-care.

The entire planning phase concludes with the formulation of the teaching plan. This teaching plan communicates the following information to all members of the nursing team:

- The nursing diagnoses that specifically relate to the patient's learning needs and the priorities of these diagnoses
- The goals of the teaching strategies
- The teaching strategies that are appropriate for goal attainment
- The expected outcomes, which identify the desired behavioral responses of the learner
- The critical time period within which each outcome is expected to be met
- The patient's behavioral responses (which are documented on the teaching plan)

The same rules that apply to writing and revising the plan of nursing care apply to the teaching plan.

Implementation

In the implementation phase of the teaching–learning process, the patient, family, and other members of the nursing and health care team carry out the activities outlined in the teaching plan. The nurse coordinates these activities.

Flexibility during the implementation phase of the teaching–learning process and ongoing assessment of patient responses to the teaching strategies support modification of the teaching plan as necessary. Creativity in promoting and sustaining the patient's motivation to learn is essential. New learning needs that may arise after discharge from the hospital or after home care visits have ended should also be taken into account.

The implementation phase ends when the teaching strategies have been completed and when the patient's responses to the actions have been recorded. This serves as the basis for evaluating how well the defined goals and expected outcomes have been achieved.

Evaluation

Evaluation of the teaching–learning process determines how effectively the patient has responded to teaching and to what extent the goals have been achieved. An evaluation must be made to determine what was effective and what needs to be changed or reinforced. It cannot be assumed that patients have learned just because teaching has occurred; learning does not automatically follow teaching. An important part of the evaluation phase addresses the question, "What can be done to improve teaching and enhance learning?" Answers to this question direct the changes to be made in the teaching plan.

Various measurement techniques can be used to identify changes in patient behavior as evidence that learning has taken place. These techniques include directly observing the behavior; using rating scales, checklists, or anecdotal notes to document the behavior; and indirectly measuring results using oral questioning and written tests. All direct measurements should be supplemented with indirect measurements whenever possible. Using more than one measuring technique enhances the reliability of the resulting data and decreases the potential for error from a measurement strategy.

In many situations, measurement of actual behavior is the most accurate and appropriate evaluation technique. Nurses often perform comparative analyses using patient admission data as the baseline: Selected data points observed when nursing care is given and self-care is initiated are compared with the patient's baseline data. In other cases, indirect measurement may be used. Some examples of indirect measurement are patient satisfaction surveys, attitude surveys, and instruments that evaluate specific health status variables.

Measurement is only the beginning of evaluation, which must be followed by data interpretation and judgments about learning and teaching. These aspects of evaluation should be conducted periodically throughout the teaching–learning program, at its conclusion, and at varying periods after the teaching has ended.

Evaluation of learning after teaching that occurs in any setting (e.g., clinics, offices, nursing centers, hospitals) is essential, because the analysis of teaching outcomes must extend into aftercare. With shortened lengths of hospital stay and with short-stay and same-day surgical procedures, follow-up evaluation is especially important. Coordination of efforts and sharing of information between hospital- and community-based nursing personnel facilitate post-discharge teaching and home care evaluation.

Evaluation is not the final step in the teaching–learning process but is the beginning of a new patient assessment. The information gathered during evaluation should be used to redirect teaching actions, with the goal of improving the patient's responses and outcomes.

Health Promotion

Health teaching and **health promotion** are linked by a common goal—to encourage people to achieve as high a level of wellness as possible so that they can live maximally healthy lives and avoid preventable illnesses. The call for health promotion has become a cornerstone in health policy because of the need to control costs and reduce unnecessary sickness and death.

Health goals for the nation are established in the publication *Healthy People 2020*. The priorities from this initiative were identified as health promotion, health protection, and the use of preventive services. *Healthy People 2020* defines the current national health promotion and disease prevention initiative for

Chart 4-2 Selected Topics for Objectives of Healthy People 2020

Access to Health Services
Adolescent Health
Arthritis, Osteoporosis, and Chronic Back Conditions
Blood Disorders and Blood Safety
Cancer
Chronic Kidney Disease
Dementias, Including Alzheimer Disease
Diabetes
Disability and Health
Educational and Community-Based Programs

the nation. Measurable goals for key health topics for the nation are shown in Chart 4-2. The overall goals are to (1) increase the quality and years of healthy life for people and (2) eliminate health disparities among various segments of the population (U.S. Department of Health and Human Services, 2010).

Definition

Health promotion may be defined as those activities that assist people in developing resources that maintain or enhance well-being and improve their quality of life. These activities involve people's efforts to remain healthy in the absence of symptoms, may not require the assistance of a health care team member, and occur within or outside of the health system (Haber, 2013; O'Donnell, 2014).

The purpose of health promotion is to focus on the person's potential for wellness and to encourage appropriate alterations in personal habits, lifestyle, and environment in ways that reduce risks and enhance health and well-being. As discussed in Chapter 1, health is viewed as a dynamic, ever-changing condition that enables people to function at an optimal potential at any given time, whereas wellness, a reflection of health, involves a conscious and deliberate attempt to maximize one's health. Health promotion is an active process—that is, it is not something that can be prescribed or dictated. It is up to each person to decide whether to make changes to promote a higher level of wellness. Only the individual can make these choices.

A significant amount of research has shown that people, by virtue of what they do or fail to do, influence their own health. Today, many of the major causes of illness are chronic diseases that have been closely related to lifestyle behaviors (e.g., diabetes, coronary artery disease, lung and colon cancer, chronic obstructive pulmonary diseases, hypertension, cirrhosis, traumatic injury, and HIV infection). To a large extent, a person's health status may be reflective of their lifestyle. Chart 4-3 summarizes a research study exploring self-care practices among individuals with dementia.

Health Promotion Models

Several health promotion models identify health-protecting behaviors and seek to explain what makes people engage in preventive behaviors. A health-protecting behavior is defined as any behavior performed by people, regardless of their actual or perceived health condition, for the purpose of promoting or maintaining their health, whether or not the behavior produces the desired outcome (Pender, Murdaugh, & Parsons, 2014).

Chart 4-3 NURSING RESEARCH PROFILE

Perception and Attitudes Toward Dementia and Dementia Risk Reduction

Kim, S., Sargent-Cox, K. A., & Anstey, K. J. (2015). A qualitative study of older and middle-aged adults' perception and attitudes towards dementia and dementia risk reduction. *Journal of Advanced Nursing*, 71(7), 1694–1703.

Purpose

The purpose of this qualitative research study was to identify and explore factors that motivate or serve as barriers to health behaviors and lifestyle changes that reduce the risk of dementia. It further addressed the knowledge of dementia and the risk and protective factors for dementia in adults without dementia.

Design

The study used a descriptive qualitative approach using the focus group methodology to facilitate discussion on dementia knowledge, risks, and attitudes. The researchers conducted six focus groups with 34 adults, ages 52 to 90 years, recruited through an advertisement in a community newspaper. All focus groups were conducted in a private conference room in a university setting. Each focus group lasted approximately 60 minutes and was audio recorded.

Findings

Findings revealed that the participants were literate about dementia risk factors. From the initial review of the data, the researcher categorized the following four themes: dementia and dementia risk factor literacy, perceived susceptibility to dementia, motivators and perceived benefits, and perceived barriers. Three themes that emerged from the data related to the participants' perceived likelihood of developing dementia were: fear of developing dementia, rationally attempting to determine how susceptible they might be to dementia, and not believing the dementia risk factors would necessarily apply to them. The fear of developing dementia and the need to acquire knowledge about dementia were the motivators influencing the adoption of healthier behaviors. An overall lack of knowledge on dementia risk factors was a barrier to lifestyle change.

Nursing Implications

Nurses must educate the community about dementia and the strategies used to reduce dementia risk in adults. Nurses must also recognize motivators and barriers that influence a person's ability to change behaviors and lifestyle to decrease dementia risk. Health care professionals must become active in motivating adults to change behaviors that place them at risk for dementia. If health promotion and education about risk and protective factors for dementia can be promoted by nurses in both community and other health care settings, then dementia literacy will increase and the prevalence of dementia may decrease.

The Health Belief Model was designed to foster understanding of why some healthy people choose actions to prevent illness while others do not. Developed by Becker (1974), the model is based on the premise that four variables influence the selection and use of health promotion behaviors. Demographic and disease factors, the first variable, include patient characteristics, such as age, gender, education, employment, severity of illness or disability, and length of illness. Barriers, the second variable, are defined as factors leading to unavailability or difficulty in gaining access to a specific health promotion alternative. Resources, the third variable, encompass such factors as financial and social support. Perceptual factors, the fourth variable, consist of how the person views his or her health status, self-efficacy, and the perceived demands of the illness. Further research has demonstrated that these four variables have a positive correlation with a person's quality of life (Becker, Stuifbergen, Oh, et al., 1993).

Another model, the Resource Model of Preventive Health Behavior, addresses the ways in which people use resources to promote health (Pender et al., 2014). It is based on social learning theory and emphasizes the importance of motivational factors in acquiring and sustaining health promotion behaviors. This model explores how cognitive-perceptual factors affect the person's view of the importance of health. It also examines perceived control of health, self-efficacy, health status, and the benefits and barriers to health-promoting behaviors. Nurse educators can use this model to assess how demographic variables, health behaviors, and social and health resources influence health promotion.

The Canadian health promotion initiative, Achieving Health for All, builds on the work of Lalonde (1977), in which four determinants of health—human biology, environment, lifestyle, and the health care delivery system—were identified. Determinants of health were defined as factors and conditions that have an influence on the health of individuals and communities. Since the 1970s, a total of 12 health determinants have been identified, and this number will continue to increase as population health research progresses. Determinants of health provide a framework for assessing and evaluating the population's health.

A model crafted to address organizational and individual health behavior change is the Awareness, Motivation, Skills and Opportunity (AMSO) Model. The four components of this model focus on empowering people, understanding their individual priorities, and assisting them to change in personal ways that promote and maintain their optimal level of health. The dimensions of optimal health are physical, emotional, social, intellectual, and spiritual. This model promotes the process of creating and maintaining a balance among these five dimensions (O'Donnell, 2014). Optimal health is a dynamic condition kept in balance by a combination of efforts to sustain awareness, maintain motivation, build skills, and have opportunities to practice positive health behaviors.

The Transtheoretical Model of Change, also known as the Stages of Change Model, is a framework that focuses on the motivation of a person to make decisions that promote healthy behavior change (DiClemente, 2007). Table 4-2 shows the six stages in the model. Research indicates that people seeking assistance from professionals or self-help groups progress through these stages of change (Chaufan, Yeh, & Sigal, 2015; Seebohm, Chaudhary, Boyce, et al., 2013). Any of the models can serve as an organizing framework for clinical work and research that support the enhancement of health. Research suggests that the application of health promotion models, concepts, and frameworks increases the nurse's understanding of the health promotion behaviors of families and

TABLE 4-2 Stages in the Transtheoretical Model of Change

Stage	Description
1. Precontemplative	The person is not thinking about making a change.
2. Contemplative	The person is only thinking about change in the near future.
3. Decision making	The person constructs a plan to change behavior.
4. Action	The person takes steps to operationalize the plan of action.
5. Maintenance	The person works to prevent relapse and to sustain the gains made from the actions taken.
6. Termination	The person has the ability to resist relapse back to unhealthy behavior(s).

Adapted from DiClemente, C. (2007). The transtheoretical model of intentional behavior change. *Drugs & Alcohol Today, 7*(1), 29–33; Miller, C. A. (2015). *Nursing for wellness in older adults* (7th ed.). Philadelphia, PA: Lippincott Williams & Wilkins.

communities (Cha, 2013; Meraviglia, Stuifbergen, Morgan, et al., 2015; Yeun, Baek, & Kim, 2013).

Components of Health Promotion

Health promotion as an active process includes the following components: self-responsibility, nutritional awareness, stress reduction and management, and physical fitness.

Self-Responsibility

Taking responsibility for oneself is the key to successful health promotion. The concept of **self-responsibility** is based on the understanding that the individual controls their life. Each person alone must make the choices that determine the health of their lifestyle. As more people recognize that lifestyle and behavior significantly affect health, they may assume responsibility for avoiding high-risk behaviors, such as smoking, alcohol and drug abuse, overeating, driving while intoxicated, risky sexual practices, and other unhealthy habits. They may also assume responsibility for adopting routines that have been found to have a positive influence on health, such as engaging in regular exercise, wearing seat belts, and eating a healthy diet.

Various techniques have been used to encourage people to accept responsibility for their health, including public service announcements, educational programs, and reward systems. No one technique has been found to be superior to any other. Instead, self-responsibility for health promotion is individualized and depends on a person's desires and inner motivations. Health promotion programs are important tools for encouraging people to assume responsibility for their health and to develop behaviors that improve health.

Nutritional Awareness

Nutrition, as a component of health promotion, has become the focus of considerable attention and publicity with the growing epidemic of obesity in the United States. A vast array of books and magazine articles address the topics of special diets; natural foods; and the hazards associated with certain substances, such as sugar, salt, cholesterol, trans fats, carbohydrates, artificial colors, and food additives. Research

suggests that good nutrition is the single most significant factor in determining health status, longevity, and weight control (U.S. Department of Agriculture and U.S. Department of Health and Human Services, 2010).

Nutritional awareness involves an understanding of the importance of a healthy diet that supplies all essential nutrients. Understanding the relationship between diet and disease is an important facet of a person's self-care. Some clinicians believe that a healthy diet is one that substitutes "natural" foods for processed and refined ones and reduces the intake of sugar, salt, fat, cholesterol, caffeine, alcohol, food additives, and preservatives.

Chapter 5 contains further information about the assessment of a person's nutritional status. It describes the physical signs indicating nutritional status, assessment of food intake (food record, 24-hour recall), the dietary guidelines presented in the MyPlate plan, and calculation of ideal body weight.

Stress Reduction and Management

Stress management and stress reduction are important aspects of health promotion. Studies suggest the negative effects of stress on health and a cause-and-effect relationship between stress and infectious diseases, traumatic injuries (e.g., motor vehicle crashes), and some chronic illnesses. Stress has become inevitable in contemporary societies in which demands for productivity have become excessive. More and more emphasis is placed on encouraging people to manage stress appropriately and to reduce the pressures that are counterproductive. Research suggests that including techniques such as relaxation training, exercise, yoga, and modification of stressful situations in health promotion programs assists patients in dealing with stress (Christaki, Kokkinos, Costarelli, et al., 2013; Hartley, Flowers, Lee, et al., 2014; Rao, Raghuram, Nagendra, et al., 2015; Smith, 2014). Further information on stress management, including health risk appraisal and stress reduction methods such as the Benson Relaxation Response, can be found in Chapter 6.

Physical Fitness

Physical fitness and exercise are important components of health promotion. Clinicians and researchers (Bruning & Sturek, 2015; Halvarsson, Franzen, & Stahle, 2015; Murimi, Chrisman, McAllister, et al., 2015; Resnick, Nahm, Zhu, et al., 2014; Yoo, Park, Yang, et al., 2014) who have examined the relationship between health and physical fitness have found that a regular exercise program can promote health in the following ways:

- Improve the function of the circulatory system and the lungs
- Decrease cholesterol and low-density lipoprotein levels
- Decrease body weight by increasing calorie expenditure
- Delay degenerative changes such as osteoporosis
- Improve flexibility and overall muscle strength and endurance

An appropriate exercise program can have a positive effect on a person's performance capacity, appearance, and level of stress and fatigue, as well as their general state of physical, mental, and emotional health (Gerber, Jonsdottir, Arvidson, et al., 2015; Groh & Urbancic, 2015; Khazaee-Pool, Sadeghi, Majlessi, et al., 2014). An exercise program should be designed specifically for a given person, with consideration to age, physical condition, and any known cardiovascular or other risk factors. Exercise can be harmful if it is not started gradually and increased slowly in accordance with a person's response.

Vincent Brody, a 67-year-old male with chronic obstructive pulmonary disease (COPD), is experiencing increased fatigue. He spends most of the day in a recliner chair watching television and smoking 1 to 2 packs per day. His nutritional intake is poor due to shortness of breath. What patient education can the nurse provide to promote self-care behaviors for symptom improvement and a healthier lifestyle? (Vincent Brody's story continues in Chapter 60.)

Care for Vincent and other patients in a realistic virtual environment: **vSim** *for Nursing* (**thepoint.lww.com/vSimMedicalSurgical**). Practice documenting these patients' care in DocuCare (**thepoint.lww.com/DocuCareEHR**).

Health Promotion Strategies Throughout the Lifespan

Health promotion is a concept and a process that extends throughout the lifespan. The health of a child can be affected either positively or negatively by the health practices of the mother during the prenatal period. Therefore, health promotion starts before birth and extends through childhood, adolescence, adulthood, and old age (Haber, 2013).

Health promotion includes health screening, counseling, immunizations, and preventive medications. The U.S. Preventive Services Task Force (2016) evaluates clinical research to assess the merits of preventive measures. Table 4-3 presents general population guidelines, including adult immunization recommendations (Centers for Disease Control and Prevention [CDC], 2016; U.S. Preventive Services Task Force, 2016).

TABLE 4-3 Selected Health Promotion Screening for Adults

Type of Screening	Suggested Time Frame
Routine health examination	Yearly
Blood chemistry profile	Baseline at age 20 years, then as mutually determined by patient and clinician
Complete blood count	Baseline at age 20 years, then as mutually determined by patient and clinician
Lipid profile	Baseline at age 20 years, then as mutually determined by patient and clinician
Hemoccult screening	Yearly after age 50 years
Electrocardiogram	Baseline at age 40 years, then as mutually determined by patient and clinician
Blood pressure	Yearly, then as mutually determined by patient and clinician
Tuberculosis skin test	Every 2 years, or as mutually determined by patient and clinician
Chest x-ray or film	For positive PPD results
Mammogram	Every other year for women older than 50 years, or earlier or more often as indicated
Clinical breast examination	Yearly
Gynecologic examination	Yearly
Papanicolaou (Pap) test	Every 3 years
Bone density screening	Based on identification of primary and secondary risk factors (prior to onset of menopause, if indicated)
Nutritional screening	As mutually determined by patient and clinician
Digital rectal examination	Yearly
Colonoscopy	Every 3–5 years after age 50 years or as mutually determined by patient and clinician
Prostate examination	Yearly
Testicular examination	Monthly
Skin examination	Yearly or as mutually determined by patient and clinician
Vision screening: Glaucoma	Every 2–3 years Baseline at age 40 years, then every 2–3 years until age 70 years, then yearly
Hearing screening	As needed
Health risk appraisal	As needed
Adult Immunizations	
Hepatitis B (if not received as a child)	Series of 3 doses (now, 1 month later, then 5 months after the second date)
Human papillomavirus (HPV)	3 doses for males up to the age of 21 years, females up to the age of 26 years; men who have sex with men between 22 and 26 years; if lacking documentation of prior immunization.
Influenza vaccine	Yearly
Meningococcal	1 or more doses after 19 years old
Td or Tdap vaccine (Tetanus, diphtheria, and pertussis)	Every 10 years
Zoster	After age 60 years
Pneumococcal conjugate vaccine (PCV13)	Given once to adults 65 years and older regardless of health status. Given to those ages 19 to 64 years if immunocompromised, asplenic, with cerebrospinal fluid (CSF) leakage or cochlear implants.
Pneumococcal polysaccharide vaccine (PPSV23)	Given routinely in a series to all adults aged 65 years and older Given in a series to adults younger than 65 years who have chronic heart, lung or liver disease; diabetes; alcoholism, and smoking.

Note: Any of these screenings may be performed more frequently if deemed necessary by the patient or recommended by the health care provider.
Adapted from U.S. Preventive Services Task Force. (2016). Recommendations. Retrieved on 8/20/2016 at: http://www.uspreventiveservicestaskforce.org/BrowseRec/Index/browse-recommendations. 2016 Adult Immunization Schedule approved by CDC Advisory Committee on Immunization Practices. (2016). Recommendations. Retrieved on 8/20/2016 at: www.cdc.gov/vaccines/schedules/hcp/adult.html

Adolescents

Health screening has traditionally been an important aspect of adolescent health care. The goal has been to detect health problems at an early age so that they can be treated at that time. Today, health promotion goes beyond the mere screening for illnesses and disabilities and includes extensive efforts to promote positive health practices at an early age. Because health habits and practices are formed early in life, adolescents should be encouraged to develop positive health attitudes. For this reason, more programs are being offered to adolescents to help them develop good health habits. Although the negative results of practices such as smoking, risky sex, alcohol and drug abuse, and poor nutrition are explained in these educational programs, emphasis is also placed on values training, self-esteem, and healthy lifestyle practices. The projects are designed to appeal to a particular age group, with emphasis on learning experiences that are fun, interesting, and relevant.

Young and Middle-Aged Adults

Young and middle-aged adults represent an age group that not only expresses an interest in health and health promotion but also responds enthusiastically to suggestions that show how lifestyle practices can improve health. Adults are frequently motivated to change their lifestyles in ways that are believed to enhance their health and wellness. Many adults who wish to improve their health turn to health promotion programs to help them make the desired changes in their lifestyles. Many have responded to programs that focus on topics such as general wellness, smoking cessation, exercise, physical conditioning, weight control, conflict resolution, and stress management. Because of the nationwide emphasis on health during the reproductive years, young adults actively seek programs that address prenatal health, parenting, family planning, and women's or men's health issues.

Programs that provide health screening, such as those that screen for cancer, high cholesterol, hypertension, diabetes, abdominal aneurysm, and visual and hearing impairments, are quite popular with young and middle-aged adults. Programs that involve health promotion for people with specific chronic illnesses such as cancer, diabetes, heart disease, and pulmonary disease are also popular. Chronic disease and disability do not preclude health and wellness; rather, positive health attitudes and practices can promote optimal health for people who must live with the limitations imposed by their chronic illnesses and disabilities.

Health promotion programs can be offered almost anywhere in the community. Common sites include local clinics, schools, colleges, recreation centers, places of worship, and even private homes. Health fairs are frequently held in civic centers and shopping malls. The outreach idea for health promotion programs has served to meet the needs of many adults who otherwise would not avail themselves of opportunities to strive toward a healthier lifestyle.

The workplace has become a center for health promotion activity for several reasons. Employers have become increasingly concerned about the rising costs of health care insurance to treat illnesses related to lifestyle behaviors, and they are also concerned about increased absenteeism and lost productivity. Some employers use health promotion specialists to develop and implement these programs, and others purchase packaged programs that have already been developed by health care agencies or private health promotion corporations.

Programs offered at the workplace usually include employee health screening and counseling, physical fitness, nutritional awareness, work safety, and stress management and stress reduction. In addition, efforts are made to promote a safe and healthy work environment. Many large businesses provide exercise facilities for their employees and offer their health promotion programs to retirees.

Gerontologic Considerations

Health promotion is as important for older adults as it is for others. Although 80% of people older than 65 years have one or more chronic illnesses and many are limited in their activity, the older adult population experiences significant gains from health promotion. Older adults are very health conscious, and most view their health positively and are willing to adopt practices that will improve their health and well-being (Touhy & Jett, 2013). Although their chronic illnesses and disabilities cannot be eliminated, these adults can benefit from activities and education that help them maintain independence and achieve an optimal level of health (Ball, Gammon, Kelly, et al., 2013; Wang, Chen, Lai, et al., 2014).

Various health promotion programs have been developed to meet the needs of older Americans. Both public and private organizations continue to be responsive to health promotion, and more programs that serve this population are emerging. Many of these programs are offered by health care agencies, places of worship, community centers, senior citizen residences, and various other organizations. The activities directed toward health promotion for older adults are the same as those for other age groups: physical fitness and exercise, nutrition, safety, and stress management (see Fig. 4-2).

Figure 4-2 • Health promotion for older adults includes physical fitness. Here, a nurse teaches simple exercises at a senior center.

Nursing Implications of Health Promotion

By virtue of their expertise in health and health care and their long-established credibility with consumers, nurses play a vital role in health promotion. In many instances, they initiate health promotion and health screening programs or participate with other health care personnel in developing and providing wellness services in various settings.

As health care professionals, nurses have a responsibility to promote activities that foster well-being, self-actualization, and personal fulfillment. Every interaction with consumers of health care must be viewed as an opportunity to promote positive health attitudes and behaviors. Health Promotion charts and tables throughout this textbook identify opportunities for promoting health.

CRITICAL THINKING EXERCISES

1 ebp A male college student goes to the nurse practitioner at the college health center to discuss his recent use of a hookah and how it has been making him feel. The student explained, "My roommates bought it and we have been mostly using it on the weekends. For the next few days after I use it, I feel like I am getting sick, but then I start to feel okay again." What health promotion factors guide the nurse practitioner in assessing the student's situation? What is the evidence base to use for providing health promotion information to help this student make appropriate health decisions and engage in positive health behaviors?

2 Four weeks after sustaining leg and arm injuries in a car accident, a woman is at the clinic for follow-up care with the nurse practitioner. The woman tells the nurse practitioner that before the accident, she used to run every day for exercise. She asks the nurse practitioner when she will be able to resume her running routine. What are the factors that will influence her ability to engage in exercise, and specifically to resume her running routine? Determine the factors that influence the relationship between health and fitness. Work with the woman to design and implement an appropriate exercise plan to promote health and fitness.

3 pg A 75-year-old woman attends a health promotion fair in the local hospital clinic. She tells the nurse coordinator, "I am only here to have my cholesterol checked as my doctor said that it is a little higher than it was at my last visit. I don't need to participate in anything else, as I'm doing just fine." What are the priorities to consider when planning a discussion on health promotion information with this older female adult? What information would be best to provide first for this older adult?

REFERENCES

*Asterisk indicates nursing research.
**Double asterisk indicates classic reference.

Books

American Nurses Association. (2015). *Nursing: Scope and standards of practice* (3rd ed.). Silver Spring, MD: ANA.

Bastable, S. B. (2014). *Nurse as educator: Principles of teaching and learning.* Sudbury, MA: Jones & Bartlett.

**Becker, M. H. (Ed.). (1974). *The health belief model and personal health behavior.* Thorofare, NJ: Charles B. Slack.

Carpenito-Moyet, L. J. (2017). *Handbook of nursing diagnosis* (15th ed.). Philadelphia, PA: Lippincott Williams & Wilkins.

Dayer-Berenson, L. (2013). *Cultural competencies for nurses: Impact on health and illness.* Sudbury, MA: Jones & Bartlett.

deChesnay, M., & Anderson, B. A. (2016). *Caring for the vulnerable: Perspectives in nursing theory, practice, and research* (2nd ed.). Sudbury, MA: Jones & Bartlett.

Edelman, C. L., Kudzma, E. C., & Mandle, C. L. (2014). *Health promotion throughout the life span* (8th ed.). Philadelphia, PA: Elsevier Health Sciences.

Haber, D. (2013). *Health promotion and aging: Practical application for health professionals* (6th ed.). New York, NY: Springer.

**Lalonde, M. (1977). *New perspectives on the health of Canadians: A working document.* Ottawa, Canada: Minister of Supply and Services.

Mauk, K. L. (2013). *Gerontological nursing: Competencies for care* (3rd ed.). Sudbury, MA: Jones & Bartlett.

McFarland, M. R., & Wehbe-Alamah, H. B. (2015). *Leininger's culture care diversity and universality: A worldwide nursing theory* (3rd ed.). Burlington, MA: Jones & Bartlett.

Miller, C. A. (2015). *Nursing for wellness in older adults* (7th ed.). Philadelphia, PA: Lippincott Williams & Wilkins.

Miller, M. A., & Stoeckel, P. R. (2016). *Client education: Theory and practice* (2nd ed.). Sudbury, MA: Jones & Bartlett.

O'Donnell, M. P. (Ed.). (2014). *Health promotion in the workplace.* Troy, MI: American Journal of Health Promotion.

Parnell, T. A. (2015). *Health literacy in nursing: Providing person-centered care.* New York, NY: Springer Publication.

Pender, N. J., Murdaugh, C. L., & Parsons, M. A. (Eds.). (2014). *Health promotion in nursing practice* (7th ed.). Upper Saddle River, NJ: Prentice-Hall Health.

Roundtable on Health Literacy & Institute of Medicine: Board on Population Health and Public Health Practice. (2014). *Health literacy and numeracy: Workshop summary.* Washington, DC: National Academies Press.

Tabloski, P. (2013). *Gerontological nursing: The essential guide to clinical practice* (3rd ed.). New York, NY: Pearson.

Touhy, T. A., & Jett, K. F. (2013). *Ebersole and Hess' gerontological nursing and healthy aging* (4th ed.). St. Louis, MO: Mosby.

U.S. Department of Agriculture and U.S. Department of Health and Human Services. (2010). *Dietary guidelines for Americans* (7th ed.). Washington, DC: U.S. Government Printing Office.

Journals and Electronic Documents

*Adam, J., & Folds, L. (2014). Depression, self-efficacy, and adherence in patients with type 2 diabetes. *Journal for Nurse Practitioners, 10*(9), 646–652.

*Ball, S., Gammon, R., Kelly, P. J., et al. (2013). Outcomes of stay strong, stay healthy in community settings. *Journal of Aging and Health, 25*(8), 1388–1397.

**Becker, H. A., Stuifbergen, A. K., Oh, H., et al. (1993). The self-rated abilities for health practices scale: A health self-efficacy measure. *Health Values, 17*, 42–50.

*Bender, C. M., Gentry, A. L., Brufsky, A. M., et al. (2014). Influence of patient and treatment factors on adherence to adjuvant endocrine therapy in breast cancer. *Oncology Nursing Forum, 41*(3), 274–285.

*Blanch-Hartigan, D., Blake, K. D., & Viswanath, K. (2014). Cancer survivors' use of numerous information sources for cancer-related information: Does more matter? *Journal of Cancer Education, 29*, 488–496.

Bruning, R. S., & Sturek, M. (2015). Benefits of exercise training on coronary blood flow in coronary artery disease patients. *Progress in Cardiovascular Diseases, 57*, 443–453.

Centers for Disease Control and Prevention (CDC). (2016). Recommended adult immunization schedule—United States, 2016. Retrieved on 8/20/2016 at: www.cdc.gov/vaccines/schedules/hcp/adult.html

*Cha, C. (2013). Health concept and health promotion process among Korean migrant women. *Health Care for Women International, 34*, 628–650.

Chaufan, C., Yeh, J., & Sigal, B. (2015). Advancing family health through the garden of eatin': On-site food gardens in early childhood. *American Journal of Public Health, 105*(4), 625–628.

*Christaki, E., Kokkinos, A., Costarelli, V., et al. (2013). Stress management can facilitate weight loss in Greek overweight and obese women: A pilot study. *Journal of Human Nutrition and Dietetics, 26*(Suppl 1), 132–139.

Claborn, K. R. (2015). A systematic review of treatment fatigue among HIV-infected patients prescribed antiretroviral therapy. *Psychology, Health and Medicine, 20*(3), 255–265.

**DiClemente, C. (2007). The transtheoretical model of intentional behavior change. *Drugs & Alcohol Today, 7*(1), 29–33.

*Fang, G., Robinson, J., Lauffenburger, J., et al. (2014). Prevalent but moderate variation across small geographic regions in patient non-adherence to evidence-based preventive therapies in older adults post myocardial infarction. *Medical Care, 52*(3), 185–193.

*Gerber, M., Jonsdottir, H., Arvidson, E., et al. (2015). Promoting grade exercise as a part of multimodal treatment in patients diagnosed with stress-related exhaustion. *Journal of Clinical Nursing, 24*, 1904–1915.

*Groh, C.F. J., & Urbancic, J. C. (2015). The impact of a lifestyle change program on the mental health of obese under-served African American women. *Archives of Psychiatric Nursing, 29*, 76–82.

*Halvarsson, A., Franzen, E., & Stahle, A. (2015). Balance training with multi-task exercises improves fall-related self-efficacy, gait, balance performance and physical function in older adults with osteoporosis: A randomized controlled study. *Clinical Rehabilitation, 29*(4), 365–375.

*Harold, L. R., Briesacher, B. A., Peterson, D., et al. (2013). Cost-related medication nonadherence in older rheumatoid arthritis patients. *Journal of Rheumatology, 40*(2), 137–143.

Harris, L., Thomas, V., & Fox, M. (2015). The influence of health care literacy on the use of PHRs among older adults. *MedSurg Nursing, 24*(4), 383–385.

*Hartley, L., Flowers, N., Lee, M. S., et al. (2014). Tai chi for primary prevention of cardiovascular disease. *The Cochrane Collection, 4*, 1–50.

*Hooper, L. M., & Huffman, L. E. (2014). Associations among depressive symptoms, well-being, patient involvement, provider cultural competency, and treatment nonadherence: An exploratory study among university student-patients. *Counseling Psychology Quarterly, 27*(3), 241–263.

*Khazaee-Pool, M., Sadeghi, R., Majlessi, F., et al. (2014). Effects of physical exercise programme on happiness among older people. *Journal of Psychiatric and Mental Health Nursing, 22*, 47–57.

*Kim, S., Sargent-Cox, K. A., & Anstey, K. J. (2015). A qualitative study of older and middle- aged adults' perception and attitudes towards dementia and dementia risk reduction. *Journal of Advanced Nursing, 71*(7), 1694–1703.

*Martins, M. M., de Souza, J., & da Silva, A. A. (2015). Children and adolescents who are substance users in the psychiatric emergency service. *Acta Paulista Enfermagem, 28*(1), 13–18.

Mehta, S., Cameron, K., & Battistella, M. (2014). Motivational interviewing: Application to end stage disease patients. *Canadian Association of Nephrology Nurses and Technologists Journal, 24*(4), 19–24.

*Meraviglia, M., Stuifbergen, A., Morgan, S., et al. (2015). Low-income cancer survivors' use of health-promoting behaviors. *MedSurg Nursing, 24*(2), 101–106.

Mitchell, J., Khoukaz, T., McNeal, D., et al. (2014). Adverse event management strategies: Optimizing treatment with regorafenib in patients with metastatic colorectal cancer. *Clinical Journal of Oncology Nursing, 18*(2), E19–E25.

*Murimi, M., Chrisman, M. S., McAllister, T., et al. (2015). Fostering healthy lifestyles in the African American population. *Health Education & Behavior, 42*(1), 109–116.

*Rao, R. M., Raghuram, N., Nagendra, H. R., et al. (2015). Effects of an integrated yoga program on self-reported depression scores in breast cancer patients undergoing conventional treatment: A randomized controlled trial. *Indian Journal of Palliative Care, 21*(2), 174–181.

*Resnick, B., Nahm, E. S., Zhu, S., et al. (2014). The impact of osteoporosis, falls, fear of falling, and efficacy expectations on exercise among community-dwelling older adults. *Orthopaedic Nursing, 35*(5), 277–286.

*Ryan, J. G., Fedders, M., Jennings, T., et al. (2014). Clinical outcomes and incremental costs from a medication adherence pilot intervention targeting low-income patients with diabetes at risk of cost-related medication nonadherence. *Clinical Therapeutics, 36*(12), 1991–2002.

*Seebohm, P., Chaudhary, S., Boyce, M., et al. (2013). The contribution of self-help/mutual aid groups to mental well-being. *Health and Social Care in the Community, 21*(4), 391–401.

*Smith, S. A. (2014). Mindfulness-based stress reduction: An intervention to enhance the effectiveness of nurses' coping with work-related stress. *International Journal of Nursing Knowledge, 25*(2), 119–130.

Tam, M. (2014). Understanding and theorizing the role of culture in the conceptualizations of successful aging and lifelong learning. *Educational Gerontology, 40*(12), 881–893.

*Theofilou, P. (2013). Medication adherence in Greek hemodialysis patients: The contribution of depression and health cognitions. *International Journal of Behavioral Medicine, 20*, 311–318.

U.S. Department of Health and Human Services. (2010). *Healthy People 2020.* Retrieved on 7/18/2015 at: www.healthypeople.gov/2020

U.S. Preventive Services Task Force. (2016). Recommendations. Retrieved on 8/20/2016 at: http://www.uspreventiveservicestaskforce. org/BrowseRec/Index/browse-recommendations

*Wang, J., Chen, C., Lai, L., et al. (2014). The effectiveness of a community-based health promotion for rural elders: A quasi-experimental design. *Applied Nursing Research, 27*, 181–185.

*Wu, J., & Moser, D. K. (2014). Type D personality predicts poor medication adherence in patients with heart failure in the USA. *International Journal of Behavioral Medicine, 21*, 833–842.

*Yeun, E. J., Baek, S., & Kim, H. (2013). Health promotion behavior in middle-aged Koreans: A cross-sectional survey. *Nursing and Health Sciences, 15*, 461–467.

*Yoo, C., Park, S., Yang, D., et al. (2014). Study of the physical condition of middle-aged office and field workers aged 50 and older. *Journal of Physical Therapy Science, 26*, 1575–1577.

Resources

Centers for Disease Control and Prevention (CDC), www.cdc.gov/nccdphp/dnpao/hwi/resources/preventative_screening.htm

Health Education Resource Exchange, Washington State Department of Health, here.doh.wa.gov

Health Promotion for Women With Disabilities, Villanova University College of Nursing, www.nurseweb.villanova.edu/WomenWithDisabilities/welcome.htm

Healthy People 2020, www.healthypeople.gov/2020/About-Healthy-People

Take Charge of Your Life by Making Healthy Choices, helpguide.org

U.S. Department of Agriculture (USDA), http://www.foodpyramid.com/myplate/

U.S. Army Public Health Command (USAPHC), phc.amedd.army.mil/topics/healthyliving/Pages/default.aspx

U.S. Department of Health and Human Services, National Institutes of Health, www.nih.gov/icd

U.S. Department of Health and Human Services, Office of Disease Prevention and Health Promotion, www.health.gov

World Health Organization, www.who.int

Adult Health and Nutritional Assessment

On completion of this chapter, the learner will be able to:

1 Describe the components of a holistic health history, physical examination, and nutritional assessment.
2 Identify modifications needed to obtain a health history and conduct a physical assessment for a person with a disability.
3 Describe the techniques of inspection, palpation, percussion, and auscultation to perform a basic physical assessment.

4 Discuss the techniques of measurement of body mass index, biochemical assessment, clinical examination, and assessment of food intake to assess a person's nutritional status.
5 Describe factors that may contribute to imbalanced nutrition in high-risk groups such as adolescents and older adults.

GLOSSARY

auscultation: listening to sounds produced within different body structures created by the movement of air or fluid
body mass index (BMI): a calculation done to estimate the amount of body fat of a person
electronic health record (EHR): computerization of health records; also referred to as electronic medical record (EMR)
ethnicity: affiliation relating to large groups of people classed according to common racial, national, tribal, religious, linguistic, or cultural background
faith: trust in God, belief in a higher power or something that a person cannot see
health history: the collection of subjective data, most often a series of questions that provides an overview of the patient's current health status

inspection: visual assessment of different aspects of the patient
palpation: examination of different organs of the body using the sense of touch
percussion: the use of sound to examine different organs of the body
physical examination: collection of objective data about the patient's health status
self-concept: a person's view of himself or herself
spirituality: connectedness with self, others, a life force, or God that allows people to find meaning in life
substance abuse: a maladaptive pattern of substance use that causes physical and emotional harm with the potential for disruption of daily life

The ability to assess patients in a holistic manner is a skill integral to nursing, regardless of the practice setting. Eliciting a complete health history, using appropriate physical assessment skills, while respecting spiritual and cultural considerations, is critical to identifying physical and psychological problems and concerns experienced by the patient. As the first step in the nursing process, a holistic patient assessment is necessary to obtain data that enable the nurse to make accurate nursing diagnoses, identify and implement appropriate interventions, and assess their effectiveness. This chapter covers health assessment, including the complete health history and basic physical assessment techniques. Because a patient's nutritional status is an important factor in overall health and well-being, nutritional assessment is addressed.

Considerations for Conducting a Health Assessment

The Role of the Nurse

All members of the health care team collaborate and use their unique skills and knowledge to contribute to the resolution of patient problems by first obtaining some level of history and assessment (Weber & Kelley, 2014). Various formats for obtaining the **health history** (the collection of subjective data about the patient's health status) and performing the **physical examination** (the collection of objective data about the patient's health status) have been developed because the focus of each member of the health care team is unique. Regardless of the format, the information obtained by the nurse complements the data obtained by other members of the health care team and focuses on nursing's unique concerns for the patient. The nurse completes a health assessment by obtaining the patient's health history and performing a physical assessment, which can be carried out in a variety of settings. These settings may include an acute care facility, a clinic or outpatient office, a long-term care facility, a school, or the patient's home. Nursing diagnoses are used to determine the appropriate plan of care for the patient and drive nursing interventions and patient outcomes. Nursing diagnoses also provide a standard nomenclature for use in the **electronic health record (EHR)**, enabling clear communication among care team members and the collection of data for continuous improvement in patient care (Herdman & Kamitsuru, 2014).

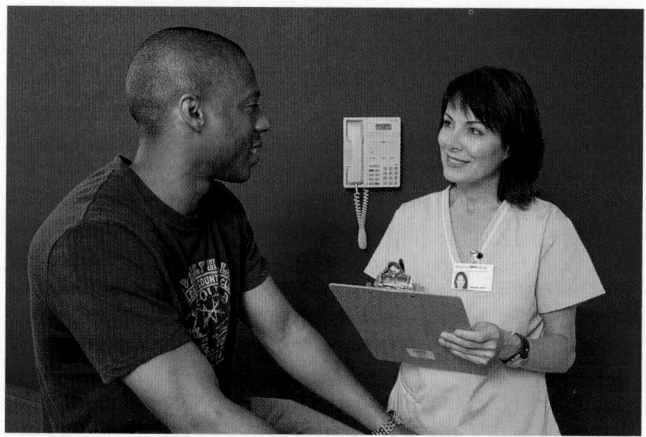

Figure 5-1 • A comfortable, relaxed atmosphere and an attentive interviewer are essential for a successful clinical interview.

Effective Communication

People who seek health care for a specific problem are often anxious. Their anxiety may be increased by fear about potential diagnoses, possible disruption of lifestyle, and other concerns. With this in mind, the nurse attempts to establish rapport, put the patient at ease, encourage honest communication, make eye contact, and listen carefully to the patient's responses to questions about health issues (see Fig. 5-1).

When obtaining a health history or performing a physical examination, the nurse must be aware of their own nonverbal communication, as well as that of the patient. The nurse should take into consideration the patient's educational and cultural background and language proficiency. Questions and instructions to the patient should be phrased so that they are easily understandable. Technical terms and medical jargon should be avoided. In addition, the nurse must consider any disabilities or impairments (hearing, vision, cognitive, and physical limitations). At the end of the assessment, the nurse summarizes and clarifies the information obtained and asks the patient whether he or she has any questions; this gives the nurse the opportunity to correct misinformation and add facts that may have been omitted.

Ethical Use of Health Assessment Data

Whenever information is elicited from a person through a health history or physical examination, the person has the right to know why the information is sought and how it will be used. For this reason, it is important to explain the purpose of the health history and physical examination, how the information will be obtained, how it will be used, and with whom it will be shared (Bickley, 2013; Weber & Kelley, 2014). It is also important that the person knows that the decision to participate is voluntary. A private setting for the history interview and physical examination should promote trust and encourage open, honest communication. After the history and examination are completed, the nurse selectively records the data pertinent to the patient's health status. This written record of the patient's history and physical examination findings is then securely maintained and made available only to those health professionals directly involved in the care of the patient. The Health Insurance Portability and Accountability Act (HIPAA), passed in

1996, established national standards to protect individuals' medical records and other personal health information and applies to health plans, health care clearinghouses, and those health care providers that conduct certain health care transactions electronically. The act requires appropriate safeguards to protect the privacy of personal health information and sets limits and conditions on the uses and disclosures that may be made of such information without patient authorization. The HIPAA outlines patients' rights over their health information, including rights to examine and obtain a copy of their health records and to request corrections (U.S. Department of Health & Human Services [HHS], 2015a).

The Role of Technology

The use of technology to augment the information-gathering process through the use of EHRs has become an increasingly important aspect of obtaining a health history and physical examination. An EHR offers convenient access to health data for the patient and for providers who can use the information more effectively to improve the quality and efficiency of patient care. Continuity of care between disciplines is also enhanced because all health providers are able to access patient information simultaneously and even remotely (HHS, 2015b). Nurses must be sensitive to the needs of older adults and others who may not be comfortable with computer technology. Nurses may need to allow extra time and provide detailed instructions or explanations. It is important to establish and maintain eye contact with the patient during the health history and to not focus solely on the computer screen for data entry.

Assessment in the Home or Community

Assessment of people in community settings, including the home, consists of collecting information specific to existing health problems, including data on the patient's physiologic and emotional status, the community and home environment, the adequacy of support systems or care given by family and other care providers, and the availability of needed resources. In addition, it is important to evaluate the ability of the individual and the family to cope with and address their respective needs. The physical assessment in the community and the home consists of similar techniques to those used in the hospital, outpatient clinic, or office setting. Privacy is provided, and the patient is made as comfortable as possible. See Chapter 2 for more information on community-based nursing practice.

Health History

The health history is a series of questions used to provide an overview of the patient's current health status. Many nurses are responsible for obtaining a detailed history of the patient's current health problems, past health history and family history, and a review of the patient's functional status. This results in a total health profile that focuses on lifestyle and health, as well as on illness.

While obtaining the health history, attention is focused on the impact of psychosocial and cultural background and ethnicity on a patient's health, illnesses, and health promotion behaviors. The interpersonal and physical environments, as well as the patient's lifestyle and activities of daily living, are explored in depth.

The format of the health history traditionally combines the medical history and the nursing assessment. Both the review of systems and the patient profile are expanded to include individual and family relationships, lifestyle patterns, health practices and nutritional assessment, and coping strategies. These components of the health history are the basis of nursing assessment and can be easily adapted to address the needs of any patient population in any setting, institution, or agency (Bickley, 2013; Weber & Kelley, 2014).

The health history format discussed in this chapter is only one approach that is useful in obtaining and organizing information about a patient's health status. Some experts consider this traditional format to be inappropriate for nurses, because it does not focus exclusively on the assessment of human responses to actual or potential health problems. Several attempts have been made to develop an assessment format and database with this focus in mind. One example is a nursing database developed by NANDA International and its 13 domains: health promotion, nutrition, elimination and exchange, activity/rest, perception/cognition, self-perception, role relationships, sexuality, coping/stress tolerance, life principles, safety/protection, comfort, and growth/development (Herdman & Kamitsuru, 2014) (see Chart 3-11 for further details) Although there is support in nursing for using this approach, no consensus for its use has been reached.

The National Information Center on Health Services Research and Health Care Technology (NICHSR) and other groups from the public and private sectors have focused on assessing not only biologic health but also other dimensions of health. These dimensions include physical, functional, emotional, mental, and social health. Efforts to assess health status have focused on the manner in which disease or disability affects a patient's functional status—that is, the ability of the patient to function normally and perform their usual physical, mental, and social activities. An emphasis on functional assessment is viewed as more holistic than the traditional medical history. Instruments to assess health status in these ways may be used by nurses along with their own clinical assessment skills to determine the impact of illness, disease, disability, and health problems on functional status (U.S. National Library of Medicine, 2015).

Regardless of the assessment format used, the focus of nurses during data collection is different from that of physicians and other health care team members. Combining the information obtained by the physician and the nurse into one health history prevents duplication of information and minimizes efforts on the part of the patient to provide this information repeatedly. This also encourages collaboration among members of the health care team who share in the collection and interpretation of the data.

The Informant

The informant, or the person providing the health history, may not always be the patient, as in the case of a developmentally delayed, mentally impaired, disoriented, confused, unconscious, or comatose patient. The interviewer should assess the reliability of the informant and the usefulness of

---

Chart 5-1 Health Assessment in the Older Adult

- Obtain the health history from older adult patients in a calm, unrushed manner.
- Consider possible vision or hearing impairments. Ensure that lighting is adequate but not glaring, and keep distracting noises to a minimum.
- Assume a position that enables the older adult patient to read lips and facial expressions. Sometimes sitting at a 90-degree angle to the patient is helpful because some visual impairments, such as macular degeneration, can limit the patient's vision to only peripheral vision. It is best to ask the patient where the interviewer should sit in relation to the patient to optimize the patient's view of the interviewer.
- Determine if the patient uses a hearing aid and ask the patient to use it during the interview. Check if the patient usually wears glasses and ensure that they are worn as well.
- Be aware that older adults often assume that new physical problems are a result of age rather than a treatable illness. Some of these problems may limit their activities of daily living and lifestyle patterns.
- Ask questions related to changes in the level of functioning. The signs and symptoms of illness in older adults are often more subtle than those in younger adults and may go unreported. A question such as "What interferes most in your daily activities?" may be useful in focusing the clinical evaluation.
- Obtain a complete history of medications used, because many older adult patients take many different kinds of prescription and over-the-counter (OTC) medications.
- Consider including a member of the family in the interview process. Although older adults may experience a decline in mental function, it should not be assumed that they are unable to provide an adequate history. Including a spouse, adult child, sibling, or caretaker may validate information and provide missing details. However, this should be done after obtaining the patient's permission. (Further details about assessment of the older adult are provided in Chapter 11.)

Adapted from Eliopoulos, C. (2018). *Gerontological nursing* (9th ed.). Philadelphia, PA: Lippincott Williams & Wilkins; Weber, J. R., & Kelley, J. H. (2014). *Health assessment in nursing* (5th ed.). Philadelphia, PA: Lippincott Williams & Wilkins.

---

the information provided. For example, a disoriented patient is often unable to provide reliable information; people who use alcohol and illicit drugs often deny using these substances. The interviewer must make a clinical judgment about the reliability of the information (based on the context of the entire interview) and include this assessment in the record. Chart 5-1 provides special considerations for obtaining a health history from an older adult.

Components of the Health History

When a patient is seen for the first time by a member of the health care team, the first requirement is that baseline information be obtained (except in emergency situations). The sequence and format of obtaining data about a patient may vary; however, the content, regardless of format, usually addresses the same general topics. A traditional health history includes the following: biographical data, chief complaint, present health concern (or history of present illness), past health history, family history, review of systems, and patient profile.

Biographical Data

Biographical information puts the patient's health history into context. This information includes the person's name, address, age, gender, marital status, occupation, and ethnic origins. Some interviewers prefer to ask more personal questions at this part of the interview, whereas others wait until more trust and confidence have been established or until a patient's immediate or urgent needs are first addressed. A patient who is in severe pain or has another urgent problem is unlikely to have a great deal of patience for an interviewer who is more concerned about marital or occupational status than with quickly addressing the problem at hand.

Chief Complaint

The chief complaint is the issue that caused the patient to seek the care of the health care provider. Questions such as "Why have you come to the health center today?" or "Why were you admitted to the hospital?" usually elicit the chief complaint. However, a statement such as "My doctor sent me" should be followed up with questions that identify and clarify the chief complaint (Bickley, 2013; Weber & Kelley, 2014). In the home setting, the initial question might be, "What is bothering you most today?" When a problem is identified, the person's exact words are usually recorded in quotation marks.

Present Health Concern or Illness

The history of the present health concern or illness is the single most important factor in helping the health care team arrive at a diagnosis or determine the patient's current needs. The physical examination is also helpful and often validates the information obtained from the history. A careful history and physical examination assist in the correct selection of appropriate diagnostic tests. Although diagnostic test results can be helpful, they often support rather than establish the diagnosis.

If the present illness is only one episode in a series of episodes, the nurse records the entire sequence of events. For example, a history from a patient whose chief complaint is an episode of chest pain should describe the entire course of their disease to put the current episode into context. The history of the present illness or problem includes information such as the date and type of onset (sudden or gradual) in which the problem occurred, the setting in which the problem occurred (at home, at work, after an argument, after exercise), manifestations of the problem, and the course of the illness or problem. This should include self-treatment (including complementary and alternative therapies), medical interventions, progress and effects of treatment, and the patient's perceptions of the cause or meaning of the problem.

Specific symptoms such as headaches, fever, or changes in bowel habits are described in detail. The interviewer should also ask whether the symptom is persistent or intermittent, what factors aggravate or alleviate it, and whether any associated manifestations exist. If the patient complains of pain, the location, quality, severity, and duration of the pain are determined. (See Chapter 12 for a more detailed discussion of pain.)

Associated manifestations are symptoms that occur simultaneously with the chief complaint. The presence or absence of such symptoms may help determine the origin or extent of the problem, as well as the diagnosis. These symptoms are referred to as significant positive or negative findings and are obtained from a review of systems directly related to the chief complaint. For example, if a patient reports a vague symptom such as fatigue or weight loss, all body systems are reviewed. On the contrary, if a patient's chief complaint is something specific, such as chest pain, then the cardiopulmonary and gastrointestinal systems will be the focus of the history of the present illness. In either situation, both positive and negative findings are recorded to further define the issue.

Past Health History

A detailed summary of a patient's past health is an important part of the health history. After determining the patient's general health status, the interviewer should inquire about immunization status and compare it with the Advisory Committee on Immunization Practices (ACIP) General Recommendations Work Group's (GRWG's) adult immunization schedule (Centers for Disease Control and Prevention [CDC], 2015a) (see Chapter 4, Table 4-3, for an adult immunization schedule) and then record the dates of immunization (if known). The interviewer should also inquire about any known allergies to medications or other substances, along with the nature of the allergy and associated adverse reactions. Other relevant material includes information, if known, about the patient's last physical examination, chest x-ray, electrocardiogram, eye examination, hearing test, dental checkup, Papanicolaou (Pap) smear and mammogram (if female), digital rectal examination of the prostate gland (if male), bone density testing, colon cancer screening, and any other pertinent tests.

The interviewer discusses previous illnesses and records negative as well as positive responses to a list of specific diseases. The dates of illnesses, or the age of the patient at the time, as well as the names of the primary providers and hospitals, the diagnoses, and the treatments, are noted. The interviewer elicits a history of the following areas:

- Childhood illnesses—rubeola, rubella, polio, whooping cough, mumps, measles, chickenpox, scarlet fever, rheumatic fever, strep throat
- Adult illnesses
- Psychiatric illnesses
- Injuries—burns, fractures, head injuries, traumatic injuries
- Hospitalizations
- Surgical and diagnostic procedures

If a particular hospitalization or major medical intervention is related to the present illness, the account of it is not repeated here; rather, the report refers to the appropriate part of the record, such as (see history of present illness) on the patient's health record.

Family History

To identify diseases that may be genetic, communicable, or possibly environmental in origin, the interviewer asks about the age and health status, or the age and cause of death, of first-order relatives (parents, siblings, spouse, children) and second-order relatives (grandparents, cousins). In general, the following conditions are included: cancer, hypertension, heart disease, diabetes, epilepsy, mental illness, tuberculosis, kidney disease, arthritis, allergies, asthma, alcoholism, and obesity. One of the easiest methods of recording such data is

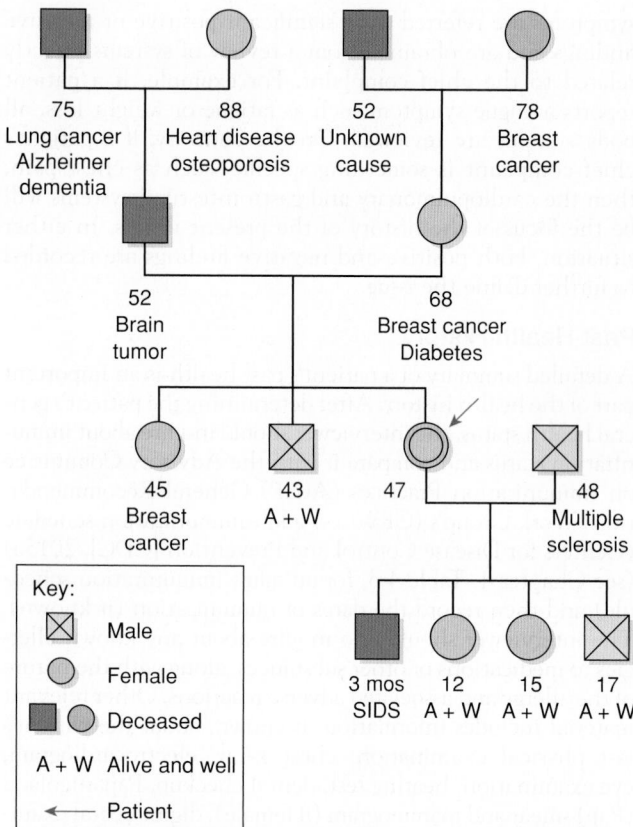

Key:

☒ Male

◯ Female

▣ ◯ Deceased

A + W Alive and well

⟵ Patient

Figure 5-2 • Diagram (called a *genogram*) used to record history of family members, including their age and cause of death or, if living, their current health status.

by using the family tree, genogram, or pedigree (see Fig. 5-2). The results of genetic testing or screening, if known, are recorded. Chart 5-2 provides genetic considerations related to health assessment. See Chapter 8 for a detailed discussion of genetics.

Review of Systems

The review of systems includes an overview of general health as well as symptoms related to each body system. Questions are asked about each of the major body systems for information about past and present symptoms. Negative and positive answers should be recorded. If a patient responds positively to questions about a particular system, the information is analyzed carefully. If any illnesses were previously mentioned or recorded, it is not necessary to repeat them in this part of the history.

A review of systems can be organized in a formal checklist, which becomes part of the health history. One advantage of a checklist is that it can be easily audited and is less subject to error than a system that relies heavily on the interviewer's memory.

Patient Profile

In the patient profile, more biographical information is gathered. A complete composite, or profile, of the patient is critical to the analysis of the chief complaint and of the patient's ability to deal with the problem. A complete patient profile is summarized in Chart 5-3.

At this point in the interview, the information elicited is highly personal and subjective. People are encouraged to express feelings honestly and to discuss significant health events. It is best to begin with general, open-ended questions and to move to direct questioning when specific facts are needed. Interviews that progress from information that is less personal (birthplace, occupation, education) to information that is more personal (sexuality, body image, coping abilities) often reduce anxiety.

A general patient profile consists of the following content areas: past life events related to health, current medications, education and occupation, financial resources, environment (physical, spiritual, interpersonal), lifestyle patterns, presence of a physical or mental disability, self-concept, sexuality, risk for abuse, and stress and coping response.

Past Life Events Related to Health

The patient profile begins with a brief life history. Questions about place of birth and past places of residence help focus attention on the earlier years of life. Personal experiences during childhood or adolescence that have special significance may be elicited by asking a question such as, "Were there any events that occurred when you were a child or adolescent that would be helpful for me to know about?" The interviewer's intent is to encourage the patient to make a quick review of their earlier life, highlighting information of particular significance. Although many patients may not recall anything significant, others may share information such as a personal achievement, a failure, a developmental crisis, or an instance of physical, emotional, or sexual abuse. The life history should include a brief medication history as appropriate for the patient.

Current Medications

A review of the patient's current medications is necessary to complete a comprehensive health history. Particular attention is given to allergies or adverse reactions to medications. The interviewer should inquire about the use of over-the-counter (OTC) medications and herbal supplements; patients often include only prescription medications when they list their current medications.

Education and Occupation

Inquiring about a patient's current occupation can reveal much about their economic status and educational preparation. A statement such as "Tell me about your job" often elicits information about role, job tasks, and satisfaction with the position. Direct questions about past employment and career goals may be asked if the person does not provide this information.

It is important to learn about a patient's educational background. Asking what kind of educational requirements were necessary for a patient to attain their present job is a more sensitive approach than asking whether he or she graduated from high school.

Financial Resources

Information about the patient's general financial status may be obtained by asking questions such as "Do you have any financial concerns at this time?" Inquiries about the person's insurance coverage and plans for health care payment are also appropriate.

Chart 5-2 GENETICS IN NURSING PRACTICE
Genetic Aspects of Health Assessment

Nursing Assessments

Family History Assessment

- Obtain information about maternal and paternal sides of family for three generations.
- Obtain history of known diseases or disorders for three generations for:
  - Clustering of diseases or disorders.
  - Early onset of disease or illness (e.g., blood clots in an active, otherwise apparently healthy 30 year old, or colon cancer in a 40 year old).
  - Similar disorder or disease in two or more close relatives.
  - History of multiple miscarriages, birth defects, or developmental delays.
  - Close biological relationship between parents.
- Assess for individual and family perceptions and beliefs around genetics topics through a cultural, social, and spiritual assessment.
- Acknowledge ethnic risk for particular genetic disorders.
- Determine whether the patient or a direct family member has had an unexpected response to medications or anesthesia.
- Recognize and evaluate for patterns of inheritance.
- Ascertain family relationships (family structure, roles, communication patterns, support system).

Patient Assessment

- Assess physical findings that may suggest a genetic condition (e.g., unusually tall stature—Marfan syndrome, low set ears and epicanthal folds—Down syndrome).
- Is there a presence of two or more dysmorphic features?
- Is there a presence of disability (physical or intellectual) or a history of developmental delay?

- Assess for conditions that occur in a less-often affected sex (e.g., stuttering in females, breast cancer in males, inguinal hernia in females).
- Presence of disease without known risk factors (e.g., hyperlipidemia).
- Acknowledge genetic-related risk related to ethnic background.
- Identify religious health, spiritual health, beliefs, and practices.

Management Issues Specific to Genetics

- Assess patient's understanding of genetic information and factors related to their health risks.
- Refer for risk assessment when a hereditary disease or disorder is suspected.
- Determine if genetic testing has been performed and if other family members are affected.
- Educate patient and family about the Genetic Information Nondiscrimination Act (GINA), passed in 2008.
- Offer appropriate genetic information and resources.
- Refer to a genetic counselor.
- Ensure that consent obtained for genetic testing is voluntary and informed.
- Provide support to patients and families with known genetic test results for hereditary disease or disorders, and refer to support groups as indicated.
- Participate in the management and coordination of risk reduction measures for those with known gene mutations.

Genetics Resources

Genetic Information Non-Discrimination Act. Retrieved on 9/2/2016 at: www.ginahelp.org
For additional genetic resources, see Chapter 8, Chart 8-7: Components of Genetic Counseling.

Environment

The concept of environment includes a person's physical environment and its potential hazards. It also includes a person's spiritual awareness, ethnicity, and support systems.

Physical Environment

Information is elicited about the type of housing (apartment, duplex, single family) in which the person lives, its location, the level of safety and comfort within the home and neighborhood, and the presence of environmental hazards (e.g., isolation, potential fire risks, inadequate sanitation). If the patient is homeless, details about available resources are important to ascertain.

Spiritual Environment

Spirituality is defined as connectedness with self, others, a life force, or God that allows people to experience self-transcendence and find meaning in life. Spirituality helps many people discover a purpose in life, understand the ever-changing qualities of life, and develop their relationship with God or a higher power. Within the framework of spirituality, people may discover truths about themselves, about the world, and their morality (O'Brien, 2013).

Spiritual behavior can be expressed through devotion, sacrifice, self-discipline, and spending time in activities that focus on the inner self or the soul. Although religion and

nature are two vehicles that people use to connect themselves with God or a higher power, bonds to religious institutions, beliefs, or dogma are not required to experience the spiritual sense of self. **Faith**, considered the foundation of spirituality, is trust in God and belief in a higher power or something that a person cannot see. The spiritual part of a person views life as a mystery that unfolds over one's lifetime, encompassing questions about meaning, hope, relatedness to a higher power, acceptance or forgiveness, and transcendence.

A person's spiritual environment refers to the degree to which he or she thinks about or contemplates their existence, accepts challenges in life, and seeks and finds answers to personal questions. Spirituality may be expressed through identification with a particular religion. Spiritual values and beliefs often direct a person's behavior and approach to health problems and can influence responses to sickness. A strong sense of spirituality or religious faith can have a positive impact on health. Spirituality is also a component of hope, and, especially during chronic, serious, or terminal illness, patients and their families often find comfort and emotional strength in their religious traditions or spiritual beliefs. At other times, illness and loss can cause a loss of faith or meaning in life and a spiritual crisis, which can place considerable stress on a person's internal resources and beliefs. It is important that the spiritual beliefs of people and families be acknowledged, valued, and respected for the

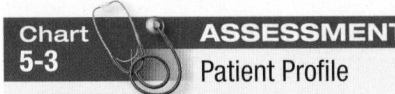

Chart 5-3 — ASSESSMENT

Patient Profile

Past Events Related to Health

Place of birth
Places lived
Significant childhood/adolescent events

Current Medications

Prescription, over-the-counter, home remedies, complementary and alternative therapies

Education and Occupation

Jobs held in past
Current position/job
Length of time at position
Educational preparation
Work satisfaction and career goals

Financial Resources

Income
Insurance coverage
Concerns

Environment

Physical—living arrangements (type of housing, neighborhood, presence of hazards)
Spiritual—extent to which religion or spirituality is a part of individual's life; religious or spiritual beliefs related to perception of health and illness; religious or spiritual practices
Interpersonal—ethnicity (language spoken, customs and values held, folk practices used to maintain health or cure illness); support systems (family relationships and friendships)

Lifestyle Patterns

Sleep (time person retires, hours per night, comfort measures, awakens rested)
Nutrition (24-hour diet recall, idiosyncrasies, restrictions)

Health promotion (exercise and recreation: type, duration, frequency; health screenings)
Caffeine (type: coffee, tea, cola, chocolate), amount
Alcohol (type, amount, pattern over past year)
Smoking (type: cigarette, pipe, cigar, marijuana; amount per day; number of years; desire to quit)
Drugs (type, amount, route of administration)

Physical or Mental Disability

Presence of a disability (physical or mental)
Effect of disability on function and health access
Accommodations needed to support functioning

Self-Concept

View of self in present
View of self in future
Body image (level of satisfaction, concerns)

Sexuality

Perception of self as a man or a woman
Quality of sexual relationships
Concerns related to sexuality or sexual functioning

Risk for Abuse

Physical injury in past
Afraid of partner, caregiver, or family member
Refusal of caregiver to provide necessary equipment or assistance

Stress and Coping Response

Major concerns or problems at present
Daily "hassles"
Past experiences with similar problems
Past coping patterns and outcomes
Present coping strategies and anticipated outcomes
Individual's expectations of family/friends and health care team in problem resolution

---

comfort and guidance they provide. Inquiring about spirituality can identify possible support systems as well as beliefs and customs that need to be considered in planning care. Information is gathered about the extent to which religion is a part of the person's life as well as religious beliefs and practices related to health and illness.

A spiritual assessment may involve asking the following questions:

- Is religion or spirituality important to you?
- If no, what is the most important thing in your life?
- If yes, in what way? For instance:
- Are there any religious or spiritual practices that are important to you?
- Do you belong to a faith community or have a place of worship?
- Do you have any religious or spiritual concerns because of your present health problem?

The nurse should assess spiritual strength further by inquiring about the patient's sense of spiritual well-being, hope, and peacefulness. It is also necessary to assess whether spiritual beliefs and values have changed in response to illness or loss. The nurse assesses current and past participation in religious or spiritual practices and notes the patient's responses

to questions regarding spiritual needs to help determine the patient's need for spiritual care. Another simple assessment technique is to inquire about the patient's and family's desire for spiritual support (O'Brien, 2013).

Interpersonal Environment

A patient's ethnicity and support system are taken into account when obtaining a health history. **Ethnicity** is defined as an affiliation relating to large groups of people classed according to common racial, national, tribal, religious, linguistic, or cultural background. Attitudes and beliefs about health, illness, health care, hospitalization, the use of medications, and the use of complementary and alternative therapies, which are derived from personal experiences, vary according to ethnicity. A person from another culture may have different views of personal health practices from those of the health care practitioner (Bickley, 2013; Weber & Kelley, 2014). See Chapter 7 for more cultural considerations.

The beliefs, customs, and practices that have been shared from generation to generation are known as ethnic patterns. The influence of these patterns on health-related behaviors and patient's perceptions of health and illness, as well as on how a patient reacts to health problems and interacts with health care providers, cannot be underestimated. Ethnic patterns can be expressed through language, dress, dietary choices, and role behaviors. The following questions may assist in obtaining relevant information:

- Where did your parents or ancestors come from? When?
- What language do you speak at home?
- Are there certain customs or values that are important to you?
- Do you have any specific practices to keep in good health or for treating illness?

Support systems are another important aspect of a patient's interpersonal environment. The evaluation of a patient's family structure (members, ages, and roles), patterns of communication, and the quality of the patient's relationships is an integral part of assessing support systems. Although the traditional family is recognized as a mother, a father, and children, many different types of living arrangements exist within our society. "Family" may mean two or more people bound by emotional ties or commitments, such as those shared by gay or lesbian partners. Live-in companions, roommates, and close friends can also play a significant role in a person's support system.

Lifestyle Patterns

The lifestyle section of the patient profile provides information about health-related behaviors. These behaviors include patterns of sleep, nutrition, and health promotion, as well as personal habits such as smoking and the use of illicit drugs, alcohol, and caffeine. Adequate sleep and nutrition are important to maintain optimal health; therefore, it is important to inquire about usual sleep habits and bedtime routines, as well as perform a nutritional assessment. Although most people readily describe their exercise patterns or recreational activities, many are unwilling to report their smoking, alcohol use, and illicit drug use, and many deny or understate the degree to which they use such substances. Questions such as "What kind of alcohol do you enjoy drinking?" may elicit more accurate information than "Do you drink?" Determining the specific type of alcohol (e.g., wine, liquor, beer) the patient drinks and the last time he or she had a drink is an important aspect of the assessment (Bickley, 2013).

The lifestyle of some people includes the use of mood-altering substances. People who engage in **substance abuse** use illegally obtained drugs, prescribed or OTC medications, and alcohol alone or in combination with other drugs in ineffective attempts to cope with the pressures, strains, and burdens of life. Over time, physiologic, emotional, cognitive, and behavioral problems develop as a result of continuous substance abuse.

If alcohol abuse is suspected, additional information may be obtained by using common alcohol screening questionnaires such as the CAGE (Cutting down, Annoyance by criticism, Guilty feeling, and Eye-openers) (Ewing, 1984), AUDIT (Alcohol Use Disorders Identification Test), or TWEAK (Tolerance, Worry about drinking, Eye-opener, Amnesia, Kut down on drinking) (Chan, Pristach, Welte, et al., 1993). The MAST (Michigan Alcohol Screening Test) has been updated to include drug use and has a geriatric version (New York State Office of Alcoholism and Substance Abuse Services [OASAS], 2015).

Similar questions can be used to elicit information about smoking and caffeine consumption. Questions about illicit drug use follow naturally after questions about smoking, caffeine consumption, and alcohol use. A nonjudgmental approach makes it easier for a person to respond truthfully and factually. If street names or unfamiliar terms are used to describe drugs, the person is asked to define the terms used.

Investigation of the patient's lifestyle patterns should also include questions about complementary and alternative medicine (CAM). Many different types of CAM practices are utilized including energy and breath work, botanical and manual healing, and mind–body therapies (Fontaine, 2014). The use of CAM therapies, in particular, special diets and/or herbal supplements, to treat illness or maintain health is an increasingly popular practice (Lindquist, 2013).

Marijuana is used for the management of symptoms, especially pain and anorexia, in several chronic conditions. Since the marijuana plant contains chemicals, called cannabinoids, that may help treat a range of illnesses or symptoms, many people argue that it should be legal for medical purposes. This has led to the legalization of marijuana for medical use in several states. The U.S. Food and Drug Administration (FDA) has not recognized or approved the marijuana plant as medicine; however, the FDA has approved two medications that contain cannabinoids in pill form. The approved drugs, dronabinol (Marinol) and nabilone (Cesamet), contain *delta-9-tetrahydrocannabinol* (THC). They are indicated specifically to treat nausea caused by chemotherapy and increase appetite in patients with extreme weight loss caused by acquired immune deficiency syndrome (AIDS) (National Institute on Drug Abuse, 2015).

The assessment of a patient's lifestyle patterns also includes questions about continuing health promotion and health-screening practices. The health history assessment should include the type, frequency, and duration of exercise and recreational activities. Inquiry should also include the types of health screenings the patient has completed. If the person has not been involved in these practices in the past, he or she should be educated about their importance and referred to the appropriate health care providers. Nurses should recognize the importance of encouraging culturally competent and health promotion activities (Shoqirat & Cameron, 2013).

Disability

The general patient profile needs to contain information about any hearing, vision, or other type of physical disability. In addition, mental, sensory, or cognitive disabilities need to be addressed. The presence of an obvious physical limitation (e.g., using crutches to walk or using a wheelchair to get around) necessitates further investigation. The initial cause or onset of the disability, as well as the impact on functional ability, should be established. Chart 5-4 presents specific issues that the nurse should consider when obtaining health histories and conducting physical assessments of patients with disabilities.

Self-Concept

Self-concept, a person's view of himself or herself, is an image that develops over many years. To assess self-concept, the interviewer might ask how a person views life, using a question such as "How do you feel about your life in general?"

Chart 5-4 ASSESSMENT
Assessing the Health of People With Disabilities

Overview

People with disabilities are entitled to the same level of health assessment and physical examination as people without disabilities. Physical and mental disabilities should be explained in the health history. Patients with mental disabilities are often marginalized from mainstream health care services because of the complexities of their disability. It is appropriate to ask the patient, or caregiver when necessary, what assistance he or she needs rather than assuming that help is needed for all activities or that, if assistance is needed, the patient will ask for it.

Health History

Communication between the nurse and the patient is essential. To ensure that the patient is able to respond to assessment questions and provide needed information, interpreters, assistive listening devices, or other alternative formats (e.g., Braille, large-print forms) may be required.

When interpreters are needed, interpretation services should be arranged. Health care facilities have a responsibility to provide these services without charge to the patient. Family members (especially children) should not be used as interpreters, because doing so violates the patient's right to privacy and confidentiality.

The nurse should speak directly to the patient and not to family members or others who have accompanied the patient. If patients have impaired hearing, they should be encouraged to use their hearing aids or hearing assistance technology during the assessment. The patient should be able to see the nurse's face clearly during the health history so that speech reading and nonverbal clues can be used to aid communication.

The health history should address general health issues that are important to all patients, including sexual history and risk for abuse. It should also address the impact of the patient's disability on health issues and access to care, as well as the effect of the patient's current health problem on their disability. An assessment of whether the patient's quality of life meets their expectations should be included in the health history.

The nurse should verify what the patient has said; if the patient has difficulty communicating verbally, the nurse should ask for clarification rather than assume that it is too difficult for the patient to do so. Most people would rather be asked to explain again than run the risk of being misunderstood.

Physical Examination

Inaccessible facilities remain a major barrier to health care for people with disabilities. Barriers include lack of ramps and grab bars, inaccessible restrooms, small examination rooms, and examination tables that cannot be lowered to allow the patient to move himself or herself onto, or be transferred easily and safely

to, the examination table. The patient may need help getting undressed for the physical examination (and dressed again), moving on and off the examination table, and maintaining positions usually required during physical examination maneuvers. It is important to ask the patient what assistance is needed.

If the patient has impaired sensory function (e.g., lack of sensation, hearing or vision loss), it is important to inform the patient that you will be touching him or her. Furthermore, it is important to explain all procedures and maneuvers.

Gynecologic examinations should not be deferred because a patient has a disability or is assumed to be sexually inactive. Explanations of the examination are important for all women, and even more so for women with disabilities, because they may have had previous negative experiences. Slow, gentle moving and positioning of the patient for the gynecologic examination and warming the speculum before attempting insertion often minimize spasticity in women with neurologically related disabilities.

Health Screenings and Testing

Many people with disabilities report that they have not been weighed for years or even decades because they are unable to stand for this measurement. Alternative methods (e.g., use of wheelchair scales) are needed to monitor weight and body mass index. This is particularly important because of the increased incidence of obesity and its effects on health status and transfer of persons with disabilities.

Patients with disabilities may require special assistance if urine specimens are to be obtained as part of the visit. They are often able to suggest strategies to obtain urine specimens based on previous experience.

If it is necessary for the nurse to wear a mask during a procedure or if the patient is unable to see the face of the nurse during a procedure, it is important to explain the procedure and the expected role of the patient ahead of time. If the patient is unable to hear or communicate with the nurse or other health care provider verbally during an examination or diagnostic test, a method of communication (e.g., signaling the patient by tapping the arm, signaling the nurse by using a bell) should be established beforehand.

People with disabilities experience difficulties related to obtaining care, challenges accessing health care facilities, perceptions that health professionals are insensitive to their needs, and concerns about the quality of care they receive. Therefore, it is important to ask about health screening and recommendations for screening. In addition, people with disabilities should be asked about their participation in health promotion activities, because inaccessible environments and other barriers may limit their participation in exercise, health programs, and other health promotion efforts such as health screenings.

Adapted from Dunkley, S. & Sales, R. (2014). The challenges of providing palliative care for people with intellectual disabilities: A literature review. *International Journal of Palliative Nursing, 20*(6), 279–284; Kelly-Campbell, R. J., & Lessoway, K. (2015). Hearing aid and hearing assistance technology use in Aotearoa/New Zealand. *International Journal of Audiology, 54*(5), 308–315; Sharts-Hopko, N. (2009). Low vision and blindness among midlife and older adults. *Holistic Nursing Practice, 23*(2), 94–100; Sharts-Hopko, N. C., Smeltzer, S. C., Ott, B. B., et al. (2010). Healthcare experiences of women with visual impairment. *Clinical Nurse Specialist, 24*(3), 149–153; Smeltzer, S. C., Sharts-Hopko, N. C., Ott, B. B., et al. (2007). Perspectives of women with disabilities on reaching those who are hard to reach. *Journal of Neuroscience Nursing, 29*(3), 163–171.

A person's self-concept can be threatened very easily by changes in physical function, appearance, or other threats to health. The impact of certain medical conditions or surgical interventions, such as a colostomy or a mastectomy, can threaten body image. The question, "Do you have any particular concerns about your body?" may elicit useful information about self-image.

Sexuality

The sexual history is an extremely personal area of assessment. Interviewers are frequently uncomfortable with such questions and ignore this area of the patient profile or conduct a very cursory interview about this subject. It is the nurse's professional and clinical responsibility to discuss issues of sexuality with patients. Effective health care for older adults requires assessment of sexual health (Kazer, Grossman, Kerins, et al., 2013). Sexual function may be affected negatively by disease (or treatment), surgery, or aging. In order for the patient to maintain sexual function and optimize quality of life, sexual issues must be addressed. During the sexual history, nurses need to recognize how their practices are influenced by assumptions about sexuality in relation to age, gender, and culture, and not make assumptions based on their own personal beliefs (Ayaz, 2013). In addition, the interviewer should project a nonjudgmental attitude related to sexual preference or toward those who are transgender.

Sexual assessment can be approached at the end of the interview or at the time interpersonal or lifestyle factors are assessed; otherwise, it may be easier to discuss sexuality as a part of the genitourinary history within the review of systems. In female patients, a discussion of sexuality could follow questions about menstruation. In male patients, a similar discussion could follow questions about the urinary system.

Obtaining the sexual history provides an opportunity to discuss sexual matters openly and gives the person permission to express sexual concerns to an informed professional. The assessment begins with an orienting sentence such as "Next, I would like to ask about your sexual health and practices." This type of opening may lead to a discussion of concerns related to sexual expression or the quality of a relationship, or to questions about contraception, risky sexual behaviors, and safer sex practices. Examples of other questions include "Do you have one or more sexual partners?" and "Are you satisfied with your sexual relationships?"

Determining whether a person is sexually active should precede any attempts to explore issues related to sexuality and sexual function. Care should be taken to initiate conversations about sexuality with older adult patients and patients with disabilities and not to treat them as asexual people. Questions are worded in such a way that the person feels free to discuss his or her sexuality regardless of marital status or sexual preference. Direct questions are usually less threatening when prefaced with such statements as "Some people feel that..." or "Many people worry about...." This suggests the normalcy of such feelings or behavior and encourages the person to share information that might otherwise be omitted because of fear of seeming "different."

If a person answers abruptly or does not wish to carry the discussion any further, then the interviewer should move to the next topic. However, introducing the subject of sexuality indicates to the person that a discussion of sexual concerns is acceptable and can be approached again in the future if so desired. (Further discussion of the sexual history is presented in Chapters 56 and 59.)

Risk for Abuse

Physical, sexual, and psychological abuse affects people of both genders and those who identify as gender fluid or nonbinary, as well as people of all ages and from all socioeconomic and ethnic groups. Patients rarely discuss this topic unless specifically asked about it. In fact, researchers report that most women in an abusive relationship have never told a health care provider (HHS, 2015c). Therefore, it is important to ask direct questions, such as:

- Is anyone physically hurting you or forcing you to engage in sexual activities?

- Has anyone ever hurt you physically or threatened to do so?
- Are you ever afraid of anyone close to you (your partner, caregiver, or other family members)?

Patients who are older or have disabilities are at increased risk for abuse and should be asked about it as a routine part of assessment (Hughes, Bellis, Jones, et al., 2012). However, when older patients are questioned directly, they rarely admit to abuse. Health care professionals should assess for risk factors, such as high levels of stress or alcoholism in caregivers, evidence of violence, and emotional outbursts, as well as financial, emotional, or physical dependency.

Two additional questions have been found to be effective in uncovering specific types of abuse that may occur only in people with disabilities:

- Does anyone prevent you from using a wheelchair, cane, respirator, or other assistive device?
- Does anyone you depend on refuse to help you with an important personal need, such as taking your medicine, getting to the bathroom, getting in or out of bed, bathing, dressing, or getting food or drink?

If a person's response indicates that abuse is a risk, further assessment is warranted, and efforts are made to ensure the patient's safety and provide access to appropriate community and professional resources and support systems. (Further discussion of domestic violence and abuse is presented in Chapters 56 and 72.)

Stress and Coping Responses

Each person handles stress differently. How well people adapt to stress depends on their ability to cope. During a health history, past coping patterns and perceptions of current stresses and anticipated outcomes are explored to identify the person's overall ability to handle stress. It is especially important to identify the expectations that a person may have related to family, friends, and caregivers in terms of providing financial, emotional, or physical support. (Further discussion of stress and coping is presented in Chapter 6.)

Physical Assessment

Physical assessment, or the physical examination (collection of objective data about the patient's health status), is an integral part of nursing assessment. The basic techniques and tools used in performing a physical examination are described in general in this chapter. The examinations of specific systems, including special maneuvers, are described in the appropriate chapters throughout the book.

Examination Considerations

The physical examination is usually performed after the health history is obtained. It is carried out in a well-lighted, warm area. The patient is asked to (or helped to) undress and is draped appropriately so that only the area to be examined is exposed. The patient's physical and psychological comfort are considered at all times. It is necessary to describe procedures to the patient and explain what sensations to expect before each part of the examination. The examiner washes his or her hands before and immediately after the examination. Fingernails are kept short to avoid injuring the patient. If there is a possibility of coming into contact with blood or other body secretions during the physical examination, gloves should be worn.

An organized and systematic examination is the key to obtaining appropriate data in the shortest time. Such an approach encourages cooperation and trust on the part of the patient. The patient's health history provides the examiner with a health profile that guides all aspects of the physical examination.

A "complete" physical examination is not routine. Many of the body systems are selectively assessed on the basis of the presenting problem. For example, if a healthy 20-year-old college student requires an examination to study abroad and reports no history of neurologic abnormality, the neurologic assessment is brief. Conversely, a history of transient numbness and diplopia (double vision) usually necessitates a complete neurologic investigation. Similarly, a patient with chest pain receives a much more intensive examination of the chest and the heart than one with an earache. In general, the health history guides the examiner in obtaining additional data for a complete picture of the patient's health.

The process of learning to perform a physical examination requires repetition and reinforcement in a simulated or clinical setting. Only after basic physical assessment techniques are mastered can the examiner tailor the routine examination to include thorough assessments of particular systems, including special maneuvers (Bickley, 2013; Weber & Kelley, 2014).

Components of the Physical Examination

The components of a physical examination include general observations and then a more focused assessment of the pertinent body systems. The tools of the physical examination are the human senses of vision, hearing, touch, and smell. These may be augmented by special tools (e.g., stethoscope, ophthalmoscope, reflex hammer) that are extensions of the human senses; they are simple tools that anyone can learn to use well. Expertise comes with practice, and sophistication comes with the interpretation of what is seen and heard.

Initial Observations

General inspection begins with the first contact with the patient. Introducing oneself and shaking hands provide opportunities for making initial observations: Is the person old or young? How old? How young? Does the person appear to be their stated age? Is the person thin or obese? Does the person appear anxious or depressed? Is the person's body structure normal or abnormal—in what way and how different from normal? It is essential to pay attention to the details in observation. Vague, general statements are not a substitute for specific descriptions based on careful observation. Consider the following examples:

- "The person appears sick." In what way does he or she appear sick? Is the skin clammy, pale, jaundiced, or cyanotic? Is the person grimacing in pain or having difficulty breathing? Does he or she have edema? What specific physical features or behavioral manifestations indicate that the person is "sick?"
- "The person appears chronically ill." In what way does he or she appear chronically ill? Does the person appear to have lost weight? People who lose weight secondary to muscle-wasting diseases (e.g., AIDS, malignancy) have a different appearance than those who are merely thin, and weight loss may be accompanied by loss of muscle

mass or atrophy. Does the skin have the appearance of chronic illness (i.e., is it pale, or does it give the appearance of dehydration or loss of subcutaneous tissue)?

These important specific observations are documented in the patient's chart or health record. Among general observations that should be noted in the initial examination of the patient are posture, body movements, nutritional status, speech pattern, and vital signs.

Posture

The posture that a person assumes often provides valuable information. Patients who have breathing difficulties (dyspnea) secondary to cardiac disease prefer to sit and may report feeling short of breath when lying flat for even a brief time. Patients with abdominal pain owing to peritonitis prefer to lie perfectly still; even slight jarring of the bed or examination table causes agonizing pain. In contrast, patients with abdominal pain owing to renal or biliary colic are often restless and may pace the room.

Body Movements

There are two kinds of abnormalities of body movement: generalized disruption of voluntary or involuntary movement and asymmetry of movement. The first category includes various tremors; some tremors may occur at rest (Parkinson disease), whereas others occur only on voluntary movement (cerebellar ataxia). Other tremors may exist during both rest and activity (alcohol withdrawal syndrome, thyrotoxicosis). Some voluntary or involuntary movements are fine and others are quite coarse. Extreme examples include the convulsive movements of generalized seizures and the choreiform (involuntary and irregular) movements of patients with rheumatic fever or Huntington disease.

Asymmetry of movement, in which only one side of the body is affected, may occur with disorders of the central nervous system (CNS), primarily in those patients who have had a cerebrovascular disease (stroke). Patients may have drooping of one side of the face, weakness or paralysis of the extremities on one side of the body, or a foot-dragging gait.

Nutritional Status

Nutritional status is important to note. Obesity may be generalized as a result of excessive intake of calories, or it may be specifically localized to the trunk in patients who have an endocrine disorder (Cushing disease) or who have been taking corticosteroids for long periods. Loss of weight may be generalized as a result of inadequate caloric intake, or it may be seen in loss of muscle mass with disorders that affect protein synthesis. Nutritional assessment is discussed in more detail later in this chapter.

Speech Pattern

Speech may be slurred because of CNS disease or because of damage to cranial nerves. Recurrent damage to the laryngeal nerve results in hoarseness, as do disorders that produce edema or swelling of the vocal cords. Speech may be halting, slurred, or interrupted in flow in patients with some CNS disorders (e.g., multiple sclerosis, stroke).

Vital Signs and Pain Assessment

The recording of vital signs is a part of every physical examination (Bickley, 2013). Blood pressure, pulse rate, respiratory rate, and body temperature measurements are obtained and recorded. Acute changes and trends over time are documented, and unexpected changes and values that deviate significantly from a patient's normal values are brought to the attention of the patient's primary provider. Pain is also assessed and documented, if indicated (see Chapter 12 for further discussion).

Focused Assessment

Following the general inspection, a more focused assessment is conducted. Although the sequence of physical examination depends on the circumstances and the patient's reason for seeking health care, the complete examination usually proceeds as follows:

- Skin
- Head and neck
- Thorax and lungs
- Breasts
- Cardiovascular system
- Abdomen
- Rectum
- Genitalia
- Neurologic system
- Musculoskeletal system

In clinical practice, all relevant body systems are tested throughout the physical examination, not necessarily in the sequence described (Weber & Kelley, 2014). For example, when the face is examined, it is appropriate to check for facial asymmetry and, thus, for the integrity of the fifth and seventh cranial nerves; the examiner does not need to repeat this as part of a neurologic examination. When systems are combined in this manner, the patient does not need to change positions repeatedly, which can be exhausting and time-consuming.

The traditional technique sequence in the focused portion of the examination is inspection, palpation, percussion, and then auscultation, except in the case of an abdominal examination (in which auscultation precedes palpation and percussion).

Inspection

The first fundamental technique is **inspection**, or observation of each relevant body system in more detail as indicated from the health history or the general inspection. Characteristics such as skin color, presence and size of lesions, edema, erythema, symmetry, and pulsations are noted. Specific body movements that are noted on inspection include spasticity, muscle spasms, and an abnormal gait (Grossman & Porth, 2014).

Palpation

Palpation, which utilizes the sense of touch, is a vital part of the physical examination. Many structures of the body, although not visible, may be assessed through the techniques of light and deep palpation (see Fig. 5-3). Examples include the superficial blood vessels, lymph nodes, thyroid gland, organs of the abdomen and the pelvis, and rectum. When the abdomen is examined, auscultation is performed before palpation and percussion to avoid altering bowel sounds (Bickley, 2013; Weber & Kelley, 2014).

Some sounds generated within the body, if within specified frequency ranges, may also be detected through touch. For example, turbulent flow in the heart or within blood

Figure 5-3 • **A.** Light palpation. **B.** Deep palpation.

vessels (thrills) may be detected. Thrills cause a sensation to the hand much like the purring of a cat. Voice sounds are transmitted along the bronchi to the periphery of the lung. These may be perceived by touch and may be altered by disorders affecting the lungs. The phenomenon is called *tactile fremitus* and is useful in assessing diseases of the chest. The significance of these findings is discussed in Chapters 20 and 25.

Percussion

The technique of **percussion** translates the application of physical force into sound. It is a skill requiring practice that yields much information about disease processes in the chest and the abdomen (Bickley, 2013; Weber & Kelley, 2014). The principle is to set the chest wall or abdominal wall into vibration by striking it with a firm object. The sound produced reflects the density of the underlying structure. Certain densities produce sounds as percussion notes. These sounds, listed in a sequence that proceeds from the least to the densest, are tympany, hyperresonance, resonance, dullness, and flatness. Tympany is the drumlike sound produced by percussing the air-filled stomach. Hyperresonance is audible when one percusses over inflated lung tissue in a person with emphysema. Resonance is the sound elicited over air-filled lungs. Percussion of the liver produces a dull sound, whereas percussion of the thigh produces a flat sound.

Percussion allows the examiner to assess such normal anatomic details as the borders of the heart and the movement of the diaphragm during inspiration. It is also possible to determine the level of a pleural effusion (fluid in the pleural cavity) and the location of a consolidated area caused by pneumonia or atelectasis (collapse of alveoli). The use of percussion is described further with disorders of the thorax and the abdomen (see Chapters 20 and 43).

 Concept Mastery Alert

Whereas auscultation involves listening to sounds produced within the body by the movement of air, percussion involves applying physical force to the body in order to discern what sounds are made, thereby assessing internal organs. Hyperresonance is audible when one percusses over inflated lung tissue in a person with emphysema.

Auscultation

Auscultation is the skill of listening to sounds produced within the body created by the movement of air or fluid (see Fig. 5-4). A stethoscope is typically used to enhance this technique. Examples include breath sounds, the spoken voice, bowel sounds, heart sounds, and cardiac murmurs. Physiologic sounds may be normal (e.g., first and second heart sounds) or pathologic (e.g., heart murmurs in diastole, crackles in the lung). Some normal sounds may be distorted by abnormalities of structures through which the sound must travel (e.g., changes in the character of breath sounds as they travel through the consolidated lung of a patient with lobar pneumonia).

Sound produced within the body, if of sufficient amplitude, may be detected with the stethoscope, which functions as an extension of the human ear and channels sound. The nurse must avoid touching the tubing or rubbing other surfaces (hair, clothing) during auscultation to minimize extraneous noises. Sounds detected by auscultation are classified according to their intensity (loud or soft), pitch (high or low), duration (length), and quality (musical, raspy, crackling) (Bickley, 2013; Weber & Kelley, 2014).

Figure 5-4 • Auscultation of the heart in forward sitting position.

Nutritional Assessment

Nutrition is important to maintain health and to prevent disease and premature death. When illness or injury occurs, optimal nutrition is essential for recovery or healing and for resisting infection and other complications. An in-depth nutritional assessment is often integrated into the health history and physical examination. Assessment of a patient's nutritional status provides information about obesity, undernutrition, and malnutrition.

Certain signs that suggest possible nutritional deficiency, such as muscle wasting, poor skin integrity, loss of subcutaneous tissue, and obesity, are easy to note because they are evident and objective. Other physical signs may be subtle, or the patient may report subjective symptoms, which must be carefully assessed. It is important to note that some signs and symptoms that appear to indicate nutritional deficiency may actually reflect other systemic conditions (e.g., endocrine disorders, infectious disease). Others may result from impaired digestion, absorption, excretion, or storage of nutrients in the body (Grossman & Porth, 2014; Weber & Kelley, 2014).

Disorders caused by nutritional deficiency, overeating, or eating unhealthy meals are among the leading causes of illness and death in the United States today. Examples of health problems associated with poor nutrition include obesity, osteoporosis, cirrhosis, diverticulitis, and eating disorders.

Obesity is a major concern for children, adolescents, and adults in the United States and globally. The World Health Organization (WHO) defines obesity as abnormal or excessive fat accumulation that may impair health. Obesity and being overweight are leading risk factors for global deaths; most of the world's population lives in countries where overweight and obesity kill more people than underweight. In addition, coronary artery disease, diabetes, musculoskeletal disorders, and certain cancers can be attributable to obesity (WHO, 2015). See Chapter 48 for a detailed discussion of obesity.

Lifespan Considerations

Adolescents

Adolescence is a time of critical growth and when lifelong eating habits are established. Nutritional assessment is particularly important during this time period. It is vital to assess for obesity in adolescents to prevent complications from obesity as they grow and develop, as well as when they enter adulthood.

Adolescent girls are at particular nutritional risk, because iron, folate, and calcium intakes frequently are below recommended levels, and they are a less physically active group than adolescent males. Adolescents with other nutritional disorders, such as anorexia and bulimia, have a better chance of recovery if these disorders are identified and treated in the adolescent years rather than in adulthood.

Older Adults

Older adults are also at risk for altered nutrition. Nutritional assessment in the older adult should include inquiry about the patient's current dietary practices as well as a nutritional screening to assess for adequate nutrition. The Mini Nutritional Assessment is a commonly used, well-validated tool developed specifically for this purpose (see Chart 5-5). Many older adults adhere to specific diets, such as those low in

Chart 5-5 Mini Nutritional Assessment

The Mini Nutritional Assessment (MNA) is a 6-item tool designed to identify adults aged 65 years and older who are either malnourished or at risk of becoming malnourished. It is available in several languages and there are several methods of delivery, including self-assessment as well as an electronic health record (EHR) version. It provides a more sensitive measure than body mass index (BMI) in identifying older adults in long-term care facilities at risk for malnutrition (Nestlé Nutrition Institute, 2011).

Mini Nutritional Assessment MNA®

Nestlé NutritionInstitute

Last name: _____ First name: _____

Sex: _____ Age: _____ Weight, kg: _____ Height, cm: _____ Date: _____

Complete the screen by filling in the boxes with the appropriate numbers. Total the numbers for the final screening score.

Screening

A Has food intake declined over the past 3 months due to loss of appetitie, digestive problems, chewing or swallowing difficulties?
0 = severe decrease in food intake
1 = moderate decrease in food intake
2 = no decrease in food intake ☐

B Weight loss during the last 3 months
0 = weight loss greater than 3 kg (6.6 lbs)
1 = does not know
2 = weight loss between 1 and 3 kg (2.2 and 6.6 lbs)
3 = no weight loss ☐

C Mobility
0 = bed or chair bound
1 = able to get out of bed / chair but does not go out
2 = goes out ☐

D Has suffered psychological stress or acute disease in the past 3 months?
0 = yes   2 = no ☐

E Neuropsychological problems
0 = severe dementia or depression
1 = mild dementia
2 = no psychological problems ☐

F1 Body Mass Index (BMI) (weight in kg) / (height in m²)
0 = BMI less than 19
1 = BMI 19 to less than 21
2 = BMI 21 to less than 23
3 = BMI 23 or greater ☐

IF BMI IS NO AVAILABLE, REPLACE QUESTION F1 WITH QUESTION F2.
DO NOT ANSWER QUESTION F2 IF QUESTION F1 IS ALREADY COMPLETED.

F2 Calf circumference (CC) in cm
0 = CC less than 31
3 = CC 31 or greater ☐

Screening score (max. 14 points)

12 - 14 points: Normal nutritional status
8 - 11 points: At risk of malnutrition
0 - 7 points: Malnourished ☐☐

References
1. Vellas B, Villars H, Abellan G, et al. Overview of MNA® - Its History and Challenges. *J Nutr Health Aging.* 2006;**10**:456-465.
2. Rubenstein LZ, Harker JO, Salva A, Guigoz Y, Vellas B. Screening for Undernutrition in Geriatric Practice: Developing the Short-Form Mini Nutritional Assessment (MNA-SF). *J Geront.* 2001;**56A**:M366-377.
3. Guigoz Y. The Mini-Nutritional Assessment (MNA®) Review of the Literature - What does it tell us? *J Nutr Health Aging.* 2006;**10**:466-487.
4. Kaiser MJ, Bauer JM, Ramsch C, et al. Validation of the Mini Nutritional Assessment Short-Form (MNA®-SF): A practical tool for identification of nutritional status. *J Nutr Health Aging.* 2009;**13**:782-788.
® Société des Produits Nestlé, S.A., Vevey, Switzerland, Trademark Owners © Nestlé, 1994, Revision 2009. N67200 12/99 10M
For more information: www.mna-elderly.com

saturated fat or sodium, for improving or maintaining health. Proper nutrition for an older adult meets daily requirements, maintains ideal body weight, and addresses specific health concerns such as cardiovascular or renal disease (Eliopoulos, 2018).

Inadequate dietary intake in older adults, which may lead to malnutrition and resultant illness and frailty, may result from physiologic changes in the gastrointestinal tract, socio-economic factors, drug interactions, disease, excessive use of alcohol, and poor dentition or missing teeth. Malnourished patients have an increased risk of morbidity and mortality; malnutrition is also linked to a poorer quality of life in older adults (Rasheed & Woods, 2014). Disorders affecting any part of the gastrointestinal tract can alter nutritional requirements and health status in people of any age; however, they are likely to occur more quickly and more frequently in older persons. Acute and chronic diseases may affect the metabolism and utilization of nutrients, which already are altered by the aging process. Even well older adults may be nutritionally at risk because of decreased odor perception, poor dental health, limited ability to shop and cook, financial hardship, and the fact that they often eat alone (Eliopoulos, 2018).

Moreover, many older adults take multiple prescribed and OTC medications; this is referred to as polypharmacy. The number of adverse reactions increases proportionately with the number of medications taken. Age-related physiologic and pathophysiologic changes may alter the metabolism and elimination of many medications (Eliopoulos, 2018). Medications can influence food intake by producing side effects such as nausea, vomiting, decreased appetite, and changes in cognition. They may also interfere with the distribution, utilization, and storage of nutrients.

Components of Nutritional Assessment

The sequence of the assessment may vary; however, evaluation of a patient's nutritional status includes the use of one or more of the following methods: measurement of body mass index (BMI) and waist circumference, biochemical assessment, clinical examination findings, and dietary data. Measurement of BMI and waist circumference is recommended to determine whether a patient is obese (CDC, 2015b).

 ### Body Mass Index, Ideal Weight, and Waist Circumference

Body mass index (BMI) is a ratio based on body weight and height (see Table 5-1). The obtained value is compared to established standards; however, trends or changes in values over time are considered more useful than isolated or one-time measurements. Body mass index is highly correlated with body fat, although increased lean body mass or a large body frame can also increase the BMI. People who have a BMI lower than 18.5 (or who are 80% or less of their desirable body weight for height) are at increased risk for problems associated with poor nutritional status. In addition, a low BMI is associated with a higher mortality rate among hospitalized patients and community-dwelling older adults. Those who have a BMI between 25 and 29.9 are considered overweight. Obesity is defined as a BMI of greater than 30 (WHO, 2015). In analyzing BMI, the nurse must be aware that cutoff scores for normal, overweight, and obese may vary for different ethnic groups.

TABLE 5-1 How Is BMI Calculated?[a]

Measurement Units	Formula and Calculation
Kilograms and meters (or centimeters)	Formula: weight (kg)/[height (m)]^2 With the metric system, the formula for BMI is weight in kilograms divided by height in meters squared. Because height is commonly measured in centimeters, divide height in centimeters by 100 to obtain height in meters. Example: Weight = 68 kg, Height = 165 cm (1.65 m) Calculation: $68 \div (1.65)^2 = 24.98$
Pounds and inches	Formula: weight (lb)/[height (in)]$^2 \times 703$ Calculate BMI by dividing weight in pounds (lb) by height in inches (in) squared and multiplying by a conversion factor of 703. Example: Weight = 150 lb, Height = 5′5″ (65″) Calculation: $[150 \div (65)^2] \times 703 = 24.96$

BMI, body mass index.
[a]BMI is calculated the same way for both adults and children. The calculation is based on formulas within this table.
Adapted from the Centers for Disease Control and Prevention (2015c). Body mass index (BMI) calculation. Retrieved on 8/18/2016 at: www.cdc.gov/healthyweight/assessing/bmi/adult_bmi

It is important to assess for usual body weight and height and to compare these values with ideal weight (see Chart 5-6). Current weight does not provide information about recent changes in weight; therefore, patients are asked about their usual body weight and any recent weight loss or gain. Loss of height may be attributable to osteoporosis—an important problem related to nutrition, especially in postmenopausal women (Bickley, 2013; Weber & Kelley, 2014).

In addition to the calculation of BMI, waist circumference measurement is a useful assessment tool. To measure waist circumference, a tape measure is placed in a horizontal plane around the abdomen at the level of the iliac crest. A waist circumference greater than 40 inches for men or 35 inches

---

Chart 5-6 — Calculating Ideal Body Weight

Women

Allow 100 lb for 5 ft of height.

- Add 5 lb for each additional inch over 5 ft.
- Subtract 10% for small frame; add 10% for large frame.

Men

- Allow 106 lb for 5 ft of height.
- Add 6 lb for each additional inch over 5 ft.
- Subtract 10% for small frame; add 10% for large frame.

Example: Ideal body weight for a 5′6″ adult:

	Female	Male
5′ of height	100 lb	106 lb
Per additional inch	6″ × 5 lb/inch = 30 lb	6″ × 6 lb/inch = 36 lb
Ideal body weight	130 lb ± 13 lb depending on frame size	142 lb ± 14 lb depending on frame size

for women indicates excess abdominal fat. Those with a high waist circumference are at an increased risk for diabetes, dyslipidemias, hypertension, heart attack, and stroke (Bickley, 2013; Weber & Kelley, 2014).

Biochemical Assessment

Biochemical measurements are applicable to a patient's nutritional assessment as they can test the level of a given nutrient and reflect abnormalities of metabolism in relation to the utilization of nutrients. Tests of serum and urine are done to determine whether the values are within an acceptable range. Some of these tests, while reflecting recent intake of the elements detected, can also identify a long-term deficiency (below-normal levels) even when there are no clinical symptoms of deficiency.

Low serum albumin and prealbumin levels are most often used as measures of protein deficit in adults. Albumin synthesis depends on normal liver function and an adequate supply of amino acids. Because the body stores a large amount of albumin, the serum albumin level may not decrease until malnutrition is severe; therefore, its usefulness in detecting recent protein depletion is limited. Decreased albumin levels may be caused by overhydration, liver or renal disease, or excessive protein loss due to burns, major surgery, infection, or cancer. Serial measurements of prealbumin levels are used to assess the effectiveness of nutritional therapy (see Chapter 44 for further discussion).

Additional laboratory data, such as levels of transferrin and retinol-binding protein, and complete blood and electrolyte counts, are used in many institutions. Transferrin is a protein that binds and carries iron from the intestine through the serum. Because of its short half-life, transferrin levels decrease more quickly than albumin levels in response to protein depletion. Low levels of transferrin can also lead to a deficiency in iron; low availability of iron in the body limits the synthesis of functioning hemoglobin causing anemia. Although measurement of retinol-binding protein is not available from many laboratories, it may be a useful

means of monitoring acute, short-term changes in protein status. The total lymphocyte count may be reduced in people who are acutely malnourished as a result of stress and low-calorie feeding, as well as in those with impaired cellular immunity. Anergy, or the absence of an immune response to injection of small concentrations of recall antigen under the skin, may also indicate malnutrition because of delayed antibody synthesis and response. Serum electrolyte levels provide information about fluid and electrolyte balance and kidney function.

A 24-hour urine collection can be utilized to calculate the creatinine/height index that assesses metabolically active tissue and indicates the degree of protein depletion. The amount of creatinine is measured and the index is calculated on the basis of the patient's height and gender. The patient's creatinine/height index is then compared to normal ranges based on the expected body weight by height. Values lower than normal may indicate loss of lean body mass and protein malnutrition (Fischbach & Dunning, 2015).

Clinical Examination

The state of nutrition is often reflected in a person's appearance. Although the most obvious physical sign of good nutrition is a normal body weight with respect to height, body frame, and age, other tissues can serve as indicators of general nutritional status and adequate intake of specific nutrients; these include the hair, skin, teeth, gums, mucous membranes, mouth and tongue, skeletal muscles, abdomen, lower extremities, and thyroid gland (Table 5-2).

Dietary Data

Commonly used methods of determining individual eating patterns include the food record, the 24-hour food recall, and a dietary interview. Each of these methods helps estimate whether food intake is adequate and appropriate. If these methods are used to obtain the dietary history, instructions must be given to the patient about measuring and recording food intake.

TABLE 5-2 Physical Indicators of Nutritional Status

Indicator	Signs of Good Nutrition	Signs of Poor Nutrition
General appearance	Alert, responsive	Listless, appears acutely or chronically ill
Hair	Shiny, lustrous; firm, healthy scalp	Dull and dry, brittle, depigmented, easily plucked; thin and sparse
Face	Skin color uniform; healthy appearance	Skin dark over cheeks and under eyes, skin flaky, face swollen or hollow/sunken cheeks
Eyes	Bright, clear, moist	Eye membranes pale, dry (xerophthalmia); increased vascularity, cornea soft (keratomalacia)
Lips	Good color (pink), smooth	Swollen and puffy; angular lesion at corners of mouth (cheilosis)
Tongue	Deep red in appearance; surface papillae present	Smooth appearance, swollen, beefy-red, sores, atrophic papillae
Teeth	Straight, no crowding, no dental caries, bright	Dental caries, mottled appearance (fluorosis), malpositioned
Gums	Firm, good color (pink)	Spongy, bleed easily, marginal redness, recession
Thyroid	No enlargement of the thyroid	Thyroid enlargement (simple goiter)
Skin	Smooth, good color, moist	Rough, dry, flaky, swollen, pale, pigmented; lack of fat under skin
Nails	Firm, pink	Spoon shaped, ridged, brittle
Skeleton	Good posture, no malformation	Poor posture, beading of ribs, bowed legs or knock knees
Muscles	Well developed, firm	Flaccid, poor tone, wasted, underdeveloped
Extremities	No tenderness	Weak and tender; edematous
Abdomen	Flat	Swollen
Nervous system	Normal reflexes	Decreased or absent ankle and knee reflexes
Weight	Normal for height, age, and body build	Overweight or underweight

Methods of Collecting Data

Food Record

The food record is used most often in nutritional status studies. A person is instructed to keep a record of food consumed over a period of time, varying from 3 to 7 days, and to accurately estimate and describe the specific foods consumed. Food records are fairly accurate if the person is willing to provide factual information and is able to estimate food quantities.

24-Hour Recall

As the name implies, the 24-hour recall method is a recall of food intake over a 24-hour period. A person is asked to recall all foods eaten during the previous day and to estimate the quantities of each food consumed. Because information does not always represent usual intake, at the end of the interview the patient is asked whether the previous day's food intake was typical. To obtain supplementary information about the typical diet, it is also necessary to ask how frequently the person eats foods from the major food groups.

Dietary Interview

The success of the interviewer in obtaining information for dietary assessment depends on effective communication, which requires that good rapport be established to promote respect and trust. The interview is conducted in a nondirective and exploratory way, allowing the respondent to express feelings and thoughts while encouraging him or her to answer specific questions. The manner in which questions are asked influences the respondent's cooperation. The interviewer must be nonjudgmental and avoid expressing disapproval by verbal comments or facial expression.

Several questions may be necessary to elicit the information needed. When attempting to elicit information about the type and quantity of food eaten at a particular time, open-ended questions should be utilized. In addition, assumptions should not be made about the size of servings; instead, questions are phrased to clearly determine the quantities. For example, to help determine the size of one hamburger, the patient may be asked, "How many servings were prepared with the pound of meat you bought?" Another approach to determining quantities is to use food models of known sizes in estimating portions of meat, cake, or pie, or to record quantities in common measurements, such as cups or spoonfuls (or the size of containers when discussing intake of bottled beverages).

In recording a particular combination dish, such as a casserole, it is useful to ask about the ingredients, recording the largest quantities first. When recording quantities of ingredients, the interviewer notes whether the food item was raw or cooked and the number of servings provided by the recipe. When a patient lists the foods for the recall questionnaire, it may help read back the list of foods and ask whether anything was forgotten, such as condiments, fruit, cake, candy, between-meal snacks, or alcoholic beverages.

Individuals' ethnicity or their personal beliefs determine to a large extent which foods are eaten and how they are prepared and served. Cultural and religious practices can determine whether certain foods are prohibited (see Chapter 7, Chart 7-2) and whether certain foods and spices are eaten on holidays or at specific family gatherings. Because of the value of food pattern choices to many individuals, it is important to be sensitive to these choices when obtaining a dietary history. It is, however,

equally important not to stereotype individuals and assume that because they are from a certain culture or religious group, they adhere to specific dietary customs. One particular area of consideration is the presence of fish and shellfish in the diet, where they come from (farmed vs. wild), and the method of preparation. Some eating patterns may put certain populations at risk for toxicity owing to contaminants or deficiencies due to food choices. Specific eating patterns, such as Mediterranean-style or vegetarian, should be explored so that appropriate dietary recommendations can be offered (U.S. Department of Agriculture & HHS, 2016). Deficiencies in certain diets may cause disorders such as anemia (see Chapter 33 for further discussion).

Evaluating Dietary Information

After obtaining basic dietary information, the nurse evaluates the patient's dietary intake and communicates the information to the dietitian and the rest of the health care team for more detailed assessment and clinical nutrition intervention. If the goal is to determine whether the patient generally eats a healthful diet, their food intake may be compared with the dietary guidelines outlined in the U.S. Department of Agriculture's Center for Nutrition Policy & Promotion's MyPlate (see Fig. 5-5). Foods are divided into five major groups (fruits, vegetables, grains, protein foods, and dairy), plus oils. Recommendations are provided related to variety in the diet, proportion of food from each food group, and moderation in eating fats, oils, and sweets. A patient's food intake is compared with recommendations based on various food groups for different age groups and activity levels (Weber & Kelley, 2014).

If nurses or dietitians are interested in knowing about the intake of specific nutrients, such as vitamin A, iron, or calcium, the patient's food intake is analyzed by consulting a list of foods and their composition and nutrient content. The diet is analyzed in terms of grams and milligrams of specific nutrients. The total nutritive value is then compared with the recommended dietary allowances specific for the patient's age

Figure 5-5 • MyPlate, a simple reminder for healthy eating. From the U.S. Department of Agriculture's Center for Nutrition Policy & Promotion. Retrieved on 1/30/2016 at: www.choosemyplate.gov/dietary-guidelines

category, gender, and special circumstances such as pregnancy or lactation.

Fat intake and cholesterol levels are additional aspects of the nutritional assessment. Trans fats are produced when hydrogen atoms are added to monounsaturated or polyunsaturated fats to produce a semisolid product, such as margarine. Partially hydrogenated oils (PHOs), the primary source of industrially produced trans fats, are found in many popular processed foods, such as baked goods and frozen foods. This is a concern because increased amounts of trans fats have been associated with increased risk for heart disease and stroke. Since 2006, the FDA has required the inclusion of trans fats information on food labels (FDA, 2014). In June 2015, the FDA announced that manufacturers must stop adding PHOs to processed food, providing a 3-year compliance period so that food manufacturers may gradually phase out the use of PHOs (FDA, 2015).

Factors Influencing Nutritional Status in Various Situations

Patients who are hospitalized may have an inadequate dietary intake because of the illness or disorder that necessitated the hospital stay. Patients who are at home may feel too sick or fatigued to shop and prepare food, or they may be unable to eat because of other physical problems or limitations. Limited or fixed incomes or the high costs of medications may result in insufficient money to buy nutritious foods. Culturally influenced food patterns can also affect nutritional status (see Chart 5-7). Because complex treatments (e.g., mechanical ventilation, intravenous infusions, chemotherapy) once

used only in the hospital setting are now being provided in the home and outpatient settings, nutritional assessment of patients in these settings is an important aspect of home and community-based care.

Many medications influence nutritional status by suppressing the appetite, irritating the oral or gastric mucosa, or causing nausea and vomiting. Others may influence bacterial flora in the intestine or directly affect nutrient absorption so that secondary malnutrition results. People who must take many medications in a single day often report feeling too full to eat. A patient's use of prescription and OTC medications and their effects on appetite and dietary intake are assessed. Many of the factors that contribute to poor nutritional status are identified in Table 5-3.

Analysis of Nutritional Status

Physical measurements (BMI, waist circumference) and biochemical and dietary data are used in combination to determine a patient's nutritional status. Often, these data provide more information about the patient's nutritional status than the clinical examination, which may not detect subclinical deficiencies unless they become so advanced that overt signs develop. A low intake of nutrients over a long period may lead to low biochemical levels and, without nutritional intervention, may result in characteristic and observable signs and symptoms. A plan of action for nutritional intervention is based on the results of the dietary assessment and the patient's clinical examination. To be effective, the plan should include a healthy diet, maintenance (or control) of weight, and compensation for increased nutritional needs.

Chart 5-7 — **NURSING RESEARCH PROFILE**
Food Patterns Among Hispanic Women

Gerchow, L., Tagliaferro, B., Squires, A., et al. (2014). Latina food patterns in the United States: A qualitative metasynthesis. *Nursing Research, 63*(3), 182–193.

Purpose

The purpose of this study was to analyze and integrate results from previous qualitative research on food patterns among immigrant Latinas residing in the United States in order to find dietary patterns across and within Latino subcultures. Only qualitative studies were included in this metasynthesis, in order to best ascertain Latina beliefs and opinions that could influence food patterns.

Design

Thirteen studies met the inclusion criteria after a systematic database search was conducted. The inclusion criteria were that qualitative studies must have been published in English between 2002 and 2013 and had to be focused upon Latinas living within the United States, and that findings had to be focused upon food patterns and their effect on weight gain. The quality of each study was assessed using the Critical Appraisal Skills Program tool and the recommendations of SQUIRES for evaluating translation methods. Themes were extracted by the researchers through content analysis, focusing upon food patterns, obesity, population breakdown, immigration, acculturation, and barriers and facilitators to healthy eating.

Findings

Findings suggest that multiple, complex factors influence food patterns among Latinas living in the United States. Two major themes emerged. The first theme revolved around the immigrant experience, with participants in these studies identifying lifestyle changes that affected food patterns since immigrating to the United States. The second theme focused upon barriers and facilitators to healthy eating, which identified more barriers than facilitators. Barriers to healthy eating included difficulties with the English language, socioeconomics, social isolation, and poor knowledge of nutrition. Family dynamics was viewed by most study participants as a facilitator to healthy eating, with some Latinas identifying that they learned healthy eating behaviors from acculturated family members. Pinpointing specific barriers and facilitators to healthy food choices is complex, however. Furthermore, it was difficult to ascertain differences in food patterns between Latinas who came from different Hispanic subcultures.

Nursing Implications

Nurses should recognize that Latinas who reside in the United States face barriers to adhering to healthy food patterns that may impact both their weight and health status. These barriers may be ameliorated through capitalizing on family networks, in particular, acculturated family members. Moreover, nurses should recognize that the influences behind eating behaviors among immigrant Latinas are complex and may be influenced by their specific Hispanic subculture.

TABLE 5-3 Factors Associated With Potential Nutritional Deficits

Factor	Possible Consequences
Dental and oral problems (missing teeth, ill-fitting dentures, impaired swallowing or chewing)	Inadequate intake of high-fiber foods
Nothing by mouth (NPO) for diagnostic testing	Inadequate caloric and protein intake; dehydration
Prolonged use of glucose and saline intravenous fluids	Inadequate caloric and protein intake
Nausea and vomiting	Inadequate caloric and protein intake; loss of fluid, electrolytes, and minerals
Diarrhea	Loss of fluid, electrolytes, and minerals; malabsorption of nutrients
Stress of illness, surgery, and/or hospitalization	Increased protein and caloric requirement; increased catabolism
Wound drainage	Loss of protein, fluid, electrolytes, and minerals
Pain	Loss of appetite; inability to shop, cook, eat
Fever	Increased caloric and fluid requirement; increased catabolism
Gastrointestinal intubation	Loss of protein, fluid, and minerals
Tube feedings	Inadequate amounts; variation of nutrients in each formula
Gastrointestinal disease	Inadequate intake and malabsorption of nutrients
Alcoholism	Inadequate intake of nutrients; increased consumption of calories without other nutrients; vitamin deficiencies
Depression	Loss of appetite; inability to shop, cook, eat
Eating disorders (anorexia, bulimia)	Inadequate caloric and protein intake; loss of fluid, electrolytes, and minerals
Medications	Inadequate intake due to medication side effects, such as dry mouth, loss of appetite, decreased taste perception, difficulty swallowing, nausea and vomiting, malabsorption of nutrients
Restricted ambulation or disability	Limited ability to shop, cook, or help self to food, liquids, other nutrients

CRITICAL THINKING EXERCISES

1 **ebp** You are conducting a pre-employment physical for a 55-year-old male. After calculating his ideal body weight, you note that his weight is well above average for his height. What standardized assessment tools would you use to determine his health risk? Identify his health risks, given his increased weight, based on the most recent evidence. Evaluate the strength of the evidence for these risks.

2 **pq** A 38-year-old woman is brought by ambulance to the emergency department after a suicide attempt, following the death of her spouse 6 months ago. What types of assessments are necessary to complete a comprehensive admission assessment? What are the priorities in this patient's care? How might your approach to this patient differ if the patient's culture viewed suicidal ideation as a sign of weakness and disrespect for the culture?

3 Your health assessment of an older adult male who has been receiving chemotherapy for lung cancer with bone metastasis reveals a decreased body mass index (BMI). You also note that the patient requires continuous oxygen and takes opioid medications routinely. Formulate a list of possible nursing diagnoses for the patient including one related to nutrition. Identify nursing interventions that would address the nursing diagnoses and determine evaluation criteria for the interventions.

REFERENCES

*Asterisk indicates nursing research.
**Double asterisk indicates classic reference.

Books

Bickley, L. S. (2013). *Bates' guide to physical examination and history taking* (11th ed.). Philadelphia, PA: Lippincott Williams & Wilkins.

Eliopoulos, C. (2018). *Gerontological nursing* (9th ed.). Philadelphia, PA: Lippincott Williams & Wilkins.

Fischbach, F., & Dunning, M. B. (2015). *A manual of laboratory and diagnostic tests* (9th ed.). Philadelphia, PA: Lippincott Williams & Wilkins.

Fontaine, K. L. (2014). *Complementary and alternative therapies for nursing practice* (4th ed.). Upper Saddle River, NJ: Prentice Hall.

Grossman, S. C., & Porth, C. M. (2014). *Porth's pathophysiology: Concepts of altered health states* (9th ed.). Philadelphia, PA: Lippincott Williams & Wilkins.

Herdman, T. H., & Kamitsura, S. (2014). *Nursing diagnoses: Definitions & classification 2015–2017.* Oxford: Wiley-Blackwell.

Lindquist, R. (2013). *Complementary & alternative therapies in nursing* (7th ed.). New York, NY: Springer.

O'Brien, M. E. (2013). *Spirituality in nursing* (5th ed.). Sudbury, MA: Jones & Bartlett.

Weber, J. R., & Kelley, J. H. (2014). *Health assessment in nursing* (5th ed.). Philadelphia, PA: Lippincott Williams & Wilkins.

Journals and Electronic Documents

*Ayaz, S. (2014). Sexuality and nursing process: A literature review. *Sexuality and Disability, 31*(1), 3–12.

Centers for Disease Control and Prevention (CDC). (2015a). General recommendations on immunization: Recommendations of the Advisory Committee on Immunization Practices (ACIP). Retrieved on 12/29/2015 at: www.cdc.gov/mmwr/preview/mmwrhtml/rr6002a1.htm

Centers for Disease Control and Prevention (CDC). (2015b). Assessing your weight. Retrieved on 12/29/2015 at: www.cdc.gov/healthyweight/assessing/index.html

Centers for Disease Control and Prevention (CDC). (2015c). About adult BMI. Retrieved on 12/29/2015 at: www.cdc.gov/healthyweight/assessing/bmi/adult_bmi/index.html

**Chan, A. W. K., Pristach, E. A., Welte, J. W., et al. (1993). Use of the TWEAK test in screening for alcoholism/heavy drinking in three populations. *Alcoholism: Clinical and Experimental Research, 17*(6), 1188–1192.

*Dunkley, S., & Sales, R. (2014). The challenges of providing palliative care for people with intellectual disabilities: A literature review. *International Journal of Palliative Nursing, 20*(6), 279–284.

**Ewing, J. A. (1984). Detecting alcoholism: The CAGE questionnaire. *JAMA, 252*(14), 1905–1907.

*Gerchow, L., Tagliaferro, B., Squires, A., et al. (2014). Latina food patterns in the United States: A qualitative metasynthesis. *Nursing Research, 63*(3), 182–193.

Hughes, K., Bellis, M. A., Jones, L., et al. (2012). Prevalence and risk of violence against adults with disabilities: A systematic review and meta-analysis of observational studies. *The Lancet, 379*(9826), 1621–1629.

*Kazer, M. W., Grossman, S., Kerins, G., et al. (2013). Validity and reliability of the geriatric sexuality inventory. *Journal of Gerontological Nursing, 39*(11), 38–45.

Kelly-Campbell, R. J., & Lessoway, K. (2015). Hearing aid and hearing assistance technology use in Aotearoa/New Zealand. *International Journal of Audiology, 54*(5), 308–315.

National Institute on Drug Abuse. (2015). DrugFacts: Is marijuana medicine? Retrieved on 12/29/2015 at: www.drugabuse.gov/publications/drugfacts/marijuana-medicine

Nestlé Nutrition Institute (2011). MNA® Mini Nutritional Assessment: Overview. Retrieved on 1/30/2016 at: www.mna-elderly.com

New York State Office of Alcoholism and Substance Abuse Services (OASAS). (2015). Elderly alcohol and substance abuse. Retrieved on 12/29/2015 at: www.oasas.ny.gov/AdMed/FYI/FYIInDepth-Elderly.cfm

Rasheed, S., & Woods, R. T. (2014) An investigation into the association between nutritional status and quality of life in older people admitted to hospital. *Journal of Human Nutrition and Dietetics, 27*(2), 142–151.

Sharts-Hopko, N. (2009). Low vision and blindness among midlife and older adults. *Holistic Nursing Practice, 23*(2), 94–100.

Sharts-Hopko, N. C., Smeltzer, S. C., Ott, B. B., et al. (2010). Healthcare experiences of women with visual impairment. *Clinical Nurse Specialist, 24*(3), 149–153.

Shoqirat, N., & Cameron, S. (2013). A qualitative study of hospital patients' understanding of health promotion.*Journal of Clinical Nursing, 22*(19–20), 2714–2722.

Smeltzer, S. C., Sharts-Hopko, N. C., Ott, B. B., et al. (2007). Perspectives of women with disabilities on reaching those who are hard to reach. *Journal of Neuroscience Nursing, 29*(3), 163–171.

U.S. Department of Agriculture. (2016). Dietary guidelines for Americans 2015–2020: Dietary guidelines and My Plate. Retrieved on 1/30/2016 at: www.choosemyplate.gov/dietary-guidelines

U.S. Department of Agriculture (USDA) & U.S. Department of Health & Human Services (HHS). (2016). Dietary guidelines for Americans 2015–2020 (8th ed.). Retrieved on 1/30/2016 at: health.gov/dietaryguidelines/2015/guidelines/

U.S. Department of Health & Human Services (HHS). (2015a). Your health information privacy rights. Retrieved on 12/29/2015 at: www.healthit.gov/patients-families/your-health-information-privacy

U.S. Department of Health & Human Services (HHS). (2015b). Privacy, security, and electronic health records. Retrieved on 12/29/2015 at: www.healthit.gov/buzz-blog/privacy-and-security-of-ehrs/privacy-security-electronic-health-records/

U.S. Department of Health & Human Services (HHS). (2015c). Violence against women. Retrieved on 12/29/2015 at: www.womenshealth.gov/violence-against-women/types-of-violence/domestic-intimate-partner-violence.html

U.S. Food and Drug Administration (FDA). (2014). Trans fat now listed with saturated fat and cholesterol. Retrieved on 12/29/2015 at: www.fda.gov/food/ingredientspackaginglabeling/labelingnutrition/ucm274590.htm

U.S. Food and Drug Administration (FDA). (2015). FDA cuts trans fat in processed foods. Retrieved on 12/29/2015 at: www.fda.gov/downloads/ForConsumers/ConsumerUpdates/UCM451467.pdf

U.S. National Library of Medicine. (2015). National Information Center on Health Services Research and Health Care Technology (NICHSR). Retrieved on 12/29/2015 at: www.nlm.nih.gov/nichsr/

World Health Organization. (2015). Obesity and overweight. Retrieved on 12/29/2015 at: www.who.int/mediacentre/factsheets/fs311/en/

Resources

Academy of Nutrition and Dietetics, www.eatright.org

Adult Children of Alcoholics World Service Organization, www.adult-children.org

Advisory Committee on Immunization Practices (ACIP), Centers for Disease Control and Prevention, National Immunization Program, Division of Epidemiology and Surveillance, www.cdc.gov/vaccines/acip/index.html

Alcoholics Anonymous, www.aa.org

Al-Anon Family Groups, www.al-anon.alateen.org

Center on Addiction and the Family, www.phoenixhouse.org

Co-Anon Family Groups, www.co-anon.org

Cocaine Anonymous, www.ca.org

Dual Recovery Anonymous World Network Central Office, www.draonline.org

American Heart Association, www.heart.org/HEARTORG/#

Genetic Alliance, www.geneticalliance.org

Healthcare Information and Management Systems Society (HIMSS), www.himss.org

Narcotics Anonymous World Services, www.na.org

National Cancer Institute, Cancer Information Service, www.nci.nih.gov or www.cancer.gov

National Council on Alcoholism and Drug Dependence, ncad.org

National Institute on Drug Abuse, /www.drugabuse.gov/

National Organization for Rare Disorders (NORD), www.rarediseases.org/

Online Mendelian Inheritance in Man (OMIM), www.ncbi.nlm.nih.gov/Omim/mimstats.html

Rational Recovery Systems, rational.org/index.php?id=1

Substance Abuse and Mental Health Services Administration (SAMHSA), www.samhsa.gov

UNIT 2

Biophysical and Psychosocial Concepts in Nursing Practice

Case Study   PROVIDING CARE FOR A PATIENT WITH A COMMUNICATION BARRIER

An 80-year-old man whose primary language is Spanish is brought into the emergency department (ED) by his grandson after slipping and falling in the garage. The grandson tells the triage nurse that his grandfather can understand a little bit of English but mainly speaks Spanish. He tells the nurse that his grandfather is allergic to morphine and to make sure that he is not given any. After his grandfather is triaged, the grandson leaves for work. A couple of hours later, the patient is in pain, and the physician orders morphine 5 mg IM. The patient becomes agitated and subsequently goes into respiratory arrest as a result of receiving the medication. He is resuscitated but suffers long-term effects of the hypoxia. A root cause analysis is requested, and the nurse who cared for the patient in the ED is part of the team.

QSEN Competency Focus: Safety

The complexities inherent in today's health care system challenge nurses to demonstrate integration of specific interdisciplinary core competencies. These competencies are aimed at ensuring the delivery of safe, quality patient care (Institute of Medicine, 2003). The Quality and Safety Education for Nurses project (QSEN, 2017; Cronenwett, Sherwood, Barnsteiner, et al., 2007) provides a framework for the knowledge, skills, and attitudes (KSA) required for nurses to demonstrate competency in these key areas, which include *patient-centered care, interdisciplinary teamwork and collaboration, evidence-based practice, quality improvement, safety,* and *informatics.*

Safety Definition: Minimize risk of harm to patients and providers through both system effectiveness and individual performance.

SELECTED PRE-LICENSURE KSAs	APPLICATION AND REFLECTION
Knowledge	
Describe processes used in understanding causes of error and allocation of responsibility and accountability (such as root cause analysis and failure mode effect analysis).	What is a root cause analysis (RCA)? What role does the nurse have as part of this process? What is the intended outcome of an effective RCA?
Skills	
Participate appropriately in analyzing errors and designing system improvements. Engage in root cause analysis rather than blaming when errors or near misses occur.	Upon review of the case it is discovered that the information from the grandson about the medication allergy was not documented in the EMR upon admission. What role could the communication barrier between the patient and staff have played in the error occurring? What processes could be put into place to ensure this documentation is not missed? What should happen to the nurse who had the knowledge and did not document it? How can this become a learning process, without placing blame, in order to improve patient outcomes in future situations?
Attitudes	
Value relationship between national safety campaign and implementation in local practices and practice settings.	Discuss national safety goals that are established to reduce medication errors and adverse drug effects. Think about the level at which these goals are identified and developed. How might a nurse in the ED be part of implementing national safety goals into local practice?

EMR, electronic medical record.

Cronenwett, L., Sherwood, G., Barnsteiner, J., et al. (2007). Quality and safety education for nurses. *Nursing Outlook, 55*(3), 122–131.

Institute of Medicine. (2003). *Health professions education: A bridge to quality.* Washington, DC: National Academies Press.

QSEN Institute. (2017). *QSEN competencies: Definitions and pre-licensure KSAs.* Retrieved on 3/1/2017 at: www.qsen.org/competencies/pre-licensure-ksas

6 Individual and Family Homeostasis, Stress, and Adaptation

LEARNING OBJECTIVES

On completion of this chapter, the learner will be able to:

1 Relate the principles of internal constancy, homeostasis, stress, and adaptation to the concept of steady state.
2 Identify the significance of the body's compensatory mechanisms in promoting adaptation and maintaining the steady state.
3 Compare physical, physiologic, and psychosocial stressors.
4 Describe the general adaptation syndrome as a theory of adaptation to biologic stress.
5 Compare the sympathetic–adrenal–medullary and hypothalamic–pituitary responses to stress.
6 Identify ways in which maladaptive responses to stress can increase the risk of illness and cause disease.
7 Describe the relationship of the process of negative feedback to the maintenance of the steady state.
8 Compare the adaptive processes of hypertrophy, atrophy, hyperplasia, dysplasia, and metaplasia.
9 Describe the inflammatory and reparative processes.
10 Assess the health patterns of a person and families; determine their effects on maintenance of the steady state.
11 Identify individual, family, and group measures that are useful in reducing stress.

GLOSSARY

adaptation: a change or alteration designed to assist in adjusting to a new situation or environment
adrenocorticotropic hormone (ACTH): a hormone produced by the anterior lobe of the pituitary gland that stimulates the secretion of cortisol and other hormones by the adrenal cortex
antidiuretic hormone (ADH): a hormone secreted by the posterior lobe of the pituitary gland that constricts blood vessels, elevates blood pressure, and reduces the excretion of urine
catecholamines: any of the group of amines (such as epinephrine, norepinephrine, or dopamine) that serve as neurotransmitters
coping: the cognitive and behavioral strategies used to manage the stressors that tax a person's resources
disease: an abnormal variation in the structure or function of any part of the body
dysplasia: bizarre cell growth resulting in cells that differ in size, shape, or arrangement from other cells of the same tissue type
family: a group whose members are related by reciprocal caring, mutual responsibilities, and loyalties
fight-or-flight response: the alarm stage in the general adaptation syndrome described by Selye
glucocorticoids: the group of steroid hormones, such as cortisol, that are produced by the adrenal cortex; they are involved in carbohydrate, protein, and fat metabolism and have anti-inflammatory properties

gluconeogenesis: the formation of glucose by the liver from noncarbohydrate sources, such as amino acids and the glycerol portion of fats
guided imagery: the mindful use of a word, phrase, or visual image to achieve relaxation or direct attention away from uncomfortable sensations or situations
homeostasis: a steady state within the body; the stability of the internal environment
hyperplasia: an increase in the number of new cells in an organ or tissue
hypoxia: inadequate supply of oxygen to the cell
inflammation: a localized reaction of tissue to injury, irritation, or infection that is manifested by pain, redness, heat, swelling, and sometimes loss of function
metaplasia: a cell transformation in which one type of mature cell is converted into another type of cell
negative feedback: response that decreases the output of a system
positive feedback: reaction that increases the output of a system
steady state: a stable condition that does not change over time, or when change in one direction is balanced by change in an opposite direction
stress: a disruptive condition that occurs in response to adverse influences from the internal or external environments
stressor: an internal or external event or situation that creates the potential for physiologic, emotional, cognitive, or behavioral changes

When the body is threatened or suffers an injury, its response may involve functional and structural changes; these changes may be adaptive (having a positive effect) or maladaptive (having a negative effect). The defense mechanisms that the body uses determine the difference between adaptation and maladaptation—health and disease. This chapter addresses individual homeostasis, stress, adaptation, health problems associated with maladaptation, and ways that nurses intervene with patients and families to reduce stress and its health-related effects.

Fundamental Concepts

Each body system performs specific functions to sustain optimal life for an organism. Compensatory mechanisms for adjusting internal conditions promote the steady state of the organism, ensure its survival, and restore balance in the body. Pathophysiologic processes result when cellular injury occurs at such a rapid rate that the body's compensatory mechanisms cannot make the adaptive changes necessary to remain healthy.

Physiologic mechanisms must be understood in the context of the body as a whole. Each person has both an internal and external environment, between which information and matter are continuously exchanged. Within the internal environment, each organ, tissue, and cell is also a system or subsystem of the whole, each with its own internal and external environment, each exchanging information and matter (see Fig. 6-1). The goal of the interaction of the body's subsystems is to produce a dynamic balance or **steady state** (even in the presence of change) so that all subsystems are in harmony with each other. Four concepts—constancy, homeostasis, stress, and adaptation—are key to the understanding of steady state.

Constancy and Homeostasis

Claude Bernard, a 19th-century French physiologist, first developed the biologic principle that for life there must be a constancy or "fixity of the internal milieu" despite changes in the external environment. The internal milieu is the fluid that bathed the cells, and the constancy the balanced internal state

maintained by physiologic and biochemical processes. His principle implies a static process.

Bernard's principle of "constancy" underpins the concept of **homeostasis**, which refers to a steady state within the body. When a change or stress occurs that causes a body function to deviate from its stable range, processes are initiated to restore and maintain dynamic balance. An example of this restorative effort is the development of rapid breathing (hyperpnea) after intense exercise in an attempt to compensate for an oxygen deficit and excess lactic acid accumulated in the muscle tissue. When these adjustment processes or compensatory mechanisms are not adequate, steady state is threatened, function becomes disordered, and dysfunctional responses occur. For example, in heart failure, the body reacts by retaining sodium and water and increasing venous pressure, which worsens the condition. Dysfunctional responses can lead to **disease** (an abnormal variation in the structure or function of any part of the body), which is a threat to steady state.

Stress and Adaptation

Stress is a state produced by a change in the environment that is perceived as challenging, threatening, or damaging to a person's dynamic balance or equilibrium. The person may feel unable to meet the demands of the new situation. The change or stimulus that evokes this state is the stressor. A person appraises and copes with changing situations. The desired goal is **adaptation** or adjustment to the change so that the person is again in equilibrium and has the energy and ability to meet new demands. This is the process of **coping** with the stress, a compensatory process that has physiologic and psychological components.

Because both stress and adaptation may exist at different levels of a system, it is possible to study these reactions at the cellular, tissue, and organ levels. Biologists are concerned mainly with subcellular components or with subsystems of the total body. Behavioral scientists, including many nurse researchers, study stress and adaptation in individuals, families, groups, and societies; they focus on how a group's organizational features are modified to meet the requirements of the social and physical environment in which the group exists. In any system, the desired goals of adaptation are survival, growth, and reproduction.

Overview of Stress

Each person operates at a certain level of adaptation and regularly encounters a certain amount of change. Such change is expected; it contributes to growth and enhances life. A stressor can upset this equilibrium. A **stressor** may be defined as an internal or external event or situation that creates the potential for physiologic, emotional, cognitive, or behavioral changes.

Types of Stressors

Stressors exist in many forms and categories. They may be described as physical, physiologic, or psychosocial. Physical stressors include cold, heat, and chemical agents; physiologic stressors include pain and fatigue. An example of a psychosocial stressor is fear (e.g., fear of failing an examination, losing

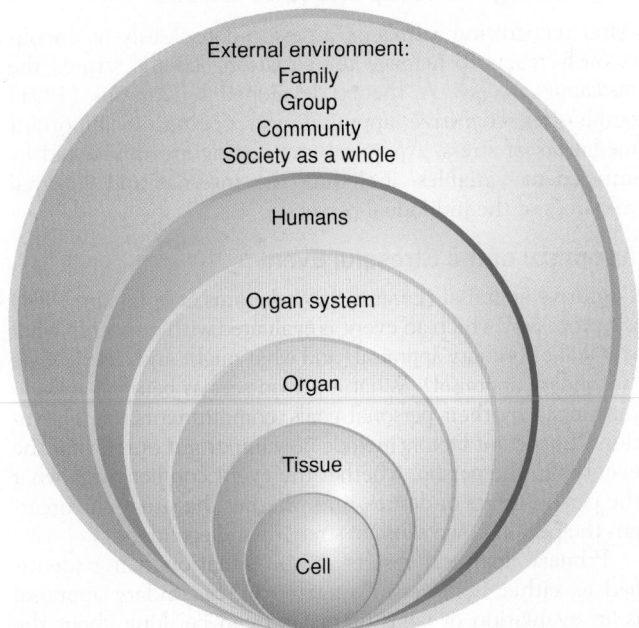

Figure 6-1 • Constellation of systems. Each system is a subsystem of the larger system (suprasystem) of which it is a part. The cells represent the smallest system and are a subsystem of all other systems.

External environment:
Family
Group
Community
Society as a whole

Humans

Organ system

Organ

Tissue

Cell

a job, waiting for a diagnostic test result). Stressors can also occur as normal life transitions that require some adjustment, such as going from childhood into puberty, getting married, or giving birth.

Stressors have also been classified as day-to-day frustrations or hassles, major complex occurrences involving large groups, and stressors that occur less frequently and involve fewer people. Day-to-day stressors include common occurrences as getting caught in a traffic jam, experiencing computer downtime, and having an argument with a spouse or roommate. These experiences vary in effect. For example, encountering a rainstorm while you are vacationing at the beach will most likely evoke a more negative response than it might at another time. These daily hassles have been shown to have a greater health impact than major life events because of the cumulative effect they have over time. They can lead to high blood pressure, palpitations, or other physiologic problems (Schonfels, Brailovskaia, Bieda, et al., 2015).

Major stressors influence larger groups of individuals, families, and sometimes even entire nations. These include events of history, such as terrorism and war, experienced either directly in the war zone or indirectly through live news coverage. The demographic, economic, and technologic changes occurring in society also serve as stressors. The tension produced by any stressor is sometimes a result not only of the change itself but also of the speed with which the change occurs.

Stressors concerning relatively infrequent situations that directly affect people have been studied extensively. This category includes the influence of life events such as death, birth, military service, marriage, divorce, and retirement. It also includes the psychosocial crises that occur in the life cycle stages of the human experience. More enduring chronic stressors may include having a permanent disability or coping with the need to provide long-term care to a developmentally disabled child or a frail older parent.

Duration may also be used to categorize stressors, as in the following:

- An acute, time-limited stressor, such as studying for final examinations
- A stressor sequence—a series of stressful events that result from an initial event such as job loss or divorce
- A chronic intermittent stressor, such as daily hassles
- A chronic enduring stressor that persists over time, such as chronic illness, a disability, or poverty

Stress as a Stimulus for Disease

Relating life events to illness (the theoretical approach that defines stress as a stimulus) has been a major focus of psychosocial studies. Research suggests that people under constant stress have a high incidence of disease (Gallo, Roesch, Fortmann, et al., 2014; Greenberg, Tanev, Marin, et al., 2014).

Holmes and Rahe (1967) developed life events scales that assign numerical values, called *life-change units*, to typical life events. Because the items in the scales reflect events that require a change in a person's life pattern, and stress is viewed as an accumulation of changes in one's life that require psychological adaptation, one can theoretically predict the likelihood of illness by checking off the number of recent events and deriving a total score. The Recent Life Changes Questionnaire (RLCQ)

(Tausig, 1982) contains 118 items such as death, birth, marriage, divorce, promotions, serious arguments, and vacations. The items include both desirable and undesirable events. Both the life events scale and the RLCQ have formed the basis for the development of two additional scales: the Positive–Negative Relationship Quality Scale (PNRQS) (Fincham & Rogge, 2010), which measures stress related to relationship quality, and the Stress Overload Scale (SOS) (Amirkhan, 2012; Amirkhan, Urizar, & Clark, 2015), which measures excessive stress. The underlying premise of the PNRQS and SOS instruments is that sources of stress such as stressful life events and an individual's personal vulnerabilities can influence and even undermine engaging in adaptive processes.

Sources of stress for people have been well researched (Lavoie, 2013; Prince, Chappelle, McDonald, et al., 2015; Shudifat & Al-Husban, 2015). People typically experience distress related to alterations in their physical and emotional health status, changes in their level of daily functioning, and decreased social support or the loss of significant others (Boland, Lee, & Bleck, 2015; Parker, Sricharoenchai, Raparla, et al., 2015; Su, Lau, Mak, et al., 2013; Taylor, 2013). Fears of immobilization, isolation, loneliness, sensory changes, financial problems, and death or disability increase a person's anxiety level. Loss of one's role or perceived purpose in life can cause intense discomfort. Any of these identified variables, plus myriad other conditions or demands, are likely to cause ineffective coping, and a lack of effective coping skills is often a source of additional distress for the person. When a person endures prolonged or unrelenting suffering, the outcome is frequently the development of a stress-related illness. Nurses have the skills to assist people to alter their distressing circumstances and manage their responses to stress, as discussed later in the chapter.

Psychological Responses to Stress

After recognizing a stressor, a person consciously or unconsciously reacts to manage the situation. This is termed the *mediating process*. A theory developed by Lazarus (1991) emphasizes cognitive appraisal and coping as important mediators of stress. Appraisal and coping are influenced by antecedent variables, including the internal and external resources of the individual person.

Appraisal of the Stressful Event

Cognitive appraisal (Lazarus, 1991; Lazarus & Folkman, 1984) is a process by which an event is evaluated with respect to what is at stake (primary appraisal) and what might and can be done (secondary appraisal). What a person sees as being at stake is influenced by their personal goals, commitments, or motivations. Important factors include how important or relevant the event is to the person, whether the event conflicts with what the person wants or desires, and whether the situation threatens the person's own sense of strength and ego identity.

Primary appraisal results in the situation being identified as either nonstressful or stressful. Secondary appraisal is an evaluation of what might and can be done about the situation. Reappraisal—a change of opinion based on new information—may occur. The appraisal process is not necessarily sequential; primary and secondary appraisal and reappraisal may occur simultaneously.

The appraisal process contributes to the development of an emotion. Negative emotions such as fear and anger accompany harm/loss appraisals, and positive emotions accompany challenge. In addition to the subjective component or feeling that accompanies a particular emotion, each emotion also includes a tendency to act in a certain way. For example, unprepared students may view an unexpected quiz as threatening. They might feel fear, anger, and resentment and might express these emotions through hostile behavior or comments.

Lazarus (1991) expanded his initial ideas about stress, appraisal, and coping into a more complex model relating emotion to adaptation. He called this model a "cognitive–motivational–relational theory," with the term *relational* "standing for a focus on negotiation with a physical and social world" (p. 13). A theory of emotion was proposed as the bridge to connect psychology, physiology, and sociology: "More than any other arena of psychological thought, emotion is an integrative, organismic concept that subsumes psychological stress and coping within itself and unites motivation, cognition, and adaptation in a complex configuration" (p. 40).

Coping With the Stressful Event

Coping consists of the cognitive and behavioral efforts made to manage the specific external or internal demands that tax a person's resources and may be emotion-focused or problem-focused. Emotion-focused coping seeks to make the person feel better by lessening the emotional distress. Problem-focused coping aims to make direct changes in the environment so that the situation can be managed more effectively. Both types of coping usually occur in a stressful situation. Even if the situation is viewed as challenging or beneficial, coping efforts may be required to develop and sustain the challenge—that is, to maintain the positive benefits of the challenge and to ward off any threats. In harmful or threatening situations, successful coping reduces or eliminates the source of stress and relieves the emotion generated.

Appraisal and coping are affected by internal characteristics such as health, energy, personal belief systems, commitments, or life goals, self-esteem, control, mastery, knowledge, problem-solving skills, and social skills. The characteristics that have been studied in nursing research are health-promoting lifestyles and resilience (Harper, Bruce, Hosek, et al., 2014; Herrick, Egan, Coulter, et al., 2014; McDonald, Jackson, Wilkes, et al., 2013). Resilience is considered both a personal trait and a process. Researchers have defined resilience as the ability of a person to function well in stressful situations such as traumatic events and other types of adverse situations (Theron, Theron, & Malindi, 2013). A resilient individual maintains flexibility even in difficult circumstances and controls strong emotional reactions using appropriate communication and problem-solving skills. Factors that play a role in building a person's resilience are having strong, supportive relationships with family members and other individuals and being exposed to positive role models. A resilient individual knows when to take action, when to step back and rely on others, and when to stop to re-energize and nurture the self. Researchers have found positive support for resilience as a significant variable that positively influences rehabilitation and overall improvement after a challenging or traumatic experience (Bertisch, Rath, Long,

et al., 2014; Guccione, 2014; Monden, Trost, Catalano, et al., 2014; Muir & Strnadova, 2014; Trief, Sandberg, Dimmock, et al., 2013; Zoellner & Feeny, 2014).

A health-promoting lifestyle buffers the effect of stressors. From a nursing practice standpoint, this outcome—buffering the effect of stressors—supports nursing's goal of promoting health. In many circumstances, promoting a healthy lifestyle is more achievable than altering the stressors.

Physiologic Response to Stress

The physiologic response to a stressor, whether it is physical, psychological, or psychosocial, is a protective and adaptive mechanism to maintain the body's homeostatic balance. When a stress response occurs, it activates a series of neurologic and hormonal processes within the brain and body systems. The duration and intensity of the stress can cause both short- and long-term effects.

Selye Theory of Adaptation

Hans Selye (1976) developed a theory of adaptation to biologic stress that profoundly influenced the scientific study of stress.

General Adaptation Syndrome

Selye theory, called the *general adaptation syndrome* (GAS), has three phases: alarm, resistance, and exhaustion. During the alarm phase, the sympathetic **fight-or-flight response** is activated with release of **catecholamines** and the onset of the **adrenocorticotropic hormone (ACTH)**–adrenal cortical response. The alarm reaction is defensive and anti-inflammatory but self-limited. Because living in a continuous state of alarm would result in death, people move into the second stage—resistance. During the resistance stage, adaptation to the noxious stressor occurs, and cortisol activity is still increased. If exposure to the stressor is prolonged, the third stage—exhaustion—occurs. During the exhaustion stage, endocrine activity increases, which has negative effects on the body systems (especially the circulatory, digestive, and immune systems) that can lead to death. Stages one and two of this syndrome are repeated, in different degrees, throughout life as the person encounters stressors.

Selye compared the GAS with the life process. During childhood, too few encounters with stress occur to promote the development of adaptive functioning, and children are vulnerable. During adulthood, numerous stressful events occur, and people develop resistance or adaptation. During the later years, the accumulation of life's stressors and wear and tear on the organism again decrease people's ability to adapt, resistance falls, and eventually death occurs.

Local Adaptation Syndrome

According to Selye, a local adaptation syndrome also occurs. This syndrome includes the inflammatory response and repair processes that occur at the local site of tissue injury. The local adaptation syndrome occurs in small, topical injuries, such as contact dermatitis. If the local injury is severe enough, the GAS is activated as well.

Selye emphasized that stress is the nonspecific response common to all stressors, regardless of whether they are physiologic, psychological, or psychosocial. The many conditioning factors in each person's environment account for why different demands are experienced by different people as stressors. Conditioning factors also account for differences in the tolerance of different people for stress: Some people may develop diseases of adaptation, such as hypertension and migraine headaches, whereas others are unaffected.

Interpretation of Stressful Stimuli by the Brain

Physiologic responses to stress are mediated by the brain through a complex network of chemical and electrical messages. The neural and hormonal actions that maintain homeostatic balance are integrated by the hypothalamus, which is located in the center of the brain, surrounded by the limbic system and the cerebral hemispheres. The hypothalamus is made up of a number of nuclei and integrates autonomic nervous system mechanisms that maintain the chemical constancy of the internal environment of the body. Together with the limbic system, which contains the amygdala, hippocampus, and septal nuclei, along with other structures, the hypothalamus regulates emotions and many visceral behaviors necessary for survival (e.g., eating, drinking, temperature control, reproduction, defense, aggression).

Each of the brain structures responds differently to stimuli. The cerebral hemispheres are concerned with cognitive functions: thought processes, learning, and memory. The limbic system has connections with both the cerebral hemispheres and the brain stem. In addition, the reticular activating system, a network of cells that forms a two-way communication system, extends from the brain stem into the midbrain and limbic system. This network controls the alert or waking state of the body.

In the stress response, afferent impulses are carried from sensory organs (eye, ear, nose, skin) and internal sensors (baroreceptors, chemoreceptors) to nerve centers in the brain. The response to the perception of stress is integrated in the hypothalamus, which coordinates the adjustments necessary to return to homeostatic balance. The degree and duration of the response vary; initially, there is a sympathetic nervous system discharge, followed by a sympathetic–adrenal–medullary discharge. If the stress persists, the hypothalamic–pituitary system is activated (see Fig. 6-2).

Sympathetic Nervous System Response

The sympathetic nervous system response is rapid and short lived. Norepinephrine is released at nerve endings that are in direct contact with their respective end organs to cause an increase in function of the vital organs and a state of general body arousal (Grossman & Porth, 2014). Heart rate increases and peripheral

Physiology/Pathophysiology

Figure 6-2 • The physiologic response to stress. The body is prepared through brain activation of the autonomic nervous system and psychoneuroendocrine system commonly referred to as the hypothalamus–pituitary–adrenal axis to cope with stress.

vasoconstriction occurs, raising the blood pressure. Blood is also shunted away from abdominal organs. The purpose of these responses is to provide better perfusion of vital organs (brain, heart, skeletal muscles). Blood glucose is increased, supplying more readily available energy. The pupils dilate, and mental activity increases; a greater sense of awareness exists. Constriction of the blood vessels of the skin limits bleeding in the event of trauma. The person is likely to experience cold feet, clammy skin and hands, chills, palpitations, and "knots" in the stomach. Typically, the person appears tense, with the muscles of the neck, upper back, and shoulders tightened; respirations may be rapid and shallow, with the diaphragm tense.

Sympathetic–Adrenal–Medullary Response

In addition to directly affecting major end organs, the sympathetic nervous system stimulates the adrenal medulla to release the hormones epinephrine and norepinephrine into the bloodstream. These hormones act similarly to the sympathetic nervous system, sustaining and prolonging its actions. Because these hormones are catecholamines, they stimulate the nervous system and produce metabolic effects that increase the blood glucose level and metabolic rate. The effect of the sympathetic–adrenal–medullary responses is summarized in Table 6-1. This effect is called the *fight-or-flight response* (Grossman & Porth, 2014).

Hypothalamic–Pituitary Response

The longest-acting phase of the physiologic response, which is more likely to occur in persistent stress, involves the hypothalamic–pituitary pathway. The hypothalamus secretes corticotropin-releasing factor, which stimulates the anterior pituitary to produce ACTH, which in turn stimulates the adrenal cortex to produce **glucocorticoids**, primarily cortisol (Grossman & Porth, 2014). Cortisol stimulates protein catabolism, releasing amino acids; stimulates liver uptake of amino acids and their conversion to glucose (**gluconeogenesis**); and inhibits glucose uptake (anti-insulin action) by many body cells but not those of the brain and the heart (Grossman & Porth, 2014). These cortisol-induced metabolic effects provide the body with a ready source of energy during a stressful situation. This effect has some important implications. For example, a person with diabetes who is under stress, such as that caused by an infection, needs more insulin than usual. Any patient who is under stress (e.g., illness, surgery, trauma,

prolonged psychological stress) catabolizes body protein and needs supplements.

The actions of the catecholamines (epinephrine and norepinephrine) and cortisol are the most important in the general response to stress. Other hormones that play a role are **antidiuretic hormone (ADH)** released from the posterior pituitary and aldosterone released from the adrenal cortex. ADH and aldosterone promote sodium and water retention, which is an adaptive mechanism in the event of hemorrhage or loss of fluids through excessive perspiration. ADH has also been shown to influence learning and may thus facilitate coping in new and threatening situations. Secretion of growth hormone and glucagon stimulates the uptake of amino acids by cells, helping to mobilize energy resources. Endorphins, which are endogenous opioids, increase during stress and enhance the threshold for tolerance of painful stimuli. They may also affect mood and have been implicated in the so-called high that long-distance runners experience. The secretion of other hormones is also affected; however, their adaptive function is less clear.

Immunologic Response

The immune system is connected to the neuroendocrine and autonomic systems. Lymphoid tissue is richly supplied by autonomic nerves capable of releasing a number of different neuropeptides that can have a direct effect on leukocyte regulation and the inflammatory response. Neuroendocrine hormones released by the central nervous system and endocrine tissues can inhibit or stimulate leukocyte function. The various stressors a person experiences may result in different alterations in autonomic activity and subtle variations in neurohormone and neuropeptide synthesis. All of these possible autonomic and neuroendocrine responses can interact to initiate, weaken, enhance, or terminate an immune response.

The study of the relationships among the neuroendocrine system, the central and autonomic nervous systems, and the immune system and the effects of these relationships on overall health outcomes is called *psychoneuroimmunology*. Because one's perception of events and one's coping styles determine whether, and to what extent, an event activates the stress response system, and because the stress response affects immune activity, one's perceptions, ideas, and thoughts can have profound neurochemical and immunologic consequences. Studies have demonstrated

TABLE 6-1 Sympathetic–Adrenal–Medullary Response to Stress or Fight-or-Flight Reaction

Effect	Purpose	Mechanism
Increased heart rate and blood pressure	More perfusion to vital organs	Increased cardiac output owing to increased myocardial contractility and heart rate; increased venous return (peripheral vasoconstriction)
Increased blood glucose level	Increased available energy	Increased liver and muscle glycogen breakdown; increased breakdown of adipose tissue triglycerides
Mental acuity	Alert state	Increase in amount of blood shunted to the brain from the abdominal viscera and skin
Dilated pupils	Increased awareness	Contraction of radial muscle of iris
Increased tension of skeletal muscles	Preparedness for activity, decreased fatigue	Excitation of muscles; increase in amount of blood shunted to the muscles from the abdominal viscera and skin
Increased ventilation (may be rapid and shallow)	Provision of oxygen for energy	Stimulation of respiratory center in medulla; bronchodilation
Increased coagulability of blood	Prevention of hemorrhage in event of trauma	Vasoconstriction of surface vessels

altered immune function in people who are under stress (Jain & Chandel, 2013; Polloni, 2015; Schwitalla, 2014). Other studies have identified certain personality traits, such as decisiveness, assertiveness, compassion, helpfulness, and conscientiousness, as having positive effects on health (Hankonen, Konttinen, & Absetz, 2014; Jokela, Pulkki-Raback, Elovaino, et al., 2014; Skodova & Lajciakova, 2013). As research continues, this field of study will likely uncover to what extent and by what mechanisms people can consciously influence their immunity.

Maladaptive Responses to Stress

The stress response, as indicated earlier, facilitates adaptation to threatening situations and is retained from humans' evolutionary past. The fight-or-flight response, for example, is an anticipatory response that mobilized the bodily resources of our ancestors to deal with predators and other harsh factors in their environment. This same mobilization comes into play in response to emotional stimuli unrelated to danger. For example, a person may get an "adrenaline rush" when competing over a decisive point in a ball game or when excited about attending a party.

When responses to stress are ineffective, they are referred to as *maladaptive*. Maladaptive responses are chronic, recurrent responses or patterns of response that do not promote the goals of adaptation. The goals of adaptation are somatic or physical health (optimal wellness); psychological health or having a sense of well-being (happiness, satisfaction with life, morale); and enhanced social functioning, which includes work, social life, and family (positive relationships). Maladaptive responses that threaten these goals include faulty appraisals and inappropriate coping (Lazarus, 1991).

The frequency, intensity, and duration of stressful situations contribute to the development of emotions and subsequent patterns of neurochemical discharge. By appraising situations adequately and coping appropriately, it is possible to anticipate and defuse some of these situations. For example, frequent stressful encounters (e.g., marital discord) might be avoided with better communication and problem solving, or a pattern of procrastination (e.g., delaying work on tasks) could be corrected to reduce stress when deadlines approach.

Coping processes that include the use of alcohol or drugs to reduce stress increase the risk of illness. Other inappropriate coping patterns may increase the risk of illness less directly. For example, people who demonstrate "type A" behaviors, including impatience, competitiveness, and achievement orientation, have an underlying aggressive approach to life and are more prone than others to develop stress-related illnesses. Type A behaviors increase the output of catecholamines, the adrenal–medullary hormones, with their attendant effects on the body. Additional forms of inappropriate coping include denial, avoidance, and distancing.

Models of illness frequently include stress and maladaptation as precursors to disease. A general model of illness, based on Selye theory, suggests that any stressor elicits a state of disturbed physiologic equilibrium. If this state is prolonged or the response is excessive, it increases the susceptibility of the person to illness. This susceptibility, coupled with a predisposition in the person (from genetic traits, health, or age), leads to illness. If the sympathetic–adrenal–medullary response is prolonged or excessive, a state of chronic arousal develops that may lead to high blood pressure, arteriosclerotic changes,

and cardiovascular disease. If the production of ACTH is prolonged or excessive, behavior patterns of withdrawal and depression are seen. In addition, the immune response is decreased and infections and tumors may develop.

Selye (1976) proposed a list of disorders known as diseases of maladaptation: high blood pressure (including hypertension of pregnancy), diseases of the heart and blood vessels, diseases of the kidney, rheumatic diseases and inflammatory diseases of the skin and eyes, infections, allergic and hypersensitivity diseases, nervous and mental diseases, sexual dysfunction, digestive diseases, metabolic diseases, and cancer. Research continues on the complex interconnections between stress, coping (adaptive and maladaptive), and disease (Akyil & Erguney, 2013; Barre, Padmaja, Saxena, et al., 2015; Cevik & Erguney, 2013; Epel, 2014; McVicar, Ravalier, & Greenwood, 2014; Smith, Fortune, Phillips, et al., 2014).

Indicators of Stress

Indicators of stress and the stress response include both subjective and objective measures. Chart 6-1 lists signs and symptoms that may be observed directly or reported by a person. They are psychological, physiologic, or behavioral and

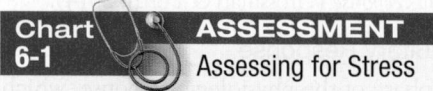

Chart 6-1	ASSESSMENT

Assessing for Stress

Be alert for the following:

Bruxism (grinding of teeth)
Changes in menstrual cycle
Change in appetite
Concentration difficulties
Diarrhea
Difficulty sleeping
Dry mouth
Emotional lability
Excessive perspiration
Fatigue
Feeling weak or dizzy
Gastrointestinal distress
Headaches
Hyperactivity
Increased substance use or abuse
Increased use of tobacco
Increased body tension
Intense or increased anxiety
Impulsive behaviors
Loss of interest in life activities
Nausea or vomiting
Nervous habits
Nervous laughter
Overpowering urge to act out
Pain in back, neck, or other parts of the body
Palpitations
Prone to injury
Restlessness
Strong startle response
Tremors
Unintentional weight loss or gain
Urinary frequency

Adapted from Rice, V. H. (Ed.). (2012). *Handbook of stress, coping, and health: Implications for theory, research, and practice* (2nd ed.). Thousand Oaks, CA: Sage; Selye, H. (1976). *The stress of life* (Rev. ed.). New York, NY: McGraw-Hill.

reflect social behaviors and thought processes. Some of these reactions may be coping behaviors. Over time, each person tends to develop a characteristic pattern of behavior during stress to warn that the system is out of balance.

Laboratory measurements of indicators of stress have helped in understanding this complex process. Blood and urine analyses can be used to demonstrate changes in hormonal levels and hormonal breakdown products. Blood levels of catecholamines, glucocorticoids, ACTH; and eosinophils are reliable measures of stress. Serum cholesterol and free fatty acid levels can be used to measure stress. When the body experiences distress, levels of adrenal hormones such as cortisol and aldosterone increase and additional cholesterol is released simultaneously into the general circulation. Both physical and psychological distress can trigger an elevated cholesterol level. In addition, the results of immunoglobulin assays are increased when a person is exposed to various stressors, especially infections and immunodeficiency conditions. With greater attention to the field of neuroimmunology, improved laboratory measures are likely to follow.

In addition to using laboratory tests, researchers have developed questionnaires to identify and assess stressors, stress, and coping strategies. The work of Rice (2012) includes a compilation of information gained from research on stress, coping, and health, and includes some of these questionnaires.

Stress at the Cellular Level

The cell exists on a continuum of function and structure, ranging from the normal cell, to the adapted cell, to the injured or diseased cell, to the dead cell (see Fig. 6-3). Changes from one state to another may occur rapidly and may not be readily detectable, because each state does not have discrete boundaries, and disease represents disruption of normal processes. The earliest changes occur at the molecular or subcellular level and are not perceptible until steady-state functions or structures are altered. With cell injury, some changes may be reversible; in other instances, the injuries are lethal. For example, tanning of the skin is an adaptive, morphologic response to exposure to the rays of the sun. However, if the exposure is continued, sunburn and injury occur, and some cells may die, as evidenced by desquamation ("peeling").

Different cells and tissues respond to stimuli with different patterns and rates of response, and some cells are more vulnerable to one type of stimulus or stressor than others. The cell involved, its ability to adapt, and its physiologic state are determinants of the response. For example, cardiac muscle cells respond to **hypoxia** (inadequate oxygenation) more quickly than do smooth muscle cells.

Other determinants of cellular response are the type or nature of the stimulus, its duration, and its severity. For example, neurons that control respiration can develop a tolerance to regular, small amounts of a barbiturate; however, one large dose may result in respiratory depression and death.

Control of the Steady State

The concept of the cell as existing on a continuum of function and structure includes the relationship of the cell to compensatory mechanisms, which occur continuously in the body to maintain the steady state. Compensatory processes are regulated primarily by the autonomic nervous system and the endocrine system, with control achieved through negative feedback.

Negative Feedback

Negative feedback mechanisms throughout the body monitor the internal environment and restore homeostasis when conditions shift out of the normal range. These mechanisms sense deviations from a predetermined set point or range of adaptability and trigger a response to offset the deviation. Functions regulated through such compensatory mechanisms include blood pressure, acid–base balance, blood glucose level, body temperature, and fluid and electrolyte balance.

Most of the human body's control systems are integrated by the brain with feedback from the nervous and endocrine systems. Control activities involve detecting deviations from the predetermined reference point and stimulating compensatory responses in the muscles and glands of the body. The major organs affected are the heart, lungs, kidneys, liver, gastrointestinal tract, and skin. When stimulated, these organs alter their rate of activity or the amount of secretions they produce. Because of this, these major organs are considered the "organs of homeostasis or adjustment" (Grossman & Porth, 2014).

In addition to the responses influenced by the nervous and endocrine systems, local responses consisting of small feedback loops in a group of cells or tissues occur. The cells detect a change in their immediate environment and initiate an action to counteract its effect. For example, the accumulation of lactic acid in an exercised muscle stimulates dilation of blood vessels in the area to increase blood flow and improve the delivery of oxygen and removal of waste products.

The net result of negative feedback loops is homeostasis. A steady state is achieved by the continuous, variable action of the organs involved in making the adjustments and by the continuous exchange of chemical substances among cells, interstitial fluid, and blood. For example, an increase in the carbon dioxide (CO_2) concentration of the extracellular fluid leads to increased pulmonary ventilation, which decreases the CO_2 level. On a cellular level, increased CO_2 raises the hydrogen ion concentration of the blood. This is detected by chemosensitive receptors in the brain's medullary respiratory control center. The chemoreceptors then stimulate an increase in the rate of discharge of the neurons that innervate

Physiology/Pathophysiology

Figure 6-3 • The cell on a continuum of function and structure. Changes in the cell are not as easily discerned as the diagram depicts, and the point at which compensation subsides and pathophysiology begins is not clearly defined.

the diaphragm and intercostal muscles, which increases the respiratory rate. Excess CO_2 is exhaled, the hydrogen ion concentration returns to normal, and the chemically sensitive neurons are no longer stimulated (Grossman & Porth, 2014).

Positive Feedback

Another type of feedback, **positive feedback**, perpetuates the chain of events set in motion by the original disturbance instead of compensating for it. As the system becomes more unbalanced, disorder and disintegration occur. There are some exceptions to this; blood clotting in humans, for example, is an important positive feedback mechanism.

Cellular Adaptation

Cells are complex units that dynamically respond to the changing demands and stresses of daily life. They possess a maintenance function and a specialized function. The maintenance function refers to the activities that the cell performs with respect to itself; specialized functions are those that the cell performs in relation to the tissues and organs of which it is a part. Individual cells may cease to function without posing a threat to the organism. However, as the number of dead cells increases, the specialized functions of the tissues are altered and health is threatened.

Cells can adapt to environmental stress through structural and functional changes. Some of these adaptations include cellular hypertrophy, atrophy, hyperplasia, dysplasia, and metaplasia. Such adaptations reflect changes in the normal cell in response to stress. If the stress is unrelenting, cellular injury and death may occur.

Hypertrophy and atrophy lead to changes in the size of cells and hence the size of the organs they form. Compensatory hypertrophy is the result of an enlarged muscle mass and commonly occurs in skeletal and cardiac muscle that experiences a prolonged, increased workload. One example is the bulging muscles of an athlete.

Atrophy can be the consequence of disease, decreased use, decreased blood supply, loss of nerve supply, or inadequate nutrition. Disuse of a body part is often associated with the aging process and immobilization. Cell size and organ size decrease, and the structures principally affected are the skeletal muscles, the secondary sex organs, the heart, and the brain.

Hyperplasia is an increase in the number of new cells in an organ or tissue. As cells multiply and are subjected to increased stimulation, the tissue mass enlarges. This mitotic response (a change occurring with mitosis) is reversible when the stimulus is removed. This distinguishes hyperplasia from neoplasia or malignant growth, which continues after the stimulus is removed. Hyperplasia may be hormonally induced. An example is the increased size of the thyroid gland caused by thyroid-stimulating hormone (secreted from the pituitary gland) when a deficit in thyroid hormone occurs.

Dysplasia is bizarre cell growth resulting in cells that differ in size, shape, or arrangement from other cells of the same tissue type. Dysplastic cells have a tendency to become malignant; dysplasia is seen commonly in epithelial cells in the bronchi of people who smoke.

Metaplasia is a cell transformation in which one type of mature cell is converted into another type of cell. This serves a protective function, because less-transformed cells are more resistant to the stress that stimulated the change. For example, the ciliated columnar epithelium lining the bronchi of people who smoke is replaced by squamous epithelium. The squamous cells can survive; loss of the cilia and protective mucus, however, can have damaging consequences.

Cellular Injury

Injury is defined as a disorder in steady-state regulation. Any stressor that alters the ability of the cell or system to maintain optimal balance of its adjustment processes leads to injury. Structural and functional damage then occurs, which may be reversible (permitting recovery) or irreversible (leading to disability or death). Homeostatic adjustments are concerned with the small changes within the body's systems. With adaptive changes, compensation occurs and a new steady state may be achieved. With injury, steady-state regulation is lost and changes in functioning ensue.

Causes of disorder and injury in the system (cell, tissue, organ, body) may arise from the external or internal environment (see Fig. 6-4) and include **hypoxia**, nutritional imbalance, physical agents, chemical agents, infectious agents, immune mechanisms, and genetic defects. The most common causes are **hypoxia** (oxygen deficiency), chemical injury, and infectious agents. In addition, the presence of one injury makes the system more susceptible to another injury. For example, inadequate oxygenation and nutritional deficiencies make the system vulnerable to infectious agents. These agents damage or destroy the integrity of the cell membrane (necessary for ionic balance) as well as the cell's ability to:

- Transform energy (aerobic respiration, production of adenosine triphosphate)
- Synthesize enzymes and other necessary proteins
- Grow and reproduce (genetic integrity)

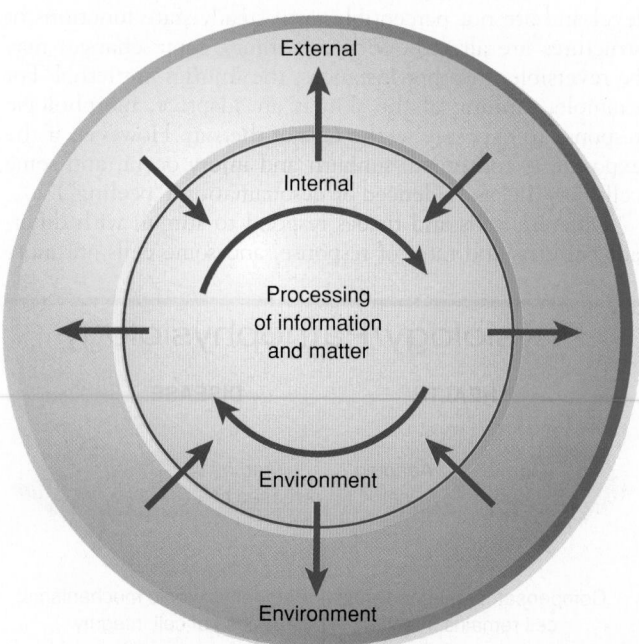

Figure 6-4 • Influences leading to disorder may arise from the internal and external environments of the system. Excesses or deficits of information and matter may occur, or there may be faulty regulation of processing.

Hypoxia

Inadequate cellular oxygenation (**hypoxia**) interferes with the cell's ability to transform energy. Hypoxia may be caused by a decrease in blood supply to an area, a decrease in the oxygen-carrying capacity of the blood (decreased hemoglobin), a ventilation–perfusion or respiratory problem that reduces the amount of arterial oxygen available, or a problem in the cell's enzyme system that makes it unable to use oxygen.

The usual cause of hypoxia is ischemia or deficient blood supply. Ischemia is commonly seen in myocardial cell injury in which arterial blood flow is decreased because of atherosclerotic narrowing of blood vessels. Ischemia also results from intravascular clots (thrombi or emboli) that may form and interfere with blood supply. Thromboemboli are common causes of cerebrovascular disease (strokes). The length of time in which different tissues can survive without oxygen varies. For example, brain cells most often succumb in 3 to 6 minutes. If the condition leading to hypoxia is slow and progressive, collateral circulation may develop, whereby blood is supplied by other blood vessels in the area. However, this mechanism is not highly reliable.

Nutritional Imbalance

Nutritional imbalance refers to a relative or absolute deficiency or excess of one or more essential nutrients. This may be manifested as undernutrition (inadequate consumption of food or calories) or overnutrition (caloric excess). Caloric excess to the point of obesity overloads cells in the body with lipids. By requiring more energy to maintain the extra tissue, obesity places a strain on the body and has been associated with the development of disease, especially pulmonary and cardiovascular disease. (See Chapter 48 for further discussion of obesity.)

Specific deficiencies arise when an essential nutrient is deficient or when a nutrient imbalance exists. Protein deficiencies and avitaminosis (deficiency of vitamins) are typical examples. An energy deficit leading to cell injury can occur if there is insufficient glucose or insufficient oxygen to transform the glucose into energy. A lack of insulin, or the inability to use insulin, may also prevent glucose from entering the cell from the blood. This occurs in diabetes, a metabolic disorder that can lead to nutritional deficiency, as well as a host of short- and long-term life-threatening complications. (See Chapter 51 for further discussion of diabetes.)

Physical Agents

Physical agents, including temperature extremes, radiation, electrical shock, and mechanical trauma, can cause injury to the cells or to the entire body. The duration of exposure and the intensity of the stressor determine the severity of damage.

Temperature

When a person's temperature is elevated, hypermetabolism occurs and the respiratory rate, heart rate, and basal metabolic rate increase. With fever induced by infections, the hypothalamic thermostat may be reset at a higher temperature and then return to normal when the fever abates. The increase in body temperature is achieved through physiologic mechanisms. Body temperatures greater than 41°C (106°F) indicate hyperthermia, because the physiologic function of the thermoregulatory center breaks down and the temperature soars (Grossman

& Porth, 2014). This physiologic condition occurs in people who have heat stroke. Eventually, the high temperature causes coagulation of cell proteins, and cells die.

The local response to burn injury is similar. Increased metabolic activity occurs, and, as heat increases, proteins coagulate and enzyme systems are destroyed. In extreme situations, charring or carbonization occurs. (See Chapter 62 for more information about burn injuries.)

Extreme low temperature, or cold, cause vasoconstriction. Blood flow becomes sluggish and clots form, leading to ischemic damage in the involved tissues. With still lower temperatures, ice crystals may form and cells may burst.

Radiation and Electrical Shock

Radiation is used for diagnosis and treatment of diseases. Ionizing forms of radiation may cause injury by their destructive action. Radiation decreases the protective inflammatory response of the cell, creating a favorable environment for opportunistic infections. Electrical shock produces burns as a result of the heat generated when electrical current travels through the body. It may also abnormally stimulate nerves, leading, for example, to fibrillation of the heart.

Mechanical Trauma

Mechanical trauma can result in wounds that disrupt the cells and tissues of the body. The severity of the wound, amount of blood loss, and extent of nerve damage are significant factors in determining the extent of injury.

Chemical Agents

Chemical injuries are caused by poisons, such as lye, that have a corrosive action on epithelial tissue, or by heavy metals, such as mercury, arsenic, and lead, each of which has its own specific destructive action. Many other chemicals are toxic in certain amounts, in certain people, and in specific tissues. For example, excessive secretion of hydrochloric acid can damage the stomach lining; large amounts of glucose can cause osmotic shifts, affecting the fluid and electrolyte balance; and too much insulin can cause subnormal levels of glucose in the blood (hypoglycemia) and can lead to coma.

Drugs, including prescribed medications, can also cause chemical poisoning. Some people are less tolerant of medications than others and manifest toxic reactions at the usual or customary dosages. Aging tends to decrease tolerance to medications. Polypharmacy (taking many medications at one time) occurs frequently in older adults, and the unpredictable effects of the resulting medication interactions can cause injury.

Alcohol (ethanol) is also a chemical irritant. In the body, alcohol is broken down into acetaldehyde, which has a direct toxic effect on liver cells that leads to various liver abnormalities, including cirrhosis in susceptible people. Disordered liver cell function leads to complications in other organs of the body.

Infectious Agents

Biologic agents known to cause disease in humans are viruses, bacteria, rickettsiae, mycoplasmas, fungi, protozoa, and nematodes. The severity of the infectious disease depends on the number of microorganisms entering the body, their virulence, and the host's defenses (e.g., health, age, immune responses).

An infection exists when the infectious agent is living, growing, and multiplying in the tissues and is able to overcome the body's normal defenses. Some bacteria, such as those that cause tetanus and diphtheria, produce exotoxins that circulate and create cell damage. Others, such as gram-negative bacteria, produce endotoxins when they die. Tubercle bacilli induce an immune reaction.

Viruses are among the smallest living organisms known and survive as parasites of the living cells they invade. Viruses infect specific cells. Through a complex mechanism, viruses replicate within cells and then invade other cells, where they continue to replicate. As the body mounts an immune response to eliminate the viruses, cells harboring the viruses can be injured in the process. Typically, an inflammatory response and immune reaction are the body's physiologic responses to viral infection.

Disordered Immune Responses

The immune system is an exceedingly complex system, the purpose of which is to defend the body from invasion by any foreign object or foreign cell type, such as cancerous cells. This is a steady-state mechanism; however, like other adjustment processes, it can become disordered and cellular injury results. The immune response detects foreign bodies by distinguishing nonself substances from self substances and destroying the nonself entities. The entrance of an antigen (foreign substance) into the body evokes the production of antibodies that attack and destroy the antigen (antigen–antibody reaction).

The immune system may function normally, or it may be hypoactive or hyperactive. When it is hypoactive, immunodeficiency diseases occur; when it is hyperactive, hypersensitivity disorders occur. A disorder of the immune system can result in damage to the body's own tissues. Such disorders are labeled autoimmune diseases (see Unit 8).

Genetic Disorders

There is intense interest in genetic defects as causes of disease and modifiers of genetic structure. Many of these defects produce mutations that have no recognizable effect, such as lack of a single enzyme; others contribute to more obvious congenital abnormalities, such as Down syndrome. (For further information on genetics, see Chapter 8.)

Cellular Response to Injury: Inflammation

Cells or tissues of the body may be injured or killed by any of the agents (physical, chemical, infectious) described earlier. When this happens, an inflammatory response (or inflammation) naturally occurs in the healthy tissues adjacent to the site of injury. **Inflammation** is a localized reaction intended to neutralize, control, or eliminate the offending agent to prepare the site for repair. It is a nonspecific response (not dependent on a particular cause) that is meant to serve a protective function. For example, inflammation may be observed at the site of a bee sting, in a sore throat, in a surgical incision, and at the site of a burn. Inflammation also occurs in cell injury events, such as stroke, deep vein thrombosis, and myocardial infarction.

Inflammation is not the same as infection. An infectious agent is only one of several agents that may trigger an inflammatory response. Regardless of the cause, a general sequence of events occurs in the local inflammatory response. This sequence involves changes in the microcirculation, includ-

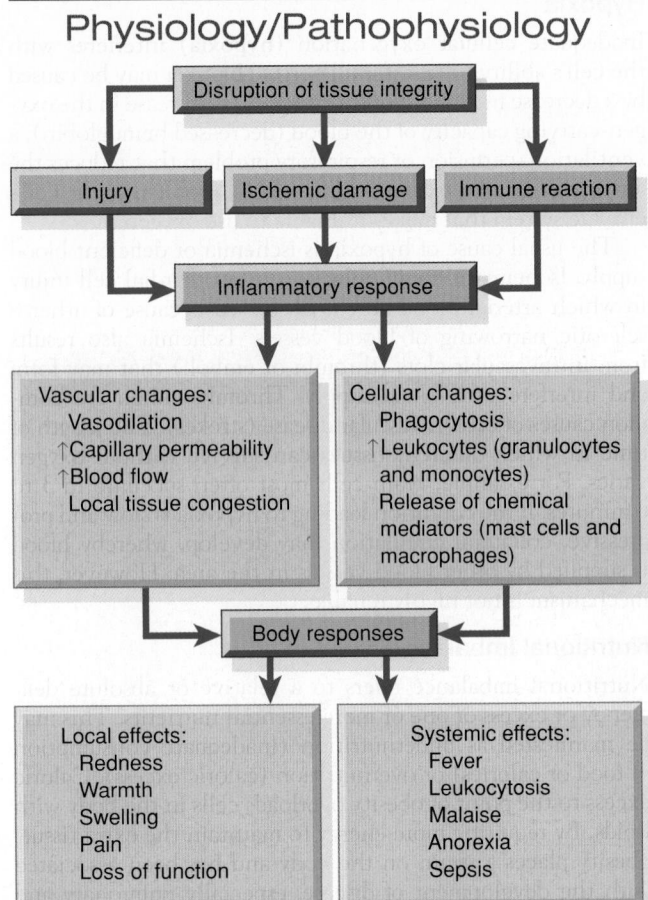

Physiology/Pathophysiology

Figure 6-5 • Inflammatory response.

ing vasodilation, increased vascular permeability, and leukocytic cellular infiltration (see Fig. 6-5). As these changes take place, five cardinal signs of inflammation are produced: redness, warmth, swelling, pain, and loss of function.

The transient vasoconstriction that occurs immediately after injury is followed by vasodilation and an increased rate of blood flow through the microcirculation to the area of tissue damage. Local warmth and redness result. Next, the structure of the microvascular system changes to accommodate the movement of plasma protein from the blood into the tissues. Following this increase in vascular permeability, plasma fluids (including proteins and solutes) leak into the inflamed tissues, producing swelling. Leukocytes migrate through the endothelium and accumulate in the tissue at the site of the injury. The pain that occurs is attributed to the pressure of fluids or swelling on nerve endings and to the irritation of nerve endings by chemical mediators released at the site. Bradykinin is one of the chemical mediators suspected of causing pain. Loss of function is most likely related to the pain and swelling; however, the exact mechanism is not completely known.

As blood flow increases and fluid leaks into the surrounding tissues, the formed elements (red blood cells, white blood cells, and platelets) remain in the blood, causing it to become more viscous. Leukocytes (white blood cells) collect in the vessels, exit, and migrate to the site of injury to engulf offending organisms and to remove cellular debris in a process called *phagocytosis*. Fibrinogen in the leaked plasma fluid coagulates, forming fibrin for clot formation, which serves to wall off the injured area and prevent the spread of infection.

Chemical Mediators of Inflammation

Injury initiates the inflammatory response; however, chemical substances released at the site induce vascular changes. Foremost among these chemicals are histamine and kinins. Histamine is present in many tissues of the body but is concentrated in the mast cells. It is released when injury occurs and is responsible for the early changes in vasodilation and vascular permeability. Kinins cause vasodilation and increased vascular permeability, and they attract neutrophils to the area. Prostaglandins—another group of chemical substances—are also suspected of causing increased vascular permeability (Grossman & Porth, 2014).

Systemic Response to Inflammation

The inflammatory response is often confined to the site, causing only local signs and symptoms. However, systemic responses can also occur. Fever is the most common sign of a systemic response to injury, and it is most likely caused by endogenous pyrogens (internal substances that cause fever) released from neutrophils and macrophages (specialized forms of leukocytes). These substances reset the hypothalamic thermostat, which controls body temperature, and produce fever. Leukocytosis, an increase in the synthesis and release of neutrophils from bone marrow, may occur, enhancing the body's ability to fight infection. During this process, general, nonspecific symptoms develop, including malaise, loss of appetite, aching, and weakness.

Types of Inflammation

Inflammation is categorized primarily by its duration and the type of exudate produced. It is most often acute or chronic. Acute inflammation is characterized by the local vascular and exudative changes described previously and usually lasts less than 2 weeks. An acute inflammatory response is immediate and serves a protective function. After the causative agent is removed, the inflammation subsides and healing takes place with the return of normal or near-normal structure and function.

Chronic inflammation develops if the injurious agent persists and the acute response is perpetuated. Symptoms are present for many months or years. Chronic inflammation may also begin insidiously and never have an acute phase. The chronic response does not serve a beneficial and protective function; on the contrary, it is debilitating and can produce long-lasting effects. As the inflammation becomes chronic, changes occur at the site of injury, and the nature of the exudate becomes proliferative. A cycle of cellular infiltration, necrosis, and fibrosis begins, with repair and breakdown occurring simultaneously. Considerable scarring may occur, resulting in permanent tissue damage.

Cellular Healing

The reparative process begins at approximately the same time as the injury. Healing proceeds after the inflammatory debris has been removed. Healing may occur by regeneration, in which the defect is gradually repaired by proliferation of the same type of cells as those destroyed, or by replacement, in which cells of another type, usually connective tissue, fill in the tissue defect and result in scar formation.

Regeneration

The ability of cells to regenerate depends on whether they are labile, permanent, or stable. Labile cells multiply constantly to replace cells worn out by normal physiologic processes; these include epithelial cells of the skin and those lining the gastrointestinal tract. Permanent cells include neurons—the nerve cell bodies, not their axons. Destruction of neurons is permanent; however, axons may regenerate. If normal activity is to return, tissue regeneration must occur in a functional pattern, especially in the growth of several axons. Stable cells in some organ systems have a latent ability to regenerate. Under normal physiologic processes, they are not shed and do not need replacement; if they are damaged or destroyed, they are able to regenerate. Examples include functional cells of the kidney, liver, and pancreas. Cells in other organs, such as the brain, for example, do not regenerate.

Replacement

The condition of the host, the environment, and the nature and severity of the injury affect the processes of inflammation, repair, and replacement. Depending on the extent of damage, repair and replacement may occur by first-, second-, or third-intention healing. In first-intention healing, the wound edges are approximated, as in a surgical wound (see Chapter 19). Little scar formation occurs, and the wound healing occurs without granulation. In second-intention healing, the edges are not approximated and the wound fills with granulation tissue. The process of repair takes longer and may result in scar formation, with loss of specialized function. For example, people who have recovered from myocardial infarction have abnormal electrocardiographic tracings because the electrical signal cannot be conducted through the connective tissue that has replaced the infarcted area. In third-intention healing, the wound edges are not approximated and healing is delayed.

Nursing Management

Stress or the potential for stress is ubiquitous—that is, it is both everywhere and anywhere. Indeed, nursing students experience stressors that can negatively affect their academic and clinical performance (Shudifat & Al-Husban, 2015) (see Chart 6-2). Anxiety, frustration, anger, and feelings of inadequacy, helplessness, or powerlessness are emotions often associated with stress. In the presence of these emotions, the customary activities of daily living may be disrupted—for example, a sleep disturbance may occur, eating and activity patterns may be altered, and family processes or role performance may be disrupted.

Nurses must know that the optimal point of intervention to promote health is during the stage when a person's own compensatory processes are still functioning effectively. A major role of nurses is the early identification of both physiologic and psychological stressors. Nurses should be able to relate the presenting signs and symptoms of distress to the physiology they represent and identify a person's position on the continuum of function, from health and compensation to pathophysiology and disease.

In the assessment of people who seek health care, both objective signs and subjective symptoms are the primary

Chart 6-2   **NURSING RESEARCH PROFILE**
Perceived Sources of Stress Among Nursing Students

Shudifat, R. M., & Al-Husban, R. Y. (2015). Perceived sources of stress among first-year nursing students in Jordan. *Journal of Psychosocial Nursing, 53*(6), 37–43.

Purpose

The main purpose of this study was to determine the most common sources of stress experienced among first-year nursing students attending a military college in the country of Jordan. An additional purpose was to examine the nature of the identified stressors.

Design

This descriptive cross-sectional study used the Student Stress Survey, a 40-item survey instrument, to obtain information on four categories of stress: interpersonal, intrapersonal, academic, and environmental. The survey was given to a convenience sample of 138 first-year nursing students who were enrolled in a college under the auspices of the Jordanian government. The students were from all the various geographical areas of Jordan. All participants lived on the college campus, wore military attire, and followed both academic and military training schedules.

Findings

All of the participants were female whose ages ranged from 18 to 22 years, with the mean age being 19 years. The identified five major sources of stress experienced were increased workload (98%), change in living environment (83%), change in social activities (78%), change in eating habits (77.5%), and change in sleeping habits (76%). The most prevalent interpersonal source

of stress was change in social activities, and the least frequent interpersonal stress reported was trouble with parents. The intrapersonal stressors reported by slightly more than 76% of the students were changes in eating and sleeping habits. Sources of intrapersonal stress least reported were financial difficulties. An increase in workload was the top academic stressor indicated, and the second most common academic stressor was receiving a grade lower grade than the one anticipated. The most frequently reported environmental stressor was the change in living environment, while the least reported was divorce between parents.

Nursing Implications

Nurse educators, administrative officers, and student support staff at the college level must recognize the extent to which stress can negatively affect a student's academic and work performance. Since stress in nursing students will consistently be present, the faculty and administrators must implement strategies to minimize it. This study revealed that academic and environmental sources of stress were the most common, thereby necessitating that the college include stress management and stress reduction strategies as a part of the orientation program. Additional reinforcement of stress management programs throughout the students' academic lives was also suggested. Furthermore, faculty and other college officials who interact with students must freely discuss how to access assistance when students experience stressful situations or other difficulties. It would also be helpful to encourage the students to integrate recreational activities into their daily lives to alleviate stress and to promote relaxation.

---

indicators of existing physiologic processes. The following questions are addressed:

- Are the heart rate, respiratory rate, and temperature normal?
- What emotional distress may be contributing to the patient's health problems?
- Are there other indicators of steady-state deviation?
- What are the patient's blood pressure, height, and weight?
- Are there any problems in movement or sensation?
- Are there any problems with affect, behavior, speech, cognitive ability, orientation, or memory?
- Are there obvious impairments, lesions, or deformities?

Objective evidence can be obtained from laboratory data, such as electrolytes, blood urea nitrogen, blood glucose, and urinalysis results. Further signs of injury are seen in diagnostic studies such as computed tomography scanning, magnetic resonance imaging, and positron emission tomography. Further information on diagnostic evaluation can be found in assessment chapters of each unit of this book. Many nursing diagnoses are possible for patients suffering from stress. One nursing diagnosis related to stress is anxiety, which is defined as a vague, uneasy feeling, the source of which may be nonspecific or not known to the person. Stress may also be manifested as ineffective coping patterns, impaired thought processes, or disrupted relationships. These human responses are reflected in the nursing diagnoses of anxiety, ineffective coping, defensive coping, and ineffective denial, all of which indicate poor adaptive responses (Herdman & Kamitsuri,

2015). Other possible nursing diagnoses include social isolation, risk for spiritual distress, readiness for enhanced family processes, decisional conflict, risk for compromised resilience, impaired resilience, readiness for enhanced resilience, and risk for powerlessness, among others. Because human responses to stress are varied, as are the sources of stress, arriving at an accurate diagnosis allows interventions and goals to be more specific and leads to improved outcomes.

Stress management is directed toward reducing and controlling stress and improving coping. The need to prevent illness, improve the quality of life, and decrease the cost of health care makes efforts to promote health essential, and stress control a significant health promotion goal. Stress reduction methods and coping enhancements can derive from either internal or external sources. For example, healthy eating habits and relaxation techniques are internal resources that help reduce stress, and a broad social network is an external resource that helps reduce stress. Goods and services that can be purchased are also external resources for stress management. It may be easier for people with adequate financial resources to cope with constraints in the environment, because their sense of vulnerability to threat is decreased compared to those without adequate financial resources.

Promoting a Healthy Lifestyle

A health-promoting lifestyle provides internal resources that aid in coping, and it buffers or cushions the impact of stressors. Lifestyles or habits that contribute to the risk of illness

---

Chart 6-3

Information Addressed in Health Risk Questionnaires

Demographic data: age, gender, race, ethnic background
Personal and family history of diseases and health problems

Lifestyle choices:

- Eating, sleeping, exercise, smoking, drinking, sexual activity, recreation activity, and driving habits
- Stressors at home and on the job
- Roles, role relationships, and associated stressors
- Living and family situation
- Social and family supports

Physical measurements:

- Blood pressure
- Height, weight, body mass index
- Laboratory analyses of blood and urine

Participation in high-risk behaviors (e.g., engaging in unprotected sexual intercourse, not using seat belts while riding in a motor vehicle, using illicit drugs)

---

can be identified through a health risk appraisal, which is an assessment method designed to promote health by examining a person's habits and recommending changes when a health risk is identified.

Health risk appraisals involve the use of health risk questionnaires to estimate the likelihood that people with a given set of characteristics will become ill. People who receive this information may be influenced to adopt healthy behaviors (e.g., stop smoking, have periodic screening examinations) to improve their health. Questionnaires typically address the information presented in Chart 6-3.

The personal information is compared with average population risk data, and the risk factors are identified and weighted. From this analysis, a person's risks and major health hazards are identified. Further comparisons with population data can estimate how many years will be added to a person's lifespan if the suggested changes are made. However, research has not yet demonstrated that providing people with such information ensures that they will change their behaviors. The single most important factor for determining health status is social class, and within a social class, research suggests that the major factor influencing health is level of education (Bastable, Gramet, Jacobs, et al., 2014).

Enhancing Coping Strategies

Bulechek, Butcher, Dochterman, and colleagues (2013) identified "coping enhancement" as a nursing intervention and defined it as "managing perceived stressors, changes, or threats that interfere with meeting life demands and roles" (p. 133) (see Chart 6-4). The nurse can build on the patient's existing coping strategies, as identified in the health appraisal, or teach new strategies for coping if necessary.

The five predominant ways of coping with illness identified in a review of 57 nursing research studies were as follows (Jalowiec, 1993):

- Trying to be optimistic about the outcome
- Using social support
- Using spiritual resources
- Trying to maintain control either over the situation or over feelings
- Trying to accept the situation

Chart 6-4

Coping Enhancement: Nursing Interventions

Definition

Facilitation of cognitive and behavioral efforts to manage perceived stressors, changes, or threats that interfere with meeting life demands and roles.

Selected Activities

Assist the patient in identifying appropriate short- and long-term goals.

Assist the patient to solve problems in a constructive manner.

Provide factual information concerning diagnosis, treatment, and prognosis.

Encourage an attitude of realistic hope as a way of dealing with feelings of helplessness.

Acknowledge the patient's spiritual/cultural background, and encourage the use of spiritual resources if desired.

Foster constructive outlets for anger and hostility.

Assist the patient in examining available resources to meet goals.

Appraise the needs and desires for social support, and assist the patient to identify available support systems.

Assist the patient to identify positive strategies to deal with limitations, manage needed lifestyle or role changes, and work through the losses of chronic illness and/or disability if appropriate.

Adapted from Bulechek, G. M., Butcher, H. K., Dochterman, J. M., & Wagner, C. M. (Eds.). (2013). *Nursing interventions classification (NIC)* (6th ed.). St. Louis, MO: Mosby-Elsevier.

Other ways of coping included seeking information, reprioritizing needs and roles, lowering expectations, making compromises, comparing oneself to others, planning activities to conserve energy, taking things one step at a time, listening to one's body, and using self-talk for encouragement.

Unfolding Patient Stories: Skyler Hansen • Part 1

Skyler Hansen is an 18-year-old male recently diagnosed with type 1 diabetes. He lives with his parents and two younger siblings and is active in high school sports. He now requires insulin injections, glucose monitoring, and a diabetic diet. Examine how the psychological, physical, and teaching needs for managing a new diagnosis can be a great source of stress to the patient and the family. How can the nurse enhance his ability to cope with and adapt to diabetes management? (Skyler Hansen's story continues in Chapter 51.)

Care for Skyler and other patients in a realistic virtual environment: **vSim *for Nursing*** (**thepoint.lww.com/vSimMedicalSurgical**). Practice documenting these patients' care in DocuCare (**thepoint.lww.com/DocuCareEHR**).

Relaxation Techniques

Relaxation techniques are a major method used to relieve stress. The goal of relaxation training is to produce a response that counters the stress response. When this goal is achieved, the action of the hypothalamus adjusts, decreasing sympathetic and parasympathetic nervous system activity. The sequence of physiologic effects and their signs and symptoms are then interrupted, thus reducing psychological stress.

This is a learned response and requires practice to achieve. Commonly used techniques include progressive muscle relaxation, the Benson relaxation response, and relaxation with **guided imagery** (all discussed later). Other relaxation techniques include meditation, breathing techniques, massage, Reiki, music therapy, biofeedback, and the use of humor.

The different relaxation techniques share four similar elements: (1) a quiet environment, (2) a comfortable position, (3) a passive attitude, and (4) a mental device (something on which to focus one's attention, such as a word, phrase, or sound).

Progressive Muscle Relaxation

Progressive muscle relaxation involves tensing and releasing the muscles of the body in sequence and sensing the difference in feeling. It is best if the person lies on a soft cushion in a quiet room, breathing easily. Someone usually reads the instructions in a low tone in a slow and relaxed manner, or a recording of the instructions may be played. The person tenses the muscles in the entire body (one muscle group at a time), holds, senses the tension, and then relaxes. As each muscle group is tensed, the person keeps the rest of the body relaxed. Each time the focus is on feeling the tension and relaxation. When the exercise is completed, the entire body should be relaxed (Benson, 1993; Benson & Stark, 1996).

The Benson Relaxation Response

The Benson relaxation response (see Chart 6-5) combines meditation with relaxation. Along with the repeated word or phrase, a passive demeanor is essential. If other thoughts or distractions (noises, pain) occur, Benson recommends not fighting the distraction but simply continuing to repeat the focus phrase. Time of day is not important; however, the exercise works best on an empty stomach (Benson, 1993; Benson & Proctor, 1984; Benson & Stark, 1996).

Guided Imagery

Simple **guided imagery** is the mindful use of a word, phrase, or visual image for the purpose of distracting oneself from distressing situations or consciously taking time to relax or re-energize. A nurse can help a person select a pleasant scene or experience, such as watching the ocean or dabbling the feet in a cool stream. The image serves as the mental device in this technique. As the person sits comfortably and quietly, the nurse guides the person to review the scene, trying to feel

and relive the imagery with all of the senses. A recording may be made of the description of the image, or commercial recordings for guided imagery and relaxation can be used.

Educating About Stress Management

Two commonly prescribed nursing educational interventions—providing sensory information and providing procedural information (e.g., preoperative education)—aim to reduce stress and improve the patient's coping ability. This preparatory education includes giving structured content, such as a lesson in childbirth preparation to expectant parents, a review of how an implantable cardioverter defibrillator works to a patient with heart disease, or a description of sensations a patient will experience during cardiac catheterization. These techniques may alter the person–environment relationship such that something that might have been viewed as harmful or a threat will now be perceived more positively. Giving patients information also reduces the emotional response so that they can concentrate and solve problems more effectively (Christaki, Kokkinos, Costarelli, et al., 2013; Kells, Rogers, Oppenheimer, et al., 2013; Miller & Stoeckel, 2016).

Promoting Family Health

In addition to individual concepts of homeostasis, stress, adaptation, and health problems associated with maladaptation, the concept of family is also important. Nurses can intervene with both individuals and families to reduce stress and its health-related effects. The **family** (group whose members are related by reciprocal caring, mutual responsibilities, and loyalties) plays a central role in the life of the patient and is a major part of the context of the patient's life. It is within families that people grow, are nurtured, acquire a sense of self, develop beliefs and values about life, and progress through life's developmental stages (see Fig. 6-6). Families are also the first source for socialization and teaching about health and illness.

Ideally, the health care team conducts a careful and comprehensive family assessment (including coping style), develops interventions tailored to handle the stressors, implements the specified treatment protocols, and facilitates the construction of social support systems. The use of existing family

---

Chart 6-5 The Benson Relaxation Response

1. Pick a brief phrase or word that reflects your basic belief system.
2. Choose a comfortable position.
3. Close your eyes.
4. Relax your muscles.
5. Become aware of your breathing and start using your selected focus word.
6. Maintain a passive demeanor.
7. Continue for a set period of time.
8. Practice the technique twice daily.

Adapted from Benson, H. (1993). The relaxation response. In D. Goleman & J. Gurin (Eds.), *Mind-body medicine: How to use your mind for better health.* Yonkers, NY: Consumer Reports Books.

Figure 6-6 • Within families, individuals progress through life's developmental stages.

strengths, resources, and education is augmented by therapeutic family interventions. The primary goals of the nurse are to maintain and improve the patient's present level of health and to prevent physical and emotional deterioration. Next, the nurse intervenes in the cycle that the illness creates: patient illness, stress for other family members, new illness in other family members, and additional patient stress.

Helping the family members manage the myriad stressors that bombard them daily involves working with family members to develop coping skills. Seven traits that enhance coping of family members under stress have been identified (Burr, Klein, Burr, et al., 1994). Communication skills and spirituality were frequently useful traits. Cognitive abilities, emotional strengths, relationship capabilities, willingness to use community resources, and individual strengths and talents were also associated with effective coping. As nurses work with families, they must not underestimate the impact of their therapeutic interactions, educational information, positive role modeling, provision of direct care, and education on promoting health. Maladaptive coping may result if health care team members are not perceived as actively supporting family members. Often, denial and blaming of others occur. Sometimes, physiologic illness, emotional withdrawal, and physical distancing are the results of severe family conflict, violent behavior, or addiction to drugs and alcohol. Substance abuse may develop in family members who feel unable to cope or solve problems. People may engage in these dysfunctional behaviors when faced with difficult or problematic situations.

Enhancing Social Support

The nature of social support and its influence on coping have been studied extensively. Social support has been demonstrated to be an effective moderator of life stress. Such support has been found to provide people with several different types of emotional information (Carpenter, Carpenter, Kimbel, et al., 2015; Cho, Jae, Choo, et al., 2014; Duax, Bohnert, Rausch, et al., 2014). The first type of information leads people to believe that they are cared for and loved. This emotional support appears most often in a relationship between two people in which mutual trust and attachment are expressed by helping one another meet their emotional needs. The second type of information leads people to believe that they are esteemed and valued. This is most effective when others in a group recognize a person's favorable position within that group, demonstrating the individual's value. Known as esteem support, this elevates the person's sense of self-worth. The third type of information leads people to feel that they belong to a network of communication and mutual obligation. Members of this network share information and make goods and services available to the members as needed.

Social support also facilitates a person's coping behaviors; however, this depends on the nature of the social support. People can have extensive relationships and interact frequently; however, the necessary support comes only when people feel a deep level of involvement and concern, not when they merely touch the surface of each other's lives. The critical qualities within a social network are the exchange of intimate communications and the presence of solidarity and trust.

Emotional support from family and significant others provides love and a sense of sharing the burden. The emotions that accompany stress are unpleasant and often increase in a spiraling fashion if relief is not provided. Being able to talk with someone and express feelings openly may help a person gain mastery of the situation. Nurses can provide this support but also must identify the person's social support system and encourage its use. People who are "loners," who are isolated, or who withdraw in times of stress have a high risk of coping failure.

Because anxiety can also distort a person's ability to process information, it helps to seek information and advice from others who can assist with analyzing the threat and developing a strategy to manage it. Again, this use of others helps people maintain mastery of a situation and self-esteem.

Thus, social networks assist with management of stress by providing people with:

- A positive social identity
- Emotional support
- Material aid and tangible services
- Access to information
- Access to new social contacts and new social roles

Recommending Support and Therapy Groups

Support groups exist especially for people in similar stressful situations. Groups have been formed by people with ostomies; women who have had mastectomies; and people with cancer or other serious diseases, chronic illnesses, and disabilities. There are groups for single parents, substance abusers and their family members, homicide bereavement, and victims of child abuse. Professional, civic, and religious support groups are active in many communities (Hundt, Robinson, Arney, et al., 2015; Wittenberg-Lyles, Goldsmith, & Reno, 2014; Wnuk, 2015). Encounter groups, assertiveness training programs, and consciousness-raising groups help people modify their usual behaviors in their transactions with their environment. Many find that being a member of a group with similar problems or goals has a releasing effect that promotes freedom of expression and exchange of ideas.

The Role of Stress in Health Patterns

As noted previously, a person's psychological and biologic health, internal and external sources of stress management, and relationships with the environment are predictors of health outcomes. These factors are directly related to the person's health patterns. The nurse has a significant role and responsibility in identifying the health patterns of patients receiving care as well as those of their families. If those patterns are not achieving physiologic, psychological, and social balance, the nurse is obligated, with the assistance and agreement of the patient, to seek ways to promote individual and family balance.

This chapter has presented some physiologic mechanisms and perspectives on health and disease, the way that one copes with stress. Nurses should keep in mind that the way that one relates to others and the values and goals held are also interwoven into those physiologic patterns. To evaluate a patient's health patterns and to intervene if a disorder exists requires a total assessment of the person. Specific disorders and their nursing management are addressed in greater depth in other chapters.

CRITICAL THINKING EXERCISES

1 `ebp` A male college student with a 3-week history of difficulty hearing in class makes an appointment with the nurse at the health center to discuss his distress and fear about losing his hearing. The student states, "I've been very stressed about this situation. What do I say to my three roommates when they have the music on very loud throughout our apartment? I've been afraid to say anything to my friends. Do you think this is serious or am I just getting a cold or an ear infection?" What is the evidence base for offering health promotion information, auditory health screening, and stress management options to help this young adult make appropriate health decisions and establish positive health behaviors? Identify the criteria used to evaluate the strength of the evidence for this practice.

2 A 40-year-old female pharmaceutical sales representative has a history of experiencing urticaria (hives) prior to giving company presentations. She tells the employee health nurse that the frequency of hives is increasing and her workload is also increasing. She is now doing bimonthly presentations and feels very anxious about these projects. What factors influence the relationship between stress and developing hives? What health promotion practices can be implemented in constructing stress management practices and a relaxation program to help decrease the patient's anxious feelings associated with giving presentations?

3 `pq` A 74-year-old man recently became a widower, stopped driving a car, and has moved from his home to a retirement community. He depends on his extended family members to provide for his transportation and shopping needs. He has hypertension and thyroid and coronary artery diseases. This patient has become increasingly sad since moving to his new home. Identify the priorities, approach, and techniques that you would use to assess this patient's health promotion needs.

REFERENCES

*Asterisk indicates nursing research.
**Double asterisk indicates classic reference.

Books

Bastable, S., Gramet, P., Jacobs, K., et al. (2014). *Health professional as educator: Principles of teaching and learning.* Sudbury, MA: Jones & Bartlett.

**Benson, H. (1993). The relaxation response. In D. Goleman & J. Gurin (Eds.), *Mind-body medicine: How to use your mind for better health.* Yonkers, NY: Consumer Reports Books.

**Benson, H., & Proctor, W. (1984). *Beyond the relaxation response.* New York, NY: Berkley Books.

**Benson, H., & Stark, M. (1996). *Timeless healing.* New York, NY: Scribner.

Bulechek, G. M., Butcher, H. K. K., Dochterman, J. M., & Wagner, C. M. (Eds.). (2013). *Nursing interventions classification (NIC)* (6th ed.). St. Louis, MO: Elsevier.

**Burr, W., Klein, S., Burr, R., et al. (1994). *Reexamining family stress: New theory and research.* Thousand Oaks, CA: Sage.

Grossman, S. C., & Porth, C. M. (2014). *Pathophysiology. Concepts of altered health status* (9th ed.). Philadelphia, PA: Lippincott Williams & Wilkins.

Herdman, T. H., & Kamitsuri, S. (2015). *NANDA International nursing diagnoses: Definitions and classification 2015–2017* (10th ed.). Oxford: Wiley-Blackwell.

**Jalowiec, A. (1993). Coping with illness: Synthesis and critique of the nursing literature from 1980–1990. In J. D. Barnfather & B. L. Lyon (Eds.), *Stress and coping: State of the science and implications for nursing theory, research, and practice.* Indianapolis, IN: Sigma Theta Tau International.

**Lazarus, R. S. (1991). *Emotion and adaptation.* New York, NY: Oxford University Press.

**Lazarus, R. S., & Folkman, S. (1984). *Stress, appraisal, and coping.* New York, NY: Springer.

Miller, M. A., & Stoeckel, P. R. (2016). *Client education: Theory and practice* (2nd ed.). Sudbury, MA: Jones & Bartlett.

Rice, V. H. (Ed.). (2012). *Handbook of stress, coping, and health: Implications for theory, research, and practice* (2nd ed.). Thousand Oaks, CA: Sage.

**Selye, H. (1976). *The stress of life* (Rev. ed.). New York, NY: McGraw-Hill.

Zoellner, L. A., & Feeny, N. C. (Eds.). (2014). *Facilitating resilience and recovery following trauma.* New York, NY: Guilford Press.

Journals and Electronic Documents

*Akyil, R. C., & Erguney, S. (2013). Roy's adaptation model-guided education for adaptation to chronic obstructive pulmonary disease. *Journal of Advanced Nursing, 69*(5), 1063–1075.

*Amirkhan, J. H. (2012). Stress overload: A new approach to the assessment of stress. *American Journal of Community Psychology, 49*(1–2), 55–71.

*Amirkhan, J. H., Urizar G. G., & Clark, S. (2015). Criterion validation of a stress measure: The Stress Overload Scale. *Psychological Assessment, 27*(3), 985–996.

*Barre, V. P., Padmaja, G., Saxena, R. K., et al. (2015). Impact of medical interventions on stress and quality of life in patients with cancer. *Indian Journal of Palliative Care, 21*(2), 203–208.

Bertisch, H., Rath, L., Long, C., et al. (2014). Positive psychology in rehabilitation: A brief report. *Neurorehabilitation and Neural Repair, 34,* 573–585.

Boland, T. A., Lee, V. H., & Bleck, T. P. (2015). Stress-induced cardiomyopathy. *Critical Care Medicine, 43*(3), 686–693.

*Carpenter, G. S., Carpenter, T. P., Kimbel, N. A., et al. (2015). Social support, stress, and suicidal ideation in professional firefighters. *American Journal of Health Behavior, 39*(2), 191–196.

*Cevik, R. C., & Erguney, S. (2013). Roy's adaptation model-guided education for adaptation to chronic obstructive pulmonary disease. *Journal of Advanced Nursing, 69*(5), 1063–1075.

Cho, J. H., Jae, S. Y., Choo, I. H., et al. (2014). Health-promoting behavior among women with abdominal obesity: A conceptual link to social support and perceived stress. *Journal of Advanced Nursing, 70*(6), 1381–1390.

*Christaki, E., Kokkinos, A., Costarelli, V., et al. (2013). Stress management can facilitate weight loss in Greek overweight and obese women: A pilot study. *Journal of Human Nutrition and Dietetics, 26*(1), 132–139.

*Duax, J. M., Bohnert, K. M., Rauch, S. A., et al. (2014). Posttraumatic stress disorder symptoms, levels of social support, and emotional hiding in returning veterans. *Journal of Rehabilitation Research and Development, 51*(4), 571–578.

Epel, E. (2014). Stress biology and aging mechanisms: Toward understanding the deep connection between adaptation to stress and longevity. *The Journal of Gerontology Series A: Biological Sciences, 69*(1), S1–S10.

Fincham, F. D., & Rogge, R. (2010). Understanding relationship quality: Theoretical challenges and new tools for assessment. *Journal of Family Theory and Review, 2,* 227–242.

*Gallo, L. C., Roesch, S. C., Fortmann, A. L., et al. (2014). Associations of chronic stress burden, perceived stress, and traumatic stress with cardiovascular disease prevalence and risk factors in the Hispanic community health study/study of Latinos sociocultural ancillary study. *Journal of Biobehavioral Medicine, 76*(6), 401–475.

*Greenberg, M. S., Tanev, K., Marin, M., et al. (2014). Stress, PTSD, and dementia. *Alzheimer's & Dementia, 10,* S155–S165.

Guccione, A. A. (2014). Resilience and self-efficacy as mediators of quality of life in geriatric rehabilitation. *Topics in Geriatric Rehabilitation, 30*(3), 164–169.

*Hankonen, N., Konttinen, H., & Absetz, P. (2014). Gender-related personality traits, self-efficacy, and social support: How do they relate to women's waist circumference change? *Journal of Health Psychology, 19*(10), 1291–1301.

*Harper, G. W., Bruce, D., Hosek, S. G., et al. (2014). Resilience processes demonstrated by gay and bisexual men living with HIV: Implications for intervention. *AIDS Patient Care and STDs, 28*(12), 666–676.

Herrick, A. L., Egan, J. E., Coulter, R. W., et al. (2014). Raising sexual minority youths' health levels by incorporating resiliencies into health promotion efforts. *American Journal of Public Health, 104*(2), 206–210.

**Holmes, T. H., & Rahe, R. H. (1967). The social readjustment rating scale. *Journal of Psychosomatic Research, 11*, 213–218.

*Hundt, N. E., Robinson, A., Arney, J., et al. (2015). Veterans' perspectives on benefits and drawbacks of peer support for posttraumatic stress disorder. *Military Medicine, 180*(8), 851–856.

Jain, M., & Chandel, N. S. (2013). Rethinking antioxidants in the intensive care unit. *American Journal of Respiratory Care Medicine, 188*(11), 1283–1285.

*Jokela, M., Pulkki-Raback, L., Elovaino, M., et al. (2014). Personality traits as risk factors for stroke and coronary heart disease mortality: Pooled analysis of three cohort studies. *Journal of Behavioral Medicine, 37*, 881–889.

Kells, M., Rogers, J., Oppenheimer, S. C., et al. (2013). The teachable moment captured: A framework for nurse-led smoking cessation interventions for parents of hospitalized children. *Public Health Nursing, 30*(5), 468–473.

*Lavoie, J. A. (2013). Eye of the beholder: Perceived stress, coping style, and coping effectiveness among discharged psychiatric patients. *Archives of Psychiatric Nursing, 27*, 185–190.

*McDonald, G., Jackson, D., Wilkes, L., et al. (2013). Personal resilience in nurses and midwives: Effects of a work-based educational intervention. *Contemporary Nurse, 45*(1), 134–143.

McVicar, A., Ravalier, J. M., & Greenwood, C. (2014). Biology of stress revisited: Intracellular mechanisms and the conceptualization of stress. *Stress and Health, 30*(4), 272–279.

*Monden, K. R., Trost, Z., Catalano, D., et al. (2014). Resilience following spinal cord injury: A phenomenological view. *Spinal Cord, 52*, 197–201.

Muir, K., & Strnadova, I. (2014). Whose responsibility? Resilience in families of children with developmental disabilities. *Disability and Society, 29*(6), 922–937.

Parker, I. M., Sricharoenchai, T., Raparla, S., et al. (2015). Posttraumatic stress disorder in critical illness survivors: A metaanalysis. *Critical Care Medicine, 43*(5), 1121–1129.

*Polloni, L. (2015). Perinatal stress and food allergy: A preliminary study on maternal reports. *Psychology, Health and Medicine, 20*(6), 732–741.

*Prince, L., Chappelle, W. L., McDonald, K. D., et al. (2015). Reassessment of psychological distress and post-traumatic stress disorder in United States Air Force distributed common ground system operators. *Military Medicine, 180*(3), 171–178.

Schonfels, P., Brailovskaia, J. Bieda, A., et al. (2015). The effects of daily stress on positive and negative mental health: Mediation through self-efficacy. *International Journal of Clinical and Health Psychology, 28*(3), 256–266.

Schwitalla, S. (2014). Tumor cell plasticity: The challenge to catch a moving target. *Journal of Gastroenterology, 49*, 618–627.

*Shudifat, R. M., & Al-Husban, R. Y. (2015). Perceived sources of stress among first-year nursing students in Jordan. *Journal of Psychosocial Nursing, 53*(6), 37–43.

*Skodova, Z., & Lajciakova, P. (2013). The effect of personality traits and psychosocial training on burnout syndrome among healthcare students. *Nurse Education Today, 33*, 1311–1315.

*Smith, A., Fortune, Z., Phillips, R., et al. (2014). UPBEAT study patients' perceptions of the effect of coronary heart disease on their lives: A cross-sectional sub-study. *International Journal of Nursing Studies, 51*, 1500–1506.

*Su, X., Lau, J. T., Mak, W. W., et al. (2013). Perceived discrimination, social support, and perceived stress among people living with HIV/AIDS in China. *AIDS Care, 25*(2), 239–248.

**Tausig, M. (1982). Measuring life events. *Journal of Health and Social Behavior, 23*(1), 52–64.

*Taylor, C. J. (2013). Physiological stress response to loss of social influence and threats to masculinity. *Social Science & Medicine, 103*, 51–59.

*Theron, L. C., Theron, A. M., & Malindi, M. J. (2013). Toward an African definition of resilience: A rural South African community's view of resilient Basotho youth. *Journal of Black Psychology, 39*(1), 63–87.

*Trief, P. M., Sandberg, J. G., Dimmock, J. A., et al. (2013). Personal and relationship challenges of adults with type 1 diabetes. *Diabetes Care, 36*, 2483–2488.

*Wittenberg-Lyles, E., Goldsmith, J., & Reno, J. (2014). Perceived benefits and challenges of an oncology nurse support group. *Clinical Journal of Oncology Nursing, 18*(4), 71–76.

*Wnuk, M. (2015). Religious-spiritual sources of hope and the meaning of life in alcohol co-dependent subjects receiving support in self-help groups. *Journal of Substance Use, 20*(3), 194–199.

Resources

A.D.A.M. Inc.: Stress, adam.about.com/reports/Stress.htm
American Holistic Nurses Association (AHNA), www.ahna.org
Anxiety and Depression Association of America (ADAA), www.adaa.org
Grief Recovery Institute, www.griefrecoverymethod.com
Help Guide: A Nonprofit Guide to Mental Health and Well Being, www.helpguide.org/articles/stress/stress-management.htm
Inflammation—The Key to Chronic Disease, www.womentowomen.com/inflammation/default.aspx
Institute of HeartMath: Connecting Hearts and Minds, www.heartmath.org
Learnthat: How to Cope With Stress—Stress Management Tutorial and Exercises, learnthat.com/2004/11/stress-management-and-relief
National Hospice and Palliative Care Organization (NHPCO), www.nhpco.org
Physiological Stress Response: Its Effects on the Body, www.stressfocus.com/stress_focus_article/physiological-stress-effects.htm
Psych Central: Tips to Decrease Stress, http://psychcentral.com/lib/20-tips-to-tame-your-stress/
Stress: The Silent Killer, holisticonline.com/stress/stress_GAS.htm
The Compassionate Friends, www.compassionatefriends.org
The Psychology of "Stress," www.guidetopsychology.com/stress.htm
Widowed Persons Service, 3950 Ferrara Dr., Silver Spring, MD; 1-301-949-7398; www.wpsgr.org/

7 Overview of Transcultural Nursing

LEARNING OBJECTIVES

On completion of this chapter, the learner will be able to:

1 Identify key components of cultural assessment.
2 Apply transcultural nursing principles, concepts, and theories when providing nursing care to individuals, families, groups, and communities.
3 Develop strategies for planning, providing, and evaluating culturally competent nursing care for patients from diverse backgrounds.

4 Critically analyze the influence of culture on nursing care decisions and actions for patients.
5 Discuss the impact of diversity and health care disparities on health care delivery.

GLOSSARY

culture: the knowledge, belief, art, morals, laws, customs, and any other capabilities and habits acquired by humans as members of society

cultural awareness or sensitivity: being alert to and having knowledge of cultural preferences, aspects, or perspectives that may impact the health care experience, including communication, personal choices, or other elements

cultural humility: acknowledging one's cultural knowledge deficits using self-reflection, continuous self-evaluation, and consultation with others (including patients) to detect barriers to culturally competent care and address bias, or lack of knowledge or skills related to a culture other than one's own, to provide culturally appropriate care

cultural nursing assessment: a systematic appraisal or examination of individuals, families, groups, and communities in terms of their cultural beliefs, values, and practices

culturally competent nursing care: effective, individualized care that demonstrates respect for the dignity, personal rights, preferences, beliefs, and practices of the person receiving care while acknowledging the biases of the caregiver and preventing these biases from interfering with the care provided

culturally congruent nursing care: nursing care that is customized to fit each person's cultural values, beliefs, traditions, practices, and lifestyle

ethnocentrism: making a value judgment on another culture from the vantage point of one's own culture

minority: a group of people whose physical or cultural characteristics differ from the dominant culture or majority of people in a society

subculture: relatively large groups of people who share characteristics that identify them as a distinct entity

transcultural nursing: providing nursing care to patients and families across cultural variations

In the health care delivery system, as in society, nurses interact with people of similar as well as diverse cultural backgrounds. People may have different frames of reference and varied preferences regarding their health and health care needs, depending on their cultures. Nurses must practice **transcultural nursing**, which is defined as providing care to patients and families across cultural variations. Acknowledging, respecting, and adapting to the cultural needs of patients, families, and communities are important components of nursing care in any health care setting. In addition, facilitating access to culturally appropriate health care is critical to ensure holistic nursing care. To plan and deliver culturally appropriate and competent care, nurses must understand the language of culture, culturally appropriate care, and cultural competence and the various aspects of culture that should be explored for each patient.

Cultural Concepts

The concept of culture and its relationship to the health care beliefs and practices of the patient and their family or significant others provide the foundation for transcultural nursing. This awareness of culture in the delivery of nursing care has been described in different terms and phrases, including respect for cultural diversity or cultural humility; cultural awareness or sensitivity; comprehensive care; or culturally congruent nursing care (Holland, 2015; Leininger, 2002; Mixer, McFarland, Andrews, et al., 2013).

Culture is commonly defined as the knowledge, belief, art, morals, laws, customs, and any other capabilities and habits acquired by humans as members of society. During the past century, many other definitions of culture have been offered that integrate these themes as well as the themes of ethnic variations of a population based on race, nationality, religion, language, physical characteristics, and geography. In particular, ethnicity, race, and minority status are words that are often used to describe key components of culture, but these words do not fully encompass the meaning of the concept of culture (Marzilli, 2014). Culture also implies that something is learned or developed, a process that occurs over time. Madeleine Leininger (2002), founder of the specialty known as transcultural nursing, writes that culture involves learned and transmitted knowledge about values, beliefs, rules of behavior, and lifestyle practices that guide designated groups in their thinking and actions in patterned ways. Culture guides each person's thinking, doing, and being, and becomes patterned expressions of who that person is and becomes.

Ethnic culture has four basic characteristics:

- It is learned from birth through language and socialization.
- It is shared by members of the same cultural group, and it includes an internal sense and external perception of distinctiveness.
- It is influenced by specific conditions related to environmental and technical factors and to the availability of resources.
- It is dynamic and ever changing.

With the exception of the first characteristic, culture related to age, physical appearance, and lifestyle, as well as other less frequently acknowledged aspects, also shares these characteristics.

Cultural diversity has also been defined in several ways. Often, differences in skin color, religion, and geographic area are the routine elements used to identify diversity, with ethnic minorities being considered the primary sources of cultural diversity. However, many other sources of cultural diversity exist. To truly acknowledge an increasingly culturally diverse population, the nurse must be prepared for and able to work with patients in a way that recognizes and respects their diversity (McClimens, Brewster, & Lewis, 2014).

Cultural humility—addressing one's cultural knowledge deficit(s) by exploring the patient's needs from the patient's cultural perspective and exploring one's own cultural beliefs and how they might conflict with the patient's beliefs—is a critical step toward becoming culturally competent. Cultural humility requires a commitment to learning that considers each individual's unique viewpoint (Isaacson, 2014). It implies that while we cannot be competent in another's culture, we may learn our own biases through self-reflection, thereby, becoming open to others' cultures. Cultural humility requires active listening and encourages self-reflection and self-awareness (Isaacson, 2014).

Subcultures

Although culture is a universal phenomenon, it takes on specific and distinctive features for a particular group because it encompasses all of the knowledge, beliefs, customs, and skills acquired by the members of that group. When such groups function within a larger cultural group, they are referred to as subcultures.

The term **subculture** is used for relatively large groups of people who share characteristics that identify them as a distinct entity (McFarland & Wehbe-Alamah, 2015). Examples of American subcultures based on ethnicity (i.e., subcultures with common traits such as physical characteristics, language, or ancestry) include African Americans, Hispanic/Latino Americans, Asian/Pacific Islanders, and Native Americans. Each of these subcultures may be further divided; for example, Native Americans consist of American Indians and Alaska Natives, who represent more than 500 federally and state-recognized tribes in addition to an unknown number of tribes that are not officially recognized.

Subcultures may also be based on religion (more than 1200 religions exist in the United States), occupation (e.g., nurses, physicians, other members of the health care team), disability (e.g., the deaf community), or illness (e.g., heart disease, cerebrovascular disease). In addition, subcultures may be based on age (e.g., infants, children, adolescents, adults, older adults), gender (e.g., male, female, transgender), sexual orientation (e.g., homosexual, bisexual, heterosexual), or geographic location (e.g., Texan, Southern, Appalachian).

Nurses should also be sensitive to interracial differences when providing care to individuals of cultures with which the nurse is unfamiliar. Differences between individuals in subcultures in a designated group add to the challenge to plan and provide culturally competent care. Cultural competence begins with cultural awareness and understanding how it influences thinking about those from other cultures. Such examination facilitates comparison of the nurse's own culture with others, so that the nurse can ultimately become sensitive to and accepting of those with different cultural backgrounds (Rew, Becker, Chontichachalalauk, et al., 2014). Nurses must refrain from culturally stereotyping patients. Instead, nurses should consult patients or significant others regarding personal values, beliefs, preferences, and cultural identification. This strategy is also applicable for members of nonethnic subcultures.

Minorities

The term **minority** refers to a group of people whose physical or cultural characteristics differ from the dominant culture or majority of people in a society. Minorities may be singled out or isolated from others in society or treated in different or unequal ways. The 2010 census identified four racial groups, as "other than White," including Blacks/African Americans, Asians, Native Hawaiians or other Pacific Islanders, and Native Americans—American Indian or Alaska Natives (Humes, Jones, & Ramerez, 2011). In addition, ethnicity in Hispanic, Latino, or Spanish origin was assessed separately from race in the 2010 census (Enis, Rios-Vargas, & Albert, 2011). Generally, persons belonging to these non-White racial groups listed or who identified themselves as of Hispanic or Latino origin are considered minorities in the United States. However, the concept of "minority" varies widely and must be understood in a cultural context. For example, men may be considered a minority in the nursing profession but constitute a majority in other fields, such as engineering. Because the term *minority* often connotes inferiority, members of many racial and ethnic groups object to being identified as minorities.

Whites/Caucasians may be in the minority in some communities; however, they are the majority group in the United States. Because most health care providers are members of this majority/Caucasian culture, health care tends to be provided from that perspective and services are often biased toward the majority group, with health care disparities noted in many minority populations. Although it has been projected that by the middle to late 21st century Caucasians may no longer represent the majority of Americans (Ortman & Guarneri, 2011), there is no evidence that this shift will change the perspective from which care is delivered or that disparities in care will be reduced.

Health Disparities

Health disparities—higher rates of morbidity, mortality, and burden of disease in a population or community than found in the overall population—are significant in ethnic and racial minorities. Key health indicators in the United States reveal a significant gap in health status between the overall American population and people of specific ethnic backgrounds (U.S. Department of Health & Human Services [HHS], 2015). Ethnic and racial minorities are disproportionately burdened with cancer, heart disease, diabetes, human immunodeficiency virus infection/acquired immunodeficiency syndrome, and other conditions. They receive a lower quality of health care than nonminorities and are at greater risk for declining health. Health disparities also occur with women, gay, lesbian, and transgender people, as well as with people who have disabilities (HHS, 2015). Many reasons are cited for these disparities, including low socioeconomic status, health behaviors, limited access to health care because of poverty or disability, environmental factors, and direct and indirect manifestations of discrimination. Other causes include lack of comprehensive health insurance; overdependence on publicly funded facilities; and barriers to health care such as insufficient transportation, geographic location (not enough providers in an area), cost of services, and the low numbers of minority health care providers (Institute of Medicine, 2003; Sullivan Commission, 2004).

Transcultural Nursing

The term *transcultural nursing* is used interchangeably with cross-cultural, intercultural, or multicultural nursing and refers to evidence-based practice that focuses on patient-centered, culturally competent nursing (Giger, 2013). Transcultural nursing addresses the differences and similarities among cultures in relation to health, health care, and illness. Furthermore, it incorporates the care (caring) values, beliefs, and practices of people and groups from a particular culture without imposing the nurse's cultural perspective on the patient. The underlying focus of transcultural nursing is to provide culturally appropriate and competent care that promotes the well-being or health of individuals, families, groups, communities, and institutions (Giger, 2013). All people, as well as the community or institution at large, benefit when culturally competent care is provided. When the care is delivered beyond a nurse's national boundaries, the term *international* or *transnational nursing* is often used.

Although many nurses, anthropologists, and others have written about the cultural aspects of nursing and health care, Leininger (2002) developed a comprehensive research-based theory—Culture Care Diversity and Universality—to promote culturally congruent nursing for people of different or similar cultures. This means promoting recovery from illness, preventing conditions that would limit the patient's health or well-being, or facilitating a peaceful death in ways that are culturally meaningful and appropriate.

Leininger theory stresses the importance of providing **culturally congruent nursing care** (i.e., meaningful and beneficial health care tailored to fit the patient's cultural values, beliefs, and lifestyles) through culture care accommodation and culture care restructuring. *Culture care accommodation* refers to professional actions and decisions that nurses make on behalf of those in their care to help people of a designated culture achieve a beneficial or satisfying health outcome. *Culture care restructuring* or repatterning refers to professional actions and decisions that help patients reorder, change, or modify their lifestyles toward new, different, or more beneficial health care patterns (see Fig. 7-1). At the same time, the patient's cultural values and beliefs are respected and a better or healthier lifestyle results. Other terms and definitions that provide further insight into culture and health care include the following:

- *Acculturation:* the process by which members of a cultural group adapt to or take on the behaviors of another group
- *Cultural blindness:* the inability of people to recognize their own values, beliefs, and practices and those of others because of strong ethnocentric tendencies (the tendency to judge others based on one's own culture)
- *Cultural imposition:* the tendency to impose one's cultural beliefs, values, and patterns of behavior on a person or people from a different culture
- *Cultural taboos:* activities or behaviors that are avoided or prohibited by a particular cultural group

Culturally Competent Nursing Care

Culturally competent nursing care is defined as effective, individualized care that demonstrates respect for the dignity, personal rights, preferences, beliefs, and practices of the person receiving care while acknowledging the biases of the caregiver and preventing these biases from interfering with the care provided. **Cultural awareness or sensitivity**, on the other hand, implies an awareness of cultural differences that might be present in the health care delivery process. The nurse should go beyond sensitivity to leverage awareness of these differences to plan appropriate culturally competent nursing care.

Culturally competent nursing care is a dynamic process that requires comprehensive knowledge of culture-specific information and an awareness of, and sensitivity to, the effect that culture has on the care situation. It requires that nurses find meaningful and useful care-delivery strategies based on knowledge of the cultural heritage, beliefs, and behaviors of those to whom they render care (Giger, 2013). Culturally competent nursing care also incorporates the delivery of interventions that are congruent with a given culture. It involves a complex integration of attitudes, knowledge, and skills (including assessment, decision making, judgments, critical thinking, and evaluation) that enables nurses to provide culturally appropriate care.

Agency policies are important to achieve culturally competent care. Policies that promote culturally competent care establish flexible regulations pertaining to visitors (number,

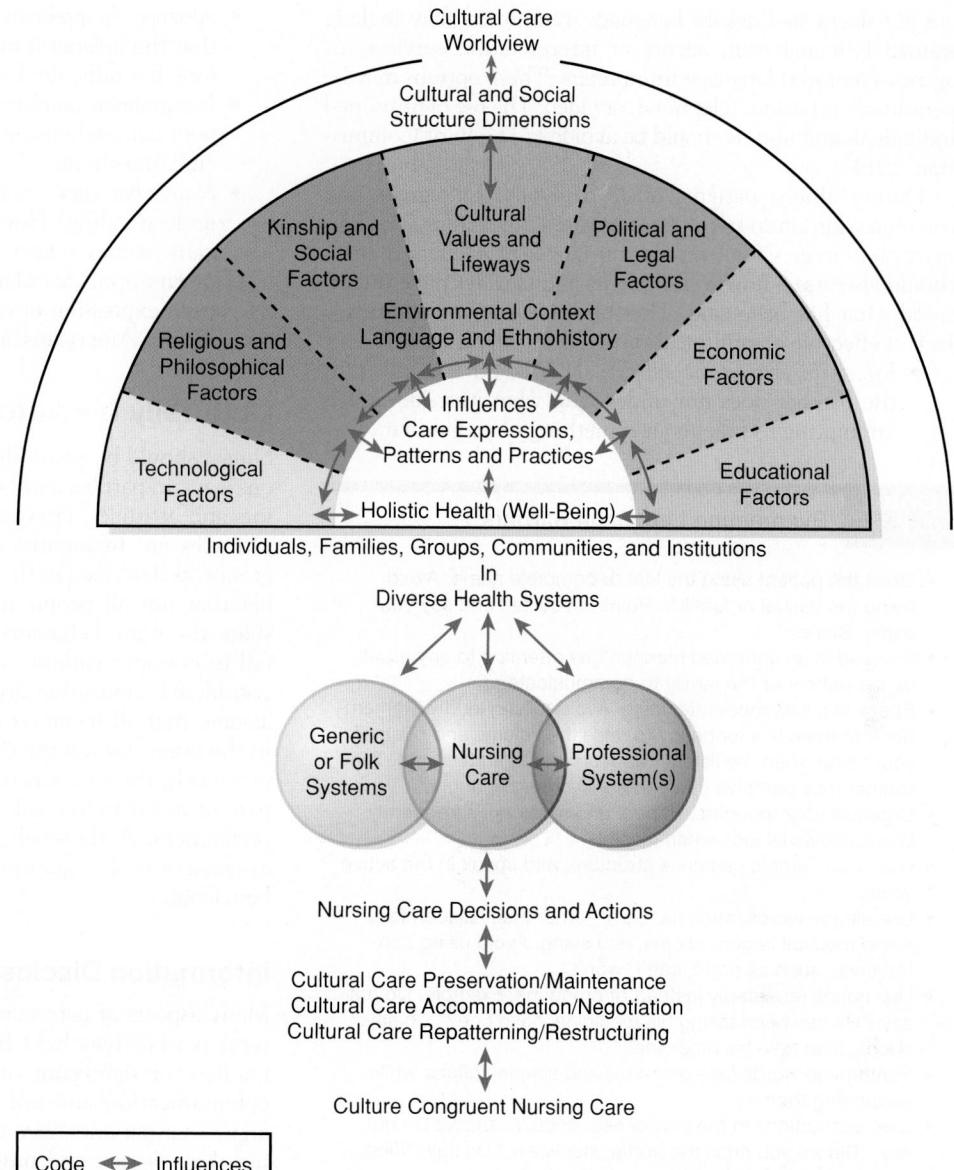

Figure 7-1 • Leininger's Sunrise Model depicts her theory of cultural care diversity and universality. Reprinted with permission from Leininger, M. M. (Ed.). (2001). *Culture care diversity and university: A theory of nursing.* New York, NY: National League for Nursing Press.

frequency, and length of visits), provide translation services for non–English-speaking patients, and train staff to provide care for patients with different cultural values (The Joint Commission, 2014). Culturally competent policies are developed to promote an environment in which the traditional healing, spiritual, and religious practices of patients are respected and encouraged and to recognize the special dietary practices of patients from selected cultural groups.

Giger and Davidhizar created the Transcultural Assessment Model to guide nurses in exploring cultural phenomena that might affect nursing care. According to the tenets of this model, in order to provide culturally appropriate and competent nursing care, nurses must recognize that each individual is culturally unique with different experiences, cultural beliefs, and cultural norms. The model identifies communication, space, time orientation, social organization, environmental control, and biologic variations as relevant phenomena. This model has been used in various patient care

settings to provide data that are essential to the provision of culturally competent care (Giger, 2013).

Cross-Cultural Communication

Establishment of an environment of culturally congruent care and respect begins with effective communication, which occurs not only through words but also through body language and other cues, such as voice, tone, and loudness. Nurse–patient interactions, as well as communication among members of a multicultural health care team, depend on the ability to understand and be understood. Communication barriers frequently exist between nurses and patients, especially when they are from different cultural backgrounds (Giger, 2013).

Approximately 150 different languages are spoken in the United States, with Spanish most common after English. Obviously, nurses cannot become fluent in all languages; however, certain strategies for fostering effective cross-cultural communication are necessary when providing care for patients who are not fluent in English. Language interpreters may include trained bilingual staff, agents of interpretation services, or agency-employed language interpreters. These options may be permitted via person, telephone, or video. The use of untrained individuals and minors should be avoided (The Joint Commission, 2014).

During illness, patients of all ages tend to regress, and the regression often involves language skills. Chart 7-1 summarizes strategies for overcoming language barriers. Nurses should also assess how well patients and families have understood what has been said. The following cues may signify a lack of effective communication:

- *Efforts to change the subject*: This could indicate that the listener does not understand what was said and is attempting to talk about something more familiar.

Chart 7-1   Overcoming Language Barriers

- Greet the patient using the last or complete name. Avoid being too casual or familiar. Point to yourself and say your name. Smile.
- Proceed in an unhurried manner. Pay attention to any effort by the patient or the family to communicate.
- Speak in a low, moderate voice. Avoid talking loudly. Remember that there is a tendency to raise the volume and pitch of your voice when the listener appears not to understand. The listener may perceive that you are shouting or angry.
- Organize your thoughts. Repeat and summarize frequently. Use audiovisual aids when feasible.
- Use short, simple sentence structure, and speak in the active voice.
- Use simple words, such as "pain" rather than "discomfort." Avoid medical jargon, idioms, and slang. Avoid using contractions, such as don't, can't, won't.
- Use nouns repeatedly instead of pronouns. *Example:* Do not say: "He has been taking his medicine, hasn't he?" Do say: "Does Juan take his medicine?"
- Pantomime words (use gestures) and simple actions while verbalizing them.
- Give instructions in the proper sequence. *Example:* Do not say: "Before you rinse the bottle, sterilize it." Do say: "First, wash the bottle. Second, rinse the bottle."
- Discuss one topic at a time and avoid giving too much information in a single conversation. Avoid using conjunctions. *Example:* Do not say: "Are you cold and in pain?" Do say (while pantomiming/gesturing): "Are you cold?" "Are you in pain?"
- Talk directly to the patient rather than to the person who accompanied him or her.
- Validate whether the person understands by having him or her repeat instructions, demonstrate the procedure, or act out the meaning.
- Use any words that you know in the person's language. This indicates that you are aware of and respect the patient's primary means of communicating.
- Be aware of culturally based gender and age differences and diverse socioeconomic, educational, and tribal or regional differences when choosing an interpreter.
- Contact hospitals for a list of language interpreters such as trained bilingual staff or interpreting services via person, telephone, or video. The use of untrained individuals and minors should be avoided.

Adapted from Jarvis, C. (2016). *Physical examination & health assessment.* (7th ed.). St. Louis, MO: Elsevier Saunders.

- *Absence of questions*: Paradoxically, this often means that the listener is not grasping the message and, therefore, has difficulty formulating questions to ask.
- *Inappropriate laughter*: A self-conscious giggle may signal poor comprehension and may be an attempt to disguise embarrassment.
- *Nonverbal cues*: A blank expression may signal poor understanding. However, among some Asian Americans, it may reflect a desire to avoid overt expression of emotion. Avoidance of eye contact may be a cultural expression of respect for the speaker among some Native Americans and Asian Americans.

Culturally Mediated Characteristics

Nurses should be aware that patients act and behave in various ways, in part because of the influence of culture on behaviors and attitudes. However, although certain attributes and attitudes are frequently associated with particular cultural groups, as described in this chapter, it is important to remember that not all people from the same cultural background share the same behaviors and views. Although nurses who fail to consider patients' cultural preferences and beliefs are considered insensitive and possibly indifferent, nurses who assume that all members of any one culture act and behave in the same way run the risk of stereotyping people. As stated previously, the best way to avoid stereotyping is to view each patient as an individual and to assess the patient's cultural preferences. A thorough culture assessment using a culture assessment tool or questionnaire (see later discussion) is very beneficial.

Information Disclosure

Many aspects of care may be influenced by the diverse cultural perspectives held by health care providers, patients, families, or significant others. One example is the issue of communication and full disclosure. In general, nurses may argue that patients have the right to full disclosure concerning their disease and prognosis and may believe that advocacy means working to provide that disclosure. However, family members in some cultural backgrounds may believe that it is their responsibility to protect and spare the patient (their loved one) knowledge about a terminal illness. In some cultures, the head of the family group, elder, or husband is expected to receive all information and make decisions. Patients may in fact not want to know about their condition and may expect their family members to "take the burden" of that knowledge and related decision making. Nurses should not decide that a family or patient is simply wrong or that a patient must know all of the details of their illness regardless of the patient's preference. Similar concerns may be noted when patients refuse pain medication or treatment because of cultural beliefs regarding pain or beliefs in divine intervention or faith healing.

Determining the most appropriate and ethical approach to patient care requires an exploration of the cultural aspects of these situations. Self-examination and recognition of one's own cultural bias and worldview, as discussed earlier, play a major part in helping the nurse resolve cultural and ethical conflicts. Nurses must promote open dialogue and work with patients, families, physicians, and other health care providers to reach the culturally appropriate solution for the individual patient.

Space and Distance

Personal space is the area that surrounds a person's body and includes the space and the objects within the space (Giger, 2013). People tend to regard the space in their immediate vicinity as an extension of themselves. The amount of space that they need between themselves and others to feel comfortable is a culturally determined phenomenon.

Because nurses and patients usually are not consciously aware of their personal space requirements, they frequently have difficulty understanding different behaviors. For example, one patient may perceive the nurse sitting close to him or her as an expression of warmth and care; another patient may perceive the nurse's act as a threatening invasion of personal space. Research reveals that people from the United States, Canada, and Great Britain require the most personal space between themselves and others, whereas those from Latin America, Japan, and the Middle East need the least amount of space and feel comfortable standing close to others (Giger, 2013).

If the patient appears to position himself or herself too close or too far away, the nurse should consider cultural preferences for space and distance. Ideally, the patient should be permitted to assume a position that is comfortable to him or her in terms of personal space and distance. The nurse should be aware that the wheelchair of a person with a disability is considered an extension of the person; therefore, the nurse should ask the person's permission before moving or touching the wheelchair. Because a significant amount of communication during nursing care requires close physical contact, the nurse should be aware that having personal space promotes self-identity by allowing opportunities for patient self-expression (Giger, 2013).

Eye Contact

Eye contact is also a culturally determined behavior. Although most nurses have been taught to maintain eye contact when speaking with patients, some people from certain cultural backgrounds may interpret this behavior differently. For example, some Asians, Native Americans, Indo-Chinese, Arabs, and Appalachians may consider direct eye contact impolite or aggressive, and they may avert their own eyes when talking with nurses and others whom they perceive to be in positions of authority. Some Native Americans stare at the floor during conversations—a cultural behavior conveying respect and indicating that the listener is paying close attention to the speaker. Some Hispanic patients maintain downcast eyes as a sign of culturally appropriate deferential behavior toward others on the basis of age, gender, social position, economic status, and position of authority (Giger, 2013). Eye contact is an important tool in a transcultural assessment and is used for both observation and to initiate interaction (Giger, 2013). The nurse who is aware that eye contact may be culturally determined can better understand the patient's behavior and provide an atmosphere in which the patient can feel comfortable.

Time

Attitudes about time vary widely among cultures and can be a barrier to effective communication between nurses and patients. Views about punctuality and the use of time are culturally determined, as is the concept of waiting. Symbols of time, such as watches, sunrises, and sunsets, represent methods for measuring the duration and passage of time (Giger, 2013).

For most health care providers, time and promptness are extremely important. For example, nurses frequently expect patients to arrive at an exact time for an appointment, although patients may be kept waiting by health care providers who are running late. Health care providers are likely to function according to an appointment system in which there are short intervals of perhaps only a few minutes. However, for patients from some cultures, time is a relative phenomenon, with little attention paid to the exact hour or minute. For example, some Hispanic people consider time in a wider frame of reference and make the primary distinction between day and night. Time may also be determined according to traditional times for meals, sleep, and other activities or events. For people from some cultures, the present is of the greatest importance, and time is viewed in broad ranges rather than in terms of a fixed hour. Being flexible in regard to schedules is the best way to accommodate these differences.

Value differences also may influence a person's sense of priority when it comes to time. For example, responding to a family matter may be more important to a patient than meeting a scheduled health care appointment. Allowing for these different views is essential in maintaining an effective nurse–patient relationship. Scolding or acting annoyed at patients for being late undermines their confidence and may result in further missed appointments or indifference to health care suggestions.

Touch

Touch is the most personal of all sensations, is central to the human communication process, and is often used as a method of communication (Giger, 2013). The meaning that people associate with touching is culturally determined to a great degree. In some cultures (e.g., Hispanic, Arab), male health care providers may be prohibited from touching or examining certain parts of the female body. Similarly, it may be inappropriate for females to care for males. Among many Asians, it is impolite to touch a person's head because the spirit is believed to reside there. Therefore, assessment of the head or evaluation of a head injury requires permission of the patient or a family member, if the patient is not able to give permission.

The patient's culturally defined sense of modesty must also be considered when providing nursing care. For example, some Jewish and Muslim women believe that modesty requires covering their head, arms, and legs with clothing. It is important for the nurse to recognize cultural variances and to understand that touch can be perceived as intrusive to some patients.

Observance of Holidays

People from all cultures observe certain civil and religious holidays. Nurses should familiarize themselves with major observances for members of the cultural groups they serve. Information about these observances is available from various sources, including religious organizations, hospital chaplains, and patients themselves. Routine health appointments, diagnostic tests, surgery, and other major procedures should be scheduled to avoid observances that patients identify as significant. If not contraindicated, efforts should also be made to accommodate patients and families or significant others who wish to perform cultural and religious rituals in the health care setting.

Diet

The cultural context of food varies widely but usually includes one or more of the following: relief of hunger; promotion of health and healing; prevention of disease or illness; expression of caring for another; promotion of interpersonal closeness among individual people, families, groups, communities, or nations; and promotion of kinship and family alliances. Food is also associated with strengthening of social ties; observance of life events (e.g., birthdays, marriages, funerals); expression of gratitude or appreciation; recognition of achievement or accomplishment; validation of social, cultural, or religious ceremonial functions; facilitation of business negotiations; and expression of affluence, wealth, or social status.

Culture determines which foods are served and when they are served, the number and frequency of meals, who eats with whom, and who receives the choicest portions. Culture determines how foods are prepared and served, how they are eaten (with chopsticks, hands, or fork, knife, and spoon), and where people shop (e.g., ethnic grocery stores, specialty food markets). Culture also determines the impact of excess weight and obesity on self-esteem and social standing. In some cultures, physical bulk is viewed as a sign of affluence and health (e.g., a chubby baby is a healthy baby).

Religious practices may include fasting (e.g., Mormons, Catholics, Buddhists, Jews, Muslims) and abstaining from selected foods at particular times (e.g., Catholics abstain from meat on Ash Wednesday and on Fridays during Lent). Practices may also include the ritualistic use of food and beverages (e.g., Passover dinner, consumption of bread and wine during religious ceremonies). Chart 7-2 summarizes some prohibited foods and beverages of selected religious groups.

Most groups feast, often in the company of family and friends, on selected holidays. For example, many Christians eat large dinners on Christmas and Easter and consume other traditional high-calorie, high-fat foods, such as seasonal cookies, pastries, and candies. These culturally based dietary practices are especially significant in the care of patients with diabetes, hypertension, gastrointestinal disorders, obesity, and other conditions in which diet plays a key role in the treatment and health maintenance regimen.

Biologic Variations

Along with psychosocial adaptations, nurses must also consider the physiologic impact of culture on patients' response to treatment, particularly medications. Data have been collected for many years regarding differences in the effect that some medications have on people of diverse ethnic or cultural origins. Genetic predispositions to different rates of metabolism cause some patients to be prone to adverse reactions to

---

Chart 7-2 Prohibited Foods and Beverages of Selected Religious Groups

Hinduism

All meats
Animal shortenings/fats

Islam

Pork
Alcoholic products and beverages (including extracts, such as vanilla and lemon)
Animal shortenings
Gelatin made from pork, marshmallow, and other confections made with gelatin
Note: *Halal* is lawful food that may be consumed according to tenets of the Koran, whereas *Haram* is food that is unlawful to consume.

Judaism

Pork
Predatory fowl
Shellfish and scavenger fish (e.g., shrimp, crab, lobster, escargot, catfish). Fish with fins and scales are permissible.
Mixing milk and meat dishes at same meal
Blood by ingestion (e.g., blood sausage, raw meat).
Note: Packaged foods will contain labels identifying kosher ("properly preserved" or "fitting") and pareve (made without meat or milk) items.

Mormonism (Church of Jesus Christ of Latter-Day Saints)

Alcohol
Beverages containing caffeine stimulants (coffee, tea, colas, and selected carbonated soft drinks)

Seventh-Day Adventism

Alcohol
Beverages containing caffeine stimulants (coffee, tea, colas, and selected carbonated soft drinks)
Pork
Certain seafood, including shellfish
Fermented beverages
Note: Optional vegetarianism is encouraged.

---

the standard dose of a medication, whereas other patients are likely to experience a greatly reduced benefit from the standard dose of the medication (Giger, 2013). For example, an antihypertensive agent may work well at reducing blood pressure to acceptable levels for a Caucasian man within a 4-week time span but may take much longer to work or not work at all for an African American man with hypertension. Future genomic research may identify genetic underpinnings of disease susceptibility, drug response, and health outcomes (Jaja, Gibson, & Quarles, 2013). Nurses must be aware that ethnicity and related factors such as values and beliefs regarding the use of herbal supplements, dietary intake, and genetic factors can affect the effectiveness of treatment and adherence to the treatment regimen (Giger, 2013).

Complementary, Alternative, and Integrative Health Therapies

Interventions for alterations in health and wellness vary among cultures. Interventions most commonly used in the

United States have been labeled as *conventional medicine*, which are also variously referred to as allopathy, Western medicine, regular medicine, mainstream medicine, and biomedicine (National Center for Complementary and Integrative Health [NCCIH], 2015). Therapy used to supplement conventional medicine is referred to as *complementary therapy*, whereas therapy used to replace conventional medicine is referred to as *alternative therapy* (NCCIH, 2015). Interest in interventions that are not an integral part of conventional medicine prompted the National Institutes of Health to create the Office of Alternative Medicine and then to establish the National Center for Complementary and Alternative Medicine, which is now called the National Center for Complementary and Integrative Health (NCCIH). Integrative health care is viewed as a comprehensive, interdisciplinary approach to preventing and treating illness and promoting health that brings together complementary, alternative, and conventional therapies. The use of an integrative approach to health wellness has grown within mainstream health care settings in the United States (NCCIH, 2015).

Integrative health therapies are classified by product or practice type into two subgroups—natural products or mind and body practices (NCCIH, 2015):

- *Natural products* include herbs (also known as botanicals), vitamins and minerals, and probiotics. These are widely marketed to consumers and often sold and used as dietary supplements.
- *Mind and body practices* include large and diverse procedures and techniques given or taught by trained practitioners or teachers and include practices such as yoga, meditation, chiropractic and osteopathic manipulation, massage therapy, acupuncture, relaxation techniques, and tai chi.

Patients may choose to seek a complementary or alternative approach to conventional medical or surgical therapies. Nurses should work with patients to develop effective, personalized health strategies that might include the use of natural products and mind and body practices to promote individual health and well-being. Nurses must assess all patients for the use of complementary therapies, be alert to the danger of natural product–drug interactions or conflicting treatments, and be prepared to provide information to patients about treatments that may be harmful or helpful, based upon best evidence from research findings. However, nurses must be accepting of patients' beliefs and right to autonomy—that is, to control their own care. As patient advocates, nurses facilitate the integration of conventional medical, complementary, and alternative therapies.

Causes of Illness

People may view illness differently. Three major views, or paradigms, attempt to explain the causes of disease and illness: the biomedical or scientific view, the naturalistic or holistic perspective, and the magico-religious view.

Biomedical or Scientific View

The biomedical or scientific worldview prevails in most health care settings and is embraced by most nurses and other health care providers. The basic assumptions underlying the biomedical perspective are that all events in life have a cause and effect, that the human body functions much like a machine, and that all of reality can be observed and measured (e.g., blood pressures, partial pressure of arterial oxygen [PaO_2] levels, intelligence tests). One example of the biomedical or scientific view is the pathogenic explanation of communicable diseases.

Naturalistic or Holistic Perspective

The naturalistic or holistic perspective is another viewpoint that explains the cause of illness and is commonly embraced by many Native Americans, Asians, and others. According to this view, the forces of nature must be kept in natural balance or harmony.

One example of a naturalistic belief, held by many Asian groups, is the yin/yang theory, the basis for Eastern or Chinese medicine, in which health is believed to exist when all aspects of a person are in perfect balance or harmony. Rooted in the ancient Chinese philosophy of Taoism (which translates as "The Way"), the yin/yang theory proposes that all organisms and objects in the universe consist of yin and yang energy. The seat of the energy forces is within the autonomic nervous system, where balance between the opposing forces is maintained during health. Yin energy represents the female and negative forces, such as emptiness, darkness, and cold, whereas the yang forces are male and positive, emitting warmth and fullness. Foods are classified as cold (yin) or hot (yang) in this theory and are transformed into yin and yang energy when metabolized by the body. Cold foods are eaten when a person has a hot illness (e.g., fever, rash, sore throat, ulcer, infection), and hot foods are eaten when a person has a cold illness (e.g., cancer, headache, stomach cramps, "a cold").

Many Hispanic, African American, and Arab groups also embrace a hot/cold theory of health and illness. The four humors of the body—blood, phlegm, black bile, and yellow bile—are believed to regulate basic bodily functions and are described in terms of temperature and moisture. The treatment of disease consists of adding or subtracting cold, heat, dryness, or wetness to restore the balance of these humors. Beverages, foods, herbs, medicines, and diseases are classified as hot or cold according to their perceived effects on the body, not their physical characteristics. According to the hot/cold theory, the person as a whole, not just a particular ailment, is significant. People who embrace hot/cold theories maintain that health consists of a positive state of total well-being, including physical, psychological, spiritual, and social aspects of the person.

According to the naturalistic worldview, breaking the laws of nature creates imbalances, chaos, and disease. People who embrace the naturalistic paradigm use metaphors such as "the healing power of nature." For example, from the perspective of many Chinese people, illness is viewed not as an intruding agent but as a part of life's rhythmic course and an outward sign of disharmony within.

Magico-Religious View

Another major way in which people view the world and explain the causes of illness is the magico-religious worldview. This view's basic premise is that the world is an arena in which supernatural forces dominate, and that the fate of the world and those in it depends on the action of supernatural forces for good or evil. Examples of magical causes of illness include belief in voodoo or witchcraft among some African Americans and people from Caribbean countries. Faith healing is based on religious beliefs and is most prevalent among selected Christian religions, including Christian Science, whereas various healing rituals may be found in many other religions, such as Roman Catholicism and Mormonism (Church of Jesus Christ of Latter-day Saints).

Of course, it is possible to hold a combination of worldviews, and many patients offer more than one explanation for the cause of their illness. As a profession, nursing largely embraces the scientific or biomedical worldview; however, some aspects of holism are popular, including various techniques for managing chronic pain, such as hypnosis, therapeutic touch, and biofeedback. Belief in spiritual power is also held by many nurses who credit supernatural forces with various unexplained phenomena related to patients' health and illness states. Regardless of the view held and whether the nurse agrees with the patient's beliefs in this regard, it is important to be aware of how the patient views illness and health and to work within this framework to promote patient care and well-being.

Folk Healers

People of some cultures believe in folk or indigenous healers. For example, nurses may find that some Hispanic patients may seek help from a *curandero* or *curandera* (spiritual healer, folk doctor, shaman), *espiritualista* (spiritualist), *yuyero* (herbalist), or *sanador* (healer who manipulates bones and muscles). Some African American patients may seek assistance from a *hougan* (voodoo priest or priestess), spiritualist, root doctor (usually a woman who uses magic rituals to treat diseases), or "old lady" (an older woman who has successfully raised a family and who specializes in child care and folk remedies). Native American patients may seek assistance from a shaman or medicine man or woman. Asian patients may mention that they have visited herbalists, acupuncturists, or bone setters. Several cultures have its own healers, most of whom speak the native tongue of that culture, make house calls, and charge significantly less than healers practicing in the conventional medical health care system.

People seeking complementary and alternative therapies have expanded the practices of folk healers beyond their traditional populations; therefore, the nurse should ask the patient about use of folk healers regardless of the patient's cultural background. Nurses should not disregard the patient's belief in folk healers or try to undermine trust in the healers, because doing so may alienate the patient and drive him or her away from receiving the prescribed care. Instead, nurses should try to accommodate the patient's beliefs while advocating the treatment indicated by the tenets of health science (see Chart 7-3).

Chart 7-3	**ETHICAL DILEMMA**

When May Folk Remedies be Considered Harmful or Complementary?

Case Scenario

You are working in an urban neighborhood health clinic. A 78-year-old woman who is a Chinese immigrant presents with a 5-day history of chills, low-grade fever, pallor, dry, nonproductive cough, and fatigue. The woman's adult daughter has brought her to the clinic, and they both insist on the daughter being present during assessment. When you begin to listen to the woman's lung sounds, you incidentally note that she has round, bruised areas in regions of her back in a symmetric pattern. A few of the marks appear to be infected at the sites where small amounts of blood were suctioned. You ask her how this happened, and her daughter interjects, "That is from cupping, but it didn't seem to work right this time, because she is still very sick. That is the reason we are here now." You have heard that in Chinese communities, wet cupping is practiced as a folk remedy and that the intent of this treatment is to remove inflammation.

Discussion

There are many folk remedies that immigrants to the United States may continue to use to treat various ailments. Some of these may be complementary to traditional Western medicine, whereas others may be considered harmful therapies in that they may result in delays to seek traditional routes to treatment or may otherwise result in harm to the patient. It is important to determine if this procedure is complementary and if the patient regularly sees a licensed primary provider to provide her with comprehensive health care. The American Nurses Association (1991) advises the professional nurse to be cognizant when their own ethnocentrism is present during interactions with patients of a different culture—that is, a belief that the nurse's culturally accepted way of practicing health care is inherently superior to another culturally acceptable health care practice.

Analysis

Describe the ethical principles that are in conflict in this case (see Chart 3-3). Which principle should have preeminence as you proceed with your assessment of this patient?

- Describe any concerns that you may have regarding preservation of the patient's autonomy. What steps might you take to assure that her autonomy is preserved?
- Cupping is a relatively common folk remedy among many people from southeastern Asian cultures. How can you determine whether the marks you find on this patient signify that she may be a victim of elder abuse rather than a willing recipient of a folk remedy? How do you ensure that the patient is not harmed (i.e., ensure nonmaleficence)? How do you ascertain if she is receiving health care to treat any existing health problems?
- Assume that you find that the patient has full capacity to make competent decisions and that she does indeed value the traditional practice of cupping. How do you professionally reconcile that she has sought to treat her illness with a folk remedy before seeking traditional care? Does her right to make an autonomous decision over her health care trump your desire that she seek traditional health care sooner (or, in this case, does the principle of autonomy outweigh the dual principles of beneficence and nonmaleficence)?

Reference

Ludwick, R., & Silva, M. C., (2000). Ethics: Nursing around the world: Cultural values and ethical conflicts. *Online Journal of Issues in Nursing,*5(3). Retrieved on 8/27/2016 at: www.nursingworld.org/MainMenuCategories/ANAMarketplace/ANAPeriodicals/OJIN/Columns/Ethics/CulturalValuesandEthicalConflicts.aspx

Resources

See Chart 3-6 for Steps of an Ethical Analysis and Ethics Resources.

Cultural Nursing Assessment

Cultural nursing assessment refers to a systematic appraisal or examination of individuals, families, groups, and communities in terms of their cultural beliefs, values, and practices. Nursing assessment instruments including tools, scales, and questionnaires may be used to measure cultural needs of patients (Shen, 2015). In an effort to establish a database for determining a patient's cultural background, nurses have developed cultural assessment tools or modified existing assessment tools (Leininger, 2002) to ensure that transcultural considerations are included in the plan of care. Giger and Davidhizar's Transcultural Assessment Model has been used to help nurses perform cultural assessments, as noted previously. Questions derived from this model may be used to direct nursing assessment of a person's ethnic, cultural, or religious beliefs and its relationship to their personal and health care traditions (see Chart 7-4) (Giger, 2013). Yet, despite the availability of tools designed to facilitate performing cultural assessments, recent research findings suggest that many nurses feel unprepared to perform cultural assessments and provide culturally competent care for ethnic minority patients (see Chart 7-5: Nursing Research Profile) (Alpers & Hanssen, 2014).

Additional Cultural Considerations: Know Thyself

Because the nurse–patient interaction is the focal point of nursing, nurses must consider their own cultural orientation when conducting assessments of patients and their families and friends. The following guidelines may prove useful to nurses who want to provide culturally appropriate care:

- Know your own cultural attitudes, values, beliefs, and practices.
- Recognize that despite "good intentions," everyone has cultural "baggage" that ultimately results in **ethnocentrism** (i.e., judging another culture based upon standards from one's own culture).
- Acknowledge that it is generally easier to understand those whose cultural heritage is similar to your own, while viewing those who are unlike you as strange and different.
- Maintain a broad, open attitude. Expect the unexpected. Enjoy surprises.
- Avoid seeing all people as alike—that is, avoid cultural stereotypes, such as "all Chinese like rice" or "all Italians eat spaghetti."
- Try to understand the reasons for any behavior by discussing commonalities and differences with representatives of ethnic groups different from your own.
- If a patient has said or done something that you do not understand, ask for clarification. Be a good listener. Most patients will respond positively to questions that arise from a genuine concern for and interest in them.
- If at all possible, speak the patient's language (even simple greetings and social courtesies are appreciated). Avoid feigning an accent or using words that are ordinarily not part of your vocabulary.
- Be yourself. There are no right ways or wrong ways to learn about cultural diversity.

Chart 7-4 ASSESSMENT

Assessing for Patients' Cultural Beliefs

Communication

Do you like communicating with friends, family, and acquaintances?

- When asked a question, do you usually respond?
- If you have something important to discuss with your family, how would you approach them?

Space

- When you talk with family members, how close do you stand?
- When you talk with acquaintances, how close do you stand?
- If a stranger touches you, how do you react or feel?
- If a loved one touches you, how do you react or feel?
- Are you comfortable with the distance between us now?

Social Organization

- What are some activities that you enjoy?
- What are your hobbies, or what do you do when you have free time?
- Do you believe in a Supreme Being?
- How do you worship that Supreme Being?
- What is your role in your family/unit system?

Time

- What kind of timepiece do you wear daily?
- If a nurse tells you that you will receive a medication "in about a half hour," how much time will you allow before calling the nurse station?

Environmental Control

- Is it acceptable for you to have visitors drop in unexpectedly?
- Do you use home remedies? Which home remedies worked? Will you use them in the future?
- What is your definition of "good health?"
- What is your definition of illness or "poor health?"

Biological Variations

- What diseases or illnesses are common in your family?
- Who usually helps you to cope during a difficult time?
- What foods do you and your family like to eat? What foods are family favorites or are considered traditional?

Nursing Process Utilization

- Note whether the patient has become culturally assimilated or observes own cultural practices.
- Incorporate data into the plan of nursing care.

Adapted from Giger, J. (2013). *Transcultural nursing: Assessment and intervention* (6th ed.). St. Louis, MO: Elsevier.

The Future of Transcultural Nursing Care

Providing culturally specific, quality nursing care for the increasingly diverse population in the United States is a looming challenge (Mareno & Hart, 2014). By the middle of the 21st century, the non–Hispanic Caucasian population is projected to proportionally decrease so that it will no longer comprise the *majority* population, and other ethnic and racial populations (i.e., *minority* populations as compared to non–Hispanic Caucasians) will collectively comprise the majority of all Americans. This projected phenomenon is called the *majority–minority* crossover (Ortman & Guarneri, 2011).

Chart 7-5 NURSING RESEARCH PROFILE

Self-Assessed Cultural Competency of Nurses

Alpers, L., & Hanssen, I. (2014). Caring for ethnic minority patients: A mixed-method study of nurses' self-assessment of cultural competency. *Nursing Education Today*, *34*(6), 999–1004.

Purpose

Research shows that nurses lack cultural competence, which may negatively affect treatment and care for ethnic minority patients. The purpose of this study was to investigate how medical unit (MU) nurses and psychiatric unit (PU) nurses assess their own cultural competency in caring for patients with minority backgrounds. The topics assessed included the following: intercultural knowledge, knowledge of medical traditions and differences in illness etiology, symptom assessment, and in-service education and availability of advice.

Design

This study used a mixed-methods study research design of nurses' self-assessment of cultural competency. Three focus group interviews were conducted with both MU and PU nurse participants to develop a Likert scale survey to learn about the participants' experiences working with ethnic minority patients. Survey items were designed to operationalize cultural competency, with an emphasis on gauging nurse participants' experience and knowledge. SPSS was used to analyze the quantitative data; hermeneutic thematic analysis was used for the qualitative data.

Findings

A total of 145 MU nurse participants and 100 PU nurse participants completed the survey. Participants lacked knowledge about a wide range of subjects, such as how to communicate well through an interpreter, how to handle nursing care with family and small children present, and how to appropriately care for a female patient who has been circumcised. They also expressed a lack of knowledge about various cultural expressions that may be important to hospitalized ethnic minority patients. Survey responses highlighted that 20% of the MU nurse participants and 28% of the PU nurse participants indicated that they had adequate intercultural knowledge, while 44% of both groups of nurse participants indicated that they had inadequate knowledge to give ethnic minority patients good treatment and care. There was no effect of years of practice experience on participants' self-rated intercultural knowledge.

Nursing Implications

Study findings suggest that experience alone is not adequate to develop cultural competency. Years of practice experience does not equip nurses with adequate knowledge to perform intercultural symptom assessment and render culturally competent treatment and care. Formal education, in-service classes, feedback, and access to relevant information are needed in order to facilitate the delivery of culturally competent nursing care.

As the population becomes more culturally diverse, efforts to increase the number of ethnic minority nurses must continue and accelerate (Sullivan Commission, 2004). As of 2013, more than 83% of all nurses are Caucasian (National Council of State Boards of Nursing, 2013). Progress toward increasing the percentage of culturally diverse nurses has been significantly slower than the increasing percentage of ethnic minorities in the United States. Greater efforts must be made to facilitate the recruitment and program completion of nursing students who are members of ethnic minorities. In addition, educational institutions must prepare nurses to deliver culturally competent care and must work to increase the number of ethnic minority providers in the nursing workforce. Nursing programs are exploring creative ways to promote cultural competence and humanistic care in nursing students, including offering multicultural health studies in their curricula. Simulation methods and role-playing could be effective methods to practice person-centered culturally competence care (McClimens et al., 2014). Through these pedagogical methods, students may develop the knowledge, skills, and attitudes needed to provide patient-centered care that is consonant with goals set through the Quality and Safety Education for Nurses (QSEN) national nursing education initiative that is funded by the Robert Wood Johnson Foundation (QSEN, 2015).

Cultural diversity remains one of the foremost issues in health care today. Nurses are expected to provide culturally competent care for patients. To do so, nurses must work effectively with the increasing number of patients, nurses, and health care team members whose ancestry reflects the multicultural complexion of contemporary society.

CRITICAL THINKING EXERCISES

1 [pq] You are assigned to care for a Filipino American patient who has degenerative joint disease of the right hip. He is scheduled for a total right hip replacement in the operating room tomorrow. You are completing a preoperative assessment for postoperative pain control as a priority goal. What biographical data in the assessment are important to identify in the preoperative assessment? What cultural beliefs should be assessed for this patient? What is your first priority for patient education? Explain why it is important to examine your own feelings about the patient's possible cultural beliefs and practices.

2 A 65-year-old Vietnamese woman who speaks little English is hospitalized with newly diagnosed congestive heart failure. You are assigned to her care and notice that the patient's blood pressure is elevated and she has a productive cough. The patient is prescribed a beta-blocker to regulate her blood pressure. The daughter shares with you that her mother does not like taking medications and chooses to take herbal remedies instead. What should be included in your initial nursing assessment? What information should you include that reflects an acceptance of the patient's health and illness beliefs and practices? What steps do you need to take to be culturally competent?

3 `ebp` You are providing care for a 78-year-old Chinese man with newly diagnosed chronic obstructive pulmonary disease who arrived in United States from China 2 years ago. During your initial assessment of the patient, you note that he speaks and understands very little English. Based on your knowledge of evidence-based guidelines, what initial assessment should be completed to determine the patient's communication needs? What language interpretation and translation services are available for you to communicate effectively with the patient and the family?

REFERENCES

*Asterisk indicates nursing research article.
**Double asterisk indicates classic reference.

Books

Giger, J. (2013). *Transcultural Nursing: Assessment and intervention* (6th ed.). St. Louis, MO: Elsevier.
**Institute of Medicine. (2003). *Unequal treatment: Confronting racial and ethnic disparities in healthcare*. Washington, DC: National Academies Press.
Jarvis, C. (2016). *Physical examination & health assessment*. (7th ed.). St. Louis, Elsevier Saunders.
**Leininger, M. M. (Ed.). (2001). *Culture care diversity and universality: A theory of nursing*. New York, NY: National League for Nursing Press.
McFarland, M. R., & Wehbe-Alamah, H. B. (2015). *Leininger's cultural care diversity and universality: A worldwide nursing theory* (3rd ed.). Burlington, MA: Jones & Bartlett.

Journals and Electronic Documents

*Alpers, L. M., & Hanssen, I. (2014). Caring for ethnic minority patients: A mixed-method study of nurses' self-assessment of cultural competency. *Nurse Education Today, 34*(6), 999–1004.
Enis, S. R., Rios-Vargas, M., & Albert, N. G. (2011). *The Hispanic population: 2010. 2010 Census Briefs*. Washington, DC: U.S. Bureau of the Census. Retrieved on 12/29/2015 at: www.census.gov/prod/cen2010/briefs/c2010br-04.pdf
Holland, A. (2015). The lived experience of teaching about race in cultural nursing education. *Journal of Transcultural Nursing Education, 26*(1), 92–100.
Humes, K. R., Jones, N. A., & Ramerez, R. R. (2011). *Overview of race and Hispanic origin: 2010. 2010 Census Briefs*. Washington, DC: U.S. Bureau of the Census. Retrieved on 12/29/2015 at: www.census.gov/prod/cen2010/briefs/c2010br-02.pdf
Isaacson, M. (2014). Clarifying concepts: Cultural humility or competency. *Journal of Professional Nursing, 30*(3), 251–258.
Jaja, C., Gibson, R., & Quarles, S. (2013). Advancing genomic research and reducing health disparities: What can nurse scholars do? *Journal of Nursing Scholarship, 45*(2), 202–209.
**Leininger, M. (2002). Culture care theory: A major contribution to advance transcultural nursing knowledge and practices. *Journal of Transcultural Nursing, 13*(3), 189–192.
Ludwick, R., & Silva, M. C. (2000). Ethics: Nursing around the world: Cultural values and ethical conflicts. *Online Journal of Issues in Nursing, 5*(3).

Retrieved on 8/27/2016 at: www.nursingworld.org/MainMenuCategories/ANAMarketplace/ANAPeriodicals/OJIN/Columns/Ethics/CulturalValuesandEthicalConflicts.aspx
Mareno, N., & Hart, P. (2014). Cultural competency among nurses with undergraduate and graduate degrees: Implications for nursing education. *Nursing Education Perspectives, 35*(2), 83–88.
Marzilli, C. (2014). Concept analysis of culture applied to nursing. *Creative Nursing, 20*(4), 227–233.
McClimens, A., Brewster, J., & Lewis, R. (2014). Recognising and respecting patients' cultural diversity. *Nursing Standard, 28*(28), 45–52.
Mixer, S. J., McFarland, M. R., Andrews, M. M., et al. (2013). Exploring faculty health and wellbeing: Creating a caring scholarly community. *Nurse Education Today, 33*(12), 1471–1476.
National Council of State Boards of Nursing. (2013). Highlights of the national workforce survey of registered nurses. Retrieved on 12/30/2015 at: www.ncsbn.org/workforce.htm
National Institutes of Health, National Center for Complementary and Integrative Health (NCCIH). (2015). Complementary, alternative, or integrative health: What's in a name? Retrieved on 10/10/2015 at: nccih.nih.gov/health/integrative-health
Ortman, J. M., & Guarneri, C. E. (2011). United States population projections: 2000 to 2050. Retrieved on 12/30/2015 at: www.census.gov/population/projections/files/analytical-document09.pdf
Quality and Safety Education for Nurses. (2015). Competency KSAs (prelicensure). Retrieved on 12/30/2015 at: qsen.org/competencies/pre-licensure-ksas/
Rew, L., Becker, H., Chontichachalalauk, J., et al. (2014). Cultural diversity among nursing students: Reanalysis of the Cultural Awareness Scale. *Journal of Nursing Education, 53*(2), 71–76.
Shen, Z. (2015). Cultural competence models and cultural competence assessment instruments in nursing: A literature review. *Journal of Transcultural Nursing, 26*(3), 308–321.
**Sullivan Commission. (2004). Missing persons: Minorities in the health professions. Retrieved on 12/30/2015 at: www.aacn.nche.edu/media-relations/SullivanReport.pdf
The Joint Commission. (2014). Crosswalk of Joint Commission Hospital Program and the National CLAS Standards. Retrieved on 10/6/2015 at: www.jointcommission.org/topics/health_equity.aspx
U.S. Department of Health & Human Services (HHS), Office of Disease Prevention and Health Promotion. (2015). Healthy People 2020: Disparities. Washington, DC. Retrieved on 12/30/2015 at: www.healthypeople.gov/2020/about/foundation-health-measures/Disparities

Resources

Asian American/Pacific Islander Nurses Association (AAPINA), aapina.org
Council on Nursing and Anthropology (CONAA), www.conaa.org
Healthy People 2020, www.healthypeople.gov/2020/default
LanguageLine Solutions, www.languageline.com (Provides written and oral translation in 140 languages.)
National Black Nurses Association (NBNA), www.nbna.org
National Center for Cultural Competence (NCCC), Georgetown University Center for Child and Human Development, nccc.georgetown.edu
National Institutes of Health, National Center for Complementary and Integrative Health (NCCIH), nccih.nih.gov
Office of Minority Health (OMH), minorityhealth.hhs.gov
Transcultural Nursing Society, www.tcns.org

8 Overview of Genetics and Genomics in Nursing

The completion of the **Human Genome Project** has had a monumental impact on the application of genetics and genomics in all sectors of health care. Some evidence of this genetic revolution is noted with the development of tests that screen and diagnose genetic alterations, so that diseases may be identified and treated earlier (e.g., certain types of breast and ovarian cancers). These advancements also have been useful in generating translational research, which has spurred advances in **pharmacogenetics**, which aims to identify the best medications that can be used to treat an individual patient with a given disease. These advancements have also spurred the development of electronic health records, which give health care providers quick access to each individual patient's comprehensive family health history and personal health risk factors (Cramer, Adjei, & Labhasetwar, 2015). Precision Medicine is a major national initiative that supports both short-term and long-term research initiatives aimed at facilitating genetic and genomic advances in health

TABLE 8-1 Transition from the Medical Era to the Genomic Era of Personalized Medicine

	Medical Era	Genomic Era of Personalized Medicine
Defining Characteristics	• Considers single genes	• Considers interaction of genes with each other and the environment
	• Waits for disease symptoms to appear	• Identifies genetic predisposition and optimizes risk reduction to prevent disease
	• Treats symptoms of presenting disease	• Treats underlying genetic cause of disease
	• Uses trial-and-error approach to treatment	• Uses personalized approach tailored to the genetic/genomic profile of the individual and the disease
	• Tailors medication administration according to clinical trials	• Adapts medication administration per clinical trials *and* personalized genetic response to medication

care (Ashley, 2015; The White House, 2015). Goals of the Precision Medicine initiative are expected to further advance personalized medicine, which tailors health care at the individual level by using a patient's genomic information, often called *genetic makeup* or *genomic profile*.

Identification of the genetic and genomic factors associated with disease, including gene–gene function and gene–environment interactions, contributes to the development of more effective therapies customized to that particular patient's genetic makeup and the genomic profile of his or her disease. The term **genetics** applies to single genes and their impact on relatively rare single gene disorders, whereas **genomics** is the study of the interaction of all genes in the human **genome**, environmental factors and their interactions with each other (Consensus Panel, 2009; National Human Genome Research Institute, 2015). The study of **epigenetics** focuses on changes in the expression of a given gene (Conley, Biesecker, Gonsalves, et al., 2013). Genetic and genomic profiles allow health care providers to prescribe individualized and effective treatment for each patient, to identify and follow individuals at high risk for disease, and to avoid adverse drug reactions (Ashley, 2015). New genomic-based strategies for disease detection, management, and treatment are being utilized, making personalized medicine a reality (see Table 8-1).

To meet the challenges of personalized medicine, nurses must understand the role of genetics as it relates to inheritance patterns, and stay abreast of new technologies and treatments of genetic- and genomic-based health care. Nurses are a vital link between the patient and health care services; patients often turn to nurses first with questions about a family history of risk factors, information regarding genetics, and genetic tests and interpretations. The incorporation of genetics and genomics is relevant to all aspects of the nursing process. For instance, genetics and genomics should be included in health assessments, in devising nursing diagnoses, as appropriate, in planning nursing interventions that are specific to the patient and based upon the patient's diagnosis and genetic makeup, in implementing interventions that support the identification of and response to genetic-related health needs, and in evaluating responses to medications based upon pharmacogenetics (Consensus Panel, 2009). This chapter offers a foundation for the clinical application of genetic and genomic principles in medical-surgical nursing; outlines the nurse's role in genetic counseling and evaluation; addresses important legal, ethical, and social issues; and provides related information and resources for nurses and patients.

Genomic Framework for Nursing Practice

The unique contribution of nursing to genomic medicine is its holistic perspective that takes into account each person's intellectual, physical, spiritual, social, cultural, biopsychologic, ethical, and aesthetic experiences. Because genomics addresses all of the genes of a given individual's human genome working together as a whole, genomics expands nursing's holistic view. Genetics and genomics are the basis of normal and pathophysiologic development, human health and disease, and health outcomes. Knowledge and interpretation of genetic and genomic information, gene-based testing, diagnosis, and treatment broaden the holistic view of nursing. Such expertise in genetics and genomics is basic to nursing practice and its holistic approach to patient care (Consensus Panel, 2009).

The *Essentials of Genetics and Genomic Nursing* (Consensus Panel, 2009) provides a framework for integrating genetics and genomics into nursing practice (see Chart 8-1). This

---

Chart 8-1 **Essential Nursing Competencies for Genetics and Genomics**

Professional Responsibilities

- Recognition of attitudes and beliefs related to genetic and genomic science
- Advocacy for genetic and genomic services
- Incorporation of genetic and genomic technologies and information into practice
- Demonstration of personalizing genetic and genomic information and services
- Providing autonomous, informed genetics- and genomics-related decision making

Professional Practice

- Integrate and apply genetic and genomic knowledge to nursing assessment.
- Identify clients who may benefit from specific genetic and genomic resources, services, or technologies.
- Facilitate referrals for genetic and genomic services.
- Provide education, care, and support related to the interpretation of genetic or genomic tests, services, interventions, or treatments.

Adapted from Consensus Panel on Genetic/Genomic Nursing Competencies. (2009). *Essentials of genetic and genomic nursing: Competencies, curricular guidelines, and outcome indicators.* (2nd ed.). Silver Spring, MD: American Nurses Association.

document includes a philosophy of care that recognizes when genetic and genomic factors play a role or could play a role in a person's health. This means assessing predictive genetic and genomic factors using family history and the results of genetic tests effectively, informing patients about genetics and genomic concepts, understanding the personal and societal impact of genetics and genomic information, and valuing the privacy and confidentiality of genetics and genomic information (Consensus Panel, 2009). In addition, there is formal consensus regarding higher-level competencies in the application of genetics and genomic for nurses with graduate degrees (Greco, Tinley, & Seibert, 2012).

A person's response to genetic and genomic information, genetic testing, or genetics-related conditions may be either empowering or disabling. Genetic and genomic information may stigmatize people if it affects how they view themselves or how others view them. Nurses help individuals and families learn how genetic traits and conditions are passed on within families as well as how genetic and environmental factors influence health and disease (Consensus Panel, 2009). Nurses facilitate communication among family members, the health care system, and community resources, and they offer valuable support to patients and families. All nurses should be able to recognize when a patient is asking a question related to genetic or genomic information and should know how to obtain genetic information by gathering family and health histories and conducting physical and developmental assessments. This enables nurses to provide appropriate genetics resources and support to patients and families (Consensus Panel, 2009).

For example, when nurses assess patients' cardiovascular risk, they can expand their assessment to include information about family history of hypertension, hypercholesterolemia, clotting disorders, or premature sudden cardiac death. Knowledge that genes are involved in the control of lipid metabolism, insulin resistance, blood pressure regulation, clotting factors, cardiac structure, and vascular lining function helps individualize care based on the patient's genetic and genomic risk profile.

Essential to a genetic and genomic framework in nursing is the awareness of one's attitudes, experience, and assumptions about genetics and genomic concepts and how these are manifested in one's own practice (Consensus Panel, 2009). To develop awareness of these attitudes, experiences, and assumptions, the nurse must examine their own:

- Beliefs or values about health as well as family, religious, or cultural beliefs about the cause of illness and how one's values or biases affect understanding of genetic conditions
- Philosophical, theologic, cultural, and ethical perspectives related to health and how these perspectives influence one's use of genetic information or services
- Level of expertise about genetics and genomics
- Experiences with birth defects, chronic illnesses, and genetic conditions, along with one's view of such conditions as disabling or empowering
- Attitudes about the right to access and other rights of individuals with genetic disorders
- View and assumptions about deoxyribonucleic acid (DNA) and beliefs about the value of information about one's risk for genetic disorders

- Beliefs about reproductive options
- View of genetic testing and engineering
- Approach to patients with disabilities

Integrating Genetic and Genomic Knowledge

Scientific developments and advances in technology have increased understanding of genetics, resulting in better understanding of relatively rare diseases, such as phenylketonuria (PKU) or hemophilia, that are related to mutations of a single inherited gene. Scientists are able to characterize inherited metabolic variations that interact over time and lead to common diseases such as cancer, heart disease, and dementia. The transition from genetics to genomics has increased understanding of how multiple genes act and control biologic processes. Most diseases are now believed to be the result of a combination of genetic and environmental influences (Roadmap Epigenomics Consortium, 2015).

Genes and Their Role in Human Variation

Genes are central components of human health and disease. The Human Genome Project has linked basic human genetics to human development, health, and disease (National Institutes of Health [NIH], 2014a). Knowledge that specific genes are associated with specific genetic conditions makes diagnosis possible, even in the unborn. Many common conditions have genetic causes, and many more associations between genetics, health, and disease continue to be identified.

Genes and Chromosomes

A person's unique genetic constitution, called a **genotype**, is made up of approximately 25,000 genes (Romanoski & Glass, 2015). A person's **phenotype**—the observable characteristics or expression of their genotype—includes physical appearance and other biologic, physiologic, and molecular traits. Environmental influences modify every person's phenotype, even phenotypes with a major genetic component. This concept of genotype and phenotype applies to a person's total genome and the respective traits of their genetic makeup.

The concepts of genotype and phenotype also apply to specific diseases. For example, in hypercholesterolemia, the genotype refers to the genes that control lipid metabolism, and the phenotype may be manifested in various corresponding ways. The genotype involves mutations in low-density lipoprotein (LDL) receptors and in one of the apolipoprotein genes. The phenotype is characterized by early onset of cardiovascular disease, high levels of LDL, skin xanthomas, and a family history of heart disease. An individual's genotype, consisting of normal functioning genes as well as some mutations, is characterized by physical and biologic traits that may predispose to disease.

Human growth, development, and disease occur as a result of both genetic and environmental influences and interactions. The contribution of genetic factors may be large or small. For example, in a person with cystic fibrosis or PKU, the genetic contribution is significant. In contrast, the genetic contribution underlying a person's response to infection may be less applicable.

Figure 8-1 • DNA is a double helix formed by base pairs attached to a sugar-phosphate backbone. DNA carries the instructions that allow cells to make proteins. DNA is made up of four chemical bases. Redrawn from Genetics Home Reference, ghr.nlm.nih.gov/handbook/illustrations/dnastructure

A single gene is conceptualized as a unit of heredity. A gene is composed of a segment of **deoxyribonucleic acid (DNA)** that contains a specific set of instructions for making the protein or proteins needed by body cells for proper functioning. Genes regulate both the types of proteins made and the rate at which proteins are produced. The structure of the DNA molecule is referred to as a double helix. The essential components of the DNA molecule are sugar–phosphate molecules and pairs of nitrogenous bases. Each nucleotide contains a sugar (deoxyribose), a phosphate group, and one of four nitrogenous bases: adenine (A), cytosine (C), guanine (G), and thymine (T). DNA is composed of two paired strands, each made up of a number of nucleotides. The strands are held together by hydrogen bonds between pairs of bases (see Fig. 8-1).

Genes are arranged in a linear order within **chromosomes**, which are located in the cell nucleus. In humans, 46 chromosomes occur in pairs in all body cells except oocytes (eggs) and sperm, which each contains only 23 unpaired chromosomes. Twenty-two pairs of chromosomes, called *autosomes*, are the same in females and males. The 23rd pair is referred to as the sex chromosomes. A female has two X chromosomes, whereas a male has one X chromosome and one Y chromosome. At conception, each parent normally gives one chromosome of each pair to their child. As a result, children receive half of their chromosomes from fathers and half from mothers (see Fig. 8-2).

Careful examination of DNA sequences from many people shows that these sequences have multiple versions in a population. The different versions of these sequences are called *alleles*. Sequences found in many forms are said to be polymorphic, meaning that there are at least two common forms of a particular gene.

Cell Division

The human body grows and develops as a result of the process of cell division. Mitosis and meiosis are two distinctly different types of cell division.

Mitosis is involved in cell growth, differentiation, and repair. During mitosis, the chromosomes of each cell duplicate. The result is two cells, called *daughter cells*, each of which contains the same number of chromosomes as the parent cell. The daughter cells are said to be diploid because they contain 46 chromosomes in 23 pairs. Mitosis occurs in all cells of the body except oocytes and sperm.

Meiosis, in contrast, occurs only in reproductive cells and is the process by which oocytes and sperm are formed. During meiosis, a reduction in the number of chromosomes takes place, resulting in oocytes or sperm that contain half the usual number, or 23 chromosomes. Oocytes and sperm are referred to as haploid because they contain a single copy of each chromosome, compared to the usual two copies in all other body cells. During meiosis, as the paired chromosomes come together in preparation for cell division, portions cross over, and an exchange of genetic material occurs before the chromosomes separate. This event, called *recombination*, creates greater diversity in the makeup of oocytes and sperm.

During the process of meiosis, a pair of chromosomes may fail to separate completely, creating a sperm or oocyte that

Figure 8-2 • Each human cell contains 23 pairs of chromosomes, which can be distinguished by their size and unique banding patterns. This set is from a male, because it contains a Y chromosome. Females have two X chromosomes. Redrawn from Genetics Home Reference, ghr.nlm.nih.gov/handbook/basics/howmanychromosomes contains either two copies or no copy of a particular chromosome. This sporadic event, called **nondisjunction**, can lead to either a trisomy or a monosomy. Down syndrome is an example of trisomy, in which people have three copies of chromosome number 21. Turner syndrome is an example of monosomy, in which girls have a single X chromosome, causing them to have short stature and infertility (U.S. National Library of Medicine [NLM], 2015a).

Gene Mutations

Within each cell, many intricate and complex interactions regulate and express human genes. Gene structure and function, transcription and translation, and protein synthesis are all involved. Alterations in gene structure and function and the process of protein synthesis may influence a person's health. Changes in gene structure, called **mutations**, permanently change the sequence of DNA, which in turn can alter the nature and type of proteins made (see Fig. 8-3).

Some gene mutations have no significant effect on the protein product, whereas others cause partial or complete changes. How a protein is altered and its importance to body functioning determines the impact of the mutation. Gene mutations may occur in hormones, enzymes, or other important protein products, with significant implications for health and disease. Sickle cell disease is a genetic condition caused by a small gene mutation that affects protein structure, producing hemoglobin S. A person who inherits two copies of the hemoglobin S gene mutation has sickle cell disease and experiences the symptoms of severe anemia and thrombotic organ damage resulting from hypoxia (NIH, 2014b).

Other gene mutations include deletion (loss), insertion (addition), duplication (multiplication), or rearrangement (translocation) of a longer DNA segment. Duchenne muscular dystrophy, myotonic dystrophy, Huntington disease, and fragile X syndrome are examples of conditions caused by gene mutations.

Gene mutations may be inherited or acquired. Inherited or germline gene mutations are present in the DNA of all body cells and are passed on in reproductive cells from parent to child.

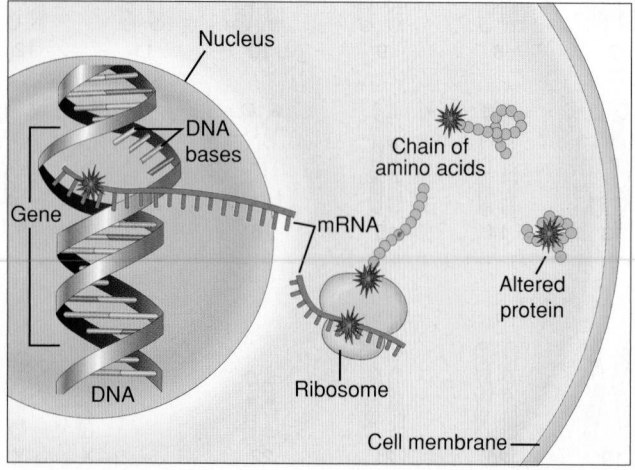

Figure 8-3 • When a gene contains a mutation, the protein encoded by that gene is likely to be abnormal. Sometimes the protein is able to function, although it does so imperfectly. In other cases, it is totally disabled. The outcome depends not only on how the mutation alters the protein's function but also on how vital that particular protein is to survival.

Figure 8-4 • Hereditary mutations are carried in the DNA of the reproductive cells. When reproductive cells containing mutations combine to produce offspring, the mutation is present in all of the offspring's body cells. Redrawn from National Cancer Institute, www.cancer.gov/cancertopics/understandingcancer/genetesting/page11

Germline or hereditary mutations are passed on to all daughter cells when body cells replicate (see Fig. 8-4). The gene that causes Huntington disease is one example of a germline mutation.

Spontaneous mutations take place in individual oocytes or sperm at the time of conception. A person who carries the new "spontaneous" mutation may pass on the mutation to his or her children. Achondroplasia, Marfan syndrome, and neurofibromatosis type 1 are examples of genetic conditions that may occur in a single family member as a result of spontaneous mutation.

Acquired mutations take place in somatic cells and involve changes in DNA that occur after conception, during a person's lifetime. Acquired mutations develop as a result of cumulative changes in body cells other than reproductive cells (see Fig. 8-5). Somatic gene mutations are passed on to the daughter cells derived from that particular cell line.

Gene mutations occur in the human body all the time. Cells have built-in mechanisms by which they can recognize mutations in DNA, and in most situations, they correct the changes before they are passed on by cell division. However, over time, body cells may lose their ability to repair damage from gene mutations, causing an accumulation of genetic changes that result in diseases such as cancer, Alzheimer disease, and other conditions of aging (Roadmap Epigenomics Consortium, 2015).

Genetic Variation

Genetic variations occur among all people. Single nucleotide polymorphisms (SNPs, referred to as "snips") is the term used to identify common genetic variations that occur most frequently throughout the human genome. SNPs are changes in a single nucleotide (an A, T, C, or G) of the DNA sequence. For example, a normal DNA sequence of AAGGT could change to ATGG; in this case, there is one single nucleotide change from A to T. Most SNPs do not alter normal cell function. Some SNPs do alter gene function and may influence disease

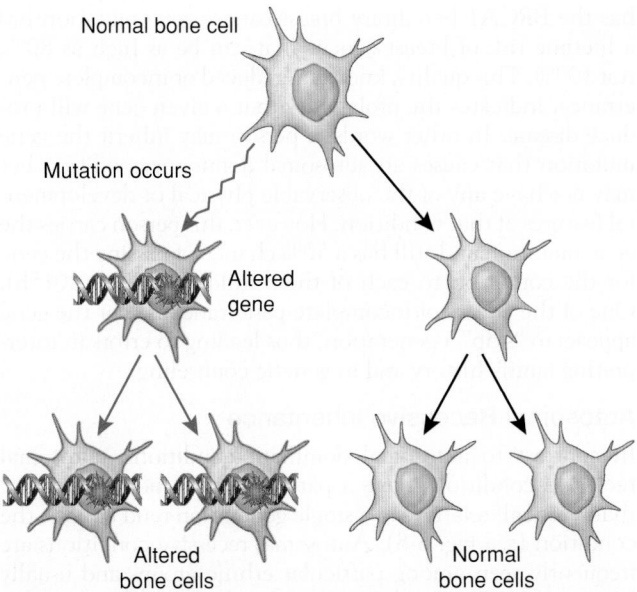

Figure 8-5 • Acquired mutations develop in DNA during a person's lifetime. If the mutation arises in a body cell, copies of the mutation will exist only in the descendants of that particular cell. Redrawn from National Cancer Institute, www.cancer.gov/cancertopics/understandingcancer/genetesting/page12

Figure 8-6 • Three-generation pedigree illustrating autosomal dominant inheritance.

development. Knowledge about SNPs that affect biologic function will help pinpoint individuals who may be more prone to common diseases such as cancer, diabetes, and heart disease. Information on SNPs has helped to clarify why some individuals metabolize drugs differently (Korf & Rehm, 2013). For example, a polymorphism or SNP can alter protein or enzyme activity of medications. If the SNP causes a variation in drug transport or drug metabolism, the drug's action, half-life, or excretion could lead to lack of drug response or drug toxicity.

Inheritance Patterns

Nursing assessment of the patient's health includes obtaining and recording family history information in the form of a **pedigree**. This is a first step in establishing the pattern of inheritance. Nurses must be familiar with mendelian patterns of inheritance and pedigree construction and analysis to help identify patients and families who may benefit from further genetic counseling, testing, and treatment (Consensus Panel, 2009).

Mendelian conditions are genetic conditions that are inherited in fixed proportions among generations. They result from gene mutations that are present on one or both chromosomes of a pair. A single gene inherited from one or both parents can cause a mendelian condition. Mendelian conditions are classified according to their pattern of inheritance: autosomal dominant, autosomal recessive, and **X-linked**. The terms **dominant** and **recessive** refer to the trait, genetic condition, or phenotype but not to the genes or alleles that cause the observable characteristics (U.S. NLM, 2015a).

Autosomal Dominant Inheritance

Autosomal dominant inherited conditions affect female and male family members equally and follow a vertical pattern of inheritance in families (see Fig. 8-6). A person who has an autosomal dominant inherited condition carries a gene mutation

for that condition on one chromosome of a pair. Each of that person's offspring has a 50% chance of inheriting the gene mutation for the condition and a 50% chance of inheriting the normal version of the gene (see Fig. 8-7). Offspring who

Figure 8-7 • In dominant genetic disorders, if one affected parent has a disease-causing allele that dominates its normal counterpart, each child in the family has a 50% chance of inheriting the disease allele and the disorder. Redrawn from Genetics Home Reference, ghr.nlm.nih.gov/handbook/illustrations/autodominant

TABLE 8-2 Patterns of Mendelian Inheritance

Characteristics	Examples
Autosomal Dominant Inherited Conditions	
Vertical transmission in families Males and females equally affected Variable expression among family members and others with condition Reduced penetrance (in some conditions) Advanced paternal age associated with sporadic cases	Hereditary breast/ovarian cancer syndrome Familial hypercholesterolemia Hereditary nonpolyposis colorectal cancer Huntington disease Marfan syndrome Neurofibromatosis
Autosomal Recessive Inherited Conditions	
Horizontal pattern of transmission seen in families Males and females equally affected Associated with consanguinity (genetic relatedness) Associated with particular ethnic groups	Cystic fibrosis Galactosemia Phenylketonuria Sickle cell disease Tay–Sachs disease Canavan disease
X-Linked Recessive Inherited Conditions	
Vertical transmission in families Males predominantly affected	Duchenne muscular dystrophy Hemophilia A and B Wiskott–Aldrich syndrome Protan and Deutran forms of color blindness
Multifactorial Inherited Conditions	
Occur as a result of combination of genetic and environmental factors May recur in families Inheritance pattern does not demonstrate characteristic pattern of inheritance seen with other mendelian conditions	Congenital heart defects Cleft lip and/or palate Neural tube defects (anencephaly and spina bifida) Diabetes mellitus Osteoarthritis High blood pressure

Adapted from Dwyer, T. M., Glaser, R. L., & Mason, T. M. (2016). Inheritance patterns in human phenotypes and types of genetic disorders. In C. E. Kasper, T. A. Schneidereith, & F. R. Lashley (Eds.), *Lashley's essentials of clinical genetics in nursing practice* (pp. 65–114). New York, NY. Springer Publishing Company; U.S. National Library of Medicine. Genetic Home Reference (NLM). (2015a). *What are the different ways in which a genetic condition can be inherited?* Retrieved on 6/30/2015 at: ghr.nlm.nih.gov/handbook/inheritance/inheritancepatterns

do not inherit the gene mutation do not develop the condition and do not have an increased chance for having children with the same condition. Table 8-2 presents characteristics and examples of different patterns of inherited conditions.

Autosomal dominant conditions often manifest with varying degrees of severity. Some affected people may have significant symptoms, whereas others may have only mild ones. This characteristic is referred to as **variable expression**; it results from the influences of genetic and environmental factors on clinical presentation.

Another phenomenon observed in autosomal dominant inheritance is penetrance, or the percentage of persons known to have a particular gene mutation who actually show the trait. Almost complete penetrance is observed in conditions such as achondroplasia, in which nearly 100% of people with the gene mutation typically display traits of the disease. However, in some conditions, the presence of a gene mutation does not invariably mean that a person has or will develop an autosomal inherited condition. For example, a woman who

has the *BRCA1* hereditary breast cancer gene mutation has a lifetime risk of breast cancer that can be as high as 80%, not 100%. This quality, known as reduced or incomplete penetrance, indicates the probability that a given gene will produce disease. In other words, a person may inherit the gene mutation that causes an autosomal dominant condition but may not have any of the observable physical or developmental features of that condition. However, this person carries the gene mutation and still has a 50% chance of passing the gene for the condition to each of their children (NLM, 2015b). One of the effects of incomplete penetrance is that the gene appears to "skip" a generation, thus leading to errors in interpreting family history and in genetic counseling.

Autosomal Recessive Inheritance

In contrast to autosomal dominant conditions, autosomal recessive conditions have a pattern that is more horizontal than vertical; relatives of a single generation tend to have the condition (see Fig. 8-8). Autosomal recessive conditions are frequently seen among particular ethnic groups and usually occur more often in children of parents who are related by blood, such as first cousins (see Table 8-2).

In autosomal recessive inheritance, each parent carries a gene mutation on one chromosome of the pair and a normal gene on the other chromosome. The parents are said to be **carriers** of the gene mutation. Unlike people with an autosomal dominant condition, carriers of a gene mutation for a recessive condition do not have symptoms of the genetic condition. When carriers have children together, there is a 25% chance that each child may inherit the gene mutation from both parents and have the condition (see Fig. 8-9). Cystic fibrosis, sickle cell disease, and PKU are examples of autosomal recessive conditions (NLM, 2015a).

X-Linked Inheritance

X-linked conditions may be inherited in recessive or dominant patterns (see Table 8-2). In both, the gene mutation is

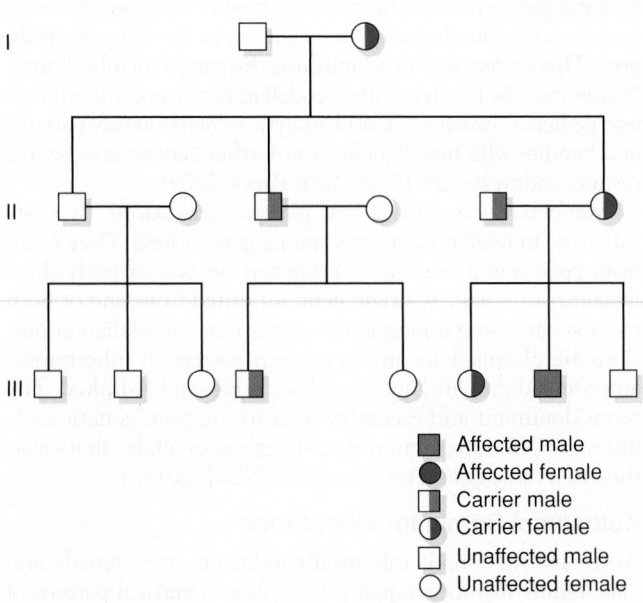

Figure 8-8 • Three-generation pedigree illustrating autosomal recessive inheritance.

■ Affected male
● Affected female
◩ Carrier male
◖ Carrier female
□ Unaffected male
○ Unaffected female

Carrier father   Carrier mother

Unaffected | Carrier | Carrier | Affected
daughter | son | daughter | son

Figure 8-9 • In diseases associated with altered recessive genes, both parents—although disease free themselves—carry one normal allele and one altered allele. Each child has one chance in four of inheriting two abnormal alleles and developing the disorder; one chance in four of inheriting two normal alleles; and two chances in four of inheriting one normal and one altered allele—therefore, being a carrier like both parents. Redrawn from Genetics Home Reference, ghr.nlm.nih.gov/handbook/illustrations/autorecessive

located on the X chromosome. All males inherit an X chromosome from mothers and a Y chromosome from fathers for a normal sex constitution of 46, XY. Because males have only one X chromosome, they do not have a counterpart for its genes, as do females. This means that a gene mutation on the X chromosome of a male is expressed even though it is present in only one copy. Females, on the contrary, inherit one X chromosome from each parent for a normal sex constitution of 46, XX A female may be an unaffected carrier of a gene mutation, or she may be affected if the condition results from a gene mutation causing an X-linked dominant condition. Either the X chromosome that she received from her mother or the X chromosome she received from her father may be passed on to each of her offspring, and this is a random occurrence.

The most common pattern of X-linked inheritance is that in which a female is a carrier for a gene mutation on one of her X chromosomes. This is referred to as X-linked recessive inheritance in which a female carrier has a 50% chance of passing on the gene mutation to a son, who would be affected, or to a daughter, who would be a carrier like her mother (see Fig. 8-10). Examples of X-linked recessive conditions include factor VIII and factor IX hemophilia, severe combined immunodeficiency, and Duchenne muscular dystrophy.

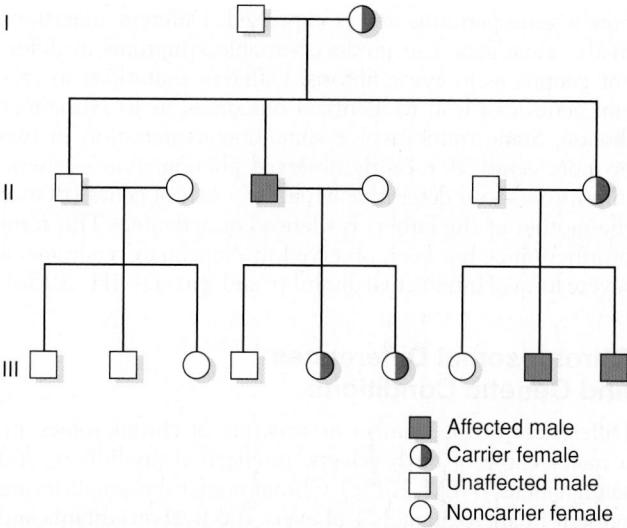

■ Affected male
◐ Carrier female
□ Unaffected male
○ Noncarrier female

Figure 8-10 • Three-generation pedigree illustrating X-linked recessive inheritance.

Multifactorial Inheritance and Complex Genetic Conditions

Many birth defects and common health conditions such as heart disease, high blood pressure, cancer, osteoarthritis, and diabetes occur as a result of interactions of multiple gene mutations and environmental influences. Thus, they are called *multifactorial* or *complex conditions* (see Table 8-2). Other examples of multifactorial genetic conditions include neural tube defects such as spina bifida and anencephaly. Multifactorial conditions may cluster in families; however, they do not always result in the characteristic pattern of inheritance seen in families who have mendelian inherited conditions (see Fig. 8-11).

Nontraditional Inheritance

Although mendelian conditions manifest with a specific pattern of inheritance in some families, many diseases and traits do not follow these simple patterns. Various factors influence

□ Unaffected male
○ Unaffected female
■ Affected male

Figure 8-11 • Three-generation pedigree illustrating multifactorial conditions.

how a gene performs and is expressed. Different mutations in the same gene can produce variable symptoms in different people, as in cystic fibrosis. Different mutations in several genes can lead to identical outcomes, as in Alzheimer disease. Some traits involve simultaneous mutation in two or more genes. A recently observed phenomenon—genetic imprinting—can determine which of a pair of genes (that of the mother or the father) is silenced or activated. This form of inheritance has been observed in Angelman syndrome, a severe form of intellectual disability and ataxia (NIH, 2015a).

Chromosomal Differences and Genetic Conditions

Differences in the number or structure of chromosomes are a major cause of birth defects, intellectual disabilities, and malignancies (NLM, 2015c). Chromosomal abnormalities are present in approximately 1 of every 160 liveborn infants and are the cause of more than 50% of all spontaneous abortions or miscarriages (Dwyer, Glaser, & Mason, 2016) Chromosomal differences most commonly involve an extra or missing chromosome; this is called *aneuploidy*. Whenever there is an extra or missing chromosome, there is always associated intellectual or physical disability to some degree.

Down syndrome, or trisomy 21, is a common chromosomal condition that occurs with greater frequency in pregnancies of women who are 35 years of age or older. A person with trisomy 21 has a complete extra chromosome 21, which causes a particular facial appearance and increased risk of congenital heart defects, thyroid and vision problems, and intellectual disability. Other examples of chromosomal differences include trisomy 13 and trisomy 18, both more severe than Down syndrome, and conditions involving extra or missing sex chromosomes, such as Turner syndrome (NIH, 2013a).

Chromosomal differences may also involve a structural rearrangement within or between chromosomes. These are less common than chromosomal conditions in which there is an extra or missing chromosome (NIH, 2015b; NLM, 2015c). People who carry "balanced" chromosome rearrangements have all of their chromosomal material; however, it is rearranged. Women with a "balanced" chromosomal rearrangement have an increased risk of spontaneous pregnancy loss and of having children with an unbalanced chromosomal arrangement that may result in physical or intellectual disabilities. Known carriers of these chromosomal differences are offered prenatal counseling and testing.

Chromosome studies may be needed at any age, depending on the indication. Two common indications are a suspected diagnosis such as Down syndrome and a history of two or more unexplained pregnancy losses. Chromosome studies are accomplished by obtaining a tissue sample (e.g., blood, skin, and amniotic fluid), preparing and staining the chromosomes, and analyzing them under a microscope. The microscopic study of chromosomes, called *cytogenetics*, is used with molecular techniques such as fluorescent in situ hybridization (FISH), which permits more detailed examination of chromosomes (Korf & Rehm, 2013). FISH is useful to detect small abnormalities and to characterize chromosomal rearrangements.

Genetic and Genomic Technologies in Practice

The application of genetics and genomics has gained significant momentum in the discovery and development of genetic tests that can be used to detect a trait, diagnose a genetic condition, and identify people who have a genetic predisposition to a disease such as cancer or heart disease (Conley et al., 2013). Pharmacogenetics uses genetic testing to identify genetic variations that relate to the safety and efficacy of medications and gene-based treatments so that individualized treatment can be developed (Johnson, 2013). Future applications may include the use of gene chips to map a person's individual genome for genetic variations that may lead to disease. Nurses are involved in caring for patients who are undergoing genetic testing and gene-based treatments. Knowledge of the clinical applications of modern genetic and genomic technologies enables nurses to inform and support patients and to provide high-quality genetics-related health care (Consensus Panel, 2009).

Genetic Testing

Genetic testing is the primary tool used to identify individuals predisposed to specific genetic diseases. Genetic tests provide information leading to the diagnosis of inherited conditions or other conditions with a known genetic contribution.

In genetic testing, approaches may be genotypic or phenotypic. Genotypic methods involve analysis of the chromosomes and genes directly, using specific laboratory techniques to learn whether a genetic alteration related to a specific disease or condition is present. This testing may be DNA based, chromosomal, or biochemical. Phenotypic methods examine the familial or biologic presentation of disease and include assessment of the patient's personal or family history and medical factors influencing their disease as well as testing for gene products such as protein markers in body fluids or diseased tissues. The family history, which is considered the first genetic test, is discussed later in this chapter (see the Family History Assessment section). It is expected that all nurses will know how to use this genetic tool.

Another phenotypic approach involves searching for gene products, such as proteins and enzymes that can clinically indicate a genetic abnormality. For example, germline mutations in the repair genes *MLH1*, *MSH2*, *MSH6*, and *PMS2* are responsible for hereditary early onset colorectal cancer. Colorectal tumors are now tested to measure the presence or absence of these proteins using immunohistochemistry, which is a routine type of pathology test. Tumors that stain negative for one of those proteins signify malfunction of the gene whose protein is missing. Patients with absent or negative protein expression in their tumors (e.g., *MLH1* protein–negative) can proceed with genetic testing for a germline *MLH1* mutation (Harkness Barrow, Newton, et al., 2015).

Genetic testing can be used for various purposes in prenatal, pediatric, and adult populations. Prenatal testing is widely used for **prenatal screening** and diagnosis of conditions such as Down syndrome. Carrier testing is used to determine if a person carries a recessive allele for an inherited condition (e.g., cystic fibrosis, sickle cell disease, Tay–Sachs disease) and, therefore, risks passing it on to their children. Genetic testing is also used widely in newborn screening.

Chart 8-2 ETHICAL DILEMMA
Can Predictive Genetic Testing Threaten Patient Autonomy?

Case Scenario

Ashley is a 34-year-old woman who is a patient in the family care clinic. Her sister just gave birth to a child who was born with fragile X syndrome (a genetic mutation associated with intellectual disabilities and impaired social development). Although her first child, a daughter, has not demonstrated any signs of this disorder, Ashley is requesting to have predictive genetic testing (PGT) on her 5-year-old daughter to determine if she is a carrier of fragile X syndrome.

Discussion

The Human Genome Project initiative has spearheaded the development of technology that can identify conditions with genetic origins in patients who have no demonstrable symptoms but may carry a mutated gene. Although not evidencing the disorder, future offspring of a patient who carries the mutation may have the disorder. PGT may be done to identify patients who may be carriers for inherited genetic disorders such as fragile X syndrome.

One of the legal and ethical concerns raised by health care providers regarding pediatric genetic screening addresses the value of testing for disorders that cannot be cured or ameliorated. In this particular case, the data obtained from this screening will not be used to medically benefit the health of Ashley's daughter. The American College of Medical Genetics contends that ultimately, the best interest of the person tested must be the focus of PGT.

Arguably, Ashley's daughter will have the right to give informed consent to this procedure as an adult, should she choose to do so.

Analysis

Describe the ethical principles that are in conflict in this case (see Chapter 3, Chart 3-3). Which principle do you believe should have preeminence in deciding whether or not parents have the right to have PGT in a child who will not medically benefit from the findings?

- Do the benefits outweigh the risks of PGT in the child? Identify the stakeholders who could benefit from the findings of PGT.
- Are there any professional guidelines that you can turn to for help in determining the ethical issues that still remain around PGT? If so, what are they, and how can they help?

References

Clayton, E. W., McCullough, L. B., Biesecker, L. G., et al. (2014). Addressing the ethical challenges in genetic testing and sequencing of children. *The American Journal of Bioethics, 14*(3), 3–9.

Porry, P., Shabani, M., & Howard, H. C. (2014). Is there a right time to know? The right not to know and genetic testing in children. *Journal of Law, Medicine, & Ethics, 42*(1), 19–27.

Resources

See Chapter 3, Chart 3-6 for ethics resources.

In the United States, genetic testing is available for more than 4000 genetic disorders (Genetests, 2015a).

Diagnostic testing is used to detect the presence or absence of a particular genetic alteration or allele to identify or confirm a diagnosis of a disease or condition (e.g., myotonic dystrophy, fragile X syndrome) (see Chart 8-2). Increasingly, genetic tests are being used to predict drug response and to design specific and individualized treatment plans or personalized medicine. For example, genetic testing is used to identify specific gene variants that can predict the effectiveness of treatments of human immunodeficiency virus infection, atherothrombosis, thrombophilia, hyperlipidemia, breast cancer, pain management, hepatitis C, rheumatoid arthritis, leukemia, depression, and bipolar disorder (Johnson, 2013; Korf & Rehm, 2013). Selected examples of current uses of genetic tests are shown in Table 8-3.

Nurses are increasingly involved in taking family histories and educating the patient about aspects of genetic testing. They contribute by ensuring informed health choices and consent, advocating for privacy and confidentiality with regard to genetic test results, and helping patients understand the complex issues involved (Consensus Panel, 2009).

Genetic Screening

Genetic screening, in contrast to genetic testing, applies to testing of populations or groups independent of a positive family history or symptom manifestation. Genetic screening, as defined in 1975 by the Committee for the Study of Inborn Errors of Metabolism of the National Academy of Sciences (Simopoulos, 2009), has several major aims. The first aim is to improve management—that is, to identify people with treatable genetic conditions that could prove dangerous to their health if left untreated. For example, newborns are screened for an increasing number of conditions, including PKU, congenital hypothyroidism, and galactosemia. The second aim is to provide reproductive options to people with a

TABLE 8-3 Selected Genetic Tests: Examples of Current Uses

Purpose of Genetic Test	Type of Genetic Test
Carrier Testing	
Cystic–fibrosis	DNA analysis
Tay–Sachs disease	Hexosaminidase A activity testing and DNA analysis
Canavan disease	DNA analysis
Sickle cell disease	Hemoglobin electrophoresis
Thalassemia	Complete blood count and hemoglobin electrophoresis
Diagnosis	
Down syndrome	Chromosomal analysis
Fragile X syndrome	DNA analysis
Myotonic dystrophy	DNA analysis
Presymptomatic Testing	
Huntington disease	DNA analysis
Myotonic dystrophy	DNA analysis
Susceptibility Testing	
Hereditary breast/ovarian cancer	DNA analysis
Hereditary nonpolyposis colorectal cancer	DNA analysis

DNA, deoxyribonucleic acid.
Adapted from U.S. National Library of Medicine. Genetics Home Reference (NLM). (2015e). *What are the types of genetic tests?* Retrieved on 11/24/2015 at: ghr.nlm.nih.gov/handbook/testing/uses

TABLE 8-4 Applications for Genetic Screening

Timing of Screening	Purpose	Examples
Preconception/ preimplantation screening	Preconception screening may be done to test for autosomal recessive inherited genetic conditions that occur with greater frequency among individuals of certain ethnic groups; furthermore, through the use of in vitro fertilization, embryos may be tested for specific genetic or chromosomal abnormalities	Cystic fibrosis—all couples, but especially northern European Caucasian and Ashkenazi Jewish Tay–Sachs disease—Ashkenazi Jewish Sickle cell disease—African American, Puerto Rican, Mediterranean, Middle Eastern Alpha-thalassemia—Southeast Asian, African American
Prenatal screening	For genetic conditions that are common and for which prenatal diagnosis is available when a pregnancy is identified at increased risk	Neural tube defects—spina bifida, anencephaly Down syndrome Other chromosomal abnormalities—trisomy 18
Newborn screening	For genetic conditions for which there is specific treatment	Phenylketonuria (PKU) Galactosemia Homocystinuria Biotinidase deficiency
Diagnostic screening	To determine whether a specific genetic mutation exists or to confirm diagnosis when phenotypic presentation exists	Hypertrophic cardiomyopathy
Carrier testing	To determine if an individual carries a mutated gene; this type of testing is useful for couples to ascertain genetic risk of having a child with a genetic disorder; particularly useful with autosomal recessive disorders	Cystic fibrosis—all couples, but especially northern European Caucasian and Ashkenazi Jewish Tay–Sachs disease—Ashkenazi Jewish Sickle cell disease—African American, Puerto Rican, Mediterranean, Middle Eastern
Predictive testing	For genetic conditions that appear later in life or for genetic disorders that have minimal phenotypic presentation	Colorectal cancer Huntington disease Hemochromatosis

Adapted from U.S. National Library of Medicine. Genetics Home Reference (NLM). (2015e). *What are the types of genetic tests?* Retrieved on 11/24/2015 at: ghr.nlm.nih.gov/handbook/testing/uses

high probability of having children with severe, untreatable diseases and for whom genetic counseling, prenatal diagnosis, and other reproductive options could be helpful and of interest. For example, people of Ashkenazi Jewish descent (Jews of eastern European origin) are screened for conditions such as Tay–Sachs disease and Canavan disease. The third aim is to screen pregnant women to detect birth defects such as neural tube defects and Down syndrome. Genetic screening may also be used for public health purposes to determine the incidence and prevalence of a birth defect or to investigate the feasibility and value of new genetic testing methods. Most commonly, genetic screening occurs in prenatal and newborn programs. Table 8-4 gives examples of types of genetic screening.

 Concept Mastery Alert

Genetic testing and genetic screening are terms that are often confused. Nurses need to remember that testing is individual; screening is population based.

Testing and Screening for Adult-Onset Conditions

Adult-onset conditions with a genetic or genomic basis are manifested in later life. Often, clinical signs or symptoms occur only in late adolescence or adulthood, and disease is clearly observed to run in families. Some of these conditions are attributed to specific genetic mutations and follow either an autosomal dominant or an autosomal recessive inheritance pattern. However, most adult-onset conditions are considered

to be genomic or multifactorial—that is, they result from a combination of genes or gene–environment interactions. Examples of multifactorial conditions include heart disease, diabetes, and arthritis. Genomic or multifactorial influences involve interactions among several genes (gene–gene interactions) and between genes and the environment (gene–environment interactions), as well as the individual's lifestyle (Waters, Muff, & Hamilton, 2014).

Nursing assessment for adult-onset conditions is based on family history, personal and medical risk factors, and identification of associated diseases or clinical manifestations (the phenotype). Knowledge of adult-onset conditions and their genetic bases (i.e., mendelian vs. multifactorial conditions) influences the nursing considerations for genetic testing and health promotion. Table 8-5 describes selected adult-onset conditions, their age of onset, patterns of inheritance, molecular genetics, and test availability.

Single Gene Conditions

If a single gene accounts for an adult-onset condition in a symptomatic person, testing is used to confirm a diagnosis to assist in the plan of care and management. Diagnostic testing for adult-onset conditions is most frequently used with autosomal dominant conditions, such as Huntington disease or factor V Leiden thrombophilia, and with autosomal recessive conditions such as hemochromatosis. Other single gene conditions are associated with a confirmed genetic mutation in an affected family member or with a family history suggestive of an inherited pattern of adult-onset disease, such as

TABLE 8-5 Selected Adult-Onset Disorders

Clinical Description	Age of Onset	Genetic Inheritance	Molecular Genetics	Test Availability
Neurologic Conditions				
Early-Onset Familial Alzheimer Disease (EOFAD)				
Progressive dementia, memory failure, personality disturbance, loss of intellectual functioning associated with cerebral cortical atrophy, beta-amyloid plaque formation, and intraneuronal neurofibrillary tangles	<60–65 years; often <55 years	A.D.	PSEN1 (14q24) mutations in presenilin 1 gene; (30–70% of pathogenic variants) APP (21q21.3); (10–15% of pathogenic variants) PSEN2 (14q24.2); (<5% of pathogenic variants)	Presymptomatic
Late-Onset Familial Alzheimer Disease				
Progressive dementia, cognitive decline	60–65 years		Apolipoprotein E (19q13) Apo E gene product	Presymptomatic
Frontotemporal Dementia With Parkinsonism-17				
Dementia and/or parkinsonism: Slowly progressive behavioral changes, language disturbances and/or extrapyramidal signs, rigidity, bradykinesia, and saccadic eye movements	40–60 years	A.D.	MAPT gene (linked to 17q21.1)	Diagnostic and presymptomatic
Huntington Disease				
Widespread degenerative brain change with progressive motor loss; both voluntary disability and involuntary disability, cognitive decline, chorea (involuntary movements) at later stage, psychiatric disturbances	Mean age, 35–44 years	A.D.	HTT HD gene (4p16)	Diagnostic and presymptomatic
Neuromuscular Disorders				
Spinocerebellar Ataxia Type 6				
Slowly progressive cerebellar ataxia, dysarthria, and nystagmus	Mean age, 43–52 years	A.D.	CACNA1A gene (19p13)	Diagnostic and presymptomatic
Spinocerebellar Ataxia Type 1				
Ataxia, dysarthria, and bulbar dysfunction	Mean age, 30–40 years	A.D.	ATXN1 gene (6p22-p23)	Diagnostic and presymptomatic
Spinocerebellar Ataxia Type 2				
Slow saccadic eye movement, peripheral neuropathy, decreased deep tendon reflexes, dementia	Mean age, 30–40 years	A.D.	ATXN2 gene (12q24.1)	Diagnostic and presymptomatic
Spinocerebellar Ataxia Type 3				
Progressive cerebellar ataxia and various other neurologic symptoms including dystonic-rigid syndrome, parkinsonian syndrome or combined dystonia, and peripheral neuropathy	Mean age onset in 30s	A.D.	ATXN3 gene (14q21)	Diagnostic and presymptomatic
Myotonic Muscular Dystrophy Type 1				
Cataracts and myotonia or muscle wasting and weakness, frontal balding and electrocardiographic changes (heart block or dysrhythmia), diabetes in 5% of all cases	20–70 years	A.D. with variable penetrance	DMPK CTG trinucleotide repeat expansion	Diagnostic
Familial Amyotrophic Lateral Sclerosis				
Progressive loss of motor function with predominantly lower motor neuron manifestations	50–70 years	Both A.D. and A.R.	ALS1 (SOD1) test for gene product superoxide/dismutase	Diagnostic
Hematologic Conditions				
Hereditary Hemochromatosis				
High absorption of iron by gastrointestinal mucosa resulting in excessive iron storage in liver, skin, pancreas, heart, joints, and testes. Abdominal pain, weakness, lethargy, and weight loss are early symptoms. Untreated individuals can present with skin pigmentation, diabetes, hepatic fibrosis or cirrhosis, congestive heart failure, dysrhythmias, or arthritis.	40–60 years in males; after menopause in females	A.R.	HFE gene (6p21) C282Y mutation	Diagnostic and presymptomatic
Factor V Leiden Thrombophilia				
Poor anticoagulant response to activated protein C with increased risk for venous thromboembolism and increased risk for fetal loss during pregnancy	30s; during pregnancy in females	A.D.	F5 (1q23) 1691G>A mutation; abnormal coagulation factor V	Diagnostic and presymptomatic

(continued on page 126)

TABLE 8-5 Selected Adult-Onset Disorders (continued)

Clinical Description	Age of Onset	Genetic Inheritance	Molecular Genetics	Test Availability
Polycystic Kidney Disease Dominant Most common genetic disease in humans. Manifests with renal cysts, liver cysts, and occasionally intracranial/aortic aneurysm and hypertension. Loss of glomerular filtration can lead to kidney failure.	Variable onset; all carriers have detectable disease by ultrasonography at age 30 years	A.D.	PKD1 (16p13) polysystin; (Approx. 85% of pathogenic variants) PKD2 (4q21-q23) polysystin2; (Approx. 15% of pathogenic variants)	Diagnostic and presymptomatic
Diabetes Type 2 Insulin resistance and impaired glucose tolerance	Variable onset most often >30 years	M.F.	Insulin promoter factor 1 (1PF); CAPN10 gene polymorphism (single nucleotide polymorphism) Interaction of $NIDDM_1$ chromosome 2 and several candidate genes on chromosomes 1, 2, 3, and 15 (CYP19)	Research Research
Cardiovascular Disease Familial hypercholesterolemia; elevated low-density lipoprotein levels leading to coronary artery disease, xanthoma, and corneal arcus.	40–50 years	A.D.	LDLR (19p13.2) (60–80% of pathogenic variants) PCSK9 (1p323) (3% of pathogenic variants) APOB (2p24.1) (1–5% of pathogenic variants)	Diagnostic
Hyperlipidemia Elevated cholesterol and triglycerides associated with premature coronary disease and peripheral vascular disease	30–40 years	A.R.	APOE gene (19q13)	Clinical testing related to Alzheimer's/research
Alpha-1 Antitrypsin Deficiency 60–70% small airway and alveolar wall destruction; emphysema, especially at base; chronic obstructive pulmonary disease	35-year-old smoker; 45-year-old non-smoker	M.F. in A.R fashion	SERPINA-1 (14q32.12)	Diagnostic and presymptomatic
Oncology Conditions				
Multiple Endocrine Neoplasia Familial medullary thyroid cancer: Medullary thyroid cancer, pheochromocytoma, and parathyroid abnormalities	Early adulthood 40–50 years	A.D.	RET gene (10q11) MEN1 (11q13.1); (80–90% of pathogenic variants)	Presymptomatic
Breast Cancer BRCA1/2 hereditary breast/ovarian cancer: Breast, ovarian, prostate, and colon (BRCA1); breast, ovarian, and other cancers (BRCA2)	30–70 years; often <50 years	A.D.	BRCA1 gene (17q21) BRCA2 (13q12 DNA analysis)	Presymptomatic Presymptomatic
Lynch Syndrome Colorectal, endometrial, bladder, gastric, biliary, and renal cell cancers as well as atypical endometrial hyperplasia and uterine leiomyosarcoma	<50 years	A.D.	MLH1 (3p21); (50% of pathogenic variants) MSH2 (2p22-p21); (40% of pathogenic variants) MSH6 (2p16); (7–10% of pathogenic variants) PMS2 (7p22); (<5% of pathogenic variants)	Presymptomatic and diagnostic
Li-Fraumeni Syndrome Soft tissue sarcoma, breast cancer, leukemia, osteosarcoma, melanoma, and other cancers often including colon, pancreas, adrenal cortex, and brain	Often <40 years	A.D.	TP53 gene (17q13); test for protein product	Presymptomatic and diagnostic
Cowden Syndrome Breast, nonmedullary (papillary or follicular) thyroid cancer; breast fibroadenomas and noncancerous thyroid modules or goiter; multiple buccal mucosa papillomas (cobblestone-line papules), facial trichilemmomas, gastrointestinal polyps; high-arched palate, thickened furrowed tongue, megalencephaly, and pectus excavatum.	40–50 years for cancer; teens—20 years for mucocutaneous lesions	A.D.	PTEN gene (10q23); gene product test	Presymptomatic and research

A.D., autosomal dominant; A.R., autosomal recessive; M.F., multifactorial.
Adapted from Genetests. (2015a). Retrieved on 7/12/2015 at: www.Genetests.org; Online Mendelian Inheritance of Man. (2013a). *Alpha-1-antitrypsin deficiency (number 613490)*. Retrieved on 11/24/15 at: www.omim.org/entry/613490?search=alpha1-antitrypsin%20deficiency&highlight=deficiency%20alpha1%20alpha1antitrypsin%20antitrypsin; Online Mendelian Inheritance of Man. (2013b). *Beta-2-adrenergic receptor; ADRB2 (number 109690)*. Retrieved on 7/02/2015 at: www.omim.org/entry/109690?search=number%3A%28109690%20OR%20600807%20OR%20605238%29&highlight=605238%20600807%20109690

a particular type of cancer. **Presymptomatic testing** provides asymptomatic people with information about the presence of a genetic mutation and about the likelihood of developing the disease. Presymptomatic testing is considered for people in families with a known adult-onset condition in which either a positive or a negative test result indicates an increased or reduced risk of developing the disease, affects medical management, or allows earlier treatment of a condition.

Huntington disease has long served as the model for presymptomatic testing because the presence of the genetic mutation predicts disease onset and progression. Although preventive measures are not yet available for Huntington disease, the genetic information enables health care providers to develop a clinical, supportive, and psychological plan of care. Indeed, the presence of a single gene mutation has implications for the risk of developing many types of cancer; therefore, presymptomatic testing has become the standard of care so that early planning and implementation of select medical measures may reduce that risk (Leoz, Carballal, Moreira, et al., 2015).

Genomic Conditions

The foremost factor that may influence the development and severity of disease is a person's genomic makeup. In the absence of a single disease-causing gene, it is thought that multiple genes and other environmental factors are related to the onset of most adult diseases. For some diseases, the interactions among several genes and other environmental or metabolic events affect disease onset and progression. Specific gene–gene interactions or SNPs can confer susceptibility to disease. Most genomic testing for gene–gene interactions and SNPs is conducted in the research setting to identify candidate genes for diseases such as Alzheimer disease, psychiatric conditions, heart disease, hypertension, and hypercholesterolemia (Conley et al., 2013; Korf & Rehm, 2013). Genomic testing helps distinguish variations within the same disease or response to treatment. For example, no single gene is associated with osteoporosis. Several polymorphisms on candidate genes related to the vitamin D receptor, estrogen and androgen receptors, and regulation of bone mineral density (BMD) have been shown to contribute to osteoporosis and fracture risk. Moreover, diet and exercise have a strong interaction with the polymorphisms regulating BMD (Cosman, de Beur, LeBoff, et al., 2014)

Some genomic tests may predict treatment response. For example, people may present with similar clinical signs and symptoms of asthma but have different responses to corticosteroid treatment. Mutations in genes that regulate glucocorticoid (i.e., corticosteroid) receptors help classify people with asthma as sensitive or resistant to treatment with corticosteroids (Online Mendelian Inheritance of Man, 2013b).

Population Screening

Population screening—the use of genetic testing for large groups or entire populations—to identify late-onset conditions is under development. For a test to be considered for population screening, there must be (1) sufficient information about gene distribution within populations, (2) accurate prediction about the development and progression of disease, and (3) appropriate medical management for asymptomatic people with a mutation. Currently, population screening is considered in some ethnic groups to identify cancer-predisposing

genes. For example, individuals of Ashkenazi Jewish ancestry have a greater chance of having a specific genetic mutation in the *BRCA1* or *BRCA2* gene. People with one of these *BRCA* mutations have approximately an 80% risk (*BRCA1* carriers) and a 45% risk (*BRCA2* carriers) of breast cancer, a 40% to 65% risk (*BRCA1* carriers) and a 20% risk (*BRCA2* carriers) of ovarian cancer, and a 16% risk of prostate cancer (GeneTests, 2015b). The identification of one of these mutations gives patients options that may include cancer screening, chemoprevention, or prophylactic mastectomy or oophorectomy. Population screening is also being explored for other adult-onset conditions such as type 2 diabetes, heart disease, and hereditary hemochromatosis (i.e., iron overload disorder).

The Nursing Role in Testing and Screening for Adult-Onset Conditions

Nurses participate in explaining risk and genetic predisposition, supporting informed health decisions and opportunities for prevention and early intervention, clarifying legal protections and risks related to genetic testing or health concerns, and protecting patients' privacy. Nurses assess family histories, which may indicate that multiple generations (autosomal dominant inheritance) or multiple siblings (autosomal recessive inheritance) are affected with the same condition or that onset of disease is earlier than expected (e.g., multiple generations with early onset hyperlipidemia). Possible adult-onset conditions are discussed with other members of the health care team for appropriate resources and referral. When a family history of disease is identified, a patient is made aware that this is a risk factor for disease; resources and referral are then provided. It is the patient's decision whether or not to pursue a genetic testing workup. For example, if a 45-year-old woman presents for her annual gynecology visit and reports a family history of colon cancer in multiple paternal relatives, including her father, the nurse should discuss the family history with the gynecologist. In addition, the woman should be alerted to the risk of colon cancer on the basis of the family history and given information about possible genetic testing and referral for a colonoscopy.

If the existence of a mutation for an adult-onset condition in a family is identified, at-risk family members can be referred for **predisposition testing**. If the patient is found to carry the mutation, the nurse provides him or her with information and referral for risk-reduction measures and information about the risk to other family members. In that discussion, the nurse assures the patient that the test results are private and confidential and will not be shared with others, including family members, without the patient's permission. If the patient is an unaffected family member, the nurse discusses inheritance and the risk of developing the disease, provides support for the decision-making process, and offers referral for genetics services.

 Concept Mastery Alert

Predisposition testing is used for at-risk family members if the existence of a mutation for an adult-onset condition in a family is identified. Presymptomatic testing provides asymptomatic people with information about the presence of a genetic mutation and about the likelihood of developing the disease.

Personalized Genomic Treatments

Information about genes and their variations helps researchers identify genetic differences that predispose certain people to more aggressive diseases and affect their responses to treatment. Genetics and genomics have revolutionized the field of oncology because genetic mutations are the basis for the development and progression of all cancers. In the medical era, individuals with cancer faced treatment based on the stage of the cancer, lymph node involvement, and spread to distant organs. Treatments of a particular type of cancer, stage for stage, were similar. Now, in the genomic era of personalized medicine, cancer is treated on the basis of genetic makeup. For example, women with early stage breast cancer (i.e., tumor diameter less than 2 cm, estrogen receptor–positive tumors, no lymph node involvement) have often received chemotherapy. In the past, deciding which of these women would benefit the most from chemotherapy was unclear. Currently, a gene tumor profile of these women's tumors can be used to predict which women are more likely to have an aggressive cancer. Genetic testing helps clinicians to provide personalized care and the most effective treatment based on the genetic signature of the tumor treatment, called *targeted therapy*, tries to match the treatment to the specific malfunctioning genes expressed in the tumor, or to selectively inhibit genetic factors that promote cancer growth (Genetests, 2015b).

Pharmacogenomics

The difference between genetics and genomics, described earlier in this chapter, corresponds to the terms *pharmacogenetics* and *pharmacogenomics*, which combine pharmacology and genetics or genomics. Pharmacogenetics refers to the study of the effect of variations in a single gene on drug response and toxicity. The field of pharmacogenetics has evolved so that it has become a broader genomic-based approach that recognizes the interaction of multiple genes and the environment on drug response. Pharmacogenomics refers to the study of the combined effect of variations in many genes on drug response and toxicity and involves methods that rapidly identify which genetic variations influence a drug's effect. Pharmacogenomics involves the search for genetic variations associated with medication metabolism and efficacy, with the goal of tailoring treatment to each individual's genomic makeup (NLM, 2015d).

It has long been known that patients differ in their response to medications. The genetic and genomic variations in drug metabolism account largely for the differences in drug response and drug-related toxicities. Drug metabolism involves genetically controlled protein/enzyme activity for absorption, distribution, drug–cell interaction, inactivation, and excretion—metabolic processes that are known as pharmacokinetics. The cytochrome *P450* (CYP) genes play a key role in the pharmacokinetic process of drug metabolism (Johnson, 2013). Once a drug reaches its target cell, other genes such as those regulating cell receptors and cell signaling control the drug's effect. This process is known as pharmacodynamics. Single genes may affect drug response. More commonly, drug response involves the interaction of multiple genes, the host, and the effects of other drugs. Figure 8-12 is a schematic display of the genetic and genomic influences on drug metabolism and treatment effect.

Figure 8-12 • Simplified schematic representation of the multiple, complex, genetic-regulated mechanisms involved in pharmacokinetics (cytochrome [CYP] dependent) and pharmacodynamics, along with other genomic and environmental factors affecting drug metabolism and treatment effect. SNPs, single nucleotide polymorphisms.

SNPs, described earlier, are common genetic variations that occur most frequently throughout the human genome and often contribute to variations in enzymatic activity that affect drug metabolism. The CYPs, a family of enzymes, play a key role in the pharmacokinetic process of drug metabolism. More than 300 variations (SNPs) of genes that control CYP activation and deactivation have been identified. Researchers have created a catalog of CYP variations because of their role in drug metabolism (HUGO Gene Nomenclature Committee, 2015).

Four classes of CYP metabolic activity levels have been identified based on a person's CYP genotype and the corresponding drug response: (1) poor metabolizers, (2) intermediate metabolizers, (3) extensive metabolizers, and (4) ultrarapid metabolizers. Poor metabolizers have a specific SNP variation in a CYP gene that causes little or no function, resulting in very little or no drug metabolism and higher blood levels of active drug because the drug cannot be absorbed or excreted. Conversely, ultrarapid metabolizers have SNP variations that cause increased enzyme activity, resulting in rapid absorption, distribution, and excretion of a drug. Ultrarapid metabolizers have lower drug blood levels, usually with inadequate therapeutic response or longer treatment time to achieve therapeutic results. Both poor metabolizers and ultrarapid metabolizers are predisposed to adverse drug reactions. Poor metabolizers may have adverse effects or toxicities from high blood levels of drugs and need a lower dose, whereas

TABLE 8-6 Examples of Clinical Effects of Cytochrome P450 Enzyme Variations

Enzyme	Drug	Effects	
		Poor Metabolizer	Ultrarapid Metabolizer
CYP2C9	Warfarin (Coumadin)	Bleeding	Longer treatment time to achieve stable dosing
	Phenytoin (Dilantin)	Ataxia	Not established
CYP2C19	Diazepam (Valium)	Sedation	Poor response
	Omeprazole (Prilosec)	Drug-induced side effects (e.g., taste perversion)	
CYP2D6	Tricyclic antidepressants	Cardiotoxicity	No response to recommended dose; need 10-fold increase in dose
	Selective serotonin reuptake inhibitors	Nausea	Not established
	Antipsychotics	Parkinson-like effects	Longer treatment time and higher drug costs

Adapted from Genetests. (2015a). Retrieved on 6/30/2015 at: www.genetests.org/; HUGO Gene Nomenclature Committee. (2015). *Cytochrome P450*. Retrieved on 7/9/2015 at: www.genenames.org/cgi-bin/search?search_type=all&search=cytochrome+P450&submit=Submit; Johnson, J. A. (2013). Pharmacogenetics in clinical practice: How far have we come and where are we going? *Pharmacogenomics*, 14(7), 835–843.

ultrarapid metabolizers have inadequate treatment response because of lower drug blood levels and may need a higher dose or more frequent dosing. Table 8-6 shows examples of differences in drug response in poor versus ultrarapid metabolizers. Intermediate metabolizers have reduced enzyme activity levels and metabolize drugs at a slower than normal rate. Because intermediate metabolizers have some enzyme activity, they may have differences in treatment response. Extensive metabolizers have normal enzyme activity levels and normal drug metabolism. Differences in metabolism of other medications occur with other genetic variations.

Nurses have traditionally monitored and reported drug response and drug adverse effects. Clinical guidelines for pharmacogenomic testing for several drugs, such as warfarin (Coumadin), abacavir (Ziagen), trastuzumab (Herceptin), mercaptopurine (Purinethol), and irinotecan (Camptosar), are currently being tested (NIH, 2014c). Pharmacogenomic testing offers patients and health care providers more information about drug dosage, time to achieve response, and risk of adverse effects. Nurses will provide education about a particular patient's genomic profile for drug metabolism and explain the rationale for the recommended dosage and likelihood of adverse effects. Nurses will continue to incorporate information about gender differences, food interactions, and drug compliance into patient education (Consensus Panel, 2009).

Ethical, Legal, and Social Issues Surrounding Genetics

The rapid application of genetics and genomics across all sectors of health care has had implications for gathering, recording, and sharing personal health information. An ethical foundation provides nurses with a holistic framework for handling these issues with integrity and provides a basis for communicating genetic and genomic information to a patient, a family, other care providers, community agencies and organizations, and society. Nurses must consider their responsibilities in handling genetic and genomic information and strive to ensure that informed decision making occurs, that patient

and family health information is kept private and confidential, and that access to and justice in health care is available to everyone (Badzek, Henaghan, Turner, et al., 2013).

Ethical Concerns

Ethical principles of beneficence (i.e., to do good) and non-maleficence (i.e., to do no harm), as well as autonomy, justice, fidelity, and veracity, are used to resolve ethical dilemmas that may arise in clinical care. Respect for people is the ethical principle underlying all nursing care. Using these principles and the values of caring, nurses can promote thoughtful discussions that are useful when patients and families are facing genetics- and genomics-related health and reproductive decisions and consequences (Consensus Panel, 2009; International Society of Nurses in Genetics [ISONG], 2014). The ethical principles of autonomy, fidelity, and veracity are also important (American Nurses Association [ANA], 2015). (Further information about ethics is included in Chapter 3.)

Ethical questions relating to genetics and genomics occur in all settings and at all levels of nursing practice. At the level of direct patient care, nurses participate in providing genetic information, testing, and gene-based therapeutics. They offer patient care based on the values of self-determination and personal autonomy. To be as fully informed as possible, patients need appropriate, accurate, and complete information given at a level and in a form so that they and their families can make well-informed personal, medical, and reproductive health decisions. Nurses can help patients clarify values and goals, assess understanding of information, protect their rights, and support their decisions. Nurses can advocate for patient autonomy in health decisions. Several resources and position statements have been developed to guide genetic-related nursing practice (Consensus Panel, 2009; ISONG, 2014).

Respecting the patient's right to self-determination—that is, supporting decisions that reflect the patient's personal beliefs, values, and interests—is a central principle in directing how nurses provide genetic and genomic information and counseling. Nurses and others participating in genetic counseling make every attempt to respect the patient's ability to make autonomous decisions. Recognizing one's own attitudes and beliefs (see Chart 8-1) and how communication of genetic and genomic information may be influenced by those attitudes and beliefs is a first step toward assuring patients' autonomous decision making.

Confidentiality of genetic and genomic information and respect for privacy are other essential principles underlying genetic counseling. Patients have the right to not have test results divulged to anyone, including insurers, physicians, employers, or family members. Some patients pay for testing themselves so that insurers will not learn of the test, and others use a different name for testing to protect their privacy.

Ethical challenges may occur for family members and health care providers when the findings of one person's test may inadvertently disclose another family member's risk or carrier status. A nurse may want to disclose genetic information to family members who could experience significant harm if they do not know such information. However, the patient may have other views and may wish to keep this information from the family, resulting in an ethical dilemma for both patient and nurse. The nurse must honor the patient's wishes, while explaining to the patient the potential benefit this information may have for other family members (ANA, 2015; ISONG, 2014).

Ethical considerations must be reviewed as part of genetic and genomic research. For example, before an individual participates in genetic and genomic clinical research, the research team must discuss how any incidental findings will be addressed. Incidental findings are genetic-related illnesses which are found secondary to the intended goals of the research project or intended testing (Christenhusz, Devriendt, & Dierickx, 2013). The American College of Medical Genetics and Genomics (ACMG, 2013) issued a policy statement that lists conditions known to be treatable and should be reported to the patient if found incidentally during clinical research.

Legal Aspects of Personalized Health Care

The Genetic Information Nondiscrimination Act (GINA), a law passed in 2008, protects individuals from genetic discrimination (Green, Lautenbach, & McGuire, 2015). Its purpose is to protect Americans against improper use of genetic and genomic information in insurance and employment decisions. GINA is particularly helpful for people who carry a gene mutation but are asymptomatic for the illness. The act prohibits health insurers from denying coverage to a healthy person or charging higher insurance rates based on a person's genetic predisposition to a disease. GINA offers legal protection with regard to health insurance and employment; however, gaps in protection exist with regard to disability, life, and long-term care insurance. The act also prevents employers from using a person's genetic and genomic information to make decisions about hiring, job placement, promotion, or firing. Protection provided by GINA does not apply to employers with less than 15 employees, to persons in the military, Veteran's Health Administration, Indian Health Services, and Federal Employees Health Benefits Programs (Lough & Seidel, 2015). As a result of GINA, most Americans are free to use genetic and genomic information in health care

without the fear of misuse; however, public awareness of this law is limited (Parkman, Foland, Anderson, et al., 2015).

While not specifically intended for genetic health-related concerns, other health care laws offer some additional protection to individuals with regard to genetics. For example, the Affordable Care Act, enacted in 2010, offers some protection for a person with a genetic illness by prohibiting health insurers from discrimination based on a preexisting condition (Green et al., 2015). The Americans with Disabilities Act offers legal protection related to employment concerns and physical or intellectual impairment as a result of a genetic disorder. Finally, the Health Insurance Portability and Accountability Act (HIPAA), enacted in 1996, places restrictions on sharing identifiable health information and places stringent requirements on maintaining the privacy of health-related content and prohibits the use of genetic information to establish insurance eligibility (Parkman, et al., 2015). However, HIPAA does not prohibit group plans from increasing premiums, excluding coverage for a specific condition, or imposing a lifetime cap on benefits.

The National Human Genome Research Institute, Policy and Program Analysis branch has a summary of each state's legislation on employment and insurance discrimination (NIH, 2015c). See also the Resources section at the end of this chapter.

Ancestry, Cultural, Social, and Spiritual Concerns Related to Genetic and Genomic Practice

Genetic assessment addresses the ancestry of patients and families, as well as their ethnicity. This information helps identify individual patients and groups who could benefit from genetic testing for carrier identification, prenatal diagnosis, and susceptibility testing. For example, as noted previously, carrier testing for sickle cell disease is routinely offered to people of African American descent, and carrier testing for Tay–Sachs disease and Canavan disease is offered to people of Ashkenazi Jewish descent. The American College of Obstetricians and Gynecologists (ACOG) recommends that members of at-risk racial and ethnic populations be offered carrier testing (ACOG Committee on Genetics, 2014a). The ACOG and the ACMG recommend that all couples, particularly those of northern European and Ashkenazi Jewish ancestry, be offered carrier screening for cystic fibrosis (ACOG, 2014b). Ideally, carrier testing is offered before conception to allow people who are carriers to make decisions about reproduction. Prenatal diagnosis is offered and discussed when both partners of a couple are found to be carriers.

It is important to inquire about the patient's ethnic backgrounds when assessing for susceptibilities to adult-onset conditions such as hereditary breast or ovarian cancer. For example, a *BRCA1* cancer-predisposing gene mutation seems to occur more frequently in women of Ashkenazi Jewish descent. Therefore, asking about ethnicity can help identify people with an increased risk of cancer gene mutations (Iqbal, Ginsburg, Rochon, et al., 2015).

Nurses should consider patients' views about the significance of a genetic condition and its effect on self-concept, as well as patients' perception of the role of genetics in health and illness, reproduction, and disability. Patients' social and

Chart 8-3	**NURSING RESEARCH PROFILE**
	Family Health History, Genetic Testing and Feasibility of Pedigree Development

Pettey, C. M., McSweeney, J. C., Stewart, K. E., et al. (2015). Perceptions of family history and genetic testing and feasibility of pedigree development among African Americans with hypertension. *European Journal of Cardiovascular Nursing, 14*(1), 8–15.

Purpose

African Americans are the largest ethnic group at risk for hypertension (HTN) and cardiovascular disease. Due to the multifactorial inheritance of these illnesses, it is challenging for health care providers to identify a person at risk for HTN prior to clinical presentation. The purpose of this research was to determine the feasibility of creating pedigrees using the *U.S. Surgeon General's My Family Health Portrait.*

Design

Twenty-nine African American adults with HTN were recruited from a faith-based urban clinic. The mixed methods research design consisted of demographic data, ethnographic interviews, and the completion of the *My Family Health Portrait* for each participant. The *My Family Health Portrait* was collected but required a moderate amount of assistance by the researchers due to the high reading level needed to complete the forms. Upon completion of the *My Family Health Portrait,* a pedigree was created based upon the information that was obtained. The pedigrees and demographic data were completed using descriptive analysis.

The pedigree was then used to guide the personal interviews (ranging from 30 to 60 minutes). Interviews were audiotaped and transcribed verbatim. Qualitative analysis was used to identify themes and code the interviews.

Findings

The use of medical terminology and overall design of the Web site was at a 12th-grade reading level and determined to be too high for the participants to comprehend. Themes from the interviews indicated that the participants were aware that family members had HTN but were not aware of specific details or did not understand the inheritance pattern. Some believed that having a family history of HTN influenced their behaviors while others believed that HTN was a matter of fate. The majority of the participants stated that they would participate in genetic testing for HTN.

Nursing Implications

It is important for nurses to be aware of genetic health literacy and offer means to assist patients in recognizing genetic health risks. The visual representation of a family pedigree, which may be developed using the *My Family Health Portrait* online tool, can aid the nurse in assessing patients' patterns of inheritance and health risks. In addition, viewing a family pedigree may motivate patients to be more engaged in health-related behaviors that will decrease their risk for familial diseases, such as HTN.

---

cultural backgrounds determine their interpretations and values about information obtained from genetic testing and evaluation and thus influence their perceptions of health, illness, and risk (see Chart 8-3). Family structure, decision making, and educational background contribute in the same way (Consensus Panel, 2009).

Assessment of the patients' beliefs, values, and expectations regarding genetic testing and genetic and genomic information helps nurses provide appropriate information about the specific genetics or genomics topic. For example, in some cultures, people believe that health means the absence of symptoms and that the cause of illness is supernatural. Patients with these beliefs may initially reject suggestions for presymptomatic or carrier testing. However, by including resources such as family and cultural and religious community leaders when providing genetics- or genomics-related health care, nurses can help ensure that patients receive information in a way that transcends social, cultural, and economic barriers (Boucher, Habin, & Underhill, 2014).

Applications of Genetics and Genomics in Nursing Practice

Nurses who provide genetics- and genomics-related health care blend the principles of human genetics with nursing care in collaboration with other professionals, including genetic specialists, to foster improvement, maintenance, and restoration of patients' health. Genetics-related nursing practice involves the care of people who have genetic conditions, those who may be predisposed to develop or pass on genetic conditions, and those who are seeking genetic information and referral for additional genetics services. The application of genomic information has been integrated into clinical practice areas of preconception, preimplantation, and prenatal testing, newborn screening, disease susceptibility, screening and diagnosis, prognosis and therapeutic decisions, and in monitoring disease recurrence (Calzone, Jenkins, Bakos, et al., 2013) (see Table 8-4). The Genomic Nursing State of the Science Advisory Panel acknowledges that genomics is a fundamental, yet critical component, to nursing practice across the health care continuum and has mapped 67 genomic nursing research topics to the National Institute of Nursing Research Strategic Plan (Calzone, Jenkins, Nikol, et al., 2013).

Nurses are positioned to support patients and families with genetics- and genomics-related health concerns by ensuring that their health choices are informed ones and by advocating for the privacy and confidentiality of genetic and genomic information and for equal access to genetic testing and treatments (Badzek, et al., 2013). Nurses are expected to attend to the genetic and genomic health care needs of the patient (Kirk & Marshallay, 2013).

Genetics and Genomics in Health Assessment

Assessment of a person's genetic and genomic health status is an ongoing process. Nurses collect information that can help identify individuals and families who have actual or potential genetics- or genomics-related health concerns or who may benefit from further genetic information, counseling, testing, and treatment. This process can begin before conception and continue throughout the lifespan. Nurses evaluate family and past medical histories, including prenatal history, childhood illnesses, developmental history, adult-onset conditions, past surgeries, treatments, and medications; this information may relate to the genetic or genomic condition at hand or to a condition being considered (see Chapter 5 for more information on assessing past medical history). Nurses also identify the patient's ethnic background and conduct a physical assessment to gather pertinent genetic information. The assessment also includes information about culture, spiritual beliefs, and ancestry. Health assessment includes determining a patient's or family's understanding of actual or potential genetics- or genomics-related health concerns and awareness of how these issues are communicated within a family (Boucher et al., 2014).

Family History Assessment

Nurses in any practice setting can assess families' genetics histories to identify a genetic trait, inherited condition, or predisposition. Targeted questions are used to identify genetic and genomic conditions for which further information, education, testing, or treatment can be offered (see Chart 8-4). After consultation and collaboration with other health care providers and specialists, further genetic testing and evaluation is offered for the trait or condition in question. The genetics family history is used to make a diagnosis, identify testing strategies, and establish a pattern of inheritance. It includes at least three generations, as well as information about the current and past health status of all family members, including the age at onset of any illness, cause of death, and age at death. Nurses can also inquire about medical conditions that are known to have a heritable component and for which genetic testing may be available. Information is obtained about the presence of birth defects, intellectual disability, familial traits, or similarly affected family members (Consensus Panel, 2009).

Nurses also consider the closeness of the relationship (genetic relatedness or consanguinity) among family members when assessing the risk of genetic conditions in couples or families. For example, when obtaining a preconception or prenatal family history, it is important for the nurse to ask if the prospective parents have common ancestors (i.e., are they first cousins?). This is important because, as noted previously, people who are related have more genes in common than those who are unrelated, thus increasing their chance of having children with an autosomal recessive inherited condition such as cystic fibrosis. Ascertaining genetic relatedness provides direction for genetic counseling and evaluation. It may also serve as an explanation for parents who have a child with a rare autosomal recessive inherited condition or for an adult who is similarly affected.

When the assessment of family history reveals that a patient has been adopted, genetic- and genomic-based health assessment becomes more challenging. Every effort is made to help the patient obtain as much information as possible about their biologic parents, including their ethnic backgrounds.

Questions about previous miscarriage or stillbirth are included in genetics health assessments to identify possible chromosomal conditions. Nurses can also inquire about any history of family members with inherited conditions or birth defects; maternal health conditions such as type 1 diabetes, seizure disorders, or PKU, which may increase the risk for birth defects in children; and about exposure to alcohol or other drugs during pregnancy. Maternal age is also noted; women who are 35 years of age or older who are considering pregnancy and childbearing or who are already pregnant should be offered prenatal diagnosis (e.g., testing through amniocentesis) because of the association between advanced maternal age and chromosomal abnormalities such as Down syndrome.

Chart 8-4   GENETICS FAMILY HISTORY
An Essential Tool for All Nurses

A well-documented family history can be used to:

- Assess risk of certain diseases
- Decide on testing strategies, such as what genetic and other diagnostic tests to order
- Establish a pattern of inheritance
- Identify other family members who are at increased risk
- Identify shared environmental risk factors
- Calculate risks
- Assess risk of passing on conditions to children
- Determine and recommend treatments that modify disease risk
- Make decisions about management or surveillance
- Develop patient rapport
- Educate patients

Key questions to ask about each family member include:

- What is the current age, or what was the age at death?
- What is the ethnic background (some genetic conditions are more common in certain ethnic groups)?

- Is there a history of:
  - Multiple pregnancy losses/stillbirths?
  - Unexplained infertility?
  - Birth defects?
  - Intellectual disability or developmental delay?
  - Learning disabilities?
  - Medical problems in children whose parents are closely related (second cousins or closer)?
  - Congenital or juvenile blindness, cataracts, hearing loss, or deafness?
  - Very short or very tall stature?
  - Several close relatives with the same or related conditions (e.g., breast or colon cancer, diabetes, heart disease, asthma, stroke, high blood pressure, kidney disease)?
  - Occurrence of a common condition with earlier age of onset than is usual (e.g., breast or colon cancer, hearing loss, dementia, heart disease)?

Adapted from Welch, B. M., Dere, W., & Schiffman, J. D. (2015). Family health history: The case for better tools. *JAMA, 313*(7) 1711–1712; Mayo Clinic. (2014). *Medical history: Compiling your medical family tree.* Retrieved on 7/12/2015 at: www.mayoclinic.org/healthy-lifestyle/adult-health/in-depth/medical-history/art-20044961; U.S. National Library of Medicine. (NLM). (2015g). Medline Plus. *Family history.* Retrieved on 7/12/2015 at: www.nlm.nih.gov/medlineplus/familyhistory.html#cat59

Chart 8-5 Indications for Making a Genetics Referral

Prepregnancy and Prenatal

- Maternal age of 35 years or older at expected time of delivery
- Previous child with a chromosome problem
- Positive alpha-fetoprotein profile screening test
- Previous child with a birth defect or family history of birth defects
- Pregnancy history of two or more unexplained miscarriages
- Maternal conditions such as diabetes, epilepsy, or alcoholism
- Exposures to certain medications or drugs during pregnancy
- Family history of intellectual disability
- Either member of the couple has a birth defect such as cleft lip or palate, spina bifida, or congenital heart defect
- Either member of the couple has a chromosome abnormality

Pediatric

- Positive newborn screening test
- One or more major birth defects
- Unusual (dysmorphic) facial features
- Developmental delay/intellectual disability
- Suspicion of a metabolic disorder
- Unusually tall or short stature, or growth delays
- Known chromosomal abnormality

Adult

- Intellectual disability without a known cause
- Unexplained infertility or multiple pregnancy losses
- A personal or family history of thrombotic events
- Adult-onset conditions such as hemochromatosis, hearing loss, and visual impairment
- Family history of an adult-onset neurodegenerative disorder (e.g., Huntington disease)
- Features of a genetic condition such as neurofibromatosis (*café-au-lait* spots, neurofibromas on the skin), Marfan syndrome (unusually tall stature, dilation of the aortic root), others
- Personal or family history of cardiovascular disorders known to be associated with genetic factors such as cardiomyopathy or long QT syndrome
- Family history of cancers known to be associated with specific genes such as hereditary breast/ovarian cancer or Lynch syndrome
- Family history of early onset cancers and familial clustering of related tumors

Adapted from Pletcher, B. A., Toriello, H. V., Noblin, S. J., et al. (2007). Indications for genetic referral: A guide for healthcare providers. *Genetics in Medicine, 9*(6), 385–389.

Physical Assessment

Physical assessment may provide clues that a particular genetic or genomic condition is present in a person and family. Family history assessment may serve as a guide to focus the physical assessment. For example, a history of familial hypercholesterolemia would alert the nurse to assess for symptoms of hyperlipidemias (xanthomas, corneal arcus, and abdominal pain of unexplained origin). A family history of neurofibromatosis type 1, an inherited condition involving tumors of the central nervous system, would prompt the nurse to carry out a detailed assessment of closely related family members. Skin findings such as *café-au-lait* spots, axillary freckling, or tumors of the skin (neurofibromas) would warrant referral for

further evaluation, including genetic evaluation and counseling (NLM, 2015f).

If a genetic or genomic condition is suspected as a result of a family history or physical assessment, the nurse, as a part of their role, and in collaboration with the health care team, may initiate further discussion of genetics and genomic information, offering and discussing genetic tests, and suggesting a referral for further genetic evaluation (see Chart 8-5).

Psychosocial Assessment

Psychosocial assessment is an essential nursing component of the genetics health assessment. The assessment findings can help identify the potential impact of new genetic and genomic information on the patient and the family and how they may cope with this information (see Chart 8-6).

Genetic Counseling and Evaluation Services

People seek genetic counseling for various reasons and at different stages of life. Some are seeking preconception or prenatal information, others are referred after the birth of a child with a birth defect or suspected genetic condition, and still others are seeking information for themselves or their families because of the presence of, or a family history of, a genetic condition. Regardless of the timing or setting, genetic counseling is offered to all people who have questions about genetics or genomics and their health.

As the contribution of genetics and genomics to the health–illness continuum is recognized, genetic counseling will become a responsibility of all health care professionals in clinical practice. Nurses are in an ideal position to assess the patient's health and genetics family history and to make

Chart 8-6 ASSESSMENT — Assessing Psychosocial Genetic Health

The nurse's assessment of psychosocial factors impacting a patient's genetic health is based on the nurse's professional responsibility to "demonstrate in practice the importance of tailoring genetic and genomic information and services to clients based on their culture, religion, knowledge level, literacy and preferred language."

The nurse assesses:

- Educational level and understanding of the genetic condition or concern in the family.
- Desired goals and health outcomes in relation to the genetic condition or concern.
- Family rules regarding disclosure of medical information (e.g., some families may not reveal a history of a disease such as cancer or mental illness during the family history assessment).
- Family rules, boundaries, and cultural practices as well as personal preference about knowing genetic information.
- Past coping mechanisms and social support.
- Ability to make an informed decision (e.g., is the patient under stress from family situations, acute or chronic illness, or medications that may impair the patient's ability to make an informed decision?).

Adapted from Consensus Panel on Genetic/Genomic Nursing Competencies. (2009). *Essentials of genetic and genomic nursing: Competencies, curricular guidelines, and outcome indicators* (2nd ed.) Silver Spring, MD: Author.

referrals for specialized diagnosis and treatment. They offer anticipatory guidance by explaining the purpose and goals of a referral. They collaborate with other health care providers in giving supportive and follow-up counseling and coordinating follow-up and case management.

Genetics Services

Genetics services provide genetic information, education, and support to patients and families. Medical geneticists, genetic counselors, and advanced practice nurses in genetics provide specific genetics services to patients and families who are referred by their primary or specialty health care providers. A team approach is often used to obtain and interpret complex family history information, evaluate and diagnose genetic conditions, interpret and discuss complicated genetic test results, support patients throughout the evaluation process, and offer professional and family support. Patients participate as team members and decision makers throughout the process. Genetics services enable patients and their families to learn and understand relevant aspects of genetics and genomics, to make informed health decisions, and to receive support as they integrate personal and family genetic and genomic information into daily living.

Genetic counseling may take place over an extended period and may entail more than one counseling session, which may include other family members. The components of genetic counseling are outlined in Chart 8-7. Although genetic counseling may be offered at any point during the lifespan, counseling issues are often relevant to the life stage in which counseling is sought (NIH, 2013b). Examples are presented in Chart 8-8.

Providing Precounseling Information

All genetic specialists, including nurses who participate in the genetic counseling process and those with access to a person's genetic information, must honor a patient's desire for confidentiality. Genetic information should not be revealed to family members, insurance companies, employers, and schools if the patient so desires, even if keeping the information confidential is difficult.

Preparing the patient and the family, promoting informed decision making, and obtaining informed consent are essential in genetic counseling. Nurses assess the patient's capacity and ability to give voluntary consent. This includes assessment of factors that may interfere with informed consent, such as hearing loss, language differences, cognitive impairment, and the effects of medication. Nurses make sure that a person's decision to undergo testing is not affected by coercion, persuasion, or manipulation. Because information may need to be repeated over time, nurses offer follow-up discussion as needed (Consensus Panel, 2009).

The genetics service to which a patient or a family is referred for genetic counseling will ask the nurse for background information for evaluation. Genetic specialists need to know the reason for referral, the patient's or family's reason for seeking genetic counseling, and potential genetics-related health concerns. For example, a nurse may refer a family with a new diagnosis of hereditary breast or ovarian cancer for counseling or to discuss the likelihood of developing the disease and the implications for other family members. The family may have concerns about confidentiality and privacy. The

---

Chart 8-7 — Components of Genetic Counseling

Information and Assessment Sources

- Reason for referral
- Family history
- Medical history/records
- Relevant test results and other medical evaluations
- Social and emotional concerns
- Relevant cultural, educational, and financial factors

Analysis of Data

- Family history
- Physical examination as needed
- Additional laboratory testing and procedures (e.g., echocardiogram, ophthalmology, or neurologic examination)

Communication of Genetic Finding

- Natural history of disorder
- Pattern of inheritance
- Reproductive and family health issues and options
- Testing options
- Management and treatment issues

Counseling and Support

- Identify individual and family questions and concerns
- Identify existing support systems
- Provide emotional and social support
- Refer for additional support and counseling as indicated

Follow-Up

- Written summary to referring primary providers and family
- Coordination of care with primary providers and specialists
- Additional discussions of test results or diagnosis

Genetics Resources

GeneTests: A registry of genetic disorders and associated genetic testing, www.genetests.org/search/disorders.php

Genetic Alliance: a directory of support groups for patients and families with genetic conditions, www.geneticalliance.org

Genetic and Rare Diseases Information Center: provides links with experienced information specialists who can answer questions in English and Spanish to patients, families, and health care providers regarding specific genetic diseases, www.genome.gov/Health/GARD/

Genetics Home Reference: provides a layman's online encyclopedic guide to understanding genetic conditions, ghr.nlm.nih.gov/BrowseConditions

National Human Genome Research Institute, Genome Statute and Legislative Database: summarizes each state's legislation on employment and insurance discrimination, www.genome.gov/PolicyEthics/LegDatabase/pubsearch.cfm

National Organization for Rare Disorders (NORD): a directory of support groups and information for patients and families with rare genetic disorders, www.rarediseases.org

Online Mendelian Inheritance in Man (OMIM): a complete listing of inherited genetic conditions, www.omim.org

Adapted from Genetics Home Reference. *Genetic consultation.* Retrieved on 8/16/2015 at: www.ghr.nlm.nih.gov/handbook/consult?show=all#consultation

Chart 8-8 Genetic Counseling Across the Lifespan

Prenatal Issues

- Understanding prenatal screening and diagnosis testing
- Implications of reproductive choices
- Potential for anxiety and emotional distress
- Effects on partnership, family, and parental–fetal bonding

Newborn Issues

- Understanding newborn screening results
- Potential for disrupted parent–newborn relationship on diagnosis of a genetic condition
- Parental guilt
- Implications for siblings and other family members
- Coordination and continuity of care

Pediatric Issues

- Caring for children with complex medical needs
- Coordination of care
- Potential for impaired parent–child relationship
- Potential for social stigmatization

Adolescent Issues

- Potential for impaired self-image and decreased self-esteem
- Potential for altered perception of family
- Implications for lifestyle and family planning

Adult Issues

- Potential for ambiguous test results
- Identification of a genetic susceptibility or diagnosis without an existing cure
- Effect on marriage, reproduction, parenting, and lifestyle
- Potential impact on insurability and employability

Adapted from Dwyer, T. M., Glaser, R. L., & Mason, T. M. (2016). Inheritance patterns in human phenotypes and types of genetic disorders. In C. E. Kasper, T. A. Schneidereith, & F. R. Lashley (Eds.), *Lashley's essentials of clinical genetics in nursing practice* (pp. 65–114). New York, NY. Springer Publishing Company.

nurse and the genetic specialist tailor the genetic counseling to respond to these concerns.

With the patient's permission, genetic specialists will request the relevant test results and medical evaluations. Nurses obtain permission from the patient and, if applicable, from other family members to provide medical records that document the genetic condition of concern. In some situations, evaluation of more than one family member may be necessary to establish a diagnosis of a genetic disorder. Nurses explain that the medical information is needed to ensure that appropriate information and counseling (including risk interpretation) are provided.

The genetics service asks nurses about the emotional and social status of the patient and the family. Genetic specialists want to know the coping skills of patients and families who have recently learned of the diagnosis of a genetic disorder as well as what type of genetic information is being sought. Nurses help identify cultural and other issues that may influence how information is provided and by whom. For example, for patients with hearing loss, a sign interpreter's services may have to be arranged. For those with vision loss, alternative forms of communication may be necessary. Genetics professionals prepare for the genetic counseling

and evaluation with these relevant issues in mind (NIH, 2013b).

Preparing Patients for Genetics Evaluation

Before a genetic counseling appointment, the nurse discusses with the patient and the family the type of family history information that will be collected during the consultation. Family history collection and analysis are comprehensive and focus on information that may be relevant to the genetics- or genomics-related concern in question. The genetic analysis always includes assessment for any other potentially inherited conditions for which testing, prevention, and treatment may be possible.

A physical examination may be performed by the medical geneticist to identify specific clinical features commonly associated with a genetic condition. The examination also helps determine if further testing is needed to diagnose a genetic disorder. This examination generally involves assessment of all body systems, with a focus on specific physical characteristics. Nurses describe the diagnostic evaluations that are part of a genetics consultation and explain their purposes.

Communicating Genetic and Genomic Information to Patients

After the family history and the physical examination are completed, the genetics team reviews the information gathered before beginning genetic counseling with the patient and the family. The genetic specialists meet with the patient and the family to discuss their findings. If information gathered confirms a genetic condition in a family, genetic specialists discuss with the patient the natural history of the condition, the pattern of inheritance, and the implications of the condition for reproductive and general health. When appropriate, specialists also discuss relevant testing and management options.

Providing Support

The genetics team provides support throughout the counseling session and identifies personal and family concerns. Genetic specialists use active listening to interpret patient concerns and emotions, seek and provide feedback, and demonstrate understanding of those concerns. They suggest referral for additional social and emotional support. In addition, genetic specialists discuss pertinent patient and family concerns and needs with nurses and primary health care teams so that they can provide additional support and guidance (Kirk & Marshallay, 2013; NIH, 2013b). Nurses assess the patient's understanding of the information given during the counseling session, clarify information, answer questions, assess patient reactions, and identify support systems.

Follow-Up After Genetic Evaluation

As a follow-up to genetic evaluation and counseling, genetic specialists prepare a written summary of the evaluation and counseling session for the patient and, with the patient's consent, send this summary to the primary provider as well as other providers identified by the patient as participants in care. The consultation summary outlines the results of the family history and physical and laboratory assessments, provides a discussion of any specific diagnosis made, reviews the inheritance and associated risk of recurrence for the patient and the family, presents reproductive and general health options, and makes recommendations for further testing and management. The nurse reviews the summary with the patient and identifies information, education, and counseling for which follow-up genetic counseling may be useful (Kirk & Marshallay, 2013).

Follow-up genetic counseling is always offered because some patients and families need more time to understand and discuss the specifics of a genetic test or diagnosis, or they may wish to review reproductive options again later, when pregnancy is being considered. Follow-up counseling is also offered to patients when further evaluation and counseling of extended family members is recommended (Kirk & Marshallay, 2013).

During follow-up sessions, nurses can educate patients about sources of information related to genetic and genomic issues. Some resources that provide the most up-to-date and reliable genetic and genomic information are available on the Internet (see the Resources section at the end of this chapter).

Genetics and Genomics Tomorrow

The pace of genetic and genomic research is transforming our understanding of the role of genetics and genomics in health and disease. In addition, it is increasing clinical opportunities for presymptomatic prediction of illness based on a patient's genetic makeup. Genetic research is now focused on identifying the genetic and environmental causes of common diseases such as diabetes, heart disease, and asthma. The studies are opening the doors for many advances in the prevention and treatment of both rare and common diseases (NIH, 2014d).

As applications of genetics and genomics to health and disease develop, genetic testing may be used to scan all of a patient's genetic material so that disease risk variants can be identified and early interventions and treatments can be determined. It is projected that the cost of testing a patient's entire genome will be less than $1000. Personalized medicine will continue to expand, and many treatments and interventions for medical conditions will be chosen on the basis of what genetic testing indicates about a patient's genetic makeup. Nurses will be on the front line in communicating genetic and genomic information to patients, families, and communities. Patients, families, and communities will also expect that health care providers, including nurses, will use new genetic and genomic information and technologies in the provision of care. It is, therefore, imperative that all nurses become fluent in the language of genetics and genomics so that they can provide effective nursing care (Consensus Panel, 2009).

CRITICAL THINKING EXERCISES

1 `ebp` A 16-year-old African American male is trying out for the football team. He has been complaining of joint pain for the past 3 days. During his last football practice, he was rushed to the hospital due to severe respiratory compromise. What immediate assessment questions should the nurse include? His parents deny any prior history of respiratory difficulty. Upon further investigation, it is learned that the patient has sickle cell disease. How does this relate to his joint pain? What is the inheritance pattern of sickle cell disease? What is unique with this type of inheritance pattern? Should the parents be treated for sickle cell disease? To help during this sickle cell crisis, how might pharmacogenetics be applied to best manage pain? What questions should the patient and his parents be asked regarding pain control? What evidence related to pain medications supports the discussion?

2 `pg` A 51-year-old man is admitted to the hospital with complaint of lower extremity pain. Upon assessment, the right calf is warm to touch and edematous. The pedal pulse is not palpable but able to be attained by Doppler. What critical questions should the nurse include in the admission assessment? The patient becomes diaphoretic and short of breath. Oxygen is applied and an x-ray is obtained. The findings from the x-ray indicate that the patient has three small blood clots in his lung. Based on these new findings, what additional questions should be asked? Hematology reports confirm that the patient has Factor V Leiden thrombophilia. What concerns should the nurse discuss with the patient? Warfarin (Coumadin) will be started according to hospital protocol for a diagnosis of deep vein thrombosis. How might principles of pharmacogenetics be applied while monitoring the effectiveness of the warfarin? Knowing that Factor V Leiden thrombosis is an autosomal dominant condition, what genetic information needs to be shared with the patient? What recommendations will be made for the patient's family?

3 A 34-year-old man is diagnosed with hypertrophic cardiomyopathy after experiencing chest pain and shortness of breath while exercising. The physician explains that this is a hereditary condition known to have an autosomal dominant pattern of inheritance. The patient has two young sons, 2 and 5 years of age. His mother is living but his father died from cardiac problems at the age of 60 years. During your assessment, you take a family history and complete a three-generation pedigree including the information that is known. Draw the pedigree illustrating autosomal dominant inheritance. What advice should be given to this patient regarding genetic testing?

REFERENCES

*Asterisk indicates nursing research.
**Double asterisk indicates classic reference.

Books

American Nurses Association. (2015). *Code of ethics for nurses with interpretive statements*. Washington, DC: American Nurses Publishing.
**Consensus Panel on Genetic/Genomic Nursing Competencies. (2009). *Essentials of genetic and genomic nursing: Competencies, curricular guidelines, and outcome indicators* (2nd ed.). Silver Spring, MD: American Nurses Association.
Dwyer, T. M., Glaser, R. L., & Mason, T. M. (2016). Inheritance patterns in human phenotypes and types of genetic disorders. In C. E. Kasper, T. A. Schneidereith, & F. R. Lashley (Eds.), *Lashley's essentials of clinical genetics in nursing practice* (pp. 65–114). New York, NY. Springer Publishing Company.

Journals and Electronic Documents

American College of Medical Genetics and Genomics Policy Statement (ACMG). (2013). ACMG recommendations for reporting of incidental findings in clinical exome and genome sequencing. *Genetics in Medicine,* *15*(7), 565–574.

American College of Obstetricians and Gynecologists Committee on Genetics (ACOG). (2014a). *Committee opinion. Committee on Genetics. Number 442 (replaces 298). Prenatal and preconceptional carrier screening for genetic diseases in individuals of eastern European Jewish descent.* Retrieved on 7/10/2015 at: www.acog.org/-/media/Committee-Opinions/Committee-on-Genetics/co442.pdf?dmc=1&ts=2015071 0T1049586049

American College of Obstetricians and Gynecologists Committee on Genetics (ACOG) (2014b). *Committee opinion. Committee on genetics. Number 486. Update on carrier screening for cystic fibrosis* (pp. 1–4). Retrieved on 7/10/2015 at: www.acog.org/-/media/Committee-Opin-ions/Committee-on-Genetics/co486.pdf?dmc=1&ts=20150710T1033 593218p

Ashley, E. A. (2015). The precision medicine initiative: A new national effort. *JAMA, 313*(21), 2119–2120.

Badzek, L., Henaghan, M., Turner, M., et al. (2013). Ethical, legal, and social issues in the translation of genomics into health care. *Journal of Nursing Scholarship, 45*(1), 15–24.

Boucher, J., Habin, K., & Underhill, M. (2014). Cancer genetics and genomics: Essentials for oncology nurses. *Clinical Journal of Oncology Nursing, 18*(3), 355–359.

Calzone, K. A., Jenkins, J., Bakos, A. D., et al. (2013). A blueprint for genomic nursing science. *Journal of Nursing Scholarship, 45*(1), 96–104.

Calzone, K. A., Jenkins, J., Nicol, N., et al. (2013). Relevance of genomics to healthcare and nursing practice. *Journal of Nursing Scholarship, 45*(1), 1–2.

Christenhusz, G. M., Devriendt, K., & Dietrickx, K. (2013). To tell or not tell? A systematic review of ethical reflections on incidental findings arising in genetics contexts. *European Journal of Human Genetics, 21*(3), 248–255.

Clayton, E. W., McCullough, L. B., Biesecker, L. G., et al. (2014). Addressing the ethical challenges in genetic testing and sequencing of children. *The American Journal of Bioethics, 14*(3), 3–9.

Conley, Y. P., Biesecker, L. G., Gonsalves, S., et al. (2013). Current and emerging technology approaches in genetics. *Journal of Nursing Scholarship, 45*(1), 5–14.

Cosman, F., de Beur, S. J., LeBoff, M. S., et al. (2014). Clinician's guide to prevention and treatment of osteoporosis. *Osteoporosis International, 25*(10), 2359–2381.

Cramer, S. A., Adjei, I. M., & Labhasetwar, V. (2015). Advancements in the delivery of epigenetic drugs. *Expert Opinion Drug Delivery, 12*(9), 1501–1512.

Genetests. (2015a). Retrieved on 6/30/2015 at: www.genetests.org/

Genetests. (2015b). Breast cancer. Retrieved on 6/30/2015 at: www.gene-tests.org/search/disorders.php?search=breast%2520cancer&submit=Search&start=0

Greco, K. E., Tinley, S., & Seibert, D. (2012). Essential genetic and genomic competencies for nurses with graduate degrees. Retrieved on 7/11/2015 at: www.nursingworld.org/MainMenuCategories/EthicsStandards/Genetics-1/Essential-Genetic-and-Genomic-Competencies-for-Nurses-With-Graduate-Degrees.pdf

Green, R. C., Lautenbach, D., & McGuire, A. L. (2015). GINA, genetic discrimination, and genomic medicine. *New England Journal of Medicine, 372*(5), 397–399.

Harkness, E. F., Barrow, E., Newton, K., et al. (2015). Lynch syndrome caused by MLH1 mutations is associated with an increased risk of breast cancer: A cohort study. *Journal of Medical Genetics, 52*(8), 553–556.

HUGO Gene Nomenclature Committee. (2015). Cytochrome P450. Retrieved on 7/9/2015 at: www.genenames.org/cgi-bin/search?search_type=all&search=cytochrome+P450&submit=Submit

International Society of Nurses in Genetics. (2014). Position statements. Retrieved on 7/9/2015 at: www.isong.org/ISONG_position_statements.php

Iqbal, J., Ginsburg, O., Rochon, P., et al. (2015). Differences in breast cancer stage at diagnosis and cancer-specific survival by race and ethnicity in the United States. *JAMA, 313*(2), 165–173.

Johnson, J. A. (2013). Pharmacogenetics in clinical practice: How far have we come and where are we going? *Pharmacogenomics, 14*(7), 835–843.

Kirk, M., & Marshallay, M. (2013). Providing nursing care and support to individuals and families with genetic / genomic healthcare needs. *Nursing Standard, 28*(16), 39–46.

Korf, B. R., & Rehm, H. L. (2013). New approaches to molecular diagnosis. *JAMA, 309*(14), 1511–1521.

Leoz, M. L., Carballal, S., Moreira, L., et al, (2015). The genetic basis of familial adenomatous polyposis and its implications for clinical practice and risk management. *The Application of Clinical Genetics, 8,* 95–107.

Lough, M. E., & Seidel, G. D. (2015). Legal and clinical issues on genetics and genomics. *Clinical Nurse Specialist, 29*(2), 68–70.

Mayo Clinic. (2014). Medical history: Compiling your medical family tree. Retrieved on 7/12/2015 at: www.mayoclinic.org/healthy-lifestyle/adult-health/in-depth/medical-history/art-20044961

National Human Genome Research Institute. (2015). Talking glossary of genetic terms. Retrieved on 11/23/2015 at: www.genome.gov/Glossary/index.cfm?id=532

National Institutes of Health. National Human Genome Research Institute (NIH). (2013a). Learning about Turner syndrome. Retrieved on 7/03/2015 at: www.genome.gov/19519119

National Institutes of Health. National Human Genome Research Institute. (NIH). (2013b). Frequently asked questions about genetic counseling. Retrieved on 7/09/2015 at: www.genome.gov/19016905

National Institutes of Health. National Human Genome Research Institute. (NIH). (2014a). All about the Human Genome Project. Retrieved on 7/05/2015 at: www.genome.gov/10001772

National Institutes of Health. National Human Genome Research Institute. (NIH). (2014b). Learning about sickle cell disease. Retrieved on 7/08/2015 at: www.genome.gov/10001219

National Institutes of Health. National Human Genome Research Institute (NIH). (2014c). Frequently asked questions about pharmacogenomics. Retrieved on 7/09/2015 at: www.genome.gov/27530645#al-3

National Institutes of Health. National Human Genome Research Institute (NIH). (2014d). New horizons and research activities. Retrieved on 12/05/2016 at: www.genome.gov/27527636

National Institutes of Health. National Human Genome Research Institute (NIH). (2015a). Talking glossary of genetic terms. Retrieved on 7/07/2015 at: www.genome.gov/Glossary/index.cfm?id=92

National Institutes of Health. National Human Genome Research Institute (NIH). (2015b). Chromosome abnormalities. Retrieved on 6/30/2015 at: www.genome.gov/11508982

National Institutes of Health. National Human Genome Research Institute (NIH). (2015c). Policy and program analysis branch. Retrieved on 7/9/2015 at: www.genome.gov/10001087

Online Mendelian Inheritance of Man. (2013a). Alpha-1-antitrypsin deficiency (number 613490). Retrieved on 11/24/15 at: www.omim.org/entry/613490?search=alpha1-antitrypsin%20deficiency&highlight=deficiency%20alpha1%20alpha1antitrypsin%20antitrypsin

Online Mendelian Inheritance of Man. (2013b). Beta-2-adrenergic receptor; ADRB2 (number 109690). Retrieved on 7/02/2015 at: www.omim.org/entry/109690?search=number%3A%28109690%20OR%20600807%20OR%20605238%29&highlight=605238%20600807%20109690

Parkman, A. A., Foland, J., Anderson, B., et al. (2015). Public awareness of genetic information laws in four states and perceived importance of life insurance protections. *Journal of Genetic Counseling, 24*(3), 512–521.

*Pettey, C. M., McSweeney, J. C., Stewart, K. E., et al. (2015). Perceptions of family history and genetic testing and feasibility of pedigree development among African Americans with hypertension. *European Journal of Cardiovascular Nursing, 14*(1), 8–15.

**Pletcher, B. A., Toriello, H. V., Noblin, S. J., et al. (2007). Indications for genetic referral: A guide for healthcare providers. *Genetics in Medicine, 9*(6), 385–389.

Porry, P., Shabani, M., & Howard, H. C. (2014). Is there a right time to know? The right not to know and genetic testing in children. *Journal of Law, Medicine & Ethics, 42*(1), 19–27.

Roadmap Epigenomics Consortium. (2015). Integrative analysis of 111 reference human epigenomes. *Nature, 518*(7539), 317–330.

Romanoski, C. E., & Glass, C. K., (2015). Roadmap for regulation: Differentiation enhanced. *Nature, 518*(7539), 314–315.

**Simopoulos, A. P. (2009) Genetic screening: Programs. Principles, and research—thirty years later. *Public Health Genomics, 12,* 105–111.

The White House. (2015). Fact sheet: President Obama's precision medicine initiative. Retrieved on 6/02/2015 at: www.whitehouse.gov/the-press-office/2015/01/30/fact-sheet-president-obama-s-precision-medicine-initiative

U.S. National Library of Medicine. Genetic Home Reference (NLM). (2015a). What are the different ways in which a genetic condition can be inherited? Retrieved on 6/30/2015 at: ghr.nlm.nih.gov/handbook/inheritance/inheritancepatterns

U.S. National Library of Medicine. Genetics Home Reference (NLM). (2015b). What are reduced penetrance and variable expressivity? Retrieved on 6/02/2015 at: ghr.nlm.nih.gov/handbook/inheritance/penetranceexpressivity

U.S. National Library of Medicine. Genetics Home Reference (NLM). (2015c). Can changes in the structure of chromosomes affect health and development? Retrieved on 6/30/2015 at: ghr.nlm.nih.gov/handbook/mutationsanddisorders/structuralchanges

U.S. National Library of Medicine. Genetics Home Reference (NLM). (2015d). What is pharmacogenomics? Retrieved on 7/9/2015 at: ghr.nlm.nih.gov/handbook/genomicresearch/pharmacogenomics

U.S. National Library of Medicine. Genetics Home Reference (NLM). (2015e). What are the types of genetic tests? Retrieved on 11/24/2015 at: ghr.nlm.nih.gov/handbook/testing/uses

U.S. National Library of Medicine. Genetics Home Reference (NLM). (2015f). Neurofibromatosis type 1. Retrieved on 7/9/2015 at: ghr.nlm.nih.gov/condition/neurofibromatosis-type-1

U.S. National Library of Medicine (NLM). (2015g). Medline Plus. Family history. Retrieved on 7/12/2015 at: www.nlm.nih.gov/medlineplus/familyhistory.html#cat59

Waters, E. A., Muff, J., & Hamilton, J. G. (2014). Multifactorial beliefs about the role of genetics and behavior in common health conditions: Prevalence and associations with participant characteristics and engagement in health behaviors. *Genetics in Medicine, 16*, 913–921.

Welch, B. M., Dere, W. & Schiffman, J. D. (2015). Family health history: The case for better tools. *JAMA, 313*(7) 1711–1712. Doi:10.1001/jama.2015.2417

Resources

Association of Women's Health, Obstetric and Neonatal Nurses (AWHONN), www.awhonn.org/awhonn

GeneTests, www.genetests.org/search/disorders.php

Genetic Alliance, www.geneticalliance.org

Genetic Home Reference: Your Guide to Understanding Genetic Conditions, ghr.nlm.nih.gov/

Genetic and Rare Diseases Information Center, www.genome.gov/Health/GARD/

Human Genome Project Information, *SNP Fact Sheet,* biophys.roma2.infn.it/members/morante/fb2_lezioni_11_12/snps_2.pdf

International Society of Nurses in Genetics (ISONG), www.isong.org

MedlinePlus Health Topics, www.nlm.nih.gov/medlineplus/healthtopics.html

National Cancer Institute (NCI), www.cancer.gov

National Center for Biotechnology Information, www.ncbi.nlm.nih.gov

National Coalition for Health Professional Education in Genetics (NCHPEG), www.nchpeg.org

National Human Genome Research Institute, Genome Statute and Legislative Database (summary of each state's legislation on employment and insurance discrimination), www.genome.gov/PolicyEthics/LegDatabase/pubsearch.cfm

National Organization for Rare Disorders (NORD), www.rarediseases.org

Oncology Nursing Society (ONS), www.ons.org

9

Chronic Illness and Disability

LEARNING OBJECTIVES

On completion of this chapter, the learner will be able to:

1. Compare and contrast the concepts of chronic illness, chronic disease, and disability.
2. Identify factors related to the increasing incidence of chronic conditions.
3. Describe characteristics of chronic conditions and implications for people with chronic conditions and for their families.
4. Specify the advantages and disadvantages of various models of disability.
5. Critically analyze the influence of disability for nursing care decisions and actions for patients.

GLOSSARY

chronic disease: medical or health problem with associated symptoms or disabilities that require long-term management; has also been referred to as noncommunicable disease, chronic condition, or chronic disorder

chronic illness: the experience of living with a chronic disease or condition; the individual's perception of the experience and the individual's and others' responses to the chronic disease or condition

disability: restriction or lack of ability to perform an activity in a normal manner; the consequences of impairment in terms of an individual's functional performance and activity—disabilities represent disturbances at the level of the person (e.g., bathing, dressing, communication, walking, grooming)

impairment: loss or abnormality of psychological, physiologic, or anatomic structure or function at the

organ level (e.g., dysphagia, hemiparesis); an abnormality of body structure, appearance, and organ or system function resulting from any cause

multiple chronic conditions (MCC): presence of more than one chronic disease or condition, which increases the complexity of care as well as morbidity and mortality rates

noncommunicable diseases: a group of conditions that are not caused by an acute infection; many are considered chronic diseases and are often due to unhealthy behaviors

secondary health conditions or disorders: any physical, mental, or social disorders resulting directly or indirectly from an initial disabling condition; a condition to which a person with a disability is more susceptible because of having a primary disabling condition

Chronic illness and disability affect people of all ages—the very young, the middle aged, older adults, and the very old. Chronic illnesses and disabilities are found in all ethnic, cultural, racial, and socioeconomic groups, although some disorders occur more frequently in some groups than in others. **Chronic diseases** may refer to noncommunicable diseases, chronic conditions, or chronic disorders. In contrast, **chronic illness** refers to the human experience of living with a chronic disease or condition. Chronic illness includes the individual's perception of the experience of having a chronic disease or condition and the individual's and others' responses to it, including health care professionals (Larsen, 2016). Individuals' and their families' values and previous experiences determine their perception and beliefs about the condition, which in turn affect their illness and wellness behaviors. Their values are influenced by a number of demographic, socioeconomic, technological, cultural, and environmental variables. Only the individual and the family really know what it is like to live with chronic illness.

Chronic diseases are the most common causes of death in the United States. The most frequently occurring chronic diseases account for 7 of the 10 leading causes of death and are responsible for more than two-thirds of the deaths that

occur globally. They include cardiovascular disease, cancers, diabetes, and chronic lung diseases (Centers for Disease Control and Prevention [CDC], 2015; World Health Organization [WHO], 2014a; 2014b). These diseases or conditions are increasing rapidly in lower-income populations and communities because of adoption of unhealthy lifestyles. Lack of physical activity, poor nutrition, tobacco use, and excessive alcohol consumption are modifiable health risk behaviors that are responsible for the high incidence of chronic disease, disability, and early death (CDC, 2015). Although many chronic diseases are a result of unhealthy lifestyles, many others are associated with nonmodifiable factors, including genetic and physiologic factors (WHO, 2014a). This chapter discusses chronic illness and disability and their implications for nursing practice. Some degree of disability is often present in severe or advanced chronic illness, limiting patient's participation in many activities.

Overview of Chronicity

Chronic diseases are long-term health conditions that affect one's well-being and function in an episodic, continuous,

Chart 9-1 Chronic Illness in the United States

- Chronic diseases are the leading causes of death and disability in the United States.
- Chronic disease and conditions (e.g., heart disease, stroke, cancer, diabetes, obesity, and arthritis) are among the most common, costly, and preventable of all health problems.
- Heart disease, cancer, stroke, chronic lower respiratory diseases, Alzheimer disease, and diabetes pose greater risks as people age.
- Chronic disease, specifically diabetes, is the leading cause of kidney failure, amputation of lower extremities, and new causes of blindness among adults.
- Obesity is a serious health concern with one-third of adults and one of five youths being obese.
- Lack of exercise or physical activity, poor nutrition, use of tobacco, and excessive alcohol use contribute to the growing prevalence of chronic diseases and resulting disability. Tobacco remains the leading cause of 6 million preventable deaths per year globally.
- Rural Americans are more likely to have chronic disease, such as high blood pressure, heart disease, and diabetes, than non-rural populations.
- Eighty-six percent of all health care spending is related to chronic disease.
- People with chronic disease may have other health problems that may or may not be related to the primary chronic disease; these include alcohol abuse and substance use or addiction disorders, mental illness, dementia or other cognitive impairments, and developmental disabilities.

Adapted from Agency for Healthcare Research and Quality. (2015). *2014 National healthcare quality and disparities report.* Rockville, MD: Agency for Healthcare Research and Quality. AHRQ Pub. No. 15-0007.
Agency for Healthcare Research and Quality. (2014). *Multiple chronic conditions chartbook: 2010 medical expenditure panel survey data.* Rockville, MD: Agency for Healthcare Research and Quality. AHRQ Pub. No. 14-0038.
Centers for Disease Control and Prevention. (2013). *The state of aging and health in America 2013.* Atlanta, GA: Author.
Centers for Disease Control and Prevention. (2015). *The four domains of chronic disease prevention. Working toward healthy people in healthy communities.* Atlanta, GA: Author. Retrieved on 7/17/2015 at: www.cdc.gov/chronicdisease/pdf/four-domains-factsheet-2015.pdf
Golics, C. J., Basra, M. K. A., Salek, M. S., et al. (2013). The impact of patients' chronic disease on family quality of life: An experience from 26 specialties. *International Journal of General Medicine, 6,* 787–798.
U.S. Department of Labor/Bureau of Labor Statistics. (2015). *Persons with a disability: Labor force characteristics—2014.* Washington, DC: Author.
World Health Organization. (2013). *Global action plan for the prevention and control of noncommunicable diseases, 2013–2020.* Geneva, Switzerland: Author.
World Health Organization. (2014a). *Global status report on noncommunicable diseases 2014.* Geneva, Switzerland: Author.
World Health Organization. (2014d). *Global health estimates: Deaths by cause, age, sex and country, 2015–2030.* Geneva, Switzerland: World Health Organization. Retrieved on 7/17/2015 at: www.who.int/gho/ncd/mortality_morbidity/en/

or progressive way over many years of life. Although each chronic disease or condition has its own specific physiologic characteristics, chronic conditions share common features. Many chronic conditions, for example, have pain and fatigue as associated symptoms. Other common symptoms are sleep disturbances and difficulty adjusting to the onset and uncertainty of a chronic condition (Lorig, Holman, Sobel, et al., 2012). Many people with chronic health conditions and disability function independently with only minor inconvenience to their everyday lives; others, however, require frequent and close monitoring or placement in long-term care facilities. Certain conditions require advanced technology for survival, as in the late stages of chronic obstructive lung disease or end-stage renal disease, or intensive care or mechanical ventilation for periods of weeks, months, or years. People with disorders such as these have been described as being chronically critically ill, although there is no consensus on a definition of chronic critical illness. An overview of chronic disease in the United States is presented in Chart 9-1.

Multiple Chronic Conditions

One of every four adults has two or more chronic health conditions, which increases the complexity of his care and requires coordination of care and services. Having **multiple chronic conditions** (MCC) puts patients at risk for conflicting medical advice, adverse effects of medications, unnecessary and duplicative tests, and preventable hospitalizations, all of which can have a negative effect on their health. The presence of various and diverse MCC often necessitates care by multiple health care specialists, a variety of treatment regimens, and prescription medications that may not be compatible (CDC, 2013; Ward, Schiller, & Goodman, 2014). Patients with MCC and their families may have to keep track of different medications with different schedules and multiple appointments with health care professionals (Agency for Healthcare Research and Quality [AHRQ], 2014). Costs of care increase with the number of chronic conditions a person has and out-of-pocket health-related expenses increase with the number of MCC. Facts about MCC are summarized in Chart 9-2.

Health Disparities and Chronic Disease

Although chronic disease occurs in all socioeconomic groups, people from low-income and disadvantaged backgrounds are more likely to report poor health. Factors such as poverty and inadequate health insurance decrease the likelihood that people with chronic illness or disability receive health care and health-screening measures such as mammography, cholesterol testing, and routine checkups (American Public Health Association, 2015). In addition, chronic conditions can lead to poverty for the patient and the family, or perhaps even for society or the nation as a whole, because chronic conditions or subsequent premature death occurs most commonly during the afflicted person's most productive years.

Chart 9-2 **Facts About Multiple Chronic Conditions (MCC)**

- About half of all adults—117 million people—have one or more chronic health conditions. One of every four adults has two or more chronic health conditions (CDC, 2015).
- The occurrence of MCC increases with age. Two out of every three older Americans have multiple chronic conditions.
- The number of people with MCC is predicted to increase substantially over the next decade, adding to the pressures on the health care system to deliver high quality of care, at optimal cost, while improving the health of this complex population.
- Women are more likely than men to have MCC.
- Non-Hispanic white adults, non-Hispanic black adults, and non-Hispanic adults of other races have a high prevalence of MCC.
- As the number of chronic conditions a person has increases, the greater the risk of dying prematurely, being hospitalized, and having poor day-to-day functioning.
- Many patients with MCC have mobility limitations and require assistance with dressing, bathing, or preparing meals.
- People with MCC account for the majority of health care visits, prescriptions, home health visits, and hospital stays in the United States.

Adapted from Agency for Healthcare Research and Quality. (2014). *Multiple chronic conditions chartbook: 2010 medical expenditure panel survey data.* Rockville, MD: Agency for Healthcare Research and Quality. AHRQ Pub. No. 14-0038.
Centers for Disease Control and Prevention. (2013). *The state of aging and health in America 2013.* Atlanta, GA: Centers for Disease Control and Prevention, U.S., Department of Health & Human Services.

Disparities in health and health outcomes are associated with social, economic, and environmental disadvantages. Although the gap between health outcomes in African Americans and Caucasians has decreased in some areas, in others (e.g., mortality due to breast cancer) the gaps have increased (McCarthy, Yang, & Armstrong, 2015). Disparities in health and health outcomes are associated with higher incidence and prevalence, earlier onset, faster progression, and poorer outcomes of disease and conditions (Dankwa-Mullan & Maddox, 2015; WHO, 2014a).

Some chronic conditions have little effect on quality of life, whereas others have a major effect because they result in disability. However, it is important to note that not all disabilities are a result of chronic illness, and not all chronic illnesses cause disability (Drum, 2014). Unlike the term *acute*, which implies a curable and relatively short disease course, the term *chronic* describes a long disease course that may be incurable. This often makes managing chronic conditions difficult for those who live with them. Although chronic conditions often cannot be cured, nurses can and do make a difference in the illness experience with quality nursing care in the absence of a cure (Larsen, 2016).

Psychological and emotional reactions of patients to acute and chronic conditions and changes in their health status are described in Chapter 6. People who develop chronic conditions or disabilities may react with shock, disbelief, anger, resentment, or other emotions. How people react to and cope with chronic illness is usually similar to how they react to other events in their lives, depending, in part, on their understanding of the condition and their perceptions of its potential impact on their own and their family's lives. Adjustment to chronic illness (and disability) is affected by various factors:

- Suddenness, extent, and duration of lifestyle changes necessitated by the illness
- Uncertainty related to the course and outcome of chronic illnesses
- Family and individual resources for dealing with stress
- Availability of support from family, friends, and the community
- Stages of individual/family life cycle
- Previous experience with illness and crises
- Underlying personality characteristics
- Unresolved anger or grief from the past

Psychological, emotional, and cognitive reactions to chronic conditions are likely to occur at the onset and to recur if symptoms worsen or recur after a period of remission. Symptoms associated with chronic health conditions are often unpredictable and may be perceived as crisis events by patients and their families, who must contend with both the uncertainty of chronic illness and the changes it brings to their lives. The possible effects of chronic conditions can guide nursing assessment and interventions for the patient who has a chronic illness.

Definition of Chronic Diseases or Conditions

Chronic diseases or conditions are often defined as medical conditions or health problems with associated symptoms or disabilities that require long-term management. No single definition for chronic disease exists, but it is generally accepted that chronic diseases are those that persist for months or years rather than days or weeks (Goodman, Posner, Huang, et al., 2013). The U.S. National Center for Health Statistics defines chronic disease as a condition lasting 3 or more months (Adams, Kirzinger, & Martinez, 2013) and the WHO (2014a) defines it as a long-lasting condition that can usually be controlled but not cured. Definitions of chronic disease or chronic illness share the characteristics of being irreversible, having a prolonged course, and unlikely to resolve spontaneously (Larsen, 2016). The specific chronic condition may be a result of illness, genetic factors, or injury; it may be a consequence of conditions or unhealthy behaviors that began during childhood and young adulthood.

Chronic diseases or disorders are one of the major health and development challenges of the 21st century because of their global human, social, and financial consequences. Although chronic diseases affect all countries, their impact is more severe in low- and middle-income countries (i.e., South American, African, and Asian countries), where the majority of premature deaths due to chronic diseases occur. Their impact is particularly devastating to poor and vulnerable populations. Chronic diseases, also referred to as **noncommunicable diseases**, cause more deaths than all other causes combined. Deaths due to chronic disease are expected to increase globally from 38 million in 2012 to 52 million per year by 2030 (WHO, 2014a).

Management of chronic conditions includes learning to live with symptoms or disabilities and coming to terms with identity changes resulting from having a chronic condition. It also consists of carrying out the lifestyle changes and regimens designed to control symptoms and prevent complications. Although some people assume what might be called a "sick role" identity, most people with chronic conditions do not consider themselves to be sick or ill and try to live as normal a life as possible. Only when complications develop or symptoms interfere with activities of daily living (ADLs) do most people with chronic health conditions think of themselves as being sick or disabled.

Prevalence and Causes of Chronic Conditions

Chronic conditions occur in people of every age group, socioeconomic level, race, and culture. Seven of the 10 leading causes of death in the United States are chronic diseases, with heart disease and cancer together accounting for nearly half of all deaths. It is predicted that by the year 2030, about half the population will have a chronic disease or disorder. One fifth of those with chronic disease also have an activity limitation. As the incidence of chronic diseases increases, the costs associated with these chronic conditions (e.g., hospital costs, equipment, medications, supportive services) also increase. Expenditures for health care for people with one chronic condition account for 86% of the $2 trillion the United States spends each year on health care (AHRQ, 2014). These costs represent four of every five health care dollars expended. The worldwide economic burden associated with chronic disease is estimated to be $47 trillion over the next two decades (Bloom, Cafiero, Jané-Llopis, et al., 2011).

Although some chronic health conditions cause little or no inconvenience, others are severe enough to cause major activity limitations. When people with activity limitations are unable to meet their needs for health care and personal services, they may be unable to carry out their therapeutic regimens or have their prescriptions filled on time, may miss appointments and office visits with their health care providers, and may be unable to carry out ADLs.

Chronic diseases are a global issue that affects both rich and poor nations. Chronic conditions have become the major cause of health-related problems in developed countries as well as in the developing countries, which are also trying to cope with new and emerging infectious diseases. In almost all countries, chronic diseases are the major cause of death among adults. Four of every five deaths occur in countries characterized as low- or middle income, where people tend to develop chronic diseases at younger ages, suffer longer, and die sooner than people in high-income countries. In contrast to common belief, the total number of people dying from chronic disease is twice that of patients dying from infectious (including human immunodeficiency virus infection), maternal, and perinatal conditions, and nutritional deficiencies combined (WHO, 2014a; 2014b). The number of people worldwide who die because of chronic disease is higher than all other diseases combined. Most of these chronic diseases and complications of chronic illness are preventable, emphasizing the importance of health promotion across the globe. Although chronic diseases or illnesses are common, people have many myths or misunderstandings about them (see Table 9-1).

TABLE 9-1 Myths and Truths About Chronic Disease

Common Misconceptions About Chronic Disease	The Reality About Chronic Disease
1. Everyone dies of something.	Chronic illnesses typically do not result in sudden death but often result in progressive illness and disability. People with chronic disease often die slowly, painfully, and prematurely.
2. People can live to old age even if they lead unhealthy lives (smoke, are obese).	While there are exceptions (some people who live unhealthy lives live to old age, and some people who live healthy lives develop chronic illnesses), most chronic illnesses can be traced to modifiable risk factors and can be prevented by eliminating these risks.
3. Solutions for chronic disease prevention and control are expensive and not feasible for low- and middle-income countries.	A full range of chronic disease interventions are very cost-effective for all regions of the world, including the poorest. Many of these interventions are inexpensive to implement. Chronic disease is increasing rapidly around the world, including in low- and middle-income countries.
4. There is nothing that can be done and chronic diseases cannot be prevented.	The major causes of chronic diseases are known, and if these risk factors were eliminated, at least more than 80% of heart disease, stroke, and type 2 diabetes and more than 40% of cancers would be prevented.
5. If individuals develop chronic disease as a result of unhealthy "lifestyles," they have only themselves to blame	Individual responsibility can have its full effect only if individuals have equal access to a healthy life and are supported to make healthy choices. Poor people often have limited choices about the food they eat, their living conditions, and access to education and health care.
6. Certain chronic diseases primarily affect men.	Chronic diseases, including heart disease, affect women and men almost equally. Almost half of all deaths attributed to chronic illness occur in women.
7. Chronic diseases primarily affect old people.	Almost half of chronic disease deaths occur prematurely in people younger than 70 years.
8. Chronic diseases mainly affect rich (affluent) people.	Poor people are much more likely than the wealthy to develop chronic diseases and as a result are more likely to die. Chronic diseases cause substantial financial burden and result in extreme poverty.
9. The priority of low- and middle-income countries should be on control of infectious diseases.	Although infectious diseases are an issue, low- and middle-income countries are experiencing a dramatic increase in chronic disease risk factors and deaths, especially in urban settings.
10. Chronic diseases affect mostly high-income countries.	Eighty percent of deaths attributed to chronic disease are in low- and middle-income countries. The prevalence of chronic diseases in low- and middle-income countries is rapidly growing.

Adapted from World Health Organization. (2005). *Widespread misunderstandings about chronic disease—and the reality. Facing the Facts #2.* Retrieved on 1/23/2016 at: www.who.int/chp/chronic_disease_report/media/Factsheet2.pdf

Causes of the increasing number of people with chronic conditions include the following:

- A decrease in mortality from infectious diseases (e.g., smallpox, diphtheria, acquired immune deficiency syndrome [AIDS]–related infections) and from acute conditions because of prompt and aggressive management of acute conditions (e.g., myocardial infarction, trauma).
- Lifestyle factors such as smoking, chronic stress, poor nutrition, and sedentary lifestyle that increase the risk of chronic health problems such as respiratory disease, hypertension, cardiovascular disease, and obesity. Although signs and symptoms of chronic illness often first appear during older age, risks typically begin earlier in life, even during fetal development.
- Obesity, often due to lifestyle issues, has become a major health issue across the lifespan and across the globe with about 2 billion people overweight and one third of them obese. Obesity is no longer limited to high-income countries but increasingly occurs in low- and middle-income countries. The proportion of adults with a body mass index (BMI) of 25 or greater increased between 1980 and 2013 from about 29% to 37% in men and about 30% to 38% in women (Seidell & Halberstadt, 2015).
- The increasing prevalence of obesity has increased the incidence of heart disease, strokes, diabetes, and hypertension. Obesity also affects one's self-esteem, achievement, and emotional state.
- Longer lifespans because of advances in technology and pharmacology, improved nutrition, safer working conditions, and greater access (for some people) to health care.
- Improved screening and diagnostic procedures enabled early detection and treatment of diseases, resulting in improved outcomes of management of cancer and other disorders.

Physiologic changes in the body often occur before the appearance of symptoms of chronic disease. Therefore, the goal of emphasizing healthy lifestyles early in life is to improve overall health status and slow the development of such disorders. Major risk factors for chronic disease, which represent a growing challenge to public health, include unhealthy eating habits, decreased energy expenditure associated with a sedentary lifestyle, increasing age, and tobacco use and alcohol consumption (WHO, 2014a). In addition, serious psychiatric or mental illness puts people at greater risk for chronic illness than the general population and leads to higher morbidity and mortality rates of chronic diseases (National Prevention Council, 2014).

Prevention of Chronic Disease

The CDC (2015) has identified risk factors for common chronic diseases and pointed out that most American adults have more than one of these risk factors:

- hypertension (high blood pressure)
- tobacco use and exposure to secondhand smoke
- overweight or obesity (high BMI)
- lack of physical activity
- excessive alcohol use

| **Chart 9-3** | **Interventions According to Risk Factors** |

Tobacco

- Reduce affordability of tobacco by increasing its costs
- Legally mandate smoke-free environments in all indoor workplaces, public places, and public transport
- Disseminate warnings about dangers of tobacco and tobacco smoke through mass media campaigns and ban all forms of tobacco advertising, promotion, and sponsorship

Harmful Use of Alcohol

- Reduce affordability of alcohol by increasing its costs
- Limit availability of alcohol
- Ban all forms of alcohol advertising and promotions

Diet and Physical Activity

- Promote reduction of dietary salt intake and replacement of trans fats with unsaturated fats
- Implement public awareness programs on diet and physical activity
- Promote and protect breast-feeding (reduces risk of obesity later in life)

Cardiovascular Disease and Diabetes

- Promote glycemic control for diabetes mellitus and control of hypertension using medication therapy
- Counsel individuals who have had a heart attack or stroke and those persons at high risk of a fatal and nonfatal cardiovascular event in the next 10 years
- Initiate acetylsalicylic acid (aspirin) use for acute myocardial infarction

Cancer

- Promote hepatitis B immunization to prevent liver cancer
- Promote screening and early treatment of precancerous lesions to prevent cervical cancer

Adapted from World Health Organization. (2013). *Global action plan for the prevention and control of noncommunicable diseases, 2013–2020*. Geneva, Switzerland: World Health Organization.

- consumption of diets low in fruits and vegetables
- consumption of food high in sodium and saturated fats

The WHO (2013) has identified high-impact, cost-effective interventions to prevent premature death due to chronic disease or chronic conditions that can be implemented even in settings with limited resources. These interventions, summarized in Chart 9-3, are consistent with the risk factors for chronic disease identified by the CDC.

Patient education to prevent chronic disease or reduce its severity or effects is another important component of the nurse's role in working with patients to identify risks for chronic disease and to identify strategies to reduce those risks. Health promotion and patient education are discussed in detail in Chapter 4 in this book.

Characteristics of Chronic Conditions

Sometimes it is difficult for people who are disease free to understand the profound effect that chronic illness often has on the lives of patients and their families. It is easy for health professionals to focus on the illness or disability itself while overlooking the person who has the disorder. In all illnesses, but even more so with chronic conditions, the illness cannot be separated from the person. People with chronic illness must contend with it daily (Lorig et al., 2012). To properly manage their chronic condition, individuals often have to find the time, and the social and financial resources, to participate in physically and psychologically beneficial activities, work with health care professionals to follow treatment guidelines, monitor their health and make decisions about their health and lifestyle and that of their family, and manage the effects of the illness on their physical, psychological, and social well-being. To relate to what people must cope with or to plan effective interventions, nurses must understand the multiple characteristics of a chronic illness.

- Psychological and social issues: Managing chronic illness involves more than treating medical problems. Associated psychological and social issues must also be addressed, because living for long periods with illness symptoms and disability can threaten identity, bring about role changes, alter body image, and disrupt lifestyles. These changes require continuous adaptation and accommodation, depending on age and situation in life. Each decline in functional ability requires physical, emotional, and social adaptation for patients and their families (Corbin, 2003).

- Phases of illness: Chronic conditions usually involve many different phases over the course of a person's lifetime. There can be acute periods, stable and unstable periods, flare-ups, and remissions. Each phase brings its own set of physical, psychological, and social problems, and each requires its own regimens and types of management.

- Therapeutic regimens: Keeping chronic conditions under control requires persistent adherence to therapeutic regimens. Failing to adhere to a treatment plan or to do so consistently increases the risks of developing complications and accelerating the disease process. However, the realities of daily life, including the impact of culture, values, and socioeconomic factors, affect the degree to which people adhere to a treatment regimen. Managing a chronic illness takes time, requires knowledge and planning, and can be uncomfortable and inconvenient. It is not unusual for patients to stop taking medications or alter dosages because of side effects that are more disturbing or disruptive than symptoms of the illness, or to cut back on regimens they consider overly time-consuming, fatiguing, or costly (Corbin, 2003).

- Development of other chronic conditions: One chronic disease can lead to the development of other chronic conditions. Diabetes, for example, can lead to neurologic and vascular changes that may result in visual, cardiac, and kidney diseases and erectile dysfunction. The presence of a chronic illness also contributes to a higher risk of morbidity and mortality in patients admitted to the intensive care unit with acute health conditions as well as greater utilization of clinical services during hospitalization.

- Family life: Chronic illness affects the entire family. Family life can be dramatically altered as a result of role reversals, unfilled roles, loss of income, time required to manage the illness, decreases in family socialization activities, and the costs of treatment. Family members often become caregivers for the person with chronic illness while trying to continue to work and keep the family intact. Stress and caretaker fatigue are common with severe chronic conditions, and the entire family may need care (Golics, Basra, Salek, et al., 2013). However, some families are able to master the treatment regimen and changes that accompany chronic illness as well as make the treatment regimen a routine part of life. Furthermore, they are able to keep the chronic illness from becoming the focal point of family life.

- Home life: The day-to-day management of illness is largely the responsibility of people with chronic disorders and their families (Lorig et al., 2012). As a result, the home, rather than the hospital, is the center of care in chronic conditions. Hospitals, clinics, physicians' offices, nursing homes, nursing centers, and community agencies (home care services, social services, and disease-specific associations and societies) are considered adjuncts or backup services to daily home management.

- Self-management: The management of chronic conditions is a process of discovery. People can be taught how to manage their conditions. However, each patient must discover how their own body reacts under varying circumstances—for example, what it is like to be hypoglycemic, what activities are likely to bring on angina, and how these or other conditions can best be prevented and managed.

- Collaborative process: Managing chronic conditions must be a collaborative process that involves many different health care professionals working together with patients and their families to provide the full range of services that are often needed for management at home. The medical, social, and psychological aspects of chronic health problems are often complex, especially in severe conditions.

- Health care costs: The management of chronic conditions is expensive. Many of the expenses incurred by an individual patient (e.g., costs for hospital stays, diagnostic tests, equipment, medications, and supportive services) may be covered by health insurance and by federal and state agencies. The Patient Protection and Affordable Care Act (ACA), passed in 2010, the most significant change to health care policy in the United States since the establishment of Medicare and Medicaid, has made available health insurance for many previously uninsured individuals who were unable to obtain health insurance. The ACA has ended lifetime and most annual limits on health care, provided patients with access to recommended preventive services, and banned the practice of denying coverage because of the presence of a preexisting health condition (Krahn, Walker, & Correa-De-Araujo, 2015). Despite the positive effects of the ACA, it has not changed the health care delivery system and how health care is delivered.

- Lost income: Direct out-of-pocket expenses represent a significant percent of income, especially in low- and middle-income families. These expenses include high copays and deductibles that must be paid out of pocket. Those with serious chronic disorders may have difficulty paying for care, resulting in bankruptcy or having to rely on family or friends to pay for health insurance or health care. People from low-income groups who do not receive adequate health care get sicker and die sooner from chronic diseases than those from groups with higher levels of education, greater financial resources, and access to care (WHO, 2014a). If a family's primary income earner becomes ill, chronic diseases can result in drastic loss in income with inadequate funds for food, education, and health care. Furthermore, affected families may become unstable and impoverished (WHO, 2014a).

- Ethical issues: Chronic conditions raise difficult ethical issues for patients, families, health care professionals, and society. Problematic questions include how to establish cost controls, how to allocate scarce resources (e.g., organs for transplantation), and what constitutes quality of life and when life support should be withdrawn.
- Living with uncertainty: Having a chronic illness means living with uncertainty. Although health care providers may be aware of the usual progression of a chronic disease such as Parkinson disease or multiple sclerosis, no one can predict with certainty a person's illness course because of individual variation. Even when a patient is in remission or symptom free, he or she often fears that the illness will reappear.

Implications of Managing Chronic Conditions

Chronic conditions have implications for everyday living and management for people and their families as well as for society at large (Lorig et al., 2012). Most importantly, individual efforts should be directed at preventing chronic conditions, because many—but not all—chronic illnesses or disorders are linked to unhealthy lifestyles or behaviors such as smoking and overeating. Therefore, changes in lifestyle can prevent some chronic disorders or at least delay onset until a later age. Because most people resist change, bringing about alterations in people's lifestyles is a major challenge for nurses today.

Once a chronic condition has occurred, the focus shifts to managing symptoms, avoiding complications (e.g., eye complications in a person with diabetes), and preventing other acute illnesses (e.g., pneumonia in a person with chronic obstructive lung disease). Quality of life—often overlooked by health care professionals in their approach to people with chronic conditions—is also important. Health-promoting behaviors, such as exercise, are essential to quality of life even in people who have chronic illnesses or disabilities, because they help maintain functional status (Larsen, 2016; Lorig et al., 2012).

Although coworkers, extended family, and health care professionals are affected by chronic illnesses, the problems of living with chronic conditions are most acutely experienced by individuals and their immediate families. They experience the greatest impact, with lifestyle changes that directly affect quality of life. Nurses provide not only direct care, especially during acute episodes, but also the education and help secure the resources and other supports that enable people to integrate their illness into their lives and to have an acceptable quality of life despite their chronic condition. To understand what nursing care is needed, it is important to recognize and appreciate the issues that people with chronic illness and their families contend with and manage, often on a daily basis

(Larsen, 2016). The challenges of living with chronic conditions include the need to accomplish the following:

- Alleviate and manage symptoms
- Psychologically adjust to and physically accommodate resulting disability
- Prevent and manage crises and complications
- Carry out regimens as prescribed
- Validate individual self-worth and family functioning
- Manage threats to identity
- Normalize personal and family life as much as possible
- Live with altered time, social isolation, and loneliness
- Establish networks of support and resources that can enhance quality of life
- Return to a satisfactory way of life after an acute debilitating episode (e.g., another myocardial infarction or stroke) or reactivation of a chronic condition
- Die with dignity and comfort

Many people with chronic disease or chronic illness must face an additional challenge: the need to deal with MCC (Ward et al., 2014). The symptoms or treatment of a second chronic condition may aggravate the first chronic condition. Patients need to be able to deal with their various chronic conditions separately as well as in combination and to coordinate the health care and directions they receive, often from more than one health care professional.

Even more challenging for many people with chronic illness is the need to hire and oversee caregivers who come into their homes to assist with ADLs and instrumental activities of daily living (IADLs), such as shopping for food, doing laundry, housekeeping, and handling financial matters. It is difficult for many people to be in a position of hiring, supervising, and sometimes firing people who may provide them with intimate physical care. The need to balance the role of recipient of care and oversight of the person providing care may lead to blurring of role boundaries.

The challenges of living with and managing a chronic illness are well known, and people with chronic illnesses often report receiving inadequate care, information, services, and counseling. This provides an opportunity for nurses to assume a more active role in addressing many of the issues experienced, coordinating care, and serving as an advocate for patients who need additional assistance to manage their illness while maintaining a quality of life that is acceptable to them.

Phases of Chronic Conditions

Several models have been developed and used to describe the continuum or phases of chronic disease and its management. The Trajectory Model of Chronic Illness, a nursing model based on many years of interdisciplinary research on chronic illness, will be used to describe the phases and the role of nurses in the trajectory of chronic illness. Table 9-2 describes the different phases of chronic illness and the focus of nursing care during different phases. In this model, the term *trajectory* refers to the path or course that the chronic illness follows. The course of an illness can be thought of as a trajectory that can be managed or shaped over time, to some extent, through proper illness management strategies (Corbin, 1998). It is important to keep in mind that the course of a patient's chronic illness may be too uncertain to predict with

TABLE 9-2 Phases in the Trajectory Model of Chronic Illness

Phase	Description	Focus of Nursing Care
Pretrajectory	Genetic factors or lifestyle behaviors that place a person or community at risk for a chronic condition.	Refer for genetic testing and counseling if indicated; provide education about prevention of modifiable risk factors and behaviors.
Trajectory onset	Appearance or onset of noticeable symptoms associated with a chronic disorder; includes period of diagnostic workup and announcement of diagnosis; may be accompanied by uncertainty as patient awaits a diagnosis and begins to discover and cope with implications of diagnosis.	Provide explanations of diagnostic tests and procedures and reinforce information and explanations given by primary provider; provide emotional support to patient and family.
Stable	Illness course and symptoms are under control as symptoms, resulting disability, and everyday life activities are being managed within limitations of illness; illness management centered in the home.	Reinforce positive behaviors and offer ongoing monitoring, provide education about health promotion, and encourage participation in health-promoting activities and health screening.
Unstable	Characterized by an exacerbation of illness symptoms, development of complications, or reactivation of an illness in remission. Period of inability to keep symptoms under control or reactivation of illness; difficulty in carrying out everyday life activities. May require more diagnostic testing and trial of new treatment regimens or adjustment of current regimen, with care usually taking place at home.	Provide guidance and support; reinforce previous patient education.
Acute	Severe and unrelieved symptoms or the development of illness complications necessitating hospitalization, bed rest, or interruption of the person's usual activities to bring illness course under control.	Provide direct care and emotional support to the patient and the family members.
Crisis	Critical or life-threatening situation requiring emergency treatment or care and suspension of everyday life activities until the crisis has passed.	Provide direct care, collaborate with other health care team members to stabilize patient's condition.
Comeback	Gradual recovery after an acute period and learning to live with or overcome disabilities and return to an acceptable way of life within the limitations imposed by the chronic condition or disability; involves physical healing, limitations stretching through rehabilitative procedures, psychosocial coming-to-terms, and biographical reengagement with adjustments in everyday life activities.	Assist in coordination of care; rehabilitative focus may require care from other health care providers; provide positive reinforcement for goals identified and accomplished.
Downward	Illness course characterized by rapid or gradual worsening of a condition; physical decline accompanied by increasing disability or difficulty in controlling symptoms; requires biographical adjustment and alterations in everyday life activities with each major downward step.	Provide home care and other community-based care to help patient and family adjust to changes and come to terms with these changes; assist patient and family to integrate new treatment and management strategies; encourage identification of end-of-life preferences and planning.
Dying	Final days or weeks before death; characterized by gradual or rapid shutting down of body processes, biographical disengagement and closure, and relinquishment of everyday life interests and activities.	Provide direct and supportive care to patients and their families through palliative care or hospice programs.

Adapted from Corbin, J. M. (1998). The Corbin and Strauss chronic illness trajectory model: An update. *Scholarly Inquiry for Nursing Practice, 12*(1), 33–41.

any degree of accuracy. Furthermore, not all phases occur in all patients; some phases do not occur at all, and some phases may recur. Each phase is characterized by different medical and psychosocial issues. For example, the needs of a patient with a stroke who is a good candidate for rehabilitation are very different from the needs of a patient with terminal cancer. By thinking in terms of phases and individual patients within a phase, nurses can target their care more specifically to each person. Not every chronic condition is necessarily life threatening, and not every patient passes through each possible phase of a chronic condition in the same order.

Using the trajectory model enables the nurse to put the present situation into the context of what might have happened to the patient in the past—that is, the life factors and understandings that might have contributed to the present state of the illness. In this way, the nurse can more readily address the underlying issues and problems.

 Gerontologic Considerations

Changes in the U.S. demographic profile are resulting in an increased number of older adults with chronic illnesses as well as increasing numbers of older adults with MCC. By 2030, older adults are expected to comprise 20% of the U.S. population (CDC, 2013). Two out of every three older Americans have MCC, and treatment for this population accounts for 66% of total US health care expenditures (AHRQ, 2014). The cost of providing health care for a person 65 years of age or older is estimated to be three to five times higher than costs for someone younger than 65 years. Chronic conditions increase the risk for death due to influenza and pneumonia among older adults, although effective vaccines for them exist (CDC, 2013).

Nursing Care of Patients With Chronic Conditions

Nursing care of patients with chronic conditions is varied and occurs in a variety of settings. Care may be direct or supportive. Direct care may be provided in the clinic or physician's office, a nurse-managed center or clinic, the hospital, long-term care facility, or the patient's home. Examples of direct care include assessing the patient's physical status, providing wound care, managing and overseeing medication regimens, and performing technical tasks. The availability of this type of nursing care may allow the patient to remain at home and return to a more normal life after an acute episode of illness.

Because much of the day-to-day responsibility for managing chronic conditions rests with the patient and the family, nurses often provide supportive care at home. Supportive care may include ongoing monitoring, education, counseling, serving as an advocate for the patient, making referrals, and case management. Giving supportive care is just as important as giving technical care. For example, through ongoing monitoring either in the home or in a clinic, a nurse might detect early signs of impending complications and make a referral (e.g., contact the primary health care clinician or consult the medical protocol in a clinic) for medical evaluation, thereby preventing a lengthy and costly hospitalization.

Working with people with chronic illness requires not only dealing with the medical aspects of their disorder but also working with the whole person—physically, emotionally, and socially. This holistic approach to care requires nurses to draw on their knowledge and skills, including knowledge from the social sciences and psychology in particular. People often respond to illness, health education, and regimens in ways that differ from the expectations of health care providers. Although quality of life is usually affected by chronic illness, especially if the illness is severe, patients' perceptions of what constitutes quality of life often drive their management behaviors or affect how they view advice about health care. Nurses and other health care professionals need to recognize this, even though it may be difficult to see patients make unwise choices and decisions about lifestyles and disease management. People have the right to receive care without fearing ridicule or refusal of treatment, even if their behaviors (e.g., smoking, substance abuse, overeating, failure to follow health care providers' recommendations) may have contributed to their chronic disorder.

Applying the Nursing Process Using the Phases of the Chronic Illness System

The focus of care for patients with chronic conditions is determined largely by the phase of the illness and is directed by the nursing process, which includes assessment, diagnosis, planning, implementation, and evaluation.

Step 1: Identifying Specific Problems and the Trajectory Phase

The first step is assessment of the patient to determine the specific problems identified by the patient, family, nurse, and other health care providers. Assessment is necessary to identify the specific medical, social, and psychological problems likely to be encountered by the patient and the family. For example, a patient with early onset Parkinson disease or emphysema is likely to have very different issues compared to a patient with advanced Parkinson disease or end-stage chronic obstructive pulmonary disease. The types of direct care, referrals, education, and emotional support needed in each situation are different as well. In addition, because complementary and alternative therapies are often used by people with chronic illness across the age spectrum (Ho, Rowland-Seymour, Frankel, et al., 2014), the assessment should address the patient's use of these therapies or regimens.

Step 2: Establishing and Prioritizing Goals

Once a patient's specific medical problems and related social and psychological problems are identified, the nurse helps prioritize these and establish the goals of care. Goals must be a collaborative effort, with the patient, family, and nurse working together, and they must be consistent with the abilities, desires, motivations, and resources of those involved.

Step 3: Defining the Plan of Action to Achieve Desired Outcomes

Next, a realistic and mutually agreed-on plan for achieving the patient's goals is identified, along with specific criteria that will be used to assess the patient's progress. Identifying the environmental, social, and psychological factors that might interfere with or facilitate achieving the desired outcome is important to guide planning.

Step 4: Implementing the Plan and Interventions

Implementation of the plan might include nursing interventions such as providing direct care, serving as an advocate for the patient, educating, counseling, making referrals, and case management (e.g., arranging for resources). These interventions should focus on enabling the patient to live with the symptoms and therapies associated with chronic conditions, while gaining or maintaining independence. The nurse works with the patient and the family to identify strategies to integrate treatment regimens into ADLs to promote (1) adherence to regimens to control symptoms and keep the illness stable and (2) healthy responses to the psychosocial issues that can hinder illness management and affect quality of life. Helping patients and their families to implement regimens and to carry out ADLs within the limits of the chronic condition is an important nursing role when caring for patients with chronic disorders and their families.

Step 5: Following Up and Evaluating Outcomes

The final step involves following up to determine if the problem is resolving or being managed and if the patient and the family are able to adhere to the treatment plan. Follow-up may uncover new problems resulting from the intervention, problems that interfere with the ability of the patient and the family to carry out the plan, or previously unexpected problems. A primary goal is to maintain the stability of the chronic condition while preserving the patient's sense of control, identity, independence, and accomplishment. Alternative strategies or revisions to the initial plan may be warranted based on evaluation and follow-up.

Helping the patient and the family to integrate changes into their lifestyle is an important part of the process. Change takes time, patience, and creativity and often requires encouragement from the nurse. Validation of the patient's progress is important for enhancing self-esteem and reinforcing behaviors. If no progress is made, or if progress toward goals seems too slow, it may be necessary to redefine the goals, the intervention, or the time frame. The nurse must realize and accept that some people will not change. Patients share responsibility for management of their conditions, and outcomes are as much related to their ability to accommodate the illness and carry out regimens as they are to nursing intervention (Lorig et al., 2012).

Home, Community-Based and Transitional Care

Educating Patients About Self-Care

Because chronic conditions are so costly to people, families, and society, two of the major goals of nursing today are the prevention of chronic conditions and the care of people with them. This requires promoting healthy lifestyles and encouraging the use of safety and disease prevention measures, such as wearing seat belts and obtaining immunizations. Prevention should also begin early in life and continue throughout life. Education on self-care may need to address interactions among the patient's chronic conditions as well as skills necessary to care for the individual diseases and their interactive effects.

Patient and family education is an important nursing role that may make the difference in the ability of the patient and the family to adapt to chronic conditions. Well-informed, educated patients are more likely than uninformed patients to be concerned about their health and do what is necessary to maintain it. They are also more likely to manage symptoms, recognize the onset of complications, and seek health care early. Knowledge is the key to making informed choices and decisions during all phases of the chronic illness trajectory.

Despite the importance of educating the patient and the family, the nurse must recognize that patients recently diagnosed with serious chronic conditions and their families may need time to understand the significance of their condition and its effect on their lives. Education must be planned carefully so that it is not acute. Furthermore, it is important to assess the impact of a new diagnosis of chronic illness on a patient's life and the meaning of self-management to the patient.

The nurse who cares for patients with chronic conditions in the hospital, clinic, home, or any other setting should assess each patient's knowledge about their illness and its management; the nurse cannot assume that patients with a long-standing chronic condition have the knowledge necessary to manage the condition. Patients' learning needs change as the chronic condition changes and their personal situations change. The nurse must also recognize that patients may know how their body responds under certain conditions and how best to manage their symptoms. Contact with patients in any setting offers nurses the ideal opportunity to reassess patients' learning needs and provide additional education about a chronic condition and its management.

Educational strategies and materials should be adapted to the individual patient so that the patient and the family can understand and follow recommendations from health care providers. For instance, educational materials should be tailored for people with low literacy levels and available in several languages and in various alternative formats (e.g., Braille, large print, audiotapes). It may be necessary to provide sign language interpreters.

Continuing and Transitional Care

Chronic illness management is a collaborative process between the patient, family, nurse, and other health care providers. Collaboration extends to all settings and throughout the illness trajectory. Keeping an illness stable over time requires careful monitoring of symptoms and attention to management regimens. Detecting problems early and helping patients develop appropriate management strategies can make a significant difference in outcomes.

Most chronic conditions are managed in the home. Therefore, care and education during hospitalization should focus on essential information about the condition so that management can continue once the patient is discharged home. Nurses in all settings should be aware of the resources and services available in a community and should make the arrangements (before hospital discharge, if the patient is hospitalized) to secure those resources and services. When appropriate, home care services are contacted directly. The home care nurse reassesses how the patient and the family are adapting to the chronic condition and its treatment and continues or revises the plan of care accordingly.

Because chronic conditions occur worldwide and the world is increasingly interconnected, nurses should think beyond the personal level to the community and global levels. In terms of illness prevention and health promotion, this entails wide-ranging efforts to assess people for risks of chronic illness (e.g., blood pressure and diabetes screening, stroke risk assessments) and group education related to illness prevention and management. Figure 9-1 provides a framework to identify and implement strategies to prevent chronic disease and promote health (CDC, 2009). In addition, nurses should remind patients with chronic illnesses or disabilities and their families about the need for ongoing health promotion and screening recommended for all people, because chronic illness and disability are often considered the main concern while other health-related issues are ignored.

Telehealth or telehomecare (use of electronic data and telecommunications technologies to support long-distance clinical health care, patient and professional health-related education, public health, and health administration) has been used effectively to provide care for patients with chronic illness. It is particularly useful in monitoring patients with

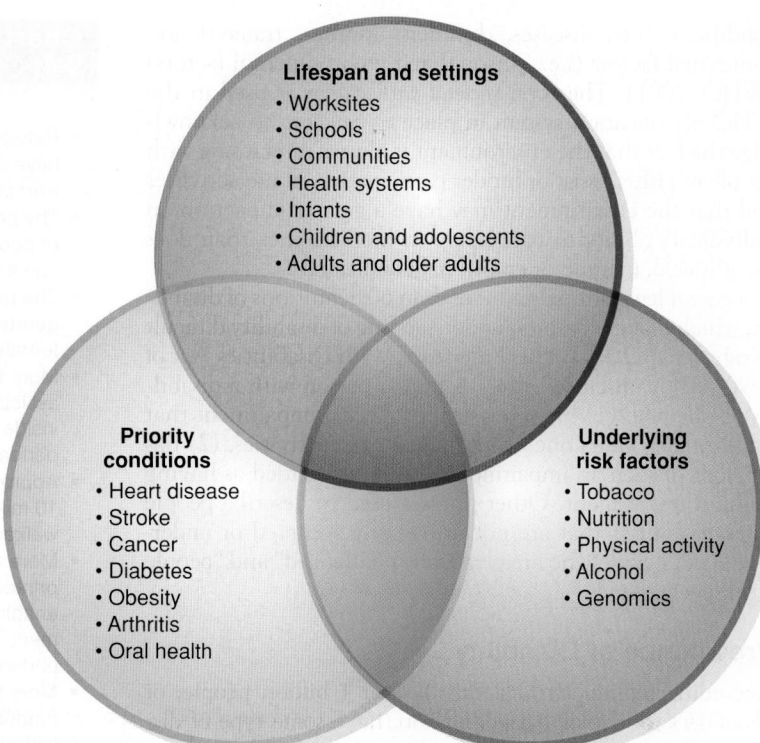

Lifespan and settings
- Worksites
- Schools
- Communities
- Health systems
- Infants
- Children and adolescents
- Adults and older adults

Priority conditions
- Heart disease
- Stroke
- Cancer
- Diabetes
- Obesity
- Arthritis
- Oral health

Underlying risk factors
- Tobacco
- Nutrition
- Physical activity
- Alcohol
- Genomics

Figure 9-1 • Framework for preventing chronic disease and promoting health. Used with permission from Centers for Disease Control and Prevention. (2009). *The power to prevent, the call to control: At a glance 2009*. Atlanta, GA: Author.

chronic conditions living in rural areas (Health Resources and Services Administration, 2013). It has also been used to deliver selected medical and nursing interventions (e.g., counseling) and provide ongoing education and support.

Transitional care, if available, should be considered and implemented when the patient has MCC, has impaired cognitive status as well as physical limitations, has complex therapies, or is frail or unstable prior to discharge from the hospital to home. The nurse trained as a transitional care nurse serves as primary coordinator of care. These nurses conduct assessments of the patient as well as the family caregivers' ability to assist in management of the patient in the home. Nurses in this role help the patient and the family set goals during hospitalization, identify the reasons for the patient's current health status, design a plan of care that addresses them, make home visits, provide telephone support, and coordinate various care providers and services (Naylor, Hirschman, Hanlon, et al., 2014; Naylor, Hirschman, O'Connor, et al., 2013; Puhr & Thompson, 2015).

Nursing Care for Special Populations With Chronic Illness

When providing care and education, the nurse must consider multiple factors (e.g., age; gender; culture and ethnicity; cognitive status; the presence of physical, sensory, and cognitive limitations; health literacy) that influence susceptibility to chronic illness and the ways patients respond to chronic disorders. Certain populations, for example, tend to be more susceptible to certain chronic conditions. Populations at high risk for specific conditions can be targeted for special education and monitoring programs; this includes those at risk because of their genetic profile (see Chapter 8 for further discussion of genetics). People of different cultures and genders may respond to illness differently, and being aware of these differences is essential. For cultures in which patients rely heavily on the support of their families, the families must be involved and made part of the nursing plan of care. As the United States becomes more multicultural and ethnically diverse, and as the general population ages, nurses need to be aware of how a person's culture and age affect chronic illness management and be prepared to adapt their care accordingly.

It is important to consider the effect of a preexisting disability, or a disability associated with recurrence of a chronic condition, on the patient's ability to manage ADLs, self-care, and the therapeutic regimen. These issues are discussed in the following section.

Overview of Disability

Definitions of Disability

A person is considered to have a **disability** (limitation in performance or function in everyday activities) if he or she has difficulty talking, hearing, seeing, walking, climbing stairs, lifting or carrying objects, performing ADLs, doing school work, or working at a job. A severe disability is present if a person is unable to perform one or more activities, uses an assistive device for mobility, or needs help from another person to accomplish basic activities. People are also considered severely disabled if they receive federal benefits because of an inability to work.

According to the WHO (2001), *disability* is an umbrella term for impairments, activity limitations, participation restrictions, and environmental factors, and **impairment** is a loss or abnormality in body structure or physiologic function, including mental function. A person's functioning or disability is viewed as a dynamic interaction between health conditions (i.e., diseases, disorders, injuries, trauma) and contextual factors (i.e., personal and environmental factors) (WHO, 2001). The term *societal participation* is used in the WHO classification system in place of *handicap* to acknowledge the fact that the environment is always interacting with people to either assist or hinder participation in life activities and that the environment may have a greater impact on an individual's ability to participate in life activities than does the physical, mental, or emotional condition.

Federal legislation uses more than 60 definitions of disability, which makes common understanding of disability difficult (Krahn et al., 2015). The Americans With Disabilities Act of 1990 (ADA; discussed later) defines a person with a disability as one who (1) has a physical or mental impairment that substantially limits one or more major life activities, (2) has a record of such an impairment, or (3) is regarded as having such an impairment. Other phrases used to describe people with disabilities that are not universally accepted or understood are "people who are physically challenged" and "people with special needs."

Prevalence of Disability

According to the WHO (2014c), over 1 billion people, or about 15% of the global population, have some type of disability. Between 110 and 190 million adults worldwide have significant difficulties in function due to disability. The number of people with disabilities is increasing and is expected to continue to climb as people with early-onset disabilities, chronic disorders, and severe trauma survive (Gostin, 2015; Iezzoni, Kurtz, & Rao, 2014).

The last U.S. Census indicates that about 20% of people have a disability and 10% have a severe disability. Approximately 60 million families have at least one family member with a disability. More than 46% of people with one disability have other disabilities. Although the prevalence of disability is higher in males than in females for people younger than 65 years, the prevalence is higher in women than in men for people older than 65 years. More than 80% of the 1 billion people worldwide with disability live in low- and middle-income countries, in which all people have limited access to basic health care and social services. However, limited access to basic health care and support services among those with disabilities has a more profound effect.

Among people 21 to 64 years of age without disabilities, the percentage of people employed in 2014 was approximately 65% compared to about 20% of people with disabilities (U.S. Department of Labor, 2015). People with a disability earn less money than people without disabilities. Chart 9-4 provides a summary of facts about the population of people with disabilities.

Characteristics of Disability

Categories and Types of Disability

Disabilities can be categorized as developmental disabilities, acquired disabilities, and age-associated disabilities. Developmental disabilities are those that occur any time from birth to 22 years of age and result in impairment of physical or mental health, cognition, speech, language, or self-care. Examples of developmental disabilities are spina bifida, cerebral palsy, Down syndrome, and muscular dystrophy. Some

---

Chart 9-4

Summary of Facts About the Population of People With Disabilities

- Between 54 million and 60 million people in the United States have a disability; this is 22.2% of the civilian noninstitutionalized population or one in every five people.
- The prevalence of disabilities in adults is approximately 10% of people 18–64 years of age and 38% of adults 65 years of age and older.
- The prevalence of disabilities varies by state and by gender, with higher prevalence in the South and among females.
- More than 11 million people with disabilities require personal assistance with everyday activities (e.g., getting around inside the home, bathing or showering, preparing meals, and performing light housework).
- Approximately 3.3 million people use a wheelchair; another 10 million use a walking aid such as cane, crutches, or walker.
- More than 1.8 million people report being unable to see printed words because of vision impairment, 1 million are unable to hear conversations because of hearing impairment, and 2.5 million have difficulty with their speech being understood.
- More than 16 million people have limitations in cognitive function or have a mental or emotional illness that interferes with daily activities, including those with Alzheimer disease and intellectual disabilities.
- Self-reported health status among adults with disabilities differs from that of people without disabilities, with fewer people with disabilities describing their health as excellent or good.
- The percentage of people with disabilities who are employed ranges from 17.8% to 23.4%; of those without disabilities, the percent ranges from 63.5% to 66.2%.
- Among all age groups, persons with a disability are much less likely to be employed than those without a disability. People with a disability who work are more likely than those without disability to work part-time. People with a disability who were not in the labor force (neither employed nor unemployed) are about 8 in 10, compared with about 3 in 10 of those without a disability.
- Many people with disabilities would like to work but are hampered in doing so by limited access, lack of accommodations in the workplace, lack of transportation, and reluctance of employers to hire them.
- The percentage of people with disabilities below the poverty level is almost twice that of people without disabilities.

Based on data from Courtney-Long, E. A., Carroll, D. D. Zhang, Q. C., et al. (2015). Prevalence of disability and disability type among adults—United States, 2013. *Morbidity and Mortality Weekly Report, 64*(29), 777–783.
Iezzoni, L. I., Kurtz, S. G., & Rao, S. R. (2014). Trends in U.S. adult chronic disability rates over time. *Disability and Health Journal, 7*(4), 402–412.
Krahn, G. L., Walker, D. K., & Correa-De-Araujo, R. (2015). Persons with disabilities as an unrecognized health disparity population. *American Journal of Public Health, 105*(S2), S198–S206.
Lagu, T., Hannon, N. S., Rothberg, M. G., et al. (2013). Access to subspecialty care for patients with mobility impairment: A survey. *Annals of Internal Medicine, 158*(6), 441–446.
U.S. Department of Labor/Bureau of Labor Statistics. (2015). *Persons with a disability: Labor force characteristics—2014.* Washington, DC: Author.
World Health Organization (2014c). *Disability and health. Fact sheet N°352.* Retrieved on 7/18/2015 at: www.who.int/mediacentre/factsheets/fs352/en/

NURSING RESEARCH PROFILE

**Chart
9-5**

Secondary Health Conditions in Individuals With Multiple Sclerosis

Newland, P., Jenson, M. P., Budhathoki, C., et al. (2015). Secondary health conditions in individuals with multiple sclerosis: A cross-sectional web-based survey analysis. *Journal of Neuroscience Nursing, 47*(3), 124–130.

Purpose

Diseases or disorders that are potentially disabling increase an individual's risk for developing other conditions because of the resulting disability. These secondary health conditions can often be predicted and as a result may be preventable. This study was undertaken to compare the rates of secondary health conditions in individuals with multiple sclerosis (MS), a neurological disorder that has the potential to produce disability.

Design

This web-based cross-sectional study surveyed individuals who were members of a Midwestern chapter of the National MS Society. Questions similar to those in the National Health Interview Survey were used to assess the presence of six health conditions in a sample of 339 individuals with MS, which represented a completion rate of 92%. Data from the Web-based sample were compared to data from the National Health Interview Survey using a one-sided *z* test. Estimates of the sample as a whole were conducted and by specific age groups.

Findings

The most commonly reported secondary health conditions in the sample of those with MS were depression, arthritis, diabetes, coronary artery disease, migraine headaches, and cancer. Furthermore, these conditions were significantly more common in the MS sample than the normative sample. The rates of some of the secondary health conditions increased with age. In addition, some of the secondary health conditions occurred at different ages for those with MS when compared to the normative sample data. Thus, those with MS may be at greater risk at a younger age than those without MS.

Nursing Implications

The results of this study indicate that nurses should be sensitive to the increased risk for secondary health conditions in patients with MS and take steps to assess them for indicators of these conditions. Nurses need to be proactive in implementing interventions to reduce the risk for the development of secondary health conditions when possible.

---

developmental disabilities occur as a result of birth trauma or severe illness or injury at a very young age, whereas many developmental disabilities are genetic in origin (see Chapter 8). Acquired disabilities may occur as a result of an acute and sudden injury (e.g., traumatic brain injury; spinal cord injury; and traumatic amputation due to traffic crashes, falls, burns, or acts of violence such as intimate partner violence and war and military conflicts), acute nontraumatic disorders (e.g., stroke, myocardial infarction), or progression of a chronic disorder (e.g., arthritis, multiple sclerosis, Parkinson disease, chronic obstructive pulmonary disease, heart disease, blindness due to diabetic retinopathy) (WHO, 2014c).

Many people with disabilities are at risk for **secondary health conditions** (e.g., pressure ulcers, urinary tract infections, low bone density, depression) because of a narrow margin of health. Therefore, attention needs to be given to assessment, prevention when possible, and management of secondary health conditions or disorders that occur (Newland, Jenson, Budhathoki, et al., 2015) (see Chart 9-5).

Types of disability include sensory disabilities that affect hearing or vision; learning disabilities that affect the ability to learn, remember, or concentrate; disabilities that affect the ability to speak or communicate; and disabilities that affect the ability to work, shop, and care for oneself, or access health care. Many disabilities are visible; however, invisible disabilities are often as disabling as those that can be seen. Some disabilities affect only IADLs, whereas others affect ADLs. People can be temporarily disabled because of an injury or acute exacerbation of a chronic disorder but later return to full functioning.

Although different impairments may result from different types of disabilities, there are some similarities across disabilities. People with disabilities are often considered by society to be dependent and needing to be cared for by others; however, many people with disabilities are highly functioning, independent, productive people who are capable of caring for themselves and others, having children and raising families, holding a full-time job, and making significant and major contributions to society. Like other people, those with disabilities often prefer to live in their own homes with family members. Most people with disabilities are able to live at home independently. Some patients live alone in their own homes and use home care services. However, alternative living arrangements may be necessary; these include assisted living facilities, long-term care facilities, and group homes.

Models of Disability

Several models of disability have been used to address or explain the issues encountered by people with disabilities (Drum, 2014; Lollar & Crews, 2003; Phelan, 2011; Smeltzer, 2007; WHO, 2001). Chart 9-6 briefly describes these models of disability. The interface model (Goodall, 1995), developed by a nurse, promotes care designed to be empowering rather than care that promotes dependency. It takes into account the disabling condition and its disabling effects. Furthermore, it promotes the view that people with disabilities are capable, responsible people who are able to function effectively despite having a disability. The interface model can serve as a basis for the role of nurses as advocates for the removal of barriers to health care and for the examination of how society and health care professionals contribute to discrimination by viewing disability as an abnormal state.

Disability Versus Disabling Disorders

Regardless of which definition or model of disability is adopted, one can understand the pathophysiology and physical changes related to a disabling condition or injury without understanding the concept of disability. The nurse caring for patients with preexisting disabilities or new disabilities must recognize the impact of a disability on current and future health and well-being, the ability to participate in self-care or self-management, and the ability to obtain required health care and health screening.

Chart 9-6 Models of Disability

Medical Model

The medical model equates people who are disabled with their disabilities and views disability as a problem of the person, directly caused by disease, trauma, or other health condition, that requires medical care provided in the form of individual treatment by professionals. Health care providers, rather than people with disabilities, are viewed as the experts or authorities. Management of the disability is aimed at cure or the person's adjustment and behavior change. The model is viewed as promoting passivity and dependency. People with disabilities are viewed as tragic.

Rehabilitation Model

The rehabilitation model emerged from the medical model. It regards disability as a deficiency that requires a rehabilitation specialist or other helping professional to fix the problem. People with disabilities are often perceived as having failed if they do not overcome the disability.

Social Model

The social model, which is also referred to as the barriers or disability model, views disability as socially constructed and as a political issue that is a result of social and physical barriers in the environment. Its perspective is that disability can be overcome by removal of these barriers.

Biopsychosocial Model

The biopsychosocial model integrates the medical and social models to address perspectives of health from a biologic, individual, and social perspective. Critiques of this model have suggested that the disabling condition, rather than the person and the experience of the person with a disability, remains the defining construct of the biopsychosocial model.

Functional Model

The functional model is driven by the World Health Organization's *International Classification of Functioning, Disability and Health* (*ICF*). Disability is considered an umbrella term for impairments, activity limitations, participation restrictions, and their interaction with environmental factors. The ICF addresses components of health rather than consequence of disease.

Interface Model

The interface model is based on the life experience of the person with a disability and views disability at the intersection (i.e., interface) of the medical diagnosis of a disability and environmental barriers. It considers rather than ignores the diagnosis. The person with a disability, rather than others, defines the problems and seeks or directs solutions.

Adapted from Drum C. F. (2014). The dynamics of disability and chronic conditions. *Disability and Health Journal, 7*(1), 2–5. Goodall, C. J. (1995). Is disability any business of nurse education? *Nurse Education Today, 15*(5), 323–327. Lollar, D. J., & Crews, J. E. (2003). Redefining the role of public health in disability. *Annual Review of Public Health, 24*, 195–208. Phelan, S. K. (2011). Constructions of disability: A call for critical reflexivity in occupational therapy. *Canadian Journal of Occupational Therapy, 78*, 164–172. Smeltzer, S. C. (2007). Improving the health and wellness of persons with disabilities: A call to action too important for nursing to ignore. *Nursing Outlook, 55*(4), 189–193. World Health Organization. (2001). *International Classification of Functioning, Disability and Health—ICF*. Geneva, Switzerland: Author.

Nursing management—from assessment through evaluation of the effectiveness of nursing interventions—must be examined to ensure that appropriate modifications have been made so that people with disabilities can receive health care equal to that of people without disabilities. Furthermore, nurses as well as other health care providers need to examine their facilities and procedures to ensure that the needs of people with various disabilities can be adequately addressed. Although the health care needs of people with disabilities generally do not differ from those of the general population, some disabilities create special needs and necessitate the use of special accommodations. Chart 9-7 reviews To questions to ask to ensure quality health care for people with disabilities.

Federal Legislation

Because of widespread discrimination against people with disabilities, the U.S. Congress enacted legislation to address health care disparities in this population. This legislation includes the Rehabilitation Act of 1973 and the ADA. In 2005, the U.S. Surgeon General called for action to improve the health and wellness of people with disabilities (Smeltzer, 2007; U.S. Department of Health & Human Services [HHS], 2005). Health care in people with disabilities has received further national attention through specific national objectives in *Healthy People 2020* (HHS, 2010).

The Rehabilitation Act of 1973 protects people from discrimination based on their disability. The act applies to employers and organizations that receive financial assistance from any federal department or agency; this includes many hospitals, long-term care facilities, mental health centers, and human service programs. It forbids organizations from excluding or denying people with disabilities equal access to program benefits and services. It also prohibits discrimination related to availability, accessibility, and delivery of services, including health care services.

The ADA of 1990 mandates that people with disabilities have access to job opportunities and to the community without discrimination based on having a disability. The ADA also requires that "reasonable accommodations" be provided for transportation and to facilitate employment of a person with a disability. Examples of reasonable accommodations in health care settings include accessible facilities and equipment (e.g., accessible restrooms, adjustable examination tables, access ramps, grab bars, elevated toilet seats) and alternative communication methods (e.g., telecommunication devices and sign language interpreters for use by people who are deaf). Failure to make reasonable accommodations can result in poor care for patients with disabilities. For example, lack of accommodation for people who are deaf can lead to failed communication and sharing of important information between them and their health care providers (McKee, McKee, Winters, et al., 2014).

Although the ADA took effect in 1992, compliance has been slow, and some facilities continue to be inaccessible although all new construction and modifications of public facilities must

Chart 9-7 To Questions to Ask to Ensure Quality Health Care for People With Disabilities

Communication Strategies

- Does the patient with a disability require or prefer accommodations (e.g., a sign language interpreter) to ensure full participation in conversations about their health care?
- Are appropriate accommodations made to communicate with the patient?
- Are efforts made to direct all conversations to the patient rather than to others who have accompanied the patient to the health care facility?

Accessibility of the Health Care Facility

- Are clinics, hospital rooms, offices, restrooms, laboratories, and imaging facilities accessible to people with disabilities, as legally required by the Americans With Disabilities Act and Rehabilitation Act?
- Has accessibility been verified by a person with a disability?
- Is a sign language interpreter other than a family member available to assist in obtaining a patient's health history and in conducting a physical assessment?
- Does the facility include appropriate equipment to permit people with disabilities to obtain health care (including mammography, gynecologic examination and care, dental care) in a dignified and safe manner?

Assessment

Usual Health Considerations

- Does the health history address the same issues that would be included when obtaining a history from a person without disabilities, including sexuality, sexual function, and reproductive health issues?

Disability-Related Considerations

- Does the health history address the patient's specific disability and the effect of disability on the patient's ability to obtain health care, manage self-care activities, and obtain preventive health screening and follow-up care?
- What physical modifications and positioning are needed to ensure a thorough physical examination, including pelvic or testicular and rectal examination?

Abuse

- Is the increased risk for abuse (physical, emotional, financial, and sexual) by various people (family, paid care providers, strangers) addressed in the assessment?
- If abuse is detected, are men and women with disabilities who are survivors of abuse directed to appropriate resources, including accessible shelters and hotlines?

Depression

- Is the patient experiencing depression? If so, is treatment offered just as it would be to a patient without a disability, without assuming that depression is normal and a result of having a disability?

Aging

- What concerns does the patient have about aging with a pre-existing disability?
- What effect has aging had on the patient's disability, and what effect has the disability had on the patient's aging?

Secondary Health Conditions

- Does the patient have secondary health conditions related to their disability or its treatment?
- Is the patient at risk for secondary health conditions because of environmental barriers or lack of access to health care or health promotion activities?
- Are strategies in place to reduce the risk for secondary health conditions or to treat existing secondary health conditions?

Accommodations in the Home

- What accommodations does the patient have at home to encourage or permit self-care?
- What additional accommodations does the patient need at home to encourage or permit self-care?

Cognitive Status

- Is it assumed that the patient is able to participate in discussion and conversation rather than assuming that he or she is unable to do so because of a disability?
- Are appropriate modifications made in written and verbal communication strategies?

Modifications in Nursing Care

- Are modifications made during hospital stays, acute illness or injury, and other health care encounters to enable a patient with disability to be as independent as he or she prefers?
- Is "people-first language" used in referring to a patient with disability, and do nurses and other staff talk directly to the patient rather than to those who accompanied the patient?
- Are all staff informed about the activities of daily living for which the patient will require assistance?
- Are accommodations made to enable the patient to use their assistive devices (hearing/visual aids, prostheses, limb support devices, ventilators, service animals)?
- If a patient with disability is immobilized because of surgery, illness, injury, or treatments, are risks of immobility addressed and strategies implemented to minimize those risks?
- Is the patient with a disability assessed for other illnesses and health issues (e.g., other acute or chronic illness, depression, psychiatric/mental health, and cognitive disorders) not related to their primary disability?

Patient Education

- Are accommodations and alternative formats of instructional materials (large print, Braille, visual materials, audiotapes) provided for patients with disabilities?
- Does patient instruction address the modifications (e.g., use of assistive devices) needed by patients with disabilities to enable them to adhere to recommendations?
- Are modifications made in educational strategies to address learning needs, cognitive changes, and communication impairment?

Health Promotion and Disease Prevention

- Are health promotion strategies discussed with people with disabilities along with their potential benefits: improving quality of life and preventing secondary health conditions (health problems that result because of preexisting disability)?
- Are patients aware of accessible community-based facilities (e.g., health care facilities, imaging centers, public exercise settings, transportation) to enable them to participate in health promotion?

Independence Versus Dependence

- Is independence, rather than dependence, of the person with a disability the focus of nursing care and interaction?
- Are care and interaction with the patient focused on empowerment rather than promoting dependence of the patient?

Insurance Coverage

- Does the patient have access to the health insurance coverage and other services for which he or she qualifies?
- Is the patient aware of various insurance and other available programs?
- Would the patient benefit from talking to a social worker about eligibility for Medicaid, Medicare, disability insurance, and other services?

address access for people with disabilities. Because courts have interpreted the definition of disability in the ADA so narrowly that few people could meet it, the ADA Amendments Act was signed into law in 2008 and enacted in January 2009 (Gostin, 2015). The act broadly defines *disability* to encompass impairments that substantially limit a major life activity. This wording states that effective use of assistive devices, auxiliary aids, accommodations, medical therapies, and supplies (other than eyeglasses and contact lenses) does not alter the determination of whether a disability qualifies under the law. The purpose of these amendments was to cover more people and to shift the attention from focusing on who has a disability to making accommodations and avoiding discrimination. Examples of modifications in nursing care that are needed to provide equal access to health care to people with disabilities are identified in Chart 9-7.

Right of Access to Health Care

People with disabilities have the right of access to health care that is equal in quality to that of other people. The United Nations Convention on the Rights of Persons with Disabilities (CRPD) (2006) identifies the rights of people with disabilities to receive the highest standard of health care, without discrimination. As of December 2016, more than 25 years after the passage of the ADA, the United States has not ratified the CRPD (Gostin, 2015). Despite the rights identified by the CRPD and the ADA in the United States, people with disabilities continue to experience health disparities (Havercamp & Scott, 2015; Krahn et al., 2015; Peacock, Iezzoni, & Harkin, 2015).

For years, people with disabilities have been discriminated against in employment, public accommodations, and public and private services, including health care (Havercamp & Scott, 2015; Krahn et al., 2015). Unmet needs of people with disabilities include but are not limited to medical, dental, and prescription medication needs (Mahmoudi & Meade, 2015). The needs of people with disabilities in health care settings present challenges to health care providers: how to communicate effectively if there are communication deficits, the additional physical requirements for mobility, and time required to provide assistance with self-care routines during hospitalization. Nurses and other clinicians need to be aware of the specific needs of people with disabilities and to provide appropriate care and services for them. People with disabilities have a legally mandated right to accessible health care facilities for all medical care and screening procedures. Furthermore, they have the right to health care provided by knowledgeable clinicians who are sensitive to the effects of disability on access to health care, including care that addresses their reproductive issues and sexuality (Baptista, Pagliuca, Sampaio, et al., 2014; Havercamp & Scott, 2015). Reasonable accommodations are mandated by law and are the financial responsibility of the health care provider or facility. People with disabilities should not be expected to provide their own accommodations (e.g., sign language interpreters, assistants). Family members should not be expected to serve as interpreters because of concern for the patient's privacy and confidentiality and the risk of errors in interpreting information by either the patient or the health care provider. Chart 9-8 identifies strategies to communicate effectively with people with disabilities. Figures 9-2(A) and 9-2(B) illustrate

inappropriate and appropriate communication with a person with a disability who uses a wheelchair or is seated.

In response to continued accessibility issues, the U.S. Surgeon General issued *Call to Action to Improve the Health and Wellness of Persons with Disabilities* (HHS, 2005). This report recognized that all persons with disabilities need to have access to comprehensive health care so that they are able to have full, engaged, and productive lives in their own communities. Among strategies to accomplish this, the call to action stipulated that health care professionals need to become knowledgeable about disability. It further recommended that schools educating health care professionals educate about disability and address the need for increased availability of methods to screen, diagnose, and treat the whole person with a disability with dignity. A recent editorial indicated that after more than 25 years after the passage of the ADA (1990), significant health status and health care disparities persist for people with disabilities (Peacock et al., 2015). Furthermore, progress has been slow in ensuring that health care professionals receive adequate education about providing quality health care to them.

Barriers to Health Care

Many people with disabilities encounter barriers to full participation in life, including health care, health screening, and health promotion (HHS, 2005). Some of these barriers are structural and make certain facilities inaccessible. Examples of structural barriers include stairs, lack of ramps, narrow doorways that do not permit entry of a wheelchair, and restroom facilities that cannot be used by people with disabilities (e.g., restrooms that lack grab bars and those that lack larger restroom stalls designed for people using wheelchairs) (Lagu et al., 2013).

Structural barriers to accessibility are most easily identified and eliminated. Other less visible barriers include negative and stereotypic attitudes (e.g., believing that all people with disabilities have a poor quality of life and are dependent and nonproductive) on the part of the public. Health care providers with similar negative attitudes make it difficult for people with disabilities to obtain health care equal in quality to that of people without disabilities. The Rehabilitation Act and the ADA were enacted more than 40 and 20 years ago, respectively, to ensure equal access to people with disabilities; however, people with disabilities continue to encounter and report multiple barriers to health care facilities and providers (Smeltzer, Avery, & Haynor, 2012). This legislation and the U.S. Surgeon General's call to action (HHS, 2005) and the ADA Amendments Act of 2008 are examples of efforts to eliminate barriers encountered by people with disabilities.

People with disabilities have also reported lack of access to information, transportation difficulties, inability to pay because of limited income, difficulty finding a health care provider knowledgeable about their particular disability, previous negative health care encounters, reliance on caregivers, and the demands of coping with the disability itself (HHS, 2005; Smeltzer, 2007; Smeltzer et al., 2012; WHO, 2014c). These issues affect both men and women with severe disabilities; however, women are at higher risk for receiving a lower level of health care than men. Women with disabilities are significantly less likely to receive pelvic examinations than women

Chart 9-8 Interacting and Communicating With People Who Have Disabilities

Patients will feel most comfortable receiving health care if you consider the following suggestions.

General Considerations

- Do not be afraid to make a mistake when interacting and communicating with someone with a disability or chronic medical condition. Keep in mind that a person with a disability is a person first and is entitled to the dignity, consideration, respect, and rights you expect for yourself.
- Treat adults as adults. Address people with disabilities by their first names only if extending the same familiarity to all others present. Never patronize people by patting them on the head or the shoulder.
- Relax. If you do not know what to do, allow the person who has a disability to identify how you may be of assistance and to put you at ease.
- If you offer assistance and the person declines, do not insist. If your offer is accepted, ask how you can best help, and follow directions. Do not take over.
- If someone with a disability is accompanied by another individual, address the person with a disability directly rather than speaking through the accompanying companion.
- Be considerate of the extra time it might take for a person with a disability to get things done or said. Let the person set the pace.
- Do not be embarrassed to use common expressions, such as "See you later" or "Got to be running," that seem to relate to the person's disability.
- Use people-first language: Refer to "a person with a disability" rather than "a disabled person" and avoid referring to people by the disability or disorder they have (e.g., "the diabetic").

Mobility Limitations

- Do not make assumptions about what a person can and cannot do.
- Do not push a person's wheelchair or grab the arm of someone walking with difficulty without first asking whether you can be of assistance and how you can assist. Personal space includes a person's wheelchair, scooter, crutches, walker, cane, or other mobility aid.
- Never move someone's wheelchair, scooter, crutches, walker, cane, or other mobility aid without permission.
- When speaking for more than a few minutes to a person who is seated in a wheelchair, try to find a seat for yourself so that the two of you are at eye level (see Figures 9-2(A) and 9-2(B)).
- When giving directions to people with mobility limitations, consider distance, weather conditions, and physical obstacles such as stairs, curbs, and steep hills.
- Shake hands when introduced to a person with a disability. People who have limited hand use or who wear an artificial limb do shake hands.

Vision Loss (Low Vision and Blindness)

- Identify yourself when you approach a person who has low vision or blindness. If a new person approaches, introduce him or her.
- Touch the person's arm lightly when you speak so that he or she knows to whom you are speaking before you begin.
- Face the person and speak directly to him or her. Use a normal tone of voice.
- Do not leave without saying that you are leaving.
- If you are offering directions, be as specific as possible and point out obstacles in the path of travel. Use specifics such as "Left about twenty feet" or "Right two yards." Use clock cues, such as "The door is at 10 o'clock."

- When you offer to assist someone with vision loss, allow the person to take your arm. This will help you guide rather than propel or lead the person. When offering seating, place the person's hand on the back or the arm of the seat.
- Alert people with low vision or blindness to posted information.
- Never pet or otherwise distract a canine companion or service animal unless the owner has given you permission.

Hearing Loss (Hard of Hearing, Deaf, Deaf–Blind)

- Ask the person how he or she prefers to communicate.
- If you are speaking through a sign language interpreter, remember that the interpreter may lag a few words behind—especially if there are names or technical terms to be finger spelled—so pause occasionally to allow the interpreter time to translate completely and accurately.
- Talk directly to the person who has hearing loss, not to the interpreter. However, although it may seem awkward to you, the person who has hearing loss will look at the interpreter and may not make eye contact with you during the conversation.
- Before you start to speak, make sure that you have the attention of the person you are addressing. A wave, a light touch on the arm or the shoulder, or other visual or tactile signals are appropriate ways of getting the person's attention.
- Speak in a clear, expressive manner. Do not overenunciate or exaggerate words. Unless you are specifically requested to do so, do not raise your voice. Speak in a normal tone; do not shout.
- To facilitate lip reading, face the person and keep your hands and other objects away from your mouth. Maintain eye contact. Do not turn your back or walk around while talking. If you look away, the person might assume that the conversation is over.
- Avoid talking while you are writing a message for someone with hearing loss, because the person cannot read your note and your lips at the same time.
- Try to eliminate background noise.
- Encourage feedback to assess clear understanding.
- If you do not understand something that is said, ask the person to repeat it or to write it down. The goal is communication; do not pretend to understand if you do not.
- If you know any sign language, try using it. It may help you communicate, and it will at least demonstrate your interest in communicating and your willingness to try.

Speech Disabilities or Speech Difficulties

- Talk to people with speech disabilities as you would talk to anyone else.
- Be friendly; start up a conversation.
- Be patient; it may take the person a while to answer. Allow extra time for communication. Do not speak for the person.
- Give the person your undivided attention.
- Ask the person for help in communicating with him or her. If the person uses a communication device such as a manual or electronic communication board, ask the person the best way to use it.
- Speak in your regular tone of voice.
- Tell the person if you do not understand what he or she is trying to say. Ask the person to repeat the message, spell it, tell you in a different way, or write it down. Use hand gestures and notes.
- Repeat what you understand. The person's reactions will clue you in and guide you to understanding.
- To obtain information quickly, ask short questions that require brief answers or a head nod. Avoid insulting the person's intelligence with oversimplification.
- Keep your manner encouraging rather than correcting.

(continued on page 156)

Chart 9-8 Interacting and Communicating With People Who Have Disabilities (continued)

Intellectual/Cognitive Disabilities

- Treat adults with intellectual/cognitive disabilities as adults.
- Be alert to the individual's responses so that you can adjust your method of communication as necessary. For example, some people may benefit from simple, direct sentences or from supplementary visual forms of communication, such as gestures, diagrams, or demonstrations.
- Use concrete rather than abstract language. Be specific, without being too simplistic. When possible, use words that relate to things you both can see. Avoid using directional terms such as right, left, east, or west.
- Be prepared to give the person the same information more than once in different ways.
- When asking questions, phrase them to elicit accurate information. People with intellectual/cognitive disabilities may be eager to please and may tell you what they think you want to hear. Verify responses by repeating the question in a different way.
- Give exact instructions. For example, "Be back for lab work at 4:30," not "Be back in 15 minutes."
- Avoid giving too many directions at one time, which may be confusing.
- Keep in mind that the person may prefer information provided in written or verbal form. Ask the person how you can best relay the information.
- Using humor is fine, but do not interpret a lack of response as rudeness. Some people may not grasp subtleties of language.
- Know that people with brain injuries may have short-term memory deficits and may repeat themselves or require information to be repeated.
- Recognize that people with auditory perceptual problems may need to have directions repeated and may take notes to help them remember directions or the sequence of tasks. They may benefit from watching a task demonstrated.
- Understand that people with perceptual or "sensory overload" problems may become disoriented or confused if there is too much to absorb at once. Provide information gradually and clearly. Reduce background noise if possible.
- Repeat information using different wording or a different communication approach if necessary. Allow time for the information to be fully understood.
- Do not pretend to understand if you do not. Ask the person to repeat what was said. Be patient, flexible, and supportive.

- Be aware that some people who have an intellectual disability are easily distracted. Try not to interpret distraction as rudeness.
- Do not expect all people to be able to read well. Some people may not read at all.

Psychiatric/Mental Health Disabilities

- Speak directly to the person. Use clear, simple communication.
- Offer to shake hands when introduced. Use the same good manners in interacting with a person who has a psychiatric/mental health disability that you would with anyone else.
- Make eye contact and be aware of your own body language. Like others, people with psychiatric/mental health disabilities will sense your discomfort.
- Listen attentively, and wait for the person to finish speaking. If needed, clarify what the person has said. Never pretend to understand.
- Treat adults as adults. Do not patronize, condescend, or threaten. Do not make decisions for the person or assume that you know the person's preferences.
- Do not give unsolicited advice or assistance. Do not panic or summon an ambulance or the police if a person appears to be experiencing a mental health crisis. Calmly ask the person how you can help.
- Do not blame the person. A person with a psychiatric disability has a complex, biomedical condition that is sometimes difficult to control. The person cannot just "shape up." It is rude, insensitive, and ineffective to tell or expect a person to do so.
- Question the accuracy of media stereotypes of psychiatric/mental health disabilities: Movies and media often sensationalize psychiatric/mental health disabilities. Most people never experience symptoms that include violent behavior.
- Relax. Be yourself. Do not be embarrassed if you happen to use common expressions that seem to relate to a psychiatric/mental health disability.
- Recognize that beneath the symptoms and behaviors of psychiatric disabilities is a person who has many of the same wants, needs, dreams, and desires as anyone else. If you are afraid, learn more about psychiatric/mental health disabilities.

This material is adapted and based in part on U.S. Department of Labor. Office of Disability Employment Policy. Retrieved 9/23/15 at: www.dol.gov/general/aboutdol/majorlaws

Sharts-Hopko, N. C., Smeltzer, S., Ott, B. B., et al. (2010). Healthcare experiences of women with visual impairment. *Clinical Nurse Specialist, 24*(3), 149–153.

without disabilities; the more severe the disability, the less frequent the examination. In particular, minority women and older women with disabilities are less likely to have regular pelvic examinations and Papanicolaou (Pap) tests. Reasons given by women for not having regular pelvic examinations are difficulty transferring on to the examination table, belief that they do not need pelvic examinations because of their disability, difficulty in accessing the office or the clinic, and difficulty finding transportation (HHS, 2005; Smeltzer, 2007). Health care providers often underestimate the effect of disabilities on women's ability to access health care, including health screening and health promotion, and they focus on women's disabilities while ignoring women's general health issues and concerns. Furthermore, women with disabilities

have reported lack of knowledge about disability and insensitivity on the part of health care providers (Smeltzer, 2007).

Race, gender, and type of disability also affect health status and receipt of health care and screening (Berman, Jo, Cumberland, et al., 2013; Horner-Johnson, Dobbertin, Lee, et al., 2013). For instance, African American women with intellectual disabilities are less likely to receive mammography than Caucasian women with intellectual disabilities (Parish, Swaine, Son, et al., 2013). Additionally, those living in rural areas are also less likely to have many types of recommended screenings (Horner-Johnson, Dobbertin, Lee, et al., 2014).

Because of the persistence of these barriers, it is essential that nurses and other health care providers take steps to ensure that clinics, offices, hospitals, and other health

Figure 9-2 • Examples of inappropriate communication by nurse with young woman with a disability in a wheelchair. The nurse stands instead of sitting at the patient's eye level (**A**) and talks to the patient's mother rather than directly to the patient (**B**).

care facilities are accessible to people with disabilities. This includes removal of structural barriers by the addition of ramps, designation of accessible parking spaces, and modification of restrooms to make them usable by people with disabilities. Alternative communication methods (e.g., sign language interpreters, teletypewriter devices, assistive listening devices) and types of patient education (e.g., audiotapes, large print, Braille) are essential to provision of appropriate health-related information to people with disabilities. Such accommodations are mandated by the ADA, which requires their provision without cost to the patient.

People with intellectual and developmental disabilities often need assistance in obtaining health care, including preventive health screening. Recent studies indicate that they often lack knowledge about cancer screening, including breast cancer screening. Educational materials and interventions modified to accommodate patients with intellectual and developmental disabilities are needed to enable them to make informed decisions about screening. Major barriers to breast cancer screening by this population of women include fear,

anxiety, and embarrassment, primarily due to lack of understanding about cancer and the importance of its early detection (Reidy, Denieffe, & Foran, 2013).

Federal Assistance Programs

Lack of financial resources, including health insurance, is an important barrier to health care for people with chronic illness and disabilities. However, several federal assistance programs provide financial assistance for health-related expenses for people with some chronic illnesses, acquired disabling acute and chronic diseases, and childhood disabilities.

Medicare is a federal health insurance program that is available to most people 65 years of age and older, people with permanent kidney injury, and qualified people with disabilities. Title II of the Social Security Disability Insurance program pays benefits to those people who meet medical criteria for disability, who have worked long enough (40 quarters of covered employment) to qualify, and who have paid Social Security taxes. Title II also provides benefits to people

Figure 9-3 • Examples of appropriate communication by nurse with young woman with a disability in a wheelchair. **A.** The nurse is sitting at patient's eye level and talks directly to the patient after asking her mother to step out of the room during the history. **B.** The nurse explains to the patient how the examination table moves up and down, which allows the patient to be as independent as possible in moving the table.

disabled since childhood (younger than 22 years), who are dependents of a deceased insured parent or a parent entitled to disability or retirement benefits, and disabled widows or widowers, 50 to 60 years of age, if their deceased spouse was insured under Social Security. Title XVI of the Social Security Disability Insurance program provides supplemental security income payments to people who are disabled and have limited income and resources.

Medicaid provides home and community-based services to people with disabilities and long-term illnesses to enable them to lead meaningful lives in their families and communities (Krahn et al., 2015). (See the Resources section for a link to information about these benefits.) The ACA has expanded insurance options for people with disabilities and made these options more affordable. Furthermore, people with preexisting chronic conditions and disabilities can no longer be dropped by insurance companies and a lifetime cap on benefits is no longer allowed (Krahn et al., 2015). (See Chapter 1, earlier discussion of the ACA in this chapter, and the Resources section at the end of this chapter.)

Despite the availability of these federal programs, people with disabilities often have health-related costs and other expenses related to disability that result in low-income status (Pumkam, Probst, Bennett, et al., 2013). Furthermore, people must undergo a disability determination process to establish eligibility for benefits, and the process can be prolonged and cumbersome for those who may need assistance in establishing their eligibility.

Nursing Care of Patients With Disabilities

As active members of society, people with disabilities are no longer an invisible minority. An increased awareness of their needs will bring about changes to improve access and accommodations. Modification of the physical environment permits access to public and private facilities and services, including health care, and nurses can serve as advocates for people with disabilities to eliminate discriminatory practices.

Nursing Considerations During Hospitalization

During hospitalization, as well as during periods of acute illness or injury or while recovering from surgery, patients with preexisting disabilities may require assistance with carrying out ADLs that they could otherwise manage at home independently and easily. Patients should be asked preferences about approaches to carrying out their ADLs, and assistive devices they require should be readily available. Careful planning with patients to ensure that the hospital room is arranged with their input enables them to manage as independently as possible. For example, patients who have paraplegia may be able to transfer independently from bed to wheelchair; however, if the bed is left in an elevated position, they may be unable to do so. If patients usually use service animals to assist them with ADLs, it is necessary to make arrangements for the accommodation of these animals. If patients with hearing loss or vision impairment are hospitalized, it is essential to establish effective communication strategies. Alternative methods for these patients to communicate with the health care team must be put in

place and used, and all staff members must be aware that some patients are not able to respond to the intercom or telephone. If patients have vision impairment, it is necessary to orient them to the environment and talk to them in a normal tone of voice (Sharts-Hopko, Smeltzer, Ott, et al., 2010). It may be necessary to obtain a referral with a speech–language therapist or communication specialist to assist in identifying alternative methods (use of sounds, gestures, eye movements) between the nurse and the patient when the patient has a severe cognitive disability that affects speech.

Health Promotion and Prevention

Health care providers often neglect health promotion concerns of people with disabilities, who may be unaware of these concerns. For example, people who have had hearing loss since childhood may lack exposure to information about AIDS through radio and television. People with lifelong disabilities may not have received information about general health issues as children, and people with new onset as well as lifelong disabilities may not receive encouragement to participate in health promotion activities. Therefore, nurses should take every opportunity to emphasize the importance of participation in health promotion activities (e.g., healthy diet, exercise, social interactions) and preventive health screening.

The management of some disabilities increases the risk of illness, and in some people, health screening (e.g., bone density testing, gynecologic examinations, mammography) may be required earlier in life or more frequently (HHS, 2005). Referrals by nurses to accessible sites for screening may be needed, because many imaging centers are inaccessible. In addition, nursing consultation with physical therapists may be needed to identify creative ways of enabling people with disabilities to exercise safely, because exercise facilities are also often inaccessible for people with disabilities.

General health promotion strategies and health-screening recommendations for all men and women also apply to those with disabilities. Although physical limitations, cognitive impairments, and structural and attitudinal barriers existing in clinical facilities may make it difficult for some men and women to obtain health care and preventive health screening, the presence of a disability should not be used as a reason or excuse to defer recommended screening. Rather, the presence of a disability may *increase* the risk of secondary health conditions or disorders that require screening and follow-up. Just as people without disabilities should have regular screening tests, such as mammography or testicular and prostate examinations, so should people with disabilities (HHS, 2005, 2015). Nurses are often in a position to influence decisions about how equipment and procedures can be adapted to meet the special needs of their patients, whether these needs are cognitive, motor, or communicative.

The effect of the disabling condition on health risks should be considered. For example, the risk of osteoporosis may be increased in women and men whose disabilities limit their ability to participate in weight-bearing exercise or who use medications that contribute to bone loss (Smeltzer, Zimmerman, & Capriotti, 2005). Although people with disabilities have an increased risk of osteoporosis at a younger age than people without disabilities, little attention is given to prevention, detection, and treatment of osteoporosis, despite the increased risk for falls associated with many disabling disorders.

Nurses can provide expert health promotion education classes that are targeted to people with disabilities and refer them to accessible online resources. Classes on nutrition and weight management are extremely important to people who are wheelchair users and need assistance with transfers. Safer sex classes are needed by adolescents and young adults who have spinal cord injury, traumatic brain injury, or developmental disabilities, because the threats of sexually transmitted infections and unplanned pregnancy exist for these populations just as they do for the population in general.

The need for health promotion in the areas of establishing relationships, sex, pregnancy, and childbearing is as great in people with disabilities, including those with intellectual and cognitive disabilities, as people without disabilities. However, societal attitudes and bias against sexual relationships and childbearing in people with disabilities often result in their exclusion from discussions about these issues as well as failure to take their interest and questions seriously. Approaching these topics at the point of interest and knowledge level of a patient with a disability is important for sexual health. Furthermore, addressing sexual issues is important to prepare people with disabilities, who are at risk of sexual and other forms of abuse, to distinguish between healthy and abusive or exploitative sexual interactions and relationships.

Other healthy behaviors about which people with neurologic disabilities need education include avoiding alcohol and nonprescription medications while taking antispasmodic and anticonvulsant medications.

Significance of "People-First" Language

It is important to all people, both those with and those without disabilities, that they not be equated with their illness or physical condition. Therefore, nurses should refer to all people using "people-first" language. That means referring to the person first: "the patient with diabetes" rather than "the diabetic" or "the diabetic patient," "the person with a disability" rather than the "disabled person," "women with disabilities" rather than "disabled women," and "people who are wheelchair users" rather than "the wheelchair bound." This simple use of language conveys the message that the person, rather than the illness or disability, is of greater importance to the nurse.

 Gerontologic Considerations

Changes in the U.S. demographic profile are resulting in an increased number of older adults with disabilities, with two thirds of Americans 85 years of age and older experiencing functional limitations. Although disability is often perceived as being associated only with old age, disability occurs across the lifespan; the majority of people with disabilities are younger than 65 years, with one third between 44 and 65 years of age (Krahn et al., 2015). Although many people with intellectual and developmental disabilities (cerebral palsy, Down syndrome) have a slightly shorter lifespan than other people from their age cohort, others live well into adulthood and old age. The number of adults with intellectual and developmental disabilities aged 60 years and older is expected to nearly double from 850,600 in 2010 to 1.4 million by 2030 (Factor, Heller, & Janicki, 2012).

Age-related disabilities are those that occur in the older adult population and are thought to be attributable to the aging process. Examples of age-related disabilities include osteoarthritis, osteoporosis, and hearing loss. Because people with disabilities, including those with severe developmental disabilities, are surviving longer than ever before, there are a growing number of young, middle-aged, and older adults with disabilities, including developmental disabilities.

Stereotypical thinking may lead to the conclusion that disability is associated only with being older. However, aging is an important issue that affects people with preexisting disabilities as they often develop changes associated with aging at a younger age than do those without disabilities. Therefore, people with preexisting disability should be evaluated for early onset of changes related to aging. The nurse must also consider the effects of aging on a preexisting disability and in turn the effects of disability on aging. The following are examples of changes that occur with aging in people with preexisting disabilities:

- People who use crutches for ambulation because of spina bifida, polio, and lower extremity amputation may experience muscle problems as they age because of longtime overuse of the upper extremities; symptoms may not occur for many years but may cause discomfort and interfere with the person's ability to perform ADLs.
- People who experienced respiratory compromise with the onset of polio decades earlier may experience increasing respiratory symptoms with aging (National Institute of Neurological Disorders and Stroke, 2015).
- Women with long-standing mobility limitations, lack of weight-bearing exercise, and issues associated with intellectual disabilities may experience bone loss and osteoporosis prior to menopause, yet their rate of screening is low (Dreyfus, Lauer, & Wilkinson, 2014; Smeltzer & Qi, 2014).

Concern about what the future holds is common in people aging with preexisting disabilities, who may have questions about what physical, financial, and emotional supports they will have as they age (Nosek, 2000). If their disability becomes more severe in the future, they may be concerned about placement in an assisted living facility or a long-term care facility. The nurse should recognize the concerns of people with disabilities about their future and encourage them to make suitable plans, which may relieve some of their fears and concerns about what will happen to them as they age.

Parents of adult children with developmental disabilities often fear what will happen when they are no longer available and able to care for their children. Limited long-term care resources, increased life expectancy for people with developmental disabilities, changing family patterns, and competition with the older adult population for similar resources increase the fears of these parents. Thus, nurses must identify needed community resources and services. Identifying these issues and concerns and assessing arrangements made by aging parents of adult children with disabilities can help reduce some of parents' fears about their children's futures.

Disability in Medical–Surgical Nursing Practice

Disability is often considered an issue that is specific or confined to rehabilitation nursing or to gerontologic nursing. However, as noted previously, disability can occur across the lifespan and is encountered in all settings. Patients with pre-existing disabilities due to conditions that have been present from birth or to illnesses or injuries experienced as an adolescent or young adult or during middle age often require health care and nursing care in medical–surgical settings. Although in the past many people with lifelong disabilities or adult onset of severe disabilities may have had shortened lifespans, today most can expect to have a normal or near-normal lifespan and to live a productive and meaningful life. They are also at risk for the same acute illnesses that can affect all people and are at increased risk for aging-related chronic diseases due to smoking, obesity, and lack of physical activity (LaPlante, 2015). In addition, they are at increased risk for unintentional injuries, with fall-related injuries the most common type of injury (Shi, Wheeler, Shi, et al., 2015).

Because of unfavorable interactions with health care providers, including negative attitudes, insensitivity, and lack of knowledge, people with disabilities may avoid seeking medical intervention or health care services (Smeltzer et al., 2012). For this reason, and because the number of people with disabilities is increasing, nurses must acquire knowledge and skills and be available to assist them in maintaining a high level of wellness. Nurses are in key positions to influence the architectural design of health care settings and the selection of equipment that promotes ease of access and health. Padded examination tables that can be raised or lowered make transfers easier for people with disabilities. Birthing chairs benefit women with disability during yearly pelvic examinations and Pap smears and during urologic evaluations. Ramps, grab bars, and raised and padded toilet seats benefit many people who have neurologic or musculoskeletal disabilities and need routine physical examination and monitoring (e.g., bone density measurements). When a patient with a disability is admitted to the hospital for any reason, the patient's needs for these modifications should be assessed and addressed (Smeltzer et al., 2012).

Men and women with disabilities may be encountered in hospitals, clinics, offices, and nursing centers when they seek health care to address a problem related to their disability. However, they may also be encountered in these settings when they seek care for a health problem that is not related in any way to their disability. For example, a woman with spina bifida, spinal cord injury, or post-polio syndrome might seek health care related to a gynecologic issue, such as vaginal bleeding. Although her disability should be considered in the course of assessment and delivery of health and nursing care, it should not be the exclusive focus of the assessment or care that she receives. Furthermore, neither a severe physical disability that affects a woman's ability to transfer to an examination table for a gynecologic examination nor a cognitive disability should be a reason to defer a complete health assessment and physical examination, including a pelvic examination. Health care, including preventive health screening and health promotion, is essential to enable people with disabilities to live the highest quality of life within the limitations imposed by their disabling conditions (Krahn et al., 2015). Men and women with disabilities have the same needs and same rights for health care and preventive health screening as others, although in some cases, the consequences of their disability increase rather than decrease their need for health screening and participation in health-promoting activities. Therefore, it is essential that medical-surgical nurses be knowledgeable about disability and how it affects people across the lifespan as well as how to provide sensitive and quality nursing care for patients with preexisting and new-onset disability. In an effort to address these issues, specific information on health care of people with disabilities has been included throughout this book.

Home, Community-Based and Transitional Care

Educating Patients About Self-Care

Chart 9-9 contains points the nurse should consider when educating patients about managing chronic illness and

---

Chart 9-9 **HOME CARE CHECKLIST**
Managing Chronic Illness and Disability at Home

At the completion of education, the patient and/or the caregiver will be able to:

- State the impact of chronic illness/disability on physiologic functioning, ADLs, IADLs, roles, relationships, and spirituality.
- State changes in lifestyle (e.g. diet, activity) necessary to maintain health.
- State the name, dose, side effects, frequency, and schedule for all medications.
- State how to carry out prescribed regimens (e.g., skin care, bladder/bowel care, daily weights).
- State how to obtain medical supplies after discharge.
- Identify durable medical equipment needs, proper usage, and maintenance necessary for safe utilization.
- Demonstrate usage of adaptive equipment for ADLs.
- Identify community resources for peer and caregiver/family support:
  - Identify sources of support (e.g., friends, relatives, faith community)
  - Identify phone numbers of support groups for people with chronic illness/disabilities and their caregivers/families
  - State meeting locations and times

- Demonstrate mobility skills and/or how to access transportation.
- Identify community resources for recreation:
  - State local recreation centers that offer programs for people with disabilities
  - Identify leisure activities that can be pursued in the community
- State how to reach health care provider with questions or complications.
- State time and date of follow-up appointments.
- Identify the need for health promotion, disease prevention, and screening activities.

Resources

See Chapter 10, Chart 10-8, for additional information on durable medical equipment, adaptive equipment, mobility skills, skin, bowel, and bladder care.

IADLs, instrumental activities of daily living; ADLs, activities of daily living.

disability at home. A major and often overlooked issue in educating patients about a health problem, a treatment regimen, or health promotion strategies is the need for alternative formats to accommodate people with various disabilities. Patients with disabilities are in need of the same information as other patients; however, they often require large print, Braille, audiotapes, or the assistance of a sign language interpreter (Berman et al., 2013). Materials may be obtained from a variety of sources for patients who need these educational strategies and for patients with cognitive impairments attributable to developmental disabilities or newly acquired disabilities.

Nurses should ensure that all people—whether or not they have disabilities—recognize the warning signs and symptoms of stroke, heart attack, and cancer, as well as how to access help. In addition, nurses should educate all patients who are stroke survivors and those with diabetes how to monitor their own blood pressure or glucose levels.

Continuing and Transitional Care

When caring for patients with disabilities and helping them plan for discharge and continuing care in the home, it is important to consider how a particular disability affects a patient's ability to adhere to recommended treatment regimens and keep follow-up appointments. Furthermore, it is important to consider how the health issue or treatment regimen affects the disability. Although many people with disabilities are independent and able to make decisions, arrangements for transportation, and appointments to accessible facilities, others may have difficulty doing so, particularly if they are experiencing a health problem. The nurse should recognize the effect that the disability has on the patient's ability to follow-up. The nurse should ask the patient whether he or she anticipates having any difficulties arranging for follow-up care. It is important for the nurse to assist the patient with disabilities to identify unmet needs and to find and use resources (community and social resources, and transportation services) that enable the patient to obtain needed services while remaining in their home, if preferred. The nurse should have a list of accessible sites and services available and share those resources with the patient and the family. In collaboration with other health care providers (occupational and physical therapists, speech therapists), the nurse can identify needed home modifications, including those that are simple and inexpensive, that will enable the patient to participate in self-care at home.

Transitional care, if available, is ideal for patients with severe disabilities being discharged home. Patients hospitalized for an acute or secondary health condition may be more vulnerable to deterioration in health status or developing other health conditions because of their narrow margin of health or deconditioning that occurs with hospitalization. Important roles of the transitional care nurse are to ensure that required services are available in the home at the time of the patient's discharge, to assess and monitor the patient through home visits, and to provide support and assistance to the patient and the family in the aftermath of hospitalization and discharge (Centeno & Kahveci, 2014; Naylor et al., 2013; Naylor et al., 2014).

CRITICAL THINKING EXERCISES

1 **ebp** A 64-year-old man is hospitalized for above-the-knee amputation because of complications of a 20-year history of uncontrolled diabetes. He indicates that he knows that he needs to take better care of himself and his diabetes and recognizes the importance of following the diabetes treatment plan. Your preoperative assessment indicates that he has decreased sensation in both of his legs and that his vision is 20/100 with correction (moderate vision impairment). In anticipating his postoperative care and eventual discharge home, what teaching will be needed for the patient? What evidence will you use to identify modifications that will be needed in teaching him about self-management and the likely new diabetes treatment plan? What are the safety implications for the patient given the postoperative change in his ability to ambulate and his impaired vision?

2 A 30-year-old woman with spina bifida uses crutches and occasionally a motorized scooter for long distance ambulation. She is being seen in an obstetrician/nurse midwifery practice because she and her partner want to explore the possibility of pregnancy and childbearing. She is a successful attorney who has had occasional hospitalizations for acute urinary tract infections with high fevers. What are the risks and benefits of pregnancy and childbearing for this woman and her partner? What nursing assessments are indicated at the time of her first visit? What are the nursing implications for her if she decides to become pregnant? What nursing care and teaching would be warranted as she progresses through a pregnancy?

3 **pq** A 25-year-old woman with mild intellectual disability has asthma, hypertension, and a history of seizures. She lives in a group home with four other individuals with intellectual disability and works 3 days a week in the cafeteria at a nearby school. She has been sent to the health clinic by her case worker for evaluation of vaginal itching and discharge. What are the priority issues that are of concern for your nursing assessment of the patient? If she has never had a gynecological examination before, how would you prepare her for such an examination? How would you address her history of chronic conditions that are reported by the case worker? What is your priority in providing health promotion information to her?

REFERENCES

*Asterisk indicates nursing research.
**Double asterisk indicates classic reference.

Books

Agency for Healthcare Research and Quality. (2014). *Multiple chronic conditions chartbook: 2010 medical expenditure panel survey Data*. Rockville, MD: Agency for Healthcare Research and Quality. AHRQ Pub. No. 14-0038.

Agency for Healthcare Research and Quality. (2015). *2014 National healthcare quality and disparities report*. Rockville, MD: Agency for Healthcare Research and Quality. AHRQ Pub. No. 15-0007.

Bloom, D. E., Cafiero, E. T., Jané-Llopis, E., et al. (2011). *The global economic burden of noncommunicable diseases*. Geneva, Switzerland: World Economic Forum.

Centers for Disease Control and Prevention (CDC). (2009). *The power to prevent, the call to control: At a glance 2009*. Atlanta, GA: Author.

Centers for Disease Control and Prevention (CDC). (2013). *The state of aging and health in America 2013*. Atlanta, GA: Author.

Larsen, P. D. (2016). *Lubkin's chronic illness—Impact and intervention* (9th ed.). Burlington, MA: Jones & Barlett Learning.

Lorig, K., Holman, H., Sobel, D., et al. (2012). *Living a healthy life with chronic conditions*. Boulder, CO: Bull Publishing Company.

Patient Protection and Affordable Care Act. (2010): S.3590, 111th Congress, 2nd Session.

United Nations Convention on the Rights of Persons with Disabilities (CRPD). (2006). *Final report of the Ad Hoc Committee on a comprehensive and integral international convention on the protection and promotion of the rights and dignity of persons with disabilities*. New York, NY: United Nations.

**U.S. Department of Health & Human Services. (2005). *Surgeon general's call to action to improve the health and wellness of people with disabilities*. Rockville, MD: Author.

U.S. Department of Health & Human Services, Office of Disease Prevention and Health Promotion. (2010). *Healthy People 2020*. Washington, DC: Author.

U.S. Department of Labor/Bureau of Labor Statistics. (2015). *Persons with a disability: Labor force characteristics—2014*. Washington, DC: Author.

**World Health Organization. (2001). *International classification of functioning, disability and health—ICF*. Geneva, Switzerland: Author.

World Health Organization. (2013). *Global action plan for the prevention and control of noncommunicable diseases, 2013–2020*. Geneva, Switzerland: Author.

World Health Organization. (2014a). *Global status report on noncommunicable diseases 2014*. Geneva, Switzerland: Author.

World Health Organization. (2014b). *Noncommunicable diseases country profiles, 2014*. Geneva, Switzerland: World Health Organization.

Journals and Electronic Documents

Adams, P. F., Kirzinger, W. K, & Martinez, M. E. (2013). Summary health statistics for the U.S. population: National Health Interview Survey, 2012. National Center for Health Statistics. *Vital Health Statistics, 10*(259), 1–95.

American Public Health Association. (2015). *Get the facts: Public health and chronic disease. Savings and return on investment*. Retrieved on 7/18/2015 at: apha.org/~/media/files/pdf/factsheets/chronicdisease fact_final.ashx

Americans with Disabilities Act of 1990. Retrieved on 7/18/2015 at: www.ada.gov/pubs/ada.htm

Americans with Disabilities Amendments Act of 2008. Retrieved on 7/18/2015 at: access-board.gov

*Baptista, R. S., Pagliuca, L. M. F., Sampaio, A. F. A., et al. (2014). Sexuality: Experience of women with physical disabilities. *Open Journal of Nursing, 4*, 920–927. http://dx.doi.org/10.4236/ojn.2014.413098.

Berman, B. A., Jo, A., Cumberland, W. G., et al. (2013). Breast cancer knowledge and practices among deaf women. *Disability and Health Journal, 6*(4), 303–316.

Centeno, M. M., & Kahveci, K. L. (2014). Transitional care models: Preventing readmissions for high-risk patient populations. *Critical Care Nursing Clinics of North America, 26*(4), 589–597.

Centers for Disease Control and Prevention (CDC). (2015). *The four domains of chronic disease prevention. Working toward healthy people in healthy communities*. Atlanta, GA: Author. Retrieved on 7/18/2015 at: www.cdc.gov/chronicdisease/pdf/four-domains- factsheet-2015.pdf

**Corbin, J. M. (1998). The Corbin and Strauss chronic illness trajectory model: An update. *Scholarly Inquiry for Nursing Practice, 12*(1), 33–41.

**Corbin, J. M. (2003). The body in health and illness. *Qualitative Health Research, 13*(2), 256–267.

Courtney-Long, E. A., Carroll, D. D., Zhang Q. C., et al. (2015). Prevalence of disability and disability type among adults—United States, 2013. *Morbidity and Mortality Weekly Report, 64*(29), 777–783.

Dankwa-Mullan, I., & Maddox, Y. T. (2015). Embarking on a science vision for health disparities research. *American Journal of Public Health, 105*(S3), S368–S369.

Dreyfus, D., Lauer, E., & Wilkinson, J. (2014). Characteristics associated with bone mineral density screening in adults with intellectual disabilities. *Journal of the American Board of Family Medicine, 27*(1), 104–114.

Drum, C. F. (2014). The dynamics of disability and chronic conditions. *Disability and Health Journal, 7*(1), 2–5.

Golics, C. J., Basra, M. K. A., Salek, M. S., et al. (2013). The impact of patients' chronic disease on family quality of life: An experience from 26 specialties. *International Journal of General Medicine, 6*, 787–798.

**Goodall, C. J. (1995). Is disability any business of nurse education? *Nurse Education Today, 15*(5), 323–327.

Goodman, R. A., Posner, S. F., Huang, E. S., et al. (2013). Defining and measuring chronic conditions: Imperatives for research, policy, program, and practice. *Preventing Chronic Disease, 10*, E66.

Gostin, L. O. (2015). The Americans with Disabilities Act at 25. The highest expression of American values. *JAMA, 313*(22), 2231–2235.

Havercamp, S. M., & Scott, H. M. (2015). National health surveillance of adults with disabilities, adults with intellectual and developmental disabilities, and adults with no disabilities. *Disability and Health Journal, 8*(2), 165–172.

Health Resources and Services Administration. (2013). *The Telehealth Network Grant Program (TNGP). A report summarizing performance of the TNGP*. Office of the Advancement of Telehealth. Office of Rural Health. HRSA. Washington, DC. Retrieved on 7/18/2015 at: www.hrsa.gov/ruralhealth/about/telehealth/telehealthnetworkgp.pdf

Ho, T. F., Rowland-Seymour, A., Frankel, E. S., et al. (2014). Generational differences in complementary and alternative medicine use in the context of chronic diseases and pain: Baby boomers versus the silent generation. *Journal of the American Board of Family Medicine, 27*(4), 465–473.

Horner-Johnson, W., Dobbertin, K., Lee, J. C., et al. (2013). Disparities in chronic conditions and health status by type of disability. *Disability and Health Journal, 6*(4), 280–286.

Horner-Johnson, W., Dobbertin, K., Lee, J. C., et al. (2014). Rural disparities in receipt of colorectal cancer screening among adults ages 50–64 with disabilities. *Disability and Health Journal, 7*(4), 394–401.

Iezzoni, L. I., Kurtz S. G., & Rao, S. R. (2014). Trends in U.S. adult chronic disability rates over time. *Disability and Health Journal, 7*(4), 402–412.

Krahn, G. L., Walker, D. K., & Correa-De-Araujo, R. (2015). Persons with disabilities as an unrecognized health disparity population. *American Journal of Public Health, 105*(S2), S198–S206.

Lagu, T., Hannon, N. S., Rothberg, M. G., et al. (2013). Access to subspecialty care for patients with mobility impairment: A survey. *Annals of Internal Medicine, 158*(6), 441–446.

LaPlante, M. P. (2015). Key goals and indicators for successful aging of adults with early-onset disability. *Disability and Health Journal, 7*(S1), S44–S50.

*Lollar, D. J., & Crews, J. E. (2003). Redefining the role of public health in disability. *Annual Review of Public Health, 24*, 195–208.

Mahmoudi, E., & Meade, M. A. (2015). Disparities in access to health care among adults with physical disabilities: Analysis of a representative national sample for a ten-year period. *Disability and Health Journal, 8*(2), 182–190.

McCarthy, A. M., Jianing Yang, J., & Armstrong, K. (2015). Increasing disparities in breast cancer mortality from 1979 to 2010 for US black women aged 20 to 49 years. *American Journal of Public Health, 105*(S3), S446–S448.

McKee, M. M., McKee, K., Winters, P., et al. (2014). Higher educational attainment but not higher income is protective of cardiovascular risk in Deaf American Sign Language (ASL) users. *Disability and Health Journal, 7*(1), 49–55.

National Institute of Neurological Disorders and Stroke. (2015). *NINDS post-polio syndrome information page*. National Institutes of Health. Retrieved on 7/18/2015 at: www.ninds.nih.gov/disorders/ post_polio/post_polio.htm

National Prevention Council. (2014). *Annual status report*. Washington, DC: U.S. Department of Health & Human Services, Office of the Surgeon General, 2014. Retrieved on 7/18/2015 at: www.surgeongeneral.gov/initiatives/prevention/about/annual_status_reports.html

*Naylor, M. D., Hirschman, K. B., Hanlon, A. L., et al. (2014). Comparison of evidence-based interventions on outcomes of hospitalized,

cognitively impaired older adults. *Journal of Comparative Effectiveness Research, 3*(3), 245–257.

*Naylor, M. D., Hirschman, K. B., O'Connor, M., et al. (2013). Engaging older adults in their transitional care: What more needs to be done? *Journal of Comparative Effectiveness Research, 2*(5), 457–468.

*Newland, P., Jensen, M. P., Budhathoki, C., et al. (2015). Secondary health conditions in individuals with multiple sclerosis: A cross-sectional web-based survey analysis. *Journal of Neuroscience Nursing, 47*(3), 124–130.

**Nosek, M. A. (2000). Overcoming the odds: The health of women with physical disabilities in the United States. *Archives of Physical Medicine and Rehabilitation, 81*(2), 135–138.

Parish S. L., Swaine, J. G., Son, E., et al. (2013). Receipt of mammography among women with intellectual disabilities: Medical record data indicate substantial disparities for African- American women. *Disability and Health Journal, 6*(1), 36–42.

Peacock, G., Iezzoni, L. I., & Harkin, T. R. (2015). Health care for Americans with disabilities—25 years after the ADA. *New England Journal of Medicine, 37*(10), 892–893.

Phelan, S. K. (2011). Constructions of disability: A call for critical reflexivity in occupational therapy. *Canadian Journal of Occupational Therapy, 78*, 164–172.

*Puhr, M. I., & Thompson, H. J. (2015). The use of transitional care models in patients with stroke. *Journal of Neuroscience Nursing, 4*(4), 223–234.

Pumkam, C., Probst, J. C., Bennett, K. J., et al. (2013). Health care expenditures among working-age adults with physical disabilities: Variations by disability spans. *Disability and Health Journal, 6*(4), 287–296.

Reidy, M., Denieffe, S., & Foran, S. (2014). Cancer screening in women with intellectual disabilities: An Irish perspective. *Journal of Intellectual Disability, 18*(1), 51–60.

Seidell, J. C., & Halberstadt, J. (2015). The global burden of obesity and the challenges of prevention. *Annals of Nutrition & Metabolism, 66*(Suppl. 2), 7–12.

*Sharts-Hopko, N. C., Smeltzer, S., Ott, B. B., et al. (2010). Healthcare experiences of women with visual impairment. *Clinical Nurse Specialist, 24*(3), 149–153.

Shi, X., Wheeler, K. K., Shi, J., et al. (2015). Increased risk of unintentional injuries in adults with disabilities: A systematic review and meta-analysis. *Disability and Health Journal, 8*(2), 153–164.

Smeltzer, S. C. (2007). Improving the health and wellness of persons with disabilities: A call to action too important for nursing to ignore. *Nursing Outlook, 55*(4), 189–193.

*Smeltzer, S. C., Avery, C., & Haynor, P. (2012). Interactions of people with disabilities with nursing staff during hospitalization. *American Journal of Nursing, 112*(4), 30–37.

Smeltzer, S. C., & Qi, B. B. (2014). The practical implications for nurses caring for patients being treated for osteoporosis. *Nursing: Research and Reviews, 4*(4), 19–33.

*Smeltzer, S. C., Zimmerman, V., & Capriotti, T. (2005). Osteoporosis risk and low bone mineral density in women with disabilities. *Archives of Physical Medicine and Rehabilitation, 86*(3), 582–586.

U.S. Department of Health & Human Services. (2015). *Multiple chronic conditions: A framework for education and training.* Washington, DC: HHS. Retrieved on 7/18/2015 at: www.hhs.gov/ash/initiatives/mcc/education-and-training/index.html

Ward, B. W., Schiller, J. S., & Goodman, R. A. (2014). Multiple chronic conditions among US adults: A 2012 update. *Preventing Chronic Disease, 11*, E62. http://dx.doi.org/10.5888/pcd11.130389

World Health Organization. (2005). Widespread misunderstandings about chronic disease—and the reality. Facing the Facts #2. Retrieved on 1/23/2016 at: www.who.int/chp/chronic_disease_report/media/Factsheet2.pdf

World Health Organization. (2014c). *Disability and health. Fact sheet N°352.* Retrieved on 7/18/2015 at: www.who.int/mediacentre/factsheets/fs352/en/

World Health Organization. (2014d). *Global health estimates: Deaths by cause, age, sex and country, 2015–2030.* Geneva, Switzerland: World Health Organization. Retrieved on 7/18/2015 at: www.who.int/gho/ncd/mortality_morbidity/en/

Resources

AbleData, www.abledata.com

Alliance for Disability in Health Care Education, Inc., ADHCE.org

American Association of the Deaf-Blind, www.aadb.org

American Association on Intellectual and Developmental Disabilities (formerly American Association on Mental Retardation), www.aaidd.org

American Foundation for the Blind, www.afb.org

American Speech-Language-Hearing Association, www.asha.org

Americans With Disabilities Act National Network, www.adata.org/

Arc of the United States, www.thearc.org

Association of Late-Deafened Adults (ALDA), www.alda.org

Center for Research on Women With Disabilities (CROWD), www.bcm.edu/crowd

Centers for Medicare & Medicaid Services (CMS), www.cms.hhs.gov

National Aphasia Association (NAA), www.aphasia.org

National Center for Learning Disabilities, www.ncld.org

People with disabilities and the Affordable Care Act (ACA), www.healthcare.gov

Through the Looking Glass, www.lookingglass.org

United Cerebral Palsy (UCP), www.ucp.org

United Spinal Association, www.unitedspinal.org

Women With Disabilities, Health Promotion for Women With Disabilities Web Site, Villanova University College of Nursing, http://nurseweb.villanova.edu/womenwithdisabilities/welcome.htm

10 Principles and Practices of Rehabilitation

LEARNING OBJECTIVES

On completion of this chapter, the learner will be able to:

1 Describe the goals of rehabilitation.
2 Discuss the interdisciplinary approach to rehabilitation.
3 Specify the components of a comprehensive assessment of functional capacity.
4 Use the nursing process as a framework for care of patients with self-care deficits, impaired physical mobility, impaired skin integrity, and altered patterns of elimination.
5 Describe the significance of continuity of care and community reentry from the health care facility to the home or extended care facility for patients who need rehabilitative assistance and services.

GLOSSARY

activities of daily living (ADLs): personal care activities, such as bathing, dressing, grooming, eating, toileting, and transferring

adaptive device: a type of assistive technology that is used to change the environment or help the person modify the environment

assistive device: a type of assistive technology that helps people with disabilities perform a given task

assistive technology: any item, piece of equipment, or product system that is used to improve the functional capabilities of individuals with disabilities; this term encompasses both assistive devices and adaptive devices

debilitated: impaired strength, weakened, injured, disabled

impairment: loss or abnormality of psychological, physiologic, or anatomic structure or function at the organ level (e.g., dysphagia, hemiparesis); an abnormality of body structure, appearance, an organ, or system function resulting from any cause

instrumental activities of daily living (IADLs): complex skills needed for independent living, such as shopping, cooking, housework, using the telephone, managing medications and finances, and being able to travel by car or public transportation

orthosis: an external appliance that provides support, prevents or corrects joint deformities, and improves function

pressure ulcer: localized area of skin breakdown due to prolonged pressure and insufficient blood supply, usually at bony prominences

prosthesis: a device used to replace a body part

rehabilitation: making able again; learning or relearning skills or abilities or adjusting existing functions to meet maximum potential

rehabilitation nursing: a branch of nursing focused on providing care to patients who have been incapacitated by illness or injury or are facing potentially life-altering health conditions throughout their lifespan

sinus tract: course or path of tissue destruction occurring in any direction from the surface or edge of a wound; results in dead space with potential for abscess formation; also called *tunneling*

slough: soft, moist avascular (devitalized) tissue; may be white, yellow, tan, gray, or green; may be loose or firmly adherent

undermining: area of destroyed tissue that extends under intact skin along the periphery of a wound; commonly seen in shear injuries; can be distinguished from sinus tract in that there is a significant portion of the wound edge involved, whereas sinus tract involves only a small portion of the wound edge

---

Rehabilitation is a goal-oriented process that enables people with acute or chronic disorders, including those with physical, mental, or emotional disabilities or impairments; activity limitations; and participation restrictions to (1) identify, reach, and maintain optimal physical, sensory, intellectual, psychological, and/or social functional levels and (2) focus on existing abilities to facilitate independence, self-determination, and social integration (Camicia, Black, Farrell, et al., 2014; Kearney & Cronin, 2014; Miller, 2014). During rehabilitation, patients adjust to disabilities by learning how to use available resources with a focus on overall health promotion (Hyde & Kautz, 2014). In rehabilitation, abilities, not disabilities, are emphasized.

Rehabilitation is an integral part of nursing because every major illness or injury carries the threat of disability or **impairment**, which involves a loss of function or an abnormality in the body structure or function. **Rehabilitation nursing** is a specialty that focuses on returning patients to optimal functionality through a holistic approach to care. The Association of Rehabilitation Nurses (ARN) has developed an *ARN Competency*

Model for Professional Rehabilitation Nurses with resources (ARN, 2014). The domains in the model (nurse-led interventions, promotion of successful living, leadership and interprofessional care) encompass all competencies needed to promote rehabilitation nursing of persons with disability and/or chronic illness (Vaughn et al., 2016). The principles of rehabilitation are basic to the care of all patients, and rehabilitation efforts should begin during the initial contact with a patient. Ultimately, the goal of rehabilitation nursing is to assist the patient to attain and maintain optimum health as defined by the patient (Bamm, Rosenbaum, Wilkins, et al., 2015a; Chang & Johnson, 2013; Dean, Siegert, & Taylor, 2012). If restoring the debilitated patient's ability to function independently or at a pre-illness or pre-injury level of functioning is not possible, the aims of rehabilitation are to maximize independence and prevent secondary disability as well as to promote a quality of life acceptable to the patient. This includes assessing and treating physical as well as psychological disorders and comorbidities after illness or injury (Craig, Perry, Guest, et al., 2015).

Rehabilitation services are required by more people than ever before because of advances in technology that save or prolong the lives of seriously ill and injured patients and patients with disabilities. Increasing numbers of patients who are recovering from serious illnesses or injuries are returning to their homes and communities with ongoing needs. Significant disability caused by war and terrorism also increases the demand for rehabilitation services. All patients, regardless of age, gender, ethnic group, socioeconomic status, or diagnosis, have a right to rehabilitation services.

A person is considered to have a disability, such as a restriction in performance or function in everyday activities, if he or she has difficulty talking, hearing, seeing, walking, climbing stairs, lifting or carrying objects, performing activities of daily living (ADLs), doing schoolwork, or working at a job. The disability is considered severe if the person cannot perform one or more activities, receives federal benefits because of an inability to work, uses an assistive device for mobility, or needs help from another person to accomplish basic activities. The purpose of **assistive technology** is to incorporate devices to improve the functional capabilities of persons with disabilities; these may include any item, piece of equipment, or product system that may be acquired commercially, off the shelf, modified, or customized. Types of assistive technology may include **adaptive devices**, which help a person with a disability to either modify or change the environment (e.g., an access ramp used in place of steps for a person who uses a wheelchair), and **assistive devices**, which help a person with a disability perform a given task (e.g., a lap board with pictures used to assist a person who cannot talk to communicate). (See Chapter 9 for further discussion on disability.)

The Rehabilitation Team

Rehabilitation is a creative, dynamic process that requires a team of professionals working together with patients and families. The interdisciplinary team members include health professionals who make unique contributions to the rehabilitation process. Communication, collaboration, understanding of roles, and educational levels of team members are all important considerations in building an effective interdisciplinary team (Papadimitriou & Cott, 2015; Strasser, Burridge, Falconer, et al., 2014; White, Gutierrez, Mclaughlin, et al., 2013). In addition to nurses, members of the rehabilitation team may include physicians, nurse practitioners, physiatrists, physical therapists, occupational therapists, recreational therapists, speech–language therapists, psychologists, psychiatric liaison nurses, spiritual advisors, social workers, vocational counselors, orthotists or prosthetists, and sex counselors.

Nurses assume an equal or, depending on the circumstances of the patient, a more critical role than other members of the health care team in the rehabilitation process. The evidence-based plan of care that nurses develop must be approved by the patient and family and is an integral part of the rehabilitation process (Clark-Wilson, Giles, & Baxter, 2014; Clark & Bassett, 2014). See Chart 10-1 for a Nursing

---

Chart 10-1 **NURSING RESEARCH PROFILE**

Understanding Interdisciplinary Teams in Rehabilitation Practice

White, M. J., Gutierrez A., Mclaughlin C., et al. (2013). A pilot study to examine interdisciplinary teams from the perspective of the rehabilitation nurse, the occupational therapist and the physiotherapist. *Rehabilitation Nursing, 38*(3), 142–152.

Purpose

The Institute of Medicine identifies interdisciplinary teams (IDTs) being able to work well together as one of five core competencies of healthcare workers. A literature review on teams identified communication, collaboration, understanding of roles, and educational levels of team members as key themes. Based on these themes, the study team developed a survey to assess perceptions of teams by rehabilitation nurses, physical therapists, and occupational therapists.

Design

A prospective pilot study of a convenience sample (*N* = 106) of 79 rehabilitation nurses, 14 physical therapists, and 13 occupational therapists was conducted to assess perceptions of IDTs and facilitators and barriers for teamwork. A survey was developed that asked about demographic characteristics of team members and open-ended questions about barriers and facilitators for effective teams.

Findings

Four major themes emerged from the pilot study: communication and collaboration, experience, education, and knowledge of roles. Education and experience levels of IDT members are facilitators in IDTs. Communication is both a barrier and a facilitator for IDT effectiveness. Understanding the roles and responsibilities of other IDT members is important to enable the team to function effectively.

Nursing Implications

Learning how to be effective team members, understanding concepts of team development, and participating in teams need to be emphasized in nursing education. Mentorship and team building support should be provided in work settings. All disciplines should come to the team understanding how to participate effectively, with good communication skills essential to develop effective IDTs.

Research Profile on multiprofessional and interdisciplinary teamwork in the rehabilitation setting. Principles that undergird the process of patient-centered rehabilitation-focused care include the following:

- Rehabilitation encompasses all domains of personhood: physical, psychosocial, emotional, cultural, spiritual, and cognitive (Chang & Johnson, 2013).
- Rehabilitation is a continuous process.
- Rehabilitation requires active patient participation.
- Rehabilitation is goal directed.
- Rehabilitation requires multiprofessional and interdisciplinary teamwork (Camicia et al., 2014; Dean et al., 2012; Kolar, 2014; O'Sullivan, Schmitz, & Fulk, 2013).

In working toward maximizing independence, nurses affirm the patient as an active participant and essential part of the health care delivery process (Bamm et al., 2015b). Indeed, the patient is a key member of the rehabilitation team, the focus of the team's effort, and the one who determines the final outcomes of the rehabilitation process. The patient participates in goal setting, in learning to function using their remaining abilities, and in adjusting to living with disabilities. Nurses also recognize the importance of informal caregivers as support team members in the rehabilitation process circle of care (Hanson, Armstrong, Green, et al., 2012; Knudson-Martin, Huenergardt, Lafontant, et al., 2015; Price & Lau, 2013). The patient's family is also incorporated into the team. Families are dynamic systems; therefore, the disability of one member affects other family members. Only by incorporating the family into the rehabilitation process can the family system adapt to the change in one of its members. The family provides ongoing support, participates in problem solving, and learns to participate in providing ongoing care.

The nurse develops a therapeutic and supportive relationship with the patient and family. The nurse emphasizes the patient's assets and strengths, positively reinforcing the patient's efforts to improve self-concept and self-care abilities. During nurse–patient interactions, the nurse actively listens, encourages, and shares patient and family successes. Using the nursing process, the nurse develops a plan of care designed to facilitate rehabilitation, restore and maintain optimal health, and prevent complications (Clarke, 2014).

Coping with the disability, fostering self-care, identifying mobility limitations, and managing skin care and bowel and bladder training are areas that frequently require nursing care. The nurse acts as a caregiver, educator, counselor, patient advocate, case manager, and consultant. The nurse is often responsible for coordinating the total rehabilitative plan and collaborating with and coordinating the services provided by all members of the health care team, including home care nurses, who are responsible for directing patient care after the patient returns home.

Areas of Specialty Rehabilitation

Although rehabilitation must be a component of every patient's care, specialty rehabilitation programs have been established in general hospitals, free-standing rehabilitation hospitals, and outpatient facilities. The Commission for the Accreditation of Rehabilitation Facilities (CARF) sets and promotes quality standards for these programs. CARF also offers a consultative accreditation and continuous improvement service for rehabilitation facilities in North and South America, Europe, Asia, and Africa (see link to CARF Web site in chapter resources). Some of these programs are described below:

- *Stroke recovery programs* and *traumatic brain injury rehabilitation* emphasize cognitive remediation, helping patients compensate for memory, perceptual, judgment, and safety deficits as well as teaching self-care and mobility skills. Other goals include helping patients swallow food safely and communicate effectively. Neurologic disorders treated in addition to stroke and brain injury include multiple sclerosis, Parkinson disease, amyotrophic lateral sclerosis, and nervous system tumors.
- *Spinal cord injury rehabilitation programs* promote understanding of the effects and complications of spinal cord injury (SCI); neurogenic bowel and bladder management; sexuality and fertility enhancement; self-care, including prevention of skin breakdown; bed mobility and transfers; and driving with adaptive equipment. The programs also focus on vocational assessment, training, and reentry into employment and the community. Model Spinal Cord Injury Centers designated by the National Institute of Disability Research and Rehabilitation (NIDRR) and SCI rehabilitation systems are operated by individual states.
- *Orthopedic rehabilitation programs* provide comprehensive services to patients with traumatic or nontraumatic amputation, patients undergoing joint replacements, and patients with arthritis. Independence with a prosthesis or new joint is a major goal of these programs. Other goals include pain management, energy conservation, and joint protection.
- *Cardiac rehabilitation* for patients who have had myocardial infarction begins during hospitalization and continues on an outpatient basis. Emphasis is placed on monitored, progressive exercise; nutritional counseling; stress management; sexuality; and risk reduction.
- *Pulmonary rehabilitation programs* may be appropriate for patients with restrictive or chronic obstructive pulmonary disease or ventilator dependency. Respiratory therapists help patients achieve more effective breathing patterns. The programs also teach energy conservation techniques, self-medication, and home ventilator management.
- *Comprehensive pain management programs* are available for people with chronic pain, especially low back pain. These programs focus on alternative pain treatment modalities, exercise, supportive counseling, and vocational evaluation.
- *Comprehensive burn rehabilitation programs* may serve as step-down units from intensive care burn units. Although rehabilitation strategies are implemented immediately in acute care, a program focused on progressive joint mobility, self-care, and ongoing counseling is imperative for burn patients.
- *Pediatric rehabilitation programs* meet the needs of children with developmental and acquired disabilities, including cerebral palsy, spina bifida, traumatic brain injuries, and spinal cord injuries.

Substance Abuse Issues in Rehabilitation

As in all areas of nursing practice, nurses practicing in the area of rehabilitation must be skilled and knowledgeable about the care of patients with substance abuse. For all people with disabilities, including adolescents, nurses must assess actual or potential substance abuse. Alcohol and drug abuse or dependence has been associated with new occurrence spinal cord and brain injury (Tétrault & Courtois, 2014). Fifty percent of spinal cord injuries are related to substance abuse, and approximately 50% of all patients with traumatic brain injury were intoxicated at the time of injury (Substance Abuse and Mental Health Services Administration, 2014).

Substance abuse is a critical issue in rehabilitation, especially for people with disabilities who are attempting to gain employment via vocational rehabilitation. The rates of substance abuse, including alcohol abuse, in people with disabilities are two to four times as high (Glazier & Kling, 2013) as in the general population, and this increased abuse is associated with numerous risks that may have an adverse impact. These risks include medication and health problems, societal enabling (i.e., acceptance and tolerance of substance abuse by key social and cultural groups), a lack of identification of potential problems, and a lack of accessible and appropriate prevention and treatment services. Treatment for alcoholism and drug dependencies includes thorough physical and psychosocial evaluations; detoxification; counseling; medical treatment; psychological assistance for patients and families; treatment of any coexisting psychiatric illness; and referral to community resources for social, legal, spiritual, or vocational assistance. The length of treatment and the rehabilitation process depends on the patient's needs. Self-help groups are also encouraged, although attendance at meetings of such groups (e.g., Alcoholics Anonymous, Narcotics Anonymous) poses various challenges for people who have neurologic disorders, are permanent wheelchair users, or must adapt to encounters with attendees without disabilities who may not understand disability.

Assessment of Functional Ability

Comprehensive assessment of functional capacity is the basis for developing a rehabilitation program. Functional capacity is a person's ability to perform ADLs and instrumental activities of daily living. **Activities of daily living (ADLs)** are those self-care activities that the patient must accomplish each day to meet personal needs; they include personal hygiene/bathing, dressing/grooming, feeding, and toileting. Many patients cannot perform such activities easily. **Instrumental activities of daily living (IADLs)** include those complex skills needed for independent living, including meal preparation, grocery shopping, household management, finances, and transportation.

The nurse observes the patient performing specific activities (e.g., eating, dressing) and notes the degree of independence; the time taken; the patient's mobility, coordination, and endurance; and the amount of assistance required. The nurse also carefully assesses joint motion, muscle strength, cardiovascular reserve, and neurologic function, because functional ability depends on these factors as well. Observations are recorded on a functional assessment tool. These tools provide a way to standardize assessment parameters and include a scale or score against which improvements may be measured. They also clearly communicate the patient's level of functioning to all members of the rehabilitation team. Rehabilitation staff members use these tools to provide an initial assessment of the patient's abilities and to monitor the patient's progress in achieving independence.

One of the most frequently used tools to assess the patient's level of independence is the Functional Independence Measure (FIM™) (Keith, Granger, Hamilton, et al., 1987). The FIM™ is a minimum data set, measuring 18 self-care items including eating, bathing, grooming, dressing upper body, dressing lower body, toileting, bladder management, and bowel management. The FIM™ addresses transfers and the ability to ambulate and climb stairs and also includes communication and social cognition items. Scoring is based on a seven-point scale, with items used to assess the patient's level of independence. The Alpha FIM™, a short version of the FIM™, is used frequently within 72 hours of admission in acute care settings to measure functional independence and the amount of assistance the patient needs to perform ADLs.

Although there are many disease-specific tools used to assess the patient's functional ability, some frequently used generic measures (Christakou, Papadopoulos, Patsaki, et al., 2013) include the following:

- The PULSES profile (Granger, Albrecht, & Hamilton, 1979) is used to assess physical condition (e.g., health/illness status), upper extremity functions (e.g., eating, bathing), lower extremity functions (e.g., transfer, ambulation), sensory function (e.g., vision, hearing, speech), bowel and bladder function (i.e., control of bowel or bladder), and situational factors (e.g., social and financial support). Each of these areas is rated on a scale from one (independent) to four (greatest dependency).
- The Barthel Index (Mahoney & Barthel, 1965) is used to measure the patient's level of independence in ADLs, continence, toileting, transfers, and ambulation (or wheelchair mobility). This scale does not address communicative or cognitive abilities.
- The Patient Evaluation Conference System (PECS) (Harvey, Hollis, & Jellinek, 1981), which contains 15 categories, is a comprehensive assessment scale that includes such areas as medications, pain, nutrition, use of assistive devices, psychological status, vocation, and recreation.
- The Disability Rating Scale (DRS) is a measure of impairment, disability, and handicap and is intended to assess general functional changes over the course of recovery (Wright, 2011).

A detailed functional evaluation of secondary conditions related to the patient's disability, such as muscle atrophy and deconditioning, skin integrity, bowel and bladder control, and sexual function, together with residual strengths unaffected by disease or disability, is necessary. In addition, the nurse assesses the patient's physical, mental, emotional, spiritual, social, and economic status, as well as cultural and familial environment. These elements may provide a context to the functional findings and influence the rehabilitation plan. For example, the patient's perception of what it means to have a disability and the implications that this might have on familial and social roles can influence the rehabilitation process.

NURSING PROCESS

The Patient With Self-Care Deficits in Activities of Daily Living

An ADL program is started as soon as the rehabilitation process begins, because the ability to perform ADLs is frequently the key to independence, return to the home, and transition into the community.

Assessment

The nurse must observe and assess the patient's ability to perform ADLs to determine the level of independence in self-care and the need for nursing intervention. Chart 10-2 depicts behaviors that may indicate struggles with function or movement and thus should be assessed. For example, bathing requires obtaining bath water and items used for bathing (e.g., soap, washcloth), washing, and drying the body after bathing. Dressing requires getting clothes from the closet, putting on and taking off clothing, and fastening the clothing. Self-feeding requires using utensils to bring food to the mouth and chewing and swallowing the food. Toileting includes removing clothing to use the toilet, cleansing

oneself, and readjusting clothing. Grooming activities include combing hair, brushing one's teeth, shaving or applying makeup, and hand washing. Patients who can sit up and raise their hands to their head can begin self-care activities. Assistive devices are often essential in achieving some level of independence in ADLs.

The nurse should also be aware of the patient's medical conditions or other health problems, the effect that they have on the ability to perform ADLs, and the family's involvement in the patient's ADLs. This information is valuable in setting goals and developing the plan of care to maximize self-care.

Nursing Diagnosis

Based on the assessment data, a major nursing diagnosis may include the following:
- Self-care deficit: bathing, dressing, feeding, toileting

Planning and Goals

The major goals include performing the following activities independently or with assistance, using adaptive or assistive devices as appropriate: bathing/hygiene, dressing/grooming, feeding, and toileting. Another goal is patient expression of satisfaction with the extent of independence achieved in self-care activities.

Nursing Interventions

Repetition, practice, and demonstrations help patients achieve maximum independence in personal care activities. The nurse's role is to provide an optimal learning environment that minimizes distractions. The nurse can identify the patient's optimal time to work on activities, encourage concentration, identify endurance issues that may affect safety, and provide cues and reminders to patients with specific disabilities (e.g., hemiparesis or hemineglect) (Hyde & Kautz, 2014). Patients with impaired mobility, sensation, strength, or dexterity may need to use assistive devices to accomplish self-care.

FOSTERING SELF-CARE ABILITIES

A patient's approach to self-care may be affected by altered or impaired mobility and influenced by family or cultural expectations. The inability to perform self-care as carried out previously may lead to ineffective coping behaviors, such as social isolation, dependency on caregivers, or depression. The nurse must motivate the patient to learn and accept responsibility for self-care. It helps to encourage an "I'd rather do it myself" attitude. The nurse must also help the patient identify the safe limits of independent activity; knowing when to ask for assistance is particularly important.

The nurse educates, guides, and supports the patient who is learning or relearning how to perform self-care activities while maintaining a focus on patient strengths and optimal level of function. Consistency in instructions and assistance given by health care providers, including rehabilitation therapists (e.g., physiotherapists, occupational therapists, recreation therapists, speech–language pathologists, and physicians) facilitates the learning process. Recording the patient's performance provides data for evaluating progress and may be used as a source for motivation and morale building. Guidelines for educating patients and families about ADLs are presented in Chart 10-3.

Chart 10-2

ASSESSMENT

Assessing Potential Struggles in Function or Movement

Be alert for the following behaviors:

- Holding onto a handrail to pull the body while going up stairs
- Holding onto a bedside rail or bedcovers to pull to a sitting position in bed
- Leaning to one side and using both hands on the handrail while going down the stairs or a ramp
- Holding onto furniture or doorways and watching the feet while walking in the house
- Lifting a leg (or arm) by using the other leg (or arm) as support or by lifting with the pants leg (or sleeve)
- Tilting the head to reach the back or side of the hair while grooming
- Pushing up, rocking forward and back, and/or leaning the body over for momentum ("nose over toes") when rising to stand from a chair
- Leaning over from the waist without bending the knees and then placing one hand on the thigh, as if it were a prop, and pushing against the thigh to assist in moving to the upright position
- Turning to reach for an object and then using the other arm or an object to support the reaching arm at the elbow or wrist
- Positioning a chair before sitting down by using the front or back of the knees and then using the back of the knees to guide sitting down; using the torso and hips to lean against a table or chair
- Reaching and leaning with the body rather than with an arm
- Walking with a lean to one side, a limp, a waddle, or other variation of a gait
- Scanning (i.e., observing or being aware of surroundings) ineffectively while eating or grooming
- Rolling or scooting the body, sliding forward in a seat, or other maneuvers to move off a bed or out of a chair

Adapted from Hoeman, S. P. (2008). *Rehabilitation nursing: Prevention, intervention, and outcomes* (4th ed.). St. Louis, MO: Mosby.

Chart 10-3

PATIENT EDUCATION
Educating Patients About Activities of Daily Living

The nurse instructs the patient to:

1. Define the goal of the activity with the patient. Be realistic. Set short-term goals that can be accomplished in the near future.
2. Identify several approaches to accomplish the task (e.g., there are several ways to put on a given garment).
3. Select the approach most likely to succeed.
4. Specify the approach on the patient's plan of care and the patient's level of accomplishment on the progress notes.
5. Identify the motions necessary to accomplish the activity (e.g., to pick up a glass, extend arm with hand open; place open hand next to glass; flex fingers around glass; move arm and hand holding glass vertically; flex arm toward body).
6. Focus on gross functional movements initially, and gradually include activities that use finer motions (e.g., buttoning clothes, eating with a fork).
7. Encourage the patient to perform the activity up to maximal capacity within the limitations of the disability.
8. Monitor the patient's tolerance.
9. Minimize frustration and fatigue.
10. Support the patient by giving appropriate praise for effort put forth and for acts accomplished.
11. Assist the patient to perform and practice the activity in real-life situations and in a safe environment.

Often, performing a simple maneuver requires the patient with a disability to concentrate intensely and exert considerable effort; therefore, self-care techniques need to be adapted to accommodate the individual patient's lifestyle. Because a self-care activity usually can be accomplished in several ways, common sense and a little ingenuity may promote increased independence. For example, a person who cannot quite reach their head may be able to do so by leaning forward. Encouraging the patient to participate in a support group may also help the patient discover creative solutions to self-care problems.

Pre-existing cultural norms may influence the degree of self-care the patient is willing to consider. Cultural and ethnic beliefs about hygiene can vary among individuals and families. The nurse must recognize these beliefs, work through any issues with the patient and family, and communicate pertinent findings to the rehabilitation team.

RECOMMENDING ADAPTIVE AND ASSISTIVE DEVICES

If the patient has difficulty performing an ADL, an adaptive or assistive device (self-help device) may be useful. Such devices may be obtained commercially or can be constructed by the nurse, occupational therapist, patient, or family. The devices may include built-up handles on toothbrushes or razors; long, curved handles on mirrors or shoe horns; suction cups to hold items in place; shower chairs; raised toilet seats; and universal cuffs to grip self-care items. Some of these are shown in Figure 10-1. To assist premenopausal women with managing menstruation, clothing adaptations (e.g., Velcro crotch flaps for ease of access), mirrors, self-sticking sanitary pads, packaged wipes, and loose underwear may be used.

 Quality and Safety Nursing Alert

To avoid injury or bleeding, people who take anticoagulant medication should be encouraged to use an electric razor. Women may wish to consider depilatory creams or electrolysis.

A wide selection of computerized devices is available, or devices can be designed to help individual patients with severe disabilities to function more independently. The Able-Data project (see Resources list at the end of this chapter)

Figure 10-1 • Adaptive and assistive devices. **A.** Raised toilet seat. **B.** Shower chair.

offers a computerized listing of commercially available aids and equipment for patients with disabilities.

The nurse should be alert to "gadgets" coming on the market and evaluate their potential usefulness. The nurse must exercise professional judgment and caution in recommending devices, because in the past, unscrupulous vendors have marketed unnecessary, overly expensive, or useless items to patients.

HELPING PATIENTS ACCEPT LIMITATIONS

If the patient has a severe disability, independent self-care may be an unrealistic goal. In this situation, the nurse educates the patient how to take charge by directing their care. The patient may require a personal attendant to perform ADLs. Family members may not be appropriate for providing bathing/hygiene, dressing/grooming, feeding, and toileting assistance, and spouses may have difficulty providing bowel and bladder care for patients and maintaining the role of sexual partners. If a personal caregiver is necessary, the patient and family members must learn how to manage an employee effectively. The nurse helps the patient accept self-care dependency. Independence in other areas, such as social interaction, should be emphasized to promote a positive self-concept.

Evaluation

Expected patient outcomes may include:
1. Demonstrates independent self-care in bathing/hygiene or with assistance, using adaptive devices as appropriate
   a. Bathes self at maximal level of independence
   b. Uses adaptive and assistive devices effectively
   c. Reports satisfaction with level of independence in bathing/hygiene
2. Demonstrates independent self-care in dressing/grooming or with assistance, using adaptive devices as appropriate
   a. Dresses/grooms self at maximal level of independence
   b. Uses adaptive devices effectively
   c. Reports satisfaction with level of independence in dressing/grooming
   d. Demonstrates increased interest in appearance
3. Demonstrates independent self-care in feeding or with assistance, using adaptive and assistive devices as appropriate
   a. Feeds self at maximal level of independence
   b. Uses adaptive and assistive devices effectively
   c. Demonstrates increased interest in eating
   d. Maintains adequate nutritional intake
4. Demonstrates independent self-care in toileting or with assistance, using adaptive and assistive devices as appropriate
   a. Toilets self at maximal level of independence
   b. Uses adaptive and assistive devices effectively
   c. Indicates positive feelings regarding level of toileting independence
   d. Experiences adequate frequency of bowel and bladder elimination
   e. Does not experience incontinence, constipation, urinary tract infection, or other complications

NURSING PROCESS
The Patient With Impaired Physical Mobility

Problems commonly associated with immobility include weakened muscles, joint contracture, and deformity. Each joint of the body has a normal range of motion; if the range is limited, the functions of the joint and the muscles that move the joint are impaired, and painful deformities may develop. The nurse must identify patients at risk for such complications. The nurse needs to assess, plan, and intervene to prevent complications of immobility.

Another problem frequently seen in rehabilitation nursing is an altered ambulatory/mobility pattern. Patients with disabilities may be either temporarily or permanently unable to walk independently and unaided. The nurse assesses the mobility of the patient and designs care that promotes independent mobility within the prescribed therapeutic limits. If a patient cannot exercise and move their joints through their full range of motion, contractures may develop. A contracture is a shortening of the muscle and tendon that leads to deformity and limits joint mobility. When the contracted joint is moved, the patient experiences pain; in addition, more energy is required to move when joints are contracted.

Assessment

Mobility may be restricted owing to pain, paralysis, loss of muscle strength, systemic disease, an immobilizing device (e.g., cast, brace), or prescribed limits to promote healing. Assessment of mobility includes positioning, ability to move, muscle strength and tone, joint function, and the prescribed mobility limits. The nurse must collaborate with physical therapists or other team members to assess mobility.

During position change, transfer, and ambulation activities, the nurse assesses the patient's abilities, the extent of disability, and residual capacity for physiologic adaptation. The nurse observes for orthostatic hypotension, pallor, diaphoresis, nausea, tachycardia, and fatigue.

In addition, the nurse assesses the patient's ability to use various assistive devices that promote mobility. If the patient cannot ambulate without assistance, the nurse assesses the patient's ability to balance, transfer, and use assistive devices (e.g., crutches, walker). Crutch walking requires high energy expenditure and produces considerable cardiovascular stress; therefore, people with reduced exercise capacity, decreased arm strength, and problems with balance because of aging or multiple diseases may be unable to use it. A walker is more stable and may be a better choice for such patients. If the patient uses an orthosis, the nurse monitors the patient for effective use and potential problems associated with its use.

Nursing Diagnosis

Based on the assessment data, major nursing diagnoses may include the following:
- Impaired physical mobility
- Activity intolerance or risk for activity intolerance
- Risk for injury
- Risk for disuse syndrome
- Impaired walking
- Impaired wheelchair mobility
- Impaired bed mobility

Planning and Goals

Major goals may include absence of contracture and deformity, maintenance of muscle strength and joint mobility, independent mobility, increased activity tolerance, and prevention of further disability.

Nursing Interventions

POSITIONING TO PREVENT MUSCULOSKELETAL COMPLICATIONS

Deformities and contractures can often be prevented by proper positioning. Maintaining correct body alignment when the patient is in bed is essential regardless of the position selected. During each patient contact, the nurse evaluates the patient's position and assists the patient to achieve and maintain proper positioning and alignment. The most common positions that patients assume in bed are supine (dorsal), side-lying (lateral), and prone. The nurse helps the patient assume these positions and uses pillows to support the body in correct alignment. At times, a splint (e.g., wrist or hand splint) may be made by the occupational therapist to support a joint and prevent deformity. The nurse must ensure proper use of the splint and provide skin care.

Preventing External Rotation of the Hip. The patient who is in bed for an extended period of time may develop external rotation deformity of the hip because the ball-and-socket joint of the hip tends to rotate outward when the patient lies on their back. A trochanter roll (i.e., a flannel sheet or bath towel folded in thirds lengthwise and rolled toward the patient or a commercially manufactured roll) extending from the crest of the ilium to the midthigh prevents this deformity; with correct placement, it serves as a mechanical wedge under the projection of the greater trochanter.

 Concept Mastery Alert

Abduction moves the body part away from the body; adduction moves the body part toward the body. External rotation occurs as the leg moves outward. To prevent external rotation deformity, the patient's hip should not be abducted or moved away from the body.

Preventing Footdrop. Footdrop is a deformity in which the foot is plantar flexed (the ankle bends in the direction of the sole of the foot). If the condition continues without correction, the patient will not be able to hold the foot in a normal position and will be able to walk only on their toes, without touching the ground with the heel of the foot. The deformity is caused by contracture of both the gastrocnemius and soleus muscles. Damage to the peroneal nerve or loss of flexibility of the Achilles tendon may also result in footdrop. To prevent this disabling deformity, the patient is positioned to sit at a 90-degree angle in a wheelchair with their feet on the footrests or flat on the floor.

When the patient is supine in bed, padded splints or protective boots are used to keep the patient's feet at right angles to the legs. Frequent skin inspection of the feet must also be performed to determine whether positioning devices have created any unwanted pressure areas.

The patient is encouraged to perform the following ankle exercises several times each hour: dorsiflexion and plantar flexion of the feet, flexion and extension (curl and stretch) of the toes, and eversion and inversion of the feet at the ankles. The nurse provides frequent passive range-of-motion exercises if the patient cannot perform active exercises.

 Quality and Safety Nursing Alert

Prolonged bed rest, lack of exercise, incorrect positioning in bed, and the weight of bedding that forces the toes into plantar flexion must be avoided to prevent footdrop. Patients should be encouraged to wear shoes for support and protection to prevent footdrop.

MAINTAINING MUSCLE STRENGTH AND JOINT MOBILITY

Optimal function depends on the strength of the muscles and joint motion, and active participation in ADLs promotes maintenance of muscle strength and joint mobility. Range-of-motion exercises and specific therapeutic exercises may be included in the nursing plan of care.

Performing Range-of-Motion Exercises. Range of motion involves moving a joint through its full range in all appropriate planes (see Chart 10-4). To maintain or increase the motion of a joint, range-of-motion exercises are initiated as soon as the patient's condition permits. The exercises are planned for individual patients to accommodate the wide variation in the degrees of motion that people of varying body builds and age groups can attain.

Range-of-motion exercises may be active (performed by the patient under the supervision of the nurse), assisted (with the nurse helping if the patient cannot do the exercise independently), or passive (performed by the nurse). Unless otherwise prescribed, a joint should be moved through its range of motion three times, at least two times a day. The joint to be exercised is supported, the bones above the joint are stabilized, and the body part distal to the joint is moved through the range of motion of the joint. For example, the humerus must be stabilized while the radius and ulna are moved through their range of motion at the elbow joint.

Chart 10-4	Range-of-Motion Terminology	

Abduction: movement away from the midline of the body
Adduction: movement toward the midline of the body
Flexion: bending of a joint so that the angle of the joint diminishes
Extension: the return movement from flexion; the joint angle is increased
Rotation: turning or movement of a part around its axis
Internal: turning inward, toward the center
External: turning outward, away from the center
Dorsiflexion: movement that flexes or bends the hand back toward the body or the foot toward the leg
Palmar flexion: movement that flexes or bends the hand in the direction of the palm
Plantar flexion: movement that flexes or bends the foot in the direction of the sole
Pronation: rotation of the forearm so that the palm of the hand is down
Supination: rotation of the forearm so that the palm of the hand is up
Opposition: touching the thumb to each fingertip on same hand
Inversion: movement that turns the sole of the foot inward
Eversion: movement that turns the sole of the foot outward

A joint should not be moved beyond its free range of motion; the joint is moved to the point of resistance and stopped at the point of pain. If muscle spasms are present, the joint is moved slowly to the point of resistance. Gentle, steady pressure is then applied until the muscle relaxes, and the motion is continued to the joint's final point of resistance.

To perform assisted or passive range-of-motion exercises, the patient must be in a comfortable supine position with the arms at the sides and the knees extended. Good body posture is maintained during the exercises. The nurse also uses good body mechanics during the exercise session.

Performing Therapeutic Exercises. Therapeutic exercises are prescribed by the primary provider and performed with the assistance and guidance of the physical therapist or nurse. The patient should have a clear understanding of the goal of the prescribed exercise. Written instructions about the frequency, duration, and number of repetitions, as well as simple line drawings of the exercise, help to ensure adherence to the exercise program. Return demonstration of the exercises also helps the patient and family to follow the instructions correctly.

When performed correctly, exercise assists in maintaining and building muscle strength, maintaining joint function, preventing deformity, stimulating circulation, developing endurance, and promoting relaxation. Exercise is also valuable in helping to restore motivation and the well-being of the patient. Weight-bearing exercises may slow the bone loss that occurs with disability. There are five types of exercise: passive, active-assistive, active, resistive, and isometric. The description, purpose, and action of each of these exercises are summarized in Table 10-1.

PROMOTING INDEPENDENT MOBILITY

When the patient's condition stabilizes, their physical condition permits, and the patient is able to stand, the patient is assisted to sit up on the side of the bed and then to stand. Tolerance of this activity is assessed. Orthostatic (postural) hypotension may develop when the patient assumes a vertical position. Because of inadequate vasomotor reflexes, blood pools in the splanchnic (visceral or intestinal) area and in the legs, resulting in inadequate cerebral circulation. If indicators of orthostatic hypotension (e.g., drop in blood pressure, pallor, diaphoresis, nausea, tachycardia, dizziness) are present, the activity is stopped, and the patient is assisted to a supine position in bed.

Some disabling conditions, such as SCI, acute brain injury, and other conditions that require extended periods in the recumbent position, prevent the patient from assuming an upright position at the bedside. Several strategies can be used to help the patient assume a 90-degree sitting position. A reclining wheelchair with elevating leg rests allows a slow and controlled progression from a supine position to a 90-degree sitting position. A tilt table (a board that can be tilted in 10-degree increments from a horizontal to a vertical position) may also be used. The tilt table promotes vasomotor adjustment to positional changes and helps patients with limited standing balance and limited weight-bearing activities avoid the decalcification of bones and low bone mass associated with disuse syndrome and lack of weight-bearing exercise. Physical therapists may use a tilt table for patients who have not been upright owing to illness or disability. Gradual elevation of the head of the bed may help. When getting patients with SCI out of bed, it is important to gradually raise the head

TABLE 10-1 Therapeutic Exercises

	Description	Purposes	Action
Passive	An exercise carried out by the therapist or the nurse without assistance from the patient	To retain as much joint range of motion as possible; to maintain circulation	Stabilize the proximal joint and support the distal part; move the joint smoothly, slowly, and gently through its full range of motion; avoid producing pain.
Active-Assistive	An exercise carried out by the patient with the assistance of the therapist or the nurse	To encourage normal muscle function	Support the distal part, and encourage the patient to take the joint actively through its range of motion; give no more assistance than is necessary to accomplish the action; short periods of activity should be followed by adequate rest periods.
Active	An exercise accomplished by the patient without assistance; activities include turning from side to side and from back to abdomen and moving up and down in bed	To increase muscle strength	When possible, active exercise should be performed against gravity; the joint is moved through full range of motion without assistance; make sure that the patient does not substitute another joint movement for the one intended.
Resistive	An active exercise carried out by the patient working against resistance produced by either manual or mechanical means	To provide resistance to increase muscle power	The patient moves the joint through its range of motion, while the therapist resists slightly at first and then with progressively increasing resistance; sandbags and weights can be used and are applied at the distal point of the involved joint; the movements should be performed smoothly.
Isometric or Muscle Setting	Alternately contracting and relaxing a muscle while keeping the part in a fixed position; this exercise is performed by the patient	To maintain strength when a joint is immobilized	Contract or tighten the muscle as much as possible without moving the joint, hold for several seconds, then let go and relax; breathe deeply.

of the bed to a 90-degree angle; this may take approximately 10 to 15 minutes.

Graduated compression stockings are used to prevent venous stasis. For some patients, a compression garment (leotard) or snug-fitting abdominal binder and elastic compression bandaging of the legs are needed to prevent venous stasis and orthostatic hypotension. When the patient is standing, the feet are protected with a pair of properly fitted shoes. Extended periods of standing are avoided because of venous pooling and pressure on the soles of the feet. The nurse monitors the patient's blood pressure and pulse and observes for signs and symptoms of orthostatic hypotension and cerebral insufficiency (e.g., the patient reports feeling faint and weak), which suggest intolerance of the upright position. If the patient does not tolerate the upright position, the nurse should return the patient to the reclining position and elevate their legs.

Assisting Patients With Transfer. A transfer is movement of the patient from one place to another (e.g., bed to chair, chair to commode, wheelchair to tub). As soon as the patient is permitted out of bed, transfer activities are started. The nurse assesses the patient's ability to participate actively in the transfer and determines, in conjunction with occupational therapists or physical therapists, the adaptive equipment required to promote independence and safety. A lightweight wheelchair with brake extensions, removable and detachable armrests, and leg rests minimize structural obstacles during the transfer. Tub seats or benches make transfers in and out of the tub easier and safer. Raised, padded commode seats may also be warranted for patients who must avoid flexing the hips greater than 90 degrees when transferring to a toilet. It is important that the nurse educate the patient about hip precautions (e.g., no adduction past the midline, no flexion greater than 90 degrees, and no internal rotation); abduction pillows can be used to keep the hip in correct alignment if precautions are warranted.

It is important that the patient maintains muscle strength and, if possible, performs push-up exercises to strengthen the arm and shoulder extensor muscles. The push-up exercises require the patient to sit upright in bed; a book is placed under each of the patient's hands to provide a hard surface, and the patient is instructed to push down on the book, raising the body. The nurse should encourage the patient to raise and move the body in different directions by means of these push-up exercises.

The nurse or physical therapist instructs the patient how to transfer. There are several methods of transferring from the bed to the wheelchair when the patient cannot stand, and the technique chosen should take into account the patient's abilities and disabilities. It is helpful to demonstrate the technique to the patient. If the physical therapist is involved in teaching the patient to transfer, the nurse and physical therapist must collaborate so that consistent instructions are given to the patient. During transfer, the nurse assists and coaches the patient. Figure 10-2 shows weight-bearing and non–weight-bearing transfers. For example, with a weight-bearing transfer from bed to chair, the patient stands up, pivots until his back is opposite the new seat, and sits down. If the patient's muscles are not strong enough to overcome the resistance of body weight, a polished lightweight board (transfer board, sliding board) may be used to bridge the gap between the bed

and the chair. The patient slides across on the board with or without assistance from a caregiver. This board may also be used to transfer the patient from the chair to the toilet or bathtub bench. It is important to avoid the effects of shear on the patient's skin while sliding across the board. The nurse should make sure that the patient's fingers do not curl around the edge of the board during the transfer, because the patient's body weight can crush the fingers as he or she moves across the board.

Safety is a primary concern during a transfer, and the following guidelines are recommended:

- Wheelchairs and beds must be locked before transfer begins.
- Detachable arm- and footrests are removed to make getting in and out of the chair easier.
- One end of the transfer board is placed under the buttocks and the other end on the surface to which the transfer is being made (e.g., the chair).
- The patient is instructed to lean forward, push up with his or her hands, and then slide across the board to the other surface.

Nurses frequently assist weak and incapacitated patients out of bed. The nurse supports and gently assists the patient during position changes, protecting the patient from injury. The nurse avoids pulling on a weak or paralyzed upper extremity to prevent dislocation of the shoulder. The patient is assisted to move toward the stronger side.

In the home setting, getting in and out of bed and performing chair, toilet, and tub transfers are difficult for patients with weak muscles and loss of hip, knee, and ankle motion. A rope attached to the headboard of the bed enables a patient to move toward the center of the bed, and the use of a rope attached to the footboard facilitates getting in and out of bed. The height of a chair can be raised with cushions on the seat or with hollowed-out blocks placed under the chair legs. Grab bars can be attached to the wall near the toilet and tub to provide leverage and stability.

Preparing for Ambulation. Regaining the ability to walk is a prime morale builder. However, to be prepared for ambulation—whether with a brace, walker, cane, or crutches—the patient must strengthen the muscles required. Therefore, exercise is the foundation of preparation. The nurse and physical therapist instruct and supervise the patient in these exercises.

For ambulation, the quadriceps muscles, which stabilize the knee joint, and the gluteal muscles are strengthened. To perform quadriceps-setting exercises, the patient contracts the quadriceps muscle by attempting to push the popliteal area against the mattress and at the same time raising the heel. The patient maintains the muscle contraction for a count of five and relaxes for a count of five. The exercise is repeated 10 to 15 times hourly. Exercising the quadriceps muscles prevents flexion contractures of the knee. In gluteal setting, the patient contracts or "pinches" the buttocks together for a count of five, relaxes for a count of five; the exercise is repeated 10 to 15 times hourly.

If assistive devices (i.e., walker, cane, crutches) will be used, the muscles of the upper extremities are exercised and strengthened. Push-up exercises are especially useful. While in a sitting position, the patient raises the body by pushing the hands against the chair seat or mattress. The patient should

A

B

C

Figure 10-2 • Methods of patient transfer from the bed to a wheelchair. The wheelchair is in a locked position. Colored areas indicate non–weight-bearing body parts. **A.** Weight-bearing transfer from bed to chair. The patient stands up, pivots until his back is opposite the new seat, and sits down. **B.** (**Left**) Non–weight-bearing transfer from chair to bed. (**Right**) With legs braced. **C.** (**Left**) Non–weight-bearing transfer, combined method. (**Right**) Non–weight-bearing transfer, pull-up method. One of the wheelchair arms is removed to make getting in and out of the chair easier.

be encouraged to do push-up exercises while in a prone position as well. Pull-up exercises done on a trapeze while lifting the body are also effective for conditioning. The patient is taught to raise the arms above the head and then lower them in a slow, rhythmic manner while holding weights. Gradually, the weight is increased. The hands are strengthened by squeezing a rubber ball.

Typically, the physical therapist designs exercises to help the patient develop sitting and standing balance, stability, and coordination needed for ambulation. After sitting and standing balance is achieved, the patient is able to use parallel bars. Under the supervision of the physical therapist, the patient practices shifting weight from side to side, lifting one leg while supporting weight on the other, and then walking between the parallel bars.

A patient who is ready to begin ambulation must be fitted with the appropriate assistive device, instructed about the prescribed weight-bearing limits (e.g., non–weight-bearing, partial weight-bearing ambulation), and taught how to use the device safely. Figure 10-3 illustrates some of the more

common assistive devices used in rehabilitation settings. The nurse continually assesses the patient for stability and adherence to weight-bearing precautions and protects the patient from falling. The nurse provides contact guarding by holding on to a gait belt that the patient wears around the waist. The patient should wear sturdy, well-fitting shoes and be advised of the dangers of wet or highly polished floors and throw rugs. The patient should also learn how to ambulate on inclines, uneven surfaces, and stairs.

AMBULATING WITH AN ASSISTIVE DEVICE: CRUTCHES, A WALKER, OR A CANE

Crutches are for partial weight-bearing or non–weight-bearing ambulation. Good balance, adequate cardiovascular reserve, strong upper extremities, and erect posture are essential for crutch walking. Ambulating a functional distance (at least the length of a room or house) or maneuvering stairs on crutches requires significant arm strength, because the arms must bear the patient's weight (see Fig. 10-4). The nurse or physical therapist determines which gait is best (see Chart 10-5).

Figure 10-3 • Mechanical aids to walking. **A.** Two types of walkers: pick-up and rolling. **B.** Three types of canes: C-cane, functional cane, and quad cane.

A walker provides more support and stability than a cane or crutches do. A pick-up walker is best for patients with poor balance and poor cardiovascular reserve, and a rolling walker, which allows automatic walking, is best for patients who cannot lift. A cane helps the patient walk with balance and support and relieves the pressure on weight-bearing joints by redistributing weight.

Before patients can be considered to be independent in walking with crutches, a walker, or a cane, they should learn to sit, stand from sitting, and go up and down stairs using the device. Table 10-2 describes how patients can ambulate and maneuver using each of the three devices and nursing actions to support using assistive devices.

Figure 10-4 • For a person walking with crutches, the tripod stance, with crutches out to the sides and in front of the toes, increases stability.

ASSISTING PATIENTS WITH AN ORTHOSIS OR PROSTHESIS

Orthoses and prostheses are designed to facilitate mobilization and to maximize the patient's quality of life. An **orthosis** is an external appliance that provides support, prevents or corrects deformities, and improves function. Orthoses include braces, splints, collars, corsets, and supports that are designed and fitted by orthotists or prosthetists. Static orthoses (no moving parts) are used to stabilize joints and prevent contractures. Dynamic orthoses are flexible and are used to improve function by assisting weak muscles. A **prosthesis** is an artificial body part that may be internal, such as an artificial knee or hip joint, or external, such as an artificial leg or arm.

In addition to learning how to apply and remove the orthosis and maneuver the affected body part correctly, patients must learn how to properly care for the skin that comes in contact with the appliance. Skin problems or pressure ulcers may develop if the device is applied too tightly or too loosely, or if it is adjusted improperly. The nurse instructs the patient to clean and inspect the skin daily, to make sure the brace fits snugly without being too tight, to check that the padding distributes pressure evenly, and to wear a cotton garment without seams between the orthosis and the skin.

If the patient has had an amputation, the nurse promotes tissue healing, uses compression dressings to promote residual limb shaping, and minimizes contracture formation. A permanent prosthetic limb cannot be fitted until the tissue has healed completely and the residual limb shape is stable and free from edema. The nurse also helps the patient cope with the emotional issues surrounding loss of a limb and encourages acceptance of the prosthesis. The prosthetist, nurse, and primary provider collaborate to provide instructions related to skin care and care of the prosthesis.

Evaluation

Expected patient outcomes may include:

1. Demonstrates improved physical mobility
   a. Maintains muscle strength and joint mobility
   b. Does not develop contractures
   c. Participates in exercise program

(*text continued on page 178*)

Chart 10-5 Crutch Gaits

Shaded areas are weight bearing. Arrow indicates advance of foot or crutch. (Read chart from bottom, starting with beginning stance.)

4-POINT GAIT	2-POINT GAIT	3-POINT GAIT	SWING-TO	SWING-THROUGH
• Partial weight bearing both feet • Maximal support provided • Requires constant shift of weight	• Partial weight bearing both feet • Provides less support • Faster than a 4-point gait	• Non–weight bearing • Requires good balance • Requires arm strength • Faster gait • Can use with walker	• Weight bearing both feet • Provides stability • Requires arm strength • Can use with walker	• Weight bearing • Requires arm strength • Requires coordination/balance • Most advanced gait
4. Advance right foot	4. Advance right foot and left crutch	4. Advance right foot	4. Lift both feet/swing forward/land feet next to crutches	4. Lift both feet/swing forward/land feet in front of crutches
3. Advance left crutch	3. Advance left foot and right crutch	3. Advance left foot and both crutches	3. Advance both crutches	3. Advance both crutches
2. Advance left foot	2. Advance right foot and left crutch	2. Advance right foot	2. Lift both feet/swing forward/land feet next to crutches	2. Lift both feet/swing forward/land feet in front of crutches
1. Advance right crutch	1. Advance left foot and right crutch	1. Advance left foot and both crutches	1. Advance both crutches	1. Advance both crutches
Beginning stance	Beginning stance	Beginning stance	Beginning stance	Beginning stance

TABLE 10-2 Nursing Actions Involved in Using Assistive Devices

	Crutches	Walker	Cane
Patient Preparation Adjusting device to fit patient	Measure patient standing or lying down: If standing, set crutch length approximately 5 cm (2 in) below axilla. If lying down, measure from anterior fold of axilla to sole of the foot and add 5 cm. If using patient's height, subtract 40 cm (16 in) to obtain crutch height. Adjust hand grip to allow 20 to 30 degrees of flexion at elbow. Use foam rubber pad on underarm piece to relieve pressure of crutch.	Adjust height to individual patient. Patient's arms should be in 20 to 30 degrees of flexion at elbows when hands are resting on hand grips.	With patient flexing elbow at 30-degree angle, hold handle of cane level with greater trochanter and place tip of cane 15 cm (6 in) lateral to base of 5th toe. Fit cane with gently flaring tip that has flexible, concentric rings to provide stability, absorb shock, and enable greater speed and less fatigue with walking.
Assessment	Assess safety. Crutches should have large rubber tips, and patients should wear firm-soled, well-fitting shoes. Assess balance by asking patient to stand on unaffected leg by a chair. Assess stability and stamina (tolerance). Sweating and shortness of breath indicate that rest is necessary.	Assess safety. Patients should wear firm-soled, well-fitting shoes. Assess stability and stamina (tolerance). Sweating and shortness of breath indicate that rest is necessary.	Assess safety. Patients should wear firm-soled, well-fitting shoes. Assess stability and stamina (tolerance). Sweating and shortness of breath indicate that rest is necessary.
Interventions and patient education	Assist with balance by using a transfer belt or holding patient near waist. Have patient practice shifting weight and maintaining balance. Protect patient from falls. To maximize stability, encourage patient to use tripod stance, with crutches to the front and sides of toes. Have patient perform prescribed preparatory exercises to strengthen shoulder girdle and upper extremity muscles.[a]	Walk with patient, holding at waist if needed for balance. Instruct patient to never pull self up using walker and to look up when walking. Discuss full, partial, or non–weight bearing as prescribed. Protect patient from falls.	Walk with patient, holding at waist if needed for balance. Have patient hold cane in hand opposite to affected extremity, if possible, to widen the base of support and reduce stress on involved extremity. Instruct patient to move opposite arm and leg together. Protect patient from falls.
Ambulation Gait/action used	Determine which gait is best (see Chart 10-5, Tripod Gait)[b] Four-point Three-point Two-point Swing-to Swing-through	Instruct patient to: Pick-up walker: lift device and move it forward with each step. Rolling walker: roll device forward and walk automatically.	Instruct patient to: Advance cane at same time that affected leg is moved forward. Keep cane fairly close to body to prevent leaning. Bear down on cane when unaffected extremity begins swing phase.
Sitting	Instruct patient to: Grasp hand piece for control. Bend forward slightly while assuming sitting position. Place affected leg forward to prevent weight bearing and flexion while sitting.	Instruct patient to hold walker on hand grips for stability.	
Standing	Instruct patient to: Move forward to edge of chair, and keep unaffected leg slightly under seat. Place both crutches on side of affected extremity. Push down on hand piece while rising to standing position.	Instruct patient to: Push off chair or bed to come to a standing position. Rolling walker: if walker has a brake, apply it before standing. Lift walker, placing it in front of self while leaning slightly forward. Walk into walker, supporting weight on hands when advancing. Balance on feet. Lift walker and place it in front of self again.	Instruct patient to: Push off chair or bed to come to a standing position. Hold cane for stability. Step forward on unaffected extremity. Swing cane and affected extremity forward in a normal walking gait.
Going down stairs	Instruct patient to: Walk forward as far as possible. Advance crutches to lower step; advance affected leg, then unaffected leg.	Continue pattern.	Instruct patient to: Step down on affected extremity. Place the cane and then unaffected extremity on down step.
Going up stairs	Instruct patient to: Advance unaffected leg first up next step. Advance crutches and affected extremity. Unaffected leg goes up first.	n/a	Instruct patient to: Step up on unaffected extremity. Place cane and affected extremity up on step.

[a]For patients who cannot support their weight through the wrist and hand because of arthritis or fracture, platform crutches that support the forearm and allow the weight to be borne through the elbow are available. If weight is borne on the axilla, the pressure of the crutch can damage the brachial plexus nerves, producing "crutch paralysis".

[b]Teach patients two gaits so that they can change from one to another to avoid fatigue. In addition, a faster gait can be used when walking an uninterrupted distance, and a slower gait can be used for shorter distances or in crowded places.

n/a, not applicable.

2. Transfers safely
   a. Demonstrates assisted transfers
   b. Performs independent transfers
3. Ambulates with maximum independence
   a. Uses ambulatory aid safely
   b. Adheres to weight-bearing prescription
   c. Requests assistance as needed
4. Demonstrates increased activity tolerance
   a. Does not experience episodes of orthostatic hypotension
   b. Reports absence of fatigue with ambulatory efforts
   c. Gradually increases distance and speed of ambulation

NURSING PROCESS

The Patient With Impaired Skin Integrity

Pressure ulcers are localized areas of necrotic soft tissue that occur when pressure applied to the skin over time is greater than normal capillary closure pressure, which is about 32 mm Hg. Critically ill patients have a lower capillary closure pressure and a greater risk of pressure ulcers. Patients who are prone to pressure ulcers include those confined to bed for long periods, those with motor or sensory dysfunction, and those who experience muscular atrophy and reduction of padding between the overlying skin and the underlying bone (Sullivan & Schoelles, 2013). The Centers for Medicare and Medicaid Services (CMS) has recently implemented an Inpatient Rehabilitation Facility quality reporting measure related to the percentage of residents with new or worsened pressure ulcers. Based on data from the 2011 International Pressure Ulcer Prevalence Survey, the facility prevalence of pressures ulcers was 11.2% among all facilities surveyed (Wang, Niewczyk, DiVita, et al., 2014). As well as significant pain and suffering, the consequences of developing a pressure ulcer include increased morbidity and mortality and higher medical costs and resource use, and lower odds of discharge to the community.

The American Nurses Association tracks hospital-acquired pressure ulcers (HAPU) quarterly as part of the National Database of Nursing Quality Indicators® (NDNQI®). Between the years 2004 and 2011, there was a decreasing trend in the HAPU rate overall, with more improvement beginning in 2008 (He, Staggs, Bergquist-Beringer, et al., 2013). This improvement corresponds to the year the Agency for Healthcare Research and Quality (AHRQ) included data on pressure ulcers as a patient safety indicator in the Healthcare Cost and Utilization Project (HCUP) hospital database. Despite this decrease in overall HAPU rates, development of a pressure ulcer still presents a significant patient safety risk, with increased rates of patient death and longer hospital lengths of stays and readmissions (He et al., 2013). The average length of stay for hospitalizations related to pressure ulcers is 13.4 days, with an average treatment cost of nearly $20,000 for each affected patient (He et al., 2013). All possible efforts to prevent skin breakdown must be made because the treatment of pressure ulcers is costly in terms of health care dollars and quality of life for patients at risk.

The initial sign of pressure is erythema (redness of the skin) caused by reactive hyperemia, which normally resolves in less than 1 hour. Unrelieved pressure results in tissue ischemia or anoxia. The cutaneous tissues become broken or destroyed, leading to progressive destruction and necrosis of underlying soft tissue, and the resulting pressure ulcer is painful and slow to heal.

Assessment

Nursing assessment involves identifying and evaluating risk for development of pressure ulcers as well as assessment of the skin.

ASSESSMENT OF RISK FACTORS

Immobility, impaired sensory perception or cognition, decreased tissue perfusion, decreased nutritional status, friction and shear forces, increased moisture, and age-related skin changes all contribute to the development of pressure ulcers (DiVita, Granger, Goldstein, et al., 2015; García-Fernández, Agreda, Verdú, et al., 2014). Chart 10-6 lists risk factors for pressure ulcers. Scales such as the Braden scale (see Table 10-3) or Norton scale (Norton, McLaren, & Exton-Smith, 1962) may be used to facilitate systematic assessment and quantification of a patient's risk for pressure ulcer, although the nurse should recognize that the reliability of these scales is not well established for all patient populations.

Specific nursing actions related to assessing risk include:
- Evaluate level of mobility.
- Note safety and assistive devices (e.g., restraints, splints).
- Assess neurovascular status.
- Evaluate circulatory status (e.g., peripheral pulses, edema).
- Note present health problems.
- Evaluate nutritional and hydration status.
- Review the results of the patient's laboratory studies, including hematocrit, hemoglobin, electrolytes, albumin, prealbumin, transferrin, and creatinine.
- Determine presence of incontinence.
- Review current medications.

Chart 10-6 ⚠️ **RISK FACTORS**
Pressure Ulcers

- Prolonged pressure on tissue
- Immobility, compromised mobility
- Loss of protective reflexes, sensory deficit/loss
- Poor skin perfusion, edema
- Malnutrition, hypoproteinemia, anemia, vitamin deficiency
- Friction, shearing forces, trauma
- Incontinence of urine or feces
- Altered skin moisture: excessively dry, excessively moist
- Advanced age, debilitation
- Equipment: casts, traction, restraints
- Skin problems on admission

Adapted from DiVita, M. A., Granger, C. V., Goldstein, R., et al. (2015). Risk factors for development of new or worsened pressure ulcers among patients in inpatient rehabilitation facilities in the United States: Data from the Uniform Data System for Medical Rehabilitation. *Physical Medicine & Rehabilitation, 7*(6), 599–612; Dunk, A. M., & Carville, K. (2015). The international clinical practice guideline for prevention and treatment of pressure ulcers/injuries. Journal of Advanced Nursing, n/a-n/a. doi: 10.1111/jan.12614; García-Fernández, F. P., Agreda, J., Verdú, J., et al. (2014). A new theoretical model for the development of pressure ulcers and other dependence-related lesions. *Journal of Nursing Scholarship, 46*(1), 28–38; Stifter, J., Yao, Y., Lodhi, M. K., et al. (2015). Nurse continuity and hospital-acquired pressure ulcers. *Nursing Research, 64*(5), 361–371.

TABLE 10-3 Braden Scale for Predicting Pressure Ulcer Risk

Patient's Name _____ Evaluator's Name _____

Date of Assessment

Sensory Perception Ability to respond meaningfully to pressure-related discomfort	**1. Completely Limited** Unresponsive (does not moan, flinch, or grasp) to painful stimuli, due to diminished level of consciousness or sedation OR limited ability to feel pain over most of body.	**2. Very Limited** Responds only to painful stimuli. Cannot communicate discomfort except by moaning or restlessness OR has a sensory impairment that limits the ability to feel pain or discomfort over half of body.	**3. Slightly Limited** Responds to verbal commands, but cannot always communicate discomfort or the need to be turned. OR has some sensory impairment that limits ability to feel pain or discomfort in one or two extremities.	**4. No Impairment** Responds to verbal commands. Has no sensory deficit that would limit ability to feel or voice pain or discomfort.				
Moisture Degree to which skin is exposed to moisture	**1. Constantly Moist** Skin is kept moist almost constantly by perspiration, urine, etc. Dampness is detected every time patient is moved or turned.	**2. Very Moist** Skin is often, but not always, moist. Linen must be changed at least once a shift.	**3. Occasionally Moist** Skin is occasionally moist, requiring an extra linen change approximately once a day.	**4. Rarely Moist** Skin is usually dry, linen only requires changing at routine intervals.				
Activity Degree of physical activity	**1. Bedfast** Confined to bed.	**2. Chairfast** Ability to walk severely limited or nonexistent. Cannot bear own weight and/or must be assisted into chair or wheelchair.	**3. Walks Occasionally** Walks occasionally during day, but for very short distances, with or without assistance. Spends majority of each shift in bed or chair.	**4. Walks Frequently** Walks outside room at least twice a day and inside room at least once every 2 hours during waking hours.				
Mobility Ability to change and control body position	**1. Completely Immobile** Does not make even slight changes in body or extremity position without assistance.	**2. Very Limited** Makes occasional slight changes in body or extremity position but unable to make frequent or significant changes independently.	**3. Slightly Limited** Makes frequent though slight changes in body or extremity position independently.	**4. No Limitation** Makes major and frequent changes in position without assistance.				
Nutrition Usual food intake pattern	**1. Very Poor** Never eats a complete meal. Rarely eats more than a 1/3 of any food offered. Eats 2 servings or less of protein (meat or dairy products) per day. Takes fluids poorly. Does not take a liquid dietary supplement OR is NPO and/or maintained on clear liquids or IVs for more than 5 days.	**2. Probably Inadequate** Rarely eats a complete meal and generally eats only about 1/2 of any food offered. Protein intake includes only 3 servings of meat or dairy products per day. Occasionally will take a dietary supplement OR receives less than optimum amount of liquid diet or tube feeding.	**3. Adequate** Eats half of most meals. Eats a total of 4 servings of protein (meat, dairy products) per day. Occasionally will refuse a meal, but will usually take a supplement when offered OR is on a tube feeding or TPN regimen, which probably meets most of nutritional needs.	**4. Excellent** Eats most of every meal. Never refuses a meal. Usually eats a total of 4 or more servings of meat and dairy products. Occasionally eats between meals. Does not require supplementation.				
Friction and Shear	**1. Problem** Requires moderate to maximum assistance in moving. Complete lifting without sliding against sheets is impossible. Frequently slides down in bed or chair, requiring frequent repositioning with maximum assistance. Spasticity, contractures, or agitation leads to almost constant friction.	**2. Potential Problem** Moves feebly or requires minimum assistance. During a move, skin probably slides to some extent against sheets, chair, restraints, or other devices. Maintains relatively good position in chair or bed most of the time but occasionally slides down.	**3. No Apparent Problem** Moves in bed and in chair independently and has sufficient muscle strength to lift up completely during move. Maintains good position in bed or chair.					
				Total Score				

NPO, nothing by mouth; TPN, total parenteral nutrition.

◢ **Quality and Safety Nursing Alert**

Pressure ulcers are associated with increased costs of treatment and length of hospital stay as well as diminished quality of life for patients. It is imperative that nurses perform a skin assessment on every patient admitted to a hospital, inpatient rehabilitation facility, or skilled nursing facility.

Immobility. When a person is immobile and inactive, pressure is exerted on the skin and subcutaneous tissue by objects on which the person rests, such as a mattress, chair seat, or cast. The development of pressure ulcers is directly related to the duration of immobility: If pressure continues long enough, small vessel thrombosis and tissue necrosis occur and a pressure ulcer results. Weight-bearing bony prominences are most susceptible to pressure ulcer development because they are covered only by skin and small amounts of subcutaneous tissue. Susceptible areas include the sacrum and coccygeal areas, ischial tuberosities (especially in people who sit for prolonged periods), greater trochanter, heel, knee, malleolus, medial condyle of the tibia, fibular head, scapula, and elbow (see Fig. 10-5).

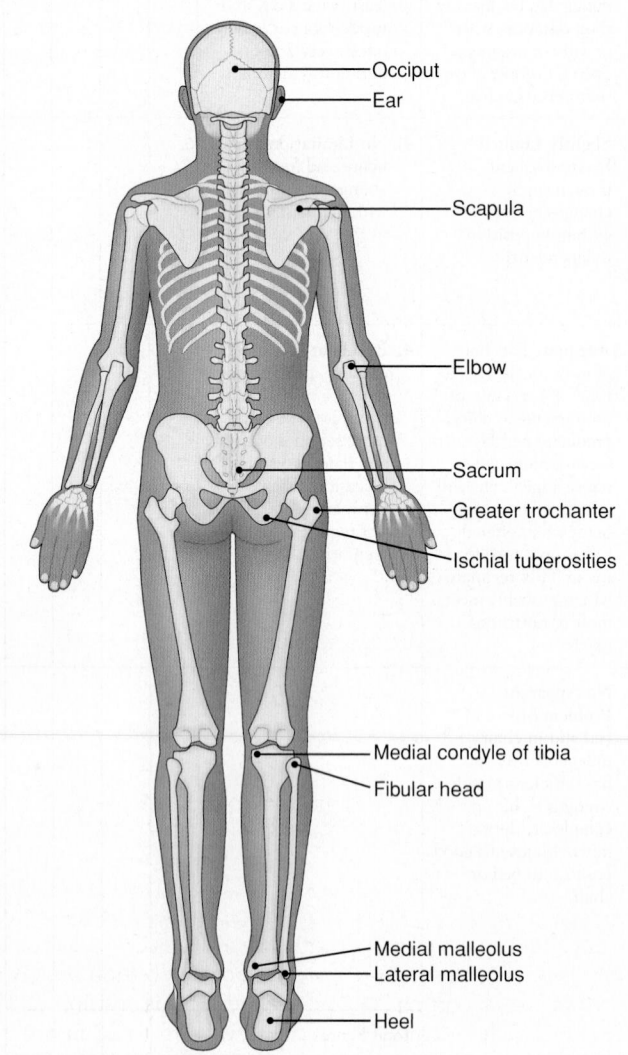

Figure 10-5 • Areas susceptible to pressure ulcers.

Impaired Sensory Perception or Cognition. Patients with sensory loss, impaired level of consciousness, or paralysis may not be aware of the discomfort associated with prolonged pressure on the skin and therefore may not change their positions to relieve the pressure. This prolonged pressure impedes blood flow, reducing nourishment of the skin and underlying tissues. A pressure ulcer may develop in a short period of time.

Decreased Tissue Perfusion. Any condition that reduces the circulation and nourishment of the skin and subcutaneous tissue (altered peripheral tissue perfusion) increases the risk of pressure ulcer development. Patients with diabetes have compromised microcirculation. Similarly, patients with edema have impaired circulation and poor nourishment of the skin tissue. Patients who are obese have large amounts of poorly vascularized adipose tissue, which is susceptible to breakdown.

Nutritional Status. Nutritional deficiencies, anemias, and metabolic disorders also contribute to the development of pressure ulcers. Anemia, regardless of its cause, decreases the blood's oxygen-carrying ability and predisposes the patient to pressure ulcers. Poor nutritional status can prolong the inflammatory phase of pressure ulcer healing and can reduce the quality and strength of wound healing (Thomas, 2015). Serum albumin and prealbumin levels are sensitive indicators of protein deficiency. Serum albumin levels of less than 3 g/dL are associated with hypoalbuminemic tissue edema and increased risk of pressure ulcers. Prealbumin levels are more sensitive indicators of protein status than albumin levels, but they are more costly to assess. The nurse should assess the patient's prealbumin and albumin values and electrolyte panel.

Friction and Shear. Mechanical forces also contribute to the development of pressure ulcers. Friction is the force of rubbing two surfaces against one another and is often caused by pulling a patient over a bed sheet (commonly known as sheet burn) or from a poorly fitted prosthetic device. Shear is the result of gravity pushing down on the patient's body and the resistance between the patient and the chair or bed (National Pressure Ulcer Advisory Panel, 2014). When shear occurs, tissue layers slide over one another, blood vessels stretch and twist, and the microcirculation of the skin and subcutaneous tissue is disrupted. Evidence of deep tissue damage may be slow to develop and may present through the development of a **sinus tract**, which is an area of destroyed tissue that extends from the edge of a wound. The sacrum and heels are most susceptible to the effects of shear. Pressure ulcers from friction and shear occur when the patient slides down in bed (see Fig. 10-6) or when the patient is positioned or moved improperly (e.g., dragged up in bed). Spastic muscles and paralysis increase the patient's vulnerability to pressure ulcers related to friction and shear.

Increased Moisture. Prolonged contact with moisture from perspiration, urine, feces, or drainage produces maceration (softening) of the skin. The skin reacts to caustic substances in the excreta or drainage and becomes irritated. Moist, irritated skin is more vulnerable to pressure breakdown. Once the skin breaks, the area is invaded by microorganisms (e.g., streptococci, staphylococci, *Pseudomonas aeruginosa*, *Escherichia coli*), and infection occurs. Foul-smelling infectious drainage is present. The lesion may enlarge and allow a continuous loss of serum, which may further deplete the body of essential protein needed for tissue repair and maintenance. The lesion may continue to enlarge and extend deep into the fascia, muscle, and bone, with multiple sinus tracts radiating from the pressure

Figure 10-6 • Mechanical forces contribute to pressure ulcer development. As the person slides down or is improperly pulled up in bed, *friction* resists this movement. *Shear* occurs when one layer of tissue slides over another, disrupting microcirculation of skin and subcutaneous tissue.

ulcer. With extensive pressure ulcers, life-threatening infections and sepsis may develop, frequently from gram-negative organisms.

Gerontologic Considerations. In older adults, the normal aging process leads to diminished epidermal thickness, dermal collagen, and tissue elasticity. The skin is drier as a result of diminished sebaceous and sweat gland activity. Cardiovascular changes result in decreased tissue perfusion. Muscles atrophy and bone structures become prominent. Diminished sensory perception and reduced ability to reposition oneself contribute to prolonged pressure on the skin. Therefore, older adults are more susceptible to pressure ulcers, which cause pain, suffering, and reduced quality of life.

Bariatric Considerations. In 2014, an international collaborative comprising members from the U.S. National Pressure Ulcer Advisory Panel (NPUAP), European Pressure Ulcer Advisory Panel (EPUAP), and the PanPacific Pressure Advisory Panel (PPPUAP) released the *Prevention and Treatment of Pressure Ulcers; Clinical Practice Guideline* (Dunk & Carville, 2015; National Pressure Ulcer Advisory Panel, 2014). These updated guidelines include recommendations for adults who are obese with specific organization-level considerations, recommendations for the bariatric individual, as well as recommendations for bed and equipment selection and repositioning. Please see the NPUAP Web site link at the end of this chapter to review the quick reference guideline.

ASSESSMENT OF SKIN AND EXISTING ULCERS

In addition to assessing risk, nursing actions to assess skin include:
- Assess total skin condition at least twice a day.
- Inspect each pressure site for erythema.
- Assess areas of erythema for blanching response.
- Palpate the skin for increased warmth.
- Inspect for dry skin, moist skin, and breaks in skin.
- Note drainage and odor.

If a pressure ulcer is seen, the nurse documents its size and location and uses a grading system to describe severity and provides a description of the site (see Chart 10-7). The appearance of purulent drainage or foul odor suggests an infection. With an extensive pressure ulcer, deep pockets of infection are often present. Drying and crusting of exudate may be present. Infection of a pressure ulcer may advance to osteomyelitis, pyarthrosis (pus formation within a joint cavity), sepsis, and septic shock.

Nursing Diagnosis

Based on the assessment data, nursing diagnoses may include the following:
- Risk for impaired skin integrity
- Impaired skin integrity related to immobility, decreased sensory perception, decreased tissue perfusion, decreased nutritional status, friction and shear forces, excessive moisture, or advanced age

Planning and Goals

The major goals may include relief of pressure, improved mobility, improved sensory perception, improved tissue perfusion, improved nutritional status, minimized friction and shear forces, dry surfaces in contact with skin, and healing of pressure ulcer, if present.

Nursing Interventions

RELIEVING PRESSURE

Frequent changes of position are needed to relieve and redistribute the pressure on the patient's skin and to promote blood flow to the skin and subcutaneous tissues. This can be accomplished by instructing the patient to change position or by turning and repositioning the patient. The patient's family members should be educated about how to position and turn the patient at home to prevent pressure ulcers. Shifting weight allows the blood to flow into the ischemic areas and helps tissues recover from the effects of pressure. Attention should be paid to patient migration (moving down in the bed) in those on bed rest, particularly when the head of the bed is elevated (Wiggermann, Kotowski, Davis, et al., 2015).

For patients who spend long periods in a wheelchair, pressure can be relieved by:
- *Push-ups:* The patient pushes down on armrests and raises buttocks off the seat of the chair (see Fig. 10-7).
- *One half push-up:* The patient repeats the push-up on the right side and then the left, pushing up on one side by pushing down on the armrest.
- *Moving side to side:* The patient moves from one side to the other while sitting in the chair.
- *Shifting:* The patient bends forward with the head down between the knees (if able) and constantly shifts in the chair.

POSITIONING THE PATIENT

The degree of ability to move independently—the comfort, fatigue, loss of sensation, overall physical and mental status, and specific disorder—influences plans for changing position. Patients should be positioned laterally, prone, and dorsally in sequence unless a position is not tolerated or is contraindicated. Generally, those who experience discomfort after 30 to 60 minutes of lying prone need to be repositioned. The recumbent position is preferred to the semi-Fowler position because of increased supporting body surface area in this position.

Patients able to shift their weight every 15 to 20 minutes and move independently may change total position every 2 to 4 hours. Indications for routine repositioning every 2 hours

Chart 10-7 Stages in the Development of Pressure Ulcers

Suspected Deep Tissue Injury

- There may be a purple or maroon localized area of discolored intact skin or blood-filled blister.
- The area may be preceded in appearance by tissue that is painful, firm, mushy, boggy, and warmer or cooler as compared to adjacent tissue.
- Evolution may include a thin blister over a dark wound bed.
- The wound may further evolve and become covered by thin eschar.
- Evolution may be rapid, exposing additional layers of tissue even with optimal treatment.

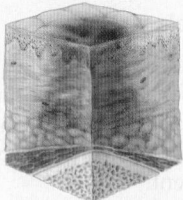

Stage I

- Intact skin
- Nonblanchable redness of a localized area, usually over a bony prominence
- Darkly pigmented skin may not have visible blanching.
- Color may differ from surrounding area.
- Area may be painful, firm, soft, and warmer or cooler as compared to adjacent tissue.

Stage II

- Partial thickness loss of dermis, presenting as a shallow open ulcer with red-pink wound bed without slough
- May present as an intact or open/ruptured serum-filled blister
- May present as a shiny or dry shallow ulcer without slough or bruising; bruising indicates suspected deep tissue injury
- Does not include skin tears, tape burns, perineal dermatitis, maceration, or excoriation

Stage III

- Full-thickness tissue loss
- Subcutaneous fat may be visible; however, bone, tendon, or muscle is not exposed.

- Slough may be present but does not obscure the depth of tissue loss.
- May include undermining and tunneling
- Depth of a stage III pressure ulcer varies by anatomic location. The bridge of the nose, ear, occiput, and malleolus do not have subcutaneous tissue; stage III ulcers can be shallow in these areas. Areas of significant adiposity can develop extremely deep stage III pressure ulcers.

Stage IV

- Ulcer presents with full-thickness tissue loss with exposed bone, tendon, or muscle.
- Slough or eschar may be present on some parts of the wound.
- Often includes undermining and tunneling
- Depth of a stage IV pressure ulcer varies by anatomic location. The bridge of the nose, ear, occiput, and malleolus do not have subcutaneous tissue; stage IV ulcers can be shallow in these areas. Stage IV ulcers can extend into muscle and/or supporting structures (e.g., fascia, tendon, or joint capsule); osteomyelitis is possible. Exposed bone/tendon is visible or directly palpable.

Unstageable

- Full-thickness tissue loss in which the base of the ulcer is covered by slough (yellow, tan, gray, green, or brown) and/or eschar (tan, brown, or black) in the wound bed
- Until enough slough and/or eschar is removed to expose the base of the wound, the true depth, and therefore stage, cannot be determined.
- Stable (dry, adherent, intact without erythema or fluctuance) eschar on the heels serves as "the body's natural (biological) cover" and should not be removed.

Adapted from Peirce, B., Dale, B., Mackey, D., & McNichol, L. (2014). Wound, Ostomy and Continence Nurses Society's Guidance on OASIS-C1 Integumentary Items: Best Practice for Clinicians. Adapted from: //c.ymcdn.com/sites/www.wocn.org/resource/resmgr/Publications/ WOCN_Guidance_on_OASIS-C1_In.pdf
NPUAP Pressure Ulcer Category/Staging Illustrations. Illustrations used with permission of the National Pressure Ulcer Advisory Panel, 2015.09.14. © NPUAP.

Figure 10-7 • Wheelchair push-up to prevent ischial pressure ulcers. These push-ups should become an automatic routine (every 15 minutes) for the person with paraplegia. The person should stay up and out of contact with the seat for several seconds. The wheels are kept in the locked position during the exercise.

or more frequently include loss of sensation, paralysis, coma, and edema.

In addition to regular turning, small shifts of body weight, such as repositioning of an ankle, elbow, or shoulder, are necessary. The skin is inspected at each position change and assessed for temperature elevation. If redness or heat is noted or if the patient complains of discomfort, pressure on the area must be relieved.

Another way to relieve pressure over bony prominences is the bridging technique, accomplished through the correct positioning of pillows. Just as a bridge is supported on pillars to allow traffic to move underneath, the body can be supported by pillows to allow for space between bony prominences and the mattress. A pillow or commercial heel protector may be used to support the heels off the bed when the patient is supine. Placing pillows superior and inferior to the sacrum relieves sacral pressure. Supporting the patient in a 30-degree side-lying position avoids pressure on the trochanter. In older adult patients, frequent small shifts of body weight may be effective. Placing a small rolled towel or sheepskin under a shoulder or hip allows a return of blood flow to the skin in the area on which the patient is sitting or lying. The towel or sheepskin is moved around the patient's pressure points in a clockwise fashion. A turning schedule can help the family keep track of the patient's turns.

Using Pressure-Relieving Devices

At times, specialty beds or alternative bed surfaces may be indicated to help relieve the pressure on the skin (Stifter, Yao, Lodhi, et al., 2015). This is particularly important for patients who cannot get out of bed and who are at high risk for pressure ulcer development. These devices are designed to provide support for specific body areas or to distribute pressure evenly.

A patient who sits in a wheelchair for prolonged periods should have wheelchair cushions fitted and adjusted on an individualized basis, using pressure measurement techniques as a guide to selection and fitting. The aim is to redistribute pressure away from areas at risk for ulcers; however, no cushion can eliminate excessive pressure completely. The patient should be reminded to shift weight frequently and to rise for a few seconds every 15 minutes while sitting in a chair.

Static support devices (e.g., high-density foam, air, or liquid mattress overlays) distribute pressure evenly by bringing more of the patient's body surface into contact with the supporting surface. Gel-type flotation pads and air-fluidized beds reduce pressure. The weight of a body floating on a fluid system is evenly distributed over the entire supporting surface. Therefore, as the body sinks into the fluid, additional surface becomes available for weight bearing, body weight per unit area is decreased, and there is less pressure on the body parts.

Soft, moisture-absorbing padding is also useful because the softness and resilience of padding provide for more even distribution of pressure and the dissipation and absorption of moisture, along with freedom from wrinkles and friction. Bony prominences may be protected by gel pads, sheepskin padding, or soft foam rubber beneath the sacrum, the trochanters, heels, elbows, scapulae, and back of the head when there is pressure on these sites. One group of researchers found that sacral pressure was reduced using a liquid-based pad that covers only the sacral area and can be applied on any bed surface (Duetzmann, Forsey, Senft, et al., 2015).

Specialized beds are designed to prevent pressure on the skin. Air-fluidized beds allow the patient to float. Dynamic support surfaces, such as low air-loss pockets, alternately inflate and deflate sections to change support pressure for very high risk patients who are critically ill and **debilitated** (i.e., impaired strength, weakened, injured, disabled) and cannot be repositioned to relieve pressure. Oscillating or kinetic beds change pressure by means of rocking movements of the bed that redistribute the patient's weight and stimulate circulation. These beds may be used with patients who have injuries attributed to multiple trauma. Specialized beds, which are more expensive than mattress overlays, are no more effective at preventing pressure ulcers than the overlays; there is insufficient evidence to support the choice of one specific bed surface over another (Qaseem, Humphrey, Forciea, et al., 2015).

Improving Mobility

The patient is encouraged to remain active and is ambulated whenever possible. When sitting, the patient is reminded to change positions frequently to redistribute weight. Active and passive exercises increase muscular, skin, and vascular tone. For patients at risk for pressure ulcers, turning and exercise schedules are essential, and repositioning must occur around the clock.

Improving Sensory Perception

The nurse helps the patient recognize and compensate for altered sensory perception. Depending on the origin of the alteration (e.g., decreased level of consciousness, spinal cord lesion), specific interventions are selected. Strategies to improve cognition and sensory perception may include stimulating the patient to increase awareness of self in the environment, encouraging the patient to participate in self-care, or supporting the patient's efforts toward active compensation for loss of sensation (e.g., a patient with paraplegia lifting up from the sitting position every 15 minutes). A patient with quadriplegia should be weight shifted every 30 minutes while sitting in a wheelchair. When decreased sensory perception exists, the patient and caregivers are taught to inspect potential pressure areas visually every morning and evening, using a mirror if necessary, for evidence of pressure ulcer development.

IMPROVING TISSUE PERFUSION

Activity, exercise, and repositioning improve tissue perfusion. Massage of erythematous areas is avoided because damage to the capillaries and deep tissue may occur (National Pressure Ulcer Advisory Panel, 2014).

 Quality and Safety Nursing Alert

The nurse should avoid massaging reddened areas because this may increase the damage to already traumatized skin and tissue.

In patients who have evidence of compromised peripheral circulation (e.g., edema), positioning and elevation of the edematous body part to promote venous return and diminish congestion improve tissue perfusion. In addition, the nurse or family must be alert to environmental factors (e.g., wrinkles in sheets, pressure of tubes) that may contribute to pressure on the skin and diminished circulation and remove the source of pressure.

IMPROVING NUTRITIONAL STATUS

The patient's nutritional status must be adequate, and a positive nitrogen balance must be maintained because pressure ulcers develop more quickly and are more resistant to treatment in patients with nutritional disorders. A high-protein diet with protein supplements may be helpful. Iron preparations may be necessary to raise the hemoglobin concentration so that tissue oxygen levels can be maintained within acceptable limits. Ascorbic acid (vitamin C) is necessary for tissue healing. Other nutrients associated with healthy skin include vitamin A, B vitamins, zinc, and sulfur. With adequate nutrition and hydration, the skin can remain healthy, and damaged tissues can be repaired (Posthauer, Banks, Dorner, et al., 2015; Saha, Smith, Totten, et al., 2013).

To assess the patient's nutritional status in response to therapeutic strategies, the nurse monitors the patient's hemoglobin, pre-albumin level, and body weight weekly. Nutritional assessment is described in further detail in Chapter 5.

REDUCING FRICTION AND SHEAR

Raising the head of the bed by even a few centimeters increases the shearing force over the sacral area; therefore, the semi-reclining position is avoided in patients at risk. Proper positioning with adequate support is also important when the patient is sitting in a chair.

 Quality and Safety Nursing Alert

To avoid shearing forces when repositioning patients, the nurse must lift and avoid dragging patients across a surface. Lift devices should be used to prevent occupational injuries.

MINIMIZING IRRITATING MOISTURE

Continuous moisture on the skin must be prevented by meticulous hygiene measures. It is important to pay special attention to skin folds, including areas under the breasts, arms, and groin, and between the toes. Perspiration, urine, stool, and drainage must be removed from the skin promptly. The soiled skin should be washed immediately with mild soap and water and blotted dry with a soft towel. The skin may be lubricated with a bland lotion to keep it soft and pliable. Drying agents and powders are avoided. Topical barrier ointments (e.g., petroleum jelly) may be helpful in protecting the skin of patients who are incontinent.

Absorbent pads that wick moisture away from the body should be used to absorb drainage. Patients who are incontinent need to be checked regularly and have their wet incontinence pads and linens changed promptly. Their skin needs to be cleansed and dried promptly.

PROMOTING PRESSURE ULCER HEALING

Regardless of the stage of the pressure ulcer, the pressure on the area must be eliminated because the ulcer will not heal until all pressure is removed. The patient must not lie or sit on the pressure ulcer, even for a few minutes. Individualized positioning and turning schedules must be written in the plan of nursing care and followed meticulously.

In addition, inadequate nutritional status and fluid and electrolyte abnormalities must be corrected to promote healing. Wounds from which body fluids and protein drain place the patient in a catabolic state and predispose to hypoproteinemia and serious secondary infections. Protein deficiency must be corrected to promote the healing of the pressure ulcer. Carbohydrates are necessary to "spare" the protein and to provide an energy source. Vitamin C and trace elements, especially zinc, are necessary for collagen formation and wound healing. (Refer to Chart 10-7 for descriptions of stages of pressure ulcers.)

Deep Tissue Injury. These tissue injuries may evolve rapidly, and immediate pressure relief to the affected area is indicated. Therefore, the nurse must be vigilant in assessing for these types of injuries (Dunk & Carville, 2015; National Pressure Ulcer Advisory Panel, 2014).

Stage I Pressure Ulcers. To permit healing of stage I pressure ulcers, the pressure is removed to allow increased tissue perfusion, nutritional and fluid and electrolyte balance is maintained, friction and shear are reduced, and moisture to the skin is avoided (Dunk & Carville, 2015; National Pressure Ulcer Advisory Panel, 2014).

Stage II Pressure Ulcers. In addition to measures listed for stage I pressure ulcers, a moist environment, in which migration of epidermal cells over the ulcer surface occurs more rapidly, should be provided to aid wound healing. The ulcer is gently cleansed with sterile saline solution. The use of a heat lamp to dry the open wound is avoided, as is the use of antiseptic solutions that damage healthy tissues and delay wound healing. Semipermeable occlusive dressings, hydrocolloid wafers, or wet saline dressings are helpful in providing a moist environment for healing and in minimizing the loss of fluids and proteins from the body (Dunk & Carville, 2015; National Pressure Ulcer Advisory Panel, 2014).

Stage III Pressure Ulcers. Stage III pressure ulcers are characterized by extensive tissue damage, including **slough** (i.e., soft, moist avascular tissue), tunneling (i.e., formation of a sinus tract), and **undermining** (i.e., extensive tunneling under wound edge), to name a few. Given the extensive damage to tissue and necrosis that characterize stage III pressure ulcers, they must be cleaned (débrided) to create an area that will heal, in addition to the measures listed for stage I pressure ulcers. Necrotic, devitalized tissue favors bacterial growth, delays granulation, and inhibits healing. Wound cleaning and dressing are uncomfortable; therefore, the nurse must prepare the patient for the procedure by explaining what will occur and administering prescribed analgesia (Dunk & Carville, 2015; National Pressure Ulcer Advisory Panel, 2014).

Stage IV Pressure Ulcers. Surgical interventions are required for these extensive pressure ulcers (National Pressure Ulcer Advisory Panel, 2014). (See the following Other Treatment Methods section.)

OTHER TREATMENT METHODS

Débridement may be accomplished by wet-to-damp dressing changes, mechanical flushing of necrotic and infective exudate, application of prescribed enzyme preparations that dissolve necrotic tissue, or surgical dissection. If eschar (dry scab) covers the ulcer, it is removed surgically to ensure the wound is clean and vitalized. Exudate may be absorbed by dressings or special hydrophilic powders, beads, or gels. Cultures of infected pressure ulcers are obtained to guide the selection of antibiotic therapy.

After the pressure ulcer is clean, a topical treatment is prescribed to promote granulation. New granulation tissue must be protected from reinfection, drying, and damage, and care should be taken to prevent pressure and further trauma to the area. Dressings, solutions, and ointments applied to the ulcer should not disrupt the healing process. For chronic, noninfected ulcers that are healing by secondary intention (healing of an open wound from the base upward by laying down new tissue), vacuum-assisted closure (VAC) or hyperbaric oxygen treatment may be used. VAC involves the use of a negative-pressure sponge dressing in the wound to increase blood flow, increasing formation of granulation tissue and nutrient uptake and decreasing bacterial load. Hyperbaric oxygen therapy involves either the application of topical oxygen at increased pressure directly to the wound or placing the patient into a hyperbaric oxygen chamber. Both methods of hyperbaric oxygen therapy promote wound healing by stimulating new vascular growth and aiding in the preservation of damaged tissue (Dauwe, Pulikkottil, Lavery, et al., 2014). In a recent systematic review, Stoekenbroek, Santema, Legemate, et al. (2014) reported that hyperbaric oxygen therapy improves healing in patients with diabetic leg ulcers; however, more studies are needed prior to routinely introducing this therapy into clinical practice.

Multiple agents and protocols are used to treat pressure ulcers; however, consistency is an important key to success. Objective evaluation of the pressure ulcer (e.g., measurement of the size and depth of the pressure ulcer, inspection for granulation tissue) for response to the treatment protocol must be made every 4 to 6 days. Taking photographs at weekly intervals is a reliable strategy for monitoring the healing process, which may take weeks to months.

Surgical intervention is necessary when the ulcer is extensive, when complications (e.g., fistula) exist, and when the ulcer does not respond to treatment. Surgical procedures include débridement, incision and drainage, bone resection, and skin grafting. Osteomyelitis is a common complication of wounds of stage IV depth. (See Chapter 41 for more information on osteomyelitis.)

PREVENTING RECURRENCE

It may take more than a year for healing tissue to regain the strength of pre-injury skin; thus, care must be taken to prevent recurrence of pressure ulcers. However, recurrence of pressure ulcers should be anticipated; therefore, active, preventive intervention and frequent continuing assessments are essential. For example, pressure ulcers are the second most comorbid problem in patients with SCI with 85% of patients with SCI developing a pressure ulcer at least once in their lifetime (Scheel-Sailer, Wyss, Boldt, et al., 2013). The patient's tolerance for sitting or lying on the healed pressure area is increased gradually by increasing the time that pressure is allowed on the area in 5- to 15-minute increments. The patient is instructed to increase mobility and to follow a regimen of turning, weight shifting, and repositioning. The patient education plan includes strategies to reduce the risk of pressure ulcers and methods to detect, inspect, and minimize pressure areas. Early recognition and intervention are keys to long-term management of potential impaired skin integrity. Gould, Olney, Nichols, et al. (2014) suggest immobility and incontinence are among modifiable risk factors that contribute to recurrent pressure ulcer development, particularly in patients with SCI; they suggest the development of structured guidelines to prevent pressure ulcers rests on the identification of factors that differ in patients with SCI who have none, one, or more pressure ulcers. Identifying potentially modifiable risk factors or protective factors may then lead to evidence-based risk assessment tools and interventions customized to patient-specific risks.

Evaluation

Expected patient outcomes may include:
1. Maintains intact skin
   a. Exhibits no areas of nonblanchable erythema at bony prominences
   b. Avoids massage of bony prominences
   c. Exhibits no breaks in skin
2. Limits pressure on bony prominences
   a. Changes position every 1 to 2 hours
   b. Uses bridging techniques to reduce pressure
   c. Uses special equipment as appropriate
   d. Raises self from seat of wheelchair every 15 minutes
3. Increases mobility
   a. Performs range-of-motion exercises
   b. Adheres to turning schedule
   c. Advances sitting time as tolerated
4. Has improved sensory and cognitive ability
   a. Demonstrates improved level of consciousness
   b. Remembers to inspect potential pressure ulcer areas every morning and evening
5. Demonstrates improved tissue perfusion
   a. Exercises to increase circulation
   b. Elevates body parts susceptible to edema
6. Attains and maintains adequate nutritional status
   a. Verbalizes the importance of protein and vitamin C in diet

b. Eats diet high in protein and vitamin C
c. Exhibits acceptable levels of hemoglobin, electrolyte, prealbumin, transferrin, and creatinine
7. Avoids friction and shear
a. Avoids semireclining position
b. Uses heel protectors when appropriate
c. Lifts body instead of sliding across surfaces
8. Maintains clean, dry skin
a. Avoids prolonged contact with wet or soiled surfaces
b. Keeps skin clean and dry
c. Uses lotion to keep skin lubricated

NURSING PROCESS

The Patient With Altered Elimination Patterns

Urinary incontinence and bowel incontinence or constipation and impaction are problems that often occur in patients with disabilities. Incontinence curtails the person's independence, causing embarrassment and isolation. Based on structured oral interviews conducted to collect data on bothersome urinary or fecal incontinence in adults aged 50 and older, 20% of women and 6.4% of men reported urinary incontinence (less than once/month, a few times/month, a few times/week or every day/night) (Gorina, Schappert, Bercovitz, et al., 2014; Roe, Flanagan, & Maden, 2015). Fecal incontinence (leakage of gas, mucus, liquid or solid stool at least monthly) was reported by 8.2% of women and 8.4% of men (Wu, Matthews, Vaughan, et al., 2015). Internationally, nearly 55% of nursing home residents will experience bowel and/or bladder incontinence at some point (Mandl, Halfens, & Lohrmann, 2015). For patients with disabilities who experience constipation, complete and predictable evacuation of the bowel is the goal. If a bowel routine is not established, the patient may experience abdominal distention; small, frequent oozing of stool; or impaction.

Assessment

Urinary incontinence may result from multiple causes, including urinary tract infection, detrusor instability, bladder outlet obstruction or incompetence, neurologic impairment, bladder spasm or contracture, and inability to reach the toilet in time. Urinary incontinence can be classified as urge, reflex, stress, functional, overflow, or total (Herdman & Kamitsuru, 2014):

- *Urge incontinence* occurs when involuntary elimination of urine is associated with a strong perceived need to void.
- *Reflex (neurogenic) incontinence* is associated with a spinal cord lesion that interrupts cerebral control, resulting in no sensory awareness of the need to void.
- *Stress incontinence* is associated with weakened perineal muscles that permit leakage of urine when intra-abdominal pressure is increased (e.g., with coughing or sneezing).
- *Functional incontinence* occurs in patients with intact urinary physiology who experience mobility impairment, environmental barriers, or cognitive problems and cannot reach and use the toilet before soiling themselves.
- *Overflow urinary incontinence* is described as the involuntary loss of urine associated with overdistention of the bladder. Reasons for overdistention and urine leakage

vary, but may be related to improper emptying of the bladder, fecal impaction, urethral obstruction, or medication side effect.
- *Total urinary incontinence* occurs in patients who cannot control urine because of physiologic or psychological impairment. Management of the urine is an essential focus of nursing care.

ELIMINATION ASSESSMENT

The health history is used to explore bladder and bowel function, symptoms associated with dysfunction, physiologic risk factors for elimination problems, perception of micturition (urination, or voiding), and functional toileting abilities. Previous and current fluid intake and voiding patterns may be helpful in designing the plan of nursing care. A record of times of voiding and amounts voided is kept for at least 48 hours. In addition, episodes of incontinence and associated activity (e.g., coughing, sneezing, lifting), fluid intake time and amount, and medications are recorded. This record is analyzed and used to determine patterns and relationships of incontinence to other activities and factors.

The ability to get to the bathroom, manipulate clothing, and use the toilet are important functional factors that may be related to incontinence. Related cognitive functioning (perception of need to void, verbalization of need to void, and ability to learn to control urination) must also be assessed. In addition, the nurse reviews the results of the diagnostic studies (e.g., urinalysis, urodynamic tests, post-voiding residual volumes).

Bowel incontinence and constipation may result from multiple causes, such as diminished or absent sphincter control, cognitive or perceptual impairment, neurogenic factors, diet, and immobility. The origin of the bowel problem must be determined. The nurse assesses the patient's normal bowel patterns, nutritional patterns, use of laxatives, gastrointestinal problems (e.g., colitis), bowel sounds, anal reflex and tone, and functional abilities. The character and frequency of bowel movements are recorded and analyzed.

Nursing Diagnosis

Based on the assessment data, major nursing diagnoses may include the following:

- Functional urinary incontinence
- Urge urinary incontinence
- Reflex urinary incontinence
- Stress urinary incontinence
- Impaired urinary elimination
- Overflow urinary incontinence
- Urinary retention
- Constipation
- Bowel incontinence

Planning and Goals

The major goals may include control of urinary incontinence or urinary retention, control of bowel incontinence, and regular elimination patterns.

Nursing Interventions

PROMOTING URINARY CONTINENCE

After the nature of the urinary incontinence has been identified, a plan of nursing care is developed based on an analysis of the assessment data. Various approaches to promote urinary continence have been developed (Roe, Flanagan, & Maden, 2015). Most approaches attempt to condition the body to control urination or to minimize the occurrence of unscheduled urination. Selection of the approach depends on the cause and type of the incontinence. For the program to be successful, participation by the patient and a desire to avoid incontinence episodes are crucial; an optimistic attitude with positive feedback for even slight gains is essential for success. Accurate recording of intake and output and of the patient's response to selected strategies is essential for evaluation.

At no time should the fluid intake be restricted to decrease the frequency of urination. Sufficient fluid intake (2,000 to 3,000 mL per day, according to patient needs) must be ensured. To optimize the likelihood of voiding as scheduled, measured amounts of fluids may be given about 30 minutes before voiding attempts. In addition, most of the fluids should be consumed before evening to minimize the need to void frequently during the night.

> ### ⚑ Quality and Safety Nursing Alert
>
> *Carbonated soft drinks, milk shakes, alcohol, tomato juice, and citrus fruit juices are alkaline-producing drinks that promote bacterial growth in the urine. Patients should be encouraged to drink more acid-producing fluids (e.g., cranberry and cranapple juice) to reduce the chance of urinary tract infection. Water is a preferred fluid because it flushes the kidneys and bladder.*

The goal of bladder training is to restore the bladder to normal function. Bladder training can be used with cognitively intact patients experiencing urge incontinence. A voiding and toileting schedule is developed based on an analysis of the assessment data. The schedule specifies times for the patient to try to empty the bladder using a bedpan, toilet, or commode. Privacy should be provided during voiding efforts. The interval between voiding times in the early phase of the bladder training period is short (90 to 120 minutes). The patient is encouraged not to void until the specified voiding time. Voiding success and episodes of incontinence are recorded. As the patient's bladder capacity and control increase, the interval is lengthened. Usually, there is a temporal relationship between drinking, eating, exercising, and voiding. Alert patients can participate in recording intake, activity, and voiding and can plan the schedule to achieve maximum continence. Barrier-free access to the toilet and modification of clothing can help patients with functional incontinence achieve self-care in toileting and continence.

Habit training is used to try to keep patients dry by strict adherence to a toileting schedule and may be successful with stress, urge, or functional incontinence. If the patient is confused, caregivers take the patient to the toilet according to the schedule before involuntary voiding occurs. Simple cuing and consistency promote success. Periods of continence and successful voiding are positively reinforced.

Biofeedback is a system through which patients learn to consciously contract urinary sphincters and control voiding cues. Cognitively intact patients who have stress or urge incontinence may gain bladder control through biofeedback.

Pelvic floor exercises (Kegel exercises) strengthen the pubococcygeus muscle. The patient is instructed to tighten the pelvic floor muscles for 4 seconds 10 times, and this is repeated 4 to 6 times a day. Stopping and starting the stream during urination is recommended to increase control. Daily practice is essential. These exercises are helpful for cognitively intact women who experience stress incontinence.

Suprapubic tapping or stroking of the inner thigh may produce voiding by stimulating the voiding reflex arc in patients with reflex incontinence. However, this method is not always effective, owing to a lack of detrusor sphincter muscle coordination. As the bladder reflexively contracts to expel urine, the bladder sphincter reflexively closes, producing a high residual urine volume and an increased incidence of urinary tract infection.

Intermittent self-catheterization is an appropriate alternative for managing reflex incontinence, urinary retention, and overflow incontinence attributed to an overdistended bladder. The nurse emphasizes regular emptying of the bladder rather than sterility. Patients with disabilities may reuse and clean catheters with bleach or hydrogen peroxide solutions or soap and water and may use a microwave oven to sterilize catheters. Aseptic intermittent catheterization technique is required in health care institutions because of the potential for bladder infection from resistant organisms. Intermittent self-catheterization may be difficult for patients with limited mobility, dexterity, or vision; however, family members can be taught the procedure.

Self-catheterization is also particularly pertinent for patients with SCI, because most of these patients do not have voluntary control of urination. Even those patients with spinal cord injuries who can voluntarily void should measure their residual urine (the amount of urine that remains in the bladder after voluntary or involuntary voiding) by self-catheterization.

Indwelling catheters are avoided if at all possible because of the high incidence of urinary tract infections associated with their use. Short-term use may be needed during treatment of severe skin breakdown due to continued incontinence. Patients with disabilities who cannot perform intermittent self-catheterization may elect to use suprapubic catheters for long-term bladder management. Suprapubic catheters are easier to maintain than indwelling catheters.

External catheters (condom catheters) and leg bags to collect spontaneous voidings are useful for male patients with reflex or total incontinence. The appropriate design and size must be chosen for maximal success, and the patient or caregiver must be taught how to apply the condom catheter and how to provide daily hygiene, including skin inspection. Instruction on emptying the leg bag must also be provided, and modifications can be made for patients with limited hand dexterity.

Incontinence pads (briefs) may be useful at times for patients with stress or total incontinence to protect clothing but should be avoided whenever possible. Incontinence pads only manage, rather than solve, the incontinence problem. In addition, they have a negative psychological effect on patients, because many people think of the pads as diapers. Every effort should be made to reduce the incidence of incontinence episodes through the other methods that have been described. When incontinence pads are used, they should wick moisture away from the body to minimize contact of moisture and excreta with the skin. Wet incontinence pads must be changed promptly, the skin cleansed, and a moisture barrier applied to protect the skin. It is important for the patient's self-esteem to avoid use of the term *diapers*.

PROMOTING BOWEL CONTINENCE

The goals of a bowel training program are to develop regular bowel habits and to prevent uninhibited bowel elimination. Regular, complete emptying of the lower bowel results in bowel continence. A bowel training program takes advantage of the patient's natural reflexes. Regularity, timing, nutrition and fluids, exercise, as well as correct positioning promote predictable defecation (Hotouras, Ribas, Allison, et al., 2014).

The nurse records defecation time, character of stool, nutritional intake, cognitive abilities, and functional self-care toileting abilities for 5 to 7 days. Analysis of this record is helpful when designing a bowel program for patients with fecal incontinence.

Consistency in implementing the plan is essential. A regular time for defecation is established, and attempts at evacuation should be made within 15 minutes of the designated time daily. Natural gastrocolic and duodenocolic reflexes occur about 30 minutes after a meal; therefore, after breakfast is one of the best times to plan for bowel evacuation. However, if the patient had a previously established habit pattern at a different time of day, it should be followed.

The anorectal reflex may be stimulated by a rectal suppository (e.g., glycerin) or by mechanical stimulation (e.g., digital stimulation with a lubricated gloved finger or anal dilator). Mechanical stimulation should be used only in patients with a disability who have no voluntary motor function and no sensation as a result of injuries above the sacral segments of the spinal cord, such as patients with quadriplegia, high paraplegia, or severe brain injuries. The technique is not effective in patients who do not have an intact sacral reflex arc (e.g., those with flaccid paralysis). Mechanical stimulation, suppository insertion, or both should be initiated about 30 minutes before the scheduled bowel elimination time, and the interval between stimulation and defecation is noted for subsequent modification of the bowel program. Once the bowel routine is well established, stimulation with a suppository may not be necessary.

The patient should assume the normal squatting position and be in a private bathroom for defecation if at all possible, although a padded commode chair or bedside toilet is an alternative. An elevated toilet seat is a simple modification that may make use of the toilet easier for the patient with a disability. Seating time is limited in patients who are at risk for skin breakdown. Bedpans should be avoided. A patient with a disability who cannot sit on a toilet should be positioned on the left side with legs flexed and the head of the bed elevated 30 to 45 degrees to increase intra-abdominal pressure. Protective padding is placed behind the buttocks. When possible, the patient is instructed to bear down and to contract the abdominal muscles. Massaging the abdomen from right to left facilitates movement of feces in the lower tract.

PREVENTING CONSTIPATION

The record of bowel elimination, character of stool, food and fluid intake, level of activity, bowel sounds, medications, and other assessment data are reviewed to develop the plan of care. Multiple approaches may be used to prevent constipation. The diet should include adequate intake of high-fiber foods (vegetables, fruits, bran) to prevent hard stools and to stimulate

peristalsis. Daily fluid intake should be 2 to 3 L unless contraindicated. Drinking prune juice (120 mL) 30 minutes before a meal once daily is helpful in some cases when constipation is a problem. Physical activity and exercise are encouraged, as is self-care in toileting. Patients are encouraged to respond to the natural urge to defecate. Privacy during toileting is provided. Stool softeners, bulk-forming agents, mild stimulants, and suppositories may be prescribed to stimulate defecation and to prevent constipation.

Evaluation

Expected patient outcomes may include:

1. Demonstrates control of bowel and bladder function
   a. Experiences no episodes of incontinence
   b. Avoids constipation
   c. Achieves independence in toileting
   d. Expresses satisfaction with level of bowel and bladder control
2. Achieves urinary continence
   a. Uses therapeutic approach that is appropriate to type of incontinence
   b. Maintains adequate fluid intake
   c. Washes and dries skin after episodes of incontinence
3. Achieves bowel continence
   a. Participates in bowel program
   b. Verbalizes need for regular time for bowel evacuation
   c. Modifies diet to promote continence
   d. Uses bowel stimulants as prescribed and needed
4. Experiences relief of constipation
   a. Uses high-fiber diet, fluids, and exercise to promote defecation
   b. Responds to urge to defecate

Promoting Home, Community-Based, and Transitional Care

An important goal of rehabilitation is to assist the patient to return to the home environment after learning to manage the disability. A referral system maintains continuity of care when the patient is transferred to the home or to a long-term care facility. The plan for discharge is formulated when the patient is first admitted to the hospital, and discharge plans are made with the patient's functional potential in mind.

 Educating Patients About Self-Care

Significant expenditures of time and resources are necessary to ensure that patients gain the skills and confidence to self-manage their health effectively after discharge from the hospital (Schmidt, 2013). Formal programs provide patients with effective strategies for interpreting and managing disease-specific issues and skills needed for problem solving, as well as building and maintaining self-awareness and self-efficacy. Self-care programs often use multifaceted approaches, including didactic teaching, group sessions, individual learning plans, and Web-based resources. When planning the approach to self-care, the nurse must consider the individual patient's knowledge, experience, social and cultural background, level of formal education, and psychological status.

The preparation for self-care must also be spread out over the course of the recovery period, and it must be monitored and updated regularly as the patient masters aspects of self-care. Preparation for self-care is also highly relevant for informal caregivers of patients in rehabilitation.

When a patient is discharged from acute care or a rehabilitation facility, informal caregivers, typically family members, often assume the care and support of the patient. Although the most obvious care tasks involve physical care (e.g., personal hygiene, dressing, meal preparation), other elements of the caregiving role include psychosocial support and a commitment to this supportive role. Thus, the nurse must assess the patient's support system (family, friends) well in advance of discharge. The positive attitudes of family and friends toward the patient, their disability, and the return home are important in making a successful transition to home. Not all families can carry out the arduous programs of exercise, physical therapy, and personal care that the patient may need. They may not have the resources or stability to care for family members with a severe disability. The physical, emotional, economic, and energy strains of a disabling condition may overwhelm even a stable family. Members of the rehabilitation team must not judge the family but rather should provide supportive interventions that help the family to attain its highest level of function.

The family members need to know as much as possible about the patient's condition and care so that they do not fear the patient's return home. The nurse develops methods to help the patient and family cope with problems that may arise. For example, the nurse may develop an ADL checklist individualized for the patient and family to ensure that the family is proficient in assisting the patient with certain tasks (see Chart 10-8).

Chart 10-8 HOME CARE CHECKLIST
Managing the Therapeutic Regimen at Home

At the completion of education, the patient and/or caregiver will be able to:

- State the impact of disability on physiologic functioning, ADLs, IADLs, roles, relationships, and spirituality.
- State changes in lifestyle (e.g., diet, activity) necessary to maintain health.
- State the name, dose, side effects, frequency, and schedule for all medications.
- State how to obtain medical supplies after discharge.
- Identify durable medical equipment needs, proper usage, and maintenance necessary for safe utilization:
  - Wheelchair—manual/power
  - Cushion
  - Grab bars
  - Sliding board
  - Mechanical lift
  - Raised padded commode seat
  - Padded commode wheelchair
  - Bedside commode
  - Crutches
  - Walker
  - Cane
  - Prosthesis
  - Orthosis
  - Shower chair
  - Specialty bed
- Demonstrate usage of adaptive equipment for activities of daily living:
  - Long-handled sponge
  - Reacher
  - Universal cuff
  - Plate mat and guard
  - Rocker-knife, spork, weighted utensils
  - Special closures for clothing
  - Other
- Demonstrate mobility skills:
  - Transfers: bed to chair; in and out of toilet and tub; in and out of car
  - Negotiate ramps, curbs, stairs
  - Assume sitting from supine position
  - Turn side to side in bed
  - Maneuver wheelchair; manage armrests and leg rests; lock brakes
  - Ambulate safely using assistive devices
  - Perform range-of-motion exercises
  - Perform muscle-strengthening exercises
- Demonstrate skin care:
  - Inspect bony prominences every morning and evening
  - Identify stage I pressure ulcer and actions to take if present
  - Change dressings for stage II to IV pressure ulcers
- State dietary requirements to promote healing of pressure ulcers
- Demonstrate pressure relief at prescribed intervals
- State sitting schedule and demonstrate weight lifts in wheelchair
- Demonstrate adherence to bed turning schedule, bed positioning, and the use of bridging techniques
- Apply and wear protective boots at prescribed times
- Demonstrate correct wheelchair sitting posture
- Demonstrate techniques to avoid friction and shear in bed
- Demonstrate proper hygiene to maintain skin integrity
- Demonstrate bladder care:
  - State schedule for voiding, toileting, and catheterization
  - Identify relationship of fluid intake to voiding and catheterization schedule
  - State how to perform pelvic floor exercises
  - Demonstrate clean self-intermittent catheterization and care of catheterization equipment
  - Demonstrate indwelling catheter care
  - Demonstrate application of external condom catheter
  - Demonstrate application, emptying, and cleaning of urinary drainage bag
  - Demonstrate application of incontinence pads and performance of perineal hygiene
  - State signs and symptoms of urinary tract infection
  - State signs and symptoms of urinary catheter blockage
- Demonstrate bowel care:
  - State optimum dietary intake to promote evacuation
  - Identify schedule for optimum bowel evacuation
  - Demonstrate techniques to increase intra-abdominal pressure; Valsalva maneuver; abdominal massage; leaning forward
  - Demonstrate techniques to stimulate bowel movements: ingesting warm liquids; digital stimulation; insertion of suppositories
  - Demonstrate optimum position for bowel evacuation: on toilet with knees higher than hips; left side in bed with knees flexed and head of bed elevated 30 to 45 degrees
  - Identify complications and corrective strategies for bowel retraining: constipation, impaction, diarrhea, hemorrhoids, rectal bleeding, anal tears

(continued on page 190)

At the completion of education, the patient and/or caregiver will be able to:

- Identify community resources for peer and caregiver/family support:
  - Identify sources of support (e.g., friends, relatives, faith community)
  - Identify phone numbers of support groups for people with disabilities and their caregivers/families
  - State meeting locations and times
- Demonstrate how to access transportation:
  - Identify locations of wheelchair accessibility for public buses or trains
  - Identify phone numbers for private wheelchair van
  - Contact Division of Motor Vehicles for handicapped parking permit
  - Contact Division of Motor Vehicles for driving test when appropriate
  - Identify resources for adapting private vehicle with hand controls or wheelchair lift

- Identify vocational rehabilitation resources:
  - State name and phone number of vocational rehabilitation counselor
  - Identify educational opportunities that may lead to future employment
- Identify community resources for recreation:
  - State local recreation centers that offer programs for people with disabilities
  - Identify leisure activities that can be pursued in the community
  - State how to reach primary provider with questions or if complications arise
  - State time and date of follow-up appointments
  - Identify the need for health promotion, disease prevention, and screening activities

ADLs, activities of daily living; IADLs, instrumental activities of daily living.

Continuing and Transitional Care

A home care or transitional care nurse may visit the patient prior to discharge, interview the patient and the family, and review the ADL sheet to learn which activities the patient can perform. This helps to ensure that continuity of care is provided and that the patient does not regress yet maintains the independence gained while in the hospital or rehabilitation setting. The family may need to purchase, borrow, or improvise needed equipment, such as safety rails, a raised toilet seat or commode, or a tub bench. Ramps may need to be built or doorways widened to allow full access.

Family members are taught how to use equipment and are given a copy of the equipment manufacturer's instruction booklet, the names of resource people, lists of equipment-related supplies, and locations where they may be obtained. A written summary of the care plan is included in family education. The patient and family members are reminded about the importance of routine health screening and other health promotion strategies.

A network of support services and communication systems may be required to enhance opportunities for independent living. The nurse uses collaborative, administrative skills to coordinate these activities and pull together the network of care. The nurse also provides skilled care, initiates additional referrals when indicated, and serves as a patient advocate and counselor when obstacles are encountered. The nurse continues to reinforce prior patient education and helps the patient to set and achieve attainable goals. The degree to which the patient adapts to the home and community environment depends on the confidence and self-esteem developed during the rehabilitation process and on the acceptance, support, and reactions of family members, employers, and community members.

There is a growing trend toward independent living by people with severe disabilities, either alone or in groups that share resources. Preparation for independent living should include training in managing a household and working with personal care attendants as well as training in mobility. The goal is integration into the community—living and working in the community with accessible housing, employment, public buildings, transportation, and recreation.

State rehabilitation administration agencies provide services to assist people with disabilities in obtaining the help they need to engage in gainful employment. These services include diagnostic, medical, and mental health services. Counseling, training, placement, and follow-up services are available to help people with disabilities select and obtain jobs.

If the patient is transferred to a long-term care facility, the transition is planned to promote continued progress. Independence gained continues to be supported, and progress is fostered. Adjustment to the facility is promoted through communication. Family members are encouraged to visit, to be involved, and to take the patient home on weekends and holidays if possible.

CRITICAL THINKING EXERCISES

1 A 74-year-old community-dwelling woman with memory impairment was admitted to your unit following a fall in which her hip was fractured. She had surgery to reduce her fracture and stabilize her hip. As a result of her injury and pre-existing memory impairment, what challenges now confront the rehabilitation nursing staff in helping this patient's recovery process? What are your priority nursing diagnoses for this patient as you plan your care for her? What strategies might you employ when caring for a patient with memory impairment? How might you involve her family in the rehabilitation and care planning process?

2 ebp You are caring for a 48-year-old male patient post lower limb amputation who is experiencing difficulty adjusting to his physical deficits, thus limiting his participation in rehabilitation sessions. You wish to create the necessary "space" for this patient so that he may practice the tasks and activities requisite to successful rehabilitation, without becoming unduly frustrated, but are unsure what approach to take. Identify a specific evidence-based question related to this patient in order to conduct a relevant and focused literature search. What key words would you use in this search, and what sources would be appropriate to search?

REFERENCES

*Asterisk indicates nursing research.
**Double asterisk indicates classic reference.

Books

Chang, E., & Johnson, A. (Eds.). (2013). *Chronic illness and disability: Principles for nursing practice* (2nd ed.). St. Louis, MO: Elsevier Health Sciences.

Dean, S. G., Siegert, R. J., & Taylor, W. J. (2012). *Interprofessional rehabilitation: A person-centred approach*. Chichester: Wiley-Blackwell.

Herdman, T. H., & Kamitsuru, S. (Eds.). (2014). *NANDA International nursing diagnoses: Definitions and classification, 2015–17*. Oxford: Wiley-Blackwell.

Hoeman, S. P. (2008). *Rehabilitation nursing: Prevention, intervention, and outcomes* (4th ed.). St. Louis, MO: Elsevier Health Sciences.

Kolar, P. (Ed.) (2014). *Clinical rehabilitation*. Prague: Alena Kobesová.

National Pressure Ulcer Advisory Panel. (2014). *Prevention and treatment of pressure ulcers: Clinical practice guideline*. Osborne Park, Western Australia: Cambridge Media.

**Norton, D., McLaren, R., & Exton-Smith, A. N. (1962). *An investigation of geriatric nursing problems in hospital*. Edinburgh: Churchill Livingstone.

O'Sullivan, S. B., Schmitz, T. J., & Fulk, G. (Eds.) (2013). *Physical rehabilitation*. Philadelphia, PA: FA Davis Company.

Substance Abuse and Mental Health Services Administration. (2014). *Results from the 2013 National Survey on Drug Use and Health: Summary of National Findings, NSDUH Series H-48, HHS Publication No. (SMA) 14–4863*. Rockville, MD: Author.

Thomas, D. R. (2015). The relationship of nutrition and pressure ulcers. In C. W. Bales & C. S. Richis. (Eds). *Handbook of clinical nutrition and aging*. New York, NY: Springer.

Wright, J. (2011). Disability rating scale. In Kreutzer, J., DeLuca, J., & Caplan, B., eds. *Encyclopedia of clinical neuropsychology*. New York, NY: Springer, 862–863.

Journals and Electronic Documents

Association of Rehabilitation Nurses. (2014). ARN competency model for professional rehabilitation nursing. Retrieved on 7/5/2015 at: www.rehabnurse.org/profresources/content/ARN-Competency-Model-for-Professional-Rehabilitation-Nursing.html.

Bamm, E. L., Rosenbaum, P., Wilkins, S., et al. (2015a). Exploring client-centered care experiences in in-patient rehabilitation settings. *Global Qualitative Nursing Research, 2*, 1–11.

Bamm, E. L., Rosenbaum, P., Wilkins, S., et al. (2015b). Performance of the measures of processes of care for adults and service providers in rehabilitation settings. *Patient Related Outcome Measures, 6*, 157–165.

*Camicia, M., Black, T., Farrell, J., et al. (2014). The essential role of the rehabilitation nurse in facilitating care transitions: A white paper by the Association of Rehabilitation Nurses. *Rehabilitation Nursing, 39*(1), 3–15.

Christakou, A., Papadopoulos, E., Patsaki, E., et al. (2013). Functional assessment scales in a general intensive care unit. *Hospital Chronicles, 8*(4), 164–170.

*Clarke, D. J. (2014). Nursing practice in stroke rehabilitation: Systematic review and meta-ethnography. *Journal of Clinical Nursing, 23*(9–10), 1201–1226.

Clark, H., & Bassett, S. (2014). An application of the health action process approach to physiotherapy rehabilitation adherence. *Physiotherapy Theory and Practice, 30*(8), 527–533.

Clark-Wilson, J., Giles, G. M., & Baxter, D. M. (2014). Revisiting the neurofunctional approach: Conceptualizing the core components for the rehabilitation of everyday living skills. *Brain Injury, 28*(13–14), 1646–1656.

Craig, A., Perry, K. N., Guest, R., et al. (2015). Prospective study of the occurrence of psychological disorders and comorbidities after spinal cord injury. *Archives of Physical Medicine and Rehabilitation, 96*(8), 1426–1434.

Dauwe, P. B., Pulikkottil, B. J., Lavery, L., et al. (2014). Does hyperbaric oxygen therapy work in facilitating acute wound healing: A systematic review. *Plastic and Reconstructive Surgery, 133*(2), 208e–215e.

DiVita, M. A., Granger, C. V., Goldstein, R., et al. (2015). Risk factors for development of new or worsened pressure ulcers among patients in inpatient rehabilitation facilities in the United States: Data from the Uniform Data System for Medical Rehabilitation. *Physical Medicine & Rehabilitation, 7*(6), 599–612.

Duetzmann, S., Forsey, L. M., Senft, C., et al. (2015). Sacral peak pressure in healthy volunteers and patients with spinal cord injury. *Nursing Research, 64*(4), 300–305.

*Dunk, A. M., & Carville, K. (2015). The international clinical practice guideline for prevention and treatment of pressure ulcers/injuries. *Journal of Advanced Nursing, 72*(2), 243–244.

*García-Fernández, F. P., Agreda, J., Verdú, J., et al. (2014). A new theoretical model for the development of pressure ulcers and other dependence-related lesions. *Journal of Nursing Scholarship, 46*(1), 28–38.

Glazier, R. E., & Kling, R. N. (2013). Recent trends in substance abuse among persons with disabilities compared to that of persons without disabilities. *Disability and Health Journal, 6*(2), 107–115.

Gorina, Y., Schappert, S., Bercovitz, A., et al. (2014). Prevalence of incontinence among older Americans. National Center for Health Statistics. *Vital & Health Statistics, 3*(36), 1–33.

Gould, L. J., Olney, C. M., Nichols, J. S., et al. (2014). Spinal cord injury survey to determine pressure ulcer vulnerability in the outpatient population. *Medical Hypotheses, 83*(5), 552–558.

**Granger, C., Albrecht, G., & Hamilton, B. (1979). Outcomes of comprehensive medical rehabilitation: Measurement by PULSES profile and the Barthel Index. *Archives of Physical and Medical Rehabilitation, 60*(4), 145–154.

Hanson, L. C., Armstrong, T. D., Green, M. A., et al. (2012). Circles of care: Development and initial evaluation of a peer support model for African Americans with advanced cancer. *Health Education & Behavior, 40*(5), 536–543.

**Harvey, R. F., Hollis, M., & Jellinek, M. (1981). Functional performance assessment: A program approach. *Archives of Physical Medicine and Rehabilitation, 62*(9), 456–461.

*He, J., Staggs, V. S., Bergquist-Beringer, S., et al. (2013). Unit-level time trends and seasonality in the rate of hospital-acquired pressure ulcers in US acute care hospitals. *Research in Nursing & Health, 36*(2), 171–180.

Hotouras, A., Ribas, Y., Allison, M. E., et al. (2014). Treatment of fecal incontinence in the era of neuromodulation: Is it time to rethink our approach? *Diseases of the Colon & Rectum, 57*(9), 1143–1144.

*Hyde, Y. M., & Kautz, D. D. (2014). Enhancing health promotion during rehabilitation through information-giving, partnership-building, and teach-back. *Rehabilitation Nursing, 39*(4), 178–182.

Kearney, P. M., & Cronin, N. (2014). Guest editorial: Rehabilitation and disability nursing: Let the cousins marry. *Journal of the Australasian Rehabilitation Nurses Association, 17*(2), 7–9.

**Keith, R. A., Granger, C. V., Hamilton, B. B., et al. (1987). The functional independence measure: A new tool for rehabilitation. *Advances in Clinical Rehabilitation, 1*, 6–18.

Knudson-Martin, C., Huenergardt, D., Lafontant, K., et al. (2015). Competencies for addressing gender and power in couple therapy: A socioemotional approach. *Journal of Marital and Family Therapy, 41*(2), 205–220.

**Mahoney, F., & Barthel, D. (1965). Functional evaluation: The Barthel Index. *Maryland State Medical Journal, 14*, 61–65.

Mandl, M., Halfens, R. J., & Lohrmann, C. (2015). Incontinence care in nursing homes: A cross-sectional study. *Journal of Advanced Nursing, 71*(9), 2142–2152.

*Miller, E. T. (2014). Ripple effect. *Rehabilitation Nursing, 39*(4), 167–168.

Papadimitriou, C., & Cott, C. (2015). Client-centred practices and work in inpatient rehabilitation teams: Results from four case studies. *Disability and Rehabilitation, 37*(13), 1135–1143.

Price, M., & Lau, F. Y. (2013). Provider connectedness and communication patterns: Extending continuity of care in the context of the circle of care. *BMC Health Services Research, 13*(1), 309.

Peirce, B., Dale, B., Mackey, D., et al. (2014). Wound, Ostomy and Continence Nurses Society's Guidance on OASIS-C1 Integumentary Items: Best Practice for Clinicians. Adapted from: //c. ymcdn.com/sites/www.wocn.org/resource/resmgr/Publications/WOCN_Guidance_on_OASIS-C1_In.pdf

Posthauer, M. E., Banks, M., Dorner, B., et al. (2015). The role of nutrition for pressure ulcer management: national pressure ulcer advisory panel, European pressure ulcer advisory panel, and pan pacific pressure injury alliance white paper. *Advances in Skin & Wound Care, 28*(4), 175–188.

Qaseem, A., Humphrey, L. L., Forciea, M. A., et al. (2015). Treatment of pressure ulcers: A clinical practice guideline from the American College of Physicians. *Annals of Internal Medicine, 162*(5), 370–379.

Roe, B., Flanagan, L., & Maden, M. (2015). Systematic review of systematic reviews for the management of urinary incontinence and promotion of continence using conservative behavioural approaches in older people in care homes. *Journal of Advanced Nursing, 71*(7), 1464–1483.

Saha, S., Smith, M. E. B., Totten, A., et al. (2013). Pressure ulcer treatment strategies: Comparative effectiveness. Comparative Effectiveness Review No. 90. (Prepared by the Oregon Evidence-based Practice Center under Contract No. 290–2007–10057-I.). Retrieved on 8/20/2015 at: ww.effectivehealthcare.ahrq.gov/reports/final.cfm

Scheel-Sailer, A., Wyss, A., Boldt, C., et al. (2013). Prevalence, location, grade of pressure ulcers and association with specific patient characteristics in adult spinal cord injury patients during the hospital stay: A prospective cohort study. *Spinal Cord, 51*(11), 828–833.

*Schmidt, A. S. (2013). Outcome trends post discharge from inpatient rehabilitation to the community. *Rehabilitation Nursing, 38*(6), 284–296.

Stoekenbroek, R. M., Santema, T. B., Legemate, D. A., et al. (2014). Hyperbaric oxygen for the treatment of diabetic foot ulcers: A systematic review. *European Journal of Vascular and Endovascular Surgery, 47*(6), 647–655.

Strasser, D. C., Burridge, A. B., Falconer, J. A., et al. (2014). Toward spanning the quality chasm: An examination of team functioning measures. *Archives of Physical Medicine and Rehabilitation, 95*(11), 2220–2223.

Stifter, J., Yao, Y., Lodhi, M.K., et al. (2015). Nurse continuity and hospital-acquired pressure ulcers. *Nursing Research, 64*(5), 361–371.

Sullivan, N., & Schoelles, K. M. (2013). Preventing in-facility pressure ulcers as a patient safety strategy: A systematic review. *Annals of Internal Medicine, 158*(5), 410–416.

Tétrault, M., & Courtois, F. (2014). Use of psychoactive substances in persons with spinal cord injury: A literature review. *Annals of Physical and Rehabilitation Medicine, 57*(9), 684–695.

Vaughn, S., Mauk, K. L., Jacelon, C. S., et al. (2016). The competency model for professional rehabilitation nursing. *Rehabilitation Nursing, 41*(1), 33–44.

Wang, H., Niewczyk, P., DiVita, M., et al. (2014). Impact of pressure ulcers on outcomes in inpatient rehabilitation facilities. *American Journal of Physical Medicine & Rehabilitation, 93*(3), 207–216.

Wiggermann, N., Kotowski, S., Davis, K., et al. (2015). The effect of patient migration in bed on torso elevation. *Nursing Research, 64*(3), 221–225.

White, M. J., Gutierrez, A., Mclaughlin C., et al. (2013). A pilot for understanding interdisciplinary teams in rehabilitation practice. *Rehabilitation Nursing, 38*(3), 142–152.

Wu, J. M., Matthews, C. A., Vaughan, C. P., et al. (2015). Urinary, fecal, and dual incontinence in older US adults. *Journal of the American Geriatrics Society, 63*(5), 947–953.

Resources

AbleData, www.abledata.com

Agency for Healthcare Research and Quality (AHRQ), www.ahrq.gov

American Association of People with Disabilities (AAPD), www.aapd.com

American Society of Addiction Medicine (ASAM), www.asam.org

Assistive Technology Industry Association (ATIA), www.atia.org

Association of Rehabilitation Nurses (ARN), www.rehabnurse.org

CARF International (CARF), www.carf.org

Canine Companions for Independence, www.caninecompanions.org

Council for Disability Rights, www.disabilityrights.org

IRF Quality Reporting Measures Information, www.cms.gov/Medicare/Quality-Initiatives-Patient-Assessment-Instruments/IRF-Quality-Reporting/IRF-Quality-Reporting-Program-Measures-Information.html

National Association on Alcohol, Drugs and Disability (NAADD), www.naadd.org

National Center for Health Statistics (NCHS), www.cdc.gov/nchs

National Center for the Dissemination of Disability Research (NCDDR), www.ncddr.org

National Council on Alcoholism and Drug Dependence, Inc. (NCADD), www.ncadd.org

National Council on Disability (NCD), www.ncd.gov

National Institute on Disability and Rehabilitation Research (NIDRR), www.acl.gov/programs/NIDILRR/

National Pressure Ulcer Advisory Panel (NPUAP), www.npuap.org

National Rehabilitation Information Center (NARIC), www.naric.com

National Spinal Cord Injury Association (NSCIA), www.spinalcord.org

Sexuality Information and Education Council of the United States (SIECUS), www.siecus.org

Stroke Engine, McGill University general information, http://strokengine.ca

Substance Abuse Resources and Disability Issues (SARDI), www.med.wright.edu/citar/sardi

U.S. Census Bureau, www.census.gov

U.S. Department of Health and Human Services, www.hhs.gov

World Health Organization, health topics: rehabilitation, www.who.int/topics/rehabilitation/en/

11 Health Care of the Older Adult

LEARNING OBJECTIVES

On completion of this chapter, the learner will be able to:

1 Specify the demographic trends and the physiologic aspects of aging in the United States.
2 Describe the significance of preventive health care and health promotion for the older adult.
3 Compare and contrast the common physical and mental health problems of aging and their effects on the functioning of older adults and their families.

4 Identify the role of the nurse in meeting the health care needs of the older patient.
5 Examine common health issues of older adults and their families in the home and the community, in the acute care setting, and in the long-term care facility.

GLOSSARY

activities of daily living (ADLs): personal care activities such as bathing, dressing, grooming, eating, toileting, and transferring

ageism: a bias that discriminates, stigmatizes, and disadvantages older adults based solely on their chronologic age

comorbidity: having more than one illness at the same time (e.g., diabetes and congestive heart failure)

delirium: an acute, confused state that begins with disorientation and if not recognized and treated early can progress to changes in level of consciousness, irreversible brain damage, and sometimes death

dementia: broad term for a syndrome characterized by a general decline in higher brain functioning, such as reasoning, with a pattern of eventual decline in the ability to perform even basic activities of daily living, such as toileting and eating

depression: the most common affective (mood) disorder of old age; results from changes in reuptake of the neurochemical serotonin in response to chronic illness and emotional stresses

durable power of attorney: a formal, legally endorsed document that identifies a proxy decision maker who can make decisions if the signer becomes incapacitated

elder abuse: the physical, emotional, or financial harm to an older person by one or more of the individual's children, caregivers, or others; includes neglect

geriatric syndromes: common conditions found in older adults that tend to be multifactorial and do not fall under

discrete disease categories; these conditions include falls, delirium, frailty, dizziness, and urinary incontinence

geriatrics: a field of practice that focuses on the physiology, pathology, diagnosis, and management of the disorders and diseases of older adults

gerontologic/geriatric nursing: the field of nursing that relates to the assessment, planning, implementation, and evaluation of older adults in all environments, including acute, intermediate, and skilled care, as well as within the community

gerontology: the combined biologic, psychological, and sociologic study of older adults within their environment

instrumental activities of daily living (IADLs): complex skills needed for independent living, such as shopping, cooking, housework, using the telephone, managing medications and finances, and being able to travel by car or public transportation

orientation: a person's ability to recognize who and where he or she is in a time continuum; used to evaluate one's basic cognitive status

polypharmacy: the use of multiple medications

presbycusis: the decreased ability to hear high-pitched tones that naturally begins in midlife as a result of irreversible inner ear changes

presbyopia: the decrease in visual accommodation that occurs with advancing age

urinary incontinence: the unplanned loss of urine

Aging, the normal process of time-related change, begins with birth and continues throughout life. Americans are living longer and healthier than any previous generation. With the baby boomers turning 65 years of age beginning in 2010, older Americans are the most rapidly expanding segment of the population. Whenever nurses work with adults, they are likely to encounter older adult patients. This chapter presents demographics of aging, normal age-related changes, health

problems associated with aging, and ways that nurses can address the health issues of older adults.

Overview of Aging

Demographics of Aging

The proportion of Americans 65 years of age and older has more than tripled in the past 100 years (4.1% in 1900 to 14.1%

of the population in 2013). As a result of the baby boomers coming of age, the older adult population increased by 8.8 million or 24.7% between 2003 and 2013 to number 44.7 million people and is expected to continue to grow to approximately 79.7 million by 2040 and then stabilize at about 20% of the population. As the older adult population increases, the number of people who live to a very old age is also dramatically increasing. The greatest growth in the older adult population is for those aged 85 years and older; this population is projected to more than double from 6 million in 2013 to grow to 14.6 million in 2040 (Administration on Aging [AoA], 2014). Life expectancy—the average number of years that a person can expect to live—varies by gender and race, with women living longer than men and white women having the longest life expectancy. Life expectancy has risen dramatically in the past 100 years. In 1900, average life expectancy was 47 years, and by 2009, that figure had increased to 78.8 years. The older adult population is becoming more diverse, reflecting changing demographics in the United States. Although this population will increase in number for all minority groups, the rate of growth is projected to be fastest in the Hispanic population, which is expected to increase by 153% by 2030. Proportionally, there will be a significant decline in the percentage of the white non-Hispanic population, which is anticipated to increase only 50% (AoA, 2014).

Health Status of the Older Adult

Although many older adults enjoy good health, most have at least one chronic illness, and many have multiple health conditions. Chronic conditions, many of which are preventable or treatable, are the major cause of disability and pain among older adults (see Fig. 11-1).

Most deaths in the United States occur in people 65 years of age and older. However, improvements in the prevention, early detection, and treatment of diseases have impacted the health of people in this age group. In the past 60 years, there has been a significant decline in overall deaths—specifically, deaths from heart disease and cancer, the two leading causes of deaths. In addition, deaths from chronic lower respiratory diseases, stroke, influenza, pneumonia, and sepsis, have declined (Kochanek, Murphy, Xu, et al., 2014). Deaths from chronic lower pulmonary diseases surpassed stroke recently,

making these diseases the third leading cause death. Deaths from Alzheimer disease (AD) among those 65 years of age and older have risen and are projected to be approximately 1.6 million annually by 2050 (Weuve, Hebert, Scherr, et al., 2014).

More than 75% of noninstitutionalized Americans aged 65 years and older rate their health as good, very good, or excellent (AoA, 2012a). Men and women report comparable levels of health; however, positive health reports decline with advancing age, even at the age of 85 years and more, the majority of Americans report good or better health. Blacks, Hispanics, and Latinos appear less likely to report good health than their white counterparts. Most Americans 75 years of age and older remain functionally independent regardless of how they perceive their health. The proportion of older Americans reporting a limitation in activities declined from 42% in 1992 to 32% in 2009 (AoA, 2012a). These declines in limitations may reflect trends in health promotion and disease prevention activities, such as improved nutrition, decreased smoking, increased exercise, and early detection and treatment of risk factors such as hypertension and elevated serum cholesterol levels.

Many chronic conditions commonly found among older people can be managed, limited, and even prevented. Older people are more likely to maintain good health and functional independence if encouraged to do so and if appropriate community-based support services are available (Miller, 2015). Nurses are challenged to promote positive lifelong health behaviors, because the impact of unhealthy behaviors and choices can result in chronic disease.

Nursing Care of the Older Adult

Gerontology, the study of the aging process, is a multidisciplinary field that draws from the biologic, psychological, and sociologic sciences. **Geriatrics** is the practice (medical or nursing) that focuses on the physiology, pathology, diagnosis, and management of the disorders and diseases of older adults. Care for older adults should not be limited to one discipline but is best provided through a cooperative effort. An interdisciplinary approach to providing care combines expertise and resources to provide comprehensive geriatric assessment and intervention. Nurses collaborate with the team to

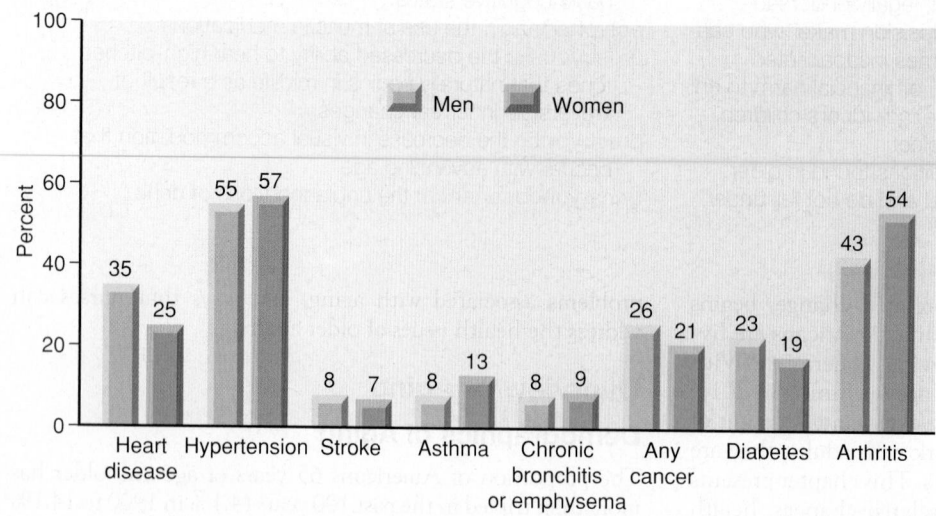

Figure 11-1 • Percentage of people 65 years of age and older who reported having selected chronic health conditions, by sex, 2013–2014. From Federal Interagency Forum on Aging-Related Statistics. (2016). *2016 older Americans: Key indicators of well-being.* Washington, DC: U.S. Government Printing Office. Retrieved at: www.agingstats.gov/docs/Latest Report/OlderAmericans2016.pdf

obtain appropriate services for patients and provide a holistic approach to care.

Gerontologic/geriatric nursing is the field of nursing that specializes in the care of older adults. The Scope and Standards of Gerontological Nursing Practice was originally developed in 1969 by the American Nurses Association (ANA) and revised in 2010 (ANA, 2010). The nurse gerontologist can be either a specialist or a generalist providing comprehensive nursing care to older adults by combining the basic nursing process with a specialized knowledge of aging. Gerontologic nursing is provided in acute care, skilled and assisted living, the community, and home settings. The goals of care include promoting and maintaining functional status as well as helping older adults identify and use their strengths to achieve optimal independence.

Nurses who are certified in geriatric nursing have specialized knowledge of the acute and chronic changes specific to older adults. The use of advanced practice nurses who have been educated in geriatric nursing concepts has proved to be very effective when dealing with the complex care needs of an older patient. When best practices are used and current scientific knowledge applied to clinical problems, there is significantly less deterioration in the overall health of aging patients (ANA, 2010).

In addition to specialists, nurses who work in all areas of adult medical-surgical nursing encounter older adult patients. Nurses must be knowledgeable and skilled in meeting the complex needs of these patients. Nurses and caregivers who work with older patients must understand that aging is not synonymous with disease and that the effects of the aging process alone are not the only or even the primary contributors to disability and disease. Aging is a highly individualized and multifaceted process (Cline, 2014).

Functional assessment is a common framework for assessing older adults. Age-related changes, as well as additional risk factors such as disease and the effects of medications, can reduce function. Assessing the functional consequences of aging and proposing practical interventions help maintain and improve the health of older adults. The goal is to help older adults sustain maximum functional level and dignity despite physical, social, and psychological losses. Early intervention can prevent complications of many health problems and help maximize the quality of life.

Theories of Aging

Aging has been defined chronologically by the passing of time—subjectively, as in how a person feels, and functionally, as in changes in physical or mental capabilities. Many theories attempt to provide a framework in which to understand aging from different perspectives. Clinicians can use each theory to gain insight into different aspects of aging.

In addition to the biologic, developmental, and sociologic theories of aging, Miller (2015) developed the Functional Consequences Theory, which encourages nurses to consider the effects of normal age-related changes as well as the damage incurred through disease or environmental and behavioral risk factors when planning care. This theory suggests that nurses can alter the outcome for patients through nursing interventions that address the consequences of these changes. Age-related changes and risk factors may negatively interfere with patient outcomes and impair patient activity and quality of life. For example, normal age-related changes in vision may increase sensitivity to glare. Alterations in the environment that reduce glare may enhance patient comfort and safety. In contrast, the development of cataracts, which is not a normal age-related change, also may increase sensitivity to glare. The nurse must differentiate between normal, irreversible age-related changes and modifiable risk factors. Doing so helps the nurse design appropriate nursing interventions that have a positive impact on outcomes for older patients—most importantly, for their quality of life.

Age-Related Changes

The well-being of older adults depends on physical, psychosocial, mental, social, economic, and environmental factors. A total assessment includes an evaluation of all major body systems, social and mental status, and the person's ability to function independently (Weber & Kelley, 2014).

Physical Aspects of Aging

Intrinsic aging (from within the person) refers to those changes caused by the normal aging process that are genetically programmed and essentially universal within a species. Universality is the major criterion used to distinguish normal aging from pathologic changes associated with illness. However, people age quite differently and at different rates; thus, chronologic age is often less predictive of obvious age characteristics than other factors, such as one's genetics (see Chart 11-1) and lifestyle. A recent longitudinal research study of almost 45,000 older US adults reported that those who participated in physical activity, had modest alcohol intake, avoided obesity, and did not smoke had a 45% lower risk of heart failure (Del Gobbo, Kalantarian, Imamura, et al., 2015).

Cellular and extracellular changes that occur with aging cause functional decline and measurable changes in physical appearance, including changes in shape and body makeup. Cellular aging and tissue deficits also diminish the body's ability to maintain homeostasis and prevent organ systems from functioning at full efficiency. As cells become less able to replace themselves, they accumulate a pigment known as lipofuscin. A degradation of elastin and collagen causes connective tissue to become stiffer and less elastic. These changes result in diminished capacity for organ function and increased vulnerability to disease and stress. Age-related changes in the hematopoietic system influence red blood cell production, leading to increased rates of anemia (Grossman & Porth, 2014).

Table 11-1 summarizes subjective and objective findings related to age-related changes in the body systems. More in-depth information about age-related changes can be found in the chapters pertaining to each organ system.

When assessing the physical aspects of aging, nurses should know that tactile sensation is reduced and changes in the ability to sense pressure, pain, and temperature all lead to a decreased ability to identify and attend to physical symptoms (Oster & Oster, 2015).

Cardiovascular System

Heart disease is the leading cause of death in older adults. Age-related changes reduce the efficiency of the heart and

Chart 11-1 GENETICS IN NURSING PRACTICE
Genetics Concepts and the Older Adult

Genetic conditions in the older adult may occur from a specific gene mutation or arise as a result of a genetic predisposition combined with other factors (multifactorial). The following are examples of some adult-onset genetic conditions:

- Colon cancer
- Hemochromatosis
- Huntington disease
- Polycystic kidney disease
- Alzheimer disease

The following are some examples of diseases with multifactorial components, which may include a genetic predisposition, in the older adult:

- Diabetes
- Emphysema
- Heart disease

Nursing Assessments

Refer to Chart 5-2: Genetics in Nursing Practice: Genetic Aspects of Health Assessment

Family History Assessment Specific to the Older Adult

- Collect and assess family history on both maternal and paternal sides of the family for three generations.
- Determine whether genetic testing has occurred with other family members.
- Assess for individual and family perceptions and beliefs around topics related to genetics.

Patient Assessment Specific to the Older Adult and Genetic Illness

- Assess older adult patient's knowledge and understanding of genetics, genetic testing, and gene-based therapies.

- Assess the patient's understanding of genetic information and decipher health literacy needs.
- Perform cultural, social, and spiritual assessment.
- Assess patient's communication capacities so that communication strategies about genetics are tailored to their needs and abilities.
- Identify patient's support system.

Management Issues Specific to Genetics and the Older Adult

- Refer for further genetic counseling and evaluation as warranted so that family members can discuss inheritance, risk to other family members, and availability of genetic testing and gene-based interventions.
- Offer appropriate genetic information and resources that take into consideration older patient's literacy needs.
- Evaluate older patient's understanding before, during, and after the introduction of genetic information and services.
- Take the time to clearly explain the concepts of genetic testing to older patients and provide written information that reinforces the topic of discussion.
- Participate in the management and coordination of care of older patients with genetic conditions and individuals predisposed to develop or pass on a genetic condition.

Genetics Resources

U.S. Department of Health and Human Services: provides information about health literacy and older adults, www.health.gov/communication/literacy/olderadults/literacy.htm

See Chapter 8, Chart 8-7: Components of Genetic Counseling for additional resources.

---

contribute to decreased compliance of the heart muscle. These changes include myocardial hypertrophy, which changes left ventricular strength and function; increased fibrosis and calcified tissues that infiltrate muscles and conductive tissues causing stenosis of the valves; and decreased pacemaker cells. As a result, the heart valves become thicker and stiffer, and the heart muscle and arteries lose their elasticity, resulting in a reduced stroke volume. Calcium and fat deposits accumulate within arterial walls, and veins become increasingly stiff and tortuous, increasing arterial resistance; this leads to hypertension and increases the workload of the heart (Capriotti & Frizzell, 2015).

It is difficult to differentiate between age- and disease-related changes in cardiovascular function because of the significant influence of behavioral factors on cardiovascular health. When cross-cultural studies are conducted, cardiovascular changes that in the past were thought to be age related do not consistently appear. For example, the higher blood pressure found in older adults in Western societies does not occur in less-developed societies and may be a result of different lifestyle behaviors rather than normal age-related changes (Miller, 2015). The cardiovascular system can adapt to many normal age-related changes and often an older person is unaware of any significant decline in cardiovascular performance. However, when challenged, for instance, during exercise or stress, the cardiovascular system of an older person is less efficient and may be unable to respond sufficiently when life-sustaining activities are needed.

Careful assessment of older adults is necessary because they often present with different symptoms than those seen in younger patients. Older adults are more likely to have dyspnea or neurologic symptoms associated with heart disease, and they may experience mental status changes or report vague symptoms such as fatigue, nausea, and syncope. Rather than the typical substernal chest pain associated with myocardial ischemia, older patients may report burning or sharp pain or discomfort in an area of the upper body. Complicating the assessment is the fact that many older patients have more than one underlying disease. When a patient complains of symptoms related to digestion and breathing and upper extremity pain, cardiac disease must be considered. The absence of chest pain in an older patient is not a reliable indicator of the absence of heart disease.

Orthostatic and postprandial hypotension may be a concern as well because of decreased baroreflex sensitivity and risk factors such as medications (Miller, 2015). Therefore, it is important to assess blood pressure in two positions. A patient experiencing hypotension should be counseled to rise slowly (from a lying, to a sitting, to a standing position), avoid straining when having a bowel movement, and consider having five or six small meals each day, rather than three, to minimize the hypotension that can occur after a large meal. Extremes

TABLE 11-1 Age-Related Changes in Body Systems and Health Promotion Strategies

Changes	Subjective and Objective Findings	Health Promotion Strategies
Cardiovascular System Decreased cardiac output; diminished ability to respond to stress; heart rate and stroke volume do not increase with maximum demand; slower heart recovery rate; increased blood pressure	Complaints of fatigue with increased activity Increased heart rate recovery time *Optimal blood pressure:* ≤120/80 mm Hg *Prehypertension:* >120–139/80–89 mm Hg *Hypertension:* ≥140/90 mm Hg	Exercise regularly; pace activities; avoid smoking; eat a low-fat, low-salt diet; participate in stress-reduction activities; check blood pressure regularly; adherence to medications; weight control (body mass index <25 kg/m²).
Respiratory System Increase in residual lung volume; decrease in muscle strength, endurance, and vital capacity; decreased gas exchange and diffusing capacity; decreased cough efficiency	Fatigue and breathlessness with sustained activity; decreased respiratory excursion and chest/lung expansion with less effective exhalation; difficulty coughing up secretions	Exercise regularly; avoid smoking; take adequate fluids to liquefy secretions; receive yearly influenza immunization and pneumonia vaccine at 65 years of age; avoid exposure to upper respiratory tract infections.
Integumentary System Decreased subcutaneous fat, interstitial fluid, muscle tone, glandular activity, and sensory receptors, resulting in atrophy and decreased protection against trauma, sun exposure, and temperature extremes; diminished secretion of natural oils and perspiration; capillary fragility	Thin, wrinkled, and dry skin; increased fragility, more easily bruised, and sunburned; complaints of intolerance to heat; prominent bone structure	Limit sun exposure to 10–15 minutes daily for vitamin D (use protective clothing and sunscreen); dress appropriately for temperature; stay hydrated; maintain a safe indoor temperature; take shower rather than hot tub bath if possible; lubricate skin with lotions that contain petroleum or mineral oil.
Reproductive System *Female:* Vaginal narrowing and decreased elasticity; decreased vaginal secretions *Male:* Gradual decline in fertility, less firm testes, and decreased sperm production *Male and female:* Slower sexual response	*Female:* Painful intercourse; vaginal bleeding following intercourse; vaginal itching and irritation; delayed orgasm *Male:* Less firm erection and delayed erection and achievement of orgasm	*Female:* May require vaginal estrogen replacement; gynecology/urology follow-up; use a lubricant with sexual intercourse.
Musculoskeletal System Loss of bone density; loss of muscle strength and size; degenerated joint cartilage	Height loss; prone to fractures; kyphosis; back pain; loss of strength, flexibility, and endurance; joint pain	Weight-bearing exercise regularly (3 times a week); recommend bone density screening; take calcium and vitamin D supplements as prescribed.
Genitourinary System Decrease in detrusor muscle contractility, bladder capacity, flow rate, ability to withhold voiding; increase in residual urine *Male:* Benign prostatic hyperplasia *Female:* Relaxed perineal muscles; detrusor instability leads to urge incontinence; urethral dysfunction (stress urinary incontinence)	Urinary retention; irritative voiding symptoms including frequency, feeling of incomplete bladder emptying, multiple nighttime voiding Urgency/frequency syndrome; decreased "warning time"; drops of urine lost with cough, laugh, position change	Drink adequate fluids but limit drinking in evening; avoid bladder irritants (e.g., caffeinated beverages, alcohol, artificial sweeteners); do not wait long periods between voiding; empty bladder completely when voiding; wear easily manipulated clothing; consider urologic workup. Women: perform pelvic floor muscle exercises, preferably learned via biofeedback
Gastrointestinal System Decreased sense of thirst, smell, and taste; decreased salivation; difficulty swallowing food; delayed esophageal and gastric emptying; reduced gastrointestinal motility	Risk of dehydration, electrolyte imbalances, and poor nutritional intake; complaints of dry mouth; complaints of fullness, heartburn, and indigestion; constipation, flatulence, and abdominal discomfort; risk for aspiration	Use ice chips, mouthwash; brush, floss, and massage gums daily; receive regular dental care; eat small, frequent meals; sit up while and after eating and avoid heavy activity after eating; limit antacids; eat a high-fiber, low-fat diet; limit laxatives; toilet regularly; drink adequate fluids.
Nervous System Decrease in brain volume and cerebral blood flow. Reduced speed in nerve conduction	Slower to respond and react; learning may take longer; increased vulnerability to delirium with illness, anesthesia, even changes in environmental cues such as a room change; increased risk of fainting and falls	Pace teaching; with hospitalization, encourage visitors; enhance sensory stimulation; with sudden confusion, look for cause; encourage slow rising from a resting position and practice fall prevention measures
Special Senses *Vision:* Presbyopia; diminished ability to focus on close objects; decreased ability to tolerate glare; pupils become more rigid and lenses more opaque; decreased contrast sensitivity; decrease in aqueous humor	Holds objects far away from face; complains of glare; poor night vision and "dry" eye; difficulty adjusting to changes in light intensity; decreased ability to distinguish colors	Wear eyeglasses and use sunglasses outdoors; avoid abrupt changes from dark to light; use adequate indoor lighting with area lights and nightlights; use large-print books; use magnifier for reading; avoid night driving; use contrasting colors for color coding; avoid glare of shiny surfaces and direct sunlight.
Hearing: Presbycusis; decreased ability to hear high-frequency sounds; tympanic membrane thinning and loss of resiliency; difficulty with sound discrimination especially in noisy environment	Gives inappropriate responses; asks people to repeat words; strains forward to hear; can result in social isolation and increases vulnerability for delirium during hospitalization	Recommend a hearing examination; reduce background noise; face person; enunciate clearly; speak with a low-pitched voice; use nonverbal cues; rephrase questions.
Taste and smell: Decreased ability to taste and smell	Decreased recognition of familiar smells including recognizing spoiled food or a gas stove left on; decreased enjoyment of food; uses excessive sugar and salt	Encourage use of lemon, spices, herbs; recommend smoking cessation.

Adapted from Carpenter, H. (2015). Summer sun safety. *American Nurse Today,* 10(7), 46. Oster, K. A., & Oster, C. A. (2015). Special needs population: Care of the geriatric patient population in the perioperative setting. *AORN Journal, 101*(4), 444–456.

in temperature, including hot showers and whirlpool baths, should be avoided.

Respiratory System

The respiratory system compensates well for the functional changes of aging. In general, healthy, nonsmoking older adults show very little decline in respiratory function; however, there are substantial individual variations and aerobic capacity declines with each decade by about 10% from peak performance in the early to mid-20s (Capriotti & Frizzell, 2015). The age-related changes that do occur are subtle and gradual, and healthy older adults are able to compensate for these changes. Diminished respiratory efficiency and reduced maximal inspiratory and expiratory force may occur as a result of calcification and weakening of the muscles of the chest wall. Lung mass decreases and residual volume increases (Grossmann & Porth, 2014).

Conditions of stress, such as illness, may increase the demand for oxygen and affect the overall function of other systems. Like cardiovascular diseases, respiratory diseases manifest more subtly in older adults than in younger adults and do not necessarily follow the typical pattern of cough, chills, and fever. Older adults may exhibit fatigue, lethargy, anorexia, dehydration, and mental status changes (Miller, 2015).

Smoking is the most significant risk factor for respiratory diseases and older adults have a higher rate of smoking, about 20%, compared to the national average of 18% (Cataldo, Peterson, Hunter, et al., 2015). Therefore, a major focus of health promotion activities should be on smoking cessation and avoidance of environmental smoke. Despite marketing by manufacturers, e-cigarettes are not an effective smoking cessation aid nor do they promote health (Cataldo et al., 2015).

Additional activities that help older adults maintain adequate respiratory function include regular exercise, appropriate fluid intake, pneumococcal vaccination, yearly influenza immunizations, and avoidance of people who are ill. Hospitalized older adults should be frequently reminded to cough and take deep breaths, particularly postoperatively, because their decreased lung capacity and decreased cough efficiency predispose them to atelectasis and respiratory infections.

Integumentary System

The functions of the skin include protection, temperature regulation, sensation, and excretion. Aging can interrupt all functions of the skin and affect appearance (Grossman & Porth, 2014). Epidermal proliferation decreases, and the dermis becomes thinner. Elastic fibers are reduced in number and collagen becomes stiffer. Subcutaneous fat diminishes, particularly in the extremities, and less vasodilation renders the body less able to produce or conserve body heat. These changes lead to lack of fever in circumstances in which fever would normally be present in younger individuals and reduced tolerance to temperature extremes, which increases the likelihood of hypothermia and hyperthermia (Capriotti & Frizzell, 2015). There is also a loss of resiliency with wrinkling and sagging of the skin. The skin becomes drier and more susceptible to burns, injury, and infection. Hair pigmentation may change and balding may occur; genetic factors strongly influence these changes. These changes in the integument reduce tolerance to temperature extremes and sun exposure.

Lifestyle practices are likely to have a large impact on skin changes. Strategies to promote healthy skin function include not smoking, avoiding exposure to the sun, using a sun protection factor of 15 or higher, wearing protective clothing, using emollient skin cream containing petrolatum or mineral oil, avoiding hot soaks in the bathtub, and maintaining optimal nutrition and hydration (Carpenter, 2015). Older adults should be encouraged to have any changes in the skin examined, because early detection and treatment of precancerous or cancerous lesions are essential for the best outcome.

Reproductive System

An outdated perception is that older adults are asexual, but older adults report that a fairly stable and active sex life is an important quality of life issue. Sexual activity declines with the loss of a partner, primarily for women as a result of widowhood and for men as a result of poor heath, erectile dysfunction, medications, and emotional factors. However, although good health is a predictor of sexual activity, older adults with chronic illnesses may be able to have a sexually active life as well. Because of the many factors that influence the ability to be sexually active, nurses and the older person need to understand the physiologic, psychological, and social factors that affect reproductive and sexual functioning as aging progresses (Miller, 2015; Mola, 2015).

Ovarian production of estrogen and progesterone declines with menopause. Changes that occur in the female reproductive system include thinning of the vaginal wall, along with a shortening of the vagina and a loss of elasticity; decreased vaginal secretions, resulting in vaginal dryness, itching, and decreased acidity; involution (atrophy) of the uterus and ovaries; and decreased pubococcygeal muscle tone, resulting in a relaxed vagina and perineum. Without the use of water-soluble lubricants, these changes may contribute to vaginal bleeding and painful intercourse.

In older men, the testes become less firm but may continue to produce viable sperm up to 90 years of age. At about 50 years of age, production of testosterone begins to diminish (Tabloski, 2013). Decreased libido and erectile dysfunction may develop but are more likely to be associated with factors other than age-related changes. These risk factors include obesity, smoking, cardiovascular disease, neurologic disorders, diabetes, respiratory disease, chronic pain, and many medications (i.e., vasodilators, antihypertensive agents, and tricyclic antidepressants) (Miller, 2015; Mola, 2015).

In both older men and women, it may take longer to become sexually aroused, longer to complete intercourse, and longer before sexual arousal can occur again. Although a less intense response to sexual stimulation and a decline in sexual activity occurs with increasing age, sexual desire does not disappear. Many couples are unaware of the causes of decreased libido or erectile dysfunction and are often reluctant to discuss decreased sexual function. In fact, one survey revealed that in men with erectile dysfunction, less than half of men had discussed the dysfunction with their primary provider (Mola, 2015). Many nonpharmacologic, pharmacologic, and surgical methods are available to improve sexual relationships. Assessment and communication require sensitivity and expert knowledge in the field of sexual dysfunction. If sexual dysfunction is present, referral to a gynecologist, urologist, or sex therapist may be warranted.

Genitourinary System

The genitourinary system continues to function adequately in older adults, although kidney mass is decreased, primarily because of a loss of nephrons. However, the loss of nephrons does not typically become significant until about 90 years of age, and changes in kidney function vary widely; approximately one third of older adults show no decrease in renal function (Tabloski, 2013). Changes in renal function may be attributable to a combination of aging and pathologic conditions such as hypertension. The changes most commonly seen include a decreased filtration rate, diminished tubular function with less efficiency in reabsorbing and concentrating the urine, and a slower restoration of acid–base balance in response to stress. In addition, older adults who take medications may experience serious consequences owing to decline in renal function because of impaired absorption, decreased ability to maintain fluid and electrolyte balance, and decreased ability to concentrate urine.

Certain genitourinary disorders are more common in older adults than in the general population. In the United States, almost 50% of women 80 years of age and older suffer from **urinary incontinence** (i.e., urine leakage or problems controlling urine flow). This condition should not be mistaken as a normal consequence of aging (Weber & Kelley, 2014). Costly and often embarrassing, it should be evaluated, because in many cases it is reversible or can be treated. (See Chapter 55 for further discussion of urinary incontinence.) Benign prostatic hyperplasia (enlarged prostate gland), a common finding in older men, causes a gradual increase in urine retention and overflow incontinence. Changes in the urinary tract increase the susceptibility to urinary tract infections. Adequate consumption of fluids is an important nursing intervention that reduces the risk of bladder infections and also helps decrease urinary incontinence.

Gastrointestinal System

Digestion of food is less influenced by changes associated with aging than by the risk of poor nutrition. Older adults can adjust to changes in the gastrointestinal system but may have difficulty purchasing, preparing, and enjoying their meals. The sense of smell diminishes as a result of neurologic changes and environmental factors such as smoking, medications, and vitamin B_{12} deficiencies. The ability to recognize sweet, sour, bitter, or salty foods diminishes over time, altering satisfaction with food. Salivary flow does not decrease in healthy adults; however, approximately 31% to 37% of older adults may experience a dry mouth as a result of medications and diseases (Miller, 2015). Difficulties with chewing and swallowing are generally associated with lack of teeth and disease.

Experts disagree on the extent of gastric changes that occur as a result of normal aging. However, gastric motility appears to slow modestly, which results in delayed emptying of stomach contents and early satiety (feeling of fullness). Diminished secretion of gastric acid and pepsin, seemingly the result of pathologic conditions rather than normal aging, reduces the absorption of iron, calcium, and vitamin B_{12}. Absorption of nutrients in the small intestine, particularly calcium and vitamin D, appears to diminish with age.

Functions of the liver, gallbladder, and pancreas are generally maintained, although absorption and tolerance to fat may decrease. The incidence of gallstones and common bile duct stones increases progressively with advancing years.

Difficulty swallowing, or dysphagia, increases with age and is a major health care problem in older patients. Normal aging alters some aspects of the swallowing function. In addition, dysphagia is a frequent complication of stroke and a significant risk factor for the development of aspiration pneumonia that can be life-threatening. Dysphagia is caused by interruption or dysfunction of neural pathways. It may also result from dysfunction of the striated and smooth muscles of the gastrointestinal tract in patients with Parkinson disease. Aspiration of food or fluid is the most serious complication and can occur in the absence of coughing or choking.

Constipation is a common pathologic condition that affects many older people as they age. Symptoms of mild constipation are abdominal discomfort and flatulence; more serious constipation leads to fecal impaction that contributes to diarrhea around the impaction, fecal incontinence, and obstruction. Predisposing factors for constipation include lack of dietary bulk, prolonged use of laxatives, some medications, inactivity, insufficient fluid intake, and excessive dietary fat. Ignoring the urge to defecate may also be a contributing factor.

Practices that promote gastrointestinal health include regular tooth brushing and flossing; receiving regular dental care; drinking sufficient fluids; eating small, frequent meals that are high in fiber and low in fat; avoiding heavy activity or lying flat after eating; and avoiding the use of laxatives and antacids. Understanding that there is a direct correlation between loss of smell and taste perception and food intake helps caregivers intervene to maintain the nutritional health of older patients.

Nutritional Health

The social, psychological, and physiologic functions of eating influence the dietary habits of older adults. Increasing age alters nutrient requirements; older adults require fewer calories and a more nutrient-rich, healthy diet in response to alterations in body mass and a more sedentary lifestyle. Recommendations include reducing fat intake while consuming sufficient protein, vitamins, minerals, and dietary fiber for health and prevention of disease. Decreased physical activity and a slower metabolic rate reduce the number of calories needed by older adults to maintain an ideal weight. As stated previously, age-related changes that alter pleasure in eating include a decrease in taste and smell. Older adults are likely to maintain a taste for sweetness but require more sugar to achieve a sweet flavor. They also may lose the ability to differentiate sour, salty, and bitter tastes. Apathy, immobility, depression, loneliness, poverty, inadequate knowledge, and poor oral health also contribute to suboptimal nutrient intake. Budgetary constraints and physical limitations may interfere with food shopping and meal preparation.

 Concept Mastery Alert

Drinking water before a meal may help curb appetite but is not recommended as a way to decrease salt intake. Replacing salt with other flavors, such as herbs and spices, pepper, and lemon, can help decrease salt intake.

MyPlate for Older Adults

20110 TUFTS UNIVERSITY

Figure 11-2 • MyPlate for older adults. Used with permission from the Jean Mayer USDA Human Nutrition Research Center on Aging (HNRCA) at Tufts University.

Health promotion for older adults is based on the individual's physiologic, pathologic, and psychosocial conditions (Cline, 2014). The goals of nutrition therapy are to maintain or restore maximal independent functioning and health and to maintain the sense of dignity and quality of life by imposing as few restrictions as possible. Dietary changes should be incorporated into the older adult's existing food pattern as much as possible. Figure 11-2 lists modified dietary guidelines for older adults.

Women older than 50 years and men older than 70 years should have a daily calcium intake of 1200 mg. To foster the absorption of calcium, adults should have 600 IU of vitamin D until 70 years of age and 800 IU after 70 years of age to maintain bone health (National Institutes of Health, 2014).

Undernutrition, which can lead to malnutrition, may be a problem for older adults. Hospitalized older adults are at particular risk of malnutrition, especially those with cognitive impairment or dementia (Oster & Oster, 2015). A recent unintentional weight loss may be a result of an illness or other factors, such as depression, that may have serious consequences and affect a person's ability to maintain health and fight illness (Grossman & Porth, 2014). Many people are unaware of dietary deficits. Nurses are in an ideal position to identify nutritional problems among their patients and to work within the patient's own framework of knowledge of their health status to improve health behaviors. (See Chapter 5 for more information on nutritional assessment.)

Sleep

Older adults have increased complaints about their sleep as they age, and as many as 50% of those living at home and 65% of those living in nursing homes complain of sleep disturbances (Daglar, Sabancoigullari, Pinar, et al., 2014). Many

factors affect sleep quality in older adults including respiratory problems during sleep, restless leg syndrome, nocturia, pain, osteoarthritis, heart failure, incontinence, prostate hypertrophy, menopause-related problems, pruritus, allergies, AD, depression, dementia, social isolation, loneliness, being bedridden, experiences of loss, drug use, and living in nursing homes (e.g., inadequate lighting, keeping light on during the night, noises). Some of the consequences of poor sleep quality in older adults include cognitive decline, increased risk of falls, daytime fatigue, and reduced physical and mental health and health-related quality of life status (Daglar et al., 2014).

The incidence of sleep apnea (a sleep disorder characterized by brief periods in which respirations are absent) increases with age. Having insomnia symptoms and a sleep-related disorder (snoring, choking, or pauses in breathing) is associated with significantly impaired daytime functioning and longer psychomotor reaction times compared with having either condition. (Sleep apnea is discussed in more detail in Chapter 22.)

The nurse often observes patients while they are sleeping and can identify problems. The nurse can provide health education on sleep hygiene behaviors such as avoiding use of the bed for activities other than sleeping (or sex), maintaining a consistent bedtime routine, avoiding or limiting daytime napping, and limiting alcohol intake to one drink a day. Additional suggestions include avoiding stimulants such as caffeine and nicotine after noon; curbing the amount of liquids in the evening to avoid nocturia; and engaging in regular physical activity, preferably in bright outside light (Daglar et al., 2014).

Musculoskeletal System

Intact musculoskeletal and neurologic systems are essential for the maintenance of safe mobility, performance of activities of daily living (ADLs) (basic personal care activities), and **instrumental activities of daily living (IADLs)** (complex skills such as shopping, cooking, housework, using the telephone, managing medications and finances, and being able to travel by car or public transportation), thus allowing older adults to remain safe and live independently in the community. Age-related changes that affect mobility include alterations in bone remodeling, leading to decreased bone density, loss of muscle mass, deterioration of muscle fibers and cell membranes, and degeneration in the function and efficiency of joints. (These factors are discussed in detail in Unit 9.)

Without exercise, a gradual, progressive decrease in bone mass begins before 40 years of age. The cartilage of joints also progressively deteriorates in middle age. Degenerative joint disease is found in most adults older than 70 years, and weight-bearing joint and back pain is a common complaint. Excessive loss of bone density results in osteoporosis, which leads to potentially life-altering hip and vertebral fractures. Osteoporosis is preventable.

The axiom "use it or lose it" is very relevant to the physical capacity of older adults. Nurses play an important role by encouraging older adults to participate in a regular exercise program. The benefits of regular exercise cannot be overstated. Aerobic exercises are the foundation of programs of cardiovascular conditioning; however, resistance and strength training and flexibility exercises are essential components of an exercise program. Even late in life, in adults who may be frail, it is believed that exercise has benefits of increasing strength, aerobic capacity, flexibility, and balance. In addition, older adults who are hospitalized benefit from getting out of bed as soon as possible and in-hospital physical activity (Oster & Oster, 2015).

Nervous System

Homeostasis is difficult to maintain with aging, but older people have a tremendous ability to adapt and function adequately, retaining their cognitive and intellectual abilities in the absence of pathologic changes. However, normal aging changes in the nervous system can affect all parts of the body. The structure, chemistry, and function of the nervous system change with advanced age. Nerve cells in the brain decrease but the decrease is compensated for by other neurons; there is high variability among individuals and the quantity of neuronal loss varies in different parts of the brain. Overall, the decreases contribute to a small loss of brain mass (Capriotti & Frizzell, 2015). Chemical changes include a decrease in the synthesis and metabolism of the major neurotransmitters. Because nerve impulses are conducted more slowly, older people take longer to respond and react (Miller, 2015). The autonomic nervous system performs less efficiently, and postural hypotension, discussed earlier, may occur. Neurologic changes can affect gait and balance, which may interfere with mobility and safety. Nurses must advise older adults to allow a longer time to respond to a stimulus and to move more deliberately. Adequate nutrition and absorption of vitamin B_{12} is important for neurologic health. Nurses should advise older adults about proper nutrition and intake of vitamin B_{12}, especially for older adults who follow a vegetarian diet.

Slowed reaction time puts older adults at risk for falls and injuries, as well as driving errors. Although older adults spend less time driving than younger people, older adults are just as likely to be involved in motor vehicle crashes that result in serious injury or death. Older adults who are driving unsafely should receive a driving fitness evaluation (Miller, 2015). The evaluation is often given by an occupational therapist in conjunction with a neuropsychologist, who conducts more detailed cognitive testing.

Mental function may be threatened by physical or emotional stresses. A sudden onset of confusion may be the first symptom of an infection or change in physical condition (e.g., pneumonia, urinary tract infection, medication interactions, and dehydration).

Sensory System

People interact with the world through their senses. Losses associated with old age affect all sensory organs, and it can be devastating not to be able to see to read or watch television, hear conversation well enough to communicate, or discriminate taste well enough to enjoy food. Nearly half of older men and one third of older women report difficulty hearing without a hearing aid. Most older adults have a decrease in visual acuity, a narrowing of the visual field, and may have trouble seeing at night (Oster & Oster, 2015). An uncompensated sensory loss negatively affects the functional ability and quality of life of the older adult. However, assistive devices such as visual and hearing aids can compensate for a sensory loss (Oster & Oster, 2015).

Sensory Loss Versus Sensory Deprivation

In contrast to sensory loss, sensory deprivation is the absence of stimuli in the environment or the inability to interpret existing stimuli (perhaps as a result of a sensory loss). Sensory deprivation can lead to boredom, confusion, irritability, disorientation, and anxiety. A decline in sensory input can mimic a decline in cognition that is in fact not present. Meaningful sensory stimulation provided to the older person is often helpful in correcting this problem. In some situations, one sense can substitute for another in observing and interpreting stimuli. Nurses can enhance sensory stimulation in the environment with colors, pictures, textures, tastes, smells, and sounds. The stimuli are most meaningful if they are appropriate for older adults and the stimuli are changed often. Cognitively impaired people tend to respond well to touch and to familiar music.

Vision

As new cells form on the outside surface of the lens of the eye, the older central cells accumulate and become yellow, rigid, dense, and cloudy, leaving only the outer portion of the lens elastic enough to change shape (accommodate) and focus at near and far distances. As the lens becomes less flexible, the near point of focus gets farther away. This common condition—**presbyopia**—usually begins in the fifth decade of life and requires the person to wear reading glasses to magnify objects (Miller, 2015). In addition, the yellowing, cloudy lens causes light to scatter and sensitivity to glare. The ability to distinguish colors decreases, particularly blue from green. The pupil dilates slowly and less completely because of increased stiffness of the muscles of the iris, thus the older person takes more time to adjust when going to and from light and dark settings and needs brighter light for close vision. Pathologic visual conditions are not a part of normal aging; however, the incidence of eye disease (most commonly cataracts, glaucoma, diabetic retinopathy, and age-related macular degeneration) increases in older adults.

Age-related macular degeneration is the primary cause of vision loss in older adults. An estimated 1.8 million Americans 40 years of age and older are affected by macular degeneration, and that number may reach 2.95 million by 2020 (Centers for Disease Control and Prevention [CDC], 2013). Macular degeneration does not affect peripheral vision, which means that it does not cause blindness. However, it affects central vision, color perception, and fine detail, greatly affecting common visual skills such as reading, driving, and seeing faces. Risk factors include sunlight exposure, cigarette smoking, and heredity. People with fair skin and blue eyes may be at increased risk. Sunglasses and hats with visors provide some protection, and stopping smoking is paramount in preventing the disease. Although there is no definitive treatment and no cure that restores vision, several treatment options are available, depending on factors such as the location of the abnormal blood vessels. Laser photocoagulation and photodynamic therapy are commonly used (CDC, 2013). The earlier this condition is diagnosed, the greater the chances of preserving sight. (See Chapter 63 for more information on altered vision.)

Hearing

Auditory changes begin to be noticed at about 40 years of age. Environmental factors, such as exposure to noise, medications, and infections, as well as genetics, may contribute to hearing loss as much as age-related changes. **Presbycusis** is a gradual sensorineural loss that progresses from the loss of the ability to hear high-frequency tones to a generalized loss of hearing. It is attributed to irreversible inner ear changes. Older adults often cannot follow conversation because tones of high-frequency consonants (the sounds *f, s, th, ch, sh, b, t, p*) all sound alike. Hearing loss may cause older adults to respond inappropriately, misunderstand conversation, and avoid social interaction. This behavior may be erroneously interpreted as confusion. Wax buildup or other correctable problems may also be responsible for hearing difficulties. A properly prescribed and fitted hearing aid may be useful in reducing some types of hearing deficits. (See Chapter 64 for discussion of alterations in hearing.)

Taste and Smell

The senses of taste and smell are reduced in older adults. Of the four basic tastes (sweet, sour, salty, and bitter), sweet tastes are particularly dulled in older adults. Blunted taste may contribute to the preference for salty, highly seasoned foods, but herbs, onions, garlic, and lemon can be used as substitutes for salt to flavor food.

Changes in the sense of smell, generally greater than the loss of taste, are related to cell loss in the nasal passages and in the olfactory bulb in the brain (Grossman & Porth, 2014). Environmental factors such as long-term exposure to toxins (e.g., dust, pollen, and smoke) contribute to the cellular damage.

Psychosocial Aspects of Aging

Successful psychological aging is reflected in the ability of older adults to adapt to physical, social, and emotional losses and to achieve life satisfaction. Because changes in life patterns are inevitable over a lifetime, older adults need resiliency and coping skills when confronting stresses and change. A positive self-image enhances risk taking and participation in new, untested roles.

Although attitudes toward older adults differ in ethnic subcultures, a subtle theme of **ageism**—prejudice or discrimination against older adults—predominates in society, and many myths surround aging. Ageism is based on stereotypes—simplified and often untrue beliefs that reinforce society's negative image of older adults. Although older adults make up an extremely heterogeneous and increasingly a racially and ethnically diverse group, these negative stereotypes are sometimes attributed to all older adults.

Fear of aging and the inability of many to confront their own aging process may trigger ageist beliefs. Retirement and perceived nonproductivity are also responsible for negative feelings, because a younger working person may falsely see older people as not contributing to society, as draining economic resources, and may actually feel that they are in competition with children for resources. Concern about the large numbers of older persons leaving the workforce (baby boomers began to turn 65 years of age in 2010) is fueling this debate.

Negative images are so common in society that older adults themselves often believe and perpetuate them. An understanding of the aging process and respect for each person as an individual can dispel the myths of aging. Nurses can facilitate successful aging by recommending health promotion strategies such as anticipatory planning for retirement, including ensuring adequate income, developing routines not associated with work, and relying on other people and groups in addition to spouse to fill leisure time (Pender, Murdaugh, & Parsons, 2014).

Stress and Coping in the Older Adult

Coping patterns and the ability to adapt to stress develop over the course of a lifetime and remain consistent later in life. Experiencing success in younger adulthood helps a person develop a positive self-image that remains solid through old age. A person's abilities to adapt to change, make decisions, and respond predictably are also determined by past experiences. A flexible, well-functioning person will probably continue as such. However, losses may accumulate within a short period of time and become acute. The older person often has fewer choices and diminished resources to deal with stressful events. Common stressors of old age include normal aging changes that impair physical function, activities, and appearance; disabilities from injury or chronic illness; social and environmental losses related to loss of income and decreased ability to perform previous roles and activities; and the deaths of significant others. Many older adults rely strongly on their families and spiritual beliefs for comfort during stressful times.

Living Arrangements

Many older adults have more than adequate financial resources and good health even until very late in life; therefore, they have many housing options. More than 90% of older adults live in the community, with a relatively small percentage (3.4%) residing in nursing homes in 2013 and a

Chart 11-2 · NURSING RESEARCH PROFILE

Care Transitions for Older Adults Discharged Home from the Emergency Department

Cadogan, M. P., Phillips, L. R. & Ziminski, C. E. (2016). A perfect storm: Care transitions for vulnerable older adults discharged home from the emergency department without a hospital admission. *The Gerontologist, 56*(2), 326–334.

Purpose

Transitions are a vulnerable time for older adults. The purpose of the study was to identify factors that influenced the quality and safety of transitions home for older adults who were discharged directly from the emergency department (ED).

Design

This qualitative descriptive study collected data through nine focus group interviews, with ED staff representing multiple interdisciplinary team members including nurses, physicians, social workers, therapists, and pharmacists. The research was conducted in a level 1 trauma center with approximately 78,000 ED visits per year. The ED is located in an ethnically and economically diverse community in California and does not have a geriatric service.

Findings

Based on the findings from the focus groups, the researchers identified a model of five overlapping concepts that influence the quality and safety for vulnerable older adults who are directly discharged home. The five concepts are the "nature of the geriatric presentation" (e.g., complex and multidimensional), "provider knowledge-base" (information about the patient including home situation), "consumer knowledge-base (ability to successfully manage the health problems), resource-base" (staff mix, time to adequately care for an older, slower patient), and "system fractures" (deficiencies and lack of connections within the health system).

Nursing Implications

Nurses need to understand the underlying factors that contribute to hospital readmission or repeat ED visits for older adult patients who visit the ED. Successful discharge to home uses interventions targeted to the needs of the patient population that clearly extend beyond the ED visit. Some recommended practices include making a follow-up appointment before the patient leaves the ED or referral for a nurse follow-up home visit.

---

comparable percentage living in some type of senior housing. Eighty-one percent of those older than 65 years own their homes. Twenty-eight percent of noninstitutionalized older people live alone and widowed women predominate. In 2014, 72% of men older than 65 years were married compared with 42% of women in the same age group. This difference in marital status increases with age and is a result of several factors: Women have a longer life expectancy than men; women tend to marry older men; and women tend to remain widowed, whereas men often remarry (AoA, 2014).

Many older adults relocate in response to changes in their lives such as retirement or widowhood, a significant deterioration in health, or disability. The type of housing they choose depends on their reason for moving. With increasing disability and illness, older adults may move to retirement facilities or assisted living communities that provide some support such as meals, transportation, and housekeeping but otherwise allow them to live somewhat independently. If they develop a serious illness or disability and can no longer live independently or semi-independently, they may need to move to a setting where additional support is available, such as a relative's home or a long-term care or assisted living facility. Often they will seek a location near an adult child's home.

Living at Home or With Family

Most older adults want to remain in their own homes; in fact, they function best in their own environment. The family home and familiar community may have strong emotional significance for them, and this should not be ignored. However, with advanced age and increasing disability, adjustments to the environment may be required to allow older adults to remain in their own homes or apartments (see Chart 11-2). Additional family support or more formal support may be necessary to compensate for declining function and mobility. Many services and organizations can assist older adults to successfully "age in place" in their own homes or in assisted living facilities (see Resources at the end of this chapter).

Sometimes older adults or couples move in with adult children. This can be a rewarding experience as the children, their parents, and the grandchildren interact and share household responsibilities (see Fig. 11-3). It can also be stressful, depending on family dynamics. Adult children and their older parents may choose to pool their financial resources by moving into a house that has an attached "in-law suite." This arrangement provides security for the older adult and privacy for both families. Many older adults and their adult children make housing decisions in times of crisis, such as during a serious illness or after the death of a spouse. Caring for an older adult may also be stressful; older adults and their families often are unaware of the emotional and physical demands of shared housing and assuming care for an increasingly dependent person, especially given the uncertain and extended length of time that may be associated with caring

Figure 11-3 • Families are an important source of psychosocial and physical support for all people. Caring interaction among grandchildren, grandparents, and other family members typically contributes to the health of all.

for a person with a chronic illness. Families can be helped by anticipatory guidance and long-term planning before a crisis occurs. Older adults should participate in decisions that affect them as much as possible.

Continuing Care Retirement Communities

Continuing care retirement communities (CCRCs) offer three levels of living arrangements and care that provide for aging in place (Miller, 2015). CCRCs consist of independent single-dwelling houses or apartments for people who can manage their day-to-day needs, assisted living apartments for those who need limited assistance with their daily living needs, and skilled nursing services when continuous nursing assistance is required. CCRCs usually contract for a large down payment before the resident moves into the community. This payment gives a person or couple the option of residing in the same community from the time of total independence through the need for assisted or skilled nursing care. Decisions about living arrangements and health care can be made before any decline in health status occurs. CCRCs also provide continuity at a time in an older adult's life when many other factors, such as health status, income, and availability of friends and family members, may be changing.

Assisted Living Facilities

Assisted living facilities are an option when an older person's physical or cognitive changes necessitate at least minimal supervision or assistance. Assisted living allows for a degree of independence while providing minimal nursing assistance with administration of medication, assistance with ADLs, or other chronic health care needs. Other services, such as laundry, cleaning, and meals, may also be included. Both assisted living and CCRCs are costly and primarily paid out-of-pocket.

Long-Term Care Facilities

Many types of nursing homes, nursing facilities, or long-term care facilities offer continuous nursing care. Contrary to the myth of family abandonment and the fear of "ending up in a nursing home," the actual percentage of long-term nursing home residents has declined, from 5.4% in 1985 to 3.4% in 2013 (AoA, 2014). However, the actual number of older people who reside in long-term care facilities has risen owing to the large increase in older adults and the use of nursing homes for short-term rehabilitation.

Short-term nursing facility care is often reimbursed by Medicare if the patient is recovering from an acute illness such as a stroke, myocardial infarction, or cancer and requires skilled nursing care or therapy for recuperation. Usually, if an older adult suffers a major health event and is hospitalized and then goes to a nursing facility, Medicare covers the cost of the first 30 to 90 days in a skilled nursing facility as long as ongoing therapy is needed. The requirement for continued Medicare coverage during this time is documentation of persistent improvement in the condition that requires therapy, most often physical therapy, occupational therapy, respiratory therapy, or cognitive therapy. Some adults choose to have long-term care insurance as a means of paying, at least in part, for the cost of these services should they become necessary. Costs of long-term care for older adults who are living in nursing homes and are medically stable, despite having multiple chronic and debilitating health issues, are primarily paid out-of-pocket by the patient. When a person's financial resources become exhausted as a result of prolonged nursing home care, the patient, the institution, or both may apply for Medicaid reimbursement. Family members are not responsible for nursing home costs.

An increasing number of skilled nursing facilities offer subacute care. This area of the facility offers a high level of nursing care that may either avoid the need for a resident to be transferred to a hospital from the nursing home or allow a hospitalized patient to be transferred back to the nursing facility sooner.

The Role of the Family

Planning for care and understanding the psychosocial issues confronting older adults must be accomplished within the context of the family. If dependency needs occur, the spouse often assumes the role of primary caregiver. In the absence of a surviving spouse, an adult child may assume caregiver responsibilities and need help in providing or arranging for care and support.

Two common myths in American society are that adult children and their aged parents are socially alienated, and that adult children abandon their parents when health and other dependency problems arise. In reality, the family has been and continues to be an important source of support for older adults; similarly, older family members provide a great deal of support to younger family members.

Although adult children are not financially responsible for their older parents, social attitudes and cultural values often dictate that adult children should provide services and assume the burden of care if their aged parents cannot care for themselves. It is estimated that in 2014, informal caregivers provided 17.9 billion hours of unpaid care (Alzheimer's Association, 2015). Caregiving, which may continue for many years, can become a source of family stress and is a well-known risk for psychiatric and physical morbidity. Evidence-based interventions to reduce distress and enhance well-being in caregivers have been identified. Three broad types of effective programs include (1) psychoeducational skill building, (2) cognitive behavioral therapy, and (3) using a combination of at least two approaches such as education, family meetings, and skill building sessions (Bakas, Clark, Kelly-Hayes, et al., 2014). Web-based programs can be effective, efficient, and a better fit for the hectic lives of caregivers (Gies, Pierce, Steiner, et al., 2014).

Cognitive Aspects of Aging

Cognition can be affected by many variables, including sensory impairment, physiologic health, environment, sleep, and psychosocial influences. Older adults may experience temporary changes in cognitive function (i.e., delirium) when hospitalized or admitted to skilled nursing facilities, rehabilitation centers, or long-term care facilities. These changes are related to differences in the environment or in medical therapy or to alteration in role performance. A commonly used assessment tool is the Mini-Mental State Examination (MMSE) (see Chart 11-3).

Good sleep hygiene can improve cognition, as can treatment of depression and anxiety. Several researchers are

Chart 11-3 — ASSESSMENT
Assessing Mental Status: Mini-Mental State Examination Sample Items

Orientation to Time

"What is the date?"

Naming

"What is this?" (Point to a pencil or pen.)

Reading

"Please read this and do what it says." (Show examinee the words on the stimulus form.) CLOSE YOUR EYES.

Reproduced by special permission of the Publisher, Psychological Assessment Resources, Inc., 16204 North Florida Avenue, Lutz, FL 33549, from the Mini-Mental State Examination, by Marshall Folstein and Susan Folstein, Copyright 1975, 1998, 2001, by Mini Mental LLC, Inc. Published 2001 by Psychological Assessment Resources, Inc. Further reproduction is prohibited without permission of PAR, Inc. The MMSE can be purchased from PAR, Inc. by calling (813) 968-3003. Used with permission.

evaluating memory enhancement programs for older adults (McDougall, Vance, Wayde, et al., 2015).

When intelligence test scores from people of all ages are compared, test scores for older adults show a progressive decline beginning in midlife. However, research has shown that environment and health have a considerable influence on scores, and that certain types of intelligence (e.g., spatial perceptions and retention of nonintellectual information) decline, whereas others (e.g., problem-solving ability based on past experiences, verbal comprehension, and mathematical ability) do not. Cardiovascular health, a stimulating environment, and high levels of education, occupational status, and income all appear to have a positive effect on intelligence scores in later life.

Significant age-related declines in intelligence, learning, and memory are not inevitable. Many factors affect the ability of older adults to learn and remember and to perform well in testing situations. Older adults who have higher levels of education, good sensory function, good nutrition, and jobs that require complex problem-solving skills continue to demonstrate intelligence, memory, and the capacity for learning. Part of the challenge in testing older adults is determining what is actually being tested (e.g., speed of response) and whether the test results are indicative of a normal age-related change, a sensory deficit, or poor health. However, age differences continue to emerge even with untimed tests and when the tests are controlled for variations in motor and sensory function. In general, fluid intelligence—the biologically determined intelligence used for flexibility in thinking and problem solving—declines. Researchers suggest this decline is related to circulatory and nervous system disorders and is not a normal age-related change (Bergman & Almkvist, 2013). Therefore, preventing or managing these diseases may positively affect the decline in fluid intelligence. Crystallized intelligence—gained through education and lifelong experiences (e.g., verbal skills)—remains intact. These differences exemplify the classic aging pattern of intelligence. Despite these slight declines, many older adults continue to learn and

participate in varied educational experiences. Good health and motivation are important influences on learning (see Chart 11-4). An important consideration for learning is allowing adequate time, particularly when new technology is involved (Harris, Thomas, & Fox, 2015).

Pharmacologic Aspects of Aging

Because an increasing number of chronic conditions affect older adults, they use more medications than any other age group. Although medications improve health and well-being by relieving pain and discomfort, treating chronic illnesses, and curing infectious processes, adverse drug reactions are common because of medication interactions, multiple medication effects, incorrect dosages, and the use of multiple medications.

Drug Interactions and Adverse Effects

Polypharmacy is the prescription, use, or administration of more medications than is clinically indicated. Over or incorrect prescribing occurs commonly in older adults (Miller, 2015). The potential for drug–drug interactions increases with increased medication use and with multiple coexisting diseases (**comorbidity**) that affect the absorption, distribution, metabolism, and elimination of the medications. Such interactions are responsible for numerous emergency department and physician visits, which cost billions of dollars annually.

Any medication is capable of altering nutritional status, and the nutritional health of an older adult may already be compromised by a marginal diet or by chronic disease and its treatment. Medications can affect the appetite, cause nausea and vomiting, irritate the stomach, cause constipation or diarrhea, and decrease absorption of nutrients. In addition, these medications may alter electrolyte balance as well as carbohydrate and fat metabolism. For example, antacids may cause thiamine deficiency; laxatives diminish absorption; antibiotics and phenytoin (Dilantin) reduce utilization of folic acid; and phenothiazines, estrogens, and corticosteroids increase appetite and cause weight gain.

Chart 11-4 — HEALTH PROMOTION
Nursing Strategies for Promoting Cognitive Function

Nurses can support the processes by which older adults learn by using the following strategies:

- Supply mnemonics to enhance recall of related data.
- Encourage ongoing learning.
- Link new information with familiar information.
- Use visual, auditory, and other sensory cues.
- Encourage learners to wear prescription glasses and hearing aids.
- Provide glare-free lighting.
- Provide a quiet, nondistracting environment.
- Set short-term goals with input from the learner.
- Prioritize the most important information and focus on the priority information.
- Keep teaching periods short.
- Pace learning tasks according to the endurance of the learner.
- Encourage verbal participation by learners.
- Reinforce successful learning in a positive manner.

Combining multiple medications with alcohol, as well as with over-the-counter and herbal medications, further complicates gastrointestinal problems. For example, St. John's wort, a common herbal supplement effective for mild depression, decreases the anticoagulant effect of warfarin (Coumadin) and interacts with many other medications metabolized in the liver (Miller, 2015).

Altered Pharmacokinetics

Alterations in absorption, metabolism, distribution, and excretion occur as a result of normal aging and may also result from drug and food interactions (Oster & Oster, 2015). Absorption may be affected by changes in gastric pH and a decrease in gastrointestinal motility. Drug distribution may be altered as a result of decrease in body water and increase in body fat. Normal age-related changes and diseases that alter blood flow, liver and renal function, or cardiac output may affect distribution and metabolism (see Table 11-2).

Nursing Implications

Principles that have been identified as appropriate for older patients include starting with a low dose, going slowly, keeping the medication regimen as simple as possible, and reconciling new and previous medication regimens at the time of discharge from an acute hospital stay (Foust & Kilbourne, 2015). A comprehensive assessment that begins with a thorough medication history, including use of alcohol, recreational drugs, and over-the-counter and herbal medications, is essential. It is best to ask the patient or reliable informants to provide all medications for review. Assessing the patient's understanding of when and how to take each medication, as well as the purpose of each medication, allows the nurse to assess the patient's health literacy and compliance with the medication regimen. The patient's beliefs and concerns about the medications should be identified, including beliefs on whether a given medication is helpful.

Nonadherence with medication regimens can lead to significant morbidity and mortality among older adults. The

TABLE 11-2 Altered Drug Responses in Older Adults

Age-Related Changes	Effect of Age-Related Change	Applicable Medications
Absorption		
Reduced gastric acid; increased pH (less acid)	Rate of drug absorption—possibly delayed	Vitamins
Reduced gastrointestinal motility; prolonged gastric emptying	Extent of drug absorption—not affected	Calcium
Distribution		
Decreased circulating plasma proteins and total body water	Serious alterations in drug binding to plasma proteins (the unbound drug gives the pharmacologic response); highly protein-bound medications have fewer binding sites, leading to increased effects and accelerated metabolism and excretion.	*Selected highly protein-binding medications:* Oral anticoagulants (warfarin) Oral hypoglycemic agents (sulfonylureas) Barbiturates Calcium channel blockers Furosemide (Lasix) Nonsteroidal anti-inflammatory drugs (NSAIDs) Sulfonamides Quinidine Phenytoin (Dilantin)
Reduced cardiac output	Decreased perfusion of many bodily organs	
Impaired peripheral blood flow	Decreased perfusion	
Increased or decreased percentage of body fat	Proportion of body fat increases with age, resulting in increased ability to store fat-soluble medications; this causes drug accumulation, prolonged storage, and delayed excretion.	*Selected fat-soluble medications:* Barbiturates Diazepam (Valium) Lidocaine Phenothiazines (antipsychotics) Ethanol Morphine
Decreased lean body mass	Decreased body volume allows higher peak levels of medications.	
Metabolism		
Decreased cardiac output; decreased size of the liver; diminished intestinal and portal vein blood flow	Decreased metabolism and delay of breakdown of medications, resulting in prolonged duration of action, accumulation, and drug toxicity	All medications metabolized by the liver
Excretion		
Decreased renal blood flow; loss of functioning nephrons; decreased renal efficiency	Decreased rates of elimination and increased duration of action; danger of accumulation and drug toxicity	*Selected medications with prolonged action:* Aminoglycoside antibiotics Cimetidine (Tagamet) Chlorpropamide (Diabinese) Digoxin Lithium Procainamide

Adapted from Comerford, K. C. (2015). *Nursing 2015 drug handbook.* Philadelphia, PA: Wolters Kluwer.

Chart 11-5	Nursing Strategies for Improving Medication Management and Adherence

The following strategies can help patients manage their medications and improve adherence:

- Assess self-management abilities, psychomotor skills, and current medication knowledge.
- Explain the purpose, adverse effects, and dosage of each medication, particularly those that are newly prescribed.
- Provide the medication schedule in writing.
- Encourage the use of standard containers without safety lids (if there are no children in the household).
- Suggest the use of a multiple-day, multiple-dose medication dispenser to help the patient adhere to the medication schedule.
- Destroy or remove old, unused medications.
- Encourage the patient to inform the primary provider about the use of over-the-counter medications and herbal agents, alcohol, and recreational drugs.
- Encourage the patient to keep a current list of all medications, including over-the-counter and herbal medications, in their purse or wallet to share with the primary provider at each visit and in case of an emergency.
- Reconcile medication schedule upon discharge from hospital or rehabilitation facility.
- Recommend using one supplier for prescriptions; pharmacies frequently track patients and are likely to notice a prescription problem such as duplication or contraindications in the medication regimen.
- If the patient's competence is doubtful, identify a reliable family member or friend who might assist the patient with adherence.

Adapted from Foust, J. B., & Kilbourne, G. A. (2015). Improving posthospital medication management for chronically ill older adults. *American Nursing Today. 10*(3), 26–29.

many contributing factors include the number of medications prescribed, the complexity of the regimen, difficulty opening containers, inadequate patient education, financial cost, and the disease or medication interfering with the patient's life. Visual and hearing problems may make it difficult to read or to hear directions. Multifaceted interventions tailored to the individual patient are the most effective strategies in improving adherence (Foust & Kilbourne, 2015) (see Chart 11-5). Allowing enough time for the older adult to learn new skills, particularly when technology is involved, is essential (Harris et al., 2015; Oster & Oster, 2015).

Mental Health Problems in the Older Adult

Severe mood swings, uncontrolled laughing or crying, changes in cognitive ability, and excessive forgetfulness are not a part of normal aging. These symptoms should not be dismissed as age-related changes; a thorough assessment may reveal a treatable, reversible condition. Changes in mental status can be related to many factors, such as alterations in diet and fluid and electrolyte balance, fever, or low oxygen levels associated with many cardiovascular and pulmonary diseases. Older adults are less likely than younger people to acknowledge or seek treatment for mental health symptoms. Changes may be reversible when the underlying condition is identified and

treated. Nurses must recognize, assess, refer, collaborate, treat, and support older adults who exhibit signs and symptoms of depression, substance abuse, delirium, or dementia.

Depression

Depression is the most common affective or mood disorder of old age. The percentage of older adults with depressive symptoms varies widely depending upon the measures used and the population studied. Modiga, Midlov, and Kristensson (2014) reported that between 7% and 29% of older adults have depressive symptoms. Depression among older adults can follow a major precipitating event or loss and is often related to chronic illness or pain. It may also be secondary to a medication interaction or an undiagnosed physical condition. Rather than obvious sadness, an older person may exhibit more subtle signs of depression such as fatigue, diminished memory and concentration, feelings of worthlessness, sleep disturbances, appetite disturbances with excessive weight loss or gain, restlessness, impaired attention span, and suicidal ideation. Mild depression with symptoms that do not meet the criteria for a major depression is often underrecognized and undertreated, which results in reduced quality of life and function (Modiga et al., 2014).

The risk of suicide is increased in older adults. There is a need for routine assessment of patients for depression and risk for suicide. Geriatric depression may be confused with dementia. However, the cognitive impairment resulting from depression is related to apathy rather than decline in brain function. When depression and medical illnesses coexist, as they often do, neglect of the depression can impede physical recovery. Assessing the patient's mental status, including depression, is vital and must not be overlooked. A commonly used assessment tool is the Geriatric Depression Scale (GDS) (see Chart 11-6).

Older adults with depression can respond appropriately to treatment. Initial management involves evaluation of the patient's medication regimen and eliminating or changing any medications that contribute to depression. Furthermore, treatment of underlying medical conditions that may produce depressive symptoms may alleviate the depression. For mild depression, nonpharmacologic measures such as exercise, bright lighting, increasing interpersonal interactions, cognitive therapy, and reminiscence therapy are effective. However, for major depression, antidepressants and short-term psychotherapy, particularly in combination, are effective in older adults. Antidepressants, such as bupropion hydrobromide (Wellbutrin), venlafaxine hydrochloride (Effexor), and mirtazapine (Remeron), as well as selective serotonin reuptake inhibitors, such as paroxetine hydrochloride (Paxil), can be effective (Comerford, 2015). Tricyclic antidepressants can be useful for treating major depression in some patients. Electroconvulsive therapy is highly effective when antidepressant medications are not tolerated, not effective, or pose a significant medical risk (Miller, 2015).

Most antidepressant medications have anticholinergic, cardiac, and orthostatic adverse effects (Comerford, 2015). They also interact with other medications and, therefore, should be used with care to avoid medication toxicity, hypotensive events, and falls. Older patients prescribed antidepressants should be carefully monitored for side effects.

Chart 11-6 Geriatric Depression Scale

Choose the best answer for how you felt this past week.

[a]1.	Are you basically satisfied with your life?	YES	NO
2.	Have you dropped many of your activities and interests?	YES	NO
3.	Do you feel that your life is empty?	YES	NO
4.	Do you often get bored?	YES	NO
[a]5.	Are you hopeful about the future?	YES	NO
6.	Are you bothered by thoughts you can't get out of your head?	YES	NO
[a]7.	Are you in good spirits most of the time?	YES	NO
8.	Are you afraid that something bad is going to happen to you?	YES	NO
[a]9.	Do you feel happy most of the time?	YES	NO
10.	Do you often feel helpless?	YES	NO
11.	Do you often get restless and fidgety?	YES	NO
12.	Do you prefer to stay at home, rather than going out and doing new things?	YES	NO
13.	Do you frequently worry about the future?	YES	NO
14.	Do you feel you have more problems with memory than most?	YES	NO
[a]15.	Do you think it is wonderful to be alive now?	YES	NO
16.	Do you often feel downhearted and blue?	YES	NO
17.	Do you feel pretty worthless the way you are now?	YES	NO
18.	Do you worry a lot about the past?	YES	NO
[a]19.	Do you find life very exciting?	YES	NO
20.	Is it hard for you to get started on new projects?	YES	NO
[a]21.	Do you feel full of energy?	YES	NO
22.	Do you feel that your situation is hopeless?	YES	NO
23.	Do you think that most people are better off than you are?	YES	NO
24.	Do you frequently get upset over little things?	YES	NO
25.	Do you frequently feel like crying?	YES	NO
26.	Do you have trouble concentrating?	YES	NO
[a]27.	Do you enjoy getting up in the morning?	YES	NO
28.	Do you prefer to avoid social gatherings?	YES	NO
[a]29.	Is it easy for you to make decisions?	YES	NO
[a]30.	Is your mind as clear as it used to be?	YES	NO

Score: _____ (Number of "depressed" answers)

Norms

Normal: 5 ± 4
Mildly depressed: 15 ± 6
Very depressed: 23 ± 5

[a]Appropriate (nondepressed) answers = yes; all others = no.
From Yesavage, J., Brink, T. L., Rose, T. L., et al. (1983). Development and validation of a geriatric screening scale: A preliminary report. *Journal of Psychiatric Research, 17*(1), 37–49. Reprinted with permission from Pergamon Press Ltd., Headington Hill Hall, Oxford OX3 OBW, UK.

Good patient education is needed to make sure older adults understand that it may take even longer than the typical 4 to 6 weeks for symptoms to diminish. During this period, nurses should offer support, encouragement, and strategies to maintain safety, such as changing positions slowly and maintaining adequate hydration (Miller, 2015).

Substance Abuse

Substance abuse caused by misuse of alcohol and drugs may be related to depression. Thirty-six percent of adults 65 years of age and older report that they are current drinkers; 2% of men and less than 1% of women meet the criteria for alcohol abuse (Miller, 2015). Moderate levels of alcohol consumption may be associated with positive health risks, such as lowering the risks for cardiovascular disease. Alcohol abuse,

while rare, is especially dangerous in older adults because of age-related changes in renal and liver function as well as the high risk of interactions with prescription medications and the resultant adverse effects. Alcohol and drug-related problems in older adults often remain hidden because many older adults deny their habit when questioned. Assessing for drug and alcohol use with direct questions in a nonaccusatory manner should be part of the routine physical assessment (AoA, 2012b). (See Chapter 5 for more information and specific assessment tools.)

Delirium

Delirium, often called *acute confusional state,* begins with disorientation and if not recognized and treated can progress to changes in level of consciousness, irreversible brain damage, and sometimes death. It is a major complication for the hospitalized older adult, costing the US health system approximately $7 billion each year for associated medical care costs (Layne et al., 2015). Patients may experience an altered level of consciousness, ranging from stupor (hypoalert–hypoactive) to excessive activity (hyperalert–hyperactive); alternatively, they may have a combination of these two types (mixed). Thinking is disorganized, and the attention span is short. Hallucinations, delusions, fear, anxiety, and paranoia may also be evident. Patients who tend to be hyperalert and hyperactive demand more attention from nurses and thus are easier to diagnose, whereas those who are hypoalert or hypoactive tend to be less problematic and pose diagnostic difficulties. Recognition of delirium can also be complicated in patients with the mixed disorders. Patients with the hypoalert–hypoactive type of delirium have higher mortality rates and even poorer outcomes of care because the delirium tends not to be recognized and treated (Layne et al., 2015).

Attentive clinical assessment is essential because delirium is sometimes mistaken for dementia; Table 11-3 compares dementia and delirium. It helps to know an individual patient's usual mental status and whether the changes noted are long term, which probably represents dementia, or are abrupt in onset, which is more likely delirium.

Delirium occurs secondary to numerous causes, including physical illness, surgery, medication or alcohol toxicity, dehydration, fecal impaction, malnutrition, infection, head trauma, lack of environmental cues, and sensory deprivation or overload. Older adults are particularly vulnerable to acute confusion because of their decreased biologic reserve and the large number of medications they may take. Nurses must recognize the symptoms of delirium and report them immediately. The Confusion Assessment Method is a commonly used screening tool (Inouye, van Dyck, Alessi, et al., 1990; Layne et al., 2015). (See Chart 11-7). Because of the acute and unexpected onset of symptoms and the unknown underlying cause, delirium is a medical emergency. If the delirium goes unrecognized and the underlying cause is not treated, permanent, irreversible brain damage or death can follow.

The most effective approach is prevention. Strategies include providing therapeutic activities for cognitive impairment, reorienting the patient as needed, ensuring early mobilization, controlling pain, minimizing the use of psychoactive drugs, preventing sleep deprivation, enhancing communication methods (particularly eye glasses and hearing aids) for vision and hearing impairment, maintaining oxygen levels and fluid and electrolyte balance, and preventing surgical complications (Layne et al., 2015; Miller, 2015).

Once delirium occurs, treatment of the underlying cause is most important. Therapeutic interventions vary depending on the cause. Delirium increases the risk of falls; therefore, management of patient safety and behavioral problems is essential. Because medication interactions and toxicity are often implicated, the nurse should alert the prescriber about any nonessential medications that could be discontinued. Nutritional and fluid intake should be supervised and monitored. The environment should be quiet and calm. To increase function and comfort, the nurse provides familiar environmental cues and encourages family members or friends to touch and talk to the patient (see Fig. 11-4). Ongoing mental status assessments using prior mental cognitive status as a baseline are helpful

Figure 11-4 • Talking to family members may increase the comfort of patients with delirium.

in evaluating responses to treatment and upon admission to a hospital or extended care facility. If the underlying problem is adequately treated, the patient often returns to baseline within several days. Several resources specific to delirium are included in the Resources section at the end of the chapter.

Dementia

The cognitive, functional, and behavioral changes that characterize dementia eventually destroy a person's ability to function. The symptoms are usually subtle in onset and often progress slowly until they are obvious and devastating. The most common type of **dementia** is AD that accounts for up to 70% of older adults with dementia (Grossman & Porth, 2014). Other non-Alzheimer dementias include degenerative, vascular, neoplastic, demyelinating, infectious, inflammatory, toxic, metabolic, and psychiatric disorders. It is important to identify reversible dementia, which occurs when pathologic conditions masquerade as dementia.

Alzheimer Disease

AD, the sixth leading cause of death for older adults, is a progressive, irreversible, degenerative neurologic disease that begins insidiously and is characterized by gradual losses of cognitive function and disturbances in behavior and affect. AD can occur in people as young as 40 years of age but is uncommon before 65 years of age. Although the prevalence of AD increases dramatically with increasing age, affecting as many as half of those 85 years and older, AD is not a normal part of aging. Without a cure or any preventive measures, it is estimated that 13.4 million Americans will have this disease by 2050 (Kochanek et al., 2014; Weuve et al., 2014).

There are numerous theories about the cause of age-related cognitive decline. Although the greatest risk factor for AD is increasing age, many environmental, dietary, and inflammatory factors also may determine whether a person suffers from this cognitive disease. AD is a complex brain disorder caused by a combination of various factors that may include genetics, neurotransmitter changes, vascular abnormalities, stress hormones, circadian changes, head trauma, and the presence of seizure disorders.

AD can be classified into two types: familial or early-onset AD and sporadic or late-onset AD (see Table 8-5). Familial

TABLE 11-3 Summary of Differences Between Dementia and Delirium

| | Dementia | | Delirium |
	Alzheimer's Disease (AD)	Vascular (Multi-Infarct) Dementia	
Etiology	Early onset (familial, genetic [chromosomes 14, 19, 21]) Late-onset sporadic—etiology unknown	Cardiovascular (CV) disease Cerebrovascular disease Hypertension	Drug toxicity and interactions; acute disease; trauma; chronic disease exacerbation Fluid and electrolyte disorders
Risk factors	Advanced age; genetics	Pre-existing CV disease	Pre-existing cognitive impairment
Occurrence	70% of dementias	10–20% of dementias	7–61% among hospitalized people
Onset	Slow	Often abrupt Follows a stroke or transient ischemic attack	Rapid, acute onset A harbinger of acute medical illness
Age of onset	Early-onset AD: 30s–65 years Late-onset AD: 65+ years Most commonly: 85+ years	Most commonly 50–70 years	Any age, although predominantly in older persons
Gender	Males and females equally	Predominantly males	Males and females equally
Course	Chronic, irreversible; progressive, regular, downhill	Chronic, irreversible Fluctuating, stepwise progression	Acute onset Hypoalert—hypoactive Hyperalert–hyperactive Mixed hypo–hyper
Duration	2–20 years	Variable; years	Lasts 1 day to 1 month
Symptom progress	Onset insidious: *Early*—mild and subtle *Middle and late*—intensified Progression to death (infection or malnutrition)	Depends on location of infarct and success of treatment; death attributed to underlying CV disease	Symptoms are fully reversible with adequate treatment; can progress to chronicity or death if underlying condition is ignored.
Mood	Depression common	Labile: mood swings	Variable
Speech/language	Speech remains intact until late in disease: *Early*—mild anomia (cannot name objects); deficits progress until speech lacks meaning; echoes and repeats words and sounds; mutism *Early*—no motor deficits	May have speech deficit/aphasia depending on location of lesion	Fluctuating; often cannot concentrate long enough to speak May be somnolent
Physical signs	*Middle*—apraxia (cannot perform purposeful movement) *Late*—Dysarthria (impaired speech) *End stage*—loss of all voluntary activity; positive neurologic signs	According to location of lesion: focal neurologic signs, seizures Commonly exhibits motor deficits	Signs and symptoms of underlying disease
Orientation	Becomes lost in familiar places (topographic disorientation) Has difficulty drawing three-dimensional objects (visual and spatial disorientation) Disorientation to time, place, and person—with disease progression		May fluctuate between lucidity and complete disorientation to time, place, and person
Memory	Loss is an early sign of dementia; loss of recent memory is soon followed by progressive decline in recent and remote memory		Impaired recent and remote memory; may fluctuate between lucidity and confusion
Personality	Apathy, indifference, irritability: *Early disease*—social behavior intact; hides cognitive deficits *Advanced disease*—disengages from activity and relationships; suspicious; paranoid delusions caused by memory loss; aggressive; catastrophic reactions		Fluctuating; cannot focus attention to converse; alarmed by symptoms (when lucid); hallucinations; paranoid
Functional status, activities of daily living	Poor judgment in everyday activities; has progressive decline in ability to handle money, use telephone, use computer and other electronic devices, function in home and workplace		Impaired
Attention span	Distractible; short attention span		Highly impaired; cannot maintain or shift attention
Psychomotor activity		Wandering, hyperactivity, pacing, restlessness, agitation	Variable; alternates between high agitation, hyperactivity, restlessness, and lethargy
Sleep–wake cycle	Often impaired; wandering and agitation at nighttime		Takes brief naps throughout day and night

Adapted from Grossman, S. C., & Porth, C. M. (2014). *Pathophysiology: Concepts of altered health states* (9th ed.). Philadelphia, PA: Lippincott Williams & Wilkins.

Chart 11-7 — ASSESSMENT: Confusion Assessment Method

Acute Onset

1. Is there evidence of an acute change in mental status from the patient's baseline?

Inattention[a]

2. **A.** Did the patient have difficulty focusing attention, for example, being easily distractible, or having difficulty keeping track of:
   What was being said?
   Not present at any time during interview.
   Present at some time during interview but in mild form.
   Present at some time during interview, in marked form.
   Uncertain.
   B. (If present or abnormal) Did this behavior fluctuate during the interview, that is, tend to come and go or increase and decrease in severity?
   Yes.
   No.
   Uncertain.
   Not applicable.
   C. (If present or abnormal) Please describe this behavior:

Disorganized Thinking

3. Was the patient's thinking disorganized or incoherent, such as rambling or irrelevant conversation, unclear or illogical flow of ideas, or unpredictable switching from subject to subject?

Altered Level of Consciousness

4. Overall, how would you rate this patient's level of consciousness?
   Alert (normal).
   Vigilant (hyperalert, overly sensitive to environmental stimuli, startled very easily).
   Lethargic (drowsy, easily aroused).
   Stupor (difficult to arouse).
   Coma (unarousable).
   Uncertain.

Disorientation

5. Was the patient disoriented at any time during the interview, such as thinking that he or she was somewhere other than the hospital, using the wrong bed, or misjudging the time of day?

Memory Impairment

6. Did the patient demonstrate any memory problems during the interview, such as inability to remember events in the hospital or difficulty remembering instructions?

Perceptual Disturbances

7. Did the patient have any evidence of perceptual disturbances, for example, hallucinations, illusions, or misinterpretations (such as thinking something was moving when it was not)?

Psychomotor Agitation

8. Part 1.
   At any time during the interview, did the patient have an unusually increased level of motor activity, such as restlessness, picking at bedclothes, tapping fingers, or making frequent sudden changes of position?

Psychomotor Retardation

8. Part 2.
   At any time during the interview, did the patient have an unusually decreased level of motor activity, such as sluggishness, staring into space, staying in one position for a long time, or moving very slowly?

Altered Sleep–Wake Cycle

9. Did the patient have evidence of disturbance of the sleep–wake cycle, such as excessive daytime sleepiness with insomnia at night?

[a]The questions listed under this topic were repeated for each topic where applicable.
From Inouye, S. K., van Dyck, C. H., Alessi, C. A., et al. (1990). Clarifying confusion: The confusion assessment method. *Annals of Internal Medicine, 113*(12), 941–948. Used with permission.

AD is rare, accounting for less than 1% of all cases, and is frequently associated with genetic mutations (Sherva & Kowall, 2015). It can occur in middle-aged adults. If family members have at least one other relative with AD, then there is a familial component, which may include both environmental triggers and genetic determinants.

Pathophysiology

The pathogenesis of AD is uncertain but the disease includes specific neuropathologic and biochemical changes that interfere with neurotransmission. These changes consist of neurofibrillary tangles (tangled masses of nonfunctioning neurons) and senile or neuritic plaques (deposits of amyloid protein, part of a larger protein called *amyloid precursor protein* in the brain) (see Fig. 11-5). The neuronal damage occurs primarily in the cerebral cortex and results in decreased brain size. Similar changes are found in the normal brain tissue of nonsymptomatic older adults, although to a lesser extent. Cells that use the neurotransmitter acetylcholine are principally affected by AD. At the biochemical level, the enzyme active in producing acetylcholine, which is specifically involved in memory processing, is decreased.

Scientists have been studying complex neurodegenerative diseases such as AD and have focused on two key issues: whether a gene might influence a person's overall risk of developing the disease, and whether a gene might influence some particular aspect of a person's risk, such as the age at which the disease begins (age at onset). There are genetic differences in early- and late-onset forms of AD (Sherva & Kowall, 2015). Researchers are investigating what predisposes people to develop the plaques and neurofibrillary tangles that can be seen at autopsy in the brains of patients with AD. Understanding the complex ways in which aging as well as genetic and nongenetic factors affect brain cells over time, eventually leading to AD, continues to increase.

Clinical Manifestations

In the early stages of AD, forgetfulness and subtle memory loss occur. Patients may experience small difficulties in work

Figure 11-5 • Healthy and diseased neurons and formation of *tau* tangles. From National Institute on Aging, National Institutes of Health, Alzheimer's Disease Education and Referral Center. Retrieved at: www.nia.nih.gov/alzheimers/scientific-images

or social activities but have adequate cognitive function to compensate for the loss and continue to function independently. With further progression of AD, the deficits can no longer be concealed. Forgetfulness is manifested in many daily actions; patients may lose their ability to recognize familiar faces, places, and objects and they may become lost in a familiar environment. They may repeat the same stories or ask the same question repeatedly. Trying to reason with people with AD and using reality **orientation** only increase their anxiety without increasing function. Conversation becomes difficult, and word-finding difficulties occur. The ability to formulate concepts and think abstractly disappears—for example, a patient can interpret a proverb only in concrete terms. Patients are often unable to recognize the consequences of their actions and, therefore, exhibit impulsive behavior—for example, on a hot day a patient may decide to wade in the city fountain fully clothed. Patients have difficulty with everyday activities, such as operating simple appliances and handling money.

Personality changes are also usually evident. Patients may become depressed, suspicious, paranoid, hostile, and even combative. Progression of the disease intensifies the symptoms: Speaking skills deteriorate to nonsense syllables, agitation and physical activity increase, and patients may wander at night. Eventually, assistance is needed for most ADLs, including eating and toileting, because dysphagia and incontinence develop. The terminal stage, in which patients are usually immobile and require total care, may last months or years. Occasionally, patients may recognize family members or caregivers. Death occurs as a result of complications such as pneumonia, malnutrition, or dehydration.

Assessment and Diagnostic Findings

A definitive diagnosis of AD can be made only at autopsy; however, an accurate clinical diagnosis can be made in the majority of cases. The most important goal is to rule out other causes of dementia that are reversible, such as depression, delirium, alcohol or drug abuse, or inappropriate drug dosage or drug toxicity. AD is a diagnosis of exclusion; a diagnosis of probable AD is made when the medical history, physical examination, and laboratory tests have excluded all known causes of other dementias.

The health history—including medical history, family history, social and cultural history, and medication history—and the physical examination, including functional and mental health status, are essential to the diagnosis of probable AD. Diagnostic tests, including complete blood count, chemistry profile, and vitamin B_{12} and thyroid hormone levels, as well as screening with electroencephalography, computed tomography (CT), magnetic resonance imaging (MRI), and examination of the cerebrospinal fluid, may all refute or support a diagnosis of probable AD.

Depression can closely mimic early-stage AD and coexists in many patients. Therefore, assessing the patient for underlying depression is important. The GDS is a useful tool to assess for depression (see Chart 11-6). Tools such as the MMSE (see Chart 11-3) are useful for assessing cognitive status and screening for AD. Both CT and MRI of the brain are useful for excluding hematoma, brain tumor, stroke, normal-pressure hydrocephalus, and atrophy but are not reliable in making a definitive diagnosis of AD. Infections and physiologic disturbances, such as hypothyroidism, Parkinson disease, and vitamin B_{12} deficiency, can cause cognitive impairment that may be misdiagnosed as AD. Biochemical abnormalities can be excluded through examination of the blood and cerebrospinal fluid.

Medical Management

In AD, the primary goal is to manage the cognitive and behavioral symptoms. Although there is no cure, several medications slow the progression of the disease. Cholinesterase inhibitors donepezil hydrochloride (Aricept) and rivastigmine tartrate (Exelon), for example, enhance acetylcholine uptake in the brain, thus maintaining memory skills for a period of time. Cognitive ability may improve within 6 to 12 months of therapy. Rivastigmine (Exelon Patch) is indicated for severe AD; It is recommended that treatment continue as long as possible (Comerford, 2015).

Behavioral problems such as agitation and psychosis can be managed by behavioral and psychosocial therapies. Associated depression and behavioral problems can also be treated pharmacologically if other interventions fail. Because symptoms change over time, all patients with AD should be reevaluated routinely, and the nurse should document and report both positive and negative responses to medications (Miller, 2015).

Nursing Management

Nurses play an important role in the recognition of dementia, particularly in hospitalized older adults, by assessing for signs (e.g., repeating or asking the same thing over and over). Nursing interventions for dementia are aimed at promoting patient function and independence for as long as possible. Other important goals include promoting the patient's physical safety, promoting independence in self-care activities, reducing anxiety and agitation, improving communication, providing for socialization and intimacy, promoting adequate nutrition, promoting balanced activity and rest, and supporting and educating family caregivers. These nursing interventions apply to all patients with dementia, regardless of cause.

Supporting Cognitive Function

Because dementia of any type is degenerative and progressive, patients display a decline in cognitive function over time. In the early phase of dementia, minimal cuing and guidance may be all that are needed for the patient to function fairly independently for a number of years. However, as the patient's cognitive ability declines, family members must provide more and more assistance and supervision. A calm, predictable environment helps people with dementia interpret their surroundings and activities. Environmental stimuli are limited, and a regular routine is established. A quiet, pleasant manner of speaking, clear and simple explanations, and the use of memory aids and cues help minimize confusion and disorientation and give patients a sense of security. Prominently displayed clocks and calendars may enhance orientation to time. Color-coding the doorway may help patients who have difficulty locating their room. Active participation may help

patients maintain cognitive, functional, and social interaction abilities for a longer period. Physical activity and communication have also been demonstrated to slow some of the cognitive decline of AD.

Promoting Physical Safety

A safe home and hospital environment allows the patient to move about as freely as possible and relieves the family of constant worry about safety. For the patient residing at home, in order to prevent falls and other injuries, all obvious hazards are removed and hand rails are installed. A hazard-free environment allows the patient maximum independence and a sense of autonomy. Adequate lighting, especially in halls, stairs, and bathrooms, is necessary. Nightlights are helpful, particularly if the patient has increased confusion at night, sometimes referred to as sundowning. Driving is prohibited, and smoking is allowed only with supervision. The patient may have a short attention span and be forgetful; therefore, the nurse and the family must be patient, repeat instructions as needed, and use reminders (i.e., post-it notes, electronic reminders) for daily activities. Doors leading from the house must be secured. Outside the home, all activities must be supervised to protect the patient, and the patient should wear some type of identification in case of separation from the caregiver.

If the patient is hospitalized, additional precautionary measures should be taken. Wandering behavior, which may be worse in the hospital due to unfamiliar surroundings, can often be reduced by gentle persuasion, distraction, or by placing the patient close to the nursing station. Restraints should be avoided because they can increase agitation and lead to injury.

Promoting Independence in Self-Care Activities

Pathophysiologic changes in the brain make it difficult for people with AD to maintain physical independence. Patients should be assisted to remain functionally independent for as long as possible. One way to do this is to simplify daily activities by organizing them into short, achievable steps so that the patient experiences a sense of accomplishment. Frequently, occupational therapists can suggest ways to simplify tasks or recommend adaptive equipment. Direct patient supervision is sometimes necessary; however, maintaining personal dignity and autonomy is important for people with AD, who should be encouraged to make choices when appropriate and to participate in self-care activities as much as possible.

Reducing Anxiety and Agitation

Despite profound cognitive losses, patients are sometimes aware of their diminishing abilities. Patients need constant emotional support that reinforces a positive self-image. When loss of skills occurs, goals are adjusted to fit the patient's declining ability.

The environment should be kept familiar and noise free. Excitement and confusion can be upsetting and may precipitate a combative, agitated state known as a catastrophic reaction (overreaction to excessive stimulation). The patient may respond by screaming, crying, or becoming abusive (physically or verbally); this may be the patient's only way of expressing an inability to cope with the environment. When this occurs, it is important to remain calm and unhurried. Forcing the patient to proceed with the activity only increases the agitation. It is better to postpone the activity until later, even to another day. Frequently, the patient quickly forgets what triggered the reaction. Measures such as moving to a familiar environment, listening to music, stroking, rocking, or distraction may quiet the patient. Research suggests that the use of activities and music therapy, both individualized and in groups, help decrease agitation (Chang, Chu, Yang, et al., 2015; Livingston, Kelly, Lewis-Holmes, et al., 2014). Becoming familiar with a particular patient's usual responses to certain stressors helps caregivers avoid stressful situations.

Patients with dementia who have progressed to the late stages of the disease often reside in nursing homes and are predominantly cared for by unlicensed assistive personnel. One systematic review found that training all staff in communication, person-centered care skills, or dementia care mapping are clinically important interventions that decreased agitation by 30% in long-term care (Livingston et al., 2014). Another study of nursing home residents with dementia suggested that adequately treating pain could reduce both physical and verbal aggression (Ahn, Garvan, & Lyon, 2015). Education for family members and caregivers is essential to minimize patient agitation and can be effectively taught by geriatric advanced nurse practitioners (Gies et al., 2014).

Improving Communication

To promote the patient's interpretation of messages, the nurse should remain unhurried and reduce noises and distractions. Use of clear, easy-to-understand sentences to convey messages is essential because patients frequently forget the meaning of words or have difficulty organizing and expressing thoughts. In the earlier stages of dementia, lists and simple written instructions that serve as reminders may be helpful. In later stages, the patient may be able to point to an object or use nonverbal language to communicate. Tactile stimuli, such as hugs or hand pats, are usually interpreted as signs of affection, concern, and security.

Providing for Socialization and Intimacy Needs

Because socialization with friends can be comforting, visits, letters, and phone calls are encouraged. Recreation is important, and people with dementia are encouraged to participate in simple activities. Realistic goals for activities that provide satisfaction are appropriate. Hobbies and activities such as walking, exercising, and socializing can improve quality of life. The nonjudgmental friendliness of a pet may provide stimulation, comfort, and contentment. Care of plants or a pet can also be satisfying and an outlet for energy.

AD does not eliminate the need for intimacy. Patients and their spouses may continue to enjoy sexual activity. Spouses should be encouraged to talk about any sexual concerns, and sexual counseling may be necessary. Simple expressions of love, such as touching and holding, are often meaningful.

Promoting Adequate Nutrition

Mealtime can be a pleasant social occasion or a time of upset and distress, and it should be kept simple and calm, without confrontations. Patients prefer familiar foods that look appetizing and taste good. Cueing may be necessary to encourage adequate nutrition and hydration. Food is cut into small pieces to prevent choking. Liquids may be easier to swallow if they are thickened. Hot food and beverages are served

Figure 11-6 • A. Assistive feeding devices make it easy for patients to grasp and get food on utensils. **B.** Assistive feeding devices may be required for patients who are weak, fatigued, or paralyzed or have neuromuscular impairment.

warm, and the temperature of the foods should be checked to prevent burns.

When lack of coordination interferes with self-feeding, adaptive equipment is helpful (see Fig. 11-6). Some patients may do well eating with a spoon or with their fingers. If this is the case, an apron or a smock, rather than a bib, is used to protect clothing. As deficits progress, it may become necessary to feed the patient. Forgetfulness, disinterest, dental problems, lack of coordination, overstimulation, and choking all serve as barriers to good nutrition and hydration.

Promoting Balanced Activity and Rest

Many patients with dementia exhibit sleep disturbances, wandering, and behaviors that may be considered inappropriate. These behaviors are most likely to occur when there are unmet underlying physical or psychological needs. Caregivers must identify the needs of patients who are exhibiting these behaviors because further health decline may occur if the source of the problem is not corrected. Adequate sleep and physical exercise are essential. If sleep is interrupted or the patient cannot fall asleep, music, warm milk, or a back rub may help the patient relax. During the day, patients should be encouraged to participate in exercise because a regular pattern of activity and rest enhances nighttime sleep. Long periods of daytime sleeping are discouraged.

Home, Community and Transitional Care

The emotional burden on the families of patients with all types of dementia is enormous. The physical health of the patient is often very stable and the decline gradual. Family members may cling to the hope that the diagnosis is incorrect and that their relative will improve with greater effort. Family members provide at least 80% of the home care that is required by patients with AD (Gies et al., 2014). They are faced with numerous difficult decisions (e.g., when the patient should stop driving, when to assume responsibility for the patient's financial affairs). Aggression and hostility exhibited by the patient are often misunderstood by caregivers, who may feel unappreciated, frustrated, and angry. Feelings of guilt, nervousness, and worry contribute to caregiver fatigue, depression, and family dysfunction. Researchers have identified that a Web-based caregiver assessment can be an effective and efficient method of identifying care needs and planning interventions that promote balance and congruence in the lives of caregivers (Gies et al., 2014).

Neglect or abuse of the patient can occur, and this has been documented in home situations as well as in institutions. If neglect or abuse of any kind—including physical, emotional, sexual, neglect, or financial abuse—is suspected, the local adult protective services agency must be notified. The responsibility of the nurse is to report the suspected abuse, not to prove it.

The Alzheimer's Association is a coalition of family members and professionals who share the goals of family support and service, education, research, and advocacy. Family support groups, respite (relief) care, and adult day care may be available through different community resources, such as the Area Agency on Aging, in which concerned volunteers are trained to provide structure to caregiver support groups (see Resource section at the end of chapter). Respite care is a commonly provided service in which caregivers can get away from the home for short periods while someone else tends to the needs of the patient.

Vascular Dementia

Vascular dementia is the second most common cause of dementia and is characterized by an uneven, stepwise downward decline in mental function (Grossman & Porth, 2014). Multi-infarct dementia, the most common form of vascular dementia, has an unpredictable course and is characterized by variable impairment depending on the affected sites in the brain. The patient may present with a deficit in only one domain such as word retrieval whereas other cognitive abilities may be intact. Diagnosis may be even more difficult if a patient has both vascular dementia and AD.

Because vascular dementia is associated with hypertension and cardiovascular disease, risk factors (e.g., hypercholesterolemia, smoking, heart disease, diabetes) are similar. Prevention and management are also similar. Measures to decrease blood pressure, control diabetes, and lower cholesterol levels may slow cognitive decline.

Additional Aspects of Health Care of the Older Adult

The nurse needs to consider other health issues of older adults. These include pseudobulbar affect, geriatric syndromes, elder neglect and abuse, as well as ethical and legal issues.

Pseudobulbar Affect

The condition known as pseudobulbar affect involves inappropriate or exaggerated emotional expression, usually episodes of laughing or crying. It is associated with brain injury (e.g., stroke, traumatic brain injury, multiple sclerosis [MS], amyotrophic lateral sclerosis [ALS], AD, and Parkinson disease). The term "pseudobulbar" refers to damage that occurs in the corticobulbar tracts in the brain (see Chapter 65). The emotional outbursts can cause embarrassment, anxiety, and depression, and often impair quality of life (Yang & Deeks, 2015).

Older adults with pseudobulbar affect can respond appropriately to treatment. Initial management involves evaluation and recognition that this condition can coexist with mood disorders, such as depression, although crying in these patients should not be considered indicative of depression. Pharmacology studies have reported effective management with Nuedexta (dextromethorphan HBr and quinidine sulfate) in patients with ALS, MS, and dementia (Yang & Deeks, 2015).

Geriatric Syndromes

Older adults tend to acquire multiple problems and illnesses as they age. The decline of physical function leads to a loss of independence and increasing frailty as well as to susceptibility to both acute and chronic health problems, which generally result from several factors rather than from a single cause. When combined with a decrease in host resistance, these factors can lead to illness or injury. Some problems commonly experienced by older adults are becoming recognized as **geriatric syndromes**. These conditions do not fit into discrete disease categories and require a multidisciplinary and comprehensive assessment to identify the underlying cause or causes. Examples include skin impairment, poor nutrition, falls or functional decline, incontinence, cognitive impairment, skin impairment, and sleep disturbances (Brown-O'Hara, 2014). Although these conditions may develop slowly, the onset of symptoms is often acute. Furthermore, the presenting symptoms may appear in other body systems before becoming apparent in the affected system. For example, an older patient may present with confusion, and the underlying disease may be a urinary tract infection, dehydration, or a heart attack (Carlson, Merel, & Yukawa, 2015).

The term *geriatric triad* includes changes in cognitive status, falls, and incontinence. This term is used to focus awareness on these three conditions, which need particular attention and the implementation of prevention measures during the hospitalization of older patients.

Impaired Mobility

The causes of decreased mobility are many and varied. Common causes include strokes, Parkinson disease, diabetic neuropathy, cardiovascular compromise, osteoarthritis, osteoporosis, and sensory deficits. To avoid immobility, older people should be encouraged to stay as active as possible. During illness, bed rest should be kept to a minimum, even with hospitalized patients, because brief periods of bed rest quickly lead to deconditioning and, consequently, to a wide range of complications. When bed rest cannot be avoided, patients should perform active range-of-motion and strengthening exercises with the unaffected extremities, and nurses or family caregivers should perform passive range-of-motion exercises on the affected extremities. Frequent position changes help offset the hazards of immobility. Both the health care staff and the patient's family can assist in maintaining the current level of mobility.

Dizziness

Older adults frequently seek help for dizziness, which presents a particular challenge because there are numerous possible causes. For many, the problem is complicated by an inability to differentiate between true dizziness (a sensation of disorientation in relation to position) and vertigo (a spinning sensation). Other similar sensations include near-syncope and disequilibrium. The causes for these sensations range in severity from minor (e.g., buildup of ear wax) to severe (e.g., dysfunction of the cerebral cortex, cerebellum, brain stem, proprioceptive receptors, or vestibular system). Even a minor reversible cause, such as ear wax impaction, can result in a loss of balance and a subsequent fall and injury. Because dizziness has many predisposing factors, nurses should seek to identify any potentially treatable factors related to the condition.

Falls and Falling

Accidental injuries rank eighth as a cause of death for older people, and falls are the most common cause of nonfatal injuries and hospital admissions. The incidence of falls rises with increasing age. One out of five falls in older adults results in serious injury such as broken bones or a head injury (CDC, 2015).

Although many falls by older adults do not result in injury, between 20% and 30% of older adults who fall sustain moderate to serious injury. Overall, older women who fall sustain a greater degree of injury than do older men; however, men are more likely to die of a fall injury (CDC, 2015). Hip fracture is a common type of fracture that can occur as a result of a fall. Many older adults who fall and sustain a hip fracture are unable to regain their prefracture ability. Causes of falls are multifactorial. Both extrinsic factors such as changes in the environment or poor lighting and intrinsic factors such as physical illness, neurologic changes, or sensory impairment play a role. Mobility difficulties, medication effects, foot problems or unsafe footwear, postural hypotension, visual problems, and tripping hazards are common and treatable causes. Polypharmacy, medication interactions, and the use of alcohol precipitate falls by causing drowsiness, decreased coordination, and postural hypotension. Falls have physical dangers as well as serious psychological and social consequences. It is not uncommon for an older person who has experienced a fall to become fearful and lose self-confidence (Miller, 2015).

Nurses can encourage older adults and their families to make lifestyle and environmental changes to prevent falls. Adequate lighting with minimal glare and shadow can be achieved through the use of small area lamps, indirect lighting, sheer curtains to diffuse direct sunlight, dull rather than shiny surfaces, and nightlights. Sharply contrasting colors can be used to mark the edges of stairs. Grab bars by the bathtub, shower, and toilet are useful. Loose clothing, improperly fitting shoes, scatter rugs, small objects, and pets create hazards and increase the risk of falls. Older adults function best in familiar settings when the arrangement of furniture and objects remains unchanged.

> ### ► Quality and Safety Nursing Alert
>
> *In hospitalized and institutionalized older adults, physical restraints (lap belts; geriatric chairs; side rails, vest, waist, and jacket restraints) and chemical restraints (medications) precipitate many of the injuries they were meant to prevent. Because of the acute negative consequences of restraint use, accrediting agencies of nursing homes and acute care facilities now maintain stringent guidelines for correct application and use.*

Urinary Incontinence

Urinary incontinence may be acute, occurring during an illness, or may develop chronically over a period of years. Older patients often do not report this very common problem unless specifically asked. Transient causes may be attributed to *d*elirium and *d*ehydration; *r*estricted mobility; *i*nflammation, *i*nfection, and *i*mpaction; and *p*harmaceuticals and *p*olyuria (the acronym *drip* may be used to remember them). Once identified, the causative factor can be eliminated.

Older patients with incontinence should be urged to seek help from appropriate health care providers because incontinence can be both emotionally devastating and physically debilitating. Nurses who specialize in behavioral approaches to urinary incontinence management can help patients regain full continence or significantly improve the level of continence. Although medications such as anticholinergics may decrease some of the symptoms of urge incontinence (detrusor instability), the adverse effects of these medications (dry mouth, slowed gastrointestinal motility, and confusion) may make them inappropriate choices for older adults. Various surgical procedures are also used to manage urinary incontinence, particularly stress urinary incontinence.

Detrusor hyperactivity with impaired contractility is a type of urge incontinence that is seen predominantly in the older adult population. In this variation of urge incontinence, patients have no warning that they are about to urinate. They often void only a small volume of urine or none at all and then experience a large volume of incontinence after leaving the bathroom. Nurses should be familiar with this form of incontinence and not show disapproval when it occurs. Many patients with dementia suffer from this type of incontinence, because both incontinence and dementia are a result of dysfunction in similar areas of the brain. Prompted, timed voiding can be of assistance in these patients, although clean intermittent catheterization may be necessary because of postvoid residual urine. (See Chapter 55 for information on management of urinary disorders.)

Increased Susceptibility to Infection

Infectious diseases present a significant threat of morbidity and mortality to older adults, in part because of the blunted response of host defenses caused by a reduction in both cell-mediated and humoral immunity (see Chapters 35 and 36). Age-related loss of physiologic reserve and chronic illnesses also contribute to increased susceptibility. Pneumonia, urinary tract infections, gastrointestinal infections, and skin infections are some of the common infections in older adults.

Because of a weakened immune response, the effects of influenza and pneumococcal infections on older adults are significant. Vaccination can help prevent both infections. There is a national goal to increase vaccination rates among persons 65 years of age and older. More than 70% of those 65 years of age and older reported receiving an influenza vaccination between January and June 2014 and 61% reported that they had received a pneumococcal vaccination (AoA, 2014).

Influenza and pneumococcal vaccinations lower the risks of hospitalization and death in older adults. The influenza vaccine, which is prepared yearly to adjust for the specific immunologic characteristics of the influenza viruses at that time, should be given annually in autumn. Recent research suggests that better protection is provided with the high-dose, trivalent, inactivated influenza vaccine versus the standard vaccine in older adults (DiazGranados, Dunning, Kimmel, et al., 2014). The pneumococcal vaccine should be given every 5 years. Both of these injections can be received at the same time in separate injection sites. Nurses should urge older adults to be vaccinated. All health care providers working with older adults or high-risk chronically ill people should also be immunized.

AIDS occurs across the age spectrum. It is increasingly recognized that AIDS does not spare the older segment of society, and many who are living with HIV/AIDS are aging.

Atypical Responses

Many altered physical, emotional, and systemic reactions to disease are attributed to age-related changes in older adults. Physical indicators of illness that are useful and reliable in young and middle-aged people cannot be relied on for the diagnosis of potential life-threatening problems in older adults. The response to pain in older adults may be lessened because of reduced acuity of touch, alterations in neural pathways, and diminished processing of sensory data.

Older adults who are experiencing a myocardial infarction may not have chest pain but present with confusion. Hiatal hernia or upper gastrointestinal distress is often the cause of chest pain. Therefore, acute abdominal conditions may go unrecognized in older adults because of atypical signs and absence of pain.

The baseline body temperature for older adults is about 1°F lower than it is for younger people (Weber & Kelley, 2014). In the event of illness, the body temperature of an older person may not be high enough to qualify as a traditionally defined fever. A temperature of 37.8°C (100°F) in combination with systemic symptoms may signal infection. A temperature of 38.3°C (101°F) almost certainly indicates a serious infection that needs prompt attention. A blunted fever in the face of an infection often indicates a poor prognosis. Temperatures rarely exceed 39.5°C (103°F). Nurses must be alert to other subtle signs of infection, such as mental confusion, increased respirations, tachycardia, and a change in skin color.

Altered Emotional Impact

The emotional component of illness in older adults may differ from that in younger people. Many older adults equate good health with the ability to perform their daily activities and believe that "you are as old as you feel." An illness that requires hospitalization or a change in lifestyle is an imminent threat to well-being. Older adults admitted to the hospital are at high risk for disorientation, confusion, change in level of consciousness, and other symptoms of delirium, as well as anxiety and fear. In addition, economic concerns and fear of becoming a burden to families often lead to high anxiety in older adults. Nurses must recognize the implications of fear, anxiety, and dependency in older patients. They should encourage autonomy, independent decision making, and early mobilization. A positive and confident demeanor in nurses and family members promotes a positive mental outlook in older patients.

Altered Systemic Response

In an older person, illness has far-reaching repercussions. The decline in organ function that occurs in every system of the aging body eventually depletes the body's ability to respond at full capacity. Illness places new demands on body systems that have little or no reserve to meet the crisis. Homeostasis is jeopardized. Older adults may be unable to respond effectively to an acute illness or, if a chronic health condition is present, they may be unable to sustain appropriate responses over a long period. Furthermore, their ability to respond to definitive treatment is impaired. The altered responses of older adults reinforce the need for nurses to monitor all body system functions closely, being alert to signs of impending systemic complication.

Elder Neglect and Abuse

Older adults are at risk for abuse and neglect both in the community setting and in nursing homes (Burnes, Phillemer, Caccamise, et al., 2015). Because of different definitions and terminology and the pattern of underreporting, a clear picture of the incidence and prevalence of abuse among older adults is lacking. Furthermore, one of the major barriers to fully understanding elder abuse is that most professionals in all professions, including law enforcement, are not equipped to recognize and report this type of abuse. Often victims are reluctant to report the abuse and clinicians are unaware of the frequency of the problems.

Neglect is the most common type of abuse. Other forms of abuse include physical, psychological or emotional, sexual, abandonment, and financial exploitation or abuse. Burnes and colleagues (2015) reported factors associated with physical and emotional abuse included being separated or divorced, living in a low income household, functional impairment, and younger age for community dwelling older adults. Neglect was associated with poor health, living below the poverty level, being separated or divorced, and younger age. Neglect was lowest in Hispanic households (Burnes et al., 2015).

Physical abuse associated with staff misconduct in long-term care facilities has received much attention in the past decade, but one study examined a less commonly investigated problem, that of resident on resident abuse (Schiamberg, von Heydrich, Chee, et al., 2015). This is a significant problem as Schiamberg and colleagues (2015) reported that the rate of this type of abuse was 17% in a sample of more than 450 family members interviewed. Factors associated with resident on resident abuse in a nursing home setting were reported as previous staff physical or emotional abuse; younger age; limitations in ADLs and IADLs; and the emotional closeness of the resident to their family (Schiamberg et al., 2015). Older adults with disabilities of all types are at increased risk for abuse from family members, paid caregivers, and staff, whether they live in the community or a long-term care facility.

Nurses should be alert to possible **elder abuse** and neglect. During the health history, the older adult should be asked about abuse during a private portion of the interview. Most states require that care providers, including nurses, report suspected abuse. Preventive action should be taken when caregiver strain is evident—before elder abuse occurs. Early detection and intervention may provide sufficient resources to the family or the person at risk to ensure patient safety. Interdisciplinary team members, including the psychologist, social worker, or chaplain, can be enlisted to help the caregiver develop self-awareness, increased insight, and an understanding of the disease or aging process. Community resources such as caregiver support groups, respite services, and local offices of Area Agencies on Aging are useful for both the older adult and the caregiver.

Social Services

Many social programs exist for older Americans, including Medicare, Medicaid, the Older Americans Act, Supplemental Security Income, Social Security amendments, Section 202 housing, and Title XX social services legislation. These federal programs have increased health care options and financial support for older Americans. The Older Americans Act mandated creation of a federal aging network, resulting in the establishment of the Area Agencies on Aging, a national system of social services and networks providing many community services for older adults. Each state has an advisory network that is charged with overseeing statewide planning and advocacy for older adults throughout the state. Among the services provided by the Area Agencies on Aging are assessment of need, information and referral, case management, transportation, outreach, homemaker services, day care, nutritional education and congregate meals, legal services, respite care, senior centers, and part-time community work. The agencies target low-income, ethnic minority, rural living, and frail older adults who are at risk for institutionalization; however, the assessment and information services are available to all older adults. Similar services such as homemaker, home health aide, and chore services can be obtained at an hourly rate through these agencies or through local community nursing services if the family does not meet the low-income criteria. Informal sources of help, such as family, friends, mail carriers, church members, and neighbors, all keep an informal watch on community-dwelling senior citizens. See Resources section at the end of the chapter.

Other community support services are available to help older adults outside the home. Senior centers have social and health promotion activities, and some provide a nutritious noontime meal. Adult day care facilities offer daily supervision and social opportunities for older adults who cannot be left alone. Adult day care services, although expensive, provide respite and enable family members to carry on daily activities while the older person is at the day care center.

Health Care Costs of Aging

Health care is a major expenditure for older adults, especially for those with chronic illness and limited financial resources. Older adults, who make up about 13% of the population, accounted for 34% of health care costs, particularly in the last year of life (Centers for Medicaid & Medicare Services [CMS], 2014).

The two major programs that finance health care in the United States are Medicare and Medicaid, both of which are overseen by the CMS. Both programs cover acute care needs such as inpatient hospitalization, physician care, outpatient care, home health services, and skilled nursing care in a nursing facility. Medicare is federally funded, whereas Medicaid is given by states; therefore, eligibility and reimbursements for Medicaid services vary from state to state. For older adults with limited incomes, even with the support of Medicare or Medicaid, paying out-of-pocket expenses can be a hardship. Out-of-pocket health care expenses represent 28% of the income of poor and near-poor older adults. Despite changes to the Medicare prescription benefit plan, out-of-pocket expenditures and prescription costs can be burdensome (AoA, 2014).

Home Health Care

The use of home care services and skilled nursing home care increases with age. Because of the rapidly growing older adult population and the availability of Medicare funding for acute care, home health care in the United States has rapidly expanded. (See Chapter 2 for more information on home health care.)

Hospice Services

Hospice is a program of supportive and palliative services for patients with advanced illness and their families. In most cases, patients are not expected to live longer than 6 months. Hospice care focuses on quality of life, and by necessity, it usually includes realistic emotional, social, spiritual, and financial preparation for death. The goal of hospice is to improve the quality of life by focusing on symptom management, pain control, and emotional support. Under Medicare and Medicaid, medical and nursing services are provided to keep patients as pain free and comfortable as possible. Hospice services may be incorporated into the care of residents in long-term care facilities and include care for end-stage dementia and other chronic diseases such as end-stage heart failure (Ersek & Carpenter, 2014). (For an in-depth discussion of end-of-life care, see Chapter 16.)

Aging With a Disability

As the life expectancy of people with all types of physical, cognitive, and mental disabilities has increased, individuals must deal with the normal changes associated with aging in addition to their preexisting disabilities. There are still large gaps in our understanding of the interaction between disabilities and aging, including how this interaction varies depending on the type and degree of disability and other factors such as socioeconomics and gender. For adults without disabilities, the changes associated with aging may be minor inconveniences. For adults with disorders such as MS, aging is associated with higher rates of secondary health conditions compared to those aging without a disability (Newland, Jenson, Budhathoki, et al., 2015). Many people with disabilities are greatly concerned about what will happen to them as they age and whether assistance will be available when they need care.

It has been proposed that nurses view people with disabilities as capable, responsible individuals who are able to function effectively despite having a disability. Both the interface and the biopsychosocial models of disability can serve as a basis for the role of nurses as advocates for removal of barriers to health care (Sharts-Hopko, Smeltzer, Ott, et al., 2010). The use of such models would also encourage public policies that support full participation of all citizens through greater availability of personal assistants and affordable and accessible transportation. (See Chapter 9 Chart 9-6 for discussion of other disability models.)

Today, children born with intellectual and physical disabilities and those who acquire them early in life are also living into middle and older age. Often, their care has been provided by the family, primarily by the parents. As parents age and can no longer provide the needed care, they seek additional help with the care or long-term care alternatives for their children. However, few services are available at present to support a smooth transition between caregiving by parents and then by others. Research and public policy must focus on supports and interventions that allow people with disabilities who are aging to increase or maintain function within their personal environment as well as in the outside community. Important questions include who will provide the care and how will it be financed. The National Institute on Aging has identified aging with a disability as a focus and is striving to provide streamlined information and access to those with a disability and their family caregivers.

Ethical and Legal Issues Affecting the Older Adult

Nurses play an important role in supporting and informing patients and families when making treatment decisions. This nursing role becomes even more important in the care of aging patients who are facing life-altering and possibly end-of-life decisions. Loss of rights, victimization, and other serious problems might occur if a patient has not made plans for personal and property management in the event of disability or death. As advocates, nurses should encourage end-of-life discussions and educate older adults to prepare advance directives before incapacitation (Miller, 2015).

An advance directive is a formal, legally endorsed document that provides instructions for care (living will) or names a proxy decision maker (**durable power of attorney**). It is to be implemented if the signer becomes incapacitated. This written document must be signed by the person and by two witnesses, and a copy should be given to the physician and placed in the medical record. The advance directive is not meant to be used only when certain (or all) types of medical treatment are withheld; rather, it allows for a description of health care preferences, including requesting full use of all available medical interventions. The health care proxy may have the authority to interpret the patient's wishes on the basis of medical circumstances and should be guided by the decisions or situations stated in the living will.

When such serious decisions are made, possibilities exist for significant conflict of values among patients, family members, health care providers, and the legal representative. Autonomy and self-determination are Western concepts, and people from different cultures may view advance directives as a method for denial of care. Older adults from some cultures may be unwilling to consider the future, or they may wish to protect relatives and not want them to be informed about a serious illness. Nurses can facilitate the decision-making process by being sensitive to the complexity of patients' values and respecting their decisions. Directives must be focused on the wishes of the patient, not those of the family or the designated proxy.

If no advance arrangement has been made and the older person appears unable to make decisions, the court may be petitioned for a competency hearing. If the court rules that an older adult is incompetent, the judge appoints a guardian—a third party who is given powers by the court to assume responsibility for making financial or personal decisions for that person.

People with communication difficulties or mild dementia tend to be viewed as incapable of self-determination. However, people with mild dementia may have sufficient cognitive capability to make some, but perhaps not all, decisions. For example, a patient may be able to identify a proxy decision maker and yet be unable to select specific treatment options. People with mild dementia may be competent to understand the nature and significance of different options for care.

In 1990, the Patient Self-Determination Act (PSDA), a federal law, was enacted to require patient education about advance directives at the time of hospital admission, as well as documentation of this education. Nursing homes are also mandated to enhance residents' autonomy by increasing their involvement in health care decision making. In both nursing homes and hospitals, the documentation and placement of advance directives in the medical record and the education of patients about advance directives vary considerably. Periodically, it is important to ensure that the directives reflect the current wishes of the patient and that all providers have a copy so that they are aware of the patient's wishes.

CRITICAL THINKING EXERCISES

1 `ebp` As a new nurse working in a busy medical-surgical unit, you notice that some of the older patients are presenting with a relatively flat affect. What do you suspect may be the cause of this flattened affect? What screening tool(s) would you recommend for these patients? Would you recommend that these tools be used for every older patient? Why? What follow-up would you recommend? What is the strength of the evidence base guiding your assessment, actions, and recommendations?

2 An 82-year-old woman has been admitted to the emergency department three times in the past 6 months for a fall without a major injury. What are some possible causes of these frequent falls? What essential assessments would you perform? What referrals would you make and why?

3 `pcc` During a posthospitalization home visit for an 81-year-old man with diabetes and an extensive cardiac history, you attempt to do medication reconciliation. The patient admits to some forgetfulness and even confusion about his complex medication schedule. How should you proceed? Identify priorities and strategies that may be helpful to the patient so that he can adhere to the regimen.

REFERENCES

*Asterisk indicates nursing research.
**Double asterisk indicates classic reference.

Books

American Nurses Association (ANA). (2010). *Gerontological nursing: Scope and standards of practice.* Silver Spring, MD: Author.

Capriotti, T., & Frizzell, J. P. (2015). *Pathophysiology: Introductory concepts and clinical perspectives.* Philadelphia, PA: FA Davis.

Comerford, K. C. (2015). *Nursing 2015 drug handbook.* Philadelphia, PA: Wolters Kluwer.

Grossman, S. C., & Porth, C. M. (2014). *Pathophysiology: Concepts of altered health states* (9th ed.). Philadelphia, PA: Lippincott Williams & Wilkins.

Miller, C. A. (2015). *Nursing for wellness in older adults* (7th ed.). Philadelphia, PA: Wolters Kluwer.

Pender, N. J., Murdaugh, C. L., & Parsons, M. A. (Eds.). (2014). *Health promotion in nursing practice* (7th ed.). Upper Saddle River, NJ: Prentice Hall Health.

Tabloski, P. A. (2013). *Gerontological nursing: The essential guide to clinical practice* (3rd ed.). Upper Saddle River, NJ: Prentice Hall Health.

Weber, J. R., & Kelley, J. H. (2014). *Health assessment in nursing* (5th ed.). Philadelphia, PA: Lippincott Williams & Wilkins.

Journals and Electronic Documents

Administration on Aging (AoA) (2012a). *Federal interagency forum on aging-related statistics-2012. Key indicators of well-being.* Retrieved on 9/23/2015 at: www.agingstats.gov/agingstatsdotnet/Main_Site/Data/Data_2012.aspx

Administration on Aging (AoA). (2012b). *Older Americans behavioral health issue brief 2: Alcohol misuse and abuse prevention.* Retrieved on 9/23/2015 at: www.aoa.acl.gov/AoA_Programs/HPW/Behavioral/docs2/Issue%20Brief%202%2 0Alcohol%20Misuse.pdf

Administration on Aging (AoA). (2014). *A profile of older Americans: 2014.* Retrieved on 9/22/2015 at: www.aoa.acl.gov/Aging_Statistics/Profile/Index.aspx

Ahn, H., Garvan, C., & Lyon, D. (2015). Pain and aggression in nursing home residents with dementia. *Nursing Research, 64*(4), 256–263.

Alzheimer's Association. (2015). *Alzheimer's disease: Facts & figures.* Retrieved on 10/14/2015 at: www.alz.org/facts/overview.asp.pdf

Bakas, T., Clark, P.C. Kelly-Hayes, M., et al. (2014). Evidence for stroke family caregiver and dyad interventions. *Stroke, 45*(7), 1–17.

Bergman, L., & Almkvist, O. (2013). The effect of age on fluid intelligence is fully mediated by physical health. *Archives of Gerontology and Geriatrics, 57*(1), 100–109

Brown-O'Hara, P. (2014). Geriatric syndromes and their implications for nursing. *Journal of Legal Nurse Consulting, 25*(2) 8–11.

Burnes, D., Phillemer, K., Caccamise, P. L., et al. (2015). Prevalence of and risk factors for elder abuse and neglect in the community: A population-based study. *Journal of the American Geriatric Society, 63*(9), 1906–1912.

Cadogan, M. P., Phillips, L. R. & Ziminski, C. E. (2016). A perfect storm: Care transitions for vulnerable older adults discharged home from the emergency department without a hospital admission. *The Gerontologist, 56*(2), 326–334.

Carlson, C., Merel, S. E, & Yukawa, M. (2015). Geriatric syndromes and geriatric assessment for the generalist. *The Medical Clinics of North America, 99*(2), 263–279.

Carpenter, H. (2015). Summer sun safety. *American Nurse Today, 10*(7), 46.

Cataldo, J. K., Peterson, A. B., Hunter, M., et al. (2015). E-cigarette marketing and older smokers: Road to renormalization. *American Journal of Health Behaviors, 39*(3), 361–371.

Centers for Disease Control and Prevention (CDC). (2013). *Vision health initiative.* Retrieved on 10/11/2015 at: www.cdc.gov/vision-health/basic_information/eye_disorders.htm

Centers for Disease Control and Prevention (CDC). (2015). *Important facts about falls.* Retrieved on 11/17/2015 at: www.cdc.gov/homeandrecreationalsafety/falls/adultfalls.html

Centers for Medicare & Medicaid Services (CMS). (2014). *National health expenditure data: Fact sheet.* Retrieved on 10/21/2015 at: www.cms.gov/Research-Statistics-Data-and- Systems/Statistics-Trends-and-Reports/NationalHealthExpendData/NHE-Fact-Sheet.html

Chang, Y., Chu, H., Yang, C., et al. (2015). The efficacy of music therapy for people with dementia: A meta-analysis of randomized controlled trials. *Journal of Clinical Nursing, 24*(23–24):3425–3440.

*Cline, D. D. (2014). A concept analysis of individualized aging. *Nursing Education Perspectives, 35*(3), 185–192.

*Daglar, G., Sabancoigullari, S., Pinar, S. E., et al. (2014). Sleep quality in the elderly either living at home or in a nursing home. *Australian Journal of Advanced Nursing, 31*(4), 6–13.

Del Gobbo, L. C., Kalantarian, S., Imamura, F., et al. (2015). Contribution of major lifestyle risk factors for incident heart failure in older adults: The cardiovascular health study. *Journal of the American College of Cardiology Heart Failure, 3*(7), 520–528.

DiazGranados, C. A., Dunning, A. J., Kimmel, M., et al. (2014). Efficacy of high-dose versus standard-dose influenza vaccine in older adults. *New England Journal of Medicine, 371*, 635–645.

Ersek, M., & Carpenter, J. G. (2014). Geriatric palliative care in long term care settings with a focus on nursing homes. *Journal of Palliative Medicine, 16*(10), 1180–1187.

Foust, J. B., & Kilbourne, G. A. (2015). Improving posthospital medication management for chronically ill older adults. *American Nursing Today, 10*(3), 26–29.

*Gies, C., Pierce, L., Steiner, V., et al. (2014). Web-based psychosocial assessment for caregivers of persons with dementia: A feasibility study. *Rehabilitation Nursing, 39*(2), 102–109.

Harris, L., Thomas, V., & Fox, M. (2015). The influence of health care literacy on the use of PHRs among older adults. *Medsurg Nursing, 24*(4), 383–385.

**Inouye, S. K., van Dyck, C. H., Alessi, C. A., et al. (1990). Clarifying confusion: The confusion assessment method. *Annals of Internal Medicine, 113*(12), 941–948.

Kochanek, K. D., Murphy, S. L., Xu, J., et al. (2014). Deaths: Preliminary data for 2013. *National Vital Statistics Report No. 178.* 1–7.

Layne, T., Haas, S. A., Davidson, J. E., et al. (2015). Postoperative delirium prevention in the older adult: An evidence-based process improvement project. *Medsurg Nursing, 24*(4), 256–263.

Livingston, G., Kelly, L., Lewis-Holmes, E., et al. (2014). Non-pharmacological interventions for agitation in dementia: Systematic review of randomized controlled trials. *The British Journal of Psychiatry, 205*, 436–442.

*McDougall, G. J., Vance, D. E., Wayde, E., et al. (2015). Memory training plus yoga for older adults. *Journal of Neuroscience Nursing, 47*(2), 178–188.

Modiga, S., Midllov, P., & Kristensson, J. (2014). Depressive symptoms among frail elderly in ordinary living: Who is affected and who is treated? *Aging & Mental Health, 18*(8), 1022–1028.

Mola, J. R. (2015). Erectile dysfunction in the older adult male. *Urologic Nursing, 35*(2), 87–93.

National Institutes of Health (NIH). (2014). *Dietary supplement fact sheet: Vitamin D.* Retrieved on 10/11/2015 at: https://ods.od.nih.gov/factsheets/VitaminD-HealthProfessional/

*Newland, P., Jensen, M. P., Budhathoki, C., et al. (2015). Secondary health conditions in individuals with multiple sclerosis: A cross-sectional web-based survey analysis. *Journal of Neuroscience Nursing, 47*(3), 124–130.

Oster, K. A., & Oster, C. A. (2015). Special needs population: Care of the geriatric patient population in the perioperative setting. *AORN Journal, 101*(4), 444–456.

Schiamberg, L. B., von Heydrich, L., Chee, G., et al. (2015). Individual and contextual determinants of resident-on-resident abuse in nursing homes: A random sample telephone survey of adults with an older family member in a nursing home. *Archives of Gerontology and Geriatrics, 61*(2), 277–284.

*Sharts-Hopko, N. C., Smeltzer, S., Ott, B. B., et al. (2010). Healthcare experiences of women with visual impairment. *Clinical Nurse Specialist, 24*(3), 149–153.

Sherva, R., & Kowall, N. W. (2015). Genetics of Alzheimer disease. In DeKosky, S. T., Raby, B. A., & Eichler, A.F. (Eds.). *UpToDate.* Retrieved on 10/7/2015 at: www.uptodate.com

Weuve, J., Hebert, L. E., Scherr, P. A., et al. (2014). Deaths in the United States among persons with Alzheimer's disease (2010–2050). *Alzheimer's & Dementia, 10*(2), e40–e46.

Yang, L. P., & Deeks, E. D. (2015). Dextromethorphan/Quinidine: A review of its use in adults with pseudobulbar affect. *Drugs, 75*, 83–90.

**Yesavage, J., Brink, T. L., Rose, T. L., et al. (1983). Development and validation of a geriatric screening scale: A preliminary report. *Journal of Psychiatric Research, 17*(1), 37–49.

Resources

Administration on Aging (AoA), www.aoa.gov

Alzheimer's Association, www.alz.org

American Association for Geriatric Psychiatry (AAGP), www.aagponline.org

American Association of Retired Persons (AARP), www.aarp.org

American Federation for Aging Research (AFAR), www.afar.org

American Geriatrics Society (AGS), www.americangeriatrics.org

Association for Gerontology in Higher Education (AGHE), www.aghe.org

Children of Aging Parents (CAPS), www.caps4caregivers.org

Family Caregiver Alliance (FCA), www.caregiver.org

Gerontological Society of America (GSA), www.geron.org

Hartford Institute for Geriatric Nursing, www.consultgerirn.org

Hospital Elder Life Program (HELP), www.hospitalelderlifeprogram.org

LeadingAge (formerly American Association of Homes and Services for the Aging), www.leadingage.org

MedicAlert + Alzheimer's Association Safe Return (program for locating lost patients), www.alz.org/care/dementia-medic-alert-safe-return.asp

National Caucus and Center on Black Aging (NCBA), www.ncba-aged.org

National Council on Aging (NCOA), www.ncoa.org

National Gerontological Nursing Association (NGNA), www.ngna.org

National Institute on Aging (NIA), Alzheimer's Disease Education and Referral (ADEAR) Center, www.nia.nih.gov/Alzheimers

UNIT 3

Concepts and Challenges in Patient Management

A patient diagnosed with end-stage lung cancer has been admitted to the inpatient hospice unit for pain control. The patient has been in a great deal of pain and discomfort. On admission the patient asked that he receive the ordered amount of pain medication as scheduled. He has since become nonverbal and difficult to arouse. Upon assessment the nurse finds that the patient is restless with slow, shallow breathing and is unable to verbalize that he has pain. The family is concerned that the use of pain medication has inhibited the patient's ability to stay alert and affected his breathing. They have requested that pain medication be held until the patient is alert and can ask for it. They have requested a case conference with the hospice team.

QSEN Competency Focus: Teamwork and Collaboration

The complexities inherent in today's health care system challenge nurses to demonstrate integration of specific interdisciplinary core competencies. These competencies are aimed at ensuring the delivery of safe, quality patient care (Institute of Medicine, 2003). The Quality and Safety Education for Nurses project (QSEN, 2017; Cronenwett, Sherwood, Barnsteiner, et al., 2007) provides a framework for the knowledge, skills, and attitudes (KSA) required for nurses to demonstrate competency in these key areas, which include ***patient-centered care, interdisciplinary teamwork and collaboration, evidence-based practice, quality improvement, safety,*** and ***informatics.***

Teamwork and Collaboration Definition: Function effectively within nursing and interprofessional teams, fostering open communication, mutual respect, and shared decision making to achieve quality patient care.

SELECTED PRE-LICENSURE KSAs	APPLICATION AND REFLECTION
Knowledge	
Describe own strengths, limitations, and values in functioning as a member of the team.	Describe the nurse's role in participating in a case conference. How does the role of the nurse differ from other members of the team?
Skills	
Function competently within own scope of practice as a member of the healthcare team.	Even though the patient is unable to verbalize his pain, what other methods of assessment can the nurse use and rely on to assess pain in this patient? What interventions for pain can a nurse implement as part of a nursing care plan?
Attitudes	
Value different styles of communication used by patients, families, and health care providers. Contribute to resolution of conflict and disagreement.	After the case conference, the hospice team agrees to give the pain medication to the patient as he has requested. The family is displeased with the decision because the patient cannot speak. How can the nurse best diffuse the conflict? Are there other members of the hospice team that may be instrumental in communicating with the family?

Cronenwett, L., Sherwood, G., Barnsteiner, J., et al. (2007). Quality and safety education for nurses. *Nursing Outlook, 55*(3), 122–131.

Institute of Medicine. (2003). *Health professions education: A bridge to quality*. Washington, DC: National Academies Press.

QSEN Institute. (2017). *QSEN competencies: Definitions and pre-licensure KSAs*. Retrieved on 3/1/2017 at: www.qsen.org/competencies/pre-licensure-ksas

12 Pain Management

LEARNING OBJECTIVES

On completion of this chapter, the learner will be able to:

1 Define the fundamental concepts of pain.
2 Distinguish between the types of pain.
3 Describe the four processes of nociception.
4 Explain underlying mechanisms of neuropathic pain.
5 Identify methods to perform a pain assessment.
6 List the first-line agents from the three groups of analgesic agents.

7 Identify the unique effects of select analgesic agents on older adults.
8 Describe practical nonpharmacologic methods that can be used in the clinical setting in patients with pain.
9 Use the nursing process as a framework for the care of patients with pain.

GLOSSARY

acute pain: recent onset of pain that abates as healing occurs; serves as a warning signal that something is wrong or needs attention

addiction: a chronic neurologic and biologic disease characterized by behaviors that include one or more of the following: impaired control over drug use, compulsive use, continued use despite harm, and craving to use the opioid for effects other than pain relief

adjuvant analgesic agent: a drug that has a primary indication other than pain (e.g., anticonvulsant, antidepressant, sodium channel blocker, or muscle relaxant) but is an analgesic agent for some painful conditions; sometimes referred to as coanalgesic

agonist–antagonist: a type of opioid (e.g., nalbuphine [Nubain] and butorphanol [Stadol]) that binds to the *kappa* opioid receptor site acting as an agonist (capable of producing analgesia) and simultaneously to the *mu* opioid receptor site acting as an antagonist (reversing *mu* agonist effects)

allodynia: pain due to a stimulus that does not normally provoke pain, such as touch; typically experienced in the skin around areas affected by nerve injury and commonly seen with many neuropathic pain syndromes

antagonist: drug that competes with agonists for opioid receptor binding sites; can displace agonists, thereby inhibiting their action

breakthrough pain: a transitory increase in pain that occurs on a background of otherwise controlled persistent pain

ceiling effect: an analgesic dose above which further dose increments produce no change in effect

central sensitization: a key central mechanism of neuropathic pain; the abnormal hyperexcitability of central neurons in the spinal cord, which results from complex changes induced by the incoming afferent barrages of nociceptors

chronic or persistent pain: pain that may or may not be time limited but that persists beyond the usual course/time of tissue healing

comfort–function goal: the pain rating identified by the individual patient above which the patient experiences interference with function and quality of life (e.g., activities the patient needs or wishes to perform)

efficacy: the extent to which a drug or another treatment "works" and can produce the effect in question—analgesia in this context

half-life: the time it takes for the plasma concentration (amount of drug in the body) to be reduced by 50% (after starting a drug, or increasing its dose, four to five half-lives are required to approach a steady-state level in the blood, irrespective of the dose, dosing interval, or route of administration; after four to five half-lives, a drug that has been discontinued generally is considered to be mostly eliminated from the body)

hydrophilic: readily absorbed in aqueous solution

intraspinal: "within the spine"; refers to the spaces or potential spaces surrounding the spinal cord into which medications can be given; synonymous with neuraxial

lipophilic: readily absorbed in fatty tissues

metabolite: the product of biochemical reactions during drug metabolism

mu agonist: any opioid that binds to the mu opioid receptor subtype and produces analgesic effects (e.g., morphine); used interchangeably with the terms *full agonist, pure agonist,* and *morphinelike drug*

neuraxial: of the central nervous system; synonymous with intraspinal

neuropathic (pathophysiologic) pain: pain sustained by injury or dysfunction of the peripheral or central nervous systems and distinctly different from nociceptive (physiologic) pain

neuroplasticity: the ability of the peripheral and central nervous systems to change both structure and function as a result of noxious stimuli

nociceptive (physiologic) pain: pain that is sustained by ongoing activation of the sensory system that conducts the perception of noxious stimuli; implies the existence of damage to somatic or visceral tissues sufficient to activate the nociceptive system

nociceptor: a type of primary afferent neuron that has the ability to respond to a noxious stimulus or to a stimulus that would be noxious if prolonged

nonopioid: refers to analgesic agents that include acetaminophen (Tylenol) and nonsteroidal anti-inflammatory drugs (NSAIDs); term is used instead of "nonnarcotic"

NSAID: an acronym for nonsteroidal anti-inflammatory drug (pronounced "en said"); also referred to as aspirinlike drugs

opioid: refers to codeine, morphine, and other natural, semisynthetic, and synthetic drugs that relieve pain by binding to multiple types of opioid receptors; term is preferred to "narcotic"

opioid dose-sparing effect: occurs when a nonopioid or adjuvant is added to an opioid, allowing the opioid dose to be lowered without diminishing analgesic effects

opioid-induced hyperalgesia: a phenomenon in which exposure to an opioid induces increased sensitivity, or a lowered threshold, to the neural activity conducting pain perception; it is the "flip side" of tolerance

opioid naïve: denotes a person who has not recently taken enough opioid on a regular enough basis to become tolerant to the opioid's effects

opioid tolerant: denotes a person who has taken opioids long enough at doses high enough to develop tolerance to many of the opioid's effects, including analgesia and sedation

peripheral sensitization: a key peripheral mechanism of neuropathic pain that occurs when there are changes in the number and location of ion channels; in particular, sodium channels abnormally accumulate in injured nociceptors, producing a lower nerve depolarization threshold, ectopic discharges, and an increase in the response to stimuli

physical dependence: the body's normal response to administration of an opioid for 2 or more weeks; withdrawal symptoms may occur if an opioid is abruptly stopped or an antagonist is given

placebo: any medication or procedure, including surgery, that produces an effect in a patient because of its implicit or explicit intent and not because of its specific physical or chemical properties

preemptive analgesic agents: preinjury pain treatments (e.g., preoperative epidural analgesia and preincision local anesthetic infiltration) to prevent the establishment of peripheral and central sensitization of pain

refractory: nonresponsive or resistant to therapeutic interventions such as analgesic agents

self-report: the ability of an individual to give a report—in this case, of pain, especially intensity; the most essential component of pain assessment

titration: upward or downward adjustment of the amount (dose) of an analgesic agent

tolerance: a process characterized by decreasing effects of a drug at its previous dose, or the need for a higher dose of drug to maintain an effect

withdrawal: result of abrupt cessation or rapid decrease in dose of a substance upon which one is physically dependent. It is not necessarily indicative of addiction

Nurses in all settings play a key role in the management of pain as experts in assessment, drug administration, and patient education. They are uniquely positioned to assume this role as the member of the health care team most consistently at the patient's bedside. These characteristics have led to their distinction as the patient's primary pain manager (Herr, St. Marie, Gordon, et al., 2015).

Fundamental Concepts

Understanding the definition, effects, and types of pain lays the foundation for proper pain assessment and management.

Definition of Pain

The American Pain Society (APS) (2008) defines pain as "an unpleasant sensory and emotional experience associated with actual or potential tissue damage, or described in terms of such damage" (p. 1). This definition describes pain as a complex phenomenon that can impact a person's psychosocial, emotional, and physical functioning. The clinical definition of pain reinforces that pain is a highly personal and subjective experience: "Pain is whatever the experiencing person says it is, existing whenever he says it does" (McCaffery, 1968, p. 8). All accepted guidelines consider the patient's report to be the most reliable indicator of pain and the most essential component of pain assessment (Sandkuhler, 2013).

Effects of Pain

Pain affects individuals of every age, sex, race, and socioeconomic class (Herr et al., 2015; International Association for the Study of Pain [IASP], 2013). It is the primary reason people seek health care and one of the most common conditions that nurses treat. Unrelieved pain has the potential to affect every system in the body and cause numerous harmful effects, some of which may last a person's lifetime (see Table 12-1). Despite many advances in the understanding of the underlying mechanisms of pain and the availability of improved analgesic agents and technology, as well as nonpharmacologic pain management methods, all types of pain continue to be undertreated (Gan, Habib, Miller, et al., 2014; Patel, Guralnik, Dansie, et al., 2013).

Types and Categories of Pain

Pain can be categorized in many ways, and clear distinctions are not always possible. Pain often is described as being acute or chronic (persistent) (MacIntyre & Schug, 2015). **Acute pain** differs from chronic pain primarily in its duration. For example, tissue damage as a result of surgery, trauma, or burns produces acute pain, which is expected to have a relatively short duration and resolve with normal healing. **Chronic pain** is subcategorized as being of cancer or noncancer origin and can be time limited (e.g., may resolve within months) or persist throughout the course of a person's life. Examples of noncancer pain include peripheral neuropathy from diabetes,

TABLE 12-1 Harmful Effects of Unrelieved Pain

Domains Affected	Specific Responses to Pain
Endocrine	↑ Adrenocorticotrophic hormone (ACTH), ↑ cortisol, ↑ antidiuretic hormone (ADH), ↑ epinephrine, ↑ norepinephrine, ↑ growth hormone (GH), ↑ catecholamines, ↑ renin, ↑ angiotensin II, ↑ aldosterone, ↑ glucagon, ↑ interleukin-1; ↓ insulin, ↓ testosterone
Metabolic	Gluconeogenesis, hepatic glycogenolysis, hyperglycemia, glucose intolerance, insulin resistance, muscle protein catabolism, ↑ lipolysis
Cardiovascular	↑ Heart rate, ↑ cardiac workload, ↑ peripheral vascular resistance, ↑ systemic vascular resistance, hypertension, ↑ coronary vascular resistance, ↑ myocardial oxygen consumption, hypercoagulation, deep vein thrombosis
Respiratory	↓ Flows and volumes, atelectasis, shunting, hypoxemia, ↓ cough, sputum retention, infection
Genitourinary	↓ Urinary output, urinary retention, fluid overload, hypokalemia
Gastrointestinal	↓ Gastric and bowel motility
Musculoskeletal	Muscle spasm, impaired muscle function, fatigue, immobility
Cognitive	Reduction in cognitive function, mental confusion
Immune	Depression of immune response
Developmental	↑ Behavioral and physiologic responses to pain, altered temperaments, higher somatization; possible altered development of the pain system, ↑ vulnerability to stress disorders, addictive behavior, and anxiety states
Future pain	Debilitating chronic pain syndromes: postmastectomy pain, postthoracotomy pain, phantom pain, postherpetic neuralgia
Quality of life	Sleeplessness, anxiety, fear, hopelessness, ↑ thoughts of suicide

Copyright 1999, Pasero C., McCaffery M. Used with permission from Pasero, C., & McCaffery, M. (2011). *Pain assessment and pharmacologic management.* St. Louis, MO: Mosby-Elsevier.

back or neck pain after injury, and osteoarthritis pain from joint degeneration. Some conditions can produce both acute and chronic pain. For example, some patients with cancer have continuous chronic pain and also experience acute exacerbations of pain periodically—called **breakthrough pain** (BTP)—or endure acute pain from repetitive painful procedures during cancer treatment (Lehne, 2013; Mantyh, 2013).

Pain is better classified by its inferred pathology as being either nociceptive pain or neuropathic pain (see Table 12-2). **Nociceptive (physiologic) pain** refers to the normal functioning of physiologic systems that leads to the perception of noxious stimuli (tissue injury) as being painful (Ringkamp, Raja, Campbell, et al., 2013). This is why nociception is described as "normal" pain transmission. **Neuropathic (pathophysiologic) pain** is pathologic and results from abnormal processing of sensory input by the nervous system as a result of damage to the peripheral or central nervous system (CNS) or both (Scadding & Koltzenburg, 2013).

Patients may have a combination of nociceptive and neuropathic pain. For example, a patient may have nociceptive pain as a result of tumor growth and also report radiating sharp and shooting neuropathic pain if the tumor is pressing against a nerve plexus. Sickle cell disease pain is usually a combination of nociceptive pain from the clumping of sickled cells and resulting perfusion deficits, and neuropathic pain from nerve ischemia.

Nociceptive Pain

Nociception includes specific processes: transduction, transmission, perception, and modulation. Figure 12-1 illustrates these processes and following is an overview of each.

Transduction

Transduction refers to the processes by which noxious stimuli, such as a surgical incision or burn, activate primary afferent neurons called **nociceptors**, which are located throughout the body in the skin, subcutaneous tissue, and visceral (organ) and somatic (musculoskeletal) structures (Smith, 2013). These neurons have the ability to respond selectively to noxious stimuli generated as a result of tissue damage from mechanical (e.g., incision, tumor growth), thermal (e.g., burn, frostbite), chemical (e.g., toxins, chemotherapy), and infectious sources. Noxious stimuli cause the release of a number of excitatory compounds (e.g., serotonin, bradykinin, histamine, substance P, and prostaglandins), which move pain along the pain pathway (Lehne, 2013) (see Fig. 12-1A).

Prostaglandins are lipid compounds that initiate inflammatory responses that increase tissue swelling and pain at the site of injury (Auriel, Regev, & Korczyn, 2014). They form when the enzyme phospholipase breaks down phospholipids into arachidonic acid. In turn, the enzyme cyclo-oxygenase (COX) acts on arachidonic acid to produce prostaglandins (see Fig. 12-2). COX-1 and COX-2 are isoenzymes of COX and play an important role in producing the effects of the **nonopioid** analgesic agents, which include the nonsteroidal anti-inflammatory drugs (**NSAIDs**) and acetaminophen (Tylenol). NSAIDs produce pain relief primarily by blocking the formation of prostaglandins in the periphery (Lehne, 2013). The nonselective NSAIDs, such as ibuprofen (Motrin, Advil), naproxen (Naprosyn), diclofenac (Voltaren), and ketorolac (Toradol), inhibit both COX-1 and COX-2, and the COX-2 selective NSAIDs, such as celecoxib (Celebrex), inhibit only COX-2. As Figure 12-2 illustrates, both types of NSAIDs produce anti-inflammation and pain relief through the inhibition of COX-2. Acetaminophen is known to be a COX inhibitor that has minimal peripheral effect, is not anti-inflammatory, and can both relieve pain and reduce fever by preventing the formation of prostaglandins in the CNS (Lehne, 2013).

Other analgesic agents work at the site of transduction by affecting the flux of ions. For example, sodium channels are closed and inactive at rest but undergo changes in response to nerve membrane depolarization. Transient channel opening leads to an influx of sodium that results in nerve conduction (King & Vetter, 2014). Local anesthetics reduce nerve conduction by blocking sodium channels. Anticonvulsants also produce pain relief by reducing the flux of other ions, such as calcium and potassium (MacIntyre & Schug, 2015).

Transmission

Transmission is another process involved in nociception. Effective transduction generates an action potential that is transmitted along the A-delta (δ) and C fibers (Ringkamp

TABLE 12-2 Classification of Pain by Inferred Pathology

	Nociceptive Pain	Neuropathic Pain	Mixed Pain
Physiologic Processes	Normal processing of stimuli that damages tissues or has the potential to do so if prolonged; can be somatic or visceral	Abnormal processing of sensory input by the peripheral or central nervous system or both	Components of both nociceptive and neuropathic pain; poorly defined
Categories and Examples	**Somatic Pain:** Arises from bone joint, muscle, skin, or connective tissue. It is usually described as aching or throbbing in quality and is well localized. *Examples:* Surgical, trauma; wound and burn pain; cancer pain (tumor growth) and pain associated with bony metastases; labor pain (cervical changes and uterine contractions); osteoarthritis and rheumatoid arthritis pain; osteoporosis pain; pain of Ehlers–Danlos syndrome; ankylosing spondylitis **Visceral Pain:** Arises from visceral organs, such as the GI tract and pancreas. This may be subdivided: <ul><li>Tumor involvement of the organ capsule that causes aching and fairly well-localized pain</li><li>Obstruction of hollow viscus, which causes intermittent cramping and poorly localized pain</li></ul> *Examples:* Organ-involved cancer pain; ulcerative colitis; irritable bowel syndrome; Crohn's disease; pancreatitis	***Centrally Generated Pain*** *Deafferentation pain:* Injury to either the peripheral or central nervous system; burning pain below the level of a spinal cord lesion reflects injury to the central nervous system. *Examples:* Phantom pain as a result of peripheral nerve damage; poststroke pain; pain following spinal cord injury *Sympathetically maintained pain:* Associated with dysregulation of the autonomic nervous system *Example:* Complex regional pain syndrome ***Peripherally Generated Pain*** *Painful polyneuropathies:* Pain is felt along the distribution of many peripheral nerves. *Examples:* Diabetic neuropathy; postherpetic neuralgia; alcohol–nutritional neuropathy; some types of neck, shoulder, and back pain; pain of Guillain–Barré syndrome *Painful mononeuropathies:* Usually associated with a known peripheral nerve injury; pain is felt at least partly along the distribution of the damaged nerve. *Examples:* Nerve root compression, nerve entrapment; trigeminal neuralgia; some types of neck, shoulder, and back pain	No identified categories *Examples:* Fibromyalgia; some types of neck, shoulder, and back pain; some headaches; pain associated with HIV; some myofascial pain; pain associated with Lyme disease
Pharmacologic Treatment	Most responsive to nonopioids, opioids, and local anesthetics	Adjuvant analgesic agents, such as antidepressants, anticonvulsants, and local anesthetics, but there is wide variability in terms of efficacy and adverse-effect profiles.	Adjuvant analgesic agents, such as antidepressants, anticonvulsants, and local anesthetics, but there is wide variability in terms of efficacy and adverse-effect profiles.

HIV, human immune deficiency virus; GI, gastrointestinal.

et al., 2013). A-δ fibers are lightly myelinated and faster conducting than the unmyelinated C fibers (see Fig. 12-1B). The endings of A-δ fibers detect thermal and mechanical injury, allow relatively quick localization of pain, and are responsible for a rapid reflex withdrawal from the painful stimulus. Unmyelinated C fibers are slow impulse conductors and respond to mechanical, thermal, and chemical stimuli. They produce poorly localized and often aching or burning pain. A-beta (β) fibers are the largest of the fibers and respond to touch, movement, and vibration but do not normally transmit pain (Todd & Koerber, 2013).

Noxious information passes through the dorsal root ganglia and synapses in the dorsal horn of the spinal cord (see Fig. 12-1B). An action potential is generated, and the impulse ascends up to the spinal cord and transmits the information to the brain, where pain is perceived. Extensive modulation occurs in the dorsal horn via complex neurochemical mechanisms (see Fig. 12-1B inset). The primary A-δ fibers and C fibers release various transmitters including glutamate, neurokinins, and substance P. Glutamate is a key neurotransmitter because it binds to the N-methyl-D-aspartate (NMDA) receptor and promotes pain transmission. The drug ketamine, an NMDA receptor **antagonist,** produces analgesia by preventing glutamate from binding to the NMDA receptor sites. Endogenous and exogenous (therapeutically given) **opioids** bind to opioid receptor sites in the dorsal horn to block substance P and thereby produce analgesia (Lehne, 2013). The opioid methadone (Dolophine) binds to opioid receptor sites and has NMDA antagonist properties (Wu, Gikas, & Connelly, 2014).

NOCICEPTION

A. Transduction

TISSUE DAMAGE
- Serotonin
- Bradykinin
- Histamine
- Prostaglandins
- Substance P

Limbic system

Thalamus

Descending pathway

Ascending pathway

Dorsal horn

A-β fiber

Dorsal root ganglion

C fiber

A-δ fiber

Spinal cord

B. Transmission

Periaqueductal gray area

Reticular formation

Descending pathway

ASCENDING PATHWAY

Dorsal horn

PRIMARY NOCICEPTIVE FIBERS (A-δ AND C FIBERS)

Spinal cord

Nociceptor terminal ending

- Norepinephrine
- Glutamate
- Substance P

Na^+

Mg^{++}

NMDA receptor

Dorsal horn

K^+

Ca^{++}

Ca^{++}

C. Perception

Limbic system

Thalamus

Periaqueductal gray area

Descending pathway

Ascending pathway

D. Modulation

Periaqueductal gray area

Reticular formation

DESCENDING PATHWAY

Ascending pathway

Figure 12-1 • Nociception. **A.** Transduction. **B.** Transmission. **C.** Perception. **D.** Modulation. Redrawn from Pasero C., & McCaffery M. (2011). *Pain assessment and pharmacologic management* (p. 5). St. Louis, MO: Mosby-Elsevier. Copyright 2011, Pasero C., McCaffery M. Used with permission.

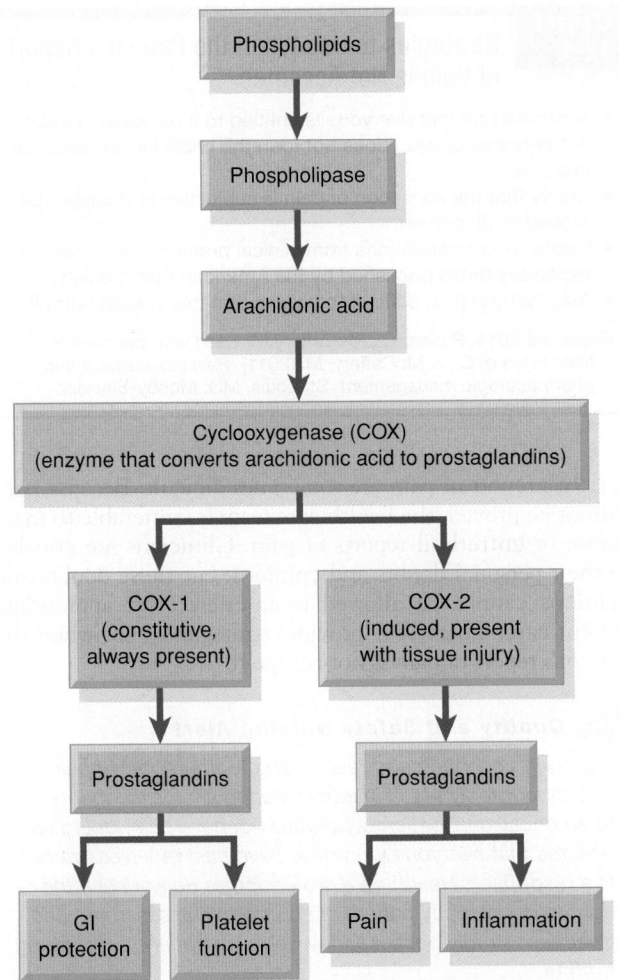

Figure 12-2 • Enzyme pathway: COX-1 and COX-2. Redrawn from Pasero, C., & McCaffery, M. (2011). *Pain assessment and pharmacologic management* (p. 6). St. Louis, MO: Mosby-Elsevier. Copyright 2004, Pasero C., McCaffery M. Used with permission.

Perception

An additional process involved in nociception is perception. Perception is the result of the neural activity associated with transmission of noxious stimuli (Apkarian, Bushnell, Schweinhardt, et al., 2013). It requires activation of higher brain structures for the occurrence of awareness, emotions, and drives associated with pain (see Fig. 12-1C). The physiology of perception of pain continues to be studied but can be targeted by mind–body therapies, such as distraction and imagery, which are based on the belief that brain processes can strongly influence pain perception (Kreitzer & Koithan, 2014).

Modulation

Modulation is another process involved in nociception. Modulation of the information generated in response to noxious stimuli occurs at every level from the periphery to the cortex and involves many different neurochemicals (Heinricher & Fields, 2013) (see Fig. 12-1D). For example, serotonin and norepinephrine are inhibitory neurotransmitters that are released in the spinal cord and the brain stem by the descending (efferent) fibers of the modulatory system. Some antidepressants provide pain relief by blocking the body's reuptake (resorption) of serotonin and norepinephrine, extending their availability to fight pain. Endogenous opioids are located throughout the peripheral and central nervous systems, and like exogenous opioids, they bind to opioid receptors in the descending system and inhibit pain transmission. Dual-mechanism analgesic agents, such as tramadol (Ultram) and tapentadol (Nucynta), bind to opioid receptor sites and block the reuptake of serotonin and/or norepinephrine (Niesters, Proto, Aarts, et al., 2014; Singh, Nag, Shetti, et al., 2013).

Neuropathic Pain

Neuropathic pain is sustained by mechanisms that are driven by damage to, or dysfunction of, the peripheral or central nervous system and is the result of abnormal processing of stimuli (Pasero & Portenoy, 2011) (see Fig. 12-3). Unlike nociceptive

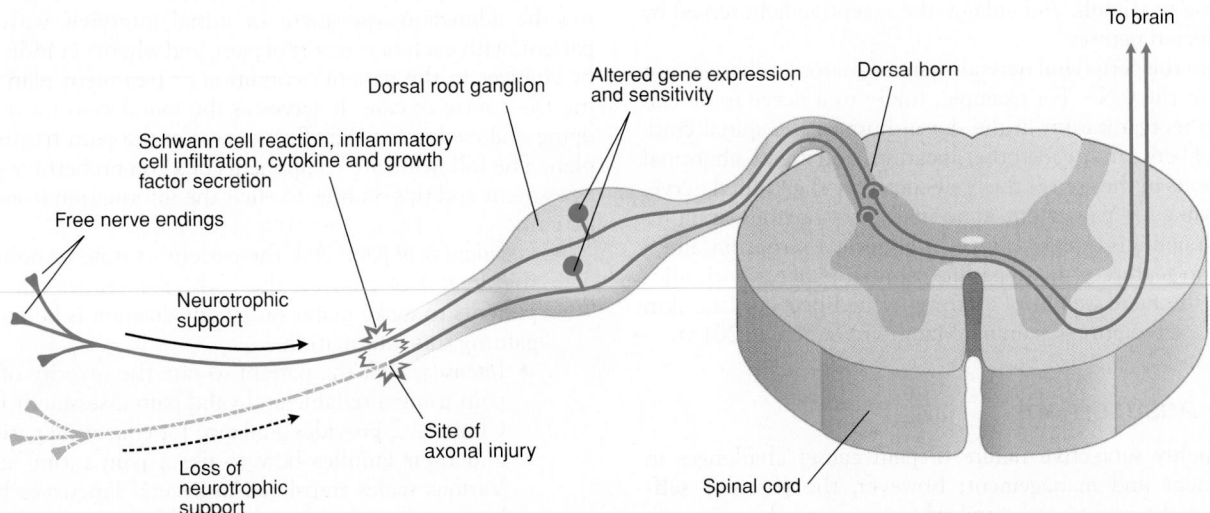

Figure 12-3 • Neuropathic pain. Nociceptive injury or inflammation may result in an altered physiologic response within the nociceptive system. These changes cause release of inflammatory cytokines that may alter gene expression and sensitivity in nociceptive fibers. In turn, these alter nociceptive activity, causing neuropathic pain. Used with permission from Golan, D. E., Tashjian, A. H., & Armstrong, E. J. (2017). *Principles of pharmacology: The pathophysiologic basis of drug therapy* (4th ed.). Baltimore, MD: Wolters Kluwer Health | Lippincott Williams & Wilkins.

pain, neuropathic pain may occur in the absence of tissue damage and inflammation, even when acute neuropathic pain serves no useful purpose. Extensive research is ongoing to better define the peripheral and central mechanisms that initiate and maintain neuropathic pain (Cohen & Mao, 2014; Hoffman, 2015; Momi, Fabiane, Lachance, et al., 2015).

Peripheral Mechanisms

At any point from the periphery to the CNS, the potential exists for the development of neuropathic pain. Hyperexcitable nerve endings in the periphery can become damaged, leading to abnormal reorganization of the nervous system called **neuroplasticity,** an underlying mechanism of some neuropathic pain states (Apkarian, 2015; MacIntyre & Schug, 2015). Changes in the number and location of ion channels can occur. For example, sodium channels abnormally accumulate in injured nociceptors, which can lower the threshold for nerve depolarization and increase response to stimuli, setting off ectopic nerve discharges (Moldovan, Alvarez, Romer Rosberg, et al., 2013). These and many other processes lead to a phenomenon called **peripheral sensitization,** which is thought to contribute to the maintenance of neuropathic pain. Topical local anesthetics, such as lidocaine patch 5% (Lidoderm), produce effects in the tissues right under the site of application by "dampening" neuropathic pain mechanisms in the peripheral nervous system (MacIntyre & Schug, 2015).

Central Mechanisms

Central mechanisms also play a role in the establishment of neuropathic pain. **Central sensitization** is defined as abnormal hyperexcitability of central neurons in the spinal cord, which results from complex changes induced by incoming afferent barrages of nociceptors (Ringkamp et al., 2013). Extensive release and binding of excitatory neurotransmitters, such as glutamate, activate the NMDA receptor and cause an increase in intracellular calcium levels into the neuron, resulting in pain. Similar to what happens in the peripheral nervous system, an increase in the influx of sodium is thought to lower the threshold for nerve activation, increase response to stimuli, and enlarge the receptive field served by the affected neuron.

As in the peripheral nervous system, anatomic changes can occur in the CNS. For example, injury to a nerve route can lead to reorganization in the dorsal horn of the spinal cord. Nerve fibers can invade other locations and create abnormal sensations in the area of the body served by the injured nerve. **Allodynia**, or pain from a normally nonnoxious stimulus (e.g., touch), is one such type of abnormal sensation and a common feature of neuropathic pain. In patients with allodynia, the mere weight of clothing or bedsheets on the skin can be excruciatingly painful (MacIntyre & Schug, 2015).

Pain Assessment

The highly subjective nature of pain causes challenges in assessment and management; however, the patient's **self-report** is the undisputed standard for assessing the existence and intensity of pain (APS, 2008; Herr, Coyne, McCaffery, et al., 2011; McCaffery, Herr, & Pasero, 2011). Self-report is considered the most reliable measure of the existence and intensity of the patient's pain. Accepting and acting on the

---

Chart 12-1 | **Strategies to Use When the Patient's Report of Pain Is Not Accepted**

- Acknowledge that everyone is entitled to a personal opinion, but personal opinion does not form the basis for professional practice.
- Clarify that the sensation of pain is subjective and cannot be proved or disproved.
- Quote recommendations from clinical practice guidelines, especially those published by the American Pain Society.
- Ask, "Why is it so difficult to believe that this person hurts?"

Copyright 2011, Pasero C., McCaffery M. Used with permission from Pasero, C., & McCaffery, M. (2011). *Pain assessment and pharmacologic management*. St. Louis, MO: Mosby-Elsevier.

---

patient's report of pain are sometimes difficult. Because pain cannot be proved, the health care team is vulnerable to inaccurate or untruthful reports of pain. Clinicians are entitled to their personal doubts and opinions, but those doubts and opinions cannot be allowed to interfere with appropriate patient care. Chart 12-1 provides strategies to use when the patient's report of pain is not accepted.

> **Quality and Safety Nursing Alert**
>
> *Although accepting and responding to the report of pain will undoubtedly result in administering analgesic agents to an occasional patient who does not have pain, doing so ensures that everyone who does have pain receives attentive responses. Health care professionals do not have the right to deprive any patient of appropriate assessment and treatment simply because they believe a patient is not being truthful.*

Performing the Comprehensive Pain Assessment: Patient Interview

A comprehensive pain assessment should be conducted during the admission assessment or initial interview with the patient, with each new report of pain, and whenever indicated by changes in the patient's condition or treatment plan during the course of care. It serves as the foundation for developing and evaluating the effectiveness of the pain treatment plan. The following are components of a comprehensive pain assessment and tips on how to elicit the information from the patient:

- *Location(s) of pain:* Ask the patient to state or point to the area(s) of pain on the body. Sometimes allowing patients to make marks on a body diagram is helpful in gaining this information.
  - *Intensity:* Ask the patient to rate the severity of the pain using a reliable and valid pain assessment tool. Chart 12-2 provides guidance for educating patients and their families how to use a pain rating scale. Various scales translated in several languages have been evaluated and made available for use in clinical practice and for educational practice. The most common include the following:
  - *Numeric Rating Scale (NRS):* The NRS is most often presented as a horizontal 0- to 10-point scale, with

Chart 12-2 · PATIENT EDUCATION
Educating Patients and Their Families How to Use a Pain Rating Scale[a]

Step 1. Show the pain rating scale to the patient and the family and explain its primary purpose.

Example: "This is a pain rating scale that many of our patients use to help us understand their pain and to set goals for pain relief. We will ask you regularly about pain, but any time you have pain you must let us know. We do not always know when you hurt."

Step 2. Explain the parts of the pain rating scale. If the patient does not like it or understand it, switch to another scale (e.g., vertical presentation, VDS, or faces).

Example: "On this pain rating scale, 0 means no pain and 10 means the worst possible pain. The middle of the scale, around 5, means moderate pain. A 2 or 3 would be mild pain, but 7 or higher means severe pain."

Step 3. Discuss pain as a broad concept that is not restricted to a severe and intolerable sensation.

Example: "Pain refers to any kind of discomfort anywhere in your body. Pain also means aching and hurting. Pain can include pulling, tightness, burning, knifelike feelings, and other unpleasant sensations."

Step 4. Verify that the patient understands the broad concept of pain. Ask the patient to mention two examples of pain he or she has experienced. If the patient is already in pain that requires treatment, use the present situation as the example.

Example: "I want to be sure that I have explained this clearly, so would you give me two examples of pain you have had recently?" If the patient's examples include various parts of the body and various pain characteristics, that indicates that he or she understands pain as a fairly broad concept. An example of what a patient might say is "I have a mild, sort of throbbing headache now, and yesterday my back was aching."

Step 5. Ask the patient to practice using the pain rating scale with the present pain or select one of the examples mentioned.

Example: "Using the scale, what is your pain right now? What is it at its worst?" OR "Using the pain rating scale and one of your examples of pain, what is that pain usually? What is it at its worst?"

Step 6. Set goals for comfort and function/recovery/quality of life. Ask patients what pain rating would be acceptable or satisfactory, considering the activities required for recovery or for maintaining a satisfactory quality of life.

Example for a surgical patient: "I have explained the importance of coughing and deep breathing to prevent pneumonia and other complications. Now we need to determine the pain rating that will not interfere with this so that you may recover quickly."

Example for patient with chronic pain or terminal illness: "What do you want to do that pain keeps you from doing? What pain rating would allow you to do this?"

[a]When a patient is obviously in pain or not focused enough to learn to use a pain rating scale, pain treatment should proceed without pain ratings. Education can be undertaken when pain is reduced to a level that facilitates understanding how to use a pain scale.

VDS, verbal descriptor scale.
Copyright 2011, McCaffery M., Pasero C. Used with permission from Pasero, C., & McCaffery, M. (2011). *Pain assessment and pharmacologic management*. St. Louis, MO: Mosby-Elsevier.

word anchors of "no pain" at one end of the scale, "moderate pain" in the middle of the scale, and "worst possible pain" at the end of the scale. It may also be put on a vertical axis, which may be helpful for patients who read from right to left.

- *Wong-Baker FACES Pain Rating Scale:* The FACES scale consists of six cartoon faces with word descriptors, ranging from a smiling face on the left for "no pain (or hurt)" to a frowning, tearful face on the right for "worst pain (or hurt)." Patients are asked to choose the face that best reflects their pain. The faces are most commonly numbered using a 0, 2, 4, 6, 8, 10 metric, although 0 to 5 can also be used. Patients are asked to choose the face that best describes their pain. The FACES scale is used in adults and children as young as 3 years (McCaffery et al., 2011). It is important to appreciate that faces scales are self-report tools; clinicians should not attempt to match a face shown on a scale to the patient's facial expression to determine pain intensity. Patients may be able to understand the tool better if it is displayed vertically with no pain as the anchor at the bottom.
- *Faces Pain Scale–Revised (FPS-R):* The FPS-R has six faces to make it consistent with other scales using the 0 to 10 metric. The faces range from a neutral facial expression to one of intense pain and are numbered 0, 2, 4, 6, 8, and 10. As with the Wong-Baker

FACES scale, patients are asked to choose the face that best reflects their pain. Faces scales have been shown to be reliable and valid measures in children as young as 3 years of age; however, the ability to optimally quantify pain (identify a number) is not acquired until approximately 8 years of age (Spagrud, Piira, & Von Baeyer, 2003). Some research shows that the FPS-R is preferred by both cognitively intact and impaired older and minority populations (Guo, Li, Liu, et al., 2015; Sayin & Akyolcu, 2014).

- *Verbal descriptor scale (VDS):* A VDS uses different words or phrases to describe the intensity of pain, such as "no pain, mild pain, moderate pain, severe pain, very severe pain, and worst possible pain." The patient is asked to select the phrase that best describes pain intensity.
- *Visual Analog Scale (VAS):* The VAS is a horizontal (sometimes vertical) 10-cm line with word anchors at the extremes, such as "no pain" on one end and "pain as bad as it could be" or "worst possible pain" on the other end. Patients are asked to make a mark on the line to indicate intensity of pain, and the length of the mark from "no pain" is measured and recorded in centimeters or millimeters. Although often used in research, the VAS is impractical for use in daily clinical practice and rarely used in that setting.

- *Quality:* Ask the patient to describe how the pain feels. Descriptors such as "sharp," "shooting," or "burning" may help identify the presence of neuropathic pain.
- *Onset and duration:* Ask the patient when the pain started and whether it is constant or intermittent.
- *Aggravating and relieving factors:* Ask the patient what makes the pain worse and what makes it better.
- *Effect of pain on function and quality of life:* The effect of pain on the ability to perform recovery activities should be regularly evaluated in the patient with acute pain. It is particularly important to ask patients with persistent pain about how pain has affected their lives, what could they do before the pain began that they can no longer do, or what they would like to do but cannot do because of the pain.
- *Comfort-function (pain intensity) goal:* For patients with acute pain, identify short-term functional goals and reinforce to the patient that good pain control will more likely lead to successful achievement of the goals. For example, surgical patients are told that they will be expected to ambulate or participate in physical therapy postoperatively. Patients with chronic pain can be asked to identify their unique functional or quality-of-life goals, such as being able to work or walk the dog. Success is measured by progress toward meeting those functional goals (Haythornwaite, 2013).
- *Other information:* The patient's culture, past pain experiences, and pertinent medical history such as comorbidities, laboratory tests, and diagnostic studies are considered when establishing a treatment plan.

Patients who are unable to report their pain are at higher risk for undertreated pain than those who can report (Gagliese & Melzack, 2013; McCaffery et al., 2011). In the adult population, this includes patients who are cognitively impaired, critically ill (intubated, unresponsive), comatose, or imminently dying. Patients who are receiving neuromuscular blocking agents or are sedated from anesthesia and other drugs given during surgery are also among this at-risk population.

The Hierarchy of Pain Measures is recommended as a framework for assessing pain in nonverbal patients (Herr et al., 2011; McCaffery et al., 2011). The key components of the hierarchy require the nurse to (1) attempt to obtain self-report, (2) consider underlying pathology or conditions and procedures that might be painful (e.g., surgery), (3) observe behaviors, (4) evaluate physiologic indicators, and (5) conduct an analgesic trial. Chart 12-3 provides detailed information on each component of the Hierarchy of Pain Measures.

Chart 12-3 Hierarchy of Pain Measures

1. Attempt to obtain the patient's self-report, the single most reliable indicator of pain. Do not assume that a patient cannot provide a report of pain; many cognitively impaired patients are able to use a self-report tool if simple actions are taken.
   - Try using standard pain assessment tools (see text).
   - Increase the size of the font and other features of the scale.
   - Present the tool in vertical format (rather than the frequently used horizontal).
   - Try using alternative words, such as "ache," "hurt," and "sore," when discussing pain.
   - Ensure eyeglasses and hearing aids are functioning.
   - Ask about pain in the present.
   - Repeat instructions and questions more than once.
   - Allow ample time to respond.
   - Remember that head nodding and eye blinking or squeezing the eyes tightly can also be used to signal presence of pain and sometimes used to rate intensity.
   - Ask awake and oriented patients who are intubated to point to a number on the numerical scale if they are able.
   - Repeat instructions and show the scale each time pain is assessed.
2. Consider the patient's condition or exposure to a procedure that is thought to be painful. If appropriate, assume pain is present and document as such when approved by institution policy and procedure. As an example, pain should be assumed to be present in a patient who is unresponsive, mechanically ventilated, and critically ill due to trauma.
3. Observe behavioral signs, for example, facial expressions, crying, restlessness, and changes in activity. A pain behavior in one patient may not be in another. Try to identify pain behaviors that are unique to the patient ("pain signature").

Many behavioral pain assessment tools are available that will yield a pain behavior score and may help determine whether pain is present. However, it is important to remember that a behavioral score is not the same as a pain intensity score. Behavioral tools are used to help identify the presence of pain, but the pain intensity is unknown if the patient is unable to provide it.
   - A surrogate who knows the patient well (e.g., parent, spouse, or caregiver) may be able to provide information about underlying painful pathology or behaviors that may indicate pain.
4. Evaluate physiologic indicators with the understanding that they are the *least* sensitive indicators of pain and may signal the existence of conditions other than pain or a lack of it (e.g., hypovolemia, blood loss). Patients quickly adapt physiologically despite pain and may have normal or below normal vital signs in the presence of severe pain. The overriding principle is that the absence of an elevated blood pressure or heart rate does not mean the absence of pain.
5. Conduct an analgesic trial to confirm the presence of pain and to establish a basis for developing a treatment plan if pain is thought to be present. An analgesic trial involves the administration of a low dose of nonopioid or opioid and observing patient response. The initial low dose may not be enough to elicit a change in behavior and should be increased if the previous dose was tolerated, or another analgesic agent may be added. If behaviors continue despite optimal analgesic doses, other possible causes should be investigated. In patients who are completely unresponsive, no change in behavior will be evident and the optimized dose of the analgesic agent should be continued.

Adapted from Pasero, C. (2009). Challenges in pain assessment. *Journal of PeriAnesthesia Nursing, 24*(1), 50–54; Pasero, C., & McCaffery, M. (2011). *Pain assessment and pharmacologic management.* St. Louis, MO: Mosby-Elsevier.

When patients cannot self-report their pain, some observational tools may be used to help with clinical decision making. Some of these assign a score by observing behaviors that tend to be associated with pain. These observational scores are not considered equivalent to a patient's self-reported pain intensity score, however. The following tools are examples of validated tools that are appropriate for different populations of patients unable to self-report their pain (Herr et al., 2011; St. Marie, 2010):

- FLACC: indicated for use in young children. Scores are assigned after assessing *Facial* expression, *Leg* movement, *Activity*, *Crying*, and *Consolability*, with each of these five categories assigned scores from 0 to 2, yielding a total composite score of 0 to 10. Scores of "0" are interpreted as reflecting that the patient is relaxed and comfortable, scores of "1" to "3" are interpreted as consistent with mild discomfort, scores from "4" to "6" are considered consistent with moderate pain, and scores from "7" to "10" are considered consistent with severe discomfort or pain.
- PAINAD (*Pain Assessment IN Advanced Dementia*): indicated for use in adults with advanced dementia who are not able to verbalize their needs. Patterned after the FLACC, this tool was developed by the U.S. Department of Veterans Affairs for patients who have dementia.
- CPOT (*Critical Care Pain Observation Tool*): indicated for use in patients in critical care units who cannot self-report pain, whether or not they may be intubated. It is also patterned after the FLACC.

Reassessing Pain

Following initiation of the pain management plan, pain is reassessed and documented on a regular basis to evaluate the effectiveness of treatment. At a minimum, pain should be reassessed with each new report of pain and before and after the administration of analgesic agents (McCaffery et al., 2011). The frequency of reassessment depends on the stability of the patient's pain and is guided by institutional policy. For example, in the postanesthesia care unit (PACU), reassessment may be necessary as often as every 10 minutes when pain is unstable during opioid **titration** but may be done every 4 to 8 hours in patients with satisfactory and stable pain 24 hours after surgery.

Pain Management

Achieving optimal pain relief is best viewed on a continuum, with the primary objective being to provide both effective and safe analgesia (Lehne, 2013). The quality of pain control should be addressed whenever patient care is passed on from one clinician to another, such as at change of shift and transfer from one clinical area to another. Optimal pain relief is the responsibility of *every* member of the health care team and begins with titration of the analgesic agent, followed by continued prompt assessment and analgesic agent administration during the course of care to safely achieve pain intensities that allow patients to meet their functional goals with relative ease.

Although it may not always be possible to achieve a patient's pain intensity goal within the short time the patient is in an area like the PACU or emergency department, this goal provides direction for ongoing analgesic care. Important information to provide during transfer report is the patient's **comfort–function goal,** how close the patient is to achieving it, what has been done thus far to achieve it (analgesic agents and doses), and how well the patient has tolerated administration of the analgesic agent (adverse effects). There is growing interest among both clinicians and researchers in linking pain management to functional goals. Pain management interventions should improve and not inhibit progress toward healing and rehabilitation (Brown & Flood, 2013; Makris, Abrams, Gurland, et al., 2014).

> **Quality and Safety Nursing Alert**
>
> *Pain control is the responsibility of every member of the health care team and begins with systematic assessment and initial analgesic titration, followed by reassessment and analgesic administration throughout the course of care to safely achieve a level of pain that allows patients to meet their functional goals with relative ease.*

Pharmacologic Management of Pain: Multimodal Analgesia

Pain is a complex phenomenon involving multiple underlying mechanisms and as such, requires more than one analgesic agent to manage it safely and effectively. The recommended approach for the treatment of all types of pain in all age groups is called *multimodal analgesia* (Manworren, 2015). A multimodal regimen combines drugs with different underlying mechanisms, which allows lower doses of each of the drugs in the treatment plan, reducing the potential for each to produce adverse effects. Furthermore, multimodal analgesia can result in comparable or greater pain relief than can be achieved with any single analgesic agent (Manworren, 2015).

Routes of Administration

The oral route is the preferred route of analgesic administration and should be used whenever feasible because it is generally the least expensive, best tolerated, and easiest to administer (MacIntyre & Schug, 2015). When the oral route is not possible, such as in patients who cannot swallow or are NPO (nothing by mouth) or nauseated, other routes of administration are used. For example, patients with cancer pain who are unable to swallow may take analgesic agents by the transdermal, rectal, or subcutaneous route of administration.

In the immediate postoperative period, the intravenous (IV) route is the first-line route of administration for analgesic delivery, and patients are transitioned to the oral route as tolerated. (See Chapter 19 for the management of postoperative pain.)

The rectal route of analgesic administration is an alternative route when oral or IV analgesic agents are not an option (e.g., for palliative purposes during end-of-life care) (MacIntyre & Schug, 2015). The rectum allows passive diffusion of medications and absorption into the systemic circulation. This route of administration can be less expensive and does not involve the skill and expertise required of the parenteral route of administration. Drawbacks are that drug absorption can be unreliable and depends on many factors including rectal tissue health and administrator technique. Some patients may be resistant to or fearful of rectal administration. The rectal route is contraindicated in patients who are neutropenic or thrombocytopenic because of potential rectal bleeding. Diarrhea, perianal abscess or fistula, and abdominoperineal resection are also relative contraindications (MacIntyre & Schug, 2015).

The topical route of administration is used for both acute and chronic pain. For example, the nonopioid diclofenac is available in patch and gel formulations for application directly over painful areas. Local anesthetic creams, such as EMLA (eutectic mixture or emulsion of local anesthetics) and L.M.X.4 (lidocaine cream 4%), can be applied directly over the injection site prior to painful needle stick procedures, and the lidocaine patch 5% is often used for well-localized types of neuropathic pain, such as postherpetic neuralgia. It is important to distinguish between topical and transdermal drug delivery. Although both routes require the drug to cross the stratum corneum to produce analgesia, transdermal drug delivery requires absorption into the systemic circulation to achieve effects; topical agents produce effects in the tissues immediately under the site of application (referred to as targeted peripheral analgesia). Compounding pharmacies may be consulted to custom blend analgesics, such as topical morphine or gabapentin (Neurontin), for topical application at the painful site.

Some of the more invasive methods used to manage pain are accomplished via catheter techniques such as **intraspinal** analgesia, sometimes referred to as **"neuraxial"** analgesia. Delivery of analgesic agents by the intraspinal routes is accomplished by inserting a needle into the subarachnoid space (for intrathecal [spinal] analgesia) or the epidural space and injecting the analgesic agent, or threading a catheter through the needle and taping it in place temporarily for bolus dosing or continuous administration (Deer, Prager, Levy, et al., 2012). Intrathecal catheters for acute pain management are used most often for providing anesthesia or a single bolus dose of an analgesic agent. Implanted intrathecal pumps deliver very small amounts of medication in a constant infusion for treatment of end-of-life pain or persistent pain (Shaparin, Sim, Pappagallo, et al., 2015). Temporary epidural catheters for acute pain management are removed after 2 to 4 days. Epidural analgesia is given by clinician-given bolus, continuous infusion (basal rate), and patient-controlled epidural analgesia (PCEA). The most common opioids given intraspinally are morphine, fentanyl, and hydromorphone (Dilaudid). These are usually combined with a local anesthetic, most often ropivacaine (Naropin) or bupivacaine (Marcaine), to improve analgesia and produce an **opioid dose-sparing effect** (Deer et al., 2012).

A pain management technique that involves the use of an indwelling catheter is the continuous peripheral nerve block (also called *perineural anesthesia*), whereby an initial local anesthetic block is established and followed by the placement of a catheter or catheters through which an infusion of local anesthetic, usually ropivacaine or bupivacaine, is infused continuously to the targeted site of innervation. The effect of local anesthetic is dose dependent: at lower doses, the smaller sensory nerve fibers are affected before the larger motor fibers.

Patients thus medicated are able to walk but are pain free (MacIntyre & Schug, 2015; Narouze, Benzon, Provenzano, et al., 2015).

Dosing Regimen

Two basic principles of providing effective pain management are preventing pain and maintaining a pain intensity that allows the patient to accomplish functional or quality-of-life goals with relative ease (MacIntyre & Schug, 2015). Accomplishment of these goals may require the mainstay analgesic agent to be given on a scheduled around-the-clock (ATC) basis, rather than PRN (as needed) to maintain stable analgesic blood levels. ATC dosing regimens are designed to control pain for patients who report pain being present 12 hours or more during a 24-hour period. PRN dosing of analgesic agents is appropriate for intermittent pain, such as prior to painful procedures and for BTP (pain that "breaks through" the pain being managed by the mainstay analgesic agent), for which supplemental doses of analgesia are provided (Lehne, 2013).

 Concept Mastery Alert

A preventive approach to pain management, also called ATC management, is designed to prevent pain from being experienced.

Patients with persistent pain in the hospital setting should be awakened to take their pain medication. Awakening postoperative patients with moderate to severe pain to take their pain medication is especially important during the first 24 to 48 hours after surgery to keep pain under control. Patients should be told that this helps avoid waking up with severe pain and that if their pain is well controlled, they are likely to go back to sleep quickly. The patient can transition gradually to PRN dosing as pain resolves. In addition to assessment of the efficacy of the pain intervention, the unintentional effects must be assessed (see the Sedation and Respiratory Depression section) (Centers for Medicare & Medicaid Services, 2014).

Patient-Controlled Analgesia

Patient-controlled analgesia (PCA) is an interactive method of pain management that allows patients to treat their pain by self-administering doses of analgesic agents. It is used to manage all types of pain by multiple routes of administration, including oral, IV, subcutaneous, epidural, and perineural (Lehne, 2013). A PCA infusion device is programmed so that the patient can press a button (pendant) to self-administer a dose of an analgesic agent (PCA dose) at a set time interval (demand or lockout) as needed. Patients who use PCAs must be able to understand the relationships between pain, pushing the PCA button or taking the analgesic agent, and pain relief and must be cognitively and physically able to use any equipment that is utilized to administer the therapy.

The use of a basal rate (continuous infusion) is commonly used for opioid tolerant patients and when PCEA is used. It is sometimes used for patients who are **opioid naïve** and receiving IV PCA to allow them to manage their pain and rest better. However, it is important to recognize that the patient has no control over the delivery of a continuous infusion. Therefore, extreme caution in using basal rates for acute pain management in opioid-naïve individuals is recommended (APS, 2008). Essential to the safe use of a basal rate with PCA is close monitoring by nurses of sedation and respiratory status and prompt decreases in opioid dose (e.g., discontinue basal rate) if increased sedation is detected (Pasero, Quinn, Portenoy, et al., 2011).

The primary benefit of PCA is that it recognizes that only the patient can feel the pain and only the patient knows how much analgesic will relieve it. This reinforces that PCA is for patient use only and that unauthorized activation of the PCA button (PCA by proxy) should be discouraged.

> ▸ **Quality and Safety Nursing Alert**
>
> Staff, family, and other visitors should be instructed to contact the nurse if they have concerns about pain control rather than pressing the PCA button for the patient.

For some patients who are candidates for PCA but unable to use the PCA equipment, the nurse or a capable family member may be authorized to manage the patient's pain using PCA equipment. This is referred to as Authorized Agent Controlled Analgesia; guidelines are available for the safe administration of this therapy (Cooney, Czarnecki, Dunwoody, et al., 2013).

Analgesic Agents

Analgesic agents are categorized into three main groups: (1) nonopioid analgesic agents, which include acetaminophen and NSAIDs; (2) opioid analgesic agents, which include, among others, morphine, hydromorphone, fentanyl, and oxycodone; and (3) **adjuvant analgesic agents** (sometimes referred to as coanalgesic agents). The adjuvant analgesic agents comprise the largest group and include various agents with unique and widely differing mechanisms of action. Examples are local anesthetics, some anticonvulsants, and some antidepressants.

Nonopioid Analgesic Agents

Acetaminophen and NSAIDs comprise the group of nonopioid analgesic agents (refer to earlier discussion of the two categories of NSAIDs; see Fig. 12-2).

Indications and Administration

Nonopioids are flexible analgesic agents used for a wide variety of painful conditions. They are appropriate alone for mild to some moderate nociceptive pain (e.g., from surgery, trauma, or osteoarthritis) and are added to opioids, local anesthetics, and/or anticonvulsants as part of a multimodal analgesic regimen for more severe nociceptive pain (Manworren, 2015). Acetaminophen and an NSAID may be given concomitantly, and there is no need for staggered doses. Unless contraindicated, all surgical patients should routinely be given acetaminophen and an NSAID in scheduled doses throughout the postoperative course, preferably initiated preoperatively (Pasero, Portenoy, & McCaffery, 2011).

The nonopioids are often combined in a single tablet with opioids, such as oxycodone (Percocet) or hydrocodone (Vicodin, Lortab), and are very popular for the treatment of mild to moderate acute pain. They are the most common choice after invasive pain management therapies are discontinued

and for pain treatment after hospital discharge and dental surgery when an opioid is prescribed. Many people with persistent pain also take a combination nonopioid–opioid analgesic agent; however, it is important to remember that these combination drugs are not appropriate for severe pain of any type because the maximum daily dose of the nonopioid limits the escalation of the opioid dose (Lehne, 2013).

Acetaminophen is versatile in that it can be given by multiple routes of administration, including oral, rectal, and IV. Oral acetaminophen has a long history of safety in recommended doses in all age groups. It is a useful addition to multimodal treatment plans for postoperative pain (Mariano, 2015). Findings from one research study suggest that patients who receive scheduled acetaminophen with as needed opioids will use less opioids than if they receive PRN acetaminophen plus opioids (Valentine, Carvalho, Lazo, et al., 2015).

IV acetaminophen (Ofirmev) is approved for the treatment of pain and fever and is given by a 15-minute infusion in single or repeated doses. It may be given alone for mild to moderate pain or in combination with opioid analgesic agents for more severe pain and has been shown to be well tolerated and to produce a significant opioid dose-sparing effect and superior pain relief compared with placebo (Enekwa, Pounds, Lovett, et al., 2014) (see later discussion of placebos). Recommended dosing is 1000 mg every 6 hours for a maximum of 4000 mg in patients weighing more than 50 kg, and 15 mg/kg every 6 hours in patients weighing less than 50 kg. Repeated doses for up to 5 days have been shown to be safe and well tolerated (Singla, Hale, Davis, et al., 2015).

A benefit of the NSAID group is the availability of a wide variety of agents for administration via noninvasive routes. Ibuprofen, naproxen, and celecoxib are the most widely used oral NSAIDs in the United States. When rectal formulations are unavailable, an intact oral tablet may be given rectally by inserting the tablet, or a crushed tablet in a gelatin capsule, into the rectum. The rectal route may require higher doses than oral route to achieve similar analgesic effects (Pasero, Quinn, et al., 2011). Diclofenac can be prescribed in patch and gel form for topical administration, and an intranasal patient-controlled formulation of ketorolac (Sprix) has been approved for the treatment of postoperative pain.

IV formulations of ketorolac (Toradol) and ibuprofen (Caldolor) are available for acute pain treatment. Both have been shown to produce excellent analgesia alone for moderate nociceptive pain and significant opioid dose-sparing effects when given as part of a multimodal analgesia plan for more severe nociceptive pain (Mariano, 2015).

Adverse Effects of Nonopioid Analgesic Agents

Acetaminophen is widely considered one of the safest and best tolerated analgesic agents (Lehne, 2013). Its most serious complication is hepatotoxicity (liver damage) as a result of overdose. In the healthy adult, a maximum daily dose below 4000 mg is rarely associated with liver toxicity. Nevertheless, one manufacturer of oral acetaminophen (Tylenol) voluntarily changed its dosing recommendations in 2011, calling for a maximum daily dose of 3000 mg (Hooten, Timming, Belgrade, et al., 2013). In 2014, the U.S. Food and Drug Administration (FDA) recommended that health care professionals stop prescribing and pharmacists to stop dispensing prescription combination drug products that contain more than 325 mg of acetaminophen per tablet, capsule, or other dosage unit in order to reduce the risk of hepatotoxicity (FDA, 2014).

Acetaminophen does not increase bleeding time and has a low incidence of gastrointestinal (GI) adverse effects, making it the analgesic agent of choice in many individuals with comorbidities.

NSAIDs have considerably more adverse effects than acetaminophen, with gastric toxicity and ulceration being the most common (Gnjidic, Blyth, LeCouteur, et al., 2014; Meara & Simon, 2013). The primary underlying mechanism of NSAID-induced gastric ulceration is the inhibition of COX-1, which leads to a reduction in GI-protective prostaglandins (see Fig. 12-2). This is a systemic (rather than local) effect and can occur regardless of the route of administration of the NSAID. Risk factors include advanced age (older than 60 years), presence of prior ulcer disease, and cardiovascular (CV) disease and other comorbidities (Lehne, 2013). In patients with elevated risks, the use of a COX-2 selective NSAID (e.g., celecoxib) or the least ulcerogenic nonselective NSAID (e.g., ibuprofen) plus a proton pump inhibitor is recommended (Lehne, 2013). GI adverse effects are also related to the dose and duration of NSAID therapy; the higher the NSAID dose and the longer the duration of NSAID use, the higher the risk of GI toxicity. A principle of nonopioid analgesic use is to administer the lowest dose for the shortest time necessary (Pasero, et al., 2011).

All NSAIDs carry a risk of CV adverse effects through prostaglandin inhibition, and the risk is increased with COX-2 inhibition, whether it is produced by a COX-2 selective NSAID (e.g., celecoxib) or by NSAIDs that are nonselective inhibitors of both COX-1 and COX-2 (e.g., ibuprofen, naproxen, and ketorolac) All patients prescribed NSAIDs should receive the lowest effective dose for the shortest time period to decrease this risk (Bello & Holt, 2014; Lehne, 2013).

The COX isoenzymes play an important role in renal function through their effects on prostaglandin formation. Overall, adverse renal effects occur in approximately 1% to 5% of long-term NSAID users (Pasero, Quinn, et al., 2011). NSAID-induced renal toxicity can occur but is relatively rare in otherwise healthy adults who are given NSAIDs for short-term pain management (e.g., in the perioperative period); however, individuals with acute or chronic volume depletion or hypotension rely on prostaglandin synthesis to maintain adequate renal blood flow, and NSAID inhibition of prostaglandin synthesis in such patients can cause acute kidney injury (Lehne, 2013). Attention to adequate hydration is essential when administering NSAIDs to prevent this complication (Pasero, et al., 2011).

Most nonselective NSAIDs increase bleeding time through inhibition of COX-1. This is both drug and dose related, so the lowest dose of nonopioids with minimal or no effect on bleeding time should be used in patients having procedures with high risk for bleeding. Options include acetaminophen, celecoxib, choline magnesium trisalicylate, salsalate (Disalcid), and nabumetone (Relafen) (Lehne, 2013).

Opioid Analgesic Agents

Although it is often used, the term *narcotic* is considered obsolete and inaccurate when discussing the use of opioids for pain management, in part because it is a term used loosely by law enforcement and the media to refer to various substances of potential abuse, which include opioids as well as cocaine and other illicit substances. Legally, controlled substances classified as narcotics include opioids, cocaine, and others. The preferred term is *opioid analgesics* when discussing these agents in the context of pain management (Lehne, 2013); patients prefer the term *pain medications* or *pain medicine* (Pasero, Quinn, et al., 2011).

Opioid analgesic agents are divided into two major groups: (1) **mu agonist** opioids (also called *morphinelike drugs*) and (2) **agonist–antagonist** opioids. The mu agonist opioids comprise the larger of the two groups and include morphine, hydromorphone, hydrocodone, fentanyl, oxycodone, and methadone, among others. The agonist–antagonist opioids include buprenorphine (Buprenex, Butrans), nalbuphine (Nubain), and butorphanol (Stadol).

Opioid analgesic agents exert their effects by interacting with opioid receptor sites located throughout the body, including in the peripheral tissues, GI system, and CNS; they are abundant in the dorsal horn of the spinal cord. There are three major classes of opioid receptor sites involved in analgesia: the mu, delta, and kappa. The pharmacologic differences in the various opioids are the result of their interaction with these opioid receptor types (Lehne, 2013; MacIntyre & Schug, 2015). When an opioid binds to the opioid receptor sites, it produces analgesia as well as unwanted effects, such as constipation, nausea, sedation, and respiratory depression.

The opioid analgesic agents that are designated as first line (e.g., morphine, hydromorphone, fentanyl, and oxycodone) belong to the mu opioid agonist class because they bind primarily to the mu-type opioid receptors. The agonist–antagonist opioids are designated as "mixed" because they bind to more than one opioid receptor site. They bind as agonists, producing analgesia, at the kappa opioid receptor sites, and as weak antagonists at the mu opioid receptor sites. Their propensity to antagonize the effects of mu opioid analgesic agents limits their usefulness in pain management (Lehne, 2013; MacIntyre & Schug, 2015). They should be avoided in patients receiving long-term mu opioid therapy because their use may trigger severe pain and opioid **withdrawal** syndrome characterized by rhinitis, abdominal cramping, nausea, agitation, and restlessness.

Antagonists (e.g., naloxone, naltrexone) are drugs that also bind to opioid receptors but produce no analgesia. If an antagonist is present, it competes with opioid molecules for binding sites on the opioid receptors and has the potential to block analgesia and other effects. Antagonists are used most often to reverse adverse effects, such as respiratory depression (Lehne, 2013).

Administration

Safe and effective use of opioid analgesic agents requires the development of an individualized treatment plan based on a comprehensive pain assessment, which includes clarifying the goals of treatment and discussing options with the patient and the family (Lehne, 2013). Goals are periodically reevaluated and changes made depending on patient response and in some cases disease progression.

Many factors are considered when determining the appropriate opioid analgesic agent for the patient with pain. These

Chart 12-4 — Use of Opioids

- Perform a comprehensive assessment that addresses pain, comorbidities, and functional status.
- Develop an individualized treatment plan that includes specific goals related to pain intensity, activities (function/quality of life), and adverse effects (e.g., pain intensity rating of 3 on a 0–10 numerical rating scale to ambulate accompanied by minimal or no sedation).
- Use multimodal analgesia (e.g., add acetaminophen and NSAID; anticonvulsant in patients at risk for persistent postsurgical pain).
- Assess for presence preoperatively of underlying persistent pain in surgical patients and optimize its treatment.
- Consider **preemptive analgesic agents** before surgery, particularly for those at risk for severe postoperative pain or a persistent postsurgical pain syndrome.
- Provide analgesic agents prior to all painful procedures.
- Drug selection
  - Consider diagnosis, condition, or surgical procedure, current or expected pain intensity, age, presence of major organ dysfunction or failure, and presence of coexisting disease.
  - Consider pharmacologic issues (e.g., accumulation of metabolites and effects of concurrent drugs).
  - Consider prior treatment outcomes and patient preference.
  - Be aware of available routes of administration (oral, transdermal, rectal, intranasal, IV subcutaneous, perineural, intraspinal) and formulations (e.g., short acting, modified release).
  - Be aware of cost differences.
- Route of administration selection
  - Use least invasive route possible.
  - Consider convenience and patient's ability to adhere to the regimen.
  - Consider staff's (or patient's or caregiver's) ability to monitor and provide care required.
- Dosing and titration
  - Consider previous dosing requirement and relative analgesic potencies when initiating therapy.
  - Use equianalgesic dose chart (see Table 12-3) to determine starting dose with consideration of patient's current status (e.g., sedation and respiratory status) and comorbidities

(e.g., medical frailty), and then titrate until adequate analgesia is achieved or dose-limiting adverse effects are encountered.
  - Use appropriate dosing schedule (e.g., around-the-clock for continuous pain; PRN for intermittent pain).
  - When dose is safe but additional analgesia is desired, titrate upward as prescribed by 25% for slight increase, 50% for moderate increase, and 100% for considerable increase in analgesia.
  - Provide supplemental doses for breakthrough pain; consider PCA if appropriate.
- Treatment of adverse effects
  - Be aware of the prevalence and impact of opioid adverse effects.
  - Remember that most opioid adverse effects are dose dependent; always consider decreasing the opioid dose as a method of treating or eliminating an adverse effect; adding nonopioid analgesic agents for additive analgesia facilitates this approach.
  - Use a preventive approach in the management of constipation, including for patients receiving short-term opioid treatment.
  - Prevent respiratory depression by monitoring sedation levels and respiratory status frequently and decreasing the opioid dose as soon as increased sedation is detected.
- Monitoring
  - Continually and consistently evaluate the plan on the basis of the specific goals identified at the outset and assess pain intensity, adverse effects, and activity levels.
  - Make necessary modifications to treatment plan to maintain efficacy and safety.
- Tapering and cessation of treatment
  - If a decrease in dose or cessation of treatment is appropriate, do so in accordance with decreased pain intensity and after evaluation of functional outcomes.
  - Be aware of the potential for withdrawal syndrome (rhinitis, abdominal cramping, diarrhea, restlessness, agitation) and need for tapering schedule in patients who have been receiving opioid therapy for more than a few days.

NSAID, nonsteroidal anti-inflammatory drug; IV, intravenous; PRN, as needed; PCA, patient-controlled analgesia.
Copyright 2011, Pasero C., McCaffery M. Modified and used with permission from Pasero, C., & McCaffery, M. (2011). *Pain assessment and pharmacologic management*. St. Louis, MO: Mosby-Elsevier.

include the unique characteristics of the various opioids and patient factors, such as pain intensity, age, coexisting disease, current drug regimen and potential drug interactions, prior treatment outcomes, and patient preference. In all cases, a multimodal approach that may rely on the selection of appropriate analgesic agents from the nonopioid, opioid, and adjuvant analgesic agent groups is recommended to manage all types of pain (Manworren, 2015; Mathiesen, Dahl, Thomsen, et al., 2013; Registered Nurses' Association of Ontario [RNAO], 2013). Chart 12-4 lists the key considerations when developing an opioid pain treatment plan.

Titration of the opioid dose is usually required at the start and throughout the course of treatment when opioids are given. Whereas patients with cancer pain most often are titrated upward over time for progressive pain, patients with acute pain, particularly postoperative pain, are eventually titrated downward as pain resolves (Smith, 2013). The dose and analgesic effect of mu agonist opioids have no **ceiling**

effect, although the dose may be limited by adverse effects. The absolute dose given is unimportant as long as a balance between pain relief and adverse effects is favorable. The goal of titration is to use the smallest dose that provides satisfactory pain relief with the fewest adverse effects. When an increase in the opioid dose is necessary and safe, this can be done by percentages. When a slight improvement in analgesia is needed, a 25% increase in the opioid dose may be sufficient and a 50% increase for moderate improvement; a 100% increase may be indicated for strong improvement, such as when treating severe pain (Smith, 2013). The time at which the dose can be increased is determined by the onset and peak effects of the opioid and its formulation. For example, the frequency of IV opioid doses during initial titration may be as often as every 5 to 15 minutes. In contrast, at least 24 hours should elapse before the dose of transdermal fentanyl is increased after the first patch application (Smith, 2013).

Equianalgesia. The term *equianalgesia* means approximately "equal analgesia." An equianalgesic chart provides a list of doses of analgesic agents, both oral and parenteral (IV, subcutaneous, and intramuscular), that are approximately equal to each other in ability to provide pain relief. Equianalgesic conversion of doses is used to help ensure that patients are not overdosed or underdosed when they are switched from one opioid or route of administration to another. It requires a series of calculations based on the daily dose of the current opioid to determine the equianalgesic dose of the opioid to which the patient is to be switched. Several excellent guidelines are available to assist in calculating equianalgesic doses (Lehne, 2013) (see Table 12-3).

Formulation Terminology. The terms *short acting, immediate release,* and *normal release* have been used interchangeably to describe oral opioids that have an onset of action of approximately 30 minutes and a relatively short duration of 3 to 4 hours. The term *immediate release* is misleading because none of the oral analgesic agents have an immediate onset of analgesia; *short acting* is preferred. The terms *modified release, extended release, sustained release, controlled release,* and *long acting* are used to describe opioids that are formulated to release over a prolonged period of time. For the purposes of this chapter, the term *modified release* will be used when discussing these opioid formulations.

Addiction, Physical Dependence, and Tolerance

The terms *physical dependence* and *tolerance* often are confused with addiction, thus clarification of definitions is important (Lehne, 2013). More than a decade ago, the American Academy of Pain Medicine, the APS, and the American Society of Addiction Medicine (2001) proposed definitions that continue to be widely accepted today:

- **Physical dependence** is a normal response that occurs with repeated administration of the opioid for 2 or more weeks and cannot be equated with addictive disease. It is manifested by the occurrence of withdrawal symptoms when the opioid is suddenly stopped or rapidly reduced or an antagonist such as naloxone is given. Withdrawal symptoms may be suppressed by the natural, gradual reduction of the opioid as pain decreases or by gradual, systematic reduction, referred to as tapering.
- **Tolerance** is also a normal response that occurs with regular administration of an opioid and consists of a decrease in one or more effects of the opioid (e.g., decreased analgesia, sedation, or respiratory depression). It cannot be equated with addictive disease. Tolerance to analgesia usually occurs in the first days to 2 weeks of opioid therapy but is uncommon after that. It may be treated with increases in dose. However, disease progression, not tolerance to analgesia, appears to be

---

TABLE 12-3   Equianalgesic Dose Chart for Common mu Opioid Analgesic Agents

- *Equianalgesic* means approximately the same pain relief.
- The equianalgesic chart is a guideline for selecting doses for opioid-naïve patients. Doses and intervals between doses are titrated according to individuals' responses.
- The equianalgesic chart is helpful when switching from one drug or route of administration to another.

Opioid	Oral	Parenteral	Comments
Morphine	30 mg	10 mg	Standard for comparison; first-line opioid via multiple routes of administration; once-daily and twice-daily oral formulations; clinically significant metabolites
Fentanyl	No formulation	100 mcg IV 100 mcg/h of transdermal fentanyl is approximately equal to 4 mg/h of IV morphine; 1 mcg/h of transdermal fentanyl is approximately equal to 2 mg/24 h of oral morphine	First-line opioid via IV, transdermal, and intraspinal routes; available in oral transmucosal and buccal formulations for breakthrough pain in opioid-tolerant patients; no clinically relevant metabolites
Hydrocodone	30 mg (not recommended)	No formulation	Available only in combination with acetaminophen (e.g., Vicodin, Lortab) and as such is appropriate only for mild to some moderate pain
Hydromorphone (Dilaudid)	7.5 mg	1.5 mg	First-line opioid via multiple routes of administration; once-daily oral formulation; clinically significant metabolites noted with long-term and high-dose infusion
Oxycodone	20 mg	No formulation in the United States	Short-acting and twice-daily oral formulations
Oxymorphone	10 mg	1 mg	Parenteral and short-acting and twice-daily oral formulations

IV, intravenous.
Adapted from Pasero, C., & McCaffery, M. (2011). *Pain assessment and pharmacologic management.* St. Louis, MO: Mosby-Elsevier.

the reason for most dose escalations. Stable pain usually results in stable opioid doses. Thus, tolerance poses very few clinical problems. With the exception of constipation, tolerance to the opioid adverse effects develops with regular daily dosing of opioids over several days (Lehne, 2013).

- Opioid **addiction**, or addictive disease, is a chronic, relapsing, treatable neurologic disease (Oliver, Coggins, Compton, et al., 2012). The development and characteristics of addiction are influenced by genetic, psychosocial, and environmental factors. No single cause of addiction, such as taking an opioid for pain relief, has been found. It is characterized by behaviors that include one or more of the following: impaired control over drug use, compulsive use, continued use despite harm, and craving to use the opioid for effects other than pain relief. This statement reinforces that taking opioids for pain relief is not addiction, no matter how long a person takes opioids or at what doses.

Pseudoaddiction is a mistaken diagnosis of addictive disease (Kwon, Tanco, Hui, et al., 2014; Weissman & Haddox, 1989). When a patient's pain is not well controlled, the patient may begin to manifest symptoms suggestive of addictive disease. In an effort to obtain adequate pain relief, the patient may respond with demanding behavior, escalating demands for more or different medications, and repeated requests for opioids on time or before the prescribed interval between doses has elapsed. Pain relief typically eliminates these behaviors and is often accomplished by increasing opioid doses or decreasing intervals between doses (MacIntyre & Schug, 2015).

The incidence of addiction as a result of taking an opioid for therapeutic reasons had been believed to be quite rare. More recently, pain specialists are realizing that the progression from opioid abuse to the disease of opioid addiction is poorly understood and complex (Hunt & Urch, 2013). National Institute on Drug Abuse (2014) estimates that the rates of addiction among patients with chronic pain may vary widely, from 3% to 40%.

The number of patients in the United States seeking treatment for dependence on prescription opioids has increased fivefold between the years 2001 and 2011 (Weiss, Sharpe Potter, Griffin, et al., 2014). Furthermore, a study of adolescents and young adults found that 20% reported misuse of prescription opioids, consisting of using too much of the medication, intentionally getting high, or using the medications to act synergistically with alcohol or other drugs. Misuse of prescription opioids is associated with higher rates of adverse health behaviors and outcomes (McCabe, West, & Boyd, 2013).

Opioid Naïve Versus Opioid Tolerant. Patients are often characterized as being either *opioid naïve* or *opioid tolerant*. Whereas an opioid naïve individual has not recently taken enough opioid on a regular basis to become tolerant to the effects of an opioid, an **opioid tolerant** individual has taken an opioid long enough at doses high enough to develop tolerance to many of the effects, including analgesia and sedation. There is no set time for the development of tolerance, and there is great individual variation with some not developing tolerance at all. By convention, most clinicians consider a patient who has taken opioids regularly for approximately 7 or more days to be opioid tolerant (Pasero, Quinn, et al., 2011).

Opioid-Induced Hyperalgesia

Hyperalgesia means increased sensitivity to pain. **Opioid-induced hyperalgesia** (OIH) is a paradoxical situation in which increasing doses of opioid result in increasing sensitivity to pain. The incidence of clinically significant OIH has not been determined; however, it appears to be a rare but serious consequence of opioid administration (Youssef, Pater, & Shehata, 2015). At this time, it is not possible to predict who will develop OIH as a result of opioid exposure, and the mechanisms underlying OIH are largely unknown. In general, OIH is thought to be the result of changes in the central and peripheral nervous systems that produce increased transmission of nociceptive signals (Youssef et al., 2015).

Some experts characterize OIH and analgesic tolerance as "opposite sides of the coin" (Pasero, Quinn, et al., 2011). In tolerance, increasing doses of opioid are needed to provide the same level of pain relief because opioid exposure induces neurophysiologic changes that reverse analgesia; in OIH, opioid exposure induces neurophysiologic changes that produce pain or increase sensitivity to noxious input (Youssef et al., 2015). In other words, tolerance may be inferred clinically when opioid treatment leads to decreased sensitivity to opioid analgesia over time (in the absence of another process that would explain this), whereas OIH may be inferred clinically when opioid treatment leads to increased pain or sensitivity to pain over time (MacIntyre & Schug, 2015). When OIH is suspected, a thorough differential assessment that rules out all other possible explanations is recommended (Schug, 2013).

Selected Opioid Analgesic Agents

Morphine is the standard against which all other opioid drugs are compared. It is the most widely used opioid worldwide, particularly for cancer pain, and its use is established by extensive research and clinical experience (Schug, 2013). It is available in a wide variety of short-acting and modified-release oral formulations and is given by multiple routes of administration. It was the first drug to be given intraspinally and remains a first-line choice for long-term intraspinal analgesia. It is the only opioid uniquely formulated to produce analgesia for up to 48 hours following epidural administration for acute pain management (extended-release epidural morphine [DepoDur]). Morphine is a **hydrophilic** drug (readily absorbed in aqueous solution), which accounts for its slow onset and long duration of action when compared with other opioid analgesic agents (see Tables 12-3 and 12-4). It has two principal, clinically significant **metabolites:** morphine-3-glucuronide (M3G) and morphine-6-glucuronide (M6G). M6G may be responsible for some of the analgesic effect of morphine; accumulation of M3G can produce neurotoxicity, which necessitates switching the patient to a different opioid (Schug, 2013).

In contrast to morphine, fentanyl (Sublimaze) is a **lipophilic** (readily absorbed in fatty tissues) opioid and as such has a fast onset and short duration of action (see Tables 12-3 and 12-4). These characteristics make it the most commonly used IV opioid when rapid analgesia is desired, such as for the treatment of severe, escalating acute pain, and for procedural pain when a short duration of action is desirable. The drug is a good choice for patients with end-organ failure because it has no clinically relevant metabolites. It also produces minimal hemodynamic adverse effects; thus, fentanyl is often preferred

TABLE 12-4 Characteristics of Selected First-Line Opioid Analgesic Agents[a]

Opioid	Onset (Minutes)	Peak (Minutes)	Duration (Hours)
Morphine	30 (PO) 5 (IV)	60–120 (PO) 20 (IV)	4–12 (PO) 4–5 (IV)
Fentanyl	5–15 (OT) 1–2 (IV)	20–30 (OT) 3–5 (IV)	2–5 (OT) 1/2–1 (IV)
Hydromorphone	15–30 (PO) 10–15 (IV)	30–60 (PO) 15–30 (IV)	4–5 (PO) 2–3 (IV)

IV, intravenous; OT, oral transmucosal; PO, oral.

[a]Characteristics do not apply to modified-release formulations.

Adapted from Pasero, C., & McCaffery, M. (2011). *Pain assessment and pharmacologic management*. St. Louis, MO: Mosby-Elsevier. Comerford, K. C. (2015). *Nursing 2015 drug handbook*. Philadelphia, PA: Wolters Kluwer.

in patients who are hemodynamically unstable, such as the critically ill (Pasero, Quinn, et al., 2011).

Its lipophilicity makes fentanyl ideal for drug delivery by transdermal patch (Duragesic) for long-term opioid administration and by the oral transmucosal (Actiq) and buccal (Fentora) routes for BTP treatment in patients who are opioid tolerant. Following application of the transdermal patch, a subcutaneous depot of fentanyl is established in the skin near the patch. After absorption from the depot into the systemic circulation, the drug distributes to fat and muscle. When the first patch is applied, 12 to 18 hours are required for clinically significant analgesia to be obtained (Weaver, 2014); attention must be paid to providing adequate supplemental analgesia during that time. The patch is changed every 48 to 72 hours depending on patient response. It is important to note that the patch is not appropriate for treating acute pain or rapidly changing pain.

⚑ Quality and Safety Nursing Alert

The application of heat (heat packs, heating pads, or hot tubs or showers) directly over the patch can cause increased absorption of transdermal fentanyl, which can lead to life-threatening respiratory depression.

Hydromorphone (Dilaudid) is less hydrophilic than morphine but less lipophilic than fentanyl, which contributes to an onset and duration of action that is intermediate between morphine and fentanyl (see Tables 12-3 and 12-4). The drug is often used as an alternative to morphine, especially for acute pain because the two drugs produce similar analgesia and have comparable adverse effect profiles (Lehne, 2013). It is a first- or second-choice opioid (after morphine) for postoperative pain management via IV PCA and is available in a once-daily modified-release oral formulation for chronic pain management. Accumulation of its neuroexcitatory metabolite hydromorphone-3-glucuronide (H3G) may occur with high-dose, long-term infusion therapy, which would necessitate a switch to another opioid (Pasero, Quinn, et al., 2011).

Oxycodone is available in the United States for administration by the oral route only and is used to treat all types of pain. In combination with acetaminophen or ibuprofen, it is appropriate for mild to some moderate pain. Single-entity short-acting (OxyIR) and modified-release (OxyContin) oxycodone formulations are used most often for moderate to severe cancer pain and in some patients with moderate to severe noncancer pain (see Table 12-3). It has been used successfully as part of a multimodal treatment plan for postoperative pain as well (Pasero, Quinn, et al., 2011).

Oxymorphone has been available for many years in parenteral formulation and more recently in short-acting (Opana IR) and modified-release (Opana ER) oral tablets for the treatment of moderate to severe chronic pain (see Table 12-3). It must be taken on an empty stomach (1 hour before or 2 hours after a meal), and coingestion of alcohol at the time of dosing must be avoided, because food and alcohol can increase the serum concentration of the drug (Lehne, 2013).

Hydrocodone is available only in combination with nonopioids (e.g., with acetaminophen in Vicodin or Lortab), which limits its use to the treatment of mild to some moderate pain (see Table 12-3). It is one of the most commonly prescribed analgesic agents in the United States; however, its prescription for the treatment of persistent pain (except for breakthrough dosing) should be carefully evaluated because of its ceiling on **efficacy** and safety inherent in the nonopioid constituent (MacIntyre & Schug, 2015). In 2014, the U.S. Drug Enforcement Agency changed hydrocodone from a schedule III to the more restrictive schedule II classification to reduce abuse of this pain medication (Federal Register, 2014).

Methadone (Dolophine) is a unique opioid analgesic agent that may have advantages over other opioids in carefully selected patients. In addition to being a mu opioid, it is an antagonist at the NMDA receptor site and thus has the potential to produce analgesic effects as a second- or third-line option for some neuropathic pain states (Wu et al., 2014). It may be used as an alternative when it is necessary to switch a patient to a new opioid because of inadequate analgesia or unacceptable adverse effects. The use of conventional equianalgesic dose conversion is not recommended when switching patients to and from methadone. Extensive guidelines on how to safely accomplish this are available elsewhere (Smith, 2013).

Methadone is usually given orally but has also been given by virtually every other route of administration. Although it has no active metabolites, methadone has a very long and highly variable **half-life** (5 to 100-plus hours; average is 20 hours), which makes it a good choice for the treatment of addictive disease; patients must be watched closely for excessive sedation, a sign of drug accumulation during this time period. (The drug is described as "long acting" because of its exceptionally long half-life.) When methadone is used to treat opioid addiction, it is dosed once daily and is not intended to manage pain; acute pain management with other analgesic medications is needed in addition to daily methadone dosing. Other limitations are its propensity to interact with a large number of medications and prolong the QTc interval on the electrocardiogram (ECG). Some drugs (e.g., clarithromycin [Cleocin] and some antifungal medications) that inhibit CYP3A4, the enzyme that metabolizes methadone, should be avoided as they can inadvertently increase methadone levels in the blood (Lehne, 2013). Despite these characteristics, methadone can be an effective and safe drug when prescribed by practitioners who have an appreciation of the drug's characteristics and experience in its use (Schug, 2013).

Dual-Mechanism Analgesic Agents

The dual-mechanism analgesic agents tramadol (Ultram) and tapentadol (Nucynta) bind weakly to the mu opioid receptor site and block the reuptake (resorption) of the inhibitory neurotransmitters serotonin and/or norepinephrine at central synapses in the spinal cord and brain stem of the modulatory descending pain pathway (MacIntyre & Schug, 2015; Niesters, Proto, et al., 2014; Singh et al., 2013). This makes these neurotransmitters more available to fight pain. Dual-mechanism analgesic agents have been described as providing automatic "built-in" multimodal analgesia because a single tablet produces an effect on more than one analgesic action site (Niesters, Proto, et al., 2014; Singh et al., 2013). The underlying mechanisms of tapentadol and tramadol differ in that tramadol blocks the reuptake of both serotonin and norepinephrine, but tapentadol blocks the reuptake of only norepinephrine. This is pertinent because norepinephrine may play a more significant role than serotonin in the endogenous analgesia pathways. A study of patients with chronic musculoskeletal pain reported deficits in pain inhibition and lower levels of plasma norepinephrine compared to patients with fibromyalgia or diabetic neuropathy (Parent, Beaudet, Daigle, et al., 2015). Serotonin may be the more powerful mediator of depression; low serotonin levels are associated with depression. This helps explain why selective serotonin reuptake inhibitors (SSRIs), such as fluoxetine (Prozac) and paroxetine (Paxil), which block only serotonin, are effective for the treatment of depression but not pain (Lehne, 2013).

Tramadol is used for both acute and chronic pain and is available in oral short-acting and modified-release (Ultram ER) formulations, including a short-acting tablet in combination with acetaminophen (Ultracet). It has demonstrated good efficacy for the treatment of neuropathic pain (Schug, 2013). The drug can lower seizure threshold and interact with other drugs that block the reuptake of serotonin, such as the SSRIs, putting the patient at risk for serotonin syndrome, characterized by agitation, diarrhea, heart and blood pressure changes, and loss of coordination (Lehne, 2013).

Tapentadol (Nucynta) is available in short-acting and modified-release oral formulations. The drug has been shown to produce dose-dependent analgesia comparable to oxycodone. In a study of patients with diabetic polyneuropathy, tapentadol appeared to potentiate the descending pain pathway to inhibit pain (Niesters, Proto, et al., 2014). Major benefits are that it has no active metabolites and a significantly more favorable adverse effect profile (particularly GI) compared with opioid analgesic agents. These characteristics make tapentadol an attractive alternative to traditional oral opioid analgesic agents for many patients with pain.

Opioids to Avoid

Codeine is a prodrug, which means it is pharmacologically inactive when given. It must be metabolized to morphine for the patient to experience pain relief. It is estimated that 8% to 10% of Caucasians of northern European heritage lack the enzyme to convert codeine to morphine via the CYP2D6 metabolic pathway (MacIntyre & Schug, 2015), meaning that in this population of patients, codeine is an ineffective analgesic agent. In contrast, codeine has been associated with overdoses in some children due to rapid metabolism of the drug to morphine. Indeed, it is estimated that 7% of Caucasians and up to 30% of persons of Asian and African descent overmetabolize codeine, resulting in higher than expected morphine blood levels (Yellon, Kenna, Cladis, et al., 2014). Because of these effects, acetaminophen or NSAIDs, rather than codeine, are recommended for the treatment of mild pain. For adults or children with moderate to severe pain, when either poor or rapid metabolism of codeine is suspected, opioids other than codeine should be selected for use (e.g., morphine, oxymorphone, buprenorphine, fentanyl, hydromorphone) (Nicholson & Formea, 2015).

Meperidine (Demerol) has either been removed from or severely restricted on hospital formularies for the treatment of pain in an effort to improve patient safety (Lehne, 2013). (It is an accepted practice to use it in low doses [12.5 to 25 mg IV] to treat shivering associated with general anesthesia.) A major drawback to the use of meperidine is its active metabolite, normeperidine, which is a CNS stimulant and can cause delirium, irritability, tremors, myoclonus, and generalized seizures.

Propoxyphene (Darvon) and propoxyphene plus acetaminophen (Darvocet) were prescribed for many years for mild to moderate pain but were withdrawn from the U.S. market in 2010.

Adverse Effects of Opioid Analgesic Agents

The most common adverse effects of opioids are constipation, nausea, vomiting, pruritus, hypotension, and sedation (Lehne, 2013). Respiratory depression, while less common, is the most serious and feared of the opioid adverse effects (Pasero, 2009). The risk of respiratory depression is increased when other medications that have depressive effects on the CNS, such as benzodiazepines (e.g., diazepam [Valium]), alcohol, and barbiturates (e.g., phenobarbital), are used concurrently with opioids (Lehne, 2013). In surgical patients, postoperative ileus can become a major complication as well. Morphine lowers blood pressure by dilating peripheral arterioles and veins. In the presence of dehydration or with concomitant use of hypotensive drugs, postural hypotension may result (Lehne, 2013). Long-term use of opioids may result in opioid-induced androgen deficiency and sleep disordered breathing (Smith, 2013).

Opioids can result in delayed gastric emptying, slowed bowel motility, and decreased peristalsis, all of which result in slow-moving, hard stool that is difficult to pass. Risk is elevated with advanced age, and immobility; however, it is an almost universal opioid adverse effect (i.e., tolerance rarely develops). Constipation is a primary reason people stop taking their pain medication, which underscores the importance of taking a preventive approach and aggressive management if symptoms are detected. Prevention includes reminding patients to take a daily stool softener plus mild peristaltic stimulant for as long as they are taking opioids (Lehne, 2013).

Postoperative nausea and vomiting (PONV) are among the most unpleasant of the adverse effects associated with surgery, and it can have a negative impact on patient outcomes and increase the need for nursing intervention (MacIntyre & Schug, 2015). Guidelines recommend that all patients be evaluated for PONV risk, baseline risk factors be reduced if possible, multimodal analgesia be provided so that no opioid or the lowest effective opioid dose can be given, and prophylactic treatment (e.g., dexamethasone [Decadron] and a serotonin receptor antagonist such as ondansetron [Zofran] at the end of surgery) be given to patients with moderate risk (American Society of PeriAnesthesia Nurses, 2006; Gan, Diemunsch, Habib, et al., 2014). More aggressive interventions should be utilized in patients with high risk (Pasero, Quinn, et al., 2011). (See Chapter 19 for further discussion of PONV.)

Pruritus is an adverse effect, not an allergic reaction, to opioids (Benson, Campbell, & Phillips, 2015). Although antihistamines such as diphenhydramine (Benadryl) are commonly used, there is no strong evidence that they relieve opioid-induced pruritus (Jannuzzi, 2015). Patients may report being less bothered by itching after taking an antihistamine, although this is likely the result of sedating effects. Sedation can be problematic in those already at risk for excessive sedation, such as postoperative patients, because this can lead to life-threatening respiratory depression (Lehne, 2013). A common clinical observation is that patients with postoperative opioid-induced pruritus usually have well-controlled pain. This may be because painful stimuli can inhibit itching, and inhibition of pain processing may enhance itching. This helps explain why the single most effective, safest, and least expensive treatment of pruritus is opioid dose reduction. In fact, simply decreasing the opioid dose is sufficient to eliminate or make most of the adverse effects tolerable for most patients (Smith, 2013). Opioid rotation is another possible treatment (Schug, 2013). Nonsedating analgesic agents can be added to facilitate this approach. A review of the literature identified the use of nalbuphine (Nubain), an agonist–antagonist opioid, to be superior to placebo, control, antihistamines, and naloxone in the treatment of pruritus caused by neuroaxial opioids (Jannuzzi, 2015).

In addition to dose reduction strategies, most opioid pain treatment plans include prescriptions for medications that can be used to treat adverse effects should they occur. Nonpharmacologic agents may also be effective, such as the application of a cool damp cloth over affected areas to help relieve the discomfort of pruritus.

As patients become opioid tolerant, tolerance to the opioid adverse effects (with the exception of constipation) develops. It is reassuring for patients receiving long-term opioid therapy to know that most of the adverse effects will subside with regular daily doses of opioids over several days.

Sedation and Respiratory Depression. Most patients experience sedation at the beginning of opioid therapy and whenever the opioid dose is increased significantly. If left untreated, excessive sedation can progress to clinically significant respiratory depression. Like other opioid adverse effects, sedation and respiratory depression are dose related. In most cases (exceptions may apply at the end of life), nurses should promptly reduce opioid doses or stop titration whenever advancing sedation is detected to prevent respiratory depression (Pasero, 2009; Pasero, Quinn, et al., 2011). In some patients (e.g., those with obstructive sleep apnea, pulmonary dysfunction), monitoring with capnography is warranted (Jarzyna, Junquist, Pasero, et al., 2011). Capnography, which reflects the adequacy of ventilation and airflow, should be used when supplemental oxygen is needed to maintain the patient's oxygen saturation; pulse oximetry may not detect hypoventilation (Buvanendran, Lubenow, & Droin, 2013).

> ► *Quality and Safety Nursing Alert*
>
> *Opioid-induced respiratory depression is dose related and preceded by increasing sedation. Prevention of clinically significant opioid-induced respiratory depression begins with the administration of the lowest effective opioid dose, careful titration, close nurse monitoring of sedation and respiratory status throughout therapy, and prompt dose reduction when advancing sedation is detected.*

The observation that excessive sedation precedes opioid-induced respiratory depression indicates that systematic sedation assessment is an essential aspect of the care of patients receiving opioid therapy (Pasero, 2009). Nursing assessment of sedation is convenient, inexpensive, and takes minimal time to perform. A simple, easy-to-understand sedation scale, developed for the assessment of *unwanted* sedation and that includes what should be done at each level of sedation, is widely recommended to enhance accuracy and consistency of assessment, monitor trends, and communicate effectively between members of the health care team (Jarzyna et al., 2011; Pasero, 2009; Pasero, Quinn, et al., 2011). Chart 12-5 presents a widely used sedation scale.

Respiratory depression is assessed on the basis of what is normal for a particular individual and is usually described as clinically significant when there is a decrease in the rate, depth, and regularity of respirations from baseline, rather than just by a specific number of respirations per minute (Pasero, Quinn, et al., 2011). There are many risk factors for opioid-induced respiratory depression, including older age

Chart 12-5 Pasero Opioid-Induced Sedation Scale With Interventions

Each level of sedation is followed by the appropriate action in italics.

S = Sleep, easy to arouse
Acceptable; no action necessary; may increase opioid dose if needed

1 = Awake and alert
Acceptable; no action necessary; may increase opioid dose if needed

2 = Slightly drowsy, easily aroused
Acceptable; no action necessary; may increase opioid dose if needed

3 = Frequently drowsy, arousable, drifts off to sleep during conversation
Unacceptable; monitor respiratory status and sedation level closely until sedation level is stable at less than 3 and respiratory status is satisfactory; decrease opioid dose 25% to 50%[1] or notify primary[2] or anesthesia provider for orders; consider administering a nonsedating, opioid-sparing nonopioid, such as acetaminophen or a NSAID, if not contraindicated; ask patient to take deep breaths every 15 to 30 minutes.

4 = Somnolent, minimal, or no response to verbal and physical stimulation
Unacceptable; stop opioid; consider administering naloxone[3,4]; call Rapid Response Team (Code Blue); stay with patient, stimulate, and support respiration as indicated by patient status; notify primary[2] or anesthesia provider; monitor respiratory status and sedation level closely until sedation level is stable at less than 3 and respiratory status is satisfactory.

[1]Opioid analgesic agent prescriptions or a hospital protocol should include the expectation that a nurse will decrease the opioid dose if a patient is excessively sedated.

[2]For example, the physician, nurse practitioner, advanced practice nurse, or physician assistant responsible for the pain management prescription.

[3]For adults experiencing respiratory depression, mix 0.4 mg of naloxone and 10 mL of normal saline in syringe and administer this dilute solution very slowly (0.5 mL over 2 minutes) while observing the patient's response (titrate to effect).

[4]Hospital protocols should include the expectation that a nurse will administer naloxone to any patient suspected of having life-threatening opioid-induced sedation and respiratory depression.

Copyright 1994, Pasero C. Used with permission from Pasero, C., & McCaffery, M. (2011). *Pain assessment and pharmacologic management.* St. Louis, MO: Mosby-Elsevier.

(65 years of age or older), obesity, obstructive sleep apnea, and pre-existing pulmonary dysfunction, or other comorbidities (Jarzyna et al., 2011; Schug, 2013). Risk is elevated during the first 24 hours following surgery and in patients who require a high dose of opioid in a short period of time (e.g., more than 10 mg of IV morphine or equivalent in the PACU).

A comprehensive respiratory assessment constitutes more than counting a patient's respiratory rate (Pasero, 2009). A proper assessment requires watching the rise and fall of the patient's chest to determine rate, depth, and regularity of respirations. Listening to the sound of the patient's respirations is critical as well—snoring indicates airway obstruction and must be attended to promptly with repositioning and, depending on severity, a request for respiratory therapy

consultation and further evaluation (Pasero, 2009; Pasero, Quinn, et al., 2011).

In most cases (exceptions may apply at the end of life), the opioid antagonist naloxone is promptly given IV to reverse clinically significant opioid-induced respiratory depression (Lehne, 2013). The goal is to reverse only the sedation and respiratory depressant effects of the opioid. To this end, it should be diluted and titrated very slowly to prevent severe pain and other adverse effects, which can include hypertension, tachycardia, ventricular dysrhythmias, pulmonary edema, and cardiac arrest (APS, 2008) (see Chart 12-5, footnote 3, for correct technique). Sometimes more than one dose of naloxone is necessary, because naloxone has a shorter duration of action (1 hour in most patients) than most opioids.

Adjuvant Analgesic Agents

The adjuvant analgesic agents comprise the largest group of analgesic agents, which is diverse and offers many options. Drug selection and dosing is based on both experience and evidence-based guideline recommendations. There is considerable variability among individuals in their response to adjuvant analgesic agents, including to agents within the same class; often a "trial and error" strategy is used in the outpatient setting. Treatment in the outpatient setting is primarily for neuropathic pain and involves the use of low initial doses and gradual dose escalation to allow tolerance to the adverse effects. Patients must be forewarned in this setting that the onset of analgesia is likely to be delayed (Pasero, Polomano, Portenoy, et al., 2011). Following is an overview of the most commonly used adjuvant analgesic agents.

Local Anesthetics

Local anesthetics have a long history of safe and effective use for all types of pain management. Local anesthetics are sodium channel blockers that affect the formation and propagation of action potentials. They are given by various routes of administration and are generally well tolerated by most individuals (Pasero, et al., 2011). Injectable and topical local anesthetics are commonly used for procedural pain treatment. Local anesthetics are added to opioid analgesic agents and other agents to be given intraspinally for the treatment of both acute and chronic pain. They are also infused for continuous peripheral nerve blocks, primarily after surgery.

The lidocaine patch 5% (Lidoderm) is placed directly over or adjacent to the painful area for absorption into the tissues directly below. The drug produces minimal systemic absorption and adverse effects. The patch is left in place for 12 hours and then removed for 12 hours (12 hours on, 12 hours off regimen). This application process is repeated as needed for continuous analgesia. The drug is approved for the neuropathic pain syndrome postherpetic neuralgia; however, research suggests that it is effective and safe for a wide variety of acute and chronic pain conditions (Pasero, et al., 2011).

Allergy to local anesthetics is rare, and adverse effects are dose related. CNS signs of systemic toxicity include ringing in the ears, metallic taste, irritability, and seizures. Signs of cardiotoxicity include circumoral tingling and numbness, bradycardia, cardiac dysrhythmias, and CV collapse (Pasero, et al., 2011).

Anticonvulsants

The anticonvulsants gabapentin (Neurontin) and pregabalin (Lyrica) are first-line analgesic agents for neuropathic pain (MacIntyre & Schug, 2015) and are increasingly being added to postoperative pain treatment plans to address the neuropathic component of surgical pain (Buvanendran et al., 2013). Although further research is needed, their addition has been shown to improve analgesia, allow lower doses of other analgesic agents, and help prevent persistent neuropathic postsurgical pain syndromes, such as phantom limb, postthoracotomy, posthernia, and postmastectomy pain (Moore, Wiffen, & Kalso, 2014). They are also effective in improving the acute pain associated with burn injuries as well as reducing the potential for subsequent neuropathic pain. Analgesic anticonvulsant therapy is initiated with low doses and titration according to patient response. Primary adverse effects of anticonvulsants are sedation and dizziness, which are usually transient and most notable during the titration phase of treatment.

Antidepressants

Antidepressant adjuvant analgesic agents are divided into two major groups: the tricyclic antidepressants (TCAs) and the serotonin and norepinephrine reuptake inhibitors (SNRIs). Evidence-based guidelines recommend the TCAs desipramine (Norpramin) and nortriptyline (Aventyl, Pamelor) and the SNRIs duloxetine (Cymbalta) and venlafaxine (Effexor) as first-line options for neuropathic pain treatment (MacIntyre & Schug, 2015). Their delayed onset of action makes them inappropriate for acute pain treatment. Analgesic antidepressant therapy is initiated with low doses and titration according to patient response.

Primary adverse effects of TCAs are dry mouth, sedation, dizziness, mental clouding, weight gain, and constipation (MacIntyre & Schug, 2015). Orthostatic hypotension is a potentially serious TCA adverse effect. The most serious adverse effect is cardiotoxicity, and patients with significant heart disease are at high risk. SNRIs are thought to have a more favorable adverse effect profile and to be better tolerated than the TCAs (MacIntyre & Schug, 2015). The most common SNRI adverse effects are nausea, headache, sedation, insomnia, weight gain, impaired memory, sweating, and tremors.

Ketamine

Ketamine (Ketalar) is a dissociative anesthetic with dose-dependent analgesic, sedative, and amnestic properties (MacIntyre & Schug, 2015). As an NMDA antagonist, it blocks the binding of glutamate at the NMDA receptors and thus prevents the transmission of pain to the brain via the ascending pathway (see Fig. 12-1B, inset). At high doses, the drug can produce psychomimetic effects (e.g., hallucinations, dreamlike feelings); however, these are minimized when low doses are given (Niesters, Martini, & Dahan, 2014). A benefit of the drug is that it does not produce respiratory depression. Ketamine is given most often by the IV route but can also be given by the oral, rectal, intranasal, and subcutaneous routes. Epidural ketamine is not approved for use in the

United States. Ketamine has been used for the treatment of persistent neuropathic pain, but its adverse effect profile makes it less favorable than other analgesic agents for long-term therapy. It is, however, increasingly used as a third-line analgesic agent for **refractory** acute pain (Porter, McClain, Howe, et al., 2015).

 ### Gerontologic Considerations

Older adults are often sensitive to the effects of the adjuvant analgesic agents that produce sedation and other CNS effects, such as antidepressants and anticonvulsants. Therapy should be initiated with low doses, and titration should proceed slowly with systematic assessment of patient response.

Older adults are also at increased risk for NSAID-induced GI toxicity. Acetaminophen should be used for mild pain. It is recommended as first line for musculoskeletal pain (e.g., osteoarthritis) in older adults but is less effective than NSAIDs for chronic inflammatory pain (e.g., rheumatoid arthritis) (Meara & Simon, 2013). If an NSAID is needed for inflammatory pain, it is recommended that a COX-2 selective NSAID (if not contraindicated by an increased CV risk) or the nonselective NSAID least likely to cause an ulcer should be used. The addition of a proton pump inhibitor to NSAID therapy, or opioid analgesic agents rather than an NSAID, is recommended for high-risk patients. The American Geriatric Society has proposed that opioids are a safer choice than NSAIDs in many older adults because of the increased risk for NSAID-induced GI adverse effects in that population (American Geriatrics Society, 2009). NSAIDs are safest when used for short-term pain flares that may occur during transient worsening in severity of chronic diseases or conditions (e.g., osteoarthritis, fibromyalgia, low back pain) (Reid, Ecclesston, & Pillemer, 2015).

Age is considered an important factor to consider when selecting an opioid dose. The starting opioid dose should be reduced by 25% to 50% in adults older than 70 years because they are more sensitive to opioid adverse effects than younger adults; the amount of subsequent doses is based on patient response (American Geriatrics Society, 2009; Lehne, 2013).

Use of Placebos

A **placebo** is defined as any medication or procedure, including surgery, that produces an effect in a patient because of its implicit or explicit intent and not because of its specific physical or chemical properties (Apkarian, 2015; MacIntyre & Schug, 2015). A saline injection is one example of a placebo. Administration of a medication at a known subtherapeutic dose (e.g., 0.10 mg of morphine in an adult) is also considered a placebo.

Placebos are appropriately used as controls in research evaluating the effects of a new medication. The new drug is compared with the effects of a placebo and must show more favorable effects than placebos to warrant further investigation or marketing of the drug (Wager & Fields, 2013). When a person responds to a placebo in accordance with its intent, it is called a *positive placebo response* (Arnstein, Broglio, Wuhrman, et al., 2011). Patients or volunteers who participate in placebo-controlled research must be able to give informed consent or have a guardian who can provide informed consent.

Occasionally, placebos may be used clinically in a deceitful manner and without informed consent. This is typically done when the clinician does not accept the patient's report of pain (see Chart 12-1). Pain relief resulting from a placebo is mistakenly believed to invalidate a patient's report of pain. This typically results in the patient being deprived of pain-relief measures, despite research showing that many patients who have obvious physical stimuli for pain (e.g., abdominal surgery) report pain relief after placebo administration (Lehne, 2013). The reason for this is a mystery, but it is one of the many reasons that pain guidelines, position papers, nurse practice acts, and hospital policies nationwide agree that there are no individuals for whom and no condition for which placebos are the recommended treatment. The deceptive use of placebos has both ethical and legal implications, violates the nurse–patient relationship, and inevitably deprives patients of more appropriate methods of assessment or treatment (Arnstein et al., 2011).

Nonpharmacologic Methods of Pain Management

Most individuals use self-management strategies to deal with their health issues and promote well-being. Recent national health survey results reveal that American adults spent $14.9 billion on complementary health practices (e.g., acupuncture, chiropractic manipulation, herbal medicines) to treat painful conditions (e.g., back pain, fibromyalgia, arthritis) (Nahin, Stussman, Herman, 2015). Nonpharmacologic complementary and alternative interventions include using natural products (e.g., herbs or botanicals, vitamins, probiotics) or using mind and body practices (e.g., acupuncture, chiropractic manipulation, massage therapy, yoga, tai chi) (National Center for Complementary and Integrative Health, 2015). Table 12-5 lists examples of select complementary and alternative therapies (see Chapter 7 for further discussion).

Nonpharmacologic therapies are usually effective alone for mild to some moderate-intensity pain, and they should complement, but not replace, pharmacologic therapies for more severe pain (Chlan & Halm, 2013). The effectiveness of nonpharmacologic methods can be unpredictable, and although not all will relieve pain, they offer many benefits to patients with pain. For example, research suggests that nonpharmacologic methods can facilitate relaxation and reduce anxiety and stress (Kreitzer & Koithan, 2014; Trail-Mahan, Mao, & Bawel-Brinkley, 2013). Many patients find that the use of nonpharmacologic methods helps them cope better with their pain and feel greater control over the pain experience.

Several nonpharmacologic methods can be used in the clinical setting to provide comfort and pain relief for all types of pain; however, time is often limited in this setting for implementation of these methods. Nurses play an important role in providing them and instructing patients about their use (Trail-Mahan et al., 2013). Many of the methods are relatively easy for nurses to incorporate into daily clinical practice and may be used individually or in combination with other nonpharmacologic therapies. A study of intubated, critically ill patients demonstrated that the use of self-initiated patient-directed music resulted in greater reduction in anxiety than usual care (Chlan, Weinert, Heidersheit, et al., 2013) (see Chart 12-6). Chart 12-7 provides points for nurses to consider before using nonpharmacologic methods.

Unfolding Patient Stories: Stan Checketts • Part 1

Stan Checketts, a 52-year-old man, is in the emergency department with severe abdominal pain. The provider has prescribed buprenorphine 0.3-mg IV push for pain. Explain the assessments performed by the nurse prior to, during, and following the administration of the medication. Also consider nonpharmacologic interventions the nurse can incorporate to assist with his pain relief. (Stan Checketts' story continues in Chapter 47.)

Care for Stan and other patients in a realistic virtual environment: *vSim for Nursing* (**thepoint.lww.com/vSimMedicalSurgical**). Practice documenting these patients' care in DocuCare (**thepoint.lww.com/DocuCareEHR**).

TABLE 12-5 Nonpharmacologic Methods of Pain Management

Type	Examples	Nursing Considerations
Physical modalities	Proper body alignment; application of heat and/or cold; massage; transcutaneous electrical nerve stimulation (TENS); acupuncture; physical therapy; and aqua therapy	Be aware that some of these methods require a prescription in the inpatient setting, as inappropriate use can cause harm (e.g., burns or frostbite from extreme temperatures and prolonged thermal application).
Cognitive and behavioral methods	Relaxation breathing; listening, singing, or rhythmic tapping to music; imagery; humor; pet therapy; prayer; meditation; hypnosis	Prior to use, evaluate patient's cognitive ability to learn and perform necessary activities.
Biologically based therapies	Taking herbs, vitamins, and proteins	Evaluate use to identify potential adverse effects.
Energy therapies	Yoga, Reiki, and T'ai chi	Prior to use, evaluate patient's physical ability to perform necessary activities.

Adapted from National Center for Complementary and Integrative Health (NCCIH). (2015). *Complementary, alternative, or integrative health: What's in a name?* Retrieved on 1/2/2016 at: nccih.nih.gov/health/integrative-health#types

Chart 12-6

NURSING RESEARCH PROFILE

Effects of Patient-Directed Music

Chlan, L. L., Weinert, C. R., Heiderscheit, A., et al. (2013). Effects of patient-directed music intervention on anxiety and sedative exposure in critically ill patients receiving mechanical ventilator support: A randomized clinical trial. *JAMA, 309*(22), 2335–2344.

Purpose

Patients who are mechanically ventilated have little control over pharmacologic interventions to decrease anxiety in the intensive care unit (ICU). Sedating medications commonly prescribed to these patients, including analgesic agents, are associated with many adverse effects such as hypotension, bradycardia, gut dysmotility, weakness, and delirium. Interventions are needed that reduce anxiety and minimize the use of sedating medications. This study tested whether listening to self-initiated, patient-directed music would reduce anxiety and use of sedating medication in patients who were critically ill and mechanically ventilated.

Design

A sample of 373 patients from twelve ICUs at five hospitals received acute mechanical ventilator support for respiratory failure. Patients who were alert and able to participate were randomized into three groups: 1. Patient-directed music (PDM), 2. Noise-canceling headphones (NCHs), and 3. Usual care in the ICU (Control)

A research nurse reviewed a starter set of six CDs, a CD player, and headphones with the PDM participants. Patients were prompted to use the music of their choice at least twice daily when feeling anxious or desiring relaxation. The NCH group was encouraged to wear headphones whenever they wanted to block out the noise in the ICU. All patients were assessed daily using a 100-mm visual analog scale to report anxiety levels. Data about the frequency and doses of sedating medications were also collected.

Findings

The PDM group listened to music for a mean of 79.8 minutes each day, while the NCH group wore noise-canceling headphones for a mean of 34 minutes each day. At any point in time, the PDM group had lower anxiety scores (19.5 points lower) than patients in the usual care group ($P = 0.003$). Over time, the PDM patients received less frequent and lower doses of sedating medications than the control group or the NCH group.

Nursing Implications

The PDM study was modeled after the concept of patient-controlled analgesia whereby patients report higher satisfaction when they can self-administer their analgesic. This unique approach that involved patients who were mechanically ventilated in self-management of anxiety launches a novel area of clinical research in the ICU. As clinicians seek to minimize the use of sedating medications in patients who are critically ill, PDM may be an appropriate complementary intervention by which patients can self-manage their anxiety and minimize the negative effects of sedating medications.

Chart 12-7

Considerations in Selecting and Using Nonpharmacologic Methods

- Does the patient, family, and health care team understand the relationship between nonpharmacologic pain management and analgesics? Patients who have been taking analgesic agents may mistakenly assume that when clinicians suggest a nonpharmacologic method, the purpose is to reduce the use or dose of analgesic agents. All involved must understand that nonpharmacologic methods are used to complement—not replace—pharmacologic methods.
- Does the patient understand the limitations of nonpharmacologic methods? Nonpharmacologic methods are valuable as comfort measures; however, not all such measures relieve pain and should not be promoted as such.
- Is the patient interested in using a nondrug method, and have any been tried previously? If so, what happened? Is the patient using nondrug methods because of unfounded fears about analgesic agents? Willingness and interest are important for successful use of nonpharmacologic methods; however, patients may fear taking analgesic agents that clearly are indicated for their pain, such as nonsteroidal anti-inflammatory drugs (NSAIDs) for an inflammatory painful condition. Such fears should be explored and accurate information and appropriate treatment provided. Alternately, the reasons a patient refuses to use a nonpharmacologic method also should be explored, but the patient's right to refuse must be respected.

- What are the patient's preferences and coping styles? Encouraging patients to choose from a variety of techniques allows them to match the technique to their individual and cultural preferences. If none of the choices appeal to the patient, the patient's right to refuse use should be respected.
- Does the patient have the physical and cognitive abilities necessary for using the nonpharmacologic method? Does the patient have sufficient energy to learn and perform any tasks involved? For example, physical and mental fatigue can interfere with the use of distraction and relaxation imagery techniques. Does the patient want to dedicate the necessary time required for the nonpharmacologic method? For example, those who do not find a 20-minute self-sustained relaxation technique appealing may be more suited for passive application of cold or heat.
- Do others (e.g., family, friends) want to be involved in helping the patient? Is the method a potential vehicle for improving relationships between the patient and others? For example, a method that patients cannot do for themselves, such as massage, may be a burden to some caregivers in the home, whereas others may welcome that opportunity to be physically close to a loved one.
- Are support materials and patient education resources available? Whenever possible, verbal, written, and in some cases, online or video education should be provided.

Adapted from McCaffery, M. (2002). What is the role of nondrug methods in the nursing care of patients with acute pain? (Guest Editorial). *Pain Management Nursing, 3*(3), 77–80; McCaffery, M., & Pasero, C. (1999). *Pain: Clinical manual.* St. Louis, MO: Mosby.

PLAN OF NURSING CARE

Chart 12-8

Care of the Patient With Acute Pain

NURSING DIAGNOSIS: Acute Pain
GOAL: Achievement and maintenance of patient's comfort-function goal

Nursing Intervention	Rationale	Expected Outcomes
1. Perform and document a comprehensive pain assessment.	1. The comprehensive pain assessment is the foundation of the pain treatment plan; documentation ensures communication between team members.	• If able, provides information about the pain • Expresses understanding of the link between function and pain control and establishes a realistic comfort-function goal • Reports a pain intensity that allows participation in important functional activities
a. Use a reliable and valid tool to determine pain intensity.	a. The use of valid and reliable tools helps ensure accuracy and consistency in assessment.	
b. Accept the patient's report of pain.	b. Accepting the patient's report of pain is the undisputed standard of pain assessment.	• If not able to report pain, demonstrates behaviors that indicate pain relief and participation in important functional activities
c. Assist the patient in establishing a comfort-function goal.	c. The comfort-function goal links function to pain control and provides direction for necessary adjustments in the treatment plan to maximize function.	• Expresses satisfaction with the use of nonpharmacologic methods • Tolerates pharmacologic and nonpharmacologic interventions without adverse effects
d. Apply the Hierarchy of Pain Measures in patients who are unable to report their pain.	d. The use of the Hierarchy of Pain Measures provides a process to ensure pain treatment in the patient who cannot report pain.	• Demonstrates an understanding of the treatment plan and goals of care
2. Administer analgesic agents as prescribed.	2. Pharmacologic interventions are the cornerstone of pain management.	
3. Offer and educate patient how to use appropriate nonpharmacologic interventions.	3. Nonpharmacologic methods are used to supplement pharmacologic interventions.	
4. Reassess for degree of pain relief and presence of adverse effects at peak effect time of intervention.	4. Reassessment permits evaluation of both the effectiveness and safety of interventions.	
5. Obtain additional prescriptions as needed.	5. Prescriptions for additional analgesic agents or adjustment in dose are often needed to maximize pain control.	
6. Prevent and treat adverse effects.	6. Adverse effects are prevented whenever possible and promptly treated to reduce patient discomfort and prevent harm.	
7. Educate patient and family about the effects of analgesic agents and the goals of care; explain how adverse effects will be prevented and treated; address fears of addiction.	7. An understanding of the treatment plan and goals of care educates patients and their families how to partner with the health care team to optimize pain control.	

Nursing Implications of Pain Management

The provision of optimal pain management requires a collaborative approach between patients with pain, their families, and members of the health care team. Everyone involved must share common goals, a common knowledge base, and a common language with regard to the analgesics and nonpharmacologic methods used to manage pain. Whether nurses provide care in the home, hospital, or any other setting, they are in a unique position to coordinate a comprehensive, evidence-based approach to meet the needs of people with pain. Chart 12-8 provides a plan of nursing care for the patient with pain.

CRITICAL THINKING EXERCISES

1 **ebp** An 82-year-old woman is admitted to the orthopedic unit posthip fracture. She is unable to answer questions about her pain history or her intensity of pain. She is crying and moaning. Her family reports that she has been very forgetful at home and recently diagnosed with dementia. What pain assessment tool would be most helpful in determining whether your pain interventions are helping? What is the strength of the evidence that supports your use of your selected tool?

2 [PQ] A 47-year-old man who is obese with chronic back pain and chronic opioid use is admitted to the medical unit with acute pancreatitis. His inpatient medications include a long-acting morphine product, intravenous hydromorphone PRN, an anxiolytic medication PRN, an antihistamine for pruritus PRN, and a hypnotic medication for sleep PRN. The patient asks you to give him all his medications at the same time so that he can get some sleep. He asserts that he has done this successfully every night at home for the past year. You are concerned that all these medications are central nervous system depressants and that given together, they could oversedate the patient. How would you prioritize the medications that he is requesting?

3 A 50-year-old woman with diabetes and bilateral neuropathic leg pain is admitted to the hospital with a leg abscess. She reports excruciating pain during dressing changes. Her only analgesic medication is an oral opioid. Using a multimodal approach, what other interventions (pharmacologic and nonpharmacologic) could be used to better manage her continuous pain as well as the procedural pain of dressing changes?

REFERENCES

*Asterisk indicates nursing research.
**Double asterisk indicates classic reference.

Books

**American Pain Society. (2008). *Principles of analgesic use in the treatment of acute and cancer pain* (6th ed.). Glenview, IL: Author.

Apkarian, A. V. (2015). *The brain adapting with pain: Contribution of neuroimaging technology to pain mechanisms.* Philadelphia, PA: International Association for the Study of Pain, Wolters Kluwer.

Apkarian, A. V., Bushnell, M. C., Schweinhardt, P., et al. (2013). Representation of pain in the brain. In S. B. McMahon, M. Koltzenburg, I. Tracey, et al. (Eds.). *Wall and Melzack's textbook of pain* (6th ed.). Philadelphia, PA: Elsevier-Saunders.

Buvanendran, A., Lubenow, T. R., & Droin, J. S. (2013). Postoperative pain and its management. In S. B. McMahon, M. Koltzenburg, I. Tracey, et al. (Eds.). *Wall and Melzack's textbook of pain* (6th ed.). Philadelphia, PA: Elsevier-Saunders.

Centers for Medicare & Medicaid Services (CMS). (2014). *Requirements for hospital medication administration, particularly intravenous (IV) medications and post-operative care of patients receiving IV opioids.* Baltimore, MD: Center for Clinical Standards and Quality/Survey & Certification Group, U.S. Department of Health & Human Services.

Comerford, K. C. (2015). *Nursing 2015 drug handbook.* Philadelphia, PA: Wolters Kluwer.

Gagliese, L., & Melzack, R. (2013). Pain in older persons. In S. B. McMahon, M. Koltzenburg, I. Tracey, et al. (Eds.). *Wall and Melzack's textbook of pain* (6th ed.). Philadelphia, PA: Elsevier-Saunders.

Golan, D. E., Tashjian, A. H., & Armstrong, E. J. (2017). *Principles of pharmacology: The pathophysiologic basis of drug therapy* (4th ed.). Baltimore, MD: Wolters Kluwer Health, Lippincott Williams & Wilkins.

Haythornwaite, J. A. (2013). Assessment of pain beliefs, coping, and function. In S. B. McMahon, M. Koltzenburg, I. Tracey, et al. (Eds.). *Wall and Melzack's textbook of pain* (6th ed.). Philadelphia, PA: Elsevier-Saunders.

Heinricher, M. M., & Fields, H. L. (2013). Central nervous system mechanisms of pain modulation. In S. B. McMahon, M. Koltzenburg, I. Tracey, et al. (Eds.). *Wall and Melzack's textbook of pain* (6th ed.). Philadelphia, PA: Elsevier-Saunders.

Hunt, S. P., & Urch, C. E. (2013). Pain, opiates and addiction. In S. B. McMahon, M. Koltzenburg, I. Tracey, et al. (Eds.). *Wall and Melzack's textbook of pain* (6th ed.). Philadelphia, PA: Elsevier-Saunders.

Kreitzer, M. J., & Koithan, M. (2014). *Integrative nursing.* Oxford, UK: Oxford University Press.

Lehne, R. A. (2013). *Pharmacology for nursing care* (8th ed.). St. Louis, MO: Elsevier Saunders.

MacIntyre, P. E., & Schug, S. A. (2015). *Acute pain management: A practical guide* (4th ed.). Boca Raton, LA: CRC Press, Taylor & Francis Group.

Mantyh, P. W. (2013). Cancer pain: Causes, consequences, and therapeutic opportunities. In S. B. McMahon, M. Koltzenburg, I. Tracey, et al. (Eds.). *Wall and Melzack's textbook of pain* (6th ed.). Philadelphia, PA: Elsevier-Saunders

**McCaffery, M. (1968). *Nursing practice theories related to cognition, bodily pain, and man-environment interactions.* Los Angeles, CA: University of California, Los Angeles.

**McCaffery, M., Herr, K., & Pasero, C. (2011). Assessment. In C. Pasero & M. McCaffery (Eds.). *Pain assessment and pharmacologic management.* St. Louis, MO: Mosby-Elsevier.

**McCaffery, M., & Pasero, C. (1999). *Pain: Clinical manual.* St. Louis, MO: Mosby.

National Institute on Drug Abuse. (2014). *Prescription drug abuse* (pp. 15–4881). Washington, DC: NIH publication.

**Pasero, C., & McCaffery, M. (2011). *Pain assessment and pharmacologic management.* St. Louis, MO: Mosby-Elsevier.

**Pasero, C., Polomano, R. C., Portenoy, R. K., et al. (2011). Adjuvant analgesics. In C. Pasero & M. McCaffery (Eds.). *Pain assessment and pharmacologic management.* St. Louis, MO: Mosby-Elsevier.

**Pasero, C., & Portenoy, R. K. (2011). Neurophysiology of pain and analgesia and the pathophysiology of neuropathic pain. In C. Pasero & M. McCaffery (Eds.). *Pain assessment and pharmacologic management.* St. Louis, MO: Mosby-Elsevier.

**Pasero, C., Portenoy, R. K., & McCaffery, M. (2011). Nonopioid analgesics. In C. Pasero & M. McCaffery (Eds.). *Pain assessment and pharmacologic management.* St. Louis, MO: Mosby-Elsevier.

**Pasero, C., Quinn, T. E., Portenoy, R. K., et al. (2011). Opioid analgesics. In C. Pasero & M. McCaffery (Eds.). *Pain assessment and pharmacologic management.* St. Louis, MO: Mosby-Elsevier.

Registered Nurses' Association of Ontario (RNAO). (2013). *Assessment and management of pain.* Washington, DC: Agency for Healthcare Research and Quality, National Guideline Clearinghouse, Guideline Summary NGC-10227.

Ringkamp, M., Raja, S. N., Campbell, J. N., et al. (2013). Peripheral mechanisms of cutaneous nociception. In S. B. McMahon, M. Koltzenburg, I. Tracey, et al. (Eds.). *Wall and Melzack's textbook of pain* (6th ed.). Philadelphia, PA: Elsevier-Saunders.

Sandkuhler, J. (2013). Spinal cord plasticity and pain. In S. B. McMahon, M. Koltzenburg, I. Tracey, et al. (Eds.). *Wall and Melzack's textbook of pain* (6th ed.). Philadelphia, PA: Elsevier-Saunders.

Scadding, J. W., & Koltzenburg, M. (2013). Painful peripheral neuropathies. In S. B. McMahon, M. Koltzenburg, I. Tracey, et al. (Eds.). *Wall and Melzack's textbook of pain* (6th ed.). Philadelphia, PA: Elsevier-Saunders.

Schug, S. A. (2013). Opioids: Clinical use. In S. B. McMahon, M. Koltzenburg, I. Tracey, et al. (Eds.). *Wall and Melzack's textbook of pain* (6th ed.). Philadelphia, PA: Elsevier-Saunders.

Smith, H.S. (Ed.). (2013). *Opioid therapy in the 21st century* (2nd ed.). Oxford, UK: Oxford University Press.

St. Marie, B. (Ed.). (2010). *Core curriculum for pain management nursing. American Society for Pain Management Nursing.* Olathe, KS: Kendall Hunt Professional.

Todd, A. J., & Koerber, H. R. (2013) Neuroanatomical substrates of spinal nociception. In S. B. McMahon, M. Koltzenburg, I. Tracey, et al. (Eds.). *Wall and Melzack's textbook of pain* (6th ed.). Philadelphia, PA: Elsevier-Saunders.

Wager, T. D., & Fields, H. L. (2013). Placebo analgesia. In S. B. McMahon, M. Koltzenburg, I. Tracey, et al. (Eds.). *Wall and Melzack's textbook of pain* (6th ed.). Philadelphia, PA: Elsevier-Saunders.

Journals and Electronic Documents

**American Geriatrics Society (AGS). (2009). Pharmacological management of persistent pain in older persons. *Journal of the American Geriatrics Society, 57*(6), 1331–1346.

**American Society of Addiction Medicine. (2001). Definitions related to the use of opioids for the treatment of pain. Retrieved on 7/12/2015 at: www.painmed.org/Workarea/DownloadAsset.aspx?id=3204

**American Society of PeriAnesthesia Nurses. (2006). ASPAN's evidence-based clinical practice guideline for the prevention and/or management of PONV/PDNV. *Journal of PeriAnesthesia Nursing*, 21(4), 230–250. Retrieved on 7/12/2015 at: aspan@aspan.org

Arnstein, P., Broglio, K., Wuhrman, E., et al. (2011). Use of placebos in pain management. *Pain Management Nursing*, 12(4), 225–229. Retrieved on 11/27/2015 at: www.aspmn.org/documents/UseofPlacebosinPainManagement.pdf

Auriel, E., Regev, K., & Korczyn, A. D. (2014). Nonsteroidal anti-inflammatory drugs exposure and the central nervous system. *Handbook of Clinical Neurology*, 119, 577–584.

Bello, A. E., & Holt, R. J. (2014). Cardiovascular risk with non-steroidal anti-inflammatory drugs: Clinical implications. *Drug Safety*, 37(11), 897–902.

Benson, J. L., Campbell, H. E., & Phillips, C. N. (2015). Opioid-induced pruritus. *The Consultant Pharmacist*, 30(4), 221–227.

Brown, C. J., & Flood, K. L. (2013). Mobility limitation in the older patient: A clinical review. *JAMA*, 310(11), 1168–1177.

Chlan, L., & Halm, M. A. (2013). Does music ease pain and anxiety in the critically ill? *American Journal of Critical Care*, 22(6). Retrieved on 11/27/2015 at: www.ajcconline.org, doi: http://dx.doi.org/10.4037/ajcc2013998

*Chlan, L. L., Weinert, C. R., Heiderscheit, A., et al. (2013). Effects of patient-directed music intervention on anxiety and sedative exposure in critically ill patients receiving mechanical ventilator support: A randomized clinical trial. *JAMA*, 309(22), 2335–2344.

Cohen, S. P., & Mao, J. (2014). Neuropathic pain mechanisms and their clinical implications. *BMJ*, 348, f7656.

Cooney, M. F., Czarnecki, M. Dunwoody, C., et al. (2013). American Society for Pain Management Nursing position statement with clinical practice guidelines: Authorized agent controlled analgesia. *Pain Management Nursing*, 14(3), 176–181.

Deer, T. R., Prager, J., Levy, R., et al. (2012). Polyanalgesic consensus conference 2012: Recommendations for the management of pain by intrathecal(intraspinal) drug delivery: Report of an interdisciplinary expert panel. *Neuromodulation*, 15, 436–466.

Enekwa, C. E., Pounds, T. I., Lovett, A., et al. (2014). Use of intravenous acetaminophen to reduce opioid use in patients undergoing bariatric surgery at a community teaching hospital. *Journal of Pharmaceutics & Pharmacology*, 2(2), 3.

Federal Register. (2014). *Schedules of controlled substances: Rescheduling of hydrocodone combination products from Schedule III to Schedule II. Final Rule. 2014.* Retrieved on 8/11/2015 at: www.gpo.gov/fdsys/pkg/FR-2014-08-22/pdf/2014-19922.pdf

Gan, T. J., Diemunsch, P., Habib, A. S., et al. (2014). Consensus guidelines for the management of postoperative nausea and vomiting. *Anesthesia & Analgesia*, 118(1), 85–113.

Gan, T. J., Habib, A. S., Miller, T. E., et al. (2014). Incidence, patient satisfaction, and perceptions of post-surgical pain: results from a US national survey. *Current Medical Research and Opinion*, 30, 1–12.

Gnjidic, D., Blyth, F. M., LeCouteur, D. G., et al. (2014). Nonsteroidal anti-inflammatory drugs(NSAIDs) in older people: Prescribing patterns according to pain prevalence and adherence to clinical guidelines. *Pain*, 155(9), 1814–1820.

*Guo, L. L., Li, L., Liu, Y. W., et al. (2015). Evaluation of two observational pain assessment scales during anesthesia recovery period in Chinese surgical older adults. *Journal of Clinical Nursing*, 24(1–2), 212–221.

**Herr, K., Coyne, P. J., McCaffery, M., et al. (2011). Pain assessment in the patient unable to self-report: Position statement with clinical practice recommendations. *Pain Management Nursing*, 12(4), 230–250.

Herr K., St. Marie, B., Gordon, D. B., et al. (2015). An interprofessional consensus of core competencies for prelicensure education in pain management: Curriculum application for nursing. *Journal of Nursing Education*, 54(6), 317–327.

Hoffman, D. (2015). Central and peripheral pain generators in women with chronic pelvic pain: Patient centered assessment and treatment. *Current Rheumatology Reviews*, 11(2), 146–166.

Hooten, W. M., Timming, R., Belgrade, M., et al. (2013). *Assessment and management of chronic pain* (p. 105). Bloomington, MN: Institute for Clinical Systems Improvement (ICSI). Retrieved on 1/1/2016 at: www.icsi.org/_asset/bw798b/ChronicPain.pdf

International Association for the Study of Pain (IASP). (2013). *Bothersome pain afflicts half of older Americans.* Retrieved on 12/31/2015

at: www.iasp-pain.org/PublicationsNews/NewsDetail.aspx?ItemNumber=919&navItemNumber=643

Jannuzzi, R. G. (2015). Nalbuphine for treatment of opioid-induced pruritus: A systematic review of literature. *The Clinical Journal of Pain*, 32(1), 87–93.

**Jarzyna, D., Junquist, C., Pasero, C., et al. (2011). American Society for Pain Management evidence-based guideline on monitoring for opioid-induced sedation and respiratory depression. *Pain Management Nursing*, 12(3), 118–145.

King, G. F., & Vetter, I. (2014). No gain, no pain: NaVI.7 as an analgesic target. *ACS Chemical Neuroscience*, 5(9), 749–751.

Kwon, J. H., Tanco, K., Hui, D., et al. (2014). Chemical coping versus pseudoaddiction in patients with cancer pain. *Palliative & Supportive Care*, 12(5), 413–417.

Makris, U. E., Abrams, R. C., Gurland, B., et al. (2014). Management of persistent pain in the older patients: A clinical review. *JAMA*, 312(8), 825–837.

Manworren, R. C. B. (2015). Multimodal pain management and the future of a personalized medicine approach to pain. *AORN Journal*, 101(3), 307–318.

Mariano, E. R. (2015). Management of acute perioperative pain. In E. W. K. Rosenquist & M. Crowley (Eds.). *Up-to-Date.* Retrieved on 8/11/2015 at: www.uptodate.com/contents/management-of-acute-perioperative-pain

Mathiesen, O., Dahl, B., Thomsen, B. A., et al. (2013). A comprehensive multimodal pain treatment reduces opioid consumption after multilevel spine surgery. *European Spine Journal*, 22(9), 2089–2096.

McCabe, S. E., West, B. T., & Boyd, C. J. (2013). Medical use, medical misuse, and nonmedical use of prescription opioids: Results from a longitudinal study. *Pain*, 154(5), 708–713.

**McCaffery, M. (2002). What is the role of nondrug methods in the nursing care of patients with acute pain? (Guest Editorial). *Pain Management Nursing*, 3(3), 77–80.

Meara, A. S., & Simon, L. S. (2013). Advice from professional societies: Appropriate use of NSAIDs. *Pain Medicine*, 14(S1), S3–S10.

Moldovan, M., Alvarez, S., Romer Rosberg, M., et al. (2013). Axonal voltage-gated ion channels as pharmacological targets for pain. *European Journal of Pharmacology*, 708(1–3), 105–112.

Momi, S. K., Fabiane, S. M., Lachance, G., et al. (2015). Neuropathic pain as part of chronic widespread pain: Environmental and genetic influences. *Pain*, 156(10), 2100–2106.

Moore, A., Wiffen, P., & Kalso, E. (2014). Antiepileptic drugs for neuropathic pain and fibromyalgia. *JAMA*, 312(2), 182–183.

Nahin, R. L., Stussman, B. J., Herman, P. M. (2015). Out-of-pocket expenditures on complementary health approaches associated with painful health conditions in a nationally representative adult sample. *Journal of Pain*, 16(11), 1147–1162.

Narouze, S., Benzon, H. T., Provenzano, D. A., et al. (2015). Interventional spine and pain procedures in patients on antiplatelet and anticoagulant medications. *Regional Anesthesia & Pain Medicine*, 40(3), 182–212.

National Center for Complementary and Integrative Health (NCCIH). (2015). *Complementary, alternative, or integrative health: What's in a name?* Retrieved on 1/2/2016 at: nccih.nih.gov/health/integrative-health#types

Nicholson, W. T., & Formea, C. M. (2015). Clinical perspective on the clinical pharmacogenetics implementation consortium updated 2014 guidelines for CYP2D6 and codeine. *Clinical Chemistry*, 61(2), 319–321.

Niesters, M., Martini, C., & Dahan, A. (2014). Ketamine for chronic pain: Risks and benefits. *British Journal of Clinical Pharmacology*, 77(2), 357–367.

Niesters, M., Proto, P. L., Aarts, L., et al. (2014). Tapentadol potentiates descending pain inhibition in chronic pain patients with diabetic polyneuropathy. *British Journal of Anaesthesia*, 113(1), 148–156. Retrieved on 11/1/2015 at: bja.oxfordjournals.org/content/early/2014/04/07/bja.aeu056.short

Oliver, J., Coggins, C., Compton, P., et al. (2012). American Society for Pain Management Nursing position statement: Pain management in patients with substance use disorders. *Pain Management Nursing*, 13(3), 169–183.

Parent, A. J., Beaudet, N., Daigle, K., et al. (2015). Relationship between blood- and cerebrospinal fluid–bound neurotransmitter concentrations and conditioned pain modulation in pain-free and chronic pain subjects. *The Journal of Pain*, 16(5), 436–444.

***Pasero, C. (2009). Assessment of sedation during opioid administration for pain management. *Journal of PeriAnesthesia Nursing, 24*(3), 186–190.

Patel, K. V., Guralnik, J. M., Dansie, E. J., et al. (2013). Prevalence and impact of pain among older adults in the United States: Findings from the 2011 National Health and Aging Trends study. *Pain, 154*(12), 2649–2657.

Porter, S. B., McClain, R. L., Howe, B. L., et al. (2015). Perioperative ketamine for acute postoperative analgesia: The Mayo Clinic—Florida experience. *Journal of PeriAnesthesia Nursing, 30*(3), 189–195.

Reid, M. C., Eccleston, C., & Pillemer, K. (2015). Management of chronic pain in older adults. *British Medical Journal, 350*, h532.

Sayin, Y. Y., & Akyolcu, N. (2014). Comparison of pain scale preferences and pain intensity according to pain scales among Turkish patients: A descriptive study. *Pain Management Nursing, 15*(1), 156–164.

Shaparin, N., Sim, A., Pappagallo, M., et al. (2015). Intrathecal analgesia: Time to consider it for your patient? *Journal of Family Practice, 64*(3), 166–172.

Singh, D. R., Nag, K., Shetti, A. N., et al. (2013). Tapentadol hydrochloride: A novel analgesic. *Saudi Journal of Anaesthesia, 7*(3), 322–326.

Singla, N, K., Hale, M. E., Davis, J. C., et al. (2015). IV acetaminophen: Efficacy of a single dose for postoperative pain after hip arthroplasty: Subset data analysis of 2 unpublished randomized clinical trials. *American Journal of Therapeutics, 22*(1), 2–10.

**Spagrud, L. J., Piira, T., & Von Baeyer, C. L. (2003). Children's self-report of pain intensity. The faces pain scale—revised. *American Journal of Nursing, 103*(12), 62–64.

Trail-Mahan, T., Mao, C. L, & Bawel-Brinkley, K. (2013). Complementary and alternative medicine: Nurses' attitudes and knowledge. *Pain Management Nursing, 14*(4), 277–286.

U.S. Food and Drug Administration (FDA). (2014). *FDA reminds health care professionals to stop dispensing prescription combination drug products with more than 325 mg of acetaminophen US Department of Health and Human Services.* Retrieved on 8/11/2015 at: www.fda.gov/Drugs/DrugSafety/ucm394916.htm

Valentine, A. R., Carvalho, B., Lazo T. A., et al. (2015). Scheduled acetaminophen with as-needed opioids compared to as-needed acetaminophen plus opioids for post-cesarean pain management. *International Journal of Obstetric Anesthesia, 24*(3), 210–216.

Weaver, J. M. (2014). Multiple risks for patients using the transdermal fentanyl patch. *Anesthesia Progress, 61*(1), 1–2.

**Weissman, D. E., & Haddox, J. D. (1989). Opioid pseudoaddiction—an iatrogenic syndrome. *Pain, 36*(3), 363–366.

Weiss, R. D., Sharpe Potter, J., Griffin, M. L., et al. (2014). Reasons for opioid use among patients with dependence on prescription opioids: The role of chronic pain. *Journal of Substance Abuse Treatment, 47*(2),140–145.

Wu, H., Gikas, P. V., & Connelly, P. (2014). Methadone: History, pharmacology, physical effects and clinical implications. *International Journal of Medical and Biological Frontiers, 20*(4), 299–323.

Yellon, R. F., Kenna, M. A., Cladis, F. P., et al. (2014). What is the best non-codeine postadenotonsillectomy pain management for children? *The Laryngoscope, 124*(8), 1737–1738.

Youssef, F., Pater, A., & Shehata, M. (2015). Opioid-induced hyperalgesia. *Journal of Pain & Relief, 4*, 183.

Resources

American Academy of Pain Management, aapainmanage.org

American Academy of Pain Medicine (AAPM), painmed.org

American Chronic Pain Association, theacpa.org

American Pain Foundation (APF), painfoundation.org

American Pain Society, ampainsoc.org

American Society for Pain Management Nursing (ASPMN), aspmn.org

City of Hope Pain & Palliative Care Resource Center, prc.coh.org/

National Center for Complementary and Integrative Health (NCCIH), nccih.nih.gov/

Pain & Policies Studies Group, www.painpolicy.wisc.edu

Pain Treatment Topics, pain-topics.org

13 Fluid and Electrolytes: Balance and Disturbance

LEARNING OBJECTIVES

On completion of this chapter, the learner will be able to:

1 Differentiate between osmosis, diffusion, filtration, and active transport.
2 Describe the role of the kidneys, lungs, and endocrine glands in regulating the body's fluid composition and volume.
3 Identify the effects of aging on fluid and electrolyte regulation.
4 Plan effective care of patients with the following imbalances: fluid volume deficit and fluid volume excess, sodium deficit (hyponatremia) and sodium excess (hypernatremia), and potassium deficit (hypokalemia) and potassium excess (hyperkalemia).
5 Describe the cause, clinical manifestations, management, and nursing interventions for the following imbalances: calcium deficit (hypocalcemia) and calcium excess (hypercalcemia), magnesium deficit (hypomagnesemia) and magnesium excess (hypermagnesemia), phosphorus deficit (hypophosphatemia) and phosphorus excess (hyperphosphatemia), and chloride deficit (hypochloremia) and chloride excess (hyperchloremia).
6 Explain the roles of the lungs, kidneys, and chemical buffers in maintaining acid–base balance.
7 Compare metabolic acidosis and alkalosis with regard to causes, clinical manifestations, diagnosis, and management.
8 Compare respiratory acidosis and alkalosis with regard to causes, clinical manifestations, diagnosis, and management.
9 Interpret arterial blood gas measurements.

GLOSSARY

acidosis: an acid–base imbalance characterized by an increase in H^+ concentration (decreased blood pH) (A low arterial pH due to reduced bicarbonate concentration is called *metabolic acidosis;* a low arterial pH due to increased PCO_2 is called *respiratory acidosis.*)

ascites: a type of edema in which fluid accumulates in the peritoneal cavity

active transport: physiologic pump that moves fluid from an area of lower concentration to one of higher concentration; active transport requires adenosine triphosphate for energy

alkalosis: an acid–base imbalance characterized by a reduction in H^+ concentration (increased blood pH) (A high arterial pH with increased bicarbonate concentration is called *metabolic alkalosis;* a high arterial pH due to reduced PCO_2 is called *respiratory alkalosis.*)

diffusion: the process by which solutes move from an area of higher concentration to one of lower concentration; does not require expenditure of energy

homeostasis: maintenance of a constant internal equilibrium in a biologic system that involves positive and negative feedback mechanisms

hydrostatic pressure: the pressure created by the weight of fluid against the wall that contains it. In the body, hydrostatic pressure in blood vessels results from the weight of fluid itself and the force resulting from cardiac contraction.

hypertonic solution: a solution with an osmolality higher than that of serum

hypotonic solution: a solution with an osmolality lower than that of serum

isotonic solution: a solution with the same osmolality as serum and other body fluids

osmolality: the number of milliosmoles (the standard unit of osmotic pressure) per kilogram of solvent; expressed as milliosmoles per kilogram (mOsm/kg). (The term *osmolality* is used more often than *osmolarity* to evaluate serum and urine.)

osmolarity: the number of milliosmoles (the standard unit of osmotic pressure) per liter of solution; expressed as milliosmoles per liter (mOsm/L); describes the concentration of solutes or dissolved particles

osmosis: the process by which fluid moves across a semipermeable membrane from an area of low solute concentration to an area of high solute concentration; the process continues until the solute concentrations are equal on both sides of the membrane

tonicity: fluid tension or the effect that osmotic pressure of a solution with impermeable solutes exerts on cell size because of water movement across the cell membrane

---

Fluid and electrolyte balance is dependent upon dynamic processes that are crucial for life and **homeostasis**. Potential and actual disorders of fluid and electrolyte balance occur in every setting, with every disorder, and with a variety of changes that affect healthy people (e.g., increased fluid and sodium loss with strenuous exercise and high environmental temperature, inadequate intake of fluid and electrolytes) as well as those who are ill.

Fundamental Concepts

Nurses need to understand the physiology of fluid and electrolyte balance and acid–base balance to anticipate, identify, and respond to possible imbalances. Nurses use effective education and communication skills to help prevent and treat various fluid and electrolyte disturbances.

Amount and Composition of Body Fluids

Approximately 60% of a typical adult's weight consists of fluid (water and electrolytes) (see Fig. 13-1). Factors that influence the amount of body fluid are age, gender, and body fat. In general, younger people have a higher percentage of body fluid than older adults, and men have proportionately more body fluid than women. People who are obese have less fluid than those who are thin, because fat cells contain little water. The skeleton also has low water content. Muscle, skin, and blood contain the highest amounts of water (Grossman & Porth, 2014).

Body fluid is located in two fluid compartments: the intracellular space (fluid in the cells) and the extracellular space (fluid outside the cells). Approximately two thirds of body fluid is in the intracellular fluid (ICF) compartment and is located primarily in the skeletal muscle mass. Approximately one third is in the extracellular fluid (ECF) compartment (Grossman & Porth, 2014).

The ECF compartment is further divided into the intravascular, interstitial, and transcellular fluid spaces:

- The intravascular space (the fluid within the blood vessels) contains plasma, the effective circulating volume. Approximately 3 L of the average 6 L of blood volume in adults is made up of plasma. The remaining 3 L is made up of erythrocytes, leukocytes, and thrombocytes.
- The interstitial space contains the fluid that surrounds the cell and totals about 11 to 12 L in an adult. Lymph is an interstitial fluid.
- The transcellular space is the smallest division of the ECF compartment and contains approximately 1 L. Examples of transcellular fluids include cerebrospinal, pericardial, synovial, intraocular, and pleural fluids, sweat, and digestive secretions.

As the next section describes, the ECF transports electrolytes; it also carries other substances, such as enzymes and hormones.

Body fluid normally moves between the two major compartments or spaces in an effort to maintain equilibrium between the spaces. Loss of fluid from the body can disrupt this equilibrium. Sometimes fluid is not lost from the body but is unavailable for use by either the ICF or ECF. Loss of ECF into a space that does not contribute to equilibrium between the ICF and the ECF is referred to as a third-space fluid shift, or third spacing (Papadakis & McPhee, 2016).

Early evidence of a third-space fluid shift is a decrease in urine output despite adequate fluid intake. Urine output decreases because fluid shifts out of the intravascular space; the kidneys then receive less blood and attempt to compensate by decreasing urine output. Other signs and symptoms of third spacing that indicate an intravascular fluid volume deficit (FVD) include increased heart rate, decreased blood pressure, decreased central venous pressure, edema, increased body weight, and imbalances in fluid intake and output (I&O). This fluid will be reabsorbed back into the extracellular space over a period of a few days to a few weeks. However, the acute volume depletion must be restored to prevent further complications. Examples of causes of third-space fluid losses include intestinal obstruction, pancreatitis, crushing traumatic injuries, bleeding (trauma or dissected aortic aneurysm), peritonitis, and major venous obstruction (Sterns, 2014a).

Electrolytes

Electrolytes in body fluids are active chemicals (cations that carry positive charges and anions that carry negative charges). The major cations in body fluid are sodium, potassium, calcium, magnesium, and hydrogen ions. The major anions are chloride, bicarbonate, phosphate, sulfate, and proteinate ions.

These chemicals unite in varying combinations. Therefore, electrolyte concentration in the body is expressed in terms of milliequivalents (mEq) per liter, a measure of chemical activity, rather than in terms of milligrams (mg), a unit of weight. More specifically, a milliequivalent is defined as being equivalent to the electrochemical activity of 1 mg of hydrogen. In a solution, cations and anions are equal in milliequivalents per liter.

Electrolyte concentrations in the ICF differ from those in the ECF, as reflected in Table 13-1. Because special techniques are required to measure electrolyte concentrations in the ICF, it is customary to measure the electrolytes in the most accessible portion of the ECF—namely, the plasma.

Sodium ions, which are positively charged, far outnumber the other cations in the ECF. Because sodium concentration affects the overall concentration of the ECF, sodium is important in regulating the volume of body fluid. Retention of sodium is associated with fluid retention, and excessive loss of sodium is usually associated with decreased volume of body fluid.

As shown in Table 13-1, the major electrolytes in the ICF are potassium and phosphate. The ECF has a low concentration of potassium and can tolerate only small changes in potassium concentrations. Therefore, the release of large

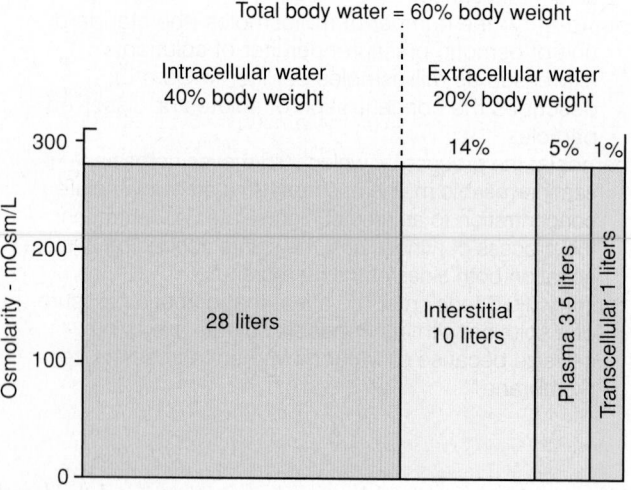

**Figure 13-1 • ** Approximate sizes of body compartments in a 70-kg adult. From Grossman, S. C., & Porth, C. M. (2014). *Porth's pathophysiology: Concepts of altered health states* (p. 1023). Philadelphia, PA: Lippincott Williams & Wilkins.

TABLE 13-1 Concentrations of Extracellular and Intracellular Electrolytes in Adults

| Electrolyte | Extracellular Concentration[a] | | Intracellular Concentration[a] | |
	Conventional Units	SI Units (mmol/L)	Conventional Units	SI Units (mmol/L)
Sodium	135–145 mEq/L	135–145	10–14 mEq/L	10–14
Potassium	3.5–5.0 mEq/L	3.5–5.0	140–150 mEq/L	140–150
Chloride	98–106 mEq/L	98–106	3–4 mEq/L	3–4
Bicarbonate	24–31 mEq/L	24–31	7–10 mEq/L	7–10
Calcium	8.5–10.5 mg/dL	2.1–2.6	<1 mEq/L	<0.25
Phosphorus	2.5–4.5 mg/dL	0.8–1.45	Variable	Variable
Magnesium	1.8–3.0 mg/dL	0.75–1.25	40 mEq/kg[b]	20

[a]Values may vary among laboratories, depending on the method of analysis used.
[b]Values vary among various tissues and with nutritional status.
Reprinted with permission from Grossman, S.C., & Porth, C. M. (2014). *Porth's pathophysiology: Concepts of altered health states* (9th ed.). Philadelphia, PA: Lippincott Williams & Wilkins.

stores of intracellular potassium, typically caused by trauma to the cells and tissues, can be extremely dangerous.

The body expends a great deal of energy maintaining the high extracellular concentration of sodium and the high intracellular concentration of potassium. It does so by means of cell membrane pumps that exchange sodium and potassium ions. Normal movement of fluids through the capillary wall into the tissues depends on **hydrostatic pressure** (the pressure exerted by the fluid on the walls of the blood vessel) at both the arterial and the venous ends of the vessel and the osmotic pressure exerted by the protein of plasma. The direction of fluid movement depends on the differences in these two opposing forces (hydrostatic vs. osmotic pressure).

Regulation of Body Fluid Compartments

Osmosis and Osmolality

When two different solutions are separated by a membrane that is impermeable to the dissolved substances, fluid shifts through the membrane from the region of low solute concentration to the region of high solute concentration until the solutions are of equal concentration. This diffusion of water caused by a fluid concentration gradient is known as **osmosis** (see Fig. 13-2A). The magnitude of this force depends on the number of particles dissolved in the solutions, not on their weights. The number of dissolved particles contained in a unit of fluid determines the osmolality of a solution, which influences the movement of fluid between the fluid compartments. **Tonicity** is the ability of all solutes to cause an osmotic driving force that promotes water movement from one compartment to another. The control of tonicity determines the normal state of cellular hydration and cell size. Sodium, mannitol, glucose, and sorbitol are effective osmoles (capable of affecting water movement). Three other terms are associated with osmosis—*osmotic pressure, oncotic pressure,* and *osmotic diuresis:*

- Osmotic pressure is the amount of hydrostatic pressure needed to stop the flow of water by osmosis. It is primarily determined by the concentration of solutes.

- Oncotic pressure is the osmotic pressure exerted by proteins (e.g., albumin).
- Osmotic diuresis is the increase in urine output caused by the excretion of substances, such as glucose, mannitol, or contrast agents in the urine.

Diffusion

Diffusion is the natural tendency of a substance to move from an area of higher concentration to one of lower concentration (see Fig. 13-2B). It occurs through the random movement of ions and molecules (Grossman & Porth, 2014). Examples of diffusion are the exchange of oxygen and carbon dioxide (CO_2) between the pulmonary capillaries and alveoli and the tendency of sodium to move from the ECF compartment, where the sodium concentration is high, to the ICF, where its concentration is low.

Filtration

Hydrostatic pressure in the capillaries tends to filter fluid out of the intravascular compartment into the interstitial fluid. Movement of water and solutes occurs from an area of high hydrostatic pressure to an area of low hydrostatic pressure. The kidneys filter approximately 180 L of plasma per day. Another example of filtration is the passage of water and electrolytes from the arterial capillary bed to the interstitial fluid; in this instance, the hydrostatic pressure results from the pumping action of the heart.

Sodium–Potassium Pump

The sodium concentration is greater in the ECF than in the ICF; because of this, sodium tends to enter the cell by diffusion. This tendency is offset by the sodium–potassium pump that is maintained by the cell membrane and actively moves sodium from the cell into the ECF. Conversely, the high intracellular potassium concentration is maintained by pumping potassium into the cell. By definition, **active transport** implies that energy must be expended for the movement to occur against a concentration gradient.

OSMOSIS

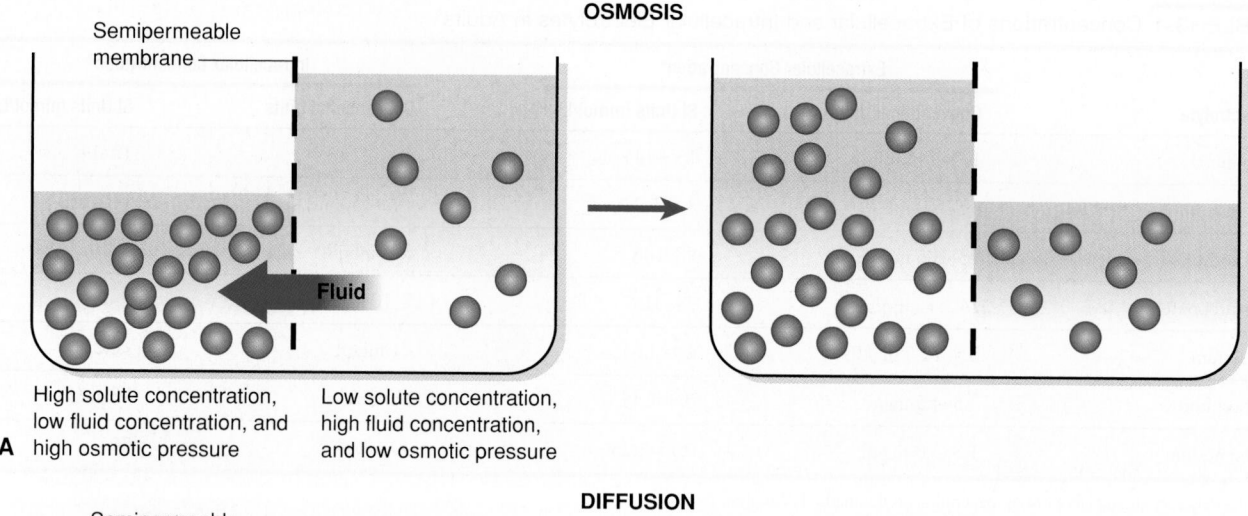

A. High solute concentration, low fluid concentration, and high osmotic pressure / Low solute concentration, high fluid concentration, and low osmotic pressure

DIFFUSION

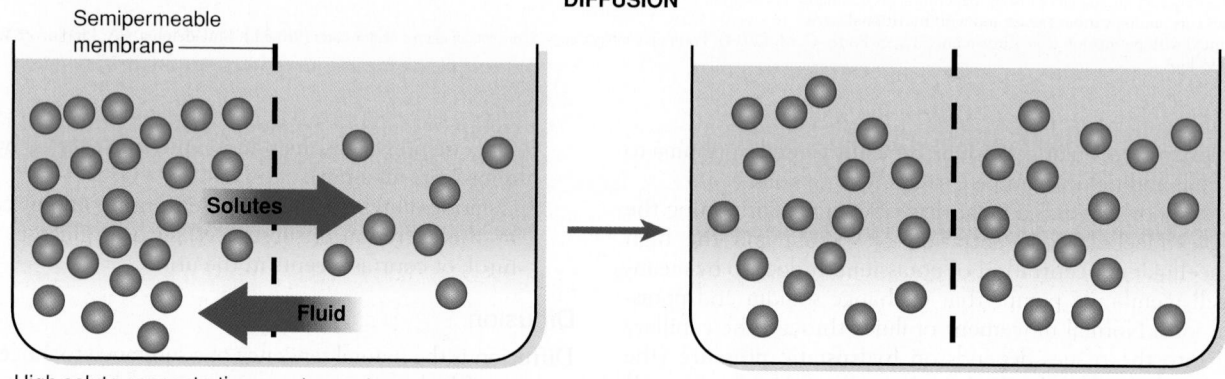

B. High solute concentration / Low solute concentration

Figure 13-2 • **A.** Osmosis: movement of fluid from an area of lower solute concentration to an area of higher solute concentration with eventual equalization of the solute concentrations. **B.** Diffusion: movement of solutes from an area of greater concentration to an area of lesser concentration, leading ultimately to equalization of the solute concentrations.

Systemic Routes of Gains and Losses

Water and electrolytes are gained in various ways. Healthy people gain fluids by drinking and eating, and their daily average I&O of water are approximately equal (see Table 13-2).

Kidneys

The usual daily urine volume in the adult is 1 to 2 L (Grossman & Porth, 2014; Sterns, 2014a). A general rule is that the output is approximately 1 mL of urine per kilogram of body weight per hour (1 mL/kg/h) in all age groups.

TABLE 13-2 Sources of Body Water Gains and Losses in the Adult

Intake (mL)		Output (mL)	
Oral intake		Urine	1500
As water	1000	Stool	200
In food	1300	Insensible	
Water of oxidation	200	Lungs	300
		Skin	500
Total gain[a]	2500	Total loss[a]	2500

[a]Approximate volumes.
Adapted with permission from Grossman, S. C., & Porth, C. M. (2014). *Porth's pathophysiology: Concepts of altered health states* (9th ed.). Philadelphia, PA: Lippincott Williams & Wilkins.

Skin

Sensible perspiration refers to visible water and electrolyte loss through the skin (sweating). The chief solutes in sweat are sodium, chloride, and potassium. Actual sweat losses can vary from 0 to 1000 mL or more every hour, depending on factors such as the environmental temperature. Continuous water loss by evaporation (approximately 500 mL/day) occurs through the skin as insensible perspiration, a nonvisible form of water loss (Grossman & Porth, 2014). Fever and exercise greatly increase insensible water loss through the lungs and the skin, as does the loss of the natural skin barrier (e.g., through major burns) (Earhart, Weiss, Rahman, et al., 2015; Sterns, 2014b).

Lungs

The lungs normally eliminate water vapor (insensible loss) at a rate of approximately 300 mL every day (Grossman & Porth, 2014). The loss is much greater with increased respiratory rate or depth, or in a dry climate.

Gastrointestinal Tract

The usual loss through the gastrointestinal (GI) tract is 100 to 200 mL daily, even though approximately 8 L of fluid circulates through the GI system every 24 hours. Because the bulk of fluid is normally reabsorbed in the small intestine, diarrhea and fistulas cause large losses.

Laboratory Tests for Evaluating Fluid Status

Osmolality is the concentration of fluid that affects the movement of water between fluid compartments by osmosis. Osmolality measures the solute concentration per kilogram in blood and urine. It is also a measure of a solution's ability to create osmotic pressure and affect the movement of water. Serum osmolality primarily reflects the concentration of sodium, although blood urea nitrogen (BUN) and glucose also play a major role in determining serum osmolality. Urine osmolality is determined by urea, creatinine, and uric acid. When measured with serum osmolality, urine osmolality is the most reliable indicator of urine concentration. Osmolality is reported as milliosmoles per kilogram of water (mOsm/kg) (Emmett, 2014).

In healthy adults, normal serum osmolality is 275 to 290 mOsm/kg (Sterns, 2014c). Sodium predominates in ECF osmolality and holds water in this compartment. Factors that increase and decrease serum and urine osmolality are identified in Table 13-3. Serum osmolality may be measured directly through laboratory tests or estimated at the bedside by doubling the serum sodium level or by using the following formula:

$$Na^+ \times 2 = \frac{Glucose}{18} + \frac{BUN}{3}$$

= Approximate value of serum osmolality

Osmolarity, another term that describes the concentration of solutions, is measured in milliosmoles per liter (mOsm/L). However, the term osmolality is used more often in clinical practice. The value of osmolarity is usually within 10 mOsm of the value of osmolality.

Urine-specific gravity measures the kidneys' ability to excrete or conserve water. The specific gravity of urine is compared to the weight of distilled water, which has a specific gravity of 1.000. The normal range of urine specific gravity is 1.010 to 1.025. Urine specific gravity can be measured by sending approximately 20 mL of urine to the laboratory for testing, or carefully assessed with dipstick. Specific gravity varies inversely with urine volume; normally, the larger the volume of urine, the lower the specific gravity is. Specific gravity is a less reliable indicator of concentration than urine osmolality; increased glucose or protein in urine can cause a falsely elevated specific gravity. Factors that increase or decrease urine osmolality are the same as those for urine specific gravity.

BUN is made up of urea, which is an end product of the metabolism of protein (from both muscle and dietary intake) by the liver. Amino acid breakdown produces large amounts of ammonia molecules, which are absorbed into the bloodstream. Ammonia molecules are converted to urea and excreted in the urine. The normal BUN is 10 to 20 mg/dL (3.6 to 7.2 mmol/L). The BUN level varies with urine output. Factors that increase BUN include decreased renal function, GI bleeding, dehydration, increased protein intake, fever, and sepsis. Those that decrease BUN include end-stage liver disease, a low-protein diet, starvation, and any condition that results in expanded fluid volume (e.g., pregnancy).

Creatinine is the end product of muscle metabolism. It is a better indicator of renal function than BUN because it does not vary with protein intake and metabolic state. The normal serum creatinine is approximately 0.7 to 1.4 mg/dL (62 to 124 mmol/L); however, its concentration depends on lean body mass and varies from person to person. Serum creatinine levels increase when renal function decreases.

Hematocrit measures the volume percentage of red blood cells (erythrocytes) in whole blood and normally ranges from

TABLE 13-3 Factors Affecting Serum and Urine Osmolality

Fluid	Factors Increasing Osmolality	Factors Decreasing Osmolality
Serum (275–290 mOsm/kg water)	Severe dehydration Free water loss Diabetes insipidus Hypernatremia Hyperglycemia Stroke or head injury Renal tubular necrosis Consumption of methanol or ethylene glycol (antifreeze) High ion gap metabolic acidosis Mannitol therapy Advanced liver disease Alcoholism Burns	Fluid volume excess Syndrome of inappropriate antidiuretic hormone (SIADH) Acute kidney injury Diuretic use Adrenal insufficiency Hyponatremia Overhydration Paraneoplastic syndrome associated with lung cancer
Urine (200–800 mOsm/kg water)	Fluid volume deficit SIADH Congestive heart failure Acidosis Prerenal failure	Fluid volume excess Diabetes insipidus Hyponatremia Aldosteronism Pyelonephritis Acute tubular necrosis

Adapted from Grossman, S. C., & Porth, C. M. (2014). *Porth's pathophysiology: Concepts of altered health states* (9th ed.). Philadelphia, PA: Lippincott Williams & Wilkins.

42% to 52% for men and 35% to 47% for women. Conditions that increase the hematocrit value are dehydration and polycythemia, and those that decrease hematocrit are overhydration and anemia.

Urine sodium values change with sodium intake and the status of fluid volume: As sodium intake increases, excretion increases; as the circulating fluid volume decreases, sodium is conserved. Normal urine sodium levels range from 75 to 200 mEq/24 hours (75 to 200 mmol/24 hours). A random specimen usually contains more than 40 mEq/L of sodium. Urine sodium levels are used to assess volume status and are useful in the diagnosis of hyponatremia and acute kidney injury.

Homeostatic Mechanisms

The body is equipped with remarkable homeostatic mechanisms to keep the composition and volume of body fluid within narrow limits of normal. Organs involved in homeostasis include the kidneys, heart, lungs, pituitary gland, adrenal glands, and parathyroid glands (Grossman & Porth, 2014).

Kidney Functions

Vital to the regulation of fluid and electrolyte balance, the kidneys normally filter 180 L of plasma every day in the adult and excrete 1 to 2 L of urine (Inker & Perrone, 2014). They act both autonomously and in response to bloodborne messengers, such as aldosterone and antidiuretic hormone (ADH) (Grossman & Porth, 2014). Major functions of the kidneys in maintaining normal fluid balance include the following:
- Regulation of ECF volume and osmolality by selective retention and excretion of body fluids
- Regulation of normal electrolyte levels in the ECF by selective electrolyte retention and excretion
- Regulation of pH of the ECF by retention of hydrogen ions
- Excretion of metabolic wastes and toxic substances (Inker & Perrone, 2014)

Given these functions, failure of the kidneys results in multiple fluid and electrolyte abnormalities.

Heart and Blood Vessel Functions

The pumping action of the heart circulates blood through the kidneys under sufficient pressure to allow for urine formation. Failure of this pumping action interferes with renal perfusion and thus with water and electrolyte regulation.

Lung Functions

The lungs are also vital in maintaining homeostasis. Through exhalation, the lungs remove approximately 300 mL of water daily in the normal adult (Sterns, 2014d). Abnormal conditions, such as hyperpnea (abnormally deep respiration) or continuous coughing, increase this loss; mechanical ventilation with excessive moisture decreases it. The lungs also play a major role in maintaining acid–base balance.

Pituitary Functions

The hypothalamus manufactures ADH, which is stored in the posterior pituitary gland and released as needed to conserve water. Functions of ADH include maintaining the osmotic pressure of the cells by controlling the retention or excretion of water by the kidneys and by regulating blood volume (see Fig. 13-3).

Adrenal Functions

Aldosterone, a mineralocorticoid secreted by the zona glomerulosa (outer zone) of the adrenal cortex, has a profound effect on fluid balance. Increased secretion of aldosterone causes sodium retention (and thus water retention) and potassium loss. Conversely, decreased secretion of aldosterone causes sodium and water loss and potassium retention.

Cortisol, another adrenocortical hormone, has less mineralocorticoid action. However, when secreted in large quantities (or given as corticosteroid therapy), it can also produce sodium and fluid retention.

Parathyroid Functions

The parathyroid glands, embedded in the thyroid gland, regulate calcium and phosphate balance by means of parathyroid hormone (PTH). PTH influences bone reabsorption, calcium absorption from the intestines, and calcium reabsorption from the renal tubules.

Other Mechanisms

Changes in the volume of the interstitial compartment within the ECF can occur without affecting body function. However, the vascular compartment cannot tolerate change as readily and must be carefully maintained to ensure that tissues receive adequate nutrients.

Baroreceptors

The baroreceptors are located in the left atrium and the carotid and aortic arches. These receptors respond to changes in the circulating blood volume and regulate sympathetic and parasympathetic neural activity as well as endocrine activities.

As arterial pressure decreases, baroreceptors transmit fewer impulses from the carotid and the aortic arches to the vasomotor center. A decrease in impulses stimulates the sympathetic nervous system and inhibits the parasympathetic nervous system. The outcome is an increase in cardiac rate, conduction, and contractility and an increase in circulating blood volume. Sympathetic stimulation constricts renal arterioles; this increases the release of aldosterone, decreases glomerular filtration, and increases sodium and water reabsorption (Hall, 2015).

Renin–Angiotensin–Aldosterone System

Renin is an enzyme that converts angiotensinogen, a substance formed by the liver, into angiotensin I (Grossman & Porth, 2014). Renin is released by the juxtaglomerular cells of the kidneys in response to decreased renal perfusion (McGloin, 2015). Angiotensin-converting enzyme (ACE) converts angiotensin I to angiotensin II. Angiotensin II, with its vasoconstrictor properties, increases arterial perfusion pressure and stimulates thirst. As the sympathetic nervous system is stimulated, aldosterone is released in response to an increased release of renin. Aldosterone is a volume regulator and is also released as serum potassium increases, serum sodium decreases, or adrenocorticotropic hormone (ACTH) increases.

Antidiuretic Hormone and Thirst

ADH and the thirst mechanism have important roles in maintaining sodium concentration and oral intake of fluids

Physiology/Pathophysiology

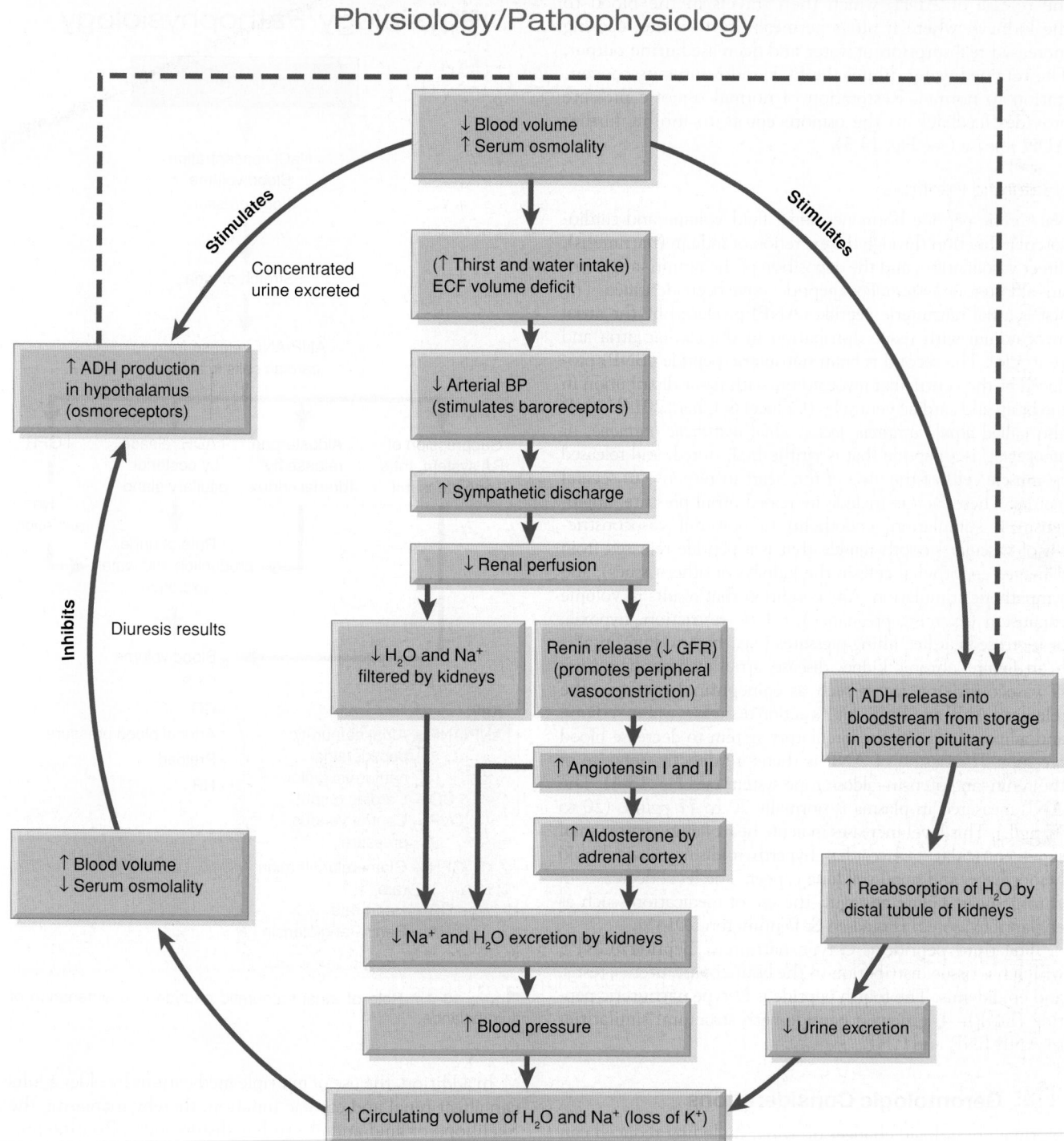

Figure 13-3 • Fluid regulation cycle. ADH, antidiuretic hormone; BP, blood pressure; ECF, extracellular fluid; GFR, glomerular filtration rate.

(Sterns, 2014e). Oral intake is controlled by the thirst center located in the hypothalamus (Grossman & Porth, 2014). As serum concentration or osmolality increases or blood volume decreases, neurons in the hypothalamus are stimulated by intracellular dehydration; thirst then occurs, and the person increases their intake of oral fluids. Water excretion is controlled by ADH, aldosterone, and baroreceptors, as mentioned previously. The presence or absence of ADH is the

most significant factor in determining whether the urine that is excreted is concentrated or dilute.

Osmoreceptors

Located on the surface of the hypothalamus, osmoreceptors sense changes in sodium concentration. As osmotic pressure increases, the neurons become dehydrated and quickly release impulses to the posterior pituitary, which increases the release of ADH, which then travels in the blood to the kidneys, where it alters permeability to water, causing increased reabsorption of water and decreased urine output. The retained water dilutes the ECF and returns its concentration to normal. Restoration of normal osmotic pressure provides feedback to the osmoreceptors to inhibit further ADH release (see Fig. 13-3).

Natriuretic Peptides

Natriuretic peptide hormones affect fluid volume and cardiovascular function through the excretion of sodium (natriuresis), direct vasodilation, and the opposition of the rennin–angiotensin–aldosterone system. Four peptides have been identified. The first is atrial natriuretic peptide (ANP) produced by the atrial myocardium with tissue distribution in the cardiac atria and ventricles. The second is brain natriuretic peptide (BNP) produced by the ventricular myocardium with tissue distribution in the brain and cardiac ventricles (Colucci & Chen, 2014). ANP, also called *atrial natriuretic factor, atrial natriuretic hormone,* or *atriopeptin,* is a peptide that is synthesized, stored, and released by muscle cells of the atria of the heart in response to several factors. These factors include increased atrial pressure, angiotensin II stimulation, endothelin (a powerful vasoconstrictor of vascular smooth muscle that is a peptide released from damaged endothelial cells in the kidneys or other tissues), and sympathetic stimulation. Any condition that results in volume expansion (exercise, pregnancy), calorie restriction, hypoxia, or increased cardiac filling pressures (e.g., high sodium intake, heart failure, chronic kidney disease, atrial tachycardia, or use of vasoconstrictor agents such as epinephrine) increases the release of ANP and BNP. ANP's action decreases water, sodium, and adipose loads on the circulatory system to decrease blood pressure. The action of ANP is therefore directly opposite of the renin–angiotensin–aldosterone system (see Fig. 13-4). The ANP measured in plasma is normally 20 to 77 pg/mL (20 to 77 ng/L). This level increases in acute heart failure, paroxysmal supraventricular tachycardia, hyperthyroidism, subarachnoid hemorrhage, and small cell lung cancer. The level decreases in chronic heart failure and with the use of medications such as enalapril (Vasotec) (Frandsen & Pennington, 2014).

The third peptide is C-type natriuretic peptide (CNP), which has tissue distribution in the brain, ovary, uterus, testis, and epididymis. The fourth peptide is D-type natriuretic peptide (DNP)—the newest peptide with structural similarities to ANP, BNP, and CNP.

🍂 Gerontologic Considerations

Normal physiologic changes of aging, including reduced cardiac, renal, and respiratory function and reserve and alterations in the ratio of body fluids to muscle mass, may alter older adults' responses to fluid and electrolyte changes and acid–base disturbances. Decreased respiratory function can cause impaired pH regulation in older adults with major illness or trauma. Renal function declines with age, as do muscle mass and daily exogenous creatinine production. Therefore, high-normal and minimally elevated serum creatinine values may indicate substantially reduced renal function in older adults. Because of a decrease in age-related muscle mass, older adults have a lower concentration of body fluid that may alter physiologic responses.

Physiology/Pathophysiology

Figure 13-4 • Role of atrial natriuretic peptide in maintenance of fluid balance.

In addition, the use of multiple medications by older adults can affect renal and cardiac function, thereby increasing the likelihood of fluid and electrolyte disturbances. Routine procedures, such as the vigorous administration of laxatives or enemas before colon x-ray studies, may produce a serious FVD, necessitating the use of intravenous (IV) fluids to prevent hypotension and other effects of hypovolemia.

Alterations in fluid and electrolyte balance that may produce minor changes in young and middle-aged adults may produce profound changes in older adults. In many older patients, the clinical manifestations of fluid and electrolyte disturbances may be subtle or atypical. For example, fluid deficit may cause delirium in the older person (see Chapter 11), whereas in the young or middle-aged person, the first sign commonly is increased thirst. Rapid infusion of an excessive volume of IV fluids may produce fluid overload and cardiac failure in older patients. These reactions are likely to occur more quickly and with the administration of smaller volumes of fluid than in healthy young and middle-aged adults because of the decreased cardiac reserve and reduced renal function that accompany aging.

Dehydration is the rapid loss of body weight owing to the loss of either water or sodium. This results in an elevated sodium concentration (Sterns, 2014d). Dehydration in older adults is common because of decreased kidney mass, decreased glomerular filtration rate, decreased renal blood flow, decreased ability to concentrate urine, inability to conserve sodium, decreased excretion of potassium, and a decrease of total-body water. Loss of subcutaneous supporting tissue and resultant thinning of the skin occurs with aging; the dermis is dehydrated and loses strength and elasticity.

FLUID VOLUME DISTURBANCES

Hypovolemia

FVD, or hypovolemia, occurs when loss of ECF volume exceeds the intake of fluid. It occurs when water and electrolytes are lost in the same proportion as they exist in normal body fluids; thus, the ratio of serum electrolytes to water remains the same. FVD should not be confused with dehydration, which refers to loss of water alone, with increased serum sodium levels. FVD may occur alone or in combination with other imbalances. Unless other imbalances are present concurrently, serum electrolyte concentrations remain essentially unchanged.

Pathophysiology

FVD results from loss of body fluids and occurs more rapidly when coupled with decreased fluid intake. FVD can also develop with a prolonged period of inadequate intake. Causes of FVD include abnormal fluid losses, such as those resulting from vomiting, diarrhea, GI suctioning, and sweating;

decreased intake, as in nausea or lack of access to fluids; and third-space fluid shifts, or the movement of fluid from the vascular system to other body spaces (e.g., with edema formation in burns, ascites with liver dysfunction). Additional causes include diabetes insipidus (a decreased ability to concentrate urine owing to a defect in the kidney tubules that interferes with water reabsorption), adrenal insufficiency, osmotic diuresis, hemorrhage, and coma.

Clinical Manifestations

FVD can develop rapidly, and its severity depends on the degree of fluid loss. Clinical signs and symptoms and laboratory findings are presented in Table 13-4.

Assessment and Diagnostic Findings

Laboratory data useful in evaluating fluid volume status include BUN and its relation to serum creatinine concentration. Normal BUN to serum creatinine concentration ratio is 10:1. A volume-depleted patient has a BUN elevated out of proportion to the serum creatinine (ratio greater than 20:1) (Sterns, 2014a).

The presence and cause of hypovolemia may be determined through the health history and physical examination. In addition, the hematocrit level is greater than normal because there is a decreased plasma volume.

Serum electrolyte changes may also exist. Potassium and sodium levels can be reduced (hypokalemia, hyponatremia) or elevated (hyperkalemia, hypernatremia).

- Hypokalemia occurs with GI and renal losses.
- Hyperkalemia occurs with adrenal insufficiency.
- Hyponatremia occurs with increased thirst and ADH release.
- Hypernatremia results from increased insensible losses and diabetes insipidus.

There may or may not be a decrease in urine (oliguria) in hypovalemia. Urine specific gravity is increased in relation to the kidneys' attempt to conserve water and is decreased with diabetes insipidus. Aldosterone is secreted when fluid volume

TABLE 13-4 Fluid Volume Disturbances

Imbalance	Contributing Factors	Signs/Symptoms and Laboratory Findings
Fluid volume deficit (hypovolemia)	Loss of water and electrolytes, as in vomiting, diarrhea, fistulas, fever, excess sweating, burns, blood loss, gastrointestinal suction, and third-space fluid shifts; and decreased intake, as in anorexia, nausea, and inability to gain access to fluid. Diabetes insipidus and uncontrolled diabetes both contribute to a depletion of extracellular fluid volume.	Acute weight loss, ↓ skin turgor, oliguria, concentrated urine, capillary filling time prolonged, low CVP, ↓ BP, flattened neck veins, dizziness, weakness, thirst and confusion, ↑ pulse, muscle cramps, sunken eyes, nausea, increased temperature; cool, clammy, pale skin *Labs indicate:* ↑ hemoglobin and hematocrit, ↑ serum and urine osmolality and specific gravity, ↓ urine sodium, ↑ BUN and creatinine, ↑ urine specific gravity and osmolality
Fluid volume excess (hypervolemia)	Compromised regulatory mechanisms, such as kidney injury, heart failure, and cirrhosis; overzealous administration of sodium-containing fluids; and fluid shifts (i.e., treatment of burns). Prolonged corticosteroid therapy, severe stress, and hyperaldosteronism augment fluid volume excess.	Acute weight gain, peripheral edema and ascites, distended jugular veins, crackles, elevated CVP, shortness of breath, ↑ BP, bounding pulse and cough, ↑ respiratory rate, ↑ urine output *Labs indicate:* ↓ hemoglobin and hematocrit, ↓ serum and urine osmolality, ↓ urine sodium and specific gravity

↑, increased; ↓, decreased; CVP, central venous pressure; BP, blood pressure; BUN, blood urea nitrogen.
Adapted from Grossman, S.C., & Porth, C. M. (2014). *Porth's pathophysiology: Concepts of altered health states* (9th ed.). Philadelphia, PA: Lippincott Williams & Wilkins.

is low causing reabsorption of sodium and chloride, resulting in decreased urinary sodium and chloride. Urine osmolality can be greater than 450 mOsm/kg because the kidneys try to compensate by conserving water. Normal values for laboratory data are listed in Appendix A on thePoint₊.

 Concept Mastery Alert

The BUN to creatinine ratio is above 20:1 in hypovolemia because of dehydration or decreased renal perfusion and function.

Gerontologic Considerations

Increased sensitivity to fluid and electrolyte changes in older patients requires careful assessment of I&O of fluids from all sources, assessment of changes in daily weight, careful monitoring of side effects and interactions of medications, and prompt reporting and management of disturbances. In most adult patients, it is useful to monitor skin turgor to detect subtle changes. However, assessment of skin turgor is not as valid in older adults because the skin has lost some of its elasticity; therefore, other assessment measures (e.g., slowness in filling of veins of the hands and feet) become more useful in detecting FVD (Cash & Glass, 2015; Weber & Kelley, 2014).

The nurse also performs a functional assessment of the older patient's ability to determine fluid and food needs and to obtain adequate intake in addition to assessments discussed earlier in this chapter. For example, is the patient cognitively intact, able to ambulate and to use both arms and hands to reach fluids and foods, and able to swallow? Results of this assessment have a direct bearing on how the patient will be able to meet their own need for fluids and foods (Kresevic, 2015). During an older patient's hospital stay, the nurse provides fluids if the patient is unable to carry out self-care activities.

The nurse should also recognize that some older patients deliberately restrict their fluid intake to avoid embarrassing episodes of incontinence. In this situation, the nurse identifies interventions to deal with the incontinence, such as encouraging the patient to wear protective clothing or devices, to carry a urinal in the car, or to pace fluid intake to allow access to toilet facilities during the day. Older adults without cardiovascular or renal dysfunction should be reminded to drink adequate fluids, particularly in very warm or humid weather.

Medical Management

When planning the correction of fluid loss for the patient with FVD, the primary provider considers the patient's maintenance requirements and other factors (e.g., fever) that can influence fluid needs. If the deficit is not severe, the oral route is preferred, provided the patient can drink. However, if fluid losses are acute or severe, the IV route is required. Isotonic electrolyte solutions (e.g., lactated Ringer solution, 0.9% sodium chloride) are frequently the first-line choice to treat the hypotensive patient with FVD because they expand plasma volume (Sterns, 2014e). As soon as the patient becomes normotensive, a hypotonic electrolyte solution (e.g., 0.45% sodium chloride) is often used to provide both electrolytes and water for renal excretion of metabolic wastes. These and additional fluids are listed in Table 13-5.

Accurate and frequent assessments of I&O, weight, vital signs, central venous pressure, level of consciousness, breath sounds, and skin color are monitored to determine when therapy should be slowed to avoid volume overload. The rate of fluid administration is based on the severity of loss and the patient's hemodynamic response to volume replacement (Sterns, 2014e).

If the patient with severe FVD is not excreting enough urine and is therefore oliguric, the primary provider needs to determine whether the depressed renal function is caused by reduced renal blood flow secondary to FVD (prerenal azotemia) or, more seriously, by acute tubular necrosis from prolonged FVD. The test used in this situation is referred to as a fluid challenge test. During a fluid challenge test, volumes of fluid are given at specific rates and intervals while the patient's hemodynamic response to this treatment is monitored (i.e., vital signs, breath sounds, orientation status, central venous pressure, urine output).

An example of a typical fluid challenge test involves administering 100 to 200 mL of normal saline solution over 15 minutes. The goal is to provide fluids rapidly enough to attain adequate tissue perfusion without compromising the cardiovascular system. The response by a patient with FVD but normal renal function is increased urine output and an increase in blood pressure and central venous pressure.

Shock can occur when the volume of fluid lost exceeds 25% of the intravascular volume or when fluid loss is rapid. (Shock and its causes and treatment are discussed in detail in Chapter 14.)

Nursing Management

To assess for FVD, the nurse monitors and measures fluid I&O at least every 8 hours, and sometimes hourly. Researchers have reported that maintaining an accurate I&O is a particular challenge with patients in critical care settings (Diacon & Bell, 2014) (see Chart 13-1). As FVD develops, body fluid losses exceed fluid intake through excessive urination (polyuria), diarrhea, vomiting, or other mechanisms. Once FVD has developed, the kidneys attempt to conserve body fluids, leading to a urine output of less than 1 mL/kg/h in an adult. Urine in this instance is concentrated and represents a healthy renal response. Daily body weights are monitored; an acute loss of 0.5 kg (1.1 lb) represents a fluid loss of approximately 500 mL (1 L of fluid weighs approximately 1 kg, or 2.2 lb).

Vital signs are closely monitored. The nurse observes for a weak, rapid pulse and orthostatic hypotension (i.e., a decrease in systolic pressure exceeding 20 mm Hg when the patient moves from a lying to a sitting position) (Weber & Kelley, 2014). A decrease in body temperature often accompanies FVD, unless there is a concurrent infection.

Skin and tongue turgor are monitored on a regular basis. In a healthy person, pinched skin immediately returns to its normal position when released (Weber & Kelley, 2014). This elastic property, referred to as turgor, is partially dependent on interstitial fluid volume. In a person with FVD, the skin flattens more slowly after the pinch is released. In a person with severe FVD, the skin may remain elevated for many seconds. Tissue turgor is best measured by pinching the skin over the sternum, inner aspects of the thighs, or forehead.

TABLE 13-5 Selected Water and Electrolyte Solutions

Solution	Considerations
Isotonic Solutions 0.9% NaCl (isotonic, also called *normal saline* [NS]) Na⁺ 154 mEq/L Cl⁻ 154 mEq/L (308 mOsm/L) Also available with varying concentrations of dextrose (a 5% dextrose concentration is commonly used)	• An isotonic solution that expands the extracellular fluid (ECF) volume; used in hypovolemic states, resuscitative efforts, shock, diabetic ketoacidosis, metabolic alkalosis, hypercalcemia, mild Na⁺ deficit • Supplies an excess of Na⁺ and Cl⁻; can cause fluid volume excess and hyperchloremic acidosis if used in excessive volumes, particularly in patients with compromised renal function, heart failure, or edema • Not desirable as a routine maintenance solution, as it provides only Na⁺ and Cl⁻ (and these are provided in excessive amounts) • When mixed with 5% dextrose, the resulting solution becomes hypertonic in relation to plasma and, in addition to the previously described electrolytes, provides 170 cal/L • Only solution that may be given with blood products • Tonicity similar to plasma
Lactated Ringer solution Na⁺ 130 mEq/L K⁺ 4 mEq/L Ca⁺⁺ 3 mEq/L Cl⁻ 109 mEq/L Lactate (metabolized to bicarbonate) 28 mEq/L (274 mOsm/L) Also available with varying concentrations of dextrose (the most common is 5% dextrose)	• An isotonic solution that contains multiple electrolytes in roughly the same concentration as found in plasma (note that solution is lacking in Mg⁺⁺); provides 9 cal/L • Used in the treatment of hypovolemia, burns, fluid lost as bile or diarrhea, and for acute blood loss replacement • Lactate is rapidly metabolized into HCO₃⁻ in the body. Lactated Ringer solution should not be used in lactic acidosis because the ability to convert lactate into HCO₃⁻ is impaired in this disorder. • Not to be given with a pH >7.5 because bicarbonate is formed as lactate breaks down, causing alkalosis • Should not be used in kidney injury because it contains potassium and can cause hyperkalemia • Tonicity similar to plasma
5% dextrose in water (D₅W) No electrolytes 50 g of dextrose	• An isotonic solution that supplies 170 cal/L and free water to aid in renal excretion of solutes • Used in treatment of hypernatremia, fluid loss, and dehydration • Should not be used in excessive volumes in the early postoperative period (when antidiuretic hormone secretion is increased due to stress reaction) • Should not be used solely in treatment of fluid volume deficit because it dilutes plasma electrolyte concentrations • Contraindicated in head injury because it may cause increased intracranial pressure • Should not be used for fluid resuscitation because it can cause hyperglycemia • Should be used with caution in patients with renal or cardiac disease because of risk of fluid overload • Electrolyte-free solutions may cause peripheral circulatory collapse, anuria in patients with sodium deficiency, and increased body fluid loss. • Converts to hypotonic solution as dextrose is metabolized by body. Over time, D₅W without NaCl can cause water intoxication (intracellular fluid volume excess [FVE]) because the solution is hypotonic. • Fluid therapy for an extended period of time without electrolytes may result in hypokalemia.
Hypotonic Solutions 0.45% NaCl (half-strength saline) Na⁺ 77 mEq/L Cl⁻ 77 mEq/L (154 mOsm/L) Also available with varying concentrations of dextrose (the most common is a 5% concentration)	• Provides Na⁺, Cl⁻, and free water • Free water is desirable to aid the kidneys in elimination of solute. • Lacking in electrolytes other than Na⁺ and Cl⁻ • When mixed with 5% dextrose, the solution becomes slightly hypertonic to plasma and in addition to the previously described electrolytes provides 170 cal/L. • Used to treat hypertonic dehydration, Na⁺ and Cl⁻ depletion, and gastric fluid loss • Not indicated for third-space fluid shifts or increased intracranial pressure • Administer cautiously, because it can cause fluid shifts from vascular system into cells, resulting in cardiovascular collapse and increased intracranial pressure
Hypertonic Solutions 3% NaCl (hypertonic saline) Na⁺ 513 mEq/L Cl⁻ 513 mEq/L (1,026 mOsm/L) 5% NaCL (hypertonic solution) Na⁺ 855 mEq/L Cl⁻ 855 mEq/L (1,710 mOsm/L)	• Used to increase ECF volume, decrease cellular swelling • Highly hypertonic solution used only in critical situations to treat hyponatremia • Must be given slowly and cautiously, because it can cause intravascular volume overload and pulmonary edema • Supplies no calories • Assists in removing intracellular fluid excess • Highly hypertonic solution used to treat symptomatic hyponatremia • Administer slowly and cautiously because it can cause intravascular volume overload and pulmonary edema. • Supplies no calories
Colloid Solutions Dextran in NS or D₅W Available in low-molecular-weight (Dextran 40) and high-molecular-weight (Dextran 70) forms	• Colloid solution used as volume/plasma expander for intravascular part of ECF • Affects clotting by coating platelets and decreasing ability to clot • Remains in circulatory system up to 24 h • Used to treat hypovolemia in early shock to increase pulse pressure, cardiac output, and arterial blood pressure • Improves microcirculation by decreasing red blood cell aggregation • Contraindicated in hemorrhage, thrombocytopenia, renal disease, and severe dehydration • Not a substitute for blood or blood products

---

Chart 13-1 **NURSING RESEARCH PROFILE**

Monitoring Intake and Output in Patients in the ICU

Diacon, A., & Bell, J. (2014). Investigating the recording and accuracy of fluid balance monitoring in critically ill patients. *South African Journal of Critical Care, 30*(2), 55–57.

Purpose

Studies suggest that an accurate I&O can have a significant impact on morbidity and mortality in critically ill patients. This study was designed to determine the current practices of fluid balance monitoring of registered nurses in intensive care units (ICUs).

Design

This was a quantitative study using an exploratory, descriptive design. The setting consisted of three ICUs within one hospital group. All three ICUs were similar in terms of patient profiles and size. An audit tool was developed and reviewed by two clinical intensive care nurse experts to determine its face validity. Medical records of patients who were admitted during a certain time frame, within age parameters, and met critical care patient classification were included for sampling purposes. The study used a simple random sampling technique to select records for inclusion. Each patient's recorded fluid balance was calculated

for a 24-hour period during the first 48 hours after admission and compared with audited calculations.

Findings

Out of 103 audited ICU patient records, 5 (2%) had a fluid deviation less than 500 mL; 71 (68.9%) had a fluid deviation within 500 mL; 14 (13.5%) were identified as deviating between 500 and 1000 mL when compared to the audited calculations; 7 (6.8%) showed a deviation between 1000 and 2000 mL; and 6 (5.8%) revealed a deviation greater than 2000 mL when compared to the audited calculations. There was a significant association between the administration of diuretics and inaccurate fluid balance documentation ($p = 0.01$), but no association with any other variables.

Nursing Implications

This study identified that I&O was not being accurately measured in the critically ill patients in the ICUs studied. It is imperative that accurate calculations of fluid balance be an integral part of nursing practice in the ICU setting. Regular outcome-driven audits may help improve practice and thus impact the mortality of patients in the ICU setting.

Tongue turgor is not affected by age (see previous Gerontologic Considerations), and evaluating this may be more valid than evaluating skin turgor (Sterns, 2014a). In a normal person, the tongue has one longitudinal furrow. In the person with FVD, there are additional longitudinal furrows and the tongue is smaller because of fluid loss. The degree of oral mucous membrane moisture is also assessed; a dry mouth may indicate either FVD or mouth breathing.

Urine concentration is monitored by measuring the urine specific gravity. In a volume-depleted patient, the urine specific gravity should be greater than 1.020, indicating healthy renal conservation of fluid.

Mental function is eventually affected, resulting in delirium in severe FVD as a result of decreasing cerebral perfusion. Decreased peripheral perfusion can result in cold extremities. In patients with relatively normal cardiopulmonary function, a low central venous pressure is indicative of hypovolemia. Patients with acute cardiopulmonary decompensation require more extensive hemodynamic monitoring of pressures in both sides of the heart to determine whether hypovolemia exists.

Preventing Hypovolemia

To prevent FVD, the nurse identifies patients at risk and takes measures to minimize fluid losses. For example, if the patient has diarrhea, measures should be implemented to control diarrhea and replacement fluids given. This includes administering antidiarrheal medications and small volumes of oral fluids at frequent intervals.

Correcting Hypovolemia

When possible, oral fluids are given to help correct FVD, with consideration given to the patient's likes and dislikes. The type of fluid the patient has lost is also considered, and fluids most likely to replace the lost electrolytes are appropriate. If

the patient is reluctant to drink because of oral discomfort, the nurse assists with frequent mouth care and provides nonirritating fluids. The patient may be offered small volumes of oral rehydration solutions (e.g., Rehydralyte, Elete, Cytomax). These solutions provide fluid, glucose, and electrolytes in concentrations that are easily absorbed. If nausea is present, an antiemetic may be needed before oral fluid replacement can be tolerated.

If the deficit cannot be corrected by oral fluids, therapy may need to be initiated by an alternative route (enteral or parenteral) until adequate circulating blood volume and renal perfusion are achieved. Isotonic fluids are prescribed to increase ECF volume (Sterns, 2014e).

Hypervolemia

Fluid volume excess (FVE), or hypervolemia, refers to an isotonic expansion of the ECF caused by the abnormal retention of water and sodium in approximately the same proportions in which they normally exist in the ECF. It is most often secondary to an increase in the total-body sodium content, which, in turn, leads to an increase in total-body water. Because there is isotonic retention of body substances, the serum sodium concentration remains essentially normal.

Pathophysiology

FVE may be related to simple fluid overload or diminished function of the homeostatic mechanisms responsible for regulating fluid balance. Contributing factors can include heart failure, kidney injury, and cirrhosis of the liver. Another contributing factor is consumption of excessive amounts of table or other sodium salts. Excessive administration of sodium-containing fluids in a patient with impaired regulatory mechanisms may predispose him or her to a serious FVE as well.

Clinical Manifestations

Clinical manifestations of FVE result from expansion of the ECF and may include edema, distended neck veins, and crackles (abnormal lung sounds). Further discussion of clinical signs and symptoms and laboratory findings can be found in Table 13-4.

Assessment and Diagnostic Findings

Laboratory data useful in diagnosing FVE include BUN and hematocrit levels. In FVE, both of these values may be decreased because of plasma dilution, low protein intake, and anemia. In chronic kidney disease, both serum osmolality and the sodium level are decreased owing to excessive retention of water. The urine sodium level is increased if the kidneys are attempting to excrete excess volume. A chest x-ray may reveal pulmonary congestion. Hypervolemia occurs when aldosterone is chronically stimulated (i.e., cirrhosis, heart failure, and nephrotic syndrome). Therefore, the urine sodium level does not increase in these conditions.

Medical Management

Management of FVE is directed at the causes, and if related to excessive administration of sodium-containing fluids, discontinuing the infusion may be all that is needed. Symptomatic treatment consists of administering diuretics and restricting fluids and sodium.

Pharmacologic Therapy

Diuretics are prescribed when dietary restriction of sodium alone is insufficient to reduce edema by inhibiting the reabsorption of sodium and water by the kidneys. The choice of diuretic is based on the severity of the hypervolemic state, the degree of impairment of renal function, and the potency of the diuretic. Thiazide diuretics block sodium reabsorption in the distal tubule, where only 5% to 10% of filtered sodium is reabsorbed. Loop diuretics, such as furosemide (Lasix) or torsemide (Demadex), can cause a greater loss of both sodium and water because they block sodium reabsorption in the ascending limb of Henle loop, where 20% to 30% of filtered sodium is normally reabsorbed. Generally, thiazide diuretics, such as hydrochlorothiazide (Microzide), are prescribed for mild to moderate hypervolemia and loop diuretics for severe hypervolemia (Comeford, 2015; Frandsen & Pennington, 2014).

Electrolyte imbalances may result from side effects of diuretics. Hypokalemia can occur with all diuretics except those that work in the last distal tubule of the nephrons. Potassium supplements can be prescribed to avoid this complication. Hyperkalemia can occur with diuretics that work in the distal tubule (e.g., spironolactone [Aldactone], a potassium-sparing diuretic), especially in patients with decreased renal function. Hyponatremia occurs with diuresis owing to increased release of ADH secondary to reduction in circulating volume. Decreased magnesium levels occur with administration of loop and thiazide diuretics due to decreased reabsorption and increased excretion of magnesium by the kidney.

Azotemia (increased nitrogen levels in the blood) can occur with FVE when urea and creatinine are not excreted owing to decreased perfusion by the kidneys and decreased excretion of wastes. High uric acid levels (hyperuricemia) can also occur from increased reabsorption and decreased excretion of uric acid by the kidneys.

Dialysis

If renal function is so severely impaired that pharmacologic agents cannot act efficiently, other modalities are considered to remove sodium and fluid from the body. Hemodialysis or peritoneal dialysis may be used to remove nitrogenous wastes and control potassium and acid–base balance, and to remove sodium and fluid. Continuous renal replacement therapy may also be required. (See Chapter 54 for a discussion of these treatment modalities.)

Nutritional Therapy

Treatment of FVE usually involves dietary restriction of sodium. An average daily diet not restricted in sodium contains 6 to 15 g of salt, whereas low-sodium diets can range from a mild restriction to as little as 250 mg of sodium per day, depending on the patient's needs. A mild sodium-restricted diet allows only light salting of food (about half the usual amount) in cooking and at the table, and no addition of salt to commercially prepared foods that are already seasoned. Foods high in sodium must be avoided. It is the sodium salt (sodium chloride) rather than sodium itself that contributes to edema. Therefore, patients are instructed to read food labels carefully to determine salt content.

Because about half of ingested sodium is in the form of seasoning, seasoning substitutes can play a major role in decreasing sodium intake. Lemon juice, onions, and garlic are excellent substitute flavorings, although some patients prefer salt substitutes. Most salt substitutes contain potassium and must therefore be used cautiously by patients taking potassium-sparing diuretics (e.g., spironolactone, triamterene, amiloride). They should not be used in conditions associated with potassium retention, such as advanced renal disease. Salt substitutes containing ammonium chloride can be harmful to patients with liver damage.

In some communities, drinking water may contain too much sodium for a sodium-restricted diet. Depending on its source, water may contain as little as 1 mg or more than 1500 mg of sodium per quart. Patients may need to use distilled water if the local water supply is very high in sodium. Bottled water can have a sodium content that ranges from 0 to 1200 mg/L; therefore, if sodium is restricted, the label must be carefully examined for sodium content before purchasing and drinking bottled water. Also, patients on sodium-restricted diets should be cautioned to avoid water softeners that add sodium to water in exchange for other ions, such as calcium. Protein intake may be increased in patients who are malnourished or who have low serum protein levels in an effort to increase capillary oncotic pressure and pull fluid out of the tissues into vessels for excretion by the kidneys.

Nursing Management

To assess for FVE, the nurse measures I&O at regular intervals to identify excessive fluid retention. The patient is weighed daily, and rapid weight gain is noted. An acute weight gain of 1 kg (2.2 lb) is equivalent to a gain of approximately 1 L of fluid. Breath sounds are assessed at regular intervals in at-risk patients, particularly if parenteral fluids are being given. The nurse monitors the degree of edema in the most dependent parts of the body, such as the feet and ankles in ambulatory patients and the sacral region in patients confined to bed. Pitting edema is assessed by pressing a finger into the affected part, creating a pit or indentation that is evaluated on a scale of 1+ (minimal) to 4+ (severe) (see Chapter 29, Fig. 29-2). Peripheral edema is monitored by measuring the circumference of the extremity with a tape marked in millimeters (Weber & Kelley, 2014).

Preventing Hypervolemia

Specific interventions vary with the underlying condition and the degree of FVE. However, most patients require sodium-restricted diets in some form, and adherence to the prescribed diet is encouraged. Patients are instructed to avoid over-the-counter (OTC) medications without first checking with a health care provider, because they may contain sodium (e.g., Alka-Seltzer). If fluid retention persists despite adherence to a prescribed diet, hidden sources of sodium, such as the water supply or use of water softeners, should be considered.

Detecting and Controlling Hypervolemia

It is important to detect FVE before the condition becomes severe. Interventions include promoting rest, restricting sodium intake, monitoring parenteral fluid therapy, and administering appropriate medications.

Regular rest periods may be beneficial, because bed rest favors diuresis of fluid. The mechanism is related to diminished venous pooling and the subsequent increase in effective circulating blood volume and renal perfusion. Sodium and fluid restriction should be instituted as indicated. Because most patients with FVE require diuretics, the patient's response to these agents is monitored. The rate of parenteral fluids and the patient's response to these fluids are also closely monitored (Frandsen & Pennington, 2014). If dyspnea or orthopnea is present, the patient is placed in a semi-Fowler position to promote lung expansion. The patient is turned and repositioned at regular intervals because edematous tissue is more prone to skin breakdown than normal tissue. Because conditions predisposing to FVE are likely to be chronic, patients are taught to monitor their response to therapy by documenting fluid I&O and body weight changes. The importance of adhering to the treatment regimen is emphasized.

 Educating Patients About Edema

Because edema is a common manifestation of FVE, patients need to recognize its symptoms and understand its importance. The nurse gives special attention to edema when instructing the patient with FVE. Edema can occur as a result of increased capillary fluid pressure, decreased capillary oncotic pressure, or increased interstitial oncotic pressure, causing expansion of the interstitial fluid compartment (Hall, 2015). Edema can be localized (e.g., in the ankle, as in rheumatoid arthritis) or generalized (as in cardiac failure and kidney injury) (Sterns, 2014c). Severe generalized edema is called *anasarca*.

Edema occurs when there is a change in the capillary membrane, increasing the formation of interstitial fluid or decreasing the removal of interstitial fluid. Sodium retention is a frequent cause of the increased ECF volume. Burns and infection are examples of conditions associated with increased interstitial fluid volume. Obstruction to lymphatic outflow, a plasma albumin level less than 1.5 to 2 g/dL, or a decrease in plasma oncotic pressure contributes to increased interstitial fluid volume. The kidneys retain sodium and water when there is decreased ECF volume as a result of decreased cardiac output from heart failure. A thorough medication history is necessary to identify any medications that could cause edema, such as nonsteroidal anti-inflammatory drugs (NSAIDs), estrogens, corticosteroids, and antihypertensive agents.

Ascites is a type of edema in which fluid accumulates in the peritoneal cavity; it results from nephrotic syndrome, cirrhosis, and some malignant tumors. The patient commonly reports shortness of breath and a sense of pressure because of pressure on the diaphragm.

The goal of treatment is to preserve or restore the circulating intravascular fluid volume. Thus, in addition to treating the cause of the edema, other treatments may include diuretic therapy, restriction of fluids and sodium, elevation of the extremities, application of antiembolism stockings, paracentesis, dialysis, and continuous renal replacement therapy in cases of kidney injury or life-threatening fluid volume overload (see Chapter 54).

ELECTROLYTE IMBALANCES

Disturbances in electrolyte balances are common in clinical practice and may need to be corrected based on history, physical examination findings, and laboratory values (with comparison to previous values).

Sodium Imbalances

Sodium (Na+) is the most abundant electrolyte in the ECF; its concentration ranges from 135 to 145 mEq/L (135 to 145 mmol/L), and it is the primary determinant of ECF volume and osmolality. Sodium has a major role in controlling water distribution throughout the body, because it does not easily cross the cell wall membrane and because of its abundance and high concentration in the body. Sodium is regulated by ADH, thirst, and the renin–angiotensin–aldosterone system. A loss or gain of sodium is usually accompanied by a loss or gain of water. Sodium also functions in establishing the electrochemical state necessary for muscle contraction and the transmission of nerve impulses (Sahay & Sahay, 2014).

The syndrome of inappropriate secretion of antidiuretic hormone (SIADH) may be associated with sodium imbalance. When there is a decrease in the circulating plasma osmolality, blood volume, or blood pressure, arginine vasopressin (AVP) is released from the posterior pituitary. Oversecretion of AVP can cause SIADH. Patients at risk are older adults, those with acquired immune deficiency syndrome (AIDS), those on mechanical ventilation, and people taking selective serotonin reuptake inhibitors (SSRIs).

Sodium imbalance can develop under simple or complex circumstances. The two most common sodium imbalances are sodium deficit and sodium excess (see Table 13-6).

TABLE 13-6 Sodium Imbalances

Imbalance	Contributing Factors	Signs/Symptoms and Laboratory Findings
Sodium deficit (hyponatremia) Serum sodium <135 mEq/L	Loss of sodium, as in use of diuretics, loss of GI fluids, renal disease, and adrenal insufficiency. Gain of water, as in excessive administration of D_5W and water supplements for patients receiving hypotonic tube feedings; disease states associated with SIADH, such as head trauma and oat-cell lung tumor; medications associated with water retention (oxytocin and certain tranquilizers); and psychogenic polydipsia. Hyperglycemia and heart failure cause a loss of sodium.	Anorexia, nausea and vomiting, headache, lethargy, dizziness, confusion, muscle cramps and weakness, muscular twitching, seizures, papilledema, dry skin, ↑ pulse, ↓ BP, weight gain, edema *Labs indicate:* ↓ serum and urine sodium, ↓ urine specific gravity and osmolality
Sodium excess (hypernatremia) Serum sodium >145 mEq/L	Fluid deprivation in patients who cannot respond to thirst, hypertonic tube feedings without adequate water supplements, diabetes insipidus, heatstroke, hyperventilation, watery diarrhea, burns, and diaphoresis. Excess corticosteroid, sodium bicarbonate, and sodium chloride administration, and saltwater near-drowning victims.	Thirst, elevated body temperature, swollen dry tongue and sticky mucous membranes, hallucinations, lethargy, restlessness, irritability, simple partial or tonic–clonic seizures, pulmonary edema, hyperreflexia, twitching, nausea, vomiting, anorexia, ↑ pulse, and ↑ BP *Labs indicate:* ↑ serum sodium, ↓ urine sodium, ↑ urine specific gravity and osmolality, ↓ CVP

↑, increased; ↓, decreased; CVP, central venous pressure; BP, blood pressure; GI, gastrointestinal; D_5W, dextrose 5% in water; SIADH, syndrome of inappropriate secretion of antidiuretic hormone.
Adapted from Grossman, S.C., & Porth, C. M. (2014). *Porth's pathophysiology: Concepts of altered health states* (9th ed.). Philadelphia, PA: Lippincott Williams & Wilkins.

Sodium Deficit (Hyponatremia)

Hyponatremia refers to a serum sodium level that is less than 135 mEq/L (135 mmol/L) (Sahay & Sahay, 2014). Hyponatremia can present as an acute or chronic form. Acute hyponatremia is commonly the result of a fluid overload in a surgical patient. Chronic hyponatremia is seen more frequently in patients outside the hospital setting, has a longer duration, and has less serious neurological sequelae. Another type of hyponatremia is exercised-associated hyponatremia, which is more frequently found in women and those of smaller stature. It can occur during extreme temperatures, because of excessive fluid intake before exercise, or prolonged exercise that results in a decrease in serum sodium (Earhart et al., 2015).

Pathophysiology

Hyponatremia primarily occurs due to an imbalance of water rather than sodium. The urine sodium value assists in differentiating renal from nonrenal causes of hyponatremia. Low urine sodium occurs as the kidney retains sodium to compensate for nonrenal fluid loss (i.e., vomiting, diarrhea, sweating). High urine sodium concentration is associated with renal salt wasting (i.e., diuretic use). In dilutional hyponatremia, the ECF volume is increased without any edema.

A deficiency of aldosterone, as occurs in adrenal insufficiency, also predisposes to sodium deficiency. In addition, the use of certain medications, such as anticonvulsants (i.e., carbamazepine [Tegretol], oxcarbazepine (Trileptal), levetiracetam [Keppra]), SSRIs (fluoxetine [Prozac], sertraline [Zoloft], paroxetine [Paxil]), or desmopressin acetate (DDAVP), increases the risk of hyponatremia (Sahay & Sahay, 2014).

SIADH is seen in hyponatremia as well as hypernatremia. The physiologic disturbances include excessive ADH activity, with water retention and dilutional hyponatremia, and inappropriate urinary excretion of sodium in the presence of hyponatremia. SIADH can be the result of either sustained secretion of ADH by the hypothalamus or production of an ADH-like substance from a tumor (aberrant ADH production). Conditions affecting the central nervous system are associated with SIADH. (SIADH is discussed in more detail in Chapter 52.)

Clinical Manifestations

Clinical manifestations of hyponatremia depend on the cause, magnitude, and speed with which the deficit occurs. Poor skin turgor, dry mucosa, headache, decreased saliva production, orthostatic fall in blood pressure, nausea, vomiting, and abdominal cramping occur. Neurologic changes, including altered mental status, status epilepticus, and coma, are probably related to the cellular swelling and cerebral edema associated with hyponatremia. As the extracellular sodium level decreases, the cellular fluid becomes relatively more concentrated and pulls water into the cells (see Fig. 13-5). In general, patients with an acute decrease in serum sodium levels have more cerebral edema and higher mortality rates than do those with more slowly developing hyponatremia. Acute decreases in sodium, developing in less than 48 hours, may be associated with brain herniation and compression of midbrain structures. Chronic decreases in sodium, developing over 48 hours or more, can occur in status epilepticus and other neurologic conditions.

Features of hyponatremia associated with sodium loss and water gain include anorexia, muscle cramps, and a feeling of exhaustion. The severity of symptoms increases with the degree of hyponatremia and the speed with which it develops. When the serum sodium level decreases to less than 115 mEq/L (115 mmol/L), signs of increasing intracranial pressure, such as lethargy, confusion, muscle twitching, focal weakness, hemiparesis, papilledema, seizures, and death, may occur.

Figure 13-5 • Effect of extracellular sodium level on cell size.

Assessment and Diagnostic Findings

Targeted assessment includes the history and physical examination with a focused neurologic examination; evaluation of signs and symptoms as well as laboratory test results; identification of current IV fluids, if applicable; and a review of all medications the patient is taking. Regardless of the cause of hyponatremia, the serum sodium level is less than 135 mEq/L; in SIADH, it may be lower than 100 mEq/L (100 mmol/L). Serum osmolality is also decreased, except in azotemia with the accumulation of toxins. When hyponatremia is due primarily to sodium loss, the urinary sodium content is less than 20 mEq/L (20 mmol/L), suggesting increased proximal reabsorption of sodium secondary to ECF volume depletion, and the specific gravity is low (1.002 to 1.004). However, when hyponatremia is due to SIADH, the urinary sodium content is greater than 20 mEq/L, and the urine specific gravity is usually greater than 1.012. Although the patient with SIADH retains water abnormally and therefore gains body weight, there is no peripheral edema; instead, fluid accumulates inside the cells. This phenomenon sometimes manifests as pitting edema.

Medical Management

The key to treating hyponatremia is an assessment that focuses on the clinical symptoms of the patient and signs of hyponatremia (including laboratory values). As a general rule, treating the underlying the condition is essential.

Sodium Replacement

The most common treatment for hyponatremia is careful administration of sodium by mouth, nasogastric tube, or a parenteral route. For patients who can eat and drink, sodium is easily replaced, because sodium is consumed abundantly in a normal diet. For those who cannot consume sodium, lactated Ringer solution or isotonic saline (0.9% sodium chlo-

ride) solution may be prescribed. Serum sodium must not be increased by more than 12 mEq/L in 24 hours to avoid neurologic damage due to demyelination (Sahay & Sahay, 2014). This condition may occur when the serum sodium concentration is overcorrected (exceeding 140 mEq/L) too rapidly or in the presence of hypoxia or anoxia. It may produce lesions that show symmetric myelin destruction affecting all fiber tracts that can present with altered cognition and decreased alertness, ataxia, paraparesis, dysarthria, horizontal gaze paralysis, pseudobulbar palsy, and coma. The usual daily sodium requirement in adults is approximately 100 mEq, provided there are not excessive losses. Selected water and electrolyte solutions are described in Table 13-5.

In SIADH, the administration of hypertonic saline solution alone cannot change the plasma sodium concentration. Excess sodium would be excreted rapidly in highly concentrated urine. With the addition of the diuretic furosemide, urine is not concentrated and isotonic urine is excreted to effect a change in water balance. In patients with SIADH, in whom water restriction is difficult, lithium (Lithobid) can antagonize the osmotic effect of ADH on the medullary collecting tubule.

Water Restriction

In patients with normal or excess fluid volume, hyponatremia is usually treated effectively by restricting fluid. However, if neurologic symptoms are severe (e.g., seizures, delirium, coma), or in patients with traumatic brain injury, it may be necessary to administer small volumes of a hypertonic sodium solution with the goal of alleviating cerebral edema (see Chapter 66). Incorrect use of these fluids is extremely dangerous, because 1 L of 3% sodium chloride solution contains 513 mEq of sodium and 1 L of 5% sodium chloride solution contains 855 mEq of sodium. The recommendation for hypertonic saline administration in patients with craniocerebral trauma is 3% saline between 0.10 and 1.0 mL/kg of body weight per hour (Sahay & Sahay, 2014; Sterns, 2014e).

> ### ⚑ Quality and Safety Nursing Alert
>
> *Highly hypertonic sodium solutions (2% to 23% sodium chloride) should be given slowly and the patient monitored closely, because only small volumes are needed to elevate the serum sodium concentration from a dangerously low level.*

Pharmacologic Therapy

AVP receptor antagonists are pharmacologic agents that treat hyponatremia by stimulating free water excretion. IV conivaptan hydrochloride (Vaprisol) use is limited to the treatment of hospitalized patients. It may be a useful therapy for those patients with moderate to severe symptomatic hyponatremia but is contraindicated in patients with seizures, delirium, or coma, which warrants the use of hypertonic saline. Tolvaptan (Samsca) is an oral medication indicated for clinically significant hypervolemic and euvolemic hyponatremia that must be initiated and monitored in the hospital setting (Comerford, 2015; Sahay & Sahay, 2014).

Nursing Management

The nurse needs to identify and monitor patients at risk for hyponatremia. The nurse monitors I&O as well as daily body weight.

The nurse needs to get a thorough history to identify if the patient is a performance athlete. Performance athletes (i.e., marathon runners) may use salt tablets to decrease sweating, thus decreasing the sodium loss during prolonged exercise. Research did not find a significant change in the sodium levels when the salt tablets were ingested; however, the safety of this practice has not been established, and it is therefore not recommended (Earhart et al., 2015).

Hyponatremia is a frequently overlooked cause of confusion in older patients, who are at increased risk because of decreased renal function and subsequent inability to excrete excess fluids. Administration of prescribed and OTC medications that cause sodium loss or water retention is the predisposing factor. A diminished sense of thirst or loss of access to food or fluids may also contribute to the problem.

Detecting and Controlling Hyponatremia

Early detection and treatment are necessary to prevent serious consequences. For patients at risk, the nurse closely monitors fluid I&O as well as daily body weight. It is also necessary to monitor laboratory values (i.e., sodium) and be alert for GI manifestations such as anorexia, nausea, vomiting, and abdominal cramping. The nurse must be alert for central nervous system changes, such as lethargy, confusion, muscle twitching, and seizures. Neurologic signs are associated with very low sodium levels that have fallen rapidly because of fluid overloading. Serum sodium is monitored very closely in patients who are at risk for hyponatremia; when indicated, urine sodium and specific gravity are also monitored.

For a patient with abnormal losses of sodium who can consume a general diet, the nurse encourages foods and fluids with high sodium content to control hyponatremia. For example, broth made with one beef cube contains approximately 900 mg of sodium; 8 oz of tomato juice contains approximately 700 mg of sodium. The nurse also needs to be familiar with the sodium content of parenteral fluids (see Table 13-5).

If the primary problem is water retention, it is safer to restrict fluid intake than to administer sodium. In normovolemia or hypervolemia, administration of sodium predisposes a patient to fluid volume overload. In severe hyponatremia, the aim of therapy is to elevate the serum sodium level only enough to alleviate neurologic signs and symptoms. It is generally recommended that the serum sodium concentration be increased to no greater than 125 mEq/L (125 mmol/L) with a hypertonic saline solution.

> ### Quality and Safety Nursing Alert
>
> *When administering fluids to patients with cardiovascular disease, the nurse assesses for signs of circulatory overload (e.g., cough, dyspnea, puffy eyelids, dependent edema, excess weight gain in 24 hours). The lungs are auscultated for crackles.*

For the patient taking lithium, the nurse observes for lithium toxicity, particularly when sodium is lost. In such

instances, supplemental salt and fluid are given. Because diuretics promote sodium loss, the patient taking lithium is instructed not to use diuretics without close medical supervision. For all patients on lithium therapy, normal salt and oral fluid intake (2.5 L/day) should be encouraged and a sodium restricted diet should be avoided (Frandsen & Pennington, 2014).

Excess water supplements are avoided in patients receiving isotonic or hypotonic enteral feedings, particularly if abnormal sodium loss occurs or water is being abnormally retained (as in SIADH). Actual fluid needs are determined by evaluating fluid I&O, urine specific gravity, and serum sodium levels.

Sodium Excess (Hypernatremia)

Hypernatremia is a serum sodium level higher than 145 mEq/L (145 mmol/L) (Sterns, 2014d). It can be caused by a gain of sodium in excess of water or by a loss of water in excess of sodium. It can occur in patients with normal fluid volume or in those with FVD or FVE. With a water loss, the patient loses more water than sodium; as a result, the serum sodium concentration increases and the increased concentration pulls fluid out of the cell. This is both an extracellular and an intracellular FVD. In sodium excess, the patient ingests or retains more sodium than water.

Pathophysiology

A common cause of hypernatremia is fluid deprivation in patients who cannot respond to thirst. Most often affected are very old, very young, and cognitively impaired patients. Administration of hypertonic enteral feedings without adequate water supplements leads to hypernatremia, as does watery diarrhea and greatly increased insensible water loss (e.g., hyperventilation, burns). In addition, diabetes insipidus can lead to hypernatremia if the patient does not experience or cannot respond to thirst, or if fluids are excessively restricted.

Less common causes of hypernatremia are heat stroke, near drowning in seawater (which contains a sodium concentration of approximately 500 mEq/L), and malfunction of hemodialysis or peritoneal dialysis systems. IV administration of hypertonic saline or excessive use of sodium bicarbonate also causes hypernatremia. Exertional dysnatremia can occur in performance athletes and can result in life-threatening encephalopathy. Hypernatremia and exercise-associated hyponatremia may manifest similarly with confusion and disorientation. On-site testing can differentiate hyponatremia from hypernatremia, assist in the assessment of the severity of the dysnatremia, and guide appropriate therapy.

Clinical Manifestations

The clinical manifestations of hypernatremia are owing to increased plasma osmolality caused by an increase in plasma sodium concentration (Sterns, 2014d). Water moves out of the cell into the ECF, resulting in cellular dehydration and a more concentrated ECF (see Fig. 13-5). Clinical signs and symptoms as well as laboratory findings can be found in Table 13-6. Dehydration (resulting in hypernatremia) is often overlooked as the cause of mental status and behavioral changes in older patients. Body temperature may increase mildly, but it returns to normal after the hypernatremia is corrected.

A primary characteristic of hypernatremia is thirst. Thirst is such a strong defender of serum sodium levels in healthy people that hypernatremia never occurs unless the person is unconscious or does not have access to water. However, those who are ill and older adults may have an impaired thirst mechanism.

Assessment and Diagnostic Findings

In hypernatremia, the serum sodium level exceeds 145 mEq/L (145 mmol/L) and the serum osmolality exceeds 300 mOsm/kg (300 mmol/L). The urine specific gravity and urine osmolality are increased as the kidneys attempt to conserve water (provided the water loss is from a route other than the kidneys). Patients with nephrogenic or central diabetes insipidus have hypernatremia and produce a dilute urine with a urine osmolality less than 250 mOsm/kg.

Medical Management

Treatment of hypernatremia consists of a gradual lowering of the serum sodium level by the infusion of a hypotonic electrolyte solution (e.g., 0.3% sodium chloride) or an isotonic nonsaline solution (e.g., dextrose 5% in water [D_5W]). D_5W is indicated when water needs to be replaced without sodium. Hypotonic sodium solution is thought to be safer than D_5W because it allows a gradual reduction in the serum sodium level, thereby decreasing the risk of cerebral edema. It is the solution of choice in severe hyperglycemia with hypernatremia. A rapid reduction in the serum sodium level temporarily decreases the plasma osmolality below that of the fluid in the brain tissue, causing dangerous cerebral edema. Diuretics also may be prescribed to treat the sodium gain.

There is no consensus about the exact rate at which serum sodium levels should be reduced. As a general rule, the serum sodium level is reduced at a rate no faster than 0.5 to 1 mEq/L/h to allow sufficient time for readjustment through diffusion across fluid compartments. Desmopressin acetate, a synthetic ADH, may be prescribed to treat diabetes insipidus if it is the cause of hypernatremia (Bichet, 2013).

Nursing Management

Fluid losses and gains are carefully monitored in patients who are at risk for hypernatremia. The nurse should assess for abnormal losses of water or low water intake and for large gains of sodium, as might occur with ingestion of OTC medications that have a high sodium content (e.g., Alka-Seltzer). In addition, the nurse obtains a medication history, because some prescription medications have a high sodium content. The nurse also notes the patient's thirst or elevated body temperature and evaluates it in relation to other clinical signs and symptoms. The nurse monitors the patient closely for changes in behavior, such as restlessness, disorientation, and lethargy.

Preventing Hypernatremia

The nurse attempts to prevent hypernatremia by providing oral fluids at regular intervals, particularly in patients who are unable to perceive or respond to thirst. If fluid intake remains inadequate or the patient is unconscious, the nurse consults with the primary provider to plan an alternative route for intake, either by enteral feedings or by the parenteral route.

If enteral feedings are used, sufficient water should be given to keep the serum sodium and BUN within normal limits. As a rule, the higher the osmolality of the enteral feeding, the greater is the need for water supplementation. Some herbal medications can also increase serum sodium levels.

For patients with diabetes insipidus, adequate water intake must be ensured. If the patient is alert and has an intact thirst mechanism, merely providing access to water may be sufficient. If the patient has a decreased level of consciousness or other disability interfering with adequate fluid intake, parenteral fluid replacement may be prescribed. This therapy can be anticipated in patients with neurologic disorders, particularly in the early postoperative period.

Correcting Hypernatremia

When parenteral fluids are necessary for managing hypernatremia, the nurse monitors the patient's response to the fluids by reviewing serial serum sodium levels and by observing for changes in neurologic signs (Maggs, 2014). With a gradual decrease in the serum sodium level, the neurologic signs should improve. Too-rapid reduction in the serum sodium level renders the plasma temporarily hypo-osmotic to the fluid in the brain tissue, causing movement of fluid into brain cells and dangerous cerebral edema.

Potassium Imbalances

Potassium (K^+) is the major intracellular electrolyte; in fact, 98% of the body's potassium is inside the cells. The remaining 2% is in the ECF and is important in neuromuscular function. Potassium influences both skeletal and cardiac muscle activity. For example, alterations in its concentration change myocardial irritability and rhythm. Under the influence of the sodium–potassium pump, potassium is constantly moving in and out of cells. The normal serum potassium concentration ranges from 3.5 to 5 mEq/L (3.5 to 5 mmol/L), and even minor variations are significant. Potassium imbalances are commonly associated with various diseases, injuries, medications (e.g., NSAIDs and ACE inhibitors), and acid–base imbalances (Mount, 2014a). The two most common potassium imbalances are potassium deficit and potassium excess (see Table 13-7).

To maintain potassium balance, the renal system must function, because 80% of the potassium excreted daily leaves the body by way of the kidneys; the other 20% is lost through the bowel and in sweat. The kidneys regulate potassium balance by adjusting the amount of potassium that is excreted in the urine. As serum potassium levels increase, so does the potassium level in the renal tubular cell. A concentration gradient occurs, favoring the movement of potassium into the renal tubule and excretion of potassium in the urine. Aldosterone also increases the excretion of potassium by the kidney. Because the kidneys do not conserve potassium as well as they conserve sodium, potassium may still be lost in urine in the presence of a potassium deficit.

Potassium Deficit (Hypokalemia)

Hypokalemia (serum potassium level below 3.5 mEq/L [3.5 mmol/L]) usually indicates a deficit in total potassium stores. However, it may occur in patients with normal

TABLE 13-7 Potassium Imbalances

Imbalance	Contributing Factors	Signs/Symptoms
Potassium deficit (hypokalemia) Serum potassium <3.5 mEq/L	Diarrhea, vomiting, gastric suction, corticosteroid administration, hyperaldosteronism, carbenicillin, amphotericin B, bulimia, osmotic diuresis, alkalosis, starvation, diuretics, and digoxin toxicity	Fatigue, anorexia, nausea and vomiting, muscle weakness, polyuria, decreased bowel motility, ventricular asystole or fibrillation, paresthesias, leg cramps, ↓ BP, ileus, abdominal distention, hypoactive reflexes. *ECG:* flattened T waves, prominent U waves, ST depression, prolonged PR interval
Potassium excess (hyperkalemia) Serum potassium >5.0 mEq/L	Pseudohyperkalemia, oliguric kidney injury, use of potassium-conserving diuretics in patients with renal insufficiency, metabolic acidosis, Addison disease, crush injury, burns, stored bank blood transfusions, rapid IV administration of potassium, and certain medications such as ACE inhibitors, NSAIDs, cyclosporine	Muscle weakness, tachycardia → bradycardia, dysrhythmias, flaccid paralysis, paresthesias, intestinal colic, cramps, abdominal distention, irritability, anxiety. *ECG:* tall tented T waves, prolonged PR interval and QRS duration, absent P waves, ST depression

↓, decreased; →, followed by; BP, blood pressure; ECG, electrocardiogram; IV, intravenous; ACE, angiotensin-converting enzyme; NSAIDs, nonsteroidal anti-inflammatory drugs.
Adapted from Grossman, S. C., & Porth, C. M. (2014). *Porth's pathophysiology: Concepts of altered health states* (9th ed.). Philadelphia, PA: Lippincott Williams & Wilkins.

potassium stores: When **alkalosis** (high blood pH) is present, a temporary shift of serum potassium into the cells occurs. (See later discussion).

Pathophysiology

Potassium-losing diuretics, such as the thiazides and loop diuretics, can induce hypokalemia (Mount, 2014a). Other medications that can lead to hypokalemia include corticosteroids, sodium penicillin, and amphotericin B. GI loss of potassium is another common cause of potassium depletion. Vomiting and gastric suction frequently lead to hypokalemia, because potassium is lost when gastric fluid is lost and because potassium is lost through the kidneys in response to metabolic alkalosis. Because relatively large amounts of potassium are contained in intestinal fluids, potassium deficit occurs frequently with diarrhea, which may contain as much potassium as 30 mEq/L. Potassium deficit also occurs from prolonged intestinal suctioning, recent ileostomy, and villous adenoma (a tumor of the intestinal tract characterized by excretion of potassium-rich mucus).

Alterations in acid–base balance have a significant effect on potassium distribution due to shifts of hydrogen and potassium ions between the cells and the ECF. Respiratory or metabolic alkalosis promotes the transcellular shift of potassium and can have a variable and unpredictable effect on serum potassium. For example, hydrogen ions move out of the cells in alkalotic states to help correct the high pH, and potassium ions move in to maintain an electrically neutral state (see later discussion of acid–base balance).

Hyperaldosteronism increases renal potassium wasting and can lead to severe potassium depletion. Primary hyperaldosteronism is seen in patients with adrenal adenomas. Secondary hyperaldosteronism occurs in patients with cirrhosis, nephrotic syndrome, heart failure, or malignant hypertension.

Because insulin promotes the entry of potassium into skeletal muscle and hepatic cells, patients with persistent insulin hypersecretion may experience hypokalemia, which is often the case in patients receiving high-carbohydrate parenteral nutrition.

Patients who are not able to eat a normal diet for a prolonged period are at risk for hypokalemia. This may occur in debilitated older adults and in patients with alcoholism or anorexia

nervosa. In addition to poor intake, people with bulimia frequently suffer increased potassium loss through self-induced vomiting and misuse of laxatives, diuretics, and enemas. Magnesium depletion causes renal potassium loss and must be corrected first; otherwise, urine loss of potassium will continue.

Clinical Manifestations

Potassium deficiency can result in widespread derangements in physiologic function. Severe hypokalemia can cause death through cardiac or respiratory arrest. Clinical signs develop when the potassium level decreases to less than 3 mEq/L (3 mmol/L) (Mount, 2014a; 2014b) Clinical signs and symptoms can be found in Table 13-7. If prolonged, hypokalemia can lead to an inability of the kidneys to concentrate urine, causing dilute urine (resulting in polyuria, nocturia) and excessive thirst. Potassium depletion suppresses the release of insulin and results in glucose intolerance.

Assessment and Diagnostic Findings

In hypokalemia, the serum potassium concentration is less than the lower limit of normal. Electrocardiographic (ECG) changes can include flat T waves or inverted T waves or both, suggesting ischemia, and depressed ST segments (see Fig. 13-6). An elevated U wave is specific to hypokalemia. Hypokalemia increases sensitivity to digitalis, predisposing the patient to digitalis toxicity at lower digitalis levels (Mount, 2014b). Metabolic alkalosis is commonly associated with hypokalemia. This is discussed further in the section on acid–base disturbances in this chapter.

The source of the potassium loss is usually evident from a careful history. However, if the cause of the loss is unclear, a 24-hour urinary potassium excretion test can be performed to distinguish between renal and extrarenal loss. Urinary potassium excretion exceeding 20 mEq/day with hypokalemia suggests that renal potassium loss is the cause.

Medical Management

If hypokalemia cannot be prevented by conventional measures such as increased intake in the daily diet or by oral

Figure 13-6 • Effect of potassium on the electrocardiogram (ECG). **A.** Normal tracing. **B.** Hypokalemia: serum potassium level below normal. **Left:** Flattening of the T wave and the appearance of a U wave. **Right:** Further flattening with prominent U wave. **C.** Hyperkalemia: serum potassium level above normal. **Left:** Moderate elevation with wide, flat P wave; wide QRS complex; and peaked T wave. **Right:** ECG changes seen with extreme potassium elevation: widening of QRS complex and absence of P wave.

potassium supplements for deficiencies, then it is treated cautiously with IV replacement therapy (Mount, 2014b). Potassium loss must be corrected daily; administration of 40 to 80 mEq/day of potassium is adequate in the adult if there are no abnormal losses of potassium.

For patients who are at risk for hypokalemia, a diet containing sufficient potassium should be provided. Dietary intake of potassium in the average adult is 50 to 100 mEq/day. Foods high in potassium include most fruits and vegetables, legumes, whole grains, milk, and meat (Dudek, 2013).

When dietary intake is inadequate for any reason, oral or IV potassium supplements may be prescribed. Many salt

substitutes contain 50 to 60 mEq of potassium per teaspoon and may be sufficient to prevent hypokalemia. If oral administration of potassium is not feasible, the IV route is indicated. The IV route is mandatory for patients with severe hypokalemia (e.g., serum level of 2 mEq/L). Although potassium chloride (KCl) is usually used to correct potassium deficits, potassium acetate or potassium phosphate may be prescribed.

Nursing Management

Because hypokalemia can be life threatening, the nurse needs to monitor for its early presence in patients at risk. Fatigue, anorexia, muscle weakness, decreased bowel motility, paresthesias, and dysrhythmias are signals that warrant assessing the serum potassium concentration. When available, the ECG may provide useful information (Mount, 2014a). For example, patients receiving digitalis who are at risk for potassium deficiency should be monitored closely for signs of digitalis toxicity, because hypokalemia potentiates the action of digitalis.

Preventing Hypokalemia

Prevention may involve encouraging the patient at risk to eat foods rich in potassium (when the diet allows). Consumption of foods high in potassium should be encouraged; examples include bananas, melon, citrus fruits, fresh and frozen vegetables (avoid canned vegetables), lean meats, milk, and whole grains (Mount, 2014c). If the hypokalemia is caused by abuse of laxatives or diuretics, patient education may help alleviate the problem. Part of the health history and assessment should be directed at identifying problems that are amenable to prevention through education. Careful monitoring of fluid I&O is necessary, because 40 mEq of potassium is lost for every liter of urine output. The ECG is monitored for changes, and arterial blood gas values are checked for elevated bicarbonate and pH levels.

Correcting Hypokalemia

The oral route is ideal to treat mild to moderate hypokalemia because oral potassium supplements are absorbed well. Care should be exercised when administering potassium, particularly in older adults, who have lower lean body mass and total-body potassium levels and therefore lower potassium requirements. In addition, because of the physiologic loss of renal function with advancing years, potassium may be retained more readily in older than in younger people.

> ▶ **Quality and Safety Nursing Alert**
>
> Oral potassium supplements can produce small bowel lesions; therefore, the patient must be assessed for and cautioned about abdominal distention, pain, or GI bleeding.

Administering Intravenous Potassium

Potassium should be given only after adequate urine output has been established. A decrease in urine volume to less than 20 mL per hour for 2 consecutive hours is an indication to stop the potassium infusion and notify the primary provider. Potassium is primarily excreted by the kidneys; when oliguria occurs, potassium administration can cause the serum potassium concentration to rise dangerously.

> ◀ *Quality and Safety Nursing Alert*
>
> *Potassium is never given by IV push or intramuscularly to avoid replacing potassium too quickly. IV potassium must be given using an infusion pump.*

Each health care facility has its own policy for the administration of potassium, which must be consulted. Administration of IV potassium is done with extreme caution using an infusion pump with the patient monitored by continuous ECG. Caution must be used when selecting a premixed solution of IV fluid containing KCl, as the concentrations range from 10 to 40 mEq/100 mL. Renal function should be monitored through BUN and creatinine levels and urine output if the patient is receiving potassium replacement. During replacement therapy, the patient is monitored for signs of worsening hypokalemia as well as hyperkalemia.

Potassium Excess (Hyperkalemia)

Hyperkalemia (serum potassium level greater than 5 mEq/L [5 mmol/L]) seldom occurs in patients with normal renal function (Mount, 2014a). In older adults, there is an increased risk of hyperkalemia due to decreases in renin and aldosterone as well as an increased number of comorbid cardiac conditions. Like hypokalemia, hyperkalemia is often caused by iatrogenic (treatment-induced) causes. Although hyperkalemia is less common than hypokalemia, it is usually more dangerous because cardiac arrest is more frequently associated with high serum potassium levels.

Pathophysiology

Major causes of hyperkalemia are decreased renal excretion of potassium, rapid administration of potassium, and movement of potassium from the ICF compartment to the ECF compartment. Hyperkalemia is commonly seen in patients with untreated kidney injury, particularly those in whom potassium levels increase as a result of infection or excessive intake of potassium in food or medications (Mount, 2014c). Patients with hypoaldosteronism or Addison disease are at risk for hyperkalemia because deficient adrenal hormones lead to sodium loss and potassium retention.

Medications have been identified as a probable contributing factor in more than 60% of hyperkalemic episodes. Medications commonly implicated are KCl, heparin, ACE inhibitors, NSAIDs, beta blockers, cyclosporine (Neoral), tacrolimus (Prograf), and potassium-sparing diuretics (Comerford, 2015). Potassium regulation is compromised in acute and chronic kidney disease, with a glomerular filtration rate less than 10% to 20% of normal (Mount, 2014c).

Improper use of potassium supplements predisposes all patients to hyperkalemia, especially if salt substitutes are used. Not all patients receiving potassium-losing diuretics require potassium supplements, and patients receiving potassium-conserving diuretics should not receive supplements.

> ◀ *Quality and Safety Nursing Alert*
>
> *Potassium supplements are extremely dangerous for patients who have impaired renal function and thus decreased ability to excrete potassium. Even more dangerous is the IV administration of potassium to such patients, because serum levels can rise very quickly. Aged (stored) blood should not be given to patients with impaired renal function, because the serum potassium concentration of stored blood increases due to red blood cell deterioration. It is possible to exceed the renal tolerance of any patient with rapid IV potassium administration, as well as when large amounts of oral potassium supplements are ingested.*

In **acidosis** (low blood pH), potassium moves out of the cells and into the ECF. This occurs as hydrogen ions enter the cells to buffer the pH of the ECF (see later discussion). An elevated ECF potassium level should be anticipated when extensive tissue trauma has occurred, as in burns, crushing injuries, or severe infections. Similarly, it can occur with lysis of malignant cells after chemotherapy (i.e., tumor lysis syndrome).

Pseudohyperkalemia (a false hyperkalemia) has several causes, including the improper collection or transport of a blood sample, a traumatic venipuncture, and use of a tight tourniquet around an exercising extremity while drawing a blood sample, producing hemolysis of the sample before analysis (Mount, 2014a). Other causes include marked leukocytosis (white blood cell count exceeding 200,000/mm^3) and thrombocytosis (platelet count exceeding 1 million/mm^3); drawing blood above a site where potassium is infusing; and familial pseudohyperkalemia, in which potassium leaks out of the red blood cells while the blood is awaiting analysis. Lack of awareness of these causes of pseudohyperkalemia can lead to aggressive treatment of a nonexistent hyperkalemia, resulting in serious lowering of serum potassium levels. Therefore, measurements of grossly elevated levels in the absence of clinical manifestations (e.g., normal ECG) should be verified by retesting.

Clinical Manifestations

Clinical signs and symptoms can be found in Table 13-7. The most important consequence of hyperkalemia is its effect on the myocardium. Cardiac effects of elevated serum potassium are usually not significant when the level is less than 7 mEq/L (7 mmol/L); however, they are almost always present when the level is 8 mEq/L (8 mmol/L) or greater. As the plasma potassium level rises, disturbances in cardiac conduction occur. The earliest changes, often occurring at a serum potassium level greater than 6 mEq/L (6 mmol/L), are peaked, narrow T waves; ST-segment depression; and a shortened QT interval. If the serum potassium level continues to increase, the PR interval becomes prolonged and is followed by disappearance of the P waves. Finally, there is decomposition and widening of the QRS complex (see Fig. 13-6). Ventricular dysrhythmias and cardiac arrest may occur (Mount, 2014c).

Assessment and Diagnostic Findings

Serum potassium levels and ECG changes are crucial to the diagnosis of hyperkalemia, as discussed previously. Arterial blood gas analysis may reveal both a metabolic and a respiratory acidosis. These are discussed further in the section on acid–base disturbances in this chapter. Correcting the acidosis helps correct the hyperkalemia.

Medical Management

An ECG should be obtained immediately to detect changes. Shortened repolarization and peaked T waves are seen initially. To verify results, a repeat serum potassium level should be obtained from a vein without an IV infusing a potassium-containing solution.

In nonacute situations, restriction of dietary potassium and potassium-containing medications may correct the imbalance. For example, eliminating the use of potassium-containing salt substitutes in a patient who is taking a potassium-conserving diuretic may be all that is needed to deal with mild hyperkalemia.

Administration, either orally or by retention enema, of cation exchange resins (e.g., sodium polystyrene sulfonate [Kayexalate]) may be necessary (Frandsen & Pennington, 2014). Cation exchange resins cannot be used if the patient has a paralytic ileus, because intestinal perforation can occur. Kayexalate binds with other cations in the GI tract and contributes to the development of hypomagnesemia and hypocalcemia; it may also cause sodium retention and fluid overload and should be used with caution in patients with heart failure.

Emergency Pharmacologic Therapy

If serum potassium levels are dangerously elevated, it may be necessary to administer IV calcium gluconate (Mount, 2014c). Within minutes after administration, calcium antagonizes the action of hyperkalemia on the heart but does not reduce the serum potassium concentration. Calcium chloride and calcium gluconate are not interchangeable; calcium gluconate contains 4.5 mEq of calcium, and calcium chloride contains 13.6 mEq of calcium. Therefore, caution is required.

Monitoring the blood pressure is essential to detect hypotension, which may result from the rapid IV administration of calcium gluconate. The ECG should be continuously monitored during administration; the appearance of bradycardia is an indication to stop the infusion. The myocardial protective effects of calcium last about 30 minutes. Extra caution is required if the patient has received an accelerated dose of a digitalis-based cardiac glycoside to reach a desired serum digitalis level rapidly as parenteral administration of calcium sensitizes the heart to digitalis and may precipitate digitalis toxicity.

IV administration of sodium bicarbonate may be necessary in severe metabolic acidosis to alkalinize the plasma, shift potassium into the cells, and furnish sodium to antagonize the cardiac effects of potassium. Effects of this therapy begin within 30 to 60 minutes and may persist for hours; however, they are temporary.

Circulatory overload and hypernatremia can occur when large amounts of hypertonic sodium bicarbonate are given. Bicarbonate therapy should be guided by the bicarbonate concentration or calculated base deficit obtained from blood gas analysis or laboratory measurement (Blevins, 2014; Burns, 2014).

IV administration of regular insulin and a hypertonic dextrose solution causes a temporary shift of potassium into the cells. Glucose and insulin therapy has an onset of action within 30 minutes and lasts for several hours. Loop diuretics, such as furosemide, increase excretion of water by inhibiting sodium, potassium, and chloride reabsorption in the ascending loop of Henle and distal renal tubule.

Beta-2 agonists, such as albuterol (Proventil, Ventolin), are highly effective in decreasing potassium; however, their use remains controversial because they can cause tachycardia and chest discomfort (Mount 2014c). Beta-2 agonists move potassium into the cells and may be used in the absence of ischemic cardiac disease. Their use is a stopgap measure that only temporarily protects the patient from hyperkalemia. If the hyperkalemic condition is not transient, actual removal of potassium from the body is required through cation exchange resins, peritoneal dialysis, hemodialysis, or other forms of renal replacement therapy.

Nursing Management

Patients at risk for potassium excess (e.g., those with kidney disease) need to be identified and closely monitored for signs of hyperkalemia. The nurse monitors I&O and observes for signs of muscle weakness and dysrhythmias. When measuring vital signs, an apical pulse should be taken. The presence of paresthesias and GI symptoms such as nausea and intestinal colic are noted. Serum potassium levels, as well as BUN, creatinine, glucose, and arterial blood gas values, are monitored for patients at risk for developing hyperkalemia.

Preventing Hyperkalemia

Measures are taken to prevent hyperkalemia in patients at risk, when possible, by encouraging the patient to adhere to the prescribed potassium restriction. Potassium-rich foods to be avoided include many fruits and vegetables, legumes, whole-grain breads, lean meat, milk, eggs, coffee, tea, and cocoa (Dudek, 2013). Conversely, foods with minimal potassium content include butter, margarine, cranberry juice or sauce, ginger ale, gumdrops or jellybeans, hard candy, root beer, sugar, and honey. Labels of cola beverages must be checked carefully because some are high in potassium and some are not.

Correcting Hyperkalemia

It is possible to exceed the tolerance for potassium if given rapidly by the IV route. Therefore, care is taken to administer and monitor potassium solutions closely. Particular attention is paid to the solution's concentration and rate of administration. IV administration is via an infusion pump (Mount 2014c).

The nurse must caution patients to use salt substitutes sparingly if they are taking other supplementary forms of potassium or potassium-conserving diuretics. In addition, potassium-conserving diuretics, potassium supplements, and salt substitutes should not be given to patients with renal dysfunction (Mount, 2014c).

Calcium Imbalances

More than 99% of the body's calcium (Ca^{++}) is located in the skeletal system; it is a major component of bones and teeth. About 1% of skeletal calcium is rapidly exchangeable with blood calcium, and the rest is more stable and only slowly

TABLE 13-8 Calcium Imbalances

Imbalance	Contributing Factors	Signs/Symptoms and Laboratory Findings
Calcium deficit (hypocalcemia) Serum calcium <8.5 mg/dL	Hypoparathyroidism (may follow thyroid surgery or radical neck dissection), malabsorption, pancreatitis, alkalosis, vitamin D deficiency, massive subcutaneous infection, generalized peritonitis, massive transfusion of citrated blood, chronic diarrhea, decreased parathyroid hormone, diuretic phase of kidney injury, ↑ PO_4, fistulas, burns, alcoholism	Numbness, tingling of fingers, toes, and circumoral region; positive Trousseau sign and Chvostek sign; seizures, carpopedal spasms, hyperactive deep tendon reflexes, irritability, bronchospasm, anxiety, impaired clotting time, ↓ prothrombin, diarrhea, ↓ BP. *ECG:* prolonged QT interval and lengthened ST *Labs indicate:* ↓ Mg^{++}
Calcium excess (hypercalcemia) Serum calcium >10.5 mg/dL	Hyperparathyroidism, malignant neoplastic disease, prolonged immobilization, overuse of calcium supplements, vitamin D excess, oliguric phase of renal failure, acidosis, corticosteroid therapy, thiazide diuretic use, increased parathyroid hormone, and digoxin toxicity	Muscular weakness, constipation, anorexia, nausea and vomiting, polyuria and polydipsia, dehydration, hypoactive deep tendon reflexes, lethargy, deep bone pain, pathologic fractures, flank pain, calcium stones, hypertension. *ECG:* shortened ST segment and QT interval, bradycardia, heart blocks

↑, increased; ↓, decreased; BP, blood pressure; ECG, electrocardiogram.
Adapted from Grossman, S. C., & Porth, C. M. (2014). *Porth's pathophysiology: Concepts of altered health states* (9th ed.). Philadelphia, PA: Lippincott Williams & Wilkins.

exchanged. The small amount of calcium located outside the bone circulates in the serum, partly bound to protein and partly ionized. Calcium plays a major role in transmitting nerve impulses and helps regulate muscle contraction and relaxation, including cardiac muscle. Calcium is instrumental in activating enzymes that stimulate many essential chemical reactions in the body, and it also plays a role in blood coagulation. Because many factors affect calcium regulation, both hypocalcemia and hypercalcemia are relatively common disturbances (see Table 13-8).

The normal total serum calcium level is 8.6 to 10.2 mg/dL (2.2 to 2.6 mmol/L) (Goltzman, 2014). Calcium exists in plasma in three forms: ionized, bound, and complex. Approximately 50% of the serum calcium exists in a physiologically active ionized form that is important for neuromuscular activity and blood coagulation; this is the only physiologically and clinically significant form. The normal ionized serum calcium level is 4.5 to 5.1 mg/dL (1.1 to 1.3 mmol/L). Less than half of the plasma calcium is bound to serum proteins, primarily albumin. The remainder is combined with nonprotein anions: phosphate, citrate, and carbonate.

Calcium is absorbed from foods in the presence of normal gastric acidity and vitamin D. It is excreted primarily in the feces, with the remainder excreted in the urine. The serum calcium level is controlled by PTH and calcitonin. As ionized serum calcium decreases, the parathyroid glands secrete PTH. This, in turn, increases calcium absorption from the GI tract, increases calcium reabsorption from the renal tubule, and releases calcium from the bone. The increase in calcium ion concentration suppresses PTH secretion. When calcium increases excessively, the thyroid gland secretes calcitonin, which inhibits calcium reabsorption from bone and decreases the serum calcium concentration.

Calcium Deficit (Hypocalcemia)

Hypocalcemia (serum calcium value lower than 8.6 mg/dL [2.15 mmol/L]) occurs in a variety of clinical situations. A patient may have a total-body calcium deficit (as in osteoporosis) but a normal serum calcium level. Older adults and those with disabilities, who spend an increased amount of

time in bed, have an increased risk of hypocalcemia, because bed rest increases bone resorption.

Pathophysiology

Several factors can cause hypocalcemia, including primary hypoparathyroidism and surgical hypoparathyroidism. The latter is far more common. Not only is hypocalcemia associated with thyroid and parathyroid surgery, but it can also occur after radical neck dissection and is most likely in the first 24 to 48 hours after surgery. Transient hypocalcemia can occur with massive administration of citrated blood (i.e., massive hemorrhage and shock), because citrate can combine with ionized calcium and temporarily remove it from the circulation.

Inflammation of the pancreas causes the breakdown of proteins and lipids. It is thought that calcium ions combine with the fatty acids released by lipolysis, forming soaps. As a result of this process, hypocalcemia occurs and is common in pancreatitis. Hypocalcemia may be related to excessive secretion of glucagon from the inflamed pancreas, which results in increased secretion of calcitonin.

Hypocalcemia is common in patients with kidney injury, because these patients frequently have elevated serum phosphate levels. Hyperphosphatemia usually causes a reciprocal drop in the serum calcium level. Other causes of hypocalcemia include inadequate vitamin D consumption, magnesium deficiency, medullary thyroid carcinoma, low serum albumin levels, alkalosis, and alcohol abuse. Medications predisposing to hypocalcemia include aluminum-containing antacids, aminoglycosides, caffeine, cisplatin, corticosteroids, mithramycin, phosphates, isoniazid, loop diuretics, and proton pump inhibitors (Goltzman, 2014).

Clinical Manifestations

Tetany, the most characteristic manifestation of hypocalcemia and hypomagnesemia, refers to the entire symptom complex induced by increased neural excitability. Clinical signs and symptoms are caused by spontaneous discharges of both sensory and motor fibers in peripheral nerves and are outlined in Table 13-8.

Figure 13-7 • A. Chvostek sign: a contraction of the facial muscles elicited in response to light tap over the facial nerve in front of the ear. **B.** Trousseau sign: a carpopedal spasm induced by inflating a blood pressure cuff above systolic blood pressure. Adapted from Bullock, B. A., & Henze, R. J. (2000). *Focus on pathophysiology* (p. 173). Philadelphia, PA: Lippincott Williams & Wilkins.

Chvostek sign (see Fig. 13-7A) consists of twitching of muscles enervated by the facial nerve when the region that is about 2 cm anterior to the earlobe, just below the zygomatic arch, is tapped. Trousseau sign (see Fig. 13-7B) can be elicited by inflating a blood pressure cuff on the upper arm to about 20 mm Hg above systolic pressure; within 2 to 5 minutes, carpal spasm (an adducted thumb, flexed wrist and metacarpophalangeal joints, extended interphalangeal joints with fingers together) will occur as ischemia of the ulnar nerve develops (Goltzman, 2015a).

Seizures may occur because hypocalcemia increases irritability of the central nervous system as well as the peripheral nervous system. Other changes associated with hypocalcemia include mental changes such as depression, impaired memory, confusion, delirium, and hallucinations. A prolonged QT interval is seen on the ECG due to prolongation of the ST segment, and torsades de pointes, a type of ventricular tachycardia, may occur. Respiratory effects with decreasing calcium include dyspnea and laryngospasm. Signs and symptoms of chronic hypocalcemia include hyperactive bowel sounds, dry and brittle hair and nails, and abnormal clotting.

Osteoporosis is associated with prolonged low intake of calcium and represents a total-body calcium deficit, even though serum calcium levels are usually normal. This disorder occurs in millions of Americans and is most common in postmenopausal women. It is characterized by loss of bone mass, which causes bones to become porous and brittle and therefore susceptible to fracture. (See Chapter 41 for further discussion of osteoporosis.)

Assessment and Diagnostic Findings

When evaluating serum calcium levels, the serum albumin level and the arterial pH must also be considered. Because abnormalities in serum albumin levels may affect interpretation of the serum calcium level, it may be necessary to

---

Chart 13-2 Calculating Corrected Serum Calcium Level

Abnormalities in serum albumin levels may affect interpretation of the serum calcium level. Below is a method for calculating the corrected serum calcium level if the serum albumin level is abnormal.

Quick Calculation Method

Measured total serum Ca^{++} level (mg/dL) + 0.8
× (4.0 − Measured albumin level [g/dL])
= Corrected total calcium concentration (mg/dL)

Example Calculation

A patient's reported serum albumin level is 2.5 g/dL; the reported serum calcium level is 10.5 mg/dL. First, the decrease in serum albumin level from normal (i.e., the difference from the normal albumin concentration of 4 g/dL) is calculated: 4 g/dL − 2.5 g/dL = 1.5 g/dL. Next, the following ratio is calculated:

0.8 mg/dL: 1 g/dL = X mg/dL: 1.5 mg/dL
X = 0.8 × 1.5 mg/dL
X = 1.2 mg/dL calcium

Finally, 1.2 mg/dL is added to 10.5 mg/dL (the reported serum calcium level) to obtain the corrected total serum calcium level: 1.2 mg/dL + 10.5 mg/dL = 11.7 mg/dL.

---

calculate the corrected serum calcium if the serum albumin level is abnormal. For every decrease in serum albumin of 1 g/dL below 4 g/dL, the total serum calcium level is underestimated by approximately 0.8 mg/dL. Chart 13-2 displays a quick method that nurses can use to calculate the corrected serum calcium level.

Clinicians often discount a low serum calcium level in the presence of a similarly low serum albumin level. The ionized calcium level is usually normal in patients with reduced total serum calcium levels and concomitant hypoalbuminemia. When the arterial pH increases (alkalosis), more calcium becomes bound to protein. As a result, the ionized portion decreases. Symptoms of hypocalcemia may occur with alkalosis. Acidosis has the opposite effect—that is, less calcium is bound to protein and therefore more exists in the ionized form. However, relatively small changes in serum calcium levels occur in these acid–base abnormalities.

Ideally, the ionized level of calcium should be measured in the laboratory. However, in many laboratories, only the total calcium level is reported; therefore, the concentration of the ionized fraction must be estimated by simultaneous measurement of the serum albumin level. PTH levels are decreased in hypoparathyroidism. Magnesium and phosphorus levels need to be assessed to identify possible causes of decreased calcium.

Medical Management

Emergency Pharmacologic Therapy

Acute symptomatic hypocalcemia is life threatening and requires prompt treatment with IV administration of a calcium salt. Parenteral calcium salts include calcium gluconate and calcium chloride (Comerford, 2015). Although calcium chloride produces a significantly higher ionized calcium level than calcium gluconate does, it is not used as often because it is more irritating and can cause sloughing of tissue if it infiltrates. IV administration of calcium is particularly dangerous in patients receiving digitalis-derived medications, because calcium ions exert an effect similar to that of digitalis and can cause digitalis toxicity, with adverse cardiac effects. The IV site must be observed often for any evidence of infiltration because of the risk of extravasation and resultant cellulitis or necrosis. A 0.9% sodium chloride solution should not be used with calcium because it increases renal calcium loss. Solutions containing phosphates or bicarbonate should not be used with calcium because they cause precipitation when calcium is added. The nurse must clarify with the primary provider and pharmacist which calcium salt to administer, because calcium gluconate yields 4.5 mEq of calcium and calcium chloride provides 13.6 mEq of calcium. Calcium replacement can cause postural hypotension; therefore, the patient is kept in bed during IV infusion, and blood pressure is monitored (Goltzman, 2015b).

> ### ▶ Quality and Safety Nursing Alert
>
> *Too rapid IV administration of calcium can cause cardiac arrest, preceded by bradycardia. Therefore, calcium should be diluted in D$_5$W and given as a slow IV bolus or a slow IV infusion using an infusion pump.*

Nutritional Therapy

Vitamin D therapy may be instituted to increase calcium absorption from the GI tract; otherwise, the amount of calcium absorbed may not satisfy the body's calcium requirement. In addition, aluminum hydroxide, calcium acetate, or calcium carbonate antacids may be prescribed to decrease elevated phosphorus levels before treating hypocalcemia in the patient with chronic kidney disease. Increasing the dietary intake of calcium to at least 1000 to 1500 mg/day in the adult is recommended (Rosen, 2015). Calcium supplements must be given in divided doses of no higher than 500 mg to promote calcium absorption. Calcium-containing foods include milk products; green, leafy vegetables; canned salmon; canned sardines; and fresh oysters. Hypomagnesemia can also cause tetany; if the tetany responds to IV calcium, then a low magnesium level is considered as a possible cause in chronic kidney injury.

Nursing Management

It is important to assess for hypocalcemia in at-risk patients. Seizure precautions are initiated if hypocalcemia is severe. The status of the airway is closely monitored, because laryngeal stridor can occur. Safety precautions are taken, as indicated, if confusion is present.

The nurse must educate the patient with hypocalcemia about foods that are rich in calcium. The nurse must also advise the patient to consider calcium supplements if sufficient calcium is not consumed in the diet. Such supplements should be taken in divided doses with meals. Alcohol and caffeine in high doses inhibit calcium absorption, and moderate cigarette smoking increases urinary calcium excretion. The patient is also cautioned to avoid the overuse of laxatives and antacids that contain phosphorus, because their use decreases calcium absorption.

Calcium Excess (Hypercalcemia)

Hypercalcemia (serum calcium value greater than 10.2 mg/dL [2.6 mmol/L]) is a dangerous imbalance when severe; in fact, hypercalcemic crisis has a mortality rate as high as 50% if not treated promptly.

Pathophysiology

The most common causes of hypercalcemia are malignancies and hyperparathyroidism (Shane, 2014). Malignant tumors can produce hypercalcemia by various mechanisms. The excessive PTH secretion associated with hyperparathyroidism causes increased release of calcium from the bones and increased intestinal and renal absorption of calcium. Calcifications of soft tissue occur when the calcium–phosphorus product (serum calcium × serum phosphorus) exceeds 70 mg/dL.

Bone mineral is lost during immobilization, and sometimes this causes elevation of total (and especially ionized) calcium in the bloodstream. However, symptomatic hypercalcemia from immobilization is rare; when it does occur, it is limited to people with high calcium turnover rates (e.g., adolescents during a growth spurt). Most cases of hypercalcemia secondary to immobility occur after severe or multiple fractures or spinal cord injury.

Thiazide diuretics can cause a slight elevation in serum calcium levels because they potentiate the action of PTH on the kidneys, reducing urinary calcium excretion. Vitamin A and D intoxication, as well as chronic lithium use and theophylline toxicity, can cause calcium excess. Calcium levels are inversely related to phosphorus levels.

Hypercalcemia reduces neuromuscular excitability because it suppresses activity at the myoneural junction. Decreased tone in smooth and striated muscle may cause symptoms such as muscle weakness, incoordination, anorexia, and constipation. Cardiac standstill can occur when the serum calcium level is about 18 mg/dL (4.5 mmol/L). Calcium enhances the inotropic effect of digitalis; therefore, hypercalcemia aggravates digitalis toxicity.

Clinical Manifestations

Clinical signs and symptoms can be found in Table 13-8. The symptoms of hypercalcemia are proportional to the degree of elevation of the serum calcium level. The more severe symptoms tend to appear when the serum calcium level is approximately 16 mg/dL (4 mmol/L) or higher. However, some patients become profoundly disturbed with serum calcium levels of only 12 mg/dL (3 mmol/L). These symptoms resolve as serum calcium levels return to normal after treatment.

Hypercalcemic crisis refers to an acute rise in the serum calcium level to 17 mg/dL (4.3 mmol/L) or higher. Severe thirst and polyuria are often present. Other findings may include muscle weakness, intractable nausea, abdominal cramps, severe constipation, diarrhea, peptic ulcer symptoms, and bone pain. Lethargy, confusion, and coma may also occur. This condition is dangerous and may result in cardiac arrest. Emergency treatment with calcitonin is indicated (see later discussion under Pharmacologic Therapy).

Assessment and Diagnostic Findings

The serum calcium level is greater than 10.2 mg/dL (2.6 mmol/L). Cardiovascular changes may include a variety of dysrhythmias (e.g., heart blocks) and shortening of the QT interval and ST segment. The PR interval is sometimes prolonged. The double-antibody PTH test may be used to differentiate between primary hyperparathyroidism and malignancy as a cause of hypercalcemia: PTH levels are increased in primary or secondary hyperparathyroidism and suppressed in malignancy. X-rays may reveal bone changes if the patient has hypercalcemia secondary to a malignancy, bone cavitations, or urinary calculi. Urine calcium can be normal or elevated in hyperparathyroidism and hypercalcemia caused by malignancy.

Medical Management

Therapeutic aims include decreasing the serum calcium level and reversing the process causing the hypercalcemia. Treating the underlying cause (e.g., chemotherapy for a malignancy, partial parathyroidectomy for hyperparathyroidism) is essential.

Pharmacologic Therapy

Measures include administering fluids to dilute serum calcium and promote its excretion by the kidneys, mobilizing the patient, and restricting dietary calcium intake. IV administration of 0.9% sodium chloride solution temporarily dilutes the serum calcium level and increases urinary calcium excretion by inhibiting tubular reabsorption of calcium. Administering IV phosphate can cause a reciprocal drop in serum calcium. Furosemide is often used in conjunction with administration of a saline solution; in addition to causing diuresis, furosemide increases calcium excretion. Although often overlooked, fluids and medications that contain calcium and dietary sources of calcium should be halted.

Calcitonin can be used to lower the serum calcium level and is particularly useful for patients with heart disease or kidney injury who cannot tolerate large sodium loads. Calcitonin reduces bone resorption, increases the deposition of calcium and phosphorus in the bones, and increases urinary excretion of calcium and phosphorus. Although several forms are available, calcitonin derived from salmon is commonly used. Skin testing for allergy to salmon calcitonin is necessary before the hormone is given. Systemic allergic reactions are possible because this hormone is a protein; resistance to the medication may develop later because of antibody formation. Calcitonin is given by intramuscular injection rather than subcutaneously, because patients with hypercalcemia have poor perfusion of subcutaneous tissue (Shane & Berenson, 2015).

For patients with cancer, treatment is directed at controlling the condition by surgery, chemotherapy, or radiation therapy. Corticosteroids may be used to decrease bone turnover and tubular reabsorption for patients with sarcoidosis, myelomas, lymphomas, and leukemias; patients with solid tumors are less responsive. Some bisphosphonates (e.g., pamidronate disodium [Aredia], and ibandronate sodium [Boniva]) inhibit osteoclast activity. IV forms can cause fever, transient leukopenia, eye inflammation, nephrotic syndrome, and jaw osteonecrosis (Shane & Berenson, 2015).

Mithramycin, a cytotoxic antibiotic, inhibits bone resorption and thus lowers the serum calcium level. This agent must be used cautiously because it has significant side effects, including thrombocytopenia, nephrotoxicity, rebound hypercalcemia when discontinued, and hepatotoxicity. Inorganic phosphate salts can be given orally or by nasogastric tube (in the form of Phospho-Soda or Neutra-Phos), rectally (as retention enemas), or IV. IV phosphate therapy is used with extreme caution in the treatment of hypercalcemia, because it can cause severe calcification in various tissues, hypotension, tetany, and acute kidney injury.

Nursing Management

The nurse must monitor for hypercalcemia in at-risk patients. Interventions such as increasing patient mobility and encouraging fluids can help prevent hypercalcemia, or at least minimize its severity. Hospitalized patients at risk should be encouraged to ambulate as soon as possible. Those who are outpatients and receive home care are educated about the importance of frequent ambulation.

When encouraging oral fluids, the nurse considers the patient's likes and dislikes. Fluids containing sodium should be given unless contraindicated, because sodium assists with calcium excretion. Patients are encouraged to drink 2.8 to 3.8 L (3 to 4 quarts) of fluid daily. Adequate fiber in the diet is encouraged to offset the tendency for constipation. Safety precautions are implemented, as necessary, when altered mental status is present. The patient and family are informed that these mental changes are reversible with treatment. Increased calcium increases the effects of digitalis; therefore, the patient is assessed for signs and symptoms of digitalis toxicity. Because ECG changes (premature ventricular contractions, paroxysmal atrial tachycardia, and heart block) can occur, the cardiac rate and rhythm are monitored for any abnormalities.

Magnesium Imbalances

Magnesium (Mg^{++}) is an abundant intracellular cation. It acts as an activator for many intracellular enzyme systems and plays a role in both carbohydrate and protein metabolism. The normal serum magnesium level is 1.3 to 2.3 mg/dL (0.62 to 0.95 mmol/L). Approximately one third of serum magnesium is bound to protein; the remaining two thirds exist as free cations—the active component (Mg^{++}). Magnesium balance is important in neuromuscular function. Because magnesium acts directly on the myoneural junction, variations in the serum level affect neuromuscular irritability and contractility. For example, an excess of magnesium diminishes the excitability of the muscle cells, whereas a deficit increases neuromuscular irritability and contractility. Magnesium produces its sedative effect at the neuromuscular junction, probably by inhibiting the release of the neurotransmitter acetylcholine. It also increases the stimulus threshold in nerve fibers. Two common magnesium imbalances are magnesium deficit and magnesium excess (see Table 13-9).

Magnesium also affects the cardiovascular system, acting peripherally to produce vasodilation and decreased peripheral resistance. Approximately one third of magnesium in the ECF is bound to protein (mostly albumin), and the other two thirds are free or ionized (Grossman & Porth, 2014).

TABLE 13-9 Magnesium Imbalances

Imbalance	Contributing Factors	Signs/Symptoms
Magnesium deficit (hypomagnesemia) Serum magnesium <1.8 mg/dL	Chronic alcoholism, hyperparathyroidism, hyperaldosteronism, diuretic phase of acute kidney injury, malabsorptive disorders, diabetic ketoacidosis, refeeding after starvation, parenteral nutrition, chronic laxative use, diarrhea, acute myocardial infarction, heart failure, decreased serum K$^+$ and Ca^{++} and certain pharmacologic agents (such as gentamicin, cisplatin, and cyclosporine)	Neuromuscular irritability, positive Trousseau sign and Chvostek sign, insomnia, mood changes, anorexia, vomiting, increased tendon reflexes, and ↑ BP. ECG: PVCs, flat or inverted T waves, depressed ST segment, prolonged PR interval, and widened QRS
Magnesium excess (hypermagnesemia) Serum magnesium >3.0 mg/dL	Oliguric phase of acute kidney injury (particularly when magnesium-containing medications are given), adrenal insufficiency, excessive IV magnesium administration, diabetic ketoacidosis, and hypothyroidism	Flushing, hypotension, muscle weakness, drowsiness, hypoactive reflexes, depressed respirations, cardiac arrest and coma, diaphoresis. ECG: tachycardia → bradycardia, prolonged PR interval and QRS, peaked T waves

↑, increased; →, followed by; BP, blood pressure; ECG, electrocardiogram; IV, intravenous; PVCs, premature ventricular contractions.
Adapted from Grossman, S. C., & Porth, C. M. (2014). *Porth's pathophysiology: Concepts of altered health states* (9th ed.). Philadelphia, PA: Lippincott Williams & Wilkins.

Magnesium Deficit (Hypomagnesemia)

Hypomagnesemia refers to a below-normal serum magnesium concentration (1.3 mg/dL [0.62 mmol/L]) and is frequently associated with hypokalemia and hypocalcemia. Magnesium is similar to calcium in two aspects: (1) it is the ionized fraction of magnesium that is primarily involved in neuromuscular activity and other physiologic processes, and (2) magnesium levels should be evaluated in combination with albumin levels. Because about 30% of magnesium is protein bound, principally to albumin, a decreased serum albumin level can reduce the measured total magnesium concentration; however, it does not reduce the ionized plasma magnesium concentration (Grossman & Porth, 2014).

Pathophysiology

An important route of magnesium loss is the GI tract; such loss can occur with nasogastric suction, diarrhea, or fistulas. Because fluid from the lower GI tract has a higher concentration of magnesium (10 to 14 mEq/L) than fluid from the upper tract (1 to 2 mEq/L), losses from diarrhea and intestinal fistulas are more likely to induce magnesium deficit than are those from gastric suction. Although magnesium losses are relatively small in nasogastric suction, hypomagnesemia occurs if losses are prolonged and magnesium is not replaced through IV infusion. Because the distal small bowel is the major site of magnesium absorption, any disruption in small bowel function (e.g., intestinal resection or inflammatory bowel disease) can lead to hypomagnesemia. Hypomagnesemia is a common yet often overlooked imbalance in acutely and critically ill patients. It may occur with withdrawal from alcohol and administration of tube feedings or parenteral nutrition.

Chronic alcohol abuse is a major cause of symptomatic hypomagnesemia in the United States (Grossman & Porth, 2014). The serum magnesium level should be measured at least every 2 or 3 days in patients undergoing withdrawal from alcohol. The level may be normal on admission but may decrease as a result of metabolic changes, such as the intracellular shift of magnesium associated with IV glucose administration.

During nutritional replacement, the major cellular electrolytes move from the serum to newly synthesized cells. Therefore, if the enteral or parenteral feeding formula is deficient in magnesium content, serious hypomagnesemia will occur. Because of this, serum magnesium levels should be measured at regular intervals in patients who are receiving parenteral or enteral feedings, especially those who have undergone a period of starvation. Other causes of hypomagnesemia include the administration of aminoglycosides, cyclosporine, cisplatin, diuretics, digitalis, and amphotericin, as well as the rapid administration of citrated blood, especially to patients with renal or hepatic disease. Magnesium deficiency often occurs in diabetic ketoacidosis, secondary to increased renal excretion during osmotic diuresis and shifting of magnesium into the cells with insulin therapy. Other causes include administration of certain oral magnesium containing medications (Grossman & Porth, 2014).

Clinical Manifestations

Clinical signs and symptoms can be found in Table 13-9. Some clinical manifestations of hypomagnesemia are due directly to the low serum magnesium level; others are due to secondary changes in potassium and calcium metabolism. Symptoms do not usually occur until the serum magnesium level has dropped to less than 1.8 mEq/L (0.75 mmol/L). Chvostek and Trousseau signs (see earlier discussion) occur, in part, because of accompanying hypocalcemia (Grossman & Porth, 2014).

Hypomagnesemia may be accompanied by marked alterations in psychological status. Apathy, depressed mood, apprehension, and extreme agitation have been noted, as well as ataxia, dizziness, insomnia, and confusion. At times, delirium, auditory or visual hallucinations, and frank psychoses may occur.

Magnesium deficiency can disturb the ECG by prolonging the QRS, depressing the ST segment, and predisposing to cardiac dysrhythmias, such as premature ventricular contractions, supraventricular tachycardia, torsades de pointes, and ventricular fibrillation. Increased susceptibility to digitalis toxicity is associated with low serum magnesium levels. This is important, because patients receiving digoxin are also likely to be receiving diuretic therapy, predisposing them to renal loss of magnesium. Concurrent hypokalemia and hypocalcemia must be addressed in addition to hypomagnesemia. These electrolyte disturbances are difficult to correct until magnesium has been repleted. Additionally, hypocalcemia can be worsened by isolated treatment of hypomagnesemia with intravenous magnesium sulfate because sulfate binds ionized calcium.

Assessment and Diagnostic Findings

On laboratory analysis, the serum magnesium level is less than 1.3 mg/dL (0.62 mmol/L). Urine magnesium may help identify the cause of magnesium depletion, and levels are measured after a loading dose of magnesium sulfate is given. Additional diagnostic techniques (nuclear magnetic resonance spectroscopy and the ion-selective electrode) are sensitive and direct means of measuring ionized serum magnesium levels.

Medical Management

Mild magnesium deficiency can be corrected by diet alone. Principal dietary sources of magnesium include green leafy vegetables, nuts, seeds, legumes, whole grains, seafood, peanut butter, and cocoa.

If necessary, magnesium salts can be given orally in an oxide or gluconate form to replace continuous losses but can produce diarrhea. Patients receiving parenteral nutrition require magnesium in the IV solution to prevent hypomagnesemia. Overt symptoms of hypomagnesemia are treated with parenteral administration of magnesium. A bolus dose of magnesium sulfate given too rapidly can produce alterations in cardiac conduction leading to heart block or asystole. Vital signs must be assessed frequently during magnesium administration to detect changes in cardiac rate or rhythm, hypotension, and respiratory distress. Monitoring urine output is essential before, during, and after magnesium administration; the physician is notified if urine volume decreases to less than 100 mL over 4 hours. Calcium gluconate must be readily available to treat hypocalcemic tetany or hypermagnesemia.

> ◤ *Quality and Safety Nursing Alert*
>
> *IV magnesium sulfate must be given by an infusion pump and at a rate not to exceed 150 mg/min, or 67 mEq over 8 hours.*

Nursing Management

The nurse should be aware of patients at risk for hypomagnesemia and observe them for its signs and symptoms. Patients receiving digitalis are monitored closely, because a deficit of magnesium can predispose them to digitalis toxicity. If hypomagnesemia is severe, seizure precautions are implemented. Other safety precautions are instituted, as indicated, if confusion is observed. Because difficulty in swallowing (dysphagia) may occur in those with magnesium depletion, these patients should be screened for dysphagia.

Patient education plays a major role in treating magnesium deficit. The patient is educated about sources of magnesium-rich foods, including green vegetables, nuts, legumes, bananas, and oranges

Magnesium Excess (Hypermagnesemia)

Hypermagnesemia (serum magnesium level higher than 3.0 mg/dL [1.25 mmol/L]) is a rare electrolyte abnormality, because the kidneys efficiently excrete magnesium (Grossman & Porth, 2014). A serum magnesium level can appear falsely elevated if blood specimens are allowed to hemolyze or are drawn from an extremity with a tourniquet that was applied too tightly.

Pathophysiology

The most common cause of hypermagnesemia is kidney injury (Yu & Gupta, 2015). In fact, most patients with advanced kidney injury have at least a slight elevation in serum magnesium levels. This condition is aggravated when such patients receive magnesium to control seizures.

Hypermagnesemia can occur in patients with untreated diabetic ketoacidosis when catabolism causes the release of cellular magnesium that cannot be excreted because of profound fluid volume depletion and resulting oliguria. A surplus of magnesium can also result from excessive magnesium given to treat hypertension of pregnancy or to treat hypomagnesemia. Increased serum magnesium levels can also occur in adrenocortical insufficiency, Addison disease, or hypothermia. Excessive use of magnesium-based antacids (e.g., Maalox, Riopan, Mylanta) or laxatives (Milk of Magnesia) and medications that decrease GI motility, including opioids and anticholinergics, can also increase serum magnesium levels. Decreased elimination of magnesium or its increased absorption due to intestinal hypomotility from any cause can contribute to hypermagnesemia. Lithium intoxication can also cause an increase in serum magnesium levels. Extensive soft tissue injury or necrosis as with trauma, shock, sepsis, cardiac arrest, or severe burns can also result in hypermagnesemia.

Clinical Manifestations

Acute elevation of the serum magnesium level depresses the central nervous system as well as the peripheral neuromuscular junction. Clinical signs and symptoms can be found in Table 13-9. The respiratory center is depressed when serum magnesium levels exceed 10 mEq/L (5 mmol/L). Coma, atrioventricular heart block, and cardiac arrest can occur when the serum magnesium level is greatly elevated and not treated. High levels of magnesium also result in platelet clumping and delayed thrombin formation.

Assessment and Diagnostic Findings

On laboratory analysis, the serum magnesium level is greater than 3.0 mg/dL (1.25 mmol/L). Increased potassium and calcium are present concurrently. As creatinine clearance decreases to less than 3.0 mL/min, the serum magnesium levels increase. ECG findings may include a prolonged PR interval, tall T waves, a widened QRS, and a prolonged QT interval, as well as an atrioventricular block (Grossman & Porth, 2014).

Medical Management

Hypermagnesemia can be prevented by avoiding the administration of magnesium to patients with kidney injury and by carefully monitoring seriously ill patients who are receiving magnesium salts. In patients with severe hypermagnesemia, all parenteral and oral magnesium salts are discontinued. In emergencies, such as respiratory depression or defective cardiac conduction, ventilatory support and IV calcium gluconate are indicated. In addition, hemodialysis with a magnesium-free dialysate can reduce the serum magnesium to a safe level within hours. Administration of loop diuretics (e.g., furosemide) and sodium chloride or lactated Ringer IV solution enhances magnesium excretion in patients with adequate renal function. IV calcium gluconate antagonizes the cardiovascular and neuromuscular effects of magnesium.

Nursing Management

Patients at risk for hypermagnesemia are identified and assessed. If hypermagnesemia is suspected, the nurse monitors the vital signs, noting hypotension and shallow respirations. The nurse also observes for decreased deep tendon reflexes (DTRs) and changes in the level of consciousness. Medications that contain magnesium are not given to patients with kidney injury or compromised renal function, and patients with kidney injury are cautioned to check with their primary providers before taking OTC medications. Caution is essential when preparing and administering magnesium-containing fluids parenterally, because available parenteral magnesium solutions (e.g., 2-mL ampules, 50-mL vials) differ in concentration.

Phosphorus Imbalances

Phosphorus (HPO_4-) is a critical constituent of all body tissues. It is essential to the function of muscle and red blood cells; the formation of adenosine triphosphate (ATP) and of 2,3-diphosphoglycerate, which facilitates the release of oxygen from hemoglobin; and the maintenance of acid–base balance, as well as the nervous system and the intermediary metabolism of carbohydrate, protein, and fat. It provides structural support to bones and teeth. Phosphorus is the primary anion of the ICF. About 85% of phosphorus is located in bones and teeth, 14% in soft tissue, and less than 1% in the ECF. The normal serum phosphorus level is 2.5 to 4.5 mg/dL (0.8 to 1.45 mmol/L) in adults. PTH assists in phosphate homeostasis by varying phosphate reabsorption in the proximal tubule of the kidney, and it allows the shift of phosphate from bone to plasma. Phosphorus deficit and phosphorus excess are two common imbalances (see Table 13-10).

Phosphorus Deficit (Hypophosphatemia)

Hypophosphatemia is indicated by a value below 2.5 mg/dL (0.8 mmol/L). Although it often indicates phosphorus deficiency, hypophosphatemia may occur under a variety of circumstances in which total-body phosphorus stores are normal. Conversely, phosphorus deficiency is an abnormally low content of phosphorus in lean tissues that may exist in the absence of hypophosphatemia. It can be caused by an intracellular shift of potassium from serum into cells, by increased urinary excretion of potassium, or by decreased intestinal absorption of potassium.

Pathophysiology

Hypophosphatemia may occur during the administration of calories to patients with severe protein–calorie malnutrition. It is most likely to result from overzealous intake or administration of simple carbohydrates. This syndrome can be induced in any person with severe protein–calorie malnutrition (e.g., patients with anorexia nervosa or alcoholism, older debilitated patients who are unable to eat).

Marked hypophosphatemia may develop in malnourished patients who receive parenteral nutrition if the phosphorus loss is not corrected. Other causes of hypophosphatemia include heat stroke, prolonged intense hyperventilation, alcohol withdrawal, poor dietary intake, diabetic ketoacidosis, respiratory alkalosis, hepatic encephalopathy, and major thermal burns. Low magnesium levels, low potassium levels, and hyperparathyroidism related to increased urinary losses of phosphorus contribute to hypophosphatemia. Loss of phosphorus through the kidneys also occurs with acute volume expansion, osmotic diuresis, the use of carbonic anhydrase inhibitors (acetazolamide [Diamox]), and some malignancies. Respiratory alkalosis can cause a decrease in phosphorus because of an intracellular shift of phosphorus.

Excess phosphorus binding by antacids may decrease the phosphorus available from the diet to an amount lower than required to maintain serum phosphorus balance. The degree of hypophosphatemia depends on the amount of phosphorus in the diet compared to the dose of antacid. Hypophosphatemia

TABLE 13-10 Phosphorus Imbalances

Imbalance	Contributing Factors	Signs/Symptoms
Phosphorus deficit (hypophosphatemia) Serum phosphorus <2.5 mg/dL	Refeeding after starvation, alcohol withdrawal, diabetic ketoacidosis, respiratory and metabolic alkalosis, ↓ magnesium, ↓ potassium, hyperparathyroidism, vomiting, diarrhea, hyperventilation, vitamin D deficiency associated with malabsorptive disorders, burns, acid–base disorders, parenteral nutrition, and diuretic and antacid use	Paresthesias, muscle weakness, bone pain and tenderness, chest pain, confusion, cardiomyopathy, respiratory failure, seizures, tissue hypoxia, and increased susceptibility to infection, nystagmus
Phosphorus excess (hyperphosphatemia) Serum phosphorus >4.5 mg/dL	Acute kidney injury and chronic kidney disease, excessive intake of phosphorus, vitamin D excess, respiratory and metabolic acidosis, hypoparathyroidism, volume depletion, leukemia/lymphoma treated with cytotoxic agents, increased tissue breakdown, rhabdomyolysis	Tetany, tachycardia, anorexia, nausea and vomiting, muscle weakness, signs and symptoms of hypocalcemia; hyperactive reflexes; soft tissue calcifications in lungs, heart, kidneys, and cornea

↓, decreased.
Adapted from Grossman, S. C., & Porth, C. M. (2014). *Porth's pathophysiology: Concepts of altered health states* (9th ed.). Philadelphia, PA: Lippincott Williams & Wilkins.

can occur with chronic diarrhea, Crohn's disease, vitamin D deficiency, anorexia, alcoholism, and malabsorption. Vitamin D regulates intestinal ion absorption; therefore, a deficiency of vitamin D may cause decreased calcium and phosphorus levels, which may lead to osteomalacia (softened and brittle bones).

Clinical Manifestations

Most of the signs and symptoms of phosphorus deficiency result from a deficiency of ATP, 2,3-diphosphoglycerate, or both (Yu & Stubbs, 2014). ATP deficiency impairs cellular energy resources; diphosphoglycerate deficiency impairs oxygen delivery to tissues, resulting in a wide range of neurologic manifestations. Clinical signs and symptoms can be found in Table 13-10. Hypoxia leads to an increase in respiratory rate and respiratory alkalosis, causing phosphorus to move into the cells and potentiating hypophosphatemia. In laboratory animals, hypophosphatemia is associated with depression of the chemotactic, phagocytic, and bacterial activity of granulocytes.

Muscle damage may develop as the ATP level in the muscle tissue declines. Clinical manifestations are muscle weakness, which may be subtle or profound and may affect any muscle group; muscle pain; and at times acute rhabdomyolysis (breakdown of skeletal muscle). Weakness of respiratory muscles may greatly impair ventilation. Hypophosphatemia also may predispose a person to insulin resistance and thus hyperglycemia. Chronic loss of phosphorus can cause bruising and bleeding from platelet dysfunction.

Assessment and Diagnostic Findings

On laboratory analysis, the serum phosphorus level is less than 2.5 mg/dL (0.80 mmol/L). When reviewing laboratory results, the nurse should keep in mind that glucose or insulin administration causes a slight decrease in the serum phosphorus level. PTH levels are increased in hyperparathyroidism. Serum magnesium may decrease due to increased urinary excretion of magnesium. Alkaline phosphatase is increased with osteoblastic activity. X-rays may show skeletal changes of osteomalacia or rickets.

Medical Management

Prevention of hypophosphatemia is the goal. In patients at risk for hypophosphatemia, serum phosphate levels should be closely monitored and correction initiated before deficits become severe. Adequate amounts of phosphorus should be added to parenteral solutions, and attention should be paid to the phosphorus levels in enteral feeding solutions.

Severe hypophosphatemia is dangerous and requires prompt attention. Aggressive IV phosphorus correction is usually limited to the patient whose serum phosphorus levels decrease to less than 1 mg/dL (0.3 mmol/L) and whose GI tract is not functioning. Possible effects of IV administration of phosphorus include tetany from hypocalcemia and calcifications in tissues (blood vessels, heart, lung, kidney, eyes) from hyperphosphatemia. IV preparations of phosphorus are available as sodium or potassium phosphate. The rate of phosphorus administration should not exceed 10 mEq/h, and the site should be carefully monitored because tissue sloughing and necrosis can occur with infiltration. In less acute situations, oral phosphorus replacement is usually adequate.

Nursing Management

The nurse identifies patients at risk for hypophosphatemia and monitors them. Because malnourished patients receiving parenteral nutrition are at risk when calories are introduced too aggressively, preventive measures involve gradually introducing the solution to avoid rapid shifts of phosphorus into the cells.

For patients with documented hypophosphatemia, careful attention is given to preventing infection, because hypophosphatemia may alter the granulocytes. In patients requiring correction of phosphorus losses, the nurse frequently monitors serum phosphorus levels and documents and reports early signs of hypophosphatemia (apprehension, confusion, change in level of consciousness). If the patient experiences mild hypophosphatemia, foods such as milk and milk products, organ meats, nuts, fish, poultry, and whole grains should be encouraged. With moderate hypophosphatemia, supplements such as Neutra-Phos capsules, K-Phos, and Fleet Phospho-Soda may be prescribed.

Phosphorus Excess (Hyperphosphatemia)

Hyperphosphatemia is a serum phosphorus level that exceeds 4.5 mg/dL (1.45 mmol/L).

Pathophysiology

Various conditions can lead to hyperphosphatemia; however, the most common is kidney injury (Stubbs & Yu, 2015). Other causes include increased intake, decreased output, or a shift from the intracellular to extracellular space. Conditions such as excessive vitamin D intake, administration of total parenteral nutrition, chemotherapy for neoplastic disease, hypoparathyroidism, metabolic or respiratory acidosis, diabetic ketoacidosis, acute hemolysis, high phosphate intake, profound muscle necrosis, and increased phosphorus absorption may also lead to this phosphorus imbalance. The primary complication of increased phosphorus is metastatic calcification (soft tissue, joints, and arteries), which occurs when the calcium–magnesium product (calcium × magnesium) exceeds 70 mg/dL.

Clinical Manifestations

Clinical signs and symptoms can be found in Table 13-10. Most symptoms result from decreased calcium levels and soft tissue calcifications. The most important short-term consequence is tetany. Because of the reciprocal relationship between phosphorus and calcium, a high serum phosphorus level tends to cause a low serum calcium concentration.

The major long-term consequence is soft tissue calcification, which occurs mainly in patients with a reduced glomerular filtration rate. High serum levels of inorganic phosphorus promote precipitation of calcium phosphate in nonosseous sites, decreasing urine output, impairing vision, and producing palpitations.

Assessment and Diagnostic Findings

On laboratory analysis, the serum phosphorus level exceeds 4.5 mg/dL (1.5 mmol/L). The serum calcium level is useful also for diagnosing the primary disorder and assessing the effects of treatments. X-rays may show skeletal changes with abnormal bone development. PTH levels are decreased in hypoparathyroidism. BUN and creatinine levels are used to assess renal function.

Medical Management

When possible, treatment is directed at the underlying disorder. For example, hyperphosphatemia may be related to volume depletion or respiratory or metabolic acidosis. In kidney injury, elevated PTH production contributes to a high phosphorus level and bone disease. Measures to decrease the serum phosphate level and bind phosphorus in the GI tract of these patients include vitamin D preparations, such as calcitriol, which is available in both oral (Rocaltrol) and parenteral (Calcijex, paricalcitol [Zemplar]) forms (Comerford, 2015; Frandsen & Pennington, 2014). IV administration of calcitriol does not increase the serum calcium unless its dose is excessive, thus permitting more aggressive treatment of hyperphosphatemia with calcium-binding antacids (calcium carbonate or calcium citrate). Administration of Amphojel with meals is effective but can cause bone and central nervous system toxicity with long-term use. Restriction of dietary phosphate, forced diuresis with a loop diuretic, volume replacement with saline, and dialysis may also lower phosphorus. Surgery may be indicated for removal of large calcium and phosphorus deposits.

Nursing Management

The nurse monitors patients at risk for hyperphosphatemia. If a low-phosphorus diet is prescribed, the patient is instructed to avoid phosphorus-rich foods, such as hard cheeses, cream, nuts, meats, whole-grain cereals, dried fruits, dried vegetables, kidneys, sardines, sweetbreads, and foods made with milk. When appropriate, the nurse instructs the patient to avoid phosphate-containing laxatives and enemas. The nurse also educates the patient about recognizing the signs of impending hypocalcemia and monitoring for changes in urine output.

Chloride Imbalances

Chloride (Cl^-), the major anion of the ECF, is found more in interstitial and lymph fluid compartments than in blood. Chloride is also contained in gastric and pancreatic juices, sweat, bile, and saliva. Sodium and chloride make up the largest electrolyte composition of the ECF and assist in determining osmotic pressure. Chloride is produced in the stomach, where it combines with hydrogen to form hydrochloric acid. Chloride control depends on the intake of chloride and the excretion and reabsorption of its ions in the kidneys. A small amount of chloride is lost in the feces.

The normal serum chloride level is 97 to 107 mEq/L (97 to 107 mmol/L). Inside the cell, the chloride level is 4 mEq/L. The serum level of chloride reflects a change in dilution or concentration of the ECF and does so in direct proportion to the sodium concentration. Serum osmolality parallels chloride levels as well. Aldosterone secretion increases sodium reabsorption, thereby increasing chloride reabsorption. The choroid plexus, which secretes cerebrospinal fluid in the brain, depends on sodium and chloride to attract water to form the fluid portion of the cerebrospinal fluid. Bicarbonate has an inverse relationship with chloride. As chloride moves from plasma into the red blood cells (called the *chloride shift*), bicarbonate moves back into the plasma. Hydrogen ions are formed, which then help the release oxygen from hemoglobin. When the level of one of these three electrolytes (sodium, bicarbonate, or chloride) is disturbed, the other two are also affected. Chloride assists in maintaining acid–base balance and works as a buffer in the exchange of oxygen and CO_2 in red blood cells (Fischbach & Dunning, 2015). Chloride is primarily obtained from the diet as table salt. The two most common chloride imbalances are chloride deficit and chloride excess (see Table 13-11).

Chloride Deficit (Hypochloremia)

Hypochloremia is a serum chloride level below 97 mEq/L (97 mmol/L).

TABLE 13-11 Chloride Imbalances

Imbalance	Contributing Factors	Signs/Symptoms and Laboratory Findings
Chloride deficit (hypochloremia) Serum chloride <96 mEq/L	Addison disease, reduced chloride intake or absorption, untreated diabetic ketoacidosis, chronic respiratory acidosis, excessive sweating, vomiting, gastric suction, diarrhea, sodium and potassium deficiency, metabolic alkalosis; loop, osmotic, or thiazide diuretic use; overuse of bicarbonate, rapid removal of ascitic fluid with a high sodium content, IV fluids that lack chloride (dextrose and water), draining fistulas and ileostomies, heart failure, cystic fibrosis	Agitation, irritability, tremors, muscle cramps, hyperactive deep tendon reflexes, hypertonicity, tetany, slow shallow respirations, seizures, dysrhythmias, coma *Labs indicate:* ↓ serum chloride, ↓ serum sodium, ↑ pH, ↑ serum bicarbonate, ↑ total carbon dioxide content, ↓ urine chloride level, ↓ serum potassium
Chloride excess (hyperchloremia) Serum chloride >108 mEq/L	Excessive sodium chloride infusions with water loss, head injury (sodium retention), hypernatremia, kidney injury, corticosteroid use, dehydration, severe diarrhea (loss of bicarbonate), respiratory alkalosis, administration of diuretics, overdose of salicylates, Kayexalate, acetazolamide, phenylbutazone and ammonium chloride use, hyperparathyroidism, metabolic acidosis	Tachypnea, lethargy, weakness, deep rapid respirations, decline in cognitive status, ↓ cardiac output, dyspnea, tachycardia, pitting edema, dysrhythmias, coma *Labs indicate:* ↑ serum chloride, ↑ serum potassium and sodium, ↓ serum pH, ↓ serum bicarbonate, normal anion gap, ↑ urinary chloride level

↑, increased; ↓, decreased; IV, intravenous.
Adapted from Grossman, S. C., & Porth, C. M. (2014). *Porth's pathophysiology: Concepts of altered health states* (9th ed.). Philadelphia, PA: Lippincott Williams & Wilkins.

Pathophysiology

Hypochloremia can occur with GI tube drainage, gastric suctioning, gastric surgery, and severe vomiting and diarrhea. Administration of chloride-deficient IV solutions, low sodium intake, decreased serum sodium levels, metabolic alkalosis, massive blood transfusions, diuretic therapy, burns, and fever may cause hypochloremia. Administration of aldosterone, ACTH, corticosteroids, bicarbonate, or laxatives decreases serum chloride levels as well. As chloride decreases (usually because of volume depletion), sodium and bicarbonate ions are retained by the kidney to balance the loss. Bicarbonate accumulates in the ECF, which raises the pH and leads to hypochloremic metabolic alkalosis.

Clinical Manifestations

The signs and symptoms of hypochloremia are outlined in Table 13-11. The signs and symptoms of hyponatremia, hypokalemia, and metabolic alkalosis may also be present. Metabolic alkalosis is a disorder that results in a high pH and a high serum bicarbonate level as a result of excess alkali intake or loss of hydrogen ions. With compensation, the partial pressure of CO_2 in arterial blood ($PaCO_2$) increases to 50 mm Hg. Hyperexcitability of muscles, tetany, hyperactive DTRs, weakness, twitching, and muscle cramps may result. Hypokalemia can cause hypochloremia, resulting in cardiac dysrhythmias. In addition, because low chloride levels parallel low sodium levels, a water excess may occur. Hyponatremia can cause seizures and coma.

Assessment and Diagnostic Findings

In addition to the chloride level, sodium and potassium levels are also evaluated, because these electrolytes are lost along with chloride. Arterial blood gas analysis identifies the acid–base imbalance, which is usually metabolic alkalosis. The urine chloride level, which is also measured, decreases in hypochloremia.

Medical Management

Treatment involves correcting the cause of hypochloremia and the contributing electrolyte and acid–base imbalances. Normal saline (0.9% sodium chloride) or half-strength saline (0.45% sodium chloride) solution is given by IV to replace the chloride. If the patient is receiving a diuretic (loop, osmotic, or thiazide), it may be discontinued or another diuretic prescribed.

Ammonium chloride, an acidifying IV agent, may be prescribed to treat metabolic alkalosis; the dosage depends on the patient's weight and serum chloride level. This agent is metabolized by the liver, and its effects last for about 3 days. Its use should be avoided in patients with impaired liver or renal function.

Nursing Management

The nurse monitors the patient's I&O, arterial blood gas values, and serum electrolyte levels. Changes in the patient's level of consciousness and muscle strength and movement are reported to the primary provider promptly. Vital signs are monitored, and respiratory assessment is carried out frequently. The nurse provides and educates the patient about foods with high chloride content, which include tomato juice, bananas, dates, eggs, cheese, milk, salty broth, canned vegetables, and processed meats. A person who drinks free water (water without electrolytes) or bottled water and excretes large amounts of chloride needs instruction to avoid drinking this kind of water.

Chloride Excess (Hyperchloremia)

Hyperchloremia exists when the serum level of chloride exceeds 107 mEq/L (107 mmol/L). Hypernatremia, bicarbonate loss, and metabolic acidosis can occur with high chloride levels.

Pathophysiology

High serum chloride levels are almost exclusively a result of iatrogenically induced hyperchloremic metabolic acidosis, stemming from excessive administration of chloride relative to sodium, most commonly as 0.9% normal saline solution, 0.45% normal saline solution, or lactated Ringer solution. This condition can also be caused by the loss of bicarbonate ions via the kidney or the GI tract with a corresponding increase in chloride ions. Chloride ions in the form of acidifying salts accumulate, and acidosis occurs with a decrease in bicarbonate ions. Head trauma, increased perspiration, excess adrenocortical hormone production, and decreased glomerular filtration can lead to a high serum chloride level.

Clinical Manifestations

The signs and symptoms of hyperchloremia are the same as those of metabolic acidosis: hypervolemia and hypernatremia. Tachypnea, weakness, lethargy, deep and rapid respirations, diminished cognitive ability, and hypertension occur. If untreated, hyperchloremia can lead to a decrease in cardiac output, dysrhythmias, and coma. A high chloride level is accompanied by a high sodium level and fluid retention.

Assessment and Diagnostic Findings

The serum chloride level is 108 mEq/L (108 mmol/L) or greater, the serum sodium level is greater than 145 mEq/L (145 mmol/L), the serum pH is less than 7.35, and the serum bicarbonate level is less than 22 mEq/L (22 mmol/L). Urine chloride excretion increases.

Medical Management

Correcting the underlying cause of hyperchloremia and restoring electrolyte, fluid, and acid–base balance are essential. Hypotonic IV solutions may be given to restore balance. Lactated Ringer solution may be prescribed to convert lactate to bicarbonate in the liver, which increases the bicarbonate level and corrects the acidosis. IV sodium bicarbonate may be given to increase bicarbonate levels, which leads to the renal excretion of chloride ions because bicarbonate and chloride compete for combination with sodium. Diuretics may be given to eliminate chloride as well. Sodium, chloride, and fluids are restricted.

Nursing Management

Monitoring vital signs, arterial blood gas values, and I&O is important to assess the patient's status and the effectiveness of treatment. Assessment findings related to respiratory, neurologic, and cardiac systems are documented, and changes are discussed with the primary provider. The nurse educates the patient about the diet that should be followed to manage hyperchloremia and maintain adequate hydration.

ACID–BASE DISTURBANCES

Acid–base disturbances are commonly encountered in clinical practice, especially in critical care units. Identification of the specific acid–base imbalance is important in ascertaining the underlying cause of the disorder and determining appropriate treatment.

Plasma pH is an indicator of hydrogen ion (H^+) concentration and measures the acidity or alkalinity of the blood

(Grossman & Porth, 2014). Homeostatic mechanisms keep pH within a normal range (7.35 to 7.45) (Emmett, 2014). These mechanisms consist of buffer systems, the kidneys, and the lungs. The H^+ concentration is extremely important: The greater the concentration, the more acidic the solution and the lower the pH. The lower the H^+ concentration, the more alkaline the solution and the higher the pH. The pH range compatible with life (6.8 to 7.8) represents a 10-fold difference in H^+ concentration in plasma (Figure 13-8).

Buffer systems prevent major changes in the pH of body fluids by removing or releasing H^+; they can act quickly to prevent excessive changes in H^+ concentration. Hydrogen ions are buffered by both intracellular and extracellular buffers. The body's major extracellular buffer system is the bicarbonate–carbonic acid buffer system, which is assessed when arterial blood gases

$$pH = 6.1 + log_{10}\ (ratio\ HCO_3^-: H_2CO_3)$$

Figure 13-8 • Normal and compensated states of pH and acid–base balance represented as a balance scale. **A.** When the ratio of bicarbonate (HCO_3^-) to carbonic acid (H_2CO_3, arterial $CO_2 \times 0.03$) = 20:1, the pH = 7.4. **B.** Metabolic acidosis with a HCO_3^-:H_3CO_3 ratio of 10:1 and a pH of 7.1. **C.** Respiratory compensation lowers the H_3CO_3 to 0.6 mEq/L and returns the HCO_3^-:H_3CO_3 ratio to 20:1 and the pH to 7.4. **D.** Respiratory alkalosis with a HCO_3^-:H_3CO_3 ratio of 40:1 and a pH of 7.7. **E.** Renal compensation eliminates HCO_3^-, reducing serum levels to 12 mEq/L, returning the HCO_3^-:H_3CO_3 ratio to 20:1 and the pH to 7.4. Normally, these compensatory mechanisms are capable of buffering large changes in pH but do not return the pH completely to normal as illustrated here. (From Rhoades R. A., & Bell D. R. (Eds.) (2009). *Medical physiology: Principles for clinical medicine* (3rd ed., p. 445). Philadelphia, PA: Lippincott Williams & Wilkins.)

are measured. Normally, there are 20 parts of bicarbonate (HCO_3^-) to 1 part of carbonic acid (H_2CO_3). If this ratio is altered, the pH will change. It is the ratio of HCO_3^- to H_2CO_3 that is important in maintaining pH, not absolute values. CO_2 is a potential acid; when dissolved in water, it becomes carbonic acid ($CO_2 + H_2O = H_2CO_3$). Therefore, when CO_2 is increased, the carbonic acid content is also increased, and vice versa. If either bicarbonate or carbonic acid is increased or decreased so that the 20:1 ratio is no longer maintained, acid–base imbalance results.

Less important buffer systems in the ECF include the inorganic phosphates and the plasma proteins. Intracellular buffers include proteins, organic and inorganic phosphates, and, in red blood cells, hemoglobin.

The kidneys regulate the bicarbonate level in the ECF; they can regenerate bicarbonate ions as well as reabsorb them from the renal tubular cells. In respiratory acidosis and most cases of metabolic acidosis, the kidneys excrete hydrogen ions and conserve bicarbonate ions to help restore balance. In respiratory and metabolic alkalosis, the kidneys retain hydrogen ions and excrete bicarbonate ions to help restore balance. The kidneys obviously cannot compensate for the metabolic acidosis created by kidney injury. Renal compensation for imbalances is relatively slow (a matter of hours or days).

The lungs, under the control of the medulla, control the CO_2 and thus the carbonic acid content of the ECF. They do so by adjusting ventilation in response to the amount of CO_2 in the blood. A rise in the partial pressure of CO_2 in arterial blood ($PaCO_2$) is a powerful stimulant to respiration. Of course, the partial pressure of oxygen in arterial blood (PaO_2) also influences respiration. However, its effect is not as marked as that produced by the $PaCO_2$.

In metabolic acidosis, the respiratory rate increases, causing greater elimination of CO_2 (to reduce the acid load). In metabolic alkalosis, the respiratory rate decreases, causing CO_2 to be retained (to increase the acid load) (Emmett, 2014).

Acute and Chronic Metabolic Acidosis (Base Bicarbonate Deficit)

Metabolic acidosis is a common clinical disturbance characterized by a low pH (increased H^+ concentration) and a low plasma bicarbonate concentration. It can be produced by a gain of hydrogen ion or a loss of bicarbonate. It can be divided clinically into two forms, according to the values of the serum anion gap: high anion gap acidosis and normal anion gap acidosis. The anion gap refers to the difference between the sum of all measured positively charged electrolytes (cations) and the sum of all negatively charged electrolytes (anions) in blood. Because the sum of measured cations is typically greater than the sum of measured anions, there normally exists a gap referred to as the anion gap. Because blood does not carry an electrical charge, the anion gap reflects normally unmeasured anions (phosphates, sulfates, and proteins) in plasma that increase the anion gap by replacing bicarbonate. Measuring the anion gap is essential in analyzing acid–base disorders. The anion gap can be calculated by either of the following equations:

$$\text{Anion gap} = Na^+ + K^+ - (Cl^- + HCO_3^-)$$
$$\text{Anion gap} = Na^+ - (Cl^- + HCO_3^-)$$

Potassium is often omitted from the equation because of its low level in the plasma; therefore, the second equation is used more often than the first (Emmett & Szerlip, 2015).

The normal value for an anion gap is 8 to 12 mEq/L (8 to 12 mmol/L) without potassium in the equation. If potassium is included in the equation, the normal value for the anion gap is 12 to 16 mEq/L (12 to 16 mmol/L). The unmeasured anions in the serum normally account for less than 16 mEq/L of the anion production. A person diagnosed with metabolic acidosis is determined to have normal anion gap metabolic acidosis if the anion gap is within this normal range. An anion gap greater than 16 mEq (16 mmol/L) suggests excessive accumulation of unmeasured anions and would indicate high anion gap metabolic acidosis as the type. An anion gap occurs because not all electrolytes are measured. More anions are left unmeasured than cations. A low or negative anion gap may be attributed to hypoproteinemia. Disorders that cause a decreased or negative anion gap are less common compared to those related to an increased or high anion gap.

Pathophysiology

Normal anion gap acidosis results from the direct loss of bicarbonate, as in diarrhea, lower intestinal fistulas, ureterostomies, and the use of diuretics; early renal insufficiency; excessive administration of chloride; and the administration of parenteral nutrition without bicarbonate or bicarbonate-producing solutes (e.g., lactate). Normal anion gap acidosis is also referred to as hyperchloremic acidosis.

High anion gap acidosis results from excessive accumulation of fixed acid. If increased to 30 mEq/L (30 mmol/L) or more, then a high anion gap metabolic acidosis is present regardless of the values of pH and HCO_3^-. High anion gap occurs in ketoacidosis, lactic acidosis, the late phase of salicylate poisoning, uremia, methanol or ethylene glycol toxicity, and ketoacidosis with starvation. The hydrogen is buffered by HCO_3^-, causing the bicarbonate concentration to fall. In all of these instances, abnormally high levels of anions flood the system, increasing the anion gap above normal limits.

 Concept Mastery Alert

Metabolic acidosis is characterized by a low pH and low plasma bicarbonate concentration. Nurses need to remember that the anion gap is calculated primarily to identify the cause (pathology) of metabolic acidosis (Grossman & Porth, 2014):

	Reduced or Negative Anion Gap	Normal Anion Gap	High Anion Gap
Anion Gap Without Potassium	<8	8–12 mEq/L	>12
Anion Gap With Potassium	<12	12–16 mEq/L	>16
Clinical Significance	Hypoproteinemia	Normal anion gap metabolic acidosis	High anion gap metabolic acidosis

Clinical Manifestations

Signs and symptoms of metabolic acidosis vary with the severity of the acidosis but include headache, confusion, drowsiness, increased respiratory rate and depth, nausea, and vomiting (Blevins, 2014; Burns, 2014). Peripheral vasodilation and decreased cardiac output occur when the pH drops to less than 7. Additional physical assessment findings include decreased blood pressure, cold and clammy skin, dysrhythmias, and shock. Chronic metabolic acidosis is usually seen with chronic kidney disease.

Assessment and Diagnostic Findings

Arterial blood gas measurements are valuable in diagnosing metabolic acidosis (Fischbach & Dunning, 2015). Expected blood gas changes include a low bicarbonate level (less than 22 mEq/L) and a low pH (less than 7.35). The cardinal feature of metabolic acidosis is a decrease in the serum bicarbonate level. Hyperkalemia may accompany metabolic acidosis as a result of the shift of potassium out of the cells. Later, as the acidosis is corrected, potassium moves back into the cells and hypokalemia may occur. Hyperventilation decreases the CO_2 level as a compensatory action. Calculation of the anion gap is helpful in determining the cause of metabolic acidosis. An ECG detects dysrhythmias caused by the increased potassium.

Medical Management

Treatment is directed at correcting the metabolic imbalance (Fischbach & Dunning, 2015). If the problem results from excessive intake of chloride, treatment is aimed at eliminating the source of the chloride. When necessary, bicarbonate is given; however, the administration of sodium bicarbonate during cardiac arrest can result in paradoxical intracellular acidosis. Hyperkalemia may occur with acidosis and hypokalemia with reversal of the acidosis and subsequent movement of potassium back into the cells. Therefore, the serum potassium level is monitored closely, and hypokalemia is corrected as acidosis is reversed.

In chronic metabolic acidosis, low serum calcium levels are treated before the chronic metabolic acidosis is treated to avoid tetany resulting from an increase in pH and a decrease in ionized calcium. Alkalizing agents may be given. Treatment modalities may also include hemodialysis or peritoneal dialysis.

Acute and Chronic Metabolic Alkalosis (Base Bicarbonate Excess)

Metabolic alkalosis is a clinical disturbance characterized by a high pH (decreased H^+ concentration) and a high plasma bicarbonate concentration. It can be produced by a gain of bicarbonate or a loss of H^+ (Grossman & Porth, 2014; Rogers & McCutcheon, 2013).

Pathophysiology

A common cause of metabolic alkalosis is vomiting or gastric suction with loss of hydrogen and chloride ions. The disorder also occurs in pyloric stenosis, in which only gastric fluid is lost. Gastric fluid has an acid pH (usually 1 to 3), and loss of this highly acidic fluid increases the alkalinity of body fluids.

Other situations predisposing to metabolic alkalosis include those associated with loss of potassium, such as diuretic therapy that promotes excretion of potassium (e.g., thiazides, furosemide), and ACTH secretion (as in hyperaldosteronism and Cushing syndrome).

Hypokalemia produces alkalosis in two ways: (1) the kidneys conserve potassium, and therefore H^+ excretion increases, and (2) cellular potassium moves out of the cells into the ECF in an attempt to maintain near-normal serum levels (as potassium ions leave the cells, hydrogen ions must enter to maintain electroneutrality). Excessive alkali ingestion from antacids containing bicarbonate or from the use of sodium bicarbonate during cardiopulmonary resuscitation can also cause metabolic alkalosis.

Chronic metabolic alkalosis can occur with long-term diuretic therapy (thiazides or furosemide), villous adenoma, external drainage of gastric fluids, significant potassium depletion, cystic fibrosis, and the chronic ingestion of milk and calcium carbonate.

Clinical Manifestations

Alkalosis is primarily manifested by symptoms related to decreased calcium ionization, such as tingling of the fingers and toes, dizziness, and hypertonic muscles. The ionized fraction of serum calcium decreases in alkalosis as more calcium combines with serum proteins. Because it is the ionized fraction of serum calcium that influences neuromuscular activity, symptoms of hypocalcemia are often the predominant symptoms of alkalosis. Respirations are depressed as a compensatory action by the lungs. Atrial tachycardia may occur. As the pH increases and hypokalemia develops, ventricular disturbances may occur. Decreased motility and paralytic ileus may also be evident.

Symptoms of chronic metabolic alkalosis are the same as for acute metabolic alkalosis, and as potassium decreases, frequent premature ventricular contractions or U waves are seen on the ECG.

Assessment and Diagnostic Findings

Evaluation of arterial blood gases reveals a pH greater than 7.45 and a serum bicarbonate concentration greater than 26 mEq/L. The $PaCO_2$ increases as the lungs attempt to compensate for the excess bicarbonate by retaining CO_2 (Emmett, 2014). This hypoventilation is more pronounced in semiconscious, unconscious, or debilitated patients than in alert patients. The former may develop marked hypoxemia as a result of hypoventilation. Hypokalemia may accompany metabolic alkalosis.

Urine chloride levels may help identify the cause of metabolic alkalosis if the patient's history provides inadequate information. Metabolic alkalosis is the setting in which urine chloride concentration may be a more accurate estimate of fluid volume than the urine sodium concentration (Emmett, 2014). Urine chloride concentrations help to differentiate between vomiting, diuretic therapy, and excessive adrenocorticosteroid secretion as the cause of the metabolic alkalosis. In patients with vomiting or cystic fibrosis, those receiving nutritional repletion, and those receiving diuretic therapy, hypovolemia and hypochloremia produce urine chloride concentrations lower than 25 mEq/L. Signs of hypovolemia are not present, and the urine chloride concentration exceeds 40 mEq/L in patients with mineralocorticoid excess or alkali loading; these patients usually have expanded fluid volume. The urine chloride concentration should be less than 15 mEq/L when decreased chloride levels and hypovolemia occur.

Medical Management

Treatment of both acute and chronic metabolic alkalosis is aimed at correcting the underlying acid–base disorder (Fischbach & Dunning, 2015). Because of volume depletion from GI loss, the patient's I&O must be monitored carefully.

Sufficient chloride must be available for the kidney to absorb sodium with chloride (allowing the excretion of excess bicarbonate). Treatment includes restoring normal fluid volume by administering sodium chloride fluids (because continued volume depletion perpetuates the alkalosis). In patients with hypokalemia, potassium is given as KCl to replace both K^+ and Cl^- losses. H_2 receptor antagonists, such as cimetidine (Tagamet), reduce the production of gastric hydrogen cloride (HCl), thereby decreasing the metabolic alkalosis associated with gastric suction. Carbonic anhydrase inhibitors are useful in treating metabolic alkalosis in patients who cannot tolerate rapid volume expansion (e.g., patients with heart failure).

Acute and Chronic Respiratory Acidosis (Carbonic Acid Excess)

Respiratory acidosis is a clinical disorder in which the pH is less than 7.35 and the $PaCO_2$ is greater than 42 mm Hg and a compensatory increase in the plasma HCO_3 occurs. It may be either acute or chronic.

Pathophysiology

Respiratory acidosis is always owing to inadequate excretion of CO_2 with inadequate ventilation, resulting in elevated plasma CO_2 concentrations and, consequently, increased levels of carbonic acid. In addition to an elevated $PaCO_2$, hypoventilation usually causes a decrease in PaO_2 (Rogers & McCutcheon, 2013). Acute respiratory acidosis occurs in emergency situations, such as acute pulmonary edema, aspiration of a foreign object, atelectasis, pneumothorax, and overdose of sedatives, as well as in nonemergent situations, such as sleep apnea associated with morbid obesity and administration of oxygen to a patient with chronic hypercapnia (excessive CO_2 in the blood), severe pneumonia, and acute respiratory distress syndrome. Respiratory acidosis can also occur in diseases that impair respiratory muscles, such as muscular dystrophy, multiple sclerosis, myasthenia gravis, and Guillain–Barré syndrome. Mechanical ventilation may be associated with hypercapnia if the rate of ventilation is inadequate and CO_2 retained.

Clinical Manifestations

Clinical signs in acute and chronic respiratory acidosis vary. Sudden hypercapnia (elevated $PaCO_2$) can cause increased pulse and respiratory rate, increased blood pressure, men-

tal cloudiness or confusion, and a feeling of fullness in the head, or a decrease in the level of consciousness. An elevated $PaCO_2$, greater than 60 mm Hg, causes cerebrovascular vasodilation and increased cerebral blood flow. Ventricular fibrillation may be the first sign of respiratory acidosis in anesthetized patients.

If respiratory acidosis is severe, intracranial pressure may increase, resulting in papilledema and dilated conjunctival blood vessels. Hyperkalemia may result as the hydrogen concentration overwhelms the compensatory mechanisms and H^+ moves into cells, causing a shift of potassium out of the cell.

Chronic respiratory acidosis occurs with pulmonary diseases such as chronic emphysema and bronchitis, obstructive sleep apnea, and obesity. As long as the $PaCO_2$ does not exceed the body's ability to compensate, the patient will be asymptomatic. However, if the $PaCO_2$ increases rapidly, cerebral vasodilation will increase the intracranial pressure, and cyanosis and tachypnea will develop. Patients with chronic obstructive pulmonary disease (COPD) who gradually accumulate CO_2 over a prolonged period (days to months) may not develop symptoms of hypercapnia because compensatory renal changes have had time to occur.

> ### Quality and Safety Nursing Alert
>
> If the $PaCO_2$ is chronically greater than 50 mm Hg, the respiratory center becomes relatively insensitive to CO_2 as a respiratory stimulant, leaving hypoxemia as the major drive for respiration. Oxygen administration may remove the stimulus of hypoxemia, and the patient develops "carbon dioxide narcosis" unless the situation is quickly reversed. Therefore, oxygen is given only with extreme caution.

Assessment and Diagnostic Findings

Arterial blood gas analysis reveals a pH less than 7.35, a $PaCO_2$ greater than 42 mm Hg, and a variation in the bicarbonate level, depending on the duration of the acute respiratory acidosis. When compensation (renal retention of bicarbonate) has fully occurred, the arterial pH is within the lower limits of normal. Depending on the cause of respiratory acidosis, other diagnostic measures include monitoring of serum electrolyte levels, chest x-ray for determining any respiratory disease, and a drug screen if an overdose is suspected. An ECG to identify any cardiac involvement as a result of COPD may be indicated as well.

Medical Management

Treatment is directed at improving ventilation; exact measures vary with the cause of inadequate ventilation (Burns, 2014; Rogers & McCutcheon, 2013). Pharmacologic agents are used as indicated. For example, bronchodilators help reduce bronchial spasm, antibiotics are used for respiratory infections, and thrombolytics or anticoagulants are used for pulmonary emboli (see Chapter 21).

Pulmonary hygiene measures are initiated, when necessary, to clear the respiratory tract of mucus and purulent drainage. Adequate hydration (2 to 3 L/day) is indicated to keep the mucous membranes moist and thereby facilitate the removal of secretions. Supplemental oxygen is given as necessary.

Mechanical ventilation, used appropriately, may improve pulmonary ventilation (Burns, 2014; Rogers & McCutcheon, 2013). Inappropriate mechanical ventilation (e.g., increased dead space, insufficient rate or volume settings, high fraction of inspired oxygen [FiO2] with excessive CO2 production) may cause such rapid excretion of CO2 that the kidneys are unable to eliminate excess bicarbonate quickly enough to prevent alkalosis and seizures. For this reason, the elevated PaCO2 must be decreased slowly. Placing the patient in a semi-Fowler position facilitates expansion of the chest wall.

Treatment of chronic respiratory acidosis is the same as for acute respiratory acidosis.

Acute and Chronic Respiratory Alkalosis (Carbonic Acid Deficit)

Respiratory alkalosis is a clinical condition in which the arterial pH is greater than 7.45 and the PaCO2 is less than 38 mm Hg. As with respiratory acidosis, acute and chronic conditions can occur (Rogers & McCutcheon, 2013).

Pathophysiology

Respiratory alkalosis is always caused by hyperventilation, which causes excessive "blowing off" of CO2 and, hence, a decrease in the plasma carbonic acid concentration. Causes include extreme anxiety, hypoxemia, early phase of salicylate intoxication, gram-negative bacteremia, and inappropriate ventilator settings.

Chronic respiratory alkalosis results from chronic hypocapnia, and decreased serum bicarbonate levels are the consequence. Chronic hepatic insufficiency and cerebral tumors are predisposing factors.

Clinical Manifestations

Clinical signs consist of lightheadedness due to vasoconstriction and decreased cerebral blood flow, inability to concentrate, numbness and tingling from decreased calcium ionization, tinnitus, and sometimes loss of consciousness. Cardiac effects of respiratory alkalosis include tachycardia and ventricular and atrial dysrhythmias.

Assessment and Diagnostic Findings

Analysis of arterial blood gases assists in the diagnosis of respiratory alkalosis (Burns, 2014; Rogers & McCutcheon, 2013). In the acute state, the pH is elevated above normal as a result of a low PaCO2 and a normal bicarbonate level (Rogers & McCutcheon, 2013). (The kidneys cannot alter the bicarbonate level quickly.) In the compensated state, the kidneys have had sufficient time to lower the bicarbonate level to a near-normal level. Evaluation of serum electrolytes is indicated to identify any decrease in potassium, as hydrogen is pulled out of the cells in exchange for potassium; decreased calcium, as severe alkalosis inhibits calcium ionization, resulting in carpopedal spasms and tetany; or decreased phosphate due to alkalosis, causing an increased uptake of phosphate by the cells. A toxicology screen should be performed to rule out salicylate intoxication.

Patients with chronic respiratory alkalosis are usually asymptomatic, and the diagnostic evaluation and plan of care are the same as for acute respiratory alkalosis.

Medical Management

Treatment depends on the underlying cause of respiratory alkalosis. If the cause is anxiety, the patient is instructed to breathe more slowly to allow CO2 to accumulate or to breathe into a closed system (such as a paper bag). An antianxiety agent may be required to relieve hyperventilation in very anxious patients. Treatment of other causes of respiratory alkalosis is directed at correcting the underlying problem.

Mixed Acid–Base Disorders

Patients can simultaneously experience two or more independent acid–base disorders. A normal pH in the presence of changes in the PaCO2 and plasma HCO3- concentration immediately suggests a mixed disorder. An example of a mixed disorder is the simultaneous occurrence of metabolic acidosis and respiratory acidosis during respiratory and cardiac arrest. The only mixed disorder that cannot occur is a mixed respiratory acidosis and alkalosis, because it is impossible to have alveolar hypoventilation and hyperventilation at the same time.

Compensation

Generally, the pulmonary and renal systems compensate for each other to return the pH to normal. In a single acid–base disorder, the system not causing the problem tries to compensate by returning the ratio of bicarbonate to carbonic acid to the normal 20:1. The lungs compensate for metabolic disturbances by changing CO2 excretion. The kidneys compensate for respiratory disturbances by altering bicarbonate retention and H+ secretion.

In respiratory acidosis, excess hydrogen is excreted in the urine in exchange for bicarbonate ions. In respiratory alkalosis, the renal excretion of bicarbonate increases, and hydrogen ions are retained. In metabolic acidosis, the compensatory mechanisms increase the ventilation rate and the renal retention of bicarbonate. In metabolic alkalosis, the respiratory system compensates by decreasing ventilation to conserve CO2 and increase the PaCO2. Because the lungs respond to acid–base disorders within minutes, compensation for metabolic imbalances occurs faster than compensation for respiratory imbalances. Table 13-12 summarizes compensation effects.

Blood Gas Analysis

Blood gas analysis is often used to identify the specific acid–base disturbance and the degree of compensation that has occurred. The analysis is usually based on an arterial blood sample; however, if an arterial sample cannot be obtained, a mixed venous sample may be used. Results of arterial blood gas analysis provide information about alveolar ventilation, oxygenation, and acid–base balance. It is necessary to evaluate the concentrations of serum electrolytes (sodium, potassium, and chloride) and CO2 along with arterial blood gas data, because they are often the first sign of an acid–base disorder. The health history, physical examination, previous blood gas results, and serum electrolytes should always be part of the assessment used

TABLE 13-12 Acid–Base Disorders and Compensation

Acid–Base Imbalance	Primary Disturbance	Respiratory Compensation and Predicted Response[a]	Renal Compensation and Predicted Response[a, b]
Metabolic acidosis	↓pH and HCO_3^- HCO_3^- <22 mEq/L	↑ventilation and ↓PCO_2 1 mEq/L ↓HCO_3^- → 1 to 1.2 mm Hg ↓PCO_2	↑H^+ excretion and ↑HCO_3^- reabsorption if no renal disease
Metabolic alkalosis	↑pH and HCO_3^- HCO_3^- >26 mEq/L	↓ventilation and ↑PCO_2 1 mEq/L ↑HCO_3^- → 0.7 mm Hg ↑PCO_2	↓H^+ excretion and ↓HCO_3^- reabsorption if no renal disease
Respiratory acidosis	↓pH and ↑PCO_2 PCO_2 >45 mm Hg	None	↑H^+ excretion and ↑HCO_3^- reabsorption *Acute: 1 mm Hg ↑PCO_2 → 0.1 mEq/L ↑HCO_3^-* *Chronic: 1 mm Hg ↑PCO_2 → 0.3 mEq/L ↑HCO_3^-*
Respiratory alkalosis	↑pH and ↓PCO_2 PCO_2 <35 mm Hg	None	↓H^+ excretion and ↓HCO_3^- reabsorption *Acute: 1 mm Hg ↓PCO_2 → 0.2 mEq/L ↓HCO_3^-* *Chronic: 1 mm Hg ↓PCO_2 → 0.4 mEq/L ↓HCO_3^-*

Note: Predicted compensatory responses are in *italics*.

[a]If blood values are the same as predicted compensatory values, a single acid–base disorder is present; if values are different, a mixed acid–base disorder is present. (Androgue H. J., Gennari F. J., Galla J. H., et al. [2009]. Assessing acid–base disorders. *Kidney International 76*, 1239–1247. doi: 10.1038/ki.2009.359.)

[b]Acute renal compensation refers to duration of minutes to several hours; chronic renal compensation refers to a duration of several days. (Androgue H. J., Gennari F. J., Galla J. H., et al. [2009]. Assessing acid–base disorders. *Kidney International 76*, 1239–1247. doi: 10.1038/ki.2009.359.)

Reprinted with permission from Grossman, S. C., & Porth, C. M. (2014). *Porth's pathophysiology: Concepts of altered health states* (9th ed.). Philadelphia, PA: Lippincott Williams & Wilkins.

to determine the cause of the acid–base disorder (Grossman & Porth, 2014). Responding to isolated sets of blood gas results without these data can lead to serious errors in interpretation. Treatment of the underlying condition usually corrects most acid–base disorders. Table 13-13 compares normal ranges of venous and arterial blood gas values. See also Chart 13-3.

PARENTERAL FLUID THERAPY

When no other route of administration is available, fluids are given by IV in hospitals, outpatient diagnostic and surgical settings, clinics, and homes to replace fluids, administer medications, and provide nutrients.

Purpose

The choice of an IV solution depends on the purpose of its administration (Gallagher & Vacchiano, 2014; McClelland,

TABLE 13-13 Normal Values for Arterial and Mixed Venous Bloods

Parameter	Arterial Blood	Mixed Venous Blood
pH	7.35–7.45	7.32–7.42
PCO_2	35–45 mm Hg	38–52 mm Hg
PO_2[a]	>80 mm Hg	24–48 mm Hg
HCO_3^-	22–26 mEq/L	19–25 mEq/L
Base excess/deficit	±2 mEq/L	±5 mEq/L
Oxygen saturation (SaO_2%)	>94%	65%–75%

[a]At altitudes of 3000 ft and higher; age dependent.

Adapted from Fischbach, F., & Dunning, M. B. (2015). *A manual of laboratory and diagnostic tests* (9th ed.). Philadelphia, PA: Lippincott Williams & Wilkins.

2014; Wunderlich, 2013). Generally, IV fluids are given to achieve one or more of the following goals:

- To provide water, electrolytes, and nutrients to meet daily requirements
- To replace water and correct electrolyte deficits
- To administer medications and blood products

IV solutions contain dextrose or electrolytes mixed in various proportions with water. Pure, electrolyte-free water can never be given by IV because it rapidly enters red blood cells and causes them to rupture.

Types of Intravenous Solutions

Solutions are often categorized as **isotonic**, **hypotonic**, or **hypertonic**, according to whether their total osmolality is the same as, less than, or greater than that of blood, respectively (see earlier discussion of osmolality). Electrolyte solutions are considered isotonic if the total electrolyte content (anions + cations) is between 250 and 375 mEq/L, hypotonic if the total electrolyte content is less than 250 mEq/L, and hypertonic if the total electrolyte content is greater than 375 mEq/L. The nurse must also consider a solution's osmolality, keeping in mind that the osmolality of plasma is approximately 300 mOsm/L (300 mmol/L). For example, a 10% dextrose solution has an osmolality of approximately 505 mOsm/L.

Isotonic Fluids

Fluids that are classified as isotonic have a total osmolality close to that of the ECF and do not cause red blood cells to shrink or swell. The composition of these fluids may or may not approximate that of the ECF. Isotonic fluids expand the ECF volume. One liter of isotonic fluid expands the ECF by 1 L; however, it expands the plasma by only 0.25 L because it is a crystalloid fluid and diffuses quickly into the ECF compartment. For the same reason, 3 L of isotonic fluid is needed to replace 1 L of blood loss. Because these fluids expand the

Chart 13-3 ASSESSMENT
Assessing for Arterial Blood Gases

The following steps are recommended to evaluate arterial blood gas values. They are based on the assumption that the average values are:

    pH = 7.4
    $PaCO_2$ = 40 mm Hg
    HCO_3^- = 24 mEq/L

1. *First, note the pH.* It can be high, low, or normal, as follows:

   A normal pH may indicate perfectly normal blood gases, *or* it may indicate a *compensated* imbalance. A compensated imbalance is one in which the body has been able to correct the pH by either respiratory or metabolic changes (depending on the primary problem). For example, a patient with primary metabolic acidosis starts out with a low bicarbonate level but a normal CO_2 level. Soon afterward, the lungs try to compensate for the imbalance by exhaling large amounts of CO_2 (hyperventilation). As another example, a patient with primary respiratory acidosis starts out with a high CO_2 level; soon afterward, the kidneys attempt to compensate by retaining bicarbonate. If the compensatory mechanism is able to restore the bicarbonate-to-carbonic acid ratio back to 20:1, full compensation (and thus normal pH) will be achieved.
   pH > 7.4 (alkalosis)
   pH < 7.4 (acidosis)
   pH = 7.4 (normal)

2. The next step is to determine the primary cause of the disturbance. This is done by evaluating the $PaCO_2$ and HCO_3^- in relation to the pH.

   Example: pH > 7.4 (alkalosis)
   a. If the $PaCO_2$ is less than 40 mm Hg, the primary disturbance is respiratory alkalosis. (This situation occurs when a patient hyperventilates and "blows off" too much CO_2. Recall that CO_2 dissolved in water becomes carbonic acid, the acid side of the "carbonic acid–bicarbonate buffer system.")
   b. If the HCO_3^- is greater than 24 mEq/L, the primary disturbance is metabolic alkalosis. (This situation occurs when the body gains too much bicarbonate, an alkaline substance. Bicarbonate is the basic or alkaline side of the "carbonic acid–bicarbonate buffer system.")

   Example: pH < 7.4 (acidosis)
   a. If the $PaCO_2$ is greater than 40 mm Hg, the primary disturbance is respiratory acidosis. (This situation occurs when a

patient hypoventilates and thus retains too much CO_2, an acidic substance.)
   b. If the HCO_3^- is less than 24 mEq/L, the primary disturbance is metabolic acidosis. (This situation occurs when the body's bicarbonate level drops, either because of direct bicarbonate loss or because of gains of acids such as lactic acid or ketones.)

3. The next step involves determining if compensation has begun. This is done by looking at the value other than the primary disorder. If it is moving in the same direction as the primary value, compensation is under way. Consider the following gases:

   The first set (1) indicates acute respiratory acidosis without compensation (the $PaCO_2$ is high, the HCO_3^- is normal). The second set (2) indicates chronic respiratory acidosis. Note that compensation has taken place—that is, the HCO_3^- has elevated to an appropriate level to balance the high $PaCO_2$ and produce a normal pH.

	pH	$PaCO_2$	HCO_3^-
(1)	7.2	60 mm Hg	24 mEq/L
(2)	7.4	60 mm Hg	37 mEq/L

4. Two distinct acid–base disturbances may occur simultaneously. These can be identified when the pH does not explain one of the changes. When the $PaCO_2$ is ↑ and the HCO_3 is ↓, respiratory acidosis and metabolic acidosis coexist. When the $PaCO_2$ is ↓ and the HCO_3 is ↑, respiratory alkalosis and metabolic alkalosis coexist.

   Example: Metabolic and respiratory acidosis

a.	pH	7.2	Decreased acid
b.	$PaCO_2$	52	Increased acid
c.	HCO_3	13	Decreased acid

5. If metabolic acidosis exists, then calculate the anion gap (AG) to determine the cause of the metabolic acidosis (AG vs. non-AG):

   $$AG = Na - (CL + HCO_3)$$
   Normal AG = 10–14 mmol/L

6. Evaluate the patient to determine if the clinical signs and symptoms are compatible with the acid–base analysis.

Adapted from Rogers, K. & McCutcheon, K. (2013). Understanding arterial blood gases. *Journal of Perioperative Practice, 23*(9), 191–197.

---

intravascular space, patients with hypertension and heart failure should be carefully monitored for signs of fluid overload.

D_5W

A solution of D_5W is unique in that it may be both isotonic and hypotonic (McClelland, 2014). Once given, the glucose is rapidly metabolized, and this initially isotonic solution (same osmolality as serum) then disperses as a hypotonic fluid—one third extracellular and two thirds intracellular. It is essential to consider this action of D_5W, especially if the patient is at risk for increased intracranial pressure. During fluid resuscitation, this solution should not be used because hyperglycemia can result. Therefore, D_5W is used mainly to supply water and to correct an increased serum osmolality. About 1 L of D_5W provides less than 170 kcal and is a minor source of the body's daily caloric requirements (McClelland, 2014).

Normal Saline Solution

Normal saline (0.9% sodium chloride) solution contains water, salt, and chloride (McClelland, 2014). Because the osmolality is entirely contributed by electrolytes, the solution remains within the ECF. For this reason, normal saline solution is often used to correct an extracellular volume deficit but is not identical to ECF. It is used with administration of blood transfusions and to replace large sodium losses, such as in burn injuries. It is not used for heart failure, pulmonary edema, renal impairment, or sodium retention. Normal saline does not supply calories.

Other Isotonic Solutions

Several other solutions contain ions in addition to sodium and chloride and are somewhat similar to the ECF in composition. Lactated Ringer solution contains potassium and calcium in addition to sodium chloride. It is used to correct dehydration and sodium depletion and replace GI losses. Lactated Ringer solution contains bicarbonate precursors as well. These solutions are marketed, with slight variations, under various trade names.

Hypotonic Fluids

One purpose of hypotonic solutions is to replace cellular fluid, because it is hypotonic compared with plasma. Another is to provide free water for excretion of body wastes. At times, hypotonic sodium solutions are used to treat hypernatremia and other hyperosmolar conditions. Half-strength saline (0.45% sodium chloride) solution is frequently used (Gallagher & Vacchiano, 2014; Wunderlich, 2013). Multiple-electrolyte solutions are also available. Excessive infusions of hypotonic solutions can lead to intravascular fluid depletion, decreased blood pressure, cellular edema, and cell damage. These solutions exert less osmotic pressure than the ECF.

Hypertonic Fluids

When normal saline solution or lactated Ringer solution contains 5% dextrose, the total osmolality exceeds that of the ECF. However, the dextrose is quickly metabolized, and only the isotonic solution remains. Therefore, any effect on the intracellular compartment is temporary. Similarly, with hypotonic multiple-electrolyte solutions containing 5% dextrose, once the dextrose is metabolized, these solutions disperse as hypotonic fluids. Higher concentrations of dextrose, such as 50% dextrose in water, are strongly hypertonic and must be given into central veins so that they can be diluted by rapid blood flow.

> ### Quality and Safety Nursing Alert
>
> *The nurse must know that solutions with higher concentrations of dextrose, such as 50% dextrose in water, are strongly hypertonic and must be given into central veins so that they can be diluted by rapid blood flow.*

Saline solutions are also available in osmolar concentrations greater than that of the ECF. These solutions draw water from the ICF to the ECF and cause cells to shrink. If given rapidly or in large quantity, they may cause an extracellular volume excess and precipitate circulatory overload and dehydration. As a result, these solutions must be given cautiously and usually only when the serum osmolality has decreased to dangerously low levels. Hypertonic solutions exert an osmotic pressure greater than that of the ECF.

Other Intravenous Therapies

When the patient is unable to tolerate food, nutritional requirements are often met using the IV route. Solutions may include high concentrations of glucose (such as 50% dextrose in water), protein, or fat to meet nutritional requirements (see Chapter 44). The IV route may also be used to administer colloids, plasma expanders, and blood products (Gallagher & Vacchiano, 2014; Wunderlich, 2013). Examples of blood products include whole blood, packed red blood cells, albumin, and cryoprecipitate (these are discussed in more detail in Chapter 33).

Many medications are also delivered by the IV route, either by continuous infusion or by intermittent bolus directly into the vein. Because IV medications enter the circulation rapidly, administration by this route is potentially hazardous. All medications can produce adverse reactions; however, medications given by the IV route can cause these reactions quickly after administration, because the medications are delivered directly into the bloodstream. Administration rates and recommended dilutions for individual medications are available in specialized texts pertaining to IV medications and in manufacturers' package inserts; these should be consulted to ensure safe IV administration of medications (Comerford, 2015).

> ### Quality and Safety Nursing Alert
>
> *The nurse must assess the patient for a history of allergic reactions to medications. Although obtaining drug allergy information is important when administering any medication, it is especially critical with IV administration, because the medication is delivered directly into the bloodstream.*

Nursing Management of the Patient Receiving Intravenous Therapy

In many settings, the ability to perform venipuncture to gain access to the venous system for administering fluids and medication is an expected nursing skill. This responsibility includes selecting the appropriate venipuncture site and type of cannula and being proficient in the technique of vein entry. The nurse should demonstrate competency in and knowledge of catheter placement according to the Nurse Practice Act applicable in their state and should follow the rules and regulations, organizational policies and procedures, and practice guidelines of that state's board of nursing (Gallagher & Vacchiano, 2014; Wunderlich, 2013).

For the procedural guidelines for starting a peripheral intravenous infusion, go to **thepoint.lww.com/Brunner14e.**

Managing Systemic Complications

Fluid Overload

Overloading the circulatory system with excessive IV fluids causes increased blood pressure and central venous pressure. Signs and symptoms of fluid overload include moist crackles on auscultation of the lungs, cough, restlessness, distended neck veins, edema, weight gain, dyspnea, and rapid, shallow respirations. Possible causes include rapid infusion of an IV solution or hepatic, cardiac, or renal disease. The risk of fluid overload and subsequent pulmonary edema is especially increased in older patients with cardiac disease; this is referred to as circulatory overload. Its treatment includes decreasing the IV rate, monitoring vital signs frequently, assessing breath sounds, and placing the patient in a high Fowler position. The primary provider is contacted immediately. This complication can be avoided by using an infusion pump and by carefully monitoring all infusions. Complications of circulatory overload include heart failure and pulmonary edema.

Air Embolism

The risk of air embolism is rare but ever-present. It is most often associated with cannulation of central veins and directly related to the size of the embolus and the rate of entry. Air entering into central veins gets to the right ventricle, where it lodges against the pulmonary valve and blocks the flow of blood from the ventricle into the pulmonary arteries. Manifestations of air embolism include palpitations, dyspnea, continued coughing, jugular venous distension, wheezing, and cyanosis; hypotension; weak, rapid pulse; altered mental status; and chest, shoulder, and low back pain. Treatment calls for immediately clamping the cannula and replacing a leaking or open infusion system, placing the patient on the left side in the Trendelenburg position, assessing vital signs and breath sounds, and administering oxygen. Air embolism can be prevented by using locking adapters on all lines, filling all tubing completely with solution, and using an air detection alarm on an IV infusion pump. Complications of air embolism include shock and death. The amount of air necessary to induce death in humans is not known; however, the rate of entry is probably as important as the actual volume of air.

Infection

Pyogenic substances in either the infusion solution or the IV administration set can cause bloodstream infections. Signs and symptoms include an abrupt temperature elevation shortly after the infusion is started, backache, headache, increased pulse and respiratory rate, nausea and vomiting, diarrhea, chills and shaking, and general malaise. Additional symptoms include erythema, edema, and induration or drainage at the insertion site. In severe sepsis, vascular collapse and septic shock may occur. (See Chapter 14 for a discussion of septic shock.)

Infection ranges in severity from local involvement of the insertion site to systemic dissemination of organisms through the bloodstream, as in sepsis. Measures to prevent infection are essential at the time the IV line is inserted and throughout the entire infusion. Prevention includes the following:

- Performing careful hand hygiene before every contact with any part of the infusion system or the patient
- Examining the IV containers for cracks, leaks, or cloudiness, which may indicate a contaminated solution
- Using strict aseptic technique
- Firmly anchoring the IV cannula to prevent to-and-fro motion (e.g., a catheter stabilization device will help). Sutureless securement devices avoid disruption around the catheter entry site and may decrease the degree of bacterial contamination
- Inspecting the IV site daily and replacing a soiled or wet dressing with a dry sterile dressing (antimicrobial agents that should be used for site care include 2% tincture of iodine, 10% povidone–iodine, alcohol, or chlorhexidine gluconate, used alone or in combination)
- Disinfecting injection/access ports with antimicrobial solution before and after each use
- Removing the IV cannula at the first sign of local inflammation, contamination, or complication
- Replacing the peripheral IV cannula according to agency policy and procedure
- Replacing the IV cannula inserted during emergency conditions (with questionable asepsis) as soon as possible
- Using a 0.2-μm air-eliminating and bacteria/particulate retentive filter with non–lipid-containing solutions that require filtration. The filter can be added to the proximal or distal end of the administration set. If added to the proximal end between the fluid container and the tubing spike, the filter ensures sterility and particulate removal from the infusate container and prevents inadvertent infusion of air. If added to the distal end of the administration set, it filters air particles and contaminants introduced from add-on devices, secondary administration sets, or interruptions to the primary system. Filters should be located as close to the catheter insertion site as possible and changed to coincide with administration set changes (Infusion Nurses Society [INS], 2011)
- Replacing the solution bag and administration set in accordance with agency policy and procedure (Wunderlich, 2013)
- Infusing or discarding medication or solution within 24 hours of its addition to an administration set
- Changing primary and secondary continuous administration sets according to agency policy and procedure, or immediately if contamination is suspected
- Using administration sets with a twist-lock design

Managing Local Complications

Local complications of IV therapy include infiltration and extravasation, phlebitis, thrombophlebitis, hematoma, and clotting of the needle (INS, 2011).

Infiltration and Extravasation

Infiltration is the unintentional administration of a nonvesicant solution or medication into surrounding tissue. This can occur when the IV cannula dislodges or perforates the wall of the vein. Infiltration is characterized by edema around the insertion site, leakage of IV fluid from the insertion site, discomfort and coolness in the area of infiltration, and a significant decrease in the flow rate. When the solution is particularly irritating, sloughing of tissue may result. Close monitoring of the insertion site is necessary to detect infiltration before it becomes severe.

Infiltration is usually easily recognized if the insertion area is larger than the same site of the opposite extremity but is not always so obvious. A common misconception is that a backflow of blood into the tubing proves that the catheter is properly placed within the vein. However, if the catheter tip has pierced the wall of the vessel, IV fluid will seep into tissues and flow into the vein. Although blood return occurs, infiltration may have occurred as well. A more reliable means of confirming infiltration is to apply a tourniquet above (or proximal to) the infusion site and tighten it enough to restrict venous flow. If the infusion continues to drip despite the venous obstruction, infiltration is present.

As soon as the nurse detects infiltration, the infusion should be stopped, the IV catheter discontinued, and a sterile dressing applied to the site after careful inspection to determine the extent of infiltration. The infiltration of any amount of blood product, irritant, or vesicant is considered the most severe.

The IV infusion should be started in a new site or proximal to the infiltration site if the same extremity must be

Chart 13-4 ASSESSMENT

Assessing for Infiltration

Grade	Clinical Criteria
0	No clinical symptoms
1	Skin blanched, edema less than 1 inch in any direction, cool to touch, with or without pain
2	Skin blanched, edema 1 to 6 inches in any direction, cool to touch, with or without pain
3	Skin blanched, translucent, gross edema greater than 6 inches in any direction, cool to touch, mild to moderate pain, possible numbness
4	Skin blanched, translucent, skin tight, leaking, skin discolored, bruised, swollen, gross edema greater than 6 inches in any direction, deep pitting tissue edema, circulatory impairment, moderate to severe pain, infiltration of any amount of blood products, irritant, or vesicant

Adapted from and Infusion Nurses Society. (2011). *Infusion nursing standards of practice.* Norwood, MA: Author.

used again. A warm compress may be applied to the site if small volumes of noncaustic solutions have infiltrated over a long period, or if the solution was isotonic with a normal pH; the affected extremity should be elevated to promote the absorption of fluid. If the infiltration is recent and the solution was hypertonic or had an increased pH, a cold compress may be applied to the area. Infiltration can be detected and treated early by inspecting the site every hour for redness, pain, edema, blood return, coolness at the site, and IV fluid leaking from the IV site. Using the appropriate size and type of cannula for the vein prevents this complication. The use of EIDs does not cause an infiltration or extravasation; however, these devices will exacerbate the problem until the infusion is turned off. The Infusion Nursing Standards of Practice state that a standardized infiltration scale should be used to document the infiltration (INS, 2011) (Chart 13-4).

Extravasation is similar to infiltration, with an inadvertent administration of vesicant or irritant solution or medication into the surrounding tissue. Medications such as vasopressors, potassium and calcium preparations, and chemotherapeutic agents can cause pain, burning, and redness at the site. Blistering, inflammation, and necrosis of tissues can occur. Older patients, comatose or anesthetized patients, patients with diabetes, and patients with peripheral vascular or cardiovascular disease are at greater risk for extravasation; other risk factors include high pressure infusion pumps, palpable cording of vein, and fluid leakage from the insertion site (INS, 2011). The extent of tissue damage is determined by the concentration of the medication, the quantity that extravasated, the location of the infusion site, the tissue response, and the duration of the process of extravasation.

When extravasation occurs, the infusion must be stopped and the provider notified promptly. The agency's protocol to treat extravasation is initiated; the protocol may specify specific treatments, including antidotes specific to the medication that extravasated, and may indicate whether the IV line should remain in place or be removed before treatment. The protocol often specifies infiltration of the infusion site with an antidote prescribed after assessment by the provider,

removal of the cannula, and application of warm compresses to sites of extravasation from alkaloids or cold compresses to sites of extravasation from alkylating and antibiotic vesicants. The affected extremity should not be used for further cannula placement. Thorough neurovascular assessments of the affected extremity must be performed frequently.

Reviewing the institution's IV policy and procedures and incompatibility charts and checking with the pharmacist before administering any IV medication, whether peripherally or centrally, are recommended to determine incompatibilities and vesicant potential to prevent extravasation. Careful, frequent monitoring of the IV site, avoiding insertion of IV devices in areas of flexion, securing the IV line, and using the smallest catheter possible that accommodates the vein help minimize the incidence and severity of this complication. In addition, when vesicant medication is given by IV push, it should be given through a side port of an infusing IV solution to dilute the medication and decrease the severity of tissue damage if extravasation occurs. Extravasation is rated as grade 4 on the infiltration scale. Complications of an extravasation may include blister formation, skin sloughing and tissue necrosis, functional or sensory loss in the injured area, and disfigurement or loss of limb (INS, 2011).

Phlebitis

Phlebitis, or inflammation of a vein, can be categorized as chemical, mechanical, or bacterial; however, two or more of these types of irritation often occur simultaneously. Chemical phlebitis can be caused by an irritating medication or solution (increased pH or high osmolality of a solution), rapid infusion rates, and medication incompatibilities. Mechanical phlebitis results from long periods of cannulation, catheters in flexed areas, catheter gauges larger than the vein lumen, and poorly secured catheters. Bacterial phlebitis can develop from poor hand hygiene, lack of aseptic technique, failure to check all equipment before use, and failure to recognize early signs and symptoms of phlebitis. Other factors include poor venipuncture technique, catheter in place for a prolonged period, and failure to adequately secure the catheter. Phlebitis is characterized by a reddened, warm area around the insertion site or along the path of the vein, pain or tenderness at the site or along the vein, and swelling (Norton, Ottoboni, Varady, et al., 2013). The incidence of phlebitis increases with the length of time the IV line is in place, the composition of the fluid or medication infused (especially its pH and tonicity), catheter material, emergency insertions, the size and site of the cannula inserted, ineffective filtration, inadequate anchoring of the line, and the introduction of microorganisms at the time of insertion. The Infusion Nurses Society (INS) has identified specific standards for assessing phlebitis (INS, 2011); these appear in Chart 13-5. Phlebitis is graded according to the most severe presenting indication.

Treatment consists of discontinuing the IV line and restarting it in another site, and applying a warm, moist compress to the affected site (INS, 2011; Norton et al., 2013). Phlebitis can be prevented by using aseptic technique during insertion, using the appropriate-size cannula or needle for the vein, considering the composition of fluids and medications when selecting a site, observing the site hourly for any complications, anchoring the cannula or needle well, and changing the IV site according to agency policy and procedures.

Grade	Clinical Criteria
0	No clinical symptoms
1	Erythema at access site with or without pain
2	Pain at access site Erythema, edema, or both
3	Pain at access site Erythema, edema, or both Streak formation Palpable venous cord (1 in or shorter)
4	Pain at access site with erythema Streak formation Palpable venous cord (longer than 1 in) Purulent drainage

Adapted from Infusion Nurses Society. (2011). *Infusion nursing standards of practice.* Norwood, MA: Author; Norton, L., Ottoboni, L. K., Varady, A., et al. (2013) Phlebitis in Amiodarone administration: Incidence, contributing factors, and clinical implications. *American Journal of Critical Care, 22*(6), 498–505.

Thrombophlebitis

Thrombophlebitis refers to the presence of a clot plus inflammation in the vein. It is evidenced by localized pain, redness, warmth, and swelling around the insertion site or along the path of the vein, immobility of the extremity because of discomfort and swelling, sluggish flow rate, fever, malaise, and leukocytosis.

Treatment includes discontinuing the IV infusion; applying a cold compress first to decrease the flow of blood and increase platelet aggregation, followed by a warm compress; elevating the extremity; and restarting the line in the opposite extremity. If the patient has signs and symptoms of thrombophlebitis, the IV line should not be flushed (although flushing may be indicated in the absence of phlebitis to ensure cannula patency and to prevent mixing of incompatible medications and solutions). The catheter should be cultured after the skin around the catheter is cleaned with alcohol. If purulent drainage exists, the site is cultured before the skin is cleaned.

Thrombophlebitis can be prevented by avoiding trauma to the vein at the time the IV line is inserted, observing the site every hour, and checking medication additives for compatibility.

Hematoma

Hematoma results when blood leaks into tissues surrounding the IV insertion site. Leakage can result if the opposite vein wall is perforated during venipuncture, the needle slips out of the vein, a cannula is too large for the vessel, or insufficient pressure is applied to the site after removal of the needle or cannula. The signs of a hematoma include ecchymosis, immediate swelling at the site, and leakage of blood at the insertion site.

Treatment includes removing the needle or cannula and applying light pressure with a sterile, dry dressing; applying ice for 24 hours to the site to avoid extension of the hematoma; elevating the extremity to maximize venous return, if tolerated; assessing the extremity for any circulatory, neurologic, or motor dysfunction; and restarting the line in the other extremity if indicated. A hematoma can be prevented by carefully inserting the needle and by using diligent care

with patients who have a bleeding disorder, are taking anticoagulant medication, or have advanced liver disease.

Clotting and Obstruction

Blood clots may form in the IV line as a result of kinked IV tubing, a very slow infusion rate, an empty IV bag, or failure to flush the IV line after intermittent medication or solution administrations. The signs are decreased flow rate and blood backflow into the IV tubing.

If blood clots in the IV line, the infusion must be discontinued and restarted in another site with a new cannula and administration set. The tubing should not be irrigated or milked. Neither the infusion rate nor the solution container should be raised, and the clot should not be aspirated from the tubing. Clotting of the needle or cannula may be prevented by not allowing the IV solution bag to run dry, taping the tubing to prevent kinking and maintain patency, maintaining an adequate flow rate, and flushing the line after intermittent medication or other solution administration. In some cases, a specially trained nurse or physician may inject a thrombolytic agent into the catheter to clear an occlusion resulting from fibrin or clotted blood.

Promoting Home, Community-Based, and Transitional Care

 Educating Patients About Self-Care

At times, IV therapy must be given in the home setting, in which case much of the daily management rests with the patient and family. Education becomes essential to ensure that the patient and family can manage the IV fluid and infusion correctly and avoid complications. Written instructions as well as demonstration and return demonstration help reinforce the key points for all of these functions.

Continuing and Transitional Care

Home infusion therapies cover a wide range of treatments, including antibiotic, analgesic, and antineoplastic medications; blood or blood component therapy; and parenteral nutrition. When direct nursing care is necessary, arrangements are made to have an infusion nurse visit the home and administer the IV therapy as prescribed. In addition to implementing and monitoring the IV therapy, the nurse carries out a comprehensive assessment of the patient's condition and continues to educate the patient and family about the skills involved in overseeing the IV therapy setup. Any dietary changes that may be necessary because of fluid or electrolyte imbalances are explained or reinforced during such sessions.

Periodic laboratory testing may be necessary to assess the effects of IV therapy and the patient's progress. Blood specimens may be obtained by a laboratory near the patient's home, or a home visit may be arranged to obtain blood specimens for analysis.

The nurse collaborates with the case manager in assessing the patient, family, and home environment; developing a plan of care in accordance with the patient's treatment plan and level of ability; and arranging for appropriate referral and follow-up if necessary. Any necessary equipment may be provided by the agency or purchased by the patient, depending on the terms of the home care arrangements. Appropriate documentation is necessary to assist in obtaining third-party payment for the service provided.

CRITICAL THINKING EXERCISES

1 **ebp** You are caring for an 84-year-old patient with chronic kidney disease. You have been given orders to start an IV on the patient after receiving lab results indicating hypocalcemia. What is the best evidence for appropriate treatment in the event of severe hypocalcemia? Which nursing interventions and precautions should you implement for this patient when administering the IV medication? Give your rationale. What will you include in discharge teaching for this patient?

2 A 72-year-old man has been admitted to the hospital. He is confused and unable to give any information. Vital signs: B/P 122/56 sitting and 102/46 standing; HR 84/min, RR 12/min. Serum sodium levels indicate that this patient has hyponatremia. What other electrolyte values will you consider? What are the causes of hyponatremia? What will you include in your assessment of this patient? Give your rationale. What special considerations are needed for this patient because he is an older adult? Give your rationale.

3 **pq** A 54-year-old man is sent to the ED by his primary provider. The patient has a history of congestive heart failure and chronic obstructive pulmonary disease. The physician has requested laboratory tests. Blood gas results are as follows: pH 7.28; HCO_3- 26; $PaCO_2$ 55 mm Hg. Blood chemistry results are as follows: potassium 4.5 mEq/L; sodium 140 mEq/L; glucose 110 mg/dL. Vital signs: B/P 140/92, HR 90/min, RR 18/min. What is your priority for this patient? Give your rationale. What further diagnostic testing is needed? Give your rationale. What is the rationale for not administering oxygen therapy to this patient immediately?

REFERENCES

*Asterisk indicates nursing research.

Books

Androgue, H. J., Gennari, F. J., Galla, J. H., et al. (2009). Assessing acid-base disorders. *Kidney International 76*, 1239–1247. doi: 10.1038/ki.2009.359

Cash, J., & Glass, C. (2015). *Adult gerontology practice guidelines*. New York, NY: Springer.

Comerford, K. C. (2015). *Nursing 2015 drug handbook*. Philadelphia, PA: Wolters Kluwer.

Dudek, S. G. (2013). *Nutrition essentials for nursing practice* (7th ed.). Philadelphia, PA: Lippincott Williams & Wilkins.

Fischbach, F., & Dunning, M. B. (2015). *A manual of laboratory and diagnostic tests* (9th ed.). Philadelphia, PA: Lippincott Williams & Wilkins.

Frandsen, G., & Pennington, S. (2014). *Abrams' clinical drug therapy: Rationales for nursing practice* (10th ed.). Philadelphia, PA: Lippincott Williams & Wilkins.

Grossman, S. C., & Porth, C. M. (2014). *Porth's pathophysiology: Concepts of altered health states* (9th ed.). Philadelphia, PA: Lippincott Williams & Wilkins.

Hall, J. E. (2015). *Guyton & Hall textbook of medical physiology* (13th ed.). Philadelphia, PA: Saunders Elsevier.

Infusion Nurses Society. (2011). *Infusion nursing standards of practice*. Norwood, MA: Author.

Papadakis, M. A., & McPhee, S. J. (Eds.). (2016). *Current medical diagnosis and treatment* (55th ed.). New York, NY: McGraw-Hill.

Weber, J., & Kelley, J. (2014). *Health assessment in nursing* (5th ed.). Philadelphia, PA: Lippincott Williams & Wilkins.

Journals and Electronic Documents

Bichet, D., (2013). Treatment of central diabetes insipidus. UpToDate. Retrieved on 02/10/2016 at: www.uptodate.com.

Blevins, S. (2014). Making ABG's simple. *MedSurg Nursing, 23*(3), 185–186.

Bullock, B. A., & Henze, R. J. (2000). *Focus on pathophysiology* (p. 173). Philadelphia, PA: Lippincott Williams & Wilkins.

Burns, G. (2014). Arterial blood gases made easy. *Clinical Medicine, 14*(1), 66–68.

Colucci, W., & Chen, H. (2014). Natriuretic peptide measurement in heart failure. UpToDate. Retrieved on 02/10/2016 at: www.uptodate.com.

*Diacon, A., & Bell, J. (2014). Investigating the recording and accuracy of fluid balance monitoring in critically ill patients. *South African Journal of Critical Care, 30*(2), 55–57.

Earhart, E., Weiss, E., Rahman, R., et al. (2015). Effects of oral sodium supplementation on thermoregulation in trained, endurance athletes. *Journal of Sports Science and Medicine, 14*(1), 172–178.

Emmett, M. (2014). Simple and mixed acid–base disorders. UpToDate. Retrieved on 02/09/2016 at: www.uptodate.com.

Emmett, M., & Szerlip, H. (2015). Approach to the adult with metabolic acidosis. UpToDate. Retrieved on 02/09/2016 at: www.uptodate.com.

Gallagher, K., & Vacchiano, C. (2014). Reexamining traditional intraoperative fluid administration: Evolving views in the age of goal-directed therapy. *AANA Journal, 82*(3), 235–242.

Goltzman, D. (2014). Etiology of hypocalcemia in adults. UpToDate. Retrieved on 02/10/2016 at: www.uptodate.com.

Goltzman, D. (2015a). Clinical manifestations of hypocalcemia. UpToDate. Retrieved on 02/10/2016 at: www.uptodate.com.

Goltzman, D. (2015b). Treatment for hypocalcemia. UpToDate. Retrieved on 02/10/2016 at: www.uptodate.com.

Inker, L., & Perrone, R., (2014). Assessment of kidney function. UpToDate. Retrieved on 02/09/2016 at: www.uptodate.com.

Kresevic, D. M. (2015). Reducing functional decline in hospitalized older adults. *American Nurse Today, 10*(5), S8–S10.

Maggs, F. (2014). The management of patients presenting with hypernatremia: Is aggressive management appropriate? *Clinical Practice, 14*(3), 260–263.

McClelland, M. (2014). IV therapies for patients with fluid and electrolyte imbalances. *MedSurg Matters, 23*(5), S4–S8.

McGloin, S. (2015). The ins and outs of fluid balance in the acutely ill patient. *British Journal of Nursing, 24*(1), 14–18.

Mount, D. B. (2014a). Causes and evaluation of hyperkalemia in adults. UpToDate. Retrieved on 02/10/2016 at: www.uptodate.com.

Mount, D. B. (2014b). Clinical manifestations and treatment of hypokalemia in adults. In R. (Ed.). *UpToDate*. Retrieved on 02/10/2016 at: www.uptodate.com.

Mount, D. B. (2014c). Treatment and prevention of hyperkalemia in adults. In R. Sterns (Ed.). *UpToDate*. Retrieved on 02/10/2016 at: www.uptodate.com.

Norton, L., Ottoboni, L. K., Varady, A., et al. (2013) Phlebitis in Amiodarone administration: Incidence, contributing factors, and clinical implications. *American Journal of Critical Care, 22*(6), 498–505.

Rhoades, R. A., & Bell, D. R. (Eds.) (2009). *Medical physiology: Principles for clinical medicine* (3rd ed., p. 445). Philadelphia, PA: Lippincott Williams & Wilkins.

Rogers, K., & McCutcheon, K. (2013). Understanding arterial blood gases. *Journal of Perioperative Practice, 23*(9), 191–197.

Rosen, H. (2015). Calcium and vitamin D supplementation in osteoporosis. UpToDate. Retrieved on 02/10/2016 at: www.uptodate.com.

Sahay, M., & Sahay, R. (2014). Hyponatremia: A practical approach. *Indian Journal of Endocrinology and Metabolism, 18*(6), 760–771.

Shane, E. (2014). Diagnostic approach to hypercalcemia. UpToDate. Retrieved on 02/10/2016 at: www.uptodate.com.

Shane, E., & Berenson, J. (2015). Treatment of hypercalcemia. UpToDate. Retrieved on 02/10/2016 at: www.uptodate.com.

Sterns, R. H. (2014a). Etiology, clinical manifestations, and diagnosis of volume depletion in adults. UpToDate. Retrieved on 02/09/2016 at: www.uptodate.com.

Sterns, R. H. (2014b). Evaluation of adults with hyponatremia. UpToDate. Retrieved on 02/09/2016 at: www.uptodate.com.

Sterns, R. H. (2014c). Clinical manifestations and diagnosis of edema in adults. UpToDate. Retrieved on 02/09/2016 at: www.uptodate.com.

Sterns, R. H. (2014d). General principles of disorders of water balance (hyponatremia and hypernatremia) and sodium balance (hypovalemia and edema). UpToDate. Retrieved on 02/09/2016 at: www.uptodate.com.

Sterns, R. H. (2014e). Maintenance and replacement fluid therapy in adults. UpToDate. Retrieved on 02/09/2016 at: www.uptodate.com.

Stubbs, J., & Yu, A. (2015). Overview of the causes and treatment of hyperphosphatemia. UpToDate. Retrieved on 02/11/2016 at: www.uptodate.com.

Yu, A., & Gupta, A. (2015). Causes and treatment of hypermagnesemia. UpToDate. Retrieved on 02/11/2016 at: www.uptodate.com.

Yu, A., & Stubbs, J. (2014). Evaluation and treatment of hypophosphatemia. UpToDate. Retrieved on 02/11/2016 at: www.uptodate.com.

Wunderlich R. (2013). Principles in the selection of intravenous solutions replacement: Sodium and water balance. *Journal of Infusion Nursing,* 36(2), 126–134.

Resources

Infusion Nurses Society (INS), www.ins1.org

14 Shock and Multiple Organ Dysfunction Syndrome

LEARNING OBJECTIVES

On completion of this chapter, the learner will be able to:

1 Describe shock and its underlying pathophysiology.
2 Compare clinical findings of the compensatory, progressive, and irreversible stages of shock.
3 Describe organ dysfunction that may occur with shock.
4 Describe similarities and differences in shock due to hypovolemic, cardiogenic, neurogenic, anaphylactic, and septic shock states.
5 Identify medical and nursing management priorities in treating patients in shock.

6 Identify vasoactive medications used in treating shock, and describe nursing implications associated with their use.
7 Discuss the importance of nutritional support in all forms of shock.
8 Discuss the role of nurses in psychosocial support of patients experiencing shock and their families.
9 Identify medical and nursing management priorities in treating patients with multiple organ dysfunction syndrome.

GLOSSARY

anaphylactic shock: distributive shock state resulting from a severe allergic reaction producing an acute systemic vasodilation and relative hypovolemia
biochemical mediators: messenger substances that may be released by a cell to create an action at that site or may be carried by the bloodstream to a distant site before being activated; also called *cytokines* or *inflammatory mediators*
cardiogenic shock: shock state resulting from impairment or failure of the myocardium
colloids: intravenous solutions that contain molecules that are too large to pass through capillary membranes
crystalloids: intravenous electrolyte solutions that move freely between the intravascular compartment and interstitial spaces
distributive shock: shock state resulting from displacement of intravascular volume creating a relative hypovolemia and inadequate delivery of oxygen to the cells

hypovolemic shock: shock state resulting from decreased intravascular volume due to fluid loss
multiple organ dysfunction syndrome: presence of altered function of two or more organs in an acutely ill patient such that interventions are necessary to support continued organ function
neurogenic shock: shock state resulting from loss of sympathetic tone causing relative hypovolemia
sepsis: life-threatening organ dysfunction caused by a dysregulated host response to infection
septic shock: a subset of sepsis in which underlying circulatory and cellular metabolism abnormalities are profound enough to substantially increase mortality
shock: physiologic condition in which there is inadequate blood flow to tissues and cells of the body
systemic inflammatory response syndrome: a syndrome resulting from a clinical insult that initiates an inflammatory response that is systemic, rather than localized to the site of the insult

Shock is a life-threatening condition that results from inadequate tissue perfusion. Many conditions may cause shock; irrespective of the cause, tissue hypoperfusion prevents adequate oxygen delivery to cells, leading to cell dysfunction and death. The progression of shock is neither linear nor predictable, and shock states, especially septic shock, comprise an area of aggressive clinical research. Nurses caring for patients with shock and those at risk for shock must understand the underlying mechanisms of the various shock states (i.e., hypovolemic, cardiogenic, obstructive (see Chapter 29), neurogenic, anaphylactic, and septic) and recognize the subtle as well as more obvious signs of each of these states. Rapid assessment with early recognition and response to shock states is essential to the patient's recovery.

Overview of Shock

Shock can best be defined as a clinical syndrome that results from inadequate tissue perfusion, creating an imbalance between the delivery of oxygen and nutrients needed to support cellular function (Maier, 2015; Moore, Dyson, Singer, et al., 2015). Adequate blood flow to the tissues and cells requires an effective cardiac pump, adequate vasculature or circulatory system, and sufficient blood volume. If one of these components is impaired, perfusion to the tissues is threatened or compromised. Without treatment, inadequate blood flow to the cells results in poor delivery of oxygen and nutrients, cellular hypoxia, and cell death that progresses to organ dysfunction and eventually death.

Shock affects all body systems. It may develop rapidly or slowly, depending on the underlying cause. During shock, the body struggles to survive, calling on all its homeostatic mechanisms to restore blood flow. Any insult to the body can create a cascade of events resulting in poor tissue perfusion. Therefore, any patient with any disease state may be at risk for developing shock. The primary underlying pathophysiologic process and underlying disorder are used to classify the shock state (e.g., hypovolemic shock, cardiogenic shock, obstructive shock, distributive shock [i.e., neurogenic, anaphylactic, septic]; all discussed later in the chapter).

Regardless of the initial cause of shock, certain physiologic responses are common to all types of shock. These physiologic responses include hypoperfusion of tissues, hypermetabolism, and activation of the inflammatory response. The body responds to shock states by activating the sympathetic nervous system and mounting a hypermetabolic and inflammatory response. Failure of compensatory mechanisms to effectively restore physiologic balance is the final pathway of all shock states and results in end-organ dysfunction and death (Dellinger, Levy, Rhodes, et al., 2013; Maier, 2015; Wacker & Winters, 2014).

Nursing care of patients with shock requires ongoing systematic assessment. Many of the interventions required in caring for patients with shock call for close collaboration with other members of the health care team and rapid implementation of prescribed therapies. Nurses are in key positions to identify early signs of shock and anticipate rapid therapy.

Normal Cellular Function

Energy metabolism occurs within the cell, where nutrients are chemically broken down and stored in the form of adenosine triphosphate (ATP). Cells use this stored energy to perform necessary functions, such as active transport, muscle contraction, and biochemical synthesis, as well as specialized cellular functions, such as the conduction of electrical impulses. ATP can be synthesized aerobically (in the presence of oxygen) or anaerobically (in the absence of oxygen). Aerobic metabolism yields far greater amounts of ATP per mole of glucose than does anaerobic metabolism; therefore, it is a more efficient and effective means of producing energy. In addition, anaerobic metabolism results in the accumulation of the toxic end product lactic acid, which must be removed from the cell and transported to the liver for conversion into glucose and glycogen.

Pathophysiology

Cellular Changes

In shock, the cells lack an adequate blood supply and are deprived of oxygen and nutrients; therefore, they must produce energy through anaerobic metabolism. This results in low-energy yields from nutrients and an acidotic intracellular environment. Because of these changes, normal cell function ceases (see Fig. 14-1). The cell swells and the cell membrane becomes more permeable, allowing electrolytes and fluids to seep out of and into the cell. The sodium–potassium pump becomes impaired; cell structures, primarily the mitochondria, are damaged, and death of the cell results.

Glucose is the primary substrate required for the production of cellular energy in the form of ATP. In stress states, catecholamines, cortisol, glucagons, and inflammatory **biochemical mediators** (i.e., cytokines) are released, causing hyperglycemia and insulin resistance to mobilize glucose for cellular metabolism. Activation of these substances promotes gluconeogenesis, which is the formation of glucose from

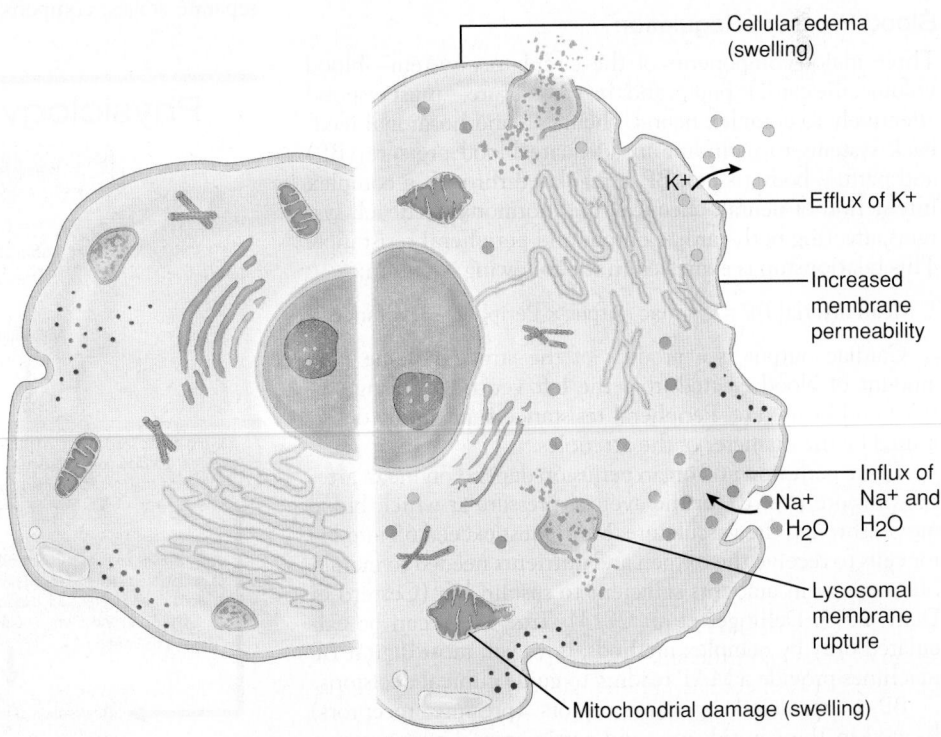

Figure 14-1 • Cellular effects of shock. The cell swells and the cell membrane becomes more permeable; fluids and electrolytes seep from and into the cell. Mitochondria and lysosomes are damaged and the cell dies.

Cellular edema (swelling)

Efflux of K⁺

Increased membrane permeability

Influx of Na⁺ and H₂O

Lysosomal membrane rupture

Mitochondrial damage (swelling)

Normal Cell   Effects of shock

noncarbohydrate sources such as proteins and fats. Glycogen that has been stored in the liver is converted to glucose through glycogenolysis to meet metabolic needs, increasing the blood glucose concentration (i.e., hyperglycemia).

Continued activation of the stress response by shock states causes a depletion of glycogen stores, resulting in increased proteolysis and eventual organ failure (Moore et al., 2015). The deficit of nutrients and oxygen for normal cellular metabolism causes a buildup of metabolic end products in the cells and interstitial spaces. The clotting cascade, also associated with the inflammatory process, becomes activated, which compounds this pathologic cycle. With significant cell injury or death caused by shock, the clotting cascade is overproductive, resulting in small clots lodging in microcirculation, further hampering cellular perfusion (Zarychanski, Abou-Setta, Kanji, et al., 2015). This upregulation of the clotting cascade further compromises microcirculation of tissues, exacerbating cellular hypoperfusion (Moore et al., 2015). Cellular metabolism is impaired, and a self-perpetuating negative situation (i.e., a positive feedback loop) is initiated.

Vascular Responses

Local regulatory mechanisms, referred to as autoregulation, stimulate vasodilation or vasoconstriction in response to biochemical mediators released by the cell, communicating the need for oxygen and nutrients (Moore et al., 2015; Zarychanski et al., 2015). A biochemical mediator is a substance released by a cell or immune cells such as macrophages; the substance triggers an action at a cell site or travels in the bloodstream to a distant site, where it triggers action. Researchers are learning more every day about the physiologic actions of numerous proinflammatory and antiinflammatory biochemical mediators that are responsible for the complex clinical presentation of shock states. (Prucha, Belligan, & Zazula, 2014).

Blood Pressure Regulation

Three major components of the circulatory system—blood volume, the cardiac pump, and the vasculature—must respond effectively to complex neural, chemical, and hormonal feedback systems to maintain an adequate blood pressure (BP) and perfuse body tissues. BP is regulated through a complex interaction of neural, chemical, and hormonal feedback systems affecting both cardiac output and peripheral resistance. This relationship is expressed in the following equation:

Mean arterial BP = Cardiac output × Peripheral resistance

Cardiac output is a product of the stroke volume (the amount of blood ejected from the left ventricle during systole) and heart rate. Peripheral resistance is primarily determined by the diameter of the arterioles.

Tissue perfusion and organ perfusion depend on mean arterial pressure (MAP), or the average pressure at which blood moves through the vasculature. MAP must exceed 65 mm Hg for cells to receive the oxygen and nutrients needed to metabolize energy in amounts sufficient to sustain life (Cestero & Dent, 2015; Dellinger et al., 2013). True MAP can be calculated only by complex methods; however, most digital BP machines provide a MAP reading to guide clinical decisions.

BP is regulated by baroreceptors (pressure receptors) located in the carotid sinus and aortic arch. These pressure receptors are responsible for monitoring the circulatory

volume and regulating neural and endocrine activities (see Chapter 31 for further description). When BP drops, catecholamines (e.g., epinephrine, norepinephrine) are released from the adrenal medulla. These increase heart rate and cause vasoconstriction, restoring BP. Chemoreceptors, also located in the aortic arch and carotid arteries, regulate BP and respiratory rate using much the same mechanism in response to changes in oxygen and carbon dioxide (CO_2) concentrations in the blood. These primary regulatory mechanisms can respond to changes in BP on a moment-to-moment basis.

The kidneys regulate BP by releasing renin, an enzyme needed for the eventual conversion of angiotensin I to angiotensin II, a potent vasoconstrictor. This stimulation of the renin–angiotensin mechanism and the resulting vasoconstriction indirectly lead to the release of aldosterone from the adrenal cortex, which promotes the retention of sodium and water (i.e., hypernatremia). Hypernatremia then stimulates the release of antidiuretic hormone (ADH) by the pituitary gland. ADH causes the kidneys to retain water further in an effort to raise blood volume and BP. These secondary regulatory mechanisms may take hours or days to respond to changes in BP. The relationship between the initiation of shock and the responsiveness of primary and secondary regulatory mechanisms that compensate for deficits in blood volume, the pumping effectiveness of the heart, or vascular tone, which may result because of the shock state, is noted in Figure 14-2.

Stages of Shock

Shock progresses along a continuum and can be identified as early or late, depending on the signs and symptoms and the overall severity of organ dysfunction. A convenient way to understand the physiologic responses and subsequent clinical signs and symptoms of shock is to divide the continuum into separate stages: compensatory (stage 1), progressive (stage 2),

Figure 14-2 • Compensatory mechanisms in shock.

and irreversible (stage 3). The earlier that interventions are initiated along this continuum, the greater the patient's chance of survival. Current research and evidence-based practice focuses on assessing patients at greatest risk for shock and implementing early and aggressive interventions to reverse tissue hypoxia (Green, 2015). Current evidence suggests that the window of opportunity that increases the likelihood of patient survival occurs when aggressive therapy begins within 3 hours of identifying a shock state, especially septic shock (Dellinger, 2015; Green, 2015; Singer, Deutschman, Seymour, et al., 2016).

Compensatory Stage

In the compensatory stage of shock, the BP remains within normal limits. Vasoconstriction, increased heart rate, and increased contractility of the heart contribute to maintaining adequate cardiac output. This results from stimulation of the sympathetic nervous system and subsequent release of catecholamines (e.g., epinephrine, norepinephrine). Patients display the often-described "fight-or-flight" response. The body shunts blood from organs such as the skin, kidneys, and gastrointestinal (GI) tract to the brain, heart, and lungs to ensure adequate blood supply to these vital organs. As a result, the skin may be cool and pale, bowel sounds are hypoactive, and urine output decreases in response to the release of aldosterone and ADH.

Clinical Manifestations

Despite a normal BP, the patient shows numerous clinical signs indicating inadequate organ perfusion (see Table 14-1). The result of inadequate perfusion is anaerobic metabolism and a buildup of lactic acid, producing metabolic acidosis. The respiratory rate increases in response to the need to increase oxygen to the cells and in compensation for metabolic acidosis. This rapid respiratory rate facilitates removal of excess CO_2 but raises the blood pH and often causes a compensatory respiratory alkalosis. The patient may experience a change in affect, feel anxious, or be confused. If treatment begins in this stage of shock, the prognosis for the patient is better than in later stages.

 Medical Management

Medical treatment is directed toward identifying the cause of the shock, correcting the underlying disorder so that shock does not progress, and supporting those physiologic processes that thus far have responded successfully to the threat. Because compensation cannot be maintained indefinitely, measures such as fluid replacement and medication therapy must be initiated to maintain an adequate BP and reestablish and maintain adequate tissue perfusion (Dellinger et al., 2013; Green, 2015).

 Nursing Management

Early intervention along the continuum of shock is the key to improving the patient's prognosis (Dellinger, 2015; Lee, 2015). The nurse must systematically assess the patient at risk for shock, recognizing subtle clinical signs of the compensatory stage before the patient's BP drops. Early interventions include identifying the cause of shock, administering intravenous (IV) fluids and oxygen, and obtaining necessary laboratory tests to rule out and treat metabolic imbalances or infection. Special considerations related to recognizing early signs of shock in the older adult patient are discussed in Chart 14-1.

Monitoring Tissue Perfusion

In assessing tissue perfusion, the nurse observes for subtle changes in level of consciousness, vital signs (including pulse pressure), urinary output, skin, respiratory rate, and laboratory values (e.g., base deficit, lactic acid levels). In the compensatory stage of shock, serum sodium and blood glucose levels are elevated in response to the release of aldosterone and catecholamines. If infection is suspected, blood cultures should be obtained prior to administration of prescribed antibiotics;

 TABLE 14-1 Clinical Findings in Stages of Shock

Finding	Stage		
	Compensatory	Progressive	Irreversible
Blood pressure	Normal	Systolic <90 mm Hg; MAP <65 mm Hg Requires fluids resuscitation to support blood pressure	Requires mechanical or pharmacologic support
Heart rate	>100 bpm	>150 bpm	Erratic
Respiratory status	>20 breaths/min $PaCO_2$ <32 mm Hg	Rapid, shallow respirations; crackles PaO_2 <80 mm Hg $PaCO_2$ >45 mm Hg	Requires intubation and mechanical ventilation and oxygenation
Skin	Cold, clammy	Mottled, petechiae	Jaundice
Urinary output	Decreased	<0.5 mL/kg/h	Anuric; requires dialysis
Mentation	Confusion and/or agitation	Lethargy	Unconscious
Acid–base balance	Respiratory alkalosis	Metabolic acidosis	Profound acidosis

MAP, mean arterial pressure; $PaCO_2$, partial pressure of arterial carbon dioxide; PaO_2, partial pressure of arterial oxygen.
Adapted from Dellinger, R. P., Levy, M. M., Rhodes, A., et al. (2013). Surviving Sepsis Campaign: International guidelines for management of severe sepsis and septic shock: 2012. *Critical Care Medicine, 41*(2), 580–637; Kleinpell, R., Aitken, L, & Schorr, C. A. (2013). Implications of the new international sepsis guidelines for nursing care. *American Journal of Critical Care, 22*(3), 212–222.

Chart 14-1 · Recognizing Shock in Older Patients

The physiologic changes associated with aging, coupled with pathologic and chronic disease states, place older adults at increased risk for developing a state of shock and possibly multiple organ dysfunction syndrome. Older adults can recover from shock if it is detected and treated early with aggressive and supportive therapies. Nurses play an essential role in assessing and interpreting subtle changes in older patients' responses to illness.

- Medications such as beta-blocking agents (metoprolol [Lopressor]) used to treat hypertension may mask tachycardia, a primary compensatory mechanism to increase cardiac output, during hypovolemic states.
- The aging immune system may not mount a truly febrile response (temperature greater than 38.3°C [101°F]); however, a lack of a febrile response (temperature less than 37°C [98.6°F]) or an increasing trend in body temperature should be addressed. The patient may also report increased fatigue and malaise in the absence of a febrile response.
- The heart does not function well in hypoxemic states, and the aging heart may respond to decreased myocardial oxygenation with dysrhythmias that may be misinterpreted as a normal part of the aging process.
- There is a progressive decline in respiratory muscle strength, maximal ventilation, and response to hypoxia. Older patients have a decreased respiratory reserve and decompensate more quickly.
- Changes in mentation may be inappropriately misinterpreted as dementia. Older adults with a sudden change in mentation should be aggressively assessed for acute delirium (hypo- and hyperdelirium states) and treated for the presence of infection and organ hypoperfusion.

Adapted from Davis, L. L. (2014). Cardiovascular issues in older adults. *Critical Care Nursing Clinics of North America, 26*(1), 61–89; Dellinger, R. P., Levy, M. M., Rhodes, A., et al. (2013). Surviving Sepsis Campaign: International guidelines for management of severe sepsis and septic shock: 2012. *Critical Care Medicine, 41*(2), 580–637; Green, J. M. (2015). Essentials of sepsis management. *Surgical Clinics of North America,95*(2), 355–365; Lineberry, C., & Stein, D. E. (2014). Infection, sepsis, and immune function in the older adult receiving critical care. *Critical Care Nursing Clinics of North America, 26*(1), 47–60; Mayr, F. B., Yende, S., & Angus, D.C. (2014). Epidemiology of severe sepsis. *Virulence, 5*(1), 4–11.

both of these interventions should be given priority in the care of the patient (Dellinger, 2015; Green, 2015).

The nurse should monitor the patient's hemodynamic status and promptly report deviations to the primary provider, assist in identifying and treating the underlying disorder by continuous in-depth assessment of the patient, administer prescribed fluids and medications, and promote patient safety. Vital signs are key indicators of hemodynamic status, and BP is an indirect measure of tissue hypoxia. The nurse should report a systolic BP lower than 90 mm Hg or a drop in systolic BP of 40 mm Hg from baseline or a MAP less than 65 mm Hg (Cestero & Dent, 2015; Dellinger et al., 2013; Green, 2015). If the patient is concurrently diagnosed with an infection or if an infection is suspected, the nurse should promptly notify the primary provider if the patient exhibits any two of the three following signs (Antonelli, DeBacker, Dorman, et al., 2016; Singer et al., 2016) (see later discussion of Septic Shock):

- Respiratory rate ≥22/min
- Altered mentation
- Systolic BP ≤100 mm Hg

Pulse pressure correlates well with stroke volume. Pulse pressure is calculated by subtracting the diastolic measurement from the systolic measurement; the difference is the pulse pressure. Normally, the pulse pressure is 30 to 40 mm Hg. Narrowing or decreased pulse pressure is an earlier indicator of shock than a drop in systolic BP (deWitt, Joshi, Meislin, et al., 2014; See, Mukhopadhyay, Lau, et al., 2015). Decreased or narrowing pulse pressure, an early indication of decreased stroke volume, is illustrated in the following example:

$$\text{Systolic BP} - \text{Diastolic BP} = \text{Pulse pressure}$$

Normal pulse pressure:

$$120 \text{ mm Hg} - 80 \text{ mm Hg} = 40 \text{ mm Hg}$$

Narrowing of pulse pressure:

$$90 \text{ mm Hg} - 70 \text{ mm Hg} = 20 \text{ mm Hg}$$

Elevation of the diastolic BP with release of catecholamines and attempts to increase venous return through vasoconstriction is an early compensatory mechanism in response to decreased stroke volume, BP, and overall cardiac output.

 Quality and Safety Nursing Alert

By the time BP drops, damage has already been occurring at the cellular and tissue levels. Therefore, the patient at risk for shock must be assessed and monitored closely before the BP falls.

Continuous central venous oximetry ($Sc\bar{v}O_2$) monitoring may be used to evaluate mixed venous blood oxygen saturation and severity of tissue hypoperfusion states. A central catheter is introduced into the superior vena cava (SVC), and a sensor on the catheter measures the oxygen saturation of the blood in the SVC as blood returns to the heart and pulmonary system for reoxygenation. A normal $Sc\bar{v}O_2$ value is 70% (Cestero & Dent, 2015; Dellinger et al., 2013). Body tissues use approximately 25% of the oxygen delivered to them during normal metabolism. During stressful events, such as shock, more oxygen is consumed and the $Sc\bar{v}O_2$ saturation is lower, indicating that the tissues are consuming more oxygen.

Interventions focus on decreasing tissue oxygen requirements and increasing perfusion to deliver more oxygen to the tissues. For instance, sedating agents may be given to lower metabolic demands, or the patient's pain may be treated with IV opioid agents to decrease metabolic demands for oxygen. Supplemental oxygen and mechanical ventilation may be required to increase the delivery of oxygen in the blood. Administration of IV fluids and medications supports BP and cardiac output, and the transfusion of packed red blood cells enhances oxygen transport. Monitoring tissue oxygen consumption with $Sc\bar{v}O_2$ is an invasive measure to more accurately assess tissue oxygenation in the compensatory stage of shock before changes in vital signs detect altered tissue perfusion (Dellinger et al., 2013).

In the patient who has an arterial line present, arterial pulse waveform analysis or pulse contour may be used to determine the patient's stroke volume and responsiveness to IV fluid replacement to meet tissue perfusion needs (Cestero & Dent, 2015). This may be used to estimate the patient's stroke volume, thus providing information to guide fluid resuscitation needs. A common limitation in using the arterial pulse waveform device is that cardiac dysrhythmias, severe peripheral vascular disease, and aortic valve regurgitation decrease its accuracy (Cestero & Dent, 2015). Other noninvasive measures that recently have been tried to monitor tissue perfusion include sublingual capnometry and near infrared spectroscopy (NIRS). Recent research has found that data from these methods are not entirely reliable; therefore, they are no longer in widespread use (Cestero & Dent, 2015).

Although treatments are prescribed and initiated by the primary provider, the nurse usually implements them, operates and troubleshoots equipment used in treatment, monitors the patient's status during treatment, and evaluates the immediate effects of treatment. In addition, the nurse assesses the response of the family to the crisis and its treatment.

Reducing Anxiety

Patients and their families often become anxious and apprehensive when they face a major threat to health and well-being and are the focus of attention of many health care providers. Providing brief explanations about the diagnostic and treatment procedures, supporting the patient during these procedures, and providing information about their outcomes are usually effective in reducing stress and anxiety and thus promoting the patient's physical and mental well-being. Speaking in a calm, reassuring voice and using gentle touch also help ease the patient's concerns. These actions may provide comfort for critically ill, frightened patients (Perrin & Kazanowski, 2015). Research suggests that family members have certain needs during a health-related crisis, including the need for honest, consistent, and thorough communication with health care providers; physical and emotional closeness to the patient; sensing that health care providers care about their patients; seeing the patient frequently; and knowing exactly what has been done for the patient (Perrin & Kazanowski, 2015).

The nurse should advocate that family members be present during procedures and while patient care is provided. The presence of family provides a necessary connection and support for the patient during a time of crisis. Research suggests that sharing decision making with the patient and the family enhances communication with the health care team, reduces patient anxiety, and improves overall satisfaction with care (Hinkle, Bosslet, & Torke, 2015).

Promoting Safety

The nurse must be vigilant for potential threats to the patient's safety, because a high anxiety level and altered mental status impair judgment. In this stage of shock, patients who were previously cooperative and followed instructions may now disrupt IV lines and catheters and complicate their condition. Close monitoring, frequent reorientation, hourly rounding, and implementing interventions to prevent falls (e.g., bed alarms) are essential.

Progressive Stage

In the second stage of shock, the mechanisms that regulate BP can no longer compensate, and the MAP falls below normal limits. Patients are clinically hypotensive; this is defined as a systolic BP of less than 90 mm Hg or a decrease in systolic BP of 40 mm Hg from baseline. The patient shows signs of declining mental status (Dellinger et al., 2013).

Pathophysiology

Although all organ systems suffer from hypoperfusion at this stage, several events perpetuate the shock syndrome. First, the overworked heart becomes dysfunctional, the body's inability to meet increased oxygen requirements produces ischemia, and biochemical mediators cause myocardial depression (Dellinger et al., 2013; Moore et al., 2015). This leads to failure of the heart, even if the underlying cause of the shock is not of cardiac origin. Second, the autoregulatory function of the microcirculation fails in response to the numerous biochemical mediators released by the cells, resulting in increased capillary permeability, with areas of arteriolar and venous constriction further compromising cellular perfusion (Moore et al., 2015). At this stage, the prognosis worsens. The relaxation of precapillary sphincters causes fluid to leak from the capillaries, creating interstitial edema and decreased return to the heart. In addition, the inflammatory response to injury is activated, and proinflammatory and anti-inflammatory mediators are released, which activate the coagulation system in an effort to reestablish homeostasis (Levi & van der Poll, 2015). The body mobilizes energy stores and increases oxygen consumption to meet the increased metabolic needs of the underperfused tissues and cells. Anaerobic metabolism ensues, resulting in a buildup of lactic acid and disruption of normal cell function (Green, 2015).

Even if the underlying cause of the shock is reversed, the sequence of compensatory responses to the decrease in tissue perfusion perpetuates the shock state, and a vicious cycle ensues. The cellular reactions that occur during the progressive stage of shock are an active area of clinical research. It is believed that the body's response to shock or lack of response in this stage of shock may be the primary factor determining the patient's survival. Early recognition of shock signs and symptoms is essential to improving morbidity and mortality.

Clinical Manifestations

Chances of survival depend on the patient's general health before the shock state as well as the amount of time it takes to restore tissue perfusion. As shock progresses, organ systems decompensate (see Table 14-1).

Respiratory Effects

The lungs, which become compromised early in shock, are affected at this stage. Subsequent decompensation of the lungs increases the likelihood that mechanical ventilation will be needed. Respirations are rapid and shallow. Crackles are heard over the lung fields. Decreased pulmonary blood flow causes arterial oxygen levels to decrease and CO_2 levels to increase. Hypoxemia and biochemical mediators cause an intense inflammatory response and pulmonary vasoconstriction, perpetuating pulmonary capillary hypoperfusion and hypoxemia. The hypoperfused alveoli stop producing surfactant and subsequently collapse. Pulmonary capillaries begin to leak, causing pulmonary edema, diffusion abnormalities (shunting), and additional alveolar collapse. This condition is called *acute lung injury* (ALI); as ALI continues, interstitial inflammation and fibrosis are common consequences, leading to acute respiratory distress syndrome (ARDS) (Silva, Pelosi, & Rocco, 2014). Further explanation of ALI and ARDS, as well as their nursing management, can be found in Chapter 23.

Cardiovascular Effects

A lack of adequate blood supply leads to dysrhythmias and ischemia. The heart rate is rapid, sometimes exceeding 150 bpm. The patient may complain of chest pain and even suffer a myocardial infarction (MI). Levels of cardiac biomarkers (e.g., cardiac troponin I [cTn-I]) increase. In addition, myocardial depression and ventricular dilation may further impair the heart's ability to pump enough blood to the tissues to meet increasing oxygen requirements.

Neurologic Effects

As blood flow to the brain becomes impaired, mental status deteriorates. Changes in mental status occur with decreased cerebral perfusion and hypoxia. Initially, the patient may exhibit subtle changes in behavior, become agitated, confused, or demonstrate signs of delirium. (See Chapter 11 for more information about delirium.) Subsequently, lethargy increases, and the patient begins to lose consciousness.

Renal Effects

When the MAP falls below 65 mm Hg (Zarbock, Gomez, & Kellum, 2014), the glomerular filtration rate of the kidneys cannot be maintained, and drastic changes in renal function occur. Acute kidney injury (AKI) is characterized by an increase in blood urea nitrogen (BUN) and serum creatinine levels, fluid and electrolyte shifts, acid–base imbalances, and a loss of the renal–hormonal regulation of BP. Urinary output usually decreases to less than 0.5 mL/kg per hour (or less than 30 mL per hour) but may vary depending on the phase of AKI. (See Chapter 54 for further information about AKI.)

Hepatic Effects

Decreased blood flow to the liver impairs the ability of liver cells to perform metabolic and phagocytic functions. Consequently, the patient is less able to metabolize medications and metabolic waste products, such as ammonia and lactic acid. Metabolic activities of the liver, including gluconeogenesis and glycogenolysis, are impaired. The patient becomes more susceptible to infection as the liver fails to filter bacteria from the blood. Liver enzymes (aspartate aminotransferase, alanine aminotransferase, lactate dehydrogenase,) and bilirubin levels are elevated, and the patient develops jaundice.

Gastrointestinal Effects

GI ischemia can cause stress ulcers in the stomach, putting the patient at risk for GI bleeding. In the small intestine, the mucosa can become necrotic and slough off, causing bloody diarrhea. Beyond the local effects of impaired perfusion, GI ischemia leads to bacterial translocation and organ dysfunction, in which bacterial toxins enter the bloodstream through the lymphatic system. In addition to causing infection, bacterial toxins can cause cardiac depression, vasodilation, increased capillary permeability, and an intense inflammatory response with activation of additional biochemical mediators. The net result is interference with healthy cellular functioning and the ability to metabolize nutrients (Dellinger et al., 2013).

Hematologic Effects

The combination of hypotension, sluggish blood flow, metabolic acidosis, coagulation system imbalance, and generalized hypoxemia can interfere with normal hemostatic mechanisms. In shock states, the inflammatory cytokines activate the clotting cascade, causing deposition of microthrombi in multiple areas of the body and consumption of clotting factors. The alterations of the hematologic system, including imbalance of the clotting cascade, are linked to the overactivation of the inflammatory response of injury (Levi & van der Poll, 2015; Moore et al., 2015). Disseminated intravascular coagulation (DIC) may occur either as a cause or as a complication of shock. In this condition, widespread clotting and bleeding occur simultaneously. Bruises (ecchymoses) and bleeding (petechiae) may appear in the skin. Coagulation times (e.g., prothrombin time, activated partial thromboplastin time) are prolonged. Clotting factors and platelets are consumed and require replacement therapy to achieve hemostasis. (Further discussion of DIC appears in Chapter 33.)

 Medical Management

Specific medical management in the progressive stage of shock depends on the type of shock, its underlying cause, and the degree of decompensation in the organ systems. Medical management specific to each type of shock is discussed later in this chapter. Although medical management in the progressive stage differs by type of shock, some medical interventions are common to all types. These include the use of appropriate IV fluids and medications to restore tissue perfusion by the following methods:

- Supporting the respiratory system
- Optimizing intravascular volume
- Supporting the pumping action of the heart
- Improving the competence of the vascular system

Other aspects of management may include early enteral nutritional support, targeted hyperglycemic control with IV insulin and use of antacids, histamine-2 (H$_2$) blockers, or antipeptic medications to reduce the risk of GI ulceration and bleeding.

Tight glycemic control (serum glucose of 80 to 100 mg/dL) is no longer recommended, as hypoglycemic events associated with regulating tight control in critically ill patients have been found to result in adverse patient outcomes (Griesdale, DeSouza, VanDam, et al., 2009; Marik & Bellomo, 2013). Current evidence suggests that maintaining serum glucose less than 180 mg/dL with insulin therapy and close monitoring is indicated in the management of the critically ill patient (Dellinger et al., 2013).

 Quality and Safety Nursing Alert

Glycemic control is linked to outcomes in the patient in shock. Although tight glycemic control is no longer indicated, evidence shows that maintaining serum glucose less than 180 mg/dL is linked to best outcomes.

 Nursing Management

Nursing care of patients in the progressive stage of shock requires expertise in assessing and understanding shock and the significance of changes in assessment data. Early interventions are essential to the survival of patients; therefore, suspecting that a patient may be in shock and reporting subtle changes in assessment are imperative. Patients in the progressive stage of shock are cared for in the intensive care setting to facilitate close monitoring (hemodynamic monitoring, electrocardiographic [ECG] monitoring, arterial blood gases, serum electrolyte levels, physical and mental status changes); rapid and frequent administration of various prescribed medications and fluids; and possibly interventions with supportive technologies, such as mechanical ventilation, dialysis (e.g., continuous renal replacement therapy), and intra-aortic balloon pump.

Working closely with other members of the health care team, the nurse carefully documents treatments, medications, and fluids that are given; recording the time; dosage or volume; and patient response. In addition, the nurse coordinates both the scheduling of diagnostic procedures that may be carried out at the bedside and the flow of health care personnel involved in the care of patients. The nurse also provides essential support through ongoing communication with the patient and the family.

Preventing Complications

The nurse helps reduce the risk of related complications and monitors the patient for early signs of complications. Monitoring includes evaluating blood levels of medications, observing invasive vascular lines for signs of infection, and checking neurovascular status if arterial lines are inserted, especially in the lower extremities. Simultaneously, the nurse promotes the patient's safety and comfort by ensuring that all procedures, including invasive procedures and arterial and venous punctures, are carried out using correct aseptic techniques and that venous and arterial puncture and infusion sites are maintained with the goal of preventing infection. Nursing interventions that reduce the incidence of ventilator-associated pneumonia (VAP) must also be implemented. These include frequent oral care, aseptic suction technique, turning, elevating the head of the bed at least 30 degrees to prevent aspiration, and implementing daily interruption of sedation as prescribed to evaluate patient readiness for extubation (Dellinger et al., 2013; Hillier, Wilson, Chamberlain, et al., 2013; Makic, Rauen, Jones, et al., 2015). See Chart 21-11 for an overview of the evidence-based ("bundled") interventions aimed at preventing VAP. Positioning and repositioning of the patient to promote comfort and maintain skin integrity are essential.

The nurse must also be vigilant in assessing for acute delirium, characterized by an acute change in mental status, inattention, disorganized thinking, and altered level of consciousness. Delirium is potentially preventable (Barr, Fraser, Puntillo, et al., 2013). Critically ill patients with delirium have longer mechanical ventilation support needs, experience higher functional decline, and have higher rates of morbidity and mortality than those without delirium. Furthermore, they are at a higher risk of developing post–intensive care syndrome, which manifests as new or worsening impairments in the patient's physical, cognitive, or mental status after a critical illness has resolved and that persists beyond the acute hospitalization (Barr et al., 2013). Delirium should be assessed at a minimum each shift using a standardized delirium assessment tool, such as the Confusion Assessment Method (CAM)-ICU (Vanderbilt University Medical Center, 2013). The CAM-ICU is a modified version of the CAM, specifically designed for use in patients who are critically ill (see Chart 11-7 for discussion of the CAM). Nursing interventions that can prevent delirium include engaging the patient in frequent reorientation activities (e.g., to date, time, place), assessing and treating pain, promoting sleep, providing early mobilization activities, and limiting sedation, especially sedation with benzodiazepines (e.g., lorazepam [Ativan]) (Makic, 2013).

Promoting Rest and Comfort

Efforts are made to minimize the cardiac workload by reducing the patient's physical activity and treating pain and anxiety. Because promoting patient rest and comfort is a priority, the nurse performs essential nursing activities in blocks of time, allowing the patient to have periods of uninterrupted rest, which may prevent acute delirium, as noted previously (Barr et al., 2013; Makic, Rauen, Watson, et al., 2014). To conserve the patient's energy, the nurse should protect the patient from temperature extremes (e.g., excessive warmth or cold, shivering), which can increase the metabolic rate and oxygen consumption and thus the cardiac workload.

Supporting Family Members

Because patients in shock receive intense attention by the health care team, families may be overwhelmed and frightened. Family members may be reluctant to ask questions or seek information for fear that they will be in the way or will interfere with the attention given to the patient. The nurse should make sure that the family is comfortably situated and kept informed about the patient's status. Often, families need encouragement from the health care team to get some rest; family members are more likely to take this advice if they feel that the patient is being well cared for and that they will be notified of any significant changes in the patient's status. A visit from the hospital chaplain may be comforting and provides some attention to the family while the nurse concentrates on the patient. Ensuring patient- and family-centered care is central to the delivery of high-quality care. This helps meet the emotional well-being as well as the physiologic needs of the patient and the family (Giles & Hall, 2013).

Irreversible Stage

The irreversible (or refractory) stage of shock represents the point along the shock continuum at which organ damage is so severe that the patient does not respond to treatment and cannot survive. Despite treatment, BP remains low. Renal and liver dysfunction, compounded by the release of biochemical mediators, creates an acute metabolic acidosis. Anaerobic metabolism contributes to a worsening lactic acidosis. Reserves of ATP are almost totally depleted, and mechanisms for storing new supplies of energy have been destroyed. Respiratory system dysfunction prevents adequate oxygenation and ventilation despite mechanical ventilatory support, and the cardiovascular system is ineffective in maintaining an adequate MAP for tissue perfusion. Multiple organ dysfunction progressing to complete organ failure has occurred, and death is imminent. Multiple organ dysfunction can occur as a progression along the shock continuum or as a syndrome unto itself and is described in more detail later in this chapter.

 ## Medical Management

Medical management during the irreversible stage of shock is similar to interventions and treatments used in the progressive stage. Although the patient may have progressed to the irreversible stage, the judgment that the shock is irreversible can be made only retrospectively on the basis of the patient's failure to respond to treatment. Strategies that may be experimental (e.g., investigational medications, such as immunomodulation therapy) may be tried to reduce or reverse the severity of shock.

 ## Nursing Management

As in the progressive stage of shock, the nurse focuses on carrying out prescribed treatments, monitoring the patient, preventing complications, protecting the patient from injury, and providing comfort. Offering brief explanations to the patient about what is happening is essential even if there is no certainty that the patient hears or understands what is being said. Simple comfort measures, including reassuring touches, should continue to be provided despite the patient's nonresponsiveness to verbal stimuli (Hinkle et al., 2015).

As it becomes obvious that the patient is unlikely to survive, the family needs to be informed about the prognosis and likely outcome. Opportunities should be provided—throughout the patient's care—for the family to see, touch, and talk to the patient. Close family friends or spiritual advisors may be of comfort to the family members in dealing with the inevitable death of their loved one. Whenever possible and appropriate, the patient's family should be approached regarding any living wills, advance directives, or other written or verbal wishes the patient may have shared in the event that he or she became unable to participate in end-of-life decisions. In some cases, ethics committees may assist families and health care teams in making difficult decisions (Hinkle et al., 2015).

During this stage of shock, the family may misinterpret the actions of the health care team. They have been told that nothing has been effective in reversing the shock and that the patient's survival is very unlikely, yet they find physicians and nurses continuing to work feverishly on the patient. Distraught, grieving families may interpret this as a chance for recovery when none exists, and family members may become angry when the patient dies. Conferences with all members of the health care team and the family promote better understanding by the family of the patient's prognosis and the purpose for management interventions. Engaging palliative care specialists can be beneficial in developing a plan of care that maximizes comfort and effective symptom management as well as assisting the family with difficult decisions (Perrin & Kazanowski, 2015). During these conferences, it is essential to explain that the equipment and treatments being provided are intended for patient comfort and do not suggest that the patient will recover. Family members should be encouraged to express their views of life-support measures (Hinkle et al., 2015; Perrin & Kazanowski, 2015).

General Management Strategies in Shock

As described previously and in the discussion of types of shock to follow, management in all types and all phases of shock includes the following:

- Support of the respiratory system with supplemental oxygen and/or mechanical ventilation to provide optimal oxygenation (see Chapter 21)
- Fluid replacement to restore intravascular volume
- Vasoactive medications to restore vasomotor tone and improve cardiac function
- Nutritional support to address the metabolic requirements that are often dramatically increased in shock

Therapies described in this section require collaboration among all members of the health care team.

Fluid Replacement

Fluid replacement, also referred to as fluid resuscitation, is given in all types of shock. The type of fluids given and the speed of delivery vary; however, fluids are given to improve cardiac and tissue oxygenation, which in part depends on flow. The fluids given may include **crystalloids** (electrolyte solutions that move freely between intravascular compartment and interstitial spaces), **colloids** (large-molecule IV solutions), and blood components (packed red blood cells, fresh frozen plasma, and platelets).

Crystalloid and Colloid Solutions

In emergencies, the "best" fluid is often the fluid that is readily available. Fluid resuscitation should be initiated early in shock to maximize intravascular volume. Isotonic crystalloid solutions are often selected because they contain the same concentration of electrolytes as the extracellular fluid and, therefore, can be given without altering the concentrations of electrolytes in the plasma. IV crystalloids commonly used for resuscitation in hypovolemic shock include 0.9% sodium chloride solution (normal saline) and lactated Ringer's solution. Ringer's lactate is an electrolyte solution containing the lactate ion, which should not be confused with lactic acid. The lactate ion is converted to bicarbonate, which helps buffer the overall acidosis that occurs in shock. A disadvantage of using isotonic crystalloid solutions is that some of the volume given is lost to the interstitial compartment and some remains in the intravascular compartment. This occurs as a consequence of cellular permeability that occurs during shock. Diffusion of crystalloids into the interstitial space means that more fluid may need to be given than the amount lost to support tissue perfusion. (Perel, Roberts, & Ker, 2013).

Care must be taken when rapidly administering isotonic crystalloids to avoid both underresuscitating and overresuscitating the patient in shock. Insufficient fluid replacement is associated with a higher incidence of morbidity and mortality from lack of tissue perfusion, whereas excessive fluid administration can cause systemic and pulmonary edema that progresses to ALI (see Chapter 23), intra-abdominal hypertension (IAH) and abdominal compartment syndrome (ACS), and multiple organ dysfunction syndrome (MODS) (see later discussion).

ACS is a serious complication that may occur when large volumes of fluid are given. It may also occur after trauma, abdominal surgery, pancreatitis, or sepsis (Holodinsky, Roberts, Ball, et al., 2013). In ACS, fluid leaks into the intra-abdominal cavity, increasing pressure that is displaced onto surrounding vessels and organs. Venous return, preload, and cardiac output are compromised. The pressure also elevates the diaphragm, making it difficult to breathe effectively. The renal and GI systems also begin to show signs of dysfunction (e.g., decreased urine output, absent bowel sounds, intolerance of tube feeding). Abdominal compartment pressure can be measured. Normally, it is 0 to 5 mm Hg, and a pressure of 12 mm Hg is considered to be indicative of IAH (Balogh, Lumsdaine, Moore, et al., 2014). If ACS is present, interventions that usually include surgical decompression are necessary to relieve the pressure.

Hypertonic crystalloid solution, often 3% sodium chloride, may be given in patients with shock and traumatic brain injury (Dubick, Shek, & Wade, 2013). These solutions exert a large osmotic force that pulls fluid from the intracellular space to the extracellular space to achieve a fluid balance (Dubick et al., 2013). This osmotic effect results in fewer fluids being given to restore intravascular volume, which is important in a patient with a head injury and cerebral swelling. Current research suggests that using hypertonic crystalloid solution does not improve patient outcomes and may result in unintended complications (Bulger, May, Kerby, et al., 2011; Dubick et al., 2013). Complications that may be associated with the use of hypertonic solutions include excessive serum osmolality, which can cause rapid fluid shifts, overwhelming the heart and leading to hypernatremia.

Generally, IV colloidal solutions are similar to plasma proteins, in that they contain molecules that are too large to pass through capillary membranes. Colloids expand intravascular volume by exerting oncotic pressure, thereby pulling fluid into the intravascular space, increasing intravascular volume. In addition, colloids have a longer duration of action than crystalloids, because the molecules remain within the intravascular compartment longer. Typically, if colloids are used to treat tissue hypoperfusion, albumin is the agent prescribed. Albumin is a plasma protein; an albumin solution is prepared from human plasma and is heated during production to reduce its potential to transmit disease. The disadvantage of albumin is its high cost compared to crystalloid solutions. Resuscitation with colloid solutions has not reduced the risk of morbidity or death compared to resuscitation with crystalloid solutions; moreover, colloids can be considerably more expensive than crystalloid solutions (Annane, Siami, Jaber, et al., 2013; Perel et al., 2013).

Quality and Safety Nursing Alert

With all colloidal solutions, side effects include the rare occurrence of anaphylactic reactions. Nurses must monitor patients closely.

Complications of Fluid Administration

Close monitoring of the patient during fluid replacement is necessary to identify side effects and complications. The most common and serious side effects of fluid replacement are cardiovascular overload, pulmonary edema, and ACS. The patient receiving fluid replacement must be monitored frequently for adequate urinary output, changes in mental status, skin perfusion, and changes in vital signs. Lung sounds are auscultated frequently to detect signs of fluid accumulation. Adventitious lung sounds, such as crackles, may indicate pulmonary edema and ALI.

Quality and Safety Nursing Alert

When administering large volumes of crystalloid solutions, the nurse must monitor the lungs for adventitious sounds, signs and symptoms of interstitial edema, and work of breathing (i.e., increasing effort required for the patient to breathe).

Often, a central venous pressure (CVP) line is inserted (typically into the subclavian or jugular vein) and is advanced until the tip of the catheter rests near the junction of the SVC and the right atrium. The CVP is used to assess preload in the right side of the heart. The CVP value assists in monitoring the patient's response to fluid replacement, especially when it is used in conjunction with additional assessment parameters (e.g., urine output, heart rate, BP response to fluid challenge) (Dellinger et al., 2013; Levy, Rhodes, Phillips, et al., 2015; Yealy, Kellum, Juang, et al., 2014). A normal CVP ranges from 4 to 12 mm Hg or cm H_2O. Several readings are obtained to determine a range, and fluid replacement is continued to achieve a CVP between 8 and 12 mm Hg (Dellinger, 2015; Dellinger et al., 2013). Interpreting blood volume on the basis of CVP readings alone has been recently challenged in the literature; therefore, CVP readings should be used in conjunction with other assessment variables to assess blood volume (Levy et al., 2015; Marik, Baram, & Vahid, 2008; Yealy et al., 2014). Some CVP catheters allow the monitoring of intravascular measures and venous oxygen levels. Assessment of venous oxygenation (venous oxygen saturation ([$S\overline{v}O_2$], or $Sc\overline{v}O_2$ with a CVP line) may be helpful in evaluating the adequacy of intravascular volume (Dellinger et al., 2013; Rivers, McIntyre, Morro, et al., 2005). Hemodynamic monitoring with arterial lines may be implemented to allow close monitoring of the patient's BP and tissue perfusion. A pulmonary artery catheter may be inserted to assist with closer monitoring of a patient's cardiac status as well as response to therapy. Advances in noninvasive or minimally invasive technology (e.g., esophageal Doppler, arterial pulse contour analysis, cardiac output devices, intrathoracic impedance monitoring) provide additional hemodynamic monitoring options (Cestero & Dent, 2015). (For additional information about hemodynamic monitoring, see Chapter 25.)

Placement of central lines for fluid administration and monitoring requires collaborative practice between the provider and the nurse to ensure that all measures to prevent central line–associated bloodstream infection (CLABSI) are implemented. Several interventions aimed at preventing CLABSI should be implemented collaboratively while the central line is being placed as well as during ongoing nursing management of the central line itself. Chart 14-2 describes the evidence-based ("bundled") interventions that have been found to reduce CLABSI.

Chart 14-2 Collaborative Practice Interventions to Prevent Central Line–Associated Bloodstream Infections (CLABSIs)

Current best practices can include the implementation of specific evidence-based bundle interventions that when used together (i.e., as a "bundle") improve patient outcomes. This chart outlines specific parameters for the central line bundled collaborative interventions that have been found to reduce central line–associated bloodstream infections (CLABSI).

What are the five key elements of the central line bundle?

- Hand hygiene
- Maximal sterile barrier precautions during line insertion (see later discussion)
- Chlorhexidine skin antisepsis
- Optimal catheter site selection with avoidance of using the femoral vein for central venous access in adult patients
- Daily review of line necessity, with prompt removal of unnecessary lines

When should hand hygiene be performed in the care of a patient with a central line?

- All clinicians who provide care to the patient should adhere to good hand hygiene practices, particularly:
  - Before and after palpating the catheter insertion site
  - With all dressing changes to the intravascular catheter access site
  - When hands are visibly soiled or contamination of hands is suspected
  - Before donning and after removing gloves

What changes can be made to improve hand hygiene?

- Implement a central line procedure checklist that requires that clinicians perform hand hygiene as an essential step in care.
- Post signage stating the importance of hand hygiene.
- Have soap and alcohol-based hand sanitizers prominently placed to facilitate hand hygiene practices.
- Model hand hygiene practices.
- Provide patient and family education and engage family in hand hygiene practices during visitation.

What are maximal sterile barrier precautions?

- These are implemented during central line insertion:
  - For the primary provider, this means strict compliance with wearing a cap, mask, sterile gown, and sterile gloves. The cap should cover all hair, and the mask should cover the nose and the mouth tightly. The nurse should also wear a cap and a mask.
  - For the patient, this means covering the patient from head to toe with a sterile drape, with a small opening for the site of insertion. If a full-size drape is not available, two drapes may be applied to cover the patient, or the operating room may be consulted to determine how to procure full-size sterile drapes, because these are routinely used in surgical settings.

- Nurses should be empowered to enforce use of a central line checklist to be sure that all processes related to central line placement are properly executed for every line placed.

Which antiseptic should be used to prepare the patient's skin for central line insertion?

- Chlorhexidine skin antisepsis has been proven to provide better skin antisepsis than other antiseptic agents, such as povidone–iodine solutions.
- An alcohol chlorhexidine antiseptic should be applied using a back-and-forth friction scrub for at least 30 seconds; this should not be wiped or blotted dry.
- The antiseptic solution should be allowed time to dry completely before the insertion site is punctured/accessed (approximately 2 minutes).

What nursing interventions are essential to reduce the risk of infection?

- Maintaining sterile technique when changing the central line dressing
- Always performing hand hygiene before manipulating or accessing the line ports
- Wearing clean gloves before accessing the line port
- Performing a 15- to 30-second "hub scrub" using chlorhexidine or alcohol and friction in a twisting motion on the access hub (reduces biofilm on the hub that may contain pathogens)
- Using chlorhexidine-containing dressings in patients older than 2 months
- Consider using antiseptic-containing port protectors to cover connectors

When should central lines be discontinued?

- Assessment for removal of central lines should be included as part of the nurse's daily goal sheets.
- The time and date of central line placement should be recorded and evaluated by staff to aid in decision making.
- The need for the central line access should be reviewed as part of multidisciplinary rounds.
- During these rounds, the "line day" should be stated to remind everyone how long the central line has been in place (e.g., "Today is line day 6").
- An appropriate time frame for regular review of the necessity for a central line should be identified, such as weekly, when central lines are placed for long-term use (e.g., chemotherapy, extended antibiotic administration).

Quality improvement processes that trend CLABSI rates and the compliance with CLABSI bundle prevention strategies have been found to effectively engage the multidisciplinary team in achieving goals to reduce infections related to central lines.

Adapted from Institute for Healthcare Improvement. (2012). *How-to guide: Prevent central line-associated bloodstream infection.* Retrieved on 11/28/2015 at: www.ihi.org/knowledge/Pages/Tools/HowtoGuidePreventCentralLineAssociatedBloodstreamInfection.aspx; Marschall, J., Mermel, L. A., Fakih, M., et al. (2014). Strategies to prevent central-line associated blood stream infections in acute care hospitals: 2014 update. *Infection Control and Hospital Epidemiology, 35*(7), 753–771; The Society for Healthcare Epidemiology of America SHEA Guideline Central. (2015). *Central line-associated bloodstream infections.* Retrieved on 11/28/2015 at: www.guidelinecentral.com/share/pocketcard/53d67314007df/#i469f5e2f

Vasoactive Medication Therapy

Vasoactive medications are given in all forms of shock to improve the patient's hemodynamic stability when fluid therapy alone cannot maintain adequate MAP. Specific medications are selected to correct the particular hemodynamic alteration that is impeding cardiac output. These medications help increase the strength of myocardial contractility, regulate the heart rate, reduce myocardial resistance, and initiate vasoconstriction.

Vasoactive medications are selected for their action on receptors of the sympathetic nervous system. These receptors are known as alpha-adrenergic and beta-adrenergic receptors. Beta-adrenergic receptors are further classified as beta-1 and beta-2 adrenergic receptors. When alpha-adrenergic receptors are stimulated, blood vessels constrict in the cardiorespiratory and GI systems, skin, and kidneys. When beta-1 adrenergic receptors are stimulated, heart rate and myocardial contraction increase. When beta-2 adrenergic receptors are stimulated, vasodilation occurs in the heart and skeletal muscles, and the bronchioles relax. The medications used in treating shock consist of various combinations of vasoactive medications to maximize tissue perfusion by stimulating or blocking the alpha- and beta-adrenergic receptors.

When vasoactive medications are given, vital signs must be monitored frequently (at least every 15 minutes until stable, or more often if indicated). Vasoactive medications should be given through a central venous line, because infiltration and extravasation of some vasoactive medications can cause tissue necrosis and sloughing (Allen, 2014). Individual medication dosages are usually titrated by the nurse, who adjusts drip rates on the basis of the prescribed dose and target outcome parameter (e.g., BP, heart rate) and the patient's response. Dosages are changed to maintain the MAP at a physiologic level that ensures adequate tissue perfusion (usually greater than 65 mm Hg).

> ### Quality and Safety Nursing Alert
>
> *Vasoactive medications should never be stopped abruptly, because this could cause severe hemodynamic instability, perpetuating the shock state.*

Dosages of vasoactive medications must be tapered. When vasoactive medications are no longer needed or are necessary to a lesser extent, the infusion should be weaned with frequent monitoring of BP (e.g., every 15 minutes). Table 14-2 presents some of the commonly prescribed vasoactive medications used in the treatment of shock. Occasionally, the patient does not respond as expected to vasoactive medications. A current topic of active research is evaluation of patients' adrenal function. Recent studies suggest that critically ill patients should be evaluated for corticosteroid insufficiency (also referred to as relative adrenal insufficiency or critical illness–related corticosteroid insufficiency) and, if this condition is present, corticosteroid replacement (e.g., hydrocortisone) should be considered (Dellinger et al., 2013).

Nutritional Support

Nutritional support is an important aspect of care for critically ill patients. Increased metabolic rates during shock increase energy requirements and therefore caloric requirements. Patients in shock may require more than 3000 calories daily. The release of catecholamines early in the shock continuum causes rapid depletion of glycogen stores. Nutritional energy requirements are then met by breaking down lean body mass. In this catabolic process, skeletal muscle mass is broken down even when the patient has large stores of fat or adipose tissue. Loss of skeletal muscle greatly prolongs the patient's recovery time.

Parenteral or enteral nutritional support should be initiated as soon as possible. Enteral nutrition is preferred, promoting GI function through direct exposure to nutrients and limiting infectious complications associated with parenteral feeding (Blaser, Starkopf, Kirsimagi, et al., 2014). Implementation of an evidence-based enteral feeding protocol that is tolerant of increased gastric residual volumes ensures the delivery of adequate nutrition to critically ill patients (Blaser et al., 2014). Gastric residual volume does not predict a patient's risk of aspiration (Blaser et al., 2014). Implementing early enteral nutrition has been found to promote gut-mediated immunity, reduce metabolic response to stress, and improve overall patient morbidity and mortality (Martindale & Warren, 2015). (See Chapter 44 for further discussion of monitoring gastric residual volumes.)

Stress ulcers occur frequently in acutely ill patients because of the compromised blood supply to the GI tract. Therefore, antacids, H_2 blockers (e.g., famotidine [Pepcid]), and proton pump inhibitors (e.g., lansoprazole [Prevacid], esomeprazole magnesium [Nexium]) are prescribed to prevent ulcer formation by inhibiting gastric acid secretion or increasing gastric pH.

TABLE 14-2 Vasoactive Agents Used in Treating Shock

Medication	Desired Action in Shock	Disadvantages
Inotropic Agents		
Dobutamine (Dobutrex) Dopamine (Intropin) Epinephrine (Adrenalin) Milrinone (Primacor)	Improve contractility, increase stroke volume, increase cardiac output	Increase oxygen demand of the heart
Vasodilators		
Nitroglycerin (Tridil) Nitroprusside (Nipride)	Reduce preload and afterload, reduce oxygen demand of heart	Cause hypotension
Vasopressor Agents		
Norepinephrine (Levophed) Dopamine (Intropin) Phenylephrine (Neo-Synephrine) Vasopressin (Pitressin) Epinephrine (Adrenalin)	Increase blood pressure by vasoconstriction	Increase afterload, thereby increasing cardiac workload; compromise perfusion to skin, kidneys, lungs, gastrointestinal tract

Adapted from Allen, J. M. (2014). Understanding vasoactive medications: Focus on pharmacology and effective titration. *Journal of Infusion Nursing, 37*(2), 82–86.

Hypovolemic Shock

Hypovolemic shock, the most common type of shock, is characterized by decreased intravascular volume. Body fluid is contained in the intracellular and extracellular compartments. Intracellular fluid accounts for about two-thirds of the total body water. The extracellular body fluid is found in one of two compartments: intravascular (inside blood vessels) or interstitial (surrounding tissues). The volume of interstitial fluid is about three to four times that of intravascular fluid. Hypovolemic shock occurs when there is a reduction in intravascular volume by 15% to 30%, which represents an approximate loss of 750 to 1,500 mL of blood in a 70-kg (154-lb) person (American College of Surgeons, 2012).

Pathophysiology

Hypovolemic shock can be caused by external fluid losses, as in traumatic blood loss, or by internal fluid shifts, as in severe dehydration, severe edema, or ascites (see Chart 14-3). Intravascular volume can be reduced by both fluid loss and fluid shifting between the intravascular and interstitial compartments.

The sequence of events in hypovolemic shock begins with a decrease in the intravascular volume. This results in decreased venous return of blood to the heart and subsequent decreased ventricular filling. Decreased ventricular filling results in decreased stroke volume (amount of blood ejected from the heart) and decreased cardiac output. When cardiac output drops, BP drops and tissues cannot be adequately perfused (see Fig. 14-3).

Medical Management

Major goals in the treatment of hypovolemic shock are to restore intravascular volume to reverse the sequence of events leading to inadequate tissue perfusion, to redistribute fluid volume, and to correct the underlying cause of the fluid loss as quickly as possible. Depending on the severity of shock and the patient's condition, often all three goals are addressed simultaneously.

Treatment of the Underlying Cause

If the patient is hemorrhaging, efforts are made to stop the bleeding. This may involve applying pressure to the bleeding site or surgical interventions to stop internal bleeding. If the cause of the hypovolemia is diarrhea or vomiting, medications

---

Physiology/Pathophysiology

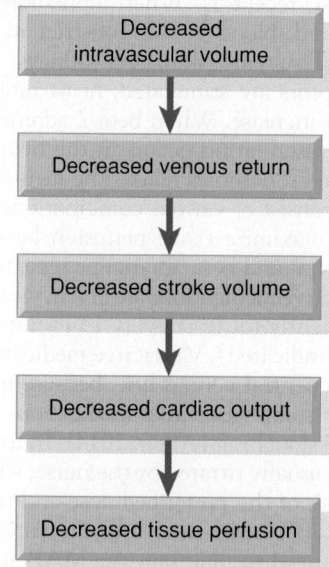

Figure 14-3 • Pathophysiologic sequence of events in hypovolemic shock.

to treat diarrhea and vomiting are given while efforts are made to identify and treat the cause. In older adult patients, dehydration may be the cause of hypovolemic shock.

Fluid and Blood Replacement

Beyond reversing the primary cause of the decreased intravascular volume, fluid replacement is of primary concern. At least two large-gauge IV lines are inserted to establish access for fluid administration. If an IV catheter cannot be quickly inserted, an intraosseous catheter may be used for access in the sternum, legs (tibia), or arms (humerus) to facilitate rapid fluid replacement (Tay, 2015). Multiple IV lines allow simultaneous administration of fluid, medications, and blood component therapy if required. Because the goal of the fluid replacement is to restore intravascular volume, it is necessary to administer fluids that will remain in the intravascular compartment to avoid fluid shifts from the intravascular compartment into the intracellular compartment. Table 14-3 summarizes the fluids commonly used in the treatment of shock.

As discussed earlier, crystalloid solutions such as lactated Ringer's solution or 0.9% sodium chloride solution are commonly used to treat hypovolemic shock, as large amounts of fluid must be given to restore intravascular volume. If hypovolemia is primarily due to blood loss, the American College of Surgeons (2012) recommends administration of 3 mL of crystalloid solution for each milliliter of estimated blood loss. This is referred to as the 3:1 rule. Colloid solutions (e.g., albumin) may also be used. Hetastarch and dextran solutions are not indicated for fluid administration because these agents interfere with platelet aggregation.

Blood products, which are also colloids, may need to be given, particularly if the cause of the hypovolemic shock is hemorrhage. The decision to give blood is based on the patient's lack of response to crystalloid resuscitation, the volume of blood lost, the need for hemoglobin to assist with oxygen transport, and the necessity to correct the patient's

---

Chart 14-3 ⚠	**RISK FACTORS**
	Hypovolemic Shock

External: Fluid Losses	**Internal: Fluid Shifts**
Trauma	Hemorrhage
Surgery	Burns
Vomiting	Ascites
Diarrhea	Peritonitis
Diuresis	Dehydration
Diabetes insipidus	Necrotizing pancreatitis

Adapted from Anderson, M. W., & Watson, G. A. (2013). Traumatic shock: The fifth shock. *Journal of Trauma Nursing, 20*(1), 37–43; Annane, D., Siami, S., Jaber, S., et al. (2013). Effects of fluid resuscitation with colloids vs crystalloids on mortality in critically ill patients presenting with hypovolemic shock: The CRISTAL randomized trial. *JAMA, 310*(17), 1809–1817.

TABLE 14-3 Fluid Replacement in Shock[a]

Fluids	Advantages	Disadvantages
Crystalloids		
0.9% Sodium chloride (normal saline solution)	Widely available, inexpensive	Requires large volume of infusion; can cause hypernatremia, pulmonary edema, abdominal compartment syndrome
Lactated Ringer's	Lactate ion that helps buffer metabolic acidosis	Requires large volume of infusion; can cause metabolic acidosis, pulmonary edema, abdominal compartment syndrome
Colloids		
Albumin (5%, 25%)	Rapidly expands plasma volume	Expensive; requires human donors; limited supply; can cause heart failure
Blood Products		
Plasma, packed red blood cells, and platelets	Rapidly replaces volume lost due to hemorrhage	Cross-match type-specific blood is desired for optimal massive transfusion protocols to reduce transfusion-related complications (e.g., transfusion-related acute lung injury, hemolytic reactions, transfusion-associated circulatory overload)

[a]Deliver a minimum of 30 mL/kg of crystalloid.
Adapted from Dellinger, R. P., Levy, M. M., Rhodes, A., et al. (2013). Surviving Sepsis Campaign: International guidelines for management of severe sepsis and septic shock: 2012. *Critical Care Medicine, 41*(2), 580–637; Kleinpell, R., Aitken, L, & Schorr, C. A. (2013). Implications of the new international sepsis guidelines for nursing care. *American Journal of Critical Care, 22*(3), 212–222; McEnvoy, M. T., & Shander A. (2013). Anemia, bleeding, and blood transfusion in the intensive care unit: Causes, risks, costs, and new strategies. *American Journal of Critical Care, 22*(6), eS1–eS13.

coagulopathy. Patients requiring massive transfusion respond better when blood products are given in a 1:1:1: ratio, meaning units of plasma, platelets, and packed red blood cells (Holcomb, Tiley, Baraniuk, et al., 2015).

Packed red blood cells are given to replenish the patient's oxygen-carrying capacity in conjunction with other fluids that will expand volume. Plasma and platelets are transfused to assist with coagulation and hemostasis. The need for transfusions is based on the patient's oxygenation needs and coagulation status, which are determined by vital signs, blood gas, chemistry, coagulation laboratory values, and clinical appearance.

Redistribution of Fluid

In addition to administering fluids to restore intravascular volume, positioning the patient properly assists fluid redistribution. A modified Trendelenburg position, also known as passive leg raising (see Fig. 14-4), is recommended in hypovolemic shock. Elevation of the legs promotes the return of venous blood and can be used as a dynamic assessment of a patient's fluid responsiveness. The nurse assesses for an improvement in the patients vital signs, specifically a rise in the BP and return of the pulse pressure to normal or near normal. A full Trendelenburg position makes breathing difficult and does not increase BP or cardiac output (Bridges & Jarquin-Valdivia, 2005; Dellinger, 2015).

Pharmacologic Therapy

If fluid administration fails to reverse hypovolemic shock, then vasoactive medications that prevent cardiac failure are given. Medications are also given to reverse the cause of the dehydration. For example, insulin is given if dehydration is secondary to hyperglycemia, desmopressin (DDAVP) is given for diabetes insipidus, antidiarrheal agents for diarrhea, and antiemetic medications for vomiting.

 Nursing Management

Primary prevention of shock is an essential focus of nursing care. Hypovolemic shock can be prevented in some instances by closely monitoring patients who are at risk for fluid deficits and assisting with fluid replacement before intravascular volume is depleted. In other circumstances, nursing care focuses on assisting with treatment targeted at the cause of the shock and restoring intravascular volume.

General nursing measures include ensuring safe administration of prescribed fluids and medications and documenting their administration and effects. Volumetric IV pumps should be used to administer vasopressor medications, if prescribed. Another important nursing role is monitoring for complications and side effects of treatment and reporting them promptly.

Administering Blood and Fluids Safely

Administering blood transfusions safely is a vital nursing role. In emergency situations, it is important to acquire blood specimens quickly, to obtain a baseline complete blood count, and to type and cross-match the blood in anticipation of blood transfusions. A patient who receives a transfusion of

Figure 14-4 • Proper positioning (modified Trendelenburg) for the patient who shows signs of shock. The lower extremities are elevated to an angle of about 20 degrees; the knees are straight, the trunk is horizontal, and the head is slightly elevated.

blood products must be monitored closely for adverse effects (see Chapter 32).

Fluid replacement complications can occur, especially when large volumes are given rapidly. Therefore, the nurse monitors the patient closely for cardiovascular overload and signs of difficulty breathing, a condition known as transfusion-associated circulatory overload. Transfusion-related acute lung injury may occur and is characterized by pulmonary edema, hypoxemia, respiratory distress, and pulmonary infiltrates, usually within hours after massive transfusion (McEnvoy & Shander, 2013). The risk of these complications is increased in older adults, in patients with preexisting cardiac disease, and with increasing number of blood products given. ACS is also a possible complication of excessive fluid resuscitation and may initially present with respiratory symptoms (difficulty breathing) and decreased urine output. Hemodynamic pressure, vital signs, arterial blood gases, serum lactate levels, hemoglobin and hematocrit levels, bladder pressure monitoring, and fluid intake and output (I&O) are among the parameters monitored. Temperature should also be monitored closely to ensure that rapid fluid resuscitation does not cause hypothermia. IV fluids may need to be warmed when large volumes are given. Physical assessment focuses on observing the jugular veins for distention and monitoring jugular venous pressure. Jugular venous pressure is low in hypovolemic shock; it increases with effective treatment and is significantly increased with fluid overload and heart failure. The nurse must monitor cardiac and respiratory status closely and report changes in BP, pulse pressure, CVP, heart rate and rhythm, and lung sounds to the primary provider.

Implementing Other Measures

Oxygen is given to increase the amount of oxygen carried by available hemoglobin in the blood. A patient who is confused may feel apprehensive with an oxygen mask or cannula in place, and frequent explanations about the need for the mask may reduce some of the patient's fear and anxiety. Simultaneously, the nurse must direct efforts to the safety and comfort of the patient.

Cardiogenic Shock

Cardiogenic shock occurs when the heart's ability to contract and to pump blood is impaired and the supply of oxygen is inadequate for the heart and the tissues. The causes of cardiogenic shock are known as either coronary or noncoronary. Coronary cardiogenic shock is more common than noncoronary cardiogenic shock and is seen most often in patients with acute MI resulting in damage to a significant portion of the left ventricular myocardium (Tharmaratnam, Nolan, & Jain, 2013). Patients who experience an anterior wall MI are at greatest risk for cardiogenic shock because of the potentially extensive damage to the left ventricle caused by occlusion of the left anterior descending coronary artery. Noncoronary causes of cardiogenic shock are related to conditions that stress the myocardium (e.g., severe hypoxemia, acidosis, hypoglycemia, hypocalcemia, tension pneumothorax) as well as conditions that result in ineffective myocardial function (e.g., cardiomyopathies, valvular damage, cardiac tamponade, dysrhythmias).

Physiology/Pathophysiology

Decreased cardiac contractility

↓

Decreased stroke volume and cardiac output

↓

Pulmonary congestion | Decreased systemic tissue perfusion | Decreased coronary artery perfusion

Figure 14-5 • Pathophysiologic sequence of events in cardiogenic shock.

Pathophysiology

In cardiogenic shock, cardiac output, which is a function of both stroke volume and heart rate, is compromised. When stroke volume and heart rate decrease or become erratic, BP falls and tissue perfusion is reduced. Blood supply for tissues and organs and for the heart muscle itself is inadequate, resulting in impaired tissue perfusion. Because impaired tissue perfusion weakens the heart and impairs its ability to pump, the ventricle does not fully eject its volume of blood during systole. As a result, fluid accumulates in the lungs. This sequence of events can occur rapidly or over a period of days (see Fig. 14-5).

Clinical Manifestations

Patients in cardiogenic shock may experience the pain of angina, develop dysrhythmias, complain of fatigue, express feelings of doom, and show signs of hemodynamic instability.

 ### Medical Management

The goals of medical management in cardiogenic shock are to limit further myocardial damage and preserve the healthy myocardium and to improve cardiac function by increasing cardiac contractility, decreasing ventricular afterload, or both (Wacker & Winters, 2014). In general, these goals are achieved by increasing oxygen supply to the heart muscle while reducing oxygen demands.

Correction of Underlying Causes

As with all forms of shock, the underlying cause of cardiogenic shock must be corrected. It is necessary first to treat the oxygenation needs of the heart muscle to ensure its continued ability to pump blood to other organs. In the case of coronary cardiogenic shock (e.g., acute coronary syndromes, acute MI), the patient may require thrombolytics (fibrinolytics) therapy, a percutaneous coronary intervention, coronary artery bypass graft surgery, intra-aortic balloon pump therapy, ventricular assist device, or some combination of these treatments (Ng & Yeghiazarians, 2013). In the case of noncoronary cardiogenic shock, interventions focus on correcting the underlying cause, such as replacement of a faulty cardiac valve, correction of a dysrhythmia, correction of acidosis and electrolyte disturbances, or treatment of a tension pneumothorax. If the cause of the cardiogenic shock was related to a cardiac arrest, once the patient is successfully resuscitated, targeted temperature management, also called *therapeutic hypothermia*, may be initiated to actively lower the body temperature to a targeted core temperature (e.g., 32°C [89.6°F] to 36°C [96.8°F]) to preserve neurologic function (American Heart Association, 2015; Subramaniam, Tiruvoipati, & Botha, 2015). (See Chapter 27 for more information regarding MI.)

Initiation of First-Line Treatment

Oxygenation

In the early stages of shock, supplemental oxygen is given by nasal cannula at a rate of 2 to 6 L/min to achieve an oxygen saturation exceeding 95%. Monitoring of arterial blood gas values, pulse oximetry values, and ventilatory effort (i.e., work of breathing) helps determine whether the patient requires a more aggressive method of oxygen delivery (including noninvasive and invasive mechanical ventilation).

Pain Control

If a patient experiences chest pain, IV morphine is given for pain relief. In addition to relieving pain, morphine dilates the blood vessels. This reduces the workload of the heart by both decreasing the cardiac filling pressure (preload) and reducing the pressure against which the heart muscle has to eject blood (afterload). Morphine may also decrease the patient's anxiety.

Hemodynamic Monitoring

Hemodynamic monitoring is initiated to assess the patient's response to treatment. In many institutions, this is performed in the intensive care unit (ICU), where an arterial line can be inserted. The arterial line enables accurate and continuous monitoring of BP and provides a port from which to obtain frequent arterial blood samples without having to perform repeated arterial punctures. A multilumen central venous and pulmonary artery catheter may be inserted to allow measurement of myocardial filling pressures, pulmonary artery pressures, cardiac output, and pulmonary and systemic resistance. (For more information, see Chapter 25.)

Laboratory Marker Monitoring

Laboratory biomarkers for ventricular dysfunction (e.g., B-type natriuretic peptide), cardiac enzyme levels and biomarkers (cTn-I), and serum lactate are measured, a transthoracic echocardiography may be performed at the bedside, and serial 12-lead electrocardiograms are obtained to assess the degree of myocardial damage (Tharmaratnam et al., 2013). Continuous ECG and ST segment monitoring is also done to closely monitor the patient for ischemic changes.

Fluid Therapy

Appropriate fluid administration is also necessary in the treatment of cardiogenic shock. Administration of fluids must be monitored closely to detect signs of fluid overload. Incremental IV fluid boluses are cautiously given to determine optimal filling pressures for improving cardiac output.

> ### Quality and Safety Nursing Alert
>
> *A fluid bolus should never be given rapidly, because rapid fluid administration in patients with cardiac failure may result in acute pulmonary edema.*

Pharmacologic Therapy

Vasoactive medication therapy consists of multiple pharmacologic strategies to restore and maintain adequate cardiac output. In coronary cardiogenic shock, the aims of vasoactive medication therapy are improved cardiac contractility, decreased preload and afterload, and stabilized heart rate and rhythm.

Because improving contractility and decreasing cardiac workload are opposing pharmacologic actions, two types of medications may be given in combination: inotropic agents and vasodilators. Inotropic medications increase cardiac output by mimicking the action of the sympathetic nervous system, activating myocardial receptors to increase myocardial contractility (inotropic action), or increasing the heart rate (chronotropic action). These agents may also enhance vascular tone, increasing preload. Vasodilators are used primarily to decrease afterload, reducing the workload of the heart and oxygen demand. Vasodilators also decrease preload. Medications commonly combined to treat cardiogenic shock include dobutamine, nitroglycerin, and dopamine (see Table 14-2).

Dobutamine

Dobutamine produces inotropic effects by stimulating myocardial beta-receptors, increasing the strength of myocardial activity and improving cardiac output. Myocardial alpha-adrenergic receptors are also stimulated, resulting in decreased pulmonary and systemic vascular resistance (decreased afterload) (Allen, 2014).

Nitroglycerin

IV nitroglycerin in low doses acts as a venous vasodilator and therefore reduces preload. At higher doses, nitroglycerin causes arterial vasodilation and therefore reduces afterload as well. These actions, in combination with dobutamine, increase cardiac output while minimizing cardiac workload. In addition, vasodilation enhances blood flow to the myocardium, improving oxygen delivery to the weakened heart muscle (Allen, 2014; Ng & Yeghiazarians, 2013).

Dopamine

Dopamine is a sympathomimetic agent that has varying vasoactive effects depending on the dosage. It may be used with dobutamine and nitroglycerin to improve tissue perfusion. Doses of 2 to 8 μg/kg/min improve contractility (inotropic action), slightly increase the heart rate (chronotropic action), and may increase cardiac output. Doses that are higher than 8 μg/kg/min predominantly cause vasoconstriction, which increases afterload and thus increases cardiac workload. Because this effect is undesirable in patients with cardiogenic shock, dopamine doses must be carefully titrated.

In severe metabolic acidosis, which occurs in the later stages of shock, metabolic acidosis must first be corrected to ensure maximum effectiveness of vasoactive medications (Allen, 2014; Dellinger et al., 2013).

Other Vasoactive Medications

Additional vasoactive agents that may be used in managing cardiogenic shock include norepinephrine, epinephrine, milrinone, vasopressin, and phenylephrine. Each of these medications stimulates different receptors of the sympathetic nervous system. A combination of these medications may be prescribed, depending on the patient's response to treatment. All vasoactive medications have adverse effects, making specific medications more useful than others at different stages of shock (see Table 14-2). Diuretics such as furosemide may be given to reduce the workload of the heart by reducing fluid accumulation.

Antiarrhythmic Medications

Multiple factors, such as hypoxemia, electrolyte imbalances, and acid–base imbalances, contribute to serious cardiac dysrhythmias in all patients with shock. In addition, as a compensatory response to decreased cardiac output and BP, the heart rate increases beyond normal limits. This impedes cardiac output further by shortening diastole and thereby decreasing the time for ventricular filling. Consequently, antiarrhythmic medications are required to stabilize the heart rate. General principles regarding the administration of vasoactive medications are discussed later in this chapter. (For a full discussion of cardiac dysrhythmias as well as commonly prescribed medications, see Chapter 26.)

Mechanical Assistive Devices

If cardiac output does not improve despite supplemental oxygen, vasoactive medications, and fluid boluses, mechanical assistive devices are used temporarily to improve the heart's ability to pump. Intra-aortic balloon counterpulsation is one means of providing temporary circulatory assistance (see Chapter 29). Other means of mechanical assistance include left and right ventricular assist devices and total temporary artificial hearts (see Chapters 28 and 29.) Another short-term means of providing cardiac or pulmonary support to the patient in cardiogenic shock is through an extracorporeal device similar to the cardiopulmonary bypass (CPB) system used in open-heart surgery (see Chapter 27). CPB is used only in emergency situations until definitive treatment, such as heart transplantation, can be initiated.

 Nursing Management

Preventing Cardiogenic Shock

Identifying at-risk patients early, promoting adequate oxygenation of the heart muscle, and decreasing cardiac workload can prevent cardiogenic shock. This can be accomplished by conserving the patient's energy, promptly relieving angina, and administering supplemental oxygen. Often, however, cardiogenic shock cannot be prevented. In such instances, nursing management includes working with other members of the health care team to prevent shock from progressing and to restore adequate cardiac function and tissue perfusion.

Monitoring Hemodynamic Status

A major role of the nurse is monitoring the patient's hemodynamic and cardiac status. Arterial lines and ECG monitoring equipment must be well maintained and functioning properly. The nurse anticipates the medications, IV fluids, and equipment that might be used and is ready to assist in implementing these measures. Changes in hemodynamic, cardiac, and pulmonary status and laboratory values are documented and reported promptly. In addition, adventitious breath sounds,

changes in cardiac rhythm, and other abnormal physical assessment findings are reported immediately.

Administering Medications and Intravenous Fluids

The nurse plays a critical role in the safe and accurate administration of IV fluids and medications. Fluid overload and pulmonary edema are risks because of ineffective cardiac function and accumulation of blood and fluid in the pulmonary tissues. The nurse documents medications and treatments that are given as well as the patient's response to treatment.

The nurse must be knowledgeable about the desired effects as well as the side effects of medications. For example, the nurse monitors the patient for decreased BP after administering morphine or nitroglycerin. Arterial and venous puncture sites must be observed for bleeding, and pressure must be applied at the sites if bleeding occurs. IV infusions must be observed closely because tissue necrosis and sloughing may occur if vasopressor medications infiltrate the tissues. When possible, vasoactive medications should be given using central IV lines (Dellinger et al., 2013). Furthermore, the need for the central IV access devices should be reviewed daily to reduce the risk of CLABSIs (Marschall, Mermel, Fakih, et al., 2014). The nurse must also monitor urine output, serum electrolytes, BUN, and serum creatinine levels to detect decreased renal function secondary to the effects of cardiogenic shock or its treatment.

Maintaining Intra-Aortic Balloon Counterpulsation

The nurse plays a critical role in caring for the patient receiving intra-aortic balloon counterpulsation (see Chapter 29). The nurse makes ongoing timing adjustments of the balloon pump to maximize its effectiveness by synchronizing it with the cardiac cycle. The patient is at risk of circulatory compromise to the leg on the side where the catheter for the balloon has been inserted; therefore, the nurse must check the neurovascular status of the lower extremities frequently.

Family presence during emergencies and procedures is becoming a more common practice. Research has explored health care provider and family member perceptions of family presence during procedures and emergent patient treatment, but few studies have explored the patient's perception of family presence. A recent qualitative research study by Twibell and colleagues (2015) found that most patients do wish to have family present during life-threatening events and procedures. An important finding in this study was that patients wish to decide who will be present; therefore, the health care team should facilitate discussions about family presence with patients before life-threatening events or emergent procedures are necessary (see Chart 14-4).

Enhancing Safety and Comfort

The nurse must take an active role in safeguarding the patient, enhancing comfort, and reducing anxiety. This includes administering medication to relieve chest pain, preventing infection at the multiple arterial and venous line insertion sites, protecting the skin, and monitoring respiratory and renal function. Proper positioning of the patient promotes effective breathing without decreasing BP and may also increase patient comfort while reducing anxiety.

Brief explanations about procedures that are being performed and the use of comforting touch often provide

Chart 14-4

NURSING RESEARCH PROFILE

Family Presence During Life-Threatening Events

Twibell, R. S., Craig, S., Siela, D., et al. (2015). Being there: Inpatients' perceptions of family presence during resuscitation and invasive cardiac procedures. *American Journal of Critical Care,* 24(6), 108–115.

Purpose

The aim of this study was to explore adult inpatients' perceptions of family presence during resuscitation, near-resuscitation, and unplanned invasive cardiac procedures within hours or days of the life-threatening event.

Design

This was a qualitative, exploratory, descriptive study that enrolled a convenience sample of physiologically stable adult hospitalized patients who had experienced a life-threatening event. Forty-eight participants were interviewed within 13 to 96 hours of the event. Participants were interviewed by one researcher who began each interview session with the same question: "Thinking of your recent life-threatening event here in the hospital, please share your thoughts on having family members present beside you as the care team intervened." All interviews were tape-recorded and transcribed. The research team analyzed the data both independently and collectively until consensus was reached on the major themes that emerged.

Findings

Approximately half of the participants experienced an unplanned cardiac procedure, one-fourth experienced resuscitation, and one-fourth experienced a near-resuscitation event. There were an equal number of men and women in the study, most were Caucasian (94%), with 33 (69%) participants between 41 and 80 years of age. More than 60% ($N = 29$) of the participants stated that they preferred family presence during these events. The four major themes that emerged from the data were labeled

with the participants' own words. The first theme was "Being there is beneficial." Participants shared the belief that having family present during these events was beneficial to both the family member and the patient. "Being there is hard" was the second theme. Participants expressed that it is hard to decide which family member should be in the room during these events, and also that it is difficult for the chosen family member to watch the events unfold. Most participants felt that the patient or families should decide who should be the family member present during these events, not the health care team. The third theme, "Families in the way" referenced participants' concerns that family members present during these events could interfere in their care because of room space constraints, or because they would likely ask questions of health care providers. The final theme, "Desire for control," referenced participants' desire for control to prevent "out of control" family members being present. None of the participants expressed concern about controlling confidentiality of information.

Nursing Implications

Findings from this study support previous research that suggests that family presence during emergencies and procedures is beneficial to the patient. Important new information that emerged from this study was that patients and their families felt that they should make the decision about family presence, not the health care professionals. Nurses should identify with the patient which family member should be present should a life-threatening event occur. These researchers suggest that this exploratory conversation could occur during the admission process with a review of the patient's advanced directives. Nurses have a key role supporting family members who are present during life-threatening events. Nurses can assist families in understanding the life-threatening events as they unfold, providing support to families during the crisis.

---

reassurance to the patient and the family. The family is usually anxious and benefits from opportunities to see and talk to the patient. Explanations of treatments and the patient's responses are often comforting to family members.

Distributive Shock

Distributive shock occurs when intravascular volume pools in peripheral blood vessels. This abnormal displacement of intravascular volume causes a relative hypovolemia because not enough blood returns to the heart, which leads to inadequate tissue perfusion. The ability of the blood vessels to constrict helps return the blood to the heart. The vascular tone is determined both by central regulatory mechanisms, as in BP regulation, and by local regulatory mechanisms, such as tissue demands for oxygen and nutrients. Therefore, distributive shock can be caused by either a loss of sympathetic tone or a release of biochemical mediators from cells that causes vasodilation.

The varied mechanisms leading to the initial vasodilation in distributive shock provide the basis for the further subclassification of shock into three types: septic shock, neurogenic shock, and anaphylactic shock. These subtypes of distributive shock cause variations in the pathophysiologic chain of events and are explained here separately. In all types of distributive shock, massive arterial and venous dilation

promotes peripheral pooling of blood. Arterial dilation reduces systemic vascular resistance. Initially, cardiac output can be high, both from the reduction in afterload (systemic vascular resistance) and from the heart muscle's increased effort to maintain perfusion despite the incompetent vasculature. Pooling of blood in the periphery results in decreased venous return. Decreased venous return results in decreased stroke volume and decreased cardiac output. Decreased cardiac output, in turn, causes decreased BP and ultimately decreased tissue perfusion. Figure 14-6 presents the pathophysiologic sequence of events in distributive shock.

Sepsis and Septic Shock

Septic shock, the most common type of distributive shock, is caused by widespread infection or sepsis. According to the Third International Consensus Definitions for Sepsis and Septic Shock (*Sepsis-3*) Task Force (2016), **sepsis** is "life-threatening organ dysfunction caused by a dysregulated host response to infection (p. 804)," and **septic shock** is "a subset of sepsis in which underlying circulatory and cellular metabolism abnormalities are profound enough to substantially increase mortality (p. 806)." Despite the increased sophistication of antibiotic therapy, the incidence of both sepsis and septic shock has continued to rise. They are the leading cause of death in noncoronary ICU patients.

Physiology/Pathophysiology

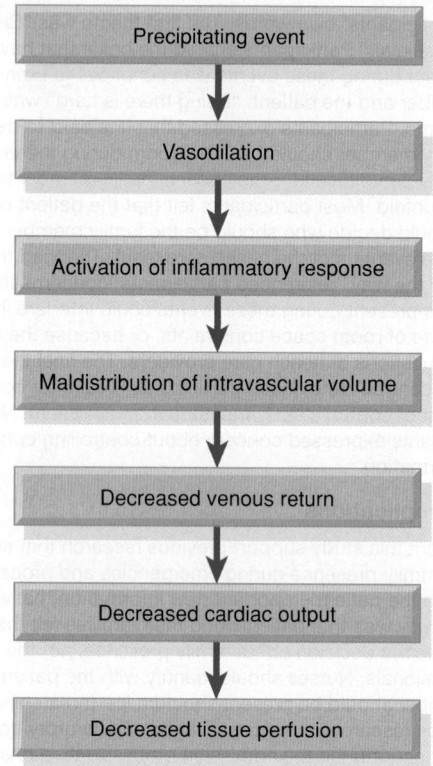

Figure 14-6 • Pathophysiologic sequence of events in distributive shock.

More than 30 million people suffer or die from sepsis worldwide (World Sepsis Day Fact Sheet, 2015), and the number of hospital admissions related to sepsis has increased threefold over the last decade (Surviving Sepsis Campaign, 2016). Finding and aggressively treating the source of infection and quickly restoring tissue perfusion are important interventions that may positively influence the clinical outcome.

Hospital-acquired conditions, which may include hospital-associated infections (i.e., infections not present at the time of admission to the health care setting) in critically ill patients that may progress to septic shock most frequently originate in the bloodstream (bacteremia), lungs (pneumonia), and urinary tract (urosepsis). Other infections include intra-abdominal infections and wound infections. Of increasing concern are bacteremias associated with intravascular catheters and indwelling urinary catheters (Centers for Medicare & Medicaid Services [CMS], 2014; Institute for Healthcare Improvement [IHI], 2012).

Additional risk factors that contribute to the growing incidence of sepsis are the increased use of invasive procedures and indwelling medical devices, the increased number of antibiotic-resistant microorganisms, and the increasingly older population (Green, 2015). Older adult patients are at particular risk for sepsis because of decreased physiologic reserves, an aging immune system, comorbid conditions and often nonspecific presentation of infection (Davis, 2014; Lineberry & Stein, 2014). Other patients at risk are those undergoing surgical and other invasive procedures, especially patients who have undergone emergency surgery or multiple surgeries (Green, 2015); those with malnutrition or immuno-

suppression; and those with chronic illness such as diabetes, hepatitis, chronic kidney disease, and immunodeficiency disorders (Lineberry & Stein, 2014) (see Chart 14-5).

The incidence of sepsis can be reduced by using strict infection control practices, beginning with thorough hand hygiene techniques (Dellinger, 2015). Other interventions include implementing programs to prevent central line infection; ensuring early removal of invasive devices that are no longer necessary (e.g., indwelling urinary catheters); implementing prevention programs to prevent ventilator associated events and pneumonia; promoting early ambulation; timely débriding of wounds to remove necrotic tissue; carrying out standard precautions and adhering to infection prevention/control practices, including the use of meticulous aseptic technique; and properly cleaning equipment and the patient environment.

Pathophysiology

Gram-negative bacteria traditionally have been the most commonly implicated microorganisms in sepsis. However, there is an increased incidence of gram-positive bacterial infections, viral infections, and fungal infections that can also cause sepsis (Wacker & Winters, 2014). Although a site

Chart 14-5

RISK FACTORS
Distributive Shock

Septic Shock

- Immunosuppression
- Extremes of age (<1 yr and >65 yrs)
- Malnourishment
- Chronic illness
- Invasive procedures
- Emergent and/or multiple surgeries

Neurogenic Shock

- Spinal cord injury
- Spinal anesthesia
- Depressant action of medications

Anaphylactic Shock

- History of medication sensitivity
- Transfusion reaction
- History of reaction to insect bites/stings
- Food allergies
- Latex sensitivity

Adapted from Anderson, M. W., & Watson, G. A. (2013). Traumatic shock: The fifth shock. *Journal of Trauma Nursing, 20*(1), 37–43; Dellinger, R. P, Levy, M. M., Rhodes, A., et al. (2013). Surviving Sepsis Campaign: International guidelines for management of severe sepsis and septic shock: 2012. *Critical Care Medicine, 41*(2), 580–637; Green, J. M. (2015). Essentials of sepsis management. *Surgical Clinics of North America, 95*(2), 355–365; Kanwar, R., Delasobera, B. E., Hudson, K., et al. (2015). Emergency department evaluation and treatment of cervical spine injuries. *Emergency Medicine Clinics of North America, 33*(2), 241–282; Lineberry, C., & Stein, D. E. (2014). Infection, sepsis, and immune function in the older adult receiving critical care. *Critical Care Nursing Clinics of North America, 26*(1), 47–60; Mayr, F. B., Yende, S., & Angus, D. C. (2014). Epidemiology of severe sepsis. *Virulence, 5*(1), 4–11; Muraro, A., Hoffmann-Sommergruber, K., Holzhauser, T., et al. (2014). EAACI food allergy and anaphylaxis guidelines: Protecting consumers with food allergies, understanding food consumption, meeting regulations and identifying unmet needs. *Allergy, 69*(11), 1464–1472.

of infection is identified in most cases, up to 30% of patients with sepsis may never have an identifiable site of infection (Surviving Sepsis Campaign, 2016).

When microorganisms invade body tissues, patients exhibit an immune response. This immune response provokes the activation of biochemical cytokines and mediators associated with an inflammatory response and produces a complex cascade of physiologic events that leads to poor tissue perfusion. Increased capillary permeability results in fluid seeping from the capillaries. Capillary instability and vasodilation interrupt the body's ability to provide adequate perfusion, oxygen, and nutrients to the tissues and cells. The widespread inflammatory response that occurs is called the **systemic inflammatory response syndrome** (SIRS). SIRS results from a clinical insult that initiates an inflammatory response that is systemic, rather than localized to the site of the insult. The insult may be a significant injury (e.g., multitrauma) or an infection (e.g., sepsis). A patient presenting with manifestations of SIRS may be exhibiting a protective inflammatory response to the initiating insult or may be exhibiting a response to infection, which may lead to sepsis. The clinical criteria used to identify SIRS, which include a temperature >38.3°C (>101°F) or <36°C (<96.8°F), tachycardia, tachypnea, and a white blood cell (WBC) count >12,000 cells/mm³, less than 4000 cells/mm³, or >10% immature WBC (bands), have been found to be not helpful in diagnosing sepsis, however (Singer et al., 2016).

In addition to SIRS, proinflammatory and anti-inflammatory cytokines released during the inflammatory response activate the coagulation system, which begins to form clots whether or not bleeding is present (Moore et al., 2015). This results not only in microvascular occlusions that further disrupt cellular perfusion but also in an inappropriate consumption of clotting factors. The imbalance of the inflammatory response and the clotting and fibrinolysis cascades are considered critical elements of the devastating physiologic progression that occurs in patients with sepsis.

Sepsis is an evolving process that may result in septic shock and life-threatening organ dysfunction if not recognized and treated early. In the early stage of septic shock, BP may remain within normal limits, or the patient may be hypotensive but responsive to fluids. The heart rate increases, progressing to tachycardia. Hyperthermia and fever, with warm, flushed skin and bounding pulses, are present. The respiratory rate is elevated. Urinary output may remain at normal levels or decrease. GI status may be compromised, as evidenced by nausea, vomiting, diarrhea, or decreased gastric motility. Hepatic dysfunction is evidenced by rising bilirubin levels and worsening coagulopathies (e.g., decreasing platelet counts). Signs of hypermetabolism include increased serum glucose and insulin resistance. Subtle changes in mental status, such as confusion or agitation, may be present. The lactate level is elevated because of the maldistribution of blood. Inflammatory markers such as WBC counts, plasma C-reactive protein (CRP), and procalcitonin levels are also elevated (Dellinger et al., 2013; Green, 2015; Moore et al., 2015; Singer et al., 2016).

As sepsis progresses, tissues become less perfused and acidotic, compensation begins to fail, and the patient begins to show signs of organ dysfunction. The cardiovascular system also begins to fail, the BP does not respond to fluid resuscitation and vasoactive agents, and signs of end-organ damage are evident

(e.g., AKI, pulmonary dysfunction, hepatic dysfunction, confusion progressing to nonresponsiveness). As sepsis progresses to septic shock, the BP drops and the skin becomes cool, pale, and mottled. Temperature may be normal or below normal. Heart and respiratory rates remain rapid. Urine production ceases, and multiple organ dysfunction progressing to death occurs.

Medical Management

A significant body of research has been conducted in the past few decades that is aimed at reducing the morbidity and mortality caused by sepsis and septic shock. In 1991, 2003, 2008, 2012, and again in 2016 (i.e., *Sepsis-3*), critical care experts systematically reevaluated the body of research and provided evidence-based recommendations for the acute management of patients with sepsis and septic shock (Dellinger et al., 2013; Singer et al., 2016; Surviving Sepsis Campaign, 2016). Developing and implementing protocols that focus on prevention and early detection and management of patients with sepsis have reduced the mortality of hospitalized patients (Dellinger, 2015; Singer et al., 2016). *Sepsis-3* provides an overview of key concepts and principles germane to sepsis that must be understood in order for physicians and nurses to be able to identify and manage patients with sepsis, including the following (Singer et al., 2016):

- As the leading cause of death from infection, sepsis must be recognized and treated promptly.
- Sepsis is different from infection in that in sepsis there is a dysregulated host response with organ dysfunction. An infection may cause specific organ dysfunction without a dysregulated host response.
- Sepsis is caused by an interplay between infectious pathogens and a myriad of patient-specific risks, including genetics, age, and the presence of other diseases/disorders.
- The organ dysfunction that occurs with sepsis may not be readily apparent; on the contrary, a new onset of organ dysfunction may be caused by an unrecognized infectious process.

Research efforts are focusing on better identification and early aggressive treatment of patients with sepsis, rapid and effective restoration of tissue perfusion, evaluation and treatment of the patient's immune response, and treatment of dysregulation of the coagulation system that occurs with sepsis (Green, 2015).

Correction of Underlying Causes

Current treatment of sepsis and septic shock involves rapid identification and elimination of the cause of infection. Current goals are to identify and treat patients in early sepsis within 3 hours to optimize patient outcome (Surviving Sepsis Campaign, 2016). Several evidence-based screening tools can be used to help identify patients for sepsis (see later discussion of assessment tools under the section Nursing Management).

In an effort to continue to reduce deaths from sepsis, CMS has launched a *Core Measure* for sepsis, requiring that hospitals demonstrate adherence to 3-hour and 6-hour timed interventions in order to receive reimbursement for services (see Chart 14-6). The focus on compliance with these evidence-based bundled interventions is to foster early recognition and interventions in patients with sepsis so that patient outcomes improve. These assessments and interventions are collectively

Chart 14-6 Surviving Sepsis Campaign Bundle

Complete within 3 hours of patient presentation/symptoms
- Obtain serum lactate level
- Obtain blood culture prior to administration of antibiotics
- Administer prescribed broad-spectrum antibiotics
- Initiate aggressive fluid resuscitation in patients with hypotension or elevated serum lactate (>4 mmol/L):
  - Minimum initial fluid bolus of 30 mL/kg using crystalloid solutions

Complete as soon as possible or within the first 6 hours of patient presentation/symptoms
- Begin vasopressor agents if hypotension is not improved (MAP < 65 mm Hg) after initial fluid resuscitation
- If hypotension persists after initial fluid administration (MAP <65 mm Hg) or initial lactate was ≥4 mmol/L, reassess intravascular volume status and tissue perfusion using two of the following assessment parameters:
  - Measure CVP (goal 8–12 mm Hg)
  - Measure $Sc\bar{v}O_2$ (goal > 70%)
  - Bedside cardiovascular ultrasound
  - Dynamic assessment of fluid responsiveness with passive leg raise or fluid challenge

Additional interventions and targets for therapy in the early management of sepsis
- Support blood pressure to achieve a urine output >0.5 mL/kg/h
- Administer vasopressor agents if fluid resuscitation does not restore an effective BP and cardiac output:
  - Norepinephrine centrally given is the initial vasopressor of choice.
  - Epinephrine, phenylephrine, or vasopressin should not be given as the initial vasopressor in septic shock.
- Obtain blood, sputum, urine, and wound cultures and administer broad-spectrum antibiotics:
  - Cultures should be obtained prior to antibiotic administration.
  - Antibiotic administration should occur within 3 hours of admission to the emergency department or within 1 hour of inpatient admission.
- Support the respiratory system with supplemental oxygen and mechanical ventilation.
- Transfuse with packed red blood cells when hemoglobin is <7 g/dL to achieve a target hemoglobin of 7–9 g/dL in adults.
- Provide adequate IV sedation and analgesia; avoid the use of neuromuscular blockade agents when possible.
- Control serum glucose <180 mg/dL with IV insulin therapy.
- Implement interventions and medications to prevent deep vein thrombosis and stress ulcer prophylaxis.
- Discuss advance care planning with patients and families.

CVP, central venous pressure; MAP, mean arterial pressure; BP, blood pressure; IV, intravenous.

Adapted from Centers for Medicare & Medicaid Services. (2014). *Improve quality of care during hospital inpatient stays.* Retrieved on 11/28/2015 at: www.cms.gov/Newsroom/MediaReleaseDatabase/Fact-sheets/2014-Fact-sheets-items/2014-08-04-2.html; Dellinger, R. P, Levy, M. M., Rhodes, A., et al. (2013). Surviving Sepsis Campaign: International guidelines for management of severe sepsis and septic shock: 2012. *Critical Care Medicine, 41*(2), 580–637; Dellinger, R. P. (2015). The future of sepsis performance improvement. *Critical Care Medicine, 43*(9), 1787–1790; Surviving Sepsis Bundle. (2015). Retrieved on 11/28/2015 at: www.survivingsepsis.org/SiteCollectionDocuments/SSC_Bundle.pdf

wound drainage, and tips of invasive catheters are collected for culture using aseptic technique. IV lines are removed and reinserted at alternate sites. If possible, urinary catheters are removed or changed. Any abscesses are drained, and necrotic areas are debrided. All cultures should be obtained prior to antibiotic administration. Current guidelines suggest that antibiotics should be initiated within the first hour of treatment of a patient with sepsis (Surviving Sepsis Campaign, 2016).

Fluid Replacement Therapy

Fluid replacement must be instituted to correct tissue hypoperfusion that results from the incompetent vasculature and the inflammatory response. Reestablishing tissue perfusion through aggressive fluid resuscitation is key to the management of sepsis and septic shock (Dellinger et al., 2013; Yealy et al., 2014). An initial fluid challenge, which includes an IV infusion of at least 30 mL/kg of crystalloids over 30 minutes, may be required to aggressively treat sepsis-induced tissue hypoperfusion. In addition to monitoring BP, CVP, fluid responsiveness with passive leg raise, urine output, and serum lactate levels are monitored to assess effectiveness of fluid resuscitation.

Pharmacologic Therapy

If the infecting organism is unknown, broad-spectrum antibiotic agents are started until culture and sensitivity reports are received (Dellinger et al., 2013; IHI, 2014a), at which time the antibiotic agents may be changed to agents that are more specific to the infecting organism and less toxic to the patient.

If fluid therapy alone does not effectively improve tissue perfusion, vasopressor agents, specifically norepinephrine or dopamine, may be initiated to achieve a MAP of 65 mm Hg or higher. Inotropic agents may also be given to provide pharmacologic support to the myocardium. Packed red blood cells may be ordered to support oxygen delivery and transport to the tissues. Neuromuscular blockade agents and sedation agents may be required to reduce metabolic demands and provide comfort to the patient. Deep vein thrombosis (DVT) prophylaxis with low-dose unfractionated heparin or low–molecular-weight heparin, in combination with mechanical prophylaxis (e.g., sequential compression devices) should be initiated, as well as medications for stress ulcer prophylaxis (e.g., H_2 blocking agents, proton pump inhibitors).

Nutritional Therapy

Aggressive nutritional supplementation should be initiated within 24 to 48 hours of ICU admission to address the hypermetabolic state present with septic shock (Martindale & Warren, 2015). Malnutrition further impairs the patient's resistance to infection. Enteral feedings are preferred to the parenteral route because of the increased risk of iatrogenic infection associated with IV catheters; however, enteral feedings may not be possible if decreased perfusion to the GI tract reduces peristalsis and impairs absorption.

 ## Nursing Management

Nurses caring for patients in any setting must keep in mind the risks of sepsis and the high mortality rate associated with sepsis and septic shock. All invasive procedures must be carried out with aseptic technique after careful hand hygiene. In addition, IV lines, arterial and venous puncture sites, surgical incisions, traumatic wounds, and urinary catheters must be monitored

referred to as the *Sepsis Bundles* (CMS, 2014). (See Chapter 1 for further discussion of *Core Measures* and *Bundles*.) (Green, 2015; IHI, 2014a; Surviving Sepsis Campaign, 2016).

Rapid identification of the infectious source is a critical element in managing sepsis. Specimens of blood, sputum, urine, for signs of infection. Nursing interventions to prevent infection need to be implemented in the care of all patients. Nurses should identify patients who are at particular risk for sepsis and septic shock (i.e., older adults and immunosuppressed patients and those with extensive trauma, burns, or diabetes), keeping in mind that these high-risk patients may not develop typical or classic signs of infection and sepsis. For example, confusion may be the first sign of infection and sepsis in older adult patients (Kleinpell, Aitken, & Schorr, 2013).

Sepsis-3 recommends that patients in the ICU setting with infection be monitored for the development of sepsis by using the *Sepsis-Related Organ Failure Assessment Score* (also known as the *Sequential Organ Failure Assessment* [SOFA] score) (Antonelli et al., 2016; Singer et al., 2016; Vincent, Moreno, Takala, et al., 1996) (see Table 14-4). The parameters that are monitored on the SOFA, which include assessment of respiratory rate, platelets, bilirubin, MAP (and use of any vasopressors), serum creatinine, urine output, and Glasgow Coma Scale (GCS) score (see Chapter 68), may all be gathered and assessed by the nurse in the ICU setting. A drop of 2 points or more in a patient's SOFA score from baseline is suggestive of organ dysfunction. In a patient with infection, the presence of organ dysfunction suggests the development of sepsis (Singer et al., 2016).

For a patient not in the ICU setting who has an infection, *Sepsis-3* recommends that the Quick SOFA (qSOFA) scale be used to screen for the development of sepsis. The qSOFA is an easy measurement tool that nurses may readily use; the presence of any two of the three parameters on this scale suggests the development of sepsis. These parameters include a respiratory rate of 22 breaths per minute or higher, a GCS score of less than 15, and a systolic BP of 100 mm Hg or less. The GCS parameter is considered positive for any score less than 15; therefore, any change in the patient's mentation status is considered positive. In order to facilitate ease of use, therefore, *Sepsis-3* recommends that any change in the patient's mentation status be used when computing the qSOFA scale score (Antonelli et al., 2016; Singer et al., 2016). Another assessment tool that is frequently used in hospital-based settings that can identify patients with sepsis is the *Modified Early Warning System* (MEWS) (IHI, 2014b). The nurse assesses the patient for changes in respiratory rate, heart rate, BP, consciousness, temperature, and urine output. Scores ranging from 0 to 3 are assigned to each assessment variable, and MEWS score is greater than 4 are suggestive of the development of sepsis (IHI, 2014b) (see Table 14-5).

When caring for a patient with sepsis or septic shock, the nurse collaborates with other members of the health care team to identify the site and source of sepsis and the specific organisms involved. The nurse often obtains appropriate specimens for culture and sensitivity. Prescribed antibiotics are not given until these specimens are obtained. Elevated body temperature (hyperthermia) is common with sepsis and raises the patient's metabolic rate and oxygen consumption. Efforts may be made to reduce the temperature by administering acetaminophen or applying a hypothermia blanket. During these therapies, the nurse monitors the patient closely for shivering, which increases oxygen consumption. Efforts to increase comfort are important if the patient experiences fever, chills, or shivering.

The nurse administers prescribed IV fluids and medications, including antibiotic agents and vasoactive medications, to restore vascular volume. Because of decreased perfusion, serum concentrations of antibiotic agents that are normally cleared by the kidneys and liver may increase and produce toxic effects. Therefore, the nurse monitors blood levels (serum levels of antibiotic agents, procalcitonin, CRP, BUN, creatinine, WBC count, hemoglobin, hematocrit, platelet levels, coagulation studies) and reports changes to the primary provider. As with other types of shock, the nurse

TABLE 14-4 The Sepsis-Related Organ Failure Assessment Score (Sequential Organ Failure Assessment [SOFA] Score)

SOFA Score	1	2	3	4
Respiration PaO_2/FiO_2, mm Hg	<400	<300	<200	<100 ——with respiratory support——
Coagulation Platelets × $10^3/mm^3$	<150	<100	<50	<20
Liver Bilirubin, mg/dL (µmol/L)	1.2–1.9 (20–32)	2.0–5.9 (33–101)	6.0–11.9 (102–204)	>12.0 (<204)
Cardiovascular Hypotension	MAP <70 mm Hg	Dopamine ≤5 or dobutamine (any dose)[a]	Dopamine >5 or epinephrine ≤0.1 or norepinephrine ≤0.1	Dopamine >15 or epinephrine >0.1 or norepinephrine >0.1
Central Nervous System Glasgow Coma Scale	13–14	10–12	6–9	<6
Renal Creatinine, mg/dL (µmol/L) or urine output	1.2–1.9 (110–170)	2.0–3.4 (171–299)	3.5–4.9 (300–440) or <500 mL/day	>5.0 (>440) or <200 mL/day

MAP, mean arterial pressure.
[a]Adrenergic agents given for at least 1 hour (doses given are in µg/kg·min).
Reprinted with permission from Vincent, J. L., Moreno, R., Takala, J., et al. (1996). The SOFA (Sepsis-related Organ Failure Assessment) score to describe organ dysfunction/failure. On behalf of the Working Group on Sepsis-Related Problems of the European Society of Intensive Care Medicine. *Intensive Care Medicine, 22*(7), 707–710.

TABLE 14-5 The MEWS (Modified Early Warning System)

	3	2	1	0	1	2	3
MEWS (Modified Early Warning System)							
Respiratory rate per minute		<8		9–14	15–20	21–29	>30
Heart rate per minute		<40	40–50	51–100	101–110	111–129	>129
Systolic blood pressure	<70	71–80	81–100	101–199		>200	
Conscious level (AVPU)	Unresponsive	Responds to **Pain**	Responds to **Voice**	Alert	New agitation; Confusion		
Temperature (°C)		<35.0	35.1–36	36.10–38	38.1–38.5	>38.6	
Hourly urine for 2 hours	<10 mL/h	<30 mL/h	<45 mL/h				

Reprinted with permission from Institute for Healthcare Improvement (IHI). (2014b). *Improving stories: Early warning systems: Scorecards that save lives.* Retrieved on 2/18/2016 at: www.ihi.org/resources/PublishingImages/Image_PatientAssessmentObservationInfusionMonitoring.jpg

monitors the patient's hemodynamic status, fluid intake and output (I&O), and nutritional status. Daily weights and close monitoring of serum albumin and prealbumin levels help determine the patient's protein requirements.

Neurogenic Shock

In **neurogenic shock,** vasodilation occurs as a result of a loss of balance between parasympathetic and sympathetic stimulation. Sympathetic stimulation causes vascular smooth muscle to constrict, and parasympathetic stimulation causes vascular smooth muscle to relax or dilate. The patient experiences a predominant parasympathetic stimulation that causes vasodilation lasting for an extended period, leading to a relative hypovolemic state. However, blood volume is adequate, because the vasculature is dilated; the blood volume is displaced, producing a hypotensive (low BP) state. The overriding parasympathetic stimulation that occurs with neurogenic shock causes a drastic decrease in the patient's systemic vascular resistance and bradycardia. Inadequate BP results in the insufficient perfusion of tissues and cells that is common to all shock states.

Neurogenic shock can be caused by spinal cord injury, spinal anesthesia, or other nervous system damage. It may also result from the depressant action of medications or from lack of glucose (e.g., insulin reaction) (see Chart 14-5). Neurogenic shock may have a prolonged course (spinal cord injury) or a short one (syncope or fainting). Normally, during states of stress, the sympathetic stimulation causes the BP and heart rate to increase. In neurogenic shock, the sympathetic system is not able to respond to body stressors. Therefore, the clinical characteristics of neurogenic shock are signs of parasympathetic stimulation. It is characterized by dry, warm skin rather than the cool, moist skin seen in hypovolemic shock. Another characteristic is hypotension with bradycardia, rather than the tachycardia that characterizes other forms of shock.

 Medical Management

Treatment of neurogenic shock involves restoring sympathetic tone, either through the stabilization of a spinal cord injury or, in the instance of spinal anesthesia, by positioning the patient properly. Specific treatment depends on the cause of the shock. (Further discussion of management of patients with a spinal cord injury is presented in Chapter 68.)

Nursing Management

It is important to elevate and maintain the head of the bed at least 30 degrees to prevent neurogenic shock when a patient receives spinal or epidural anesthesia. Elevation of the head helps prevent the spread of the anesthetic agent up the spinal cord. In suspected spinal cord injury, neurogenic shock may be prevented by carefully immobilizing the patient to prevent further damage to the spinal cord (Kanwar, Delasobera, Hudson, et al., 2015). Nursing interventions are directed toward supporting cardiovascular and neurologic function until the usually transient episode of neurogenic shock resolves.

Patients with neurogenic shock have a higher risk for venous thromboembolism (VTE) formation because of increased pooling of blood from vascular dilation; this risk is greater in patients with neurogenic shock related to spinal cord injury (Zhang, Wadhwa, Haydel, et al., 2013). The nurse must check the patient daily for any lower extremity pain, redness, tenderness, and warmth. If the patient complains of pain and objective assessment of the calf is suspicious, the patient should be evaluated for DVT. Passive range of motion of the immobile extremities helps promote circulation. Early interventions to prevent VTE include the application of pneumatic compression devices often combined with antithrombotic agents (e.g., low–molecular-weight heparin).

A patient who has experienced a spinal cord injury may not report pain caused by internal injuries. Therefore, in the immediate postinjury period, the nurse must monitor the patient closely for signs of internal bleeding that could lead to hypovolemic shock.

Anaphylactic Shock

Anaphylactic shock is caused by a severe allergic reaction when patients who have already produced antibodies to a foreign substance (antigen) develop a systemic antigen–antibody reaction; specifically, an immunoglobulin E (IgE)-mediated response. This antigen–antibody reaction provokes mast cells to release potent vasoactive substances, such as histamine or bradykinin, and activates inflammatory cytokines, causing widespread vasodilation and capillary permeability. The most common triggers are foods (especially peanuts), medications, and insects (Muraro, Hoffmann-Sommergruber, Holzhauser, et al., 2014) (see Chart 14-5). Anaphylaxis has three defining characteristics (Muraro et al., 2014; Triggiani, Montagni, Parente, et al., 2014):

- Acute onset of symptoms
- Presence of two or more symptoms that include respiratory compromise, reduced BP, GI distress, and skin or mucosal tissue irritation
- Cardiovascular compromise from minutes to hours after exposure to the antigen

Signs and symptoms of anaphylaxis may present within 2 to 30 minutes of exposure to the antigen; however, occasionally some reactions may not develop for several hours (Triggiani et al., 2014). The patient may complain of headache, lightheadedness, nausea, vomiting, acute abdominal pain or discomfort, pruritus, and feeling of impending doom. Assessment may reveal diffuse erythema and generalized flushing, difficulty breathing (laryngeal edema), bronchospasm, cardiac dysrhythmias, and hypotension. Characteristics of severe anaphylaxis usually include rapid onset of hypotension, neurologic compromise, respiratory distress, and cardiac arrest (Triggiani et al., 2014). Anaphylactoid reactions present similarly to anaphylaxis but are not mediated by IgE responses. Anaphylaxis and anaphylactoid reactions are often clinically indistinguishable (Muraro et al., 2014).

 Medical Management

Treatment of anaphylactic shock requires removing the causative antigen (e.g., discontinuing an antibiotic agent), administering medications that restore vascular tone, and providing emergency support of basic life functions. Fluid management is critical, as massive fluid shifts can occur within minutes due to increased vascular permeability (Muraro et al., 2014). Intramuscular epinephrine is given for its vasoconstrictive action. Diphenhydramine (Benadryl) is given intravenously to reverse the effects of histamine, thereby reducing capillary permeability. Nebulized medications, such as albuterol (Proventil), may be given to reverse histamine-induced bronchospasm.

If cardiac arrest and respiratory arrest are imminent or have occurred, cardiopulmonary resuscitation (CPR) is performed. Endotracheal intubation may be necessary to establish an airway. IV lines are inserted to provide access for administering fluids and medications. (See Chapter 37 for further discussion of anaphylaxis and specific chemical mediators.)

 Nursing Management

The nurse has an important role in prevention and early recognition of anaphylactic shock. The nurse must assess all patients for allergies or previous reactions to antigens (e.g., medications, blood products, foods, contrast agents, latex) and communicate the existence of these allergies or reactions to others. In addition, the nurse assesses the patient's understanding of previous reactions and steps taken by the patient and the family to prevent further exposure to antigens. When new allergies are identified, the nurse advises the patient to wear or carry identification that names the specific allergen or antigen.

When administering any new medication, the nurse observes all patients for allergic reactions. This is especially important with antibiotics, beta-blockers, angiotensin inhibitors (angiotensin-converting enzyme inhibitors, angiotensin receptor blockers), aspirin, and nonsteroidal anti-inflammatory drugs (Triggiani et al., 2014). Previous adverse drug reactions increase the risk that the patient will develop a reaction to a new medication. If the patient reports an allergy to a medication, the nurse must be aware of the risks involved in the administration of similar medications.

At hospital and outpatient diagnostic testing sites, the nurse must identify patients who are at risk for anaphylactic reactions to contrast agents (radiopaque, dye-like substances that may contain iodine) used for diagnostic tests. The nurse must be knowledgeable about the clinical signs of anaphylaxis, must take immediate action if signs and symptoms occur, and must be prepared to begin CPR if cardiorespiratory arrest occurs.

 Quality and Safety Nursing Alert

Patients with a known allergy to iodine or fish and those who have had previous allergic reactions to contrast agents are at high risk for anaphylactic reactions. This information must be communicated to the staff at the diagnostic testing site, including x-ray personnel.

Community health and home care nurses who administer medications, including antibiotic agents, in the patient's home or other settings, must be prepared to administer epinephrine intramuscularly in the event of an anaphylactic reaction.

After recovery from anaphylaxis, the patient and the family require an explanation of the event. Furthermore, the nurse provides education about avoiding future exposure to antigens and administering emergency medications to treat anaphylaxis (see Chapter 37).

Multiple Organ Dysfunction Syndrome

Multiple organ dysfunction syndrome (MODS) is altered organ function in acutely ill patients that requires medical intervention to support continued organ function. It is another phase in the progression of shock states. The actual incidence of MODS is difficult to determine, because it develops with acute illnesses that compromise tissue perfusion. Dysfunction of one organ system is associated with 20% mortality, and if more than four organs fail, the mortality is at least 60% (Rossaint & Zarbock, 2015).

Pathophysiology

MODS may be a complication of any form of shock, but it is most commonly seen in patients with sepsis and is a result of inadequate tissue perfusion. The precise mechanism by which MODS occurs remains unknown. However, MODS frequently occurs toward the end of the continuum of septic shock when tissue perfusion cannot be effectively restored. It is not possible to predict which patients who experience shock will develop MODS, partly because much of the organ damage occurs at the cellular level and, therefore, cannot be directly observed or measured.

The clinical presentation of MODS is insidious; tissues become hypoperfused at both a microcellular and macrocellular level, eventually causing organ dysfunction that requires mechanical and pharmacologic intervention to support organ function. Organ failure usually begins in the lungs, and cardiovascular instability, as well as failure of the hepatic, GI, renal, immunologic, and central nervous systems, follows (Anderson & Watson, 2013; Guirgis, Khadpe, Kuntz, et al., 2014).

Clinical Manifestations

While it is not possible to predict MODS, clinical severity assessment tools may be used to anticipate patient risk of organ dysfunction and mortality. These clinical assessment tools include APACHE (Acute Physiology and Chronic Health Evaluation); SAPS (Simplified Acute Physiology Score); PIRO (Predisposing factors, the Infection, the host Response, and Organ dysfunction); and SOFA score (see Table 14-4) (Gustot, 2011).

In MODS, the sequence of organ dysfunction varies depending on the patient's primary illness and comorbidities before experiencing shock. Advanced age, malnutrition, and coexisting disease appear to increase the risk of MODS in acutely ill patients. For simplicity of presentation, the classic pattern is described. Typically, the lungs are the first organs to show signs of dysfunction. The patient experiences progressive dyspnea and respiratory failure that are manifested as ALI or ARDS, requiring intubation and mechanical ventilation (see Chapters 21 and 23). The patient usually remains hemodynamically stable but may require increasing amounts of IV fluids and vasoactive agents to support BP and cardiac output. Signs of a hypermetabolic state, characterized by hyperglycemia (elevated blood glucose level), hyperlactic acidemia (excess lactic acid in the blood), and increased BUN, are present. The metabolic rate may be 1.5 to 2 times the basal metabolic rate. At this time, there is a severe loss of skeletal muscle mass (autocatabolism) to meet the high energy demands of the body.

After approximately 7 to 10 days, signs of hepatic dysfunction (e.g., elevated bilirubin and liver function tests) and renal dysfunction (e.g., elevated creatinine and anuria) are evident. As the lack of tissue perfusion continues, the hematologic system becomes dysfunctional, with worsening immunocompromise, increasing the risk of bleeding. The cardiovascular system becomes unstable and unresponsive to vasoactive agents, and the patient's neurologic response progresses to a state of unresponsiveness or coma.

The goal of all shock states is to reverse the tissue hypoperfusion and hypoxia. If effective tissue perfusion is restored before organs become dysfunctional, the patient's condition stabilizes. Along the septic shock continuum, the onset of organ dysfunction is an ominous prognostic sign; the more organs that fail, the worse the outcome.

 ## Medical Management

Prevention remains the top priority in managing MODS. Older adult patients are at increased risk for MODS because of the lack of physiologic reserve and the natural degenerative process, especially immune compromise (Guirgis et al., 2014). Early detection and documentation of initial signs

of infection are essential in managing MODS in older adult patients. Subtle changes in mentation and a gradual rise in temperature are early warning signs. Other patients at greater risk for MODS are those with chronic illness, malnutrition, immunosuppression, or surgical or traumatic wounds.

If preventive measures fail, treatment measures to reverse MODS are aimed at (1) controlling the initiating event, (2) promoting adequate organ perfusion, (3) providing nutritional support, and (4) maximizing patient comfort.

 ## Nursing Management

The general plan of nursing care for patients with MODS is the same as that for patients with shock. Primary nursing interventions are aimed at supporting the patient and monitoring organ perfusion until primary organ insults are halted. Providing information and support to family members is a critical role of the nurse. The health care team must address end-of-life decisions to ensure that supportive therapies are congruent with the patient's wishes (see Chapter 16).

Promoting Communication

Nurses should encourage frequent and open communication about treatment modalities and options to ensure that the patient's wishes regarding medical management are met. Patients who survive MODS must be informed about the goals of rehabilitation and expectations for progress toward these goals, because massive loss of skeletal muscle mass makes rehabilitation a long, slow process. A strong nurse–patient relationship built on effective communication provides needed encouragement during this phase of recovery.

Promoting Home, Community-Based, and Transitional Care

Educating Patients About Self-Care

Patients who experience and survive shock may have been unable to get out of bed for an extended period of time and are likely to have a slow, prolonged recovery. The patient and the family are educated about strategies to prevent further episodes of shock by identifying the factors implicated in the initial episode (Kleinpell et al., 2013). In addition, the patient and the family require education about assessments needed to identify the complications that may occur after the patient is discharged from the hospital. Depending on the type of shock and its management, the patient or the family may require education about treatment modalities such as emergency administration of medications, IV therapy, parenteral or enteral nutrition, skin care, exercise, and ambulation. The patient and the family are also educated about the need for gradual increases in ambulation and other activity. The need for adequate nutrition is another crucial aspect of education.

Continuing and Transitional Care

Because of the physical toll associated with recovery from shock, patients may be cared for in a long-term care facility or rehabilitation setting after hospital discharge. Alternatively, a referral may be made for home, community-based, or transitional care. The nurse assesses the patient's physical status and monitors recovery. The adequacy of treatments continued at home and the ability of the patient and the family to cope with these treatments are also assessed. The patient is likely to require close medical supervision until complete recovery occurs. The nurse reinforces the importance of continuing medical care and helps the patient and the family identify and mobilize community resources.

CRITICAL THINKING EXERCISES

1 **pq** A patient arrives in the preoperative day surgery waiting room. The patient has a sensitivity to peanuts. The waiting room does not have a "no food or drink policy" and several family members are observed eating. The patient's significant other approaches the secretary in the waiting room stating that the patient has a peanut allergy and he is complaining of increasing anxiety, shortness of breath, and chest discomfort. He is flushed, anxious, tachypneic, and visibly uncomfortable. The secretary comments that it is common for preoperative surgery patients to be anxious and encourages the family member to engage in distracting behaviors with the patient. Three minutes later, the patient's significant other approaches the secretary stating that the patient is in extreme distress with worsening shortness of breath and chest discomfort. The secretary calls the preoperative intake nurse to immediately assess the patient. What are the immediate nursing priorities in providing care to this patient? What assessment data are needed to determine whether this patient is experiencing shock? What type of shock do you anticipate the patient may be experiencing and why? What nursing interventions and medical treatments should be anticipated? What additional nursing interventions should be implemented to prevent future adverse medication events for this patient? What follow-up might the nurse provide to the secretary and/or the leadership team related to food and drink in the preoperative waiting areas? Are there quality and safety interventions the nurse can lead to prevent future adverse events associated with food and drink in the preoperative day surgery waiting room?

2 **ebp** A community-dwelling older woman is admitted to the hospital with a hip fracture after falling at home. Her past medical history includes hypertension and depression; both are well-controlled by medications. She is also hard of hearing but does not wear hearing aids. She is now 72 hours post–hip fracture repair. Initial shift assessment reveals the patient to be confused and somewhat combative in behavior. Should you assess the patient for acute delirium? Why or why not? You know that changes in mental status may be an early sign of sepsis in older adults. How would you assess this patient for the possibility of sepsis? What risk factors place an older patient at higher risk for sepsis? What risk factors does this patient have that placed her at increased risk for sepsis? How would you ensure the accuracy of vital signs and interpretation of vital signs in the older patient experiencing sepsis? What is the evidence base for these risk factors? How would the management of the older adult patient differ from that of a younger patient? What objective assessment data should

you convey to the primary provider to support your assessment of possible sepsis? If the patient is thought to have sepsis, what interventions need to be initiated within the next 3- and 6-hour time frames?

3 A 34-year-old patient fell from his roof while doing home repairs. He was found down in his front yard by a passing neighbor. Upon admission to the hospital, he is not responsive to questions. He does not spontaneously move his lower extremities. Vital signs are: BP 92/60, HR 88 bpm, RR 28/min, and temperature 38.0°C (100.4°F). What types of shock do you think that this patient could be experiencing? What risk factors does this patient have for developing a shock state? What therapy and treatments would you anticipate? Describe the rationale for the therapies that you have identified. How would you use the patient's history, assessment, and symptom presentation to help you identify shock states? Describe likely symptoms and the underlying pathophysiology of the shock state.

4 A 47-year-old woman presents to the ED complaining of generalized fatigue, indigestion, uncomfortable chest pain, and shortness of breath. What clinical condition(s) do you believe the patient may be experiencing? If cardiogenic shock is suspected, what nursing interventions do you anticipate initiating in the care of this patient? What vasopressor and inotropic agents may need to be started? What laboratory analysis will be required in the care of this patient? What risk factors can be identified for this patient related to her presenting condition and subsequent shock state? What educational interventions may be incorporated into the patient's plan of care to optimize her health after hospital discharge? If the primary provider plans to insert a central venous catheter, what essential care is required of the nurse to reduce the risk of CLABSI for the patient?

REFERENCES

*Asterisk indicates nursing research.
**Double asterisk indicates classic reference.

Books

American College of Surgeons, Committee on Trauma. (2012). *Advanced trauma life support for doctors: Instructors course manual* (9th ed.). Chicago, IL: American College of Surgeons.

Maier, R. V. (2015). Approach to the patient with shock. In D. Kasper, J. Loscalzo, S. Hauser, et al. (Eds.). *Harrison's principles of internal medicine* (19th ed.). New York: McGraw-Hill Medical.

Journals and Electronic Documents

Allen, J. M. (2014). Understanding vasoactive medications: Focus on pharmacology and effective titration. *Journal of Infusion Nursing, 37*(2), 82–86.

American Heart Association. (2015). *Highlights of the 2015 American Heart Association Guidelines update for CPR and ECC.* Retrieved on 2/15/2016 at: eccguidelines.heart.org/wp-content/uploads/2015/10/2015-AHA-Guidelines-Highlights-English.pdf

Anderson, M. W., & Watson, G. A. (2013). Traumatic shock: The fifth shock. *Journal of Trauma Nursing, 20*(1), 37–43.

**Annane, D., Siami, S., Jaber, S., et al. (2013). Effects of fluid resuscitation with colloids vs crystalloids on mortality in critically ill patients presenting with hypovolemic shock: The CRISTAL randomized trial. *JAMA, 310*(17), 1809–1817.

Antonelli, M., DeBacker, D., Dorman, T., et al. (2016). *Surviving Sepsis Campaign responds to Sepsis-3*. Retrieved on 3/24/2016 at: www.survivingsepsis.org/SiteCollectionDocuments/SSC-Statements-Sepsis-Definitions-3-2016.pdf

Balogh, Z., Lumsdaine, W., Moore, E. E., et al. (2014). Post-injury abdominal compartment syndrome: From recognition to prevention. *Lancet, 384*(9952), 1466–1475.

**Barr, J., Fraser, G. L., Puntillo, K., et al. (2013). Clinical practice guidelines for the management of pain, agitation, and delirium in adult patients in the intensive care unit. *Critical Care Medicine, 41*(1), 263–306.

Blaser, A. R., Starkopf, J., Kirsimagi, U., et al. (2014). Definition, prevalence, and outcome of feeding intolerance in intensive care: A systematic review an meta-analysis. *Acta Anaesthesiologica Scandinavica, 58*(8), 914–922.

**Bridges, N., & Jarquin-Valdivia, A. A. (2005). Use of the Trendelenburg position as the resuscitation position: To T or not to T? *American Journal of Critical Care, 14*(3), 364–367.

**Bulger, E. M., May, S., Kerby, J. D., et al. (2011). Out of hospital hypertonic resuscitation after traumatic hypovolemic shock: A randomized, placebo, controlled trial. *Annals of Surgery, 253*(3), 431–441.

Centers for Medicare & Medicaid Services. (2014). *Improve quality of care during hospital inpatient stays*. Retrieved on 11/28/2015 at: www.cms.gov/Newsroom/MediaReleaseDatabase/Fact-sheets/2014-Fact-sheets-items/2014-08-04-2.html

Cestero, R. F., & Dent, D. L. (2015). Endpoints of resuscitation. *Surgical Clinics of North America, 95*(2), 319–336.

Davis, L. L. (2014). Cardiovascular issues in older adults. *Critical Care Nursing Clinics of North America, 26*(1), 61–89.

Dellinger, R. P. (2015). The future of sepsis performance improvement. *Critical Care Medicine, 43*(9), 1787–1790.

**Dellinger, R. P., Levy, M. M., Rhodes, A., et al. (2013). Surviving Sepsis Campaign: International guidelines for management of severe sepsis and septic shock: 2012. *Critical Care Medicine, 41*(2), 580–637.

deWitt, B., Joshi, R., Meislin, H., et al. (2014). Optimizing oxygen delivery in the critically ill: Assessment of volume responsiveness in the septic patient. *The Journal of Emergency Medicine, 47*(5), 608–615.

Dubick, M. A., Shek, P., & Wade, C. E. (2013). ROC trials update on prehospital hypertonic saline resuscitation in the aftermath of the US-Canadian trials. *Clinics, 68*(6), 883–886.

*Giles, T. M, & Hall, K. L. (2013). Qualitative systematic review: The unique experiences of the nurse-family member when a loved one is admitted with a critical illness. *Journal of Advanced Nursing, 70*(7), 1451–1464.

Green, J. M. (2015). Essentials of sepsis management. *Surgical Clinics of North America, 95*(2), 355–365.

**Griesdale, D. E., DeSouza, R. J., VanDam, R. M., et al. (2009). Intensive insulin therapy and mortality among critically ill patients: A meta-analysis including NICE-Sugar study data. *Canadian Medical Association Journal, 180*(8), 821–827.

Guirgis, F. W., Khadpe, J. D., Kuntz, G. M., et al. (2014). Persistent organ dysfunction after severe sepsis: A systematic review. *Journal of Critical Care, 29*(3), 320–326.

**Gustot, T. (2011). Multiple organ failure in sepsis: Prognosis and role of systemic inflammatory response. *Current Opinion in Critical Care, 17*(2), 153–159.

Hillier, B., Wilson, C., Chamberlain, D., et al. (2013). Preventing ventilator-associated pneumonia through oral care, product selection, and application method: A literature review. *AACN Advanced Critical Care, 24*(1), 38–58.

Hinkle, L. J., Bosslet, G. T., & Torke, A. M. (2015). Factors associated with family satisfaction with end of life care in the ICU: A systematic review. *Chest, 147*(1), 82–93.

Holcomb, J. B., Tiley, B. C., Baraniuk, S., et al. (2015). Transfusion of plasma, platelets, and red blood cells in a 1:1:1: vs a 1:1:2 ration and mortality in patients with severe trauma. *JAMA, 313*(5), 471–482.

Holodinsky J. K., Roberts, D. J., Ball, C. G., et al. (2013). Risk factors for intra-abdominal hypertension and abdominal compartment syndrome among adult intensive care unit patients: A systematic review and meta-analysis. *Critical Care, 17*(5), R249.

Institute for Healthcare Improvement. (2012). *How-to guide: Prevent central line–associated bloodstream infection*. Retrieved on 11/28/2015 at: www.ihi.org/knowledge/Pages/Tools/HowtoGuidePreventCentralLineAssociatedBloodstreamInfection.aspx

Institute for Healthcare Improvement. (2014a). *Implement the sepsis resuscitation bundle*. Retrieved on 11/29/2015 at: www.ihi.org/resources/Pages/Tools/SevereSepsisBundles.aspx

Institute for Healthcare Improvement (IHI). (2014b). *Improving stories: Early warning systems: Scorecards that save lives*. Retrieved on 2/18/2016 at: www.ihi.org/resources/PublishingImages/Image_PatientAssessmentObservationInfusionMonitoring.jpg

Kanwar, R., Delasobera, B. E., Hudson, K., et al. (2015). Emergency department evaluation and treatment of cervical spine injuries. *Emergency Medicine Clinics of North America, 33*(2), 241–282.

Kleinpell, R., Aitken, L, & Schorr, C. A. (2013). Implications of the new international sepsis guidelines for nursing care. *American Journal of Critical Care, 22*(3), 212–222.

Lee, R. (2015). Ask the experts: Time frames for sepsis screening criteria. *Critical Care Nurse, 35*(3), 74–75.

Levi, M., & van der Poll, T., (2015). Coagulation in patients with severe sepsis. *Seminars in Thrombosis and Hemostasis, 41*(1), 9–15.

Levy, M. M., Rhodes, A., Phillips, G. S., et al. (2015). Surviving Sepsis Campaign: Association between performance metrics and outcomes in a 7.5 year study. *Critical Care Medicine, 43*(1), 3–12.

Lineberry, C., & Stein, D. E. (2014). Infection, sepsis, and immune function in the older adult receiving critical care. *Critical Care Nursing Clinics of North America, 26*(1), 47–60.

Makic, M. B. F. (2013). Preventing delirium in postoperative patients. *Journal of PeriAnesthesia Nursing, 28*(6), 404–408.

Makic, M. B. F., Rauen, C. A., Jones, K., et al. (2015). Continuing to challenge practice to be evidence-based. *Critical Care Nurse, 35*(2), 39–50.

Makic, M. B. F., Rauen, C. A., Watson, R., et al. (2014). Examining the evidence to guide practice: Challenging practice habits. *Critical Care Nurse, 34*(2), 28–45.

**Marik, P. E., Baram, M., & Vahid, B. (2008). Does central venous pressure predict fluid responsiveness? A systematic review of the literature and the tale of seven mares. *Chest, 134*(1), 172–178.

Marik P. E., & Bellomo, R. (2013). Stress hyperglycemia: An essential survival response. *Critical Care, 17*(2), 305. Retrieved on 11/29/2015 at: ccforum.com/content/17/2/305

Marschall, J., Mermel, L. A., Fakih, M., et al., (2014). Strategies to prevent central-line associated blood stream infections in acute care hospitals: 2014 update. *Infection Control and Hospital Epidemiology, 35*(7), 753–771.

Martindale, R. G., & Warren, M. (2015). Should enteral nutrition be started in the first week of critical illness? *Current Opinion in Clinical Nutrition & Metabolic Care, 18*(2), 202–206.

Mayr, F. B., Yende, S., & Angus, D.C. (2014). Epidemiology of severe sepsis. *Virulence, 5*(1), 4–11.

McEnvoy, M. T., & Shander A. (2013). Anemia, bleeding, and blood transfusion in the intensive care unit: Causes, risks, costs, and new strategies. *American Journal of Critical Care, 22*(6), eS1–eS13.

Moore, J. P. R., Dyson, A., Singer M., et al. (2015). Microcirculatory dysfunction and resuscitations: Why when, and how. *British Journal of Anaesthesia, 115*(3), 366–375.

Muraro, A., Hoffmann-Sommergruber, K., Holzhauser, T., et al., (2014). EAACI food allergy and anaphylaxis guidelines: Protecting consumers with food allergies, understanding food consumption, meeting regulations and identifying unmet needs. *Allergy, 69*(11), 1464–1472.

Ng, R., & Yeghiazarians, Y. (2013). Post myocardial infarction cardiogenic shock: A review of current therapies. *Journal of Intensive Care Medicine, 28*(3), 151–165.

Perel, P., Roberts, I., & Ker, K. (2013). Colloids versus crystalloids for fluid resuscitation in critically ill patients (review). *Cochrane Database of Systematic Reviews, 2*, CD000567.

Perrin, K. O., & Kazanowski, M. (2015). Overcoming barriers to palliative care consultation. *Critical Care Nurse, 35*(5), 44–52.

Prucha, M., Belligan, G., & Zazula, R. (2014). Sepsis biomarkers. *Clinica Chimica Acta, 440*(2), 97–103.

**Rivers, E. P., McIntyre, L., Morro, D. C., et al. (2005). Early and innovative interventions for severe sepsis and septic shock: Taking advantage of a window of opportunity. *Canadian Medical Association Journal, 173*(9), 1054–1065.

Rossaint, J., & Zarbock, A. (2015). Pathogenesis of multiple organ failure in sepsis. *Critical Reviews in Immunology, 35*(4), 277–291.

See, K. C., Mukhopadhyay, A., Lau, S. C., et al. (2015). Shock in the first 24 hours of intensive care unit stay: Observational study of protocol-based fluid management. *Shock, 43*(5), 456–462.

Silva, P. L., Pelosi, P., & Rocco, P. R. M. (2014). Fluids in acute respiratory distress syndrome: Pros and cons. *Current Opinion in Critical Care, 20*(1), 104–112.

Singer, M., Deutschman, C. S., Seymour, C. W., et al. (2016). The third international consensus definitions for sepsis and septic shock (sepsis-3). *JAMA, 315*(8), 801–810.

Society for Healthcare Epidemiology of America. (2015) SHEA Guideline Central. Retrieved on 11/28/2015 at: www.guidelinecentral.com/share/pocketcard/53d67314007df/#i469f5e2f

Subramaniam, S., Tiruvoipati, R., & Botha, J. (2015). Current advances in the use of therapeutic hypothermia. *Therapeutic Hypothermia and Temperature Management, 5*(1), 13–16.

Surviving Sepsis Bundle. (2015). Retrieved on 11/28/2015 at: www.survivingsepsis.org/SiteCollectionDocuments/SSC_Bundle.pdf

Surviving Sepsis Campaign. (2016). Retrieved on 3/24/2016 at: www.survivingsepsis.org

Tay, E. T. (2015). Intraosseous access. Medscape. Retrieved on 11/29/2015 at: reference.medscape.com/article/80431-overview

Tharmaratnam, D., Nolan, J., & Jain, A. (2013). Management of cardiogenic shock complicating acute coronary syndromes. *Heart, 99*(3), 1614–1623.

Triggiani, M., Montagni, M., Parente, R., et al. (2014). Anaphylaxis and cardiovascular diseases: A dangerous liaison. *Current Opinion in Allergy and Clinical Immunology, 14*(4), 309–315.

*Twibell, R. S., Craig., S., Siela, D., et al. (2015). Being there: Inpatients' perceptions of family presence during resuscitation and invasive cardiac procedures. *American Journal of Critical Care, 24*(6), 108–115.

Vanderbilt University Medical Center. (2013). *ICU delirium and cognitive impairment study group.* Retrieved on 2/15/2016 at: www.icudelirium.org/delirium/monitoring.html

**Vincent, J. L., Moreno, R., Takala, J., et al. (1996). The SOFA (Sepsis-related Organ Failure Assessment) score to describe organ dysfunction/failure. On behalf of the Working Group on Sepsis-Related Programs of the European Society of Intensive Care Medicine. *Intensive Care Medicine, 22*(7), 707–710.

Wacker, D. A., & Winters, M. E. (2014). Shock. *Emergency Medicine Clinics of North America, 32*(4), 747–758.

World Sepsis Day: Sepsis Fact Sheet. (2015). *World Sepsis Day.* Retrieved on 11/29/2015 at: www.world-sepsis-day.org/CONTENTPIC/2015_WSD_FactSheet_long_English.pdf

Yealy, D. M., Kellum J. A., Juang, D. T., et al. (2014). A randomized trial of protocol-based care for early septic shock. *New England Journal of Medicine, 370*(18), 1683–1693.

Zarbock, A., Gomez, H., & Kellum, J. A. (2014). Sepsis-induced acute kidney injury revisited: Pathophysiology, prevention and future therapies. *Current Opinion in Critical Care, 20*(6), 588–595.

Zarychanski, R., Abou-Setta, A. M., Kanji S., et al. (2015). The efficacy and safety of heparin in patients with sepsis: A systematic review and meta-analysis. *Critical Care Medicine, 43*(3), 511–518.

Zhang, S., Wadhwa, R., Haydel, J., et al. (2013). Spine and spinal cord trauma: Diagnosis and management. *Neurologic Clinics, 31*(1), 183–206.

Resources

Institute for Healthcare Improvement, www.ihi.org
Surviving Sepsis, www.survivingsepsis.org

15

Management of Patients With Oncologic Disorders

On completion of this chapter, the learner will be able to:

1 Compare the function and behavior of normal and cancer cells.
2 Differentiate between the different malignant processes that occur in oncologic disorders.
3 Identify agents and factors that are carcinogenic.
4 Describe the role of nurses in health education and prevention of oncologic disorders.
5 Differentiate among the goals of cancer care: prevention, diagnosis, cure, control, and palliation.

6 Describe the roles of surgery, radiation therapy, chemotherapy, hematopoietic stem cell transplantation, hyperthermia, targeted therapy, and symptom management in treating cancer.
7 Use the nursing process as a framework for the care of patients with cancer.
8 Identify assessment parameters and nursing management of patients with oncologic emergencies.
9 Discuss the role of nurses in cancer survivorship care.

GLOSSARY

alopecia: hair loss

anaplasia: pattern of growth in which cells lack normal characteristics and differ in shape and organization with respect to their cells of origin; usually, anaplastic cells are malignant

angiogenesis: growth of new blood vessels that allow cancer cells to grow

apoptosis: a normal cell mechanism of programmed cell death

benign: not cancerous; benign tumors may grow but are unable to spread to other organs or body parts

brachytherapy: delivery of radiation therapy through internal implants placed inside or adjacent to the tumor

cancer: a group of disorders characterized by abnormal cell proliferation, in which cells ignore growth-regulating signals in the surrounding environment

carcinogenesis: process of transforming normal cells into malignant cells

carcinogens: chemicals, physical factors, and other agents that cause cancer

chemotherapy: the use of medications to kill tumor cells by interfering with cellular functions and reproduction

cytokines: substances produced primarily by cells of the immune system to enhance production and functioning of components of the immune system

extravasation: leakage of intravenous medication from the veins into the subcutaneous tissues

grading: identification of the type of tissue from which the tumor originated and the degree to which the tumor cells retain the functional and structural characteristics of the tissue of origin

graft-versus-host disease (GVHD): an immune response initiated by T lymphocytes of donor tissue against the recipient's tissues (skin, gastrointestinal tract, liver); an undesirable response

graft-versus-tumor effect: the donor immune cell response against the malignancy; a desirable response

malignant: having cells or processes that are characteristic of cancer

metastasis: spread of cancer cells from the primary tumor to distant sites

mucositis: inflammation of the lining of the mouth, throat, and gastrointestinal tract often associated with cancer therapies

myelosuppression: suppression of the blood cell–producing function of the bone marrow

nadir: lowest point of white blood cell depression after therapy that has toxic effects on the bone marrow

neoplasia: uncontrolled cell growth that follows no physiologic demand; cancer

neutropenia: abnormally low absolute neutrophil count

oncology: field or study of cancer

palliation: relief of symptoms and promotion of comfort and quality of life regardless of the disease stage

precision medicine: using advances in research, technology, and policies to develop individualized plans of care to prevent and treat disease

radiation therapy: the use of ionizing radiation to kill malignant cells

staging: process of determining the extent of disease, including tumor size and spread or metastasis to distant sites

stomatitis: inflammation of the oral tissues, often associated with some chemotherapeutic agents and radiation therapy to the head and neck region

targeted therapies: cancer treatments that seek to minimize the negative effects on healthy tissues by disrupting specific cancer cell functions (such as malignant transformation), metabolism, communication pathways, processes for growth and metastasis, and genetic coding

thrombocytopenia: decrease in the number of circulating platelets; associated with the potential for bleeding

vesicant: substance that can cause inflammation, damage, and necrosis with extravasation from blood vessels and contact with tissues

Cancer is a large group of disorders with different causes, manifestations, treatments, and prognoses. Because cancer can involve any organ system and treatment approaches have the potential for multisystem effects, cancer nursing practice overlaps with numerous nursing specialties. Cancer nursing practice covers all age groups and is carried out in various settings, including acute care institutions, outpatient centers, physician offices, rehabilitation facilities, the home, and long-term care facilities. The scope, responsibilities, and goals of cancer nursing, also called **oncology** nursing, are as diverse and complex as those of any nursing specialty. Nursing management of the patient with oncologic disorders includes care of patients throughout the cancer trajectory from prevention through end-of-life care (see Fig. 15-1).

Precision medicine is now possible because of the recent development of biologic databases (e.g., human genome sequencing), technological advances that can identify unique characteristics of individual persons (e.g., genomics, cellular assay tests), and computer-driven systems that can mine and analyze datasets (see Chapter 1). This is an exciting time for oncology as the immediate goal of the precision medicine initiative is to focus on preventing and curing cancers (Collins & Varmus, 2015).

Epidemiology

In 2015, nearly 700,000 new cancer cases were diagnosed. In the same year, nearly 600,000 Americans died as a result of cancer. Despite significant advances in science and technology, cancer is the second leading cause of death in the United States (Siegel, Miller, & Jemal, 2015). Currently, one in four deaths is caused by cancer. The leading causes of cancer death in the United States in order of frequency and location are lung, prostate, and colorectal cancer in men and lung, breast, and colorectal cancer in women. Most cancer occurs in older adults; according to the American Cancer Society (ACS), 78% of all cancer diagnoses are in people 55 years of age or older (2015a). Overall, the incidence of cancer is higher in men than in women.

Although the overall rate of cancer deaths has declined, cancer death rates in African American men remain substantially higher than those among Caucasian men and two times those of Hispanic men (Siegel et al., 2015). While African American women have a lower risk of cancer overall than white women, they have 14% higher death rates for all cancers compared with white women and women in general (ACS, 2016a). Racial disparities may be attributed to the burdens of comorbid conditions, such as cardiovascular disease, and poverty experienced more often in the African American population than in others (ACS, 2016a; DeNavas-Walt, Proctor, & Smith, 2013).

Cancer incidence and death rates also vary by geography. In states where the prevalence of tobacco use is high, the incidence of lung cancer tends to be greater than in states where smoking is not as common. In locations where there is greater socioeconomic disparity, the incidence of advanced cancer and overall cancer death rates are higher than in regions where there is not such disparity (Kohler, Sherman, Howlader, et al., 2015).

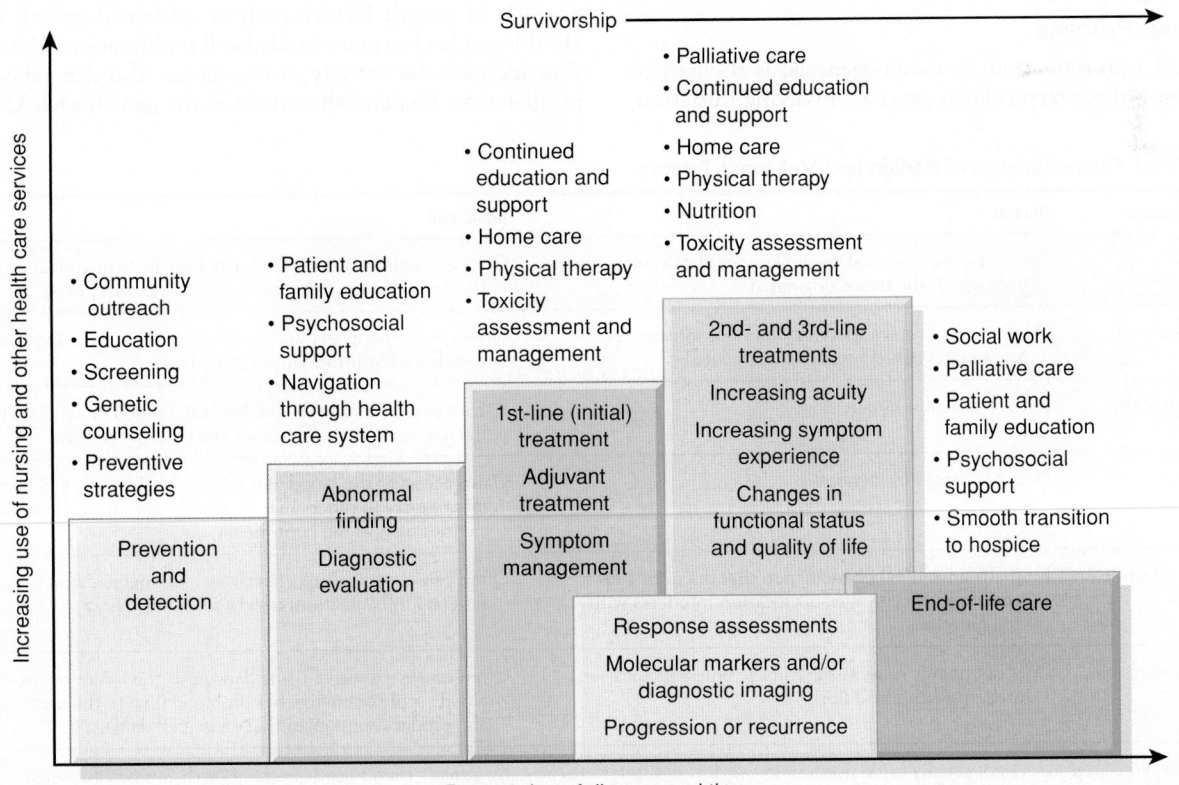

Figure 15-1 • Cancer care trajectory. The cancer care trajectory reflects the phases and care required during the continuum of the cancer experience from prevention and early detection through end-of-life care. Specialized nursing care is provided throughout the entire trajectory.

Pathophysiology of the Malignant Process

Cancer is a disease process that begins when a cell is transformed by genetic mutations of the cellular deoxyribonucleic acid (DNA). Genetic mutations may be inherited and/or acquired, leading to abnormal cell behavior (Grossman & Porth, 2014). The initial genetically altered cell forms a clone and begins to proliferate abnormally, evading normal intracellular and extracellular growth-regulating processes or signals as well as the immune system defense mechanisms of the body. Genetic mutations may lead to abnormalities in cell signaling transduction processes (signals from outside and within cells that turn cell activities either on or off) that can in turn lead to cancer development. Ultimately cells acquire a variety of capabilities that allow them to invade surrounding tissues and/or gain access to lymph and blood vessels, which carry the cells to other areas of the body resulting in **metastasis** or spread of the cancer (Acharyya, Matrisian, Welch, et al., 2015).

Characteristics of Malignant Cells

Benign and malignant cells differ in many cellular growth characteristics, including the method and rate of growth, ability to metastasize or spread, destruction of tissue, and ability to cause death. These differences are summarized in Table 15-1. The degree of **anaplasia** (a pattern of growth in which cells lack normal characteristics and differ in shape and organization with respect to their cells of origin) is associated with increased malignant potential.

Carcinogenesis

Molecular Process

Malignant transformation, or **carcinogenesis,** is thought to be at least a three-step cellular process, involving initiation, promotion, and progression. Agents that initiate or promote malignant transformation are referred to as **carcinogens.**

During *initiation*, carcinogens (substances that can cause cancer), such as chemicals, physical factors, or biologic agents, cause mutations in the cellular DNA. Normally, these alterations are reversed by DNA repair mechanisms or the changes initiate programmed cellular death (**apoptosis**) or cell senescence. Cells can escape these protective mechanisms with permanent cellular mutations occurring, but these mutations usually are not significant to cells until the second step of carcinogenesis.

During *promotion*, repeated exposure to promoting agents (co-carcinogens) causes proliferation and expansion of initiated cells with increased expression or manifestations of abnormal genetic information, even after long latency periods. Promoting agents are not mutagenic and do not need to interact with the DNA. Latency periods for the promotion of cellular mutations vary with the type of agent, the dosage of the promoter, and the innate characteristics and genetic stability of the target cell. The promotion phase generally leads to the formation of a preneoplastic or **benign** (noncancerous) lesion.

During *progression*, the altered cells exhibit increasingly malignant behavior. These cells acquire the ability to stimulate **angiogenesis** (growth of new blood vessels that allow cancer cells to grow), to invade adjacent tissues, and to metastasize. Cellular oncogenes are responsible for vital cell functions, including proliferation and differentiation. Cellular proto-oncogenes, such as those for the epidermal growth factor receptor (EGFR), transcription factors such as *c-Myc*, or cell signaling proteins such as *Kirsten ras* (*KRAS*), act as "on switches" for cellular growth. Amplification of proto-oncogenes or overexpression of growth factors, such as epidermal growth factor (EGF), can lead to uncontrolled cell proliferation. Mutations that increase the activity of oncogenes also deregulate cell proliferation. Genetic alterations in the gene for *KRAS* have

TABLE 15-1 Characteristics of Benign and Malignant Tumors

Characteristics	Benign	Malignant
Cell	Well-differentiated cells resemble normal cells of the tissue from which the tumor originated.	Cells are undifferentiated and may bear little resemblance to the normal cells of the tissue from which they arose.
Mode of growth	Tumor grows by expansion and does not infiltrate the surrounding tissues; usually encapsulated.	Grows at the periphery and overcomes contact inhibition to invade and infiltrate surrounding tissues
Rate of growth	Rate of growth is usually slow.	Rate of growth is variable and depends on level of differentiation; the more anaplastic the tumor, the faster its growth.
Metastasis	Does not spread by metastasis	Gains access to the blood and lymphatic channels and metastasizes to other areas of the body or grows across body cavities such as the peritoneum
General effects	Is usually a localized phenomenon that does not cause generalized effects unless its location interferes with vital functions	Often causes generalized effects, such as anemia, weakness, systemic inflammation, weight loss, and CACS
Tissue destruction	Does not usually cause tissue damage unless its location interferes with blood flow	Often causes extensive tissue damage as the tumor outgrows its blood supply or encroaches on blood flow to the area; may also produce substances that cause cell damage
Ability to cause death	Does not usually cause death unless its location interferes with vital functions	Eventually causes death unless growth can be controlled

CACS, cancer-related anorexia-cachexia syndrome.
Adapted from Grossman, S. C., & Porth, C. M. (2014). *Porth's pathophysiology: Concepts of altered health states* (9th ed.). Philadelphia, PA: Lippincott Williams & Wilkins.

Chart 15-1	**GENETICS IN NURSING PRACTICE**

Genetics Concepts and Oncologic Disorders

Cancer is a genetic disease. Every phase of carcinogenesis is affected by multiple gene mutations. Some of these mutations are inherited (present in germ-line cells) and present a greater risk for a person to develop oncologic disorders; however, most (90%) are somatic mutations that are acquired mutations in specific cells. Examples of cancers influenced by genetics include:

Autosomal dominant:

- Breast and ovarian cancer
- Colorectal cancer
- Familial adenomatous polyposis
- Cowden syndrome
- Li-Fraumeni syndrome
- Lynch Syndrome (Hereditary nonpolyposis colon cancer)
- Multiple endocrine neoplasia types 1 and 2
- Neurofibromatosis types 1 and 2
- Prostate cancer
- Retinoblastoma
- Von Hippel–Lindau syndrome
- Wilm's tumor

Autosomal recessive:

- Ataxia telangiectasis
- Endometrial cancer
- Gastrointestinal stromal tumor
- Familial melanoma syndrome
- Xeroderma pigmentosum

Nursing Assessments

Refer to Chart 5-2: Genetics in Nursing Practice: Genetic Aspects of Health Assessment

Family History Assessment Specific to Oncologic Disorders

- Obtain information about both maternal and paternal sides of family for three generations.
- Obtain cancer history for at least three generations.
- Look for clustering of cancers that occur at young ages, multiple primary cancers in one individual, cancer in paired organs, and two or more close relatives with the same type of cancer suggestive of hereditary cancer syndromes.

Patient Assessment

- Assess for the following:
  - Physical findings that may predispose the patient to cancer, such as multiple colon polyps or the presence of more than one tumor. If a tumor was previously diagnosed, inquire about the age of the patient when the first tumor was noted.
  - Skin findings, such as atypical moles, that may be related to familial melanoma syndrome.
  - Multiple café-au-lait spots, axillary freckling, and two or more neurofibromas associated with neurofibromatosis type 1.
  - Facial trichilemmomas, mucosal papillomatosis, multinodular thyroid goiter or thyroid adenomas, macrocephaly, fibrocystic breasts, and other fibromas or lipomas related to Cowden syndrome.
- Assess for lifestyle risks (e.g., smoking, obesity, alcohol use).
- Determine potential occupational or environmental hazards that may generate exposure to inhaled chemicals, gases, or other irritants (e.g., toxic metals, asbestos, radon).

Management Issues Specific to Oncologic Disorders

- Assess patient's understanding of genetics factors related to their cancer.
- Offer appropriate genetics information and resources.
- Refer for cancer risk assessment when a hereditary cancer syndrome is suspected so that patient and family can discuss inheritance risk with other family members and availability of genetic testing.
- Provide support to patients and families with known genetic test results for hereditary cancer syndromes. Refer to support groups as appropriate.
- Participate in the management and coordination of risk reduction measures for those with known gene mutations.

Genetics Resources Specific to Oncologic Disorders

American Cancer Society: www.cancer.org
National Cancer Institute: www.cancer.gov
See also Chapter 8, Chart 8-7 for additional components of genetic counseling.

---

been associated with pancreatic, lung, and colorectal cancers (http://www.mycancergenome.org/content/disease/lung-cancer/kras/Lovly, Horn, & Pao, 2015). Just as proto-oncogenes "turn on" cellular growth, cancer suppressor genes "turn off," or regulate, unneeded cellular proliferation. When suppressor genes are mutated, resulting in loss of function or expression, the cells begin to produce mutant cell populations that are different from their original cellular ancestors. See Chart 15-1 for further discussion of genetics concepts and cancer.

Proliferative Patterns

During the lifespan, various body tissues normally undergo periods of rapid or proliferative growth that must be distinguished from malignant growth activity. Several patterns of cell growth exist: hyperplasia, dysplasia, and metaplasia (see Chapter 6). Cancerous cells, described as **malignant** neoplasms, demonstrate uncontrolled cell growth that follows no physiologic demand (**neoplasia**). Although both benign and malignant growths are classified and named by tissue of origin, the *International Classification of Diseases for Oncology* (Fritz, Percy, Jack, et al., 2013) is used by scientists and clinicians around the world as the nomenclature for malignant disease (see Table 15-2).

Etiology

Factors implicated or known to induce carcinogenesis include viruses and bacteria, physical agents, chemicals, genetic or familial factors, lifestyle factors, and hormones. Additional research is needed for a better understanding of the relationships between etiologic factors and cancer.

Viruses and Bacteria

It is estimated that about 11% of all cancers worldwide are linked to viral infections (Schiller & Lowy, 2014). After infecting individuals, DNA viruses insert a part of their own DNA near the infected cell genes causing cell division. The newly formed cells that now carry viral DNA lack normal controls on growth. Examples of these viruses that are known

TABLE 15-2   Classification of Cancer by Tissue of Origin

Classification	Tissue of Origin	Characteristics	Term	Examples
Carcinoma	Epithelial	Account for 80–90% of all cancers		
	• Glandular epithelium	Organs or glands capable of secretion	Adenocarcinoma	Adenocarcinoma of the breast, lung, prostate
	• Squamous epithelium	Covers or lines all external and internal body surfaces	Squamous cell carcinoma	Squamous cell cancer of the skin, lung, esophagus
Sarcoma	Connective or Supportive			
	• Bone	Most common form of cancer of the bone	Osteosarcoma	Osteosarcoma of the femur, humerus
	• Cartilage	Rare, arises from within bones	Chondrosarcoma	Chondrosarcoma of the femur, pelvis
	• Adipose	Arises from deep soft tissue	Liposarcoma	Liposarcoma of the retroperitoneum, thigh
	• Smooth muscle	Very rare	Leiomyosarcoma	Leiomyosarcoma of the uterus, intestines, stomach
	• Skeletal muscle	Most common in young children	Rhabdosarcoma	Rhabdosarcoma of the head and neck, limbs
	• Fibrous tissue	Often involves long or flat bones	Fibrosarcoma	Fibrosarcoma of the femur, tibia, mandible
	• Membranes lining body cavities	Most often related to asbestos exposure	Mesothelial sarcoma or mesothelioma	Mesothelioma of the pleura or peritoneum
	• Blood vessels	With liver involvement may be related to occupational exposure to vinyl chloride monomer	Angiosarcoma	Angiosarcoma of the liver, heart
Myeloma	Plasma cells	Produced by B-cell lymphocytes; plasma cells produce antibodies	Not applicable (N/A)	N/A
Lymphoma	Lymphocytes	Two main classifications; may involve lymph nodes and/or body organs	Non-Hodgkin lymphoma	B-cell lymphoma, T-cell lymphoma
			Hodgkin lymphoma	N/A
Leukemia	Hematopoietic cells in the bone marrow	May involve various cell lines produced in the bone marrow		
	• White blood cells (WBCs)	N/A	Myelogenous	Acute myelogenous leukemia
	• Lymphocytes	N/A	Lymphocytic	Acute lymphocytic leukemia
	• Red blood cells (RBCs)	Involves overproduction of RBCs and is associated with increased levels of WBCs and platelets; also risk of additional bone marrow disease	Erythremia	Polycythemia vera

Adapted from Fritz, A., Percy, C., Jack, A., et al. (2013). World Health Organization. (2013). *International classification of diseases for oncology (ICD-O)–3rd edition, 1st revision.* Retrieved on 2/25/2016 at: apps.who.int/iris/bitstream/10665/96612/1/9789241548496_eng.pdf?ua=1

to cause cancer include human papillomavirus (HPV) (cervical and head and neck cancers), hepatitis B virus (HBV) (liver cancer), and Epstein-Barr virus (EBV) (Burkitt lymphoma and nasopharyngeal cancer) (Chen, Hsu, Yang, et al., 2014).

There is little evidence to support the link of most bacteria to cancer, although chronic inflammatory reactions to bacteria and the production of carcinogenic metabolites are possible mechanisms that continue to be investigated. *Helicobacter pylori* is one bacterium identified as a significant cause of gastric cancer (Bessede, Dubus, Megraud, et al., 2014).

Physical Agents

Physical factors associated with carcinogenesis include exposure to sunlight, radiation, chronic irritation or inflammation, tobacco carcinogens, industrial chemicals and asbestos.

Excessive exposure to the ultraviolet rays of the sun, especially in fair-skinned people, increases the risk of skin cancers. Factors such as clothing styles (sleeveless shirts or shorts), the use of sunscreens, occupation, recreational habits, and environmental variables, including humidity, altitude, and latitude, all play a role in the amount of exposure to ultraviolet light.

Exposure to ionizing radiation can occur with repeated diagnostic x-ray procedures or with radiation therapy used to treat disease. Improved x-ray equipment minimizes the risk of extensive radiation exposure. Radiation therapy used in cancer treatment and exposure to radioactive materials at nuclear weapon manufacturing sites or nuclear power plants in the past have been associated with a higher incidence of leukemia, multiple myeloma, and cancers of the lung, bone, breast, thyroid, and other tissues. Background radiation from the natural decay processes that produce radon has also been associated with lung cancer. Ventilation is advised in homes with high levels of trapped radon to allow the gas to disperse into the atmosphere.

Chemical Agents

Many cancers are thought to be related to environmental factors (ACS, 2015a). Most hazardous chemicals produce their toxic effects by altering DNA structure. This can occur in body sites distant from that of initial chemical exposure.

Tobacco smoke, thought to be the single most lethal chemical carcinogen, accounts for about one third of cancer deaths (ACS, 2015a). Smoking is strongly associated with cancers of the lung, head and neck, esophagus, stomach, pancreas, cervix, kidney, and bladder and with acute myeloblastic leukemia (U.S. Department of Health and Human Services [HHS], 2014).

Passive smoke (i.e., secondhand smoke) has been linked to lung cancer; nonsmokers who live with a smoker have about a 20% to 30% greater risk of developing lung cancer (HHS, 2014). There is evidence that passive smoke may be linked with childhood leukemia and cancers of the larynx, pharynx, brain, bladder, rectum, stomach, and breast (HHS, 2014).

Other combustible forms of tobacco such as cigars, pipes, roll-your-own products, and water pipes (or hookah) are also associated with increased cancer risk (ACS, 2015a). Electronic nicotine delivery systems referred to as electronic cigarettes have gained increased popularity as an alternative to tobacco. Although there are no data regarding the safety of these products, there is great concern about potential negative health effects.

Smokeless tobacco products, such as chewing tobacco and snuff, used most often by young adults aged 18 to 24 years, are associated with an increased risk of oral, pancreatic, and esophageal cancer (ACS, 2015a).

Many chemical substances found in the workplace are carcinogens or co-carcinogens. In the United States, carcinogens are classified by two federal agencies: the National Toxicology Program of the Department of Health and Human Services (HHS) and the Environmental Protection Agency's (EPA) Integrated Risk Information System (IRIS). The Centers for Disease Control and Prevention (CDC) established the National Institute for Occupational Safety and Health (NIOSH) to provide occupational exposure limits and guidelines for protection of the workforce as regulated by the Occupational Safety and Health Act of 1970. The extensive list of suspected chemical substances continues to grow and includes aromatic amines and aniline dyes; pesticides and formaldehydes; arsenic, soot, and tars; asbestos; benzene; cadmium; chromium compounds; nickel and zinc ores; wood dust; beryllium compounds; and polyvinyl chloride. Betel nut and lime, which are chewed as stimulants in some cultures, are also included.

Genetics and Familial Factors

Almost every cancer type has been shown to run in families. This may be due to genetics, shared environments, cultural or lifestyle factors. Genetic factors play a fundamental role in cancer cell development. Cancer has been associated with extra chromosomes, too few chromosomes, or translocated chromosomes. Cancers with these underlying genetic abnormalities include chronic myelogenous leukemia, meningiomas, acute leukemia, retinoblastomas, and Wilms tumor. In addition, certain syndromes represent a cluster of cancers identified by a specific genetic alteration that is inherited across generations. In these families, the associated genetic mutation is found in all cells (it is germline and somatic) and represents an inherited susceptibility to cancer for all family members who carry the mutation.

Approximately 5% to 10% of cancers in adults display a pattern of cancers suggestive of a familial predisposition (NCI, 2016). The hallmarks of families with a hereditary cancer syndrome include cancer in two or more first-degree relatives (the parent, sibling, or child of an individual), onset of cancer in family members younger than 50 years, the same type of cancer in several family members, individual family members with more than one type of cancer, and a rare cancer in one or more family members (NCI, 2016). There is also evidence of an autosomal dominant inheritance pattern of cancers affecting several generations of a family.

There have been considerable advances in the recognition of inherited cancer susceptibility syndromes and in the ability to isolate and identify the inherited genetic mutations responsible for cancer. These advances have enabled the appropriate identification of families at risk for certain syndromes. Examples include hereditary breast and ovarian cancer syndrome (*BRCA1* and *BRCA2*) and multiple endocrine **neoplasia** syndrome (*MEN1* and *MEN2*) (see Chart 15-1). Other cancers associated with familial inheritance syndromes include nephroblastomas, pheochromocytomas, and colorectal, stomach, thyroid, renal, prostate, and lung cancers (NCI, 2016).

Life Style Factors

Approximately one quarter to one third of all cancers in the United States have been linked to lifestyle factors, such as diet, obesity, and insufficient physical activity. These factors are second only to tobacco use as major risk factors associated with cancer development (ACS, 2015a).

The risk of cancer increases with long-term ingestion of carcinogens or co-carcinogens or the absence of protective substances in the diet. Dietary substances that appear to increase the risk of cancer include fats, alcohol, salt-cured or smoked meats, nitrate- and nitrite-containing foods, and red and processed meats. Heavy alcohol use increases the risk of cancers of the mouth, pharynx, larynx, esophagus, liver, colon, rectum, and breast (ACS, 2015a).

Poor diet and obesity have been identified as contributing factors to the development of cancers of the breast (in postmenopausal women), colon, endometrium, esophagus, and kidney. Obesity is also associated with an increased risk for cancers of the pancreas, gallbladder, thyroid, ovary, and cervix, and for multiple myeloma, Hodgkin lymphoma, and an aggressive form of prostate cancer. Multiple studies have long linked sedentary lifestyles and lack of regular exercise to cancer development (Lu, Clague, & Bernstein, 2015; Thomson, McCullough, Wertheim, et al., 2014).

Hormonal Agents

Tumor growth may be promoted by disturbances in hormonal balance, either by the body's own (endogenous) hormone production or by administration of exogenous hormones. Cancers of the breast, prostate, and uterus are thought to depend on endogenous hormonal levels for growth. Prenatal exposure to diethylstilbestrol (a synthetic form of the female hormone estrogen) has long been recognized as a risk factor for clear cell adenocarcinoma of the lower genital tract.

Hormonal changes related to the female reproductive cycle are also associated with cancer incidence. Early onset of menses before age 12 and delayed onset of menopause after age 55, null parity (never giving birth), and delayed childbirth after age 30 are all associated with an increased risk of breast cancer. Increased numbers of pregnancies are associated with a decreased incidence of breast, endometrial, and ovarian cancers.

Women who take estrogen after menopause appear to have an increased risk of ovarian cancer. Combination estrogen and progesterone therapy is linked to a higher risk of breast cancer. The longer the combined therapy is used, the higher the risk. However, within 3 years of stopping the hormones, the risk returns to that of a woman who never used this therapy. Women who have taken hormonal therapy appear to have a lower risk of getting colorectal cancer, but when cancers are found it may be more advanced (more likely to have spread to lymph nodes or distant sites) than the cancers found in women not taking hormones (ACS, 2015b).

Role of the Immune System

In humans, transformed cells arise on a regular basis, but are recognized by surveillance cells of the immune system that destroy them before cell growth becomes uncontrolled (immune surveillance). When the immune system fails to identify and stop the growth of transformed cells, a tumor can develop and progress.

Patients who are immunocompromised have an increased incidence of cancer. Transplant recipients who receive immunosuppressive therapy to prevent rejection of the transplanted organ have an increased incidence of cancer (Grossman & Porth, 2014). Patients with acquired immune deficiency syndrome (AIDS) have an increased incidence of Kaposi sarcoma and other cancers. Patients who were previously treated for one cancer are at increased risk for secondary cancers (Grossman & Porth, 2014).

Normal Immune Responses

Through the process of immune surveillance, an intact immune system usually has the ability to recognize and combat cancer cells through multiple, interacting cells and actions of the innate, humoral, and cellular components of the immune system. Tumor-associated antigens (TAAs; also called *tumor cell antigens*) are found on the membranes of many cancer cells. TAAs are processed by antigen-presenting cells (APCs) (e.g., macrophages and dentritic cells [very specialized cells of the immune system] that present antigens to both T- and B lymphocytes) and are presented to T lymphocytes that recognize the antigen-bearing cells as foreign. Multiple TAAs have been identified—some are found in many types of cancer, some exist in the normal tissues of origin as well as the cancer cells, some exist in both normal and cancer cells but are overexpressed (exist in higher concentrations) in cancer cells, and others are very specific to certain cancer types (Kasper, Fauci, Hauser, et al., 2015).

In response to recognizing TAAs as foreign, T-cell lymphocytes release several cytokines that elicit various immune system actions, including (1) proliferation of cytotoxic (cell-killing) T lymphocytes capable of direct destruction of cancer cells, (2) induction of cancer cell apoptosis, and (3) recruitment of additional immune system cells (B-cell lymphocytes that produce antibodies, natural killer cells, and macrophages) that contribute to the destruction and degradation of cancer cells.

Immune System Evasion

Several theories postulate how malignant cells survive and proliferate, evading the elaborate immune system defense mechanisms (Grossman & Porth, 2014). If the body fails to recognize the TAAs on cancer cells or the function of the APCs is impaired, the immune response is not stimulated. Some cancer cells have been found to have altered cell membranes that interfere with APC binding and presentation to T lymphocytes. Tumors can also express molecules that induce T-lymphocyte anergy or tolerance such as PD-1 ligand. These molecules bind to PD-1 proteins on T lymphocytes and either block the killing of the tumor or induce cell death in the lymphocyte. In addition, cancer cells have been found to release cytokines that inhibit APCs as well as other cells of the immune system. When tumors do not possess TAAs that label them as foreign, the immune response is not alerted. This allows the tumor to grow too large to be managed by normal immune mechanisms.

The immunogenicity (immunologic appearance) of cancer cells can be altered through genetic mutations, allowing the cells to evade immune cell recognition. Conversely, mutations are the source for some TAAs. Tumor antigens may combine with the antibodies produced by the immune system and hide or disguise themselves from normal immune defense mechanisms. The tumor antigen–antibody complexes that evade recognition lead to a false message to decrease further production of antibodies as well as other immune system components.

Overexpression (abnormally high concentrations) of host suppressor T lymphocytes induced through the release of cytokines by malignant cells is thought to down-regulate the immune response, thus permitting uncontrolled cell growth (Kasper et al., 2015). Suppressor T lymphocytes normally assist in regulating lymphocyte production and diminishing immune responses (i.e., antibody production) when they are no longer required. Low levels of antibodies and high levels of suppressor cells have been found in patients with multiple myeloma, which is a cancer associated with hypogammaglobulinemia (low amounts of serum antibodies). Conversely, there is evidence that proliferation of helper T lymphocytes, which promote the immune response, is impaired by cytokines produced by cancer cells (Kasper et al., 2015). Without helper T lymphocytes, the immune system response is limited and the cancer cells continue to proliferate. Understanding the role of the immune system and identification of the ways in which cancer evades the body's natural defenses provide the foundation for therapeutic approaches that seek to support and enhance the immune system's role in combating cancer (see Chapter 35).

Detection and Prevention of Cancer

Nurses in all settings play a key role in cancer detection and prevention. Primary, secondary, and tertiary prevention of cancer are all important.

Chart 15-2	**HEALTH PROMOTION**
	American Cancer Society Guidelines on Nutrition and Physical Activity for Cancer Prevention

Individual Choices

Achieve and Maintain a Healthy Weight Throughout Life

- Be as lean as possible throughout life without being underweight.
- Avoid excessive weight gain at all ages. For those who are currently overweight or obese, losing even a small amount of weight has health benefits and is a good place to start.
- Engage in regular physical activity and limit consumption of high-calorie foods and beverages as key strategies for maintaining a healthy weight.

Adopt a Physically Active Lifestyle

- Adults should engage in at least 150 minutes of moderate-intensity or 75 minutes of vigorous-intensity physical activity each week, or an equivalent combination, preferably spread throughout the week.
- Children and adolescents should engage in at least 1 hour of moderate- or vigorous-intensity physical activity each day, with vigorous-intensity activity at least 3 days each week.
- Limit sedentary behavior such as sitting, lying down and watching television, and other forms of screen-based entertainment.
- Doing any intentional physical activity above usual activities, no matter what one's level of activity, can have many health benefits.

Consume a Healthy Diet, With an Emphasis on Plant Sources

- Choose foods and beverages in amounts that help achieve and maintain a healthy weight.
- Limit consumption of processed meat and red meats.
- Eat at least 2½ cups of vegetables and fruits each day.
- Choose whole grains in preference to processed (refined) grains.

If You Drink Alcoholic Beverages, Limit Consumption

- Drink no more than one drink per day for women or two per day for men.

Community Action

Public, private, and community organizations should work collaboratively at national, state, and local levels to implement policy environmental changes that:

- Increase access to affordable, healthy foods in communities, worksites, and schools, and decrease access to and marketing of foods and beverages of low nutritional value, particularly to youth.
- Provide safe, enjoyable, and accessible environments for physical activity in schools and worksites, and for transportation and recreation in communities.

Primary Prevention

Primary prevention is about reducing the risks of disease through health promotion and risk reduction strategies. Guidelines on nutrition and physical activity for cancer prevention can be found in Chart 15-2.

An example of primary prevention is the use of immunization to reduce the risk of cancer through prevention of infections associated with cancer. The HPV vaccine is recommended to prevent cervical and head and neck cancers (Chen et al., 2014). The vaccine to prevent HBV infection is recommended by the CDC (2015) to reduce the risk of hepatitis and subsequent development of liver cancer.

Secondary Prevention

Secondary prevention involves screening and early detection activities that seek to identify precancerous lesions and early-stage cancer in individuals who lack signs and symptoms of cancer. ACS screening is advocated for many types of cancer (See Table 15-3) (ACS, 2016b). Detection of cancer at an early stage may reduce costs, use of resources, and the morbidity associated with advanced stages of cancer and their associated complex treatment approaches. Many screening and detection programs target people who do not regularly practice health-promoting behaviors or lack access to health care. Nurses continue to develop community-based screening and detection programs that address barriers to health care or reflect the socioeconomic and cultural beliefs of the target population (Benito, Binefa, Lluch, et al., 2014; Brittain & Murphy, 2015; Shackelford, Weyhenmeyer, & Mabus, 2015).

The evolving understanding of the role of genetics in cancer cell development has contributed to prevention and screening efforts. Many centers offer cancer risk evaluation programs that provide interdisciplinary in-depth assessment,

screening, education, and counseling as well as follow-up monitoring for people at high risk for cancer (National Comprehensive Cancer Network [NCCN] 2015a; NCCN 2015b). The NCI provides guidance for cancer risk assessment, counseling, education, and genetic testing (NCI, 2016).

Unfolding Patient Stories: Doris Bowman • Part 1

Doris Bowman, a 39-year-old diagnosed with uterine fibroids, dysmenorrhea, and menorrhagia, is scheduled for a total abdominal hysterectomy with bilateral salpingooopherectomy. She has a family history of uterine and ovarian cancer. She asks the nurse what she can do to further reduce her risk for cancer and is also concerned for her family members. What patient and family education should the nurse present on risk reduction strategies, health promotion, and cancer screening? (Doris Bowman's story continues in Chapter 57.)

Care for Doris and other patients in a realistic virtual environment: **vSim** *for Nursing* (**thepoint.lww. com/vSimMedicalSurgical**). Practice documenting these patients' care in DocuCare (**thepoint.lww.com/ DocuCareEHR**).

Tertiary Prevention

Improved screening, diagnosis, and treatment approaches have led to an estimated 14.5 million cancer survivors in the United States (ACS, 2014). Tertiary prevention efforts focus on monitoring for and preventing recurrence of the primary cancer as well as screening for the development of second malignancies in cancer survivors. Survivors are assessed for

TABLE 15-3 American Cancer Society Screening Guidelines for the Early Detection of Cancer in Average-Risk Asymptomatic People[a]

Cancer Site	Population	Test or Procedure	Recommendation
Breast	Women, ages 40–54	Mammography	Women should undergo regular screening mammography starting at age 45 years. Women ages 45–54 should be screened annually. Women should have the opportunity to begin annual screening between the ages of 40 and 44.
	Women age 55 and over	Mammography	Transition to biennial screening, or have the opportunity to continue annual screening. Continue screening as long as overall health is good and life expectancy is 10+ years.
Cervix	Women, ages 21–29	Pap test	Screening should be done every 3 years with conventional or liquid-based Pap tests. Screening should be done every 5 years with both the HPV test and the Pap test (preferred), or every 3 years with the Pap test alone (acceptable).
	Women ages 30–65 Women ages 66+	Pap test & HPV DNA test Pap test & HPV DNA test	Women ages 66+ who have had ≥3 consecutive negative Pap tests or ≥2 consecutive negative HPV and Pap tests within the past 10 years, with the most recent test occurring in the past 5 years should stop cervical cancer screening. Women who have had a total hysterectomy should stop cervical cancer screening.
Colorectal[b]	Men and women, ages 50+	Guaiac-based fecal occult blood test (gFOBT) with at least 50% sensitivity or fecal immunochemical test (FIT) with at least 50% sensitivity, or	Annual testing of spontaneously passed stool specimens. Single stool testing during a clinician office visit is not recommended, nor are "throw in the toilet bowl" tests. In comparison with guaiac-based tests for the detection of occult blood, immunochemical tests are more patient-friendly and are likely to be equal or better in sensitivity and specificity. There is no justification for repeating FOBT in response to an initial positive finding.
		Stool DNA test, or	Every 3 years
		Flexible sigmoidoscopy (FSIG), or	Every 5 years. FSIG can be performed alone, or consideration can be given to combining FSIG performed every 5 years with a highly sensitive guaiac-based gFOBT or FIT performed annually.
		Double-contrast barium enema (DCBE), or	Every 5 years
		Colonoscopy, or	Every 10 years
		CT Colonography	Every 5 years
Endometrial	Women, at menopause	At the time of menopause, women at average risk should be informed about risks and symptoms of endometrial cancer and encouraged to report any unexpected bleeding or spotting to their physicians.	N/A
Lung	Current or former smokers (quit within past 15 years) ages 55–74 in good health with at least a 30 pack-year history	Low-dose helical CT (LDCT)	Clinicians with access to high-volume, high-quality lung cancer screening and treatment centers should initiate a discussion about lung cancer screening with apparently healthy patients aged 55–74 who have at least a 30 pack-year smoking history, and who currently smoke or have quit within the past 15 years. A process of informed and shared decision making with a clinician related to the potential benefits, limitations, and harms associated with screening for lung cancer with LDCT should occur before any decision is made to initiate lung cancer screening. Smoking cessation counseling remains a high priority for clinical attention in discussions with current smokers, who should be informed of their continuing risk of lung cancer. Screening should not be viewed as an alternative to smoking cessation.

TABLE 15-3 American Cancer Society Screening Guidelines for the Early Detection of Cancer in Average-Risk Asymptomatic People[a] (continued)

Cancer Site	Population	Test or Procedure	Recommendation
Prostate	Men, age 50+	Digital rectal examination (DRE) and prostate-specific antigen (PSA) test	Men who have at least a 10-year life expectancy should have an opportunity to make an informed decision with their health care provider about whether to be screened for prostate cancer, after receiving information about the potential benefits, risks, and uncertainties associated with prostate cancer screening. Prostate cancer screening should not occur without an informed decision-making process.
Cancer-related checkup	Men and women, age 20+	On the occasion of a periodic health examination, the cancer-related checkup should include examination for cancers of the thyroid, testicles, ovaries, lymph nodes, oral cavity, and skin, as well as health counseling about tobacco, sun exposure, diet and nutrition, risk factors, sexual practices, and environmental and occupational exposures.	N/A

HPV, human papillomavirus; DNA, deoxyribonucleic acid; CT, computed tomography.
[a]All individuals should become familiar with the potential benefits, limitations, and harms associated with cancer screening.
[b]All positive tests (other than colonoscopy) should be followed up with colonoscopy.
Adapted with permission from American Cancer Society. Cancer Facts and Figures 2016. Atlanta: American Cancer Society, Inc.

the development of second malignancies such as lymphoma and leukemia, which have been associated with certain chemotherapy agents and the use of radiation therapy (ACS, 2014). Survivors may also develop second malignancies not related to treatment but genetic mutations related to inherited cancer syndromes, environmental exposures, and lifestyle factors.

Diagnosis of Cancer

A cancer diagnosis is based on assessment of physiologic and functional changes and results of the diagnostic evaluation. Patients with suspected cancer undergo extensive testing to (1) determine the presence and extent of cancer, (2) identify possible disease metastasis, (3) evaluate the function of involved and uninvolved body systems and organs, and (4) obtain tissue and cells for analysis, including evaluation of tumor stage and grade. The diagnostic evaluation includes a review of systems; physical examination; imaging studies; laboratory tests of blood, urine, and other body fluids; procedures; and pathologic analysis. A selection of diagnostic tests is found in Table 15-4.

Patients undergoing extensive testing may be fearful of the procedures and anxious about possible test results. Nurses help address the patient's fear and anxiety by explaining the tests to be performed, the sensations likely to be experienced, and the patient's role in the test procedures. The nurse encourages the patient and family to voice their fears about the test results, supports the patient and family throughout the diagnostic evaluation, and reinforces and clarifies information conveyed by the physician. The nurse also encourages the patient and family to communicate, share their concerns, and discuss their questions and concerns with one another.

Tumor Staging and Grading

A complete diagnostic evaluation includes identifying the stage and grade of the tumor. This is accomplished prior to treatment to provide baseline data for evaluating outcomes of therapy and to maintain a systematic and consistent approach to ongoing diagnosis and treatment. Treatment options and prognosis are based on tumor stage and grade.

Staging provides a common language used by health care providers and scientists to accurately communicate about cancer across clinical settings and in research. These systems also provide a convenient shorthand notation that condenses lengthy descriptions into manageable terms for comparisons of treatments and prognoses.

Staging determines the size of the tumor, the existence of local invasion, lymph node involvement, and distant metastasis. Several systems exist for classifying the anatomic extent of disease. The tumor, nodes, and metastasis (TNM) system (see Chart 15-3) is one system used to describe many solid tumors (Acharyya et al., 2015; ACS, 2015a).

Grading is the pathologic classification of tumor cells. Grading systems seek to define the type of tissue from which the tumor originated and the degree to which the tumor cells retain the functional and histologic characteristics of the tissue of origin (differentiation). Samples of cells used to establish the tumor grade may be obtained from tissue scrapings, body fluids, secretions, washings, biopsy, or surgical excision. This information helps providers predict the behavior and prognosis of various tumors. The grade corresponds with a numeric value ranging from I to IV. Grade I tumors, also known as well-differentiated tumors, closely resemble the tissue of origin in structure and function. Tumors that do not clearly resemble the tissue of origin in structure or function are described as poorly differentiated or undifferentiated and are assigned grade IV. These tumors tend to be more aggressive, less responsive to

TABLE 15-4 Selected Diagnostic Tests Used to Detect Cancer

Test	Description	Examples of Diagnostic Uses
Tumor marker identification	Analysis of substances found in tumor tissue, blood, or other body fluids that are indicative of cancer cells or specific characteristics of cancer cells. These substances may also be found in some normal body tissues	Breast, colon, lung, ovarian, testicular, prostate cancers
Genetic tumor markers (Also called prognostic indicators)	Analysis for the presence of mutations (alterations) in genes found in tumors or body tissues. Assists in diagnosis, selection of treatment, prediction of response to therapy, and risk of progression or recurrence	Breast, lung, kidney, ovarian, brain cancers; leukemia; and lymphoma. Many uses of genetic profiling are considered investigational
Mammography	Use of x-ray images of the breast	Breast cancer
Magnetic resonance imaging (MRI)	Use of magnetic fields and radiofrequency signals to create sectioned images of various body structures	Neurologic, pelvic, abdominal, thoracic, breast cancers
Computed tomography (CT) scan	Use of narrow-beam x-ray to scan successive layers of tissue for a cross-sectional view	Neurologic, pelvic, skeletal, abdominal, thoracic cancers
Fluoroscopy	Use of x-rays that identify contrasts in body tissue densities; may involve the use of contrast agents	Skeletal, lung, gastrointestinal cancers
Ultrasonography (ultrasound)	High-frequency sound waves echoing off body tissues are converted electronically into images; used to assess tissues deep within the body	Abdominal and pelvic cancers
Endoscopy	Direct visualization of a body cavity or passageway by insertion of an endoscope into a body cavity or opening; allows tissue biopsy, fluid aspiration, and excision of small tumors. Used for diagnostic and therapeutic purposes	Bronchial, gastrointestinal cancers
Nuclear medicine imaging	Uses IV injection or ingestion of radioisotope substances followed by imaging of tissues that have concentrated the radioisotopes	Bone, liver, kidney, spleen, brain, thyroid cancers
Positron emission tomography (PET)	Through the use of a tracer, provides black-and-white or color-coded images of the biologic activity of a particular area, rather than its structure. Used in detection of cancer or its response to treatment	Lung, colon, liver, pancreatic, head and neck cancers; Hodgkin and non-Hodgkin lymphoma and melanoma
PET fusion	Use of a PET scanner and a CT scanner in one machine to provide an image combining anatomic detail, spatial resolution, and functional metabolic abnormalities	See PET
Radioimmunoconjugates	Monoclonal antibodies are labeled with a radioisotope and injected IV into the patient; the antibodies that aggregate at the tumor site are visualized with scanners	Colorectal, breast, ovarian, head and neck cancers; lymphoma and melanoma
Vascular imaging	Use of contrast agents that are injected into veins or arteries and monitored by fluoroscopy, CT, or MRI imaging in order to assess tumor vasculature. Used to assess tumor vascularity prior to surgical procedures. Use in assessing the efficacy of antiangiogenesis (preventing new blood vessel formation) drugs is largely investigational	Liver and brain cancers

treatment, and associated with a poorer prognosis as compared to well-differentiated, grade I tumors. Various staging and grading systems are used to characterize cancers.

Anatomic Stage Group

Once the diagnosis, clinical stage, and histologic grade have been determined, the anatomic stage group, designated by I through IV (representing increasing severity of disease), is assigned to facilitate communication, treatment decisions, and estimation of prognosis. The anatomic stage group is also useful for comparing clinical outcomes.

Management of Cancer

Treatment options offered to patients with cancer are based on treatment goals for each specific type, stage, and grade of cancer. The range of possible treatment goals includes

complete eradication of malignant disease (cure), prolonged survival and containment of cancer cell growth (control), or relief of symptoms associated with the disease and improvement of quality of life (**palliation**). Treatment approaches are not initiated until the diagnosis of cancer has been confirmed and staging and grading have been completed.

The health care team and the patient and family must have a clear understanding of the treatment options and goals. Open communication and support are vital as those involved periodically reassess treatment plans and goals when complications of therapy develop or disease progresses.

Multiple modalities are commonly used in cancer treatment. Various approaches, including surgery, radiation therapy, chemotherapy, hematopoietic stem cell transplantation (HSCT), hyperthermia, and targeted therapy, may be used together or at different times throughout treatment. Understanding the principles of each and how they

TNM Classification System

T   The extent of the primary tumor

N   The absence or presence and extent of regional lymph
node metastasis

M   The absence or presence of distant metastasis

The use of numerical subsets of the TNM components
indicates the progressive extent of the malignant disease.

Primary Tumor (T)

Tx   Primary tumor cannot be assessed

T0   No evidence of primary tumor

Tis   Carcinoma in situ

T1, T2, T3, T4   Increasing size and/or local extent of the
primary tumor

Regional Lymph Nodes (N)

Nx   Regional lymph nodes cannot be assessed

N0   No regional lymph node metastasis

N1, N2, N3   Increasing involvement of regional lymph nodes

Distant Metastasis (M)

Mx   Distant metastasis cannot be assessed

M0   No distant metastasis

M1   Distant metastasis

Adapted from American Cancer Society (ACS). (2015a). Cancer facts
and figures 2015. Retrieved on 2/22/2016 at: www.cancer.org/acs/
groups/content/@editorial/documents/document/acspc-044552.pdf

interrelate is important in understanding the rationale and goals of treatment.

Surgery

Surgical removal of the entire cancer remains the ideal and most frequently used treatment method. However, the specific surgical approach may vary for several reasons. Diagnostic surgery is the definitive method for obtaining tissue to identify the cellular characteristics that influence all treatment decisions. Surgery may be the primary method of treatment, or it may be prophylactic, palliative, or reconstructive.

Diagnostic Surgery

Diagnostic surgery, or biopsy, is performed to obtain a tissue sample for histologic analysis of cells suspected to be malignant. In most instances, the biopsy is taken from the actual tumor; however, in some situations, it is necessary to take a sample of lymph nodes near a suspicious tumor. Many cancers can metastasize from the primary site to other areas of the body through the lymphatic circulation. Knowing whether adjacent lymph nodes contain tumor cells helps the health care team plan the best therapeutic approach to combat cancer that has spread beyond the primary tumor site. The use of injectable dyes and nuclear medicine imaging can help identify the sentinel lymph node or the initial lymph node to which the primary tumor and surrounding tissue drain. Sentinel lymph node biopsy (SLNB), also known as sentinel lymph node mapping, is a minimally invasive surgical approach that in many instances has replaced more invasive lymph node dissections (lymphadenectomy) and the associated complications such

as lymphedema and delayed healing. SLNB has been widely adopted for regional lymph node **staging** in selected cases of melanoma and breast cancer (NCCN, 2015c).

Biopsy Types

Biopsy methods include excisional, incisional, and needle biopsy. The biopsy type is determined by the size and location of the tumor, the type of treatment anticipated if the cancer diagnosis is confirmed, and the need for surgery and general anesthesia. The biopsy method that allows for the least invasive approach while permitting the most representative tissue sample is chosen. Diagnostic imaging techniques can be used to assist in locating the suspicious lesion and to facilitate accurate tissue sampling. The patient and family are provided the opportunity and time to discuss the options before definitive plans are made.

Excisional biopsy is used for small, easily accessible tumors of the skin, upper or lower gastrointestinal and upper respiratory tracts. In many cases, the surgeon can remove the entire tumor as well as the surrounding marginal tissues. The removal of normal tissue beyond the tumor area decreases the possibility that residual microscopic malignant cells may lead to a recurrence of the tumor. This approach not only provides the pathologist with the entire tissue specimen for the determination of stage and grade but also decreases the chance of seeding tumor cells (disseminating cancer cells throughout surrounding tissues).

Incisional biopsy is performed if the tumor mass is too large to be removed. In this case, a wedge of tissue from the tumor is removed for analysis. The cells of the tissue wedge must be representative of the tumor mass so that the pathologist can provide an accurate diagnosis. If the specimen does not contain representative tissue and cells, negative biopsy results do not guarantee the absence of cancer.

Excisional and incisional approaches are often performed through endoscopy. However, a surgical procedure may be required to determine the anatomic extent or stage of the tumor. For example, a diagnostic or staging laparotomy (the surgical opening of the abdomen to assess malignant abdominal disease) may be necessary to assess malignancies such as gastric or colon cancer.

Needle biopsy is performed to sample suspicious masses that are easily and safely accessible, such as some masses in the breasts, thyroid, lung, liver, and kidney. Needle biopsies are most often performed on an outpatient basis. They are fast, relatively inexpensive, easy to perform, and may require only local anesthesia. In general, the patient experiences slight and temporary physical discomfort. In addition, the surrounding tissues are minimally disturbed, thus decreasing the likelihood of seeding cancer cells (disseminating cancer cells to adjacent tissue). Fine-needle aspiration (FNA) biopsy involves aspirating cells rather than intact tissue through a needle that is guided into a suspected diseased area. This type of specimen can only be analyzed by cytological examination (viewing only cells, not tissue). Often, x-ray, computed tomography (CT) scanning, ultrasonography, or magnetic resonance imaging (MRI) is used to help locate the suspicious area and guide placement of the needle. FNA does not always yield enough material to permit accurate diagnosis, necessitating additional biopsy procedures. A core needle biopsy uses a specially designed needle to obtain a small core of tissue that permits histologic analysis. Most often, this specimen is sufficient to permit accurate diagnosis.

Surgery as Primary Treatment

When surgery is the primary approach in treating cancer, the goal is to remove the entire tumor or as much as is feasible (a procedure sometimes called *debulking*) as well as any involved surrounding tissue, including regional lymph nodes.

Two common surgical approaches used for treating primary tumors are local and wide excisions. Local excision, often performed on an outpatient basis, is warranted when the mass is small. It includes removal of the mass and a small margin of normal tissue that is easily accessible. Wide or radical excisions (en bloc dissections) include removal of the primary tumor, lymph nodes, adjacent involved structures, and surrounding tissues that may be at high risk for tumor spread. This surgical method may result in disfigurement and altered functioning, necessitating rehabilitation, reconstructive procedures, or both. However, wide excisions are considered if the tumor can be removed completely and the chances of cure or control are good.

Minimally invasive surgical techniques are increasingly replacing traditional surgery associated with large incisions for a variety of cancers. The advantages of minimally invasive approaches include minimization of surgical trauma, decreased blood loss, decreased incidence of wound infection and other complications associated with surgery, decreased surgical time and requirement for anesthesia, decreased postoperative pain and limited mobility, and shorter periods of recovery (Nguyen, Summers, & Finkelstein, 2015).

Video-assisted endoscopic surgery, an example of minimally invasive surgery, uses an endoscope with intense lighting and an attached multichip mini-camera that is inserted into the body through a small incision. The surgical instruments are inserted into the surgical field through one or two additional small incisions, each about 3 cm in length. The camera transmits the image of the involved area to a monitor so that the surgeon can manipulate the instruments to perform the necessary procedure. Such surgery is used for many thoracic and abdominal procedures. The use of robotics during laparoscopic procedures permits the removal of tumors with more precision and dexterity than could be accomplished by laparoscopic surgery alone (Niklas, Saar, Berg, et al., 2016). Laparoscopic robotic-assisted surgery has been used for prostate and gynecologic cancers. Transoral robotic-assisted surgery is being used for certain types of oral and laryngeal cancers (Chung, Rosenthal, Magnuson, et al., 2015).

Salvage surgery is an additional treatment option that uses an extensive surgical approach to treat the local recurrence of cancer after the use of a less extensive primary approach. Mastectomy to treat recurrent breast cancer after primary lumpectomy and radiation is an example of salvage surgery.

Surgery may completely excise limited areas of metastatic disease (referred to as oligometastatic disease) as well. An example would be colon cancer with one to three small areas of liver metastasis and no evidence of cancer elsewhere. In the past, patients with recurrent or metastatic disease were treated with palliation only as their disease was considered incurable. However, evidence suggests possible cure or prolonged disease-free survival for patients with controlled or completely removed primary cancer and completely removed, limited, metastatic disease (Corbin, Hellman, & Weichselbaum, 2013; Di Lascio & Pagani, 2014).

In addition to surgery that uses surgical blades or scalpels to excise the mass and surrounding tissues, several other types of techniques are available. Table 15-5 provides examples of these techniques.

A multidisciplinary approach to patient care is essential for the patient undergoing cancer-related surgery. The effects of surgery on the patient's body image, self-esteem, and functional abilities are addressed. If necessary, a plan for postoperative rehabilitation is made before the surgery is performed. The growth and dissemination of cancer cells may have produced distant micrometastases by the time the patient seeks treatment. Therefore, attempting to remove wide margins of tissue in the hope of "getting all the cancer" may not be feasible. This reality substantiates the need for a coordinated multidisciplinary approach to cancer therapy.

Once the surgery has been completed, one or more additional (or adjuvant) modalities may be chosen to increase the likelihood of eradicating the remaining microscopic cancer cells that are undetectable by available diagnostic procedures.

TABLE 15-5 Selected Techniques Used for Localized Destruction of Tumor Tissue

Type of Procedure	Description	Examples of Use
Chemosurgery	Use of chemicals or chemotherapy applied directly to tissue to cause destruction	Intraperitoneal chemotherapy for ovarian cancer involving the abdomen and peritoneum
Cryoablation	Use of liquid nitrogen or a very cold probe to freeze tissue and cause cell destruction	Cervical, prostate, and rectal cancers
Electrosurgery	Use of an electric current to destroy tumor cells	Basal and squamous cell skin cancers
Laser surgery	Use of light and energy aimed at an exact tissue location and depth to vaporize cancer cells (also referred to as photocoagulation or photoablation)	Dyspnea associated with endobronchial obstructions
Photodynamic therapy	IV administration of a light-sensitizing agent (hematoporphyrin derivative [HPD]) that is taken up by cancer cells, followed by exposure to laser light within 24–48 hours; causes cancer cell death	Palliative treatment of dysphagia associated with esophageal and dyspnea associated with endobronchial obstructions
Radiofrequency ablation (RFA)	Uses localized application of thermal energy that destroys cancer cells through heat: temperatures exceed 50°C (122°F)	Nonresectable liver tumors, pain control with bone metastasis

However, some cancers that are treated surgically in the very early stages (e.g., skin and testicular cancers) are considered to be curable without additional therapy.

Prophylactic Surgery

Prophylactic or risk reduction surgery involves removing nonvital tissues or organs that are at increased risk of developing cancer. The following factors are considered when discussing possible prophylactic surgery:

- Family history and genetic predisposition
- Presence or absence of signs and symptoms
- Potential risks and benefits
- Ability to detect cancer at an early stage
- Alternative options for managing increased risk
- The patient's acceptance of the postoperative outcome

Colectomy, mastectomy, and oophorectomy are examples of prophylactic surgeries. Identification of genetic markers indicative of inherited cancer syndromes or a predisposition to develop some types of cancer plays a role in decisions concerning prophylactic surgeries. However, what is adequate justification for prophylactic surgery remains controversial. For example, several factors are considered when deciding to proceed with a prophylactic mastectomy, including a strong family history of breast cancer; positive *BRCA1* or *BRCA2* findings; an abnormal physical finding on breast examination, such as progressive nodularity and cystic disease; a proven history of breast cancer in the opposite breast; abnormal mammography findings; abnormal biopsy results; and individual factors that may influence the patient's decision-making process (Mahon, 2014). Prophylactic surgery is discussed with patients and families along with other approaches for managing increased risk of cancer development. Preoperative education and counseling, as well as long-term follow-up, are provided.

Palliative Surgery

When surgical cure is not possible, the goals of surgical interventions are to relieve symptoms, make the patient as comfortable as possible, and promote quality of life as defined by the patient and family. Palliative surgery is performed in an attempt to relieve symptoms, such as ulceration, obstruction, hemorrhage, pain, and malignant effusions (see Table 15-6). Honest and informative communication with the patient and family about the goal of surgery is essential to avoid false hope and disappointment.

Reconstructive Surgery

Reconstructive surgery may follow curative or extensive surgery in an attempt to improve function or obtain a more desirable cosmetic effect. It may be performed in one operation or in stages. The surgeon who will perform the surgery discusses possible reconstructive surgical options with the patient before the primary surgery is performed. Reconstructive surgery may be indicated for breast, head and neck, and skin cancers.

The nurse assesses the patient's needs and the impact that altered functioning and body image may have on quality of life. Nurses provide patients and families with opportunities to discuss these issues. The individual needs of the patient undergoing reconstructive surgery and their families must be accurately recognized and addressed.

TABLE 15-6 Types of Palliative Surgery and Interventions

Procedure	Indications
Abdominal shunt placement	Ascites
Biliary stent placement	Biliary obstruction
Bone stabilization	Displaced bone fracture related to metastatic disease
Colostomy or ileostomy	Bowel obstruction
Cordotomy	Pain
Epidural catheter placement (for administering epidural analgesics)	Pain
Excision of solitary metastatic lesion	Metastatic lung, liver, or brain lesion
Gastrostomy, jejunostomy tube placement	Upper gastrointestinal tract obstruction
Hormone manipulation (removal of ovaries, testes, adrenals, pituitary)	Tumors that depend on hormones for growth
Nerve block	Pain
Percutaneous enteral gastrostomy (PEG) tube placement	Enteral nutrition
Pericardial drainage tube placement	Pericardial effusion
Peritoneal drainage tube placement	Ascites
Pleural drainage tube placement	Pleural effusion
Ureteral stent placement	Ureteral obstruction
Venous access device placement (for administering parenteral analgesics)	Pain

Nursing Management

Patients undergoing surgery for cancer require general perioperative nursing care (see Chapter 18). Surgical care is individualized according to age, organ impairment, specific deficits, comorbidities, cultural implications, and altered immunity. Combining other treatment methods, such as radiation and chemotherapy, with surgery also contributes to postoperative complications, such as infection, impaired wound healing, altered pulmonary or renal function, and the development of venous thromboembolism (VTE). The nurse completes a thorough preoperative assessment for factors that may affect the patient undergoing the surgical procedure.

Preoperatively, the nurse provides the patient and family with verbal and written information about the surgical procedure as well as other interventions that may take place intraoperatively (i.e., radiation implants). Instructions concerning prophylactic antibiotic requirements, diet, and bowel preparation are also provided.

Patients who are undergoing surgery for the diagnosis or treatment of cancer may be anxious about the surgical procedure, possible findings, postoperative limitations, changes in normal body functions, and prognosis. The patient and family require time and assistance to process this information, possible changes, and expected outcomes resulting from the surgery.

The nurse serves as the patient advocate and liaison and encourages the patient and family to take an active role in decision making when possible. If the patient or family asks about the results of diagnostic testing and surgical procedures, the nurse's response is guided by the information that was conveyed previously. The nurse may be asked to explain and clarify information for patients and families that was provided initially but was not grasped because of intense anxiety. It is important that the nurse, as well as other members of the health care team, provide information that is consistent.

Postoperatively, the nurse assesses patient responses to surgery and monitors the patient for possible complications, such as infection, bleeding, thrombophlebitis, wound dehiscence, fluid and electrolyte imbalance, and organ dysfunction. The nurse also provides for the patient's comfort. Postoperative education addresses wound care, pain management, activity, nutrition, and medication information.

Plans for discharge, follow-up, home care, and subsequent treatment and rehabilitation are initiated as early as possible to ensure continuity of care from hospital to home or from a cancer referral center to the patient's local hospital and health care provider. Patients and families are encouraged to use community resources such as the ACS for support and information (see the Resources section at the end of this chapter).

Radiation Therapy

Approximately 60% of patients with cancer receive **radiation therapy** at some point during treatment (Halperin, Wazer, Perez, et al., 2013). Radiation may be used to cure cancer, as in thyroid carcinomas, localized cancers of the head and neck, and cancers of the cervix. Radiation therapy may also be used to control cancer when a tumor cannot be removed surgically or when local nodal metastasis is present. Neoadjuvant (prior to local definitive treatment) radiation therapy, with or without chemotherapy, is used to reduce tumor size in order to facilitate surgical resection. Radiation therapy may be given prophylactically to prevent local recurrence or spread of microscopic cells from the primary tumor to a distant area (e.g., irradiating the breast and axilla following lumpectomy or mastectomy for breast cancer). Palliative radiation therapy is used to relieve the symptoms of locally advanced or metastatic disease, especially when the cancer has spread to the brain, bone, or soft tissue, or to treat oncologic emergencies, such as superior vena cava syndrome, bronchial airway obstruction, or spinal cord compression.

Two types of ionizing radiation—electromagnetic radiation (x-rays and gamma rays) and particulate radiation (electrons, beta particles, protons, neutrons, and alpha particles)—can be used to kill cells. The most lethal damage is the direct alteration of the DNA molecule within the cells of both malignant and normal tissues. Ionizing radiation can directly break the strands of the DNA helix, leading to cell death. It can also indirectly damage DNA through the formation of free radicals. If the DNA cannot be repaired, the cell may die immediately or may initiate apoptosis (Datta, Kundu, Ghosh, et al., 2104; Montezano, Dulak-Lis, Tsiropoulou, et al., 2015).

Replicating cells are most vulnerable to the disruptive effects of radiation (during DNA synthesis and mitosis, i.e., early S, G₂, and M phases of the cell cycle; see Fig. 15-2). Therefore, those body tissues that undergo frequent cell division are most sensitive to radiation therapy. These tissues include bone marrow, lymphatic tissue, epithelium of the gastrointestinal tract, hair follicles, and gonads. Slower-growing tissues

Figure 15-2 • Cell cycle. The cell cycle's four steps are illustrated beginning with G₁ and proceeding to M. The first growth phase (G₁), DNA synthesis phase (S), second growth phase (G₂), and mitosis (M) are illustrated. Reprinted with permission from Grossman, S. G., & Porth, C.M. (2014). *Porth's pathophysiology: Concepts of altered health states* (9th ed.). Philadelphia, PA: Lippincott Williams & Wilkins.

and tissues at rest (e.g., muscle, cartilage, nervous system, and connective tissues) are relatively radioresistant (less sensitive to the effects of radiation). However, it is important to remember that radiation therapy is localized treatment, and only the tissues that are within the treatment field are affected.

A radiosensitive tumor is one that can be destroyed by a dose of radiation that still allows for cell repair and regeneration in the surrounding normal tissue. If the radiation is delivered when most tumor cells are cycling through the cell cycle, the number of cancer cells destroyed (cell kill) is maximal. Radiation sensitivity is enhanced in tumors that are smaller in size and that contain cells that are rapidly dividing (highly proliferative) and poorly differentiated (no longer resembling the tissue of origin).

Radiation Dosage

The radiation dosage depends on the sensitivity of the target tissues to radiation, the size of the tumor, radiation tolerance of the surrounding normal tissues, and critical structures adjacent to the tumor target. The lethal tumor dose is defined as the dose that will eradicate 95% of the tumor yet preserve normal tissue. In external-beam radiation therapy (EBRT), the total radiation dose is delivered over several weeks in daily doses called *fractions*. This allows healthy tissue to repair and achieves greater cell kill by exposing more cells to the radiation as they begin active cell division. Repeated radiation treatments over time (fractionated doses) also allow for the periphery of the tumor to be reoxygenated repeatedly, because tumors shrink from the outside inward. This increases the radiosensitivity of the tumor, thereby increasing tumor cell death (Morgan, Ten Haken, & Lawrence, 2015). Newer approaches take advantage of increased radiation beam conformality (better tumor targeting) to administer radiation in fewer doses with larger fractions sizes (hypo-fractionation and stereotactic body radiotherapy [SBRT]).

Administration of Radiation

Radiation therapy can be given in various ways depending on the source of radiation used, the location of the tumor, and the type of cancer. The primary radiotherapy modalities include EBRT, **brachytherapy** (a form of internal radiation), systemic (radioisotopes), and contact or surface molds.

External Radiation

EBRT is the most commonly used form of radiation therapy. The energy utilized in EBRT is generated either from a linear accelerator or from a unit that generates energy directly from a core source of radioactive material such as a GammaKnife™ unit. Through computerized software programs, both approaches are able to shape an invisible beam of highly charged photons or gamma rays to penetrate the body and target the tumor with pinpoint accuracy.

Advances in computer technology allow multiple imaging modalities (CT, MRI, and PET scans) to be used to provide three-dimensional images of the tumor, neighboring tissues at risk for microscopic spread, and surrounding normal tissues or organs at risk for radiation-induced toxicity. These images, referred to as volumetric images, allow the radiation oncologist to plan for multiple radiation beams directed from different angles and different planes so that the beams conform

precisely around the tumor (referred to as conformal radiation). The dose of radiation that reaches the surrounding normal tissues is reduced, leading to much less toxicity than in older forms of radiation therapy (Halperin et al., 2013). Treatment enhancements in EBRT include the ability to control different intensity or energy levels of radiation beams at different angles directed at the tumor, a process known as intensity-modulated radiation therapy (IMRT), which enables higher doses to be delivered to the tumor while sparing the important healthy structures surrounding the tumor (Halperin et al., 2013). IMRT can be given as standard daily fractions or as "hyperfractionated" twice-daily fractions, which shortens the duration of the patient's treatment schedule. Image-guided radiation therapy (IGRT) uses continuous monitoring of the tumor with ultrasound, x-ray, or CT scans during the treatment to allow for automatic adjustment of the beams as the tumor changes shape or position in an effort to spare the healthy surrounding tissue and reduce side effects. Additional treatment enhancements include respiratory gating, where the treatment delivery is actually synchronized with the patient's respiratory cycle, enabling the beam to be adjusted as the tumor or organ moves. These treatment advancements improve tumor destruction while reducing acute and long-term toxicities (Halperin et al., 2013).

Gamma rays generated from the spontaneous decay of naturally occurring solid source of radioactivity, such as cobalt-60, are one of the oldest forms of EBRT. With the advent of modern linear accelerators, the use of solid radioactive elements is confined primarily to the GammaKnife™ stereotactic radiosurgery unit, which is used as a one-time, high-dose delivery of EBRT for treatment of both benign and malignant intracranial lesions.

Stereotactic body radiotherapy (SBRT) is another form of EBRT that uses higher doses of radiation to penetrate very deeply into the body to control deep-seated tumors that cannot be treated by other approaches such as surgery. SBRT is delivered with considerably higher treatment fraction doses over a short span of time, usually 1 to 5 treatment days, in contrast to daily treatments for 5 days per week for 6 to 8 weeks for conventional EBRT. Specialized linear accelerators with the capability of robotically moving around the patient are used to deliver SBRT, such as the CyberKnife™, Trilogy™, and TomoTherapy™ delivery systems, which are now more commonly available.

Proton therapy is another approach to EBRT. Proton therapy utilizes high linear energy transfer (LET) in the form of charged protons generated by a large magnetic unit called a *cyclotron*. The advantage of proton therapy is that it is capable of delivering its high-energy dose to a deep-seated tumor, with decreased doses of radiation to the tissues in front of the tumor while virtually no energy exits through the patient's healthy tissue behind the tumor (Halperin et al., 2013). Proton therapy permits treatment of deep tumors in close proximity to critical structures, such as the heart or major blood vessels.

Internal Radiation

Internal radiation includes localized implantation or systemic radionuclide administration. Brachytherapy delivers the dose of radiation to a localized area while systemic radiotherapy relies on strategies for getting the radionuclides closer to the tumor. The specific radioisotope used is selected on the basis of its half-life, which is the time it takes for half of its radioactivity to decay, and the depth of penetration of the radiation.

Brachytherapy

Brachytherapy is the placement of radioactive sources within or immediately next to the cancer site in order to provide a highly targeted, intense dose of radiation beyond a dose that is usually provided by EBRT. In addition, this form of radiation delivery helps to spare exposure to normal surrounding tissue. The radiation source can be implanted by means of needles or rods, seeds, beads, ribbons, or catheters placed into body cavities (vagina, abdomen, pleura), lumens within organs, or interstitial tissue compartments (breast, prostate). Multiple imaging techniques such as ultrasound, CT, or MRI are used to guide placement of radiation sources. Patients may have many fears or concerns about internal radiation, and the nurse explains the various approaches and safety precautions that will be used to protect the patient, family, and health care staff.

Brachytherapy may be delivered as a temporary or a permanent implant. Temporary applications are delivered as high-dose radiation (HDR) for short periods of time, while low-dose radiation (LDR) is delivered over a more extended period of time. The primary advantage of HDR brachytherapy is that treatment time is shorter, there is reduced exposure to personnel, and the procedure can be performed on an outpatient basis over several days. HDR brachytherapy can be used for intraluminal, surface, interstitial, and intra-cavitary lesions. Intraluminal HDR brachytherapy involves the insertion of catheters or hollow tubes into the lumens of organs so that the radioisotope can be delivered as close to the tumor bed as possible. Lesions in the bronchus, esophagus, rectum, or bile duct can be treated with this approach. Contact or surface application is used for treatment of tumors of the eye, such as retinoblastoma in children or ocular melanoma in adults.

Interstitial HDR implants, used in treating such malignancies as prostate, pancreatic, or breast cancer, may be temporary or permanent, depending on the site and radioisotope used. Based on the dose to be delivered (LDR or HDR), the implants may consist of seeds, needles, wires, strands, or small catheters positioned to provide a local radiation source. Prostate HDR therapy is one form of interstitial brachytherapy, in which radioactive strands or wires are placed, while the patient is under anesthesia, into hollow catheters that have been inserted in the perineum close to the prostate gland (Halperin et al., 2013).

Intracavitary radioisotopes are used to treat gynecologic cancers. In these malignancies, the radioisotopes are inserted into specially positioned applicators within the vagina. The applicator placement is verified by x-ray. Treatment can be achieved with either HDR or LDR brachytherapy sources, depending on the extent of disease. LDR therapy requires hospitalization because the patient is treated over several days. HDR intraoperative radiotherapy (IORT) has been used as a treatment approach for advanced gynecologic cancer that has spread to the para-aortic area or pelvic wall (Lukens, Gamez, Hu, et al., 2014).

Systemic radiotherapy (radiopharmaceutical therapy) involves the intravenous (IV) administration of a therapeutic radioactive isotope targeted to a specific tumor. Radioactive iodine (I-131) is a widely used form of systemic brachytherapy that is the primary treatment for thyroid cancer (Beck, 2015). Radium-223 dichloride selectively targets prostate cancer bone metastases with high-energy, short-range alpha particles and is approved for the treatment of patients with symptomatic bone metastases and no known visceral metastatic disease (NCCN, 2015d). Radioisotopes are also used as a form of radioimmunotherapy for the treatment of refractory non-Hodgkin lymphoma. (See Chapter 34 for more information on lymphoma.)

Toxicity

Toxicities associated with radiation therapy are most often localized in the region being irradiated and may be increased if concomitant chemotherapy is given. Acute or early toxicities most often begin within 2 weeks of the initiation of treatment occur when normal cells within the treatment area are damaged and cellular death exceeds regeneration. Body tissues most affected are those that normally proliferate rapidly, such as the skin, the epithelial lining of the gastrointestinal tract, and the bone marrow.

Altered skin integrity is common and can include **alopecia** (hair loss) associated with whole brain radiation. Other skin reactions, referred to as radiation dermatitis, occur along a continuum ranging from erythema and dry desquamation (flaking of skin) to moist or wet desquamation (dermis exposed, skin oozing serous fluid) to, potentially, ulceration. Factors that contribute to the severity of radiation dermatitis include the dose and form of radiation, inclusion of skin folds in the irradiated area, increased age and the presence of medical comorbidities (Fogh & Yom, 2014). Symptoms of radiation dermatitis may necessitate treatment interruption, delays, or cessation of therapy. Re-epithelialization occurs after treatments have been completed. Hyperpigmentation, a less severe radiation-associated skin reaction, may develop about 2 to 4 weeks after the initiation of treatment.

Alterations in oral mucosa secondary to radiation therapy in the head and neck region include stomatitis (inflammation of the oral tissues), decreased salivation and xerostomia (dryness of the mouth), and change in or loss of taste. Depending on the targeted region, any portion of the gastrointestinal mucosa may be involved, causing mucositis (inflammation of the lining of the mouth, throat, and gastrointestinal tract). For example, patients receiving thoracic irradiation for lung cancer may experience acute esophageal irritation—associated chest pain and dysphagia. Anorexia, nausea, vomiting, and diarrhea may occur if the stomach or colon is in the radiation field. Symptoms subside and gastrointestinal re-epithelialization occurs after treatments have been completed. Bone marrow cells proliferate rapidly, and if sites containing bone marrow (e.g., the iliac crest or sternum) are included in the radiation field, anemia, leukopenia (decreased white blood cells [WBCs]), and thrombocytopenia (a decrease in platelets) may result. The patient is then at increased risk for infection and bleeding until blood cell counts return to normal. One medication, amifostine (Ethyol), is occasionally used in patients with head and neck cancers to reduce acute and chronic xerostomia while preserving antitumor efficacy of the necessary radiation doses (Citrin & Mitchell, 2014).

Systemic side effects are commonly experienced by patients receiving radiation therapy. These include fatigue, malaise, and anorexia that may be secondary to substances released when tumor cells are destroyed. Early effects tend to be temporary and most often subside within 6 months of the cessation of treatment.

Late effects (approximately 6 months to years after treatment) of radiation therapy may occur in body tissues that were in the field of radiation. These effects are chronic, usually a result of permanent damage to tissues, loss of elasticity, and changes secondary to a decreased vascular supply. Severe late effects include fibrosis, atrophy, ulceration, and necrosis and may affect the lungs, heart, central nervous system, and bladder. With advances in treatment planning and the accuracy of treatment delivery, the occurrence of late toxicities has diminished. However, late or chronic symptoms, such as dysphagia, incontinence, cognitive impairment, and sexual dysfunction, may persist for several years with implications for survivors' overall health and quality of life (Oeffinger, 2013).

Nursing Management

Nurses anticipate, prevent, and work collaboratively with other providers to manage symptoms associated with radiation therapy in order to promote healing, patient comfort, and quality of life. Symptoms that are not appropriately managed may lead to poor outcomes as a result of interruptions, decreased doses, or early cessation of treatment (Fogh & Yom, 2014). Ideally, nurses consider factors that may be predictive of radiation toxicities or radiosensitivity of tissues. In particular, diminished body mass index (BMI) and elevated radiation doses have been associated with greater toxicity and symptoms (O'Gorman, Sasiadek, Denieffe, et al., 2015). The area of the body being irradiated partially guides the focus of nursing assessments.

In patients receiving EBRT, the nurse assesses the patient's skin regularly throughout the course of treatment. In addition, nutritional status and general feelings of well-being are assessed throughout the course of treatment. Evidence-based protocols for nursing management of the toxicities associated with radiation therapy are used. If systemic symptoms, such as weakness and fatigue, occur, the nurse explains that these symptoms are a result of the treatment and do not represent deterioration or progression of the disease.

Protecting Caregivers

When the patient has a radioactive implant in place, the nurse and other health care providers need to protect themselves, as well as the patient, from the effects of radiation. Patients receiving internal radiation emit radiation while the implant is in place; therefore, contact with the health care team is guided by principles of time, distance, and shielding to minimize exposure of personnel to radiation. Specific instructions are provided by the radiation safety officer from the radiology department and specify the maximum time that can be spent safely in the patient's room, the shielding equipment to be used, and special precautions and actions to be taken if the implant is dislodged (Halperin et al., 2013). Safety precautions used in caring for a patient receiving brachytherapy include assigning the patient to a private room, posting appropriate notices about radiation safety precautions, having staff members wear dosimeter badges, making sure that pregnant staff members are not assigned to the patient's care, prohibiting visits by children or pregnant visitors, limiting visits from others to 30 minutes daily, and seeing that visitors maintain a 6-foot distance from the radiation source.

Patients with seed implants typically are able to return home; radiation exposure to others is minimal. Information about any precautions, if needed, is provided to the patient and family members to ensure safety. Depending on the dose and energy emitted by a systemic radionuclide, patients may or may not require special precautions or hospitalization (Halperin et al., 2013). The nurse should explain the rationale for these precautions to keep the patient from feeling unduly isolated.

Chemotherapy

Chemotherapy involves the use of antineoplastic drugs in an attempt to destroy cancer cells by interfering with cellular functions, including replication and DNA repair (Grossman & Porth, 2014). Chemotherapy is used primarily to treat systemic disease rather than localized lesions that are amenable to surgery or radiation. Chemotherapy may be combined with surgery, radiation therapy, or both to reduce tumor size preoperatively (neoadjuvant), to destroy any remaining tumor cells postoperatively (adjuvant), or to treat some forms of leukemia or lymphoma (primary). The goals of chemotherapy (cure, control, or palliation) must be realistic because they will determine the medications that are used and the aggressiveness of the treatment plan.

Cell Kill and the Cell Cycle

Each time a tumor is exposed to chemotherapy, a percentage of the tumor cells (20% to 99%, depending on dosage and agent) are destroyed. Repeated doses of chemotherapy are necessary over a prolonged period to achieve regression of the tumor. Eradication of 100% of the tumor is almost impossible; the goal of treatment is eradication of enough of the tumor so that the remaining malignant cells can be destroyed by the body's immune system (Grossman & Porth, 2014)

Actively proliferating cells within a tumor are the most sensitive to chemotherapy (the ratio of dividing cells to resting cells is referred to as the growth fraction). Non-dividing cells capable of future proliferation are the least sensitive to antineoplastic medications and consequently are potentially dangerous. However, the non-dividing cells must be destroyed to eradicate the disease. Repeated cycles of chemotherapy or sequencing of multiple chemotherapeutic agents is used to achieve more tumor cell destruction by destroying the non-dividing tumor cells as they begin active cell division.

Reproduction of both healthy and malignant cells follows the cell cycle pattern (see Fig. 15-2). The cell cycle time is the time required for one cell to divide and reproduce two identical daughter cells. The cell cycle of any cell has four distinct phases, each with a vital underlying function (Grossman & Porth, 2014):

- G_1 phase—RNA and protein synthesis occurs
- S phase—DNA synthesis occurs
- G_2 phase—premitotic phase; DNA synthesis is complete, mitotic spindle forms
- Mitosis—duplicated chromosomes separate and cell division occurs

Classification of Chemotherapeutic Agents

Chemotherapeutic agents may be classified by their mechanism of action in relation to the cell cycle. Agents that exert their maximal effect during specific phases of the cell cycle are termed *cell cycle–specific agents*. These agents destroy cells that are actively reproducing by means of the cell cycle; most affect cells in the S phase by interfering with DNA and RNA synthesis. Other agents, such as plant alkaloids, are specific to the M phase, where they halt mitotic spindle formation. Chemotherapeutic agents that act independently of the cell cycle phases are termed *cell cycle–nonspecific agents*. These agents usually have a prolonged effect on cells, leading to cellular damage or death. Many treatment plans combine cell cycle–specific and cell cycle–nonspecific agents to increase the number of vulnerable tumor cells killed during a treatment period (Neuss, Polovich, McNiff, et al., 2013).

Chemotherapeutic agents are also classified by chemical group, each with a different mechanism of action. These include the alkylating agents, nitrosoureas, antimetabolites, antitumor antibiotics, topoisomerase inhibitors, plant alkaloids (also referred to as mitotic inhibitors), hormonal agents, and miscellaneous agents. The classification, mechanism of action, cell cycle specificity, and common side effects of selected antineoplastic agents are listed in Table 15-7.

Chemotherapeutic agents from multiple categories may be used together to maximize cell destruction. Combination chemotherapy relies on agents with varying mechanisms, potential synergistic actions, and differing toxicities. The use of combination therapy also helps prevent the development of drug-resistant cells.

Adjunct Chemotherapeutic Agents

In certain regimens, additional medications are given with chemotherapy agents to enhance activity or protect normal cells from injury. For example, leucovorin (Wellcovorin) is often given with fluorouracil (5-FU) to treat colorectal cancer. Leucovorin, a compound similar to folic acid, helps fluorouracil bind with an enzyme inside of cancer cells and enhances the ability of fluorouracil to remain in the intracellular environment. Leucovorin also rescues normal cells from the toxic effects of high doses of methotrexate (Trexall). When given at certain doses for the treatment of some forms of leukemia or lymphoma, methotrexate causes a folic acid deficiency in cells, resulting in cell death. Significant toxicity, including severe bone marrow suppression, mucositis, diarrhea and liver, and lung and kidney damage, can occur. Leucovorin helps to prevent or lessen these toxicities.

Administration of Chemotherapeutic Agents

Chemotherapy may be given in the hospital, outpatient center, or home setting by multiple routes. The route of administration depends on the type of agent; the required dose; and the type, location, and extent of malignant disease being treated. Standards for the safe administration of chemotherapy have been developed by the Oncology Nursing Society (ONS) and the American Society of Clinical Oncology (ASCO) (Neuss et al., 2013). Patient education is essential to maximize safety when chemotherapy is given in the home.

Dosage

The dosage of chemotherapeutic agents is based primarily on the patient's total body surface area, weight, previous exposure and response to chemotherapy or radiation therapy, and function of major organ systems. Dosages are determined to maximize cell kill while minimizing impact on healthy tissues and subsequent toxicities. The therapeutic effect may be compromised if modified and inadequate dosing is required due to toxicities. Modification of dosage is often required if critical laboratory values or the patient's symptoms indicate unacceptable or dangerous toxicities. Chemotherapy treatment regimens include standard-dose therapy, dose-dense regimens (giving chemotherapy more frequently than standard treatment regimens), and myeloablative therapy for HSCT. For certain chemotherapeutic agents, there is a maximum lifetime dose limit that must be adhered to because of the danger of long-term irreversible organ complications (e.g., because of the risk of cardiomyopathy, doxorubicin [Adriamycin] has a cumulative lifetime dose limit of 550 mg/m^2).

Extravasation

Intravenously given chemotherapy agents are additionally classified by their potential to damage tissue if they inadvertently leak from a vein into surrounding tissue (**extravasation**). The consequences of extravasation range from mild discomfort to severe tissue destruction, depending on whether the agent is classified as a nonvesicant, irritant, or vesicant. The pH levels of irritant agents (<5 or >9) induce inflammatory reactions but usually cause no permanent tissue damage (Schulmeister, 2014).

Vesicants are those agents that, if deposited into the subcutaneous or surrounding tissues (extravasation), cause inflammation; tissue damage; and possibly necrosis of tendons, muscles, nerves, and blood vessels. Although the mechanism of vesicant actions varies with each drug, some agents bind to cell DNA and cause cell death that progresses to involve neighboring cells, whereas other agents are metabolized into cells and cause a localized, painful reaction that usually improves over time (Schulmeister, 2014). Sloughing and ulceration of the tissue may progress to tissue necrosis that is so severe that skin grafting becomes necessary. The full extent of tissue damage may take several weeks to become apparent. Examples of commonly used agents classified as vesicants include dactinomycin (Cosmegen), daunorubicin (DaunoXome), doxorubicin (Adriamycin), nitrogen mustard (Mustargen), mitomycin (Mutamycin), vinblastine (Velban), and vincristine (Oncovin). Chemotherapy administration safety standards require the availability of defined extravasation management procedures, including antidote order sets and accessibility of antidotes in all settings where vesicant chemotherapy is given (Neuss et al., 2013; Schulmeister, 2014).

Chemotherapy is given only by those who have the knowledge and established competencies for vesicant and extravasation management (Schulmeister, 2014). Prevention and management of extravasation are essential. Vesicant chemotherapy should never be given in peripheral veins involving the hand or wrist. Peripheral administration is permitted for short-duration infusions only, and placement of the venipuncture site should be on the forearm area using a soft, plastic catheter. For any frequent or prolonged administration of

TABLE 15-7 Select Antineoplastic Agents

Drug Class and Examples	Mechanism of Action	Cell Cycle Specificity	Common Side Effects
Alkylating Agents			
Busulfan (Busulfex, Myleran), carboplatin (Paraplatin), chlorambucil (Leukeran), cisplatin (Platinol-AQ), cyclophosphamide (Cytoxan), dacarbazine (DTIC-Dome), altretamine (Hexalen), ifosfamide (Ifex), melphalan (Alkeran), nitrogen mustard (Mustargen), oxaliplatin (Eloxatin), thiotepa (Thioplex)	Bond with DNA, RNA, and protein molecules leading to impaired DNA replication, RNA transcription, and cell functioning; all resulting in cell death	Cell cycle—non-specific	Bone marrow suppression, nausea, vomiting, cystitis (cyclophosphamide, ifosfamide), stomatitis, alopecia, gonadal suppression, renal toxicity (cisplatin), and development of secondary malignancies
Nitrosoureas			
Carmustine (BCNU [BiCNU, Gliadel]), lomustine or CCNU (CeeNU), semustine (methyl-CCNU [MeCCNU]), streptozocin (Zanosar)	Similar to alkylating agents; cross the blood–brain barrier	Cell cycle—non-specific	Delayed and cumulative myelosuppression, especially thrombocytopenia; nausea, vomiting, pulmonary, hepatic and renal damage
Topoisomerase I Inhibitors			
Irinotecan (Camptosar) Topotecan (Hycamtin)	Induce breaks in the DNA strand by binding to enzyme topoisomerase, preventing cells from dividing	Cell cycle—specific (S phase)	Bone marrow suppression, diarrhea, nausea, vomiting, flulike symptoms (topotecan), rash (etoposide), hepatotoxicity (teniposide)
Topoisomerase II Inhibitors Etoposide (Etopophos, VePesid) Teniposide (Vumon, VM-26)			
Antimetabolites			
5-Azacytidine (Vidaza), capecitabine (Xeloda), cytarabine (DepoCyt, Tarabine), edatrexate fludarabine (Fludara), 5-fluorouracil (5-FU), gemcitabine (Gemzar), hydroxyurea (Droxia, Hydrea), cladribine (Leustatin), 6-mercaptopurine (Purinethol), methotrexate (Trexall, Rheumatrex), pentostatin (Nipent), 6-thioguanine (Tabloid)	Interferes with the biosynthesis of metabolites or nucleic acids necessary for RNA and DNA synthesis; inhibits DNA replication and repair	Cell cycle—specific (S phase)	Nausea, vomiting, diarrhea, bone marrow suppression, stomatitis, renal toxicity (methotrexate), hepatotoxicity (6-thioguanine), hand-foot syndrome (capecitibine)
Antitumor Antibiotics			
Bleomycin (BLM, Blenoxane), dactinomycin (Cosmegen), daunorubicin (DaunoXome), doxorubicin (Adriamycin), epirubicin, idarubicin (Idamycin), mitomycin (Mutamycin), mitoxantrone (Novantrone), plicamycin (Mithracin)	Interfere with DNA synthesis by binding DNA; prevent RNA synthesis	Cell cycle—non-specific	Bone marrow suppression, nausea, vomiting, alopecia, anorexia, cardiac toxicity (daunorubicin, doxorubicin), red urine (doxorubicin, idarubicin, epirubicin), pulmonary fibrosis (bleomycin)
Mitotic Spindle Inhibitors			
Plant alkaloids: vinblastine (Velban), vincristine (VCR [Oncovin]), vinorelbine (Navelbine)	Arrest metaphase by inhibiting mitotic tubular formation (spindle); inhibit DNA and protein synthesis	Cell cycle—specific (M phase)	Bone marrow suppression (mild with VCR), peripheral neuropathies, nausea and vomiting
Taxanes: paclitaxel (Taxol), docetaxel (Taxotere)	Arrest metaphase by inhibiting tubulin depolymerization	Cell cycle—specific (M phase)	Hypersensitivity reactions, bone marrow suppression, alopecia, peripheral neuropathies, **mucositis**
Epothilones: ixabepilone (Ixempra)	Alters microtubules and inhibits mitosis	Cell cycle—specific (M phase)	Peripheral neuropathies, bone marrow suppression, hypersensitivity reactions, hepatic impairment
Hormonal Agents			
Androgens and antiandrogens, estrogens and antiestrogens, progestins and antiprogestins, aromatase inhibitors, luteinizing hormone-releasing hormone analogues, steroids	Bind to hormone receptor sites that alter cellular growth; block binding of estrogens to receptor sites (antiestrogens); inhibit RNA synthesis; suppress cytochrome P450 system	Cell cycle—non-specific	Hypercalcemia, jaundice, increased appetite, masculinization, feminization, sodium and fluid retention, nausea, vomiting, hot flashes, vaginal estrogen dryness
Miscellaneous Agents			
Asparaginase (Elspar), procarbazine (Matulane)	Inhibits protein, DNA, and RNA synthesis	Varies	Anorexia, nausea, vomiting, bone marrow suppression, hepatotoxicity, hypersensitivity reaction, pancreatitis
Arsenic trioxide (Trisenox)	Causes fragmentation of DNA resulting in cell death; in acute promyelocytic leukemia, it corrects protein changes and changes malignant cells into normal white blood cells.		Nausea, vomiting, electrolyte imbalances, fever, headache, cough, dyspnea, electrocardiogram abnormalities

DNA, deoxyribonucleic acid; RNA, ribonucleic acid.
Adapted from Comerford, K. C. (2015). *Nursing 2015 drug handbook*. Philadelphia: Wolters Kluwer; Neuss, M. N., Polovich, M., McNiff, K., et al. (2013). 2013 Updated American Society of Clinical Oncology/Oncology Nursing Society chemotherapy administration safety standards including standards for the safe administration and management of oral chemotherapy. *Oncology Nursing Forum, 40*(3), 225–233.

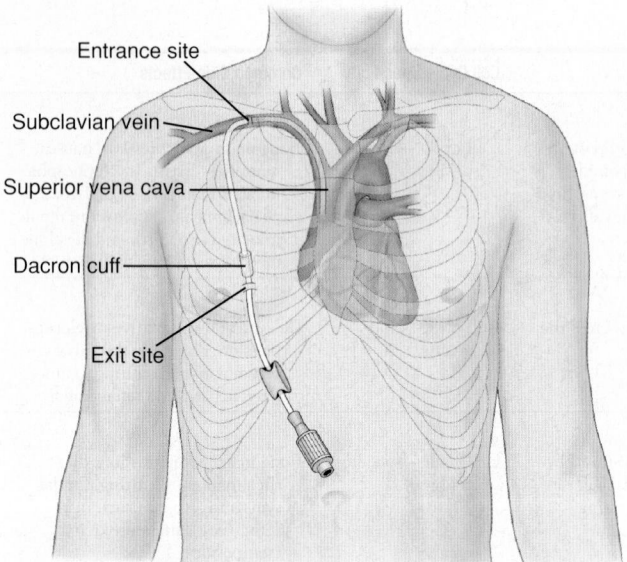

Figure 15-3 • Right atrial catheter. The right atrial catheter is inserted into the subclavian vein and advanced until its tip lies in the superior vena cava just above the right atrium. The proximal end is then tunneled from the entry site through the subcutaneous tissue of the chest wall and brought out through an exit site on the chest. The Dacron cuff anchors the catheter in place and serves as a barrier to infection.

antineoplastic vesicants, right atrial silastic catheters, implanted venous access devices, or peripherally inserted central catheters (PICCs) should be inserted to promote safety during medication administration and reduce problems with access to the circulatory system (Figs. 15-3 and 15-4).

Hypersensitivity Reactions

Although hypersensitivity reactions (HSRs) can occur with any medication, many chemotherapy agents pose a high risk and have been associated with life-threatening outcomes. HSRs are a subgroup of adverse drug reactions that are unexpected and associated with mild or progressively worsening signs and symptoms, such as rash, urticaria, fever, hypotension, cardiac instability, dyspnea, wheezing, throat tightness, and syncope (Braskett & Cohen, 2014). Immediate HSRs appear within 1 hour of an infusion, while delayed HSRs may occur hours afterward. Although patients may or may not react to the first infusion of a chemotherapy agent, repeated exposure increases the likelihood of a reaction.

Most immediate HSRs are immunoglobulin E (IgE)-mediated reaction—an allergic reaction. Examples of agents that may cause an allergic, IgE-mediated response include carboplatin, oxaliplatin (Eloxatin), and L-asparaginase. However, some HSRs, such as anaphylactoid reactions, are non–IgE-mediated (nonallergic) and a result of cytokine release syndrome (Braskett & Cohen, 2014; Castells, 2015). Rituximab and cetuximab are examples of agents associated with non-IgE-mediated (nonallergic) HSRs. When signs and symptoms of HSR occur, the medication should be discontinued immediately and emergency procedures initiated. Many institutions have developed specific protocols for responding to HSRs, including standing orders for administration of emergency medications (Castells, 2015). (Chapter 38 presents further discussion of allergic reactions.)

For some chemotherapeutic agents, especially if they are essential in the treatment plan, desensitization procedures may be possible, and the patient is retreated with the agent at reduced dosages or slower infusion rates. Premedication regimens are used for certain chemotherapy agents to prevent or minimize reactions.

Toxicity

Toxicity associated with chemotherapy can be acute or chronic. Cells with rapid growth rates (e.g., epithelium, bone marrow, hair follicles, sperm) are very susceptible to damage, and the effects may manifest in virtually any body system.

Gastrointestinal System

The most common side effects of chemotherapy are nausea and vomiting, which may persist for 24 to 48 hours; delayed nausea and vomiting may occur up to 1 week after administration.

Figure 15-4 • Implanted vascular access device. **A.** A schematic diagram of an implanted vascular access device used for administration of medications, fluids, blood products, and nutrition. The self-sealing septum permits repeated puncture by Huber needles without damage or leakage. **B.** Two Huber needles used to enter the implanted vascular port. The 90-degree needle is used for top-entry ports for continuous infusions.

The experience of chemotherapy-induced nausea and vomiting (CINV) may affect quality of life, psychological status, nutrition, fluid and electrolyte status, functional ability, compliance with treatment, and utilization of health care resources (Gonella & Di Giulio, 2015). Comorbidities, the underlying malignancy, other treatment approaches, and medications, as well as symptoms (i.e., pain), may contribute to CINV. Acute CINV is experienced in the first 24 hours after chemotherapy with a maximal intensity after 5–6 hours; delayed CINV occurs 24 hours posttreatment and may last as many as 7 days with a maximal intensity 48–72 hours after drug administration (Gonella & Di Giulio, 2015). Anticipatory nausea and vomiting, occurring prior to administration of chemotherapy, may be a conditioned response triggered by a stimulus such as the smell of the infusion setting, the sight of the nurse, or the outpatient center waiting room.

Several mechanisms are responsible for the occurrence of nausea and vomiting, including activation of multiple receptors found in the vomiting center of the medulla, the chemoreceptor trigger zone, the gastrointestinal tract, the pharynx, and the cerebral cortex. Activation of neurotransmitter receptors in these areas is thought to induce CINV. Stimulation may originate through peripheral, autonomic, vestibular, or cognitive pathways. The primary neuroreceptors known to be implicated in CINV are 5-hydroxytryptamine (5-HT or serotonin) and dopamine receptors (NCCN, 2015e).

The approach for managing CINV is based on the knowledge of the probability of emesis of the chemotherapy agents used. Algorithms are used to prevent and treat CINV based on national guidelines that consider this classification of chemotherapy agents (NCCN, 2015e).

Corticosteroids, phenothiazines, sedatives, and histamines are helpful, especially when used in combination with serotonin blockers to provide antiemetic protection (NCCN, 2015e). In order to manage delayed nausea and vomiting, antiemetic medications may be combined and are given for the first week at home after chemotherapy. Nonpharmacologic approaches such as relaxation techniques, imagery, acupressure, or acupuncture can help decrease stimuli contributing to symptoms and may be most helpful for patients with anticipatory nausea and vomiting. Small, frequent meals, bland foods, and comfort foods may reduce the frequency or severity of symptoms.

Stomatitis is commonly associated with some chemotherapy agents because of the rapid turnover of epithelium that lines the oral cavity. The entire gastrointestinal tract is susceptible to **mucositis** (inflammation of the mouth, throat, and gastrointestinal tract) with diarrhea. Antimetabolites and antitumor antibiotics are the major culprits in mucositis and other gastrointestinal symptoms, which can be severe in some patients.

Hematopoietic System

Many chemotherapy agents cause some degree of **myelosuppression** (depression of bone marrow function), resulting in decreased WBCs (leukopenia), granulocytes (**neutropenia**), red blood cells (RBCs) (anemia), and platelets (thrombocytopenia) and increased risk of infection and bleeding. Depression of these cells is the usual reason for limiting the dose of the chemotherapy. Myelosuppression is predictable; for most agents, patients usually reach the point at which blood counts are lowest 7 to 14 days after chemotherapy has been given. During these 2 weeks, nurses anticipate associated toxicities, especially a fever associated with neutrophil count less than 1,500 cells/mm^3. Frequent monitoring of blood cell counts is essential, and patients are educated about strategies to protect against infection, injury, and blood loss, particularly while counts are low (Manea, 2014).

Other agents—colony-stimulating factors (granulocyte colony-stimulating factor [G-CSF] and granulocyte-macrophage colony-stimulating factor [GM-CSF])—can be given after chemotherapy to stimulate the bone marrow to produce WBCs, especially neutrophils, at an accelerated rate, thus decreasing the duration of neutropenia. G-CSF and GM-CSF decrease the episodes of infection and the need for antibiotics and allow for more timely treatment cycles of chemotherapy with less need to reduce the dosage. Erythropoietin (EPO) stimulates RBC production, thus decreasing the symptoms of treatment-induced chronic anemia and reducing the need for blood transfusions. Interleukin 11 (IL-11) (oprelvekin [Neumega]) stimulates the production of megakaryocytes (precursors to platelets) and can be used to prevent and treat severe thrombocytopenia but has had limited use because of toxicities, such as HSR; capillary leak syndrome; pulmonary edema; atrial dysrhythmias; and nausea, vomiting, and diarrhea (Kuter, 2015).

Renal System

Some chemotherapy agents damage the kidneys because they impair water secretion, leading to syndrome of inappropriate secretion of antidiuretic hormone (SIADH), decrease renal perfusion, precipitate end products after cell lysis, and cause interstitial nephritis (Comerford, 2015). Cisplatin (Platinol), methotrexate, and mitomycin (Mutamycin) are particularly toxic to the kidneys. Rapid tumor cell lysis after chemotherapy results in increased urinary excretion of uric acid, which can cause renal damage. In addition, intracellular contents are released into the circulation, resulting in hyperkalemia, hyperphosphatemia, and hypocalcemia and obstructive nephropathy. (See later discussion of tumor lysis syndrome.)

Monitoring laboratory values of blood urea nitrogen (BUN), serum creatinine, creatinine clearance, and serum electrolytes is essential (Comerford, 2015). Adequate hydration, diuresis, alkalinization of the urine to prevent formation of uric acid crystals, and administration of allopurinol (Zyloprim) may be used to prevent renal toxicity. Amifostine has demonstrated an ability to minimize renal toxicities associated with cisplatin, cyclophosphamide (Cytoxan), and ifosfamide (Ifex) therapy.

Hemorrhagic cystitis is a bladder toxicity that can result from cyclophosphamide and ifosfamide therapy. Hematuria can range from microscopic to frank bleeding with symptoms ranging from transient irritation during urination, dysuria, and suprapubic pain to life-threatening hemorrhage. Protection of the bladder focuses on aggressive IV hydration, frequent voiding, and diuresis. Mesna (Mesnex) is a cytoprotectant agent that binds with the toxic metabolites of cyclophosphamide or ifosfamide in the kidneys to prevent hemorrhagic cystitis.

Cardiopulmonary System

Several agents are associated with cardiac toxicity. Anthracyclines (e.g., daunorubicin, doxorubicin) are known to cause irreversible cumulative cardiac toxicities, especially when total dosage reaches 300 mg/m^2 and 550 mg/m^2, respectively (Comerford, 2015). If these agents are given in the presence of thoracic radiation therapy or other agents with cardiotoxicity potential, the cumulative dose limit is lower. Patients at increased risk for the development of cardiopulmonary toxicities include those older than 70 years, those with a history of preexisting cardiac disease, hypertension, tobacco use, renal or hepatic dysfunction, and longer survival time. Dexrazoxane (Zinecard) has been used on a limited basis as a cardioprotectant when doxorubicin is needed in individuals who have already received a cumulative dose limit and continuation of therapy is deemed beneficial. Patients with known cardiac disease (e.g., heart failure) are treated with lower doses or agents not known to be associated with cardiac toxicity. Cardiac ejection fraction (volume of blood ejected from the heart with each beat) and other signs of heart failure must be monitored closely.

Bleomycin (Blenoxane), carmustine (BCNU), busulfan (Busulfex, Myleran), mitomycin, and paclitaxel/docetaxel, among other agents, have toxic effects on lung function, such as alveolar damage, bronchospasm, pneumonitis, and pulmonary fibrosis. Therefore, patients are monitored closely for changes in pulmonary function, including pulmonary function test results. Patients with known lung disease are treated with alternative agents not known to cause pulmonary toxicity. When pulmonary toxicity occurs, the agent is stopped and patients are treated with steroids and other supportive therapies (Schulmeister, 2014).

Capillary leak syndrome with resultant pulmonary edema is an effect of cytarabine (DepoCyt, Tarabine, Ara-C), mitomycin C, cyclophosphamide, and carmustine. Subtle onset of dyspnea and cough may progress rapidly to acute respiratory distress and subsequent respiratory failure. Patients who are at significant risk for capillary leak syndrome are monitored closely.

Reproductive System

Testicular and ovarian function can be affected by chemotherapeutic agents, resulting in possible sterility. Women may develop problems with ovulation or early menopause, whereas men may develop temporary or permanent azoospermia (absence of spermatozoa). Because treatment may damage reproductive cells, banking of sperm is often recommended for men before treatment is initiated (Frankel Kelvin, 2015). Options available for women prior to initiation of chemotherapy include freezing (cryopreservation) of oocytes, embryos, or ovarian tissue (Frankel Kelvin, 2015). Patients and their partners are informed about potential changes in reproductive function resulting from chemotherapy. In addition, many chemotherapy agents are known or thought to be teratogenic. Therefore, patients are advised to use reliable methods of birth control while receiving chemotherapy and not to assume that sterility has resulted.

Neurologic System

Chemotherapy-induced neurotoxicity, a potentially dose-limiting toxicity, can affect the central nervous system, peripheral nervous system, and/or the cranial nerves. Neurotoxicity characterized by metabolic encephalopathy can occur with ifosfamide, high-dose methotrexate, and cytarabine. With repeated doses, the taxanes and plant alkaloids, especially vincristine, can cause cumulative peripheral nervous system damage with sensory alterations in the feet and hands. These sensations can be described as tingling, pricking, or numbness of the extremities; burning or freezing pain; sharp, stabbing, or electric shock–like pain; and extreme sensitivity to touch. If unreported by patients or undetected, progressive motor axon damage can lead to loss of deep tendon reflexes, with muscle weakness, loss of balance and coordination, and paralytic ileus.

Severe peripheral neuropathies may lead to diminished quality of life and functional abilities and result in dose reductions, a change in chemotherapy regimen, or early cessation of treatment (Tofthagen, Visovsky, & Hopgood, 2013). Although often reversible, these side effects may take many months to resolve or persist indefinitely. Along with the usual paresthesias of the hands and feet, oxaliplatin has a unique and frightening neurotoxicity presentation that is often precipitated by exposure to cold and is characterized by pharyngolaryngeal dysesthesia consisting of lip paresthesia, discomfort or tightness in the back of the throat, inability to breathe, and jaw pain.

> ### ▶ Quality and Safety Nursing Alert
>
> *Patients receiving oxaliplatin must be instructed to avoid drinking cold fluids or going outside with hands and feet exposed to cold temperatures to avoid exacerbation of these symptoms. Cisplatin may cause peripheral neuropathies and hearing loss due to damage to the acoustic nerve.*

Cognitive Impairment

Many patients with cancer experience difficulty with remembering dates, multitasking, managing numbers and finances, organization, face or object recognition, inability to follow directions, feeling easily distracted, and motor and behavioral changes. Although not completely understood, these are viewed as symptoms of cognitive impairment, defined as a decline in the information-handling processes of attention and concentration, executive function, information processing speed, language, visual-spatial skill, psychomotor ability, learning, and memory (Von Ah, 2015). Commonly referred to by patients as "chemo brain," cognitive impairment has been associated with both cancer and cancer treatments, including surgery, radiation, chemotherapy, and targeted agents (Bender & Thelen, 2013). The symptoms may be subtle or profound with potential negative effects on functional abilities, employment, independence, quality of life, and psychosocial status. Comorbidities, age, medications, pain, impaired nutrition, anemia, fatigue, fluid and electrolyte disturbances, organ dysfunction, infection, and hormonal imbalances are factors that may contribute to the experience of cognitive impairment and make it difficult to fully understand. Underlying mechanisms of cognitive impairment in patients with cancer being explored include neurotoxic effects, oxidative stress, hormonal changes, immune dysregulation, cytokine release, clotting, genetic predisposition, and accelerated aging processes (Merriman, Von Ah, Miaskowski, et al., 2013; Von Ah, 2015).

Fatigue

Cancer-related fatigue has been defined as an unusual, persistent, and subjective sense of tiredness that is not proportional to recent activity and interferes with usual functioning (NCCN, 2015f). Fatigue is a distressing side effect for most patients that greatly affects quality of life, during treatment and for months after treatment. The health care team works together to identify effective pharmacologic and nonpharmacologic approaches for fatigue management.

Nursing Management

Nurses play an important role in assessing and managing many of the problems experienced by patients receiving chemotherapy. Chemotherapy agents affect both normal and malignant cells; therefore, their effects are often widespread, affecting many body systems.

Laboratory and physical assessments of metabolic indices and the dermatologic, hematologic, hepatic, renal, cardiovascular, neurologic, and pulmonary systems are critical in evaluating the body's response to chemotherapy. These assessments are performed prior to, during, and after a course of chemotherapy to determine optimal treatment options, evaluate the patient's response, and monitor toxicity. Patients are monitored for long-term effects of chemotherapy after active treatment has been completed during the period of survivorship (see Chart 15-4).

Assessing Fluid and Electrolyte Status

Anorexia, nausea, vomiting, altered taste, mucositis, and diarrhea put patients at risk for nutritional and fluid and electrolyte disturbances. Therefore, it is important for the nurse to assess the patient's nutritional and fluid and electrolyte status on an ongoing basis and to identify creative ways to encourage an adequate fluid and dietary intake.

Assessing Cognitive Status

Nurses should assess patients routinely for indications of cognitive impairment. Prior to the initiation of treatment, patients and families should be informed about the possibility of cognitive impairment. Nursing assessment plays an important role in determining the need for referral for neurocognitive evaluation and intervention (Jansen, 2013).

Modifying Risks for Infection and Bleeding

Suppression of the bone marrow and immune system is expected and frequently serves as a guide in determining appropriate chemotherapy dosage but increases the risk of anemia, infection, and bleeding disorders. Nursing assessment and care address factors that would further increase the patient's risk. The nurse's role in decreasing the risk of infection and bleeding is discussed further in the Nursing Care of Patients With Cancer section (see Chart 15-7).

Administering Chemotherapy

Nurses must be aware of chemotherapy and other agents most associated with HSRs, strategies for prevention, signs and symptoms characteristic of HSRs, and the appropriate early and time-sensitive interventions for preventing progression to anaphylaxis. Nurses provide patient and family education that emphasizes two key points: the importance of adhering to prescribed self-administered premedication before presenting to the infusion center, and recognizing and reporting the signs and symptoms to the nurse once the infusion has started. Patients and families are also educated about signs and symptoms that may occur at home following discharge from the infusion area that may warrant medication administration or immediate transport to the emergency department for further assessment and treatment.

The local effects of the chemotherapeutic agent are also of concern. The patient is observed closely during administration of the agent because of the risk and consequences of extravasation. Prevention of extravasation is essential and relies on vigilant nursing care (Neuss et al., 2013). Selection of peripheral veins, skilled venipuncture, and careful administration of medications are essential. Peripheral administration is limited to short duration (less than 1 hour; IV push or bolus) infusions using only a soft, plastic catheter placed in the forearm area. Continuous infusion of vesicants that takes longer than 1 hour or are given frequently are given only via a central line, such as a right atrial silastic catheter, implanted venous access device, or PICC. These long-term venous access devices promote safety during medication administration and reduce problems with repeated access to the circulatory system (see Figs. 15-3 and 15-4). Indwelling or subcutaneous venous access devices require consistent nursing care. Complications include infection and thrombosis (Cotogni, Barbero, Garrino, et al., 2015).

Chart 15-4

Potential Long-Term Complications of Cancer Chemotherapy

Abnormalities in senses of taste, smell, and touch
Abnormal balance, tremors, or weakness
Avascular necrosis
Cardiovascular toxicity (coronary artery disease, myocardial infarction, congestive heart failure, valvular heart disease, peripheral arterial disease)
Decreased libido
Dental caries
Dry mouth
Dysphagia
Dyspnea on exertion
Growth retardation in children
Herpes infections (zoster and varicella)
Hypothyroidism
Immune dysfunction
Infertility
Osteoporosis
Pericarditis (acute or chronic)
Pneumococcal sepsis
Pneumonitis (acute or chronic)
Secondary cancers:
    Acute myeloid leukemia
    Myelodysplastic syndromes
    Non-Hodgkin lymphoma
    Solid tumors (especially bone and soft tissue, lung, breast)
    Thyroid cancer
    Thymic hyperplasia

Indications of extravasation during administration of vesicant agents include the following:
- Absence of blood return from the IV catheter
- Resistance to flow of IV fluid
- Burning or pain, swelling, or redness at the site

 Quality and Safety Nursing Alert

If extravasation is suspected, the medication administration is stopped immediately.

An extravasation kit should be readily available with emergency equipment and antidote medications, as well as a quick reference for how to properly manage an extravasation of the specific vesicant agent used (although evidence-based data regarding effective antidotes are limited) (Gonzalez, 2013). Nurses should refer to their organization's policy and procedures for reporting, managing, and documenting extravasation. Safety standards require the availability of defined extravasation management procedures, including antidote order sets and accessibility of antidotes in all settings where vesicant chemotherapy is given (Neuss et al., 2013). Recommendations and guidelines for managing vesicant extravasation, which vary with each agent, have been issued by individual medication manufacturers, pharmacies, and the ONS (Neuss et al., 2013; Schulmeister, 2014).

Difficulties or problems with administration of chemotherapeutic agents are brought to the attention of the primary provider promptly so that corrective measures can be taken to minimize local tissue damage.

The nurse evaluates the patient receiving neurotoxic chemotherapy, communicates findings with the medical oncologist, provides education to patients and families, and makes appropriate referrals for complete neurologic evaluation and occupational or rehabilitative therapies (Coyle, Griffie, & Czaplewski, 2014).

Preventing Nausea and Vomiting

Nurses are integral to the prevention and management of CINV. They collaborate with other members of the oncology care team to identify factors contributing to the experience of CINV and select effective antiemetic regimens that maximize currently available therapies. Nurses provide education for patients and families regarding antiemetic regimens and care for delayed CINV that may continue at home after the chemotherapy infusion has completed (NCCN, 2015e).

Managing Cognitive Changes

Although several approaches have been explored, no evidence-based guidelines for the prevention, treatment, or management of cognitive impairment have been established. Examples of nonpharmacologic approaches that nurses recommend to patients include exercise, natural restorative environmental intervention (walking in nature or gardening), and cognitive training programs (Merriman, et al., 2013; Von Ah, 2015). Nurses should assist patients to address factors, such as fluid and electrolyte imbalances, nutrition deficits, fatigue, pain, and infection to minimize their contribution to cognitive impairment.

Managing Fatigue

Fatigue is a common side effect of chemotherapy. Nurses assist patients to explore the role that the underlying disease processes, combined treatments, other symptoms, and psychosocial distress play in the patient's experience of fatigue. In addition, nurses work with the patient and other team members to identify effective approaches for fatigue management (NCCN, 2015f).

Protecting Caregivers

Nurses involved in handling chemotherapeutic agents may be exposed to low doses of the agents by direct contact, inhalation, or ingestion. Studies suggest that nurses and others preparing chemotherapy agents or handling linens and other materials that are contaminated with body fluids of patients receiving chemotherapy have been unknowingly exposed (Leduc-Souville, Bertrand, & Schlatter, 2013). Skin and eye irritation, nausea, vomiting, nasal mucosal ulcerations, infertility, low-birth-weight babies, congenital anomalies, spontaneous abortions, and mutagenic substances in urine have been reported in nurses preparing and handling chemotherapy agents (Leduc-Souville et al., 2013). The Occupational and Safety Health Administration (OSHA), the ONS, hospitals, and other health care agencies have developed specific precautions for health care providers involved in the preparation and administration of chemotherapy and for handling materials exposed to body fluids of those who have received these hazardous agents (see Chart 15-5) (Neuss et al., 2013; Schulmeister, 2014). Nurses must be familiar with their institutional policies and procedures regarding personal protective equipment, handling and disposal of chemotherapy agents and supplies, and management of accidental spills or exposures. Emergency spill kits should be readily available in any treatment area where chemotherapy is prepared or given. Precautions must also be taken when handling any bodily fluids or excreta from the patient, as many agents are excreted unaltered in urine and feces. Nurses in all treatment settings have a responsibility to educate patients, families, caregivers, assistive personnel, and housekeepers concerning precautions.

Hematopoietic Stem Cell Transplantation

HSCT has been used to treat several malignant and nonmalignant diseases for many years. The use of HSCT for solid tumors is limited to clinical trials (Maziarz & Schubach-Slater, 2015). However, the use of HSCT in the treatment of certain adult hematologic malignancies (i.e., malignant myeloma, acute leukemia, and non-Hodgkin lymphoma) is considered standard of care.

The process of obtaining hematopoietic stem cells (HSCs) has evolved over the years. Historically, HSCs were obtained in the operating room by harvesting large amounts of bone marrow tissue from a donor under general anesthesia. However, peripheral blood stem cell collection using the process of apheresis has gained widespread use. The cells collected are specially processed and ultimately reinfused into the patient. This method of collecting HSCs is a safe and a more cost-effective means of collection than the process of harvesting

Chart 15-5

Safety in Handling Chemotherapy for Health Care Providers

- When preparing (compounding, reconstituting) chemotherapy for administration, use the following safety equipment to prevent exposure through inhalation, direct contact, and ingestion:
  - Class II or III biological safety cabinet (BSC)
  - Closed system transfer devices
  - Puncture and leak-proof containers, IV bags
  - Needleless systems (i.e., IV tubing and syringes)
- If BSC is not available when preparing chemotherapy for administration, use the following safety equipment to minimize exposure:
  - Surgical N-95 respirator to provide respiratory and splash protection
  - Eye and face protection (both face shield and goggles) working at or above eye level or cleaning a spill
- When preparing or administering chemotherapy or handling linens and other materials contaminated with chemotherapy or blood and body fluids of patients receiving chemotherapy, wear the following for personal protection:
  - Double layer of powder-free gloves specifically designated for chemotherapy handling (the inner glove is worn under the gown cuff and the outer glove is worn over the cuff)
  - Long sleeve, disposable gowns (without seams or closures that can allow drugs to pass through) made of polyethylene-coated polypropylene or other laminate materials
- Linens contaminated with chemotherapy or blood and body fluids of patients receiving chemotherapy should be placed in the following:
  - Closed-system, puncture- and leak-proof containers labeled "hazardous: chemotherapy contaminated linens"

- Above referenced container maintained in the infusion center soiled utility room for outpatient settings
- Above referenced container maintained in the patient room and/or soiled utility room for inpatient settings
- Chemotherapy preparation equipment (i.e., syringes, tubing, empty vials, etc.), gowns, and gloves should be disposed of in:
  - Closed-system, puncture- and leak-proof containers labeled "hazardous: chemotherapy contaminated waste"
- Wash hands with soap and water after removing gloves used to prepare or administer chemotherapy or clean contaminated linens and other materials.
- "Spill kits" with the appropriate gowns, gloves, disposable absorbent materials for cleansing large areas, and hazard sign should be kept in all areas where chemotherapy is prepared and given.
- Implement a quality improvement program addressing safe chemotherapy handling that includes the following:
  - Standard operating policies and procedures for:
  - Chemotherapy handling, preparation, and disposal
  - Handling and disposal of chemotherapy spills
  - Handling and disposal of blood and body fluids and contaminated materials of patients receiving chemotherapy
  - Conduct competency-based education, training, and performance evaluations regarding chemotherapy safety procedures at orientation and at subsequent regular intervals.
  - Medical monitoring program to identify indicators of exposure
  - Root cause analysis for all chemotherapy spills and exposure incidents

Adapted from National Institute for Occupational Safety and Health. (2010). Personal protective equipment for health care workers who work with hazardous drugs. Available at: www.cdc.gov/niosh/docs/wp-solutions/2009–106/pdfs/2009–106.pdf

---

of marrow (Maziarz & Schubach-Slater, 2015). Stem cells can also be collected from umbilical cord blood harvested from the placenta of newborns at birth.

Types of Hematopoietic Stem Cell Transplantation

Types of HSCT are based on the source of donor cells and the treatment (conditioning) regimen used to prepare the patient for stem cell infusion and eradicate malignant cells. These include:

- *Allogeneic HSCT (AlloHSCT)*: From a donor other than the patient (may be a related donor such as a family member or a matched unrelated donor from the National Bone Marrow Registry or Cord Blood Registry)
- *Autologous*: From the patient
- *Syngeneic*: From an identical twin
- *Myeloablative*: Consists of giving patients high-dose chemotherapy and, occasionally, total-body irradiation
- *Nonmyeloablative*: Also called *mini-transplants*; does not completely destroy bone marrow cells

AlloHSCTs are used primarily for diseases of the bone marrow and are dependent on the availability of a human leukocyte antigen–matched donor, which greatly limits the number of possible transplants. An advantage of AlloHSCT is that the transplanted cells should not be immunologically tolerant of a patient's malignancy and should cause a lethal

graft-versus-tumor effect in which the donor cells recognize the malignant cells and act to eliminate them.

AlloHSCT may involve either myeloablative (high-dose) or nonmyeloablative (mini-transplant) chemotherapy. In ablative AlloHSCT, the recipient receives high doses of chemotherapy and possibly total-body irradiation to completely eradicate (ablate) the bone marrow and any malignant cells and help prevent rejection of the donor stem cells. The collected HSCs that are infused IV into the recipients travel to sites in the body where they produce bone marrow and establish themselves through the process of engraftment. Once engraftment is complete (2 to 4 weeks, sometimes longer), the new bone marrow becomes functional and begins producing RBCs, WBCs, and platelets. In nonablative AlloHSCT, the chemotherapy doses are lower and are aimed at destroying malignant cells (without completely eradicating the bone marrow), thus suppressing the recipient's immune system to allow engraftment of donor stem cells. The lower doses of chemotherapy, associated with less organ toxicity and infection, can be used for older patients or those with underlying organ dysfunction for whom high-dose chemotherapy would be prohibitive. After engraftment, it is hoped that the donor cells will create a graft-versus-tumor effect. Before engraftment, patients are at high risk for infection, sepsis, and bleeding. Side effects of the high-dose chemotherapy and total-body irradiation can be acute and chronic. Acute side effects include alopecia, hemorrhagic cystitis, nausea, vomiting, diarrhea, encephalopathy, pulmonary edema, acute kidney injury, fluid and electrolyte imbalances, and severe mucositis (Maziarz & Schubach-Slater, 2015). Chronic side effects include sterility; pulmonary, cardiac, renal, neurologic, and hepatic dysfunction; osteoporosis; avascular bone necrosis; diabetes; and secondary malignancy (Maziarz & Schubach-Slater, 2015).

During the first 30 days after the conditioning regimen, AlloHSCT patients are at risk for developing hepatic sinusoidal obstructive syndrome (HSOS) (previously referred to as veno-oclusive disease) related to chemotherapy-induced inflammation of the sinusoidal epithelium. Inflammation causes embolization of RBCs, resulting in destruction, fibrosis, and occlusion of the sinusoids (Maziarz & Schubach-Slater, 2015). Signs and symptoms of HSOS may include weight gain, hepatomegaly, increased bilirubin, and ascites. Although various approaches have been used to treat HSOS, evidence-based strategies have not emerged. The use of peripheral stem cells, specific chemotherapy dosing, and nonmyeloablative regimens have been associated with a decreased incidence (Maziarz & Schubach-Slater, 2015).

Graft-versus-host disease (GVHD), a major cause of morbidity and mortality in 30% to 50% of the allogeneic transplant population, occurs when the donor lymphocytes initiate an immune response against the recipient's tissues (skin, gastrointestinal tract, liver) during the beginning of engraftment (Maziarz & Schubach-Slater, 2015). The donor cells view the recipient's tissues as foreign or immunologically different from what they recognize as "self" in the donor. To prevent GVHD, patients receive immunosuppressant drugs, such as cyclosporine (Sandimmune), methotrexate, tacrolimus (Prograf), or mycophenolate mofetil (MMF).

GVHD may be acute, occurring within the first 100 days, or chronic, occurring after 100 days (Barbarotta, 2015). Clinical manifestations of acute GVHD include diffuse rash progressing to blistering and desquamation similar to second-degree burns; mucosal inflammation of the eyes and the entire gastrointestinal tract with subsequent diarrhea that may exceed 2 L per day; and biliary stasis with abdominal pain, hepatomegaly, and elevated liver enzymes progressing to obstructive jaundice. The first 100 days or so after AlloHSCT is crucial for patients; the immune system and blood-making capacity (hematopoiesis) must recover sufficiently to prevent infection and hemorrhage. Most acute side effects, such as nausea, vomiting, and mucositis, resolve during this period of time. However, there are some complications that may occur, such as encephalopathy, hemolytic uremia syndrome, hemolytic anemia, and thrombotic thrombocytopenia purpura (Maziarz & Schubach-Slater, 2015).

Autologous HSCT (AuHSCT) is considered for patients with disease of the bone marrow who do not have a suitable donor for AlloHSCT or for patients who have healthy bone marrow but require bone marrow–ablative doses of chemotherapy to cure an aggressive malignancy. The most common malignancies treated with AuHSCT include lymphoma and multiple myeloma. However, the use of AuHSCT has gained increasing acceptance in treating neuroblastoma, Ewing sarcoma, and germ cell tumors (Maziarz & Schubach-Slater, 2015). Stem cells are collected from the patient and preserved for reinfusion; if necessary, they are treated to kill any malignant cells within the marrow, called *purging*. The patient is then treated with ablative chemotherapy and, possibly, total-body irradiation to eradicate any remaining tumor. Stem cells are then reinfused. Until engraftment occurs in the bone marrow sites of the body, there is a high risk of infection, sepsis, and bleeding. Acute and chronic toxicities from chemotherapy and radiation therapy may be severe. The risk of HSOS is also present after autologous transplantation. No immunosuppressant medications are necessary after AuHSCT, because the patient does not receive foreign tissue. A disadvantage of AuHSCT is the risk that tumor cells may remain in the bone marrow despite high-dose chemotherapy (conditioning regimens).

Syngeneic transplants result in less incidence of GVHD and graft rejection; however, there is also less graft-versus-tumor effect to fight the malignancy. Syngeneic transplant is associated with transmission of genetic defects (Maziarz & Schubach-Slater, 2015). For this reason, even when an identical twin is available for marrow donation, another matched sibling or even an unrelated donor may be the most suitable donor to combat an aggressive malignancy.

Nursing Management

Nursing care of patients undergoing HSCT is complex and demands a high level of skill. The success of HSCT is greatly influenced by nursing care throughout the transplantation process.

Implementing Care Before Treatment

All patients must undergo extensive evaluations before the transplant to assess the current clinical status of the disease. Nutritional assessments, extensive physical examinations, organ function tests, and psychological evaluations are conducted. Blood work includes assessing past infectious antigen exposure (e.g., hepatitis virus, cytomegalovirus, herpes simplex virus, human immunodeficiency virus, and syphilis). The patient's social support systems and financial and insurance resources are also evaluated. Informed consent and patient education about the procedure and care before and after HSCT are vital.

Providing Care During Treatment

Skilled nursing care is required during the treatment phase of HSCT when high-dose chemotherapy (conditioning regimen) and total-body irradiation are given. The acute toxicities of nausea, diarrhea, mucositis, and hemorrhagic cystitis require close monitoring and symptom management by the nurse.

Nursing management during stem cell infusion consists of monitoring the patient's vital signs and blood oxygen saturation; assessing for adverse effects, such as fever, chills, shortness of breath, chest pain, cutaneous reactions, nausea, vomiting, hypotension or hypertension, tachycardia, anxiety, and taste changes; and providing strategies for symptom control, ongoing support, and patient education. During stem cell infusion, patients may experience adverse reactions to the cryoprotectant dimethylsulfoxide (DMSO) used to preserve the harvested stem cells. These reactions may include nausea, vomiting, chills, dyspnea, cardiac dysrhythmias, and hypotension progressing to cardiac or respiratory arrest. Less common toxicities include neurologic and renal impairment (Maziarz & Schubach-Slater, 2015).

A cluster of symptoms referred to as engraftment syndrome may occur during the neutrophil recovery phase in both allogeneic and autologous transplants. Clinical features of this syndrome vary widely but may include noninfectious fever associated with skin rash, weight gain, diarrhea, and pulmonary infiltrates, with improvement noted after the initiation of corticosteroid therapy rather than antibiotic therapy (Maziarz & Schubach-Slater, 2015). Until engraftment is well established, the patient requires support with blood products and hematopoietic growth factors.

Potential infections may be bacterial, viral, fungal, or protozoan in origin. During the first 30 days following transplant, the patient is most at risk for developing reactivations of viral infections, including herpes simplex, EBV, cytomegalovirus, and varicella zoster. Mucosal denudement poses a risk for *Candida* (yeast) infection locally and systemically. Pulmonary toxicities offer the opportunity for fungal infections such as *Aspergillus*. Renal complications arise from the nephrotoxic chemotherapy agents used in the conditioning regimen or those used to treat infection (amphotericin B, aminoglycosides). A neutropenic diet is usually prescribed for patients to decrease the risk of exposure to foodborne infections from bacteria, yeast, molds, viruses, and parasites (Lassiter & Schneider, 2015). Whether a neutropenic diet decreases rates of infection is currently in question; see the nursing research profile in Chart 15-6.

Tumor lysis syndrome and acute tubular necrosis are also risks after HSCT. Nursing assessment for signs of these complications is essential for early identification and treatment. GVHD requires skillful nursing assessment to detect early effects on the skin, liver, and gastrointestinal tract. HSOS resulting from the conditioning regimens used can result in fluid retention, jaundice, abdominal pain, ascites, tender and enlarged liver, and encephalopathy. Pulmonary complications, such as pulmonary edema, interstitial pneumonia, and other pneumonias, often complicate recovery.

Providing Care After Treatment

Caring for Recipients

Ongoing nursing assessment during follow-up visits is essential to detect late effects of therapy after HSCT, which may occur 100 days or more after the procedure. Late effects include infections (e.g., varicella-zoster infection), restrictive pulmonary abnormalities, and recurrent pneumonias. Sterility often results due to total-body irradiation, chemotherapy, or both as components of the ablative regimen. Chronic GVHD can involve the skin, liver, intestine, esophagus, eyes, lungs, joints, and vaginal mucosa. Cataracts may also develop after total-body irradiation.

The potential psychological impact of HSCT has been described as unique and unlike other experiences (Miceli, Lilleby, Noonan, et al., 2013). Psychosocial assessments by nursing staff must be ongoing and a priority. In addition to the multiple physical and psychological stressors affecting patients at each phase of the transplantation experience, the nature of the treatment and patient experience can place extreme emotional, social, financial, and physical demands on family, friends, and donors. Nurses assess the family and other caregivers' needs and provide education, support, and information about resources.

Caring for Donors

Like HSCT recipients, donors also require nursing care. They may experience mood alterations, decreased self-esteem, and guilt from feelings of failure if the transplantation fails. Family members must be educated and supported to reduce anxiety and promote coping during this difficult time. In addition, they must also be assisted to maintain realistic expectations of themselves as well as of the patient.

Chart 15-6 — NURSING RESEARCH PROFILE

Do Neutropenic Diets Prevent Infection?

Lassiter, M., & Schneider, S. M. (2015). A pilot study comparing the neutropenic diet to a non-neutropenic diet in the allogeneic hematopoietic stem cell transplantation population. *Oncology Nursing Forum, 19*(3), 273–278.

Purpose

Despite years of implementation on oncology units, there is little evidence to support the use of a neutropenic diet. The purpose of this pilot study was to determine whether a neutropenic diet compared to a diet without restrictions made a difference in the incidence of infections and nutritional status of patients receiving myeloablative allogeneic hematopoietic stem cell transplantation (HSCT).

Design

This was a prospective randomized pilot study. A variety of laboratory measurements were collected for indications of infection (blood cultures) and to assess nutritional status. Laboratory measurements were compared between the control (neutropenic diet) and experimental (regular diet) arms using the two-sided Wilcoxon rank-sum test. Chi square was used to compare the percentage of patients with positive blood cultures in the two groups.

Findings

No significant differences between the control group ($n = 21$) and experimental group ($n = 25$) were found for demographic variables or patients who required total parenteral nutrition. Across all time points, no significant differences were found in any of the laboratory values with the exception of the total protein level. The median in the total protein level across all time points was 20% in the control arm and 16% in the experimental group, a significant difference ($p = 0.023$). Analysis of positive blood cultures failed to demonstrate any significant difference between the experimental and control groups.

Nursing Implications

Nurses should know that this pilot study provides beginning evidence that the neutropenic diet does not contribute to differences in infection rates or nutrition when compared to unrestricted diets in patients undergoing HSCT. Nurses need to conduct additional research with larger samples and multi-institutional involvement before the safety of changing this long-standing practice can be established.

Hyperthermia

The use of hyperthermia (thermal therapy), which is the generation of temperatures greater than physiologic fever range (greater than 41.5°C [106.7°F]), has been used for many years to destroy cancerous tumors. Hyperthermia is most effective when combined with radiation therapy, chemotherapy, or biologic therapy. Hyperthermia and radiation therapy are thought to work well together because hypoxic tumor cells and cells in the S phase of the cell cycle are more sensitive to heat than radiation, and the addition of heat damages tumor cells so that they cannot repair themselves after radiation therapy. Hyperthermia preferentially damages tumor blood vessels, partly because these vessels are of inadequate size to dissipate the heat generated by hyperthermia.

Hyperthermia is thought to alter cellular membrane permeability when used with chemotherapy, allowing for an increased uptake of the chemotherapeutic agent. Hyperthermia may enhance the function of immune system cells, such as macrophages and T cells, to assist in combating malignant cells. Resistance to hyperthermia may develop during the treatment because cells adapt to repeated thermal insult.

Heat can be produced by using radio waves, ultrasound, microwaves, magnetic waves, hot-water baths, or even hot-wax immersions. Hyperthermia may be local or regional, or it may include the whole body. Local or regional hyperthermia may be delivered into a tumor, on the skin, into a body orifice, or by regional perfusion (i.e., an extremity affected by melanoma). Heated intraperitoneal chemotherapy has been used (in combination with surgery) to treat abdominal malignancies (Damsky-Dell, Held-Warmkessel, Jakubek, et al., 2014). Side effects of hyperthermia treatments include burns, fatigue, hypotension, peripheral neuropathies, thrombophlebitis, nausea, vomiting, diarrhea, and electrolyte imbalances. Cardiovascular stress may develop in patients receiving hyperthermia to a large area or whole body due to changes in pulse and blood pressure.

Nursing Management

Although hyperthermia has been used for years, patients and their families may be unfamiliar with this cancer treatment. Consequently, they need explanations about the procedure, its goals, and its effects. The nurse assesses the patient for adverse effects. Local skin care at the site of the implanted probes is necessary.

Targeted Therapies

Normal cell growth is regulated by well-defined communication pathways between the environment surrounding the cell and the internal cell environment, the nucleus, and the intracellular cytoplasm. The cell membrane contains important protein receptors that respond to signals transmitted from the external cell environment and transmit that signal to the internal cell environment using enzymatic pathways called *signal transduction pathways*. Although normal cells have transduction pathways, scientific advances have led to the recognition that cancer, at the cellular level, is characterized by deregulated cell signaling transduction pathways (both intra- and extracellular pathways), and receptors and proteins as well as altered cell membrane receptors and proteins play an important role in tumor initiation, growth, and spread (Caruana, Diaconu,

& Dottia, 2014). This improved understanding of cancer cell behavior has allowed scientists to develop molecular-based therapies, called **targeted therapies.** These specifically target (like a lock and key mechanism) receptors, proteins, signal transduction pathways, and other processes to prevent the continued growth of cancer cells. Targeted therapies seek to work against cancer cell capabilities, such as malignant transformation, uncontrolled reproduction, growth and metastasis, blocking apoptosis, and altered genetic coding. Examples of targeted therapies include biologic response modifiers (BRMs) (such as monoclonal antibodies [MoAbs], growth factors and cytokines) and some types of gene therapy (Caruana et al., 2014).

Biologic Response Modifiers

BRM therapy involves the use of naturally occurring or recombinant (reproduced through genetic engineering) agents or treatment methods that can alter the immunologic relationship between the tumor and the patient with cancer (host) to provide a therapeutic benefit. Although the mechanisms of action vary with each type of BRM, the goal is to destroy or stop the malignant growth. The basis of BRM treatment lies in the restoration, modification, stimulation, or augmentation of the body's natural immune defenses against cancer (Blix, 2014).

Nonspecific Biologic Response Modifiers

Early investigations of the stimulation of the immune system involved nonspecific agents, such as bacille Calmette-Guérin (BCG) and *Corynebacterium parvum*. When injected into the patient, these agents serve as antigens that stimulate an immune response. The hope is that the stimulated immune system will then eradicate malignant cells. Extensive animal and human investigations with BCG have shown promising results, especially in treating localized malignant melanoma. In addition, BCG bladder instillation is a standard form of treatment for localized bladder cancer (Blix, 2014). However, the use of nonspecific agents in advanced cancer remains limited, and research is ongoing to identify other uses and agents.

Monoclonal Antibodies (MoAbs)

MoAbs, another type of BRM, have become available through technologic advances, enabling investigators to grow and produce targeted antibodies for specific malignant cells. Theoretically, this type of specificity allows MoAbs to destroy the cancer cells and spare normal cells. The specificity of MoAbs is dependent on identifying key antigen proteins on the surface of tumors that are not present on normal tissues. When the MoAb attaches to the cell surface antigen, an important signal transduction pathway for communication between the malignant cells and the extracellular environment is blocked. The results may include an inability to initiate apoptosis, reproduce, or invade surrounding tissues.

The production of MoAbs involves injecting tumor cells that act as antigens into mice. B-cell lymphocytes in the spleen of the mouse produce immunoglobulin (antibodies) made in response to the injected antigens. Antibody-producing B cells are combined with a cancer cell that has the ability to grow indefinitely in culture medium and continue producing more antibodies.

The combination of spleen cells and the cancer cells is referred to as a hybridoma. From hybridomas that continue to

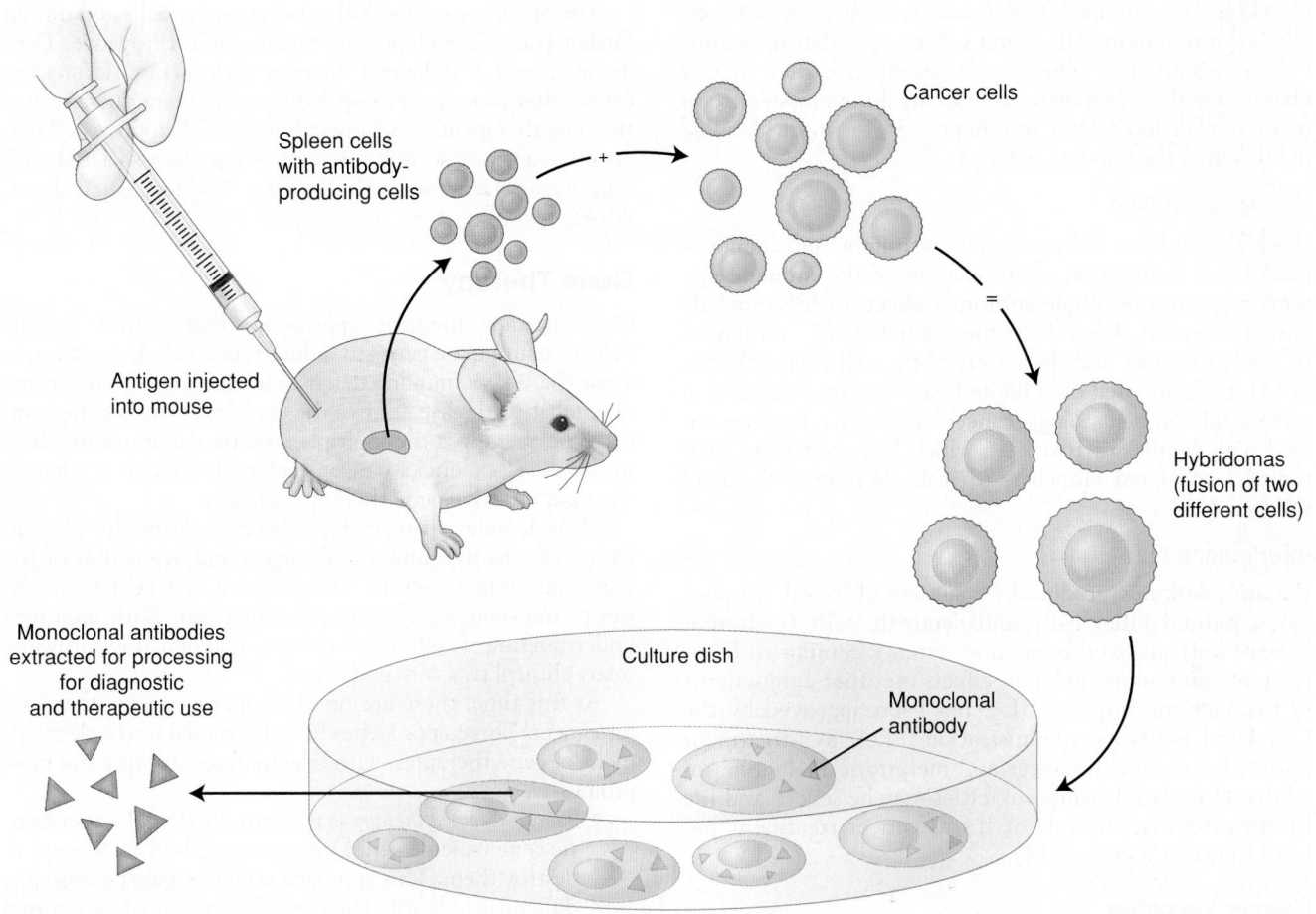

Cancer cells

Spleen cells
with antibody-
producing cells

Antigen injected
into mouse

Hybridomas
(fusion of two
different cells)

Monoclonal antibodies
extracted for processing
for diagnostic
and therapeutic use

Culture dish

Monoclonal
antibody

Hybridomas multiply in culture medium

Figure 15-5 • Antibody-producing spleen cells are fused with cancer cells. This process produces cells called *hybridomas*. These cells, which can grow indefinitely in a culture medium, produce antibodies that are harvested, purified, and prepared for diagnostic or treatment purposes.

grow in the culture medium, the desired antibodies are harvested, purified, and prepared for diagnostic or therapeutic use (see Fig. 15-5). Advances in genetic engineering have led to the production of MoAbs with combinations of mouse and human components (*chimeric MoAbs*) or all-human components (*human MoAbs*). MoAbs made with human genes have greater immunologic properties and are less likely to cause allergic reactions (Grossman & Porth, 2014).

Several MoAbs are used for treatment in cancer using various extracellular (on the cell membrane) and intracellular targets. Trastuzumab (Herceptin) has the ability to target the HER2 protein, an error of gene overexpression found in breast and other cancers (Comerford, 2015). Rituxumab (Rituxin) is a MoAb that binds specifically with the CD20 antigen expressed by non-Hodgkin lymphoma and B-cell chronic lymphocytic leukemia (Comerford, 2015).

Some MoAbs are used alone, whereas others are used in combination with agents that facilitate their antitumor actions. Ibritumomab tiuxetan (Zevalin), a MoAb conjugated with a radioactive isotope, is used in the treatment of certain types of lymphoma (Mack, Ritchie, & Sapra, 2014). MoAbs are also used as aids in diagnostic evaluation of both primary and metastatic tumors through radiologic imaging and labo-

ratory techniques. For example, the process of immunohistochemistry uses a MoAb tagged with a stain that binds with the protein of interest, providing a visual stain for the presence or absence of the protein (Mack et al., 2014). This type of test is used to identify the presence of estrogen and progesterone receptors on breast cancer cells to see if the cells will be responsive to hormonal agents. Immunohistochemistry testing is also used to detect several proteins associated with hereditary nonpolyposis colon cancer (Mack et al., 2014). MoAbs are used to assist in the diagnosis of ovarian, colorectal, breast, and prostate cancers and some types of leukemia and lymphoma. MoAbs are also used in purging residual tumor cells from peripheral stem cell collections for patients who are undergoing HSCT after high-dose cytotoxic therapy. Researchers continue to explore the development and use of MoAbs, either alone or in combination with other substances such as radioactive materials, chemotherapy agents, toxins, hormones, or other BRMs.

Cytokines

Cytokines, substances produced primarily by cells of the immune system to enhance or suppress the production and functioning of components of the immune system, are used to treat cancer or the adverse effects of some cancer treatments.

Cytokines are grouped into families, such as interferons (IFNs), interleukins (ILs), and colony-stimulating factors. Colony-stimulating factors were described earlier in this chapter for their supportive role in myelosuppressive treatment modalities. (Refer to Chapter 35 for more detailed discussion of the immune system.)

Interferons (IFNs)

IFNs are cytokines with antiviral, antitumor, and immuno-modulatory (inhibition or stimulation of the immune system) properties. Multiple antitumor effects of IFNs include antiangiogenesis, direct destruction of tumor cells, inhibition of growth factors, and disruption of the cell cycle (Weber, 2014). IFNs are used on a limited basis for the treatment of some solid and hematologic cancers. IFNs have been associated with significant toxicities, which have restricted their use and prompted clinicians to seek alternative therapies (Weber, 2014).

Interleukins (ILs)

ILs are cytokines produced by subsets of T-cell lymphocytes, natural killer cells, and dendritic cells (cells that present antigens to the immune system). Similar to IFNs, ILs have immunomodulatory effects on other components of the immune response. IL-2 has been approved by the U.S. Food and Drug Administration (FDA) as a treatment option for renal cell cancer and metastatic melanoma in adults. However, because toxicities may be severe and life-threatening, the role of ILs as cancer treatment has been limited (Weber, 2014).

Cancer Vaccines

Cancer vaccines mobilize the body's immune response to prevent or treat cancer. These vaccines contain either portions of cancer cells alone or portions of cells in combination with other substances (adjuvants) that can augment or boost immune responses. *Autologous* vaccines are made from the patient's own cancer cells, which are taken from tumor tissue obtained during biopsy or surgical intervention. The cancer cells are killed and prepared for injection back into the patient. *Allogeneic* vaccines are made from cancer cell lines that are immortalized cells that were originally obtained from other people who had a specific type of cancer. These cancer cells are grown in a laboratory and eventually killed and prepared for injection.

Prophylactic vaccines prevent disease. Three vaccines have been approved by the FDA for the prevention of HPV. HPV2 (Cervarix), recommended for use in females only, protects against HPV types 16 and 18 that are responsible for about 70% of all cervical cancers (ACS, 2015a). HPV4 (Gardasil) provides protection against four HPV types (6, 11, 16, and 18) and is recommended for use in both males and females. HPV9 (Gardasil-9), recommended for both males and females, protects against nine HPV types associated with cervical, anal, vaginal, and vulvar cancers. HPV9 also protects against genital warts. All of the HPV vaccines are given as a series of three doses over 6 months. Although the role of HPV vaccines in prevention of oropharyngeal cancers related to HPV 16 has not been fully established, there are preliminary data to suggest effectiveness (Herrero, Quint, Hildesheim, et al., 2015).

Therapeutic vaccines kill existing cancer cells and inhibit further cancer development. Sipuleucel-T (Provenge, Dendreon Corp.) is indicated for men with metastatic prostate cancer that is no longer responding to hormone therapy. It is the only therapeutic vaccine currently FDA approved. Therapeutic vaccines do not cure cancer but are associated with improved patient survival (Kannan, Madden, & Andrews, 2014).

Gene Therapy

Gene therapy includes approaches that correct genetic defects, manipulate genes to induce tumor cell destruction, or assist the body's immune defenses in the hope of preventing or combating disease. One of the challenges confronting cancer gene therapy is the multiple somatic mutations involved in the development of cancer, making it difficult to identify the most effective gene therapy approach.

Considerable advances have been made in the identification of effective tumor cell targets and evaluation of the most appropriate vectors. Vectors serve as a vehicle or carrier to transport a gene into the target cell. With improved understanding of cell surface proteins and signaling pathways, many clinical trials are under way.

At this time, there are no FDA-approved gene therapies for cancer. Three approaches have been used in the development of gene therapies, with adenoviruses showing the most promise in each:

*   *Tumor-directed therapy* is the introduction of a therapeutic gene (suicide gene) into tumor cells in an attempt to destroy them. This approach is challenging because it is difficult to identify the gene that would cause optimal tumor destruction, and patients with widespread disease would require multiple injections to treat every site of disease.
*   *Active immunotherapy* is the administration of genes that will invoke the antitumor responses of the immune system.
*   *Adoptive immunotherapy* is the administration of genetically altered lymphocytes that are programmed to cause tumor destruction.

Nursing Management

Patients receiving targeted therapies have many of the same needs as patients undergoing other cancer treatments. However, manipulation and stimulation of the immune system create unique challenges. Consequently, the nurse must assess the need for education, support, and additional resources for both the patient and the family and assist in planning and evaluating patient care. Patient education is important, as many of the toxicities associated with targeted therapies are not only a source of physical discomfort, but they also impact the quality of life, and potentially impact patient adherence to oral drug regimens (Vioral, Leslie, Best, et al., 2014; Yagasaki & Komatsu, 2013).

Monitoring Therapeutic and Adverse Effects

The nurse must become familiar with each agent given and its potential effects. Adverse effects such as fever, myalgia, nausea, and vomiting, as seen with IFN therapy, may not be life-threatening. Other adverse effects (e.g., capillary leak syndrome, pulmonary edema, hypotension) that may become life-threatening can occur with BRM approaches such as high-dose IL-2 therapy. MoAbs are associated with both common and unique adverse effects. Although mild to moderate infusion reactions are more commonly associated with chimeric MoAbs, severe HSRs have been seen with MoAb infusions. Nurses must be aware of the adverse effects of BRMs and recognize the signs and symptoms of serious reactions to emergently institute appropriate interventions and supportive care. Nurses monitor patients for the impact of adverse effects on performance status and quality of life so that appropriate measures can be implemented to improve patient outcomes.

Promoting Home, Community-Based, and Transitional Care

The nurse educates patients about self-care and assists in providing for continuing care. Some targeted therapies can be given subcutaneously by the patient or family members at home. As needed, the home care nurse educates the patient and family how to administer these agents and monitors the use of appropriate technique as well as safe disposal of sharps and contaminated materials. The nurse also provides instructions about side effects and helps the patient and family identify strategies to manage many of the common side effects of BRM therapy, such as fatigue, anorexia, and flulike symptoms.

The use of oral medications to treat cancer has risen greatly in the past several years, especially with advances in targeted therapies, many of which are given by mouth. It has been estimated that almost half of the new antineoplastic drugs are oral agents (IMS, 2014). Of over 700 drugs in development, 80% are based on targeted approaches and about 35% are oral agents. The rising use of oral therapies shifts the responsibility for delivery of treatment to patients and families in the home setting. Treatment approaches with newer mechanisms of action and associated toxicities, as well as the transition of responsibility to patients and families, increase the need for nurses to identify factors affecting adherence and develop strategies to address adherence barriers (see Table 15-8).

The nurse collaborates with physicians, social workers, third-party payers, and pharmaceutical companies to help the patient obtain reimbursement or support for the cost of oral targeted therapies and other required medications. The nurse also reminds the patient about the importance of keeping follow-up appointments with the physician and assesses the patient's need for symptom management related to the underlying diseases and/or adverse effects of treatment. Home care nurses maintain communication with the physician regarding patient adherence and tolerance of treatment so that changes in care can be implemented in a timely fashion.

Complementary, Alternative, and Integrative Health Therapies

Integrative healthcare is viewed as a comprehensive, interdisciplinary approach to preventing and treating illness and promoting health that brings together complementary, alternative, and conventional therapies. The use of an integrative approach to health wellness has grown within mainstream healthcare settings in the United States, particularly within oncology care (National Center for Complementary and Integrative Health [NCCIH], 2015).

Individuals use complementary approaches to prevent and treat cancer, although there are no data to support efficacy. Patients also use complementary approaches to manage symptoms related to cancer and associated treatments; some approaches are supported by clinical research while others are not. The NCCIH suggests that as many as 65% of people diagnosed with cancer have used some form of complementary medicine. The use of complementary strategies is influenced by age, race, ethnicity, and geography (Clarke, Black, Stussman, et al., 2015). However, patients do not routinely communicate complementary practices to their health care providers because they usually are not asked about its use; they withhold the information, fearing that their physicians would not approve, or they feel that the use of these approaches will not affect the conventional treatment they are receiving

Although many complementary modalities can be a source of comfort and emotional support for patients, assessment of complementary therapy use is important for patient safety. Patients often perceive vitamins and dietary supplements as harmless, natural products that have no side effects or potential toxicities. In patients receiving any conventional therapies, the use of herbs or botanicals may interfere with drug metabolism, decrease or increase desired effects, or contain elements of uncertain pharmacologic capacities (NCCIH, 2015). Deep tissue massage and other manipulative therapies are contraindicated in patients with open wounds, radiation dermatitis, thrombocytopenia, VTE, and coagulation disorders, and in those taking anticoagulants. See Chapter 7 for more information on complementary, alternative, and integrative health therapies.

Nursing Care of Patients With Cancer

The outlook for patients with cancer has greatly improved because of scientific and technologic advances. However, as a result of the underlying disease or various treatment modalities, patients with cancer may experience a variety of secondary problems such as reduced WBC counts, infection, bleeding, skin and nutritional problems, pain, fatigue, and psychological stress. Chart 15-7 provides a nursing care plan for patients with cancer.

Maintaining Tissue Integrity

Some of the most frequently encountered disturbances of tissue integrity include stomatitis, skin and tissue reactions to radiation therapy, cutaneous toxicities associated with targeted therapy, alopecia, and metastatic skin lesions.

Stomatitis

Mucositis, a common side effect of radiation and some types of chemotherapy, refers to an inflammatory process involving the mucous membranes of the oral cavity and the gastrointestinal tract. **Stomatitis,** a form of mucositis, is an inflammatory process of the mouth, including the mucosa and tissues surrounding the teeth. Stomatitis is characterized by changes in sensation, mild redness (erythema), and edema or, if severe, by painful ulcerations, bleeding, and secondary infection. Stomatitis commonly develops 5 to 14 days

TABLE 15-8 Strategies for Promoting Adherence to Oral Antineoplastic Agents

Assess for factors that may interfere with adherence to oral antineoplastic agents; develop plan of care that addresses specific assessment findings.

Barriers to Adherence	Strategies for Promoting Adherence
Sociodemographic Factors • Limited financial resources • Competing priorities for financial resources • Joblessness • Limited or no insurance • Racial or ethnic disparities • Lower level of education • Poor health literacy • Illiteracy • Non–English speaking • Lack of transportation • Lack of or limited social support • Rural residence	• Refer to financial counseling through health care facility, local nonprofit health/oncology support/advocacy, or other nonprofit community advocacy organizations. • Refer to social worker for referrals as described above and/or for disability applications through employer or Social Security Administration, Medicaid, or Medicare applications. • Explore patient assistance programs for costs of health care, copays, medications, household costs, transportation services (costs or availability), and home care available through nonprofit organizations, oncology support/advocacy or other nonprofit community advocacy organizations, religious institutions, philanthropic organizations, pharmaceutical industry–sponsored programs, health care institution–specific programs; assist with financial documentation and application procedures as needed. • Explore assistance programs for other priorities competing for financial resources (i.e., for utility costs, gas, child care, food). • Assist patient to identify family, friends, or other available supports to assist with activities of daily living, household responsibilities, errands, shopping, meals, transportation or other responsibilities; assist with delegation of needs and schedules of availability if needed. • Assess preferred method of learning (i.e., verbal, visual, written materials); tailor instructional materials to patient needs, including language. • Include family, significant other, and friends in education whenever feasible. • Use return demonstration of behaviors and devices used to support adherence. • Provide contact information that spans 24 hours for questions or problems. • Contact patient by phone or other means (e-mail) to assess for concerns in between follow-up visits to physician. • Encourage patient to use adherence reminders, such as pill boxes, medication calendars, checklists, medication diaries, alarms on cell phone or other devices/timers; explore availability of programmed telephone reminder services, text messages from family member, friend, or other caregiver; review diary at each visit. • Instruct patient to bring pill bottles to each follow-up visit; perform pill counts to monitor adherence. • Send postcard reminder to patient weekly (or less often) or 1 week prior to due date for medication refill. • Refer to home care for continued education, and follow up on adherence. • Identify local pharmacies that supply oral cancer therapies. Instruct patients to contact nurse if the pharmacy cannot fill the prescription within 24 hours. • Remind patients to anticipate need for adequate supply of medications prior to travel or vacation.
Age • Older adults; especially those >75 years	• Ensure that printed education materials and instructions are printed in black using at least 14-point sans serif font such as Arial or Calibri. • Use illustrated education materials. • Review and revise adherence strategies if patient status declines or changes. • Explore availability of alarmed medication box.
Beliefs • Oral medications less effective or important than IV treatments • Fatalism about disease outcomes	• Provide education regarding oral versus IV medications. • Discuss goals of care and ongoing assessment of response to treatment.
Comorbidities • Preexisting chronic disease • Vision or hearing impairments	• Communicate with primary care and other providers involved in care of patient regarding current cancer disease status and treatment; collaborate with other providers for ongoing management of nononcology issues or exacerbation of issues that may impact cancer treatment adherence. • Collaborate with appropriate resources to assist with special needs and assistive devices for vision or hearing impairments.
Polypharmacy • Multiple medications for comorbidities and/or cancer treatment and symptom management	• Review all medications prescribed by oncology physicians and other providers involved in care of patient for preexisting chronic disease. • Assess patient use of over-the-counter medications and other agents. • Consult with pharmacist to identify medications and other agents that may be contraindicated or that may interfere with antineoplastic regimen. • Collaborate with all providers prescribing medications in order to simplify and/or reduce number of required medications if possible. • Provide patient, family, or other caregiver education regarding specific instructions when multiple medications are required. • Provide written checklist for patient to utilize daily to check off each medication when taken. • Do not give patients prescriptions that allow for refills; prescriptions should be for a finite period of time that concludes with next scheduled visit.

TABLE 15-8 Strategies for Promoting Adherence to Oral Antineoplastic Agents (continued)

Barriers to Adherence	Strategies for Promoting Adherence
Psychiatric, Psychological, or Cognitive Concerns • Psychiatric disease • Depression • Cognitive impairments • Anxiety	• Avoid initial education regarding oral medications at the same time of first physician visit; have patient and other learners return for another appointment to see nurse for education, and follow up with subsequent visit if deemed to be at high risk for adherence challenges. • Discuss with physician the necessity for referral to psychiatrist to evaluate need for psychotropic medications. • Refer patient for professional mental health counseling as needed. • Identify additional supports for care and education as discussed earlier.
Disease Factors • Symptoms such as pain, nausea, fatigue, skin rashes, etc. • Impaired mobility	• Proactively assess and manage symptoms related to underlying disease and/or treatments. • Provide patient, family, or other caregivers education about expected side effects and management strategies. • Instruct patient to premedicate with antiemetic as prescribed 30 minutes prior to taking oral antineoplastic agent if needed for nausea and/or vomiting. • Identify additional supports for care as discussed earlier. • Assess need for referral to home physical and/or occupational therapy to address impaired mobility and need for assistive devices.
Communication Issues • Patient–Clinician • Clinician—Clinician	• Establish rapport and allow patients, families, and other caregivers time and opportunity to ask questions. • Do not assume adherence to oral antineoplastic agents; assess potential barriers consistently throughout course of treatment at each follow-up visit. • Communicate with primary provider regarding current cancer disease status, treatment and information regarding antineoplastic agents, such as drug–drug interactions, expected toxicities, and toxicities requiring prompt intervention.

Adapted from Vioral, A., Leslie, M., Best, R., et al. (2014). Patient adherence with oral oncolytic therapies. *Seminars in Oncology Nursing, 30*(3), 190–199.

after patients receive certain chemotherapeutic agents, such as doxorubicin and 5-fluorouracil; immunotherapies, such as IL-2 and IFN; and molecular targeted drugs, such as temsirolimus and everolimus. Stomatitis affects up to 100% of patients undergoing high-dose chemotherapy with HSCT, 80% of patients with malignancies of the head and neck receiving radiotherapy, and up to 40% of patients receiving standard-dose chemotherapy (Gibson, Keefe, Lalla, et al., 2013). Stomatitis may be worse in patients with head and neck cancers who receive combined modality therapy of both radiation and chemotherapy. When severe, stomatitis can lead to interruptions, delays, and modifications in the course of treatment, all of which may contribute to less desirable patient outcomes. Severe oral pain can significantly affect swallowing, nutritional intake, speech, quality of life, coping abilities, and willingness to adhere to treatment regimens. In addition, stomatitis may lead to more frequent health care visits, hospitalizations, and increased health care costs (Eilers, Harris, Henry, et al., 2014). Stomatitis and mucositis are attributed to a cascade of molecular processes and submucosal endothelial cell destruction that begin almost immediately after the initiation of radiation and certain types of chemotherapy, prior to the development of signs and symptoms. Mucositis develops as a consequence of a sequence of related and interacting biologic events, culminating in injury and apoptosis of basal epithelial cells, leading to the loss of epithelial renewal, atrophy, and ulceration. Gram-positive and gram-negative organisms can invade the ulcerated tissue and result in infection.

Nursing assessment begins with an understanding of the patient's usual practices for oral hygiene and identification of individuals at risk for stomatitis. Oral cavity assessment is performed daily or at each patient visit (Tipian, 2014). Risk factors and comorbidities associated with stomatitis include poor oral hygiene, general debilitation, existing dental disease, prior irradiation to the head and neck region, impaired salivary gland function, the use of other medications that dry mucous membranes, **myelosuppression** (bone marrow depression), advanced age, tobacco use, previous stomatoxic chemotherapy, diminished renal function, and impaired nutritional status (Eilers et al., 2014). The patient is also assessed for dehydration, infection, pain, and nutritional impairment resulting from mucositis.

Optimal evidence-based prevention and treatment approaches for stomatitis remain limited but continue to be studied across disciplines (Eilers et al., 2014). Most clinicians agree that maintenance of good oral hygiene, including brushing, flossing, rinsing, and dental care, is necessary to minimize the risk of oral complications associated with cancer therapies.

Palifermin (Kepivance), an IV-administered synthetic form of human keratinocyte growth factor, is beneficial in the prevention of stomatitis in patients with hematologic malignancies who are preparing for HSCT (Vadhan-Raj, Goldberg, Perales, et al., 2013). Palifermin promotes epithelial cell repair and accelerated replacement of cells in the mouth and gastrointestinal tract. Careful timing of administration and monitoring are essential for effectiveness and to detect adverse effects. Other approaches recommended for practice include cryotherapy (topical application of oral ice during infusions), consistent oral hygiene, low-level laser therapy, and sodium bicarbonate mouth rinses (Eilers et al., 2014; Tayyem, 2014). Additional aspects of care are discussed in Chart 15-7: nursing care plan for patients with cancer.

(text continued on page 370)

Chart 15-7

PLAN OF NURSING CARE

The Patient With Cancer

NURSING DIAGNOSIS: Risk for infection related to inadequate defenses related to myelosuppression secondary to radiation or antineoplastic agents
GOAL: Prevention of infection

Nursing Interventions	Rationale	Expected Outcomes

1. Assess patient for evidence of infection.
  a. Check vital signs every 4 hours.
  b. Monitor white blood cell (WBC) count and differential each day.
  c. Inspect all sites that may serve as entry ports for pathogens (IV sites, wounds, skin folds, bony prominences, perineum, and oral cavity).
	1. Signs and symptoms of infection may be diminished in the immunocompromised host. Prompt recognition of infection and subsequent initiation of therapy will reduce morbidity and mortality associated with infection.	• Demonstrates normal temperature and vital signs
		• Exhibits absence of signs of inflammation: local edema, erythema, pain, and warmth
		• Exhibits normal breath sounds on auscultation
		• Takes deep breaths and coughs every 2 hours to prevent respiratory dysfunction and infection.
		• Exhibits absence of pathogens on cultures
		• Avoids contact with others with infections
		• Avoids crowds

2. Report fever (≥38.3°C [101°F] or ≥38°C [100.4°F] for >1 hour) (see Table 15-10), chills, diaphoresis, swelling, heat, pain, erythema, exudate on any body surfaces. Also report change in respiratory or mental status, urinary frequency or burning, malaise, myalgias, arthralgias, rash, or diarrhea.	2. Early detection of infection facilitates early intervention.	
3. Obtain cultures and sensitivities as indicated before initiation of antimicrobial treatment (wound exudate, sputum, urine, stool, blood).	3. Tests identify the organism and indicate the most appropriate antimicrobial therapy. The use of inappropriate antibiotics enhances proliferation of additional flora and encourages growth of antibiotic-resistant organisms.	• All personnel carry out hand hygiene after each voiding and bowel movement. • Excoriation and trauma of skin are avoided. • Trauma to mucous membranes is avoided (avoidance of rectal thermometers, suppositories, vaginal tampons, perianal trauma).

4. Initiate measures to minimize infection.
  a. Discuss with patient and family:
    1. Placing patient in private room if absolute WBC count <1000/mm³.
    2. Importance of patient avoiding contact with people who have known or recent infection or recent vaccination.
	4. Exposure to infection is reduced.
	  a. Preventing contact with pathogens helps prevent infection.
		• Uses evidence-based procedures and techniques if participating in management of invasive lines or catheters
		• Uses electric razor
		• Is free of skin breakdown and stasis of secretions

b. Instruct all personnel in careful hand hygiene before and after entering room.	b. Hands are significant source of contamination.	• Adheres to dietary and environmental precautions • Exhibits no signs of sepsis or septic shock
c. Avoid rectal or vaginal procedures (rectal temperatures, examinations, suppositories; vaginal tampons).	c. Incidence of rectal and perianal abscesses and subsequent systemic infection is high. Manipulation may cause disruption of membrane integrity and enhance progression of infection.	• Exhibits normal vital signs, cardiac output, and arterial pressures when monitored
d. Use stool softeners to prevent constipation and straining.	d. Minimizes trauma to tissues	• Demonstrates ability to administer colony-stimulating factor
e. Assist patient in practice of meticulous personal hygiene.	e. Prevents skin irritation	• Has bowel movements at regular intervals without constipation or straining

f. Instruct patient to use electric razor.
  g. Encourage patient to ambulate in room unless contraindicated.
	f. Minimizes skin trauma
	  g. Minimizes chance of skin breakdown and stasis of pulmonary secretions
		• Patient hygiene is maintained.
		• Absence of IV catheter–related infection

h. Provide patient and family education on food hygiene and safe food handling.	h. No evidence supports dietary restrictions of avoiding raw or fresh fruit and vegetables for patients who are neutropenic. General precautions regarding food handling and storage are recommended.	• Absence of skin abcesses • Absence of urinary catheter–related infection
i. Each day, change water pitcher, denture cleaning fluids, and respiratory equipment containing water.	i. Stagnant water is a source of infection.	

5. Assess IV sites every day for evidence of infection.
  a. Change peripheral short-term IV sites every other day.
  b. Cleanse skin with povidone–iodine before arterial puncture or venipuncture.
	5. Nosocomial staphylococcal septicemia is closely associated with IV catheters.
	  a. Incidence of infection is increased when catheter is in place >72 hours.
	  b. Povidone–iodine is effective against many gram-positive and gram-negative pathogens.	

Chart 15-7

PLAN OF NURSING CARE (Continued)

The Patient With Cancer

Nursing Interventions	Rationale	Expected Outcomes

c. Change central venous catheter dressings every 48 hours.
d. Change all solutions and infusion sets every 72–96 hours.
e. Follow Infusion Nursing Society guidelines for care of peripheral and central venous access devices.

6. Avoid intramuscular injections.
7. Avoid insertion of urinary catheters; if catheters are necessary, use aseptic technique.
8. Educate patient or family member to administer granulocyte (or granulocyte-macrophage) colony-stimulating factor when prescribed.
9. Advise patient to avoid exposure to animal excreta, discuss dental procedures with primary provider, avoid vaginal douche, and avoid vaginal or rectal manipulation during sexual contact during the period of neutropenia.

c. Allows observation of site and removes source of contamination
d. Once introduced into the system, microorganisms are capable of growing in infusion sets despite replacement of container and high flow rates.
e. Infusion Nursing Society collaborates with other nursing subspecialties in determining guidelines for IV access care.

6. Reduces risk for skin abscesses.
7. Rates of infection greatly increase after urinary catheterization.
8. Granulocyte colony-stimulating factor decreases the duration of neutropenia and the potential for infection.
9. Minimizes exposure to potential sources of infection and disruption of skin integrity

---

NURSING DIAGNOSIS: Risk for impaired skin integrity: erythematous and wet desquamation reactions to radiation therapy
GOAL: Maintenance of skin integrity

Nursing Intervention	Rationale	Expected Outcomes
1. In erythematous areas:	1. Care to the affected areas must focus on preventing further skin irritation, drying, and damage.	• Avoids use of soaps, powders, and other cosmetics on site of radiation therapy
a. Avoid the use of soaps, cosmetics, perfumes, powders, lotions, and ointments; non–aluminum-based deodorant may be used on intact skin.	a. These substances may cause pain and additional skin irritation and damage.	• States rationale for special care of skin
b. Use only lukewarm water to bathe the area.	b. Avoiding water of extreme temperatures and soap minimizes additional skin damage, irritation, and pain.	• Exhibits minimal change in skin • Avoids trauma to affected skin region (avoids shaving, constricting and irritating clothing, extremes of temperature, and the use of adhesive tape)
c. Avoid rubbing or scratching the area.	c. Rubbing, scratching, or both will lead to additional skin irritation, damage, and increased risk of infection.	• Reports change in skin promptly • Demonstrates proper care of blistered or open areas
d. Avoid shaving the area with a straight-edged razor.	d. The use of razors may lead to additional irritation and disruption of skin integrity and increased risk of infection.	• Exhibits absence of infection of blistered and opened areas. • Wound is free of development of eschar.
e. Avoid applying hot-water bottles, heating pads, ice, and adhesive tape to the area.	e. Avoiding extreme temperatures minimizes additional skin damage, irritation, burns, and pain.	
f. Avoid exposing the area to sunlight or cold weather.	f. Sun exposure or extreme cold weather may lead to additional skin damage and pain.	
g. Avoid tight clothing in the area. Use cotton clothing.	g. Allows air circulation to affected area	
h. Topical agents such as Aquaphor, Radiacare gel, aloe vera, or Biafine (Valeant may be used, and low- or medium-potency corticosteroid cream may be given if pruritus is present.)	h. May aid healing; however, evidence supporting the benefits of topical agents is lacking.	

(continued on page 360)

Chart 15-7 **PLAN OF NURSING CARE** (Continued)

The Patient With Cancer

Nursing Interventions	Rationale	Expected Outcomes
2. If wet desquamation occurs:	2. Open weeping areas are susceptible to bacterial infection. Care must be taken to prevent introduction of pathogens.	
a. Do not disrupt any blisters that have formed.	a. Disruption of skin blisters disrupts skin integrity and may lead to increased risk of infection.	
b. Avoid frequent washing of the area.	b. Frequent washing may lead to increased irritation and skin damage, with increased risk of infection.	
c. Report any blistering.	c. Blistering of skin represents progression of skin damage.	
d. Use *prescribed* creams or ointments; topical antibacterial creams may help to dry a wet wound (e.g., Silvadene cream)	d. Anecdotally believed to decrease irritation and inflammation of the area and promote healing; although a variety of products are used in many settings, there are few randomized controlled trials with evidence to support one product or intervention over another.	
e. If area weeps, apply a nonadhesive absorbent dressing.	e. Easier to remove and associated with less pain and trauma when drainage dries and adheres to dressing.	
f. If the area is without drainage, moisture and vapor-permeable dressings, such as hydrocolloids and hydrogels on noninfected areas, have been used in many settings.	f. May promote healing; however, randomized controlled clinical trial support is lacking in the setting of moist desquamation. Hydrocolloid dressings may enhance comfort.	
g. Consult with wound-ostomy-continence nurse (WOCN) and primary provider if eschar forms.	g. Eschar must be removed to promote healing and prevent infection. WOCNs have expertise in the care of wounds.	

NURSING DIAGNOSIS: Impaired oral mucous membrane: stomatitis
GOAL: Maintenance of intact oral mucous membranes

Nursing Intervention	Rationale	Expected Outcomes
1. Assess oral cavity daily using the same assessment criteria or rating scale.	1. Provides baseline for later evaluation; maintains consistency in assessment findings	• States rationale for frequent oral assessment and hygiene • Factors associated with the incidence, severity, and complications are identified prior to initiation of cancer treatment
2. Identify individuals at increased risk for stomatitis and related complications.	2. Patient and treatment variables are associated with the incidence and severity of stomatitis as well as related complications such as delayed healing and infection.	• Oral mucosal assessment is conducted at baseline and on an ongoing basis.
3. Instruct patient to report oral burning, pain, areas of redness, open lesions on oropharyngeal mucosa and lips, pain associated with swallowing, or decreased tolerance to temperature extremes of food.	3. Identification of initial stages of stomatitis will facilitate prompt interventions, including modification of treatment as prescribed by primary provider.	• Oral hygiene practices are initiated prior to development of stomatitis. • Identifies signs and symptoms of stomatitis to report to nurse or primary provider
4. Encourage and assist as needed in oral hygiene.	4. Patients who are having discomfort or pain, or other symptoms related to the disease and treatment, may require encouragement and assistance in performing oral hygiene. Oral hygiene is maintained to prevent complications of stomatitis, such as infection.	• Participates in recommended oral hygiene regimen • Avoids mouthwashes with alcohol • Brushes teeth and mouth with soft toothbrush • Uses lubricant to keep lips soft and nonirritated • Avoids hard-to-chew, spicy, hot foods or other irritating foods • Maintains adequate hydration

Chart 15-7

PLAN OF NURSING CARE (Continued)

The Patient With Cancer

Nursing Interventions	Rationale	Expected Outcomes
Preventive		
1. Advise patient to avoid irritants such as commercial mouthwashes, alcoholic beverages, and tobacco.	1. Alcohol content of mouthwashes and tobacco smoke will dry oral tissues and potentiate breakdown.	• Exhibits clean, intact oral mucosa
2. Brush with soft toothbrush using non-abrasive toothpaste for 90 seconds after meals and at bedtime; allow toothbrush to air dry before storing; floss at least once daily or as advised by the clinician; patients who have not previously flossed regularly should not initiate flossing during stomatoxic treatment; rinse mouth four times a day with a bland rinse (normal saline, sodium bicarbonate, or saline and sodium bicarbonate); avoid irritating foods (acidic, hot, rough, and spicy); use water-based moisturizers to protect lips.	2. Limits trauma and removes debris. Patients who have not previously flossed regularly do initiate flossing during stomatoxic treatment due to potential for injury to the oral mucosa and increased susceptibility to infection.	• Exhibits no ulcerations or infections of oral cavity • Exhibits no evidence of bleeding • Reports absent or decreased oral pain • Reports no difficulty swallowing • Exhibits healing (reepithelialization) of oral mucosa within 5–7 days (mild stomatitis)
3. Consider use of oral ice chips during stomatoxic chemotherapy infusions.	3. Oral cryotherapy has demonstrated reduced oral mucositis incidence, severity, and pain; improved quality of life; and minimizes chances of complications of oral mucositis	
4. Consider use of low level laser therapy.	4. Low energy level laser therapy has demonstrated decreased severity, duration, and pain associated with stomatitis.	
5. Consider administration of Palifermin as prescribed for patients receiving high-dose chemotherapy.	5. Palifermin, a recombinant keratinocyte growth factor (KGF) that stimulates the growth of cells lining the mouth and intestinal tract, has been shown to decrease the severity and duration of stomatitis.	
6. Maintain adequate hydration.	6. Maintenance of hydration prevents mucosal drying and breakdown.	
7. Provide written instruction and education to patients on the above items.	7. Written information reinforces patient education and provides the patient and family with a source.	
Mild stomatitis (generalized erythema, limited ulcerations, small white patches: *Candida*)		
1. Use normal saline mouth rinses every 1–4 hours.	1. Assists in removing debris, thick secretions, and bacteria	• Exhibits healing of oral tissues within 10–14 days (severe stomatitis)
2. Use soft toothbrush or toothette.	2. Minimizes trauma	• Exhibits no bleeding or oral ulceration
3. Remove dentures except for meals; be certain that dentures fit well.	3. Minimizes friction and discomfort	• Consumes adequate fluid and food
4. Apply water-soluble lip lubricant.	4. Promotes comfort	• Exhibits absence of dehydration and weight loss
5. Avoid foods that are spicy or hard to chew and those with extremes of temperature.	5. Prevents local trauma	• Exhibits no evidence of infection
Severe stomatitis (confluent ulcerations with bleeding and white patches covering >25% of oral mucosa)		
1. Obtain tissue samples for culture and sensitivity tests of areas of infection.	1. Assists in identifying need for antimicrobial therapy	a. Adheres to oral care regimen
2. Assess ability to chew and swallow; assess gag reflex.	2. Patient may be in danger of aspiration	b. Exhibits healing of oral tissues within 10–14 days (severe stomatitis) • Consumes adequate fluid and food
3. Use oral rinses (may combine in solution saline, anti-*Candida* agent, such as Mycostatin, and topical anesthetic agent [described later] as prescribed, or place patient on side and irrigate mouth; have suction available.	3. Facilitates cleansing and provides for safety and comfort	• Exhibits absence of dehydration and weight loss • Exhibits no evidence of infection • Reports absent or decreased discomfort or pain

(continued on page 362)

Chart 15-7   **PLAN OF NURSING CARE** (Continued)
The Patient With Cancer

Nursing Interventions	Rationale	Expected Outcomes
4. Remove dentures.	4. Prevents trauma from ill-fitting dentures	
5. Use toothette or gauze soaked with solution for cleansing.	5. Limits trauma and promotes comfort	
6. Use water-soluble lip lubricant.	6. Promotes comfort and minimizes loss of skin integrity	
7. Provide liquid or pureed diet.	7. Ensures intake of easily digestible foods without chewing	
8. Monitor for dehydration.	8. Decreased oral intake and ulcerations potentiate fluid deficits.	
9. Minimize discomfort.		
a. Consult primary provider for use of topical anesthetic, such as dyclonine and diphenhydramine, or viscous lidocaine.	a. Alleviates pain and increases sense of well-being; promotes participation in oral hygiene and nutritional intake	
b. Administer systemic analgesics as prescribed.	b. Adequate management of pain related to severe stomatitis can facilitate improved quality of life, participation in other aspects of activities of daily living, oral intake, and verbal communication.	
c. Perform mouth care as described.	c. Promotes removal of debris, healing, and comfort	

NURSING DIAGNOSIS: Impairment of skin integrity related to rash
GOALS: Maintenance of skin integrity

Nursing Intervention	Rationale	Expected Outcomes
Prevention		
1. Instruct patients to avoid sunlight through use of protective clothing, use of sun screen with SPF of 30 with physical blockers (zinc oxide, titanium dioxide), or avoidance of direct sun exposure.	1. Many agents are associated with photosensitivity; sunburn would intensify inflammation associated with rash and potentiate loss of skin integrity	• Sun exposure will be limited; no development of sun burn • Absence of dehydration • Participates in skin care regimen as instructed • Absence of dryness, flaking
2. Maintain adequate oral hydration.	2. Prevents skin dryness related to dehydration	
3. Avoid long hot showers or baths, harsh soaps and laundry detergents, perfumes, and non-hypoallergenic cosmetics.	3. Prevents skin irritation, dryness, flaking, and inflammation	
4. Apply emollients; apply hydrocortisone 1% cream with moisturizer at least twice daily; administer doxycycline 100 mg twice per day or minocycline, as prescribed	4. Minimizes dryness, flaking, and disruption of skin integrity.	
Treatment		
1. Apply topical treatment as prescribed: clindamycin 1%, fluocinonide 0.05% cream twice a day, or alclometasone 0.05% cream twice a day	1. Recommended as treatment to minimize skin disruption and prevent infection by Multinational Association of Supportive Care in Cancer (MSACC)	• Rash severity does not interfere with level of comfort and adherence to targeted therapy as prescribed; absence of local or systemic infection
2. For severe papulopustular rash: Administer systemic treatment as prescribed: doxycycline 100 mg twice per day; minocycline 100 mg daily; or isotretinion at low doses of 20–30 mg per day	2. Recommended as treatment to minimize skin disruption and prevent infection by Multinational Association of Supportive Care in Cancer (MSACC)	• Rash severity does not interfere with level of comfort and adherence to targeted therapy as prescribed; absence of local or systemic infection
3. Assess for development of infection: obtain cultures of pustules and administer appropriate antibiotics as prescribed by the physician	3. Prompt recognition and treatment of infection are necessary to prevent bacteremia, sepsis, and further patient compromise	• Local infection is controlled; absence of bacteremia and sepsis

Chart 15-7

PLAN OF NURSING CARE (Continued)

The Patient With Cancer

NURSING DIAGNOSIS: Impaired tissue integrity: alopecia
GOAL: Maintenance of tissue integrity; coping with hair loss

Nursing Intervention	Rationale	Expected Outcomes
1. Discuss potential hair loss and regrowth with patient and family; advise that hair loss may occur on body parts other than the head.	1. Provides information so that patient and family can begin to prepare cognitively and emotionally for loss	• Identifies alopecia as potential side effect of treatment
2. Explore potential impact of hair loss on self-image, interpersonal relationships, and sexuality.	2. Facilitates coping and maintenance of interpersonal relationships	• Identifies positive and negative feelings and threats to self-image
3. Prevent or minimize hair loss through the following:	3. Retains hair as long as possible.	• Verbalizes meaning that hair and possible hair loss have for him or her
a. Use scalp hypothermia and scalp tourniquets, if appropriate.	a. Decreases hair follicle uptake of chemotherapy (not used for patients with leukemia or lymphoma because tumor cells may be present in blood vessels or scalp tissue)	• States rationale for modifications in hair care and treatment
b. Cut long hair before treatment.	b. Minimizes hair loss due to the weight and manipulation of hair	• Uses mild shampoo and conditioner, and shampoos hair only when necessary
c. Use mild shampoo and conditioner, gently pat dry, and avoid excessive shampooing.		• Avoids hair dryer, curlers, sprays, and other stresses on hair and scalp
d. Avoid electric curlers, curling irons, dryers, clips, barrettes, hair sprays, hair dyes, and permanent waves.		• Wears hat or scarf over hair when exposed to sun
e. Avoid excessive combing or brushing; use wide-toothed comb.		• Takes steps to deal with possible hair loss before it occurs; purchases wig or hairpiece if desired
4. Prevent trauma to scalp.	4. Preserves tissue integrity	• Maintains hygiene and grooming
a. Lubricate scalp with vitamin A and D ointment to decrease itching.	a. Assists in maintaining skin integrity	• Interacts and socializes with others
b. Use sunscreen or wear hat when in the sun.	b. Prevents ultraviolet light exposure	
5. Suggest ways to assist in coping with hair loss.	5. Minimizes change in appearance	
a. Purchase wig or hairpiece before hair loss.	a. Wig that closely resembles hair color and style is more easily selected if hair loss has not begun.	
b. If hair loss has occurred, take photograph to wig shop to assist in selection.	b. Facilitates adjustment	
c. Begin to wear wig before hair loss.	c. Enables patient to be prepared for loss and facilitates adjustment	
d. Contact the American Cancer Society for donated wigs or a store that specializes in this product.	d. Provides options to patient and assists with financial burden if necessary	
e. Wear hat, scarf, or turban.	e. Conceals loss and protects scalp	
6. Encourage patient to wear own clothes and retain social contacts.	6. Assists in maintaining personal identity	
7. Explain that hair growth usually begins again once therapy is completed.	7. Reassures patient that hair loss is usually temporary	

NURSING DIAGNOSIS: Imbalanced nutrition: less than body requirements, related to nausea and vomiting
GOAL: Patient experiences less nausea and vomiting associated with chemotherapy; weight loss is minimized

Nursing Intervention	Rationale	Expected Outcomes
1. Assess the patient's previous experiences and expectations of nausea and vomiting, including causes and interventions used.	1. Identifies patient concerns, misinformation, and potential strategies for intervention; also gives patient sense of empowerment and control	• Identifies previous triggers of nausea and vomiting
2. Adjust diet before and after drug administration according to patient preference and tolerance.	2. Each patient responds differently to food after chemotherapy. A diet containing foods that relieve or prevent nausea or vomiting is most helpful.	• Exhibits decreased apprehension and anxiety
		• Identifies previously used successful interventions for nausea and vomiting

(continued on page 364)

Chart 15-7

PLAN OF NURSING CARE (Continued)

The Patient With Cancer

Nursing Interventions	Rationale	Expected Outcomes
3. Prevent unpleasant sights, odors, and sounds in the environment.	3. Unpleasant sensations can stimulate the nausea and vomiting center.	• Reports decrease in nausea
4. Use distraction, music therapy, bio-feedback, self-hypnosis, relaxation techniques, and guided imagery before, during, and after chemotherapy.	4. Decreases anxiety, which can contribute to nausea and vomiting. Psychological conditioning may also be decreased.	• Reports decrease in incidence of vomiting • Consumes adequate fluid and food when nausea subsides • Demonstrates use of distraction, relaxation, and imagery when indicated
5. Administer prescribed antiemetics, sedatives, and corticosteroids before chemotherapy and afterward as needed.	5. Administration of antiemetic regimen before onset of nausea and vomiting limits the adverse experience and facilitates control. Combination drug therapy reduces nausea and vomiting through various triggering mechanisms.	• Exhibits normal skin turgor and moist mucous membranes • No additional weight loss
6. Ensure adequate fluid hydration before, during, and after drug administration; assess intake and output.	6. Adequate fluid volume dilutes drug levels, decreasing stimulation of vomiting receptors.	
7. Encourage frequent oral hygiene.	7. Reduces unpleasant taste sensations	
8. Provide pain-relief measures, if necessary.	8. Increased comfort increases physical tolerance of symptoms.	
9. Consult with dietician as needed.	9. Interdisciplinary collaboration is essential in addressing complex patient needs.	
10. Assess and address other contributing factors to nausea and vomiting, such as other symptoms, constipation, gastrointestinal irritation, electrolyte imbalance, radiation therapy, medications, and central nervous system metastasis.	10. Multiple factors may contribute to nausea and vomiting.	

NURSING DIAGNOSIS: Imbalanced nutrition: less than body requirements, related to anorexia, cachexia, or malabsorption
GOAL: Maintenance of nutritional status and of weight within 10% of pretreatment weight

Nursing Intervention	Rationale	Expected Outcomes
1. Assess and address factors that interfere with oral intake or are associated with increased risk of decreased nutritional status.	1. Multiple patient or treatment-related factors are associated with increased risk of impaired nutritional intake, such as radiation to the head, neck, and thorax; stomatoxic or emetogenic chemotherapy; prior oral, head, and neck surgery; mucositis; impaired swallowing or dysphagia; poor dentition; cough or shortness of breath.	• Factors associated with increased risk for impaired nutritional intake are identified. • Factors associated with increased risk of impaired nutritional intake are identified and addressed, whenever possible, through interdisciplinary collaboration.
2. Initiate appropriate referrals for inter-disciplinary collaboration to manage factors that interfere with oral intake.	2. Other disciplines may be more appropriate for assessment and management of issues such as swallowing impairments (speech therapy), fatigue and decreased physical ability (physical and occupational therapy), nutritional assessment and determination of patient needs (nutritionist), cough and shortness of breath (respiratory therapy), poor dentition (dental medicine), depression/anxiety (social worker, psychologist, or psychiatrist).	• Patient and family identify minimal nutritional requirements • Maintains or increases weight and body cell mass as per goals identified by nutritionist • Reports decreasing anorexia and increased interest in eating • Demonstrates normal skin turgor • Identifies rationale for dietary modifications; patient and family verbalize strategies to minimize nutritional deficits • Participates in calorie counts and diet histories • Uses relaxation techniques and guided imagery before meals
3. Educate patient to avoid unpleasant sights, odors, and sounds in the environment during mealtime.	3. Anorexia can be stimulated or increased with noxious stimuli.	
4. Suggest foods that are preferred and well tolerated by the patient, preferably high-calorie and high-protein foods. Respect ethnic and cultural food preferences.	4. Foods preferred, well tolerated, and high in calories and protein maintain nutritional status during periods of increased metabolic demand.	

Chart 15-7

PLAN OF NURSING CARE (Continued)

The Patient With Cancer

Nursing Interventions	Rationale	Expected Outcomes
5. Encourage adequate fluid intake, but limit fluids at mealtime.	5. Fluids are necessary to eliminate wastes and prevent dehydration. Increased fluids with meals can lead to early satiety.	• Exhibits laboratory and clinical findings indicative of adequate nutritional intake: normal serum levels of protein, albumin, transferrin, iron, blood urea nitrogen (BUN), creatinine, vitamin D, electrolytes, hemoglobin, hematocrit, and lymphocytes; normal urinary creatinine levels
6. Suggest smaller, more frequent meals.	6. Smaller, more frequent meals are better tolerated because early satiety is less likely to occur.	
7. Promote relaxed, quiet environment during mealtime with increased social interaction as desired.	7. A quiet environment promotes relaxation. Social interaction at mealtime may foster appetite, divert focus on food, and promote enjoyment of eating.	• Consumes diet containing required nutrients • Carries out oral hygiene before meals • Reports decreased pain and/or other symptoms; symptoms do not interfere with oral intake
8. If patient desires, serve wine at mealtime with foods.	8. Wine may stimulate appetite and add calories.	• Reports decreasing episodes of nausea and vomiting
9. Consider cold foods, if desired.	9. Cold, high-protein foods are often more tolerable and less odorous than hot foods.	• Participates in increasing levels of activity as measured by assessment of performance status
10. Encourage nutritional supplements and high-protein foods between meals.	10. Supplements and snacks add protein and calories to meet nutritional requirements.	• Family and friends do not focus efforts on encouraging food intake
11. Encourage frequent oral hygiene, particularly prior to meals.	11. Oral hygiene may stimulate appetite and increase saliva production.	• States rationale for use of tube feedings or parenteral nutrition
12. Address pain and other symptom management needs.	12. Pain and other symptoms impair appetite and nutritional intake.	• Demonstrates ability to manage enteral feedings or parenteral nutrition, if prescribed
13. Increase activity level as tolerated.	13. Increased activity promotes appetite.	• Maintains body position and alignment needed to facilitate chewing and swallowing
14. Decrease anxiety by encouraging verbalization of fears and concerns; use relaxation techniques and guided imagery at mealtime.	14. Relief of anxiety may increase appetite.	
15. Instruct patient and family about body alignment and proper positioning at mealtime.	15. Proper body position and alignment are necessary to aid chewing and swallowing.	
16. Collaborate with dietician to provide nutritional counseling; instruct patient and family regarding enteral tube feedings of commercial liquid diets, elemental diets, or other foods as prescribed.	16. Nutritional counseling may improve outcomes. Tube feedings may be necessary in the severely debilitated patient who has a functioning gastrointestinal system but is unable to maintain adequate oral intake.	
17. Collaborate with dietician or nutrition support team to instruct patient and family regarding home parenteral nutrition with lipid supplements as prescribed.	17. Parenteral nutrition with supplemental fats supplies needed calories and proteins to meet nutritional demands, especially in the nonfunctional gastrointestinal system.	
18. Administer appetite stimulants as prescribed by primary provider.	18. Although the mechanism is unclear, medications such as megestrol acetate (Megace) have been noted to improve appetite in patients with cancer and human immunodeficiency virus infection.	
19. Encourage family and friends not to nag or cajole patient about eating.	19. Pressuring patient to eat may cause conflict and unnecessary stress.	
20. Assess and address other contributing factors to nausea, vomiting, and anorexia such as electrolyte imbalance, radiation therapy, medications, and central nervous system metastasis.	20. Multiple factors contribute to anorexia and nausea.	

(continued on page 366)

Chart 15-7   **PLAN OF NURSING CARE** (Continued)

The Patient With Cancer

NURSING DIAGNOSIS: Fatigue
GOAL: Decreased fatigue level

Nursing Intervention	Rationale	Expected Outcomes
1. Assess patient and treatment factors that are associated with or increase fatigue (e.g., anemia, fluid and electrolyte imbalances, pain, anxiety, etc.)	1. Multiple factors are associated with or contribute to cancer-related fatigue. Although fatigue is common in patients receiving chemotherapy or radiation therapy, there are several factors that can be modified or addressed, such as dehydration, electrolye abnormalities, organ impairment, anemia, impaired nutrition, pain and other symptoms, depression, anxiety, impaired mobility, and shortness of breath.	• Factors contributing to fatigue are assessed and managed whenever possible. • Exhibits acceptable serum value levels for nutritional indices (See Imbalanced Nutrition) • Reports decreased pain and/or other symptoms • Consumes diet with recommended nutritional intake • Achieves or maintains appropriate weight and body mass • Maintains adequate hydration • Reports decreasing levels of fatigue • Adopts healthy lifestyle practices • Rests when fatigued • Reports adequate sleep • Requests assistance with activities appropriately • Uses relaxation exercises and imagery to decrease anxiety and promote rest • Reports no breathlessness during activities • Reports improved ability to relax and rest • Exhibits improved mobility and decreased fatigue Fatigue does not interfere with ability to participate in activities of daily living or pleasure
2. Institute interventions to address factors contributing to fatigue (e.g., correct electrolyte imbalance, manage pain, collaborative management of anemia, administer prescribed antidepressants, anxiolytics, hypnotics, or psychostimulants, as indicated)	2. Addressing factors contributing to fatigue assists in managing fatigue (i.e., lowered hemoglobin and hematocrit predispose patient to fatigue due to decreased oxygen availability especially in a setting of impaired mobility that requires increased energy expenditure).	
3. Encourage balance of rest and exercise; avoiding extended periods of inactivity. At minimum, promote patient's normal sleep habits.	3. Sleep helps to restore energy levels. Prolonged napping during the day may interfere with sleep habits.	
4. During active treatment, rearrange daily schedule and organize activities to conserve energy expenditure; encourage patient to ask for others' assistance with necessary chores, such as housework, child care, shopping, and cooking. During periods of profound fatigue, consider reduced job workload, if necessary and possible, by reducing number of hours worked per week.	4. Reorganization of activities can reduce energy losses and stressors.	
5. Encourage protein, fat, and calorie intake at least equal to that recommended for the general public.	5. Protein and calorie depletion decreases activity tolerance; preventing malnutrition, achieving and maintaining recommended weight and body mass assist in management of fatigue	
6. Encourage the use of relaxation techniques and guided imagery.	6. Promotion of relaxation and psychological rest limits contribution to physical fatigue.	
7. Encourage participation in planned exercise programs involving aerobic, resistance, and flexibility training based on individual limitations and safety measures. a. Minimum exercise for survivors depending on individual capabilities ranges from 10 minutes of light exercise, yoga, or stretching daily to 30 minutes of moderate to vigorous of activity	7. Various approaches to exercise programs have demonstrated increases in endurance and stamina and lower fatigue.	
8. Collaborate with other cancer providers to encourage them to give patients a prescription to exercise and explain role of exercise in cancer treatment.	8. Many providers fail to discuss the role of exercise and healthy lifestyle practices for patients during and after cancer treatment. Patients maybe more likely to utilize the benefits of exercise in addressing fatigue if they receive a formal prescription.	

Chart 15-7

PLAN OF NURSING CARE (Continued)

The Patient With Cancer

Nursing Interventions	Rationale	Expected Outcomes
9. Partner with community organizations (i.e., YMCA) to develop and offer cancer survivor specific rehab/exercise programs.	9. Creates community partnerships, a non-clinical environment of support, fosters increased awareness of survivorship needs, and provides referral sources that can reach more survivors.	
10. Collaborate with physical and occupational therapy and/or refer to American College of Sports Medicine (ACSM) Certified Cancer Exercise Trainer (CET) to identify safe and appropriate activities.	10. A CET designs and administers fitness assessments and exercise programs specific to an individual's cancer diagnosis, treatment, current recovery status; possesses basic understanding of cancer diagnoses, treatments, and potential adverse effects.	

NURSING DIAGNOSIS: Chronic pain
GOAL: Relief of pain and discomfort

Nursing Intervention	Rationale	Expected Outcomes
1. Use pain scale to assess pain and discomfort characteristics: location, quality, frequency, duration, etc., at baseline and on an ongoing basis.	1. Provides baseline for assessing changes in pain level and evaluation of interventions	• Reports decreased level of pain and discomfort on pain scale
2. Assure patient that you know the pain is real and will assist him or her in reducing it.	2. Fear that pain will not be considered real increases anxiety and reduces pain tolerance.	• Reports less disruption in activity and quality of life from pain and discomfort
3. Assess prior pain experiences and previous management strategies the patient found successful.	3. Helps to individualize pain management approaches and identify potential challenges or approaches that should not be utilized because of safety or other issues	• Reports decrease in other symptoms and psychosocial distress • Adheres to analgesic regimen as prescribed
4. Assess other factors contributing to patient's pain: fear, fatigue, other symptoms, psychosocial distress, etc.	4. Provides data about factors that decrease the patient's ability to tolerate pain and increase pain level	• Barriers to adequately addressing pain do not interfere with strategies for managing pain.
5. Provide education to patient and family about prescribed analgesic regimen.	5. Analgesics tend to be more effective when given early in pain cycle, around the clock at regular intervals, or when given in long-acting forms; breaks the pain cycle; premedication with analgesics is used for activities that cause increased pain or breakthrough pain.	• Takes an active role in administration of analgesia • Identifies additional effective pain-relief strategies • Uses previously employed successful pain-relief strategies appropriately
6. Address myths or misconceptions and lack of knowledge about the use of opioid analgesics.	6. Barriers to adequate pain management involve patients' fear of side effects, fatalism about the possibility of achieving pain control, fear of distracting providers from treating the cancer, belief that pain is indicative of progressive disease, and fears about addiction. Professional health providers also have demonstrated limited knowledge about evidence-based approaches to pain.	• Identifies and/or utilizes nonpharmacologic pain-relief strategies and reports successful decrease in pain • Reports that decreased level of pain permits participation in other activities and events and quality of life
7. Collaborate with patient, primary provider, and other health care team members when changes in pain management are necessary.	7. New methods of administering analgesia must be acceptable to patient, primary provider, and health care team to be effective; patient's participation decreases the sense of powerlessness.	
8. Consult with palliative care providers or team throughout the cancer continuum.	8. Palliative care specialists provide expertise and contribute to symptom management regardless of stage of disease or treatment within the cancer continuum, not only during end-stage disease. Palliative care can improve quality of life, length of survival, symptom burden, mood, and efficient utilization of health services.	
9. Explore nonpharmacologic and complementary strategies to relieve pain and discomfort: distraction, imagery, relaxation, cutaneous stimulation, acupuncture, etc.	9. Increases the number of options and strategies available to patient that serve as adjuncts to pharmacologic interventions.	

(continued on page 368)

Chart 15-7

PLAN OF NURSING CARE (Continued)

The Patient With Cancer

NURSING DIAGNOSIS: Grieving related to loss; altered role functioning
GOAL: Appropriate progression through grieving process

Nursing Intervention	Rationale	Expected Outcomes
1. Encourage verbalization of fears, concerns, and questions regarding disease, treatment, and future implications.	1. An increased and accurate knowledge base decreases anxiety and dispels misconceptions.	The patient and family: • Progress through the phases of grief as evidenced by increased verbalization and expression of grief.
2. Explore previous successful coping strategies.	2. Provides frame of reference and examples of coping.	• Identify resources available to aid coping strategies during grieving.
3. Encourage active participation of patient or family in care and treatment decisions.	3. Active participation maintains patient independence and control.	• Use resources and supports appropriately.
4. Visit family and friends to establish and maintain relationships and physical closeness.	4. Frequent contacts promote trust and security and reduce feelings of fear and isolation.	• Discuss the future openly with each other.
5. Encourage ventilation of negative feelings, including projected anger and hostility, within acceptable limits.	5. This allows for emotional expression without loss of self-esteem.	• Discuss concerns and feelings openly with each other. • Use nonverbal expressions of concern for each other.
6. Allow for periods of crying and expression of sadness.	6. These feelings are necessary for separation and detachment to occur.	• Develop positive or adaptive coping mechanisms for processing of grief.
7. Involve spiritual advisor as desired by the patient and family.	7. This facilitates the grief process and spiritual care.	
8. Refer patient and family to professional counseling as indicated to alleviate pathologic or nonadaptive grieving.	8. Goal is to facilitate the grief process or adaptive methods of coping.	
9. Allow for progression through the grieving process at the individual pace of the patient and family.	9. Grief work is variable. Not every person uses every phase of the grief process, and the time spent in dealing with each phase varies with every person. To complete grief work, this variability must be allowed.	

NURSING DIAGNOSIS: Disturbed body image and situational low self-esteem related to changes in appearance, function, and roles
GOAL: Improved body image and self-esteem

Nursing Intervention	Rationale	Expected Outcomes
1. Assess patient's feelings about body image and level of self-esteem.	1. Provides baseline assessment for evaluating changes and assessing effectiveness of interventions	• Identifies concerns of importance • Takes active role in activities • Maintains participation in decision making
2. Identify potential threats to patient's self-esteem (e.g., altered appearance, decreased sexual function, hair loss, decreased energy, role changes). Validate concerns with patient.	2. Anticipates changes and permits patient to identify importance of these areas to him or her	• Verbalizes feelings and reactions to losses or threatened losses • Participates in self-care activities • Permits others to assist in care when he or she is unable to be independent
3. Encourage continued participation in activities and decision making.	3. Encourages and permits continued control of events and self	• Exhibits interest in appearance, maintains grooming, and uses aids (cosmetics, scarves, etc.) appropriately if desired
4. Encourage patient to verbalize concerns.	4. Identifying concerns is an important step in coping with them.	
5. Individualize care for the patient.	5. Prevents or reduces depersonalization and emphasizes patient's self-worth	
6. Assist patient in self-care when fatigue, lethargy, nausea, vomiting, and other symptoms prevent independence.	6. Physical well-being improves self-esteem.	• Participates with others in conversations and social events and activities
7. Assist patient in selecting and using cosmetics, scarves, hair pieces, hats, and clothing that increase their sense of attractiveness.	7. Promotes positive body image.	• Verbalizes concern about sexual partner and/or significant others
8. Encourage patient and partner to share concerns about altered sexuality and sexual function and to explore alternatives to their usual sexual expression.	8. Provides opportunity for expressing concern, intimacy, affection, and acceptance.	• Explores alternative ways of expressing concern and affection • The patient and significant other are able to maintain level of intimacy and express affection and acceptance.
9. Refer to collaborating specialists as needed.	9. Interdisciplinary collaboration is essential in meeting patient needs.	

Chart 15-7

PLAN OF NURSING CARE (Continued)

The Patient With Cancer

COLLABORATIVE PROBLEM: Potential complication: risk for bleeding problems
GOAL: Prevention of bleeding

Nursing Intervention	Rationale	Expected Outcomes
1. Monitor for factors increasing risk of bleeding (thrombocytopenia, elevated INR/PT/PTT, decreased fibrinogen or other clotting factors, use of medications affecting platelets or other clotting indices)	1. The underlying cancer, antineoplastic agents or other medications may interfere with normal mechanisms of clotting.	• Signs and symptoms of bleeding are identified.
2. Assess for and instruct patient/family about signs and symptoms of bleeding:	2. Early detection promotes early intervention.	• Exhibits no blood in feces, urine, or emesis
a. Petechiae or ecchymosis (bruising)	a. Petechiae and ecchymosis indicate injury to microcirculation and larger vessels.	• Exhibits no bleeding of gums or injection/venipuncture sites
b. Decrease in hemoglobin or hematocrit	b. Decreased hemoglobin or hematocrit may indicate blood loss.	• Exhibits no ecchymosis (bruising) or petechiae
c. Prolonged bleeding from invasive procedures, venipunctures, minor cuts or scratches	c. Prolonged bleeding may indicate abnormal clotting indices.	• Patient and family identify ways to prevent bleeding.
d. Frank or occult blood in any body fluids	d. Occult blood in body fluids indicates bleeding.	• Uses recommended measures to reduce risk of bleeding (uses soft toothbrush, shaves with electric razor only)
e. Bleeding from any body orifice	e. Indicates blood loss	• Exhibits normal vital signs
f. Altered mental status	f. Altered mental status may indicate decreased cerebral tissue oxygenation or bleeding.	• Reports that environmental hazards have been reduced or removed
g. Hypotension; tachycardia	g. Hypotension or tachycardia may indicate blood loss.	• Maintains hydration
3. Instruct patient and family about ways to minimize risk of bleeding.	3. Patient can participate in self-protection.	• Reports absence of constipation
a. Use soft toothbrush or toothette for mouth care.	a. Prevents trauma to oral tissues	• Avoids substances interfering with clotting
b. Avoid commercial mouthwashes.	b. Contain high alcohol content that will dry oral tissues	• Absence of tissue destruction
c. Use electric razor for shaving.	c. Prevents trauma to skin	• Exhibits normal mental status and absence of signs of intracranial bleeding
d. Use emery board for nail care.	d. Reduces risk of trauma to nail beds	• Avoids medications that interfere with clotting (e.g., aspirin)
e. Avoid foods that are difficult to chew.	e. Prevents oral tissue trauma	• Absence of epistaxis and cerebral bleeding
f. Keep lips moisturized with water-based lubricant	f. Prevents skin from drying	
g. Maintain fluid intake of at least 3 L per 24 hours unless contraindicated	g. Prevents skin and oral tissue membranes from drying	
h. Use stool softeners or increase bulk in diet.	h. Prevents trauma to rectal mucosa from straining	
i. Recommend use of water-based lubricant before sexual intercourse.	i. Prevents friction and tissue trauma	
4. Initiate measures to minimize bleeding. Draw all blood for lab work with one daily venipuncture for hospitalized patients.	4. Measures are taken to minimize bleeding.	
a. Avoid taking temperature rectally or administering suppositories and enemas.	a. Minimizes blood loss	
b. Avoid intramuscular injections; use smallest needle possible.	b. Bleeding may occur from intramuscular injection sites, particularly if large bore needles are used.	
c. Apply direct pressure to injection and venipuncture sites for at least 5 minutes.	c. Bleeding may occur if direct pressure is not applied for a long enough time period.	
d. Avoid bladder catheterizations; use smallest catheter if catheterization is necessary.	d. Prevents trauma to urethra	
e. Avoid medications that will interfere with clotting (e.g., aspirin).	e. Minimizes risk of bleeding	

(continued on page 370)

Chart 15-7 PLAN OF NURSING CARE (Continued)
The Patient With Cancer

Nursing Interventions	Rationale	Expected Outcomes
f. Recommend use of water-based lubricant before sexual intercourse. g. Platelet transfusions as prescribed; administer prescribed diphenhydramine hydrochloride (Benadryl) or hydrocortisone sodium succinate (Solu-Cortef) to prevent reaction to platelet transfusion. h. Supervise activity when out of bed. i. Caution against forceful nose blowing.	f. Helps prevent bleeding from small skin tears. g. Platelet count <20,000/mm³ (0.02 × 1,012/L) is associated with increased risk of spontaneus bleeding. Allergic reactions to blood products are associated with antigen–antibody reaction that causes platelet destruction. h. Reduces risk of falls i. Prevents trauma to nasal mucosa and increased intracranial pressure	

Adapted from Eaton, L. H., Mitchell, D. H., & Doorenbos, A. Z. (2015). Evidence-based practice beliefs and behaviors of nurses providing cancer pain management: A mixed-methods approach. *Oncology Nursing Forum, 42*(2), 165–173; Eilers, J., Harris, D., Henry, K., et al. (2014). Evidence-based interventions for cancer treatment– related mucositis: Putting evidence into practice. *Clinical Journal of Oncology Nursing, 18*(6), 80–96; Fogh, S., & Yom, S. S. (2014). Symptom management during the radiation oncology treatment course: A practical guide for the oncology clinician. *Seminars in Oncology, 41*(6), 764–775; Heston, A. H., Schwartz, A. L., Justice-Gardiner, H., et al. (2015). Addressing physical activity needs of survivors by developing a community-based exercise program: LIVESTRONG® at the YMCA. *Clinical Journal of Oncology Nursing, 19*(2), 213–217; Mazanec, P., & Prince-Paul, M. (2014). Integrating palliative care into active cancer treatment. *Seminars in Oncology Nursing, 30*(4), 203–211.

Radiation-Associated Impairment of Skin Integrity

Although advances in radiation therapy have resulted in decreased incidence and severity of skin impairments, patients may still develop radiation dermatitis associated with pain, irritation, pruritus, burning, skin sloughing without drainage (dry desquamation) or with drainage (wet desquamation), and diminished quality of life. Nursing care for patients with radiation dermatitis includes maintenance of skin integrity, cleansing, promotion of comfort, pain reduction, prevention of additional trauma, prevention and management of infection, and promotion of a moist wound-healing environment (Fogh & Yom, 2014). In order to prevent impaired skin integrity, patients are advised to use moisturizer on the skin, avoid sun exposure to the area of treatment, and avoid tape or bandages and other sources of irritation or trauma. Although a variety of methods and products are used in clinical practice for patients with radiation-induced skin impairment, there is limited evidence to support their value. Patients with skin and tissue reactions to radiation therapy require careful skin care to prevent further skin irritation, drying, and damage, as discussed in the nursing care plan (see Chart 15-7, Risk for impaired skin integrity: erythematous and wet desquamation reactions to radiation therapy).

Alopecia

The temporary or permanent thinning or complete loss of hair is a potential adverse effect of whole brain radiation therapy, various chemotherapies and targeted agents. Alopecia usually begins 2 to 3 weeks after the initiation of chemotherapy and radiation therapy; regrowth most often begins within 8 weeks after the last treatment. Some patients who undergo radiation to the head may sustain permanent hair loss. The onset of gradually progressing alopecia and body hair loss associated with targeted therapies generally occurs 1 to 3 months after the start of treatment and may be patchy appearing as temporal or frontal hair loss. This type of hair loss is usually reversible after the end of therapy and in some cases beginning sooner. Several targeted agents are associated with changes in hair growth rate, curliness, texture, and pigmentation. Although health care providers may view hair loss as a minor issue, for many patients it is a major assault on body image, challenging to self-esteem, and resulting in psychosocial distress and depression. Despite the significant psychosocial impact of alopecia, few studies have addressed methods to prevent or minimize the impact of alopecia. The use of cryotherapy to the head during the administration of chemotherapy has been explored but is not consistently used because of concern about later development of scalp metastasis. When cryotherapy is offered, its use avoided in patients with hematologic malignancies. Nurses provide information about hair loss and support the patient and family in coping with changes in body image. Patients are assisted to identify proactive choices that may empower them to improve responses to cancer and perceived lack of control as discussed in the nursing care plan (see Chart 15-7, Impaired tissue integrity: alopecia).

Malignant Skin Lesions

Skin lesions may occur with local extension or metastasis of the tumor into the epithelium and its surrounding lymph and blood vessels. Either locally invasive or metastatic cancer to the skin may result in redness (erythema), discolored nodules, or progression to wounds involving edema, exudates, and tissue necrosis. The most extensive lesions involve ulceration (referred to as fungating lesions) with an overgrowth of malodorous microorganisms. These lesions are a source of considerable pain, discomfort, and embarrassment. Although skin lesions occur in various malignancies, they are most commonly associated with breast cancer.

Ulcerating skin lesions usually indicate advanced or disseminated disease that is unlikely to be eradicated but may be controlled or palliated through systemic treatment (chemotherapy and targeted therapy) or radiation therapy. Local care of these lesions is a nursing priority. Nurses carefully assess malignant skin lesions for the size, appearance, condition of surrounding tissue, odor, bleeding, drainage, and associated pain or other symptoms, including evidence of infection. The potential for serious complications such as hemorrhage, vessel compression/obstruction, or airway obstruction, especially in head and neck cancer, should be noted so that the caregiver can be instructed in palliative measures to maintain patient comfort.

Nursing care (see Chart 15-7) also includes wound cleansing, reduction of superficial bacteria, control of bleeding, odor reduction, protection from further skin trauma, and pain management. The patient and family require emotional support, assistance, and guidance in providing wound care and addressing comfort measures at home.

Promoting Nutrition

Nutritional Impairment

Most patients with cancer experience some weight loss during their illness. Anorexia, malabsorption, and cancer-related anorexia-cachexia syndrome (CACS) are some common nutritional problems. Impaired nutritional status may contribute to both physical and psychosocial consequences (see Chart 15-8). Nutritional concerns include decreased protein and caloric intake, metabolic or mechanical effects of the cancer, systemic disease, side effects of the treatment, or the patient's emotional status.

Anorexia

Among the many causes of anorexia in patients with cancer are alterations in taste, manifested by increased salty, sour, and metallic taste sensations, and altered responses to sweet and bitter flavors. Taste changes contribute to decreased appetite and nutritional intake and subsequently protein–calorie malnutrition. Taste alterations may result from mineral (e.g., zinc) deficiencies, increases in circulating amino acids and cellular metabolites, or the administration of chemotherapeutic agents. Patients undergoing radiation therapy to the head and neck may experience "mouth blindness," which is a severe impairment of taste.

Anorexia may occur because patients develop early satiety after eating only a small amount of food. This sense of fullness occurs secondary to a decrease in digestive enzymes, abnormalities in the metabolism of glucose and triglycerides, and prolonged stimulation of gastric volume receptors, which convey the feeling of being full. Psychological distress (e.g., fear, pain, depression, and isolation) throughout illness

may also have a negative impact on appetite. Patients may develop an aversion to food because of nausea and vomiting associated with treatment.

Malabsorption

Some patients with cancer are unable to absorb nutrients from the gastrointestinal system as a result of tumor activity, cancer treatments, or both. Malignancy can affect gastrointestinal activity in several ways (i.e., impaired enzyme production, interference with both protein and fat digestion) that can lead to increased gastrointestinal irritation, peptic ulcer disease, and fistula formation.

Chemotherapy and radiation associated with mucositis cause damage to mucosal cells of the bowel, resulting in impaired nutrient absorption. Abdominal irradiation has been associated with sclerosis of intestinal blood vessels and fibrotic changes in the gastrointestinal tissue, both impacting nutrient absorption. Surgical intervention may change peristaltic patterns, alter gastrointestinal secretions, and reduce the absorptive surfaces of gastrointestinal mucosa, all of which contribute to malabsorption.

Cancer-Related Anorexia-Cachexia Syndrome

CACS is a complex biologic process that results from a combination of increased energy expenditure and decreased intake (Alt-Epping & Nauck, 2015; Bozzetti, 2013). This syndrome can occur in both the curative and palliative stages of treatment and care. Combined immunologic, neuroendocrine, and metabolic processes give rise to anorexia, unintentional weight loss, and increased metabolic demand with impaired metabolism of glucose and lipids. As this syndrome continues, altered metabolic processes and tumor responses lead to cytokine release, causing generalized systemic inflammation. The patient experiences continued weight loss and malnutrition characterized by loss of adipose tissue, visceral protein, and skeletal muscle mass. Patients with CACS complain of loss of appetite, early satiety, and fatigue. As many as 80% of all patients with cancer experience some degree of cachexia (Alt-Epping & Nauck, 2015; Bozzetti, 2013). Protein losses are associated with the development of anemia, peripheral edema, and progressive debilitation. The signs and symptoms of cancer cachexia and progressive debilitation appear to result in decreased quality of life, psychological distress, and anxiety for both patient and family as they respond to actual and perceived impending losses, fear, lack of control, and helplessness.

Nursing care is integral to an interdisciplinary approach that addresses the multiple factors contributing to impaired nutritional status in patients with cancer (see Chart 15-7).

General Nutrition Considerations

Assessment of the patient's nutritional status is conducted at diagnosis and monitored throughout the course of treatment and follow-up. Early identification of patients at risk for problems with intake, absorption, and cachexia, particularly during the early stages of disease, can facilitate timely implementation of specifically targeted interventions that attempt to improve quality of life, treatment outcomes, and survival (Bozzetti, 2013). Current weight, weight loss, diet and medication history, patterns of anorexia, nausea and vomiting, diarrhea, and situations and foods that aggravate or relieve symptoms are assessed and addressed.

Chart 15-8

Potential Consequences of Impaired Nutrition in Patients With Cancer

- Anemia
- Decreased survival
- Immune incompetence and increased incidence of infection
- Delayed tissue and wound healing
- Fatigue
- Diminished functional ability
- Decreased capacity to continue antineoplastic therapy
- Increased hospital admissions
- Increased length of hospital stay
- Impaired psychosocial functioning

The type of cancer, stage, and treatment approaches are considered so that proactive measures to support nutrition can be identified. For example, patients with head and neck cancers who are treated with radiation therapy, or some combination of surgery, radiation, chemotherapy and/or targeted agents, are at high risk for inadequate oral intake and nutritional deficits. In many centers, these patients have a percutaneous endoscopic gastrostomy (PEG) tube placed for enteral nutrition prior to initiation of treatment and the onset of mucositis, weight loss, and other consequences of impaired oral intake (Bozzetti, 2013). A speech therapy consult may be helpful for patients with oropharyngeal or laryngeal tumors or surgical interventions that are anticipated to effect swallowing, secretion management, speech, or respiratory function.

Whenever possible, every effort is made to maintain adequate nutrition through the oral route. Prokinetic agents such as metoclopramide (Reglan) are used to increase gastric emptying in patients with early satiety and delayed gastric emptying. Other pharmacologic interventions such as megestrol acetate (Megace) or corticosteroids (on a short term basis) may be used to improve appetite. Oral nutritional supplements are encouraged to meet nutritional needs and to maintain or improve weight gain and physical functioning. Supplements containing n-3 polyunsaturated fatty acids (omega-3), arginine, and nucleotides are suggested to decrease the inflammatory response and improve oxygen metabolism and intestinal function (Bozzetti, 2013). Approaches incorporate nutritional counseling, exercise, pharmacological interventions to combat anorexia, and symptom management when feasible (Alesi & del Fabbro, 2014). If adequate nutrition cannot be maintained by oral intake, nutritional support via the enteral route may be necessary as discussed previously. When needed, the patient and family are taught to administer enteral nutrition in the home. Home care nurses assist with patient education and monitor the patient's symptoms and response to enteral nutrition.

When malabsorption is a problem, enzyme and vitamin replacement may be instituted. Additional strategies include changing the feeding schedule, using simple diets, and relieving diarrhea. If malabsorption is severe, or the cancer involves the upper gastrointestinal tract, parenteral nutrition may be necessary. However, patients receiving parenteral nutrition are at increased risk for complications, including catheter-related and systemic infection. The use of parenteral nutrition in patients with advanced or end-stage cancer is seldom used and controversial (Bozzett, 2013). Parenteral nutrition can be given in several ways: by a long-term venous access device such as a right atrial catheter (see Fig. 15-3), implanted venous port (see Fig. 15-4), or PICC (see Fig. 15-6). The nurse educates the patient and family to care for the venous access device and to administer parenteral nutrition. Home care nurses provide education and assist with or supervise parenteral nutrition administration in the home.

Relieving Pain

More than half of patients with cancer experience pain throughout the cancer trajectory. Moderate to severe pain is reported by approximately 30% to 70% of patients with cancer during treatment and as many as 80% of those with advanced disease (Eaton, Mitchell, & Doorenbos, 2015). Although cancer pain may be acute, it is more frequently

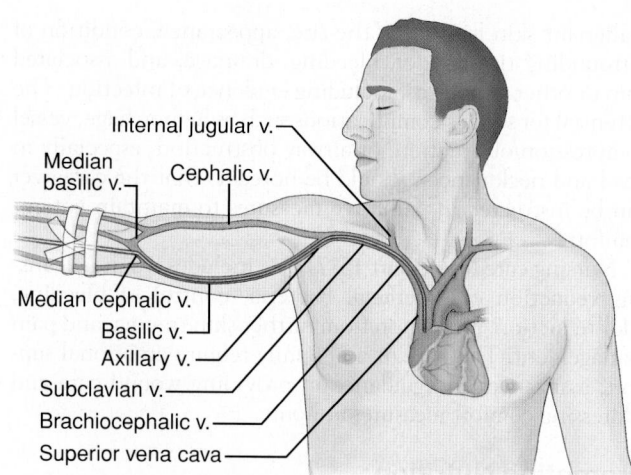

Figure 15-6 • A peripherally inserted central catheter is advanced through the cephalic or basilic vein to the axillary, subclavian, or brachiocephalic vein or the superior vena cava.

characterized as chronic. (See Chapter 12 for more information on pain.) As in other situations involving pain, the experience of cancer pain is influenced by physical, psychosocial, cultural, and spiritual factors.

Cancer can cause pain in various ways (see Table 15-9). Initially, pain is most often related to the underlying cancer process. Pain is also associated with various cancer treatments. Acute pain is linked with trauma from surgery. Occasionally, chronic pain syndromes, such as postsurgical neuropathies (pain related to nerve tissue injury), occur. Some chemotherapeutic agents cause tissue necrosis, peripheral neuropathies, and stomatitis—all potential sources of pain—whereas radiation therapy can cause pain secondary to skin, nervous tissue, or organ inflammation. Patients with cancer may have other sources of pain, such as arthritis or migraine headaches, that are unrelated to the underlying cancer or its treatment.

The nurse assesses the patient for the source and site of pain as well as those factors that influence the patient's perception and experience of pain, such as fear and apprehension,

TABLE 15-9 Examples of Sources of Cancer Pain

Source	Descriptions	Underlying Cancer
Bone metastasis	Throbbing, aching	Breast, prostate, myeloma
Ischemia	Sharp, throbbing	Kaposi's sarcoma
Lymphatic or venous obstruction	Dull, aching, tightness	Lymphoma, breast, Kaposi's sarcoma
Nerve compression, infiltration	Burning, sharp, tingling	Breast, prostate, lymphoma
Organ obstruction	Dull, crampy, gnawing	Colon, gastric
Organ infiltration	Distention, crampy	Liver, pancreatic
Skin inflammation, ulceration, infection, necrosis	Burning, sharp	Breast, head and neck, Kaposi's sarcoma

Freedom from cancer pain

Opioid for moderate
to severe pain
+/– Nonopioid
+/– Adjuvant — Step 3

Pain persisting or increasing

Opioid for mild to
moderate pain
+/– Nonopioid
+/– Adjuvant — Step 2

Pain persisting or increasing

Nonopioid
+/– Adjuvant — Step 1

Figure 15-7 • Adapted from the World Health Organization three-step ladder approach to relieving cancer pain. Various opioid (narcotic) and nonopioid medications may be combined with other medications to control pain.

fatigue, anger, and social isolation. Pain assessment scales (see Chapter 12) are useful for assessing the patient's pain before and after pain-relieving interventions are instituted to assess the effectiveness of interventions. Other symptoms that contribute to the pain experience, such as nausea and fatigue, are assessed and addressed as well.

In today's society, most people expect pain to disappear or resolve quickly. Although it is often controllable, advanced cancer pain is commonly irreversible and not quickly resolved. For many patients, pain is often seen as a signal that cancer is advancing and that death is approaching. As patients anticipate pain and anxiety increases, pain perception heightens, producing fear and further pain. Thus, chronic cancer pain can lead to a cycle progressing from pain to anxiety to fear and back to pain, especially when the pain is not adequately managed. Inadequate pain management is most often the result of misconceptions and insufficient knowledge about pain assessment and management on the part of patients, families, and health care providers (Eaton et al., 2015). Chapter 12 provides information regarding factors contributing to the pain experience, pain perception, and tolerance as well as pharmacologic and nonpharmacologic nursing interventions addressing pain. The nursing care plan (see Chart 15-7) also provides strategies for nursing assessment and management of chronic pain.

The World Health Organization advocates a three-step approach to treat cancer pain (see Fig. 15-7). Analgesics are given based on the patient's reported level of pain. A cancer pain algorithm, developed as a set of analgesic guiding principles, is given in Figure 15-8.

Pharmacologic and nonpharmacologic approaches, even those that may be invasive, are considered in managing cancer-related pain regardless of the patient's status along the cancer trajectory. The nurse assists the patient and family to take an active role in managing pain. The nurse provides education

and support to correct fears and misconceptions about opioid use. Inadequate pain management leads to a diminished quality of life characterized by distress, suffering, anxiety, fear, immobility, isolation, and depression.

Decreasing Fatigue

Fatigue is one of the most frequent and distressing symptoms experienced by patients receiving cancer therapy. Patients report that fatigue persists and interferes with activities of daily living for months to years after the completion of treatment (Pachman, Price, & Carey, 2014). Fatigue rarely exists in isolation; patients typically experience other symptoms concurrently, such as pain, dyspnea, anemia, sleep disturbances, or depression.

In assessing fatigue, the nurse distinguishes between *acute fatigue*, which occurs after an energy-demanding experience, and *cancer-related fatigue*, which is defined as "a distressing persistent, subjective sense of physical, emotional and/or cognitive tiredness or exhaustion related to cancer or cancer treatment that is not proportional to recent activity and interferes with usual functioning" (NCCN, 2015f). Acute fatigue serves a protective function, whereas cancer-related fatigue does not. The exact mechanisms of fatigue are not well understood and are multifactorial in nature.

Despite the commonly occurring experience of fatigue in patients with cancer, a reliable assessment tool has not been identified. The experience of fatigue is highly subjective, with patient descriptors varying greatly (NCCN, 2015f). The nurse assesses physiologic and psychological factors that can contribute to fatigue (see Chart 15-9).

Exercise and physical activity are effective approaches to the management of cancer-related fatigue (Pachman et al., 2014). Psychoeducational approaches, cognitive-behavioral therapy to address sleep, progressive muscle relaxation, yoga

---

Chart 15-9 | **Sources of Fatigue in Patients With Cancer**

- Pain, pruritus
- Imbalanced nutrition related to nausea, vomiting, cancer-related anorexia-cachexia syndrome
- Electrolyte imbalance related to vomiting, diarrhea
- Ineffective protection related to neutropenia, thrombocytopenia, anemia
- Impaired tissue integrity related to stomatitis, mucositis
- Impaired physical mobility related to neurologic impairments, surgery, bone metastasis, pain, and analgesic use
- Uncertainty and deficient knowledge related to disease process, treatment
- Anxiety related to fear, diagnosis, role changes, uncertainty of future
- Ineffective breathing patterns related to cough, shortness of breath, and dyspnea
- Disturbed sleep pattern related to cancer therapies, anxiety, and pain

Adapted from Bryant, A. L., Walton, A. L., & Phillips, B. (2015). Cancer-related fatigue: Scientific progress has been made in 40 years. *Clinical Journal of Oncology Nursing, 19*(2), 137–139; National Comprehensive Cancer Network. (2015f). NCCN guidelines for supportive care: Cancer related fatigue. Retrieved on 3/24/2016 at: www.nccn.org/professionals/physician_gls/f_guidelines.asp#fatigue

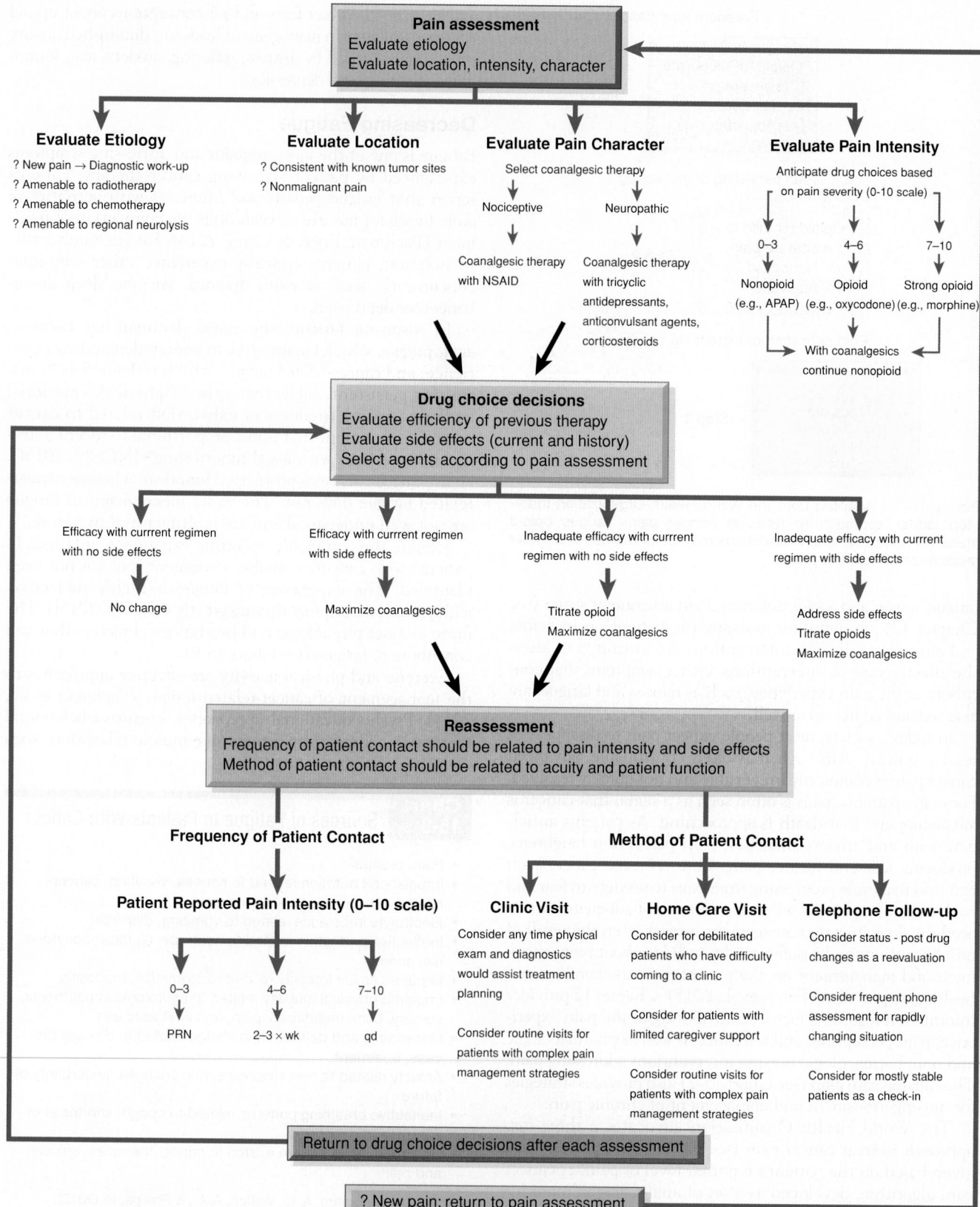

Figure 15-8 • The cancer pain algorithm (highest-level view) is a decision-tree model for pain treatment. Redrawn with permission from DuPen, A. R., DuPen, S., Hansberry, J., et al. (2000). An educational implementation of a cancer pain algorithm for ambulatory care. *Pain Management Nursing, 1*(4), 118.

and mindfulness meditation maybe effective measures to facilitate fatigue management (Mitchell, Hoffman, Clark, et al., 2014). Nurses assist patients with strategies to minimize fatigue or help the patient cope with fatigue as described in the nursing care plan (see Chart 15-7, Fatigue). Occasionally, pharmacologic interventions are utilized, including antidepressants for patients with depression, anxiolytics for those with anxiety, hypnotics for patients with sleep disturbances, and psychostimulants for some patients with advanced cancer or fatigue that does not respond to other interventions (NCCN, 2015f).

Improving Body Image and Self-Esteem

The nurse identifies potential threats to the patient's body image and assesses the patient's ability to cope with the many bodily changes that may be experienced throughout the course of disease and treatment. Entry into the health care system is often accompanied by depersonalization. Threats to self-concept occur as the patient faces the realization of illness, disfigurement, possible disability, and death. To accommodate treatments or because of the disease, many patients with cancer are forced to alter their lifestyles. Priorities and values change when body image is threatened. Disfiguring surgery, hair loss, cachexia, skin changes, altered communication patterns, and sexual dysfunction can threaten the patient's self-esteem and body image.

A creative and positive approach is essential when caring for patients with altered body image. Nursing strategies for addressing issues related to body image and self-esteem are included in the nursing care plan (see Chart 15-7). The nurse serves as a listener and counselor to both the patient and the family. Possible influences of the patient's culture and age are considered when discussing concerns and potential interventions.

Addressing Sexuality

The physiologic processes associated with cancer; potential short- and long-term effects of cancer treatments; and psychosocial, emotional, and spiritual responses to the entire experience may lead patients to confront a variety of sexuality-based issues. Patients at the greatest risk of sexual dysfunction are those with tumors that involve the sexual or pelvic organs and those whose treatment affects the hormonal systems mediating sexual function (Goldfarb, Mulhall, Nelson, et al., 2013). Although sexuality is an important component of overall health, many nurses and other health professionals are hesitant to include sexuality in their discussions with patients (Kelvin, Steed, & Jarrett, 2014). Workshops have been developed to help nurses overcome barriers to discussing sexuality (Smith, 2015). In offering a holistic approach to the care of patients with cancer, nurses should initiate discussions about sexuality and assess sexual health.

Infertility, a common consequence of cancer and cancer treatments, can be of concern to patients and their partners. The potential for impaired fertility is discussed and options reviewed for fertility preservation (Frankel Kelvin, 2015). Fertility plans are discussed and determined prior to the initiation of any therapy that may compromise reproductive abilities.

Referrals are made as needed for specialized evaluation and interventions that are beyond the scope of nursing intervention.

Assisting in the Grieving Process

A cancer diagnosis need not indicate a fatal outcome. Many forms of cancer are curable, and others may be controlled for long periods of time similar to the course of other chronic diseases. Despite the tremendous advances in cancer, many patients and their families still view cancer as a fatal disease that is inevitably accompanied by pain, suffering, debilitation, and emaciation. Grieving is a normal response to these fears and to actual or potential losses: loss of health, normal sensations, body image, social interaction, intimacy, independence, and usual social roles. Patients, families, and friends may grieve for the loss of quality time to spend with others, the loss of future and unfulfilled plans, and the loss of control over the patient's body and emotional reactions. Nurses continue to assess the patient and family for positive or maladaptive coping behaviors, interpersonal communication, and evidence of the need for additional psychosocial support or interventions such as referral for professional counseling.

If the patient enters the terminal phase of disease, the nurse may assess that the patient and family members are at different stages of grief. In such cases, the nurse assists the patient and family to acknowledge and cope with their reactions and feelings. The nurse also empowers the patient and family to explore preferences for issues related to end-of-life care, such as withdrawal of active disease treatment, desire for the use of life-support measures, and symptom management approaches. Oncology nurses respectfully support the patient's spiritual or religious views and facilitate contact with their preferred clergy member, if desired. In addition, nurses consider the patient's cultural beliefs and practices when addressing issues related to grief. After the death of a patient with cancer, home care and/or hospice nurses follow up with surviving family members for bereavement counseling to facilitate expression and coping with feelings of loss and grief. (See Chapter 16 for further discussion of end-of-life issues.)

Management of Psychosocial Distress

Despite advances in cancer care, patients experience varying levels of psychosocial distress related to actual or potential losses, fear of the unknown, symptoms due to cancer or cancer treatments, changes in usual family and social roles, financial concerns, and a sense of loss of control. Psychosocial distress is defined as a multifactorial unpleasant emotional experience of a psychological (cognitive, behavioral, emotional), social, and/or spiritual nature that may interfere with the ability to cope effectively with cancer, its physical symptoms and its treatment (NCCN, 2015g). Distress occurs along a continuum, ranging from common normal feelings of vulnerability, sadness, and fears to problems that can become disabling, such as depression, anxiety, panic, social isolation, and existential and spiritual crisis. Distress that is not addressed can have a significant impact on the overall well-being, interpersonal relationships, cognitive abilities, and adherence to treatment regimens, leading to poor outcomes.

Nurses need to screen patients for psychosocial distress during the course of the cancer experience. Patients are supported in managing various sources and levels of distress. Referral to mental health providers may be helpful to address specific concerns (Schilli, 2014).

Monitoring and Managing Potential Complications

Infection

For patients in all stages of cancer, the nurse assesses factors associated with the development of infection. Although infection-associated morbidity and mortality have greatly decreased, prevention and prompt treatment of infection are essential in patients with cancer. Often, more than one predisposing factor is present in patients with cancer. The nurse monitors laboratory studies to detect early changes in WBC counts. Common sites of infection, such as the pharynx, skin, perianal area, urinary, and respiratory tracts, are assessed on a regular basis. However, the typical signs of infection (swelling, redness, drainage, and pain) may not occur in myelosuppressed patients because of decreased circulating WBCs and a diminished local inflammatory response. Fever may be the only sign of infection (NCCN, 2015h). The nurse monitors the patient for sepsis, particularly if invasive catheters or long-term IV catheters are in place.

WBC function is often impaired in patients with cancer. Among the five types of WBCs, (neutrophils [granulocytes], lymphocytes, monocytes, basophils, and eosinophils), neutrophils serve as the body's primary initial defense against invading organisms. Comprising 60% to 70% of the body's WBCs, neutrophils act by engulfing and destroying infective organisms through phagocytosis. Both the total WBC count and the concentration of neutrophils are important in determining the patient's ability to fight infection. A decrease in circulating WBCs is referred to as leukopenia. Granulocytopenia is a decrease in neutrophils.

A differential WBC count identifies the relative numbers of WBCs and permits tabulation of polymorphonuclear neutrophils (PMNs) or segmented neutrophils (mature neutrophils, reported as "polys," PMNs, or "segs") and immature forms of neutrophils (reported as bands, metamyelocytes, and "stabs"). The absolute neutrophil count (ANC) is calculated by the following formula:

$$ANC = (\text{segmented neutrophils [\%]} + \text{bands [\%]}) \times \text{WBC count (cells/mm}^3)$$

$$\text{Example: } (25\% \text{ segs} + 25\% \text{ bands}) \times 6000 \text{ WBC cells/mm}^3 = 3000 \text{ ANC}$$

Neutropenia, an abnormally low ANC, is associated with an increased risk of infection. The risk of infection rises as the ANC decreases. As the ANC declines below 1,500 cells/mm^3, the risk of infection rises. An ANC less than 500 cells/mm^3 reflects a severe risk of infection (NCCN, 2015h; Segal, Walsh, Gea-Banacloche, et al., 2015). The nadir is the lowest ANC following chemotherapy, targeted therapy, or radiation therapy that suppresses bone marrow function. Severe neutropenia may necessitate delays in administration of myelosuppressive therapies or treatment dose adjustments, although the use of the hematopoietic growth factors (i.e., colony-stimulating factors; see previous discussion) has reduced the severity and duration of treatment-associated neutropenia as well as infection-related morbidity and early death (Smith, Bohlke, Lyman, et al., 2015). The administration of these growth factors assists in maintaining treatment schedules, drug dosages, treatment effectiveness, and quality of life.

Febrile patients who are neutropenic are assessed for factors that increase the risk of infection and for sources of infection through cultures of blood, sputum, urine, stool, IV and urinary or other catheters, and wounds, if appropriate (see Table 15-10). In addition, a chest x-ray is usually obtained to assess for pulmonary infection.

Defense against infection is compromised in many different ways. The integrity of the skin and mucous membranes is challenged by multiple invasive diagnostic procedures, by the adverse effects of all cancer treatment modalities, and by the detrimental effects of immobility. Impaired nutrition as a result of CACS, nausea, vomiting, diarrhea, and the underlying disease alters the body's ability to combat invading organisms. Medications such as antibiotics disturb the balance of normal flora, allowing the overgrowth of normal flora and pathogenic organisms. Other medications can also alter the immune response (see Chapter 35). Cancer itself may lead to defects in cellular and humoral immunity. Advanced cancer may cause obstruction of hollow viscera (e.g., intestines), blood, and lymphatic vessels, creating a favorable environment for proliferation of pathogenic organisms. In some patients, tumor cells infiltrate bone marrow and prevent normal production of WBCs.

Nurses are in a key position to assist in preventing and identifying symptoms of infection, as discussed in the nursing care plan (see Chart 15-7). Clinical practice guidelines developed by the ONS, the Infusion Nurses Society (INS), the NCCN, and the ASCO are used to guide prevention and management of infection. Interventions to prevent infection and alternative patient education formats for infection-related instruction are high nursing research priorities.

Gram-positive bacteria (*Streptococcus*, enterococci, and *Staphylococcus* species) and gram-negative organisms (*Escherichia coli*, *Klebsiella pneumoniae*, *Enterobacter*, and *Pseudomonas aeruginosa*) are the most frequently isolated causes of infection. Fungal organisms, such as *Candida albicans*, also contribute to the incidence of serious infection. Viral infections in immunocompromised patients are caused most often by herpes simplex, respiratory syncytial, parainfluenza, and influenza A and B viruses.

Fever is reported promptly as it is an important sign of infection in patients when associated with neutropenia. Patients with neutropenic fever (see Table 15-10) are assessed for infection and reported promptly (NCCN, 2015h). Antibiotics may be prescribed after cultures of wound drainage, exudates, sputum, urine, stool, or blood are obtained. Careful consideration is given to the underlying malignancy, prior antineoplastic treatment, ANC, comorbidities, and other patient-related factors prior to the identification of the most appropriate antibiotic therapy. Evidence-based guidelines are available for prevention and treatment of cancer-related infections (NCCN, 2015h). Patients with neutropenia are treated with broad-spectrum antibiotics before the infecting organism is identified because of the increased risk of mortality associated with untreated infection. Broad-spectrum antibiotic therapy targets the most likely major pathogenic organisms. It is important for these medications to be given and taken promptly as scheduled to achieve adequate blood levels. Once the offending organism is identified, more specific antimicrobial therapy is prescribed as appropriate. Nurses provide education for patients and families regarding prevention of

TABLE 15-10 Assessment of Neutropenic Fever in Patients With Cancer

Fever Criteria	Neutropenia Criteria
• Any one-time temperature of 38.3°C (101°F) or • Any temperature of ≥38°C (100.4°F) or ≥1 h	• <500 neutrophils/mcL or • <1000 neutrophils/mcL and predicted to decline to ≤500 neutrophils/mcL over the next 48 hours

Assessment Targets for Neutropenic Fever Evaluation

Infection Risk Factors	Physical Assessment	Diagnostic Procedures	Microbiologic Cultures
• Chronic comorbid illnesses • Underlying hematologic malignancies • Immunosuppression related to factors other than neutropenia (i.e., immunosuppressive therapy following allogeneic HSCT or hypogammaglobulinemia [decreased gammaglobulin production]) • Solid tumors causing obstructions of the bronchial tree, ureters, colon, or biliary ducts • Advanced or refractory underlying malignancy • Prolonged duration of neutropenia • Age ≥65 years • Limited mobility and/or debilitation • Medications (e.g., corticosteroids such as prednisone) • Antibiotic therapy or prophylaxis • Recent surgery for diagnosis or treatment • Chemotherapy or targeted therapy received within the last 7–10 days • Prior treatment with multiple types of chemotherapy regimens • Recent radiation therapy; especially to areas associated with bone marrow reserves • Prior documented infections • Impaired skin integrity • Invasive drainage or urinary catheters • Peripheral or central venous access devices • Exposures (travel, others with infection, blood administration, pets) • Diarrhea • Poor nutritional status • Recent lumbar puncture or indwelling Ommaya reservoir™ (long-term intraventricular catheter for administration of chemotherapy into CSF and ventricles)	• Skin, pressure points, wounds • Surgical or biopsy incision sites • IV access or reservoir sites • Drainage catheter sites • Tracheostomy site • Lungs and sinuses • Perivaginal and peri-rectal area • Alimentary canal, abdomen • Neurologic assessment • Vital signs	• Diagnostic imaging as appropriate to identify abscesses, fistulas, pneumonia, obstruction, etc. • Complete blood count/differential • Serum chemistries, liver function tests • Renal function tests • Pulse oximetry or arterial blood gases • Lumbar puncture for CSF analysis	• Blood (peripheral and central venous access if applicable) • Urine (especially with indwelling catheter) • Skin wounds, lesions, incision sites, catheter exit sites • Catheter tips when feasible • Drainage from catheters • Stool, diarrhea • Sputum • CSF

CSF, cerebrospinal fluid.
Adapted from National Comprehensive Cancer Network. (2015h). Clinical practice guidelines: Prevention and treatment of cancer related infections (v2.2015). Available at: www.nccn.org/professionals/physician_gls/pdf/infections.pdf; Segal, B. H., Walsh, T. J., Gea-Banacloche, J. C., et al. (2015). Infections in the cancer patient. In V. T., DeVita, T. S., Lawrence, & S. A., Rosenberg, SA (Eds.). *Cancer: Principles & practice of oncology.* Philadelphia: Lippincott Williams & Wilkins.

infection, signs and symptoms to report, and the importance of adherence to prescribed antimicrobial therapy.

 Septic Shock

The nurse assesses the patient frequently for signs and symptoms of infection and inflammation throughout the trajectory of cancer care. Sepsis and septic shock are life-threatening complications that must be prevented or detected and treated promptly. Although all patients with cancer are at risk, patients who are neutropenic or who have hematologic malignancies are at the greatest risk. Patients with signs and symptoms of impending sepsis and septic shock require immediate hospitalization and aggressive treatment in the intensive care setting. (See Chapter 14 for discussion of sepsis and septic shock.)

Bleeding and Thrombocytopenia

Platelets are essential for normal blood clotting and coagulation (hemostasis). **Thrombocytopenia**, a decrease in the circulating platelet count, is the most common cause of bleeding in patients with cancer and is usually defined as a platelet count less than 100,000/mm³ (0.1 × 10¹²/L). The risk of bleeding increases when the platelet count decreases below 50,000/mm³ (0.05 × 10¹²/L). At platelet counts lower than 10,000/mm³ (0.02 × 10¹²/L), the risk for spontaneous bleeding is increased (Barbarotta, 2015).

Thrombocytopenia often results from bone marrow depression after certain types of chemotherapy and radiation therapy and with tumor infiltration of the bone marrow. In some cases, platelet destruction is associated with an enlarged spleen (hypersplenism) and abnormal antibody function, which occur with leukemia and lymphoma. Bacterial and viral infections may lead to early platelet destruction or impaired bone marrow production of platelets and subsequent thrombocytopenia. Some medications (i.e., heparin, vancomycin) may cause bone marrow toxicity leading to decreases in circulating platelets. Less commonly, posttransfusion complications may lead to antibody destruction of platelets causing profound thrombocytopenia. Lastly, coagulopathies associated with infection or malignancies, such as gastric and pancreatic cancer, may result in thrombocytopenia (Kuter, 2015). The nursing care plan addresses nursing assessment parameters and interventions for patients at risk for bleeding (see Chart 15-7).

> ▶ *Quality and Safety Nursing Alert*
>
> *Although laboratory test results confirm the diagnosis of thrombocytopenia, the patient who is developing thrombocytopenia may display early signs and symptoms. Thus, nurses need to observe keenly for petechiae and ecchymoses, which are early indicators of decreasing platelet levels. Early detection promotes early intervention.*

Additional medications may be prescribed to address bleeding or thrombocytopenia based on the underlying etiology. (Refer to Chapter 33 for further discussion of assessment and treatment of thrombocytopenia and coagulopathies.)

Venous thromboembolism (VTE), a common problem for patients with cancer, includes deep venous thrombosis (DVT), pulmonary embolism (PE), superficial venous thrombosis (SVT), and thrombosis in other abdominal or thoracic venous tributaries such as the mesenteric veins or the superior vena cava. The incidence of VTE has been linked to an increased likelihood of death in patients with cancer (NCCN, 2015i). Factors associated with risk for VTEs in cancer patients include pre-existing underlying or cancer-related coagulopathies, medications including chemotherapy, hospitalizations, surgical procedures, increased age, debilitation, immobility, infection, and peripheral and central venous catheters (NCCN, 2015i). Patients with cancer are monitored for associated risk factors and are assessed on an ongoing basis for VTE. Nurses provide patient and

family education regarding symptoms of VTE to report to the provider. Recommendations for prophylaxis are based on national guidelines and patient risk factors. Nursing assessment findings associated with VTE are reported promptly so that VTE evaluation and treatment can be initiated expeditiously.

Promoting Home, Community-Based, and Transitional Care

 Educating Patients About Self-Care

Most commonly, patients with cancer are diagnosed and treated in the outpatient setting. Nurses in outpatient settings often have the responsibility for patient education and helping coordinate care in the home (see Chart 15-10). The shift of care from acute care facilities to the home or outpatient settings as well as the increasing use of oral antineoplastic agents places significant responsibility for care on the patient and family. In order to maintain optimal patient outcomes and quality of life, patients and families require support and information that will prepare them to engage in self-care. Education initially focuses on the most immediate care needs likely to be encountered at home.

Approaches to preparing patients for self-care responsibilities are chosen with consideration of the patient's preferred learning strategies, level of education, and health literacy. Knobf (2013) suggests that patient education is best achieved through a nurse–patient relationship that involves an exchange of information to support patient needs that can vary across time points of the cancer continuum. Easily understood, concrete, objective information that assists patients to understand what to expect and includes sensory and temporal components is important. Symptoms, side

---

Chart 15-10 🏠 **HOME CARE CHECKLIST**

The Patient Receiving Care for an Oncologic Disorder

At the completion of education, the patient and/or caregiver will be able to:

- State the impact of cancer treatment on physiologic functioning, ADLs, IADLs, roles, relationships, and spirituality.
- State changes in lifestyle (e.g., diet, activity) necessary to maintain health.
- State the name, dose, side effects, frequency, and schedule for all medications.
- Demonstrate how to administer the chemotherapy agent in the home:
  - Describe safe storage and handling of oral chemotherapy/targeted agents in the home.
  - Demonstrate safe disposal of needles, syringes, IV supplies, or unused chemotherapy medications.
  - List possible side effects of chemotherapeutic agents and suggested management approaches.
- List possible side effects of radiation therapy and suggested management approaches.
- List complications of medications/therapeutic regimen necessitating a call to the nurse or primary provider.
- List complications of medications/therapeutic regimen necessitating a visit to the emergency department.

- Locate list of names and telephone numbers of resource personnel involved in care (e.g., home care nurse, infusion services, IV vendor, equipment company, radiation therapy department).
- Explain treatment plan and importance of upcoming visits to the primary provider.
- State how to obtain medical supplies after discharge.
- Identify durable medical equipment needs, proper usage, and maintenance necessary for safe utilization.
- Demonstrate usage of adaptive equipment for ADLs.
- Identify community resources for peer and caregiver/family support:
  - Identify sources of support (e.g., friends, relatives, faith community)
  - Identify phone numbers of support groups for people with cancer and their caregivers/families
  - State meeting locations and times
- Identify the need for health promotion, disease prevention, and screening activities

ADL, activities of daily living; IADL, independent activities of daily living.

effects of treatment, and changes in the patient's status that should be reported are discussed and reinforced with printed materials that can be referred to in the home. Nurses help to empower patients by sharing strategies to manage side effects or other symptoms. Additional learning needs are based on the priorities conveyed by the patient and family as well as on the complexity of care required.

Technologic advances allow home administration of IV chemotherapy, blood products, and antibiotics; enteral or parenteral nutrition; and parenteral analgesics. Patients and families are taught to care for vascular access devices, infusion pumps, various types of drainage catheters, and on occasion complex wounds. The importance of patient safety and infection control is included in patient and family education. Although nurses are often available to provide some assistance with cancer care in the home, patients and families need information that will enable them to have a sense of comfort, decrease distress, improve coping, foster self-management, promote adherence, and enhance quality of life (Knobf, 2013).

Continuing and Transitional Care

Referral for home or transitional care is often indicated for patients with cancer. The responsibilities of the nurse include assessing the home environment and suggesting modifications in the home or in care to help address the patient's physical and safety needs. Home care nurses also assess the psychosocial impact of cancer on the patient and family so that appropriate interventions can be identified and/or referrals for support services are instituted.

Ongoing nursing visits and/or phone contact from the home or transitional care nurse assist in prevention, early identification, prompt reporting, and management of patient problems. Timely modifications in therapy to manage symptoms and adverse effects of treatment may decrease patient suffering and decrease emergency department visits or hospital admissions. Continued contact facilitates evaluation of the patient's progress, responses to treatment, and assessment of the ongoing needs of the patient and family. It is necessary to assess the patient's and family's understanding of the treatment plan and management strategies and to reinforce previous education. The nurse facilitates coordination of patient care by maintaining close communication with all involved health care providers. The nurse may make referrals and coordinate available community resources (e.g., local office of the ACS, home aides, church groups, faith community nurses, support groups) to assist patients and caregivers.

Gerontologic Considerations

Approximately 53% of cancer incidence and 69% of cancer deaths occur in persons aged 65 years or older (ACS, 2015a). The rising number of individuals over age 65 with cancer has led to the emergence of geriatric oncology, a multidimensional and multidisciplinary approach to treating growing numbers of older adults with cancer.

Nurses working with older adults must understand the normal physiologic changes that occur with aging and the implications for the patient with cancer (see Table 15-11). These changes that affect all body systems may ultimately influence older patients' responses to cancer treatment. In addition, many older patients have other chronic diseases requiring multiple medications. The existence of comorbidities and multiple medications may contribute to drug interactions and toxicities in older patients.

The understanding of the effects and tolerance of chemotherapy, targeted therapies, and radiation in the older adult is limited, as older adults have been underrepresented in oncology clinical trials. Potential chemotherapy-related toxicities, such as renal impairment, myelosuppression, fatigue, and cardiomyopathy, may increase as a result of declining organ function and diminished physiologic reserves. The recovery of normal tissues after radiation therapy may be delayed, and older adult patients may experience more severe adverse effects, such as mucositis, nausea and vomiting, and myelosuppression. Because of impaired healing and declining pulmonary and cardiovascular functioning, older patients are slower to recover from surgery. Older patients are also at increased risk for complications, such as atelectasis, pneumonia, and wound infections.

Cancer Survivorship

In the United States, there are currently about 14.5 million adult cancer survivors with estimates of 19 million by the year 2024 (ACS, 2014). Advances in cancer screening, treatment, and management of complications have contributed to a lengthened survival period for many, with long-term survival becoming possible for many patients. *Cancer survivorship* has been defined as the period from cancer diagnosis through the remaining years of life and focuses on the health and life of a person beyond diagnostic and treatment phases. Although individuals vary and many types of cancers and treatments exist, the acute, long-term, and late effects of cancer and its treatment may have multiple long-term physical, cognitive, psychological, social, and financial consequences that can impact activities of daily living, ultimately affecting quality of life (Given, 2015).

Survivorship care is often based on expert opinion and experience rather than on evidence-based practices. Knowledge regarding survivorship concerns continues to evolve. The Institute of Medicine has identified four components of survivorship care, the period that follows primary treatment for cancer and lasts until end of life. In addition to a summary of prior diagnosis and treatment, survivorship care includes monitoring and treatment for late effects related to disease and prior treatments, physical and vocational rehabilitation, psychosocial support and counseling as necessary, and surveillance and screening for new and recurrent cancer (Hewitt, Greenfield, & Stovall, 2006) (see Table 15-12). Advocacy organizations across the country have recommended that a survivorship care plan be provided to all patients with cancer and their primary provider at the completion of treatment. The survivorship care plan includes a summary of cancer diagnosis and treatment and recommendations for follow-up and care, including approaches to treat symptoms, rehabilitative needs, monitoring for late effects, and surveillance and screening for new and recurrent cancer. Referrals for specific services such as lymphedema therapy, chronic pain management, and genetic counseling are also provided. Nurses assist in the development of the survivorship care plan and provide education and care for cancer survivors. Nurses, other health

TABLE 15-11 Age-Related Changes and Their Effects on Patients With Cancer

Age-Related Changes	Implications
Impaired immune system	Use special precautions to avoid infection; monitor for atypical signs and symptoms of infection.
Altered drug absorption, distribution, metabolism, and elimination	Mandates careful calculation of chemotherapy and frequent assessment for drug response and side effects; dose adjustments may be necessary.
Increased prevalence of other chronic diseases	Monitor for effect of cancer or its treatment on patient's other chronic diseases; monitor patient's tolerance for cancer treatment; monitor for interactions with medications used to treat chronic diseases.
Diminished renal, respiratory, and cardiac reserve	Be proactive in prevention of decreased renal function, atelectasis, pneumonia, and cardiovascular compromise; monitor for side effects of cancer treatment.
Decreased skin and tissue integrity; reduction in body mass; delayed healing	Prevent pressure ulcers secondary to immobility; monitor skin and mucous membranes for changes related to radiation or chemotherapy; monitor nutritional status.
Decreased musculoskeletal strength	Prevent falls; assess support for performing activities of daily living in home setting; encourage safe use of assistive mobility devices.
Decreased neurosensory functioning: loss of vision, hearing, and distal extremity tactile senses	Provide instruction modified for patient's hearing and vision changes; provide instruction concerning safety and skin care for distal extremities; assess home for safety.
Altered social and economic resources	Assess for financial concerns, living conditions, and resources for support.
Potential changes in cognitive and emotional capacity	Provide education and support modified for patient's level of functioning and safety.

care providers, public health professionals, and patient advocates design and conduct research to identify needs of cancer survivors and evidence-based approaches to care.

TABLE 15-12 Components of Survivorship Care

Component	Examples of Care
Prevention and detection of new and recurrent cancer	• Mammography (per ACS guidelines) • Papanicolaou (Pap) smears (per ACS guidelines) • Smoking cessation programs • Nutrition counseling
Surveillance for cancer spread, recurrence, or second cancers	• Colonoscopy post colon cancer • Mammography post breast cancer • Liver function tests post colon cancer • Prostate-specific antigen post prostate cancer
Intervention for consequences of cancer and its treatments	• Lymphedema therapy • Pain management • Enterostomal therapy • Fertility care • Psychosocial support or counseling • Reconstructive surgery
Coordination between specialists and primary providers to meet health needs	• Care for comorbidities (e.g., diabetes) • Influenza vaccination • Bone densitometry • Monitoring for chemotherapy induced cardiotoxicity

ACS, American Cancer Society.
Adapted from Hewitt, M., Greenfield, S., & Stovall, E. (Eds.). (2006). *From cancer patient to cancer survivor.* Washington, DC: Institute of Medicine and National Research Council, National Academies Press. Components of survivorship care provided by the Institute of Medicine report on cancer survivorship.

Providing Care to the Patient With Advanced Cancer

Providing Care in Oncologic Emergencies

Table 15-13 discusses selected nursing and medical care of oncologic emergencies.

As a result of advances in all aspects of cancer care, it is more common that individuals are living with cancer that has advanced beyond the original site of development to regional or distant sites. Patients with advanced cancer are likely to experience many of the problems described previously, although more often and to a greater degree. Symptoms of pain, anorexia, weight loss, CACS, fatigue, and impaired functional status and mobility make patients more susceptible to depressive symptoms, skin breakdown, fluid and electrolyte imbalances, and infection.

Treatment for the patient with advanced cancer is likely to be palliative rather than curative, with an emphasis on prevention and appropriate management of pain. The use of long-acting analgesic agents at set intervals, rather than on an "as needed" basis, is recommended in addressing pain management. Working with the patient and family, as well as with other health care providers, to manage pain is essential to increase the patient's comfort and offer some sense of control. Other medications (e.g., sedatives, tranquilizers, muscle relaxants, antiemetics) are added to assist in palliating additional symptoms and promoting quality of life.

If the patient is a candidate for radiation therapy or surgical interventions to relieve pain or other symptoms, the potential benefits and risks of these procedures (e.g., percutaneous nerve block, cordotomy) are explained to the patient and family. Measures are taken to prevent complications that result from altered sensation, immobility, and changes in bowel and bladder function.

TABLE 15-13 Oncologic Emergencies: Manifestations and Management

Emergency	Clinical Manifestations and Diagnostic Findings	Management
Superior Vena Cava Syndrome (SVCS) Compression or invasion of the superior vena cava by tumor; enlarged lymph nodes; intraluminal thrombus that obstructs venous circulation; or drainage of the head, neck, arms, and thorax. Most often associated with lung cancer, SVCS is also associated with lymphoma, thymoma, and testicular cancers and mediastinal metastases from breast cancer. If untreated, SVCS may lead to cerebral anoxia (because not enough oxygen reaches the brain), laryngeal edema, bronchial obstruction, and death.	**Clinical** Gradually or suddenly impaired venous drainage giving rise to: • Progressive shortness of breath (dyspnea), cough, hoarseness, chest pain, and facial swelling • Edema of the neck, arms, hands, and thorax and reported sensation of skin tightness, difficulty swallowing, and stridor • Possibly engorged and distended jugular, temporal, and arm veins • Dilated thoracic vessels causing prominent venous patterns on the chest wall • Increased intracranial pressure, associated visual disturbances, headache, and altered mental status **Diagnostic** Diagnosis is confirmed by: • Clinical findings • Chest x-ray • Thoracic computed tomography (CT) scan • Thoracic magnetic resonance imaging (MRI) • Venogram if intraluminal thrombosis is suspected	**Medical** • Radiation therapy to shrink tumor or enlarged lymph nodes and relieve symptoms • Chemotherapy for sensitive cancers (e.g., lymphoma, small cell lung cancer) or when the mediastinum has been irradiated to maximum tolerance • Anticoagulant or thrombolytic therapy for central venous catheter related intraluminal thrombosis • Percutaneously placed intravascular stents may be priority consideration rather than surgery unless symptoms are rapidly progressing. • Supportive measures such as oxygen therapy, corticosteroids, and diuretics (in cases of fluid overload) **Nursing** • Identify patients at risk for SVCS. • Provide patient education regarding signs and symptoms to report • Monitor and report clinical manifestations of SVCS. • Monitor cardiopulmonary and neurologic status. • Avoid upper extremity venipuncture and blood pressure measurement; instruct patient to avoid tight or restrictive clothing and jewelry on fingers, wrist, and neck. • Facilitate breathing and drainage from upper portion of body by instructing patient to maintain some elevation of head and upper body with semi-Fowler position; avoid completely supine or prone position (this helps to promote comfort and reduce anxiety associated with dependent and progressive edema). • Promote energy conservation to minimize shortness of breath. • Monitor the patient's fluid volume status; administer fluids cautiously to minimize edema. • Assess for thoracic radiation-related problems such as mucositis with resultant dysphagia (difficulty swallowing) and esophagitis. • Monitor for chemotherapy-related problems, such as myelosuppression. • Provide postoperative care as appropriate.
Spinal Cord Compression Most commonly caused by compression of the cord and its nerve roots by a metastatic paravertebral tumor that extends into the epidural space; vertebral bone metastasis leading to bone collapse and displacement impinging on the spinal cord or nerve roots; and less commonly, primary malignancy of the cord. May potentially lead to significant and permanent neurologic impairment associated with multiple physical, psychosocial consequences. Most often associated with cancers that metastasize to the bone such as breast, lung, and prostate cancers and lymphoma. Also seen in nasopharyngeal cancer and multiple myeloma. About 70% of compressions occur at the thoracic level, 20% in the lumbosacral level, and 10% in the cervical and sacral regions. The prognosis depends on the severity and rapidity of onset.	**Clinical** • Local inflammation, edema, venous stasis, and impaired blood supply to nerve tissues • Local or radicular back or neck pain along the dermatomal areas innervated by the affected nerve root (e.g., thoracic radicular pain extends in a band around the chest or abdomen) • Pain exacerbated by movement, supine recumbent position, coughing, sneezing, or the Valsalva maneuver • Neurologic dysfunction and related motor and sensory deficits (numbness, tingling, feelings of coldness in the affected area, inability to detect vibration, loss of positional sense) • Motor loss ranging from subtle weakness to flaccid paralysis • Bladder and/or bowel dysfunction depending on level of compression (above S2, overflow incontinence; from S3 to S5, flaccid sphincter tone and bowel incontinence).	**Medical** • Radiation therapy to reduce tumor size and halt progression; corticosteroid therapy to decrease inflammation and swelling at the compression site • Surgery to debulk tumor and stabilize the spine if symptoms progress despite radiation therapy or if vertebral fracture or bone fragments lead to additional nerve damage; surgery is also an option when the tumor is not radiosensitive or is located in an area that was previously irradiated. • Minimally invasive surgical procedures, referred to as vertebral augmentation, may be used for patients with vertebral fractures to attain stability of the bone, prevent nerve compression, and decrease pain. Procedures include: • Vertebroplasty: involves percutaneous injection of polymethyl methacrylate (PMMA), a bone cement filler, into the vertebral body • Kyphoplasty: a balloon is inserted into the damaged vertebral body and then inflated to create a cavity within the bone that can be filled with bone cement. The balloon helps to compress the fracture fragments together as the cavity is created.

(continued on page 382)

TABLE 15-13 Oncologic Emergencies: Manifestations and Management (continued)

Emergency	Clinical Manifestations and Diagnostic Findings	Management
	Diagnostic • Percussion tenderness at the level of compression • Abnormal reflexes • Sensory and motor abnormalities • MRI is a preferred diagnostic tool; may also utilize x-rays, bone scans, and CT scan.	• Radiofrequency vertebral augmentation: similar to kyphoplasty; instead of the balloon, a small navigational canula is inserted into the vertebra to create small pathways for cement. The cement is heated with radiofrequency to create an ultra high viscosity that is thought to promote bone stability • Chemotherapy as adjuvant to other local therapies for patients with chemosensitive cancers such as lymphoma or small cell lung cancer *Note:* Despite treatment, patients with poor neurologic function before treatment are less likely to regain complete motor and sensory function; patients who develop complete paralysis usually do not regain all neurologic function. **Nursing** • Perform ongoing assessment of neurologic function to identify existing and progressing dysfunction. • Control pain with pharmacologic and nonpharmacologic measures. • Prevent complications of immobility resulting from pain and decreased function (e.g., skin breakdown, urinary stasis, thrombophlebitis, decreased clearance of pulmonary secretions). • Maintain muscle tone by assisting with range-of-motion exercises in collaboration with physical and occupational therapists; patients with unstable vertebral fractures do not initiate physical therapy until spine stabilization procedures have been completed. • Institute intermittent urinary catheterization and bowel training programs for patients with bladder or bowel dysfunction. • Provide encouragement and support to patient and family coping with pain and altered functioning, lifestyle, roles, and independence. • Institute appropriate referrals for home care and physical and occupational therapy.
Hypercalcemia Hypercalcemia is a potentially life-threatening metabolic abnormality resulting when the calcium released from the bones is more than the kidneys can excrete or the bones can reabsorb. • It may result from production of cytokines, hormonal substances, and growth factors by cancer cells, or by the body in response to substances produced by cancer cells, which lead to bone breakdown and calcium release. • Most commonly seen in breast, lung, and renal cancers; myeloma; and some types of leukemia	**Clinical** Fatigue, weakness, confusion, decreased level of responsiveness, hyporeflexia, nausea, vomiting, constipation, ileus, polyuria (excessive urination), polydipsia (excessive thirst), dehydration, and dysrhythmias **Diagnostic** Total serum calcium level >10.5 mg/dL (2.74 mmol/L) Ionized serum calcium >1.29 mmol/L	**Medical** • Identify patients at risk for hypercalcemia and assess for signs and symptoms of hypercalcemia. • Educate patient and family; prevention and early detection can prevent fatality. • Educate at-risk patients to recognize and report signs and symptoms of hypercalcemia. • Provide patient and family education regarding: • Need to consume 2–4 L of fluid daily unless contraindicated by existing renal or cardiac disease • Use of dietary and pharmacologic interventions such as stool softeners and laxatives for constipation • Maintenance of nutritional intake without restricting normal calcium intake • Antiemetic therapy for nausea and vomiting • Promotion of mobility and emphasis on importance in preventing demineralization and breakdown of bones • Safety precautions for patients with impaired mental and mobility status

TABLE 15-13 Oncologic Emergencies: Manifestations and Management (continued)

Emergency	Clinical Manifestations and Diagnostic Findings	Management
Tumor Lysis Syndrome (TLS) Potentially fatal complication that occurs spontaneously or more commonly following radiation, biotherapy, or chemotherapy-induced cell destruction of large or rapidly growing cancers such as leukemia, lymphoma, and small cell lung cancer. The release of tumor intracellular contents (nuclei acids, electrolytes, and debris) leads to rapidly induced electrolyte imbalances—hyperkalemia, hyperphosphatemia (leading to hypocalemia), and hyperuricemia—that can have life-threatening end-organ effects on the myocardium, kidneys, and central nervous system	**Clinical** Clinical manifestations depend on the extent of metabolic abnormalities. Clinical TLS is diagnosed when ≥1 of 3 conditions arise either 3 days prior to or 7 days after cytotoxic cancer therapy: acute kidney injury (defined as a rise in creatinine to ≥1.5 times the upper limit of normal that is not attributable to medications), dysrhythmias (including sudden cardiac death), and seizures. • *Neurologic:* Fatigue, weakness, memory loss, altered mental status, muscle cramps, tetany, paresthesias (numbness and tingling), seizures • *Cardiac:* Elevated blood pressure, shortened QT complexes, widened QRS waves, altered T waves, dysrhythmias, cardiac arrest • *GI:* Anorexia, nausea, vomiting, abdominal cramps, diarrhea, increased bowel sounds • *Renal:* Flank pain, oliguria, anuria, kidney injury, acidic urine pH • *Other:* Gout, malaise, pruritis **Diagnostic** • Electrolyte imbalances identified by serum electrolyte measurement and urinalysis (see Chapter 13); electrocardiogram to detect cardiac dysrhythmias	**Medical** • To prevent kidney injury and restore electrolyte balance, aggressive fluid hydration is initiated 24–48 hours before and after the initiation of cytotoxic therapy to increase urine volume and eliminate uric acid and electrolytes; urine is alkalinized by adding sodium bicarbonate to IV fluid to maintain a urine pH of 7–7.5; this prevents kidney injury secondary to uric acid precipitation in the kidneys. • Diuresis with a loop diuretic or osmotic diuretic if urine output is not sufficient • Allopurinol (Zyloprim) therapy to inhibit the conversion of nucleic acids to uric acid; rasburicase (Elitek) may be used to convert already formed uric acid to allantoin, which is highly water soluble and eliminated in urine. • Administration of a cation-exchange resin, such as sodium polystyrene sulfonate (Kayexalate), to treat hyperkalemia by binding and eliminating potassium through the bowel • Administration of IV sodium bicarbonate, hypertonic dextrose, and regular insulin temporarily shifts potassium into cells and lowers serum potassium levels if a rapid decrease in potassium is necessary. • Administration of phosphate-binding gels, such as aluminum hydroxide, to treat hyperphosphatemia by promoting phosphate excretion in the feces • Hemodialysis when patients are unresponsive to the standard approaches for managing uric acid and electrolyte abnormalities. • Identify at-risk patients. • Institute essential preventive measures (e.g., fluid hydration, medications) as prescribed. • Assess patient for signs and symptoms of electrolyte imbalances. • Assess urine pH to confirm alkalization. • Monitor serum electrolyte and uric acid levels for evidence of fluid volume overload secondary to aggressive hydration. • Instruct patients to monitor for and report symptoms indicating electrolyte disturbances.

MRI, magnetic resonance imaging; CT, computed tomography.

Adapted from Baehring, Y. (2015). Oncologic emergencies: Spinal cord compression. In V. T. DeVita, T. S. Lawrence, & S. A. Rosenberg (Eds.). *Cancer: Principles & practice of oncology.* Philadelphia, PA: Lippincott Williams & Wilkins; Wallace, A., Robinson, C., Myer, J., et al. (2015). The metastatic spine disease multidisciplinary working group algorithms. *The Oncologist, 20* (9), 1—11; Wang, L., Jian, Y., Yang, G., et al. (2015). Management of tumor lysis syndrome in patients with multiple myeloma during bortezomib treatment. *Clinical Journal of Oncology Nursing. 19*(1), E4–E7; Yahalom, J. (2015). Oncologic emergencies: Superior vena cava syndrome. In V. T. DeVita, T. S. Lawrence, & S. A. Rosenberg (Eds.). *Cancer: Principles & Practice of Oncology.* Philadelphia, PA: Lippincott Williams & Wilkins.

Weakness, altered mobility, fatigue, and inactivity typically increase with advanced cancer as a result of the disease, treatment, inadequate nutritional intake, or dyspnea. The nurse works with the patient and family to identify realistic goals and promote comfort. Measures include use of energy conservation methods to accomplish tasks and activities that the patient values most.

Efforts are made to provide the patient with as much control and independence as desired but with assurance that support and assistance are available when needed. In addition, health care teams work with the patient and family to ascertain and comply with the patient's wishes about treatment methods and care as the terminal phase of illness and death approach.

Hospice

The needs of patients with end-stage illness are best met by a comprehensive interdisciplinary specialty program that focuses on quality of life; palliation of symptoms; and provision of physical, psychosocial, and spiritual support for patients and families when cure and control of the disease are no longer possible. The concept of hospice best addresses these needs.

Hospice care is often delivered through coordination of specialty services provided by hospitals, home care programs, and the community. Patients need to be referred to hospice services in a timely fashion so that complex patient and family needs can be addressed. (See Chapter 16 for detailed discussion of end-of-life care.)

CRITICAL THINKING EXERCISES

1 pq A 63-year-old man previously treated for stage III prostate cancer with HDR brachytherapy and androgen deprivation therapy returns to the cancer center for a follow-up visit. While you are assessing his vital signs, he tells you that he has been having back pain for the last 3 weeks that he attributes to sleeping on an old mattress. What are the priorities to include in your nursing assessment of this patient? Identify the diagnostic procedures that you anticipate will be required to further evaluate this patient's back pain. What are your priorities for care of this patient?

2 An 80-year-old woman, who lives alone, was just recently diagnosed with stage IV colon cancer. She is being discharged from the hospital following a palliative colon resection. What will be the focus of educating this patient for self-care? Describe at least three age-related implications that will be important to consider. What type of referrals might be appropriate for this woman?

3 ebp You are caring for a 32-year-old woman who is a breast cancer survivor. The patient takes tamoxifen 20 mg orally once daily and this will continue for the next 5 years. Are there any preventive measures that should be considered to address survivorship needs? What is the evidence for these interventions and education that you identified? How strong is that evidence, and what criteria did you use to assess the strength of that evidence?

REFERENCES

*Asterisk indicates nursing research.
**Double asterisk indicates classic reference.

Books

Acharyya, S., Matrisian, L., Welch, D. R., et al. (2015). Invasion and metastasis. In J. Mendelsohn, P. M. Howley, M. A. Israel, et al. (Eds.). *The molecular basis of cancer*. Philadelphia, PA: Elsevier-Saunders.

Alt-Epping, B., & Nauck, F. (Eds.). (2015). *Palliative care in oncology*. Berlin: Springer.

Baehring, Y. (2015). Oncologic emergencies: Spinal cord compression. In V.T. DeVita, T. S. Lawrence, & S. A. Rosenberg (Eds.). *Cancer: Principles & practice of oncology*. Philadelphia, PA: Lippincott Williams & Wilkins.

Barbarotta, L. M. (2015). Oncologic emergencies in critical care. In Booker, K. J. *Critical care nursing: Monitoring and treatment for advanced nursing practice*. Oxford, UK: Wiley Blackwell.

Comerford, K. C. (2015). *Nursing 2015 drug handbook*. Philadelphia, PA: Wolters Kluwer.

DeNavas-Walt, C., Proctor, B. D., & Smith, J. C. (2013). *Income, poverty, and health insurance coverage in the United States: 2012*. Washington, DC: U.S. Government Printing Office, Report # P60–245.

Grossman, S. C., & Porth, C. M. (2014). *Porth's pathophysiology: Concepts of altered health states* (9th ed.). Philadelphia, PA: Lippincott Williams & Wilkins.

**Hewitt, M., Greenfield, S., & Stovall, E. (Eds.). (2006). *From cancer patient to cancer survivor*. Washington, DC: Institute of Medicine and National Research Council, National Academies Press.

Halperin, E. C., Wazer, D. E, Perez, C. A., et al. (Eds.). (2013). *Perez and Brady's principles and practice of radiation oncology* (6th ed.). Philadelphia, PA: Lippincott Williams and Wilkins.

Kasper, D. L., Fauci, A. S., Hauser, S. L., et al. (Eds.). (2015). *Harrison's principles of internal medicine* (19th ed.). New York: McGraw Hill Education.

Lu, Y., Clague, J., & Bernstein, L. (2015). Cancer etiology: Obesity and physical activity. In V. T. DeVita, T. S. Lawrence, & S. A. Rosenberg (Eds.). *Cancer: Principles & practice of oncology*. Philadelphia, PA: Lippincott Williams & Wilkins.

Maziarz, R. T., & Schubach-Slater, S. (Eds.). (2015). *Blood and marrow transplant handbook: Comprehensive guide for patient care*. New York: Springer.

Morgan, M. A., Ten Haken, R. K., & Lawrence, T. S. (2015). Essentials of radiation therapy In V. T. DeVita, T. S. Lawrence, & S. A. Rosenberg (Eds.). *Cancer: Principles & practice of oncology*. Lippincott Williams & Wilkins: Philadelphia.

Nguyen, D. M., Summers, R. M., & Finkelstein, S. E. (2015). Cancer diagnosis: Respiratory tract. In V. T. DeVita, T. S. Lawrence, & S. A. Rosenberg (Eds.). *Cancer: Principles & practice of oncology*. Philadelphia, PA: Lippincott Williams & Wilkins.

Schulmeister, L. (2014). Safe management of chemotherapy: Infusion-related complications. In M. Polovich, M. Olsen, & M. LeFebvre (Eds.). *Chemotherapy and biotherapy guideline and recommendations for practice* (4th ed.). Pittsburgh: Oncology Nursing Society.

Segal, B. H., Walsh, T. J., Gea-Banacloche, J. C., et al. (2015). Infections in the cancer patient. In V. T. DeVita, T. S. Lawrence, & S. A. Rosenberg (Eds.). *Cancer: Principles & practice of oncology*. Philadelphia, PA: Lippincott Williams & Wilkins.

U.S. Department of Health and Human Services. (2014). *The health consequences of smoking-50 years of progress: A report from the Surgeon General*. Atlanta, GA: Author.

Yahalom, J. (2015). Oncologic emergencies: Superior vena cava syndrome. In V. T. DeVita, T. S. Lawrence, & S. A. Rosenberg (Eds.). *Cancer: Principles & practice of oncology*. Philadelphia, PA: Lippincott Williams & Wilkins.

Journals and Electronic Documents

Alesi E. R., & del Fabbro, E. (2014). Opportunities for targeting the fatigue-anorexia-cachexia symptom cluster. *The Cancer Journal, 20*(5), 325–329.

American Cancer Society (ACS). (2014). Cancer treatment and survivorship: Facts and figures 2014–2015. Retrieved on 3/22/2016 at: www.cancer.org/acs/groups/content/@research/documents/document/acspc- 042801.pdf

American Cancer Society (ACS). (2015a). Cancer facts and figures 2015. Retrieved on 2/22/2016 at: www.cancer.org/acs/groups/content/@editorial/documents/document/acspc-044552.pdf

American Cancer Society (ACS). (2015b). Menopausal hormone therapy and cancer risk. Retrieved on 3/4/2016 at: www.cancer.org/cancer/cancercauses/othercarcinogens/medicaltreatments/menopausal- hormone-replacement-therapy-and-cancer-risk

American Cancer Society (ACS). (2016a). Cancer facts and figures for African Americans 2016–2018. Retrieved on 12/01/2016 at: www.cancer.org/acs/groups/content/@editorial/documents/document/acspc-047403.pdf

American Cancer Society (ACS). (2016b). Cancer facts and figures 2016. Retrieved 12/1/16 at: www.cancer.org/acs/groups/content/@research/documents/document/acspc-047079.pdf

Braskett, M., & Cohen, M. (2014). Diagnosis and management of chemotherapy induced hypersensitivity reactions. American College of Physicians Hospitalist, Retrieved on 3/11/2016 at: www.acphospitalist.org/archives/2014/06/expert_analysis.htm.

Beck, M. (2015). Radiation safety in the management of patients undergoing radioactive iodine ablation therapy. *Clinical Journal of Oncology Nursing, 19*(1), 44–46.

Bender, C. M., & Thelen, B. D. (2013). Cancer and cognitive changes: The complexity of the problem. *Seminars in Oncology Nursing, 29*(4), 232–237.

Benito, L., Binefa, G., Lluch, T., et al. (2014). Defining the role of the nurse in population-based cancer screening programs: A literature review. *Oncology Nursing Forum, 18*(2), 77–83.

Bessede, E., Dubus, P., Megraud, F., et al. (2014). Helicobacter pylori infection and stem cells at the origin of gastric cancer. *Oncogene, 34*(20), 2547–2555.

Blix, A. (2014). Personalized medicine, genomics, and pharmacogenomics: A primer for nurses. *Clinical Journal of Oncology Nursing, 18*(4), 437–441.

Bozzetti, F. (2013). Nutritional support of the oncology patient. *Critical Reviews in Oncology & Hematology, 87*(2), 172–200.

Brittain, K., & Murphy, V. P. (2015). Sociocultural and health correlates related to colorectal cancer screening adherence among urban African Americans. *Cancer Nursing, 38*(2), 118–124.

Bryant, A. L., Walton, A. L., & Phillips, B. (2015). Cancer-related fatigue: Scientific progress has been made in 40 years. *Clinical Journal of Oncology Nursing, 19*(2), 137–139.

Caruana, I., Diaconu, I., & Dottia, G. (2014). From monoclonal antibodies to chimeric antigen receptors for the treatment of human malignancies. *Seminars in Oncology, 41*(5), 661–666.

Castells, M. C. (2015). Anaphylaxis to chemotherapy and monoclonal antibodies in anapylaxis. *Immunology and allergy clinics of North America, 35*(2), 335–348.

Centers for Disease Control and Prevention (CDC). (2015). Hepatitis B FAQs for health professionals. Retrieved 3/7/16 at: www.cdc.gov/hepatitis/hbv/hbvfaq.htm#D4

Chen, C. J., Hsu, W. L., Yang, H. I., et al. (2014). Epidemiology of virus infection and human cancer. *Recent Results in Cancer Research, 193*, 11–32.

Citrin, D. E., & Mitchell, J. B. (2014). Altering the response to radiation: Sensitizers and protectors. *Seminars in Oncology, 41*(6), 848–859.

Chung, T. K., Rosenthal, E. L., Magnuson, J. S., et al. (2015). Transoral robotic surgery for oropharyngeal and tongue cancer in the United States. *Laryngoscope, 125*(1), 140–145.

Clarke, T. C., Black, L. I., Stussman, B. J., et al. (2015). Trends in the use of complementary health approaches among adults: United States, 2002–2012. *National Health Statistics Reports, 79*, 1–16.

Collins, F. S., & Varmus, H., (2015). A new initiative on precision medicine. *New England Journal of Medicine, 372*(9), 793–795.

Corbin, K. S., Hellman, S., & Weichselbaum, R. R. (2013). Extracranial oligometastases: A subset of metastases curable with stereotactic radiotherapy. *Journal of Clinical Oncology, 31*(11), 1384–1390.

Cotogni, P., Barbero, C., Garrino C., et al. (2015). Peripherally inserted central catheters in non-hospitalized cancer patients: 5-year results of a prospective study. *Supportive Care in Cancer, 23*(2), 403–409.

Coyle, C. E., Griffie, J., & Czaplewski, L. M. (2014). Eliminating extravasation events: A multidisciplinary approach. *Journal of Infusion Nursing, 37*(3), 157–164.

Damsky-Dell, D., Held-Warmkessel, J., Jakubek, P., et al. (2014). Care of the open abdomen after cytoreductive surgery and hyperthermic intraperitoneal chemotherapy for peritoneal surface malignancies. *Oncology Nursing Forum, 41*(4), 438–441.

Datta, S., Kundu, S., Ghosh, P., et al. (2014). Correlation of oxidant status with oxidative tissue damage in patients with rheumatoid arthritis. *Clinical Rheumatology, 33*(11), 1557–1564.

Di Lascio, S., & Pagani, O. (2014). Oligometastatic breast cancer: A shift from palliative to potentially curative treatment? *Breast Care, 9*(1), 7–14.

**DuPen, A. R., DuPen, S., Hansberry, J., et al. (2000). An educational implementation of a cancer pain algorithm for ambulatory care. *Pain Management Nursing, 1*(4), 118.

*Eaton, L. H., Mitchell, D. H., & Doorenbos, A. Z. (2015). Evidence-based practice beliefs and behaviors of nurses providing cancer pain management: A mixed-methods approach. *Oncology Nursing Forum, 42*(2), 165–173.

Eilers, J., Harris, D., Henry, K., et al (2014). Evidence-based interventions for cancer treatment-related mucositis: Putting evidence into practice. *Clinical Journal of Oncology Nursing, 18*(6), 80–96.

Fogh, S., & Yom, S. S. (2014). Symptom management during the radiation oncology treatment course: A practical guide for the oncology clinician. *Seminars in Oncology, 41*(6), 764–775.

Frankel Kelvin, J. (2015) Sperm banking: Fertility preservation for male patients with cancer. *Clinical Journal of Oncology Nursing, 19*(1), 108–110.

Fritz, A., Percy, C., Jack, A., et al. (2013). International classification of diseases for oncology (ICD-O)–3rd edition, 1st revision. Retrieved on 2/25/2016 at: apps.who.int/iris/bitstream/10665/96612/1/9789241548496_eng.pdf?ua=1

Gibson, R. J., Keefe, D. M., Lalla, R. V., et al. (2013). Systematic review of agents for the management of gastrointestinal mucositis in cancer patients. *Supportive Care in Cancer, 21*(1), 313–326.

Given, B. (2015). Prevention, identification, and management of late effects through risk reduction. *Seminars in Oncology Nursing, 31*(1), 31–41.

Goldfarb, S., Mulhall, J., Nelson, C., et al. (2013). Sexual and reproductive health in cancer survivors. *Seminars in Oncology, 40*(6), 726–744.

Gonella, S., & Di Giulio, P. (2015). Delayed chemotherapy-induced nausea and vomiting in the hematology population: A review of the literature. *Clinical Journal of Oncology Nursing, 19*(4), 438–443.

Gonzalez, T. (2013). Chemotherapy extravasations: Prevention, identification, management and documentation. *Clinical Journal of Oncology Nursing, 17*(1), 61–66.

Herrero, R., Quint, W., Hildesheim, S., et al. (2015). Reduced prevalence of oral human papillomavirus (HPV) 4 years after bivalent HPV vaccination in a randomized clinical trial in Costa Rica. *PLoS ONE, 8*(7), 1–9.

Heston, A. H., Schwartz, A. L., Justice-Gardiner, H., et al. (2015). Addressing physical activity needs of survivors by developing a community-based exercise program: LIVESTRONG® at the YMCA. *Clinical Journal of Oncology Nursing, 19*(2), 213–217.

IMS Institute. (2014). Innovation in cancer care and implications for health systems: Global oncology trend report. Retrieved 3/7/16 at: www.imshealth.com/vgn- ext-templating/v/index.jsp?vgnextoid=f8d4df7a5e8b5410VgnVCM10000076192ca2RCRD

Jansen, C. E. (2013). Cognitive changes associated with cancer and cancer therapy: Patient assessment and education. *Seminars in Oncology Nursing, 29*(4), 270–279.

Kannan, R., Madden, K., & Andrews, S. (2014). Primer on immuno-oncology and immune Response. *Clinical Journal of Oncology Nursing, 18*(3), 311–317, 326.

Kelvin, J. F., Steed, R., & Jarrett, J. (2014). Discussing safe sexual practices during cancer treatment. *Clinical Journal of Oncology Nursing, 18*(4), 449–453.

Knobf, M. (2013). Being prepared: Essential to self-care and quality of life for the person with cancer. *Clinical Journal of Oncology Nursing, 17*(3), 255–261.

Kohler, B. A., Sherman, R. L., Howlader N., et al. (2015). Annual report to the nation on the status of cancer, 1975–2011. *Journal of the National Cancer Institute, 107*(6), 1–25.

Kuter, D. J. (2015). Managing thrombocytopenia associated with cancer chemotherapy. *Oncology, 29*(4), 282–294.

*Lassiter, M., & Schneider, S. M. (2015). A pilot study comparing the neutropenic diet to a non-neutropenic diet in the allogeneic hematopoietic stem cell transplantation population. *Oncology Nursing Forum, 19*(3), 273–278.

Lovly, C. M., Horn, L., & Pao, W. (2015). KRAS in non-small cell lung cancer (NSCLC). My cancer genome. Retrieved on 2/25/2016 at: www.mycancergenome.org/content/disease/lung-cancer/kras/

Leduc-Souville, B., Bertrand, E., & Schlatter, J. (2013). Risk management of excreta in a cancer unit. *Clinical Journal of Oncology Nursing, 17*(3), 248–252.

Mack, F., Ritchie, M., & Sapra, P., (2014). The next generation of antibody drug conjugates. *Seminars in Oncology, 41*(5), 637–652.

Lukens, N. J., Gamez, M., Hu, K., et al. (2014). Modern brachytherapy. *Seminars in Oncology, 41*(6), 831–847.

Mahon, S. M. (2014). Providing care for previvors: Implications for oncology nurses. *Clinical Journal of Oncology Nursing, 18*(1), 21–24.

Manea, P. (2014). Optimizing the management of patients with myelofibrosis. *Clinical Journal of Oncology Nursing, 18*(3), 330–337.

Mazanec, P., & Prince-Paul, M. (2014). Integrating palliative care into active cancer treatment. *Seminars in Oncology Nursing, 30*(4), 203–211.

Merriman, J. D., Von Ah, D., Miaskowski, C., et al. (2013). Proposed mechanisms for cancer and treatment-related cognitive changes. *Seminars in Oncology Nursing, 29*(4), 260–269.

Miceli, T, Lilleby, T., Noonan, K., et al. (2013). Autologous hematopoietic stem cell transplantation for patients with multiple myeloma: An overview for nurses in community practice. *Clinical Journal of Oncology Nursing, 17*(6), 13–24.

Mitchell, S. A., Hoffman, A. J., Clark, J. C., et al. (2014). Putting evidence into practice: An update of evidence-based interventions for cancer-related fatigue during and following treatment. *Clinical Journal of Oncology Nursing, 18*(6), S38–S58.

Montezano A. C., Dulak-Lis, M., Tsiropoulou S., et al. (2015). Oxidative stress and human hypertension: Vascular mechanisms, biomarkers, and novel therapies. *Journal of Canadian Cardiology, 31*(5), 631–641.

National Cancer Institute (NCI). (2016). Cancer genetics overview for health professionals. Retrieved on 3/2/2016 at: www.cancer.gov/cancertopics/pdq/genetics/overview/healthprofessional

National Comprehensive Cancer Network (NCCN). (2015a). Clinical practice guidelines in oncology: Genetic/familial high risk assessment:

Breast and ovarian. Retrieved on 3/7/2016 at: www.nccn.org/professionals/physician_gls/pdf/genetics_screening.pdf

National Comprehensive Cancer Network (NCCN). (2015b). Clinical practice guidelines in oncology: Genetic/familial high risk assessment: Colorectal. Retrieved on 3/7/2016 at:www.nccn.org/professionals/physician_gls/pdf/genetics_colon.pdf

National Comprehensive Cancer Network (NCCN). (2015c). Clinical practice guidelines: Breast. Retrieved on 3/7/2016 at: www.nccn.org/professionals/physician_gls/PDF/infections.pdf

National Comprehensive Cancer Network (NCCN). (2015d). NCCN clinical practice guidelines in oncology: Prostate cancer. Retrieved on 3/10/2016 at: www.nccn.org/professionals/physician_gls/pdf/prostate.pdf

National Comprehensive Cancer Network (NCCN). (2015e). NCCN clinical practice guidelines in oncology: Antiemesis. Retrieved on 3/11/2016 at: www.nccn.org/professionals/physician_gls/pdf/antiemesis.pdf

National Comprehensive Cancer Network (NCCN). (2015f). NCCN guidelines for supportive care: Cancer related fatigue. Retrieved on 3/24/2016 at: www.nccn.org/professionals/physician_gls/f_guidelines.asp#fatigue

National Comprehensive Cancer Network (NCCN). (2015g). NCCN clinical practice guidelines in oncology: Distress [v.2.2015]. Retrieved on 3/28/2016 at: http://www.nccn.org/professionals/physician_gls/pdf/distress.pdf

National Comprehensive Cancer Network (NCCN). (2015h). NCCN clinical practice guidelines in oncology: Prevention and treatment of cancer-related infection [v.2.2015]. Retrieved on 3/28/2016 at: http://www.nccn.org/professionals/physician_gls/pdf/infections.pdf

National Comprehensive Cancer Network (NCCN). (2015i). NCCN clinical practice guidelines in oncology: Cancer-associated thromboembolic disease [v.1.2015]. Retrieved on 4/24/2016 at: http://www.nccn.org/professionals/physician_gls/pdf/vte.pdf

National Institutes of Health, National Center for Complementary and Integrative Health (NCCIH). (2015). Complementary, alternative, or integrative health: What's in a name? Retrieved on 10/10/2015 at: nccih.nih.gov/health/integrative-health

Neuss, M. N., Polovich. M., McNiff, K., et al. (2013). 2013 Updated American Society of Clinical Oncology/Oncology Nursing Society chemotherapy administration safety standards including standards for the safe administration and management of oral chemotherapy. *Oncology Nursing Forum, 40*(3), 225–233.

Niklas, C., Saar, M., Berg, B., et al. (2016). da Vinci and open radical prostatectomy: Comparison of clinical outcomes and analysis of insurance costs. *Urologia International, 96*(3), 287–294.

Oeffinger, K. C. (Ed.). (2013). Science of survivorship: Moving from risk to risk reduction. *Seminars in Oncology, 40*(6), 659–812, S1–S4

O'Gorman, C., Sasiadek, W., Denieffe, S., et al. (2015). Predicting radiotherapy-related clinical toxicities in cancer: A literature review. *Clinical Journal of Oncology Nursing, 18*(3), 37–44.

Pachman, D., Price, K. A., & Carey, E. C. (2014). Nonpharmacologic approach to fatigue in patients with cancer. *The Cancer Journal, 20*(5), 313–318.

Schiller, J. T., & Lowy, D. R. (2014). Virus infection and human cancer: An overview. *Recent Results in Cancer Research. 193,*1–10.

Schilli, S. M. (2014). Screening for distress in patients with cancer. *Clinical Journal of Oncology Nursing, 18*(6), E103–E106.

Shackelford, J. A., Weyhenmeyer, D. P., & Mabus, L. K. (2015). Fostering early breast cancer detection: Faith community nurses reaching at-risk populations. *Oncology Nursing Forum, 18*(6), 113–118.

Siegel, R. L., Miller, K. D., & Jemal, A. (2015). Cancer statistics, 2015. *Cancer Journal for Clinicians, 65*(1), 5–29.

Tayyem, A. Q. (2014). Cryotherapy effect on oral mucositis severity among recipients of bone marrow transplantation: A literature review. *Clinical Journal of Oncology Nursing, 18*(4), E84–E87.

Tipian, C. (2014). Brushing up on mouth care for cancer patients with mucositis. *American Nurse Today, 9*(11), 38–40.

Thomson, C. A., McCullough, M. L., Wertheim, B., et al. (2014). Nutrition and physical activity cancer prevention guidelines, cancer risk, and mortality in the Women's Health Initiative. *Cancer Prevention Research, 7*(1), 42–53.

Tofthagen, C., Visovsky, C. M., & Hopgood, R. (2013). Chemotherapy-induced peripheral neuropathy: An algorithm to guide nursing management. *Clinical Journal of Oncology Nursing, 17*(2), 138–144.

Smith, A. (2015). A workshop for educating nurses to address sexual health in patients with breast cancer. *Clinical Journal of Oncology Nursing, 19*(3), 248–250.

Smith, T. J., Bohlke, K., Lyman, G. H., et al. (2015). Recommendations for the use of WBC growth factors: American Society of Clinical Oncology clinical practice guideline update. *Journal of Clinical Oncology, 33*(28), 3199–3212.

Vadhan-Raj, S., Goldberg, J. D., Perales, M. A., et al. (2013). Clinical applications of palifermin: Amelioration of oral mucositis and other potential indications. *Journal of Cell & Molecular Medicine. 17*(11), 1371–1384.

Vioral, A., Leslie, M., Best, R., et al. (2014). Patient adherence with oral oncolytic therapies. *Seminars in Oncology Nursing, 30*(3), 190–199.

**Vogel, V. G., Costantino, J. P., Wickerham, D. L., et al. (2010). Update of the national surgical adjuvant breast and bowel project study of Tamoxifen and Raloxifene (STAR) P- 2 Trial: Preventing breast cancer. *Cancer Prevention Research, 3*(6), 696–706.

Von Ah, D. (2015). Cognitive changes associated with cancer and cancer treatment: State of the science. *Clinical Journal of Oncology Nursing, 19*(1), 47–56.

Wallace, A., Robinson, C., Myer, J., et al. (2015). The metastatic spine disease multidisciplinary working group algorithms. *The Oncologist, 20*(9), 1–11.

Wang, L., Jian,Y., Yang, G., et al. (2015). Management of tumor lysis syndrome in patients with multiple myeloma during bortezomib treatment. *Clinical Journal of Oncology Nursing, 19*(1), E4–E7.

Weber, J. S. (2014). Immuno-oncology comes of age. *Seminars in Oncology, 41*(5), S1–S2.

Yagasaki, K., & Komatsu, H. (2013). The need for a nursing presence in oral chemotherapy. *Clinical Journal of Oncology Nursing, 17*(5), 512–516.

Resources

American Association of Cancer Research (AACR), www.aacr.org
American Cancer Society (ACS), www.cancer.org/
American College of Surgeons Commission on Cancer (CoC), https://www.facs.org/quality-programs/cancer/coc
American Pain Society (APS), www.ampainsoc.org
American Society of Clinical Oncology (ASCO), www.asco.org
American Society for Radiation Oncology (ASTRO), www.astro.org
Association of Oncology Social Work (AOSW), http://www.aosw.org
Cancer Care, http://www.cancercare.org/
Centers for Disease Control and Prevention (CDC): Cancer Control and Prevention: http://www.cdc.gov/cancer/
Hospice and Palliative Nurses Association (HPNA), www.hpna.org
LIVESTRONG Survivorship Centers of Excellence, www.livestrong.org
National Cancer Institute (NCI), www.cancer.gov
National Institutes of Health, National Center for Complementary and Integrative Health (NCCIH), nccih.nih.gov
National Coalition for Cancer Survivorship, www.canceradvocacy.org
National Comprehensive Cancer Network (NCCN), www.nccn.org
National Hospice and Palliative Care Organization, www.nhpco.org
OncoLink (cancer resources), www.oncolink.org
Oncology Nursing Society (ONS), www.ons.org
Quackwatch, www.quackwatch.org
The Bone Marrow Foundation, http://bonemarrow.org/
The Cancer Support Community, http://www.cancersupportcommunity.org/
The Leukemia and Lymphoma Society, www.lls.org

16 End-of-Life Care

On completion of this chapter, the learner will be able to:

1 Discuss the historical, legal, and sociocultural perspectives of palliative and end-of-life care in the United States.
2 Define palliative and end-of-life care.
3 Compare and contrast the settings where palliative care and end-of-life care are provided.
4 Describe the principles and components of hospice care.
5 Identify barriers to improving care at the end of life.
6 Reflect on personal experience with and attitudes toward death and dying.

7 Apply skills for communicating with seriously ill patients and their families.
8 Provide culturally and spiritually sensitive care to seriously ill patients and their families.
9 Implement nursing measures to manage physiologic responses to terminal illness.
10 Support imminently dying patients and their families.
11 Identify components of uncomplicated grief and mourning and implement nursing measures to support patients and families.

GLOSSARY

assisted suicide: providing another person the means to end their own life
autonomy: self-determination; in the health care context, the right of the individual to make choices about the use and discontinuation of medical interventions
bereavement: period during which mourning for a loss takes place
euthanasia: Greek for "good death"; has evolved to mean the intentional killing by act or omission of a dependent human being for their alleged benefit
grief: personal feelings that accompany an anticipated or actual loss
hospice: a coordinated program of interdisciplinary care and services for terminally ill patients and their families that in the United States is provided primarily in the home
interdisciplinary collaboration: communication and cooperation among members of diverse health care disciplines jointly to plan, implement, and evaluate care
Medicare Hospice Benefit: a Medicare Part A entitlement that provides for comprehensive, interdisciplinary palliative care and services for eligible beneficiaries who have a terminal illness and a life expectancy of less than 6 months

mourning: individual, family, group, and cultural expressions of grief and associated behaviors
palliative care: philosophy of and system for delivering care that expands on traditional medical care for serious, progressive illness to include a focus on quality of life, function, decision making, and opportunities for personal growth
palliative sedation: the use of pharmacologic agents, at the request of the terminally ill patient or the patient's legal proxy, to induce sedation, or near-sedation, when symptoms have not responded to other management measures; the purpose is not to hasten the patient's death but to relieve intractable symptoms
prognosis: the expected course of an illness and the chance for recovery
spirituality: personal belief systems that focus on a search for meaning and purpose in life, intangible elements that impart meaning and vitality to life, and a connectedness to a higher or transcendent dimension
terminal illness: progressive, irreversible illness that despite cure-focused medical treatment will result in the patient's death

Nurses can have a significant and lasting effect on the way patients live until they die, the manner in which the death occurs, and the enduring memories of that death for the families. The contemporary definition of nursing includes "…the diagnosis and treatment of human responses, and advocacy in the care of individuals, families, groups, communities, and populations" (American Nurses Association [ANA], 2015, p. 1). There may be no group more important than seriously ill and dying patients.

Knowledge about palliative and end-of-life principles of care and patients' and families' unique responses to illness is essential to supporting their unique values and goals. Nurses

have an opportunity to bring research, education, and practice together to impact the culture of dying, bringing much-needed improvement to care that is relevant across practice settings, age groups, cultural backgrounds, and illnesses. The National Institute of Nursing Research established the Office of End-of-Life and Palliative Care Research (OEPCR) to further advance the science and coordinate research-related to end-of-life care within the National Institutes of Health (NIH). Nurses in all settings are likely to encounter seriously ill patients and families who can benefit from palliative care during advanced illness and at end of life. This chapter presents concepts about death and dying in the United States, settings for end-of-life care of the dying, and ways that nurses can address the health issues of terminally ill patients.

Nursing and End-of-Life Care

Death and Dying in America

Focus on care of the dying is motivated by the aging of the population, the prevalence of and publicity surrounding life-threatening illnesses, and the increasing likelihood of a prolonged period of chronic illness prior to death (e.g., cancer and noncancer diagnoses such as heart failure, chronic obstructive pulmonary disease (COPD), and Alzheimer's disease). By 2030, the number of persons older than 85 years is expected to double. Although there are more opportunities than ever before to support peaceful death, the technologies that are often applied in advanced illness and at end of life continue to make the process of dying anything but peaceful. Patients, families, and clinicians may view death as what happens when medicine fails. This attitude places death and improvement of the dying process outside the focus of modern medicine and health care. Numerous initiatives aimed at improving end-of-life care have been launched in recent years, spurred by a widespread call for substantive change in the way Americans deal with death.

The National Consensus Project for Quality Palliative Care (NCP, 2013) identified the following eight key domains underlying a more comprehensive and humane approach to care of the dying. These include:

- *Structure and processes of care:* The timely plan of care is based on a comprehensive interdisciplinary assessment of the patient and the family.
- *Physical aspects of care:* Pain, other symptoms, and side effects are managed based on the best available evidence, with attention to disease-specific pain and symptoms, which is skillfully and systematically applied.
- *Psychological and psychiatric aspects of care:* Psychological status is assessed and managed based on the best available evidence, which is skillfully and systematically applied. When necessary, psychiatric issues are addressed and treated.
- *Social aspects of care:* Comprehensive interdisciplinary assessment identifies the social needs of patients and their families, and a plan of care is developed to respond to these needs as effectively as possible.
- *Spiritual, religious, and existential aspects of care:* Spiritual and existential dimensions are assessed and responded to based on the best available evidence, which is skillfully and systematically applied.
- *Cultural aspects of care:* The palliative care program assesses and attempts to meet the needs of the patient, family, and community in a culturally sensitive manner.
- *Care of the patient at the end of life:* Signs and symptoms of impending death are recognized and communicated in developmentally appropriate language for children and patients with cognitive disabilities with respect to family preferences. Care appropriate to this phase of illness is provided to the patient and the family.
- *Ethical and legal aspects of care:* The patient's goals, preferences, and choices are respected within the limits of applicable state and federal law, within current accepted standards of medical care, and form the basis for the plan of care.

The practice guidelines specified under each of these domains have been endorsed by more than 50 national organizations such as the AARP (formerly known as the American Association for Retired Persons), American Cancer Society (ACS), Hospice and Palliative Nurses Association (HPNA), and the National Hospice and Palliative Care Organization (NHPCO) to structure and evaluate quality palliative and end-of-life programs.

In 2014, the Institute of Medicine (IOM) released a consensus report titled *Dying in America: Improving Quality and Honoring Individual Preferences Near the End of Life.* The report presents a summary of findings from a review of the evidence and recommendations for improving palliative and end-of-life care. The authors noted that patients experienced many transitions in settings, frequent and potentially avoidable hospital readmission, and inconsistent referral to palliative care. Recommendations include widespread and timely access to, and comprehensive coverage for palliative care services, improved communication between providers, greater emphasis on advance care planning, professional education and development, and stronger public education and engagement (IOM, 2014a).

Technology and End-of-Life Care

In the 20th century, chronic, degenerative diseases replaced communicable diseases as the major causes of death. In the earlier part of the 20th century, most deaths occurred at home and most families had direct experience with death, providing care to family members at the end of life and then mourning their losses. As the place of death shifted from home to hospitals, families became increasingly distanced from the death experience.

The application of technology to prolong life raises numerous ethical issues. One major question is: Because we *can* prolong life through increasingly sophisticated technology, does it necessarily follow that we *must* do so? In the latter half of the 20th century, a "technologic imperative" practice pattern among health care professionals emerged, along with an expectation among patients and families that every available means to extend life must be tried. By the early 1970s, when hospice care was just beginning in the United States, technology had become an expected companion of the critically and terminally ill.

In the 21st century, technological intervention at the end of life continues to have profound implications, affecting how clinicians care for the dying, how family and friends participate in care, how patients and families understand and choose among end-of-life care options, how families prepare for terminal illness and death, and how they heal after the death of a loved one.

Sociocultural Context

Although **terminal illness**, a progressive, irreversible illness that despite cure-focused medical treatment will result in the patient's death, is experienced uniquely by each person, it is also shaped by the broader social and cultural contexts in which it occurs. The approach in the United States to serious illness has been described as "death denying"—that is, the health care system has been built on management of acute illness and the use of technology to cure (when possible) and to extend life. As a result, life-threatening illness, life-sustaining treatment decisions, dying, and death occur in a social environment in which illness is largely considered an enemy. Many common expressions reflect this dominant sociocultural view. For example, people talk about the "war" against cancer or "fighting" illness, and when patients choose not to pursue the most aggressive course of medical treatment available, many health care providers and indeed patients and families perceive this as "giving up." A care/cure dichotomy has persisted in which health care providers may view cure as the ultimate good and care as second best, a good only when cure is no longer possible. In such a model, alleviating suffering is not as valued as curing disease. Patients who cannot be cured feel distanced from the health care team, and when curative treatments have failed, they may feel that they too have failed. Patients and families may fear that any shift from curative goals to comfort-focused care will result in no care or lower-quality care, and that the clinicians on whom they have come to rely will abandon them if they withdraw from a focus on cure.

The statement in late-stage illness that exemplifies this care versus cure dichotomy is "nothing more can be done." This all-too-frequently used statement communicates the belief of many clinicians that there is nothing of value to offer patients beyond cure; however, in a care-focused perspective, there is always more that can be done. This expanded notion of healing implies that healing can take place throughout life. There are many opportunities for physical, spiritual, emotional, and social healing, even as body systems begin to fail at the end of life.

Clinicians' Attitudes Toward Death

Clinicians' attitudes toward the terminally ill and dying remain the greatest barrier to improving care at the end of life. Kübler-Ross illuminated the concerns of the seriously ill and dying in her seminal work, *On Death and Dying*, first published in 1969. At that time, it was common for patients to be kept uninformed about life-threatening diagnoses, particularly cancer, and for physicians and nurses to avoid open discussion of death and dying with their patients. Kübler-Ross's work revealed that, given open discussion, adequate time, and some help in working through the process, patients could reach a stage of acceptance in which they were neither angry nor depressed about their fate (see later discussion).

Clinicians' reluctance to discuss disease and death openly with patients stems from their own anxieties about death as well as misconceptions about what and how much patients want to know about their illnesses. In an early study of care of the dying in hospital settings, sociologists Glaser and Strauss (1965) discovered that health care professionals in hospital settings avoided direct communication about dying in the hope that the patient would discover it on their own. They identified four "awareness contexts":

1. *Closed awareness:* The patient is unaware of their terminal state, whereas others are aware. Closed awareness may be characterized as a conspiracy between the family and the health care professionals to guard the "secret," fearing that the patient may not be able to cope with full disclosure about their status and the patient's acceptance of others' accounts of their "future biography" as long as the others give him or her no reason to be suspicious.

2. *Suspected awareness:* The patient suspects what others know and attempts to find out details about their condition. Suspected awareness may be triggered by inconsistencies in the family's and the clinician's communication and behavior, discrepancies between clinicians' accounts of the seriousness of the patient's illness, or a decline in the patient's condition or other environmental cues.

3. *Mutual pretense awareness:* The patient, the family, and the health care professionals are aware that the patient is dying, but all pretend otherwise.

4. *Open awareness:* The patient, the family, and the health care professionals are aware that the patient is dying and openly acknowledge that reality.

Glaser and Strauss (1965) also identified a pattern of clinician behavior in which those clinicians who feared or were uncomfortable discussing death developed and substituted "personal mythologies" for appraisals of what level of disclosure their patients actually wanted. For example, clinicians avoided direct communication with patients about the seriousness of their illness based on their beliefs that (1) patients already knew the truth or would ask if they wanted to know, or (2) patients would subsequently lose all hope, give up, or be psychologically harmed by disclosure.

Although Glaser and Strauss's findings were published decades ago, their observations remain valid today. The growth of palliative and hospice care programs has led to greater numbers of health care providers becoming comfortable with and skilled in assessing patients' and families' information needs and disclosing honest information about the seriousness of illness (Bernacki & Block, 2014). However, in many settings, clinicians still avoid the topic of death in the hope that patients will ask or find out on their own. Despite progress on many health care fronts, many who work with seriously ill and dying patients recognize a persistent conspiracy of silence about dying.

How to communicate truthfully with patients and encourage patient **autonomy** (the right of the individual to make choices) in a way that acknowledges where they are on the continuum of acceptance is a challenge. Despite continued reluctance of health care providers to engage in open discussion about end-of-life issues, patients want information about their illness and end-of-life choices and are not harmed by open discussion about death (The Conversation Project, 2013; Hoff & Hermeren, 2014). Timing of sensitive discussion takes experience, but speaking the truth can be a relief to patients and families, enhancing their autonomy by making way for truly informed consent as the basis for decision making. (See later section for detailed discussion of communication skills.)

Patient and Family Concerns

Patient and family denial about the seriousness of terminal illness has also been cited as a barrier to discussion about end-of-life treatment options. Yet, research demonstrates that denial can be a useful coping mechanism that enables the patient to gain temporary emotional distance from a situation that is too painful to contemplate fully (Benkel, Wijk, & Molander, 2010). Denial may become a *barrier* to care if patients or families refuse to acknowledge a diagnosis or refuse to hear about treatment options. Nurses must accept patients regardless of the degree to which they are in denial about their illness and work with other health care providers to present a consistent message.

Patient and family awareness of **prognosis** is a key factor in acceptance of and planning for death. Even patients and families who have received clear and honest information may not fully accept the situation. For patients who have been informed about terminal illness, their understanding of treatment goals and prognosis is dynamic and may sometimes require reinforcement.

Another concern is that patients' and their caregivers' understanding of treatment goals and prognosis can differ dramatically. In a study of patients receiving palliative radiation therapy for metastases, researchers found that 25% of patients believed that radiation therapy would cure the cancer and prolong their lives (Mitera, Zhang, Sahgal, et al., 2012). Such misunderstandings can complicate both delivery of effective care and informed consent for care.

Patients with noncancer diagnoses, such as heart failure, COPD, kidney injury, dementia, or neurodegenerative diseases such as amyotrophic lateral sclerosis, frequently do not receive adequate information and support to fully understand their prognosis, yet they often desire clear and honest information. For example, they may have troublesome symptoms and reduced quality of life paralleling or exceeding that of patients with cancer. Patients may want but are unlikely to receive clear information about disease progression, advance care planning, and prognosis. Research is needed to examine the complex interactions between patients' misconceptions about advanced illness, their underlying psychological states, and barriers to clinicians' explanations of treatment expectations and prognosis.

Assisted Suicide

The assisted suicide debate has aimed a spotlight on the adequacy and quality of end-of-life care in the United States. **Assisted suicide** refers to providing another person the means to end their own life. Physician-assisted suicide involves the prescription by a physician of a lethal dose of medication for the purpose of ending someone's life (not to be confused with the ethically and legally supported practice of withholding or withdrawing medical treatment in accordance with the wishes of the terminally ill person).

Although assisted suicide is expressly prohibited under statutory or common law in the majority of states, calls for legalized assisted suicide have highlighted inadequacies in the care of the dying. Public support for physician-assisted suicide has resulted in numerous state ballot initiatives. In 1994, Oregon voters approved the Oregon Death With Dignity Act, the first and—until 2008—only such legislative initiative to pass. This law provides for access to physician-assisted suicide by terminally ill patients under very controlled circumstances. After numerous challenges, the law was enacted in 1997. Of 1327 Oregonians who have received written prescriptions under the terms of the law since it was passed in 1997, 859 have self-administered physician-prescribed lethal medication and have died (Oregon Public Health Division, 2015).

In November 2008, voters approved the Washington Death With Dignity Act. Modeled after the Oregon Death With Dignity law, the act contains the same safeguards and is given through the Washington State Department of Health (Washington State Department of Health, 2015). In 2009, Montana's Supreme Court ruled that physician aid in dying is not a crime, making this the third state to legalize assisted suicide. In 2013, Vermont became the next state to enact assisted suicide legislation (Vermont Department of Health, 2015). In 2014, 29-year-old California resident Brittany Maynard learned that she had terminal brain cancer and moved to Oregon, so that she could establish residence and end her life under Oregon's law. In 2015, California's governor signed the End of Life Options Act, modeled after Oregon's law. Numerous other states have considered and rejected assisted suicide ballot initiatives. A Gallup Poll (2015) reflected an increase in support for assisted suicide (68%), an increase of nearly 20 points in the prior 2 years. It is likely that the issue will continue to be pursued in the courts and through ballot measures in other states.

Proponents of physician-assisted suicide argue that terminally ill people should have a legally sanctioned right to make independent decisions about the value of their lives and the timing and circumstances of their deaths, and its opponents argue for greater access to symptom management and psychosocial support for people approaching the end of life.

In its 2010 position statement on *Registered Nurses' Roles and Responsibilities in Providing Expert Care and Counseling at the End of Life*, the ANA acknowledges the complexity of the assisted suicide debate but clearly states that nursing participation in assisted suicide is a violation of the Code for Nurses. The ANA position statement further stresses the important role of the nurse in supporting effective symptom management, contributing to the creation of environments for care that honor the patient's and family's wishes, as well as identifying their concerns and fears (ANA, 2010). In its position statement on *Euthanasia, Assisted Suicide and Aid in Dying*, the ANA clearly prohibits nurses' participation in assisted suicide and euthanasia

> because these acts are in direct violation of (*the Code of Ethics*), the ethical traditions and goals of the profession, and its covenant with society. Nurses have an obligation to provide humane, comprehensive, and compassionate care that respects the rights of patients but upholds the standards of the profession in the presence of chronic, debilitating illness and at end-of-life (ANA, 2013, p. 1).

Similarly, the HPNA opposes the legalization of assisted suicide and affirms the value of comprehensive end-of-life care (HPNA, 2011). The Oncology Nursing Society has endorsed the HPNA position, and this organization also calls for quality palliative care (ONS, 2014). The American Academy of Hospice and Palliative Medicine (AAHPM, 2007) has taken a position of "studied neutrality" on assisted death, recommending that clinicians carefully assess the fear and suffering that have led patients to request assisted suicide and to address these without hastening death (see Chart 16-1).

Settings for End-of-Life Care

Palliative Care

Palliative care is an approach to care for the seriously ill that has long been a part of cancer care. More recently, it has

Chart 16-1   ETHICAL DILEMMA
What If a Patient Asks You to Help Her End Her Life?

Case Scenario

You are a hospice nurse making a first home visit to a 54-year-old woman, a registered nurse, with stage IV ovarian cancer with metastases to her lungs and liver. She now reports severe dyspnea and chest and abdominal pain that is increasing and unrelieved by any of the pharmacologic and nonpharmacologic interventions that have been tried. In addition, she appears grossly jaundiced and cachectic. Prior to her illness, she worked as a staff nurse in an oncology unit at a local hospital. She is married, with three children, one of whom is in college and studying nursing, and two of whom are in high school. The patient tells you "My oldest daughter is ready to enter her senior year of nursing school. She has told me she is going to drop out of school so she can take care of me and I don't want her to do that." She then tells you "I know what is in store for me and I don't want to go through that, and I do not want to ruin my daughter's career and her life. I want you to help me end things and if you do not, I will take care of ending things myself, on my own terms."

Discussion

Assisted suicide remains a highly controversial topic—is it a matter of personal choice (i.e., does it preserve the autonomy of those who are dying), or does it constitute homicide by health care professionals who should "first do no harm" (i.e., nonmaleficence)? At this time, five states in the United States (Oregon, Washington, Montana, Vermont, and California) legally permit physician-assisted suicide. However, the laws in these states include highly prescriptive criteria that must be present before a patient may be given a lethal prescription to end their own life.

The American Nurses Association, in its *Euthanasia, Assisted Suicide, and Aid in Dying Position Statement* (ANA, 2013), acknowledges the importance of the patient's right to self-determination, advocates that nurses must deliver optimal, compassionate care but avows that the nurse must never deliberately end a patient's life by euthanasia or physician-assisted suicide.

Analysis

How might you proceed with providing further consultation or follow-up with this patient? Would this follow-up be based upon whether or not she resided in a state where physician-assisted suicide is legal? Would her state of residence have any effect on your personal decision-making process?

Further describe the ethical principles that are in conflict in this case and in other cases that surround requests for assisted suicide (see Chart 3-3). Which principle do you believe should have preeminence in deciding whether or not patients have the right to request assistance in suicide at the end of life? Identify other resources or referrals that could be made to assist this patient in her end-of-life care.

Reference

American Nurses Association (2013). *Euthanasia, assisted suicide, and aid in dying position statement.* Retrieved on 8/27/2016 at: www.nursingworld.org/MainMenuCategories/EthicsStandards/Ethics-Position-Statements/Euthanasia-Assisted-Suicide-and-Aid-in-Dying.pdf

Resources

See Chapter 3, Chart 3-6 for ethics resources.

---

been expanded to address the comprehensive symptom management, psychosocial care, and spiritual support needed to enhance the quality of life for any person with advanced illness. Although hospice care is considered by many to be the gold standard for palliative care, the term **hospice** is generally associated with palliative care that is delivered at home or in special facilities to patients who are approaching the end of life (see later discussion). Palliative care and hospice care have been recognized as important bridges between cure-oriented treatment and the needs of terminally ill patients and their families for comprehensive care in the final years, months, or weeks of life. Advocates for improved care for the dying have stated that acceptance, management, and understanding of death should become fully integrated concepts in mainstream health care.

Palliative care, which is conceptually broader than hospice care, is both an approach to care and a structured system for care delivery that aims to optimize "quality of life by anticipating, preventing and treating suffering" (NCP, 2013, p. 9). Palliative care is characterized by interdisciplinary communication and coordination across the trajectory of serious illness, emphasizing management of psychological, social, and spiritual problems in addition to control of pain and other physical symptoms. As the definition suggests, palliative care does not begin when cure-focused treatment ends but instead is offered "concurrently with or independent of curative or life-prolonging care" (NCP, 2013, p. 9). The goal of palliative care is to improve the patient's and family's quality of life, and indeed many aspects of this type of

comprehensive, comfort-focused approach to care are applicable earlier in the process of life-threatening disease and in conjunction with cure-focused treatment.

In palliative care, **interdisciplinary collaboration** is necessary to bring about the desired outcomes for patients and their families. Interdisciplinary collaboration, which is different from multidisciplinary practice, is based on communication and cooperation among the various disciplines, with each member of the team contributing to a single integrated care plan that addresses the needs of the patient and the family. In contrast, multidisciplinary care refers to participation of clinicians with varied backgrounds and skill sets but without coordination and integration.

Palliative Care at the End of Life

The broadening of the application of palliative care in the United States actually *followed* the development of hospice programs. All hospice care is palliative care; however, not all palliative care is hospice care. The difference is that hospice care is an application of palliative care delivered at the end of life. Hospice care focuses on quality of life, and by necessity, it usually includes realistic emotional, social, spiritual, and financial preparation for death. After hospice care was recognized as a distinct program of services under Medicare in the early 1980s, organizations providing hospice care were able to receive Medicare reimbursement if they could demonstrate that the hospice program met the Medicare "conditions of participation," or regulations, for hospice providers.

Hospice providers endeavor to make the services available to all persons with advanced illness, regardless of diagnosis. Many chronic progressive diseases do not have a predictable "end stage" that fits hospice eligibility criteria, and as a result, many patients die after a long, slow, and often painful decline, without the benefit of the coordinated palliative care that is unique to hospice programs. The palliative approach to care could benefit many more patients if it were available across care settings and earlier in the disease process. Palliative care programs are now being developed in other settings for patients who are either not eligible for hospice or who do not choose to enroll in a formal hospice program. At this time, there is no dedicated reimbursement to providers for palliative care services when they are delivered outside the hospice setting, making the sustainability of such programs challenging.

Palliative Care in the Hospital Setting

Hospitals have a financial incentive to transfer patients with terminal illnesses who are no longer in need of acute care to receive care in other settings, such as long-term care facilities and home. Despite the economic and human costs associated with death in the hospital setting, approximately 30% of all deaths occur in acute care settings. While hospital deaths declined in the 10 years between 2000 and 2010, 25% of deaths are accounted for by persons older than 85 years (Hall, Levant, & DeFrances, 2013). The landmark Study to Understand Prognoses and Preferences for Outcomes and Risks of Treatments (SUPPORT) documented troubling deficiencies in the care of the dying in hospital settings (SUPPORT Principal Investigators, 1995). The Patient Protection and Affordable Care Act (PPACA) required the development of a Measures Application Partnership (MAP), which was convened by the National Quality Forum and reports directly to the Department of Health & Human Services (HHS). Importantly, the MAP workgroup responsible for hospice and palliative care measures has recommended "cross cutting" quality measures that would "follow the patient and their full set of experiences" (NCP, 2013, p. 7). This move will help ensure that standards of care for patients with advanced illness and at end of life will apply regardless of where the patients are receiving care, ensuring quality of care for persons receiving care or dying in settings other than their preferred location.

Many patients will continue to opt for hospital care or will by default find themselves in hospital settings at the end of life. Increasingly, hospitals are conducting system-wide assessments of end-of-life care practices and outcomes and are developing innovative models for delivering high-quality, person-centered care to patients approaching the end of life. A growing body of evidence supports the role of palliative care that is delivered *concurrently* with standard medical treatment. For example, in a landmark study of referral to palliative care for patients newly diagnosed with metastatic non–small cell lung cancer (a disease with very poor prognosis), researchers found that those patients randomized to the palliative care plus standard oncology care arm of the trial not only showed improved quality of life and mood but also had longer median survival than those who received standard oncology care alone (Temel, Greer, Muzikansky, et al., 2010).

This study underscores the value of palliative care and undercuts one of the principal objections to palliative care, which equates it with "giving up."

In 2011, The Joint Commission launched an advanced certification program for palliative care to recognize hospitals that provide exceptional patient and family-centered care. Despite early financial barriers to providing high-quality palliative care in acute care settings (Connor, 2007–2008), palliative care services in hospitals have grown significantly; in 2015, almost all large hospitals (90%) had a palliative care program (Center to Advance Palliative Care [CAPC], 2015a). Public policy changes have been called for that would reimburse hospitals for care delivered via designated hospital-wide palliative care beds, clustered palliative care units, or palliative care consultation services in acute care settings. Resources are available for developing hospital–hospice partnerships to provide high-quality palliative care for hospitalized patients and for addressing the palliative care needs of other specialized populations, such as patients receiving such care in intensive care units (ICUs), pediatric patients, residents of long-term care facilities, and patients receiving care in community settings (CAPC, 2015b). In 2013, the state of Maryland passed legislation that requires hospitals with more than 50 beds to have an accredited palliative care program by 2016. In a statewide survey of hospitals, researchers found that although 89% of Maryland providers already had a palliative care program in place, 41% indicated that they did not have procedures in place for ensuring timely delivery of services (Gibbs, Mahon, Truss, et al., 2015). This action by the Maryland legislature is an example of state policy that can contribute to wider adoption of palliative care.

Palliative Care in Skilled Nursing Facilities

Experts estimate that the number of people who will need some form of short- or long-term skilled nursing care in their lifetimes, whether in the community or in a residential care facility, will double by the year 2050 (Centers for Disease Control and Prevention, 2013). As a result, the likely place of death for a growing number of Americans after the age of 65 years will be a skilled nursing facility. For those Americans younger than 65 years, the most common place for death remains the hospital (38%), although the proportion that die at home has increased steadily over the years. Similarly, for those older than 65 years, death at home has become more common (24%); however, the hospital (35%) and nursing home (28%) as the location of death still exceed the number of deaths at home, and although hospital death is decreasing, nursing home death is increasing (National Center for Health Statistics, 2010).

Residents of skilled nursing facilities typically have poor access to palliative care. Regulations that govern how care in these facilities is organized and reimbursed tend to emphasize restorative measures and serve as a disincentive to palliative care. Since 1989, home hospice programs have been permitted to enroll long-term care facility residents in hospice programs and to provide interdisciplinary services to residents who qualify for hospice care. Of the more than 1.7 million Medicare beneficiaries who received hospice services in 2014, 14.5% resided in long-term care facilities, a decrease from 17.9% in 2013 (NHPCO, 2014). Because hospices provide some services that may overlap with services provided by the skilled nursing provider, payment models have been developed to define and reconcile duplication of services. In 1997, the Office of Inspector General (OIG), an oversight arm of the federal government, questioned whether hospice services in nursing homes were an unnecessary duplication of services already provided by long-term care facility staff. In 2011, the OIG reported on the inappropriateness of payments for hospice patients in nursing homes who did not meet eligibility, plan of care, and certification of terminal illness requirements. Hospice/skilled nursing facility contracts continue to be scrutinized by federal regulators. Meanwhile, facilities are under increasing public pressure to improve care of the dying and are beginning to develop palliative care units or services; continuing to contract with home hospice programs to provide palliative care consultations and hospice care in the facilities; and to educate staff, residents, and their families about pain and symptom management and end-of-life care. Many skilled nursing providers have implemented "culture change" innovations such as resident-centered care plans and consistent staff assignments to change the experience of long-term skilled nursing care. Researchers have observed that well-developed culture change practices could provide a strong implementation platform for palliative care (Tyler, Shield, & Miller, 2015). Further research is needed to test models for providing palliative and end-of-life care in skilled nursing facilities (Ersek & Carpenter, 2013).

Outpatient Palliative Care

As palliative care has become more prevalent in hospitals, skilled nursing settings, and in home hospice programs, outpatient palliative care has emerged as an approach to providing services and support to patients and families who opt not to or are not eligible for home hospice but could benefit from comprehensive palliative care in the community. Outpatient palliative care benefits both patients and their families and other providers by providing expert consultation and management of symptoms and other needs. Studies demonstrate that outpatient palliative care increases patient satisfaction with care, improves symptom management and quality of life, reduces utilization of other health care services (such as avoidable acute care admissions), and may lengthen survival for some patients (Rabow, Kvale, Barbour, et al., 2013).

Hospice Care

Hospice is a coordinated program of interdisciplinary services provided by professional caregivers and trained volunteers to patients with serious, progressive illnesses that are not responsive to cure. The root of the word *hospice* is *hospes*, meaning "host." According to Cicely Saunders, who founded the world-renowned St. Christopher's Hospice in London, the principles underlying hospice are as follows:

- Death must be accepted.
- The patient's total care is best managed by an interdisciplinary team whose members communicate regularly with one another.
- Pain and other symptoms of terminal illness must be managed.
- The patient and the family should be viewed as a single unit of care.

- Home care of the dying is necessary.
- Bereavement care must be provided to family members.
- Research and education should be ongoing.

Hospice Care in the United States

Hospice in the United States is not a place but a concept of care in which the end of life is viewed as a developmental stage. The hospice movement in the United States is based on the belief that meaningful living is achievable during terminal illness and that it is best supported in the home, free of technologic interventions to prolong physiologic dying. The concept of hospice care as an alternative to depersonalized death in institutions began in the early 1970s as a grassroots, volunteer-based, and spiritually centered movement. In 2014, there were more than 6100 hospice programs in operation across all 50 states, serving an estimated 1.7 million patients (NHPCO, 2014).

Despite more than 40 years of existence in the United States, hospice remains an option for end-of-life care that has not been fully integrated into mainstream health care. Physicians are reluctant to refer patients to hospice, and patients are reluctant to accept this form of care. Reasons include the difficulties in making a terminal prognosis (especially for those patients with noncancer diagnoses), the strong association of hospice with death, advances in "curative" treatment options in late-stage illness, and financial pressures on health care providers that may cause them to retain rather than refer hospice-eligible patients. As a result, many patients and families do not fully benefit from the comprehensive, interdisciplinary support offered by hospice programs; the median length of stay in a hospice program is just a little greater than 2 weeks, at 17.4 days (NHPCO, 2014).

The goal of hospice is to enable the patient to remain at home, surrounded by the people and objects that have been important to him or her throughout life. The patient and the family comprise the unit of care. Hospice care does not seek to hasten death or encourage the prolongation of life through artificial means. Hospice care hinges on the competent patient's full or "open" awareness of dying; it embraces realism about death and helps patients and families understand the dying process so that they can live each moment as fully as possible. Approximately 30% of hospice programs have developed inpatient facilities or residences (NHPCO, 2014) where terminally ill patients without family support and those who desire inpatient care may receive hospice services.

Hospice Care Eligibility and Benefits

Since 1983, the **Medicare Hospice Benefit** has covered costs of hospice care for Medicare beneficiaries. State Medical Assistance (Medicaid) also provides coverage for hospice care, as do most commercial insurers. To receive Medicare payment for hospice services, programs are required to comply with rules known as "conditions of participation," which are enforced by the Centers for Medicare & Medicaid Services (CMS, 2015). In many aspects, Medicare standards have come to largely define hospice philosophy and services.

Eligibility criteria for hospice vary depending on the hospice program, but generally patients must have a progressive, irreversible illness and limited life expectancy and must

---

Chart 16-2 Eligibility Criteria for Hospice Care

General

- Serious, progressive illness
- Limited life expectancy
- Informed choice of palliative care over cure-focused treatment

Hospice Specific

- Presence of a family member or other caregiver continuously in the home when the patient is no longer able to safely care for himself or herself (some hospices have created special services within their programs for patients who live alone, although this varies widely).

Medicare and Medicaid Hospice Benefits

- Medicare Part A; Medical Assistance eligibility
- Waiver of traditional Medicare/Medicaid benefits for the terminal illness
- Life expectancy of ≤6 months
- Physician certification of terminal illness
- Care must be provided by a Medicare-certified hospice program

---

Chart 16-3 Home Hospice Services Covered Under the Medicare/Medicaid Hospice Benefit Routine Home Care Level

- Nursing care provided by or under the supervision of a registered nurse, available 24 hours a day
- Medical social services
- Physician's services
- Counseling services, including dietary counseling
- Home health aide/homemaker
- Physical/occupational/speech therapists
- Volunteers
- Bereavement follow-up (for up to 13 months after the death of the patient)
- Medical supplies for the palliation of the terminal illness
- Medical equipment for the palliation of the terminal illness
- Medications for the palliation of the terminal illness

---

opt for palliative care rather than cure-focused treatment. Chart 16-2 presents the eligibility criteria for hospice coverage under the Medicare Hospice Benefit. The patient who wishes to use their Medicare Hospice Benefit must be certified by a physician as terminally ill, with a life expectancy of 6 months or less if the disease follows its natural course. Thus, hospice has come to be defined as palliative care provided to terminally ill persons and their families in the last 6 months of the patient's life. Because of additional Medicare rules concerning a palliative focus for medical treatment under the Medicare Hospice Benefit, many patients delay enrollment in hospice programs until very close to the end of life.

Federal rules for hospices require that eligibility be reviewed periodically. Patients who live longer than 6 months under hospice care are *not* discharged, provided that their physician and the hospice medical director continue to certify that they are terminally ill with a life expectancy of 6 months or less (assuming that the disease continues its expected course). Once a patient meets eligibility criteria and elects to use the benefit, the Medicare-certified hospice program assumes responsibility for providing and paying for the care and treatment to palliate the terminal illness for which hospice care was elected. The Medicare-certified hospice is paid a predetermined dollar amount for each day of hospice care that each patient receives. Four levels of hospice care are covered under Medicare and Medicaid hospice benefits:

- *Routine home care:* All services provided are included in the daily rate to the hospice.
- *Inpatient respite care:* A 5-day inpatient stay, provided on an occasional basis to relieve the family caregivers.
- *Continuous care:* Continuous nursing care provided in the home for the management of a medical crisis. Care reverts to the routine home care level after the crisis is resolved. (For example, seizure activity develops and a nurse is placed in the home continuously to monitor the patient and administer medications. After 72 hours, the seizure activity is under control, the family has been

instructed how to care for the patient, and the continuous nursing care is discontinued.)
- *General inpatient care:* Inpatient stay for symptom management that cannot be provided in the home. This is not subject to the guidelines for a standard hospital inpatient stay.

Most hospice care is provided at the "routine home care" level and includes the services described in Chart 16-3. According to federal guidelines, hospices may provide no more than 20% of the aggregate annual patient-days at the inpatient level. Patients may "revoke" their hospice benefits at any time, resuming traditional coverage under Medicare or Medicaid for the terminal illness. Those who revoke their benefits may also reelect to use them at a later time.

Hospice Care Utilization

Hospice programs are reaching out to patients with very advanced illness and seeking ways to provide them with hospice services while they are completing courses of treatment that many programs previously defined as "life prolonging," such as disease-modifying therapies for dementia, enteral or parenteral nutritional support, and certain types of chemotherapy. Hospice providers frequently refer to more flexible policies concerning disease-modifying medical treatment at the time of admission as "open access." The NHPCO acknowledges the concept of open access, stating that palliative care is "treatment that enhances comfort and improves the quality of an individual's life during the last phase of life. No specific therapy is excluded from consideration" (NHPCO, 2010, p. 1). The Medicare Hospice Benefit requirement that beneficiaries make a choice between palliative care (to enroll in hospice) and cure-focused treatment has long been a barrier to earlier hospice enrollment. A Medicare beneficiary could not receive BOTH palliative care and cure-focused care under their hospice benefit. The PPACA authorized a study of concurrent palliative and curative care services. Under this federally funded study, titled Medicare Care Choices, CMS will evaluate whether beneficiaries would choose palliative care under hospice guidelines while they *continue to receive* cure-focused care (CMS, 2015). The model will be tested for 3 to 5 years with more than 140 Medicare-certified hospices. It is projected to reach 150,000 Medicare beneficiaries with advanced cancer and complex chronic illnesses such as heart failure and COPD (CMS, 2016).

Hospice use has increased steadily since the inception of the Medicare Hospice Benefit. In 2012, approximately 46.7% of Medicare beneficiaries who died used hospice services compared to 22.9% in 2000 (Medicare Payment Advisory Commission [MedPAC], 2014). The most common primary hospice diagnoses among Medicare patients are dementia, heart disease, and lung disease. Whereas most patients who enrolled in hospice in previous decades had cancer diagnoses, just 36.6% of hospice enrollees in 2014 had cancer diagnoses (NHPCO, 2014).

Although hospice utilization continues to increase, many patients who could benefit from hospice care do not receive it. Most terminally ill patients who are not enrolled in hospice die in hospitals and long-term care facilities.

Nursing Care of Terminally Ill Patients

Many patients suffer unnecessarily when they do not receive adequate attention for the symptoms accompanying serious illness. Careful evaluation of the patient should include not only the physical problems but also the psychosocial and spiritual dimensions of the patient's and family's experience of serious illness. This approach contributes to a more comprehensive understanding of how the patient's and family's life has been affected by illness and leads to nursing care that addresses their needs in every dimension.

Psychosocial and Regulatory Issues

Nurses are responsible for educating patients and their caregivers and for supporting them as they adapt to life with the illness. Nurses can assist patients and families with life review, values clarification, treatment decision making, and end-of-life goals. The only way to do this effectively is to try to appreciate and understand the illness from the patient's perspective.

Nurses should be both culturally aware and sensitive in their approaches to communication with patients and families about death. Attitudes toward open disclosure about terminal illness vary widely among different cultures, and direct communication with patients about such matters may be viewed as harmful (Sarafis, Tsounis, Malliarou, et al., 2014). To provide effective patient- and family-centered care at the end of life, nurses must be willing to set aside their own assumptions and attitudes so that they can discover what type and amount of disclosure is most meaningful to each patient and family within their unique belief systems (see Table 16-1).

The social and legal evolution of advance directive documents represents some progress in people's willingness to both contemplate and communicate their wishes concerning the end of life (see Chart 16-4). Now legally sanctioned in every state and federally sanctioned through the Patient Self-Determination Act of 1991, advance directives are written documents that allow competent people to document their preferences regarding the use or abatement of medical treatment at the end of life, specify their preferred setting for care, and communicate other valuable insights into their values and beliefs. The proxy directive (appointment and authorization of another person to make medical decisions on behalf

of the person who created the advance directive when he or she can no longer speak for himself or herself) is an important addition to the living will or medical directive that specifies the signer's preferences. These documents are widely available from health care providers, community organizations, bookstores, and the Internet. However, their underuse reflects society's continued discomfort with openly confronting the subject of death. Furthermore, the existence of a properly executed advance directive does not reduce the complexity of end-of-life decisions.

The Patient Self-Determination Act requires that health care entities receiving Medicare or Medicaid reimbursement must ask whether patients have advance directives, provide information about advance directives, and incorporate advance directives into the medical record. However, advance directives should not be considered a substitute for ongoing communication among the health care provider, patient, and family as the end of life approaches.

 Concept Mastery Alert

An advance directive states a patient's wishes for treatment. A proxy directive appoints another person to make medical decisions on behalf of the patient and is added to the advance directive.

Communication

Remarkable strides have been made in the ability to prolong life; however, attention to care for the dying lags behind. On one level, this should come as no surprise. Each of us will eventually face death, and most would agree that one's own demise is a subject that he or she would prefer not to contemplate. Confronting death in our patients often uncovers our own deeply rooted fears.

To develop a level of comfort and expertise in communicating with seriously and terminally ill patients and their families, nurses must first consider their own experiences with and values concerning illness and death. Reflection, reading, and talking with family members, friends, and colleagues can help nurses examine beliefs about death and dying. Talking with people from different cultural and religious backgrounds can help nurses view personally held beliefs through a different lens and can increase their sensitivity to death-related beliefs and practices in other cultures. Discussion with nursing and nonnursing colleagues can also be useful; it may reveal the values shared by many health care professionals and may also identify diversity in the values of patients in their care. Values clarification and personal death awareness exercises can provide a starting point for self-discovery and discussion.

Skills for Communicating With the Seriously Ill

Nurses need to develop skill and comfort in assessing patients' and families' responses to serious illness and planning interventions that support their values and choices throughout the continuum of care (Wittenberg-Lyles, Goldmith, Ferrell, et al., 2013). Throughout the course of a serious illness, patients and their families encounter complicated treatment options and bad news about disease progression. They may have to make difficult decisions at the time of diagnosis, when disease-focused treatment fails, when the effectiveness of a

TABLE 16-1 Overview of Religious and Cultural Beliefs and Views on Death and Dying

Religion	General Religious/Cultural Beliefs	Views About Death/Preparing for Death
Hinduism	• Each caste has a different view of death. • This life is a transition between the previous life and the next. • Postdeath rituals are important. Bodies are cremated. During the first 10 days after death, relatives must create a new ethereal body. • Karma is the manner through which one reaps benefits and penalties of past actions. "Good karma" leads to good rebirth or release, and "bad karma" leads to bad rebirth. • Astrological timing of birth and death is important	• No firmly established medical ethics, principles, or codes to guide decision making/care. • Many older adults withdraw into their homes, where they prepare for death through prayer and meditation. • Family is very important; health care decisions may be made communally with senior family member as final authority. Deference to spouse and family may be especially prevalent among women (acquiescing autonomy to a family member). • A "good death" is timely, in the right place (on the ground at home), conscious and prepared, with the mind on God. All affairs should be in order. • A "bad death" is untimely, violent, and unprepared. The worst death is suicide. • Pain and suffering may be viewed as consequence of past actions, "bad karma".
Judaism	• Central tenet is the sanctity of human life. • Human beings are mortal, and their bodies belong to God. • Although the primary provider has the authority to determine the appropriate course of treatment, ultimately the patient has the right to choose, as long as the medical regimen follows Jewish law. • Disclosure is important. Most patients want to know the truth. • Jews are obligated to visit the sick.	• Traditional criteria for death are cessation of breathing and heartbeat. Conservative rabbis have accepted brain death as fulfilling these criteria. • Advance directives for health care are permissible. • Life-extending measures for the terminally ill are not mandated. • Views on the use of artificial nutrition and hydration vary, depending on the particular sect/movement. • Most rabbis maintain that Jews may enroll in hospice.
Buddhism	• There is no central authority in the Buddhist religion. • Taboo and religious purity play little, if any, role, and religious law imposes no special requirements for medical treatment. • Treatment by someone of the same gender is preferable. • Cremation is the most common way of disposing of the dead. • Some Buddhists may be unwilling to take pain-relieving medications or strong sedatives. It is believed that an unclouded mind can lead to a better rebirth. • Buddhists believe that after death there is either rebirth or nirvana—the latter being enlightenment that frees the soul from the cycle of death and rebirth.	• Life is basically good and preserving it is important. Enlightenment can only be achieved through living. • Teachings emphasize the inevitability of death; therefore, Buddhists tend to be psychologically prepared to accept impending death with calmness and dignity. • Death occurs when a body is bereft of vitality, heat, and sentiency. Brain death is disputed as meeting the requirements for death. • It is often appropriate to decide that the patient is beyond medical help and to allow events to take their course. In these cases, it is justifiable to refuse or withdraw treatment in light of the overall prognosis. • Buddhism supports the use of hospice.
Islam	• Muslims believe in one God. • God revealed the message of God to Muhammad, the prophet, in the Qur'an (Koran), which states that Muslims should maintain a balanced diet and exercise. • Muslim patients may wish to engage in ritual prayer, practiced five times during the day. • Fasting during the month of Ramadan is a pillar of Islam. • Completion of the pilgrimage (*hajj*) to Mecca (money and health permitting), at least once, is also a pillar of Islam.	• Everyone will face death, and the way a person dies is of great individual importance. • Death cannot happen except by God's permission. However, it is recognized that diseases and trauma cause death. • There is a belief that God is the one who cures and primary providers are a means to enact God's will. • Decisions are made within families, and disclosure of diagnosis and prognosis must be considered in this context. • Pain is a cleansing instrument of God. Pain can also be viewed as having an educational purpose (pain can compensate for sin). • The killing of a terminally ill person is an act of disobedience against God. However, pain relief or withholding or withdrawing of life support when there is no doubt that the person's disease is causing untreatable suffering is permissible as long as there is formal agreement among all parties concerned. • Withholding and withdrawing artificial nutrition and hydration (ANH) at the end of life raises concerns. Nutritional support is considered basic care and not medical treatment and should be continued unless it would hasten death or cause more harm than benefit.

TABLE 16-1 Overview of Religious and Cultural Beliefs and Views on Death and Dying (continued)

Religion	General Religious/Cultural Beliefs	Views About Death/Preparing for Death
Traditional Christianity	• Christians believe in one God. • The belief in eternal salvation sets Christianity apart. • Beliefs vary. Some Christians hope to attain eternal salvation. • Even within family, religious views can differ. Some family members may not follow the religion at all.	• Each human life has inherent and equal dignity. • Intentionally bringing about death by either omission or commission is prohibited. • The appropriateness of analgesia and sedation to avoid terminal suffering and despair is acceptable, if it does not, by clouding consciousness, take away the final opportunity for repentance. • Christians are not obligated to postpone death; it is forbidden to try to save life at all costs. • However, there could be a duty to use high-technology medicine to gain a last opportunity for repentance. • ANH is obligatory for most patients except when the means to provide ANH cause complications, the patient has progressive illness, or clearly refuses ANH. • Impending death offers a final chance to become reconciled with those whom one has harmed and to ask God's forgiveness. • Liturgical (ceremonial) Christians generally regard last rites as integral to the relationship with God. Repentance can include confessing formally and receiving Communion and final anointing. This often involves particular ministers. • Christians who follow the religion at a cultural level are likely to have secular approaches to end-of-life decisions. • Advance directives allow patients to appoint decision makers and to provide instructions that ensure that their wishes are followed.

Adapted from Alsolamy, S. (2014). Islamic views on artificial nutrition and hydration in terminally ill patients. *Bioethics, 28,* 96–99. Dewar, R., Cahners, N., Mitchell, C., & Forrow, L. (2015). Hinduism and death with dignity: Historic and contemporary case examples. *Journal of Clinical Ethics, 26*(1), 40–47.
Linzer, R. D. (2013). Treatment of terminally ill patients according to Jewish law. *The Virtual Mentor, 15,* 1081–1087.
McCormick, A. J. (2013). Buddhist ethics and end-of-life care decisions. *Journal of Social Work in End-of-Life & Palliative Care, 9,* 209–225.
Zientek, D. M. (2013). Artificial nutrition and hydration in Catholic healthcare: Balancing tradition, recent teaching, and law. *HEC Forum, 25,* 145–159.

particular intervention is being discussed, and when decisions about hospice care are presented. These critical points on the treatment continuum demand patience, empathy, and honesty from nurses. Discussing sensitive issues such as serious illness, hopes for survival, and fears associated with death is never easy. However, the art of therapeutic communication can be learned and, like other skills, must be practiced to gain expertise. Like other skills, communication should be practiced in a "safe" setting, such as a classroom or clinical skills laboratory with other students and clinicians.

Chart 16-4 Methods of Stating End-of-Life Preferences

Advance directives: written documents that allow the individual of sound mind to document preferences regarding end-of-life care that should be followed when the signer is terminally ill and unable to verbally communicate their wishes. The documents are generally completed in advance of serious illness but may be completed after a diagnosis of serious illness if the signer is still of sound mind. The most common types are the durable power of attorney for health care and the living will.

Do Not Resuscitate: A medical order to withhold cardiopulmonary resuscitation (CPR) in the event of cardiac arrest. In some settings, the term "allow natural death" (AND) is used in place of do not resuscitate (DNR).

Durable power of attorney for health care: a legal document through which the signer appoints and authorizes another individual to make medical decisions on their behalf when he or she is no longer able to speak for himself or herself. This is also known as a health care power of attorney, medical power of attorney, or a proxy directive.

Living will: a type of advance directive in which the individual documents treatment preferences. It provides instructions for care in the event that the signer is terminally ill and not able to communicate their wishes directly and often is accompanied by a durable power of attorney for health care. This is also known as a medical directive or treatment directive.

Physician orders for life-sustaining treatment (POLST): a form that translates patient preferences expressed in advance directives to medical "orders" that are transferable across settings and readily available to all health care providers, including emergency medical personnel. The POLST form is a brightly colored form that specifies preferences related to CPR and use of IV medications or fluids, antibiotics, artificial nutrition, and other medical interventions. The form is signed by the patient or surrogate and the physician, advanced practice nurse, or physician assistant. The use of the POLST is subject to state laws and regulations. Numerous states have endorsed the POLST or a similar form.

Information about the advance care planning and state-specific advance directive documents and instructions is available at www.caringinfo.org. Information about the POLST is available at www.polst.org

In practice, communication with each patient and family should be tailored to their particular level of understanding and values concerning disclosure. Before disclosing any health information about a patient to family members, nurses should follow their agency's policy for obtaining patient consent in accordance with Health Insurance Portability and Accountability Act rules.

Nursing Interventions When Patients and Families Receive Bad News

Communicating about a life-threatening diagnosis or disease progression is best accomplished in any setting by the interdisciplinary team: A physician, nurse, social worker, and chaplain should be present whenever possible to provide information, facilitate discussion, and address concerns. Most important, the presence of the team conveys caring and respect for the patient and the family. If the patient wishes to have family present for the discussion, arrangements should be made to have the discussion at a time that is best for everyone. Creating the right setting is particularly important. A quiet area with a minimum of disturbances should be used. All clinicians present should turn off pagers, cell phones, and other communication devices for the duration of the meeting and should allow sufficient time for the patient and the family to absorb and respond to the news. Finally, the space in which the meeting takes place should be conducive to seating all participants at eye level. It is difficult enough for the patient and the family to be the recipients of bad news without having an array of clinicians standing uncomfortably over them at the foot of the patient's bed (see Chart 16-5).

After the initial discussion of a life-threatening illness or progression of a disease, the patient and the family will probably have many questions and may need to be reminded of factual information. Coping with news about a serious diagnosis or poor prognosis is an ongoing process. The nurse should be sensitive to these ongoing needs and may need to repeat previously provided information or simply be present while the patient and the family react emotionally. The most important intervention the nurse can provide is listening empathetically. Seriously ill patients and their families need time and support to cope with the changes brought about by serious illness and the prospect of impending death. The nurse who is able to listen without judging and without trying to solve the patient's and family's problems provides an invaluable intervention. Keys to effective listening include the following:

- Resist the impulse to fill the "empty space" in communication with talk.
- Allow the patient and the family sufficient time to reflect and respond after asking a question.
- Prompt gently: "Do you need more time to think about this?"
- Avoid distractions (noise, interruptions).
- Avoid the impulse to give advice.
- Avoid canned responses: "I know just how you feel."
- Ask questions.
- Assess understanding—your own and the patient's—by restating, summarizing, and reviewing.

(See the Nursing Research Profile in Chart 16-6.)

Responding With Sensitivity to Difficult Questions

Patients often direct questions or concerns to nurses before they have been able to fully discuss the details of their diagnosis and prognosis with their physicians or the entire health care team. Using open-ended questions allows the nurse to

---

Chart 16-5 COMFORT: A Framework for Communication in Palliative Care

Communication (C)

- Narrative clinical practice: Elicit and be fully present for the patient's and family's story.
- Verbal clarity: Use compassionate, nonambiguous language.
- Nonverbal immediacy: Use eye contact, body position, and self-awareness to show attentiveness.

Orientation (O)

- Support health literacy.
- Acknowledge vulnerability.
- Express cultural sensitivity.

Mindfulness (M)

- Stay in the moment: Avoid scripted responses.
- Avoid prejudgment: Do not have expectations that this patient and family will or should respond as others have in the past.
- Adapt to rapid changes: Be ready to shift to new topics and concerns that are revealed.

Family (F)

- Think of the family as a "second-order" patient: The family and the patient comprise the unit of care.
- Know that the family is a bridge to the patient: You must gain the family's trust to work effectively.

- Use family meetings (patient included) to clarify goals for treatment.

Openings (O)

- Address essential transitions in care or status.
- Seek a higher level of understanding of the disease process.
- Engage spiritual concerns.

Relating (R)

- Prioritize the turning point in illness.
- Understand that communication should be nonlinear: The patient and the family may need to revisit topics multiple times and on multiple occasions.
- Know that the patient's and family's acceptance must drive communication.

Team (T)

- The interdisciplinary team includes members trained in various aspects of palliative care.
- Assure the patient and the family that they will not be abandoned.
- Ensure continuity of care across settings: Goals and plans should be clearly communicated to other providers.

Adapted with permission from Wittenberg-Lyles, E., Goldsmith, J., & Ragan, S. L. (2010). The COMFORT initiative: Palliative nursing and the centrality of communication. *Journal of Hospice and Palliative Nursing, 12*(5), 282–292.

NURSING RESEARCH PROFILE

Chart 16-6

Perceptions of Helpful Interventions During End-of-Life Care

Cronin, C., Arnstein, P., & Flanagan, J. (2015). Family members' perceptions of most helpful interventions during end-of-life care. *Journal of Hospice & Palliative Nursing, 17*(3), 223–228.

Purpose

Hospice care and support is directed not just to the patient but to those whom the patient considers family, as well. Numerous studies have provided insight to nurses' perceptions of priorities for as well as barriers to and facilitators of end-of-life care. Better understanding of families' needs could improve their experience of hospice care. This study aimed to explore the needs of family members and friends while their loved ones received end-of-life care in a hospital setting.

Design

This was a qualitative study in which the researchers used semi-structured interviews to collect data from a family member or close friend of a patient enrolled in hospice in a hospital setting. Nine potential study participants were identified through convenience sampling on an 18-bed gynecologic oncology unit in a large academic medical center; seven of the nine agreed to participate. Interview questions focused on perceived helpfulness of nurses' and other staff members' activities, perceptions of communication, and adequacy and helpfulness of referred services (e.g., chaplaincy). Data were compiled as transcripts from handwritten interview notes and analyzed using content analysis techniques.

Findings

Importantly, the principal investigator observed that although she had anticipated that participants might be uncomfortable being interviewed at such a difficult time, she found that participants were not only comfortable, they appreciated the chance to tell their stories and would have been willing to share even more than was requested. Researchers identified four principal themes from the data analysis: (1) family/friend awareness of nursing vigilance provided them with a sense of being cared for, (2) nursing presence enhanced mutual connectedness and appreciation, (3) when death was imminent, family/friends wanted to understand the process, be included in discussions, and be validated after decisions were made, and (4) attention to the environment of care provided peace and relaxation at a difficult time.

Nursing Implications

Nurses working in end-of-life care need to keep in mind that support for family members and validation of difficult decisions are vital components of their communication. Furthermore, this communication is essential to increase family members' levels of comfort and trust in the entire health care team.

---

elicit the patient's and family's concerns, explore misconceptions and needs for information, and form the basis for collaboration with physicians and other team members.

For example, a seriously ill patient might ask the nurse, "Am I dying?" The nurse should avoid making unhelpful responses that dismiss the patient's real concerns or defer the issue to another care provider. Nursing assessment and intervention are always possible, even when a need for further discussion with a physician is clearly indicated. Whenever possible, discussions in response to a patient's concerns should occur when the patient expresses a need, although that may be the least convenient time for the nurse. Creating an uninterrupted space of just 5 minutes can do much to identify the source of the concern, allay anxieties, and plan for follow-up.

In response to the question "Am I dying?" the nurse could establish eye contact and follow with a statement acknowledging the patient's fears ("This must be very difficult for you") and an open-ended statement or question ("Tell me more about what is on your mind"). The nurse then needs to listen intently, ask additional questions for clarification, and provide reassurance only when it is realistic. In this example, the nurse might quickly ascertain that the patient's question emanates from a need for specific information—about diagnosis and prognosis from the physician, about the physiology of the dying process from the nurse, or perhaps about financial implications for the family from the social worker. The chaplain may also be called to talk with the patient about existential concerns.

As a member of the interprofessional team caring for the patient at the end of life, the nurse plays an important role in facilitating the team's understanding of the patient's values and preferences, family dynamics concerning decision making, and the patient's and the family's response to treatment and changing health status. Many dilemmas in patient care at the end of life are related to poor communication between team members and the patient and the family, as well as to failure of team members to communicate with one another effectively. Regardless of the care setting, the nurse can ensure a proactive approach to the psychosocial care of the patient and the family. Periodic, structured assessments provide an opportunity for all parties to consider their priorities and plan for an uncertain future. The nurse can help the patient and the family clarify their values and preferences concerning end-of-life care by using a structured approach. Sufficient time must be devoted to each step so that the patient and the family have time to process new information, formulate questions, and consider their options. The nurse may need to plan several meetings to facilitate communication to accomplish the steps described in Chart 16-5.

Providing Culturally Sensitive Care at the End of Life

Although death, grief, and mourning are universally accepted aspects of living, the values, expectations, and practices during serious illness as death approaches and after death are culturally bound and expressed. Health care providers may share similar values concerning end-of-life care and may find that they are inadequately prepared to assess for and implement care plans that support culturally diverse perspectives. Historical mistrust of the health care system and unequal access to even basic medical care may underlie the beliefs and attitudes among ethnically diverse populations (see Table 16-1). In addition, lack of education or knowledge about end-of-life care treatment options and language barriers influence decisions among many socioeconomically disadvantaged groups.

The nurse's role is to assess the values, preferences, and practices of every patient, regardless of ethnicity, socioeconomic status, or background. The nurse can share knowledge about a patient's and family's cultural beliefs and practices with the health care team and facilitate the adaptation of the care plan to accommodate these practices. For example, a nurse may find that a male patient prefers to have his eldest son make all of his care decisions. Institutional practices and laws governing informed consent are also rooted in the Western notion of autonomous decision making and informed consent. If a patient wishes to defer decisions to his son, the nurse can work with the team to negotiate informed consent, respecting the patient's right not to participate in decision making and honoring his family's cultural practice.

The nurse should assess and document the patient's and family's specific beliefs, preferences, and practices regarding end-of-life care, preparation for death, and after-death rituals. Chart 16-7 identifies topics that the nurse should cover and questions the nurse may use to elicit the information.

The nurse must use judgment and discretion about the timing and setting for eliciting this information. Some patients may wish to have a family member speak for them or may be unable to provide information because of advanced illness. The nurse should give the patient and the family a context for the discussion, such as

It is very important to us to provide care that addresses your needs and the needs of your family. We want to honor and support your wishes, and want you to feel free to tell us how we are doing, and what we could do to better meet your needs. I'd like to ask you some questions; what you tell me will help me to understand and support what is most important to you at this time. You don't need to answer anything that makes you uncomfortable. Is it all right to ask some questions?

The assessment of end-of-life beliefs, preferences, and practices should be carried out in short segments over a period of time (e.g., across multiple days of an inpatient hospital stay or in conjunction with multiple patient visits to an outpatient setting or over several home care visits). The discomfort of novice nurses with asking questions and discussing this type of sensitive content can be reduced by prior practice in a classroom or clinical skills laboratory, observation of interviews conducted by experienced nurses, and partnering with experienced nurses during the first few assessments.

Goal Setting in Palliative Care at the End of Life

As treatment goals begin to shift to emphasize comfort care with or in lieu of aggressive disease-focused treatment, symptom relief and patient/family-defined quality of life assume greater prominence in treatment decision making. Throughout the course of the illness, and especially as the patient's

---

Chart 16-7   **ASSESSMENT**

Assessing End-of-Life Care Beliefs, Preferences, and Practices

Disclosure/truth telling: "Tell me how you/your family talk about very sensitive or serious matters."
- Content: "Are there any topics that you or your family are uncomfortable discussing?"
- Person responsible for disclosure: "Is there one person in the family who assumes responsibility for obtaining and sharing information?"
- Disclosure practices regarding children: "What kind of information may be shared with children in your family, and who is responsible for communicating with the children?"
- Sharing of information within the family or community group: "What kind/how much information should be shared with your immediate family? Your extended family? Others in the community (e.g., members of a religious community)?"

Decision-making style: "How are decisions made in your family? Who would you like to be involved in decisions about your treatment or care?"
- Individual
- Family centered
- Family elder or patriarch/matriarch
- Deference to authority (such as the physician)

Symptom management: "How would you like us to help you to manage the physical effects of your illness?"
- Acceptability of medications used for symptom relief
- Beliefs regarding expression of pain and other symptoms
- Degree of symptom management desired

Life-sustaining treatment expectations: "Have you thought about what type of medical treatment you or your loved one would want as the end of life is nearing? Do you have an advance directive (living will and/or durable power of attorney)?"

- Nutrition/hydration at the end of life
- Cardiopulmonary resuscitation
- Ventilator
- Dialysis
- Antibiotics
- Medications to treat infection

Desired location of dying: "Do you have a preference about being at home or in some other location when you die?"
- Desired role for family members in providing care: "Who do you want to be involved in caring for you at the end of life?"
- Gender-specific prohibitions: "Are you uncomfortable having either males or females provide your care or your loved one's personal care?"

Spiritual/religious practices and rituals: "Is there anything that we should know about your spiritual or religious beliefs about death? Are there any practices that you would like us to observe as death is nearing?"

Care of the body after the death: "Is there anything that we should know about how a body/your body should be treated after death?"

Expression of grief: "What types of losses have you and your family experienced? How do you and your family express grief?"

Funeral and burial practices: "Are there any rituals or practices associated with funerals or burial that are especially important to you?"

Mourning practices: "How have you and your family carried on after a loss in the past? Are particular behaviors or practices expected or required?"

functional status and symptoms indicate approaching death, the clinician should help the patient and the family weigh the benefits of continued diagnostic testing and disease-focused medical treatment in the context of their goals for care. The patient and the family may be extremely reluctant to forego monitoring that has become routine throughout the illness (e.g., blood testing, x-rays) but that may contribute little to a primary focus on comfort. Likewise, health care providers may have difficulty discontinuing such diagnostic testing or medical treatment.

Specifically, the nurse should collaborate with other members of the interdisciplinary team to share assessment findings, develop a coordinated plan of care, and make decisions about diagnostic testing at the end of life (see Fig. 16-1). In addition, the nurse should help the patient and the family clarify their goals, expected outcomes, and values as they consider treatment options (see Chart 16-8). The nurse should work with colleagues in other disciplines to ensure that the patient and the family are referred for continuing psychosocial support, symptom management, and assistance with other care-related challenges (e.g., arrangements for home care or hospice support, referrals for financial assistance).

Chart 16-8

ASSESSMENT

Assessing the Patient and Family Perspective: Goal Setting in Palliative Care

- **Awareness of diagnosis, illness stage, and prognosis:** "Tell me your understanding of your illness right now."
- **Values:** "Tell me what is most important to you as you are thinking about the treatment options available to you/your loved one."
- **Preferences:** "You've said that being comfortable and pain free is most important to you right now. Where would you like to receive care (home, hospital, long-term care facility, doctor's office), and how can I help?"
- **Expected/desired outcomes:** "What are your hopes and expectations for this (diagnostic test [e.g., CT scan] or treatment)?"
- **Benefits and burdens:** "Is there a point at which you would say that the testing or treatment is outweighed by the burdens it is causing you (e.g., getting from home to the hospital, pain, nausea, fatigue, interference with other important activities)?"

CT, computed tomography.

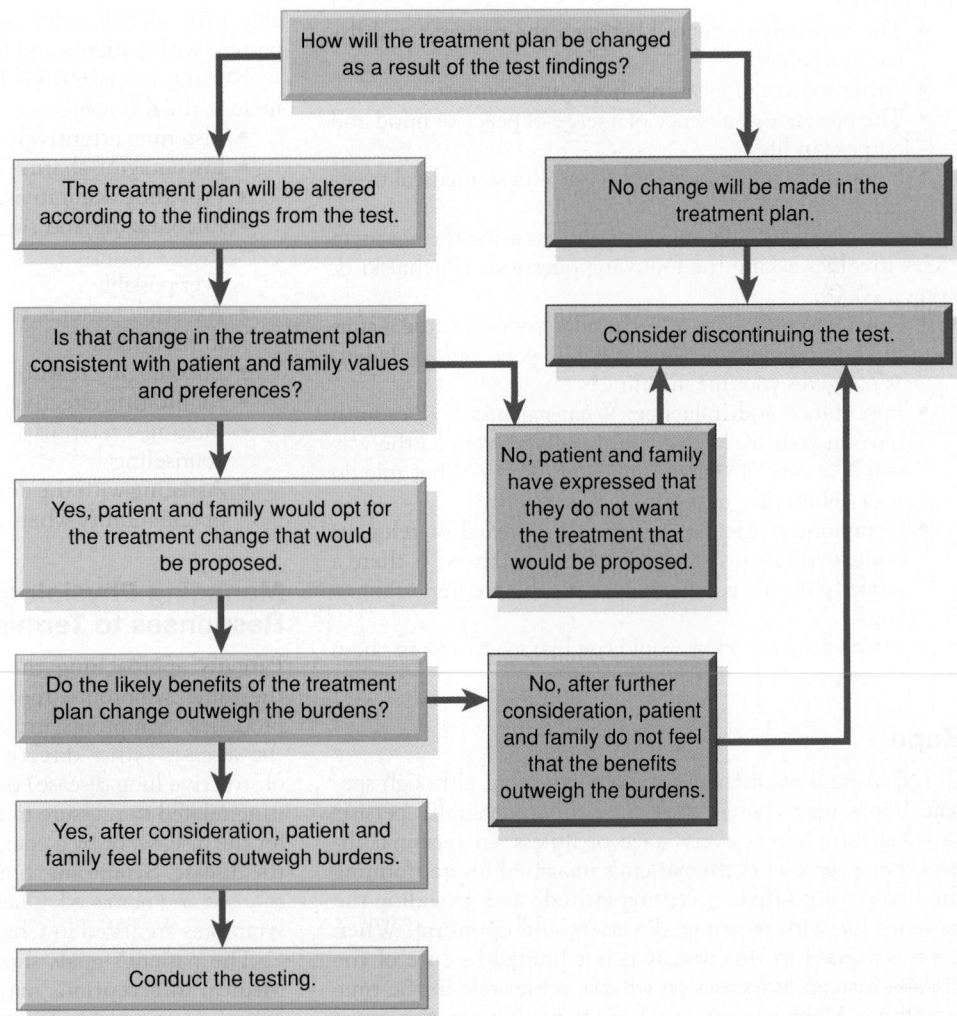

Figure 16-1 • An algorithm for decision making about diagnostic testing at the end of life.

Spiritual Care

Attention to the spiritual component of the illness experienced by the patient and the family is not new within the context of nursing care, yet many nurses lack the comfort or skills to assess and intervene in this dimension. Spirituality contains features of religiosity; however, the two concepts are not interchangeable. **Spirituality** includes domains such as how a person derives meaning and purpose from life, one's beliefs and faith, sources of hope, and attitudes toward death (Puchalski, Vitillo, Hull, et al., 2014). For most people, contemplating one's own death raises many issues, such as the meaning of existence, the purpose of suffering, and the existence of an afterlife. A survey on end-of-life issues conducted by the Pew Research Center (2013) revealed that personal attitudes and preferences concerning end-of-life treatment are related to religious affiliation, race, and ethnicity. The spiritual assessment is a key component of comprehensive nursing assessment for terminally ill patients and their families. Although the nursing assessment should include religious affiliation, spiritual assessment is conceptually much broader than religion and, therefore, is relevant regardless of a patient's expression of religious preference or affiliation. In addition to the assessment of the role of religious faith and practices, important religious rituals, and connection to a religious community (see Table 16-1), the nurse should further explore:

*   The harmony or discord between the patient's and the family's beliefs
*   Other sources of meaning, hope, and comfort
*   The presence or absence of a sense of peace of mind and purpose in life
*   Spiritual or religious beliefs about illness, medical treatment, and care of the sick

A four-step spiritual assessment process using the acronym FICA involves asking the following questions (Puchalski & Romer, 2000):

*   Faith and belief: Do you consider yourself to be a spiritual or religious person? What is your *faith* or belief? What gives your life meaning?
*   Importance and Influence: What *importance* does faith have in your life? Have your beliefs influenced the way you take care of yourself and your illness? What role do your beliefs play in regaining your health?
*   Community: Are you a part of a spiritual or religious *community*? Is this of support to you and how? Is there a group of people you really love or who are important to you?
*   Address in care: How would you like me to *address* these issues in your health care?

Hope

Clinicians and researchers have observed that although specific hopes may change over time, hope generally persists in some form across every stage of illness. In terminal illness, hope represents the patient's imagined future, forming the basis of a positive, accepting attitude and providing the patient's life with meaning, direction, and optimism. When hope is viewed in this way, it is not limited to cure of the disease; instead, it focuses on what is achievable in the time remaining. Many patients find hope in working on important

relationships and creating legacies. Terminally ill patients can be extremely resilient, reconceptualizing hope repeatedly as they approach the end of life.

Numerous nurse researchers have studied the concept of hope, and they have related its presence to spirituality, quality of life, and transcendence (Knabe, 2013). Hope is a multidimensional construct that provides comfort as a person endures life threats and personal challenges. The following are hope-fostering and hope-hindering activities among terminally ill hospice patients with various diagnoses:

*   *Hope-fostering categories:* Love of family and friends, spirituality/faith, setting goals and maintaining independence, positive relationships with clinicians, humor, personal characteristics, and uplifting memories
*   *Hope-hindering categories:* Abandonment and isolation, uncontrollable pain/discomfort, and devaluation of personhood

Nurses can support hope for the patient and the family by using effective listening and communication skills, thus encouraging realistic hope that is specific to their needs for information, expectations for the future, and values and preferences concerning the end of life. Nurses must engage in self-reflection and identify their own biases and fears concerning illness, life, and death. As nurses become more skilled in working with seriously ill patients, they can become less determined to "fix" and more willing to listen; more comfortable with silence, grief, anger, and sadness; and more fully present with patients and their families.

Nursing interventions for enabling and supporting hope include the following:

*   Listening attentively
*   Encouraging sharing of feelings
*   Providing accurate information
*   Encouraging and supporting the patients' control over their circumstances, choices, and environment whenever possible
*   Assisting patients to explore ways for finding meaning in their lives
*   Encouraging realistic goals
*   Facilitating effective communication within families
*   Making referrals for psychosocial and spiritual counseling
*   Assisting with the development of supports in the home or community when none exist

Managing Physiologic Responses to Terminal Illness

Patients approaching the end of life experience many of the same symptoms, regardless of their underlying disease processes. Symptoms in terminal illness may be caused by the disease, either directly (e.g., dyspnea owing to chronic obstructive lung disease) or indirectly (e.g., nausea and vomiting related to pressure in the gastric area), by the treatment for the disease, or by a coexisting disorder that is unrelated to the disease. Symptoms should be carefully and systematically assessed and managed. Questions that guide the assessment of symptoms are listed in Chart 16-9.

The patient's goals should guide symptom management. Medical interventions may be aimed at treating the underlying causes of the symptoms or reducing the impact of

Chart 16-9

ASSESSMENT

Assessing Symptoms Associated With Terminal Illness

- How is this symptom affecting the patient's life?
- What is the meaning of the symptom to the patient? To the family?
- How does the symptom affect physical functioning, mobility, comfort, sleep, nutritional status, elimination, activity level, and relationships with others?
- What makes the symptom better?
- What makes it worse?
- Is it worse at any particular time of the day?
- What are the patient's expectations and goals for managing the symptom? The family's expectations?
- How is the patient coping with the symptom?
- What is the economic effect of the symptom and its management?

Adapted from Jacox, A., Carr, D. B., & Payne, R. (1994). *Management of cancer pain*. Rockville, MD: Agency for Health Care Policy and Research.

symptoms. For example, a medical intervention such as thoracentesis (an invasive procedure in which fluid is drained from the pleural space) may be performed to temporarily relieve dyspnea in a patient with pleural effusion secondary to lung cancer. Pharmacologic and nonpharmacologic methods of symptom management may be used in combination with medical interventions to modify the physiologic causes of symptoms. For example, pharmacologic management with low-dose oral morphine effectively relieves dyspnea (Kamal, McGuire, Wheeler, et al., 2012), and mindful breathing can relive distress for patients and families receiving palliative care (Beng, Ahmad, Loong, et al., 2015). As is true with pain, the principles of pharmacologic symptom management are the use of the smallest dose of the medication to achieve the desired effect, avoidance of polypharmacy, anticipation and management of adverse effects, and creation of a therapeutic regimen that is acceptable to the patient based on their goals for maximizing quality of life.

The patient's goals take precedence over the clinicians' goals. Although clinicians may believe that symptoms must be completely relieved whenever possible, the patient might choose instead to decrease symptoms to a tolerable level rather than to relieve them completely if the side effects of medications are unacceptable to him or her. This often allows the patient to have greater independence, mobility, and alertness and to devote attention to issues that he or she considers of higher priority and greater importance.

Anticipating and planning interventions for symptoms is a cornerstone of both palliative and end-of-life care. Patients and family members cope more effectively with new symptoms and exacerbations of existing symptoms when they know what to expect and how to manage them. At the end of life, hospice programs typically provide "emergency kits" containing ready-to-administer doses of various medications that are useful to treat symptoms in advanced illness. For example, a kit might contain small doses of oral morphine liquid for pain or shortness of breath, a benzodiazepine for restlessness, and an acetaminophen suppository for fever. Family members can be instructed to administer a prescribed dose from the emergency kit, often avoiding prolonged

suffering for the patient as well as rehospitalization for symptom management.

Pain

In the final stages of illnesses such as cancer, heart disease, COPD, and renal disease, pain and other symptoms are common. Pain results from the diseases as well as the modalities used to treat them. The Worldwide Palliative Care Alliance and World Health Organization (2014) called attention to the continuing, worldwide high prevalence of pain at the end of life and the inadequate supply of opioids, particularly in developing nations. Pain at the end of life is preventable or treatable in most cases: it is every nurse's role to ensure that pain is assessed, prevented where possible, and managed. Chapter 12 presents the importance of pain assessment, assessment principles for pain that include identifying the effect of the pain on the patient's life, and the importance of believing the patient's report of the pain and its effect. Although the means to relieve pain have existed for many years, the continued, pervasive undertreatment of pain has been well documented (Reynolds, Drew, & Dunwoody, 2013). Poorly managed pain affects the psychological, emotional, social, and financial well-being of patients. Despite studies demonstrating the negative effects of inadequate pain management, practice has been slow to change. Every clinician should be able to assess and oversee the basic management of pain (IOM, 2014b).

Patients who are receiving an established regimen of analgesics should continue to receive those medications as they approach the end of life. Inability to communicate pain should not be equated with the absence of pain (McGuire, Reifsnyder, Soeken, et al., 2011). Although most pain can be managed effectively using the oral route, as the end of life nears, patients may be less able to swallow oral medications due to somnolence or nausea. Patients who have been receiving opioids should continue to receive equianalgesic doses via rectal or sublingual routes. Concentrated morphine solution can be effectively delivered by the sublingual route, because the small liquid volume is well tolerated even if swallowing is not possible. As long as the patient continues to receive opioids, a regimen to combat constipation must be implemented. If the patient cannot swallow laxatives or stool softeners, rectal suppositories or enemas may be necessary.

The nurse should educate the family about continuation of comfort measures as the patient approaches the end of life, how to administer analgesics via alternative routes, and how to assess for pain when the patient cannot verbally report pain intensity. Because the analgesics given orally or rectally are short acting and typically scheduled as frequently as every 3 to 4 hours around the clock, there is always a strong possibility that a patient approaching the end of life will die in close proximity to the time of analgesic administration. If the patient is at home, family members administering analgesics should be prepared for this possibility. They need reassurance that they did not "cause" the death of the patient by administering a dose of analgesic medication.

Dyspnea

Dyspnea, an uncomfortable awareness of breathing, is one of the most prevalent symptoms at the end of life and can be challenging to manage (Kamal et al., 2012). A highly subjective symptom, dyspnea often is not associated with visible signs of distress, such as tachypnea, diaphoresis, or cyanosis. Although the underlying cause of the dyspnea can be identified and treated in some cases, the burdens of additional diagnostic evaluation and treatment aimed at the physiologic problem may outweigh the benefits. The treatment of dyspnea varies depending on the underlying cause, the patient's general physical condition, and imminence of death. For example, a blood transfusion may provide temporary symptom relief for a patient with anemia earlier in the disease process; however, as the patient approaches the end of life, the benefits are typically short-lived or absent.

Nursing Assessment

As with assessment of pain, reports of dyspnea by patients must be believed. As is true for physical pain, the meaning of dyspnea to an individual patient may increase their suffering. For example, the patient may interpret increasing dyspnea as a sign that death is approaching. For some patients, sensations of breathlessness may invoke frightening images of drowning or suffocation, and the resulting cycle of fear and anxiety may increase the sensation of breathlessness. Therefore, the nurse should conduct a careful assessment of the psychosocial and spiritual components of the dyspnea. Physical assessment parameters include symptom intensity, distress, and interference with activities; auscultation of lung sounds; assessment of fluid balance, including measurement of dependent edema (circumference of lower extremities) and abdominal girth; temperature; skin color; sputum quantity and character; and cough.

To determine the intensity of dyspnea and its interference with daily activities, the patient can be asked to report the severity of the dyspnea using a scale of 0 to 10, where 0 is no dyspnea and 10 is the worst imaginable dyspnea. The nurse should assess the patient's baseline rating before treatment and should elicit subsequent measurements taken during exacerbation of the symptom, periodically during treatment, and whenever the treatment plan changes; these parameters provide ongoing objective evidence for the efficacy of the treatment plan. In addition, physical assessment findings may assist in locating the source of the dyspnea and selecting nursing interventions to relieve the symptom. The components of the assessment change as the patient's condition changes. For example, when the patient who has been on daily weights can no longer get out of bed, the goal of comfort may outweigh the benefit of continued weights. Like other symptoms at the end of life, dyspnea can be managed effectively in the absence of assessment and diagnostic data (e.g., arterial blood gases) that are standard when a patient's illness or symptom is acute and considered reversible. A numeric rating scale similar to one that is used for assessing pain can provide objective evidence of the severity of the patient's dyspnea.

Nursing Management

Nursing management of dyspnea at the end of life is directed toward administering medical treatment for the underlying pathology, monitoring the patient's response to treatment, helping the patient and the family manage anxiety (which exacerbates dyspnea), altering the perception of the symptom, and conserving energy (see Chart 16-10). Pharmacologic intervention is aimed at modifying lung physiology and

---

Chart 16-10 Palliative Nursing Interventions for Dyspnea

Decrease Anxiety

- Administer prescribed anxiolytic medications as indicated for anxiety or panic associated with dyspnea.
- Assist with relaxation techniques, guided imagery.
- Provide patient with a means to call for assistance (call bell/light within reach in a hospital or long-term care facility; handheld bell or other device for home).

Treat Underlying Pathology

- Administer prescribed bronchodilators and corticosteroids (obstructive pathology).
- Administer blood products, erythropoietin as prescribed (typically not beneficial in advanced disease).
- Administer prescribed diuretics and monitor fluid balance.

Alter Perception of Breathlessness

- Administer prescribed oxygen therapy via nasal cannula, if tolerated; masks may not be well tolerated.
- Administer prescribed low-dose opioids via oral route (morphine sulfate is used most commonly).
- Provide air movement in the patient's environment with a portable fan.

Reduce Respiratory Demand

- Educate patient and family to implement energy conservation measures.
- Place needed equipment, supplies, and nourishment within reach.
- For home or hospice care, offer bedside commode, electrical bed (with head that elevates).

---

improving performance as well as altering the perception of the symptom. Bronchodilators and corticosteroids are used to treat underlying obstructive pathology, thereby improving overall lung function. Low doses of opioids effectively relieve dyspnea, although the mechanism of relief is not entirely clear. Although dyspnea in terminal illness is typically not associated with diminished blood oxygen saturation, low-flow oxygen often provides psychological comfort to both patients and families, particularly in the home setting.

As mentioned previously, dyspnea may be exacerbated by anxiety, and anxiety may trigger episodes of dyspnea, setting off a respiratory crisis in which the patient and the family may panic. For patients receiving care at home, patient and family education should include anticipation and management of crisis situations and a clearly communicated emergency plan. The patient and the family should be instructed about medication administration, condition changes that should be reported to the physician and the nurse, and strategies for coping with diminished reserves and increasing symptomatology as the disease progresses. The patient and the family require reassurance that the symptom can be effectively managed at home without the need for activation of the emergency medical services or hospitalization and that a nurse will be available at all times via telephone and to make a visit.

Nutrition and Hydration at the End of Life

Anorexia and cachexia are common in the seriously ill. The profound changes in the patient's appearance and a lack of interest in the socially important rituals of mealtime

TABLE 16-2 Measures for Managing Anorexia

Nursing Interventions	Patient and Family Education Tips
Initiate measures to ensure adequate dietary intake without adding stress to the patient at mealtimes.	Reduce the focus on "balanced" meals; offer the same food as often as the patient desires it.
Assess the impact of medications (e.g., chemotherapy, antiretrovirals) or other therapies (radiation therapy, dialysis) that are being used to treat the underlying illness.	Increase the nutritional value of meals. For example, add dry milk powder to milk, and use this fortified milk to prepare cream soups, milkshakes, and gravies.
Administer and monitor effects of prescribed treatment of nausea, vomiting, and delayed gastric emptying.	
Encourage patient to eat when effects of medications have subsided.	Allow and encourage the patient to eat when hungry, regardless of usual mealtimes.
Assess and modify environment to eliminate unpleasant odors and other factors that cause nausea, vomiting, and anorexia.	Eliminate or reduce noxious cooking odors, pet odors, or other odors that may precipitate nausea, vomiting, or anorexia.
Remove items that may reduce appetite (soiled tissues, bedpans, emesis basins, clutter).	Keep patient's environment clean, uncluttered, and comfortable.
Assess and manage anxiety and depression to the extent possible.	Make mealtime a shared experience away from the "sick" room whenever possible. Reduce stress at mealtimes. Avoid confrontations about the amount of food consumed. Reduce or eliminate routine weighing of the patient.
Position to enhance gastric emptying.	Encourage patient to eat in a sitting position; elevate the head of the patient's bed. Plan meals (food selection and portion size) that the patient desires. Provide small frequent meals if they are easier for patient to eat.
Assess for constipation and/or intestinal obstruction.	Ensure that patient and family understand that prevention of constipation is essential, even when the patient's intake is minimal.
Prevent and manage constipation on an ongoing basis, even when the patient's intake is minimal.	Encourage adequate fluid intake, dietary fiber, and the use of a bowel program to prevent constipation.
Provide frequent mouth care, particularly following nourishment.	Assist the patient to rinse after every meal. Avoid mouthwashes that contain alcohol or glycerine, which dry mucous membranes.
Ensure that dentures fit properly.	Weight loss may cause dentures to loosen and cause irritation. Remove them to inspect the gums and to provide oral care.
Administer and monitor effects of topical and systemic treatment for oropharyngeal pain.	The patient's comfort may be enhanced if medications for pain relief given on an as-needed basis for breakthrough pain are given before mealtimes.

are particularly disturbing to families. The approach to the problem varies depending on the patient's stage of illness, level of disability associated with the illness, and desires. The anorexia–cachexia syndrome is characterized by disturbances in carbohydrate, protein, and fat metabolism; endocrine dysfunction; and anemia. The syndrome results in severe asthenia (loss of energy).

Anorexia and cachexia differ from starvation (simple food deprivation) in several important ways. Appetite is lost early in the process, the body becomes catabolic in a dysfunctional way, and supplementation by gastric feeding (tube feeding) or parenteral nutrition in advanced disease does not replenish lean body mass that has been lost.

Anorexia

Although causes of anorexia may be controlled for a period of time, progressive anorexia is an expected and natural part of the dying process. Anorexia may be related to or exacerbated by situational variables (e.g., the ability to have meals with the family vs. eating alone in the "sick room"), progression of the disease, treatment of the disease, or psychological distress. The patient and the family should be instructed in strategies to manage the variables associated with anorexia (see Table 16-2).

Use of Pharmacologic Agents to Stimulate Appetite

Several pharmacologic agents are commonly used to stimulate appetite in patients with anorexia, although only progestational agents (e.g., megestrol acetate [Megace]) and glucocorticoids (e.g., dexamethasone [Dexpak]) have been found to stimulate appetite when examined in well-controlled research studies (Bondly & Jatoi, 2015). However, these agents have not been found to improve survival or quality in life in patients approaching end of life (Arensmeyer, 2012). Dexamethasone initially increases appetite and may provide short-term weight gain in some patients. It should be considered for those patients whose life expectancy is limited because the beneficial effects may be limited to the first few weeks of therapy and side effects increase over time (Del Fabbro, 2015). Therapy may need to be discontinued in patients with a longer life expectancy; after 3 to 4 weeks, corticosteroids interfere with the synthesis of muscle protein.

Megestrol acetate produces temporary weight gain of primarily fatty tissue, with little effect on protein balance. This agent carries risk of serious side effects, including thromboembolism, and risk increases with prolonged use (Del Fabbro, 2015).

Dronabinol is a psychoactive compound found in cannabis that may be helpful in reducing nausea and vomiting, appetite loss, pain, and anxiety, thereby improving food and fluid intake in some patients. However, in most patients, it is not as effective as other agents for appetite stimulation. Although dronabinol may have beneficial effects on appetite in patients with advanced cancer, it has not been shown to be more effective than megestrol. In addition, it possesses undesirable central nervous system side effects (Del Fabbro, 2015).

Cachexia

Cachexia refers to severe lean muscle loss with or without fat loss that cannot be reversed by traditional nutritional interventions (Fearon, Strasser, Anker, et al., 2011). Although anorexia may exacerbate cachexia, it is not the primary cause. Cachexia is associated with anabolic and catabolic changes in metabolism that relate to activity of neurohormones and proinflammatory cytokines, resulting in profound protein loss. These processes appear to be similar at the end stages of both cancer and some noncancerous illnesses, such as AIDS (Del Fabbro, 2015). However, the pathophysiology of cachexia in terminal illness is not well understood. In terminal illness, the severity of tissue wasting is greater than would be expected from reduced food intake alone, and typically increasing appetite or food intake does not reverse cachexia.

At one time, it was believed that patients with cancer with rapidly growing tumors developed cachexia because the tumor created an excessive nutritional demand and diverted nutrients from the rest of the body. Research links cytokines produced by the body in response to a tumor to a complex inflammatory-immune response present in patients whose tumors have metastasized, leading to anorexia, weight loss, and altered metabolism. An increase in cytokines occurs not only in cancer but also in AIDS and many other chronic diseases (Del Fabbro, 2015).

Artificial Nutrition and Hydration

Along with breathing, eating and drinking are essential to survival throughout life. Near the end of life, the body's nutritional needs change, and the desire for food and fluid may diminish. People may no longer be able to use, eliminate, or store nutrients and fluids adequately. Eating and sharing meals are important social activities in families and communities, and food preparation and enjoyment are linked to happy memories, strong emotions, and hope for survival. For patients with serious illness, food preparation and mealtimes often become battlegrounds in which well-meaning family members argue, plead, and cajole to encourage ill people to eat. Seriously ill patients often lose their appetites entirely, develop strong aversions to foods that they have enjoyed in the past, or crave a particular food to the exclusion of all other foods.

Although nutritional supplementation may be an important part of the treatment plan in early or chronic illness, unintended weight loss and dehydration are expected characteristics of progressive illness. As illness progresses, patients, families, and clinicians may believe that without artificial nutrition and hydration, terminally ill patients will "starve," causing profound suffering and hastened death. However, starvation should not be viewed as the failure to insert tubes for nutritional supplementation or hydration of terminally ill patients with irreversible progression of disease. Research has demonstrated that terminally ill patients with cancer who were hydrated did not have improved biochemical parameters and exhibited lower serum albumin levels, leading to fluid retention. The use of artificial nutrition and hydration (tube and intravenous [IV] fluids and feeding) carries considerable risks and generally does not contribute to comfort at the end of life (Casarett, Kapo, & Kaplan, 2005). Similarly, survival is not increased when terminally ill patients with advanced dementia receive enteral feeding, and no data support an association between tube feeding and improved quality of life in these patients (Mitchell, Black, Ersek, et al., 2012). Furthermore, in patients who are close to death, symptoms associated with dehydration such as dry mouth, confusion, and diminished alertness are common and typically do not respond to artificial nutrition (Danis, Arnold, & Savarese, 2015). Dry mouth can generally be managed through nursing measures such as mouth care and environmental changes with medications to diminish confusion.

As the patient approaches the end of life, the family and the health care providers should offer the patient what he or she prefers and can most easily tolerate. The nurse should instruct the family how to separate feeding from caring and how to demonstrate love, sharing, and caring by being with the loved one in other ways. Preoccupation with appetite, feeding, and weight loss diverts energy and time that the patient and the family could use in other meaningful activities. In addition to those given in Table 16-2, the following are the tips to promote nutrition for terminally ill patients:

- Offer small portions of favorite foods.
- Be aware that cool foods may be better tolerated than hot foods.
- Offer cheese, eggs, peanut butter, mild fish, chicken, or turkey. Meat (especially beef) may taste bitter and unpleasant.
- Add milk shakes, meal replacement drinks, or other liquid supplements.
- Place nutritious foods at the bedside (fruit juices, milk shakes in insulated drink containers with straws).
- Schedule meals when family members can be present to provide company and stimulation.
- Offer ice chips made from frozen fruit juices.
- Allow the patient to refuse foods and fluids.

Delirium

Many patients remain alert, arousable, and able to communicate until very close to death. Others sleep for long intervals and awaken only intermittently, with eventual somnolence until death. Delirium refers to concurrent disturbances in the level of consciousness, attention, awareness, and cognitive capability that develop over a relatively short period of time (Wright, Brajtman, & Macdonald, 2014). In some patients, a period of agitated delirium precedes death, sometimes causing families to be hopeful that suddenly active patients may be getting better. Confusion may be related to underlying, treatable conditions such as medication side effects or interactions, pain or discomfort, hypoxia or dyspnea, or a full bladder or impacted stool. In patients with cancer, confusion may be secondary to brain metastases. Delirium may also be related to metabolic changes, infection, and organ failure.

Patients with delirium may become hypoactive or hyperactive, restless, irritable, and fearful. Sleep deprivation and hallucinations may occur. If treatment of the underlying factors contributing to these symptoms brings no relief, a combination of pharmacologic intervention with neuroleptics or benzodiazepines may be effective in decreasing distressing symptoms for some patients. There have been few randomized clinical trials to establish evidence for practice, nor are there current clinical guidelines for delirium management (Lawlor & Bush, 2014). The neuroleptic drug haloperidol (Haldol) is the most frequently used drug to treat delirium in palliative care settings and may reduce hallucinations and agitation at the end of life. Newer (atypical) neuroleptics, such as olanzapine (Zyprexa), quetiapine (Seroquel), and risperidone (Risperdal) have been less well studied (Lawlor & Bush, 2014). Benzodiazepines (e.g., lorazepam [Ativan]) can reduce anxiety but may contribute to worsening cognitive impairment if used alone.

Nursing interventions are aimed at identifying the underlying causes of delirium; acknowledging the family's distress over its occurrence; reassuring family members about what is normal; educating family members how to interact with and ensure safety for the patient with delirium; and monitoring the effects of medications used to treat severe agitation, paranoia, and fear. Confusion may mask the patient's unmet spiritual needs and fears about dying. Spiritual intervention, music therapy, gentle massage, and therapeutic touch may provide some relief. Reduction of environmental stimuli, avoidance of harsh lighting or very dim lighting (which may produce disturbing shadows), presence of familiar faces, and gentle reorientation and reassurance are also helpful.

Depression

Clinical depression should neither be accepted as an inevitable consequence of dying nor confused with sadness and anticipatory grieving, which are normal reactions to the losses associated with impending death. Emotional and spiritual support and control of disturbing physical symptoms are appropriate interventions for situational depression associated with terminal illness. Researchers have linked the psychological effects of cancer pain to suicidal thought and, less frequently, to carrying out a planned suicide (Robson, Scrutton, Wilkinson, et al., 2010). Patients and their families must be given space and time to experience sadness and to grieve; however, patients should not have to endure untreated depression at the end of their lives. An effective combined approach to clinical depression includes relief of physical symptoms, attention to emotional and spiritual distress, psychotherapy, and pharmacologic intervention with psychostimulants and antidepressants (Marks & Heinrich, 2013).

Palliative Sedation at the End of Life

Effective control of symptoms can be achieved under most conditions; however, some patients may experience distressing, intractable symptoms. Although **palliative sedation** remains controversial, it is offered in some settings to patients who are close to death or who have symptoms that do not respond to conventional pharmacologic and nonpharmacologic approaches, resulting in unrelieved suffering. Palliative sedation is distinguished from **euthanasia** and physician-assisted suicide in that the intent of palliative sedation is to relieve symptoms, not to hasten death. Palliative sedation is most commonly used when the patient exhibits intractable pain, dyspnea, seizures, or delirium, and it is generally considered appropriate in only the most difficult situations. Before implementing palliative sedation, the health care team should assess for the presence of underlying and treatable causes of suffering, such as depression or spiritual distress. Finally, the patient and the family should be fully informed about the use of this treatment and alternatives. Whereas proportionate palliative sedation uses the minimum drug necessary to relieve the symptom while preserving consciousness, palliative sedation induces unconsciousness, which is more controversial.

Palliative sedation is accomplished through an infusion of one or more pharmacologic agents in doses adequate to eliminate signs of discomfort and, in some cases, induce sleep. In a review of published guidelines for pharmacologic management of palliative sedation, researchers reported that although most published guidelines varied considerably, most mentioned the use of midazolam (Versed), a short-acting hypnotic sedative (Schildmann, Schildmann, & Kiesewetter, 2015). Nurses act as collaborating members of the interdisciplinary health care team, providing emotional support to patients and families, facilitating clarification of values and preferences, and providing comfort-focused physical care. Once sedation has been induced, the nurse should continue to comfort the patient, monitor the physiologic effects of the sedation, support the family during the final hours or days of their loved one's life, and ensure communication within the health care team and between the team and the family.

Nursing Care of Patients Who Are Close to Death

Providing care to patients who are close to death and being present at the time of death can be one of the most rewarding experiences a nurse can have. Patients and their families are understandably fearful of the unknown, and the approach of death may prompt new concerns or cause previous fears or issues to resurface. Family members who have always had difficulty communicating or who are part of families in which there are old resentments and hurts may experience heightened difficulty as their loved one nears death. However, the time at the end of life can also afford opportunities to resolve old hurts and learn new ways of being a family. Regardless of the setting, skilled practitioners can make dying patients comfortable, make space for their loved ones to remain present if they wish, and can give family members the opportunity to experience growth and healing. Likewise, patients and family members may be less apprehensive near the time of death if they know what to expect and how to respond.

Expected Physiologic Changes

As death approaches and organ systems begin to fail, observable, expected changes in the body take place. Nursing care

Chart 16-11 · EDUCATING THE FAMILY
Signs of Approaching Death

The person shows less interest in eating and drinking. For many patients, refusal of food is an indication that they are ready to die. Fluid intake may be limited to that which will keep their mouths from feeling too dry.

- *What you can do:* Offer, but do not force, fluids and medication. Sometimes pain or other symptoms that have required medication in the past may no longer be present. For most patients, pain medications are still needed, and they can be provided by concentrated oral solutions placed under the tongue or by rectal suppository.

Urinary output may decrease in amount and frequency.

- *What you can do:* No response is needed unless the patient expresses a desire to urinate and cannot. Call the hospice nurse for advice if you are not sure.

As the body weakens, the patient will sleep more and begin to detach from the environment. He or she may refuse your attempts to provide comfort.

- *What you can do:* Allow your loved one to sleep. You may wish to sit with him or her, play soft music, or hold hands. Your loved one's withdrawal is normal and is not a rejection of your love.

Mental confusion may become apparent. This occurs because less oxygen is available to supply the brain. The patient may report strange dreams or visions.

- *What you can do:* As he or she awakens from sleep, remind him or her of the day and time, where he or she is, and who is present. This is best done in a casual, conversational way.

Vision and hearing may become somewhat impaired, and speech may be difficult to understand.

- *What you can do:* Speak clearly but no more loudly than necessary. Keep the room as light as the patient wishes, even at night. Carry on all conversations as if they can be heard, because hearing may be the last of the senses to cease functioning.
- Many patients are able to talk until minutes before death and are reassured by the exchange of a few words with a loved one.

Secretions may collect in the back of the throat and rattle or gurgle as the patient breathes through the mouth. He or she may try to cough, and their mouth may become dry and encrusted with secretions.

- *What you can do:* If the patient is trying to cough up secretions and is experiencing choking or vomiting, call the hospice nurse for assistance.
- Secretions may drain from the mouth if you place the patient on their side and provide support with pillows.

- Cleansing the mouth with moistened mouth swabs will help relieve the dryness that occurs with mouth breathing.
- Offer water in small amounts to keep the mouth moist. A straw with one finger placed over the end can be used to transfer sips of water to the patient's mouth.

Breathing may become irregular with periods of no breathing (apnea). The patient may be working very hard to breathe and may make a moaning sound with each breath. As the time of death nears, the breathing remains irregular and may become more shallow and mechanical.

- *What you can do:* Raising the head of the bed may help the patient to breathe more easily. The moaning sound does not mean that the patient is in pain or other distress; it is the sound of air passing over very relaxed vocal cords.

As the oxygen supply to the brain decreases, the patient may become restless. It is not unusual to pull at the bed linens, to have visual hallucinations, or even to try to get out of bed at this point.

- *What you can do:* Reassure the patient in a calm voice that you are there. Prevent him or her from falling by trying to get out of bed. Soft music or a back rub may be soothing.

The patient may feel hot one moment and cold the next as the body loses its ability to control temperature. As circulation slows, the arms and legs may become cool and bluish. The underside of the body may darken. It may be difficult to feel a pulse at the wrist.

- *What you can do:* Provide and remove blankets as needed. Avoid using electrical blankets, which may cause burns because the patient cannot tell you if he or she is too warm.
- Sponge the patient's head with a cool cloth if this provides comfort.

Loss of bladder and bowel control may occur around the time of death.

- *What you can do:* Protect the mattress with waterproof padding, and change the padding as needed to keep the patient comfortable.

As people approach death, many times they report seeing gardens, libraries, or family or friends who have died. They may ask you to pack their bags and find tickets or a passport. Sometimes they may become insistent and attempt to do these chores themselves. They may try getting out of bed (even if they have been confined to bed for a long time) so that they can "leave."

- *What you can do:* Reassure the patient that it is all right; he or she can "go" without getting out of bed. Stay close, share stories, and be present.

Used with permission from the Hospice of Philadelphia. (2015). *Signs of approaching death*. Philadelphia, PA: Author.

---

measures aimed at patient comfort, such as pain medications (given rectally or sublingually), turning, mouth care, eye care, positioning to facilitate draining of secretions, and measures to protect the skin from urine or feces (if the patient is incontinent), should be continued. The nurse should consult with the interprofessional team about discontinuing measures that no longer contribute to patient comfort, such as drawing blood, administering tube feedings, suctioning (in most cases), and invasive monitoring. The nurse should prepare the family for the normal, expected changes that accompany the period immediately preceding death. Although the exact

time of death cannot be predicted, it is often possible to identify when the patient is very close to death. Hospice programs frequently provide written information for families so that they know what to expect and what to do as death nears (see Chart 16-11).

If family members have been prepared for the time of death, they are less likely to panic and are better able to be with their loved one in a meaningful way. Noisy, gurgling breathing or moaning is generally most distressing to family members. In most cases, the sounds of breathing at the end of life are related to oropharyngeal relaxation and diminished awareness. Family members may have difficulty believing that the patient is not in pain or that the patient's breathing could not be improved by suctioning secretions. Patient positioning and family reassurance are the most helpful responses to these symptoms.

When death is imminent, patients may become increasingly somnolent and unable to clear sputum or oral secretions, which may lead to further impairment of breathing from pooled or dried and crusted secretions. The sound (terminal bubbling) and appearance of the secretions are often more distressing to family members than is the presence of the secretions to the patient. Family distress over the changes in the patient's condition may be eased by supportive nursing care. Continuation of comfort-focused interventions and reassurance that the patient is not in any distress can do much to ease family concerns. Gentle mouth care with a moistened swab or very soft toothbrush helps maintain the integrity of the patient's mucous membranes. In addition, gentle oral suctioning, positioning to enhance drainage of secretions, and sublingual or transdermal administration of anticholinergic drugs (see Table 16-3) reduce the production of secretions and provide comfort to the patient and support to the family. Deeper suctioning may cause significant discomfort to the dying patient and is rarely of any benefit because secretions reaccumulate rapidly.

The Death Vigil

Although each death is unique, it is often possible for experienced clinicians to assess that the patient is "actively" or imminently dying and to prepare the family in the final days or hours leading to death. As death nears, the patient may withdraw, sleep for longer intervals, or become somnolent. Death is generally preceded by a period of gradual diminishment of bodily functions, increased intervals between respirations, a weakened and irregular pulse, diminished blood pressure, and skin color changes or mottling. Family members

TABLE 16-3 Secretions and Terminal Respiratory Congestion Table

Medication	Suggested Initial Dosing
Atropine 1% ophthalmic (Isopto-Atropine®)	1 to 2 drops PO/SL every 4 hours, scheduled or PRN
Atropine injection[a]	0.4 mg IV/SC/IM every 4 hours, scheduled or PRN
Glycopyrrolate[a] (Robinul®)	1 mg PO TID, scheduled or PRN, up to 6 mg/d, or 0.1 mg SC/IM/IV TID PRN or
Hyoscyamine[a] (Levsin®)	0.125 mg PO/SL every 4 hours PRN, up to 1.5 mg/d
Hyoscyamine extended-release[a] (Levbid®)	0.375 mg PO every 12 hours, up to 1.5 mg/d
Scopolamine (Transderm Scop®)	Apply 1 patch topically behind the ear every 72 hours, up to 3 patches/72 hours

IM, intramuscularly; IV, intravenously; PO, by mouth; PRN, as needed; SC, subcutaneously; SL, sublingually; TID, twice a day.
[a]Preferred agent(s).
Reprinted with permission from Enclara Pharmacia, Inc. (2015). *Enclara Pharmacia Medication Use Guidelines* (1st ed.). Philadelphia, PA: Author.

should be encouraged to be with the patient, to speak and reassure the patient of their presence, to stroke or touch the patient, or to lie alongside the patient (even in the hospital or long-term care facility) if the family members are comfortable with this degree of closeness and can do so without causing discomfort to the patient.

The family may go to great lengths to ensure that their loved one will not die alone. However, despite the best intentions and efforts of the family and clinicians, the patient may die at a time when no one is present. In any setting, it is unrealistic for family members to be at the patient's bedside 24 hours a day. Experienced hospice clinicians have observed and reported that some patients appear to "wait" until family members are away from the bedside to die, perhaps to spare their loved ones the pain of being present at the time of death. Nurses can reassure family members throughout the death vigil by being present intermittently or continuously, modeling behaviors (such as touching and speaking to the patient), providing encouragement in relation to family caregiving, providing reassurance about normal physiologic changes, and encouraging family rest breaks. If a patient dies while family members are away from the bedside, they may express feelings of guilt and profound grief and may need emotional support.

After-Death Care

For patients who have received adequate management of symptoms and for families who have received adequate preparation and support, the actual time of death is commonly peaceful and occurs without struggle. Nurses may or may not be present at the time of a patient's death. In many states, nurses are authorized to make the pronouncement of death and sign the death certificate when death is expected. Death is defined as the permanent cessation of respiratory and circulatory functions (Bernat, 2009). The determination of death is made through a physical examination that includes auscultation for the absence of breathing and heart sounds. Home care or hospice programs in which nurses make the time-of-death visit and pronounce death have policies and procedures to guide the nurse's actions during this visit. Immediately on cessation of vital functions, the body begins to change. It becomes dusky or bluish, waxen appearing, and cool; blood darkens and pools in dependent areas of the body (e.g., the back and the sacrum if the body is in a supine position); and urine and stool may be evacuated.

Immediately after death, family members should be allowed and encouraged to spend time with the deceased. Normal responses of family members at the time of death vary widely and range from quiet expressions of grief to overt expressions that include wailing and prostration. The family members' desire for privacy during their time with the deceased should be honored. Family members may wish to independently manage or assist with care of the body after death. In the home, after-death care of the body frequently includes culturally specific rituals such as bathing the body. Home care agencies and hospices vary in the policies surrounding removal of tubes. In the absence of specific guidance from the organization, the nurse should shut off infusions of any kind (IV or tube feeding) and leave IV access devices, feeding tubes, catheters, and wound dressings in place. When an expected death occurs in the home setting, the family generally will have received assistance with funeral arrangements in advance of the death. The funeral home has often been prearranged, and the funeral director will transport the body directly to the funeral home. In the hospital or long-term care facility, nurses follow the facility's procedure for preparation of the body and transportation to the facility's morgue. However, the needs of families to remain with the deceased, to wait until other family members arrive before the body is moved, and to perform after-death rituals should be honored.

Some patients may have elected to donate tissue such as corneas, bone, veins, or heart valves for transplant. Typically, this information would be known to the care team before the patient dies. In some cases, such as late referral or an unexpectedly rapid progression, the patient's wishes with respect to donation might be unknown. If the patient died at home or in a nursing home and the deceased's wishes are known, a team member should contact the organ procurement organization through which the deceased had arranged to donate tissue. That organization will ordinarily transport the body for tissue procurement and to the funeral home.

Grief, Mourning, and Bereavement

A wide range of feelings and behaviors are normal, adaptive, and healthy reactions to the loss of a loved one. **Grief** refers to the personal feelings that accompany an anticipated or actual loss. **Mourning** refers to individual, family, group, and cultural expressions of grief and associated behaviors. **Bereavement** refers to the period of time during which mourning for a loss takes place. Both grief reactions and mourning behaviors change over time as people learn to live with the loss. Although the pain of the loss may be tempered by the passage of time, loss is an ongoing developmental process, and time does not heal the bereaved individual completely. That is, the bereaved do not get over a loss entirely, nor do they return to who they were before the loss. Rather, they develop a new sense of who they are and where they fit in a world that has changed dramatically and permanently.

Anticipatory Grief and Mourning

Denial, sadness, anger, fear, and anxiety are normal grief reactions in people with life-threatening illness and those close to them. Kübler-Ross (1969) described five common emotional reactions to dying that are applicable to the experience of any loss (see Table 16-4). Not every patient or family member experiences every stage; many patients never reach a stage of acceptance, and patients and families sometimes fluctuate on a daily basis in their emotional responses. Furthermore, although impending loss stresses the patient, the people who are close to him or her, and the functioning of the family unit, awareness of dying also provides a unique opportunity for family members to reminisce, resolve relationships, plan for the future, and say goodbye.

Individual and family coping with the anticipation of death is complicated by the varied and conflicting trajectories that grief and mourning may assume in families. For example, the patient may be experiencing sadness while contemplating role changes that have been brought about by the illness, and the patient's spouse or partner may be expressing or suppressing feelings of anger about the current changes in role and impending loss of the relationship. Others in the family may be engaged in denial (e.g., "Dad will get better. He just needs to eat more"), fear ("Who will take care of us?" or "Will I get sick, too?"), or profound sadness and withdrawal. Although each of these behaviors is normal, tension may arise when

TABLE 16-4 Kübler-Ross's Five Stages of Grief

Stage	Nursing Implications
Denial: "This cannot be true." Feelings of isolation. May search for another health care professional who will give a more favorable opinion. May seek unproven therapies.	Denial can be an adaptive response, providing a buffer after bad news. It allows time to mobilize defenses but can be maladaptive when it prevents the patient or the family from seeking help or when denial behaviors cause more pain or distress than the illness or interfere with everyday functions. Nurses should assess the patient's and family's coping style, information needs, and understanding of the illness and treatment to establish a basis for empathetic listening, education, and emotional support. Rather than confronting the patient with information that he or she is not ready to hear, the nurse can encourage him or her to share fears and concerns. Open-ended questions or statements such as "Tell me more about how you are coping with this new information about your illness" can provide a springboard for expression of concerns.
Anger: "Why me?" Feelings of rage, resentment, or envy directed at God, health care professionals, family, others.	Anger can be very isolating, and loved ones or clinicians may withdraw. Nurses should allow the patient and family to express anger, treating them with understanding, respect, and knowledge that the root of the anger is grief over impending loss.
Bargaining: "I just want to see my grandchild's birth, then I'll be ready...." Patient and/or family plead for more time to reach an important goal. Promises are sometimes made with God.	Terminally ill patients are sometimes able to outlive prognoses and achieve some future goal. Nurses should be patient, allow expression of feelings, and support realistic and positive hope.
Depression: "I just don't know how my kids are going to get along after I'm gone." Sadness, grief, mourning for impending losses.	Normal and adaptive response. Clinical depression should be assessed and treated when present. Nurses should encourage the patient and the family to fully express their sadness. Insincere reassurance or encouragement of unrealistic hopes should be avoided.
Acceptance: "I've lived a good life, and I have no regrets." Patient and/or family are neither angry nor depressed.	The patient may withdraw as their circle of interest diminishes. The family may feel rejected by the patient. Nurses need to support the family's expression of emotions and encourage them to continue to be present for the patient.

Adapted from Kübler-Ross, E. (1969). *On death and dying.* New York, NY: Macmillan.

one or more family members perceive that others are less caring, too emotional, or too detached.

The nurse should assess the characteristics of the family system and intervene in a manner that supports and enhances the cohesion of the family unit. Parameters for assessing the family facing life-threatening illness are identified in Chart 16-12. The nurse can suggest that family members talk about their feelings and understand them in the broader context of anticipatory grief and mourning. Acknowledging and expressing feelings, continuing to interact with the patient in meaningful ways, and planning for the time of death and bereavement are adaptive family behaviors. Professional support provided by grief counselors, whether in the community, at a local hospital, in the long-term care facility, or associated with a hospice program, can help both the patient and the family sort out and acknowledge feelings and make the end of life as meaningful as possible.

Grief and Mourning After Death

When a loved one dies, family members enter a new phase of grief and mourning as they begin to accept the loss, feel the pain of permanent separation, and prepare to live a life without the deceased. Even if the loved one died after a long illness, preparatory grief experienced during the terminal illness does not preclude the grief and mourning that follow the death. With a death after a long or difficult illness, family members may experience conflicting feelings of relief that the loved one's suffering has ended, compounded by guilt and grief related to unresolved issues or the circumstances of death. Grief work may be especially difficult if a patient's death was painful, prolonged, accompanied by unwanted interventions, or unattended. Families that had no preparation or support during the period of imminent death may have a more difficult time finding a place for the painful memories.

Although some family members may experience prolonged or complicated mourning, most grief reactions fall within a "normal" range. The feelings are often profound; however, bereaved people eventually reconcile the loss and find a way to reengage with their lives. Grief and mourning are affected by several factors, including individual characteristics, coping skills, and experiences with illness and death; the nature of the relationship to the deceased; factors surrounding the illness and the death; family dynamics; social support; and cultural expectations and norms. Uncomplicated grief and mourning are characterized by a range of emotions and behaviors from sadness and yearning to thoughts about or preoccupation with the deceased and for many, a temporary withdrawal from the activities of living in which they engaged before the death (Shear, 2012).

After-death rituals, including preparation of the body, funeral practices, and burial rituals, are socially and culturally significant ways in which family members begin to accept the reality and finality of death. Preplanning of funerals is becoming increasingly common, and hospice professionals in particular help the family make plans for death, often involving the patient, who may wish to play an active role. Preplanning of the funeral relieves the family of the burden of making decisions in the intensely emotional period after a death.

In general, the period of mourning is an adaptive response to loss during which mourners come to accept the loss as real and permanent, acknowledge and experience the painful emotions that accompany the loss, experience life without the deceased, overcome impediments to adjustment, and find a new way of living in a world without the loved one. Particularly immediately after the death, mourners begin to recognize the reality and permanence of the loss by talking about the deceased and telling and retelling the story of the illness and death. Societal norms in the United States are frequently at odds with the normal grieving processes of people; time excused from work obligations is typically measured in days, and mourners are often expected to get over the loss quickly and get on with life.

In reality, the work of grief and mourning takes time, and avoiding grief work after the death often leads to long-term adjustment difficulties. According to Rando (2000), mourning for a loss involves the "undoing" of psychosocial ties that bind mourners to the deceased, personal adaptation to the loss, and learning to live in the world without the deceased. Six key processes of mourning allow people to accommodate to the loss in a healthy way (Rando, 2000):

1. Recognition of the loss
2. Reaction to the separation and experiencing and expressing the pain of the loss

Chart 16-12 — ASSESSMENT

Assessing for Anticipatory Mourning in the Family Facing Life-Threatening Illness

Family Constellation

- Identify the members who constitute the patient's family. Who is important to the patient?
- Identify roles and relationships among the family members:
- Who is the primary caregiver?
- By what authority is this person the primary caregiver?

Cohesion and Boundaries

- How autonomous/interdependent are family members?
  - Degree of involvement with each other as individuals and as a family
  - Degree of bonding between family members
  - Degree of "teamwork" in the family
  - Degree of reliance on individual family members for specific tasks/roles
- How do family members differ in:
  - Personality?
  - Worldview?
  - Priorities?
- What are the implicit and explicit expectations or "rules" for behavior within the family?

Flexibility and Adaptability

- What is the family's ability to integrate new information?
- How does the family manage change?
- How able are the family members to assume new roles and responsibilities?

Communication

- What is the style of communication in the family, in terms of:
  - Openness?
  - Directness?
  - Clarity?
- What are the constraints on communication?
- What topics are avoided?

Chart 16-13 Nursing Interventions for Grief and Mourning

Support the Expression of Feelings

- Encourage the telling of the story using open-ended statements or questions (e.g., "Tell me about your husband").
- Assist the mourner to find an outlet for their feelings: talking, attending a support group, keeping a journal, finding a safe outlet for angry feelings (writing letters that will not be mailed, physical activity).
- Assess emotional affect and reinforce the normalcy of feelings.
- Assess for guilt and regrets:
  - "Are you especially troubled by a certain memory or thought?"
  - "How do you manage those memories?"

Assess for the Presence of Social Support

- "Do you have someone to whom you can talk about your husband?"
- "May I help you find someone you can talk to?"

Assess Coping Skills

- "How are you managing day to day?"
- "Have you experienced other losses? How did you manage those?"
- "Are there things that you are having trouble doing?"
- "Do you have/need help with specific tasks?"

Assess for Signs of Complicated Grief and Mourning and Offer Professional Referral

- Are you preoccupied with thoughts of the deceased that interfere with your ability to care for yourself?
- Do you have frequent and prolonged intense emotional pain?

---

3. Recollection and reexperiencing the deceased, the relationship, and the associated feelings
4. Relinquishing old attachments to the deceased
5. Readjustment to adapt to the new world without forgetting the old
6. Reinvestment

Although many people complete the work of mourning with the informal support of families and friends, many find that talking with others who have had a similar experience, such as in formal support groups, normalizes the feelings and experiences and provides a framework for learning new skills to cope with the loss and create a new life. Hospitals, hospices, religious organizations, and other community organizations often sponsor bereavement support groups. Groups for parents who have lost a child, children who have lost a parent, widows, widowers, and gay men and lesbians who have lost a life partner are some examples of specialized support groups available in many communities. Nursing interventions for those experiencing grief and mourning are identified in Chart 16-13.

Complicated Grief and Mourning

Complicated grief and mourning are characterized by prolonged feelings of sadness and feelings of general worthlessness or hopelessness that persist long after the death, prolonged symptoms that interfere with activities of daily living (anorexia, insomnia, fatigue, panic), or self-destructive behaviors such as alcohol or substance abuse and suicidal ideation or attempts (Howarth, 2011). Complicated grief and mourning require professional assessment and can be treated with psychological interventions and, in some cases, with medications.

Coping With Death and Dying: Professional Caregiver Issues

Whether practicing in a trauma center, ICU, or other acute care setting, home care, hospice, long-term care, or the many locations where patients and their families receive ambulatory services, nurses are closely involved with complex and emotionally laden issues surrounding loss of life. To be most effective and satisfied with the care they provide, nurses should attend to their own emotional responses to the losses witnessed every day. Well before exhibiting symptoms of stress or burnout, nurses should acknowledge the difficulty of coping with others' pain on a daily basis and establish healthy practices that guard against emotional exhaustion. In hospice settings, where death, grief, and loss are expected outcomes of patient care, interdisciplinary colleagues rely on one another for support, using meeting time to express frustration, sadness, anger, and other emotions; to learn coping skills from one another; and to speak about how they were affected by the lives of those patients who have died since the last meeting. In many settings, staff members organize or attend memorial services to support families and other caregivers, who find comfort in joining one another to remember and celebrate the lives of patients. Finally, healthy personal habits, including diet, exercise, stress reduction activities (e.g., dance, yoga, T'ai chi, meditation), and sleep, help guard against the detrimental effects of stress.

CRITICAL THINKING EXERCISES

1 Your patient is a 46-year-old man who is hospitalized for complications associated with advanced colon cancer. He has metastases to the liver and the bone, exhibits anorexia and cachexia, and reports that his pain is controlled but he feels that he cannot catch his breath. He has three young children with his same sex partner of 15 years. He will be discharged home on hospice care. You note that his breathing does not appear labored, nor is he tachypneic. Does he have dyspnea? What would your comprehensive dyspnea assessment include?

2 ebp Your patient is a 65-year-old woman with Class IV heart failure. She lives with her husband and two adult daughters in a mobile home park near the outpatient practice where you are seeing her today. She tells you that she feels so tired that she does not even want to get out of bed or eat most days, and that she thinks she is losing weight. What is the evidence base about anorexia and cachexia care? How will you evaluate the evidence?

3 pq You are a new hospice nurse in your third week of night shift in a freestanding hospice inpatient unit.

> Your patient, a 55-year-old woman with advanced ovarian cancer was admitted 3 days prior. When you enter her room at the beginning of your shift, you note that she is not arousable and is having periods of apnea. It is 11 pm and the nurse who reported off told you that the patient's family left at approximately 9 pm. You are not sure but you think that your patient might be imminently dying. You have four other patients you have not seen yet. What should you do first? Why? What additional actions should be taken?

REFERENCES

*Asterisk indicates nursing research.
**Double asterisk indicates classic reference.

Books

American Nurses Association. (2015). *Nursing scope and standards of practice* (3rd ed.). Silver Spring, MD: Author.
Bondly, C., & Jatoi, A. (2015). Overview of the management of the anorexia/weight loss syndrome. In E. Bruera, I. Higginson, D. F. von Gunten, & T. Morita (Eds.). *Textbook of palliative medicine and supportive care* (2nd ed.). Boston, MA: CRC.
Center to Advance Palliative Care. (2015a). *America's care of serious illness: 2015 state by state report card on access to palliative care in our nation's hospitals.* New York, NY: Author.
Del Fabbro, E. (2015). *Current and future care of patients with the anorexia-cachexia syndrome.* 2015 ASCO Educational Book. Alexandria, VA: American Society of Clinical Oncology.
**Glaser, B. G., & Strauss, A. (1965). *Awareness of dying.* Chicago, IL: Aldine.
Hospice of Philadelphia. (2015). *Signs of approaching death.* Philadelphia, PA: Author.
**Jacox, A., Carr, D. B., & Payne, R. (1994). *Management of cancer pain.* Rockville, MD: Agency for Health Care Policy and Research.
**Kübler-Ross, E. (1969). *On death and dying.* New York, NY: Macmillan.
National Center for Health Statistics. (2010). *Health, United States, 2010: With special feature on death and dying.* Hyattsville, MD: Author.
National Hospice and Palliative Care Organization. (2014). *NHPCO facts and figures: Hospice care in America* (2014 ed.). Alexandria, VA: Author.
**Rando, T. A. (2000). Promoting healthy anticipatory mourning in intimates of the life-threatened or dying person. In T. A. Rando (Ed.): *Clinical dimensions of anticipatory mourning.* Champaign, IL: Research Press.
Wittenberg-Lyles, E., Goldmith, G., Ferrell, B. R., et al. (2013). *Communication in palliative nursing.* New York, NY: Oxford.

Journals and Electronic Documents

Alsolamy S. (2014). Islamic views on artificial nutrition and hydration in terminally ill patients. *Bioethics, 28,* 96–99.
American Academy of Hospice and Palliative Medicine. (2007). *Position statements: Physician-assisted death.* Retrieved on 10/5/2015 at: www.aahpm.org/positions/default/suicide.html
**American Nurses Association. (2010). *Position statement: Registered nurses' roles and responsibilities in providing expert care and counseling at the end of life.* Retrieved on 10/5/2015 at: gm6.nursingworld.org/MainMenuCategories/EthicsStandards/Ethics-Position-Statements/etpain14426.pdf
American Nurses Association. (2013). *Position statement: Euthanasia, assisted suicide, and aid in dying.* Retrieved on 12/12/2015 at: www.nursingworld.org/MainMenuCategories/EthicsStandards/Ethics-Position-Statements/Euthanasia-Assisted-Suicide-and-Aid-in-Dying.pdf
Arensmeyer, K. (2012). *Nursing management of patients with cancer-related anorexia.* Retrieved on 11/12/2015 at: www.oncolink.org/resources/article.cfm?id=1006
*Benkel, I., Wijk, H., & Molander, U. (2010). Using coping strategies is not denial: Helping loved ones to adjust to living with a patent with

a palliative diagnosis. *Journal of Hospice and Palliative Medicine, 13*(9), 1119–1123.
Beng, T. S., Ahmad, F., Loong, L. C., et al. (2015). Distress reduction for palliative care patients and families with 5-minute mindful breathing: A pilot study. *American Journal of Hospice and Palliative Medicine.* Epub ahead of print, pii: 1049909115569048
Bernacki, R. E., & Block, S. D. (2014). Communication about serious illness goals: A review and synthesis of best practices. *JAMA Internal Medicine, 174*(12), 1994–2003.
Bernat, J. L. (2009). Contemporary controversies in the definition of death. *Progress in Brain Research, 177,* 21–23.
**Casarett, D. J., Kapo, J., & Kaplan, A. (2005). Appropriate use of artificial nutrition and hydration—fundamental principles and recommendations. *New England Journal of Medicine, 353*(24), 2607–2612.
Center to Advance Palliative Care. (2015b). *Member resources.* Retrieved on 11/12/2015 at: www.capc.org/providers/member-resources/
Centers for Disease Control and Prevention. (2013). *Long term care services in the United States: 2013 overview.* Retrieved on 11/21/2015 at: www.cdc.gov/nchs/data/nsltcp/long_term_care_services_2013.pdf
Centers for Medicare & Medicaid Services (CMS). (2015). *Medicare Care Choices model awards.* Retrieved on 11/21/2015 at: www.cms.gov/Newsroom/MediaReleaseDatabase/Fact-sheets/2015-Fact-sheets-items/2015-07-20.html
Centers for Medicare & Medicaid Services (CMS). (2016). *Medicare Care Choices model.* Retrieved on 3/15/2016 at: innovation.cms.gov/initiatives/Medicare-Care-Choices/
Connor, S. R. (2007–2008). Development of hospice and palliative care in the United States. *Omega, 56*(1), 89–99.
Cronin, C., Arnstein, P., & Flanagan, J. (2015). Family members' perceptions of most helpful interventions during end-of-life care. *Journal of Hospice & Palliative Nursing, 17*(3), 223–228.
Danis, R., Arnold, R. M., & Savarese, D. M. F. (2015). *Stopping artificial nutrition and hydration at the end of life.* Retrieved on 11/21/2015 at: www.uptodate.com/contents/stopping-artificial- nutrition-and-hydration-at-the-end-of-life
Dewar, R., Cahners, N., Mitchell, C., et al. (2015). Hinduism and death with dignity: Historic and contemporary case examples. *Journal of Clinical Ethics, 26*(1), 40–47.
Enclara Pharmacia, Inc. (2015). *Enclara Pharmacia Medication Use Guidelines* (1st ed.). Philadelphia, PA: Author.
Ersek, M., & Carpenter, J. G. (2013). Geriatric palliative care in long term care settings with a focus on nursing homes. *Journal of Palliative Medicine, 16*(10), 1180–1187.
Fearon, K., Strasser, F., Anker, S. D., et al. (2011). Definition and classification of cancer cachexia: An international consensus. *Lancet Oncology, 12,* 489–495.
Gallup Poll. (2015). In *U.S., support up for doctor-assisted suicide.* Retrieved on 11/21/2015 at: www.gallup.com/poll/183425/support-doctor-assisted-suicide.aspx
Gibbs, K. D., Mahon, M. M., Truss, M., et al. (2015). An assessment of hospital-based palliative care in Maryland: Infrastructure, barriers, and opportunities. *Journal of Pain and Symptom Management, 49*(6), 1102–1108.
Hall, M. J., Levant, S., & DeFrances, C. J. (2013). *Trends in inpatient hospital deaths: National hospice discharge survey, 2000–2010.* NCHS Data Brief, Number 118. Hyattsville, MD: National Center for Health Statistics.
Hoff, L., & Hermeren, G. (2014). Identifying challenges to communicating with patients about their imminent death. *The Journal of Clinical Ethics, 25*(4), 296–306.
Hospice and Palliative Nurses Association. (2011). *HPNA position statement: Legalization of assisted suicide.* Retrieved on 11/21/2015 at: www.hpna.org/DisplayPage.aspx?Title=Position%20Statements
Howarth, R. A. (2011). Concepts and controversies in grief and loss. *Journal of Mental Health Counseling, 33*(1), 4–10.
Institute of Medicine. (2014a). *Dying in America: Improving quality and honoring individual preferences near the end of life.* Retrieved on 11/21/2015 at: iom.nationalacademies.org/Reports/2014/Dying-In-America-Improving-Quality-and-Honoring-Individual-Preferences-Near-the-End-of-Life.aspx
Institute of Medicine. (2014b). *Dying in America: IOM Committee's proposed core components of quality end-of-life care.* Retrieved on 11/21/2015 at: iom.nationalacademies.org/~/media/Files/Report%20Files/2014/

EOL/Table%20-%20Core%20Components%20of%20Quality%20Care.pdf

The Joint Commission. (2011). *Facts about the advanced certification program for palliative care.* Retrieved on 10/5/2015 at: www.jointcommission.org/assets/1/18/Palliative_Care.pdf

Kamal, A. H., Maguire, J. M., Wheeler, J. L., et al. (2012). Dyspnea review for the palliative care professional: Treatment goals and therapeutic options. *Journal of Palliative Medicine, 15*(1), 106–114.

Knabe, H. E. (2013). The meaning of hope for patients coping with a terminal illness: A review of the literature. *Journal of Palliative Care in Medicine.* Retrieved on 12/12/2015 at: www.omicsgroup.org/journals/the-meaning-of-hope-for-patients-coping-with-a-terminal-illness-a%20review-of-literature-2165-7386.S2-004.pdf

Lawlor, P. G., & Bush, S. H. (2014). Delirium diagnosis, screening and management. *Current Opinion in Supportive and Palliative Care, 8*(3), 286–295.

Linzer RD. (2013). Treatment of terminally ill patients according to Jewish law. *The Virtual Mentor, 15*, 1081–1087.

Marks, S., & Heinrich, T. (2013). Assessing and treating depression in palliative care patients. *Current Psychiatry, 12*(8), 35–40.

McCormick, A. J. (2013). Buddhist ethics and end-of-life care decisions. *Journal of Social Work in End-Of-Life & Palliative Care, 9*, 209–225.

McGuire, D. B., Reifsnyder, J., Soeken, K., et al. (2011). Assessing pain in non-responsive hospice patients: Development and preliminary testing of the Multidimensional Objective Pain Assessment Tool. *Journal of Palliative Medicine, 14*(3), 287–292.

Medicare Payment Advisory Commission (MedPAC). (2014). *Hospice services.* Retrieved on 11/21/2015 at: www.medpac.gov/documents/reports/mar14_ch12.pdf?sfvrsn=0

Mitchell, S. L., Black, B. S., Ersek, M., et al. (2012). Advanced dementia: State of the art and priorities for the next decade. *Annals of Internal Medicine, 156*(1), 45–51.

Mitera, G., Zhang, L., Sahgal, A., et al. (2012). A survey of expectations and understanding of palliative radiotherapy from patients with advanced cancer. *Clinical Oncology, 24*(2), 134–138.

National Consensus Project for Quality Palliative Care. (2013). *Clinical practice guidelines for quality palliative care* (3rd ed.). Retrieved on 10/14/2015 at: www.nationalconsensusproject.org

National Hospice and Palliative Care Organization. (2010). *Preamble and philosophy.* Retrieved on 10/14/2015 at: www.nhpco.org/i4a/pages/index.cfm?pageid=5308

Oncology Nursing Society. (2014). *Role of the nurse when hastened death is requested (endorsed position statement Hospice and Palliative Nurses Association).* Retrieved on 11/18/2015 at: www.ons.org/advocacy-policy/positions/ethics/hastened-death

Oregon Public Health Division. (2015). *Oregon's Death with Dignity Act—2014.* Retrieved on 11/18/2015 at: public.health.oregon.gov/ProviderPartnerResources/EvaluationResearch/DeathwithDignityAct/Documents/year17.pdf

Pew Research Center. (2013). *Views on end-of-life medical treatments.* Retrieved on 12/11/2015 at: www.pewforum.org/files/2013/11/end-of-life-survey-report-full-pdf.pdf

**Puchalski, C., & Romer, A. L. (2000). Taking a spiritual history allows clinicians to understand patients more fully. *Journal of Palliative Medicine, 3*(1), 129–137.

Puchalski, C. M., Vitillo, R., Hull, S. K., et al. (2014). Improving the spiritual dimension of whole person care: Reaching national and international consensus. *Journal of Palliative Medicine, 17*(6), 642–656.

Rabow, M., Kvale, E., Barbour, L., et al. (2013). Moving upstream: A review of the evidence of the impact of outpatient palliative care. *Journal of Palliative Medicine, 16*(12), 1540–1549.

Reynolds, R., Drew, D., & Dunwoody, C. (2013). American Society for Pain Management Nursing position statement: Pain management at the end of life. *Pain Management Nursing, 14*(3), 172–175.

Robson, A., Scrutton, F., Wilkinson, L., et al. (2010). The risk of suicide in cancer patients: A review of the literature. *Psychooncology, 19*(12),1250–1258.

Sarafis, P., Tsounis, A., Malliarou, M., et al. (2014). Disclosing the truth: A dilemma between instilling hope and respecting patient autonomy in everyday clinical practice. *Global Journal of Health Science, 6*(2), 128–137.

Schildmann, E. K., Schildmann, J., & Kiesewetter, I. (2015). Medication and monitoring in palliative sedation therapy: A systematic review and quality assessment of published guidelines. *Journal of Pain and Symptom Management, 49*(4), 734–746.

Shear, M. K. (2012). Grief and mourning gone awry: Pathway and course of complicated grief. *Dialogues in Clinical Neuroscience, 14*(2), 119–128.

**SUPPORT Principal Investigators. (1995). A controlled trial to improve care for seriously ill hospitalized patients. *JAMA, 274*(20), 1591–1598.

**Temel, J. S., Greer, J. A., Muzikansky, A., et al. (2010). Early palliative care for patients with metastatic non-small-cell lung cancer. *New England Journal of Medicine, 363*(8), 733–742.

The Conversation Project. (2013). *New survey reveals "conversation disconnect."* Retrieved on 12/11/2015 at: theconversationproject.org/wp-content/uploads/2013/09/TCP-Survey-Release_FINAL-9-18-13.pdf

Tyler, D. A., Shield, R. R., & Miller, S. C. (2015). Diffusion off palliative care in nursing homes: Lessons from the culture change movement. *Journal of Pain and Symptom Management, 49*(5), 846–852.

Vermont Department of Health. (2015). Patient choice and control at end of life. Retrieved on 11/18/2015 at: healthvermont.gov/family/end_of_life_care/patient_choice.aspx

Washington State Department of Health. (2015). *Death with Dignity Act.* Retrieved on 11/18/2015 at: www.doh.wa.gov/YouandYourFamily/IllnessandDisease/DeathwithDignityAct

**Wittenberg-Lyles, E., Goldsmith, J., & Ragan, S. L. (2010). The COMFORT initiative: Palliative nursing and the centrality of communication. *Journal of Hospice and Palliative Nursing, 12*(5), 282–292.

World Palliative Care Alliance. (2014). *Global atlas of palliative care at the end of life.* Retrieved on 12/11/2015 at: www.who.int/nmh/Global_Atlas_of_Palliative_Care.pdf

Wright, D. K., Brajtman, S., & Macdonald, M. E. (2014). A relational ethical approach to end-of-life delirium. *Journal of Pain and Symptom Management, 48*(2), 191–198.

Zientek, D. M. (2013). Artificial nutrition and hydration in Catholic healthcare: Balancing tradition, recent teaching, and law. *HEC Forum, 25*, 145–159.

Resources

American Academy of Hospice and Palliative Medicine (AAHPM), www.aahpm.org/

American Hospice Foundation, www.americanhospice.org/

Americans for Better Care of the Dying (ABCD), www.abcd-caring.org/

Association for Death Education and Counseling (ADEC), www.adec.org/

Caring Connections: a program of the National Hospice and Palliative Care Organization, www.caringinfo.org/i4a/pages/index.cfm?pageid=1

Center to Advance Palliative Care, www.capc.org/

Children's Hospice International, www.chionline.org/

Compassion & Choices, www.compassionandchoices.org/

Directory of State Hospice Organizations, www.hospicedirectory.org/cm/about/state_hospice

End-of-Life Nursing Education Consortium (ELNEC), www.aacn.nche.edu/elnec

Family Caregiver Alliance (FCA), caregiver.org/

Get Palliative Care (Blog and resources for palliative care), getpalliativecare.org/resources/

Growth House, Inc., provides information and referral services for agencies working with death and dying issues, www.growthhouse.org/

Harvard Medical School Center for Palliative Care, Dana Farber Cancer Institute, www.hms.harvard.edu/pallcare/

Hospice and Palliative Credentialing Corporation (HPCC), hpcc.advancingexpertcare.org/

Hospice and Palliative Nurses Association (HPNA), www.hpna.org

Hospice Association of America, National Association for Home Care, www.nahc.org/haa/

Hospice Education Institute, www.hospiceworld.org/

Hospice Foundation of America (HFA), www.hospicefoundation.org/

Hospice Net, provides information and support to patients and families facing life-threatening illnesses, www.hospicenet.org/

International Association for Hospice & Palliative Care (IAHPC), hospicecare.com/home/

National Consensus Project for Quality Palliative Care (national guidelines), www.nationalconsensusproject.org

National Hospice and Palliative Care Organization (NHPCO), www.nhpco.org

National Palliative Care Research Center (NPCRC), Brookdale Department of Geriatrics and Adult Development, www.npcrc.org

National Prison Hospice Association, www.npha.org

Office of End of Life and Palliative Care Research (OEPCR), www.ninr.nih.gov/reasearchandfunding/dea/desp/oepcr#.VhO5YCjnOLO

Palliative Care Fast Facts and Concepts, www.capc.org/fast-facts/

POLST (Physician Orders for Life-Sustaining Treatment Paradigm), www.polst.org/

Promoting Excellence in End-of-Life Care, www.promotingexcellence.org/

Supportive Care Coalition, www.supportivecarecoalition.org/

TIME: Toolkit of Instruments to Measure End-of-Life Care (Brown University), www.chcr.brown.edu/pcoc/toolkit.htm

We Honor Veterans (Partnership Between Veterans Administration and NHPCO), www.wehonorveterans.org/

World health Organization (WHO) Palliative Care, www.who.int/cancer/palliative/en/

UNIT

UNIT 4

Perioperative Concepts and Nursing Management

Case Study   EMPOWERING THROUGH INFORMED CONSENT

Last week a patient recently diagnosed with lymphoma had a lymph node removed from his right groin area to stage the lymphoma. He is now admitted to the hospital with fever and sepsis from infection of the wound. He is drowsy but easily awakened. The patient is scheduled for surgery tomorrow to débride the wound. The surgeon visits the patient to describe the procedure and the risks and benefits of the surgery. He then asks the nurse to have the informed consent signed by the patient.

QSEN Competency Focus: Patient-Centered Care

The complexities inherent in today's health care system challenge nurses to demonstrate integration of specific interdisciplinary core competencies. These competencies are aimed at ensuring the delivery of safe, quality patient care (Institute of Medicine, 2003). The Quality and Safety Education for Nurses project (QSEN, 2017; Cronenwett, Sherwood, Barnsteiner, et al., 2007) provides a framework for the knowledge, skills, and attitudes (KSA) required for nurses to demonstrate competency in these key areas, which include *patient-centered care, interdisciplinary teamwork and collaboration, evidence-based practice, quality improvement, safety,* and *informatics.*

Patient-Centered Care Definition: Recognize the patient or designee as the source of control and full partner in providing compassionate and coordinated care based on respect for patient's preferences, values, and needs.

SELECTED PRE-LICENSURE KSAs	APPLICATION AND REFLECTION
Knowledge	
Explore ethical and legal implications of patient-centered care.	How would you define ethical patient-centered care? Compare and contrast ethical and legal implications of patient-centered care.
Skills	
Facilitate informed consent.	What is the responsibility of the nurse in obtaining an informed consent? What is within the scope of practice for a nurse in obtaining an informed consent? If the patient has questions about the procedure, how should the nurse respond? Discuss how the nurse would advocate for the patient so that he receives the care that is best for him.
Attitudes	
Acknowledge the tension that may exist between patient rights and the organizational responsibility for professional, ethical care.	Think about your own experience and training with patient rights and informed consent. Why is it important for nurses to demonstrate respect for the principles of informed consent?

Cronenwett, L., Sherwood, G., Barnsteiner, J., et al. (2007). Quality and safety education for nurses. *Nursing Outlook, 55*(3), 122–131.
Institute of Medicine (2003). *Health professions education: A bridge to quality.* Washington, DC: National Academies Press.
QSEN Institute. (2017). *QSEN competencies: Definitions and pre-licensure* KSAs. Retrieved on 3/1/2017 at: www.qsen.org/competencies/pre-licensure-ksas

17 Preoperative Nursing Management

As techniques to perform surgery change with improved technology and expertise, surgery becomes less invasive and less debilitating. The increased use of **minimally invasive surgery** (procedures that use specialized instruments inserted into the body either through natural orifices or through small incisions) enables many procedures to be performed on an outpatient basis. Surgery remains a complex, stressful experience, whether minimally invasive, elective, or emergent. Even healthy patients having elective outpatient surgery may experience unanticipated complications during otherwise benign procedures. Many patients enter the hospital 90 minutes prior to surgery and have necessary medical assessments and analyses preceding the surgical intervention. The surgery is followed by a limited recovery period in the postanesthesia care unit (PACU). Later that day the patient goes home. When comorbidities exist or procedures are more complex, the patient may have laboratory studies completed prior to admission, and may be admitted to the hospital for postoperative recovery.

Traumatic and emergency surgery most often results in prolonged hospital stays. Patients who are acutely ill or undergoing

major surgery and patients with concurrent medical disorders may require supportive supplementary care from other medical disciplines, which can be coordinated more easily within the hospital setting. The high acuity level of surgical inpatients and the greater complexity of procedures have placed greater demands on the practice of nursing in this setting.

Although each setting (ambulatory, outpatient, or inpatient) offers its own unique advantages for the delivery of patient care, all patients require a comprehensive preoperative nursing assessment, patient education, and nursing interventions to prepare for surgery.

Perioperative Nursing

Communication, teamwork, and patient assessment are crucial to ensure good patient outcomes in the perioperative setting. Professional perioperative and perianesthesia nursing standards encompass the domains of behavioral response, physiologic response, and patient safety and are used as guides toward development of nursing diagnoses, interventions, and plans.

Perioperative nursing, which spans the entire surgical experience, consists of three phases that begin and end at particular points in the sequence of surgical experience events. The **preoperative phase** begins when the decision to proceed with surgical intervention is made and ends with the transfer of the patient onto the operating room (OR) bed. The **intraoperative phase** begins when the patient is transferred onto the OR bed and ends with admission to the PACU. Intraoperative nursing responsibilities involve acting as scrub nurse, circulating nurse, or registered nurse first assistant (see Chapter 18 for the description of these roles). The **postoperative phase** begins with the admission of the patient to the PACU and ends with a follow-up evaluation in the clinical setting or home (see Chapter 19).

Each perioperative phase includes the many diverse activities a nurse performs, using the nursing process, and is based on the recommended practice standards of the Association of periOperative Registered Nurses, formerly known as the Association of Operating Room Nurses (still abbreviated AORN) (AORN, 2014) and the American Society of PeriAnesthesia Nurses (ASPAN, 2015). Chart 17-1 presents nursing activities characteristic of the three perioperative phases of care. The phases of the surgical experience are reviewed in more detail in this chapter and in the other chapters in this unit.

A conceptual model of patient care, published by AORN, helps delineate the relationships between various components of nursing practice and patient outcomes into four domains: safety, physiologic responses, behavioral responses, and health care systems. The first three domains reflect phenomena of concern to perioperative nurses and are composed of nursing diagnoses, interventions, and outcomes. The fourth domain—the health care system—consists of structural data elements and focuses on clinical processes and outcomes. The model is used to depict the relationship of nursing process components to the achievement of optimal patient outcomes (Rothrock, 2014).

Technology and Anesthesia

Technologic advancements continue to lead health care industry providers toward performing more complex procedures that are less invasive, and therefore cause less morbidity during the recovery phase of surgery (Rothrock, 2014). Innovative high-definition microsurgical and laser technology enable increasingly minute repairs of tissue resulting in accelerated tissue regeneration. Sophisticated bypass equipment and minimally invasive techniques (i.e., robot-assisted technology) have changed many surgeries, such as abdominal aortic aneurysm bypass surgery, into outpatient procedures (Finkelstein, Rabino, Mashiach, et al., 2014).

Enhanced anesthesia methodology complements advances in surgical technology. Modern methods of achieving airway patency, sophisticated monitoring devices, and new pharmacologic agents, such as short-acting anesthetics, have created a safer atmosphere in which to operate. Effective antiemetics have reduced postoperative nausea and vomiting. Improved postoperative pain management and shortened procedure and recovery times have improved the operative experience for surgical patients.

Surgical Classifications

The decision to perform surgery may be based on facilitating a diagnosis (a diagnostic procedure such as biopsy, exploratory laparotomy, or laparoscopy), a cure (e.g., excision of a tumor or an inflamed appendix), or repair (e.g., multiple wound repair). It may be reconstructive or cosmetic (such as mammoplasty or a facelift) or palliative (to relieve pain or correct a problem—such as debulking a tumor to achieve comfort, or removal of a dysfunctional gallbladder). In addition, surgery might be rehabilitative (e.g., total joint replacement surgery to correct crippling pain or progression of degenerative osteoarthritis.) Surgery can also be classified based upon the degree of urgency involved: emergent, urgent, required, elective, and optional (see Table 17-1).

Preadmission Testing

Concurrent with the increase in **ambulatory surgeries** (surgery that does not require an overnight hospital stay) have been changes in the delivery of and payment for health care. Incentives to reduce hospital stays and contain costs have resulted in diagnostic preadmission testing (PAT) and preoperative preparation prior to admission. Many facilities have a presurgical services department to facilitate PAT and to initiate the nursing assessment process, which focuses on admission data such as patient demographics, health history, and other information pertinent to the surgical procedure (i.e., appropriate consent forms, diagnostic and laboratory tests) (Rothrock, 2014). The increasing use of ambulatory, outpatient, or short-stay surgery means that patients leave the hospital sooner and recuperate quicker. These changes increase the need for patient education, discharge planning, preparation for self-care, and referral for home care and rehabilitation services (ASPAN, 2015; Allison & George, 2014).

Special Considerations During the Perioperative Period

In an effort to reduce surgical complications, the Surgical Care Improvement Project (SCIP) was instituted as a national partnership of the Joint Commission and the Center for Medicare and Medicaid Services (CMS). The SCIP identifies performance measures aimed at preventing surgical complications, including venous thromboembolism (VTE) and surgical site infections (SSIs) (Joint Commission, 2016). In addition, if the surgical patient is currently using beta-blockers, particular attention is given to ensure timely administration of the beta-blocker and appropriate monitoring of vital signs. If the patient has not taken the usual dosage of this medication, the anesthesiologist or certified registered nurse anesthetist (CRNA) must evaluate whether or not it should be administered prior to surgery or during the perioperative period. The nurse in the perioperative area needs to be alert for appropriate preoperative prescriptions aimed at preventing VTE and SSI. If these are not present, they should be requested so that appropriate treatment begins before the start of surgery.

 Gerontologic Considerations

The hazards of surgery for older adults are proportional to the number and severity of comorbidities and the nature and duration of the operative procedure. The underlying principle that guides the preoperative assessment, surgical care, and postoperative care is that older adult patients have

---

Chart 17-1   Examples of Nursing Activities in the Perioperative Phases of Care

Preoperative Phase

Preadmission Testing

1. Initiates initial preoperative assessment
2. Initiates education appropriate to patient's needs
3. Involves family in interview
4. Verifies completion of preoperative diagnostic testing
5. Verifies understanding of surgeon-specific preoperative orders (e.g., bowel preparation, preoperative shower)
6. Discusses and reviews advance directive document
7. Begins discharge planning by assessing patient's need for postoperative transportation and care

Admission to Surgical Center

1. Completes preoperative assessment
2. Assesses for risks for postoperative complications
3. Reports unexpected findings or any deviations from normal
4. Verifies that operative consent has been signed
5. Coordinates patient education and plan of care with nursing staff and other health team members
6. Reinforces previous education
7. Explains phases in perioperative period and expectations
8. Answers patient's and family's questions

In the Holding Area

1. Identifies patient
2. Assesses patient's status, baseline pain, and nutritional status
3. Reviews medical record
4. Verifies surgical site and that it has been marked per institutional policy
5. Establishes IV line
6. Administers medications if prescribed
7. Takes measures to ensure patient's comfort
8. Provides psychological support
9. Communicates patient's emotional status to other appropriate members of the health care team

Intraoperative Phase

Maintenance of Safety

1. Maintains aseptic, controlled environment
2. Effectively manages human resources, equipment, and supplies for individualized patient care
3. Transfers patient to operating room bed or table
4. Positions patient based on functional alignment and exposure of surgical site
5. Applies grounding device to patient
6. Ensures that the sponge, needle, and instrument counts are correct
7. Completes intraoperative documentation

Physiologic Monitoring

1. Calculates effects on patient of excessive fluid loss or gain
2. Distinguishes normal from abnormal cardiopulmonary data
3. Reports changes in patient's vital signs
4. Institutes measures to promote normothermia

IV, intravenous.

Psychological Support (Before Induction and When Patient is Conscious)

1. Provides emotional support to patient
2. Stands near or touches patient during procedures and induction
3. Continues to assess patient's emotional status

Postoperative Phase

Transfer of Patient to Postanesthesia Care Unit

1. Communicates intraoperative information:
   a. Identifies patient by name
   b. States type of surgery performed
   c. Identifies type and amounts of anesthetic and analgesic agents used
   d. Reports patient's vital signs and response to surgical procedure and anesthesia
   e. Describes intraoperative factors (e.g., insertion of drains or catheters, administration of blood, medications during surgery, or occurrence of unexpected events)
   f. Describes physical limitations
   g. Reports patient's preoperative level of consciousness
   h. Communicates necessary equipment needs
   i. Communicates presence of family or significant others

Postoperative Assessment Recovery Area

1. Determines patient's immediate response to surgical intervention
2. Monitors patient's vital signs and physiologic status
3. Assesses patient's pain level and administers appropriate pain-relief measures
4. Maintains patient's safety (airway, circulation, prevention of injury)
5. Administers medications, fluid, and blood component therapy, if prescribed
6. Provides oral fluids if prescribed for ambulatory surgery patient
7. Assesses patient's readiness for transfer to in-hospital unit or for discharge home based on institutional policy (e.g., Aldrete score, see Chapter 19)

Surgical Nursing Unit

1. Continues close monitoring of patient's physical and psychological response to surgical intervention
2. Assesses patient's pain level and administers appropriate pain-relief measures
3. Provides education to patient during immediate recovery period
4. Assists patient in recovery and preparation for discharge home
5. Determines patient's psychological status
6. Assists with discharge planning

Home or Clinic

1. Provides follow-up care during office or clinic visit or by telephone contact
2. Reinforces previous education and answers patient's and family's questions about surgery and follow-up care
3. Assesses patient's response to surgery and anesthesia and their effects on body image and function
4. Determines family's perception of surgery and its outcome IV, intravenous.

---

less physiologic reserve (i.e., the ability of an organ to return to normal after a disturbance in its equilibrium) than younger patients (Oster & Oster, 2015). Respiratory and cardiac complications are the leading causes of postoperative morbidity and mortality in older adults (Thanavaro, 2015). Cardiac

reserves are lower, renal and hepatic functions are depressed, and gastrointestinal activity is likely to be reduced. See Table 11-1 for additional age-related changes.

As the body ages, the ability to perspire decreases, leading to dry itchy skin that can become fragile and easily abraded

TABLE 17-1 Categories of Surgery Based on Urgency

Classification	Indications for Surgery	Examples
I. Emergent—Patient requires immediate attention; disorder may be life-threatening	Without delay	Severe bleeding Bladder or intestinal obstruction Fractured skull Gunshot or stab wounds Extensive burns
II. Urgent—Patient requires prompt attention	Within 24–30 h	Acute gallbladder infection Kidney or ureteral stones
III. Required—Patient needs to have surgery	Plan within a few weeks or months	Prostatic hyperplasia without bladder obstruction Thyroid disorders Cataracts
IV. Elective—Patient should have surgery	Failure to have surgery not catastrophic	Repair of scars Simple hernia Vaginal repair
V. Optional—Decision rests with patient	Personal preference	Cosmetic surgery

(Meiner, 2014). Precautions are taken when moving an older adult. Decreased subcutaneous fat makes older adults more susceptible to temperature changes. A lightweight cotton blanket is an appropriate cover when an older patient is moved to and from the OR but never replaces asking patients if they feel sufficiently warm and attending to their needs.

Because the older patient may have greater perioperative risks, the following factors are critical: (1) skillful preoperative assessment and treatment (Tabloski, 2013), (2) proficient anesthesia and surgical care, and (3) meticulous and competent postoperative and postanesthesia management. Nurses must educate patients about appropriate pain management and encourage good communication to obtain greater postoperative pain relief. Older adults may need more time and multiple explanations to understand and retain what is communicated (see Providing Patient Education section).

Bariatric Patients

Bariatrics is a specialty that revolves around diagnosing, treating, and managing patients who are obese. Obesity is defined as a body mass index of greater than 30 kg/m^2 (Centers for Disease Control and Prevention [CDC], 2015). Approximately one-third (34.9% or 78.6 million) of U.S. adults are obese (Ogden, Carroll, Kit, et al., 2014). Obesity increases the risk and severity of complications associated with surgery. During surgery, fatty tissues are especially susceptible to infection. Wound infections are more common in patients that are obese (Edmiston & Spencer, 2014). Obesity also increases technical and mechanical problems related to surgery, such as dehiscence (wound separation). It may be more challenging to provide care for the patient who is obese owing to the excessive weight and possible restrictions in movement. It is estimated that about 25 additional miles of blood vessels are needed for every 30 pounds of excess weight; this results in increased cardiac demand (Rider, Cox, Tyler, et al., 2013). The patient with obesity tends to have shallow respirations when supine, increasing the risk of hypoventilation and postoperative pulmonary complications.

Certain physical characteristics found in patients who are obese impede intubation, such as short thick necks, large tongues, recessed chins, and redundant pharyngeal tissue. These characteristics are associated with increased oxygen demand and decreased pulmonary reserves. The preoperative assessment looks for these characteristics as well as the presence of obstructive sleep apnea, frequently diagnosed in patients who are obese. Sleep apnea is treated with continuous positive airway pressure (CPAP). The use of CPAP should be incorporated throughout the perioperative period (Barash, Cullen, Stoelting, et al., 2013).

Patients With Disabilities

Special considerations for patients with mental or physical disabilities include the need for appropriate assistive devices, modifications in preoperative education, and additional assistance with and attention to positioning or transferring. Assistive devices include hearing aids, eyeglasses, braces, prostheses, and other devices. People who are hearing impaired may need and are entitled by law to a sign interpreter or some alternative communication system perioperatively. If the patient relies on signing or speech (lip) reading and their eyeglasses or contact lenses are removed or the health care staff wears surgical masks, an alternative method of communication will be needed. These needs must be identified in the preoperative evaluation and clearly communicated to personnel. Specific strategies for accommodating the patient's needs must be identified in advance. Ensuring the security of assistive devices is important, because these devices are expensive and require time to replace if lost.

Most patients are directed to move from the stretcher to the OR bed prior to surgery and back again following the procedure. In addition to being unable to see or hear instructions, the patient with a disability may be unable to move without special devices or a great deal of assistance (Lagu, Hannon, Rothberg, et al., 2013). The patient with a disability that affects body position (e.g., cerebral palsy, postpolio syndrome, and other neuromuscular disorders) may need special positioning during surgery to prevent pain and injury. Patients with disabilities may be unable to sense painful positioning if their extremities are incorrectly adjusted, or they may be unable to communicate their discomfort.

Patients with respiratory problems related to a disability (e.g., multiple sclerosis, muscular dystrophy) may experience difficulties unless the problems are made known to the anesthesiologist or CRNA and adjustments are made (Barash et al., 2013). These factors need to be clearly identified in the preoperative period and communicated to the appropriate personnel.

Patients Undergoing Ambulatory Surgery

Ambulatory surgery includes outpatient, same-day, or short-stay surgery not requiring admission for an overnight hospital stay but may entail observation in a hospital setting for 23 hours or less. During the brief time the patient and family spend in the ambulatory setting, the nurse must quickly and comprehensively assess and anticipate the needs of the patient and at the same time begin planning for discharge and follow-up home care.

The nurse needs to be sure that the patient and family understand that the patient will first go to the preoperative holding area before going to the OR for the surgical procedure and then will spend some time in the PACU before being discharged home with the family member later that day. Other preoperative education content should also be verified and reinforced as needed (see later discussion). The nurse should ensure that any plans for follow-up home care or new assistive devices are in place if needed.

Patients Undergoing Emergency Surgery

Emergency surgeries are unplanned and occur with little time for preparation of the patient or the perioperative team. The unpredictable nature of trauma and emergency surgery poses unique challenges throughout the perioperative period. It is important for the nurse to communicate with the patient and team members as calmly and effectively as possible in these situations. (See Chapter 18 for the duties of the members of the perioperative team.)

Factors that affect patients preparing to undergo surgery also apply to patients undergoing emergency surgery, although usually in a very condensed time frame. The only opportunity for preoperative assessment may take place at the same time as resuscitation in the emergency department. A quick visual survey of the patient is essential to identify all sites of injury if the emergency surgery is due to trauma (see Chapters 68 and 72 for more information). The patient, who may have undergone a traumatic experience, may need extra support and explanation of the surgery. For the unconscious patient, informed consent and essential information, such as pertinent past medical history and allergies, need to be obtained from a family member, if one is available.

Informed Consent

Informed consent is the patient's autonomous decision about whether to undergo a surgical procedure. Voluntary and written informed consent from the patient is necessary before nonemergent surgery can be performed to protect the patient from unsanctioned surgery and protect the surgeon from claims of an unauthorized operation or battery. Consent is a legal mandate, but it also helps the patient to prepare psychologically, because it helps to ensure that the patient understands the surgery to be performed (Rothrock, 2014).

The nurse may ask the patient to sign the consent form and witness the signature; however, it is the surgeon's responsibility to provide a clear and simple explanation of what the surgery will entail prior to the patient giving consent. The surgeon must also inform the patient of the benefits, alternatives, possible risks, complications, disfigurement, disability, and removal of body parts as well as what to expect in the early and late postoperative periods. The nurse clarifies the information provided, and if the patient requests additional information, the nurse notifies the physician. The nurse ascertains that the consent form has been signed before administering psychoactive premedication, because consent is not valid if it is obtained while the patient is under the influence of medications that can affect judgment and decision-making capacity.

> ▶ **Quality and Safety Nursing Alert**
>
> *The signed consent form is placed in a prominent place on the patient's medical record and accompanies the patient to the OR.*

Many ethical principles are integral to informed consent. Informed consent is necessary in the following circumstances:
- Invasive procedures, such as a surgical incision, a biopsy, a cystoscopy, or paracentesis
- Procedures requiring sedation and/or anesthesia (see Chapter 18 for a discussion of anesthesia)
- A nonsurgical procedure, such as an arteriography, that carries more than a slight risk to the patient
- Procedures involving radiation
- Blood product administration

The patient personally signs the consent if of legal age and mentally capable. Permission is otherwise obtained from a surrogate, who most often is a responsible family member (preferably next of kin) or legal guardian. (See Chart 17-2 for criteria for valid informed consent.) State regulations and agency policy must be followed. In an emergency, it may be necessary for the surgeon to operate as a lifesaving measure without the patient's informed consent. However, every effort must be made to contact the patient's family. In such a situation, contact can be made by telephone, fax, or other electronic means and consent obtained.

If the patient has doubts and has not had the opportunity to investigate alternative treatments, a second opinion may be requested. No patient should be urged or coerced to give informed consent. Refusing to undergo a surgical procedure is a person's legal right and privilege. Such information must be documented and relayed to the surgeon so that other arrangements can be made. Additional explanations may be provided to the patient and family, or the surgery may be rescheduled. Consents for specific procedures such as sterilization, therapeutic abortion, disposal of severed body parts, organ donation, and blood product administration provide additional protection for the patient (Rothrock, 2014). States and regions may vary in their mandates.

Discussion with patients and their family members may be supplemented with audiovisual materials. Consent forms should be written in easily understandable words and concepts to facilitate the consent process and should use other strategies and resources as needed to help the patient understand the content (see Chart 17-2). Asking patients to describe in

Chart 17-2	Valid Informed Consent

Voluntary Consent

Valid consent must be freely given, without coercion. Patient must be at least 18 years of age (unless an emancipated minor), a physician must obtain consent, and a professional staff member must witness patient's signature.

Incompetent Patient

Legal definition: individual who is *not* autonomous and cannot give or withhold consent (e.g., individuals who are cognitively impaired, mentally ill, or neurologically incapacitated).

Informed Subject

Informed consent should be in writing. It should contain the following:

- Explanation of procedure and its risks
- Description of benefits and alternatives
- An offer to answer questions about procedure
- Instructions that the patient may withdraw consent
- A statement informing the patient if the protocol differs from customary procedure

Patient Able to Comprehend

If the patient is non-English speaking, it is necessary to provide consent (written and verbal) in a language that is understandable to the client. A trained medical interpreter may be consulted. Alternative formats of communication (e.g., Braille, large print, sign interpreter) may be needed if the patient has a disability that affects vision or hearing. Questions must be answered to facilitate comprehension if material is confusing.

Chart 17-3 ⚠	SELECTED RISK FACTORS Surgical Complications

- Arthritis
- Cardiovascular disease:
  - Coronary artery disease or previous myocardial infarction
  - Cardiac failure
  - Cerebrovascular disease
  - Dysrhythmias
  - Hemorrhagic disorders
  - Hypertension
  - Prosthetic heart valve
  - Venous thromboembolism (VTE)
- Dehydration or electrolyte imbalance
- Endocrine dysfunction:
  - Adrenal disorders
  - Diabetes
  - Thyroid malfunction
- Extremes of age (very young, very old)
- Extremes of weight (emaciation, obesity)
- Hepatic disease:
  - Cirrhosis
  - Hepatitis
- Hypovolemia
- Immunologic abnormalities
- Infection and sepsis
- Low socioeconomic status
- Medications
- Nicotine use
- Nutritional deficits
- Pregnancy:
  - Diminished maternal physiologic reserve
- Preexisting mental or physical disability
- Pulmonary disease:
  - Obstructive disease
  - Restrictive disorder
  - Respiratory infection
- Renal or urinary tract disease:
  - Decreased kidney function
  - Urinary tract infection
  - Obstruction
  - Toxic conditions

their own words the surgery they are about to have promotes nurses' understanding of patients' comprehension.

Preoperative Assessment

The goal in the preoperative period is for the patient to be as healthy as possible. Every attempt is made to assess for and address risk factors that may contribute to postoperative complications and delay recovery (see Chart 17-3). A plan of action is designed so that potential complications are averted. Before any surgical treatment is initiated, a health history is obtained, a physical examination is performed during which vital signs are noted, and a baseline is established for future comparisons (Alvarex, Brodsky, Lemmens, et al., 2014). The nurse should ask about any allergies and comorbid conditions that may affect anesthesia (Bourdon, 2015). During the physical examination, many factors that have the potential to affect the patient undergoing surgery are considered, such as joint mobility. Genetic considerations are also taken into account during assessment to prevent complications with anesthesia (see Chart 17-4).

Asking the patient about use of prescription and over-the-counter (OTC) medications, including herbal and other supplements provides useful information. Activity and functional levels should be determined, including that involving regular aerobic exercise. Known allergies to drugs, foods, and latex could avert an anaphylactic response (Barash et al., 2013). Patients may have early manifestations of a latex allergy and be unaware of this. If a patient states that he or she is allergic to kiwi, avocado, or banana, or cannot blow up balloons, there may be an association with an allergy to latex.

Latex, the milky fluid from the rubber tree, is found in many everyday products, and repeated exposure may cause some people to develop the allergy as an immune response to the protein (Australasian Society of Clinical Immunology and Allergy [ASCIA], 2015). Most hospital products today are latex free, especially in ORs; however, even the rubber stopper on a medication vial can trigger a deadly reaction following injection from that vial.

⚑ Quality and Safety Nursing Alert

A latex allergy can manifest as a rash, asthma, or anaphylactic shock.

Health care providers also should be alert for signs of abuse, which can occur at any age, in either sex, and in any socioeconomic, ethnic, and cultural group. Findings need to be reported accordingly (see Chapter 5 for further discussion of signs of abuse). Laboratory tests and other diagnostic tests are prescribed when indicated by information obtained from the history and physical examination. Autologous blood donation or patient self-donation is discussed as needed for

GENETICS IN NURSING PRACTICE
Genetics Concepts and Perioperative Nursing

Nurses who are caring for patients undergoing surgery need to take various genetic considerations into account when assessing patients throughout the operative experience. Genetic disorders can impact pre-, intra- and postoperative surgical outcomes. In particular, consideration must be given to genetic disorders associated with the delivery of anesthesia as well as other genetic disorders that may increase the risk of postoperative complications. Examples of genetic conditions that may cause complications with anesthesia include the following:

Autosomal Dominant:

- Central core disease
- Hyperkalemic periodic paralysis
- Malignant hyperthermia

Examples of other genetic conditions that must be evaluated and that are associated with perioperative risks include the following:

- Cystic fibrosis (autosomal recessive)
- Duchenne muscular dystrophy (X-linked recessive)
- Ehlers–Danlos syndrome
- Factor V Leiden (autosomal dominant)
- Hemophilia (X-linked)
- Scleroderma

Nursing Assessments

Refer to Chart 5-2: Genetics in Nursing Practice: Genetic Aspects of Health Assessment

Family History Assessment Specific to Genetics and Perioperative Nursing

- Obtain a thorough assessment of personal and family history for three generations, inquiring about prior problems with surgery or anesthesia with specific attention to complications, such as fever, rigidity, dark urine, and unexpected reactions.
- Inquire about any history of musculoskeletal complaints, history of heat intolerance, fevers of unknown origin, or unusual drug reactions.

DNA, deoxyribonucleic acid.

- Assess for family history of any sudden or unexplained death, especially during participation in athletic events.
- Assess whether any family members have been diagnosed with King–Denborough syndrome, as this is a form of congenital myopathy that places the patient at risk for malignant hyperthermia.

Patient Assessment Specific to Genetics and Perioperative Nursing

- Identify the presence of other inherited genetic disorders that may impact surgical outcomes (e.g., inherited connective tissue, metabolic, bleeding, or neurologic disorders).
- Assess for subclinical muscle weakness.
- Assess for other physical features suggestive of an underlying genetic condition, such as contractures, kyphoscoliosis, and pterygium with progressive weakness.

Management Issues Specific to Genetics and Perioperative Nursing

- Inquire as to whether DNA mutation or other genetic testing has been performed on an affected family member.
- If indicated, refer for further genetic counseling and evaluation so that family members can discuss inheritance, risk to other family members, and availability of diagnostic/genetic testing.
- Provide support to families of patients with newly diagnosed malignant hyperthermia.
- Participate in management and coordination of care of patients with genetic conditions and individuals predisposed to develop or pass on a genetic condition.

Genetics Resources

Malignant Hyperthermia Association, www.mhaus.org
See Chart 8-7: Components of Genetic Counseling for genetics resources.

---

the type of surgical procedure planned. See Chapter 32 for further discussion of autologous blood donation.

Nutritional and Fluid Status

Optimal nutrition is an essential factor in promoting healing and resisting infection and other surgical complications. Assessment of a patient's nutritional status identifies factors that can affect the patient's surgical course, such as obesity, weight loss, malnutrition, deficiencies in specific nutrients, metabolic abnormalities, and the effects of medications on nutrition. Nutritional needs may be determined by measurement of body mass index and waist circumference. (See Chapter 5 for further discussion of nutritional assessment.)

Any nutritional deficiency should be corrected before surgery to provide adequate protein for tissue repair. The nutrients needed for wound healing are summarized in Table 17-2.

Assessment of a patient's hydration status is also essential. Dehydration, hypovolemia, and electrolyte imbalances can lead to significant problems in patients with comorbid medical conditions or in older adults (Oster & Oster, 2015). The depletion of fluids and electrolytes following bowel preparation, especially

when combined with prolonged fasting, can result in dehydration and chemical imbalances, even among healthy surgical patients. Any identified fluid and electrolyte imbalances should be corrected prior to surgery.

Dentition

The condition of the mouth is an important health factor to assess. Dental caries, dentures, and partial plates are particularly significant to the anesthesiologist or CRNA, because decayed teeth or dental prostheses may become dislodged during intubation and occlude the airway. This is especially important for older patients as well as those who may not have regular dental care. The condition of the mouth is also important because any bodily infection, even in the mouth, can be a source of postoperative infection.

Drug or Alcohol Use

Ingesting even moderate amounts of alcohol prior to surgery can weaken a patient's immune system and increase the likelihood of developing postoperative complications (Rubinsky, Bishop, Maynard, et al., 2013). In addition, the use of illicit

TABLE 17-2 Nutrients Important for Wound Healing

Nutrient	Rationale for Increased Need	Possible Deficiency Outcome
Protein	To allow collagen deposition and wound healing to occur	Collagen deposition leading to impaired/delayed wound healing Decreased skin and wound strength Increased wound infection rates
Arginine (amino acid)	To provide necessary substrate for collagen synthesis and nitric oxide (crucial for wound healing) at wound site To increase wound strength and collagen deposition To stimulate T-cell response Associated with various essential reactions of intermediary metabolism	Impaired wound healing
Carbohydrates and fats	Primary source of energy in the body and consequently in the wound-healing process To meet the demand for increased essential fatty acids needed for cellular function after an injury To spare protein To restore normal weight	Signs and symptoms of protein deficiency due to the use of protein to meet energy requirements Extensive weight loss
Water	To replace fluid lost through vomiting, hemorrhage, exudates, fever, drainage, diuresis To maintain homeostasis	Signs, symptoms, and complications of dehydration, such as poor skin turgor, dry mucous membranes, oliguria, anuria, weight loss, increased pulse rate, decreased central venous pressure
Vitamin C	Important for capillary formation, tissue synthesis, and wound healing through collagen formation Needed for antibody formation	Impaired/delayed wound healing related to impaired collagen formation and increased capillary fragility and permeability Increased risk for infection related to decreased antibodies
Vitamin B complex	Indirect role in wound healing through their influence on host resistance	Decreased enzymes available for energy metabolism
Vitamin A	Increases inflammatory response in wounds, reduces anti-inflammatory effects of corticosteroids on wound healing	Impaired/delayed wound healing related to decreased collagen synthesis; impaired immune function Increased risk for infection
Vitamin K	Important for normal blood clotting Impaired intestinal synthesis associated with the use of antibiotics	Prolonged prothrombin time Hematomas contributing to impaired healing and predisposition to wound infections
Magnesium	Essential cofactor for many enzymes that are involved in the process of protein synthesis and wound repair	Impaired/delayed wound healing (impaired collagen production)
Copper	Required cofactor in the development of connective tissue	Impaired wound healing
Zinc	Involved in DNA synthesis, protein synthesis, cellular proliferation needed for wound healing Essential to immune function	Impaired immune response

DNA, deoxyribonucleic acid.
Adapted from Porth, C. M. (2015). *Essentials of pathophysiology: Concepts of altered states* (4th ed.). Philadelphia, PA: Lippincott Williams & Wilkins.

drugs and alcohol may impede the effectiveness of some medications. Because acutely intoxicated people are susceptible to injury, surgery is postponed if possible. If emergency surgery is required, local, spinal, or regional block anesthesia is used for minor surgery (Porth, 2015). In an emergency, to prevent vomiting and potential aspiration, a nasogastric tube is inserted before general anesthesia is given.

The person with a history of alcohol abuse often suffers from malnutrition and other systemic problems or metabolic imbalances that increase surgical risk. Research suggests that patients who have more than two drinks of alcohol per day in the 2 weeks prior to surgery have more complications, longer hospital stays, and more days in ICU postoperatively

(Rubinsky et al., 2013). People who have a substance abuse problem may deny or attempt to hide it. In such situations, the nurse who is obtaining the patient's health history needs to ask frank questions with patience, care, and a nonjudgmental attitude. Such questions should include asking whether the patient has had two drinks per day or more on a regular basis in the 2 weeks prior to surgery. (See Chapter 5 for an assessment of alcohol and drug use.)

Respiratory Status

The patient is educated about breathing exercises and the use of an incentive spirometer, if indicated, to achieve optimal respiratory function prior to surgery. The potential compromise of ventilation during all phases of surgical treatment necessitates a proactive response to respiratory infections. Surgery is usually postponed for elective cases if the patient has a respiratory infection. Patients with underlying respiratory disease (e.g., asthma, chronic obstructive pulmonary disease) are assessed carefully for current threats to their pulmonary status. Patients also need to be assessed for comorbid conditions and age-related changes that may affect respiratory function (Oster & Oster, 2015).

Patients who smoke are urged to stop 30 days before surgery to significantly reduce pulmonary and wound healing complications (Allison & George, 2014). Preoperative smoking cessation interventions can be effective in changing smoking behavior and reducing the incidence of postoperative complications. Patients who smoke are more likely to experience poor wound healing, a higher incidence of SSI, and complications that include VTE and pneumonia.

Cardiovascular Status

Patient preparation for surgical intervention includes ensuring that the cardiovascular system can support the oxygen, fluid, and nutritional needs of the perioperative period. If the patient has uncontrolled hypertension, surgery may be postponed until the blood pressure is under control. At times, surgical treatment can be modified to meet the cardiac tolerance of the patient. For example, in a patient with obstruction of the descending colon and coronary artery disease, a temporary simple colostomy may be performed rather than a more extensive colon resection that would require a prolonged period of anesthesia.

Hepatic and Renal Function

The presurgical goal is optimal function of the liver and urinary systems so that medications, anesthetic agents, body wastes, and toxins are adequately metabolized and removed from the body. The liver, lungs, and kidneys are the routes for elimination of drugs and toxins.

The liver is important in the biotransformation of anesthetic compounds. Disorders of the liver may substantially affect how anesthetic agents are metabolized. Acute liver disease is associated with high surgical mortality; preoperative improvement in liver function is a goal. Careful assessment may include various liver function tests (see Chapter 49).

The kidneys are involved in excreting anesthetic medications and their metabolites; therefore, surgery is contraindicated if a patient has acute nephritis, acute renal insufficiency with oliguria or anuria, or other acute renal problems (see Chapter 54). Exceptions include surgeries performed as lifesaving measures, surgery to enable easier access for dialysis, or those necessary to improve urinary function (e.g., obstructive uropathy or hydronephrosis).

Endocrine Function

The patient with diabetes who is undergoing surgery is at risk for both hypoglycemia and hyperglycemia. Hypoglycemia may develop during anesthesia or postoperatively from inadequate carbohydrates or excessive administration of insulin. Hyperglycemia, which can increase the risk of surgical wound infection, may result from the stress of surgery, which can trigger increased levels of catecholamine. Other risks are acidosis and glucosuria.

Although the surgical risk in the patient with controlled diabetes is no greater than in the patient without diabetes, strict glycemic control (80 to 110 mg/dL) leads to better outcomes (Alvarex et al., 2014). Frequent monitoring of blood glucose levels is important before, during, and after surgery. (See Chapter 51 for a discussion of the patient with diabetes.)

Patients who have received corticosteroids are at risk for adrenal insufficiency. The use of corticosteroids for any purpose during the preceding year must be reported to the anesthesiologist or CRNA and surgeon. The patient is monitored for signs of adrenal insufficiency (see Chapter 52).

Patients with uncontrolled thyroid disorders are at risk for thyrotoxicosis (with hyperthyroid disorders) or respiratory failure (with hypothyroid disorders). The patient with an associated history of a thyroid disorder is assessed preoperatively (see Chapter 52).

Immune Function

An important function of the preoperative assessment is to determine the presence of infection or allergies. Routine laboratory tests used to detect infection include the white blood count (WBC) and the urinalysis. Surgery may be postponed in the presence of infection.

It is important to identify and document any sensitivity to medications and past adverse reactions (ASPAN, 2015). The patient is asked to identify any substances that precipitated previous allergic reactions, including medications, blood transfusions, contrast agents, latex, and food products, and to describe the signs and symptoms produced by these substances. A sample latex allergy screening questionnaire is shown in Figure 17-1.

Immunosuppression is common with corticosteroid therapy, organ transplantation, radiation therapy, chemotherapy, and disorders affecting the immune system, such as acquired immunodeficiency syndrome and leukemia. The mildest symptoms or slightest temperature elevation must be investigated.

Previous Medication Use

A medication history is obtained because of the possible interactions with medications that might be given during surgery and the effects of any of these medications on the patient's perioperative course. Any medications the patient is using or has used in the past are documented, including OTC preparations and herbal agents, as well as the frequency with which they are used. Many medications have an effect on physiologic functions; interactions of such medications with anesthetic agents can cause serious problems, such as hypotension and circulatory collapse. Medications that cause particular concern are listed in Table 17-3.

Aspirin, a common OTC medication that inhibits platelet aggregation, should be prudently discontinued 7 to 10 days before surgery; otherwise, the patient may be at increased risk for bleeding (Rothrock, 2014). Any use of aspirin or other OTC medications is noted in the patient's medical record and conveyed to the anesthesiologist or CRNA and surgeon. The anesthesia provider evaluates the potential effects of prior medication therapy, considering the length of time the patient has used the medication, the physical condition of the patient, and the nature of the proposed surgery.

Latex Allergy Assessment

Ask the patient the following questions. Check "Yes" or "No" in the box.	YES	NO
1. Has a doctor ever told you that you are allergic to latex?		
2. Do you have on-the-job exposure to latex?		
3. Were you born with problems involving your spinal cord?		
4. Have you ever had allergies, asthma, hay fever, eczema, or problems with rashes?		
5. Have you ever had respiratory distress, rapid heart rate, or swelling?		
6. Have you ever had swelling, itching, hives, or other symptoms after contact with a balloon?		
7. Have you ever had swelling, itching, hives, or other symptoms after a dental examination or procedure?		
8. Have you ever had swelling, itching, hives, or other symptoms following a vaginal or rectal examination or after contact with a diaphragm or condom?		
9. Have you ever had swelling, itching, hives, or other symptoms during or within 1 hour after wearing rubber gloves?		
10. Have you ever had a rash on your hands that lasted longer than 1 week?		
11. Have you ever had swelling, itching, hives, runny nose, eye irritation, wheezing, or asthma after contact with any latex or rubber product?		
12. Have you ever had swelling, itching, hives, or other symptoms after being examined by someone wearing rubber or latex gloves?		
13. Are you allergic to bananas, avocados, kiwi, or chestnuts?		
14. Have you ever had an unexplained anaphylactic episode?		

Preop RN Signature: _____

Patient Name: _____

Procedure: _____

Scheduled Date / Time: _____

Surgeon: _____

Figure 17-1 • Example of a latex allergy assessment form. Courtesy of Inova Fair Oaks Hospital, Fairfax, VA.

> **Quality and Safety Nursing Alert**
>
> *The possible adverse interactions of some medications require the nurse to assess and document the patient's use of prescription medications, OTC medications (especially aspirin), herbal agents, and the frequency with which medications are used. The nurse must clearly communicate this information to the anesthesiologist or CRNA.*

The use of medications is widespread among patients; approximately 40% of Americans report taking some form of OTC supplements (Allison & George, 2014). Commonly used herbal medications may include echinacea, garlic (*Allium sativum*), ginkgo biloba, ginseng, kava kava (*Piper methysticum*), St. John's wort (*Hypericum perforatum*), licorice extract (*Glycyrrhizic acid*), and valerian (*Valeriana officinalis*). Many patients fail to report the use of herbal medicines to health care service providers; therefore, the nurse must ask surgical patients specifically about the use of these agents. It is recommended that patients anticipating surgery discontinue the use of herbal medicines at least 2 weeks before surgery, because many herbal agents can adversely affect surgical outcomes (Allison & George, 2014).

Psychosocial Factors

The nurse anticipates that most patients have emotional reactions prior to surgery—obvious or veiled, normal or abnormal. Fear may be related to the unknown, lack of control, or of death and may be influenced by anesthesia, pain, complications, cancer, or prior surgical experience. Preoperative anxiety can be a preemptive response to a threat to the patient's role in life, a permanent incapacity or body integrity, increased responsibilities or burden on family members, or life itself. Less obvious concerns may occur because of previous experiences with the health care system and people the patient has known with the same condition. Psychological distress directly influences body functioning. Identification of anxiety by the health care team using supportive guidance at every juncture of the perioperative process helps to ease anxiety.

People express fear in different ways. Some patients may ask repeated questions, regardless of information already shared with them. Others may withdraw, deliberately avoiding communication by reading, watching television, or talking about trivialities. Consequently, the nurse must be empathetic, listen well, and provide information that helps alleviate concerns.

An important outcome of the psychosocial assessment is the determination of the extent and role of the patient's support network. The value and reliability of available support systems are assessed. Other information, such as knowledge of the usual level of functioning and typical daily activities, may assist in the patient's care and recovery. Assessing the patient's readiness to learn and determining the best approach to maximize comprehension provide the basis for preoperative patient education. This is of particular importance in patients who are developmentally delayed and those who are cognitively impaired, where the approach to patient education and consent will include the legal guardian.

Spiritual and Cultural Beliefs

Spiritual beliefs play an important role in how people cope with fear and anxiety. Regardless of the patient's religious affiliation, adhering to spiritual beliefs can be therapeutic. Every attempt must be made to help the patient obtain the spiritual support that he or she requests. Therefore, the nurse must respect and support the beliefs of each patient. Some nurses may avoid the subject of a clergy visit lest the suggestion alarm the patient. Asking whether the patient's spiritual advisor knows about the impending surgery is a caring, nonthreatening approach.

Showing respect for a patient's cultural values and beliefs facilitates rapport and trust. Assessment includes identifying

TABLE 17-3 Examples of Medications With the Potential to Affect the Surgical Experience

Agent	Effect of Interaction With Anesthetics
Corticosteroids Dexamethasone (Dexpak)	Cardiovascular collapse can occur if discontinued suddenly. Therefore, a bolus of corticosteroid may be administered IV immediately before and after surgery.
Diuretics Hydrochlorothiazide (Microxide)	During anesthesia, may cause excessive respiratory depression resulting from an associated electrolyte imbalance.
Phenothiazines Chlorpromazine hydrochloride	May increase the hypotensive action of anesthetics.
Tranquilizers Diazepam (Valium)	May cause anxiety, tension, and even seizures if withdrawn suddenly.
Insulins Insulin (Humalog)	Interaction between anesthetics and insulin must be considered when a patient with diabetes is undergoing surgery. IV insulin may need to be given to keep the blood glucose within the normal range.
Anticoagulants Warfarin (Coumadin)	Can increase the risk of bleeding during the intraoperative and postoperative periods; should be discontinued in anticipation of elective surgery. The surgeon will determine how long before the elective surgery the patient should stop taking an anticoagulant, depending on the type of planned procedure and the medical condition of the patient.
Anticonvulsant Medications Carbamazepine (Tegretol)	IV administration of medication may be needed to keep the patient seizure free in the intraoperative and postoperative periods.
Thyroid Hormone Levothyroxine sodium (Synthroid)	IV administration may be needed during the postoperative period to maintain thyroid levels.
Opioids Morphine sulfate (MS Contin)	Long-term use of opioids for chronic pain (≥6 mo) in the preoperative period may alter the patient's response to analgesic agents.

IV, intravenous.
Adapted from Comerford, K. C. (2015). *Nursing 2015 drug handbook*. Philadelphia, PA: Wolters Kluwer.

the ethnic group to which the patient relates and the customs and beliefs the patient holds about illness and health care providers. The Amish culture, for example, with its strong work ethic and unique social structure, has better outcomes following a traumatic injury. Researchers have reported decreased mortality rates and shorter lengths of stay compared to non-Amish patients (Rogers, Horst, Rogers, et al., 2013).

Certain ethnic groups are unaccustomed to expressing feelings openly with strangers and nurses need to consider this pattern of communication when assessing pain. In some cultural groups, it is seen as impolite to make direct eye contact with others and doing so is seen as disrespectful. The nurse should know that this lack of eye contact is not avoidance nor does it reflect a lack of interest. Other ethnicities view the top of the head as sacred; therefore, a nurse would not put the surgical cap on the patient but would ask the patient to don the cap.

Perhaps the most valuable skill at the nurse's disposal is listening carefully to the patient and observing body language, especially when obtaining the history. Invaluable information and insights may be gained through effective communication and interviewing skills. An unhurried, understanding, and caring nurse promotes confidence on the part of the patient.

Preoperative Nursing Interventions

A wide range of interventions are used to prepare the patient physically and psychologically and to maintain safety. Beginning with the nursing history and physical examination, listing of medications taken routinely, history of allergies, and surgical and anesthetic histories, the patient's overall health status and level of experience and understanding may be established.

 Providing Patient Education

Nurses have long recognized the value of preoperative instruction (Rothrock, 2014). Each patient's education is individualized, with consideration for any unique concerns or learning needs. Multiple education strategies should be used (e.g., verbal, written, return demonstration), depending on the patient's needs and abilities.

Preoperative education is initiated as soon as possible, beginning in the physician's office, in the clinic, or at the time of PAT when diagnostic tests are performed. During PAT, the nurse or health care provider makes resources available related to patient education, such as written instructions (designed to be copied and given to patients), audiovisual resources, and telephone numbers, to ensure that education continues until the patient arrives for the surgical intervention. When possible, instruction is spaced over a period of time to allow the patient to assimilate information and ask questions as they arise.

Frequently, education sessions are combined with various preparation procedures to allow for an easy and timely flow of information. The nurse should guide the patient through the experience and allow ample time for questions. Education should go beyond descriptions of the procedure and should include explanations of the sensations the patient will experience. Telling the patient that preoperative medication will cause relaxation before the operation is not as effective as also noting that the medication will act quickly and may result in lightheadedness, dizziness, and drowsiness. Knowing what to expect will help the patient anticipate these reactions and attain a superior degree of relaxation. Overly detailed descriptions may increase anxiety in some patients; therefore, the nurse should be sensitive to this, by watching and listening, and provide less detail based on the individual patient's needs.

Unfolding Patient Stories: Vernon Watkins • Part 1

Vernon Watkins, a 69-year-old male, came to the emergency department with severe abdominal pain, and a bowel perforation was diagnosed. He is being prepared for surgery. Significant medical history includes controlled hypertension and smoking for 50 years. What preoperative education should the nurse discuss with Mr. Watkins prior to his emergent surgery? (Vernon Watkins' story continues in Chapter 63.)

Care for Vernon and other patients in a realistic virtual environment: *vSim for Nursing* (**thepoint.lww.com/vSimMedicalSurgical**). Practice documenting these patients' care in DocuCare (**thepoint.lww.com/DocuCareEHR**).

Deep Breathing, Coughing, and Incentive Spirometry

One goal of preoperative nursing care is to educate the patient how to promote optimal lung expansion and resulting blood oxygenation after anesthesia. The patient assumes a sitting position to enhance lung expansion. The nurse then demonstrates how to take a deep, slow breath and how to exhale slowly. After practicing deep breathing several times, the patient is instructed to breathe deeply, exhale through the mouth, take a short breath, and cough deeply in the lungs (see Chart 17-5). The nurse or respiratory therapist also demonstrates how to use an incentive spirometer, a device that provides measurement and feedback related to breathing effectiveness (see Chapter 21). In addition to enhancing respiration, these exercises may help the patient relax.

If a thoracic or abdominal incision is anticipated, the nurse demonstrates how to splint the incision to minimize pressure and control pain. The patient should put the palms of both hands together, interlacing the fingers snugly. Splinting or placing the hands across the incision site acts as an effective support when coughing. The patient is informed that medications are available to relieve pain and should be taken regularly for pain relief so that effective deep-breathing and coughing exercises can be performed comfortably. The goal in promoting coughing is to mobilize secretions so that they can be removed. Deep breathing before coughing stimulates the cough reflex. If the patient does not cough effectively, atelectasis (collapse of the alveoli), pneumonia, or other lung complications may occur.

Mobility and Active Body Movement

The goals of promoting mobility postoperatively are to improve circulation, prevent venous stasis, and promote optimal respiratory function. The patient should be taught that early and frequent ambulation postoperatively, as tolerated, will help prevent complications.

The nurse explains the rationale for frequent position changes after surgery and then shows the patient how to turn from side to side and how to assume the lateral position without causing pain or disrupting intravenous (IV) lines, drainage tubes, or other equipment. Any special position the patient needs to maintain after surgery (e.g., adduction or elevation of an extremity) is discussed, as is the importance of maintaining as much mobility as possible despite restrictions. Reviewing the process before surgery is helpful, because the patient may be too uncomfortable or drowsy after surgery to absorb new information.

Exercise of the extremities includes extension and flexion of the knee and hip joints (similar to bicycle riding while lying on the side) unless contraindicated by type of surgical procedure (e.g., hip replacement). The foot is rotated as though tracing the largest possible circle with the great toe (see Chart 17-5). The elbow and shoulder are also put through their range of motion. At first, the patient is assisted and reminded to perform these exercises. Later, the patient is encouraged to do them independently. Muscle tone is maintained so that ambulation will be easier. The nurse should remember to use proper body mechanics and to instruct the patient to do the same. Whenever the patient is positioned, their body needs to be properly aligned.

Pain Management

A pain assessment should include differentiation between acute and chronic pain. A pain intensity scale should be introduced and explained to the patient to promote more effective postoperative pain management. (See Chapter 12 for examples of pain scales.) Preoperative patient education also needs to include the difference between acute and chronic pain so that the patient is prepared to differentiate acute postoperative pain from a chronic condition such as back pain. Preoperative pain assessment and education for the older patient may require additional attention (see Chart 17-6).

Postoperatively, medications are given to relieve pain and maintain comfort without suppressing respiratory function. The patient is instructed to take the medication as frequently as prescribed during the initial postoperative period for pain relief. Anticipated methods of administration of analgesic agents for inpatients include patient-controlled analgesia (PCA), epidural catheter bolus or infusion, or patient-controlled epidural analgesia (PCEA). (See Chapter 12 for discussion of PCA and PCEA.) A patient who is expected to go home will likely receive oral analgesic agents. These methods are discussed with the patient before surgery, and the patient's interest and willingness to use them are assessed.

Chart 17-5

PATIENT EDUCATION

Preoperative Instructions to Prevent Postoperative Complications

Diaphragmatic Breathing

Diaphragmatic breathing refers to a flattening of the dome of the diaphragm during inspiration, with resultant enlargement of the upper abdomen as air rushes in. During expiration, the abdominal muscles contract.

1. Practice in the same position you would assume in bed after surgery: a semi-Fowler's position, propped in bed with the back and shoulders well supported with pillows.
2. Feel the movement with your hands resting lightly on the front of the lower ribs and fingertips against the lower chest.

Diaphragmatic breathing

3. Breathe out gently and fully as the ribs sink down and inward toward midline.
4. Then take a deep breath through your nose and mouth, letting the abdomen rise as the lungs fill with air.
5. Hold this breath for a count of five.
6. Exhale and let out *all* the air through your nose and mouth.
7. Repeat this exercise 15 times with a short rest after each group of five.
8. Practice this twice a day preoperatively.

Coughing

1. Lean forward slightly from a sitting position in bed, interlace your fingers together, and place your hands across the incision site to act as a splint for support when coughing.

Splinting of chest when coughing

2. Breathe with the diaphragm as described under "Diaphragmatic Breathing."
3. With your mouth slightly open, breathe in fully.

4. "Hack" out sharply for three short breaths.
5. Then, keeping your mouth open, take in a quick deep breath and immediately give a strong cough once or twice. This helps clear secretions from your chest. It may cause some discomfort but will not harm your incision.

Leg Exercises

1. Lie in a semi-Fowler's position and perform the following simple exercises to improve circulation.
2. Bend your knee and raise your foot—hold it a few seconds, then extend the leg and lower it to the bed.

Straighten · Flex · Down

Leg exercises

3. Do this five times with one leg and then repeat with the other leg.
4. Then trace circles with the feet by bending them down, in toward each other, up, and then out.
5. Repeat these movements five times.

Turning to the Side

1. Turn on your side with the uppermost leg flexed most and supported on a pillow.
2. Grasp the side rail as an aid to maneuver to the side.
3. Practice diaphragmatic breathing and coughing while on your side.

Foot exercises

Getting Out of Bed

1. Turn on your side.
2. Push yourself up with one hand as you swing your legs out of bed.

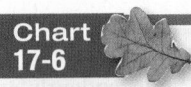

Chart 17-6 Preoperative Assessment and Education for Older Adults

Assessment

- Assess for allergies and medical comorbidities.
- Assess the patient's cognitive and sensory function before the surgeon begins the informed consent process.
- Determine the need for a designated support person or power of attorney to complete the informed consent process.
- Review medications to identify potential polypharmaceutical risks to include the following:
  - multiple medications,
  - multiple prescribers,
  - several filling pharmacies,
  - too many forms of medications,
  - over-the-counter medications, or
  - multiple dosing schedules.
- Document baseline physical assessment parameters, including pain, anxiety, cardiac rhythm, and oxygen saturation level
- Document a detailed skin assessment with notation of areas of dryness, lesions, or bruising
- Document preoperative fasting status and assess for dehydration, malnutrition, and hypoglycemia
- Identify social support to determine whether the patient has home assistance to complete ADLs

Education

- Discuss advanced directives and code status to identify the patient's wishes.
- Educate the patient about the benefits of controlling pain.
- Be prepared to spend additional time, increase the amount of therapeutic touch utilized, and encourage family members to be present to decrease anxiety.

ADLs, activities of daily living.
Adapted from Bourdon, L. (2015). Care of the patient receiving local anesthesia. *AORN Journal, 101*(3), 10–12; Oster, K.A., & Oster, C.A. (2015). Special needs population: Care of the geriatric patient population in the perioperative setting. *AORN Journal, 101*(4), 444–456.

Cognitive Coping Strategies

Cognitive strategies may be useful for relieving tension, overcoming anxiety, decreasing fear, and achieving relaxation. Examples of general strategies include:

- *Imagery:* The patient concentrates on a pleasant experience or restful scene.
- *Distraction:* The patient thinks of an enjoyable story or recites a favorite poem or song.
- *Optimistic self-recitation:* The patient recites optimistic thoughts ("I know all will go well").
- *Music:* The patient listens to soothing music (an easy-to-administer, inexpensive, noninvasive intervention).

Several researchers have reported that individualized nurse-delivered interventions reduce anxiety levels and are highly valued by patients (Renouf, Leary, & Wiseman, 2014; Thompson, Moe, & Lewis, 2014). Interventions may include teaching positive thinking, relaxation techniques, or guided imagery.

Education for Patients Undergoing Ambulatory Surgery

Preoperative education for the same-day or ambulatory surgical patient comprises all previously discussed patient education as well as collaborative planning with the patient and family for discharge and follow-up home care. The major difference in outpatient preoperative education is the environment.

Preoperative education content may be presented in a group class, in a media presentation, at PAT, or by telephone in conjunction with the preoperative interview. In addition to answering questions and describing what to expect, the nurse tells the patient when and where to report, what to bring (insurance card, list of medications and allergies), what to leave at home (jewelry, watch, medications, contact lenses), and what to wear (loose-fitting, comfortable clothes; flat shoes). The nurse in the surgeon's office may initiate education before the perioperative telephone contact.

During the final preoperative telephone call, education is completed or reinforced as needed and last-minute instructions are given. The patient is reminded not to eat or drink for a specified period of time preoperatively.

Providing Psychosocial Interventions

Reducing Anxiety and Decreasing Fear

Perioperative nurses in the preoperative department have a limited amount of time to acquire information and establish trust. Nurses must introduce themselves, giving their title and a brief synopsis of their professional role and background. Each preoperative patient should be acknowledged as an individual, and each patient's needs and desires must be assessed. The patient should be thanked for choosing that particular hospital or surgical center. These methods facilitate establishing a positive nurse–patient relationship. Discussion of the surgical experience, its length, and explanation of what will happen may diminish the patient's anxiety.

During the preoperative assessment of psychological factors and spiritual and cultural beliefs, the nurse assists the patient to identify coping strategies that he or she has previously used to decrease fear. Discussions with the patient to help determine the source of fears can help with expression of concerns. The patient benefits from knowing when family and friends will be able to visit after surgery and that a spiritual advisor will be available if desired. The preoperative education and cognitive coping strategies addressed earlier help decrease preoperative anxiety in many patients (Renouf et al., 2014). Knowing ahead of time about the possible need for a ventilator, drainage tubes, or other types of equipment helps decrease anxiety related to the postoperative period.

Respecting Cultural, Spiritual, and Religious Beliefs

Psychosocial interventions include identifying and showing respect for cultural, spiritual, and religious beliefs (Rogers et al., 2013). In some cultures, for example, people are stoic in regard to pain, whereas in others they are more expressive. These responses should be recognized as normal for those patients and families and should be respected by perioperative personnel. If patients decline blood transfusions for religious reasons (Jehovah's Witnesses), this information needs to be clearly identified in the preoperative period, documented, and communicated to the appropriate personnel. Although minimally invasive surgery has significantly lowered blood loss, any surgical procedure has the potential for hemorrhage.

Chart 17-7 Summary of the 2016 National Patient Safety Goals

- Identify patients correctly
- Improve staff communication
- Use medicines safely
- Use alarms safely
- Prevent infection
- Identify patient safety risks
- Prevent mistakes in surgery

Adapted from Joint Commission (2016). 2016 National Patient Safety Goals. Retrieved on 12/9/15 at: www.jointcommission.org/standards_information/npsgs.aspx

Maintaining Patient Safety

Protecting patients from injury is one of the major roles of the perioperative nurse. Adherence to AORN-recommended practices and the Joint Commission's National Patient Safety Goals (see Chart 17-7) are crucial (Rothrock, 2014). These apply to hospitals as well as to ambulatory surgery centers and office-based surgery facilities (Joint Commission, 2016).

Managing Nutrition and Fluids

The purpose of withholding food and fluid before surgery is to prevent aspiration. Until recently, fluid and food were restricted preoperatively overnight and often longer. The American Society of Anesthesiologists reviewed this practice and made new recommendations for people undergoing elective surgery who are otherwise healthy. Specific recommendations depend on the age of the patient and the type of food eaten. For example, adults may be advised to fast for 8 hours after eating fatty food and 4 hours after ingesting milk products. Healthy patients are allowed clear liquids up to 2 hours before an elective procedure. One study reported that the safety of administering preoperative oral carbohydrate-rich fluids was supported, but researchers were unable to confirm or refute the benefit of this fluid regimen for shortening the length of hospital stay after elective colorectal surgery (Webster, Osborne, Gill, et al., 2014).

Preparing the Bowel

Enemas are not commonly prescribed preoperatively unless the patient is undergoing abdominal or pelvic surgery. In this case, a cleansing enema or laxative may be prescribed the evening before surgery and may be repeated the morning of surgery. The goals of this preparation are to allow satisfactory visualization of the surgical site and to prevent trauma to the intestine or contamination of the peritoneum by fecal material. Unless the condition of the patient presents some contraindication, the toilet or bedside commode, rather than the bedpan, is used for evacuating the enema if the patient is hospitalized during this time. In addition, antibiotics may be prescribed to reduce intestinal flora.

Preparing the Skin

The goal of preoperative skin preparation is to decrease bacteria without injuring the skin. If the surgery is not performed as an emergency, most health care facilities and ambulatory surgical centers have implemented antiseptic skin cleansing protocols. There is an ongoing debate as to the efficacy of skin protocols in preventing SSIs, particularly when the patient is instructed to carry out the preparation independently at home prior to surgery (Chlebicki, Safdar, O'Horo, et al., 2013; Edmiston & Spencer, 2014).

Generally, hair is not removed preoperatively unless the hair at or around the incision site is likely to interfere with the operation. If hair must be removed, electric clippers are used for safe hair removal before transferring the patient to the OR (Edmiston & Spencer, 2014). To ensure the correct site, the surgical site is typically marked by the patient and the surgeon prior to the procedure.

Immediate Preoperative Nursing Interventions

Immediately prior to the procedure, the patient changes into a hospital gown that is left untied and open in the back. The patient with long hair may braid it, remove hairpins, and cover the head completely with a disposable paper cap. The mouth is inspected, and dentures or plates are removed. If left in the mouth, these items could easily fall to the back of the throat during induction of anesthesia and cause respiratory obstruction.

Jewelry is not worn to the OR; wedding rings and jewelry or body piercings should be removed to prevent injury. If a patient objects to removing a ring, some institutions allow the ring to be securely fastened to the finger with tape. All articles of value, including assistive devices, dentures, glasses, and prosthetic devices, are given to family members or are labeled clearly with the patient's name and stored in a safe and secure place according to the institution's policy.

All patients (except those with urologic disorders) should void immediately before going to the OR. This is particularly important in promoting visibility of anatomy and continence during low abdominal surgery. Urinary catheterization is performed in the OR only as necessary.

Administering Preanesthetic Medication

The use of preanesthetic medication is minimal with ambulatory or outpatient surgery. If prescribed, it is usually given in the preoperative holding area. If a preanesthetic medication is given, the patient is kept in bed with the side rails raised, because the medication can cause lightheadedness or drowsiness. During this time, the nurse observes the patient for any untoward reaction to the medications. The immediate surroundings are kept quiet to promote relaxation, and some facilities use soft classical music (Thompson et al., 2014).

Often, surgery is delayed or schedules change, and it becomes impossible to request that a medication be given at a specific time. In these situations, the preoperative medication is prescribed "on call to OR." The nurse can have the medication ready to administer as soon as a call is received from the OR staff. It usually takes 15 to 20 minutes to prepare the patient for the OR. If the nurse gives the medication before attending to the other details of preoperative preparation, the patient will have at least partial benefit from the preoperative medication and will have a smoother anesthetic and operative course.

Preoperative Checklist

1. Patient's name: _____ Date: _____ Height: _____ Weight: _____
   Identification band present: _____
2. Informed consent signed: _____ Special permits signed: _____
3. Surgical site: _____ (Ex: Sterilization)
4. History & physical examination report present: _____ Date: _____
5. Laboratory records present: _____
   CBC: _____ Hgb: _____ Urinalysis: _____ Hct: _____

6. | Item | Present | Removed |
|------|---------|---------|
| a. Natural teeth | _____ | _____ |
| Dentures; upper, lower, partial | _____ | _____ |
| Bridge, fixed; crown | _____ | _____ |
| b. Contact lenses | _____ | _____ |
| c. Other prostheses—type: _____ | _____ | _____ |
| d. Jewelry: | | |
| Wedding band (taped/tied) | _____ | _____ |
| Rings | _____ | _____ |
| Earrings: pierced, clip-on | _____ | _____ |
| Neck chains | _____ | _____ |
| Any other body piercings | _____ | _____ |
| e. Make-up | _____ | _____ |
| Nail polish | _____ | _____ |
| 7. Clothing | | |
| a. Clean patient gown | _____ | _____ |
| b. Cap | _____ | _____ |
| c. Sanitary pad, etc. | _____ | _____ |

8. Family instructed where to wait? _____
9. Valuables secured? _____
10. Blood available? _____ Ordered? _____ Where? _____
11. Preanesthetic medication given: _____
    Type: _____ Time: _____
12. Voided: _____ Amount: _____ Time: _____ Catheter: _____
    Mouth care given: _____
13. Vital signs: Temperature: _____ Pulse: _____ Resp: _____ Blood Pressure: _____
14. Special problems/precautions: (Allergies, deafness, etc.): _____
15. Area of skin preparation: _____
16. _____ Date: _____ Time: _____
    Signature: Nurse releasing patient

Figure 17-2 • Example of a preoperative checklist.

Maintaining the Preoperative Record

Preoperative checklists contain critical elements that must be checked and verified preoperatively (Rothrock, 2014). The nurse completes the preoperative checklist (see Fig. 17-2). The completed medical record (with the preoperative checklist and verification form) accompanies the patient to the OR with the surgical consent form attached, along with all laboratory reports and nurses' records. Any unusual last-minute observations that may have a bearing on anesthesia or surgery are noted prominently at the front of the medical record.

Transporting the Patient to the Presurgical Area

The patient is brought to the holding area or presurgical suite about 30 to 60 minutes before the anesthetic is to be given. The stretcher should be as comfortable as possible, with a sufficient number of blankets to prevent chilling in an air-conditioned room. Evidence supports the use of preoperative warming to increase patient reports of being warm during the perioperative period (Erdling & Johansson, 2015). The time period and settings (i.e., holding area, surgical suite or both) for warming are subjects of ongoing investigation (Adriani & Moriber, 2013; Erdling & Johansson, 2015; Fettes, Mulvaine, & Van Doren, 2013; Roberson, Dieckmann, Rodriguez, et al., 2013). A small head pillow is usually provided for patient comfort.

The patient is taken to the preoperative holding area, greeted by name, and positioned comfortably on the stretcher or bed. The surrounding area should be kept quiet if the preoperative medication is to have maximal effect. Unpleasant sounds or conversation should be avoided, because a sedated patient may misinterpret them.

Patient safety in the preoperative area is a priority. The use of a standard process or procedure to verify patient identification, the surgical procedure, and the surgical site is imperative to maximize patient safety (Huang, Kim, & Berry, 2013). This allows for prompt intervention if any discrepancies are identified.

Chart 17-8   Expected Patient Activities in the Preoperative Phase of Care

Relief of anxiety, evidenced when the patient:

- Discusses with the anesthesiologist, or CRNA concerns related to types of anesthesia and induction
- Verbalizes an understanding of the preanesthetic medication and general anesthesia
- Discusses last-minute concerns with the nurse or physician
- Discusses financial concerns with the social worker, when appropriate
- Requests visit with spiritual advisor, when appropriate
- Appears relaxed when visited by health care team members

Decreased fear, evidenced when the patient:

- Discusses fears with health care professionals or a spiritual advisor, or both
- Verbalizes an understanding of any expected bodily changes, including expected duration of bodily changes

Understanding of the surgical intervention, evidenced when the patient:

- Participates in preoperative preparation as appropriate (i.e., bowel preparation, shower)
- Demonstrates and describes exercises that he or she is expected to perform postoperatively
- Reviews information about postoperative care
- Accepts preanesthetic medication, if prescribed
- Remains in bed once premedicated
- Relaxes during transportation to the operating room or unit
- States rationale for use of side rails
- Discusses postoperative expectations

CRNA, certified registered nurse anesthetist.

Attending to Family Needs

Most hospitals and ambulatory surgery centers have a waiting room where family members and significant others can wait while the patient is undergoing surgery. This room may be equipped with comfortable chairs, televisions, telephones, and light refreshments. Volunteers may remain with the family, offer them coffee, and keep them informed of the patient's progress. After surgery, the surgeon may meet the family in the waiting room and discuss the outcome.

The family and significant others should never judge the seriousness of an operation by the length of time the patient is in the OR. A patient may be in the OR much longer than the actual operating time for several reasons:

- Patients are routinely transported well in advance of the actual operating time.
- The anesthesiologist or CRNA often makes additional preparations that may take 30 to 60 minutes.
- The surgeon may take longer than expected with the preceding case, which delays the start of the next surgical procedure.

After surgery, the patient is taken to the PACU to ensure safe emergence from anesthesia. Family members and significant others waiting to see the patient after surgery should be informed that the patient may have certain equipment or devices (e.g., IV lines, indwelling urinary catheter, nasogastric tube, oxygen lines, monitoring equipment, blood transfusion lines) in place when he or she returns from surgery. When the patient returns to the room, the nurse provides explanations regarding the frequent postoperative observations that will be made. However, it is the responsibility of the surgeon, not the nurse, to relay the surgical findings and the prognosis, even when the findings are favorable.

Expected Patient Outcomes

Expected patient activities to decrease anxiety, and fear, as well as increase knowledge in the preoperative phase of care are summarized in Chart 17-8. Nurse-sensitive outcomes often include central line-associated bloodstream infections (CLABSI), catheter-associated urinary tract infections (CAUTI), hospital-acquired pressure ulcers and unit-acquired pressure ulcers. Researchers have reported some patient outcomes are influenced by the level of nurse certification. (See Chart 17-9.)

Chart 17-9   NURSING RESEARCH PROFILE

The Relationship Between Certification of Nurses and Surgical Outcomes.

Boyle, D. K., Cramer, E., Potter, C., et al. (2014). The relationship between direct-care RN specialty certification and surgical patient outcomes. *AORN Journal,100*(11), 511–528.

Purpose

Specialty certification is thought to enhance the safety of patients by validating that standards of practice are met. The purpose of this study was to explore the relationship between specialty-certified nurses in perioperative units and surgical intensive care units (SICUs) and nurse-sensitive patient outcomes. The nurse-sensitive outcomes included central line-associated bloodstream infections (CLABSI), catheter-associated urinary tract infections (CAUTI), hospital-acquired pressure ulcers and unit-acquired pressure ulcers.

Design

This was a retrospective, repeated measures analysis of secondary data from the National Database of Nursing Quality Indicators. Outcomes were examined by unit types and included four specific specialty certifications commonly held by perioperative nurses (CAPA [certified postanesthesia nurse], CPAN [certified postanesthesia nurse], CNOR [certified nurse operating room], CRNFA [certified RN first assistant]). The data were analyzed using an autoregressive generalized linear regression model at the unit level. Patient outcome variables were collected concurrently with the other predictor variables.

Findings

Lower rates of CLABSI in SICUs were significantly associated with higher proportions of CPAN ($\beta = -0.09$, $p = 0.05$) and CNOR/CRNFA ($\beta = -0.17$, $p = 0.00$) certifications in perioperative units. Interestingly, higher proportions of CNOR/CRNFA certification in perioperative units were associated with higher proportions of hospital-acquired pressure ulcers ($\beta = 0.08$, $p = 0.03$) and unit-acquired pressure ulcers ($\beta = 0.13$, $p = 0.00$), possibly because of a higher risk of pressure ulcers in the patient population.

Nursing Implications

Nurses should know that at least in this one study higher rates of nurse certifications were associated with lower rates of CLABSI in SICUs. These findings lend credence to perioperative, SICU, and surgical nurses participating in lifelong learning and continuous professional development, including achievement of specialty certification.

CRITICAL THINKING EXERCISES

1 `pq` A 55-year-old man with intractable pain of his lower back is unable to lie flat on the stretcher while waiting for his spinal surgery. He assesses his pain at 10 on a scale of 0 being no pain and 10 being the worst pain imaginable. What are the priorities of the perioperative nurse? What further assessments are priorities? What nursing interventions are warranted?

2 `ebp` A morbidly obese 60-year-old woman has been admitted for a minimally invasive hysterectomy. Her medical history includes high blood pressure as well as diabetes controlled with insulin and diet. The patient also takes antihypertensive medication, aspirin, and several herbal supplements daily. What resources would you use to identify evidence-based practices for prevention of complications during the perioperative period? Identify the evidence, as well as the criteria used to evaluate the strength of the evidence, for the practices identified.

3 A 38-year-old man is admitted for knee surgery following a horse riding accident. He is in good physical condition but the electrocardiogram (ECG) is showing an abnormal cardiac rhythm. What is your next step? What is your nursing plan of care?

REFERENCES

*Asterisk indicates nursing research.

Books

American Society of PeriAnesthesia Nurses (ASPAN). (2015). *2015–2017 Perianesthesia nursing standards, practice recommendations and interpretive statements.* Cherry Hill, NJ: Author.
Association of PeriOperative Registered Nurses (AORN). (2014). *Association of PeriOperative Registered Nurses (AORN) standards, recommended practice, and guidelines.* Denver, CO: Author.
Alvarex, A., Brodsky, J. B., Lemmens, H. J., et al. (2014). *PeriAnesthesia Nursing Core Curriculum: Preprocedure, phase I and phase II PACU nursing* (2nd ed.). St. Louis, MO: Elsevier.
Barash, P. G., Cullen, B. F., Stoelting, R. K., et al. (2013). *Clinical anesthesia* (7th ed.). Philadelphia, PA: Lippincott Williams & Wilkins.
Comerford, K. C. (2015). *Nursing 2015 drug handbook.* Philadelphia, PA: Wolters Kluwer.
Meiner, S. E. (2014). *Gerontologic nursing* (5th ed.). St. Louis, MO: Elsevier Mosby.
Porth, C. M. (2015). *Essentials of pathophysiology: Concepts of altered states* (4th ed.). Philadelphia, PA: Lippincott Williams & Wilkins.
Rothrock, J. C. (2014). *Alexander's care of the patient in surgery* (14th ed.). St. Louis, MO: Mosby Jones & Bartlett.
Tabloski, P. A. (2013). *Gerontological nursing: The essential guide to clinical practice* (3rd ed.). Upper Saddle River, NJ: Prentice Hall.

Journals and Electronic Documents

*Adriani, M. B., & Moriber, N. (2013). Preoperative forced-air warming combined with intraoperative warming versus intraoperative warming alone in the prevention of hypothermia during gynecologic surgery. *American Anesthesia Nursing Journal, 81*(6), 446–451.
Allison, J., & George, M. (2014). Using preoperative assessment and patient instruction to improve patient safety. *AORN Journal, 99*(3), 364–375.
Australasian Society of Clinical Immunology and Allergy. (2015). Latex allergy. Retrieved on 12/9/15 at: www.allergy.org.au

Bourdon, L. (2015). Care of the patient receiving local anesthesia. *AORN Journal, 101*(3), 10–12.
*Boyle, D. K., Cramer, E., Potter, C., et al. (2014). The relationship between direct-care RN specialty certification and surgical patient outcomes. *AORN Journal, 100*(5), 511–528.
Centers for Disease Control and Prevention. (2015). About BMI for adults. Retrieved on 10/20/15 at: www.cdc.gov/healthyweight/assessing/bmi/adult_bmi/index.html
*Chlebicki, M. P., Safdar, N., O'Höro, J. C., et al. (2013). Preoperative chlorhexidine shower or bath for prevention of surgical site infection: A meta-analysis. *American Journal of Infection Control, 41,* 167–173.
Edmiston, C. E., & Spencer, M. (2014.) Patient care interventions to help reduce the risk of surgical site infections. *AORN Journal, 100*(6), 590–602.
*Erdling, A., & Johansson, A. (2015). Core temperature: The intraoperative difference between esophageal versus nasopharyngeal temperatures and the impact of prewarming, age, and weight: A randomized clinical trial. *AANA Journal, 83*(2), 99–105.
*Fettes, S., Mulvaine, M., & Van Doren, E. (2013). Effect of preoperative forced-air warming on postoperative temperature and postanesthesia care unit length of stay. *AORN Journal, 97*(3), 323–328.
Finkelstein, R., Rabino, G., Mashiach, T., et al. (2014). Effect of preoperative antibiotic prophylaxis on surgical site infections complicating cardiac surgery. *Infection Control & Hospital Epidemiology, 35*(1), 69–74.
Huang, L., Kim, R., & Berry, W. (2013). Creating a culture of safety by using checklists. *AORN Journal, 97*(3), 365–368
Joint Commission. (2016). 2016 National Patient Safety Goals. Retrieved on 12/9/15 at: www.jointcommission.org/standards_information/npsgs.aspx
Lagu, T., Hannon, N. S., Rothberg, M. G., et al. (2013). Access to subspecialty care for patients with mobility impairment: A survey. *Annals of Internal Medicine, 158*(6), 441–446.
Ogden, C.L., Carroll, M.D., Kit, B.K., et al. (2014). Prevalence of childhood and adult obesity in the United States, 2011–2012. *JAMA, 311*(8), 806–814.
Oster, K.A., & Oster, C.A. (2015). Special needs population: Care of the geriatric patient population in the perioperative setting. *AORN Journal, 101*(4), 444–456.
Renouf, T., Leary, A., & Wiseman, T. (2014). Do psychological interventions reduce preoperative anxiety? *British Journal of Nursing, 23*(22), 1208–1212.
Rider, O. J., Cox, P., Tyler, D., et al. (2013). Myocardial substrate metabolism in obesity. *International Journal of Obesity, 37,* 972–979.
*Roberson, M.C., Dieckmann, L. S., Rodriguez, R. E., et al. (2013). A review of the evidence for active preoperative warming of adults undergoing general anesthesia. *American Anesthesia Nursing Journal, 81*(5), 351–356.
Rogers, A., Horst, M., Rogers, F., et al. (2013). From the barn to the operating room and back: The Amish way of life leads to improved throughput and outcomes following trauma. *Journal of Trauma and Acute Care Surgery, 75,* 916–918.
Rubinsky, A.D., Bishop, M. J., Maynard, C., et al. (2013). Postoperative risks associated with alcohol screening depend on documented drinking at the time of surgery. *Drug and Alcohol Dependence, 132,* 521–527.
Thanavaro, J. L. (2015). Cardiac risk assessment: Decreasing postoperative complications. *AORN Journal, 101*(2), 201–212.
Thompson, M., Moe, K., & Lewis, C. P. (2014). The effects of music on diminishing anxiety among preoperative patients. *Journal of Radiology Nursing, 33*(4), 199–202.
Webster, J., Osborne, S.R., Gill, R., et al. (2014). Does preoperative oral carbohydrate reduce hospital stay? A randomized trial. *AORN Journal, 99*(2), 233–242.

Resources

American Academy of Ambulatory Care Nursing (AACN), www.aaacn.org
American Association of Gynecologic Laparoscopy (AAGL), www.aagl.org
American Society for Metabolic and Bariatric Surgery (ASMBS), www.asbs.org
American Society of PeriAnesthesia Nurses (ASPAN), www.aspan.org
Association of periOperative Registered Nurses (AORN), www.aorn.org
Centers for Medicare and Medicaid Services (CMS), www.cms.hhs.gov
Joint Commission, www.jointcommission.org

18

Intraoperative Nursing Management

LEARNING OBJECTIVES

On completion of this chapter, the learner will be able to:

1 Describe the interdisciplinary approach to the care of the patient during surgery.
2 Specify the principles of surgical asepsis.
3 Describe the roles of the surgical team members during the intraoperative phase of care.
4 Identify adverse effects of surgery and anesthesia.
5 Identify the surgical risk factors related to age-specific populations and nursing interventions to reduce those risks.
6 Compare types of anesthesia with regard to uses, advantages, disadvantages, and nursing responsibilities.
7 Use the nursing process to optimize patient outcomes during the intraoperative period.

GLOSSARY

anesthesia: a state of narcosis or severe central nervous system depression produced by pharmacologic agents

anesthesiologist: physician trained to deliver anesthesia and to monitor the patient's condition during surgery

anesthetic agent: the substance, such as a chemical or gas, used to induce anesthesia

circulating nurse (or circulator): registered nurse who coordinates and documents patient care in the operating room

laparoscope: a thin endoscope inserted through a small incision into a cavity or joint using fiber-optic technology to project live images of structures onto a video monitor; other small incisions allow additional instruments to be inserted to facilitate laparoscopic surgery

malignant hyperthermia: a rare life-threatening condition triggered by exposure to most anesthetic agents inducing a drastic and uncontrolled increase in skeletal muscle oxidative metabolism that can overwhelm the body's capacity to supply oxygen, remove carbon dioxide, and regulate body temperature, eventually leading to circulatory collapse and death if untreated; often inherited as an autosomal dominant disorder

moderate sedation: previously referred to as conscious sedation, involves the use of sedation to depress the level of consciousness without altering the patient's ability

to maintain a patent airway and to respond to physical stimuli and verbal commands

monitored anesthesia care: moderate sedation given by an anesthesiologist or certified registered nurse anesthetist (CRNA)

registered nurse first assistant: a member of the operating room team whose responsibilities may include handling tissue, providing exposure at the operative field, suturing, and maintaining hemostasis

restricted zone: area in the operating room where scrub attire and surgical masks are required; includes operating room and sterile core areas

scrub role: registered nurse, licensed practical nurse, or surgical technologist who scrubs and dons sterile surgical attire, prepares instruments and supplies, and hands instruments to the surgeon during the procedure

semirestricted zone: area in the operating room where scrub attire is required; may include areas where surgical instruments are processed

surgical asepsis: absence of microorganisms in the surgical environment to reduce the risk of infection

unrestricted zone: area in the operating room that interfaces with other departments; includes patient reception area and holding area

The intraoperative experience has undergone many changes and advances that make it safer and less disturbing to patients. Even with these advances, anesthesia and surgery still place the patient at risk for several complications or adverse events. Consciousness or full awareness, mobility, protective biologic functions, and personal control are totally or partially relinquished by the patient when entering the operating room (OR). Staff from the departments of anesthesia, nursing, and surgery work collaboratively to implement professional standards of care, to control iatrogenic and individual risks, to prevent complications, and to promote high-quality patient outcomes.

The Surgical Team

The surgical team consists of the patient, the anesthesiologist (physician) or certified registered nurse anesthetist (CRNA), the surgeon, nurses, surgical technicians, and registered nurse first assistants (RFNAs) or certified surgical technologists (assistants). The anesthesiologist or CRNA administers the **anesthetic agent** (substance used to induce anesthesia) and monitors the patient's physical status throughout the surgery. The surgeon, nurses, technicians, and assistants scrub and perform the surgery. The person in the scrub role, either a nurse or a surgical technician, provides sterile instruments and supplies to the surgeon during the procedure by anticipating the surgical needs as the surgical case progresses. The circulating nurse coordinates the care of the patient in the OR. Care provided by the circulating nurse includes planning for and assisting with patient positioning, preparing the site for surgery, managing surgical specimens, anticipating the needs of the surgical team, and documenting intraoperative events. Collaboration of the core surgical team using evidence-based practices tailored to the specific case results in optimum patient care and improved outcomes.

The Patient

As the patient enters the OR, he or she may feel either relaxed and prepared or fearful and highly stressed. These feelings depend to a large extent on the amount and timing of preoperative sedation, preoperative education, and the individual patient. Fears about loss of control, the unknown, pain, death, changes in body structure, appearance, or function, and disruption of lifestyle all contribute to anxiety. These fears can increase the amount of anesthetic medication needed, the level of postoperative pain, and overall recovery time. (See Chapter 6 for more information on stress.)

The patient is subject to several risks. Infection, failure of the surgery to relieve symptoms or correct a deformity, temporary or permanent complications related to the procedure or the anesthetic agent, and death are uncommon but potential outcomes of the surgical experience (see Chart 18-1). In addition to fears and risks, the patient undergoing sedation and anesthesia temporarily loses both cognitive function and biologic self-protective mechanisms. Loss of the sense of pain, reflexes, and the ability to communicate subjects the intraoperative patient to possible injury. The OR nurse is the patient's advocate while surgery proceeds.

Gerontologic Considerations

Approximately one third of surgical patients are 65 years of age or older (Oster & Oster, 2015). Older adult patients are at higher risk for complications from anesthesia and surgery compared with younger adult patients due to several factors (Rothrock, 2014). There is a progressive loss of skeletal muscle mass in conjunction with an increase in adipose tissue (Tabloski, 2013). Comorbidities, advanced systemic disease, and increased susceptibility to illness, even in the healthiest older adults, can complicate perioperative management. Age alone confers enough surgical risk that it is a clinical predictor of cardiovascular complications (Meiner, 2014).

Biologic variations of particular importance include age-related cardiovascular and pulmonary changes. The aging heart and blood vessels have decreased the ability to respond to stress. Reduced cardiac output and limited cardiac reserve make the older adult vulnerable to changes in circulating volume and blood oxygen levels (Meiner, 2014). Excessive or rapid administration of intravenous (IV) solutions can cause pulmonary edema. A sudden or prolonged decline in blood pressure may lead to cerebral ischemia, thrombosis, embolism, infarction, and anoxia. Reduced gas exchange can result in cerebral hypoxia.

Lower doses of anesthetic agents are required in older adults due to decreased tissue elasticity (lung and cardiovascular systems) and reduced lean tissue mass. Older patients

---

Chart 18-1

Potential Adverse Effects of Surgery and Anesthesia

Anesthesia and surgery disrupt all major body systems. Although most patients can compensate for surgical trauma and the effects of anesthesia, all patients are at risk during the operative procedure. These risks include the following:

- Allergic reactions
- Anesthesia awareness
- Cardiac dysrhythmia from electrolyte imbalance or adverse effect of anesthetic agents
- Myocardial depression, bradycardia, and circulatory collapse
- Central nervous system agitation, seizures, and respiratory arrest
- Oversedation or undersedation
- Agitation or disorientation, especially in older adult patients
- Hypoxemia or hypercarbia from hypoventilation and inadequate respiratory support during anesthesia
- Laryngeal trauma, oral trauma, and broken teeth from difficult intubation
- Hypothermia from cool operating room temperatures, exposure of body cavities, and impaired thermoregulation secondary to anesthetic agents
- Hypotension from blood loss or adverse effect of anesthesia
- Infection
- Thrombosis from compression of blood vessels or stasis
- Malignant hyperthermia secondary to adverse effect of anesthesia
- Nerve damage and skin breakdown from prolonged or inappropriate positioning
- Electrical shock or burns
- Laser burns
- Drug toxicity, faulty equipment, and other types of human error

Adapted from Association of PeriOperative Registered Nurses (AORN). (2014). *Association of PeriOperative Registered Nurses (AORN) standards, recommended practice, and guidelines*. Denver, CO: Author; Spruce, L. (2015). Back to basics: Procedural sedation. *AORN Journal, 101*(3), 345–353.

---

often experience an increase in the duration of clinical effects of medications. With decreased plasma proteins, more of the anesthetic agent remains free or unbound, and the result is more potent action (Barash, Cullen, Stoelting, et al., 2013).

In addition, body tissues of the older adult are made up predominantly of water, and those tissues with a rich blood supply, such as skeletal muscle, liver, and kidneys, shrink as the body ages. Reduced liver size decreases the rate at which the liver can inactivate many anesthetic agents, and decreased kidney function slows the elimination of waste products and anesthetic agents. Other factors that affect the older surgical patient in the intraoperative period include the following:

- Impaired ability to increase metabolic rate and impaired thermoregulatory mechanisms increase susceptibility to hypothermia.
- Bone loss (25% in women, 12% in men) necessitates careful manipulation and positioning during surgery.
- Reduced ability to adjust rapidly to emotional and physical stress influences surgical outcomes and requires meticulous observation of vital functions.

All of these factors lead to a higher likelihood of perioperative mortality and morbidity in older adult patients

(Oster & Oster, 2015; Penprase & Johnson, 2015). (Further discussion of age-related physiologic changes can be found in Chapter 11.)

Nursing Care

Throughout surgery, nursing responsibilities include providing for the safety and well-being of the patient, coordinating the OR personnel, and performing scrub and circulating activities. Because the patient's emotional state remains a concern, the intraoperative nursing staff provides the patient with information and reassurance, continuing the care initiated by preoperative nurses. The nurse supports coping strategies and reinforces the patient's ability to influence outcomes by encouraging active participation in the plan of care, incorporating cultural, ethnic, and religious considerations as appropriate. The establishment of an environment of trust and relaxation through visualization techniques is another method of patient reassurance that can be used as the patient is anesthetically induced.

As patient advocates, intraoperative nurses monitor factors that have the potential to cause injury, such as patient position, equipment malfunction, and environmental hazards. Nurses also protect the patient's dignity and interests while the patient is under anesthesia. Additional nursing responsibilities include maintaining surgical standards of care, identifying risks, and minimizing complications.

Cultural Diversity

Cultural, ethnic, and religious diversities are important considerations for all health care professionals. Nurses in the perioperative area should be aware of medications that may be prohibited by certain groups (e.g., Muslims and those of the Jewish faith may not wish to use porcine-based products [heparin (porcine or bovine)]; Buddhists may choose not to use bovine products). In certain cultures, the head is a sacred area, and staff should allow patients to apply their own surgical cap in this case. When English is the second language of the patient having surgery under local anesthesia, certified medical translators can be provided to maintain understanding and comprehension by the patient. Translator phones are also available at most hospitals. Family members may have the ability to translate but should not be used as medical translators, as they may wish to save the patient anxiety and not provide an accurate translation, resulting in the patient not receiving complete information.

The Circulating Nurse

The **circulating nurse (or circulator)**, a qualified registered nurse, works in collaboration with surgeons, anesthesia providers, and other health care providers to plan the best course of action for each patient (Rothrock, 2014). In this leadership role, the circulating nurse manages the OR and protects the patient's safety and health by monitoring the activities of the surgical team, checking the OR conditions, and continually assessing the patient for signs of injury and implementing appropriate interventions. A foremost responsibility includes verifying consent; if not obtained, surgery may not commence. The team is coordinated by the circulating nurse, who ensures cleanliness, proper temperature, humidity, appropriate lighting, safe function of equipment, and the availability of supplies and materials.

The circulating nurse monitors aseptic practices to avoid breaks in technique while coordinating the movement of related personnel (medical, x-ray, and laboratory), as well as implementing fire safety precautions (Seifert, Peterson, & Graham, 2015). The circulating nurse also monitors the patient and documents specific activities throughout the operation to ensure the patient's safety and well-being.

In addition, the circulating nurse is responsible for ensuring that the second verification of the surgical procedure and site takes place and is documented (see Fig. 18-1). In some institutions, this is referred to as a time out, surgical pause, or universal protocol that takes place among the surgical team prior to induction of anesthesia with a briefing about anticipated problems, potential complications, allergies, and comorbidities. Every member of the surgical team verifies the patient's name, procedure, and surgical site using objective documentation and data before beginning the surgery. Identifying patients correctly is a 2016 National Patient Safety Goal (see Chart 17-8 in Chapter 17). Research suggests that the use of surgical checklists (see Fig. 18-1) help create a culture of safety and reduce morbidity and mortality (Huang, Kim & Berry, 2013). A team debriefing session, led by the circulating nurse, often follows the completion of surgery to identify potential problems with the postsurgical care of the patient and potential areas for improvement (American Society of PeriAnesthesia Nurses [ASPAN], 2015).

> ### Quality and Safety Nursing Alert
>
> It is imperative that the correct patient identity, surgical procedure, and surgical site be verified prior to surgery. The surgical site should be marked by the patient and physician prior to coming to the OR suite during the consent process.

The Scrub Role

The registered nurse, licensed practical nurse, or surgical technologist (or assistant) performs the activities of the **scrub role**, including performing hand hygiene; setting up the sterile equipment, tables and sterile field; preparing sutures, ligatures, and special equipment (e.g., a **laparoscope**, which is a thin endoscope inserted through a small incision into a cavity or joint using fiber-optic technology to project live images of structures onto a video monitor); and assisting the surgeon and the surgical assistants during the procedure by anticipating the instruments and supplies that will be required, such as sponges, drains, and other equipment. As the surgical incision is closed, the scrub person and the circulating nurse count all needles, sponges, and instruments to be sure that they are accounted for and not retained as a foreign body in the patient (Association of PeriOperative Registered Nurses [AORN], 2014; Rothrock, 2014). Standards call for all sponges used in surgery to be visible on x-ray and for sponge counts to take place at the beginning of surgery and twice at the end (when wound closure begins and again as the skin is being closed). Tissue specimens obtained during surgery are labeled by the person in the scrub role and sent to the laboratory by the circulating nurse.

The Surgeon

The surgeon performs the surgical procedure, heads the surgical team, and is a licensed physician (MD or DO), oral

Surgical Safety Checklist

World Health Organization | Patient Safety
A World Alliance for Safer Health Care

Before induction of anaesthesia →

(with at least nurse and anaesthetist)

Has the patient confirmed his/her identity, site, procedure, and consent?
☐ Yes

Is the site marked?
☐ Yes
☐ Not applicable

Is the anaesthesia machine and medication check complete?
☐ Yes

Is the pulse oximeter on the patient and functioning?
☐ Yes

Does the patient have a:

Known allergy?
☐ No
☐ Yes

Difficult airway or aspiration risk?
☐ No
☐ Yes, and equipment/assistance available

Risk of >500ml blood loss (7ml/kg in children)?
☐ No
☐ Yes, and two IVs/central access and fluids planned

Before skin incision →

(with nurse, anaesthetist and surgeon)

☐ **Confirm all team members have introduced themselves by name and role.**

☐ **Confirm the patient's name, procedure, and where the incision will be made.**

Has antibiotic prophylaxis been given within the last 60 minutes?
☐ Yes
☐ Not applicable

Anticipated Critical Events

To Surgeon:
☐ What are the critical or non-routine steps?
☐ How long will the case take?
☐ What is the anticipated blood loss?

To Anaesthetist:
☐ Are there any patient-specific concerns?

To Nursing Team:
☐ Has sterility (including indicator results) been confirmed?
☐ Are there equipment issues or any concerns?

Is essential imaging displayed?
☐ Yes
☐ Not applicable

Before patient leaves operating room

(with nurse, anaesthetist and surgeon)

Nurse Verbally Confirms:
☐ The name of the procedure
☐ Completion of instrument, sponge and needle counts
☐ Specimen labelling (read specimen labels aloud, including patient name)
☐ Whether there are any equipment problems to be addressed

To Surgeon, Anaesthetist and Nurse:
☐ What are the key concerns for recovery and management of this patient?

This checklist is not intended to be comprehensive. Additions and modifications to fit local practice are encouraged.   Revised 1 / 2009   © WHO, 2009

Figure 18-1 • Surgical safety checklist. Used with permission from World Health Organization. (2015). New checklist to help make surgery safer. *WHO Bulletin, 86*(7), 496–576. Retrieved on 8/12/2016 at: http://apps.who.int/iris/bitstream/10665/44186/2/9789241598590_eng_Checklist.pdf

surgeon (DDS or DMD), or podiatrist (DPM) who is specially trained and qualified. Qualifications and training must adhere to Joint Commission standards, hospital standards, and local and state admitting practices and procedures (Rothrock, 2014).

The Registered Nurse First Assistant

The **registered nurse first assistant** (RNFA) is another member of the OR team. Although the scope of practice of the RNFA depends on each state's nurse practice act, the RNFA practices under the direct supervision of the surgeon. RNFA responsibilities may include handling tissue, providing exposure at the operative field, suturing, and maintaining hemostasis (Rothrock, 2014). The role requires a thorough understanding of anatomy and physiology, tissue handling, and the principles of surgical asepsis. The RNFA must be aware of the objectives of the surgery, must have the knowledge and ability to anticipate needs and to work as a skilled member of a team, and must be able to handle any emergency situation in the OR.

The Anesthesiologist and CRNA

An **anesthesiologist** is a physician specifically trained in the art and science of anesthesiology. A CRNA is a qualified and specifically trained health care professional who administers anesthetic agents, has graduated from an accredited nurse anesthesia master's program, and has passed examinations sponsored by the American Association of Nurse Anesthetists. The anesthesiologist or CRNA assesses the patient before surgery, selects the anesthesia, administers it, intubates the patient if necessary, manages any technical problems related to the administration of the anesthetic agent, and supervises the patient's condition throughout the surgical procedure. Before the patient enters the OR, often at preadmission testing, the anesthesiologist or CRNA visits the patient to perform an assessment, supply information, and answer questions. The type of anesthetic agent to be given, previous reactions to anesthetic medications, and known anatomic abnormalities that would make airway management difficult are among topics addressed.

The anesthesiologist or CRNA uses the American Society of Anesthesiologists (ASA) Physical Status Classification System to determine the patient's status. A patient who is classified as P2, P3, or P4 has a systemic disease that may or may not be related to the cause of surgery. If a patient with a classification of P1, P2, P3, P4, or P5 requires emergency surgery, an E is added to the physical status designation (e.g., P1E, P2E). P6 refers to a patient who is brain dead and is undergoing surgery as an organ donor. The abbreviations ASA1 through ASA6 are often used interchangeably with P1 to P6 to designate physical status (Rothrock, 2014).

> ### Chart 18-2 NURSING RESEARCH PROFILE
> #### Comparing Methods of Intraoperative Temperature Monitoring
>
> Erdling, A., & Johansson, A. (2015). Core temperature—The intraoperative difference between esophageal versus nasopharyngeal temperatures and the impact of prewarming, age, and weight: A randomized clinical trial. *AANA Journal, 83*(2), 99–105.
>
> **Purpose**
>
> Unplanned hypothermia can occur in perioperative practice. The purpose of this study was to compare two methods of temperature monitoring (esophageal and nasopharyngeal) and to investigate the impact of prewarming, age, and weight on intraoperative temperature.
>
> **Design**
>
> The study had two design aspects. The first aspect was that both esophageal and nasopharyngeal temperature were prospectively measured for a period of 210 minutes of anesthesia and compared in 43 patients. The second aspect was that patients undergoing colorectal surgery, once they gave consent, were randomly assigned to two groups. One group of patients received prewarming ($n = 21$), while the other group received no prewarming ($n = 22$).
>
> BMI, body mass index.
>
> **Findings**
>
> Demographics were similar in both groups. Mean temperatures at 210 minutes were statistically different between the groups at both sites of measurement. Esophageal temperature in prewarmed patients was 36.5 ± 0.6 compared to 35.8 ± 0.7 in those without prewarming ($p = 0.001$). The nasopharyngeal temperature was 36.7 ± 0.6 and 36.0 ± 0.6 in those prewarmed and those without prewarming, respectively ($p = 0.002$). A negative correlation was found between esophageal temperature and age ($r^2 = -0.381, p < 0.012$). Esophageal temperature was different with respect to BMI below or above 25. The temperatures were 35.81 ± 0.66 in the lower BMI group compared to 36.46 ± 0.59 in the higher BMI group ($p < 0.001$).
>
> **Nursing Implications**
>
> Nurses should know that in the perioperative period in this small study, esophageal temperature measurement was more accurate. This study adds to the evidence that prewarming can prevent hypothermia in the perioperative period, particularly in older adult patients and those with a lower BMI.

When the patient arrives in the OR, the anesthesiologist or CRNA reassesses the patient's physical condition immediately prior to initiating anesthesia. The anesthetic agent is given, and the patient's airway is maintained through an intranasal intubation (if the surgeon is using an oral approach to surgery), intubation with an endotracheal tube (ETT), or a laryngeal mask airway (LMA). During surgery, the anesthesiologist or CRNA monitors the patient's blood pressure, pulse, and respirations, as well as the electrocardiogram (ECG), blood oxygen saturation level, tidal volume, blood gas levels, blood pH, alveolar gas concentrations, and body temperature. Monitoring by electroencephalography (EEG) is sometimes required. Levels of anesthetic medications in the body can also be determined; a mass spectrometer can provide instant readouts of critical concentration levels on display terminals. This information is used to assess the patient's ability to breathe unassisted or the need for mechanical assistance if ventilation is poor and the patient is not breathing well independently.

The Surgical Environment

The surgical environment is known for its stark appearance and cool temperature. The surgical suite is behind double doors, and access is limited to authorized, appropriately clad personnel. Precautions include adherence to principles of surgical asepsis; strict control of the OR environment is required, including use of laminar airflow rooms as indicated for the surgical procedure, and decreasing noise as well as the number of operating theater door openings (Pada & Perl, 2015). Policies governing this environment address such issues as the health of the staff; the cleanliness of the rooms; the sterility of equipment and surfaces; processes for scrubbing, gowning, and gloving; and OR attire (AORN, 2014).

Warming the patient, which may begin in the preoperative phase of surgery, is continued or initiated during the perioperative stage (Erdling & Johansson, 2015). Maintaining normothermia has been linked to improved patient outcomes, such as enhanced healing, lower infection rates, decreased pain intensity, and reduced malaise (Sobczak, 2014) (see Chart 18-2).

To provide the best possible conditions for surgery, the OR is situated in a location that is central to all supporting services (e.g., pathology, x-ray, and laboratory). The OR has special air filtration devices to screen out contaminating particles, dust, and pollutants.

Many National Patient Safety Goals pertain to the perioperative areas (see Chart 17-8 in Chapter 17); however, the one with the most direct relevance to the OR is to identify patient safety risks. A unique risk is the risk of fire in the OR due to three factors: a source of fuel, an oxygen source, and a mechanism to ignite a fire (AORN, 2014; ASPAN, 2015). All surgical services personnel must familiarize themselves with the department fire emergency response plan and be competent in the use and safeguards of all combustible materials and equipment in the surgical environment (Guglielmi, 2014; Seifert et al., 2015). Surgical drapes provide an opportunity for oxygen to concentrate; a stray spark could more easily ignite a fire. This occurs most commonly in ambulatory surgery settings (Joint Commission, 2016). To further improve safety, electrical hazards, emergency exit clearances, and storage of equipment and anesthetic gases are monitored periodically by official agencies, such as the respective state Department of Health and the Joint Commission.

To help decrease microbes, the surgical area is divided into three zones: the **unrestricted zone,** where street clothes are allowed; the **semirestricted zone,** where attire consists of scrub clothes and caps; and the **restricted zone,** where scrub clothes, shoe covers, caps, and masks are worn. The surgeons and other surgical team members wear additional sterile clothing and protective devices during surgery.

The AORN recommends specific practices for personnel wearing surgical attire to promote a high level of cleanliness in a particular practice setting (AORN, 2014). OR attire includes close-fitting cotton dresses, pantsuits, jumpsuits, gowns, and jackets. Knitted cuffs on sleeves prevent organisms from shedding and being released into the immediate surroundings. Shirts and waist drawstrings should be tucked inside the pants to prevent accidental contact with sterile areas and to contain skin shedding. Wet or soiled garments should be changed.

Masks are worn at all times in the restricted zone of the OR. High-filtration masks decrease the risk of postoperative wound infection by containing and filtering microorganisms from the oropharynx and nasopharynx. Masks should fit tightly; should cover the nose and mouth completely; and should not interfere with breathing, speech, or vision. Masks must be adjusted to prevent venting from the sides. Disposable masks have a filtration efficiency exceeding 95%. Masks are changed between patients and should not be worn outside the surgical department. The mask must be either on or off; it must not be allowed to hang around the neck.

Headgear should completely cover the hair (head and neckline, including beard) so that hair, bobby pins, clips, and particles of dandruff or dust do not fall on the sterile field.

Shoes designated for use inside the OR (not worn home) should be comfortable and supportive. Shoe covers are used when spills or splashes are anticipated. If worn, the covers should be changed whenever they become wet, torn, or soiled (AORN 2014; Rothrock, 2014).

Barriers such as scrub attire and masks do not entirely protect the patient from microorganisms. Upper respiratory tract infections, sore throats, and skin infections in staff and patients are sources of pathogens and must be reported.

Because artificial fingernails harbor microorganisms and can cause nosocomial infections, a ban on artificial nails by OR personnel is supported by the Centers for Disease Control and Prevention (CDC), AORN, and the Association for Professionals in Infection Control and Epidemiology (APIC). Research provides support for policies prohibiting artificial nails for health care workers (AORN, 2014). Short, natural fingernails are encouraged.

Principles of Surgical Asepsis

Surgical asepsis prevents the contamination of surgical wounds. The patient's natural skin flora or a previously existing infection may cause postoperative wound infection. Rigorous adherence to the principles of surgical asepsis by OR personnel is basic to preventing surgical site infections.

All surgical supplies, instruments, needles, sutures, dressings, gloves, covers, and solutions that may come in contact with the surgical wound or exposed tissues must be sterilized before use (Rothrock, 2014). Traditionally, the surgeon, surgical assistants, and nurses prepared themselves by scrubbing their hands and arms with antiseptic soap and water; however, this practice is being challenged by research investigating the optimal length of time to scrub and the best preparation to use. In some institutions, various alcohol-based products or scrub less soaps are used to prepare the patient for surgery (Rothrock, 2014) but are only effective when no gross contaminants are present.

Surgical team members wear long-sleeved, sterile gowns and gloves. Head and hair are covered with a cap, and a mask is worn over the nose and mouth to minimize the possibility that bacteria from the upper respiratory tract will enter the wound.

During surgery, only personnel who have scrubbed, gloved, and gowned touch sterilized objects. Nonscrubbed personnel refrain from touching or contaminating anything sterile.

An area of the patient's skin larger than that requiring exposure during the surgery is meticulously cleansed, and an antiseptic solution is applied (Rothrock, 2014). If hair removal needs to take place and this was unable to be performed before the patient arrived in the OR suite, this is done immediately before the procedure with electric clippers (not shaved) to minimize the risk of infection (AORN, 2014). The remainder of the patient's body is covered with sterile drapes.

Environmental Controls

In addition to the protocols described previously, surgical asepsis requires meticulous cleaning and maintenance of the OR environment. Floors and horizontal surfaces are cleaned between cases with detergent, soap, and water or a detergent-germicide. Sterilized equipment is inspected regularly to ensure optimal operation and performance.

All equipment that comes into direct contact with the patient must be sterile. Sterilized linens, drapes, and solutions are used. Instruments are cleaned and sterilized in a unit near the OR. Individually wrapped sterile items are used when additional individual items are needed.

Airborne bacteria are a concern. To decrease the amount of bacteria in the air, standard OR ventilation provides 15 air exchanges per hour, at least 3 of which are fresh air (AORN, 2014; Rothrock, 2014). A room temperature of 20°C to 24°C (68°F to 73°F), humidity between 30% and 60%, and positive pressure relative to adjacent areas are maintained. Staff members shed skin scales, resulting in about 1000 bacteria-carrying particles (or colony-forming units [CFUs]) per cubic foot per minute. With the standard air exchanges, air counts of bacteria are reduced to 50 to 150 CFUs per cubic foot per minute. Systems with high-efficiency particulate air (HEPA) filters are needed to remove particles larger than 0.3 µm (Rothrock, 2014). Unnecessary personnel and physical movement may be restricted to minimize bacteria in the air and achieve an OR infection rate no greater than 3% to 5% in clean, infection-prone surgery.

Some ORs have laminar airflow units. These units provide 400 to 500 air exchanges per hour (Rothrock, 2014). When used appropriately, laminar airflow units result in fewer than 10 CFUs per cubic foot per minute during surgery. The goal for a laminar airflow–equipped OR is an infection rate of less than 1%. An OR equipped with a laminar airflow unit is frequently used for total joint replacement or organ transplant surgery.

Even using all precautions, wound contamination may inadvertently occur. Constant surveillance and conscientious technique in carrying out aseptic practices are necessary to reduce the risk of contamination and infection.

Basic Guidelines for Maintaining Surgical Asepsis

All practitioners involved in the intraoperative phase have a responsibility to provide and maintain a safe environment. Adherence to aseptic practice is part of this responsibility. The basic principles of aseptic technique follow (AORN, 2014):

- All materials in contact with the surgical wound or used within the sterile field must be sterile. Sterile surfaces or articles may touch other sterile surfaces or articles

Figure 18-2 • Proper draping exposes only the surgical site, which decreases the risk of infection.

and remain sterile; contact with unsterile objects at any point renders a sterile area contaminated.

- Gowns of the surgical team are considered sterile in front from the chest to the level of the sterile field. The sleeves are also considered sterile from 2 in above the elbow to the stockinette cuff.
- Sterile drapes are used to create a sterile field (see Fig. 18-2). Only the top surface of a draped table is considered sterile. During draping of a table or patient, the sterile drape is held well above the surface to be covered and is positioned from front to back.
- Items are dispensed to a sterile field by methods that preserve the sterility of the items and the integrity of the sterile field. After a sterile package is opened, the edges are considered unsterile. Sterile supplies, including solutions, are delivered to a sterile field or handed to a scrubbed person in such a way that the sterility of the object or fluid remains intact.
- The movements of the surgical team are from sterile to sterile areas and from unsterile to unsterile areas. Scrubbed people and sterile items contact only sterile areas; circulating nurses and unsterile items contact only unsterile areas.
- Movement around a sterile field must not cause contamination of the field. Sterile areas must be kept in view during movement around the area. At least a 1-ft distance from the sterile field must be maintained to prevent inadvertent contamination.
- Whenever a sterile barrier is breached, the area must be considered contaminated. A tear or puncture of the drape permitting access to an unsterile surface underneath renders the area unsterile. Such a drape must be replaced.
- Every sterile field is constantly monitored and maintained. Items of doubtful sterility are considered unsterile. Sterile fields are prepared as close as possible to the time of use.
- The routine administration of hyperoxia (high levels of oxygen) is *not* recommended to reduce surgical site infections.

Robotics

Robot-assisted technology is increasingly part of the intraoperative environment for cardiac, colorectal, general, gynecologic,

head and neck, thoracic, and urologic surgeries (Finkelstein, Rabino, Mashiach, et al., 2014). Several types of robotic-driven tools assist in making surgery more precise and less invasive for patients. All practitioners have a responsibility to be knowledgeable about equipment as well as related policies and procedures for its safe use.

Health Hazards Associated With the Surgical Environment

Faulty equipment, improper use of equipment, exposure to toxic substances, surgical plume (smoke generated by electrosurgical cautery), as well as infectious waste, cuts, needle stick injuries, and lasers are some of the associated hazards in the surgical environment (Rothrock, 2014). Internal monitoring of the OR includes the analysis of surface swipe samples and air samples for infectious and toxic agents. In addition, policies and procedures for minimizing exposure to body fluids and reducing the dangers associated with lasers and radiation are identified in AORN standards (AORN, 2014).

Regardless of the size or location of an incision, unintentional retention of an object (e.g., sponge, instrument) can occur. A retained object can cause wound infection or disruption, an abscess can form, and fistulas may develop between organs (Rothrock, 2014).

Laser Risks

The AORN has recommended practices for laser safety (AORN, 2014). When lasers are in use, warning signs must be clearly posted to alert personnel. Safety precautions are implemented to reduce the possibility of exposing the eyes and skin to laser beams, to prevent inhalation of the laser plume (smoke and particulate matter), and to protect the patient and personnel from the risk of surgical fire and electrical hazards (Guglielmi, 2014; Norton, Gorgone, & Belanger, 2014). Several types of lasers are available for clinical use; perioperative personnel should be familiar with the unique features, specific operation, and safety measures for each type of laser used in the practice setting and wear appropriate laser goggles for the type of laser beam in use. Registered nurses trained and certified in laser safety maintain the established standards in the OR (AORN, 2014).

Smoke evacuators are used in some procedures to remove the laser plume from the operative field. In recent years, this technology has been extended to all surgical cases to protect the surgical team from the potential hazards associated with the generalized smoke plume generated by standard electric cautery units.

Exposure to Blood and Body Fluids

OR attire has changed dramatically since the advent of acquired immune deficiency syndrome (AIDS). Double-gloving is routine in trauma and other types of surgery where sharp bone fragments are present. In addition to the routine scrub suit and double gloves, some surgical personnel wear rubber boots, a waterproof apron, and sleeve protectors. Goggles, or a wraparound face shield, are worn to protect against splashing when the surgical wound is irrigated or when bone drilling is performed. In hospitals where numerous total joint procedures are performed, a complete bubble mask may be used. This mask provides full-barrier protection from bone fragments and splashes. Ventilation is accomplished through an accompanying hood with a separate air filtration system.

The Surgical Experience

During the surgical procedure, the patient will need sedation, anesthesia, or some combination of these. There are many low-risk anesthesia agents to choose from.

Types of Anesthesia and Sedation

Research estimates anesthesia-related death rates in the United States to be less than 1 per 10,000 surgeries (Barash et al., 2013). For the patient, the anesthesia experience consists of having an IV line inserted, if it was not inserted earlier; receiving a sedating agent prior to induction with an anesthetic agent; losing consciousness; being intubated, if indicated; and then receiving a combination of anesthetic agents. Typically, the experience is a smooth one, and the patient has no recall of the events. The main types of anesthesia are general anesthesia (inhalation, IV), regional anesthesia (epidural, spinal, and local conduction blocks), moderate sedation (monitored anesthesia care [MAC]), and local anesthesia.

General Anesthesia

Anesthesia is a state of narcosis (severe central nervous system depression produced by pharmacologic agents), analgesia, relaxation, and reflex loss. Patients under general anesthesia are not arousable, not even to painful stimuli. They lose the ability to maintain ventilatory function and require assistance in maintaining a patent airway. Cardiovascular function may be impaired as well.

The Joint Commission has issued an alert regarding the phenomenon of patients being partially awake while under general anesthesia (referred to as anesthesia awareness). Patients at greatest risk of anesthesia awareness are cardiac, obstetric, and major trauma patients. The entire surgical team must be aware of this phenomenon and help prevent or manage it (Joint Commission, 2011).

General anesthesia consists of four stages, each associated with specific clinical manifestations (Rothrock, 2014). Understanding of these stages is necessary for nurses because of the emotional support that the patient might need as anesthesia progresses. These stages occur in reverse as the patient wakes up at the end of surgery, so the nurse must be aware of the need for appropriate patient support.

- *Stage I: beginning anesthesia.* Dizziness and a feeling of detachment may be experienced during induction. The patient may have a ringing, roaring, or buzzing in the ears and, although still conscious, may sense an inability to move the extremities easily. These sensations can result in agitation. During this stage, noises are exaggerated; even low voices or minor sounds seem loud and unreal. For these reasons, unnecessary noises and motions are avoided when anesthesia begins.
- *Stage II: excitement.* The excitement stage, characterized variously by struggling, shouting, talking, singing, laughing, or crying, is often avoided if IV anesthetic agents are given smoothly and quickly. The pupils dilate, but they constrict if exposed to light; the pulse rate is rapid, and respirations may be irregular. Because of the possibility

of uncontrolled movements of the patient during this stage, the anesthesiologist or CRNA must always be assisted by someone ready to help restrain the patient or to apply cricoid pressure in the case of vomiting to prevent aspiration. Manipulation increases circulation to the operative site and thereby increases the potential for bleeding.
- *Stage III: surgical anesthesia.* Surgical anesthesia is reached by administration of anesthetic vapor or gas and supported by IV agents as necessary. The patient is unconscious and lies quietly on the table. The pupils are small but constrict when exposed to light. Respirations are regular, the pulse rate and volume are normal, and the skin is pink or slightly flushed. With proper administration of the anesthetic agent, this stage may be maintained for hours in one of several planes, ranging from light (1) to deep (4), depending on the depth of anesthesia needed.
- *Stage IV: medullary depression.* This stage is reached if too much anesthesia has been given. Respirations become shallow, the pulse is weak and thready, and the pupils become widely dilated and no longer constrict when exposed to light. Cyanosis develops and, without prompt intervention, death rapidly follows. If this stage develops, the anesthetic agent is discontinued immediately and respiratory and circulatory support is initiated to prevent death. Stimulants, although rarely used, may be given; narcotic antagonists can be used if the overdose is due to opioids. It is not a planned stage of surgical anesthesia.

When opioid agents (narcotics) and neuromuscular blockers (relaxants) are given, several of the stages are absent. During smooth administration of an anesthetic agent, there is no sharp division between stages. The patient passes gradually from one stage to another, and it is through close observation of the signs exhibited by the patient that an anesthesiologist or CRNA controls the situation. The responses of the pupils, the blood pressure, and the respiratory and cardiac rates are among the most reliable guides to the patient's condition.

Anesthetic medications produce anesthesia because they are delivered to the brain at a high partial pressure that enables them to cross the blood–brain barrier. Relatively large amounts of anesthetic medication must be given during induction and the early maintenance phases because the anesthetic agent is recirculated and deposited in body tissues. As these sites become saturated, smaller amounts of the anesthetic agent are required to maintain anesthesia because equilibrium or near-equilibrium has been achieved between brain, blood, and other tissues. When possible, the anesthesia induction (initiation) begins with IV anesthesia and is then maintained at the desired stage by inhalation methods, achieving a smooth transition and eliminating the obvious stages of anesthesia (see Table 18-1). All are given in combination with oxygen and usually nitrous oxide as well.

Any condition that diminishes peripheral blood flow, such as vasoconstriction or shock, may reduce the amount of anesthetic medication required. Conversely, when peripheral blood flow is unusually high, as in a muscularly active or apprehensive patient, induction is slower, and greater quantities of anesthetic agents are required because the brain receives a smaller quantity of anesthetic agent.

TABLE 18-1 Inhalation Anesthetic Agents

Agent	Administration	Advantages	Disadvantages	Implications/Considerations
Volatile Liquids				
Halothane (Fluothane)	Inhalation; special vaporizer	Not explosive or flammable Induction rapid and smooth Useful in almost every type of surgery Low incidence of postoperative nausea and vomiting	Requires skillful administration to prevent overdose May cause liver damage May produce hypotension Requires special vaporizer for administration	In addition to observation of pulse and respiration postoperatively, blood pressure must be monitored frequently
Enflurane (Ethrane)	Inhalation	Rapid induction and recovery Potent analgesic agent Not explosive or flammable	Respiratory depression may develop rapidly, along with electrocardiogram abnormalities Not compatible with epinephrine	Observe for possible respiratory depression. Administration with epinephrine may cause ventricular fibrillation
Isoflurane (Forane)	Inhalation	Rapid induction and recovery Muscle relaxants are markedly potentiated	A profound respiratory depressant	Monitor respirations closely, support when necessary, and monitor for malignant hyperthermia
Sevoflurane[a] (Ultane)	Inhalation	Rapid induction and excretion; minimal side effects	Coughing and laryngospasm; trigger for malignant hyperthermia	Monitor for malignant hyperthermia
Desflurane (Suprane)	Inhalation	Rapid induction and emergence; rare organ toxicity	Respiratory irritation; trigger for malignant hyperthermia	Monitor for malignant hyperthermia and dysrhythmias
Gases				
Nitrous oxide (N$_2$O)	Inhalation (semiclosed method)	Induction and recovery rapid Nonflammable Useful with oxygen for short procedures Useful with other agents for all types of surgery	Poor relaxant Weak anesthetic May produce hypoxia	Most useful in conjunction with other agents with longer action Monitor for chest pain, nausea and vomiting, hypertension, and stroke
Oxygen (O$_2$)	Inhalation	Can increase O$_2$ available to tissues	High concentrations are hazardous	Increased fire risk when used with lasers

[a]Currently most popular choice.

Adapted from Association of PeriOperative Registered Nurses (AORN). (2014). *Association of PeriOperative Registered Nurses (AORN) standards, recommended practice, and guidelines*. Denver, CO: Author.

Inhalation

Inhaled anesthetic agents include volatile liquid agents and gases. Volatile liquid anesthetic agents produce anesthesia when their vapors are inhaled. Some commonly used inhalation agents are included in Table 18-1. All are given in combination with oxygen and usually nitrous oxide as well.

Gas anesthetic agents are given by inhalation and are always combined with oxygen. Nitrous oxide is the most commonly used gas anesthetic agent. When inhaled, the anesthetic agents enter the blood through the pulmonary capillaries and act on cerebral centers to produce loss of consciousness and sensation. When anesthetic administration is discontinued, the vapor or gas is eliminated through the lungs.

The vapor from inhalation anesthetic agents can be given to the patient by several methods. The inhalation anesthetic agent may be given through an LMA—a flexible tube with an inflatable silicone ring and cuff that can be inserted into the larynx (see Fig. 18-3A). The endotracheal technique for administering anesthetic medications consists of introducing a soft rubber or plastic ETT into the trachea, usually by means of a laryngoscope. The ETT may be inserted through either the nose (see Fig. 18-3B) or mouth (see Fig. 18-3C). When in place, the tube seals off the lungs from the esophagus so that if the patient vomits, stomach contents do not enter the lungs.

Intravenous Administration

General anesthesia can also be produced by the IV administration of various anesthetic and analgesic agents, such as barbiturates, benzodiazepines, nonbarbiturate hypnotics, dissociative agents, and opioid agents. Table 18-2 lists commonly used IV anesthetic and analgesic agents, including IV medications used as muscle relaxants in the intraoperative period. These medications may be given to induce or maintain anesthesia. Although they are often used in combination with inhalation anesthetic agents, they may be used alone. They may also be used to produce moderate sedation, as discussed later in this chapter.

An advantage of IV anesthesia is that the onset of anesthesia is pleasant; there is none of the buzzing, roaring, or dizziness known to follow administration of an inhalation anesthetic agent. The duration of action is brief, and the patient awakens with little nausea or vomiting.

The IV anesthetic agents are nonexplosive, require little equipment, and are easy to administer. The low incidence of postoperative nausea and vomiting makes the method useful in eye surgery, because in this setting vomiting would increase intraocular pressure and endanger vision in the operated eye. IV anesthesia is useful for short procedures but is used less often for the longer procedures of abdominal surgery. It is not indicated for those who require intubation because of their

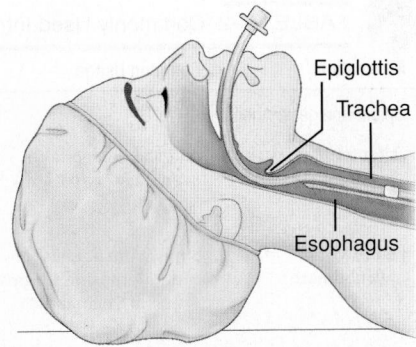

A. Laryngeal Mask Airway (LMA)   **B.** Intranasal intubation   **C.** Oral intubation

Figure 18-3 • Anesthetic delivery methods. **A.** Laryngeal mask airway (LMA). **B.** Nasal endotracheal catheter used when oral access will be required by the surgeon (in position with cuff inflated). **C.** Oral endotracheal intubation (tube is in position with cuff inflated).

susceptibility to respiratory obstruction. The combination of IV and inhaled anesthetic agents produces an effective and smooth experience for the patient, with a controlled emergence following surgery.

IV neuromuscular blockers (muscle relaxants) block the transmission of nerve impulses at the neuromuscular junction of skeletal muscles. Muscle relaxants are used to relax muscles in abdominal and thoracic surgery, relax eye muscles in certain types of eye surgery, facilitate endotracheal intubation, treat laryngospasm, and assist in mechanical ventilation.

Regional Anesthesia

In regional anesthesia, an anesthetic agent is injected around nerves so that the region supplied by these nerves is anesthetized. The effect depends on the type of nerve involved. Motor fibers are the largest fibers and have the thickest myelin sheath. Sympathetic fibers are the smallest and have a minimal covering. Sensory fibers are intermediate. A local anesthetic agent blocks motor nerves least readily and sympathetic nerves most readily. An anesthetic agent is not considered metabolized until all three systems (motor, sensory, and autonomic) are no longer affected.

The patient receiving regional anesthesia is awake and aware of their surroundings unless medications are given to produce mild sedation or to relieve anxiety. The health care team must avoid careless conversation, unnecessary noise, and unpleasant odors; these may be noticed by the patient in the OR and may contribute to a negative response to the surgical experience. A quiet environment is therapeutic. The diagnosis must not be stated aloud if the patient is not to know it at this time.

Epidural Anesthesia

Epidural anesthesia is achieved by injecting a local anesthetic agent into the epidural space that surrounds the dura mater of the spinal cord (see Fig. 18-4). The given medication diffuses across the layers of the spinal cord to provide anesthesia and pain relief (AORN, 2014; ASPAN, 2015). In contrast, spinal anesthesia involves injection through the dura mater into the subarachnoid space surrounding the spinal cord. Epidural anesthesia blocks sensory, motor, and autonomic functions; it differs from spinal anesthesia by the site of the injection and

the amount of anesthetic agent used. Epidural doses are much higher because the epidural anesthetic agent does not make direct contact with the spinal cord or nerve roots (AORN, 2014; ASPAN, 2015).

An advantage of epidural anesthesia is the absence of headache that can result from spinal anesthesia. A disadvantage is the greater technical challenge of introducing the anesthetic agent into the epidural space rather than the subarachnoid space. If inadvertent puncture of the dura occurs during epidural anesthesia and the anesthetic agent travels toward the head, high spinal anesthesia can result; this can produce severe hypotension and respiratory depression and arrest. Treatment of these complications includes airway support, IV fluids, and the use of vasopressors.

Spinal Anesthesia

Spinal anesthesia is an extensive conduction nerve block that is produced when a local anesthetic agent is introduced into the subarachnoid space at the lumbar level, usually between L4 and L5 (see Fig. 18-4). It produces anesthesia of the lower extremities, perineum, and lower abdomen. For the lumbar puncture procedure, the patient usually lies on the side in a knee–chest position. Sterile technique is used as a spinal puncture is made and the medication is injected through the needle. As soon as the injection has been made, the patient is positioned on their back. If a relatively high level of block is sought, the head and shoulders are lowered.

The spread of the anesthetic agent and the level of anesthesia depend on the amount of agent injected, the speed with which it is injected, the positioning of the patient after the injection, and the specific gravity of the agent. If the specific gravity is greater than that of cerebrospinal fluid (CSF), the agent moves to the dependent position of the subarachnoid space. If the specific gravity is less than that of CSF, the anesthetic agent moves away from the dependent position. The anesthesiologist or CRNA controls the administration of the agent. Table 18-3 presents selected regional anesthesia agents.

A few minutes after induction of a spinal anesthetic agent, anesthesia and paralysis affect the toes and perineum and then gradually the legs and abdomen. Nausea, vomiting, and pain may occur during surgery when spinal anesthesia is used.

TABLE 18-2 Commonly Used Intravenous Medications

Medication	Common Usage	Advantages	Disadvantages	Comments
Opioid Analgesic Agents				
Alfentanil (Alfenta)	Surgical analgesia in ambulatory patients	Ultra–short-acting (5–10 min) analgesic agent; duration of action 0.5 h; bolus or infusion	—	Potency: 750 µg; half-life 1.6 h
Fentanyl (Sublimaze)	Surgical analgesia: epidural infusion for postoperative analgesia; add to SAB	Good cardiovascular stability; duration of action 0.5 h	May cause muscle or chest wall rigidity	Most commonly used opioid; potency: 100 µg = 10 mg morphine sulfate; elimination half-life 3.6 h
Morphine sulfate (MS-Contin)	Preoperative pain; premedication; postoperative pain	Inexpensive; duration of action 4–5 h; euphoria; good cardiovascular stability	Nausea and vomiting; histamine release; postural ↓ BP and ↓ SVR	Epidural and intrathecal administration for postoperative pain; elimination half-life 3 h
Remifentanil (Ultiva)	IV infusion for surgical analgesia; small boluses for brief, intense pain	Easily titrated; very short duration; good cardiovascular stability. Ultiva is rapidly metabolized by hydrolysis of the propanoic acid–methyl ester linkage by nonspecific blood and tissue esterases.	Expensive; requires mixing; may cause muscle rigidity	Potency: 25 µg = 10 mg morphine sulfate; 20–30 times potency of alfentanil; elimination half-life 3–10 min
Sufentanil (Sufenta)	Surgical analgesia	Duration of action 0.5 h; prolonged analgesia exceptionally potent (5–10 times more than fentanyl); provides good stability in cardiovascular surgery	Prolonged respiratory depression	Potency: 15 µg = 10 mg morphine sulfate; elimination half-life 2.7 h
Depolarizing Muscle Relaxants				
Succinylcholine	Relax skeletal muscles for surgery and orthopedic manipulations; short procedures; intubation	Short duration; rapid onset	No known effect on consciousness, pain threshold, or cerebration; fasciculations, postoperative myalgias, dysrhythmias; raises serum K⁺ in tissue trauma, muscular disease, paralysis, burns; histamine release is slight; requires refrigeration	Prolonged muscle relaxation with serum cholinesterase deficiency and some antibiotics; may trigger malignant hyperthermia
Nondepolarizing Muscle Relaxants—Intermediate Onset and Duration				
Atracurium besylate (Tracrium)	Intubation; maintenance of skeletal muscle relaxation	No significant cardiovascular or cumulative effects; good with kidney injury	Requires refrigeration; slight histamine release; pregnancy risk category C; do not mix with lactated Ringer's solution or alkaline solutions such as barbiturates	Rapid IV bolus; use cautiously with geriatric and debilitated patients
Cisatracurium besylate (Nimbex)	Intubation; maintenance of skeletal muscle relaxation	Similar to atracurium	No histamine release	Similar to atracurium
Mivacurium (Mivacron)	Intubation; maintenance of skeletal muscle relaxation	Short acting; rapid metabolism by plasma cholinesterase; used as bolus or infusion	Expensive in longer cases	Competes with acetylcholine for receptor sites at the motor end plate, blocking neuromuscular transmission; new; rarely need to reverse; prolonged effect with plasma cholinesterase deficiency
Rocuronium (Zemuron)	Intubation; maintenance of relaxation	Rapid onset (dose dependent); elimination via kidney and liver	No known effect on consciousness, pain threshold, or cerebration; vagolytic; may ↑ HR	Duration similar to atracurium and vecuronium
Vecuronium (Norcuron)	Intubation; maintenance of relaxation	No significant cardiovascular or cumulative effects; no histamine release	Requires mixing	Mostly eliminated in bile, some in urine

TABLE 18-2 Commonly Used Intravenous Medications (continued)

Medication	Common Usage	Advantages	Disadvantages	Comments
Nondepolarizing Muscle Relaxants—Longer Onset and Duration				
d-Tubocurarine	Adjunct to anesthesia; maintenance of relaxation	—	No known effect on consciousness, pain threshold, or cerebration; might cause histamine release and transient ganglionic blockade	Mostly used for pretreatment with succinylcholine
Metocurine (Metubine)	Maintenance of relaxation	Good cardiovascular stability	Slight histamine release	Most commonly used opioid; potency: 100 μg = 10 mg morphine sulfate; elimination half-life 3.6 h
Pancuronium (Pavulon)	Maintenance of relaxation	—	May cause ↑ HR and ↑ BP	Used intrathecally and epidurally for postoperative pain; elimination half-life 3 h
Intravenous Anesthetic Agents				
Diazepam (Valium, Dizac)	Amnesia; hypnotic; relieves anxiety; preoperative	Good sedation	Long acting	Residual effects for 20–90 h; increased effect with alcohol
Etomidate (Amidate)	Induction of general anesthesia; indicated to supplement low-potency anesthetic agents	Short-acting hypnotic; good cardiovascular stability; fast, smooth induction and recovery	May cause brief period of apnea; pain with injection and myotonic movements	—
Ketamine (Ketalar)	Induction; occasional maintenance (IV or IM)	Short acting; profound analgesia; patient maintains airway; good in small children and burn patients	Large doses may cause hallucinations and respiratory depression; chest wall rigidity; laryngeal spasm	Need darkened, quiet room for recovery; often used in trauma cases
Midazolam (Versed)	Hypnotic; anxiolytic; sedation; often used as adjunct to induction	Excellent amnesia; water soluble (no pain with IV injection); short acting	Slower induction than thiopental	Often used for amnesia with insertion of invasive monitors or regional anesthesia; depresses all levels of CNS, including limbic and reticular formation, probably through increased action of GABA, which is major inhibitory neurotransmitter in brain
Propofol (Diprivan)	Induction and maintenance; sedation with regional anesthesia or MAC	Rapid onset; awakening in 4–8 min; produces sedation/hypnosis rapidly (within 40 s) and smoothly with minimal excitation; decreases intraocular pressure and systemic vascular resistance; rarely is associated with malignant hyperthermia and histamine release	May cause pain when injected; suppresses cardiac output and respiratory drive	Short elimination half-life (34–64 min)
Methohexital sodium (Brevital)	Induction; methohexital slows the activity of brain and nervous system	Ultra–short-acting barbiturate	May cause hiccups	Can be given rectally
Thiopental sodium (Pentothal)	Induction; stops seizures	—	May cause laryngospasm	Large doses may cause apnea and cardiovascular depression; can be given rectally

SAB, subarachnoid block; BP, blood pressure; SVR, stroke volume ratio; IV, intravenous; K⁺, potassium; HR, heart rate; IM, intramuscular; CNS, central nervous system; GABA, gamma-aminobutyric acid; MAC, monitored anesthesia care.

Adapted from Association of PeriOperative Registered Nurses (AORN). (2014). *Association of PeriOperative Registered Nurses (AORN) standards, recommended practice, and guidelines.* Denver, CO: Author; Spruce, L. (2015). Back to basics: Procedural sedation. *AORN Journal, 101*(3), 345–353.

Comerford, K. C. (2015). *Nursing 2015 drug handbook.* Philadelphia, PA: Wolters Kluwer.

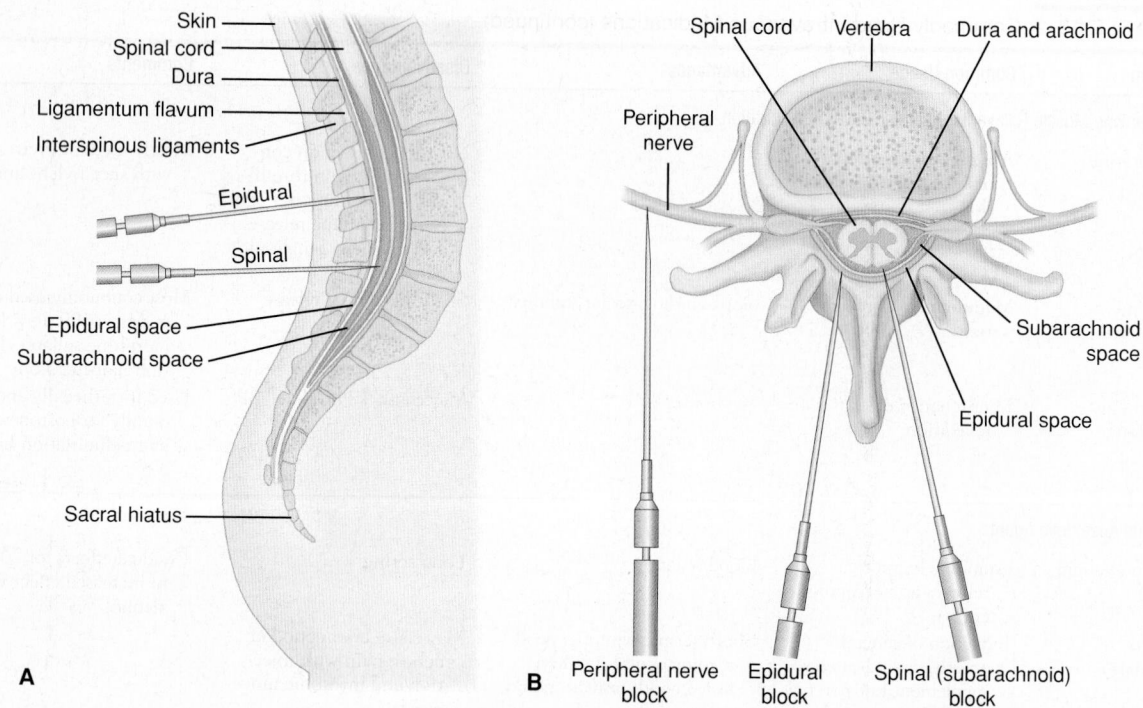

Figure 18-4 • A. Injection sites for spinal and epidural anesthesia. **B.** Cross-section of injection sites for peripheral nerve, epidural, and spinal blocks.

Headache may be an aftereffect of spinal anesthesia. Several factors are related to the incidence of headache: the size of the spinal needle used, the leakage of fluid from the subarachnoid space through the puncture site, and the patient's hydration status. Measures that increase cerebrospinal pressure are helpful in relieving headache. These include maintaining a quiet environment, keeping the patient lying flat, and keeping the patient well hydrated.

In continuous spinal anesthesia, the tip of a plastic catheter remains in the subarachnoid space during the surgical procedure so that more anesthetic medication may be injected as needed. This technique allows greater control of the dosage; however, there is greater potential for postanesthetic headache because of the large-gauge needle used.

Local Conduction Blocks

Examples of common local conduction blocks include:
- Brachial plexus block, which produces anesthesia of the arm
- Paravertebral anesthesia, which produces anesthesia of the nerves supplying the chest, abdominal wall, and extremities
- Transsacral (caudal) block, which produces anesthesia of the perineum and, occasionally, the lower abdomen

Moderate Sedation

Moderate sedation, previously referred to as conscious sedation, is a form of anesthesia that involves the IV administration of sedatives or analgesic medications to reduce patient

TABLE 18-3 Selected Regional and Local Anesthetic Agents

Agent	Administration	Advantages	Disadvantages	Implications/Considerations
Lidocaine (Xylocaine)	Epidural, spinal, peripheral IV anesthesia, and local infiltration	Rapid Longer duration of action (compared with procaine) Free of local irritative effect	Occasional allergic reaction	Useful topically for cystoscopy Observe for untoward reactions—drowsiness, depressed respiration, seizures
Bupivacaine (Marcaine, Sensorcaine)	Epidural, spinal, peripheral IV anesthesia, and local infiltration	Duration is 2–3 times longer than lidocaine	Use cautiously in patients with known drug allergies or sensitivities.	A period of analgesia persists after return of sensation; therefore, the need for strong analgesic agents is reduced Greater potency and longer action than lidocaine
Tetracaine (Pontocaine)	Topical, infiltration, and nerve block	Long acting, produces good relaxation	Occasional allergic reaction	>10 times as potent as procaine (Novocaine)
Procaine (Novocaine)	Local infiltration	—	Occasional allergic reaction	Commonly used in oral or dental surgery

IV, intravenous.

anxiety and control pain during diagnostic or therapeutic procedures. It is being used increasingly for specific short-term surgical procedures in hospitals and ambulatory care centers (Rothrock, 2014). The goal is to depress a patient's level of consciousness to a moderate level to enable surgical, diagnostic, or therapeutic procedures to be performed while ensuring the patient's comfort during and cooperation with the procedures. With moderate sedation, the patient is able to maintain a patent airway, retain protective airway reflexes, and respond to verbal and physical stimuli.

Moderate sedation can be given by an anesthesiologist, CRNA, or other specially trained and credentialed physician or nurse. The patient receiving moderate sedation is never left alone and is closely monitored by a physician or nurse who is knowledgeable and skilled in detecting dysrhythmias, administering oxygen, and performing resuscitation (Spruce, 2015). The continual assessment of the patient's vital signs, level of consciousness, and cardiac and respiratory function is an essential component of moderate sedation. Pulse oximetry, a continuous ECG monitor, and frequent measurement of vital signs are used to monitor the patient. Regulations for the use and administration of moderate sedation differ from state to state, and its administration is addressed by standards issued by the Joint Commission and by institutional policies and nursing specialty organizations, including the ASPAN, 2015 (Spruce, 2015).

Monitored Anesthesia Care

Monitored anesthesia care (MAC), also referred to as monitored sedation, is moderate sedation given by an anesthesiologist or CRNA who must be prepared and qualified to convert to general anesthesia if necessary. The skills of an anesthesiologist or CRNA may be necessary to manage the effects of a level of deeper sedation to return the patient to the appropriate level of sedation (Barash et al., 2013). MAC may be used for healthy patients undergoing relatively minor surgical procedures and for some critically ill patients who may be unable to tolerate anesthesia without extensive invasive monitoring and pharmacologic support (Rothrock, 2014).

Local Anesthesia

Local anesthesia is the injection of a solution containing the anesthetic agent into the tissues at the planned incision site. Often it is combined with a local regional block by injecting around the nerves immediately supplying the area. It is given directly to the surgical field, and the circulating nurse observes and monitors the patient for possible side effects (Bourdon, 2015). Advantages of local anesthesia are as follows:

- It is simple, economical, and nonexplosive.
- Equipment needed is minimal.
- Postoperative recovery is brief.
- Undesirable effects of general anesthesia are avoided.
- It is ideal for short and minor surgical procedures.

Local anesthesia is often given in combination with epinephrine. Epinephrine constricts blood vessels, which prevents rapid absorption of the anesthetic agent and thus prolongs its local action and prevents seizures. Selected local anesthetic agents are listed in Table 18-3; some of the same agents used in regional anesthesia are used as local anesthetic agents.

Local anesthesia is the preferred anesthetic method in any surgical procedure. However, contraindications include high preoperative levels of anxiety as the thought of surgery with local anesthesia may increase anxiety in some patients. For some surgical procedures, local anesthesia is impractical because of the number of injections and the amount of anesthetic medication that would be required (e.g., breast reconstruction) and might result in doses that would be toxic to the patient.

The skin is prepared as for any surgical procedure, and a small-gauge needle is used to inject a modest amount of the anesthetic medication into the skin layers. This produces blanching or a wheal. Additional anesthetic medication is then injected into the skin until an area the length of the proposed incision is anesthetized. A larger, longer needle then is used to infiltrate deeper tissues with the anesthetic agent. The action of the agent is almost immediate, so surgery may begin shortly after the injection is complete. The anesthetic may be mixed with a fast-acting analgesic of short duration to circumvent the burning felt when the longer-acting anesthetics are injected.

Potential Intraoperative Complications

The surgical patient is subject to several risks. Potential intraoperative complications include anesthesia awareness, nausea and vomiting, anaphylaxis, hypoxia, hypothermia, and malignant hyperthermia. The Surgical Care Improvement Project (SCIP) set a national goal to reduce surgical complications. Targeted areas include surgical site infections as well as cardiac, respiratory, and venous thromboembolic complications (Joint Commission, 2016).

Anesthesia Awareness

It is important to discuss concerns about intraoperative awareness with patients preoperatively so that they realize that only general anesthesia is meant to create a state of oblivion. All other forms of anesthesia will eliminate pain, but sensation of pushing and pulling tissues may still be recognized and they may hear conversations among the operative team. In many cases, patients may be able to respond to questions and involve themselves in the discussion. This is normal and is not what is referred to as anesthesia awareness.

Unintended intraoperative awareness refers to a patient becoming cognizant of surgical interventions while under general anesthesia and then recalling the incident. Neuromuscular blocks, sometimes required for surgical muscle relaxation, intensify the fear of the patient experiencing awareness because they are then unable to communicate during the episode. The frequency of anesthesia awareness is 0.1% to 0.2% of general anesthesia patients, equivalent to about 30,000 cases per year in the United States (Oster & Oster, 2015).

Indications of the occurrence of anesthesia awareness include an increase in the blood pressure, rapid heart rate, and patient movement. However, hemodynamic changes can be masked by paralytic medication, beta-blockers, and calcium channel blockers, thus the awareness may remain undetected. Premedication with amnesic agents and avoidance of muscle paralytics except when essential help to preclude its occurrence.

Nausea and Vomiting

Nausea and vomiting, or regurgitation, may affect patients during the intraoperative period. If gagging occurs, the patient is turned to the side, the head of the table is lowered, and a basin is provided to collect the vomitus. Suction is used to remove saliva and vomited gastric contents. The advent of new anesthetic agents has reduced the incidence; however, there is no single way to prevent nausea and vomiting. An interdisciplinary approach involving the surgeon, anesthesiologist or CRNA, and nurse is best (Crosson, 2015).

In some cases, the anesthesiologist or CRNA administers antiemetics preoperatively or intraoperatively to counteract possible aspiration. If the patient aspirates vomitus, an attack with severe bronchial spasms and wheezing is triggered. Pneumonitis and pulmonary edema can subsequently develop, leading to extreme hypoxia. Increasing medical attention is being paid to silent regurgitation of gastric contents (not related to preoperative fasting times), which occurs more frequently than previously realized. The volume and acidity of the aspirate determine the extent of damage to the lungs. Patients may be given citric acid and sodium citrate (Bicitra), a clear, nonparticulate antacid to increase gastric fluid pH or a histamine-2 (H_2) receptor antagonist such as cimetidine (Tagamet), ranitidine (Zantac), or famotidine (Pepcid) to decrease gastric acid production (Rothrock, 2014).

Anaphylaxis

Any time the patient comes into contact with a foreign substance, there is potential for an anaphylactic reaction. Because medications are the most common cause of anaphylaxis, intraoperative nurses must be aware of any patient allergies as well as the type and method of anesthesia used including specific agents (Bourdon, 2015). An anaphylactic reaction can occur in response to many medications, latex, or other substances. The reaction may be immediate or delayed. Anaphylaxis can be a life-threatening reaction.

Latex allergy—the sensitivity to natural rubber latex products—has become more prevalent, creating the need for alert responsiveness among health care professionals. The allergy exhibits with urticaria, asthma, rhinoconjunctivitis, and anaphylaxis (Australasian Society of Clinical Immunology and Allergy [ASCIA], 2015). If patients state that they have allergies to latex, even if they are wearing latex in their clothing, treatment must be latex free. In the OR, many products are latex free with the notable exception of softer latex catheters. Surgical cases should use latex-free gloves in anticipation of a possible allergy, and if no allergy is present, then personnel can switch to other gloves after the case starts if desired.

Fibrin sealants are used in various surgical procedures, and cyanoacrylate tissue adhesives are used to close wounds without the use of sutures. These sealants have been implicated in allergic reactions and anaphylaxis (Rothrock, 2014). Although these reactions are rare, the nurse must be alert to the possibility and observe the patient for changes in vital signs and symptoms of anaphylaxis when these products are used. (Chapters 14 and 37 provide more details about the signs, symptoms, and treatment of anaphylaxis and anaphylactic shock.)

Hypoxia and Other Respiratory Complications

Inadequate ventilation, occlusion of the airway, inadvertent intubation of the esophagus, and hypoxia are significant potential complications associated with general anesthesia. Many factors can contribute to inadequate ventilation. Respiratory depression caused by anesthetic agents, aspiration of respiratory tract secretions or vomitus, and the patient's position on the operating table can compromise the exchange of gases. Anatomic variation can make the trachea difficult to visualize and result in insertion of the artificial airway into the esophagus rather than into the trachea. In addition to these dangers, asphyxia caused by foreign bodies in the mouth; spasm of the vocal cords; relaxation of the tongue; or aspiration of vomitus, saliva, or blood can occur. Brain damage from hypoxia occurs within minutes; therefore, vigilant monitoring of the patient's oxygenation status is a primary function of the anesthesiologist or CRNA and the circulating nurse. Peripheral perfusion is checked frequently, and pulse oximetry values are monitored continuously.

Hypothermia

During anesthesia, the patient's temperature may fall. Glucose metabolism is reduced, and as a result, metabolic acidosis may develop. This condition is called *hypothermia* and is indicated by a core body temperature that is lower than normal (36.6°C [98°F] or less). Inadvertent hypothermia may occur as a result of a low temperature in the OR, infusion of cold fluids, inhalation of cold gases, open body wounds or cavities, decreased muscle activity, advanced age, or the pharmaceutical agents used (e.g., vasodilators, phenothiazines, general anesthetic medications). Hypothermia can depress neuronal activity and decrease cellular oxygen requirements below the minimum levels normally required for continued cell viability. As a result, it is used to protect function during some surgical procedures (e.g., carotid endarterectomy, cardiopulmonary bypass) (Barash et al., 2013).

Unintentional hypothermia needs to be avoided. If it occurs, it must be minimized or reversed. If hypothermia is intentional, the goal is safe return to normal body temperature. Environmental temperature in the OR can temporarily be set at 25°C to 26.6°C (78°F to 80°F). IV and irrigating fluids are warmed to 37°C (98.6°F). Wet gowns and drapes are removed promptly and replaced with dry materials, because wet materials promote heat loss. Warm air blankets and thermal blankets can also be used on the areas not exposed for surgery, and minimizing the area of the patient that is exposed will help maintain core temperature. Whatever methods are used to rewarm the patient, warming must be accomplished gradually, not rapidly. Conscientious monitoring of core temperature, urinary output, ECG, blood pressure, arterial blood gas levels, and serum electrolyte levels is required. There are many products on the market (i.e., blankets, forced air devices) used during perioperative care to maintain normothermia (Erdling & Johansson, 2015; Sobczak, 2014).

Malignant Hyperthermia

Malignant hyperthermia is a rare inherited muscle disorder that is chemically induced by anesthetic agents

(Rothrock, 2014). This disorder can be triggered by myopathies, emotional stress, heatstroke, neuroleptic malignant syndrome, strenuous exercise exertion, and trauma. It occurs in 1 in 50,000 to 100,000 adults. Mortality from malignant hyperthermia had been reported to be as high as 70%; however, with prompt recognition and rapid treatment, it has fallen to less than 10% (Isaak & Steigler, 2015). Susceptible people include those with strong and bulky muscles, a history of muscle cramps or muscle weakness and unexplained temperature elevation, and an unexplained death of a family member during surgery that was accompanied by a febrile response (Isaak & Steigler, 2015).

Pathophysiology

During anesthesia, potent agents such as inhalation anesthetic agents (i.e., halothane, enflurane, isoflurane) and muscle relaxants (succinylcholine) may trigger the symptoms of malignant hyperthermia (Rothrock, 2014). Stress and some medications, such as sympathomimetics (epinephrine), theophylline, aminophylline, anticholinergics (atropine), and cardiac glycosides (digitalis), can induce or intensify a reaction.

The pathophysiology of malignant hyperthermia is related to a hypermetabolic condition that involves altered mechanisms of calcium function in skeletal muscle cells. This disruption of calcium causes clinical symptoms of hypermetabolism, which in turn increases muscle contraction (rigidity) and causes hyperthermia and subsequent damage to the central nervous system.

Clinical Manifestations

The initial symptoms of malignant hyperthermia are often cardiovascular, respiratory, and abnormal musculoskeletal activity. Tachycardia (heart rate greater than 150 bpm) may be an early sign. Sympathetic nervous stimulation also leads to ventricular dysrhythmia, hypotension, decreased cardiac output, oliguria, and, later, cardiac arrest. Hypercapnia, an increase in carbon dioxide (CO_2), may be an early respiratory sign. With the abnormal transport of calcium, rigidity or tetanus-like movements occur, often in the jaw. Generalized muscle rigidity is one of the earliest signs. The rise in temperature is actually a late sign that develops rapidly; body temperature can increase 1°C to 2°C (2°F to 4°F) every 5 minutes, and core body temperature can exceed 42°C (107°F) (Rothrock, 2014).

Medical Management

Recognizing symptoms early and discontinuing anesthesia promptly are imperative (Isaak & Steigler, 2015). Goals of treatment are to decrease metabolism, reverse metabolic and respiratory acidosis, correct dysrhythmias, decrease body temperature, provide oxygen and nutrition to tissues, and correct electrolyte imbalance. The Malignant Hyperthermia Association of the United States (MHAUS) publishes a treatment protocol that should be posted in the OR and be readily available on a malignant hyperthermia cart (see Resource section).

Anesthesia and surgery should be postponed. However, if end-tidal CO_2 monitoring and dantrolene sodium (Dantrium) are available and the anesthesiologist is experienced in managing malignant hyperthermia, the surgery may continue using a different anesthetic agent (Barash et al., 2013). Although malignant hyperthermia usually manifests about 10 to 20 minutes after induction of anesthesia, it can also occur during the first 24 hours after surgery.

Nursing Management

Although malignant hyperthermia is uncommon, the nurse must identify patients at risk, recognize the signs and symptoms, have the appropriate medication and equipment available, and be knowledgeable about the protocol to follow. Preparation may be lifesaving for the patient.

NURSING PROCESS

The Patient During Surgery

Intraoperative nurses focus on nursing diagnoses, interventions, and outcomes that surgical patients and their families experience. Additional priorities include collaborative problems and expected goals.

Assessment

Nursing assessment of the intraoperative patient involves obtaining data from the patient and the patient's medical record to identify factors that can affect care. These serve as guidelines for an individualized plan of patient care. The intraoperative nurse uses the focused preoperative nursing assessment documented on the patient record. This includes assessment of physiologic status (e.g., health–illness level, level of consciousness), psychosocial status (e.g., anxiety level, verbal communication problems, coping mechanisms), physical status (e.g., surgical site, skin condition, and effectiveness of preparation; mobility of joints), and ethical concerns.

Diagnosis

NURSING DIAGNOSES

Based on the assessment data, major nursing diagnoses may include the following:

- Anxiety related to surgical or environmental concerns
- Risk of latex allergy response due to possible exposure to latex in OR environment
- Risk for perioperative positioning injury related to positioning in the OR
- Risk for injury related to anesthesia and surgical procedure
- Risk for compromised human dignity related to general anesthesia or sedation

COLLABORATIVE PROBLEMS/POTENTIAL COMPLICATIONS

Based on the assessment data, potential complications may include the following:

- Anesthesia awareness
- Nausea and vomiting
- Anaphylaxis
- Hypoxia
- Unintentional hypothermia
- Malignant hyperthermia
- Infection

Planning and Goals

The major goals for care of the patient during surgery include reduced anxiety, absence of latex exposure, absence of positioning injuries, freedom from injury, maintenance of the patient's dignity, and absence of complications.

Nursing Interventions

REDUCING ANXIETY

The OR environment can seem cold, stark, and frightening to the patient, who may be feeling isolated and apprehensive. Introducing yourself, addressing the patient by name warmly and frequently, verifying details, providing explanations, and encouraging and answering questions provide a sense of professionalism and friendliness that can help the patient feel safe and secure. When discussing what the patient can expect in surgery, the nurse uses basic communication skills, such as touch and eye contact, to reduce anxiety. Attention to physical comfort (warm blankets, padding, and position changes) helps the patient feel more comfortable. Telling the patient who else will be present in the OR, how long the procedure is expected to take, and other details helps the patient prepare for the experience and gain a sense of control.

The circulating nurse may assist to decrease anxiety during induction by using techniques such as guided imagery by talking about the patient's favorite place, or walking down a beach, or through a forest, in a soft voice and using eye contact, if culturally appropriate.

REDUCING LATEX EXPOSURE

Patients with latex allergies require early identification and communication to all personnel about the presence of the allergy according to standards of care for patients with latex allergy (AORN, 2014). In most ORs, there are few latex items currently in use, but because there still remain some instances of latex use, maintenance of latex allergy precautions throughout the perioperative period must be observed. For safety, manufacturers and hospital materials managers need to take responsibility for identifying the latex content in items used by patients and health care personnel. (See Chapters 17 and 37 for assessment for latex allergy.)

> ### ◀ Quality and Safety Nursing Alert
>
> *It is the responsibility of all nurses, and particularly perianesthesia and perioperative nurses, to be aware of latex allergies, necessary precautions, and products that are latex free. Hospital staff are also at risk for development of a latex allergy secondary to repeated exposure to latex products.*

PREVENTING PERIOPERATIVE POSITIONING INJURY

The patient's position on the operating table depends on the surgical procedure to be performed as well as the patient's physical condition (see Fig. 18-5). One type of injury, peripheral nerve injury, is defined as the interruption of electrical activity that affects either the sensory, motor, or both nerve functions resulting in a deficit. The incidence of this type of injury to upper and lower extremities has a widely reported range of 0.02% to 21% in surgical patients because of the absence of standardized methods to document injury (Bouyer-Ferullo, Androwitch, & Dykes, 2015). The potential for transient discomfort or permanent injury is present

because many surgical procedures require awkward anatomical positions. Hyperextending joints, compressing arteries, or pressing on nerves and bony prominences usually results in discomfort simply because the position must be sustained for a long period of time (Oster & Oster, 2015; Rothrock, 2014). Factors to consider include the following:

- The patient should be in as comfortable a position as possible, whether conscious or unconscious.
- The operative field must be adequately exposed.
- An awkward anatomical position, undue pressure on a body part, or the use of stirrups or traction should not obstruct the vascular supply.
- Respiration should not be impeded by pressure of arms on the chest or by a gown that constricts the neck or chest.
- Nerves must be protected from undue pressure. Improper positioning of the arms, hands, legs, or feet can cause serious injury or paralysis. Shoulder braces must be well padded to prevent irreparable nerve injury, especially when the Trendelenburg position is necessary.
- Precautions for patient safety must be observed, particularly with older adults, patients who are thin or obese, and those with a physical deformity.
- The patient may need light restraint before induction in case of excitement.

The usual position for surgery, called the *dorsal recumbent position,* is flat on the back. Both arms are positioned at the side of the table: one with the hand placed palm down and the other carefully positioned on an armboard to facilitate IV infusion of fluids, blood, or medications. This position is used for most abdominal surgeries, except for surgery of the gallbladder or pelvis (see Fig. 18-5A).

The Trendelenburg position usually is used for surgery on the lower abdomen and pelvis to obtain good exposure by displacing the intestines into the upper abdomen. In this position, the head and body are lowered. The patient is supported in position by padded shoulder braces (see Fig. 18-5B), bean bags, and foam padding. Reverse Trendelenburg position provides the space to operate on the upper abdomen by shifting the intestines into the pelvis. A padded footboard and other supportive cushioning preserve a safe environment for the patient.

The lithotomy position is used for nearly all perineal, rectal, and vaginal surgical procedures (see Fig. 18-5C). The patient is positioned on the back with the legs and thighs flexed. The position is maintained by placing the feet in stirrups.

The Sims or lateral position is used for renal surgery. The patient is placed on the nonoperative side with an air pillow 12.5 to 15 cm (5 to 6 in) thick under the loin, or on a table with a kidney or back lift (see Fig. 18-5D).

PROTECTING THE PATIENT FROM INJURY

Various activities are used to address the diverse patient safety issues that arise in the OR. The nurse protects the patient from injury by providing a safe environment. Verifying information, checking the medical record for completeness, and maintaining surgical asepsis and an optimal environment are critical nursing responsibilities. Verification that all the required documentation is completed is an important function of the intraoperative nurse. A surgical checklist is used prior to induction of anesthesia, before the skin incision is

A. Patient in position on the operating table for a laparotomy. Note the strap above the knees.

B. Patient in Trendelenburg position on operating table. Note padded shoulder braces in place. Be sure that brace does not press on brachial plexus.

C. Patient in lithotomy position. Note that the hips extend over the edge of the table.

D. Patient lies on unaffected side for kidney surgery. Table is spread apart to provide space between the lower ribs and the pelvis. The upper leg is extended; the lower leg is flexed at the knee and hip joints; a pillow is placed between the legs.

Figure 18-5 • Patient positions on the operating table. Captions call attention to safety and comfort features. All surgical patients wear caps to cover the hair completely.

made, and before the patient leaves the OR (see Fig. 18-1). It is important to review the patient's record for the following:

- Allergies (including latex)
- Correct informed surgical consent, with patient's signature
- Completed records for health history and physical examination
- Results of diagnostic studies

In addition to checking that all necessary patient data are complete, the perioperative nurse obtains the necessary equipment specific to the procedure. The need for nonroutine medications, blood components, instruments, and other equipment and supplies is assessed, and the readiness of the room, completeness of physical setup, and completeness of instrument, suture, and dressing setups are determined. Any aspects of the OR environment that may negatively affect the patient are identified. These include physical features, such as room temperature and humidity; electrical hazards; potential contaminants (dust, blood, and discharge on floor or surfaces; uncovered hair; nonsterile attire of personnel; jewelry worn by personnel; chipped or artificial fingernails); and unnecessary traffic. The circulating nurse also sets up and maintains suction equipment in working order, sets up invasive monitoring equipment, assists with insertion of vascular access and monitoring devices (arterial, pulmonary arterial, and central venous pressure; IV lines), and initiates appropriate physical comfort measures for the patient.

Preventing physical injury includes using safety straps and side rails and not leaving the sedated patient unattended. Transferring the patient from the stretcher to the OR table requires safe transferring practices. Other safety measures include properly positioning a grounding pad under the patient to prevent electrical burns and shock, removing excess antiseptic solution from the patient's skin, and promptly and completely draping exposed areas after the sterile field has been created to decrease the risk of hypothermia.

Nursing measures to prevent injury from excessive blood loss include blood conservation using equipment such as a cell saver (a device for recirculating the patient's own blood cells) and administration of blood products (Rothrock, 2014). Fewer patients undergoing an elective procedure require blood transfusion, but those undergoing high-risk procedures (such as orthopedic or cardiac surgeries) may require an intraoperative transfusion. The circulating nurse anticipates this need, checks that blood has been cross-matched and held in reserve, and is prepared to administer blood.

SERVING AS PATIENT ADVOCATE

The patient undergoing general anesthesia or moderate sedation experiences temporary sensory or perceptual alteration or loss, and has an increased need for protection and advocacy. Patient advocacy in the OR entails maintaining the patient's physical and emotional comfort, privacy, rights, and dignity. Patients, whether conscious or unconscious, should not be subjected to excess noise, inappropriate conversation, or, most of all, derogatory comments. Banter in the OR should not include comments about the patient's physical appearance, job, personal history, and so forth. Cases have been reported in which seemingly deeply anesthetized patients recalled the entire surgical experience, including disparaging personal remarks made by OR personnel. As an advocate, the nurse never engages in such conversation and discourages others from doing so. Other advocacy activities include minimizing the clinical, dehumanizing aspects of being a surgical patient by making sure that the patient is treated as a person, respecting cultural and spiritual values, providing physical privacy, and maintaining confidentiality.

MONITORING AND MANAGING POTENTIAL COMPLICATIONS

It is the responsibility of the surgeon and the anesthesiologist or CRNA to monitor and manage complications. However, intraoperative nurses also play an important role. Being alert to and reporting changes in vital signs, cardiac dysrhythmias, symptoms of nausea and vomiting, anaphylaxis, hypoxia, hypothermia, and malignant hyperthermia and assisting with their management are important nursing functions. Each of these complications was discussed earlier. Maintaining asepsis and preventing infection are responsibilities of all members of the surgical team (Rothrock, 2014). Evidence-based interventions to decrease surgical site infections include appropriate skin preparation and antibiotic administration. Using clippers to remove hair from the surgical site as needed instead of shaving the site is recommended (AORN, 2014).

Evaluation

Expected patient outcomes may include:

1. Exhibits low level of anxiety while awake during the intraoperative phase of care
2. Has no symptoms of latex allergy
3. Remains free of perioperative positioning injury
4. Experiences no unexpected threats to safety
5. Has dignity preserved throughout OR experience
6. Is free of complications (e.g., nausea and vomiting, anaphylaxis, hypoxia, hypothermia, malignant hyperthermia, or deep vein thrombosis) or experiences successful management of adverse effects of surgery and anesthesia should they occur

CRITICAL THINKING EXERCISES

1 **ebp** A 48-year-old man is scheduled to have robotic-assisted abdominal surgery under general anesthesia. Is there evidence that supports that his intraoperative positioning will have any effect on his vital signs? What is the best evidence for how his vital signs should be monitored? What are the best practices that the OR nurse should implement to support the patient and OR team during this minimally invasive surgery?

2 A 66-year-old woman with chronic obstructive pulmonary disease (COPD) is scheduled for an elective procedure on her face. She is having problems breathing, is agitated, and cannot lie flat on the surgical bed. What actions should the circulating nurse take to improve the patient's breathing and relieve her agitation? What complications may occur? What safety measures should be implemented?

3 **pq** Identify the priorities, assessments, and nursing interventions you would implement for a 76-year-old woman who is hard of hearing and is having spinal anesthesia for total knee replacement surgery. How would your priorities, approach, and techniques differ if the patient is having general anesthesia?

REFERENCES

*Asterisk indicates nursing research.

Books

American Society of PeriAnesthesia Nurses (ASPAN). (2015). *2015–2017 Perianesthesia nursing standards, practice recommendations and interpretive statements.* Cherry Hill, NJ: Author.

Association of PeriOperative Registered Nurses (AORN). (2014). *Association of PeriOperative Registered Nurses (AORN) standards, recommended practice, and guidelines.* Denver, CO: Author.

Barash, P. G., Cullen, B. F., Stoelting, R. K., et al. (2013). *Clinical anesthesia* (7th ed.). Philadelphia, PA: Lippincott Williams & Wilkins.

Comerford, K. C. (2015). *Nursing 2015 drug handbook.* Philadelphia, PA: Wolters Kluwer.

Meiner, S. E. (2014). *Gerontologic nursing* (5th ed.). St. Louis, MO: Elsevier Mosby.

Rothrock, J. C. (Ed.). (2014). *Alexander's care of the patient in surgery* (15th ed.). St. Louis, MO: Mosby.

Tabloski, P. A. (2013). *Gerontological nursing: The essential guide to clinical practice* (2nd ed.). Upper Saddle River, NJ: Prentice Hall Health.

Journals and Electronic Documents

Australasian Society of Clinical Immunology and Allergy. (2015). Latex allergy. Retrieved on 12/9/2015 at: www.allergy.org.au

Bourdon, L. (2015). Care of the patient receiving local anesthesia. *AORN Journal, 101*(3), 10–12.

Bouyer-Ferullo, S., Androwitch, I. M., & Dykes, P. C. (2015). Clinical decision support and perioperative peripheral nerve injury. *Computers Informatics Nursing, 33*(6), 238–248.

Crosson, J. A. (2015). Keeping patients safe: The importance of collaboration. *AORN Journal, 101*(2), 279–281.

*Erdling, A., & Johansson, A. (2015). Core temperature—The intraoperative difference between esophageal versus nasopharyngeal temperatures and the impact of prewarming, age, and weight: A randomized clinical trial. *AANA Journal, 83*(2), 99–105.

Finkelstein, R., Rabino, G., Mashiach, T., et al. (2014). Effect of preoperative antibiotic prophylaxis on surgical site infections complicating cardiac surgery. *Infection Control & Hospital Epidemiology*, 35(1), 69–74.

Guglielmi, C. L. (2014). Empowering providers to eliminate surgical fires. *AORN Journal, 100*(4), 412–413.

Huang, L., Kim, R., & Berry, W. (2013). Creating a culture of safety by using checklists. *AORN Journal, 97*(3), 365–368.

Isaak, E. S., & Steigler, M. P. (2015). Review of crisis resource management (CRM) principles in the setting of intraoperative malignant hyperthermia. *Journal of Anesthesiology, 30*(2), 298–306.

Joint Commission. (2011). Sentinel alert: Patient alert under anesthesia. Retrieved on 3/24/2016 at: www.jointcommission.org/sentinel_event_alert_issue_32_preventing_and_managing_the_impact_of_anesthesia_awareness/

Joint Commission. (2016). 2016 National Patient Safety Goals. Retrieved on 12/9/2015 at: www.jointcommission.org/standards_information/npsgs.aspx

Norton, E., Gorgone, P., & Belanger, B. (2014). In focus: Surgical fire risk reduction strategies. *AORN Journal, 99*(1), 5–6.

Oster, K. A., & Oster, C. A. (2015). Special needs population: Care of the geriatric patient population in the perioperative setting. *AORN Journal, 101*(6), 444–456.

Pada, S., & Perl, T. M. (2015). Operating room myths: What is the evidence for common practices? *Current opinion in infectious diseases, 28*(4), 369–374.

Penprase, B., & Johnson, C. (2015). Optimizing the perioperative nursing role for the older adult surgical patient. *OR Nurse, 8*(4), 26–33.

Seifert, P. C., Peterson, E., & Graham, K. (2015). Crisis management of fire in the OR. *AORN Journal, 101*(2), 250–263.

*Sobczak, K. (2014). Complications of perioperative hypothermia. *OR Nurse, 8*(5), 33–39.

Spruce, L. (2015). Back to basics: Procedural sedation. *AORN Journal, 101*(3), 345–353.

World Health Organization. (2015). New checklist to help make surgery safer. *WHO Bulletin, 86*(7), 496–576. Retrieved on 8/12/2016 at: http://apps.who.int/iris/bitstream/10665/44186/2/9789241598590_eng_Checklist.pdf

Resources

American Latex Allergy Association (ALAA), latexallergyresources.org

American Society of Anesthesiologists (ASA), www.asahq.org

American Society of PeriAnesthesia Nurses (ASPAN), www.aspan.org

Association of PeriOperative Registered Nurses, www.aorn.org

Centers for Disease Control and Prevention, Injury and Violence Prevention and Control, www.cdc.gov/injury

Joint Commission, www.jointcommission.org

Malignant Hyperthermia Association of the United States (MHAUS), www.mhaus.org

National SCIP Partnership, www.leapfroggroup.org/news/leapfrog_news/144968

World Health Organization (WHO), www.who.int/en/

19

Postoperative Nursing Management

LEARNING OBJECTIVES

On completion of this chapter, the learner will be able to:

1 Describe the responsibilities of the postanesthesia care nurse in the prevention of immediate postoperative complications.
2 Compare postoperative care of the ambulatory surgery patient with that of the hospitalized surgery patient.
3 Identify common postoperative problems and their management.

4 Describe the gerontologic considerations related to postoperative management.
5 Describe variables that affect wound healing.
6 Demonstrate postoperative dressing techniques.
7 Identify assessment parameters appropriate for the early detection of postoperative complications.

GLOSSARY

dehiscence: partial or complete separation of wound edges
evisceration: protrusion of organs through the surgical incision
first-intention healing: method of healing in which wound edges are surgically approximated and integumentary continuity is restored without granulation
phase I PACU: area designated for care of surgical patients immediately after surgery and for patients whose condition warrants close monitoring
phase II PACU: area designated for care of surgical patients who have been transferred from a phase I PACU because their condition no longer requires the close monitoring provided in a phase I PACU

phase III PACU: setting in which the patient is cared for in the immediate postoperative period and then prepared for discharge from the facility
postanesthesia care unit (PACU): area where postoperative patients are monitored as they recover from anesthesia; formerly referred to as the recovery room or postanesthesia recovery room
second-intention healing: method of healing in which wound edges are not surgically approximated and integumentary continuity is restored by the process known as granulation
third-intention healing: method of healing in which surgical approximation of wound edges is delayed and integumentary continuity is restored by opposing areas of granulation

---

The postoperative period extends from the time the patient leaves the operating room (OR) until the last follow-up visit with the surgeon. This may be as short as a day or two or as long as several months. During the postoperative period, nursing care focuses on reestablishing the patient's physiologic equilibrium, alleviating pain, preventing complications, and educating the patient about self-care (Rodriguez, 2015). Careful assessment and immediate intervention assist the patient in returning to optimal function quickly, safely, and as comfortable as possible. Ongoing care in the community through home care, clinic visits, office visits, or telephone follow-up facilitates an uncomplicated recovery.

Care of the Patient in the Postanesthesia Care Unit

The **postanesthesia care unit** (PACU), formerly referred to as the recovery room or postanesthesia recovery room, is located adjacent to the OR suite. Patients still under anesthesia or recovering from anesthesia are placed in this unit for

easy access to experienced, highly skilled nurses, anesthesia providers, surgeons, advanced hemodynamic and pulmonary monitoring and support, special equipment, and medications.

Phases of Postanesthesia Care

In some hospitals and ambulatory surgical centers, postanesthesia care is divided into three phases (Rothrock, 2014). In the **phase I PACU**, used during the immediate recovery phase, intensive nursing care is provided. After this phase, the patient transitions to the next phase of care as either an inpatient to a nursing unit or phase II PACU. In the **phase II PACU**, the patient is prepared for self-care or an extended care setting. In phase **III PACU**, the patient is prepared for discharge. Recliners rather than stretchers or beds are standard in many phase III units, which may also be referred to as step-down, sit-up, or progressive care units. In many hospitals, phase II and phase III units are combined. Patients may remain in a PACU for as long as 4 to 6 hours, depending on the type of surgery and any preexisting conditions or comorbidities. In facilities without separate phase I, II, and III units, the patient remains in the PACU and may be discharged home directly from this unit.

Admitting the Patient to the Postanesthesia Care Unit

Transferring the postoperative patient from the OR to the PACU is the responsibility of the anesthesiologist or certified registered nurse anesthetist (CRNA) and other licensed members of the OR team. During transport from the OR to the PACU, the anesthesia provider remains at the head of the stretcher (to maintain the airway), and a surgical team member remains at the opposite end. Transporting the patient involves special consideration of the incision site, potential vascular changes, and exposure. The surgical incision is considered every time the postoperative patient is moved; many wounds are closed under considerable tension, and every effort is made to prevent further strain on the incision. The patient is positioned so that he or she is not lying on and obstructing drains or drainage tubes. Orthostatic hypotension may occur when a patient is moved too quickly from one position to another (e.g., from a lithotomy position to a horizontal position or from a lateral to a supine position), so the patient must be moved slowly and carefully. As soon as the patient is placed on the stretcher or bed, the soiled gown is removed and replaced with a dry gown. The patient is covered with lightweight blankets and warmed. Only three side rails may be raised to prevent falls because in many states raising all side rails constitutes restraint.

The nurse who admits the patient to the PACU reviews essential information with the anesthesiologist or CRNA (see Chart 19-1) and the circulating nurse. Oxygen is applied, monitoring equipment is attached, and an immediate physiologic assessment is conducted.

Nursing Management in the Postanesthesia Care Unit

The nursing management objectives for the patient in the PACU are to provide care until the patient has recovered

---

Chart 19-1	Anesthesia Provider-to-Nurse Report and Nurse-to-Nurse Report: Information to Convey

Patient name, gender, age
Allergies
Surgical procedure
Length of time in the operating room
Anesthetic agents and reversal agents used
Estimated blood loss/fluid loss
Fluid/blood replacement
Last set of vital signs and any problems during the procedure (e.g., nausea and/or vomiting)
Any complications encountered (anesthetic or surgical)
Medical comorbidities (e.g., diabetes, hypertension)
Considerations for immediate postoperative period (pain management, reversals, ventilator settings)
Language barrier
Location of patient's family

Ideally, the anesthesia provider should not leave the patient until the nurse is satisfied with the patient's airway and immediate condition.

---

from the effects of anesthesia (e.g., until resumption of motor and sensory functions), is oriented, has stable vital signs, and shows no evidence of hemorrhage or other complications (Helvig, Minick, & Patrick, 2014; Noble & Pasero, 2014; Penprase & Johnson, 2015).

Assessing the Patient

Frequent, skilled assessments of the patient's airway, respiratory function, cardiovascular function, skin color, level of consciousness, and ability to respond to commands are the cornerstones of nursing care in the PACU (Liddle, 2013a & 2013b). Vital signs are observed and recorded, as well as level of consciousness. The nurse performs and documents a baseline assessment, then checks the surgical site for drainage or hemorrhage and makes sure that all drainage tubes and monitoring lines are connected and functioning. The nurse checks any intravenous (IV) fluids with the goal of maintaining a euvolumic state (Gallagher & Vacchiano, 2014). Medications currently infusing are checked, verifying that they are infusing at the correct dosage and rate.

After the initial assessment, vital signs are monitored and the patient's general physical status is assessed and documented at least every 15 minutes (Liddle, 2013a; Thanavaro, 2015). The nurse must be aware of any pertinent information from the patient's history that may be significant (e.g., patient is deaf or hard of hearing, has a history of seizures, has diabetes, or is allergic to certain medications or to latex). Administration of the patient's postoperative analgesic medications is a top priority in order to provide pain relief before it becomes severe (Ward, 2014) and facilitate early ambulation (Liddle, 2013b).

 Concept Mastery Alert

Following surgery, patients who had ketamine as anesthesia must be placed in a quiet, darkened area of the PACU. See Table 18-2 for more information about anesthetic agents.

Maintaining a Patent Airway

The primary objective in the immediate postoperative period is to maintain ventilation and thus prevent hypoxemia (reduced oxygen in the blood) and hypercapnia (excess carbon dioxide in the blood). Both can occur if the airway is obstructed and ventilation is reduced (hypoventilation). Besides administering supplemental oxygen as prescribed, the nurse assesses respiratory rate and depth, ease of respirations, oxygen saturation, and breath sounds.

Patients who have experienced prolonged anesthesia usually are unconscious, with all muscles relaxed. This relaxation extends to the muscles of the pharynx. When the patient lies on their back, the lower jaw and the tongue fall backward and the air passages become obstructed (Fig. 19-1A). This is called *hypopharyngeal obstruction*. Signs of occlusion include choking; noisy and irregular respirations; decreased oxygen saturation scores; and, within minutes, a blue, dusky color (cyanosis) of the skin. Because movement of the thorax and the diaphragm does not necessarily indicate that the patient is breathing, the nurse needs to place the palm of the hand at the patient's nose and mouth to feel the exhaled breath.

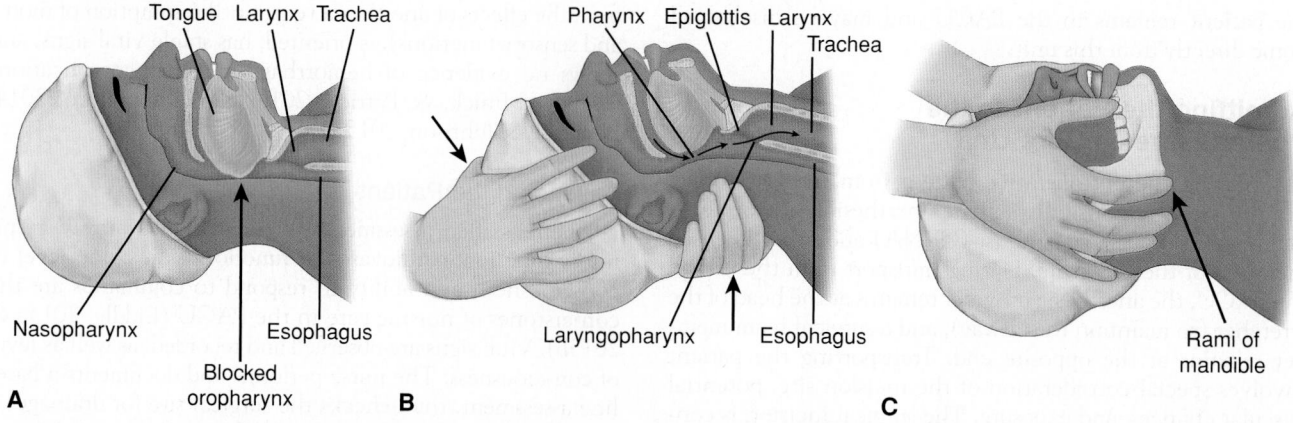

Figure 19-1 • A. A hypopharyngeal obstruction occurs when neck flexion permits the chin to drop toward the chest; obstruction almost always occurs when the head is in the midposition. **B.** Tilting the head back to stretch the anterior neck structure lifts the base of the tongue off the posterior pharyngeal wall. The direction of the *arrows* indicates the pressure of the hands. **C.** Opening the mouth is necessary to correct a valvelike obstruction of the nasal passage during expiration, which occurs in about 30% of unconscious patients. Open the patient's mouth (separate lips and teeth) and move the lower jaw forward so that the lower teeth are in front of the upper teeth. To regain backward tilt of the neck, lift with both hands at the ascending rami of the mandible.

> **▶ Quality and Safety Nursing Alert**
>
> *The treatment of hypopharyngeal obstruction involves tilting the head back and pushing forward on the angle of the lower jaw, as if to push the lower teeth in front of the upper teeth (see Fig. 19-1B,C). This maneuver pulls the tongue forward and opens the air passages.*

The anesthesiologist or CRNA may leave a hard rubber or plastic airway in the patient's mouth to maintain a patent airway (see Fig. 19-2). Such a device should not be removed until signs such as gagging indicate that reflex action is returning. Alternatively, the patient may enter the PACU with an endotracheal tube still in place and may require continued mechanical ventilation. The nurse assists in initiating the use of the ventilator as well as the weaning and

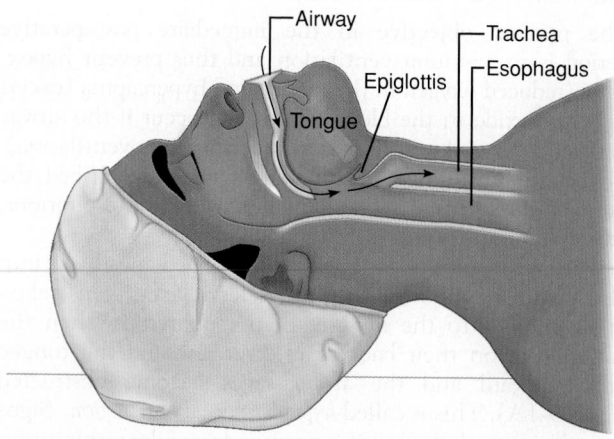

Figure 19-2 • The use of an airway to maintain a patent airway after anesthesia. The airway passes over the base of the tongue and permits air to pass into the pharynx in the region of the epiglottis. Patients often leave the operating room with an airway in place. The airway should remain in place until the patient recovers sufficiently to breathe normally. As the patient regains consciousness, the airway usually causes irritation and should be removed.

extubation processes. Some patients, particularly those who have had extensive or lengthy surgical procedures, may be transferred from the OR directly to the intensive care unit (ICU) or from the PACU to the ICU while still intubated and receiving mechanical ventilation. In most facilities, the patient is awakened and extubated in the OR (except in cases of trauma or critical illness) and arrives in the PACU breathing without support.

If the teeth are clenched, the mouth may be opened manually but cautiously with a padded tongue depressor. The head of the bed is elevated 15 to 30 degrees unless contraindicated, and the patient is closely monitored to maintain the airway as well as to minimize the risk of aspiration. If vomiting occurs, the patient is turned to the side to prevent aspiration and the vomitus is collected in the emesis basin. Mucus or vomitus obstructing the pharynx or the trachea is suctioned with a pharyngeal suction tip or a nasal catheter introduced into the nasopharynx or oropharynx to a distance of 15 to 20 cm (6 to 8 in). Caution is necessary in suctioning the throat of a patient who has had a tonsillectomy or other oral or laryngeal surgery because of the risk of bleeding and discomfort.

Maintaining Cardiovascular Stability

To monitor cardiovascular stability, the nurse assesses the patient's level of consciousness; vital signs; cardiac rhythm; skin temperature, color, and moisture; and urine output. The nurse also assesses the patency of all IV lines. The primary cardiovascular complications seen in the PACU include hypotension and shock, hemorrhage, hypertension, and dysrhythmias.

In patients who are critically ill, have significant comorbidity, or have undergone riskier procedures, additional monitoring may have been done in the OR and will continue in the PACU. These may include central venous pressure, pulmonary artery pressure, pulmonary artery wedge pressure, and cardiac output.

Hypotension and Shock

Hypotension can result from blood loss, hypoventilation, position changes, pooling of blood in the extremities, or side effects of medications and anesthetics. The most common cause is loss of circulating volume through blood and plasma loss. If the amount of blood loss exceeds 500 mL (especially if the loss is rapid), replacement is usually indicated.

> ▶ *Quality and Safety Nursing Alert*
>
> *A systolic blood pressure of less than 90 mm Hg is usually considered immediately reportable. However, the patient's preoperative or baseline blood pressure is used to make informed postoperative comparisons. A previously stable blood pressure that shows a downward trend of 5 mm Hg at each 15-minute reading should also be reported.*

Shock, which is one of the most serious postoperative complications, can result from hypovolemia and decreased intravascular volume (Gallagher & Vacchiano, 2014). Types of shock are classified as hypovolemic, cardiogenic, neurogenic, anaphylactic, and septic. The classic signs of hypovolemic shock (the most common type of shock) are pallor; cool, moist skin; rapid breathing; cyanosis of the lips, gums, and tongue; rapid, weak, thready pulse; narrowing pulse pressure; low blood pressure; and concentrated urine. (See Chapter 14 for a detailed discussion of shock.)

Hypovolemic shock can be avoided largely by the timely administration of IV fluids, blood, blood products, and medications that elevate blood pressure. The primary intervention for hypovolemic shock is volume replacement, with an infusion of lactated Ringer solution, 0.9% sodium chloride solution, colloids, or blood component therapy (see Table 14-3 in Chapter 14). Oxygen is given by nasal cannula, facemask, or mechanical ventilation. If fluid administration fails to reverse hypovolemic shock, then various cardiac, vasodilator, and corticosteroid medications may be prescribed to improve cardiac function and reduce peripheral vascular resistance.

The PACU bed provides easy access to the patient; is easily movable; can readily be positioned to facilitate the use of measures to counteract shock; and has features that facilitate care, such as IV poles, side rails, and wheel brakes. The patient is placed flat with the legs elevated, usually with a pillow. Respiratory rate, pulse rate, blood pressure, blood oxygen concentration, urinary output, and level of consciousness are monitored to provide information on the patient's respiratory and cardiovascular status. Vital signs are monitored continuously until the patient's condition has stabilized.

Other factors can contribute to hemodynamic instability, such as body temperature and pain. The PACU nurse implements measures to manage these factors. The nurse keeps the patient warm (while avoiding overheating to prevent cutaneous vessels from dilating and depriving vital organs of blood), avoids exposure, and maintains normothermia (to prevent vasodilation). Pain control measures are implemented, as discussed later in this chapter.

Hemorrhage

Hemorrhage is an uncommon yet serious complication of surgery that can result in hypovolemic shock and death. It can present insidiously or emergently at any time in the immediate postoperative period or up to several days after surgery (see Table 19-1). The patient presents with hypotension; rapid, thready pulse; disorientation; restlessness; oliguria; and

TABLE 19-1 Types of Hemorrhage

Classification	Defining Characteristic
Time Frame	
Primary	Hemorrhage occurs at the time of surgery.
Intermediary	Hemorrhage occurs during the first few hours after surgery when the rise of blood pressure to its normal level dislodges insecure clots from untied vessels.
Secondary	Hemorrhage may occur sometime after surgery if a suture slips because a blood vessel was not securely tied, became infected, or was eroded by a drainage tube.
Type of Vessel	
Capillary	Hemorrhage is characterized by slow, general ooze.
Venous	Darkly colored blood flows quickly.
Arterial	Blood is bright red and appears in spurts with each heartbeat.
Visibility	
Evident	Hemorrhage is on the surface and can be seen.
Concealed	Hemorrhage is in a body cavity and cannot be seen.

cold, pale skin. The early phase of shock will manifest in feelings of apprehension, decreased cardiac output, and vascular resistance. Breathing becomes labored, and "air hunger" will be exhibited; the patient will feel cold (hypothermia) and may experience tinnitus. Laboratory values may show a sharp drop in hemoglobin and hematocrit levels. If shock symptoms are left untreated, the patient will continually grow weaker but can remain conscious until near death (Rothrock, 2014).

Transfusing blood or blood products and determining the cause of hemorrhage are the initial therapeutic measures. The surgical site and incision should always be inspected for bleeding. If bleeding is evident, a sterile gauze pad and a pressure dressing are applied, and the site of the bleeding is elevated to heart level if possible. The patient is placed in the shock position (flat on back; legs elevated at a 20-degree angle; knees kept straight). If hemorrhage is suspected but cannot be visualized, the patient may be taken back to the OR for emergency exploration of the surgical site.

If hemorrhage is suspected, the nurse should be aware of any special considerations related to blood loss replacement. Certain patients may decline blood transfusions for religious or cultural reasons and may identify this request on their advance directives or living will.

Hypertension and Dysrhythmias

Hypertension is common in the immediate postoperative period secondary to sympathetic nervous system stimulation from pain, hypoxia, or bladder distention. Dysrhythmias are associated with electrolyte imbalance, altered respiratory function, pain, hypothermia, stress, and anesthetic agents. Both hypertension and dysrhythmias are managed by treating the underlying causes.

Relieving Pain and Anxiety

The nurse in the PACU monitors the patient's physiologic status, manages pain, and provides psychological support in an effort to relieve the patient's fears and concerns. The nurse checks the medical record for special needs and concerns of

TABLE 19-2 Medications Used to Control Postoperative Nausea and Vomiting

Drug Classes	Name	Nursing Implications
GI stimulant	Metoclopramide (Reglan)	Acts by stimulating gastric emptying and increasing GI transit time. Administration recommended at the end of procedure. Available in oral, IM, and IV forms.
Phenothiazine antiemetic	Prochlorperazine (Compazine)	Indicated for control of severe nausea and vomiting. Available in oral, SR, rectal, IM, and IV forms.
Phenothiazine antiemetic antimotion sickness	Promethazine (Phenergan)	Recommended every 4–6 hrs for nausea and vomiting associated with anesthesia and surgery. Available in oral, IM, and IV forms.
Antimotion sickness	Dimenhydrinate (Dramamine)	Indicated for prevention of nausea, vomiting, or vertigo of motion sickness. Available in oral, IM, and IV forms.
Antiemetic	Hydroxyzine (Vistaril, Atarax)	Control of nausea and vomiting and as adjunct to analgesia preoperatively and postoperatively to allow decreased opioid dosage. Available in oral and IM forms.
Antiemetic antimotion sickness	Scopolamine (Transderm Scop)	Used to prevent and control of nausea and vomiting associated with motion sickness and recovery from surgery. Available in oral, transdermal SC, and IM forms.
Antiemetic	Ondansetron (Zofran)	Prevention of postoperative nausea and vomiting. Available in oral, IM, and IV forms. With few side effects, frequently the drug of choice.

GI, gastrointestinal; IM, intramuscular; IV, intravenous; SR, sustained release; SC, subcutaneous.
Adapted from Comerford, K. C. (2015). *Nursing 2015 drug handbook.* Philadelphia, PA: Wolters Kluwer.

the patient. Opioid analgesic medications are given mostly by IV in the PACU (Rothrock, 2014). IV opioids provide immediate pain relief and are short acting, thus minimizing the potential for drug interactions or prolonged respiratory depression while anesthetics are still active in the patient's system (Barash, Cullen, Stoelting, et al., 2013). (See Chapter 12 for more information about pain management.) When the patient's condition permits, a close member of the family may visit in the PACU to decrease the family's anxiety and make the patient feel more secure.

Controlling Nausea and Vomiting

Nausea and vomiting occur in about 10% of patients in the PACU. The nurse should intervene at the patient's first report of nausea to control the problem rather than wait for it to progress to vomiting (Tinsley & Barone, 2013).

 Quality and Safety Nursing Alert

At the slightest indication of nausea, the patient is turned completely to one side to promote mouth drainage and prevent aspiration of vomitus, which can cause asphyxiation and death.

Many medications are available to control postoperative nausea and vomiting (PONV) without over-sedating the patient; they are commonly given during surgery as well as in the PACU (Tinsley & Barone, 2013). Table 19-2 contains selected medications prescribed to control PONV. A variety of alternative techniques have been suggested to help control PONV, including deep breathing and aromatherapy (Hodge, McCarthy, & Peirce, 2014; Sites, Johnson, Miller, et al., 2014). (See Chart 19-2).

Chart 19-2 **NURSING RESEARCH PROFILE**

The Effectiveness of Aromatherapy for Relief of Postoperative Nausea and Vomiting

Hodge, N. S., McCarthy, M. S., & Peirce, R. M. (2014). A prospective randomized study of the effectiveness of aromatherapy for relief of postoperative nausea and vomiting. *Journal of PeriAnesthesia Nursing, 29*(1), 5–11.

Purpose

Postoperative nausea and vomiting (PONV) is a major concern for patients having surgery under general anesthesia. The purpose of this study was to compare the effectiveness of a placebo unscented inhaler to an aromatherapy inhaler in relieving PONV.

Design

The study used a prospective two-group design. The 121 patients who experienced PONV were randomized into a control group that received a placebo inhaler or another group that received the treatment with aromatics. Patients in both groups evaluated and ranked their nausea before and after therapy using

a descriptive scale with 0 equal to "no nausea" and 10 equal to "the worst nausea ever". The patients self-administered the inhalers.

Findings

The initial and follow-up nausea assessment scores in both the placebo and treatment groups decreased significantly ($p < 0.01$), and there was a significant difference between the two groups ($p = 0.03$). Perceived effectiveness of aromatherapy was significantly higher in the treatment group ($p < 0.001$).

Nursing Implications

Nurses working with postoperative patients should be aware that alternatives to pharmacologic intervention are available to control PONV. An aromatherapy inhaler is patient controlled, and it appears to present an effective postoperative nausea treatment.

The risk of PONV ranges from approximately 10% in the PACU to 30% in the first 24 hours of postoperative care (Tinsley & Barone, 2013). Risks include general anesthesia, female gender, nonsmoker, history of PONV, and history of motion sickness (Tinsley & Barone, 2013). Surgical risks are increased with PONV due to an increase in intra-abdominal pressure, elevated central venous pressure, the potential for aspiration, increased heart rate, and systemic blood pressure, which increase the risk of myocardial ischemia and dysrhythmias. Patients are at increased risk of dehydration, electrolyte disturbances, aspiration, and wound dehiscence (Hodge et al., 2014). Postoperative pain is increased as well (McGuire & Bolyanatz, 2014; Rodriguez, 2015).

Gerontologic Considerations

The older patient, like all patients, is transferred from the OR table to the bed or stretcher slowly and gently. The effects of this action on blood pressure and ventilation are monitored. Special attention is given to keeping the patient warm, because older adults are more susceptible to hypothermia. The patient's position is changed frequently to stimulate respirations as well as promote circulation and comfort.

Immediate postoperative care for the older adult is the same as for any surgical patient; however, additional support is given if cardiovascular, pulmonary, or renal function is impaired. With careful monitoring, it is possible to detect cardiopulmonary deficits before signs and symptoms are apparent. Changes associated with the aging process, the prevalence of chronic diseases, alteration in fluid and nutrition status, and the increased use of medications result in the need for postoperative vigilance (Oster & Oster, 2015). Nurses should keep in mind that older adults may have slower recovery from anesthesia due to the prolonged time it takes to eliminate sedatives and anesthetic agents (Tabloski, 2013).

Postoperative confusion and delirium may occur in up to half of all older patients. Acute confusion may be caused by pain, altered pharmacokinetics of analgesic agents, hypotension, fever, hypoglycemia, fluid loss, fecal impaction, urinary retention, or anemia (Hayes & Gordon, 2015; Meiner, 2014). Providing adequate hydration, reorienting to the environment, and reassessing the doses of sedative, anesthetic, and analgesic agents may reduce the risk of confusion. Hypoxia can present as confusion and restlessness, as can blood loss and electrolyte imbalances. Exclusion of all other causes of confusion must precede the assumption that confusion is related to age, circumstances, and medications.

Dehydration, constipation, and malnutrition may occur postoperatively. Sensory limitations, such as impaired vision or hearing and reduced tactile sensitivity, frequently interact with the unfamiliar postoperative environment, so falls are more likely to occur (Meiner, 2014). Maintaining a safe environment for older adults requires alertness and planning. Arthritis is a common condition among older patients, and it affects mobility, creating difficulty turning from one side to the other or ambulating without discomfort.

Determining Readiness for Postanesthesia Care Unit Discharge

A patient remains in the PACU until fully recovered from the anesthetic agent. Indicators of recovery include stable blood pressure, adequate respiratory function, and adequate oxygen saturation level compared with baseline.

The Aldrete score is used to determine the patient's general condition and readiness for transfer from the PACU (Aldrete & Wright, 1992). Throughout the recovery period, the patient's physical signs are observed and evaluated by means of a scoring system based on a set of objective criteria. This evaluation guide allows an objective assessment of the patient's condition in the PACU (see Fig. 19-3). The patient is assessed at regular intervals, and a total score is calculated and recorded on the assessment record. The Aldrete score is usually between 7 and 10 before discharge from the PACU. Patients with a score of less than 7 must remain in the PACU until their condition improves or until they are transferred to an ICU, depending on their preoperative baseline score (Rothrock, 2014).

The patient is discharged from the phase I PACU by the anesthesiologist or CRNA to the critical care unit, the medical-surgical unit, the phase II PACU, or home with a responsible adult. In some hospitals and ambulatory care centers, patients are discharged to a phase III PACU, where they are prepared for discharge.

Preparing the Postoperative Patient for Direct Discharge

Ambulatory surgical centers frequently have a step-down PACU similar to a phase II PACU. Patients seen in this type of unit are usually healthy, and the plan is to discharge them directly to home. Prior to discharge, the patient will require verbal and written instructions and information about follow-up care.

Promoting Home, Community-Based, and Transitional Care

To ensure patient safety and recovery, expert patient education and discharge planning are necessary when a patient undergoes same-day or ambulatory surgery (Association of PeriOperative Registered Nurses [AORN], 2014; American Society of PeriAnesthesia Nurses [ASPAN], 2015). Because anesthetics cloud memory for concurrent events, verbal and written instructions should be given to both the patient and the adult who will be accompanying the patient home. Alternative formats (e.g., large print, Braille) of instructions or the use of a sign language interpreter may be required to ensure patient and family understanding. A translator may be required if the patient and family members do not understand English.

Discharge Preparation

The patient and caregiver (e.g., family member, friend) are informed about expected outcomes and immediate postoperative changes anticipated (AORN, 2014; ASPAN, 2015). Chart 19-3 identifies important educational points; before discharging the patient, the nurse provides written instructions covering each of those points. Prescriptions are given to the patient. The nursing unit or surgeon's telephone number is provided, and the patient and caregiver are encouraged to call with questions and to schedule follow-up appointments.

Although recovery time varies depending on the type and extent of surgery and the patient's overall condition,

Post Anesthesia Care Unit
MODIFIED ALDRETE SCORE

Patient: _____ Final score: _____

Room: _____ Surgeon: _____

Date: _____ PACU nurse: _____

Area of Assessment	Point Score	Upon Admission	After			
			15 min	30 min	45 min	60 min
Activity						
(Able to move spontaneously or on command)						
• Ability to move all extremities	2					
• Ability to move 2 extremities	1					
• Unable to control any extremity	0					
Respiration						
• Ability to breathe deeply and cough	2					
• Limited respiratory effort (dyspnea or splinting)	1					
• No spontaneous effort	0					
Circulation						
• BP 20% of preanesthetic level	2					
• BP 20% –49% of preanesthetic level	1					
• BP 50% of preanesthetic level	0					
Consciousness						
• Fully awake	2					
• Arousable on calling	1					
• Not responding	0					
O_2 Saturation						
• Able to maintain O_2 sat >92% on room air	2					
• Needs O_2 inhalation to maintain O_2 sat >90%	1					
• O_2 sat <90% even with O_2 supplement	0					
Totals:						

Required for discharge from Post Anesthesia Care Unit: 7–8 points

_____ _____
Time of release   Signature of nurse

Figure 19-3 • Postanesthesia care unit record; modified Aldrete score. O_2 sat, oxygen saturation; BP, blood pressure. Adapted from Aldrete, A., & Wright, A. (1992). Revised Aldrete score for discharge. *Anesthesiology News*, *18*(1), 17.

instructions usually advise limited activity for 24 to 48 hours. During this time, the patient should not drive a vehicle, drink alcoholic beverages, or perform tasks that require high levels of energy or skill. Fluids may be consumed as desired and smaller than normal amounts may be eaten at mealtime. Patients are cautioned not to make important decisions at this time because the medications, anesthesia, and surgery may affect their decision-making ability.

Continuing and Transitional Care

Although most patients who undergo ambulatory surgery recover quickly and without complications, some patients require referral for some type of continuing or transitional care. These may be older or frail patients, those who live alone, and patients with other health care problems or disabilities that might interfere with self-care or resumption of

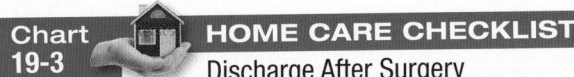

HOME CARE CHECKLIST

Chart 19-3

Discharge After Surgery

At the completion of education, the patient and/or caregiver will be able to:

- Name the procedure that was performed and identify any permanent changes in anatomic structure or function as well as changes in ADLs, IADLs, roles, relationships, and spirituality.
- Identify interventions and strategies (e.g., durable medical equipment, adaptive equipment) used in adapting to any permanent changes in structure or function.
- Describe ongoing postoperative therapeutic regimen, including diet and activities to perform (e.g., walking and breathing exercises) and to limit or avoid (e.g., lifting weights, driving a car, contact sports).
- State the name, dose, side effects, frequency, and schedule for all medications.
- State how to obtain medical supplies and carry out dressing changes, wound care, and other prescribed regimens.

ADLs, activities of daily living; IADLs, instrumental activities of daily living.

- Describe signs and symptoms of complications.
- State time and date of follow-up appointments.
- Relate how to reach health care provider with questions or complications.
- State understanding of community resources and referrals (if any).
- Identify the need for health promotion (e.g., weight reduction, smoking cessation, stress management), disease prevention, and screening activities.

Resources

See Chapter 10, Chart 10-8 for additional information related to durable medical equipment, adaptive equipment, mobility skills, skin, bowel, and bladder care.

---

usual activities. The home, community, or transitional care nurse assesses the patient's physical status (e.g., respiratory and cardiovascular status, adequacy of pain management, the surgical incision, surgical complications) and the patient's and family's ability to adhere to the recommendations given at the time of discharge. Previous education is reinforced as needed. Nursing interventions may include changing surgical dressings, monitoring the patency of a drainage system, or administering medications. The patient and family are reminded about the importance of keeping follow-up appointments with the surgeon. Follow-up phone calls from the nurse are also used to assess the patient's progress and to answer any questions.

Care of the Hospitalized Postoperative Patient

Most surgeries are now performed in ambulatory care centers, but there are unanticipated transfers of some patients for hospitalization (Allison & George, 2014). However, the majority of surgical patients who require hospital stays are trauma patients, acutely ill patients, patients undergoing major surgery, patients who require emergency surgery, and patients with a concurrent medical disorder. Seriously ill patients and those who have undergone major cardiovascular, pulmonary, or neurologic surgery may be admitted to specialized ICUs for close monitoring and advanced interventions and support. The care required by these patients in the immediate postoperative period is discussed in specific chapters of this book.

Patients admitted to the clinical unit for postoperative care have multiple needs and stay for a short period of time. Postoperative care for those surgical patients returning to the general medical-surgical unit is discussed later in this chapter.

Receiving the Patient in the Clinical Unit

The patient's room is readied by assembling the necessary equipment and supplies: IV pumps, drainage receptacle holder, suction equipment, oxygen, emesis basin, tissues, disposable pads, blankets, and postoperative documentation forms. When the call comes to the unit about the patient's transfer from the PACU, the need for any additional items is communicated. The PACU nurse reports relevant data about the patient to the receiving nurse (see Chart 19-1).

Usually, the surgeon speaks to the family after surgery and relates the general condition of the patient. The receiving nurse gets a report about the patient's condition, reviews the postoperative orders, admits the patient to the unit, performs an initial assessment, and attends to the patient's immediate needs (see Chart 19-4).

Nursing Management After Surgery

During the first 24 hours after surgery, nursing care of the hospitalized patient on the medical-surgical unit involves continuing to help the patient recover from the effects of anesthesia (Barash et al., 2013), frequently assessing the patient's physiologic status, monitoring for complications, managing pain, and implementing measures designed to achieve the long-range goals of independence with self-care, successful management of the therapeutic regimen, discharge to home, and full recovery (Liddle, 2013a & 2013b; Penprase & Johnson, 2015 ; Rosen, Bergh, Schwartz-Barcott, et al., 2014). In the initial hours after admission to the clinical unit, adequate ventilation, hemodynamic stability, incisional pain, surgical site integrity, nausea and vomiting, neurologic status, and spontaneous voiding are primary concerns. The pulse rate, blood pressure, and respiration rate are recorded at least every 15 minutes for the first hour and every 30 minutes for the next 2 hours. Thereafter, they are measured less frequently if they remain stable. The temperature is monitored every 4 hours for the first 24 hours (ASPAN, 2015).

Patients usually begin to return to their usual state of health several hours after surgery or after awaking the next morning. Although pain may still be intense, many patients feel more alert, less nauseous, and less anxious. They have begun their breathing and leg exercises as appropriate for the type of surgery, and most will have dangled their legs over the edge of the bed, stood, and ambulated a few feet or been assisted out of

Chart 19-4 Immediate Postoperative Nursing Interventions

Nursing Interventions	Rationale
1. Assess breathing and administer supplemental oxygen, if prescribed.	1. Assessment provides a baseline and helps identify signs and symptoms of respiratory distress early.
2. Monitor vital signs and note skin warmth, moisture, and color.	2. A careful baseline assessment helps identify signs and symptoms of shock early.
3. Assess the surgical site and wound drainage systems. Connect all drainage tubes to gravity or suction as indicated and monitor closed drainage systems.	3. Assessment provides a baseline and helps identify signs and symptoms of hemorrhage early.
4. Assess level of consciousness, orientation, and ability to move extremities.	4. These parameters provide a baseline and help identify signs and symptoms of neurologic complications.
5. Assess pain level; pain characteristics (location, quality); and timing, type, and route of administration of the last dose of analgesic.	5. Assessment provides a baseline of current pain level and assesses effectiveness of pain management strategies.
6. Administer analgesic medications as prescribed and assess their effectiveness in relieving pain.	6. Administration of analgesic agents helps decrease pain.
7. Place the call light, emesis basin, ice chips (if allowed), and bedpan or urinal within reach.	7. Attending to these needs provides for comfort and safety.
8. Position the patient to enhance comfort, safety, and lung expansion.	8. This promotes safety and reduces risk of postoperative complications.
9. Assess IV sites for patency and infusions for correct rate and solution.	9. Assessing IV sites and infusions helps detect phlebitis and prevents errors in rate and solution type.
10. Assess urine output in closed drainage system or use bladder scanner to detect distention.	10. Assessment provides a baseline and helps identify signs of urinary retention.
11. Reinforce the need to begin deep breathing and leg exercises.	11. These activities help prevent complications related to immobility (e.g., atelectasis, VTE).
12. Provide information to the patient and family.	12. Patient education helps decrease the patient's and family's anxiety.

VTE, venous thromboembolism.
Adapted from Association of PeriOperative Registered Nurses (AORN). (2014). *Association of PeriOperative Registered Nurses (AORN) standards, recommended practice, and guidelines*. Denver, CO: Author.

---

bed to the chair at least once. Many will have tolerated a light meal and had IV fluids discontinued. The focus of care shifts from intense physiologic management and symptomatic relief of the adverse effects of anesthesia to regaining independence with self-care and preparing for discharge.

NURSING PROCESS

The Hospitalized Patient Recovering From Surgery

Nursing care of the hospitalized patient recovering from surgery takes place in a compressed time frame, with much of the healing and recovery occurring after the patient is discharged to home or to a rehabilitation center.

Assessment

Assessment of the hospitalized postoperative patient includes monitoring vital signs and completing a review of systems upon the patient's arrival to the clinical unit (see Chart 19-4) and at regular intervals thereafter.

Respiratory status is important because pulmonary complications are among the most frequent and serious problems encountered by the surgical patient. The nurse monitors for airway patency and any signs of laryngeal edema. The quality of respirations, including depth, rate, and sound, is assessed regularly.

Chest auscultation verifies that breath sounds are normal (or abnormal) bilaterally, and the findings are documented as a baseline for later comparisons. Often, because of the effects of analgesic and anesthetic medications, respirations are slow. Shallow and rapid respirations may be caused by pain, constricting dressings, gastric dilation, abdominal distention, or obesity. Noisy breathing may be due to obstruction by secretions or the tongue. Another possible complication is flash pulmonary edema that occurs when protein and fluid accumulate in the alveoli unrelated to elevated pulmonary artery occlusive pressure. Signs and symptoms include agitation; tachypnea; tachycardia; decreased pulse oximetry readings; frothy, pink sputum; and crackles on auscultation.

The nurse assesses the patient's pain level using a verbal or visual analog scale and assesses the characteristics of the pain. The patient's appearance, pulse, respirations, blood pressure, skin color (adequate or cyanotic), and skin temperature (cold and clammy, warm and moist, or warm and dry) are clues to cardiovascular function. When the patient arrives in the clinical unit, the surgical site is assessed for bleeding, type and integrity of dressings, and drains.

The nurse also assesses the patient's mental status and level of consciousness, speech, and orientation and compares them with the preoperative baseline. Although a change in mental status or postoperative restlessness may be related to anxiety, pain, or medications, it may also be a symptom of oxygen deficit or hemorrhage. These serious causes must be investigated and excluded before other causes are pursued.

General discomfort that results from lying in one position on the operating table, the handling of tissues by the surgical team, the body's reaction to anesthesia, and anxiety are also common causes of restlessness. These discomforts may be relieved by administering the prescribed analgesic medication, changing the patient's position frequently, and assessing and alleviating the cause of anxiety. If tight, drainage-soaked bandages are causing discomfort, reinforcing or changing the dressing completely as prescribed by the provider may make the patient more comfortable. The bladder is assessed for distention (usually with a bladder scanner) because urinary retention can also cause restlessness (AORN, 2014).

Diagnosis

NURSING DIAGNOSES

Based on the assessment data, major nursing diagnoses may include the following:

- Risk for ineffective airway clearance related to depressed respiratory function, pain, and bed rest
- Acute pain related to surgical incision
- Decreased cardiac output related to shock or hemorrhage
- Risk for activity intolerance related to generalized weakness secondary to surgery
- Impaired skin integrity related to surgical incision and drains
- Ineffective thermoregulation related to surgical environment and anesthetic agents
- Risk for imbalanced nutrition, less than body requirements related to decreased intake and increased need for nutrients secondary to surgery
- Risk for constipation related to effects of medications, surgery, dietary change, and immobility
- Risk for urinary retention related to anesthetic agents
- Risk for injury related to surgical procedure/positioning or anesthetic agents
- Anxiety related to surgical procedure
- Deficient knowledge related to wound care, dietary restrictions, activity recommendations, medications, follow-up care, or signs and symptoms of complications in preparation for discharge

COLLABORATIVE PROBLEMS OR POTENTIAL COMPLICATIONS

Based on the assessment data, potential complications may include the following:

- Pulmonary infection/hypoxia
- Venous thromboembolism (VTE) (e.g., deep vein thrombosis [DVT], pulmonary embolism [PE])
- Hematoma or hemorrhage
- Infection
- Wound dehiscence or evisceration

Planning and Goals

The major goals for the patient include optimal respiratory function, relief of pain, optimal cardiovascular function, increased activity tolerance, unimpaired wound healing, maintenance of body temperature, and maintenance of nutritional balance (Dudek, 2013). Further goals include resumption of usual pattern of bowel and bladder elimination, identification of any perioperative positioning injury, acquisition of sufficient knowledge to manage self-care after discharge, and absence of complications.

Nursing Interventions

PREVENTING RESPIRATORY COMPLICATIONS

Respiratory depressive effects of opioid medications, decreased lung expansion secondary to pain, and decreased mobility combine to put the patient at risk for respiratory complications, particularly atelectasis (alveolar collapse; incomplete expansion of the lung), pneumonia, and hypoxemia (Rothrock, 2014). Atelectasis remains a risk for the patient who is not moving well or ambulating or who is not performing deep-breathing and coughing exercises or using an incentive spirometer. Signs and symptoms include decreased breath sounds over the affected area, crackles, and cough. Pneumonia is characterized by chills and fever, tachycardia, and tachypnea. Cough may or may not be present and may or may not be productive. Hypostatic pulmonary congestion, caused by a weakened cardiovascular system that permits stagnation of secretions at lung bases, may develop; this condition occurs most frequently in older patients who are not mobilized effectively (Tabloski, 2013). The symptoms are often vague, with perhaps a slight elevation of temperature, pulse, and respiratory rate as well as a cough. Physical examination reveals dullness and crackles at the base of the lungs. If the condition progresses, the outcome may be fatal.

The types of hypoxemia that can affect postoperative patients are subacute and episodic. Subacute hypoxemia is a constant low level of oxygen saturation when breathing appears normal. Episodic hypoxemia develops suddenly, and the patient may be at risk for cerebral dysfunction, myocardial ischemia, and cardiac arrest. Risk for hypoxemia is increased in patients who have undergone major surgery (particularly abdominal), are obese, or have preexisting pulmonary problems. Hypoxemia is detected by pulse oximetry, which measures blood oxygen saturation (Liddle, 2013a). Factors that may affect the accuracy of pulse oximetry readings include cold extremities, tremors, atrial fibrillation, acrylic nails, and black or blue nail polish (these colors interfere with the functioning of the pulse oximeter; other colors do not).

Preventive measures and timely recognition of signs and symptoms help avert pulmonary complications. Crackles indicate static pulmonary secretions that need to be mobilized by coughing and deep-breathing exercises. When a mucus plug obstructs one of the bronchi entirely, the pulmonary tissue beyond the plug collapses, resulting in atelectasis.

To clear secretions and prevent pneumonia, the nurse encourages the patient to turn frequently, take deep breaths, cough, and use the incentive spirometer at least every 2 hours. These pulmonary exercises should begin as soon as the patient arrives on the clinical unit and continue until the patient is discharged. Even if he or she is not fully awake from anesthesia, the patient can be asked to take several deep breaths. This helps expel residual anesthetic agents, mobilize secretions, and prevent atelectasis. Careful splinting of abdominal or thoracic incision sites helps the patient overcome the fear that the exertion of coughing might open the incision (see Chapter 17, Chart 17-6). Analgesic agents are given to permit more effective coughing, and oxygen is given as prescribed to prevent or relieve hypoxia. To encourage lung expansion, the patient is encouraged to yawn or take sustained maximal inspirations to create a negative intrathoracic pressure of −40 mm Hg and expand lung volume to total capacity. Chest physical therapy may be prescribed if indicated (see Chapter 21).

Coughing is contraindicated in patients who have head injuries or who have undergone intracranial surgery (because of the risk for increasing intracranial pressure), as well as in patients who have undergone eye surgery (because of the risk for increasing intraocular pressure) or plastic surgery (because of the risk for increasing tension on delicate tissues).

Early ambulation increases metabolism and pulmonary aeration and, in general, improves all body functions. The patient is encouraged to be out of bed as soon as possible (i.e., on the day of surgery or no later than the first postoperative day) (Harrington, 2013). This practice is especially valuable in preventing pulmonary complications in older patients (Oster & Oster, 2015).

RELIEVING PAIN

Most patients experience some pain after a surgical procedure. Complete absence of pain in the area of the surgical incision may not occur for a few weeks, depending on the site and nature of the surgery, but the intensity of postoperative pain gradually subsides on subsequent days. About one-third of patients report severe pain, one third moderate pain, and one third little or no pain (Grossman & Porth, 2014; Rodriguez, 2015). This does not mean that the patients in the last group have no pain; rather, they appear to activate psychodynamic mechanisms that impair the registering of pain (nociceptive transmission). (See Chapter 12 for a more detailed discussion of pain.)

Many factors (motivational, affective, cognitive, emotional, and cultural) influence the pain experience (Rodriguez, 2015). The degree and severity of postoperative pain and the patient's tolerance for pain depend on the incision site, the nature of the surgical procedure, the extent of surgical trauma, the type of anesthesia, and the route of administration. The preoperative preparation received by the patient (including information about what to expect, reassurance, psychological support, and educating specific communication techniques related to pain) is a significant factor in decreasing anxiety, apprehension, the amount of postoperative pain, and PONV (Tinsley & Barone, 2013; Ward, 2014).

Intense pain stimulates the stress response, which adversely affects the cardiac and immune systems. When pain impulses are transmitted, both muscle tension and local vasoconstriction increase, further stimulating pain receptors. This increases myocardial demand and oxygen consumption. The hypothalamic stress response also results in an increase in blood viscosity and platelet aggregation, increasing the risk of thrombosis and PE.

In some states, providers may prescribe different medications or dosages to cover various levels of pain. The nurse discusses these options with the patient to determine the best medication and dosage regimen. The nurse assesses the effectiveness of the medication periodically, beginning 30 minutes after administration, or sooner if the medication is being delivered by patient-controlled analgesia (PCA) (Ward, 2014).

Opioid Analgesic Medications. Opioid analgesic agents are commonly prescribed for pain and immediate postoperative restlessness. A preventive approach, rather than an "as needed" (PRN) approach, is more effective in relieving pain. With a preventive approach, the medication is given at prescribed intervals rather than when the pain becomes severe or unbearable. Many patients (and some health care providers) are overly concerned about the risk of drug addiction in the postoperative patient. However, this risk is negligible with the use of opioid medications for short-term pain control (McGuire & Bolyanatz, 2014).

Patient-Controlled Analgesia. The goal is pain prevention rather than sporadic pain control. Patients recover more quickly when adequate pain relief measures are used, and PCA permits patients to administer their own pain medication when needed. Most patients are candidates for PCA. The two requirements for PCA are an understanding of the need to self-dose and the physical ability to self-dose. The amount of medication delivered by the IV or epidural route and the time span during which the opioid medication is released are controlled by the PCA device. PCA promotes patient participation in care; eliminates delayed administration of analgesic medications; maintains a therapeutic drug level; and enables the patient to move, turn, cough, and take deep breaths with less pain, thus reducing postoperative pulmonary complications (Rothrock, 2014).

Epidural Infusions and Intrapleural Anesthesia. Patients undergoing many types of procedures and surgeries benefit from the use of epidural infusion of opioids (Hayes & Gordon, 2015; Rodriguez, 2015). Epidural infusions are used with caution in chest procedures because the analgesic may ascend along the spinal cord and affect respiration. Intrapleural anesthesia involves the administration of a local anesthetic by a catheter between the parietal and visceral pleura. It provides sensory anesthesia without affecting motor function to the intercostal muscles. This anesthesia allows more effective coughing and deep breathing in conditions such as cholecystectomy, renal surgery, and rib fractures, in which pain in the thoracic region would interfere with these exercises.

A local opioid or a combination anesthetic (opioid plus local anesthetic agent) is used in the epidural infusion.

Other Pain Relief Measures. For pain that is difficult to control, a subcutaneous pain management system may be used. In this system, a nylon catheter is inserted at the site of the affected area. The catheter is attached to a pump that delivers a continuous amount of local anesthetic at a specific amount determined and prescribed by the primary provider (see Fig. 19-4).

Nonpharmacologic measures, such as guided imagery, music, and the implementation of healing touch, have been successful clinical adjuncts used to decrease pain and anxiety (Anderson, Suchicital, Lang, et al., 2015). Changing the patient's position, using distraction, applying cool washcloths to the face, and providing back massage may be useful in relieving general discomfort temporarily, promoting relaxation, and rendering medication more effective when it is given.

PROMOTING CARDIAC OUTPUT

If signs and symptoms of shock or hemorrhage occur, treatment and nursing care are implemented as described in the discussion of care in the PACU and in Chapter 14.

Although most patients do not hemorrhage or go into shock, changes in circulating volume, the stress of surgery, and the effects of medications and preoperative preparations all affect

Clip to patient's gown or dressing

ON-Q pump

Clamp

In-line filter

Catheter

Flow restrictor

Figure 19-4 • Subcutaneous pain management system consists of a pump, filter, and catheter that delivers a specific amount of prescribed local anesthetic at the rate determined by the physician. Redrawn with permission from Kimberly-Clark Corporation, Neenah, WI.

cardiovascular function. IV fluid replacement may be prescribed for up to 24 hours after surgery or until the patient is stable and tolerating oral fluids. Close monitoring is indicated to detect and correct conditions, such as fluid volume deficit, altered tissue perfusion, and decreased cardiac output, all of which can increase the patient's discomfort, place him or her at risk of complications, and prolong the hospital stay. Some patients are at risk for fluid volume excess secondary to existing cardiovascular or renal disease, advanced age, and other factors (Grossman & Porth, 2014). Consequently, fluid replacement must be carefully managed, and intake and output records must be accurate.

Nursing management includes assessing the patency of the IV lines and ensuring that the correct fluids are given at the prescribed rate. Intake and output, including emesis and output from wound drainage systems, are recorded separately and totaled to determine fluid balance. If the patient has an indwelling urinary catheter, hourly outputs are monitored and should not be less than 0.5 mL/kg/h; oliguria is reported immediately (Liddle, 2013a). Electrolyte levels and hemoglobin and hematocrit levels are monitored. Decreased hemoglobin and hematocrit levels can indicate blood loss or dilution of circulating volume by IV fluids. If dilution is contributing to the decreased levels, the hemoglobin and hematocrit will rise as the stress response abates and fluids are mobilized and excreted.

Venous stasis from dehydration, immobility, and pressure on leg veins during surgery put the patient at risk for VTE. Leg exercises and frequent position changes are initiated early in the postoperative period to stimulate circulation. Patients should avoid positions that compromise venous return, such as raising the bed's knee gatch, placing a pillow under the knees, sitting for long periods, and dangling the legs with pressure at the back of the knees. Venous return is promoted by antiembolism stockings and early ambulation.

ENCOURAGING ACTIVITY

Early ambulation has a significant effect on recovery and the prevention of complications (e.g., atelectasis, hypostatic pneumonia, gastrointestinal [GI] discomfort, circulatory problems) (Rothrock, 2014). Postoperative activity orders are checked before the patient is assisted to get out of bed, in many instances, on the evening following surgery. Sitting up at the edge of the bed for a few minutes may be all that the patient who has undergone a major surgical procedure can tolerate at first.

Ambulation reduces postoperative abdominal distention by increasing GI tract and abdominal wall tone and stimulating peristalsis. Early ambulation prevents stasis of blood, and thromboembolic events occur less frequently. Pain is often decreased when early ambulation is possible, and the hospital stay is shorter and less costly.

Despite the advantages of early ambulation, patients may be reluctant to get out of bed on the evening of surgery. Reminding them of the importance of early mobility in preventing complications may help patients overcome their fears. When a patient gets out of bed for the first time, orthostatic hypotension, also called *postural hypotension*, is a concern. Orthostatic hypotension is an abnormal drop in blood pressure that occurs as the patient changes from a supine to a standing position. It is common after surgery because of changes in circulating blood volume and bed rest. Signs and symptoms include a decrease of 20 mm Hg in systolic blood pressure or 10 mm Hg in diastolic blood pressure, weakness, dizziness, and fainting (Weber & Kelley, 2013). Older adults are at increased risk for orthostatic hypotension secondary to age-related changes in vascular tone. To detect orthostatic hypotension, the nurse assesses the patient's blood pressure first in the supine position, after the patient sits up, again after the patient stands, and 2 to 3 minutes later. Gradual position change gives the circulatory system time to adjust. If the patient becomes dizzy, he or she is returned to the supine position, and ambulation is delayed for several hours.

To assist the postoperative patient in getting out of bed for the first time after surgery, the nurse:

1. Helps the patient move gradually from the lying position to the sitting position by raising the head of the bed and encourages the patient to splint the incision when applicable.
2. Positions the patient completely upright (sitting) and turned so that both legs are hanging over the edge of the bed.
3. Helps the patient stand beside the bed.

After becoming accustomed to the upright position, the patient may start to walk. The nurse should be at the patient's side to give physical support and encouragement. Care must be taken not to tire the patient; the extent of the first few periods of ambulation varies with the type of surgical procedure and the patient's physical condition and age.

Whether or not the patient can ambulate early in the postoperative period, bed exercises are encouraged to improve circulation. Bed exercises consist of the following:

- Arm exercises (full range of motion, with specific attention to abduction and external rotation of the shoulder)
- Hand and finger exercises
- Foot exercises to prevent VTE, footdrop, and toe deformities and to aid in maintaining good circulation

- Leg flexion and leg-lifting exercises to prepare the patient for ambulation
- Abdominal and gluteal contraction exercises

Hampered by pain, dressings, IV lines, or drains, many patients cannot engage in activity without assistance. Helping the patient increase their activity level on the first postoperative day is important to prevent complications related to prolonged inactivity. One way to increase the patient's activity is to have the patient perform as much routine hygiene care as possible. Setting up the patient to bathe with a bedside wash basin or, if possible, assisting the patient to the bathroom to sit in a chair at the sink not only gets the patient moving but helps restore a sense of self-control and prepares the patient for discharge.

For a safe discharge to home, patients need to be able to ambulate a functional distance (e.g., length of the house or apartment), get in and out of bed unassisted, and be independent with toileting. Patients can be asked to perform as much as they can and then to call for assistance. The patient and the nurse can collaborate on a schedule for progressive activity that includes ambulating in the room and hallway and sitting out of bed in a chair. Assessing the patient's vital signs

before, during, and after a scheduled activity helps the nurse and patient determine the rate of progression. By providing physical support, the nurse maintains the patient's safety; by communicating a positive attitude about the patient's ability to perform the activity, the nurse promotes the patient's confidence. The nurse encourages the patient to continue to perform bed exercises, wear pneumatic compression or prescribed anti-embolism stockings when in bed, and rest as needed. If the patient has had orthopedic surgery of the lower extremities or will require a mobility aid (i.e., walker, crutches) at home, a physical therapist may be involved the first time the patient gets out of bed to educate him or her to ambulate safely or to use the mobility aid correctly.

CARING FOR WOUNDS

Wound Healing. Wounds heal by different mechanisms, depending on the condition of the wound. Surgical wound healing may occur in three ways, by **first-intention, second-intention**, and **third-intention wound healing** (Rothrock, 2014) (see Chart 19-5). With shorter hospital stays, much of

---

Chart 19-5 — Wound-Healing Mechanisms

First-Intention Healing

Wounds made aseptically with a minimum of tissue destruction that are properly closed heal with little tissue reaction by first intention (primary union). When wounds heal by first-intention healing, granulation tissue is not visible and scar formation is minimal. Postoperatively, many of these wounds are covered with a dry sterile dressing. If a cyanoacrylate tissue adhesive (LiquiBand) has been used to close the incision without sutures, a dressing is contraindicated.

Second-Intention Healing

Second-intention healing (granulation) occurs in infected wounds (abscess) or in wounds in which the edges have not been approximated. When an abscess is incised, it collapses partly, but the dead and dying cells forming its walls are still being released into the cavity. For this reason, a drainage tube or gauze packing is inserted into the abscess pocket to allow drainage to escape easily. Gradually, the necrotic material disintegrates and escapes, and the abscess cavity fills with a red, soft, sensitive tissue that bleeds easily. This tissue is composed of minute, thin-walled capillaries and buds that later form connective tissue. These buds, called *granulations,* enlarge until they fill the area left by the destroyed tissue. The cells surrounding the capillaries change their round shape to become long, thin, and intertwined to form a scar (cicatrix). Healing is complete when skin cells (epithelium) grow over these granulations. This method of repair is referred to as healing by granulation, and it takes place whenever pus is formed or when loss of tissue has occurred for any reason. When the postoperative wound is to be allowed to heal by secondary intention, it is usually packed with saline-moistened sterile dressings and covered with a dry sterile dressing.

Third-Intention Healing

Third-intention healing (secondary suture) is used for deep wounds that either have not been sutured early or break down and are resutured later, thus bringing together two opposing granulation surfaces. This results in a deeper and wider scar.

These wounds are also packed postoperatively with moist gauze and covered with a dry sterile dressing.

A. FIRST INTENTION

Clean incision — Early suture — Hairline scar

B. SECOND INTENTION

Gaping irregular wound — Granulation — Epithelium grows over scar

C. THIRD INTENTION

Wound — Increased granulation — Late suturing with wide scar the healing takes place at home, and both the hospital and the transitional or home care nurse should be informed about the principles of wound healing.

Ongoing assessment of the surgical site involves inspection for approximation of wound edges, integrity of sutures or staples, redness, discoloration, warmth, swelling, unusual tenderness, or drainage. The area around the wound should also be inspected for a reaction to tape or trauma from tight bandages. Many factors, such as adequate nutrition, glycemic control (Klinkner & Murray, 2014), cleanliness, rest, and position determine how quickly healing occurs. These factors are influenced by nursing interventions. Specific nursing assessments and interventions that address these factors and help promote wound healing are presented in Table 19-3.

Caring for Surgical Drains. Nursing interventions to promote wound healing also include management of surgical drains. Drains are tubes that exit the peri-incisional area, either into a portable wound suction device (closed) or into the dressings (open). The principle involved is to allow the escape of fluids that could otherwise serve as a culture medium for bacteria. In portable wound suction, the use of gentle, constant suction enhances drainage of these fluids and collapses the skin flaps against the underlying tissue, thus removing "dead space." Types of wound drains include the Penrose, Hemovac, and Jackson-Pratt drains (see Fig. 19-5). Output (drainage) from wound systems is recorded. The amount of bloody drainage on the surgical dressing is assessed frequently. Spots of drainage on the dressings are outlined with a pen, and the date and time of the outline are recorded on the dressing so that increased drainage can be easily seen. A certain amount of bloody drainage in a wound drainage system or on the dressing is expected, but excessive amounts should be reported to the surgeon. Increasing amounts of fresh blood on the dressing should be reported immediately. Some wounds are irrigated heavily before closure in the OR, and open drains exiting the wound may be embedded in the dressings. These wounds may drain large amounts of blood-tinged fluid that saturate the dressing. The dressing can be reinforced with sterile gauze bandages; the time at which they were reinforced should be documented. If drainage continues, the surgeon should be notified so that the dressing can be changed. Multiple similar drains are numbered or otherwise labeled (e.g., left lower quadrant, left upper quadrant) so that output measurements can be reliably and consistently recorded.

Changing the Dressing. Although the first postoperative dressing is usually changed by a member of the surgical team, subsequent dressing changes in the immediate postoperative period are usually performed by the nurse. A dressing is applied to a wound for one or more of the following reasons: (1) to provide a proper environment for wound healing; (2) to absorb drainage; (3) to splint or immobilize the wound; (4) to protect the wound and new epithelial tissue from mechanical injury; (5) to protect the wound from bacterial contamination and from soiling by feces, vomitus, and urine; (6) to promote hemostasis, as in a pressure dressing; and (7) to provide mental and physical comfort for the patient.

The patient is told that the dressing is to be changed and that changing the dressing is a simple procedure associated with little discomfort. The dressing change is performed at a suitable time (e.g., not at mealtimes or when visitors are present). Privacy is provided, and the patient is not unduly exposed. The nurse should avoid referring to the incision as a *scar* because the term may have negative connotations for the patient. Assurance is given that the incision will shrink as it heals and that the redness will fade.

The nurse performs hand hygiene before and after the dressing change and wears disposable gloves (sterile or clean as needed) for the dressing change itself. Most dressing changes following surgery are sterile. In accordance with standard precautions, dressings are never touched by ungloved hands because of the danger of transmitting pathogenic organisms. The tape or adhesive portion of the dressing is removed by pulling it parallel with the skin surface and in the direction of hair growth rather than at right angles. Alcohol wipes or nonirritating solvents aid in removing adhesive painlessly and quickly. The soiled dressing is removed and deposited in a container designated for disposal of biomedical waste.

Gloves are changed, and a new dressing is applied. If the patient is sensitive to adhesive tape, the dressing may be held in place with hypoallergenic tape. Many tapes are porous to prevent skin maceration. Some wounds become edematous after having been dressed, causing considerable tension on the tape. If the tape is not flexible, the stretching bandage will also cause a shear injury to the skin. This can result in denuded areas or large blisters and should be avoided. An elastic adhesive bandage (Elastoplast, 3M Microfoam) may be used to hold dressings in place over mobile areas, such as the neck or the extremities, or where pressure is required.

While changing the dressing, the nurse has an opportunity to educate the patient in how to care for the incision and change the dressings at home. The nurse observes for indicators of the patient's readiness to learn, such as looking at the incision, expressing interest, or assisting in the dressing change. Information on self-care activities and possible signs of infection is summarized in Chart 19-6.

MAINTAINING NORMAL BODY TEMPERATURE

The patient is still at risk for malignant hyperthermia and hypothermia in the postoperative period. Efforts are made to identify malignant hyperthermia and to treat it early and promptly (Rothrock, 2014). (See the discussion of malignant hyperthermia in Chapter 18.)

Patients who have received anesthesia are susceptible to chills and drafts. Hypothermia management, begun in the intraoperative period, extends into the postoperative period to prevent significant nitrogen loss and catabolism (Liddle, 2013a). Low body temperature is reported to the primary provider. The room is maintained at a comfortable temperature, and blankets are provided to prevent chilling. Treatment includes oxygen administration, adequate hydration, and proper nutrition including glycemic control. The patient is also monitored for cardiac dysrhythmias. The risk of hypothermia is greater in older adults and in patients who were in the cool OR environment for a prolonged period.

MANAGING GASTROINTESTINAL FUNCTION AND RESUMING NUTRITION

Discomfort of the GI tract (nausea, vomiting, and hiccups) and resumption of oral intake are issues for the patient and affect their outcome following surgery. See the earlier discussion of PONV in the PACU.

TABLE 19-3 Factors Affecting Wound Healing

Factors	Rationale	Nursing Interventions
Age of patient	The older the patient, the less resilient the tissues.	Handle all tissues gently.
Handling of tissues	Rough handling causes injury and delayed healing.	Handle tissues carefully and evenly.
Hemorrhage	Accumulation of blood creates dead spaces as well as dead cells that must be removed. The area becomes a growth medium for organisms.	Monitor vital signs. Observe incision site for evidence of bleeding and infection.
Hypovolemia	Insufficient blood volume leads to vasoconstriction and reduced oxygen and nutrients available for wound healing.	Monitor for volume deficit (circulatory impairment). Correct by fluid replacement as prescribed.
Local Factors		
Edema	Reduces blood supply by exerting increased interstitial pressure on vessels.	Elevate part; apply cool compresses.
Inadequate dressing technique:		
Too small	Permits bacterial invasion and contamination.	Follow guidelines for proper dressing technique.
Too tight	Reduces blood supply carrying nutrients and oxygen.	
Nutritional deficits	Protein–calorie depletion may occur. Insulin secretion may be inhibited, causing blood glucose to rise.	Correct deficits; this may require parenteral nutritional therapy. Monitor blood glucose levels. Administer vitamin supplements as prescribed.
Foreign bodies	Foreign bodies retard healing.	Keep wounds free of dressing threads and talcum powder from gloves.
Oxygen deficit (tissue oxygenation insufficient)	Insufficient oxygen may be due to inadequate lung and cardiovascular function as well as localized vasoconstriction.	Encourage deep breathing, turning, and controlled coughing.
Drainage accumulation	Accumulated secretions hamper healing process.	Monitor closed drainage systems for proper functioning. Institute measures to remove accumulated secretions.
Medications		
Corticosteroids	May mask presence of infection by impairing normal inflammatory response	Be aware of action and effect of medications patient is receiving.
Anticoagulants	May cause hemorrhage	
Broad-spectrum and specific antibiotics	Effective if given immediately before surgery for specific pathology or bacterial contamination. If given after wound is closed, ineffective because of intravascular coagulation.	
Patient overactivity	Prevents approximation of wound edges. Resting favors healing.	Use measures to keep wound edges approximated: taping, bandaging, splints. Encourage rest.
Systemic Disorders		
Hemorrhagic shock	These depress cell functions that directly affect wound healing.	Be familiar with the nature of the specific disorder. Administer prescribed treatment. Cultures may be indicated to determine appropriate antibiotic.
Acidosis		
Hypoxia		
Kidney injury		
Hepatic disease		
Sepsis		
Immunosuppressed state	Patient is more vulnerable to bacterial and viral invasion; defense mechanisms are impaired.	Provide maximum protection to prevent infection. Restrict visitors with colds; institute mandatory hand hygiene by all staff.
Wound Stressors		
Vomiting	Produce tension on wounds, particularly of the torso.	Encourage frequent turning and ambulation, and administer antiemetic medications as prescribed. Assist patient in splinting incision.
Valsalva maneuver		
Heavy coughing		
Straining		

Adapted from Edmiston, C. E., & Spencer, M. (2014.) Patient care interventions to help reduce the risk of surgical site infections. *AORN Journal, 100*(6), 590–602.

A

Drain sponge

Loose stitch keeps drain from slipping into wound

B

C

Figure 19-5 • Types of surgical drains: **A.** Penrose. **B.** Jackson–Pratt. **C.** Hemovac.

If the risk of vomiting is high due to the nature of surgery, a nasogastric tube is inserted preoperatively and remains in place throughout the surgery and the immediate postoperative period. A nasogastric tube also may be inserted before surgery if postoperative distention is anticipated. In addition, a nasogastric tube may be inserted if a patient who has food in the stomach requires emergency surgery.

Hiccups, produced by intermittent spasms of the diaphragm secondary to irritation of the phrenic nerve, can occur after surgery. The irritation may be direct, such as from stimulation of the nerve by a distended stomach, subdiaphragmatic abscess, or abdominal distention; indirect, such as from toxemia or uremia that stimulates the nerve; or reflexive, such as from irritation from a drainage tube or obstruction of the intestines. These occurrences usually are mild, transitory attacks that cease spontaneously. If hiccups persist, they may produce considerable distress and serious effects, such as vomiting, exhaustion, and wound dehiscence. The physician may prescribe phenothiazine medications (e.g., chlorpromazine [Thorazine]) for intractable hiccups (Thanavaro, 2015).

> ⚑ **Quality and Safety Nursing Alert**
>
> *Any condition that is persistent or considered intractable, such as hiccups, should be reported to the primary provider so that appropriate measures can be implemented.*

Once PONV have subsided and the patient is fully awake and alert, the sooner he or she can tolerate a usual diet, the more quickly normal GI function will resume. Taking food by mouth stimulates digestive juices and promotes gastric function and intestinal peristalsis. The return to normal dietary

---

Chart 19-6

PATIENT EDUCATION
Wound Care Instructions

Until Sutures Are Removed

1. Keep the wound dry and clean.
   - If there is no dressing, ask your nurse or physician if you can bathe or shower.
   - If a dressing or splint is in place, do not remove it unless it is wet or soiled.
   - If wet or soiled, change dressing yourself if you have been taught to do so; otherwise, call your nurse or physician for guidance.
   - If you have been taught, instruction might be as follows:
     - Cleanse area *gently* with sterile normal saline once or twice daily.
     - Cover with a sterile Telfa pad™ or gauze square large enough to cover wound.
     - Apply hypoallergenic tape (Dermicel™ or paper). Adhesive is not recommended because it is difficult to remove without possible injury to the incisional site.
2. Immediately report any of these signs of infection:
   - Redness, marked swelling exceeding 0.5 in (2.5 cm) from incision site; tenderness; or increased warmth around wound
   - Red streaks in skin near wound
   - Pus or discharge, foul odor
   - Chills or temperature higher than 37.7°C (100°F)
3. If soreness or pain causes discomfort, apply a dry cool pack (containing ice or cold water) or take prescribed

acetaminophen tablets every 4–6 h. Avoid using aspirin without direction or instruction because bleeding can occur with its use.
4. Swelling after surgery is common. To help reduce swelling, elevate the affected part to the level of the heart.
   - Hand or arm:
     - Sleep—elevate arm on pillow at side
     - Sitting—place arm on pillow on adjacent table
     - Standing—rest affected hand on opposite shoulder; support elbow with unaffected hand
   - Leg or foot:
     - Sitting—place a pillow on a facing chair; provide support underneath the knee
     - Lying—place a pillow under affected leg

After Sutures Are Removed

Although the wound appears to be healed when sutures are removed, it is still tender and will continue to heal and strengthen for several weeks.
1. Follow recommendations of physician or nurse regarding extent of activity.
2. Keep suture line clean; do not rub vigorously; pat dry. Wound edges may look red and may be slightly raised. This is normal.
3. If the site continues to be red, thick, and painful to pressure after 8 wks, consult the health care provider. (This may be due to excessive collagen formation and should be checked.)

intake should proceed at a pace set by the patient. The nature of the surgery and the type of anesthesia directly affect the rate at which normal gastric activity resumes. Research suggests patients undergoing colon surgery have more energy and higher protein levels when nutritional supplements are started in the PACU compared with patients who did not receive supplements (Grode & Sogaard, 2014).

Clear liquids are typically the first substances desired and tolerated by the patient after surgery. Water, juice, and tea may be given in increasing amounts. Cool fluids are tolerated more easily than those that are ice cold or hot. Soft foods (gelatin, custard, milk, and creamed soups) are added gradually after clear fluids have been tolerated. As soon as the patient tolerates soft foods well, solid food may be given.

Assessment and management of GI function are important after surgery because the GI tract is subject to uncomfortable or potentially life-threatening complications. Any postoperative patient may suffer from distention. Postoperative distention of the abdomen results from the accumulation of gas in the intestinal tract. Manipulation of the abdominal organs during surgery may produce a loss of normal peristalsis for 24 to 48 hours, depending on the type and extent of surgery. Even though nothing is given by mouth, swallowed air and GI tract secretions enter the stomach and intestines; if not propelled by peristalsis, they collect in the intestines, producing distention and causing the patient to complain of fullness or pain in the abdomen. Most often, the gas collects in the colon. Abdominal distention is further increased by immobility, anesthetic agents, and the use of opioid medications.

After major abdominal surgery, distention may be avoided by having the patient turn frequently, exercise, and ambulate as early as possible. This also alleviates distention produced by swallowing air, which is common in anxious patients. A nasogastric tube inserted before surgery may remain in place until full peristaltic activity (indicated by the passage of flatus) has resumed. The nurse detects bowel sounds by listening to the abdomen with a stethoscope. Bowel sounds are documented so that diet progression can occur.

Paralytic ileus and intestinal obstruction are potential postoperative complications that occur more frequently in patients undergoing intestinal or abdominal surgery. (Refer to Chapter 47 for discussion of treatment.)

PROMOTING BOWEL FUNCTION

Constipation can occur after surgery as a minor or a serious complication. Decreased mobility, decreased oral intake, and opioid analgesic medications can contribute to difficulty having a bowel movement. In addition, irritation and trauma to the bowel during surgery may inhibit intestinal movement for several days. The combined effect of early ambulation, improved dietary intake, and a stool softener (if prescribed) promotes bowel elimination. Research suggests that chewing gum, particularly following laprascopic surgery, can help restore bowel function and prevent paralytic ileus by promoting peristalsis (Keenahan, 2014). The nurse should assess the abdomen for distention and the presence and frequency of bowel sounds. If the patient does not have a bowel movement by the second or third postoperative day, the primary provider should be notified and a laxative or other test or intervention may be needed.

MANAGING VOIDING

Urinary retention after surgery can occur for various reasons. Anesthetics, anticholinergic agents, and opioids interfere with the perception of bladder fullness and the urge to void and inhibit the ability to initiate voiding and completely empty the bladder. Abdominal, pelvic, and hip surgery may increase the likelihood of retention secondary to pain. In addition, some patients find it difficult to use the bedpan or urinal in the recumbent position.

Bladder distention and the urge to void should be assessed at the time of the patient's arrival on the unit and frequently thereafter. The patient is expected to void within 8 hours after surgery (this includes time spent in the PACU). If the patient has an urge to void and cannot, or if the bladder is distended and no urge is felt or the patient cannot void, catheterization is not delayed solely on the basis of the 8-hour time frame. All methods to encourage the patient to void should be tried (e.g., letting water run, applying heat to the perineum). The bedpan should be warm; a cold bedpan causes discomfort and automatic tightening of muscles (including the urethral sphincter). If the patient cannot void on a bedpan, it may be possible to use a commode or a toilet (if there is one in the PACU). Male patients are often permitted to sit up or stand beside the bed to use the urinal; however, safeguards should be taken to prevent the patient from falling or fainting due to loss of coordination from medications or orthostatic hypotension. If the patient has not voided within the specified time frame, an ultrasound bladder scan or bladder ultrasonography is performed to check for urinary retention (see Chapter 53 Fig. 53-8). The patient is catheterized, and the catheter is removed after the bladder has emptied. Straight intermittent catheterization is preferred over indwelling catheterization because the risk of infection is increased with an indwelling catheter.

Even if the patient voids, the bladder may not necessarily be empty. The nurse notes the amount of urine voided and palpates the suprapubic area for distention or tenderness. Postvoid residual urine may be assessed by using either straight catheterization or an ultrasound bladder scanner and is considered diagnostic of urinary retention. Intermittent catheterization may be prescribed every 4 to 6 hours until the patient can void spontaneously and the postvoid residual is less than 50 mL in the middle-aged adult and less than 50 to 100 mL in the older adult (Weber & Kelley 2013).

MAINTAINING A SAFE ENVIRONMENT

During the immediate postoperative period, the patient recovering from anesthesia should have three side rails up, and the bed should be in the low position. The nurse assesses the patient's level of consciousness and orientation and determines whether the patient can resume wearing assistive devices as needed (e.g., eyeglasses, hearing aid). Impaired vision, inability to hear postoperative instructions, or inability to communicate verbally places the patient at risk for injury. All objects the patient may need should be within reach, especially the call light. Any immediate postoperative orders concerning special positioning, equipment, or interventions should be implemented as soon as possible. The patient is instructed to ask for assistance with any activity. Although restraints are occasionally necessary for the disoriented patient, they should be avoided if at all possible.

Agency policy on the use of restraints must be consulted and followed.

Any surgical procedure has the potential for injury due to disrupted neurovascular integrity resulting from prolonged awkward positioning in the OR, manipulation of tissues, inadvertent severing of nerves or blood vessels, or tight bandages. Any orthopedic or neurologic surgery or surgery involving the extremities carries a risk of peripheral nerve damage. Vascular surgeries, such as replacement of sections of diseased peripheral arteries or insertion of an arteriovenous graft, put the patient at risk for thrombus formation at the surgical site and subsequent ischemia of tissues distal to the thrombus. Assessment includes having the patient move the hand or foot distal to the surgical site through a full range of motion, assessing all surfaces for intact sensation, and assessing peripheral pulses (Rothrock, 2014).

PROVIDING EMOTIONAL SUPPORT TO THE PATIENT AND FAMILY

Although patients and families are undoubtedly relieved that surgery is over, stress and anxiety levels may remain high in the immediate postoperative period. Many factors contribute to this stress and anxiety, including pain, being in an unfamiliar environment, inability to control one's circumstances or care for oneself, fear of the long-term effects of surgery, fear of complications, fatigue, spiritual distress, altered role responsibilities, ineffective coping, and altered body image, and all are potential reactions to the surgical experience. The nurse helps the patient and family work through their stress and anxieties by providing reassurance and information and by spending time listening to and addressing their concerns. The nurse describes hospital routines and what to expect in the time until discharge and explains the purpose of nursing assessments and interventions. Informing patients when they will be able to drink fluids or eat, when they will be getting out of bed, and when tubes and drains will be removed helps them gain a sense of control and participation in recovery and engages them in the plan of care. Acknowledging family members' concerns and accepting and encouraging their participation in the patient's care assist them in feeling that they are helping their loved one. The nurse can modify the environment to enhance rest and relaxation by providing privacy, reducing noise, adjusting lighting, providing enough seating for family members, and encouraging a supportive atmosphere.

MANAGING POTENTIAL COMPLICATIONS

The postoperative patient is at risk for complications as outlined next and summarized in Table 19-4.

Venous Thromboembolism. Serious potential VTE complications of surgery include DVT and PE (Rothrock, 2014).

Prophylactic treatment is common for patients at high risk for VTE. Low-molecular-weight or low-dose heparin and low-dose warfarin (Coumadin) are other anticoagulants that may be used (Harrington, 2013). External pneumatic compression and anti-embolism stockings can be used alone or in combination with low-dose heparin. The stress response that is initiated by surgery inhibits the thrombolytic (fibrinolytic) system, resulting in blood hypercoagulability. Dehydration, low cardiac output, blood pooling in the extremities, and bed rest add to the risk of thrombosis formation. Although all postoperative patients are at some risk, factors such as a history of thrombosis, malignancy, trauma, obesity, indwelling

TABLE 19-4 Selected Postoperative Complications

Body System/Type	Complications
Respiratory	Atelectasis, pneumonia, pulmonary embolism, aspiration
Cardiovascular	Shock, thrombophlebitis
Neurologic	Delirium, stroke
Skin/wound	Breakdown, infection, dehiscence, evisceration, delayed healing, hemorrhage, hematoma
Gastrointestinal	Constipation, paralytic ileus, bowel obstruction
Urinary	Acute urine retention, urinary tract infection
Functional	Weakness, fatigue, functional decline
Thromboembolic	Deep vein thrombosis, pulmonary embolism

venous catheters, and hormone use (e.g., estrogen) increase the risk. The first symptom of DVT may be a pain or cramp in the calf although many patients are asymptomatic. Initial pain and tenderness may be followed by a painful swelling of the entire leg, often accompanied by fever, chills, and diaphoresis (Harrington, 2013).

The benefits of early ambulation and leg exercises in preventing DVT cannot be overemphasized, and these activities are recommended for all patients, regardless of their risk. It is important to avoid the use of blanket rolls, pillow rolls, or any form of elevation that can constrict vessels under the knees. Even prolonged "dangling" (having the patient sit on the edge of the bed with legs hanging over the side) can be dangerous and is not recommended in susceptible patients because pressure under the knees can impede circulation. Adequate hydration is also encouraged; the patient can be offered juices and water throughout the day to avoid dehydration. (Refer Chapter 30 for discussion of DVT and Chapter 23 for discussion of PE.)

Hematoma. At times, concealed bleeding occurs beneath the skin at the surgical site. This hemorrhage usually stops spontaneously but results in clot (hematoma) formation within the wound. If the clot is small, it will be absorbed and need not be treated. If the clot is large, the wound usually bulges somewhat, and healing will be delayed unless the clot is removed. Several sutures are removed by the surgeon, the clot is evacuated, and the wound is packed lightly with gauze. Healing occurs usually by granulation, or a secondary closure may be performed.

Infection (Wound Sepsis). The creation of a surgical wound disrupts the integrity of the skin, bypassing the body's primary defense and protection against infection. Exposure of deep body tissues to pathogens in the environment places the patient at risk for infection of the surgical site, and a potentially life-threatening complication such as infection can increase the length of hospital stay, costs of care, and risk of further complications.

Joint Commission-approved hospitals measure surgical site infections (SSIs) for the first 30 or 90 days following surgical procedures based on national standards. Overall there

TABLE 19-5 Wound Classification and Associated Surgical Site Infection Risk

Surgical Category	Determinants of Category	Expected Risk of Postsurgical Infection (%)
Clean	Nontraumatic site Uninfected site No inflammation No break in aseptic technique No entry into respiratory, alimentary, genitourinary, or oropharyngeal tracts	1–3
Clean contaminated	Entry into respiratory, alimentary, genitourinary, or oropharyngeal tracts without unusual contamination Appendectomy Minor break in aseptic technique Mechanical drainage	3–7
Contaminated	Open, newly experienced traumatic wounds Gross spillage from gastrointestinal tract Major break in aseptic technique Entry into genitourinary or biliary tract when urine or bile is infected	7–16
Dirty	Traumatic wound with delayed repair, devitalized tissue, foreign bodies, or fecal contamination Acute inflammation and purulent drainage encountered during procedure	16–29

Adapted from Edmiston, C. E., & Spencer, M. (2014.) Patient care interventions to help reduce the risk of surgical site infections. *AORN Journal, 100*(6), 590–602.

has been a 20% decrease in SSIs for a number of surgical procedures (Edmiston & Spencer, 2014). Reduction of SSIs remains an important national safety goal (see Chart 17-8) (Joint Commission, 2016).

Multiple factors, including the type of wound, place the patient at potential risk for infection. Surgical wounds are classified according to the degree of contamination. Table 19-5 defines the classification of surgical wounds and SSI rates per category. Patient-related factors include age, nutritional status, diabetes, smoking, obesity, remote infections, endogenous mucosal microorganisms, altered immune response, length of preoperative stay, and severity of illness (Rothrock, 2014). Factors related to the surgical procedure include the method of preoperative skin preparation, surgical attire of the team, method of sterile draping, duration of surgery, antimicrobial prophylaxis, aseptic technique, factors related to surgical technique, drains or foreign material, OR ventilation, length of procedure, and exogenous microorganisms (Edmiston & Spencer, 2014; Pada & Perl, 2015). Other risk factors for wound sepsis include wound contamination, foreign body, faulty suturing technique, devitalized tissue, hematoma, debilitation, dehydration, malnutrition, anemia, obesity, shock, duration of surgical procedure, and associated disorders (e.g., diabetes) (Gadler, Gardiner & Martinez, 2014). Efforts to prevent wound infection are directed at reducing risks. (Preoperative and intraoperative risks and interventions are discussed in Chapters 17 and 18.) Postoperative care of the wound centers on assessing the wound, preventing contamination and infection before wound edges have sealed, and enhancing healing.

Wound infection may not be evident until at least postoperative day 5. Most patients are discharged before that time, and more than half of wound infections are diagnosed after discharge, highlighting the importance of patient education regarding wound care (Liddle, 2013a; Penprase & Johnson, 2015). Signs and symptoms of wound infection include increased pulse rate and temperature; an elevated white blood cell count; wound swelling, warmth, tenderness, or discharge; and increased incisional pain. Local signs may be absent if the infection is deep. *Staphylococcus aureus* accounts for many postoperative wound infections. Other infections may result from *Escherichia coli, Proteus vulgaris, Aerobacter aerogenes, Pseudomonas aeruginosa,* and other organisms. Although they are rare, beta-hemolytic streptococcal or clostridial infections can be rapid and deadly and need strict infection control practices to prevent the spread of infection to others. Intensive medical and nursing care is essential if the patient is to survive (Ackley & Ladwig, 2013).

When a wound infection is diagnosed in a surgical incision, the surgeon may remove one or more sutures or staples and, using aseptic precautions, separate the wound edges with a pair of blunt scissors or a hemostat. Once the incision is opened, a drain is inserted. If the infection is deep, an incision and drainage procedure may be necessary. Antimicrobial therapy and a wound care regimen are also initiated.

Wound Dehiscence and Evisceration. Wound **dehiscence** (disruption of surgical incision or wound) and **evisceration** (protrusion of wound contents) are serious surgical complications (see Fig. 19-6). Dehiscence and evisceration are especially serious when they involve abdominal incisions or wounds. These complications result from sutures giving way, from infection, or, more frequently, from marked distention or strenuous cough. They may also occur because of increasing age, anemia, poor nutritional status, obesity, malignancy, diabetes, the use of steroids, and other factors in patients undergoing abdominal surgery (Meiner, 2014).

When the wound edges separate slowly, the intestines may protrude gradually or not at all, and the earliest sign may be a gush of bloody (serosanguineous) peritoneal fluid from the wound. When a wound ruptures suddenly, coils of intestine may push out of the abdomen. The patient may report that "something gave way." The evisceration causes pain and may be associated with vomiting.

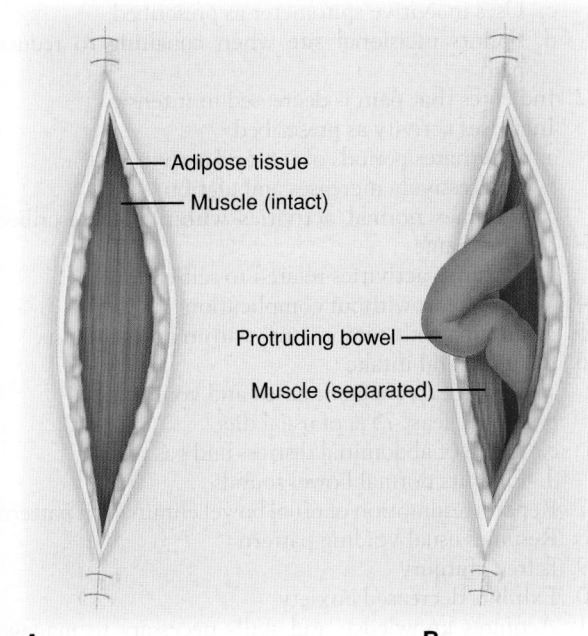

Figure 19-6 • A. Wound dehiscence. **B.** Wound evisceration.

> ▶ *Quality and Safety Nursing Alert*
>
> *If disruption of a wound occurs, the patient is placed in the low Fowler's position and instructed to lie quietly. These actions minimize protrusion of body tissues. The protruding coils of intestine are covered with sterile dressings moistened with sterile saline solution, and the surgeon is notified at once.*

An abdominal binder can provide support and guard against dehiscence and may be used along with the primary dressing, especially in patients with weak or pendulous abdominal walls or when rupture of a wound has occurred.

Gerontologic Considerations. Older patients recover more slowly, have longer hospital stays, and are at greater risk for development of postoperative complications. Delirium, pneumonia, decline in functional ability, exacerbation of comorbid conditions, pressure ulcers, decreased oral intake, GI disturbance, and falls are all threats to recovery in the older adult (Tabloski, 2013). Expert nursing care can help the older adult avoid these complications or minimize their effects (Rothrock, 2014).

Postoperative delirium, characterized by confusion, perceptual and cognitive deficits, altered attention levels, disturbed sleep patterns (Makic, 2014), and impaired psychomotor skills, is a significant problem for older adults (Meiner, 2014). Causes of delirium are multifactorial (see Chart 19-7). Skilled and frequent assessment of mental status and of all physiologic factors influencing mental status helps the nurse plan for care because delirium may be the initial or only indicator of infection, fluid and electrolyte imbalance, or deterioration of respiratory or hemodynamic status in the older adult patient. Factors that determine whether a patient is at risk for delirium include age, history of alcohol abuse, preoperative cognitive function, physical function, serum chemistries, and type of surgery.

| Chart 19-7 | Potential Causes of Postoperative Delirium |

- Acid–base disturbances
- Acute myocardial infarction
- Age >80 years
- Alcohol withdrawal
- Blood loss
- Cerebral hypoxia
- Decreased cardiac output
- Dehydration
- Emergent surgery
- Fecal impaction
- Fluid and electrolyte imbalance
- Heart failure
- High stress or anxiety levels
- History of dementia like symptoms
- Hypercarbia
- Hypothermia or hyperthermia
- Hypoxia
- Infection (urinary tract, wound, respiratory)
- Medications (anticholinergics, benzodiazepines, central nervous system depressants)
- Polypharmacy
- Presence of multiple diseases
- Sensory impairments
- Unfamiliar surroundings and sensory deprivation
- Unrelieved pain
- Urinary retention

Recognizing postoperative delirium and identifying and treating its underlying cause are the goals of care. Postoperative delirium is sometimes mistaken for preexisting dementia or is attributed to age. In addition to monitoring and managing identifiable causes, the nurse implements supportive interventions. Keeping the patient in a well-lit room and in close proximity to staff can reduce sensory deprivation. At the same time, distracting and unfamiliar noises should be minimized. Because pain can contribute to postoperative delirium, adequate pain control without oversedation is essential (Rothrock, 2014).

The patient is reoriented as often as necessary, and staff should introduce themselves each time they come in contact with the patient. Engaging the patient in conversation and care activities and placing a clock and calendar nearby may improve cognitive function. Physical activity should not be neglected while the patient is confused because physical deterioration can worsen delirium and place the patient at increased risk for other complications. Restraints should be avoided because they can worsen confusion. A staff member is asked to stay with the patient instead. Medications may be given during episodes of acute confusion but should be discontinued as soon as possible to avoid side effects.

Other problems confronting the older postoperative patient, such as pneumonia, altered bowel function, DVT, weakness, and functional decline, often can be prevented by early and progressive ambulation. Prolonged sitting positions are avoided at they promote venous stasis in the lower extremities. A physical therapy referral may be indicated to promote safe, regular exercise for the older adult.

Urinary incontinence can be prevented by providing easy access to the call bell and the commode and by prompting voiding. Early ambulation and familiarity with the room help the patient become self-sufficient sooner.

Optimal nutritional status (including control of hyperglycemia) is important for wound healing (Klinkner & Murray, 2014), return of normal bowel function, and fluid and electrolyte balance. The nurse and patient can consult with the dietitian to plan appealing, high-protein meals that provide sufficient fiber, calories, and vitamins. Nutritional supplements, such as Ensure™ or Sustacal™, may be recommended. Multivitamins, iron, and vitamin C supplements may be prescribed to aid in tissue healing, formation of new red blood cells, and overall nutritional status.

In addition to monitoring and managing physiologic recovery of the older adult, the nurse identifies and addresses psychosocial needs. The older adult may require much encouragement and support to resume activities, and the pace may be slow. Sensory deficits may require frequent repetition of instructions, and decreased physiologic reserve may necessitate frequent rest periods. The older adult may require extensive discharge planning to coordinate both professional and family care providers, and the nurse, social worker, or nurse case manager may institute the plan for continuing and transitional care.

PROMOTING HOME, COMMUNITY-BASED, OR TRANSITIONAL CARE

Patient Self-Care. Patients often need detailed discharge instructions to become proficient in self-care needs and prevent readmission after surgery (Gadler et al., 2014). Although needs are specific to individual patients and the procedures they have undergone, general patient education needs prior to discharge have been identified (see Chart 19-3).

Continuing and Transitional Care. Community-based and transitional care services are frequently necessary after surgery. Older patients, patients who live alone, patients without family support, and patients with preexisting chronic illness or disabilities are often in greatest need. Planning for discharge involves arranging for necessary services early in the acute care hospitalization for wound care, drain management, catheter care, infusion therapy, and physical or occupational therapy. The home, community-based, or transitional care nurse coordinates these activities and services.

During home visits, the nurse assesses the patient for postoperative complications by assessment of the surgical incision, respiratory and cardiovascular status, adequacy of pain management, fluid and nutritional status, and the patient's progress in returning to preoperative status. The nurse evaluates the patient's and family's ability to manage dressing changes and drainage systems and other devices and to administer prescribed medications. The nurse may change dressings or catheters if needed. The nurse identifies any additional services that are needed and assists the patient and family to arrange for them. Previous education is reinforced, and the patient is reminded to keep follow-up appointments. The patient and family are instructed about signs and symptoms to be reported to the surgeon. In addition, the nurse provides information about how to obtain needed supplies and suggests resources or support groups.

Evaluation

Expected patient outcomes may include the following:

1. Maintains optimal respiratory function
   a. Performs deep-breathing exercises
   b. Displays clear breath sounds
   c. Uses incentive spirometer as prescribed
   d. Splints incisional site when coughing to reduce pain
2. Indicates that pain is decreased in intensity
3. Increases activity as prescribed
   a. Alternates periods of rest and activity
   b. Progressively increases ambulation
   c. Resumes normal activities within the prescribed time frame
   d. Performs activities related to self-care
4. Wound heals without complication
5. Maintains body temperature within normal limits
6. Resumes oral intake
   a. Reports absence of nausea and vomiting
   b. Eats at least 75% of usual diet
   c. Is free of abdominal distress and gas pains
   d. Exhibits normal bowel sounds
7. Reports resumption of usual bowel elimination pattern
8. Resumes usual voiding pattern
9. Is free of injury
10. Exhibits decreased anxiety
11. Acquires knowledge and skills necessary to manage regimen after discharge
12. Experiences no complications

CRITICAL THINKING EXERCISES

1 A 38-year-old woman is admitted to the PACU following open abdominal surgery for excision of a benign tumor and lysis of adhesions. The patient has been a smoker for many years and begins coughing as soon as she is transferred from the OR stretcher to the bed in PACU. Identify the initial assessments that need to be done on this patient. Develop a nursing plan of care that addresses her care from admission to the unit until discharge home. How will you modify the plan of care if the patient needs wound care after discharge? What would be the signs and symptoms you would assess this patient for and why? What would you do differently if the surgery had been done using minimally invasive methods?

2 **pq** A 60-year-old man who is morbidly obese and has a history of diabetes is admitted to the PACU following a laparoscopic procedure and is scheduled to be discharged home. Identify the essential information you would need reported from the OR team. What are the immediate priorities in delivering care to this patient? He is transferred to Phase II PACU. What are the priorities for discharge instructions and education for this patient?

3 **ebp** An 80-year-old man has had a right total knee replacement. The anesthesia given was a spinal anesthetic. What signs and symptoms might he exhibit as he awakens from the surgery? What complications should the PACU nurse observe the patient for as he recovers? Describe an evidence-based nursing care plan for the patient during his hospital stay.

REFERENCES

*Asterisk indicates nursing research.
**Double asterisk indicates classic reference.

Books

Ackley, B. J., & Ladwig, G. B. (2013). *Nursing diagnosis handbook: An evidence-based guide to planning care* (10th ed.). St. Louis, MO: Mosby.

American Society of PeriAnesthesia Nurses (ASPAN). (2015). *2015–2017 Perianesthesia nursing standards, practice recommendations and interpretive statements.* Cherry Hill, NJ: Author.

Association of PeriOperative Registered Nurses (AORN). (2014). *Association of PeriOperative Registered Nurses (AORN) standards, recommended practice, and guidelines.* Denver, CO: Author.

Barash, P. G., Cullen, B. F., Stoelting, R. K., et al. (2013). *Clinical anesthesia* (7th ed.). Philadelphia, PA: Lippincott Williams & Wilkins.

Comerford, K. C. (2015). *Nursing 2015 drug handbook.* Philadelphia, PA: Wolters Kluwer.

Dudek, S. G. (2013). *Nutrition essentials for nursing practice* (7th ed.). Philadelphia, PA: Lippincott Williams & Wilkins.

Grossman, S. C., & Porth, C. M. (2014). *Pathophysiology: Concepts of altered health states* (9th ed.). Philadelphia, PA: Lippincott Williams & Wilkins.

Meiner, S. E. (2014). *Gerontologic nursing* (5th ed.). St. Louis, MO: Elsevier Mosby.

Rothrock, J. C. (Ed.). (2014). *Alexander's care of the patient in surgery* (15th ed.). St. Louis, MO: Mosby.

Tabloski, P. A. (2013). *Gerontological nursing: The essential guide to clinical practice* (2nd ed.). Upper Saddle River, NJ: Prentice Hall Health.

Weber, J., & Kelley, J. H. (2013). *Health assessment in nursing* (5th ed.). Philadelphia, PA: Lippincott Williams & Wilkins.

Journals and Electronic Documents

**Aldrete, A., & Wright, A. (1992). Revised Aldrete score for discharge. *Anesthesiology News, 18*(1), 17.

Allison, J., & George, M. (2014). Using preoperative assessment and patient instruction to improve patient safety. *AORN Journal, 99*(3), 364–375.

*Anderson, J. G., Suchicital, L., Lang, M., et al. (2015). The effects of healing touch on pain, nausea, and anxiety following bariatric surgery: A pilot study. *The Journal of Science and Healing, 11*(3), 208–216.

Edmiston, C. E., & Spencer, M. (2014.) Patient care interventions to help reduce the risk of surgical site infections. *AORN Journal, 100*(6), 590–602.

Gadler, T., Gardiner, A., & Martinez, N. (2014). Caring for the postoperative patient with complications presenting to the emergency department. *Advanced Emergency Nursing Journal, 36*(2), 134–144.

Gallagher, K., & Vacchiano, C. (2014). Reexamining traditional intraoperative fluid administration: Evolving views in the age of goal-directed therapy. *AANA Journal, 82*(3), 235–242.

*Grode, L. B., & Sogaard, A. (2014). Improvement of nutritional care after colon surgery: The impact of early oral nutrition in the postanesthesia care unit. *Journal of PeriAnesthesia Nursing, 29*(4), 266–274.

Keenahan, M. (2014). Does gum chewing prevent postoperative paralytic ileus? *Nursing, 44*(6), 1–2.

Harrington, D. (2013). Preventing and recognizing venous thromboembolism after obstetric and gynecologic surgery. *Nursing for Women's Health Journal, 17*(4), 325–329.

Hayes, K., & Gordon, D. B. (2015). Delivering quality pain management: The challenge for nurses. *AORN Journal, 101*(3), 335–337.

Helvig, A. W., Minick, P., & Patrick, D. (2014). Postoperative management of patients with obstructive sleep apnea: Implications for the medical-surgical nurse. *Medsurg Nursing, 2*(3), 171–177.

*Hodge, N. S., McCarthy, M. S., & Peirce, R. M. (2014). A prospective randomized study of the effectiveness of aromatherapy for relief of postoperative nausea and vomiting. *Journal of PeriAnesthesia Nursing, 29*(1), 5–11.

Joint Commission. (2016). 2016 National Patient Safety Goals. Retrieved on 12/9/2015 at: www.jointcommission.org/standards_information/npsgs.aspx

Klinkner, G., & Murray, M. (2014). Clinical nurse specialists lead teams to impact glycemic control after cardiac surgery. *Clinical nurse specialist, 28*(4), 240–246.

Liddle, C. (2013a). Principles of monitoring postoperative patients. *Nursing Times, 109*(22), 24–26.

Liddle, C. (2013b). How to reduce the risk of deterioration after surgery. *Nursing Times, 109*(23), 16–17.

Makic, M. B. F. (2014). Enhancing sleep in critically ill perianesthesia patients. *Journal of PeriAnesthesia Nursing, 29*(2), 140–142.

McGuire, L., & Bolyanatz, P. (2014). Dispelling pain myths. *American Nurse Today, 9*(7), 8–10.

Noble, K. A., & Pasero, C. (2014). Opioid-induced ventilatory impairment (OIVI). *Journal of PeriAnesthesia Nursing, 29*(2), 143–151.

Oster, K. A., & Oster, C. A. (2015). Special needs population: Care of the geriatric patient population in the perioperative setting. *AORN Journal, 101*(6), 444–456.

Penprase, B., & Johnson, C. (2015). Optimizing the perioperative nursing role for the older adult surgical patient. *OR Nurse, 8*(4), 26–33.

Pada, S., & Perl, T.M. (2015). Operating room myths: What is the evidence for common practices? *Current opinion in infectious diseases, 28*(4), 369–374.

Rodriguez, L. (2015). Pathophysiology of pain: Implications for perioperative nursing. *AORN Journal, 101*(3), 338–344.

Rosen, H. I., Bergh, I. H. E., Schwartz-Barcott, D., et al. (2014). The recovery process after day surgery within the symptom management theory. *Nursing Forum, 49*(2), 100–110.

*Sites, D. S., Johnson, N. T., Miller, J. A., et al. (2014). Controlled breathing with or without peppermint aromatherapy for postoperative nausea and/or vomiting symptom relief: A randomized controlled trial. *Journal of PeriAnesthesia Nursing, 29*(1) 12–19.

Thanavaro, J. L. (2015). Cardiac risk assessment: Decreasing postoperative complications. *AORN Journal, 101*(2), 201–212.

Tinsley, M. H., & Barone, C. P. (2013). Preventing postoperative nausea and vomiting. *Nursing, 43*(12), 42–50.

Ward, C. W. (2014). Procedure-specific postoperative pain management. *MedSurg Nursing, 23*(2), 107–110.

Resources

American Academy of Ambulatory Care Nursing (AAACN), www.aaacn.org

American Society of PeriAnesthesia Nurses (ASPAN), www.aspan.org

Association of PeriOperative Registered Nurses (AORN), www.aorn.org

Malignant Hyperthermia Association of the United States (MHAUS), www.mhaus.org

UNIT 5

Gas Exchange and Respiratory Function

Case Study

PREVENTING READMISSIONS IN PATIENTS WITH COPD

A 55-year-old woman is admitted to the medical unit for an exacerbation of chronic obstructive pulmonary disease (COPD). The nurse notes that this patient was on the unit two weeks ago and has experienced several hospital admissions in the past year for exacerbations. The nurse manager observes that recently the unit has had an increase in 30-day hospital readmissions of patients with exacerbations of COPD. The manager then asks the nurse to chair a task force to examine how to decrease the rate of 30-day hospital readmissions among patients with COPD.

QSEN Competency Focus: Quality Improvement (QI)

The complexities inherent in today's health care system challenges nurses to demonstrate integration of specific inter-disciplinary core competencies. These competencies are aimed at ensuring the delivery of safe, quality patient care (Institute of Medicine, 2003). The Quality and Safety Education for Nurses project (QSEN, 2017; Cronenwett, Sherwood, Barnsteiner, et al., 2007) provides a framework for the knowledge, skills, and attitudes (KSA) required for nurses to demonstrate competency in these key areas, which include **patient-centered care, interdisciplinary teamwork and collaboration, evidence-based practice, quality improvement, safety,** and **informatics.**

Quality Improvement Definition: Use data to monitor the outcomes of care processes and use improvement methods to design and test changes to continuously improve the quality and safety of health care systems.

SELECTED PRE-LICENSURE KSAs	APPLICATION AND REFLECTION
Knowledge	
Describe strategies for learning about the outcomes of care in the setting in which one is engaged in clinical practice.	Identify why patients with COPD may be at risk for hospital readmissions. Describe how you, as the task force chairperson, could verify whether 30-day hospital readmissions have increased. What data would provide benchmarks for 30-day hospital readmissions?
Skills	
Seek information about outcomes of care for populations served in care setting.	As you analyze the data, you find that there appears to be a higher rate of 30-day hospital readmissions of patients with COPD discharged from the hospital to skilled nursing facilities compared to those discharged to home. Describe how you can use this information to develop interventions to decrease 30-day hospital readmissions among patients with COPD.
Attitudes	
Appreciate that continuous quality improvement is an essential part of the daily work of all health professionals.	Reflect on your role in decreasing the rates of 30-day readmission of patients with COPD. How do you feel this will impact your unit, the hospital, local long term care facilities, home care services, and the quality of life for the patients you provide care for?

Cronenwett, L., Sherwood, G., Barnsteiner, J., et al. (2007). Quality and safety education for nurses. *Nursing Outlook, 55*(3), 122–131.
Institute of Medicine. (2003). *Health professions education: A bridge to quality.* Washington, DC: National Academies Press.
QSEN Institute. (2017). *QSEN Competencies: Definitions and pre-licensure KSAs.* Retrieved on 3/1/2017 at: www.qsen.org/competencies/pre-licensure-ksas.

20 Assessment of Respiratory Function

LEARNING OBJECTIVES

On completion of this chapter, the learner will be able to:

1 Describe the structures and functions of the upper and lower respiratory tracts.
2 Describe ventilation, diffusion, perfusion, and ventilation–perfusion imbalances.
3 Explain proper techniques utilized to perform a comprehensive respiratory assessment.

4 Discriminate between normal and abnormal assessment findings identified by inspection, palpation, percussion, and auscultation of the respiratory system.
5 Recognize and evaluate the major symptoms of respiratory dysfunction by applying concepts from the patient's health history and physical assessment findings.
6 Identify the diagnostic tests used to evaluate respiratory function and related nursing implications.

GLOSSARY

apnea: temporary cessation of breathing
bronchophony: abnormal increase in clarity of transmitted voice sounds heard when auscultating the lungs
bronchoscopy: direct examination of the larynx, trachea, and bronchi using an endoscope
cilia: short, fine hairs that provide a constant whipping motion that serves to propel mucus and foreign substances away from the lung toward the larynx
compliance: measure of the force required to expand or inflate the lungs
crackles: soft, high-pitched, discontinuous popping sounds during inspiration caused by delayed reopening of the airways
dyspnea: subjective experience that describes difficulty breathing; shortness of breath
egophony: abnormal change in tone of voice that is heard when auscultating the lungs
fremitus: vibrations of speech felt as tremors of the chest wall during palpation
hemoptysis: expectoration of blood from the respiratory tract
hypoxemia: decrease in arterial oxygen tension in the blood
hypoxia: decrease in oxygen supply to the tissues and cells
obstructive sleep apnea: temporary absence of breathing during sleep secondary to transient upper airway obstruction

orthopnea: shortness of breath when lying flat; relieved by sitting or standing
oxygen saturation: percentage of hemoglobin that is bound to oxygen
physiologic dead space: portion of the tracheobronchial tree that does not participate in gas exchange
pulmonary diffusion: exchange of gas molecules (oxygen and carbon dioxide) from areas of high concentration to areas of low concentration
pulmonary perfusion: blood flow through the pulmonary vasculature
respiration: gas exchange between atmospheric air and the blood and between the blood and cells of the body
rhonchi: low-pitched wheezing or snoring sound associated with partial airway obstruction, heard on chest auscultation
stridor: harsh high-pitched sound heard on inspiration, usually without need of a stethoscope, secondary to upper airway obstruction
tachypnea: abnormally rapid respirations
tidal volume: volume of air inspired and expired with each breath during normal breathing
ventilation: movement of air in and out of the airways
wheezes: continuous musical sounds associated with airway narrowing or partial obstruction
whispered pectoriloquy: whispered sounds heard loudly and clearly upon thoracic auscultation

Disorders of the respiratory system are common and are encountered by nurses in every setting, from the community to the intensive care unit. Expert assessment skills must be developed and used to provide the best care for patients with acute and chronic respiratory problems. Alterations in respiratory status have been identified as important predictors of clinical deterioration in hospitalized patients (Helling, Martin, Martin, et al., 2014; Kirkland, Malinchoc, O'Byrne, et al., 2013). To differentiate between normal and abnormal assessment findings and recognize subtle changes that may negatively impact patient outcomes, nurses require an understanding of respiratory function and the significance of abnormal diagnostic test results.

Anatomic and Physiologic Overview

The respiratory system is composed of the upper and lower respiratory tracts. Together, the two tracts are responsible for ventilation (movement of air in and out of the airways). The upper respiratory tract, known as the upper airway, warms and filters inspired air so that the lower respiratory tract (the lungs) can accomplish gas exchange or diffusion. Gas exchange involves delivering oxygen to the tissues through the bloodstream and expelling waste gases, such as carbon dioxide, during expiration. The respiratory system depends on the cardiovascular system for perfusion, or blood flow through the pulmonary system (Porth, 2015).

Anatomy of the Respiratory System

Upper Respiratory Tract

Upper airway structures consist of the nose; paranasal sinuses; pharynx, tonsils, and adenoids; larynx; and trachea.

Nose

The nose serves as a passageway for air to pass to and from the lungs. It filters impurities and humidifies and warms the air as it is inhaled. The nose is composed of an external and an internal portion. The external portion protrudes from the face and is supported by the nasal bones and cartilage. The anterior nares (nostrils) are the external openings of the nasal cavities.

The internal portion of the nose is a hollow cavity separated into the right and left nasal cavities by a narrow vertical divider, the septum. Each nasal cavity is divided into three passageways by the projection of the turbinates from the lateral walls. The turbinate bones are also called *conchae* (the name suggested by their shell-like appearance). Because of their curves, these bones increase the mucous membrane surface of the nasal passages and slightly obstruct the air flowing through them (see Fig. 20-1).

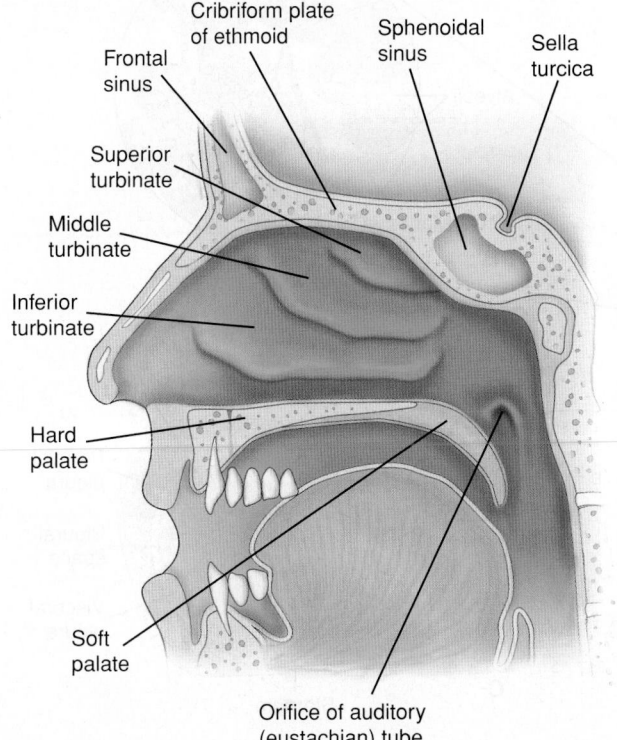

Figure 20-1 • Cross-section of nasal cavity.

Labels: Cribriform plate of ethmoid; Sphenoidal sinus; Sella turcica; Frontal sinus; Superior turbinate; Middle turbinate; Inferior turbinate; Hard palate; Soft palate; Orifice of auditory (eustachian) tube

Figure 20-2 • The paranasal sinuses.

Labels: Frontal; Ethmoid; Sphenoid; Maxillary

Air entering the nostrils is deflected upward to the roof of the nose, and it follows a circuitous route before it reaches the nasopharynx. It comes into contact with a large surface of moist, warm, highly vascular, ciliated mucous membrane (called *nasal mucosa*) that traps practically all of the dust and organisms in the inhaled air. The air is moistened, warmed to body temperature, and brought into contact with sensitive nerves. Some of these nerves detect odors; others provoke sneezing to expel irritating dust. Mucus, secreted continuously by goblet cells, covers the surface of the nasal mucosa and is moved back to the nasopharynx by the action of the **cilia** (short, fine hairs).

Paranasal Sinuses

The paranasal sinuses include four pairs of bony cavities that are lined with nasal mucosa and ciliated pseudostratified columnar epithelium. These air spaces are connected by a series of ducts that drain into the nasal cavity. The sinuses are named by their location: frontal, ethmoid, sphenoid, and maxillary (see Fig. 20-2). A prominent function of the sinuses is to serve as a resonating chamber in speech. The sinuses are a common site of infection.

Pharynx, Tonsils, and Adenoids

The pharynx, or throat, is a tubelike structure that connects the nasal and oral cavities to the larynx. It is divided into three regions: nasal, oral, and laryngeal. The nasopharynx is located posterior to the nose and above the soft palate. The oropharynx houses the faucial, or palatine, tonsils. The laryngopharynx extends from the hyoid bone to the cricoid cartilage. The epiglottis forms the entrance to the larynx.

The adenoids, or pharyngeal tonsils, are located in the roof of the nasopharynx. The tonsils, the adenoids, and other lymphoid tissue encircle the throat. These structures are important links in the chain of lymph nodes guarding the body from invasion by organisms entering the nose and the throat. The pharynx functions as a passageway for the respiratory and digestive tracts.

Larynx

The larynx, or voice box, is a cartilaginous epithelium-lined organ that connects the pharynx and the trachea and consists of the following:

- *Epiglottis*: a valve flap of cartilage that covers the opening to the larynx during swallowing
- *Glottis*: the opening between the vocal cords in the larynx

- *Thyroid cartilage:* the largest of the cartilage structures; part of it forms the Adam's apple
- *Cricoid cartilage:* the only complete cartilaginous ring in the larynx (located below the thyroid cartilage)
- *Arytenoid cartilages:* used in vocal cord movement with the thyroid cartilage
- *Vocal cords:* ligaments controlled by muscular movements that produce sounds; located in the lumen of the larynx

Although the major function of the larynx is vocalization, it also protects the lower airway from foreign substances and facilitates coughing; it is, therefore, sometimes referred to as the "watchdog of the lungs" (Porth, 2015).

Trachea

The trachea, or windpipe, is composed of smooth muscle with C-shaped rings of cartilage at regular intervals. The cartilaginous rings are incomplete on the posterior surface and give firmness to the wall of the trachea, preventing it from collapsing. The trachea serves as the passage between the larynx and the right and left main stem bronchi, which enter the lungs through an opening called the *hilus.*

Lower Respiratory Tract

The lower respiratory tract consists of the lungs, which contain the bronchial and alveolar structures needed for gas exchange.

Lungs

The lungs are paired elastic structures enclosed in the thoracic cage, which is an airtight chamber with distensible walls (see Fig. 20-3). Each lung is divided into lobes. The right lung has upper, middle, and lower lobes, whereas the left lung consists of upper and lower lobes (see Fig. 20-4). Each lobe is further subdivided into two to five segments separated by fissures, which are extensions of the pleura.

Pleura

The lungs and wall of the thoracic cavity are lined with a serous membrane called the *pleura.* The visceral pleura covers the lungs; the parietal pleura lines the thoracic cavity, lateral wall of the mediastinum, diaphragm, and inner aspects of the ribs. The visceral and parietal pleura and the small amount of pleural fluid between these two membranes serve to lubricate the thorax and the lungs and permit smooth motion of the lungs within the thoracic cavity during inspiration and expiration.

Mediastinum

The mediastinum is in the middle of the thorax, between the pleural sacs that contain the two lungs. It extends from the sternum to the vertebral column and contains all of the thoracic tissue outside the lungs (heart, thymus, the aorta and vena cava, and esophagus).

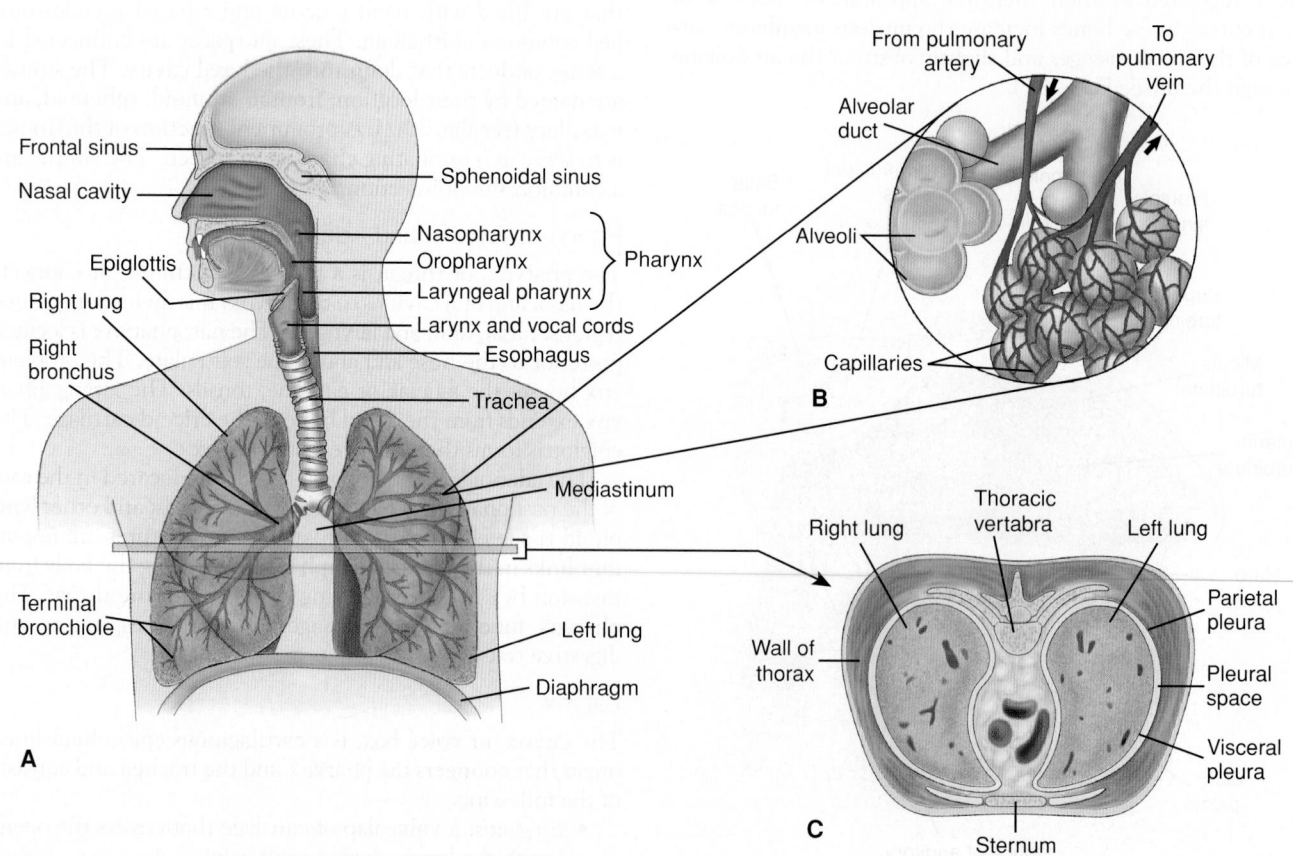

Figure 20-3 • The respiratory system. A. Upper respiratory structures and the structures of the thorax. **B.** Alveoli. **C.** A horizontal cross-section of the lungs.

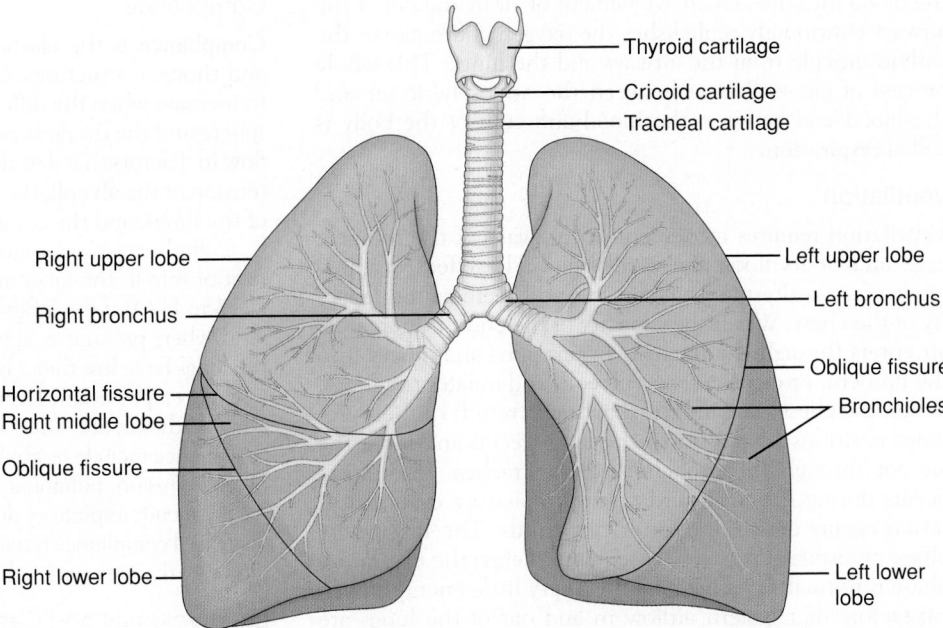

Figure 20-4 • Anterior view of the lungs. The lungs consist of five lobes. The right lung has three lobes (upper, middle, lower); the left has two (upper and lower). The lobes are further subdivided by fissures. The bronchial tree, another lung structure, inflates with air to fill the lobes.

Thyroid cartilage
Cricoid cartilage
Tracheal cartilage
Right upper lobe
Left upper lobe
Right bronchus
Left bronchus
Oblique fissure
Horizontal fissure
Right middle lobe
Bronchioles
Oblique fissure
Right lower lobe
Left lower lobe

Bronchi and Bronchioles

There are several divisions of the bronchi within each lobe of the lung. First are the lobar bronchi (three in the right lung and two in the left lung). Lobar bronchi divide into segmental bronchi (10 on the right and 8 on the left); these structures facilitate effective postural drainage in the patient. Segmental bronchi then divide into subsegmental bronchi. These bronchi are surrounded by connective tissue that contains arteries, lymphatics, and nerves.

The subsegmental bronchi then branch into bronchioles, which have no cartilage in their walls. Their patency depends entirely on the elastic recoil of the surrounding smooth muscle and on the alveolar pressure. The bronchioles contain submucosal glands, which produce mucus that covers the inside lining of the airways. The bronchi and bronchioles are also lined with cells that have surfaces covered with cilia. These cilia create a constant whipping motion that propels mucus and foreign substances away from the lungs toward the larynx.

The bronchioles branch into terminal bronchioles, which do not have mucous glands or cilia. Terminal bronchioles become respiratory bronchioles, which are considered to be the transitional passageways between the conducting airways and the gas exchange airways. Up to this point, the conducting airways contain about 150 mL of air in the tracheobronchial tree that does not participate in gas exchange, known as **physiologic dead space.** The respiratory bronchioles then lead into alveolar ducts and sacs and then alveoli (see Fig. 20-3). Oxygen and carbon dioxide exchange takes place in the alveoli.

Alveoli

The lung is made up of about 300 million alveoli, constituting a total surface area between 50 and 100 m² (Porth, 2015). There are three types of alveolar cells. Type I and type II cells make up the alveolar epithelium. Type I cells account for 95% of the alveolar surface area and serve as a barrier between the air and the alveolar surface; type II cells account for only

5% of this area but are responsible for producing type I cells and surfactant. Surfactant reduces surface tension, thereby improving overall lung function. Alveolar macrophages, the third type of alveolar cells, are phagocytic cells that ingest foreign matter and, as a result, provide an important defense mechanism.

Function of the Respiratory System

The cells of the body derive the energy they need from the oxidation of carbohydrates, fats, and proteins. This process requires oxygen. Vital tissues, like the brain and the heart, cannot survive long without a continuous supply of oxygen. As a result of oxidation, carbon dioxide is produced and must be removed from the cells to prevent the buildup of acid waste products. The respiratory system performs this function by facilitating life-sustaining processes such as oxygen transport, respiration, ventilation, and gas exchange.

Oxygen Transport

Oxygen is supplied to, and carbon dioxide is removed from, cells by way of the circulating blood through the thin walls of the capillaries. Oxygen diffuses from the capillary through the capillary wall to the interstitial fluid. At this point, it diffuses through the membrane of tissue cells, where it is used by mitochondria for cellular respiration. The movement of carbon dioxide occurs by diffusion in the opposite direction—from cell to blood.

Respiration

After these tissue capillary exchanges, blood enters the systemic venous circulation and travels to the pulmonary circulation. The oxygen concentration in blood within the capillaries of the lungs is lower than that in the lungs' alveoli. Because of this concentration gradient, oxygen diffuses from the alveoli to the blood. Carbon dioxide, which has a higher concentration in the blood than in the alveoli, diffuses from the blood into the alveoli. Movement of air in and out of the airways continually replenishes the oxygen and removes the carbon dioxide from the airways and the lungs. This whole process of gas exchange between the atmospheric air and the blood and between the blood and cells of the body is called **respiration.**

Ventilation

Ventilation requires movement of the walls of the thoracic cage and of its floor, the diaphragm. The effect of these movements is alternately to increase and decrease the capacity of the chest. When the capacity of the chest is increased, air enters through the trachea (inspiration) and moves into the bronchi, bronchioles, and alveoli, and inflates the lungs. When the chest wall and the diaphragm return to their previous positions (expiration), the lungs recoil and force the air out through the bronchi and the trachea. Inspiration occurs during the first third of the respiratory cycle; expiration occurs during the latter two thirds. The inspiratory phase of respiration normally requires energy; the expiratory phase is normally passive, requiring very little energy. Physical factors that govern airflow in and out of the lungs are collectively referred to as the mechanics of ventilation and include air pressure variances, resistance to airflow, and lung compliance.

Air Pressure Variances

Air flows from a region of higher pressure to a region of lower pressure. During inspiration, movements of the diaphragm and intercostal muscles enlarge the thoracic cavity and thereby lower the pressure inside the thorax to a level below that of atmospheric pressure. As a result, air is drawn through the trachea and the bronchi into the alveoli. During expiration, the diaphragm relaxes and the lungs recoil, resulting in a decrease in the size of the thoracic cavity. The alveolar pressure then exceeds atmospheric pressure, and air flows from the lungs into the atmosphere.

Airway Resistance

Resistance is determined by the radius, or size of the airway through which the air is flowing, as well as by lung volumes and airflow velocity. Any process that changes the bronchial diameter or width affects airway resistance and alters the rate of airflow for a given pressure gradient during respiration (see Chart 20-1). With increased resistance, greater-than-normal respiratory effort is required to achieve normal levels of ventilation.

Chart 20-1	Causes of Increased Airway Resistance

Common phenomena that may alter bronchial diameter, which affects airway resistance, include the following:

- Contraction of bronchial smooth muscle—as in asthma
- Thickening of bronchial mucosa—as in chronic bronchitis
- Obstruction of the airway—by mucus, a tumor, or a foreign body
- Loss of lung elasticity—as in emphysema, which is characterized by connective tissue encircling the airways, thereby keeping them open during both inspiration and expiration

Compliance

Compliance is the elasticity and expandability of the lungs and thoracic structures. Compliance allows the lung volume to increase when the difference in pressure between the atmosphere and the thoracic cavity (pressure gradient) causes air to flow in. Factors that determine lung compliance are the surface tension of the alveoli, the connective tissue and water content of the lungs, and the compliance of the thoracic cavity.

Compliance is determined by examining the volume–pressure relationship in the lungs and the thorax. Compliance is normal (1 L/cm H_2O) if the lungs and the thorax easily stretch and distend when pressure is applied. Increased compliance occurs if the lungs have lost their elastic recoil and become overdistended (e.g., in emphysema). Decreased compliance occurs if the lungs and the thorax are "stiff." Conditions associated with decreased compliance include morbid obesity, pneumothorax, hemothorax, pleural effusion, pulmonary edema, atelectasis, pulmonary fibrosis, and acute respiratory distress syndrome (ARDS). Lungs with decreased compliance require greater-than-normal energy expenditure by the patient to achieve normal levels of ventilation.

Lung Volumes and Capacities

Lung function, which reflects the mechanics of ventilation, is viewed in terms of lung volumes and lung capacities. Lung volumes are categorized as tidal volume, inspiratory reserve volume, expiratory reserve volume, and residual volume. Lung capacity is evaluated in terms of vital capacity, inspiratory capacity, functional residual capacity, and total lung capacity. These terms are explained in Table 20-1.

Pulmonary Diffusion and Perfusion

Pulmonary diffusion is the process by which oxygen and carbon dioxide are exchanged from areas of high concentration to areas of low concentration at the air–blood interface. The alveolar–capillary membrane is ideal for diffusion because of its thinness and large surface area. In the normal healthy adult, oxygen and carbon dioxide travel across the alveolar–capillary membrane without difficulty as a result of differences in gas concentrations in the alveoli and capillaries.

Pulmonary perfusion is the actual blood flow through the pulmonary vasculature. The blood is pumped into the lungs by the right ventricle through the pulmonary artery. The pulmonary artery divides into the right and left branches to supply both lungs. Normally, about 2% of the blood pumped by the right ventricle does not perfuse the alveolar capillaries. This shunted blood drains into the left side of the heart without participating in alveolar gas exchange. Bronchial arteries extending from the thoracic aorta also support perfusion but do not participate in gas exchange, further diluting oxygenated blood exiting through the pulmonary vein (Porth, 2015).

The pulmonary circulation is considered a low-pressure system because the systolic blood pressure in the pulmonary artery is 20 to 30 mm Hg and the diastolic pressure is 5 to 15 mm Hg. Because of these low pressures, the pulmonary vasculature normally can vary its capacity to accommodate the blood flow it receives. However, when a person is in an upright position, the pulmonary artery pressure is not great enough to supply blood to the apex of the lung against the force of gravity. Thus, when a person is upright, the lung may be considered to be divided into three sections: an upper part with poor blood supply, a lower part with maximal blood

TABLE 20-1 Lung Volumes and Lung Capacities

Term	Symbol	Description	Normal Value[a]	Significance
Lung Volumes				
Tidal volume	VT or TV	The volume of air inhaled and exhaled with each breath	500 mL or 5–10 mL/kg	The tidal volume may not vary, even with severe disease.
Inspiratory reserve volume	IRV	The maximum volume of air that can be inhaled after a normal inhalation	3000 mL	
Expiratory reserve volume	ERV	The maximum volume of air that can be exhaled forcibly after a normal exhalation	1100 mL	Expiratory reserve volume is decreased with restrictive conditions, such as obesity, ascites, pregnancy.
Residual volume	RV	The volume of air remaining in the lungs after a maximum exhalation	1200 mL	Residual volume may be increased with obstructive disease.
Lung Capacities				
Vital capacity	VC	The maximum volume of air exhaled from the point of maximum inspiration: VC = TV + IRV + ERV	4600 mL	A decrease in vital capacity may be found in neuromuscular disease, generalized fatigue, atelectasis, pulmonary edema, COPD, and obesity.
Inspiratory capacity	IC	The maximum volume of air inhaled after normal expiration: IC = TV + IRV	3500 mL	A decrease in inspiratory capacity may indicate restrictive disease. It may also be decreased in obesity.
Functional residual capacity	FRC	The volume of air remaining in the lungs after a normal expiration: FRC = ERV + RV	2300 mL	Functional residual capacity may be increased with COPD and decreased in ARDS and obesity.
Total lung capacity	TLC	The volume of air in the lungs after a maximum inspiration TLC = TV + IRV + ERV + RV	5800 mL	Total lung capacity may be decreased with restrictive disease such as atelectasis and pneumonia and increased in COPD.

[a]Values for healthy men; women are 20% to 25% less.
ARDS, acute respiratory distress syndrome; COPD, chronic obstructive pulmonary disease; ERV, expiratory reserve volume; FRC, functional residual capacity; IRV, inspiratory reserve volume.
Adapted from West, J. B., & Luks, A. M. (2016). *West's respiratory physiology: The essentials* (10th ed.). Philadelphia, PA: Wolters Kluwer Health Lippincott Williams & Wilkins.

supply, and a section between the two with an intermediate supply of blood. When a person who is lying down turns to one side, more blood passes to the dependent lung.

Perfusion is also influenced by alveolar pressure. The pulmonary capillaries are sandwiched between adjacent alveoli. If the alveolar pressure is sufficiently high, the capillaries are squeezed. Depending on the pressure, some capillaries completely collapse, whereas others narrow.

Pulmonary artery pressure, gravity, and alveolar pressure determine the patterns of perfusion. In lung disease, these factors vary, and the perfusion of the lung may become abnormal.

Ventilation and Perfusion Balance and Imbalance

Adequate gas exchange depends on an adequate ventilation–perfusion $(\dot{V}/\dot{Q})$ ratio. In different areas of the lung, the $(\dot{V}/\dot{Q})$ ratio varies. Airway blockages, local changes in compliance, and gravity may alter ventilation. Alterations in perfusion may occur with a change in the pulmonary artery pressure, alveolar pressure, or gravity.

$\dot{V}/\dot{Q}$ imbalance occurs as a result of inadequate ventilation, inadequate perfusion, or both. There are four possible $(\dot{V}/\dot{Q})$ states in the lung: normal $(\dot{V}/\dot{Q})$ ratio, low $(\dot{V}/\dot{Q})$ ratio (shunt), high $(\dot{V}/\dot{Q})$ ratio (dead space), and absence of ventilation and perfusion (silent unit) (see Chart 20-2). $\dot{V}/\dot{Q}$ imbalance causes shunting of blood, resulting in **hypoxia** (low level of cellular oxygen). Shunting appears to be the main cause of hypoxia after thoracic or abdominal surgery and most types of respiratory failure. Severe hypoxia results when the amount of shunting exceeds 20%. Supplemental oxygen may eliminate hypoxia, depending on the type of $(\dot{V}/\dot{Q})$ imbalance.

Gas Exchange
Partial Pressure of Gases

The air we breathe is a gaseous mixture consisting mainly of nitrogen (78.6%) and oxygen (20.8%), with traces of carbon dioxide (0.04%), water vapor (0.05%), helium, and argon. The atmospheric pressure at sea level is about 760 mm Hg. Partial pressure is the pressure exerted by each type of gas in a mixture of gases. The partial pressure of a gas is proportional to the concentration of that gas in the mixture. The total pressure exerted by the gaseous mixture, whether in the atmosphere or in the lungs, is equal to the sum of the partial pressures.

Based on these facts, the partial pressures of nitrogen and oxygen can be calculated. The partial pressure of nitrogen in the atmosphere at sea level is 78.6% of 760, or 597 mm Hg; that of oxygen is 20.8% of 760, or 158 mm Hg (Grossman & Porth, 2014). Chart 20-3 identifies and defines terms and abbreviations related to partial pressure of gases.

Once the air enters the trachea, it becomes fully saturated with water vapor, which displaces some of the other gases. Water vapor exerts a pressure of 47 mm Hg when it fully saturates a mixture of gases at the body temperature of 37°C (98.6°F). Nitrogen and oxygen are responsible for almost all of the remaining 713 mm Hg pressure. Once this mixture enters the alveoli, it is further diluted by carbon dioxide. In the alveoli, the water vapor continues to exert a pressure of 47 mm Hg. The remaining 713 mm Hg pressure is now exerted as follows: nitrogen, 569 mm Hg (74.9%); oxygen, 104 mm Hg (13.6%); and carbon dioxide, 40 mm Hg (5.3%).

When a gas is exposed to a liquid, the gas dissolves in the liquid until equilibrium is reached. The dissolved gas also

<table>
<tr><td>**Chart 20-2**</td><td>Ventilation–Perfusion Ratios</td></tr>
</table>

Normal Ratio (A)

In the healthy lung, a given amount of blood passes an alveolus and is matched with an equal amount of gas **(A)**. The ratio is 1:1 (ventilation matches perfusion).

Low Ventilation–Perfusion Ratio: Shunts (B)

Low ventilation–perfusion states may be called *shunt-producing disorders.* When perfusion exceeds ventilation, a shunt exists **(B)**. Blood bypasses the alveoli without gas exchange occurring. This is seen with obstruction of the distal airways, such as with pneumonia, atelectasis, tumor, or a mucus plug.

High Ventilation–Perfusion Ratio: Dead Space (C)

When ventilation exceeds perfusion, dead space results **(C)**. The alveoli do not have an adequate blood supply for gas exchange to occur. This is characteristic of a variety of disorders, including pulmonary emboli, pulmonary infarction, and cardiogenic shock.

Silent Unit (D)

In the absence of both ventilation and perfusion or with limited ventilation and perfusion, a condition known as a silent unit occurs **(D)**. This is seen with pneumothorax and severe acute respiratory distress syndrome.

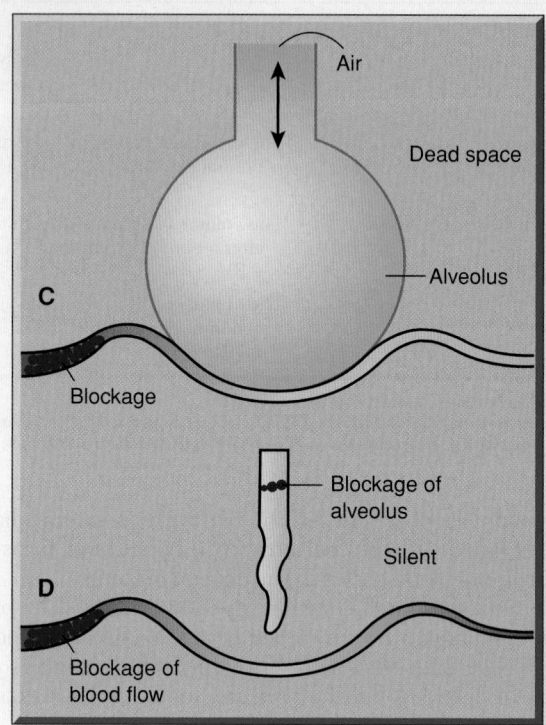

exerts a partial pressure. At equilibrium, the partial pressure of the gas in the liquid is the same as the partial pressure of the gas in the gaseous mixture. Oxygenation of venous blood in the lung illustrates this point. In the lung, venous blood and alveolar oxygen are separated by a very thin alveolar membrane. Oxygen diffuses across this membrane to dissolve in the blood until the partial pressure of oxygen in the blood is the same as that in the alveoli (104 mm Hg). However, because carbon dioxide is a by-product of oxidation in the cells, venous blood contains carbon dioxide at a higher partial pressure than that in the alveolar gas. In the lung, carbon dioxide diffuses out of venous blood into the alveolar gas. At equilibrium, the partial pressure of carbon dioxide in the blood and in alveolar gas is the same (40 mm Hg). The changes in partial pressure are shown in Figure 20-5.

<table>
<tr><td>**Chart 20-3**</td><td>Partial Pressure Abbreviations</td></tr>
</table>

P = Pressure
PO_2 = Partial pressure of oxygen
PCO_2 = Partial pressure of carbon dioxide
PAO_2 = Partial pressure of alveolar oxygen
$PACO_2$ = Partial pressure of alveolar carbon dioxide
PaO_2 = Partial pressure of arterial oxygen
$PaCO_2$ = Partial pressure of arterial carbon dioxide
PvO_2 = Partial pressure of venous oxygen
$PvCO_2$ = Partial pressure of venous carbon dioxide
P_{50} = Partial pressure of oxygen when the hemoglobin is 50% saturated

Effects of Pressure on Oxygen Transport

Oxygen and carbon dioxide are transported simultaneously, either dissolved in blood or combined with hemoglobin in red blood cells. Each 100 mL of normal arterial blood carries 0.3 mL of oxygen physically dissolved in the plasma and 20 mL of oxygen in combination with hemoglobin. Large amounts of oxygen can be transported in the blood because oxygen combines easily with hemoglobin to form oxyhemoglobin:

$$O_2 + Hgb \leftrightarrow HgbO_2$$

Figure 20-5 • Changes occur in the partial pressure of gases during respiration. These values vary as a result of the exchange of oxygen and carbon dioxide and the changes that occur in their partial pressures as venous blood flows through the lungs.

The volume of oxygen physically dissolved in the plasma is measured by the partial pressure of oxygen in the arteries (PaO_2). The higher the PaO_2, the greater the amount of oxygen dissolved. For example, at a PaO_2 of 10 mm Hg, 0.03 mL of oxygen is dissolved in 100 mL of plasma. At PaO_2 of 20 mm Hg, twice this amount is dissolved in plasma, and at PaO_2 of 100 mm Hg, 10 times this amount is dissolved. Therefore, the amount of dissolved oxygen is directly proportional to the partial pressure, regardless of how high the oxygen pressure becomes.

The amount of oxygen that combines with hemoglobin depends on both the amount of hemoglobin in the blood and on PaO_2, although only up to a PaO_2 of about 150 mm Hg. This is measured as O_2 saturation (SaO_2), the percentage of the O_2 that could be carried if all the hemoglobin held the maximum possible amount of O_2. When the PaO_2 is 150 mm Hg, hemoglobin is 100% saturated and does not combine with any additional oxygen. When hemoglobin is 100% saturated, 1 g of hemoglobin combines with 1.34 mL of oxygen. Therefore, in a person with 14 g/dL of hemoglobin, each 100 mL of blood contains about 19 mL of oxygen associated with hemoglobin. If the PaO_2 is less than 150 mm Hg, the percentage of hemoglobin saturated with oxygen decreases. For example, at a PaO_2 of 100 mm Hg (normal value), saturation is 97%; at a PaO_2 of 40 mm Hg, saturation is 70%.

Oxyhemoglobin Dissociation Curve

The oxyhemoglobin dissociation curve (see Chart 20-4) shows the relationship between the partial pressure of oxygen (PaO_2) and the percentage of saturation of oxygen (SaO_2). The percentage of saturation can be affected by carbon dioxide, hydrogen ion concentration, temperature, and 2,3-diphosphoglycerate. An increase in these factors shifts the curve to the right, thus less oxygen is picked up in the lungs, but more oxygen is released to the tissues, if PaO_2 is unchanged. A decrease in these factors causes the curve to shift to the left, making the bond between oxygen and hemo-

---

Chart 20-4

Oxyhemoglobin Dissociation Curve

The oxyhemoglobin dissociation curve is marked to show three oxygen levels:

1. Normal levels—PaO_2 >70 mm Hg
2. Relatively safe levels—PaO_2 45–70 mm Hg
3. Dangerous levels—PaO_2 <40 mm Hg

The normal (middle) curve (N) shows that 75% saturation occurs at a PaO_2 of 40 mm Hg. If the curve shifts to the right (R), the same saturation (75%) occurs at the higher PaO_2 of 57 mm Hg. If the curve shifts to the left (L), 75% saturation occurs at a PaO_2 of 25 mm Hg.

globin stronger. If the PaO_2 is still unchanged, more oxygen is picked up in the lungs, but less oxygen is given up to the tissues. The unusual shape of the oxyhemoglobin dissociation curve is a distinct advantage to the patient for two reasons:

1. If the PaO_2 decreases from 100 to 80 mm Hg as a result of lung disease or heart disease, the hemoglobin of the arterial blood remains almost maximally saturated (94%), and the tissues do not suffer from hypoxia.
2. When the arterial blood passes into tissue capillaries and is exposed to the tissue tension of oxygen (about 40 mm Hg), hemoglobin gives up large quantities of oxygen for use by the tissues.

With a normal value for PaO_2 (80 to 100 mm Hg) and SaO_2 (95% to 98%), there is a 15% margin of excess oxygen available to the tissues. With a normal hemoglobin level of 15 mg/dL and a PaO_2 level of 40 mm Hg (SaO_2 75%), there is adequate oxygen available for the tissues but no reserve for physiologic stresses that increase tissue oxygen demand. If a serious incident occurs (e.g., bronchospasm, aspiration, hypotension, or cardiac dysrhythmias) that reduces the intake of oxygen from the lungs, tissue hypoxia results.

An important consideration in the transport of oxygen is cardiac output, which determines the amount of oxygen delivered to the body and affects lung and tissue perfusion. If the cardiac output is normal (5 L/min), the amount of oxygen delivered to the body per minute is normal. Under normal conditions, only 250 mL of oxygen is used per minute, which is approximately 25% of available oxygen. The rest of the oxygen returns to the right side of the heart, and the PaO_2 of venous blood drops from 80 to 100 mm Hg to about 40 mm Hg. If cardiac output falls, however, the amount of oxygen delivered to the tissues also falls and may be inadequate to meet the body's needs.

Carbon Dioxide Transport

At the same time that oxygen diffuses from the blood into the tissues, carbon dioxide diffuses from tissue cells to blood and is transported to the lungs for excretion. The amount of carbon dioxide in transit is one of the major determinants of the acid–base balance of the body. Normally, only 6% of the venous carbon dioxide is removed in the lungs and enough remains in the arterial blood to exert a pressure of 40 mm Hg. Most of the carbon dioxide (90%) is carried by red blood cells; the small portion (5%) that remains dissolved in the plasma (partial pressure of carbon dioxide [PCO_2]) is the critical factor that determines carbon dioxide movement in or out of the blood.

Although the many processes involved in respiratory gas transport seem to occur in intermittent stages, the changes are rapid, simultaneous, and continuous.

Neurologic Control of Ventilation

Resting respiration is the result of cyclic excitation of the respiratory muscles by the phrenic nerve. The rhythm of breathing is controlled by respiratory centers in the brain. The inspiratory and expiratory centers in the medulla oblongata and pons control the rate and depth of ventilation to meet the body's metabolic demands.

The apneustic center in the lower pons stimulates the inspiratory medullary center to promote deep, prolonged inspirations. The pneumotaxic center in the upper pons is thought to control the pattern of respirations.

Several groups of receptor sites assist in the brain's control of respiratory function. The central chemoreceptors, located in the medulla, respond to chemical changes in the cerebrospinal fluid, which result from chemical changes in the blood. These receptors respond to an increase or decrease in the pH and convey a message to the lungs to change the depth and then the rate of ventilation to correct the imbalance. The peripheral chemoreceptors are located in the aortic arch and the carotid arteries and respond first to changes in PaO_2, then to partial pressure of carbon dioxide ($PaCO_2$) and pH.

Mechanoreceptors in the lung include stretch, irritant, and juxtacapillary receptors, and respond to changes in resistance by altering breathing patterns to support optimal lung function. For example, the Hering–Breuer reflex is activated by stretch receptors in the alveoli. When the lungs are distended, inspiration is inhibited; as a result, the lungs do not become overdistended.

Proprioceptors in the muscles and chest wall respond to body movements, causing an increase in ventilation. Thus, range-of-motion exercises in an immobile patient stimulate breathing. Finally, baroreceptors, also located in the aortic and carotid bodies, respond to an increase or decrease in arterial blood pressure and cause reflex hypoventilation or hyperventilation.

Gerontologic Considerations

A gradual decline in respiratory function begins in early to middle adulthood and affects the structure and function of the respiratory system. The vital capacity of the lungs and the strength of the respiratory muscles peak between 20 and 25 years of age and decrease thereafter. With aging (40 years and older), changes occur in the alveoli that reduce the surface area available for the exchange of oxygen and carbon dioxide. At approximately 50 years of age, the alveoli begin to lose elasticity. A decrease in vital capacity occurs with the loss of chest wall mobility, which restricts the tidal flow of air. The amount of respiratory dead space increases with age. These changes result in a decreased diffusion capacity for oxygen with increasing age, producing lower oxygen levels in the arterial circulation. Older adults have a decreased ability to rapidly move air in and out of the lungs.

Gerontologic changes in the respiratory system are summarized in Table 20-2. Despite these changes, in the absence of chronic pulmonary disease, older adults are able to carry out activities of daily living, but they may have decreased tolerance for, and require additional rest after, prolonged or vigorous activity.

Assessment

Health History

The health history initially focuses on the patient's presenting problem and associated symptoms. In conducting the history, the nurse should explore the onset, location, duration, character, aggravating and alleviating factors, radiation (if relevant), and timing of the presenting problem and associated signs and symptoms. The nurse should also explore how these factors impact the patient's activities of daily living, usual work and family activities, and quality of life.

Common Symptoms

The major signs and symptoms of respiratory disease are dyspnea, cough, sputum production, chest pain, wheezing, and hemoptysis. During the health history, the nurse should also consider nonpulmonary diseases when evaluating symptoms, as these symptoms may occur with a variety of other illnesses.

Dyspnea

Dyspnea (subjective feeling of difficult or labored breathing, breathlessness, shortness of breath) is a multidimensional symptom common to many pulmonary and cardiac disorders, particularly when there is decreased lung compliance or increased airway resistance. Dyspnea may also be associated with allergic reactions, anemia, neurologic or neuromuscular disorders, trauma, and advanced disease, and is common at the end of life. Dyspnea predicts adverse clinical outcomes, including increased mortality (Baker, Barsamian, Leone, et al., 2013). Dyspnea can also occur after exercise in people without disease (Porth, 2015).

In general, acute diseases of the lungs produce a more severe grade of dyspnea than do chronic diseases. Sudden dyspnea in a healthy person may indicate pneumothorax (air in the pleural cavity), acute respiratory obstruction, allergic reaction, or myocardial infarction. In immobilized patients, sudden dyspnea may denote pulmonary embolism (PE). Dyspnea and **tachypnea** (abnormally rapid respirations) accompanied by progressive **hypoxemia** (low blood oxygen level) in a person who has recently experienced lung trauma, shock, cardiopulmonary bypass, or multiple blood transfusions may

TABLE 20-2 Age-Related Changes in the Respiratory System

	Structural Changes	Functional Changes	History and Physical Findings
Defense Mechanisms (Respiratory and Nonrespiratory)	↓ Number of cilia and ↓ mucus ↓ Cough and gag reflex Loss of surface area of the capillary membrane Lack of a uniform or consistent ventilation and/or blood flow	↓ Protection against foreign particles ↓ Protection against aspiration ↓ Antibody response to antigens ↓ Response to hypoxia and hypercapnia (chemoreceptors)	↓ Cough reflex and mucus ↑ Infection rate History of respiratory infections, chronic obstructive pulmonary disease (COPD), pneumonia. Risk factors: smoking, environmental exposure, exposure to tuberculosis (TB)
Lung	↓ Size of airway ↑ Diameter of alveolar ducts ↑ Collagen of alveolar walls ↑ Thickness of alveolar membranes ↓ Elasticity of alveolar sacs	↑ Airway resistance ↑ Pulmonary compliance ↓ Expiratory flow rate ↓ Oxygen diffusion capacity ↑ Dead space Premature closure of airways ↑ Air trapping ↓ Expiratory flow rates Ventilation–perfusion mismatch ↓ Exercise capacity ↑ Anteroposterior (AP) diameter	Unchanged total lung capacity (TLC) ↑ Residual volume (RV) ↓ Inspiratory reserve volume (IRV) ↓ Expiratory reserve volume (ERV) ↓ Forced vital capacity (FVC) and vital capacity (VC) ↑ Functional residual capacity (FRC) ↓ PaO_2 ↑ CO_2
Chest Wall and Muscles	Calcification of intercostal cartilages Arthritis of costovertebral joints ↓ Continuity of diaphragm Osteoporotic changes ↓ Muscle mass Muscle atrophy	↑ Rigidity and stiffness of thoracic cage ↓ Respiratory muscle strength ↑ Work of breathing ↓ Capacity for exercise ↓ Peripheral chemosensitivity ↑ Risk for inspiratory muscle fatigue	Kyphosis, barrel chest Skeletal changes ↑ AP diameter Shortness of breath ↑ Abdominal and diaphragmatic breathing ↓ Maximum expiratory flow rates

Adapted from Ramly, E., Kaafarani, H. M. A., & Velmahos, G. C. (2015). The effect of aging on pulmonary function: Implications for monitoring and support of the surgical and trauma patient. *Surgical Clinics of North America*, 95(1), 53–69. doi:http://dx.doi.org/10.1016/j.suc.2014.09.009

signal ARDS. **Orthopnea** (shortness of breath when lying flat, relieved by sitting or standing) may be found in patients with heart disease and occasionally in patients with chronic obstructive pulmonary disease (COPD); dyspnea with an expiratory wheeze occurs with COPD. Dyspnea associated with noisy breathing may result from a narrowing of the airway or localized obstruction of a major bronchus by a tumor or foreign body. The high-pitched sound heard (usually on inspiration) when someone is breathing through a partially blocked upper airway is called **stridor.** To help determine the cause of dyspnea, the nurse should ask the following questions:

- Is the shortness of breath related to other symptoms? Is a cough present?
- Was the onset of shortness of breath sudden or gradual?
- At what time of day or night does the shortness of breath occur?
- Is the shortness of breath worse when lying flat?
- How much exertion triggers shortness of breath? Does it occur with exercise? Climbing stairs? At rest?
- How severe is the shortness of breath? On a scale of 1 to 10, if 1 is not at all breathless and 10 is very breathless, how hard is it to breathe?

Because patients use a variety of terms to describe breathlessness, the nurse must explore what these terms mean to each patient. Patients experiencing dyspnea frequently experience fear and anxiety (Dudgeon, 2015; Yorke, 2014). It is especially important to assess the patient's rating of the intensity or distress of breathlessness, what breathing feels like, and its impact on the patient's general health, function, and quality of life. A variety of valid and reliable instruments including various Likert scale-types of quality of life tools, the visual analogue scale

(see Table 20-3), and the modified Borg scale are available to assist the nurse in measuring dyspnea. The modified Borg scale is a type of numeric rating scale. The patient is asked to self-rate the difficulty breathing is causing him/her at the present time, with 0 corresponding to no difficulty at all and 10 corresponding to maximal breathing difficulty (Dudgeon, 2015; Parshall, Schwartzstein, Adams, et al., 2012).

Cough

Cough is a reflex that protects the lungs from the accumulation of secretions or the inhalation of foreign bodies. Its presence or absence can be a diagnostic clue because some disorders cause coughing and others suppress it. The cough reflex may be impaired by weakness or paralysis of the respiratory muscles, prolonged inactivity, the presence of a nasogastric tube, or depressed function of the brain's medullary centers (e.g., anesthesia, brain disorders).

Cough results from irritation or inflammation of the mucous membranes anywhere in the respiratory tract and

TABLE 20-3 Visual Analogue Scale[a]

Patient Instructions—*Rate the difficulty of your breathing. Draw a line on this scale that matches how short of breath you are feeling right now.*

No shortness of breath	Shortness of breath as bad as can be

[a]The scale is 100 mm in length. Alternatively, a vertical line can be used.
Reprinted with permission from the Registered Nurses' Association of Ontario. (2013). *Nursing best practice guidelines: Visual analogue scale as a measure of clinical dyspnea.* Retrieved on 2/19/2016 at: pda.rnao.ca/content/visual-analogue-scale-measure-clinical-dyspnea

is associated with multiple pulmonary disorders. Mucus, pus, blood, or an airborne irritant, such as smoke or a gas, may stimulate the cough reflex. Common causes of cough include asthma, gastrointestinal reflux disease, infection, and side effects of medications, such as angiotensin-converting enzyme (ACE) inhibitors (Poot, 2014).

To help determine the cause of the cough, the nurse inquires about the onset and time of coughing. Coughing at night may indicate the onset of left-sided heart failure or bronchial asthma. A cough in the morning with sputum production may indicate bronchitis. A cough that worsens when the patient is supine suggests postnasal drip (rhinosinusitis). Coughing after food intake may indicate aspiration of material into the tracheobronchial tree. A cough of recent onset is usually from an acute infection.

The nurse assesses the character of the cough and associated symptoms. A dry, irritative cough is characteristic of an upper respiratory tract infection of viral origin, or it may be a side effect of ACE inhibitor therapy. An irritative, high-pitched cough can be caused by laryngotracheitis. A brassy cough is the result of a tracheal lesion, and a severe or changing cough may indicate bronchogenic carcinoma. Pleuritic chest pain that accompanies coughing may indicate pleural or chest wall (musculoskeletal) involvement. Violent coughing causes bronchial spasm, obstruction, and further irritation of the bronchi and may result in syncope (fainting).

 Concept Mastery Alert

> A nurse interviewing a patient who says he has a dry, irritating cough that is not "bringing anything up" should ask whether he is taking ACE inhibitors.

A persistent cough may affect a patient's quality of life and may produce embarrassment, exhaustion, inability to sleep, and pain. Therefore, the nurse should explore how a chronic cough impacts all aspects of the patient's life.

Sputum Production

Sputum production is the reaction of the lungs to any constantly recurring irritant and often results from persistent coughing. It may also be associated with a nasal discharge. The nature of the sputum is often indicative of its cause. A profuse amount of purulent sputum (thick and yellow, green, or rust colored) or a change in color of the sputum is a common sign of a bacterial infection. Thin, mucoid sputum frequently results from viral bronchitis. A gradual increase of sputum over time may occur with chronic bronchitis or bronchiectasis. Pink-tinged mucoid sputum suggests a lung tumor. Profuse, frothy, pink material, often welling up into the throat, may indicate pulmonary edema. Foul-smelling sputum and bad breath point to the presence of a lung abscess, bronchiectasis, or an infection caused by fusospirochetal or other anaerobic organisms.

Chest Pain

Chest pain or discomfort may be associated with pulmonary, cardiac, gastrointestinal, or musculoskeletal disease or anxiety. Chest pain associated with pulmonary conditions may be sharp, stabbing, and intermittent, or it may be dull, aching, and persistent. The pain usually is felt on the side where

the pathologic process is located, although it may be referred elsewhere—for example, to the neck, back, or abdomen.

Chest pain may occur with pneumonia, pulmonary infarction, or pleurisy, or as a late symptom of bronchogenic carcinoma. In carcinoma, the pain may be dull and persistent because the cancer has invaded the chest wall, mediastinum, or spine.

Lung disease does not always cause thoracic pain because the lungs and the visceral pleura lack sensory nerves and are insensitive to pain stimuli. However, the parietal pleura have a rich supply of sensory nerves that are stimulated by inflammation and stretching of the membrane. Pleuritic pain from irritation of the parietal pleura is sharp and seems to "catch" on inspiration; patients often describe it as being "like the stabbing of a knife." Patients are more comfortable when they lay on the affected side because this position splints the chest wall, limits expansion and contraction of the lung, and reduces the friction between the injured or diseased pleurae on that side. Pain associated with cough may be reduced manually by splinting the rib cage.

The nurse assesses the quality, intensity, and radiation of pain and identifies and explores precipitating factors and their relationship to the patient's position. In addition, the nurse must assess the relationship of pain to the inspiratory and expiratory phases of respiration. (See Chapter 12 for further discussion on assessment of pain.)

Wheezing

Wheezing is a high-pitched, musical sound heard on either expiration (asthma) or inspiration (bronchitis). It is often the major finding in a patient with bronchoconstriction or airway narrowing. **Rhonchi** are low-pitched continuous sounds heard over the lungs in partial airway obstruction. Depending on their location and severity, these sounds may be heard with or without a stethoscope.

Hemoptysis

Hemoptysis is the expectoration of blood from the respiratory tract. It can present as small to moderate blood-stained sputum to a large hemorrhage and always warrants further investigation. The onset of hemoptysis is usually sudden, and it may be intermittent or continuous. The most common causes are:

- Pulmonary infection
- Carcinoma of the lung
- Abnormalities of the heart or blood vessels
- Pulmonary artery or vein abnormalities
- PE or infarction

The nurse must determine the source of the bleeding, as the term *hemoptysis* is reserved for blood coming from the respiratory tract. Potential sources of bleeding include the gums, nasopharynx, lungs, or stomach. The nurse may be the only witness to the episode, and when evaluating the bleeding episode, the following points should be considered:

- Bloody sputum from the nose or the nasopharynx is usually preceded by considerable sniffing, with blood possibly appearing in the nose.
- Blood from the lung is usually bright red, frothy, and mixed with sputum. Initial symptoms include a tickling sensation in the throat, a salty taste, a burning or bubbling sensation in the chest, and perhaps chest pain, in

which case, the patient tends to splint the bleeding side. This blood has an alkaline pH (greater than 7).
- Blood from the stomach is vomited rather than expectorated, may be mixed with food, and is usually much darker and often referred to as "coffee ground emesis." This blood has an acid pH (less than 7).

Past Health, Social, and Family History

In addition to the presenting problem and associated symptoms, the history should also focus on the patient's health,

personal, and social history, and the family health history. Specific questions are asked about childhood illnesses, immunizations (including the most recent influenza and pneumonia vaccinations), medical conditions, injuries, hospitalizations, surgeries, allergies, and current medications (including over-the-counter medications and herbal remedies). Personal and social history addresses issues such as diet, exercise, sleep, recreational habits, and religion. Psychosocial factors that may affect the patient are also explored (see Chart 20-5).

The nurse assesses for risk factors and genetic factors that may contribute to the patient's lung condition (see Charts 20-6 and 20-7). Many lung disorders are related to or exacerbated

Figure 20-6 • Clubbed finger. In clubbing, the distal phalanx of each finger is rounded and bulbous. The nail plate is more convex, and the angle between the plate and the proximal nail fold increases to 180° or more. The proximal nail fold, when palpated, feels spongy or floating. Among the many causes are chronic hypoxia and lung cancer.

by tobacco smoke; therefore, smoking history (including exposure to secondhand smoke) is also obtained. Smoking history is usually expressed in pack-years, which is the number of packs of cigarettes smoked per day times the number of years the patient has smoked. It is important to find out whether the patient is still smoking or when the patient quit smoking. The nurse should also ask patients whether they use electronic nicotine delivery systems (ENDS) including e-cigarettes, e-pens, e-pipes, e-hookah and e-cigars, or new or traditional smokeless tobacco products. These agents, which are currently not regulated by the U.S. Food and Drug Administration (FDA), are being marketed as safer alternatives to cigarettes, and sometimes, in the case of ENDS, as an option to facilitate smoking cessation. The American Lung Association currently views these products as a potential public health threat and calls for additional research to better understand potential risks (American Lung Association, 2015). Finally, socioeconomic differences rooted in race and ethnicity may predispose certain groups to greater burdens related to lung disease and should also be considered (see Chart 20-8).

If the patient is experiencing severe dyspnea, the nurse may need to modify the questions asked and the timing of the health history to avoid increasing the patient's breathlessness and anxiety. Once the history is complete, the nurse conducts a comprehensive assessment. Data obtained from both the history and the assessment guide the development of a nursing care plan and patient education.

Physical Assessment of the Respiratory System

General Appearance

The patient's general appearance may give clues to respiratory status. In particular, the nurse inspects for clubbing of the fingers and notes skin color.

Clubbing of the Fingers

Clubbing of the fingers is a change in the normal nail bed. It appears as sponginess of the nail bed and loss of the nail bed angle (see Fig. 20-6). It is a sign of lung disease that is found in patients with chronic hypoxic conditions, chronic lung infections, or malignancies of the lung. Clubbing can also be seen in congenital heart disease and other chronic infections or inflammatory conditions, such as endocarditis or inflammatory bowel disease (Bickley, 2013; Rutherford, 2013).

Cyanosis

Cyanosis, a bluish coloring of the skin, is a very late indicator of hypoxia. The presence or absence of cyanosis is determined by the amount of unoxygenated hemoglobin in the blood. Cyanosis appears when there is at least 5 g/dL of unoxygenated hemoglobin. A patient with a hemoglobin level of 15 g/dL does not demonstrate cyanosis until 5 g/dL of that hemoglobin becomes unoxygenated, reducing the effective circulating hemoglobin to two thirds of the normal level.

A patient with anemia rarely manifests cyanosis, and a patient with polycythemia may appear cyanotic even if adequately oxygenated. Therefore, cyanosis is *not* a reliable sign of hypoxia.

Assessment of cyanosis is affected by room lighting, the patient's skin color, and the distance of the blood vessels from the surface of the skin. In the presence of a pulmonary condition, central cyanosis is assessed by observing the color of the tongue and lips. This indicates a decrease in oxygen tension in the blood. Peripheral cyanosis results from decreased blood flow to the body's periphery (fingers, toes, or earlobes), as in vasoconstriction from exposure to cold, and does not necessarily indicate a central systemic problem.

Upper Respiratory Structures

For a routine examination of the upper airway, only a simple light source, such as a penlight, is necessary. A more thorough examination requires the use of a nasal speculum.

Nose and Sinuses

The nurse inspects the external nose for lesions, asymmetry, or inflammation and then asks the patient to tilt the head backward. Gently pushing the tip of the nose upward, the nurse examines the internal structures of the nose, inspecting the mucosa for color, swelling, exudate, or bleeding. The nasal mucosa is normally redder than the oral mucosa. It may appear swollen and hyperemic if the patient has a common cold; however, in allergic rhinitis, the mucosa appears pale and swollen.

Next, the nurse inspects the septum for deviation, perforation, or bleeding. Most people have a slight degree of septal deviation; such deviation usually causes no symptoms. However, actual displacement of the cartilage into either the right or left side of the nose may produce nasal obstruction.

While the head is still tilted back, the nurse inspects the inferior and middle turbinates. In chronic rhinitis, nasal polyps may develop between the inferior and middle turbinates; they are distinguished by their gray appearance. Unlike the turbinates, they are gelatinous and freely movable.

Next, the nurse may palpate the frontal and maxillary sinuses for tenderness (see Fig. 20-7). Using the thumbs, the nurse applies gentle pressure in an upward fashion at the supraorbital ridges (frontal sinuses) and in the cheek area adjacent to the nose (maxillary sinuses). Tenderness in either area suggests inflammation. The frontal and maxillary sinuses can be inspected by transillumination (passing a strong light through a bony area, such as the sinuses, to inspect the cavity; see Fig. 20-8). If the light fails to penetrate, the cavity likely contains fluid or pus.

Mouth and Pharynx

After the nasal inspection, the nurse assesses the mouth and the pharynx, instructing the patient to open the mouth wide and take a deep breath. Usually, this flattens the posterior tongue and briefly allows a full view of the anterior and posterior pillars, tonsils, uvula, and posterior pharynx (see Fig. 45-2 in Chapter 45). The nurse inspects these structures for color, symmetry, and evidence of exudate, ulceration, or enlargement. If a tongue blade is needed to depress the tongue to visualize the pharynx, it is pressed firmly beyond the midpoint of the tongue to avoid a gagging response.

Figure 20-8 • At left, the nurse positions the light source for transillumination of the frontal sinus. At right, the nurse shields the patient's brow and shines the light. In normal conditions (a darkened room), the light should shine through the tissues and appear as a reddish glow (above the nurse's hand) over the sinus.

Trachea

Next, the position and mobility of the trachea are noted by direct palpation. This is performed by placing the thumb and the index finger of one hand on either side of the trachea just above the sternal notch. The trachea is highly sensitive, and palpating too firmly may trigger a coughing or gagging response. The trachea is normally in the midline as it enters the thoracic inlet behind the sternum; however, it may be deviated by masses in the neck or the mediastinum. Pulmonary disorders such as a pneumothorax or pleural effusion may also displace the trachea.

Lower Respiratory Structures and Breathing

Assessment of the lower respiratory structures includes inspection, palpation, percussion, and auscultation of the thorax. The patient should be positioned as necessary prior to the assessment.

Positioning

To assess the posterior thorax and the lungs, the patient should be in a sitting position with arms crossed in front of the chest and hands placed on the opposite shoulders (Bickley, 2013). This position separates the scapulae widely and exposes more lung area for assessment. If the patient is unable to sit, with the patient supine, the nurse should roll the patient from side to side to complete the posterior examination. To assess the anterior thorax and lungs, the patient should be either supine or sitting. The supine position allows easier displacement of the patient's breast tissue, improving the nurse's ability to perform the chest examination.

Thoracic Inspection

Inspection of the thorax provides information about the respiratory system, the musculoskeletal structure, and the patient's nutritional status. The nurse observes the skin over the thorax for color and turgor and for evidence of loss of subcutaneous tissue. It is important to note asymmetry, if present. In documenting or reporting the findings, anatomic landmarks are used as points of reference (see Chart 20-9).

Figure 20-7 • Technique for palpating the frontal sinuses at left and the maxillary sinuses at right.

Chart 20-9 Locating Thoracic Landmarks

With respect to the thorax, location is defined both horizontally and vertically. With respect to the lungs, location is defined by lobe.

Horizontal Reference Points

Horizontally, thoracic locations are identified according to their proximity to the rib or the intercostal space under the examiner's fingers. On the anterior surface, identification of a specific rib is facilitated by first locating the angle of Louis. This is where the manubrium joins the body of the sternum in the midline. The second rib joins the sternum at this prominent landmark.

Other ribs may be identified by counting down from the second rib. The intercostal spaces are referred to in terms of the rib immediately above the intercostal space; for example, the fifth intercostal space is directly below the fifth rib.

Locating ribs on the posterior surface of the thorax is more difficult. The first step is to identify the spinous process. This is accomplished by finding the seventh cervical vertebra (*vertebra prominens*), which is the most prominent spinous process. When the neck is slightly flexed, the seventh cervical spinous process stands out. Other vertebrae are then identified by counting downward.

Vertical Reference Points

Several imaginary lines are used as vertical referents or landmarks to identify the location of thoracic findings. The *midsternal line* passes through the center of the sternum. The *midclavicular line* is an imaginary line that descends from the middle of the clavicle. The *point of maximal impulse* of the heart normally lies along this line on the left thorax.

When the arm is abducted from the body at 90°, imaginary vertical lines may be drawn from the anterior axillary fold, from the middle of the axilla, and from the posterior axillary fold. These lines are called, respectively, the *anterior axillary line,* the *midaxillary line,* and the *posterior axillary line.* A line drawn vertically through the superior and inferior poles of the scapula is called the *scapular line,* and a line drawn down the center of the vertebral column is called the *vertebral line.* Using these landmarks, for example, the examiner communicates findings by referring to an area of dullness extending from the vertebral to the scapular line between the seventh and tenth ribs on the right.

Lobes of the Lungs

The lobes of the lung may be mapped on the surface of the chest wall in the following manner. The line between the upper and lower lobes on the left begins at the fourth thoracic spinous process posteriorly, proceeds around to cross the fifth rib in the midaxillary line, and meets the sixth rib at the sternum. This line on the right divides the right middle lobe from the right lower lobe. The line dividing the right upper lobe from the middle lobe is an incomplete one that begins at the fifth rib in the midaxillary line, where it intersects the line between the upper and lower lobes and traverses horizontally to the sternum. Thus, the upper lobes are dominant on the anterior surface of the thorax, and the lower lobes are dominant on the posterior surface. There is no presentation of the right middle lobe on the posterior surface of the chest.

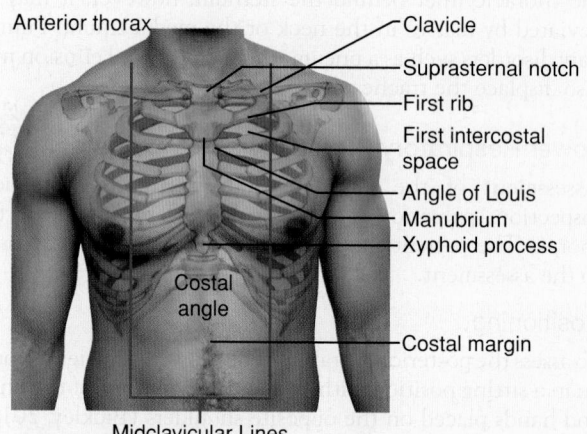

Anterior thorax — Clavicle, Suprasternal notch, First rib, First intercostal space, Angle of Louis, Manubrium, Xyphoid process, Costal angle, Costal margin, Midclavicular Lines

Posterior thorax — C7, T1, Scapula, Spinous process, T12, Midscapular lines

Anterior view of lungs — Midsternal line, Midclavicular line, Right upper lobe, Right middle lobe, Right lower lobe, Left upper lobe, Left lower lobe

Lateral view of lungs — Midaxillary line, Anterior axillary line, Right upper lobe, Right middle lobe, Right lower lobe, Posterior axillary line

Chest Configuration

Normally, the ratio of the anteroposterior diameter to the lateral diameter is 1:2. However, there are four main deformities of the chest associated with respiratory disease that alter this relationship: barrel chest, funnel chest (pectus excavatum), pigeon chest (pectus carinatum), and kyphoscoliosis.

Barrel Chest. Barrel chest occurs as a result of overinflation of the lungs, which increases the anteroposterior diameter of the thorax. It occurs with aging and is a hallmark sign of emphysema and COPD. In a patient with emphysema, the ribs are more widely spaced and the intercostal spaces tend to bulge on expiration. The appearance of the patient with advanced emphysema is thus quite characteristic, allowing the nurse to detect its presence easily, even from a distance.

Funnel Chest (Pectus Excavatum). Funnel chest occurs when there is a depression in the lower portion of the sternum. This may compress the heart and great vessels, resulting in murmurs. Funnel chest may occur with rickets or Marfan syndrome.

Pigeon Chest (Pectus Carinatum). A pigeon chest occurs as a result of the anterior displacement of the sternum, which also increases the anteroposterior diameter. This may occur with rickets, Marfan syndrome, or severe kyphoscoliosis.

Kyphoscoliosis. Kyphoscoliosis is characterized by elevation of the scapula and a corresponding S-shaped spine. This deformity limits lung expansion within the thorax. It may occur with osteoporosis and other skeletal disorders that affect the thorax.

Breathing Patterns and Respiratory Rates

Observing the rate and depth of respiration is a simple but important aspect of assessment. The normal adult who is resting comfortably takes 14 to 20 breaths per minute (Bickley, 2013). Except for occasional sighs, respirations are quiet and regular in depth and rhythm. This normal pattern is described as eupnea. Certain patterns of respiration are characteristic of specific disease states. Changes in respiratory rate and rhythm may be the first sign of clinical deterioration in patients who are acutely ill (Philip, Richardson, & Cohen, 2013). The rate and depth of various patterns of respiration are presented in Table 20-4.

Concept Mastery Alert

There are subtle differences between Cheyne–Stokes and Biot's respiration patterns. Between regularly cycled periods of apnea, Cheyne–Stokes respirations demonstrate a regular pattern with the rate and depth of breathing increasing and then decreasing. In Biot's respiration, irregularly cycled periods of apnea are interspersed with cycles of normal rate and depth.

Temporary pauses of breathing, or **apnea**, may be noted. When apneas occur repeatedly during sleep, secondary to transient upper airway blockage, the condition is called **obstructive sleep apnea**. In thin people, it is quite normal to note a slight retraction of the intercostal spaces during quiet breathing. Bulging of the intercostal spaces during expiration implies obstruction of expiratory airflow, as in emphysema. Marked retraction on inspiration, particularly if asymmetric, implies blockage of a branch of the respiratory tree.

Asymmetric bulging of the intercostal spaces, on either side of the thorax, is created by an increase in pressure within the hemithorax. This may be a result of air trapped under pressure within the pleural cavity, where it is not normally present (pneumothorax), or the pressure of fluid within the pleural space (pleural effusion).

Use of Accessory Muscles

In addition to breathing patterns and respiratory rates, the nurse should observe for the use of accessory muscles, such as the sternocleidomastoid, scalene, and trapezius muscles during inspiration, and the abdominal and internal intercostal muscles during expiration. These muscles provide additional support to assist the breathing effort during times of exertion as seen in exercise or certain disease states (Bickley, 2013).

Thoracic Palpation

The nurse palpates the thorax for tenderness, masses, lesions, respiratory excursion, and vocal fremitus. If the patient has reported an area of pain or if lesions are apparent, the nurse performs direct palpation with the fingertips (for skin lesions and subcutaneous masses) or with the ball of the hand (for deeper masses or generalized flank or rib discomfort).

Respiratory Excursion

Respiratory excursion is an estimation of thoracic expansion and may disclose significant information about thoracic movement during breathing. The nurse assesses the patient for range and symmetry of excursion. For anterior assessment, the nurse places the thumbs along the costal margin of the chest wall and instructs the patient to inhale deeply. The nurse observes movement of the thumbs during inspiration and expiration. This movement is normally symmetric (Bickley, 2013).

Posterior assessment is performed by placing the thumbs adjacent to the spinal column at the level of the 10th rib (see Fig. 20-9). The hands lightly grasp the lateral rib cage. Sliding the thumbs medially about 2.5 cm (1 in) raises a small skin fold between the thumbs. The patient is instructed to take a full inspiration and to exhale fully. The nurse observes for normal flattening of the skin fold and feels the symmetric movement of the thorax.

Decreased chest excursion may be caused by chronic fibrotic disease. Asymmetric excursion may be due to splinting secondary to pleurisy, fractured ribs, trauma, or unilateral bronchial obstruction.

Tactile Fremitus

Tactile **fremitus** describes vibrations of the chest wall that result from speech detected on palpation. Normally, sounds generated by the larynx travel distally along the bronchial tree to set the chest wall in resonant motion. This is most pronounced with consonant sounds.

Normal fremitus varies on the basis of numerous factors. It is influenced by the thickness of the chest wall, especially muscle, and the subcutaneous tissue associated with obesity. It is also influenced by pitch; lower-pitched sounds travel better through the normal lung and produce greater vibration of the chest wall. Therefore, fremitus is more pronounced in men than in women because of the deeper male voice. Normally, fremitus is most pronounced where the large bronchi are closest to the chest wall, is more prominent on the right

TABLE 20-4 Rates and Depths of Respiration

Type	Description
Eupnea Inspiration Expiration	Normal, breathing at 14–20 breaths/min
Bradypnea	Slower than normal rate (<10 breaths/min), with normal depth and regular rhythm Associated with increased intracranial pressure, brain injury, and drug overdose
Tachypnea	Rapid, shallow breathing >24 breaths/min Associated with pneumonia, pulmonary edema, metabolic acidosis, septicemia, severe pain, or rib fracture
Hypoventilation	Shallow, irregular breathing
Hyperpnea	Increase depth of respirations
Hyperventilation	Increased rate and depth of breathing that results in decreased $PaCO_2$ level Inspiration and expiration nearly equal in duration Associated with exertion, anxiety, and metabolic acidosis Called *Kussmaul's respiration* if associated with diabetic ketoacidosis or renal origin
Apnea	Period of cessation of breathing; time duration varies; apnea may occur briefly during other breathing disorders, such as with sleep apnea; life-threatening if sustained
Cheyne–Stokes	Regular cycle where the rate and depth of breathing increase, then decrease until apnea (usually about 20 seconds) occurs Duration of apnea may vary and progressively lengthen; therefore, it is timed and reported. Associated with heart failure and damage to the respiratory center (drug induced, tumor, trauma)
Biot's respiration	Periods of normal breathing (3–4 breaths), followed by a varying period of apnea (usually 10–60 seconds) Also called *ataxic breathing*; associated with complete irregularity Associated with respiratory depression resulting from drug overdose and brain injury, normally at the level of the medulla
Obstructive Prolonged expiration	Prolonged expiratory phase of respiration Associated with airway narrowing and seen in asthma, chronic obstructive pulmonary disease, and bronchitis

Adapted from Bickley, L. S. (2013). *Bates' guide to physical examination and history taking* (11th ed.). Philadelphia, PA: Wolters Kluwer Health Lippincott Williams & Wilkins.

side, and is least palpable over the lower lung fields (Bickley, 2013).

The patient is asked to repeat "ninety-nine" or "one, one, one" as the nurse's hands move down the patient's thorax (Bickley, 2013). The vibrations are detected with the palmar surfaces of the hands, or the ulnar aspect of the extended hands, on the thorax. The hand or hands are moved in sequence down the thorax. Corresponding areas of the thorax are compared (see Fig. 20-10). Bony areas are not assessed.

Air does not conduct sound well; however, a solid substance such as tissue does, provided that it has elasticity and is not compressed. Therefore, an increase in solid tissue per unit volume of lung enhances fremitus, and an increase in air per unit volume of lung impedes sound. Patients with emphysema exhibit almost no tactile fremitus. A patient with consolidation of a lobe of the lung from pneumonia has increased tactile fremitus over that lobe.

Figure 20-9 • Method for assessing posterior respiratory excursion. Place both hands posteriorly at the level of T9 or T10. Slide hands medially to pinch a small amount of skin between your thumbs. Observe for symmetry as the patient exhales fully following a deep inspiration.

Thoracic Percussion

Percussion produces audible and tactile vibration and allows the nurse to determine whether underlying tissues are filled with air, fluid, or solid material. Healthy lung tissue is resonant.

Dullness over the lung occurs when air-filled lung tissue is replaced by fluid or solid tissue. Table 20-5 reviews percussion sounds and their characteristics. Percussion is also used to estimate the size and location of certain structures within the thorax (e.g., diaphragm, heart, liver).

Percussion usually begins with the posterior thorax. The nurse percusses across each shoulder top, locating the 5-cm width of resonance overlying the lung apices (see Fig. 20-11). Then the nurse proceeds down the posterior thorax, percussing symmetric areas at intervals of 5 to 6 cm (2 to 2.5 in). To perform percussion, the middle finger of the nondominant hand is firmly placed against the area of the chest wall to be percussed. The distal interphalangeal joint of this finger is struck with the tip of the middle finger of the dominant hand. This finger is partially flexed and percussion occurs in a smooth, dartlike fashion. Bony structures (scapulae or ribs) are not percussed.

To perform percussion over the anterior chest, the nurse begins in the supraclavicular area and proceeds downward, from one intercostal space to the next. Dullness noted to the left of the sternum between the third and fifth intercostal spaces is a normal finding, because that is the location of the heart. Similarly, there is a normal span of liver dullness below the lung at the right costal margin (Bickley, 2013).

Diaphragmatic Excursion

The normal resonance of the lung stops at the diaphragm. The position of the diaphragm is different during inspiration and expiration.

To assess the position and motion of the diaphragm, the nurse instructs the patient to take a deep breath and hold it while the maximal descent of the diaphragm is percussed. The point at which the percussion note at the midscapular line changes from resonance to dullness is marked with a pen. The patient is then instructed to exhale fully and hold

Figure 20-10 • Palpation sequence for tactile fremitus: posterior thorax (**left**) and anterior thorax (**right**).

TABLE 20-5 • Characteristics of Percussion Sounds

Sound	Relative Intensity	Relative Pitch	Relative Duration	Location Example	Examples
Flatness	Soft	High	Short	Thigh	Large pleural effusion
Dullness	Medium	Medium	Medium	Liver	Lobar pneumonia
Resonance	Loud	Low	Long	Normal lung	Simple chronic bronchitis
Hyperresonance	Very loud	Lower	Longer	None normally	Emphysema, pneumothorax
Tympany	Loud	High[a]	Medium	Gastric air bubble or puffed-out cheek	Large pneumothorax

[a]Distinguished mainly by its musical timbre.
Adapted from Bickley, L. S. (2013). *Bates' guide to physical examination and history taking* (11th ed.). Philadelphia, PA: Wolters Kluwer Health Lippincott Williams & Wilkins.

it while the nurse again percusses downward to the dullness of the diaphragm. This point is also marked. The distance between the two markings indicates the range of motion of the diaphragm.

Maximal excursion of the diaphragm may be as much as 8 to 10 cm (3 to 4 in) in healthy, tall young men, but for most people, it is usually 5 to 7 cm (2 to 2.75 in). Normally, the diaphragm is about 2 cm (0.75 in) higher on the right because of the location of the liver. Decreased diaphragmatic excursion may occur with pleural effusion. Atelectasis, diaphragmatic paralysis, or pregnancy may account for a diaphragm that is positioned high in the thorax (Bickley, 2013).

Thoracic Auscultation

Assessment concludes with auscultation of the anterior, posterior, and lateral thorax. Auscultation helps the nurse assess

the flow of air through the bronchial tree and evaluate the presence of fluid or solid obstruction in the lung. The nurse auscultates for normal breath sounds, adventitious sounds, and voice sounds.

The nurse places the diaphragm of the stethoscope firmly against the bare skin of the chest wall as the patient breathes slowly and deeply through the mouth. Corresponding areas of the chest are auscultated in a systematic fashion from the apices to the bases and along midaxillary lines. The sequence of auscultation is similar to that used for percussion. The nurse may need to listen to two full inspirations and expirations at each anatomic location for valid interpretation of the sound heard. Repeated deep breaths may result in symptoms of hyperventilation (e.g., lightheadedness); this is avoided by having the patient rest and breathe normally periodically during the examination.

Breath Sounds

Normal breath sounds are distinguished by their location over a specific area of the lung and are identified as vesicular, bronchovesicular, and bronchial (tubular) breath sounds (see Table 20-6).

The location, quality, and intensity of breath sounds are determined during auscultation. When airflow is decreased by bronchial obstruction (atelectasis) or when fluid (pleural effusion) or tissue (obesity) separates the air passages from the stethoscope, breath sounds are diminished or absent. For example, the breath sounds of the patient with emphysema are faint or often completely inaudible. When they are heard, the expiratory phase is prolonged. In the patient who is obese, breath sounds may be inaudible. Bronchial and bronchovesicular sounds that are audible anywhere except over the main bronchus in the lungs signify pathology, usually indicating consolidation in the lung (e.g., pneumonia, heart failure). This finding requires further evaluation.

Adventitious Sounds

An abnormal condition that affects the bronchial tree and alveoli may produce adventitious (additional) sounds. Some adventitious sounds are divided into two categories: discrete, discontinuous sounds (**crackles**) and continuous musical sounds (**wheezes**) (see Table 20-7). The duration of the sound is the important distinction to make in identifying the sound as discontinuous or continuous. Friction rubs may be either discontinuous or continuous.

Figure 20-11 • Percussion of the posterior thorax. With the patient in a sitting position, symmetric areas of the lungs are percussed at 5-cm intervals. This progression starts at the apex of each lung and concludes with percussion of each lateral chest wall.

TABLE 20-6 **Breath Sounds**

	Duration of Sounds	Intensity of Expiratory Sound	Pitch of Expiratory Sound	Locations Where Heard Normally
Vesicular[a]	Inspiratory sounds last longer than expiratory ones.	Soft	Relatively low	Entire lung field except over the upper sternum and between the scapulae
Bronchovesicular	Inspiratory and expiratory sounds are about equal.	Intermediate	Intermediate	Often in the 1st and 2nd interspaces anteriorly and between the scapulae (over the main bronchus)
Bronchial	Expiratory sounds last longer than inspiratory ones.	Loud	Relatively high	Over the manubrium, if heard at all
Tracheal	Inspiratory and expiratory sounds are about equal.	Very loud	Relatively high	Over the trachea in the neck

[a]The thickness of the bars indicates intensity of breath sounds: The steeper their incline, the higher the pitch of the sounds.
Adapted from Bickley, L. S. (2013). *Bates' guide to physical examination and history taking* (11th ed.). Philadelphia, PA: Wolters Kluwer Health Lippincott Williams & Wilkins.

TABLE 20-7 **Abnormal (Adventitious) Breath Sounds**

Breath Sound	Description	Etiology
Crackles		
Crackles in general	Soft, high-pitched, discontinuous popping sounds that occur during inspiration (while usually heard on inspiration, they may also be heard on expiration); may or may not be cleared by coughing	Secondary to fluid in the airways or alveoli or to delayed opening of collapsed alveoli Associated with heart failure and pulmonary fibrosis
Coarse crackles	Discontinuous popping sounds heard in early inspiration; harsh, moist sound originating in the large bronchi	Associated with obstructive pulmonary disease
Fine crackles	Discontinuous popping sounds heard in late inspiration; sounds like hair rubbing together; originates in the alveoli	Associated with interstitial pneumonia, restrictive pulmonary disease (e.g., fibrosis); fine crackles in early inspiration are associated with bronchitis or pneumonia
Wheezes		
Wheezes in general	Usually heard on expiration but may be heard on inspiration depending on the cause	Associated with bronchial wall oscillation and changes in airway diameter Associated with chronic bronchitis or bronchiectasis
Sonorous wheezes (rhonchi)	Deep, low-pitched rumbling sounds heard primarily during expiration; caused by air moving through narrowed tracheobronchial passages	Associated with secretions or tumor
Sibilant wheezes	Continuous, musical, high-pitched, whistle-like sounds heard during inspiration and expiration caused by air passing through narrowed or partially obstructed airways; may clear with coughing	Associated with bronchospasm, asthma, and buildup of secretions
Friction Rubs		
Pleural friction rub	Harsh, crackling sound, like two pieces of leather being rubbed together (sound imitated by rubbing thumb and finger together near the ear) Heard during inspiration alone or during both inspiration and expiration May subside when patient holds breath; coughing will not clear sound Best heard over the lower lateral anterior surface of the thorax Sound can be enhanced by applying pressure to the chest wall with the diaphragm of the stethoscope.	Secondary to inflammation and loss of lubricating pleural fluid

Adapted from Bickley, L. S. (2013). *Bates' guide to physical examination and history taking* (11th ed.). Philadelphia, PA: Wolters Kluwer Health Lippincott Williams & Wilkins.

Voice Sounds

The sound heard through the stethoscope as the patient speaks is known as vocal resonance. The nurse should assess voice sounds when abnormal breath sounds are auscultated. The vibrations produced in the larynx are transmitted to the chest wall as they pass through the bronchi and alveolar tissue. Voice sounds are evaluated by having the patient repeat "ninety-nine" or "eee" while the nurse listens with the stethoscope in corresponding areas of the chest from the apices to the bases. With normal physiology, the sounds are faint and indistinct. Pathology that increases lung density, such as pneumonia and pulmonary edema, alters this normal physiologic response and may result in the following sounds:

- **Bronchophony** describes vocal resonance that is more intense and clearer than normal.
- **Egophony** describes voice sounds that are distorted. It is best appreciated by having the patient repeat the letter E. The distortion produced by consolidation transforms the sound into a clearly heard A rather than E.
- **Whispered pectoriloquy** describes the ability to clearly and distinctly hear whispered sounds that should not normally be heard.

Whenever an abnormality is detected on examination, it should be evident using more than one assessment method. A change in tactile fremitus is more subtle and can be missed, but bronchophony can be noted loudly and clearly.

Interpreting Findings

The physical findings for the most common respiratory diseases are summarized in Table 20-8.

Assessment of Respiratory Function in the Acutely or Critically Ill Patient

Assessment of respiratory status is essential for the well-being of the patient who is acutely or critically ill. Often, such a patient is intubated and receiving mechanical ventilation. In addition to expertise in physical assessment, the nurse should be skilled in monitoring techniques and knowledgeable about possible ventilator-associated events and evidenced-based interventions to prevent these events (Klompas, 2013). The nurse analyzes findings from the health history and assessment while considering laboratory and diagnostic test results. After checking the ventilator settings to make sure that they are set as prescribed and that alarms are always in the "on" position, the nurse must assess for patient–ventilator synchrony and for agitation, restlessness, and other signs of respiratory distress (nasal flaring, excessive use of intercostals and accessory muscles, uncoordinated movement of the chest and abdomen, and a report by the patient of shortness of breath). The nurse must note changes in the patient's vital signs and evidence of hemodynamic instability and report them to the primary provider, because they may indicate that the mechanical ventilation is ineffective or that the patient's status has deteriorated. The patient's position must be assessed to ensure that the head of the bed is elevated to prevent aspiration, especially if the patient is receiving enteral feedings. In addition, the patient's mental status should be assessed and compared to previous status. Lethargy and somnolence may be signs of increasing carbon dioxide levels and should not be considered insignificant, even if the patient is receiving sedation or analgesic agents.

Chest auscultation, percussion, and palpation are essential and routine parts of the evaluation of the critically ill patient with or without mechanical ventilation. A recumbent patient must be turned to assess all lung fields. Dependent areas must be assessed for normal breath sounds and adventitious sounds. Failure to examine the dependent areas of the lungs can result in missing the findings associated with disorders such as atelectasis or pleural effusion.

Tests of the patient's respiratory status are easily performed at the bedside by measuring the respiratory rate, tidal volume, minute ventilation, vital capacity, inspiratory force, and compliance. These tests are particularly important for patients who are at risk for pulmonary complications, including those who have undergone chest or abdominal surgery, have had prolonged anesthesia, or have preexisting pulmonary disease, and those who are older or obese. These tests are also used routinely for mechanically ventilated patients. Although

TABLE 20-8 Assessment Findings in Common Respiratory Disorders

Disorder	Tactile Fremitus	Percussion	Auscultation
Consolidation (e.g., pneumonia)	Increased	Dull	Bronchial breath sounds, crackles, bronchophony, egophony, whispered pectoriloquy
Bronchitis	Normal	Resonant	Normal to decreased breath sounds; possible scattered coarse crackles, rhonchi, or wheezes
Emphysema	Decreased	Hyperresonant	Absent or decreased breath sounds; possible crackles, wheezes, or rhonchi
Asthma	Decreased	Resonant to hyperresonant	Wheezes, occasional crackles
Pulmonary edema	Normal	Resonant	Crackles at lung bases, possibly wheezes
Pleural effusion	Decreased to absent but may be increased over large effusion	Dull to flat	Decreased to absent breath sounds, bronchial breath sounds sometimes heard atop of large effusion, possible pleural rub
Pneumothorax	Decreased to absent	Hyperresonant	Absent breath sounds, possible pleural rub
Atelectasis	Absent	Dull	Decreased to absent breath sounds; may be increased in right upper lobe atelectasis

Adapted from Bickley, L. S. (2013). *Bates' guide to physical examination and history taking* (11th ed.). Philadelphia, PA: Wolters Kluwer Health Lippincott Williams & Wilkins.

some of these tests are performed by respiratory therapists, it is useful for nurses to understand the significance of these test results.

The patient whose chest expansion is limited by external restrictions such as obesity or abdominal distention, or who cannot breathe deeply because of postoperative pain or sedation will inhale and exhale a low volume of air (referred to as low tidal volumes). Prolonged hypoventilation at low tidal volumes can produce alveolar collapse (atelectasis). Consequently, when the forced residual capacity decreases, compliance is reduced, and the patient must breathe faster to maintain the same degree of tissue oxygenation. These events can be exaggerated in patients who have preexisting pulmonary diseases; in older adult patients whose airways are less compliant because the small airways may collapse during expiration; or in patients who are obese, who have relatively low tidal volumes even when healthy. (More details of the assessment of the patient with lung disease are described in subsequent chapters in this unit.)

> ### ◤ Quality and Safety Nursing Alert
>
> *The nurse should not rely only on visual inspection of the rate and depth of a patient's respiratory excursions to determine the adequacy of ventilation. Respiratory excursions may appear normal or exaggerated due to an increased work of breathing, but the patient may actually be moving only enough air to ventilate the dead space. If there is any question regarding adequacy of ventilation, the nurse should use auscultation or pulse oximetry (or both) for additional assessment of respiratory status.*

Tidal Volume

The volume of each breath is referred to as the **tidal volume** (see Table 20-1 to review lung capacities and volumes). A spirometer is an instrument that can be used at the bedside to measure volumes. If the patient is breathing through an endotracheal tube or tracheostomy, the spirometer is directly attached to it and the exhaled volume is obtained from the reading on the gauge. In other patients, the spirometer is attached to a face mask or a mouthpiece positioned so that it is airtight, and the exhaled volume is measured.

The tidal volume may vary from breath to breath. To ensure that the measurement is reliable, it is important to measure the volumes of several breaths and to note the range of tidal volumes, together with the average tidal volume.

Minute Ventilation

Because respiratory rates and tidal volumes vary widely from breath to breath, these data alone are unreliable indicators of adequate ventilation. However, the tidal volume multiplied by the respiratory rate provides what is called *minute ventilation* or *minute volume*, the volume of air exchanged per minute. This value is useful in detecting respiratory failure. In practice, the minute volume is not calculated but is measured directly using a spirometer. In a patient receiving mechanical ventilation, minute volume is often monitored by the ventilator and can be viewed on the monitoring screen.

Minute ventilation may be decreased by a variety of conditions that result in hypoventilation. When the minute

---

Chart 20-10 ⚠ RISK FACTORS
Hypoventilation

- Limited neurologic impulses transmitted from the brain to the respiratory muscles, as in spinal cord trauma, cerebrovascular accidents, tumors, myasthenia gravis, Guillain–Barré syndrome, polio, and drug overdose.
- Depressed respiratory centers in the medulla, as with anesthesia, sedation, and drug overdose.
- Limited thoracic movement (kyphoscoliosis), limited lung movement (pleural effusion, pneumothorax), or reduced functional lung tissue (chronic pulmonary diseases, severe pulmonary edema).

Adapted from Bulbul, Y., Ayik, S., Ozlu, T., et al. (2014). Frequency and predictors of obesity hypoventilation in hospitalized patients at a tertiary health care institution. *Annals of Thoracic Medicine*, 9(2), 87–91; Karez, M., & Papadakos, P. J. (2013). Respiratory complications in the postanesthesia care unit: A review of pathophysiological mechanisms. *Canadian Journal of Respiratory Therapy*, 49(4), 21–29.

---

ventilation falls, alveolar ventilation in the lungs also decreases and the $PaCO_2$ increases. Risk factors for hypoventilation are listed in Chart 20-10.

Vital Capacity

Vital capacity is measured by having the patient take in a maximal breath and exhale fully through a spirometer. The normal value depends on the patient's age, gender, body build, and weight.

> ### ◤ Quality and Safety Nursing Alert
>
> *Most patients can generate a vital capacity twice the volume they normally breathe in and out (tidal volume). If the vital capacity is less than 10 mL/kg, the patient will be unable to sustain spontaneous ventilation and will require respiratory assistance.*

When the vital capacity is exhaled at a maximal flow rate, the forced vital capacity (FVC) is measured. Most patients can exhale at least 80% of their vital capacity in 1 second (forced expiratory volume in 1 second, or FEV_1) and almost all of it in 3 seconds (FEV_3). A reduction in FEV_1 suggests abnormal pulmonary airflow. If the patient's FEV_1 and FVC are proportionately reduced, maximal lung expansion is restricted in some way. If the reduction in FEV_1 greatly exceeds the reduction in FVC (FEV_1/FVC less than 85%), the patient may have some degree of airway obstruction.

Inspiratory Force

Inspiratory force evaluates the effort the patient is making during inspiration. It does not require patient cooperation and, therefore, is a useful measurement in the patient who is unconscious. The equipment needed for this measurement includes a manometer that measures negative pressure and adapters that are connected to an anesthesia mask or a cuffed endotracheal tube. The manometer is attached, and the airway is completely occluded for 10 to 20 seconds while the inspiratory efforts of the patient are registered on the manometer. The normal inspiratory pressure is about 100 cm H_2O.

If the negative pressure registered after 15 seconds of occluding the airway is less than about 25 cm H_2O, mechanical ventilation is usually required because the patient lacks sufficient muscle strength for deep breathing or effective coughing.

Diagnostic Evaluation

A wide range of diagnostic studies may be performed in patients with respiratory conditions. The nurse should educate the patient on the purpose of the studies, what to expect, and any possible side effects related to these examinations prior to testing. The nurse should note trends in results because they provide information about disease progression as well as the patient's response to therapy.

Pulmonary Function Tests

Pulmonary function tests (PFTs) are routinely used in patients with chronic respiratory disorders to aid diagnosis. They are performed to assess respiratory function and to determine the extent of dysfunction, response to therapy, and as screening tests in potentially hazardous industries, such as coal mining and those that involve exposure to asbestos and other noxious irritants. PFTs are also used prior to surgery to screen patients who are scheduled for thoracic and upper abdominal surgical procedures, patients who are obese, and symptomatic patients with a history suggesting high risk. Such tests include measurements of lung volumes, ventilatory function, and the mechanics of breathing, diffusion, and gas exchange.

PFTs generally are performed by a technician using a spirometer that has a volume-collecting device attached to a recorder that demonstrates volume and time simultaneously. Several tests are carried out because no single measurement provides a complete picture of pulmonary function. The most frequently used PFTs are described in Table 20-9. Technology is available that allows for more complex assessment of pulmonary function. Methods include exercise tidal flow–volume loops, negative expiratory pressure, nitric oxide, forced oscillation, and diffusing capacity for helium or carbon monoxide. These assessment methods allow for detailed evaluation of expiratory flow limitations and airway inflammation.

PFT results are interpreted on the basis of the degree of deviation from normal, taking into consideration the patient's height, weight, age, gender, and ethnicity. Because there is a wide range of normal values, PFTs may not detect early localized changes. The patient with respiratory symptoms usually undergoes a complete diagnostic evaluation, even if the results of PFTs are "normal." Patients with respiratory disorders may be taught how to measure their peak flow rate (which reflects maximal expiratory flow) at home using a spirometer. This allows them to monitor the progress of therapy, to alter medications and other interventions as needed on the basis of caregiver guidelines, and to notify the primary provider if there is inadequate response to their own interventions. (Instructions for home care education are described in Chapter 24, which discusses asthma.)

Arterial Blood Gas Studies

Arterial blood gas (ABG) studies aid in assessing the ability of the lungs to provide adequate oxygen and remove carbon dioxide, which reflects ventilation, and the ability of the kidneys to reabsorb or excrete bicarbonate ions to maintain normal body pH, which reflects metabolic states. ABG levels are obtained through an arterial puncture at the radial, brachial, or femoral artery or through an indwelling arterial catheter. Pain (related to nerve injury or noxious stimulation), infection, hematoma, and hemorrhage are potential complications that may be associated with obtaining ABGs (Perry, Potter, & Ostendorf, 2014). (See Chapter 13 for discussion of ABG analysis.)

Venous Blood Gas Studies

Venous blood gas (VBG) studies provide additional data on oxygen delivery and consumption. VBG levels reflect the balance between the amount of oxygen used by tissues and

TABLE 20-9 Pulmonary Function Tests

Term Used	Symbol	Description	Remarks
Forced vital capacity	FVC	Vital capacity performed with a maximally forced expiratory effort	Forced vital capacity is often reduced in chronic obstructive pulmonary disease because of air trapping
Forced expiratory volume (qualified by subscript indicating the time interval in seconds)	FEV_t (usually FEV_1)	Volume of air exhaled in the specified time during the performance of forced vital capacity; FEV_1 is volume exhaled in 1 second	A valuable clue to the severity of the expiratory airway obstruction
Ratio of timed forced expiratory volume to forced vital capacity	$FEV_t/FVC\%$, usually $FEV_1/FVC\%$	FEV_t expressed as a percentage of the forced vital capacity	Another way of expressing the presence or absence of airway obstruction
Forced expiratory flow	$FEF_{200-1,200}$	Mean forced expiratory flow between 200 and 1200 mL of the FVC	An indicator of large airway obstruction
Forced midexpiratory flow	$FEF_{25-75\%}$	Mean forced expiratory flow during the middle half of the FVC	Slowed in small airway obstruction
Forced end expiratory flow	$FEF_{75-85\%}$	Mean forced expiratory flow during the terminal portion of the FVC	Slowed in obstruction of smallest airways
Maximal voluntary ventilation	MVV	Volume of air expired in a specified period (12 seconds) during repetitive maximal effort	An important factor in exercise tolerance

organs and the amount of oxygen returning to the right side of the heart in the blood. Mixed venous oxygen saturation ($S\bar{v}O_2$) levels, the most accurate indicator of this balance, can be obtained only from blood samples drawn from a pulmonary artery catheter. Central venous oxygen saturation ($Sc\bar{v}O_2$) levels, which are measured using blood drawn from a central venous catheter, closely approximate $S\bar{v}O_2$ levels and are, therefore, used more frequently (Reid, 2013). VBG analysis is recommended to guide goal-directed therapy in postoperative patients at risk for hemodynamic instability or in patients with septic shock and may decrease morbidity and mortality in these groups (Davis, Walsh, Sittig, et al., 2013).

Pulse Oximetry

Pulse oximetry, or SpO_2, is a noninvasive method of continuously monitoring the **oxygen saturation** of hemoglobin (SaO_2). Although pulse oximetry does not replace blood gas analysis, it is an effective tool to monitor for subtle or sudden changes in SaO_2 and can easily be used in the home and various health care settings.

A probe or sensor is attached to the fingertip (see Fig. 20-12), forehead, earlobe, or bridge of the nose. The sensor detects changes in oxygen saturation levels by monitoring light signals generated by the oximeter and reflected by blood pulsing through the tissue at the probe. Normal SpO_2 values are more than 95%. Values less than 90% indicate that the tissues are not receiving enough oxygen, in which case further evaluation is needed. SpO_2 values are unreliable in cardiac arrest, shock, and other states of low perfusion (e.g., sepsis, peripheral vascular disease, hypothermia), and when vasoconstrictor medications have been used (Chan, Chan, & Chan, 2013). Additional causes of inaccurate pulse oximetry results include anemia, abnormal hemoglobin, high carbon monoxide level, the use of dyes (e.g., methylene blue), or if the patient has dark skin or is wearing nail polish. Bright light, particularly sunlight, fluorescent and xenon lights, and patient movement (including shivering) also affect accuracy. SpO_2 values cannot reliably detect hypoventilation when supplemental oxygen is in use (Chan et al., 2013).

Cultures

Throat, nasal, and nasopharyngeal cultures can identify pathogens responsible for respiratory infections, such as pharyngitis. Throat cultures are performed in adults with severe or ongoing sore throats accompanied by fever and lymph node enlargement and are most useful in detecting streptococcal infection. Rapid strep tests are now available that can provide results within 15 minutes, often replacing the need for throat cultures. Other sources of infection, such as *Staphylococcus aureus* or *Influenza*, are detected via nasal or nasopharyngeal cultures. Ideally, all cultures should be obtained prior to the initiation of antibiotic therapy. Results usually take between 48 and 72 hours, with preliminary reports available usually within 24 hours. Cultures may be repeated to assess a patient's response to therapy (Pagana & Pagana, 2013).

Sputum Studies

Sputum is obtained for analysis to identify pathogenic organisms and to determine whether malignant cells are present. Periodic sputum examinations may be necessary for patients

A

B

Figure 20-12 • Measuring blood oxygenation with pulse oximetry reduces the need for invasive procedures, such as drawing blood for analysis of oxygen levels. **A.** Self-contained digital fingertip pulse oximeter, which incorporates the sensor and the display into one unit. **B.** Tabletop model with sensor attached. Memory permits tracking heart rate and oxygen saturation over time.

receiving antibiotics, corticosteroids, and immunosuppressive medications for prolonged periods because these agents are associated with opportunistic infections.

Sputum samples ideally are obtained early in the morning before the patient has had anything to eat or drink. The patient is instructed to clear the nose and the throat and rinse the mouth to decrease contamination of the sputum and not to simply spit saliva into the container. Rather, after taking a few deep breaths, the patient coughs deeply and expectorates sputum from the lungs into a sterile container.

If the patient cannot expel an adequate sputum sample following the above techniques, coughing can be induced by administering an aerosolized hypertonic solution via a nebulizer. Other methods of collecting sputum specimens include endotracheal or transtracheal aspiration or bronchoscopic removal. The nurse should label the specimen and send it to the laboratory as soon as possible to avoid contamination.

Imaging Studies

Imaging studies, including x-rays, computed tomography (CT), magnetic resonance imaging (MRI), and radioisotope or nuclear scanning may be part of any diagnostic workup, ranging from a determination of the extent of infection in sinusitis to tumor growth in cancer.

Chest X-Ray

Normal pulmonary tissue is radiolucent because it consists mostly of air and gases; therefore, densities produced by fluid, tumors, foreign bodies, and other pathologic conditions can be detected by x-ray examination. In the absence of symptoms, a chest x-ray may reveal an extensive pathologic process in the lungs. The routine chest x-ray consists of two views: the posteroanterior projection and the lateral projection. Chest x-rays are usually obtained after full inspiration because the lungs are best visualized when they are well aerated. In addition, the diaphragm is at its lowest level and the largest expanse of lung is visible. Patients, therefore, need to be able to take a deep breath and hold it without discomfort. Chest x-rays are contraindicated in pregnant women.

Nursing Interventions

The nurse should notify the patient that chest x-rays do not require fasting, nor typically cause pain. However, in order to best visualize the lungs, the patient must be able to take a deep breath and hold it without discomfort, while the technician takes the images. The patient will be positioned in a standing, sitting, or recumbent position, in order to obtain the appropriate view of the chest (posterior–anterior, lateral, oblique, or decubitus position). The patient will be asked to wear a gown, remove metal objects from the chest, such as necklaces, and may be given a lead shield to minimize radiation exposure to the thyroid gland, ovaries, or testicles (Pagana & Pagana, 2013).

Computed Tomography

A CT is an imaging method in which the lungs are scanned in successive layers by a narrow-beam x-ray. The images produced provide a cross-sectional view of the chest. Whereas a chest x-ray shows major contrasts between body densities such as bone, soft tissue, and air, a CT scan can distinguish fine tissue density. A CT scan may be used to define pulmonary nodules and small tumors adjacent to pleural surfaces that are not visible on routine chest x-rays and to demonstrate mediastinal abnormalities and hilar adenopathy, which are difficult to visualize with other techniques. Contrast agents are useful when evaluating the mediastinum and its contents, particularly its vasculature. Advancements in CT scanning technology, referred to as multidetection, spiral, or helical CT, enable the chest to be scanned quickly while generating an extensive number of images that can generate a three-dimensional analysis (Pagana & Pagana, 2013). CT pulmonary angiography is now used routinely in place of catheter angiography to diagnose PE (York, Kane, Smith, et al., 2015). Contraindications include allergy to dye, pregnancy, claustrophobia, and morbid obesity, whereas potential complications include acute kidney injury and acidosis secondary to contrast (Pagana & Pagana, 2013).

Nursing Interventions

The nurse should inform patients preparing for CT scans that they will be required to remain supine and still for a short period, typically less than 30 minutes, while a body scanner surrounds them and takes multiple images. Patients typically do not experience claustrophobia during CT scanning but can be given antianxiety medications preprocedure if this is a concern. If contrast dye is required, patients will need to stay *nil per os* (NPO) for 4 hours prior to the examination. In this case, the nurse should also assess for allergies to iodine or shellfish (Pagana & Pagana, 2013).

Magnetic Resonance Imaging

MRI is similar to a CT scan except that magnetic fields and radiofrequency signals are used instead of radiation. MRI is able to better distinguish between normal and abnormal tissues than CT and, therefore, yields a much more detailed diagnostic image. MRI is used to characterize pulmonary nodules; to help stage bronchogenic carcinoma (assessment of chest wall invasion); and to evaluate inflammatory activity in interstitial lung disease, acute PE, and chronic thrombolytic pulmonary hypertension. Contraindications for MRI include morbid obesity, claustrophobia, confusion and agitation, and having implanted metal or metal support devices that are considered unsafe (Pagana & Pagana, 2013). Various labels and icons are used to indicate whether a medical device is safe or unsafe for use during MRI. Recent improvements in technology have contributed to the design of certain medical devices, such as infusion pumps and ventilators, deemed safe for the MRI room. The nurse should consult with specially trained MRI personnel to clarify the safety of various devices (Wells & Murphy, 2014). Gadolinium-based contrast agents used during MRI may potentially lead to nephrogenic systemic fibrosis in patients with reduced kidney function (Pagana & Pagana, 2013).

Nursing Interventions

Patients scheduled for MRI should be instructed to remove all metal items such as hearing aids, hair clips, and medication patches with metallic foil components (e.g., nicotine patches). Prior to the MRI, the nurse should assess for the presence of implanted metal devices, such as aneurysm clips or a cardiac pacemaker/defibrillator. The nurse should inform patients preparing for MRI that they will need to lie flat and remain still for between 30 to 90 minutes, while the table that they are on moves into a large tubular magnet. Patients should be notified that they will hear a loud humming or thumping noise. Earplugs are typically offered to patients to minimize this noise. Patients will be able to communicate with the MRI staff via a microphone and earphones. The nurse should clarify with the physician or the technologist if the ordered test requires the use of dye or the patient should remain NPO pre-examination. Patients who experience claustrophobia should be offered antianxiety medications preprocedure or be scheduled at a facility that uses an open MRI system (Pagana & Pagana, 2013).

Fluoroscopic Studies

Fluoroscopy, which allows live x-ray images to be generated via a camera to a video screen, is used to assist with invasive procedures, such as a chest needle biopsy or transbronchial biopsy, that are performed to identify lesions. It also may be used to study the movement of the chest wall, mediastinum, heart, and diaphragm; to detect diaphragm paralysis; and to locate lung masses. The specific procedure performed under fluoroscopy will guide those respective nursing interventions (e.g., see nursing interventions described in the Lung Biopsy Procedures section).

Pulmonary Angiography

Pulmonary angiography is used to investigate congenital abnormalities of the pulmonary vascular tree, and less frequently PE, when less invasive tests are inconclusive, but there is a high clinical suspicion for PE (Ma, Yan, Zhou, et al., 2016). To visualize the pulmonary vessels, a radiopaque agent is injected through a catheter, which has been initially inserted into a vein (e.g., jugular, subclavian, brachial, or femoral vein) and then threaded into the pulmonary artery. Contraindications include allergy to the radiopaque dye, pregnancy, and bleeding abnormalities, whereas potential complications include acute kidney injury, acidosis, cardiac dysrhythmias, and bleeding (Pagana & Pagana, 2013).

Nursing Interventions

Prior to the angiography, the nurse should verify that informed consent has been obtained; assess for known allergies that may suggest allergies to radiopaque dye (e.g., iodine and shellfish); assess anticoagulation status and renal function; ensure that the patient has not eaten or had anything to drink preprocedurally as prescribed (normally for 6 to 8 hours); and administer preprocedure medications that may include antianxiety medications, secretion-reducing agents, and antihistamines. The nurse should instruct patients that they may experience a warm flushing sensation or chest pain during the injection of the dye. If an arterial puncture is necessary, the affected extremity will need to be immobilized for a certain amount of time depending on the size of the sheath that was used and the type of arterial closure device employed. Following the procedure, the nurse should closely monitor vital signs, level of consciousness, oxygen saturation, and the vascular access site for bleeding or hematoma, and perform frequent assessment of neurovascular status (Perry et al., 2014).

Radioisotope Diagnostic Procedures (Lung Scans)

Several types of lung scans—$\dot{V}/\dot{Q}$ scan, gallium scan, and positron emission tomography (PET)—are performed to assess normal lung functioning, pulmonary vascular supply, and gas exchange. Pregnancy is a contraindication for these scans.

A $\dot{V}/\dot{Q}$ lung scan is performed by injecting a radioactive agent into a peripheral vein and then obtaining a scan of the chest to detect radiation. The isotope particles pass through the right side of the heart and are distributed into the lungs in proportion to the regional blood flow, making it possible to trace and measure blood perfusion through the lung. This procedure is used clinically to measure the integrity of the pulmonary vessels relative to blood flow and to evaluate blood flow abnormalities, as seen in PE. The imaging time is 20 to 40 minutes, during which the patient lies under the camera with a mask fitted over the nose and the mouth. This is followed by the ventilation component of the scan.

The patient takes a deep breath of a mixture of oxygen and radioactive gas, which diffuses throughout the lungs. A scan is performed to detect ventilation abnormalities in patients who have regional differences in ventilation. It may be helpful in the diagnosis of bronchitis, asthma, inflammatory fibrosis, pneumonia, emphysema, and lung cancer. Ventilation without perfusion is seen with PE.

A gallium scan is a radioisotope lung scan used to detect inflammatory conditions, abscesses, adhesions, and the presence, location, and size of tumors. It is used to stage bronchogenic cancer and to document tumor regression after chemotherapy or radiation. Gallium is injected intravenously, and scans are obtained at intervals (e.g., 6, 24, and 48 hours) to evaluate gallium uptake by the pulmonary tissues.

PET is a radioisotope study with advanced diagnostic capabilities that is used to evaluate lung nodules for malignancy. PET can detect and display metabolic changes in tissue, distinguish normal tissue from diseased tissue (such as in cancer), differentiate viable from dead or dying tissue, show regional blood flow, and determine the distribution and fate of medications in the body. PET is more accurate in detecting malignancies than CT and has equivalent accuracy in detecting malignant nodules when compared with invasive procedures such as thoracoscopy. Images from PET scans are now being superimposed on CT and MRI images to enhance the accuracy of diagnosis (Pagana & Pagana, 2013).

Nursing Interventions

For each of these nuclear scans, the nurse should educate the patient on what to expect. Intravenous access is required. Sometimes, an enema is prescribed prior to a gallium scan to decrease its uptake in the gastrointestinal tract. Chest x-ray should be performed prior to a $\dot{V}/\dot{Q}$ scanning. Patients should be told that $\dot{V}/\dot{Q}$ and gallium scans require only a small amount of radioisotopes; therefore, radiation safety measures are not indicated. Normally, the patient may eat or drink prior to $\dot{V}/\dot{Q}$ or gallium scans. Multiple factors can hinder the uptake of radioactive agents used for a PET scan. The nurse should instruct the patient to avoid caffeine, alcohol, and tobacco for 24 hours prior to the PET scan and abstain from food and fluids for 4 hours prior to the scan. Accurate results depend on an empty bladder; thus, a Foley catheter may be indicated. The nurse should encourage fluid intake postprocedure to facilitate the elimination of radioisotopes in the urine (Pagana & Pagana, 2013).

Endoscopic Procedures

Endoscopic procedures include bronchoscopy, thoracoscopy, and thoracentesis.

Bronchoscopy

Bronchoscopy is the direct inspection and examination of the larynx, trachea, and bronchi through either a flexible fiberoptic bronchoscope or a rigid bronchoscope (see Fig. 20-13). The fiberoptic scope is used more frequently in current practice.

Procedure

The purposes of diagnostic bronchoscopy are (1) to visualize tissues and determine the nature, location, and extent of the pathologic process; (2) to collect secretions for analysis and to obtain a tissue sample for diagnosis; (3) to determine whether

Fiberoptic bronchoscopy

Rigid bronchoscopy

Figure 20-13 • Endoscopic bronchoscopy permits visualization of bronchial structures. The bronchoscope is advanced into bronchial structures orally. Bronchoscopy permits the clinician to not only diagnose but also treat various lung problems.

a tumor can be resected surgically; and (4) to diagnose sources of hemoptysis.

Therapeutic bronchoscopy is used to (1) remove foreign bodies or secretions from the tracheobronchial tree, (2) control bleeding, (3) treat postoperative atelectasis, (4) destroy and excise lesions, and (5) provide brachytherapy (endobronchial radiation therapy). It has also been used to insert stents to relieve airway obstruction that is caused by tumors or miscellaneous benign conditions or that occurs as a complication of lung transplantation.

The fiberoptic bronchoscope is a thin, flexible bronchoscope that can be directed into the segmental bronchi. Because of its small size, its flexibility, and its excellent optical system, it allows increased visualization of the peripheral airways and is ideal for diagnosing pulmonary lesions. Fiberoptic bronchoscopy allows biopsy of previously inaccessible tumors and can be performed at the bedside. It also can be performed through endotracheal or tracheostomy tubes of patients on ventilators. Cytologic examinations can be performed without surgical intervention.

The rigid bronchoscope is a hollow metal tube with a light at its end. It is used mainly for removing foreign substances, investigating the source of massive hemoptysis, or performing endobronchial surgical procedures. Rigid bronchoscopy is performed in the operating room, not at the bedside.

Possible complications of bronchoscopy include a reaction to the local anesthetic, oversedation, prolonged fever, infection, aspiration, vasovagal response, laryngospasm, bronchospasm, hypoxemia, pneumothorax, and bleeding (Pagana & Pagana, 2013; Perry et al., 2014).

Nursing Interventions

Before the procedure, the nurse should verify that informed consent has been obtained. Food and fluids are withheld for 4 to 8 hours before the test to reduce the risk of aspiration when the cough reflex is blocked by anesthesia. The nurse explains the procedure to the patient to reduce fear and decrease anxiety and then administers preoperative medications (usually atropine and a sedative or opioid) as prescribed to inhibit vagal stimulation (thereby guarding against bradycardia, dysrhythmias, and hypotension), suppress the cough reflex, sedate the patient, and relieve anxiety.

> ⚑ **Quality and Safety Nursing Alert**
>
> Sedation given to patients with respiratory insufficiency may precipitate respiratory arrest.

The patient must remove dentures and other oral prostheses. The examination is usually performed under local anesthesia or moderate sedation; however, general anesthesia may be used for rigid bronchoscopy. A topical anesthetic such as lidocaine (Xylocaine) is normally sprayed on the pharynx or dropped on the epiglottis and vocal cords and into the trachea to suppress the cough reflex and minimize discomfort.

After the procedure, the patient must take nothing by mouth until the cough reflex returns, because the preoperative sedation and local anesthesia impair the protective laryngeal reflex and swallowing. Once the patient demonstrates a cough reflex, the nurse may offer ice chips and eventually fluids. In the older adult patient, the nurse assesses for confusion and lethargy, which may be owing to the large doses of lidocaine given during the procedure. The nurse also monitors the patient's respiratory status and observes for hypoxia, hypotension, tachycardia, dysrhythmias, hemoptysis, and dyspnea. Any abnormality is reported promptly. A small amount of blood-tinged sputum and fever may be expected within the first 24 hours (Pagana & Pagana, 2013). The patient is not discharged from the recovery area until adequate cough reflex and respiratory status are present. The nurse instructs the patient and caregivers to report any shortness of breath or bleeding immediately.

Thoracoscopy

Thoracoscopy is a diagnostic procedure in which the pleural cavity is examined with an endoscope and fluid and tissues can be obtained for analysis (see Fig. 20-14).

Procedure

This procedure is performed in the operating room, normally under anesthesia. Small incisions are made into the pleural cavity in an intercostal space at the location indicated by clinical and diagnostic findings. The fiberoptic mediastinoscope is inserted into the pleural cavity, any fluid present is aspirated, and the pleural cavity is inspected through the instrument. After the procedure, a chest tube may be inserted to facilitate re-expansion of the lung.

Thoracoscopy is primarily indicated in the diagnostic evaluation and treatment of pleural effusions, pleural disease, and tumor staging. Biopsies of the lesions and resection of tissues can be performed under visualization for diagnosis.

Thoracoscopic procedures have expanded with the availability of video monitoring, which permits improved visualization of

Figure 20-14 • Endoscopic thoracoscopy. Like bronchoscopy, thoracoscopy uses fiber-optic instruments and video cameras for visualizing thoracic structures. Unlike bronchoscopy, thoracoscopy usually requires the surgeon to make a small incision before inserting the endoscope. A combined diagnostic–treatment procedure, thoracoscopy includes excising tissue for biopsy.

the lung. Video-assisted thoracoscopy (VATS) may be used in the diagnosis and treatment of empyema, pleural effusion, pulmonary and pleural masses, and pneumothorax. Although VATS does not replace the need for thoracotomy in the treatment of some lung cancers, its use continues to grow, because it is less invasive than open surgical procedures, and hospitalization and recovery are shorter.

Nursing Interventions

The nurse should follow routine preoperative practices, such as ensuring that informed consent is obtained and that the patient remains NPO (has nothing by mouth) prior to the procedure. Postoperatively, the nurse should monitor vital signs, pain level, and respiratory status, and should look for signs of bleeding and infection at the incisional site. Shortness of breath may indicate a pneumothorax and should be reported immediately. If a chest tube was inserted during the procedure, monitoring of the chest drainage system and chest tube insertion site is essential (see Chapter 21).

Thoracentesis

In some respiratory disorders, pleural fluid may accumulate. Thoracentesis (aspiration of fluid and air from the pleural space) is performed for diagnostic or therapeutic reasons. Purposes of the procedure include removal of fluid and, very rarely, air from the pleural cavity; aspiration of pleural fluid for analysis; pleural biopsy; and instillation of medication into the pleural space. Studies of pleural fluid include Gram stain culture and sensitivity, acid-fast staining and culture, differential cell count, cytology, pH, total protein, lactic dehydrogenase, glucose, amylase, triglycerides, and cancer markers such as carcinoembryonic antigen.

For the procedural guidelines for assisting with a thoracentesis, go to **thepoint.lww.com/Brunner14e**.

Biopsy

Biopsy—the excision of a small amount of tissue—may be performed to permit examination of cells from the upper and lower respiratory structures and adjacent lymph nodes. Local, topical, or moderate sedation, or general anesthesia, may be given, depending on the site and the procedure.

Pleural Biopsy

Pleural biopsy is accomplished by needle biopsy of the pleura, thoracoscopy, or pleuroscopy, a visual exploration through a fiberoptic pleuroscope inserted into the pleural space or through a thoracotomy. Pleural biopsy is performed when there is pleural exudate of undetermined origin or when there is a need to culture or stain the tissue to identify tuberculosis or fungi.

Lung Biopsy Procedures

Lung biopsy is performed to obtain tissue for examination when other diagnostic testing indicates potential interstitial lung disease, such as cancer, infection, or sarcoidosis. Several nonsurgical lung biopsy techniques are used because they yield accurate information with low morbidity: transbronchial brushing or needle aspiration, transbronchial lung biopsy, and percutaneous (through-the-skin) needle biopsy. Possible complications for all methods include pneumothorax, pulmonary hemorrhage, and empyema (Pagana & Pagana, 2013).

Procedure

In transbronchial brushing, a fiberoptic bronchoscope is introduced into the bronchus under fluoroscopy. A small brush attached to the end of a flexible wire is inserted through the bronchoscope. Under direct visualization, the area under suspicion is brushed back and forth, causing cells to slough off and adhere to the brush. The catheter port of the bronchoscope may be used to irrigate the lung tissue with saline solution to secure material for additional studies. The brush is removed from the bronchoscope, and a slide is made for examination under the microscope. The brush may be cut off and sent to the pathology laboratory for analysis. This procedure is especially useful in the immunologically compromised patient.

In transbronchial needle aspiration, a catheter with a needle is inserted into the tissue through the bronchoscope and aspirated, whereas in transbronchial lung biopsy, biting or cutting forceps are introduced by a fiberoptic bronchoscope to excise the tissue.

In percutaneous needle biopsy, a cutting needle or a spinal-type needle is used to obtain a tissue specimen for histologic study under fluoroscopic or CT guidance. Analgesia may be given before the procedure. The skin over the biopsy site is cleansed and anesthetized and a small incision is made. The biopsy needle is inserted through the incision into the pleura with the patient holding their breath in midexpiration. The surgeon guides the needle into the periphery of the lesion and obtains a tissue sample from the mass.

Nursing Interventions

After the procedure, recovery and home care are similar to those for bronchoscopy and thoracoscopy. Nursing care involves monitoring the patient for complications such as shortness of breath, bleeding, or infection. In preparation for discharge, the patient and the family are instructed to report pain, shortness of breath, visible bleeding, redness of the biopsy site, or purulent drainage (pus) to the primary provider immediately. Patients who have undergone biopsy are often anxious because of the need for the biopsy and the potential findings; the nurse must consider this in providing postbiopsy care and patient education.

Lymph Node Biopsy

The scalene lymph nodes, which are enmeshed in the deep cervical pad of fat overlying the scalenus anterior muscle, drain the lungs and mediastinum and may show histologic changes from intrathoracic disease. If these nodes are palpable on physical examination, a scalene node biopsy may be performed. A biopsy of these nodes may be performed to detect spread of pulmonary disease to the lymph nodes and to establish a diagnosis or prognosis in such diseases as Hodgkin lymphoma, sarcoidosis, fungal disease, tuberculosis, and carcinoma.

Procedure

Mediastinoscopy is the endoscopic examination of the mediastinum for exploration and biopsy of mediastinal lymph nodes that drain the lungs; this examination does not require a thoracotomy. Biopsy is usually performed through a suprasternal incision. Mediastinoscopy is carried out to detect mediastinal involvement of pulmonary malignancy and to obtain tissue for diagnostic studies of other conditions (e.g., sarcoidosis).

An anterior mediastinotomy is thought to provide better exposure and diagnostic possibilities than a mediastinoscopy. An incision is made in the area of the second or third costal cartilage. The mediastinum is explored, and biopsies are performed on any lymph nodes found. Chest tube drainage is required after the procedure. Mediastinotomy is particularly valuable to determine whether a pulmonary lesion is resectable.

Nursing Interventions

Postprocedure care focuses on providing adequate oxygenation, monitoring for bleeding, and providing pain relief. The patient may be discharged a few hours after the chest drainage system is removed. The nurse should instruct the patient and the family about monitoring for changes in respiratory status, taking into consideration the impact of anxiety about the potential findings of the biopsy on their ability to remember those instructions.

CRITICAL THINKING EXERCISES

1 **ebp** You are caring for a 73-year-old woman who was transferred 4 hours ago to your unit from the postanesthesia care unit (PACU), status post–open reduction internal fixation (ORIF) of the right hip after sustaining a hip fracture from a fall. On arrival, the patient's vital signs are as follows: BP 130/88, HR 74 bpm, RR 20/min, temperature 37°C (98.6°F), and SaO2 96% on 4 L/min via nasal cannula. On reassessment, you note an increased RR of 26/min and decreased SaO$_2$ of 90% on current oxygen therapy. To better assess the changes in your patient's condition, what additional questions will you ask her? In performing a focused respiratory assessment, what components of a comprehensive respiratory assessment will you include and why? You notify your charge nurse of your findings, but he does not seem concerned. What evidenced-based tools are available to help you assess the significance of these changes in vital signs and to more effectively communicate your concerns to the charge nurse? Evaluate the strength of the evidence supporting available tools to determine which would be the most helpful.

2 A patient is admitted to a medical surgical unit for increasing shortness of breath. He states that over the last few days, he does not seem to be able to catch his breath. When conducting his health history, what pulmonary risk factors will you assess for? What other signs and symptoms will you ask him about? The patient tells you that he has a history of chronic obstructive pulmonary disease (COPD) and was recently treated for pneumonia. To better assess whether either of these conditions are contributing to his shortness of breath, what additional questions will you ask about his dyspnea? What physical assessment findings will help you differentiate between these two potential diagnoses?

3 **pq** A 65-year-old man, who was recently diagnosed with lung cancer, has developed a pleural effusion. The patient is scheduled for a thoracentesis. He asks whether you can explain to him what to expect before, during, and after this procedure. What do you tell him? What will the priority nursing assessments be after the procedure? What potential complications could occur as a result of this procedure and how would you know if they were occurring?

4 A 69-year-old African American man was admitted to have his pacemaker battery changed. He tolerated the surgery well, without any complications. You are in the process of discharging him when you realize that he has not had an influenza vaccination this year. You mention the importance of him receiving this vaccine prior to discharge, since it has been an exceptionally bad year for the flu. He states that he is afraid to receive the vaccine prior to leaving the hospital because he understands that it can cause the flu and he lives over 60 miles away from the hospital in a very rural area. What will you teach this patient about the influenza vaccine? What resources can you use to support your teaching? What other factors will you assess to better understand this patient's risk of influenza and complications that could result from influenza?

REFERENCES

*Asterisk indicates nursing research.

Books

Bickley, L. S. (2013). *Bates' guide to physical examination and history taking* (11th ed.). Philadelphia, PA: Wolters Kluwer Health Lippincott Williams & Wilkins.

Dudgeon, D. (2015). Dyspnea, terminal secretions, and cough. In B. R. Ferrel, N. Coyle, & J. A. Pace (Eds.). *Oxford textbook of palliative nursing* (4th ed.). Oxford: Oxford University Press.

Grossman, S., & Porth, C. M. (2014). *Porth's pathophysiology: Concepts of altered health states* (9th ed.). Philadelphia, PA: Wolters Kluwer Health Lippincott Williams & Wilkins.

Pagana, K. S., & Pagana, T. J. (2013). *Mosby's diagnostic and laboratory test reference* (11th ed.). St. Louis, MO: Mosby Elsevier.

Perry, A. G., Potter, P. A., & Ostendorf, W. (2014). *Clinical nursing skills and techniques* (8th ed.). St. Louis, MO: Mosby Elsevier.

Porth, C. M. (2015). *Essentials of pathophysiology* (4th ed.). Philadelphia, PA: Wolters Kluwer Health Lippincott Williams & Wilkins.

West, J. B., & Luks, A. M. (2016). *West's respiratory physiology: The essentials.* (10th ed.). Philadelphia, PA: Wolters Kluwer Health Lippincott Williams & Wilkins.

Journals and Electronic Documents

American Lung Association. (2015). *Tobacco: Statement on e-cigarettes.* Retrieved on 2/19/2016 at: www.lung.org/our-initiatives/tobacco/oversight-and-regulation/statement-on-e-cigarettes.html

*Baker, K., Barsamian, J., Leone, D., et al., (2013). Routine dyspnea assessment on unit admission. *American Journal of Nursing, 113*(11), 42–49.

Bulbul, Y., Ayik, S., Ozlu, T., et al. (2014). Frequency and predictors of obesity hypoventilation in hospitalized patients at a tertiary health care institution. *Annals of Thoracic Medicine, 9*(2), 87–91.

Chan, E. D., Chan, M. M., & Chan, M. M. (2013). Pulse oximetry: Understanding its basic principles facilitates appreciation of its limitations. *Respiratory Medicine, 107*(6), 789–799.

Davis, M. D., Walsh, B. K., Sittig, S. E., et al. (2013). AARC clinical practice guideline: Blood gas analysis and hemoximetry: 2013. *Respiratory Care, 58*(10), 1694–1703.

Ferkol, T., & Schraufnagel, D. (2014). The global burden of respiratory disease. *Annals of the American Thoracic Society, 11*(3), 404–406.

Helling, T. S., Martin, L. C., Martin, M., et al. (2014). Failure events in transition of care for surgical patients. *Journal of the American College of Surgeons, 218*(4), 723–733.

Karez, M., & Papadakos, P. J. (2013). Respiratory complications in the postanesthesia care unit: A review of pathophysiological mechanisms. *Canadian Journal of Respiratory Therapy, 49*(4), 21–29.

Kirkland, L. L., Malinchoc, M., O'Byrne, M., et al. (2013). A clinical deterioration prediction tool for internal medicine patients. *American Journal of Medical Quality, 28*(2), 135–142.

Klompas, M. (2013). Ventilator-associated events surveillance: A patient safety opportunity. *Current Opinions in Critical Care, 19*(5), 424–431.

Ma, Y., Yan, S., Zhou, L., et al. (2016). Competitive assessments of pulmonary embolism: Noninvasiveness versus the golden standard. *Vascular, 24*(2), 217–224.

Parshall, M. P., Schwartzstein, R. M., Adams, L., et al. (2012). An official American Thoracic Society statement: Update on the mechanisms, assessment, and management of dyspnea. *American Journal of Respiratory Critical Care Medicine, 185*(4), 432–452.

*Philip, K., Richardson, R., & Cohen, M. (2013). Staff perceptions of respiratory rate measurement in a general hospital. *British Journal of Nursing, 22*(10), 570–574.

*Poot, B. (2014). Nurse-led chronic cough clinic: What is the impact on patient waiting times? *Kai Tiaki Nursing Research, 5*(1), 17–20.

Ramly, E., Kaafarani, H. M. A., & Velmahos, G. C. (2015). The effect of aging on pulmonary function: Implications for monitoring and support of the surgical and trauma patient. *Surgical Clinics of North America, 95*(1), 53–69. doi: http://dx.doi.org/10.1016/j.suc.2014.09.009.

Registered Nurses' Association of Ontario. (2013). *Nursing best practice guidelines: Visual analogue scale as a measure of clinical dyspnea.* Retrieved on 2/19/2016 at: pda.rnao.ca/content/visual-analogue-scale-measure-clinical-dyspnea

Reid, M. (2013). Central venous oxygen saturation: Analysis, clinical use and effects on mortality. *British Association of Critical Care Nurses, 18*(5), 245–250.

Rutherford, J. D. (2013). Digital clubbing. *Circulation, 127*(19), 1997–1999.

Wells, J. L., & Murphy, P. S. (2014). Clearing the runway: An innovative approach to preparing the intensive care unit patient for a magnetic resonance imaging scan. *Journal of Radiology Nursing, 33*(3), 147–151.

York, N. L., Kane, C. J., Smith, C., et al. (2015). Care of the patient with an acute pulmonary embolism. *Dimensions of Critical Care Nursing, 34*(1), 3–9.

Yorke, J. (2014).Breathlessness in the community: Part 1—assessment. *Journal of Community Nursing, 28*(5), 83–90.

Resources

American Association for Respiratory Care (AARC), www.aarc.org
American Lung Association, www.lung.org
Cystic Fibrosis Foundation, www.cff.org
Genetic Alliance, www.geneticalliance.org
National Heart, Lung, and Blood Institute, National Institutes of Health, www.nhlbi.nih.gov
National Organization for Rare Disorders (NORD), www.rarediseases.org
OMIM: Online Mendelian Inheritance in Man, www.omim.org

21

Respiratory Care Modalities

On completion of this chapter, the learner will be able to:

1. Describe the nursing management of patients receiving oxygen therapy, incentive spirometry, flutter valve therapy, small-volume nebulizer therapy, chest physiotherapy, and breathing retraining.
2. Discuss the patient education and transitions in care considerations for patients receiving oxygen therapy.
3. Identify the nursing care of a patient with an endotracheal tube and a patient with a tracheostomy.
4. Use the nursing process as a framework for care of patients who are mechanically ventilated.
5. Describe the process of weaning the patient from mechanical ventilation.
6. Examine the significance of preoperative nursing assessment and patient education for the patient who is going to have thoracic surgery.
7. Explain the principles of chest drainage and the nursing responsibilities related to the care of the patient with a chest drainage system.
8. Use the nursing process as a framework for care of a patient who has had a thoracotomy.

GLOSSARY

airway pressure release ventilation (APRV): mode of mechanical ventilation that allows unrestricted, spontaneous breaths throughout the ventilatory cycle; on inspiration the patient receives a preset level of continuous positive airway pressure, and pressure is periodically released to aid expiration

bilevel positive airway pressure (BiPAP): noninvasive spontaneous breath mode of mechanical ventilation that allows for the separate control of inspiratory and expiratory pressures; given via a mask

chest drainage system: the use of a chest tube and closed drainage system to re-expand the lung and to remove excess air, fluid, and/or blood

chest percussion: manually cupping hands over the chest wall and using vibration to mobilize secretions by mechanically dislodging viscous or adherent secretions in the lungs

chest physiotherapy (CPT): therapy used to remove bronchial secretions, improve ventilation, and increase the efficiency of the respiratory muscles; types include postural drainage, chest percussion, and vibration

continuous mandatory (volume or pressure) ventilation (CMV): also referred to as assist–control (A/C) ventilation; mode of mechanical ventilation in which the patient's breathing pattern may trigger the ventilator to deliver a preset tidal volume or set pressure; in the absence of spontaneous breathing, the machine delivers a controlled breath at a preset minimum rate and tidal volume or set pressure

continuous positive airway pressure (CPAP): positive pressure applied throughout the respiratory cycle to a spontaneously breathing patient to promote alveolar and airway stability and increase functional residual capacity; may be given with endotracheal or tracheostomy tube or by mask

endotracheal intubation: insertion of a breathing tube (type of artificial airway) through the nose or mouth into the trachea

flutter valve: portable handheld mucous clearance device; consisting of a tube with an oscillating steel ball inside; upon expiration high frequency oscillations facilitate mucous expectoration

fraction of inspired oxygen (FiO_2): concentration of oxygen delivered (1.0 = 100% oxygen)

hypoxemia: decrease in arterial oxygen tension in the blood

hypoxia: decrease in oxygen supply to the tissues and cells

incentive spirometry: method of deep breathing that provides visual feedback to help the patient inhale deeply and slowly and achieve maximum lung inflation

Intermittent mandatory (volume or pressure) ventilation (IMV): mode of mechanical ventilation that provides a combination of mechanically assisted breaths at a preset volume or pressure and rate and spontaneous breaths

mechanical ventilator: a positive- or negative-pressure breathing device that supports ventilation and oxygenation

pneumothorax: partial or complete collapse of the lung due to positive pressure in the pleural space

positive end-expiratory pressure (PEEP): positive pressure maintained by the ventilator at the end of exhalation (instead of a normal zero pressure) to increase functional residual capacity and open collapsed alveoli; improves oxygenation with lower fraction of inspired oxygen

postural drainage: positioning the patient to allow drainage from all lobes of the lungs and airways

pressure support ventilation (PSV): mode of mechanical ventilation in which preset positive pressure is delivered with spontaneous breaths to decrease work of breathing

proportional assist ventilation (PAV): mode of mechanical ventilation that provides partial ventilatory support in proportion to the patient's inspiratory efforts; decreases the work of breathing

respiratory weaning: process of gradual, systematic withdrawal or removal of ventilator, breathing tube, and oxygen

synchronized intermittent mandatory ventilation (SIMV): mode of mechanical ventilation in which the ventilator allows the patient to breathe spontaneously while providing a preset number of breaths to ensure adequate ventilation; ventilated breaths are synchronized with spontaneous breathing

thoracotomy: surgical opening into the chest cavity

tidal volume: volume of air inspired and expired with each breath

tracheostomy tube: indwelling tube inserted directly into the trachea to assist with ventilation

tracheotomy: surgical opening into the trachea

vibration: a type of massage given by quickly tapping the chest with the fingertips or alternating the fingers in a rhythmic manner, or by using a mechanical device to assist in mobilizing lung secretions

---

Numerous treatment modalities are used when caring for patients with respiratory conditions. The choice of modality is based on the oxygenation disorder and whether there is a problem with gas ventilation, diffusion, or both. Therapies range from simple and noninvasive (oxygen and nebulizer therapy, chest physiotherapy [CPT], breathing retraining) to complex and highly invasive treatments (intubation, mechanical ventilation, surgery). Assessment and management of the patient with respiratory disorders are best accomplished when the approach is multidisciplinary and collaborative.

NONINVASIVE RESPIRATORY THERAPIES

Oxygen Therapy

Oxygen therapy is the administration of oxygen at a concentration greater than that found in the environmental atmosphere. At sea level, the concentration of oxygen in room air is 21%. The goal of oxygen therapy is to provide adequate transport of oxygen in the blood while decreasing the work of breathing and reducing stress on the myocardium.

Oxygen transport to tissues depends on factors such as cardiac output, arterial oxygen content, concentration of hemoglobin, and metabolic requirements. These factors must be kept in mind when oxygen therapy is considered. (Respiratory physiology and oxygen transport are discussed in Chapter 20.)

Indications

A change in the patient's respiratory rate or pattern may be one of the earliest indicators of the need for oxygen therapy. These changes may result from hypoxemia or hypoxia. **Hypoxemia**, a decrease in the arterial oxygen tension in the blood, is manifested by changes in mental status (progressing through impaired judgment, agitation, disorientation, confusion, lethargy, and coma), dyspnea, increase in blood pressure, changes in heart rate, dysrhythmias, central cyanosis (late sign), diaphoresis, and cool extremities. Hypoxemia usually leads to **hypoxia**, a decrease in oxygen supply to the tissues and cells that can also be caused by problems outside the respiratory system. Severe hypoxia can be life threatening.

The signs and symptoms signaling the need for oxygen may depend on how suddenly this need develops. With rapidly developing hypoxia, changes occur in the central nervous system because the neurologic centers are very sensitive to oxygen deprivation. The clinical picture may resemble that of alcohol intoxication, with the patient exhibiting lack of coordination and impaired judgment. With long-standing hypoxia (as seen in chronic obstructive pulmonary disease [COPD] and chronic heart failure), fatigue, drowsiness, apathy, inattentiveness, and delayed reaction time may occur. The need for oxygen is assessed by arterial blood gas analysis, pulse oximetry, and clinical evaluation. More information about hypoxia is presented in Chart 21-1.

Chart 21-1 | **Types of Hypoxia**

Hypoxia can occur from either severe pulmonary disease (inadequate oxygen supply) or from extrapulmonary disease (inadequate oxygen delivery) affecting gas exchange at the cellular level. The four general types of hypoxia are hypoxemic hypoxia, circulatory hypoxia, anemic hypoxia, and histotoxic hypoxia.

Hypoxemic Hypoxia

Hypoxemic hypoxia is a decreased oxygen level in the blood resulting in decreased oxygen diffusion into the tissues. It may be caused by hypoventilation, high altitudes, ventilation–perfusion mismatch that may include disorders of dead space (e.g., pulmonary embolism) and shunts in which the alveoli are collapsed and cannot provide oxygen to the blood (e.g., atelectasis), and pulmonary diffusion defects. It is corrected by increasing alveolar ventilation or providing supplemental oxygen.

Circulatory Hypoxia

Circulatory hypoxia is hypoxia resulting from inadequate capillary circulation. It may be caused by decreased cardiac output, local vascular obstruction, low-flow states such as shock, or cardiac arrest. Although tissue partial pressure of oxygen (PO_2) is reduced, arterial oxygen (PaO_2) remains normal. Circulatory hypoxia is corrected by identifying and treating the underlying cause.

Anemic Hypoxia

Anemic hypoxia is a result of decreased effective hemoglobin concentration, which causes a decrease in the oxygen-carrying capacity of the blood. It is rarely accompanied by hypoxemia. Carbon monoxide poisoning, because it reduces the oxygen-carrying capacity of hemoglobin, produces similar effects but is not strictly anemic hypoxia, because hemoglobin levels may be normal.

Histotoxic Hypoxia

Histotoxic hypoxia occurs when a toxic substance, such as cyanide, interferes with the ability of tissues to use available oxygen. The defect in the use of oxygen leads to a reduction in adenosine triphosphate (ATP) production by the mitochondria.

Complications

Oxygen is a medication, and except in emergency situations it is given only when prescribed by a provider with prescriptive authority. As with other medications, the nurse administers oxygen with caution and carefully assesses its effects on each patient.

In general, patients with respiratory disorders are given oxygen therapy only to increase the partial pressure of oxygen (PaO_2) back to the patient's normal baseline, which may vary from 60 to 95 mm Hg. In terms of the oxyhemoglobin dissociation curve (see Chapter 20), arterial hemoglobin at these levels is 80% to 98% saturated with oxygen; higher **fraction of inspired oxygen (FiO_2)** flow values add no further significant amounts of oxygen to the red blood cells or plasma. Instead of helping, increased amounts of oxygen may produce toxic effects on the lungs and central nervous system or may depress ventilation (see later discussion).

It is important to observe for subtle indicators of inadequate oxygenation when oxygen is given by any method. Therefore, the nurse assesses the patient frequently for confusion, restlessness progressing to lethargy, diaphoresis, pallor, tachycardia, tachypnea, and hypertension. Intermittent or continuous pulse oximetry is used to monitor oxygen levels.

Oxygen Toxicity

Oxygen toxicity may occur when too high concentration of oxygen (greater than 50%) is given for an extended period (generally longer than 24 hours) (Urden, Stacy, & Lough, 2014). It is caused by overproduction of oxygen free radicals, which are by-products of cell metabolism.

If oxygen toxicity is untreated, these radicals can severely damage the alveolar capillary membrane leading to pulmonary edema and progressing to cell death. Clinical manifestations of oxygen toxicity causing lung damage are similar to acute respiratory distress syndrome (ARDS) (see Chapter 23).

Signs and symptoms of oxygen toxicity include substernal discomfort, paresthesias, dyspnea, restlessness, fatigue, malaise, progressive respiratory difficulty, refractory hypoxemia, alveolar atelectasis, and alveolar infiltrates evident on chest x-rays.

Using the lowest amount of oxygen needed to maintain an acceptable PaO_2 level and treating the underlying condition aids in the prevention of oxygen toxicity. If high concentrations of oxygen are necessary, it is important to minimize the duration of administration and reduce its concentration as soon as possible. Often, **positive end-expiratory pressure (PEEP)** applied at the end of expiration of ventilator breaths or continuous positive airway pressure (CPAP) used with oxygen therapy reverses or prevents microatelectasis, thus allowing a lower percentage of oxygen to be used. The level of PEEP that allows the best oxygenation without hemodynamic compromise is known as "best PEEP" or optimal PEEP (Cairo, 2014).

Absorption Atelectasis

An additional adverse effect of the administration of high concentrations of oxygen (greater than 50%) to patients who are sedated and breathing small **tidal volumes** of air (volume of air inspired and expired with each breath) is absorption atelectasis. Normally, 79% of room air is comprised of nitrogen. During inhalation, nitrogen, in addition to other gases, fills the alveoli and helps keep the alveoli open. With the administration of high concentrations of oxygen, nitrogen is diluted and replaced with oxygen. Oxygen in the alveoli is absorbed quickly into the bloodstream and not replaced rapidly enough in the alveoli to maintain patency. The alveoli collapse, causing atelectasis (Kacmarek, Stroller, & Huer, 2017).

Suppression of Ventilation

For many years, it was assumed the stimulus for respiration in patients with COPD, unlike those without COPD, is a decrease in blood oxygen rather than an elevation in carbon dioxide levels, commonly referred to as the hypoxic drive. The hypoxic drive theory posited that the administration of a high concentration of oxygen removes the respiratory drive that has been created largely by the patient's chronic low oxygen tension. The resulting decrease in alveolar ventilation would then cause a progressive increase in partial pressure of arterial carbon dioxide ($PaCO_2$) and in rare cases, lead to acute respiratory failure secondary to carbon dioxide narcosis, acidosis, and death.

The hypoxic drive is a real phenomenon; however, research reports it accounts for only 10% of the stimulus to breathe (Makic, Martin, Burns, et al., 2013). Although patients with COPD are at risk for hypoxemia and hypercapnia, many also do require supplemental oxygen therapy to improve oxygenation. Therefore, it is important to closely monitor the respiratory rate and the oxygen saturation as measured by pulse oximetry (SpO_2) in order to maintain an oxygen saturation between 90% and 93% on the lowest liter flow of oxygen (Makic et al., 2013; Urden et al., 2014).

Other Complications

Because oxygen supports combustion, there is always a danger of fire when it is used. It is important to post "No Smoking" signs when oxygen is in use. Oxygen therapy equipment is also a potential source of bacterial contamination; therefore, the nurse (or respiratory therapist) changes the tubing according to infection prevention policy, manufacturer's recommendations, and the type of oxygen delivery equipment.

Methods of Oxygen Administration

Oxygen is dispensed from a cylinder or a piped-in system. A reduction gauge is necessary to reduce the pressure to a working level, and a flow meter regulates the flow of oxygen in liters per minute (L/min). When oxygen is used at high flow rates, it should be moistened by passing it through a humidification system to prevent it from drying the mucous membranes of the respiratory tract.

The use of oxygen concentrators is another means of providing varying amounts of oxygen, especially in the home setting. These devices are relatively portable, easy to operate, and cost-effective but require more maintenance than tank or liquid systems. These models can deliver oxygen flows from 1 to 10 L/min and provide an FiO_2 of about 40% (Cairo, 2014).

Many different oxygen devices are used (see Table 21-1). The amount of oxygen delivered is expressed as a percentage concentration (e.g., 70%). The appropriate form of oxygen therapy is best determined by arterial blood gas levels (see Chapter 13), which indicate the patient's oxygenation status.

TABLE 21-1 Oxygen Administration Devices

Device	Suggested Flow Rate (L/min)	O₂ Percentage Setting	Advantages	Disadvantages
Low-Flow Systems				
Cannula	1—2 3–5 6	24–28 32–40 44	Lightweight, comfortable, inexpensive, continuous use with meals and activity	Easily dislodged, from nares, skin breakdown over ears or nares, nasal mucosal drying, variable FiO_2
Nasal catheter	1–6	24–44	Inexpensive, does not require a tracheostomy	Nasal mucosa irritation; catheter should be changed frequently to alternate nostril
Mask, simple	5–8	40–60	Simple to use, inexpensive	Poor fitting, variable FiO_2, must remove to eat
Mask, partial rebreathing	8–11	50–75	Moderate O_2 concentration	Warm, poorly fitting, must remove to eat
Mask, nonrebreathing	10–15	80–95	High O_2 concentration	Poorly fitting, must remove to eat
High-Flow Systems				
Transtracheal catheter	¼–4	60–100	More comfortable, concealed by clothing, less oxygen liters per minute needed than nasal cannula	Requires frequent and regular cleaning, requires surgical intervention, with associated risk for surgical complications
Mask, Venturi	4–6 6–8	24, 26, 28 30, 35, 40	Provides low levels of supplemental O_2 Precise FiO_2, additional humidity available	Must remove to eat
Mask, aerosol	8–10	30–100	Good humidity, accurate FiO_2	Uncomfortable for some
Tracheostomy collar	8–10	30–100	Good humidity, comfortable, fairly accurate FiO_2	
T-piece	8–10	30–100	Same as tracheostomy collar	Heavy with tubing
Face tent	8–10	30–100	Good humidity, fairly accurate FiO_2	Bulky and cumbersome
Oxygen-Conserving Devices				
Pulse dose (or demand)	10–40 mL/ breath		Deliver O_2 only on inspiration, conserve 50–75% of O_2 used	Must carefully evaluate function individually

Oxygen delivery systems are classified as low-flow (variable performance) or high-flow (fixed performance) delivery systems. Low-flow systems contribute partially to the inspired gas the patient breathes, which means that the patient breathes some room air along with the oxygen. These systems do not provide a constant or precise concentration of inspired oxygen. The amount of inspired oxygen changes as the patient's breathing changes. Examples of low-flow systems are included in Table 21-1. In contrast, high-flow systems provide the total inspired air. A specific percentage of oxygen is delivered independent of the patient's breathing. High-flow systems are indicated for patients who require a constant and precise amount of oxygen. Examples of these systems can also be found in Table 21-1 (Cairo, 2014).

A nasal cannula is used when the patient requires a low-to-medium concentration of oxygen for which precise accuracy is not essential. This method allows the patient to move about in bed, talk, cough, and eat without interrupting oxygen flow. Flow rates in excess of 4 L/min may lead to swallowing of air or may cause irritation and drying of the nasal and pharyngeal mucosa.

The nasal (oropharyngeal) catheter is rarely used but may be prescribed for short-term therapy to administer low-to-moderate concentrations of oxygen. The catheter should be changed frequently (e.g., every 8 hours), alternating nostrils to prevent nasal irritation and infection.

When oxygen is given via cannula or catheter, the percentage of oxygen reaching the lungs varies with the depth and rate of respirations, particularly if the nasal mucosa is swollen or if the patient is a mouth breather.

Oxygen masks come in several forms. Each is used for different purposes (see Fig. 21-1). *Simple masks* are used to administer low-to-moderate concentrations of oxygen. The body of the mask itself gathers and stores oxygen between breaths. The patient exhales directly through openings or ports in the body of the mask. If oxygen flow ceases, the patient can draw air in through these openings around the mask edges. Although widely used, these masks cannot be used for controlled oxygen concentrations and must be adjusted for proper fit. They should not press too tightly against the skin, because this can cause a sense of claustrophobia as well as skin breakdown; adjustable elastic bands are provided to ensure comfort and security.

Partial rebreathing masks have a reservoir bag that must remain inflated during both inspiration and expiration. The nurse adjusts the oxygen flow to ensure that the bag does not collapse during inhalation. A moderate concentration of oxygen can be delivered because both the mask and the bag serve as reservoirs for oxygen. Oxygen enters the mask through small-bore tubing that connects at the junction of the mask and bag. As the patient inhales, gas is drawn from the mask, from the bag, and potentially from room air through the

Figure 21-1 • Types of oxygen masks used to deliver varying concentrations of oxygen. **A.** Venturi mask. **B.** Nonrebreathing mask. **C.** Partial rebreathing mask.

exhalation ports. As the patient exhales, the first third of the exhalation fills the reservoir bag. This is mainly dead space and does not participate in gas exchange in the lungs. Therefore, it has a high oxygen concentration. The remainder of the exhaled gas is vented through the exhalation ports. The actual percentage of oxygen delivered is influenced by the patient's ventilatory pattern (Cairo, 2014).

Nonrebreathing masks are similar in design to partial rebreathing masks except that they have additional valves. A one-way valve located between the reservoir bag and the base of the mask allows gas from the reservoir bag to enter the mask on inhalation but prevents gas in the mask from flowing back into the reservoir bag during exhalation. One-way valves located at the exhalation ports prevent room air from entering the mask during inhalation. They also allow the patient's exhaled gases to exit the mask on exhalation. As with the partial rebreathing mask, it is important to adjust the oxygen flow so that the reservoir bag does not completely collapse on inspiration. In theory, if the nonrebreathing mask fits the patient snugly and both side exhalation ports have one-way valves, it is possible for the patient to receive 100% oxygen, making the nonrebreathing mask a high-flow oxygen system. However, because it is difficult to get an exact fit from the mask on every patient, and some nonrebreathing masks have only one one-way exhalation valves, it is almost impossible to ensure 100% oxygen delivery, making it a low-flow oxygen system.

The *Venturi mask* is the most reliable and accurate method for delivering precise concentrations of oxygen through noninvasive means. The mask is constructed in a way that allows a constant flow of room air blended with a fixed flow of oxygen. It is used primarily for patients with COPD because it can accurately provide appropriate levels of supplemental oxygen, thus avoiding the risk of suppressing the hypoxic drive.

The Venturi mask uses the Bernoulli principle of air entrainment (trapping the air like a vacuum), which provides a high airflow with controlled oxygen enrichment. For each liter of oxygen that passes through a jet orifice, a fixed proportion of room air is entrained. Varying the size of the jet orifice and adjusting the flow of oxygen can deliver a precise volume of oxygen. Excess gas leaves the mask through the two exhalation ports, carrying with it the exhaled carbon dioxide. This method allows a constant oxygen concentration to be inhaled regardless of the depth or rate of respiration.

The mask should fit snugly enough to prevent oxygen from flowing into the patient's eyes. The nurse checks the patient's skin for irritation. It is necessary to remove the mask so that the patient can eat, drink, and take medications, at which time supplemental oxygen is provided through a nasal cannula.

 Concept Mastery Alert

Oxygen delivery systems are classified as either low-flow or high-flow systems. Whereas a low-flow oxygen delivery system may imprecisely deliver high concentrations of oxygen (e.g., up to 100% via a nonrebreathing mask), the Venturi mask, which is a high-flow system, is specifically designed to deliver precise but lower concentrations of oxygen (less than 30% oxygen).

The *transtracheal oxygen catheter* requires minor surgery, to insert a catheter through a small incision directly into the trachea. It is indicated for patients with chronic oxygen therapy needs. These catheters are more comfortable, less dependent on breathing patterns, and less obvious than other oxygen delivery methods. Because no oxygen is lost into the surrounding environment, the patient achieves adequate oxygenation at lower rates, making this method less expensive and more efficient.

Figure 21-2 • T-pieces and tracheostomy collars are devices used when weaning patients from mechanical ventilation.

The *T-piece* is a special adaptor used to deliver oxygen, which connects to the endotracheal or tracheostomy tube and is useful in weaning patients from mechanical ventilation (see Fig. 21-2).

Other oxygen devices include *aerosol masks, tracheostomy collars* (see Fig. 21-2), and *face tents*, all of which are used with aerosol devices (nebulizers) that can be adjusted for oxygen concentrations from 27% to 100% (0.27 to 1.00). If the gas mixture flow falls below patient demand, room air is pulled in, diluting the concentration. The aerosol mist must be available for the patient during the entire inspiratory phase.

Although most oxygen therapy is given as continuous flow oxygen, methods of oxygen conservation continue to be investigated. The *demand oxygen delivery system* (DODS) interrupts the flow of oxygen during exhalation, when it is otherwise mostly wasted. Several versions of the DODS are being evaluated for their effectiveness. Studies show that DODS models conserve oxygen and maintain oxygen saturation better than continuous flow oxygen systems when the respiratory rate increases (Langenhof & Fichter, 2005).

Hyperbaric oxygen therapy is the administration of 100% oxygen, either intermittently or continuously, at pressures greater than atmospheric pressure. As a result, the amount of oxygen dissolved in plasma is increased, which increases oxygen levels in the tissues. During therapy, the patient is placed in a small (single patient use) or large (multiple patient use) cylinder chamber. Hyperbaric oxygen therapy is used to treat conditions such as decompression sickness, air embolism, carbon monoxide poisoning, cyanide poisoning, smoke inhalation, gangrene, tissue necrosis, wound healing, skin grafts, refractory anaerobic infections, and refractory osteomyelitis (Cairo, 2014). Potential side effects include ear trauma, central nervous system disorders, oxygen toxicity, and anxiety in patients with claustrophobia.

Gerontologic Considerations

The respiratory system changes throughout the aging process, and it is important for nurses to be aware of these changes when assessing older adult patients who are receiving oxygen therapy. As the respiratory muscles weaken and the large bronchi and alveoli become enlarged, the available surface area of the lungs decreases, resulting in reduced ventilation and respiratory gas exchange. The number of functional cilia is also reduced, decreasing ciliary action and the cough reflex. As a result of osteoporosis and calcification of the costal cartilages, chest wall compliance is decreased. Patients may display increased chest rigidity and respiratory rate and decreased PaO$_2$ and lung expansion. The older adult is at risk for aspiration and infection related to these changes. In addition, patient education regarding adequate nutrition is essential because appropriate dietary intake can help diminish the excess buildup of carbon dioxide and maintain optimal respiratory functioning (Meiner, 2015).

Nursing Management

Promoting Home, Community-Based, and Transitional Care

Educating Patients About Self-Care

At times, oxygen must be given to the patient at home. The nurse instructs the patient or family in the methods for administering oxygen safely and informs the patient and family that oxygen is available in gas, liquid, and concentrated forms. The gas and liquid forms come in portable devices so that the patient can leave home while receiving oxygen therapy. Humidity must be provided while oxygen is used (except with portable devices) to counteract the dry, irritating effects of compressed oxygen on the airway (see Chart 21-2).

Continuing and Transitional Care

Home visits by a nurse or respiratory therapist may be arranged based on the patient's status and needs. It is important to assess the patient's home environment, the patient's physical and psychological status, and the need for further education. The nurse reinforces educational points on how to use oxygen safely and effectively, including fire safety tips. To maintain a consistent quality of care and to maximize the patient's financial reimbursement for home oxygen therapy, the nurse ensures that the prescription given by the primary provider includes the diagnosis,

HOME CARE CHECKLIST
Oxygen Therapy

At the completion of education, the patient and/or caregiver will be able to:

- State proper care of and administration of oxygen to patient:
  - State primary provider's prescription for oxygen and the manner in which it is to be used.
  - Indicate when a humidifier should be used.
  - Identify signs and symptoms indicating the need for change in oxygen therapy.
  - Describe precautions and safety measures to be used when oxygen is in use:
    - Know NOT to smoke or be around people who are smoking while using oxygen.
    - Post "No Smoking—Oxygen In Use" signs on doors.
    - Notify local fire department and electric company of oxygen use in home.
    - Never use paint thinners, cleaning fluids, gasoline, aerosol sprays, and other flammable materials while using oxygen.
    - Keep all methods of oxygen delivery at least 15 ft away from matches, candles, gas stove, or other source of flame, and 5 ft away from television, radio, and other appliances.
    - Keep oxygen tank out of direct sunlight.
    - When traveling in automobile, place oxygen tank on floor behind front seat.

- If traveling by airplane, notify air carrier of need for oxygen at least 2 weeks in advance.
- State how and when to place an order for more oxygen.
- Maintain and use equipment properly:
  - Identify when a portable oxygen delivery device should be used.
  - Demonstrate safe and appropriate use of and how to change from one oxygen delivery system to another (e.g., from oxygen concentrator to portable oxygen delivery)
  - Demonstrate correct adjustment of prescribed flow rate.
  - Describe how to clean and when to replace oxygen tubing.
  - Identify causes of malfunction of equipment and when to call for the replacement of equipment.
  - Describe the importance of determining that all electrical outlets are working properly.

Resources

See Chapter 10, Chart 10-8 for additional information related to durable medical equipment, adaptive equipment, mobility skills, skin, bowel, and bladder care.

---

the prescribed oxygen flow, and conditions for use (e.g., continuous use and nighttime use only). Because oxygen is a medication, the nurse reminds the patient receiving long-term oxygen therapy and the family about the importance of keeping follow-up appointments with the patient's primary provider. The patient is instructed to see their primary provider every 6 months or more often, if indicated. Arterial blood gas measurements and laboratory tests are repeated annually or more often if the patient's condition changes.

Incentive Spirometry (Sustained Maximal Inspiration)

Incentive spirometry is a method of deep breathing that provides visual feedback to encourage the patient to inhale slowly and deeply to maximize lung inflation and prevent or reduce atelectasis. The purpose of an incentive spirometer is to ensure that the volume of air inhaled is increased gradually as the patient takes deeper and deeper breaths.

Incentive spirometers are available in two types: volume or flow. In the volume type, the tidal volume is set using the manufacturer's instructions. The patient takes a deep breath through the mouthpiece, pauses at peak lung inflation, and then relaxes and exhales. Taking several normal breaths before attempting another with the incentive spirometer helps avoid fatigue. The volume is periodically increased as tolerated.

In the flow type, the volume is not preset. The spirometer contains a number of movable balls that are pushed up by the force of the breath and held suspended in the air while the patient inhales. The amount of air inhaled and the flow of the air are estimated by how long and how high the balls are suspended.

Indications

Incentive spirometry is used after surgery, especially thoracic and abdominal surgery, to promote the expansion of the alveoli and to prevent or treat atelectasis.

Nursing Management

Nursing management of the patient using incentive spirometry includes placing the patient in the proper position, educating the patient on the technique for using the incentive spirometer, setting realistic goals for the patient, and recording the results of the therapy (see Chart 21-3). Ideally, the patient assumes a sitting or semi-Fowler's position to enhance diaphragmatic excursion; however, this procedure may be performed with the patient in any position.

PATIENT EDUCATION
Performing Incentive Spirometry

The inspired air helps inflate the lungs. The ball or weight in the spirometer rises in response to the intensity of the intake of air. The higher the ball rises, the deeper the breath.

The nurse instructs the patient to:

- Assume a semi-Fowler position or an upright position before initiating therapy.
- Use diaphragmatic breathing.
- Place the mouthpiece of the spirometer firmly in the mouth, breathe air in (inspire) slowly through the mouth, and hold the breath at the end of inspiration for about 3 seconds to maintain the ball/indicator between the lines. Exhale slowly through the mouthpiece.
- Cough during and after each session. Splint the incision when coughing postoperatively.
- Perform the procedure approximately 10 times in succession, repeating the 10 breaths with the spirometer each hour during waking hours.

Chart
21-4
PATIENT EDUCATION
Breathing Exercises

General Instructions

The nurse instructs the patient to:
- Breathe slowly and rhythmically to exhale completely and empty the lungs completely.
- Inhale through the nose to filter, humidify, and warm the air before it enters the lungs.
- If you feel out of breath, breathe more slowly by prolonging the exhalation time.
- Keep the air moist with a humidifier.

Diaphragmatic Breathing

Goal: To use and strengthen the diaphragm during breathing
   The nurse instructs the patient to:

- Place one hand on the abdomen (just below the ribs) and the other hand on the middle of the chest to increase the awareness of the position of the diaphragm and its function in breathing.
- Breathe in slowly and deeply through the nose, letting the abdomen protrude as far as possible.
- Breathe out through pursed lips while tightening (contracting) the abdominal muscles.
- Press firmly inward and upward on the abdomen while breathing out.
- Repeat for 1 minute; follow with a rest period of 2 minutes.

- Gradually increase duration up to 5 minutes, several times a day (before meals and at bedtime).

Pursed-Lip Breathing

Goal: To prolong exhalation and increase airway pressure during expiration, thus reducing the amount of trapped air and the amount of airway resistance
   The nurse instructs the patient to:

- Inhale through the nose while slowly counting to 3—the amount of time needed to say "Smell a rose."
- Exhale slowly and evenly against pursed lips while tightening the abdominal muscles. (Pursing the lips increases intratracheal pressure; exhaling through the mouth offers less resistance to expired air.)
- Count to 7 slowly while prolonging expiration through pursed lips—the length of time to say "Blow out the candle."
- While sitting in a chair:
  Fold arms over the abdomen.
  Inhale through the nose while counting to 3 slowly.
  Bend forward and exhale slowly through pursed lips while counting to 7 slowly.
- While walking:
  Inhale while walking two steps.
  Exhale through pursed lips while walking four or five steps.

Small-Volume Nebulizer (Mini-Nebulizer) Therapy

The small-volume nebulizer is a handheld apparatus that disperses a moisturizing agent or medication, such as a bronchodilator or mucolytic agent, into microscopic particles and delivers it to the lungs as the patient inhales. The small-volume nebulizer is usually air driven by means of a compressor through connecting tubing. In some instances, the nebulizer is oxygen driven rather than air driven. To be effective, a visible mist must be available for the patient to inhale.

Indications

Indications for the use of a small-volume nebulizer include difficulty in clearing respiratory secretions, reduced vital capacity with ineffective deep breathing and coughing, and unsuccessful trials of simpler and less costly methods for clearing secretions, delivering aerosol, or expanding the lungs (Cairo, 2014). The patient must be able to generate a deep breath. Diaphragmatic breathing (see Chart 21-4) is a helpful technique to prepare for proper use of the small-volume nebulizer. Small-volume nebulizers are frequently used for patients with COPD to dispense inhaled medications, and they are commonly used at home on a long-term basis.

Nursing Management

The nurse instructs the patient to breathe through the mouth, taking slow, deep breaths, and then to hold the breath for a few seconds at the end of inspiration to increase intrapleural pressure and reopen collapsed alveoli, thereby increasing functional residual capacity. The nurse encourages the patient to cough and to monitor the effectiveness of the therapy. The nurse instructs the patient and family about the purpose of the treatment, equipment setup, medication additive, and proper cleaning and storage of the equipment.

Chest Physiotherapy

Chest physiotherapy (CPT) includes postural drainage, chest percussion and vibration, and breathing retraining. In addition, educating the patient about effective coughing technique is an important part of CPT. The goals of CPT are to remove bronchial secretions, improve ventilation, and increase the efficiency of the respiratory muscles.

Postural Drainage (Segmented Bronchial Drainage)

Postural drainage allows the force of gravity to assist in the removal of bronchial secretions. The secretions drain from the affected bronchioles into the bronchi and trachea and are removed by coughing or suctioning. Postural drainage is used to prevent or relieve bronchial obstruction caused by accumulation of secretions.

   Because the patient usually sits in an upright position, secretions are likely to accumulate in the lower parts of the lungs. Several other positions (see Fig. 21-3) are used so that the force of gravity helps move secretions from the smaller bronchial airways to the main bronchi and trachea. Each position contributes to effective drainage of a different lobe of the lungs; lower and middle lobe bronchi drain more effectively when the head is down, whereas the upper lobe bronchi drain more effectively when the head is up. The secretions then are removed by coughing. The nurse instructs the patient to inhale bronchodilators and mucolytic agents, if prescribed, before postural drainage, because these medications improve drainage of the bronchial tree.

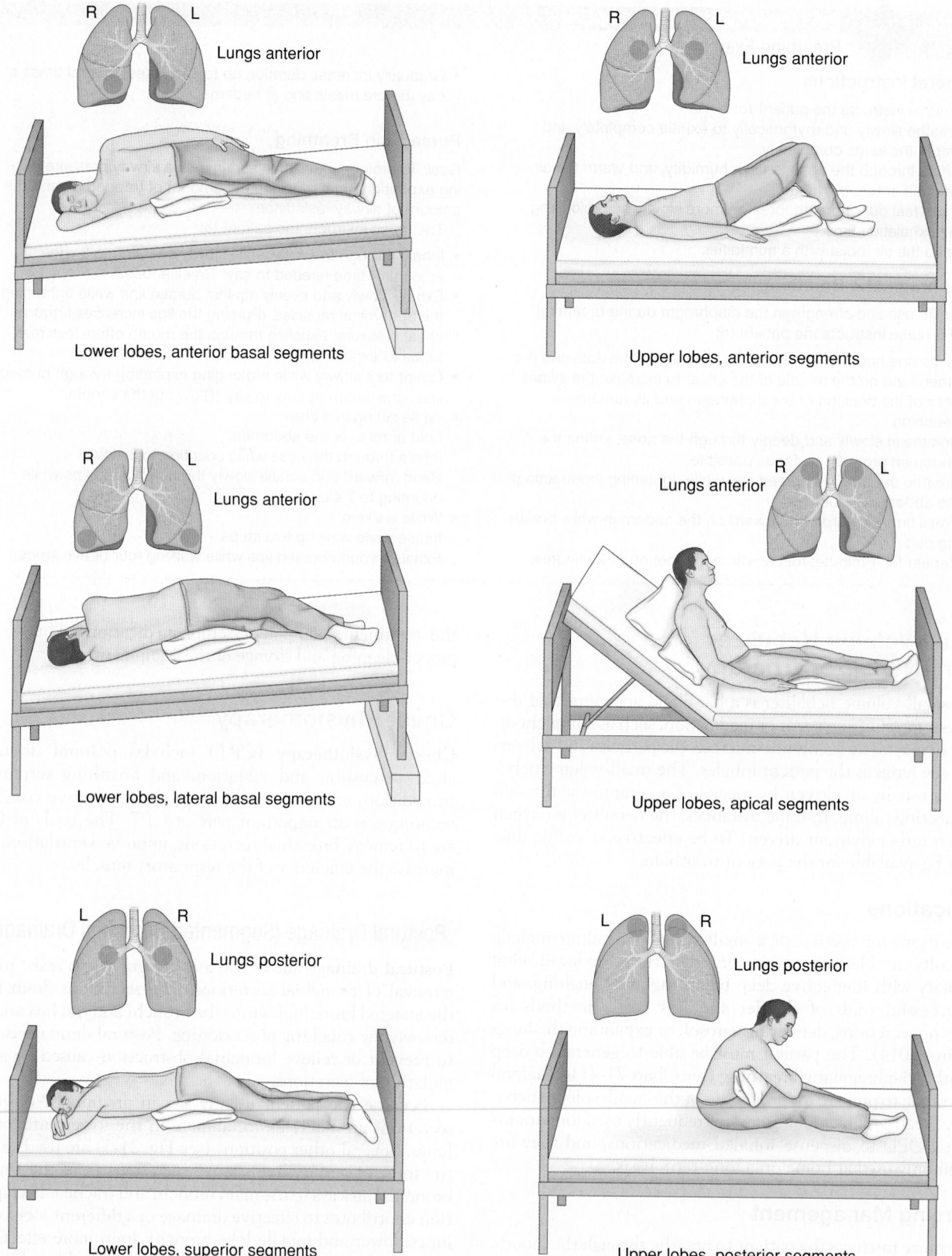

R L Lungs anterior

Lower lobes, anterior basal segments

R L Lungs anterior

Upper lobes, anterior segments

R L Lungs anterior

Lower lobes, lateral basal segments

R L Lungs anterior

Upper lobes, apical segments

L R Lungs posterior

Lower lobes, superior segments

L R Lungs posterior

Upper lobes, posterior segments

Figure 21-3 • Postural drainage positions and the areas of lung drained by each position.

Nursing Management

The nurse should keep in mind the medical diagnosis, the lung lobes or segments involved, the cardiac status, and any structural deformities of the chest wall and spine. Auscultation of the chest before and after the procedure is used to identify the areas that need drainage and assess the effectiveness of treatment. The nurse educates family members who will assist the patient at home to evaluate breath sounds before and after treatment. The nurse explores strategies that will enable the patient to assume the indicated positions at home. This may require the creative use of objects readily available at home, such as pillows, cushions, or cardboard boxes.

Postural drainage is usually performed two to four times daily, before meals (to prevent nausea, vomiting, and aspiration) and at bedtime. Prescribed bronchodilators, water, or saline may be nebulized and inhaled before postural drainage to dilate the bronchioles, reduce bronchospasm, decrease the thickness of mucus and sputum, and combat edema of the bronchial walls. The recommended sequence starts with positions to drain the lower lobes, followed by positions to drain the upper lobes.

The nurse makes the patient as comfortable as possible in each position and provides an emesis basin, sputum cup, and paper tissues. The nurse instructs the patient to remain in each position for 10 to 15 minutes and to breathe in slowly through the nose and out slowly through pursed lips to help keep the airways open so that secretions can drain. If a position cannot be tolerated, the nurse helps the patient assume a modified position. When the patient changes position, the nurse explains how to cough and remove secretions (see Chart 21-5).

If the patient cannot cough, the nurse may need to suction the secretions mechanically. It also may be necessary to use chest percussion and vibration or a high-frequency chest wall oscillation (HFCWO) vest to loosen bronchial secretions and mucus plugs that adhere to the bronchioles and bronchi and to propel sputum in the direction of gravity drainage (see later discussion). If suctioning is required at home, the nurse instructs caregivers in safe suctioning technique and care of the suctioning equipment.

After the procedure, the nurse or family caregivers note the amount, color, viscosity, and character of the expelled sputum. The nurse evaluates the patient's skin color and pulse the first few times the procedure is performed. It may be necessary to administer oxygen during postural drainage.

If the sputum is foul smelling, postural drainage is performed in a room away from other patients or family members. (Deodorizers may be used to counteract the odor. Because aerosol sprays can cause bronchospasm and irritation, they should be used sparingly and with caution.) After the procedure, the patient may find it refreshing to brush the teeth and use a mouthwash before resting.

Chest Percussion and Vibration

Thick secretions that are difficult to cough up may be loosened by tapping (percussing) and vibrating the chest or through the use of an HFCWO vest. Chest percussion and vibration help dislodge mucus adhering to the bronchioles and bronchi. A scheduled program of coughing and clearing sputum, together with hydration, reduces the amount of sputum in most patients.

Chest percussion is carried out by cupping the hands and lightly striking the chest wall in a rhythmic fashion over the lung segment to be drained. The wrists are alternately flexed and extended so that the chest is cupped or clapped in a painless manner (see Fig. 21-4). A soft cloth or towel may be placed over the segment of the chest that is being cupped to prevent skin irritation and redness from direct contact. Percussion, alternating with vibration, is performed for 3 to 5 minutes for each position. The patient uses diaphragmatic breathing during this procedure to promote relaxation (see later discussion). As a precaution, percussion over chest drainage tubes and the sternum, spine, liver, kidneys, spleen, or breasts (in women) is avoided. Percussion is performed cautiously in older adult patients because of their increased incidence of osteoporosis and risk of rib fracture.

Vibration is the technique of applying manual compression and tremor to the chest wall during the exhalation phase of respiration (see Fig. 21-4). This helps increase the velocity of the air expired from the small airways, thus freeing mucus. After 3 or 4 vibrations, the patient is encouraged to cough, contracting the abdominal muscles to increase the effectiveness of the cough.

The number of times the percussion and coughing cycle is repeated depends on the patient's tolerance and clinical response. The nurse evaluates breath sounds before and after the procedures.

An inflatable HFCWO vest (see Fig. 21-5) may be used to provide chest therapy. The vest uses air pulses to compress the chest wall 8 to 18 times/sec, causing secretions to detach from the airway wall and enabling the patient to expel them by coughing. Patients prescribed vest therapy are generally more satisfied with this mode of treatment delivery than patients who receive manual CPT. Furthermore, research suggests that the vest is equally effective to manual CPT; however, the mode of therapy selected should consider the patient's specific needs and preferences (Hanlon, 2015). Recent technological advances to the HFCWO vest include a portable version, the AffloVest®, which allows users to move about freely during therapy, thus improving patient adherence and satisfaction (Pedersen, 2013). In addition, chest therapy may also be delivered using specialized beds. These beds feature programmable mattresses that deliver vibropercussion and

---

Chart 21-5 **PATIENT EDUCATION**

Effective Coughing Technique

The nurse instructs the patient to:

- Assume a sitting position and bend slightly forward. This upright position permits a stronger cough.
- Flex the knees and hips to promote relaxation and reduce the strain on the abdominal muscles while coughing.
- Inhale slowly through the nose and exhale through pursed lips several times.
- Cough twice during each exhalation while contracting (pulling in) the abdomen sharply with each cough.
- Splint the incisional area, if any, with firm hand pressure or support it with a pillow or rolled blanket while coughing (see Fig. 21-12). (This can be demonstrated by placing the patient's hands.)

Figure 21-4 • Percussion and vibration. **A.** Proper hand position for vibration. **B.** Proper technique for vibration. The wrists and elbows remain stiff; the vibrating motion is produced by the shoulder muscles. **C.** Proper hand position for percussion.

may rotate the upper torso up to 45° to help mobilize pulmonary secretions.

To increase the effectiveness of coughing, a flutter valve may be used, which is especially useful for patients who have cystic fibrosis. The **flutter valve** looks like a pipe but has a cap covering the bowl, which contains a steel ball. When the patient exhales actively into the device, movement of the ball causes pressure oscillations, thereby decreasing viscosity of the mucus, facilitating mucous clearance.

Nursing Management

When performing CPT, the nurse ensures that the patient is comfortable, is not wearing restrictive clothing, and has not just eaten. The nurse gives medication for pain, as prescribed, before percussion and vibration and splints any incision and provides pillows for support as needed. The positions are varied, but focus is placed on the affected areas. On completion of the treatment, the nurse assists the patient to assume a comfortable position.

If an HFCWO vest is being used, the patient may assume whatever position is most comfortable and may even continue

Figure 21-5 • High-frequency chest wall oscillation (HFCWO) vest. © 2013 Hill-Rom Services, Inc. Reprinted with permission—all rights reserved.

to perform light activity during therapy. The patient does not need to assume specific positions for the vest to be effective.

Treatment should be stopped if any of the following occur: increased pain, increased shortness of breath, weakness, light-headedness, or hemoptysis. Therapy is indicated until the patient has normal respirations, can mobilize secretions, and has normal breath sounds, and until the chest x-ray findings are normal.

Nursing management of the patient using flutter valve therapy includes ensuring that the patient assumes the proper position, educating the patient on the technique for using the flutter valve, and setting realistic goals for the patient.

Promoting Home, Community-Based, and Transitional Care

Educating Patients About Self-Care

CPT is frequently indicated at home for patients with COPD, bronchiectasis, or cystic fibrosis. The techniques are the same as described previously; however, gravity drainage is achieved by placing the hips over a box, a stack of magazines, or pillows (unless a hospital bed is available). The nurse instructs the patient and family in the positions and techniques of percussion and vibration so that therapy can be continued in the home. In addition, the nurse instructs the patient to maintain an adequate fluid intake and air humidity to prevent secretions from becoming thick and tenacious. It also is important to educate the patient to recognize early signs of infection, such as fever and a change in the color or character of sputum.

Continuing and Transitional Care

CPT may be carried out during visits by a home or transitional care nurse. The patient's physical status, understanding of the treatment plan, adherence with recommended therapy, and the effectiveness of therapy are assessed. Patient and family education is reinforced during these visits. The nurse reports to the patient's primary provider any deterioration in the patient's physical status or inability to clear secretions.

Breathing Retraining

Breathing retraining consists of exercises and breathing practices that are designed to achieve more efficient and controlled ventilation and to decrease the work of breathing. Breathing retraining is especially indicated in patients with COPD and dyspnea. These exercises promote maximal alveolar inflation and muscle relaxation; relieve anxiety; eliminate ineffective, uncoordinated patterns of respiratory muscle activity; slow the respiratory rate; and decrease the work of breathing (Kacmarek et al., 2017). Slow, relaxed, rhythmic breathing also helps to control the anxiety that occurs with dyspnea. Specific breathing exercises include diaphragmatic and pursed-lip breathing (see Chart 21-4).

Diaphragmatic breathing can become automatic with sufficient practice and concentration. Pursed-lip breathing, which improves oxygen transport, helps induce a slow, deep breathing pattern and assists the patient to control breathing, even during periods of stress. This type of breathing helps prevent airway collapse secondary to loss of lung elasticity in emphysema. The nurse instructs the patient in diaphragmatic breathing and pursed-lip breathing, as described in Chart 21-4. Breathing exercises should be practiced in several positions because air distribution and pulmonary circulation vary with the position of the chest.

Many patients require additional oxygen, using a low-flow method, while performing breathing exercises. Emphysema-like changes in the lung occur as part of the natural aging process of the lung; therefore, breathing exercises are appropriate for all older adult patients, whether hospitalized or not, who are sedentary, even without primary lung disease.

Nursing Management

The nurse instructs the patient to breathe slowly and rhythmically in a relaxed manner and to exhale completely to empty the lungs. The patient is instructed to always inhale through the nose because this filters, humidifies, and warms the air. If short of breath, the patient should be instructed to concentrate on prolonging the length of exhalation; this helps avoid initiating a cycle of increasing shortness of breath and panic.

The nurse instructs the patient that an adequate dietary intake promotes gas exchange and increases energy levels. It is important to obtain adequate nutrition without overeating by consuming small, frequent meals and snacks. Having ready-prepared meals and favorite foods available helps encourage nutrient consumption. Gas-producing foods such as beans, legumes, broccoli, cabbage, and Brussels sprouts should be avoided to prevent gastric distress. Because many patients lack the energy to eat, they should be instructed to rest before and after meals to conserve energy.

AIRWAY MANAGEMENT

Adequate ventilation depends on free movement of air through the upper and lower airways. In many disorders, the airway becomes narrowed or blocked as a result of disease, bronchoconstriction (narrowing of the airway by contraction of muscle fibers), a foreign body, or secretions. Maintaining a patent (open) airway is achieved through meticulous airway management, whether in an emergency situation, such as airway obstruction, or in long-term management, as in caring for a patient with an endotracheal or a tracheostomy tube.

Emergency Management of Upper Airway Obstruction

Upper airway obstruction has a variety of causes. Acute upper airway obstruction may be caused by food particles, vomitus, blood clots, or anything that obstructs the larynx or trachea. It also may occur from enlargement of tissue in the wall of the airway, as in epiglottitis, obstructive sleep apnea, laryngeal edema, laryngeal carcinoma, or peritonsillar abscess, or from thick secretions. Pressure on the walls of the airway, as occurs in retrosternal goiter, enlarged mediastinal lymph nodes, hematoma around the upper airway, and thoracic aneurysm, also may result in upper airway obstruction.

The patient with an altered level of consciousness from any cause is at risk for upper airway obstruction because of loss of the protective reflexes (cough and swallowing) and loss of the tone of the pharyngeal muscles, which causes the tongue to fall back and block the airway.

The nurse makes the following rapid observations to assess for signs and symptoms of upper airway obstruction:

- *Inspection:* Is the patient conscious? Is there any inspiratory effort? Does the chest rise symmetrically? Is there use or retraction of accessory muscles? What is the skin color? Are there any obvious signs of deformity or obstruction (trauma, food, teeth, vomitus)? Is the trachea midline?
- *Palpation:* Do both sides of the chest rise equally with inspiration? Are there any specific areas of tenderness, fracture, or subcutaneous emphysema (crepitus)?
- *Auscultation:* Is there any audible air movement, stridor (inspiratory sound), or wheezing (expiratory sound)? Are breath sounds present over the lower trachea and all lobes?

As soon as an upper airway obstruction is identified, the nurse takes emergency measures (see Chart 21-6). (See Chapter 22 or Chapter 72 for more details on managing a foreign body airway obstruction.)

Endotracheal Intubation

Endotracheal intubation involves passing an endotracheal tube through the nose or mouth into the trachea (see Fig. 21-6). The oral route is preferred since oral intubation is associated with less trauma and lesser rates of infection; furthermore, the oral route can typically accommodate a larger diameter endotracheal tube than may be passed when the nasal route is used. Intubation provides a patent airway when the patient is having respiratory distress that cannot be treated with simpler methods and is the method of choice in emergency care. Endotracheal intubation is a means of providing an airway for patients who cannot maintain an adequate airway on their own (e.g., patients who are comatose and patients with upper airway obstruction), for patients needing mechanical ventilation, and for suctioning secretions from the pulmonary tree.

An endotracheal tube usually is passed with the aid of a laryngoscope by specifically trained medical, nursing, or respiratory therapy personnel. Once the tube is inserted and positioned about 2 cm above the carina, a cuff at the distal end of

Chart 21-6 Clearing an Upper Airway Obstruction

Attempt to Open the Airway

Perform the head-tilt/chin-lift maneuver by placing one hand on the forehead and placing the fingers of the other hand underneath the jaw and lifting upward and forward. This action pulls the tongue away from the back of the pharynx.

Attempt to Clear the Airway

- Assess the patient by observing the chest and listening and feeling for the movement of air.
- Use a cross-finger technique to open the mouth and observe for obvious obstructions such as secretions, blood clots, or food particles.
- If no passage of air is detected, begin cardiopulmonary resuscitation (CPR).

Bag and Mask Resuscitation

- Apply the mask to the patient's face and create a seal by pressing the thumb of the nondominant hand on the bridge of the nose and the index finger on the chin.
- Using the rest of the fingers on that hand, pull on the chin and the angle of the mandible to maintain the head in extension.
- Use the dominant hand to inflate the lungs by squeezing the bag to its full volume.

Adapted from American Heart Association. (2015). Basic life support for healthcare providers: Student manual. Dallas, TX: Author.

---

the endotracheal tube is inflated with the use of a pilot balloon. Inflation of the cuff prevents air from leaking around the outer part of the tube in order to minimize the possibility of aspiration and secure the tube. The position of the endotracheal tube is verified by checking end-tidal carbon dioxide levels and confirmed with chest x-ray. Chart 21-7 discusses the nursing care of the patient with an endotracheal tube.

Figure 21-6 • Endotracheal tube in place. The tube has been inserted using the oral route. The cuff has been inflated to maintain the tube's position and to minimize the risk of aspiration.

Complications can occur from pressure exerted by the cuff on the tracheal wall. Cuff pressures should be maintained between 20 and 25 mm Hg (24 to 30 cm H_2O) because high cuff pressure can cause tracheal bleeding, ischemia, and pressure necrosis, whereas low cuff pressure can increase the risk of aspiration pneumonia. Routine deflation of the cuff is not recommended because of the increased risk of aspiration and hypoxia (Urden et al., 2014). Tracheobronchial secretions are suctioned through the tube. Warmed, humidified oxygen should always be introduced through the tube, whether the patient is breathing spontaneously or is receiving ventilatory support. Endotracheal intubation may be used for no longer than 14 to 21 days, by which time a tracheostomy must be considered to decrease irritation of and trauma to the tracheal lining, to reduce the incidence of vocal cord paralysis (secondary to laryngeal nerve damage), and to decrease the work of breathing (Wiegand, 2011).

Endotracheal and tracheostomy tubes have several disadvantages. The tubes cause discomfort. The cough reflex is depressed because glottis closure is hindered. Secretions tend to become thicker because the warming and humidifying effect of the upper respiratory tract has been bypassed. The swallowing reflexes (glottic, pharyngeal, and laryngeal reflexes) are depressed because of prolonged disuse and the

Chart 21-7 — Care of the Patient With an Endotracheal Tube

Immediately After Intubation

1. Check symmetry of chest expansion.
2. Auscultate breath sounds of anterior and lateral chest bilaterally.
3. Obtain capnography or end-tidal CO_2 as indicated
4. Ensure chest x-ray obtained to verify proper tube placement.
5. Check cuff pressure every 6–8 hours.
6. Monitor for signs and symptoms of aspiration.
7. Ensure high humidity; a visible mist should appear in the T-piece or ventilator tubing.
8. Administer oxygen concentration as prescribed by the primary provider.
9. Secure the tube to the patient's face with tape, and mark the proximal end for position maintenance.
   a. Cut proximal end of tube if it is longer than 7.5 cm (3 in) to prevent kinking.
   b. Insert an oral airway or mouth device if orally intubated to prevent the patient from biting and obstructing the tube.
10. Use sterile suction technique and airway care to prevent iatrogenic contamination and infection.
11. Continue to reposition patient every 2 hours and as needed to prevent atelectasis and to optimize lung expansion.
12. Provide oral hygiene and suction the oropharynx whenever necessary.

Extubation (Removal of Endotracheal Tube)

1. Explain procedure.
2. Have self-inflating bag and mask ready in case ventilatory assistance is required immediately after extubation.
3. Suction the tracheobronchial tree and oropharynx, remove tape, and then deflate the cuff.
4. Give 100% oxygen for a few breaths, then insert a new, sterile suction catheter inside tube.
5. Have the patient inhale. At peak inspiration, remove the tube, suctioning the airway through the tube as it is pulled out.

Note: In some hospitals, this procedure can be performed by respiratory therapists; in others, by nurses. Check hospital policy.

Care of Patient Following Extubation

1. Give heated humidity and oxygen by facemask and maintain the patient in a sitting or high Fowler's position.
2. Monitor respiratory rate and quality of chest excursions. Note stridor, color change, and change in mental alertness or behavior.
3. Monitor the patient's oxygen level using a pulse oximeter.
4. Keep patient NPO (nothing by mouth), or give only ice chips for next few hours.
5. Provide mouth care.
6. Educate the patient about how to perform coughing and deep-breathing exercises.

---

mechanical trauma produced by the endotracheal or tracheostomy tube, increasing the risk of aspiration as well as microaspiration and subsequent ventilator-associated pneumonia (VAP) (Urden et al., 2014). In addition, ulceration and stricture of the larynx or trachea may develop. Of great concern to the patient is the inability to talk and to communicate needs.

Unintentional or premature removal of the tube is a potentially life-threatening complication of endotracheal intubation. Removal of the tube is a frequent problem in intensive care units (ICUs) and occurs mainly during nursing care or by the patient. Nurses must instruct and remind patients and family members about the purpose of the tube and the dangers of removing it. Baseline and ongoing assessment of the patient and of the equipment ensures effective care. Providing comfort measures, including opioid analgesia and sedation, can improve the patient's tolerance of the endotracheal tube.

> **Quality and Safety Nursing Alert**
>
> Inadvertent removal of an endotracheal tube can cause laryngeal swelling, hypoxemia, bradycardia, hypotension, and even death. Measures must be taken to prevent premature or inadvertent removal.

To prevent tube removal by the patient, the nurse should explain to the patient and family the purpose of the tube, distract the patient through one-to-one interaction or with television, and maintain comfort measures. If the patient cannot move the arms and hands to the endotracheal tube, restraints are not needed. If the patient is alert, oriented, able to follow directions, and cooperative to the point that it is highly unlikely that he or she will remove the endotracheal

tube, restraints are not needed. However, if the nurse determines there is a risk that the patient may try to remove the tube, the least invasive method of restraints (e.g., soft wrist restraints and hand mitts) may be appropriate as prescribed by the primary provider (check agency policy) (The Joint Commission [TJC], 1998). The rationale for use of restraints should be documented, and the patient's significant others should receive explanations why restraints are necessary. Close monitoring of the patient is essential to ensure safety and prevent harm. The use of restraints is generally limited to no more than 24 hours (Sole, Klein, & Moseley, 2013).

Tracheostomy

A **tracheotomy** is a surgical procedure in which an opening is made into the trachea. The indwelling tube inserted into the trachea is called a **tracheostomy tube** (see Fig. 21-7). A tracheostomy (the stoma that is the product of the tracheotomy) may be either temporary or permanent.

A tracheotomy is used to bypass an upper airway obstruction, to allow removal of tracheobronchial secretions, to permit the long-term use of mechanical ventilation, to prevent aspiration of oral or gastric secretions in the unconscious or paralyzed patient (by closing off the trachea from the esophagus), and to replace an endotracheal tube. Many disease processes and emergency conditions make a tracheotomy necessary.

Procedure

The surgical procedure is usually performed in the operating room or in an ICU, where the patient's ventilation can be well controlled and optimal aseptic technique can be maintained. A surgical opening is made between the second and

A

B

Figure 21-7 • Tracheostomy tubes. **A.** Fenestrated tube, which allows patient to talk. **B.** Double-cuffed tube. Inflating the two cuffs alternately can help prevent tracheal damage.

third tracheal rings. After the trachea is exposed, a cuffed tracheostomy tube of an appropriate size is inserted. The cuff is an inflatable attachment to the tracheostomy tube that is designed to occlude the space between the tracheal walls and the tube, to permit effective mechanical ventilation, and to minimize the risk of aspiration. See Figure 21-7 for the different types of tracheostomy tubes.

The tracheostomy tube is held in place by twill tape ties or a tube holder fastened around the patient's neck. Usually, a square of sterile gauze is placed between the tube and the skin to absorb drainage and reduce the risk of infection.

Complications

Complications may occur early or late in the course of tracheostomy tube management. They may even occur years after the tube has been removed. Early complications include tube dislodgement, accidental decannulation, bleeding, pneumothorax, air embolism, aspiration, subcutaneous or mediastinal emphysema, recurrent laryngeal nerve damage, and posterior tracheal wall penetration. Long-term complications include airway obstruction from accumulation of secretions or protrusion of the cuff over the opening of the tube, infection, rupture of the innominate artery, dysphagia, tracheoesophageal fistula, tracheal dilation, tracheal ischemia, and necrosis. Tracheal

stenosis may develop after the tube is removed. Chart 21-8 outlines measures nurses can take to prevent complications.

Nursing Management

The patient requires continuous monitoring and assessment. The newly made opening must be kept patent by proper suctioning of secretions. After the vital signs are stable, the patient is placed in a semi-Fowler's position to facilitate ventilation, promote drainage, minimize edema, and prevent strain on the suture lines. Analgesia and sedative agents must be given with caution because of the risk of suppressing the cough reflex.

Major objectives of nursing care are to ensure a patent airway, monitor the patient's respiratory status, assess for complications, alleviate the patient's apprehension, and provide an effective means of communication. The nurse keeps paper and pencil or a Magic Slate® and the call light within the patient's reach at all times to ensure a means of communication.

 For the procedural guidelines for nursing care of a patient with a tracheostomy tube, go to **thepoint.lww.com/Brunner14e**.

Suctioning the Tracheal Tube (Tracheostomy or Endotracheal Tube)

When a tracheostomy or endotracheal tube is in place, it is usually necessary to suction the patient's secretions because of the decreased effectiveness of the cough mechanism. Tracheal suctioning is performed when adventitious breath sounds are detected or whenever secretions are obviously present. Unnecessary suctioning can initiate bronchospasm and cause mechanical trauma to the tracheal mucosa.

All equipment that comes into direct contact with the patient's lower airway must be sterile to prevent sepsis.

 For the procedural guidelines for suctioning a patient with a tracheostomy tube, go to **thepoint.lww.com/Brunner14e**.

In patients who are mechanically ventilated, an in-line suction catheter may be used to allow rapid suction when needed and to minimize cross-contamination by airborne pathogens. An in-line suction device allows the patient to be suctioned without being disconnected from the ventilator circuit. In-line suctioning (also called *closed suctioning*) decreases hypoxemia, sustains PEEP, and can decrease patient anxiety associated with suctioning (Sole et al., 2013). Because in-line suctioning protects staff from patient secretions, it can be performed without using personal protective gear.

Managing the Cuff

The cuff on an endotracheal or tracheostomy tube should be inflated if the patient requires mechanical ventilation or is at high risk for aspiration. The pressure within the cuff should be the lowest possible pressure (20 to 25 mm Hg) that allows delivery of adequate tidal volumes and prevents pulmonary aspiration (Urden et al., 2014). Cuff pressure must be monitored by the respiratory therapist or nurse at least every 8 hours by attaching a handheld pressure gauge to the pilot balloon of the tube or by using the minimal leak volume or minimal occlusion volume technique.

Promoting Home, Community-Based, and Transitional Care

 Educating Patients About Self-Care

If the patient is pending discharge to the home setting with a tracheostomy tube, the nurse should ensure that suction and other appropriate equipment is in place in the home prior to discharge. The nurse also instructs the patient and family about daily care, including techniques to prevent infection, as well as measures to take in an emergency. The nurse provides the patient and family with a list of community contacts for education and support needs.

Continuing and Transitional Care

A referral for home, community-based, or transitional care is indicated for ongoing assessment of the patient and of the ability of the patient and family to provide appropriate and safe care. The nurse assesses the patient's and family's ability to cope with the physical changes and psychological issues associated with having a tracheostomy. Minimizing the amount of dust or particles in the air and providing adequate humidification may make it easier for the patient to breathe. Dust and particles in the air can be decreased by removing drapes and upholstered furniture; using air filters; and washing floors, dusting, and vacuuming frequently. The nurse identifies resources and makes referrals for appropriate services to assist the patient and family to manage the tracheostomy tube at home.

 ## Mechanical Ventilation

Mechanical ventilation may be required for a variety of reasons: to control the patient's respirations during surgery or treatment, to oxygenate the blood when the patient's ventilatory efforts are inadequate, and to rest the respiratory muscles, among others. Many patients placed on a ventilator can breathe spontaneously, although the effort needed to do so may be exhausting.

A **mechanical ventilator** is a positive- or negative-pressure breathing device that can maintain ventilation and oxygen delivery for a prolonged period. Caring for a patient on mechanical ventilation has become an integral part of nursing care in critical care or general medical-surgical units, extended care facilities, and the home. Nurses, physicians, and respiratory therapists must understand each patient's specific pulmonary needs and work together to set realistic goals. Positive patient outcomes depend on an understanding of the principles of mechanical ventilation and the patient's care needs as well as open communication among members of the health care team about the goals of therapy, weaning plans, and the patient's tolerance of changes in ventilator settings.

Indications

If a patient has evidence of respiratory failure or a compromised airway, endotracheal intubation and mechanical ventilation are indicated. This clinical evidence may be corroborated by a continuous decrease in oxygenation (PaO_2), an increase in arterial carbon dioxide levels ($PaCO_2$), and a persistent acidosis (decreased pH); however, if the patient's status appears emergent, then waiting for these laboratory results prior to ensuring these ventilator support measures is imprudent (Amitai & Sinert, 2015). Conditions such as thoracic or abdominal surgery, drug overdose, neuromuscular disorders, inhalation injury, COPD, multiple trauma, shock, multisystem failure, and coma may lead to respiratory failure and the need for mechanical ventilation. General indications for mechanical ventilation are displayed in Chart 21-9.

Classification of Ventilators

Mechanical ventilators were traditionally classified according to the method by which they supported ventilation. The two general categories are negative-pressure and positive-pressure ventilators. Figure 21-8 displays commonly used positive-pressure ventilators. Negative-pressure ventilators (e.g., "iron lungs," chest cuirass) are older modes of ventilatory support that are rarely utilized today.

Chart 21-9 Indications for Mechanical Ventilation

Laboratory Values

PaO_2 <55 mm Hg
$PaCO_2$ >50 mm Hg and pH <7.32
Vital capacity <10 mL/kg
Negative inspiratory force <25 cm H_2O
FEV_1 <10 mL/kg

Clinical Manifestations

Apnea or bradypnea
Respiratory distress with confusion
Increased work of breathing not relieved by other interventions
Confusion with need for airway protection
Circulatory shock
Controlled hyperventilation (e.g., patient with a severe head injury)

Adapted from Amitai, A. & Sinert, R. H. (2015). Introduction to ventilator management. *Medscape.* Retrieved on 5/7/2016 at: emedicine.medscape.com/article/810126-overview#a3

Figure 21-8 • Positive-pressure ventilators. **A.** The AVEA can be used to both ventilate and monitor neonatal, pediatric, and adult patients. It can also deliver noninvasive ventilation with Heliox to adult and pediatric patients. Courtesy of Vyaire Medical Inc., Yorba Linda, CA. **B.** The Puritan-Bennett 840 Ventilator System has volume, pressure, and mixed modes designed for adult, pediatric, and infant ventilation. Courtesy of Tyco Healthcare/Nellcor Puritan Bennett, Pleasanton, CA.

Positive-Pressure Ventilators

Positive-pressure ventilators inflate the lungs by exerting positive pressure on the airway, pushing air in, similar to a bellows mechanism, and forcing the alveoli to expand during inspiration. Expiration occurs passively. Endotracheal intubation or tracheostomy is usually necessary. These ventilators are widely used in the hospital setting and are increasingly used in the home for patients with primary lung disease. Three types of positive-pressure ventilators are classified by the method of ending the inspiratory phase of respiration: volume cycled, pressure cycled, and high-frequency oscillatory support. The fourth type, noninvasive positive-pressure ventilation (NIPPV), does not require intubation (Cairo, 2014).

Volume-Cycled Ventilators

Volume-cycled ventilators deliver a preset volume of air with each inspiration. Once this preset volume is delivered to the patient, the ventilator cycles off and exhalation occurs passively. From breath to breath, the volume of air delivered by the ventilator is relatively constant, ensuring consistent, adequate breaths despite varying airway pressures. A major disadvantage to using volume-cycled ventilators is that patients may experience barotrauma because the pressures required to deliver the breaths may be excessive. This trauma causes damage to the alveolar capillary membrane and air to leak into the surrounding tissues (Urden et al., 2014).

Pressure-Cycled Ventilators

When the pressure-cycled ventilator cycles on, it delivers a flow of air (inspiration) until it reaches a preset pressure, and then cycles off, and expiration occurs. The major limitation is the volume of air or oxygen can vary as the patient's airway resistance or compliance changes. As a result, the tidal volume delivered may be inconsistent, possibly compromising ventilation.

High-Frequency Oscillatory Support Ventilators

These types of ventilators deliver very high respiratory rates (i.e., 180 to 900 breaths/min) that are accompanied by very low tidal volumes and high airway pressures (hence the name *high-frequency oscillatory support*). These small pulses of oxygen-enriched air move down the center of the airways, allowing alveolar air to exit the lungs along the margins of the airways. This ventilatory mode is used to open the alveoli in situations characterized by closed small airways, such as atelectasis and ARDS (see Chapter 23), and it is also thought to protect the lung from pressure injury (Cairo, 2014).

Noninvasive Positive-Pressure Ventilation

NIPPV is a method of positive-pressure ventilation that can be given via facemasks that cover the nose and mouth, nasal masks, or other oral or nasal devices such as the nasal pillow (a small nasal cannula that seals around the nares to maintain the prescribed pressure). NIPPV eliminates the need for endotracheal intubation or tracheostomy and decreases the risk of nosocomial infections such as pneumonia. The most comfortable mode for the patient is pressure-controlled ventilation with pressure support. This eases the work of breathing and enhances gas exchange. The ventilator can be set with a minimum backup rate for patients with periods of apnea.

Patients are candidates for NIPPV if they have acute or chronic respiratory failure, acute pulmonary edema, COPD, chronic heart failure, or a sleep-related breathing disorder. The technique also may be used at home to improve tissue oxygenation and to rest the respiratory muscles while patients sleep at night. NIPPV is contraindicated for those who have experienced respiratory arrest, serious dysrhythmias, cognitive impairment, or head or facial trauma. NIPPV may also be used for obstructive sleep apnea, for patients at the end of life, and for those who do not want endotracheal intubation but may need short- or long-term ventilatory support (Amitai & Sinert, 2015).

CPAP provides positive pressure to the airways throughout the respiratory cycle. Although it can be used as an adjunct to mechanical ventilation with a cuffed endotracheal tube or tracheostomy tube to open the alveoli, it is also used with a leak-proof mask to keep alveoli open, thereby preventing respiratory failure. CPAP is an effective treatment of obstructive sleep apnea because the positive pressure acts as a splint, keeping the upper airway and trachea open during sleep. To use CPAP, the patient must be breathing independently.

Bilevel positive airway pressure (BiPAP) ventilation offers independent control of inspiratory and expiratory pressures while providing **pressure support ventilation (PSV)**. It delivers two levels of positive airway pressure provided via a nasal or oral mask, nasal pillow, or mouthpiece with a tight seal and a portable ventilator. Each inspiration can be initiated either by the patient or by the machine if it is programmed with a backup rate. The backup rate ensures that the patient receives a set number of breaths per minute. BiPAP is most often used for patients who require ventilatory assistance at night, such as those with severe COPD or sleep apnea. Tolerance is variable; BiPAP usually is most successful with highly motivated patients.

Ventilator Modes

Ventilator mode refers to how breaths are delivered to the patient. The most commonly used modes are controlled mechanical ventilation, continuous mandatory ventilation, also known as assist–control (A/C), intermittent mandatory ventilation (IMV), synchronized intermittent mandatory ventilation (SIMV), PSV, and airway pressure release ventilation (APRV) (see Fig. 21-9).

Controlled mechanical ventilation provides full ventilator support by delivering a preset tidal volume and respiratory rate. This mode of ventilation is indicated for patients who are apneic. In A/C ventilation, more commonly called **continuous mandatory (volume or pressure) ventilation (CMV)**, the ventilator delivers a preset tidal volume or pressure at a preset rate of respirations. However, if the patient initiates a breath between the machine's breaths, the ventilator delivers at the preset volume or pressure (assisted breath). Therefore,

A. Controlled mechanical ventilation

B. Continuous mandatory ventilation (assist control ventilation)

C. Synchronized intermittent mandatory ventilation (SIMV)

D. Positive end expiratory pressure (PEEP)

E. Continuous positive airway pressure (CPAP)

F. Pressure support with SIMV

G. Airway pressure release ventilation (APRV)

H. High-frequency jet ventilation

Figure 21-9 • Modes of mechanical ventilation with airflow waveforms. Inhalations marked with an asterisk (*) are spontaneous.

every breath is the preset volume or pressure, regardless of whether it is initiated by the patient or the ventilator.

IMV provides a combination of mechanically assisted breaths and spontaneous breaths. Mechanical breaths are delivered at preset intervals and a preselected tidal volume, regardless of the patient's efforts. Although the patient can increase the respiratory rate by initiating inspiration between ventilator-delivered breaths, these spontaneous breaths are limited to the tidal volume generated by the patient. IMV allows patients to use their own muscles for ventilation to help prevent muscle atrophy. It lowers mean airway pressure, which can assist in preventing barotrauma. However, "fighting the ventilator" or "bucking the ventilator" (i.e., trying to exhale when the ventilator is delivering a breath) may be increased.

SIMV also delivers a preset tidal volume and number of breaths per minute. Between ventilator-delivered breaths, the patient can breathe spontaneously with no assistance from the ventilator on those extra breaths. Because the ventilator senses patient breathing efforts and does not initiate a breath in opposition to the patient's efforts, fighting the ventilator is reduced. As the patient's ability to breathe spontaneously increases, the preset number of ventilator breaths is decreased and the patient does more of the work of breathing. Like IMV, SIMV can be used to provide full or partial ventilatory support. Nursing interventions for patients receiving IMV or SIMV include monitoring progress by recording respiratory rate, minute volume, spontaneous and machine-generated tidal volume, FiO_2, and arterial blood gas levels.

PSV applies a pressure plateau to the airway throughout the patient-triggered inspiration to decrease resistance within the tracheal tube and ventilator tubing. Pressure support is reduced gradually as the patient's strength increases. An SIMV backup rate may be added for extra support. The nurse must closely observe the patient's respiratory rate and tidal volumes on initiation of PSV. It may be necessary to adjust the pressure support to avoid tachypnea or large tidal volumes.

APRV is a time-triggered, pressure-limited, time-cycled mode of mechanical ventilation that allows unrestricted, spontaneous breathing throughout the ventilatory cycle. The inflation period is long, and breaths may be initiated spontaneously as well as by the ventilator. APRV allows alveolar gas to be expelled through the lungs' natural recoil. APRV has the important advantages of causing less ventilator-induced lung injury and fewer adverse effects on cardiocirculatory function and being associated with lower need for sedation and neuromuscular blockade (Cairo, 2014).

Proportional assist ventilation (PAV) provides partial ventilatory support in which the ventilator generates pressure in proportion to the patient's inspiratory efforts. With every breath, the ventilator synchronizes with the patient's ventilatory efforts. The more inspiratory pressure the patient generates, the more pressure the ventilator generates, amplifying the patient's inspiratory effort without any specific preselected target pressure or volume. It generally adds "additional muscle" to the patient's effort; the depth and frequency of breaths are controlled by the patient (Cairo, 2014).

Other modes of mechanical ventilation that incorporate computerized control of ventilation are being developed. In some of these modes, the ventilator constantly monitors many variables and adjusts gas delivery during individual breaths; these within-breath adjustment systems include automatic tube compensation, volume-ensured pressure support, and proportional support ventilation. In other modes, the ventilator evaluates gas delivery during one breath and uses that information to adjust the next breath; these between-breath adjustment systems can be made to ensure a preset tidal volume by adjusting pressure, up to a preset maximum, and include pressure volume support, pressure-regulated volume control, and adaptive support ventilation.

Adjusting the Ventilator

The ventilator is adjusted so that the patient is comfortable and breathes synchronously (i.e., "in sync") with the machine. Minimal alteration of the normal cardiovascular and pulmonary dynamics is desired. If the volume ventilator is adjusted appropriately, the patient's arterial blood gas values will be satisfactory and there will be little or no cardiovascular compromise. Chart 21-10 describes initial ventilator settings.

Chart 21-10 | **Initial Ventilator Settings**

The following guide is an example of the steps involved in operating a mechanical ventilator. The nurse, in collaboration with the respiratory therapist, always reviews the manufacturer's instructions, which vary according to the equipment, before beginning mechanical ventilation.

1. Set the machine to deliver the tidal volume required (6–10 mL/kg) or (4–8 mL/kg for patients with ARDS).
2. Adjust the machine to deliver the lowest concentration of oxygen to maintain normal PaO_2 (greater than 60 mm Hg) or an SpO_2 level greater than 92%. This setting may be high initially but will gradually be reduced based on arterial blood gas (ABG) results.
3. Record peak inspiratory pressure.
4. Set mode (continuous mandatory ventilation [also known as assist–control], or synchronized intermittent mandatory ventilation) and rate as prescribed by the primary provider. (See the glossary for definitions of modes of mechanical ventilation.) Set positive end-expiratory pressure (PEEP) and pressure support if prescribed.
5. Set sigh settings (usually set at 1.5 times the tidal volume and ranging from 1 to 3 per hour), if applicable.
6. Adjust sensitivity so that the patient can trigger the ventilator with a minimal effort (usually 2 mm Hg negative inspiratory force).
7. Record minute volume and obtain ABGs to measure carbon dioxide partial pressure ($PaCO_2$), pH, and PaO_2 after 20 minutes of continuous mechanical ventilation.
8. Adjust setting (FiO_2 and rate) according to results of ABG analysis to provide normal values or those set by the primary provider.
9. If there is poor coordination between the breathing rhythms of the patient and the ventilator (i.e., if the patient is "fighting" or "bucking the ventilator"), assess for hypoxia and manually ventilate on 100% oxygen with a resuscitation bag.

Adapted from Amitai, A. & Sinert, R. H. (2015). Introduction to ventilator management. *Medscape.* Retrieved on 5/7/2016 at: emedicine.medscape.com/article/810126-overview#a3.

Monitoring the Equipment

The ventilator needs to be monitored to make sure that it is functioning properly and that the settings are appropriate. Although the nurse may not be primarily responsible for adjusting the settings on the ventilator or measuring ventilator parameters (these are usually responsibilities of the respiratory therapist), the nurse is responsible for the patient and therefore needs to evaluate how the ventilator affects the patient's overall status.

When monitoring the ventilator, the nurse notes the following:

- Controlling mode (e.g., A/C ventilation and SIMV).
- Tidal volume and rate settings (tidal volume is usually set at 6 to 10 mL/kg [ideal body weight] or 4 to 8 mL/kg for the patient with ARDS [ideal body weight]; rate is usually set at 12 to 16 breaths/min).
- FiO_2 setting may be set between 21% and 100% to maintain an optimal PaO_2 level (e.g., greater than 60 mm Hg) or SpO_2 level greater than 92%.
- Peak inspiratory pressure (PIP) (Normal is 15 to 20 cm H_2O; this increases if there is increased airway resistance or decreased compliance).
- Sensitivity (A 2-cm H_2O inspiratory force should trigger the ventilator).
- Inspiratory-to-expiratory ratio (usually 1:2 [1 second of inspiration to 2 seconds of expiration] unless inverse ratio is ordered).
- Minute volume (tidal volume × respiratory rate).
- Sigh settings (usually set at 1.5 times the tidal volume and ranging from 1 to 3 per hour), if applicable.
- Water in the tubing, disconnection or kinking of the tubing.
- Humidification (humidifier filled with water) and temperature.
- Alarms (turned on and functioning properly at all times per the Joint Commission Alarm Safety Goal) (TJC, 2016).
- PEEP and pressure support level, if applicable.

As is true with any type of patient-sensitive life support equipment, mechanical ventilators have multiple alarms that are set to alert the health care team of potential patient problems. With the increased number of alarms and their high sensitivity to subtle changes, members of the health care team, including nurses, are at risk for experiencing alarm fatigue, which means that they may become desensitized to alarms and not respond to them with sufficient speed. According to the National Patient Safety Goals (TJC, 2016), measures must be instituted to prevent alarm fatigue.

> ▶ **Quality and Safety Nursing Alert**
>
> *To prevent alarm fatigue associated with mechanical ventilators, nurses can manage the physical layout of the critical care unit (e.g., avoid locating patients on mechanical ventilators in close proximity); devise protocols for setting of alarms based upon best practices; and educate staff on how to set alarms and when and how to respond to them.*

NURSING PROCESS

The Patient Receiving Mechanical Ventilation

Assessment

The nurse plays a vital role in assessing the patient's status and the functioning of the ventilator. In assessing the patient, the nurse evaluates the patient's physiologic status and how he or she is coping with mechanical ventilation. Physical assessment includes systematic assessment of all body systems, with an in-depth focus on the respiratory system. Respiratory assessment includes vital signs, respiratory rate and pattern, breath sounds, evaluation of spontaneous ventilatory effort, and potential evidence of hypoxia (e.g., skin color). Increased adventitious breath sounds may indicate a need for suctioning. The nurse maintains the patient's head of the bed so that it is elevated 30° or higher unless contraindicated to prevent the risk of aspiration and VAP. The nurse evaluates the settings and functioning of the mechanical ventilator, as described previously, and verifies endotracheal tube position as applicable.

Assessment also addresses the patient's neurologic status and effectiveness of coping with the need for assisted ventilation and the changes that accompany it. The nurse assesses the patient's comfort level and ability to communicate as well. Because weaning from mechanical ventilation requires adequate nutrition, it is important to assess the patient's gastrointestinal system and nutritional status.

Diagnosis

NURSING DIAGNOSES

Based on the assessment data, major nursing diagnoses may include:

- Impaired gas exchange related to underlying illness, ventilator setting adjustments, or weaning
- Ineffective airway clearance related to increased mucus production associated with presence of the tube in trachea or continuous positive-pressure mechanical ventilation
- Risk for trauma and infection related to endotracheal intubation or tracheostomy
- Impaired physical mobility related to ventilator dependency
- Impaired verbal communication related to endotracheal tube or tracheostomy tube
- Defensive coping and powerlessness related to ventilator dependency

COLLABORATIVE PROBLEMS/POTENTIAL COMPLICATIONS

Based on the assessment data, potential complications may include the following (see Table 21-2):

- Ventilator problems (increase in peak airway pressure or decrease in pressure or loss of volume)
- Alterations in cardiac function
- Barotrauma (trauma to the trachea or alveoli secondary to positive pressure) and pneumothorax
- Pulmonary infection and sepsis (e.g., VAP; see Chart 21-11)
- Delirium

TABLE 21-2 Troubleshooting Problems With Mechanical Ventilation

Problem	Cause	Solution
Ventilator Problems		
Increase in peak airway pressure	Coughing or plugged airway tube	Suction airway for secretions; empty condensation fluid from circuit.
	Patient "fighting" ventilator	Adjust sensitivity; consider administering sedatives as prescribed
	Decreasing lung compliance	Manually ventilate patient. Assess for hypoxia or bronchospasm. Check arterial blood gas values. Sedate only if necessary.
	Tubing kinked	Check tubing; reposition patient; insert oral airway if necessary.
	Pneumothorax	Manually ventilate patient; notify primary provider.
	Atelectasis or bronchospasm	Clear secretions.
Decrease in pressure or loss of volume	Increase in compliance	None
	Leak in ventilator or tubing; cuff on tube/humidifier not tight	Check entire ventilator circuit for patency. Correct leak.
Patient Problems		
Cardiovascular compromise	Decrease in venous return due to application of positive pressure to lungs	Assess for adequate volume status by measuring heart rate, blood pressure, central venous pressure, pulmonary capillary wedge pressure, and urine output; notify primary provider if values are abnormal.
Barotrauma/ pneumothorax	Application of positive pressure to lungs; high mean airway pressures lead to alveolar rupture	Notify primary provider. Prepare patient for chest tube insertion. Avoid high pressure settings for patients with COPD, ARDS, or history of pneumothorax.
Pulmonary infection	Bypass of normal defense mechanisms; frequent breaks in ventilator circuit; decreased mobility; impaired cough reflex	Use strict aseptic technique. Provide frequent mouth care. Optimize nutritional status.

COPD, chronic obstructive pulmonary disease; ARDS, acute respiratory distress syndrome.

Chart 21-11

Collaborative Practice Interventions to Prevent Ventilator-Associated Pneumonia

Current best practices can include the implementation of specific evidence-based bundle interventions that, when used together (i.e., as a "bundle"), improve patient outcomes. This chart outlines specific parameters for the ventilator-bundled collaborative interventions that have been found to reduce ventilator-associated pneumonia (VAP).

What are the five key elements of the VAP bundle?
- Elevation of the head of the bed (30° to 45°)
- Daily "sedation vacations" and assessment of readiness to extubate (see below)
- Peptic ulcer disease prophylaxis
- Deep venous thrombosis (DVT) prophylaxis (see below)
- Daily oral care with chlorhexidine (0.12% oral rinses)

What is meant by daily "sedation vacations," and how does this tie into assessing readiness to extubate?
- Protocols should be developed so that sedative doses are purposely decreased at a time of the day when it is possible to assess the patient's neurologic readiness for extubation.
- Vigilance must be employed during the time that sedative doses are lower to ensure that the patient does not self-extubate.

What effect does DVT prophylaxis have on preventing VAP?
- The exact relationship is unclear. However, when appropriate, evidence-based methods to ensure DVT prophylaxis are applied (see Chapter 30), then the rates of VAP also drop.

Adapted from Institute for Healthcare Improvement. (2012). *How-to guide: Prevent ventilator-associated pneumonia.* Cambridge, MA: Institute for Healthcare Improvements. Retrieved on 5/7/2016 at: www.ihi.org/resources/Pages/Tools/HowtoGuidePreventVAP.aspx

Planning and Goals

The major goals for the patient may include achievement of optimal gas exchange, maintenance of a patent airway, absence of trauma or infection, attainment of optimal mobility, adjustment to nonverbal methods of communication, acquisition of successful coping measures, and absence of complications.

Nursing Interventions

Nursing care of the patient who is mechanically ventilated requires expert technical and interpersonal skills. Nursing interventions are similar regardless of the setting; however, the frequency of interventions and the stability of the patient vary from setting to setting. Nursing interventions for the patient who is mechanically ventilated are not uniquely different from those for patients with other pulmonary disorders, but astute nursing assessment and a therapeutic nurse–patient relationship are critical. The specific interventions used by the nurse are determined by the underlying disease process and the patient's response.

Two general nursing interventions that are important in the care of the patient who is mechanically ventilated are pulmonary auscultation and interpretation of arterial blood gas measurements. The nurse is often the first to note changes in physical assessment findings or significant trends in blood gases that signal the development of a serious problem (e.g., pneumothorax, tube displacement, and pulmonary embolus).

ENHANCING GAS EXCHANGE

The purpose of mechanical ventilation is to optimize gas exchange by maintaining alveolar ventilation and oxygen delivery. The alteration in gas exchange may be caused by the underlying illness or by mechanical factors related to adjustment of the machine to the patient. The health care team, including the nurse, physician, and respiratory therapist, continually assesses the patient for adequate gas exchange, signs and symptoms of hypoxia, and response to treatment. Therefore, the nursing diagnosis of impaired gas exchange is, by its complex nature, multidisciplinary and collaborative. The team members must share goals and information freely. All other goals directly or indirectly relate to this primary goal.

Nursing interventions to promote optimal gas exchange include judicious administration of analgesic agents to relieve pain without suppressing the respiratory drive and frequent repositioning to diminish the pulmonary effects of immobility. The nurse also monitors for adequate fluid balance by assessing for the presence of peripheral edema, calculating daily intake and output, and monitoring daily weights. The nurse administers medications prescribed to control the primary disease and monitors for their side effects.

PROMOTING EFFECTIVE AIRWAY CLEARANCE

Continuous positive-pressure ventilation increases the production of secretions regardless of the patient's underlying condition. The nurse assesses for the presence of secretions by lung auscultation at least every 2 to 4 hours. Measures to clear the airway of secretions include suctioning, CPT, frequent position changes, and increased mobility as soon as possible. Frequency of suctioning should be determined by patient assessment. If excessive secretions are identified by inspection or auscultation techniques, suctioning should be performed. Sputum is not produced continuously or every 1 to 2 hours but as a response to a pathologic condition. Therefore, there is no rationale for routine suctioning of all patients every 1 to 2 hours. Although suctioning is used to aid in the clearance of secretions, it can damage the airway mucosa and impair cilia action.

The sigh mechanism on the ventilator may be adjusted to deliver at least 1 to 3 sighs per hour at 1.5 times the tidal volume if the patient is receiving A/C ventilation. Periodic sighs prevent atelectasis and the further retention of secretions. Because of the risk for hyperventilation and trauma to pulmonary tissue from excess ventilator pressure (barotrauma, pneumothorax), the sigh feature is not used frequently. If the SIMV mode is being used, the mandatory ventilations act as sighs because they are of greater volume than the patient's spontaneous breaths.

Humidification of the airway via the ventilator is maintained to help liquefy secretions so that they are more easily removed. Bronchodilators may be indicated to dilate the bronchioles in patients with acute lung injury or COPD and are classified as adrenergic or anticholinergic. Adrenergic bronchodilators (see Chapter 24, Table 24-3) are mostly inhaled and work by stimulating the beta-receptor sites, mimicking the effects of epinephrine in the body. The desired effect is smooth muscle relaxation, which dilates the constricted bronchial tubes. Anticholinergic bronchodilators (see Chapter 24, Table 24-3) produce airway relaxation by blocking cholinergic-induced bronchoconstriction. Patients receiving bronchodilator therapy of either type should be monitored for adverse effects, including dizziness, nausea, decreased oxygen saturation, hypokalemia, increased heart rate, and urine retention. Mucolytic agents (e.g., acetylcysteine [Mucomyst]) may also be indicated in these patients to liquefy secretions so that they are more easily mobilized. Nursing management of patients receiving mucolytic therapy includes assessment of an adequate cough reflex, sputum characteristics, and (in patients not receiving mechanical ventilation) improvement in incentive spirometry. Side effects include nausea, vomiting, bronchospasm, stomatitis (oral ulcers), urticaria, and rhinorrhea (runny nose) (Karch, 2013).

PREVENTING TRAUMA AND INFECTION

Maintaining the endotracheal or tracheostomy tube is an essential part of airway management. The nurse positions the ventilator tubing so that there is minimal pulling or distortion of the tube in the trachea, reducing the risk of trauma to the trachea. Cuff pressure is monitored every 8 hours to maintain the pressure at 20 to 25 mm Hg (Urden et al., 2014). The nurse assesses for the presence of a cuff leak at the same time.

Patients with an endotracheal or tracheostomy tube do not have the normal defenses of the upper airway. In addition, these patients frequently have multiple additional body system disturbances that lead to immunocompromise. Tracheostomy care is performed at least every 8 hours, and more frequently if needed, because of the increased risk of infection. The ventilator circuit tubing and in-line suction tubing are replaced periodically, according to infection prevention guidelines, to decrease the risk of infection.

The nurse administers oral hygiene frequently because the oral cavity is a primary source of contamination of the lungs in the patient who is intubated (El-Rabbany, Zaghlol, Bhandari, et al., 2015). The presence of a nasogastric tube in the patient who is intubated can increase the risk of aspiration, leading to nosocomial pneumonia. The nurse positions the patient with the head elevated above the stomach as much as possible. Chart 21-11 provides an overview of strategies to prevent VAP.

PROMOTING OPTIMAL LEVEL OF MOBILITY

Being connected to a ventilator limits the patient's mobility. Immobility in patients who are mechanically ventilated is associated with decreases in muscle strength and increases length of hospital stay, as well as increased mortality rates (Campbell, Fisher, Anderson, et al., 2015). The nurse helps the patient whose condition has become stable to get out of bed and move to a chair as soon as possible. If the patient is unable to get out of bed, the nurse encourages performance of active range-of-motion exercises at least every 6 to 8 hours. If the patient cannot perform these exercises, the nurse performs passive range-of-motion exercises at least every 8 hours to prevent contractures and venous stasis.

PROMOTING OPTIMAL COMMUNICATION

It is important to develop alternative methods of communication for the patient who is receiving mechanical ventilation. The nurse assesses the patient's communication abilities to evaluate for limitations. Questions to consider when assessing

Chart 21-12 — NURSING RESEARCH PROFILE
The Patient Receiving Mechanical Ventilation

Fink, R. M., Makic, M. B. F., Poteet, A. W. et al. (2015). The ventilation patient's experience. *Dimensions of Critical Care Nursing, 34*(5), 301–308.

Purpose

Patients experience a variety of emotions while mechanically ventilated in the intensive care unit. Some patients have little or no recall of events while others have total recall. Limited studies have explored family recall of events or how these recollections correlate with the patient's experience. The purpose of this study was threefold: (1) to explore patient and family memories of pain, anxiety, distress, and dyspnea following mechanical ventilation, (2) to identify if a correlation exists among nurse documented pain assessment and patient-family reports of pain, and, (3) to explore patient and family satisfaction with mechanical ventilation care.

Design

This study was conducted using a mixed methods approach. Qualitative data were collected through individual semistructured interviews with each patient and family member or significant other. Quantitative data were collected from the medical record, and included patient demographics, medications given, and nurses' assessment of pain and sedation. The convenience sample consisted of 85 patients and 77 family members (32% were spouses); the mean ventilation time was 100.2 hours. Quantitative data were analyzed using descriptive statistics and tests of difference and association. Qualitative data were analyzed through qualitative content analysis, which gave rise to categories.

Findings

Findings from quantitative data revealed most patient and family members reported memories of symptom distress. Patients' memories of pain did not correlate with the nurses' assessment of pain; however, family members' memories of patients' pain did correlate. Both patients and family members were satisfied with the care they received. Through qualitative analysis, the researchers uncovered three main categories: pain/discomfort, sedation/sleeping, and communication difficulties. A source of major distress for patients was the lack of effective communication during the period of mechanical ventilation. Trying to talk and lack of a mechanism to communicate needs affected their pain management and sleeping schedule. Patients remembered being in pain.

Nursing Implications

These findings provide insight for nurses caring for patients who require mechanical ventilation and their families. These findings stress the importance of incorporating the input of family members in the plan of care. Moreover, nurses should strive to optimize communication techniques with patients requiring mechanical ventilation. Patients can benefit from frequent reorientation, use of communication boards, and a calming presence. These findings suggest that nurses should treat pain first and implement effective sedation management protocols second, in order to promote optimal patient outcomes and prevent complications.

---

the ability of the patient who is ventilator dependent to communicate include the following:

- Is the patient conscious and able to communicate? Can the patient nod or shake their head?
- Is the patient's mouth unobstructed by the tube so that words can be mouthed?
- Is the patient's dominant hand strong and available for writing? For example, if the patient is right-handed, the intravenous (IV) line should be placed in the left arm if possible so that the right hand is free.
- Is the patient a candidate for a fenestrated tracheostomy tube or a one-way speaking valve (such as Passy-Muir valve® or Olympic Trach-Talk®) that permits talking?

Once the patient's limitations are known, the nurse offers several appropriate communication approaches: lip or speech reading (use single key words), pad and pencil or Magic Slate®, iPad ® or tablet, communication board, gesturing, sign language, or electric larynx. The use of a "talking" or fenestrated tracheostomy tube or one-way valve may be suggested to the primary provider, which would allow the patient to talk while on the ventilator. The nurse makes sure that the patient's eyeglasses, hearing aid, sign interpreter, and language translator are available if needed to enhance the patient's ability to communicate.

Some communication methods may be frustrating to the patient, family, and nurse; these need to be identified and minimized. A speech therapist can assist in determining the most appropriate method.

PROMOTING COPING ABILITY

Dependence on a ventilator is frightening to both the patient and the family and disrupts even the most stable families. Encouraging the family to verbalize their feelings about the ventilator, the patient's condition, and the environment in general is beneficial. Explaining procedures every time they are performed helps reduce anxiety and familiarizes the patient with ventilator procedures. To restore a sense of control, the nurse encourages the patient to use alternative methods of communication in order to participate in decisions about care, schedules, and treatment when possible (see Nursing Research Profile Chart 21-12: The Patient Receiving Mechanical Ventilation). The patient may become withdrawn or depressed while receiving mechanical ventilation, especially if its use is prolonged. To promote effective coping, the nurse informs the patient about progress when appropriate. It is important to provide diversions such as watching television, playing music, or taking a walk (if appropriate and possible). Stress reduction techniques (e.g., a back rub, relaxation measures) relieve tension and help the patient deal with anxieties and fears about both the condition and the dependence on the ventilator.

MONITORING AND MANAGING POTENTIAL COMPLICATIONS

Alterations in Cardiac Function. Alterations in cardiac output may occur as a result of positive-pressure ventilation. The positive intrathoracic pressure during inspiration compresses the heart and great vessels, thereby reducing venous return and cardiac output. This is usually corrected during exhalation when the positive pressure is off. The patient may have decreased cardiac output and resultant decreased tissue perfusion and oxygenation.

To evaluate cardiac function, the nurse first observes for signs and symptoms of hypoxia (restlessness, apprehension, confusion, tachycardia, tachypnea, pallor progressing to cyanosis, diaphoresis, transient hypertension, and decreased urine output). If a pulmonary artery catheter is in place, cardiac output, cardiac index, and other hemodynamic values can be used to assess the patient's status (see Chapter 25).

Barotrauma and Pneumothorax. Excessive positive pressure can cause lung damage, or barotrauma, which may result in a spontaneous pneumothorax, which may quickly develop into a tension pneumothorax, further compromising venous return, cardiac output, and blood pressure (see Chapter 23 for discussion of pneumothorax). The nurse considers any sudden changes in oxygen saturation or the onset of respiratory distress to be a life-threatening emergency requiring immediate action.

Pulmonary Infection. The patient is at high risk for infection, as described earlier. The nurse reports fever or a change in the color or odor of sputum to the primary provider for follow-up. (See Chapter 23 for discussion of pneumonia.) Subglottic secretions may increase the patients' risk for the development of VAP. Patients expected to be intubated for longer than 72 hours may benefit from the use of an endotracheal tube with a subglottic suction port. This extra port that is connected to continuous suction (20 to 30 cm H_2O) allows for the removal of secretions above the cuff (Urden et al., 2014).

Delirium. Patients who are critically ill are at risk for delirium. The Awakening and Breathing Coordination, Delirium monitoring and management, Early mobility bundle (ABCDE) proposes an interdisciplinary process using evidence based practice to manage delirium and weakness in the critically ill patient. The goal of this bundle is to (1) improve communication among members of the health care team, (2) standardize care related to the assessment and use of sedation, (3) provide nonpharmacologic interventions in the management of delirium, and (4) provide early exercise and ambulation (see Chart 21-13) (Balas, Vasilevskis, Burke, et al., 2012).

PROMOTING HOME, COMMUNITY-BASED, AND TRANSITIONAL CARE

Increasingly, patients are being cared for in extended care facilities or at home while receiving mechanical ventilation, with a tracheostomy tube, or receiving oxygen therapy. Patients receiving home ventilator care usually have a chronic neuromuscular condition or COPD. Providing the opportunity for ventilator-dependent patients to return home to live with their families in familiar surroundings can be a positive experience. The ultimate goal of home ventilator therapy is to enhance the patient's quality of life, not simply to support or prolong life.

Educating Patients About Self-Care. Caring for the patient with mechanical ventilator support at home can be accomplished successfully. A home or transitional care team consisting of the nurse, physician, respiratory therapist, social service or home care agency, and equipment supplier is needed. The home is evaluated to determine whether the electrical equipment needed can be operated safely. Chart 21-14 summarizes the basic assessment criteria needed for successful home care.

Once the decision to initiate mechanical ventilation at home is made, the nurse prepares the patient and family for

---

Chart 21-13 The ABCDE Bundle

The *Awakening and Breathing Coordination, Delirium monitoring and management, Early mobility bundle*

Overview: Typically, patients on mechanical ventilators require some form of sedation or analgesia during their hospital stay. Recent studies suggest a correlation between the use of potent sedatives and analgesia and ICU acquired delirium, oversedation, and prolonged mechanical ventilation.

Key components of each of the three categories of the ABCDE Bundle include:

1. *Awakening and spontaneous breathing trials*
   Using predefined criteria:
   - The nurse determines if it is safe to stop sedation.
   - If determined safe, the nurse will determine if patient tolerated the sedation interruption.
   - If the patient tolerated the interruption, the respiratory therapist will determine if the patient is a candidate for a breathing trial.
   - If the patient is a candidate for a breathing trial, the respiratory therapist and nurse will evaluate the patient's response.
2. *Monitoring and management of delirium*
   - The patient will be assessed at least every 2 to 4 hours using a sedation assessment scale (e.g., the CAM-ICU, see Chapter 14).
3. *Early Mobility*
   The patient will be assessed using the following criteria for mobility:
   - The patient is able to respond to verbal stimuli.
   - The patient is receiving less than 60% FiO_2 and less than 10 cm of PEEP.
   - The patient has no circulatory or central catheters or injuries that may contraindicate mobility.

ICU, intensive care unit; PEEP, positive end-expiratory pressure.
Adapted from Balas, M. C., Vasilevskis, E. E., Burke, W. J., et al. (2012). Critical care nurse's role in implementing the "ABCDE Bundle" into practice. *Critical Care Nurse, 32*(2), 35–48.

---

home care. The nurse educates the patient and family about the ventilator, suctioning, tracheostomy care, signs of pulmonary infection, cuff inflation and deflation, and assessment of vital signs. Education begins in the hospital and continues at home. Nursing responsibilities include evaluating the patient's and family's understanding of the information presented.

The nurse educates the family about cardiopulmonary resuscitation, including mouth-to-tracheostomy tube (instead of mouth-to-mouth) breathing. The nurse also explains how to handle a power failure, which usually involves converting the ventilator from an electrical power source to a battery power source. Conversion is automatic in most types of home ventilators and lasts approximately 1 hour. The nurse instructs the family on the use of a manual self-inflation bag should it be necessary. Chart 21-15 lists some of the patient's and family's responsibilities.

Continuing and Transitional Care. A home or transitional care nurse monitors and evaluates how well the patient and family are adapting to providing care in the home. The nurse assesses the adequacy of the patient's ventilation and oxygenation as well as airway patency. The nurse addresses any unique adaptation problems that the patient may have and listens to the patient's and family's anxieties and frustrations, offering support and encouragement where possible.

Chart 21-14 Criteria for Successful Home Ventilator Care

The decision to proceed with home ventilation therapy is usually based on the following parameters.

Patient Criteria

- The patient has a chronic underlying pulmonary or neuromuscular disorder.
- The patient's clinical pulmonary status is stable.
- The patient is willing to go home on mechanical ventilation.

Home Criteria

- The home environment is conducive to care of the patient.
- The electrical facilities are adequate to operate all equipment safely.
- The home environment is controlled, without drafts in cold weather and with proper ventilation in warm weather.
- Space is available for cleaning and storing ventilator equipment.

Family Criteria

- Family members are competent, dependable, and willing to spend the time required for proper training as primary caregivers.
- Family members understand the diagnosis and prognosis.
- Family has sufficient financial and supportive resources and can obtain professional support if necessary.

The nurse helps identify and contact community resources that may assist in home management of the patient with mechanical ventilation.

The technical aspects of the ventilator are managed by vendor follow-up. A respiratory therapist usually is assigned to the patient and makes home visits to evaluate the patient and perform a maintenance check of the ventilator as needed.

Transportation services are identified in case the patient requires transportation in an emergency. These arrangements must be made before an emergency arises.

Evaluation

Expected patient outcomes may include the following:

1. Exhibits adequate gas exchange, as evidenced by normal breath sounds, acceptable arterial blood gas levels, and vital signs
2. Demonstrates adequate ventilation with minimal mucus accumulation
3. Is free of injury or infection, as evidenced by normal temperature, white blood cell count, and clear sputum
4. Is mobile within limits of ability
   a. Gets out of bed to chair, bears weight, or ambulates as soon as possible
   b. Performs range-of-motion exercises every 6 to 8 hours
5. Communicates effectively through written messages, gestures, or other communication strategies
6. Copes effectively
   a. Verbalizes fears and concerns about condition and equipment
   b. Participates in decision making when possible
   c. Uses stress reduction techniques when necessary

Chart 21-15 HOME CARE CHECKLIST
Ventilator Care

At the completion of education, the patient and/or caregiver will be able to:

- Name the procedure that was performed, as indicated, and how the patient's present status impacts physiologic functioning, ADLs, IADLs, relationships, and spirituality.
- State the name, dose, side effects, frequency, and schedule for all medications.
- State what types of changes are needed (if any) to maintain a clean home environment and prevent infection.
- State how to contact the primary provider, the team of home care professionals overseeing care, respiratory vendor and obtain supplies.
- Complete CPR training program for caregivers.
- Identify a plan for operation of ventilator and other devices during a power outage or other emergency.
- State proper care of patient on ventilator:
  - Observe physical signs such as color, secretions, breathing pattern, and state of consciousness.
  - Perform physical care such as suctioning, postural drainage, and ambulation.
  - Observe the tidal volume and pressure manometer regularly. Intervene when they are abnormal (i.e., suction if airway pressure increases).
  - Provide a communication method for the patient (e.g., pad and pencil, electric larynx, talking tracheostomy tube, and sign language).
  - Monitor vital signs as directed.

- Use a predetermined signal to indicate when feeling short of breath or in distress.
- Care for and maintain equipment properly:
  - Check the ventilator settings twice each day and whenever the patient is removed from the ventilator.
  - Adjust the volume and pressure alarms if needed.
  - Fill humidifier as needed and check its level three times a day.
  - Empty water in tubing as needed.
  - Use a clean humidifier when circuitry is changed.
  - Keep exterior of ventilator clean and free of any objects.
  - Change external circuitry once a week or more often as indicated.
  - Report malfunction or strange noises immediately.
- Identify caregiver support resources (e.g., backup caregivers, respite services, and support groups).

Resources

See Chapter 21, Figure 21-3 for additional information on postural drainage positions.

For the procedural guidelines for caring for a patient with a tracheostomy tube and performing tracheal suction, go to **thepoint.lww.com/Brunner14e.**

ADL, activities of daily living; IADL, independent activities of daily living.

7. Absence of complications
   a. Absence of cardiac compromise, as evidenced by stable vital signs and adequate urine output
   b. Absence of pneumothorax, as evidenced by bilateral chest excursion, normal chest x-ray, and adequate oxygenation
   c. Absence of pulmonary infection, as evidenced by normal temperature, clear pulmonary secretions, and negative sputum cultures
   d. Absence of delirium, as evidenced by not "fighting" the ventilator, and being oriented to person, place, and time

Weaning the Patient from the Ventilator

Respiratory weaning, the process of withdrawing the patient from dependence on the ventilator, takes place in three stages: the patient is gradually removed from the ventilator, then from either the endotracheal or tracheostomy tube, and finally from oxygen. Weaning from mechanical ventilation is performed at the earliest possible time consistent with patient safety. The decision must be made from a physiologic rather than a mechanical viewpoint. A thorough understanding of the patient's clinical status is required in making this decision. Weaning is started when the patient is physiologically and hemodynamically stable, demonstrates spontaneous breathing capability, recovering from the acute stage of medical and surgical problems, and when the cause of respiratory failure is sufficiently reversed (Kacmarek et al. 2017). Chart 21-16 presents information about patient care during weaning from mechanical ventilation.

Successful weaning involves collaboration among the primary provider, respiratory therapist, and nurse. Each health care provider must understand the scope and function of other team members in relation to patient weaning to conserve the patient's strength, use resources efficiently, and maximize successful outcomes.

Criteria for Weaning

Careful assessment is required to determine whether the patient is ready to be removed from mechanical ventilation. If the patient is stable and showing signs of improvement or reversal of the disease or condition that caused the need for mechanical ventilation, weaning indices should be assessed (see Chart 21-16).

Stable vital signs and arterial blood gases are also important predictors of successful weaning. Once readiness has been determined, the nurse records baseline measurements of weaning indices to monitor progress.

Patient Preparation

To maximize the chances of success of weaning, the nurse must consider the patient as a whole, taking into account factors that impair the delivery of oxygen and elimination of carbon dioxide as well as those that increase oxygen demand (e.g., sepsis, seizures, and thyroid imbalances) or decrease the patient's overall strength (e.g., inadequate nutrition and neuromuscular disease). Adequate psychological preparation is necessary before and during the weaning process.

Chart 21-16

Care of the Patient Being Weaned from Mechanical Ventilation

1. Assess patient for weaning criteria:
   a. Vital capacity: 10–15 mL/kg
   b. Maximum inspiratory pressure (MIP) at least –20 cm H_2O
   c. Tidal volume: 7–9 mL/kg
   d. Minute ventilation: 6 L/min
   e. Rapid/shallow breathing index: Below 100 breaths/min/L; PaO_2 >60 mm Hg with FiO_2 <40%
2. Monitor activity level, assess dietary intake, and monitor results of laboratory tests of nutritional status. Reestablishing independent spontaneous ventilation can be physically exhausting. It is crucial that the patient have enough energy reserves to succeed.
3. Assess the patient's and family's understanding of the weaning process and address any concerns about the process. Explain that the patient may feel short of breath initially and provide encouragement as needed. Reassure the patient that he or she will be attended closely and that if the weaning attempt is not successful, it can be tried again later.
4. Implement the weaning method as prescribed (e.g., continuous positive airway pressure [CPAP] and T-piece).
5. Monitor vital signs, pulse oximetry, electrocardiogram, and respiratory pattern constantly for the first 20–30 minutes and every 5 minutes after that until weaning is complete. Monitoring the patient closely provides ongoing indications of success or failure.
6. Maintain a patent airway; monitor arterial blood gas levels and pulmonary function tests. Suction the airway as needed.
7. In collaboration with the primary provider, terminate the weaning process if adverse reactions occur. These include a heart rate increase of 20 bpm, systolic blood pressure increase of 20 mm Hg, a decrease in oxygen saturation to <90%, respiratory rate <8 or >20 breaths/min, ventricular dysrhythmias, fatigue, panic, cyanosis, erratic or labored breathing, paradoxical chest movement.
8. If the weaning process continues, measure tidal volume and minute ventilation every 20–30 minutes; compare with the patient's desired values, which have been determined in collaboration with the primary provider.
9. Assess for psychological dependence if the physiologic parameters indicate that weaning is feasible and the patient still resists. Possible causes of psychological dependence include fear of dying and depression from chronic illness. It is important to address this issue before the next weaning attempt.

Adapted from Wiegand, D. J. L. (2011). *AACN Procedure Manual for Critical Care* (6th ed.). St. Louis: Elsevier Saunders.

Methods of Weaning

Successful weaning depends on the combination of adequate patient preparation, available equipment, and an interdisciplinary approach to solve patient problems (see Chart 21-16). All usual modes of ventilation can be used for weaning.

CPAP (also known as spontaneous mode ventilation in this context) allows the patient to breathe spontaneously while applying positive pressure throughout the respiratory cycle to keep the alveoli open and promote oxygenation. Providing CPAP during spontaneous breathing also offers the advantage of an alarm system and may reduce patient anxiety if the patient has been taught that the machine is keeping track of breathing. It also maintains lung volumes and improves the patient's oxygenation status. CPAP is often used in conjunction with PSV. Nurses should carefully assess for tachypnea, tachycardia, reduced tidal volumes, decreasing oxygen saturations, and increasing carbon dioxide levels.

SIMV can also be used as a weaning method. The patient is placed on SIMV mode of ventilation and the rate is slowly decreased by 1 to 3 breaths per minute until the patient is fully breathing on their own (Urden et al., 2014).

Furthermore, T-piece trials can also be used. When the patient can breathe spontaneously, weaning trials using a T-piece for the patient with an endotracheal tube or tracheostomy mask for the patient with a tracheostomy tube (see Fig. 21-2) are normally conducted with the patient disconnected from the ventilator, receiving humidified oxygen only and performing all work of breathing. Because patients do not have to overcome the resistance of the ventilator, they may find this mode more comfortable, or they may become anxious as they breathe with no support from the ventilator. During these trial periods, the nurse monitors the patient closely and provides encouragement. This method of weaning is usually used when the patient is awake and alert, is breathing without difficulty, has good gag and cough reflexes, and is hemodynamically stable. During the weaning process, the patient is maintained on the same or a higher oxygen concentration than when receiving mechanical ventilation. While the patient is using the T-piece or tracheostomy mask, he or she is observed for signs and symptoms of hypoxia, increasing respiratory muscle fatigue, or systemic fatigue. These include restlessness, increased respiratory rate (greater than 35 breaths/min), the use of accessory muscles, tachycardia with premature ventricular contractions, and paradoxical chest movement (asynchronous breathing, chest contraction during inspiration and expansion during expiration). Fatigue or exhaustion is initially manifested by an increased respiratory rate associated with a gradual reduction in tidal volume; later there is a slowing of the respiratory rate.

If the patient appears to be tolerating the T-piece/tracheostomy mask trial, a second set of arterial blood gas measurements is drawn 20 minutes after the patient has been on spontaneous ventilation at a constant FiO_2 PSV. (Alveolar–arterial equilibration takes 15 to 20 minutes to occur.)

Signs of exhaustion and hypoxia correlated with deterioration in the blood gas measurements indicate the need for ventilatory support. The patient is placed back on the ventilator each time signs of fatigue or deterioration develop.

If clinically stable, the patient usually can be extubated within 2 or 3 hours after weaning and allowed spontaneous ventilation by means of a mask with humidified oxygen. Patients who have had prolonged ventilatory assistance usually require more gradual weaning; it may take days or even weeks. They are weaned primarily during the day and placed back on the ventilator at night to rest.

Because patients respond in different manners to weaning methods, there is no definitive way to assess which method is best. Regardless of the weaning method being used, ongoing assessment of respiratory status is essential to monitor patient progress.

Successful weaning from the ventilator is supplemented by intensive pulmonary care. The following methods are used: oxygen therapy; arterial blood gas evaluation; pulse oximetry; bronchodilator therapy; CPT; adequate nutrition, hydration,

and humidification; blood pressure measurement; and incentive spirometry. Daily spontaneous breathing trials may be used to evaluate the patient's ability to breathe without ventilatory support. If the patient is receiving IV sedatives (e.g., propofol and midazolam), current guidelines recommend that the patient's sedative dose be decreased by 25% to 50% prior to weaning, called a *sedation vacation*. In order to decrease agitation in patients who do not tolerate withdrawal of sedation, dexmedetomidine (Precedex) may be initiated for spontaneous breathing trials without causing significant respiratory depression (Gupta, Singh, Sood, et al., 2015). A patient may still have borderline pulmonary function and need vigorous supportive therapy before their respiratory status returns to a level that supports activities of daily living.

Removal of the Tracheostomy Tube

Removal of the tracheostomy tube is considered when the patient can breathe spontaneously; maintain an adequate airway by effectively coughing up secretions, swallow, and move the jaw. Secretion clearance and aspiration risks are assessed to determine whether active pharyngeal and laryngeal reflexes are intact.

Once the patient can clear secretions adequately, a trial period of mouth breathing or nose breathing is conducted. This can be accomplished by several methods. The first method requires changing to a smaller size tube to increase the resistance to airflow or plugging the tracheostomy tube (deflating the cuff first). The smaller tube is sometimes replaced by a cuffless tracheostomy tube, which allows the tube to be plugged at lengthening intervals to monitor patient progress. A second method involves changing to a fenestrated tube (a tube with an opening or window in its bend). This permits air to flow around and through the tube to the upper airway and enables talking. A third method involves switching to a smaller tracheostomy button (stoma button). A tracheostomy button is a plastic tube approximately 1 inch long that helps keep the windpipe open after the larger tracheostomy tube has been removed. Finally, when the patient demonstrates the ability to maintain a patent airway, the tube can be removed. An occlusive dressing is placed over the stoma, which heals in several days to weeks.

Weaning from Oxygen

The patient who has been successfully weaned from the ventilator, cuff, and tube and has adequate respiratory function is then weaned from oxygen. The FiO_2 is gradually reduced until the PaO_2 is in the range of 70 to 100 mm Hg while the patient is breathing room air. If the PaO_2 is less than 70 mm Hg on room air, supplemental oxygen is recommended. To be eligible for financial reimbursement from the Centers for Medicare and Medicaid Services (CMS) for in-home oxygen, the patient must have a PaO_2 at or less than 55 mm Hg while awake and at rest or arterial oxygen saturation at or below 88%, breathing room air (American Association of Respiratory Care, 2007; CMS, 1993).

Nutrition

Success in weaning the patient who is long-term ventilator dependent requires early and aggressive but judicious nutritional support. The respiratory muscles (diaphragm and especially intercostals) become weak or atrophied after just a few days of mechanical ventilation and may be catabolized for energy, especially if nutrition is inadequate. Compensation for inadequate nutrition must be undertaken with care; excessive intake can increase the production of carbon dioxide and the demand for oxygen and lead to prolonged ventilator dependence and difficulty in weaning. Because the metabolism of fat produces less carbon dioxide than the metabolism of carbohydrates, it was long presumed that a high-fat and limited carbohydrate diet would be most therapeutic; however, evidence-based findings do not support its efficacy (McClave, Taylor, Martindale, et al., 2016). Adequate protein intake is important in increasing respiratory muscle strength. Protein intake should be approximately 25% of total daily kilocalories, or 1.2 to 1.5 g/kg/day. Daily nutrition should be closely monitored.

Soon after the patient is admitted, a consultation with a dietitian or nutrition support team should be arranged to plan the best form of nutritional replacement. Adequate nutrition may decrease the duration of mechanical ventilation and prevent other complications, especially sepsis. Sepsis can occur if bacteria enter the bloodstream and release toxins that, in turn, cause vasodilation and hypotension, fever, tachycardia, increased respiratory rate, and coma. Aggressive treatment of sepsis is essential to reverse this threat to survival and to promote weaning from the ventilator when the patient's condition improves.

THE PATIENT UNDERGOING THORACIC SURGERY

Respiratory care modalities are particularly important for the patient undergoing thoracic surgery. Frequently, patients undergoing such surgery have obstructive pulmonary disease or other chronic disease. Careful preoperative preparation, assessment, and postoperative management are crucial for successful patient outcomes because these patients may have a narrow range between their physical tolerance for certain activities and their limitations, which, if exceeded, can lead to distress. Various types of thoracic surgical procedures are performed to relieve disease conditions such as lung abscesses, lung cancer, cysts, benign tumors, and emphysema (see Chart 21-17). An exploratory **thoracotomy** (creation of a surgical opening into the thoracic cavity) may be performed to diagnose lung or chest disease. A biopsy may be performed in this procedure with a small amount of lung tissue removed for analysis; the chest incision is then closed.

The objectives of preoperative assessment and care for the patient undergoing thoracic surgery are to ascertain the patient's functional reserve, to determine whether the patient is likely to survive and recover from the surgery, and to ensure that the patient is in optimal condition for surgery.

Preoperative Management

Assessment and Diagnostic Findings

The nurse performs chest auscultation to assess breath sounds in all regions of the lungs (see Chapter 20). It is important to note whether breath sounds are normal, indicating a free flow of air in and out of the lungs. (In the patient with emphysema, the breath sounds may be markedly decreased or even absent on auscultation.) The nurse notes crackles

and wheezes and assesses for hyperresonance and decreased diaphragmatic motion. Unilateral diminished breath sounds and rhonchi can be the result of occlusion of the bronchi by mucus plugs. The nurse assesses for retained secretions during auscultation by asking the patient to cough. It is important to note any signs of rhonchi or wheezing. The patient history and assessment should include the following questions:

- What signs and symptoms (cough, sputum expectorated [amount and color], hemoptysis, chest pain, dyspnea) are present?
- If there is a smoking history, how long has the patient smoked? Does the patient smoke or use e-cigarettes currently? How many packs or e-cigarettes a day?
- What is the patient's cardiopulmonary tolerance while resting, eating, bathing, and walking?
- What is the patient's breathing pattern? How much exertion is required to produce dyspnea?
- Does the patient need to sleep in an upright position or with more than two pillows?
- What is the patient's general physiologic status (e.g., general appearance, mental alertness, behavior, and nutritional status)?
- What other medical conditions exist (e.g., allergies, cardiac disorders, and diabetes)?

Numerous tests are performed to determine the patient's preoperative status and to assess the patient's physical assets and limitations. Many patients are seen by their surgeons in the office, and many diagnostic tests and examinations are performed on an outpatient basis. The decision to perform any pulmonary resection is based on the patient's cardiovascular status and pulmonary reserve. Pulmonary function studies (especially lung volume and vital capacity) are performed to determine whether the planned resection will leave sufficient functioning lung tissue. Arterial blood gas values are assessed to provide a more complete picture of the functional capacity of the lung. Exercise tolerance tests are useful to determine whether the patient who is a candidate for pneumonectomy can tolerate removal of one of the lungs.

Preoperative studies provide a baseline for comparison during the postoperative period and detect additional abnormalities. Studies may include a bronchoscopic examination (a lighted scope is inserted into the airways to examine the bronchi), chest x-ray, magnetic resonance imaging, electrocardiogram (ECG) (for arteriosclerotic heart disease, conduction defects), nutritional assessment, determination of blood urea nitrogen and serum creatinine levels (to assess renal function), determination of glucose tolerance or blood glucose level (to check for diabetes), serum electrolytes and protein levels, blood volume determinations, and complete blood cell count.

Preoperative Nursing Management

Improving Airway Clearance

The underlying lung condition often is associated with increased respiratory secretions. Before surgery, the airway is cleared of secretions to reduce the possibility of postoperative atelectasis or infection. Chart 21-18 lists the risk factors for postoperative atelectasis and pneumonia. Strategies to reduce the risk of atelectasis and infection include humidification, postural drainage, and chest percussion after

Chart 21-17 Thoracic Surgeries and Procedures

Pneumonectomy

The removal of an entire lung (pneumonectomy) is performed chiefly for cancer when the lesion cannot be removed by a less extensive procedure. It also may be performed for lung abscesses, bronchiectasis, or extensive unilateral tuberculosis. The removal of the right lung is more dangerous than the removal of the left, because the right lung has a larger vascular bed and its removal imposes a greater physiologic burden.

A posterolateral or anterolateral thoracotomy incision is made, sometimes with resection of a rib. The pulmonary artery and the pulmonary veins are ligated and severed. The main bronchus is divided and the lung removed. The bronchial stump is stapled, and usually no drains are used because the accumulation of fluid in the empty hemithorax prevents mediastinal shift.

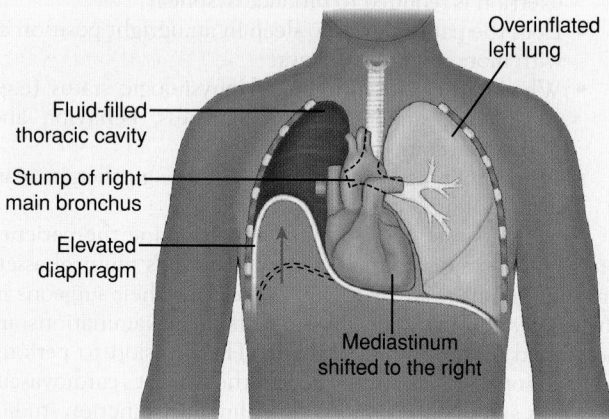

Fluid-filled thoracic cavity
Stump of right main bronchus
Elevated diaphragm
Overinflated left lung
Mediastinum shifted to the right

Pneumonectomy

Lobectomy

When the pathology is limited to one area of a lung, a lobectomy (removal of a lobe of a lung) is performed. Lobectomy, which is more common than pneumonectomy, may be carried out for bronchogenic carcinoma, giant emphysematous blebs or bullae, benign tumors, metastatic malignant tumors, bronchiectasis, and fungal infections.

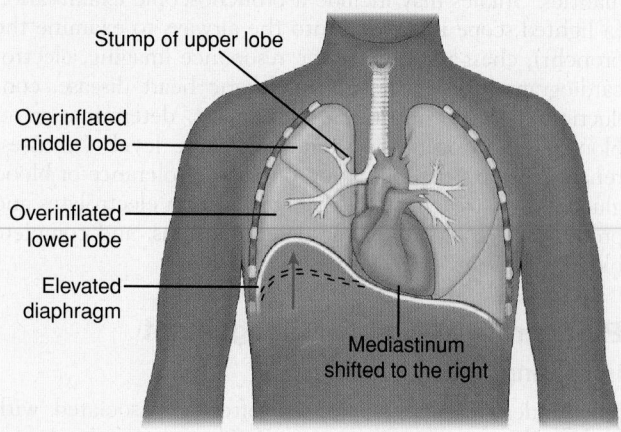

Stump of upper lobe
Overinflated middle lobe
Overinflated lower lobe
Elevated diaphragm
Mediastinum shifted to the right

Lobectomy

The surgeon makes a thoracotomy incision. Its exact location depends on the lobe to be resected. When the pleural space is entered, the involved lung collapses and the lobar vessels and the bronchus are ligated and divided. After the lobe is removed, the remaining lobes of the lung are re-expanded. Usually, two chest catheters are inserted for drainage. The upper tube is for air removal; the lower one is for fluid drainage. Sometimes, only one catheter is needed. The chest tube is connected to a chest drainage apparatus for several days.

Segmentectomy (Segmental Resection)

Some lesions are located in only one segment of the lung. Bronchopulmonary segments are subdivisions of the lung that function as individual units. They are held together by delicate connective tissue. Disease processes may be limited to a single segment. Care is used to preserve as much healthy and functional lung tissue as possible, especially in patients who already have limited cardiopulmonary reserve. Single segments can be removed from any lobe; the right middle lobe, which has only two small segments, invariably is removed entirely. On the left side, corresponding to a middle lobe, is a "lingular" segment of the upper lobe. This can be removed as a single segment or by lingulectomy. This segment frequently is involved in bronchiectasis.

Wedge Resection

A wedge resection of a small, well-circumscribed lesion may be performed without regard to the location of the intersegmental planes. The pleural cavity usually is drained because of the possibility of an air or blood leak. This procedure is performed for diagnostic lung biopsy and for the excision of small peripheral nodules.

Bronchoplastic or Sleeve Resection

Bronchoplastic resection is a procedure in which only one lobar bronchus, together with a part of the right or left bronchus, is excised. The distal bronchus is reanastomosed to the proximal bronchus or trachea.

Lung Volume Reduction

Lung volume reduction is a surgical procedure involving the removal of 20–30% of a patient's lung through a midsternal incision or video thoracoscopy. The diseased lung tissue is identified on a lung perfusion scan. This surgery leads to significant improvements in dyspnea, exercise capacity, quality of life, and survival of a subgroup of people with end-stage emphysema.

Video Thoracoscopy

A video thoracoscopy is an endoscopic procedure that allows the surgeon to look into the thorax without making a large incision. The procedure is performed to obtain specimens of tissue for biopsy, to treat recurrent spontaneous pneumothorax, and to diagnose either pleural effusions or pleural masses. Thoracoscopy has also been found to be an effective diagnostic and therapeutic alternative for the treatment of mediastinal disorders. Some advantages of video thoracoscopy are rapid diagnosis and treatment of some conditions, a decrease in postoperative complications, and a shortened hospital stay.

Adapted from Urden, L. D., Stacy, K. M., & Lough, M. E. (2014). *Critical care nursing: Diagnosis and management* (7th ed.). St. Louis: Elsevier Mosby.

bronchodilators are given, if prescribed. The nurse estimates the volume of sputum if the patient expectorates large amounts of secretions. Such measurements are carried out to determine whether and when the amount decreases. Antibiotics are given as prescribed for infection, which can cause excessive secretions.

 Educating the Patient

Increasingly, patients are admitted on the day of surgery, which does not provide much time for preoperative assessment or education. Nurses in all settings must take an active role in educating the patient and relieving anxiety. The nurse informs the patient about what to expect, from administration of anesthesia to thoracotomy and the likely use of chest tubes and a drainage system in the postoperative period. The patient is also informed about the usual postoperative administration of oxygen to facilitate breathing and the possible use of a ventilator. It is essential to explain the importance of frequent turning to promote drainage of lung secretions. Instruction in the use of incentive spirometry begins before surgery to familiarize the patient with its correct use. The nurse educates the patient on the use of diaphragmatic and pursed-lip breathing, and the patient should begin practicing these techniques (see Charts 21-3 and 21-4).

Because a coughing schedule is necessary in the postoperative period to promote the clearance or removal of secretions, the nurse instructs the patient in the technique of coughing and warns the patient that the coughing routine may be uncomfortable. The nurse educates the patient about how to splint the incision with the hands, a pillow, or a folded towel (see Chart 21-5).

Encouraging the use of forced expiratory technique (FET) may be helpful for the patient with diminished expiratory flow rates or for the patient who refuses to cough because of severe pain. FET is the expulsion of air through an open glottis. This technique stimulates pulmonary expansion and assists in alveolar inflation (Kacmarek et al., 2017). The nurse instructs the patient as follows:

- Take a deep diaphragmatic breath and exhale forcefully against the hand in a quick, distinct pant, or huff.
- Practice doing small huffs and progress to one strong huff during exhalation.

Patients should be informed preoperatively that blood and other fluids may be given, oxygen will be given, and vital signs will be checked often for several hours after surgery. If a chest tube is needed, the patient should be informed that it will drain the fluid and air that normally accumulate after chest surgery. The patient and family are informed that the patient may be admitted to the ICU for 1 to 2 days after surgery, that the patient may experience pain at the incision site, and that medication is available to relieve pain and discomfort.

Relieving Anxiety

The nurse listens to the patient to evaluate their feelings about the illness and proposed treatment. The nurse also determines the patient's motivation to return to normal or baseline function. The patient may reveal significant concerns: fear of hemorrhage because of bloody sputum, fear of discomfort from a chronic cough and chest pain, fear of ventilator dependence, or fear of death because of dyspnea and the underlying disease (e.g., tumor).

The nurse helps the patient to address fears and to cope with the stress of surgery by correcting any misconceptions, supporting the patient's decision to undergo surgery, reassuring the patient that the incision will "hold," and dealing honestly with questions about pain and discomfort and the patient's treatment. The management and control of pain begin before surgery, when the nurse informs the patient that many postoperative problems can be overcome by following certain routines related to deep breathing, coughing, turning, and moving. Nonopioid preemptive analgesic agents (e.g., acetaminophen and nonsteroidal anti-inflammatory drugs [NSAIDs]) may also be prescribed to help decrease the dose of postoperative opioid agents. This also helps to facilitate deep-breathing techniques and return to normal respiratory function. If patient-controlled analgesia (PCA) or patient-controlled epidural analgesia (PCEA) is to be used after surgery, the nurse instructs the patient in its use.

 Postoperative Management

After surgery, the vital signs are checked frequently. Oxygen is given by a mechanical ventilator, nasal cannula, or mask for as long as necessary. A reduction in lung capacity requires a period of physiologic adjustment, and fluids may be given at a low hourly rate to prevent fluid overload and pulmonary edema. After the patient is conscious and the vital signs have stabilized, the head of the bed may be elevated 30° to 45°. Careful positioning of the patient is important. After pneumonectomy, a patient is usually turned every hour from the back to the operative side and should not be completely

TABLE 21-3 Comparison of Chest Drainage Systems[a]

Types of Chest Drainage Systems	Description	Comments
Traditional Water Seal		
Also referred to as wet suction	Has three chambers: a collection chamber, water seal chamber (middle chamber), and wet suction control chamber	Requires that sterile fluid be instilled into water seal and suction chambers Has positive- and negative-pressure release valves Intermittent bubbling indicates that the system is functioning properly. Additional suction can be added by connecting system to a suction source.
Dry Suction Water Seal		
Also referred to as dry suction	Has three chambers: a collection chamber, water seal chamber (middle chamber), and suction regulator dial	Requires that sterile fluid be instilled in water seal chamber at 2-cm level No fluid-filled suction chamber Suction pressure is set with a suction regulator dial Has positive- and negative-pressure release valves Has an indicator to signify that the suction pressure is adequate Quieter than traditional water seal systems
Dry Suction		
Also referred to as one-way valve system	Has a one-way mechanical valve that allows air to leave the chest and prevents air from moving back into the chest	No need to fill suction chamber with fluid; thus, can be set up quickly in an emergency Works even if knocked over, making it ideal for patients who are ambulatory

[a]If no fluid drainage is expected, a drainage collection device may not be needed.

turned to the unoperated side. This allows the fluid left in the space to consolidate and prevents the remaining lung and the heart from shifting (mediastinal shift) toward the operative side. The patient with a lobectomy may be turned to either side, and a patient with a segmental resection usually is not turned onto the operative side unless the surgeon prescribes this position.

Medication for pain is needed for several days after surgery; it is usually a combination of epidural analgesia, PCA, and scheduled or as-needed oral analgesics. Because coughing can be painful, the patient should be encouraged to splint the chest as taught in the preoperative period. Exercises are resumed early in the postoperative period to facilitate lung ventilation. The nurse assesses for signs of complications, including cyanosis, dyspnea, and acute chest pain. These may indicate atelectasis and should be reported immediately. Increased temperature or white blood cell count may indicate an infection, and pallor and increased pulse may indicate internal hemorrhage. Dressings are assessed for fresh bleeding.

Mechanical Ventilation

Depending on the nature of the surgery, the patient's underlying condition, the intraoperative course, and the depth of anesthesia, the patient may require mechanical ventilation after surgery. The primary provider is responsible for determining and ordering the ventilator settings and modes, as well as determining the overall method and pace of weaning. It is important to assess the patient's tolerance and weaning progress. Early extubation from mechanical ventilation can lead to earlier removal of arterial lines.

Chest Drainage

A crucial intervention for improving gas exchange and breathing in the postoperative period is the proper management of chest drainage and the chest drainage system. After thoracic surgery, chest tubes and a closed drainage system are used to re-expand the involved lung and to remove excess air,

fluid, and blood. Chest drainage systems also are used in the treatment of spontaneous pneumothorax and trauma resulting in pneumothorax. Table 21-3 describes and compares the main features of these systems.

For the procedural guidelines for setting up and managing chest drainage systems, go to **thepoint.lww.com/Brunner14e.**

Chart 21-19 discusses actions that may prevent cardiopulmonary complications after thoracic surgery.

The normal breathing mechanism operates on the principle of negative pressure. The pressure in the chest cavity normally is lower than the pressure of the atmosphere, causing air to move into the lungs during inspiration. Whenever the chest is opened, there is a loss of negative pressure, which results in collapse of the lung. The collection of air, fluid, or other substances in the chest can compromise cardiopulmonary function and can also cause the lung to collapse. Pathologic substances that collect in the pleural space include fibrin or clotted blood, liquids (serous fluids, blood, pus, chyle), and gases (air from the lung, tracheobronchial tree, or esophagus).

Chest tubes may be inserted to drain fluid or air from any of the three compartments of the thorax (the right and left pleural spaces and the mediastinum). The pleural space, located between the visceral and parietal pleura, normally contains 20 mL or less of fluid, which helps lubricate the visceral and parietal pleura (Grossman & Porth, 2014). Surgical incision of the chest wall almost always causes some degree of **pneumothorax** (air accumulating in the pleural space) or hemothorax (buildup of serous fluid or blood in the pleural space). Air and fluid collect in the pleural space, restricting lung expansion and reducing gas exchange. Placement of a chest tube in the pleural space restores the negative intrathoracic pressure needed for lung re-expansion after surgery or trauma.

Preventing Postoperative Cardiopulmonary Complications After Thoracic Surgery

Patient Management

- Auscultate lung sounds and assess for rate, rhythm, and depth.
- Monitor oxygenation with pulse oximetry.
- Monitor electrocardiogram for rate and rhythm changes.
- Assess capillary refill, skin color, and status of the surgical dressing.
- Encourage and assist the patient to turn, cough, and take deep breaths.

Chest Drainage Management

- Verify that all connection tubes are patent and connected securely.
- Assess that the water seal is intact when using a wet suction system, and assess the regulator dial and water seal chamber in dry suction systems.
- Monitor characteristics of drainage, including color, amount, and consistency. Assess for significant increases or decreases in drainage output.
- Note fluctuations in the water seal chamber for wet suction systems and the air leak indicator in dry suction systems.
- Keep system below the patient's chest level.
- Assess suction control chamber for bubbling in wet suction systems.
- Keep suction at prescribed level.
- Maintain appropriate fluid in water seal in wet suction systems.
- Keep air vent open when suction is off.

The mediastinal space is an extrapleural space that lies between the right and left thoracic cavities and contains the large blood vessels, heart, mainstem bronchus, and thymus gland. If fluid accumulates here, the heart can become compressed and stop beating, causing death. Mediastinal chest tubes can be inserted either anteriorly or posteriorly to the heart to drain blood after surgery.

There are two types of chest tubes: small-bore and large-bore catheters. Small-bore catheters (7 Fr to 12 Fr) have a one-way valve apparatus to prevent air from moving back into the chest. They can be inserted through a small skin incision. Large-bore catheters, which range in size up to 40 Fr, are usually connected to a chest drainage system to collect any pleural fluid and monitor for air leaks. After the chest tube is positioned, it is sutured to the skin and connected to a drainage apparatus to remove the residual air and fluid from the pleural or mediastinal space. This results in the re-expansion of remaining lung tissue.

Chest Drainage Systems

Chest drainage systems have a suction source, a collection chamber for pleural drainage, and a mechanism to prevent air from reentering the chest with inhalation (see Fig. 21-10). Various types of **chest drainage systems** are available for use in the removal of air and fluid from the pleural space and re-expansion of the lungs. Chest drainage systems come with either wet (water seal) or dry suction control. In wet suction systems, the amount of suction is determined by the amount of water instilled in the suction chamber. The amount of bubbling in the suction chamber indicates the strength of the

Figure 21-10 • Chest drainage systems. **A.** The Atrium Ocean is an example of a water seal chest drain system composed of a drainage chamber and water seal chamber. The suction control is determined by the height of the water column in that chamber (usually 20 cm). *A,* suction control chamber; *B,* water seal chamber; *C,* air leak zone; *D,* collection chamber. **B.** The Atrium Oasis is an example of a dry suction water seal system that uses a mechanical regulator for vacuum control, a water seal chamber, and a drainage chamber. *A,* dry suction regulator; *B,* water seal chamber; *C,* air leak monitor; *D,* collection chamber; *E,* suction monitor bellows. Photos used with permission from Atrium Medical Corporation, Hudson, NH.

suction. Wet systems use a water seal to prevent air from moving back into the chest on inspiration. Dry systems use a one-way valve and may have a suction control dial in place of the water. Both systems can operate by gravity drainage, without a suction source.

Quality and Safety Nursing Alert

When the wall vacuum is turned off, the drainage system must be open to the atmosphere so that intrapleural air can escape from the system. This can be done by detaching the tubing from the suction port to provide a vent.

Water Seal Systems

The traditional water seal system (or wet suction) for chest drainage has three chambers: a collection chamber, a water seal chamber, and a wet suction control chamber. The collection chamber acts as a reservoir for fluid draining from the chest tube. It is graduated to permit easy measurement of drainage. Suction may be added to create negative pressure and promote drainage of fluid and removal of air. The suction control chamber regulates the amount of negative pressure applied to the chest. The amount of suction is determined by the water level. It is usually set at 20 cm H_2O; adding more fluid results in more suction. After the suction is turned on, bubbling appears in the suction chamber. A positive-pressure valve is located at the top of the suction chamber that automatically opens with increases in positive pressure within the system. Air is automatically released through a positive-pressure relief valve if the suction tubing is inadvertently clamped or kinked.

The water seal chamber has a one-way valve or water seal that prevents air from moving back into the chest when the patient inhales. There is an increase in the water level with inspiration and a return to the baseline level during exhalation; this is referred to as tidaling. Intermittent bubbling in the water seal chamber is normal, but continuous bubbling can indicate an air leak. Bubbling and tidaling do not occur when the tube is placed in the mediastinal space; however, fluid may pulsate with the patient's heartbeat. If the chest tube is connected to gravity drainage only, suction is not used. The pressure is equal to the water seal only. Two-chamber chest drainage systems (water seal chamber and collection chamber) are available for use with patients who need only gravity drainage.

The water level in the water seal chamber reflects the negative pressure present in the intrathoracic cavity. A rise in the water level indicates negative pressure in the pleural or mediastinal space. Excessive negative pressure can cause trauma to tissue. Most chest drainage systems have an automatic means to prevent excessive negative pressure. By pressing and holding a manual high-negativity vent (usually located on the top of the chest drainage system) until the water level in the water seal chamber returns to the 2-cm mark, excessive negative pressure is avoided, preventing damage to tissue.

> ▶ **Quality and Safety Nursing Alert**
>
> *If the chest tube and drainage system become disconnected, air can enter the pleural space, producing a pneumothorax. To prevent pneumothorax if the chest tube is inadvertently disconnected from the drainage system, a temporary water seal can be established by immersing the chest tube's open end in a bottle of sterile water.*

Dry Suction Water Seal Systems

Dry suction water seal systems, also referred to as dry suction, have a collection chamber for drainage, a water seal chamber, and a dry suction control regulator. The water seal chamber is filled with water to the 2-cm level. Bubbling in this area can indicate an air leak. The dry suction control regulator provides a dial that conveniently regulates vacuum to the chest drain. The system does not contain a suction control chamber

filled with water. Without a water-filled suction chamber, the machine is quieter. However, if the container is knocked over, the water seal may be lost.

Once the tube is connected to the suction source, the regulator dial allows the desired level of suction to be set; the suction is increased until an indicator appears. The indicator has the same function as the bubbling in the traditional water seal system—that is, it indicates that the vacuum is adequate to maintain the desired level of suction. Some drainage systems use a bellows (a chamber that can be expanded or contracted) or an orange-colored float device as an indicator of when the suction control regulator is set.

When the water in the water seal rises above the 2-cm level, intrathoracic pressure increases. Dry suction water seal systems have a manual high-negativity vent located on top of the drain. The manual high-negativity vent is pressed until the indicator appears (either a float device or bellows) and the water level in the water seal returns to the desired level, indicating that the intrathoracic pressure is decreased.

> ▶ **Quality and Safety Nursing Alert**
>
> *The manual vent should not be used to lower the water level in the water seal when the patient is on gravity drainage (no suction) because intrathoracic pressure is equal to the pressure in the water seal.*

Dry Suction Systems With a One-Way Valve

A third type of chest drainage system is dry suction with a one-way mechanical valve. This system has a collection chamber, a one-way mechanical valve, and a dry suction control chamber. The valve permits air and fluid to leave the chest but prevents their movement back into the pleural space. This model lacks a water seal chamber and therefore can be set up quickly in emergency situations, and the dry control drain still works even if it is knocked over. This makes the dry suction systems useful for the patient who is ambulating or being transported. However, without the water seal chamber, there is no way to tell by inspection whether the pressure in the chest has changed, even though an air leak indicator is present so that the system can be checked. If an air leak is suspected, 30 mL of water is injected into the air leak indicator or the container is tipped so that fluid enters the air leak detection chamber. Bubbles will appear if a leak is present.

If the chest tube has been inserted to re-expand a lung after pneumothorax, or if very little fluid drainage is expected, a one-way valve (Heimlich valve) may be connected to the chest tube. This valve may be attached to a collection bag (see Fig. 21-11) or covered with a sterile dressing if no drainage is expected.

Postoperative Nursing Management

Postoperative nursing care of the patient who has undergone thoracic surgery involves close monitoring of the patient's respiratory and cardiovascular status, as well as interventions to prevent complications. The psychological reactions that occur in response to this major surgical procedure and the fears that it often engenders in patients and their families are also addressed. For a detailed plan of

Figure 21-11 • One-way (Heimlich) valve, a disposable, single-use chest drainage system with 30-mL collection volume. Used when minimal volume of chest drainage is expected.

Chest tube

One-way seal valve

Air leak well

Stepped connector

Stepped connector with tube

30-mL collection chamber

Needleless luer port

nursing care for the patient who has had a thoracotomy (see Chart 21-20).

Monitoring Respiratory and Cardiovascular Status

The nurse monitors the heart rate and rhythm by auscultation and ECG because episodes of major dysrhythmias are common after thoracic and cardiac surgery. In the immediate postoperative period, an arterial line may be maintained to allow frequent monitoring of arterial blood gases, serum electrolytes, hemoglobin and hematocrit values, and arterial pressure. Central venous pressure may be monitored to detect early signs of fluid volume disturbances; however, central venous pressure monitoring devices are being used less than in the past. Early extubation from mechanical ventilation can also lead to earlier removal of arterial lines (Urden et al., 2014). Another important component of postoperative assessment is to note the results of the preoperative evaluation of the patient's lung reserve by pulmonary function testing. A preoperative FEV_1 (the volume of air that the patient can forcibly exhale in 1 second) of more than 2 L or more than 70% of predicted value indicates a good lung reserve. Patients who have a postoperative FEV_1 of less than 40% of predicted value have decreased tidal volume, which places them at risk for respiratory failure, other morbidity, and death.

Improving Gas Exchange and Breathing

Gas exchange is determined by evaluating oxygenation and ventilation. In the immediate postoperative period, this is achieved by measuring vital signs (blood pressure, pulse, and respirations) at least every 15 minutes for the first 1 to 2 hours and then less frequently as the patient's condition stabilizes.

Pulse oximetry is used for continuous monitoring of the adequacy of oxygenation. Arterial blood gas measurements are obtained early in the postoperative period to establish a baseline to assess the adequacy of oxygenation and ventilation and the possible retention of carbon dioxide. The frequency with which postoperative arterial blood gases are measured depends on whether the patient is mechanically ventilated and whether he or she exhibits signs of respiratory distress; these measurements can help determine appropriate therapy. It also is common practice for patients to have an arterial line in place to obtain blood for blood gas measurements and to monitor blood pressure closely. Hemodynamic monitoring may be used to assess hemodynamic stability (Urden et al., 2014).

Breathing techniques, such as diaphragmatic and pursed-lip breathing, taught prior to surgery should be performed by the patient every 2 hours to expand the alveoli and prevent atelectasis. Sustained maximal inspiration therapy or incentive spirometry promotes lung inflation, improves the cough mechanism, and allows early assessment of acute pulmonary changes. See Charts 21-3 and 21-4 for more information.

If the patient is oriented and blood pressure is stabilized, the head of the bed is elevated 30° to 40° during the immediate postoperative period. This position facilitates ventilation, promotes chest drainage from the lower chest tube, and helps residual air to rise in the upper portion of the pleural space, where it can be removed through the upper chest tube.

The nurse consults with the surgeon about patient positioning to determine the best side-lying position. In general, the patient should be repositioned from back to side frequently and moved from a flat to a semi-upright position as soon as tolerated. Most commonly, the patient is instructed to lie on the operative side. However, the patient with unilateral lung pathology may not be able to turn well onto that side because of pain. In addition, positioning the patient with the "good lung" (the nonoperated lung) down allows a better match of ventilation and perfusion and therefore may actually improve oxygenation. The patient's position is changed from flat to semi-upright as soon as possible because remaining in one position tends to promote the retention of secretions in the dependent portion of the lungs, and the upright position increases diaphragmatic excursion, enhancing lung expansion. After a pneumonectomy, the operated side should be dependent so that fluid in the pleural space remains below the level of the bronchial stump and the other lung can fully expand.

Improving Airway Clearance

Retained secretions are a threat to the patient after thoracotomy surgery. Trauma to the tracheobronchial tree during surgery, diminished lung ventilation, and diminished cough reflex all result in the accumulation of excessive secretions. If the secretions are retained, airway obstruction occurs. This, in turn, causes the air in the alveoli distal to the obstruction to become absorbed and the affected portion of the lung to collapse. Atelectasis, pneumonia, and respiratory failure may result.

To maintain a patent airway, secretions are suctioned from the tracheobronchial tree before the endotracheal tube is discontinued. Secretions continue to be removed by suctioning until the patient can cough up secretions effectively.

(*text continued on page 546*)

Chart 21-20 — PLAN OF NURSING CARE
Care of the Patient After Thoracotomy

NURSING DIAGNOSIS: Impaired gas exchange related to lung impairment and surgery
GOAL: Improvement of gas exchange and breathing

Nursing Interventions	Rationale	Expected Outcomes

1. Monitor pulmonary status as directed and as needed.
  a. Auscultate breath sounds.
  b. Check rate, depth, and pattern of respirations.
  c. Assess blood gases for signs of hypoxemia or CO_2 retention.
  d. Evaluate patient's color for cyanosis.
	1. Changes in pulmonary status indicate improvement or onset of complications.	• Lungs are clear on auscultation.
		• Respiratory rate is within acceptable range with no episodes of dyspnea.
		• Vital signs are stable.
		• Dysrhythmias are not present or are treated effectively.
		• Demonstrates deep, controlled, effective breathing to allow maximal lung expansion
		• Uses incentive spirometer every 2 hours while awake
		• Demonstrates deep, effective coughing technique
		• Lungs are expanded to capacity (evidenced by chest x-ray).

2. Monitor and record blood pressure, apical pulse, and temperature every 2–4 hours, and central venous pressure (if indicated) every 2 hours.	2. Vital signs aid in evaluating effect of surgery on cardiac status.	
3. Monitor continuous electrocardiogram for pattern and dysrhythmias.	3. Dysrhythmias (especially atrial fibrillation and atrial flutter) are more frequently seen after thoracic surgery. A patient with total pneumonectomy is especially prone to cardiac irregularity.	
4. Elevate head of bed 30° to 40° when patient is oriented and hemodynamic status is stable.	4. Maximum lung excursion is achieved when patient is as close to upright as possible.	
5. Encourage deep-breathing exercises (see Breathing Retraining section) and effective use of incentive spirometer (sustained maximal inspiration).	5. Helps to achieve maximal lung inflation and to open closed airways	
6. Encourage and promote an effective cough routine to be performed every hour during first 24 hours.	6. Coughing is necessary to remove retained secretions.	

7. Assess and monitor the chest drainage system.[a]
  a. Assess for leaks and patency as needed (see procedural guidelines for setting up and managing chest drainage systems at thepoint.lww.com/Brunner14e).
  b. Monitor amount and character of drainage and document every 2 hours. Notify primary provider if drainage is ≥150 mL per hour.
	7. System is used to eliminate any residual air or fluid after thoracotomy.	

NURSING DIAGNOSIS: Ineffective airway clearance related to lung impairment, anesthesia, and pain
GOAL: Improvement of airway clearance and achievement of a patent airway

Nursing Interventions	Rationale	Expected Outcomes
1. Maintain an open airway.	1. Provides for adequate ventilation and gas exchange	• Airway is patent. • Coughs effectively • Splints incision while coughing • Sputum is clear or colorless. • Lungs are clear on auscultation.
2. Perform endotracheal suctioning until patient can cough effectively.	2. Endotracheal secretions are present in excessive amounts in postthoracotomy patients due to trauma to the tracheobronchial tree during surgery, diminished lung ventilation, and cough reflex.	
3. Assess and medicate for pain. Encourage deep-breathing and coughing exercises. Help splint incision during coughing.	3. Helps to achieve maximal lung inflation and to open closed airways. Coughing is painful; incision needs to be supported.	
4. Monitor amount, viscosity, color, and odor of sputum. Notify primary provider if sputum is excessive or contains bright-red blood.	4. Changes in sputum suggest presence of infection or change in pulmonary status. Colorless sputum is not unusual; opacification or coloring of sputum may indicate dehydration or infection.	

Chart 21-20

PLAN OF NURSING CARE (Continued)

Care of the Patient After Thoracotomy

Nursing Interventions	Rationale	Expected Outcomes
5. Administer humidification and small-volume nebulizer therapy as prescribed.	5. Secretions must be moistened and thinned if they are to be raised from the chest with the least amount of effort.	
6. Perform postural drainage, percussion, and vibration as prescribed. Do not percuss or vibrate directly over operative site.	6. Chest physiotherapy uses gravity to help remove secretions from the lung.	
7. Auscultate both sides of chest to determine changes in breath sounds.	7. Indications for tracheal suctioning are determined by chest auscultation.	

NURSING DIAGNOSIS: Acute pain related to incision, drainage tubes, and the surgical procedure
GOAL: Relief of pain and discomfort

Nursing Interventions	Rationale	Expected Outcomes
1. Evaluate location, character, quality, and severity of pain. Administer analgesic medication as prescribed and as needed. Observe for respiratory effect of opioid. Note if patient seems too somnolent to cough or if respirations are depressed.	1. Pain limits chest excursions and thereby decreases ventilation.	• Asks for pain medication but verbalizes that he or she expects some discomfort while deep breathing and coughing • Verbalizes that he or she is comfortable and not in acute distress • No signs of incisional infection evident
2. Maintain care postoperatively in positioning the patient. a. Place patient in semi-Fowler position. b. Patients with limited respiratory reserve may not be able to turn on unoperated side. c. Assist or turn patient every 2 hours.	2. The patient who is comfortable and free of pain will be less likely to splint the chest while breathing. A semi-Fowler position permits residual air in the pleural space to rise to upper portion of pleural space and be removed via the upper chest catheter.	
3. Assess incision area every 8 hours for redness, heat, induration, swelling, separation, and drainage.	3. These signs indicate possible infection.	
4. Request order for patient-controlled analgesia pump if appropriate for patient.	4. Allowing patient control over frequency and dose improves comfort and adherence with treatment regimen.	

NURSING DIAGNOSIS: Anxiety related to outcomes of surgery, pain, technology
GOAL: Reduction of anxiety to a manageable level

Nursing Interventions	Rationale	Expected Outcomes
1. Explain all procedures in understandable language.	1. Explaining what can be expected in understandable terms decreases anxiety and increases cooperation.	• States that anxiety is at a manageable level • Participates with health care team in treatment regimen • Uses appropriate coping skills (verbalization; pain relief strategies; the use of support systems such as family, clergy) • Demonstrates basic understanding of technology used in care
2. Assess for pain and medicate, especially before potentially painful procedures.	2. Premedication before painful procedures or activities improves comfort and minimizes undue anxiety.	
3. Silence all *unnecessary* alarms on technology (monitors, ventilators).	3. *Unnecessary* alarms increase the risk of sensory overload and may increase anxiety. *Essential* alarms must be turned on at all times.	
4. Encourage and support patient while increasing activity level.	4. Positive reinforcement improves patient motivation and independence.	
5. Mobilize resources (family, clergy, social worker) to help patient cope with outcomes of surgery (diagnosis, change in functional abilities).	5. A multidisciplinary approach promotes the patient's strengths and coping mechanisms.	

(continued on page 546)

Chart 21-20

PLAN OF NURSING CARE (Continued)

Care of the Patient After Thoracotomy

NURSING DIAGNOSIS: Impaired physical mobility of the upper extremities related to thoracic surgery
GOAL: Increased mobility of the affected shoulder and arm

Nursing Interventions	Rationale	Expected Outcomes

1. Assist patient with normal range of motion and function of shoulder and trunk.
  a. Educate about use of breathing exercises to mobilize thorax.
  b. Encourage skeletal exercises to promote abduction and mobilization of shoulder (see Chart 21-21).
  c. Assist out of bed to chair as soon as pulmonary and circulatory systems are stable (usually by evening of surgery).
2. Encourage progressive activities according to level of fatigue.
	1. Necessary to regain normal mobility of arm and shoulder and to speed recovery and minimize discomfort
	
	2. Increases patient's use of affected shoulder and arm
		• Demonstrates arm and shoulder exercises and verbalizes intent to perform them on discharge
		• Regains previous range of motion in shoulder and arm

NURSING DIAGNOSIS: Risk for imbalanced fluid volume related to the surgical procedure
GOAL: Maintenance of adequate fluid volume

Nursing Interventions	Rationale	Expected Outcomes
• Monitor and record hourly intake and output. Urine output should be at least 0.5 mL/kg/hr after surgery. • Administer blood component therapy and parenteral fluids and/or diuretics as prescribed to restore and maintain fluid volume.	1. Fluid management may be altered before, during, and after surgery, and patient's response to and need for fluid management must be assessed. 2. Pulmonary edema due to transfusion or fluid overload is an ever-present threat; after pneumonectomy, the pulmonary vascular system has been greatly reduced.	• Patient is adequately hydrated, as evidenced by: • Urine output >0.5 mL/kg/hr • Vital signs stable, heart rate, and central venous pressure approaching normal • No excessive peripheral edema

NURSING DIAGNOSIS: Deficient knowledge of home care procedures
GOAL: Increased ability to carry out care procedures at home

Nursing Interventions	Rationale	Expected Outcomes
1. Encourage patient to practice arm and shoulder exercises 5 times daily at home. 2. Instruct patient to practice assuming a functionally erect position in front of a full-length mirror. 3. Instruct patient about home care (see Chart 21-22).	1. Exercise accelerates recovery of muscle function and reduces long-term pain and discomfort. 2. Practice will help restore normal posture. 3. Knowing what to expect facilitates recovery.	• Demonstrates arm and shoulder exercises • Verbalizes need to try to assume an erect posture • Verbalizes the importance of relieving discomfort, alternating walking and rest, performing breathing exercises, avoiding heavy lifting, avoiding undue fatigue, avoiding bronchial irritants, preventing colds or lung infections, getting influenza vaccine, keeping follow-up visits, and stopping smoking

[a] A patient with a pneumonectomy usually does not have water seal chest drainage because it is desirable that the pleural space fill with an effusion, which eventually obliterates this space. Some surgeons do use a modified water seal system.

Nasotracheal suctioning may be needed to stimulate a deep cough and aspirate secretions that the patient cannot clear by coughing. However, it should be used only after other methods to raise secretions have been unsuccessful.

For the procedural guidelines for nasotracheal suctioning, go to **thepoint.lww.com/ Brunner14e.**

The patient is encouraged to cough effectively to maintain a patent airway; ineffective coughing results in exhaustion and retention of secretions (see Chart 21-5). To be effective, the cough must be low-pitched, deep, and controlled. Because it is difficult to cough in a supine position, the patient is helped to a sitting position on the edge of the bed, with the feet resting on a chair. The patient should cough at least every hour during the first 24 hours and when necessary thereafter. If audible crackles are present, it may be necessary to use chest percussion

A. Nurse's hands should support the chest incision anteriorly and posteriorly. The patient is instructed to take several deep breaths, inhale, and then cough forcibly.

B. With one hand, the nurse exerts downward pressure on the soulder of the affected side while firmly supporting the area beneath the wound. The patient is instructed to take several deep breaths, inhale, and then cough forcibly.

C. The nurse can wrap a towel or sheet around the patient's chest and hold the ends together, pulling slightly as the patient coughs, and releasing during deep breaths.

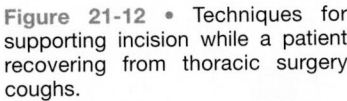

Figure 21-12 • Techniques for supporting incision while a patient recovering from thoracic surgery coughs.

D. The patient can be taught to hold a pillow firmly against the incision while coughing. This can be done while lying down or sitting in an upright position.

with the cough routine until the lungs are clear. Aerosol therapy is helpful in humidifying and mobilizing secretions so that they can easily be cleared with coughing. To minimize incisional pain during coughing, the nurse supports the incision or encourages the patient to do so (see Fig. 21-12). If a patient is identified as being at high risk for postoperative pulmonary complications, then CPT is started immediately (perhaps even before surgery). The techniques of postural drainage, vibration, and percussion help loosen and mobilize the secretions so that they can be coughed up or suctioned.

Following the use of these measures, the nurse listens to both lungs, anteriorly and posteriorly, to determine whether there are any changes in breath sounds. Diminished breath sounds may indicate collapsed or hypoventilated alveoli.

Relieving Pain and Discomfort

Pain after a thoracotomy may be severe, depending on the type of incision and the patient's reaction and ability to cope with pain. Pain can impair the patient's ability to breathe deeply and cough. Preoperatively or postoperatively, an anesthesiologist or anesthetist can perform paravertebral blocks with a long-acting local anesthetic such as bupivacaine (Marcaine) or ropivacaine (Bottiger, Esper, & Stafford, 2014). A thoracic epidural catheter may be placed for continuous analgesia or PCEA using a combination of a long-acting local anesthetic and an opioid. As an alternative, a continuous epidural infusion may be combined with IV PCA using an opioid. Bupivacaine or ropivacaine is titrated in the epidural catheter to relieve postoperative pain, improving the patient's mobility and ability to deep breathe and cough. Opioid analgesic agents such as morphine are commonly used in PCA, which allows the patient to control the frequency and total dosage. Preset limits on the pump avoid overdosage.

With proper instruction, PCA and PCEA are well tolerated and allow earlier mobilization and cooperation with the treatment regimen. (See Chapter 12 for a more extensive discussion of PCA and pain management.)

It is important to avoid depressing the respiratory system with excessive opioid analgesia. The patient should not be so sedated as to be unable to cough. Incorporating a multimodal approach to pain management with PCEAs and NSAIDs can help to alleviate this problem. Inadequate treatment of pain, however, may also lead to hypoventilation and decreased coughing.

Lidocaine (Xylocaine) and prilocaine (Citanest) are local anesthetic agents that may be used to treat pain at the site of the chest tube insertion. These medications are given as topical transdermal analgesics that penetrate the skin; they have also been found to be effective when used together. EMLA cream, which is a mixture of the two medications, may be effective in treating pain from chest tube removal. However, analgesia is not typically indicated when removing chest tubes, because the pain, although severe, is of short duration (usually less than a few minutes) and the analgesia might interfere with respiratory effort.

Promoting Mobility and Shoulder Exercises

Because large shoulder girdle muscles are transected during a thoracotomy, the arm and shoulder must be mobilized by full range of motion of the shoulder. As soon as physiologically possible, usually within 8 to 12 hours, the patient is helped to get out of bed. Although this may be painful initially, the earlier the patient moves, the sooner the pain will subside. In addition to getting out of bed, the patient begins arm and shoulder exercises to restore movement and prevent painful stiffening of the affected arm and shoulder, as approved and prescribed by the surgeon (see Chart 21-21).

Chart 21-21	**PATIENT EDUCATION**

Performing Arm and Shoulder Exercises

Arm and shoulder exercises are performed after thoracic surgery to restore movement, prevent painful stiffening of the shoulder, and improve muscle power.

Hold hand of the affected side with the other hand, palms facing in. Raise the arms forward, upward, and then overhead, while taking a deep breath. Exhale while lowering the arms. Repeat five times.

Raise arm sideward, upward, and downward in a waving motion

Place arm at side. Raise arm sideward, upward, and then overhead. Repeat five times. These exercises can also be performed while lying in bed.

Extend the arm up and back, out to the side and back, down at the side, and back.

Place hands in small of back. Push elbows as far back as possible.

Sit erect in an armchair; place the hands on arms of the chair. Press down on hands, consciously pulling the abdomen in and stretching up from the waist. Inhale while raising the body until elbows are extended completely. Hold this position a moment, and begin exhaling while lowering the body slowly to the original position.

A scheduled regimen of 3 to 4 g of acetaminophen daily can help relieve shoulder pain.

Maintaining Fluid Volume and Nutrition

During the surgical procedure or immediately after, the patient may receive a transfusion of blood products if required (see Chapter 32), followed by a continuous IV infusion. Because a reduction in lung capacity often occurs after thoracic surgery, a period of physiologic adjustment is needed. Fluids should be given at a low hourly rate and titrated (as prescribed) to prevent overloading the vascular system and precipitating pulmonary edema. The nurse performs careful respiratory and cardiovascular assessments and monitors intake and output, vital signs, and jugular vein distention. The nurse also monitors the infusion site for signs of infiltration, including swelling, tenderness, and redness.

Patients undergoing thoracotomy may have poor nutritional status before surgery because of dyspnea, sputum production, and poor appetite. Therefore, it is especially important that adequate nutrition be provided. A liquid diet is provided as soon as bowel sounds return, and the patient is progressed to a full diet as soon as possible. Small, frequent meals are better tolerated and are crucial to the recovery and maintenance of lung function.

Monitoring and Managing Potential Complications

Complications after thoracic surgery are always a possibility and must be identified and managed early. The nurse monitors the patient at regular intervals for signs of respiratory distress or developing respiratory failure, dysrhythmias, bronchopleural fistula, hemorrhage and shock, atelectasis, and incisional or pulmonary infection.

Respiratory distress is treated by identifying and eliminating its cause while providing supplemental oxygen. If the patient progresses to respiratory failure, intubation and mechanical ventilation are necessary.

Dysrhythmias are often related to the effects of hypoxia or the surgical procedure. They are treated with antiarrhythmic medication and supportive therapy (see Chapter 26). Pulmonary infections or effusion, often preceded by atelectasis, may occur a few days into the postoperative course.

Pneumothorax may occur after thoracic surgery if there is an air leak from the surgical site to the pleural cavity or from the pleural cavity to the environment. Failure of the chest drainage system prevents return of negative pressure in the pleural cavity and results in pneumothorax. In the postoperative patient, pneumothorax is often accompanied by hemothorax. The nurse maintains the chest drainage system and monitors the patient for signs and symptoms of pneumothorax: increasing shortness of breath, tachycardia, increased respiratory rate, and increasing respiratory distress.

Bronchopleural fistula is a serious but rare complication that prevents the return of negative intrathoracic pressure and lung re-expansion. Depending on its severity, it is treated with closed chest drainage, mechanical ventilation, and possibly pleurodesis (described in Chapter 23).

Hemorrhage and shock are managed by treating the underlying cause, whether by reoperation or by administration of blood products or fluids. Pulmonary edema from overinfusion of IV fluids is a significant danger. Early symptoms are dyspnea; crackles; tachycardia; and pink, frothy sputum. This constitutes an emergency and must be reported and treated immediately (see Chapter 29 for further discussion).

Promoting Home, Community-Based, and Transitional Care

Educating Patients About Self-Care

The nurse instructs the patient and family about postoperative care that will be continued at home. The nurse explains signs and symptoms that should be reported to the primary provider. These include the following:

- Change in respiratory status, such as increasing shortness of breath, fever, increased restlessness or other changes in mental or cognitive status, increased respiratory rate, change in respiratory pattern, change in amount or color of sputum

---

Chart 21-22

HOME CARE CHECKLIST
The Patient With a Thoracotomy

At the completion of education, the patient and/or caregiver will be able to:

- Name the procedure that was performed and identify any permanent changes in anatomic structure or function as well as changes in ADLs, IADLs, roles, relationships, and spirituality.
- State the name, dose, side effects, frequency, and schedule for all medications.
- Identify interventions and strategies (e.g., durable medical equipment, oxygen, and adaptive equipment) used in adapting to any permanent changes in structure or function.
- Describe ongoing postoperative therapeutic regimen, including diet and activities to perform (e.g., walking and breathing exercises) and to limit or avoid (e.g., lifting weights, driving a car, and contact sports).
  - Alternate walking and other activities with frequent rest periods, expecting weakness and fatigue for the first 3 weeks.
  - Walk at a moderate pace, gradually and persistently extending walking time and distance.
  - Perform arm and shoulder exercises as prescribed
  - Perform breathing exercises several times daily for the first few weeks at home.
  - Avoid lifting >20 lb until complete healing has taken place; the chest muscles and incision may be weaker than normal for 3–6 months after surgery.
  - Use local heat and oral analgesia to relieve intercostal pain.

- Immediately stop any activity that causes undue fatigue, increased shortness of breath, or chest pain.
- Avoid bronchial irritants (smoke, fumes, air pollution, aerosol sprays).
- Avoid others with known colds or lung infections.
- Describe signs and symptoms of complications (e.g., increased shortness of breath, fever, restlessness, mental status changes, change in rate or pattern of respiration, increased pain, or bleeding from incision).
- Relate how to reach primary provider with questions or complications.
- State time and date of follow-up appointments.
- Obtain an annual influenza vaccine, and discuss vaccination against pneumonia with the primary provider.
- State understanding of community resources and referrals (if any).
- Identify the need for health promotion (e.g., weight reduction, smoking cessation, and stress management), disease prevention and screening activities

Resources

See Chapter 21, Chart 21-2 for additional information on oxygen therapy at home and Chart 21-21 or additional information on performing arm and shoulder exercises.

ADL, activities of daily living; IADL, independent activities of daily living.

- Bleeding or other drainage from the surgical incision or chest tube exit sites
- Increased chest pain

In addition, respiratory care and other treatment modalities (oxygen; incentive spirometry; CPT; and oral, inhaled, or IV medications) may be continued at home. Therefore, the nurse needs to instruct the patient and family in their correct and safe use.

The nurse emphasizes the importance of progressively increased activity. The nurse instructs the patient to ambulate within limits and explains that return of strength is likely to be very gradual. Another important aspect of patient education addresses shoulder exercises. The patient is instructed to do these exercises five times daily. Additional patient education is described in Chart 21-22.

Continuing and Transitional Care

Depending on the patient's physical status and the availability of family assistance, a referral for home, community-based, or transitional care may be indicated. The home care nurse assesses the patient's recovery from surgery, with special attention to respiratory status, the surgical incision, chest drainage, pain control, ambulation, and nutritional status. The patient's use of respiratory modalities is assessed to ensure that they are being used correctly and safely. In addition, the nurse assesses the patient's adherence to the postoperative treatment plan and identifies acute or late postoperative complications.

The recovery process may take longer than the patient had expected, and providing support to the patient is an important task for the nurse. Because of shorter hospital stays, follow-up appointments with the primary provider are essential. The nurse educates the patient about the importance of keeping follow-up appointments and completing laboratory tests as prescribed to assist the primary provider in evaluating recovery. The nurse provides continuous encouragement and education to the patient and family during the process. As recovery progresses, the nurse also reminds the patient and family about the importance of participating in health promotion activities and recommended health screening.

CRITICAL THINKING EXERCISES

1 **pq** A 56-year-old man is admitted to a cardiopulmonary unit following a transbronchial lung biopsy for lung cancer. Shortly after arrival to the unit, the patient complains of excruciating pain in his upper right back, shortness of breath, and feeling anxious. Physical examination reveals tachycardia at 112 bpm, tachypnea at 28 breaths/min, and hypotension at 90/46 mm Hg. Auscultation reveals absence of breath sounds in the right mid and lower lobes. The patient is diaphoretic with a SpO$_2$ on room air of 88%. The physician prescribes emergent chest tube insertion with dry suction water seal chest drainage set up. What is the likely cause of the patient's clinical manifestations? What are your priority interventions?

What is the primary difference between a traditional water seal chest drainage system and a dry suction water seal chest drainage system? Describe nursing responsibilities following chest tube insertion.

2 **ebp** An 82-year-old man is admitted to an orthopedic unit following a total hip replacement for a right hip fracture, which occurred 2 days ago. Four hours after arrival to the unit, the patient complains of increasing shortness of breath and tachypnea with a respiratory rate of 38 breaths/min. Physical examination reveals tachycardia at 122 bpm, hypotension at 96/56 mm Hg, and SpO$_2$ of 84% on 4 L/min via nasal cannula. The nurse places the patient on a nonrebreather mask and notifies the physician. Arterial blood gases reveal pH 7.22, PO$_2$ 48 mm Hg, PCO$_2$ 52 mm Hg, and HCO$_3$ 24 mEq/L. The patient's respiratory status continues to deteriorate and the physician emergently places an endotracheal tube. The patient is sedated and placed on mechanical ventilation. What is the likely cause of the patient's respiratory distress? How do you interpret the patient's blood gas values? Outline the nursing care of the patient on a mechanical ventilator. Describe the essential components of the VAP bundle of evidence-based practice.

3 **pq** A 32-year-old woman is admitted to a general surgery unit following a thyroidectomy. Upon assessment of the patient, the nurse observes bleeding at the incision site, swelling of the neck, and harsh, high-pitched respiratory sounds. The nurse calls a rapid response and an emergent tracheostomy is performed at the bedside. The patient is transferred to the ICU. What are the priority nursing diagnoses for patients requiring a tracheostomy? Discuss nursing interventions to prevent complications following tracheostomy procedure. Describe the technique to suction an artificial airway.

REFERENCES

*Asterisk indicates nursing research.
**Double asterisk indicates classic reference.

Books

American Heart Association. (2015). *Basic life support for healthcare providers: Student manual.* Dallas, TX: Author.

Cairo, J. M. (2014). *Mosby's respiratory care equipment* (9th ed.). St. Louis, MO: Elsevier Mosby.

Grossman, S., & Porth, C. M. (2014). *Pathophysiology: Concepts of altered health states* (9th ed.). Philadelphia, PA: Lippincott Williams & Williams.

Kacmarek, R. M., Stroller, J. K., & Huer, A. (2017). *Egan's fundamentals of respiratory care* (11th ed.). St. Louis, MO: Elsevier.

Karch, A. M, (2013). *Focus on nursing pharmacology* (6th ed.). Philadelphia, PA: LWW.

Meiner, S. E. (2015). *Gerontologic nursing* (5th ed.). St. Louis, MO: Elsevier Mosby.

Sole, M. L., Klein, D. G., & Moseley, M. J. (2013). *Introduction to critical care nursing* (6th ed.). St. Louis, MO: Elsevier Saunders.

Urden, L. D., Stacy, K. M., & Lough, M. E. (2014). *Critical care nursing: Diagnosis and management* (7th ed.). St. Louis, MO: Elsevier Mosby.

Wiegand, D. J. L. (2011). *AACN procedure manual for critical care* (6th ed.). St. Louis, MO: Elsevier Saunders.

Journals and Electronic Documents

American Association for Respiratory Care. (2007). Clinical practice guideline: Oxygen therapy in the home or alternate site health care facility. *Respiratory Care, 52*(1), 1063–1068.

Amitai, A., & Sinert, R. H. (2015). Introduction to ventilator management. *Medscape*. Retrieved on 5/7/2016 at: emedicine.medscape.com/article/810126-overview#a3

Balas, M. C., Vasilevskis, E. E., Burke, W. J., et al. (2012). Critical care nurse's role in implementing the "ABCDE Bundle" into practice. *Critical Care Nurse, 32*(2), 35–48.

Bottiger, B., Esper S., & Stafford-Smith, M. (2014). Pain management strategies for thoracotomy and thoracic pain syndromes. *Seminars in Cardiothoracic and Vascular Anesthesia, 18*(1), 45–56.

Campbell, M. R., Fisher, J., Anderson, L., et al. (2015). Implementation of early exercise and progressive mobility: Steps to success. *Critical Care Nurse, 35*(1), 82–88. doi:10.4037/ccn2015701

**Centers for Medicare and Medicaid Services. (1993). National coverage determination (NCD) for home use of oxygen (240.2). Retrieved on 5/3/2016 at: www.cms.gov/medicare-coverage-database/details/ncddetails.aspx?NCDId=169&ncdver=1&DocID=240.2&SearchType=Advanced&bc=IAAAABAAAAAA&

El-Rabbany, M., Zaghlol, N., Bhandari, M., et al. (2015). Prophylactic oral health procedures to prevent hospital-acquired and ventilator-associated pneumonia: A systematic review. *International Journal of Nursing Studies, 52*(1), 452–464. doi:10.1016/j.ijnurstu.2014.07.010

*Fink, R. M., Makic, M. B. F., Poteet, A. W. (2015). The ventilated patient's experience. *Dimensions of Critical Care Nursing, 34*(5), 301–308.

Gupta, S., Singh, D., Sood, D., et al. (2015). Role of dexmedetomidine in early extubation of the intensive care unit patients. *Journal of Anaesthesiology Clinical Pharmacology, 31*(1), 92–98. doi:10.4103/0970–9185.150554

Hanlon, P. (2015). Secretion and airway clearance: Techniques and devices offer a range of treatment options. *RT: The Journal for Respiratory Care Practitioners, 28*(8), 11–14.

Institute for Healthcare Improvement. (2012). *How-to guide: Prevent ventilator-associated pneumonia*. Cambridge, MA: Institute for Healthcare Improvements. Retrieved on 5/7/2016 at: www.ihi.org/resources/Pages/Tools/HowtoGuidePreventVAP.aspx

**Langenhof, S., & Fichter, J. (2005). Comparison of two demand oxygen delivery devices for administration of oxygen in COPD. *Chest, 128*(4), 2082–2087.

Makic, M. B. F., Martin, S. A., Burns S., et al. (2013). Putting evidence into practice: Four traditional practices not supported by the evidence. *Critical Care Nurse, 33*(2), 28–43.

McClave, S. A., Taylor, B. E., Martindale, R. G., et al., (2016). Guidelines for the provision and assessment of nutrition support therapy in the adult critically ill patient: Society of Critical Care Medicine (SCCM) and American Society for Parenteral and Enteral Nutrition (A.S.P.E.N.). *Journal of Parenteral and Enteral Nutrition, 40*(2), 159–211.

Pedersen, A. (2013). New HFCWO vest offers patients more freedom. *Medical Device Daily, 17*(94), 1–10.

** The Joint Commission (TJC). (1998). Hospital Accreditation Standards. Provision of Care, Treatment and Services. Standards PC.03.05.01 through PC.03.05.19. 2010.

The sentinel event alert: Preventing restraint deaths, Issue 8. Retrieved on 6/26/2016 at: www.jointcommission.org/assets/1/18/SEA_8.pdf.

The Joint Commission (TJC). (2016). *Hospital National Patient Safety Goals*. Retrieved on 6/22/2016 at: www.jointcommission.org/assets/1/6/2016_NPSG_HAP_ER.pdf

Resources

American Association for Respiratory Care (AARC), www.aarc.org

American Lung Association, www.lung.org

American Thoracic Society (ATS), www.thoracic.org

Institute for Healthcare Improvement (IHI), www.ihi.org/Pages/default.aspx

National Institutes of Health, National Heart, Lung, and Blood Institute, www.nhlbi.nih.gov/

National Lung Health Education Program (NLHEP), www.nlhep.org/Pages/default.aspx

22

Management of Patients With Upper Respiratory Tract Disorders

LEARNING OBJECTIVES

On completion of this chapter, the learner will be able to:

1 Describe nursing management of patients with upper airway disorders.
2 Compare and contrast the upper respiratory tract infections according to cause, incidence, clinical manifestations, management, and the significance of preventive health care.

3 Use the nursing process as a framework for care of patients with upper airway infection.
4 Describe nursing management of the patient with epistaxis.
5 Use the nursing process as a framework for care of patients undergoing laryngectomy.

GLOSSARY

alaryngeal communication: alternative modes of speaking that do not involve the normal larynx; used by patients whose larynx has been surgically removed
aphonia: impaired ability to use one's voice due to disease or injury to the larynx
apnea: cessation of breathing
dysphagia: difficulties in swallowing
epistaxis: hemorrhage from the nose due to rupture of tiny, distended vessels in the mucous membrane of any area of the nose
herpes simplex (cold sore): a cutaneous viral infection with painful vesicles and erosions on the tongue, palate, gingiva, buccal membranes, or lips
laryngectomy: surgical removal of all or part of the larynx and surrounding structures
laryngitis: inflammation of the larynx; may be caused by voice abuse, exposure to irritants, or infectious organisms

nuchal rigidity: stiffness of the neck or inability to bend the neck
pharyngitis: inflammation of the throat; usually viral or bacterial in origin
rhinitis: inflammation of the mucous membranes of the nose; may be infectious, allergic, or inflammatory in origin
rhinitis medicamentosa: rebound nasal congestion commonly associated with overuse of over-the-counter nasal decongestants
rhinorrhea: drainage of a large amount of fluid from the nose
rhinosinusitis: inflammation of the nares and paranasal sinuses, including frontal, ethmoid, maxillary, and sphenoid sinuses; replaces the term *sinusitis*
tonsillitis: inflammation of the tonsils, usually due to an acute infection
xerostomia: dryness of the mouth from a variety of causes

Upper respiratory tract disorders are those that involve the nose, paranasal sinuses, pharynx, larynx, trachea, or bronchi. Many of these conditions are relatively minor, and their effects are limited to mild and temporary discomfort and inconvenience for the patient. However, others are acute, severe, and life threatening and may require permanent alterations in breathing and speaking. Therefore, the nurse must have expert assessment skills, an understanding of the wide variety of disorders that may affect the upper airway, and an awareness of the impact of these alterations on patients. Patient education is an important aspect of nursing care because many of these disorders are treated outside the hospital or at home by patients themselves. When caring for patients with acute, life-threatening disorders, the nurse needs highly developed assessment and clinical management skills, along with a focus on rehabilitation needs.

UPPER AIRWAY INFECTIONS

Upper airway infections (otherwise known as upper respiratory infections or URIs) are the most common cause of illness and affect most people on occasion. Some infections are acute, with symptoms that last several days; others are chronic, with symptoms that may last for weeks or months or recur. The American Academy of Family Physicians defines a URI as an infection of the mucous membranes from the nose down to the respiratory tree or bronchi (Fashner, Erickson, & Werner, 2012).

The common cold is the most frequently occurring example of a URI. URIs occur when microorganisms such as viruses and bacteria are inhaled. There are many causative organisms, and people are susceptible throughout life. Viruses, the most common cause of URIs, affect the upper respiratory passages and lead to subsequent mucous membrane inflammation (Fashner et al., 2012). URIs are the most common reason for seeking health care and for absences from school and work.

URIs affect the nasal cavity; ethmoidal air cells; and frontal, maxillary, and sphenoid sinuses; as well as the pharynx, larynx, and trachea. On average, adults typically develop 2 to 4 URIs per year because of the wide variety of respiratory viruses that circulate in the community. Although patients are rarely hospitalized for the treatment of URIs, nurses working in community settings or long-term care facilities may encounter patients who have these infections. It is important for nurses to recognize the signs and symptoms of URIs and provide appropriate care. Nurses in these settings also can influence patient outcomes through patient education. Special considerations with regard to URIs in older adults are summarized in Chart 22-1.

Rhinitis

Rhinitis is a group of disorders characterized by inflammation and irritation of the mucous membranes of the nose. These conditions can have a significant impact on quality of life and contribute to sinus, ear, and sleep problems and learning disorders. Rhinitis often coexists with other respiratory disorders, such as asthma. It affects between 10% and 30% of the population worldwide annually. Viral rhinitis, especially the common cold, affects approximately one billion individuals yearly (Krouse & Krouse, 2014).

Rhinitis may be acute or chronic, and allergic or nonallergic. Allergic rhinitis is further classified as seasonal or perennial rhinitis and is commonly associated with exposure to airborne particles such as dust, dander, or plant pollens in people who are allergic to these substances. Seasonal rhinitis occurs during pollen seasons, and perennial rhinitis occurs throughout the year. See Chapter 37 for detailed descriptions of allergic disorders, including allergic rhinitis.

Pathophysiology

Rhinitis may be caused by a variety of factors, including changes in temperature or humidity; odors; infection; age; systemic disease; use of over-the-counter (OTC) and prescribed nasal decongestants; and the presence of a foreign body. Allergic rhinitis may occur with exposure to allergens such as foods (e.g., peanuts, walnuts, Brazil nuts, wheat, shellfish, soy, cow's milk, and eggs), medications (e.g., penicillin, sulfa medications, and aspirin), and particles in the indoor and outdoor environment (see Chart 22-2). The most common cause of nonallergic rhinitis is the common cold (Seidman, Gurgel, Lin, et al., 2015).

Drug-induced rhinitis may occur with antihypertensive agents, such as angiotensin-converting enzyme (ACE) inhibitors and beta-blockers; "statins," such as atorvastatin (Lipitor) and simvastatin (Zocor); antidepressants and antipsychotics such as risperidone (Risperdal); aspirin; and some

---

Chart 22-1 — Upper Respiratory Tract Disorders in Older Adults

- Upper respiratory infections in older adults may have more serious consequences if patients have concurrent medical problems that compromise their respiratory or immune status.
- Influenza causes exacerbations of chronic obstructive pulmonary disease and reduced pulmonary function.
- Antihistamines and decongestants used to treat upper respiratory disorders must be used cautiously in older adults because of their side effects and potential interactions with other medications.
- Of Americans 65 years and older, approximately 14.1% have chronic rhinosinusitis (CRS). With anticipated future growth in the older adult population, the need for endoscopic sinus surgery will increase. Older patients with CRS present with symptoms similar to those of younger adults and experience a similar degree of improvement and quality of life after endoscopic sinus surgery.
- The structure of the nose changes with aging; it lengthens and the tip droops from loss of cartilage. This can cause restriction in airflow and predispose older adult patients to geriatric rhinitis, characterized by increased thin, watery sinus drainage. These structural changes may also adversely affect the sense of smell.
- Laryngitis in older adults is common and may be secondary to gastroesophageal reflux disease (GERD). Older adults are more likely to have impaired esophageal peristalsis and a weaker esophageal sphincter. Treatment measures include sleeping with the head of the bed elevated and the use of medications such as histamine-2 receptor blockers (e.g., famotidine [Pepcid], ranitidine [Zantac]) or proton pump inhibitors (omeprazole [Prilosec]).
- Age-related loss of muscle mass and thinning of the mucous membranes can cause structural changes in the larynx that may change characteristics of the voice. In general, the pitch of voice becomes higher in older adult men and lower in older adult women. The voice also "thins" (decreased projection) and may sound tremulous. These changes should be discriminated from signs that could indicate pathologic conditions.

Adapted from American Academy of Otolaryngology. (2015). *Fact sheet: Sinusitis: Special considerations for aging patients.* Retrieved on 10/8/2015 at: www.entnet.org/content/sinusitis-special-considerations-aging-patients

---

Chart 22-2 — Examples of Common Indoor and Outdoor Allergens

Common Indoor Allergens

- Dust mite feces
- Dog dander
- Cat dander
- Cockroach droppings
- Molds

Common Outdoor Allergens

- Trees (e.g., oak, elm, western red cedar, ash, birch, sycamore, maple, walnut, and cypress)
- Weeds (e.g., ragweed, tumbleweed, sagebrush, pigweed, cockle weed, and Russian thistle)
- Grasses (e.g., timothy, orchard, sweet vernal, bermuda, sour dock, redtop, and bluegrass)
- Molds (*Alternaria, Cladosporium, Aspergillus*)

Adapted from Aljubran, S. & Lockey, R. F. (2014) *Aeroallergens.* Retrieved on 3/9/2016 at www.emedicine.medscape.com/article/137911-overview

A. Rhinitis

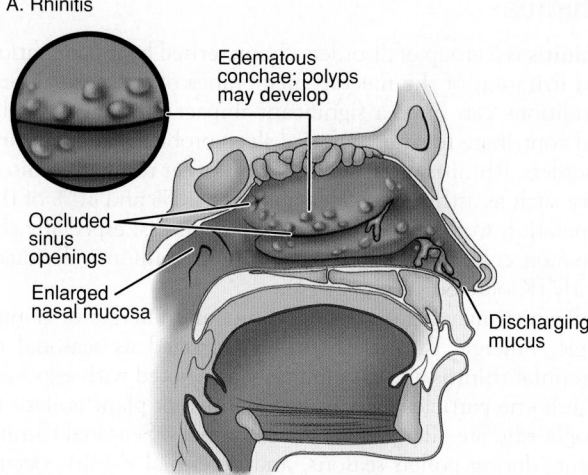

Edematous
conchae; polyps
may develop

Occluded
sinus
openings

Enlarged
nasal mucosa

Discharging
mucus

B. Rhinosinusitis

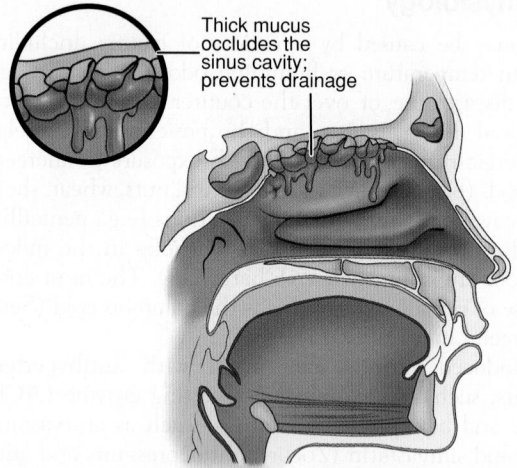

Thick mucus
occludes the
sinus cavity;
prevents drainage

Figure 22-1 • Pathophysiologic processes in rhinitis and rhinosinusitis. Although pathophysiologic processes are similar in rhinitis and rhinosinusitis, they affect different structures. **A.** In rhinitis, the mucous membranes lining the nasal passages become inflamed, congested, and edematous. The swollen nasal conchae block the sinus openings, and mucus is discharged from the nostrils. **B.** Rhinosinusitis is also marked by inflammation and congestion, with thickened mucous secretions filling the sinus cavities and occluding the openings.

antianxiety medications. Figure 22-1 shows the pathologic processes involved in rhinitis and rhinosinusitis. Other causes of rhinovirus are identified in Table 22-1.

Clinical Manifestations

The signs and symptoms of rhinitis include **rhinorrhea** (excessive nasal drainage, runny nose); nasal congestion; nasal discharge (purulent with bacterial rhinitis); sneezing; and pruritus of the nose, roof of the mouth, throat, eyes, and ears. Headache may occur, particularly if rhinosinusitis is also present. Nonallergic rhinitis can occur throughout the year.

TABLE 22-1 Causes of Rhinosinusitis

Category	Causes
Vasomotor	Idiopathic
	Abuse of nasal decongestants (rhinitis medicamentosa)
	Psychological stimulation (anger, sexual arousal)
	Irritants (smoke, air pollution, exhaust fumes, cocaine)
Mechanical	Tumor
	Deviated septum
	Crusting
	Hypertrophied turbinates
	Foreign body
	Cerebrospinal fluid leak
Chronic inflammatory	Polyps (in cystic fibrosis)
	Sarcoidosis
	Wegener granulomatosis
	Midline granuloma
Infectious	Acute viral infection
	Acute or chronic rhinosinusitis
	Rare nasal infections (syphilis, tuberculosis)
Hormonal	Pregnancy
	Use of oral contraceptives
	Hypothyroidism

Adapted from Peters, A. (2015). *Rhinosinusitis: Synopsis*. Retrieved on 10/8/2015 at: www.worldallergy.org/professional/allergic_diseases_center/rhinosinusitis/sinusitissynopsis.php

Medical Management

The management of rhinitis depends on the cause, which may be identified through the history and physical examination. The nurse asks the patient about recent symptoms as well as possible exposure to allergens in the home, environment, or workplace. If viral rhinitis is the cause, medications may be prescribed to relieve the symptoms. In allergic rhinitis, allergy tests may be performed to identify possible allergens. Depending on the severity of the allergy, desensitizing immunizations and corticosteroids may be required (see Chapter 37 for more details). If symptoms suggest a bacterial infection, an antimicrobial agent is used (see later discussion of rhinosinusitis). Patients with nasal septal deformities or nasal polyps may be referred to an ear, nose, and throat specialist.

Pharmacologic Therapy

Medication therapy for allergic and nonallergic rhinitis focuses on symptom relief. Antihistamines and corticosteroid nasal sprays may be useful. Antihistamines remain the most common treatment and are given for sneezing, pruritus, and rhinorrhea. (Examples of commonly prescribed antihistamines are discussed in more detail in Chapter 37.) Brompheniramine/pseudoephedrine (Dimetapp) is an example of combination antihistamine/decongestant medications. Cromolyn (Nasal-Crom), a mast cell stabilizer that inhibits the release of histamine and other chemicals, is also used in the treatment of rhinitis. Oral decongestant agents may be used for nasal obstruction. The use of saline nasal spray can act as a mild decongestant and can liquefy mucus to prevent crusting. Two inhalations of intranasal ipratropium (Atrovent) can be given in each nostril two to three times per day for symptomatic relief of rhinorrhea. In addition, intranasal corticosteroids may be used for severe congestion, and ophthalmic agents (cromolyn ophthalmic solution 4%) may be used to relieve irritation, itching, and redness of the eyes. Appropriate allergy treatments may include leukotriene modifiers (e.g., montelukast [Singulair], zafirlukast [Accolate], zileuton [Zyflo]), and immunoglobulin E modifiers (omalizumab [Xolair]), which are also components of asthma treatment guidelines (discussed further in Chapter 24). The choice of medications depends on the symptoms, adverse reactions, adherence factors, risk of drug interactions, and cost to the patient.

Nursing Management

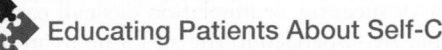

Educating Patients About Self-Care

The nurse instructs the patient with allergic rhinitis to avoid or reduce exposure to allergens and irritants, such as dusts, molds, animals, fumes, odors, powders, sprays, and tobacco smoke. Patient education is essential when assisting the patient in the use of all medications. To prevent possible drug interactions, the patient is cautioned to read drug labels before taking any OTC medication.

The nurse instructs the patient about the importance of controlling the environment at home and at work. Saline nasal sprays or aerosols may be helpful in soothing mucous membranes, softening crusted secretions, and removing irritants. The nurse instructs the patient in correct administration of nasal medications. To achieve maximal relief, the patient is instructed to blow the nose before applying any medication into the nasal cavity. In addition, the patient is taught to keep the head upright; spray quickly and firmly into each nostril away from the nasal septum; and wait at least 1 minute before administering the second spray. The container should be cleaned after each use and should never be shared with other people to avoid cross-contamination.

In the case of infectious rhinitis, the nurse reviews hand hygiene technique with the patient as a measure to prevent transmission of organisms. This is especially important for those in contact with vulnerable populations such as the very young, older adults, or people who are immunosuppressed (e.g., patients with human immune deficiency virus [HIV] infection, those taking immunosuppressive medications). In older adults and other high-risk populations, the nurse reviews the importance of receiving an influenza vaccination each year to achieve immunity before the beginning of the flu season.

Viral Rhinitis (Common Cold)

Viral rhinitis is the most frequent viral infection in the general population (Krouse & Krouse, 2014). The term *common cold* often is used when referring to a URI that is self-limited and caused by a virus. The term *cold* refers to an infectious, acute inflammation of the mucous membranes of the nasal cavity characterized by nasal congestion, rhinorrhea, sneezing, sore throat, and general malaise. More broadly, the term refers to an acute URI, whereas terms such as *rhinitis, pharyngitis,* and *laryngitis* distinguish the sites of the symptoms. The term is also used when the causative virus is influenza (the flu). Colds are highly contagious because virus is shed for

about 2 days before the symptoms appear and during the first part of the symptomatic phase.

Colds caused by rhinoviruses tend to occur in the early fall and spring. Other viruses tend to cause winter colds (Centers for Disease Control and Prevention [CDC], 2015). Seasonal changes in relative humidity may affect the prevalence of colds. The most common cold-causing viruses survive better when humidity is low, in the colder months of the year.

Colds are caused by as many as 200 different viruses (National Institute of Allergy and Infectious Diseases, 2015). Rhinoviruses are the most likely causative organisms. Other viruses implicated in the common cold include coronavirus, adenovirus, respiratory syncytial virus, influenza virus, and parainfluenza virus. Each virus may have multiple strains; as a result, people are susceptible to colds throughout life. Development of a vaccine against the multiple strains of virus is almost impossible. Immunity after recovery is variable and depends on many factors, including a person's natural host resistance and the specific virus that caused the cold. Despite popular belief, cold temperatures and exposure to cold rainy weather do not increase the incidence or severity of the common cold.

Clinical Manifestations

Signs and symptoms of viral rhinitis may include low-grade fever, nasal congestion, rhinorrhea and nasal discharge, halitosis, sneezing, tearing watery eyes, "scratchy" or sore throat, general malaise, chills, and often headache and muscle aches. As the illness progresses, cough usually appears. In some people, the virus exacerbates **herpes simplex,** commonly called a *cold sore* (see Chart 22-3).

The symptoms of viral rhinitis may last from 1 to 2 weeks. If severe systemic respiratory symptoms occur, it is no longer considered viral rhinitis but one of the other acute URIs. Allergic conditions can affect the nose, mimicking the symptoms of a cold.

Medical Management

Management consists of symptomatic therapy that includes adequate fluid intake, rest, prevention of chilling, and the use of expectorants as needed. Warm salt-water gargles soothe the sore throat, and nonsteroidal anti-inflammatory drugs (NSAIDs), such as aspirin or ibuprofen, relieve aches and pains. Antihistamines are used to relieve sneezing, rhinorrhea, and nasal congestion. Petroleum jelly can soothe irritated, chapped, and raw skin around the nares (National Institute of Allergy and Infectious Diseases, 2015).

Guaifenesin (Mucinex), an expectorant, is available without a prescription and is used to promote removal of secretions. Antimicrobial agents (antibiotics) should not be used, because they do not affect the virus or reduce the incidence of bacterial complications. In addition, their inappropriate use has been implicated in the development of organisms resistant to therapy.

Topical nasal decongestants (e.g., phenylephrine nasal [Neo-Synephrine] and oxymetazoline nasal [Afrin]) should be used with caution. Topical therapy delivers medication directly to the nasal mucosa, and its overuse can produce **rhinitis medicamentosa,** or rebound rhinitis. Most patients treat the common cold with OTC medications that produce moderate clinical benefits, such as relief of symptoms.

Chart 22-3

Colds and Cold Sores (Herpes Simplex Virus)

Herpes labialis is an infection that is caused by herpes simplex virus type 1 (HSV-1). It is characterized by an eruption of small, painful blisters on the skin of the lips, mouth, gums, tongue, or the skin around the mouth. The blisters are commonly referred to as cold sores or fever blisters. Once the person is infected with this virus, it can lie latent in the cells for a period of time. The incubation period is about 2 to 12 days. Between 50% and 80% of Americans are infected by age 30 years, because HSV-1 is typically transmitted during childhood through non-sexual contact. Herpes labialis is extremely contagious and can be spread through contaminated razors, towels, and dishes. It is activated by overexposure to sunlight or wind, colds, influenza and similar infections, heavy alcohol use, and physical or emotional stress.

Although herpes simplex virus type 2 (HSV-2) typically causes painful vesicular and ulcerative lesions in the genital and anal areas, HSV-1 may also cause genital herpes. Oral–genital contact can spread oral herpes to the genitals (and vice versa). People with active herpetic lesions should avoid oral sex. It is extremely important for patients to understand that the virus can be transmitted by asymptomatic people. Estimates suggest that 80% of people infected are asymptomatic.

Early symptoms of herpes labialis include burning, itching, and increased sensitivity or tingling sensation. These symptoms may occur several days before the appearance of lesions. The lesions appear as macules or papules, progressing to small blisters (vesicles) filled with clear, yellowish fluid. They are raised, red, and painful and can break and ooze. The lesions typically extend through the epidermis and penetrate into the underlying dermis, consistent with a partial-thickness wound. Eventually, yellow crusts slough to reveal pink, healing skin. Typically, the virus is no longer detectable in the lesion or wound 5 days after the vesicle has developed.

Medications used in the management of herpes labialis include acyclovir (Zovirax) and valacyclovir (Valtrex), which help to minimize the symptoms and the duration or length of flare-up. Acetaminophen may be given for analgesia. Topical anesthetics such as lidocaine (Xylocaine) can help in the control of discomfort. Occlusive dressings have been shown to speed the healing process. Not only do such dressings prevent desiccation and scab formation but they also maintain an aqueous wound environment rich in growth factors and matrix materials. However, occlusive dressings are not practical for lip and mucosal lesions. In this case, alternatives include occlusive ointments such as Herpecin-L or docosanol (Abreva).

Adapted from Salvaggio, M. R. (2014). *Herpes simplex*. Retrieved on 10/12/2015 at: www.emedicine.medscape.com/article/218580-overview

In addition, alternative medicines (e.g., echinacea, zinc lozenges, and zinc nasal spray) are frequently used to treat the common cold; however, evidence regarding their effectiveness in shortening the symptomatic phase is limited (Karsch-Volk, Barrett, Keifer, et al., 2014). The inhalation of steam or heated, humidified air has been a mainstay of home remedies to treat the common cold; however, the value of this therapy has not been demonstrated.

Nursing Management

Educating Patients About Self-Care

Most viruses can be transmitted in several ways: direct contact with infected secretions, inhalation of large particles from others' coughing or sneezing, or inhalation of small particles (aerosol) that may be suspended in the air for up to an hour. Implementation of appropriate hand hygiene measures (see Chart 71-1 for further information on hand hygiene methods) remains the most effective measure to prevent transmission of organisms. The nurse educates the patient about how to break the chain of infection with appropriate hand hygiene and the use of tissues to avoid the spread of the virus with coughing and sneezing, and to cough or sneeze into the upper arm if tissues are not readily available. The nurse instructs the patient about methods to treat symptoms of the common cold and provides both verbal and written information to assist in the prevention and management of URIs.

Rhinosinusitis

Rhinosinusitis, formerly called *sinusitis*, is an inflammation of the paranasal sinuses and nasal cavity. The American Academy of Otolaryngology–Head and Neck Surgery Foundation (Rosenfeld, Andes, Bhattacharyya, et al., 2015) recommends the use of the term *rhinosinusitis* because sinusitis is almost always accompanied by inflammation of the nasal mucosa. Rhinosinusitis affects 1 in 8 Americans; about 30 million people in the United States are diagnosed with this condition each year, resulting in direct annual health care costs of $11 billion, with $5.8 billion in ambulatory and emergency services alone (Rosenfeld et al., 2015).

Uncomplicated rhinosinusitis occurs without extension of inflammation outside of the paranasal sinuses and nasal cavity. Rhinosinusitis is classified by duration of symptoms as acute (less than 4 weeks), subacute (4 to 12 weeks), and chronic (more than 12 weeks). Rhinosinusitis can be caused by a bacterial or viral infection.

Acute Rhinosinusitis

Acute rhinosinusitis is classified as acute bacterial rhinosinusitis (ABRS) or acute viral rhinosinusitis (AVRS). Recurrent acute rhinosinusitis is characterized by four or more acute episodes of ABRS per year (Rosenfeld et al., 2015) and is discussed with chronic rhinosinusitis (CRS).

Pathophysiology

Acute rhinosinusitis usually follows a viral URI or cold, such as an unresolved viral or bacterial infection, or an exacerbation of allergic rhinitis. Normally, the sinus openings into the nasal passages are clear and infections resolve promptly. However, if their drainage is obstructed by a deviated septum or by hypertrophied turbinates, spurs, or nasal polyps or tumors, sinus infection may persist as a smoldering (persistent) secondary infection or progress to an acute suppurative process (causing purulent discharge).

Nasal congestion, caused by inflammation, edema, and transudation of fluid secondary to URI, leads to obstruction of the sinus cavities (see Fig. 22-1). This provides an excellent medium for bacterial growth. Other conditions and activities that can block the normal flow of sinus secretions include abnormal structures of the nose, enlarged adenoids, diving and swimming, tooth infection, trauma to the nose, tumors, and the pressure of foreign objects. Some people are more prone to rhinosinusitis because exposure to environmental hazards such as paint, sawdust, and chemicals may result in chronic inflammation of the nasal passages.

Bacterial organisms account for more than 60% of the cases of acute rhinosinusitis. Typical pathogens include *Streptococcus pneumoniae*, *Haemophilus influenzae*, and less commonly *Staphylococcus aureus*, and *Moraxella catarrhalis* (Brook, 2015). Biofilms, which consist of organized, heterogeneous communities of bacteria, have been found to be 10 to 1000 times more resistant to antibiotic treatment and more likely to contribute to host resistance when compared with other bacteria. They serve as bacterial reservoirs that can cause systemic illness when released into the circulation. Although antibiotics kill bacteria in the biofilm margin, cells deep in the biofilm are not affected, allowing for regrowth once antibiotic therapy has been discontinued. Pathogens in the upper respiratory tract that form biofilms include those species listed earlier as well as *Pseudomonas aeruginosa*.

Other organisms that are occasionally isolated include *Chlamydia pneumoniae*, *Streptococcus pyogenes*, viruses, and fungi (*Aspergillus fumigatus*). Fungal infections occur most often in immunosuppressed patients (Brook, 2015).

Clinical Manifestations

Symptoms of ABRS include purulent nasal drainage (anterior, posterior, or both) accompanied by nasal obstruction or a combination of facial pain, pressure, or a sense of fullness (referred to collectively as facial pain–pressure–fullness), or both (Rosenfeld et al., 2015). The facial pain–pressure–fullness may involve the anterior face or the periorbital region. The patient may also report cloudy or colored nasal discharge congestion, blockage, or stuffiness as well as a localized or diffuse headache. Patients with ABRS may present with a high fever (i.e., 39°C [102°F] or higher). In addition, the occurrence of symptoms for 10 days or more after the initial onset of upper respiratory symptoms indicates ABRS (Brook, 2015).

The symptoms of AVRS are similar to those of ABRS, except the patient does not present with a high fever, nor with the same intensity of symptoms (e.g., there tends to be an absence of facial pain–pressure–fullness), nor with symptoms that persist for as long a period of time. Symptoms of AVRS occur for fewer than 10 days after the onset of upper respiratory symptoms and do not worsen (Tierney, McPhee, & Papadakis, 2015).

Assessment and Diagnostic Findings

A careful history and physical examination are performed. The head and neck, particularly the nose, ears, teeth, sinuses, pharynx, and chest, are examined. There may be tenderness to palpation over the infected sinus area. The sinuses are percussed using the index finger, tapping lightly to determine whether the patient experiences pain. Although less frequently performed, transillumination of the affected area may reveal a decrease in the transmission of light with rhinosinusitis (see Chapter 20). Diagnostic imaging (x-ray, computed tomography [CT], magnetic resonance imaging [MRI]) is not recommended and generally not needed for the diagnosis of acute rhinosinusitis if the patient meets clinical diagnostic criteria (Rosenfeld et al., 2015). When a complication or alternative diagnosis is suspected, CT scans may be indicated because these scans are sensitive to inflammatory changes and bone destruction and identify anatomic variations that can guide sinus surgery if indicated.

To confirm the diagnosis of maxillary and frontal rhinosinusitis and identify the pathogen, sinus aspirates may be obtained. Flexible endoscopic culture techniques and swabbing of the sinuses have been used for this purpose (Krouse & Krouse, 2015).

Complications

If untreated, acute rhinosinusitis may lead to severe complications. Local complications include osteomyelitis and mucocele (cyst of the paranasal sinuses). Osteomyelitis requires prolonged antibiotic therapy and at times removal of necrotic bone. Intracranial complications, although rare, include cavernous sinus thrombosis, meningitis, brain abscess, ischemic brain infarction, and severe orbital cellulitis (Tierney et al., 2015). Mucoceles may require surgical treatment to establish intranasal drainage or complete excision with ablation of the sinus cavity. Brain abscesses occur by direct spread and can be life threatening. Frontal epidural abscesses are usually quiescent but can be detected by CT scan.

Medical Management

Treatment of acute rhinosinusitis depends on the cause; a 5- to 7-day course of antibiotics is prescribed for bacterial cases (Tewfik, 2015). The goals of treatment for acute rhinosinusitis are to shrink the nasal mucosa, relieve pain, and treat infection. Because of the inappropriate use of antibiotics for nonbacterial illness, including AVRS, and the resulting resistance that has occurred, oral antibiotics are only prescribed when there is sufficient empiric evidence that the patient has ABRS (e.g., high fever or symptoms that persist for at least 10 days or worsening symptoms following a viral respiratory illness).

Antibiotics should be given as soon as the diagnosis of ABRS is established. Amoxicillin–clavulanic acid (Augmentin) is the antibiotic of choice. For patients who are allergic to penicillin, doxycycline (Vibramycin) or respiratory quinolones such as levofloxacin (Levaquin) or moxifloxacin (Avelox) can be used. Other antibiotics prescribed previously to treat ABRS, including cephalosporins such as cephalexin (Keflex), cefuroxime (Ceftin), cefaclor (Ceclor), and cefixime (Suprax), trimethoprim–sulfamethoxazole (Bactrim, Septra), and macrolides such as clarithromycin (Biaxin) and azithromycin (Zithromax), are no longer recommended because they are not effective in treating antibiotic-resistant organisms that are now more commonly implicated in ABRS (Tewfik, 2015). Intranasal saline lavage is an effective adjunct therapy to antibiotics in that it may relieve symptoms, reduce inflammation, and help clear the passages of stagnant mucus. Neither decongestants nor antihistamines are recommended adjunctive medications for treating ABRS (Tewfik, 2015).

Treatment of AVRS typically involves nasal saline lavage and decongestants (guaifenesin/pseudoephedrine [Entex PSE]). Decongestants or nasal saline sprays can increase patency of the ostiomeatal unit and improve drainage of the sinuses. Topical decongestants should not be used for longer than 3 or 4 days. Oral decongestants must be used cautiously in patients with hypertension. OTC antihistamines, such as diphenhydramine (Benadryl) and cetirizine (Zyrtec), and prescription antihistamines, such as fexofenadine (Allegra), are used if an allergic component is suspected.

Intranasal corticosteroids have been shown to produce complete or marked improvement in acute symptoms of either bacterial or viral rhinosinusitis; however, they are only recommended for use in patients with a previous history of allergic rhinitis (Krouse & Krouse, 2014; Rosenfeld et al., 2015). Examples of intranasal corticosteroids, side effects, and contraindications are presented in Table 22-2.

Nursing Management

Educating Patients About Self-Care

Patient education is an important aspect of nursing care for the patient with acute rhinosinusitis. The nurse instructs the patient about symptoms of complications that require immediate follow-up. Referral to the primary provider is indicated if periorbital edema and severe pain on palpation occur. The nurse instructs the patient about methods to promote drainage of the sinuses, including humidification of the air in the home and the use of warm compresses to relieve pressure. The patient is advised to avoid swimming, diving, and air travel during the acute infection. Patients using tobacco are instructed to immediately stop smoking or using any form of tobacco. Most patients use nasal sprays incorrectly, which can lead to several side effects that include nasal irritation, nasal

burning, bad taste, and drainage in the throat or even epistaxis. Therefore, if an intranasal corticosteroid is prescribed, it is important to instruct the patient about the correct use of prescribed nasal sprays through demonstration, explanation, and return demonstration to evaluate the patient's understanding of the correct method of administration. The nurse also educates the patient about the side effects of prescribed and OTC nasal sprays and about rebound congestion (rhinitis medicamentosa). Once the decongestant is discontinued, the nasal passages close and congestion results. Appropriate medications to use for pain relief include acetaminophen (Tylenol) and NSAIDs such as ibuprofen (Advil), naproxen sodium (Aleve), and aspirin for adults older than 20 years.

The nurse tells patients with recurrent rhinosinusitis to begin decongestants, such as pseudoephedrine (Sudafed), at the first sign of rhinosinusitis. This promotes drainage and decreases the risk of bacterial infection. Patients should also check with their primary provider or pharmacist before using OTC medications because many cold medications can worsen symptoms or other health problems, specifically hypertension.

The nurse stresses the importance of following the recommended antibiotic regimen because a consistent blood level of the medication is critical to treat the infection. The nurse educates the patient about the early signs of a sinus infection and recommends preventive measures such as following healthy practices and avoiding contact with people with URIs.

The nurse explains to the patient that fever, severe headache, and **nuchal rigidity** (stiffness of the neck or inability to bend the neck) are signs of potential complications. Patients with chronic symptoms of rhinosinusitis who do not have marked improvement in 4 weeks with continuous medical treatment may be candidates for functional endoscopic sinus surgery (FESS, see later discussion) (Krings, Kallogjeri, Wineland, et al., 2014).

> ### ◣ Quality and Safety Nursing Alert
>
> *Patients with nasotracheal and nasogastric tubes in place are at the risk for development of sinus infections. Thus, accurate assessment of patients with these tubes is critical. Removal of the nasotracheal or nasogastric tube as soon as the patient's condition permits allows the sinuses to drain, possibly avoiding septic complications.*

TABLE 22-2 Selected Nasal Corticosteroids and Common Side Effects

Nasal Corticosteroids	Side Effects	Contraindications (for all nasal corticosteroids)
Beclomethasone (Beconase AQ)	Nasal irritation, headache, nausea, lightheadedness, epistaxis, rhinorrhea, watering eyes, sneezing, dry nose and throat	Avoid in patients with recurrent epistaxis, glaucoma, and cataracts. Patients who have been exposed to measles/varicella or who have adrenal insufficiency should avoid these medications.
Budesonide (Rhinocort)	Epistaxis, pharyngitis, cough, nasal irritation, bronchospasm	
Mometasone (Nasonex)	Headache, viral infection, pharyngitis, epistaxis, cough, dysmenorrhea, musculoskeletal pain, arthralgia	
Triamcinolone (Nasacort AQ)	Pharyngitis, epistaxis, cough, headache	

Adapted from Peters, A. (2015). *Rhinosinusitis: Synopsis.* Retrieved on 10/8/2015 at: www.worldallergy.org/professional/allergic_diseases_center/rhinosinusitis/sinusitissynopsis.php

Chronic Rhinosinusitis and Recurrent Acute Rhinosinusitis

CRS affects about 13% of the U.S. population and occurs most commonly in young and middle-aged adults (Brook, 2015). It is diagnosed when the patient has experienced 12 weeks or longer of two or more of the following symptoms: mucopurulent drainage, nasal obstruction, facial pain–pressure–fullness, or hyposmia (decreased sense of smell). It is estimated that in about 40% of patients, CRS is accompanied by nasal polyps (Rosenfeld et al., 2015). Recurrent acute rhinosinusitis is diagnosed when four or more episodes of ABRS occur per year with no signs or symptoms of rhinosinusitis between the episodes. The use of antibiotics in patients with recurrent acute rhinosinusitis is higher than in patients with CRS. Both CRS and recurrent acute rhinosinusitis affect quality of life as well as physical and social function (Rosenfeld et al., 2015).

Pathophysiology

Mechanical obstruction in the ostia of the frontal, maxillary, and anterior ethmoid sinuses (known collectively as the ostiomeatal complex) is the usual cause of CRS and recurrent acute rhinosinusitis. Obstruction prevents adequate drainage of the nasal passages, resulting in accumulation of secretions and an ideal medium for bacterial growth. Persistent blockage in an adult may occur because of infection, allergy, or structural abnormalities. Other associated conditions and factors may include cystic fibrosis, ciliary dyskinesia, neoplastic disorders, gastroesophageal reflux disease, tobacco use, and environmental pollution (Rosenfeld et al., 2015).

Both aerobic and anaerobic bacteria have been implicated in CRS and recurrent rhinosinusitis. Common aerobic bacteria include alpha-hemolytic streptococci, microaerophilic streptococci, and *S. aureus*. Common anaerobic bacteria include gram-negative bacilli, *Peptostreptococcus*, and *Fusobacterium*.

In addition, immunodeficiency should be considered in patients with CRS or acute recurrent rhinosinusitis. Acute fulminant/invasive rhinosinusitis is a life-threatening illness and is commonly attributed to *Aspergillus* in immunocompromised patients. Chronic fungal sinusitis also poses a risk. Chronic invasive fungal sinusitis occurs in immunocompromised patients along with fungus ball/mycetoma and allergic fungal sinusitis—the more common forms of chronic fungal sinusitis—which are considered noninvasive conditions in immunocompromised patients. The fungus ball is characterized by the presence of a noninvasive accumulation of a dense conglomeration of fungal hyphae in one sinus cavity, usually the maxillary sinus. The fungus generally remains contained in the fungus ball, which consists of mucopurulent cheesy or claylike materials within the sinus, but can become invasive when immunosuppression occurs, leading to encephalopathy (Lal, 2015). Symptoms include nasal stuffiness, nasal discharge, and facial pain. Vision loss, headache, and cranial nerve palsies have been identified in patients with a sphenoid sinus fungal ball (Lal, 2015).

Clinical Manifestations

Clinical manifestations of CRS include impaired mucociliary clearance and ventilation, cough (because the thick discharge constantly drips backward into the nasopharynx), chronic hoarseness, chronic headaches in the periorbital area, periorbital edema, and facial pain. As a result of chronic nasal congestion, the patient is usually required to breathe through the mouth. Snoring, sore throat, and, in some situations, adenoidal hypertrophy may also occur. Symptoms are generally most pronounced on awakening in the morning. Fatigue and nasal congestion are also common. Many patients experience a decrease in smell and taste and a sense of fullness in the ears.

Assessment and Diagnostic Findings

The health assessment focuses on onset and duration of symptoms. It addresses the quantity and quality of nasal discharge and cough, the presence of pain, factors that relieve or aggravate the pain, and allergies. It is essential to obtain any history of comorbid conditions, including asthma and history of tobacco use. A history of fever, fatigue, previous episodes and treatments and previous response to therapies is also obtained.

In the physical assessment, the external nose is evaluated for any evidence of anatomic abnormality. A crooked-appearing external nose may imply septal deviation internally. The nasal mucous membranes are assessed for erythema, pallor, atrophy, edema, crusting, discharge, polyps, erosions, and septal perforations or deviations. Appropriate lighting improves visualization of the nasal cavity and should be used in every examination. Pain on examination of the teeth, with tapping with a tongue blade, suggests tooth infection (Bickley & Szilagyi, 2013).

Assessment of the posterior oropharynx may reveal purulent or mucoid discharge, which is indicative of an infection caused by CRS. The patient's eyes are examined for conjunctival erythema, tearing, photophobia, and edema of the lids. Additional assessment techniques include transillumination of the sinuses and palpation of the sinuses. The frontal and maxillary sinuses are palpated, and the patient is asked whether this produces tenderness. The pharynx is inspected for erythema and discharge and palpated for cervical node adenopathy (Rosenfeld et al., 2015).

Imaging studies such as x-ray, sinoscopy, ultrasound, CT scanning, and MRI may be used in the diagnosis of CRS. X-ray is an inexpensive and readily available tool to assess disorders of the paranasal sinuses. A CT scan of the paranasal sinuses can identify mucosal abnormalities, sinus ostial obstruction, anatomic variants, sinonasal polyposis, and neoplastic disease. In addition, nasal endoscopy allows for visualization of the posterior nasal cavity, nasopharynx, and sinus drainage pathways and can identify posterior septal deviation and polyps. Osseous destruction, extrasinus extension of the disease process, and local invasion suggest malignancy (Rosenfeld et al., 2015). (See Chapter 21 for further discussion of CT, MRI, and x-ray.)

Complications

Complications of CRS, although uncommon, include severe orbital cellulitis, subperiosteal abscess, cavernous sinus thrombosis, meningitis, encephalitis, and ischemic infarction. CRS can lead to intracranial infection either by direct spread through bone or via venous channels, resulting in epidural abscess, subdural empyema, meningitis, and brain abscess. Clinical sequelae can include personality changes with frontal lobe abscesses, headache, symptoms of elevated intracranial pressure to include alterations of consciousness, visual changes, focal neurologic deficits, seizures, and, ultimately, coma and death.

Frontal rhinosinusitis can lead to osteomyelitis of the frontal bones. Patients typically present with headache, fever, and a characteristic doughy edema over the involved bone. Ethmoid rhinosinusitis may result in orbital cellulitis, which usually begins with edema of the eyelids and rapidly progresses to ptosis (droopy eyelid), proptosis (bulging eye), chemosis (edema of the bulbar conjunctiva), and diminished extraocular movements. Patients are usually febrile and acutely ill and require immediate attention, because pressure on the optic nerve can lead to loss of vision and spread of infection can lead to intracranial infection. Cavernous sinus thrombophlebitis can result from extension of infection along venous channels from the orbit, ethmoid or frontal sinuses, or nose. Symptoms may include altered consciousness, lid edema, and proptosis, as well as third, fourth, and sixth cranial nerve palsies.

Medical Management

Medical management of CRS and recurrent acute rhinosinusitis is similar to that of acute rhinosinusitis. General measures include encouraging adequate hydration and recommending the use of OTC nasal saline sprays, analgesics such as acetaminophen or NSAIDs, and decongestants such as oxymetazoline and pseudoephedrine (Tewfik, 2015; Brook, 2015). Patients are instructed to sleep with the head of the bed elevated and to avoid exposure to cigarette smoke and fumes. Patients are cautioned to avoid caffeine and alcohol, which can cause dehydration.

Prescribed antibiotics may include amoxicillin-clavulanic acid, erythromycin–sulfisoxazole (Eryzole), second- or third-generation cephalosporins such as cefuroxime or cefixime, or newer fluoroquinolones such as moxifloxacin (Avelox) (Brook, 2015). The course of antibiotic treatment for CRS and recurrent ABRS is typically as long as 2 to 4 weeks to effectively eradicate the offending organism, and may be indicated for up to 12 months in some cases (Brook, 2015). Corticosteroid nasal sprays such as fluticasone (Flonase) or beclomethasone (Beconase AQ) may be indicated in patients with concomitant allergic rhinitis or nasal polyps. Patients with allergic rhinitis may also benefit from the addition of a mast cell stabilizer such as cromolyn. For patients with concomitant asthma, leukotriene inhibitors such as montelukast and zafirlukast may be used (Brook, 2015).

Surgical Management

If standard medical therapy fails and symptoms persist, FESS may be indicated to correct structural deformities that obstruct the ostia (openings) of the sinuses. FESS is a minimally invasive surgical procedure that is associated with reduced postoperative discomfort and improvement in the patient's quality of life. In particular, FESS is associated with either complete or moderate relief of symptoms in more than 85% to 91% of patients (Patel, 2014). Some of the specific procedures performed include excising and cauterizing nasal polyps, correcting a deviated septum, incising and draining the sinuses, aerating the sinuses, and removing tumors.

Antimicrobial agents may be given before and after surgery. Computer-assisted or computer-guided surgery is used to increase the precision of the surgical procedure and to minimize complications (Patel, 2014).

Surgical intervention may be required in acute invasive fungal rhinosinusitis to excise the fungus ball and necrotic tissue and drain the sinuses. Patients require aggressive surgical débridement and drainage as well as systemic antifungal medications.

Nursing Management

Patients usually perform care measures for rhinosinusitis at home; therefore, nursing management consists of good patient education.

 ### Educating Patients About Self-Care

Many people with sinus infections tend to blow their nose frequently and with force to clear their nasal passages. Doing so often increases the symptoms; therefore, the patient is instructed to blow the nose gently and to use tissue to remove the nasal drainage. Increasing fluid intake, applying local heat (hot wet packs), and elevating the head of the bed promote drainage of the sinuses. The nurse also instructs the patient about the importance of following the prescribed medication regimen. Instructions on the early signs of a sinus infection are provided, and preventive measures are reviewed. The nurse instructs the patient about signs and symptoms that require follow-up and provides these instructions verbally and in writing. Instructions in alternate formats (e.g., large font, patient's language) may be needed to increase the patient's understanding and adherence to the treatment plan. The nurse encourages the patient to follow up with their primary provider if symptoms persist.

 Quality and Safety Nursing Alert

URIs, specifically CRS and recurrent acute rhinosinusitis, may be linked to primary or secondary immune deficiency or treatment with immunosuppressive therapy (e.g., for cancer or organ transplantation). Typical symptoms may be blunted or absent due to immunosuppression. Immuno-compromised patients are at the increased risk for acute or chronic fungal infections; these infections can progress rapidly and become life threatening. Thus, assessment, early reporting of symptoms to the patient's primary provider and immediate initiation of treatment are essential.

Pharyngitis
Acute Pharyngitis

Acute **pharyngitis** is a sudden painful inflammation of the pharynx, the back portion of the throat that includes the posterior third of the tongue, soft palate, and tonsils. It is commonly referred to as a sore throat. In the United States, approximately 15 million health care visits are due to pharyngitis each year (Randel, 2013). Because of environmental exposure to viral agents and poorly ventilated rooms, the incidence of viral pharyngitis peaks during winter and early spring in regions that have warm summers and cold winters. Viral pharyngitis spreads easily in the droplets of coughs and sneezes, as well as from unclean hands that have been exposed to the contaminated fluids.

Pathophysiology

Viral infection causes most cases of acute pharyngitis. Responsible viruses include the adenovirus, influenza virus, Epstein–Barr virus, and herpes simplex virus. Bacterial infection accounts for the remainder of cases. Ten percent of adults with pharyngitis have group A beta-hemolytic streptococcus (GABHS), which is commonly referred to as group A streptococcus (GAS) or streptococcal pharyngitis. Streptococcal pharyngitis warrants the use of antibiotic treatment. When GAS causes acute pharyngitis, the condition is known as strep throat. The body responds by triggering an inflammatory response in the pharynx. This results in pain, fever, vasodilation, edema, and tissue damage, manifested by redness and swelling in the tonsillar pillars, uvula, and soft palate. A creamy exudate may be present in the tonsillar pillars (see Fig. 22-2). Other bacterial organisms implicated in acute pharyngitis include groups B and G streptococci, *Neisseria gonorrhoeae*, *Mycoplasma pneumoniae*, *C. pneumoniae*, *Arcanobacterium haemolyticum*, and HIV (Randel, 2013).

Uncomplicated viral infections usually subside promptly, within 3 to 10 days after onset. However, pharyngitis caused by more virulent bacteria, such as GAS, is a more severe illness. If left untreated, the complications can be severe and life threatening. Complications include rhinosinusitis, otitis media, peritonsillar abscess, mastoiditis, and cervical adenitis. In rare cases, the infection may lead to bacteremia, pneumonia, meningitis, rheumatic fever, and nephritis.

Clinical Manifestations

The signs and symptoms of acute pharyngitis include a fiery-red pharyngeal membrane and tonsils, lymphoid follicles that are swollen and flecked with white-purple exudate, enlarged and tender cervical lymph nodes, and no cough. Fever (higher than 38.3°C [101°F]), malaise, and sore throat also may be present. Occasionally, patients with GAS pharyngitis exhibit vomiting, anorexia, and a scarlatina-form rash with urticaria known as scarlet fever.

People who have streptococcal pharyngitis suddenly develop a painful sore throat 1 to 5 days after being exposed to the streptococcus bacteria. They usually report malaise, fever (with or without chills), headache, myalgia, painful cervical adenopathy, and nausea. The tonsils appear swollen and

erythematous, and they may or may not have an exudate. The roof of the mouth is often erythematous and may demonstrate petechiae. Bad breath is common.

Assessment and Diagnostic Findings

Accurate diagnosis of pharyngitis is essential to determine the cause (viral or bacterial) and to initiate treatment early. Rapid antigen detection testing (RADT) uses swabs that collect specimens from the posterior pharynx and tonsil. RADT is reported to be 90% to 95% sensitive, thus facilitating earlier treatment and earlier symptom improvement and reductions in pathogen transmission. Negative results should be confirmed by a throat culture (Randel, 2013). In most communities, preliminary culture reports are available in 24 hours. Once a definitive diagnosis of GAS is made, administration of appropriate antibiotics hastens symptom resolution and reduces the transmission of the illness.

Medical Management

Viral pharyngitis is treated with supportive measures because antibiotics have no effect on the causal organism. Bacterial pharyngitis is treated with a variety of antimicrobial agents.

Pharmacologic Therapy

If the cause of pharyngitis is bacterial, penicillin is usually the treatment of choice. Penicillin V potassium given orally for 5 days is the regimen of choice. Penicillin injections are recommended only if there is a concern that the patient will not adhere to therapy (Tierney et al., 2015).

For patients who are allergic to penicillin or have organisms that are resistant to erythromycin (one fifth of GAS and most *S. aureus* organisms are resistant to penicillin and erythromycin), cephalosporins and macrolides (clarithromycin and azithromycin) may be used. Once-daily azithromycin may be given for only 3 days due to its long half-life (Tierney et al., 2015). A 5- or 10-day course of cephalosporin may be prescribed. Five-day administration of cefpodoxime and cefuroxime has also been successful in producing bacteriologic cures.

Severe sore throats can also be relieved by analgesic medications, as prescribed. For example, aspirin or acetaminophen can be taken at 4- to 6-hour intervals; if required, acetaminophen with codeine can be taken three or four times daily. In severe cases, gargles with benzocaine may relieve symptoms.

Nutritional Therapy

A liquid or soft diet is provided during the acute stage of the disease, depending on the patient's appetite and the degree

Figure 22-2 • Pharyngitis—inflammation without exudate. **A.** Redness and vascularity of the pillars and uvula are mild to moderate. **B.** Redness is diffuse and intense. Each patient would probably complain of a sore throat. From the Wellcome Trust, National Medical Slide Bank, London, UK.

of discomfort that occurs with swallowing. Cool beverages, warm liquids, and flavored frozen desserts such as ice pops are often soothing. Occasionally, the throat is so sore that liquids cannot be taken in adequate amounts by mouth. In severe situations, intravenous (IV) fluids may be needed. Otherwise, the patient is encouraged to drink as much fluid as possible (at least 2 to 3 L/day).

Nursing Management

Nursing care for patients with viral pharyngitis focuses on symptomatic management. For patients who demonstrate signs of strep throat and have a history of rheumatic fever, who have scarlet fever, or who have symptoms suggesting peritonsillar abscess, nursing care focuses on prompt initiation and correct administration of prescribed antibiotic therapy. The nurse instructs the patient about signs and symptoms that warrant prompt contact with the primary provider. These include dyspnea, drooling, inability to swallow, and inability to fully open the mouth.

The nurse instructs the patient to stay in bed during the febrile stage of illness and to rest frequently once up and about. Used tissues should be disposed of properly to prevent the spread of infection. The nurse (or the patient or family member, if the patient is not hospitalized) should examine the skin once or twice daily for possible rash, because acute pharyngitis may precede some other communicable diseases (e.g., rubella).

Depending on the severity of the pharyngitis and the degree of pain, warm saline gargles or throat irrigations are used. The benefits of this treatment depend on the degree of heat that is applied. The nurse educates the patient about these procedures and about the recommended temperature of the solution, which should be high enough to be effective and as warm as the patient can tolerate, usually 40.6°C to 43.3°C (105°F to 110°F). Irrigating the throat may reduce spasm in the pharyngeal muscles and relieve soreness of the throat.

An ice collar also can relieve severe sore throats. Mouth care may promote the patient's comfort and prevent the development of fissures (cracking) of the lips and oral inflammation when bacterial infection is present. The nurse instructs the patient to resume activity gradually and to delay returning to work or school until after 24 hours of antibiotic therapy. A full course of antibiotic therapy is indicated in patients with strep infection because of the potential complications such as nephritis and rheumatic fever, which may have their onset 2 or 3 weeks after the pharyngitis has subsided. The nurse instructs the patient and family about the importance of taking the full course of therapy and informs them about the symptoms to watch for that may indicate complications.

In addition, the nurse instructs the patient about preventive measures that include not sharing eating utensils, glasses, napkins, food, or towels; cleaning telephones after use; using a tissue to cough or sneeze; disposing of used tissues appropriately; coughing or sneezing into the upper arm if tissues are not readily available; and avoiding exposure to tobacco and secondhand smoke. The nurse also instructs the patient with pharyngitis, especially streptococcal pharyngitis, to replace their toothbrush with a new one.

Chronic Pharyngitis

Chronic pharyngitis is a persistent inflammation of the pharynx. It is common in adults who work in dusty surroundings, use their voice to excess, suffer from chronic cough, or habitually use alcohol and tobacco.

There are three types of chronic pharyngitis:
- Hypertrophic—characterized by general thickening and congestion of the pharyngeal mucous membrane
- Atrophic—probably a late stage of the first type (the membrane is thin, whitish, glistening, and at times wrinkled)
- Chronic granular—characterized by numerous swollen lymph follicles on the pharyngeal wall

Clinical Manifestations

Patients with chronic pharyngitis complain of a constant sense of irritation or fullness in the throat, mucus that collects in the throat and can be expelled by coughing, and difficulty swallowing. This is often associated with intermittent postnasal drip that causes minor irritation and inflammation of the pharynx. A sore throat that is worse with swallowing in the absence of pharyngitis suggests the possibility of thyroiditis, and patients with this symptom are referred for the evaluation of possible thyroiditis.

Medical Management

Treatment of chronic pharyngitis is based on relieving symptoms; avoiding exposure to irritants; and correcting any upper respiratory, pulmonary, gastrointestinal, or cardiac condition that might be responsible for a chronic cough.

Nasal congestion may be relieved by short-term use of nasal sprays or medications containing ephedrine sulfate or phenylephrine. For a patient with a history of allergy, one of the antihistamine decongestant medications, such as pseudoephedrine or brompheniramine/pseudoephedrine, is prescribed orally every 4 to 6 hours. Aspirin (for patients older than 20 years) or acetaminophen is recommended for its analgesic properties.

For adults with chronic pharyngitis, tonsillectomy may be an effective option. For further information, see the Tonsillitis and Adenoiditis section.

Nursing Management

 Educating Patients About Self-Care

The nurse recommends avoidance of alcohol, tobacco, secondhand smoke, and exposure to cold or to environmental or occupational pollutants. The patient may minimize exposure to pollutants by wearing a disposable facemask. The nurse encourages the patient to drink plenty of fluids. Gargling with warm saline solution may relieve throat discomfort. Lozenges keep the throat moistened.

Tonsillitis and Adenoiditis

The tonsils are composed of lymphatic tissue and are situated on each side of the oropharynx. The faucial or palatine tonsils and lingual tonsils are located behind the pillars of fauces and tongue, respectively. They frequently serve as the site of acute infection (**tonsillitis**). Acute tonsillitis can be confused with pharyngitis. Chronic tonsillitis is less common and may be mistaken for other disorders such as allergy, asthma, and rhinosinusitis.

The adenoids or pharyngeal tonsils consist of lymphatic tissue near the center of the posterior wall of the nasopharynx. Infection of the adenoids frequently accompanies acute tonsillitis. Frequently occurring bacterial pathogens include GABHS, the most common organism. The most common viral pathogen is Epstein–Barr virus, although cytomegalovirus may also cause tonsillitis and adenoiditis. Often thought of as a childhood disorder, tonsillitis can occur in adults.

Clinical Manifestations

The symptoms of tonsillitis include sore throat, fever, snoring, and difficulty swallowing. Enlarged adenoids may cause mouth breathing, earache, draining ears, frequent head colds, bronchitis, foul-smelling breath, voice impairment, and noisy respiration. Unusually enlarged adenoids fill the space behind the posterior nares, making it difficult for the air to travel from the nose to the throat and resulting in nasal obstruction. Infection can extend to the middle ears by way of the auditory (eustachian) tubes and may result in acute otitis media, which can lead to spontaneous rupture of the tympanic membranes (eardrums) and further extension of the infection into the mastoid cells, causing acute mastoiditis. The infection also may reside in the middle ear as a chronic, low-grade, smoldering process that eventually may cause permanent deafness.

Assessment and Diagnostic Findings

The diagnosis of acute tonsillitis is primarily clinical, with attention given to whether the illness is viral or bacterial in nature. As in acute pharyngitis, RADT is quick and convenient; however, it is less sensitive than the throat swab culture.

A thorough physical examination is performed and a careful history is obtained to rule out related or systemic conditions. The tonsillar site is cultured to determine the presence of bacterial infection. When cytomegalovirus infection is present, the differential diagnosis should include HIV, hepatitis A, and rubella. In adenoiditis, if recurrent episodes of suppurative otitis media result in hearing loss, comprehensive audiometric assessment is warranted (see Chapter 64).

Medical Management

Tonsillitis is treated with supportive measures that include increased fluid intake, analgesics, salt-water gargles, and rest. Bacterial infections are treated with penicillin (first-line therapy) or cephalosporins. Viral tonsillitis is not effectively treated with antibiotic therapy.

Tonsillectomy (with or without adenoidectomy) continues to be a commonly performed surgical procedure and remains the treatment of choice for patients with chronic tonsillitis (Shah, 2015). Adults who have undergone a tonsillectomy to treat recurrent streptococcal infections experience a decrease in the number of episodes of streptococcal or other throat infections or days with throat pain.

Tonsillectomy is indicated if the patient has had repeated episodes of tonsillitis despite antibiotic therapy; hypertrophy of the tonsils and adenoids that could cause obstruction and

obstructive sleep apnea (OSA); repeated attacks of purulent otitis media; and suspected hearing loss due to serous otitis media that has occurred in association with enlarged tonsils and adenoids. Indications for adenoidectomy include chronic nasal airway obstruction, chronic rhinorrhea, obstruction of the eustachian tube with related ear infections, and abnormal speech. Surgery is also indicated if the patient has developed a peritonsillar abscess that occludes the pharynx, making swallowing difficult and endangering the patency of the airway (particularly during sleep). The presence of persistent tonsillar asymmetry should prompt an excisional biopsy to rule out lymphoma (Tierney et al., 2015). Antibiotic therapy may be initiated for patients undergoing tonsillectomy or adenoidectomy. Therapy may include oral penicillin or a cephalosporin (e.g., cefdinir [Omnicef] or moxifloxacin).

Nursing Management

Providing Postoperative Care

Continuous nursing observation is required in the immediate postoperative and recovery periods because of the risk of hemorrhage, which may also compromise the patient's airway (Seshamani, Vogtmann, Gattwood, et al., 2014). In the immediate postoperative period, the most comfortable position is prone, with the patient's head turned to the side to allow drainage from the mouth and pharynx. The nurse must not remove the oral airway until the patient's gag and swallowing reflexes have returned. The nurse applies an ice collar to the neck, and a basin and tissues are provided for the expectoration of blood and mucus.

Symptoms of postoperative complications include fever, throat pain, ear pain, and bleeding. Pain can be effectively controlled with analgesic medications. Postoperative bleeding may be seen as bright red blood if the patient expectorates it before swallowing it. If the patient swallows the blood, it becomes brown because of the action of the acidic gastric juice. If the patient vomits large amounts of dark blood or bright-red blood at frequent intervals, or if the pulse rate and temperature rise and the patient is restless, the nurse notifies the surgeon immediately. The nurse should have the following items ready for the examination of the surgical site for bleeding: a light, a mirror, gauze, curved hemostats, and a waste basin.

Occasionally, suture or ligation of a bleeding vessel is required. In such cases, the patient is taken to the operating room and given general anesthesia. After ligation, continuous nursing observation and postoperative care are required, as in the initial postoperative period. If there is no bleeding, water and ice chips may be given to the patient as soon as desired. The patient is instructed to refrain from too much talking and coughing, because these activities can produce throat pain. (See Chapter 19 for further discussion of postoperative nursing care.)

Educating Patients About Self-Care

Tonsillectomy and adenoidectomy are usually performed as outpatient surgery, and the patient is sent home from the recovery room once awake, oriented, and able to drink liquids and void. The patient and family must understand the signs and symptoms of hemorrhage. Bleeding may occur up to 8 days after surgery. The nurse instructs the patient about the use of liquid acetaminophen with or without codeine for pain control and explains that the pain will subside during the first 3 to 5 days. The nurse informs the patient about the need to take the full course of any prescribed antibiotic for the first postoperative week (Drake & Carr, 2015).

Alkaline mouthwashes and warm saline solutions are useful in coping with the thick mucus and halitosis that may be present after surgery. The nurse should explain to the patient that a sore throat, stiff neck, minor ear pain, and vomiting may occur in the first 24 hours. The patient should eat an adequate diet with soft foods, which are more easily swallowed than hard foods. The patient should avoid spicy, hot, acidic, or rough foods. Milk and milk products (ice cream and yogurt) may be restricted because they make removal of mucus more difficult for some patients. The nurse instructs the patient about the need to maintain good hydration. The patient is advised to avoid vigorous tooth brushing or gargling because these activities can cause bleeding. The nurse encourages the use of a cool-mist vaporizer or humidifier in the home postoperatively. The patient should avoid smoking and heavy lifting or exertion for 10 days.

Peritonsillar Abscess

Peritonsillar abscess (also called *quinsy*) is the most common major suppurative complication of sore throat accounting for roughly 30% of soft tissue head and neck abscesses. It most commonly afflicts adults between the ages of 20 to 40 years, with the incidence roughly the same between men and women (Flores, 2015). This collection of purulent exudate between the tonsillar capsule and the surrounding tissues, including the soft palate, may develop after an acute tonsillar infection that progresses to a local cellulitis and abscess. Several bacteria are typically implicated in the pathogenesis of these abscesses, including *S. pyogenes*, *S. aureus*, *Neisseria* species, and *Corynebacterium* species (Flores, 2015; Shah, 2015). In more severe cases, the infection can spread over the palate and to the neck and chest. Edema can cause airway obstruction, which can be life threatening and is a medical emergency. Peritonsillar abscess can be life threatening with mediastinitis, intracranial abscess, and empyemas resulting from spread of infection. Early detection and aggressive management are essential (Flores, 2015).

Clinical Manifestations

The patient with a peritonsillar abscess is acutely ill with a severe sore throat, fever, trismus (inability to open the mouth), and drooling. Inflammation of the medial pterygoid muscle that lies lateral to the tonsil results in spasm, severe pain, and difficulty in opening the mouth fully. The pain may be so intense that the patient has difficulty swallowing saliva. The patient's breath often smells rancid. Other symptoms include a raspy voice, odynophagia (a severe sensation of burning, squeezing pain while swallowing), **dysphagia** (difficulty swallowing), and otalgia (pain in the ear). Odynophagia is caused by the inflammation of the superior constrictor muscle of the pharynx that forms the lateral wall of the tonsil. This causes pain on lateral movement of the head. The patient may also have tender and enlarged cervical lymph nodes. Examination of the oropharynx reveals erythema of the anterior pillar and soft palate as well as a purulent tonsil on the side of the peritonsillar abscess. The tonsil is pushed inferomedially, and the uvula is shifted contralaterally (Flores, 2015).

Assessment and Diagnostic Findings

Emergency department (ED) physicians frequently are the providers who diagnose patients with peritonsillar abscesses. When this occurs in the ED setting, the ED physician decides whether aspiration—an invasive procedure—should be carried out based on the patient's clinical picture. Intraoral ultrasound and transcutaneous cervical ultrasound are used in the diagnosis of peritonsillar cellulitis and abscesses.

Medical Management

Antimicrobial agents and corticosteroid therapy are used for the treatment of peritonsillar abscess. Antibiotics (usually penicillin) are extremely effective in controlling the infection, and if they are prescribed early in the course of the disease, the abscess may resolve without needing to be incised. However, if the abscess does not resolve, treatment choices include needle aspiration, incision and drainage under local or general anesthesia, and drainage of the abscess with simultaneous tonsillectomy. Following needle aspiration (discussed later) intramuscular administration of clindamycin (Cleocin) can be used in the outpatient setting, thus reducing both antibiotic and hospital costs. The use of topical anesthetic agents and throat irrigations may be prescribed to promote comfort along with administration of prescribed analgesic agents.

Patients with complications require hospitalization for IV antibiotics, imaging studies, observation, and proper airway management. Rarely, the patient with a peritonsillar abscess presents with acute airway obstruction and requires immediate airway management. Procedures may include intubation, cricothyroidotomy, or tracheotomy (Flores, 2015).

Surgical Management

Needle aspiration may be preferred over a more extensive procedure due to its high efficacy, low cost, and patient tolerance. The mucous membrane over the swelling is first sprayed with a topical anesthetic and then injected with a local anesthetic. Single or repeated needle aspirations are performed to decompress the abscess. Alternatively, the abscess may be incised and drained. These procedures are performed best with the patient in the sitting position to make it easier to expectorate the pus and blood that accumulate in the pharynx. The patient experiences almost immediate relief. Incision and drainage is also an effective option but is more painful than needle aspiration.

Tonsillectomy is considered for patients who are poor candidates for needle aspiration or incision and drainage. The risk of hemorrhage following tonsillectomy to treat peritonsillar abscess is higher than that of elective tonsillectomy and may be due to the patient's previous use of aspirin for pain relief.

Nursing Management

If the patient requires intubation, cricothyroidotomy, or tracheotomy to treat airway obstruction, the nurse assists with the procedure and provides support to the patient before, during, and after the procedure. The nurse also assists with the needle aspiration when indicated.

The nurse encourages the patient to use prescribed topical anesthetic agents and assists with throat irrigations or the frequent use of mouthwashes or gargles, using saline or alkaline solutions at a temperature of 40.6°C to 43.3°C (105°F to 110°F). Gentle gargling after the procedure with a cool normal saline gargle may relieve discomfort. The patient must be upright and clearly expectorate forward. The nurse instructs the patient to gargle *gently* at intervals of 1 or 2 hours for 24 to 36 hours. Liquids that are cool or at room temperature are usually well tolerated. Adequate fluids must be provided to treat dehydration and prevent its recurrence.

The nurse also observes the patient for complications and instructs the patient about signs and symptoms of complications that require prompt attention by the patient's primary provider. At discharge, the nurse provides verbal and written instructions regarding foods to avoid, when to return to work, and the need to refrain from or cease smoking. The need for continuation of good oral hygiene is also reinforced.

Laryngitis

Laryngitis, an inflammation of the larynx, often occurs as a result of voice abuse or exposure to dust, chemicals, smoke, and other pollutants or as part of a URI. It also may be caused by isolated infection involving only the vocal cords. Laryngitis is also associated with gastroesophageal reflux (referred to as reflux laryngitis).

Laryngitis is very often caused by the pathogens that cause the common cold and pharyngitis; the most common cause is a virus, and laryngitis is often associated with allergic rhinitis or pharyngitis. Bacterial invasion may be secondary. The onset of infection may be associated with exposure to sudden temperature changes, dietary deficiencies, malnutrition, or an immunosuppressed state. Viral laryngitis is common in the winter and is easily transmitted to others.

Clinical Manifestations

Signs of acute laryngitis include hoarseness or **aphonia** (loss of voice) and severe cough. Chronic laryngitis is marked by persistent hoarseness. Other signs of acute laryngitis include sudden onset made worse by cold dry wind. The throat feels worse in the morning and improves when the patient is indoors in a warmer climate. At times, the patient presents with a dry cough and a dry, sore throat that worsens in the evening hours. If allergies are present, the uvula will be visibly edematous. Many patients also complain of a "tickle" in the throat that is made worse by cold air or cold liquids.

Medical Management

Management of acute laryngitis includes resting the voice, avoiding irritants (including smoking), resting, and inhaling cool steam or an aerosol. If the laryngitis is part of a more extensive respiratory infection caused by a bacterial organism or if it is severe, appropriate antibacterial therapy is instituted. The majority of patients recover with conservative treatment; however, laryngitis tends to be more severe in older adult patients and may be complicated by pneumonia.

For chronic laryngitis, the treatment includes resting the voice, eliminating any primary respiratory tract infection, eliminating smoking, and avoiding secondhand smoke.

Corticosteroids, such as beclomethasone, may be given. These preparations have few systemic or long-lasting effects and may reduce local inflammatory reactions. Treatment of reflux laryngitis typically involves use of proton pump inhibitors such as omeprazole (Prilosec) given once daily.

Nursing Management

The nurse instructs the patient to rest the voice and to maintain a well-humidified environment. If laryngeal secretions are present during acute episodes, expectorant agents are suggested, along with a daily fluid intake of 2 to 3 L to thin secretions. The nurse instructs the patient about the importance of taking prescribed medications, including proton pump inhibitors, and using continuous positive airway therapy at bedtime, if prescribed for OSA. In cases involving infection, the nurse informs the patient that the symptoms of laryngitis often extend a week to 10 days after completion of antibiotic therapy. The nurse instructs the patient about signs and symptoms that require contacting the primary provider. These signs and symptoms include loss of voice with sore throat that makes swallowing saliva difficult, hemoptysis, and noisy respirations. Continued hoarseness after voice rest or laryngitis that persists for longer than 5 days must be reported because of the possibility of malignancy.

NURSING PROCESS

The Patient With Upper Airway Infection

Assessment

A health history may reveal signs and symptoms of headache, sore throat, pain around the eyes and on either side of the nose, difficulty in swallowing, cough, hoarseness, fever, stuffiness, and generalized discomfort and fatigue. Determining when the symptoms began, what precipitated them, what if anything relieves them, and what aggravates them is part of the assessment. The nurse should also determine any history of allergy or the existence of a concomitant illness. Inspection may reveal swelling, lesions, or asymmetry of the nose as well as bleeding or discharge. The nurse inspects the nasal mucosa for abnormal findings such as increased redness, swelling, exudate, and nasal polyps, which may develop in chronic rhinitis. The mucosa of the nasal turbinates may also be swollen (boggy) and pale bluish-gray. The nurse palpates the frontal and maxillary sinuses for tenderness, which suggests inflammation and then inspects the throat by having the patient open the mouth wide and take a deep breath. Redness, asymmetry, or evidence of drainage, ulceration, or enlargement of the tonsils and pharynx is abnormal. Palpation of the neck lymph nodes for enlargement and tenderness is necessary.

Diagnosis

Nursing Diagnoses

Based on the assessment data, major nursing diagnoses may include the following:

- Ineffective airway clearance related to excessive mucus production secondary to retained secretions and inflammation

- Acute pain related to upper airway irritation secondary to an infection
- Impaired verbal communication related to physiologic changes and upper airway irritation secondary to infection or swelling
- Deficient fluid volume related to decreased fluid intake and increased fluid loss secondary to diaphoresis associated with a fever
- Deficient knowledge regarding prevention of URIs, treatment regimen, surgical procedure, or postoperative self care

COLLABORATIVE PROBLEMS/POTENTIAL COMPLICATIONS

Based on the assessment data, potential complications include:
- Sepsis
- Meningitis or brain abscess
- Peritonsillar abscess, otitis media, or rhinosinusitis

Planning and Goals

The major goals for the patient may include maintenance of a patent airway, relief of pain, maintenance of effective means of communication, normal hydration, knowledge of how to prevent upper airway infections, and absence of complications.

Nursing Interventions

MAINTAINING A PATENT AIRWAY

An accumulation of secretions can block the airway in patients with an upper airway infection. As a result, changes in the respiratory pattern occur and the work of breathing increases to compensate for the blockage. The nurse can implement several measures to loosen thick secretions or to keep the secretions moist so that they can be easily expectorated. Increasing fluid intake helps thin the mucus. The use of room vaporizers or steam inhalation also loosens secretions and reduces inflammation of the mucous membranes. To enhance drainage from the sinuses, the nurse instructs the patient about positioning; this depends on the location of the infection or inflammation. For example, drainage for rhinosinusitis or rhinitis is achieved in the upright position. In some conditions, topical or systemic medications, when prescribed, help relieve nasal or throat congestion.

PROMOTING COMFORT

URIs usually produce localized discomfort. In rhinosinusitis, pain may occur in the area of the sinuses, or a general headache may be produced. In pharyngitis, laryngitis, or tonsillitis, a sore throat occurs. The nurse encourages the patient to take analgesics, such as acetaminophen with codeine, as prescribed, to relieve this discomfort. A pain intensity rating scale (see Chapter 12) may be used to assess effectiveness of pain relief measures. Other helpful measures include topical anesthetic agents for symptomatic relief of herpes simplex blisters (see Chart 22-3) and sore throats, hot packs to relieve the congestion of rhinosinusitis and promote drainage, and warm water gargles or irrigations to relieve the pain of a sore throat. The nurse encourages rest to relieve the generalized discomfort and fever that accompany many upper airway conditions (especially rhinitis, pharyngitis, and laryngitis). For postoperative care after tonsillectomy and adenoidectomy, an ice collar may reduce swelling and decrease bleeding.

PROMOTING COMMUNICATION

Upper airway infections may result in hoarseness or loss of speech. The nurse instructs the patient to refrain from speaking as much as possible and, if possible, to communicate in writing instead. Additional strain on the vocal cords may delay full return of the voice. The nurse encourages the patient and family to use alternative forms of communication, such as a memo pad or a bell to signal for assistance.

ENCOURAGING FLUID INTAKE

Upper airway infections lead to fluid loss. Sore throat, malaise, and fever may interfere with a patient's willingness to eat and drink. The nurse provides a list of easily ingested foods to increase caloric intake during the acute phase of illness. These include soups, gelatin, pudding, yogurt, cottage cheese, high-protein drinks, water, ice, and ice pops. The nurse encourages the patient to drink 2 to 3 L of fluid per day during the acute stage of airway infection, unless contraindicated, to thin the secretions and promote drainage. Liquids (hot or cold) may be soothing, depending on the disorder.

PROMOTING HOME, COMMUNITY-BASED, AND TRANSITIONAL CARE

Educating Patients About Self-Care. Prevention of most upper airway infections is challenging because of the many potential causes. But because most URIs are transmitted by hand-to-hand contact, the nurse educates the patient and family about techniques to minimize the spread of infection to others, including implementing hand hygiene measures. The nurse advises the patient to avoid exposure to people who are at the risk for serious illness if respiratory infection is transmitted (older adults, immunosuppressed people, and those with chronic health problems).

The nurse instructs patients and their families about strategies to relieve symptoms of URIs and reinforces the need to complete the treatment regimen, particularly when antibiotics are prescribed.

Continuing and Transitional Care. Referral for home, community-based, or transitional care is rare. However, it may be indicated for people whose health status was compromised before the onset of the respiratory infection and for those who cannot manage self-care without assistance. In such circumstances, the home care nurse assesses the patient's respiratory status and progress in recovery. The nurse may advise older adult patients and those at increased risk from a respiratory infection to consider annual influenza and pneumococcal vaccination. A follow-up appointment with the primary provider may be indicated for patients with compromised health status to ensure that the respiratory infection has resolved.

MONITORING AND MANAGING POTENTIAL COMPLICATIONS

Although major complications of URIs are rare, the nurse must be aware of them and assess the patient for them. Because most patients with URIs are managed at home, patients and their families must be instructed to monitor for signs and symptoms and to seek immediate medical care if the patient's condition does not improve or if the patient's physical status appears to be worsening.

Sepsis or meningitis may occur in patients with compromised immune status or in those with an acute bacterial infection. The patient and caregiver are instructed to seek medical care if the patient's condition fails to improve within several days after the onset of symptoms, if unusual symptoms develop, or if the patient's condition deteriorates. They are instructed about signs and symptoms that require further attention: persistent or high fever, increasing shortness of breath, confusion, and increasing weakness and malaise. The patient with sepsis requires expert care to treat the infection, stabilize vital signs, and prevent or treat septic shock (see Chapter 14). Deterioration of the patient's condition necessitates intensive care measures (e.g., hemodynamic monitoring and administration of vasoactive medications, IV fluids, nutritional support, and corticosteroids) to monitor the patient's status and to support the patient's vital signs. High doses of antibiotics may be given to treat the causative organism. The nurse's role is to monitor the patient's vital signs, hemodynamic status, and laboratory values; administer needed treatment; alleviate the patient's physical discomfort; and provide explanations, education, and emotional support to the patient and family.

Peritonsillar abscess may develop after an acute infection of the tonsils. The patient requires treatment to drain the abscess and receives antibiotics for infection and topical anesthetic agents and throat irrigations to relieve pain and sore throat. Follow-up is necessary to ensure that the abscess resolves; tonsillectomy may be required. The nurse assists the patient in administering throat irrigations and instructs the patient and family about the importance of adhering to the prescribed treatment regimen and recommended follow-up appointments.

In some severe situations, peritonsillar abscess may progress to meningitis or brain abscess. The nurse assesses for changes in mental status ranging from subtle personality changes through drowsiness to coma, nuchal rigidity, and focal neurologic signs that signal increasing cerebral edema around the abscess (see Chapter 69). Seizures, typically tonic–clonic, occur in this setting. Intensive care measures are necessary. High doses of antibiotics may be used to treat the causative organism. The nurse's role is similar to caring for the patient with sepsis in an intensive care setting. The nurse monitors the patient's neurologic status and reports changes immediately.

Otitis media and rhinosinusitis may develop with URI. The patient and family are instructed about the signs and symptoms of otitis media and rhinosinusitis and about the importance of follow-up with the primary provider to ensure adequate evaluation and treatment of these conditions.

Evaluation

Expected patient outcomes may include the following:

1. Maintains a patent airway by managing secretions
   a. Reports decreased congestion
   b. Assumes best position to facilitate drainage of secretions
   c. Uses self-care measures appropriately and consistently to manage secretions during the acute phase of illness
2. Reports relief of pain and discomfort using pain intensity scale
   a. Uses comfort measures: analgesics, hot packs, gargles, rest
   b. Demonstrates adequate oral hygiene

3. Demonstrates ability to communicate needs, wants, level of comfort
4. Maintains adequate fluid and nutrition intake
5. Utilizes strategies to prevent upper airway infections and allergic reactions
   a. Demonstrates hand hygiene technique
   b. Identifies the value of the influenza vaccine
6. Demonstrates an adequate level of knowledge and performs self-care adequately
7. Becomes free of signs and symptoms of infection
   a. Exhibits normal vital signs (temperature, pulse, respiratory rate)
   b. Absence of purulent drainage
   c. Free of pain in ears, sinuses, and throat
   d. Absence of signs of inflammation
8. Absence of complications
   a. No signs of sepsis: fever, hypotension, deterioration of cognitive status
   b. Vital signs and hemodynamic status normal
   c. No evidence of neurologic involvement
   d. No signs of development of peritonsillar abscess
   e. Resolution of URI without development of otitis media or rhinosinusitis
   f. No signs and symptoms of brain abscess

OBSTRUCTION AND TRAUMA OF THE UPPER RESPIRATORY AIRWAY

Obstructive Sleep Apnea

OSA is a disorder characterized by recurrent episodes of upper airway obstruction and a reduction in ventilation. It is defined as cessation of breathing (**apnea**) during sleep usually caused by repetitive upper airway obstruction. The estimated prevalence of OSA is approximately 26% of adults between the ages of 30 and 70 years (Peppard, Young, Barnet, et al., 2013). It is believed that between 4% and 9% of women and 9% and 24% of men in the United States have OSA, and that up to 90% are not diagnosed; these increased rates have been linked to the increase in rates of obesity (Downey, 2015) (see Chapter 48). OSA interferes with people's ability to obtain adequate rest, thus affecting memory, learning, and decision making.

Risk factors for OSA include obesity, male gender, postmenopausal status, and advanced age. The major risk factor is obesity; a larger neck circumference and increased amounts of peripharyngeal fat narrow and compress the upper airway. Other associated factors include alterations in the upper airway, such as structural changes (e.g., tonsillar hypertrophy, abnormal posterior positioning of one or both jaws, and variations in craniofacial structures) that contribute to the collapsibility of the upper airway (Downey, 2015).

Pathophysiology

The pharynx is a collapsible tube that can be compressed by the soft tissues and structures surrounding it. The tone of the muscles of the upper airway is reduced during sleep. Mechanical factors such as reduced diameter of the upper airway or dynamic changes in the upper airway during sleep may result in obstruction. These sleep-related changes may predispose to upper airway collapse when small amounts of negative pressure are generated during inspiration.

Repetitive apneic events result in hypoxia (decreased oxygen saturation) and hypercapnia (increased concentration of carbon dioxide), which triggers a sympathetic response. As a consequence, patients with OSA have a high prevalence of hypertension. In addition, OSA is associated with an increased risk of myocardial infarction and stroke (cerebrovascular accident), which may be mitigated with appropriate treatment (Downey, 2015).

Clinical Manifestations

OSA is characterized by frequent and loud snoring with breathing cessation for 10 seconds or longer, for at least five episodes per hour, followed by awakening abruptly with a loud snort as the blood oxygen level drops. Patients with sleep apnea may have anywhere from five apneic episodes per hour to several hundred per night.

Classic signs and symptoms of OSA include the "3S's"—namely, snoring, sleepiness, and significant-other report of sleep apnea episodes. Common signs and symptoms of OSA are presented in Chart 22-4. Symptoms typically progress with increases in weight and aging (Downey, 2015). Patients are typically unaware of nocturnal upper airway obstruction during sleep. They frequently complain of insomnia, including difficulty in going to sleep, nighttime awakenings, and early morning awakenings with an inability to go back to sleep, as well as chronic fatigue and hypersomnolence (daytime sleepiness). When obtaining the health history, the nurse asks the patient about sleeping during normal activities such as eating or talking. Patients with this symptom are considered to have pathologic hypersomnolence (Downey, 2015).

Assessment and Diagnostic Findings

The diagnosis of sleep apnea is based on clinical features plus a polysomnographic finding (i.e., sleep study), which is the definitive test for OSA. The test is an overnight study,

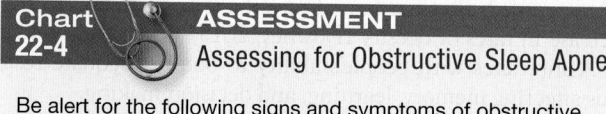

Chart 22-4 ASSESSMENT

Assessing for Obstructive Sleep Apnea

Be alert for the following signs and symptoms of obstructive sleep apnea:
- Excessive daytime sleepiness
- Frequent nocturnal awakening
- Insomnia
- Loud snoring
- Morning headaches
- Intellectual deterioration
- Personality changes, irritability
- Impotence
- Systemic hypertension
- Dysrhythmias
- Pulmonary hypertension, cor pulmonale
- Polycythemia
- Enuresis

Adapted from Downey, R. (2015). *Obstructive sleep apnea.*
Retrieved on 10/12/2015 at: www.emedicine.medscape.com/article/295807-overview

performed in a specialized sleep disorders center, which continuously measures multiple physiologic signals while the patient sleeps. These signals are analyzed as they are related to stages of sleep; measures include those taken by electroencephalogram (EEG), electro-oculogram, and chin electromyogram (EMG). In addition, cardiac rhythms and dysrhythmias are monitored with a single-lead electrocardiogram (ECG) and leg movements are recorded by an anterior tibialis EMG. Airflow at the nose and mouth is monitored using both a thermal sensor and a nasal pressure transducer, breathing effort is monitored using inductance plethysmography, and hemoglobin oxygen saturation is monitored by oximetry. The breathing pattern is analyzed for the presence of apneas and hypopneas. Characteristic findings consistent with OSA include apneic episodes occurring in the presence of respiratory muscle effort, clinically significant apneic episodes lasting 10 seconds or longer, and apneic episodes most prevalent during the rapid eye movement (REM) stage of sleep. Sleep disruption from automated patient arousal is usually seen at the termination of an episode of apnea (Downey, 2105).

Medical Management

Patients usually seek medical treatment because their sleeping partners express concern or because they experience excessive sleepiness at inappropriate times or settings (e.g., while driving a car). A variety of treatments are used. Weight loss, avoidance of alcohol, positional therapy (using devices that prevent patients from sleeping on their backs), and oral appliances such as mandibular advancement devices (MADs) are the first steps (American Sleep Apnea Association, 2015; Downey, 2015). When applied correctly, an MAD advances the mandible so that it is slightly anterior to the upper front teeth, preventing airway obstruction by the tongue and soft tissue during sleep. A randomized controlled trial that compared the effectiveness of these devices among patients with OSA with the more conventional therapy, continuous positive airway pressure (CPAP), found no difference in short-term outcomes between MAD and CPAP, including daytime sleepiness and quality of life, suggesting that MAD is as effective a treatment as CPAP in patients with mild-to-moderate OSA (White & Shafazan, 2013). In more severe cases involving hypoxemia and severe hypercapnia, the treatment includes CPAP or bilevel positive airway pressure (BiPAP) therapy with supplemental oxygen via nasal cannula. CPAP is used to prevent airway collapse, whereas BiPAP makes breathing easier and results in a lower average airway pressure. (The use of CPAP and BiPAP is discussed in more detail in Chapter 21.)

Surgical Management

Surgical procedures also may be performed to correct OSA. Simple tonsillectomy may be effective for patients with larger tonsils when deemed clinically necessary, or when other options have failed or are refused by patients (Morgan, 2015). Uvulopalatopharyngoplasty is the resection of pharyngeal soft tissue and removal of approximately 15 mm of the free edge of the soft palate and uvula. Effective in about 50% of patients, it is more effective in eliminating snoring than apnea. Nasal septoplasty may be performed for gross anatomic nasal septal deformities. Maxillomandibular surgery may be performed to advance the maxilla and mandible forward in order to enlarge the posterior pharyngeal region (Morgan, 2015). Tracheostomy relieves upper airway obstruction but has numerous adverse effects, including speech difficulties and increased risk of infections. These procedures, as well as other maxillofacial surgeries, are reserved for patients with concomitant cardiovascular disease and life-threatening dysrhythmias or severe disability who have not responded to conventional therapy (Tierney et al., 2015).

Pharmacologic Therapy

Some medications are useful in managing symptoms associated with OSA. Modafinil (Provigil) has been used to reduce daytime sleepiness (Downey, 2015). Protriptyline (Triptil) given at bedtime may increase the respiratory drive and improve upper airway muscle tone. Medroxyprogesterone acetate (Provera) and acetazolamide (Diamox) have been used for sleep apnea associated with chronic alveolar hypoventilation; however, their benefits have not been well established. The patient must understand that these medications are not a substitute for CPAP, BiPAP, or MAD. Administration of low-flow nasal oxygen at night can help relieve hypoxemia in some patients but has little effect on the frequency or severity of apnea.

Nursing Management

The patient with OSA may not recognize the potential consequences of the disorder. Therefore, the nurse explains the disorder in terms that are understandable to the patient and relates symptoms (daytime sleepiness) to the underlying disorder. The nurse also instructs the patient and family about treatments, including the correct and safe use of CPAP, BiPAP, MAD, and oxygen therapy, if prescribed. The nurse educates the patient about the risk of untreated OSA and the benefits of treatment approaches.

Epistaxis (Nosebleed)

Epistaxis, a hemorrhage from the nose, is caused by the rupture of tiny, distended vessels in the mucous membrane of any area of the nose. Rarely does epistaxis originate in the densely vascular tissue over the turbinates. Most commonly, the site is the anterior septum, where three major blood vessels enter the nasal cavity: (1) the anterior ethmoidal artery on the forward part of the roof (Kiesselbach plexus), (2) the sphenopalatine artery in the posterosuperior region, and (3) the internal maxillary branches (the plexus of veins located at the back of the lateral wall under the inferior turbinate).

Several risk factors are associated with epistaxis (see Chart 22-5).

Medical Management

Management of epistaxis depends on its cause and the location of the bleeding site. A nasal speculum, penlight, or headlight may be used to identify the site of bleeding in the nasal cavity. Most nosebleeds originate from the anterior portion of the nose. Initial treatment may include applying direct pressure. The patient sits upright with the head tilted forward to prevent swallowing and aspiration of blood and is directed

---

Chart 22-5 · RISK FACTORS — Epistaxis

- Local infections (vestibulitis, rhinitis, rhinosinusitis)
- Systemic infections (scarlet fever, malaria)
- Drying of nasal mucous membranes
- Nasal inhalation of corticosteroids (e.g., beclomethasone) or illicit drugs (e.g., cocaine)
- Trauma (digital trauma, blunt trauma, fracture, forceful nose blowing)
- Arteriosclerosis
- Hypertension
- Tumor (sinus or nasopharynx)
- Thrombocytopenia
- Use of aspirin
- Liver disease
- Rendu–Osler–Weber syndrome (hereditary hemorrhagic telangiectasia)

Adapted from Nguyen, Q. A. (2015). *Epistaxis*. Retrieved on 10/12/2015 at: www.emedicine.medscape.com/article/863220-overview

---

to pinch the soft outer portion of the nose against the midline septum for 5 or 10 minutes continuously. Application of nasal decongestants (phenylephrine, one or two sprays) to act as vasoconstrictors may be necessary. If these measures are unsuccessful in stopping the bleeding, the nose must be examined using good illumination and suction to determine the site of bleeding. Visible bleeding sites may be cauterized with silver nitrate or electrocautery (high-frequency electrical current). A supplemental patch of Surgicel or Gelfoam may be used (Tierney et al., 2015).

Alternatively, a cotton tampon may be used to try to stop the bleeding. Suction may be used to remove excess blood and clots from the field of inspection. The search for the bleeding site should shift from the anteroinferior quadrant to the anterosuperior, then to the posterosuperior, and finally to the posteroinferior area. The field is kept clear by using suction and by shifting the cotton tampon.

If the origin of the bleeding cannot be identified, the nose may be packed with gauze impregnated with petrolatum jelly or antibiotic ointment; a topical anesthetic spray and decongestant agent may be used before the gauze packing is inserted, or a balloon-inflated catheter may be used (see Fig. 22-3). Alternatively, a compressed nasal sponge may be used. Once the sponge becomes saturated with blood or is moistened with a small amount of saline, it will expand and produce tamponade to halt the bleeding. The packing may remain in place for 3 to 4 days if necessary to control bleeding (Nguyen, 2015). Antibiotics may be prescribed because of the risk of iatrogenic rhinosinusitis and sepsis.

Nursing Management

The nurse monitors the patient's vital signs, assists in the control of bleeding, and provides tissues and an emesis basin to allow the patient to expectorate any excess blood. It is common for patients to be anxious in response to a nosebleed. Blood loss on clothing and handkerchiefs can be frightening, and the nasal examination and treatment are uncomfortable. Assuring the patient in a calm, efficient manner that bleeding can be controlled can help reduce anxiety. The nurse

Figure 22-3 • Packing to control bleeding from the posterior nose. **A.** Catheter is inserted and packing is attached. **B.** Packing is drawn into position as the catheter is removed. **C.** Strip is tied over a bolster to hold the packing in place with an anterior pack installed "accordion pleat" style. **D.** Alternative method, using a balloon catheter instead of gauze packing.

continuously assesses the patient's airway and breathing as well as vital signs. On rare occasions, a patient with significant hemorrhage requires IV infusions of crystalloid solutions (normal saline) as well as cardiac and pulse oximetry monitoring.

Educating Patients About Self-Care

Once the bleeding is controlled, the nurse instructs the patient to avoid vigorous exercise for several days and to avoid hot or spicy foods and tobacco, because this may cause vasodilation and increase the risk of rebleeding. Discharge education includes reviewing ways to prevent epistaxis: avoiding forceful nose blowing, straining, high altitudes, and nasal trauma (including nose picking). Adequate humidification may prevent drying of the nasal passages. The nurse explains how to apply direct pressure to the nose with the thumb and the index finger for 15 minutes in the case of a recurrent nosebleed. If recurrent bleeding cannot be stopped, the patient is instructed to seek additional medical attention.

Nasal Obstruction

The passage of air through the nostrils is frequently obstructed by a deviation of the nasal septum, hypertrophy of the turbinate bones, or the pressure of nasal polyps. Chronic nasal congestion forces the patient to breathe through the mouth, thus producing dryness of the oral mucosa and associated problems including persistent dry, cracked lips. Patients with chronic nasal congestion often suffer from sleep deprivation due to difficulty maintaining an adequate airway while lying flat and during sleep.

Persistent nasal obstruction also may lead to chronic infection of the nose and result in frequent episodes of nasopharyngitis. Frequently, the infection extends to the nasal sinuses.

When rhinosinusitis develops and the drainage from these cavities is obstructed by deformity or swelling within the nose, pain is experienced in the region of the affected sinus.

Medical Management

The treatment of nasal obstruction requires the removal of the obstruction, followed by measures to treat whatever chronic infection exists. In many patients, an underlying allergy also requires treatment. Measures to reduce or alleviate nasal obstruction include nonsurgical as well as surgical techniques. Commonly used medications include nasal corticosteroids (see Table 22-2) as well as oral leukotriene inhibitors, such as montelukast. Treatment with nasal corticosteroids for 1 to 3 months is usually successful for the treatment of small polyps and may even reduce the need for surgical intervention. A short course of oral corticosteroids (6-day course of prednisone) may be beneficial in the treatment of nasal obstruction due to polyps (Tierney et al., 2015). Additional medications may include antibiotics for the treatment of underlying infection or antihistamines for the management of allergies. Hypertrophied turbinates may be treated by applying an astringent agent to shrink them.

A more aggressive approach in treating nasal obstruction caused by turbinate hypertrophy involves surgical reduction in the hypertrophy. Surgical procedures used to treat obstructive nasal conditions are collectively known as functional rhinoplasty. Technical advances with newer techniques provide a number of options for reconstruction and reshaping of the nose.

Nursing Management

When a surgical procedure is indicated, most often it is performed on an outpatient basis. The nurse explains the procedure to the patient. Postoperatively, the nurse elevates the head of the bed to promote drainage and to alleviate discomfort from edema. Frequent oral hygiene is encouraged to overcome dryness caused by breathing through the mouth. Before discharge from the outpatient or same-day surgical unit, the patient is instructed to avoid blowing the nose with force during the postoperative recovery period. The patient is also instructed about the signs and symptoms of bleeding and infection and when to contact the primary provider. The patient is provided with written postoperative instructions, including emergency phone numbers.

Fractures of the Nose

The location of the nose makes it susceptible to injury. Nasal fracture is the most common facial fracture and the most common fracture in the body (Becker, 2014). Fractures of the nose usually result from a direct assault. Nasal fractures may affect the ascending process of the maxilla and the septum. The torn mucous membrane results in a nosebleed. Complications include hematoma, infection, abscess, and avascular or septic necrosis. However, as a rule, serious consequences usually do not occur.

Clinical Manifestations

The signs and symptoms of a nasal fracture are pain, bleeding from the nose externally and internally into the pharynx, swelling of the soft tissues adjacent to the nose, periorbital ecchymosis, nasal obstruction, and deformity. The patient's nose may have an asymmetric appearance that may not be obvious until the edema subsides.

Assessment and Diagnostic Findings

The nose is examined internally to rule out the possibility that the injury may be complicated by a fracture of the nasal septum and a submucosal septal hematoma. Intranasal examination is performed in all cases to rule out septal hematoma (Tierney et al., 2015). Because of the swelling and bleeding that occur with a nasal fracture, an accurate diagnosis can be made only after the swelling subsides.

Clear fluid draining from either nostril suggests a fracture of the cribriform plate with leakage of cerebrospinal fluid. Usually, careful inspection or palpation discloses any deviations of the bone or disruptions of the nasal cartilages. An x-ray may reveal displacement of the fractured bones and may help rule out extension of the fracture into the skull.

Medical Management

A nasal fracture very often produces bleeding from the nasal passage. As a rule, bleeding is controlled with the use of packing. Cold compresses are used to prevent or reduce edema. For the patient who has sustained enough trauma to break the nose or any facial bone, the emergency medical team must consider the possibility of a cervical spine fracture. Therefore, it is essential to ensure a patent airway and to rule out a cervical spine fracture (see Chapter 68). Uncomplicated nasal fractures may be treated initially with antibiotics, analgesic agents, and a decongestant nasal spray.

Treatment of nasal fractures is aimed at restoring nasal function and returning the appearance of the nose to baseline. The patient is referred to a specialist to evaluate the need to realign the bones. Although improved outcomes are obtained when reduction in the fracture is performed during the first 3 hours after the injury, this is often not possible because of the edema. If immediate reduction in the fracture is not possible, it is performed within 3 to 7 days. Timing is important when treating nasal fractures because further delay in treatment may result in significant bone healing, which ultimately may require surgical intervention that includes rhinoplasty to reshape the external appearance of the nose. A septorhinoplasty is performed when the nasal septum needs to be repaired. In patients who develop a septal hematoma, the physician drains the hematoma through a small incision. A septal hematoma that is not drained can lead to permanent deformity of the nose.

Nursing Management

Immediately after the fracture, the nurse applies ice and encourages the patient to keep the head elevated. The nurse instructs the patient to apply ice packs to the nose to decrease swelling. The patient who experiences bleeding from the nose (epistaxis) is usually frightened and anxious and needs reassurance. The packing inserted to stop the bleeding may be uncomfortable and unpleasant, and obstruction of the nasal passages by the packing forces the patient to breathe through the mouth. This in turn causes the oral mucous membranes to become dry. Mouth rinses help to moisten the mucous membranes and to reduce the odor and taste of dried blood in the oropharynx and nasopharynx. The use of analgesic agents such as acetaminophen or NSAIDs (i.e., ibuprofen or naproxen) is encouraged. When removing the cotton pledgets, the nurse carefully inspects the mucosa for lacerations or a septal hematoma. The nurse instructs the patient to avoid sports activities for 6 weeks.

Laryngeal Obstruction

Obstruction of the larynx because of edema is a serious condition that may be fatal without swift, decisive intervention. The larynx is a stiff box that will not stretch. It contains a narrow space between the vocal cords (glottis), through which air must pass. Swelling of the laryngeal mucous membranes may close off the opening tightly, leading to life-threatening hypoxia or suffocation. Edema of the glottis occurs rarely in patients with acute laryngitis, occasionally in patients with urticaria, and more frequently in patients with severe inflammation of the throat, as in scarlet fever. It is an occasional cause of death in severe anaphylaxis (angioedema).

Hereditary angioedema is also characterized by episodes of life-threatening laryngeal edema. Laryngeal edema in people with hereditary angioedema can occur at any age, although young adults are at greatest risk. Some causes of laryngeal obstruction appear in Table 22-3.

Foreign bodies frequently are aspirated into the pharynx, the larynx, or the trachea and cause a twofold problem. First, they obstruct the air passages and cause difficulty in breathing, which may lead to asphyxia; later, they may be drawn farther down, entering the bronchi or a bronchial branch

TABLE 22-3 **Causes of Laryngeal Obstruction**

Precipitating Event	Mechanism of Obstruction
History of allergies; exposure to medications, latex, foods (peanuts, tree nuts [e.g., walnuts, pecans]), bee stings	Anaphylaxis
Foreign body	Inhalation/ingestion of meat or other food items, coin, chewing gum, balloon fragments, drug packets (ingested to avoid criminal arrest)
Heavy alcohol consumption; heavy tobacco use	Obstruction from tumor
Family history of airway problems	Suggests angioedema (type I hypersensitivity reaction)
Use of angiotensin-converting enzyme inhibitor	Increased risk of angioedema of the mucous membranes
Recent throat pain or recent fever	Infectious process
History of surgery or previous tracheostomy	Possible subglottic stenosis

Adapted from Reardon, R. F., Mason, P. E., & Clinton, J. E. (2014). Basic airway management and decision-making. In J. D. Roberts (Ed.). *Roberts & Hedges' clinical procedures in emergency medicine* (6th ed.). Philadelphia, PA: Elsevier Saunders.

and causing symptoms of irritation, such as a croupy cough, expectoration of blood or mucus, or labored breathing.

Clinical Manifestations

The patient's clinical presentation and x-ray findings confirm the diagnosis of laryngeal obstruction. The patient may demonstrate lowered oxygen saturation; however, normal oxygen saturation should not be interpreted as a sign that the obstruction is not significant. The use of accessory muscles to maximize airflow may occur and is often manifested by retractions in the neck or abdomen during inspirations. Patients who demonstrate these symptoms are at an immediate risk of collapse, and respiratory support (i.e., mechanical ventilation or positive-pressure ventilation) is considered.

Assessment and Diagnostic Findings

A thorough history can be very useful in diagnosing and treating the patient with a laryngeal obstruction. However, emergency measures to secure the patient's airway should not be delayed to obtain a history or perform tests. If possible, the nurse obtains a history from the patient or family about heavy alcohol or tobacco consumption, current medications, history of airway problems, recent infections, pain or fever, dental pain or poor dentition, and any previous surgeries, radiation therapy, or trauma.

Medical Management

Medical management is based on the initial evaluation of the patient and the need to ensure a patent airway. If the airway is obstructed by a foreign body and signs of asphyxia are apparent, immediate treatment is necessary. Emergent maneuvers to clear an airway obstruction were presented in Chart 21-6 in Chapter 21. If all efforts are unsuccessful, an immediate tracheotomy is necessary (see Chapter 21 for further discussion). If the obstruction is caused by edema resulting from an allergic reaction, treatment may include immediate administration of subcutaneous epinephrine and a corticosteroid (see Chapter 37). Ice may be applied to the neck in an effort to reduce edema. Continuous pulse oximetry is essential in the patient who has experienced acute upper airway obstruction.

Cancer of the Larynx

Cancer of the larynx accounts for approximately half of all head and neck cancers. The American Cancer Society (ACS, 2015) estimates that about 13,560 new cases and 3,640 deaths occur annually, with a 5-year relative survival rate that ranges from 32% to 90%, depending upon the location of the tumor and its stage at the time of diagnosis (ACS, 2015). Cancer of the larynx is most common in people older than 65 years and is four times more common in men (ACS, 2015) (see Chart 22-6).

Almost all malignant tumors of the larynx arise from the surface epithelium and are classified as squamous cell carcinoma. Approximately 55% of patients with laryngeal cancer present with involved lymph nodes at the time of diagnosis, with bilateral lesions present in 16% of patients (De Vita, Hellman, & Rosenberg, 2014). Recurrence occurs usually within the first 2 to 3 years after diagnosis. The presence

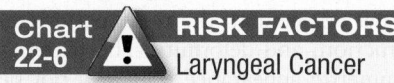

Chart 22-6 **RISK FACTORS**
Laryngeal Cancer

Carcinogens

- Tobacco (smoke, smokeless, e-cigarettes, hookahs)
- Combined effects of alcohol and tobacco
- Asbestos
- Secondhand smoke
- Paint fumes
- Wood dust
- Cement dust
- Chemicals
- Tar products
- Mustard gas
- Leather and metals

Other Factors

- Nutritional deficiencies (vitamins)
- History of alcohol abuse
- Genetic predisposition
- Age (higher incidence after 65 years of age)
- Gender (more common in men)
- Race (more prevalent in African Americans and Caucasians)
- Weakened immune system

Adapted from American Cancer Society. (2015). *What are the risk factors for laryngeal and hypopharyngeal cancers?* Retrieved on 3/9/2016 at: www.cancer.org/Cancer/LaryngealandHypopharyngealCancer/DetailedGuide/laryngeal-and-hypopharyngeal-cancer-risk-factors

of disease after 5 years is often secondary to a new primary malignancy. The incidence of distant metastasis with squamous cell carcinoma of the head and neck (including larynx cancer) is relatively low.

Clinical Manifestations

Hoarseness of more than 2 weeks' duration occurs in the patient with cancer in the glottic area because the tumor impedes the action of the vocal cords during speech. The voice may sound harsh, raspy, and lower in pitch. Affected voice sounds are not always early signs of subglottic or supraglottic cancer, however. The patient may complain of a persistent cough or sore throat and pain and burning in the throat, especially when consuming hot liquids or citrus juices. A lump may be felt in the neck. Later symptoms include dysphagia, dyspnea (difficulty breathing), unilateral nasal obstruction or discharge, persistent hoarseness, persistent ulceration, and foul breath. Cervical lymph adenopathy, unintentional weight loss, a general debilitated state, and pain radiating to the ear may occur with metastasis.

Assessment and Diagnostic Findings

An initial assessment includes a complete history and physical examination of the head and neck. This includes identification of risk factors, family history, and any underlying medical conditions. An indirect laryngoscopy, using a flexible endoscope, is initially performed in the otolaryngologist's office to visually evaluate the pharynx, larynx, and possible tumor. Mobility of the vocal cords is assessed; if normal movement is limited, the growth may affect muscle, other tissue, and even the airway. The lymph nodes of the neck and the thyroid gland are palpated for enlargement.

Diagnostic procedures that may be used include fine-needle aspiration (FNA) biopsy, a barium swallow, endoscopy, CT or MRI scan, and a positron emission tomography (PET) scan (ACS, 2015). FNA biopsy may be done as an initial screening procedure to obtain samples of any enlarged lymph nodes in the neck. A barium swallow may be done if the patient initially presents with a chief complaint of difficulty in swallowing, to outline any structural anomalies of the neck that could pinpoint a tumor. However, if a tumor of the larynx is suspected on an initial examination, a direct laryngoscopic examination is indicated. Laryngoscopy is performed under local or general anesthesia to evaluate all areas of the larynx. In some cases, intraoperative examination obtained by direct microscopic visualization and palpation of the vocal folds may yield a more accurate diagnosis. Samples of the suspicious tissue are obtained for analysis. It is rare for human papillomavirus (HPV) to be implicated with laryngeal cancers, although it is frequently implicated in oral cancers. Whether or not the tumor is positive for HPV does not have an effect on the course of treatment (ACS, 2015).

The classification, including stage of the tumor (i.e., size and histology of the tumor, presence and extent of cervical lymph node involvement) and location of the tumor serve as a basis for treatment. CT scanning and MRI are used to assess regional adenopathy and soft tissues and to stage and determine the extent of a tumor. MRI is also helpful in post-treatment follow-up to detect a recurrence. PET scanning may also be used to detect recurrence of the laryngeal tumor after treatment.

Medical Management

The goals of treatment of laryngeal cancer include cure; preservation of safe, effective swallowing; preservation of useful voice; and avoidance of permanent tracheostoma (Tierney et al., 2015). Treatment options include surgery, radiation therapy, and adjuvant chemoradiation therapy. The prognosis depends on the tumor location (i.e., supraglottic, glottis, and subglottic), as well as the tumor grade and stage (i.e., using the TNM system; see Chapter 15). The treatment plan also depends on whether the cancer is an initial diagnosis or a recurrence. In addition, before treatment begins, a complete dental examination is performed to rule out any oral disease. A consultation with a dental oncologist may be warranted. Any dental problems are resolved, if possible, before surgery and radiotherapy (ACS, 2015).

For patients with early-stage tumors (i.e., stages I and II) and lesions without lymph node involvement, external-beam radiation therapy or conservation surgery (i.e., less invasive surgery, such as vocal cord stripping or cordectomy) may be effective. Other indicated surgical procedures may include transoral endoscopic laser excision or partial laryngectomy (NCI, 2015). Patients with stage III and IV tumors that are resectable may be advised to have either total laryngectomies with or without postoperative radiation therapy or radiation therapy with concurrent adjuvant chemotherapy (with single-agent cisplatin) and surgical resection aimed at preserving some of the larynx (i.e., organ preservation surgery). Patients with late-stage tumors that extend through cartilage and into soft tissues are generally advised to have total laryngectomies with postoperative radiation therapy (NCI, 2015).

Patients should be educated so that they carefully consider the various side effects and complications associated with the different treatment modalities. The presence of lymph node involvement in the neck can affect the outcome. Supraglottic tumors metastasize early and bilaterally even when there appears to be no lymph node involvement at the time of diagnosis. When the neck lymph nodes are involved, the treatment includes surgery, chemoradiation, or both (Tierney et al., 2015).

Surgical Management

The overall goals for the patient undergoing surgical treatment include minimizing the effects of surgery on speech, swallowing, and breathing while maximizing the cure of the cancer. Several different curative procedures are available that can offer voice-sparing results while achieving a positive cure rate for the patient who has an early laryngeal carcinoma. Surgical options include vocal cord stripping, cordectomy, laser surgery, partial laryngectomy, or total laryngectomy (NCI, 2015).

Vocal Cord Stripping

Stripping of the vocal cord is used to treat dysplasia, hyperkeratosis, and leukoplakia and is often curative for these lesions. The procedure involves removal of the mucosa of the edge of the vocal cord, using an operating microscope. Early vocal cord lesions are initially treated with radiation therapy.

Cordectomy

Cordectomy, which is an excision of the vocal cord, is usually performed via transoral laser. This procedure is used for lesions limited to the middle third of the vocal cord. The resulting voice quality is related to the extent of tissue removed.

Laser Surgery

Laser microsurgery is well known to have several advantages for the treatment of early glottic cancers. Treatment and recovery are shorter, with fewer side effects, and treatment may be less costly than for other forms of therapy. Microelectrodes are useful for surgical resection of smaller laryngeal carcinomas. The carbon dioxide (CO_2) laser can be used for the treatment of many laryngeal tumors, with the exception of large vascular tumors. When compared with the results of other treatments for early laryngeal cancer, laser microsurgery is considered to be the method of choice based on patient outcomes (NCI, 2015).

Partial Laryngectomy

A partial laryngectomy (laryngofissure–thyrotomy) is often used for patients in the early stages of cancer in the glottic area when only one vocal cord is involved. The surgery is associated with a very high cure rate. It may also be performed for recurrence when high-dose radiation has failed. A portion of the larynx is removed, along with one vocal cord and the tumor; all other structures remain. The airway remains intact, and the patient is expected to have no difficulty swallowing. The voice quality may change, or the patient may sound hoarse.

Total Laryngectomy

Complete removal of the larynx (total **laryngectomy**) can provide a cure in most advanced laryngeal cancers, when the tumor extends beyond the vocal cords, or for cancer that recurs or persists after radiation therapy. In a total laryngectomy, the laryngeal structures are removed, including the hyoid bone, epiglottis, cricoid cartilage, and two or three rings of the trachea. The tongue, pharyngeal walls, and most of the trachea are preserved. A total laryngectomy results in permanent loss of the voice and a change in the airway, requiring a permanent tracheostomy (see Fig. 22-4). Occasionally, patients continue to have a laryngectomy tube in the stoma. Laryngectomy tubes are similar in appearance to tracheostomy tubes; however, a laryngectomy tube can be distinguished from a tracheostomy tube because the patient is unable to speak or breathe when the laryngectomy tube is occluded. Patients who have a total

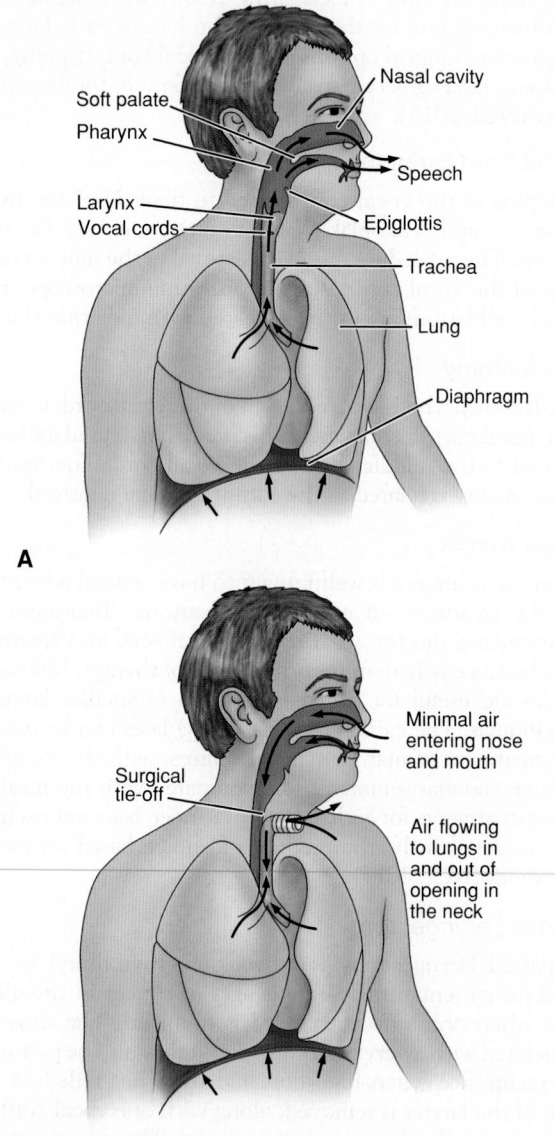

laryngectomy require alternatives to normal speech; these may include a prosthetic device, such as a Blom-Singer valve, to speak without aspirating (see later discussion).

Surgery is more difficult when the lesion involves the midline structures or both vocal cords. With or without neck dissection, a total laryngectomy requires a permanent tracheal stoma because the larynx that provides the protective sphincter is no longer present. The tracheal stoma prevents the aspiration of food and fluid into the lower respiratory tract. The patient has no voice but has normal swallowing. A total laryngectomy changes the manner in which airflow is used for breathing and speaking, as depicted in Figure 22-4. The patient has significant loss of the natural voice and the need to breathe through an opening (stoma) created in the lower neck. Complications that may occur include a salivary leak, wound infection from the development of a pharyngocutaneous fistula, stomal stenosis, and dysphagia secondary to esophageal stricture. In some cases, the patient may be a candidate for a near-total laryngectomy. In this situation, the patient would be a candidate for chemoradiation therapy regimens postoperatively. Voice preservation can be achieved in most cases and tends to be associated with overall improved quality of life (Aalia, 2014). Advances in surgical techniques for treating laryngeal cancer may minimize the cosmetic and functional deficits previously seen with total laryngectomy. Some microlaryngeal surgery can be performed endoscopically.

Radiation Therapy

The goal of radiation therapy is to eradicate the cancer and preserve the function of the larynx. The decision to use radiation therapy is based on several factors, including the staging of the tumor and the patient's overall health status, lifestyle (including occupation), and personal preference. Excellent results have been achieved with radiation therapy in patients with early-stage glottic tumors when only one vocal cord is involved and there is normal mobility of the cord (i.e., with phonation), as well as in small supraglottic lesions. One of the benefits of radiation therapy is that patients retain a near-normal voice. A few may develop chondritis (inflammation of the cartilage) or stenosis; a small number may later require laryngectomy.

Radiation therapy may also be used preoperatively to reduce the tumor size. Radiation therapy is combined with surgery in advanced laryngeal cancer as adjunctive therapy to surgery or chemotherapy and as a palliative measure.

Complications from radiation therapy are a result of external radiation to the head and neck area, which may also include the parotid gland, which is responsible for mucus production. Symptoms may include acute mucositis, ulceration of the mucous membranes, pain, **xerostomia** (dry mouth), loss of taste, dysphasia, fatigue, and skin reactions. Later complications may include laryngeal necrosis, edema, and fibrosis (see Chapter 15).

Speech Therapy

The patient who undergoes a laryngectomy and the patient's family face potentially complex challenges, including significant changes in the ability to communicate. To minimize anxiety and frustration on the part of the patient and family, the loss or alteration of speech is discussed with them.

Figure 22-4 • Total laryngectomy produces a change in airflow for breathing and speaking. **A.** Normal airflow. **B.** Airflow after total laryngectomy.

To plan postoperative communication strategies and speech therapy, the speech therapist or pathologist conducts a preoperative evaluation (ACS, 2015). During this time, the nurse discusses with the patient and family the methods of communication that will be available in the immediate postoperative period. These include writing, lip speaking and reading, and communication or word boards. A system of communication is established with the patient, family, nurse, and primary provider and is implemented consistently after surgery.

In addition, a long-term postoperative communication plan for **alaryngeal communication** is developed. The three most common techniques of alaryngeal communication are esophageal speech, artificial larynx (electric larynx), and tracheoesophageal puncture. Training in these techniques begins once medical clearance is obtained from the primary provider.

Esophageal Speech

The patient needs the ability to compress air into the esophagus and expel it, setting off a vibration of the pharyngeal esophageal segment for esophageal speech. The technique can be taught once the patient begins oral feedings, approximately 1 week after surgery. First, the patient learns to belch and is reminded to do so an hour after eating. Then, the technique is practiced repeatedly. Later, this conscious belching action is transformed into simple explosions of air from the esophagus for speech purposes. The speech therapist continues to work with the patient to make speech intelligible and as close to normal as possible. Because it takes a long time to become proficient, the success rate is low (ACS, 2015).

Artificial Larynx

If esophageal speech is not successful, or until the patient masters the technique, an electric larynx may be used for communication. This battery-powered apparatus projects sound into the oral cavity. When the mouth forms words (articulation), the sounds from the electric larynx become audible words. The voice that is produced sounds mechanical, and some words may be difficult to understand. The advantage is that the patient is able to communicate with relative ease while working to become proficient at either esophageal or tracheoesophageal puncture speech.

Tracheoesophageal Puncture

The third technique of alaryngeal speech is tracheoesophageal puncture (see Fig. 22-5). This technique for voice restoration is simple and has few complications. It is associated with high phonation success, good phonation quality, and steady long-term results. This technique is the most widely used because the speech associated with it most resembles normal speech (the sound produced is a combination of esophageal speech and voice), and it is easily achieved either during the initial surgery to treat the tumor or at a later date (ACS, 2015). A valve is placed in the tracheal stoma to divert air into the esophagus and out the mouth. Once the puncture is surgically created and has healed, a voice prosthesis (Blom-Singer) is fitted over the puncture site. A speech therapist teaches the patient how to produce sounds. Moving the tongue and lips to form the sound into words produces speech as before. To prevent airway obstruction, the prosthesis is removed and cleaned when mucus builds up.

Figure 22-5 • Schematic representation of tracheoesophageal puncture speech. Air travels from the lung through a puncture in the posterior wall of the trachea into the esophagus and out the mouth. A voice prosthesis is fitted over the puncture site.

NURSING PROCESS

The Patient Undergoing Laryngectomy

Assessment

The nurse obtains a health history and assesses the patient's physical, psychosocial, and spiritual domains. The health history focuses on the following symptoms: hoarseness, sore throat, dyspnea, dysphagia, and pain or burning in the throat. The physical assessment includes a thorough head and neck examination with an emphasis on the patient's airway. In addition, the neck and thyroid are palpated for swelling, nodularity, or adenopathy.

The nurse also assesses the patient's general state of nutrition, including height and weight and body mass index and reviews laboratory values that assist in determining the patient's nutritional status (albumin, protein, glucose, and electrolyte levels). If treatment includes surgery, the nurse must know the nature of the surgery to plan appropriate care. If the patient is expected to have no voice as a result of the surgical procedure, a preoperative evaluation by the speech therapist is essential. The patient's ability to hear, see, read, and write is assessed. Visual impairment and functional illiteracy may create additional problems with communication and may require creative approaches to ensure that the patient is able to communicate any needs. Because alcohol abuse is a risk factor for cancer of the larynx, the patient's pattern of alcohol intake must be assessed. Patients who are accustomed to daily consumption of alcohol are at the risk for alcohol withdrawal syndrome (delirium tremens) when alcohol intake is stopped suddenly. It is also not uncommon that patients are active smokers at the time of diagnosis; assessment of readiness for smoking cessation should be done, and nicotine replacements prescribed to avoid nicotine withdrawal, as indicated (NCI, 2015) (see Chapter 27: Promoting Cessation of Tobacco Use).

In addition, the nurse assesses the psychological readiness of the patient and family. The fear of a diagnosis of cancer is compounded by the possibility of permanent voice loss and, in some cases, some degree of disfigurement. The nurse evaluates the patient's and family's knowledge of the planned surgical procedure and expected postoperative course and assesses their coping methods and support systems. The nurse assesses the patient's spirituality needs based on the patient's individual preferences, beliefs, and culture.

Diagnosis

NURSING DIAGNOSES

Based on the assessment data, major nursing diagnoses may include the following:

- Deficient knowledge about the surgical procedure and postoperative course
- Anxiety related to the diagnosis of cancer and impending surgery
- Ineffective airway clearance related to excess mucus production secondary to surgical alterations in the airway
- Impaired verbal communication related to anatomic deficit secondary to removal of the larynx and to edema
- Imbalanced nutrition: less than body requirements, related to inability to ingest food secondary to swallowing difficulties
- Disturbed body image and low self-esteem secondary to major neck surgery, change in appearance, and altered structure and function
- Self-care deficit related to pain, weakness, fatigue, musculoskeletal impairment related to surgical procedure and postoperative course

COLLABORATIVE PROBLEMS/POTENTIAL COMPLICATIONS

Based on the assessment data, potential complications may include the following:

- Respiratory distress (hypoxia, airway obstruction, tracheal edema)
- Hemorrhage, infection, and wound breakdown
- Aspiration
- Tracheostomal stenosis

Planning and Goals

The major goals for the patient may include attainment of an adequate level of knowledge, reduction in anxiety, maintenance of a patent airway (patient is able to handle own secretions), effective use of alternative means of communication, attainment of optimal levels of nutrition and hydration, improvement in body image and self-esteem, improved self-care management, and absence of complications.

Nursing Interventions

PROVIDING PREOPERATIVE PATIENT EDUCATION

The diagnosis of laryngeal cancer often produces misconceptions and fears. Many people assume that loss of speech and disfigurement are inevitable with this condition. Once the primary provider explains the diagnosis and discusses treatment options with the patient and family, the nurse clarifies any misconceptions by identifying the location of the larynx, its function, the nature of the planned surgical procedure, and its effect on speech. Further, the patient's ability to sing, laugh, and whistle will be lost. Informational materials (written and audiovisual) about the surgery are given to the patient and family for review and reinforcement. If a complete laryngectomy is planned, the patient must understand that the natural voice will be lost, but that special training can provide a means for communicating. The patient needs to know that until training is started, communication will be possible by using the call light, by writing, or by using a communication device. The interdisciplinary team conducts an initial assessment of the patient and family. In addition to the nurse in charge of the patient's care and the primary provider, the team might include an advanced practice nurse (e.g., nurse practitioner), speech therapist, respiratory therapist, social worker, dietitian, and home care nurse. The services of a spiritual advisor are made available to the patient and family, as appropriate.

The nurse also reviews equipment and treatments for postoperative care with the patient and family, teaches important coughing and deep-breathing exercises, and helps the patient perform return demonstrations. The nurse clarifies the patient's role in the postoperative and rehabilitation periods. The family's needs must also be addressed because family members are often responsible for complex care of the patient in the home.

REDUCING ANXIETY

Because surgery of the larynx is performed most often for a malignant tumor, the patient may have many questions: Will the surgeon be able to remove all of the tumor? Is it cancer? Will I die? Will I choke? Will I suffocate? Will I ever speak again? What will I look like? Because of these and other questions, the psychological preparation of the patient is as important as the physical preparation.

Any patient undergoing surgery may have many fears. In laryngeal surgery, these fears may relate to the diagnosis of cancer and the possibility of permanent loss of the voice and disfigurement. The nurse provides the patient and family with opportunities to ask questions, verbalize feelings, and discuss perceptions. The nurse should address any questions and misconceptions the patient and family have. During the preoperative or postoperative period, a visit from someone who has had a laryngectomy may reassure the patient that people are available to assist and that rehabilitation is possible.

In the immediate postoperative period, the nurse attempts to build trust and reduce the patient's anxiety. Active listening provides an environment that promotes open communication and allows the patient to verbalize feelings. Clear instructions and explanations are given to the patient and family in a calm, reassuring manner. The nurse listens attentively, encourages the patient, and identifies and reduces environmental stressors. The nurse seeks to learn from the patient what activities promote feelings of comfort and assists the patient in such activities (e.g., listening to music, reading). Relaxation techniques such as guided imagery and meditation are often helpful. The nurse remains with the patient during episodes of severe anxiety and includes the patient in decision making.

MAINTAINING A PATENT AIRWAY

The nurse helps maintain a patent airway by positioning the patient in the semi-Fowler or Fowler position after recovery from anesthesia. This position decreases surgical edema and promotes lung expansion. Observing the patient for restlessness, labored breathing, apprehension, and increased pulse rate helps identify possible respiratory or circulatory problems. The nurse assesses the patient's lung sounds and reports changes that may indicate impending complications. Medications that depress respiration, particularly opioids, should be used cautiously. However, adequate use of analgesic medications is essential for pain relief because postoperative pain can result in shallow breathing and an ineffective cough (see Chapter 12 for discussion of pain management). The nurse encourages the patient to turn, cough, and take deep breaths. If necessary, suctioning may be performed to remove secretions, but disruption of suture lines must be avoided. The nurse also encourages and assists the patient with early ambulation to prevent atelectasis, pneumonia, and venous thromboemboli formation (e.g., pulmonary embolism and deep vein thrombosis). Pulse oximetry is used to monitor the patient's oxygen saturation level.

If a total laryngectomy was performed, a laryngectomy tube will most likely be in place. In some instances a laryngectomy tube is not used; in others it is used temporarily; and in many it is used permanently. The laryngectomy tube, which is shorter than a tracheostomy tube but has a larger diameter, is the patient's only airway. The care of this tube is similar to that for a tracheostomy tube (see Chapter 21). The nurse changes the inner cannula (if present) every 8 hours if it is disposable. Although nondisposable tubes are used infrequently, if one is used, the nurse cleans the inner cannula every 8 hours or more often as needed. If a tracheostomy tube without an inner cannula is used, humidification and suctioning of this tube are essential to prevent formation of mucus plugs. If a T-shaped laryngectomy tube is used, both sides of the T-tube should be suctioned to prevent obstruction due to copious secretions. The nurse should also use secure tracheostomy ties to prevent tube dislodgement. The nurse cleans the stoma daily with soap and water or another prescribed solution and a soft cloth or gauze, taking care to prevent water and soap or solution from entering the stoma. If a non–oil-based antibiotic ointment is prescribed, it is applied around the stoma and suture line. If crusting appears around the stoma, the crusts are removed with sterile tweezers and additional ointment is applied.

Wound drains, inserted during surgery, may be in place to assist in removal of fluid and air from the surgical site. Suction also may be used, but cautiously, to avoid trauma to the surgical site and incision. The nurse observes, measures, and records drainage. When drainage is less than 30 mL/day for 2 consecutive days, the surgeon usually removes the drains.

Frequently, the patient coughs up large amounts of mucus through this opening. Because air passes directly into the trachea without being warmed and moistened by the upper respiratory mucosa, the tracheobronchial tree compensates by secreting excessive amounts of mucus. Therefore, the patient has frequent coughing episodes and may develop a brassy-sounding, mucus-producing cough. The nurse reassures the patient that these problems will diminish in time as the tracheobronchial mucosa adapts to the altered physiology.

After the patient coughs, the tracheostomy opening must be wiped clean and clear of mucus. A simple gauze dressing, washcloth, or even paper towel (because of its size and absorbency) worn below the tracheostomy may serve as a barrier to protect the clothing from the copious mucus that the patient may initially expel.

One of the most important factors in decreasing cough, mucus production, and crusting around the stoma is adequate humidification of the environment. Mechanical humidifiers and aerosol generators (nebulizers) increase the humidity and are important for the patient's comfort. The laryngectomy tube may be removed when the stoma is well healed, within 3 to 6 weeks after surgery. The nurse teaches the patient how to clean and change the tube (see Chapter 21) and remove secretions.

PROMOTING ALTERNATIVE COMMUNICATION METHODS

Establishing an effective means of communication is usually the ultimate goal in the rehabilitation of the laryngectomy patient. To understand and anticipate the patient's postoperative needs, the nurse works with the patient, speech therapist, and family to encourage the use of alternative communication methods. These means of communication are established preoperatively and must be used consistently by all personnel who come in contact with the patient postoperatively. The patient is now unable to use an intercom system. A call bell or hand bell must be placed within easy reach of the patient. In the immediate postoperative period, a handheld communication device like a Magic Slate can be used for communication; as alternatives, electronic tablets, notebooks, and smart phones can be used if the patient has any of these devices. If the patient cannot write, a picture-word-phrase board or hand signals can be used. The nurse documents which hand is the patient's dominant hand (e.g., used for writing) so that the opposite arm can be used for IV infusions. (To ensure the patient's privacy, the nurse discards notes used for communication.)

Writing everything or communicating through gestures can be very time consuming and frustrating. The patient must be given adequate time to communicate their needs. The patient may become impatient and angry when not understood.

PROMOTING ADEQUATE NUTRITION AND HYDRATION

Postoperatively, the patient may not be permitted to eat or drink for at least 7 days (Kishikova & Fleming, 2014). Alternative sources of nutrition and hydration include IV fluids, enteral feedings through a nasogastric or gastrostomy tube, and parenteral nutrition (see Chapter 44).

When the patient is ready to start oral feedings, a speech therapist or radiologist may conduct a swallow study (a video fluoroscopy radiology procedure) to evaluate the patient's risk of aspiration. Once the patient is cleared for oral feedings, the nurse explains that thick liquids will be used first because they are easy to swallow. Different swallowing maneuvers are attempted with various food consistencies. Once the patient is cleared for food intake, the nurse stays with the patient during initial oral feedings and keeps a suction setup at the bedside for needed suctioning. The nurse instructs the patient to avoid sweet foods, which increase salivation and suppress the appetite. Solid foods are introduced as tolerated. The patient is instructed to rinse the mouth with warm water or mouthwash after oral feedings and to brush the teeth frequently.

Because taste and smell are so closely related, taste sensations are altered for a while after surgery because inhaled air passes directly into the trachea, bypassing the nose and the olfactory end organs. In time, however, the patient usually accommodates to this change and olfactory sensation adapts, often with return of interest in eating. The nurse observes the patient for any difficulty in swallowing, particularly when eating resumes, and reports its occurrence to the primary provider.

The patient's weight and laboratory data are monitored to ensure that nutritional and fluid intake are adequate. In addition, skin turgor and vital signs are assessed for signs of decreased fluid volume.

PROMOTING POSITIVE BODY IMAGE AND SELF-ESTEEM

Disfiguring surgery and an altered communication pattern are threats to a patient's body image and self-esteem. The reaction of family members and friends is a major concern for the patient. The nurse encourages the patient to express feelings about the changes brought about by surgery, particularly feelings related to fear, anger, depression, and isolation. Encouraging the use of previous effective coping strategies may be helpful. Referral to a support group, such as the International Association of Laryngectomees (IAL), WebWhispers, and I Can Cope (through the ACS) may help the patient and family deal with the changes in their lives. Information about these support groups can be found in the Resource section at the end of the chapter.

PROMOTING SELF-CARE MANAGEMENT

A positive approach along with promotion of self-care activities is important when caring for the patient. The patient should begin participating in self-care activities as soon as possible. The nurse assesses the patient's readiness for decision making and encourages the patient to participate actively in performing care. The nurse provides positive reinforcement when the patient makes an effort in self-care. The nurse needs to be a good listener and a support to the family, especially when explaining the tubes, dressings, and drains that are in place postoperatively.

MONITORING AND MANAGING POTENTIAL COMPLICATIONS

The potential complications after laryngectomy include respiratory distress and hypoxia, hemorrhage, infection, wound breakdown, aspiration, and tracheostomal stenosis.

Respiratory Distress and Hypoxia. The nurse monitors the patient for signs and symptoms of respiratory distress and hypoxia, particularly restlessness, irritation, agitation, confusion, tachypnea, the use of accessory muscles, and decreased oxygen saturation on pulse oximetry (SpO_2). Any change in respiratory status requires immediate intervention. Hypoxia may cause restlessness and an initial rise in blood pressure; this is followed by hypotension and somnolence. Cyanosis is a late sign of hypoxia. Obstruction needs to be ruled out immediately by suctioning and by having the patient cough and breathe deeply. Hypoxia and airway obstruction, if not treated immediately, are life threatening.

Other nursing measures include repositioning of the patient to ensure an open airway and administering oxygen as prescribed. Oxygen is used with caution in patients with chronic obstructive pulmonary disease. The nurse should always be prepared for possible intubation and mechanical ventilation. The nurse must be knowledgeable about the hospital's emergency code protocols and skilled in the use of emergency equipment. The nurse must remain with the patient at all times during respiratory distress and initiate a call to the rapid response team as necessary.

Hemorrhage. Bleeding from the drains at the surgical site or with tracheal suctioning may signal the occurrence of hemorrhage. The nurse promptly notifies the surgeon of any active bleeding, which can occur at a variety of sites, including the surgical site, drains, and trachea. Rupture of the carotid artery is especially dangerous. Should this occur, the nurse must apply direct pressure over the artery, summon assistance, and provide emotional support to the patient until the vessel is ligated. The nurse monitors vital signs for changes, particularly increased pulse rate, decreased blood pressure, and rapid deep respirations. Cold, clammy, pale skin may indicate active bleeding. IV fluids and blood components may be given and other measures implemented to prevent or treat hemorrhagic shock. (Management of the patient with shock is discussed in detail in Chapter 14.)

Infection. The nurse monitors the patient for signs of postoperative infection. These include an increase in temperature and pulse, a change in the type of wound drainage, and increased areas of redness or tenderness at the surgical site. Other signs include purulent drainage, odor, and increased wound drainage. The nurse monitors the patient's white blood cell (WBC) count; a rise in WBCs may indicate the body's effort to combat infection. In older adult patients, infection can be present without an increase in the patient's WBC count; therefore, the nurse must monitor the patient for more subtle signs, such as lethargy, weakness, and decreased appetite. WBCs are suppressed in the patient with decreased immune function (e.g., patients receiving chemotherapy or radiation therapy); this predisposes the patient to a severe infection and sepsis. Antimicrobial (antibiotic) medications must be given as scheduled. All suspicious drainage is cultured, and the patient may be placed on the appropriate infection prevention precautions. Strategies are implemented to minimize the exposure of the patient to microorganisms and their spread to others. The nurse reports any significant change in the patient's status to the surgeon.

Wound Breakdown. Wound breakdown caused by infection, poor wound healing, development of a fistula, radiation therapy, or tumor growth can create a life-threatening emergency. The carotid artery, which is close to the stoma, may rupture from erosion if the wound does not heal properly. The nurse observes the stoma area for wound breakdown, hematoma, and bleeding and reports their occurrence to the surgeon. If wound breakdown occurs, the patient must be monitored carefully and identified as at high risk for carotid hemorrhage.

Aspiration. The patient who has undergone a laryngectomy is at the risk for aspiration and aspiration pneumonia due to depressed cough, the sedating effects of anesthetic and analgesic medications, alteration in the airway, impaired swallowing, and the administration of tube feedings. The nurse assesses for the presence of nausea and administers antiemetic medications, as prescribed. The nurse keeps a suction setup available in the hospital and instructs the family to do so at home for use if needed. Patients receiving tube feedings are positioned with the head of the bed at 30° or higher during feedings and for 30 to 45 minutes after tube feedings. Patients receiving oral feedings are positioned with the head of the bed in an upright position for 30 to 45 minutes after feedings. For patients with a nasogastric or gastrostomy tube, the placement of the tube and residual gastric volume must be checked before each feeding. High amounts of residual volume (greater than 50% of previous intake) indicate delayed gastric emptying; this can lead to reflux and aspiration (Tierney, et al., 2015). Signs or symptoms of aspiration are reported to the primary provider immediately.

Tracheostomal Stenosis. Tracheostomal stenosis is an abnormal narrowing of the trachea or the tracheostomy stoma. Infection at the stoma site, excessive traction on the tracheostomy tube by the connecting tubing, and persistent high tracheostomy cuff pressure are risk factors for tracheostomal stenosis. The incidence of this condition varies widely, and it is often preventable. The nurse assesses the patient's stoma for signs and symptoms of infection and reports any evidence of this to the primary provider immediately. Tracheostomy care is performed routinely. The nurse assesses the connecting tubing (e.g., ventilation tubing) and secures the tubing to avoid excessive traction on the patient's tracheostomy. The nurse ensures that the tracheostomy cuff is deflated (for a patient with a cuffed tube) except for short periods, such as when the patient is eating or taking medications.

PROMOTING HOME, COMMUNITY-BASED, AND TRANSITIONAL CARE

Educating Patients About Self-Care. The nurse has an important role in the recovery and rehabilitation of the patient who has had a laryngectomy. To facilitate the patient's ability to manage self-care, discharge instruction begins as soon as the patient is able to participate. Nursing care and patient education in the hospital, outpatient setting, and rehabilitation or long-term care facility must take into consideration the many emotions, physical changes, and lifestyle changes experienced by the patient. In preparing the patient to go home, the nurse assesses the patient's readiness to learn and the level of knowledge about self-care management. The nurse also reassures the patient and family that most self-care management strategies can be mastered. The patient needs to learn a variety of self-care behaviors, including tracheostomy and stoma care, wound care, and oral hygiene. The nurse also instructs the patient about the need for adequate dietary intake, safe hygiene, and recreational activities.

Tracheostomy and Stoma Care. The nurse provides specific instructions to the patient and family about what to expect with a tracheostomy and its management. The nurse instructs the patient and caregiver how to perform suctioning and emergency measures and tracheostomy and stoma care. The nurse stresses the importance of humidification at home and instructs the family to obtain and set up a humidification system before the patient returns home. (See Chapter 21 for details about tracheostomy care.)

Hygiene and Safety Measures. The nurse instructs the patient and family about safety precautions that are needed because of the changes in structure and function resulting from the surgery. Special precautions are needed in the shower to prevent water from entering the stoma. Wearing a loose-fitting plastic bib over the tracheostomy or simply holding a hand over the opening is effective. Swimming is not recommended because a person with a laryngectomy can drown without submerging their face. Barbers and beauticians need to be alerted so that hair sprays, loose hair, and powder do not get near the stoma, because they can block or irritate the trachea and possibly cause infection. These self-care points are summarized in Chart 22-7.

The nurse educates the patient and caregiver about the signs and symptoms of infection and identifies indications that require contacting the primary provider after discharge. A discussion regarding cleanliness and infection control behaviors is essential. The nurse educates the patient and family to use hand hygiene before and after caring for the tracheostomy, to use tissues to remove mucus, and to dispose of soiled dressings and equipment properly. If the patient's surgery included cervical lymph node dissection, the nurse instructs the patient about how to perform exercises to strengthen the shoulder and neck muscles.

Recreation and exercise are important for the patient's well-being and quality of life, and all but very strenuous exercise can be enjoyed safely. Avoidance of strenuous exercise and fatigue is important because the patient will have more difficulty speaking when tired, which can be discouraging. Additional safety points to address include the need for the patient to wear or carry medical identification, such as a bracelet or card, to alert medical personnel to the special requirements for resuscitation should this need arise. If resuscitation is needed, direct mouth-to-stoma ventilation should be performed. For home emergency situations, prerecorded emergency messages for police, the fire department, or other rescue services can be kept near the phone to be used quickly.

The nurse instructs and encourages the patient to perform oral care frequently to prevent halitosis and infection. If the patient is receiving radiation therapy, synthetic saliva may be required because of decreased saliva production. Patients receiving radiation therapy frequently report dry mouth, change in taste, lack of appetite, and mouth sores (Haisfield-Wolfe, Brown, Richardson, et al., 2015) (see Chart 22-8). The nurse instructs the patient to drink water or sugar-free liquids throughout the day and to use a humidifier at home. Brushing the teeth or dentures and rinsing the mouth several times a day will assist in maintaining proper oral hygiene.

Continuing and Transitional Care. Referral for home, community-based, or transitional care is an important aspect of postoperative care for the patient who has had a laryngectomy and will assist the patient and family in the discharge home. The nurse assesses the patient's general health status and the ability of the patient and family to care for the stoma and tracheostomy. The surgical incisions, nutritional and respiratory status, and adequacy of pain management are also assessed. The nurse assesses for signs and symptoms of complications and the patient's and family's knowledge of signs and symptoms to be reported to the physician. During the home visit, the nurse identifies and addresses other learning needs and concerns of the patient and family, such as adaptation to physical, lifestyle, and functional changes, as well as the patient's progress with learning and using new communication strategies. The nurse assesses the patient's psychological status, reinforces previous instructions, and provides reassurance and support to the patient and family caregivers as needed.

Chart 22-7 HOME CARE CHECKLIST
The Patient With a Laryngectomy

At the completion of education, the patient and/or caregiver will be able to:

- Name the procedure that was performed and identify any permanent changes in anatomic structure or function as well as changes in ADLs, IADLs, communication, roles, relationships, and spirituality.
- State the name, dose, side effects, frequency, and schedule for all medications.
- Identify interventions and strategies (e.g., durable medical equipment, oxygen, nebulizer, humidifier) used in adapting to any permanent changes in structure or function.
- Describe ongoing postoperative therapeutic regimen, including stoma care, diet, and activities to perform (e.g., shoulder and neck exercises if a node dissection was performed) and to limit or avoid (e.g., swimming and contact sports).
  - Demonstrate tracheostomy care and tracheal suctioning to clear the airway and handle secretions.
  - Explain the rationale for maintaining adequate humidification with a humidifier or nebulizer.
  - Demonstrate how to clean the skin around the stoma and how to use ointments and tweezers to remove encrustations.
  - State the rationale for wearing a loose-fitting protective cloth at the stoma and covering the stoma when showering or bathing.
  - Discuss the need to avoid sprays, powders, particulates, and cold air from air-conditioning and the environment to prevent irritation of the airway.
  - Demonstrate safe technique in changing the laryngectomy/tracheostomy tube.
  - Identify fluid and caloric needs.

- Describe mouth care and discuss its importance.
- Identify the signs and symptoms of wound infection and state what to do about them.
- Describe safety or emergency measures to implement in case of breathing difficulty or bleeding.
- State the rationale for wearing or carrying special medical identification and ways to obtain help in an emergency.
- Demonstrate alternative communication methods.
- Relate how to reach primary provider with questions or to report complications.
- State time and date of follow-up appointments.
- Obtain an annual influenza vaccine, and discuss vaccination against pneumonia with the primary provider.
- State understanding of community resources, support groups and referrals (if any).
- Identify the need for health promotion (e.g., weight reduction, smoking cessation, and stress management), disease prevention and screening activities.

Resources

In student resources for Chapter 21 at thepoint.lww.com/Brunner 14e, see Procedural Guidelines: Care of the Patient With a Tracheostomy Tube and Procedural Guidelines: Performing Tracheal Suction.

See Chapter 10, Chart 10-8 for additional information related to durable medical equipment, adaptive equipment, mobility skills, skin, bowel, and bladder care.

ADL, activities of daily living; IADL, independent activities of daily living.

The person who has had a laryngectomy should have regular physical examinations and seek advice concerning any problems related to recovery and rehabilitation. The nurse reminds the patient to participate in health promotion activities and health screening and about the importance of keeping scheduled appointments with the physician, speech therapist, and other health care providers.

Evaluation

Expected patient outcomes may include the following:

1. Demonstrates an adequate level of knowledge, verbalizing an understanding of the surgical procedure and performing self-care adequately
2. Demonstrates less anxiety
   a. Expresses a sense of hope
   b. Is aware of available community organizations and agencies that provide patient education and support groups
   c. Participates in support group for people with a laryngectomy
3. Maintains a clear airway and handles own secretions; also demonstrates practical, safe, and correct technique for cleaning and changing the tracheostomy or laryngectomy tube
4. Acquires effective communication techniques
   a. Uses assistive devices and strategies for communication (Magic Slate, call bell, picture board, sign language, speech reading, handheld electronic devices)

   b. Follows the recommendations of the speech therapist
   c. Demonstrates ability to communicate with new communication strategy
   d. Reports availability of prerecorded messages to summon emergency assistance by telephone
5. Maintains adequate nutrition and adequate fluid intake
6. Exhibits improved body image, self-esteem, and self-concept
   a. Expresses feelings and concerns
   b. Participates in self-care and decision making
   c. Accepts information about support group
7. Adheres to rehabilitation and home care program
   a. Practices recommended speech therapy
   b. Demonstrates proper methods for caring for stoma and laryngectomy or tracheostomy tube (if present)
   c. Verbalizes understanding of symptoms that require medical attention
   d. States safety measures to take in emergencies
   e. Performs oral hygiene as prescribed
8. Absence of complications
   a. Demonstrates a patent airway
   b. No bleeding from surgical site and minimal bleeding from drains; vital signs (blood pressure, temperature, pulse, respiratory rate) are normal
   c. No redness, tenderness, or purulent drainage at surgical site
   d. No wound breakdown

Chart 22-8

NURSING RESEARCH PROFILE

Patterns of Symptom Severity of Patients With Cancer of the Head and Neck

Haisfield-Wolfe, M. E., Brown, C., Richardson, M. et al. (2015). Variations in symptom severity patterns among oropharyngeal and laryngeal cancer outpatients during radiation treatment: A pilot study. *Cancer Nursing, 38*(4), 279–287.

Purpose

Patients diagnosed with laryngeal and oropharyngeal cancer (head and neck cancer [HNC]) commonly receive radiotherapy (RT) treatment on an outpatient basis. Patients with HNC who receive RT treatment commonly experience disturbing symptoms that include pain, difficulty swallowing, dry mouth, change in taste, lack of appetite, and mouth sores. While it is known that these patients tend to experience these symptoms, the patterns and severity of these symptoms are unknown. This pilot study aimed to identify the individual symptom patterns that patients with HNC experience over the course of 6 weeks of RT treatment.

Design

This was a secondary study derived from a parent study that examined symptoms patients with HNC experience when RT therapy is initiated. The study sites included two university-affiliated outpatient cancer centers located in the eastern United States. There were 21 patients with HNC who consented to participate in this study. Eligible participants were at least 18 years of age, with a new diagnosis of HNC, receiving RT treatment, and able to speak and write English. Sampling yielded 21 participants, 5 with laryngeal cancer, and 16 with oropharyngeal cancer. The Memorial Symptom Assessment Scale, a validated and reliable Likert scale survey that measures 32 symptoms associated with cancer treatment, was used to measure participants' symptoms during RT treatment at the time of midtreatment (week 5), end of treatment (week 9), and 6 weeks post-treatment

(week 12). Visual graphical analysis was performed to find patterns of symptoms.

Findings

Participants reported variability in symptoms they experienced over time. The most common symptom experienced was pain; peak pain severity was commonly reported by participants, with no detectable pattern based upon study time points. Difficulty swallowing frequently accompanied pain. The other four symptoms of dry mouth, mouth sores, change in taste, and lack of appetite, along with difficulty swallowing, were commonly experienced during midtreatment and at treatment completion. Three patterns were identified. The first pattern noted increase in symptom severity after RT treatment initiation and declined in severity by midtreatment. The second pattern revealed increase in severity of symptoms post-treatment. The last pattern revealed symptom severity that persisted from RT treatment initiation to the post-treatment period. The small sample size precluded conducting inferential statistical analysis.

Nursing Implications

Findings from this study confirm that patients diagnosed with HNC and who receive RT treatment commonly experience the symptoms of pain, difficulty swallowing, dry mouth, change in taste, lack of appetite, and mouth sores. However, patients' symptoms varied in this pilot both in terms of intensity and patterns over the course of RT treatment. Therefore, nurses should assess patients' symptoms and provide individualized plans of care. In particular, participants in this study reported peak pain intensity at different time points during RT treatment, suggesting that patients with HNC require frequent pain assessment, reassessment, and implementation of proactive preventive pain management strategies.

---

e. Clear breath sounds; oxygen saturation level within acceptable range; chest x-ray clear
f. No indications of infection, stenosis, or obstruction of tracheal stoma

CRITICAL THINKING EXERCISES

1 **pq** A 20-year-old female college student comes to the student health clinic with complaints of a terrible sore throat with difficulty swallowing and opening her mouth; in addition, she appears to be drooling. She states that she has had a fever lasting several days. What further questions do you have regarding her symptoms? What is your priority focus for your physical examination? What diagnostic tests and treatments may you anticipate?

2 **ebp** A 65-year-old man presents to the family health clinic for a follow-up visit to check his blood pressure (BP), which has been generally high and difficult to control with antihypertensive medications. The patient is obese, with a body mass index of 38. In addition to his elevated BP, he also reports falling asleep during the day and not feeling like he has slept when he wakes up. You

suspect that this patient may have OSA. What risk factors for OSA will your health history focus on? What are the common signs and symptoms of OSA? Describe how a patient with OSA is diagnosed and the treatment(s) that might be prescribed. What is the strength of the evidence that commonly prescribed therapies (such as CPAP) may be effective in alleviating symptoms and improving quality of life for patients with OSA?

3 **pq** You are attending a family reunion where a lively game of soccer is taking place. Two players collide and one falls to the ground holding his nose. You suspect that the injured player on the ground has a fractured nose. Briefly describe what you would do in this situation. What are your priority assessments? What are the signs and symptoms of a fractured nose? What are your priority interventions?

4 At the family practice clinic where you work, you are assessing a patient who reports having had a cold about ten days ago. Most of her symptoms have abated, but she is now complaining of a severe headache over the front of her face and a fever of 38.9^0 C (102^0 F). She states that the pain increases when she bends over to pick up something off the floor. What further questions do you have regarding her symptoms? What will you focus on during your physical assessment? Briefly, describe the treatment you anticipate could be prescribed for this patient.

REFERENCES

*Asterisk indicates nursing research.

Books

Bickley, L. S., & Szilagyi, P. G. (2013). *Bates' guide to physical examination and history taking* (11th ed.). Philadelphia, PA: Lippincott Williams & Wilkins.

De Vita, V., Hellman, S., & Rosenberg, S. (Eds.). (2014). *Cancer: Principles and practice of oncology* (10th ed.). Philadelphia, PA: Lippincott Williams & Wilkins.

Reardon, R. F., Mason, P. E., & Clinton, J. E. (2014). Basic airway management and decision-making. In J. D. Roberts (Ed.): *Roberts & Hedges' clinical procedures in emergency medicine* (6th ed.). Philadelphia, PA: Elsevier Saunders.

Tierney, L., McPhee, S. J., & Papadakis, M. (Eds.). (2015). *Current medical diagnosis and treatment* (54th ed.). New York: McGraw-Hill.

Journals and Electronic Documents

Aalia, E. (2014). *Total laryngectomy.* Retrieved on 10/12/2015 at: www.emedicine.medscape.com/article/2051731-overview

Aljubran, S., & Lockey, R. F. (2014). *Aeroallergens.* Retrieved on 3/9/2016 at www.emedicine.medscape.com/article/137911-overview

American Academy of Otolaryngology. (2015). *Fact sheet: Sinusitis: Special considerations for aging patients.* Retrieved on 10/8/2015 at: www.entnet.org/content/sinusitis-special-considerations-aging-patients

American Cancer Society. (2015). *What are the risk factors for laryngeal and hypopharyngeal cancers?* Retrieved on 3/9/2016 at: www.cancer.org/Cancer/LaryngealandHypopharyngealCancer

American Sleep Apnea Association. (2015). *Obstructive sleep apnea.* Available at: www.sleepapnea.org/learn/sleep-apnea/obstructive-sleep-apnea.html

Becker, D. (2014). *Nasal and septal fractures.* Retrieved on 10/12/2015 at: www.emedicine.medscape.com/article/878595-overview

Brook, I. (2015). *Chronic sinusitis.* Retrieved on 10/12/2015 at: www.emedicine.medscape.com/article/232791-overview

Centers for Disease Control and Prevention. (2015). *Common colds: Protect yourself and others.* Retrieved on 10/12/2015 at: www.cdc.gov/Features/Rhinoviruses/index.html

Downey, R. (2015). *Obstructive sleep apnea.* Retrieved on 10/12/2015 at: www.emedicine.medscape.com/article/295807-overview

Drake, A. F., & Carr, M. M. (2015). *Tonsillectomy.* Retrieved on 3/4/2016 at: reference.medscape.com/article/872119-overview#showall

Fashner, J. Erickson, K., & Werner, S. (2012). Treatment of the common cold in children and adults. *American Family Physician, 86*(2), 153–159.

Flores, J. (2015). *Peritonsillar abscess in emergency medicine.* Retrieved on 10/12/2015 at: www.emedicine.medscape.com/article/764188-overview

*Haisfield-Wolfe, M. E., Brown, C., Richardson, M., et al. (2015). Variations in symptom severity patterns among oropharyngeal and laryngeal cancer outpatients during radiation treatment: A pilot study. *Cancer Nursing, 38*(4), 279–287.

Karsch-Völk, M., Barrett, B., Kiefer, D., et al. (2014). Echinacea for preventing and treating the common cold. *Cochrane Database of Systematic Reviews, Issue 2,* CD000530. DOI: 10.1002/14651858.CD000530.pub3

Kishikova, L., & Fleming, J. (2014). Oral feeding following laryngectomy: Early or delayed. *International Journal of Surgery, 42*(11), 1137–1140.

Krings, J., Kallogjeri, D., Wineland, A., et al. (2014). Complications of primary and revision functional endoscopic sinus surgery for chronic rhinosinusitis. *The Laryngoscope, 124*(4), 838–845.

Krouse, H., & Krouse, J. (2014). Allergic rhinitis: Diagnosis through management. *The Nurse Practitioner, 39*(4), 20–28.

Lal, D. (2015). Fungal sinusitis. *The American Rhinologic Society.* Retrieved on 2/28/2016 at: www.care.american-rhinologic.org/fungal_sinusitis

Morgan, C. (2015). *Surgical approach to snoring and sleep apnea.* Retrieved on 10/12/2015 at: www.emedicine.medscape.com/article/868770-overview

National Cancer Institute. (2015). *Laryngeal cancer treatment (PDQR).* Retrieved on 3/9/2016 at: www.cancer.gov/types/head-and-neck/patient/laryngeal-treatment-pdq

National Institute of Allergy and Infectious Diseases. (2015). *Common cold.* Retrieved on 10/12/2015 at: www.niaid.nih.gov/topics/common-cold/Pages/default.aspx

Nguyen, Q. A. (2015). *Epistaxis.* Retrieved on 10/12/2015 at: www.emedicine.medscape.com/article/863220-overview

Patel, A. (2014). *Functional endoscopic sinus surgery.* Retrieved on 10/12/2015 at: www.emedicine.medscape.com/article/863420-overview

Peppard, P. E., Young, T., Barnet, J. H., et al. (2013). Increased prevalence of sleep-disordered breathing in adults. *American Journal of Epidemiology, 177*(9),1006–1014.

Peters, A. (2015). *Rhinosinusitis: Synopsis.* Retrieved on 10/8/2015 at: www.worldallergy.org/professional/allergic_diseases_center/rhinosinusitis/sinusitissynopsis.php

Randel, A. (2013) IDSA updates: Guideline for managing Group A Streptococcal Pharyngitis. *American Family Physician, 88*(5), 338–340.

Rosenfeld, R. M., Andes, D., Bhattacharyya, M., et al. (2015). Clinical practice guideline update: Adult sinusitis executive summary. *Otolaryngology Head & Neck Surgery, 152*(4), 598–609.

Salvaggio, M. R. (2014). *Herpes simplex.* Retrieved on 10/12/2015 at: www.emedicine.medscape.com/article/218580-overview

Seidman, M., Gurgel, R. K., Lin, S. Y., et al. (2015). Clinical practice guideline: Allergic Rhinitis: Executive summary. *Otolaryngology Head and Neck Surgery, 152*(2), 197–206.

Seshamani, M., Vogtmann, E., Gatwood, J., et al. (2014). Prevalence of complications from adult tonsillectomy and impact on health care expenditures. *Otolaryngology-Head and Neck Surgery, 150*(4), 574–581.

Shah, U. K. (2015). *Tonsillitis and peritonsillar abscess: Treatment and management.* Retrieved on 3/4/2016 at: emedicine.medscape.com/article/871977-overview#showall

Tewfik, T. (2015). *Medical treatment for acute sinusitis.* Retrieved on 10/12/2015 at: www.emedicine.medscape.com/article/861646-overview

White, D. P., & Shafazand, S. (2013). Mandibular advancement device vs. CPAP in the treatment of obstructive sleep apnea: Are they equally effective in short term health outcomes? *Journal of Clinical Sleep Medicine, 9*(9), 971–972.

Resources

American Academy of Allergy, Asthma & Immunology (AAAAI), www.aaaai.org

American Academy of Family Physicians, www.aafp.org/home.html

American Academy of Otolaryngology–Head and Neck Surgery, www.entnet.org

American Cancer Society, www.cancer.org

American Lung Association, www.lung.org

American Sleep Apnea Association (ASAA), www.sleepapnea.org/info/index.html

International Association of Laryngectomees (IAL), www.theial.com/ial/

National Cancer Institute (NCI), www.cancernet.nci.nih.gov

National Comprehensive Cancer Network (NCCN), www.nccn.org/about/contact.asp

National Heart, Lung, and Blood Institute (NHBLI), www.nhlbi.nih.gov

National Institute of Allergy and Infectious Diseases (NIAID), www.niaid.nih.gov/Pages/default.aspx

National Sleep Foundation, www.sleepfoundation.org

WebWhispers, www.webwhispers.org

23

Management of Patients With Chest and Lower Respiratory Tract Disorders

LEARNING OBJECTIVES

On completion of this chapter, the learner will be able to:

1 Identify patients at risk for atelectasis and the nursing interventions related to its prevention and management.
2 Compare the various pulmonary infections with regard to causes, clinical manifestations, nursing management, complications, and prevention.
3 Use the nursing process as a framework for care of the patient with pneumonia.
4 Describe nursing measures to prevent aspiration.
5 Relate pleurisy, pleural effusion, and empyema to pulmonary infection.

6 Relate the therapeutic management techniques of acute respiratory distress syndrome to the underlying pathophysiology of the syndrome.
7 Specify risk factors and measures appropriate for prevention and management of pulmonary embolism.
8 Describe preventive measures appropriate for controlling and eliminating occupational lung disease.
9 Discuss the modes of therapy and related nursing management of patients with lung cancer.
10 Describe the complications of chest trauma and their clinical manifestations and nursing management.

GLOSSARY

acute lung injury: an umbrella term for hypoxemic respiratory failure; acute respiratory distress syndrome is a severe form of acute lung injury

acute respiratory distress syndrome (ARDS): nonspecific pulmonary response to a variety of pulmonary and nonpulmonary insults to the lung; characterized by interstitial infiltrates, alveolar hemorrhage, atelectasis, decreased compliance, and refractory hypoxemia

asbestosis: diffuse lung fibrosis resulting from exposure to asbestos fibers

aspiration: inhalation of either oropharyngeal or gastric contents into the lower airways

atelectasis: collapse or airless condition of the alveoli caused by hypoventilation, obstruction to the airways, or compression

central cyanosis: bluish discoloration of the skin or mucous membranes due to hemoglobin carrying reduced amounts of oxygen

consolidation: lung tissue that has become more solid in nature due to collapse of alveoli or infectious process (pneumonia)

cor pulmonale: "heart of the lungs;" enlargement of the right ventricle from hypertrophy or dilation or as a secondary response to disorders that affect the lungs

empyema: accumulation of purulent material in the pleural space

fine-needle aspiration: insertion of a needle through the chest wall to obtain cells of a mass or tumor; usually performed under fluoroscopy or chest computed tomography guidance

hemoptysis: the coughing up of blood from the lower respiratory tract

hemothorax: partial or complete collapse of the lung due to blood accumulating in the pleural space; may occur after surgery or trauma

induration: an abnormally hard lesion or reaction, as in a positive tuberculin skin test

open lung biopsy: biopsy of lung tissue performed through a limited thoracotomy incision

orthopnea: shortness of breath when reclining or in the supine position

pleural effusion: abnormal accumulation of fluid in the pleural space

pleural friction rub: localized grating or creaking sound caused by the rubbing together of inflamed parietal and visceral pleurae

pleural space: the area between the parietal and visceral pleurae; a potential space

pneumothorax: partial or complete collapse of the lung due to positive pressure in the pleural space

pulmonary edema: increase in the amount of extravascular fluid in the lung

pulmonary embolism: obstruction of the pulmonary vasculature with an embolus; embolus may be due to blood clot, air bubbles, or fat droplets

purulent: consisting of, containing, or discharging pus

restrictive lung disease: disease of the lung that causes a decrease in lung volumes

tension pneumothorax: pneumothorax characterized by increasing positive pressure in the pleural space with each breath; this is an emergency situation, and the positive pressure needs to be decompressed or released immediately

thoracentesis: insertion of a needle into the pleural space to remove fluid that has accumulated and decrease pressure on the lung tissue; may also be used diagnostically to identify potential causes of a pleural effusion

transbronchial: through the bronchial wall, as in a transbronchial lung biopsy

ventilation–perfusion ratio (V̇/Q̇): the ratio between ventilation and perfusion in the lung; matching of ventilation to perfusion optimizes gas exchange

Conditions affecting the chest and lower respiratory tract range from acute problems to chronic disorders. Many of these disorders are serious and often life threatening. Patients with lower respiratory tract disorders require care from nurses with astute assessment and clinical management skills as well as knowledge of evidence-based practice. Nurses must also understand the impact of the particular disorder on the patient's quality of life and ability to carry out usual activities of daily living. Patient and family education is an important nursing intervention in the management of all lower respiratory tract disorders.

ATELECTASIS

Atelectasis refers to closure or collapse of alveoli and often is described in relation to chest x-ray findings and/or clinical signs and symptoms. It is one of the most commonly encountered abnormalities seen on a chest x-ray (Stark, 2015). Atelectasis may be acute or chronic and may cover a broad range of pathophysiologic changes, from microatelectasis (which is not detectable on chest x-ray) to macroatelectasis with loss of segmental, lobar, or overall lung volume. The most commonly described atelectasis is acute atelectasis, which occurs most often in the postoperative setting or in people who are immobilized and have a shallow, monotonous breathing pattern (Conde & Adams, 2015; Smetana, 2015). Excess secretions or mucus plugs may also cause obstruction of airflow and result in atelectasis in an area of the lung. Atelectasis also is observed in patients with a chronic airway obstruction that impedes or blocks the flow of air to an area of the lung (e.g., obstructive atelectasis in the patient with lung cancer that is invading or compressing the airways). This type of atelectasis is more insidious and slower in onset (Conde & Adams, 2015; Stark, 2015).

Pathophysiology

Atelectasis may occur in adults as a result of reduced ventilation (nonobstructive atelectasis) or any blockage that obstructs passage of air to and from the alveoli (obstructive atelectasis), thus reducing alveolar ventilation (Stark, 2015). Obstructive atelectasis is the most common type and results from reabsorption of gas (trapped alveolar air is absorbed into the bloodstream); no additional air can enter into the alveoli because of the blockage. As a result, the affected portion of the lung becomes airless and the alveoli collapse. Causes of atelectasis include foreign body, tumor or growth in an airway, altered breathing patterns, retained secretions, pain, alterations in small airway function, prolonged supine positioning, increased abdominal pressure, reduced lung volumes due to musculoskeletal or neurologic disorders, restrictive defects, and specific surgical procedures (e.g., upper abdominal, thoracic, or open heart surgery) (Conde & Adams, 2015).

Patients are at high risk for atelectasis postoperatively because of several factors. A monotonous, low tidal breathing pattern may cause small airway closure and alveolar collapse. This can result from the effects of anesthesia or analgesic agents, supine positioning, splinting of the chest wall because of pain, or abdominal distention. Secretion retention, airway obstruction, and an impaired cough reflex may also occur, or patients may be reluctant to cough because of pain (Conde & Adams, 2015). Figure 23-1 shows the mechanisms and consequences of acute atelectasis in postoperative patients.

Atelectasis resulting from bronchial obstruction by secretions may also occur in patients with impaired cough mechanisms (e.g., musculoskeletal or neurologic disorders) as well as in those who are debilitated and bedridden. In addition, atelectasis may develop because of excessive pressure on the lung tissue (i.e., compressive atelectasis), which restricts normal lung expansion on inspiration (Stark, 2015). Such pressure can be produced by fluid accumulating within the pleural space (**pleural effusion**), air in the pleural space (**pneumothorax**), or blood in the pleural space (**hemothorax**). The **pleural space** is the area between the parietal and the visceral pleurae. Pressure may also be produced by a pericardium distended with fluid (pericardial effusion), tumor growth within the thorax, or an elevated diaphragm.

Clinical Manifestations

The development of atelectasis usually is insidious. Signs and symptoms include increasing dyspnea, cough, and sputum production.

In acute atelectasis involving a large amount of lung tissue (lobar atelectasis), marked respiratory distress may be observed. In addition to the previously mentioned signs and symptoms, tachycardia, tachypnea, pleural pain, and **central cyanosis** (a bluish skin hue that is a late sign of hypoxemia) may be anticipated. Patients characteristically have difficulty breathing in the supine position and are anxious.

In chronic atelectasis, signs and symptoms are similar to those of acute atelectasis. The chronic nature of the alveolar collapse predisposes patients to infection distal to the obstruction. Therefore, the signs and symptoms of a pulmonary infection also may be present.

Assessment and Diagnostic Findings

When clinically significant atelectasis develops, it is generally characterized by increased work of breathing and hypoxemia. Decreased breath sounds and crackles are heard over the affected area. A chest x-ray may suggest a diagnosis of atelectasis before clinical symptoms appear; the x-ray may reveal patchy infiltrates or consolidated areas. Depending on the degree of hypoxemia, pulse oximetry (SpO_2) may demonstrate a low saturation of hemoglobin with oxygen (less than 90%) or a lower-than-normal partial pressure of arterial oxygen (PaO_2).

> ### Quality and Safety Nursing Alert
>
> *Tachypnea, dyspnea, and mild-to-moderate hypoxemia are hallmarks of the severity of atelectasis.*

Prevention

Nursing measures to prevent atelectasis include frequent turning, early mobilization, and strategies to expand the lungs and to manage secretions. Voluntary deep-breathing maneuvers (at least every 2 hours) assist in preventing and treating atelectasis. The performance of these maneuvers requires the patient to be alert and cooperative. Patient education and reinforcement are key elements to the success of these interventions. The use of incentive spirometry or voluntary deep

Physiology/Pathophysiology

Figure 23-1 • Relationship of risk factors, pathogenic mechanisms, and consequences of acute atelectasis in the postoperative patient. ASA, acetylsalicylic acid; COPD, chronic obstructive pulmonary disease; BMI, body mass index; (V̇/Q̇), ventilation–perfusion ratio. From the work of Jo Ann Brooks, PhD, RN, FAAN, FCCP, Indiana University Health, Indianapolis.

breathing enhances lung expansion, decreases the potential for airway closure, and may generate a cough. Secretion management techniques include directed cough, suctioning, aerosol nebulizer treatments followed by chest physiotherapy (postural drainage and chest percussion), and bronchoscopy. In some settings, a pressurized metered-dose inhaler is used to dispense a bronchodilator rather than an aerosol nebulizer. Chart 23-1 summarizes measures used to prevent atelectasis.

Management

The goal of the treatment is to improve ventilation and remove secretions. Strategies to prevent atelectasis, which include frequent turning, early ambulation, lung volume expansion maneuvers (e.g., deep-breathing exercises and incentive spirometry), and coughing, also serve as the first-line measures to minimize or treat atelectasis by improving ventilation. Multidisciplinary, evidence-based standardized intervention programs, such as ICOUGH^SM (see Chart 23-2), hold promise in preventing atelectasis (Cassidy, Rosenkranz, McCade, et al., 2013; Smetana, 2015).

In patients who do not respond to first-line measures or who cannot perform deep-breathing exercises, other treatments such as positive end-expiratory pressure (PEEP; a simple mask and one-way valve system that provides varying

---

Chart 23-1 Preventing Atelectasis

- Change patient's position frequently, especially from supine to upright position, to promote ventilation and prevent secretions from accumulating.
- Encourage early mobilization from bed to chair followed by early ambulation.
- Encourage appropriate deep breathing and coughing to mobilize secretions and prevent them from accumulating.
- Educate/reinforce appropriate technique for incentive spirometry.
- Administer prescribed opioids and sedatives judiciously to prevent respiratory depression.
- Perform postural drainage and chest percussion, if indicated.
- Institute suctioning to remove tracheobronchial secretions, if indicated.

amounts of expiratory resistance, usually 10 to 15 cm H$_2$O), continuous positive airway breathing (CPAB), or bronchoscopy may be used. Before initiating more complex, costly, and labor-intensive therapies, the nurse should ask several questions:

- Has the patient been given an adequate trial of deep-breathing exercises?
- Has the patient received adequate education, supervision, and coaching to carry out the deep-breathing exercises?
- Have other factors been evaluated that may impair ventilation or prevent a good patient effort (e.g., lack of turning, mobilization; excessive pain; excessive sedation)?

If the cause of atelectasis is bronchial obstruction from secretions, the secretions must be removed by coughing or suctioning to allow air to reenter that portion of the lung. Chest physiotherapy (chest percussion and postural drainage) may also be used to mobilize secretions. Nebulizer treatments with a bronchodilator or sodium bicarbonate may be used to assist patients in the expectoration of secretions. If respiratory care measures fail to remove the obstruction, a bronchoscopy is performed. Although bronchoscopy is an excellent measure to acutely remove secretions and increase ventilation, it is imperative for the nurse to assist the patient with maintaining the patency of the airways after bronchoscopy, using the traditional techniques of deep breathing, coughing, and suctioning. Severe or massive atelectasis may lead to acute respiratory failure, especially in patients with underlying lung disease. Endotracheal intubation and mechanical ventilation may be necessary.

If the cause of atelectasis is compression of lung tissue, the goal is to decrease the compression. With a large pleural effusion that is compressing lung tissue and causing alveolar collapse, treatment may include **thoracentesis** (removal of the fluid by needle aspiration) or insertion of a chest tube. The measures to increase lung expansion described previously also are used.

Management of chronic atelectasis focuses on removing the cause of the obstruction of the airways or the compression of the lung tissue. For example, bronchoscopy may be used to open an airway obstructed by lung cancer or a nonmalignant lesion, and the procedure may involve cryotherapy or laser therapy. If the atelectasis is a result of obstruction caused by lung cancer, an airway stent or radiation therapy to shrink a tumor may be used to open the airways and provide ventilation to the collapsed area. However, reopening the airways and reaerating the area of the lung may not be possible in patients who have experienced chronic, long-term collapse. In some cases, surgical management may be indicated.

RESPIRATORY INFECTIONS

Acute Tracheobronchitis

Acute tracheobronchitis, an acute inflammation of the mucous membranes of the trachea and the bronchial tree, often follows infection of the upper respiratory tract (see Chapter 22). Patients with viral infections have decreased resistance and can readily develop a secondary bacterial infection. Adequate treatment of upper respiratory tract infection is one of the major factors in the prevention of acute bronchitis.

Pathophysiology

In acute tracheobronchitis, the inflamed mucosa of the bronchi produces mucopurulent sputum, often in response to infection by *Streptococcus pneumoniae*, *Haemophilus influenzae*, or *Mycoplasma pneumoniae*. In addition, a fungal infection (e.g., *Aspergillus*) may also cause tracheobronchitis. A sputum culture is essential to identify the specific causative organism. In addition to infection, inhalation of physical and chemical irritants, gases, or other air contaminants can also cause acute bronchial irritation. A subcategory of tracheobronchitis is ventilator-associated tracheobronchitis, which is a common illness in chronically ventilated patients. If managed appropriately, ventilator-associated pneumonia (VAP) may be prevented (Kollef, 2015).

 Concept Mastery Alert

Remember that *Streptococcus pneumoniae* is not a fungal organism. An infection with a fungal organism such as *Aspergillus* can cause tracheobronchitis.

Clinical Manifestations

Initially, the patient has a dry, irritating cough and expectorates a scanty amount of mucoid sputum. The patient may report sternal soreness from coughing and have fever or chills, night sweats, headache, and general malaise. As the infection progresses, the patient may be short of breath, have noisy inspiration and expiration (inspiratory stridor and expiratory wheeze), and produce **purulent** (pus-filled) sputum. In severe tracheobronchitis, blood-streaked secretions may be expectorated as a result of the irritation of the mucosa of the airways.

Medical Management

Antibiotic treatment may be indicated depending on the symptoms, sputum purulence, and results of the sputum culture and sensitivity. Antihistamines usually are not prescribed, because they can cause excessive drying and make secretions more difficult to expectorate. Fluid intake is increased to thin viscous and tenacious secretions. Copious, purulent secretions that cannot be cleared by coughing place patients at risk for increasing airway obstruction and the development of more severe lower respiratory tract infections, such as pneumonia. Suctioning and bronchoscopy may be needed to remove secretions. Rarely, endotracheal intubation may be necessary in cases of acute tracheobronchitis leading to acute respiratory failure, such as in patients who are severely debilitated or who have coexisting diseases that also impair the respiratory system.

In most cases, treatment of tracheobronchitis is largely symptomatic. Increasing the vapor pressure (moisture content) in the air reduces airway irritation. Cool vapor therapy or steam inhalations may help relieve laryngeal and tracheal irritation. Moist heat to the chest may relieve the soreness and pain, and mild analgesics may be prescribed.

Nursing Management

Acute tracheobronchitis is usually treated in the home setting. A primary nursing function is to encourage bronchial hygiene, such as increased fluid intake and directed coughing to remove secretions. The nurse encourages and assists the patient to sit up frequently to cough effectively and to prevent retention of mucopurulent sputum. If the patient is taking antibiotics for an underlying infection, the need to complete the full course of antibiotics prescribed is emphasized. Fatigue is a consequence of tracheobronchitis; therefore, the nurse cautions the patient against overexertion, which can induce a relapse or exacerbation of the infection. The patient is advised to rest.

Pneumonia

Pneumonia is an inflammation of the lung parenchyma caused by various microorganisms, including bacteria, mycobacteria, fungi, and viruses. *Pneumonitis* is a more general term that describes an inflammatory process in the lung tissue that may predispose or place the patient at risk for microbial invasion. Pneumonia and influenza are the most common causes of death from infectious diseases in the United States. Pneumonia and influenza accounted for 50,636 deaths in the U. S. in 2012 and 1.1 million discharges from hospitals (Centers for Disease Control and Prevention [CDC], 2015a; CDC, 2015b). Together these diseases were the eighth leading cause of death in the United States in 2012 (CDC, 2015a).

Classification

Pneumonia can be classified into four types: community-acquired pneumonia (CAP), health care–associated pneumonia (HCAP), hospital-acquired pneumonia (HAP), and VAP (American Thoracic Society & Infectious Diseases Society of America, 2005; File, 2016). HCAP was added as a category in 2005 to identify patients at increased risk for multidrug-resistant (MDR) pathogens versus community-acquired pathogens (File, 2016). Chart 23-3 describes the different classifications and definitions of pneumonias. Other subcategories of HCAPs are those in the immunocompromised host and aspiration pneumonia. There is overlap in how specific pneumonias are classified, because they may occur in differing settings. Risk factors associated for specific pathogens are shown in Chart 23-4.

Community-Acquired Pneumonia

CAP, a common infectious disease, occurs either in the community setting or within the first 48 hours after

---

Chart 23-3

Classifications and Definitions of Pneumonias

- *Community-acquired pneumonia (CAP):* Pneumonia occurring in the community or ≤48 hours after hospital admission or institutionalization of patients who do not meet the criteria for health care–associated pneumonia (HCAP)
- *Health care–associated pneumonia (HCAP):* Pneumonia occurring in a nonhospitalized patient with extensive health care contact with one or more of the following:
  - Hospitalization for ≥2 days in an acute care facility within 90 days of infection
  - Residence in a nursing home or long-term care facility
  - Antibiotic therapy, chemotherapy, or wound care within 30 days of current infection
  - Hemodialysis treatment at a hospital or clinic
  - Home infusion therapy or home wound care
  - Family member with infection due to multidrug-resistant bacteria
- *Hospital-acquired pneumonia (HAP):* Pneumonia occurring ≥48 hours after hospital admission that did not appear to be incubating at the time of admission
- *Ventilator-associated pneumonia (VAP):* A type of HAP that develops ≥48 hours after endotracheal tube intubation

Adapted from File, T. (2016). Risk factors and prevention of hospital-acquired, ventilator-associated and healthcare-associated pneumonia in adults. *UpToDate.* Last updated January 29, 2016. Retrieved on 4/23/2016 at: www.uptodate.com/contents/treatment-of-hospital-acquired-ventilator-associated-and-healthcare-associated-pneumonia-in-adults?source=search_result&search=Treatment+of+hospital-acquired%2C+ventilator-associated+and+healthcare-associated+pneumonia+in+adults&selectedTitle=1~150

---

hospitalization or institutionalization. The need for hospitalization for CAP depends on the severity of the pneumonia. The causative pathogens for CAP by site of care are shown in Table 23-1. The specific etiologic pathogen is identified in about 50% of cases. The overall rate of CAP in

---

Chart 23-4 **RISK FACTORS**
Pneumonia Based Upon Pathogen Type

Risk Factors for Infection With Penicillin-Resistant and Drug-Resistant Pneumococci

- Age >65 years
- Alcoholism
- Beta-lactam therapy (e.g., cephalosporins) in past 3 months
- Immunosuppressive disorders
- Multiple medical comorbidities
- Exposure to a child in a day care facility

Risk Factors for Infection With Enteric Gram-Negative Bacteria

- Residency in a long-term care facility
- Underlying cardiopulmonary disease
- Multiple medical comorbidities
- Recent antibiotic therapy

Risk Factors for Infection With *Pseudomonas aeruginosa*

- Structural lung disease (e.g., bronchiectasis)
- Corticosteroid therapy
- Broad-spectrum antibiotic therapy (>7 days in the past month)
- Malnutrition

TABLE 23-1 Community-Acquired Pneumonia Microbial Causes by Site of Care[a]

Outpatients	Hospitalized Patients	
	Non-ICU	ICU
Streptococcus pneumonia	S. pneumoniae	S. pneumoniae
Mycoplasma pneumonia	M. pneumoniae	Staphylococcus aureus
Haemophilus influenza	Chlamydophila pneumoniae	Legionella
C. pneumonia	H. influenzae	Gram-negative bacilli
Respiratory viruses	Legionella	H. influenzae

ICU, intensive care unit.

[a]Listed in descending order of frequency at each site.

Adapted from File, T. M. (2016). Treatment of hospital-acquired, ventilator associated and healthcare-associated pneumonia in adutls. UpToDate. Last updated January 29, 2016. Retrieved on 4/23/2016 at: www.uptodate.com/contents/treatment-of-hospital-acquired-ventilator-associated-and-healthcare-associated-pneumonia-in-adults?source=search_result&search=Treatment+of+hospital-acquired%2C+ventilator-associated+and+healthcare-associated+pneumonia+in+adults&selectedTitle=1~150

Marrie, T. J. (2015). Epidemiology, pathogenesis, and microbiology of community-acquired pneumonia in adults. UpToDate. Last updated August 13, 2015. Retrieved on 4/23/2016 at: www.uptodate.com/contents/epidemiology-pathogenesis-and-microbiology-of-community-acquired-pneumonia-in-adults?source=search_result&search=Epidemiology%2C+pathogenesis%2C+and+microbiology+of+community-acquired+pneumonia+in+adults&selectedTitle=1~145

adults is approximately 5.16 to 6.11 cases per 1000 persons per year; the rate of CAP increases with age (Marrie, 2015). More than five million cases of CAP are reported each year, with the greatest number in those 65 years and older (CDC, 2014a; Marrie, 2015).

S. pneumoniae (pneumococcus) is the most common cause of CAP in people younger than 60 years without comorbidity and in those 60 years and older with comorbidity (Cunha, 2015; Marrie, 2015). S. pneumoniae, a gram-positive organism that resides naturally in the upper respiratory tract, colonizes the upper respiratory tract and can cause disseminated invasive infections, pneumonia and other lower respiratory tract infections, and upper respiratory tract infections such as otitis media and rhinosinusitis. It may occur as a lobar or bronchopneumonic form in patients of any age and may follow a recent respiratory illness.

H. influenzae causes a type of CAP that frequently affects older adults and those with comorbid illnesses (e.g., chronic obstructive pulmonary disease [COPD], alcoholism, and diabetes). The presentation is indistinguishable from that of other forms of bacterial CAP and may be subacute, with cough or low-grade fever for weeks before diagnosis.

Mycoplasma pneumonia is caused by M. pneumoniae. Mycoplasma pneumonia is spread by infected respiratory droplets through person-to-person contact. Patients can be tested for mycoplasma antibodies. The inflammatory infiltrate is primarily interstitial rather than alveolar. It spreads throughout the entire respiratory tract, including the bronchioles, and has the characteristics of a bronchopneumonia. Earache and bullous myringitis are common. Impaired ventilation and diffusion may occur.

Viruses are the most common cause of pneumonia in infants and children but are relatively uncommon causes of CAP in adults. In immunocompromised adults, cytomegalovirus is the most common viral pathogen, followed by herpes simplex virus, adenovirus, and respiratory syncytial virus. The acute stage of a viral respiratory infection occurs within the ciliated cells of the airways, followed by infiltration of the tracheobronchial tree. With pneumonia, the inflammatory process extends into the alveolar area, resulting in edema and exudation. The clinical signs and symptoms of a viral pneumonia are often difficult to distinguish from those of a bacterial pneumonia.

Health Care–Associated Pneumonia

An important distinction of HCAP is that the causative pathogens are often MDR. Consequently, identifying this type of pneumonia in areas such as the emergency department is crucial. Because HCAP is often difficult to treat, initial antibiotic treatment must not be delayed. Initial antibiotic treatment of HCAP is often different from that for CAP due to the possibility of MDR bacteria (File, 2016).

Hospital-Acquired Pneumonia

HAP develops 48 hours or more after admission and does not appear to be incubating at the time of admission. VAP can be considered a subtype of HAP, as the only differentiating factor is the presence of an endotracheal tube (see later discussion of VAP). Certain factors may predispose patients to HAP because of impaired host defenses (e.g., severe acute or chronic illness), a variety of comorbid conditions, supine positioning and aspiration, coma, malnutrition, prolonged hospitalization, hypotension, and metabolic disorders. Hospitalized patients are also exposed to potential bacteria from other sources (e.g., respiratory therapy devices and equipment, and transmission of pathogens by the hands of health care personnel). Numerous intervention-related factors also may play a role in the development of HAP (e.g., therapeutic agents leading to central nervous system depression with decreased ventilation, impaired removal of secretions, or potential aspiration; prolonged or complicated thoracoabdominal procedures, which may impair mucociliary function and cellular host defenses; endotracheal intubation (VAP); prolonged or inappropriate use of antibiotics; the use of nasogastric tubes). In addition, immunocompromised patients are at particular risk. HAP is associated with a high mortality rate, in part because of the virulence of the organisms, the resistance to antibiotics, and the patient's underlying disorder. It is the most common cause of death among all patients with hospital-acquired infections, with mortality rates up to 33% (Cunha, 2015).

The common organisms responsible for HAP include the Enterobacter species, Escherichia coli, H. influenzae, Klebsiella species, Proteus, Serratia marcescens, Pseudomonas aeruginosa, methicillin-sensitive or methicillin-resistant Staphylococcus aureus (MRSA), and S. pneumoniae. Most patients with HAP are colonized by multiple organisms. Pseudomonal pneumonia occurs in patients who are debilitated, those with altered mental status, and those with prolonged intubation or with tracheostomy. Staphylococcal pneumonia can occur through inhalation of the organism or spread through the hematogenous route. It is often accompanied by bacteremia and positive blood cultures. Its mortality rate is high. Specific strains of staphylococci are resistant to all available antimicrobial agents except vancomycin (File, 2016). Overuse and misuse of antimicrobial agents are major risk factors for the emergence of these resistant pathogens. Because MRSA is highly virulent, steps must be taken to prevent its spread. Patients with MRSA are isolated in a private room, and contact precautions (gown, mask, gloves, and antibacterial soap) are used. The number of people in contact with affected patients is minimized, and appropriate precautions must be taken when transporting these patients within or between facilities.

The usual presentation of HAP is a new pulmonary infiltrate on chest x-ray combined with evidence of infection such as fever, respiratory symptoms, purulent sputum, or leukocytosis. Pneumonias from *Klebsiella* or other gram-negative organisms (*E. coli*, *Proteus*, *Serratia*) are characterized by the destruction of lung structure and alveolar walls, **consolidation** (tissue that solidifies as a result of collapsed alveoli or infectious process such as pneumonia), and bacteremia. Older adult patients and those with alcoholism, chronic lung disease, or diabetes are at particular risk (File, 2016). Development of a cough or increased cough and sputum production are common presentations, along with low-grade fever and general malaise. In debilitated or dehydrated patients, sputum production may be minimal or absent. Pleural effusion, high fever, and tachycardia are common.

 ### Ventilator-Associated Pneumonia

As noted earlier, VAP can be thought of as a subtype of HAP; however, in such cases, the patient has been endotracheally intubated and has received mechanical ventilatory support for at least 48 hours. VAP is a complication in as many as 28% of patient who require mechanical ventilation (Amanullah, 2015). The incidence of VAP increases with the duration of mechanical ventilation. The estimated rates are 3% per day for the first 5 days, 2% per day for days 6 through 10, and 1% per day thereafter (Amanullah, 2015). The crude mortality for VAP is 27% to 76%, with an estimated attributable mortality rate of 8% to 15% (Amanullah, 2015; File, 2016). The etiologic bacteriologic agents associated with VAP typically differ based on the timing of the occurrence of the infection relative to the start of mechanical ventilation. VAP occurring within 96 hours of the onset of mechanical ventilation is usually due to antibiotic-sensitive bacteria that colonize the patient prior to hospital admission, whereas VAP developing after 96 hours of ventilatory support is more often associated with MDR bacteria. Prevention remains the key to reducing the burden of VAP (Amanullah, 2015). See Chart 21-11 in Chapter 21 for overview of bundled interventions aimed at preventing VAP.

Pneumonia in the Immunocompromised Host

Pneumonia in immunocompromised hosts includes *Pneumocystis* pneumonia (PCP), fungal pneumonias, and *Mycobacterium tuberculosis*. The organism that causes PCP is now known as *Pneumocystis jiroveci* instead of *Pneumocystis carinii*. The acronym PCP still applies because it can be read "**P**neumocystis **p**neumonia."

Pneumonia in the immunocompromised host occurs with the use of corticosteroids or other immunosuppressive agents, chemotherapy, nutritional depletion, the use of broad-spectrum antimicrobial agents, acquired immune deficiency syndrome (AIDS), genetic immune disorders, and long-term advanced life support technology (mechanical ventilation). It is seen with increasing frequency because affected patients constitute a growing portion of the population; however, pneumonias that typically occur in immunocompromised people may also occur in immunocompetent people. Pneumonia carries a higher morbidity and mortality rate in immunocompromised patients than in those who are immunocompetent (Augenbraun, 2014). Patients with compromised immune systems commonly develop pneumonia from organisms of low virulence. In addition, increasing numbers of patients with impaired defenses develop HAP from gram-negative bacilli (*Klebsiella*, *Pseudomonas*, *E. coli*, Enterobacteriaceae, *Proteus*, *Serratia*) (Augenbraun, 2014).

Pneumonia in immunocompromised hosts may be caused by the organisms also observed in CAP or HAP (*S. pneumoniae*, *S. aureus*, *H. influenzae*, *P. aeruginosa*, *M. tuberculosis*). PCP is rarely observed in immunocompetent hosts and is often an initial AIDS-defining complication. Whether patients are immunocompromised or immunocompetent, the clinical presentation of pneumonia is similar. PCP has a subtle onset, with progressive dyspnea, fever, and a nonproductive cough.

Aspiration Pneumonia

Aspiration pneumonia refers to the pulmonary consequences resulting from entry of endogenous or exogenous substances into the lower airway. The most common form of aspiration pneumonia is bacterial infection from aspiration of bacteria that normally reside in the upper airways. Aspiration pneumonia may occur in the community or hospital setting. Common pathogens are anaerobes, *S. aureus*, *Streptococcus* species, and gram-negative bacilli (Bartlett, 2015). Substances other than bacteria may be aspirated into the lung, such as gastric contents, exogenous chemical contents, or irritating gases. This type of aspiration or ingestion may impair the lung defenses, cause inflammatory changes, and lead to bacterial growth and a resulting pneumonia. (See later discussion of aspiration.)

Pathophysiology

Normally, the upper airway prevents potentially infectious particles from reaching the sterile lower respiratory tract. Pneumonia arises from normal flora present in patients whose resistance has been altered or from aspiration of flora present in the oropharynx; patients often have an acute or chronic underlying disease that impairs host defenses. Pneumonia may also result from bloodborne organisms that enter the pulmonary circulation and are trapped in the pulmonary capillary bed.

Pneumonia affects both ventilation and diffusion. An inflammatory reaction can occur in the alveoli, producing an exudate that interferes with the diffusion of oxygen and carbon dioxide. White blood cells, mostly neutrophils, also migrate into the alveoli and fill the normally air-filled spaces. Areas of the lung are not adequately ventilated because of secretions and mucosal edema that cause partial occlusion of the bronchi or alveoli, with a resultant decrease in alveolar

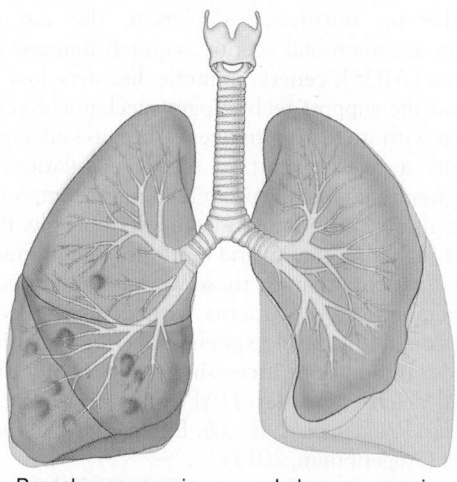

Bronchopneumonia   Lobar pneumonia

Figure 23-2 • Distribution of lung involvement in bronchial and lobar pneumonia. In bronchopneumonia (*left*), patchy areas of consolidation occur. In lobar pneumonia (*right*), an entire lobe is consolidated.

oxygen tension. Bronchospasm may also occur in patients with reactive airway disease. Because of hypoventilation, a ventilation–perfusion ($\dot{V}/\dot{Q}$) mismatch occurs in the affected area of the lung. Venous blood entering the pulmonary circulation passes through the underventilated area and travels to the left side of the heart poorly oxygenated. The mixing of oxygenated and unoxygenated or poorly oxygenated blood eventually results in arterial hypoxemia.

If a substantial portion of one or more lobes is involved, the disease is referred to as lobar pneumonia. The term *bronchopneumonia* is used to describe pneumonia that is distributed in a patchy fashion, having originated in one or more localized areas within the bronchi and extending to the adjacent surrounding lung parenchyma. Bronchopneumonia is more common than lobar pneumonia (see Fig. 23-2).

Risk Factors

Being knowledgeable about the factors and circumstances that commonly predispose people to pneumonia helps identify patients at high risk for the disease (Bartlett, 2015). Table 23-2 describes risk factors for pneumonia; additional risk factors are travel or exposure to certain environments and residence in a long-term care facility. Increasing numbers of patients who have compromised defenses against infections are susceptible to pneumonia. Some types of pneumonia, such as those caused by viral infections, occur in previously healthy people, often after a viral illness.

Pneumonia occurs in patients with certain underlying disorders such as heart failure, diabetes, alcoholism, COPD, and AIDS (Cunha, 2015; File, 2016). Certain diseases also have been associated with specific pathogens. For example, staphylococcal pneumonia has been noted after epidemics of influenza, and patients with COPD are at increased risk for development of pneumonia caused by pneumococci or *H. influenzae*. In addition, cystic fibrosis is associated with respiratory infection caused by pseudomonal and staphylococcal organisms, and PCP has been associated with AIDS. Pneumonias occurring in hospitalized patients often involve organisms not usually found in CAP, including enteric gram-negative bacilli and *S. aureus*.

Clinical Manifestations

Pneumonia varies in its signs and symptoms depending on the type, causal organism, and presence of underlying disease. However, it is not possible to diagnose a specific form or classification of pneumonia by clinical manifestations alone. The patient with streptococcal (pneumococcal) pneumonia usually has a sudden onset of chills, rapidly rising fever (38.5° to 40.5°C [101° to 105°F]), and pleuritic chest pain that is aggravated by deep breathing and coughing. The patient is severely ill, with marked tachypnea (25 to 45 breaths/min), accompanied by other signs of respiratory distress (e.g., shortness of breath and the use of accessory muscles in respiration) (Weinberger, Cockrill & Mandel, 2014). A relative bradycardia (a pulse–temperature deficit in which the pulse is slower than that expected for a given temperature) may suggest viral infection, mycoplasma infection, or infection with a *Legionella* organism.

Some patients exhibit an upper respiratory tract infection (nasal congestion, sore throat), and the onset of symptoms of pneumonia is gradual and nonspecific. The predominant symptoms may be headache, low-grade fever, pleuritic pain, myalgia, rash, and pharyngitis. After a few days, mucoid or mucopurulent sputum is expectorated. In severe pneumonia, the cheeks are flushed and the lips and nail beds demonstrate central cyanosis (a late sign of poor oxygenation [hypoxemia]).

The patient may exhibit **orthopnea** (shortness of breath when reclining or in the supine position), preferring to be propped up or sitting in bed leaning forward (orthopneic position) in an effort to achieve adequate gas exchange without coughing or breathing deeply. Appetite is poor, and the patient is diaphoretic and tires easily. Sputum is often purulent; however, this is not a reliable indicator of the etiologic agent. Rusty, blood-tinged sputum may be expectorated with streptococcal (pneumococcal), staphylococcal, and *Klebsiella* pneumonia.

Signs and symptoms of pneumonia may also depend on a patient's underlying condition. Different signs occur in patients with conditions such as cancer, and in those who are undergoing treatment with immunosuppressant medications, which decrease the resistance to infection. Such patients have fever, crackles, and physical findings that indicate consolidation of lung tissue, including increased tactile fremitus (vocal vibration detected on palpation), percussion dullness, bronchial breath sounds, egophony (when auscultated, the spoken "E" becomes a loud, nasal-sounding "A"), and whispered pectoriloquy (whispered sounds are easily auscultated through the chest wall). These changes occur because sound is transmitted better through solid or dense tissue (consolidation) than through normal air-filled tissue; these sounds are described in Chapter 20.

Purulent sputum or slight changes in respiratory symptoms may be the only sign of pneumonia in patients with COPD. Determining whether an increase in symptoms is an exacerbation of the underlying disease process or an additional infectious process may be difficult.

Assessment and Diagnostic Findings

The diagnosis of pneumonia is made by history (particularly of a recent respiratory tract infection), physical examination,

TABLE 23-2 Risk Factors and Preventive Measures for Pneumonia

Risk Factor	Preventive Measure
Conditions that produce mucus or bronchial obstruction and interfere with normal lung drainage (e.g., cancer, cigarette smoking, chronic obstructive pulmonary disease)	Promote coughing and expectoration of secretions. Encourage smoking cessation
Immunosuppressed patients and those with a low neutrophil count (neutropenic)	Initiate special precautions against infection
Smoking (cigarette smoke disrupts both mucociliary and macrophage activity)	Encourage smoking cessation
Prolonged immobility and shallow breathing pattern	Reposition frequently and promote lung expansion exercises and coughing. Initiate suctioning and chest physical therapy if indicated
Depressed cough reflex (due to medications, a debilitated state, or weak respiratory muscles); aspiration of foreign material into the lungs during a period of unconsciousness (head injury, anesthesia, depressed level of consciousness), or abnormal swallowing mechanism	Reposition frequently to prevent aspiration and administer medications judiciously, particularly those that increase risk for aspiration. Perform suctioning and chest physical therapy if indicated
Nothing-by-mouth (NPO) status; placement of nasogastric, orogastric, or endotracheal tube	Promote frequent oral hygiene. Minimize risk for aspiration by checking placement of tube and proper positioning of patient
Supine positioning in patients unable to protect their airway	Elevate head of bed at least 30 degrees
Antibiotic therapy (in very ill people, the oropharynx is likely to be colonized by gram-negative bacteria)	Monitor patients receiving antibiotic therapy for signs and symptoms of pneumonia
Alcohol intoxication (because alcohol suppresses the body's reflexes, may be associated with aspiration, and decreases white cell mobilization and tracheobronchial ciliary motion)	Encourage reduced or moderate alcohol intake (in case of alcohol stupor, position patient to prevent aspiration)
General anesthetic, sedative, or opioid preparations that promote respiratory depression, which causes a shallow breathing pattern and predisposes to the pooling of bronchial secretions and potential development of pneumonia	Observe the respiratory rate and depth during recovery from general anesthesia and before giving medications. If respiratory depression is apparent, withhold the medication and contact the primary provider
Advanced age, because of possible depressed cough and glottic reflexes and nutritional depletion	Promote frequent turning, early ambulation and mobilization, effective coughing, breathing exercises, and nutritious diet
Respiratory therapy with improperly cleaned equipment	Make sure that respiratory equipment is cleaned properly; participate in continuous quality improvement monitoring with the respiratory care department
Transmission of organisms from health care providers	Use strict hand hygiene and gloves. Implement health care provider education

chest x-ray, blood culture (bloodstream invasion [bacteremia] occurs frequently), and sputum examination. The sputum sample is obtained by having patients do the following: (1) rinse the mouth with water to minimize contamination by normal oral flora, (2) breathe deeply several times, (3) cough deeply, and (4) expectorate the raised sputum into a sterile container.

More invasive procedures may be used to collect specimens. Sputum may be obtained by nasotracheal or orotracheal suctioning with a sputum trap or by fiberoptic bronchoscopy (see Chapter 20). Bronchoscopy is often used in patients with acute severe infection, in patients with chronic or refractory infection, in immunocompromised patients when a diagnosis cannot be made from an expectorated or induced specimen, and in mechanically ventilated patients. Bronchoscopic techniques may include a protected brush specimen or bronchoalveolar lavage.

Unfolding Patient Stories: Kenneth Bronson • Part 1

Kenneth Bronson, a 27-year-old man, has a history of fatigue, high fever, and a productive cough for a week and arrives in the emergency department with difficulty breathing. A chest x-ray reveals a right lower lobe pneumonia. What are the clinical manifestations and assessment findings associated with a right lower lobe pneumonia that the nurse should investigate when evaluating the patient? (Kenneth Bronson's story continues in Chapter 26.)

Care for Kenneth and other patients in a realistic virtual environment: *vSim for Nursing* (**thepoint.lww.com/vSimMedicalSurgical**). Practice documenting these patients' care in DocuCare (**thepoint.lww.com/DocuCareEHR**).

Prevention

Pneumococcal vaccination reduces the incidence of pneumonia, hospitalizations for cardiac conditions, and deaths in the older adult population. About 1 million adults in the United States get pneumococcal pneumonia every year and about 18,000 will die from it (CDC, 2015b). There are two types of pneumococcal vaccine recommended for adults: a pneumococcal conjugate vaccine (PCV13) and a pneumococcal polysaccharide vaccine (PPSV23).

PCV13 protects against 13 types of pneumococcal bacteria. PCV13 is recommended for all adults 65 years of age or older as well as adults 19 years or older with conditions that weaken the immune system, such as HIV infection, organ transplantation, leukemia, lymphoma, and severe kidney disease (CDC, 2015c). PPSV23 is a newer vaccine and protects against 23 types of pneumococcal bacteria. It is recommended for all adults 65 years of age or older and for those adults 19 through 64 years of age who smoke cigarettes or who have asthma (CDC, 2015c). Most patients who have previously received PCV13 should receive PPSV23. In particular, all adults 65 years of age or older should receive both PCV13 and PPSV23. For immunocompetent adults age 65 or older who have not received PCV13, a dose of PCV13 should be given followed by PPSV23 at least 1 year later. These two vaccines should not be co-administered (Kobayashi, Bennett & Gierke, 2015). As pneumococcal vaccination guidelines may change from year to year, it is important to consult the CDC website for the most current recommendations. Other preventive measures are summarized in Table 23-2.

Medical Management

Pharmacologic Therapy

The treatment of pneumonia includes administration of the appropriate antibiotic as determined by the results of a culture and sensitivity. However, the causative organism is not identified in half of CAP cases when therapy is initiated (Marrie, 2015). Guidelines are used to guide antibiotic choice; however, the resistance patterns, prevalence of causative organisms, patient risk factors, treatment setting (inpatient vs. outpatient), and costs and availability of newer antibiotic agents must all be considered. See Table 23-3 for the treatment of patients with pneumonia due to specific pathogens.

Inpatients should be switched from intravenous (IV) to oral therapy when they are hemodynamically stable, are improving clinically, are able to take medications/fluids by mouth, and have a normally functioning gastrointestinal tract. As soon as patients are clinically stable, have no medical problems, and have a safe environment for continued care, they should be discharged from the hospital. Clinical stability is defined as temperature less than or equal to 37.8°C (100°F), heart rate less than or equal to 100 bpm, respiratory rate less than or equal to 24 breaths/min, systolic blood pressure greater than or equal to 90 mm Hg, and oxygen saturation greater than or equal to 90%, with ability to maintain oral intake and normal (baseline) mental status.

In suspected HAP, treatment is usually initiated with a broad-spectrum IV antibiotic and may be monotherapy or combination therapy. For patients with no known multidrug resistance, monotherapy with ceftriaxone (Rocephin), ampicillin/sulbactam (Unasyn), levofloxacin (Levaquin), or ertapenem (Invanz) is used. With known multidrug resistance, a three-drug combination therapy may be used; this drug regimen may include an antipseudomonal cephalosporin or ceftazidime (Fortaz) or antipseudomonal carbapenem or piperacillin/tazobactam (Zosyn) plus antipseudomonal fluoroquinolone or aminoglycoside plus linezolid (Zyvox) or vancomycin (Vancocin). The patient's status must be assessed 72 hours after the initiation of therapy, and antibiotics should be discontinued or modified based on the culture results. Of concern is the rampant rise in respiratory pathogens that are resistant to available antibiotics. Examples include vancomycin-resistant enterococcus (VRE), MRSA, and drug-resistant *S. pneumoniae*. Clinicians tend to use antibiotics aggressively; broad-spectrum agents may be used when narrow-spectrum agents are more appropriate. Mechanisms to monitor and minimize the inappropriate use of antibiotics are in place. In 2014, the CDC recommended all acute care hospitals participate in an antibiotic stewardship program (Fridkin, Baggs, Fagan, et al., 2014). Antibiotic stewardship refers to a set of coordinated strategies to improve the use of antimicrobial medications with the goal of enhancing patient health outcomes, reducing resistance to antibiotics, and decreasing unnecessary costs. Education of clinicians about the use of evidence-based guidelines in the treatment of respiratory infection is important, and some institutions have implemented algorithms to assist clinicians in choosing the appropriate antibiotics. Monitoring and surveillance of susceptibility patterns for pathogens are also important.

Other Therapeutic Regimens

Antibiotics are ineffective in viral upper respiratory tract infections and pneumonia, and their use may be associated with adverse effects. Treatment of viral infections with antibiotics is a major reason for the overuse of these medications in the United States. Antibiotics are indicated with a viral respiratory infection *only* if a secondary bacterial pneumonia, bronchitis, or rhinosinusitis is present. With the exception of the use of antimicrobial therapy, treatment of viral pneumonia is the same as that for bacterial pneumonia.

Treatment of viral pneumonia is primarily supportive. Hydration is a necessary part of therapy, because fever and tachypnea may result in insensible fluid losses. Antipyretics may be used to treat headache and fever; antitussive medications may be used for the associated cough. Warm, moist inhalations are helpful in relieving bronchial irritation. Antihistamines may provide benefit with reduced sneezing and rhinorrhea. Nasal decongestants may also be used to treat symptoms and improve sleep; however, excessive use can cause rebound nasal congestion. Bed rest is prescribed until the infection shows signs of clearing. If hospitalized, the patient is observed carefully until the clinical condition improves.

If hypoxemia develops, oxygen is given. Pulse oximetry or arterial blood gas analysis is used to determine the need for oxygen and to evaluate the effectiveness of the therapy. Arterial blood gases may be used to obtain a baseline measure of the patient's oxygenation and acid–base status; however, pulse oximetry is used to continuously monitor the patient's oxygen saturation and response to therapy. More aggressive respiratory support measures include administration of high concentrations of oxygen (fraction of inspired

(*text continued on page 596*)

TABLE 23-3 Commonly Encountered Pneumonias

Type (Causal Organism)	Epidemiology	Clinical Features	Treatment	Complications/ Comments
Community-Acquired Pneumonia				
Streptococcal pneumonia (*Streptococcus pneumoniae*)	Most prevalent in winter months More frequent occurrence in African Americans	Abrupt onset, toxic appearance, pleuritic chest pain; usually involves ≥1 lobes	Severity determines type of antibiotic and route (IV vs. oral) PCN sensitive: PCN, amoxicillin (Amoxil), ceftriaxone (Rocephin), cefotaxime (Claforan), cefprozil (Cefzil) or a macrolide PCN resistant: levofloxacin (Levaquin), moxifloxacin (Avelox), vancomycin (Vancocin) or linezolid (Zyvox)	Shock, pleural effusion, superinfections, pericarditis, and otitis media
	Incidence greatest in older adults and in patients with COPD, heart failure, alcoholism, asplenia, diabetes, and after influenza Leading infectious cause of illness worldwide among young children, people with underlying chronic health conditions, and older adults Mortality rate (in hospitalized adults with invasive disease): 14%	Lobar infiltrate common on chest x-ray or bronchopneumonia pattern		
Haemophilus influenzae (*Haemophilus influenzae*)	Incidence greatest in alcoholics, older adults, patients in long-term care facilities and nursing homes, patients with diabetes or COPD, and children <5 years of age Accounts for 5–20% of community-acquired pneumonias *Mortality rate: 30%*	Frequently insidious onset associated with upper respiratory tract infection 2–6 wks before onset of illness; fever, chills, productive cough; usually involves ≥1 lobes Bacteremia is common. Infiltrate, occasional bronchopneumonia pattern on chest x-ray	Severity determines type of antibiotic and route (IV vs. oral) Doxycycline (Vibramycin), second- or third-generation cephalosporin or a fluoroquinolone	Lung abscess, pleural effusion, meningitis, arthritis, pericarditis, epiglottitis
Legionnaires disease (*Legionella pneumophila*)	Highest occurrence in summer and fall May cause disease sporadically or as part of an epidemic Incidence greatest in middle-aged and older men, smokers, patients with chronic diseases, those receiving immunosuppressive therapy, and those in close proximity to excavation sites Accounts for 15% of community-acquired pneumonias *Mortality rate: 15–50%*	Flulike symptoms; high fevers, mental confusion, headache, pleuritic pain, myalgias, dyspnea, productive cough, hemoptysis, leukocytosis Bronchopneumonia, unilateral or bilateral disease, lobar consolidation	Severity determines type of antibiotic and route (IV vs. oral) Azithromycin (Zithromax), moxifloxacin (Avelox) or a fluoroquinolone	Hypotension, shock, and acute renal failure
Mycoplasma pneumoniae (*Mycoplasma pneumoniae*)	Increase in fall and winter Responsible for epidemics of respiratory illness Most common type of atypical pneumonia Accounts for 20% of community-acquired pneumonias; more common in children and young adults Mortality rate: <0.1%	Onset is usually insidious. Patients not usually as ill as in other pneumonias. Sore throat, nasal congestion, ear pain, headache, low-grade fever, pleuritic pain, myalgias, diarrhea, erythematous rash, pharyngitis. Interstitial infiltrates on chest x-ray	Severity determines type of antibiotic and route (IV vs. oral) Macrolides, combination drugs (macrolide plus ampicillin and sulbactam [Unasyn]) or tetracyclines (doxycycline)	Aseptic meningitis, meningoencephalitis, transverse myelitis, cranial nerve palsies, pericarditis, myocarditis

(continued on page 594)

TABLE 23-3 Commonly Encountered Pneumonias (continued)

Type (Causal Organism)	Epidemiology	Clinical Features	Treatment	Complications/ Comments
Viral pneumonia (influenza viruses types A, B adenovirus, parainfluenza, cytomegalovirus, coronavirus, varicella-zoster)	Incidence greatest in winter months Epidemics occur every 2–3 years. Most common causative organisms in adults; other organisms in children (e.g., cytomegalovirus and respiratory syncytial virus) Accounts for 20% of community-acquired pneumonias	Patchy infiltrate, small pleural effusion on chest x-ray In most patients, influenza begins as an acute upper respiratory infection; others have bronchitis, pleurisy, and so on, and still others develop gastrointestinal symptoms	Treated symptomatically; treat in high-risk patients; oseltamivir (Tamiflu) or zanamivir (Relenza) (+ other agents depending upon dominant strain [type of virus]) Does not respond to treatment with currently available antimicrobials	Superimposed bacterial infection, bronchopneumonia
Chlamydial pneumonia (*Chlamydophila pneumoniae*)	Reported mainly in college students, military recruits, and older adults May be a common cause of community-acquired pneumonia or observed in combination with other pathogens Mortality rate is low because the majority of cases are relatively mild. Older adults with coexistent infections, comorbidities, and reinfections may require hospitalization.	Hoarseness, fever, chills, pharyngitis, rhinitis, nonproductive cough, myalgias, arthralgias Single infiltrate on chest x-ray; pleural effusion possible	Macrolide or doxycycline	Reinfection and acute respiratory failure

Hospital-Acquired and Health Care–Associated Pneumonias

Type (Causal Organism)	Epidemiology	Clinical Features	Treatment	Complications/ Comments
Pseudomonas pneumonia (*Pseudomonas aeruginosa*)	Incidence greatest in those with preexisting lung disease, cancer (particularly leukemia); those with homograft transplants, burns; debilitated people; and patients receiving antimicrobial therapy and treatments such as tracheostomy, suctioning, and in postoperative settings. Almost always of nosocomial origin Accounts for 15% of hospital-acquired pneumonias Mortality rate: 40–60%	Diffuse consolidation on chest x-ray; toxic appearance: fever, chills, productive cough, relative bradycardia, leukocytosis	Sensitivity tests guide choice and severity determines type of antibiotic and route (IV vs. oral): ceftazidime (Fortaz), ciprofloxacin (Cipro), cefepime (Maxipime), aztreonam (Azactam), imipenem/cilastatin (Primaxin), meropenem (Merrem), piperacillin (Pipracil), +/– an aminoglycoside	Lung cavitation; has capacity to invade blood vessels, causing hemorrhage and lung infarction; usually requires hospitalization
Staphylococcal pneumonia (*Staphylococcus aureus*)	Incidence greatest in immunocompromised patients, IV drug users, and as a complication of epidemic influenza Commonly nosocomial in origin Accounts for 10–30% of hospital-acquired pneumonias Mortality rate: 25–60% MRSA may also cause community-based infection	Severe hypoxemia, cyanosis, necrotizing infection. Bacteremia is common	Severity determines type of antibiotic and route (IV vs. oral) MSSA: oxacillin or nafcillin MRSA or PCN allergy: vancomycin or linezolid	Pleural effusion/ pneumothorax, lung abscess, empyema, meningitis, endocarditis Frequently requires hospitalization. Treatment must be vigorous and prolonged because disease tends to destroy lung tissue

TABLE 23-3 Commonly Encountered Pneumonias (continued)

Type (Causal Organism)	Epidemiology	Clinical Features	Treatment	Complications/ Comments
Klebsiella pneumonia (*Klebsiella pneumoniae* [Friedländer's bacillus-encapsulated gram-negative aerobic bacillus])	Incidence greatest in older adults; alcoholics; patients with chronic disease, such as diabetes, heart failure, COPD; patients in chronic care facilities and nursing homes Accounts for 2–5% of community-acquired and 10–30% of hospital-acquired pneumonias Mortality rate: 40–50%	Tissue necrosis occurs rapidly. Toxic appearance: fever, cough, sputum production, bronchopneumonia, lung abscess. Lobar consolidation, bronchopneumonia pattern on chest x-ray	Severity determines type of antibiotic and route (IV vs. oral) Hospital acquired: cefepime, ceftazidime, imipenem, meropenem, or piperacillin/tazobactam plus an aminoglycoside or a fluoroquinolone; Community acquired: a levofloxacin plus ciprofloxacin or nitrofurantoin (Macrodantin) or nitrofurantoin macrocrystals	Multiple lung abscesses with cyst formation, empyema, pericarditis, pleural effusion; may be fulminating, progressing to fatal outcome
Pneumonia in the Immunocompromised Host				
Pneumocystis pneumonia (*Pneumocystis jiroveci*)	Incidence greatest in patients with AIDS and patients receiving immunosuppressive therapy for cancer, organ transplantation, and other disorders Frequently seen with cytomegalovirus infection Mortality rate 15–20% in hospitalized patients and fatal if not treated	Pulmonary infiltrates on chest x-ray; nonproductive cough, fever, dyspnea	Severity determines type of antibiotic and route (IV vs. oral) Trimethoprim/sulfamethoxazole (TMP-SMZ)	Respiratory failure
Fungal pneumonia (*Aspergillus fumigatus*)	Incidence greatest in immunocompromised and neutropenic patients Mortality rate: 15–20%	Cough, hemoptysis, infiltrates, fungus ball on chest x-ray	Severity determines type of antibiotic and route (IV vs. oral) Voriconazole (Vfend); for invasive disease: amphotericin B or liposomal amphotericin B (L-AMB) or caspofungin (Cancidas) Lobectomy for fungus ball	Dissemination to brain, myocardium, and thyroid gland
Tuberculosis (*Mycobacterium tuberculosis*)	Incidence increased in indigent, immigrant, and prison populations; people with AIDS; and the homeless Mortality rate: <1% (depending on comorbidity)	Weight loss, fever, night sweats, cough, sputum production, hemoptysis, nonspecific infiltrate (lower lobe), hilar node enlargement, pleural effusion on chest x-ray	Isoniazid (INH) + rifampin (Rifadin) + ethambutol (Myambutol) + pyrazinamide (PZA) (see section on TB and Table 23-4)	Reinfection and acute respiratory infection
Pneumonia From Aspiration				
Anaerobic bacteria (*S. pneumoniae, H. influenzae, S. aureus*)	Risk: reduced consciousness, dysphagia, disorders of upper GI tract; mechanical disruption of glottic closure (endotracheal tube, tracheostomy, nasogastric feeding)	Abrupt onset of dyspnea, low-grade fever, cough, predisposing condition for aspiration	Severity determines type of antibiotic and route (IV vs. oral) Clindamycin (Cleocin) +/– a fluoroquinolone	Identification of potential aspirate is important for treatment

PCN, penicillin; COPD, chronic obstructive pulmonary disease; IV, intravenous; MSSA, methicillin-sensitive *Staphylococcus aureus*; MRSA, methicillin resistant *Staphylococcus aureus*; AIDS, acquired immunodeficiency syndrome; TB, tuberculosis; GI, gastrointestinal.
Adapted from Gilbert, D. N., Chambers, H. F., Eliopoulos, G. M., et al. (2015). *The Sanford guide to antimicrobial therapy 2015* (45th ed.). Sperryville, VA: Antimicrobial Therapy, Inc.

oxygen [FiO$_2$]), endotracheal intubation, and mechanical ventilation. Different modes of mechanical ventilation may be required (see Chapter 21).

Gerontologic Considerations

Pneumonia in older adult patients may occur as a primary diagnosis or as a complication of a chronic disease. Pulmonary infections in older adults frequently are difficult to treat and result in a higher mortality rate than in younger people. Jain and colleagues (2015) studied approximately 2500 adults in a population-based surveillance project. They estimated the incidence of hospitalization for pneumonia among adults aged 50 to 64 was four times the incidence as compared to adults 18 to 49 years. For patients between 65 and 79 years, the estimated incidence was nine times the younger population. And, for those at least 80 years of age, the estimated incidence was 25 times higher (Jain, Self, Wunderink, et al., 2015). General deterioration, weakness, abdominal symptoms, anorexia, confusion, tachycardia, and tachypnea may signal the onset of pneumonia. The diagnosis of pneumonia may be missed because the classic symptoms of cough, chest pain, sputum production, and fever may be absent or masked in older adult patients. In addition, the presence of some signs may be misleading. Abnormal breath sounds, for example, may be caused by microatelectasis that occurs as a result of decreased mobility, decreased lung volumes, or other respiratory function changes. Chest x-rays may be needed to differentiate chronic heart failure, which is often seen in older adults, from pneumonia as the cause of clinical signs and symptoms.

Supportive treatment includes hydration (with caution and with frequent assessment because of the risk of fluid overload in older adults); supplemental oxygen therapy; and assistance with deep breathing, coughing, frequent position changes, and early ambulation. All of these are particularly important in the care of older adult patients with pneumonia. To reduce or prevent serious complications of pneumonia in older adults, vaccination against pneumococcal and influenza infections is recommended.

Complications

Shock and Respiratory Failure

Severe complications of pneumonia include hypotension and septic shock and respiratory failure (especially with gram-negative bacterial disease in older adult patients). These complications are encountered chiefly in patients who have received no specific treatment or inadequate or delayed treatment. These complications are also encountered when the infecting organism is resistant to therapy, when a comorbid disease complicates the pneumonia, or when the patient is immunocompromised. (See Chapter 14 for further discussion of management of the patient with septic shock.)

Pleural Effusion

A pleural effusion is an accumulation of pleural fluid in the pleural space (space between the parietal and visceral pleurae of the lung). A parapneumonic effusion is any pleural effusion associated with bacterial pneumonia, lung abscess, or bronchiectasis. After the pleural effusion is detected on a chest x-ray, a thoracentesis may be performed to remove the fluid, which is sent to the laboratory for analysis. There are three stages of parapneumonic pleural effusions based on pathogenesis: uncomplicated, complicated, and thoracic empyema. An **empyema** occurs when thick, purulent fluid accumulates within the pleural space, often with fibrin development and a loculated (walled-off) area where the infection is located (see later discussion). A chest tube may be inserted to treat pleural infection by establishing proper drainage of the empyema. Sterilization of the empyema cavity requires 4 to 6 weeks of antibiotics, and sometimes surgical management is required.

NURSING PROCESS

The Patient With Pneumonia

Assessment

Nursing assessment is critical in detecting pneumonia. Fever, chills, or night sweats in a patient who also has respiratory symptoms should alert the nurse to the possibility of bacterial pneumonia. Respiratory assessment further identifies the clinical manifestations of pneumonia: pleuritic-type pain, fatigue, tachypnea, the use of accessory muscles for breathing, bradycardia or relative bradycardia, coughing, and purulent sputum. The nurse monitors the patient for the following: changes in temperature and pulse; amount, odor, and color of secretions; frequency and severity of cough; degree of tachypnea or shortness of breath; changes in physical assessment findings (primarily assessed by inspecting and auscultating the chest); and changes in the chest x-ray findings.

In addition, it is important to assess older adult patients for unusual behavior, altered mental status, dehydration, excessive fatigue, and concomitant heart failure.

Diagnosis

NURSING DIAGNOSES

Based on the assessment data, major nursing diagnoses may include the following:

- Ineffective airway clearance related to copious tracheobronchial secretions
- Fatigue and activity intolerance related to impaired respiratory function
- Risk for deficient fluid volume related to fever and a rapid respiratory rate
- Imbalanced nutrition: less than body requirements
- Deficient knowledge about the treatment regimen and preventive measures

COLLABORATIVE PROBLEMS/POTENTIAL COMPLICATIONS

Based on the assessment data, collaborative problems or potential complications that may occur include the following:

- Continuing symptoms after initiation of therapy
- Sepsis and septic shock
- Respiratory failure
- Atelectasis
- Pleural effusion
- Delirium

Planning and Goals

The major goals may include improved airway patency, increased activity, maintenance of proper fluid volume, maintenance of adequate nutrition, an understanding of the treatment protocol and preventive measures, and absence of complications.

Nursing Interventions

IMPROVING AIRWAY PATENCY

Removing secretions is important because retained secretions interfere with gas exchange and may slow recovery. The nurse encourages hydration (2 to 3 L/day), because adequate hydration thins and loosens pulmonary secretions. Humidification may be used to loosen secretions and improve ventilation. A high-humidity facemask (using either compressed air or oxygen) delivers warm, humidified air to the tracheobronchial tree, helps liquefy secretions, and relieves tracheobronchial irritation. Coughing can be initiated either voluntarily or by reflex. Lung expansion maneuvers, such as deep breathing with an incentive spirometer, may induce a cough. To improve airway patency, the nurse encourages the patient to perform an effective, directed cough, which includes correct positioning, a deep inspiratory maneuver, glottic closure, contraction of the expiratory muscles against the closed glottis, sudden glottic opening, and an explosive expiration. In some cases, the nurse may assist the patient by placing both hands on the lower rib cage (either anterior or posterior) to focus the patient on a slow deep breath, and then manually assisting the patient by applying constant, external pressure during the expiratory phase.

Chest physiotherapy (percussion and postural drainage) is important in loosening and mobilizing secretions (see Chapter 21). Indications for chest physiotherapy include sputum retention not responsive to spontaneous or directed cough, a history of pulmonary problems previously treated with chest physiotherapy, continued evidence of retained secretions (decreased or abnormal breath sounds, change in vital signs), abnormal chest x-ray findings consistent with atelectasis or infiltrates, and deterioration in oxygenation. The patient is placed in the proper position to drain the involved lung segments, then the chest is percussed and vibrated either manually or with a mechanical percussor. The nurse may consult the respiratory therapist for volume expansion protocols and secretion management protocols that help direct the respiratory care of the patient and match the patient's needs with appropriate treatment schedules.

After each position change, the nurse encourages the patient to breathe deeply and cough. If the patient is too weak to cough effectively, the nurse may need to remove the mucus by nasotracheal suctioning (see Chapter 21). It may take time for secretions to mobilize and move into the central airways for expectoration. Therefore, it is important for the nurse to monitor the patient for cough and sputum production after the completion of chest physiotherapy.

The nurse also administers and titrates oxygen therapy as prescribed or via protocols. The effectiveness of oxygen therapy is monitored by improvement in clinical signs and symptoms, patient comfort, and adequate oxygenation values as measured by pulse oximetry or arterial blood gas analysis.

PROMOTING REST AND CONSERVING ENERGY

The nurse encourages the debilitated patient to rest and avoid overexertion and possible exacerbation of symptoms. The patient should assume a comfortable position to promote rest and breathing (e.g., semi-Fowler's position) and should change positions frequently to enhance secretion clearance and pulmonary ventilation and perfusion. Outpatients must be instructed to avoid overexertion and to engage in only moderate activity during the initial phases of treatment.

PROMOTING FLUID INTAKE

The respiratory rate of patients with pneumonia increases because of the increased workload imposed by labored breathing and fever. An increased respiratory rate leads to an increase in insensible fluid loss during exhalation and can lead to dehydration. Therefore, unless contraindicated, increased fluid intake (at least 2 L/day) is encouraged. Hydration must be achieved more slowly and with careful monitoring in patients with preexisting conditions such as heart failure (see Chapter 29).

MAINTAINING NUTRITION

Many patients with shortness of breath and fatigue have a decreased appetite and consume only fluids. Fluids with electrolytes (commercially available drinks, such as Gatorade) may help provide fluid, calories, and electrolytes. Other nutritionally enriched drinks such as oral nutritional supplements may be used to supplement calories. Small, frequent meals may be advisable. In addition, IV fluids and nutrients may be given if necessary.

PROMOTING PATIENTS' KNOWLEDGE

The patient and family are instructed about the cause of pneumonia, management of symptoms, signs and symptoms that should be reported to the primary provider or nurse, and the need for follow-up. The patient also needs information about factors (both patient risk factors and external factors) that may have contributed to the development of pneumonia and strategies to promote recovery and prevent recurrence. If the patient is hospitalized, he or she is instructed about the purpose and importance of management strategies that have been implemented and about the importance of adhering to them during and after the hospital stay. Explanations should be given simply and in language that the patient can understand. If possible, written instructions and information should be provided, and alternative formats should be provided for patients with hearing or vision loss, if necessary. Because of the severity of symptoms, the patient may require that instructions and explanations be repeated several times.

MONITORING AND MANAGING POTENTIAL COMPLICATIONS

Continuing Symptoms After Initiation of Therapy. The patient is observed for response to antibiotic therapy; patients usually begin to respond to treatment within 24 to 48 hours after antibiotic therapy is initiated. If the patient started taking antibiotics before evaluation by culture and sensitivity of the causative organisms, antibiotics may need to be changed once the results are available. The patient is monitored for changes in physical status (deterioration of condition or resolution of symptoms) and for persistent recurrent fever, which may be a result of medication allergy (signaled possibly by a rash); medication resistance or slow response (greater than 48 hours) of the susceptible organism to therapy; pleural effusion; or pneumonia caused by an unusual organism, such as *P. jiroveci* or *Aspergillus fumigatus*. Failure of the pneumonia to resolve or persistence of symptoms despite changes on the chest x-ray raises the suspicion of other underlying disorders, such as lung cancer. As described previously, lung cancers may invade or compress airways, causing an obstructive atelectasis that may lead to pneumonia.

In addition to monitoring for continuing symptoms of pneumonia, the nurse also monitors for other complications, such as septic shock and multiple organ dysfunction syndrome (MODS) and atelectasis, which may develop during the first few days of antibiotic treatment.

Shock and Respiratory Failure. The nurse assesses for signs and symptoms of septic shock and respiratory failure by evaluating the patient's vital signs, pulse oximetry values, and hemodynamic monitoring parameters. The nurse reports signs of deteriorating patient status and assists in administering IV fluids and medications prescribed to combat shock. Intubation and mechanical ventilation may be required if respiratory failure occurs. (Sepsis and septic shock are described in detail in Chapter 14, and care of the patient receiving mechanical ventilation is described in Chapter 21.)

Pleural Effusion. If pleural effusion develops and thoracentesis is performed to remove fluid, the nurse assists in the procedure and explains it to the patient. After thoracentesis, the nurse monitors the patient for pneumothorax or recurrence of pleural effusion. If a chest tube needs to be inserted, the nurse monitors the patient's respiratory status. (See Chapter 21 for more information on care of patients with chest tubes.)

Delirium. A patient with pneumonia is assessed for delirium and other more subtle changes in cognitive status; this is especially true in the older adult. The Confusion Assessment Method (CAM) is a commonly used screening tool (see Chapter 11, Chart 11-7). Confusion, suggestive of delirium, and other changes in cognitive status resulting from pneumonia are poor prognostic signs (File, 2016). Delirium may be related to hypoxemia, fever, dehydration, sleep deprivation, or developing sepsis. The patient's underlying comorbid conditions may also play a part in the development of confusion. Addressing and correcting underlying factors as well as ensuring patient safety are important nursing interventions.

PROMOTING HOME, COMMUNITY-BASED, AND TRANSITIONAL CARE

Educating Patients About Self-Care. Depending on the severity of the pneumonia, treatment may occur in the hospital or in the outpatient setting. Patient education is crucial regardless of the setting, and the proper administration of antibiotics is important. In some instances, the patient may be treated initially with IV antibiotics as an inpatient and then discharged to continue the IV antibiotics at home. A seamless system of care must be maintained for the patient from hospital to home; this includes communication between the nurses caring for the patient in both settings.

If oral antibiotics are prescribed, the nurse educates the patient about their proper administration and potential side effects. The patient should be instructed about symptoms that require contacting the primary provider: difficulty breathing, worsening cough, recurrent/increasing fever, and medication intolerance.

After the fever subsides, the patient may gradually increase activities. Fatigue and weakness may be prolonged after pneumonia, especially in older adults. The nurse encourages breathing exercises to promote secretion clearance and volume expansion. A patient who is being treated as an outpatient should be contacted by the health care team or instructed to contact the primary provider 24 to 48 hours after starting therapy. The patient is also instructed to return to the clinic or primary provider's office for a follow-up chest x-ray and physical examination. Often, improvement in chest x-ray findings lags behind improvement in clinical signs and symptoms.

The nurse encourages the patient who smokes to stop smoking. Smoking inhibits tracheobronchial ciliary action, which is the first line of defense of the lower respiratory tract. Smoking also irritates the mucous cells of the bronchi and inhibits the function of alveolar macrophage (scavenger) cells. The patient is instructed to avoid stress, fatigue, sudden changes in temperature, and excessive alcohol intake, all of which lower resistance to pneumonia. The nurse reviews with the patient the principles of adequate nutrition and rest, because one episode of pneumonia may make a patient susceptible to recurring respiratory tract infections.

Continuing and Transitional Care. A patient who is severely debilitated or who cannot care for him- or herself may require referral for home, transitional, or community-based care. During home visits, the nurse assesses the patient's physical status, monitors for complications, assesses the home environment, and reinforces previous education. The nurse evaluates the patient's adherence to the therapeutic regimen (i.e., taking medications as prescribed; performing breathing exercises; consuming adequate fluid and dietary intake; and avoiding smoking, alcohol, and excessive activity). The nurse stresses to the patient and family the importance of monitoring for complications or exacerbation of the pneumonia. The nurse encourages the patient to obtain an influenza vaccination at the prescribed times, because influenza increases susceptibility to secondary bacterial pneumonia, especially that caused by staphylococci, *H. influenzae,* and *S. pneumoniae.* The nurse also urges the patient to receive the pneumococcal vaccine(s) according to CDC recommendations (see previous discussion).

Evaluation

Expected patient outcomes may include the following:

1. Demonstrates improved airway patency, as evidenced by adequate oxygenation by pulse oximetry or arterial blood gas analysis, normal temperature, normal breath sounds, and effective coughing
2. Rests and conserves energy by limiting activities and remaining in bed while symptomatic and then slowly increasing activities
3. Maintains adequate hydration, as evidenced by an adequate fluid intake and urine output and normal skin turgor
4. Consumes adequate dietary intake, as evidenced by maintenance or increase in body weight without excess fluid gain
5. Verbalizes increased knowledge about management strategies
6. Complies with management strategies
7. Exhibits no complications
   a. Exhibits acceptable vital signs, pulse oximetry, and arterial blood gas measurements
   b. Reports productive cough that diminishes over time
   c. Has absence of signs or symptoms of sepsis, septic shock, respiratory failure, or pleural effusion
   d. Remains oriented and aware of surroundings
8. Maintains or increases weight
9. Adheres to treatment protocol and prevention strategies

Chart 23-5 ⚠️ RISK FACTORS
Aspiration

- Seizure activity
- Brain injury
- Decreased level of consciousness from trauma, drug or alcohol intoxication, excessive sedation, or general anesthesia
- Flat body positioning
- Stroke
- Swallowing disorders
- Cardiac arrest

Adapted from American Association of Critical-Care Nurses. (2016). AACN practice alert: Prevention of aspiration in adults. *Critical Care Nurse*, 36(1), e20–e24; Bartlett, J. (2015). Aspiration pneumonia in adults. *UpToDate*. Last updated June 6, 2015. Retrieved on 3/19/16 at: www.uptodate.com/contents/aspiration-pneumonia-in-adults

Aspiration

Aspiration is inhalation of foreign material (e.g., oropharyngeal or stomach contents) into the lungs. It is a serious complication that can cause pneumonia and result in the following clinical picture: tachycardia, dyspnea, central cyanosis, hypertension, hypotension, and potentially death. It can occur when the protective airway reflexes are decreased or absent due to a variety of factors (see Chart 23-5). Aspiration pneumonia represents 5% to 15% of pneumonias in the hospitalized population (DiBardino & Wunderink, 2015).

Pathophysiology

The primary factors responsible for death and complications after aspiration are the volume and character of the aspirated contents. Aspiration pneumonia develops after inhalation of colonized oral or pharyngeal material. The pathologic process involves an acute inflammatory response to bacteria and bacterial products. Most commonly, the bacteriologic findings include gram-positive cocci, gram-negative rods, and occasionally anaerobic bacteria (Bartlett, 2015).

A full stomach contains solid particles of food. If these are aspirated, the problem then becomes one of mechanical blockage of the airways and secondary infection. During periods of fasting, the stomach contains acidic gastric juice, which, if aspirated, can be very destructive to the alveoli and capillaries. Fecal contamination (more likely seen in intestinal obstruction) increases the likelihood of death, because the endotoxins produced by intestinal organisms may be absorbed systemically, or the thick proteinaceous material found in the intestinal contents may obstruct the airway, leading to atelectasis and secondary bacterial invasion.

Esophageal conditions may also be associated with aspiration pneumonia. These include dysphagia, esophageal strictures, neoplasm or diverticula, tracheoesophageal fistula, and gastroesophageal reflux disease.

Prevention

The risk of aspiration is indirectly related to the level of consciousness of the patient. Aspiration of small amounts of material from the buccal (oral) cavity is not uncommon, particularly during sleep; however, disease as a result of aspiration does not occur in healthy persons because the material is cleared by the mucociliary tree and the macrophages. Witnessed aspiration of large volumes occurs occasionally; however, small-volume clinically silent aspiration is more common. Prevention is the primary goal when caring for patients at risk for aspiration (AACN, 2016).

> **Quality and Safety Nursing Alert**
>
> *When a nonfunctioning nasogastric tube allows the gastric contents to accumulate in the stomach, a condition known as silent aspiration may result. Silent aspiration often occurs unobserved and may be more common than suspected. If untreated, massive inhalation of gastric contents develops in a period of several hours.*

Compensating for Absent Reflexes

Aspiration may occur if the patient cannot adequately coordinate protective glottic, laryngeal, and cough reflexes. This hazard is increased if the patient has a distended abdomen, is supine, has the upper extremities immobilized in any manner, receives local anesthetic agents to the oropharyngeal or laryngeal area for diagnostic procedures, has been sedated, or has had long-term intubation. Clinical interventions are key to preventing aspiration (see Chart 23-6).

For patients with known swallowing dysfunction or those recently extubated following prolonged endotracheal intubation, a swallowing assessment is necessary. Patients deemed at risk are then assessed by a speech therapist. Besides positioning the patient semirecumbent or upright prior to eating, other helpful techniques may include suggesting a soft diet and encouraging the patient to take small bites. The patient should be instructed to keep the chin tucked and the head turned with repeated swallowing. Straws should not be used.

When vomiting, people can normally protect their airway by sitting up or turning on the side and coordinating

Chart 23-6 Clinical Practice to Prevent Aspiration

- Maintain head-of-bed elevation at an angle of 30–45 degrees, unless contraindicated
- Use sedatives as sparingly as possible
- Before initiating enteral tube feeding, confirm the tip location
- For patients receiving tube feedings, assess placement of the feeding tube at 4-hour intervals, assess for gastrointestinal residuals (<150 mL before next feeding) to the feedings at 4-hour intervals
- For patients receiving tube feedings, avoid bolus feedings in those at high risk for aspiration
- Consult with primary provider about obtaining a swallowing evaluation before oral feedings are started for patients who were recently extubated but were previously intubated for >2 days
- Maintain endotracheal cuff pressures at an appropriate level, and ensure that secretions are cleared from above the cuff before it is deflated.

Adapted from American Association of Critical-Care Nurses. (2016). AACN practice alert: Prevention of aspiration in adults. *Critical Care Nurse*, 36(1), e20–e24; Swaminathan, A. (2015). Aspiration pneumonitis and pneumonia. *Medscape*, Updated April 2, 2–2015. Retrieved on 6/8/2016 at: emedicine.medscape.com/article/296198-overview breathing, coughing, gag, and glottic reflexes. If these reflexes are active, an oral airway should not be inserted. If an airway is in place, it should be pulled out the moment the patient gags so as not to stimulate the pharyngeal gag reflex and promote vomiting and aspiration. Suctioning of oral secretions with a catheter should be performed with minimal pharyngeal stimulation.

For patients with an endotracheal tube and feeding tube, the endotracheal cuff pressure should be maintained at greater than 20 cm H_2O (but less than 30 cm H_2O to minimize injury) to prevent leakage of secretions from around the cuff into the lower respiratory tract. In addition, hypopharyngeal suctioning is recommended before the cuff is deflated (AACN, 2016).

Assessing Feeding Tube Placement

Tube feedings must be given only when it is certain that the feeding tube is positioned correctly in the stomach. Many patients receive enteral feeding directly into the duodenum through a small-bore flexible feeding tube or surgically implanted tube. (See Chapter 44 for discussion of confirming placement of enteral tubes and administration of tube feedings.)

Identifying Delayed Stomach Emptying

A full stomach can cause aspiration because of increased intragastric or extragastric pressure. The following may delay emptying of the stomach: intestinal obstruction; increased gastric secretions in gastroesophageal reflux disease; increased gastric secretions during anxiety, stress, or pain; and abdominal distention due to paralytic ileus, ascites, peritonitis, the use of opioids or sedatives, severe illness, or vaginal delivery. (See Chapter 44 for discussion of management of patients receiving gastric tube feedings.)

Managing Effects of Prolonged Intubation

Prolonged endotracheal intubation or tracheostomy can depress the laryngeal and glottic reflexes because of disuse. Patients with prolonged tracheostomies are encouraged to phonate and exercise their laryngeal muscles. For patients who have had long-term intubation or tracheostomies, it may be helpful to have a speech therapist experienced in swallowing disorders work with the patient to address swallowing problems, as noted previously.

Pulmonary Tuberculosis

Tuberculosis (TB) is an infectious disease that primarily affects the lung parenchyma. It also may be transmitted to other parts of the body, including the meninges, kidneys, bones, and lymph nodes. The primary infectious agent, *M. tuberculosis*, is an acid-fast aerobic rod that grows slowly and is sensitive to heat and ultraviolet light. *Mycobacterium bovis* and *Mycobacterium avium* have rarely been associated with the development of a TB infection.

TB is a worldwide public health problem that is closely associated with poverty, malnutrition, overcrowding, substandard housing, and inadequate health care. Mortality and morbidity rates continue to rise; *M. tuberculosis* infects an estimated one third of the world's population and remains the leading cause of death from infectious disease in the world. In

2014, 9.6 million people were sick with TB throughout the world and there were 1.5 million TB-related deaths (CDC, 2015d).

In the United States, 9,421 cases of TB were reported in 2014 (CDC, 2015d). Factors that prevent elimination of TB in the United States include the prevalence of TB among foreign-born residents, delays in detecting and reporting cases of TB, the lack of protection of contacts of people with infectious cases of TB, the presence of a substantial number of people with latent TB, and maintaining clinical and public health expertise in this disease (CDC, 2015d).

Transmission and Risk Factors

TB spreads from person to person by airborne transmission. An infected person releases droplet nuclei (usually particles 1 to 5 mcm in diameter) through talking, coughing, sneezing, laughing, or singing. Larger droplets settle; smaller droplets remain suspended in the air and are inhaled by a susceptible person. Chart 23-7 lists risk factors for TB. Chart 23-8 summarizes the CDC's recommendations for the prevention of TB transmission in health care settings.

Pathophysiology

TB begins when a susceptible person inhales mycobacteria and becomes infected. The bacteria are transmitted through the airways to the alveoli, where they are deposited and begin

---

Chart 23-7 ⚠ **RISK FACTORS**
Tuberculosis

- Close contact with someone who has active TB. Inhalation of airborne nuclei from an infected person is proportional to the amount of time spent in the same air space, the proximity of the person, and the degree of ventilation.
- Immunocompromised status (e.g., those with HIV infection, cancer, transplanted organs, and prolonged high-dose corticosteroid therapy).
- Substance abuse (IV/injection drug users and alcoholics).
- Any person without adequate health care (the homeless; impoverished; minorities, particularly children <15 years and young adults between ages 15 and 44 years).
- Preexisting medical conditions or special treatment (e.g., diabetes, chronic kidney injury, malnourishment, selected malignancies, hemodialysis, transplanted organ, gastrectomy, and jejunoileal bypass).
- Immigration from or recent travel to countries with a high prevalence of TB (southeastern Asia, Africa, Latin America, Caribbean).
- Institutionalization (e.g., long-term care facilities, psychiatric institutions, prisons).
- Living in overcrowded, substandard housing.
- Being a health care worker performing high-risk activities: administration of aerosolized pentamidine and other medications, sputum induction procedures, bronchoscopy, suctioning, coughing procedures, caring for the immunosuppressed patient, home care with the high-risk population, and administering anesthesia and related procedures (e.g., intubation, suctioning).

TB, tuberculosis.
Adapted from Centers for Disease Control and Prevention. (2012). *TB fact sheets-infection control and prevention; TB in specific populations.* Last updated September 1, 2012. Retrieved on 3/26/16 at: www.cdc.gov/tb/publications/factsheets/specpop.htm

Chart 23-8	Centers for Disease Control and Prevention Recommendations for Preventing Transmission of Tuberculosis in Health Care Settings

1. Early identification and treatment of persons with active TB
   a. Maintain a high index of suspicion for TB to identify cases rapidly.
   b. Promptly initiate effective multidrug anti-TB therapy based on clinical and drug-resistance surveillance data.
2. Prevention of spread of infectious droplet nuclei by source control methods and by reduction of microbial contamination of indoor air
   a. Initiate AFB isolation precautions immediately for all patients who are suspected or confirmed to have active TB and who may be infectious. AFB isolation precautions include the use of a private room with negative pressure in relation to surrounding areas and a minimum of six air exchanges per hour. Air from the room should be exhausted directly to the outside. The use of ultraviolet lamps and/or high-efficiency particulate air filters to supplement ventilation may be considered.
   b. Persons entering the AFB isolation room should use disposable particulate respirators that fit snugly around the face.
   c. Continue AFB isolation precautions until there is clinical evidence of reduced infectiousness (i.e., cough has substantially decreased and the number of organisms on sequential sputum smears is decreasing). If drug resistance is suspected or confirmed, continue AFB precautions until the sputum smear is negative for AFB.
   d. Use special precautions during cough-inducing procedures.
3. Surveillance for TB transmission
   a. Maintain surveillance for TB infection among health care workers (HCWs) by routine, periodic tuberculin skin testing. Recommend appropriate preventive therapy for HCWs when indicated.
   b. Maintain surveillance for TB cases among patients and HCWs.
   c. Promptly initiate contact investigation procedures among HCWs, patients, and visitors exposed to an untreated, or ineffectively treated, patient with infectious TB for whom appropriate AFB procedures are not in place. Recommend appropriate therapy or preventive therapy for contacts with disease or TB infection without current disease. Therapeutic regimens should be chosen based on the clinical history and local drug-resistance surveillance data.

TB, tuberculosis; AFB, acid-fast bacilli.
Adapted from Centers for Disease Control and Prevention. (2012). *TB fact sheet-infection control and prevention*. Retrieved on 3/26/16 at www.cdc.gov/tb/publications/factsheets/prevention.htm.

to multiply. The bacilli also are transported via the lymph system and bloodstream to other parts of the body (kidneys, bones, cerebral cortex) and other areas of the lungs (upper lobes). The body's immune system responds by initiating an inflammatory reaction. Phagocytes (neutrophils and macrophages) engulf many of the bacteria, and TB-specific lymphocytes lyse (destroy) the bacilli and normal tissue. This tissue reaction results in the accumulation of exudate in the alveoli, causing bronchopneumonia. The initial infection usually occurs 2 to 10 weeks after exposure.

Granulomas, new tissue masses of live and dead bacilli, are surrounded by macrophages, which form a protective wall.

They are then transformed to a fibrous tissue mass, the central portion of which is called a *Ghon tubercle*. The material (bacteria and macrophages) becomes necrotic, forming a cheesy mass. This mass may become calcified and form a collagenous scar. At this point, the bacteria become dormant, and there is no further progression of active disease.

After initial exposure and infection, active disease may develop because of a compromised or inadequate immune system response. Active disease also may occur with reinfection and activation of dormant bacteria. In this case, the *Ghon tubercle* ulcerates, releasing the cheesy material into the bronchi. The bacteria then become airborne, resulting in the further spread of the disease. Then, the ulcerated tubercle heals and forms scar tissue. This causes the infected lung to become more inflamed, resulting in the further development of bronchopneumonia and tubercle formation.

Unless this process is arrested, it spreads slowly downward to the hilum of the lungs and later extends to adjacent lobes. The process may be prolonged and is characterized by long remissions when the disease is arrested, followed by periods of renewed activity. Approximately 10% of people who are initially infected develop active disease (Pozniak, 2016). Some people develop reactivation TB (also called *adult-type progressive TB*). The reactivation of a dormant focus occurring during the primary infection is the cause.

Clinical Manifestations

The signs and symptoms of pulmonary TB are insidious. Most patients have a low-grade fever, cough, night sweats, fatigue, and weight loss. The cough may be nonproductive, or mucopurulent sputum may be expectorated. Hemoptysis also may occur. Both the systemic and the pulmonary symptoms are chronic and may have been present for weeks to months. Older adult patients usually present with less pronounced symptoms than younger patients. Extrapulmonary disease occurs in up to 21% of cases in the United States (Bernardo, 2014). In patients infected with HIV, extrapulmonary disease is more prevalent.

Assessment and Diagnostic Findings

Once a patient presents with a positive skin test, blood test, or sputum culture for acid-fast bacilli (AFB; see later discussion on these), additional assessments must be done. These tests include a complete history, physical examination, tuberculin skin test, chest x-ray, and drug susceptibility testing.

Clinical manifestations of fever, anorexia, weight loss, night sweats, fatigue, cough, and sputum production prompt a more thorough assessment of respiratory function—for example, assessing the lungs for consolidation by evaluating breath sounds (diminished, bronchial sounds; crackles), fremitus, and egophony. If the patient is infected with TB, the chest x-ray usually reveals lesions in the upper lobes. For all patients, the initial M. *tuberculosis* isolate should be tested for drug resistance. Drug susceptibility patterns should be repeated at 3 months for patients who do not respond to therapy (Sterling, 2016).

Tuberculin Skin Test

The Mantoux method is used to determine whether a person has been infected with the TB bacillus and is used widely in

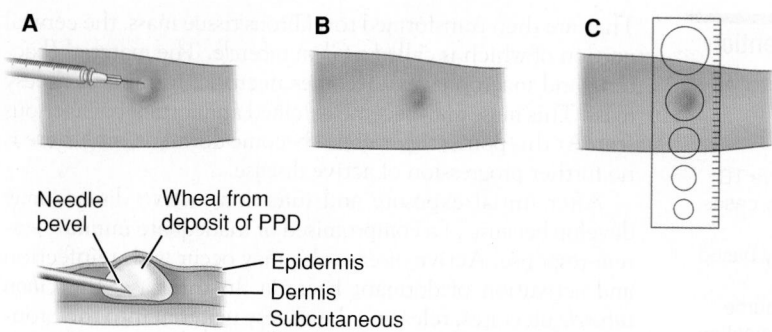

Needle bevel
Wheal from deposit of PPD
Epidermis
Dermis
Subcutaneous tissue

Figure 23-3 • The Mantoux test for tuberculosis. **A.** Correct technique for inserting the needle involves depositing the purified protein derivative (PPD) subcutaneously with the needle bevel facing upward. **B.** The reaction to the Mantoux test usually consists of a wheal, a hivelike, firm welt. **C.** To determine the extent of the reaction, the wheal is measured using a commercially prepared gauge. Interpretation of the Mantoux test is discussed in the text.

screening for latent *M. tuberculosis* infection. The Mantoux method is a standardized, intracutaneous injection procedure and should be performed only by those trained in its administration and reading. Tubercle bacillus extract (tuberculin), purified protein derivative (PPD), is injected into the intradermal layer of the inner aspect of the forearm, approximately 4 inches below the elbow (see Fig. 23-3). Intermediate-strength PPD, in a tuberculin syringe with a half-inch 26- or 27-gauge needle, is used. The needle, with the bevel facing up, is inserted beneath the skin. Then, 0.1 mL of PPD is injected, creating an elevation in the skin, a well-demarcated wheal 6 to 10 mm in diameter. The site, antigen name, strength, lot number, date, and time of the test are recorded. The test result is read 48 to 72 hours after injection. Tests read after 72 hours tend to underestimate the true size of induration (raised hard area or swelling). A delayed localized reaction indicates that the person is sensitive to tuberculin.

A reaction occurs when both induration and erythema (redness) are present. After the area is inspected for induration, it is lightly palpated across the injection site, from the area of normal skin to the margins of the induration. The diameter of the induration (not erythema) is measured in millimeters at its widest part (see Fig. 23-3), and the size of the induration is documented. Erythema without induration is not considered significant.

The size of the induration determines the significance of the reaction. A reaction of 0 to 4 mm is considered not significant. A reaction of 5 mm or greater may be significant in people who are considered to be at risk. It is defined as positive in patients who are HIV positive or have HIV risk factors and are of unknown HIV status, in those who are close contacts of someone with active TB, and in those who have chest x-ray results consistent with TB. An induration of 10 mm or greater is usually considered significant in people who have normal or mildly impaired immunity. A significant reaction indicates past exposure to *M. tuberculosis* or vaccination with bacille Calmette-Guérin (BCG) vaccine. The BCG vaccine is given to produce a greater resistance to development of TB. BCG has between 60% and 80% protective efficacy against severe forms of TB; its overall efficacy is variable (Roy, Eisenhut, Harris, et al., 2014). The BCG vaccine is used in Europe and Latin America but not routinely in the United States.

A significant (positive) reaction does not necessarily mean that active disease is present in the body. More than 90% of people who are tuberculin-significant reactors do not develop clinical TB (CDC, 2014b). However, all significant reactors are candidates for active TB. In general, the more intense the reaction, the greater the likelihood of an active infection.

Additional testing is needed to determine if the person has latent TB infection or active TB.

A nonsignificant (negative) skin test means the person's immune system did not react to the test and that latent TB infection or TB disease is not likely. It does not exclude TB infection or disease, because patients who are immunosuppressed cannot develop an immune response that is adequate to produce a positive skin test. This is referred to as anergy.

QuantiFERON-TB Gold® In-Tube and T-SPOT®

There are two TB blood tests (called interferon–gamma release assays or IGRAs) available in the United States: the QuantiFERON-TB Gold® In-Tube (QFT-GIT) test and the T-SPOT®. TB blood tests are the preferred diagnostic tests for patients who have received the BCG vaccine and for patients who are not likely to return for a second appointment to look for a reaction to the tuberculin skin test. The results of both of these tests are available within 24 to 36 hours. A positive IGRA signifies that the patient has been infected with TB bacteria and additional tests are needed. A negative IGRA means that the patient's blood did not react to the test and a latent or active TB infection is not likely (CDC, 2015d).

Sputum Culture

A sputum specimen may be used to screen for TB. The presence of AFB on a sputum smear may indicate disease but does not confirm the diagnosis of TB because some AFB are not *M. tuberculosis*. A culture is done to confirm the diagnosis. For all patients, the initial *M. tuberculosis* isolate should be tested for drug resistance (Sterling, 2016).

 Gerontologic Considerations

TB may have atypical manifestations in older adult patients, whose symptoms may include unusual behavior and altered mental status, fever, anorexia, and weight loss. In many older adult patients, the tuberculin skin test produces no reaction (loss of immunologic memory) or delayed reactivity for up to 1 week (recall phenomenon). A second skin test is performed in 1 to 2 weeks. Older adults who live in long-term care facilities are at increased risk for primary and reactivation TB as compared to those in the community (Pagali, Verdoom, Wieland, et al., 2014).

Medical Management

Pulmonary TB is treated primarily with anti-TB agents for 6 to 12 months. A prolonged treatment duration is necessary to ensure eradication of the organisms and to prevent relapse.

The continuing and increasing resistance of *M. tuberculosis* to TB medications is a worldwide concern and challenge in TB therapy. Several types of drug resistance must be considered when planning effective therapy:

- *Primary drug resistance:* Resistance to one of the first-line anti-TB agents in people who have not had previous treatment
- *Secondary or acquired drug resistance:* Resistance to one or more anti-TB agents in patients undergoing therapy
- *Multidrug resistance:* Resistance to two agents, isoniazid (INH) and rifampin. The populations at greatest risk for multidrug resistance are those who are HIV positive, institutionalized, or homeless.

The increasing prevalence of drug resistance points out the need to begin TB treatment with four or more medications, to ensure completion of therapy, and to develop and evaluate new anti-TB medications.

In current TB therapy, four first-line medications are used (see Table 23-4): INH, rifampin (Rifadin), pyrazinamide (PZA),

and ethambutol (Myambutol). Combination medications, such as INH and rifampin (Rifamate) or INH, pyrazinamide, and rifampin (Rifater) and medications given twice a week (e.g., rifapentine [Priftin]) are available to help improve patient adherence. However, these medications are more costly.

Multidrug-resistant TB is difficult to treat. Treatment is guided by sputum specimen culture and sensitivity testing as the patient typically is resistant to INH and/or rifampin. Usually three to five drugs are identified as appropriate to prescribe. Examples of these second-line drugs include: aminoglycosides, fluoroquinolones, capreomycin (Capastat), ethionamide (Trecator), para-aminosalicylate sodium, and cycloserine (Seromycin) (Gilbert, Chambers, Eliopoulos, et al., 2015).

Recommended treatment guidelines for newly diagnosed cases of pulmonary TB have two phases: an initial treatment phase and a continuation phase (CDC, 2015d; Gilbert et al., 2015). The initial phase consists of a multiple-medication

TABLE 23-4 First-Line Antituberculosis Medications for Active Disease

Commonly Used Agents	Adult Daily Dosage[a]	Most Common Side Effects	Drug Interactions[b]	Nursing Considerations[a]
Isoniazid (INH)	5 mg/kg (300 mg maximum daily)	Peripheral neuritis, hepatic enzyme elevation, hepatitis, hypersensitivity	Phenytoin—synergistic Antabuse Alcohol	Bactericidal Pyridoxine is used as prophylaxis for neuritis. Monitor AST and ALT
Rifampin (Rifadin)	10 mg/kg (600 mg maximum daily)	Hepatitis, febrile reaction, purpura (rare), nausea, vomiting	Rifampin increases metabolism of oral contraceptives, quinidine, corticosteroids, coumarin derivatives and methadone, digoxin, oral hypoglycemics. PAS may interfere with absorption of rifampin	Bactericidal Orange urine and other body secretions Discoloring of contact lenses Monitor AST and ALT
Rifabutin (Mycobutin)	5 mg/kg (300 mg maximum daily)		Avoid protease inhibitors.	
Rifapentine (Priftin)	10 mg/kg (600 mg twice weekly)	Hepatotoxicity, thrombocytopenia		Orange-red coloration of body secretions, contact lenses, dentures Use with caution in older adults or in those with renal disease
Pyrazinamide	15–30 mg/kg (2 g maximum daily)[a]	Hyperuricemia, hepatotoxicity, skin rash, arthralgias, GI distress		Bactericidal Monitor uric acid, AST, and ALT
Ethambutol (Myambutol)	15–25 mg/kg (1.6 g maximum daily dose)[a]	Optic neuritis (may lead to blindness; very rare at 15 mg/kg), skin rash		Bacteriostatic Use with caution with renal disease or when eye testing is not feasible. Monitor visual acuity, color, and discrimination[c]
Combinations: INH + rifampin (e.g., Rifamate)	150-mg and 300-mg caps (2 caps daily)			

AST, aspartate transaminase; ALT, alanine transaminase; PAS, para-aminosalicylic acid; GI, gastrointestinal.
[a]Check product labeling for detailed information on dose, contraindications, drug interactions, adverse reactions, and monitoring.
[b]Refer to current literature, particularly on rifampin, because it increases hepatic microenzymes and therefore interacts with many drugs.
[c]Initial examination should be performed at start of treatment.
Adapted from Gilbert, D. N., Chambers, H. F., Eliopoulos, G. M., et al. (2015). *The Sanford guide to antimicrobial therapy 2015* (45th ed.). Sperryville, VA: Antimicrobial Therapy, Inc.

regimen of INH, rifampin, pyrazinamide, and ethambutol plus vitamin B_6 50 mg. All are taken once a day and are oral medications (Gilbert et al., 2015). This initial intensive-treatment regimen is given daily for 8 weeks, after which options for the continuation phase of treatment include INH and rifampin or INH and rifapentine. The continuation regimen lasts for an additional 4 or 7 months. The 4-month period is used for the large majority of patients (Gilbert et al., 2015). The 7-month period is recommended for patients with cavitary pulmonary TB whose sputum culture after the initial 2 months of treatment is positive, for those whose initial phase of treatment did not include PZA, and for those being treated once weekly with INH and rifapentine whose sputum culture is positive at the end of the initial phase of treatment. People are considered noninfectious after 2 to 3 weeks of continuous medication therapy. The total number of doses taken, not simply the duration of treatment, more accurately determines whether a course of therapy has been completed.

INH also may be used as a prophylactic (preventive) measure for people who are at risk for significant disease, including:

- Household family members of patients with active disease
- Patients with HIV infection who have a PPD test reaction with 5 mm of induration or more
- Patients with fibrotic lesions suggestive of old TB detected on a chest x-ray and a PPD reaction with 5 mm of induration or more
- Patients whose current PPD test results show a change from former test results, suggesting recent exposure to TB and possible infection (skin test converters)
- Users of IV/injection drugs who have PPD test results with 10 mm of induration or more
- Patients with high-risk comorbid conditions and a PPD result with 10 mm of induration or more

Other candidates for preventive INH therapy are those 35 years or younger who have PPD test results with 10 mm of induration or more and one of the following criteria:

- Foreign-born individuals from countries with a high prevalence of TB
- High-risk, medically underserved populations
- Institutionalized patients

Prophylactic INH treatment involves taking daily doses for 6 to 12 months. Liver enzymes, blood urea nitrogen (BUN), and creatinine levels are monitored monthly. Sputum culture results are monitored for AFB to evaluate the effectiveness of treatment and the patient's adherence to the treatment regimen.

Nursing Management

Nursing management includes promoting airway clearance, advocating adherence to the treatment regimen, promoting activity and nutrition, and preventing transmission.

Promoting Airway Clearance

Copious secretions obstruct the airways in many patients with TB and interfere with adequate gas exchange. Increasing the fluid intake promotes systemic hydration and serves as an effective expectorant. The nurse instructs the patient about correct positioning to facilitate airway drainage (postural drainage; described in Chapter 21).

Promoting Adherence to Treatment Regimen

Adherence to the prescribed treatment regimen is key in treating the disease and controlling the spread of infection (Reichman & Lardizabal, 2015). The multiple-medication regimen that the patient must follow can be quite complex. Understanding of the medications, schedule, and side effects is important. The nurse educates the patient that TB is a communicable disease and that taking medications is the most effective means of preventing transmission. The major reason treatment fails is that patients do not take their medications regularly and for the prescribed duration. This may be due to side effects or the complexity of the treatment regimen. Risk factors for nonadherence to the drug regimen include patients who have previously failed to complete the course of therapy; patients who are physically, emotionally or mentally challenged; patients unable to pay for medication; patients actively abusing illicit substances; and patients who do not understand the importance of treatment (Reichman & Lardizabal, 2015).

The nurse educates the patient to take the medication either on an empty stomach or at least 1 hour before meals, because food interferes with medication absorption (although taking medications on an empty stomach frequently results in gastrointestinal upset). Patients taking INH should avoid foods that contain tyramine and histamine (tuna, aged cheese, red wine, soy sauce, yeast extracts), because eating them while taking INH may result in headache, flushing, hypotension, lightheadedness, palpitations, and diaphoresis. Patients should also avoid alcohol because of the high potential for hepatotoxic effects.

In addition, rifampin can alter the metabolism of certain other medications, making them less effective. These medications include beta-blockers, oral anticoagulants such as warfarin (Coumadin), digoxin, quinidine, corticosteroids, oral hypoglycemic agents, oral contraceptives, theophylline, and verapamil (Calan, Isoptin). This issue should be discussed with the primary provider and pharmacist so that medication dosages can be adjusted accordingly. The nurse informs the patient that rifampin may discolor contact lenses and that the patient may want to wear eyeglasses during treatment. The nurse monitors for other side effects of anti-TB medications, including hepatitis, neurologic changes (hearing loss, neuritis), and rash. Liver enzymes, BUN, and serum creatinine levels are monitored to detect changes in liver and kidney function. Sputum culture results are monitored for AFB to evaluate the effectiveness of the treatment regimen and adherence to therapy.

The nurse instructs the patient about the risk of drug resistance if the medication regimen is not strictly and continuously followed. The nurse carefully monitors vital signs and observes for spikes in temperature or changes in the patient's clinical status. Caregivers of patients who are not hospitalized are taught to monitor the patient's temperature and respiratory status. Changes in the patient's respiratory status are reported to the primary provider.

For patients at risk of nonadherence, programs used in the community setting may include comprehensive case management and directly observed therapy (DOT). In case management, each patient with TB is assigned a case manager who coordinates all aspects of the patient's care. DOT consists of a health care provider or other responsible person who directly observes that the patient ingests the prescribed medications. Although successful, DOT is a resource intensive program (Reichman & Lardizabal, 2015).

Promoting Activity and Adequate Nutrition

Patients with TB are often debilitated from prolonged chronic illness and impaired nutritional status. The nurse plans a progressive activity schedule that focuses on increasing activity tolerance and muscle strength. Anorexia, weight loss, and malnutrition are common in patients with TB. The patient's willingness to eat may be altered by fatigue from excessive coughing; sputum production; chest pain; generalized debilitated state; or cost, if the patient has few resources. Identifying facilities (e.g., shelters, soup kitchens, and Meals on Wheels) that provide meals in the patient's neighborhood may increase the likelihood that the patient with limited resources and energy will have access to a more nutritious intake. A nutritional plan that allows for small, frequent meals may be required. Liquid nutritional supplements may assist in meeting basic caloric requirements.

Preventing Transmission of Tuberculosis Infection

To prevent transmission of TB to others, the nurse carefully instructs the patient about important hygiene measures, including mouth care, covering the mouth and nose when coughing and sneezing, proper disposal of tissues, and hand hygiene. TB is a disease that must be reported to the health department so that people who have been in contact with the affected patient during the infectious stage can undergo screening and possible treatment, if indicated.

In addition to the risk of transmission of TB infection to other people, it can also be spread to other parts of the body of affected patients. Spread or dissemination of TB infection to nonpulmonary sites of the body is known as miliary TB. It is the result of invasion of the bloodstream by the tubercle bacillus. Usually, it results from late reactivation of a dormant infection in the lung or elsewhere. The origin of the bacilli that enter the bloodstream is either a chronic focus that has ulcerated into a blood vessel or multitudes of miliary tubercles lining the inner surface of the thoracic duct. The organisms migrate from these foci into the bloodstream, are carried throughout the body, and disseminate throughout all tissues, with tiny miliary tubercles developing in the lungs, spleen, liver, kidneys, meninges, and other organs.

The clinical course of miliary TB may vary from an acute, rapidly progressive infection with high fever to a slowly developing process with low-grade fever, anemia, and debilitation. At first, there may be no localizing signs except an enlarged spleen and a reduced number of leukocytes. However, within a few weeks, the chest x-ray reveals small densities scattered diffusely throughout both lung fields; these are the miliary tubercles, which gradually grow.

The possibility of spread to nonpulmonary sites in the body requires careful monitoring for this very serious form of TB. The nurse monitors vital signs and observes for spikes in temperature as well as changes in renal and cognitive function. Few physical signs may be elicited on physical examination of the chest, but at this stage, the patient has a severe cough and dyspnea. Treatment of miliary TB is the same as for pulmonary TB.

Lung Abscess

A lung abscess is a localized collection of pus caused by microbial infection (Weinberger et al., 2014). It is generally caused by aspiration of anaerobic bacteria. By definition, in a lung abscess, the chest x-ray demonstrates a cavity of at least 2 cm. Patients who are at risk for aspiration of foreign material and development of a lung abscess include those with impaired cough reflexes who cannot close the glottis and those with swallowing difficulties. Other at-risk patients include those with central nervous system disorders (e.g., seizure and stroke), drug addiction, alcoholism, esophageal disease, or compromised immune function; patients without teeth and those receiving nasogastric tube feedings; and patients with an altered state of consciousness due to anesthesia.

Pathophysiology

Most lung abscesses are a complication of bacterial pneumonia or are caused by aspiration of oral anaerobes into the lung. Abscesses also may occur secondary to mechanical or functional obstruction of the bronchi by a tumor, foreign body, or bronchial stenosis, or from necrotizing pneumonias, TB, pulmonary embolism (PE), or chest trauma.

Most lung abscesses are found in areas of the lung that may be affected by aspiration. The site of the lung abscess is related to gravity and is determined by position. For patients who are confined to bed, the posterior segment of an upper lobe and the superior segment of the lower lobe are the most common areas. However, atypical presentations may occur, depending on the position of the patient when the aspiration occurred.

Initially, the cavity in the lung may or may not extend directly into a bronchus. Eventually, the abscess becomes surrounded, or encapsulated, by a wall of fibrous tissue. The necrotic process may extend until it reaches the lumen of a bronchus or the pleural space and establishes communication with the respiratory tract, the pleural cavity, or both. If the bronchus is involved, the purulent contents are expectorated continuously in the form of sputum. If the pleura is involved, the result is an empyema. A communication or connection between the bronchus and pleura is known as a bronchopleural fistula.

The organisms frequently associated with lung abscesses are anaerobic; however aerobic organisms may be involved as well. The organisms vary depending on the underlying predisposing factors (Weinberger et al., 2014).

Clinical Manifestations

The clinical manifestations of a lung abscess may vary from a mild productive cough to acute illness. Most patients have a fever and a productive cough with moderate to copious amounts of foul-smelling, sometimes bloody, sputum. The fever and cough may develop insidiously and may have been present for several weeks before diagnosis. Leukocytosis may be present. Pleurisy or dull chest pain, dyspnea, weakness, anorexia, and weight loss are common.

Assessment and Diagnostic Findings

Physical examination of the chest may reveal dullness on percussion and decreased or absent breath sounds with an intermittent **pleural friction rub** (grating or creaking sound) on auscultation. Crackles may be present. Confirmation of the diagnosis is made by chest x-ray, sputum culture, and, in some cases, fiberoptic bronchoscopy. The chest x-ray reveals an infiltrate with an air–fluid level. A computed tomography (CT) scan of the chest may be required to provide more detailed images of different cross-sectional areas of the lung.

Prevention

The following measures reduce the risk of lung abscess:

- Appropriate antibiotic therapy before any dental procedures in patients who must have teeth extracted while their gums and teeth are infected
- Adequate dental and oral hygiene, because anaerobic bacteria play a role in the pathogenesis of lung abscess
- Appropriate antimicrobial therapy for patients with pneumonia

Medical Management

The findings of the history, physical examination, chest x-ray, and sputum culture indicate the type of organism and the treatment required. Adequate drainage of the lung abscess may be achieved through postural drainage and chest physiotherapy. Patients should be assessed for an adequate cough. Some patients require insertion of a percutaneous chest catheter for long-term drainage of the abscess. Therapeutic use of bronchoscopy to drain an abscess is uncommon. A diet high in protein and calories is necessary, because chronic infection is associated with a catabolic state, necessitating increased intake of calories and protein to facilitate healing. Surgical intervention is rare, but pulmonary resection (lobectomy) is performed if massive **hemoptysis** (coughing up of blood) occurs or if there is little or no response to medical management.

IV antimicrobial therapy depends on the results of the sputum culture and sensitivity and is given for an extended period. Standard treatment of an anaerobic lung infection is clindamycin (Cleocin), ampicillin-sulbactam (Unasyn) or carbapenem (Gilbert et al., 2015). Large IV doses are usually required, because the antibiotic must penetrate the necrotic tissue and the fluid in the abscess. The duration of treatment with IV antibiotics is controversial (Bartlett, 2014). Treatment with IV antibiotics may continue for 3 weeks and longer, depending upon the clinical severity and organism involved. Improvement is demonstrated by normal temperature, decreased white blood cell count, and improvement on chest x-ray (resolution of surrounding infiltrate, reduction in cavity size, and absence of fluid). Once improvement is demonstrated, IV antibiotics are discontinued and oral administration of antibiotic therapy is continued for an additional 4 to 12 weeks and sometimes longer. If treatment is stopped too soon, a relapse may occur (Bartlett, 2014).

Nursing Management

The nurse administers antibiotics and IV treatments as prescribed and monitors for adverse effects. Chest physiotherapy is initiated as prescribed to facilitate drainage of the abscess. The nurse educates the patient to perform deep-breathing and coughing exercises to help expand the lungs. To ensure proper nutritional intake, the nurse encourages a diet that is high in protein and calories. The nurse also offers emotional support, because the abscess may take a long time to resolve.

Promoting Home, Community-Based, and Transitional Care

 Educating Patients About Self-Care

A patient who has had surgery may return home before the wound closes entirely or with a drain or tube in place. In these cases, the nurse educates the patient or caregivers about how to change the dressings to prevent skin excoriation and odor, how to monitor for signs and symptoms of infection, and how to care for and maintain the drain or tube. The nurse also reminds the patient to perform deep-breathing and coughing exercises every 2 hours during the day and shows caregivers how to perform chest percussion and postural drainage to facilitate expectoration of lung secretions.

Continuing and Transitional Care

A patient whose condition requires therapy at home may need referral for home, transitional, or community-based care. During home visits, the nurse assesses the patient's physical condition, nutritional status, and home environment, as well as the ability of the patient and family to carry out the therapeutic regimen. Patient education is reinforced, and nutritional counseling is provided with the goal of attaining and maintaining an optimal state of nutrition. To prevent relapses, the nurse emphasizes the importance of completing the antibiotic regimen and of following suggestions for rest and appropriate activity. If IV antibiotic therapy is to continue at home, the services of home care nurses may be arranged to initiate IV therapy and to evaluate its administration by the patient or family.

Although most outpatient IV therapy is given in the home setting, the patient may visit a nearby clinic or provider's office for this treatment. In some cases, patients with lung abscess may have ignored their health. Therefore, the nurse should use this opportunity to address health promotion strategies and health screening with the patient.

PLEURAL CONDITIONS

Pleural conditions are disorders that involve the membranes covering the lungs (visceral pleura) and the surface of the chest wall (parietal pleura) or disorders affecting the pleural space.

Pleurisy

Pathophysiology

Pleurisy (pleuritis) refers to inflammation of both layers of the pleurae (parietal and visceral). Pleurisy may develop in conjunction with pneumonia or an upper respiratory tract infection, TB, or collagen disease; after trauma to the chest, pulmonary infarction, or PE; in patients with primary or metastatic cancer; and after thoracotomy. The parietal pleura has nerve endings, and the visceral pleura does not. When the inflamed pleural membranes rub together during respiration (intensified on inspiration), the result is severe, sharp, knife-like pain.

Clinical Manifestations

The key characteristic of pleuritic pain is its relationship to respiratory movement. Taking a deep breath, coughing, or sneezing worsens the pain. Pleuritic pain is limited in distribution rather than diffuse; it usually occurs only on one side. The pain may become minimal or absent when the breath is held. It may be localized or radiate to the shoulder or abdomen. Later, as pleural fluid develops, the pain decreases (Weinberger et al., 2014).

Assessment and Diagnostic Findings

In the early period, when little fluid has accumulated, a pleural friction rub can be heard with the stethoscope, only to disappear later as more fluid accumulates and separates the inflamed pleural surfaces. Diagnostic tests may include chest x-rays, sputum analysis, thoracentesis to obtain a specimen of pleural fluid for examination, and, less commonly, a pleural biopsy.

Medical Management

The objectives of treatment are to discover the underlying condition causing the pleurisy and to relieve the pain. As the underlying disease (pneumonia, infection) is treated, the pleuritic inflammation usually resolves. At the same time, the patient must be monitored for signs and symptoms of pleural effusion, such as shortness of breath, pain, assumption of a position that decreases pain, and decreased chest wall excursion.

Prescribed analgesic agents and topical applications of heat or cold provide symptomatic relief. A nonsteroidal anti-inflammatory drug may provide pain relief while allowing the patient to take deep breaths and cough more effectively. If the pain is severe, an intercostal nerve block may be required (Weinberger et al., 2014).

Nursing Management

Because the patient has pain on inspiration, the nurse offers suggestions to enhance comfort, such as turning frequently onto the affected side to splint the chest wall and reduce the stretching of the pleurae. The nurse also educates the patient to use the hands or a pillow to splint the rib cage while coughing.

Pleural Effusion

Pleural effusion, a collection of fluid in the pleural space, is rarely a primary disease process; it is usually secondary to other diseases. Normally, the pleural space contains a small amount of fluid (5 to 15 mL), which acts as a lubricant that allows the pleural surfaces to move without friction (see Fig. 23-4). Pleural effusion may be a complication of heart failure, TB, pneumonia, pulmonary infections (particularly viral infections), nephrotic syndrome, connective tissue disease, PE and neoplastic tumors. The most common malignancy associated with a pleural effusion is bronchogenic carcinoma.

Pathophysiology

In certain disorders, fluid may accumulate in the pleural space to a point at which it becomes clinically evident. This

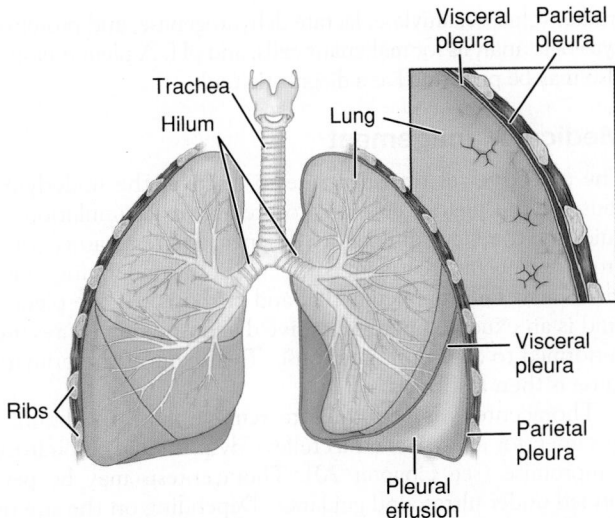

Figure 23-4 • In pleural effusion, an abnormal volume of fluid collects in the pleural space, causing pain and shortness of breath. Pleural effusion is usually secondary to other disease processes.

almost always has pathologic significance. The effusion can be a relatively clear fluid, or it can be bloody or purulent. An effusion of clear fluid may be a transudate or an exudate. A transudate (filtrate of plasma that moves across intact capillary walls) occurs when factors influencing the formation and reabsorption of pleural fluid are altered, usually by imbalances in hydrostatic or oncotic pressures. The finding of a transudative effusion generally implies that the pleural membranes are not diseased. A transudative effusion most commonly results from heart failure. An exudate (extravasation of fluid into tissues or a cavity) usually results from inflammation by bacterial products or tumors involving the pleural surfaces (Heffner, 2015a).

Clinical Manifestations

Usually, the clinical manifestations are caused by the underlying disease. Pneumonia causes fever, chills, and pleuritic chest pain, whereas a malignant effusion may result in dyspnea, difficulty lying flat, and coughing. The severity of symptoms is determined by the size of the effusion, the speed of its formation, and the underlying lung disease. A large pleural effusion causes dyspnea (shortness of breath). A small-to-moderate pleural effusion causes minimal or no dyspnea.

Assessment and Diagnostic Findings

Assessment of the area of the pleural effusion reveals decreased or absent breath sounds; decreased fremitus; and a dull, flat sound on percussion. In the case of an extremely large pleural effusion, the assessment reveals a patient in acute respiratory distress. Tracheal deviation away from the affected side may also be apparent.

Physical examination, chest x-ray, chest CT, and thoracentesis confirm the presence of fluid. In some instances, a lateral decubitus x-ray is obtained. For this x-ray, the patient lies on the affected side in a side-lying position. A pleural effusion can be diagnosed because this position allows for the "layering out" of the fluid, and an air–fluid line is visible.

Pleural fluid is analyzed by bacterial culture, Gram stain, AFB stain (for TB), red and white blood cell counts, chemistry studies (glucose, amylase, lactate dehydrogenase, and protein), cytologic analysis for malignant cells, and pH. A pleural biopsy also may be performed as a diagnostic tool.

Medical Management

The objectives of treatment are to discover the underlying cause of the pleural effusion; to prevent reaccumulation of fluid; and to relieve discomfort, dyspnea, and respiratory compromise. Specific treatment is directed at the underlying cause (e.g., heart failure, pneumonia, and cirrhosis). If the pleural fluid is an exudate, more extensive diagnostic procedures are performed to determine the cause. Treatment of the primary cause is then instituted.

Thoracentesis is performed to remove fluid, to obtain a specimen for analysis, and to relieve dyspnea and respiratory compromise (see Chapter 20). Thoracentesis may be performed under ultrasound guidance. Depending on the size of the pleural effusion, the patient may be treated by removing the fluid during the thoracentesis procedure or by inserting a chest tube connected to a water-seal drainage system or suction to evacuate the pleural space and re-expand the lung.

However, if the underlying cause is a malignancy, the effusion tends to recur within a few days or weeks. Repeated thoracenteses result in pain, depletion of protein and electrolytes, and sometimes pneumothorax. Once the pleural space is adequately drained, a chemical pleurodesis may be performed to obliterate the pleural space and prevent reaccumulation of fluid. Pleurodesis may be performed using either a thoracoscopic approach or a chest tube. A chemically irritating agent (e.g., talc or another chemical irritant) is instilled or aerosolized into the pleural space. With the chest tube approach, after the agent is instilled, the chest tube is clamped for 60 to 90 minutes and the patient is assisted to assume various positions to promote uniform distribution of the agent and to maximize its contact with the pleural surfaces (Heffner, 2015b). The tube is unclamped as prescribed, and chest drainage may be continued several days longer to prevent reaccumulation of fluid and to promote the formation of adhesions between the visceral and parietal pleurae.

Other treatments for pleural effusions caused by malignancy include surgical pleurectomy, insertion of a small catheter attached to a drainage bottle for outpatient management (e.g., PleurX® catheter [CareFusion]), or implantation of a pleuroperitoneal shunt. A pleuroperitoneal shunt consists of two catheters connected by a pump chamber containing two one-way valves. Fluid moves from the pleural space to the pump chamber and then to the peritoneal cavity. The patient manually pumps on the reservoir daily to move fluid from the pleural space to the peritoneal space.

Nursing Management

The nurse's role in the care of patients with a pleural effusion includes supporting the medical regimen. The nurse prepares and positions the patient for thoracentesis and offers support throughout the procedure. The nurse is responsible for making sure the thoracentesis fluid amount is recorded and sent for appropriate laboratory testing. If a chest tube drainage and water-seal system is used, the nurse is responsible for monitoring the system's function and recording the amount of drainage at prescribed intervals. Nursing care related to

the underlying cause of the pleural effusion is specific to the underlying condition. (See Chapter 21 for a discussion of care of the patient with a chest tube.)

If a chest tube is inserted for talc instillation, pain management is a priority and the nurse helps the patient assume positions that are the least painful. However, frequent turning and movement are important to facilitate adequate spreading of the talc over the pleural surface. The nurse evaluates the patient's pain level and administers analgesic agents as prescribed and as needed.

If the patient is to be managed as an outpatient with a pleural catheter for drainage, the nurse educates the patient and family about management and care of the catheter and drainage system.

Empyema

An empyema is an accumulation of thick, purulent fluid within the pleural space, often with fibrin development and a loculated (walled-off) area where infection is located (Strange, 2016).

Pathophysiology

Most empyemas occur as complications of bacterial pneumonia or lung abscess. They also result from penetrating chest trauma, hematogenous infection of the pleural space, nonbacterial infections, and iatrogenic causes (after thoracic surgery or thoracentesis). At first the pleural fluid is thin, with a low leukocyte count, but it frequently progresses to a fibropurulent stage and, finally, to a stage where it encloses the lung within a thick exudative membrane (loculated empyema).

Clinical Manifestations

The patient is acutely ill and has signs and symptoms similar to those of an acute respiratory infection or pneumonia (fever, night sweats, pleural pain, cough, dyspnea, anorexia, weight loss). If the patient is immunocompromised, the symptoms may be vague. If the patient has received antimicrobial therapy, the clinical manifestations may be less obvious.

Assessment and Diagnostic Findings

Chest auscultation demonstrates decreased or absent breath sounds over the affected area, and there is dullness on chest percussion as well as decreased fremitus. The diagnosis is established by chest CT. Usually, a diagnostic thoracentesis is performed, often under ultrasound guidance.

Medical Management

The objectives of treatment are to drain the pleural cavity and to achieve complete expansion of the lung. The fluid is drained, and appropriate antibiotics (usually begun by the IV route) in large doses are prescribed based on the causative organism. Sterilization of the empyema cavity requires 4 to 6 weeks of antibiotics (Strange, 2016). Drainage of the pleural fluid depends on the stage of the disease and is accomplished by one of the following methods:

- Needle aspiration (thoracentesis) with a thin percutaneous catheter, if the volume is small and the fluid is not too purulent or too thick

- Tube thoracostomy (chest drainage using a large-diameter intercostal tube attached to water-seal drainage [see Chapter 21]) with fibrinolytic agents instilled through the chest tube in patients with loculated or complicated pleural effusions
- Open chest drainage via thoracotomy, including potential rib resection, to remove the thickened pleura, pus, and debris and to remove the underlying diseased pulmonary tissue

With long-standing inflammation, an exudate can form over the lung, trapping it and interfering with its normal expansion. This exudate must be removed surgically (decortication). The drainage tube is left in place until the pus-filled space is obliterated completely. The complete obliteration of the pleural space is monitored by serial chest x-rays, and the patient should be informed that treatment may be long term (weeks to months). Patients are frequently discharged from the hospital with a chest tube in place, with instructions to monitor fluid drainage at home.

Nursing Management

Resolution of empyema is a prolonged process. The nurse helps the patient cope with the condition and instructs the patient in lung-expanding breathing exercises to restore normal respiratory function. The nurse also provides care specific to the method of drainage of the pleural fluid (e.g., needle aspiration, closed chest drainage, rib resection, and drainage). When the patient is discharged home with a drainage tube or system in place, the nurse instructs the patient and family on care of the drainage system and drain site, measurement and observation of drainage, signs and symptoms of infection, and how and when to contact the primary provider. (See The Patient Undergoing Thoracic Surgery section in Chapter 21.)

 ## Pulmonary Edema (Noncardiogenic)

Pulmonary edema is defined as abnormal accumulation of fluid in the lung tissue, the alveolar space, or both. It is a severe, life-threatening condition. Pulmonary edema can be classified as cardiogenic or noncardiogenic. (See Chapter 29 for further discussion of cardiogenic pulmonary edema.) Noncardiogenic pulmonary edema occurs due to damage of the pulmonary capillary lining. It may be due to direct injury to the lung (e.g., chest trauma, aspiration, and smoke inhalation), hematogenous injury to the lung (e.g., sepsis, pancreatitis, multiple transfusions, and cardiopulmonary bypass), or injury plus elevated hydrostatic pressures. Management of noncardiogenic pulmonary edema mirrors that of cardiogenic pulmonary edema (see Chapter 29); however, hypoxemia may persist despite high concentrations of supplemental oxygen, due to the intrapulmonary shunting of blood.

 ## Acute Respiratory Failure

Respiratory failure is a sudden and life-threatening deterioration of the gas exchange function of the lung and indicates failure of the lungs to provide adequate oxygenation or ventilation for the blood. Acute respiratory failure is defined as a decrease in arterial oxygen tension (PaO_2) to less than 60 mm Hg (hypoxemia) and an increase in arterial carbon dioxide tension ($PaCO_2$) to greater than 50 mm Hg (hypercapnia), with an arterial pH of less than 7.35 (Fournier, 2014).

It is important to distinguish between acute and chronic respiratory failure. Chronic respiratory failure is defined as deterioration in the gas exchange function of the lung that has developed insidiously or has persisted for a long period after an episode of acute respiratory failure. The absence of acute symptoms and the presence of a chronic respiratory acidosis suggest the chronicity of the respiratory failure. Two causes of chronic respiratory failure are COPD (discussed in Chapter 24) and neuromuscular diseases (discussed in Chapter 70). Patients with these disorders develop a tolerance to the gradually worsening hypoxemia and hypercapnia. However, patients with chronic respiratory failure can develop acute failure. For example, a patient with COPD may develop an exacerbation or infection that causes additional deterioration of gas exchange. The principles of management of acute versus chronic respiratory failure are different; the following discussion is limited to acute respiratory failure.

Pathophysiology

In acute respiratory failure, the ventilation or perfusion mechanisms in the lung are impaired. Ventilatory failure mechanisms leading to acute respiratory failure include impaired function of the central nervous system (i.e., drug overdose, head trauma, infection, hemorrhage, and sleep apnea), neuromuscular dysfunction (i.e., myasthenia gravis, Guillain–Barré syndrome, amyotrophic lateral sclerosis, and spinal cord trauma), musculoskeletal dysfunction (i.e., chest trauma, kyphoscoliosis, and malnutrition), and pulmonary dysfunction (i.e., COPD, asthma, and cystic fibrosis).

Oxygenation failure mechanisms leading to acute respiratory failure include pneumonia, acute respiratory distress syndrome (ARDS), heart failure, COPD, PE, and **restrictive lung diseases** (diseases that cause decrease in lung volumes).

In the postoperative period, especially after major thoracic or abdominal surgery, inadequate ventilation and respiratory failure may occur because of several factors. During this period, for example, acute respiratory failure may be caused by the effects of anesthetic, analgesic, and sedative agents, which may depress respiration (as described earlier) or enhance the effects of opioids and lead to hypoventilation. Pain may interfere with deep breathing and coughing. A $\dot{V}/\dot{Q}$ mismatch is the usual cause of respiratory failure after major abdominal, cardiac, or thoracic surgery.

Clinical Manifestations

Early signs are those associated with impaired oxygenation and may include restlessness, fatigue, headache, dyspnea, air hunger, tachycardia, and increased blood pressure. As the hypoxemia progresses, more obvious signs may be present, including confusion, lethargy, tachycardia, tachypnea, central cyanosis, diaphoresis, and finally respiratory arrest. Physical findings are those of acute respiratory distress, including the use of accessory muscles, decreased breath sounds if the patient cannot adequately ventilate, and other findings related specifically to the underlying disease process and cause of acute respiratory failure.

Concept Mastery Alert

In the early phase of acute respiratory failure, vague signs and symptoms such as restlessness, anxiety, fatigue, and headache make it difficult to determine what the patient is experiencing. However, as oxygenation becomes more impaired, hypoxemia increases and leads to more obvious signs such as tachycardia, tachypnea, circumoral cyanosis, diaphoresis, accessory muscle use, inability to speak in full sentences, and altered mental status. Pain usually is not present. Some patients may progress through these phases over several hours, whereas others may progress within seconds.

Medical Management

The objectives of treatment are to correct the underlying cause and to restore adequate gas exchange in the lung. Endotracheal intubation and mechanical ventilation may be required to maintain adequate ventilation and oxygenation while the underlying cause is corrected.

Nursing Management

Nursing management of patients with acute respiratory failure includes assisting with intubation and maintaining mechanical ventilation (described in Chapter 21). Patients are usually managed in the intensive care unit (ICU). The nurse assesses the patient's respiratory status by monitoring the level of responsiveness, arterial blood gases, pulse oximetry, and vital signs. In addition, the nurse assesses the entire respiratory system and implements strategies (e.g., turning schedule, mouth care, skin care, and range of motion of extremities) to prevent complications. The nurse also assesses the patient's understanding of the management strategies that are used and initiates some form of communication to enable the patient to express concerns and needs to the health care team.

Finally, the nurse addresses the problems that led to the acute respiratory failure. As the patient's status improves, the nurse assesses the patient's knowledge of the underlying disorder and provides education as appropriate to address the disorder.

 ## Acute Respiratory Distress Syndrome

ARDS can be thought of as a spectrum of disease, from its milder form (**acute lung injury**) to its most severe form of fulminate, life-threatening ARDS. This clinical syndrome is characterized by a severe inflammatory process causing diffuse alveolar damage that results in sudden and progressive pulmonary edema, increasing bilateral infiltrates on chest x-ray, hypoxemia unresponsive to oxygen supplementation regardless of the amount of PEEP, and the absence of an elevated left atrial pressure (Siegel, 2015a). Patients often demonstrate reduced lung compliance. A wide range of factors are associated with the development of ARDS (see Chart 23-9), including direct injury to the lungs (e.g., smoke inhalation) or indirect insult to the lungs (e.g., shock). ARDS has been associated with a mortality rate ranging from 26% to 58% (Siegel, 2015b). The major cause of death in ARDS is nonpulmonary MODS, often with sepsis.

Chart 23-9 ⚠️ **RISK FACTORS**
Acute Respiratory Distress Syndrome

- Aspiration (gastric secretions, drowning, hydrocarbons)
- Drug ingestion and overdose
- Hematologic disorders (disseminated intravascular coagulopathy, massive transfusions, cardiopulmonary bypass)
- Prolonged inhalation of high concentrations of oxygen, smoke, or corrosive substances
- Localized infection (bacterial, fungal, viral pneumonia)
- Metabolic disorders (pancreatitis, uremia)
- Shock (any cause)
- Trauma (pulmonary contusion, multiple fractures, head injury)
- Major surgery
- Fat or air embolism
- Sepsis

Pathophysiology

Inflammatory triggers initiate the release of cellular and chemical mediators, causing injury to the alveolar capillary membrane in addition to other structural damage to the lungs. Severe $\dot{V}/\dot{Q}$ mismatching occurs. Alveoli collapse because of the inflammatory infiltrate, blood, fluid, and surfactant dysfunction. Small airways are narrowed because of interstitial fluid and bronchial obstruction. Lung compliance may markedly decrease, resulting in decreased functional residual capacity and severe hypoxemia. The blood returning to the lung for gas exchange is pumped through the nonventilated, nonfunctioning areas of the lung, causing shunting. This means that blood is interfacing with nonfunctioning alveoli and gas exchange is markedly impaired, resulting in severe, refractory hypoxemia. Figure 23-5 shows the sequence of pathophysiologic events leading to ARDS.

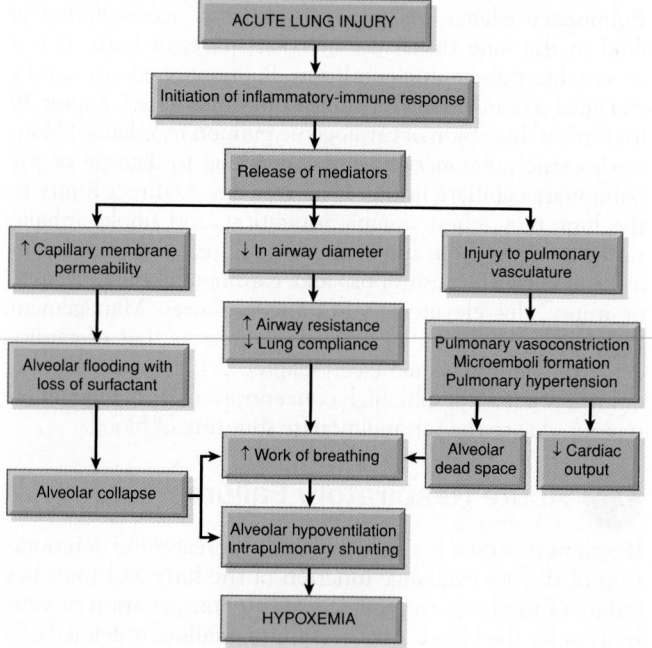

Figure 23-5 • Pathogenesis and pathophysiology of acute respiratory distress syndrome.

Clinical Manifestations

Initially, ARDS closely resembles severe pulmonary edema. The acute phase of ARDS is marked by a rapid onset of severe dyspnea that usually occurs less than 72 hours after the precipitating event (Siegel, 2015a). Arterial hypoxemia that does not respond to supplemental oxygen is characteristic. Findings on chest x-ray are similar to those seen with cardiogenic pulmonary edema and are visible as bilateral infiltrates that quickly worsen. The acute lung injury then progresses to fibrosing alveolitis with persistent, severe hypoxemia. The patient also has increased alveolar dead space (ventilation to alveoli but poor perfusion) and decreased pulmonary compliance ("stiff lungs," which are difficult to ventilate). Clinically, the patient is thought to be in the recovery phase if the hypoxemia gradually resolves, the chest x-ray improves, and the lungs become more compliant.

Assessment and Diagnostic Findings

On physical examination, intercostal retractions and crackles may be present as the fluid begins to leak into the alveolar interstitial space. Common diagnostic tests performed in patients with potential ARDS include plasma brain natriuretic peptide (BNP) levels, echocardiography, and pulmonary artery catheterization. The BNP level is helpful in distinguishing ARDS from cardiogenic pulmonary edema. Transthoracic echocardiography may be used if the BNP is not conclusive.

Medical Management

The primary focus in the management of ARDS includes identification and treatment of the underlying condition. Aggressive, supportive care must be provided to compensate for the severe respiratory dysfunction. This supportive therapy almost always includes endotracheal intubation and mechanical ventilation. In addition, circulatory support, adequate fluid volume, and nutritional support are important. Supplemental oxygen is used as the patient begins the initial spiral of hypoxemia. As the hypoxemia progresses, intubation and mechanical ventilation are instituted. The concentration of oxygen and ventilator settings and modes are determined by the patient's status. This is monitored by arterial blood gas analysis, pulse oximetry, and bedside pulmonary function testing.

Providing ventilatory PEEP support is a critical part of the treatment of ARDS. PEEP usually improves oxygenation, but it does not influence the natural history of the syndrome. The use of PEEP helps increase functional residual capacity and reverse alveolar collapse by keeping the alveoli open, resulting in improved arterial oxygenation and a reduction in the severity of the $\dot{V}/\dot{Q}$ imbalance. By using PEEP, a lower FiO_2 may be required. The goal is a PaO_2 greater than 60 mm Hg or an oxygen saturation level of greater than 90% at the lowest possible FiO_2. (See Chapter 21 for a discussion of PEEP and modes of mechanical ventilation.)

Systemic hypotension may occur in ARDS as a result of hypovolemia secondary to leakage of fluid into the interstitial spaces and depressed cardiac output from high levels of PEEP therapy. Hypovolemia must be carefully treated without causing further overload. Inotropic or vasopressor agents may

be required. Additional supportive treatments may include prone positioning, sedation, paralysis, and nutritional support (Siegel, 2015b).

Pharmacologic Therapy

There is no specific pharmacologic treatment of ARDS except supportive care. Neuromuscular blocking agents, sedatives, and analgesics may be used to improve patient–ventilator synchronization and help to decrease severe hypoxemia (see later discussion in Ventilator Considerations section). Inhaled nitric oxide (an endogenous vasodilator) may help to reduce $\dot{V}/\dot{Q}$ mismatch and improve oxygenation. Multiple therapies are undergoing clinical evaluation but are not yet approved or supported for widespread clinical use (Siegel, 2015a; Siegel, 2015b).

Nutritional Therapy

Adequate nutritional support is vital in the treatment of ARDS. Patients with ARDS require 35 to 45 kcal/kg/day to meet caloric requirements. Enteral feeding is the first consideration; however, parenteral nutrition also may be required.

Nursing Management
General Measures

A patient with ARDS is critically ill and requires close monitoring in an ICU. Most of the respiratory modalities discussed in Chapter 21 are used in this situation (oxygen administration, nebulizer therapy, chest physiotherapy, endotracheal intubation or tracheostomy, mechanical ventilation, suctioning, bronchoscopy). Frequent assessment of the patient's status is necessary to evaluate the effectiveness of treatment.

In addition to supporting the medical plan of care, the nurse considers other needs of the patient. Positioning is important. The nurse turns the patient frequently to improve ventilation and perfusion in the lungs and enhance secretion drainage. However, the nurse must closely monitor the patient for deterioration in oxygenation with changes in position. Oxygenation in patients with ARDS is sometimes improved in the prone position. This position may be evaluated for improvement in oxygenation and used in special circumstances. Devices and specialty beds are available to assist the nurse in placing the patient in a prone position.

The patient is extremely anxious and agitated because of the increasing hypoxemia and dyspnea. It is important to reduce the patient's anxiety because anxiety increases oxygen expenditure by preventing rest. Rest is essential to limit oxygen consumption and reduce oxygen needs.

Ventilator Considerations

If the patient is intubated and receiving mechanical ventilation with PEEP, several considerations must be addressed. PEEP, which causes increased end-expiratory pressure, is an unnatural pattern of breathing and feels strange to the patient. The patients may be anxious and "fight" the ventilator. Nursing assessment is important to identify problems with ventilation that may be causing the anxiety reaction: tube blockage by kinking or retained secretions, other acute respiratory problems (e.g., pneumothorax and pain), a sudden decrease in the oxygen level, the level of dyspnea, or ventilator malfunction. In some cases, sedation may be required to

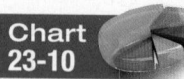

Chart 23-10

NURSING RESEARCH PROFILE

Nurses' Knowledge About Neuromuscular Blocking Agents

Frazee, E. N., Personett, H. A., Bauer, S. R., et al. (2015). Intensive care nurses' knowledge about use of neuromuscular blocking agents in patients with respiratory failure. *American Journal of Critical Care, 24*(5), 431–439.

Purpose

The purpose of this study was to describe critical care nurses' knowledge of neuromuscular blocking agents (NMBAs). Areas evaluated were the therapeutic properties, adverse effects and monitoring parameters for patients on NMBAs.

Design

Five academic medical centers were utilized for data collection; medical intensive care nurses' knowledge was evaluated using a web-based survey between May 2012 and May 2013. To be eligible for the study, a nurse must have had more than 25% of his/her clinical practice in an intensive care unit (ICU) with a patient population of more than 50% medical patients. A 16 question survey was designed for this study. The survey had two sections: general knowledge about NMBAs and perceptions of the role of NMBAs in patients with acute respiratory distress syndrome (ARDS).

Findings

Responses were received from 160 nurses, which was 22% of the eligible participants identified by unit leaders at the five academic medical centers. Most of the participants (92%) were able to correctly identify the NMBAs vecuronium and cisatracurium as nonanalgesics. Most of the participants (82%) correctly identified the NMBAs pancuronium and atracurium as nonanxiolytics. Of 6 different NMBAs, nurses identified the elimination properties of these drugs correctly ranging from 28% to 64% of the time. The nurses had variable responses to NMBAs' specific adverse events. Over 75% of nurses identified the relationship between foot drop and NMBAs; however, only 34% identified the independent association of NMBAs and consciousness. The perceived durations of action of NMBAs varied widely.

Nursing Implications

NMBAs are used in patients with ARDS and improve oxygenation, inflammation, and mortality. The ICU nurse is responsible for the safe and effective use of these agents in patients who are critically ill. It is crucial that ICU nurses understand the properties and adverse effects of these drugs. This study demonstrates that focused education and demonstrated competence is necessary for ICU nurses to safely care for this patient population.

decrease the patient's oxygen consumption, allow the ventilator to provide full support of ventilation, and decrease the patient's anxiety. Sedatives that may be used are lorazepam (Ativan), midazolam (Versed), dexmedetomidine (Precedex), propofol (Diprivan), and short-acting barbiturates.

If the PEEP level cannot be maintained despite the use of sedatives, neuromuscular blocking agents (paralytic agents) may be given to paralyze the patient. Examples of these agents include pancuronium (Pavulon), vecuronium (Norcuron), atracurium (Tracrium), and rocuronium (Zemuron). The resulting paralysis allows the patient to be ventilated more easily. With paralysis, the patient appears to be unconscious; loses motor function; and cannot breathe, talk, or blink independently. However, the patient retains sensation and is awake and able to hear. The nurse must reassure the patient that the paralysis is a result of the medication and is temporary. Paralysis should be used for the shortest possible time and never without adequate sedation and pain management.

Peripheral nerve stimulators are used to assess nerve impulse transmissions at the neuromuscular junction of select skeletal muscles when neuromuscular blocking agents are used. A "train-of-four" test may be used to measure the level of neuromuscular blockade. With this test, four consecutive stimuli are delivered along the path of a nerve, and the response of the muscle is measured in order to evaluate whether or not stimuli are effectively blocked. Four equal muscle contractions, seen as "twitches," will result if there is no neuromuscular blockade. However, if neuromuscular blockade is present, there will be a loss of twitch height and number, which will indicate the degree of blockade. If all four stimulations result in an absence of twitches, it is estimated that 100% of the receptors are blocked (Saenz, 2015).

The use of neuromuscular blocking agents has many dangers and side effects. The nurse must be sure the patient does not become disconnected from the ventilator, because respiratory muscles are paralyzed and the patient will be apneic. Consequently, the nurse ensures that the patient is closely monitored; all ventilator and patient alarms must be on at all times. Eye care is important as well, because the patient cannot blink, increasing the risk of corneal abrasions. Neuromuscular blockers predispose the patient to venous thromboembolism (VTE), muscle atrophy, foot drop, peptic ulcer disease, and skin breakdown (see Chart 23-10).

 Quality and Safety Nursing Alert

Nursing assessment is essential to minimize the complications related to neuromuscular blockade. The patient may have discomfort or pain but cannot communicate these sensations. In addition, frequent oral care and suctioning may be needed.

Analgesia must be given concurrently with neuromuscular blocking agents (Saenz, 2015). The nurse must anticipate the patient's needs regarding pain and comfort. The nurse checks the patient's position to ensure it is comfortable without excessive pressure points and in normal alignment. Talking to and not about the patient while in the patient's presence is important.

In addition, the nurse must describe the purpose and effects of the neuromuscular blocking agents to the patient's family. If family members are unaware that these agents have been given, they may become distressed by the change in the patient's status.

Pulmonary Hypertension

Pulmonary hypertension (PH) is characterized by elevated pulmonary arterial pressure and secondary right heart ventricular failure (Rubin & Hopkins, 2016). It may be suspected in a patient with dyspnea with exertion without other clinical manifestations. Unlike systemic blood pressure, the pulmonary pressures cannot be measured indirectly. In the absence of these measurements, clinical recognition becomes the only indicator of PH. However, PH is a condition that is often not clinically evident until late in its progression. Patients are classified by the World Health Organization (WHO) into five groups based upon the mechanism of PH (Rubin & Hopkins, 2016) (see Chart 23-11).

Pathophysiology

Conditions such as collagen vascular disease, congenital heart disease, anorexigens (specific appetite depressants), chronic use of stimulants, portal hypertension, and HIV infection increase the risk of PH in susceptible patients. Vascular injury occurs with endothelial dysfunction and vascular smooth muscle dysfunction, which leads to disease progression (vascular smooth muscle hypertrophy, adventitial and intimal proliferation [thickening of the wall], and advanced vascular lesion formation). Normally, the pulmonary vascular bed can handle the blood volume delivered by the right ventricle. It has a low resistance to blood flow and compensates for increased blood volume by dilation of the vessels in the pulmonary circulation. However, if the pulmonary vascular bed is destroyed or obstructed, as in PH, the ability to handle whatever flow or volume of blood it receives is impaired, and the increased blood flow then increases the pulmonary artery pressure. As the pulmonary arterial pressure increases, the pulmonary vascular resistance also increases. Both pulmonary artery constriction (as in hypoxemia or hypercapnia) and a reduction of the pulmonary vascular bed (which occurs with PE) result in increased pulmonary vascular resistance and pressure. This increased workload affects right ventricular function. The myocardium ultimately cannot meet the increasing demands imposed on it, leading to right ventricular hypertrophy (enlargement and dilation) and failure. Passive hepatic congestion may also develop.

Clinical Manifestations

Dyspnea, the main symptom of PH, occurs at first with exertion and eventually at rest. Substernal chest pain also is common. Other signs and symptoms include weakness, fatigue, syncope, occasional hemoptysis, and signs of right-sided heart failure (peripheral edema, ascites, distended neck veins, liver engorgement, crackles, heart murmur). Anorexia and abdominal pain in the right upper quadrant may also occur.

Assessment and Diagnostic Findings

Diagnostic testing is used to confirm that PH exists, determine its severity, and identify its causes. Initial diagnostic evaluation includes a history, physical examination, chest x-ray, pulmonary function studies, electrocardiogram (ECG), and echocardiogram. Echocardiography can be used to estimate the pulmonary artery systolic pressure and to assess right ventricular size, thickness, and function. It can also evaluate the right atrial size, left ventricular system, and diastolic function as well as valve function. Right heart catheterization is necessary to confirm the diagnosis of PH and to accurately assess the hemodynamic abnormalities. PH is confirmed with a mean pulmonary artery pressure greater than 25 mm Hg. If left heart disease is identified via echocardiography and correlates with the degree of estimated PH, then exercise testing and both a right and left heart catheterization may be done to determine the functional severity of the disease and the abnormalities in pressures (left heart filling, pulmonary vascular resistance, transpulmonary gradient) (Rubin & Hopkins, 2016).

Pulmonary function studies may be normal or show a slight decrease in vital capacity and lung compliance, with a mild decrease in the diffusing capacity. The PaO_2 also is decreased (hypoxemia). The ECG reveals right ventricular hypertrophy, right axis deviation, and tall peaked P waves in inferior leads; tall anterior R waves; and ST-segment depression, T-wave inversion, or both anteriorly. An echocardiogram can assess the progression of the disease and rule out other conditions with similar signs and symptoms. A $\dot{V}/\dot{Q}$ scan or pulmonary angiography detects defects in pulmonary vasculature, such as PE.

Chart 23-11 Clinical Classification of Pulmonary Hypertension (PH)

Group 1: Pulmonary Arterial Hypertension (PAH)

- Sporadic idiopathic PAH
- Heritable idiopathic PAH
- Drug and toxin-induced PAH
- PAH due to diseases such as connective tissues disorders, HIV infection, portal hypertension, congenital heart disease

Group 2: PH due to left heart disease

- Systolic dysfunction
- Diastolic dysfunction
- Valvular heart disease

Group 3: PH due to chronic lung diseases and/or hypoxemia

- Chronic obstructive pulmonary disease
- Interstitial lung disease
- Mixed restrictive and obstructive lung disease
- Sleep disordered breathing

Group 4: Chronic thromboembolic pulmonary hypertension (CTEPH)

- Due to thromboembolic occlusion of the proximal or distal pulmonary vasculature

Group 5: PH with unclear multifactorial mechanisms

- Hematologic disorders
- Systemic disorders (e.g., sarcoidosis)
- Metabolic disorders

Adapted from Rubin, L., & Hopkins, W. (2016). Overview of pulmonary hypertension in adults. *UpToDate*. Last updated February 5, 2016. Retrieved on 4/23/2016 at: www.uptodate.com/contents/overview-of-pulmonary-hypertension-in-adults?source=search_result&search=Overview+of+pulmonary+hypertension+in+adults&selectedTitle=1~15

Medical Management

The primary goal of treatment is to manage the underlying condition related to PH if the cause is known. Recommendations regarding therapy are tailored to the patient's individual situation, functional New York Heart Association class, and specific needs (Rubin & Hopkins, 2016). All patients with PH should be considered for the following therapies: diuretics, oxygen, anticoagulation, digoxin, and exercise training. Diuretics and oxygen should be added as needed. Appropriate oxygen therapy (see Chapter 21) reverses the vasoconstriction and reduces the PH in a relatively short time. Most patients with PH do not have hypoxemia at rest but require supplemental oxygen with exercise. Anticoagulation should be considered for patients at risk for intrapulmonary thrombosis. Digoxin may improve right ventricular ejection fraction in some patients and may help to control heart rate; however, patients must be monitored closely for potential complications (Rubin & Hopkins, 2016).

Pharmacologic Therapy

Different classes of medications are used to treat PH; these include calcium channel blockers, prostanoids, endothelin antagonists, and phosphodiesterase-5 inhibitors. The choice of therapeutic agents is based on many facets, including the classification group status of the patient with PH (see Chart 23-11), as well as the cost and the patient's tolerance of the agents (Hopkins & Rubin, 2016). In addition, a vasoreactivity test may be done to identify which medication is best suited for the patient with PH; this is done during cardiac catheterization using vasodilating medications such as nitric oxide. A positive vasoreactivity test occurs when there is a decrease of at least 10 mm Hg in the pulmonary artery pressure with an overall pressure that is less than 40 mm Hg in the presence of both an increased or unchanged cardiac output and a minimally decreased or unchanged systemic blood pressure (Hopkins & Rubin, 2016).

Patients with a positive vasoreactivity test may be prescribed calcium channel blockers. Calcium channel blockers have a significant advantage over other medications taken to treat PH in that they may be taken orally and are generally less costly; however, because calcium channel blockers are indicated in only a small percentage of patients, other treatment options, including prostanoids, are often necessary (Hopkins & Rubin, 2016).

Prostanoids mimic the effect of the prostaglandin prostacyclin. Prostacyclin relaxes vascular smooth muscle by stimulating the production of cyclic 3',5'-adenosine monophosphate (AMP) and inhibits the growth of smooth muscle cells. Prostanoids used to treat PH include epoprostenol (Flolan), treprostinil (Remodulin), and iloprost (Ventavis). Limitations of the prostanoids include their short half-life (epoprostenol's half-life is less than 3 minutes) and variable patient responses to therapy (Hopkins & Rubin, 2016). IV epoprostenol (Flolan) is the most widely studied advanced therapy for PH. It is continuously delivered through a permanently implanted central venous catheter using a portable infusion pump. Although a useful therapy, it requires extensive patient education and caregiver support. Treprostinil can be delivered IV or subcutaneously, although the subcutaneous method causes severe pain at the injection site. A benefit of iloprost (Ventavis) is that it is an inhaled preparation; however, it needs to be given six to nine times daily. Clinical trials comparing epoprostenol and treprostinil have not been performed (Hopkins & Rubin, 2016).

Endothelin receptor antagonists are vasodilators. Bosentan (Tracleer), an endothelin receptor antagonist, causes vasodilation and is prescribed for its antihypertensive effects in patients with PH. It is given orally twice a day. Liver function must be monitored in patients using bosentan. An additional selective endothelin receptor antagonist includes ambrisentan (Letairis).

The oral medications sildenafil (Revatio, Viagra), tadalafil (Cialis, Adcirca), and vardenafil (Levitra) are potent, specific phosphodiesterase-5 inhibitors that degrade cyclic 3',5'-guanosine monophosphate (cGMP) and promotes pulmonary vasodilation. These drugs are also prescribed to treat erectile dysfunction (Hopkins & Rubin, 2016).

Surgical Management

Lung transplantation remains an option for a select group of patients with PH who are refractory to medical therapy. Bilateral lung or heart–lung transplantation is the procedure of choice. Atrial septostomy may be considered for selected patients with severe disease (Hopkins & Rubin, 2016); this procedure results in shunting of blood from the right side of the heart to the left, decreasing the strain on the right side of the heart and maintaining left ventricular output.

Nursing Management

The major nursing goal is to identify patients at high risk for PH, such as those with COPD, PE, congenital heart disease, and mitral valve disease so that early treatment can commence. The nurse must be alert for signs and symptoms, administer oxygen therapy appropriately, and instruct the patient and family about the use of home oxygen therapy. In patients treated with prostanoids (e.g., epoprostenol or treprostinil), education about the need for central venous access (epoprostenol), subcutaneous infusion (treprostinil), proper administration and dosing of the medication, pain at the injection site, and potential severe side effects is extremely important. Emotional and psychosocial aspects of this disease must be addressed. Formal and informal support groups for patients and families are extremely valuable.

Pulmonary Heart Disease (Cor Pulmonale)

Cor pulmonale is a condition that results from PH, which causes the right side of the heart to enlarge because of the increased work required to pump blood against high resistance through the pulmonary vascular system. This causes right-sided heart failure (Klings, 2014). (See Chapter 29 for further discussion of management of right-sided heart failure.)

Pulmonary Embolism

PE refers to the obstruction of the pulmonary artery or one of its branches by a thrombus (or thrombi) that originates somewhere in the venous system or in the right side of the heart. Deep vein thrombosis (DVT), a related condition, refers to thrombus formation in the deep veins, usually in the calf or thigh, but sometimes in the arm, especially in patients with peripherally inserted central catheters. VTE is a term that includes both DVT and PE. (DVT is discussed in detail in Chapter 30.)

PE can be associated with trauma, surgery (orthopedic, major abdominal, pelvic, gynecologic), pregnancy, heart failure, age older than 50 years, hypercoagulable states, and prolonged immobility. It also may occur in apparently healthy people. In the United States, the precise number of people impacted by VTE is unknown; as many as 900,000 people could be affected each year (CDC, 2015e). One-third of people with a VTE will have a recurrence within 10 years. Estimates range that from 60,000 to 100,000 Americans die of VTE; 10% to 30% of people will die within the first month of diagnosis, and sudden death is the first clinical sign in about 25% of people who experience a PE (CDC, 2015e). The outcome in acute PE depends on the presence of preexisting comorbidities and the extent of hemodynamic compromise. (Risk factors for PE are identified in Chart 30-7 in Chapter 30.)

Pathophysiology

Most commonly, PE is due to a blood clot or thrombus. However, there are other types of emboli: air, fat, amniotic fluid, and septic (from bacterial invasion of the thrombus).

When a thrombus completely or partially obstructs a pulmonary artery or its branches, the alveolar dead space is increased. The area, although continuing to be ventilated, receives little or no blood flow. Therefore, gas exchange is impaired or absent in this area. In addition, various substances are released from the clot and surrounding area that cause regional blood vessels and bronchioles to constrict. This results in an increase in pulmonary vascular resistance—a reaction that compounds the $\dot{V}/\dot{Q}$ imbalance.

The hemodynamic consequences are increased pulmonary vascular resistance due to the regional vasoconstriction and reduced size of the pulmonary vascular bed. This results in an increase in pulmonary arterial pressure and, in turn, an increase in right ventricular work to maintain pulmonary blood flow. When the work requirements of the right ventricle exceed its capacity, right ventricular failure occurs, leading to a decrease in cardiac output followed by a decrease in systemic blood pressure and the development of shock. Atrial fibrillation can also cause PE. An enlarged right atrium in fibrillation causes blood to stagnate and form clots in this area. These clots are prone to travel into the pulmonary circulation.

A massive PE is best defined by the degree of hemodynamic instability rather than the percentage of pulmonary vasculature occlusion. It is described as an occlusion of the outflow tract of the main pulmonary artery or of the bifurcation of the pulmonary arteries. Multiple small emboli can lodge in the terminal pulmonary arterioles, producing multiple small infarctions of the lungs. A pulmonary infarction causes ischemic necrosis of part of the lung.

Clinical Manifestations

Symptoms of PE depend on the size of the thrombus and the area of the pulmonary artery occluded by the thrombus; they may be nonspecific. Dyspnea is the most frequent symptom; the duration and intensity of the dyspnea depend on the extent of embolization. Chest pain is common and is usually sudden and pleuritic in origin. It may be substernal and may mimic angina pectoris or a myocardial infarction. Other symptoms include anxiety, fever, tachycardia, apprehension, cough, diaphoresis, hemoptysis, and syncope. The most frequent sign is tachypnea (very rapid respiratory rate).

The clinical picture may mimic that of bronchopneumonia or heart failure. In atypical instances, PE causes few signs and symptoms, whereas in other instances, it mimics various other cardiopulmonary disorders. Obstruction of the pulmonary artery results in pronounced dyspnea, sudden substernal pain, rapid and weak pulse, shock, syncope, and sudden death.

Assessment and Diagnostic Findings

Death from acute PE commonly occurs within 1 hour after the onset of symptoms; therefore, early recognition and diagnosis are priorities. Initially, a clinical assessment will focus on the clinical probability of risk, clinical history, symptoms, signs, and testing. Because the symptoms of PE can vary from few to severe, a diagnostic workup is performed to rule out other diseases. The initial diagnostic workup may include chest x-ray, ECG, pulse oximetry, arterial blood gas analysis, and $\dot{V}/\dot{Q}$ scan. The chest x-ray is usually normal but may show infiltrates, atelectasis, elevation of the diaphragm on the affected side, or a pleural effusion. The chest x-ray is most helpful in excluding other possible causes. In addition to sinus tachycardia, the most frequent ECG abnormality is nonspecific ST-T wave abnormalities. If an arterial blood gas analysis is performed, it may show hypoxemia and hypocapnia (from tachypnea); however, arterial blood gas measurements may be normal even in the presence of PE.

Multidetector-row computed tomography angiography (MDCTA) is the criterion standard for diagnosing PE. The MDCTA can be performed quickly and provides the advantage of high-quality visualization of the lung parenchyma (Weinberger et al., 2014). If MDCTA is not available, pulmonary angiography is considered a reasonable alternative diagnostic method (Ouellette, 2015). The pulmonary angiogram allows for direct visualization under fluoroscopy of the arterial obstruction and accurate assessment of the perfusion deficit. A specially trained team must be available to perform the procedure, in which a catheter is threaded through the vena cava to the right side of the heart to inject dye, similar to a cardiac catheterization.

The $\dot{V}/\dot{Q}$ scan continues to be used to diagnose PE, especially in facilities that do not use pulmonary angiography or do not have access to MDCTA. The $\dot{V}/\dot{Q}$ scan is minimally invasive, involving the IV administration of a contrast agent. This scan evaluates different regions of the lung (upper, middle, lower) and allows comparisons of the percentage of $\dot{V}/\dot{Q}$ in each area. This test has a high sensitivity but can be more cumbersome than a CT scan and is not as accurate as a pulmonary angiogram.

A high suspicion of PE may warrant a MDCTA, D-dimer assay (blood test for evidence of blood clots), or pulmonary arteriogram. This allows for a more accurate visualization of a PE. However, CT has limitations. It cannot be performed at the bedside, so unstable patients must be transported to a CT scanner. In addition, IV infusion of contrast agent is necessary for visualization.

Prevention

For patients at risk for PE, the most effective approach is prevention. Active leg exercises to avoid venous stasis, early ambulation, and the use of anti-embolism stockings are general preventive measures. Guidelines for prevention and treatment of VTE and PE are available (Kearon, Aki, Omelas, et al., 2016). (See Chapter 30 for discussion of VTE prevention.)

Medical Management

Because PE is often a medical emergency, emergency management is of primary concern. After emergency measures have been initiated and the patient is stabilized, the treatment goal is to dissolve (lyse) the existing emboli and prevent new ones from forming. Treatment may include a variety of modalities: general measures to improve respiratory and vascular status, anticoagulation therapy, thrombolytic therapy, and surgical intervention.

 Emergency Management

Massive PE is a life-threatening emergency. The immediate objective is to stabilize the cardiopulmonary system. A sudden increase in pulmonary resistance increases the work of the right ventricle, which can cause acute right-sided heart failure with cardiogenic shock. Emergency management consists of the following actions:

- Nasal oxygen is given immediately to relieve hypoxemia, respiratory distress, and central cyanosis; severe hypoxemia may necessitate emergent endotracheal intubation and mechanical ventilatory support.
- IV infusion lines are inserted to establish routes for medications or fluids that will be needed.
- For hypotension that does not resolve with IV fluids, prompt initiation of vasopressor therapy is recommended, with agents that may include dobutamine, dopamine, or norepinephrine.
- Hemodynamic measurements and evaluation for hypoxemia (pulse oximetry or arterial blood gas) are performed. If available, MDCTA will be performed.
- The ECG is monitored continuously for dysrhythmias and right ventricular failure, which may occur suddenly.
- Blood is drawn for serum electrolytes, complete blood count, and coagulation studies.
- If the patient has suffered massive embolism and is hypotensive, an indwelling urinary catheter is inserted to monitor urinary output.
- Small doses of IV morphine or sedatives are given to relieve patient anxiety, to alleviate chest discomfort, to improve tolerance of the endotracheal tube, and to ease adaptation to the mechanical ventilator, if necessary.

General Management

Measures are initiated to improve respiratory and vascular status. Oxygen therapy is given to correct the hypoxemia, relieve the pulmonary vascular vasoconstriction, and reduce the PH. The use of anti-embolism stockings or intermittent pneumatic leg compression devices reduces venous stasis. These measures compress the superficial veins and increase the velocity of blood in the deep veins by redirecting the blood through the deep veins. Elevating the leg (above the level of the heart) also increases venous flow. However, increasing flow may cause a volume challenge to a hemodynamically unstable patient.

Pharmacologic Therapy
Anticoagulation Therapy

In patients with suspected PE, immediate anticoagulation is indicated to prevent a reoccurrence or extension of the thrombus and may continue up to 10 days (Tapson, 2016). Long-term anticoagulation is also indicated from 10 days to 3 months following the PE and is critical in the prevention of recurrence of VTE. This duration may be extended indefinitely in patients who are at high risk for recurrence (Tapson, 2016).

In patients with proven PE and who are hemodynamically stable, the initial anticoagulant selected may include a low molecular weight heparin (e.g., enoxaparin [Lovenox]), unfractionated heparin, or one of the new oral anticoagulants (NOACs), such as a direct thrombin inhibitor (e.g., dabigatran [Pradaxa]), or a Factor Xa inhibitor (e.g., fondaparinux [Arixtra], rivaroxaban [Xarelto], apixaban [Eliquis], or edoxaban [Savaysa]) (Kearon et al., 2016). The NOACs are contraindicated in patients who may receive thrombolytic therapy because their safety and efficacy are unknown in hemodynamically significant PE. Unfractionated heparin is preferred in patients who are hemodynamically unstable in anticipation of a potential need for thrombolysis or embolectomy.

In very select patients with PE, outpatient therapy can be started by administering the first dose in the emergency department or urgent care center and the remaining doses given at home. Although there are not specific selection criteria for outpatient treatment, the patient is usually at low risk of death, has no respiratory or hemodynamic compromise, does not require narcotics for pain control, has no risk factors for bleeding, has no serious comorbid conditions, and has normal mental status with a good understanding of the benefits and risks (Tapson, 2016). The ideal agent for outpatient administration is unknown, although the NOACs are often used.

Long-term treatment options include warfarin (Coumadin) and the NOACs. Low molecular weight heparin may also be indicated but is usually not prescribed for long-term therapy since it is given via a subcutaneous injection. Warfarin dosing requires regular blood draws for international normalized ratio (INR) monitoring and has a higher bleeding risk, but has long been the standard of care prior to the development of NOACs. An antidote (Vitamin K) is available if the INR is high and there is a risk of bleeding. Warfarin does have interactions with several medications and has dietary restrictions (see Chapter 33-12 in Chapter 33). A NOAC may be prescribed. These drugs do not require regular monitoring; however, they are more costly than warfarin, and antidotes are not available for most of these NOACs at this time. The choice of warfarin versus a NOAC is dependent upon risk of bleeding, cost, presence of comorbidities and provider preference (Hull & Lip, 2016; Kearon et al., 2016).

Thrombolytic Therapy

Thrombolytic therapy is used in patients with an acute PE who have hypotension and do not have a contraindication or potential bleeding risk (Ouellette, 2015). Thrombolytic therapy with recombinant tissue plasminogen activator (Activase) or other thrombolytic agents like kabikinase (Streptase) are used in treating massive PE, particularly in patients who are severely compromised (e.g., those who are hypotensive and have significant hypoxemia despite oxygen supplementation) (Ouellette, 2015). Thrombolytic therapy resolves the thrombi or emboli quickly and restores more normal hemodynamic functioning of the pulmonary circulation, thereby reducing pulmonary hypertension and improving perfusion, oxygenation, and cardiac output. However, the risk of bleeding is significant. Contraindications to thrombolytic therapy include a cerebrovascular disease (stroke) within the past 2 months, other active intracranial processes, active bleeding, surgery within 10 days of the thrombotic event, recent labor and delivery, trauma, or severe hypertension. Consequently, thrombolytic agents are advocated only for PE affecting a significant area of blood flow to the lung and causing hemodynamic instability.

Before thrombolytic therapy is started, INR, partial thromboplastin time (PTT), hematocrit, and platelet counts are obtained. An anticoagulant is stopped prior to administration of a thrombolytic agent. During therapy, all but essential invasive procedures are avoided because of potential bleeding. If necessary, fresh whole blood, packed red cells, cryoprecipitate, or frozen plasma is given to replace blood loss and reverse the bleeding tendency. After the thrombolytic infusion is completed (which varies in duration according to the agent used), maintenance anticoagulation therapy is initiated.

Surgical Management

A surgical embolectomy is rarely performed but may be indicated if the patient has a massive PE or hemodynamic instability or if there are contraindications to thrombolytic (fibrinolytic) therapy. Embolectomy can be performed using catheters or surgically. Surgical removal must be performed by a cardiovascular surgical team with the patient on cardiopulmonary bypass (Ouellette, 2015).

For patients who have an absolute contraindication to therapeutic anticoagulation or when recurrent PE occurs despite therapeutic anticoagulation, an inferior vena cava (IVC) filter may be inserted (Kearson et al. 2016; Tapson, 2016). IVC filters are not recommended for the initial treatment of patients with PE and should not be used in patients receiving anticoagulants (Kearon et al. 2016). The IVC filter provides a screen in the IVC, allowing blood to pass through while large emboli from the pelvis or lower extremities are blocked or fragmented before reaching the lung. Numerous catheters have been developed since the introduction of the original Greenfield filter (see Fig. 23-6). Sometimes, newer filters may be removed if the patient may begin to take anticoagulants and evidences therapeutic anticoagulation, although this tends to occur infrequently (Fedullo & Roberts, 2015).

Nursing Management

Minimizing the Risk of Pulmonary Embolism

A key role of the nurse is to identify the patient at high risk for PE and to minimize the risk of PE in all patients. The nurse must have a high degree of suspicion for PE in all patients, but particularly in those with conditions predisposing to a slowing of venous return.

Figure 23-6 • An umbrella filter is in place in the inferior vena cava to prevent PE. The filter (compressed within an applicator catheter) is inserted through an incision in the right internal jugular vein. The applicator is withdrawn when the filter fixes itself to the wall of the inferior vena cava after ejection from the applicator.

Preventing Thrombus Formation

Preventing thrombus formation is a major nursing responsibility. The nurse encourages ambulation and active and passive leg exercises to prevent venous stasis in patients prescribed bed rest. The nurse instructs the patient to move the legs in a "pumping" exercise so that the leg muscles can help increase venous flow. The nurse also advises the patient not to sit or lie in bed for prolonged periods, not to cross the legs, and not to wear constrictive clothing. Intermittent pneumatic compression (IPC) devices may be used to prevent venous thrombosis by enhancing blood flow in the deep veins of the legs. These include sleeves placed on the legs that inflate with sequential compression. The nurse must pay attention to optimal fitting of the compression sleeves and adherence to keeping the sleeves on when the patient is in a seated or supine position. Legs should not be dangled or feet placed in a dependent position while the patient sits on the edge of the bed; instead, feet should rest on the floor or on a chair. In addition, IV catheters (for parenteral therapy or measurements of central venous pressure) should not be left in place for prolonged periods.

Assessing Potential for Pulmonary Embolism

All patients are evaluated for risk factors for thrombus formation and PE. The nurse conducts a careful assessment of the patient's health history, family history, and medication record. On a daily basis, the patient is asked about pain or discomfort in the extremities. In addition, the extremities are evaluated for warmth, redness, and inflammation.

Monitoring Thrombolytic Therapy

The nurse is responsible for monitoring thrombolytic and anticoagulant therapy. Thrombolytic therapy (urokinase, tissue plasminogen activator) causes lysis of deep vein thrombi and PE, which helps dissolve the clots. During thrombolytic infusion, while the patient remains on bed rest, vital signs are assessed every 2 hours and invasive procedures are avoided. Tests to determine INR or PTT are performed 3 to 4 hours after the thrombolytic infusion is started to confirm that the fibrinolytic systems have been activated. (See Chapter 30 for nursing management for the patient receiving anticoagulant or thrombolytic therapy.)

> **▶ Quality and Safety Nursing Alert**
>
> *Because of the prolonged clotting time, only essential arterial punctures or venipunctures are performed in patients who have received thrombolytics and manual pressure is applied to any puncture site for at least 30 minutes. Pulse oximetry is used to monitor changes in oxygenation. The thrombolytic infusion is discontinued immediately if uncontrolled bleeding occurs.*

Managing Pain

Chest pain, if present, is usually pleuritic rather than cardiac in origin. A semi-Fowler's position provides a more comfortable position for breathing. However, the nurse must continue to turn patients frequently and reposition them to improve the V̇/Q̇ in the lung. The nurse administers opioid analgesic agents as prescribed for severe pain.

Managing Oxygen Therapy

Careful attention is given to the proper use of oxygen. The patient must understand the need for continuous oxygen therapy. The nurse assesses the patient frequently for signs of hypoxemia and monitors the pulse oximetry values to evaluate the effectiveness of the oxygen therapy. Deep breathing and incentive spirometry are indicated for all patients to minimize or prevent atelectasis and improve ventilation. Nebulizer therapy or percussion and postural drainage may be used for management of secretions.

Relieving Anxiety

The nurse encourages the stabilized patient to talk about any fears or concerns related to this frightening episode, answers the patient's and family's questions concisely and accurately, explains the therapy, and describes how to recognize untoward effects early.

Monitoring for Complications

When caring for a patient who has had PE, the nurse must be alert for the potential complication of cardiogenic shock or right ventricular failure subsequent to the effect of PE on the cardiovascular system. (Nursing activities for managing shock are found in Chapter 14; see Chapter 29 for nursing management of right ventricular failure.)

Providing Postoperative Nursing Care

If the patient has undergone surgical embolectomy, the nurse measures the patient's pulmonary arterial pressure and urinary output. The nurse also assesses the insertion site of the arterial catheter for hematoma formation and infection. Maintaining the blood pressure at a level that supports perfusion of vital organs is crucial. To prevent peripheral venous stasis and edema of the lower extremities, the nurse elevates the foot of the bed and encourages isometric exercises, the use of IPC devices, and walking when the patient is permitted out of bed. Sitting for long periods is discouraged, because hip flexion compresses the large veins in the legs.

Promoting Home, Community-Based, and Transitional Care

 Educating Patients About Self-Care

Before hospital discharge and at follow-up visits to the clinic, the nurse educates the patient about preventing recurrence and reporting signs and symptoms. Patient education instructions, presented in Chart 23-12, are intended to help prevent recurrences and side effects of treatment.

Continuing and Transitional Care

During follow-up or home visits, the nurse monitors the patient's adherence to the prescribed management plan and reinforces previous instructions. The nurse also monitors the patient for residual effects of the PE and recovery. The patient is reminded about the importance of keeping follow-up appointments for coagulation tests and appointments with the primary provider. The nurse also reminds the patient about the importance of participation in health promotion activities (e.g., immunizations) and health screening.

Sarcoidosis

Sarcoidosis is a type of interstitial lung disease. It is a multisystem, granulomatous disease of unknown etiology (King, 2016). Although 90% of patients demonstrate thoracic involvement, any organ may be affected. Sarcoidosis usually presents between 20 and 40 years of age and is slightly more common in women than men (Weinberger et al., 2014). In the United States, the disease is more common in African Americans, and the estimated prevalence is 10 to 20 per 100,000 persons (King, 2016).

Pathophysiology

Sarcoidosis is thought to be a hypersensitivity response to one or more exogenous agents (bacteria, fungi, virus, chemicals) in people with an inherited or acquired predisposition to the disorder. The hypersensitivity response and inflammation result in the formation of a noncaseating granuloma, which is a noninfectious organized collection of macrophages that appear as a nodule. In the lung, granuloma infiltration and fibrosis may occur, resulting in low lung compliance, impaired diffusing capacity, and reduced lung volumes (King, 2016).

Clinical Manifestations

Hallmarks of sarcoidosis are its insidious onset and lack of prominent clinical signs or symptoms. The clinical picture depends on the systems affected. The lung is most commonly involved; signs and symptoms may include dyspnea, cough, hemoptysis, and congestion. Generalized symptoms include anorexia, fatigue, and weight loss. Other signs include uveitis; joint pain; fever; and granulomatous lesions of the skin, liver, spleen, kidney, and central nervous system. The granulomas may disappear or gradually convert to fibrous tissue. With multisystem involvement, patients may also have fatigue, fever, anorexia, and weight loss.

Chart 23-12 **HOME CARE CHECKLIST**
Prevention of Recurrent Pulmonary Embolism

At the completion of education, the patient and/or caregiver will be able to:

- State the impact of pulmonary embolism on physiologic functioning, ADLs, IADLs, roles, relationships, and spirituality.
- State changes in lifestyle (e.g., diet, activity) necessary to restore health.
- State the name, dose, side effects, frequency, and schedule for all medications.
  - Name the anticoagulant prescribed and identify dosage and schedule of administration.
  - Describe the need for continued anticoagulant therapy after the initial embolism.
  - Describe the importance of follow-up appointments for coagulation tests and appointments with providers.
- Describe potential side effects of coagulation such as bruising and bleeding and identify ways to prevent bleeding:
  - Avoid the use of sharps (razors, knives, etc.) to prevent cuts; shave with an electric shaver.
  - Use a toothbrush with soft bristles to prevent gum injury.
  - Do not take aspirin or antihistamines while taking warfarin sodium (Coumadin).
  - Always check with the primary provider before taking any medicine, including over-the-counter medications.
  - Avoid laxatives, because they may affect vitamin K absorption.
  - Report the occurrence of dark, tarry stools to the primary provider immediately.

- Wear an identification bracelet or carry a medicine card stating that you are taking anticoagulants.
- Describe strategies to prevent recurrent deep venous thrombosis and pulmonary emboli:
  - Continue to wear anti-embolism stockings (compression hose) as long as directed.
  - Avoid sitting with legs crossed or sitting for prolonged periods of time.
  - When traveling, change position regularly, walk occasionally, and do active exercises of moving the legs and ankles while sitting.
  - Drink fluids, especially while traveling and in warm weather, to avoid hemoconcentration due to fluid deficit.
- Describe the signs and symptoms of lower extremity circulatory compromise and potential deep venous thrombosis: calf or leg pain, swelling, pedal edema.
- Describe the signs and symptoms of pulmonary compromise related to recurrent pulmonary embolism (e.g., dyspnea, chest pain, anxiety, fever, tachycardia, apprehension, cough, syncope, diaphoresis, hemoptysis).
- Describe how and when to contact the primary provider if symptoms of circulatory compromise or pulmonary compromise are identified.
- Identify the need for health promotion, disease prevention and screening activities

ADL, activities of daily living; IADL, independent activities of daily living.

Assessment and Diagnostic Findings

Chest x-rays and CT scans are used to assess pulmonary adenopathy. These may show hilar adenopathy and disseminated miliary and nodular lesions in the lungs. A mediastinoscopy or **transbronchial** biopsy (in which a tissue specimen is obtained through the bronchial wall) may be used to confirm the diagnosis. In rare cases, an **open lung biopsy** is performed. Diagnosis is confirmed by a biopsy that shows noncaseating granulomas. Pulmonary function test results are abnormal if there is restriction of lung function (reduction in total lung capacity). Arterial blood gas measurements may be normal or may show reduced oxygen levels (hypoxemia) and increased carbon dioxide levels (hypercapnia).

Medical Management

Many patients undergo remission without specific treatment. Corticosteroids may be beneficial because of their anti-inflammatory effects. Oral corticosteroids have been the most commonly used agents for the relief of symptoms and control of potentially disabling respiratory impairment from pulmonary sarcoidosis. Once begun, corticosteroid therapy is usually continued in tapering doses for 12 months, and longer if the patient has recurrence of symptoms and chest x-ray indications (i.e., continued pulmonary adenopathy) (King, 2014). Corticosteroids have been shown to be useful in patients with ocular and myocardial involvement, skin involvement, extensive pulmonary disease that compromises pulmonary function, hepatic involvement, and hypercalcemia. However, it is not known if steroids alter the long-term course of the disease (King, 2014). When there is inadequate response

to prednisone or the dose cannot be decreased, an immune modulator may be added (e.g., methotrexate [Trexall], azathioprine [Imuran], leflunomide [Arava], and mycophenolate [CellCept]). No single test monitors the progression or recurrence of sarcoidosis; multiple tests are used to monitor involved systems.

OCCUPATIONAL LUNG DISEASES: PNEUMOCONIOSES

Pneumoconiosis is a general term given to any lung disease caused by dusts that are breathed in and then deposited deep in the lungs causing damage. Pneumoconiosis is usually considered an occupational lung disease, and includes **asbestosis**, silicosis and coal workers' pneumoconiosis, also known as "Black Lung Disease" (ALA, 2016) (see Table 23-5). Pneumoconiosis refers to a non-neoplastic alteration of the lung resulting from inhalation of mineral or inorganic dust (e.g., "dusty lung"). This alteration results in pulmonary fibrosis and parenchymal changes. Usually, extended exposure to irritating or toxic substances accounts for these changes, although severe single exposures may also lead to chronic lung disease. Occupational lung disease is the number one work-related illness in the United States based on its frequency, severity, and preventability (American Lung Association [ALA], 2016). Many people with early pneumoconiosis are asymptomatic, but advanced disease often is accompanied by disability and premature death.

Diseases of the lungs occur in numerous occupations as a result of exposure to several different types of agents,

TABLE 23-5 Occupational Lung Diseases: Pneumoconioses

Disease (Source)	Pathophysiology	Clinical Manifestations
Silicosis (glass manufacturing, foundry work, stone cutting)	Inhaled silica dust produces nodular lesions in the lungs. Nodules enlarge and coalesce. Dense masses form on upper portion of lungs, resulting in loss of pulmonary volume. Fibrotic destruction of pulmonary tissue can lead to restrictive lung disease, emphysema, pulmonary hypertension, and cor pulmonale	*Acute silicosis:* dyspnea, fever, cough, weight loss *Chronic silicosis:* progressive symptoms indicative of hypoxemia, severe airflow obstruction, and right-sided heart failure
Asbestosis (shipbuilding, building demolition)	Inhaled asbestos fibers enter alveoli and are surrounded by fibrous tissue. Fibrous changes can also affect the pleura, which thicken and develop plaque. These changes lead to restrictive lung disease, with a decrease in lung volume, diminished exchange of oxygen and carbon dioxide, hypoxemia, cor pulmonale, and respiratory failure. It also increases risk of lung cancer, mesothelioma, and pleural effusion	Progressive dyspnea; persistent, dry cough; mild-to-moderate chest pain; anorexia; weight loss; malaise; clubbing of the fingers
Coal worker's pneumoconiosis	Encompasses a variety of lung diseases; is also known as black lung disease. Inhaled dusts that are mixtures of coal, kaolin, mica, and silica are deposited in the alveoli and respiratory bronchioles. When macrophages that engulf the dust can no longer be cleared, they aggregate and fibroblasts appear. The bronchioles and alveoli become clogged with dust, dying macrophages, and fibroblasts, leading to formation of coal macules. Fibrotic lesions develop and subsequently localized emphysema develops, with cor pulmonale and respiratory failure	Chronic cough, dyspnea, and expectoration of black or gray sputum, especially in miners who are smokers with cavitation in the lungs

Adapted from American Lung Association. (2016). *Lung health & diseases: Pneumoconiosis.* Retrieved on 3/27/16 at: www.lung.org/lung-health-and-diseases/lung-disease-lookup/pneumoconiosis

such as mineral dusts, metal dusts, biologic dusts, and toxic fumes. Smoking may compound the problem and may increase the risk of lung cancers in people exposed to the mineral asbestos and other potential carcinogens (ALA, 2016). The effects of inhaling these materials depend on the composition of the substance, its concentration, its ability to initiate an immune response, its irritating properties, the duration of exposure, and the individual's response or susceptibility to the irritant.

These diseases are not treatable once they develop; however, they are preventable. Therefore, a major role for nurses, especially occupational health nurses, is that of advocate for employees. Nurses need to make every effort to promote measures to reduce the exposure of workers to industrial products. Strategies to control exposure should be identified and encouraged; these strategies include the use of protective devices (facemasks, hoods, industrial respirators) to minimize exposure and screening/monitoring of individuals at risk.

Key aspects of any assessment of patients with a potential occupational respiratory history include job and job activities, exposure levels, general hygiene, time frame of exposure, smoking history, effectiveness of respiratory protection used, and direct versus indirect exposures (Goldman, 2015). Specific information that should be obtained includes the following:

- Exposure to an agent known to cause an occupational disorder
- Length of time from exposure of agent to onset of symptoms
- Congruence of symptoms with those of known exposure-related disorder
- Lack of other more likely explanations of the signs and symptoms

More than one million workers are exposed to silica each year. Symptoms rarely develop in less than 5 years; however, progression of the disease results in extreme shortness of breath, loss of appetite, chest pains, and potentially respiratory failure (ALA, 2016). Asbestosis is progressive and causes severe scarring of the lung, which leads to fibrosis. The lungs become stiff, making it difficult to breathe or to oxygenate well. The disease may not evidence manifestations until 10 to 40 years after exposure (ALA, 2016). Coal worker's pneumoconiosis is a collection of lung disease caused by exposure to inhaled dusts.

The nurse provides education about preventive measures to patients and their families, assesses patients for a history of exposure to environmental agents, and makes referrals so that pulmonary function can be evaluated and the patient can be treated early in the course of the disease. These diseases have no effective treatment because damage is irreversible. Supportive therapy is aimed at preventing infections and managing complications.

CHEST TUMORS

Tumors of the lung may be benign or malignant. A malignant chest tumor can be primary, arising within the lung, chest wall, or mediastinum or it can be a metastasis from a primary tumor site elsewhere in the body.

Lung Cancer (Bronchogenic Carcinoma)

Lung cancer is the leading cancer killer among men and women in the United States, with about 1 out of 4 cancer deaths from lung cancer; almost 158,000 deaths were estimated in 2016. Each year, more people die of lung cancer than of colon, breast, and prostate cancers combined. Approximately 225,000 new cases of lung cancer are diagnosed annually; 13% to 14% of new cancers for men and women involve the lung or bronchus. In approximately 57% of patients with lung cancer, the disease has spread to regional lymphatics and other sites by the time of diagnosis (Siegel, Miller, & Jemal, 2015). As a result, the long-term survival rate is low. Overall, the 5-year survival rate is 17% (Siegel et al., 2015).

Pathophysiology

The most common cause of lung cancer is inhaled carcinogens, most often cigarette smoke (>85%); other carcinogens include radon gas and occupational and environmental agents (Weinberger et al. 2014). Lung cancers arise from a single transformed epithelial cell in the tracheobronchial airways, in which the carcinogen binds to and damages the cell's DNA. This damage results in cellular changes, abnormal cell growth, and eventually a malignant cell. As the damaged DNA is passed on to daughter cells, the DNA undergoes further changes and becomes unstable. With the accumulation of genetic changes, the pulmonary epithelium undergoes malignant transformation from normal epithelium eventually to invasive carcinoma. Carcinoma tends to arise at sites of previous scarring (TB, fibrosis) in the lung.

Classification and Staging

For purposes of staging and treatment, most lung cancers are classified into one of two major categories: small cell lung cancer (SCLC) and non-small cell lung cancer (NSCLC). SCLC represents approximately 15% of tumors; NSCLC represents approximately 85% of tumors, including squamous cell (20%), large cell (5%), adenocarcinoma (38%), others which cannot be classified (18%) and others (6%) (American Cancer Society [ACS], 2016; Midthun, 2015). In SCLC, the two general cell types include small cell and combined small cell.

NSCLC is further classified by cell type. Squamous cell cancer is usually more centrally located and arises more commonly in the segmental and subsegmental bronchi. Adenocarcinoma is the most prevalent carcinoma of the lung in both men and women; it occurs peripherally as peripheral masses or nodules and often metastasizes. Large cell carcinoma (also called *undifferentiated carcinoma*) is a fast-growing tumor that tends to arise peripherally. Bronchoalveolar cell cancer is found in the terminal bronchi and alveoli and is usually slower growing compared with other bronchogenic carcinomas.

In addition to classification according to cell type, lung cancers are staged. The stage of the tumor refers to the size of the tumor, its location, whether lymph nodes are involved, and whether the cancer has spread (ACS, 2016). NSCLC is staged as I to IV. Stage I is the earliest stage and has the highest cure rate, whereas stage IV designates metastatic spread. Survival rates for NSCLC are shown in Table 23-6. (Diagnostic tools and further information on staging are described in Chapter 15.)

Risk Factors

Environmental factors (i.e., tobacco smoke, secondhand (passive) smoke, environmental and occupational exposures)

TABLE 23-6 Five-Year Survival Rates for Lung Cancer

Stage	5-Year Survival Rate (%)
NSCLC	
IA	49
IB	45
IIA	30
IIB	31
IIIA	14
IIIB	5
IV	1
SCLC	
I	31
II	19
III	8
IV	2

NSCLC, non–small cell lung cancer; SCLC, small cell lung cancer.
Adapted from American Cancer Society (ACS). (2016). *Learn about cancer: Lung cancer*. Last updated 2/8/2016. Retrieved on 3/27/2016 at: www.cancer.org/cancer/lungcancer/index

account for an estimated 75% to 80% of cancer cases and deaths in the United States (ACS, 2016). Other factors that have been associated with lung cancer include genetic predisposition, dietary deficits, and underlying respiratory diseases, such as COPD and TB. Some familial predisposition to lung cancer exists, as the incidence of lung cancer in close relatives of patients with lung cancer is two to three times that in the general population regardless of smoking status.

Tobacco Smoke

The risk of developing lung cancer is about 23 times higher in male smokers and 13 times higher in female smokers compared to lifelong nonsmokers (ACS, 2016). Risk is determined by the pack-year history (number of packs of cigarettes used each day, multiplied by the number of years smoked), the age of initiation of smoking, the depth of inhalation, and the tar and nicotine levels in the cigarettes smoked. The younger a person is when he or she starts smoking, the greater the risk of developing lung cancer. Smokers who use smokeless products as a supplemental source of nicotine will increase their risk of lung cancer (ACS, 2016).

Almost all cases of SCLC are due to cigarette smoking. SCLC is rare in people who have never smoked. It is the most aggressive form of lung cancer, grows quickly, and usually starts in the airways in the center of the chest (ACS, 2016).

Electronic Cigarettes

Electronic cigarettes are a form of electronic nicotine delivery system. Per the ACS, there are questions about how safe it is to inhale some substances in the vapor. The amounts of nicotine and other substances a person gets from each cartridge are also unclear and have been found to vary greatly even when comparing same brand cartridges from the same manufacturer (ACS, 2016).

Secondhand Smoke

Passive smoking has been identified as a cause of lung cancer in nonsmokers. People who are involuntarily exposed to tobacco smoke in a closed environment (house, automobile, building) have an increased risk of lung cancer when compared with unexposed nonsmokers.

Environmental and Occupational Exposure

Various carcinogens have been identified in the atmosphere, including motor vehicle emissions and pollutants from refineries and manufacturing plants. Evidence suggests that the incidence of lung cancer is greater in urban areas as a result of the buildup of pollutants and motor vehicle emissions.

Radon is a colorless, odorless gas found in soil and rocks. For many years, it has been associated with uranium mines, but it is now known to seep into homes through ground rock. High levels of radon have been associated with the development of lung cancer, especially when combined with cigarette smoking. Homeowners are advised to have radon levels checked in their houses and to arrange for special venting if the levels are high.

Chronic exposure to industrial carcinogens, such as arsenic, asbestos, mustard gas, chromates, coke oven fumes, nickel, oil, and radiation, has been associated with the development of lung cancer. Laws have been passed to control exposure to these carcinogens in the workplace.

Genetic Mutations

Genetic mutations may be one of the risk factors for lung cancer and can cause certain changes in the DNA of lung cells. These changes can lead to abnormal cell growth and, sometimes, cancer. There are inherited gene changes and acquired gene changes. Inherited gene changes probably do not play a large role in lung cancer. Acquired mutations in lung cells often result from exposure to factors in the environment, such as cancer-causing chemicals in tobacco smoke (ACS, 2016). Acquired changes in certain genes, such as the *TP53* or *p16* tumor suppressor genes and the *K-RAS* or *ALK* oncogenes, are thought to be important in the development of NSCLC. Ongoing research will help to both identify additional changes in genes and develop targeted therapies for lung cancer (ACS, 2016) (see Chapter 8).

Clinical Manifestations

Often, lung cancer develops insidiously and is asymptomatic until late in its course. The signs and symptoms depend on the location and size of the tumor, the degree of obstruction, and the existence of metastases to regional or distant sites.

The most frequent symptom of lung cancer is cough or change in a chronic cough. People frequently ignore this symptom and attribute it to smoking or a respiratory infection. The cough may start as a dry, persistent cough, without sputum production. When obstruction of airways occurs, the cough may become productive due to infection.

> ### Quality and Safety Nursing Alert
>
> *A cough that changes in character should arouse suspicion of lung cancer.*

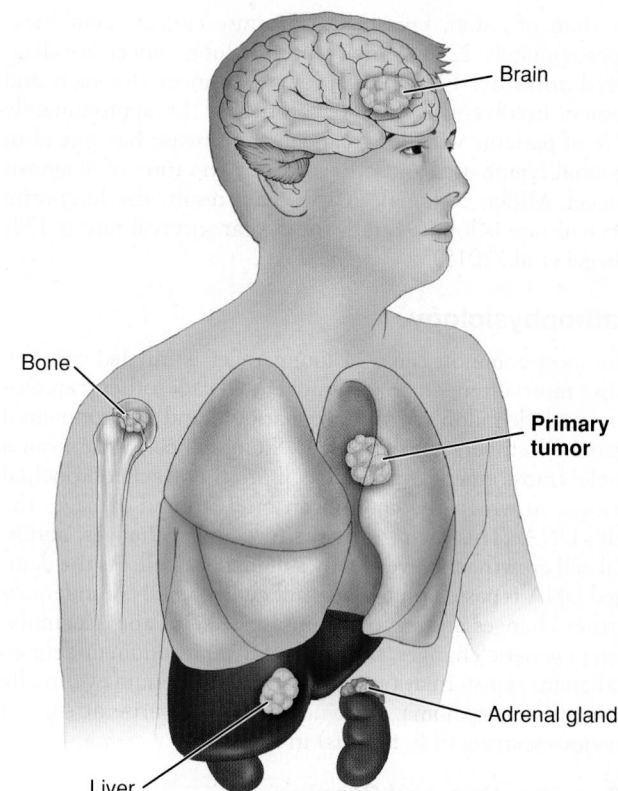

Figure 23-7 • Frequent sites of lung cancer metastasis.

Dyspnea is prominent in patients early in their disease. Causes of dyspnea may include tumor occlusion of the airway or lung parenchyma, pleural effusion, pneumonia, or complications of treatment. Hemoptysis or blood-tinged sputum may be expectorated. Chest or shoulder pain may indicate chest wall or pleural involvement by a tumor. Pain also is a late manifestation and may be related to metastasis to the bone.

In some patients, a recurring fever is an early symptom in response to a persistent infection in an area of pneumonitis distal to the tumor. In fact, cancer of the lung should be suspected in people with repeated unresolved upper respiratory tract infections. If the tumor spreads to adjacent structures and regional lymph nodes, the patient may present with chest pain and tightness, hoarseness (involving the recurrent laryngeal nerve), dysphagia, head and neck edema, and symptoms of pleural or pericardial effusion. The most common sites of metastases are lymph nodes, bone, brain, contralateral lung, adrenal glands, and liver (see Fig. 23-7). Nonspecific symptoms of weakness, anorexia, and weight loss also may be present.

Assessment and Diagnostic Findings

If pulmonary symptoms occur in heavy smokers, cancer of the lung should always be considered. A chest x-ray is performed to search for pulmonary density, a solitary pulmonary nodule (coin lesion), atelectasis, and infection. CT scans of the chest are used to identify small nodules not easily visualized on the chest x-ray and also to serially examine areas for lymphadenopathy.

Sputum cytology is rarely used to make a diagnosis of lung cancer. Fiberoptic bronchoscopy is commonly used; it provides a detailed study of the tracheobronchial tree and allows for brushings, washings, and biopsies of suspicious areas. For peripheral lesions not amenable to bronchoscopic biopsy, a transthoracic **fine-needle aspiration** may be performed under CT guidance to aspirate cells from a suspicious area.

A variety of scans may be used to assess for metastasis of the cancer. These may include bone scans, abdominal scans, positron emission tomography (PET) scans, and liver ultrasound. CT scan of the brain, magnetic resonance imaging (MRI), and other neurologic diagnostic procedures are used to detect central nervous system metastases. Mediastinoscopy or mediastinotomy may be used to obtain biopsy samples from lymph nodes in the mediastinum. Endobronchial ultrasound biopsy of mediastinal nodes is also used. In some circumstances, an endoscopy with esophageal ultrasound may be used to obtain a transesophageal biopsy of enlarged subcarinal lymph nodes.

If surgery is a potential treatment, the patient is evaluated to determine whether the tumor is resectable and whether the patient can tolerate the physiologic impairment resulting from such surgery. Pulmonary function tests, arterial blood gas analysis, $\dot{V}/\dot{Q}$ scans, and exercise testing may all be used as part of the preoperative assessment.

Medical Management

The objective of management is to provide a cure, if possible. Treatment depends on the cell type, the stage of the disease, and the patient's physiologic status (particularly cardiac and pulmonary status). In general, treatment may involve surgery, radiation therapy, or chemotherapy—or a combination of these. Newer and more specific and targeted therapies to modulate the immune system (gene therapy, therapy with defined tumor antigens) are becoming available. Drugs such as crizotinib (Xalkori®) and ceritinib (Zykadia™) target genetic alterations (National Comprehensive Cancer Network [NCCN] Guidelines, 2016).

SCLC treatment includes surgery (but only if the cancer is in one lung and there is no metastasis), radiation therapy, laser therapy to open airways blocked by tumor growth, and endoscopic stent placement (to open an airway). Although the cancer cells are small, they grow very quickly and create large tumors. These tumors often spread rapidly (metastasize) to other parts of the body, including the brain, liver, and bone. By the time a patient presents with SCLC, it is late in the course of the disease and metastasis has occurred.

Surgical Management

Surgical resection is the preferred method of treating patients with localized non-small cell tumors, no evidence of metastatic spread, and adequate cardiopulmonary function. If the patient's cardiovascular status, pulmonary function, and functional status are satisfactory, surgery is generally well tolerated. However, coronary artery disease, pulmonary insufficiency, and other comorbidities may contraindicate surgical intervention. The cure rate of surgical resection depends on the type and stage of the cancer. Surgery is primarily used for NSCLCs, because small cell cancer of the lung grows rapidly and metastasizes early and extensively. Lesions of many patients with bronchogenic cancer are inoperable at the time of diagnosis. Several different types of lung resection may be performed (see Chart 23-13). The most common surgical procedure for a small, apparently curable tumor of the lung is lobectomy (removal of a lobe of the lung). In some cases, an

---

> **Chart 23-13**
>
> ## Types of Lung Resection
>
> - Lobectomy: a single lobe of the lung is removed
> - Bilobectomy: two lobes of the lung are removed
> - Sleeve resection: cancerous lobe(s) is removed and a segment of the main bronchus is resected
> - Pneumonectomy: removal of entire lung
> - Segmentectomy: a segment of the lung is removed[a]
> - Wedge resection: removal of a small, pie-shaped area of the segment
> - Chest wall resection with removal of cancerous lung tissue: for cancers that have invaded the chest wall
>
> [a]Not recommended as curative resection for lung cancer.

---

entire lung may be removed (pneumonectomy) (see Chapter 21 for further details).

Radiation Therapy

Radiation therapy may offer cure in a small percentage of patients. It is useful in controlling neoplasms that cannot be surgically resected but are responsive to radiation. Irradiation also may be used to reduce the size of a tumor, to make an inoperable tumor operable, or to relieve the pressure of the tumor on vital structures. It can reduce symptoms of spinal cord metastasis and superior vena caval compression. In addition, prophylactic brain irradiation is used in certain patients to treat microscopic metastases to the brain. Radiation therapy may help relieve cough, chest pain, dyspnea, hemoptysis, and bone and liver pain. Relief of symptoms may last from a few weeks to many months and is important in improving the quality of the remaining period of life.

Radiation therapy usually is toxic to normal tissue within the radiation field, and this may lead to complications such as esophagitis, pneumonitis, and radiation lung fibrosis, although the incidence of these complications have decreased over time with improvements in delivery of radiation therapy (ACS, 2016). These complications may impair ventilatory and diffusion capacity and significantly reduce pulmonary reserve. The patient's nutritional status, psychological outlook, fatigue level, and signs of anemia and infection are monitored throughout the treatment. (See Chapter 15 for management of the patient receiving radiation therapy.)

Chemotherapy

Chemotherapy is used to alter tumor growth patterns, to treat distant metastases or small cell cancer of the lung, and as an adjunct to surgery or radiation therapy. Chemotherapy may provide relief, especially of pain, but it does not usually cure the disease or prolong life to any great degree. Chemotherapy is also accompanied by side effects. It is valuable in reducing pressure symptoms of lung cancer and in treating brain, spinal cord, and pericardial metastasis. (See Chapter 15 for a discussion of chemotherapy for the patient with cancer.)

The choice of agent depends on the growth of the tumor cell and the specific phase of the cell cycle that the medication affects. In combination with surgery, chemotherapy may be given before surgery (neoadjuvant therapy) or after surgery (adjuvant therapy). Over 40 medications have been approved by the U.S. Food and Drug Administration (FDA) to treat NSCLC. Often, combinations of 2 or more medications may be more beneficial than single-dose regimens. Specific guidelines are available for the treatment of differing states of NSCLC through the National Comprehensive Cancer Network (NCCN Guidelines, 2016). To date, fewer than 20 medications have been approved to treat SCLC. Numerous new agents are being investigated for various types of lung cancer.

Palliative Therapy

Palliative care, concurrent with standard oncologic care for lung cancer, should be considered early in the course of illness for any patient with metastatic cancer or high symptom burden. In lung cancer, palliative therapy may include radiation therapy to shrink the tumor to provide pain relief, a variety of bronchoscopic interventions to open a narrowed bronchus or airway, and pain management and other comfort measures. Evaluation and referral for hospice care are important in planning for comfortable and dignified end-of-life care for the patient and family (see Chapter 16 for further discussion).

Treatment-Related Complications

A variety of complications may occur as a result of treatment of lung cancer. Surgical resection may result in respiratory failure, particularly if the cardiopulmonary system is compromised before surgery. Surgical complications and prolonged mechanical ventilation are potential outcomes. Radiation therapy may result in diminished cardiopulmonary function and other complications, such as pulmonary fibrosis, pericarditis, myelitis, and cor pulmonale. Chemotherapy, particularly in combination with radiation therapy, can cause pneumonitis. Pulmonary toxicity is a potential side effect of chemotherapy.

Nursing Management

Nursing care of patients with lung cancer is similar to that for other patients with cancer (see Chapter 15) and addresses the physiologic and psychological needs of the patient. The physiologic problems are primarily due to the respiratory manifestations of the disease. Nursing care includes strategies to ensure relief of pain and discomfort and to prevent complications.

Managing Symptoms

The nurse educates the patient and family about the potential side effects of the specific treatment and strategies to manage them. Strategies for managing such symptoms as dyspnea, fatigue, nausea and vomiting, and anorexia help the patient and family cope with therapeutic measures.

Relieving Breathing Problems

Airway clearance techniques are key to maintaining airway patency through the removal of excess secretions. This may be accomplished through deep-breathing exercises, chest physiotherapy, directed cough, suctioning, and in some instances bronchoscopy. Bronchodilator medications may be prescribed to promote bronchial dilation. As the tumor enlarges or spreads, it may compress a bronchus or involve a large area of lung tissue, resulting in an impaired breathing pattern and poor gas exchange. At some stage of the disease, supplemental oxygen will probably be necessary.

Nursing measures focus on decreasing dyspnea by encouraging the patient to assume positions that promote lung expansion and to perform breathing exercises for lung expansion and relaxation. Patient education about energy conservation and airway clearance techniques is also necessary. Many of the techniques used in pulmonary rehabilitation can be applied to patients with lung cancer. Depending on the severity of disease and the patient's wishes, a referral to a pulmonary rehabilitation program may be helpful in managing respiratory symptoms.

Reducing Fatigue

Fatigue is a devastating symptom that affects quality of life in patients with cancer. It is commonly experienced by patients with lung cancer and may be related to the disease itself, the cancer treatment and complications (e.g., anemia), sleep disturbances, pain and discomfort, hypoxemia, poor nutrition, or the psychological ramifications of the disease (e.g., anxiety and depression) (see Chapter 15 for nursing strategies to reduce fatigue.)

Providing Psychological Support

Another important part of the nursing care of patients with lung cancer is provision of psychological support and identification of potential resources for the patient and family (see Chart 23-14). Often, the nurse must help the patient and family deal with the following:

- The poor prognosis and relatively rapid progression of this disease
- Informed decision making regarding the possible treatment options
- Methods to maintain the patient's quality of life during the course of this disease
- End-of-life treatment options

 Gerontologic Considerations

At the time of diagnosis of lung cancer, most patients are older than 65 years and have stage III or IV disease (Gajra & Jatoi, 2014). In older patients, the management of a cancer is complex and challenging. Although age is not a significant prognostic factor for overall survival and response to treatment of either NSCLC or SCLC, older patients have specific needs. The presence of comorbidities and the patient's cognitive, functional, nutritional, and social status are important issues to consider with the patient of advanced age. Depending on the comorbidities and functional status of older adult patients, chemotherapy agents, doses, and cycles may need to be adjusted to maintain quality of life.

Tumors of the Mediastinum

Tumors of the mediastinum include neurogenic tumors, tumors of the thymus, lymphomas, germ cell tumors, cysts, and mesenchymal tumors. These tumors may be malignant or benign. They are usually described in relation to location: anterior, middle, or posterior masses or tumors.

Clinical Manifestations

Nearly all symptoms of mediastinal tumors result from the pressure of the mass against important intrathoracic organs. Symptoms may include cough, wheezing, dyspnea, anterior chest or neck pain, bulging of the chest wall, heart palpitations, angina,

Chart 23-14 ETHICAL DILEMMA
Who Makes Difficult Health Care Decisions for Patients Who Lack Capacity?

Case Scenario

As a nurse working on a medical-surgical unit, you are caring for an 84-year-old woman with a history of emphysema and a new diagnosis of adenocarcinoma of the lung. She is a widow with two adult daughters, one of whom she resides with. The surgeon recommends a lobectomy for this patient to better control the disease. The patient has mild-to-moderate Alzheimer's disease and has recently lost 10 lb. She appears debilitated and frail. She has a history of tobacco abuse, and although she no longer smokes, the daughter she resides with smokes two packs of cigarettes per day. Because of her dementia, the patient is not considered to have mental capacity to sign informed consent for the lobectomy. The patient's daughter with whom she resides has informed the surgeon that she will not agree to sign surgical consent for a lobectomy. The daughter has asked to speak with you regarding her concerns. She tells you that she knows for certain that her mother would not want this surgery and would want to continue to live at home and not in a skilled nursing facility. She asks, "Who will take care of Mom after this? I have been told I need to stop smoking if she is going to continue to live with me after the surgery, but I don't see why I need to change my lifestyle. And she always said she would not want to go to a nursing home." The patient's other daughter agrees with the recommendation for a lobectomy and is willing to sign surgical consent. However, this daughter is estranged from her sister and has not had contact with her mother since she moved in with her sister 2 years ago. The patient does not have a designated health care surrogate or a medical power of attorney.

Discussion

This patient has been diagnosed with a life-threatening illness and needs surgical intervention for the control of the disease. She is unable to make medical decisions due to her dementia and lack of mental capacity. The patient's decision-making capacity is determined by the physician on the basis of a clinical assessment. End of life decision making in patients who are terminally ill is complicated because ongoing quality of life must be examined. Although the lobectomy may prolong the patient's life, her loss of the ability to talk and care for herself may compromise her integrity. In the absence of a spouse, her adult daughters are now responsible to

function as her health care surrogates since she has no advanced directive and has not appointed a medical power of attorney. She will be unable to care for herself at home postoperatively. Her daughters disagree regarding the recommended treatment plan. Yet, the patient is entitled to receive adequate and timely treatment of her illness and appropriate physical, psychological, and home care should she undergo this procedure.

Analysis

- Describe the ethical principles that are in conflict in this case (see Chart 3-3). Which principle should have preeminence in recommending the best treatment plan for the patient?
- What resources might be available in your hospital/community to help you, your professional colleagues (e.g., the multidisciplinary health care team), and the patient and her family determine what is in the patient's best interests?
- How can you advocate for a patient's autonomy when dementia is present? Is it possible to determine what the patient's wishes would be in this particular situation? Of those involved, who would be best able to make this type of determination?
- Compare and contrast the legal ramifications of an advanced directive and designated power of attorney in a situation where the patient is mentally competent and in a situation where the patient is mentally incompetent.
- For whom do you feel an obligation to advocate for in this situation—the patient, the daughter with whom the patient resides, the other daughter, or perhaps the surgeon? Does any one of these people merit your primary focus of concern, according to the American Nurses Association (2015) Code of Ethics?

Reference

American Nurses Association. (2015). *Code of ethics for nurses with interpretive statements*. Washington, DC: American Nurses Publishing, American Nurses Foundation/American Nurses Association.
Kepple, A. L., Azzam, P. N., Gopalan, P., et al. (2015). Decision-making capacity at the end of life. *Progress in Palliative Care*, 23(3), 133–136.

Resources

See Chapter 3, Chart 3-6 for ethics resources.

---

other circulatory disturbances, central cyanosis, superior vena cava syndrome (i.e., swelling of the face, neck, and upper extremities), marked distention of the veins of the neck and the chest wall (evidence of the obstruction of large veins of the mediastinum by extravascular compression or intravascular invasion), and dysphagia and weight loss from pressure or invasion into the esophagus (Berry, 2015).

Assessment and Diagnostic Findings

Chest x-rays are the major method used initially to diagnose mediastinal tumors and cysts. A CT scan is the standard diagnostic test for the assessment of the mediastinum and surrounding structures. MRI, as well as PET, may be used in some circumstances (Berry, 2015; Thomas & Gould, 2015).

Medical Management

If the tumor is malignant and has infiltrated the surrounding tissue and complete surgical removal is not feasible, radiation therapy, chemotherapy, or both are used.

Many mediastinal tumors are benign and operable. The location of the tumor (anterior, middle, or posterior compartment) in the mediastinum dictates the type of incision. The common incision used is a median sternotomy; however, a thoracotomy may be used, depending on the location of the tumor. Additional approaches include a bilateral anterior thoracotomy (clamshell incision) and video-assisted thoracoscopic surgery (see Chapter 21). The care is the same as for any patient undergoing thoracic surgery. Major complications include hemorrhage, injury to the phrenic or recurrent laryngeal nerve, and infection.

CHEST TRAUMA

Thoracic injuries occurred in over 183,000 patients and accounted for 21% of the types of trauma recently recorded in a national trauma database (American College of Surgeons, 2015). Thoracic trauma also accounts for 20% to 25% of deaths due to trauma and contributed to 25% to 50% of the remaining deaths. Four of the top 10 complications in trauma patients were related to the respiratory system: pneumonia, DVT/PE, unplanned extubation, and acute lung injury/ARDS (American College of Surgeons, 2015). Major chest trauma may occur alone or in combination with multiple other injuries. Chest trauma is classified as either blunt or penetrating. Blunt chest trauma results from sudden compression or positive pressure inflicted to the chest wall. Penetrating trauma occurs when a foreign object penetrates the chest wall.

Blunt Trauma

Overall, blunt thoracic injuries are directly responsible for 20% to 25% of all trauma deaths (Mancini, 2014). Although blunt chest trauma is more common than penetrating trauma, it is often difficult to identify the extent of the damage because the symptoms may be generalized and vague. In addition, patients may not seek immediate medical attention, which may complicate the problem.

Pathophysiology

The most common causes of blunt chest trauma are motor vehicle crashes (trauma from steering wheel, seat belt), falls, and bicycle crashes (trauma from handlebars). Types of blunt chest trauma include chest wall fractures, dislocations, and barotraumas (including diaphragmatic injuries); injuries of the pleura, lungs, and aerodigestive tracts; and blunt injuries of the heart, great arteries, veins, and lymphatics (Mancini, 2014). Injuries to the chest are often life threatening and result in one or more of the following pathologic states:

- Hypoxemia from disruption of the airway; injury to the lung parenchyma, rib cage, and respiratory musculature; massive hemorrhage; collapsed lung; and pneumothorax
- Hypovolemia from massive fluid loss from the great vessels, cardiac rupture, or hemothorax
- Cardiac failure from cardiac tamponade, cardiac contusion, or increased intrathoracic pressure

These pathologic states frequently result in impaired $\dot{V}/\dot{Q}$ leading to acute kidney injury, hypovolemic shock, and death.

Assessment and Diagnostic Findings

Because time is critical in treating chest trauma, the patient must be assessed immediately to determine the following: time elapsed since injury occurred, mechanism of injury, level of responsiveness, specific injuries, estimated blood loss, recent drug or alcohol use, and prehospital treatment. Initial assessment of thoracic injuries includes assessment of airway obstruction, tension pneumothorax, open pneumothorax, massive hemothorax, flail chest, and cardiac tamponade. These injuries are life threatening and require immediate treatment. Secondary assessment includes assessment of simple pneumothorax, hemothorax, pulmonary contusion, traumatic aortic rupture, tracheobronchial disruption, esophageal perforation, traumatic diaphragmatic injury, and penetrating wounds to the mediastinum. Although listed as secondary, these injuries may be life threatening as well.

The physical examination includes inspection of the airway, thorax, neck veins, and breathing difficulty. Specifics include assessing the rate and depth of breathing for abnormalities such as stridor, cyanosis, nasal flaring, the use of accessory muscles, drooling, and overt trauma to the face, mouth, or neck. The chest is assessed for symmetric movement, symmetry of breath sounds, open chest wounds, entrance or exit wounds, impaled objects, tracheal shift, distended neck veins, subcutaneous emphysema, and paradoxical chest wall motion. In addition, the chest wall is assessed for bruising, petechiae, lacerations, and burns. The vital signs and skin color are assessed for signs of shock. The thorax is palpated for tenderness and crepitus, and the position of the trachea is also assessed.

The initial diagnostic workup includes a chest x-ray, CT scan, complete blood count, clotting studies, type and crossmatch, electrolytes, oxygen saturation, arterial blood gas analysis, and ECG. The patient is completely undressed to avoid missing additional injuries that may complicate care. Many patients with injuries involving the chest have associated head and abdominal injuries that require attention. Ongoing assessment is essential to monitor the patient's response to treatment and to detect early signs of clinical deterioration.

Medical Management

The goals of treatment are to evaluate the patient's condition and to initiate aggressive resuscitation. An airway is immediately established with oxygen support and, in some cases, endotracheal intubation and ventilatory support. Reestablishing fluid volume and negative intrapleural pressure and draining intrapleural fluid and blood are essential.

The potential for massive blood loss and exsanguination with blunt or penetrating chest injuries is high because of injury to the great blood vessels. Many patients die at the scene of the injury or are in shock by the time help arrives. Agitation and irrational and combative behavior are signs of decreased oxygen delivery to the cerebral cortex. Strategies to restore and maintain cardiopulmonary function include ensuring an adequate airway and ventilation; stabilizing and reestablishing chest wall integrity; occluding any opening into the chest (open pneumothorax); and draining or removing any air or fluid from the thorax to relieve pneumothorax, hemothorax, or cardiac tamponade. Hypovolemia and low cardiac output must be corrected. Many of these treatment efforts, along with the control of hemorrhage, are carried out simultaneously at the scene of the injury or in the emergency department. Depending on the success of efforts to control the hemorrhage in the emergency department, the patient may be taken immediately to the operating room. Principles of management are essentially those pertaining to care of the postoperative thoracic patient (see Chapter 21).

Sternal and Rib Fractures

Sternal fractures are most common in motor vehicle crashes with a direct blow to the sternum via the steering wheel. Rib fractures are the most common type of chest trauma with blunt chest injury (Mancini, 2014). Most rib fractures are benign and are treated conservatively; ribs 4 through 10 are most frequently involved. Fractures of the first three ribs are rare but can result in a high mortality rate because they are associated with laceration of the subclavian artery or vein. Fractures of the lower ribs are associated with injury to the spleen and liver, which may be lacerated by fragmented sections of the rib. Older adult patients with three or more rib fractures have been shown to have a fivefold increased mortality rate and a fourfold increased incidence of pneumonia (Mancini, 2014).

Clinical Manifestations

Patients with sternal fractures have anterior chest pain, overlying tenderness, ecchymosis, crepitus, swelling, and possible chest wall deformity. For patients with rib fractures, clinical manifestations are similar: severe pain, point tenderness, and muscle spasm over the area of the fracture that are aggravated by coughing, deep breathing, and movement. The area around the fracture may be bruised. To reduce the pain, the patient splints the chest by breathing in a shallow manner and avoids sighs, deep breaths, coughing, and movement. This reluctance to move or breathe deeply results in diminished ventilation, atelectasis (collapse of unaerated alveoli), pneumonitis, and hypoxemia. Respiratory insufficiency and failure can be the outcomes of such a cycle.

Assessment and Diagnostic Findings

The patient must be closely evaluated for underlying cardiac injuries. A crackling, grating sound in the thorax (subcutaneous crepitus) may be detected with auscultation. The diagnostic workup may include a chest x-ray, rib films of a specific area, ECG, continuous pulse oximetry, and arterial blood gas analysis.

Medical Management

Medical management is directed toward relieving pain, avoiding excessive activity, and treating any associated injuries. Surgical fixation is rarely necessary unless fragments are grossly displaced and pose a potential for further injury.

The goals of treatment of rib fractures are to control pain and to detect and treat the injury. Sedation is used to relieve pain and to allow deep breathing and coughing. Care must be taken to avoid oversedation and suppression of respiratory drive. Alternative strategies to relieve pain include an intercostal nerve block and ice over the fracture site. A chest binder may be used as supportive treatment to provide stability to the chest wall and may decrease pain. The patient is instructed to apply the binder snugly enough to provide support, but not to impair respiratory excursion. Usually, the pain abates in 5 to 7 days, and discomfort can be relieved with epidural analgesia, patient-controlled analgesia (PCA), or nonopioid analgesia.

Most rib fractures heal in 3 to 6 weeks. The patient is monitored closely for signs and symptoms of associated injuries.

Flail Chest

Flail chest is frequently a complication of blunt chest trauma from a steering wheel injury. It occurs when three or more adjacent ribs (multiple contiguous ribs) are fractured at two or more sites, resulting in free-floating rib segments. It may also result as a combination fracture of ribs and costal cartilages or sternum. As a result, the chest wall loses stability, causing respiratory impairment and usually severe respiratory distress.

Pathophysiology

During inspiration, as the chest expands, the detached part of the rib segment (flail segment) moves in a paradoxical manner (pendelluft movement) in that it is pulled inward during inspiration, reducing the amount of air that can be drawn into the lungs. On expiration, because the intrathoracic pressure exceeds atmospheric pressure, the flail segment bulges outward, impairing the patient's ability to exhale. The mediastinum then shifts back to the affected side (see Fig. 23-8). This paradoxical action results in increased dead space, a reduction in alveolar ventilation, and decreased compliance. Retained airway secretions and atelectasis frequently accompany flail chest. The patient has hypoxemia, and if gas exchange is greatly compromised, respiratory acidosis develops as a result of carbon dioxide retention. Hypotension, inadequate tissue perfusion, and metabolic acidosis often follow as the paradoxical motion of the mediastinum decreases cardiac output.

Medical Management

As with rib fracture, treatment of flail chest is usually supportive. Management includes providing ventilatory support, clearing secretions from the lungs, and controlling pain. Specific management depends on the degree of respiratory dysfunction. If only a small segment of the chest is involved, the objectives are to clear the airway through positioning, coughing, deep breathing, and suctioning to aid in the expansion of the lung, and to relieve pain by intercostal nerve blocks, high thoracic epidural blocks, or cautious use of IV opioids.

For mild-to-moderate flail chest injuries, the underlying pulmonary contusion is treated by monitoring fluid intake

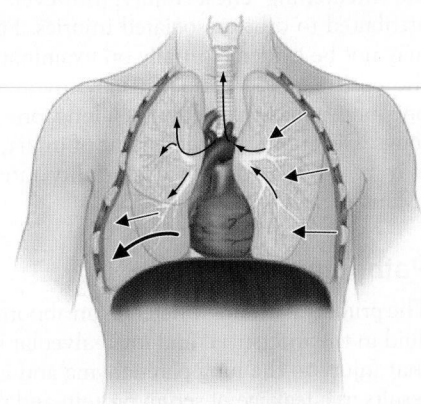

Figure 23-8 • Flail chest is caused by a free-floating segment of rib cage resulting from multiple rib fractures. **A.** Paradoxical movement on inspiration occurs when the flail rib segment is sucked inward and the mediastinal structures shift to the unaffected side. The amount of air drawn into the affected lung is reduced. **B.** On expiration, the flail segment bulges outward and the mediastinal structures shift back to the affected side.

A. Inspiration

B. Expiration

and appropriate fluid replacement while relieving chest pain. Pulmonary physiotherapy focusing on lung volume expansion and secretion management techniques is performed. The patient is closely monitored for further respiratory compromise.

For severe flail chest injuries, endotracheal intubation and mechanical ventilation are required to provide internal pneumatic stabilization of the flail chest and to correct abnormalities in gas exchange. This helps to treat the underlying pulmonary contusion, serves to stabilize the thoracic cage to allow the fractures to heal, and improves alveolar ventilation and intrathoracic volume by decreasing the work of breathing. This treatment modality requires endotracheal intubation and ventilator support. Differing modes of ventilation are used depending on the patient's underlying disease and specific needs (see Chapter 21).

In rare circumstances, surgery may be required to more quickly stabilize the flail segment. This may be used for patients who are difficult to ventilate or for patients who are at high risk with underlying lung disease who may be difficult to wean from mechanical ventilation. Other countries utilize internal rib fixation—a surgical procedure that places clips, bars, or plates on the broken ribs to stabilize the flail segments—however, it is not widely used in the United States because there is insufficient clinical evidence to support its effectiveness (Bulger, 2016).

Regardless of the type of treatment, the patient is carefully monitored by serial chest x-rays, arterial blood gas analysis, pulse oximetry, and bedside pulmonary function monitoring. Pain management is key to successful treatment. PCA, intercostal nerve blocks, epidural analgesia, and intrapleural administration of opioids may be used to relieve or manage thoracic pain.

Pulmonary Contusion

Pulmonary contusion is a common thoracic injury and is frequently associated with flail chest. It is defined as damage to the lung tissues resulting in hemorrhage and localized edema. It is associated with chest trauma when there is rapid compression and decompression to the chest wall (i.e., blunt trauma). Pulmonary contusion represents a spectrum of lung injury characterized by the development of infiltrates and various degrees of respiratory dysfunction and sometimes respiratory failure. It is often cited as the most common potentially life-threatening chest injury; however, mortality is often attributed to other associated injuries. Pulmonary contusion may not be evident initially on examination but develops in the posttraumatic period; it may involve a small portion of one lung, a massive section of a lung, one entire lung, or both lungs. Depending on the extent of injury, this type of trauma may be associated with a mortality rate greater than 50% (Mancini, 2014).

Pathophysiology

The primary pathologic defect is an abnormal accumulation of fluid in the interstitial and intra-alveolar spaces. It is thought that injury to the lung parenchyma and its capillary network results in a leakage of serum protein and plasma. The leaking serum protein exerts an osmotic pressure that enhances loss of fluid from the capillaries. Blood, edema, and cellular debris (from cellular response to injury) enter the lung and accumulate in the bronchioles and alveoli, where they interfere with gas exchange. An increase in pulmonary vascular resistance and pulmonary artery pressure occurs. The patient has hypoxemia and carbon dioxide retention.

Clinical Manifestations

Pulmonary contusion may be mild, moderate, or severe. The clinical manifestations vary from decreased breath sounds, tachypnea, tachycardia, chest pain, hypoxemia, and blood-tinged secretions to more severe tachypnea, tachycardia, crackles, frank bleeding, severe hypoxemia (cyanosis), and respiratory acidosis. Changes in sensorium, including increased agitation or combative irrational behavior, may be signs of hypoxemia.

In addition, patients with moderate pulmonary contusion have a large amount of mucus, serum, and frank blood in the tracheobronchial tree; patients often have a constant cough but cannot clear the secretions. Patients with severe pulmonary contusion have signs and symptoms that mirror ARDS, which may include central cyanosis; agitation; combativeness; and productive cough with frothy, bloody secretions.

Assessment and Diagnostic Findings

The efficiency of gas exchange is determined by pulse oximetry and arterial blood gas measurements. Pulse oximetry is also used to measure oxygen saturation continuously. The initial chest x-ray may show no changes; changes may not appear for 1 or 2 days after the injury and appear as pulmonary infiltrates on chest x-ray.

Medical Management

Treatment priorities include maintaining the airway, providing adequate oxygenation, and controlling pain. In mild pulmonary contusion, adequate hydration via IV fluids and oral intake is important to mobilize secretions. However, fluid intake must be closely monitored to avoid hypervolemia. Volume expansion techniques, postural drainage, physiotherapy including coughing, and endotracheal suctioning are used to remove the secretions. Pain is managed by intercostal nerve blocks or by opioids via PCA or other methods. Usually, antimicrobial therapy is given because the damaged lung is susceptible to infection. Supplemental oxygen is usually given by mask or cannula for 24 to 36 hours.

In patients with moderate pulmonary contusion, bronchoscopy may be required to remove secretions. Intubation and mechanical ventilation with PEEP (see Chapter 21) may also be necessary to maintain the pressure and keep the lungs inflated. A nasogastric tube is inserted to relieve gastrointestinal distention.

In patients with severe contusion, who may develop respiratory failure, aggressive treatment with endotracheal intubation and ventilatory support, diuretics, and fluid restriction may be necessary. Antimicrobial medications may be prescribed for the treatment of pulmonary infection. This is a common complication of pulmonary contusion (especially pneumonia in the contused segment) because the fluid and blood that extravasate into the alveolar and interstitial spaces serve as an excellent culture medium.

Penetrating Trauma

Any organ or structure within the chest is potentially susceptible to traumatic penetration. These organs include the chest wall, lung and pleura, tracheobronchial system, esophagus, diaphragm, and major thoracic blood vessels, as well as heart and other mediastinal structures. The clinical consequence of penetrating trauma to the chest depends on the mechanism of injury, location, associated injuries, and underlying illnesses (Shahani, 2015). Common injuries include pneumothorax and cardiac tamponade.

Medical Management

The objective of immediate management is to restore and maintain cardiopulmonary function. After an adequate airway is ensured and ventilation is established, examination for shock and intrathoracic and intra-abdominal injuries is necessary. The patient is undressed completely so that additional injuries are not missed. (See Chapter 72 for discussion of primary and secondary survey.) There is a high risk of associated intra-abdominal injuries with stab wounds below the level of the fifth anterior intercostal space. Death can result from exsanguinating hemorrhage or intra-abdominal sepsis.

The diagnostic workup includes a chest x-ray, chemistry profile, arterial blood gas analysis, pulse oximetry, and ECG. The patient's blood is typed and cross-matched in case blood transfusion is required. After the status of the peripheral pulses is assessed, a large-bore IV line is inserted. An indwelling catheter is inserted to monitor urinary output. A nasogastric tube is inserted and connected to low suction to prevent aspiration, minimize leakage of abdominal contents, and decompress the gastrointestinal tract.

Hemorrhagic shock is treated simultaneously with colloid solutions, crystalloids, or blood, as indicated by the patient's condition. Diagnostic procedures are carried out as dictated by the needs of the patient (e.g., CT scans of chest or abdomen, flat plate x-ray of the abdomen, and abdominal tap to check for bleeding) (see Chapter 14).

A chest tube is inserted into the pleural space in most patients with penetrating wounds of the chest to achieve rapid and continuing re-expansion of the lungs. The insertion of the chest tube frequently results in a complete evacuation of the blood and air. The chest tube also allows early recognition of continuing intrathoracic bleeding, which would make surgical exploration necessary. If the patient has a penetrating wound of the heart or great vessels, the esophagus, or the tracheobronchial tree, surgical intervention is required.

Pneumothorax

Pneumothorax occurs when the parietal or visceral pleura is breached and the pleural space is exposed to positive atmospheric pressure. Normally, the pressure in the pleural space is negative or subatmospheric; this negative pressure is required to maintain lung inflation. When either pleura is breached, air enters the pleural space, and the lung or a portion of it collapses.

Types of Pneumothorax

Types of pneumothorax include simple, traumatic, and tension pneumothorax.

Simple Pneumothorax

A simple, or spontaneous, pneumothorax occurs when air enters the pleural space through a breach of either the parietal or visceral pleura. Most commonly, this occurs as air enters the pleural space through the rupture of a bleb or a bronchopleural fistula. A spontaneous pneumothorax may occur in an apparently healthy person in the absence of trauma due to rupture of an air-filled bleb, or blister, on the surface of the lung, allowing air from the airways to enter the pleural cavity. It may be associated with diffuse interstitial lung disease and severe emphysema.

Traumatic Pneumothorax

A traumatic pneumothorax occurs when air escapes from a laceration in the lung itself and enters the pleural space or from a wound in the chest wall. It may result from blunt trauma (e.g., rib fractures), penetrating chest or abdominal trauma (e.g., stab wounds or gunshot wounds), or diaphragmatic tears. Traumatic pneumothorax may occur during invasive thoracic procedures (i.e., thoracentesis, transbronchial lung biopsy, and insertion of a subclavian line) in which the pleura is inadvertently punctured, or with barotrauma from mechanical ventilation.

A traumatic pneumothorax resulting from major injury to the chest is often accompanied by hemothorax (collection of blood in the pleural space resulting from torn intercostal vessels, lacerations of the great vessels, or lacerations of the lungs). Often both blood and air are found in the chest cavity (hemopneumothorax) after major trauma. Chest surgery can be classified as a traumatic pneumothorax as a result of the entry into the pleural space and the accumulation of air and fluid in the pleural space.

Open pneumothorax is one form of traumatic pneumothorax. It occurs when a wound in the chest wall is large enough to allow air to pass freely in and out of the thoracic cavity with each attempted respiration. Because the rush of air through the wound in the chest wall produces a sucking sound, such injuries are termed *sucking chest wounds*. In such patients, not only does the lung collapse, but the structures of the mediastinum (heart and great vessels) also shift toward the uninjured side with each inspiration and in the opposite direction with expiration. This is termed *mediastinal flutter* or *swing*, and it produces serious circulatory problems.

> ◤ *Quality and Safety Nursing Alert*
>
> *Traumatic open pneumothorax calls for emergency interventions. Stopping the flow of air through the opening in the chest wall is a lifesaving measure.*

Tension Pneumothorax

A **tension pneumothorax** occurs when air is drawn into the pleural space from a lacerated lung or through a small opening or wound in the chest wall. It may be a complication of other types of pneumothorax. In contrast to open pneumothorax, the air that enters the chest cavity with each inspiration is trapped; it cannot be expelled during expiration through the air passages or the opening in the chest wall. In effect, a one-way valve or ball valve mechanism occurs where air enters the pleural space but cannot escape. With each breath,

Open pneumothorax

Inspiration   Expiration

Tension pneumothorax

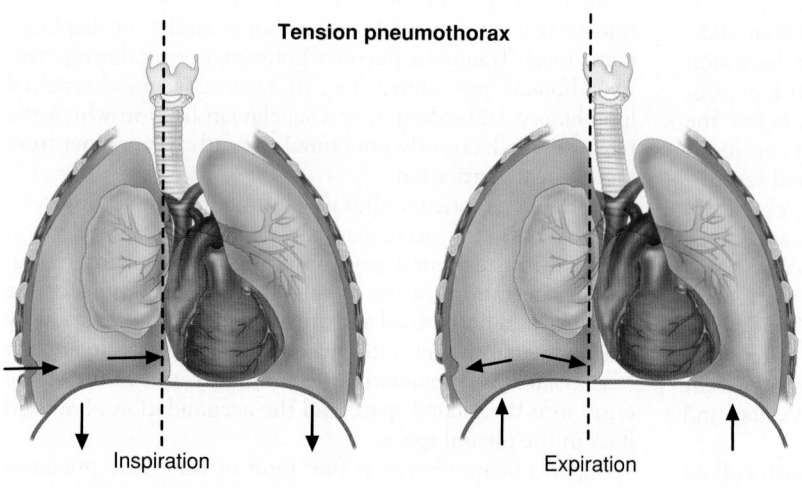

Inspiration   Expiration

Figure 23-9 • Open pneumothorax (**top**) and tension pneumothorax (**bottom**). In open pneumothorax, air enters the chest during inspiration and exits during expiration. A slight shift of the affected lung may occur because of a decrease in pressure as air moves out of the chest. In tension pneumothorax, air enters but cannot leave the chest. As the pressure increases, the heart and great vessels are compressed and the mediastinal structures are shifted toward the opposite side of the chest. The trachea is pushed from its normal midline position toward the opposite side of the chest, and the unaffected lung is compressed.

tension (positive pressure) is increased within the affected pleural space. This causes the lung to collapse and the heart, the great vessels, and the trachea to shift toward the unaffected side of the chest (mediastinal shift). Both respiration and circulatory function are compromised because of the increased intrathoracic pressure, which decreases venous return to the heart, causing decreased cardiac output and impairment of peripheral circulation. In extreme cases, the pulse may be undetectable—this is known as pulseless electrical activity.

Clinical Manifestations

The signs and symptoms associated with pneumothorax depend on its size and cause. Pain is usually sudden and may be pleuritic. The patient may have only minimal respiratory distress with slight chest discomfort and tachypnea with a small simple or uncomplicated pneumothorax. If the pneumothorax is large and the lung collapses totally, acute respiratory distress occurs. The patient is anxious, has dyspnea and air hunger, has increased use of the accessory muscles, and may develop central cyanosis from severe hypoxemia.

In assessing the chest for any type of pneumothorax, the nurse assesses tracheal alignment, expansion of the chest, breath sounds, and percussion of the chest. In a simple pneumothorax, the trachea is midline, expansion of the chest is decreased, breath sounds may be diminished or absent, and

percussion of the chest may reveal normal sounds or hyperresonance depending on the size of the pneumothorax. In a tension pneumothorax, the trachea is shifted away from the affected side, chest expansion may be decreased or fixed in a hyperexpansion state, breath sounds are diminished or absent, and percussion to the affected side is hyperresonant. The clinical picture is one of air hunger, agitation, increasing hypoxemia, central cyanosis, hypotension, tachycardia, and profuse diaphoresis. Figure 23-9 compares open and tension pneumothorax.

Medical Management

Medical management of pneumothorax depends on its cause and severity. The goal of treatment is to evacuate the air or blood from the pleural space. A small chest tube (28 Fr) is inserted near the second intercostal space; this space is used because it is the thinnest part of the chest wall, minimizes the danger of contacting the thoracic nerve, and leaves a less visible scar. If a patient also has a hemothorax, a large-diameter chest tube (32 Fr or greater) is inserted, usually in the fourth or fifth intercostal space at the midaxillary line. The tube is directed posteriorly to drain the fluid and air. Once the chest tube or tubes are inserted and suction is applied (usually to 20 mm Hg suction), effective decompression of the pleural cavity (drainage of blood or air) occurs.

If an excessive amount of blood enters the chest tube in a relatively short period, an autotransfusion may be needed. This technique involves taking the patient's own blood that has been drained from the chest, filtering it, and then transfusing it back into the vascular system.

In such an emergency, anything may be used that is large enough to fill the chest wound—a towel, a handkerchief, or the heel of the hand. If conscious, the patient is instructed to inhale and strain against a closed glottis. This action assists in re-expanding the lung and ejecting the air from the thorax. In the hospital, the opening is plugged by sealing it with gauze impregnated with petrolatum. A pressure dressing is applied. Usually, a chest tube connected to water-seal drainage is inserted to remove air and fluid. Antibiotics usually are prescribed to combat infection from contamination.

The severity of open pneumothorax depends on the amount and rate of thoracic bleeding and the amount of air in the pleural space. The pleural cavity can be decompressed by needle aspiration (thoracentesis) or by chest tube drainage of the blood or air. The lung is then able to re-expand and resume the function of gas exchange. As a rule of thumb, the chest wall is opened surgically (thoracotomy) if more than 1,500 mL of blood is aspirated initially by thoracentesis (or is the initial chest tube output) or if chest tube output continues at greater than 200 mL per hour (Shahani, 2015). The urgency with which the blood must be removed is determined by the degree of respiratory compromise. An emergency thoracotomy may also be performed in the emergency department if a cardiovascular injury secondary to chest or penetrating trauma is suspected. The patient with a possible tension pneumothorax should immediately be given a high concentration of supplemental oxygen to treat the hypoxemia, and pulse oximetry should be used to monitor oxygen saturation. In an emergency situation, a tension pneumothorax can be decompressed or quickly converted to a simple pneumothorax by inserting a large-bore needle (14-gauge) at the second intercostal space, midclavicular line on the affected side. This relieves the pressure and vents the positive pressure to the external environment. A chest tube is then inserted and connected to suction to remove the remaining air and fluid, reestablish the negative pressure, and re-expand the lung. If the lung re-expands and air leakage from the lung parenchyma stops, further drainage may be unnecessary. If a prolonged air leak continues despite chest tube drainage to underwater seal, surgery may be necessary to close the leak.

Cardiac Tamponade

Cardiac tamponade is compression of the heart resulting from fluid or blood within the pericardial sac. It usually is caused by blunt or penetrating trauma to the chest. A penetrating wound of the heart is associated with a high mortality rate. Cardiac tamponade also may follow diagnostic cardiac catheterization, angiographic procedures, and pacemaker insertion, which can produce perforations of the heart and great vessels. Pericardial effusion with fluid compressing the heart also may develop from metastases to the pericardium from malignant tumors of the breast, lung, or mediastinum and may occur with lymphomas and leukemias, kidney injury, TB, and high-dose radiation to the chest. (See Chapter 29 for a detailed discussion of cardiac tamponade.)

Subcutaneous Emphysema

No matter what kind of chest trauma a patient has, when the lung or the air passages are injured, air may enter the tissue planes and pass for some distance under the skin (e.g., neck and chest). The tissues give a crackling sensation when palpated, and the subcutaneous air produces an alarming appearance as the face, neck, body, and scrotum become misshapen by subcutaneous air. Subcutaneous emphysema is of itself usually not a serious complication. The subcutaneous air is spontaneously absorbed if the underlying air leak is treated or stops spontaneously. In severe cases in which there is widespread subcutaneous emphysema, a tracheostomy is indicated if airway patency is threatened by pressure of the trapped air on the trachea.

CRITICAL THINKING EXERCISES

1 **PQ** A 25-year-old white woman reports to the emergency department because of sharp left sided chest pain and shortness of breath of 1 day duration. The patient was in excellent health until yesterday. She was awakened from her sleep by sharp left sided chest pain. The pain worsened with motion and deep breathing. The pain has been progressively increasing in severity and she now has severe left shoulder pain. She complains of shortness of breath and is very apprehensive about dying. She denies any cough, fever, sputum production, or hemoptysis. She is married and had one normal vaginal delivery 3 years ago. She is currently taking oral contraceptives. She has never been hospitalized except for her previous labor and delivery. Review of systems is negative. She denies any past history of venous problems. Describe your priorities of care. What respiratory conditions may be associated with this type of presentation? How would you help this patient be more comfortable and less apprehensive?

2 A 38-year-old man presents with an 11-month history of rhinitis, followed by cough, shortness of breath, and chest tightness. He takes no environmental (seasonal) medications. He is an ex-smoker with a 10 pack-year history and occasional marijuana intake. He has been an automobile painter for 3 years. He states his symptoms are worse at the end of the work day and improve on the weekends and on vacations. His chest examination is unremarkable. What are your initial thoughts about this patient's symptoms? What additional questions would you ask and why?

3 A 56-year-old man presents to the surgical floor following a colon resection. He is obese and a smoker. He has a PCA pump running and appears to be comfortable. He is receiving O_2 by nasal cannula at 2 L/min. With some difficulty, you can awake him and he can tell you his name and where he is. His vital signs are BP, 145/92; heart rate, 75 bpm; respiratory rate, 16 breaths/min. Soon after you finish your postop check, he falls back asleep. During rounds an hour later, you have difficulty awakening him. His BP is 110/78, heart rate 70 bpm; respiratory rate, 12 breaths/min. You get a pulse oximetry and it is 62%. What are the potential causes of his respiratory problem and what nursing interventions are important?

4 ebp You are on a surgical unit caring for a 66-year-old man who has undergone a right middle lobectomy for lung cancer. The patient is an active smoker. When you assess his readiness to stop smoking, he says to you "What difference does it make now? I already have lung cancer." What strategies would you consider to encourage the patient to stop smoking? What is the evidence base for the strategies that you consider? How would you evaluate the strength of the evidence?

REFERENCES

*Asterisk indicates nursing research.
**Double asterisk indicates classic reference.

Books

Gilbert, D. N., Chambers, H. F., Eliopoulos, G. M., et al. (2015). *The Sanford guide to antimicrobial therapy 2015* (45th ed.). Sperryville, VA: Antimicrobial Therapy, Inc.

Weinberger, S. E., Cockrill, B. A., & Mandel, J. (2014). *Principles of pulmonary medicine* (6th ed.). Philadelphia, PA: Elsevier Saunders.

Journals and Electronic Documents

Amanullah, S. (2015). Ventilator-associated pneumonia overview of nosocomial pneumonias. Medscape. Last updated December 31, 2015. Retrieved on 3/27/2016 at: emedicine.medscape.com/article/304836overview

American Association of Critical Care Nurses (AACN) (2016). AACN practice alert: Prevention of aspiration in adults. *Critical Care Nurse,* 36(1), e20-e24.

American Cancer Society (ACS). (2016). *Learn about cancer: lung cancer.* Last updated 2/8/2016. Retrieved on 3/27/2016 at: www.cancer.org/cancer/lungcancer/index

American College of Surgeons (2015). *National trauma data bank 2015-annual report.* Retrieved on 3/27/2016 at: www.facs.org/quality-programs/trauma/ntdb/docpub

American Lung Association (ALA). (2016). Lung health & diseases: Pneumoconiosis. Retrieved on 3/27/16 at: www.lung.org/lung-health-and-diseases/lung-disease-lookup/pneumoconiosis

**American Thoracic Society & Infectious Diseases Society of America. (2005). Guidelines for the management of adults with hospital-acquired, ventilator-associated, and healthcare-associated pneumonia. *American Journal of Respiratory and Critical Care Medicine,* 171(4), 388–416.

Augenbraun, M. H. (2014). Pneumonia in immunocompromised patients. *Emedicine/Medscape.* Last updated November 13, 2014. Retrieved on 3/27/2016 at: emedicine.medscape.com/article/807846-overview

Bartlett, J. (2015). Aspiration pneumonia in adults. UpToDate. Last updated July 6, 2015. Retrieved on 4/23/2016 at: www.uptodate.com/contents/aspiration-pneumonia-in-adults

Bartlett, J. G. (2014). Lung abscess. UpToDate. Last updated July 8, 2014. Retrieved on 6/7/2016 at: www.uptodate.com/contents/lung-abscess

Bernardo, J. (2014). Epidemiology and pathology of miliary and extrapulmonary tuberculosis. UpToDate. Last updated February 7, 2014. Retrieved on 6/6/2016 at: www.uptodate.com/contents/epidemiology-and-pathology-of-miliary-and-extrapulmonary-tuberculosis

Berry, M. F. (2015). Evaluation of mediastinal masses. UpToDate. Last updated November 9, 2015. Retrieved on 6/8/2016 at: www.uptodate.com/contents/evaluation-of-mediastinal-masses

Boston University School of Medicine. ICOUGH^SM. Retrieved on 12/1/16 at: https://www.bumc.bu.edu/surgery/quality-safety/i-cough/

Bulger, E. M. (2016). Inpatient management of traumatic rib fractures. UpToDate. Last updated February 18, 2016. Retrieved on 4/23/2016 at: www.uptodate.com/contents/inpatient-management-of-traumatic-rib-fractures?source=search_result&search=inpatient+management+of+traumatic+rib+fractures&selectedTitle=1~150

Cassidy, M. R., Rosenkranz, P., McCade, K., et al. (2013). ICOUGH reduction postoperative pulmonary complications with a multidisciplinary patient care program. *JAMA Surgery,* 148(8), 740–745.

Centers for Disease Control and Prevention (CDC). (2012). TB fact sheets-infection control and prevention; TB in specific populations.

Last updated September 1, 2012. Retrieved on 3/26/2016 at: www.cdc.gov/tb/publications/factsheets/specpop.htm

Centers for Disease Control and Prevention (CDC). (2014a). National Center for Health Statistics CDC Wonder On-line database, compiled from compressed mortality file 1999–2013 Series 20(2S), 2014. Retrieved on 6/8/2016 at: www.cdc.gov/nchs/data_access/cmf.htm

Centers for Disease Control and Prevention (CDC). (2014b). TB fact sheets- the difference between latent TB infection and TB disease. Last updated November 21, 2014. Retrieved on 1/13/2017 at: www.cdc.gov/tb/publications/factsheets/general/ltbiandactivetb.htm

Centers for Disease Control and Prevention (CDC). (2015a). *National vital statistics reports,* 64(10). Retrieved on 6/8/2016 at: www.cdc.gov/nchs/data/nvsr/nvsr64/nvsr64_10.pdf

Centers for Disease Control and Prevention (CDC). (2015b). *Faststats pneumonia.* Retrieved on 7/8/2016 at: www.cdc.gov/nchs/fastats/pneumonia.htm

Centers for Disease Control and Prevention (CDC). (2015c). Pneumococcal disease: Pneumococcal vaccination. Last updated December 10, 2015. Retrieved on 4/23/2016 at: www.cdc.gov/pneumococcal/vaccination.html

Centers for Disease Control and Prevention (CDC). (2015d). Tuberculosis: Data and statistics. Last updated September 24, 2015. Retrieved on 3/27/2016 at: www.cdc.gov/tb/statistics/

Centers for Disease Control and Prevention (CDC). (2015e). Venous thromboembolism (blood clots). Last updated June 22, 2015. Retrieved on 3/27/2016 at: www.cdc.gov/ncbddd/dvt/data.html

Conde, M. V., & Adams, S. G. (2015). Overview of the management of postoperative pulmonary complications. *UpToDate.* Last updated October 13, 2015. Retrieved on 4/23/2016 at: www.uptodate.com/contents/overview-of-the-management-of-postoperative-pulmonary-complications?source=search_result&search=Overview+of+the+management+of+postoperative+pulmonary+complications&selectedTitle=1~150

Cunha, B. A. (2015). Community-acquired pneumonia. Emedicine/Medscape. Updated August 13, 2015. Retrieved on 4/23/2016 at: emedicine.medscape.com/article/234240-overview

DeBardino, D. M., & Wunderink, R. G. (2015). Aspiration pneumonia: A review of modern trends. *Journal of Critical Care,* 30(1), 40–48.

Fedullo, P. F., & Roberts, A. (2015). Placement of vena cava filters and their complications. UpToDate. Last updated September 29, 2015. Retrieved on 6/7/2016 at: www.uptodate.com/contents/placement-of-vena-cava-filters-and-their-complications?source=search_result&search=Placement+of+vena+cava+filters+and+their+complications&selectedTitle=1~150

File, T. M. (2016). Treatment of hospital-acquired, ventilator-associated and healthcare-associated pneumonia in adults. UpToDate. Last updated January 29, 2016. Retrieved on 4/23/2016 at: www.uptodate.com/contents/treatment-of-hospital-acquired-ventilator-associated-and-healthcare-associated-pneumonia-in-adults?source=search_result&search=Treatment+of+hospital-acquired%2C+ventilator-associated+and+healthcare-associated+pneumonia+in+adults&selectedTitle=1~150

Fournier, M. (2014). Caring for patients in respiratory failure. *American Nurse Today,* 9(11), 18–23.

*Frazee, E. N., Personett, H. A., Bauer, S. R, et al. (2015). Intensive care nurses' knowledge about use of neuromuscular blocking agents in patients with respiratory failure. *American Journal of Critical Care,* 24(5), 431–439.

Fridkin, S. K., Baggs J., Fagan R., et al. (2014). Vital signs: Improving antibiotic use among hospitalized patients. *Morbidity and Mortality Weekly Report,* 63(9), 194–200.

Garja, A., & Jatoi, A. (2014). Non-small-cell lung cancer in elderly patients: A discussion of treatment options. *Journal of Clinical Oncology,* 32(24), 2562–2569.

Goldman, R. H. (2015). Overview of occupational and environmental health. *UpToDate.* Last updated April 2, 2015. Retrieved on 4/23/2016 at: www.uptodate.com/contents/overview-of-occupational-and-environmental-health?source=search_result&search=Overview+of+occupational+and+environmental+health&selectedTitle=1~150

Heffner, J. E. (2015a). Diagnostic evaluation of pleural effusion in adults: Initial testing. *UpToDate.* Last updated December 2, 2015. Retrieved on 4/23/2016 at: www.uptodate.com/contents/diagnostic-evaluation-of-a-pleural-effusion-in-adults-initial-testing?source=search_result&search=Diagnostic+evaluation+of+pleural+effusion+in+adults%3A+Initial+testing&selectedTitle=1~150

Heffner, J. E. (2015b). Chemical pleurodesis. UpToDate. Last updated April 7, 2015. Retrieved on 6/7/2016 at: www.uptodate.com/contents/chemical-pleurodesis?source=search_result&search=Heffner+Chemical+Pleurodesis&selectedTitle=1~56

Hopkins, W., & Rubin, L. (2016). Treatment of pulmonary hypertension in adults. UpToDate. Last updated January 12, 2016. Retrieved on 4/23/2016: www.uptodate.com/contents/treatment-of-pulmonary-hypertension-in-adults?source=search_result&search=Overview+of+pulmonary+hypertension+in+adults&selectedTitle=2~150

Hull, R. D., & Lip G. Y. H. (2016). Venous thromboembolism: Anticoagulation after initial management. UpToDate. Last updated April 12, 2016. Retrieved on 6/7/2016 at: www.uptodate.com/contents/venous-thromboembolism-anticoagulation-after-initial-management/?source=search_result&search=Venous+thromboembolism%3A+Anticoagulation+after+initial+management&selectedTitle=1~150

Jain, S., Self, W. H., Wunderink, R. G., et al. (2015). CDC EPIC Study Team. Community-acquired pneumonia requiring hospitalization among US adults. *New England Journal of Medicine, 373*(5), 415–427.

Kearon, C., Aki, E. A., Omelas, J, et al. (2016). Antithrombotic therapy for VTE diseases: Chest guideline, *Chest,* 2015.11.026

King, T. (2014). Treatment of pulmonary sarcoidosis with glucosteroids. *UpToDate.* Last updated December 15, 2014. Retrieved on 4/23/2016 at: www.uptodate.com/contents/treatment-of-pulmonary-sarcoidosis-with-glucocorticoids?source=search_result&search=Treatment+of+pulmonary+sarcoidosis+with+glucosteroids&selectedTitle=2~98

King, T. (2016). Clinical manifestations and diagnosis of sarcoidosis. *UpToDate.* Last updated February 12, 2016. Retrieved on 4/23/2016 at: www.uptodate.com/contents/clinical-manifestations-and-diagnosis-of-pulmonary-sarcoidosis?source=search_result&search=Clinical+manifestations+and+diagnosis+of+sarcoidosis&selectedTitle=1~150

Klings, E. S., (2014). Cor pulmonale. UpToDate. Last updated February 24, 2014. Retrieved on 4/23/2016 at: www.uptodate.com/contents/cor-pulmonale?source=search_result&search=cor+pulmonale&selectedTitle=1~102

Kobayashi, M., Bennett, N., Gierke, R., et al. (2015). Intervals between PCV13 and PPSV23 vaccines: recommendations of the Advisory Committee on Immunization Practices (ACIP). *Morbidity and Mortality Weekly Report, 64*(34), 944–947.

Kollef, M. H. (2015). Clinical presentation and diagnosis of ventilator-associated pneumonia. UpToDate. Last updated December 3, 2015. Retrieved on 4/23/2016 at: www.uptodate.com/contents/clinical-presentation-and-diagnosis-of-ventilator-associated-pneumonia?source=search_result&search=Clinical+presentation+and+diagnosis+of+VAP&selectedTitle=1~72

Mancini, M. C. (2014). Blunt chest trauma. Emedicine/Medscape. Last updated October 3, 2014. Retrieved on 3/27/2016 at: emedicine.medscape.com/article/428723-overview

Marrie, T. J. (2015). Epidemiology, pathogenesis, and microbiology of community-acquired pneumonia in adults. UpToDate. Last updated August 13, 2015. Retrieved on 4/23/2016 at: www.uptodate.com/contents/epidemiology-pathogenesis-and-microbiology-of-community-acquired-pneumonia-in-adults?source=search_result&search=Epidemiology%2C+pathogenesis%2C+and+microbiology+of+community-acquired+pneumonia+in+adults&selectedTitle=1~145

Midthun, D. E. (2015). Overview of risk factors, pathology and clinical manifestations of lung cancer. UpToDate. Last updated February 23, 2015. Retrieved on 6/8/2016 at: www.uptodate.com/contents/overview-of-the-risk-factors-pathology-and-clinical-manifestations-of-lung-cancer

National Comprehensive Cancer Network (NCCN) Guidelines. (2016). Non-small cell lung cancer Version 4.2016. Retrieved on 6/8/2016 at: www.nccn.org/professionals/physician_gls/pdf/nscl.pdf

Ouellette, D. R. (2015). Pulmonary embolism. Emedicine/ Medscape. Last updated January 30, 2015. Retrieved on 3/27/2016 at: www.emedicine.medscape.com/article/300901-overview

Pagali, S. R., Verdoom, B. P., Wieland, M. L., et al. (2014). Infection control and managing tuberculosis at long term care facility: A case report. *The Journal of Post-Acute and Long-Term Care Medicine, 15*(3), B6.

Pozniak, A. (2016) Clinical manifestations and complications of pulmonary tuberculosis. UpToDate. Last updated January 12, 2016. Retrieved on 4/23/2016 at: www.uptodate.com/contents/clinical-manifestations-and-complications-of-pulmonary-tuberculosis?source=search_result&search=Clinical+manifestations+and+complications+of+pulmonary+tuberculosis&selectedTitle=1~150

Reichman, L. E., & Lardizabal, A. (2015) Adherence to tuberculosis treatment. UpToDate. Last updated December 9, 2015. Retrieved on 6/7/2016 at: www.uptodate.com/contents/adherence-to-tuberculosis-treatment/contributors

Roy, A., Eisenhut, M., Harris, R. J., et al. (2014). Effect of BCG vaccination against Mycobacterium tuberculosis infection in children: Systematic review and meta-analysis. *British Medical Journal, 349*, g4643 doi: http://dx.doi.org/10.1136/bmj.g4643

Rubin, L., & Hopkins, W. (2016). Overview of pulmonary hypertension in adults. UpToDate. Last updated February 5, 2016. Retrieved on

4/23/2016 at: www.uptodate.com/contents/overview-of-pulmonary-hypertension-in-adults?source=search_result&search=Overview+of+pulmonary+hypertension+in+adults&selectedTitle=1~150

Saenz, A. D. (2015). Peripheral nerve stimulator-train of four monitoring. Emedicine/ Medscape. Updated September 17, 2015. Retrieved on 3/27/2017 at: emedicine.medscape.com/article/2009530-overview

Shahani, R. (2015). Penetrating chest trauma. Emedicine/Medscape. Updated November 8, 2015. Retrieved on 3/27/2016 at: emedicine.medscape.com/article/425698-overview

Siegel, M. D. (2015a). Acute respiratory distress syndrome: Epidemiology, pathophysiology, pathology and etiology in adults. UpToDate. Last updated October 14, 2015. Retrieved on 4/23/2016 at: www.uptodate.com/contents/acute-respiratory-distress-syndrome-epidemiology-pathophysiology-pathology-and-etiology-in-adults?source=search_result&search=Acute+respiratory+distress+syndrome%3A+epidemiology%2C+pathophysiology%2C+pathology+and+etiology+in+adults&selectedTitle=1~150

Siegel, M. D. (2015b). Acute respiratory distress syndrome: Prognosis and outcomes in adults. UpToDate. Last updated February 4, 2016. Retrieved on 4/23/2016 at: www.uptodate.com/contents/acute-respiratory-distress-syndrome-prognosis-and-outcomes-in-adults?source=search_result&search=Acute+respiratory+distress+syndrome%3A+Prognosis+and+outcomes+in+adults&selectedTitle=1~150

Siegel, R. L., Miller, K. D., & Jemal, A. (2015). Cancer statistics 2016. *CA A Cancer Journal for Clinicians, 66*(1), 7–30.

Smetana, G. W. (2015). Strategies to reduce postoperative pulmonary complications. UpToDate. Last updated August 11, 2015. Retrieved on 4/23/2016 at: www.uptodate.com/contents/strategies-to-reduce-postoperative-pulmonary-complications?source=search_result&search=Strategies+to+reduce+postoperative+pulmonary+complications&selectedTitle=1~150

Stark, P. (2015). Atelectasis: Types and pathogenesis in adults. UpToDate. Last updated May 28, 2015. Retrieved on 4/23/2016 at: www.uptodate.com/contents/atelectasis-types-and-pathogenesis-in-adults?source=search_result&search=Atelectasis%3A+Types+and+pathogenesis+in+adults&selectedTitle=1~150

Sterling, T. R. (2016). Treatment of pulmonary tuberculosis in HIV-noninfected adults. UpToDate. Last updated May 2, 2016. Retrieved on 6/6/2106 at: www.uptodate.com/contents/treatment-of-pulmonary-tuberculosis-in-hiv-uninfected-adults

Strange, C. (2016). Parapneumonic effusion and empyema in adults. UpToDate. Last updated May 17, 2016. Retrieved on 6/7/2016 at: www.uptodate.com/contents/parapneumonic-effusion-and-empyema-in-adults?source=search_result&search=Parapneumonic+effusion+and+empyema+in+adults&selectedTitle=1~150

Swaminathan, A. (2015). Aspiration pneumonitis and pneumonia. Medscape, Updated April 2, 2–2015. Retrieved on 6/8/2016 at: emedicine.medscape.com/article/296198-overview

Tapson, V. F. (2016). Overview of the treatment, prognosis, and follow-up of acute pulmonary embolism in adults. UpToDate. Last updated April 7, 2016. Retrieved on 6/7/2016 at: www.uptodate.com/contents/overview-of-the-treatment-prognosis-and-follow-up-of-acute-pulmonary-embolism-in-adults?source=search_result&search=Tapson+Overview+of+the+treatment%2C+prognosis%2C+and+follow-up+of+acute+pulmonary+embolism+in+adults&selectedTitle=1~150

Thomas, K. W., & Gould, M. K. (2015). Overview of the initial evaluation, diagnosis, and staging of patient with suspected lung cancer. UpToDate. Last updated December 4, 2015. Retrieved on 4/23/2016 at: www.uptodate.com/contents/overview-of-the-initial-evaluation-diagnosis-and-staging-of-patients-with-suspected-lung-cancer?source=search_result&search=Overview+of+the+initial+evaluation%2C+diagnosis%2C+and+staging+of+patient+with+suspected+lung+cancer&selectedTitle=1~150

Resources

Agency for Healthcare Quality and Research (AHRQ), www.ahrq.gov
American Association for Respiratory Care (AARC), www.aarc.org
American Cancer Society, www.cancer.org
American College of Chest Physicians (ACCP), www.chestnet.org
American Lung Association, www.lung.org
American Thoracic Society (ATS), www.thoracic.org
Centers for Disease Control and Prevention (CDC), National Institute for Occupational Safety and Health and Safety (NIOSH), www.cdc.gov/niosh/
National Cancer Institute (NCI), www.cancer.gov
National Heart, Lung, and Blood Institute (NHLBI), www.nhlbi.nih.gov
Occupational Safety and Health Administration (OSHA), www.osha.gov
Pulmonary Hypertension Association (PHA), www.phassociation.org
Respiratory Nursing Society (RNS), www.respiratorynursingsociety.org

24 Management of Patients With Chronic Pulmonary Disease

LEARNING OBJECTIVES

On completion of this chapter, the learner will be able to:

1. Describe the pathophysiology, clinical manifestations, and treatment of chronic obstructive pulmonary disease (COPD).
2. Discuss the major risk factors for developing COPD and nursing interventions to minimize or prevent these risk factors.
3. Use the nursing process as a framework for care of patients with COPD.

4. Develop an education plan for patients with COPD.
5. Describe the pathophysiology, clinical manifestations, and treatment of bronchiectasis.
6. Identify medical and nursing management of bronchiectasis.
7. Describe the pathophysiology, clinical manifestations, and treatment of asthma
8. Describe asthma self-management strategies.
9. Describe the pathophysiology, clinical manifestations, and treatment of cystic fibrosis.

GLOSSARY

air trapping: incomplete emptying of alveoli during expiration due to loss of lung tissue elasticity (emphysema), bronchospasm (asthma), or airway obstruction

alpha₁-antitrypsin deficiency: genetic disorder resulting from deficiency of alpha₁-antitrypsin, a protective agent for the lung; increases patient's risk for developing panacinar emphysema even in the absence of smoking

asthma: a heterogeneous disease, usually characterized by chronic airway inflammation; defined by history of symptoms such as wheeze, shortness of breath, chest tightness, and cough that vary over time and in intensity

bronchiectasis: chronic, irreversible dilation of the bronchi and bronchioles that results from the destruction of muscles and elastic connective tissue; dilated airways become saccular and are a medium for chronic infection

chronic bronchitis: a disease of the airways defined as the presence of cough and sputum production for at least a combined total of 3 months in each of 2 consecutive years

chronic obstructive pulmonary disease: disease state characterized by airflow limitation that is not fully reversible; sometimes referred to as chronic airway obstruction or chronic obstructive lung disease

desaturate: a precipitous drop in the saturation of hemoglobin with oxygen

emphysema: a disease of the airways characterized by destruction of the walls of overdistended alveoli

polycythemia: increase in the red blood cell concentration in the blood; in COPD, the body attempts to improve oxygen carrying capacity by producing increasing amounts of red blood cells

pressurized metered-dose inhaler: patient-activated medication canister that provides aerosolized medication that the patient inhales into the lungs

spirometry: pulmonary function tests that measure specific lung volumes (e.g., FEV_1, FVC) and rates (e.g., $FEF_{25-75\%}$); may be measured before and after bronchodilator administration

Chronic pulmonary disorders are a leading cause of morbidity and mortality in the United States. Nurses care for patients with chronic pulmonary disease across the spectrum of care, from outpatient and home care to emergency department (ED), critical care, and hospice settings. To care for these patients, nurses not only need to have astute assessment and clinical management skills, but they also need knowledge of how these disorders can affect quality of life. In addition, the nurse's knowledge of palliative and end-of-life care is important for applicable patients. Patient and family education is an important nursing intervention to enhance self-management in patients with any chronic pulmonary disorder.

Chronic Obstructive Pulmonary Disease

Chronic obstructive pulmonary disease (COPD) is a preventable and treatable slowly progressive respiratory disease of airflow obstruction involving the airways, pulmonary parenchyma, or both (Global Initiative for Chronic Obstructive Lung Disease [GOLD], 2015). The parenchyma includes any form of lung tissue, including bronchioles, bronchi, blood vessels, interstitium, and alveoli. The airflow limitation or obstruction in COPD is not fully reversible. Most patients with COPD present with overlapping signs and symptoms of emphysema and chronic bronchitis, which are two distinct disease processes.

COPD may include diseases that cause airflow obstruction (e.g., emphysema, chronic bronchitis) or any combination of these disorders. Other diseases such as cystic fibrosis (CF), bronchiectasis, and asthma are classified as chronic pulmonary disorders. Asthma is considered a distinct, separate disorder and is classified as an abnormal airway condition characterized primarily by reversible inflammation. COPD can coexist with asthma. Both of these diseases have the same major symptoms; however, symptoms are generally more variable in asthma than in COPD. This chapter discusses COPD as a disease and describes chronic bronchitis and emphysema as distinct disease states, providing a foundation for understanding the pathophysiology of COPD. Bronchiectasis, asthma, and CF are discussed separately.

COPD and lower respiratory diseases are the third leading cause of death in the United States, with heart disease and cancer being number one and two (Centers for Disease Control and Prevention [CDC], 2015a). In 2012, approximately 144,000 Americans died from chronic lower respiratory diseases (CDC, 2015a). Whereas mortality from other major causes of death has been decreasing, deaths from COPD have continued to rise. COPD affects more than 5% of the adult population in the United States. An estimated 27 million adults have COPD, including 14 million diagnosed and more than 12 million undiagnosed adults. There are approximately 700,000 hospitalizations with the principal diagnosis of COPD each year in the United States; of these, 1 in 5 are readmitted within 30 days (Agency for Health Care Research and Quality [AHRQ], 2014). COPD has estimated annual direct costs of $29.5 billion and indirect costs of $20.4 billion (GOLD, 2015). COPD exacerbations account for the greatest proportion of COPD burden.

Pathophysiology

People with COPD commonly become symptomatic during the middle adult years, and the incidence of the disease increases with age. Although certain aspects of lung function normally decrease with age—for example, vital capacity and forced expiratory volume in 1 second (FEV_1)—COPD accentuates and accelerates these physiologic changes as described later. In COPD, the airflow limitation is both progressive and associated with the lungs' abnormal inflammatory response to noxious particles or gases. The inflammatory response occurs throughout the proximal and peripheral airways, lung parenchyma, and pulmonary vasculature (GOLD, 2015). Because of the chronic inflammation and the body's attempts to repair it, changes and narrowing occur in the airways. In the proximal airways (trachea and bronchi greater than 2 mm in diameter), changes include increased numbers of goblet cells and enlarged submucosal glands, both of which lead to hypersecretion of mucus. In the peripheral airways (bronchioles less than 2 mm diameter), inflammation causes thickening of the airway wall, peribronchial fibrosis, exudate in the airway, and overall airway narrowing (obstructive bronchiolitis). Over time, this ongoing injury-and-repair process causes scar tissue formation and narrowing of the airway lumen (GOLD, 2015). Inflammatory and structural changes also occur in the lung parenchyma (respiratory bronchioles and alveoli). Alveolar wall destruction leads to loss of alveolar attachments and a decrease in elastic recoil. Finally, the chronic inflammatory process affects the pulmonary vasculature and causes thickening of the lining of the vessel and hypertrophy of smooth muscle, which may lead to pulmonary hypertension (GOLD, 2015).

Processes related to imbalances of substances (proteinases and antiproteinases) in the lung may also contribute to airflow limitation. When activated by chronic inflammation, proteinases and other substances may be released, damaging the parenchyma of the lung. These parenchymal changes may also occur as a consequence of inflammation or environmental or genetic factors (e.g., alpha$_1$-antitrypsin deficiency).

Chronic Bronchitis

Chronic bronchitis, a disease of the airways, is defined as the presence of cough and sputum production for at least 3 months in each of 2 consecutive years. Although *chronic bronchitis* is a clinically and epidemiologically useful term, it does not reflect the major impact of airflow limitation on morbidity and mortality in COPD (GOLD, 2015). In many cases, smoke or other environmental pollutants irritate the airways, resulting in inflammation and hypersecretion of mucus. Constant irritation causes the mucus-secreting glands and goblet cells to increase in number, leading to increased mucus production. Mucus plugging of the airway reduces ciliary function. Bronchial walls also become thickened, further narrowing the bronchial lumen (see Fig. 24-1). Alveoli adjacent to the bronchioles may become damaged and fibrosed, resulting in altered function of the alveolar macrophages. This is significant because the macrophages play an important role in destroying foreign particles, including bacteria. As a result, the patient becomes more susceptible to respiratory infection. A wide range of viral, bacterial, and mycoplasma infections can produce acute episodes of bronchitis. Exacerbations of chronic bronchitis

Physiology/Pathophysiology

Figure 24-1 • Pathophysiology of chronic bronchitis as compared to a normal bronchus. The bronchus in chronic bronchitis is narrowed and has impaired airflow due to multiple mechanisms: inflammation, excess mucus production, and potential smooth muscle constriction (bronchospasm).

NORMAL BRONCHUS

CHRONIC BRONCHITIS

Smooth muscle

Open airway

Mucous gland

Inflammation

Increased number of mucous glands

Excess mucus causing chronic cough

are most likely to occur during the winter when viral and bacterial infections are more prevalent.

Emphysema

In **emphysema,** impaired oxygen and carbon dioxide exchange results from destruction of the walls of overdistended alveoli. *Emphysema* is a pathologic term that describes an abnormal distention of the airspaces beyond the terminal bronchioles and destruction of the walls of the alveoli (GOLD, 2015). In addition, a chronic inflammatory response may induce disruption of the parenchymal tissues. This end-stage process progresses slowly for many years. As the walls of the alveoli are destroyed (a process accelerated by recurrent infections), the alveolar surface area in direct contact with the pulmonary capillaries continually decreases. This causes an increase in dead space (lung area where no gas exchange can occur) and impaired oxygen diffusion, which leads to hypoxemia. In the later stages of disease, carbon dioxide elimination is impaired, resulting in increased carbon dioxide tension in arterial blood (hypercapnia) leading to respiratory acidosis. As the alveolar walls continue to break down, the pulmonary capillary bed is reduced in size. Consequently, resistance to pulmonary blood flow is increased, forcing the right ventricle to maintain a higher blood pressure in the pulmonary artery. Hypoxemia may further increase pulmonary artery pressures (pulmonary hypertension). Cor pulmonale, one of the complications of emphysema, is right-sided heart failure brought on by long-term high blood pressure in the pulmonary arteries. This high pressure in the pulmonary arteries and right ventricle lead to back up of blood in the venous system, resulting in dependent edema, distended neck veins, or pain in the region of the liver (see Chapter 29 for further discussion).

There are two main types of emphysema, based on the changes taking place in the lung (see Fig. 24-2). Both types may occur in the same patient. In the panlobular (panacinar) type of emphysema, there is destruction of the respiratory bronchiole, alveolar duct, and alveolus. All airspaces within the lobule are essentially enlarged, but there is little inflammatory disease. A hyperinflated (hyperexpanded) chest, marked dyspnea on exertion, and weight loss typically occur. To move air into and out of the lungs, negative pressure is required during inspiration, and an adequate level of positive pressure must be attained and maintained during expiration. Instead of being an involuntary passive act, expiration becomes active and requires muscular effort.

In the centrilobular (centroacinar) form, pathologic changes take place mainly in the center of the secondary lobule, preserving the peripheral portions of the acinus (i.e., the terminal airway unit where gas exchange occurs). Frequently, there is a derangement of ventilation–perfusion ratios, producing chronic hypoxemia, hypercapnia, **polycythemia** (i.e., an increase in red blood cells), and episodes of right-sided heart failure. This leads to central cyanosis and respiratory failure. The patient also develops peripheral edema.

Risk Factors

Risk factors for COPD include environmental exposures and host factors (see Chart 24-1). The most important environmental risk factor for COPD worldwide is cigarette smoking. A dose–response relationship exists between the intensity of smoking (pack-year history) and the decline in pulmonary function. Other environmental risk factors include smoking pipes, cigars, and other types of tobacco. Passive smoking (i.e., secondhand smoke) also contributes to respiratory symptoms and COPD (GOLD, 2015). Smoking depresses the activity of scavenger cells and affects the respiratory tract's ciliary cleansing mechanism, which keeps breathing passages free of inhaled irritants, bacteria, and other foreign matter. When smoking damages this cleansing mechanism, airflow is obstructed and air becomes trapped behind the obstruction. The alveoli greatly distend, which diminishes lung capacity. Smoking also irritates the goblet cells and mucous glands, causing an increased accumulation of mucus, which in turn produces more irritation, infection, and damage to the lung (U.S. Department of Health and Human Services [HHS], 2014a; HHS, 2014b). In addition, carbon monoxide (a by-product of smoking) combines with hemoglobin to form carboxyhemoglobin. Hemoglobin that is bound by carboxyhemoglobin cannot carry oxygen efficiently.

Physiology/Pathophysiology

Panlobular emphysema
(PLE)

Normal

Centrilobular
emphysema (CLE)

Figure 24-2 • Changes in alveolar structure in centrilobular and panlobular emphysema. In panlobular emphysema, the bronchioles, alveolar ducts, and alveoli are destroyed, and the airspaces within the lobule are enlarged. In centrilobular emphysema, the pathologic changes occur in the lobule, whereas the peripheral portions of the acinus are preserved.

Chart 24-1	**RISK FACTORS** Chronic Obstructive Pulmonary Disease

- Exposure to tobacco smoke accounts for an estimated 80% to 90% of cases of chronic obstructive pulmonary disease
- Passive smoking (i.e., secondhand smoke)
- Increased age
- Occupational exposure—dust, chemicals
- Indoor and outdoor air pollution
- Genetic abnormalities, including a deficiency of alpha$_1$-antitrypsin, an enzyme inhibitor that normally counteracts the destruction of lung tissue by certain other enzymes

Adapted from Global Initiative for Chronic Obstructive Disease. (2015). *Global strategy for the diagnosis, management and prevention of COPD*. Retrieved on 4/18/2016 at: www.goldcopd.org/uploads/users/files/GOLD_Report_2015.pdf

Cigarette smoking is the best-studied COPD risk factor; however, it is not the only risk factor and studies have demonstrated nonsmokers may also develop chronic airflow obstruction. Other environmental risk factors for COPD include prolonged and intense exposure to occupational dusts and chemicals, indoor air pollution, and outdoor air pollution (GOLD, 2015).

Host risk factors include a person's genetic makeup. One well-documented genetic risk factor is a deficiency of **alpha$_1$-antitrypsin**, an enzyme inhibitor that protects the lung parenchyma from injury. This deficiency may lead to lung and liver disease. Worldwide, alpha$_1$-antitrypsin deficiency impacts between 1/1700 and 1/5000 people (American Liver Foundation, 2015). Of patients with COPD, 1% to 2% are found to have severe alpha$_1$-antitrypsin deficiency. This deficiency predisposes young people to rapid development of lobular emphysema, even in the absence of smoking. Among Caucasians, alpha$_1$-antitrypsin deficiency is one of the most commonly genetically linked lethal diseases. COPD may also result from gene–environment interactions (GOLD, 2015). Genetically susceptible people are sensitive to environmental factors (e.g., smoking, air pollution, infectious agents, and allergens) and eventually develop chronic obstructive symptoms. Carriers must be identified so that they can modify environmental risk factors to delay or prevent overt symptoms of disease. Genetic counseling should be offered. Alpha-protease inhibitor replacement therapy, which slows the progression of the disease, is available for patients with this genetic defect and for those with severe disease. However, this infusion therapy is costly and is required on an ongoing basis.

Other genetic risk factors may predispose a patient to COPD. Work is ongoing to identify specific variants of genes hypothesized to be involved in the development of COPD. These may include specific phenotypes to several chromosomal regions in families with multiple members developing early-onset COPD.

Age is often identified as a risk factor for COPD, but it is unclear whether healthy aging is an independent risk or whether the risk is related to cumulative exposures to risks over time (GOLD, 2015). There is a strong inverse relationship between COPD and lower socioeconomic status. However, perhaps it is not the lower socioeconomic status but how the socioeconomic status places the person at risk of increased patterns of exposure (indoor and outdoor pollutants, crowding, poor nutrition, infections and increased smoking).

Clinical Manifestations

Although the natural history of COPD is variable, it is generally a progressive disease characterized by three primary symptoms: chronic cough, sputum production, and dyspnea (GOLD, 2015). These symptoms often worsen over time. Chronic cough and sputum production often precede the development of airflow limitation by many years. However, not all people with cough and sputum production develop COPD. The cough may be intermittent and may be unproductive in some patients (GOLD, 2015). Dyspnea may be severe and interfere with the patient's activities and quality of life. It is usually progressive, is worse with exercise, and is persistent. As COPD progresses, dyspnea may occur at rest. Weight loss is common, because dyspnea interferes with eating and the work of breathing is energy depleting. As the

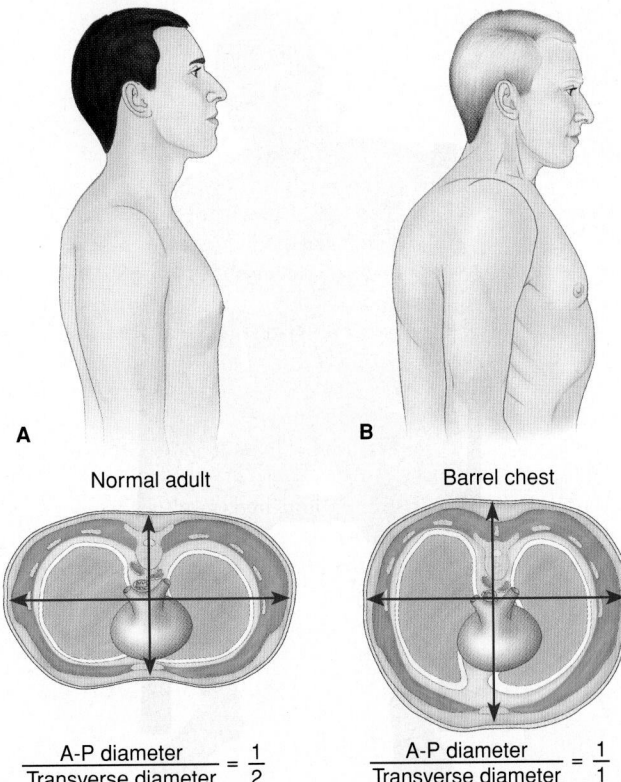

$$\frac{\text{A-P diameter}}{\text{Transverse diameter}} = \frac{1}{2} \qquad \frac{\text{A-P diameter}}{\text{Transverse diameter}} = \frac{1}{1}$$

Figure 24-3 • Characteristics of normal chest wall and chest wall in emphysema. **A.** The normal chest wall and its cross-section. **B.** The barrel-shaped chest of emphysema and its cross-section.

work of breathing increases over time, the accessory muscles are recruited in an effort to breathe. Patients with COPD are at risk for respiratory insufficiency and respiratory infections or COPD exacerbation, which in turn increase the risk of acute and chronic respiratory failure.

In patients with COPD who have a primary emphysematous component, chronic hyperinflation leads to the "barrel chest" thorax configuration. This configuration results from a more fixed position of the ribs in the inspiratory position (due to hyperinflation) and from loss of lung elasticity (see Fig. 24-3). Retraction of the supraclavicular fossae occurs on inspiration, causing the shoulders to heave upward (see Fig. 24-4). In advanced emphysema, the abdominal muscles may also contract on inspiration.

There are systemic or extrapulmonary manifestations of COPD. These include musculoskeletal wasting (see Chapter 5 for discussion of nutrition assessment and Chapter 44 for discussion of nutrition therapy), metabolic syndrome (see Chapter 27), and depression (a frequent comorbidity that accompanies chronic debilitating illnesses). These clinical manifestations beyond the lungs must also be assessed and treated in order to decrease the morbidity and improve the quality of life of the patient with COPD.

Assessment and Diagnostic Findings

The nurse obtains a thorough health history from patients with known or potential COPD. Chart 24-2 lists the key factors to assess for patients with known or suspected COPD. Pulmonary function studies are used to help confirm the

Figure 24-4 • Typical posture of a person with chronic obstructive pulmonary disease—primarily emphysema. The person tends to lean forward and uses the accessory muscles of respiration to breathe, forcing the shoulder girdle upward and causing the supraclavicular fossae to retract on inspiration.

diagnosis of COPD, determine disease severity, and monitor disease progression. **Spirometry** is used to evaluate airflow obstruction, which is determined by the ratio of FEV_1 to forced vital capacity (FVC). Spirometric results are expressed as an absolute volume and as a percentage of the predicted value using appropriate normal values for gender, age, and height. With obstruction, the patient either has difficulty exhaling or cannot forcibly exhale air from the lungs, reducing the FEV_1. Spirometry is also used to determine reversibility of obstruction after the use of bronchodilators (GOLD, 2015). Spirometry is initially performed, the patient is given an inhaled bronchodilator treatment according to a standard protocol, and then spirometry is repeated. The patient demonstrates a degree of reversibility if the pulmonary function values improve after administration of the bronchodilator.

Arterial blood gas measurements may also be obtained to assess baseline oxygenation and gas exchange and are especially important in advanced COPD. A chest x-ray may be obtained to exclude alternative diagnoses. A computed tomography (CT) chest scan is not routinely obtained in the diagnosis of COPD, but a high-resolution CT scan may help in the differential diagnosis. Lastly, screening for alpha₁-antitrypsin deficiency may be performed for patients younger than 45 years and for those with a family history of COPD, particularly if they have a family history of blood relatives with alpha₁-antitrypsin deficiency or COPD that is primarily emphysematous in nature.

COPD is classified into four grades depending on the severity measured by pulmonary function tests, as shown in Table 24-1 (GOLD, 2015). However, pulmonary function is not the only way to assess or classify COPD; pulmonary function is evaluated in conjunction with symptoms, health status impairment with COPD, and the potential for exacerbations. Factors that determine the clinical course and survival of patients with COPD include history of cigarette smoking, passive smoking exposure, age, rate of decline of FEV_1, hypoxemia, pulmonary artery pressure, resting heart rate, weight loss, reversibility of airflow obstruction, and comorbidities.

In diagnosing COPD, several differential diagnoses must be ruled out. The primary differential diagnosis is asthma. It may be difficult to differentiate between a patient with COPD and one with chronic asthma. Other diseases that must be considered in the differential diagnosis include heart failure, bronchiectasis, tuberculosis, obliterative bronchiolitis, and diffuse panbronchiolitis (GOLD, 2015). Key factors in determining the diagnosis are the patient's history, severity of symptoms, and responsiveness to bronchodilators.

Complications

Respiratory insufficiency and failure are major life-threatening complications of COPD. The acuity of the onset and the severity of respiratory failure depend on baseline pulmonary function, pulse oximetry or arterial blood gas values, comorbid conditions, and the severity of other complications of COPD. Respiratory insufficiency and failure may be chronic (with severe COPD) or acute (with severe bronchospasm or pneumonia in a patient with severe COPD). Acute respiratory insufficiency and failure may necessitate ventilatory support until other acute complications, such as infection, can be treated. (See Chapter 21 for the management of the patient requiring ventilatory support.) Other complications of COPD include pneumonia, chronic atelectasis, pneumothorax, and pulmonary arterial hypertension (cor pulmonale).

Medical Management

Therapeutic strategies for the patient with COPD include promoting smoking cessation as appropriate, prescribing medications that typically include bronchodilators and may include corticosteroids, managing exacerbations, and providing supplemental oxygen therapy as indicated.

Risk Reduction

For patients with stable disease, treatment aims to reduce risk and symptoms. The major risk factor associated with COPD is environmental exposure and it is modifiable. The most important environmental exposure is smoking. Approximately 8 million people in the United States have chronic illnesses related to smoking. Smoking kills more than 500,000 each year and costs the nation more than $300 billion in health care expenses and lost productivity each year (HHS, 2015a). Smoking cessation is the single most cost-effective intervention to reduce the risk of developing COPD and to stop its progression (GOLD, 2015). However, smoking cessation is difficult to achieve and even more difficult to sustain in the long term. Factors associated with continued smoking vary among patients and may include the strength of the nicotine addiction, continued exposure to smoking-associated stimuli (at work or in social settings), stress, depression, and habit.

Chart 24-2 ASSESSMENT
Assessing Patients With Chronic Obstructive Pulmonary Disease

Health History

- Has the patient been exposed to risk factors (types, intensity, duration)?
- Does the patient have a past medical history of respiratory diseases/problems, including asthma, allergy, sinusitis, nasal polyps, or respiratory infections?
- Does the patient have a family history of chronic obstructive pulmonary disease or other chronic respiratory diseases?
- How long has the patient had respiratory difficulty?
- What is the pattern of symptom development?
- Does exertion increase the dyspnea? What type of exertion?
- What are the limits of the patient's tolerance for exercise?
- At what times during the day does the patient complain most of fatigue and shortness of breath?
- Does the patient describe any discomfort or pain in any part of the body? If so, where does it occur, how intense is this pain, when does it occur, and does it interfere with activities of daily living? Is there any intervention that helps to alleviate the pain or discomfort?
- Which eating and sleeping habits have been affected?
- What is the impact of respiratory disease on quality of life?
- What does the patient know about the disease and their condition?
- What is the patient's smoking history (primary and secondary)?
- Is there occupational exposure to smoke or other pollutants?
- What are the triggering events (e.g., exertion, strong odors, dust, exposure to animals)?
- Does the patient have a history of exacerbations or previous hospitalizations for respiratory problems?
- Are comorbidities present?

- How appropriate are current medical treatments?
- Does the patient have available social and family support?
- What is the potential for reducing risk factors (e.g., smoking cessation)?

Physical Assessment

- What position does the patient assume during the interview?
- What are the pulse and the respiratory rates?
- What is the character of respirations? Even and without effort? Other?
- Can the patient complete a sentence without having to take a breath?
- Does the patient contract the abdominal muscles during inspiration?
- Does the patient use accessory muscles of the shoulders and neck when breathing?
- Does the patient take a long time to exhale (prolonged expiration)?
- Is central cyanosis evident?
- Are the patient's neck veins engorged?
- Does the patient have peripheral edema?
- Is the patient coughing?
- What are the color, amount, and consistency of the sputum?
- Is clubbing of the fingers present?
- What types of breath sounds (i.e., clear, diminished or distant, crackles, and wheezes) are heard? Describe and document findings and locations.
- Are there any sensory deficits?
- Is there short- or long-term memory impairment?
- Is there increasing stupor?
- Is the patient apprehensive?

Because multiple factors are associated with continued smoking, successful cessation often requires multiple strategies. Health care providers should promote cessation by explaining the risks of smoking and personalizing the "at-risk" message to the patient. After giving a strong warning about smoking, health care providers should work with the patient to set a definite "quit date." Referral to a smoking cessation program may be helpful. Follow-up within 3 to 5 days after the quit date to review progress and to address any problems is associated with an increased rate of success; this should be repeated as needed. Continued reinforcement with a modality that is individualized to the patient and their lifestyle (e.g., telephone calls, texting, e-mail, or clinic visits) is beneficial. Relapses should be analyzed, and the patient and health care provider should jointly identify possible solutions to prevent future backsliding. It is important to emphasize successes rather than failures. Nicotine replacement—a first-line pharmacotherapy that reliably increases long-term smoking abstinence rates—comes in a variety of forms (gum, inhaler, nasal spray, transdermal patch, sublingual tablet, or lozenge). Bupropion SR (Wellbutrin, Zyban) and nortriptyline (Aventyl), both antidepressants, may also increase long-term quit rates. Other pharmacologic agents include the antihypertensive agent clonidine (Catapres); however, its side effects limit its use. Varenicline (Chantix), a nicotinic acetylcholine receptor partial agonist, may assist in smoking cessation (GOLD, 2015). Patients who are not appropriate candidates for such pharmacotherapy include those with medical contraindications, light smokers (fewer than 10 cigarettes per day), pregnant women, and adolescent smokers.

Smoking cessation can begin in a variety of health care settings—outpatient clinic, nursing center, pulmonary rehabilitation center, community, hospital, and in the home. Regardless of the setting, nurses have the opportunity to educate patients about the risks of smoking and the benefits of

TABLE 24-1 Grades of Chronic Obstructive Pulmonary Disease

Grade	Severity	Pulmonary Function
Grade I	Mild	FEV$_1$/FVC <70% FEV$_1$ ≥80% predicted
Grade II	Moderate	FEV$_1$/FVC <70% FEV$_1$ 50–80% predicted
Grade III	Severe	FEV$_1$/FVC <70% FEV$_1$ <30–50% predicted
Grade IV	Very severe	FEV$_1$/FVC <70% FEV$_1$ <30% predicted

FEV$_1$, forced expiratory volume in 1 second; FVC, forced vital capacity.
Adapted from Global Initiative for Chronic Obstructive Disease. (2015). *Global strategy for the diagnosis, management and prevention of COPD.* Retrieved on 4/18/2016 at: www.goldcopd.org/uploads/users/files/GOLD_Report_2015.pdf

smoking cessation. Various materials, resources, and programs developed by several organizations (e.g., Agency for Healthcare Research and Quality, Centers for Disease Control and Prevention [CDC], National Cancer Institute, American Lung Association, American Cancer Society) are available to assist with this effort.

Pharmacologic Therapy

Medication regimens used to manage COPD are based on disease severity. For grade I (mild) COPD, a short-acting bronchodilator may be prescribed. For grade II or III COPD, a short-acting bronchodilator and regular treatment with one or more long-acting bronchodilators may be used. For grade III or IV (severe or very severe) COPD, medication therapy includes regular treatment with one or more bronchodilators and/or inhaled corticosteroids for repeated exacerbations.

Bronchodilators

Bronchodilators are key for symptom management in stable COPD (GOLD, 2015). Inhaled therapy is preferred, and the choice of bronchodilator depends on availability and individual response in terms of symptom relief and side effects. Inhaled therapy may be prescribed on an as-needed or regular basis to reduce symptoms. Long-acting bronchodilators are more convenient for patients to use, and combining bronchodilators with different durations of action and different mechanisms may optimize symptom management (GOLD, 2015). Even patients who do not show a significant response to a short-acting bronchodilator test may benefit symptomatically from long-term bronchodilator treatment.

Bronchodilators relieve bronchospasm by improving expiratory flow through widening of the airways and promoting lung emptying with each breath. These medications alter smooth muscle tone and reduce airway obstruction by allowing increased oxygen distribution throughout the lungs and improving alveolar ventilation. Although regular use of bronchodilators that act primarily on the airway smooth muscle does not modify the decline of function or the prognosis of COPD, their use is central in the management of COPD (GOLD, 2015). These agents can be delivered through a pressurized metered-dose inhaler (pMDI) or other type of inhaler, by nebulization, or via the oral route in pill or liquid form. Bronchodilators are often given regularly throughout the day as well as on an as-needed basis. They may also be used prophylactically to prevent breathlessness by having the patient use them before participating in or completing an activity, such as eating or walking.

Several devices are available to deliver medication via the inhaled route. These include pMDIs, breath-actuated pMDIs, dry powder inhalers, spacer or valved-holding chambers, and nebulizers (also called wet nebulizers; nebulization of liquid medication via an air compressor) (Gardenhire, Ari, Hess et al., 2013). Attention to effective drug delivery and training in proper inhaler technique is essential. A respiratory therapist is an excellent health care provider to consult on appropriate inhaler technique. The choice of an inhaler device will depend on availability, cost, prescribing physician, insurance coverage and the skills and ability of the patient (GOLD, 2015). Key aspects of each are described in Table 24-2. A pMDI is a pressurized device that contains an aerosolized powder of medication. A precise amount of medication is released with each activation of the canister. Patients must be instructed in the correct use of the device. A spacer or valved-holding chamber may also be used to enhance deposition of the medication in the lung and help the patient coordinate activation of the pMDI with inspiration. Spacers come in several designs, but all are attached to the pMDI and have a mouthpiece on the opposite end (see Fig. 24-5).

A new breath-actuated multidose, dry powder inhaler was approved by the U.S. Food and Drug Administration (FDA) in 2015, albuterol (ProAir RespiClick). Although this inhaler is prescribed primarily for asthma at this time, it is indicated for treatment or prevention of reversible bronchospasm. COPD may have a component of bronchospasm that can be treated with this drug. In addition, the newly introduced breath-actuated mechanism seems a promising method of delivery. The breath-actuated method minimizes the patient coordination necessary to activate the inhaler on inspiration (Teva Respiratory, 2016).

Several classes of bronchodilators are used that include beta-adrenergic agonists, muscarinic antagonists (anticholinergics) and combination agents. Beta-adrenergic agonists include short-acting beta$_2$-agonists (SABA) and long-acting beta$_2$-agonists (LABA). The anticholinergic agents include short-acting muscarinic (anticholinergic) antagonists (SAMA) and long-acting muscarinic antagonists (LAMA) (Bellinger & Peters, 2015; GOLD, 2015). Inhaled corticosteroids may also be combined with bronchodilators. These medications may be used in combination to optimize bronchodilation. Long-acting beta$_2$-agonist bronchodilators are more convenient for patient use as compared to short-acting beta$_2$-agonist bronchodilators. Examples of these medications are described in Table 24-3. Nebulized medications also known as wet nebulizers (nebulization of medication via an air compressor) may also be effective in patients who cannot use a pMDI properly or who prefer this method of administration. However, wet nebulizers are more expensive than other devices and require appropriate cleaning and maintenance (GOLD, 2015).

Corticosteroids

Although inhaled and systemic corticosteroids may improve the symptoms of COPD, they do not slow the decline in lung function. Their effects are less dramatic than in asthma. A short trial course of oral corticosteroids may be prescribed for patients to determine whether pulmonary function improves and symptoms decrease. Long-term treatment with oral corticosteroids is not recommended in COPD and can cause steroid myopathy, leading to muscle weakness, decreased ability to function, and, in advanced disease, respiratory failure (GOLD, 2015). Inhaled corticosteroids are frequently prescribed in COPD.

Combination long-term beta$_2$-agonists plus corticosteroids in one inhaler may be appropriate; examples include formoterol/budesonide (Symbicort), vilanterol/fluticasone furoate (Breo Ellipta) and salmeterol/fluticasone (Advair) (Bellinger & Peters, 2015; GOLD, 2015).

Other Medications

Other pharmacologic treatments that may be used in COPD include alpha$_1$-antitrypsin augmentation therapy, antibiotic agents, mucolytic agents, antitussive agents, vasodilators,

TABLE 24-2 • Aerosol Delivery Devices

Devices/Drugs	Optimal Technique	Therapeutic Issues
Pressurized metered-dose inhaler (pMDI) Beta$_2$-agonists Corticosteroids Cromolyn sodium Anticholinergics	Actuation[a] during a slow (30 L/min or 3–5 s) deep inhalation, followed by 10-s breath-hold	Slow inhalation and coordination of actuation may be difficult for some patients. Patients may incorrectly stop inhalation at actuation. Deposition of 50–80% of actuated dose in the oropharynx. Mouth washing and spitting is effective in reducing the amount of drug swallowed and absorbed systemically
Breath-actuated MDI Beta$_2$-agonists	Tight seal around mouthpiece and slightly more rapid inhalation than standard pMDI (see above) followed by 10-s breathhold	May be particularly useful for patients unable to coordinate inhalation and actuation. May also be useful for older patients. Patients may incorrectly stop inhalation at actuation. Cannot be used with currently available spacer/valved-holding chamber (VHC) devices
Dry powder inhaler Beta$_2$-agonists Corticosteroids Anticholinergics	Rapid (1–2 s) deep inhalation. Minimally effective inspiratory flow is device dependent	Dose is lost if patient exhales through device after actuating. Delivery may be greater or lesser than pMDIs, depending on device and technique. Delivery is more flow dependent in devices with highest internal resistance. Rapid inhalation promotes greater deposition in larger central airways. Mouth washing and spitting are effective in reducing amount of drug swallowed and absorbed systemically
Spacer or VHC	Slow (30 L/min or 3–5 s) deep inhalation, followed by 10-s breathhold immediately following actuation. Actuate only once into spacer/VHC per inhalation. Rinse plastic VHCs once a month with low concentration of liquid household dishwashing detergent (1:5000 or 1–2 drops per cup of water) and let drip dry	Indicated for patients who have difficulty performing adequate pMDI technique. May be bulky. Simple tubes do not obviate coordinating actuation and inhalation. VHCs are preferred. Spacers or VHCs may increase delivery of inhalational corticosteroids to the lungs
Nebulizer Beta$_2$-agonists Corticosteroids Cromolyn sodium Anticholinergics	Slow tidal breathing with occasional deep breaths. Tightly fitting facemask for those unable to use mouthpiece	Less dependent on patient's coordination and cooperation. May be expensive, time consuming, and bulky; output depends on device and operating parameters (fill volume, driving gas flow); internebulizer and intranebulizer output variances are significant. The use of a facemask reduces delivery to lungs by 50%. Choice of delivery system depends on resources, availability, and clinical judgment of clinician caring for patient. There is potential for infections if device is not cleaned properly

[a]Actuation refers to release of dose of medication with inhalation.
Gardenhire, D. S., Ari, A., Hess, D., et al. (2013). *A guide to aerosol delivery devices for respiratory therapists* (3rd ed.). Dallas, TX: American Association for Respiratory Care.

and narcotics. Vaccines are also effective in that they prevent exacerbations by preventing respiratory infections. For instance, influenza vaccines can reduce serious morbidity and death in patients with COPD by approximately 50% (GOLD, 2015). It is recommended that people limit their risk through influenza vaccination and smoking cessation. Pneumococcal vaccination also reduces the incidence of pneumonia, hospitalizations for cardiac conditions, and deaths in the general

Figure 24-5 • A. Examples of pressurized metered-dose inhalers and spacers. **B.** A pressurized metered-dose inhaler and spacer in use.

TABLE 24-3 Common Types of Bronchodilator Medications for Chronic Obstructive Pulmonary Disease

Class/Drug (Trade Name)	Inhaler[a]	Nebulizer	Oral	Duration of Action[b]
Beta$_2$-Adrenergic Agonist Agents				
fenoterol (Berotec N)	X	X	X	SABA
salbutamol, albuterol (Ventolin)	X	X	X	SABA
albuterol (ProAir RespiClick)	X			SABA
levalbuterol (Xopenex HFA)				SABA
terbutaline (Brethine, Brethaire)	X		X	SABA
arformoterol (Brovana)		X		LABA
formoterol (Foradil)	X	X		LABA
salmeterol (Serevent Diskus)	X			LABA
indacaterol (Arcapta, Onbrez)	X			LABA
Anticholinergic Agents				
ipratropium bromide (Atrovent, Ipraxa)	X	X		SAMA
tiotropium bromide	X			LAMA
(Spiriva) umeclidinium (Incruse Ellipta)	X			LAMA
Combination Short-Acting Beta$_2$-Adrenergic Agonist and Anticholinergic Agents				
fenoterol/ipratropium (Beodual N)	X	X		SABA/SAMA
salbutamol/ipratropium (Combivent, DuoNeb)	X			SABA/SAMA
Inhaled Corticosteroids (ICS)				
beclomethasone propionate (Qvar)	X	X		
budesonide (Pulmicort Flexhaler)	X	X		
fluticasone propionate (Flovent)	X	X		
Combination Inhaled Corticosteroids and Long Acting Beta$_2$-Adrenergic Agonist				
budesonide/formoterol (Symbicort)	X			ICS/LABA
mometasone/formoterol/(Dulera)	X			ICS/LABA
fluticasone/salmetereol/(Advair Discus)	X			ICS/LABA
fluticasone furoate/vilanterol (Breo Ellipta)	X			ICS/LABA

[a]Inhaler may include pressurized metered-dose inhaler, dry powdered inhalation with inhaler, or discus.
[b]Short acting, 4–6 h; long acting, 12+ h.
SABA, short acting beta$_2$-agonist; LABA, long acting beta$_2$-agonist; SAMA, short acting anticholinergic; LAMA, long acting anticholinergic; ICS, inhaled corticosteroid.
Adapted from Global Initiative for Chronic Obstructive Lung Disease (GOLD). (2015). *Global strategy for the diagnosis, management and prevention of COPD.* Retrieved on 4/18/2016 at: www.goldcopd.org/uploads/users/files/GOLD_Report_2015.pdf

older adult population (GOLD, 2015) (see Chapter 23 for further discussion of pneumococcal vaccination).

Management of Exacerbations

An exacerbation of COPD is defined as an event in the natural course of the disease characterized by acute changes (worsening) in the patient's respiratory symptoms beyond the normal day-to-day variations. An exacerbation also leads to change in medication (GOLD, 2015). Primary causes of an acute exacerbation include tracheobronchial infection and air pollution. However, the cause of approximately one third of severe exacerbations cannot be identified (GOLD, 2015). Roflumilast (Daliresp) may be used as a treatment to reduce the risk of exacerbations in patients with severe COPD associated with chronic bronchitis and a history of exacerbations. Roflumilast is a selective phosphodiesterase-4 (PDE4) inhibitor and is taken as a tablet once daily.

Treatment of an exacerbation requires identifying the primary cause (if possible) and administering the specific treatment. Optimization of bronchodilator medications is first-line therapy and involves identifying the best medication or combinations of medications taken on a regular

schedule for a specific patient. Depending on the signs and symptoms, corticosteroids, antibiotic agents, oxygen therapy, and intensive respiratory interventions may also be used. Indications for hospitalization for acute exacerbation of COPD include severe dyspnea that does not respond adequately to initial therapy, confusion or lethargy, respiratory muscle fatigue, paradoxical chest wall movement, peripheral edema, worsening or new onset of central cyanosis, persistent or worsening hypoxemia, and the need for noninvasive or invasive assisted mechanical ventilation (GOLD, 2015). The outcome from an exacerbation of COPD is closely related to the development of respiratory acidosis, the presence of significant comorbidities, and the need for noninvasive or invasive positive pressure ventilatory support.

The GOLD guidelines (2015) provide indications for assessment, hospital admission, and possible critical care admission for patients with exacerbations of COPD. Indications for hospitalization include marked increase in intensity of symptoms, severe underlying COPD, onset of new physical signs (e.g., the use of accessory muscles, paradoxical chest wall movement, worsening or new onset of central cyanosis, peripheral edema, signs of right heart failure, and reduced alertness), failure to respond to initial medical management, older age, and insufficient home support.

When the patient arrives in an ED, the first line of treatment is supplemental oxygen therapy and rapid assessment to determine if the exacerbation is life threatening (GOLD, 2015). A short-acting inhaled bronchodilator may be used to assess response to treatment. Oral or intravenous (IV) corticosteroids, in addition to bronchodilators, are recommended in the hospital management of a COPD exacerbation. Antibiotics also benefit patients with COPD because bacterial infections often follow viral infections.

General Principles of Oxygen Therapy

Oxygen therapy can be given as long-term continuous therapy, during exercise, or to prevent acute dyspnea during an exacerbation. The goal of supplemental oxygen therapy is to increase the baseline resting partial pressure of arterial oxygen (PaO_2) to at least 60 mm Hg at sea level and an arterial oxygen saturation (SaO_2) to at least 90% (GOLD, 2015). Long-term oxygen therapy (more than 15 hours per day) has also been shown to improve quality of life, reduce pulmonary arterial pressure and dyspnea, and improve survival (GOLD, 2015). Long-term oxygen therapy is usually introduced in very severe COPD, and indications generally include a PaO_2 of 55 mm Hg or less or evidence of tissue hypoxia and organ damage such as cor pulmonale, secondary polycythemia, edema from right-sided heart failure, or impaired mental status (GOLD, 2015). For patients with exercise-induced hypoxemia, oxygen supplementation during exercise may improve performance. No evidence supports the idea that short bursts of oxygen before or after exercise provide any symptomatic relief (GOLD, 2015). Patients who are hypoxemic while awake are likely to be so during sleep. Therefore, nighttime oxygen therapy is recommended as well, and the prescription for oxygen therapy is for continuous, 24-hour use. Intermittent oxygen therapy is indicated for patients who **desaturate** (i.e., experience a precipitous drop in hemoglobin molecule saturation with oxygen) only during activities of daily living, exercise, or sleep.

The main objective in treating patients with hypoxemia and hypercapnia is to give sufficient oxygen to improve oxygenation. Patients with COPD who require oxygen may have respiratory failure that is caused primarily by a ventilation–perfusion mismatch. These patients respond to oxygen therapy and should be treated to keep the resting oxygen saturation at or above 90%, which is associated with a PaO_2 of 60 mm Hg or higher (Hooley, 2015). Although the hypoxic drive is often cited as a concern in administering supplemental oxygen to patients with COPD, in actuality it is a very small part of the overall stimulus driving the respiratory system. However, a small subset of patients with COPD and chronic hypercapnia (elevated partial pressure of arterial carbon dioxide [$PaCO_2$] levels) may be more oxygen sensitive; their respiratory failure is caused more by alveolar hypoventilation (hypoxic drive). Administering too much oxygen can result in the retention of carbon dioxide. Patients with alveolar hypoventilation cannot increase ventilation to adjust for this increased load, and increasing hypercapnia occurs. Monitoring and assessment are essential in the care of patients with COPD on supplemental oxygen. Pulse oximetry is helpful in assessing response to therapy but does not assess $PaCO_2$

levels. In addition, the nurse must evaluate for other factors and medications which could further decrease the respiratory drive—neurologic impairment, fluid and electrolyte issues, and narcotics or sedatives. Optimal oxygenation of patients is important while monitoring for any possible complications of oxygen supplementation.

Quality and Safety Nursing Alert

Oxygen therapy is variable in patients with COPD; its aim in COPD is to achieve an acceptable oxygen level without a fall in the pH (increasing hypercapnia).

Surgical Management

Surgical options might be necessary for patients who do not demonstrate symptom improvement with nonsurgical therapies.

Bullectomy

A bullectomy is a surgical option for select patients with bullous emphysema. Bullae are enlarged airspaces that do not contribute to ventilation but occupy space in the thorax; these areas may be surgically excised. These bullae compress areas of the lung and may impair gas exchange. Bullectomy may help reduce dyspnea and improve lung function. It can be performed via a video-assisted thoracoscope or a limited thoracotomy incision (see Chapter 21).

Lung Volume Reduction Surgery

Treatment options for patients with advanced or end-stage COPD (grade IV) with a primary emphysematous component are limited, although lung volume reduction surgery is a palliative surgical option that is approved by Medicare in selected patients. This includes patients with homogenous disease or disease that is focused in one area and not widespread throughout the lungs. Lung volume reduction surgery involves the removal of a portion of the diseased lung parenchyma. This reduces hyperinflation and allows the functional tissue to expand, resulting in improved elastic recoil of the lung and improved chest wall and diaphragmatic mechanics. This type of surgery does not cure the disease but may improve life expectancy, decrease dyspnea, improve lung function and exercise tolerance, and improve the patient's overall quality of life (GOLD, 2015).

Bronchoscopic lung volume reduction therapies are under investigation in clinical research protocols. These bronchoscopic procedures were developed to collapse areas of emphysematous lung and thus improve aeration of the functional lung tissue. Techniques include endobronchial placement of a one-way valve that allows air and mucus to exit the treated area but does not allow air to reenter. Another technique achieves biologic lung volume reduction through bronchoscopic instillation of a sealant or gel, valves or coils into the airway of the hyperinflated lung tissue. Because air can no longer enter the airway, the lung tissue beyond the sealed airway collapses over time. There is insufficient evidence to determine the benefit–risk ratios, cost-effectiveness, and possible roles of these procedures in care of the patient with severe emphysema (GOLD, 2015).

Lung Transplantation

Lung transplantation is a viable option for definitive surgical treatment of severe COPD in selected patients. It has been shown to improve quality of life and functional capacity in a select group of patients with COPD. Limited not only by the shortage of donor organs, it is also a costly procedure with financial implications for months to years because of complications and the need for costly immunosuppressive medication regimens (GOLD, 2015).

Pulmonary Rehabilitation

Pulmonary rehabilitation for patients with COPD is well established and widely accepted as a means to alleviate symptoms and optimize functional status. (McCarthy, Casey, Murphy, et al., 2015). The primary goals of rehabilitation are to reduce symptoms, improve quality of life, and increase physical and emotional participation in everyday activities (GOLD, 2015). The benefits of this therapy include improvement of exercise capacity, reduction in the perceived intensity of breathlessness, improvement in health-related quality of life, reduction in the number of hospitalizations and days in the hospital, and reduction in the anxiety and depression associated with COPD (GOLD, 2015). Pulmonary rehabilitation services are multidisciplinary and include assessment, education, smoking cessation, physical reconditioning, nutritional counseling, skills training, and psychological support. Patients are taught methods to alleviate symptoms. Breathing exercises, as well as retraining and exercise programs, are used to improve functional status.

Pulmonary rehabilitation is appropriate for patients with grades II through IV COPD (GOLD, 2015). The minimum length of an effective program is 6 weeks; the longer the program, the more effective the results (GOLD, 2015). Programs vary in duration and may be conducted in inpatient, outpatient, or home settings. Program selection depends on the patient's physical, functional, and psychosocial status; insurance coverage; availability of programs; and preference. Pulmonary rehabilitation may also be used therapeutically in other disorders besides COPD, including asthma, CF, lung cancer, interstitial lung disease, thoracic surgery, and lung transplantation. Despite their proven efficacy, it was only in the past decade that these services were approved for coverage by Medicare and other payers. Medicare covers a comprehensive program, but specific criteria must be met.

Patient Education

Nurses play a key role in identifying potential candidates for pulmonary rehabilitation and in facilitating and reinforcing the material learned in the rehabilitation program. Not all patients have access to a formal rehabilitation program. However, nurses can be instrumental in educating patients and families as well as facilitating specific services, such as respiratory therapy education, physical therapy for exercise and breathing retraining, occupational therapy for conserving energy during activities of daily living, and nutritional counseling. Patient education is a major component of pulmonary rehabilitation and includes a broad variety of topics.

Depending on the length and setting of the educational program, topics may include normal anatomy and physiology of the lung, pathophysiology and changes with COPD, medications and home oxygen therapy, nutrition, respiratory therapy treatments, symptom alleviation, smoking cessation, sexuality and COPD, coping with chronic disease, communicating with the health care team, and planning for the future (advance directives, living wills, informed decision making about health care alternatives). Education, including that relating to smoking cessation, should be incorporated into all aspects of care for COPD and in many settings (physicians' offices, clinics, hospitals, home and community health care settings, and comprehensive rehabilitation programs).

Breathing Exercises

The breathing pattern of most people with COPD is shallow, rapid, and inefficient; the more severe the disease, the more inefficient the breathing pattern. With practice, this type of upper chest breathing can be changed to diaphragmatic breathing, which reduces the respiratory rate, increases alveolar ventilation, and sometimes helps expel as much air as possible during expiration (see Chapter 21 for technique). Pursed-lip breathing helps slow expiration, prevents collapse of small airways, and helps the patient control the rate and depth of respiration. It also promotes relaxation, enabling the patient to gain control of dyspnea and reduce feelings of panic.

Activity Pacing

People with COPD have decreased exercise tolerance during specific periods of the day, especially in the morning on arising, because bronchial secretions have collected in the lungs during the night while the patient was lying down. The patient may have difficulty bathing or dressing and may become fatigued. Activities that require the arms to be supported above the level of the thorax may produce fatigue or respiratory distress but may be tolerated better after the patient has been up and moving around for an hour or more. The nurse can help the patient reduce these limitations by planning self-care activities and determining the best times for bathing, dressing, and other daily activities.

Self-Care Activities

As gas exchange, airway clearance, and the breathing pattern improve, the patient is encouraged to assume increasing participation in self-care activities. The patient is taught to coordinate diaphragmatic breathing with activities such as walking, bathing, bending, or climbing stairs. The patient should bathe, dress, and take short walks, resting as needed to avoid fatigue and excessive dyspnea. Fluids should always be readily available, and the patient should begin to drink fluids without having to be reminded. If management of secretions is a problem and some type of postural drainage or airway clearance maneuver is to be performed at home, the nurse or respiratory therapist instructs and supervises the patient before discharge or in an outpatient setting.

Physical Conditioning

People with COPD of all grades may benefit from exercise training programs. These benefits may include increased exercise tolerance and decreased dyspnea and fatigue (GOLD, 2015). Physical conditioning techniques include breathing exercises and general exercises intended to conserve energy and increase pulmonary ventilation. Graded exercises and physical conditioning programs using treadmills, stationary bicycles, and measured level walks can improve symptoms and increase work capacity and exercise tolerance. Any physical activity that can be performed regularly is helpful. Walking aids may be beneficial (GOLD, 2015). Lightweight portable oxygen systems are available for ambulatory patients who require oxygen therapy during physical activity.

Oxygen Therapy

Oxygen supplied to the home comes in compressed gas, liquid, or concentrator systems. Portable oxygen systems allow the patient to exercise, work, and travel. To help the patient adhere to the oxygen prescription, the nurse explains the proper flow rate and required number of hours for oxygen use as well as the dangers of arbitrary changes in flow rate or duration of therapy. The nurse also reassures the patient that oxygen is not "addictive" and explains the need for regular evaluations of blood oxygenation by pulse oximetry or arterial blood gas analysis.

 Quality and Safety Nursing Alert

The nurse should caution the patient that smoking with or near oxygen is extremely dangerous.

Nutritional Therapy

Nutritional assessment and counseling are important for patients with COPD. Nutritional status is reflected in severity of symptoms, degree of disability, and prognosis. Significant weight loss is often a major problem; however, excessive weight can also be problematic, although it occurs less often. Most patients with COPD have difficulty gaining and maintaining weight. A thorough assessment of caloric needs and counseling about meal planning and supplementation is part of the rehabilitation process. Continual monitoring of weight and interventions as necessary are important parts of the care of patients with COPD.

Coping Measures

Any factor that interferes with normal breathing quite naturally induces anxiety, depression, and changes in behavior. Constant shortness of breath and fatigue may make the patient irritable and apprehensive to the point of panic. Restricted activity (and reversal of family roles due to loss of employment), the frustration of having to work to breathe, and the realization that the disease is prolonged and unrelenting may cause the patient to become angry, depressed, and demanding. Sexual function may be compromised, which also diminishes self-esteem. The nurse should provide education and support to spouses or significant others and families, because the caregiver role in end-stage COPD can be challenging.

Palliative Care

Palliative care is integral for the patient with advanced COPD. Unfortunately, palliative care is often not considered until the disease is far advanced. The overall goals of palliative care are to manage symptoms and improve the quality of life for patients and families with advanced disease (GOLD, 2015; Rocker, Simpson & Horton, 2015). Areas addressed in palliative care include effective and empathetic communication with patients and families; close attention to pain and other symptoms; psychosocial, spiritual and bereavement support; and coordination of the wide range of medical and social services required with this disease. Palliative care should be considered complementary to hospice and end-of-life care (Rocker et al. 2015) (see Chapter 16).

Nursing Management

Assessing the Patient

Assessment involves obtaining information about current symptoms as well as previous disease manifestations. See Chart 24-2 for sample questions that may be used to obtain a clear history of the disease process. In addition to the history, the nurse reviews the results of available diagnostic tests.

Achieving Airway Clearance

Bronchospasm, which occurs in many pulmonary diseases, reduces the caliber of the small bronchi and may cause dyspnea, static secretions, and infection. Bronchospasm can sometimes be detected on auscultation with a stethoscope when wheezing or diminished breath sounds are heard. Increased mucus production, along with decreased mucociliary action, contributes to further reduction in the caliber of the bronchi and results in decreased airflow and decreased gas exchange. This is further aggravated by the loss of lung elasticity that occurs with COPD (GOLD, 2015). These changes in the airway require that the nurse monitor the patient for dyspnea and hypoxemia. If bronchodilators or corticosteroids are prescribed, the nurse must administer the medications properly and be alert for potential side effects. The relief of bronchospasm is confirmed by measuring improvement in expiratory flow rates and volumes (the force of expiration, how long it takes to exhale, and the amount of air exhaled) as well as by assessing the dyspnea and making sure that it has lessened.

Diminishing the quantity and viscosity of sputum can clear the airway and improve pulmonary ventilation and gas exchange. All pulmonary irritants should be eliminated or reduced, particularly cigarette smoke, which is the most persistent source of pulmonary irritation. The nurse instructs the patient in directed or controlled coughing, which is more effective and reduces the fatigue associated with undirected forceful coughing. Directed coughing consists of a slow, maximal inspiration followed by breath-holding for several seconds and then two or three coughs. "Huff" coughing may also be effective. The technique consists of one or two forced exhalations (huffs) from low to medium lung volumes with the glottis open.

Chest physiotherapy with postural drainage, intermittent positive pressure breathing, increased fluid intake, and bland aerosol mists (with normal saline solution or water) may be useful for some patients with COPD. The use of these measures must be based on the response and tolerance of each patient.

Improving Breathing Patterns

Ineffective breathing patterns and shortness of breath are due to the modified respiratory mechanics of the chest wall and lung resulting from **air trapping** (i.e., incomplete emptying of alveoli during expiration), ineffective diaphragmatic movement, airway obstruction, the metabolic cost of breathing, and stress. Inspiratory muscle training and breathing retraining may help improve breathing patterns. Training in diaphragmatic breathing reduces the respiratory rate, increases alveolar ventilation, and sometimes helps expel as much air as possible during expiration. Pursed-lip breathing helps slow expiration, prevent collapse of small airways, and control the rate and depth of respiration. It also promotes relaxation, which allows patients to gain control of dyspnea and reduce feelings of panic.

Improving Activity Tolerance

Patients with COPD experience progressive activity and exercise intolerance that may lead to disability. Education is focused on rehabilitative therapies to promote independence in executing activities of daily living. These may include pacing activities throughout the day or using supportive devices to decrease energy expenditure. The nurse evaluates the patient's activity tolerance and limitations and uses education strategies to promote independent activities of daily living. The patient may be a candidate for exercise training to strengthen the muscles of the upper and lower extremities and to improve exercise tolerance and endurance. The use of walking aids may be recommended to improve activity levels and ambulation (GOLD, 2015). Other health care professionals (rehabilitation therapist, occupational therapist, physical therapist) may be consulted as additional resources.

Monitoring and Managing Potential Complications

The nurse must assess for various complications of COPD, such as life-threatening respiratory insufficiency and failure, as well as respiratory infection and chronic atelectasis, which may increase the risk of respiratory failure. The nurse monitors for cognitive changes (personality and behavioral changes, memory impairment), increasing dyspnea, tachypnea, and tachycardia, which may indicate increasing hypoxemia and impending respiratory failure.

The nurse monitors pulse oximetry values to assess the patient's need for oxygen and administers supplemental oxygen as prescribed. The nurse also instructs the patient about signs and symptoms of respiratory infection that may worsen hypoxemia and reports changes in the patient's physical and cognitive status to the primary provider.

Bronchopulmonary infections must be controlled to diminish inflammatory edema and to permit recovery of normal ciliary action. Minor respiratory infections that are of no consequence to people with normal lungs can be life threatening to people with COPD. Infection compromises lung function and is a common cause of respiratory failure in people with COPD. In COPD, infection may be accompanied by subtle changes. The nurse instructs the patient to report any signs of infection, such as a fever or change in sputum color, character, consistency, or amount. Any worsening of symptoms (increased tightness of the chest, increased dyspnea, fatigue) also suggests infection and must be reported. Viral infections are hazardous to the patient because they are often followed by infections caused by bacterial organisms, such as *Streptococcus pneumoniae*, *Moraxella catarrhalis*, and *Haemophilus influenzae* (Bartlett & Sethi, 2016).

To prevent infection, the nurse encourages the patient with COPD to be immunized against influenza and pneumococcal pneumonia, because the patient is prone to respiratory infection. In addition, because each patient reacts differently to external exposures (significant air pollution, high or low temperatures, high humidity, strong smells), the nurse must assess the patient's actual and potential triggers that cause bronchospasm so that avoidance or a treatment plan can be established.

Pneumothorax is a potential complication of COPD and can be life threatening in patients with COPD who have minimal pulmonary reserve. Patients with severe emphysematous changes can develop large bullae, which may rupture and cause a pneumothorax. Development of a pneumothorax may be spontaneous or related to an activity such as severe coughing or large intrathoracic pressure changes. If a rapid onset of shortness of breath occurs, the nurse should quickly evaluate the patient for potential pneumothorax by assessing the symmetry of chest movement, differences in breath sounds, and pulse oximetry.

Over time, pulmonary hypertension may occur as a result of chronic hypoxemia, which causes the pulmonary arteries to constrict and thus leads to this complication. Pulmonary hypertension may be prevented by maintaining adequate oxygenation through an adequate hemoglobin level, improved ventilation–perfusion of the lungs, or continuous administration of supplemental oxygen (if needed).

Promoting Home, Community-Based, and Transitional Care

 Educating Patients About Self-Care

When providing education about self-management, the nurse must assess the knowledge of patients and family members about self-care and the therapeutic regimen. The nurse should also consider whether they are comfortable with this knowledge. Familiarity with prescribed medications' potential side effects is essential. In addition, patients and family members need to learn the early signs and symptoms of infection and other complications so that they seek appropriate health care promptly. Nurses are key in promoting smoking cessation and educating patients about its importance. Patients diagnosed with COPD who continue to smoke must be encouraged and assisted to quit.

A major area of patient education involves setting and accepting realistic short-term and long-range goals. If the COPD is mild (i.e., grade I), the objectives of treatment are to increase exercise tolerance and prevent further loss of pulmonary function. If the COPD is severe (i.e., grade III), the objectives are to preserve current pulmonary function and relieve symptoms as much as possible. It is important to plan and share the goals and expectations of treatment with the patient. Both the patient and the care provider need patience to achieve these goals.

The nurse instructs the patient to avoid extremes of heat and cold. Heat increases the body temperature, thereby raising oxygen requirements, and cold tends to promote bronchospasm. Air pollutants such as fumes, smoke, dust, and even talcum, lint, and aerosol sprays may initiate bronchospasm. High altitudes aggravate hypoxemia.

A patient with COPD should adopt a lifestyle of moderate activity, ideally in a climate with minimal shifts in temperature

NURSING RESEARCH PROFILE

Chart 24-3

Sleep and Quality of Life in Chronic Obstructive Pulmonary Disease

Geiger-Brown, J., Lindberg, S., Krachman, S., et al. (2015). Self-reported sleep quality and acute exacerbations of chronic obstructive pulmonary disease. *International Journal of COPD, 10*(1), 389–397.

Purpose

The purpose of this secondary analysis study was to characterize sleep quality in patients with clinically stable COPD; describe relationships between sleep quality, concomitant medical conditions and medications; and determine if sleep quality during the clinically stable period was predictive of health-related quality of life or was an independent predictor of exacerbation.

Design

This secondary analysis was from a randomized trial of 1117 patients with moderate to severe COPD. Measures of quality of life included the Medical Outcomes Study 36-item Short Form Survey and the St. Georges Respiratory Questionnaire. Self-reported sleep quality was measured using the Pittsburgh Sleep Quality Index (PSQI). Higher scores reflect poorer sleep quality (range 0–21). Outcomes were measured as time to first exacerbation and exacerbation rate.

Findings

In 53% of participants, sleep quality was rated as low (score >5). This finding was not related to age or severity of airflow obstruction.

COPD, chronic obstructive pulmonary disease.

"Poor" sleepers had worse quality of life measures as compared to "good" sleepers. Comorbidities were more common in the "poor" sleepers. In comparing "poor" and "good" sleepers, unadjusted time to first exacerbation was shorter (190 days vs. 239 days) and exacerbation rate was higher in the "poor" sleepers (1.7 vs. 1.37 per year). Once these data were adjusted for more medications and comorbid conditions, there were no significant differences between the two groups.

Nursing Implications

Sleep quality is an issue in the patient with COPD that has received little attention. Results from this study suggest that sleep quality is related to quality of life. Sleep quality was poor in 53% of the patients at the beginning and end of this clinical trial despite receiving therapy that reduced exacerbations. The nurse should assess sleep quality in the patient with COPD in both the inpatient and outpatient setting. In the outpatient setting, it may be helpful to evaluate patients' self-reported sleep quality, duration of sleep, use of sleep aids and any daytime dysfunction over time to evaluate changes in sleep. In the inpatient setting, the nurse should work closely with the patient to plan care that may improve sleep while in the hospital. At this time it is unknown whether therapy directed at improving sleep can also lead to improved prognosis of COPD.

---

and humidity. As much as possible, the patient should avoid emotional disturbances and stressful situations that might trigger a coughing episode. Self-management also includes getting sufficient rest and sleep (see Chart 24-3). The medication regimen can be quite complex; patients receiving aerosol medications by a pMDI or other type of inhaler may be particularly challenged. The nurse must review educational information and have the patient demonstrate correct pMDI use before discharge, during follow-up visits to a caregiver's office or clinic, and during home visits (see Chart 24-4).

Smoking cessation goes hand in hand with lifestyle changes, and reinforcing the patient's efforts is a key nursing activity. Smoking cessation is the single most important therapeutic intervention for patients with COPD. There are many strategies, including prevention, cessation with or without oral or topical patch medications, and behavior modification techniques.

Numerous educational materials are available to assist nurses in educating patients with COPD (see Resources at the end of the chapter).

Continuing and Transitional Care

Referral for home, community-based, or transitional care is important to enable assessment of the patient's home environment and physical and psychological status, to evaluate the patient's adherence to a prescribed regimen, and to assess the patient's ability to cope with changes in lifestyle and physical status. Home visits provide an opportunity to reinforce the information and activities learned in the inpatient or outpatient pulmonary rehabilitation program and to have the patient and family demonstrate correct administration of medications and oxygen, if indicated, and performance of exercises. If the patient does not have access to a formal

PATIENT EDUCATION

Chart 24-4

Use of Pressurized Metered-Dose Inhaler (pMDI)

The nurse instructs the patient to:
- Remove the cap and hold the inhaler upright.
- Shake the inhaler.
- Sit upright or stand upright. Breathe out slowly and all the way.
- Use one of two techniques: open-mouth technique or closed-mouth technique.
  - *Open-mouth technique*
    - Place the pMDI 2 finger widths away from lips.
    - With mouth open and tongue flat, tilt outlet of the pMDI so that it is pointed toward the upper back of the mouth.
    - Actuate the pMDI and begin to breathe in slowly. Breathe slowly and deeply through the mouth and try to hold breath for 10 seconds.
  - *Closed-mouth technique*
    - Place the pMDI between the teeth and make sure the tongue is flat under the mouth-piece and does not block pMDI.
    - Seal lips around mouthpiece and actuate the pMDI. Breathe in slowly through the mouth and try to hold breath for 10 seconds.
- Repeat puffs as directed, allowing 1 minute between puffs. There is no need to wait for other medications.
- Apply the cap to the pMDI for storage.
- After inhalation, rinse mouth with water when using a corticosteroid-containing pMDI.

The pMDI mouthpiece should be cleaned on a regular basis as should the nozzle of the canister based on the manufacturer's recommendations. As there are many types of inhalers, it is important to follow the manufacturer's instructions for use and care of the inhaler.

From Gardenhire, D. S., Ari, A., Hess, D., et al. (2013). *A guide to aerosol delivery devices for respiratory therapists* (3rd ed.). Dallas, TX: American Association for Respiratory Care.

pulmonary rehabilitation program, the nurse provides the education and breathing retraining necessary to optimize the patient's functional status.

The nurse directs patients to community resources, such as pulmonary rehabilitation programs and smoking cessation programs, to help improve patients' ability to cope with their chronic condition and the therapeutic regimen and to provide a sense of worth, hope, and well-being. In addition, the nurse reminds the patient and family about the importance of participating in general health promotion activities and health screening.

Patients with COPD have indicated that information about their end-of-life needs is limited. Areas to discuss regarding end of life care may include symptom management, quality of life, satisfaction with care, information/communication, use of care professionals, use of differing care facilities, hospital admission, and place of death. It is crucial that patients know what to expect as the disease progresses. In addition, they should have information about their role in decisions regarding aggressiveness of care near the end of life and access to specialists who may help them and their families. As the disease course progresses, a holistic assessment of physical and psychological needs should be undertaken at each hospitalization, clinic visit, or home visit. This helps gauge the patient's assessment of the progression of the disease and its impact on quality of life and guides planning for future interventions and management (see Chapter 16 for additional information).

Chart 24-5 provides further information on providing nursing care for the patient with COPD.

Bronchiectasis

Bronchiectasis is a chronic, irreversible dilation of the bronchi and bronchioles that results from destruction of muscles and elastic connective tissue. In the United States, it is estimated that 110,000 people have bronchiectasis; it is more common in women than men (Barker, 2015a). It is considered a disease process separate from COPD (GOLD, 2015). Numerous factors can induce or contribute to the development of bronchiectasis. Some of these include recurrent respiratory infections, CF, rheumatic and other systemic diseases, primary ciliary dysfunction, tuberculosis, or immunodeficiency disorders (Barker, 2015a).

Pathophysiology

The inflammatory process associated with pulmonary infections damages the bronchial wall, causing a loss of its supporting structure and resulting in thick sputum that ultimately obstructs the bronchi. The walls become permanently distended and distorted, impairing mucociliary clearance. In saccular bronchiectasis, each dilated peribronchial tube amounts to a lung abscess, the exudate of which drains freely through the bronchus. Bronchiectasis is usually localized, affecting a segment or lobe of a lung, most frequently the lower lobes.

The retention of secretions and subsequent obstruction ultimately cause the alveoli distal to the obstruction to collapse (atelectasis). Inflammatory scarring or fibrosis replaces functioning lung tissue. In time, the patient develops respiratory insufficiency with reduced vital capacity, decreased ventilation,

and an increased ratio of residual volume to total lung capacity. There is impairment in the match of ventilation to perfusion (ventilation–perfusion imbalance) and hypoxemia.

Clinical Manifestations

Characteristic symptoms of bronchiectasis include chronic cough and the production of purulent sputum in copious amounts. Many patients with this disease have hemoptysis. Clubbing of the fingers also is common because of respiratory insufficiency. Patients usually have repeated episodes of pulmonary infection.

Assessment and Diagnostic Findings

Bronchiectasis is not readily diagnosed because the symptoms can be mistaken for those of chronic bronchitis. A definite sign is a prolonged history of productive, chronic cough, with sputum consistently negative for tubercle bacilli. The diagnosis is established by a CT scan, which reveals bronchial dilation. The advent of high-resolution CT scanning makes it possible to diagnose this disease during its earlier stages.

Medical Management

Treatment objectives are to promote bronchial drainage, to clear excessive secretions from the affected portion of the lungs, and to prevent or control infection. Postural drainage is part of all treatment plans, because draining of the bronchiectatic areas by gravity reduces the amount of secretions and the degree of infection. Sometimes, mucopurulent sputum must be removed by bronchoscopy. Chest physiotherapy, including percussion and postural drainage, is important in the management of secretions. Smoking cessation is important, because smoking impairs bronchial drainage by paralyzing ciliary action, increasing bronchial secretions, and causing inflammation of the mucous membranes, resulting in hyperplasia of the mucous glands.

Antibiotics are the cornerstone therapy for management of a bronchiectatic exacerbation. Antimicrobial therapy choice is based on the results of sensitivity studies on organisms cultured from sputum; however, empiric coverage (i.e., broad-spectrum antibiotics that are effective in treating commonly implicated pathogens) is often prescribed initially, pending results of sputum cultures. The most commonly implicated pathogens include *Haemophilus influenza*, which may be treated with amoxicillin-clavulanate (Augmentin), *M. catarrhalis*, which can be treated with gemifloxacin (Factive) or levofloxacin (Levaquin), *Staphylococcus aureus*, which responds to clindamycin (Cleocin), and *Pseudomonas aeruginosa*, which may be treated with ciprofloxacin (Cipro) (Barker, 2015b). Because infection with *P. aeruginosa* is associated with a greater rate of lung function deterioration, more aggressive oral or IV antibiotic therapy may be used for a longer duration. For patients with recurrent exacerbations (usually 2 or more during the past year), a low dose macrolide antibiotic may be used as preventative, ongoing therapy (Barker, 2015b). In addition, patients should be vaccinated against influenza and pneumococcal pneumonia.

Secretion management is an issue for patients with bronchiectasis. Bronchodilators, which may be prescribed for

(*text continued on page 654*)

Chart 24-5

PLAN OF NURSING CARE

Care of the Patient With Chronic Obstructive Pulmonary Disease

NURSING DIAGNOSIS: Impaired gas exchange and Ineffective airway clearance due to chronic inhalation of toxins
GOAL: Improvement in gas exchange

Nursing Interventions	Rationale	Expected Outcomes
1. Evaluate current smoking status, educate regarding smoking cessation, and facilitate efforts to quit. a. Evaluate current smoking habits of patient and family. b. Educate regarding hazards of smoking and relationship to COPD. c. Evaluate previous smoking cessation attempts. d. Provide educational materials. e. Refer to a smoking cessation program or resource. 2. Evaluate current exposure to occupational toxins or pollutants and indoor/outdoor pollution. a. Evaluate current exposures to occupational toxins, indoor and outdoor air pollution (e.g., smog, toxic fumes, chemicals). b. Emphasize primary prevention to occupational exposures. This is best achieved by elimination or reduction in exposures in the workplace. c. Educate regarding types of indoor and outdoor air pollution (e.g., biomass fuel burned for cooking and heating in poorly ventilated buildings, outdoor air pollution). d. Advise patient to monitor public announcements regarding air quality.	1. Smoking causes permanent damage to the lungs and diminishes the lungs' protective mechanisms. Airflow is obstructed, secretions are increased, and lung capacity is reduced. Continued smoking increases morbidity and mortality in COPD and is also a risk factor for lung cancer. 2. Chronic inhalation of both indoor and outdoor toxins causes damage to the airways and impairs gas exchange.	• Identifies the hazards of cigarette smoking • Identifies resources for smoking cessation • Enrolls in smoking cessation program • Reports success in stopping smoking • Verbalizes types of inhaled toxins • Minimizes or eliminates exposures • Monitors public announcements regarding air quality and minimizes or eliminates exposures during episodes of severe pollution

NURSING DIAGNOSIS: Impaired gas exchange related to ventilation–perfusion inequality
GOAL: Improvement in gas exchange

Nursing Interventions	Rationale	Expected Outcomes
1. Administer bronchodilators as prescribed. a. Inhalation is the preferred route. b. Observe for side effects: tachycardia, dysrhythmias, central nervous system excitation, nausea, and vomiting. c. Assess for correct technique of pressurized metered-dose inhaler (pMDI) or other type of administration. 2. Evaluate effectiveness of nebulizer or pMDI treatments. a. Assess for decreased shortness of breath, decreased wheezing or crackles, loosened secretions, and decreased anxiety. b. Ensure that treatment is given before meals to avoid nausea and to reduce fatigue that accompanies eating.	1. Bronchodilators dilate the airways. The medication dosage is carefully adjusted for each patient, in accordance with clinical response. 2. Combining medication with aerosolized bronchodilators is typically used to control bronchoconstriction in an acute exacerbation. Generally, however, the pMDI with spacer is the preferred route (less cost and time to treatment).	• Verbalizes need for bronchodilators and for taking them as prescribed • Evidences minimal side effects; heart rate near normal, absence of dysrhythmias, normal mentation • Reports a decrease in dyspnea • Shows an improved expiratory flow rate • Uses and cleans respiratory therapy equipment as applicable • Demonstrates diaphragmatic breathing and coughing • Uses oxygen equipment appropriately when indicated • Evidences improved arterial blood gases or pulse oximetry • Demonstrates correct technique for use of pMDI

(continued on page 650)

Chart 24-5

PLAN OF NURSING CARE (Continued)

Care of the Patient With Chronic Obstructive Pulmonary Disease

Nursing Interventions	Rationale	Expected Outcomes
3. Instruct and encourage patient in diaphragmatic breathing and effective coughing.	3. These techniques improve ventilation by opening airways to facilitate clearing the airways of sputum. Gas exchange is improved, and fatigue is minimized.	

4. Administer oxygen by the method prescribed.
  a. Explain rationale and importance to patient.
  b. Evaluate effectiveness; observe for signs of hypoxemia. Notify primary provider if restlessness, anxiety, somnolence, cyanosis, or tachycardia is present.
  c. Analyze arterial blood gases and compare with baseline values. When arterial puncture is performed and a blood sample is obtained, hold puncture site for 5 minutes to prevent arterial bleeding and development of ecchymoses.
  d. Initiate pulse oximetry to monitor oxygen saturation.
  e. Explain that no smoking is permitted by patient or visitors while oxygen is in use.
	4. Oxygen will correct the hypoxemia. Careful observation of the liter flow or the percentage given and its effect on the patient is important. These patients generally require low-flow oxygen rates of 1–2 L/min. Monitor and titrate to achieve desired PaO_2. Periodic arterial blood gases and pulse oximetry help evaluate adequacy of oxygenation. Smoking may render pulse oximetry inaccurate because the carbon monoxide from cigarette smoke also saturates hemoglobin.	

NURSING DIAGNOSIS: Ineffective airway clearance related to bronchoconstriction, increased mucus production, ineffective cough, bronchopulmonary infection, and other complications

GOAL: Achievement of airway clearance

Nursing Interventions	Rationale	Expected Outcomes
1. Adequately hydrate the patient.	1. Systemic hydration keeps secretions moist and easier to expectorate. Fluids must be given with caution if right- or left-sided heart failure is present.	• Verbalizes need to drink fluids • Demonstrates diaphragmatic breathing and coughing • Performs postural drainage correctly • Coughing is minimized. • Does not smoke • Verbalizes that pollens, fumes, gases, dusts, and extremes of temperature and humidity are irritants to be avoided • Identifies signs of early infection • Is free of infection (no fever, no change in sputum, lessening of dyspnea) • Verbalizes need to notify primary provider at the earliest sign of infection • Verbalizes need to stay away from crowds or people with colds in flu season • Discusses flu and pneumonia vaccines with clinician to help prevent infection
2. Instruct in and encourage the use of diaphragmatic breathing and coughing techniques.	2. These techniques help to improve ventilation and mobilize secretions without causing breathlessness and fatigue.	
3. Assist in administering nebulizer or pMDI.	3. This ensures adequate delivery of medication to the airways.	
4. If indicated, perform postural drainage with percussion and vibration in the morning and at night as prescribed.	4. This uses gravity to help raise secretions so they can be more easily expectorated or suctioned.	
5. Instruct patient to avoid bronchial irritants such as cigarette smoke, aerosols, extremes of temperature, and fumes.	5. Bronchial irritants cause bronchoconstriction and increased mucus production, which then interfere with airway clearance.	

6. Educate about early signs of infection that are to be reported to the clinician immediately:
  a. Increased sputum production
  b. Change in color of sputum
  c. Increased thickness of sputum
  d. Increased shortness of breath, tightness in chest, or fatigue
  e. Increased coughing
  f. Fever or chills
	6. Minor respiratory infections that are of no consequence to the person with normal lungs can produce fatal disturbances in the lungs of the person with emphysema. Early recognition is crucial.	

7. Administer antibiotics as prescribed.	7. Antibiotics may be prescribed to prevent or treat infection.	
8. Encourage patient to be immunized against influenza and *Streptococcus pneumoniae*.	8. Patients with respiratory conditions are prone to respiratory infections and are encouraged to be immunized.	

Chart 24-5

PLAN OF NURSING CARE (Continued)

Care of the Patient With Chronic Obstructive Pulmonary Disease

NURSING DIAGNOSIS: Ineffective breathing pattern related to shortness of breath, mucus, bronchoconstriction, and airway irritants
GOAL: Improvement in breathing pattern

Nursing Interventions	Rationale	Expected Outcomes
1. Instruct patient in diaphragmatic and pursed-lip breathing. 2. Encourage alternating activity with rest periods. Allow patient to make some decisions (bath, shaving) about care based on tolerance level. 3. Encourage the use of an inspiratory muscle trainer if prescribed.	1. This helps patient prolong expiration time and decreases air trapping. With these techniques, patient will breathe more efficiently and effectively. 2. Pacing activities permits patient to perform activities without excessive distress. 3. This strengthens and conditions the respiratory muscles.	• Practices pursed-lip and diaphragmatic breathing and uses them when short of breath and with activity • Shows signs of decreased respiratory effort and paces activities • Uses inspiratory muscle trainer as prescribed

NURSING DIAGNOSIS: Self-care deficits related to fatigue secondary to increased work of breathing and insufficient ventilation and oxygenation
GOAL: Independence in self-care activities

Nursing Interventions	Rationale	Expected Outcomes
1. Educate patient to coordinate diaphragmatic breathing with activity (e.g., walking, bending). 2. Encourage patient to begin to bathe self, dress self, walk, and drink fluids. Discuss energy conservation measures. 3. Educate patient about postural drainage if appropriate.	1. This will allow the patient to be more active and to avoid excessive fatigue or dyspnea during activity. 2. As condition resolves, patient will be able to do more but needs to be encouraged to avoid increasing dependence. 3. This encourages patient to become involved in own care and prepares patient to manage at home.	• Uses controlled breathing while bathing, bending, and walking • Paces activities of daily living to alternate with rest periods to reduce fatigue and dyspnea • Describes energy conservation strategies • Performs same self-care activities as before • Performs postural drainage correctly

NURSING DIAGNOSIS: Activity intolerance due to fatigue, hypoxemia, and ineffective breathing patterns
GOAL: Improvement in activity tolerance

Nursing Interventions	Rationale	Expected Outcomes
1. Support patient in establishing a regular regimen of exercise using treadmill and exercise bicycle, walking, or other appropriate exercises, such as mall walking. a. Assess the patient's current level of functioning, and develop exercise plan based on baseline functional status. b. Suggest consultation with a physical therapist or pulmonary rehabilitation program to determine an exercise program specific to the patient's capability. Have portable oxygen unit available if oxygen is prescribed for exercise.	1. Muscles that are deconditioned consume more oxygen and place an additional burden on the lungs. Through regular, graded exercise, these muscle groups become more conditioned, and the patient can do more without getting as short of breath. Graded exercise breaks the cycle of debilitation.	• Performs activities with less shortness of breath • Verbalizes need to exercise daily and demonstrates an exercise plan to be carried out at home • Walks and gradually increases walking time and distance to improve physical condition • Exercises both upper and lower body muscle groups

NURSING DIAGNOSIS: Ineffective coping related to reduced socialization, anxiety, depression, lower activity level, and the inability to work
GOAL: Attainment of an optimal level of coping

Nursing Interventions	Rationale	Expected Outcomes
1. Help the patient develop realistic goals. 2. Encourage activity to level of symptom tolerance.	1. Developing realistic goals will promote a sense of hope and accomplishment rather than defeat and hopelessness. 2. Activity reduces tension and decreases degree of dyspnea as patient becomes conditioned.	• Expresses interest in the future • Participates in the discharge plan • Discusses activities or methods that can be performed to ease shortness of breath • Uses relaxation techniques appropriately

(continued on page 652)

Chart 24-5

PLAN OF NURSING CARE (Continued)

Care of the Patient With Chronic Obstructive Pulmonary Disease

Nursing Interventions	Rationale	Expected Outcomes
3. Educate the patient about relaxation techniques or provide a relaxation recording on audiotape, CD, or digital audio available on smart phones or tablets. 4. Enroll patient in pulmonary rehabilitation program where available.	3. Relaxation reduces stress, anxiety, and dyspnea and helps patient to cope with disability. 4. Pulmonary rehabilitation programs have been shown to promote a subjective improvement in a patient's status and self-esteem as well as increased exercise tolerance and decreased hospitalizations.	• Expresses interest in a pulmonary rehabilitation program

NURSING DIAGNOSIS: Deficient knowledge about self-management to be performed at home
GOAL: Adherence to therapeutic program and home care

Nursing Interventions	Rationale	Expected Outcomes

1. Help patient identify/develop short- and long-term goals.
  a. Educate the patient about disease, medications, procedures, and how and when to seek help.
  b. Refer patient to pulmonary rehabilitation.
2. Give strong message to stop smoking. Discuss smoking cessation strategies. Provide information about resource groups (e.g., SmokEnders, American Cancer Society, American Lung Association).
	1. Patient needs to be a partner in developing the plan of care and needs to know what to expect. Education about the condition is one of the most important aspects of care; it will prepare the patient to live and cope with the condition and improve quality of life.
	2. Smoking causes permanent damage to the lung and diminishes the lungs' protective mechanisms. Airflow is obstructed, and lung capacity is reduced. Smoking increases morbidity and mortality and is also a risk factor for lung cancer.
		• Understands disease and what affects it
		• Verbalizes the need to preserve existing lung function by adhering to the prescribed program
		• Understands purposes and proper administration of medications
		• Stops smoking or enrolls in a smoking cessation program
		• Identifies when and whom to call for assistance

COLLABORATIVE PROBLEM: Atelectasis
GOAL: Absence of atelectasis on x-ray and physical examination

Nursing Interventions	Rationale	Expected Outcomes
1. Monitor respiratory status, including rate and pattern of respirations, breath sounds, signs and symptoms of respiratory distress, and pulse oximetry. 2. Instruct in and encourage diaphragmatic breathing and effective coughing techniques. 3. Promote the use of lung expansion techniques (e.g., deep-breathing exercises, incentive spirometry) as prescribed.	1. A change in respiratory status, including tachypnea, dyspnea, and diminished or absent breath sounds, may indicate atelectasis. 2. These techniques improve ventilation and lung expansion and ideally improve gas exchange. 3. Deep-breathing exercises and incentive spirometry promote maximal lung expansion.	• Normal (baseline for patient) respiratory rate and pattern • Normal breath sounds for patient • Demonstrates diaphragmatic breathing and effective coughing • Performs deep-breathing exercises, incentive spirometry as prescribed • Pulse oximetry ≥90%

COLLABORATIVE PROBLEM: Pneumothorax
GOAL: Absence of signs and symptoms of pneumothorax

Nursing Interventions	Rationale	Expected Outcomes
1. Monitor respiratory status, including rate and pattern of respirations, symmetry of chest wall movement, breath sounds, signs and symptoms of respiratory distress, and pulse oximetry. 2. Assess pulse. 3. Assess for chest pain and precipitating factors.	1. Dyspnea, tachypnea, tachycardia, acute pleuritic chest pain, tracheal deviation away from the affected side, absence of breath sounds on the affected side, and decreased tactile fremitus may indicate pneumothorax. 2. Tachycardia is associated with pneumothorax and anxiety. 3. Pain may accompany pneumothorax.	• Normal respiratory rate and pattern for patient • Normal breath sounds bilaterally • Normal pulse for patient • Normal tactile fremitus • Absence of pain • Tracheal position is midline • Pulse oximetry ≥90% • Maintains normal oxygen saturation and arterial blood gas measurements

PLAN OF NURSING CARE (Continued)

Chart 24-5

Care of the Patient With Chronic Obstructive Pulmonary Disease

Nursing Interventions	Rationale	Expected Outcomes
4. Palpate for tracheal deviation/shift away from the affected side. 5. Monitor pulse oximetry and, if indicated, arterial blood gases. 6. Administer supplemental oxygen therapy, as indicated. 7. Administer analgesic agents, as indicated, for chest pain. 8. Assist with chest tube insertion and use pleural drainage system, as prescribed.	4. Early detection of pneumothorax and prompt intervention will prevent other serious complications. 5. Recognition of deterioration in respiratory function will prevent serious complications. 6. Oxygen will correct hypoxemia; administer it with caution. 7. Pain interferes with deep breathing, resulting in decreased lung expansion. 8. Removal of air from the pleural space will re-expand the lung.	• Exhibits no hypoxemia and hypercapnia (or returns to baseline values) • Absence of pain • Symmetric chest wall movement • Lungs fully expanded bilaterally on chest x-ray

COLLABORATIVE PROBLEM: Respiratory failure
GOAL: Absence of signs and symptoms of respiratory failure; no evidence of respiratory failure on laboratory tests

Nursing Interventions	Rationale	Expected Outcomes
1. Monitor respiratory status, including rate and pattern of respirations, breath sounds, and signs and symptoms of acute respiratory distress. 2. Monitor pulse oximetry and arterial blood gases. 3. Administer supplemental oxygen and initiate mechanisms for mechanical ventilation, as prescribed.	1. Early recognition of deterioration in respiratory function will avert further complications, such as respiratory failure, severe hypoxemia, and hypercapnia. 2. Recognition of changes in oxygenation and acid–base balance will guide in correcting and preventing complications. 3. Acute respiratory failure is a medical emergency. Hypoxemia is a hallmark sign. Administration of oxygen therapy and mechanical ventilation (if indicated) are critical to survival.	• Normal respiratory rate and pattern for patient with no acute distress • Recognizes symptoms of hypoxemia and hypercapnia • Maintains normal arterial blood gases/pulse oximetry or returns to baseline values

COLLABORATIVE PROBLEM: Pulmonary arterial hypertension
GOAL: Absence of evidence of pulmonary arterial hypertension on physical examination or laboratory tests

Nursing Interventions	Rationale	Expected Outcomes
1. Monitor respiratory status, including rate and pattern of respirations, breath sounds, pulse oximetry, and signs and symptoms of acute respiratory distress. 2. Assess for signs and symptoms of right-sided heart failure, including peripheral edema, ascites, distended neck veins, crackles, and heart murmur. 3. Administer oxygen therapy, as prescribed.	1. Dyspnea is the primary symptom of pulmonary arterial hypertension. Other symptoms include fatigue, angina, near-syncope, edema, and palpitations. 2. Right-sided heart failure is a common clinical manifestation of pulmonary arterial hypertension due to increased right ventricular workload. 3. Continuous oxygen therapy is a major component of management of pulmonary arterial hypertension; it prevents hypoxemia, thereby reducing pulmonary vascular constriction (resistance) secondary to hypoxemia.	• Normal respiratory rate and pattern for patient • Exhibits no signs and symptoms of right-sided failure • Maintains baseline pulse oximetry values and arterial blood gases

patients who also have reactive airway disease, may also assist with secretion management. In addition, nebulized mucolytics may help to clear airway secretions. Ensuring adequate hydration and employing chest physiotherapy may also be of help in loosening and thinning secretions (Barker, 2015b).

Surgical intervention, although used infrequently, may be indicated for patients who continue to expectorate large amounts of sputum and have repeated bouts of pneumonia and hemoptysis despite adherence to treatment regimens. The disease must involve only one or two areas of the lung that can be removed without producing respiratory insufficiency. The goals of surgical treatment are to conserve normal pulmonary tissue and to avoid infectious complications. Diseased tissue is removed, provided that postoperative lung function will be adequate. It may be necessary to remove a segment of a lobe (segmental resection), a lobe (lobectomy), or, rarely, an entire lung (pneumonectomy). (See Chapter 21 for further information.) Segmental resection is the removal of an anatomic subdivision of a pulmonary lobe. In select cases, video-assisted surgery (VATS) segmentectomy or lobectomy may be performed, which is associated with fewer complications and decreased length of stay. The chief advantage is that only diseased tissue is removed, and healthy lung tissue is conserved.

The surgery is preceded by a period of careful preparation. The objective is to obtain a dry (free of infection) tracheobronchial tree to prevent complications (atelectasis, pneumonia, bronchopleural fistula, and empyema). This is accomplished by postural drainage or, depending on the location, by direct suction through a bronchoscope. A course of antibacterial therapy may be prescribed. After surgery, care is the same as for any patient who has undergone chest surgery (see Chapter 21).

Nursing Management

Nursing management focuses on alleviating symptoms and helping patients clear pulmonary secretions. Patient education targets eliminating smoking and other factors that increase the production of mucus and hamper its removal. Patients and families are taught to perform postural drainage and to avoid exposure to people with upper respiratory or other infections. If the patient experiences fatigue and dyspnea, he or she is informed about strategies to conserve energy while maintaining as active a lifestyle as possible. The patient is educated about the early signs of respiratory infection and the progression of the disorder so that appropriate treatment can be implemented promptly. The presence of a large amount of mucus may decrease the patient's appetite and result in an inadequate dietary intake; therefore, the patient's nutritional status is assessed and strategies are implemented to ensure an adequate diet.

Asthma

Asthma is a heterogeneous disease, usually characterized by chronic airway inflammation (GINA [Global Initiative for Asthma], 2015). This chronic inflammatory disease of the airways causes airway hyperresponsiveness, mucosal edema, and mucus production. This inflammation ultimately leads to recurrent episodes of asthma symptoms: cough, chest tightness, wheezing, and dyspnea (see Fig. 24-6). In the United States, asthma affects more than 18.7 million adults and accounts

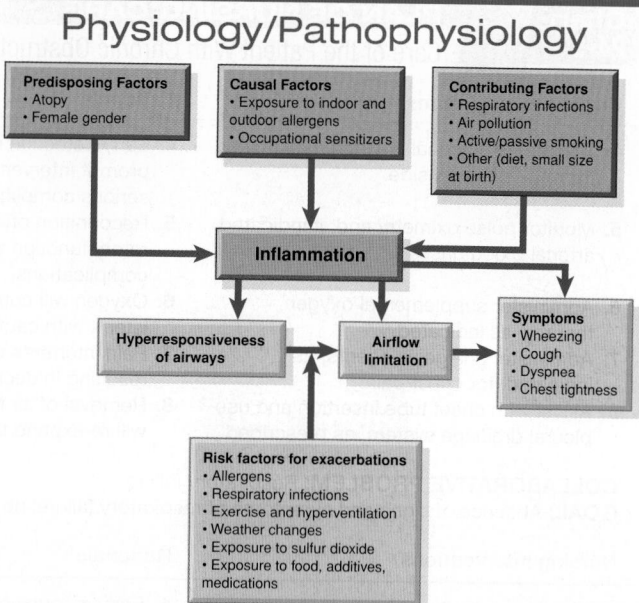

Figure 24-6 • Pathophysiology of asthma. Adapted from materials developed for the Global Initiative for Asthma (2015). Global strategy for asthma management and prevention. Available at: www.ginasthma.org.

for approximately 3,500 deaths per year (CDC, 2015b). Of these adults, 35.2% have intermittent severity and 64.8% have persistent severity of asthma symptoms (CDC, 2015c). Twenty-one percent of patients with asthma smoke even though cigarette smoke is known to trigger an attack, while nearly 17% of people without asthma smoke (CDC 2015c). Asthma accounts for 1.8 million ED visits per year and close to 440,000 hospital admissions (CDC, 2015b). Although asthma is the most common chronic disease of childhood, it can occur at any age. For most patients, asthma is a disruptive disease, affecting school and work attendance, occupational choices, physical activity, and general quality of life.

Despite increased knowledge regarding the pathology of asthma and the development of improved medications and management plans, the death rate from the disease continues to rise. Ethnic and racial disparities affect morbidity and mortality in asthma, which are higher in inner-city African Americans and Latinos (CDC, 2015c). Contributing to these disparities are epidemiology and risk factors, genetics and molecular aspect, inner-city environments, limited community assets, health care access/delivery/and quality, and insufficient health insurance coverage.

Unlike other obstructive lung diseases, asthma is largely reversible, either spontaneously or with treatment. Patients with asthma may experience symptom-free periods alternating with acute exacerbations that last from minutes to hours or days.

Allergy is the strongest predisposing factor for asthma. Chronic exposure to airway irritants or allergens also increases the risk of asthma. Common allergens can be seasonal (e.g., grass, tree, and weed pollens) or perennial (e.g., mold, dust, roaches, animal dander). Common triggers for asthma symptoms and exacerbations include airway irritants (e.g., air pollutants, cold, heat, weather changes, strong odors or perfumes, smoke, occupational exposure), foods (e.g., shellfish, nuts), exercise, stress, hormonal factors, medications, viral respiratory tract infections, and gastroesophageal reflux. Most people who have asthma are sensitive to a variety of triggers.

Pathophysiology

The underlying pathology in asthma is reversible diffuse airway inflammation that leads to long-term airway narrowing. This narrowing, which is exacerbated by various changes in the airway, includes bronchoconstriction, airway edema, airway hyperresponsiveness, and airway remodeling. The interaction of these factors determines the clinical manifestations and severity of asthma (GINA, 2015). Over the course of a lifetime, the impact of increasing pathophysiologic changes and environmental susceptibility lead to an irreversible disease process.

Asthma is a complex disease process that involves numerous inflammatory and structural cells as well as mediators that lead to the disorder's effects. Mast cells, macrophages, T lymphocytes, neutrophils, and eosinophils all play a key role in the inflammation of asthma. When activated, mast cells release several chemicals called *mediators*. These chemicals, which include histamine, bradykinin, prostanoids, cytokines, leukotrienes, and other mediators, perpetuate the inflammatory response, causing increased blood flow, vasoconstriction, fluid leak from the vasculature, attraction of white blood cells to the area, mucus secretion, and bronchoconstriction (GINA, 2015).

During acute exacerbations of asthma, bronchial smooth muscle contraction or bronchoconstriction occurs quickly to narrow the airway in response to an exposure. Acute bronchoconstriction due to allergens results from an immunoglobulin E (IgE)-dependent release of mediators from mast cells; these mediators include histamine, tryptase, leukotrienes, and prostaglandins that directly contract the airway. There are also non–IgE-mediated responses and proinflammatory cytokines (GINA, 2015). In addition, alpha- and beta$_2$-adrenergic receptors of the sympathetic nervous system located in the bronchi play a role. When the alpha-adrenergic receptors are stimulated, bronchoconstriction occurs. The balance between alpha- and beta$_2$-adrenergic receptors is controlled primarily by cyclic 3',5'-adenosine monophosphate (cAMP). Beta$_2$-adrenergic stimulation results in increased levels of cAMP, which inhibits the release of chemical mediators and causes bronchodilation.

As asthma becomes more persistent, the inflammation progresses and other factors may be involved in airflow limitation. These include airway edema, mucus hypersecretion, and the formation of mucus plugs. In addition, airway "remodeling" (i.e., structural changes) may occur in response to chronic inflammation, causing further airway narrowing.

Clinical Manifestations

The three most common symptoms of asthma are cough, dyspnea, and wheezing. In some instances, cough may be the only symptom. An asthma attack often occurs at night or early in the morning, possibly because of circadian variations that influence airway receptor thresholds.

An asthma exacerbation may begin abruptly but most frequently is preceded by increasing symptoms over the previous few days. There is cough, with or without mucus production. At times, the mucus is so tightly wedged in the narrowed airway that the patient cannot cough it up. There may be generalized wheezing (the sound of airflow through narrowed airways), first on expiration and then possibly during inspiration as well. Generalized chest tightness and dyspnea occur. Expiration requires effort and becomes prolonged. As the exacerbation progresses, diaphoresis, tachycardia, and a widened pulse pressure may occur along with hypoxemia and central cyanosis (a late sign of poor oxygenation). Although severe, life-threatening hypoxemia can occur in asthma, it is relatively uncommon. The hypoxemia is secondary to a ventilation–perfusion mismatch and readily responds to supplemental oxygenation.

Symptoms of exercise-induced asthma include maximal symptoms during exercise, absence of nocturnal symptoms, and sometimes only a description of a "choking" sensation during exercise.

Assessment and Diagnostic Findings

To establish the diagnosis, the clinician must determine that episodic symptoms of airflow obstruction are present, airflow is at least partially reversible, and other causes have been excluded. A positive family history and environmental factors, including seasonal changes, high pollen counts, mold, pet dander, climate changes (particularly cold air), and air pollution, are primarily associated with asthma. In addition, asthma is associated with a variety of occupation-related chemicals, foods, and compounds. Comorbid conditions that may accompany asthma include viral infections, gastroesophageal reflux disease, drug-induced asthma, and allergic bronchopulmonary aspergillosis. Other possible allergic reactions that may accompany asthma include eczema, rashes, and temporary edema. Specific in the assessment that may help to evaluate the patient's asthma control include:

- Have your symptoms awakened you at night or in the early morning?
- Have you needed your quick-acting relief medication more than usual?
- Have you needed unscheduled care for your asthma—a call to the primary provider's office, office visit, ED?
- Have your symptoms impacted your normal activities at school/work/sports?

During acute episodes, sputum and blood tests may disclose eosinophilia (elevated levels of eosinophils). Serum levels of IgE may be elevated if allergy is present. Arterial blood gas analysis and pulse oximetry reveal hypoxemia during acute attacks. Initially, hypocapnia and respiratory alkalosis are present. As the patient's condition worsens and he or she becomes more fatigued, the PaCO$_2$ may increase. Because carbon dioxide is 20 times more diffusible than oxygen, it is rare for PaCO$_2$ to be normal or elevated in a person who is breathing very rapidly.

> ### Quality and Safety Nursing Alert
>
> Normal PaCO$_2$ during an asthma attack may be a signal of impending respiratory failure.

During an exacerbation, the FEV$_1$ and FVC are markedly decreased but improve with bronchodilator administration (demonstrating reversibility). Pulmonary function is usually normal between exacerbations. The occurrence of a severe, continuous reaction is referred to as status asthmaticus and is considered life threatening (see later discussion).

Asthma severity is considered in the selection of the initial type, amount, and schedule of treatments (GINA, 2015; National Heart Lung and Blood Institute [NHLBI], 2012). Disease severity is classified by current impairment and future risk of adverse events. Impairment is defined by the following factors: nighttime awakenings, the need for short-acting bronchodilators for symptom relief, work/school days missed, ability to engage in normal activities, and quality of life. Lung function is evaluated by spirometry. Assessment of risk of future adverse events is evaluated by numbers of exacerbations, the need for ED care or hospitalizations in the past year, demographic data (gender, ethnicity, nonuse of prescribed inhaled corticosteroid therapy, existing smoking), psychosocial factors and attitudes, and beliefs about taking medication (GINA, 2015; NHLBI, 2012).

Prevention

Patients with recurrent asthma should undergo tests to identify the substances that precipitate the symptoms. Possible causes are dust, dust mites, roaches, certain types of cloth, pets, horses, detergents, soaps, certain foods, molds, and pollens. If the attacks are seasonal, pollens can be strongly suspected. Patients are instructed to avoid the causative agents whenever possible. Knowledge is the key to quality asthma care. Evaluation of impairment and risk are primary methods that help ensure control.

Occupational asthma refers to asthma induced by exposure in the work environment to dusts, vapors, or fumes, with or without a preexisting diagnosis of asthma. An estimated 15% of new asthma cases in the United States are related to workplace exposures (American Academy of Allergy, Asthma and Immunology [AAAAI], 2016a; GINA, 2015). Work-related asthma should be part of the differential diagnosis of every case of adult-onset asthma. A detailed work history evaluation is key to identifying occupational asthma. Immediate treatment is aimed at removing or decreasing the exposure in the patient's environment and following the patient on an ongoing basis. Standard asthma medications may be prescribed to minimize bronchoconstriction and airway inflammation. In certain cases, patients may be impaired or disabled from the disease. Compensation systems are in place to protect a worker; however, these systems are often slow and complex to navigate.

Complications

Complications of asthma may include status asthmaticus, respiratory failure, pneumonia, and atelectasis. Airway obstruction, particularly during acute asthmatic episodes, often results in hypoxemia, requiring the administration of oxygen and the monitoring of pulse oximetry and arterial blood gases. Fluids are given because people with asthma are frequently dehydrated from diaphoresis and insensible fluid loss with hyperventilation.

Medical Management

Immediate intervention may be necessary because continuing and progressive dyspnea leads to increased anxiety,

aggravating the situation. The NHLBI (2012) and GINA (2015) recommendations are based on the concept of severity and control of asthma along with the domains of reducing impairment and reducing risk as keys to improving care. Primary treatment concerns are impairment of lung function and normal life and risk of exacerbations, decline in lung function, and adverse effects from medications (NHLBI, 2012).

Pharmacologic Therapy

Figure 24-7 shows the pharmacologic treatment of asthma using a stepwise approach. There are two general classes of asthma medications: quick-relief medications for immediate treatment of asthma symptoms and exacerbations and long-acting medications to achieve and maintain control of persistent asthma (see Tables 24-4 and 24-5). Because the underlying pathology of asthma is inflammation, control of persistent asthma is accomplished primarily with regular use of anti-inflammatory medications. These medications have systemic side effects when used over the long term. The route of choice for administration of these medications is a pMDI or other type of inhaler, because it allows for topical administration (see Chart 24-4 and Table 24-2).

Quick-Relief Medications

Short-acting beta₂-adrenergic agonists (SABA) (e.g., albuterol [AccuNeb, Proventil, Ventolin, ProAir RespiClick], levalbuterol [Xopenex HFA], and pirbuterol [Maxair]) are the medications of choice for relief of acute symptoms and prevention of exercise-induced asthma. They are used to relax smooth muscle.

Anticholinergics (e.g., ipratropium [Atrovent]) inhibit muscarinic cholinergic receptors and reduce intrinsic vagal tone of the airway. These may be used in patients who do not tolerate short-acting beta₂-adrenergic agonists.

Long-Acting Control Medications

Corticosteroids are the most potent and effective anti-inflammatory medications currently available. They are broadly effective in alleviating symptoms, improving airway function, and decreasing peak flow variability. Initially, an inhaled form is used. A spacer should be used with inhaled corticosteroids, and patients should rinse their mouth after administration to prevent thrush, a common complication associated with the use of inhaled corticosteroids. A systemic preparation may be used to gain rapid control of the disease; to manage severe, persistent asthma; to treat moderate to severe exacerbations; to accelerate recovery; and to prevent recurrence.

Cromolyn sodium (Crolom, NasalCrom) and *nedocromil* (Alocril, Tilade) are mild to moderate anti-inflammatory agents and are considered alternative medications for treatment. These medications stabilize mast cells. They also are effective on a prophylactic basis to prevent exercise-induced asthma or in unavoidable exposure to known triggers. These medications are contraindicated in acute asthma exacerbations.

Long-acting beta₂-agonists (LABA) are used with anti-inflammatory medications to control asthma symptoms, particularly those that occur during the night. These agents are also effective in the prevention of exercise-induced asthma. Long-acting beta₂-agonists are not indicated for

(*text continued on page 660*)

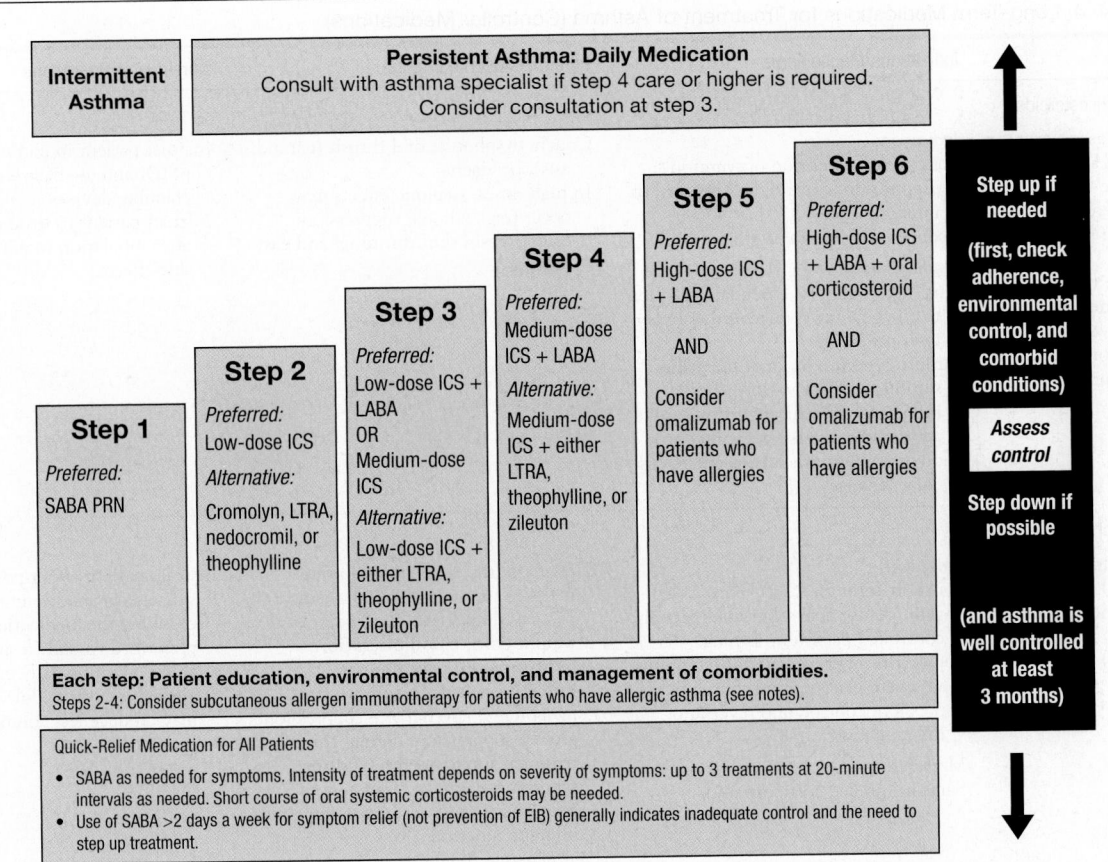

Persistent Asthma: Daily Medication
Consult with asthma specialist if step 4 care or higher is required.
Consider consultation at step 3.

Intermittent Asthma

Step 1

Preferred:
SABA PRN

Step 2

Preferred:
Low-dose ICS

Alternative:
Cromolyn, LTRA, nedocromil, or theophylline

Step 3

Preferred:
Low-dose ICS + LABA
OR
Medium-dose ICS

Alternative:
Low-dose ICS + either LTRA, theophylline, or zileuton

Step 4

Preferred:
Medium-dose ICS + LABA

Alternative:
Medium-dose ICS + either LTRA, theophylline, or zileuton

Step 5

Preferred:
High-dose ICS + LABA

AND

Consider omalizumab for patients who have allergies

Step 6

Preferred:
High-dose ICS + LABA + oral corticosteroid

AND

Consider omalizumab for patients who have allergies

Step up if needed

(first, check adherence, environmental control, and comorbid conditions)

Assess control

Step down if possible

(and asthma is well controlled at least 3 months)

Each step: Patient education, environmental control, and management of comorbidities.
Steps 2-4: Consider subcutaneous allergen immunotherapy for patients who have allergic asthma (see notes).

Quick-Relief Medication for All Patients
- SABA as needed for symptoms. Intensity of treatment depends on severity of symptoms: up to 3 treatments at 20-minute intervals as needed. Short course of oral systemic corticosteroids may be needed.
- Use of SABA >2 days a week for symptom relief (not prevention of EIB) generally indicates inadequate control and the need to step up treatment.

Key: **Alphabetical order is used when more than one treatment option is listed within either preferred or alternative therapy.** EIB, exercise-induced bronchospasm; ICS, inhaled corticosteroid; LABA, inhaled long-acting beta$_2$-agonist; LTRA, leukotriene receptor antagonist; SABA, inhaled short-acting beta$_2$-agonist

Notes:

■ The stepwise approach is meant to assist, not replace, the clinical decision making required to meet individual patient needs.

■ If alternative treatment is used and response is inadequate, discontinue it and use the preferred treatment before stepping up.

■ Zileuton is a less desirable alternative due to limited studies as adjunctive therapy and the need to monitor liver function. Theophylline requires monitoring of serum concentration levels.

■ In step 6, before oral systemic corticosteroids are introduced, a trial of high-dose ICS + LABA + either LTRA, theophylline, or zileuton may be considered, although this approach has not been studied in clinical trials.

■ Steps 1, 2, and 3 preferred therapies are based on evidence A; step 3 alternative therapy is based on evidence A for LTRA, evidence B for theophylline, and evidence D for zileuton. Step 4 preferred therapy is based on evidence B, and alternative therapy is based on evidence B for LTRA and theophylline and evidence D for zileuton. Step 5 preferred therapy is based on evidence B. Step 6 preferred therapy is based on (EPR−2 1997) and evidence B for omalizumab.

■ Immunotherapy for steps 2-4 is based on evidence B for house-dust mites, animal danders, and pollens; evidence is weak or lacking for molds and cockroaches. Evidence is strongest for immunotherapy with single allergens. The role of allergy in asthma is greater in children than in adults.

■ Clinicians who administer immunotherapy or omalizumab should be prepared and equipped to identify and treat anaphylaxis that may occur.

Figure 24-7 • Stepwise approach for managing asthma in youths 12 years and older and adults. Redrawn and adapted from Expert Panel Report 3. (2007). *Guidelines for the diagnosis and management of asthma.* National Asthma Education and Prevention Program. NIH Publication Number 08–5846. Bethesda, MD: U.S. Department of Health and Human Services, National Heart, Lung and Blood Institute; National Heart, Lung and Blood Institute (NHLBI) (2012). Asthma care quick reference: diagnosing and managing asthma. NIH Publication No. 12–5075. Revised September 2012.

TABLE 24-4 Long-Term Medications for Treatment of Asthma (Controller Medications)

Medication	Indications/Mechanisms	Potential Adverse Effects	Nursing Considerations
Inhaled Corticosteroids			
beclomethasone propionate (QVAR) budesonide (Pulmicort Flexhaler) ciclesonide (Alvesco) flunisolide (AeroBid) fluticasone (Flovent) mometasone furoate (Asmanex) triamcinolone acetonide (Azmacort)	*Indications* Long-term prevention of symptoms; suppression, control, and reversal of inflammation Reduce need for oral corticosteroid *Mechanisms* Anti-inflammatory; block late reaction to allergen and reduce airway hyperresponsiveness Inhibit cytokine production, adhesion protein activation, and inflammatory cell migration and activation; reverse beta$_2$-receptor down-regulation; inhibit microvascular leakage	Cough, dysphonia, oral thrush (candidiasis), headache In high doses, systemic effects may occur (e.g., adrenal suppression, osteoporosis, skin thinning, and easy bruising)	Instruct patient in correct use of pMDI and use of spacer/holding chamber devices. Instruct patient to rinse mouth after inhalation to reduce local side effects.
Systemic Corticosteroids			
methylprednisolone (Medrol) prednisolone (Prelone) prednisone (Deltasone, Orasone)	*Indications* For short-term (3–10 d) "burst": to gain prompt control of inadequately controlled persistent asthma For long-term prevention of symptoms in severe persistent asthma: suppression, control, and reversal of inflammation *Mechanisms* Same as inhaled corticosteroids	*Short-term use:* reversible abnormalities in glucose metabolism, increased appetite, fluid retention, weight gain, mood alteration, hypertension, peptic ulcer, and rarely aseptic necrosis *Long-term use:* adrenal axis suppression, growth suppression, dermal thinning, hypertension, diabetes, Cushing syndrome, cataracts, muscle weakness, and, in rare instances, impaired immune function Consideration should be given to comorbidities that could be worsened by systemic corticosteroids	Instruct patient about possible side effects and the importance of taking the medication as prescribed (usually a single dose in the morning daily or on an alternate-day schedule, which may produce less adrenal suppression).
Long-Acting Beta$_2$-Agonists			
Inhaled salmeterol (Serevent Diskus) formoterol (Foradil Aerolizer)	*Indications* Long-term prevention of symptoms, added to ICS Prevention of exercise-induced bronchospasm *Mechanisms* Bronchodilation; smooth muscle relaxation following adenylate cyclase activation and increase in cAMP, producing functional antagonism of bronchoconstriction Compared to SABA, salmeterol (but not formoterol) has slower onset of action (15–30 min). Both salmeterol and formoterol have longer duration (>12 h) compared to SABA	Should *not* be used to treat acute symptoms or exacerbations Decreased protection against exercise-induced bronchospasm may occur with regular use Tachycardia, muscle tremor, hypokalemia, ECG changes with overdose. A diminished bronchoprotective effect may occur within 1 week of chronic therapy. Potential risk of uncommon, severe, life-threatening, or fatal exacerbation	Reinforce to patient that these medications should *not* be used to treat acute asthma symptoms or exacerbations. Instruct patient about correct use of pMDI or aerolizer inhaler.
Oral albuterol (Proventil) sustained release		Inhaled route is preferred to oral route because LABAs are longer acting and have fewer side effects than oral sustained-release agents	
Methylxanthines			
theophylline (Slo-Bid, Theo-Dur) sustained-release tablets and capsules	*Indications* Long-term control and prevention of symptoms in mild persistent asthma or as adjunctive with ICS, in moderate or persistent asthma	Dose-related acute toxicities include tachycardia, nausea and vomiting, tachyarrhythmias (SVT), central nervous system stimulation, headache, seizures, hematemesis, hyperglycemia, and hypokalemia	Maintain steady-state serum concentrations between 5 and 15 mcg/mL.

TABLE 24-4 Long-Term Medications for Treatment of Asthma (Controller Medications) (continued)

Medication	Indications/Mechanisms	Potential Adverse Effects	Nursing Considerations
	Mechanisms Bronchodilation; smooth muscle relaxation from phosphodiesterase inhibition and possibly adenosine antagonism May affect eosinophilic infiltration into bronchial mucosa as well as decreased T-lymphocyte numbers in epithelium Increases diaphragm contractility and mucociliary clearance	Adverse effects at usual therapeutic doses include insomnia, gastric upset, aggravation of ulcer or reflux, and difficulty in urination in older males who have prostatism Not generally recommended for exacerbations. There is minimal evidence for added benefit to optimal doses of SABA. Serum concentration monitoring is mandatory Available as sustained-release tablets and capsules	Be aware that absorption and metabolism may be affected by numerous factors that can produce significant changes in steady-state serum theophylline concentrations. Instruct patients to discontinue if they experience toxicity. Inform patients about the importance of blood tests to monitor serum concentration. Instruct patient to check with primary provider before taking any new medication.
Combined Medication (corticosteroid/long acting beta agonist)			
fluticasone/salmeterol (Advair)	*DPI* 100 mcg/50 mcg 250 mcg/50 mcg 500 mcg/50 mcg *HFA* 45 mcg/21 mcg 115 mcg/21 mcg 230 mcg/21 mcg	Lowest dose of DPI or HFA used for patients whose asthma is not controlled on low- to medium-dose ICS Higher doses of DPI or HFA used for patients whose asthma is not controlled on medium- to high-dose ICS	
budesonide/formoterol (Symbicort)	*HFA pMDI* 80 mcg/4.5 mcg 160 mcg/4.5 mcg	Lower dose used for patients who have asthma not controlled on low- to medium-dose ICS Higher dose used for patients who have asthma not controlled on medium- to high-dose ICS	
fluticasone furoate/ vilanterol (Breo Ellipta)	100 mcg/25 mcg	Used if asthma not controlled on long term asthma control medication. Do not use with other long acting beta agonist drugs	
Cromolyn and Nedocromil			
cromolyn sodium (Crolom, NasalCrom, Intal) nedocromil (Alocril, Tilade)	*Indications* Long-term prevention of symptoms in mild persistent asthma; may modify inflammation Preventive treatment prior to exposure to exercise or known allergen *Mechanisms* Anti-inflammatory; blocks *early* and late reaction to allergen Stabilizes mast cell membranes and inhibits activation and release of mediators from eosinophils and epithelial cells Inhibits acute response to exercise, cold dry air, and SO$_2$	Cough and irritation 15–20% of patients complain of an unpleasant taste from nedocromil. Dose of cromolyn by pMDI may be inadequate to affect airway hyperresponsiveness. Nebulizer delivery may be preferred for some patients Safety is the primary advantage of these agents. One dose before exercise or exposure to allergen provides effective prophylaxis for 1–2 h. Not as effective for exercise-induced bronchospasm as short-acting beta$_2$-agonist	Inform patient that 4–6-wk trial may be needed to determine maximum benefit. Instruct patient about correct use of inhaler.
Leukotriene Modifiers			
Leukotriene Receptor Antagonists montelukast (Singulair)	*Mechanism* Selective competitive inhibitor of CysLT1 receptor *Indications* Long-term control and prevention of symptoms in mild persistent asthma for patients ≥1 y of age May also be used with ICS as combination therapy in moderate persistent asthma	May attenuate EIB in some patients, but less effective than ICS therapy LTRA + LABA should not be used as a substitute for ICS + LABA. No specific adverse effects have been identified. Available in tablets and granules	Instruct patient to take at least 1 h before meals or 2 h after meals. Inform patient that zafirlukast can inhibit the metabolism of warfarin. INRs should be monitored if patient is taking both medications.
zafirlukast (Accolate)	Long-term control and prevention of symptoms in mild persistent asthma; may also be used with ICS as combination therapy in moderate persistent asthma	Cases of reversible hepatitis have been reported along with rare cases of irreversible hepatic failure resulting in death and liver transplantation Available in tablets	Instruct patients to discontinue use if they experience signs and symptoms of liver dysfunction (right upper quadrant pain, pruritus, lethargy, jaundice, nausea), and to notify their primary provider.

(continued on page 660)

TABLE 24-4 Long-Term Medications for Treatment of Asthma (Controller Medications) (continued)

Medication	Indications/Mechanisms	Potential Adverse Effects	Nursing Considerations
5-Lipoxygenase Inhibitor			
zileuton (Zyflo)	*Mechanism* Inhibits the production of leukotrienes from arachidonic acid, both LTB and the cysteinyl leukotrienes *Indications* Long-term control and prevention of symptoms in mild persistent asthma for patients May be used with ICS as combination therapy in moderate persistent asthma in patients	Elevation of liver enzymes has been reported. Limited case reports of reversible hepatitis and hyperbilirubinemia	Inform patient that zileuton can inhibit the metabolism of warfarin and theophylline. Therefore, the doses of these medications should be monitored accordingly. Educate patient about the importance of monitoring medication levels and tests of liver function.
Immunomodulators			
omalizumab (Xolair)	*Indications* Long-term control and prevention of symptoms in adults with moderate or severe persistent allergic asthma inadequately controlled with ICS *Mechanisms* Monoclonal antibody (anti-IgE) that binds to circulating IgE, preventing it from binding to the high-affinity receptors on basophils and mast cells Decreases mast cell mediator release from allergen exposure	Given by subcutaneous injection Anaphylaxis has been reported in 0.2% of treated patients Pain, bruising, and skin reactions (itching, redness, stinging) at injection sites Dose is given either every 2 or 4 wks and depends on the patient's body weight and IgE level before therapy A maximum of 150 mg can be given in 1 injection Medication needs to be stored under refrigeration at 2–8°C (35.6–46.4°F) It is unknown if patients will develop significant antibody titers to the drug with long-term administration	Monitor patients for allergic reactions or anaphylaxis following administration. Be prepared to initiate emergency treatment if anaphylaxis occurs. Instruct patient about signs and symptoms that indicate allergic reaction and immediate action to take. Remind patient to continue to take other medications prescribed for treatment of asthma.

pMDI, pressurized metered-dose inhaler; ICS, inhaled corticosteroid; cAMP, cyclic 3′, 5′-adenosine monophosphate; ECG, electrocardiogram; SABA, inhaled short-acting beta₂-agonist; LABA, long-acting beta₂-agonist; SVT, supraventricular tachycardia; DPI, dry powder inhaler; HFA, hydrofluoroalkane; SO₂, sulfur dioxide; CysLT1, cysteinyl leukotriene receptor 1; EIB, exercise-induced bronchospasm; LTRA, leukotriene receptor antagonist; INR, international normalized ratio; LTB, leukotriene B; IgE, immunoglobulin E.
Adapted from Global Strategy for Asthma Management and Prevention, Global Initiative for Asthma (GINA) 2015. Retrieved on 1/25/2015 at: www.ginasthma.org/local/uploads/files/GINA_Report_2015_Aug11.pdf

immediate relief of symptoms. Theophylline (Slo-Bid, Theo-Dur) is a mild to moderate bronchodilator that is usually used in addition to inhaled corticosteroids, mainly for relief of nighttime asthma symptoms. Salmeterol (Serevent Diskus) and formoterol (Foradil Aerolizer) have duration of bronchodilation of at least 12 hours. They are used with other medications in long-term control of asthma.

Leukotriene modifiers (inhibitors), or *antileukotrienes*, are a class of medications that include montelukast (Singulair), zafirlukast (Accolate), and zileuton (Zyflo). Leukotrienes, which are synthesized from membrane phospholipids through a cascade of enzymes, are potent bronchoconstrictors that also dilate blood vessels and alter permeability. Leukotriene inhibitors act either by interfering with leukotriene synthesis or by blocking the receptors where leukotrienes exert their action. They may provide an alternative to inhaled corticosteroids for mild persistent asthma, or they may be added to a regimen of inhaled corticosteroids in more severe asthma to attain further control.

Immunomodulators prevent binding of IgE to the high-affinity receptors of basophils and mast cells. Omalizumab (Xolair) is a monoclonal antibody and may be used for patients with allergies and severe persistent asthma.

Numerous asthma biologic agents are in development. Most of these target a specific cell or mediator and may only be appropriate for a small subset of patients. The future of asthma may be stratification of specific pathway-selective phenotypes in patients; thus, treatment in the future may include individually tailored medications (Choby & Lee, 2015; GINA, 2015).

Management of Exacerbations

Asthma exacerbations are best managed by early treatment and education, including the use of written action plans as part of any overall effort to educate patients about self-management techniques, especially those with moderate or severe persistent asthma or with a history of severe exacerbations (GINA, 2015; NHLBI, 2012). Quick-acting beta₂-adrenergic agonist medications are first used for prompt relief of airflow obstruction. Systemic corticosteroids may be necessary to decrease airway inflammation in patients who fail to respond to inhaled beta-adrenergic medications. In some patients, oxygen supplementation may be required to relieve

TABLE 24-5 Quick-Relief Medications for Treatment of Asthma

Medication	Indications/Mechanisms	Potential Adverse Effects	Nursing Considerations
Inhaled Short-Acting Beta₂-Agonists albuterol (AccuNeb, Proventil HFA, Ventolin HFA, ProAir RespiClick) levalbuterol HFA (Xopenex HFA) metaproterenol sulfate (Alupent)	*Indications* Relief of acute symptoms; quick-relief medication Preventive treatment for exercise-induced bronchospasm *Mechanisms* Bronchodilation; binds to the beta₂-adrenergic receptor, producing smooth muscle relaxation and decreased bronchoconstriction	Tachycardia, muscle tremor, hypokalemia, increased lactic acid, headache, and hyperglycemia. Inhaled route causes few systematic adverse effects. Patients with preexisting cardiovascular disease, especially older adults, may have adverse cardiovascular reactions with inhaled therapy Lack of effect or need for regular use indicates inadequate asthma control	Instruct patient in correct use of inhaled agents and how to evaluate amount of remaining medication in pressurized metered-dose inhaler. Recommend periodic cleaning of device. Inform patient about possible adverse effects and need to inform primary provider about increased use of medication to control symptoms.
Anticholinergics ipratropium (Atrovent)	*Indications* Relief of acute bronchospasm *Mechanisms* Bronchodilation; inhibition of muscarinic cholinergic receptors Reduction in vagal tone of airways May decrease mucous gland secretion	Dryness of mouth and respiratory secretions; may cause increased wheezing in some patients Does not block exercise-induced bronchospasm Is not effective in long-term control of asthma	Instruct patient in correct use of inhaled agents. Ensure adequate fluid intake. Assess patient for hypersensitivity to atropine, soybeans, peanuts; glaucoma; prostatic hypertrophy.
Corticosteroids *Systemic* methylprednisolone (Medrol) prednisolone (Prelone) prednisone (Deltasone, Orasone)	*Indications* For moderate or severe exacerbations to prevent progression of exacerbation, reverse inflammation, speed recovery, and reduce rate of relapse *Mechanisms* Anti-inflammatory; block reaction to allergen and reduce hyperresponsiveness; inhibit cytokine production, adhesion protein activation, and inflammatory cell migration and activation; reverses beta₂-receptor down-regulation	Blood glucose abnormalities, increased appetite, fluid retention, weight gain, mood alteration, hypertension, peptic ulcer Consideration must be given to comorbidities that may be worsened by systemic corticosteroids	Explain to patient that action is often rapid in onset, although resolution of symptoms may take 3–10 d. Instruct patient about possible side effects and the importance of taking the medication as prescribed.

HFA, hydrofluoroalkane.
Adapted from Global Strategy for Asthma Management and Prevention, Global Initiative for Asthma (GINA) 2015. Retrieved on 1/25/2015 at: www.ginasthma.org/local/uploads/files/GINA_Report_2015_Aug11.pdf

hypoxemia associated with moderate to severe exacerbations. In addition, response to treatment may be monitored by serial measurements of lung function.

Evidence from clinical trials suggests that antibiotic therapy, whether given routinely or when suspicion of bacterial infection is low, is not beneficial for asthma exacerbations (GINA, 2015). Antibiotics may be appropriate in the treatment of acute asthma exacerbations in patients with comorbid conditions (e.g., fever and purulent sputum, evidence of pneumonia, suspected bacterial sinusitis).

Despite insufficient data supporting or refuting the benefits of using a written asthma action plan as compared to medical management alone, it is recommended to use a written asthma action plan to educate patients about

self-management (Fig. 24-8). Plans can be based on either symptoms or peak flow measurements. They should focus on daily management as well as the recognition and handling of worsening symptoms. Patient self-management and early recognition of problems lead to more efficient communication with health care providers about asthma exacerbations (GINA, 2015; NHLBI, 2012).

Peak Flow Monitoring

Peak flow meters measure the highest airflow during a forced expiration (see Fig. 24-9). Daily peak flow monitoring is recommended for patients who meet one or more of the following criteria: have moderate or severe persistent asthma, have poor perception of changes in airflow or worsening symptoms,

Asthma Action Plan

For: _____ Doctor: _____ Date: _____

Doctor's Phone Number _____ Hospital/Emergency Department Phone Number _____

GREEN ZONE

Doing Well
- No cough, wheeze, chest tightness, or shortness of breath during the day or night
- Can do usual activites

And, if a peak flow meter is used,
Peak flow: more than _____
(80% or more of my best peak flow)
My best peak flow is: _____

Take these long-term-control medicines each day (include an anti-inflammatory).

Medicine	How much to take	When to take it
_____	_____	_____
_____	_____	_____

Identify and avoid and control the things that make your asthma worse, like (list here):

_____ _____
_____ _____

Before exercise, if prescribed, take: ☐ 2 or ☐ 4 puffs _____ 5 to 60 minutes before exercise

YELLOW ZONE

Asthma Is Getting Worse
- Cough, wheeze, chest tightness, or shortness of breath, or
- Waking at night due to asthma, or
- Can do some, but not all, usual activites

-Or-
Peak flow: _____ to _____
(50% to 79% of my best peak flow)

First Add: quick-relief medicine—and keep taking your GREEN ZONE medicine.

_____ ☐ 2 or ☐ 4 puffs, every 20 minutes for up to 1 hour
(short-acting beta₂-agonist) ☐ Nebulizer, once

If applicable, remove yourself from the thing that made your asthma worse.

Second If your symptoms (and peak flow, if used) return to GREEN ZONE after 1 hour of above treatment:
  Continue monitoring to be sure you stay in the green zone.
-Or-
If your symptoms (and peak flow, if used) do not return to GREEN ZONE after 1 hour of above treatment:
☐ Take: _____ ☐ 2 or ☐ 4 puffs or ☐ Nebulizer
(short-acting beta₂-agonist)
☐ Add: _____ mg per day For _____ (3-10) days
(oral corticosteroid)
☐ Call the doctor: _____ , ☐ before/☐ within _____ hours after taking the oral corticosteroid.
(phone)

RED ZONE

Medical Alert!
- Very short of breath, or
- Quick-relief medicines have not helped, or
- Cannot do usual activites, or
- Symptoms are same or get worse after 24 hours in Yellow Zone

-Or-
Peak flow: less than _____
(50% of my best peak flow)

Take this medicine:

☐ _____ ☐ 4 or ☐ 6 puffs or ☐ Nebulizer
(short-acting beta₂-agonist)
☐ _____ mg
(oral corticosteroid)

Then call your doctor NOW. Go to the hospital or call an ambulance if:
- You are still in the red zone after 15 minutes AND
- You have not reached your doctor.

DANGER SIGNS
- Trouble walking and talking due to shortness of breath
- Lips or fingernails are blue

- Take ☐ 4 or ☐ 6 puffs of your quick-relief medicine AND
- Go to the hospital or call for an ambulance _____ NOW!
(phone)

Figure 24-8 • Asthma action plan. Adapted from National Heart, Lung and Blood Institute (NHLBI). (2012). Asthma care quick reference: diagnosing and managing asthma. NIH Publication No. 12-5075. Revised September 2012.

Figure 24-9 • Peak flow meters measure the highest volume of airflow during a forced expiration. The patient takes a deep breath and places lips around the mouthpiece (**A**), and then exhales hard and fast (**B**). Volume may be measured in color-coded zones: the green zone signifies 80% to 100% of personal best; yellow, 60% to 80%; and red, less than 60%. If peak flow falls below the red zone, the patient should take the appropriate actions prescribed by their primary provider.

Chart 24-6	**HOME CARE CHECKLIST**
	Use of Peak Flow Meter in Asthma Management

At the completion of education, the patient and/or caregiver will be able to:

- Describe the rationale for using a peak flow meter in asthma management.
- Explain how peak flow monitoring is used along with symptoms to determine severity of asthma.
- Demonstrate steps for using the peak flow meter correctly.
  - Move the indicator to the bottom of the numbered scale.
  - Stand up.
  - Take a deep breath, and fill the lungs completely.
  - Place mouthpiece in mouth, and close lips around mouthpiece. (Do not put tongue inside opening.)
  - Blow out hard and fast with a single blow.

- Record the number achieved on the indicator. If patient coughs or a mistake is made in the process, do it again.
- Repeat steps 1–5 two more times, and write the highest number in the asthma diary.
- Explain how to determine the "personal best" peak flow reading.
- Describe the significance of the color zones for peak flow monitoring.
- Demonstrate how to clean the peak flow meter.
- Discuss how and when to contact the primary provider about changes or decreases in peak flow values.

have unexplained response to environmental or occupational exposures, or at the discretion of the clinician and patient (GINA, 2015). Peak flow monitoring helps measure asthma severity and, when added to symptom monitoring, indicates the current degree of asthma control.

The patient is instructed in the proper technique (see Chart 24-6), particularly about using maximal effort; peak flows are monitored for 2 or 3 weeks after receipt of optimal asthma therapy. Then, the patient's "personal best" value is measured. The green (80% to 100% of personal best), yellow (60% to 80%), and red (less than 60%) zones are determined, and specific actions are delineated for each zone, enabling the patient to monitor and manipulate their own therapy after careful instruction (GINA, 2015; NHLBI, 2012).

GINA (2015) recommends that peak flow monitoring be considered an adjunct to asthma management for patients with moderate to severe persistent asthma. Peak flow monitoring plans may enhance communication between the patient and health care providers and may increase the patient's awareness of disease status and control.

Nursing Management

The immediate nursing care of patients with asthma depends on the severity of symptoms. The patient may be treated successfully as an outpatient if asthma symptoms are relatively mild or may require hospitalization and intensive care if symptoms are acute and severe. The patient and family are often frightened and anxious because of the patient's dyspnea. Therefore, a calm approach is an important aspect of care. The nurse assesses the patient's respiratory status by monitoring the severity of symptoms, breath sounds, peak flow, pulse oximetry, and vital signs.

The nurse generally performs the following interventions:
- Obtains a history of allergic reactions to medications before administering medications.
- Identifies medications the patient is taking.
- Administers medications as prescribed and monitors the patient's responses to those medications. These medications may include an antibiotic if the patient has an underlying respiratory infection.
- Administers fluids if the patient is dehydrated.

If the patient requires intubation because of acute respiratory failure, the nurse assists with the intubation procedure,

continues close monitoring of the patient, and keeps the patient and family informed about procedures. (See Chapter 21 for discussion of intubation and mechanical ventilation.)

Promoting Home, Community-Based, and Transitional Care

Educating Patients About Self-Care

Implementation of basic asthma management principles at the community level is a major challenge. Strategies include education of health care providers, establishment of programs for asthma education (for patients and providers), the use of outpatient follow-up care for patients, and a focus on chronic management versus acute episodic care. Nurses are pivotal to achievement of these objectives.

Patient education is a critical component of care for patients with asthma. Multiple inhalers, different types of inhalers, antiallergy therapy, antireflux medications, and avoidance measures are essential for long-term control. This complex therapy requires a partnership between the patient and the health care providers to determine the desired outcomes and to formulate a plan to achieve those outcomes. The patient then carries out daily therapy as part of self-care management, with input and guidance by their health care providers. Before a partnership can be established, the patient must understand the following:
- Nature of asthma as a chronic inflammatory disease
- Definitions of inflammation and bronchoconstriction
- Purpose and action of each medication
- Triggers to avoid and how to avoid them
- Proper inhalation technique
- How to perform peak flow monitoring (see Chart 24-6)
- How to implement an asthma action plan (see Fig. 24-8)
- When to seek assistance, and how to do so

An assortment of excellent educational materials is available from the NHLBI and other sources (GINA, 2015). The nurse should obtain current educational materials for the patient based on the patient's diagnosis, causative factors, educational level, and cultural background. If a patient has a coexisting sensory impairment (i.e., vision loss or hearing impairment), materials should be provided in an alternative format.

Continuing and Transitional Care

Nurses who have contact with patients in the hospital, clinic, school, or office use the opportunity to assess the patient's respiratory status and ability to manage self-care to prevent serious exacerbations. Nurses emphasize adherence to the prescribed therapy, preventive measures, and the need to keep follow-up appointments with health care providers. Home visits to assess the home environment for allergens may be indicated for patients with recurrent exacerbations. Nurses refer patients to community support groups. In addition, nurses remind patients and families about the importance of health promotion strategies and recommended health screening.

Unfolding Patient Stories: Jennifer Hoffman • Part 1

Jennifer Hoffman is a 33-year-old woman diagnosed with asthma in childhood. She has come to the clinic multiple times over the last 2 months complaining of continued symptoms. Her asthma action plan was adjusted by her primary provider last month.

What measures can the nurse take to determine areas needing education reinforcement? How can the nurse ensure that Jennifer is accurately following the prescribed asthma regimen and monitoring medication effectiveness? (Jennifer Hoffman's story continues in Chapter 37.)

Care for Jennifer and other patients in a realistic virtual environment: **vSim** *for Nursing* (**thepoint.lww.com/vSimMedicalSurgical**). Practice documenting these patients' care in DocuCare (**thepoint.lww.com/DocuCareEHR**).

 ## Status Asthmaticus

An asthma exacerbation can range from mild to severe with potential respiratory arrest (GINA, 2015). The term *status asthmaticus* is sometimes used to describe rapid onset, severe, and persistent asthma that does not respond to conventional therapy. The attacks can occur with little or no warning and can progress rapidly to asphyxiation. Infection, anxiety, nebulizer abuse, dehydration, increased adrenergic blockage, and nonspecific irritants may contribute to these episodes. An acute episode may be precipitated by hypersensitivity to medications, such as aspirin, beta blockers, and nonsteroidal anti-inflammatory drugs (NSAIDs) (AAAAI, 2016b).

Pathophysiology

The basic characteristics of asthma (inflammation of bronchial mucosa, constriction of the bronchiolar smooth muscle, and thickened secretions) decrease the diameter of the bronchi and occur in status asthmaticus. The most common scenario is severe bronchospasm, with mucus plugging leading to asphyxia. A ventilation–perfusion abnormality results in hypoxemia. There is a reduced PaO_2 and initial respiratory alkalosis, with a decreased $PaCO_2$ and an increased pH. As status asthmaticus worsens, the $PaCO_2$ increases and the pH decreases, reflecting respiratory acidosis.

Clinical Manifestations

The clinical manifestations are the same as those seen in severe asthma; signs and symptoms include labored breathing, prolonged exhalation, engorged neck veins, and wheezing. However, the extent of wheezing does not indicate the severity of the attack. As the obstruction worsens, the wheezing may disappear; this is frequently a sign of impending respiratory failure.

Assessment and Diagnostic Findings

The severity of an exacerbation may be evaluated by a general assessment of the patient (degree of breathlessness, ability to talk, positioning of patient, level of alertness or cognitive function), physical assessment (respiratory rate, the use of accessory muscles, presence of central cyanosis, auscultatory findings, pulse, and pulsus paradoxus), and laboratory evaluation (peak expiratory flow after a bronchodilator, PaO_2 and $PaCO_2$, and pulse oximetry). Pulmonary function studies are the most accurate means of assessing an acute, severe airway obstruction, though not practical to obtain during this type of an emergent situation. Arterial blood gas measurement and/or pulse oximetry are obtained if the patient cannot perform pulmonary function maneuvers because of severe obstruction or fatigue, or if the patient does not respond to treatment. Respiratory alkalosis (low $PaCO_2$) is the most common finding in patients with an ongoing asthma exacerbation and is due to hyperventilation.

 Quality and Safety Nursing Alert

In status asthmaticus, increasing $PaCO_2$ (to normal levels or levels indicating respiratory acidosis) is a danger sign signifying impending respiratory failure.

Medical Management

Close monitoring of the patient and objective reevaluation for response to therapy are key in status asthmaticus. In the emergency setting, the patient is treated initially with a short-acting $beta_2$-adrenergic agonist and subsequently a short course of systemic corticosteroids, especially if the patient does not respond to the short-acting $beta_2$-adrenergic agonist. Corticosteroids are critical in the therapy of status asthmaticus and are used to decrease the intense airway inflammation and swelling. Short-acting inhaled $beta_2$-adrenergic agonists provide the most rapid relief from bronchospasm. A pMDI with or without a spacer may be used for nebulization of the medications. However, more commonly, short-acting bronchodilators will be given via a nebulizer. A mouthpiece or face mask can be used and the bronchodilator is continuously given to the patient. The patient does not have to work to coordinate their breathing pattern, which can otherwise cause additional anxiety in this acute situation. The patient requires supplemental oxygen and IV fluids for hydration. Oxygen therapy is initiated to treat dyspnea, central cyanosis, and hypoxemia. High-flow supplemental oxygen is best delivered using a partial or complete non-rebreathing mask. Sedatives are contraindicated. Magnesium sulfate, a calcium antagonist, may be given to induce smooth muscle relaxation; the magnesium can relax smooth muscle and hence cause bronchodilation by competing with calcium at calcium-mediated smooth muscle binding sites. IV magnesium sulfate is not recommended for routine use in asthma exacerbations; however, when given as a single 2 g infusion over 20 minutes, it may be helpful in treating patients who present with severely compromised pulmonary function, who have not responded to initial therapy, and with persistent hypoxemia (GINA, 2015). Adverse effects of magnesium sulfate may include facial warmth, flushing, tingling, nausea, central nervous system depression, respiratory depression, and hypotension.

If there is no response to repeated treatments, hospitalization is required. Other criteria for hospitalization include poor pulmonary function test results and deteriorating blood gas levels (respiratory acidosis), which may indicate that the patient is tiring and will require mechanical ventilation. Most patients do not need mechanical ventilation, but it is used for patients in respiratory failure, for those who tire and are too fatigued by the attempt to breathe, and for those whose condition does not respond to initial treatment.

For a very select group of patients with uncontrolled severe asthma, bronchial thermoplasty may be considered. Bronchial thermoplasty is the first nondrug therapy for the treatment of severe, uncontrolled asthma. It consists of controlled radiofrequency heating of the central airways through a bronchoscope. The thermal energy reduces the amount of smooth muscle involved in bronchospasm and potentially decreases the severity and frequency of symptoms. This therapy is invasive and relatively new; therefore, only select centers have the ability to perform this procedure, and it should only be considered in a select group of patients (GINA, 2015).

Death from asthma is associated with several risk factors, including the following (GINA, 2015:

- Past history of severe exacerbation (e.g., intubation or intensive care unit admission)
- Two or more hospitalizations for asthma within the past year
- Three or more emergency care visits for asthma in the past year
- Hospitalization or emergency care visit for asthma in the past month
- Use of more than two canisters of short-acting beta-agonist inhalers per month
- Difficulty in perceiving asthma symptoms or severity of exacerbations
- Lack of written asthma action plan
- Concurrent cardiovascular disease, COPD, or chronic psychiatric disease
- Low socioeconomic status or inner-city residence
- Illicit drug use

Nursing Management

The main focus of nursing management is to actively assess the airway and the patient's response to treatment. The nurse should be prepared for the next intervention if the patient does not respond to treatment.

The nurse vigilantly monitors the patient for the first 12 to 24 hours, or until the severe exacerbation resolves. The nurse also assesses the patient's skin turgor for signs of dehydration. Fluid intake is essential to combat dehydration, to loosen secretions, and to facilitate expectoration. Nurses administer IV fluids as prescribed, up to 3 to 4 L/day, unless contraindicated. Blood pressure and cardiac rhythm should be monitored continuously during the acute phase and until the patient stabilizes and responds to therapy. The patient's energy needs to be conserved, and his or her room should be quiet and free of respiratory irritants, including flowers, tobacco smoke, perfumes, or odors of cleaning agents. Non-allergenic pillows should be used. An asthma attack may also be precipitated or aggravated by exposure to latex if the patient has a latex allergy; therefore, this type of hypersensitivity must be identified and latex-free products used, as warranted. Once the exacerbation is resolved, the factors that precipitated the exacerbation should be identified and strategies for their future avoidance implemented. In addition, the patient's medication plan should be reviewed.

Cystic Fibrosis

CF is the most common fatal autosomal recessive disease among Caucasians. It is less frequently found among Hispanic-, Asian-, and African Americans. A person must inherit a defective copy of the CF gene (one from each parent) to have CF. Each year, 1000 new cases of CF are diagnosed, and more than 75% of patients are diagnosed by 2 years of age (Cystic Fibrosis Foundation [CFF], 2015). Approximately 30,000 children and adults in the United States have CF and nearly half are over the age of 18. CF was once a fatal childhood disease; however, the median expected survival age is now in the late 30s (CFF, 2015).

Although most patients are diagnosed by age 2 years, this disease may not be diagnosed until later in life (CFF, 2015). Respiratory symptoms are frequently the major manifestation of CF when it is diagnosed later in life. However, many patients will not demonstrate the classic symptoms of CF, which may potentially cause a diagnostic dilemma.

Pathophysiology

CF is caused by mutations or dysfunction in the protein cystic fibrosis transmembrane conductance regulator (CFTR), which normally transports chloride ions across epithelial cell membranes. Gene mutations affect transport of these ions, leading to CF, which is characterized by thick, viscous secretions in the lungs, pancreas, liver, intestine, and reproductive tract as well as increased salt content in sweat gland secretions. The most common mutation is deltaF508; however, more than 1,800 mutations have been identified (Nakano, 2014; Pittman & Ferkol, 2015). The numerous mutations of the *CFTR* gene create multiple variations in the presentation and progression of the disease.

The ability to detect the common mutations of this gene allows for routine screening for CF and the detection of carriers of the disease. Genetic counseling is an important part of health care for couples at risk (see Chapter 8). People who are heterozygous for CF (i.e., have one defective gene and one normal gene) do not have the disease but can be carriers and pass the defective gene on to their children. If both parents are carriers, their risk of having a child with CF is one in four (25%) with each pregnancy. Genetic testing should be offered to adults with a positive family history of CF and to partners of people with CF who are planning a pregnancy or seeking prenatal counseling. The hallmark pathology of CF is bronchial mucus plugging, inflammation, and eventual bronchiectasis. Commonly, the bronchiectasis begins in the upper lobes and progresses to involve all lobes.

Clinical Manifestations

The pulmonary manifestations of CF include a productive cough, wheezing, hyperinflation of the lung fields on chest x-ray, and pulmonary function test results consistent with obstructive disease of the airways. Chronic respiratory inflammation and infection are caused by impaired mucus clearance. Colonization of the airways with pathogenic bacteria usually occurs early in life. *S. aureus* and *H. influenzae* are common organisms during early childhood. As the disease progresses, *P. aeruginosa* is ultimately isolated from the sputum of most patients (Katkin, 2016). Upper respiratory manifestations of the disease include sinusitis and nasal polyps.

Nonpulmonary manifestations include gastrointestinal problems (e.g., pancreatic insufficiency, recurrent abdominal pain, biliary cirrhosis, vitamin deficiencies, recurrent pancreatitis, and weight loss), CF-related diabetes, and genitourinary problems (male and female infertility). (See Chapter 50 for a discussion of pancreatitis.)

Assessment and Diagnostic Findings

The diagnosis of CF requires a clinical picture consistent with the CF phenotype and laboratory evidence of CFTR dysfunction. Key assessment findings in adults include (Katkin, 2016):

- Chronic sinopulmonary disease as manifested by chronic cough and sputum production, persistent infection consistent with typical CF pathogens, and x-ray evidence of bronchiectasis and chronic sinusitis, often with nasal polyps
- Gastrointestinal tract and nutritional abnormalities (pancreatic insufficiency, recurrent pancreatitis, biliary cirrhosis and portal hypertension, CF-related diabetes)
- Male urogenital problems as manifested by congenital bilateral absence of the vas deferens; reduced female fertility

Medical Management

CF requires both acute and chronic therapy. Because chronic bacterial infection of the airways occurs in CF, control of infections is essential to treatment. For acute airway exacerbations, aggressive therapy involves airway clearance and antibiotics based on results of sputum cultures. The majority of patients are colonized with *P. aeruginosa*; however *S. aureus*, *methicillin-resistant S. aureus*, and *Burkholderia cepacia complex* may be found.

Chronic infection with *P. aeruginosa* is an independent risk factor for accelerated loss of lung function and decreased survival (Simon, 2016a). Routine cultures of respiratory secretions are used to identify organisms and guide antibiotic selection. Two IV antibiotics typically are chosen to treat a severe exacerbation of *P. aeruginosa*. Tobramycin (Nebcin), along with piperacillin-tazobactam (Zosyn), a third-generation cephalosporin (e.g., ceftizoxime [Cefizox], ceftazidime [Fortaz]),

a carbapenem (e.g., meropenem [Merrem]), or aztreonam (Azactam) may be prescribed (Simon, 2016a). Dosing of antibiotics is determined on a case-by-case basis; some patients may require higher doses or an extended IV infusion. Careful monitoring is always required to minimize any side effects of the antibiotics.

Oral antibiotics such as dicloxacillin (Dynapen), amoxicillin-clavulanate or cephalexin (Keflex) may be appropriate to treat mild methicillin-sensitive *S. aureus* infection. For more serious exacerbations, oral linezolid (Zyvox) may be used (Simon, 2016a). Treatment is continued until the exacerbation has resolved and is usually a minimum of 10 days to as long as 3 weeks or more. Inhaled antibiotics may be used in severe exacerbations, bacterial resistance to all orally given antibiotics, or failure of oral antibiotics to resolve an exacerbation (Simon, 2016a).

In an acute exacerbation, airway clearance treatments may be used three to four times per day. The therapeutic options for chronic disease management of CF have undergone tremendous changes. Cornerstones of treatment include airway clearance measures, the mucolytic dornase alfa (Pulmozyme), nebulized antibiotics, antibiotic inhalation powder (tobramycin sulfate [TOBI Podhaler]), oral antibiotics, inhaled hypertonic saline, nutritional support, and exercise (Pittman & Ferkol, 2015).

Airway clearance is a key intervention, and various pulmonary techniques are used to enhance secretion clearance. Examples include manual postural drainage and chest physiotherapy; high-frequency chest wall oscillation; autogenic drainage (a combination of breathing techniques at different lung volume levels to move the secretions to where they can be huff-coughed out); and other devices that assist in airway clearance, such as masks that generate positive expiratory pressure (PEP masks) and "flutter devices" (devices that provide an oscillatory expiratory pressure pattern with PEP and assist with expectoration of secretions).

Dornase alfa is a nebulized medication given to degrade the large amount of deoxyribonucleic acid (DNA) that accumulates within CF mucus. This agent helps decrease the viscosity of the sputum and promotes expectoration of secretions. It is recommended for patients with moderate to severe disease (severity of lung disease classification is based on predicted FEV_1 percentage). In addition, inhaled hypertonic saline may be used in the chronic treatment of CF. Inhalations increase hydration of the airway surface liquid in patients with CF and improve airway clearance.

Nebulized and IV antibiotics or a combination may be used to treat chronic colonization of the lung. Nebulization provides high intrapulmonary drug concentrations and minimal systemic absorption. Inhaled tobramycin (TOBI) or aztreonam (AZLI) have been shown to decrease the frequency of pulmonary exacerbations. Acute infections are treated with a variety of IV antibiotics. Such infections remain a major cause of mortality related to pulmonary exacerbations in adults with CF.

Other therapeutic measures may be necessary as well. Anti-inflammatory agents may be used to treat inflammatory response in the airways. The CFF states that there is insufficient evidence for the use of routine inhaled or oral corticosteroids. IV corticosteroids are used during acute exacerbations and only for those patients with asthma-like symptoms (Simon, 2016b). Long-term use of high-dose non-steroidal anti-inflammatory agents (ibuprofen) is recommended in children ages 6 to 17 years to slow the loss of lung function, but is not recommended for patients older than 13 years of age as there is no evidence to support this practice (Pittman & Ferkol, 2015; Simon, 2016b). Inhaled bronchodilators (e.g., salmeterol [Serevent Diskus], tiotropium bromide [Spiriva]) may be used in patients who have a significant bronchoconstrictive component; this is confirmed by spirometry before and after therapy is instituted. (Simon, 2016b).

Nearly 90% of patients with CF have pancreatic exocrine insufficiency and require oral pancreatic enzyme supplementation with meals (CFF, 2015). Given the fat malabsorption in CF and increased caloric needs due to the work of breathing, nutritional counseling and weight monitoring are extremely important. Supplements of fat-soluble vitamins A, D, E, and K are also used.

CFTR modulators are a new class of drugs and help to improve function of the defective CFTR protein (Simon, 2016b). Ivacaftor (Kalydeco) was recently FDA-approved for adults and children ages 6 years of age and older. Ivacaftor is an oral CFTR potentiator designed to keep the proteins at the cell surface open more often to improve salt and water movement across the membrane (thus improving hydration and clearing of mucus from the airways). Only one gene mutation, G551D, is addressed by ivacaftor and this gene mutation occurs in approximately 4.4% of patients with CF (Simon, 2016b). The drug does not correct the gene mutation; it only helps in the movement of salt and water across the membrane.

Another CFTR drug, lumacaftor 200 mg/ivacaftor 125 mg (Orkambi) was FDA-approved to treat CF in patients 12 years and older, who have the deltaF508 mutation, which is present in approximately half of patients with CF in the United States (Cystic Fibrosis NewsToday, 2015). These newer drugs for CF are extremely costly with some insurance companies reluctant to pay for these treatments.

As the pulmonary deterioration advances, supplemental oxygen is used to treat the progressive hypoxemia that occurs with CF. It helps correct the hypoxemia and may minimize the complications seen with chronic hypoxemia (pulmonary hypertension). Lung transplantation is an option for a small, selected population of patients with CF. A double-lung transplantation technique is used because of chronic infection of both lungs in end-stage CF. Because there is a long waiting list for lung transplants, many patients die while waiting for suitable lungs for transplantation.

Nursing Management

Nursing management is crucial to the interdisciplinary approach required for care of adults with CF. Nursing care includes helping patients manage pulmonary symptoms and prevent complications. Specific measures include strategies that promote removal of pulmonary secretions, chest physiotherapy (including postural drainage, chest percussion, and vibration), and breathing exercises (which are implemented and taught to the patient and family when the patient is very young). The patient is reminded of the need to reduce risk factors associated with respiratory infections (e.g., exposure to crowds or to people with known infections). In addition, the patient is taught the early signs and symptoms of respiratory infection and disease progression that indicate the need to notify a primary provider.

The nurse emphasizes the importance of an adequate fluid and dietary intake to promote removal of secretions and to ensure an adequate nutritional status. Because CF is a lifelong disorder, patients often have learned to modify their daily activities to accommodate their symptoms and treatment modalities. As the disease progresses, periodic reassessment of the home environment may be warranted to identify modifications required to address changes in the patient's needs, increasing dyspnea and fatigue, and nonpulmonary symptoms.

As with any chronic disease, palliative care and end-of-life issues and concerns need to be addressed with the patient when warranted. For the patient whose disease is progressing and who is developing increasing hypoxemia, preferences for end-of-life care should be discussed, documented, and honored (see Chapter 16). Patients and family members require support as they face a shortened lifespan and an uncertain future.

CRITICAL THINKING EXERCISES

1 **PQ** In the ED, a 60-year-old man tells the triage nurse that he has limited insurance and does not have a primary provider because he lost his job 3 years ago. He presents with a chief complaint of increased shortness of breath and a change in the quantity and color of his sputum. He says he was diagnosed with COPD 6 years ago, but continues to smoke 2 packs per day. He says he usually has little sputum in the morning and that it is clear, but in the last week it has become yellow in color, continues all day, and is difficult to cough out. He is dyspneic at rest while sitting on the examination table and has difficulty completing a sentence without taking a breath. When asked if he has been on any medications, he told the nurse that he received an inhaler "for breathing" at the free clinic but that ran out a month ago. He does not know the name of the medication but it did help him breathe better. What are your focused priorities with this patient? For instance, what additional questions would you ask him? What are some of the physical examination findings you might observe or assess? What other tests might be ordered to continue to evaluate this patient and why? What resources might be appropriate for this patient before he leaves the hospital?

2 A 37-year-old African American woman with a history of asthma presents to the clinic with tachypnea and acute shortness of breath with audible wheezing. She says that she has continued to take her prescribed inhaler with no relief in symptoms and symptoms have gotten worse over time. She admits she was taking her inhaler more frequently than she was supposed to do. She called her doctor a week ago but could not get an appointment until today. Physical examination reveals tachycardia at 110 bpm and tachypnea at 30 breaths/min with signs of accessory muscle use. Auscultation reveals decreased breath sounds with inspiratory and expiratory wheezes. Her SaO_2 is 92% on room air. When you ask her what type of inhaler she uses, she says she has one for fast relief but did not bring it. She also could not afford the other one that that was prescribed 3 months ago. She never got it filled. The clinic is not equipped to give nebulizer treatments. What do you think the next step of care that may be needed with this patient? What type of education and resources would benefit this patient? What type of follow-up is needed for this patient?

3 **ebp** A 31-year-old woman with CF is admitted to your unit from the ED. She has been relatively free from exacerbations and started working about 3 months ago in an office setting. She obtains her CF care in a CF Center that is about 150 miles away from her home. She presently does not have a primary provider since she just moved to this city about 6 months ago. She lives alone. She has become progressively short of breath over the past week and has tried to manage her shortness of breath but finally came to the ED out of desperation. In short and choppy phrases, she tells you that she is extremely short of breath and that it has been getting worse; she is having paroxysms of coughing. You note that the cough is productive, with thick, yellow sputum, and that she is febrile. She does not know if she has lost any weight, but has not been able to eat. She is extremely anxious and wants to see her "regular CF doctor" who is 150 miles away. She says he is the only one that understands CF. What are the pathophysiologic mechanisms that have caused these clinical manifestations? What evidence-based medical and nursing interventions might be used to decrease or alleviate these signs and symptoms? What is the strength of the evidence? How might you help in decreasing the anxiety and fear she has about not being seen by her CF specialist? What members of the health care team would you consult and why?

REFERENCES

*Asterisk indicates nursing research.
**Double asterisk indicates classic reference.

Books

Gardenhire, D. S., Ari, A., Hess, D., et al. (2013). *A guide to aerosol delivery devices for respiratory therapists* (3rd ed.). Dallas, TX: American Association for Respiratory Care.

National Heart, Lung and Blood Institute (NHLBI). (2012). Asthma care quick reference: Diagnosing and managing asthma. NIH Publication No. 12–5075. Revised September 2012.

U.S. Department of Health and Human Services (HHS). (2014a). The Health Consequences of Smoking—50 Years of Progress: A Report of the Surgeon General. Atlanta, GA: U.S. Department of Health and Human Services, Centers for Disease Control and Prevention, National Center for Chronic Disease Prevention and Health Promotion, Office of Smoking and Health, 2014.

U.S. Department of Health and Human Services (HHS). (2014b). *Ending the tobacco epidemic: A tobacco control strategic action plan for the U.S. Department of Health and Human Services.* Washington, DC: Office of the Assistant Secretary for Health.

Journals and Electronic Documents

Agency for Healthcare Research and Quality. (2014). HCUPnet: Online query system based on data from the Healthcare Cost and Utilization Project. HCUPnet website. Retrieved on 5/19/2016 at: hcupnet.ahrq.gov/hcupnet/

American Academy of Allergy, Asthma and Immunology (AAAAI). (2016a). Occupational asthma. Retrieved on 1/10/2016 at: www.aaaai.org/conditions-and-treatments/library/at-a-glance/occupational-asthma

American Academy of Allergy, Asthma, and Immunology (AAAAI). (2016b). Medications that may trigger asthma symptoms. Retrieved on 5/18/2016 at: www.aaaai.org/conditions-and-treatments/library/asthma-library/medications-that-can-trigger-asthma-symptoms

American Liver Foundation. (2015). Alpha-1 antitrypsin deficiency. Retrieved on 12/1/2015 at: www.liverfoundation.org/abouttheliver/info/alphaone/

Barker, A. F. (2015a). Clinical manifestations and diagnosis of bronchiectasis in adults. UpToDate. Last updated December 10, 2015. Retrieved on 5/18/2016 at: www.uptodate.com/contents/clinical-manifestations-and-diagnosis-of-bronchiectasis-in-adults

Barker, A. F. (2015b). Treatment of bronchiectasis in adults. UpToDate. Last updated December 15, 2015. Retrieved on 5/18/2016 at: www.uptodate.com/contents/treatment-of-bronchiectasis-in-adults

Bartlett, J. G., & Sethi, S. (2016). Management of infection in exacerbations of chronic obstructive pulmonary disease. UpToDate. Last updated March 17, 2016. Retrieved on 5/18/2016 at: www.uptodate.com/contents/management-of-infection-in-exacerbations-of-chronic-obstructive-pulmonary-disease

Bellinger, C. R, & Peters, S. P. (2015). Outpatient COPD management: Going for the GOLD. *Journal of Allergy and Clinical Immunology Practice, 3*(4), 471–478.

Centers for Disease Control and Prevention (CDC). (2015a). FAST-STATS: Deaths: Final data for 2013, Table A. CDC/ National Center for Health Statistics. Last updated September 30, 2015. Retrieved on 4/18/2016 at: www.cdc.gov/nchs/fastats/deaths.htm

Centers for Disease Control and Prevention (CDC). (2015b). *Faststats sheet: Asthma.* Atlanta, GA: National Center for Health Statistics. Retrieved on 1/25/2016 at: www.cdc.gov/nchs/fastats/asthma.htm

Centers for Disease Control and Prevention (CDC). (2015c). *Asthma: data, statistics and surveillance.* Atlanta, GA: National Center for Health Statistics. Retrieved on 1/25/2016 at: www.cdc.gov/asthma/asthmadata.htm

Choby, G. W., & Lee, S. (2015). Pharmacotherapy for the treatment of asthma: current treatment options and future directions. *International Forum of Allergy and Rhinology, 5*(S1), S35–S40.

Cystic Fibrosis Foundation. (2015). About cystic fibrosis. Retrieved on 1/25/2016 at: www.cff.org/AboutCF/

Cystic Fibrosis News Today. (2015). Ivacaftor/lumacaftor (Orkambi). Retrieved on 5/19/18 at: cysticfibrosisnewstoday.com/orkambi-lumacaftor-ivacaftor-vertex/

*Geiger-Brown, J., Lindberg, S., Krachman, S., et al. (2015). Self-reported sleep quality and acute exacerbations of chronic obstructive pulmonary disease. *International Journal of COPD, 10*(1), 389–397.

Global Initiative for Chronic Obstructive Lung Disease (GOLD). (2015). Global strategy for the diagnosis, management and prevention of COPD. Retrieved on 4/18/2016 at: www.goldcopd.org/uploads/users/files/GOLD_Report_2015.pdf

Global Strategy for Asthma Management and Prevention, Global Initiative for Asthma (GINA). (2015). Retrieved on 1/25/2015 at: www.ginasthma.org/local/uploads/files/GINA_Report_2015_Aug11.pdf

Hooley, J. (2015). Decoding the oxyhemoglobin dissociation curve. *American Nurse Today, 10*(1), 18–23.

Katkin, J. P. (2016). Cystic fibrosis: clinical manifestations and diagnosis. UpToDate. Last updated March 28, 2016. Retrieved on 5/18/16 at: www.uptodate.com/contents/cystic-fibrosis-clinical-manifestations-of-pulmonary-disease/contributors

McCarthy, B., Casey, D., Murphy, K., et al. (2015). Pulmonary rehabilitation for chronic obstructive pulmonary disease. *Cochrane Database Systematic Review, 23*(2), CD003793.

Nakano, S. J. (2014). Genomic breakthroughs in the diagnosis and treatment of cystic fibrosis. *American Journal of Nursing, 114*(6), 36–44.

Pittman, J. E., & Ferkol, T. W. (2015). The evolution of cystic fibrosis care. *Chest, 148*(2), 533–542.

Rocker, G. M., Simpson, A. C., & Horton, R. (2015). Palliative care in advanced lung disease: The challenge of integrating palliation into everyday care. *Chest, 143*(3), 801–809.

Simon, R. H. (2016a). Cystic fibrosis: Antibiotic therapy for lung disease. UpToDate. Last updated April 12, 2016. Retrieved on 5/19/2016 at: www.uptodate.com/contents/cystic-fibrosis-antibiotic-therapy-for-lung-disease

Simon. R. H. (2016b). Cystic fibrosis: Overview of the treatment of lung disease. UpToDate. Last updated April 14, 2016. Retrieved on 5/19/2016 at: www.uptodate.com/contents/cystic-fibrosis-overview-of-the-treatment-of-lung-disease

Teva Respiratory. (2016). ProAir Respiclick: Highlights of prescribing information. Retrieved on 5/18/16 at: www.myproair.com/respiclick/library/docs/PI.pdf

Resources

Agency for Healthcare Research and Quality (AHRQ), www.ahrq.gov

Alpha-1 Foundation, www.alpha1.org

American Academy of Allergy, Asthma, and Immunology (AAAAI), www.aaaai.org

American Association for Respiratory Care (AARC), www.aarc.org

American Association of Cardiovascular and Pulmonary Rehabilitation (AACVPR), www.aacvpr.org

American Cancer Society, www.cancer.org

American College of Chest Physicians (ACCP), www.chestnet.org

American Lung Association, www.lungusa.org

American Thoracic Society (ATS), www.thoracic.org

Centers for Disease Control and Prevention (CDC), www.cdc.gov

COPD Foundation, www.copdfoundation.org

Cystic Fibrosis Foundation, www.cff.org

National Heart, Lung, and Blood Institute (NHLBI), www.nhlbi.nih.gov

SmokEnders, www.smokenders.org

U.S. Department of Health and Human Services (HHS), www.hhs.gov or healthfinder.gov

UNIT 6

Cardiovascular and Circulatory Function

AVOIDING A NEAR MISS WITH ANTICOAGUALTION THERAPY

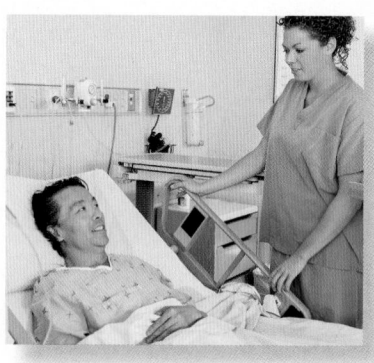

A 45-year-old patient is brought to the emergency department (ED) complaining of pain in his left lower leg, which is swollen and painful. Ultrasound reports reveal that he has a deep vein thrombosis (DVT). He is admitted to a general medical/surgical unit for anticoagulation therapy. He is begun on a weight-based heparin intravenous (IV) drip, with concomitant oral doses of warfarin (Coumadin). When the IV heparin arrives on the unit, the nurse notes that the prescribed order dose does not match the dose on the IV bag sent from the pharmacy. The nurse sends the bag back to the pharmacy, requesting that the correct dose be sent as soon as possible. The patient is anxious to begin the heparin therapy and asks the nurse why there is a delay in starting the heparin drip.

QSEN Competency Focus: Safety

The complexities inherent in today's health care system challenges nurses to demonstrate integration of specific interdisciplinary core competencies. These competencies are aimed at ensuring the delivery of safe, quality patient care (Institute of Medicine, 2003). The Quality and Safety Education for Nurses project (QSEN, 2017; Cronenwett, Sherwood, Barnsteiner, et al., 2007) provides a framework for the knowledge, skills, and attitudes (KSA) required for nurses to demonstrate competency in these key areas, which include *patient-centered care, interdisciplinary teamwork and collaboration, evidence-based practice, quality improvement, safety,* and *informatics.*

Safety Definition: Minimize risk of harm to patients and providers through both system effectiveness and individual performance.

SELECTED PRE-LICENSURE KSAs	APPLICATION AND REFLECTION
Knowledge	
Describe the factors that create a culture of safety (such as open communication strategies and organizational error reporting systems).	Identify how medication errors may occur in hospitals. Identify the different points during the process, from the time a medication is prescribed to the time it is given to a patient, that an error may occur. What system designs are in place in hospitals to prevent medication errors from occurring?
Skills	
Communicate observations or concerns related to hazards and errors to patients, families, and the health care team.	How and to whom should the nurse report this type of "near miss" event? Although a medication error was averted, the patient's treatment is delayed; describe how treatment delays such as these may also cause harm to patients. How should the nurse respond to the patient's question regarding his treatment delay? Should the nurse disclose that the wrong dose was sent to the unit by the pharmacy? Should others be involved in disclosing this "near miss" event to the patient?
Attitudes	
Value own role in preventing errors.	Reflect on how you would feel in this type of situation. Would you be pleased with yourself for discovering the error and inclined to blame the pharmacist? Or would you feel concerned that a flaw in the hospital's system design allowed this type of "near miss" event to occur, and frightened that you could have administered the wrong dose of medication to this patient? How could you engage in system-design advocacy so that this type of safety-design flaw is rectified? How comfortable would you be in disclosing an error or potential error to a patient?

Cronenwett, L., Sherwood, G., Barnsteiner, J., et al. (2007). Quality and safety education for nurses. *Nursing Outlook, 55*(3), 122–131.
Institute of Medicine. (2003). *Health professions education: A bridge to quality.* Washington, DC: National Academies Press.
QSEN Institute. (2017). *QSEN Competencies: Definitions and pre-licensure KSAs.* Retrieved on 3/1/2017 at: www.qsen.org/competencies/pre-licensure-ksas.

Assessment of Cardiovascular Function

LEARNING OBJECTIVES

On completion of this chapter, the learner will be able to:

1 Describe the relationship between the anatomic structures and the physiologic function of the cardiovascular system.
2 Incorporate assessment of cardiac risk factors into the health history and physical assessment of the patient with cardiovascular disease.
3 Explain the proper techniques to perform a comprehensive cardiovascular assessment.
4 Discriminate between normal and abnormal assessment findings identified by inspection, palpation, percussion, and auscultation of the cardiovascular system.

5 Recognize and evaluate the major manifestations of cardiovascular dysfunction by applying concepts from the patient's health history and physical assessment findings.
6 Discuss the clinical indications, patient preparation, and other related nursing implications for common tests and procedures used to assess cardiovascular function and diagnose cardiovascular diseases.
7 Compare the various methods of hemodynamic monitoring (e.g., central venous pressure, pulmonary artery pressure, and arterial pressure monitoring) with regard to indications for use, potential complications, and nursing responsibilities.

GLOSSARY

acute coronary syndrome: a constellation of signs and symptoms due to the rupture of atherosclerotic plaque and resultant partial or complete thrombosis within a diseased coronary artery; leads to unstable angina or acute myocardial infarction

afterload: the amount of resistance to ejection of blood from the ventricle

apical impulse: impulse normally palpated at the fifth intercostal space, left midclavicular line; caused by contraction of the left ventricle; also called the *point of maximal impulse*

atrioventricular (AV) node: secondary pacemaker of the heart, located in the right atrial wall near the tricuspid valve

baroreceptors: nerve fibers located in the aortic arch and carotid arteries that are responsible for control of the blood pressure

cardiac catheterization: an invasive procedure used to measure cardiac chamber pressures and assess patency of the coronary arteries

cardiac conduction system: specialized heart cells strategically located throughout the heart that are responsible for methodically generating and coordinating the transmission of electrical impulses to the myocardial cells

cardiac output: amount of blood pumped by each ventricle in liters per minute

cardiac stress test: a test used to evaluate the functioning of the heart during a period of increased oxygen demand; test may be initiated by exercise or medications

contractility: ability of the cardiac muscle to shorten in response to an electrical impulse

depolarization: electrical activation of a cell caused by the influx of sodium into the cell while potassium exits the cell

diastole: period of ventricular relaxation resulting in ventricular filling

ejection fraction: percentage of the end-diastolic blood volume ejected from the ventricle with each heartbeat

hemodynamic monitoring: the use of pressure monitoring devices to directly measure cardiovascular function

hypertension: blood pressure that is persistently greater than 140/90 mm Hg

hypotension: a decrease in blood pressure to less than 100/60 mm Hg that compromises systemic perfusion

murmurs: sounds created by abnormal, turbulent flow of blood in the heart

myocardial ischemia: condition in which heart muscle cells receive less oxygen than needed

myocardium: muscle layer of the heart responsible for the pumping action of the heart

normal heart sounds: sounds produced when the valves close; normal heart sounds are S_1 (atrioventricular valves) and S_2 (semilunar valves)

opening snaps: abnormal diastolic sound generated during opening of a rigid atrioventricular valve leaflet

postural (orthostatic) hypotension: a significant drop in blood pressure (20 mm Hg systolic or more or 10 mm Hg diastolic or more) after an upright posture is assumed

preload: degree of stretch of the cardiac muscle fibers at the end of diastole

pulmonary vascular resistance: resistance to blood flow out of the right ventricle created by the pulmonary circulatory system

pulse deficit: the difference between the apical and radial pulse rates

radioisotopes: unstable atoms that give off small amounts of energy in the form of gamma rays as they decay; used in cardiac nuclear medicine studies

repolarization: return of the cell to resting state, caused by reentry of potassium into the cell while sodium exits the cell

S_1: the first heart sound produced by closure of the atrioventricular (mitral and tricuspid) valves

S_2: the second heart sound produced by closure of the semilunar (aortic and pulmonic) valves

S_3: an abnormal heart sound detected early in diastole as resistance is met to blood entering either ventricle; most often due to volume overload associated with heart failure

S_4: an abnormal heart sound detected late in diastole as resistance is met to blood entering either ventricle during atrial contraction; most often caused by hypertrophy of the ventricle

sinoatrial (SA) node: primary pacemaker of the heart, located in the right atrium

stroke volume: amount of blood ejected from one of the ventricles per heartbeat

summation gallop: abnormal sounds created by the presence of an S_3 and S_4 during periods of tachycardia

systemic vascular resistance: resistance to blood flow out of the left ventricle created by the systemic circulatory system

systole: period of ventricular contraction resulting in ejection of blood from the ventricles into the pulmonary artery and aorta

systolic click: abnormal systolic sound created by the opening of a calcified aortic or pulmonic valve during ventricular contraction

telemetry: the process of continuous electrocardiographic monitoring by the transmission of radio waves from a battery-operated transmitter worn by the patient

More than 85.6 million Americans have one or more types of cardiovascular disease (CVD), including hypertension, coronary artery disease (CAD), heart failure (HF), stroke, and congenital cardiovascular defects (American Heart Association [AHA], 2016). Because of the prevalence of CVD, nurses practicing in any setting across the continuum of care, whether in the home, office, hospital, long-term care facility, or rehabilitation facility, must be able to assess the cardiovascular system. Key components of assessment include a health history, physical assessment, and monitoring of a variety of laboratory and diagnostic test results. This assessment provides the information necessary to identify nursing diagnoses, formulate an individualized plan of care, evaluate the response of the patient to the care provided, and revise the plan as needed.

Anatomic and Physiologic Overview

An understanding of the structure and function of the heart in health and in disease is essential to develop cardiovascular assessment skills.

Anatomy of the Heart

The heart is a hollow, muscular organ located in the center of the thorax, where it occupies the space between the lungs (mediastinum) and rests on the diaphragm. It weighs approximately 300 g (10.6 oz); the weight and size of the heart are influenced by age, gender, body weight, extent of physical exercise and conditioning, and heart disease. The heart pumps blood to the tissues, supplying them with oxygen and other nutrients.

The heart is composed of three layers (see Fig. 25-1). The inner layer, or endocardium, consists of endothelial tissue and lines the inside of the heart and valves. The middle layer, or **myocardium,** is made up of muscle fibers and is responsible for the pumping action. The exterior layer of the heart is called the *epicardium*.

The heart is encased in a thin, fibrous sac called the *pericardium*, which is composed of two layers. Adhering to the epicardium is the visceral pericardium. Enveloping the visceral pericardium is the parietal pericardium, a tough fibrous tissue that attaches to the great vessels, diaphragm, sternum, and vertebral column and supports the heart in the mediastinum. The space between these two layers (pericardial space) is normally filled with about 20 mL of fluid, which lubricates the surface of the heart and reduces friction during systole.

Heart Chambers

The pumping action of the heart is accomplished by the rhythmic relaxation and contraction of the muscular walls of its two top chambers (atria) and two bottom chambers (ventricles). During the relaxation phase, called **diastole**, all four chambers relax simultaneously, which allows the ventricles to fill in preparation for contraction. Diastole is commonly referred to as the period of ventricular filling. **Systole** refers to the events in the heart during contraction of the atria and the ventricles. Unlike diastole, atrial and ventricular systole are not simultaneous events. Atrial systole occurs first, just at the end of diastole, followed by ventricular systole. This synchronization allows the ventricles to fill completely prior to ejection of blood from these chambers.

The right side of the heart, made up of the right atrium and right ventricle, distributes venous blood (deoxygenated blood) to the lungs via the pulmonary artery (pulmonary circulation) for oxygenation. The pulmonary artery is the only artery in the body that carries deoxygenated blood. The right atrium receives venous blood returning to the heart from the superior vena cava (head, neck, and upper extremities), inferior vena cava (trunk and lower extremities), and coronary sinus (coronary circulation). The left side of the heart, composed of the left atrium and left ventricle, distributes oxygenated blood to the remainder of the body via the aorta (systemic circulation). The left atrium receives oxygenated blood from the pulmonary circulation via four pulmonary veins. The flow of blood through the four heart chambers is shown in Figure 25-1.

The varying thicknesses of the atrial and ventricular walls are due to the workload required by each chamber. The myocardial layer of both atria is much thinner than that of the ventricles because there is little resistance as blood flows out of the atria and into the ventricles during diastole. In contrast, the ventricular walls are much thicker than the atrial walls.

Superior vena cava
Right pulmonary artery
Interatrial septum
Pulmonary veins
Pulmonic valve
Right atrium
Tricuspid valve
Inferior vena cava
Right ventricle
Papillary muscle
Interventricular septum

Aortic arch
Left pulmonary artery
Descending aorta
Pulmonary veins
Left atrium
Aortic valve
Mitral valve
Left ventricle
Chordae tendinae
Papillary muscle

Visceral pericardium
Parietal pericardium
Endocardium
Myocardium
Epicardium
Pericardial space

→ Unoxygenated blood
→ Oxygenated blood

Figure 25-1 • Structure of the heart. *Arrows* show course of blood flow through the heart chambers.

During ventricular systole, the right and left ventricles must overcome resistance to blood flow from the pulmonary and systemic circulatory systems, respectively. The left ventricle is two to three times more muscular than the right ventricle. It must overcome high aortic and arterial pressures, whereas the right ventricle contracts against a low-pressure system within the pulmonary arteries and capillaries (Woods, Froelicher,

Motzer, et al., 2009). Figure 25-2 identifies the pressures in each of these areas.

The heart lies in a rotated position within the chest cavity. The right ventricle lies anteriorly (just beneath the sternum), and the left ventricle is situated posteriorly. As a result of this close proximity to the chest wall, the pulsation created during normal ventricular contraction, called the

Superior vena cava
Right pulmonary artery
Interatrial septum
Pulmonary veins
Pulmonic valve
Right atrium
Tricuspid valve
Inferior vena cava
Right ventricle
Papillary muscle
Interventricular septum

Aortic arch
Left pulmonary artery
Descending aorta
Pulmonary veins
Left atrium
Aortic valve
Mitral valve
Left ventricle
Chordae tendinae
Papillary muscle

8–10   110–130 / 70–90
15–25 / 8–15
0–8   4–12
110–130 / 4–12
15–25 / 0–8

Figure 25-2 • Great vessel and chamber pressures. Pressures are identified in millimeters of mercury (mm Hg) as mean pressure or systolic over diastolic pressure.

apical impulse (also called the *point of maximal impulse* [PMI]), is easily detected. In the normal heart, the PMI is located at the intersection of the midclavicular line of the left chest wall and the fifth intercostal space (Bickley, 2014).

Heart Valves

The four valves in the heart permit blood to flow in only one direction. The valves, which are composed of thin leaflets of fibrous tissue, open and close in response to the movement of blood and pressure changes within the chambers. There are two types of valves: atrioventricular (AV) and semilunar.

Atrioventricular Valves

The AV valves separate the atria from the ventricles. The tricuspid valve, so named because it is composed of three cusps or leaflets, separates the right atrium from the right ventricle. The mitral or bicuspid (two cusps) valve lies between the left atrium and the left ventricle (see Fig. 25-1).

During diastole, the tricuspid and mitral valves are open, allowing the blood in the atria to flow freely into the relaxed ventricles. As ventricular systole begins, the ventricles contract and blood flows upward into the cusps of the tricuspid and mitral valves, causing them to close. As the pressure against these valves increases, two additional structures, the papillary muscles and the chordae tendineae, maintain valve closure. The papillary muscles, located on the sides of the ventricular walls, are connected to the valve leaflets by the chordae tendineae, which are thin fibrous bands. During ventricular systole, contraction of the papillary muscles causes the chordae tendineae to become taut, keeping the valve leaflets approximated and closed. This action prevents backflow of blood into the atria (regurgitation) as blood is ejected out into the pulmonary artery and aorta.

Semilunar Valves

The two semilunar valves are composed of three leaflets, which are shaped like half-moons. The valve between the right ventricle and the pulmonary artery is called the *pulmonic valve*. The valve between the left ventricle and the aorta is called the *aortic valve*. The semilunar valves are closed during diastole. At this point, the pressure in the pulmonary artery and aorta decreases, causing blood to flow back toward the semilunar valves. This action fills the cusps with blood and closes the valves. The semilunar valves are forced open during ventricular systole as blood is ejected from the right and left ventricles into the pulmonary artery and aorta, respectively.

Coronary Arteries

The left and right coronary arteries and their branches supply arterial blood to the heart. These arteries originate from the aorta just above the aortic valve leaflets. The heart has high metabolic requirements, extracting approximately 70% to 80% of the oxygen delivered (other organs extract, on average, 25%) (Woods et al., 2009). Unlike other arteries, the coronary arteries are perfused during diastole. With a normal heart rate of 60 to 80 bpm, there is ample time during diastole for myocardial perfusion. However, as heart rate increases, diastolic time is shortened, which may not allow adequate time for myocardial perfusion. As a result, patients are at risk for **myocardial ischemia** (inadequate oxygen supply) during tachycardia (heart rate greater than 100 bpm), especially patients with CAD.

The left coronary artery has three branches. The artery from the point of origin to the first major branch is called the *left main coronary artery*. Two branches arise from the left main coronary artery: the left anterior descending artery, which courses down the anterior wall of the heart, and the circumflex artery, which circles around to the lateral left wall of the heart.

The right side of the heart is supplied by the *right coronary artery*, which travels to the inferior wall of the heart. The posterior wall of the heart receives its blood supply by an additional branch from the right coronary artery called the *posterior descending artery* (see Fig. 27-2 in Chapter 27).

Superficial to the coronary arteries are the coronary veins. Venous blood from these veins returns to the heart primarily through the coronary sinus, which is located posteriorly in the right atrium.

Myocardium

The myocardium is the middle, muscular layer of the atrial and ventricular walls. It is composed of specialized cells called *myocytes*, which form an interconnected network of muscle fibers. These fibers encircle the heart in a figure-of-eight pattern, forming a spiral from the base (top) of the heart to the apex (bottom). During contraction, this muscular configuration facilitates a twisting and compressive movement of the heart that begins in the atria and moves to the ventricles. The sequential and rhythmic pattern of contraction, followed by relaxation of the muscle fibers, maximizes the volume of blood ejected with each contraction. This cyclical pattern of myocardial contraction is controlled by the conduction system.

Function of the Heart

Cardiac Electrophysiology

The **cardiac conduction system** generates and transmits electrical impulses that stimulate contraction of the myocardium. Under normal circumstances, the conduction system first stimulates contraction of the atria and then the ventricles. The synchronization of the atrial and ventricular events allows the ventricles to fill completely before ventricular ejection, thereby maximizing cardiac output. Three physiologic characteristics of two types of specialized electrical cells, the nodal cells and the Purkinje cells, provide this synchronization:

- *Automaticity*: ability to initiate an electrical impulse
- *Excitability*: ability to respond to an electrical impulse
- *Conductivity*: ability to transmit an electrical impulse from one cell to another

Both the **sinoatrial (SA) node** (the primary pacemaker of the heart) and the **atrioventricular (AV) node** (the secondary pacemaker of the heart) are composed of nodal cells. The SA node is located at the junction of the superior vena cava and the right atrium (see Fig. 25-3). The SA node in a normal resting adult heart has an inherent firing rate of 60 to 100 impulses per minute; however, the rate changes in response to the metabolic demands of the body (Weber & Kelley, 2014).

The electrical impulses initiated by the SA node are conducted along the myocardial cells of the atria via specialized tracts called *internodal pathways*. The impulses cause electrical stimulation and subsequent contraction of the atria.

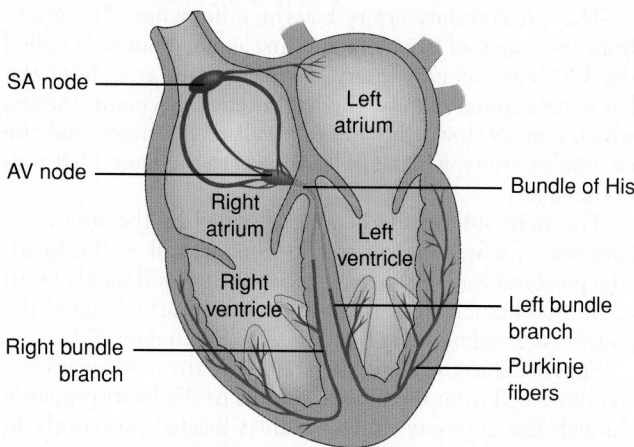

Figure 25-3 • Cardiac conduction system. AV, atrioventricular; SA, sinoatrial.

The impulses are then conducted to the AV node, which is located in the right atrial wall near the tricuspid valve (see Fig. 25-3). The AV node coordinates the incoming electrical impulses from the atria and after a slight delay (allowing the atria time to contract and complete ventricular filling) relays the impulse to the ventricles.

Initially, the impulse is conducted through a bundle of specialized conducting tissue, referred to as the bundle of His, which then divides into the right bundle branch (conducting impulses to the right ventricle) and the left bundle branch (conducting impulses to the left ventricle). To transmit impulses to the left ventricle—the largest chamber of the heart—the left bundle branch divides into the left anterior and left posterior bundle branches. Impulses travel through the bundle branches to reach the terminal point in the conduction system, called the *Purkinje fibers*. These fibers are composed of Purkinje cells that rapidly conduct impulses throughout the thick walls of the ventricles. This action stimulates the ventricular myocardial cells to contract (Weber & Kelley, 2014).

The heart rate is determined by the myocardial cells with the fastest inherent firing rate. Under normal circumstances, the SA node has the highest inherent rate (60 to 100 impulses per minute), the AV node has the second-highest inherent rate (40 to 60 impulses per minute), and the ventricular pacemaker sites have the lowest inherent rate (30 to 40 impulses per minute) (Woods et al., 2009). If the SA node malfunctions, the AV node generally takes over the pacemaker function of the heart at its inherently lower rate. Should both the SA and the AV nodes fail in their pacemaker function, a pacemaker site in the ventricle will fire at its inherent bradycardic rate of 30 to 40 impulses per minute.

Cardiac Action Potential

The nodal and Purkinje cells (electrical cells) generate and transmit impulses across the heart, stimulating the cardiac myocytes (working cells) to contract. Stimulation of the myocytes occurs due to the exchange of electrically charged particles, called *ions*, across channels located in the cell membrane. The channels regulate the movement and speed of specific ions—namely, sodium, potassium, and calcium—as they enter and exit the cell. Sodium rapidly enters into the cell

through sodium fast channels, in contrast to calcium, which enters the cell through calcium slow channels. In the resting or polarized state, sodium is the primary extracellular ion, whereas potassium is the primary intracellular ion. This difference in ion concentration means that the inside of the cell has a negative charge compared with the positive charge on the outside. The relationship changes during cellular stimulation, when sodium or calcium crosses the cell membrane into the cell and potassium ions exit into the extracellular space. This exchange of ions creates a positively charged intracellular space and a negatively charged extracellular space that characterizes the period known as **depolarization**. Once depolarization is complete, the exchange of ions reverts to its resting state; this period is known as **repolarization**. The repeated cycle of depolarization and repolarization is called the *cardiac action potential*.

As shown in Figure 25-4, the cardiac action potential has five phases:

- *Phase 0:* Cellular depolarization is initiated as positive ions influx into the cell. During this phase, the atrial and ventricular myocytes rapidly depolarize as sodium moves into the cells through sodium fast channels. The myocytes have a fast response action potential. In contrast, the cells of the SA and AV node depolarize when calcium enters these cells through calcium slow channels. These cells have a slow response action potential.
- *Phase 1:* Early cellular repolarization begins during this phase as potassium exits the intracellular space.
- *Phase 2:* This phase is called the *plateau phase* because the rate of repolarization slows. Calcium ions enter the intracellular space.
- *Phase 3:* This phase marks the completion of repolarization and return of the cell to its resting state.
- *Phase 4:* This phase is considered the resting phase before the next depolarization.

Refractory Periods

Myocardial cells must completely repolarize before they can depolarize again. During the repolarization process, the cells are in a refractory period. There are two phases of the refractory period: the effective (or absolute) refractory period and the relative refractory period. During the effective refractory period, the cell is completely unresponsive to any electrical stimulus; it is incapable of initiating an early depolarization.

Figure 25-4 • Cardiac action potential of a fast-response Purkinje fiber. The *arrows* indicate the approximate time and direction of movement of each ion influencing membrane potential. Ca++ movement out of the cell is not well defined but is thought to occur during phase 4.

The effective refractory period corresponds with the time in phase 0 to the middle of phase 3 of the action potential. The relative refractory period corresponds with the short time at the end of phase 3. During the relative refractory period, if an electrical stimulus is stronger than normal, the cell may depolarize prematurely. Early depolarizations of the atrium or ventricle cause premature contractions, placing the patient at risk for dysrhythmias. Premature ventricular contractions in certain situations, such as the presence of myocardial ischemia, are of concern because these early ventricular depolarizations can trigger life-threatening dysrhythmias, including ventricular tachycardia or ventricular fibrillation. Several circumstances make the heart more susceptible to early depolarization during the relative refractory period, thus increasing the risk for serious dysrhythmias. (These dysrhythmias and others are discussed in detail in Chapter 26.)

Cardiac Hemodynamics

An important determinant of blood flow in the cardiovascular system is the principle that fluid flows from a region of higher pressure to one of lower pressure (see Fig. 25-2). The pressures responsible for blood flow in the normal circulation are generated during systole and diastole.

Cardiac Cycle

The cardiac cycle refers to the events that occur in the heart from the beginning of one heartbeat to the next. The number of cardiac cycles completed in a minute depends on the heart rate. Each cardiac cycle has three major sequential events: diastole, atrial systole, and ventricular systole. These events cause blood to flow through the heart due to changes in chamber pressures and valvular function during diastole and systole. During diastole, all four heart chambers are relaxed. As a result, the AV valves are open and the semilunar valves are closed. Pressures in all of the chambers are the lowest during diastole, which facilitates ventricular filling. Venous blood returns to the right atrium from the superior and inferior vena cava, then into the right ventricle. On the left side, oxygenated blood returns from the lungs via the four pulmonary veins into the left atrium and ventricle.

Toward the end of this diastolic period, atrial systole occurs as the atrial muscles contract in response to an electrical impulse initiated by the SA node. Atrial systole increases the pressure inside the atria, ejecting the remaining blood into the ventricles. Atrial systole augments ventricular blood volume by 15% to 25% and is sometimes referred to as the atrial kick (Woods et al., 2009). At this point, ventricular systole begins in response to propagation of the electrical impulse that began in the SA node some milliseconds earlier.

Beginning with ventricular systole, the pressure inside the ventricles rapidly increases, forcing the AV valves to close. As a result, blood ceases to flow from the atria into the ventricles, and regurgitation (backflow) of blood into the atria is prevented. The rapid increase in pressure inside the right and left ventricles forces the pulmonic and aortic valves to open, and blood is ejected into the pulmonary artery and aorta, respectively. The exit of blood is at first rapid; then, as the pressure in each ventricle and its corresponding artery equalizes, the flow of blood gradually decreases. At the end of systole, pressure within the right and left ventricles rapidly decreases. As a result, pulmonary arterial and aortic pressures decrease, causing

closure of the semilunar valves. These events mark the onset of diastole, and the cardiac cycle is repeated.

Chamber pressures can be measured with the use of special monitoring catheters and equipment. This technique is called *hemodynamic monitoring*. Methods of hemodynamic monitoring are covered in more detail at the end of this chapter.

Cardiac Output

Cardiac output refers to the total amount of blood ejected by one of the ventricles in liters per minute. The cardiac output in a resting adult is 4 to 6 L/min but varies greatly depending on the metabolic needs of the body. Cardiac output is computed by multiplying the stroke volume by the heart rate. **Stroke volume** is the amount of blood ejected from one of the ventricles per heartbeat. The average resting stroke volume is about 60 to 130 mL (Woods et al., 2009).

Effect of Heart Rate on Cardiac Output

The cardiac output responds to changes in the metabolic demands of the tissues associated with stress, physical exercise, and illness. To compensate for these added demands, the cardiac output is enhanced by increases in both stroke volume and heart rate. Changes in heart rate are due to inhibition or stimulation of the SA node mediated by the parasympathetic and sympathetic divisions of the autonomic nervous system. The balance between these two reflex control systems normally determines the heart rate. Branches of the parasympathetic nervous system travel to the SA node by the vagus nerve. Stimulation of the vagus nerve slows the heart rate. The sympathetic nervous system increases heart rate by innervation of the beta-1 receptor sites located within the SA node. The heart rate is increased by the sympathetic nervous system through an increased level of circulating catecholamines (secreted by the adrenal gland) and by excess thyroid hormone, which produces a catecholamine-like effect.

In addition, the heart rate is affected by central nervous system and baroreceptor activity. **Baroreceptors** are specialized nerve cells located in the aortic arch and in both right and left internal carotid arteries (at the point of bifurcation from the common carotid arteries). The baroreceptors are sensitive to changes in blood pressure (BP). During significant elevations in BP (**hypertension**), these cells increase their rate of discharge, transmitting impulses to the cerebral medulla. This action initiates parasympathetic activity and inhibits sympathetic response, lowering the heart rate and the BP. The opposite is true during **hypotension** (low BP). Less baroreceptor stimulation during periods of hypotension prompts a decrease in parasympathetic activity and enhances sympathetic responses. These compensatory mechanisms attempt to elevate the BP through vasoconstriction and increased heart rate.

Effect of Stroke Volume on Cardiac Output

Stroke volume is primarily determined by three factors: preload, afterload, and contractility.

Preload refers to the degree of stretch of the ventricular cardiac muscle fibers at the end of diastole. The end of diastole is the period when filling volume in the ventricles is the highest and the degree of stretch on the muscle fibers is the greatest. The volume of blood within the ventricle at the end of diastole determines preload, which directly affects stroke volume. Therefore, preload is commonly referred to as left ventricular end-diastolic pressure. As the volume of blood returning to the heart increases, muscle fiber stretch also increases (increased preload), resulting in stronger contraction and a greater stroke volume. This relationship, referred to as the Frank–Starling (or Starling) law of the heart, is maintained until the physiologic limit of the muscle is reached.

The Frank–Starling law is based on the fact that, within limits, the greater the initial length or stretch of the cardiac muscle cells (sarcomeres), the greater the degree of shortening that occurs. This result is caused by increased interaction between the thick and thin filaments within the cardiac muscle cells. Preload is decreased by a reduction in the volume of blood returning to the ventricles. Diuresis, venodilating agents (e.g., nitrates), excessive loss of blood, or dehydration (excessive loss of body fluids from vomiting, diarrhea, or diaphoresis) reduce preload. Preload is increased by increasing the return of circulating blood volume to the ventricles. Controlling the loss of blood or body fluids and replacing fluids (i.e., blood transfusions and intravenous [IV] fluid administration) are examples of ways to increase preload.

Afterload, or resistance to ejection of blood from the ventricle, is the second determinant of stroke volume. The resistance of the systemic BP to left ventricular ejection is called **systemic vascular resistance**. The resistance of the pulmonary BP to right ventricular ejection is called **pulmonary vascular resistance**. There is an inverse relationship between afterload and stroke volume. For example, afterload is increased by arterial vasoconstriction, which leads to decreased stroke volume. The opposite is true with arterial vasodilation, in which case afterload is reduced because there is less resistance to ejection, and stroke volume increases.

Contractility refers to the force generated by the contracting myocardium. Contractility is enhanced by circulating catecholamines, sympathetic neuronal activity, and certain medications (e.g., digoxin [Lanoxin], dopamine, or dobutamine). Increased contractility results in increased stroke volume. Contractility is depressed by hypoxemia, acidosis, and certain medications (e.g., beta-adrenergic blocking agents such as metoprolol [Lopressor]).

The heart can achieve an increase in stroke volume (e.g., during exercise) if preload is increased (through increased venous return), if contractility is increased (through sympathetic nervous system discharge), and if afterload is decreased (through peripheral vasodilation with decreased aortic pressure).

The percentage of the end-diastolic blood volume that is ejected with each heartbeat is called the **ejection fraction.** The ejection fraction of the normal left ventricle is 55% to 65% (Woods et al., 2009). The right ventricular ejection fraction is rarely measured. The ejection fraction is used as a measure of myocardial contractility. An ejection fraction of less than 40% indicates that the patient has decreased left ventricular function and likely requires treatment of HF (refer to Chapter 29 for further discussion).

Gerontologic Considerations

Changes in cardiac structure and function occur with age. A loss of function of the cells throughout the conduction system leads to a slower heart rate. The size of the heart increases due to hypertrophy (thickening of the heart walls), which reduces the volume of blood that the chambers can hold. Hypertrophy also changes the structure of the myocardium, reducing the strength

of contraction. Both of these changes negatively affect cardiac output. The valves, due to stiffening, no longer close properly. The resulting backflow of blood creates heart murmurs, a common finding in older adults (Bickley, 2014; Woods et al., 2009).

As a result of these age-related changes, the cardiovascular system takes longer to compensate from increased metabolic demands due to stress, exercise, or illness. In these situations, older adults may become symptomatic with fatigue, shortness of breath, or palpitations and present with new physical examination findings (Bickley, 2014; Woods et al., 2009). The structural and functional changes with aging and associated history and physical examination findings are summarized in Table 25-1.

Gender Considerations

Structural differences between the hearts of men and women have significant implications. The heart of a woman tends to be smaller than that of a man. The coronary arteries of a woman are also narrower in diameter than a man's arteries. When atherosclerosis occurs, these differences make procedures such as cardiac catheterization and angioplasty technically more difficult.

Women typically develop CAD 10 years later than men, as women have the benefit of the female hormone estrogen and its cardioprotective effects. The three major effects of estrogen are (1) an increase in high-density lipoprotein (HDL) that transports cholesterol out of arteries; (2) a reduction in low-density lipoprotein (LDL) that deposits cholesterol in the artery; and (3) dilatation of the blood vessels, which enhance blood flow to the heart. As women reach menopause, around 50 years of age, estrogen levels slowly disappear and place women at higher risk for CAD. By age 45 years for men and 55 years of age for women, the risk for CAD is equivalent (McSweeney, Rosenfeld, Abel, et al., 2016).

In the past, hormone therapy (HT) was routinely prescribed for postmenopausal women with the belief that it would deter the onset and progression of CAD. However, the AHA no longer recommends its use due to strong evidence that HT is not a beneficial CAD preventative strategy for women (McSweeney et al., 2016). In fact, recent studies report that HT after menopause can be harmful to women by putting them at increased risk for stroke and venous thromboembolic events (Boardman, Hartley, Eisinga, et al., 2015).

Assessment of the Cardiovascular System

The frequency and extent of the nursing assessment of cardiovascular function are based on several factors, including the severity of the patient's symptoms, the presence of risk factors, the practice setting, and the purpose of the assessment. An acutely ill patient with CVD who is admitted to the emergency department (ED) or intensive care unit (ICU) requires a very different assessment than a person who is being examined for a chronic stable condition. Although the key components of the cardiovascular assessment remain the same, the assessment priorities vary according to the needs of the patient. For example, an ED nurse performs a rapid and focused assessment of a patient in which **acute coronary syndrome** (ACS), signs and symptoms caused by

TABLE 25-1 Age-Related Changes of the Cardiac System

Cardiovascular Structure	Structural Changes	Functional Changes	History and Physical Findings
Atria	↑ Size of left atrium Thickening of the endocardium	↑ Atrial irritability	Irregular heart rhythm from atrial dysrhythmias
Left ventricle	Endocardial fibrosis Myocardial thickening (hypertrophy) Infiltration of fat into myocardium	Left ventricle stiff and less compliant Progressive decline in cardiac output ↑ Risk for ventricular dysrhythmias Prolonged systole	Fatigue ↓ Exercise tolerance Signs and symptoms of heart failure or ventricular dysrhythmias Point of maximal impulse palpated lateral to the midclavicular line ↓ Intensity S_1, S_2; split S_2 S_4 may be present
Valves	Thickening and rigidity of AV valves Calcification of aortic valve	Abnormal blood flow across valves during cardiac cycle	Murmurs may be present Thrill may be palpated if significant murmur is present
Conduction system	Connective tissue collects in SA node, AV node, and bundle branches ↓ Number of SA node cells ↓ Number of AV, bundle of His, and right and left bundle branch cells	Slower SA node rate of impulse discharge Slowed conduction across AV node and ventricular conduction system	Bradycardia Heart block ECG changes consistent with slowed conduction (↑ PR interval, widened QRS complex)
Sympathetic nervous system	↓ Response to beta-adrenergic stimulation	↓ Adaptive response to exercise: contractility and heart rate slower to respond to exercise demands Heart rate takes more time to return to baseline	Fatigue Diminished exercise tolerance ↓ Ability to respond to stress
Aorta and arteries	Stiffening of vasculature ↓ Elasticity and widening of aorta Elongation of aorta, displacing the brachiocephalic artery upward	Left ventricular hypertrophy	Progressive increase in systolic BP; slight ↑ in diastolic BP Widening pulse pressure Pulsation visible above right clavicle
Baroreceptor response	↓ Sensitivity of baroreceptors in the carotid artery and aorta to transient episodes of hypertension and hypotension	Baroreceptors unable to regulate heart rate and vascular tone, causing slow response to postural changes in body position	Postural BP changes and reports of feeling dizzy, fainting when moving from lying to sitting or standing position

AV, atrioventricular; SA, sinoatrial; ECG, electrocardiographic; BP, blood pressure.
Adapted from Bickley, L. S. (2014). *Bates' guide to physical examination and history taking* (11th ed.). Philadelphia, PA: Lippincott Williams & Wilkins.

ruptured atheromatous plaque in a diseased coronary artery, is suspected. Diagnosis and treatment must be started within minutes of arrival to the ED. The physical assessment is ongoing and concentrates on evaluating the patient for ACS complications, such as dysrhythmias and HF, and determining the effectiveness of medical treatment.

Health History

The patient's ability to recognize cardiac symptoms and to know what to do when they occur is essential for effective self-care management. All too often, a patient's new symptoms or those of progressing cardiac dysfunction go unrecognized. This results in prolonged delays in seeking lifesaving treatment. Major barriers to seeking prompt medical care include lack of knowledge about the symptoms of heart disease, attributing symptoms to a benign source, denying symptom significance, and feeling embarrassed about having symptoms (Gillis, Arslanian-Engoren, & Struble, 2014). Therefore, during the health history, the nurse determines if the patient and involved family members are able to recognize symptoms of an acute cardiac problem, such as ACS or HF, and seek timely treatment of these symptoms. Responses

to this level of inquiry will help the nurse individualize the plan for patient and family education.

Common Symptoms

The signs and symptoms experienced by people with CVD are related to dysrhythmias and conduction problems (see Chapter 26); CAD (see Chapter 27); structural, infectious, and inflammatory disorders of the heart (see Chapter 28); and complications of CVD such as HF and cardiogenic shock (see Chapters 29 and 14, respectively). These disorders have many signs and symptoms in common; therefore, the nurse must be skillful at recognizing these signs and symptoms so that patients are given timely and often lifesaving care.

The following are the most common signs and symptoms of CVD, with related medical diagnoses in parentheses:

- Chest pain or discomfort (angina pectoris, ACS, dysrhythmias, valvular heart disease)
- Pain or discomfort in other areas of upper body, including one or both arms, back, neck, jaw, or stomach (ACS)
- Shortness of breath or dyspnea (ACS, cardiogenic shock, HF, valvular heart disease)
- Peripheral edema, weight gain, abdominal distention due to enlarged spleen and liver or ascites (HF)

- Palpitations (tachycardia from a variety of causes, including ACS, caffeine or other stimulants, electrolyte imbalances, stress, valvular heart disease, ventricular aneurysms)
- Unusual fatigue, sometimes referred to as vital exhaustion (an early warning symptom of ACS, HF, or valvular heart disease, characterized by feeling unusually tired or fatigued, irritable, and dejected)
- Dizziness, syncope, or changes in level of consciousness (cardiogenic shock, cerebrovascular disorders, dysrhythmias, hypotension, postural hypotension, vasovagal episode)

Symptoms of ACS can differ between men and women. Although chest pain or discomfort can occur in both men and women, it is more likely to be experienced by men. On the contrary, women can experience more atypical symptoms including fatigue, nausea, neck pain, right arm pain, jaw pain, dizziness, and syncope (McSweeney et al., 2016).

Chest Pain

Chest pain and chest discomfort are common symptoms that may be caused by a number of cardiac and noncardiac problems. Table 25-2 summarizes the characteristics and patterns of common causes of chest pain or discomfort. To differentiate among these causes of pain, the nurse asks the patient to identify the quantity (0 = no pain to 10 = worst pain), location, and quality of pain. The nurse assesses for radiation of the pain to other areas of the body and determines if associated signs and symptoms are present, such as diaphoresis or nausea. It is important to identify the events that precipitate the onset of symptoms, the duration of the symptoms, and measures that aggravate or relieve the symptoms.

The nurse keeps the following important points in mind when assessing patients reporting chest pain or discomfort:

- The location of chest symptoms is not well correlated with the cause of the pain. For example, substernal chest pain can result from a number of causes as outlined in Table 25-2.
- The severity or duration of chest pain or discomfort does not predict the seriousness of its cause. For example, when asked to rate pain using a 0 to 10 scale, patients experiencing esophageal spasm may rate their chest pain as a 10. In contrast, patients having an acute myocardial infarction (MI), which is a potentially life-threatening event, may report having moderate pain rated as a 4 to 6 on the pain scale.
- More than one clinical cardiac condition may occur simultaneously. During an MI, patients may report chest pain from myocardial ischemia, shortness of breath from HF, and palpitations from dysrhythmias. Both HF and dysrhythmias can be complications of an acute MI. (See Chapter 27 for discussion of clinical manifestations of ACS, including MI.)

Past Health, Family, and Social History

The health history provides an opportunity for the nurse to assess patients' understanding of their personal risk factors for peripheral vascular, cerebrovascular, and CADs (see Chart 27-1 in Chapter 27) and any measures that they are taking to modify these risks. Some risk factors, such as increasing age, male sex, and heredity, including race are not modifiable.

However, there are a number of risk factors, such as smoking, hypertension, high cholesterol, diabetes, obesity, and physical inactivity that can be modified by lifestyle changes or medications (Goff, Lloyd-Jones, Bennett, et al., 2013). There is a tool available on the internet from the National Institute of Health (NIH) that is used to assess an individual's 10 year risk for having an acute MI. It takes into consideration all of these risk factors (NIH, 2014) (see tool in Resources section at end of chapter).

In an effort to determine how patients perceive their current health status, the nurse asks the following questions:

- How is your health? Have you noticed any changes from last year? From 5 years ago?
- Do you have a cardiologist or primary provider? How often do you go for checkups?
- What health concerns do you have?
- Do you have a family history of genetic disorders that place you at risk for CVD (see Chart 25-1)?
- What are your risk factors for CAD (see Chart 27-1 in Chapter 27)?
- What do you do to stay healthy and take care of your heart?

Patients who do not understand the connection between risk factors and CAD may be unwilling to make recommended lifestyle changes or manage their illness effectively. On the contrary, patients who have this understanding may be more motivated to alter their lifestyle to avoid the risk of future cardiac events. The AHA has published lifestyle management guidelines that identify interventions and treatment goals for each of these risk factors (Eckel, Jakicic, Ard, et al., 2014). Chapter 27 provides an overview of this information.

Medications

Nurses collaborate with other health care providers, including pharmacists, to obtain a complete list of the patient's medications, including dose and frequency. Vitamins, herbals, and other over-the-counter medications are included on this list. During this aspect of the health assessment, the nurse asks the following questions to ensure that the patient is safely and effectively taking the prescribed medications.

- What are the names and doses of your medications?
- What is the purpose of each of these medications?
- How and when are these medications taken? Do you ever skip a dose or forget to take them?
- Are there any special precautions associated with any of these medications?
- What symptoms or problems do you need to report to your primary provider?

Aspirin, a nonprescription medication, is an important antithrombotic therapy for secondary prevention in patients recovering from ACS (Amsterdam, Wenger, Brindis, et al., 2014). However, patients who are not aware of this benefit may be inclined to stop taking aspirin if they think it is a trivial medication. A careful medication history often uncovers common medication errors and causes for nonadherence to the medication regimen.

Nutrition

Dietary modifications, exercise, weight loss, and careful monitoring are important strategies for managing three major cardiovascular risk factors: hyperlipidemia, hypertension, and

TABLE 25-2 Assessing Chest Pain

Location	Character	Duration	Precipitating Events and Aggravating Factors	Alleviating Factors
Angina Pectoris, ACS (unstable angina, MI) Usual distribution of pain with myocardial ischemia Jaw Epigastrium Right side Back Less common sites of pain with myocardial ischemia	*Angina:* Uncomfortable pressure, squeezing, or fullness in substernal chest area Can radiate across chest to the medial aspect of one or both arms and hands, jaw, shoulders, upper back, or epigastrium Radiation to arms and hands, described as numbness, tingling, or aching	*Angina:* 5–15 min	*Angina:* Physical exertion, emotional upset, eating large meal, or exposure to extremes in temperature	*Angina:* Rest, nitroglycerin, oxygen
	ACS: Same as angina pectoris Pain or discomfort ranges from mild to severe Associated with shortness of breath, diaphoresis, palpitations, unusual fatigue, and nausea or vomiting	ACS: >15 min	ACS: Emotional upset or unusual physical exertion occurring within 24 h of symptom onset Can occur at rest or while asleep	ACS: Morphine, reperfusion of coronary artery with thrombolytic (fibrinolytic) agent or percutaneous coronary intervention
Pericarditis	Sharp, severe substernal or epigastric pain Can radiate to neck, arms, and back Associated symptoms include fever, malaise, dyspnea, cough, nausea, dizziness, and palpitations	Intermittent	Sudden onset Pain increases with inspiration, swallowing, coughing, and rotation of trunk	Sitting upright, analgesia, anti-inflammatory medications
Pulmonary Disorders (pneumonia, pulmonary embolism)	Sharp, severe substernal or epigastric pain arising from inferior portion of pleura (referred to as pleuritic pain) Patient may be able to localize the pain	≥30 min	Follows an infectious or noninfectious process (MI, cardiac surgery, cancer, immune disorders, uremia) Pleuritic pain increases with inspiration, coughing, movement, and supine positioning Occurs in conjunction with community- or hospital-acquired lung infections (pneumonia) or venous thromboembolism (pulmonary embolism)	Treatment of underlying cause

(continued on page 682)

TABLE 25-2 Assessing Chest Pain (continued)

Location	Character	Duration	Precipitating Events and Aggravating Factors	Alleviating Factors
Esophageal Disorders (hiatal hernia, reflux esophagitis or spasm)	Substernal pain described as sharp, burning, or heavy. Often mimics angina. Can radiate to neck, arm, or shoulders	5–60 min	Recumbency, cold liquids, exercise	Food or antacid Nitroglycerin
Anxiety and Panic Disorders	Pain described as stabbing to dull ache. Associated with diaphoresis, palpitations, shortness of breath, tingling of hands or mouth, feeling of unreality, or fear of losing control	Peaks in 10 min	Can occur at any time including during sleep. Can be associated with a specific trigger	Removal of stimulus, relaxation, medications to treat anxiety or underlying disorder
Musculoskeletal Disorders (costochondritis)	Sharp or stabbing pain localized in anterior chest. Most often unilateral. Can radiate across chest to epigastrium or back	Hours to days	Most often follows respiratory tract infection with significant coughing, vigorous exercise, or posttrauma. Some cases are idiopathic. Exacerbated by deep inspiration, coughing, sneezing, and movement of upper torso or arms	Rest, ice, or heat. Analgesic or anti-inflammatory medications

ACS, acute coronary syndrome; MI, myocardial infarction.
Adapted from Bickley, L. S. (2014). *Bates' guide to physical examination and history taking* (11th ed.). Philadelphia, PA: Lippincott Williams & Wilkins; King, J. E., & Magdic, K. S. (2014). Chest pain: A time for concern? *AACN Advanced Critical Care, 25*(3), 279–283; Woods, S. L., Froelicher, E. S., Motzer, S. A., et al. (2009). *Cardiac nursing* (6th ed.). Philadelphia, PA: Lippincott Williams & Wilkins.

diabetes. Diets that are restricted in sodium, fat, cholesterol, or calories are commonly prescribed. The nurse obtains the following information:

- The patient's current height and weight (to determine body mass index [BMI]); waist measurement (assessment for obesity); BP; and any laboratory test results such as blood glucose, glycosylated hemoglobin (diabetes), total blood cholesterol, HDL and LDL levels, and triglyceride levels (hyperlipidemia)
- How often the patient self-monitors BP, blood glucose, and weight as appropriate to the medical diagnoses
- The patient's level of awareness regarding their target goals for each of the risk factors and any problems achieving or maintaining these goals

Chart 25-1 GENETICS IN NURSING PRACTICE
Cardiovascular Disorders

Several cardiovascular disorders are associated with genetic abnormalities. Some examples are:

- Arrhythmogenic right ventricular dysplasia (ARVD)
- Brugada syndrome
- Familial hypercholesterolemia
- Hypertrophic cardiomyopathy
- Long QT syndrome
  - Jervell and Lange-Nielsen syndrome (autosomal recessive form)
  - Romano–Ward syndrome (autosomal dominant form)

Genetic connective tissue disorders that impact the cardiovascular system:

- Ehlers–Danlos syndrome
- Loeys–Dietz syndrome
- Marfan syndrome

Genetic blood disorders that can impair the function of the cardiovascular system:

- Factor V Leiden
- Hemochromatosis
- Sickle cell disease

Nursing Assessments

Refer to Chart 5-2: Genetics in Nursing Practice: Genetic Aspects of Health Assessment

Family History Assessment Specific to Cardiovascular Disorders

- Assess all patients with cardiovascular symptoms for coronary artery disease, regardless of age.

- Inquire about a family history of sudden death or unexplained death.
- Ask about other family members with biochemical or neuromuscular conditions (e.g., hemochromatosis or muscular dystrophy).

Patient Assessment Specific to Cardiovascular Disorders

- Assess for signs and symptoms of hyperlipidemias (xanthomas, corneal arcus, or abdominal pain of unexplained origin).
- Obtain an electrocardiogram and an echocardiogram
- Assess for muscular weakness
- Assess for episodes of shortness of breath, dizziness, or palpitations.
- Review laboratory data for abnormal values.
- Gather dietary history.
- Assess for secondary risk factors (e.g., diet, smoking, overweight, high stress, and alcohol use)

Genetics Resources

American Heart Association, www.heart.org
Hypertrophic Cardiomyopathy Association, www.4hcm.org
Familial Hypercholesterolemia Foundation, www.thefhfoundation.org
Sudden Arrhythmia Death Syndromes, www.sads.org
See Chapter 8, Chart 8-7 for additional components of genetic counseling.

- What the patient normally eats and drinks in a typical day and any food preferences (including cultural or ethnic preferences)
- Eating habits (canned or commercially prepared foods vs. fresh foods, restaurant meals vs. home cooking, assessing for high-sodium foods, dietary intake of fats)
- Who shops for groceries and prepares meals

Elimination

Typical bowel and bladder habits need to be identified. Nocturia (awakening at night to urinate) is common in patients with HF. Fluid collected in gravity-dependent tissues (extremities) during the day (i.e., edema) redistributes into the circulatory system once the patient is recumbent at night. The increased circulatory volume is excreted by the kidneys (increased urine production).

When straining during defecation, the patient bears down (the Valsalva maneuver), which momentarily increases pressure on the baroreceptors. This triggers a vagal response, causing the heart rate to slow and resulting in syncope in some patients. Straining during urination can produce the same response.

Because many cardiac medications can cause gastrointestinal side effects or bleeding, the nurse asks about bloating, diarrhea, constipation, stomach upset, heartburn, loss of appetite, nausea, and vomiting. Screening for bloody urine or stools should be done for patients taking platelet-inhibiting medications such as aspirin and clopidogrel (Plavix); platelet aggregation inhibitors such as abciximab (ReoPro), eptifibatide (Integrilin), and tirofiban (Aggrastat); anticoagulants, such as low–molecular-weight heparin (e.g., dalteparin [Fragmin], enoxaparin [Lovenox]), heparin, or oral anticoagulants such as warfarin (Coumadin), rivaroxaban (Xarelto), or apixaban (Eliquis).

Activity and Exercise

Changes in the patient's activity tolerance are often gradual and may go unnoticed. The nurse determines if there are recent changes by comparing the patient's current activity level with that performed in the past 6 to 12 months. New symptoms or a change in the usual symptoms during activity is a significant finding. Activity-induced angina or shortness of breath may indicate CAD. These CAD-related symptoms occur when myocardial ischemia is present, due to an inadequate arterial blood supply to the myocardium, in the setting of increased demand (e.g., exercise, stress, or anemia). Patients experiencing these kinds of symptoms need to seek medical attention. Fatigue, associated with a low left ventricular ejection fraction (less than 40%) and certain medications (e.g., beta-adrenergic blocking agents), can result in activity intolerance. Patients with fatigue may benefit from having their medications adjusted and learning energy conservation techniques.

Additional areas to explore include the presence of architectural barriers in the home (stairs, multilevel home); the patient's participation in cardiac rehabilitation; and his or her current exercise pattern including intensity, duration, and frequency.

Sleep and Rest

Clues to worsening cardiac disease, especially HF, can be revealed by sleep-related events. Patients with worsening HF often experience *orthopnea*, a term used to indicate the need to sit upright or stand to avoid feeling short of breath. Patients experiencing orthopnea will report that they need to sleep upright in a chair or add extra pillows to their bed. Sudden awakening with shortness of breath, called *paroxysmal nocturnal dyspnea,* is an additional symptom of worsening HF. This nighttime symptom is caused by the reabsorption of fluid from dependent areas of the body (arms and legs) back into the circulatory system within hours of lying in bed. This sudden fluid shift increases preload and places increased demand on the heart of patients with HF, causing sudden pulmonary congestion.

There is mounting evidence of the cardiac consequences associated with sleep-disordered breathing (SDB). Often also called obstructive sleep apnea (OSA), SDB is an abnormal respiratory pattern due to intermittent episodes of upper airway obstruction causing apnea and hypopnea (shallow respirations) during sleep. These abnormal sleep events cause intermittent hypoxemia, sympathetic nervous system activation, and increased intrathoracic pressure that puts mechanical stress on the heart and large artery walls. Untreated SDB has been linked to CAD, hypertension, HF and dysrhythmias. SDB is treated by the use of continuous positive airway pressure (CPAP) and mandibular advancement devices (MAD) (see Chapter 22). These devices maintain an open airway during sleep, preventing hypoxemia and resulting abnormal elevations in BP. The cardinal signs of SBD are loud disruptive snoring and apnea lasting 10 seconds or more. Obesity and large neck circumference are two important risk factors for SDB (Ayas, Owens, & Kheirandish-Gozal, 2015).

During the health history, the nurse assesses for SDB by asking patients at high risk if they snore loudly, have frequent bouts of awaking from sleep, awaken with a headache, or experience severe daytime sleepiness (hypersomnolence). For patients with a diagnosis of SDB, the nurse determines if the patient has been prescribed a CPAP or MAD and the frequency of its use. Patients who are being admitted to the hospital or going for an ambulatory surgical procedure should be instructed to bring their sleep aid devices with them.

Self-Perception and Self-Concept

Self-perception and self-concept are both related to the cognitive and emotional processes that people use to formulate their beliefs and feelings about themselves. Having a chronic cardiac illness, such as HF, or experiencing an acute cardiac event, such as an MI, can alter an individual's self-perception and self-concept. Patients' beliefs and feelings about their health are key determinants of adherence to self-care recommendations and recovery after an acute cardiac event. To reduce the risk of future cardiovascular-related health problems, patients are asked to make difficult lifestyle changes, such as quitting smoking. Patients who have misperceptions about the health consequences of their illness are at risk for nonadherence to these recommended lifestyle changes. The health history is used to discover how patients perceive their health by asking questions that may include the following:

- What is your cardiac condition?
- How has this illness changed your feelings about your health?

- What do you think caused this illness?
- What consequences do you think this illness will have on your physical activity, work, social relationships, and role in your family?
- How much of an influence do you think you have on controlling this illness?

The patient's responses to these questions can guide the nurse in planning interventions to ensure that the patient is prepared to manage the illness and that adequate services are in place to support the patient's recovery and self-care needs.

Roles and Relationships

Patients with CVD are being managed with complex medical regimens and sophisticated technology, such as implantable cardioverter defibrillators (ICDs) and left ventricular assist devices. Hospital stays for cardiac disorders have shortened. Many invasive diagnostic cardiac procedures, such as cardiac catheterization, are being performed in the ambulatory setting. Support from family members helps to lessen the patient's burden of managing self-care for cardiac illnesses. A recent Scientific Statement from the AHA highlights the importance of social support. Based on findings from recent studies, social support has been found to be closely linked to CVD outcomes. In fact, patients with lower levels of social support have an increased risk for cardiac-related mortality and stroke, compared with others having higher levels of support (Havranek, Mujahid, Barr, et al., 2015).

To assess patients' roles in their families and their relationships, both components of social support, the nurse asks each patient: Who do you live with? Who is your primary caregiver at home? Who helps you manage your health? The nurse also assesses for any significant effects that the cardiac illness has had on the patient's role in the family. Are there adequate finances and health insurance? The answers to these questions help the nurse determine if consultation with social services or others is necessary to tailor the plan of care to meet the patient's self-care needs.

Sexuality and Reproduction

Sexual dysfunction affects twice as many people with CVD compared with the general population. In men, erectile dysfunction may develop as a side effect of cardiac medications (e.g., beta-blockers); some men will stop taking their medication as a result. Few patients with sexual dysfunction or concerns about resuming sexual activity seek medical care (Steinke, Jaarsma, Barnason, et al., 2013). The nurse can help patients by initiating discussions about sexuality and encouraging them to discuss problems with their primary provider or cardiologist.

A common reason for decreasing sexual activity is due to concerns that people have about the effects of physical exertion on the heart. They are worried that sexual activity may cause another heart attack, sudden death, or untoward symptoms such as angina, dyspnea, or palpitations. Often couples lack adequate information about the physical demands related to sexual activity and ways in which these demands can be modified. The physiologic demands associated with sexual activity range between 3 and 5 metabolic equivalents (METs), which is similar to the METs expended during mild to moderate activity. Sharing this information may make patients and their partners more comfortable about resuming sexual activity (Steinke et al., 2013).

A reproductive history is necessary for women of child-bearing age, particularly those with seriously compromised cardiac function. The reproductive history includes information about previous pregnancies, plans for future pregnancies, oral contraceptive use (especially in women older than 35 years who smoke), menopausal status, and the use of HT.

Coping and Stress Tolerance

Anxiety, depression, and stress are known to influence both the development of and recovery from CAD and HF. High levels of anxiety are associated with an increased incidence of CAD and in-hospital complication rates after MI. Patients with a diagnosis of an acute MI and depression have an increased risk of rehospitalization, death, more frequent angina, more physical limitations, and poorer quality of life compared with patients without depression (Lichtman, Froelicher, Blumenthal, et al., 2014). Although the association between depression and CAD is not completely understood, both biologic factors (e.g., platelet abnormalities, inflammatory responses) and lifestyle factors may contribute to the development of CAD. Patients who are depressed are less motivated to adhere to recommended lifestyle changes and medical regimens necessary to prevent future cardiac events, such as an MI (Havranek et al., 2015; Lichtman et al., 2014).

Patients with CAD or HF should be assessed for depression. Patients who have depression exhibit common signs and symptoms, such as feelings of worthlessness or guilt, problems falling asleep or staying asleep, having little interest or pleasure in doing things that they usually enjoy, having difficulty concentrating, restlessness, and recent changes in appetite or weight. A quick and simple screening tool recommended by the AHA is the two-question Patient Health Questionnaire (PHQ-2) (Bigger & Glassman, 2010). The nurse asks the patient the following:

Over the past 2 weeks, how often have you been bothered by either of the following problems?
- *Little interest or pleasure in doing things*
- *Feeling down, depressed, or hopeless*

The nurse scores the patient's responses to each question by assigning 0 for "not at all," 1 for "several days," 2 for "more than half the days," or 3 for "nearly every day." The PHQ-2 score ranges from 0 to 6. Patients with a score of 3 or higher may be experiencing major depression and should be referred to their primary providers for further evaluation and treatment.

Stress initiates a variety of responses, including increased levels of catecholamines and cortisol, and has been strongly linked to cardiovascular events, such as an MI. Therefore, patients need to be assessed for sources of stress; the nurse asks about recent or ongoing stressors, previous coping styles and effectiveness, and the patient's perception of their current mood and coping ability. A widely used tool used to measure life stress is the Social Readjustment Rating Scale (Homes & Rahe, 1967). Examples of items on this scale include death of a spouse, divorce, and change in responsibilities at work. Each item is assigned a score of 11 to 100. Patients identify the items that happened to them in the previous year. Patients with a score less than 150 have a slight risk for future illness, whereas a score of 150 to 299 indicates a moderate risk. A score of 300 or higher indicates a high risk for future illness. Consultation with a psychiatric advanced practice nurse,

psychologist, psychiatrist, or social worker is indicated for patients who are anxious or depressed or for patients who are having difficulty coping with their cardiac illness.

Physical Assessment

Physical assessment is conducted to confirm information obtained from the health history, to establish the patient's current or baseline condition, and, in subsequent assessments, to evaluate the patient's response to treatment. Once the initial physical assessment is completed, the frequency of future assessments is determined by the purpose of the encounter and the patient's condition. For example, a focused cardiac assessment may be performed each time the patient is seen in the outpatient setting, whereas patients in the acute care setting may require a more extensive assessment at least every 8 hours. During the physical assessment, the nurse evaluates the cardiovascular system for any deviations from normal with regard to the following (examples of abnormalities are in parentheses):
- The heart as a pump (reduced pulse pressure, displaced PMI from fifth intercostal space midclavicular line, gallop sounds, murmurs)
- Atrial and ventricular filling volumes and pressures (elevated jugular venous distension, peripheral edema, ascites, crackles, postural changes in BP)
- Cardiac output (reduced pulse pressure, hypotension, tachycardia, reduced urine output, lethargy, or disorientation)
- Compensatory mechanisms (peripheral vasoconstriction, tachycardia).

General Appearance

This part of the assessment evaluates the patient's level of consciousness (alert, lethargic, stuporous, comatose) and mental status (oriented to person, place, time; coherence). Changes in level of consciousness and mental status may be attributed to inadequate perfusion of the brain from a compromised cardiac output or thromboembolic event (stroke). Patients are observed for signs of distress, which include pain or discomfort, shortness of breath, or anxiety.

The nurse notes the size of the patient (normal, overweight, underweight, or cachectic). The patient's height and weight are measured to calculate BMI (weight in kilograms/square of the height in meters), as well as the waist circumference (see Chapter 5). These measures are used to determine if obesity (BMI greater than 30 kg/m^2) and abdominal fat (males: waist greater than 40 in; females: waist greater than 35 in) are placing the patient at risk for CAD.

Assessment of the Skin and Extremities

Examination of the skin includes all body surfaces, starting with the head and finishing with the lower extremities. Skin color, temperature, and texture are assessed for acute and chronic problems with arterial or venous circulation. Table 25-3 summarizes common skin and extremity assessment findings in patients with CVD. The most noteworthy changes include the following:
- Signs and symptoms of acute obstruction of arterial blood flow in the extremities, referred to as the 6 *P*'s, are *p*ain, *p*allor, *p*ulselessness, *p*aresthesia, *p*oikilothermia (coldness), and *p*aralysis. During the first few hours

TABLE 25-3 Common Assessment Findings Associated With Cardiovascular Disease

Assessment Findings	Associated Causes and Conditions
Clubbing of the fingers or toes (thickening of the skin under the fingers or toes)	Chronic hemoglobin desaturation most often due to congenital heart disease, advanced pulmonary diseases
Cool/cold skin and diaphoresis	Low cardiac output (e.g., cardiogenic shock, acute myocardial infarction) causing sympathetic nervous system stimulation with resultant vasoconstriction
Cold, pain, pallor of the fingertips or toes	Intermittent arteriolar vasoconstriction (Raynaud disease). Skin may change in color from white, blue, and red accompanied by numbness, tingling, and burning pain
Cyanosis, central (a bluish tinge observed in the tongue and buccal mucosa)	Serious cardiac disorders (pulmonary edema, cardiogenic shock, congenital heart disease) result in venous blood passing through the pulmonary circulation without being oxygenated
Cyanosis, peripheral (a bluish tinge, most often of the nails and skin of the nose, lips, earlobes, and extremities)	Peripheral vasoconstriction, allowing more time for the hemoglobin molecules to become desaturated. It can be caused by exposure to cold environment, anxiety, or ↓ cardiac output
Ecchymosis or bruising (a purplish-blue color fading to green, yellow, or brown)	Blood leaking outside of the blood vessels Excessive bruising is a risk for patients on anticoagulants or platelet-inhibiting medications
Edema, lower extremities (collection of fluid in the interstitial spaces of the tissues)	Heart failure and vascular problems (PAD, chronic venous insufficiency, deep vein thrombosis, thrombophlebitis)
Hematoma (localized collection of clotted blood in the tissue)	Bleeding after catheter removal/tissue injury in patients on anticoagulant/antithrombotic agents
Pallor (↓ skin color in fingernails, lips, oral mucosa, and lower extremities)	Anemia or ↓ arterial perfusion. Suspect PAD if feet develop pallor after elevating legs 60° from a supine position
Rubor (a reddish-blue discoloration of the legs, seen within 20 s to 2 min after placing in a dependent position)	Filling of dilated capillaries with deoxygenated blood, indicative of PAD
Ulcers, feet and ankles: Superficial, irregular ulcers at medial malleolus. Red to yellow granulation tissue	Rupture of small skin capillaries from chronic venous insufficiency
Ulcers, feet and ankles: Painful, deep, round ulcers on feet or from exposure to pressure. Pale to black wound base	Prolonged ischemia to tissues due to PAD. Can lead to gangrene
Thinning of skin around a pacemaker or an implantable cardioverter defibrillator	Erosion of the device through the skin
Xanthelasma (yellowish, raised plaques observed along nasal portion of eyelids)	Elevated cholesterol levels (hypercholesterolemia)

PAD, peripheral arterial disease.
Adapted from Bickley, L. S. (2014). *Bates' guide to physical examination and history taking* (11th ed.). Philadelphia, PA: Lippincott Williams & Wilkins; Woods, S. L., Froelicher, E. S., Motzer, S. A., et al. (2009). *Cardiac nursing* (6th ed.). Philadelphia, PA: Lippincott Williams & Wilkins.

after invasive cardiac procedures (e.g., cardiac catheterization, percutaneous coronary intervention [PCI], or cardiac electrophysiology testing), affected extremities should be assessed frequently for these acute vascular changes.

- Major blood vessels of the arms and legs may be used for catheter insertion. During these procedures, systemic anticoagulation with heparin is necessary, and bruising or small hematomas may occur at the catheter access site. However, large hematomas are a serious complication that can compromise circulating blood volume and cardiac output. Patients who have undergone these procedures must have catheter access sites frequently observed until hemostasis is adequately achieved.

- Edema of the feet, ankles, or legs is called *peripheral edema*. Edema can be observed in the sacral area of patients on bed rest. The nurse assesses the patient for edema by using the thumb to place firm pressure over the dorsum of each foot, behind each medial malleolus, over the shins or sacral area for 5 seconds. *Pitting edema* is the term used to describe an indentation in the skin created by this pressure (see Fig. 29-2 in Chapter 29). The degree of pitting edema relies on the clinician's judgment of depth of edema and time the indentation remains after release of pressure. Pitting edema is graded as absent (0) or as present on a scale from slight (1+ = up to 2 mm) to very marked (4+ = more than 8 mm) (Weber & Kelley, 2014). It is important that clinicians use a consistent scale in order to ensure reliable clinical measurements and management. Peripheral edema is a common finding in patients with HF and peripheral vascular diseases, such as deep vein thrombosis or chronic venous insufficiency.

- Prolonged capillary refill time indicates inadequate arterial perfusion to the extremities. To test capillary refill time, the nurse compresses the nail bed briefly to occlude perfusion and the nail bed blanches. Then, the nurse releases pressure and determines the time it takes to restore perfusion. Normally, reperfusion occurs within 2 seconds, as evidenced by the return of color to the nail bed. Prolonged capillary refill time indicates compromised arterial perfusion, a problem associated with cardiogenic shock and HF.
- Clubbing of the fingers and toes indicates chronic hemoglobin desaturation and is associated with congenital heart disease.
- Hair loss, brittle nails, dry or scaling skin, atrophy of the skin, skin color changes, and ulcerations are indicative of chronically reduced oxygen and nutrient supply to the skin observed in patients with arterial or venous insufficiency (see Chapter 30 for a complete description of these conditions) (Weber & Kelley, 2014).

Blood Pressure

Systemic arterial BP is the pressure exerted on the walls of the arteries during ventricular systole and diastole. It is affected by factors such as cardiac output; distention of the arteries; and the volume, velocity, and viscosity of the blood. A normal BP in adults is considered a systolic BP less than 120 mm Hg over a diastolic BP less than 80 mm Hg. High BP, called hypertension, is defined by having a systolic BP that is consistently greater than 140 mm Hg or a diastolic BP greater than 90 mm Hg (Weber, Schiffrin, White, et al., 2014). Hypotension refers to an abnormally low systolic and diastolic BP that can result in lightheadedness or fainting. (See Chapter 31 for additional definitions, measurement, and management.)

Pulse Pressure

The difference between the systolic and the diastolic pressures is called the *pulse pressure*. It is a reflection of stroke volume, ejection velocity, and systemic vascular resistance. Pulse pressure, which normally is 30 to 40 mm Hg, indicates how well the patient maintains cardiac output. The pulse pressure increases in conditions that elevate the stroke volume (anxiety, exercise, bradycardia), reduce systemic vascular resistance (fever), or reduce distensibility of the arteries (atherosclerosis, aging, hypertension). Decreased pulse pressure reflects reduced stroke volume and ejection velocity (shock, HF, hypovolemia, mitral regurgitation) or obstruction to blood flow during systole (mitral or aortic stenosis). A pulse pressure of less than 30 mm Hg signifies a serious reduction in cardiac output and requires further cardiovascular assessment (Woods et al., 2009).

Postural (Orthostatic) Blood Pressure Changes

There is a gravitational redistribution of approximately 300 to 800 mL of blood into the lower extremities and the gastrointestinal system immediately upon standing. These changes reduce venous return to the heart, compromising

preload that ultimately reduces stroke volume and cardiac output. As a consequence, the autonomic nervous system is activated. The sympathetic nervous system increases heart rate and enhances peripheral vasoconstriction, whereas parasympathetic activity of the heart via the vagus nerve is decreased. These compensatory mechanisms stabilize arterial BP (Arnold & Shibao, 2013).

Normal postural responses that occur when a person moves from a lying to a standing position include (1) a heart rate increase of 5 to 20 bpm above the resting rate; (2) an unchanged systolic pressure, or a slight decrease of up to 10 mm Hg; and (3) a slight increase of 5 mm Hg in diastolic pressure.

Postural (orthostatic) hypotension is a sustained decrease of at least 20 mm Hg in systolic BP or 10 mm Hg in diastolic BP within 3 minutes of moving from a lying or sitting to a standing position. It is usually accompanied by dizziness, lightheadedness, or syncope (Arnold & Shibao, 2013).

Postural hypotension in patients with CVD is most often due to a significant reduction in preload, which compromises cardiac output. Reduced preload, which is reflective of intravascular volume depletion, is caused by dehydration from overdiuresis, bleeding (due to antiplatelet or anticoagulant medications or post intravascular procedures), or medications that dilate the blood vessels (e.g., nitrates and antihypertensive agents). In these situations, the usual mechanisms needed to maintain cardiac output (increased heart rate and peripheral vasoconstriction) cannot compensate for the significant loss in intravascular volume. As a result, the BP drops and heart rate increases with changes from lying or sitting to upright positions (see Chart 25-2).

The following is an example of BP and heart rate measurements in a patient with postural hypotension:

Supine: BP 120/70 mm Hg, heart rate 70 bpm
Sitting: BP 100/55 mm Hg, heart rate 90 bpm
Standing: BP 98/52 mm Hg, heart rate 94 bpm

Chart 25-2   **ASSESSMENT**
Assessing Patients for Postural Hypotension

The following steps are recommended when assessing patients for postural hypotension:

- Position the patient supine for 10 minutes before taking the initial blood pressure (BP) and heart rate measurements.
- Reposition the patient to a sitting position with legs in the dependent position, wait 2 minutes, then reassess both BP and heart rate measurements.
- If the patient is symptom free or has no significant decreases in systolic or diastolic BP, assist the patient into a standing position, obtain measurements immediately, and recheck in 2 minutes; continue measurements every 2 min for a total of 10 minutes to rule out postural hypotension.
- Return the patient to a supine position if postural hypotension is detected or if the patient becomes symptomatic.
- Document heart rate and BP measured in each position (e.g., supine, sitting, and standing) and any signs or symptoms that accompany the postural changes.

Adapted from Woods, S. L., Froelicher, E. S., Motzer, S. A., et al. (2009). *Cardiac nursing* (6th ed.). Philadelphia, PA: Lippincott Williams & Wilkins.

Arterial Pulses

The arteries are palpated to evaluate the pulse rate, rhythm, amplitude, contour, and obstruction to blood flow.

Pulse Rate

The normal pulse rate varies from a low of 50 bpm in healthy, athletic young adults to rates well in excess of 100 bpm after exercise or during times of excitement. Anxiety frequently raises the pulse rate during the physical examination. If the rate is higher than expected, the nurse should reassess the pulse near the end of the physical examination, when the patient may be more relaxed.

Pulse Rhythm

The rhythm of the pulse is normally regular. Minor variations in regularity of the pulse may occur with respirations. The pulse rate may increase during inhalation and slow during exhalation due to changes in blood flow to the heart during the respiratory cycle. This phenomenon, called *sinus arrhythmia*, occurs most commonly in children and young adults.

For the initial cardiac examination, or if the pulse rhythm is irregular, the heart rate should be counted by auscultating the apical pulse, located at the PMI, for a full minute while simultaneously palpating the radial pulse. Any discrepancy between contractions heard and pulses felt is noted. Disturbances of rhythm (dysrhythmias) often result in a **pulse deficit**, which is a difference between the apical and radial pulse rates. Pulse deficits commonly occur with atrial fibrillation, atrial flutter, and premature ventricular contractions. These dysrhythmias stimulate the ventricles to contact prematurely, before diastole is finished. As a result, these early ventricular contractions produce a smaller stroke volume, which can be heard during auscultation but do not produce a palpable pulse (see Chapter 26 for a detailed discussion of these dysrhythmias).

Pulse Amplitude

The pulse amplitude, indicative of the BP in the artery, is used to assess peripheral arterial circulation. The nurse assesses pulse amplitude bilaterally and describes and records the amplitude of each artery. The simplest method characterizes the pulse as absent, diminished, normal, or bounding. Scales are also used to rate the strength of the pulse. The following is an example of a 0-to-4 scale:

0: Not palpable or absent
+1: Diminished—weak, thready pulse; difficult to palpate; obliterated with pressure
+2: Normal—cannot be obliterated
+3: Moderately increased—easy to palpate, full pulse; cannot be obliterated
+4: Markedly increased—strong, bounding pulse; may be abnormal

The numerical classification is subjective; therefore, when documenting the pulse amplitude, specify location of the artery and scale range (e.g., "left radial +3/+4") (Weber & Kelley, 2014).

If the pulse is absent or difficult to palpate, the nurse can use a continuous wave Doppler. This portable ultrasound device has a transducer that is placed over the artery. The transducer emits and receives ultrasound beams. Rhythmic changes are heard as blood cells flow through patent arteries, whereas obstruction to blood flow is evidenced by no changes in sound. (Ultrasound techniques are discussed in more detail in Chapter 30.)

Pulse Contour

The contour of the pulse conveys important information. In patients with stenosis of the aortic valve, the valve opening is narrowed, reducing the amount of blood ejected into the aorta. The pulse pressure is narrow, and the pulse feels feeble. In aortic insufficiency, the aortic valve does not close completely, allowing blood to flow back from the aorta into the left ventricle. The rise of the pulse wave is abrupt and strong, and its fall is precipitous—a "collapsing" or "water hammer" pulse. The true contour of the pulse is best appreciated by palpating over the carotid artery rather than the distal radial artery, because the dramatic characteristics of the pulse wave may be distorted when the pulse is transmitted to smaller vessels.

Palpation of Arterial Pulses

To assess peripheral circulation, the nurse locates and evaluates all arterial pulses. Arterial pulses are palpated at points where the arteries are near the skin surface and are easily compressed against bones or firm musculature. Pulses are detected over the right and left temporal, common carotid, brachial, radial, femoral, popliteal, dorsalis pedis, and posterior tibial arteries (see Fig. 30-2 in Chapter 30). A reliable assessment of the pulses depends on accurate identification of the location of the artery and careful palpation of the area. Light palpation is essential; firm finger pressure can obliterate the temporal, dorsalis pedis, and posterior tibial pulses and confuse the examiner. In approximately 10% of patients, the dorsalis pedis pulses are not palpable (Woods et al., 2009). In such circumstances, both are usually absent and the posterior tibial arteries alone provide adequate blood supply to the feet. Arteries in the extremities are often palpated simultaneously to facilitate comparison of quality.

> **Quality and Safety Nursing Alert**
>
> Do not simultaneously palpate both the temporal and carotid arteries, because it is possible to decrease the blood flow to the brain.

Jugular Venous Pulsations

Right-sided heart function can be estimated by observing the pulsations of the jugular veins of the neck, which reflects central venous pressure (CVP). CVP is the pressure in the right atria or the right ventricle at the end of diastole. If the internal jugular pulsations are difficult to see, pulsations of the external jugular veins may be noted. These veins are more superficial and are visible just above the clavicles, adjacent to the sternocleidomastoid muscles.

In patients who have normal blood volume (euvolemia), the jugular veins are normally visible in the supine position with the head of the bed elevated to 30° (Bickley, 2014). Obvious distention of the veins with the patient's head elevated 45° to 90° indicates an abnormal increase in CVP. This abnormality is observed in patients with right-sided HF, due to hypervolemia, pulmonary hypertension, and pulmonary stenosis; less commonly with obstruction of blood

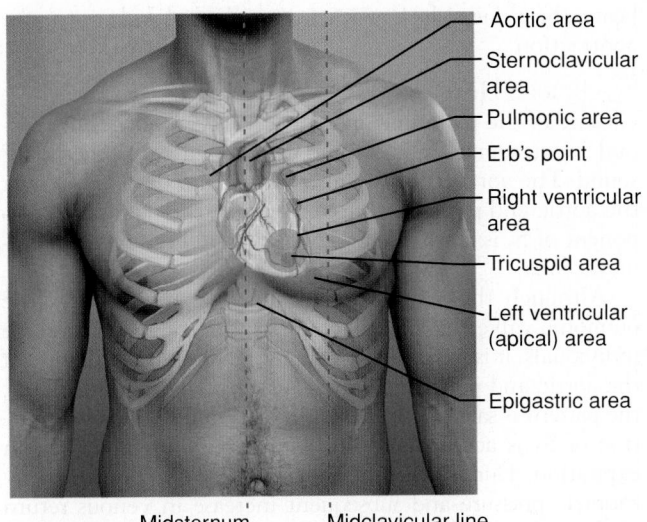

- Aortic area
- Sternoclavicular area
- Pulmonic area
- Erb's point
- Right ventricular area
- Tricuspid area
- Left ventricular (apical) area
- Epigastric area

Midsternum   Midclavicular line

Figure 25-5 • Areas of the precordium to be assessed when evaluating heart function.

flow in the superior vena cava; and rarely with acute massive pulmonary embolism.

Heart Inspection and Palpation

The heart is examined by inspection, palpation, and auscultation of the precordium or anterior chest wall that covers the heart and lower thorax. A systematic approach is used to examine the precordium in the following six areas. Figure 25-5 identifies these important landmarks:

1. *Aortic area*—second intercostal space to the right of the sternum. To determine the correct intercostal space, the nurse first finds the angle of Louis by locating the bony ridge near the top of the sternum, at the junction of the sternum and the manubrium. From this angle, the second intercostal space is located by sliding one finger to the left or right of the sternum. Subsequent intercostal spaces are located from this reference point by palpating down the rib cage.

2. *Pulmonic area*—second intercostal space to the left of the sternum
3. *Erb point*—third intercostal space to the left of the sternum
4. *Tricuspid area*—fourth and fifth intercostal spaces to the left of the sternum
5. *Mitral (apical) area*—left fifth intercostal space at the midclavicular line
6. *Epigastric area*—below the xiphoid process

For most of the examination, the patient lies supine, with the head of the bed or the examination table slightly elevated. A right-handed examiner stands at the right side of the patient, a left-handed examiner at the left side.

Each area of the precordium is inspected for pulsations and is then palpated. An apical impulse is a normal finding observed in young patients and adults who have thin chest walls.

The apical impulse may be felt as a light pulsation, 1 to 2 cm in diameter. It is felt at the onset of the first heart sound and lasts for only half of ventricular systole (see the next section for a discussion of heart sounds). The nurse uses the palm of the hand to locate the apical impulse initially and the finger pads to assess its size and quality. Palpation of the apical pulse may be facilitated by repositioning the patient to the left lateral position, which puts the heart in closer contact with the chest wall (see Fig. 25-6).

There are several abnormalities that the nurse may find during palpation of the precordium. Normally, the apical impulse is palpable in only one intercostal space; palpability in two or more adjacent intercostal spaces indicates left ventricular enlargement. An apical impulse below the fifth intercostal space or lateral to the midclavicular line usually denotes left ventricular enlargement from left ventricular heart failure. If the apical impulse can be palpated in two distinctly separate areas and the pulsation movements are paradoxical (not simultaneous), a ventricular aneurysm may be suspected. A broad and forceful apical impulse is known as a left ventricular heave or lift because it appears to lift the hand from the chest wall during palpation.

A vibration or purring sensation may be felt over areas where abnormal, turbulent blood flow is present. It is best

Figure 25-6 • Palpating the apical impulse. **A.** Remain on the patient's right side, and ask the patient to remain supine. Use the finger pads to palpate the apical impulse in the mitral area (fifth intercostal space at the midclavicular line). **B.** You may ask the patient to roll to the left side to better feel the impulse using the palmar surfaces of your hand. Photos from Weber, J. R., & Kelley, J. H. (2014). *Health assessment in nursing* (5th ed.). Philadelphia, PA: Lippincott Williams & Wilkins.

detected by using the palm of the hand. This vibration is called a *thrill* and is associated with a loud murmur. Depending on the location of the thrill, it may be indicative of serious valvular heart disease; an atrial or ventricular septal defect (abnormal opening); or stenosis of a large artery, such as the carotid artery.

Heart Auscultation

A stethoscope is used to auscultate each of the locations identified in Figure 25-5, with the exception of the epigastric area. The purpose of cardiac auscultation is to determine heart rate and rhythm and evaluate heart sounds. The apical area is auscultated for 1 minute to determine the apical pulse rate and the regularity of the heartbeat. Normal and abnormal heart sounds detected during auscultation are described next.

Normal Heart Sounds

Normal heart sounds, referred to as S_1 and S_2, are produced by closure of the AV valves and the semilunar valves, respectively. The period between S_1 and S_2 corresponds with ventricular systole (see Fig. 25-7). When the heart rate is within the normal range, systole is much shorter than the period between S_2 and S_1 (diastole). However, as the heart rate increases, diastole shortens.

Normally, S_1 and S_2 are the only sounds heard during the cardiac cycle (Bickley, 2014).

S_1—First Heart Sound

Tricuspid and mitral valve closure creates the first heart sound (S_1). The word "lub" is used to replicate its sound. S_1 is usually heard the loudest at the apical area. S_1 is easily identifiable and serves as the point of reference for the remainder of the cardiac cycle.

The intensity of S_1 increases during tachycardias or with mitral stenosis. In these circumstances, the AV valves are wide open during ventricular contraction. The accentuated S_1 occurs as the AV valves close with greater force than normal. Similarly, dysrhythmias can vary the intensity of S_1 from

beat to beat due to lack of synchronized atrial and ventricular contraction.

S_2—Second Heart Sound

Closure of the pulmonic and aortic valves produces the second heart sound (S_2), commonly referred to as the "dub" sound. The aortic component of S_2 is heard the loudest over the aortic and pulmonic areas. However, the pulmonic component of S_2 is a softer sound and is heard best over the pulmonic area.

Although these valves close almost simultaneously, the pulmonic valve lags slightly behind the aortic valve. In some individuals, it is possible to distinguish between the closure of the aortic and pulmonic valves. When this situation occurs, the patient is said to have a split S_2. Normal physiologic splitting of S_2 is accentuated on inspiration and disappears on expiration. During inspiration, there is a decrease in intrathoracic pressure and subsequent increase in venous return to the right atrium and ventricle. The right ventricle takes a little longer to eject this extra volume, which causes the pulmonic valve to close a little later than normal. Splitting of S_2 that remains constant during inspiration and expiration is an abnormal finding. Abnormal splitting of the second heart sound can be caused by a variety of disease states (valvular heart disease, septal defects, bundle branch blocks). Splitting of S_2 is best heard over the pulmonic area.

Abnormal Heart Sounds

Abnormal sounds develop during systole or diastole when structural or functional heart problems are present. These sounds are called S_3 or S_4 gallops, opening snaps, systolic clicks, and murmurs. S_3 and S_4 gallop sounds are heard during diastole. These sounds are created by the vibration of the ventricle and surrounding structures as blood meets resistance during ventricular filling. The term *gallop* evolved from the cadence that is produced by the addition of a third or fourth heart sound, similar to the sound of a galloping horse. Gallop sounds are very low-frequency sounds and are heard with the bell of the stethoscope placed very lightly against the chest.

Figure 25-7 • Normal heart sounds. The first heart sound (S_1) is produced by closure of the mitral and tricuspid valves ("lub"). The second heart sound (S_2) is produced by closure of the aortic and pulmonic valves ("dub"). *Arrows* represent the direction of blood flow.

Figure 25-8 • Gallop sounds. An S_3 ("DUB") is an abnormal sound heard immediately following S_2 (closure of semilunar valves). This sound is generated very early in diastole as blood flowing into the right or left ventricle is met with resistance. S_4 ("LUB") is an abnormal sound created during atrial systole as blood flowing into the right or left ventricle is met with resistance. *Arrows* represent the direction of blood flow.

S_3—Third Heart Sound

An S_3 ("DUB") is heard early in diastole during the period of rapid ventricular filling as blood flows from the atrium into a noncompliant ventricle. It is heard immediately after S_2. "Lub-dub-DUB" is used to imitate the abnormal sound of a beating heart when an S_3 is present. It represents a normal finding in children and adults up to 35 or 40 years of age. In these cases, it is referred to as a physiologic S_3 (see Fig. 25-8). In older adults, an S_3 is a significant finding, suggesting HF. It is best heard with the bell of the stethoscope. If the right ventricle is involved, a right-sided S_3 is heard over the tricuspid area with the patient in a supine position. A left-sided S_3 is best heard over the apical area with the patient in the left lateral position.

S_4—Fourth Heart Sound

S_4 ("LUB") occurs late in diastole (see Fig. 25-8). S_4 heard just before S_1 is generated during atrial contraction as blood forcefully enters a noncompliant ventricle. This resistance to blood flow is due to ventricular hypertrophy caused by hypertension, CAD, cardiomyopathies, aortic stenosis, and numerous other conditions. "LUB lub-dub" is the mnemonic used to imitate this gallop sound. S_4, produced in the left ventricle, is auscultated using the bell of the stethoscope over the apical area with the patient in the left lateral position. A right-sided S_4, although less common, is heard best over the tricuspid area with the patient in supine position. There are times when both S_3 and S_4 are present, creating a quadruple rhythm, which sounds like "LUB lub-dub DUB." During tachycardia, all four sounds combine into a loud sound, referred to as a **summation gallop**.

Opening Snaps and Systolic Clicks

Normally, no sound is produced when valves open. However, diseased valve leaflets create abnormal sounds as they open during diastole or systole. **Opening snaps** are abnormal diastolic sounds heard during opening of an AV valve. For example, mitral stenosis can cause an opening snap, which is an unusually high-pitched sound very early in diastole. This sound is caused by high pressure in the left atrium that abruptly displaces or "snaps" open a rigid valve leaflet. Timing helps to distinguish an opening snap from the other gallop

sounds. It occurs too long after S_2 to be mistaken for a split S_2 and too early in diastole to be mistaken for an S_3. The high-pitched, snapping quality of the sound is another way to differentiate an opening snap from an S_3. Hearing a murmur or the sound of turbulent blood flow is expected following the opening snap. An opening snap is heard best using the diaphragm of the stethoscope placed medial to the apical area and along the lower left sternal border.

In a similar manner, stenosis of one of the semilunar valves creates a short, high-pitched sound in early systole, immediately after S_1. This sound, called a **systolic click**, is the result of the opening of a rigid and calcified aortic or pulmonic valve during ventricular contraction. Mid- to late systolic clicks may be heard in patients with mitral or tricuspid valve prolapse as the malfunctioning valve leaflet is displaced into the atrium during ventricular systole. Murmurs are expected to be heard following these abnormal systolic sounds. These sounds are the loudest in the areas directly over the malfunctioning valve.

Murmurs

Murmurs are created by turbulent flow of blood in the heart. The causes of the turbulence may be a critically narrowed valve, a malfunctioning valve that allows regurgitant blood flow, a congenital defect of the ventricular wall, a defect between the aorta and the pulmonary artery, or an increased flow of blood through a normal structure (e.g., with fever, pregnancy, and hyperthyroidism). Murmurs are characterized and consequently described by several characteristics, including their timing in the cardiac cycle, location on the chest wall, intensity, pitch, quality, and pattern of radiation (see Chart 25-3).

Friction Rub

A harsh, grating sound that can be heard in both systole and diastole is called a *friction rub*. It is caused by abrasion of the inflamed pericardial surfaces from pericarditis. Because a friction rub may be confused with a murmur, care should be taken to identify the sound and to distinguish it from murmurs that may be heard in both systole and diastole. A pericardial friction rub can be heard best using the diaphragm of the stethoscope, with the patient sitting up and leaning forward.

Chart 25-3 Characteristics of Heart Murmurs

Heart murmurs are described in terms of location, timing, intensity, pitch, quality, and radiation. These characteristics provide information needed to determine the cause of the murmur and its clinical significance.

Location

Pinpointing the location of the murmur helps to determine the underlying structures that are involved in generating the abnormal sounds. The locations described in Figure 25-5 are used to identify where the loudest sounds are detected. The description should include the exact location from which the sound emanates, such as the location of the intercostal space and other important landmarks (right or left sternal border; midsternal, midclavicular, anterior axillary, or midaxillary lines). For example, a ventricular septal defect can be located at the left sternal border in the third and fourth intercostal spaces.

Timing

A murmur is described in terms of when it occurs during the cardiac cycle (systole or diastole). Murmurs are further differentiated by identifying exactly when during systole or diastole they are heard. A skilled clinician can detect that the murmur is occurring during early, mid-, or late systole or diastole. Some murmurs have sounds that occur in both systole and diastole.

Intensity

A grading system is used to describe the intensity or loudness of a murmur.

Grade 1: Very faint and difficult for the inexperienced clinician to hear

Grade 2: Quiet but readily perceived by the experienced clinician
Grade 3: Moderately loud
Grade 4: Loud and may be associated with a thrill
Grade 5: Very loud; heard when stethoscope is partially off the chest; associated with a thrill
Grade 6: Extremely loud; detected with the stethoscope off the chest; associated with a thrill

Pitch

Pitch describes the sound frequency, identified as high, medium, or low pitched. High-pitched murmurs are heard best with the stethoscope's diaphragm, whereas low-pitched sounds are detected using the bell of the stethoscope placed lightly on the chest wall.

Quality

Quality describes the sound that the murmur resembles. Murmurs can produce a rumbling, blowing, whistling, harsh, or musical sound. For example, murmurs caused by mitral or tricuspid regurgitation have a blowing quality, whereas mitral stenosis generates a rumbling sound.

Radiation

Radiation refers to the transmission of the murmur from the point of maximal intensity to other areas in the upper chest. The examiner determines if radiation is present by listening carefully to areas of the heart adjacent to the point where the murmur is the loudest. If radiation is present, the exact location is described. A murmur associated with aortic stenosis, for example, can radiate into the neck, down the left sternal border, and into the apical area.

Auscultation Procedure

During auscultation, the patient remains supine and the examining room is as quiet as possible. A stethoscope with both diaphragm and bell functions is necessary for accurate auscultation of the heart.

Using the diaphragm of the stethoscope, the examiner starts at the apical area and progresses upward along the left sternal border to the pulmonic and aortic areas. Alternatively, the examiner may begin the examination at the aortic and pulmonic areas and progress downward to the apex of the heart. Initially, S_1 is identified and evaluated with respect to its intensity and splitting. Next, S_2 is identified, and its intensity and any splitting are noted. After concentrating on S_1 and S_2, the examiner listens for extra sounds in systole and then in diastole.

Sometimes it helps to ask the following questions: Do I hear snapping or clicking sounds? Do I hear any high-pitched blowing sounds? Is this sound in systole, or diastole, or both? The examiner again proceeds to move the stethoscope to all of the designated areas of the precordium, listening carefully for these sounds. Finally, the patient is turned on the left side and the stethoscope is placed on the apical area, where an S_3, an S_4, and a mitral murmur are more readily detected.

Once an abnormality is heard, the entire chest surface is reexamined to determine the exact location of the sound and its radiation. The patient may be concerned about the prolonged examination and must be supported and reassured. The auscultatory findings, particularly murmurs, are documented by identifying the following characteristics

(see Chart 25-3): location on chest wall, timing, intensity, pitch, quality, and radiation.

Interpretation of Heart Sounds

Interpreting heart sounds requires detailed knowledge of cardiac physiology and pathophysiology. However, all nurses should have adequate knowledge and skill to recognize normal heart sounds (S_1, S_2) and the presence of abnormal sounds. When assessment is at this very basic level of practice, abnormal findings are reported for further evaluation and treatment. More advanced skills are required of nurses caring for critically ill patients with CVD or those nurses functioning in advanced practice roles. Nurses in these roles readily identify abnormal heart sounds, recognize the diagnostic significance of their findings, and use their assessment skills to evaluate patients' responses to medical interventions. For example, these highly skilled nurses monitor heart sounds in patients with HF to detect the resolution of an S_3 after treatment with a diuretic.

Assessment of Other Systems

Lungs

The details of respiratory assessment are described in Chapter 20. Findings frequently exhibited by patients with cardiac disorders include the following:

Hemoptysis: Pink, frothy sputum is indicative of acute pulmonary edema.

Cough: A dry, hacking cough from irritation of small airways is common in patients with pulmonary congestion from HF.

Crackles: HF or atelectasis associated with bed rest, splinting from ischemic pain, or the effects of analgesic, sedative, or anesthetic agents often results in the development of crackles. Typically, crackles are first noted at the bases (because of gravity's effect on fluid accumulation and decreased ventilation of basilar tissue), but they may progress to all portions of the lung fields.

Wheezes: Compression of the small airways by interstitial pulmonary edema may cause wheezing. Beta-adrenergic blocking agents (beta-blockers), particularly noncardioselective beta-adrenergic blocking agents such as propranolol (Inderal), may cause airway narrowing, especially in patients with underlying pulmonary disease.

Abdomen

For the patient with a cardiovascular disorder, several components of the abdominal examination are relevant:

Abdominal distension: A protuberant abdomen with bulging flanks indicates ascites. Ascites develops in patients with right ventricular or biventricular HF (both right- and left-sided HF). In the failing right heart, abnormally high chamber pressures impede the return of venous blood. As a result, the liver and spleen become engorged with excessive venous blood (hepatosplenomegaly). As pressure in the portal system rises, fluid shifts from the vascular bed into the abdominal cavity. Ascitic fluid, found in the dependent or lowest points in the abdomen, will shift with position changes.

Hepatojugular reflux: This test is performed when right ventricular or biventricular HF is suspected. The patient is positioned so that the jugular venous pulse is visible in the lower part of the neck. While observing the jugular venous pulse, firm pressure is applied over the right upper quadrant of the abdomen for 30 to 60 seconds. An increase of 1 cm or more in jugular venous pressure is indicative of a positive hepatojugular reflux. This positive test aids in confirming the diagnosis of HF.

Bladder distention: Urine output is an important indicator of cardiac function. Reduced urine output may indicate inadequate renal perfusion or a less serious problem such as one caused by urinary retention. When urine output is decreased, the patient must be assessed for a distended bladder or difficulty voiding. The bladder may be assessed with an ultrasound scanner (see Fig. 53-8 in Chapter 53) or the suprapubic area palpated for an oval mass and percussed for dullness, indicative of a full bladder.

 Gerontologic Considerations

When performing a cardiovascular examination on an older patient, the nurse may note such differences as more readily palpable peripheral pulses because of decreased elasticity of the arteries and a loss of adjacent connective tissue. Palpation of the precordium in older adults is affected by the changes in the shape of the chest. For example, a cardiac impulse may not be palpable in patients with chronic obstructive pulmonary disease, because these patients usually have an increased anterior–posterior chest diameter. Kyphoscoliosis, a spinal deformity that occurs in many older adult patients, may move the cardiac apex downward so that palpation of the apical impulse is obscured.

Isolated systolic hypertension is directly correlated to the aging process, affecting more than 50% of people 65 years of age or older. By middle age, those without hypertension have a 90% lifetime risk of developing this problem. Untreated hypertension is associated with significant cardiovascular morbidity and mortality, including stroke (Rosendorff, Lackland, Allison, et al., 2015). Another common BP problem in the older adult is postural (orthostatic) hypotension. It is a result of impaired baroreceptor function, which is necessary to regulate BP. Other factors that heighten the risk for postural hypotension include prolonged bed rest, dehydration, and many cardiovascular medications (e.g., beta-blockers, angiotensin-converting enzyme inhibitors, angiotensin receptor blockers, diuretics, nitrates). Postural hypotension, regardless of the cause, places older adults at risk for falls (Weber & Kelley, 2014).

An S_4 that is associated with hypertension is common in older adults. It is thought to be due to a decrease in compliance of the left ventricle. The S_2 is usually split. At least 60% of older patients have murmurs, the most common being a soft systolic ejection murmur resulting from sclerotic changes of the aortic leaflets (Bickley, 2014) (see Table 25-1).

Diagnostic Evaluation

A wide range of diagnostic studies may be performed in patients with cardiovascular conditions. The nurse should educate the patient on the purpose, what to expect, and any possible side effects related to these examinations prior to testing. The nurse should note trends in results because they provide information about disease progression as well as the patient's response to therapy.

Laboratory Tests

Samples of the patient's blood are sent to the laboratory for the following reasons:
- To assist in making a diagnosis
- To screen for risk factors associated with CAD
- To establish baseline values before initiating other diagnostic tests, procedures, or therapeutic interventions
- To monitor response to therapeutic interventions
- To assess for abnormalities in the blood that affect prognosis

Normal values for laboratory tests may vary depending on the laboratory and the health care institution. This variation is due to the differences in equipment and methods of measurement across organizations.

Cardiac Biomarker Analysis

The diagnosis of MI is made by evaluating the history and physical examination, the 12-lead electrocardiogram (ECG), and the results of laboratory tests that measure serum cardiac biomarkers. Myocardial cells that become necrotic from prolonged ischemia or trauma release specific enzymes (creatine kinase [CK]), CK isoenzymes (CK-MB), and proteins (myoglobin, troponin T, and troponin I). These substances leak into the interstitial spaces of the myocardium and are carried by the lymphatic system into general circulation. As a result, abnormally high levels of these substances can be detected in serum blood samples. (See Chapter 27 for further discussion of cardiac biomarker analysis.)

Blood Chemistry, Hematology, and Coagulation Studies

Table 25-4 provides information about some common serum laboratory tests and the implications for patients with CVD.

TABLE 25-4 Common Serum Laboratory Tests and Implications for Patients With Cardiovascular Disease

Laboratory Test Reference Range	Implications
Blood Chemistries	
Blood urea nitrogen (BUN): 10–20 mg/dL	BUN and creatinine are end products of protein metabolism excreted by the kidneys. Elevated BUN reflects reduced renal perfusion from decreased cardiac output or intravascular fluid volume deficit as a result of diuretic therapy or dehydration.
Calcium (Ca^{++}): 8.5–10.5 mg/dL	Calcium is necessary for blood coagulability, neuromuscular activity, and automaticity of the nodal cells (sinus and atrioventricular nodes). *Hypocalcemia:* Decreased calcium levels slow nodal function and impair myocardial contractility. The latter effect increases the risk for heart failure. *Hypercalcemia:* Increased calcium levels can occur with the administration of thiazide diuretics because these medications reduce renal excretion of calcium. Hypercalcemia potentiates digitalis toxicity, causes increased myocardial contractility, and increases the risk for varying degrees of heart block and sudden death from ventricular fibrillation.
Creatinine: 0.7–1.4 mg/dL	Both BUN and creatinine are used to assess renal function, although creatinine is a more sensitive measure. Renal impairment is detected by an increase in both BUN and creatinine. A normal creatinine level and an elevated BUN suggest an intravascular fluid volume deficit.
Magnesium (Mg^{++}): 1.8–3.0 mg/dL	Magnesium is necessary for the absorption of calcium, maintenance of potassium stores, and metabolism of adenosine triphosphate. It plays a major role in protein and carbohydrate synthesis and muscular contraction. *Hypomagnesemia:* Decreased magnesium levels are due to enhanced renal excretion of magnesium from the use of diuretic or digitalis therapy. Low magnesium levels predispose patients to atrial or ventricular tachycardias. *Hypermagnesemia:* Increased magnesium levels are commonly caused by the use of cathartics or antacids containing magnesium. Increased magnesium levels depress contractility and excitability of the myocardium, causing heart block and, if severe, asystole.
Potassium (K^+): 3.5–5 mEq/L	Potassium has a major role in cardiac electrophysiologic function. *Hypokalemia:* Decreased potassium levels due to administration of potassium-excreting diuretics can cause many forms of dysrhythmias, including life-threatening ventricular tachycardia or ventricular fibrillation, and predispose patients taking digitalis preparations to digitalis toxicity. *Hyperkalemia:* Increased potassium levels can result from an increased intake of potassium (e.g., foods high in potassium or potassium supplements), decreased renal excretion of potassium, the use of potassium-sparing diuretics (e.g., spironolactone), or the use of angiotensin-converting enzyme inhibitors that inhibit aldosterone function. Serious consequences of hyperkalemia include heart block, asystole, and life-threatening ventricular dysrhythmias.
Sodium (Na^+): 135–145 mEq/L	Low or high serum sodium levels do not directly affect cardiac function. *Hyponatremia:* Decreased sodium levels indicate fluid excess and can be caused by heart failure or administration of thiazide diuretics. *Hypernatremia:* Increased sodium levels indicate fluid deficits and can result from decreased water intake or loss of water through excessive sweating or diarrhea.
Coagulation Studies	Injury to a vessel wall or tissue initiates the formation of a thrombus. This injury activates the coagulation cascade, the complex interactions among phospholipids, calcium, and clotting factors that convert prothrombin to thrombin. The coagulation cascade has two pathways: the intrinsic and extrinsic pathways. Coagulation studies are routinely performed before invasive procedures, such as cardiac catheterization, electrophysiology testing, and cardiac surgery.
Partial thromboplastin time (PTT): 60–70 s Activated partial thromboplastin time (aPTT): 20–39 s	PTT or aPTT measures the activity of the intrinsic pathway and is used to assess the effects of unfractionated heparin. A therapeutic range is 1.5–2.5 times baseline values. Adjustment of heparin dose is required for aPTT <50 s (↑ dose) or >100 s (↓ dose).
Prothrombin time (PT): 9.5–12 s	PT measures the extrinsic pathway activity and is used to monitor the level of anticoagulation with warfarin (Coumadin).
International normalized ratio (INR): 1	The INR, reported with the PT, provides a standard method for reporting PT levels and eliminates the variation of PT results from different laboratories. The INR, rather than the PT alone, is used to monitor the effectiveness of warfarin. The therapeutic range for INR is 2–3.5, although specific ranges vary based on diagnosis.
Hematologic Studies	
Complete blood count (CBC)	The CBC identifies the total number of white and red blood cells and platelets, and measures hemoglobin and hematocrit. The CBC is carefully monitored in patients with cardiovascular disease.
Hematocrit *Male:* 42–52% *Female:* 35–47% Hemoglobin *Male:* 13–18 g/dL *Female:* 12–16 g/dL	The hematocrit represents the percentage of red blood cells found in 100 mL of whole blood. The red blood cells contain hemoglobin, which transports oxygen to the cells. Low hemoglobin and hematocrit levels have serious consequences for patients with cardiovascular disease, such as more frequent angina episodes or acute myocardial infarction.
Platelets: 150,000–450,000 (mm^3)	Platelets are the first line of protection against bleeding. Once activated by blood vessel wall injury or rupture of atherosclerotic plaque, platelets undergo chemical changes that form a thrombus. Several medications inhibit platelet function, including aspirin, clopidogrel (Plavix), and intravenous glycoprotein IIb/IIIa inhibitors (abciximab [ReoPro], eptifibatide [Integrilin], and tirofiban [Aggrastat]). When these medications are given, it is essential to monitor for thrombocytopenia (low platelet counts).
White blood cell (WBC) count: 4500–110,00 (mm^3)	WBC counts are monitored in immunocompromised patients, including patients with heart transplants or in situations where there is concern for infection (e.g., after invasive procedures or surgery).

Adapted from Woods, S. L., Froelicher, E. S., Motzer, S. A., et al. (2009). *Cardiac nursing* (6th ed.). Philadelphia, PA: Lippincott Williams & Wilkins.

Discussion of lipid, brain (B-type) natriuretic peptide (BNP), C-reactive protein (CRP), and homocysteine measurements follows.

Lipid Profile

Cholesterol, triglycerides, and lipoproteins are measured to evaluate a person's risk of developing CAD, especially if there is a family history of premature heart disease, or to diagnose a specific lipoprotein abnormality. Cholesterol and triglycerides are transported in the blood by combining with plasma proteins to form lipoproteins called LDL and HDL. Although cholesterol levels remain relatively constant over 24 hours, the blood specimen for the lipid profile should be obtained after a 12-hour fast.

Cholesterol Levels

Cholesterol is a lipid required for hormone synthesis and cell membrane formation. It is found in large quantities in brain and nerve tissue. Two major sources of cholesterol are diet (animal products) and the liver, where cholesterol is synthesized. Factors that contribute to variations in cholesterol levels include age, gender, diet, exercise patterns, genetics, menopause, tobacco use, and stress levels. Total cholesterol level is calculated by adding the HDL, LDL, and 20% of the triglyceride level.

New CAD prevention guidelines no longer focus on achieving specific cholesterol levels as there is inadequate evidence to support this practice. The mainstay of cholesterol lowering therapy is lifestyle changes. Medical management focuses on determining an individual's 10-year risk for atherosclerotic vascular disease to identify those most likely to benefit from taking prescribed statins, a class of cholesterol-lowering medications (Stone, Robinson, Lichtenstein, et al., 2014) (see Chapter 27 for more details).

LDL is the primary transporter of cholesterol and triglycerides into the cell. One harmful effect of LDL is the deposition of these substances in the walls of arterial vessels. HDL has a protective action because it transports cholesterol away from the tissue and cells of the arterial wall to the liver for excretion (Stone et al., 2014).

Triglycerides

Triglycerides, composed of free fatty acids and glycerol, are stored in the adipose tissue and are a source of energy. Triglyceride levels increase after meals and are affected by stress. Diabetes, alcohol use, and obesity can elevate triglyceride levels. These levels have a direct correlation with LDL and an inverse one with HDL.

Brain (B-Type) Natriuretic Peptide

BNP is a neurohormone that helps regulate BP and fluid volume. It is primarily secreted from the ventricles in response to increased preload with resulting elevated ventricular pressure. The level of BNP in the blood increases as the ventricular walls expand from increased pressure, making it a helpful diagnostic, monitoring, and prognostic tool in the setting of HF. Because this serum laboratory test can be quickly obtained, BNP levels are useful for prompt diagnosis of HF in settings such as the ED. Elevations in BNP can occur from a number of other conditions such as pulmonary embolus, MI, and ventricular hypertrophy. Therefore, the clinician correlates BNP levels with abnormal physical assessment findings and other diagnostic tests before making a definitive diagnosis of HF. A BNP level greater than 100 pg/mL is suggestive of HF.

C-Reactive Protein

CRP is a protein produced by the liver in response to systemic inflammation. Inflammation is thought to play a role in the development and progression of atherosclerosis. The high-sensitivity CRP (hs-CRP) test is used as an adjunct to other tests to predict CVD risk. People with high hs-CRP levels (3 mg/L or greater) may be at greatest risk for CVD compared to people with moderate (1 to 3 mg/L) or low (less than 1 mg/L) hs-CRP levels (Woods et al., 2009).

Homocysteine

Homocysteine, an amino acid, is linked to the development of atherosclerosis because it can damage the endothelial lining of arteries and promote thrombus formation. Therefore, an elevated blood level of homocysteine is thought to indicate a high risk for CAD, stroke, and peripheral vascular disease, although it is not an independent predictor of CAD. Genetic factors and a diet low in folate, vitamin B_6, and vitamin B_{12} are associated with elevated homocysteine levels. A 12-hour fast is necessary before drawing a blood sample for an accurate serum measurement. Test results are interpreted as optimal (less than 12 mcmol/L), borderline (12 to 15 mcmol/L), and high risk (greater than 15 mcmol/L) (Woods et al., 2009).

Chest X-Ray and Fluoroscopy

A chest x-ray is obtained to determine the size, contour, and position of the heart. It reveals cardiac and pericardial calcifications and demonstrates physiologic alterations in the pulmonary circulation. Although it does not help diagnose acute MI, it can help diagnose some complications (e.g., HF). Correct placement of pacemakers and pulmonary artery catheters is also confirmed by chest x-ray.

Fluoroscopy is an x-ray imaging technique that allows visualization of the heart on a screen. It shows cardiac and vascular pulsations and unusual cardiac contours. This technique uses a movable x-ray source, which makes it a useful aid for positioning transvenous pacing electrodes and for guiding the insertion of arterial and venous catheters during cardiac catheterization and other cardiac procedures.

Electrocardiography

The ECG is a graphic representation of the electrical currents of the heart. The ECG is obtained by placing disposable electrodes in standard positions on the skin of the chest wall and extremities (see Chapter 26 for electrode placement). Recordings of the electrical current flowing between two electrodes is made on graph paper or displayed on a monitor. Several different recordings can be obtained by using a variety of electrode combinations, called *leads*. Simply stated, a lead is a specific view of the electrical activity of heart. The standard ECG is composed of 12 leads or 12 different views, although it is possible to record 15 or 18 leads.

The 12-lead ECG is used to diagnose dysrhythmias, conduction abnormalities, and chamber enlargement, as well as myocardial ischemia, injury, or infarction. It can also suggest cardiac effects of electrolyte disturbances (high or low calcium and potassium levels) and the effects of antiarrhythmic medications. A 15-lead ECG adds three additional chest leads across the right precordium and is used for early diagnosis of right ventricular and left posterior (ventricular) infarction. The 18-lead ECG adds three posterior leads to the 15-lead ECG and is useful for early detection of myocardial ischemia and injury. To enhance interpretation of the ECG, the patient's age, gender, BP, height, weight, symptoms, and medications (especially digitalis and antiarrhythmic agents) are noted on the ECG requisition. (See Chapter 26 for a more detailed discussion of ECG.)

Continuous Electrocardiographic Monitoring

Continuous ECG monitoring is the standard of care for patients who are at high risk for dysrhythmias. This form of cardiac monitoring detects abnormalities in heart rate and rhythm. Many systems have the capacity to monitor for changes in ST segments, which are used to identify the presence of myocardial ischemia or injury (see Chapter 27). Two types of continuous ECG monitoring techniques are used in health care settings: hardwire cardiac monitoring, found in EDs, critical care units, and progressive care units; and telemetry, found in general nursing care units or outpatient cardiac rehabilitation programs. Hardwire cardiac monitoring and telemetry systems vary in sophistication; however, most systems have the following features in common:

- Monitor more than one ECG lead simultaneously
- Monitor ST segments (ST-segment depression is a marker of myocardial ischemia; ST-segment elevation provides evidence of an evolving MI)
- Provide graded visual and audible alarms (based on priority, asystole merits the highest grade of alarm)
- Interpret and store alarms
- Trend data over time
- Print a copy of rhythms from one or more specific ECG leads over a set time (called a *rhythm strip*)

> **▶ Quality and Safety Nursing Alert**
>
> *Patients placed on continuous ECG monitoring must be informed of its purpose and cautioned that it does not detect shortness of breath, chest pain, or other ACS symptoms. Thus, patients are instructed to report new or worsening symptoms immediately.*

 ### Hardwire Cardiac Monitoring

Hardwire cardiac monitoring is used to continuously observe the heart for dysrhythmias and conduction disorders using 1 or 2 ECG leads. A real-time ECG is displayed on a bedside monitor and at a central monitoring station. In critical care units, additional components can be added to the bedside monitor to continuously monitor hemodynamic parameters (noninvasive BP, arterial pressures, pulmonary artery pressures), respiratory parameters (respiratory rate, oxygen saturation), and ST segments for myocardial ischemia.

Telemetry

In addition to hardwire cardiac monitoring, the ECG can be continuously observed by **telemetry**—the transmission of radio waves from a battery-operated transmitter to a central bank of monitors. The primary benefit of using telemetry is

that the system is wireless, which allows patients to ambulate while one or two ECG leads are monitored. The patient has electrodes placed on the chest with a lead cable that connects to the transmitter. The transmitter can be placed in a disposable pouch and worn around the neck, or simply secured to the patient's clothing. Most transmitter batteries are changed every 24 to 48 hours.

Lead Systems

The number of electrodes needed for hardwire cardiac monitoring and telemetry is dictated by the lead system used in the clinical setting. Electrodes need to be securely and accurately placed on the chest wall. Chart 25-4 provides helpful hints on how to apply these electrodes. There are three-, four-, or five-lead systems available for ECG monitoring. The type of lead system used determines the number of lead options for monitoring. For example, the five-lead system provides up to seven different lead selections. Unlike the other two systems, the 5-lead system can monitor the activity of the anterior wall of the left ventricle. Figure 25-9 presents diagrams of electrode placement.

The two ECG leads most often selected for continuous ECG monitoring are leads II and V_1. Lead II provides the best visualization of atrial depolarization (represented by the P wave). Lead V_1 best records ventricular depolarization and is most helpful when monitoring for certain dysrhythmias (e.g., premature ventricular contractions, tachycardias, bundle branch blocks) (see Chapter 26).

Ambulatory Electrocardiography

Ambulatory electrocardiography is a form of continuous or intermittent ECG home monitoring. It is used to identify the etiology of syncope or palpitation caused by dysrhythmias, detect episodes of myocardial ischemia, evaluate effectiveness of treatment of HF and dysrhythmias, as well as evaluate the

---

Chart 25-4 | **Applying Electrodes**

The monitoring system requires an adequate electrical signal to analyze the patient's cardiac rhythm. When applying electrodes, the recommendations below should be followed to optimize skin adherence and conduction of the heart's electrical current:

- Débride the skin surface of dead cells with soap and water; dry well using a wash cloth or gauze
- Clip (do not shave) hair from around the electrode site, if needed.
- Connect the electrodes to the lead wires prior to placing them on the chest (connecting lead wires when electrodes are in place may be uncomfortable for some patients).
- Peel the backing off the electrode, and check to make sure the center is moist with electrode gel.
- Locate the appropriate lead placement, and apply the electrode to the skin, securing it in place with light pressure.
- Change the electrodes every 24 hours, examine the skin for irritation, and apply the electrodes to different locations.
- If the patient is sensitive to the electrodes, use hypoallergenic electrodes.

Adapted from Sendelbach, S., & Jepsen, S. (2013). *AACN practice alert: Alarm management*. Retrieved on 1/25/2016 at www.aacn.org/wd/practice/content/practicealerts/alarm-management-practice-alert.pcms?menu=practice

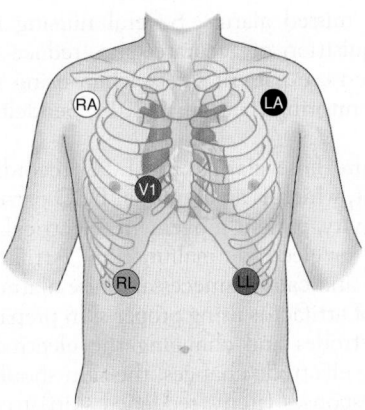

RA – Right arm (white)
LA – Left arm (black)
RL – Right leg (green)
LL – Left leg (red)
V1 – Chest or precordium (brown)

Figure 25-9 • Electrode placement used in continuous electrocardiographic monitoring for three-lead system, placement on RA, LA, and LL; four-lead system, placement on RA, LA, RL, and LL; five-lead system, placement on RA, LA, RL, LL, and V1.

functioning of ICDs and pacemakers. Several types of devices are available and are worn either externally or implanted under the skin. The ECG is transmitted to a centralized monitoring station via telephone. Newer devices transmit ECGs through the use of wireless technology to a secure website (Leahy & Davenport, 2015; Romero, 2013; Walsh, Topol, & Steinhubl, 2014).

Continuous Monitors

Commonly called Holter monitors, these small portable recorders are connected to chest electrodes (number varies based on model used) that record the ECG using several leads onto a digital memory device. The patient wears the recorder for 24 to 48 hours and in certain cases up to 2 weeks. If the patient experiences symptoms they are instructed to activate the event marker. The patient is also asked to keep a diary to note the date and time of symptoms or performance of unusual activities. The diary is used by the primary provider to correlate symptoms with detected dysrhythmias. Once monitoring is completed the patient returns the device to the primary provider's office. Data from the digital memory device are then uploaded into a computer for analysis, and rhythms that need further evaluation by the primary provider are identified. The effectiveness of this form of monitoring is dependent upon the patient's adherence with keeping a diary and marking events. Holter monitors do not provide real-time ECG recordings, which is another limitation.

A novel alternative to the use of the Holter monitor is ECG patch monitoring, which uses blue-tooth technology. An ECG patch with adhesive backing is placed over the left pectoral area, eliminating the need for multiple ECG electrodes, wires, and recorders. The patch is single use, waterproof, and easily concealed under clothing. The patient wears the patch for up to 14 days and then returns it to the manufacturer for analysis. These devices, which are available from several manufactures, have one major limitation. The ECG

patch is capable of monitoring just one ECG lead, which makes it less sensitive to dysrhythmia detection (Walsh et al., 2014).

Continuous Real-Time Monitors

This technology allows the ECG to be monitored continuously at a remote central monitoring station. The patient has three electrodes applied to the chest or wears an electrode belt that is attached to a small sensor. The sensor transmits each heartbeat to a small monitor. When a dysrhythmia is detected, the system automatically transmits the ECG to a monitoring center either through the patient's telephone line when at home or through wireless communications systems when outside of the home. The patient can also trigger activation of ECG transmissions. The ECG is analyzed real time by technicians who communicate abnormal findings to the patient's primary provider. This method of monitoring enhances detection and early treatment of dysrhythmias that might otherwise be diagnosed only after the patient develops serious symptoms (Walsh et al., 2014).

Cardiac Event Recorders

Cardiac event recorders allow patients to record the electrical activity of the heart when they experience symptoms, such as palpitations, dizziness, or lightheadedness. Patients may need to record events for several days to a month. The recorded ECGs are transmitted to the primary provider by telephone. Newer technology has the capability of wireless transmission of the events automatically through the use of cellular networks. There are three main forms of recorders.

The symptom event monitor is used to record and store the ECG during only during times when the patient is experiencing symptoms. Patients activate the symptom event monitor by pressing a button for devices that are worn on the wrist or by placing a hand held device over the chest. The recorded event is then transmitted to the primary provider by telephone.

The continuous looping memory monitor, a small battery operated device, can record and store the ECG for short periods of time. The monitor is attached to the patient with chest electrodes or a wrist band. Patients are instructed to activate ECG recordings by the push of a button. The device records the patient's ECG for a predetermined time before and after the device activation. Some of these devices are programmable to detect bradycardia, tachycardia, and irregular rhythms and do not require patient interaction. It is a preferred method over the symptom event monitor because it has more monitoring capabilities.

Real-time smart phone monitoring is a novel approach to cardiac event recording. An adaptor, attached to the smart phone, converts the phone into a monitoring device. The patient places a finger in the device that digitally records lead I of the ECG. The ECG can be viewed immediately and also be sent as a PDF file via a secure server to the patient's primary provider (Walsh et al., 2014).

Cardiac Implantable Electronic Devices

Cardiac implantable electronic devices include pacemakers and ICDs. These lifesaving devices are used to manage patients with serious cardiac illnesses. The technology available today allows for remote wireless monitoring of these devices to determine battery life, pacing parameters and therapies, and occurrence of serious atrial and ventricular dysrhythmias. A transmitter, which is placed in the patient's home, sends device data to a secure data repository on a secure web portal. A unique feature of these implantable devices is that they have programmable alerts that automatically detect and transmit dysrhythmias without the need for patient interaction (see Chapter 26 for further discussion) (Leahy & Davenport, 2015).

An implantable loop recorder is another type of a cardiac implantable electronic device. This small device, composed of a battery and microchips, is injected under the skin. Compared with event recorders described above, this device offers several advantages It can record ECGs continuously for up to 3 years. It also can eliminate the patient's need to change electrodes and wear or carry the monitoring device. This type of monitoring is recommended for patients who have infrequent symptoms or require longer term ECG monitoring (Romero, 2013).

Nursing Interventions for Inpatient Cardiac Monitoring

A body of evidence indicates that most alarms occurring during inpatient ECG monitoring are false alarms. Nurses dealing with excessive alarms become desensitized to these sounds and develop alarm fatigue. Alarm fatigue delays response time or results in missed alarms. Several nursing interventions facilitate acquisition of accurate data, reduce risk of alarm fatigue, and ensure patient safety when using various forms of cardiac monitoring (Hannibal, 2014; Sendelbach & Funk, 2013).

To minimize false alarms, the ECG recordings must be free of artifact, which is an abnormal ECG pattern caused by muscular activity, patient movement, electrical interference, or lead cable or electrode malfunction. Artifact can mimic dysrhythmias and cause unnecessary false alarms. Key to the elimination of artifact is using proper skin preparation before applying electrodes and changing the electrodes every 24 hours. During electrode changes, the skin should be assessed for allergic responses (itchy, reddened skin) to the adhesive or electrode gel. If present, the electrodes are replaced with hypoallergenic electrodes. Rotation of electrode placement on the skin will reduce the risk for skin breakdown (see Fig. 25-9). See Chart 25-5 for a Nursing Research Profile on electrode placement, skin preparation, and alarm fatigue.

Electrodes and lead connections need to be positioned correctly. Improper positioning can result in artifact that mimics ischemia or dysrhythmias. Two leads should be selected that provide the best tracing for dysrhythmia monitoring, which are usually lead II and the chest lead V_1. Electrical equipment in use around the patient should be inspected to be certain that it is functioning properly and has been recently checked

---

Chart 25-5 | **NURSING RESEARCH PROFILE**
Electrode Placement, Skin Preparation, and Alarm Fatigue

Walsh-Irwin, C. & Jurgens, C. Y. (2015). Proper skin preparation and electrode placement decreases alarms on a telemetry unit. *Dimensions of Critical Care Nursing, 34*(3), 134–139.

Purpose

Electrocardiographic (ECG) monitoring in the inpatient setting is a common practice for patients at risk for cardiac dysrhythmias, ST-segment changes, or prolongation of the QT interval. It is used for the early detection and notification of an abnormality in the patient's ECG. When this situation occurs, the monitor sounds an alarm, which can vary in intensity and duration based on its clinical significance. Unfortunately, many things can cause the monitor to alarm inappropriately. Muscle tremors, patient movement, artifact from inadequate skin preparation, and improper ECG electrode placement are the most common reasons for these false alarms.

Nurses faced with excessive alarms become desensitized to these sounds, causing alarm fatigue. Alarm fatigue results in delayed responses to alarms and missing alarms, which may have serious life-threatening consequences for the patient. The Joint Commission has set a goal for 2017 that no patient should be harmed by false alarms. Therefore, the purpose of this study was to evaluate the effect of proper skin preparation and ECG electrode placement on alarm rates. The nurse researchers hypothesized that using proper techniques would reduce alarms on a telemetry unit.

Design

The conceptual framework for this study was the American Association of Critical Care Nurses *Synergy Model for Patient Care*. This model links competent nursing practice with positive patient outcomes. A prospective descriptive design was used to test the effect that proper skin preparation and ECG electrode placement had on the number of alarms on a telemetry unit in a suburban

Veterans Affairs Medical Center. The hospital's Institutional Review Board ruled that the study was quality improvement and subjects were not required to provide consent to participate. After admission, the number of alarms was counted for 24 hours on 25 patients who had ECG electrodes placed using usual care. After 24 hours, the ECG electrodes were removed, the skin prepared (clipping hair if necessary, cleansing skin with soap and water, drying the skin with a wash cloth that causes mild skin abrasions), and reapplying the electrode using proper anatomic locations. The number of alarms was then recounted for 24 hours.

Findings

After the reapplication of ECG electrodes, nine patients were discharged before 24 hours and one patient refused to have his leads changes. Therefore, the final sample was composed of 15 men; the majority were white (93%) and had a mean age of 71.2 (±12.7) years. The initial alarm count for the first 24 hours was between 2 and 1341, compared with 1 and 992 alarms in the second 24 hours period. The mean number of alarms was significantly lower in patients after the second 24 hours, as compared with the first 24 hours. The use of proper skin preparation and lead placement was associated with a 44% reduction in the mean number of alarms.

Nursing Implications

The results of this study demonstrate that the use of guidelines for skin preparation and electrode placement recommended by the American Association of Critical Care Nurses results in safer and more effective ECG monitoring practices. The use of evidence-based ECG monitoring practices by nurses results in fewer false alarms and minimizes the risks to patients associated with alarm fatigue.

by the medical engineering department per organization policy, because improperly functioning equipment may cause false alarms from artifact.

An effort should be made to individualize the ECG alarm parameters to meet the patient's monitoring needs. For example, if the patient has atrial fibrillation, it is appropriate to turn off the irregular heart rate alarm. Keeping it on will create unnecessary alarms, contributing to alarm fatigue. Similarly, the bradycardia and tachycardia alarms should be adjusted, slightly below or above the patient's underlying heart rate (Drew, Harris, Ze'gre-Hemsey, et al., 2014).

The nurse's role is to respond to and correct all monitor alarms immediately. Inoperative (inop) monitoring alarms—used to communicate that electrodes have fallen off, that leads are loose, or that the system's battery power is low (e.g., telemetry)—are just as significant as dysrhythmia alarms indicating that the patient is tachycardic, bradycardic, or experiencing another potentially life-threatening dysrhythmia. Timely responses to all alarms can prevent serious consequences, including death.

Hospital-acquired infections may be prevented by keeping lead wire cables and transmitter equipment clean, per organizational policy. A patient should never be connected to monitoring equipment that has not been thoroughly cleaned between patients. If a patient is scheduled for a device implant, such as a pacemaker, electrodes should not be placed over the planned incision site. Likewise, electrodes should never be placed over an incision, implanted device, open wounds, or inflamed skin.

Electrodes should be removed once monitoring is discontinued and skin cleansed to remove excess electrode gel and adhesive. Metal-containing electrodes must be removed before sending a patient for any magnetic resonance scan, including magnetic resonance angiography (MRA).

Telemetry transmitters and other monitoring equipment should be maintained according to the manufacturer's recommendations. Monitoring devices of any type should not be submerged in water. A monitoring device may break if dropped; therefore, it should be secured to the patient's gown or clothing.

Cardiac Stress Testing

Normally, the coronary arteries dilate to four times their usual diameter in response to increased metabolic demands for oxygen and nutrients. However, coronary arteries affected by atherosclerosis dilate less, compromising blood flow to the myocardium and causing ischemia. Therefore, abnormalities in cardiovascular function are more likely to be detected during times of increased demand, or "stress." The **cardiac stress test** procedures—the exercise stress test and the pharmacologic stress test—are noninvasive ways to evaluate the response of the cardiovascular system to stress. The stress test helps determine the following: (1) presence of CAD, (2) cause of chest pain, (3) functional capacity of the heart after an MI or heart surgery, (4) effectiveness of antianginal or antiarrhythmic medications, (5) occurrence of dysrhythmias, and (6) specific goals for a physical fitness program. Contraindications to stress testing include acute MI within 48 hours, unstable angina, uncontrolled dysrhythmias with hemodynamic compromise, severe aortic stenosis, acute myocarditis or pericarditis, and

decompensated HF (Fletcher, Ades, Kligfield, et al., 2013). Because complications of stress testing can be life threatening (MI, cardiac arrest, HF, and bradycardia and tachycardia with hemodynamic compromise), testing facilities must have staff and equipment ready to provide treatment, including advanced cardiac life support.

Stress testing is often combined with echocardiography or radionuclide imaging, techniques used to capture images of the heart. Cardiac imaging is performed during the resting state and immediately after stress testing.

Exercise Stress Testing

Procedure

During an exercise stress test, the patient walks on a treadmill (most common) or pedals a stationary bicycle. Exercise intensity progresses according to established protocols. The protocol selected for the test is based on the purpose of the test and the physical fitness level and health of the patient (Fletcher et al. 2013). During the test, the following are monitored: 2 or more ECG leads for heart rate, rhythm, and ischemic changes; BP; skin temperature; physical appearance; perceived exertion; and symptoms, including chest pain, dyspnea, dizziness, leg cramping, and fatigue. The test is terminated when the target heart rate is achieved or if the patient experiences signs of myocardial ischemia. Further diagnostic testing, such as a cardiac catheterization, may be warranted if the patient develops chest pain, extreme fatigue, a decrease in BP or pulse rate, serious dysrhythmias, or ST-segment changes on the ECG during the stress test.

Nursing Interventions

In preparation for the exercise stress test, the patient is instructed to fast for at least 3 hours before the test and to avoid stimulants such as tobacco and caffeine. Medications may be taken with sips of water. The primary provider may instruct the patient not to take certain cardiac medications, such as beta-adrenergic blocking agents, before the test. Clothes and sneakers or rubber-soled shoes suitable for exercising are to be worn. The nurse prepares the patient for the stress test by describing how the stress test is performed, the type of monitoring equipment used, the rationale for insertion of an IV catheter, and what symptoms to report. The exercise method is reviewed, and patients are asked to put forth their best exercise effort. If the test is to be performed with echocardiography or radionuclide imaging (described in the next section), this information is reviewed as well. After the test, the patient is monitored for 10 to 15 minutes. Once stable, patients may resume their usual activities.

Pharmacologic Stress Testing

Procedure

Patients who are cognitively impaired and unable to follow directions or physically disabled or deconditioned will not be able to achieve their target heart rate by exercising on a treadmill or bicycle. Vasodilating agents such as dipyridamole (Persantine), adenosine (Adenocard), or regadenoson (Lexiscan) given as an IV infusion are used to mimic the effects of exercise by maximally dilating normal coronary arteries. The side effects of these agents are related to the vasodilating action and include chest pain, headache, flushing, nausea, heart block and dyspnea. If necessary the effects of these drugs can be reversed with IV aminophylline. Adenosine has an extremely short half-life (less than 10 seconds), so any severe effects subside rapidly. These vasodilating medications are the agents used in conjunction with radionuclide imaging techniques. Patients undergoing pharmacologic stress tests must avoid xanthine derivatives including theophylline, aminophylline, and caffeine as they block the effects of the vasodilating agents.

Dobutamine is another option for use during a pharmacologic stress test. This medication is a synthetic sympathomimetic agent that increases heart rate, myocardial contractility, and BP, thereby increasing the metabolic demands of the heart. It is the agent of choice when echocardiography is used because of its effects on altering myocardial wall motion (due to enhanced contractility). Dobutamine is also used for patients who have bronchospasm or pulmonary disease and cannot tolerate having doses of theophylline withheld.

Nursing Interventions

In preparation for the pharmacologic stress test, the patient is instructed not to eat or drink anything for at least 3 hours before the test. The patient must also be told to refrain from eating any liquids or food that contain chocolate or caffeine for 24 hours. This restriction also includes caffeine-free coffee, tea, carbonated beverages, as well as medications containing caffeine (e.g., Anacin). If caffeine is ingested before a stress test using vasodilating agents, the test will have to be rescheduled. Patients taking aminophylline, theophylline, or dipyridamole are instructed to stop taking these medications for 24 to 48 hours before the test (if tolerated). The patient is informed about the transient sensations that may occur during infusion of the vasodilating agent, such as flushing or nausea, which will disappear quickly. The patient is instructed to report the occurrence of any other symptoms during the test to the cardiologist or nurse. The stress test may take about 1 hour, or up to 3 hours if imaging is performed.

Radionuclide Imaging

Radionuclide imaging studies are noninvasive tests that use radioisotopes to evaluate coronary artery perfusion, detect myocardial ischemia and infarction, and/or assess left ventricular function. **Radioisotopes** are unstable atoms that give off small amounts of energy in the form of gamma rays as they decay. When radioisotopes are injected into the bloodstream, the energy emitted can be detected by a gamma scintillation camera positioned over the body. These radioisotopes are called tracers.

Myocardial Perfusion Imaging

Myocardial perfusion imaging is performed using two types of techniques: single photon emission computed tomography (SPECT) or positron emission tomography (PET). It is commonly performed after an acute MI to determine if arterial perfusion to the heart is compromised during activity and to evaluate the extent of myocardial damage. It is also used to evaluate if myocardial ischemia from CAD is the cause of chest pain or other CAD-related symptoms.

These imaging techniques are performed in combination with stress testing to compare images obtained when the heart is resting to images of the heart in a stressed state resulting from exercise or medications. An area of the myocardium

that shows no perfusion or reduced perfusion is said to have a "defect" present. Comparing resting images with images taken after the stress test help differentiate ischemic myocardium from infarct-related myocardium. A defect that does not change in size before and after stress is called a fixed defect. Fixed defects indicate that there is no perfusion in that area of the myocardium, which is the case after an MI. Defects that appear or that get larger after the stress test images are taken indicate reduced perfusion to that area of the heart. Because the defect disappears with rest, it is called a reversible defect. Reversible defects constitute positive stress test findings. Typically, cardiac catheterization is recommended after a positive test result to determine the severity of obstructions to blood flow caused by CAD.

The patient undergoing myocardial perfusion imaging with stress testing should be prepared for the type of stressor to be used (exercise or medication) and provided with details of what to expect during imaging. The imaging is performed in two stages. Usually, the resting images are taken first. An IV is inserted to administer the radioisotope, and electrodes are placed on the chest to monitor the heart rate and rhythm. Women who are nursing, pregnant or think they are pregnant should not undergo myocardial perfusion imaging. The nurse alerts the primary provider if any of these conditions are present.

Single Photon Emission Computed Tomography

SPECT is used most often because it is more widely available and is technically easier to perform than PET. In addition, the diagnostic and prognostic value of SPECT is better established than PET (Fletcher et al., 2013).

Procedure

SPECT is a painless, noninvasive procedure that involves the injection of one of three commercially available tracers (technetium [Tc]-99m sestamibi, Tc-99m-tetrofosmin, or thallium-201).

During SPECT, patients are positioned supine on the table with their arms over their heads. The gamma camera circles around the chest area converting the signals from the traces into pictures of the heart. The procedure takes approximately 30 minutes. The second scan is repeated following the exercise or pharmacologic stress test.

Nursing Interventions

The nurse's primary role is to prepare the patient for SPECT and insert an IV catheter or assess an existing IV for patency and suitability. The IV is used to inject the tracer. The patient may be concerned about receiving a radioactive substance and needs to be reassured that these tracers are safe—the radiation exposure is similar to that of other diagnostic x-ray studies. No postprocedure radiation precautions are necessary.

Positron Emission Tomography

PET produces better pictures than SPECT, is faster, and uses lower doses of radiation. However, its use is limited because not all facilities have a PET scanner and the technical equipment needed to produce the tracers (Fletcher et al., 2013).

Procedure

During PET, tracers are given by injection; one compound is used to determine blood flow in the myocardium, and another determines the metabolic function. The PET camera provides detailed three-dimensional images of the distributed compounds. The viability of the myocardium is determined by comparing the extent of glucose metabolism in the myocardium to the degree of blood flow. For example, ischemic but viable tissue will show decreased blood flow and elevated metabolism. For a patient with this finding, revascularization through surgery or angioplasty will probably be indicated to improve heart function. Restrictions of food intake before the test vary among institutions, but because PET evaluates glucose metabolism, the patient's blood glucose level should be within the normal range before testing.

Nursing Interventions

The nurse instructs the patient to refrain from using alcohol and caffeine for 24 hours before undergoing PET because of the stimulating effects they may have on the heart. For patients with diabetes and who are taking insulin, the nurse needs to discuss insulin doses and food restrictions with the primary provider. The nurse assesses patients for fear of closed spaces or claustrophobia. Patients who have this condition are reassured that medications can be given to help them relax. The nurse also reassures patients that radiation exposure is at safe and acceptable levels, similar to those of other diagnostic x-ray studies.

To prepare the patient for PET, the nurse inserts an IV or assesses the existing IV catheter for patency and suitability, and then describes the procedure to the patient. The patient is positioned on a table with hands above the head. The table then slides into a donut shaped scanner. While in the scanner, the patient must lie still so that clear images of the heart can be obtained. A baseline scan is performed, which takes about 30 minutes. Then a tracer is injected into the IV and the scan is repeated. The patient's glucose level is monitored throughout the procedure. The scan takes from 1 to 3 hours to complete.

Test of Ventricular Function and Wall Motion

Equilibrium radionuclide angiocardiography (ERNA), also known as multiple-gated acquisition (MUGA) scanning, is a common noninvasive technique that uses a conventional scintillation camera interfaced with a computer to record images of the heart during several hundred heartbeats. The computer processes the data and allows for sequential viewing of the functioning heart. The sequential images are analyzed to evaluate left ventricular function, wall motion, and ejection fraction.

The patient is reassured that there is no known radiation danger and is instructed to remain motionless during the scan.

Additional Imaging

Computed Tomography

Procedure

Cardiac CT scanning is a form of cardiac imaging that uses x-rays to provide accurate cross-sectional "virtual" slices of specific areas of the heart and surrounding structures. Complex mathematical and computer algorithms are used to analyze the slices to create three-dimensional images. Multidetector CT (MDCT) is a fast form of CT scanning that takes multiple slices at the same time. This technology helps to produce clear images by eliminating artifact created by the beating heart and respirations (Stone et al., 2014). There are two types of cardiac CT scanning that include coronary CT angiography and electron beam CT (EBCT) (for coronary calcium scoring).

Coronary CT angiography requires the use of an IV contrast agent to enhance the x-rays and improve visualization of cardiac structures. This test is used to evaluate coronary arteries for stenosis, the aorta for aneurisms or dissections, graft patency after coronary artery bypass grafting (CABG), pulmonary veins in patients with atrial fibrillation, and cardiac structures for congenital anomalies. Patients may receive beta-blockers prior to the scan to control heart rate and rhythm and reduce artifact. Another way to minimize artifact is to have patients hold their breath periodically throughout the scan. Coronary CT angiography is used with caution in patients with renal insufficiency. The contrast agent used during the CT scan is excreted through the kidneys; therefore, renal function should be assessed prior to the scan. It may be necessary to administer IV hydration before and after the scan to minimize the effect of the contrast on renal function. Patients will require premedication with corticosteroids and antihistamines if they experienced a reaction to a contrast agent in the past (Mervak, Davenport, Ellis, et al., 2015).

EBCT is used to calculate a coronary artery calcium score that is based on the amount of calcium deposits in the coronary arteries. This score is used to predict the likelihood of cardiac events, such as MI, or the need for a revascularization procedure in the future. Coronary artery calcium scoring is used for the evaluation of individuals without known CAD and offers limited incremental prognostic value for individuals with known CAD, such as those with stents and bypass grafts. Currently, EBCT is thought to be a reasonable test to consider in patients with low to intermediate risk for future CAD-related events. Results of the test may help to reclassify them to higher risk and thus intensify primary prevention measures (Lloyd-Jones, 2015).

Nursing Interventions

The nurse provides details of the procedure to help prepare the patient for the test. Patients need to be prepared to hold their breath at certain time during the procedure, so it is important for the nurse to practice with the patient before going for CT scan. The patient is positioned on a table, and the scanner rotates around the table during the test. The procedure is noninvasive and painless. However, to obtain adequate images, the patient must lie completely still during the scanning process. An IV is necessary if contrast is to be used to enhance the images. The patient should be told to expect transient flushing, metallic taste, nausea, or bradycardia during the contrast infusion.

Magnetic Resonance Angiography

Procedure

MRA is a noninvasive, painless technique that is used to examine both the physiologic and anatomic properties of the heart. MRA uses a powerful magnetic field and computer-generated pictures to image the heart and great vessels. It is valuable in diagnosing diseases of the aorta, heart muscle, and pericardium, as well as congenital heart lesions. The application of this technique to the evaluation of coronary artery anatomy is limited because the quality of the images are distorted by respirations, the beating heart, and certain implanted devices (stents and surgical clips). In addition, this technique cannot adequately visualize the small distal coronary arteries as accurately as conventional angiography performed during a cardiac catheterization.

Nursing Interventions

Because of the magnetic field used during MRA, patients must be screened for contraindications for its use. MRA cannot be performed on patients who have a pacemaker, metal plates, prosthetic joints, or other metallic implants that can become dislodged if exposed to MRA. Patients are instructed to remove any jewelry, watches, or other metal items (e.g., ECG leads). Transdermal patches that contain a heat-conducting aluminized layer (e.g., NicoDerm, Androderm, Transderm Nitro, Transderm Scop, Catapres-TTS) must be removed before MRA to prevent burning of the skin. During MRA, the patient is positioned supine on a table that is placed into an enclosed imager or tube containing the magnetic field. A patient who is claustrophobic may need to receive a mild sedative before undergoing an MRA. An intermittent clanking or thumping that can be annoying is generated by the magnetic coils, so the patient may be offered a headset to listen to music. The scanner is equipped with a microphone so that the patient can communicate with the staff. The patient is instructed to remain motionless during the scan.

Echocardiography

Transthoracic Echocardiography

Echocardiography is a noninvasive ultrasound test that is used to measure the ejection fraction and examine the size, shape, and motion of cardiac structures. It is particularly useful for diagnosing pericardial effusions; determining chamber size and the etiology of heart murmurs; evaluating the function of heart valves, including prosthetic heart valves; and evaluating ventricular wall motion.

Procedure

Echocardiography involves transmission of high-frequency sound waves into the heart through the chest wall and the recording of the return signals. With the traditional transthoracic approach, the ultrasound is generated by a handheld transducer applied to the front of the chest. The transducer picks up the echoes and converts them to electrical impulses that are recorded and displayed on a monitor. It creates sophisticated, spatially correct images of the heart. An ECG is recorded simultaneously to assist in interpretation of the echocardiogram.

With the use of Doppler techniques, an echocardiogram can also show the direction and velocity of the blood flow through the heart. These techniques are used to assess for "leaking valves," conditions referred to as valvular regurgitation, and will also detect abnormal blood flow between the septum of the left and right heart.

Echocardiography may be performed with an exercise or pharmacologic stress test. Images are obtained at rest and then immediately after the target heart rate is reached. Myocardial ischemia from decreased perfusion during stress causes abnormalities in ventricular wall motion and is easily detected by echocardiography. A stress test using echocardiography is considered positive if abnormalities in ventricular wall motion are detected during stress but not during rest. These findings are highly suggestive of CAD and require further evaluation, such as a cardiac catheterization.

Nursing Interventions

Before transthoracic echocardiography, the nurse informs the patient about the test, explaining that it is painless. Echocardiographic monitoring is performed while a transducer that emits sound waves is moved over the surface of the chest wall. Gel applied to the skin helps transmit the sound waves. Periodically, the patient is asked to turn onto the left side or hold a breath. The test takes about 30 to 45 minutes. If the patient is to undergo an exercise or pharmacologic stress test with echocardiography, information on stress testing is also reviewed with the patient.

Transesophageal Echocardiography
Procedure

A significant limitation of transthoracic echocardiography is the poor quality of the images produced. Ultrasound loses its clarity as it passes through tissue, lung, and bone. An alternate technique involves threading a small transducer through the mouth and into the esophagus. This technique, called *transesophageal echocardiography* (TEE), provides clearer images because ultrasound waves pass through less tissue. A topical anesthetic agent and moderate sedation are used during TEE because of the discomfort associated with the positioning of the transducer in the esophagus (refer to Chapter 18 for further discussion of moderate sedation). Once the patient is comfortable, the transducer is inserted into the mouth and the patient is asked to swallow several times until it is positioned in the esophagus.

The high-quality imaging obtained during TEE makes this technique an important first-line diagnostic tool for evaluating patients with many types of CVD, including HF, valvular heart disease, dysrhythmias, and many other conditions that place the patient at risk for atrial or ventricular thrombi. Pharmacologic stress testing using dobutamine and TEE can also be performed. It is frequently used during cardiac surgery to continuously monitor the response of the heart to the surgical procedure (e.g., valve replacement or coronary artery bypass). Complications are uncommon during TEE; however, if they do occur, they are serious. These complications are caused by sedation and impaired swallowing resulting from the topical anesthesia (respiratory depression and aspiration) and by insertion and manipulation of the transducer into the esophagus and stomach (vasovagal response or esophageal perforation). The patient must be assessed before TEE for a history of dysphagia or radiation therapy to the chest, which increases the likelihood of complications.

Nursing Interventions

Prior to the test, the nurse provides preprocedure education and ensures that the patient has a clear understanding of what the test entails and why it is being performed, instructs the patient not to eat or drink anything for 6 hours prior to the study, and checks to make sure that informed consent has been obtained. The nurse also inserts an IV line or assesses an existing IV for patency and suitability and asks the patient to remove full or partial dentures. During the test, the nurse provides emotional support and monitors level of consciousness, BP, ECG, respiration, and oxygen saturation (SpO_2). During the recovery period, the patient must maintain bed rest with the head of the bed elevated to 45°. Following the moderate sedation policy of the agency, the nurse monitors the patient for dyspnea and assesses vital signs, SpO_2, level of consciousness, and gag reflex as recommended. Food and oral fluids are withheld until the patient is fully alert and the effects of the topical anesthetic agent are reversed, usually 2 hours after the procedure; if the gag reflex is intact, the nurse begins feeding with sips of water, then advances to the preprocedure diet. Patients are informed that a sore throat may be present for the next 24 hours; they are instructed to report the presence of a persistent sore throat, shortness of breath, or difficulty swallowing to the medical staff. If the procedure is performed in an outpatient setting, a family member or friend must be available to transport the patient home from the test site.

Cardiac Catheterization

Cardiac catheterization is a common invasive procedure used to diagnose structural and functional diseases of the heart and great vessels. The results guide treatment decisions including the need for revascularization (PCI or CABG) and other interventions to manage structural defects of the valves or septum (see Chapter 27).

This procedure involves the percutaneous insertion of radiopaque catheters into a large vein and an artery. Fluoroscopy is used to guide the advancement of the catheters through the right and left heart, referred to as right and left heart catheterization, respectively. In most situations, patients undergo both right and left heart catheterizations. However, right heart catheterization is performed without a left heart catheterization when patients only need myocardial biopsies or measurement of pulmonary artery pressures. Of note, left heart catheterization involves the use of a contrast agent. These agents are necessary to visualize patency of the coronary arteries and evaluate left ventricular function.

In preparation for the procedure, patients have blood tests performed to evaluate metabolic function (electrolytes and glucose) and renal function (blood urea nitrogen and creatinine level). Baseline coagulation studies (activated partial thromboplastin time [aPTT], international normalized ratio [INR] and prothrombin time [PT]) are obtained to guide dosing of anticoagulation during the procedure. Because bleeding and hematoma formation are procedural risks, a complete blood cell count (CBC; includes the hematocrit, hemoglobin, and platelets) is necessary to establish baseline values. Later these results are compared with postprocedure results to monitor for blood loss.

A health history is obtained to assess for previous reactions to a contrast agent and determine if the patient has any risk factors for contrast-induced nephropathy (CIN). This uncommon complication is a form of acute kidney injury that is usually reversible. Patients with chronic kidney disease or renal insufficiency, diabetes, HF, hypotension, dehydration, use of nephrotoxic medications, and advanced age are at risk for CIN. CIN is defined as an increase in the baseline serum creatinine by 25% or more or an absolute increase of 0.5 mg/dL within 48 to 72 hours after the procedure (Jorgensen, 2013). See Chart 53-5 for further discussion of nursing care of patient undergoing imaging study with the use of a contrast agent.

During a cardiac catheterization, the patient has one or more IV catheters for administration of fluids, sedatives, heparin, and other medications. The patient is continuously monitored for chest pain or dyspnea and for changes in BP and ECG, which are indicative of myocardial ischemia, hemodynamic instability, or dysrhythmias. Resuscitation equipment must be readily available, and staff must be prepared to provide advanced cardiac life support measures as necessary.

Postprocedure, patients remain on bed rest for 2 to 6 hours before they are permitted to ambulate. Variations in time to ambulation are related to the size of the catheters used during the procedure, the site of catheter insertion (femoral or radial artery), the patient's anticoagulation status, and other factors (e.g., advanced age, obesity, and bleeding disorder). The use of smaller (4 or 6 Fr) arterial catheters is associated with shorter bed rest restrictions.

Cardiac catheterization may be performed in the ambulatory setting. Unless the results demonstrate the need for immediate treatment, patients are discharged home. Hospitalized patients undergoing cardiac catheterization for diagnostic and interventional purposes (PCI, valvuloplasty) are returned to their hospital rooms for recovery (see Chapter 27).

Right Heart Catheterization

Right heart catheterization usually precedes left heart catheterization. It is performed to assess the function of the right ventricle and tricuspid and pulmonary valves. The procedure involves the passage of a catheter from an antecubital or femoral vein into the right atrium, right ventricle, pulmonary artery, and pulmonary arterioles. Pressures and oxygen saturations from each of these areas are obtained and recorded. The pulmonary artery pressures are used to diagnose pulmonary hypertension. A biopsy of a small piece of myocardial tissue can also be obtained during a right heart catheterization. The results of the biopsy are used to diagnose the etiology of a cardiomyopathy (abnormality of myocardium) or heart transplant rejection. At the completion of the procedure, the venous catheter is removed and hemostasis of the affected vein is achieved using manual pressure. Although right heart catheterization is considered relatively safe, potential complications include dysrhythmias (from contact of the catheter with the endocardium), venous spasm, infection at the insertion site, and right heart perforation.

Left Heart Catheterization

Prior to left heart catheterization, patients who have previously experienced a reaction to a contrast agent are premedicated with antihistamines (e.g., diphenhydramine [Benadryl]) and corticosteroids (e.g., prednisone). Patients at risk for CIN receive pre- and postprocedure preventive strategies. IV hydration increases vascular volume and facilitates removal of contrast from the kidneys. Administration of sodium bicarbonate and the antioxidant acetylcysteine (Mucomyst), both urine alkalizing agents, aids in protecting the renal tubules from an acidic environment (Jorgensen, 2013).

Left heart catheterization is performed to evaluate the aortic arch and its major branches, patency of the coronary arteries, and the function of the left ventricle and mitral and aortic valves. Left heart catheterization is performed by retrograde catheterization of the left ventricle. In this approach, the interventional cardiologist usually inserts the catheter into the right brachial artery or a femoral artery and advances it into the aorta and left ventricle. Potential complications include dysrhythmias, MI, perforation of the left heart or great vessels, and systemic embolization.

During a left heart catheterization, angiography is performed. Angiography is an imaging technique that involves the injection of the contrast agent into the arterial catheter. The contrast agent is filmed as it passes through the chambers of the left heart, aortic arch, and its major arteries. Coronary angiography is another technique used to observe the coronary artery anatomy and evaluate the degree of stenosis from atherosclerosis. To perform this test, a catheter is positioned into one of the coronary arteries. Once in position, the contrast agent is injected directly into the artery and images are obtained. The procedure is then repeated using the opposite coronary artery. Ventriculography is also performed to evaluate the size and function of the left ventricle. For this test, a catheter is positioned in the left ventricle and a large amount of contrast agent (30 mL) is rapidly injected into the ventricle.

The manipulation of catheters in the coronary arteries and left ventricle as well as injection of the contrast agent can cause intermittent myocardial ischemia. Vigilant monitoring throughout left heart catheterization is needed to detect myocardial ischemia, which can trigger chest pain and life-threatening dysrhythmias.

Once the procedure is completed, the arterial catheter is withdrawn. There are several options available to achieve arterial hemostasis, including applying manual pressure and hemostatic devices available from numerous vendors. For the radial artery, a compression device, such as the Termuo TR Band™, is positioned over the artery. It has a mechanism that is inflated with air to put pressure against the artery. It remains in place for about 2 hours.

For the femoral approach, manual pressure may be used alone or in combination with mechanical compression devices such as the FemoStop™ (placed over the puncture site for 30 minutes). Many types of percutaneously deployed vascular closure devices are also available. These devices are positioned at the femoral arterial puncture site after completion of the procedure. They deploy a saline-soaked gelatin sponge (Quick-Seal), collagen (VasoSeal), sutures (Perclose, Techstar), or a combination of both collagen and sutures (Angio-Seal). Other products that expedite arterial hemostasis include external patches (Syvek Patch, Clo-Sur P.A.D). These products are placed over the puncture site as the catheter is removed and manual pressure is applied for 4 to 10 minutes. Once hemostasis is achieved, the patch is covered with a dressing that remains in place for 24 hours. The interventional cardiologist determines which closure device, if any, will be deployed based on the artery used to insert the catheter, patient's condition, device availability, and personal preference.

Major benefits of the vascular closure devices include reliable, immediate hemostasis and a shorter time on bed rest without a significant increase in bleeding or other complications. Rare complications associated with these devices include bleeding around the closure device, infection, and arterial obstruction.

Nursing Interventions

Nursing responsibilities before cardiac catheterization include:

- Instructing the patient to fast, usually for 8 to 12 hours, before the procedure
- Informing the patient that if catheterization is to be performed as an outpatient procedure, a friend, family member, or other responsible person must transport the patient home
- Informing the patient about the expected duration of the procedure and advising that it will involve lying on a hard table for less than 2 hours
- Reassuring the patient that IV medications are given to maintain comfort
- Informing the patient about sensations that will be experienced during the catheterization. Knowing what to expect can help the patient cope with the experience. The nurse explains that an occasional pounding sensation (palpitation) may be felt in the chest because of extra heartbeats that almost always occur, particularly when the catheter tip touches the endocardium. The patient may be asked to cough and to breathe deeply, especially after the injection of the contrast agent. Coughing may help disrupt a dysrhythmia and clear the contrast agent from the arteries. Breathing deeply and holding the breath help lower the diaphragm for better visualization of heart structures. The injection of a contrast agent into either side of the heart may produce a flushed feeling throughout the body and a sensation similar to the need to void, which subsides in 1 minute or less.
- Encouraging the patient to express fears and anxieties. The nurse provides education and reassurance to reduce apprehension.

Nursing responsibilities after cardiac catheterization are dictated by hospital policy and primary provider preferences and may include:

- Observing the catheter access site for bleeding or hematoma formation and assessing peripheral pulses in the affected extremity (dorsalis pedis and posterior tibial pulses in the lower extremity, radial pulse in the upper extremity) every 15 minutes for 1 hour, every 30 minutes for 1 hour, and hourly for 4 hours or until discharge. BP and heart rate are also assessed during these same time intervals.
- Evaluating temperature, color, and capillary refill of the affected extremity during these same time intervals. The patient is assessed for affected extremity pain, numbness, or tingling sensations that may indicate arterial insufficiency. The best technique to use is to compare the examination findings between the affected and unaffected extremities. Any changes are reported promptly.
- Screening carefully for dysrhythmias by observing the cardiac monitor or by assessing the apical and peripheral pulses for changes in rate and rhythm. A vasovagal reaction, consisting of bradycardia, hypotension, and nausea, can be precipitated by a distended bladder or by discomfort from manual pressure that is applied during removal of an arterial or venous catheter. The vasovagal response

is reversed by promptly elevating the lower extremities above the level of the heart, infusing a bolus of IV fluid, and administering IV atropine to treat the bradycardia.

- Maintaining bed rest for 2 to 6 hours after the procedure. Duration of bed rest is dependent upon location of arterial approach, size of the catheter used during the procedure, and method used to maintain hemostasis. If manual pressure or a mechanical device was used during a femoral artery approach, the patient remains on bed rest for up to 6 hours with the affected leg straight and the head of the bed elevated no greater than 30°. For comfort, the patient may be turned from side to side with the affected extremity straight. If a percutaneous vascular closure device or patch was deployed, the nurse checks local nursing care standards and anticipates that the patient will have fewer activity restrictions. The patient may be permitted to ambulate within 2 hours. If the radial artery was accessed, the patient remains on bed rest for 2 hours or until the effects of sedation have dissipated. The patient may sit up in bed. A hemostasis band or pressure dressing may be applied over the catheter access site. Patients are instructed to avoid sleeping on the affected arm for 24 hours and to avoid repetitive movement of the affected extremity for 24 to 48 hours (Rosendorff, 2013). Analgesic medication is given as prescribed for discomfort.
- Instructing the patient to report chest pain and bleeding or sudden discomfort from the catheter insertion sites promptly.
- Monitoring the patient for contrast-induced nephropathy by observing for elevations in serum creatinine levels. IV hydration is used to increase urinary output and flush the contrast agent from the urinary tract; accurate oral and IV intake and urinary output are recorded.
- Ensuring patient safety by instructing the patient to ask for help when getting out of bed the first time after the procedure. The patient is monitored for bleeding from the catheter access site and for orthostatic hypotension, indicated by complaints of dizziness or lightheadedness.

For patients being discharged from the hospital on the same day as the procedure, additional instructions are provided (see Chart 25-6).

Electrophysiologic Testing

The electrophysiology study (EPS) is an invasive procedure that plays a major role in the diagnosis and management of serious dysrhythmias. EPS may be indicated for patients with syncope, palpitations, or both, and for survivors of cardiac arrest from ventricular fibrillation (sudden cardiac death) (Woods et al., 2009). EPS is used to distinguish atrial from ventricular tachycardias when the determination cannot be made from the 12-lead ECG; to evaluate how readily a life-threatening dysrhythmia (e.g., ventricular tachycardia, ventricular fibrillation) can be induced; to evaluate AV node function; to evaluate the effectiveness of antiarrhythmic medications in suppressing the dysrhythmia; or to determine the need for other therapeutic interventions, such as a pacemaker, ICD, or radiofrequency ablation. (See Chapter 26 for a detailed discussion of EPS.)

Chart 25-6 ◆ **PATIENT EDUCATION**

Self-Management After Cardiac Catheterization

After discharge from the hospital for cardiac catheterization, patients should follow these guidelines for self-care:

- *If the artery in your arm or wrist artery was used:* For the next 48 hours, avoid lifting anything heavier than 5 lb and avoid repetitive movement of your affected hand and wrist.
- *If the artery in your groin was used:* For the next 24 hours, do not bend at the waist, strain, or lift heavy objects.
- Do not submerge the puncture site in water. Avoid tub baths, but shower as desired.
- Talk with your primary provider about when you may return to work, drive, or resume strenuous activities.
- If bleeding occurs, sit (arm or wrist approach) or lie down (groin approach) and apply firm pressure to the puncture site for 10 minutes. Notify your primary provider as soon as possible and follow instructions. If there is a large amount of bleeding, call 911. Do not drive to the hospital.
- Call your primary provider if any of the following occur: swelling, new bruising or pain from your procedure puncture site, temperature of 101°F or more.
- If test results show that you have coronary artery disease, talk with your primary provider about options for treatment, including cardiac rehabilitation programs in your community.
- Talk with your primary provider about lifestyle changes to reduce your risk for further or future heart problems, such as quitting smoking, lowering your cholesterol level, initiating dietary changes, beginning an exercise program, or losing weight.
- Your primary provider may prescribe one or more new medications depending on your risk factors (medications to lower your blood pressure or cholesterol; aspirin or clopidogrel to prevent blood clots). Take all of your medications as instructed. If you feel that any of them are causing side effects, call your primary provider immediately. Do not stop taking any medications before talking to your primary provider.

Adapted from Woods, S. L., Froelicher, E. S., Motzer, S. A., et al. (2009). *Cardiac nursing* (6th ed.). Philadelphia, PA: Lippincott Williams & Wilkins.

Hemodynamic Monitoring

Critically ill patients require continuous assessment of their cardiovascular system to diagnose and manage their complex medical conditions. This type of assessment is achieved by the use of direct pressure monitoring systems, referred to as hemodynamic monitoring. Common forms include CVP, pulmonary artery pressure, and intra-arterial BP monitoring. Patients requiring hemodynamic monitoring are cared for in critical care units. Some progressive care units also admit stable patients with CVP or intra-arterial BP monitoring. To perform hemodynamic monitoring, a CVP, pulmonary artery, or arterial catheter is introduced into the appropriate blood vessel or heart chamber. It is connected to a pressure monitoring system that has several components, including:

- A disposable flush system, composed of IV normal saline solution (which may include heparin), tubing, stopcocks, and a flush device, which provides continuous and manual flushing of the system.
- A pressure bag placed around the flush solution that is maintained at 300 mm Hg of pressure. The pressurized flush system delivers 3 to 5 mL of solution per hour

through the catheter to prevent clotting and backflow of blood into the pressure monitoring system.

- A transducer to convert the pressure coming from the artery or heart chamber into an electrical signal
- An amplifier or monitor, which increases the size of the electrical signal for display on an oscilloscope

Nurses caring for patients who require hemodynamic monitoring receive training prior to using this sophisticated technology. The nurse helps ensure safe and effective care by adhering to the following guidelines:

- Ensuring that the system is set up and maintained properly. For example, the pressure monitoring system must be kept patent and free of air bubbles.
- Checking that the stopcock of the transducer is positioned at the level of the atrium before the system is used to obtain pressure measurements. This landmark is referred to as the phlebostatic axis (see Fig. 25-10). The nurse uses a marker to identify this level on the chest wall, which provides a stable reference point for subsequent pressure readings.
- Establishing the zero reference point in order to ensure that the system is properly functioning at atmospheric pressure. This process is accomplished by placing the stopcock of the transducer at the phlebostatic axis, opening the transducer to air, and activating the zero function key on the bedside monitor. Measurements of CVP, BP, and pulmonary artery pressures can be made with the head of the bed elevated up to 60°; however, the system must be repositioned to the phlebostatic axis to ensure an accurate reading (Urden, Stacy, & Lough, 2014).

Complications from the use of hemodynamic monitoring systems are uncommon and can include pneumothorax, infection, and air embolism. The nurse observes for signs of pneumothorax during the insertion of catheters using a central venous approach (CVP and pulmonary artery catheters). The longer any of these catheters are left in place (after 72 to 96 hours), the greater the risk of infection. Air emboli can be introduced into the vascular system if the stopcocks attached to the pressure transducers are mishandled during blood drawing, administration of medications, or other procedures that require opening the system to air. Therefore, nurses handling this equipment must demonstrate competence prior to caring independently for a patient requiring hemodynamic monitoring.

Catheter-related bloodstream infections are the most common preventable complication associated with hemodynamic monitoring systems. Comprehensive guidelines for the prevention of these infections have been published by Centers for Disease Control and Prevention (CDC) (O'Grady, Alexander, Burns, et al., 2011). To minimize the risk of infection, a group of evidence-based interventions, called a care *bundle*, should be implemented (see Chart 14-2).

The CDC has additional infection control guidelines that pertain to the ongoing care of these patients, including skin care, dressing changes, and pressure monitoring systems that are outlined in Table 25-5.

Central Venous Pressure Monitoring

CVP is a measurement of the pressure in the vena cava or right atrium. The pressure in the vena cava, right atrium, and right ventricle are equal at the end of diastole; thus, the CVP also reflects the filling pressure of the right ventricle (preload). The normal CVP is 2 to 6 mm Hg. It is measured by positioning a catheter in the vena cava or right atrium and connecting it to a pressure monitoring system. The CVP is most valuable when it is monitored over time and correlated with the patient's clinical status. A CVP greater than 6 mm Hg indicates an elevated right ventricular preload. There are many problems that can cause an elevated CVP, but the most common problem is hypervolemia (excessive fluid circulating in the body) or right-sided HF. In contrast, a low CVP (less than 2 mm Hg) indicates reduced right ventricular preload, which is most often from hypovolemia. Dehydration, excessive blood loss, vomiting or diarrhea, and overdiuresis can result in hypovolemia and a low CVP. This diagnosis can be substantiated when a rapid IV infusion of fluid causes the CVP to increase.

Before insertion of a CVP catheter, the site is prepared as recommended by the CDC (see Chart 14-2). The preferred site is the subclavian vein; the femoral vein is generally avoided (O'Grady et al., 2011). A local anesthetic agent is used. During this sterile procedure, the physician threads a single-lumen or multilumen catheter through the vein into the vena cava just above or within the right atrium. Once the CVP catheter is inserted, it is secured and a dry sterile dressing is applied. Position of the catheter is confirmed by a chest x-ray.

Figure 25-10 • A. The phlebostatic axis is the reference point for the atrium when the patient is positioned supine. It is the intersection of two lines on the chest wall: (*1*) the midaxillary line drawn between the anterior and posterior surfaces of the chest and (*2*) the line drawn through the fourth intercostal space. Its location is identified with a skin marker. The stopcock of the transducer used in hemodynamic monitoring is "leveled" at this mark prior to taking pressure measurements. **B.** Measurements can be taken with the head of the bed (HOB) elevated up to 60°. Note the phlebostatic axis changes as the HOB is elevated; thus, the stopcock and transducer must be repositioned after each position change.

TABLE 25-5 Nursing Interventions to Prevent Intravascular Catheter-Related Bloodstream Infections

Topic	Intervention
Hand hygiene	• Wash hands with soap and water or use alcohol-based hand rubs before and after contact with the catheter for any reason.
Dressing	• Wear clean or sterile gloves when changing the dressing. • Cleanse the skin during dressing changes with a >0.5% chlorhexidine preparation with alcohol. • Dress the site with sterile gauze or sterile, transparent, semipermeable dressing to cover the catheter site. If the patient is diaphoretic or if the site is bleeding or oozing, use a gauze dressing until it is resolved. • Change gauze dressings every 2 days or transparent dressings at least every 7 days and whenever dressings become damp, loosened, or visibly soiled. • Do not use topical antibiotic ointment or creams on insertion sites.
Catheter site	• Assess the site regularly—visually when changing the dressing or by palpation through an intact dressing. Remove the dressing for a thorough assessment if the patient has tenderness at the insertion site, fever without obvious source, or other signs of local or bloodstream infection.
Pressure monitoring system	• Keep all components of the pressure monitoring system sterile. • Replace transducers, tubing, continuous-flush device, and flush solution every at 96-hour intervals. • Do not infuse dextrose containing solutions through the monitoring system.
Bathing	• Do not submerge the catheter or catheter site in water. • Showering is permitted if the catheter and related tubing are placed in an impermeable cover.
Patient education	• Ask patients to report any new discomforts from the catheter site.

Adapted from O'Grady, N. P., Alexander, A., Burns, L., et al. (2011). 2011 guidelines for the prevention of intravascular catheter-related infections. Retrieved on 1/25/2016 at: www.cdc.gov/hicpac/bsi/bsi-guidelines-2011.html

Nursing Interventions

The frequency of CVP measurements is dictated by the patient's condition and the treatment plan. In addition to obtaining pressure readings, the CVP catheter is used for infusing IV fluids, administering IV medications, and drawing blood specimens. Nursing care of the patient with a CVP catheter is outlined in Table 25-5.

Pulmonary Artery Pressure Monitoring

Pulmonary artery pressure monitoring is used in critical care for assessing left ventricular function, diagnosing the etiology of shock, and evaluating the patient's response to medical interventions (e.g., fluid administration, vasoactive medications). A pulmonary artery catheter and a pressure monitoring system are used. A variety of catheters are available for cardiac pacing, oximetry, cardiac output measurement, or a combination of functions. Pulmonary artery catheters are balloon-tipped, flow-directed catheters that have distal and proximal lumens (see Fig. 25-11). The distal lumen has a port that opens into the pulmonary artery. Once connected by its hub to the pressure monitoring system, it is used to continuously measure pulmonary artery pressures. The proximal lumen has a port that opens into the right atrium. It is used to administer IV medications and fluids or to monitor right atrial pressures (i.e., CVP). Each catheter has a balloon inflation hub and valve. A syringe is connected to the hub, which is used to inflate or deflate the balloon with air (1.5-mL capacity). The valve opens and closes the balloon inflation lumen.

Figure 25-11 • The pulmonary artery catheter used for obtaining pressure measurements and cardiac output. **A.** The pressure monitoring system is connected to the distal lumen hub. **B.** Intravenous solutions are infused through the proximal infusion and injectate lumen hubs. **C.** An air-filled syringe connected to the balloon inflation valve is used for balloon inflation during catheter insertion and pulmonary artery wedge pressure measurements. **D.** To obtain cardiac output, the thermistor connector is inserted into the cardiac output component of the bedside cardiac monitor, and 5 to 10 mL of normal saline is injected in 4 seconds into the proximal injectate port. **E.** The thermistor located near the balloon is used to calculate the cardiac output. Redrawn courtesy of Baxter Healthcare Corporation, Edwards Critical Care Division, Santa Ana, California.

A pulmonary artery catheter with specialized capabilities has additional components. For example, the thermodilution catheter has three additional features that enable it to measure cardiac output: a thermistor connector attached to the cardiac output computer of the bedside monitor, a proximal injectate port used for injecting fluids when obtaining the cardiac output, and a thermistor (positioned near the distal port) (see Fig. 25-11).

The pulmonary artery catheter, covered with a sterile sleeve, is inserted into a large vein, preferably the subclavian, through a sheath. As noted previously, the femoral vein

is avoided; insertion techniques and protocols mirror those used for inserting a CVP catheter (see previous discussion) (O'Grady et al., 2011). The sheath is equipped with a side port for infusing IV fluids and medications. The catheter is then passed into the vena cava and right atrium. In the right atrium, the balloon tip is inflated, and the catheter is carried rapidly by the flow of blood through the tricuspid valve into the right ventricle, through the pulmonic valve, and into a branch of the pulmonary artery. When the catheter reaches the pulmonary artery, the balloon is deflated and the catheter is secured with sutures (see Fig. 25-12). Fluoroscopy

Figure 25-12 • Pulmonary artery (PA) catheter and pressure monitoring systems. Bedside monitor that connects with cables (**A**) to the pressure monitoring systems (includes intravenous [IV] solution in a pressure bag, IV tubing, and two transducers with stopcocks and flush devices) (**B**). This system connects to the proximal infusion port that opens in the right atria (**C**) and is used to infuse fluids or medications and monitor central venous pressures and the distal infusion port (**D**). This port opens in the PA and is used to monitor PA pressures. **E.** The thermistor connector is attached to the bedside cardiac monitor to obtain cardiac output. **F.** An air-filled syringe is attached to the balloon inflation valve during catheter insertion and measurement of PA wedge pressure. **G.** PA catheter positioned in the pulmonary artery. Note the sterile sleeve over the PA catheter. The PA catheter is threaded through the sheath until it reaches the desired position in the PA. The side port on the sheath is used to infuse medications or fluids. ECG, electrocardiogram; RA, right atrium.

may be used during insertion to visualize the progression of the catheter through the right heart chambers to the pulmonary artery. This procedure can be performed in the operating room, in the cardiac catheterization laboratory, or at the bedside in the critical care unit. During insertion of the pulmonary artery catheter, the bedside monitor is observed for pressure and waveform changes, as well as dysrhythmias, as the catheter progresses through the right heart to the pulmonary artery.

Once the catheter is in position, the following are measured: right atrial, pulmonary artery systolic, pulmonary artery diastolic, mean pulmonary artery, and pulmonary artery wedge pressures (see Fig. 25-2 for normal chamber pressures). Monitoring of the pulmonary artery diastolic and pulmonary artery wedge pressures is particularly important in critically ill patients because they are used to evaluate left ventricular filling pressures (i.e., left ventricular preload).

It is important to note that the pulmonary artery wedge pressure is achieved by inflating the balloon tip, which causes it to float more distally into a smaller portion of the pulmonary artery until it is wedged into position. This is an occlusive maneuver that impedes blood flow through that segment of the pulmonary artery. Therefore, the wedge pressure is measured immediately and the balloon deflated promptly to restore blood flow.

> ◤ **Quality and Safety Nursing Alert**
>
> *After measuring the pulmonary artery wedge pressure, the nurse ensures that the balloon is deflated and that the catheter has returned to its normal position. This important intervention is verified by evaluating the pulmonary artery pressure waveform displayed on the bedside monitor.*

Nursing Interventions

Catheter site care is essentially the same as for a CVP catheter. Similar to CVP measurement, the transducer must be positioned at the phlebostatic axis to ensure accurate readings (see Fig. 25-10). Serious complications include pulmonary artery rupture, pulmonary thromboembolism, pulmonary infarction, catheter kinking, dysrhythmias, and air embolism.

Intra-Arterial Blood Pressure Monitoring

Intra-arterial BP monitoring is used to obtain direct and continuous BP measurements in critically ill patients who have severe hypertension or hypotension. Arterial catheters are also useful when arterial blood gas measurements and blood samples need to be obtained frequently.

The radial artery is the usual site selected. However, placement of a catheter into the radial artery can further impede perfusion to an area that has poor circulation. As a result, the tissue distal to the cannulated artery can become ischemic or necrotic. Patients with diabetes, peripheral vascular disease, or hypotension, receiving IV vasopressors, or having had previous surgery are at highest risk for this complication. Traditionally, collateral circulation to the involved extremity was assessed by using the Allen test. To perform the Allen test, the hand is elevated and the patient is asked to make a fist for 30 seconds. The nurse compresses the radial and ulnar arteries simultaneously, causing the hand to blanch. After the patient opens the fist, the nurse releases the pressure on the ulnar artery. If blood flow is restored (hand turns pink) within 6 seconds, the circulation to the hand may be adequate enough to tolerate placement of a radial artery catheter. Evidence suggests that pulse oximetry and plethysmography are additional reliable methods for assessing circulation to the hand (Rosendorff, 2013).

Nursing Interventions

Site preparation and care are the same as for CVP catheters. The catheter flush solution is the same as for pulmonary artery catheters. A transducer is attached, and pressures are measured in millimeters of mercury (mm Hg). The nurse monitors the patient for complications, which include local obstruction with distal ischemia, external hemorrhage, massive ecchymosis, dissection, air embolism, blood loss, pain, arteriospasm, and infection.

Minimally Invasive Cardiac Output Monitoring Devices

Monitoring cardiac output using the pulmonary artery catheter has been the standard of practice in critical care since its inception almost 50 years ago. Its use has diminished recently with the availability of new, less invasive devices. Several types of devices are commercially available. Selection of a specific device for clinical use is determined by availability, provider preferences, and the patient's clinical condition (Urden et al., 2014).

Pulse pressure analysis uses an arterial pressure waveform to continuously estimate the patient's stroke volume. One such device, the Edwards Lifesciences Vigileo monitoring system, is connected to an existing radial or femoral arterial line via its FloTrac transducer. Using age, gender, body surface area, and BP of the patient, this device calculates continuous cardiac output and other parameters used in the management of critically ill patients. The major drawback to this device is that in order for it to capture accurate data, it must first capture optimal arterial waveforms. Therefore, this type of device has limited usefulness in patients with poor waveform signals, various dysrhythmias, hemodynamic instability, and those who may be concomitantly using an intra-aortic balloon pump (see Chapter 29).

Esophageal Doppler probes are used to noninvasively estimate cardiac output. The esophageal probe measures blood flow velocity within a cross-sectional area of the descending aorta to calculate cardiac output. The use of this device in the perioperative setting has been shown to improve patient outcomes, including decreased lengths of hospital stay and an overall decrease in rates of complications (Urden et al., 2014).

In patients who are sedated, intubated, and on mechanical ventilation, the Fick principle, which uses carbon dioxide (CO_2) measures, is an additional method used to estimate cardiac output. To obtain cardiac output in this select patient population, a rebreathing loop is attached to the ventilator along with an infrared CO_2 sensor, an airflow sensor, and pulse oximeter. Continuous readings of cardiac output may be updated every 3 minutes with the use of this device.

CRITICAL THINKING EXERCISES

1 Your patient is being admitted to the cardiac ICU directly from the chronic HF clinic with acute decompensated HF. He is a 74-year-old man with a history of several MIs and an ejection fraction of 28%. The clinic nurse tells you that he is not responding to diuretics due to poor renal function. The cardiologist is planning to insert a pulmonary artery catheter to monitor the patient's response to IV dobutamine, prescribed to strengthen myocardial contractility. What information will you need to gather during the admission history and physical assessment? What laboratory results will you review to determine the patient's renal function? Why is a pulmonary artery catheter indicated for monitoring this patient? What parameters will you monitor to determine the patient's response to dobutamine? How will you determine that the catheter remains in a stable position in the pulmonary artery?

2 `ebp` After working on a medical nursing unit for a year, you are transferring to a new position in the diagnostic imaging department. As part of your responsibilities you provide preprocedure telephone calls to patients undergoing diagnostic cardiac catheterizations. How will you determine if patients are at risk for contrast agent allergies or contrast-induced nephropathy? What information will you include in your conversation with patients regarding what to expect during the procedure? What information will you teach the patient about pre- and postprocedure care? What is the strength of the evidence that guides your teaching strategies? How will you know your teaching was effective?

3 `pq` During morning cardiology rounds, the team tells your patient that he will be scheduled for a stress test with imaging the following day. As they leave the patient's bedside, the cardiologist asks you to prepare the patient for the stress test. What additional information do you need to discuss with the team before they leave the unit? What priority health history and physical assessment findings of the patient will be used to determine if a pharmacologic or exercise stress test is appropriate for this patient? Discuss the differences between these two stress tests. How do these differences affect patient preparation and education?

REFERENCES

*Asterisk indicates nursing research.
**Double asterisk indicates classic reference.

Books

Bickley, L. S. (2014). *Bates' guide to physical examination and history taking* (11th ed.). Philadelphia, PA: Wolters Kluwer Health/Lippincott Williams & Wilkins.
Rosendorff, C. (2013). *Essential cardiology: Principles and practice* (3rd ed.). New York: Springer.
Urden, L. D., Stacy, K. M., & Lough, M. E. (2014). *Critical care nursing: Diagnosis and management (Thelans critical care nursing diagnosis)* (7th ed.). St. Louis, MO: Elsevier Mosby.
Weber, J. R., & Kelley, J. H. (2014). *Health assessment in nursing* (5th ed.). Philadelphia, PA: Lippincott Williams & Wilkins.

*Woods, S. L., Froelicher, E. S., Motzer, S. A., et al. (2009). *Cardiac nursing* (6th ed.). Philadelphia, PA: Lippincott Williams & Wilkins.

Journals and Electronic Documents

Amsterdam, E. A., Wenger, N. K., Brindis, R. G., et al. (2014). 2014 AHA/ACC Guideline for the management of patients with non–ST-elevation acute coronary syndromes: Executive summary a report of the American College of Cardiology/American Heart Association Task Force on Practice. *Circulation, 130*(25), 2354–2394.
American Heart Association. (2016). *Heart disease and stroke statistics—2016 update*. Retrieved on 3/12/2016 at: circ.ahajournals.org/content/early/2015/12/16/CIR.0000000000000350.long
Arnold, A. C., & Shibao, C. (2013). Current concepts in orthostatic hypotension management. *Current Hypertension Reports, 15*(4), 304–312.
Ayas, N. T., Owens, R. L., & Kheirandish-Gozal, L. (2015). Update in sleep medicine 2014. *American Journal of Respiratory Critical Care Medicine, 192*(4), 415–420.
**Bigger, J. T., & Glassman, A. H. (2010). The American Heart Association science advisory on depression and coronary heart disease: An exploration of the issues raised. *Cleveland Clinic Journal of Medicine, 77*(Suppl 3), S12–S19.
Boardman, H. M., Hartley, L., Eisinga, A., et al. (2015). Hormone therapy for preventing cardiovascular disease in post-menopausal women. *Cochrane Database of Systematic Review, (3), CD002229.
Drew, B. J., Harris, P., Ze'gre-Hemsey, J. K., et al. (2014) Insights into the problem of alarm fatigue with physiologic monitor devices: A comprehensive observational study of consecutive intensive care unit patients. *PLoS ONE, 9*(10), e110274.
Eckel, R. H., Jakicic, J. M., Ard, J. D., et al. (2014). 2013 AHA/ACC Guideline on lifestyle management to reduce cardiovascular risk: A report of the American College of Cardiology/American Heart Association Task Force on Practice Guidelines. *Circulation, 129*(25 Suppl 2), S1–S45.
Fletcher, G. F., Ades, P. A., Kligfield, P., et al. (2013). Exercise standards for testing and training: A scientific statement from the American Heart Association. *Circulation, 128*(8), 873–934.
Gillis, N. K., Arslanian-Engoren, C., & Struble, L. (2014). Acute coronary syndromes in older adults: A review of literature. *Journal of Emergency Nursing, 40*(3), 270–275.
Goff, D. C., Lloyd-Jones, D. M., Bennett, G., et al. (2014). 2013 ACC/AHA Guideline on the assessment of cardiovascular risk: A report of the American College of Cardiology/American Heart Association Task Force on Practice Guidelines. *Circulation, 129*(suppl 2), S49–S73.
Hannibal, G. B. (2014). Cardiac monitoring and electrode placement revisited. *AACN Advanced Critical Care, 25*(2), 188–192.
Havranek, E. P., Mujahid, M. S., Barr, D. A., et al. (2015). Social determinants of risk and outcomes for cardiovascular disease: A scientific statement from the American Heart Association. *Circulation, 132*(9), 873–898.
**Homes, T. H., & Rahe, R. H. (1967). The Social Readjustment Rating Scale. *Journal of Psychosomatic Research, 11*(2), 213–218.
Jorgensen, A. L. (2013). Contrast-induced nephropathy: Pathophysiology and preventive strategies. *Critical Care Nurse, 33*(1), 37–47.
King, J. E., & Magdic, K. S. (2014). Chest pain: a time for concern? *AACN Advanced Critical Care, 25*(3), 279–283.
Leahy, R. A., & Davenport, E. E. (2015). Home monitoring for cardiovascular implantable electronic devices: Benefits to patients and to their follow-up clinic. *AACN Advanced Critical Care, 26*(4), 343–355.
Lichtman, J. H., Froelicher, E. S., Blumenthal, J. A., et al. (2014). Depression as a risk factor for poor prognosis among patients with acute coronary syndrome: Systematic review and recommendations: A scientific statement from the American Heart Association. *Circulation, 129*(12), 1350–1369.
Lloyd-Jones, D. M. (2015). Coronary artery calcium scoring. Are we there yet? *Journal of the American College of Cardiology, 66*(15), 1654–1656.
*Mervak, B. M., Davenport, M. S., Ellis, J. H., et al. (2015). Rates of breakthrough reactions in inpatients at high risk receiving premedication before contrast-enhanced CT. *American Journal of Roentgenology, 205*(1), 77–84.
McSweeney, J. C., Rosenfeld, A. G., Abel, W. M., et al. (2016). Preventing and experiencing ischemic heart disease as a woman: State of the science: A scientific statement from the American Heart Association, *Circulation, 133*(10), 949–1048.

National Institute of Health. (2014). *Risk assessment tool for estimating your 10-year risk of having a heart attack.* Retrieved on 1/25/2016 at: cvdrisk.nhlbi.nih.gov/

O'Grady, N. P., Alexander, A., Burns, L., et al. (2011). *2011 guidelines for the prevention of intravascular catheter-related infections.* Retrieved on 1/25/2016 at: www.cdc.gov/hicpac/bsi/bsi-guidelines-2011.html

Romero, I. (2013). Ambulatory electrocardiology. *Cardiology in Review, 21*(5), 239–248.

Rosendorff, C., Lackland, D. T., Allison, M., et al. (2015). Treatment of hypertension in patients with coronary artery disease: A scientific statement from the American Heart Association, American College of Cardiology, and American Society of Hypertension. *Hypertension, 65*(6), 1372–1407.

Sendelbach, S., & Funk, M. (2013). Alarm fatigue: A patient safety concern. *AACN Advanced Critical Care, 24*(4), 378–386.

Sendelbach, S., & Jepsen, S. (2013). *AACN practice alert: Alarm management.* Retrieved on 1/25/2016 at www.aacn.org/wd/practice/content/practicealerts/alarm-management-practice-alert.pcms?menu=practice

Steinke, E. E., Jaarsma, T., Barnason, S. A., et al. (2013). Sexual counseling for individuals with cardiovascular disease and their partners: A consensus document from the American Heart Association and the ESC Council on Cardiovascular Nursing and Allied Professions (CCNAP). *Circulation, 128*(18), 2075–2096.

Stone, N. J., Robinson, J., Lichtenstein, A. H., et al. (2014). 2013 ACC/AHA guideline on the treatment of blood cholesterol to reduce atherosclerotic cardiovascular risk in adults: A report of the American College of Cardiology/American Heart Association Task Force on Practice Guidelines. *Circulation, 129*(25 Suppl 2), S1–S45.

Walsh, J. A., Topol, E. J., & Steinhubl, R. S. (2014). Novel wireless devices for cardiac monitoring. *Circulation, 130*(7), 573–581.

*Walsh-Irwin, C., & Jurgens, C. Y. (2015). Proper skin preparation and electrode placement decreases alarms on a telemetry unit. *Dimensions of Critical Care Nursing, 34*(3), 134–139.

Weber, M. A, Schriffrin, E. L., White, W. B., et al. (2014). Clinical Practice Guidelines from the Management of Hypertension in the Community: A Statement by the American Society of Hypertension and the International Society of Hypertension. *Journal of Clinical Hypertension, 32*(1), 3–15.

Resources

American Association of Critical Care Nurses (AACN), www.aacn.org

American College of Cardiology (ACC), www.acc.org

American Heart Association (AHA), www.heart.org/HEARTORG/

National Institutes of Health (NIH), National Heart, Lung, and Blood Institute (NHLBI), www.nhlbi.nih.gov

NIH NHLBI Risk Assessment Tool, cvdrisk.nhlbi.nih.gov/

Management of Patients With Dysrhythmias and Conduction Problems

LEARNING OBJECTIVES

On completion of this chapter, the learner will be able to:

1 Correlate the components of the normal electrocardiogram (ECG) with physiologic events of the heart.
2 Define the ECG as a waveform that represents the cardiac electrical event in relation to the lead (placement of electrodes).
3 Analyze elements of an ECG rhythm strip: ventricular and atrial rate, ventricular and atrial rhythm, QRS complex and shape, QRS duration, P wave and shape, PR interval, and P:QRS ratio.

4 Identify the ECG criteria, causes, and management of several dysrhythmias, including conduction disturbances.
5 Use the nursing process as a framework for care of patients with dysrhythmias.
6 Compare the different types of pacemakers, their uses, possible complications, and nursing implications.
7 Describe the key points of using a defibrillator.
8 Identify the purpose of an implantable cardioverter defibrillator, the types available, and the nursing implications.
9 Describe the nursing management of patients with implantable cardiac devices.

GLOSSARY

ablation: removal of material, by mechanical means, from the surface of an object; in the context of cardiology, it is the purposeful destruction of heart muscle cells, usually in an attempt to correct or eliminate a dysrhythmia

artifact: distorted, irrelevant, and extraneous electrocardiographic (ECG) waveforms

automaticity: ability of the cardiac cells to initiate an electrical impulse

cardiac resynchronization therapy (CRT): biventricular pacing used to correct interventricular, intraventricular, and atrioventricular conduction disturbances that occur in patients with heart failure

cardioversion: electrical current given in synchrony with the patient's own QRS complex to stop a dysrhythmia

chronotropy: rate of impulse formation

conduction: transmission of electrical impulses from one cell to another

defibrillation: electrical current given to stop a dysrhythmia, not synchronized with the patient's QRS complex

depolarization: process by which cardiac muscle cells change from a more negatively charged to a more positively charged intracellular state

dromotropy: conduction velocity

dysrhythmia: disorder of the formation or conduction (or both) of the electrical impulse within the heart, altering the heart rate, heart rhythm, or both and potentially causing altered blood flow (also referred to as arrhythmia)

elective replacement indicator (ERI): a signal produced by a pacemaker when it is interrogated to indicate a near-depleted battery

electrocardiogram (ECG): a record of a test that graphically measures the electrical activity of the heart, including each phase of the cardiac cycle

implantable cardioverter defibrillator (ICD): a device implanted into the chest wall to treat dysrhythmias

inotropy: force of myocardial contraction

P wave: the part of an ECG that reflects conduction of an electrical impulse through the atrium; atrial depolarization

paroxysmal: a dysrhythmia that has a sudden onset and terminates spontaneously; usually of short duration, but may recur

PP interval: the duration between the beginning of one P wave and the beginning of the next P wave; used to calculate atrial rate and rhythm

PR interval: the part of an ECG that reflects conduction of an electrical impulse from the sinoatrial node through the atrioventricular node

QRS complex: the part of an ECG that reflects conduction of an electrical impulse through the ventricles; ventricular depolarization

QT interval: the part of an ECG that reflects the time from ventricular depolarization through repolarization

repolarization: process by which cardiac muscle cells return to a more negatively charged intracellular condition, their resting state

RR interval: the duration between the beginning of one QRS complex and the beginning of the next QRS complex; used to calculate ventricular rate and rhythm

sinus rhythm: electrical activity of the heart initiated by the sinoatrial node

ST segment: the part of an ECG that reflects the end of the QRS complex to the beginning of the T wave

T wave: the part of an ECG that reflects repolarization of the ventricles

TP interval: the part of an ECG that reflects the time between the end of the T wave and the beginning of the next P wave; used to identify the isoelectric line

U wave: the part of an ECG that may reflect Purkinje fiber repolarization; usually, it is not seen unless a patient's serum potassium level is low

Without a regular rate and rhythm, the heart may not perform efficiently as a pump to circulate oxygenated blood and other life-sustaining nutrients to all of the body's tissues and organs (including the heart itself). With an irregular or erratic rhythm, the heart is considered to be dysrhythmic (also called *arrhythmic*). This is a potentially dangerous condition.

Nurses may encounter patients with dysrhythmias in all health care settings, including primary care settings, skilled nursing facilities, rehabilitation settings, and hospitals. Some dysrhythmias are acute and others chronic; some require emergent interventions, while others may not. Because patients with dysrhythmias are frequently encountered in many different types of settings, nurses must be able to identify and provide appropriate first-line treatment of dysrhythmias.

DYSRHYTHMIAS

Dysrhythmias are disorders of the formation or conduction (or both) of the electrical impulse within the heart. These disorders can cause disturbances of the heart rate, the heart rhythm, or both. Dysrhythmias may initially be evidenced by the hemodynamic effect they cause (e.g., a change in conduction may change the pumping action of the heart and cause decreased blood pressure), and are diagnosed by analyzing the electrocardiographic (ECG) waveform. Their treatment is based on the frequency and severity of symptoms produced. Dysrhythmias are named according to the site of origin of the electrical impulse and the mechanism of formation or conduction involved. For example, an impulse that originates in the sinoatrial (SA) node and at a slow rate is called *sinus bradycardia*.

Normal Electrical Conduction

The electrical impulse that stimulates and paces the cardiac muscle normally originates in the SA node, also called the *sinus node*, an area located near the superior vena cava in the right atrium. In the adult, the electrical impulse usually occurs at a rate of 60 to 100 times a minute. The electrical impulse quickly travels from the SA node through the atria to the atrioventricular (AV) node (see Fig. 26-1); this process is known as **conduction**. The electrical stimulation of the muscle cells of the atria causes them to contract. The structure of the AV node slows the electrical impulse, giving the atria time to contract and fill the ventricles with blood. This part of atrial contraction is frequently referred to as the atrial kick and accounts for nearly one third of the volume ejected during ventricular contraction (Fuster, Walsh, & Harrington, 2011). The electrical impulse then travels very quickly through the bundle of His to the right and left bundle branches and the Purkinje fibers, located in the ventricular muscle.

The electrical stimulation is called **depolarization**, and the mechanical contraction is called *systole*. Electrical relaxation is called **repolarization**, and mechanical relaxation is called *diastole*. The process from sinus node electrical impulse generation through ventricular repolarization completes the electromechanical circuit, and the cycle begins again. (See Chapter 25 for a more complete explanation of cardiac function.)

Influences on Heart Rate and Contractility

The heart rate is influenced by the autonomic nervous system, which consists of sympathetic and parasympathetic fibers. Sympathetic nerve fibers (also referred to as adrenergic fibers) are attached to the heart and arteries as well as several other areas in the body. Stimulation of the sympathetic system increases heart rate (positive **chronotropy**), conduction through the AV node (positive **dromotropy**), and the force of myocardial contraction (positive **inotropy**). Sympathetic stimulation also constricts peripheral blood vessels, therefore increasing blood pressure. Parasympathetic nerve fibers are also attached to the heart and arteries. Parasympathetic stimulation reduces the heart rate (negative chronotropy), AV conduction (negative dromotropy), and the force of atrial myocardial contraction. The decreased sympathetic stimulation results in dilation of arteries, thereby lowering blood pressure.

Manipulation of the autonomic nervous system may increase or decrease the incidence of dysrhythmias. Increased sympathetic stimulation (e.g., caused by exercise, anxiety, fever, or administration of catecholamines, such as dopamine [Intropin], aminophylline, or dobutamine [Dobutrex]) may increase the incidence of dysrhythmias. Decreased sympathetic stimulation (e.g., with rest, anxiety reduction methods such as therapeutic communication or meditation, or administration of beta-adrenergic blocking agents) may decrease the incidence of dysrhythmias.

The Electrocardiogram

The electrical impulse that travels through the heart can be viewed by means of electrocardiography, the end product of which is an **electrocardiogram (ECG)**. Each phase of the cardiac cycle is reflected by specific waveforms on the screen of a cardiac monitor or on a strip of ECG graph paper.

Obtaining an Electrocardiogram

An ECG is obtained by placing electrodes on the body at specific areas. Biomonitoring electrodes come in various shapes and sizes, but all have two components: (1) an adhesive substance that attaches to the skin to secure the electrode in place and (2) a substance that reduces the skin's electrical impedance, facilitating the transfer of ions from the tissue to electrons in the electrode, enhancing conductivity. Gently abrading the skin with a clean dry gauze pad helps to expose the inner conductive layer of epidermis, which will reduce skin impedance. Although cleansing the skin with alcohol removes any oily residue from the skin, it also increases the skin's electrical impedance and hinders detection of the cardiac electrical signal. If the amount of chest hair prevents the electrode from having good contact with the skin, the hair may need to be clipped (Sendelbach & Jepsen, 2013) (see Chapter 25, Chart 25-4: Applying Electrodes). Poor electrode adhesion will cause significant **artifact** (distorted, irrelevant, and extraneous ECG waveforms), which may distort capturing an accurate ECG waveform.

The number and placement site of the electrodes depend on the type of ECG being obtained. Most continuous

Figure 26-1 • Relationship of electrocardiographic (ECG) complex, lead system, and electrical impulse. The heart conducts electrical activity, which the ECG measures and shows. The configurations of electrical activity displayed on the ECG vary depending on the lead (or view) of the ECG and on the rhythm of the heart. Therefore, the configuration of a normal rhythm tracing from lead I will differ from the configuration of a normal rhythm tracing from lead II, lead II will differ from lead III, and so on. The same is true for abnormal rhythms and cardiac disorders. To make an accurate assessment of the heart's electrical activity or to identify where, when, and what abnormalities occur, the ECG needs to be evaluated from every lead, not just from lead II. Here the different areas of electrical activity are identified by color. RA, right arm; LA, left arm; SA, sinoatrial; AV, atrioventricular; LL, left leg.

monitors use 2 to 5 electrodes, usually placed on the limbs and the chest. These electrodes create an imaginary line, called a *lead,* which serves as a reference point from which the electrical activity is viewed. A lead is like an eye of a camera—it has a narrow peripheral field of vision, looking only at the electrical activity directly in front of it. Therefore, the ECG waveforms that appear on the ECG paper and cardiac monitor represent the electrical impulse in relation to the lead (see Fig. 26-1). A change in the waveform can be caused by a change in the electrical impulse (where it originates or how it is conducted) or by a change in the lead. Electrodes are attached to cable wires, which are connected to one of the following:

- An ECG machine placed at the patient's side for an immediate recording (standard 12-lead ECG)

- A cardiac monitor at the patient's bedside for continuous reading; this kind of monitoring, usually called *hardwire monitoring,* is used in intensive care units
- A small box that the patient carries and that continuously transmits the ECG information by radiowaves to a central monitor located elsewhere (called *telemetry*)
- A small, lightweight tape recorder–like machine (called *ambulatory ECG monitoring* or a *Holter monitor*) that the patient wears and that continuously records the ECG, which is later viewed and analyzed with a scanner (see Chapter 25 for further discussion of ECG monitoring systems).

A patient may undergo an electrophysiology (EP) study in which electrodes are placed inside the heart in order to obtain an intracardiac ECG. This is used not only to diagnose the dysrhythmia but also to determine the most effective treatment plan. However, because an EP study is invasive, it is performed in the hospital and may require that the patient be admitted. (A more in-depth discussion is found later in this chapter.)

During open heart surgery, temporary pacemaker wires may be lightly sutured to the epicardium and brought through the chest wall. These wires may be used not only for temporary pacing but also, when connected to the V lead cable, to obtain an atrial ECG, which can be helpful in the differential diagnosis of tachydysrhythmias (see Chapter 27 for further discussion).

The placement of electrodes for monitoring varies with the type of technology, the purpose of monitoring, and the standards of the health care facility. For a standard 12-lead ECG, 10 electrodes (6 on the chest and 4 on the limbs) are placed on the body (see Fig. 26-2). To prevent interference from the

electrical activity of skeletal muscle, the limb electrodes are placed on areas that are not bony and that do not have significant movement. The limb electrodes provide the first six leads: leads I, II, III, aVR (augmented voltage right arm), aVL (augmented voltage left arm), and aVF (augmented voltage left leg/foot). The 6 chest electrodes are applied to the chest at very specific areas. The chest electrodes provide the V or precordial leads, V_1 through V_6. To locate the fourth intercostal space and the placement of V_1, the sternal angle and then the sternal notch, which is about 1 or 2 inches below the sternal angle, are located. When the fingers are moved to the patient's immediate right, the second rib can be palpated. The second intercostal space is the indentation felt just below the second rib. Locating the specific intercostal space is critical for the correct placement of each chest electrode. Errors in diagnosis can occur if electrodes are incorrectly placed. Sometimes, when a patient in the hospital needs to be monitored more closely for ECG changes, the chest electrodes are left in place to ensure the same placement for follow-up 12-lead ECGs.

A standard 12-lead ECG reflects the electrical activity primarily in the left ventricle. Placement of additional electrodes for other leads may be needed to obtain more complete information. For example, in patients with suspected right-sided heart damage, right-sided precordial leads are required to evaluate the right ventricle (see Fig. 26-2).

Components of the Electrocardiogram

The ECG waveform reflects the function of the heart's conduction system in relation to the specific lead. The ECG offers important information about the electrical activity of the heart and is useful in diagnosing dysrhythmias. ECG waveforms are printed on graph paper that is divided by vertical and horizontal lines at standard intervals (see Fig. 26-3). Time and rate are measured on the horizontal axis of the graph, and amplitude or voltage is measured on the vertical axis. When an ECG waveform moves toward the top of the paper, it is called a *positive deflection*. When it moves toward the bottom of the paper, it is called a *negative deflection*. When reviewing an ECG, each waveform should be examined and compared with the others.

Waves, Complexes, and Intervals

The ECG is composed of waveforms (including the P wave, the QRS complex, the T wave, and possibly a U wave) and of segments and intervals (including the PR interval, the ST segment, and the QT interval) (see Fig. 26-3).

The **P wave** represents the electrical impulse starting in the SA node and spreading through the atria. Therefore, the P wave represents atrial depolarization. It is normally 2.5 mm or less in height and 0.11 seconds or less in duration.

The **QRS complex** represents ventricular depolarization. Not all QRS complexes have all three waveforms. The Q wave is the first negative deflection after the P wave. The Q wave is normally less than 0.04 seconds in duration and less than 25% of the R-wave amplitude. The R wave is the first positive deflection after the P wave, and the S wave is the first negative deflection after the R wave. When a wave is less than 5 mm in height, small letters (q, r, s) are used; when a wave is taller than 5 mm, capital letters (Q, R, S) are used to label the waves. The QRS complex is normally less than 0.12 seconds in duration.

Figure 26-2 • ECG electrode placement. The standard left precordial leads are V_1—fourth intercostal space, right sternal border; V_2—fourth intercostal space, left sternal border; V_3—diagonally between V_2 and V_4; V_4—fifth intercostal space, left midclavicular line; V_5—same level as V_4, anterior axillary line; V_6 (not illustrated)—same level as V_4 and V_5, midaxillary line. The right precordial leads, placed across the right side of the chest, are the mirror opposite of the left leads. RA, right arm; LA, left arm; RL, right leg; LL, left leg.

Labels in figure: Supplemental right precordial leads; V_5R V_3R V_1R; V_4R V_2R; Mid-clavicle; Anterior axillary line; Horizontal plane of V_4–V_6; RA; LA; V_1 V_2 V_3 V_4 V_5; RL; LL; ECG machine; ECG strip

Figure 26-3 • ECG graph and commonly measured components. Each small box represents 0.04 seconds on the horizontal axis and 1 mm or 0.1 millivolt on the vertical axis. The PR interval is measured from the beginning of the P wave to the beginning of the QRS complex, the QRS complex is measured from the beginning of the Q wave to the end of the S wave, the QT interval is measured from the beginning of the Q wave to the end of the T wave, and the TP interval is measured from the end of the T wave to the beginning of the next P wave.

The **T wave** represents ventricular repolarization (when the cells regain a negative charge; also called the *resting state*). It follows the QRS complex and is usually the same direction (deflection) as the QRS complex. Atrial repolarization also occurs but is not visible on the ECG because it occurs at the same time as ventricular depolarization (i.e., the QRS).

The **U wave** is thought to represent repolarization of the Purkinje fibers; although this wave is rare, it sometimes appears in patients with hypokalemia (low potassium levels), hypertension, or heart disease. If present, the U wave follows the T wave and is usually smaller than the P wave. If larger in amplitude, it may be mistaken for an extra P wave.

The **PR interval** is measured from the beginning of the P wave to the beginning of the QRS complex and represents the time needed for sinus node stimulation, atrial depolarization, and conduction through the AV node before ventricular depolarization. In adults, the PR interval normally ranges from 0.12 to 0.20 seconds in duration.

The **ST segment,** which represents early ventricular repolarization, lasts from the end of the QRS complex to the beginning of the T wave. The beginning of the ST segment is usually identified by a change in the thickness or angle of the terminal portion of the QRS complex. The end of the ST segment may be more difficult to identify because it merges into the T wave. The ST segment is normally isoelectric (see later discussion of TP interval). It is analyzed to identify whether it is above or below the isoelectric line, which may be, among other signs and symptoms, a sign of cardiac ischemia (see Chapter 27).

The **QT interval,** which represents the total time for ventricular depolarization and repolarization, is measured from the beginning of the QRS complex to the end of the T wave. The QT interval varies with heart rate, gender, and age; therefore, the measured interval needs to be corrected (QT_c) for these variables through specific calculations. The QT_c may be automatically calculated by the ECG technology, or a nurse may manually calculate or use a resource that

contains a chart of these calculations. The QT interval is usually 0.32 to 0.40 seconds in duration if the heart rate is 65 to 95 bpm. Many medications commonly given in the hospital can cause prolongation of the QT interval (QT_c), placing the patient at risk for a lethal ventricular dysrhythmia called *torsades de pointes*. However, studies demonstrate that patients with an indication for QT_c monitoring rarely have a QT_c calculated and documented (Sandau, Sendelbach, Fletcher, et al., 2015). Best practice recommends, at a minimum, documentation of the patient's QT interval, QTc interval, the lead in which the measurement was made, correction formula used, and patient assessment for administration of proarrhythmic medications be completed once a shift (Pickham, 2013).

The **TP interval** is measured from the end of the T wave to the beginning of the next P wave—an isoelectric period (see Fig. 26-3). When no electrical activity is detected, the line on the graph remains flat; this is called the *isoelectric line*. The ST segment is compared with the TP interval to detect ST segment changes. The PR segment is sometimes used to determine the isoelectric line. However, because that sometimes is altered due to ischemic conditions, the TP interval is the preferred reference for the isoelectric line.

The **PP interval** is measured from the beginning of one P wave to the beginning of the next P wave. The PP interval is used to determine atrial rate and rhythm. The **RR interval** is measured from one QRS complex to the next QRS complex. The RR interval is used to determine ventricular rate and rhythm (see later discussion).

Analyzing the Electrocardiogram Rhythm Strip

The ECG rhythm strip must be analyzed in a systematic manner to determine the patient's cardiac rate and rhythm, and to detect dysrhythmias and conduction disorders, as well as evidence of myocardial ischemia, injury, and infarction.

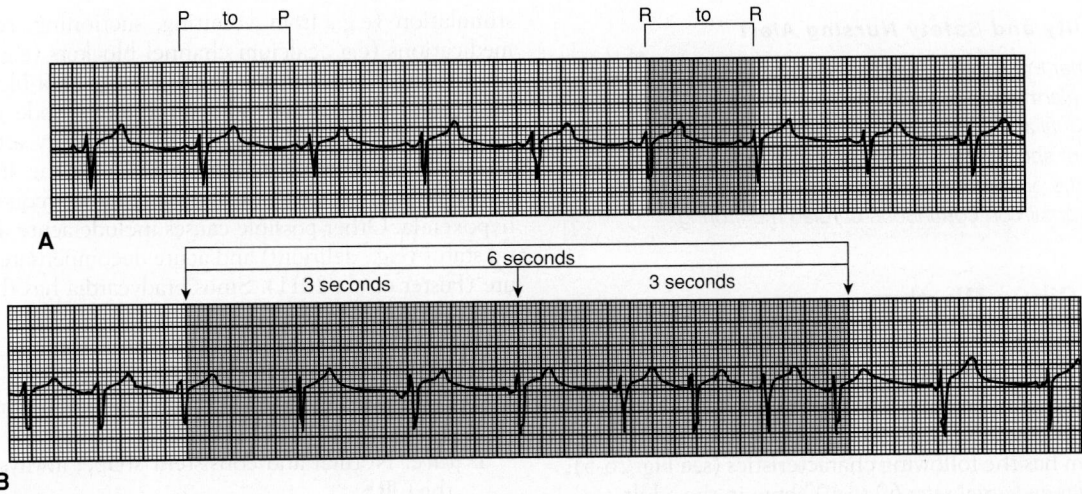

Figure 26-4 • **A.** Ventricular and atrial heart rate determination with a regular rhythm: 1,500 divided by the number of small boxes between two P waves (atrial rate) or between two R waves (ventricular rate). In this example, there are 25 small boxes between both the R waves and the P waves, so the heart rate is 60 bpm. **B.** Heart rate determination if the rhythm is irregular. There are approximately 7 RR intervals in 6 seconds, so there are about 70 RR intervals in 60 seconds (7 × 10 = 70). The ventricular heart rate is 70 bpm.

Determining Heart Rate from the Electrocardiogram

Heart rate can be obtained from the ECG rhythm strip by several methods. A 1-minute rhythm strip contains 300 large boxes and 1,500 small boxes. Therefore, an easy and accurate method of determining heart rate with a regular rhythm is to count the number of small boxes within an RR interval and divide 1,500 by that number. If, for example, there are 10 small boxes between two R waves, the heart rate is 1,500/10, or 150 bpm; if there are 25 small boxes, the heart rate is 1,500/25, or 60 bpm (see Fig. 26-4A).

An alternative but less accurate method for estimating heart rate, which is usually used when the rhythm is irregular, is to count the number of RR intervals in 6 seconds and multiply that number by 10. The top of the ECG paper is usually marked at 3-second intervals, which is 15 large boxes horizontally (see Fig. 26-4B). The RR intervals are counted, rather than QRS complexes, because a computed heart rate based on the latter might be inaccurately high.

The same methods may be used for determining atrial rate, using the PP interval instead of the RR interval.

Determining Heart Rhythm from the Electrocardiogram

The rhythm is often identified at the same time the rate is determined. Chart 26-1 provides an example of a method that can be used to analyze the patient's rhythm. The RR interval is used to determine ventricular rhythm and the PP interval to determine atrial rhythm. If the intervals are the same or if the difference between the intervals is less than 0.8 seconds throughout the strip, the rhythm is called *regular*. If the intervals are different, the rhythm is called *irregular*.

Once the rhythm has been analyzed, the findings are compared with and matched to the ECG criteria for dysrhythmias to determine a diagnosis. It is important for the nurse not only to identify the dysrhythmia, but also to assess the patient

to determine the physiologic effect of the dysrhythmia and identify possible causes. Treatment of a dysrhythmia is based on clinical evaluation of the patient with identification of the dysrhythmia's etiology and physiologic effect, not on its presence alone.

Most cardiac monitoring has functionality that includes that ability to continuously monitor the rhythm and alert health care personnel with an auditory and visual alarm when a clinically significant change in the rhythm occurs. However, a high rate of triggered, clinically insignificant alarms may lead to alarm fatigue, which has been linked to nurses ignoring, disabling, or silencing alarms (Sendelbach & Jepsen, 2013)—putting patients at increased risk of adverse events.

Chart 26-1

Interpreting Dysrhythmias: Systematic Analysis of the Electrocardiogram

When examining an electrocardiogram (ECG) rhythm strip to learn more about a patient's dysrhythmia:

1. Determine the ventricular rate.
2. Determine the ventricular rhythm.
3. Determine the QRS duration.
4. Determine whether the QRS duration is consistent throughout the strip. If not, identify other duration.
5. Identify the QRS shape; if not consistent, then identify other shapes.
6. Identify P waves; is there a P in front of every QRS?
7. Identify the P-wave shape; identify whether it is consistent or not.
8. Determine the atrial rate.
9. Determine the atrial rhythm.
10. Determine each PR interval.
11. Determine if the PR intervals are consistent, irregular but with a pattern to the irregularity, or just irregular.
12. Determine how many P waves for each QRS (P:QRS ratio).

In many cases, the nurse may use a checklist and document the findings next to the appropriate ECG criterion.

> **Quality and Safety Nursing Alert**
>
> *It is vital that the nurse assesses the cause(s) of a cardiac monitor's alarm and then adjusts the alarm default settings and individualizes the alarm parameter limits and levels. The assessment should also include an evaluation and discussion with the primary provider to validate that the patient needs to remain on continuous cardiac monitoring.*

Normal Sinus Rhythm

Electrical conduction that begins in the SA node generates a **sinus rhythm.** Normal sinus rhythm occurs when the electrical impulse starts at a regular rate and rhythm in the SA node and travels through the normal conduction pathway. Normal sinus rhythm has the following characteristics (see Fig. 26-5):

Ventricular and atrial rate: 60 to 100 bpm in the adult

Ventricular and atrial rhythm: Regular

QRS shape and duration: Usually normal, but may be regularly abnormal

P wave: Normal and consistent shape; always in front of the QRS

PR interval: Consistent interval between 0.12 and 0.20 seconds

P:QRS ratio: 1:1

Although normal sinus rhythm is generally indicative of good cardiovascular health, patients with an average resting heart rate that exceeds 90 bpm over a 24-hour period should receive a full medical workup for potential underlying causes (Sheldon, Grubb, Olshansky, et al., 2015).

Types of Dysrhythmias

Dysrhythmias include sinus, atrial, junctional, and ventricular dysrhythmias and their various subcategories, as well as conduction abnormalities.

Sinus Node Dysrhythmias

Sinus node dysrhythmias originate in the SA node; these include sinus bradycardia, sinus tachycardia, and sinus arrhythmia.

Sinus Bradycardia

Sinus bradycardia occurs when the SA node creates an impulse at a slower-than-normal rate. Causes include lower metabolic needs (e.g., sleep, athletic training, hypothyroidism), vagal stimulation (e.g., from vomiting, suctioning, severe pain), medications (e.g., calcium channel blockers (e.g., nifedipine [Procardia]), amiodarone [Cordarone], beta-blockers (e.g., metoprolol [Lopressor]), idiopathic sinus node dysfunction, increased intracranial pressure, and coronary artery disease, especially myocardial infarction (MI) of the inferior wall. Unstable and symptomatic bradycardia is frequently due to hypoxemia. Other possible causes include acute altered mental status (e.g., delirium) and acute decompensated heart failure (Fuster et al., 2011). Sinus bradycardia has the following characteristics (see Fig. 26-6):

Ventricular and atrial rate: Less than 60 bpm in the adult

Ventricular and atrial rhythm: Regular

QRS shape and duration: Usually normal, but may be regularly abnormal

P wave: Normal and consistent shape; always in front of the QRS

PR interval: Consistent interval between 0.12 and 0.20 seconds

P:QRS ratio: 1:1

All characteristics of sinus bradycardia are the same as those of normal sinus rhythm, except for the rate. The patient is assessed to determine the hemodynamic effect and the possible cause of the dysrhythmia. If the decrease in heart rate results from stimulation of the vagus nerve, such as with bearing down during defecation or vomiting, attempts are made to prevent further vagal stimulation. If the bradycardia is caused by a medication such as a beta-blocker, the medication may be withheld. If the slow heart rate causes significant hemodynamic changes resulting in shortness of breath, acute alteration of mental status, angina, hypotension, ST-segment changes, or premature ventricular complexes (PVCs), treatment is directed toward increasing the heart rate. Slow heart rate may be due to sinus node dysfunction (previously known as *sick sinus syndrome*), which has a number of risk factors including increased age; white race; obesity; hypertension; lower heart rate; and a history of a cardiovascular event, such as myocardial infarction, heart failure, or stroke (Jensen, Gronroos, Chen, et al., 2014). *Tachy-brady syndrome* is the term used when bradycardia alternates with tachycardia.

Medical Management

Management depends on the cause and symptoms. Resolving the causative factors may be the only treatment needed. If the bradycardia produces signs and symptoms of clinical instability (e.g., acute alteration in mental status, chest discomfort, or hypotension), 0.5 mg of atropine may be given rapidly as

Figure 26-5 • Normal sinus rhythm in lead II.

Figure 26-6 • Sinus bradycardia in lead II.

an intravenous (IV) bolus and repeated every 3 to 5 minutes until a maximum dosage of 3 mg is given. Rarely if the bradycardia is unresponsive to atropine, emergency transcutaneous pacing can be instituted, or catecholamines, such as dopamine or epinephrine, are given (Link, Berkow, Kudenchuk, et al., 2015) (see later discussion in Pacemaker Therapy).

Sinus Tachycardia

Sinus tachycardia occurs when the sinus node creates an impulse at a faster-than-normal rate. Causes may include the following:

- Physiologic or psychological stress (e.g., acute blood loss, anemia, shock, hypervolemia, hypovolemia, heart failure, pain, hypermetabolic states, fever, exercise, anxiety)
- Medications that stimulate the sympathetic response (e.g., catecholamines, aminophylline, atropine), stimulants (e.g., caffeine, nicotine), and illicit drugs (e.g., amphetamines, cocaine, Ecstasy)
- Enhanced automaticity of the SA node and/or excessive sympathetic tone with reduced parasympathetic tone that is out of proportion to physiologic demands, a condition called *inappropriate sinus tachycardia*
- Autonomic dysfunction, which results in a type of sinus tachycardia referred to as postural orthostatic tachycardia syndrome (POTS). POTS is characterized by tachycardia (increase in heart rate greater than 30 bpm) without hypotension when moving to a standing position, or with frequent symptoms such as palpitations, light-headedness, weakness, and blurred vision that occur with standing (Sheldon et al., 2015).

Sinus tachycardia has the following characteristics (see Fig. 26-7):

Ventricular and atrial rate: Greater than 100 bpm in the adult, but usually less than 120 bpm

Ventricular and atrial rhythm: Regular

QRS shape and duration: Usually normal, but may be regularly abnormal

P wave: Normal and consistent shape; always in front of the QRS, but may be buried in the preceding T wave

PR interval: Consistent interval between 0.12 and 0.20 seconds

P:QRS ratio: 1:1

All aspects of sinus tachycardia are the same as those of normal sinus rhythm, except for the rate. Sinus tachycardia does not start or end suddenly (i.e., it is nonparoxysmal). As the heart rate increases, the diastolic filling time decreases, possibly resulting in reduced cardiac output and subsequent symptoms of syncope and low blood pressure. If the rapid rate persists and the heart cannot compensate for the decreased ventricular filling, the patient may develop acute pulmonary edema.

Medical Management

Medical management of sinus tachycardia is determined by the severity of symptoms and directed at identifying and abolishing its cause. If the tachycardia is persistent and causing hemodynamic instability, synchronized cardioversion is the treatment of choice (see later discussion). Otherwise, vagal maneuvers, such as carotid sinus massage, gagging, bearing down against a closed glottis (as if having a bowel movement), forceful and sustained coughing, and applying a cold stimulus to the face (such as immersing the face in ice water), or administration of adenosine (Adenocard) may be considered

Figure 26-7 • Sinus tachycardia in lead II.

to interrupt the tachycardia. These increase parasympathetic stimulation, causing slower conduction through the AV node and blocking the reentry of the rerouted impulse (Smith, Fry, Taylor, et al., 2015). Beta-blockers (Class II antiarrhythmic) and calcium channel blockers (Class IV antiarrhythmic) (see Table 26-1), although rarely used, may also be considered in a narrow-QRS tachycardia. If the tachycardia has a wide QRS, then adenosine is considered only if the QRS is monomorphic (uniform shape) and the ventricular rhythm is regular. Otherwise, procainamide (Pronestyl), amiodarone, and sotalol (Betapace) are the options in wide QRS tachycardia (see later discussion of all of these medications). Catheter ablation (see later discussion in Atrial Fibrillation) of the SA node may be used in cases of persistent inappropriate sinus tachycardia unresponsive to other treatments. Treatment for POTS often involves a combination of approaches, with treatment targeted at the underlying problem. For example, patients with hypovolemia may be advised to increase their fluid and sodium intake, or use salt tablets if necessary (Sheldon et al., 2015).

Sinus Arrhythmia

Sinus arrhythmia occurs when the sinus node creates an impulse at an irregular rhythm; the rate usually increases with inspiration and decreases with expiration. Nonrespiratory causes include heart disease and valvular disease, but these are rare. Sinus arrhythmia has the following characteristics (see Fig. 26-8):

Ventricular and atrial rate: 60 to 100 bpm in the adult
Ventricular and atrial rhythm: Irregular
QRS shape and duration: Usually normal, but may be regularly abnormal
P wave: Normal and consistent shape; always in front of the QRS
PR interval: Consistent interval between 0.12 and 0.20 seconds
P:QRS ratio: 1:1

Medical Management

Sinus arrhythmia does not cause any significant hemodynamic effect and therefore is not typically treated.

Atrial Dysrhythmias

Atrial dysrhythmias originate from foci within the atria and not the SA node. These include aberrancies such as premature atrial complexes (PACs) as well as atrial fibrillation and atrial flutter.

Premature Atrial Complex

A premature atrial complex (PAC) is a single ECG complex that occurs when an electrical impulse starts in the atrium before the next normal impulse of the sinus node. The PAC may be caused by caffeine, alcohol, nicotine, stretched atrial myocardium (e.g., as in hypervolemia), anxiety, hypokalemia (low potassium level), hypermetabolic states (e.g., with pregnancy), or atrial ischemia, injury, or infarction. PACs are often seen with sinus tachycardia. PACs have the following characteristics (see Fig. 26-9):

Ventricular and atrial rate: Depends on the underlying rhythm (e.g., sinus tachycardia)
Ventricular and atrial rhythm: Irregular due to early P waves, creating a PP interval that is shorter than the others. This

is sometimes followed by a longer-than-normal PP interval, but one that is less than twice the normal PP interval. This type of interval is called a *noncompensatory pause.*
QRS shape and duration: The QRS that follows the early P wave is usually normal, but it may be abnormal (aberrantly conducted PAC). It may even be absent (blocked PAC).
P wave: An early and different P wave may be seen or may be hidden in the T wave; other P waves in the strip are consistent.
PR interval: The early P wave has a shorter-than-normal PR interval, but still between 0.12 and 0.20 seconds.
P:QRS ratio: Usually 1:1

PACs are common in normal hearts. The patient may say, "My heart skipped a beat." A pulse deficit (a difference between the apical and radial pulse rate) may exist.

Medical Management

If PACs are infrequent, no treatment is necessary. If they are frequent (more than six per minute), this may herald a worsening disease state or the onset of more serious dysrhythmias, such as atrial fibrillation. Medical management is directed toward treating the underlying cause (e.g., reduction of caffeine intake, correction of hypokalemia).

Atrial Fibrillation

Atrial fibrillation is the most common sustained dysrhythmia, affecting as many as 6.1 million Americans (Mozaffarian, Benjamin, Go, et al., 2015). Hospitalizations in the United States for atrial fibrillation increased by 23% between 2000 and 2010, and represented a significant source of increased costs to the health care system (Patel, Deshmukh, Pant, et al., 2014). Atrial fibrillation causes electrophysiologic changes in the atrial myocardium (remodeling of the atrial electrical circuit) and structural remodeling (fibrosis), which provides the basis for continuance of the dysrhythmia (January, Wann, Alpert, et al., 2014; Stavrakis, Nakagawa, Po, et al., 2015). Atrial fibrillation can result from diverse pathophysiologic etiologies and risks (see Chart 26-2).

Atrial fibrillation results from abnormal impulse formation that occurs when structural or electrophysiological abnormalities alter the atrial tissue causing a rapid, disorganized, and uncoordinated twitching of the atrial musculature (January et al., 2014). Both the extrinsic (central) and intrinsic cardiac autonomic nervous systems (CANS) are thought to play an important role in the initiation and continuance of atrial fibrillation (Stavrakis et al., 2015). Separate from the extrinsic (central) nervous system, which includes the brain and spinal cord, the CANS consists of a highly interconnected network of autonomic ganglia and nerve cell bodies embedded within the epicardium, largely within the atrial myocardium and great vessels (pulmonary veins). Hyperactive autonomic ganglia in the CANS are thought to play a critical role in atrial fibrillation, resulting in impulses that are initiated from the pulmonary veins and conducted through to the AV node. The ventricular rate of response depends on the conduction of atrial impulses through the AV node, presence of accessory electrical conduction pathways, and therapeutic effect of medications.

Lack of consistency in describing patterns or types of atrial fibrillation has led to the use of numerous labels (e.g., **paroxysmal** [i.e., it has a sudden onset and terminates spontaneously],

TABLE 26-1 Summary of Antiarrhythmic Medications[a]

Class[a]	Action	Drug Names	Side Effects	Nursing Interventions
IA	Moderate depression of depolarization; prolongs repolarization Treats and prevents atrial and ventricular dysrhythmias	quinidine (Quinaglute, Quinidex, Cardioquin) procainamide (Pronestyl, Procanbid, disopyramide (Norpace)	Decreased cardiac contractility Prolonged QRS, QT Proarrhythmic Hypotension with IV administration Diarrhea with quinidine, constipation with disopyramide Cinchonism with quinidine Lupuslike syndrome with procainamide Anticholinergic effects: dry mouth, urinary hesitancy with disopyramide	Observe for HF. Monitor BP with IV administration. Monitor QRS duration for increase >50% from baseline. Monitor for prolonged QT. Monitor N-acetyl procainamide (NAPA) laboratory values during procainamide therapy. If given for atrial fibrillation, ensure that the patient has been pretreated with a medication to control AV conduction.
IB	Minimal depression of depolarization; shortened repolarization Treats ventricular dysrhythmias	lidocaine (Xylocaine, LidoPen)	CNS changes (e.g., confusion, lethargy) Bradycardia GI distress Tremors	Monitor for CNS changes and tremors. Discuss with the primary provider decreasing lidocaine dose in older adult patients and patients with cardiac/liver dysfunction.
IC	Marked depression of depolarization; little effect on repolarization Treats atrial and ventricular dysrhythmias	flecainide (Tambocor) propafenone (Rythmol)	Proarrhythmic HF Dizziness, visual disturbances, dyspnea	Decrease dose with renal dysfunction and strict vegetarian diets. Avoid use in patients with structural heart disease (e.g., coronary artery disease and heart failure).
II	Decreases automaticity and conduction Treats atrial and ventricular dysrhythmias	acebutolol (Sectral)[c] atenolol (Tenormin) bisoprolol/HCTZ (Ziac, Zebeta) esmolol (Brevibloc)[c] labetalol (Trandate) metoprolol (Lopressor, Toprol-XL) nadolol (Corgard) nebivolol (Bystolic) propranolol (Inderal, InnoPran XL)[c] sotalol (Betapace; Sorine; Sotylize also has class III actions)[c] timolol (Blocadren)	Bradycardia, AV block Decreased contractility Bronchospasm Nausea Asymptomatic and symptomatic hypotension Masks hypoglycemia and thyrotoxicosis CNS disturbances (e.g., confusion, dizziness, fatigue, depression)	Monitor heart rate, PR interval, signs and symptoms of HF, especially in those also taking calcium channel blockers. Monitor blood glucose level in patients with type 2 diabetes. Caution the patient about abrupt withdrawal to avoid tachycardia, hypertension, and myocardial ischemia.
III	Prolongs repolarization Amiodarone treats and prevents ventricular and atrial dysrhythmias, especially in patients with ventricular dysfunction. Dofetilide and ibutilide treat and prevent atrial dysrhythmias.	amiodarone (Cordarone, Pacerone) dofetilide (Tikosyn) Dronedarone (MULTAQ) ibutilide (Corvert)	Pulmonary toxicity (amiodarone) Corneal microdeposits (amiodarone) Photosensitivity (amiodarone) Bradycardia Hypotension, especially with IV administration Polymorphic ventricular dysrhythmias (rare with amiodarone) Nausea and vomiting Potentiates digoxin (amiodarone) See beta-blockers above (sotalol).	Make sure that the patient is sent for baseline pulmonary function tests (amiodarone). Closely monitor the patient. Assess for contraindications prior to administration. Monitor QT duration. Continuous ECG monitoring with initiation of dofetilide and ibutilide. Monitor renal function.
IV	Blocks calcium channel Treats and prevents paroxysmal atrial dysrhythmias[b]	verapamil (Calan, Covera-HS, Isoptin) diltiazem (Cardizem, Dilacor, Tiazac, Diltia, Cartia)	Bradycardia, AV blocks Hypotension with IV administration HF, peripheral edema Constipation, dizziness, headache, nausea	Monitor heart rate, PR interval. Monitor blood pressure closely with IV administration. Monitor for signs and symptoms of HF. Do not crush sustained-release medications.

IV, intravenous; HF, heart failure; BP, blood pressure; AV, atrioventricular; CNS, central nervous system; GI, gastrointestinal; HCTZ, hydrochlorothiazide; ECG, electrocardiogram.
[a]Based on Vaughan–Williams classification.
[b]There are other calcium channel blockers, but they are not approved or used for dysrhythmias.
[c]Beta-blocker with labeled use for dysrhythmias.
Adapted from the American Society of Health System Pharmacists. (2012). *AHFS drug information* Bethesda, MD: Author; Fuster, V., Walsh, R., & Harrington, R. A. (Eds.). (2011). *Hurst's the heart* (13th ed.). New York: McGraw-Hill.

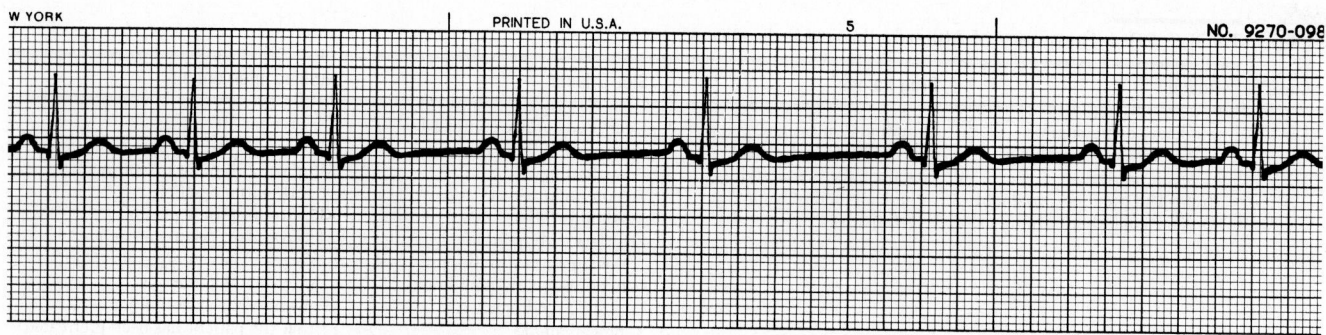

Figure 26-8 • Sinus arrhythmia in lead II. Note irregular RR and PP intervals.

persistent, and permanent). The recommended classification system is noted in Chart 26-3. The use of the term "chronic atrial fibrillation" is no longer included in the classification system, due to a lack of consensus on what constitutes chronicity (January et al., 2014).

Atrial fibrillation has the following characteristics (Fig. 26-10):

Ventricular and atrial rate: Atrial rate is 300 to 600 bpm; ventricular rate is usually 120 to 200 bpm in untreated atrial fibrillation.

Ventricular and atrial rhythm: Highly irregular

QRS shape and duration: Usually normal, but may be abnormal

P wave: No discernible P waves; irregular undulating waves that vary in amplitude and shape are seen and referred to as fibrillatory or f waves

PR interval: Cannot be measured

P:QRS ratio: Many:1

Patients with atrial fibrillation are at increased risk of heart failure, myocardial ischemia, and embolic events such as stroke (January et al., 2014). A rapid and irregular ventricular response reduces the time for ventricular filling, resulting in a smaller stroke volume. Because atrial fibrillation causes a loss in AV synchrony (the atria and ventricles contract at different times), the atrial kick (the last part of diastole and ventricular filling, which accounts for 25% to 30% of the cardiac output)

is also lost. As a consequence, although some patients with atrial fibrillation are asymptomatic, others experience palpitations and clinical manifestations of heart failure (e.g., shortness of breath, hypotension, dyspnea on exertion, fatigue; see Chapter 29). In addition, a high ventricular rate of response during atrial fibrillation (greater than 80 bpm) can eventually lead to mitral valve dysfunction, mitral regurgitation, intraventricular conduction delays, and dilated ventricular cardiomyopathy.

Patients with atrial fibrillation may exhibit a pulse deficit—a numeric difference between apical and radial pulse rates. The shorter time in diastole reduces the time available for coronary artery perfusion, thereby increasing the risk of myocardial ischemia with the onset of anginal symptoms (see Chapter 27). Decreasing the ventricular rate may avoid and correct these effects.

The erratic nature of atrial contraction, alterations in ventricular ejection, and atrial myocardial dysfunction promote the formation of thrombi, especially within the left atrium, increasing the risk of an embolic event. The origin of embolisms resulting in stroke for patients with nonvalvular atrial fibrillation is most often the left atrial appendage (LAA) (Masoudi, Calkins, Kavinsky, et al., 2015). A therapeutic approach to addressing the role of the LAA in atrial fibrillation, left atrial appendage occlusion (LAAO), is discussed later in this chapter.

Figure 26-9 • Premature atrial complexes (PACs) in lead II. Note that the pause following the PAC is longer than the normal PP interval but shorter than twice the normal PP interval.

Chart 26-2 · RISK FACTORS
Atrial Fibrillation

- Increasing age
- Hypertension
- Diabetes
- Obesity
- Valvular heart disease
- Heart failure
- Obstructive sleep apnea
- Alcohol consumption—moderate (1–3 drinks/day) and high (>3 drinks/day)
- Hyperthyroidism
- Cardiac ischemia
- Cardiac inflammatory disease (pericarditis, myocarditis, amyloidosis)
- Myocardial hypertrophy, fibrosis, or dilation
- Atrial remodeling
- Postoperative cardiac surgery

Adapted from LaPar, D. J., Speir, A. M., Crosby, I. K., et al. (2014). Postoperative atrial fibrillation significantly increases mortality, hospital readmission, and hospital costs. *Annals of Thoracic Surgery*, 98(2), 527–533; Larsson, S.C., Drca, N., & Wolk, A. (2014). Alcohol consumption and risk of atrial fibrillation: A prospective study and dose-response meta-analysis. *Journal of the American College of Cardiology*, 64(3), 282–289; January, C. T., Wann, L. S., Alpert, J. S., et al. (2014). 2014 AHA/ACC/HRS guideline for the management of patients with atrial fibrillation: A report of the ACC/AHA Task Force on practice guidelines and the Heart Rhythm Society. *Circulation*, 130(23), e199–e267; Shukla, A., Aizer, A., Holmes, D., et al. (2015). Effect of obstructive sleep apnea treatment on atrial fibrillation recurrence. *JACC: Clinical Electrophysiology*, 1(1–2), 41–51.

Chart 26-3 Atrial Fibrillation Classification System

Type	Description
Paroxysmal	Sudden onset with termination that occurs spontaneously or after an intervention; lasts ≤7 days, but may recur
Persistent	Continuous, lasting >7 days
Long-standing persistent	Continuous, lasting >12 months
Permanent	Persistent, but decision has been made not to restore or maintain sinus rhythm
Nonvalvular	Absence of mitral stenosis, valve replacement or repair

Adapted from January, C. T., Wann, L. S., Alpert, J. S., et al. (2014). 2014 AHA/ACC/HRS guideline for the management of patients with atrial fibrillation: A report of the ACC/AHA Task Force on practice guidelines and the Heart Rhythm Society. *Circulation*, 130(23), e199–e267.

Assessment and Diagnostic Findings

The clinical evaluation of atrial fibrillation should include a history and physical examination that identifies the onset and nature of signs and symptoms, including their frequency, duration and any precipitating factors, and any response to medications. Whether or not the patient has a known history of heart disease or other risks is identified (see Chart 26-2). A 12-lead ECG is performed to verify the atrial fibrillation rhythm, as well as to identify the presence (or absence) of left ventricular hypertrophy, bundle branch block, prior myocardial ischemia, or other dysrhythmias. The RR, QRS, and QT intervals are analyzed to verify the effectiveness of any prescribed antiarrhythmic medications (January et al., 2014). A transthoracic echocardiogram (TEE) can identify the presence of valvular heart disease, provide information about left ventricular (LV) and right ventricular (RV) size and function,

RV pressures (to identify pulmonary hypertension, which may exist concomitant with atrial fibrillation), LV hypertrophy, and presence of left atrial thrombi (January et al., 2014).

Blood tests to screen for diseases that are known risks for atrial fibrillation (see Chart 26-2), including thyroid, renal, and hepatic function, are assessed in the patient with a new onset of atrial fibrillation, as well as when the ventricular rate is difficult to control (January et al., 2014). Additional tests may include a chest x-ray (to evaluate pulmonary vasculature in a patient suspected of having pulmonary hypertension), exercise stress test (to exclude myocardial ischemia or reproduce exercise-induced atrial fibrillation), Holter or event monitoring (see Chapter 25), and an EP study (January et al., 2014) (see later discussion).

Medical Management

Treatment of atrial fibrillation depends on the cause, pattern, and duration of the dysrhythmia, the ventricular response rate, as well as the presence of structural or valvular heart disease and other cardiac conditions such as coronary artery disease or heart failure. Strategies for both rhythm control (i.e., conversion to sinus rhythm) and rate control are dependent on shared clinical decision making between the patient and primary provider. In some cases, atrial fibrillation spontaneously converts to sinus rhythm within 24 to 48 hours and without treatment. However, in instances where atrial fibrillation is concomitant with significant other morbid conditions

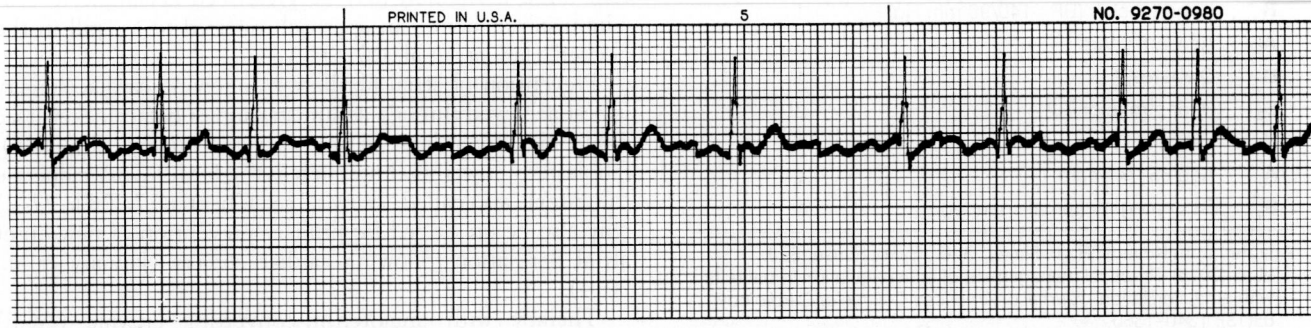

Figure 26-10 • Atrial fibrillation in lead II.

(e.g., severe heart failure), the atrial fibrillation may be classified as "permanent," meaning that the patient and primary provider have made a joint decision to stop further attempts to restore or maintain sinus rhythm. Therefore, management of atrial fibrillation may not only be different in different patients, but it also may change over time for any one patient.

Medical management revolves around preventing embolic events such as stroke with antithrombotic drugs, controlling the ventricular rate of response with antiarrhythmic agents, and treating the dysrhythmia as indicated so that it is converted to a sinus rhythm (i.e., *cardioversion*).

Pharmacologic Therapy

Antithrombotic Medications. Antithrombotic drugs may include anticoagulants and antiplatelet drugs. Oral antithrombotic therapy is indicated for most patients with nonvalvular atrial fibrillation because it reduces the risk of stroke (Kovacs, Flaker, Saxonhouse, et al., 2015). Atrial fibrillation guidelines (January et al., 2014) recommend use of a scoring system to assist in assessment of stroke risk. Antithrombotic therapy is then selected based on risk factors outlined in the mnemonic CHA_2DS_2-VAS_C (see Chart 26-4) with each risk factor assigned points tallied for a total score that indicates an overall risk of stroke (Kovacs et al., 2015).

According to pharmacologic treatment guidelines (Kovacs et al., 2015):

- Patients with low stroke risk (i.e., CHA_2DS_2-VAS_C score of zero) may choose the option of no antithrombotic therapy or may be placed on aspirin therapy dosed at 75 to 325 mg daily.
- Patients with at least moderate risk (i.e., CHA_2DS_2-VAS_C score of one of higher) may choose either warfarin (Coumadin) or a direct-acting oral anticoagulant or Factor Xa inhibitor (e.g., dabigatran [Pradaxa], rivaroxaban [Xarelto], apixaban [Eliquis], edoxaban [Savaysa]).

Medication selection depends on patient characteristics, primary provider and patient preference, current medication regimen, and cost, as well as time required for therapeutic drug monitoring (Kovacs et al., 2015). For instance, treatment

with warfarin will require weekly international normalized ratio (INR) testing during initiation of therapy, as well as ongoing monitoring (see Chapters 25 and 30 for further discussion). Home monitoring of therapy is an option in selected patients. Direct-acting oral anticoagulants and Factor Xa inhibitors require baseline assessment of hemoglobin and hematocrit, as well as liver and renal function, along with INR. Advantages of these medications include fewer drug–drug interactions and dietary limitations, as well as the elimination of frequent INR testing (Kovacs et al., 2015). For patients with mechanical heart valves, warfarin is recommended (January et al., 2014). If immediate or short-term anticoagulation is necessary, the patient may be placed on IV or low–molecular-weight heparin until warfarin therapy can be started and the INR level reaches a therapeutic range consistent with antithrombosis, usually defined as an INR between 2.0 and 3.0 (see Chapter 30 for further discussion).

Medications That Control the Heart Rate. A strategy to control the ventricular rate of response so that the resting heart rate is less than 80 bpm is recommended in order to manage symptoms of atrial fibrillation (January et al., 2014). To decrease the ventricular rate in patients with paroxysmal, persistent, or permanent atrial fibrillation, a beta-blocker (Class II antiarrhythmic, see Table 26-1) or non-dihydropyridine calcium channel blocker (Class IV antiarrhythmic, see Table 26-1) is generally recommended (January et al., 2014).

Medications That Convert the Heart Rhythm or Prevent Atrial Fibrillation. For patients with atrial fibrillation lasting 48 hours or longer, anticoagulation is recommended prior to attempts to restore sinus rhythm, which may be achieved through pharmacological or electrical cardioversion (January et al., 2014). In the absence of therapeutic anticoagulation, TEE may be performed prior to cardioversion to identify left atrial thrombus formation, including in the LAA (January et al., 2014). If no thrombus is identified, cardioversion can proceed.

Medications that may be given to achieve pharmacologic cardioversion to sinus rhythm include flecainide (Tambocor), dofetilide (Tikosyn), propafenone (Rythmol), amiodarone, and IV ibutilide (Corvert) (January et al., 2014). These medications are most effective if given within 7 days of the onset of atrial fibrillation. It is recommended that patients who were prescribed dofetilide be hospitalized so that the QT interval and renal function both may be monitored. Despite a degree of risk, dofetilide is a preferred medication because it is highly effective at converting atrial fibrillation to sinus rhythm, has fewer drug-to-drug interactions, and is better tolerated by patients than other medications. Some patients with recurrent atrial fibrillation may be prescribed flecainide to self-administer at home, an approach referred to as "pill in the pocket" (January et al., 2014).

Prevention of atrial fibrillation following cardiac surgery is best achieved through administration of beta-blockers (see Table 26-1) for at least 24 hours prior to surgery (Shi, 2016). Cholesterol-lowering drugs such as the HMG-CoA reductase inhibitors (also called "statins," see Chapter 27, Table 27–2) may also be prescribed for primary prevention of new-onset atrial fibrillation following cardiac surgery (January et al., 2014).

Therapy with angiotensin-converting enzyme (ACE) inhibitors and angiotensin receptor blockers (ARBs) (see

Chart 26-4	Stroke Risk Assessment for the Patient With Atrial Fibrillation: The CHA_2DS_2-VAS_C Scoring System	
	Risk Factor	**Points**
C	Congestive Heart Failure (left ventricular systolic dysfunction)	1
H	Hypertension (BP >140/90 mm Hg)	1
A$_2$	Age ≥75 years	2
D	Diabetes	1
S$_2$	Prior stroke or TIA	2
V	Vascular disease	1
A	Age 65–74 years	1
S$_c$	Sex category (female gender)	1

Adapted from Kovacs, R. J., Flaker, G. C., Saxonhouse, S. J., et al. (2015). Practical management of anticoagulation in patients with atrial fibrillation. *Journal of American College of Cardiology*, 65(13), 1340–1360.

Chapter 31, Table 31-4) may decrease the incidence of atrial fibrillation for patients with concomitant hypertension, although the use of these drugs is not found to be beneficial as a primary prevention strategy for patients without hypertension (January et al., 2014).

If symptomatic, paroxysmal atrial fibrillation is refractory to at least one Class I or Class III antiarrhythmic medication (see Table 26-1), and rhythm control is desired, catheter ablation may be indicated (January et al., 2014) (see later discussion).

Electrical Cardioversion for Atrial Fibrillation

Electrical cardioversion is indicated for patients with atrial fibrillation that is hemodynamically unstable (e.g., acute alteration in mental status, chest discomfort, hypotension) and does not respond to medications (January et al., 2014). Flecainide, propafenone, amiodarone, dofetilide, or sotalol may be given prior to cardioversion to enhance the success of cardioversion and maintain sinus rhythm (January et al., 2014).

> ◣ *Quality and Safety Nursing Alert*
>
> *The patient with atrial fibrillation is at high risk for thrombus formation. When electrical cardioversion is indicated, the nurse may anticipate that a transesophageal echocardiogram may be performed to evaluate for possible atrial thrombi.*

Because atrial function may be impaired for several weeks after cardioversion, warfarin is indicated for at least 4 weeks after the procedure (January et al., 2014). Repeated attempts at electrical cardioversion may be made, following administration of an antiarrhythmic medication (see later discussion on Electrical Cardioversion).

Cardiac Rhythm Therapies

Atrial fibrillation that does not respond to medications or electrical cardioversion may be treated by cardiac rhythm therapies, including catheter ablation, maze or mini-maze procedure, or convergent procedure.

Catheter Ablation Therapy

Catheter **ablation** destroys specific cells that are the cause of a tachydysrhythmia. Catheter ablation is performed most often today for atrial fibrillation, although it may also be useful in treating atrioventricular nodal reentry tachycardia (AVNRT) and recurrent ventricular tachycardia (VT) (see later discussion of these dysrhythmias).

Recent evidence demonstrates that the pathogenesis of atrial fibrillation is associated with intrinsic cardiac autonomic nervous system activity to the pulmonary veins (Stavrakis et al., 2015). Ablation involves a procedure similar to a cardiac catheterization (see Chapter 25); however, in this instance, a special catheter is advanced at or near the origin of the dysrhythmia, where high-frequency, low-energy sound waves are passed through the catheter, causing thermal injury, localized cell destruction, and scarring. The tissue damage is more specific to the dysrhythmic tissue, with less trauma to the surrounding cardiac tissue. Ablation may also be accomplished using a special catheter to apply extremely cold temperature to destroy selected cardiac cells, called *cryoablation*. The goal of each of these ablation procedures is to eliminate the dysrhythmia, by preventing the ectopic activity arising from the pulmonary veins from reaching the atria, thereby stopping fibrillation (Stavrakis et al., 2015).

An EP study (see later discussion) may be performed to induce the dysrhythmia prior to the catheter ablation. During the ablation procedure, defibrillation pads, an automatic blood pressure cuff, and a pulse oximeter are used. The patient is usually given moderate sedation (see Chapter 18) and IV heparin to reduce the risk of periprocedural thromboembolism. Immediately postablation, the patient is monitored for another 30 to 60 minutes and then retested to ensure that the dysrhythmia does not recur. Successful ablation is achieved when the dysrhythmia cannot be induced. Major risks of catheter ablation include AV block, pericardial tamponade, phrenic nerve injury, stroke, hematoma, retroperitoneal bleeding, pulmonary vein stenosis, and atrioesophageal fistulas (January et al., 2014; Mann, Zipes, Libby, et al., 2015). Obstructive sleep apnea is one known risk factor associated with the recurrence of atrial fibrillation after catheter ablation (Shukla, Aizer, Holmes, et al., 2015).

Nursing Management. Postprocedural care on a stepdown unit for the patient who has had ablation is similar to the nursing management of a patient who has had a cardiac catheterization (see Chapter 25); the patient is monitored closely to ensure recovery from sedation. Postprocedural nursing interventions include frequent monitoring for dysrhythmias and for signs and symptoms of a stroke, vascular access site complications (see Chapter 25), and fluid imbalance (Hoke & Steletsky, 2015). Because of the prolonged time required for the procedure as well as the time needed in bed to obtain hemostasis at the vascular access site, it is not unusual for the patient to have back discomfort. In addition to administering any pain medications, the nurse may help to alleviate this pain by placing rolled towels under the patient's knees and waist.

Maze and Mini-Maze Procedures

The maze procedure is an open heart surgical procedure for refractory atrial fibrillation. Small transmural incisions are made throughout the atria. The resulting formation of scar tissue prevents reentry conduction of the aberrant electrical impulse. Because the procedure requires significant time and cardiopulmonary bypass, its use is reserved only for those patients undergoing cardiac surgery for another reason (e.g., coronary artery bypass, see Chapter 27) (January et al., 2014). Some patients may need a permanent pacemaker after this surgery because of subsequent injury to the SA node.

A modification of the maze procedure, minimally invasive maze surgery, or mini-maze, may be performed by making small incisions between the ribs, through which video-guided instruments are inserted. The pulmonary veins are encircled with surgical incisions within the left atrium. This surgery eliminates the need for opening the sternum, heart-lung bypass, and the use of cardioplegia (see Chapter 27 for further discussion of cardiac surgery). This results in a shorter recovery time and a lower risk of infection (January et al., 2014).

Convergent Procedure

The convergent procedure utilizes a hybrid approach to ablation, requiring the skills of both a cardiothoracic surgeon and an electrophysiologist. The surgeon creates a few small incisions in the abdomen so that a special catheter that allows visualization can be inserted through the diaphragm and toward the posterior wall of the heart (Elrod, 2014). The surgeon performs ablation of the epicardial wall in the area around the pulmonary veins and the electrophysiologist performs ablation around the endocardial area of the pulmonary veins. Because of the incisions, the patient usually has a 3-day hospital length of stay (Elrod, 2014). The patient may experience mild dull chest pain that is caused by the resulting inflammation from the ablation that usually resolves within a few days (Elrod, 2014). This pain is usually alleviated by treatment with acetaminophen as needed. In addition, if the phrenic nerve was affected, the patient may experience shortness of breath that may take days to weeks to resolve (Elrod, 2014).

Left Atrial Appendage Occlusion (LAAO)

Left atrial appendage occlusion (LAAO) has been recently approved in the United States by the Food and Drug Administration (FDA) as an alternative to warfarin for stroke prevention in patients with nonvalvular atrial fibrillation (Masoudi et al., 2015). As noted previously, the LAA is the area where the majority of stroke-causing blood clots form in patients with nonvalvular atrial fibrillation. However, concerns about the risk of long-term anticoagulant use and the risk of bleeding can complicate effective management (Alli, Asirvatham, & Holmes, 2015).

Candidates for LAAO include those patients with increased risk of stroke based on CHA_2DS_2-VAS_C scores of one or higher (see Chart 26-4) and those patients seeking a nonpharmacological alternative to warfarin (Masoudi et al., 2015). The device most commonly used is the WATCHMAN device; this device is typically inserted while the patient is under general anesthesia. Similar to a percutaneous coronary intervention (PCI) procedure (see Chapter 27), a small incision is made in the femoral area and a catheter is then inserted that guides the device into position. The parachute-shaped device is threaded through to the opening of the LAA, sealing it off and preventing it from releasing clots (see Fig. 26-11).

Patients typically stay in the hospital overnight after placement of a WATCHMAN device. The nursing management of patients who received this device is similar to that of patients postcardiac catheterization (see Chapter 25). Patients are prescribed aspirin and warfarin postprocedure; approximately 6 weeks postprocedure, they should return to the cardiology clinic for a TEE to confirm that the device has effectively occluded the LAA. If LAAO has occurred, then the patient may stop taking warfarin and is prescribed clopidogrel (Plavix), an antiplatelet medication. After 6 months, the patient may stop taking clopidogrel but must continue taking daily aspirin indefinitely.

Wolff–Parkinson–White Syndrome

In the patient with atrial fibrillation, if the QRS is wide and the ventricular rhythm is very fast and irregular, an accessory pathway should be suspected. An accessory pathway is typically congenital tissue between the atria, bundle of His, AV node, Purkinje fibers, or ventricular myocardium. This anomaly is known as Wolff–Parkinson–White (WPW) syndrome.

Figure 26-11 • The WATCHMAN device in place over the left atrial appendage. Image provided courtesy of Boston Scientific. © 2016 Boston Scientific Corporation or its affiliates. All rights reserved.

Electrical cardioversion is the treatment of choice for atrial fibrillation in the presence of WPW syndrome that causes hemodynamic instability. Medications that block AV conduction (e.g., digoxin, diltiazem [Cardizem], and verapamil [Calan]) should be avoided in WPW because they can increase the ventricular rate. If the patient is hemodynamically stable, procainamide, propafenone, flecainide, and amiodarone are recommended to restore sinus rhythm (January et al., 2014). Catheter ablation is performed for long-term management (see previous discussion on Catheter Ablation Therapy).

Atrial Flutter

Atrial flutter occurs because of a conduction defect in the atrium and causes a rapid, regular atrial impulse at a rate between 250 and 400 bpm. Because the atrial rate is faster than the AV node can conduct, not all atrial impulses are conducted into the ventricle, causing a therapeutic block at the AV node. This is an important feature of this dysrhythmia. If all atrial impulses were conducted to the ventricle, the ventricular rate would also be 250 to 400 bpm, which would result in ventricular fibrillation, a life-threatening dysrhythmia. Atrial flutter risk factors mirror those for atrial fibrillation (Fuster et al., 2011) (see Chart 26-2).

Atrial flutter has the following characteristics (see Fig. 26-12):

Ventricular and atrial rate: Atrial rate ranges between 250 and 400 bpm; ventricular rate usually ranges between 75 and 150 bpm.

Ventricular and atrial rhythm: The atrial rhythm is regular; the ventricular rhythm is usually regular but may be irregular because of a change in the AV conduction.

QRS shape and duration: Usually normal, but may be abnormal or may be absent.

Figure 26-12 • Atrial flutter in lead II.

P wave: Saw-toothed shape; these waves are referred to as
  F waves.
PR interval: Multiple F waves may make it difficult to
  determine the PR interval.
P:QRS ratio: 2:1, 3:1, or 4:1

Medical Management

Atrial flutter can cause serious signs and symptoms, such
as chest pain, shortness of breath, and low blood pressure.
Medical management involves the use of vagal maneuvers
(see previous discussion under Sinus Tachycardia) or a trial
administration of adenosine, which causes sympathetic
block and slowing of conduction through the AV node. This
may terminate the tachycardia; optimally, it will facilitate
visualization of flutter waves for diagnostic purposes. Adenosine is given intravenously by rapid administration, and
immediately followed by a 20-mL saline flush and elevation
of the arm with the IV line to promote rapid circulation of
the medication.

Atrial flutter is treated with antithrombotic therapy, rate
control, and rhythm control in the same manner as atrial
fibrillation (January et al., 2014). Electrical cardioversion is
often successful in converting atrial flutter to sinus rhythm
(see later discussion of Electrical Cardioversion).

Junctional Dysrhythmias

Junctional dysrhythmias originate within AV nodal tissue,
and may include premature junctional complexes, junctional
rhythms, nonparoxysmal junctional tachycardia, and AV
nodal reentry tachycardia.

Premature Junctional Complex

A premature junctional complex is an impulse that starts
in the AV nodal area before the next normal sinus impulse
reaches the AV node. Premature junctional complexes are
less common than PACs. Causes include digitalis toxicity,
heart failure, and coronary artery disease. The ECG criteria
for premature junctional complex are the same as for PACs,
except for the P wave and the PR interval. The P wave may
be absent, may follow the QRS, or may occur before the QRS
but with a PR interval of less than 0.12 seconds. This dysrhythmia rarely produces significant symptoms. Treatment for
frequent premature junctional complexes is the same as for
frequent PACs.

Junctional Rhythm

Junctional or idionodal rhythm occurs when the AV node,
instead of the sinus node, becomes the pacemaker of the
heart. When the sinus node slows (e.g., from increased vagal
tone) or when the impulse cannot be conducted through the
AV node (e.g., because of complete heart block), the AV
node automatically discharges an impulse. Junctional rhythm
not caused by complete heart block has the following characteristics (see Fig. 26-13):

Ventricular and atrial rate: Ventricular rate 40 to 60 bpm;
  atrial rate also 40 to 60 bpm if P waves are discernible
Ventricular and atrial rhythm: Regular
QRS shape and duration: Usually normal, but may be
  abnormal
P wave: May be absent, after the QRS complex, or before
  the QRS; may be inverted, especially in lead II

Figure 26-13 • Junctional rhythm in lead II; note short PR intervals and inverted P wave.

PR interval: If the P wave is in front of the QRS, the PR interval is less than 0.12 seconds.

P:QRS ratio: 1:1 or 0:1

Medical Management

Junctional rhythm may produce signs and symptoms of reduced cardiac output. If this occurs, the treatment is the same as for sinus bradycardia. Emergency pacing may be needed (see later discussion under Pacemaker Therapy).

Nonparoxysmal Junctional Tachycardia

Junctional tachycardia is caused by enhanced automaticity in the junctional area, resulting in a rhythm similar to junctional rhythm, except at a rate of 70 to 120 bpm. Although this rhythm generally does not have any detrimental hemodynamic effect, it may indicate a serious underlying condition, such as digitalis toxicity, myocardial ischemia, hypokalemia, or chronic obstructive pulmonary disease. Because junctional tachycardia is caused by increased automaticity, cardioversion is not an effective treatment (Mann et al., 2015).

Atrioventricular Nodal Reentry Tachycardia

Atrioventricular nodal reentry tachycardia (AVNRT) is a common dysrhythmia that occurs when an impulse is conducted to an area in the AV node that causes the impulse to be rerouted back into the same area over and over again at a very fast rate. Each time the impulse is conducted through this area, it is also conducted down into the ventricles, causing a fast ventricular rate. AVNRT that has an abrupt onset and an abrupt cessation with a QRS of normal duration has frequently been called *paroxysmal atrial tachycardia (PAT)*. AVNRT also occurs when the duration of the QRS complex is 0.12 seconds or greater and a block in the bundle branch is known to be present. This dysrhythmia may last for seconds or several hours. Factors associated with the development of AVNRT include caffeine, nicotine, hypoxemia, and stress. Underlying pathologies include coronary artery disease and cardiomyopathy; however, it occurs more often in females and not in association with underlying structural heart disease. AVNRT has the following characteristics (see Fig. 26-14):

Ventricular and atrial rate: Atrial rate usually 150 to 250 bpm; ventricular rate usually 120 to 200 bpm

Ventricular and atrial rhythm: Regular; sudden onset and termination of the tachycardia

QRS shape and duration: Usually normal, but may be abnormal

P wave: Usually very difficult to discern

PR interval: If the P wave is in front of the QRS, the PR interval is less than 0.12 seconds.

P:QRS ratio: 1:1, 2:1

The clinical symptoms vary with the rate and duration of the tachycardia and the patient's underlying condition. The tachycardia usually is of short duration, resulting only in palpitations. A fast rate may also reduce cardiac output, resulting in significant signs and symptoms such as restlessness, chest pain, shortness of breath, pallor, hypotension, and loss of consciousness.

Medical Management

Because AVNRT is generally a benign dysrhythmia, the goal of medical management is to alleviate symptoms and improve quality of life. Patients who become significantly symptomatic and require emergency department visits to terminate the rhythm may want to initiate therapy immediately. However, those with minimum symptoms with an AVRNT that terminates spontaneously or with minimal treatment may choose just to be monitored and self-treat.

The aim of therapy is to break the reentry of the impulse. Catheter ablation is the initial treatment of choice and is used to eliminate the area that permits the rerouting of the impulse that causes the tachycardia (Mann et al., 2015) (see previous discussion of Atrial Fibrillation: Catheter Ablation Therapy). Vagal maneuvers (see previous discussion under Sinus Tachycardia) may be used to interrupt AVNRT. These techniques increase parasympathetic stimulation, causing slower conduction through the AV node and blocking the reentry of the rerouted impulse. Some patients use some of these methods to terminate the episode on their own. Because of the risk of a cerebral embolic event, carotid sinus massage, which may be performed by physicians, is contraindicated in patients with carotid artery disease.

Pharmacologic Therapy

If the vagal maneuvers are ineffective, the patient may then receive a bolus of adenosine to correct the rhythm; this is nearly 100% effective in terminating AVNRT (Mann et al., 2015). Because the effect of adenosine is so short, AVNRT may recur; the first dose may be followed with a larger dose or with a calcium channel blocker, such as verapamil (Calan), followed by one or two additional boluses. If the patient is unstable or does not respond to the medications, electrical cardioversion is the treatment of choice (see later discussion). The patient who is unstable may be given adenosine while preparations for cardioversion are being made. For recurrent

Figure 26-14 • AV nodal reentry tachycardia in lead II.

sustained AVNRT, treatment with calcium channel blockers such as verapamil and diltiazem, class Ia antiarrhythmic agents such as procainamide and disopyramide (Norpace), class Ic antiarrhythmic agents such as flecainide and propafenone, and class III agents such as sotalol and amiodarone may prevent a recurrence. If the rhythm is infrequent and there is no underlying cardiac structural disorder, a single oral dose of flecainide or a combination of diltiazem and propranolol (Inderal) during an episode of tachycardia may be effective (Mann et al., 2015).

If P waves cannot be identified, the rhythm may be called supraventricular tachycardia (SVT), or paroxysmal supraventricular tachycardia (PSVT) if it has an abrupt onset, until the underlying rhythm and resulting diagnosis is determined. SVT and PSVT indicate only that the rhythm is not VT. SVT could be atrial fibrillation, atrial flutter, or AVNRT, among others. Vagal maneuvers and adenosine may be used to convert the rhythm or at least slow conduction in the AV node to allow visualization of the P waves. If the ECG does not assist in the differentiation of the dysrhythmia, EP studies may be necessary to make the diagnosis (Mann et al., 2015) (see later discussion).

Ventricular Dysrhythmias

Ventricular dysrhythmias originate from foci within the ventricles; these may include premature ventricular complexes, VT, ventricular fibrillation, and idioventricular rhythms. Technically, ventricular asystole is characterized by an absence of rhythm formation.

Premature Ventricular Complex

A PVC is an impulse that starts in a ventricle and is conducted through the ventricles before the next normal sinus impulse. PVCs can occur in healthy people, especially with intake of caffeine, nicotine, or alcohol. PVCs may be caused by cardiac ischemia or infarction, increased workload on the heart (e.g., heart failure and tachycardia), digitalis toxicity, hypoxia, acidosis, or electrolyte imbalances, especially hypokalemia.

In a rhythm referred to as bigeminy, every other complex is a PVC. In trigeminy, every third complex is a PVC, and in quadrigeminy, every fourth complex is a PVC. PVCs have the following characteristics (see Fig. 26-15):

Ventricular and atrial rate: Depends on the underlying rhythm (e.g., sinus rhythm)
Ventricular and atrial rhythm: Irregular due to early QRS, creating one RR interval that is shorter than the others. The PP interval may be regular, indicating that the PVC did not depolarize the sinus node.

QRS shape and duration: Duration is 0.12 seconds or longer; shape is bizarre and abnormal.
P wave: Visibility of the P wave depends on the timing of the PVC; may be absent (hidden in the QRS or T wave) or in front of the QRS. If the P wave follows the QRS, the shape of the P wave may be different.
PR interval: If the P wave is in front of the QRS, the PR interval is less than 0.12 seconds.
P:QRS ratio: 0:1; 1:1

The patient may feel nothing or may say that the heart "skipped a beat." The effect of a PVC depends on its timing in the cardiac cycle and how much blood was in the ventricles when they contracted. Initial treatment is aimed at correcting the cause.

Medical Management

PVCs usually are not serious. PVCs that are frequent and persistent may be treated with amiodarone or sotalol, but long-term pharmacotherapy for only PVCs is not usually indicated. In patients with an acute MI, studies have found that PVCs are not associated with sudden cardiac death and do not warrant more aggressive therapy (Mann et al., 2015). PVCs are not considered a warning for ensuing VT. However, a recent study reported a higher frequency of PVCs preceded the development of cardiomyopathy, with an increased incidence of heart failure and increased mortality (Dukes, Dewland, Vittinghoff, et al., 2015).

Unfolding Patient Stories: Kenneth Bronson • Part 2

Recall from Chapter 23 Kenneth Bronson, who came to the Emergency Department with difficulty breathing after a week of flu-like symptoms, productive cough, and high fever. He was diagnosed with a right lower lobe pneumonia. Sinus tachycardia with occasional unifocal premature ventricular contractions (PVCs) is seen on the cardiac monitor. What are potential causes for the tachycardia and PVCs that the nurse should investigate when considering his age of 27 years, symptoms experienced over the last week, and the clinical manifestations associated with his diagnosis?

Care for Kenneth and other patients in a realistic virtual environment: *vSim for Nursing* (**thepoint.lww.com/vSimMedicalSurgical**). Practice documenting these patients' care in DocuCare (**thepoint.lww.com/DocuCareEHR**).

Figure 26-15 • Multifocal premature ventricular complexes (PVCs) in quadrigeminy in lead V₁. Note regular PP interval (P wave within PVC).

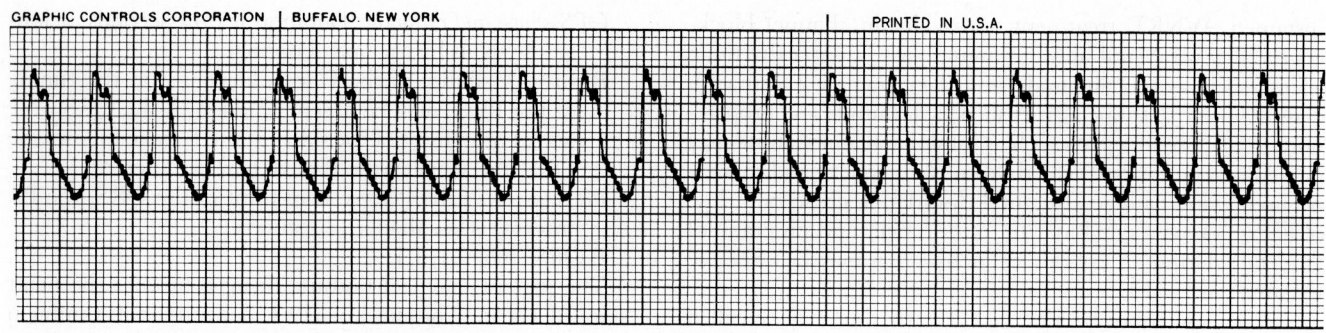

Figure 26-16 • Ventricular tachycardia in lead V₁.

 ## Ventricular Tachycardia

VT is defined as three or more PVCs in a row, occurring at a rate exceeding 100 bpm. The causes are similar to those of PVC. Patients with larger MIs and lower ejection fractions are at higher risk of lethal VT. VT is an emergency because the patient is nearly always unresponsive and pulseless. VT has the following characteristics (see Fig. 26-16):

Ventricular and atrial rate: Ventricular rate is 100 to 200 bpm; atrial rate depends on the underlying rhythm (e.g., sinus rhythm).

Ventricular and atrial rhythm: Usually regular; atrial rhythm may also be regular.

QRS shape and duration: Duration is 0.12 seconds or more; bizarre, abnormal shape.

P wave: Very difficult to detect, so the atrial rate and rhythm may be indeterminable.

PR interval: Very irregular, if P waves are seen

P:QRS ratio: Difficult to determine, but if P waves are apparent, there are usually more QRS complexes than P waves.

The patient's tolerance or lack of tolerance for this rapid rhythm depends on the ventricular rate and severity of ventricular dysfunction. However, hemodynamic stability does not predict mortality risk (Mann et al., 2015).

Medical Management

Several factors determine the initial treatment, including the following: identifying the rhythm as monomorphic (having a consistent QRS shape and rate) or polymorphic (having varying QRS shapes and rhythms), determining the existence of a prolonged QT interval before the initiation of VT, any comorbidities, and ascertaining the patient's heart function (normal or decreased). If the patient is stable, continuing the assessment, especially obtaining a 12-lead ECG, may be the only action necessary.

However, the patient may need antiarrhythmic medications, antitachycardia pacing, or direct cardioversion or defibrillation. Procainamide may be used for monomorphic stable VT in patients who do not have acute MI or severe HF (Link et al., 2015). IV amiodarone is the medication of choice for a patient with impaired cardiac function or acute MI. Sotalol may also be considered for stable monomorphic VT. Although lidocaine had been the medication most commonly used for immediate, short-term therapy, especially for patients with impaired cardiac function, it has no proven short- or long-term efficacy in cardiac arrest (Link et al., 2015).

Cardioversion is the treatment of choice for monophasic VT in a symptomatic patient. Defibrillation is the treatment of choice for pulseless VT. Any type of VT in a patient who is unconscious and without a pulse is treated in the same manner as ventricular fibrillation: immediate defibrillation is the action of choice (see later discussion on Cardioversion and Defibrillation).

For long-term management, patients with an ejection fraction less than 35% should be considered for an implantable cardioverter defibrillator (ICD) (see later discussion). Those with an ejection fraction greater than 35% may be managed with amiodarone. A small percentage of patients with VT have structurally normal hearts and respond well to medications and catheter ablation, and they have an excellent prognosis (Russo, Stainback, Bailey, et al., 2013). If the ventricular rate is above 200 bpm, then the presence of an accessory pathway should be suspected. If the ventricular rhythm is irregular, atrial fibrillation should be suspected and treated appropriately (Mann et al., 2015).

Torsades de pointes is a polymorphic VT preceded by a prolonged QT interval, which could be congenital or acquired. Common causes include central nervous system disease; certain medications (e.g., ciprofloxacin [Cipro], erythromycin [Zmax, Zithromax, Biaxin], haloperidol [Haldol], lithium (Eskalith, Lithobid), methadone [Dolophine, Methadose]); or low levels of potassium, calcium, or magnesium. Congenital QT prolongation is another cause. Because this rhythm is likely to cause the patient to deteriorate and become pulseless, immediate treatment is required and includes correction of any electrolyte imbalance, such as administration of IV magnesium, and with IV isoproterenol (Isuprel) or pacing if associated with bradycardia (Link et al., 2015).

 ## Ventricular Fibrillation

The most common dysrhythmia in patients with cardiac arrest is ventricular fibrillation, which is a rapid, disorganized ventricular rhythm that causes ineffective quivering of the ventricles. No atrial activity is seen on the ECG. The most common cause of ventricular fibrillation is coronary artery disease and resulting acute MI. Other causes include untreated or unsuccessfully treated VT, cardiomyopathy, valvular heart disease, several proarrhythmic medications, acid–base and electrolyte abnormalities, and electrical shock. Another cause is Brugada syndrome, in which the patient (frequently of Asian descent) has a structurally normal heart, few or no

Figure 26-17 • Ventricular fibrillation in lead II.

risk factors for coronary artery disease, and a family history of sudden cardiac death (Aizawa, Takatsuki, Sano, et al., 2013; Tokioka, Kusano, Morita, et al., 2014). Ventricular fibrillation has the following characteristics (see Fig. 26-17):

Ventricular rate: Greater than 300 bpm

Ventricular rhythm: Extremely irregular, without a specific pattern

QRS shape and duration: Irregular, undulating waves with changing amplitudes. There are no recognizable QRS complexes

Medical Management

Ventricular fibrillation is always characterized by the absence of an audible heartbeat, a palpable pulse, and respirations. Because there is no coordinated cardiac activity, cardiac arrest and death are imminent if the dysrhythmia is not corrected. Early defibrillation is critical to survival, with administration of immediate bystander cardiopulmonary resuscitation (CPR) until defibrillation is available. For refractory ventricular fibrillation, administration of amiodarone and epinephrine may facilitate the return of a spontaneous pulse after defibrillation (Link et al., 2015) (see Chapter 29 for further discussion on interventions during Cardiac Arrest).

Idioventricular Rhythm

Idioventricular rhythm, also called *ventricular escape rhythm,* occurs when the impulse starts in the conduction system below the AV node. When the sinus node fails to create an impulse (e.g., from increased vagal tone) or when the impulse is created but cannot be conducted through the AV node (e.g., due to complete AV block), the Purkinje fibers automatically discharge an impulse. When idioventricular rhythm is not caused by AV block, it has the following characteristics (see Fig. 26-18):

Ventricular rate: Between 20 and 40 bpm; if the rate exceeds 40 bpm, the rhythm is known as accelerated idioventricular rhythm.

Ventricular rhythm: Regular

QRS shape and duration: Bizarre, abnormal shape; duration is 0.12 seconds or more.

Medical Management

Idioventricular rhythm commonly causes the patient to lose consciousness and experience other signs and symptoms of reduced cardiac output. In such cases, the treatment is the same as for asystole and pulseless electrical activity (PEA) (see Chapter 29) if the patient is in cardiac arrest or for bradycardia if the patient is not in cardiac arrest. Interventions include identifying the underlying cause; administering IV epinephrine, atropine, and vasopressor medications; and initiating emergency transcutaneous pacing. In some cases, idioventricular rhythm may cause no symptoms of reduced cardiac output.

Ventricular Asystole

Commonly called *flatline,* ventricular asystole (see Fig. 26-19) is characterized by absent QRS complexes confirmed in two different leads, although P waves may be apparent for a short duration. There is no heartbeat, no palpable pulse, and no respiration. Without immediate treatment, ventricular asystole is fatal.

Medical Management

Ventricular asystole is treated the same as PEA, focusing on high-quality CPR with minimal interruptions and identifying underlying and contributing factors. The key to successful treatment is a rapid assessment to identify a possible cause, which is known as the Hs and Ts: hypoxia, hypovolemia,

Figure 26-18 • Idioventricular rhythm in lead V₁.

Figure 26-19 • Asystole. Always check two different leads to confirm rhythm.

hydrogen ion (acid–base imbalance), hypo- or hyperglycemia, hypo- or hyperkalemia, hyperthermia, trauma, toxins, tamponade (cardiac), tension pneumothorax, or thrombus (coronary or pulmonary) (Link et al., 2015). After the initiation of CPR, intubation and establishment of IV access are the next recommended actions, with no or minimal interruptions in chest compressions (see Chapter 29 for interventions during Cardiac Arrest).

Conduction Abnormalities

When assessing the rhythm strip, the underlying rhythm is first identified (e.g., sinus rhythm, sinus arrhythmia). Then, the PR interval is assessed for the possibility of an AV block. AV blocks occur when the conduction of the impulse through the AV nodal or bundle of His area is decreased or stopped. These blocks can be caused by medications (e.g., digitalis, calcium channel blockers, beta-blockers), Lyme disease, myocardial ischemia and infarction, valvular disorders, cardiomyopathy, endocarditis, or myocarditis (Mann et al., 2015). If the AV block is caused by increased vagal tone (e.g., long-term athletic training, sleep, coughing, suctioning, pressure above the eyes or on large vessels, anal stimulation), it is commonly accompanied by sinus bradycardia. AV block may be temporary and resolve on its own, or it may be permanent and require permanent pacing.

The clinical signs and symptoms of a heart block vary with the resulting ventricular rate and the severity of any underlying disease processes. Whereas first-degree AV block rarely causes any hemodynamic effect, the other blocks may result in decreased heart rate, causing a decrease in perfusion

to vital organs, such as the brain, heart, kidneys, lungs, and skin. A patient with third-degree AV block caused by digitalis toxicity may be stable; another patient with the same rhythm caused by acute MI may be unstable. Health care providers must always keep in mind the need to treat the patient, not the rhythm. The treatment is based on the hemodynamic effect of the rhythm.

First-Degree Atrioventricular Block

First-degree AV block occurs when all the atrial impulses are conducted through the AV node into the ventricles at a rate slower than normal. This conduction disorder has the following characteristics (see Fig. 26-20):

Ventricular and atrial rate: Depends on the underlying rhythm

Ventricular and atrial rhythm: Depends on the underlying rhythm

QRS shape and duration: Usually normal, but may be abnormal

P wave: In front of the QRS complex; shows sinus rhythm, regular shape

PR interval: Greater than 0.20 seconds; PR interval measurement is constant.

P:QRS ratio: 1:1

Second-Degree Atrioventricular Block, Type I (Wenckebach)

Second-degree AV block, type I, occurs when there is a repeating pattern in which all but one of a series of atrial impulses are conducted through the AV node into the ventricles

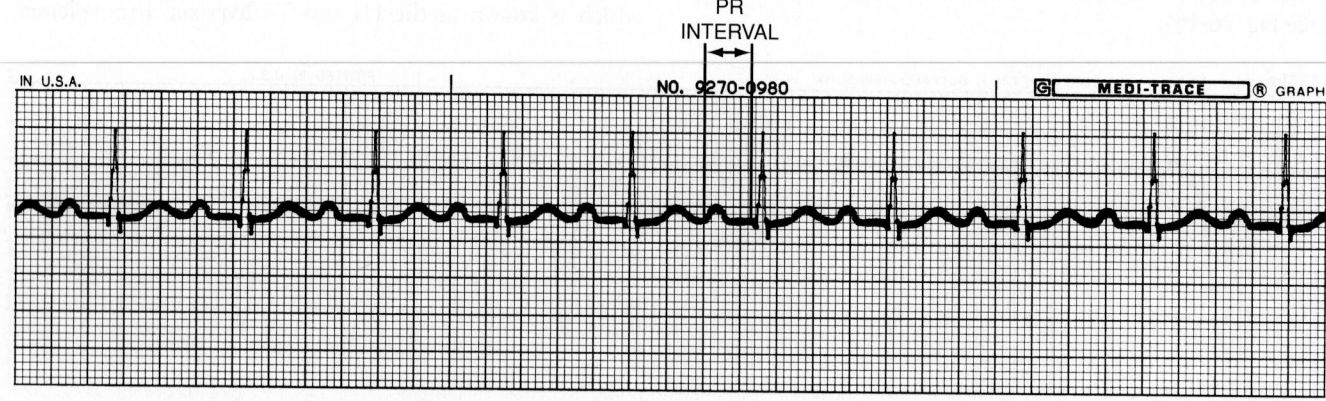

Figure 26-20 • Sinus rhythm with first-degree atrioventricular block in lead II. Note that PR is constant but greater than 0.20 seconds.

Figure 26-21 • Sinus rhythm with second-degree atrioventricular block, type I, in lead II. Note progressively longer PR durations until there is a nonconducted P wave, indicated by the *asterisk* (*).

(e.g., every four of five atrial impulses are conducted). Each atrial impulse takes a longer time for conduction than the one before, until one impulse is fully blocked. Because the AV node is not depolarized by the blocked atrial impulse, the AV node has time to fully repolarize so that the next atrial impulse can be conducted within the shortest amount of time. Second-degree AV block, type I, has the following characteristics (see Fig. 26-21):

Ventricular and atrial rate: Depends on the underlying rhythm, but the ventricular rate is lower than the atrial rate.

Ventricular and atrial rhythm: The PP interval is regular if the patient has an underlying normal sinus rhythm; the RR interval characteristically reflects a pattern of change. Starting from the RR that is the longest, the RR interval gradually shortens until there is another long RR interval.

QRS shape and duration: Usually normal, but may be abnormal

P wave: In front of the QRS complex; shape depends on underlying rhythm.

PR interval: The PR interval becomes longer with each succeeding ECG complex until there is a P wave not followed by a QRS. The changes in the PR interval are repeated between each "dropped" QRS, creating a pattern in the irregular PR interval measurements.

P:QRS ratio: 3:2, 4:3, 5:4, and so forth

Second-Degree Atrioventricular Block, Type II

Second-degree AV block, type II, occurs when only some of the atrial impulses are conducted through the AV node into the ventricles. Second-degree AV block, type II, has the following characteristics (see Fig. 26-22):

Ventricular and atrial rate: Depends on the underlying rhythm, but the ventricular rate is lower than the atrial rate.

Ventricular and atrial rhythm: The PP interval is regular if the patient has an underlying normal sinus rhythm. The RR interval is usually regular but may be irregular, depending on the P:QRS ratio.

QRS shape and duration: Usually abnormal, but may be normal

P wave: In front of the QRS complex; shape depends on underlying rhythm.

Figure 26-22 • Sinus rhythm with second-degree atrioventricular block, type II, in lead V₁. Note constant PR interval and presence of more P waves than QRS complexes.

Regular PP intervals   Regular RR intervals

PR   PR   PR   ★ = P-wave hidden in the t-wave

Figure 26-23 • Sinus rhythm with third-degree atrioventricular block and idioventricular rhythm in lead V₁. Note irregular PR intervals.

PR interval: The PR interval is constant for those P waves just before QRS complexes.

P:QRS ratio: 2:1, 3:1, 4:1, 5:1, and so forth

Third-Degree Atrioventricular Block

Third-degree AV block occurs when no atrial impulse is conducted through the AV node into the ventricles. In third-degree AV block, two impulses stimulate the heart: one stimulates the ventricles, represented by the QRS complex, and one stimulates the atria, represented by the P wave. P waves may be seen, but the atrial electrical activity is not conducted down into the ventricles to cause the QRS complex, the ventricular electrical activity. Having two impulses stimulate the heart results in a condition referred to as AV dissociation, which may also occur during VT. Complete block (third-degree AV block) has the following characteristics (see Fig. 26-23):

Ventricular and atrial rate: Depends on the escape rhythm (idionodal or idioventricular) and underlying atrial rhythm, but the ventricular rate is lower than the atrial rate.

Ventricular and atrial rhythm: The PP interval is regular and the RR interval is regular, but the PP interval is not equal to the RR interval.

QRS shape and duration: Depends on the escape rhythm; with junctional rhythm, QRS shape and duration are usually normal; with idioventricular rhythm, QRS shape and duration are usually abnormal.

P wave: Depends on underlying rhythm

PR interval: Very irregular

P:QRS ratio: More P waves than QRS complexes

Medical Management of Conduction Abnormalities

Based on the cause of the AV block and the stability of the patient, treatment is directed toward increasing the heart rate to maintain a normal cardiac output. If the patient is stable and has no symptoms, no treatment may be indicated or it may simply consist of decreasing or eliminating the cause (e.g., withholding the medication or treatment). If the causal medication is necessary for treating other conditions and no effective alternative is available, pacemaker implantation may be indicated. The initial treatment of choice is an IV bolus of atropine, although it is not effective in second-degree AV block, type II, or third-degree AV block. If the patient does not respond to atropine, has advanced AV block, or has had an acute MI, temporary transcutaneous pacing may be started. If the patient has no pulse, treatment is the same as for ventricular asystole (Link et al., 2015). A permanent pacemaker may be necessary if the block persists (see later discussion).

NURSING PROCESS
The Patient With a Dysrhythmia
Assessment

Major areas of assessment include possible causes of the dysrhythmia, contributing factors, and the dysrhythmia's effect on the heart's ability to pump an adequate blood volume. When cardiac output is reduced, the amount of oxygen reaching the tissues and vital organs is diminished. This diminished oxygenation produces the signs and symptoms associated with dysrhythmias. If these signs and symptoms are severe or if they occur frequently, the patient may experience significant distress and disruption of daily life.

A health history is obtained to identify any previous occurrences of decreased cardiac output, such as syncope (fainting), lightheadedness, dizziness, fatigue, chest discomfort, and palpitations. Possible causes of the dysrhythmia (e.g., heart disease, chronic obstructive pulmonary disease) need to be identified. All medications, prescribed and over-the-counter (including herbs and nutritional supplements), as well as the route of administration, are reviewed. If a patient is taking an antiarrhythmic medication, assessment for treatment adherence, side effects, adverse reactions, and potential contraindications is necessary. For example, some medications (e.g., digoxin) can cause dysrhythmias. Laboratory results are reviewed to assess levels of medications as well as factors that could contribute to the dysrhythmia (e.g., anemia). A thorough psychosocial assessment is performed to identify the possible effects of the dysrhythmia, the patient's perception and understanding of the dysrhythmia and its treatment, and whether anxiety is a significant contributing factor.

The nurse conducts a physical assessment to confirm the data obtained from the history and to observe for signs of diminished cardiac output during the dysrhythmic event, especially changes in level of consciousness. The nurse assesses the patient's skin, which may be pale and cool. Signs of fluid retention, such as neck vein distention and crackles and wheezes auscultated in the lungs, may be detected. The rate and rhythm of apical and peripheral pulses are also assessed, and any pulse deficit is noted. The nurse auscultates for extra heart sounds (especially S_3 and S_4) and for heart murmurs, measures blood pressure, and determines pulse pressures. A declining pulse pressure indicates reduced cardiac output. One assessment may not disclose significant changes in cardiac output; therefore, the nurse compares multiple assessment findings over time, especially those that occur with and without the dysrhythmia.

Diagnosis

Nursing Diagnoses

Based on the assessment data, major nursing diagnoses may include:

- Decreased cardiac output related to inadequate ventricular filling or altered heart rate
- Anxiety related to fear of the unknown outcome of altered health state
- Deficient knowledge about the dysrhythmia and its treatment

Collaborative Problems/Potential Complications

Potential complications may include the following:

- Cardiac arrest (see Chapter 29)
- Heart failure (see Chapter 29)
- Thromboembolic event, especially with atrial fibrillation (see Chapter 29)

Planning and Goals

The major goals for the patient may include eliminating or decreasing the occurrence of the dysrhythmia (by decreasing contributory factors) to maintain cardiac output; verbalizing reduction in anxiety; verbalizing an understanding about the dysrhythmia, tests used to diagnose the problem, and its treatment; and developing or maintaining self-management skills.

Nursing Interventions

Monitoring and Managing the Dysrhythmia to Maintain Cardiac Output

The nurse evaluates the patient's blood pressure, pulse rate and rhythm, rate and depth of respirations, and breath sounds on an ongoing basis to determine the dysrhythmia's hemodynamic effect. The nurse also asks the patient about possible symptoms of the dysrhythmia (e.g., episodes of lightheadedness, dizziness, or fainting) as part of the ongoing assessment. If a patient with a dysrhythmia is hospitalized, the nurse may obtain a 12-lead ECG, continuously monitor the patient, and analyze rhythm strips to track the dysrhythmia.

Control of the occurrence or the effect of the dysrhythmia, or both, is often achieved with antiarrhythmic medications. The nurse assesses and observes for the benefits and adverse effects of each medication. The nurse, in collaboration with the primary provider, also manages medication administration carefully so that a constant serum level of the medication is maintained. The nurse may also conduct a 6-minute walk test as prescribed, which is used to identify the patient's ventricular rate in response to exercise. The patient is asked to walk for 6 minutes, covering as much distance as possible (Zielińska, Bellwon, Rynkiewicz, et al., 2013). The nurse monitors the patient for symptoms. At the end, the nurse records the distance covered and the pre- and postexercise heart rate as well as the patient's response.

The nurse assesses for factors that contribute to the dysrhythmia (e.g., oxygen deficits, acid–base and electrolyte imbalances, caffeine, or nonadherence to the medication regimen). The nurse also monitors for ECG changes (e.g., widening of the QRS, prolongation of the QT interval, increased heart rate) that increase the risk of a dysrhythmic event.

Reducing Anxiety

When the patient experiences episodes of dysrhythmia, the nurse stays with the patient and provides assurance of safety and security while maintaining a calm and reassuring attitude. This assists in reducing anxiety (reducing the sympathetic response) and fosters a trusting relationship with the patient. The nurse seeks the patient's view of the events and discusses the emotional response to the dysrhythmia, encouraging verbalization of feelings and fears, providing supportive or empathetic statements, and assisting the patient to recognize feelings of anxiety, anger, or sadness. The nurse emphasizes successes with the patient to promote a sense of self-management of the dysrhythmia. For example, if a patient is experiencing episodes of dysrhythmia and a medication is given that begins to reduce the incidence of the dysrhythmia, the nurse communicates that information to the patient and explores the patient's response to this information. In addition, the nurse can help the patient develop a system to identify possible causative, influencing, and alleviating factors (e.g., keeping a diary). The nursing goal is to maximize the patient's control and to make the episode less threatening.

Promoting Home, Community-Based, and Transitional Care

Educating Patients About Self-Care. When educating patients about dysrhythmias, the nurse first assesses the patient's understanding, clarifies misinformation, and then shares needed information in terms that are understandable and in a manner that is not frightening or threatening. Research findings suggest that uncertainty about the cause of a dysrhythmia and when recurrence may occur is particularly disturbing among family members (Dalteg, Benzein, Sandgren, et al., 2014) (see Chart 26-5). The nurse clearly explains the etiology of the dysrhythmia and treatment options to the patient and family. If necessary, the nurse explains the importance of maintaining therapeutic serum levels of antiarrhythmic medications so that the patient understands why medications should be taken regularly each day and the importance of regular blood testing. If the medication has the potential to alter the heart rate, the patient should be taught how to take their pulse before each dose and to notify the primary provider if the pulse is abnormal. In addition, the relationship between a dysrhythmia and cardiac output is explained so that the patient recognizes symptoms of the dysrhythmia and the rationale for the treatment regimen. The patient and family need to be educated about measures to take to decrease the risk of recurrence of the dysrhythmia. If the patient has a potentially lethal dysrhythmia, the nurse establishes with the patient and family a plan of action to take in case of an emergency and, if appropriate, encourages a family member to obtain CPR training.

Chart 26-5

NURSING RESEARCH PROFILE

Uncertainty Among Couples With Atrial Fibrillation

Dalteg, T., Benzein, E., Sandgren, A., et al. (2014). Managing uncertainty in couples living with atrial fibrillation. *Journal of Cardiovascular Nursing, 29*(3), e1–e10.

Purpose

Atrial fibrillation is a common dysrhythmia that has many root causes and morbid consequences. Patients diagnosed with atrial fibrillation have higher rates of morbidity and mortality than the general population. Atrial fibrillation is associated with symptoms that can include palpitations, chest pain, dizziness, and dyspnea, to name a few. Furthermore, patients with atrial fibrillation report diminished quality of life. Yet, little is known about the impact atrial fibrillation has on couples and their relationship. Therefore, the purpose of this study was to explore the main concerns that couples have when they live with atrial fibrillation.

Design

Classical grounded theory was chosen to discover couples' concerns relative to a diagnosis of atrial fibrillation. This study was conducted in a hospital in the south of Sweden among couples in a relationship where one member was admitted to the hospital with atrial fibrillation. Both members of the couple had to be at least 18 years of age and agreed to participate in the research. Twelve couples agreed to participate in the

research and data collection process, which was conducted through interviews.

Findings

Participant couples living with atrial fibrillation voiced a common main concern that they lived with uncertainty. This uncertainty was grounded in not understanding what caused the atrial fibrillation and anxiety over its recurrence. Participant couples managed uncertainty through explicitly sharing their concerns with each other. They also managed uncertainty through implicitly sharing, which was conceptualized as keeping distance from each other as needed and through tacit understanding, or appreciating times when they would prefer to not talk through their feelings.

Nursing Implications

Findings from this study suggest that atrial fibrillation can have a profound effect on a couple's relationship because uncertainty becomes a part of their daily experience. Nurses can help alleviate stress experienced from uncertainty by explicitly sharing information with both members of couples confronted with a diagnosis of atrial fibrillation. Assessing their educational needs and providing them with information on the cause and rationale for treatment of atrial fibrillation can be helpful management strategies. Encouraging couples to give each other distance as needed may also be therapeutic.

The patient and family should also be educated about potential risks of the dysrhythmia and their signs and symptoms. For example, the patient with chronic atrial fibrillation should be educated about the possibility of an embolic event.

Continuing and Transitional Care. A referral for home, community-based, or transitional care usually is not necessary for the patient with a dysrhythmia unless the patient is hemodynamically unstable and has significant symptoms of decreased cardiac output. Home, community-based, or transitional care may be warranted if the patient has significant comorbidities, socioeconomic issues, or limited self-management skills that could increase the risk of nonadherence to the therapeutic regimen. A referral may also be indicated if the patient has had an electronic device implanted recently.

Evaluation

Expected patient outcomes may include:

1. Maintains cardiac output
   a. Demonstrates heart rate, blood pressure, respiratory rate, and level of consciousness within normal ranges
   b. Demonstrates no or decreased episodes of dysrhythmia
2. Experiences reduced anxiety
   a. Expresses a positive attitude about living with the dysrhythmia
   b. Expresses confidence in ability to take appropriate actions in an emergency
3. Expresses understanding of the dysrhythmia and its treatment
   a. Explains the dysrhythmia and its effects
   b. Describes the medication regimen and its rationale

   c. Explains the need to maintain a therapeutic serum level of the medication
   d. Describes a plan to eliminate or limit factors that contribute to the dysrhythmia
   e. States actions to take in the event of an emergency

ADJUNCTIVE MODALITIES AND MANAGEMENT

Dysrhythmia treatments depend on whether the disorder is acute or chronic, as well as on the cause of the dysrhythmia and its actual or potential hemodynamic effects.

Acute dysrhythmias may be treated with medications or with external electrical therapy (emergency defibrillation, cardioversion, or pacing). Many antiarrhythmic medications are used to treat atrial and ventricular tachydysrhythmias (see Table 26-1). The choice of medication depends on the specific dysrhythmia and its duration, the presence of structural heart disease (e.g., heart failure), and the patient's response to previous treatment. The nurse is responsible for monitoring and documenting the patient's responses to the medication and for ensuring that the patient has the knowledge and ability to manage the medication regimen.

If medications alone are ineffective in eliminating or decreasing the dysrhythmia, certain adjunctive mechanical therapies are available. The most common therapies are elective cardioversion and defibrillation for acute tachydysrhythmia, and implantable devices (pacemakers for bradycardias and ICDs for chronic tachydysrhythmias). Surgical treatments, although less common, are also available. The nurse is responsible for assessing the patient's understanding of and response to mechanical therapy, as well as the patient's self-management abilities. The nurse explains that the purpose of the device is to help the patient lead a life that is as active and productive as possible.

Cardioversion and Defibrillation

Cardioversion and defibrillation are used to treat tachydysrhythmias by delivering an electrical current that depolarizes a critical mass of myocardial cells. When the cells repolarize, the SA node is usually able to recapture its role as the heart's pacemaker.

Concept Mastery Alert

One major difference between cardioversion and defibrillation is the timing of the delivery of electrical current. In **cardioversion**, the delivery of the electrical current is synchronized with the patient's electrical events; in **defibrillation**, the delivery of the current is immediate and unsynchronized.

The same type of device, called a *defibrillator*, is used for both cardioversion and defibrillation. The electrical voltage required to defibrillate the heart is usually greater than that required for cardioversion and may cause more myocardial damage. Only biphasic types of defibrillators are now manufactured; these deliver an electrical charge from one paddle that then automatically redirects its charge back to the originating paddle. Because the delivery of the electrical charge varies among devices, the manufacturer's recommended dose should be followed for the first and subsequent defibrillations (Link et al., 2015)

The electrical current may be delivered externally through the skin with the use of paddles or with conductor pads. The paddles or pads may be placed on the front of the chest (see Fig. 26-24) (standard placement), or one pad may be placed on the front of the chest and the other pad placed under the patient's back just left of the spine (anteroposterior placement) (see Fig. 26-25)

Defibrillator multifunction conductor pads contain a conductive medium and are connected to the defibrillator to allow for hands-off defibrillation. This method reduces the risk of touching the patient during the procedure and increases electrical safety. Automated external defibrillators (AEDs), which are now found in many public areas, use this type of delivery for the electrical current.

Figure 26-24 • Standard paddle placement for defibrillation.

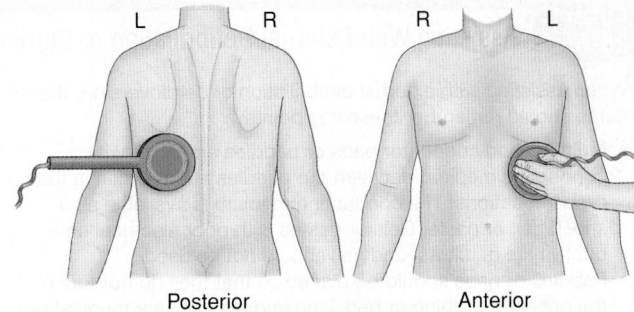

Posterior   Anterior

Figure 26-25 • Anteroposterior paddle placement for defibrillation.

► Quality and Safety Nursing Alert

When using paddles, the appropriate conductant is applied between the paddles and the patient's skin. Any other type of conductant, such as ultrasound gel, should not be substituted.

Whether using pads or paddles, the nurse must observe two safety measures. First, good contact must be maintained between the pads or paddles and the patient's skin (with a conductive medium between them) to prevent electrical current from leaking through the air (arcing) when the defibrillator is discharged. Second, no one is to be in contact with the patient or with anything that is touching the patient when the defibrillator is discharged, to minimize the chance that electrical current is conducted to anyone other than the patient. Chart 26-6 provides a review of nursing responsibility when a patient is cardioverted or defibrillated.

Electrical Cardioversion

Electrical cardioversion involves the delivery of a "timed" electrical current to terminate a tachydysrhythmia. In cardioversion, the defibrillator is set to synchronize with the ECG on a cardiac monitor so that the electrical impulse discharges during ventricular depolarization (QRS complex). The synchronization prevents the discharge from occurring during the vulnerable period of repolarization (T wave), which could result in VT or ventricular fibrillation. The ECG monitor connected to the external defibrillator usually displays a mark or line that indicates sensing of a QRS complex. Sometimes the lead and the electrodes must be changed for the monitor to recognize the patient's QRS complex. When the synchronizer is on, no electrical current is delivered if the defibrillator does not discern a QRS complex. Therefore, it is important to ensure that the patient is connected to the monitor and to select a lead (not "paddles") that has the most appropriate sensing of the QRS. Because there may be a short delay until recognition of the QRS, the discharge buttons of an external manual defibrillator must be held down until the shock has been delivered. In most monitors, the synchronization mode must be reactivated if the initial cardioversion was ineffective and another cardioversion is needed (i.e., the device defaults to unsynchronized defibrillation mode).

If the cardioversion is elective and the dysrhythmia has lasted longer than 48 hours, anticoagulation for a few weeks before cardioversion may be indicated (January et al., 2014). Digoxin is usually withheld for 48 hours before cardioversion

---

Chart 26-6 Assisting With External Defibrillation or Cardioversion

When assisting with external defibrillation or cardioversion, the nurse should remember these key points:

- Multifunction conductor pads or paddles are used, with a conducting medium between the paddles and the skin in the proper locations. The conducting medium is available as a sheet, gel, or paste. Gels or pastes with poor electrical conductivity (e.g., ultrasound gel) should not be used.
- Paddles or pads should be placed so that they do not touch the patient's clothing or bed linen and are not near medication patches or in the direct flow of oxygen.
- Women with large breasts should have the left pad or paddle placed underneath or lateral to the left breast.
- During cardioversion, the monitor leads must be attached to the patient in order to set the defibrillator to the synchronized mode ("in sync"). If defibrillating, the defibrillator must *not* be in the synchronized mode (most machines default to the "not-sync" mode).
- When using paddles, 20–25 lb of pressure must be used in order to ensure good skin contact.
- When using a manual discharge device, it must not be charged until it is ready to shock; then thumbs and fingers must be kept off the discharge buttons until paddles or pads are on the chest and ready to deliver the electrical charge.
- When it is time to defibrillate, whomever is delivering the charge should announce, "charging to (number of joules)" prior to discharging.

- "Clear!" must be called three times before discharging: As "Clear" is called the first time, the discharger must visually check that he or she is not touching the patient, bed, or equipment; as "Clear" is called the second time, the discharger must visually check that no one else is touching the bed, the patient, or equipment, including the endotracheal tube or adjuncts; and as "Clear" is called the third time, the discharger must perform a final visual check to ensure that everyone is clear of the patient and anything touching the patient.
- The delivered energy and resulting rhythm are recorded.
- Cardiopulmonary resuscitation (CPR) is immediately resumed after the defibrillation charge is delivered, if appropriate, starting with chest compressions.
- If CPR is warranted, after five cycles (about 2 minutes) of CPR, the cardiac rhythm is checked again and another shock is delivered, if warranted. A vasoactive or antiarrhythmic medication is given as soon as possible after the rhythm check to facilitate a positive response to defibrillation.
- After the event is complete, the skin under the pads or paddles is inspected for burns; if any are detected, the primary provider or a wound care nurse is consulted about appropriate treatment.
- The defibrillator is plugged back into an outlet, and supplies are restocked as needed.

Adapted from Link, M. S., Berkow, L. C., Kudenchuk, P. J., et al. (2015). Part 7: Adult advanced cardiovascular life support: 2015 American Heart Association guidelines update for cardiopulmonary resuscitation and emergency cardiovascular care. *Circulation, 132*(18 supp 2), S444–S464.

---

to ensure the resumption of sinus rhythm with normal conduction. The patient is instructed not to eat or drink for at least 4 hours before the procedure. Gel-covered paddles or conductor pads are positioned front and back (anteroposteriorly) for cardioversion. Before cardioversion, the patient receives moderate sedation IV as well as an analgesic medication or anesthesia. Respiration is then supported with supplemental oxygen delivered by a bag-valve mask device with suction equipment readily available. Although patients rarely require intubation, equipment is nearby in case it is needed. The amount of voltage used varies from 50 to 360 joules, depending on the defibrillator's technology, the type and duration of the dysrhythmia, and the size and hemodynamic status of the patient (Link et al., 2015).

Indications of a successful response are conversion to sinus rhythm, adequate peripheral pulses, and adequate blood pressure. Because of the sedation, airway patency must be maintained and the patient's state of consciousness assessed. Vital signs and oxygen saturation are monitored and recorded until the patient is stable and recovered from sedation and analgesic medications or anesthesia. ECG monitoring is required during and after cardioversion (Link et al., 2015).

Defibrillation

Defibrillation is used in emergency situations as the treatment of choice for ventricular fibrillation and pulseless VT, the most common cause of abrupt loss of cardiac function and sudden cardiac death. Defibrillation is not used for patients who are conscious or have a pulse. The energy setting for the initial and subsequent shocks using a monophasic defibrillator should be set at 360 joules (Link et al., 2015). The energy setting for the initial shock using a biphasic defibrillator may be set at 150 to 200 joules, with the same or an increasing dose with subsequent shocks (Link et al., 2015). The sooner defibrillation is used, the better the survival rate (Kronick, Kurz, Lin, et al., 2015; Link et al., 2015). Several studies have demonstrated that early defibrillation performed by lay people in a community setting can increase the survival rate (Kronick et al., 2015). If immediate CPR is provided and defibrillation is performed within 5 minutes, more adults in ventricular fibrillation may survive with intact neurologic function (Link et al., 2015). The availability and the use of AEDs in public places, especially exercise facilities, shorten the interval from collapse to rhythm recognition and defibrillation, which can significantly increase survival (Page, Husain, White, et al., 2013).

Epinephrine is given after initial unsuccessful defibrillation to make it easier to convert the dysrhythmia to a normal rhythm with the next defibrillation. This medication may also increase cerebral and coronary artery blood flow. Antiarrhythmic medications such as amiodarone, lidocaine, or magnesium may be given if ventricular dysrhythmia persists (see Table 26-1). This treatment with continuous CPR, medication administration, and defibrillation continues until a stable rhythm resumes or until it is determined that the patient cannot be revived.

Electrophysiology Studies

An EP study is an invasive procedure used to evaluate and treat various chronic dysrhythmias that have caused cardiac arrest or significant symptoms. It also is indicated for patients with symptoms that suggest a dysrhythmia that has gone undetected and undiagnosed by other methods. Because an EP study is invasive, it is performed in the hospital and may require that the patient be admitted. An EP study is used to do the following:

- Identify the impulse formation and propagation through the cardiac electrical conduction system
- Assess the function or dysfunction of the SA and AV nodal areas
- Identify the location (called *mapping*) and mechanism of the dysrhythmogenic foci (the exact site where the dysrhythmia originates)
- Assess the effectiveness of antiarrhythmic medications and devices for the patient with a dysrhythmia
- Treat certain dysrhythmias through the destruction of the causative cells (ablation)

An EP procedure is a type of cardiac catheterization that is performed in a specially equipped cardiac catheterization laboratory by an electrophysiologist, who is a cardiologist with specialized training, assisted by other EP laboratory personnel. The patient is conscious but lightly sedated. Usually, a catheter with multiple electrodes is inserted through a small incision in the femoral vein, threaded through the inferior vena cava, and advanced into the heart; however, depending on the type of study and the information needed, a second catheter may be inserted into the femoral artery. The electrodes are positioned within the heart at specific locations—for instance, in the right atrium near the sinus node, in the coronary sinus, near the tricuspid valve, and at the apex of the right ventricle. The number and placement of electrodes depend on the type of study being conducted. These electrodes allow the electrical signal to be recorded from within the heart (intracardiogram).

The electrodes also allow the clinician to introduce a pacing stimulus to the intracardiac area at a precisely timed interval and rate, thereby stimulating the area (programmed stimulation). An area of the heart may be paced at a rate much faster than the normal rate of **automaticity**, the rate at which impulses are spontaneously formed (e.g., in the sinus node). This allows the pacemaker to become an artificial focus of automaticity and to assume control (overdrive suppression). Then, the pacemaker is stopped suddenly, and the time it takes for the sinus node to resume control is assessed. A prolonged time indicates dysfunction of the sinus node.

One of the main purposes of programmed stimulation is to assess the ability of the area surrounding the electrode to cause a reentry dysrhythmia. One or a series of premature impulses is delivered to an area in an attempt to cause the tachydysrhythmia. Because the precise location of the suspected area and the specific timing of the pacing needed are unknown, the electrophysiologist uses many different techniques to cause the dysrhythmia during the study. If the dysrhythmia can be reproduced by programmed stimulation, it is called *inducible*. Once a dysrhythmia is induced, a treatment plan is determined and implemented. If, on the follow-up EP study, the tachydysrhythmia cannot be induced, then the treatment is determined to be effective. Different medications may be given and combined with electrical devices (pacemaker, ICD) to determine the most effective treatment to suppress the dysrhythmia.

Patient care, patient education, and associated complications of an EP study are similar to those associated with cardiac catheterization (see Chapter 25). The study is usually about 2 hours in length; however, if the electrophysiologist conducts not only a diagnostic procedure but also treatment, the study can take up to 6 hours. During the procedure, patients benefit from a calm, reassuring approach.

Patients who are to undergo an EP study may be anxious about the procedure and its outcome. A detailed discussion involving the patient, the family, and the electrophysiologist usually occurs to ensure that the patient can give informed consent and to reduce the patient's anxiety about the procedure. Before the procedure, the patient should receive instructions about the procedure and its usual duration, the environment where the procedure is performed, and what to expect. Although an EP study is not painful, it does cause discomfort and can be tiring. It may also cause feelings that were experienced when the dysrhythmia occurred in the past. In addition, patients are educated about what will be expected of them (e.g., lying very still during the procedure, reporting symptoms or concerns).

The patient should also know that the dysrhythmia may occur during the procedure. It often stops on its own; if it does not, treatment is given to restore the patient's normal rhythm. The dysrhythmia may have to be terminated using cardioversion or defibrillation, but this is performed under more controlled circumstances than if performed in an emergency.

Postprocedural care is similar to that for cardiac catheterization, including restriction of activity to promote hemostasis at the insertion site (see Chapter 25). To identify any complications and to ensure healing, the patient's vital signs and the appearance of the insertion site are assessed frequently. Because an artery is not always used, there is a lower incidence of vascular complications than with other catheterization procedures. Cardiac arrest may occur, but the incidence is low (less than 1%) (Mann et al., 2015).

Pacemaker Therapy

A pacemaker is an electronic device that provides electrical stimuli to the heart muscle. Pacemakers are usually used when a patient has a permanent or temporary slower-than-normal impulse formation, or a symptomatic AV or ventricular conduction disturbance. They may also be used to control some tachydysrhythmias that do not respond to medication. Biventricular (both ventricles) pacing, also called **cardiac resynchronization therapy (CRT)**, may be used to treat advanced heart failure. Pacemaker technology also may be used in an ICD (e.g., in patients with coronary artery disease and a reduced ejection fraction). (See Chapter 29 for further discussion of heart failure.)

Pacemakers can be permanent or temporary. Temporary pacemakers are used to support patients until they improve or receive a permanent pacemaker (e.g., after acute MI or during open heart surgery). Temporary pacemakers are used only in hospital settings.

Pacemaker Design and Types

Pacemakers consist of two components: an electronic pulse generator and pacemaker electrodes, which are located on leads or wires. The generator contains the circuitry and batteries that determine the rate (measured in beats per minute) and the strength or output (measured in milliamperes [mA]) of the electrical stimulus delivered to the heart. The generator also has circuitry that can detect the intracardiac electrical activity to cause an appropriate response; this component of pacing is called *sensitivity* and is measured in millivolts (mV). Sensitivity is set at the level that the intracardiac electrical activity must exceed to be sensed by the device. Leads, which carry the impulse created by the generator to the heart, can be threaded by fluoroscopy through a major vein into the heart, usually the right atrium and ventricle (endocardial leads), or they can be lightly sutured onto the outside of the heart and brought through the chest wall during open heart surgery (epicardial wires). The epicardial wires are always temporary and are removed by a gentle tug a few days after surgery. The endocardial leads may be temporarily placed with catheters through a vein (usually the femoral, subclavian, or internal jugular vein [transvenous wires]), usually guided by fluoroscopy. The leads may also be part of a specialized pulmonary artery catheter (see Chapter 25). However, obtaining a pulmonary artery wedge pressure may cause the leads to move out of pacing position. The endocardial and epicardial wires are connected to a temporary generator, which is about the size of a small paperback book. The energy source for a temporary generator is a common household battery. Monitoring for pacemaker malfunctioning and battery failure is a nursing responsibility.

The endocardial leads also may be placed permanently, passed into the heart through the subclavian, axillary, or cephalic vein, and connected to a permanent generator. Most current leads have a fixation mechanism (e.g., a screw) at the end of the lead that allows precise positioning and avoidance of dislodgement. The permanent generator, which often weighs less than 1 oz and is the size of a large book of matches, is usually implanted in a subcutaneous pocket created in the pectoral region, below the clavicle, or behind the breast, especially in young women (see Fig. 26-26). This procedure usually

takes about 1 hour, and it is performed in a cardiac catheterization laboratory using a local anesthetic and moderate sedation. Close monitoring of the respiratory status is needed until the patient is fully awake.

Permanent pacemaker generators are insulated to protect against body moisture and warmth and have filters that protect them from electrical interference from most household devices, motors, and appliances. Lithium cells are most commonly used; they last approximately 6 to 12 years, depending on the type of pacemaker, how it is programmed, and how often it is used. Most pacemakers have an **elective replacement indicator (ERI)**, which is a signal that indicates when the battery is approaching depletion. The pacemaker continues to function for several months after the appearance of ERI to ensure that there is adequate time for a battery replacement. Although some batteries are rechargeable, most are not. Because the battery is permanently sealed in the pacemaker, the entire generator must be replaced. To replace a failing generator, the leads are disconnected, the old generator is removed, and a new generator is reconnected to the existing leads and reimplanted in the already existing subcutaneous pocket. Sometimes the leads are also replaced. Battery replacement is usually performed using a local anesthetic. Hospitalization is necessary for implantation or battery replacement; the patient usually can be discharged that day or the next day.

If a patient suddenly develops a bradycardia, is symptomatic but has a pulse, and is unresponsive to atropine, emergency pacing may be started with transcutaneous pacing, which most defibrillators are now equipped to perform. Some AEDs are able to do both defibrillation and transcutaneous pacing. Large pacing ECG electrodes (sometimes the same conductive pads used for cardioversion and defibrillation) are placed on the patient's chest and back. The electrodes are connected to the defibrillator, which is the temporary pacemaker generator (see Fig. 26-27). Because the impulse must travel through the patient's skin and tissue before reaching the heart, transcutaneous pacing can cause significant discomfort (burning sensation and involuntary muscle contraction) and is intended to be used only in emergencies for short periods of time. This type of pacing necessitates hospitalization. If the

Pacemaker lead enters external jugular vein

Pacemaker lead tunneled subcutaneously between pacemaker and external jugular vein

Pacemaker generator placed beneath skin in pectoral region

Tip of lead (electrode) lodged in apex of right ventricle

Figure 26-26 • Implanted transvenous pacing lead (with electrode) and pacemaker generator.

Figure 26-27 • Transcutaneous pacemaker with electrode pads connected to the anterior and posterior chest walls.

patient is alert, sedation and analgesia may be given. After transcutaneous pacing, the skin under the electrode should be inspected for erythema and burns. Transcutaneous pacing is not indicated for pulseless bradycardia (Link et al., 2015).

Pacemaker Generator Functions

Because of the sophistication and wide use of pacemakers, a universal code has been adopted to provide a means of safe communication about their function. The coding is referred to as the NASPE-BPEG code because it is sanctioned by the North American Society of Pacing and Electrophysiology and the British Pacing and Electrophysiology Group. The complete code consists of five letters; the fourth and fifth letters are used only with permanent pacemakers (Bernstein, Daubert, Fletcher, et al., 2002; Tracy, Epstein, Darbar, et al., 2012) (see Chart 26-7).

The pacemaker paces the atrium and then the ventricle when no ventricular activity is sensed for a period of time (the time is individually programmed into the pacemaker for each patient). A straight vertical line usually can be seen on the ECG when pacing is initiated. The line that represents pacing is called a *pacemaker spike*. The appropriate ECG complex should immediately follow the pacing spike; therefore, a P wave should follow an atrial pacing spike and a QRS complex should follow a ventricular pacing spike. Because the impulse starts in a different place than the patient's normal rhythm, the QRS complex or P wave that responds to pacing looks different from the patient's normal ECG complex. *Capture* is a term used to denote that the appropriate complex followed the pacing spike.

The type of pacemaker generator and the settings selected depend on the patient's dysrhythmia, underlying cardiac function, and age. Pacemakers are generally set to sense and respond to intrinsic activity, which is called *on-demand pacing* (see Fig. 26-28). If the pacemaker is set to pace but not to sense, it is called a *fixed* or *asynchronous pacemaker* (see Fig. 26-29); this is written in pacing code as AOO or VOO. The pacemaker paces at a constant rate, independent of the patient's intrinsic rhythm. VOO pacing may indicate battery failure.

VVI (V, paces the ventricle; V, senses ventricular activity; I, paces only if the ventricles do not depolarize) pacing causes loss of AV synchrony and atrial kick, which may cause a decrease in cardiac output and an increase in atrial distention and venous congestion. Pacemaker syndrome, causing symptoms such as chest discomfort, shortness of breath, fatigue, activity intolerance, and postural hypotension, is most common with VVI pacing (Tracy et al., 2012). Atrial pacing and dual-chamber (right atrial and right ventricular) pacing have been found to reduce the incidence of atrial fibrillation, ventricular dysfunction, and heart failure (Tracy et al., 2012).

Single-chamber atrial pacing (AAI) or dual-chamber pacing (DDD) is recommended over VVI in patients with sinus node dysfunction (formerly called *sick sinus syndrome*), the most common cause of bradycardias requiring a pacemaker, and a functioning AV node (Tracy et al., 2012). AAI pacing ensures synchrony between atrial and ventricular stimulation (and therefore contraction), as long as the patient has no conduction disturbances in the AV node. Dual-chamber pacemakers are recommended as the treatment for patients with AV conduction disturbances (Tracy et al., 2012).

Chart 26-7	**North American Society of Pacing and Electrophysiology and the British Pacing and Electrophysiology Group Code (NASPE-BPEG Code) for Pacemaker Generator Function**

- The first letter of the code identifies the chamber or chambers being paced (i.e., the chamber containing a pacing electrode). The letter characters for this code are A (atrium), V (ventricle), or D (dual, meaning both A and V).
- The second letter identifies the chamber or chambers being sensed by the pacemaker generator. Information from the electrode within the chamber is sent to the generator for interpretation and action by the generator. The letter characters are A (atrium), V (ventricle), D (dual), and O (indicating that the sensing function is turned off).
- The third letter of the code describes the type of response that will be made by the pacemaker to what is sensed. The letter characters used to describe this response are I (inhibited), T (triggered), D (dual—inhibited and triggered), and O (none). Inhibited response means that the response of the pacemaker is controlled by the activity of the patient's heart—that is, when the patient's heart beats, the pacemaker does not function, but when the heart does not beat, the pacemaker does function. In contrast, a triggered response means that the pacemaker responds (paces the heart) when it senses intrinsic heart activity.
- The fourth letter of the code is related to a permanent generator's ability to vary the heart rate. This ability is available in most current pacemakers. The possible letters are O, indicating no

rate responsiveness, or R, indicating that the generator has rate modulation (i.e., the pacemaker has the ability to automatically adjust the pacing rate from moment to moment based on parameters, such as QT interval, physical activity, acid–base changes, body temperature, rate and depth of respirations, or oxygen saturation). A pacemaker with rate-responsive ability is capable of improving cardiac output during times of increased cardiac demand, such as exercise and decreasing the incidence of atrial fibrillation. All contemporary pacemakers have some type of sensor system that enables them to provide rate-adaptive pacing.

- The fifth letter of the code has two different indications: (1) that the permanent generator has multisite pacing capability with the letters A (atrium), V (ventricle), D (dual), and O (none); or (2) that the pacemaker has an antitachycardia function.
- Commonly, only the first three letters are used for a pacing code. An example of an NASPE-BPEG code is DVI:
  - **D:** Both the atrium and the ventricle have a pacing electrode in place.
  - **V:** The pacemaker is sensing the activity of the ventricle only.
  - **I:** The pacemaker's stimulating effect is inhibited by ventricular activity—in other words, it does not create an impulse when the pacemaker senses that the patient's ventricle is active.

Adapted from Bernstein, A. D., Daubert, J-C., Fletcher, R. D., et al. (2002). The revised NASPE/BPEG generic code for antibradycardia, adaptive-rate, and multisite pacing. *Journal of Pacing and Clinical Electrophysiology, 25*(2), 260–264; Gillis, A. M., Russo, A. M., Ellenbogen, K.A., et al. (2012). HRS/ACCF expert consensus statement on pacemaker device and mode selection. *Journal of American College of Cardiology, 60*(7), 682–703.

Figure 26-28 • Pacing with appropriate sensing (on-demand pacing) in lead V₁. *Arrows* denote pacing spike. *Asterisk* (*) denotes intrinsic (patient's own) beats; therefore, no pacing. F denotes a fusion beat, which is a combination of an intrinsic beat and a paced beat occurring at the same time.

Synchronized biventricular pacing, also called *cardiac resynchronization therapy (CRT)*, has been found to modify the intraventricular, interventricular, and AV conduction defects identified with symptomatic moderate to severe left ventricular dysfunction and heart failure (New York Heart Association [NYHA] functional classes III and IV) (Cooper, 2015) (see Table 29-1 in Chapter 29). CRT has also been implemented in patients with heart failure and atrial fibrillation and is associated with improved mortality rates (Gasparini, Leclercq, Lunati, et al., 2013). The generator for biventricular pacing has three leads: one for the right atrium; one for the right ventricle, as with most standard pacemaker generators; and one for the left ventricle, usually placed in the left lateral wall. This therapy improves cardiac function, resulting in decreased heart failure symptoms and an improved quality of life. Biventricular pacing may be used with an ICD.

Complications of Pacemaker Use

Complications associated with pacemakers relate to their presence within the body and improper functioning (see Chart 26-8). In the initial hours after a temporary or permanent pacemaker is inserted, the most common complication is dislodgment of the pacing electrode. Minimizing patient activity can help prevent this complication. If a temporary electrode is in place, the extremity through which the catheter has been advanced is immobilized. With a permanent pacemaker, the patient is instructed initially to restrict activity on the side of the implantation.

The ECG is monitored very carefully to detect pacemaker malfunction. Improper pacemaker function, which can arise from failure in one or more components of the pacing system, is outlined in Table 26-2. The following data should be noted on the patient's record: model of pacemaker, type of generator, date and time of insertion, location of pulse generator, stimulation threshold, and pacer settings (e.g., rate, energy output [mA], sensitivity [mV], and duration of interval between atrial and ventricular impulses [AV delay]). This information is important for identifying normal pacemaker function and diagnosing pacemaker malfunction.

A patient experiencing pacemaker malfunction may develop bradycardia as well as signs and symptoms of decreased cardiac output (e.g., diaphoresis, postural hypotension, syncope). The degree to which these symptoms become apparent depends on the severity of the malfunction, the patient's level of dependency on the pacemaker, and the patient's underlying condition. Pacemaker malfunction is diagnosed by analyzing the ECG. Manipulating the electrodes, changing the generator's settings, or replacing the pacemaker generator or leads (or both) may be necessary.

Inhibition of permanent pacemakers or reversion to asynchronous fixed rate pacing can occur with exposure to strong electromagnetic fields (electromagnetic interference [EMI]). However, recent pacemaker technology allows patients to safely

Figure 26-29 • Fixed pacing or total loss of sensing pacing in lead V₁. *Arrows* denote pacing spikes.

Chart 26-8 Potential Complications from Insertion of a Pacemaker

- Local infection at the entry site of the leads for temporary pacing, or at the subcutaneous site for permanent generator placement. Prophylactic antibiotic and antibiotic irrigation of the subcutaneous pocket prior to generator placement has decreased the rate of infection to a minimal rate.
- Pneumothorax; the use of sheaths marketed as "safe" reduces this risk.
- Bleeding and hematoma at the lead entry sites for temporary pacing, or at the subcutaneous site for permanent generator placement. This usually can be managed with cold compresses and discontinuation of antiplatelet and antithrombotic medications.
- Hemothorax from puncture of the subclavian vein or internal mammary artery.
- Ventricular ectopy and tachycardia from irritation of the ventricular wall by the endocardial electrode.

- Movement or dislocation of the lead placed transvenously (perforation of the myocardium).
- Phrenic nerve, diaphragmatic (hiccuping may be a sign), or skeletal muscle stimulation if the lead is dislocated or if the delivered energy (mA) is set high. The occurrence of this complication is avoided by testing during device implantation.
- Cardiac perforation resulting in pericardial effusion and, rarely, cardiac tamponade, which may occur at the time of implantation or months later. This condition can be recognized by the change in QRS complex morphology, diaphragmatic stimulation, or hemodynamic instability.
- Twiddler syndrome may occur when the patient manipulates the generator, causing lead dislodgement or fracture of the lead.
- Pacemaker syndrome (hemodynamic instability caused by ventricular pacing and the loss of AV synchrony).

Adapted from Link, M. S., Berkow, L. C., Kudenchuk, P. J., et al. (2015). Part 7: Adult advanced cardiovascular life support: 2015 American Heart Association guidelines update for cardiopulmonary resuscitation and emergency cardiovascular care. *Circulation, 132*(18 supp. 2), S444–S464; Tracy, C. M., Epstein, A. E., Darbar, D., et al. (2012). ACCF/AHA/HRS focused update of the 2008 guidelines for device-based therapy of cardiac rhythm abnormalities: A report of the American College of Cardiology Foundation/American Heart Association Task Force on Practice Guidelines. *Journal of the American College of Cardiology, 60*(14), 1297–1313.

use most household electronic appliances and devices (e.g., microwave ovens, electric tools). Gas-powered engines should be turned off before working on them. Objects that contain magnets (e.g., the earpiece of a phone, large stereo speakers, jewelry) should not be near the generator for longer than a few seconds. Patients are advised to place digital cellular phones at least 6 to 12 inches away from (or on the side opposite of) the pacemaker generator and not to carry them in a shirt pocket. Large electromagnetic fields, such as those produced by magnetic resonance imaging, radio and television transmitter towers

TABLE 26-2 Assessing Pacemaker Malfunction

Problem	Possible Cause	Nursing Considerations
Loss of capture—complex does *not* follow pacing spike	Inadequate stimulus Lead dislodgement Lead wire fracture Catheter malposition Battery depletion Electronic insulation break Medication change Myocardial ischemia	Check security of all connections; increase milliamperage. Reposition extremity; turn patient to left side. Change battery. Change generator.
Undersensing—pacing spike occurs at preset interval despite the patient's intrinsic rhythm	Sensitivity too high Electrical interference (e.g., by a magnet) Faulty generator	Decrease sensitivity. Eliminate interference. Replace generator.
Oversensing—loss of pacing artifact; pacing does not occur at preset interval despite the lack of intrinsic rhythm	Sensitivity too low Electrical interference Battery depletion Change in medication	Increase sensitivity. Eliminate interference. Change battery.
Loss of pacing—total absence of pacing spikes	Oversensing Battery depletion Loose or disconnected wires Perforation	Change battery. Check security of all connections. Apply magnet over permanent generator. Obtain 12-lead ECG and portable chest x-ray. Assess for murmur. Contact physician.
Change in pacing QRS shape	Septal perforation	Obtain 12-lead ECG and portable chest x-ray. Assess for murmur. Contact physician.
Rhythmic diaphragmatic or chest wall twitching or hiccuping	Output too high Myocardial wall perforation	Decrease milliamperage. Turn pacer off. Contact physician at once. Monitor closely for decreased cardiac output.

ECG, electrocardiogram.

and lines, transmission power lines (not the distribution lines that bring electricity into a home), and electrical substations may cause EMI. Patients should be cautioned to avoid such situations or to simply move farther away from the area if they experience dizziness or a feeling of rapid or irregular heartbeats (palpitations). Welding and the use of a chain saw should be avoided. If such tools are used, precautionary steps such as limiting the welding current to a 60- to 130-ampere range or using electric rather than gasoline-powered chain saws are advised.

In addition, the metal of the pacemaker generator may trigger store and library antitheft devices as well as airport and building security alarms; however, these alarm systems generally do not interfere with the pacemaker function. Patients should walk through them quickly and avoid standing in or near these devices for prolonged periods of time. The handheld screening devices used in airports may interfere with the pacemaker. Patients should be advised to ask security personnel to perform a hand search instead of using the handheld screening device. Patients also should be educated to wear or carry medical identification to alert personnel to the presence of the pacemaker.

Pacemaker Surveillance

Remote monitoring technology can now be embedded in the device that not only replaces the need for in-person follow up cardiologist visits, but it also is associated with improved survival (Varma, Piccini, Snell, et al., 2015). In addition, with the ability to obtain ECG recordings with phone applications, which can then be sent to the primary provider at the cardiology clinic, the frequency of the in-person pacemaker checks varies significantly. Transtelephonic transmission of the generator's information is a commonly utilized follow-up method. Special equipment is used to transmit information about the patient's pacemaker over the telephone to a receiving system at the cardiology clinic. The information is converted into tones; equipment at the clinic converts these tones to an electronic signal and records them on an ECG strip. The pacemaker rate and other data concerning pacemaker function (e.g., generator setting, battery status, sensing function, lead integrity, pacing data, such as number of pacing events) are obtained and evaluated by a cardiologist. This simplifies the diagnosis of a failing generator, reassures the patient, and improves management when the patient is physically remote from pacemaker testing facilities. A typical follow-up schedule is every 2 weeks during the first month, every 4 to 8 weeks for 3 years, and every 4 weeks thereafter.

Implantable Cardioverter Defibrillator

The **implantable cardioverter defibrillator (ICD)** is an electronic device that detects and terminates life-threatening episodes of tachycardia or fibrillation, especially those that are ventricular in origin. Patients at high risk of VT or ventricular fibrillation and who would benefit from an ICD are those who have survived sudden cardiac death syndrome, which usually is caused by ventricular fibrillation, or have experienced spontaneous, symptomatic VT (syncope secondary to VT) not due to a reversible cause (called a *secondary*

prevention intervention). Patients with coronary artery disease who are 40 days postacute MI with moderate to severe left ventricular dysfunction (ejection fraction less than or equal to 35%) are at risk of sudden cardiac death and therefore an ICD is indicated (called a *primary prevention intervention*) (Wilkoff, Fauchier, Stiles, et al., 2015). An ICD implantation is also recommended in patients who have been diagnosed with nonischemic dilated cardiomyopathy for at least 9 months and have functional NYHA Class II or III heart failure (Wilkoff et al., 2015) (see Table 29-1 in Chapter 29). The American College of Cardiology, American Heart Association, and Society for Critical Care Medicine, in conjunction with other key clinical societies, developed appropriate use criteria (AUC) to be used as guides for cost-effective use of ICDs, with the caveat that AUC guidelines do not supersede clinical judgment (Russo et al., 2013). Indications for the use of ICDs continue to be refined (Kusumoto, Calkins, Boehmer, et al., 2014). In particular, use of ICDs for internal defibrillation in patients with symptomatic, recurrent, medication-refractory atrial fibrillation continues to be explored (Gerstenfeld & Everett, 2014).

Because there may be a waiting period for ICD implantation, especially those postacute MI, patients who are at risk for sudden cardiac death may be prescribed a wearable vestlike automated defibrillator, which works just like an AED in that a shock is delivered less than a minute after a life-threatening rhythm is detected (Epstein, Abraham, Bianco, et al., 2013) (see Fig. 26-30). Prior to the delivery of the shock, the vest vibrates and issues an alarm to announce that a shock is imminent. The vest weighs about a pound, is worn under the patient's clothing, and is attached to a monitor with a battery that is worn in a holster or on a shoulder strap. The monitor automatically downloads information once a day, usually in the

Figure 26-30 • The wearable automatic cardioverter defibrillator vest. Courtesy of ZOLL LifeVest.

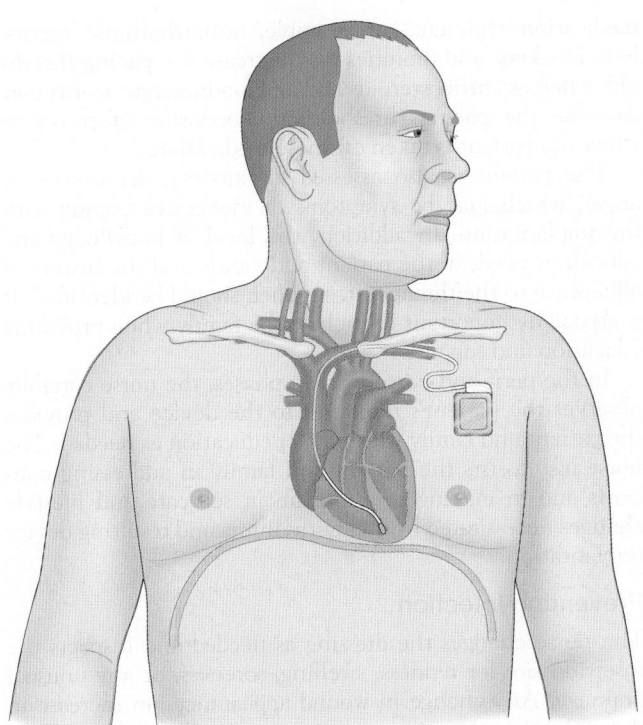

Figure 26-31 • The implantable cardioverter defibrillator consists of a generator and a sensing/pacing/defibrillating electrode.

middle of the night. The vest must be worn at all times, even if the patient is admitted to the hospital and placed on an ECG monitor, and removed only when showering or bathing. The battery needs to be changed every day. Education is provided to the patient by the device manufacturer. However, the nurse should assess the patient's understanding of the education provided and explore any issues that may prevent the patient from wearing it.

An ICD has a generator about the size of a book of matches that is implanted in a subcutaneous pocket, usually in the upper chest wall. An ICD also has at least a right ventricular lead that is implanted transvenously and can sense intrinsic electrical activity and deliver an electrical impulse. The implantation procedure, postimplantation care, and length of hospital stay are much like those for insertion of a pacemaker (see Fig. 26-31).

ICDs are designed to respond to two criteria: a rate that exceeds a predetermined level and a change in the isoelectric line segments. When a dysrhythmia occurs, rate sensors require a set duration of time to sense the dysrhythmia. Then, the device automatically charges; after a second "look" confirms the dysrhythmia, it delivers the programmed charge through the lead to the heart. The time from dysrhythmia detection to electrical discharge depends on the charging time, which depends on the programmed energy level (Mann et al., 2015). However, in an ICD that has the capability of providing atrial therapies, the device can be programmed to be activated by the patient, giving the patient time to activate the charge at a time and place of their choosing. The life of the lithium battery is about 9 years but varies depending on the use of the ICD. ICD surveillance is similar to that of the pacemaker; however, it includes stored endocardial ECGs

as well as information about the number and frequency of shocks that have been delivered.

Antiarrhythmic medication may be given with this technology to minimize the occurrence of a tachydysrhythmia and to reduce the frequency of ICD discharge.

Several types of devices are available. ICD, the generic name, is used as the abbreviation for these various devices. Each device offers a different delivery sequence, but all are capable of delivering high-energy (high-intensity) defibrillation to treat a tachycardia (atrial or ventricular). The device may deliver up to six shocks if necessary.

Some ICDs can respond with (1) antitachycardia pacing, in which the device delivers electrical impulses at a fast rate in an attempt to disrupt the tachycardia, (2) low-energy (low-intensity) cardioversion, or (3) defibrillation; others may use all three techniques. Pacing is used to terminate tachycardias caused by a conduction disturbance called *reentry*, which is repetitive restimulation of the heart by the same impulse. An impulse or a series of impulses is delivered to the heart by the device at a fast rate to collide with and stop the heart's reentry conduction impulses, and therefore to stop the tachycardia. Some ICDs also have pacemaker capability if the patient develops bradycardia, which sometimes occurs after treatment of the tachycardia. Usually, the mode is VVI. Subcutaneous ICDs are now available; the generator is implanted in a subcutaneous pocket over the fifth intercostal space and the lead is implanted subcutaneously to the left and parallel to the sternum (Burke, Gold, Knight, et al., 2015). However, this technology does not include bradycardia or anti-tachycardia pacing and so currently has limited utility (Aziz, Leon, & El-Chami, 2014).

Which device is used and how it is programmed depend on the patient's dysrhythmia(s). The device may be programmed differently for different dysrhythmias (e.g., ventricular fibrillation, VT with a fast ventricular rate, and VT with a slow ventricular rate). As with pacemakers, there is an NASPE-BPEG code for communicating the functions of the ICDs (Bernstein et al., 2002; Wilkoff et al., 2015). The first letter represents the chamber or chambers shocked (O, none; A, atrium; V, ventricle; D, both atrium and ventricle). The second letter represents the chamber that can be antitachycardia paced (O, A, V, D, meaning the same as the first letter). The third letter indicates the method used by the generator to detect a tachycardia (E, electrogram; H, hemodynamics). The last letter represents the chambers that have antibradycardia pacing (O, A, V, D, meaning the same as the first and second letters of the ICD code).

Complications of ICD implantation are similar to those associated with pacemaker insertion. The primary complication is surgery-related infection; its risk increases with battery or lead replacement. Postimplantation mortality rates are higher when the procedure is done for reasons other than generator replacement, when the patient has advanced heart failure or renal dysfunction, and when it is performed as a consequence of an emergency admission (Dodson, Reynolds, Bao, et al., 2014). A few complications are associated with the technical aspects of the equipment, like those of pacemakers, such as premature battery depletion and dislodged or fractured leads. Inappropriate delivery of ICD therapy, usually due to oversensing or atrial and sinus tachycardias with a rapid ventricular rate response, is the most frequent long-term complication. This requires reprogramming of the device.

Nursing Management

After a permanent electronic device (pacemaker or ICD) is inserted, the patient's heart rate and rhythm are monitored by ECG. The device's settings are noted and compared with the ECG recordings to assess the device's function. For example, pacemaker malfunction is detected by examining the pacemaker spike and its relationship to the surrounding ECG complexes (see Fig. 26-32). In addition, cardiac output and hemodynamic stability are assessed to identify the patient's response to pacing and the adequacy of pacing. The appearance or increasing frequency of dysrhythmia is observed and reported to the primary provider. If the patient has an ICD implanted and develops VT or ventricular fibrillation, the ECG should be recorded to note the time between the onset of the dysrhythmia and the onset of the device's shock or antitachycardia pacing.

The incision site where the generator was implanted is observed for bleeding, hematoma formation, or infection, which may be evidenced by swelling, unusual tenderness, drainage, and increased warmth. The patient may complain of continuous throbbing or pain. These symptoms are reported to the primary provider.

A chest x-ray is usually taken after the procedure and prior to discharge to document the position of leads in addition to ensuring that the procedure did not cause a pneumothorax. It is necessary to assess the function of the device throughout its lifetime and especially after changes in the patient's medication regimen. For example, antiarrhythmic agents, beta-blockers, and diuretics may increase the pacing threshold, whereas corticosteroids and alpha-adrenergic agents may decrease the pacing threshold; the opposite effect occurs when the patient is taken off these medications.

The patient is also assessed for anxiety, depression, or anger, which may be symptoms of ineffective coping with the implantation. In addition, the level of knowledge and education needs of the patient and family and the history of adherence to the therapeutic regimen should be identified. It is especially important to include the family when providing education and support.

In the peri- and postoperative phases, the nurse carefully observes the patient's responses to the device and provides the patient and family with further education as needed. The nurse also assists the patient and family in addressing concerns and in making decisions about self-care and lifestyle changes necessitated by the dysrhythmia and resulting device implantation.

Preventing Infection

The nurse changes the dressing as needed and inspects the insertion site for redness, swelling, soreness, or any unusual drainage. Any change in wound appearance, an increase in the patient's temperature, or an increase in the patient's white blood count should be reported to the primary provider.

Promoting Effective Coping

The patient treated with an electronic device experiences not only lifestyle and physical changes but also emotional changes. At different times during the healing process, the patient may

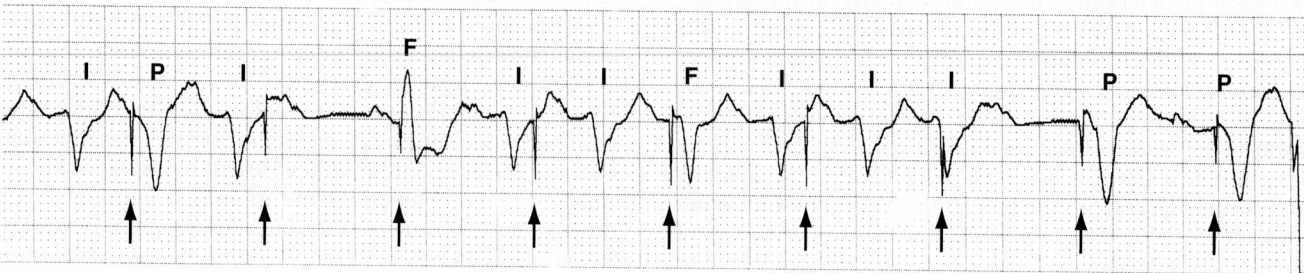

Figure 26-32 • A. Ventricular pacing in lead V₁ with intermittent loss of capture (a pacing spike not followed by a QRS complex). **B.** Ventricular pacing with loss of sensing (a pacing spike occurring at an inappropriate time). ↑, pacing spike; *, loss of capture; P, pacemaker-induced QRS complex; I, patient's intrinsic QRS complex; F, fusion (a QRS complex formed by a merging of the patient's intrinsic QRS complex and the pacemaker-induced QRS complex).

Chart 26-9 HOME CARE CHECKLIST
Educating the Patient With an Implantable Cardiac Device

At the completion of education, the patient and/or caregiver will be able to:

- State the impact of device implantation on physiologic functioning, ADLs, IADLs, self-image and roles, relationships (including sexuality), and spirituality.
- State changes in lifestyle (e.g., diet, activity, mobility/driving restrictions) necessary to maintain health.
- State the name, dose, side effects, frequency, and schedule for all medications.
- For patients with pacemakers, check pulse daily. Report *immediately* any sudden slowing or increasing of the pulse rate. This may indicate pacemaker malfunction.
- Avoid infection at the insertion site of the device:
  - Leave the incision uncovered and observe it daily for redness, increased swelling, and heat.
  - Take temperature at same time each day; report any increase.
  - Avoid wearing tight, restrictive clothing that may cause friction over the insertion site.
  - Initially avoid soaking in the tub and lotion, creams, or powders in the area of the device.
- Adhere to activity restrictions:
  - Restrict movement of arm until incision heals; do not raise arm above head for 2 weeks.
  - Avoid heavy lifting for a few weeks.
  - Discuss safety of activities (e.g., driving) with a primary provider.
  - Recognize that although it may take up to 2–3 weeks to resume normal activities, physical activity does not usually have to be curtailed, with the exception of contact sports.
- Electromagnetic interference: Understand the importance of the following:
  - Avoid large magnetic fields, such as those created by magnetic resonance imaging, large motors, arc welding, and electrical substations. Magnetic fields may deactivate the device, negating its effect on a dysrhythmia.
  - At security gates at airports, government buildings, or other secured areas, show identification card and request a hand (not handheld device) search. Obtain and carry a letter from the primary provider about this requirement.
  - Some electrical and small motor devices, as well as products that contain magnets (e.g., cellular phones), may interfere

with the functioning of the cardiac device if the electrical device is placed very close to it. Avoid leaning directly over large electrical devices or motors, or ensure that contact is of brief duration; place cellular phone on opposite side of cardiac device.
  - Household appliances (e.g., microwave ovens) should not cause any concern.
- Describe precautions and safety measures to be used:
  - Describe what to do if symptoms occur, and notify the primary provider if any discharges seem unusual.
  - Maintain a log that records discharges of an implantable cardioverter defibrillator (ICD). Record events that precipitate the sensation of shock. This provides important data for the primary provider to use in readjusting the medical regimen.
  - Encourage family members to attend a cardiopulmonary resuscitation class.
  - Call 911 for emergency assistance if feeling of dizziness occurs.
  - Wear medical identification (e.g., Medic-Alert) that includes primary provider information.
  - Avoid frightening family or friends with unexpected shocks from an ICD, which will not harm them. Inform family and friends that in the event they are in contact with the patient when a shock is delivered, they may also feel the shock. It is especially important to warn sexual partners that this may occur.
  - Carry medical identification with the primary provider's name, type and model number of the device, manufacturer's name, and hospital where device was inserted.
- Identify community resources for peer and caregiver/family support.
- Adhere to appointments for follow-up care that are scheduled to monitor the electronic performance of the cardiac device. This is especially important during the first month after implantation and near the end of the battery life. Remember to take log of ICD discharges to review with the primary provider.
- Identify the need for health promotion, disease prevention, and screening activities.

ADL, activities of daily living; IADL, independent activities of daily living, ICD, implantable cardioverter defibrillator.

---

feel angry, depressed, fearful, anxious, or a combination of these emotions. Although each patient uses individual coping strategies (e.g., humor, prayer, communication with a significant other) to manage emotional distress, some strategies may work better than others. Signs that may indicate ineffective coping include social isolation, increased or prolonged irritability or depression, and difficulty in relationships.

To promote effective coping strategies, the nurse must recognize both the patient's and family's perceptions of the situation and their resulting emotional state and assist them to explore their reactions and feelings. Because of the unpredictable and possibly painful ICD discharge, patients with ICDs are most vulnerable to feelings of helplessness, leading to depression. The nurse can help the patient identify positive methods to deal with the actual or perceived limitations and manage any lifestyle changes needed. The nurse may help the patient identify changes (e.g., loss of

ability to participate in contact sports), the emotional responses to the change (e.g., anger), and how the patient responds to that emotion (e.g., quickly becomes angry when talking with spouse). The nurse reassures the patient that these responses are normal and helps the patient identify realistic goals (e.g., develop interest in another activity) and develop a plan to attain these goals. The patient and family should be encouraged to talk about their experiences and emotions with each other and the health care team. The nurse may refer the patient and family to a hospital, community, or online support group. The nurse may also encourage the use of spiritual resources. Based on the patient's interest, the nurse also may educate the patient about easy-to-use stress reduction techniques (e.g., deep-breathing exercises, relaxation) to facilitate coping. Instructing the patient about the ICD may help the patient cope with changes that occur as a result of device implantation.

Promoting Home, Community-Based, and Transitional Care

After device insertion, the patient's hospital stay may be 1 day or less, and follow-up in an outpatient clinic, office, or device clinic is common. The patient's anxiety and feelings of vulnerability may interfere with the ability to learn information provided. The nurse needs to include caregivers in the education and provide printed materials for use by the patient and caregiver. The nurse establishes priorities for learning with the patient and caregiver. Education may include the importance of periodic device monitoring, promoting safety, surgical site care, and avoiding EMI (see Chart 26-9). In addition, the educational plan should include information about activities that are safe and those that may be dangerous. The nurse discusses with the patient and family what they have to do when a shock is delivered. The nurse may facilitate CPR training for the family.

CRITICAL THINKING EXERCISES

1 **ebp** Your aunt, who has a history of heart failure, calls to tell you that her primary provider told her that she has atrial fibrillation. She says that she has been prescribed warfarin and that she really doesn't want to take it because she knows it will stop her from clotting, and she is afraid of bleeding. What is the strength of the evidence that supports your aunt's continued adherence to warfarin therapy? What are the risks involved should she decide she will not take this drug as prescribed?

2 **pq** You answer a patient's call light on the medical/surgical unit where you work. The patient complains of a sudden onset of "palpitations" and "lightheadedness." Reviewing the bedside cardiac monitor, you see that the patient has a new onset of atrial flutter with a heart rate of 145 bpm. Prior to contacting the primary provider, what other assessment information would you obtain? What interventions do you anticipate?

3 A 35-year-old mother of two grade school-aged children who is in the middle of a contentious divorce presents to the clinic where you work. She tells you that yesterday when she got home from work, she was bending over to put laundry in the washer and she suddenly felt her "heart racing, pounding" in her chest. She also tells you that her skin was cool and clammy. She rested and eventually her symptoms resolved. What are some possible causes of these symptoms? Identify other key factors that you would want to include in your assessment to help identify the cause of the dysrhythmia. What nursing interventions are needed?

REFERENCES

*Asterisk indicates nursing research.
**Double asterisk indicates classic reference.

Book

American Society of Health System Pharmacists (2012). *AHFS drug information.* Bethesda, MD: Author.
Fuster, V., Walsh, R. A., & Harrington, R. A. (Eds.). (2011). *Hurst's the heart* (13th ed.). New York: McGraw-Hill.

Mann, D. L., Zipes, D. P., Libby, P., et al. (2015) *Braunwald's heart disease: A textbook of cardiovascular medicine* (10th ed.). Philadelphia, PA: Elsevier.

Journals and Electronic Documents

Aizawa, Y., Takatsuki, S., Sano, M., et al. (2013). Brugada syndrome behind complete right bundle-branch block. *Circulation, 128*(10), 1048–1054.
Alli, O., Asirvatham, S., & Holmes, D. R. (2015). Strategies to incorporate left atrial appendage occlusion into clinical practice. *Journal of the American College of Cardiology, 65*(21), 2337–44.
Aziz, S., Leon, A. R., & El-Chami, M. R. (2014). The subcutaneous debrillator. *Journal of American College of Cardiology, 63*(15), 1473–1479.
**Bernstein, A. D., Daubert, J-C., Fletcher, R. D., et al. (2002). The revised NASPE/BPEG generic code for antibradycardia, adaptive-rate, and multisite pacing. *Journal of Pacing and Clinical Electrophysiology, 25*(2), 260–264.
Burke M. C., Gold, M. R., Knight, B. P., et al., (2015). Safety and efficacy of the totally subcutaneous implantable defibrillator. 2-year results from a pooled analysis of the IDE study and EFFORTLESS Registry. *Journal of American College of Cardiology, 65*(16), 1605–1615.
Cooper, K. L. (2015). Biventricular pacemakers in patients with heart failure. *Critical Care Nurse, 35*(2), 20–27.
*Dalteg, T., Benzein, E., Sandgren, A., et al. (2014). Managing uncertainty in couples living with atrial fibrillation. *Journal of Cardiovascular Nursing, 29*(3), e1-e10.
Dodson, J. A., Reynolds, M. R., Bao, H., et al. (2014). Developing a risk model for in-hospital adverse events following implantable cardioverter-defibrillator implantation. A report from the NCDR, National Cardiovascular Data Registry. *Journal of American College of Cardiology, 63*(8), 788–796.
Dukes, J. W., Dewland, T. A., Vittinghoff, E., et al. (2015). Ventricular ectopy as a predictor of heart failure and death. *Journal of American College of Cardiology, 66*, 101–109.
Elrod, J. (2014). The convergent procedure: The CONVERGE IDE Clinical Trial. *EP Lab Digest, 14*(5), Retrieved on 7/10/2016 at: www.eplabdigest.com/articles/Convergent-Procedure-CONVERGE-IDE-Clinical-Trial
Epstein, A. E., Abraham, W. T., Bianco, N. R., et al. (2013). Wearable cardioverter-defibrillator use in patients perceived to be at high risk early post-myocardial infarction. *Journal of American College of Cardiology, 62*(21), 2000–2007.
Gasparini, M., Leclercq, C., Lunati, M., et al. (2013). Cardiac resynchronization therapy in patients with atrial fibrillation. The CERTIFY study (Cardiac Resynchronization Therapy in Atrial Fibrillation Patients Multinational Registry). *Journal of American College of Cardiology, 1*(6), 500–507.
Gerstenfeld, E. P., & Everett, T. H. (2014). Internal atrial defibrillation revisited. How long can we go? *Journal of American College of Cardiology, 62*(1), 49–51.
Gillis, A. M., Russo, A. M., Ellenbogen, K.A., et al. (2012). HRS/ACCF expert consensus statement on pacemaker device and mode selection. *Journal of American College of Cardiology, 60*(7), 682–703.
Hoke, L. M., & Steletsky, Y. (2015). Catheter ablations of atrial fibibrillation, *American Journal of Nursing, 115*(10), 32–43.
January, C. T., Wann, L. S., Alpert, J. S., et al. (2014). 2014 AHA/ACC/HRS guideline for the management of patients with atrial fibrillation: A report of the ACC/AHA Task Force on practice guidelines and the Heart Rhythm Society. *Circulation, 130*(23), e199–e267.
Jensen, P. N., Gronroos, N. N., Chen, L. Y., et al. (2014). Incidence of and risk factors for sick sinus syndrome in the general population. *Journal of the American College of Cardiology, 64*(6), 531–538.
Kovacs, R. J., Flaker, G. C., Saxonhouse, S. J., et al. (2015). Practical management of anticoagulation in patients with atrial fibrillation. *Journal of American College of Cardiology, 65*(13), 1340–1360.
Kronick, S. L., Kurz, M. C., Lin, S., et al. (2015). Part 4: Systems of Care and Continuous Quality Improvement: 2015 American Heart Association Guidelines Update for Cardiopulmonary Resuscitation and Emergency Cardiovascular Care. *Circulation, 132*(18), S397–S413.
Kusumoto, F. M., Calkins, H., Boehmer, J., et al. (2014). HRS/ACC/AHA expert consensus statement on the use of implantable cardioverter-defibrillator therapy in patients who are not included or not well represented in clinical trials. *Journal of American College of Cardiology, 64*(11), 1143–1177.

LaPar, D. J., Speir, A. M., Crosby, I. K., et al. (2014). Postoperative atrial fibrillation significantly increases mortality, hospital readmission, and hospital costs. *Annals of Thoracic Surgery, 98*(2), 527–533.

Larsson, S.C., Drca, N., & Wolk, A. (2014). Alcohol consumption and risk of atrial fibrillation: A prospective study and dose-response meta-analysis. *Journal of the American College of Cardiology, 64*(3), 282–289.

Link, M. S., Berkow, L. C., Kudenchuk, P. J., et al. (2015). Part 7: Adult advanced cardiovascular life support: 2015 American Heart Association guidelines update for cardiopulmonary resuscitation and emergency cardiovascular care. *Circulation, 132*(18 supp 2), S444–S464.

Masoudi, F. A., Calkins, H., Kavinsky, C. J., et al. (2015). 2015 ACC/HRS/SCAI left atrialappendage occlusion device societal overview: A professional society overview from the American College of Cardiology, Heart Rhythm Society, and the Society for Cardiovascular Angiography and Interventions. *Heart Rhythm, 12*(10), e122–e136. Retrieved on 2/28/2016 at: dx.doi.org/10.1016/j.hrthm.2015.06.034

Mozaffarian D., Benjamin E. J., Go A. S., et al. (2015). Heart disease and stroke statistics—2015update: A report from the American Heart Association. *Circulation, 131*(1), e29–e322.

Page, R. L., Husain, S., White, L. Y., et al. (2013). Cardiac arrest at exercise facilities. Implications for placement of automated external defibrillators. *Journal of American College of Cardiology, 62*(22), 2102–2109.

Patel, N. J., Deshmukh, A., Pant, S., et al. (2014) Contemporary trends of hospitalization for atrial fibrillation in the United States, 2000 through 2010: Implications for healthcare planning. *Circulation, 129*(23), 2371–2379.

Pickham, D. (2013). Understanding and documenting QT intervals. *Critical Care Nurse, 33*(4), 73–75.

Russo, A. M., Stainback, R. F., Bailey, S. R, et al. (2013). ACCF/HRS/AHA/ASE/HFSA/SCAI/SCCT/SCMR 2013 appropriate use criteria for implantable cardioverter-defibrillators and cardiac resynchronization therapy. A report of the American College of Cardiology Foundation Appropriate Use Criteria Task Force, Heart Failure Society, American Heart Association, American Society of Echocardiography, Heart Failure Society of America, Society for Cardiovascular Angiography and Interventions, Society of Cardiovascular Computed Tomography and Society for Cardiovascular Magnetic Resonance. *Journal of American College of Cardiology, 61*(12), 1318–1368.

Sandau, K. E., Sendelbach, S., Fletcher, L., et al. (2015). Computer-assisted interventions to improve QTc documentation in patients receiving QT-prolonged drugs. *American Journal of Critical Care, 24*(2), 6–14.

Sendelbach, S., & Jepsen, S. (2013). American Association of Critical Care Nurses practice alert: Alarm management. Retrieved 9/22/2015 at: www.aacn.org/wd/practice/docs/practicealerts/alarm-management-practice-alert.pdf

Sheldon, R. S., Grubb, B. P., Olshansky, B., et al. (2015). 2015 Heart Rhythm Society Expert Consensus Statement on the diagnosis and treatment of postural tachycardia syndrome, inappropriate sinus tachycardia, and vasovagal syncope. *Heart Rhythm, 12*(6), e41–e63.

Shi, X. (2016). Preventing postoperative atrial fibrillation. *Nursing Critical Care, 11*(1), 5.

Shukla, A., Aizer, A., Holmes, D., et al. (2015). Effect of obstructive sleep apnea treatment on atrial fibrillation recurrence. *JACC: Clinical Electrophysiology, 1*(1–2), 41–51.

Smith, G. D., Fry, M. M., Taylor, D., et al. (2015). Effectiveness of the valsalva manoeuvre for reversion of supraventricular tachycardia. *Cochrane Database of Systematic Reviews,* CD009502(2).

Stavrakis, S., Nakagawa, H., Po, S. S., et al. (2015). The role of the autonomic ganglia in atrial fibrillation. *JACC: Clinical Electrophysiology, 1*(1–2), 1–13.

Tokioka, K., Kusano, K. F., Morita, H., et al. (2014). Electrocardiographic parameters and fatal arrhythmic evens in patients with Brugada syndrome. *Journal of American College of Cardiology, 63*(20), 2131–2138.

Tracy, C. M., Epstein, A. E., Darbar, D., et al. (2012). ACCF/AHA/HRS focused update of the 2008 guidelines for device-based therapy of cardiac rhythm abnormalities: A report of the American College of Cardiology Foundation/American Heart Association Task Force on Practice Guidelines. *Journal of the American College of Cardiology, 60*(14), 1297–1313.

Varma, N., Piccini, J. P., Snell, J., et al. (2015). Relationship between level of adherence to automatic wireless remote monitoring and survival in pacemaker and defibrillator patients. *Journal of American College of Cardiology, 65*(24), 2601–2610.

Wilkoff, B. L., Fauchier, L., Stiles, M. K., et al. (2015). 2015 HRS/EHRA/APHRS/SOLAECE expert consensus statement on optimal implantable cardioverter-defibrillator programming and testing. *Journal of Arrhythmia, 32*(1), 1–28.

Zielińska, D., Bellwon, J., Rynkiewicz, A., et al. (2013). Prognostic value of the six-minute walk test in heart failure patients undergoing cardiac surgery: A literature review. *Rehabilitation Research and Practice,* Article ID 965494, 5 pages. doi:10.1155/2013/965494.

Resources

American Association of Critical-Care Nurses, www.aacn.org

American Association of Heart Failure Nurses (AAHFN), aahfn.org

American College of Cardiology (ACC), www.acc.org

American Heart Association, National Center, www.americanheart.org/HEARTORG/

Heart Rhythm Society, www.hrsonline.org

National Institutes of Health, National Heart, Lung, Blood Institute, Health Information Center, www.nhlbi.nih.gov

27

Management of Patients With Coronary Vascular Disorders

LEARNING OBJECTIVES

On completion of this chapter, the learner will be able to:

1 Describe the pathophysiology, clinical manifestations, and treatment of coronary atherosclerosis.
2 Discuss the pathophysiology, clinical manifestations, and treatment of angina pectoris.
3 Use the nursing process as a framework for care of patients with angina pectoris.
4 Describe the pathophysiology, clinical manifestations, and treatment of myocardial infarction.

5 Use the nursing process as a framework for care of a patient with acute coronary syndrome.
6 Describe percutaneous coronary interventional and coronary artery revascularization procedures.
7 Identify the nursing care of a patient who has had a percutaneous coronary interventional procedure for treatment of coronary artery disease.
8 Apply the nursing process as a framework for care of a patient who has undergone cardiac surgery.

GLOSSARY

acute coronary syndrome (ACS): signs and symptoms that indicate unstable angina or acute myocardial infarction
angina pectoris: chest pain brought about by myocardial ischemia
atheroma: fibrous cap composed of smooth muscle cells that forms over lipid deposits within arterial vessels and protrudes into the lumen of the vessel, narrowing the lumen and obstructing blood flow; also called plaque
atherosclerosis: abnormal accumulation of lipid deposits and fibrous tissue within arterial walls and the lumen
contractility: ability of the cardiac muscle to shorten in response to an electrical impulse
coronary artery bypass graft (CABG): a surgical procedure in which a blood vessel from another part of the body is grafted onto the occluded coronary artery below the occlusion in such a way that blood flow bypasses the blockage
high-density lipoprotein (HDL): a protein-bound lipid that transports cholesterol to the liver for excretion in the bile; composed of a higher proportion of protein to lipid than low-density lipoprotein; exerts a beneficial effect on the arterial wall
ischemia: insufficient tissue oxygenation
low-density lipoprotein (LDL): a protein-bound lipid that transports cholesterol to tissues in the body;

composed of a lower proportion of protein to lipid than high-density lipoprotein; exerts a harmful effect on the arterial wall
metabolic syndrome: a cluster of metabolic abnormalities including insulin resistance, obesity, dyslipidemia, and hypertension that increase the risk of cardiovascular disease
myocardial infarction (MI): death of heart tissue caused by lack of oxygenated blood flow
percutaneous coronary intervention (PCI): a procedure in which a catheter is placed in a coronary artery, and one of several methods is employed to reduce blockage within the artery
percutaneous transluminal coronary angioplasty (PTCA): a type of percutaneous coronary intervention in which a balloon is inflated within a coronary artery to break an atheroma and open the vessel lumen, improving coronary artery blood flow
stent: a metal mesh that provides structural support to a coronary vessel, preventing its closure
sudden cardiac death: abrupt cessation of effective heart activity
thrombolytic: a pharmacologic agent that breaks down blood clots; alternatively referred to as a fibrinolytic
troponin: a cardiac muscle biomarker; measurement is used as an indicator of heart muscle injury

Cardiovascular disease is the leading cause of death in the United States for men and women of all racial and ethnic groups (Mozaffarian, Benjamin, Go, et al., 2016). Research related to the identification of and treatment for cardiovascular disease includes all segments of the population affected by cardiac conditions, including women, children, and people of diverse racial and ethnic backgrounds. The results of ongoing research are used by nurses

to identify specific prevention and treatment strategies in these populations.

Coronary Artery Disease

Coronary artery disease (CAD) is the most prevalent type of cardiovascular disease in adults. For this reason, nurses must recognize various manifestations of coronary artery conditions and evidence-based methods for assessing, preventing, and treating these disorders.

Coronary Atherosclerosis

The most common cause of cardiovascular disease in the United States is **atherosclerosis**, an abnormal accumulation of lipid, or fatty substances, and fibrous tissue in the lining of arterial blood vessel walls. These substances block and narrow the coronary vessels in a way that reduces blood flow to the myocardium. Atherosclerosis involves a repetitious inflammatory response to injury of the artery wall and subsequent alteration in the structural and biochemical properties of the arterial walls. New information that relates to the development of atherosclerosis has increased the understanding of treatment and prevention of this progressive and potentially life-threatening process.

Pathophysiology

The inflammatory response involved with the development of atherosclerosis begins with injury to the vascular endothelium and progresses over many years (McCance, Huether, Brashers, et al., 2014). The injury may be initiated by smoking, hypertension, hyperlipidemia, and other factors. The endothelium undergoes changes and stops producing the normal antithrombotic and vasodilating agents. The presence of inflammation attracts inflammatory cells, such as monocytes (macrophages). The macrophages ingest lipids, becoming "foam cells" that transport the lipids into the arterial wall. Some of the lipid is deposited on the arterial wall, forming fatty streaks. Activated macrophages also release biochemical substances that can further damage the endothelium by contributing to the oxidation of low-density lipoprotein (LDL). The oxidized LDL is toxic to the endothelial cells and fuels progression of the atherosclerotic process (Grossman & Porth, 2014).

Following the transport of lipid into the arterial wall, smooth muscle cells proliferate and form a fibrous cap over a core filled with lipid and inflammatory infiltrate. These deposits, called **atheromas**, or plaques, protrude into the lumen of the vessel, narrowing it and obstructing blood flow (see Fig. 27-1). Plaque may be stable or unstable, depending on the degree of inflammation and thickness of the fibrous cap. If the fibrous cap over the plaque is thick and the lipid pool remains relatively stable, it can resist the stress of blood flow and vessel movement. If the cap is thin and inflammation is ongoing, the lesion becomes what is called *vulnerable plaque*. At this point, the lipid core may grow, causing the fibrous plaque to rupture. A ruptured plaque attracts platelets and causes thrombus formation. A thrombus may then obstruct blood flow, leading to acute coronary syndrome (ACS), which may result in an acute **myocardial infarction (MI)**. When an MI occurs, a portion of the heart muscle no longer receives blood flow and becomes necrotic.

The anatomic structure of the coronary arteries makes them particularly susceptible to atherosclerosis. As Figure 27-2 shows, the three major coronary arteries have multiple branches. Atherosclerotic lesions most often form where the vessels branch, suggesting a hemodynamic component that favors their formation (Grossman & Porth, 2014). Although

Figure 27-1 • A, B. Atherosclerosis begins as monocytes and lipids enter the intima of an injured vessel. Smooth muscle cells proliferate within the vessel wall (**C**), contributing to the development of fatty accumulations and atheroma (**D**). As the plaque enlarges, the vessel narrows and blood flow decreases (**E**). The plaque may rupture and a thrombus might form, obstructing blood flow.

heart disease is most often caused by atherosclerosis of the coronary arteries, other phenomena may also decrease blood flow to the heart. Examples include vasospasm (sudden constriction or narrowing) of a coronary artery and profound hypotension.

Clinical Manifestations

CAD produces symptoms and complications according to the location and degree of narrowing of the arterial lumen, thrombus formation, and obstruction of blood flow to the myocardium. This impediment to blood flow is usually progressive, causing an inadequate blood supply that deprives the cardiac muscle cells of oxygen needed for their survival. The condition is known as **ischemia**. **Angina pectoris** refers to chest pain that is brought about by myocardial ischemia. Angina pectoris usually is caused by significant coronary atherosclerosis. If the decrease in blood supply is great enough, of long enough duration, or both, irreversible damage and death

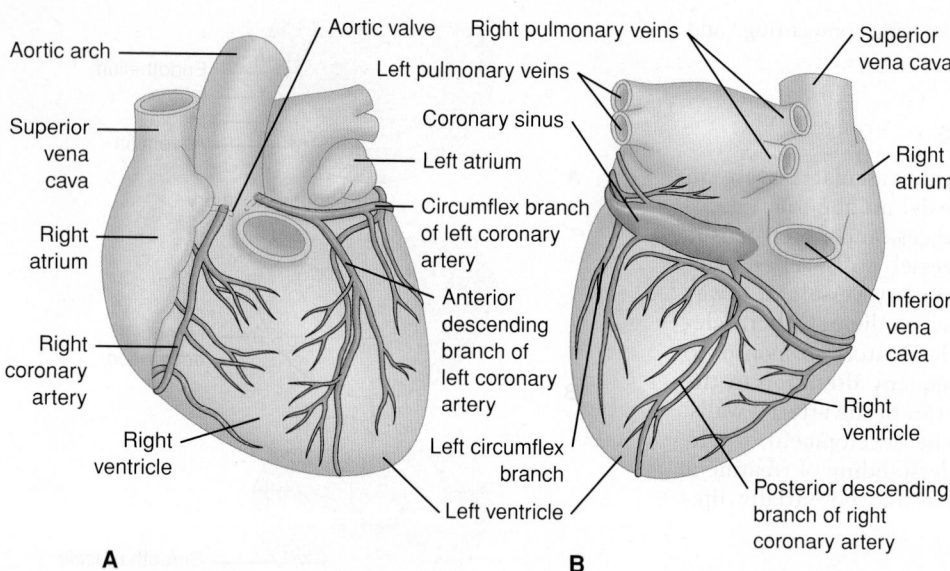

Figure 27-2 • The coronary arteries supply the heart muscle with oxygenated blood, adjusting the flow according to metabolic needs. **A.** Anterior view of the heart. **B.** Posterior view of heart.

of myocardial cells may result. Over time, irreversibly damaged myocardium undergoes degeneration and is replaced by scar tissue, causing various degrees of myocardial dysfunction. Significant myocardial damage may result in persistently low cardiac output and heart failure where the heart cannot support the body's needs for blood. A decrease in blood supply from CAD may cause the heart to abruptly stop beating; this is known as **sudden cardiac death** (see Chapter 29 for further discussion on CPR).

The most common manifestation of myocardial ischemia is the onset of chest pain. However, the classic epidemiologic study of the people in Framingham, Massachusetts, showed that nearly 15% of men and women who had coronary events, which included unstable angina, MIs, or sudden cardiac death events, were totally asymptomatic prior to the coronary event (Kannel, 1986). Patients with myocardial ischemia may present to an emergency department (ED) or clinic with a variety of symptoms other than chest pain. Some complain of epigastric distress and pain that radiates to the jaw or left arm. Patients who are older or have a history of diabetes or heart failure may report shortness of breath. Many women have been found to have atypical symptoms, including indigestion, nausea, palpitations, and numbness (Canto, Canto, & Goldberg, 2014). Prodromal symptoms may occur (i.e., angina a few hours to days before the acute episode), or a major cardiac event may be the first indication of coronary atherosclerosis.

Risk Factors

Epidemiologic studies point to several factors that increase the probability that a person will develop heart disease. Major risk factors are listed in Chart 27-1. Although many people with CAD have one or more risk factors, some do not have classic risk factors. Elevated **low-density lipoprotein (LDL)** cholesterol, also known as bad cholesterol, is a well-known risk factor and the primary target of cholesterol-lowering therapy. People at the highest risk for having a cardiac event are those with known CAD or those with diabetes, peripheral arterial disease, abdominal aortic aneurysm, or carotid artery disease. The latter diseases are referred to as CAD risk equivalents, because

patients with these diseases have the same risk for a cardiac event as patients with CAD. The likelihood of having a cardiac event is also affected by factors, such as age, gender, systolic blood pressure, smoking history, level of total cholesterol, and level of **high-density lipoprotein (HDL)**, also known as good cholesterol. The Framingham Risk Calculator is a tool

---

Chart 27-1 ⚠ **RISK FACTORS**
Coronary Artery Disease

A nonmodifiable risk factor is a circumstance over which a person has no control. A modifiable risk factor is one over which a person may exercise control, such as by changing a lifestyle or personal habit or by using medication. A risk factor may operate independently or in tandem with other risk factors. The more risk factors a person has, the greater the likelihood of coronary artery disease (CAD). Those at risk are advised to seek regular medical examinations and to engage in heart-healthy behavior (a deliberate effort to reduce the number and extent of risks).

Nonmodifiable Risk Factors

Family history of CAD (first-degree relative with cardiovascular disease at 55 years of age or younger for men and at 65 years of age or younger for women)
  Increasing age (more than 45 years for men; more than 55 years for women)
  Gender (men develop CAD at an earlier age than women)
  Race (higher incidence of heart disease in African Americans than in Caucasians)

Modifiable Risk Factors

Hyperlipidemia
Cigarette smoking, tobacco use
Hypertension
Diabetes
Metabolic syndrome
Obesity
Physical inactivity

Adapted from Mozaffarian, D., Benjamin, E. J., Go, A. S., et al. (2016). Heart disease and stroke statistics—2016 update: A report from the American Heart Association. *Circulation, 133*(4) e38–e360.

commonly used to estimate the risk for having a cardiac event within the next 10 years (Goff, Lloyd-Jones, Bennett, et al., 2014). This tool is designed for adults 20 years and older. The calculation is performed using the individual's risk factor data, including age, gender, total cholesterol, HDL cholesterol, smoking status, systolic blood pressure, and need for antihypertensive medication.

In addition, a cluster of metabolic abnormalities known as **metabolic syndrome** has emerged as a major risk factor for cardiovascular disease (Kim, Park, & Kang, 2015). A diagnosis of this syndrome includes three of the following conditions:

- Insulin resistance (fasting plasma glucose more than 100 mg/dL or abnormal glucose tolerance test)
- Central obesity (waist circumference more than 35 inches in females, more than 40 inches in males)
- Dyslipidemia (triglycerides more than 150 mg/dL, HDL less than 50 mg/dL in females, less than 40 mg/dL in males)
- Blood pressure persistently greater than 130/85 mm Hg
- Proinflammatory state (high levels of C-reactive protein [CRP])
- Prothrombotic state (high fibrinogen level)

Many people with type 2 diabetes fit this clinical picture. Theories suggest that in patients who are obese, excessive adipose tissue may secrete mediators that lead to metabolic changes. Adipokines (adipose tissue cytokines), free fatty acids, and other substances are known to modify insulin action and contribute to atherogenic changes in the cardiovascular system (see Fig. 27-3).

Physiology/Pathophysiology

Figure 27-3 • Pathophysiology of cardiovascular disease in metabolic syndrome. Central adiposity plays a major role in the development of metabolic syndrome. Adipokines released from fat cells along with other hormones and metabolites are thought to contribute to the development of metabolic abnormalities. The eventual effect of these processes is the promotion of atherosclerosis.

CRP is known to be an inflammatory marker for cardiovascular risk, including acute coronary events and stroke. The liver produces CRP in response to a stimulus such as tissue injury, and high levels of this protein may occur in people with diabetes and those who are likely to have an acute coronary event (Institute for Clinical Systems Improvement [ICSI], 2013a). To determine overall cardiovascular risk, clinicians may view high sensitivity C-reactive protein (hs-CRP) test results together with other screening tools such as measurements of lipid levels.

Prevention

Four modifiable risk factors—cholesterol abnormalities, tobacco use, hypertension, and diabetes—are established risk factors for CAD and its complications. As a result, they receive much attention in health promotion programs.

Controlling Cholesterol Abnormalities

The association of a high blood cholesterol level with heart disease is well established, and the metabolism of fats is known to be an important contributor to the development of heart disease. Fats, which are insoluble in water, are encased in water-soluble lipoproteins that allow them to be transported within the circulatory system. The various lipoproteins are categorized by their protein content, which is measured in density. The density increases when more protein is present. Four elements of fat metabolism—total cholesterol, LDL, HDL, and triglycerides—are known to affect the development of heart disease. Cholesterol is processed by the gastrointestinal (GI) tract into lipoprotein globules called *chylomicrons*. These are reprocessed by the liver as lipoproteins (see Fig. 27-4). This is a physiologic process necessary for the formation of lipoprotein-based cell membranes and other important metabolic processes. When an excess of LDL is produced, LDL particles adhere to receptors in the arterial endothelium. Here, macrophages ingest them, contributing to plaque formation.

The American College of Cardiology and the American Heart Association (ACC/AHA) have developed clinical practice guidelines on the treatment of blood cholesterol to reduce cardiovascular risk in adults based on the recommendations from the Adult Treatment Panel (ATP IV) (Stone, Robinson, Lichtenstein, et al., 2014). These guidelines address primary prevention (preventing the occurrence of CAD) and secondary prevention (preventing the progression of CAD). All adults 20 years and older should have a fasting lipid profile (total cholesterol, LDL, HDL, and triglycerides) performed at least once every 5 years, and more often if the profile is abnormal. Patients who have had an acute event (e.g., MI), a percutaneous coronary intervention (PCI), or a coronary artery bypass graft (CABG) require assessment of their LDL cholesterol level within a few months of the event or procedure, because LDL levels may be low immediately after the acute event or procedure. Subsequently, lipids should be monitored every 6 weeks until the desired level is achieved and then every 4 to 6 months. A fasting lipid profile should demonstrate the following values (ICSI, 2013a):

- LDL cholesterol less than 100 mg/dL (less than 70 mg/dL for very high-risk patients)
- Total cholesterol less than 200 mg/dL

Physiology/Pathophysiology

Stomach

Chylomicrons

Liver

Chylomicrons remnants

Macrophage injesting LDLs

VLDLs

LDLs

HDLs

Foam cell

Lipid debris

Smooth muscle cells

Figure 27-4 • Lipoproteins and the development of atherosclerosis. As dietary cholesterol and saturated fat are processed by the gastrointestinal tract, chylomicrons enter the blood. They are broken down into chylomicron remnants in the capillaries. The liver processes them into lipoproteins. When these are released into the circulation, excess low-density lipoproteins (LDLs) adhere to receptors on the intimal wall. Macrophages also ingest LDLs and transport them into the vessel wall, beginning the process of plaque formation. HDLs, high-density lipoproteins; VLDLs, very-low-density lipoproteins.

- HDL cholesterol greater than 40 mg/dL for males and greater than 50 mg/dL for females
- Triglyceride less than 150 mg/dL

LDL is the target of current therapy because of its strong association with advancing CAD. The total cholesterol level is also a clear predictor of coronary events. HDL is known as good cholesterol because it transports other lipoproteins such as LDL to the liver, where they can be degraded and excreted. Because of this, a high HDL level is a strong negative risk factor for heart disease (i.e., it protects against heart disease).

Triglyceride is made up of fatty acids and is transported through the blood by a lipoprotein. Although an elevated triglyceride level (more than 200 mg/dL) may be genetic in origin, it also can be caused by obesity, physical inactivity, excessive alcohol intake, high-carbohydrate diets, diabetes, kidney disease, and certain medications, such as oral contraceptives and corticosteroids.

 Concept Mastery Alert

It is important to remember the different types of cholesterol and the role of each as a risk factor for heart disease. HDL is the "good cholesterol," and higher levels are better; LDL is the "bad cholesterol," and lower levels are better.

Dietary Measures

Table 27-1 provides recommendations of the Therapeutic Lifestyle Changes (TLC) diet, a diet low in saturated fat and high in soluble fiber (ICSI, 2013a). These general recommendations may need to be adjusted for the individual patient who has other nutritional needs, such as the patient who has diabetes. In addition, referral to a dietitian can help the patient in following the appropriate TLC diet. Other TLC recommendations include weight loss, cessation of tobacco use, and increased physical activity.

TABLE 27-1 Nutrient Content of the Therapeutic Lifestyle Changes (TLC) Diet

Nutrient	Recommended Intake
Total calories[a]	Balance intake and expenditure to maintain desirable weight.
Total fat	25–35% of total calories
Saturated fat[b]	<7% of total calories
Polyunsaturated fat	Up to 10% of total calories
Monounsaturated fat	Up to 20% of total calories
Carbohydrate[c]	50–60% of total calories
Dietary fiber	20–30 g/day
Protein	Approximately 15% of total calories
Cholesterol	<200 mg/day

[a]Daily energy expenditure should include at least moderate physical activity (contributing approximately 200 kcal/day).

[b]Trans fatty acids are formed from the processing (manufacturing, hydrogenation) of vegetable oils into a more solid form. The effects of trans fatty acids are similar to saturated fats (i.e., raising low-density lipoprotein and lowering high-density lipoprotein). Intake of trans-fatty acids should be minimized.

[c]Carbohydrates should be derived predominantly from foods rich in complex carbohydrates, including grains, especially whole grains, fruits, and vegetables.

Adapted from the TLC Diet Regimen. Retrieved on 11/18/2015 at: tlcdiet.org/tlc-diet-regime/

The Mediterranean diet, another diet that promotes vegetables and fish and restricts red meat, is also reported to reduce mortality from cardiovascular disease (Martinez-Gonzalez, Salas-Salvado, Estruch, et al., 2015). People who adopt strict vegetarian diets can significantly reduce blood lipids, blood glucose, body mass index, and blood pressure. However, very intensive dietary programs such as these may not be acceptable to all patients who need to modify risk factors.

Many resources are available to assist people in controlling their cholesterol levels. The National Heart, Lung, and Blood Institute (NHLBI) and its National Cholesterol Education Program (NCEP), the AHA, and the American Diabetes Association (ADA), as well as CAD support groups and reliable Internet sources, are a few examples of the available resources. Cookbooks and recipes that include the nutritional contents of foods can be included as resources for patients. Dietary control has been made easier because food manufacturers are required to provide nutritional data on product labels. The label information of interest to a person attempting to eat a heart-healthy diet is as follows: serving size (expressed in household measures), amount of total fat per serving, amount of saturated fat and trans fat per serving, amount of cholesterol per serving, and amount of fiber per serving.

Physical Activity

Management of an elevated triglyceride level focuses on weight reduction and increased physical activity. Regular, moderate physical activity increases HDL levels and reduces triglyceride levels, decreasing the incidence of coronary events and reducing overall mortality risk. According to the Centers for Disease Control and Prevention (CDC) (2015), the goal for most adults is to engage in moderate-intensity aerobic activity of at least 150 minutes per week or vigorous-intensity aerobic activity of at least 75 minutes per week, or an equivalent combination. In addition, adults should engage in muscle-strengthening activities on 2 or more days each week that work all major muscle groups. The nurse helps the patient to set realistic goals for physical activity. For example, inactive patients can start with activity that lasts 3 minutes, such as parking farther from a building to increase daily walking time. Patients should be instructed to engage in an activity or variety of activities that interest them to maintain motivation. They should also be taught to exercise to an intensity that does not preclude their ability to talk; if they cannot have a conversation while exercising, they should slow down or switch to a less intensive activity. When the weather is hot and humid, patients should exercise during the early morning, or indoors, and wear loose-fitting clothing. When the weather is cold, they should layer clothing and wear a hat. Patients should stop any activity if chest pain, unusual shortness of breath, dizziness, lightheadedness, or nausea occurs.

Medications

If diet alone cannot normalize serum cholesterol levels, medications can have a synergistic effect with the prescribed diet and control cholesterol levels (see Table 27-2). Lipid-lowering medications can reduce CAD mortality in patients with elevated lipid levels and in at-risk patients with normal lipid levels (ICSI, 2013a). The various types of lipid-lowering agents affect the lipid components somewhat differently; these types include 3-hydroxy-3-methylglutaryl coenzyme A (HMG-CoA) (or statins), fibric acids (or fibrates), bile acid sequestrants (or resins), cholesterol absorption inhibitors, and omega-3-acid ethyl esters. A new class of lipid-lowering medications known as proprotein convertase subtilisin-kexin type 9 (PCSK9) agents has recently been approved by the U.S. Food and Drug Administration (FDA). Because of limited clinical trial evidence and their high cost, these PCSK9 agents are prescribed on a limited basis, but may be considered for more patients in the future (White, 2015).

Promoting Cessation of Tobacco Use

Cigarette smoking contributes to the development and severity of CAD in at least three ways:

- Nicotinic acid in tobacco triggers the release of catecholamines, which raise the heart rate and blood pressure (McCance et al., 2014). Nicotinic acid can also cause the coronary arteries to constrict. These effects lead to an increased risk of CAD and sudden cardiac death.
- Smoking can increase the oxidation of LDL, damaging the vascular endothelium (Grossman & Porth, 2014). This increases platelet adhesion and leads to a higher probability of thrombus formation.
- Inhalation of smoke increases the blood carbon monoxide level and decreases the supply of oxygen to the myocardium (Grossman & Porth, 2014). Hemoglobin, the oxygen-carrying component of blood, combines more readily with carbon monoxide than with oxygen. Myocardial ischemia and reduced contractility can result.

A person at increased risk for heart disease is encouraged to stop tobacco use through any means possible: educational programs, counseling, consistent motivation and reinforcement messages, support groups, and medications. Some people have found complementary therapies (e.g., acupuncture, guided imagery, hypnosis) to be helpful. People who stop smoking reduce their risk of heart

TABLE 27-2 Commonly Prescribed Medications That Affect Lipoprotein Metabolism

Medications	Therapeutic Effects	Considerations
HMG-CoA Reductase Inhibitors (Statins)		
Atorvastatin (Lipitor) Simvastatin (Zocor)	↓ Total cholesterol ↓ LDL ↑ HDL ↓ TGs Inhibit enzyme involved in lipid synthesis (HMG-CoA) Favorable effects on vascular endothelium, including anti-inflammatory and antithrombotic effects	Frequently given as initial therapy for significantly elevated cholesterol and LDL levels Myalgia and arthralgia are common adverse effects Myopathy and possible rhabdomyolysis are potential serious effects Monitor liver function tests Contraindicated in liver disease Check for drug interactions Indication for use now includes ACS and stroke Administer in evening
Fibric Acids (Fibrates)		
Fenofibrate (TriCor) Gemfibrozil (Lopid)	↑ HDL ↓ TGs ↓ Synthesis of TGs and other lipids	Adverse effects include diarrhea, flatulence, rash, myalgia Serious adverse effects include pancreatitis, hepatotoxicity, and rhabdomyolysis Contraindicated in severe renal and liver disease Use with caution in patients who are also taking statins
Bile Acid Sequestrants		
Cholestyramine (Questran) Colestipol (Colestid)	↓ LDL Slight ↑ HDL Oxidize cholesterol into bile acids, which ↓ fat absorption	Most often used as adjunct therapy when statins alone have not been effective in controlling lipid levels Side effects include constipation, abdominal pain, GI bleeding May decrease absorption of other drugs Taken before meals
Cholesterol Absorption Inhibitor		
Ezetimibe (Zetia)	↓ LDL Inhibits absorption of cholesterol in small intestine	Better tolerated than bile acid sequestrants Used in combination with other agents, such as statins Side effects include abdominal pain, arthralgia, myalgia Contraindicated in liver disease
Omega-3-Acid Ethyl Esters		
Fish oil capsules	↓ TGs Inhibit TG production in liver	May be used alone or in combination with other agents Side effects include GI distress, taste perversion, rash, and back pain

HMG-CoA, 3-hydroxy-3-methylglutaryl coenzyme A; ↓ decrease, ↑ increase; LDL, low-density lipoprotein; HDL, high-density lipoprotein; TGs, triglycerides; ACS, acute coronary syndrome; GI, gastrointestinal.

Adapted from Institute for Clinical Systems Improvement (ICSI). (2013a). *Lipid management in adults*. Retrieved on 11/18/2015 at: www.guideline.gov/content.aspx?id=47783&search=lipid+management+in+adult

disease within the first year, and the risk continues to decline as long as they refrain from smoking (Office of the U.S. Surgeon General, 2014).

The use of medications such as the nicotine patch (Nico-Derm CQ, Habitrol), varenicline (Chantix), or bupropion (Zyban) may assist with stopping the use of tobacco (FDA, 2015). Products containing nicotine have some of the same effects as smoking: catecholamine release (increasing heart rate and blood pressure) and increased platelet adhesion. These medications should be used for a short time and at the lowest effective doses.

Exposure to other smokers' smoke (passive or secondhand smoke) is believed to cause cardiovascular disease in nonsmokers. Secondhand smoke also increases the risk for stroke by an estimated 20% to 30% (Office of the U.S. Surgeon General, 2014). Other tobacco products such as electronic cigarettes (e-cigarettes or vapor cigarettes) and waterpipes (hookahs) are also thought to lead to health problems, but scant research exists on the effects of these alternative smoking methods. There is concern that because these products expose people to tobacco and its toxins, they also may carry risk of lung disease, cancer, and cardiovascular disease (American Society of Clinical Oncology, 2016).

Managing Hypertension

Hypertension is defined as blood pressure measurements that repeatedly exceed 140/90 mm Hg. The risk of cardiovascular disease increases as blood pressure increases, and current guidelines support treating hypertension with a goal of keeping the blood pressure under 150/90 in those age 60 and over, and a goal of less than 140/90 in others (James, Oparil, Carter et al., 2014). Long-standing elevated blood pressure may result in increased stiffness of the vessel walls, leading to vessel injury and a resulting inflammatory response within the intima. Inflammatory mediators then lead to the release of growth-promoting factors that cause vessel hypertrophy and hyperresponsiveness. These changes result in acceleration and aggravation of atherosclerosis. Hypertension also increases the work of the left ventricle, which must pump harder to eject blood into the arteries. Over time, the increased workload causes the heart to enlarge and thicken (i.e., hypertrophy) and may eventually lead to heart failure.

Early detection of high blood pressure and adherence to a therapeutic regimen can prevent the serious consequences associated with untreated elevated blood pressure, including CAD. A recent study confirmed that intensive management of hypertension lowers the risk of cardiovascular events, including heart attack and stroke, and lowers the risk of death (Wright, Williamson, & Whelton et al., 2015). See Chapter 31 for a detailed discussion of hypertension.

Controlling Diabetes

Diabetes is known to accelerate the development of heart disease. Hyperglycemia fosters dyslipidemia, increased platelet aggregation, and altered red blood cell function, which can lead to thrombus formation. These metabolic alterations may impair endothelial cell–dependent vasodilation and smooth muscle function, promoting the development of atherosclerosis. Treatment with insulin, metformin (Glucophage), and other therapeutic interventions that lower plasma glucose levels can lead to improved endothelial function and patient outcomes. See Chapter 51 for a detailed discussion of diabetes.

Gender

Heart disease has long been recognized as a cause of morbidity and mortality in men, but it has not always been as readily recognized in women. Cardiovascular events in women occur an average of 10 years later in life than they do in men. The male-to-female ratio is approximately 3-to-2 (Amsterdam, Wenger, Brinidis, et al., 2014). Women also tend to have a higher incidence of complications from cardiovascular disease and a higher mortality. In addition, women tend to not recognize the symptoms of CAD as early as men, and they wait longer to report their symptoms and seek medical assistance (Canto et al., 2014).

The age difference between women and men who were newly diagnosed with CAD was traditionally thought to be related to estrogen. Menopause is now recognized as a milestone in the aging process, during which risk factors tend to accumulate. Cardiovascular disease may be well developed by the time of menopause despite the supposed protective effects of estrogen (AHA, 2015). Although hormone therapy (HT) (formerly referred to as hormone replacement therapy) for menopausal women was once promoted as preventive therapy for CAD, research does not support HT as an effective means of prevention. HT decreases menopausal symptoms and the risk of osteoporosis-related bone fractures; however, it also has been associated with an increased incidence of CAD, breast cancer, deep vein thrombosis, stroke, and pulmonary embolism. Current guidelines do not recommend HT for primary or secondary prevention of CAD (AHA, 2015) (see Chapter 25 for further discussion).

In the past, women who possibly had coronary vascular events were less likely than men to be referred for coronary artery diagnostic procedures such as heart catheterization or treatment with invasive interventions (e.g., PCI). However, as a result of better education of health care professionals and the general public, gender differences now have less influence on diagnosis and treatment (Canto et al., 2014).

Angina Pectoris

Angina pectoris is a clinical syndrome usually characterized by episodes or paroxysms of pain or pressure in the anterior chest. The cause is insufficient coronary blood flow, resulting in a decreased oxygen supply when there is increased myocardial demand for oxygen in response to physical exertion or emotional stress. In other words, the need for oxygen exceeds the supply.

Pathophysiology

Angina is usually caused by atherosclerotic disease. Almost invariably, angina is associated with a significant obstruction of at least one major coronary artery. Normally, the myocardium extracts a large amount of oxygen from the coronary circulation to meet its continuous demands. When demand increases, flow through the coronary arteries needs to be increased. When there is a blockage in a coronary artery, flow cannot be increased and ischemia results. The types of angina are listed in Chart 27-2. Several factors are associated with typical anginal pain:

- Physical exertion, which precipitates an attack by increasing myocardial oxygen demand
- Exposure to cold, which causes vasoconstriction and elevated blood pressure, with increased oxygen demand
- Eating a heavy meal, which increases the blood flow to the mesenteric area for digestion, thereby reducing the

Chart 27-2   Types of Angina

- **Stable angina:** predictable and consistent pain that occurs on exertion and is relieved by rest and/or nitroglycerin
- **Unstable angina** (also called *preinfarction angina* or *crescendo angina*): symptoms increase in frequency and severity; may not be relieved with rest or nitroglycerin
- **Intractable or refractory angina:** severe incapacitating chest pain
- **Variant angina** (also called *Prinzmetal's angina*): pain at rest with reversible ST-segment elevation; thought to be caused by coronary artery vasospasm
- **Silent ischemia:** objective evidence of ischemia (such as electrocardiographic changes with a stress test), but patient reports no pain

blood supply available to the heart muscle; in a severely compromised heart, shunting of blood for digestion can be sufficient to induce anginal pain
- Stress or any emotion-provoking situation, causing the release of catecholamines, which increases blood pressure, heart rate, and myocardial workload

Unstable angina is not closely associated with these listed factors. It may occur at rest. See the later discussion of unstable angina in Acute Coronary Syndrome and Myocardial Infarction section.

Clinical Manifestations

Ischemia of the heart muscle may produce pain or other symptoms, varying from mild indigestion to a choking or heavy sensation in the upper chest. The severity ranges from discomfort to agonizing pain. The pain may be accompanied by severe apprehension and a feeling of impending death. It is often felt deep in the chest behind the sternum (retrosternal area). Typically, the pain or discomfort is poorly localized and may radiate to the neck, jaw, shoulders, and inner aspects of the upper arms, usually the left arm. The patient often feels tightness or a heavy choking or strangling sensation that has a viselike, insistent quality. The patient with diabetes may not have severe pain with angina because diabetic neuropathy can blunt nociceptor transmission, dulling the perception of pain (McCance et al., 2014).

A feeling of weakness or numbness in the arms, wrists, and hands, as well as shortness of breath, pallor, diaphoresis, dizziness or lightheadedness, and nausea and vomiting, may accompany the pain. An important characteristic of angina is that it subsides with rest or administering nitroglycerin. In many patients, anginal symptoms follow a stable, predictable pattern.

Unstable angina is characterized by attacks that increase in frequency and severity and are not relieved by rest and administering nitroglycerin. Patients with unstable angina require medical intervention.

Gerontologic Considerations

The older adult with angina may not exhibit a typical pain profile because of the diminished pain transmission that can occur with aging. Often the presenting symptom in older adults is dyspnea. Sometimes there are no symptoms ("silent" CAD), making recognition and diagnosis a clinical challenge. Older patients should be encouraged to recognize their chest pain–like symptom (e.g., weakness) as an indication that they should rest or take prescribed medications. Pharmacologic stress testing and cardiac catheterization may be used to diagnose CAD in older patients. Medications used to manage angina are given cautiously in older adults because they are associated with an increased risk of adverse reactions (Burchum & Rosenthal, 2016). Invasive procedures (e.g., PCI) that were once considered too risky in older adults may be considered; when these procedures are performed, many older adults benefit from symptom relief and longer survival (Shan, Saxena, & McMahon, 2014).

Assessment and Diagnostic Findings

The diagnosis of angina begins with the patient's history related to the clinical manifestations of ischemia. A 12-lead

electrocardiogram (ECG) may show changes indicative of ischemia, such as T-wave inversion, ST-segment elevation, or the development of an abnormal Q wave (Grossman & Porth, 2014). Laboratory studies are performed; these generally include cardiac biomarker testing to rule out ACS (refer to the Acute Coronary Syndrome and Myocardial Infarction section). The patient may undergo an exercise or pharmacologic stress test in which the heart is monitored continuously by an ECG, echocardiogram, or both. The patient may also be referred for a nuclear scan or invasive procedure (e.g., cardiac catheterization, coronary angiography).

Medical Management

The objectives of the medical management of angina are to decrease the oxygen demand of the myocardium and to increase the oxygen supply. Medically, these objectives are met through pharmacologic therapy and control of risk factors. Alternatively, reperfusion procedures may be used to restore the blood supply to the myocardium. These include PCI procedures (e.g., percutaneous transluminal coronary angioplasty [PTCA] and intracoronary stents) and CABG. (See later discussion.)

Pharmacologic Therapy

Table 27-3 summarizes drug therapy.

TABLE 27-3 Summary of Medications Used to Treat Angina

Medications	Major Indications
Nitrates	
Nitroglycerin (Nitrostat, Nitro-Bid)	Short- and long-term reduction of myocardial oxygen consumption through selective vasodilation
Beta-Adrenergic Blocking Agents (Beta-Blockers)	
Metoprolol (Lopressor) Atenolol (Tenormin)	Reduction of myocardial oxygen consumption by blocking beta-adrenergic stimulation of the heart
Calcium Ion Antagonists (Calcium Channel Blockers)	
Amlodipine (Norvasc) Diltiazem (Cardizem, Tiazac)	Negative inotropic effects; indicated in patients not responsive to beta-blockers; used as primary treatment for vasospasm
Antiplatelet Medications	
Aspirin Clopidogrel (Plavix) Prasugrel (Effient)	Prevention of platelet aggregation
Anticoagulants	
Heparin (unfractionated) Low–molecular-weight heparins: Enoxaparin (Lovenox) Dalteparin (Fragmin)	Prevention of thrombus formation

Adapted from Amsterdam, E. A., Wenger, N. K., Brindis, R. G., et al. (2014). 2014 AHA/ACC guideline for the management of patients with non-ST-elevation acute coronary syndromes. *Circulation, 130*(25), e344–e426.

Nitroglycerin

Nitrates are a standard treatment for angina pectoris. Nitroglycerin is a potent vasodilator that improves blood flow to the heart muscle and relieves pain. Nitroglycerin dilates primarily the veins and, to a lesser extent, the arteries. Dilation of the veins causes venous pooling of blood throughout the body. As a result, less blood returns to the heart, and filling pressure (preload) is reduced. If the patient is hypovolemic (does not have adequate circulating blood volume), the decrease in filling pressure can cause a significant decrease in cardiac output and blood pressure (Burchum & Rosenthal, 2016).

Nitrates also relax the systemic arteriolar bed, lowering blood pressure and decreasing afterload. These effects decrease myocardial oxygen requirements, bringing about a more favorable balance between supply and demand.

Nitroglycerin may be given by several routes: sublingual tablet or spray, oral capsule, topical agent, and intravenous (IV) administration. Sublingual nitroglycerin is generally placed under the tongue or in the cheek (buccal pouch) and ideally alleviates the pain of ischemia within 3 minutes. Chart 27-3 provides more information on self-administration of sublingual nitroglycerin. Oral preparations and topical patches are used to provide sustained effects. A regimen in which the patches are applied in the morning and removed at bedtime allows for a nitrate-free period to prevent the development of tolerance.

A continuous or intermittent IV infusion of nitroglycerin may be given to the hospitalized patient with recurring signs and symptoms of ischemia or after a revascularization procedure. The rate of infusion is titrated to the patient's pain level and blood pressure. It usually is not given if the systolic blood pressure is less than 90 mm Hg. Generally, after the patient is symptom-free, the nitroglycerin may be switched to an oral or topical preparation within 24 hours. A common adverse effect of nitroglycerin is headache, which may limit the use of this drug in some patients.

Beta-Adrenergic Blocking Agents

Beta-blockers such as metoprolol (Lopressor) reduce myocardial oxygen consumption by blocking beta-adrenergic sympathetic stimulation to the heart. The result is a reduction in heart rate, slowed conduction of impulses through the conduction system, decreased blood pressure, and reduced myocardial **contractility** (force of contraction). Because of these effects, beta-blockers balance the myocardial oxygen needs (demands) and the amount of oxygen available (supply). This helps control chest pain and delays the onset of ischemia during work or exercise. Beta-blockers reduce the incidence of recurrent angina, infarction, and cardiac mortality. The dose can be titrated to achieve a resting heart rate of 50 to 60 bpm (Burchum & Rosenthal, 2016).

Cardiac side effects and possible contraindications include hypotension, bradycardia, advanced atrioventricular block, and acute heart failure. If a beta-blocker is given IV for an acute cardiac event, the ECG, blood pressure, and heart rate are monitored closely after the medication has been given. Side effects include depressed mood, fatigue, decreased libido, and dizziness. Patients taking beta-blockers are cautioned not to stop taking them abruptly, because angina may worsen and MI may develop. Beta-blocker therapy should be decreased gradually over several days before being discontinued. Patients with diabetes who take beta-blockers are instructed to monitor their blood glucose levels as prescribed because beta-blockers can mask signs of hypoglycemia. Beta-blockers that are not cardioselective also affect the beta-adrenergic receptors in the bronchioles, causing bronchoconstriction, and therefore are contraindicated in patients with significant chronic pulmonary disorders, such as asthma.

Calcium Channel Blocking Agents

Calcium channel blockers have a variety of effects on the ischemic myocardium. These agents decrease sinoatrial node automaticity and atrioventricular node conduction, resulting in a slower heart rate and a decrease in the strength of myocardial contraction (negative inotropic effect). These effects decrease the workload of the heart. Calcium channel blockers also increase myocardial oxygen supply by dilating the smooth muscle wall of the coronary arterioles; they decrease myocardial oxygen demand by reducing systemic arterial pressure and the workload of the left ventricle (Burchum & Rosenthal, 2016).

The calcium channel blockers most commonly used are amlodipine (Norvasc) and diltiazem (Cardizem). In addition to their use to treat angina, they are commonly prescribed for hypertension. Hypotension may occur after the administration of any of the calcium channel blockers, particularly when administered IV. Other side effects may include atrioventricular block, bradycardia, and constipation.

Chart 27-3 | PHARMACOLOGY
Self-Administration of Nitroglycerin

Most patients with angina pectoris self-administer nitroglycerin on an as-needed basis. A key nursing role in such cases is educating patients about the medication and how to take it. Sublingual nitroglycerin comes in tablet and spray forms.

- Instruct the patient to make sure that the mouth is moist, the tongue is still, and saliva is not swallowed until the nitroglycerin tablet dissolves. If the pain is severe, the patient can crush the tablet between the teeth to hasten sublingual absorption.
- Advise the patient to carry the medication at all times as a precaution. However, because nitroglycerin is very unstable, it should be carried securely in its original container (e.g., capped dark glass bottle); tablets should never be removed and stored in metal or plastic pillboxes.
- Explain that nitroglycerin is volatile and is inactivated by heat, moisture, air, light, and time. Instruct the patient to renew the nitroglycerin supply every 6 months.
- Inform the patient that the medication should be taken in anticipation of any activity that may produce pain. Because nitroglycerin increases tolerance for exercise and stress when taken prophylactically (i.e., before angina-producing activity, such as exercise, stair-climbing, or sexual intercourse), it is best taken before pain develops.
- Recommend that the patient note how long it takes for the nitroglycerin to relieve the discomfort. Advise the patient that if pain persists after taking three sublingual tablets at 5-minute intervals, emergency medical services should be called.
- Discuss possible side effects of nitroglycerin, including flushing, throbbing headache, hypotension, and tachycardia.
- Advise the patient to sit down for a few minutes when taking nitroglycerin to avoid hypotension and syncope.

Adapted from Burchum, J. R., & Rosenthal, L. D. (2016). *Lehne's pharmacology for nursing care* (9th ed.). St. Louis, MO: Elsevier.

Antiplatelet and Anticoagulant Medications

Antiplatelet medications are given to prevent platelet aggregation and subsequent thrombosis, which impedes blood flow through the coronary arteries.

Aspirin

Aspirin prevents platelet aggregation and reduces the incidence of MI and death in patients with CAD (Bobadilla, 2016). A 162- to 325-mg dose of aspirin should be given to the patient with a new diagnosis of angina and then continued with 81 to 325 mg daily. Patients should be advised to continue aspirin even if they concurrently take other analgesics such as acetaminophen (Tylenol). Because aspirin may cause GI upset and bleeding, the use of histamine-2 (H_2) blockers (e.g., famotidine [Pepcid]) or proton pump inhibitors (e.g., omeprazole [Prilosec]) should be considered concomitant with continued aspirin therapy (Burchum & Rosenthal, 2016).

Adenosine Diphosphate Receptor Antagonists ($P2Y_{12}$)

These medications act on different pathways than aspirin to block platelet activation. However, unlike aspirin, these agents may take a few days to achieve antiplatelet effects. Clopidogrel (Plavix) is commonly prescribed in addition to aspirin in patients at high risk for MI. Newer agents such as prasugrel (Effient) may be used in place of clopidogrel during coronary events and interventions (Schnapf, 2013). Both carry the risk of bleeding from the GI tract or other sites.

Heparin

Unfractionated IV heparin prevents the formation of new blood clots (i.e., it is an anticoagulant). Treating patients with unstable angina with heparin reduces the occurrence of MI. If the patient's signs and symptoms indicate a significant risk for a cardiac event, the patient is hospitalized and may be given an IV bolus of heparin and started on a continuous infusion. The dose of heparin given is based on the results of the activated partial thromboplastin time (aPTT). Heparin therapy is usually considered therapeutic when the aPTT is 2 to 2.5 times the normal aPTT value.

A subcutaneous injection of low–molecular-weight heparin (LMWH; enoxaparin [Lovenox] or dalteparin [Fragmin]) may be used instead of IV unfractionated heparin to treat patients with unstable angina or non–ST-segment elevation myocardial infarction (NSTEMI) (Amsterdam et al., 2014). LMWH provides effective and stable anticoagulation, potentially reducing the risk of rebound ischemic events, and eliminating the need to monitor aPTT results. LMWHs may be beneficial before and during PCIs as well as for ACS.

Because unfractionated heparin and LMWH increase the risk of bleeding, the patient is monitored for signs and symptoms of external and internal bleeding, such as low blood pressure, increased heart rate, and decreased serum hemoglobin and hematocrit. The patient receiving heparin is placed on bleeding precautions, which include:

- Applying pressure to the site of any needle puncture for a longer time than usual
- Avoiding intramuscular (IM) injections
- Avoiding tissue injury and bruising from trauma or use of constrictive devices (e.g., continuous use of an automatic blood pressure cuff)

A decrease in platelet count or evidence of thrombosis may indicate heparin-induced thrombocytopenia (HIT), an antibody-mediated reaction to heparin that may result in thrombosis. Patients who have received heparin within the past 3 months and those who have been receiving unfractionated heparin for 5 to 10 days are at high risk for HIT (Greinacher, 2015). (See Chapter 33 for further discussion of HIT.)

Glycoprotein IIb/IIIa Agents

IV administration of glycoprotein (GP) IIb/IIIa agents, such as abciximab (ReoPro) or eptifibatide (Integrilin), is indicated for hospitalized patients with unstable angina and as adjunct therapy for PCI. These agents prevent platelet aggregation by blocking the GP IIb/IIIa receptors on the platelets, preventing adhesion of fibrinogen and other factors that crosslink platelets to each other and thus form intracoronary clots (Urden, Stacy, & Lough, 2014). As with heparin, bleeding is the major side effect, and bleeding precautions should be initiated.

Oxygen Administration

Oxygen therapy is usually initiated at the onset of chest pain in an attempt to increase the amount of oxygen delivered to the myocardium and to decrease pain. The therapeutic effectiveness of oxygen is determined by observing the rate and rhythm of respirations and the color of skin and mucous membranes. Blood oxygen saturation is monitored by pulse oximetry; the normal oxygen saturation (SpO_2) level is greater than 95% on room air (Urden et al., 2014).

NURSING PROCESS

The Patient With Angina Pectoris

Assessment

The nurse gathers information about the patient's symptoms and activities, especially those that precede and precipitate attacks of angina pectoris. Appropriate questions are listed in Chart 27-4. The answers to these questions form the basis for designing an effective program of treatment and prevention. In addition to assessing angina pectoris or its equivalent, the nurse also assesses the patient's risk factors for CAD, the patient's response to angina, the patient's and family's understanding of the diagnosis, and adherence to the current treatment plan.

Chart 27-4 | **ASSESSMENT**
Assessing Angina

Ask the following:

- "Where is the pain (or prodromal symptoms)? Can you point to it?"
- "Can you feel the pain anywhere else?"
- "How would you describe the pain?"
- "Is it like the pain you had before?"
- "Can you rate the pain on a 0–10 scale, with 10 being the most pain?"
- "When did the pain begin?"
- "How long does it last?"
- "What brings on the pain?"
- "What helps the pain go away?"
- "Do you have any other symptoms with the pain?"

Diagnosis

NURSING DIAGNOSES

Based on the assessment data, major nursing diagnoses may include:

- Risk for decreased cardiac tissue perfusion
- Anxiety related to cardiac symptoms and possible death
- Deficient knowledge about the underlying disease and methods for avoiding complications
- Noncompliance, ineffective management of therapeutic regimen related to failure to accept necessary lifestyle changes

COLLABORATIVE PROBLEMS/POTENTIAL COMPLICATIONS

Potential complications may include the following:

- ACS and/or MI (described later in this chapter)
- Dysrhythmias and cardiac arrest (see Chapters 26 and 29)
- Heart failure (see Chapter 29)
- Cardiogenic shock (see Chapter 14)

Planning and Goals

Major patient goals include immediate and appropriate treatment when angina occurs, prevention of angina, reduction of anxiety, awareness of the disease process and understanding of the prescribed care, adherence to the self-care program, and absence of complications.

Nursing Interventions

TREATING ANGINA

If the patient reports pain (or cardiac ischemia is suggested by prodromal symptoms, which may include sensations of indigestion or nausea, choking, heaviness, weakness or numbness in the upper extremities, dyspnea, or dizziness), the nurse takes immediate action. The patient experiencing angina is directed to stop all activities and sit or rest in bed in a semi-Fowler's position to reduce the oxygen requirements of the ischemic myocardium. The nurse assesses the patient's angina, asking questions to determine whether the angina is the same as the patient typically experiences. A change may indicate a worsening of the disease or a different cause. The nurse then continues to assess the patient, measuring vital signs and observing for signs of respiratory distress. If the patient is in the hospital, a 12-lead ECG is usually obtained and assessed for ST-segment and T-wave changes. If the patient has been placed on cardiac monitoring with continuous ST-segment monitoring, the ST segment is assessed for changes.

Nitroglycerin is given sublingually, and the patient's response is assessed (relief of chest pain and effect on blood pressure and heart rate). If the chest pain is unchanged or is lessened but still present, nitroglycerin administration is repeated up to three doses. Each time blood pressure, heart rate, and the ST segment (if the patient is on a monitor with ST-segment monitoring capability) are assessed. The nurse administers oxygen therapy if the patient's respiratory rate is increased or if the oxygen saturation level is decreased. Oxygen is usually given at 2 L/min by nasal cannula, even without evidence of desaturation, although there is no current evidence of a positive effect on patient outcome. If the pain is significant and continues after these interventions, the patient is further evaluated for acute MI and may be transferred to a higher-acuity nursing unit (Amsterdam et al., 2014).

REDUCING ANXIETY

Patients with angina often fear loss of their roles within society and the family. They may also fear that the pain (or the prodromal symptoms) may lead to an MI or death. Exploring the implications that the diagnosis has for the patient and providing information about the illness, its treatment, and methods of preventing its progression are important nursing interventions. Various stress reduction methods, such as guided imagery or music therapy, should be explored with the patient (Ackley & Ladwig, 2014). Addressing the spiritual needs of the patient and family may also assist in allaying anxieties and fears.

PREVENTING PAIN

The nurse reviews the assessment findings, identifies the level of activity that causes the patient's pain or prodromal symptoms, and plans the patient's activities accordingly. If the patient has pain frequently or with minimal activity, the nurse alternates the patient's activities with rest periods. Balancing activity and rest is an important aspect of the educational plan for the patient and family.

PROMOTING HOME, COMMUNITY-BASED, AND TRANSITIONAL CARE

Educating Patients About Self-Care. The program for educating the patient with angina is designed so that the patient and family understand the illness, identify the symptoms of myocardial ischemia, state the actions to take when symptoms develop, and discuss methods to prevent chest pain and the advancement of CAD. The goals of education are to reduce the frequency and severity of anginal attacks, to delay the progress of the underlying disease if possible, and to prevent complications. The factors outlined in Chart 27-5 are important in educating the patient with angina pectoris.

The self-care program is prepared in collaboration with the patient and family or friends. Activities should be planned to minimize the occurrence of anginal episodes. The patient needs to understand that any pain unrelieved within 15 minutes by the usual methods, including nitroglycerin (see Chart 27-3), should be treated at the closest ED; the patient should call 911 for assistance.

Continuing and Transitional Care. For patients with disabilities or special needs, arrangements are made for transitional, home, or community care when appropriate. A home or transitional care nurse can assist the patient with scheduling and keeping follow-up appointments. The patient may need reminders about follow-up monitoring, including periodic laboratory testing. In addition, the home care nurse may monitor the patient's adherence to dietary restrictions and to prescribed antianginal medications, including nitroglycerin. If the patient has severe anginal symptoms, the nurse may assess the home environment and recommend modifications that diminish the occurrence of anginal episodes. For instance, if a patient cannot climb stairs without experiencing ischemia, the home care nurse may help the patient plan daily activities that minimize stair-climbing.

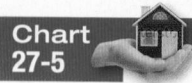

Chart 27-5	HOME CARE CHECKLIST

Managing Angina Pectoris

At the completion of education, the patient and/or caregiver will be able to:

- State the impact of angina pectoris on physiologic functioning, ADLs, IADLs, roles, relationships, and spirituality.
- State changes in lifestyle (e.g., diet, activity) or home environment necessary to maintain health.
- Follow a diet low in saturated fat, high in fiber, and, if indicated, lower in calories.
- Reduce the probability of an episode of anginal pain by balancing rest with regular daily activities that do not produce chest discomfort, shortness of breath, or undue fatigue.
- Follow the prescribed exercise regimen.
  - Recognize that temperature extremes (particularly cold) may induce anginal pain; therefore, avoid exercise in temperature extremes.
- State the name, dose, side effects, frequency, and schedule for all medications.
- Take medications, especially aspirin and beta-blockers, as prescribed.
- Carry nitroglycerin at all times; state when and how to use it; identify its side effects.

- Avoid using medications or any over-the-counter substances (e.g., diet pills, nasal decongestants) that can increase the heart rate and blood pressure without first discussing with the primary provider.
- Use appropriate resources for support during emotionally stressful times (e.g., counselor, nurse, clergy, physician).
- Stop smoking and the use of other forms of tobacco, and avoid secondhand smoke (because smoking increases the heart rate, blood pressure, and blood carbon monoxide levels).
- Achieve and maintain normal blood pressure.
- Achieve and maintain normal blood glucose levels.
- State how to reach primary provider with questions or complications.
  - Report increase in symptoms to the primary provider.
  - State time and date of follow-up appointments and testing.
- Identify the need for health promotion (e.g., weight reduction, smoking cessation, stress management), disease prevention, and screening activities.

ADL, activities of daily living; IADL, independent activities of daily living.

Evaluation

Expected patient outcomes may include:

1. Reports that pain is relieved promptly
   a. Recognizes symptoms
   b. Takes immediate action
   c. Seeks medical assistance if pain persists or changes in quality
2. Reports decreased anxiety
   a. Expresses acceptance of diagnosis
   b. Expresses control over choices within medical regimen
   c. Does not exhibit signs and symptoms that indicate a high level of anxiety
3. Understands ways to avoid complications and is free of complications
   a. Describes the process of angina
   b. Explains reasons for measures to prevent complications
   c. Exhibits stable ECG
   d. Experiences no signs and symptoms of acute MI
4. Adheres to self-care program
   a. Takes medications as prescribed
   b. Keeps health care appointments
   c. Implements plan to reduce risk factors

Acute Coronary Syndrome and Myocardial Infarction

Acute coronary syndrome (ACS) is an emergent situation characterized by an acute onset of myocardial ischemia that results in myocardial death (i.e., MI) if definitive interventions do not occur promptly. (Although the terms *coronary occlusion, heart attack,* and *myocardial infarction* are used synonymously, the preferred term is *myocardial infarction.*)

The spectrum of ACS includes unstable angina, NSTEMI, and ST-segment elevation myocardial infarction (STEMI).

Pathophysiology

In unstable angina, there is reduced blood flow in a coronary artery, often due to rupture of an atherosclerotic plaque. A clot begins to form on top of the coronary lesion, but the artery is not completely occluded. This is an acute situation that can result in chest pain and other symptoms that may be referred to as preinfarction angina because the patient will likely have an MI if prompt interventions do not occur.

In an MI, plaque rupture and subsequent thrombus formation result in complete occlusion of the artery, leading to ischemia and necrosis of the myocardium supplied by that artery. Vasospasm (sudden constriction or narrowing) of a coronary artery, decreased oxygen supply (e.g., from acute blood loss, anemia, or low blood pressure), and increased demand for oxygen (e.g., from a rapid heart rate, thyrotoxicosis, or ingestion of cocaine) are other causes of MI. In each case, a profound imbalance exists between myocardial oxygen supply and demand.

The area of infarction develops over minutes to hours. As the cells are deprived of oxygen, ischemia develops, cellular injury occurs, and the lack of oxygen results in infarction, or the death of cells. The expression "time is muscle" reflects the urgency of appropriate treatment to improve patient outcomes. Approximately every 43 seconds, an American will have an MI (Mozaffarian et al., 2016), and many of these people will die as a result. Early recognition and treatment of patients presenting with an MI will improve their chances of survival.

Various descriptions are used to further identify an MI: the type (NSTEMI, STEMI), the location of the injury to the ventricular wall (anterior, inferior, posterior, or lateral wall), and the point in time within the process of infarction (acute, evolving, or old). The differentiation between NSTEMI and STEMI is determined by diagnostic tests and is explained later in this chapter.

The 12-lead ECG identifies the type and location of the MI, and other ECG indicators, such as a Q wave and patient history, identify the timing. Regardless of the location, the goals of medical therapy are to relieve symptoms, prevent or minimize myocardial tissue death, and prevent complications. The pathophysiology of CAD and the risk factors involved were discussed earlier in this chapter.

Clinical Manifestations

Chest pain that occurs suddenly and continues despite rest and medication is the presenting symptom in most patients with ACS. Some of these patients have prodromal symptoms or a previous diagnosis of CAD, but others report no previous symptoms. Patients may present with a combination of symptoms, including chest pain, shortness of breath, indigestion, nausea, and anxiety. They may have cool, pale, and moist skin. Their heart rate and respiratory rate may be faster than normal. These signs and symptoms, which are caused by stimulation of the sympathetic nervous system, may be present for only a short time or may persist. In many cases, the signs and symptoms of MI cannot be distinguished from those of unstable angina; hence, the evolution of the term *acute coronary syndrome*.

Assessment and Diagnostic Findings

The diagnosis of ACS is generally based on the presenting symptoms (see Chart 27-6); the 12-lead ECG and laboratory tests (e.g., serial cardiac biomarkers) are performed to clarify whether the patient has unstable angina, NSTEMI, or STEMI (Amsterdam et al., 2014). The prognosis depends on the severity of coronary artery obstruction and the presence and extent of myocardial damage. Physical examination is always conducted, but the examination alone does not confirm the diagnosis.

Patient History

The patient history includes the description of the presenting symptom (e.g., pain), the history of previous cardiac and other illnesses, and the family history of heart disease. The history should also include information about the patient's risk factors for heart disease.

Electrocardiogram

The 12-lead ECG provides information that assists in ruling out or diagnosing an acute MI. It should be obtained within 10 minutes from the time a patient reports pain or arrives in the ED. By monitoring serial ECG changes over time, the location, evolution, and resolution of an MI can be identified and monitored.

The ECG changes that occur with an MI are seen in the leads that view the involved surface of the heart. The expected ECG changes are T-wave inversion, ST-segment elevation, and development of an abnormal Q wave (see Fig. 27-5). Because infarction evolves over time, the ECG also changes over time. The first ECG signs of an acute MI are usually seen in the T wave and ST segment (Amsterdam et al., 2014). As the area of injury becomes ischemic, myocardial repolarization is altered and delayed, causing the T wave

Chart 27-6 **ASSESSMENT**

Assessing for Acute Coronary Syndrome or Acute Myocardial Infarction

Be alert for the following signs and symptoms:

Cardiovascular

- Chest pain or discomfort not relieved by rest or nitroglycerin; palpitations. Heart sounds may include S_3, S_4, and new onset of a murmur.
- Increased jugular venous distention may be seen if the myocardial infarction (MI) has caused heart failure.
- Blood pressure may be elevated because of sympathetic stimulation or decreased because of decreased contractility, impending cardiogenic shock, or medications.
- Irregular pulse may indicate atrial fibrillation.
- In addition to ST-segment and T-wave changes, the electrocardiogram may show tachycardia, bradycardia, or other dysrhythmias.

Respiratory

Shortness of breath, dyspnea, tachypnea, and crackles if MI has caused pulmonary congestion. Pulmonary edema may be present.

Gastrointestinal

Nausea, indigestion, and vomiting.

Genitourinary

Decreased urinary output may indicate cardiogenic shock.

Skin

Cool, clammy, diaphoretic, and pale appearance due to sympathetic stimulation may indicate cardiogenic shock.

Neurologic

Anxiety, restlessness, and lightheadedness may indicate increased sympathetic stimulation or a decrease in contractility and cerebral oxygenation. The same symptoms may also herald cardiogenic shock.

Psychological

Fear with feeling of impending doom, or denial that anything is wrong.

to invert. Myocardial injury also causes ST-segment changes. The ST segment is normally flat on the ECG tracing. The injured myocardial cells depolarize normally but repolarize more rapidly than normal cells, causing the ST segment to rise at least 1 mm above the isoelectric line (the area between the T wave and the next P wave is used as the reference for the isoelectric line). This change is measured 0.06 to 0.08 seconds after the end of the QRS—a point called the *J point* (Urden et al., 2014) (see Fig. 27-6). An elevation in the ST segment in two contiguous leads is a key diagnostic indicator for MI (i.e., STEMI).

The appearance of abnormal Q waves is another indication of MI. Q waves develop within 1 to 3 days because there is no depolarization current conducted from necrotic tissue (Urden et al., 2014). A new and significant Q wave is 0.04 seconds or longer and 25% of the R wave depth. An acute MI may also cause a significant decrease in the height of

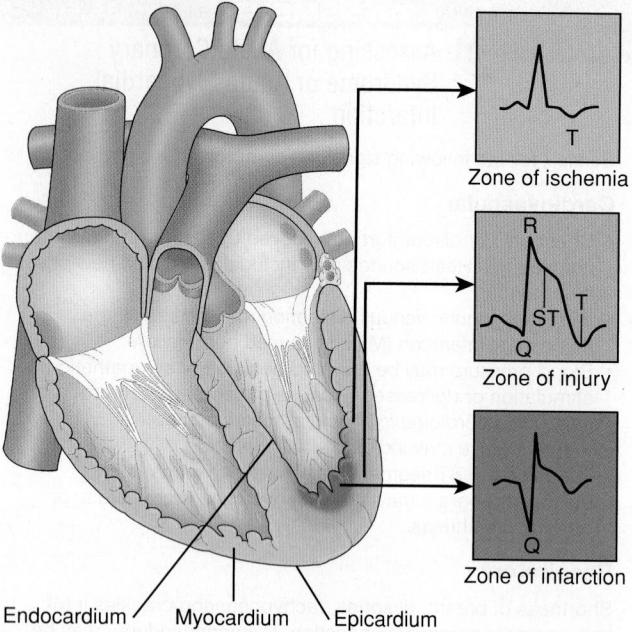

Figure 27-5 • Effects of ischemia, injury, and infarction on an electrocardiogram recording. Ischemia causes inversion of the T wave because of altered repolarization. Cardiac muscle injury causes elevation of the ST segment. Later, Q waves develop because of the absence of depolarization current from the necrotic tissue and opposing currents from other parts of the heart.

the R wave. During an acute MI, injury and ischemic changes are usually present. An abnormal Q wave may be present without ST-segment and T-wave changes, which indicates an old, not acute, MI. For some patients, there is no persistent ST elevation or other ECG changes; therefore, an NSTEMI is diagnosed by blood levels of cardiac biomarkers.

Using the information presented, patients are diagnosed with one of the following forms of ACS:

- *Unstable angina:* The patient has clinical manifestations of coronary ischemia, but ECG and cardiac biomarkers show no evidence of acute MI.

Figure 27-6 • Using the electrocardiogram to diagnose acute myocardial infarction (MI). (ST-segment elevation is measured 0.06 to 0.08 seconds after the J point. An elevation of more than 1 mm in contiguous leads is indicative of acute MI.)

- *STEMI:* The patient has ECG evidence of acute MI with characteristic changes in two contiguous leads on a 12-lead ECG. In this type of MI, there is a significant damage to the myocardium.
- *NSTEMI:* The patient has elevated cardiac biomarkers (e.g., troponin) but no definite ECG evidence of acute MI. In this type of MI, there may be less damage to the myocardium.

During recovery from an MI, the ST segment often is the first ECG indicator to return to normal. Q-wave alterations are usually permanent. An old STEMI is usually indicated by an abnormal Q wave or decreased height of the R wave without ST-segment and T-wave changes.

Echocardiogram

The echocardiogram is used to evaluate ventricular function. It may be used to assist in diagnosing an MI, especially when the ECG is nondiagnostic. The echocardiogram can detect hypokinetic and akinetic wall motion and can determine the ejection fraction (see Chapter 25).

Laboratory Tests

Cardiac enzymes and biomarkers, which include troponin, creatine kinase (CK), and myoglobin, are used to diagnose an acute MI. Cardiac biomarkers can be analyzed rapidly, expediting an accurate diagnosis. These tests are based on the release of cellular contents into the circulation when myocardial cells die. Figure 27-7 shows the time courses of cardiac enzymes and biomarkers.

Troponin

Troponin, a protein found in myocardial cells, regulates the myocardial contractile process. There are three isomers of troponin: C, I, and T. Troponins I and T are specific for cardiac muscle, and these biomarkers are currently recognized as reliable and critical markers of myocardial injury (Amsterdam et al., 2014). An increase in the level of troponin in the serum can be detected within a few hours during acute MI. It remains elevated for a long period, often as long as 2 weeks, and it therefore can be used to detect recent myocardial damage. It should be noted that cardiac troponin levels may rise during inflammation and other forms of mechanical stress on the myocardium. These include sepsis, heart failure, and respiratory failure (Liu, Shehu, Herrold, et al., 2015).

Creatine Kinase and Its Isoenzymes

There are three CK isoenzymes: CK-MM (skeletal muscle), CK-MB (heart muscle), and CK-BB (brain tissue). CK-MB is the cardiac-specific isoenzyme; it is found mainly in cardiac cells and therefore increases when there has been damage to these cells. Elevated CK-MB is an indicator of acute MI; the level begins to increase within a few hours and peaks within 24 hours of an infarct.

Myoglobin

Myoglobin is a heme protein that helps transport oxygen. Like the CK-MB enzyme, myoglobin is found in cardiac and skeletal muscle. The myoglobin level starts to increase within 1 to 3 hours and peaks within 12 hours after the onset of symptoms. An increase in myoglobin is not very specific in indicating an acute cardiac event; however, negative results can be used to rule out an acute MI.

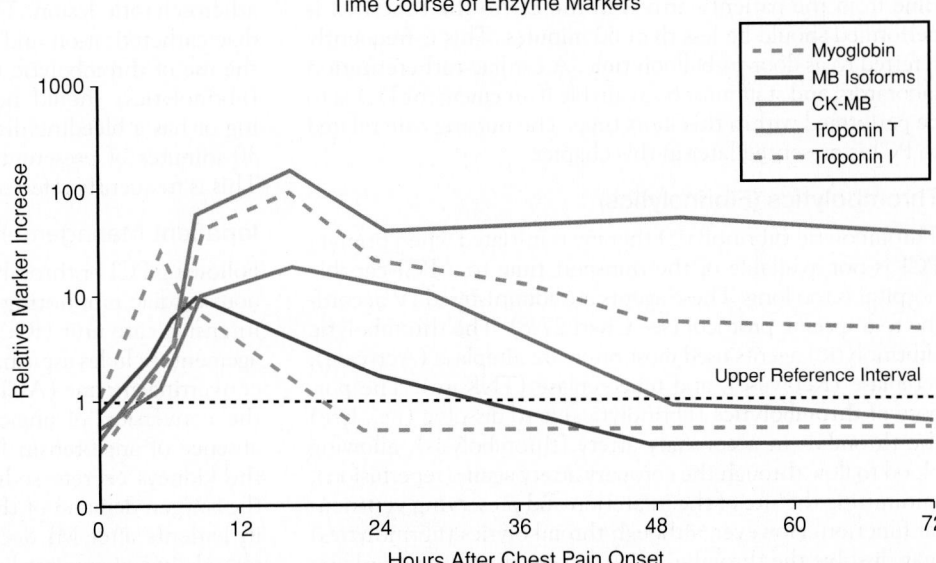

Time Course of Enzyme Markers

Figure 27-7 • Peak elevation and duration of serum enzymes and biomarkers after acute myocardial infarction. From Morton, P. G., & Fontaine, D. K. (2013). *Critical care nursing* (10th ed.). Philadelphia, PA: Lippincott Williams & Wilkins.

Medical Management

The goals of medical management are to minimize myocardial damage, preserve myocardial function, and prevent complications. These goals are facilitated by the use of guidelines developed by the American College of Cardiology (ACC) and the AHA (see Chart 27-7).

The goals for treating patients with acute MI may be achieved by interventions that reestablish coronary flow. Minimizing myocardial damage is also accomplished by reducing myocardial oxygen demand and increasing oxygen supply with medications, oxygen administration, and bed rest. The resolution of pain and ECG changes indicate that demand and supply are in equilibrium; they may also indicate reperfusion. Visualization of blood flow through an open vessel in the catheterization laboratory is evidence of reperfusion.

Initial Management

The patient with suspected MI should immediately receive supplemental oxygen, aspirin, nitroglycerin, and morphine. Morphine is the drug of choice to reduce pain and anxiety. It also reduces preload and afterload, decreasing the work of the heart. The response to morphine is monitored carefully to assess for hypotension or decreased respiratory rate. A beta-blocker may also be used if dysrhythmias occur. If a beta-blocker is not needed in the initial management period, it should be introduced within 24 hours of admission, once hemodynamics have stabilized and it is confirmed that the patient has no contraindications (Amsterdam et al., 2014). Unfractionated heparin or LMWH may also be prescribed along with platelet-inhibiting agents to prevent further clot formation.

Emergent Percutaneous Coronary Intervention

The patient with STEMI is taken directly to the cardiac catheterization laboratory for an immediate PCI (if a cardiac catheterization laboratory is on site). The procedure is used to open the occluded coronary artery and promote reperfusion to the area that has been deprived of oxygen. Superior outcomes have been reported with the use of PCI when compared to thrombolytic (Amsterdam et al., 2014) (also called *fibrinolytic*) agents; see the Thrombolytics (Fibrinolytics) section. Early PCI can be effective in patients of all ages, including those older than 75 years (Brenes-Salazar & Forman, 2014). The procedure treats the underlying atherosclerotic lesion. Because the duration of oxygen deprivation determines the number of myocardial cells that die, the time from the patient's arrival in the ED to the time PCI is performed should be less than 60 minutes. This is frequently referred to as door-to-balloon time. A cardiac catheterization laboratory and staff must be available if an emergent PCI is to be performed within this short time. The nursing care related to PCI is presented later in this chapter.

Thrombolytics (Fibrinolytics)

Thrombolytic (fibrinolytic) therapy is initiated when primary PCI is not available or the transport time to a PCI-capable hospital is too long. These agents are administered IV according to a specific protocol (see Chart 27-8). The thrombolytic (fibrinolytic) agents used most often are alteplase (Activase), reteplase (Retavase), and tenecteplase (TNKase). The purpose of **thrombolytics** (fibrinolytics) is to dissolve (i.e., lyse) the thrombus in a coronary artery (thrombolysis), allowing blood to flow through the coronary artery again (reperfusion), minimizing the size of the infarction and preserving ventricular function. However, although thrombolytics (fibrinolytics) may dissolve the thrombus, they do not affect the underlying

---

Chart 27-8 · PHARMACOLOGY

Administration of Thrombolytic (Fibrinolytic) Therapy

Indications

- Chest pain lasting more than 20 minutes, unrelieved by nitroglycerin
- ST-segment elevation in at least two leads that face the same area of the heart
- Less than 6 hours from onset of pain

Absolute Contraindications

- Active bleeding
- Known bleeding disorder
- History of hemorrhagic stroke
- History of intracranial vessel malformation
- Recent major surgery or trauma
- Uncontrolled hypertension
- Pregnancy

Nursing Considerations

- Minimize the number of times the patient's skin is punctured.
- Avoid intramuscular injections.
- Draw blood for laboratory tests when starting the IV line.
- Start IV lines before thrombolytic (fibrinolytic) therapy; designate one line to use for blood draws.
- Avoid continual use of noninvasive blood pressure cuff.
- Monitor for acute dysrhythmias and hypotension.
- Monitor for reperfusion: resolution of angina or acute ST-segment changes.
- Check for signs and symptoms of bleeding: decrease in hematocrit and hemoglobin values, decrease in blood pressure, increase in heart rate, oozing or bulging at invasive procedure sites, back pain, muscle weakness, changes in level of consciousness, complaints of headache.
- Treat major bleeding by discontinuing thrombolytic (fibrinolytic) therapy and any anticoagulants; apply direct pressure and notify the primary provider immediately.
- Treat minor bleeding by applying direct pressure if accessible and appropriate; continue to monitor.

Adapted from Urden, L. D., Stacy, K. M., & Lough, M.E. (2014). *Critical care nursing* (7th ed.). St. Louis, MO: Elsevier.

---

atherosclerotic lesion. The patient may be referred for a cardiac catheterization and other invasive procedures following the use of thrombolytic (fibrinolytic) therapy. Thrombolytics (fibrinolytics) should not be used if the patient is bleeding or has a bleeding disorder. They should be given within 30 minutes of presentation to the hospital (ICSI, 2013b). This is frequently referred to as door-to-needle time.

Inpatient Management

Following PCI or thrombolytic (fibrinolytic) therapy, continuous cardiac monitoring is indicated, preferably in a cardiac intensive care unit (ICU). Continuing pharmacologic management includes aspirin, a beta-blocker, and an angiotensin-converting enzyme (ACE) inhibitor. ACE inhibitors prevent the conversion of angiotensin I to angiotensin II. In the absence of angiotensin II, the blood pressure decreases and the kidneys excrete sodium and fluid (diuresis), decreasing the oxygen demand of the heart. The use of ACE inhibitors in patients after MI decreases mortality rates and prevents remodeling of myocardial cells that is associated with the onset of heart failure. Blood pressure, urine output, and serum sodium, potassium, and creatinine levels need to be monitored closely. If an ACE inhibitor is not suitable, an angiotensin receptor blocker (ARB) should be prescribed (Amsterdam et al., 2014). Nicotine replacement therapy and smoking cessation counseling should also be initiated for smokers.

Cardiac Rehabilitation

After the patient with an MI is in a stable condition, an active rehabilitation program is initiated. Cardiac rehabilitation is an important continuing care program for patients with CAD that targets risk reduction by providing patient and family education, offering individual and group support, and encouraging physical activity and physical conditioning. The goals of rehabilitation for the patient who has had an MI are to extend life and improve the quality of life. The immediate objectives are to limit the effects and progression of atherosclerosis, return the patient to work and a pre-illness lifestyle, enhance the patient's psychosocial and vocational status, and prevent another cardiac event. Cardiac rehabilitation programs increase survival, reduce recurrent events and the need for interventional procedures, and improve quality of life (Amsterdam et al., 2014).

Physical conditioning is achieved gradually over time. Many times, patients will "overdo it" in an attempt to achieve their goals too rapidly. Patients are observed for chest pain, dyspnea, weakness, fatigue, and palpitations and are instructed to stop exercise if any of these occur. Patients may also be monitored for an increase in heart rate above the target heart rate, an increase in systolic or diastolic blood pressure of more than 20 mm Hg, a decrease in systolic blood pressure, onset or worsening of dysrhythmias, or ST-segment changes on the ECG.

Cardiac rehabilitation programs are categorized into three phases (Fletcher, Ades, Kligfield, et al., 2013). Phase I begins with the diagnosis of atherosclerosis, which may occur when the patient is admitted to the hospital for ACS. Because of brief hospital lengths of stay, mobilization occurs early and patient education focuses on the essentials of self-care rather than instituting behavioral changes for risk reduction. Priorities for in-hospital education include the signs and symptoms that indicate the need to call 911 (seek emergency assistance), the medication regimen, rest–activity balance, and follow-up appointments with the primary provider. The patient is reassured that although CAD is a lifelong disease and must be treated as such, he or she can likely resume a normal life after an MI. The amount and type of activity recommended at discharge depend on the patient's age, his or her condition before the cardiac event, the extent of the disease, the course of the hospital stay, and the development of any complications.

Phase II occurs after the patient has been discharged. The patient attends sessions three times a week for 4 to 6 weeks but may continue for as long as 6 months. The outpatient program consists of supervised, often ECG-monitored, exercise training that is individualized. At each session, the patient is assessed for the effectiveness of and adherence to the treatment. To prevent complications and another hospitalization, the cardiac rehabilitation staff alerts the referring primary provider to any problems. Phase II cardiac rehabilitation also includes educational sessions for patients and families that are given by cardiologists, exercise physiologists, dietitians, nurses, and other health care professionals. These sessions may take place outside a traditional classroom setting. For instance, a dietitian may take a group of patients to a grocery store to examine labels and meat selections or to a restaurant to discuss menu offerings for a heart-healthy diet.

Phase III is a long-term outpatient program that focuses on maintaining cardiovascular stability and long-term conditioning. The patient is usually self-directed during this phase and does not require a supervised program, although it may be offered. The goals of each phase build on the accomplishments of the previous phase.

NURSING PROCESS
The Patient With Acute Coronary Syndrome

Assessment

One of the most important aspects of care of the patient with ACS is the assessment. It establishes the patient's baseline, identifies the patient's needs, and helps determine the priority of those needs. Systematic assessment includes a careful history, particularly as it relates to symptoms: chest pain or discomfort, difficulty breathing (dyspnea), palpitations, unusual fatigue, faintness (syncope), or other possible indicators of myocardial ischemia. Each symptom must be evaluated with regard to time, duration, and the factors that precipitate the symptom and relieve it, and in comparison with previous symptoms. A focused physical assessment is critical to detect complications and any change in patient status. Chart 27-6 identifies important assessments and possible findings.

Two IV lines are typically placed for any patient with ACS to ensure that access is available for administering emergency medications. Medications are administered IV to achieve rapid onset and to allow for timely adjustment. After the patient's condition stabilizes, IV lines may be changed to a saline lock to maintain IV access.

Diagnosis

NURSING DIAGNOSES

Based on the clinical manifestations, history, and diagnostic assessment data, major nursing diagnoses may include:

- Acute pain related to increased myocardial oxygen demand and decreased myocardial oxygen supply
- Risk for decreased cardiac tissue perfusion related to reduced coronary blood flow
- Risk for imbalanced fluid volume
- Risk for ineffective peripheral tissue perfusion related to decreased cardiac output from left ventricular dysfunction
- Anxiety related to cardiac event and possible death
- Deficient knowledge about post-ACS self-care

COLLABORATIVE PROBLEMS/POTENTIAL COMPLICATIONS

Potential complications may include the following:

- Acute pulmonary edema (see Chapter 29)
- Heart failure (see Chapter 29)
- Cardiogenic shock (see Chapter 14)
- Dysrhythmias and cardiac arrest (see Chapters 26 and 29)
- Pericardial effusion and cardiac tamponade (see Chapter 29)

Planning and Goals

The major goals for the patient include relief of pain or ischemic signs (e.g., ST-segment changes) and symptoms, prevention of myocardial damage, maintenance of effective respiratory function, maintenance or attainment of adequate tissue perfusion, reduced anxiety, adherence to the self-care program, and early recognition of complications. Care of the patient with ACS who has an uncomplicated MI is summarized in the Plan of Nursing Care (see Chart 27-9).

Nursing Interventions

RELIEVING PAIN AND OTHER SIGNS AND SYMPTOMS OF ISCHEMIA

Balancing myocardial oxygen supply with demand (e.g., as evidenced by the relief of chest pain) is the top priority in the care of the patient with an ACS. Although administering medications as described previously is required to accomplish this goal, nursing interventions are also important. Collaboration among the patient, nurse, and primary provider is critical in evaluating the patient's response to therapy and in altering the interventions accordingly.

Oxygen should be given along with medication therapy to assist with relief of symptoms. Administration of oxygen raises the circulating level of oxygen to reduce pain associated with low levels of myocardial oxygen. The route of administration (usually by nasal cannula) and the oxygen flow rate are documented. A flow rate of 2 to 4 L/min is usually adequate to maintain oxygen saturation levels of at least 95% unless chronic pulmonary disease is present.

Vital signs are assessed frequently as long as the patient is experiencing pain and other signs or symptoms of acute ischemia. Physical rest in bed with the head of the bed elevated or in a supportive chair helps decrease chest discomfort and dyspnea. Elevation of the head and torso is beneficial for the following reasons:

- Tidal volume improves because of reduced pressure from abdominal contents on the diaphragm and better lung expansion.

Chart 27-9

PLAN OF NURSING CARE

Care of the Patient With an Uncomplicated Myocardial Infarction

NURSING DIAGNOSIS: Risk for decreased cardiac tissue perfusion related to reduced coronary blood flow
GOAL: Relief of chest pain/discomfort

Nursing Interventions	Rationale	Expected Outcomes

1. Initially assess, document, and report to the primary provider the following:
 	
  a. The patient's description of chest discomfort, including location, intensity, radiation, duration, and factors that affect it; other symptoms such as nausea, diaphoresis, or complaints of unusual fatigue
  b. The effect of coronary ischemia on perfusion to the heart (e.g., change in blood pressure, heart rhythm), to the brain (e.g., changes in level of consciousness), to the kidneys (e.g., decrease in urine output), and to the skin (e.g., color, temperature)
2. Obtain a 12-lead ECG recording during symptomatic events, as prescribed, to assess for ongoing ischemia.
3. Administer oxygen as prescribed.
 	
4. Administer medication therapy as prescribed, and evaluate the patient's response continuously.
 	
5. Ensure physical rest: head of bed elevated to promote comfort; diet as tolerated; the use of bedside commode; the use of stool softener to prevent straining at stool. Provide a restful environment, and allay fears and anxiety by being calm and supportive. Individualize visitation, based on patient response.
	1. These data assist in determining the cause and effect of the chest discomfort and provide a baseline with which post-therapy symptoms can be compared.
	  a. There are many conditions associated with chest discomfort. There are characteristic clinical findings of ischemic pain and symptoms.
	
	  b. Myocardial infarction (MI) decreases myocardial contractility and ventricular compliance and may produce dysrhythmias. Cardiac output is reduced, resulting in reduced blood pressure and decreased organ perfusion.
	
	2. An ECG during symptoms may be useful in the diagnosis of ongoing ischemia.
	3. Oxygen therapy increases the oxygen supply to the myocardium.
	4. Medication therapy (nitroglycerin, morphine, beta-blocker, aspirin) is the first line of defense in preserving myocardial tissue.
	5. Physical rest reduces myocardial oxygen consumption. Fear and anxiety precipitate the stress response; this results in increased levels of endogenous catecholamines, which increase myocardial oxygen consumption.
		• Reports beginning relief of chest discomfort and symptoms
		• Appears comfortable and is free of pain and other signs or symptoms
		• Respiratory rate, cardiac rate, and blood pressure return to prediscomfort level
		• Skin warm and dry
		• Adequate cardiac output as evidenced by:
		  • Stable/improving electrocardiogram (ECG)
		  • Heart rate and rhythm
		  • Blood pressure
		  • Mentation
		  • Urine output
		  • Serum blood urea nitrogen (BUN) and creatinine
		  • Skin color and temperature
		• No adverse effects from medications

NURSING DIAGNOSIS: Risk for decreased cardiac output related to left ventricular failure
GOAL: Absence of respiratory distress

Nursing Interventions	Rationale	Expected Outcomes
1. Initially, every 4 hours, and with chest discomfort or symptoms, assess, document, and report to the primary provider abnormal heart sounds (S_3 and S_4 gallop or new murmur), abnormal breath sounds (particularly crackles), decreased oxygenation, and activity intolerance.	1. These data are useful in diagnosing left ventricular failure. Diastolic filling sounds (S_3 and S_4) result from decreased left ventricular compliance associated with MI. Papillary muscle dysfunction (from infarction of the papillary muscle) can result in mitral regurgitation and a reduction in stroke volume. The presence of crackles (usually at the lung bases) may indicate pulmonary congestion from increased left heart pressures. The association of symptoms and activity can be used as a guide for activity prescription and a basis for patient education.	• No shortness of breath, dyspnea on exertion, orthopnea, or paroxysmal nocturnal dyspnea • Respiratory rate <20 breaths/min with physical activity and 16 breaths/min with rest • Skin color and temperature normal • SpO_2, PaO_2, and $PaCO_2$ within normal limits • Heart rate <100 bpm and >60 bpm, with blood pressure within patient's normal limits • Chest x-ray unchanged • Appears comfortable and rested

PLAN OF NURSING CARE (Continued)

Chart 27-9

Care of the Patient With an Uncomplicated Myocardial Infarction

NURSING DIAGNOSIS: Risk for ineffective peripheral tissue perfusion related to decreased cardiac output
GOAL: Maintenance/attainment of adequate tissue perfusion

Nursing Interventions	Rationale	Expected Outcomes
1. Initially, every 4 hours, and with chest discomfort, assess, document, and report to the primary provider the following: a. Hypotension b. Tachycardia and other dysrhythmia c. Activity intolerance d. Mentation changes (use family input) e. Reduced urine output (<0.5 mL/kg/h) f. Cool, moist, cyanotic extremities, decreased peripheral pulses, prolonged capillary refill	1. These data are useful in determining a low cardiac output state.	• Blood pressure within the patient's normal range • Ideally, normal sinus rhythm without dysrhythmia is maintained, or patient's baseline rhythm is maintained between 60 and 100 bpm without further dysrhythmia. • Prescribed activity is well tolerated. • Remains alert and oriented and without cognitive or behavioral change • Appears comfortable • Urine output >0.5 mL/kg/h • Extremities warm and dry with normal color

NURSING DIAGNOSIS: Anxiety related to cardiac event
GOAL: Reduction of anxiety

Nursing Interventions	Rationale	Expected Outcomes
1. Assess, document, and report to the primary provider the patient's and family's level of anxiety and coping mechanisms.	1. These data provide information about psychological well-being. Causes of anxiety are variable and individual, and may include acute illness, hospitalization, pain, disruption of activities of daily living at home and at work, changes in role and self-image due to illness, and financial concerns. Because anxious family members can transmit anxiety to the patient, the nurse must also identify strategies to reduce the family's fear and anxiety.	• Reports less anxiety • The patient and family discuss their anxieties and fears about illness and death. • The patient and family appear less anxious. • Appears restful, respiratory rate <16 breaths/min, heart rate <100 bpm without ectopic beats, blood pressure within patient's normal limits, skin warm and dry • Participates actively in a progressive rehabilitation program • Practices stress reduction techniques
2. Assess the need for spiritual counseling and refer as appropriate.	2. If a patient finds support in a religion, spiritual counseling may assist in reducing anxiety and fear.	
3. Assess the need for social service referral.	3. Social services can assist with posthospital care and financial concerns.	

NURSING DIAGNOSIS: Deficient knowledge about post-MI self-care
GOAL: Adheres to the home health care program; chooses lifestyle consistent with heart-healthy recommendations See Chart 27-10.

• Drainage of the upper lung lobes improves.
• Venous return to the heart (preload) decreases, reducing the work of the heart.

The pain associated with an acute MI reflects an imbalance in myocardial oxygen supply and demand or ineffective myocardial tissue perfusion. The pain also results in increases in heart rate, respiratory rate, and blood pressure. Promptly relieving the pain helps to reestablish this balance, thus decreasing the workload of the heart and minimizing damage to the myocardium. Relief of pain also helps to reduce the patient's anxiety level, which in turn reduces the sympathetic stress response, leading to a decrease in workload of the already stressed heart.

IMPROVING RESPIRATORY FUNCTION

Regular and careful assessment of respiratory function detects early signs of pulmonary complications. The nurse monitors fluid volume status to prevent fluid overload and encourages

the patient to breathe deeply and change position frequently to maintain effective ventilation throughout the lungs. Pulse oximetry guides the use of oxygen therapy.

PROMOTING ADEQUATE TISSUE PERFUSION

Bed or chair rest during the initial phase of treatment helps reduce myocardial oxygen consumption. This limitation on mobility should remain until the patient is pain free and hemodynamically stable. Skin temperature and peripheral pulses must be checked frequently to monitor tissue perfusion.

REDUCING ANXIETY

Alleviating anxiety and decreasing fear are important nursing functions that reduce the sympathetic stress response. Less sympathetic stimulation decreases the workload of the heart, which may relieve pain and other signs and symptoms of ischemia.

Chart 27-10

HEALTH PROMOTION

Promoting Health After Myocardial Infarction and Other Acute Coronary Syndromes

To extend and improve the quality of life, a patient who has had a myocardial infarction (MI) must make lifestyle adjustments to promote heart-healthy living. With this in mind, the nurse and patient develop a program to help achieve desired outcomes.

Making Lifestyle Modifications During Convalescence and Healing

Adaptation to an MI is an ongoing process and usually requires some modification of lifestyle. Educate patients to make the following specific modifications:

- Avoid any activity that produces chest pain, extreme dyspnea, or undue fatigue.
- Avoid extremes of heat and cold and walking against the wind.
- Lose weight, if indicated.
- Stop smoking and the use of tobacco; avoid secondhand smoke.
- Develop heart-healthy eating patterns, and avoid large meals and hurrying while eating.
- Modify meals to align with the Therapeutic Lifestyle Changes (TLC) or other recommended diets.
- Adhere to medical regimen, especially in taking medications.
- Follow recommendations that ensure that blood pressure and blood glucose are in control.
- Pursue activities that relieve and reduce stress.

Adopting an Activity Program

In addition, the patient needs to undertake a structured program of activity and exercise for long-term rehabilitation. Advise patients to:

- Engage in a regimen of physical conditioning with a gradual increase in activity duration and then a gradual increase in activity intensity.
- Enroll in a cardiac rehabilitation program.
- Walk daily, increasing distance and time as prescribed.
- Monitor pulse rate during physical activity.
- Avoid physical exercise immediately after a meal.
- Alternate activity with rest periods (some fatigue is normal and expected during convalescence).
- Participate in a daily program of exercise that develops into a program of regular exercise for a lifetime.

Managing Symptoms

The patient must learn to recognize and take appropriate action for recurrent symptoms. Make sure that patients know to do the following:

- Call 911 if chest pressure or pain (or prodromal symptoms) is not relieved in 15 minutes by taking 3 nitroglycerin tablets at 5-minute intervals.
- Contact the primary provider if any of the following occur: shortness of breath, fainting, slow or rapid heartbeat, swelling of feet and ankles.

The development of a trusting and caring relationship with the patient is critical in reducing anxiety. Providing information to the patient and family in an honest and supportive manner encourages the patient to be a partner in care and greatly assists in developing a positive relationship. Other interventions that can be used to reduce anxiety include ensuring a quiet environment, preventing interruptions that disturb sleep, and providing spiritual support consistent with the patient's beliefs. The nurse provides frequent opportunities for the patient to privately share concerns and fears. An atmosphere of acceptance helps the patient know that these concerns and fears are both realistic and normal. Alternative therapies such as pet therapy can help certain patients relax and reduce anxiety (Sehr, Eisele-Hlubocky, Junker, et al., 2013). Many hospitals have developed infection control and safety procedures pertaining to the animals, their handlers, and the patients eligible for pet therapy.

MONITORING AND MANAGING POTENTIAL COMPLICATIONS

Complications that can occur after acute MI are caused by the damage that occurs to the myocardium and to the conduction system from reduced coronary blood flow. Because these complications can be life-threatening, close monitoring for and early identification of their signs and symptoms are critical (see Chart 27-9).

The nurse monitors the patient closely for changes in cardiac rate and rhythm, heart sounds, blood pressure, chest pain, respiratory status, urinary output, skin color and temperature, mental status, ECG changes, and laboratory values. Any changes in the patient's condition must be reported promptly to the primary provider and emergency measures instituted when necessary.

PROMOTING HOME, COMMUNITY-BASED, AND TRANSITIONAL CARE

Educating Patients About Self-Care. The most effective way to increase the probability that the patient will implement a self-care regimen after discharge is to identify the patient's priorities, provide adequate education about heart-healthy living, and facilitate the patient's involvement in a cardiac rehabilitation program (Amsterdam et al., 2014). Patient participation in the development of an individualized program enhances the potential for an effective treatment plan (see Chart 27-10).

Continuing and Transitional Care. Depending on the patient's condition and the availability of family assistance, home, community-based, or transitional, care may be indicated. The nurse making a home visit can assist the patient with scheduling and keeping follow-up appointments and with adhering to the prescribed cardiac rehabilitation regimen. The patient may need reminders about follow-up monitoring, including periodic laboratory testing, as well as ongoing assessment of cardiac status. In addition, the home care nurse monitors the patient's adherence to dietary restrictions and to prescribed medications. If the patient is receiving home oxygen, the nurse ensures that the patient is using the oxygen as prescribed and that appropriate home safety measures are maintained. If the patient has evidence of heart failure secondary to an MI, appropriate home care guidelines for the patient with heart failure are followed (see Chapter 29).

Evaluation

Expected patient outcomes may include:

1. Experiences relief of angina
2. Has stable cardiac and respiratory status
3. Maintains adequate tissue perfusion

4. Exhibits decreased anxiety
5. Adheres to a self-care program
6. Has no complications

INVASIVE CORONARY ARTERY PROCEDURES

Methods to reperfuse ischemic myocardial tissue when patients are refractory to more conservative management methods include PCIs and CABG surgery, as noted previously. The following sections discuss specific indications for each of these and the nursing management of patients who are having either PCIs or CABGs.

Percutaneous Coronary Interventions

Types of Procedures

Invasive interventional procedures to treat CAD include PTCA and intracoronary stent implantation. These procedures are classified as **percutaneous coronary interventions (PCIs),** as they are performed through a skin puncture rather than a surgical incision.

Percutaneous Transluminal Coronary Angioplasty

In **percutaneous transluminal coronary angioplasty (PTCA)**, a balloon-tipped catheter is used to open blocked coronary vessels and resolve ischemia. It is used in patients with angina and as an intervention for ACS. Catheter-based interventions can also be used to open blocked CABGs (see later discussion). The purpose of PTCA is to improve blood flow within a coronary artery by compressing the atheroma. The procedure is attempted when the interventional cardiologist believes that PTCA can improve blood flow to the myocardium.

PTCA is carried out in the cardiac catheterization laboratory. Hollow catheters called *sheaths* are inserted, usually in the femoral artery (and sometimes the radial artery), providing a conduit for other catheters. Catheters are then threaded through the femoral artery, up through the aorta, and into the coronary arteries. Angiography is performed using injected radiopaque contrast agents (commonly called *dye*) to identify the location and extent of the blockage. A balloon-tipped dilation catheter is passed through the sheath and positioned over the lesion. The physician determines the catheter position by examining markers on the balloon that can be seen with fluoroscopy. When the catheter is properly positioned, the balloon is inflated with high pressure for several seconds and then deflated. The pressure compresses and often "cracks" the atheroma (see Fig. 27-8). The media and adventitia of the coronary artery are also stretched.

Several inflations with different balloon sizes may be required to achieve the goal, usually defined as an improvement in blood flow and a residual stenosis of less than 30% (Urden et al., 2014). Other measures of the success of PTCA are an increase in the artery's lumen and no clinically obvious arterial trauma. Because the blood supply to the coronary artery decreases while the balloon is inflated, the patient may complain of chest pain and the ECG may display ST-segment changes. Intracoronary stents are usually positioned in the intima of the vessel to maintain patency of the artery after the balloon is withdrawn.

Coronary Artery Stent

After PTCA, the area that has been treated may close off partially or completely—a process called *restenosis*. The intima of the coronary artery has been injured and responds

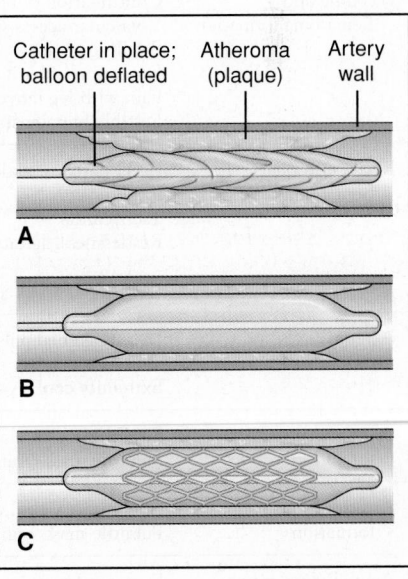

Figure 27-8 • Percutaneous transluminal coronary angioplasty. **A.** A balloon-tipped catheter is passed into the affected coronary artery and placed across the area of the atheroma (plaque). **B.** The balloon is then rapidly inflated and deflated with controlled pressure. **C.** A stent is placed to maintain patency of the artery, and the balloon is removed.

by initiating an acute inflammatory process. This process may include release of mediators that leads to vasoconstriction, clotting, and scar tissue formation. A coronary artery stent may be placed to overcome these risks. A **stent** is a metal mesh that provides structural support to a vessel at risk of acute closure. The stent is initially positioned over the angioplasty balloon. When the balloon is inflated, the mesh expands and presses against the vessel wall, holding the artery open. The balloon is withdrawn, but the stent is left permanently in place within the artery (see Fig. 27-8). Eventually, endothelium covers the stent and it is incorporated into the vessel wall. The original stents do not contain medications and are known as bare metal stents. Some stents are coated with medications, such as sirolimus (Rapamune) or paclitaxel (Taxol), which may minimize the formation of thrombi or scar tissue within the coronary artery lesion. These drug-eluting stents have increased the success of PCI (Palmerini, Benedetto, Biondi-Zoccai, et al., 2015). Because of the risk of thrombus formation within the stent, the patient receives antiplatelet medications, usually aspirin and clopidogrel. Aspirin should be continued indefinitely and clopidogrel is continued for 1 year following stent placement (Amsterdam et al., 2014).

Complications

Complications that can occur during a PCI procedure include coronary artery dissection, perforation, abrupt closure, or vasospasm. Additional complications include acute MI, serious dysrhythmias (e.g., ventricular tachycardia), and cardiac arrest. Some of these complications may require emergency surgical treatment. Complications after the procedure may include abrupt closure of the coronary artery and a variety of vascular complications, such as bleeding at the insertion site, retroperitoneal bleeding, hematoma, and arterial occlusion (Douglas & Applegate, 2013). In addition, there is a risk of acute kidney injury from the contrast agent used during the procedure (see Table 27-4).

Postprocedure Care

Patient care is similar to that for a diagnostic cardiac catheterization (see Chapter 25). Patients who are not already hospitalized are admitted the day of the PCI. Those with no complications go home the next day. When the PCI is performed emergently to treat ACS, patients typically go to a critical care unit and stay in the hospital for a few days. During the PCI, patients receive IV heparin or a thrombin inhibitor (e.g., bivalirudin [Angiomax]) and are monitored closely for signs of bleeding. Patients may also receive a GP IIb/IIIa agent (e.g., eptifibatide) for several hours following the PCI to prevent platelet aggregation and thrombus formation in the coronary artery (Amsterdam et al., 2014). Hemostasis is achieved, and femoral sheaths may be removed at the end of the procedure by using a vascular closure device

TABLE 27-4 Complications After Percutaneous Coronary Interventions

Complication	Clinical Manifestations	Possible Causes	Nursing Actions
Myocardial ischemia	Chest pain Ischemic changes on ECG Dysrhythmias	Thrombosis Restenosis of coronary artery	Administer oxygen and nitroglycerin. Obtain 12-lead ECG. Notify cardiologist.
Bleeding and hematoma formation	Continuation of bleeding from vascular access site Swelling at site Formation of hard lump Pain with leg movement Possible hypotension and tachycardia	Anticoagulant therapy Vascular trauma Inadequate hemostasis Leg movement	Keep patient on bed rest. Apply manual pressure over sheath insertion site. Outline hematoma with marking pen. Notify primary provider if bleeding continues.
Retroperitoneal hematoma	Back, flank, or abdominal pain Hypotension Tachycardia Restlessness, agitation	Arterial leak of blood into the retroperitoneal space	Notify primary provider. Stop anticoagulants. Administer IV fluids. Anticipate diagnostic testing (e.g., computed tomography scan). Prepare patient for intervention.
Arterial occlusion	Lost/weakened pulse distal to sheath insertion site Extremity cool, cyanotic, painful	Arterial thrombus or embolus	Notify primary provider. Anticipate intervention.
Pseudoaneurysm formation	Swelling at vascular access site Pulsatile mass, bruit	Vessel trauma during the procedure	Notify primary provider. Anticipate intervention.
Arteriovenous fistula formation	Swelling at vascular access site Pulsatile mass, bruit	Vessel trauma during the procedure	Notify primary provider. Anticipate intervention.
Acute kidney injury	Decreased urine output Elevated BUN, serum creatinine	Nephrotoxic contrast agent	Monitor urine output, BUN, creatinine, electrolytes. Provide adequate hydration. Administer renal protective agents (acetylcysteine) before and after procedure as prescribed.

ECG, electrocardiogram; IV, intravenous; BUN, blood urea nitrogen.
Adapted from Urden, L. D., Stacy, K. M., & Lough, M.E. (2014). *Critical care nursing* (7th ed.). St. Louis, MO: Elsevier.

(e.g., Angio-Seal, VasoSeal) or a device that sutures the vessels. Hemostasis after sheath removal may also be achieved by direct manual pressure, a mechanical compression device (e.g., C-shaped clamp), or a pneumatic compression device (e.g., FemoStop).

Patients may return to the nursing unit with the large peripheral vascular access sheaths in place. The sheaths are then removed after blood studies (e.g., activated clotting time) indicate that the heparin is no longer active and the clotting time is within an acceptable range. This usually takes a few hours, depending on the amount of heparin given during the procedure. The patient must remain flat in bed and keep the affected leg straight until the sheaths are removed and then for a few hours afterward to maintain hemostasis. Because immobility and bed rest may cause discomfort, treatment may include analgesics and sedation. Nonpharmacologic interventions include repositioning and heat application for back pain. Sheath removal and the application of pressure on the vessel insertion site may cause the heart rate to slow and the blood pressure to decrease (vasovagal response). A dose of IV atropine is usually given to treat this response.

Some patients with unstable lesions and at high risk for abrupt vessel closure are restarted on heparin after sheath removal, or they receive an IV infusion of a GP IIb/IIIa inhibitor. These patients are monitored closely and may have a delayed recovery period.

After hemostasis is achieved, a pressure dressing is applied to the site. Patients resume self-care and ambulate unassisted within a few hours of the procedure. The duration of immobilization depends on the size of the sheath inserted, the type of anticoagulant given, the method of hemostasis, the patient's condition, and the physician's preference. On the day after the procedure, the site is inspected and the dressing removed. The patient is instructed to monitor the site for bleeding or development of a hard mass indicative of hematoma.

Surgical Procedures: Coronary Artery Revascularization

Advances in diagnostics, medical management, and surgical and anesthesia techniques, as well as the care provided in critical care and surgical units, home care, and rehabilitation programs, have continued to make surgery an effective treatment option for patients with CAD. CAD has been treated by myocardial revascularization since the 1960s, and the most common CABG techniques have been performed for more than 40 years. **Coronary artery bypass graft (CABG)** is a surgical procedure in which a blood vessel is grafted to an occluded coronary artery so that blood can flow beyond the occlusion; it is also called a *bypass graft*.

The major indications for CABG are:
- Alleviation of angina that cannot be controlled with medication or PCI
- Treatment for left main coronary artery stenosis or multivessel CAD
- Prevention of and treatment for MI, dysrhythmias, or heart failure
- Treatment for complications from an unsuccessful PCI

The recommendation for CABG is determined by a number of factors, including the number of diseased coronary vessels, the degree of left ventricular dysfunction, the presence of other health problems, the patient's symptoms, and any previous treatment. CABG and PCI have shown similar results in outcomes, such as MI rate, mortality, and improvement of angina post-intervention. However, the requirement of a second reperfusion intervention has been shown to be lower with CABG compared to PCI therapy (Bravo, Rondon Clavo, Oliva, et al., 2014).

CABG is performed less frequently in women (Ferrari, Abergel, Ford, et al., 2013). Compared with men, women referred for this surgery tend to be older and have more comorbidities such as diabetes. In addition, they have a higher risk of surgical complications and increased mortality (Pollock, Hamman, Sass, et al., 2015). Although some women have good outcomes following CABG, men generally have a better rate of graft patency and symptom relief.

For a patient to be considered for CABG, the coronary arteries to be bypassed must have at least a 70% occlusion, or at least a 50% occlusion if in the left main coronary artery (Hillis, Smith, Anderson, et al., 2011). If significant blockage is not present, flow through the artery will compete with flow through the bypass, and circulation to the ischemic area of myocardium may not improve. The artery also must be patent beyond the area of blockage or the flow through the bypass will be impeded.

Current guidelines recommend that the internal mammary artery should be used for CABG, if possible. Recent studies demonstrate increased survival when using bilateral internal mammary artery grafting (Yi, Shine, Rehman, et al., 2014). Arterial grafts are preferred to venous grafts because they do not develop atherosclerotic changes as quickly and remain patent longer. The surgeon leaves the proximal end of the mammary artery intact and detaches the distal end of the artery from the chest wall. This end of the artery is then grafted to the coronary artery distal to the occlusion. The internal mammary arteries may not be long enough to use for multiple bypasses. Because of this, many CABG procedures are performed with a combination of venous and arterial grafts.

A vein commonly used for CABG is the greater saphenous vein, followed by the lesser saphenous vein (see Fig. 27-9). The vein is removed from the leg and grafted to the ascending aorta and to the coronary artery distal to the lesion. Traditionally, a skin incision was made over the length of vein segment, but new techniques allow small leg incisions. Endovascular methods of vein harvesting have reduced complications such as infection and wound dehiscence, which are associated with longer leg incisions (Raja & Sarang, 2013). Lower extremity edema continues to be a common adverse effect of vein removal. The degree of edema varies and usually diminishes over time. The patency of vein grafts can be limited. Within 5 to 10 years, atherosclerotic changes often develop in saphenous vein grafts.

Traditional Coronary Artery Bypass Graft

CABG procedures are performed with the patient under general anesthesia. In the traditional CABG procedure, the surgeon performs a median sternotomy and connects the patient

Figure 27-9 • The greater and lesser saphenous veins are commonly used in bypass graft procedures.

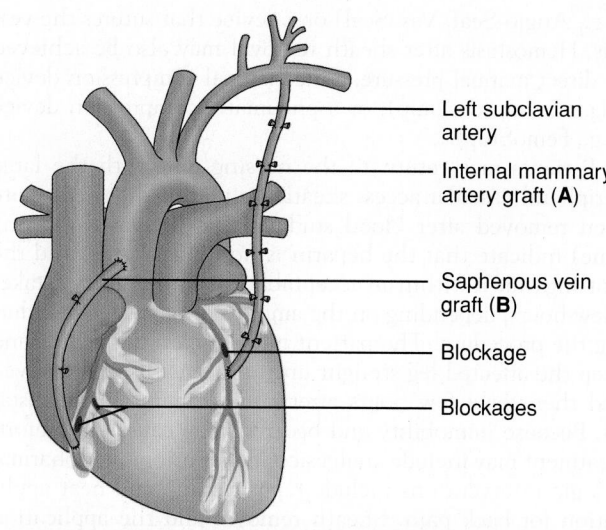

Figure 27-10 • Coronary artery bypass grafts. One or more procedures may be performed using various veins and arteries. **A.** Left internal mammary artery, used frequently because of its functional longevity. **B.** Saphenous vein, also used as bypass graft.

to the cardiopulmonary bypass (CPB) machine. Next, a blood vessel from another part of the patient's body (e.g., saphenous vein, left internal mammary artery) is grafted distal to the coronary artery lesion, bypassing the obstruction (see Fig. 27-10). CPB is then discontinued, chest tubes and epicardial pacing wires are placed, and the incision is closed. The patient is then admitted to a critical care unit.

Cardiopulmonary Bypass

Many cardiac surgical procedures are possible because of CPB (i.e., extracorporeal circulation). The procedure mechanically circulates and oxygenates blood for the body while bypassing the heart and lungs. CPB maintains perfusion to body organs and tissues and allows the surgeon to complete the anastomoses in a motionless, bloodless surgical field.

CPB is accomplished by placing a cannula in the right atrium, vena cava, or femoral vein to withdraw blood from the body. The cannula is connected to tubing filled with an isotonic crystalloid solution. Venous blood removed from the body by the cannula is filtered, oxygenated, cooled or warmed by the machine, and then returned to the body. The cannula used to return the oxygenated blood is usually inserted in the ascending aorta, or it may be inserted in the femoral artery (see Fig. 27-11). The heart is stopped by the injection of a potassium-rich cardioplegia solution into the coronary arteries. The patient receives heparin to prevent clotting and thrombus formation in the bypass circuit when blood comes

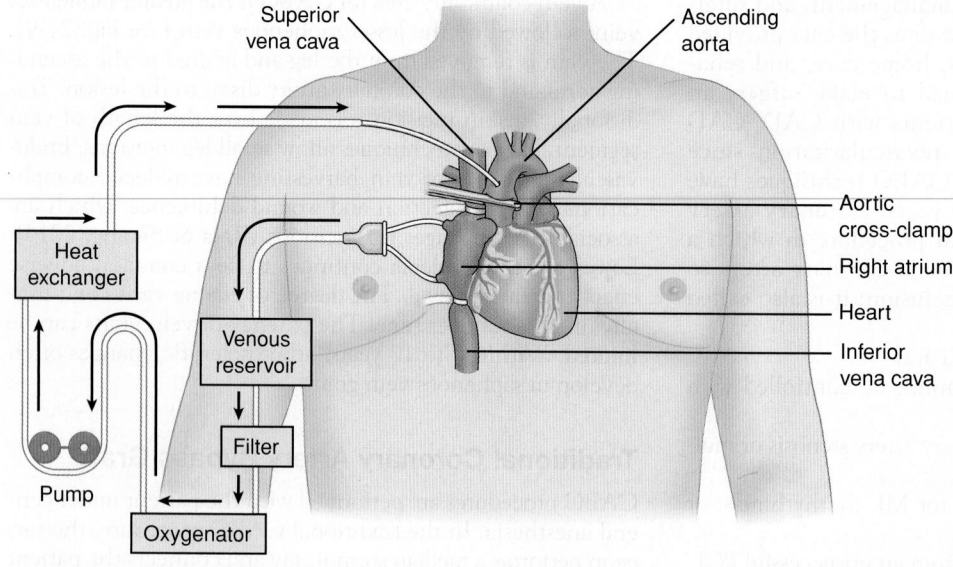

Figure 27-11 • The cardiopulmonary bypass system, in which cannulas are placed through the right atrium into the superior and inferior vena cavae to divert blood from the body and into the bypass system. The pump system creates a vacuum, pulling blood into the venous reservoir. The blood is cleared of air bubbles, clots, and particulates by the filter and then is passed through the oxygenator, releasing carbon dioxide and obtaining oxygen. Next, the blood is pulled to the pump and pushed out to the heat exchanger, where its temperature is regulated. The blood is then returned to the body via the ascending aorta.

in contact with the surfaces of the tubing. At the end of the procedure when the patient is disconnected from the bypass machine, protamine sulfate is given to reverse the effects of heparin.

During the procedure, hypothermia is maintained at a temperature of about 28°C (82.4°F) (Urden et al., 2014). The blood is cooled during CPB and returned to the body. The cooled blood slows the body's basal metabolic rate, thereby decreasing the demand for oxygen. Cooled blood usually has a higher viscosity, but the crystalloid solution used to prime the bypass tubing dilutes the blood. When the surgical procedure is completed, the blood is rewarmed as it passes through the CPB circuit. Urine output, arterial blood gases, electrolytes, and coagulation studies are monitored to assess the patient's status during CPB.

Alternative Coronary Artery Bypass Graft Techniques

A number of alternative CABG techniques have been developed that may have fewer complications for some groups of patients. Off-pump coronary artery bypass (OPCAB) surgery has been used successfully in many patients. OPCAB involves a standard median sternotomy incision, but the surgery is performed without CPB. A beta-adrenergic blocker may be used to slow the heart rate. The surgeon also uses a myocardial stabilization device to hold the site still for the anastomosis of the bypass graft into the coronary artery while the heart continues to beat (see Fig. 27-12). Research suggests that OPCAB is associated with reduced short-term postoperative morbidity, including stroke and other complications. However, with on-pump CABG, graft patency rate is higher and long-term mortality may be lower (Kim, Yun, Lim, et al., 2014).

Minimally invasive surgical techniques that eliminate median sternotomy have also been developed. These endoscopic techniques use smaller incisions and a robotic system

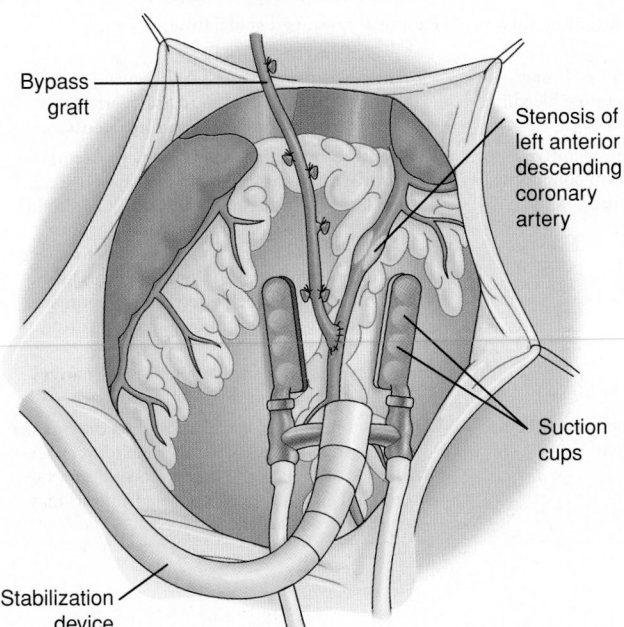

Bypass graft

Stenosis of left anterior descending coronary artery

Suction cups

Stabilization device

Figure 27-12 • Stabilizer device for off-pump coronary artery bypass surgery.

to place bypass grafts. The patient is placed on CPB via the femoral vessels. Minimally invasive heart surgery is developing into a high-quality alternative to conventional CABG. It has allowed patients to recover earlier, require fewer blood transfusions, and experience fewer infections (Ruel, Une, Bonatti, et al., 2013).

Complications of Coronary Artery Bypass Graft

CABG may result in complications such as hemorrhage, dysrhythmias, and MI (see Table 27-5). The patient may require interventions for more than one complication at a time. Collaboration among nurses, physicians, pharmacists, respiratory therapists, and dietitians is necessary to achieve the desired patient outcomes. Although most patients improve symptomatically following surgery, CABG is not a cure for CAD, and angina, exercise intolerance, or other symptoms experienced before CABG may recur. Medications required before surgery may need to be continued. Lifestyle modifications recommended before surgery remain important to treat the underlying CAD and for the continued viability of the newly implanted grafts.

 Nursing Management

Cardiac surgery patients have many of the same needs and require the same perioperative care as other surgical patients (see Chapters 17 through 19), as well as some special needs.

Preoperative Management

Comprehensive preoperative medical management prevents complications and improves outcomes. This is particularly important because patients undergoing CABG surgery tend to be older and often have multiple comorbidities. The use of aspirin, beta-blockers, and statins during the preoperative period, along with the assessment of hematocrit and glucose levels, is among the interventions associated with better outcomes (Chaisson, Sanford, Boss, et al., 2014). Preoperative use of aspirin is associated with a reduction in perioperative morbidity and mortality. Beta-blockers, when given at least 24 hours before CABG, reduce the incidence of postoperative atrial fibrillation. Perioperative use of statins has been shown to reduce the rates of postoperative MI, atrial fibrillation, neurological dysfunction, renal dysfunction, infection, and death (Hillis et al., 2011).

Assessing the Patient

Patients are frequently admitted to the hospital the day of the procedure. Therefore, most of the preoperative evaluation is completed in the physician's office and during preadmission testing.

Nursing and medical personnel perform a history and physical examination. Preoperative testing consists of a chest x-ray; ECG; laboratory tests, including coagulation studies; and blood typing and cross-matching. The preoperative history and health assessment should be thorough and well documented because they provide a basis for postoperative comparison. The nurse assesses the patient for disorders that could complicate or affect the postoperative course, such as diabetes, hypertension, and lung disease.

The health assessment focuses on obtaining baseline physiologic, psychological, and social information. Cognitive status

TABLE 27-5 Potential Complications of Cardiac Surgery

Complication	Cause	Assessment and Management
Cardiac Complications		
Hypovolemia (most common cause of decreased cardiac output after cardiac surgery)	Net loss of blood and intravascular volume Vasodilation due to postoperative rewarming Intravascular fluid loss to the interstitial spaces because surgery and anesthesia increase capillary permeability	Arterial hypotension, tachycardia, low CVP, and low PAWP are often seen. Fluid replacement may be prescribed. Replacement fluids include colloid (albumin), packed red blood cells, or crystalloid solution (normal saline, lactated Ringer's solution).
Persistent bleeding	Cardiopulmonary bypass causes platelet dysfunction, and hypothermia alters clotting mechanisms. Surgical trauma causes tissues and blood vessels to ooze bloody drainage. Intraoperative anticoagulant (heparin) therapy Postoperative coagulopathy may also result from liver dysfunction and depletion of clotting components.	Accurate measurement of wound bleeding and chest tube blood is essential. Drainage should not exceed 200 mL/h for the first 4–6 hours. Drainage should decrease and stop within a few days, while progressing from serosanguinous to serous. Serial hemoglobin, hematocrit, and coagulation studies guide therapy. Administration of blood products: packed red blood cells, fresh frozen plasma, platelet concentrate, recombinant factor VII Protamine sulfate may be given to neutralize unfractionated heparin. Administration of desmopressin acetate (DDAVP) to enhance platelet function If bleeding persists, the patient may return to the operating room.
Cardiac tamponade	Fluid and clots accumulate in the pericardial sac, which compress the heart, preventing blood from filling the ventricles.	Signs and symptoms include arterial hypotension, tachycardia, decreased urine output, and ↑ CVP. Arterial pressure waveform may show pulsus paradoxus (decrease of >10 mm Hg systolic blood pressure during inspiration). The chest drainage system is checked to eliminate possible kinks or obstructions in the tubing. Chest x-ray may show a widening mediastinum. Emergency medical management is required; may include return to surgery.
Fluid overload	IV fluids and blood products increase circulating volume.	High CVP and pulmonary artery pressures, as well as crackles, indicate fluid overload. Diuretics are prescribed, and the rate of IV fluid administration is reduced. Alternative treatments include continuous renal replacement therapy and dialysis.
Hypothermia	Low body temperature leads to vasoconstriction, shivering, and arterial hypertension.	Patient is rewarmed gradually after surgery, decreasing vasoconstriction.
Hypertension	Results from postoperative vasoconstriction. It may stretch suture lines and cause postoperative bleeding. The condition is usually transient.	Vasodilators (nitroglycerin [Tridil], nitroprusside [Nipride]) may be used to treat hypertension. Administer cautiously to avoid hypotension.
Tachydysrhythmias	Increased heart rate is common with perioperative volume changes. Rapid atrial fibrillation commonly occurs during the first few days postoperatively.	If a tachydysrhythmia is the primary problem, the heart rhythm is assessed and medications (e.g., amiodarone [Cordarone], diltiazem [Cardizem]) may be prescribed. Antidysrhythmic agents (e.g., beta-blockers) are often given before coronary artery bypass graft to minimize the risk. Carotid massage may be performed by a primary provider to assist with diagnosing or treating the dysrhythmia. Cardioversion and defibrillation are alternatives for symptomatic tachydysrhythmias.
Bradycardias	Decreased heart rate due to surgical trauma and edema affecting the cardiac conduction system	Many postoperative patients have temporary pacer wires that can be attached to an external pacemaker to stimulate the heart to beat faster. Less commonly, atropine or other medications may be used to increase heart rate.

TABLE 27-5 Potential Complications of Cardiac Surgery (continued)

Complication	Cause	Assessment and Management
Cardiac failure	Myocardial contractility may be decreased perioperatively.	The nurse observes for and reports signs of heart failure, including hypotension, ↑ CVP, ↑ PAWP, venous distention; labored respirations; and edema. Medical management includes diuretics and IV inotropic agents.
MI (may occur intraoperatively or postoperatively)	Portion of the cardiac muscle dies; therefore, contractility decreases. Impaired ventricular wall motion further decreases cardiac output. Symptoms may be masked by the postoperative surgical discomfort or the anesthesia–analgesia regimen.	Careful assessment to determine the type of pain the patient is experiencing; MI is suspected if the mean blood pressure is low with normal preload. Serial electrocardiograms and cardiac biomarkers assist in making the diagnosis (alterations may be due to the surgical intervention).
Pulmonary Complications		
Impaired gas exchange	During and after anesthesia, patients require mechanical assistance to breathe. Anesthetic agents stimulate production of mucus, and chest incision pain may decrease the effectiveness of ventilation. Potential for postoperative atelectasis	Pulmonary complications are detected during assessment of breath sounds, oxygen saturation levels, arterial blood gases, and ventilator readings. Extended periods of mechanical ventilation may be required while complications are treated.
Neurologic Complications		
Neurologic changes; stroke	Thrombi and emboli may cause cerebral infarction, and neurologic signs may be evident when patients recover from anesthesia.	Inability to follow simple commands within 6 hours of recovery from anesthetic; weakness on one side of body or other neurologic changes may indicate stroke. Patients who are older or who have renal or hepatic failure may take longer to recover from anesthesia.
Kidney Injury and Electrolyte Imbalance		
Acute kidney injury	May result from hypoperfusion of the kidneys or from injury to the renal tubules by nephrotoxic drugs	May respond to diuretics or may require continuous renal replacement therapy or dialysis Fluids, electrolytes, and urine output are monitored frequently. May result in chronic kidney injury and require ongoing dialysis
Electrolyte imbalance	Postoperative imbalances in potassium, magnesium, sodium, calcium, and blood glucose are related to surgical losses, metabolic changes, and the administration of medications and IV fluids.	Monitor electrolytes and basic metabolic studies frequently. Implement treatment to correct electrolyte imbalance promptly (see Chart 27-11).
Other Complications		
Hepatic failure	Surgery and anesthesia stress the liver. Most common in patients with cirrhosis, hepatitis, or prolonged right-sided heart failure.	The use of medications metabolized by the liver must be minimized. Bilirubin and albumin levels are monitored, and nutritional support is provided.
Infection	Surgery and anesthesia alter the patient's immune system. Multiple invasive devices used to monitor and support the patient's recovery may serve as a source of infection.	Monitor for signs of possible infection: body temperature, white blood cell and differential counts, incision and puncture sites, urine (clarity, color, and odor), bilateral breath sounds, sputum (color, odor, amount). Antibiotic therapy may be instituted or modified as necessary. Invasive devices are discontinued as soon as they are no longer required. Institutional protocols for maintaining and replacing invasive lines and devices are followed to minimize the risk of infection.

CVP, central venous pressure; PAWP, pulmonary artery wedge pressure; ↑, increased; IV, intravenous; MI, myocardial infarction.
Adapted from Urden, L. D., Stacy, K. M., & Lough, M.E. (2014). *Critical care nursing* (7th ed.). St. Louis, MO: Elsevier.

is carefully assessed, as patients with impaired cognitive status will need more assistance after surgery and may require subacute care prior to returning home. Older adults are at a high risk for suffering adverse cognitive outcomes following cardiac surgery (Bartels, McDonagh, Newman, et al., 2013). The patient's and family's learning needs are identified and addressed. Of particular importance are the patient's usual functional level, coping mechanisms, and available support systems. These affect the patient's postoperative course, discharge plans, and rehabilitation.

The status of the cardiovascular system is determined by reviewing the patient's symptoms, including past and present experiences with chest pain, palpitations, dyspnea, leg pain that occurs with walking (intermittent claudication), and peripheral edema. The patient's history of major illnesses; previous surgeries; medication; and the use of illicit and over-the-counter drugs, herbal supplements, alcohol, and tobacco is also obtained. Particular attention is paid to blood glucose control in patients with diabetes because there is a higher incidence of postoperative complications when glycemic control is poor (Engoren, Schwann, & Habib, 2014).

The psychosocial assessment and the assessment of the patient's and family's learning needs are also important. Anticipation of cardiac surgery is a source of great stress to the patient and family, and patients with high anxiety levels have poorer outcomes (Feuchtinger, Burbaum, Heilmann, et al., 2013). However, some anxiety is expected, and the work of worrying can help patients identify priorities and find coping strategies that help them face the threat of surgery. Questions may be asked to obtain the following information:

- Knowledge and understanding of the surgical procedure, postoperative course, and recovery
- Fears and concerns regarding the surgery and future health status
- Coping mechanisms helpful to the patient
- Support systems available during and following hospitalization

Reducing Fear and Anxiety

The nurse gives the patient and family time and opportunity to express their fears. Topics of concern may be pain, changes in body image, fear of the unknown, and fear of disability or death. It may be helpful to describe the sensations that the patient can expect, including the preoperative sedation, surgical anesthesia, and postoperative pain management. The nurse reassures the patient that the fear of pain is normal, that some pain will be experienced, that medication to relieve pain will be provided, and that the patient will be closely monitored. In addition, the nurse instructs the patient to request analgesic medication before the pain becomes severe. If the patient has concerns about scarring from surgery, the nurse encourages him or her to discuss this issue and corrects any misconceptions. The patient and family may want to discuss their fear of the patient dying. After the fear is expressed, the nurse can assure the patient and family that this fear is normal and further explore their feelings. For patients with extreme anxiety or fear and for whom emotional support and education are not successful, antianxiety medication such as lorazepam (Ativan) may be helpful.

Monitoring and Managing Potential Complications

Angina may occur because of increased stress and anxiety related to the forthcoming surgery. The patient who develops angina usually responds to typical therapy for angina, most commonly nitroglycerin. Some patients require oxygen and IV nitroglycerin infusions. Physiologically unstable patients may require preoperative management in a critical care unit.

 Providing Patient Education

Prior to surgery, patients and their families are given specific instructions. This includes information on how the patient should take or stop specific medications, including anticoagulant agents, antihypertensive medications, and medications that control diabetes. The patient is instructed to shower with an antiseptic solution such as chlorhexidine gluconate. Hair removal with an electric clipper rather than a razor is used when indicated (Hillis et al., 2011) (see Chapter 17 for further discussion of preoperative preparation).

Education also includes information about the hospitalization and surgery. The nurse informs the patient and family about the equipment, tubes, and lines that will be present after surgery and their purposes. They should expect monitors, several IV lines, chest tubes, and a urinary catheter. Explaining the purpose and the approximate time that these devices will be in place helps reassure the patient. Most patients remain intubated and on mechanical ventilation for several hours after surgery. It is important for patients to know that this will prevent them from talking, and the nurse should reassure them that the staff will be able to assist them with other means of communication.

The nurse takes care to answer the patient's questions about postoperative care and procedures. After the nurse explains deep breathing and coughing, the use of the incentive spirometer, and foot exercises, the nurse practices these procedures with the patient. The benefit of early and frequent ambulation is discussed. The family's questions at this time usually focus on the length of the surgery, who will discuss the results of the procedure with them after surgery, where to wait during the surgery, the visiting procedures for the critical care unit, and how they can support the patient before surgery and in the critical care unit.

Intraoperative Management

The perioperative nurse performs assessments and prepares the patient as described in Chapters 17 and 18. In addition to assisting with the surgical procedure, perioperative nurses are responsible for the comfort and safety of the patient.

Possible intraoperative complications include low cardiac output, dysrhythmias, hemorrhage, MI, organ failure from shock, and thromboembolic events including stroke (Urden et al., 2014). Astute intraoperative nursing assessment is critical to prevent, detect, and initiate prompt intervention for these complications. Before the chest incision is closed, chest tubes are inserted to evacuate air and drainage from the mediastinum and the thorax. Temporary epicardial pacemaker electrodes may be implanted on the surface of the right atrium and the right ventricle. These epicardial electrodes can be connected to an external pacemaker if the patient has persistent bradycardia perioperatively (see Chapter 26 for a discussion of pacemakers).

Postoperative Nursing Management

Initial postoperative care focuses on achieving or maintaining hemodynamic stability and recovery from general anesthesia. Care may be provided in the postanesthesia care unit (PACU) or ICU. The immediate postoperative period for the patient who has undergone cardiac surgery presents many challenges to the health care team. All efforts are made to facilitate the transition from the operating room to the ICU or PACU with minimal risk. Specific information about the surgical procedure and important factors about postoperative management are communicated by the surgical team and anesthesia personnel to the critical care or PACU nurse, who then assumes responsibility for the patient's care. Figure 27-13 presents an overview of the many aspects of postoperative care of the cardiac surgical patient.

After the patient's cardiac status and respiratory status are stable, the patient is transferred to a surgical progressive care unit with telemetry. Care in both the ICU and progressive care unit focuses on monitoring of cardiopulmonary status, pain management, wound care, progressive activity, and nutrition. Education about medications and risk factor modification is emphasized.

A typical plan of postoperative nursing care is presented in Chart 27-11.

(*text continued on page 784*)

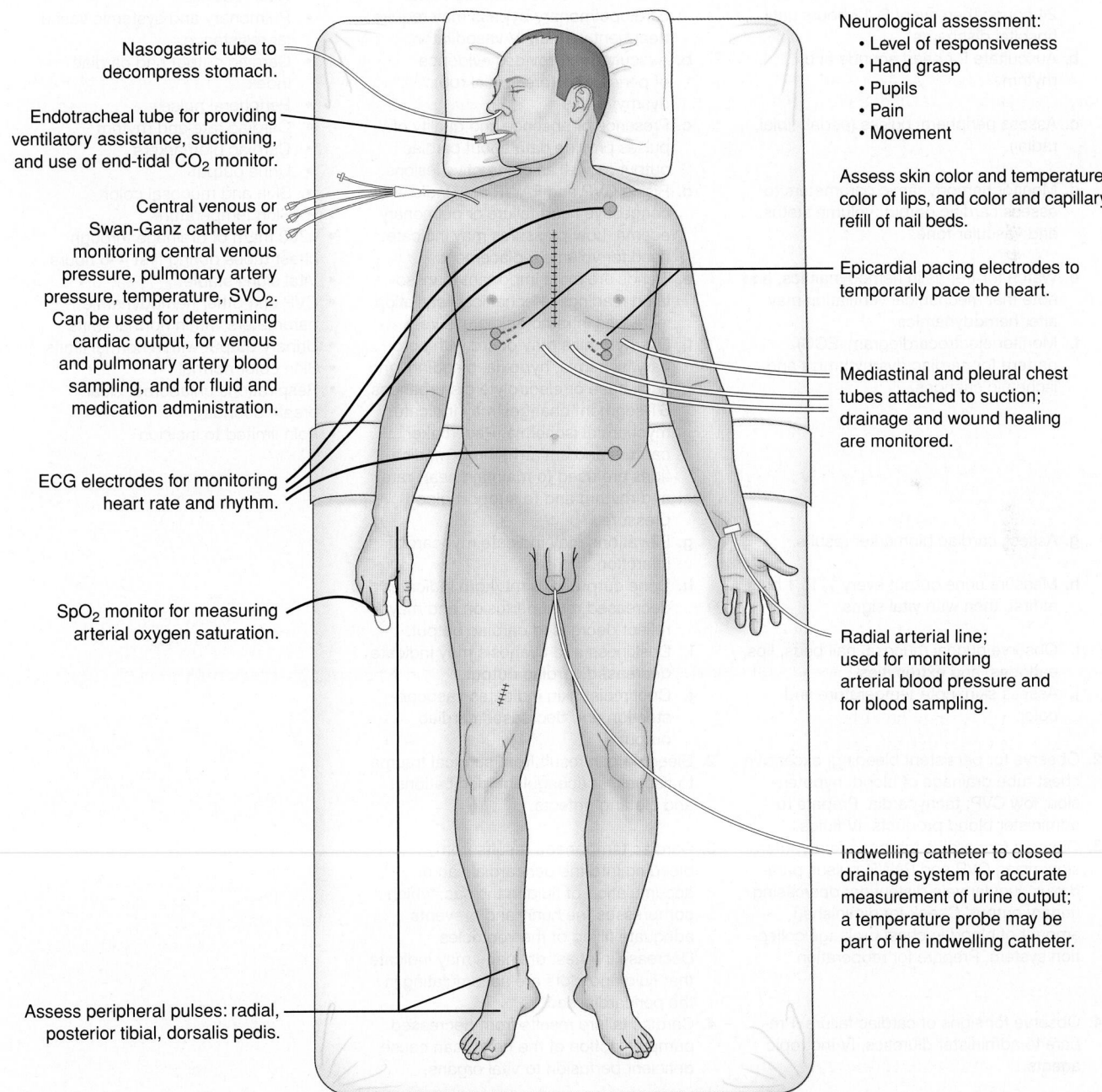

Nasogastric tube to decompress stomach.

Endotracheal tube for providing ventilatory assistance, suctioning, and use of end-tidal CO_2 monitor.

Central venous or Swan-Ganz catheter for monitoring central venous pressure, pulmonary artery pressure, temperature, SVO_2. Can be used for determining cardiac output, for venous and pulmonary artery blood sampling, and for fluid and medication administration.

ECG electrodes for monitoring heart rate and rhythm.

SpO$_2$ monitor for measuring arterial oxygen saturation.

Assess peripheral pulses: radial, posterior tibial, dorsalis pedis.

Neurological assessment:
• Level of responsiveness
• Hand grasp
• Pupils
• Pain
• Movement

Assess skin color and temperature, color of lips, and color and capillary refill of nail beds.

Epicardial pacing electrodes to temporarily pace the heart.

Mediastinal and pleural chest tubes attached to suction; drainage and wound healing are monitored.

Radial arterial line; used for monitoring arterial blood pressure and for blood sampling.

Indwelling catheter to closed drainage system for accurate measurement of urine output; a temperature probe may be part of the indwelling catheter.

Figure 27-13 • Postoperative care of the cardiac surgical patient requires the nurse to be proficient in interpreting hemodynamics, correlating physical assessment data with laboratory results, sequencing interventions, and evaluating progress toward desired outcomes.

Chart 27-11

PLAN OF NURSING CARE

Care of the Patient After Cardiac Surgery

NURSING DIAGNOSIS: Decreased cardiac output related to blood loss and compromised myocardial function
GOAL: Restoration of cardiac output to maintain organ and tissue perfusion

Nursing Interventions	Rationale	Expected Outcomes

1. Monitor cardiovascular status. Serial readings of blood pressure, other hemodynamic parameters, and cardiac rhythm and rate are obtained, recorded, and correlated with the patient's overall condition.
 	
a. Assess arterial blood pressure every 15 minutes until stable; then arterial or cuff blood pressure every 1–4 hours × 24 hours; then every 8–12 hours until hospital discharge.
 	
b. Auscultate for heart sounds and rhythm.
 	
c. Assess peripheral pulses (pedal, tibial, radial).
 	
d. Monitor hemodynamic parameters to assess cardiac output, volume status, and vascular tone.
 	
e. Watch for trends in hemodynamics, and note that mechanical ventilation may alter hemodynamics.
 	
f. Monitor electrocardiogram (ECG) pattern for cardiac dysrhythmias and ischemic changes.
 	
g. Assess cardiac biomarker results.
 	
h. Measure urine output every ½ to 1 hour at first, then with vital signs.
 	
i. Observe buccal mucosa, nail beds, lips, earlobes, and extremities.
j. Assess skin; note temperature and color.
	1. Effectiveness of cardiac output is evaluated by continuous monitoring.
	
	a. Blood pressure is one of the most important physiologic parameters to monitor; vasoconstriction after cardiopulmonary bypass may require treatment with an IV vasodilator.
	
	b. Auscultation provides evidence of pericarditis (precordial rub), dysrhythmias.
	c. Presence or absence and quality of pulses provide data about cardiac output as well as obstructive lesions.
	d. Rising CVP and PAWP may indicate congestive heart failure or pulmonary edema. Low pressures may indicate need for volume replacement.
	e. Trends are more important than isolated readings. Mechanical ventilation increases intrathoracic pressure.
	f. Dysrhythmias may occur with coronary ischemia, hypoxia, bleeding, and acid–base or electrolyte disturbances. ST-segment changes may indicate myocardial ischemia. Pacemaker capture and antiarrhythmic medications are used to maintain heart rate and rhythm and to support blood pressure.
	g. Elevations may indicate myocardial infarction.
	h. Urine output <0.5 mL/kg/h indicates decreased renal perfusion and may reflect decreased cardiac output.
	i. Duskiness and cyanosis may indicate decreased cardiac output.
	j. Cool moist skin indicates vasoconstriction and decreased cardiac output.
		• The following parameters are within the patient's normal ranges:
		  • Arterial pressure
		  • Central venous pressure (CVP)
		  • Pulmonary artery pressures
		  • Pulmonary artery wedge pressure (PAWP)
		  • Heart sounds
		  • Pulmonary and systemic vascular resistance
		  • Cardiac output and cardiac index
		  • Peripheral pulses
		  • Cardiac rate and rhythm
		  • Cardiac biomarkers
		  • Urine output
		  • Skin and mucosal color
		  • Skin temperature
		• <200 mL/h of drainage through chest tubes during first 4–6 hours
		• Vital signs stable
		• CVP and other hemodynamic parameters within normal limits
		• Urinary output within normal limits
		• Skin color normal
		• Respirations unlabored, clear breath sounds
		• Pain limited to incision

2. Observe for persistent bleeding: excessive chest tube drainage of blood; hypotension; low CVP; tachycardia. Prepare to administer blood products, IV fluids.	2. Bleeding can result from surgical trauma to tissues, anticoagulant medications, and clotting defects.	
3. Observe for cardiac tamponade: hypotension; rising CVP and PAWP, pulsus paradoxus; jugular vein distention; decreasing urinary output. Check for diminished amount of blood in chest drainage collection system. Prepare for reoperation.	3. Cardiac tamponade results from bleeding into the pericardial sac or accumulation of fluid in the sac, which compresses the heart and prevents adequate filling of the ventricles. Decrease in chest drainage may indicate that fluid and clots are accumulating in the pericardial sac.	
4. Observe for signs of cardiac failure. Prepare to administer diuretics, IV inotropic agents.	4. Cardiac failure results from decreased pumping action of the heart; can cause deficient perfusion to vital organs.	

Chart 27-11

PLAN OF NURSING CARE (Continued)

Care of the Patient After Cardiac Surgery

NURSING DIAGNOSIS: Impaired gas exchange related to chest surgery
GOAL: Adequate gas exchange

Nursing Interventions	Rationale	Expected Outcomes
1. Maintain mechanical ventilation until the patient is able to breathe independently.	1. Ventilatory support is used to decrease work of the heart, to maintain effective ventilation, and to provide an airway in the event of complications.	• Airway patent • Arterial blood gases (ABGs) within normal range • Endotracheal tube correctly placed, as evidenced by x-ray
2. Monitor ABGs, tidal volume, peak inspiratory pressure, and extubation parameters.	2. ABGs and ventilator parameters indicate effectiveness of ventilator and changes that need to be made to improve gas exchange.	• Breath sounds clear bilaterally • Ventilator synchronous with respirations
3. Auscultate chest for breath sounds.	3. Crackles indicate pulmonary congestion; decreased or absent breath sounds may indicate pneumothorax, hemothorax, dislodgement of tube.	• Breath sounds clear after suctioning/coughing • Nail beds and mucous membranes pink
4. Sedate patient adequately, as prescribed, and monitor respiratory rate and depth.	4. Sedation helps the patient to tolerate the endotracheal tube and to cope with mechanical ventilation.	• Mental acuity consistent with amount of sedatives and analgesics received
5. Suction tracheobronchial secretions as needed, using strict aseptic technique.	5. Retention of secretions leads to hypoxia and possible infection.	• Oriented to person; able to respond "yes" and "no" appropriately
6. Assist in weaning and endotracheal tube removal.	6. Extubation decreases risk of pulmonary infections and enhances ability of patient to communicate.	• Able to be weaned successfully from ventilator
7. After extubation, promote deep breathing, coughing, and turning. Encourage the use of the incentive spirometer and compliance with breathing treatments. Instruct about incisional splinting with a "cough pillow" to decrease discomfort.	7. Aids in keeping airway patent, preventing atelectasis, and facilitating lung expansion	

NURSING DIAGNOSIS: Risk for imbalanced fluid volume and electrolyte imbalance related to alterations in blood volume
GOAL: Fluid and electrolyte balance

Nursing Interventions	Rationale	Expected Outcomes
1. Monitor fluid and electrolyte balance.	1. Adequate circulating blood volume is necessary for optimal cellular activity; fluid and electrolyte imbalance can occur after surgery.	• Fluid intake and output balanced • Hemodynamic assessment parameters negative for fluid overload or hypovolemia
a. Accurately document intake and output; record urine volume every half hour to 4 hours while in critical care unit; then every 8–12 hours while hospitalized.	a. Provides a method to determine positive or negative fluid balance and fluid requirements	• Normal blood pressure with position changes • Absence of dysrhythmia • Stable weight
b. Assess blood pressure, hemodynamic parameters, weight, electrolytes, hematocrit, jugular venous pressure, breath sounds, urinary output, and nasogastric tube drainage.	b. Provides information about state of hydration	• Arterial blood pH 7.35–7.45 • Serum potassium 3.5–5 mEq/L (3.5–5 mmol/L) • Serum magnesium 1.8–3.0 mg/dL (0.75–1.25 mmol/L)
c. Measure postoperative chest drainage; cessation of drainage may indicate kinked or blocked chest tube. Ensure patency and integrity of the drainage system.	c. Excessive blood loss from chest cavity can cause hypovolemia.	• Serum sodium 135–145 mEq/L (135–145 mmol/L) • Serum calcium 8.5–10.5 mg/dL (2.1–2.6 mmol/L)
d. Weigh daily and correlate with intake and output.	d. Indicator of fluid balance	• Serum glucose < 160 g/dL

(continued on page 782)

Chart 27-11

PLAN OF NURSING CARE (Continued)

Care of the Patient After Cardiac Surgery

Nursing Interventions	Rationale	Expected Outcomes
2. Be alert to changes in serum electrolyte levels. a. Hypokalemia (low potassium) *Effects:* Dysrhythmias: premature ventricular contractions, ventricular tachycardia. Observe for specific ECG changes. Administer IV potassium replacement as prescribed. b. Hyperkalemia (high potassium) *Effects:* ECG changes, tall peaked T waves, wide QRS, bradycardia. Be prepared to administer diuretic or an ion-exchange resin (sodium polystyrene sulfonate [Kayexalate]); or IV insulin and glucose. c. Monitor serum magnesium, sodium, and calcium. d. Hyperglycemia (high blood glucose) *Effects:* Increased urine output, thirst, impaired healing. Administer insulin as prescribed.	2. A specific concentration of electrolytes is necessary in both extracellular and intracellular body fluids to sustain life. a. *Causes:* Inadequate intake, diuretics, vomiting, excessive nasogastric drainage, perioperative stress response b. *Causes:* Increased intake, hemolysis from cardiopulmonary bypass/mechanical assist devices, acidosis, renal insufficiency. The resin binds potassium and promotes intestinal excretion of it. Insulin assists the cells with glucose and potassium absorption. c. Low levels of magnesium are associated with dysrhythmias. Low levels of sodium are associated with weakness and neurological symptoms. Low levels of calcium can lead to dysrhythmias and muscle spasm. d. *Cause:* Stress response to surgery. Affects both patients with diabetes and those without diabetes.	

NURSING DIAGNOSIS: Risk for acute confusion related to alteration in sleep–wake cycle, impaired metabolic functioning, use of multiple medications

GOAL: Prevention of acute confusion/postcardiotomy delirium

Nursing Interventions	Rationale	Expected Outcomes
1. Use measures to prevent postcardiotomy delirium: a. Explain all procedures and the need for patient cooperation. b. Plan nursing care to provide for periods of uninterrupted sleep with patient's normal day–night pattern. c. Promote continuity of care. d. Orient to time and place frequently. Encourage family to visit. e. Assess for medications that may contribute to delirium. 2. Observe for perceptual distortions, hallucinations, disorientation, and paranoid delusions.	1. Postcardiotomy delirium may result from alterations in sleep–wake cycle, impaired metabolic functioning, and use of multiple medications. Normally, sleep cycles are at least 50 minutes long. The first cycle may be as long as 90–120 minutes and then shorten during successive cycles. Sleep deprivation results when the sleep cycles are interrupted or are inadequate in number. 2. Delirium can indicate a serious medical condition such as hypoxia, acid–base imbalance, metabolic abnormalities, and cerebral infarction.	• Cooperates with procedures • Sleeps for long, uninterrupted intervals • Oriented to person, place, time • Experiences no perceptual distortions, hallucinations, disorientation, delusions

NURSING DIAGNOSIS: Acute pain related to surgical trauma and pleural irritation caused by chest tubes

GOAL: Relief of pain

Nursing Interventions	Rationale	Expected Outcomes
1. Record nature, type, location, intensity, and duration of pain. 2. Encourage routine pain medication dosing for the first 24–72 hours, and observe for side effects of lethargy, hypotension, tachycardia, respiratory depression.	1. Pain and anxiety increase pulse rate, oxygen consumption, and cardiac workload. 2. Analgesia promotes rest, decreases oxygen consumption caused by pain, and aids patient in performing deep-breathing and coughing exercises; pain medication is more effective when taken before pain is severe.	• States pain is decreasing in severity • Restlessness decreased • Vital signs stable • Participates in deep-breathing and coughing exercises • Verbalizes fewer complaints of pain each day • Positions self; participates in care activities • Gradually increases activity

Chart 27-11

PLAN OF NURSING CARE (Continued)
Care of the Patient After Cardiac Surgery

NURSING DIAGNOSIS: Risk for ineffective renal perfusion related to decreased cardiac output, hemolysis, or vasopressor drug therapy
GOAL: Maintenance of adequate renal perfusion

Nursing Interventions	Rationale	Expected Outcomes
1. Assess renal function: a. Measure urine output every half hour to 4 hours in critical care, then every 8–12 hours until hospital discharge. b. Monitor and report lab results: BUN, serum creatinine, serum electrolytes. 2. Prepare to administer rapid-acting diuretics or inotropic drugs (e.g., dobutamine). 3. Prepare patient for dialysis or continuous renal replacement therapy if indicated.	1. Renal injury can be caused by deficient perfusion, hemolysis, low cardiac output, and the use of vasopressor agents to increase blood pressure. a. <0.5 mL/kg/h indicates decreased renal function. b. These tests indicate the kidneys' ability to excrete waste products. 2. These agents promote renal function and increase cardiac output and renal blood flow. 3. Provides patient with the opportunity to ask questions and prepare for the procedure	• Urine output consistent with fluid intake; >0.5 mL/kg/h • Urine specific gravity 1.003–1.030 • Blood urea nitrogen (BUN), creatinine, electrolytes within normal limits

NURSING DIAGNOSIS: Ineffective thermoregulation related to infection or postpericardiotomy syndrome
GOAL: Maintenance of normal body temperature

Nursing Interventions	Rationale	Expected Outcomes
1. Assess temperature every hour. 2. Use aseptic technique when changing dressings, suctioning endotracheal tube; maintain closed systems for all IV and arterial lines and for indwelling urinary catheter. 3. Observe for symptoms of postpericardiotomy syndrome. 4. Obtain cultures and other lab work (CBC, ESR); administer antibiotic agents as prescribed. 5. Administer anti-inflammatory agents as directed.	1. Fever can indicate infectious or inflammatory process. 2. Decreases risk of infection 3. Occurs in 10% of patients after cardiac surgery. 4. Antibiotic agents treat documented infection. 5. Anti-inflammatory agents relieve symptoms of inflammation.	• Normal body temperature • Incisions are free of infection and are healing. • Absence of symptoms of postpericardiotomy syndrome: fever, malaise, pericardial effusion, pericardial friction rub, arthralgia

NURSING DIAGNOSIS: Deficient knowledge about self-care activities
GOAL: Ability to perform self-care activities

Nursing Interventions	Rationale	Expected Outcomes
1. Develop education plan for patient and family. Provide specific instructions for the following: • Diet and daily weights • Activity progression • Exercise • Deep breathing, coughing, lung expansion exercises • Temperature and pulse monitoring • Medication regimen • Incision care • Access to the emergency medical system 2. Provide verbal and written instructions; provide several education sessions for reinforcement and answering questions. 3. Involve family in education sessions. 4. Provide contact information for surgeon and cardiologist and instructions about follow-up visit with surgeon. 5. Make appropriate referrals: home care agency, cardiac rehabilitation program, community support groups.	1. Each patient has unique learning needs. 2. Repetition promotes learning by allowing for questions and clarification of misinformation. 3. Family members responsible for home care are usually anxious and require adequate time for learning. 4. Arrangements for contacts with health care personnel help to allay anxieties. 5. Learning, recovery, and lifestyle changes continue after discharge from the hospital.	• Patient and family members explain and comply with therapeutic regimen. • Patient and family members identify necessary lifestyle changes. • Has copy of discharge instructions (in the patient's primary language and at appropriate reading level; has an alternate format if indicated) • Keeps follow-up appointments

Assessing the Patient

When the patient is admitted to the critical care unit or PACU, nursing and medical personnel perform a complete assessment of all systems at least every 4 hours. It is necessary to assess the following parameters:

Neurologic status: level of responsiveness, pupil size and reaction to light, facial symmetry, movement of the extremities, and hand grip strength

Cardiac status: heart rate and rhythm, heart sounds, pacemaker status, arterial blood pressure, central venous pressure (CVP); in selected patients, hemodynamic parameters: pulmonary artery pressure, pulmonary artery wedge pressure (PAWP), cardiac output and index, systemic and pulmonary vascular resistance, mixed venous oxygen saturation ($Sv-O_2$). A pulmonary artery catheter is often used to monitor these parameters. Alternatively, minimally invasive monitoring of stroke volume, systemic vascular resistance, and cardiac output are calculated through pressures obtained in the arterial line (e.g., Vigileo monitor with FloTrac sensor). (See Chapter 25 for a detailed description of hemodynamic monitoring.)

Respiratory status: chest movement, breath sounds, ventilator settings (e.g., rate, tidal volume, oxygen concentration, mode such as assist-control, positive end-expiratory pressure, pressure support), respiratory rate, peak inspiratory pressure, percutaneous oxygen saturation (SpO_2), end-tidal carbon dioxide (CO_2), pleural chest tube drainage, arterial blood gases. (See Chapters 20 and 21 for detailed descriptions of respiratory assessment and ventilatory management.)

Peripheral vascular status: peripheral pulses; color of skin, nail beds, mucosa, lips, and earlobes; skin temperature; edema; condition of dressings and invasive lines

Renal function: urinary output; serum creatinine and electrolytes

Fluid and electrolyte status: strict intake and output, including all IV fluids and blood products, output from all drainage tubes; clinical and laboratory indicators of imbalance

Pain: nature, type, location, and duration; apprehension; response to analgesics

Assessment also includes checking all equipment and tubes to ensure that they are functioning properly: endotracheal tube, ventilator, end-tidal CO_2 monitor, SpO_2 monitor, pulmonary artery catheter, $Sv-O_2$ monitor, arterial and IV lines, IV infusion devices and tubing, cardiac monitor, pacemaker, chest tubes, and urinary drainage system.

As the patient regains consciousness and progresses through the postoperative period, the nurse also assesses indicators of psychological and emotional status. The patient may exhibit behavior that reflects denial or depression or may experience postoperative delirium. Characteristic signs of delirium include transient perceptual illusions, visual and auditory hallucinations, disorientation, and paranoid delusions. Patients who have delirium after cardiac surgery have poorer outcomes than do similar patients without this complication (Mangusan, Hooper, Denslow, et al., 2015).

The family's needs also must be assessed. The nurse ascertains how family members are coping with the situation; determines their psychological, emotional, and spiritual needs; and finds out whether they are receiving adequate information about the patient's condition.

Monitoring for Complications

The patient is continuously assessed for impending complications (see Table 27-5). The nurse and the surgical team function collaboratively to prevent complications, to identify early signs and symptoms of complications, and to institute measures to reverse their progression.

Decreased Cardiac Output

A decrease in cardiac output is always a threat to the patient who has had cardiac surgery, and it can have a variety of causes. Preload alterations occur when too little blood volume returns to the heart as a result of persistent bleeding and hypovolemia. Excessive postoperative bleeding can lead to decreased intravascular volume, hypotension, and low cardiac output. Bleeding problems are common after cardiac surgery because of the effects of CPB, trauma from the surgery, and anticoagulation. Preload can also decrease if there is a collection of fluid and blood in the pericardium (cardiac tamponade), which impedes cardiac filling. Cardiac output is also altered if too much volume returns to the heart, causing fluid overload.

Afterload alterations occur when the arteries are constricted as a result of postoperative hypertension or hypothermia, increasing the workload of the heart. Heart rate alterations from bradycardia, tachycardia, and dysrhythmias can lead to decreased cardiac output, and contractility can be altered in cardiac failure, MI, electrolyte imbalances, and hypoxia.

Fluid Volume and Electrolyte Imbalance

Fluid and electrolyte imbalance may occur after cardiac surgery. Nursing assessment for these complications includes monitoring of intake and output, weight, hemodynamic parameters, hematocrit levels, neck vein distention, edema, breath sounds (e.g., fine crackles, wheezing), and electrolyte levels. The nurse reports changes in serum electrolytes promptly so that treatment can be instituted. Especially important are dangerously high or dangerously low levels of potassium, magnesium, sodium, and calcium. Elevated blood glucose levels are common in the postoperative period. Administration of IV insulin is recommended in patients both with and without diabetes to achieve the glycemic control necessary to promote wound healing, decrease infection, and improve survival after surgery (Engoren et al., 2014). Implementing an insulin infusion protocol that targets moderate glycemic control has been demonstrated as effective in treating acute hyperglycemia following cardiac surgery while also decreasing the incidence of hypoglycemia (Hargraves, 2014) (see Chart 27-12).

Impaired Gas Exchange

Impaired gas exchange is another possible complication after cardiac surgery. All body tissues require an adequate supply of oxygen for survival. To achieve this after surgery, an endotracheal tube with ventilator assistance may be used for hours to days. The assisted ventilation is continued until the patient's blood gas values are acceptable and the patient demonstrates the ability to breathe independently. Patients who are stable after surgery may be extubated as early as 2 to 4 hours after surgery, which reduces their discomfort and anxiety and facilitates patient–nurse communication.

While receiving mechanical ventilation, the patient is continuously assessed for signs of impaired gas exchange: restlessness,

Chart 27-12

NURSING RESEARCH PROFILE
Glycemic Control in Patients Post-Cardiac Surgery

Hargraves, J. D. (2014). Glycemic control in cardiac surgery: Implementing an evidence-based insulin infusion protocol. *American Journal of Critical Care, 23*(3), 250–258.

Purpose

Acute hyperglycemia following cardiac surgery increases the risk of sternal wound infections. However, insulin infusion protocols that target tight glycemic control to treat hyperglycemia are linked to hypoglycemia and increased mortality. Therefore, recent studies support moderate glycemic control following cardiac surgery. The first purpose of this study was to measure critical care nurses' knowledge of glycemic control in cardiac surgery before and after education. The second purpose was to evaluate the safety and effectiveness of an evidence-based insulin infusion protocol targeting moderate glycemic control in cardiac surgery patients.

Design

The Iowa Model of Evidence-based Practice to Promote Quality Care provided the framework for this project. Nurses completed a questionnaire to measure knowledge of glycemic control before and after education was provided. Blood glucose data were retrospectively collected on 76 cardiac surgery patients from anesthesia end time through 11:59 PM on postoperative day 2. Glucose levels were compared between 2 months before to 2 months after the new insulin infusion protocol was instituted. The new protocol identified a blood glucose goal of 120–160 mg/dL.

Findings

Nurses' knowledge increased significantly after education, based upon improved test scores. Mean pretest scores were 53% ($n = 29$) and posttest mean scores were 79% ($n = 27$). The mean blood glucose level after implementation of the protocol was 148 mg/dL. Furthermore, the incidence of hypoglycemia, defined as a blood glucose of less than 70 mg/dL, was significantly reduced with the new protocol. The percentage of blood glucose levels less than 180 mg/dL was 88.30%.

Nursing Implications

Nurses' knowledge of glycemic control improves when nurses are educated on the use of the best evidence. Furthermore, when nurses implement evidence-based insulin infusion protocols that target moderate glycemic control, patient outcomes improve.

---

anxiety, cyanosis of mucous membranes and peripheral tissues, tachycardia, and fighting the ventilator. Breath sounds are assessed often to detect pulmonary congestion and monitor lung expansion. Arterial blood gases, SpO_2, and end-tidal CO_2 are assessed for decreased oxygen and increased CO_2. Following extubation, aggressive pulmonary interventions such as turning, coughing, deep breathing, and early ambulation are necessary to prevent atelectasis and pneumonia.

Impaired Cerebral Circulation

Hypoperfusion or microemboli during or following cardiac surgery may produce injury to the brain. Brain function depends on a continuous supply of oxygenated blood. The brain does not have the capacity to store oxygen and must rely on adequate continuous perfusion by the heart. The nurse observes the patient for signs and symptoms of cerebral hypoxia: restlessness, confusion, dyspnea, hypotension, and cyanosis. An assessment of the patient's neurologic status includes the level of consciousness, response to verbal commands and painful stimuli, pupil size and reaction to light, facial symmetry, movement of the extremities, and hand grip strength. The nurse documents any indication of a change in status and reports abnormal findings to the surgeon because they may signal the onset of a complication such as a stroke.

Maintaining Cardiac Output

Ongoing evaluation of the patient's cardiac status continues as the nurse monitors the effectiveness of cardiac output through clinical observations and routine measurements: serial readings of blood pressure, heart rate, CVP, arterial pressure, and pulmonary artery pressures.

Renal function is related to cardiac function, as blood pressure and cardiac output drive glomerular filtration; therefore, urinary output is measured and recorded. Urine output less than 0.5 mL/kg/h may indicate a decrease in cardiac output or inadequate fluid volume.

Body tissues depend on adequate cardiac output to provide a continuous supply of oxygenated blood to meet the changing demands of the organs and body systems. Because the buccal mucosa, nail beds, lips, and earlobes are sites with rich capillary beds, they are observed for cyanosis or duskiness as possible signs of reduced cardiac output. Distention of the neck veins when the head of the bed is elevated to 30 degrees or more may signal right-sided heart failure.

Dysrhythmias may develop due to decreased perfusion to or irritation of the myocardium from surgery. The most common dysrhythmias encountered during the postoperative period are atrial fibrillation, bradycardias, tachycardias, and ectopic beats (Urden et al., 2014). Continuous observation of the cardiac monitor for dysrhythmias is essential.

The nurse reports any indications of decreased cardiac output promptly. The assessment data are used to determine the cause of the problem. After a diagnosis has been made, the primary provider and the nurse work collaboratively to restore cardiac output and prevent further complications. When indicated, blood components; fluids; and antidysrhythmics, diuretics, vasodilators, or vasopressors are prescribed. If additional interventions are necessary, such as the placement of an intra-aortic balloon pump, the patient and family are prepared for the procedure.

Promoting Adequate Gas Exchange

To ensure adequate gas exchange, the patency of the endotracheal tube is assessed and maintained. The tube must be secured to prevent it from slipping out or down into the right mainstem bronchus. Suctioning is necessary when crackles or coughing is present. Arterial blood gas determinations are compared with baseline data, and changes are reported to the primary provider promptly.

When the patient's hemodynamic parameters stabilize, body position is changed every 1 to 2 hours. Frequent changes of patient position provide for optimal pulmonary ventilation and perfusion, allowing the lungs to expand more fully.

Physical assessment and arterial blood gas results guide the process of weaning the patient from the ventilator. The nurse assists with the weaning process and eventually with the removal of the endotracheal tube. After extubation, the nurse encourages deep breathing and coughing at least every 1 to 2 hours to clear secretions, open the alveolar sacs, and promote effective ventilation. See Chapter 21 for discussion of weaning the patient from the ventilator.

Maintaining Fluid and Electrolyte Balance

To promote fluid and electrolyte balance, the nurse carefully assesses the intake and output to determine positive or negative fluid balance. It is necessary to record all fluid intake, including IV, nasogastric tube, and oral fluids, as well as all output, including urine, nasogastric drainage, and chest drainage.

Hemodynamic parameters (e.g., blood pressure, CVP, cardiac output) are correlated with intake, output, and weight to determine the adequacy of hydration and cardiac output. Serum electrolytes are monitored, and the patient is observed for signs of potassium, magnesium, sodium, or calcium imbalance (see Chapter 13).

Indications of dehydration, fluid overload, or electrolyte imbalance are reported promptly, and the primary provider and nurse work collaboratively to restore fluid and electrolyte balance and monitor the patient's response to therapies.

Minimizing Confusion

Some patients exhibit abnormal behaviors and acute confusion that occur with varying intensity and duration. The risk of delirium is high in cardiac surgery patients and increases with patients' age (Mangusan et al., 2015). Clinical manifestations of postoperative delirium include restlessness, agitation, visual and auditory hallucinations, and paranoia. The delirium typically appears after a 2- to 5-day stay in an ICU. Patients are assessed for this problem with tools such as the Confusion Assessment Method for the ICU (CAM-ICU) (Brooks, Spillane, Dick, et al., 2014) (see Chart 11-7 for discussion of CAM). The CAMU-ICU scale assesses for key indicators of delirium such as disorganized thinking and inattention. When this testing is positive, further assessment of the patient's physiologic and psychological status is required. Presumed causes of postoperative delirium include anxiety, sleep deprivation, increased sensory input, medications, and physiologic problems such as hypoxemia and metabolic imbalance (Mangusan et al., 2015). Treatment includes correction of identified physiologic problems such as metabolic and electrolyte imbalances. In addition, behavioral interventions are used (e.g., frequent reorientation). Sedative medications such as haloperidol (Haldol) may help reduce agitation. The delirium often resolves after the patient is transferred from the unit, but nonetheless can be associated with negative outcomes including cognitive and functional decline, longer lengths of hospital stay, and higher mortality (Mangusan et al., 2015).

For all postoperative patients, basic comfort measures are used in conjunction with prescribed analgesics and sedatives to promote rest. Invasive lines and tubes are discontinued as soon as possible. Patient care is coordinated to provide undisturbed periods of rest. As the patient's condition stabilizes and the patient is disturbed less frequently for monitoring and therapeutic procedures, rest periods can be extended. Uninterrupted sleep is provided as much as possible, especially during the patient's normal hours of sleep.

Careful explanations of all procedures and of the patient's role in facilitating them help keep the patient positively involved throughout the postoperative course. Continuity of care is desirable; a familiar face and a nursing staff with a consistent approach help the patient feel safe. The patient's family should be welcomed at the bedside. A well-designed and individualized plan of nursing care can assist the nursing team in coordinating its efforts for the emotional well-being of the patient.

Relieving Pain

Patients who have had cardiac surgery may have pain in the peri-incisional area or throughout the chest, shoulders, and back. Pain results from trauma to the chest wall and irritation of the pleura by the chest tubes as well as incisional pain from peripheral vein or artery graft harvest sites.

The nurse assesses patients for verbal and nonverbal indicators of pain and records the nature, type, location, and duration of the pain. To reduce the amount of pain, the nurse encourages the patient to accept medication on a regular basis. The addition of adjunctive pain relievers (anti-inflammatory agents, muscle relaxants) to opioids decreases the amount of opioids required for pain relief and increases patient comfort. Patients report the most pain during coughing, turning, and moving. Physical support of the incision with a folded bath blanket or small pillow during deep breathing and coughing helps minimize pain. The patient should then be able to participate in respiratory exercises and to progressively increase self-care. Patient comfort improves after removal of the chest tubes.

Pain produces distress, which may stimulate the central nervous system to release catecholamines, resulting in constriction of the arterioles and increased heart rate. This can cause increased afterload and decreased cardiac output. Opioids alleviate pain and induce sleep and feelings of well-being, which reduce the metabolic rate and oxygen demands. After the administration of opioids, it is necessary to document observations indicating relief of apprehension and pain in the patient's record. The nurse observes the patient for any adverse effects of opioids, including respiratory depression, hypotension, constipation, ileus, or urinary retention. If respiratory depression occurs, an opioid antagonist (e.g., naloxone [Narcan]) may be required (see Chapter 12 for further discussion of nonpharmacologic pain interventions).

Maintaining Adequate Tissue Perfusion

The nurse routinely palpates peripheral pulses (e.g., pedal, tibial, femoral, radial, brachial) to assess for arterial obstruction. If a pulse is absent in any extremity, the cause may be prior catheterization of that extremity, chronic peripheral vascular disease, or a thromboembolic obstruction. The nurse immediately reports newly identified absence of any pulse.

Thromboembolic events can result from vascular injury, dislodgment of a clot from a damaged valve, loosening of mural thrombi, or coagulation problems. Air embolism can result from CPB or central venous cannulation. Symptoms of embolization vary according to site. The usual embolic sites are the lungs, coronary arteries, mesentery, spleen, extremities, kidneys, and brain. The patient is observed for the onset of the following:

- Acute onset of chest pain and respiratory distress, as occur in pulmonary embolus or MI
- Abdominal or back pain, as occur in mesenteric emboli
- Pain, cessation of pulses, blanching, numbness, or coldness in an extremity
- One-sided weakness and pupillary changes, as occur in stroke

The nurse promptly reports any of these symptoms.

Venous stasis, which can cause venous thromboembolism (e.g., deep vein thrombosis, pulmonary embolism), may occur after surgery. It can be prevented by using the following measures:

- Apply sequential pneumatic compression devices as prescribed.
- Discourage crossing of legs.
- Avoid elevating the knees on the bed.
- Omit pillows in the popliteal space.
- Begin passive exercises followed by active exercises to promote circulation and prevent venous stasis.

Inadequate renal perfusion can occur as a complication of cardiac surgery. One possible cause is low cardiac output. Trauma to blood cells during CPB can cause hemolysis of red blood cells, which then occlude the renal glomeruli. The use of vasopressor agents to increase blood pressure may constrict the renal arterioles and reduce blood flow to the kidneys.

Nursing management includes accurate measurement of urine output. An output less than 0.5 mL/kg/h may indicate hypovolemia or renal insufficiency. The primary provider may prescribe fluids to increase cardiac output and renal blood flow, or IV diuretics may be given to increase urine output. The nurse should be aware of the patient's blood urea nitrogen, serum creatinine, glomerular filtration rate, and serum electrolyte levels. The nurse should report abnormal levels promptly, because it may be necessary to adjust fluids and the dose or type of medication given. If efforts to maintain renal perfusion are ineffective, the patient may require continuous renal replacement therapy or dialysis (see Chapter 54).

Maintaining Normal Body Temperature

Patients are usually hypothermic when admitted to the critical care unit following the cardiac surgical procedure. Because induced hypothermia from CPB and anesthesia lower the patient's core temperature, the patient must be gradually warmed to a normal temperature. This is accomplished partially by the patient's own basal metabolic processes and often with the assistance of heated air blanket systems. While the patient is hypothermic, shivering and hypertension are common. Lowering the blood pressure with a vasodilator such as nitroprusside (Nipride) may be necessary. These problems typically resolve as warming occurs.

After cardiac surgery, the patient is at risk for developing elevated body temperature as a result of tissue inflammation or infection. The inflammatory/immune response to surgery includes the release of cytokines that cause fever (Grossman

& Porth, 2014). The resultant increase in metabolic rate increases tissue oxygen demands and increases cardiac workload. Antipyretics and other measures are used to lower body temperature.

Common sites of postoperative infection include the lungs, urinary tract, incisions, and intravascular catheters. Meticulous care is used to prevent contamination at the sites of catheter and tube insertions. Aseptic technique is used when changing dressings and when providing endotracheal tube and catheter care. Clearance of pulmonary secretions is accomplished by frequent repositioning of the patient, suctioning, and chest physical therapy, as well as educating and encouraging the patient to breathe deeply and cough. All invasive lines and tubes are discontinued as soon as possible after surgery to avoid infection.

Postpericardiotomy syndrome may occur in patients who undergo cardiac surgery. The syndrome is characterized by fever, pericardial pain, pleural pain, dyspnea, pericardial effusion, pericardial friction rub, and arthralgia. These signs and symptoms may occur days to weeks after surgery, often after the patient has been discharged from the hospital.

Postpericardiotomy syndrome must be differentiated from other postoperative complications (e.g., infection, incisional pain, MI, pulmonary embolus, bacterial endocarditis, pneumonia, atelectasis). Treatment depends on the severity of the signs and symptoms. Anti-inflammatory agents may produce an improvement in symptoms (Imazio, Brucato, Ferrazzi, et al., 2014).

Promoting Home, Community-Based, and Transitional Care

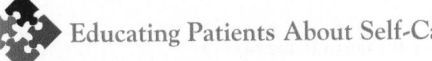 **Educating Patients About Self-Care**

Depending on the type of surgery and postoperative progress, the patient may be discharged from the hospital 3 to 5 days after surgery. Following recovery from the surgery, patients can expect fewer symptoms from CAD and an improved quality of life. CABG has been shown to increase the lifespan of high-risk patients, including those with left main artery blockages and left ventricular dysfunction with multivessel blockages (Hlatky, Boothroyd, Baker, et al., 2013).

Although the patient may be eager to return home, the patient and family usually are apprehensive about this transition. Family members often express the fear that they are not capable of caring for the patient at home or that they are unprepared to handle complications that may occur.

The nurse helps the patient and family set realistic, achievable goals. An education plan that meets the patient's individual needs is developed with the patient and family. Specific instructions are provided about incision care; signs and symptoms of infection; diet; activity progression and exercise; deep breathing, incentive spirometry, and tobacco use cessation; weight and temperature monitoring; the medication regimen; and follow-up visits with home care nurses, the rehabilitation personnel, the surgeon, and the cardiologist or internist.

Some patients have difficulty learning and retaining information after cardiac surgery. The patient may experience recent memory loss, short attention span, difficulty with simple math, poor handwriting, and visual disturbances. Patients with these difficulties often become frustrated when they try to resume normal activities. The patient and family are

Chart 27-13

HOME CARE CHECKLIST

Discharge After Cardiac Surgery

At the completion of education, the patient and/or caregiver will be able to:

- Name the procedure that was performed and identify any permanent changes in anatomic structure or function as well as changes in ADLs, IADLs, roles, relationships, and spirituality.
- Identify interventions and strategies (e.g., durable medical equipment, adaptive equipment) used in recovery period.
- Describe ongoing postoperative therapeutic regimen, including diet and activities to perform (e.g., walking and breathing exercises) and to limit or avoid (e.g., lifting weights, driving a car, contact sports).
- State the name, dose, side effects, frequency, and schedule for all medications.
- State how to obtain medical supplies and carry out dressing changes, wound care, and other prescribed regimens.

- Identify durable medical equipment needs, proper usage, and maintenance necessary for safe utilization.
- Describe signs and symptoms of complications.
- State time and date of follow-up appointments.
- Relate how to reach the primary provider with questions or complications.
- Identify community resources for peer and caregiver/family support:
  - Identify sources of support (e.g., friends, relatives, faith community)
  - Identify phone numbers, meeting locations/times of support groups for people and their caregivers/families
- Identify the need for health promotion (e.g., weight reduction, smoking cessation, stress management), disease prevention, and screening activities

ADL, activities of daily living; IADL, independent activities of daily living.

---

reassured that the difficulty is almost always temporary and will subside, usually in 6 to 8 weeks. In the meantime, instructions are given to the patient at a slower pace than normal, and a family member assumes responsibility for making sure that the prescribed regimen is followed.

Continuing and Transitional Care

Arrangements are made for home, community-based, or transitional care when appropriate. Because the hospital stay is relatively short, it is particularly important for the nurse to assess the patient's and family's ability to manage care in the home. The nurse making a home visit continues the education process (see Chart 27-13), monitors vital signs and incisions, assesses for signs and symptoms of complications, and provides support for the patient and family. Additional interventions may include dressing changes, diet counseling, and tobacco use cessation strategies. Patients and families need to know that cardiac surgery did not cure the patient's underlying heart disease process. Lifestyle changes for risk factor reduction are essential, and medications taken before surgery to control problems such as blood pressure and hyperlipidemia will still be necessary.

The nurse encourages the patient to contact the surgeon, cardiologist, or office nurse with problems or questions. This provides the patient and family with reassurance that professional support is available. The patient is expected to have at least one follow-up visit with the surgeon.

Education does not end at the time of discharge from the hospital, transitional, or home health care. Many patients and families benefit from supportive programs, including cardiac rehabilitation. These programs provide monitored exercise; instructions about diet and stress reduction; information about resuming work, driving, and sexual activity; assistance with tobacco use cessation; and support groups for patients and families. Hospital or community-based support groups provide information as well as an opportunity for families to share experiences.

CRITICAL THINKING EXERCISES

1 A 68-year-old patient just had his fasting lipid panel drawn with the following results: Total cholesterol 267 mg/dL, LDL 177 mg/dL, HDL 38 mg/dL, and triglyceride 459 mg/dL. He is asking for more information about hypercholesterolemia and how to improve his lipid profile. What are the normal values of a fasting cholesterol panel? What lifestyle modifications could this patient make to improve his cholesterol levels? What medications may be prescribed? In addition to the patient's primary provider, are there any other members of the healthcare team who should be involved in the treatment plan?

2 **ebp** An 80-year-old man was admitted to your hospital unit yesterday with chest pain. He was reported to be stable during the last shift. As you begin your assessment, he tells you that his chest pain is worse and he feels short of breath. Based on your knowledge of evidence-based guidelines, what would be your initial interventions? Which diagnostic tests may be performed? What types of interventions are available if the diagnosis of acute myocardial infarction is determined?

3 **pq** You are in the ICU and caring for a 75-year-old female who underwent coronary artery bypass grafting 2 days ago. She is pulling at her chest tubes and trying to get out of bed by herself. You are concerned she may have delirium. What interventions are your priorities to keep this patient safe? Identify what parameters need to be assessed immediately. What diagnostic testing should be done to rule out physiological problems? Which types of medications may be contributing to her delirium?

REFERENCES

*Asterisk indicates nursing research.
**Double asterisk indicates classic reference.

Books

Ackley, B. J., & Ladwig, G. B. (2014). *Nursing diagnosis handbook* (10th ed.). Maryland Heights, MO: Elsevier.

Burchum, J. R., & Rosenthal, L. D. (2016).*Lehne's pharmacology for nursing care* (9th ed.). St. Louis, MO: Elsevier.

Grossman, S. C., & Porth, C. M. (2014). *Porth's pathophysiology* (9th ed.). Philadelphia, PA: Lippincott Williams & Wilkins.

McCance, K. L., Huether, S. E., Brashers, V. L., et al. (2014). *Pathophysiology: The biologic basis for disease in adults and children* (7th ed.). St. Louis, MO: Elsevier.

Morton, P.G., & Fontaine, D.K. (2013). *Critical care nursing* (10th ed.). Philadelphia, PA: Lippincott Williams & Wilkins

Urden, L. D., Stacy, K. M., & Lough, M. E. (2014). *Critical care nursing* (7th ed.). St. Louis, MO: Elsevier.

Journals and Electronic Documents

American Heart Association (2015). *Menopause and heart disease.* Retrieved on 11/18/2015 at: www.heart.org/HEARTORG/Conditions/More/MyHeartandStrokeNews/Menopause-and-Heart-Disease_UCM_448432_Article.jsp

American Society of Clinical Oncology (2016). *Health risks of e-cigarettes, smokeless tobacco, and waterpipes.* Retrieved on 2/26/2016 at: www.cancer.net/navigating-cancer-care/prevention-and-healthy-living/tobacco-use

Amsterdam, E. A., Wenger, N. K., Brindis, R. G., et al. (2014). 2014 AHA/ACC guideline for the management of patients with non-ST-elevation acute coronary syndromes. *Circulation, 130*(25), e344–e426.

Bartels, K., McDonagh, D. L., Newman, M. F., et al. (2013). Neurocognitive outcomes after cardiac surgery. *Current Opinion in Anesthesiology, 26*(1), 91–97.

Bobadilla, R.V. (2016) Acute coronary syndrome: Focus on antiplatelet therapy. *Critical Care Nurse 30*(1), 15–27.

Bravo, C., Rondon Clavo, C. M., Oliva, P., et al. (2014). Percutaneous coronary intervention versus coronary artery bypass grafting for adults with diabetes and multivessel coronary artery disease. *Cochrane Database of Systematic Reviews, 3*(CD011012). doi: 10.1002/14651858.CD011012.

Brenes-Salazar, J. A., & Forman, D. E. (2014). Advances in percutaneous coronary interventions for elderly patients. *Progress in Cardiovascular Diseases, 57*(2), 176–186.

Brooks, P., Spillane, J. J., Dick, K., et al. (2014). Developing a strategy to identify and treat older patients with postoperative delirium. *AORN Journal, 99*(2), 256–276.

Canto, J. G., Canto, E. A., & Goldberg, R. J. (2014). Time to standardize and broaden the criteria of acute coronary syndrome symptom presentations in women. *Canadian Journal of Cardiology, 30*(7), 721–728.

Centers for Disease Control and Prevention (CDC). (2015). How much physical activity do adults need? Retrieved on 10/18/2015 at: www.cdc.gov/physicalactivity/basics/adults/index.htm.

*Chaisson, K., Sanford, M., Boss, R. A., et al. (2014) Improving patients' readiness for coronary artery bypass graft surgery. *Critical Care Nurse, 30*(6), 29–38.

Douglas, C. J., & Applegate, R. J. (2013). Minimizing complications following stent implantation: Outcomes and follow-up. *Interventional Cardiology, 5*(3), 301.

Engoren, M., Schwann, T. A., & Habib, R. H. (2014). Hyperglycemia, hypoglycemia and glycemic complexity are associated with worse outcomes after surgery. *Journal of Critical Care, 29*(4), 611–617.

Ferrari, R., Abergel, H., Ford, I., et al. (2013). Gender- and age-related differences in clinical presentation and management of outpatients with stable coronary artery disease. *International Journal of Cardiology, 167*(6), 2938–2943.

Feuchtinger, J., Burbaum, C., Heilmann, C., et al. (2013). Anxiety and fear in patients with short waiting times before coronary artery bypass surgery—a qualitative study. *Journal of Clinical Nursing, 23*(13–14), 1900–1907. doi: 10.1111/jocn.12467.

Fletcher, G. F., Ades, P. A., Kligfield, P., et al. (2013) Exercise standards for testing and training: A scientific statement from the American Heart Association. *Circulation, 128*(8), 873–934.

Goff, D. C., Lloyd-Jones, D. M., Bennett, G., et al. (2014). 2013 ACC/AHA guideline on the assessment of cardiovascular risk: A report of the American College of Cardiology/American Heart Association Task Force on Practice Guidelines. *Circulation, 129*(suppl 2), S49–S73. doi: 10.1161/01.cir.0000437741.48606.98.

Greinacher, A. (2015). Heparin-induced thrombocytopenia. *New England Journal of Medicine, 373*(3), 252–261.

*Hargraves, J. D. (2014). Glycemic control in cardiac surgery: Implementing an evidence-based insulin infusion protocol. *American Journal of Critical Care, 23*(3), 250–258.

Hillis, L. D., Smith, P. K., Anderson, J. L., et al. (2011). 2011 ACCF/AHA guideline for coronary artery bypass graft surgery: A report of the American College of Cardiology Foundation/American Heart Association Task Force on Practice Guidelines. *Circulation, 124*(23), e652–e735.

Hlatky, M. A., Boothroyd, D. B., Baker, L., et al. (2013). Comparative effectiveness of multivessel coronary bypass surgery and multivessel percutaneous coronary intervention. *Annals of Internal Medicine, 158*(10), 727–734.

Imazio, M., Brucato, A., Ferrazzi, P., et al. (2014). Colchicine for prevention of postpericardiotomy syndrome and postoperative atrial fibrillation: The COPPS-2 randomized clinical trial. *JAMA, 312*(10), 1016–1023. doi: 10.1001/jama.2014.11026.

Institute for Clinical Systems Improvement (ICSI). (2013a). Lipid management in adults. Retrieved on 11/18/2015 at: www.guideline.gov/content.aspx?id=47783&search=lipid+management+in+adults

Institute for Clinical Systems Improvement (ICSI). (2013b). Myocardial infarction with ST-segment elevation. The acute management of myocardial infarction with ST-segment elevation. Retrieved on 11/18/2015 at: www.guideline.gov/content.aspx?id=47019&search=myocardial+in farction

Institute for Clinical Systems Improvement (ICSI). (2013c). 2013 ACCF/AHA guideline for the management of ST-elevation myocardial infarction. A report of the American College of Cardiology Foundation/American Heart Association Task Force on Practice Guidelines. Retrieved on 11/18/2015 at: www.guideline.gov/content.aspx?id=39429&search=myocardial+infarction

James, P. A., Oparil, S., Carter, B. L., et al. (2014) 2014 Evidence-based guidelines for the management of high blood pressure in adults. Report from the panel members appointed to the Eighth Joint National Committee (JNC 8). *JAMA, 311*(5), 507–520.

**Kannel, W. B. (1986). Silent myocardial ischemia and infarction: Insights from the Framingham Study. *Cardiology Clinics, 4*(4), 583–591.

Kim, C., Park, J., & Kang, S. (2015). Prevalence of metabolic syndrome and cardiovascular risk level in a vulnerable population. *International Journal of Nursing Practice, 21*, 175–183.

Kim, J. B., Yun, S., Lim, J. W., et al. (2014). Long-term survival following coronary artery bypass grafting: Off-pump versus on-pump strategies. *Journal of the American College of Cardiology, 63*(21), 2280–2288.

Liu, M., Shehu, M., Herrold, E., et al. (2015) Prognostic value of initial elevation in cardiac troponin I level in critically ill patients without acute coronary syndrome. *Critical Care Nurse 35*(2), e1–e10.

Mangusan, R. F., Hooper, V., Denslow, S. A., et al. (2015). Outcomes associated with postoperative delirium after cardiac surgery. *American Journal of Critical Care, 24*(2), 156–164. doi: 10.4037/ajcc2015137.

Martinez-Gonzalez, M. A., Salas-Salvado, J., Estruch, R., et al. (2015). Benefits of the Mediterranean Diet: Insights from the PREDIMED study. *Progress In Cardiovascular Disease, 58*(1), 50–60.

Mozaffarian, D., Benjamin, E. J., Go, A. S., et al. (2016). Heart disease and stroke statistics—2016 update: A report from the American Heart Association. *Circulation, 133*(4), e38–e360.

Office of the U.S. Surgeon General. (2014). The health consequences of smoking—50 years of progress. Rockville, MD. Retrieved on 10/18/2015 at: www.surgeongeneral.gov/library/reports/50-years-of-progress/exec-summary.pdf

Palmerini, T., Benedetto, U., Biondi-Zoccai, G., et al. (2015) Long-term safety of drug-eluting and bare-metal stents. *Journal of the American College of Cardiology, 65*(23), 2496–2507.

Pollock, B., Hamman, B. L., Sass, D. M., et al., (2015). Effect of gender and race on operative mortality after isolated coronary artery bypass grafting. *The American Journal of Cardiology, 115*(5), 614–618.

Raja, S. G., & Sarang, Z. (2013). Endoscopic vein harvesting: Technique, outcomes, concerns & controversies. *Journal of Thoracic Disease, 5*(S6), S630–S637.

Ruel, M., Une, D., Bonatti, J., et al. (2013). Minimally invasive coronary artery bypass grafting: Is it time for the robot? *Current Opinion in Cardiology, 28*(6), 639–645. doi: 10.1097/HCO.0b013e3283653fd1.

Schnapf, A. J. (2013). Prasugrel versus clopidogrel: New management strategies for acute coronary syndrome. *Journal of Cardiovascular Nursing, 28*(5), 483–494. doi: 10.1097/JCN.0b013e31826173ba

Sehr, J., Eisele-Hlubocky, L., Junker, R., et al., (2013). Family pet visitation. *American Journal of Nursing, 113*(12), 54–59.

Shan, L., Saxena A., & McMahon, R. (2014). A systematic review on the quality of life benefits after percutaneous coronary intervention in the elderly. *Cardiology, 129*(1), 46–54. doi: 10.1159/000360603.

Stone, N. J., Robinson, J. G., Lichtenstein, A. H., et al. (2014). Treatment of blood cholesterol to reduce atherosclerotic cardiovascular disease risk in adults: Synopsis of the 2013 American College of Cardiology/American Heart Association Cholesterol Guideline. *Annals of Internal Medicine, 160*(5), 339–343.

TLC Diet Regimen. Retrieved on 11/18/2015 at: tlcdiet.org/tlc-diet-regime/

U.S. Food and Drug Administration (FDA). (2015). FDA 101: Smoking cessation products. Retrieved on 10/18/2015 at: www.fda.gov/forconsumers/consumerupdates/ucm198176.htm

White, C. M. (2015) Therapeutic potential and critical analysis of the PCSK9 monoclonal antibodies evolocumab and alirocumab. *Annals of Pharmacology, 49*(12), 1327–1335.

Wright, J. T., Williamson, J. D., & Whelton, P. K., et al; the SPRINT Research Group. (2015). A randomized trial of intensive versus standard blood-pressure control. *New England Journal of Medicine, 373*(22), 2103–2116.

Yi, G., Shine, B., Rehman, S. M., et al., (2014). Effect of bilateral internal mammary artery grafts on long-term survival. *Circulation, 130*(7), 539–545.

Resources

American Heart Association, www.heart.org/HEARTORG/

National Institutes of Health, National Heart, Lung, and Blood Institute, www.nhlbi.nih.gov

Therapeutic Lifestyles Changes (TLC) Diet, TLCdiet.org

28

Management of Patients With Structural, Infectious, and Inflammatory Cardiac Disorders

LEARNING OBJECTIVES

On completion of this chapter, the learner will be able to:

1 Define valvular disorders of the heart and describe the pathophysiology, clinical manifestations, as well as the medical and nursing management of patients with mitral and aortic disorders.
2 Describe types of cardiac valve repair and replacement procedures used to treat valvular problems and care needed by patients who undergo these procedures.
3 Identify the pathophysiology, clinical manifestations, as well as the medical and nursing management of patients with cardiomyopathies.
4 Describe the pathophysiology, clinical manifestations, as well as the medical and nursing management of patients with infections of the heart.
5 Use the nursing process as a framework of care for the patient with a cardiomyopathy and the patient with pericarditis.

GLOSSARY

allograft: heart valve replacement made from a human heart valve (*synonym:* homograft)
annuloplasty: repair of a cardiac valve's outer ring
aortic valve: semilunar valve located between the left ventricle and aorta
autograft: heart valve replacement made from the patient's own heart valve (e.g., pulmonic valve excised and used as an aortic valve)
bioprosthesis: heart valve replacement made of tissue from an animal heart valve (*synonym:* heterograft)
cardiomyopathy: disease of the heart muscle
chordae tendineae: nondistensible fibrous strands connecting papillary muscles to atrioventricular (mitral, tricuspid) valve leaflets
chordoplasty: repair of chordae tendineae
commissurotomy: splitting or separating fused cardiac valve leaflets
heterograft: heart valve replacement made of tissue from an animal heart valve (*synonym:* bioprosthesis)
homograft: heart valve replacement made from a human heart valve (*synonym:* allograft)
leaflet repair: repair of a cardiac valve's movable "flaps" (leaflets)

mitral valve: atrioventricular valve located between the left atrium and left ventricle
orthotopic transplantation: the recipient's heart is removed and a donor heart is grafted into the same site
prolapse (of a valve): stretching of an atrioventricular heart valve leaflet into the atrium during systole
pulmonic valve: semilunar valve located between the right ventricle and pulmonary artery
regurgitation: backward flow of blood through a heart valve
stenosis: narrowing or obstruction of a cardiac valve's orifice
total artificial heart: mechanical device used to aid a failing heart, assisting the right and left ventricles
tricuspid valve: atrioventricular valve located between the right atrium and right ventricle
valve replacement: insertion of a device at the site of a malfunctioning heart valve to restore blood flow in one direction through the heart
valvuloplasty: repair of a stenosed or regurgitant cardiac valve by commissurotomy, annuloplasty, leaflet repair, or chordoplasty (or a combination of procedures)
ventricular assist device: mechanical device used to aid a failing right or left ventricle

Structural, infectious, and inflammatory disorders of the heart present many challenges for the patient, family, and health care team. Problems with heart valves, cardiomyopathies, and infectious diseases of the heart alter cardiac output. Treatments for these disorders may be noninvasive, such as medication therapy and activity or dietary modification. Invasive treatments also may be used, such as valve repair or replacement, ventricular assist devices (VADs), total artificial hearts, cardiac transplantation, and other procedures. Nurses have an integral role in the care of patients with structural, infectious, and inflammatory cardiac conditions.

VALVULAR DISORDERS

Valves of the heart control the flow of blood through the heart into the pulmonary artery and aorta by opening and closing in response to blood pressure changes during each cardiac cycle (heart contraction and relaxation).

Atrioventricular valves separate the atria from the ventricles and include the **tricuspid valve**, which separates the right atrium from the right ventricle, and the **mitral valve**, which separates the left atrium from the left ventricle. The tricuspid valve has three leaflets; the mitral valve has two.

Aortic (semilunar) valve

Tricuspid valve

Mitral valve

Figure 28-1 • Valves of the heart (aortic or semilunar, tricuspid, and mitral) in closed positions.

Both valves have **chordae tendineae** that anchor valve leaflets to papillary muscles of the ventricles.

Semilunar valves are located between the ventricles and their corresponding arteries. The **pulmonic valve** lies between the right ventricle and the pulmonary artery; the aortic valve lies between the left ventricle and the aorta. Figure 28-1 shows valves in the closed position. (Also refer to Fig. 25-1 in Chapter 25 to review the structure of a normal heart.)

When any heart valve does not close or open properly, blood flow is affected. When valves do not close completely, blood flows backward through the valve, a condition called **regurgitation**. When valves do not open completely, a condition called **stenosis**, blood flow through the valve is reduced.

Regurgitation and stenosis affect all heart valves. The mitral valve may also **prolapse** (i.e., stretching of the valve leaflet into the atrium during systole). Depending on the severity of symptoms, patients with valve disorders may not require treatment, or they may need to make lifestyle changes, take medications, or require surgical repair or replacement of the valve. Disorders of the mitral and aortic valve cause more symptoms, require treatment, and cause more complications than disorders of the tricuspid and pulmonic valves. Regurgitation and stenosis may occur at the same time in the same or different valves (see Fig. 28-2).

Mitral Valve Prolapse

Mitral valve prolapse is a deformity that usually produces no symptoms. Rarely, it progresses and can result in sudden death. This condition occurs in up to 2.5% of the general population and twice as frequently in women than in men (Delling & Vassan, 2014; Mann, Zipes, Bonow, et al., 2015). The cause may be an inherited connective tissue disorder resulting in enlargement of one or both of the mitral valve leaflets, but in many cases the cause is unknown. The annulus often dilates; chordae tendineae and papillary muscles may elongate or rupture.

Pathophysiology

In mitral valve prolapse, a portion of one or both mitral valve leaflets balloons back into the atrium during systole. Rarely, ballooning stretches the leaflet to the point that the valve does not remain closed during systole. Blood then regurgitates from the left ventricle back into the left atrium. About 15% of patients who develop murmurs eventually experience heart enlargement, atrial fibrillation, pulmonary hypertension, or heart failure (Fuster, Walsh, Harrington, et al., 2011).

Clinical Manifestations

Most people with mitral valve prolapse never have symptoms. A few have fatigue, shortness of breath, lightheadedness, dizziness, syncope, palpitations, chest pain, or anxiety. Fatigue may occur regardless of activity level and amount of rest or sleep. Shortness of breath is not correlated with activity levels or pulmonary function. Atrial or ventricular dysrhythmias may produce the sensation of palpitations, but palpitations have been reported while the heart has been beating normally. Pain, which is often localized to the chest, is not correlated with activity and may last for days. Anxiety may be a response to symptoms; however, some patients

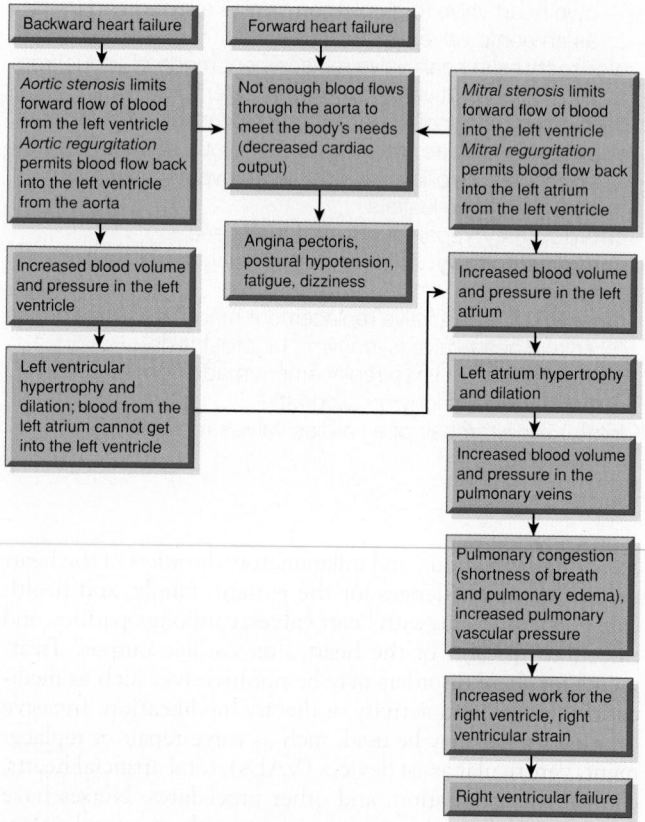

Physiology/Pathophysiology

Backward heart failure	Forward heart failure

Aortic stenosis limits forward flow of blood from the left ventricle
Aortic regurgitation permits blood flow back into the left ventricle from the aorta

Not enough blood flows through the aorta to meet the body's needs (decreased cardiac output)

Mitral stenosis limits forward flow of blood into the left ventricle
Mitral regurgitation permits blood flow back into the left atrium from the left ventricle

Increased blood volume and pressure in the left ventricle

Angina pectoris, postural hypotension, fatigue, dizziness

Increased blood volume and pressure in the left atrium

Left ventricular hypertrophy and dilation; blood from the left atrium cannot get into the left ventricle

Left atrium hypertrophy and dilation

Increased blood volume and pressure in the pulmonary veins

Pulmonary congestion (shortness of breath and pulmonary edema), increased pulmonary vascular pressure

Increased work for the right ventricle, right ventricular strain

Right ventricular failure

Figure 28-2 • Pathophysiology. Left-sided heart failure as a result of aortic and mitral valvular heart disease and development of right ventricular failure.

report anxiety as the only symptom. Some clinicians speculate that symptoms may be explained by dysautonomia (a dysfunction of the autonomic nervous system that results in increased excretion of catecholamines). No consensus exists about the cause of symptoms (Mann et al., 2015; Runge, Stouffer, & Patterson, 2011).

Assessment and Diagnostic Findings

Often the first and only sign of mitral valve prolapse is an extra heart sound, referred to as a mitral click. A systolic click is an early sign that a valve leaflet is ballooning into the left atrium. In addition to the mitral click, a murmur of mitral regurgitation may be heard if the valve opens during systole and blood flows back into the left atrium. If mitral regurgitation exists, a patient may experience signs and symptoms of heart failure. Echocardiography is used to diagnose and monitor progression of mitral valve prolapse (Mann et al., 2015).

Medical Management

Medical management is directed at controlling symptoms. If dysrhythmias are documented and cause symptoms, the patient is advised to eliminate caffeine and alcohol from the diet and to stop the use of tobacco products. Most patients do not require medication, but some are prescribed antiarrhythmic medications. Prophylactic antibiotics are not recommended prior to dental or invasive procedures (Nishimura, Otto, Bonow, et al., 2014).

Chest pain that does not respond to nitrates may respond to calcium channel blockers or beta-blockers. Heart failure is treated the same as it would be for any other case of heart failure (see Chapter 29). Patients with severe mitral regurgitation and symptomatic heart failure may require mitral valve repair or replacement (discussed later in this chapter).

Nursing Management

The nurse educates the patient about the diagnosis and the possibility that the condition is hereditary. First-degree relatives (e.g., parents, siblings) may be advised to have echocardiograms. Patients with mitral valve prolapse may be at risk for infective endocarditis from bacteria entering the bloodstream and adhering to abnormal valve structures. The nurse educates the patient how to minimize this risk (see discussion of Infective Endocarditis later in this chapter).

Because most patients with mitral valve prolapse are asymptomatic, the nurse explains the need to inform the patient's primary provider about any symptoms that may develop. To minimize symptoms, the nurse instructs the patient to avoid caffeine and alcohol. The nurse encourages the patient to read product labels, particularly on over-the-counter products such as cough medicine, because these products may contain alcohol, caffeine, ephedrine, and epinephrine, which may produce dysrhythmias and other symptoms. The nurse also explores diet, activity, sleep, and other lifestyle factors that may correlate with symptoms. Treatment of dysrhythmias, chest pain, heart failure, or other complications of mitral valve prolapse is described in Chapters 26 and 29. Women diagnosed with mitral valve prolapse without mitral regurgitation or other complications may complete pregnancies with vaginal deliveries.

Mitral Regurgitation

Mitral regurgitation involves blood flowing back from the left ventricle into the left atrium during systole. Often, edges of mitral valve leaflets do not close completely during systole because leaflets and chordae tendineae have thickened and fibrosed, resulting in their contraction. The most common causes of mitral valve regurgitation in developed countries are degenerative changes of the mitral valve (e.g., mitral valve prolapse) and ischemia of the left ventricle (Fuster et al., 2011; Mann et al., 2015). The most common cause in developing countries is rheumatic heart disease and its sequelae (Fuster et al., 2011).

Other conditions that lead to mitral regurgitation include myxomatous changes, which enlarge and stretch the left atrium and ventricle, causing leaflets and chordae tendineae to stretch or rupture. Infective endocarditis may cause perforation of a leaflet, or scarring following the infection may cause retraction of leaflets or chordae tendineae. Collagen vascular diseases (e.g., systemic lupus erythematosus), cardiomyopathy, and ischemic heart disease also may result in changes in the left ventricle, causing papillary muscles, chordae tendineae, or leaflets to stretch, shorten, or rupture.

Pathophysiology

Mitral regurgitation may result from problems with one or more leaflets, chordae tendineae, annulus, or papillary muscles. A mitral valve leaflet may shorten or tear, and chordae tendineae may elongate, shorten, or tear. The annulus may be stretched by heart enlargement or deformed by calcification. A papillary muscle may rupture, stretch, or be pulled out of position by changes in the ventricular wall (e.g., scar from a myocardial infarction, ventricular dilation). Papillary muscles may be unable to contract because of ischemia. Regardless of the cause, blood regurgitates into the atrium during systole.

With each beat of the left ventricle, some blood is forced back into the left atrium, adding to blood flowing in from the lungs. This causes the left atrium to stretch and eventually hypertrophy (i.e., thicken), then dilate. Backward flow of blood from the ventricle decreases blood flow from the lungs into the atrium. As a result, the lungs become congested, eventually adding extra strain to the right ventricle. During diastole, the increased blood volume from the atrium fills the ventricle. The volume overload causes ventricular hypertrophy. Eventually, the ventricle dilates and systolic heart failure develops.

Clinical Manifestations

Chronic mitral regurgitation is often asymptomatic, but acute mitral regurgitation (e.g., resulting from a myocardial infarction) usually manifests as severe congestive heart failure. Dyspnea, fatigue, and weakness are the most common symptoms. Palpitations, shortness of breath on exertion, and cough from pulmonary congestion also occur.

Assessment and Diagnostic Findings

A systolic murmur is a high-pitched, blowing sound at the apex that may radiate to the left axilla (Mann et al., 2015; Weber & Kelley, 2014). The pulse may be regular and of good volume, or it may be irregular as a result of extrasystolic beats or atrial fibrillation. Echocardiography is used to diagnose and monitor the progression of mitral regurgitation (Mann et al., 2015).

Medical Management

Management of mitral regurgitation is the same as for heart failure (see Chapter 29). Patients with mitral regurgitation and heart failure benefit from afterload reduction (arterial dilation) by treatment with angiotensin-converting enzyme (ACE) inhibitors such as captopril (Capoten), enalapril (Vasotec), lisinopril (Prinivil, Zestril) or ramipril (Altace), or hydralazine (Apresoline); or angiotensin receptor blockers (ARBs) such as losartan (Cozaar) or valsartan (Diovan); and beta-blockers, such as carvedilol (Coreg) (see Table 29-3). Once symptoms of heart failure develop, the patient needs to restrict their activity level to minimize symptoms. Symptoms also are an indicator for surgical intervention by mitral valvuloplasty (i.e., surgical repair of the valve) or valve replacement (discussed later) (Nishimura et al., 2014).

Mitral Stenosis

Mitral stenosis is an obstruction to blood flowing from the left atrium into the left ventricle. It most often is caused by rheumatic endocarditis, which progressively thickens mitral valve leaflets and chordae tendineae. Leaflets often fuse together. Eventually, the mitral valve orifice narrows and progressively obstructs blood flow into the ventricle.

Pathophysiology

Normally, the mitral valve orifice is as wide as the diameter of three fingers. In cases of severe stenosis, the orifice narrows to the width of a pencil. The left atrium has difficulty moving blood into the ventricle because of increased resistance by the narrowed orifice. Poor left ventricular filling can cause decreased cardiac output. Increased blood volume in the left atrium causes it to dilate and hypertrophy. Because there is no valve to protect pulmonary veins from backward flow of blood from the atrium, the pulmonary circulation becomes congested. As a result, the right ventricle must contract against abnormally high pulmonary arterial pressure and is subjected to excessive strain. The right ventricle hypertrophies, eventually dilates, and fails. If the heart rate increases, diastole is shortened; thus, the amount of time for forward flow of blood is less, and more blood backs into the pulmonary veins. Therefore, as the heart rate increases, cardiac output decreases and pulmonary pressures increase.

Clinical Manifestations

The first symptom of mitral stenosis often is dyspnea on exertion (DOE) as a result of pulmonary venous hypertension. Symptoms usually develop after the valve opening is reduced by one third to one half its usual size. Patients may experience progressive fatigue and decreased exercise tolerance as a result of low cardiac output. An enlarged left atrium may create pressure on the left bronchial tree, resulting in a dry cough or wheezing. Patients may expectorate blood (i.e., hemoptysis) or experience palpitations, orthopnea, paroxysmal nocturnal dyspnea (PND), and repeated respiratory infections. As a result of increased blood volume and pressure, the atrium

dilates, hypertrophies, and becomes electrically unstable (patients experience atrial dysrhythmias).

Assessment and Diagnostic Findings

The pulse is weak and irregular in the presence of atrial fibrillation (caused by strain on the atrium). A low-pitched, rumbling diastolic murmur is heard at the apex and the patient may have signs or symptoms of heart failure (Mann et al., 2015; Weber & Kelley, 2014). Echocardiography is used to diagnose and quantify the severity of mitral stenosis. Electrocardiography (ECG), exercise testing, and cardiac catheterization with angiography may be used to help determine the severity of mitral stenosis.

Prevention

Prevention of mitral stenosis primarily is minimizing risk of and treatment for bacterial infections (see prevention of endocarditis later in this chapter). Prevention of acute rheumatic fever depends on effective antibiotic treatment of group A streptococcal infection (Nishimura et al., 2014). Antibiotic prophylaxis for recurrent rheumatic fever with rheumatic carditis may require 10 or more years of antibiotic coverage (e.g., penicillin G intramuscularly every 4 weeks, penicillin V orally twice daily, sulfadiazine orally daily, or erythromycin orally twice daily) (Fuster et al., 2011; Mann et al., 2015; Nishimura et al., 2014).

Medical Management

Congestive heart failure is treated as described in Chapter 29. Patients with mitral stenosis may benefit from anticoagulants to decrease the risk of developing atrial thrombus and may require treatment for angina. If atrial fibrillation develops, cardioversion is attempted to restore normal sinus rhythm. If unsuccessful, the ventricular rate is controlled with beta-blockers, digoxin, or calcium channel blockers; furthermore, patients require anticoagulation for thromboembolism prevention. Patients with mitral stenosis are advised to avoid strenuous activities, competitive sports, and pregnancy, all of which increase heart rate. Surgical intervention consists of valvuloplasty, usually a commissurotomy to open or rupture the fused commissures of the valve. Percutaneous transluminal valvuloplasty or valve replacement may be performed.

Aortic Regurgitation

Aortic regurgitation is flow of blood back into the left ventricle from the aorta during diastole. It may be caused by inflammatory lesions that deform aortic valve leaflets or dilation of the aorta, preventing complete closure of the aortic valve. This valvular defect also may result from infective or rheumatic endocarditis, congenital abnormalities, diseases such as syphilis, a dissecting aneurysm that causes dilation or tearing of the ascending aorta, blunt chest trauma, or deterioration of a surgically replaced aortic valve (Cohn, 2012; Fuster et al., 2011; Mann et al., 2015).

Pathophysiology

Blood from the aorta returns to the left ventricle during diastole, in addition to blood normally delivered by the left atrium. The left ventricle dilates in an attempt to accommodate the increased volume of blood. It also hypertrophies in an attempt to increase muscle strength to expel more blood with above-normal force, thus increasing systolic blood pressure. Arteries attempt to compensate for higher pressures by reflex vasodilation; peripheral arterioles relax, reducing peripheral resistance and diastolic blood pressure.

Clinical Manifestations

Aortic insufficiency develops without symptoms in most patients. Some patients are aware of a forceful heartbeat, especially in the head or neck. Marked arterial pulsations visible or palpable at carotid or temporal arteries may be present as a result of increased force and volume of blood ejected from a hypertrophied left ventricle. Exertional dyspnea and fatigue follow. Signs and symptoms of progressive left ventricular failure include breathing difficulties (e.g., orthopnea, PND).

Assessment and Diagnostic Findings

A high-pitched, blowing diastolic murmur is heard at the third or fourth intercostal space at the left sternal border (Weber & Kelley, 2014). The pulse pressure (i.e., difference between systolic and diastolic pressures) is considerably widened in patients with aortic regurgitation. One characteristic sign is the water hammer (Corrigan's) pulse, in which the pulse strikes a palpating finger with a quick, sharp stroke and then suddenly collapses. The diagnosis may be confirmed by echocardiography (preferably transesophageal), cardiac magnetic resonance imaging (MRI), and cardiac catheterization (Mann et al., 2015; Pennell, Baksi, Kilner, et al., 2014). Patients with symptoms usually have echocardiograms every 6 months, and those without symptoms have echocardiograms every 2 to 5 years (Nishimura et al., 2014; Otto & Bonow, 2013).

Prevention

Prevention of aortic regurgitation is primarily based on prevention of and treatment for bacterial infections (see prevention of endocarditis later in this chapter). The same strategies aimed at preventing acute and recurrent rheumatic fever previously described for the patient with mitral stenosis apply to patients with aortic regurgitation.

Medical Management

The symptomatic patient, or patient with decreased left ventricular function, is advised to avoid physical exertion, competitive sports, and isometric exercise (Mann et al., 2015). Dysrhythmias and heart failure are treated as described in Chapters 26 and 29. There is no strong indication for medical therapy based on findings from clinical trials. Patients with aortic regurgitation and also hypertension should be treated with dihydropyridine calcium channel blockers (e.g., felodipine [Plendil], nifedipine [Adalat, Procardia]) or ACE inhibitors (e.g., captopril, enalapril, lisinopril, ramipril) to provide afterload reduction (Nishimura et al., 2014). Symptomatic patients should be instructed to restrict sodium intake to avoid volume overload (Mann, et al., 2015; Nishimura et al., 2014).

> ▶ **Quality and Safety Nursing Alert**
>
> *The calcium channel blockers diltiazem (Cardizem) and verapamil (Calan, Isoptin) are contraindicated for patients with aortic regurgitation because they decrease ventricular contractility and may cause bradycardia.*

The treatment of choice is aortic valve replacement or valvuloplasty (described later), preferably performed before left ventricular failure occurs. Surgery is recommended for any patient with left ventricular dilation, regardless of the presence or absence of symptoms (Mann et al., 2015; Nishimura et al., 2014; Otto & Bonow, 2013). Surgery is also recommended for any patient who is symptomatic (Grossman & Porth, 2014).

Aortic Stenosis

Aortic valve stenosis is narrowing of the orifice between the left ventricle and aorta. In adults, stenosis often is a result of degenerative calcifications. Calcifications may be caused by proliferative and inflammatory changes that occur in response to years of normal mechanical stress, similar to changes that occur in atherosclerotic arterial disease. Age, diabetes, hypercholesterolemia, hypertension, smoking, and elevated levels of low-density lipoprotein cholesterol may be risk factors for degenerative calcific changes of the valve (Mann et al., 2015). Congenital leaflet malformations or an abnormal number of leaflets (i.e., one or two rather than three) may be involved. Rheumatic endocarditis may cause adhesions or fusion of the commissures and valve ring, stiffening of the cusps, and calcific nodules on the cusps.

Pathophysiology

Progressive narrowing of the valve orifice occurs, usually over several years to several decades. The left ventricle overcomes obstruction to emptying by contracting more slowly but with more power than normal, forcibly squeezing blood through the smaller orifice. Obstruction to left ventricular outflow increases pressure on the left ventricle, so the ventricular wall hypertrophies. When these compensatory mechanisms of the heart begin to fail, clinical signs and symptoms develop (Otto & Bonow, 2013).

Clinical Manifestations

Many patients with aortic stenosis are asymptomatic. When symptoms develop, patients usually first have exertional dyspnea, caused by increased pulmonary venous pressure due to left ventricular failure. Orthopnea, PND, and pulmonary edema also may occur. Reduced blood flow to the brain may cause dizziness and syncope. Angina pectoris is a frequent symptom; it results from increased oxygen demand of the hypertrophied left ventricle with decreased blood supply due to decreased blood flow into the coronary arteries and decreased time in diastole for myocardial perfusion. Blood pressure is usually normal but may be low. Pulse pressure may be low (30 mm Hg or less) because of diminished blood flow.

Assessment and Diagnostic Findings

On physical examination, a loud, harsh systolic murmur may be heard over the aortic area (i.e., right second intercostal space) and may radiate to the carotid arteries and apex of the left ventricle. The murmur is low pitched, crescendo–decrescendo, rough, rasping, and vibrating (Weber & Kelley, 2014). An S_4 sound may be heard. If the examiner rests a hand over the base of the heart (second intercostal space next to the sternum and above the suprasternal notch) and up along the carotid arteries, a vibration may be felt. The vibration is caused by turbulent blood flow across the narrowed valve orifice. By having the patient lean forward during auscultation and palpation, especially during exhalation, it is possible to accentuate sounds of aortic stenosis (Weber & Kelley, 2014).

Echocardiography, cardiac MRI, and computed tomography (CT) scanning are used to diagnose and monitor progression of aortic stenosis. Patients with symptoms usually have echocardiograms every 6 to 12 months, and those without symptoms have echocardiograms every 1 to 5 years (Fuster et al., 2011; Nishimura et al., 2014). Evidence of left ventricular hypertrophy may be seen on a 12-lead ECG and an echocardiogram. After stenosis progresses to the point that surgical intervention is considered, left-sided heart catheterization is necessary to measure the severity of the valvular abnormality and to evaluate the coronary arteries. Pressure tracings are taken from the left ventricle and base of the aorta. The systolic pressure in the left ventricle is considerably higher than that in the aorta during systole. Graded exercise studies (stress tests) to assess exercise capacity are performed with caution for patients with aortic stenosis because of the high risk of precipitating ventricular tachycardia or fibrillation, and should not be performed on symptomatic patients (Cohn, 2012; Mann et al., 2015; Nishimura et al., 2014).

Prevention

Prevention of aortic stenosis is primarily focused on controlling risk factors for proliferative and inflammatory responses—namely, through treating diabetes, hypertension, hypercholesterolemia, and elevated triglycerides and avoiding tobacco products. (See prevention of endocarditis later in this chapter.)

Medical Management

Medications are prescribed to treat dysrhythmia or left ventricular failure (see Chapters 26 and 29). Definitive treatment for aortic stenosis is surgical replacement of the aortic valve. Patients who are symptomatic and are not surgical candidates may benefit from one- or two-balloon percutaneous valvuloplasty procedures with or without transcatheter aortic valve implantation (TAVI) as described later in the chapter.

Nursing Management: Valvular Heart Disorders

The nurse educates the patient with valvular heart disease about the diagnosis, progressive nature of the disease, and treatment plan. The patient is instructed to report new symptoms or changes in symptoms to the primary provider. The nurse also educates the patient that an infectious agent, usually a bacterium, is able to adhere to a diseased heart valve more readily than to a normal valve. Once attached to the valve, the infectious agent multiplies, resulting in endocarditis and further damage to the valve. In addition, the nurse educates the patient about how to minimize the risk of developing infective endocarditis (discussed later in this chapter).

The nurse measures the patient's heart rate, blood pressure, and respiratory rate, compares these results with previous data, and notes any changes. Heart and lung sounds are auscultated and peripheral pulses palpated. The nurse assesses the patient with valvular heart disease for the following:

- Signs and symptoms of heart failure, such as fatigue, DOE, decreased activity tolerance, an increase in coughing, hemoptysis, multiple respiratory infections, orthopnea, and PND (see Chapter 29)
- Dysrhythmias, by palpating the patient's pulse for strength and rhythm (i.e., regular or irregular) and asking whether the patient has experienced palpitations or felt forceful heartbeats (see Chapter 26)
- Symptoms such as dizziness, syncope, increased weakness, or angina pectoris (see Chapter 27)

The nurse collaborates with the patient to develop a medication schedule and provides education about the name, dosage, actions, adverse effects, and any drug–drug or drug–food interactions of prescribed medications for heart failure, dysrhythmias, angina pectoris, or other symptoms. Specific precautions are emphasized, such as the risk to patients with aortic stenosis who experience angina pectoris and take nitroglycerin. The venous dilation that results from nitroglycerin use decreases blood return to the heart, thus decreasing cardiac output and increasing the risk of syncope and decreased coronary artery blood flow. The nurse instructs the patient about the importance of attempting to relieve the symptoms of angina with rest and relaxation before taking nitroglycerin and to anticipate the potential adverse effects.

In addition, the nurse educates the patient to take a daily weight and report sudden weight gain, as defined by the primary provider (American Heart Association, 2015). For example, in the past patients were instructed to call their primary providers if they gained 3 lb in 1 day or 5 lb in 1 week. Now weight gain parameters are more individualized to each patient. The nurse may assist the patient with planning activity and rest periods to achieve an acceptable lifestyle. Patients who experience symptoms of pulmonary congestion are advised to rest and sleep sitting in a chair or bed with the head elevated. Care of patients treated with valvuloplasty or surgical valve replacement is described later in this chapter.

SURGICAL MANAGEMENT: VALVE REPAIR AND REPLACEMENT PROCEDURES

Valvuloplasty

Repair, rather than replacement, of a cardiac valve is referred to as **valvuloplasty**. Patients who undergo valvuloplasty do not require continuous anticoagulation (Mann et al., 2015; Cohn, 2012; Otto & Bonow, 2013). The type of valvuloplasty depends on the cause and type of valve dysfunction. Repair may be made to commissures between the leaflets in a procedure known as **commissurotomy**, to the annulus of the valve by annuloplasty, to leaflets, or to chordae by chordoplasty. Transesophageal echocardiogram (TEE) usually is performed at the conclusion of a valvuloplasty to evaluate the effectiveness of the procedure.

Most valvuloplasty procedures require general anesthesia and often require cardiopulmonary bypass. However, some procedures do not require general anesthesia or cardiopulmonary bypass and can be performed in a cardiac catheterization laboratory or hybrid room. A hybrid room is an operating room with imaging capability (e.g., fluoroscopy, CT, MRI) and interventional devices for open, minimally invasive, image-guided and catheter-based procedures (Kaneko & Davidson, 2014). Percutaneous partial cardiopulmonary bypass is used in some cardiac catheterization laboratories and hybrid rooms. (Cardiopulmonary Bypass is described in Chapter 27.)

Commissurotomy

The most common valvuloplasty procedure is commissurotomy. Each valve has leaflets; the site where the leaflets meet is called the *commissure*. Leaflets may adhere to one another and close the commissure (i.e., stenosis). Less commonly, leaflets fuse in such a way that in addition to stenosis, the leaflets also are prevented from closing completely, resulting in backward flow of blood (i.e., regurgitation). A commissurotomy is the procedure performed to separate the fused leaflets.

Closed Commissurotomy/Balloon Valvuloplasty

Closed commissurotomies do not require cardiopulmonary bypass. The valve is not directly visualized. Closed commissurotomy is more commonly performed in developing nations; it is a surgical technique performed in the operating room with the patient under general anesthesia. It is the preferred technique for patients with congenital mitral stenosis, severe calcified mitral stenosis, left atrial thrombus, moderate-to-severe coexisting mitral regurgitation, or in patients with coexisting moderate-to-severe tricuspid regurgitation who would also benefit from tricuspid valve repair (Nishimura et al., 2014). A midsternal incision is made, a small hole is cut into the heart, and a dilator is used to open the commissure.

Percutaneous balloon valvuloplasty is the technique most commonly performed in the United States as a bridge to surgical valve replacement or transfemoral aortic valve replacement for closed commissurotomy (Badheka, Patel, Singh, et al., 2014; Kapadia, Stewart, Anderson, et al., 2015). Balloon valvuloplasty is beneficial for mitral valve stenosis in younger patients and for patients with complex medical conditions that place them at high risk for complications of more extensive surgical procedures. Most often used for mitral and aortic valve stenosis, balloon valvuloplasty has been used for tricuspid and pulmonic valve stenosis. The procedure is contraindicated for patients with left atrial or ventricular thrombus, severe aortic root dilation, significant mitral valve regurgitation, severe valvular calcification, thoracolumbar scoliosis, rotation of the great vessels, and other cardiac conditions that require open heart surgery (Cohn, 2012; Fuster et al., 2011).

Balloon valvuloplasty (see Fig. 28-3) is performed in the cardiac catheterization laboratory. The patient may receive light or moderate sedation or a local anesthetic. Mitral balloon valvuloplasty involves advancing one or two catheters into the right atrium, through the atrial septum into the left

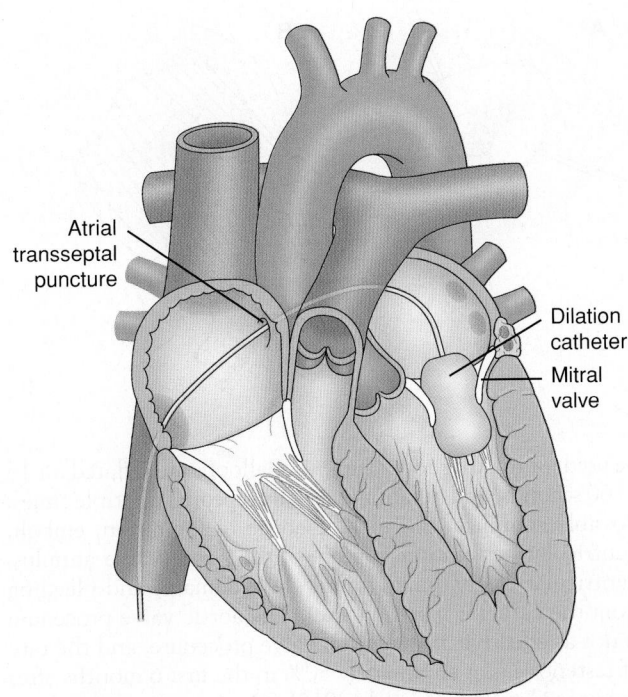

Figure 28-3 • Balloon valvuloplasty. Cross-section of heart illustrating the dilation catheter placed through an atrial transseptal puncture and across the mitral valve. The Inoue balloon inflates in three stages: first below the valve, then above, and finally in the valve orifice (this diagram shows the first two sections inflated).

atrium, across the mitral valve, and into the left ventricle. A guidewire is placed through each catheter, and the original catheter is removed. Most often a specially designed balloon catheter is placed over the guidewire and positioned with the balloon across the mitral valve. The balloon has three sections with progressively greater resistance to inflation. The balloon first expands in the ventricle to help position the catheter at the valve. The second section of the balloon expands above the valve, holding the catheter across the valve. Finally, the middle section of the balloon expands in the valve orifice opening the commissures. Alternately, two balloons are used. Guidewires may be advanced into the aorta to stabilize the balloons' positions. These single-section balloons are inflated simultaneously and expand their entire length. The advantage of two balloons is that each is smaller than the one large balloon, making smaller atrial septal defects. As the two balloons are inflated, they usually do not completely occlude the valve, thereby permitting some forward flow of blood during the inflation period. Balloons are inflated with a dilute angiographic solution for 10 to 30 seconds. Multiple inflations usually are required to achieve the desired results.

All patients have some degree of mitral regurgitation after the procedure. Other possible complications include bleeding from the catheter insertion sites, emboli resulting in complications such as strokes, and, rarely, left-to-right atrial shunts through the atrial septal defect created during the procedure.

Aortic balloon valvuloplasty is performed most commonly by introducing a catheter through the aorta, across the aortic valve, and into the left ventricle, although it also may be performed by passing the balloon or balloons through the atrial septum. The one- or two-balloon technique can

Figure 28-4 • Annuloplasty ring insertion. **A.** Mitral valve regurgitation; leaflets do not close. **B.** Insertion of an annuloplasty ring. **C.** Completed valvuloplasty; leaflets close.

be used for treating aortic stenosis. Balloons are inflated for 15 to 60 seconds, and inflation is usually repeated multiple times. Possible complications include aortic regurgitation, emboli, ventricular perforation, rupture of the aortic valve annulus, ventricular dysrhythmia, mitral valve damage, and bleeding from the catheter insertion sites. The aortic valve procedure is not as effective as the mitral valve procedure, and the rate of restenosis is approximately 50% in the first 6 months after the procedure (Mann et al., 2015).

Open Commissurotomy

Open commissurotomies are performed with direct visualization of the valve. The patient is under general anesthesia. A midsternal or left thoracic incision is made. Cardiopulmonary bypass is initiated, and an incision is made into the heart. The valve is exposed, and a scalpel, finger, balloon, or dilator is used to open the commissures.

An added advantage of directly visualizing the valve is that thrombus and calcifications may be identified and removed. If the valve has chordae or papillary muscles, they may be inspected and surgically repaired as necessary.

Annuloplasty

Annuloplasty is repair of the valve annulus (i.e., junction of valve leaflets and muscular heart wall). General anesthesia and cardiopulmonary bypass are required for most annuloplasties. The procedure narrows the diameter of the valve's orifice and is a useful treatment for valvular regurgitation.

There are two annuloplasty techniques. One technique uses an annuloplasty ring (see Fig. 28-4), which may be preshaped (rigid/semirigid) or flexible. Leaflets of the valve are sutured to a ring, creating an annulus of the desired size. When the ring is in place, tension created by moving blood and the contracting heart is borne by the ring rather than

by the valve or a suture line. The repair prevents progressive regurgitation.

A second technique to tighten the annulus involves folding elongated tissue over onto itself (i.e., taking tucks) in leaflets or tacking leaflets to the atrium or each other with sutures. Because the valve's leaflets and suture lines are subjected to direct forces of the blood and heart muscle movement, the repair may degenerate more quickly than one using an annuloplasty ring.

Leaflet Repair

Damage to cardiac valve leaflets may result from stretching, shortening, or tearing. **Leaflet repair** for elongated, ballooning, or other excess tissue leaflets is removal of the extra tissue. Elongated tissue may be tucked and sutured (i.e., leaflet plication). A wedge of tissue may be cut from the middle of the leaflet and the gap sutured closed (i.e., leaflet resection) (see Fig. 28-5). Short leaflets are most often repaired by chordoplasty. After short chordae are released, leaflets often unfurl and resume their normal function (closing the valve during systole). A leaflet may be extended by suturing a piece of pericardium to it. A pericardial or synthetic patch may be used to repair holes in the leaflets.

Chordoplasty

Chordoplasty is repair of chordae tendineae. The mitral valve is most often involved with chordoplasty. The tricuspid valve seldom requires chordoplasty because tricuspid valve disease is often a result of mitral or aortic valve disease or left ventricular dysfunction (Fuster et al., 2011). Stretched, torn, or shortened chordae tendineae may cause regurgitation. Stretched chordae tendineae can be shortened, transposed to the other leaflet, or replaced with synthetic chordae.

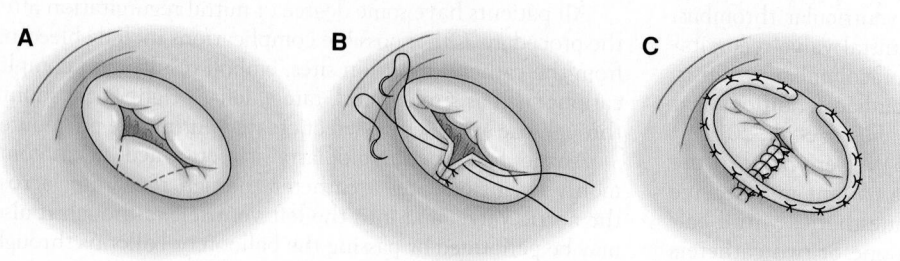

Figure 28-5 • Valve leaflet resection and repair with a ring annuloplasty. **A.** Mitral valve regurgitation; the section indicated by *dashed lines* is excised. **B.** Approximation of edges and suturing. **C.** Completed valvuloplasty, leaflet repair, and annuloplasty ring.

Torn chordae can be reattached to the leaflet, and shortened chordae can be elongated. Stretched papillary muscles, which may also cause regurgitation, can be shortened or relocated.

Valve Replacement

When valvuloplasty is not a viable alternative (e.g., when the annulus or leaflets of the valve are immobilized by calcifications, severe fibrosis or fusion of leaflets, chordae tendineae, or papillary muscles), **valve replacement** is performed. Ideally, a multidisciplinary team (e.g., cardiologists, cardiac thoracic surgeons, structural valve interventionalists, anesthesiologists, and nurses) work together with the patient to determine candidacy for surgical versus more minimally invasive replacement (Nishimura et al., 2014). General anesthesia and cardiopulmonary bypass are used for most valve replacements. The standard surgical procedure is performed through a median sternotomy (i.e., incision through the sternum), although the mitral valve may be approached through a right thoracotomy incision.

Mitral, and more rarely aortic, valve replacements may be performed with minimally invasive techniques that do not involve cutting through the length of the sternum. Instead, a 2- to 4-in incision is made in only the upper or lower half of the sternum or between ribs, or performed percutaneously. Some minimally invasive procedures are robot assisted; surgical instruments are connected to a robot, and the surgeon, watching a video display, uses a joystick to control the robot and surgical instruments. With these procedures, patients have less bleeding, pain, risk of infection, and scarring. Hospital length of stay averages 5 days, and recovery may be as short as 3 to 4 weeks (Cohn, 2012; Holmes, Mack, Kaul, et al., 2012).

After the valve is visualized, leaflets of the aortic or pulmonic valve are removed, but some or all of the mitral valve structures (leaflets, chordae, and papillary muscles) are left in place to help maintain the shape and function of the left ventricle after mitral valve replacement. Sutures are placed around the annulus and then through the valve prosthesis. The replacement valve is slid down the suture into position and tied into place (see Fig. 28-6). The patient is weaned from cardiopulmonary bypass, the quality of the surgical repair is often assessed with color flow Doppler TEE, and then surgery is completed.

TAVI, a minimally invasive aortic valve replacement procedure, may be performed in a catheterization laboratory or hybrid room. It does not involve cardiopulmonary bypass or sternotomy (Hong, Hong, Ko, et al., 2014). TAVI is indicated for patients with aortic stenosis who are not candidates for surgical valve replacement or have a high surgical risk (Fuster et al., 2011; Holmes et al., 2012; Mann et al., 2015). With the patient under general anesthesia, a balloon valvuloplasty is performed. Then, a bioprosthetic (tissue) replacement valve (see Fig. 28-7A,B) attached to a catheter is inserted percutaneously, positioned at the aortic valve, and implanted (deployed). The MitraClip (see Fig. 28-7C) has been approved as a transcatheter procedure to treat degenerative forms of mitral regurgitation (Mann et al., 2015). This procedure is most beneficial for patients with severe symptomatic mitral regurgitation who have high surgical risk. The procedure creates a mechanical bridge between two leaflets; it has demonstrated decreased regurgitant flow, improvement of symptoms, and decreased rates of hospitalization for heart failure (Mann et al., 2015; Munkholm-Larsen, Wan, Tian, et al., 2014).

Before surgery, the heart gradually adjusted to the pathology; however, surgery abruptly "corrects" the way blood flows through the heart. Complications unique to valve replacement are related to the sudden changes in intracardiac blood pressures. All prosthetic valve replacements create a degree of stenosis when they are implanted in the heart. Usually, the stenosis is mild and does not affect heart function. If valve replacement was for a stenotic valve, blood flow through the heart is often improved. The signs and symptoms of backward heart failure resolve in a few hours or days. If valve replacement was for a regurgitant valve, it may take months for the chamber into which blood had been regurgitating to achieve its optimal postoperative function. Signs and symptoms of heart failure resolve gradually as heart function improves. Patients are at risk for many postoperative complications, such as bleeding, thromboembolism, infection, heart failure, hypertension, dysrhythmias, hemolysis, and mechanical obstruction of the valve.

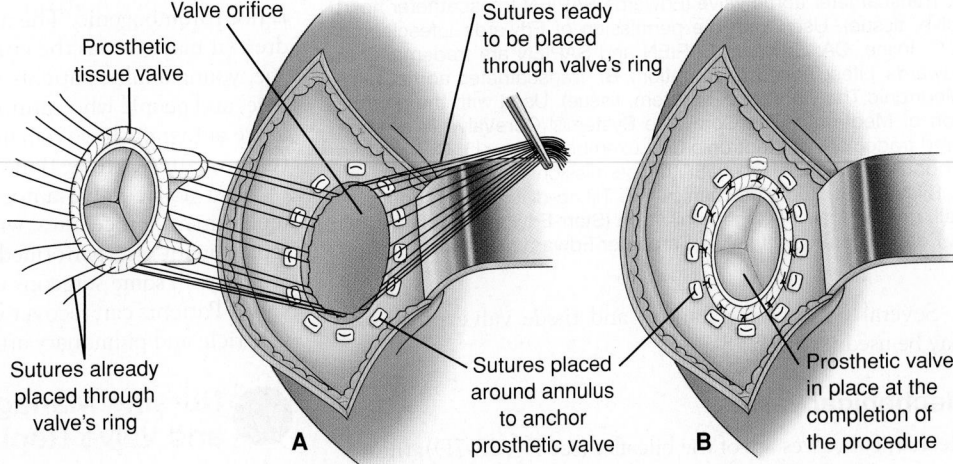

Figure 28-6 • Valve replacement. **A.** The native valve is trimmed, and the prosthetic valve is sutured in place. **B.** Once all sutures are placed through the ring, the surgeon slides the prosthetic valve down the sutures and into the natural orifice. Sutures are then tied off and trimmed.

Valve orifice

Prosthetic tissue valve

Sutures ready to be placed through valve's ring

Sutures already placed through valve's ring

Sutures placed around annulus to anchor prosthetic valve

Prosthetic valve in place at the completion of the procedure

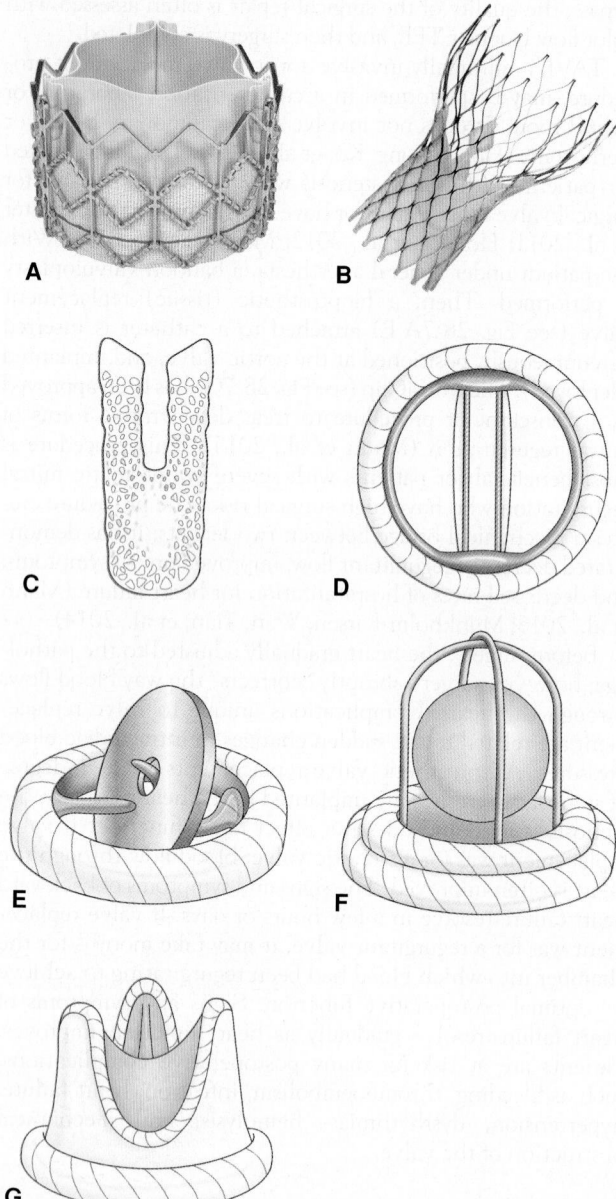

Figure 28-7 • Common mechanical and tissue valve replacements. **A.** Transcatheter aortic valve (Edwards SAPIEN transcatheter heart valve, tissue). Used with the permission of Edwards Lifesciences LLC, Irvine, CA; Edwards SAPIEN and SAPIEN are trademarks of Edwards Lifesciences Corporation. **B.** Transcatheter aortic valve (Medtronic The CoreValve® system, tissue). Used with the permission of Medtronic. The CoreValve System® CoreValve is a registered trademark of Medtronic CV Luxembourg S.a.r.l.). **C.** MitraClip (Abbott Vascular). Used with the permission of Abbott Vascular. **D.** Bileaflet (St. Jude, mechanical). **E.** Tilting-disc valve (Medtronic-Hall, mechanical). **F.** Caged ball valve (Starr-Edwards, mechanical). **G.** Porcine heterograft valve (Carpenter-Edwards, tissue).

Several types of mechanical and tissue valve prostheses may be used (see Fig. 28-7).

Mechanical Valves

Mechanical valves are of the bileaflet (see Fig. 28-7D), tilting-disc (see Fig. 28-7E), or ball-and-cage (see Fig. 28-7F) design and are thought to be more durable than tissue prosthetic

valves (see Fig. 28-7G); therefore, they often are used for younger patients. These valves also are used for patients with kidney injury, hypercalcemia, endocarditis, or sepsis who require valve replacement. For patients with these conditions, mechanical valves do not deteriorate or become infected as easily as tissue valves. Significant complications associated with mechanical valves are thromboemboli and long-term use of required anticoagulants (Mann et al., 2015).

Tissue Valves

Tissue valves are of three types: bioprostheses, homografts, and autografts. Tissue valves are less likely than mechanical valves to generate thromboemboli, and long-term anticoagulation is not required. Tissue valves are not as durable as mechanical valves and require replacement more frequently.

Bioprostheses

Bioprostheses are tissue valves (e.g., **heterografts**) used for aortic, mitral, and tricuspid valve replacement. They are not thrombogenic; therefore, patients do not need long-term anticoagulation therapy. They are used for women of childbearing age because potential complications of long-term anticoagulation associated with menses, placental transfer to a fetus, and delivery of a child are avoided. They also are used for patients older than 70 years and others who cannot tolerate long-term anticoagulation. Most bioprostheses are from pigs (porcine), but some are from cows (bovine) or horses (equine). They may be stented or nonstented. Viability is 7 to 15 years (Cohn, 2012; Fuster et al., 2011).

Homografts

Homografts, or **allografts** (i.e., human valves), are obtained from cadaver tissue donations and are used for aortic and pulmonic valve replacement. The aortic valve and a portion of aorta or the pulmonic valve and a portion of pulmonary artery are harvested and stored cryogenically. Homografts are not always available and are very expensive. They last for about 10 to 15 years (Cohn, 2012; Otto & Bonow, 2013).

Autografts

Autografts (i.e., autologous valves) are obtained by excising the patient's own pulmonic valve and a portion of the pulmonary artery for use as the aortic valve. Anticoagulation is unnecessary because the valve is the patient's own tissue and is not thrombogenic. The autograft is an alternative for children (it may grow as the child grows), women of childbearing age, young adults, patients with a history of peptic ulcer disease, and people who cannot tolerate anticoagulation. Aortic valve autografts have remained viable for more than 20 years (Cohn, 2012; Otto & Bonow, 2013).

Most aortic valve autograft procedures are double valve replacement procedures with a homograft pulmonic valve replacement also performed. If pulmonary vascular pressures are normal, some surgeons elect not to replace the pulmonic valve. Patients can recover without a valve between the right ventricle and pulmonary artery.

● Nursing Management: Valvuloplasty and Valve Replacement

The nurse assists the patient and family to prepare for the procedure, reinforces and supplements explanations provided by the physician, and provides psychosocial support. (See Chapters 17 through 19 for care of the surgical patient.)

Patients who have undergone percutaneous balloon valvuloplasty with or without percutaneous valve replacement may be admitted to a telemetry unit or intensive care unit (ICU). The nurse assesses for signs and symptoms of heart failure and emboli (see Chapter 29), auscultates the chest for changes in heart sounds at least every 4 hours, and provides the patient with the same care as for postprocedure cardiac catheterization or percutaneous transluminal coronary angioplasty (see Chapter 27). After undergoing percutaneous balloon valvuloplasty, the patient usually remains in the hospital for 24 to 48 hours.

Patients who have undergone surgical valvuloplasty or valve replacements are admitted to the ICU. Care focuses on recovery from anesthesia and hemodynamic stability. Vital signs are assessed every 5 to 15 minutes and as needed until the patient recovers from anesthesia or sedation and then are assessed according to unit protocol (American Society of Perianesthesia Nurses, 2014). Intravenous (IV) medications to increase or decrease blood pressure and to treat dysrhythmias or altered heart rates are given and their effects monitored. Medications are gradually decreased until they are no longer required or the patient takes the needed medication by another route (e.g., oral, topical). Patient assessments are conducted every 1 to 4 hours and as needed, with particular attention to neurologic, respiratory, and cardiovascular systems (see Chapter 27, Chart 27-12).

After the patient has recovered from anesthesia and sedation, is hemodynamically stable without IV medications, and has stable physical assessment parameters, he or she usually is transferred to a telemetry unit, typically within 24 to 72 hours of surgery. Nursing care continues as for most postoperative patients, including wound care and patient education regarding diet, activity, medications, and self-care. The patient usually is discharged from the hospital in 3 to 7 days.

The nurse educates the patient about anticoagulant therapy, explaining the need for frequent follow-up appointments and blood laboratory studies. Patients who take warfarin (Coumadin) have individualized target international normalized ratios, usually between 2 and 3.5 for mitral valve replacement and 1.8 and 2.2 for aortic valve replacement. Patients who have been treated with an annuloplasty ring or a tissue valve replacement usually require anticoagulation for only 3 months unless there are other risk factors such as atrial fibrillation or a history of thromboembolism. Aspirin is prescribed with warfarin for patients with bioprostheses or at high risk for embolic events (e.g., history of embolic event or having two or more preexisting conditions: diabetes, hypertension, coronary artery disease, congestive heart failure, older than 75 years) (Nishimura et al., 2014; Otto & Bonow, 2013). The nurse provides education about all prescribed medications, including the name of medication, dosage, actions, prescribed schedule, potential adverse effects, and any drug–drug or drug–food interactions.

Patients with a mechanical valve prosthesis (including annuloplasty rings and other prosthetic materials used in valvuloplasty) require education to prevent infective endocarditis. Patients may be at risk for infective endocarditis that results from bacteria entering the bloodstream and adhering to abnormal valve structures or prosthetic devices.

The nurse educates the patient about how to minimize the risk of developing infective endocarditis (see prevention of endocarditis later in this chapter). Antibiotic prophylaxis is necessary before dental procedures involving manipulation of gingival tissue, the periapical area of the teeth, or perforation of the oral mucosa (not including routine anesthetic injections, placement of orthodontic brackets, or loss of deciduous teeth). Antibiotic therapy should also be used before invasive procedures involving the respiratory tract (e.g., biopsy of respiratory mucosa, tonsillectomy, and adenectomy).

Transitional, home care, office, or clinic nurses help reinforce all new information and self-care instructions with patients and families for 4 to 8 weeks after the procedure. Echocardiograms often are performed 3 to 4 weeks after hospital discharge to further evaluate the effects and results of surgery. The echocardiogram also provides a baseline for future comparison if cardiac symptoms or complications develop. Echocardiograms usually are repeated every 1 to 2 years.

Cardiomyopathy

Cardiomyopathy is disease of the heart muscle that is associated with cardiac dysfunction. It is classified according to the structural and functional abnormalities of the heart muscle: dilated cardiomyopathy (DCM), hypertrophic cardiomyopathy (HCM), restrictive or constrictive cardiomyopathy (RCM), arrhythmogenic right ventricular cardiomyopathy/dysplasia (ARVC/D), and unclassified cardiomyopathy (Mann et al., 2015). A patient may have pathology representing more than one of these classifications, such as a patient with HCM developing dilation and symptoms of DCM. *Ischemic cardiomyopathy* is a term frequently used to describe an enlarged heart caused by coronary artery disease, which is usually accompanied by heart failure (see Chapter 29). In 2006, the American Heart Association proposed a set of Contemporary Classifications. Under this classification system, cardiomyopathies are divided into two major groups based on predominant organ involvement. These include *primary cardiomyopathies* (genetic, nongenetic, and acquired), which are focused primarily on the heart muscle, and *secondary cardiomyopathies*, which show myocardial involvement secondary to the influence of a vast list of disease processes that include, but are not limited to, amyloidosis, Fabry disease, sarcoidosis, and scleroderma (Maron, Towbin, Thiene, et al., 2006). This chapter focuses on the primary cardiomyopathies.

Pathophysiology

The pathophysiology of all cardiomyopathies is a series of events that culminate in impaired cardiac output. Decreased stroke volume stimulates the sympathetic nervous system and the renin–angiotensin–aldosterone response, resulting in increased systemic vascular resistance and increased sodium and fluid retention, which place an increased workload on the heart. These alterations can lead to heart failure (see Chapter 29).

 Concept Mastery Alert

Sodium is the major electrolyte involved with cardiomyopathy. Cardiomyopathy often leads to heart failure, which develops, in part, from fluid overload. Fluid overload is often associated with elevated sodium levels.

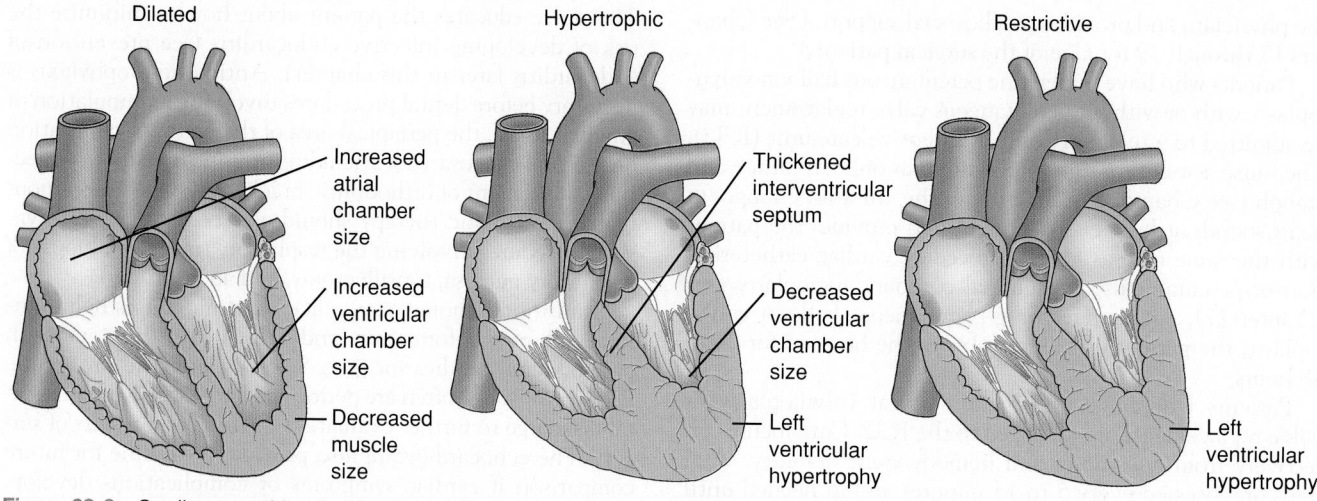

Figure 28-8 • Cardiomyopathies that lead to congestive heart failure. Adapted from Anatomical Chart Company. (2010). *Atlas of pathophysiology* (3rd ed.). Ambler, PA: Lippincott Williams & Wilkins.

Dilated Cardiomyopathy

DCM is the most common form of cardiomyopathy, with an incidence of five to eight cases per 100,000 people per year (Mann & Felker, 2016). DCM is distinguished by significant dilation of the ventricles without simultaneous hypertrophy (i.e., increased muscle wall thickness) and systolic dysfunction (see Fig. 28-8). The ventricles have elevated systolic and diastolic volumes but a decreased ejection fraction.

More than 75 conditions and diseases may cause DCM, including pregnancy, heavy alcohol intake, viral infection (e.g., influenza), chemotherapeutic medications (e.g., daunorubicin [Cerubidine], doxorubicin [Adriamycin]), thyrotoxicosis, myxedema, persistent tachycardia, and Chagas disease. When the causative factor cannot be identified, the diagnosis is idiopathic DCM, which accounts for the largest subset of patients with DCM (Bennett, 2014; Mann & Felker, 2016). Approximately 30% of all idiopathic DCM can be linked to familial genetics, and as diagnostic testing continues to improve, it is thought that this estimate may increase (Mann & Felker, 2016). Because genetic factors may be involved, echocardiography and ECG should be used to screen all first-degree blood relatives (e.g., parents, siblings, and children) for DCM (Bennett, 2014; Mann et al., 2015).

Microscopic examination of the muscle tissue shows diminished contractile elements (actin and myosin filaments) of the muscle fibers and diffuse necrosis of myocardial cells. The result is poor systolic function. The structural changes decrease the amount of blood ejected from the ventricle with systole, increasing the amount of blood remaining in the ventricle after contraction. Less blood is then able to enter the ventricle during diastole, increasing end-diastolic pressure and eventually increasing pulmonary and systemic venous pressures. Altered valve function, usually regurgitation, can result from an enlarged stretched ventricle. Poor blood flow through the ventricle may also cause ventricular or atrial thrombi, which may embolize to other locations in the body. Early diagnosis and treatment can prevent or delay significant symptoms and sudden death from DCM.

Restrictive Cardiomyopathy

RCM is characterized by diastolic dysfunction caused by rigid ventricular walls that impair diastolic filling and ventricular stretch (see Fig. 28-8). Systolic function is usually normal. RCM may be associated with amyloidosis (amyloid, a protein substance, is deposited within cells) and other such infiltrative diseases. However, the cause is idiopathic in most cases. Signs and symptoms are similar to constrictive pericarditis and include dyspnea, nonproductive cough, and chest pain. Echocardiography, as well as measurement of pulmonary artery systolic pressure, pulmonary artery wedge pressure, and central venous pressure is used to differentiate the two conditions.

Hypertrophic Cardiomyopathy

HCM is an autosomal dominant condition, occurring in men, women, and children (often detected after puberty) with an estimated prevalence rate of 0.2% of the population in the United States (Gersh, Maron, Bonow, et al., 2011; Mann et al., 2015; Sheffle & Bowden, 2014). Echocardiograms, 12-lead ECGs, and complete history and physical examinations are typically performed every 12 to 18 months from age 12 to 18 years. These screenings may extend to every 5 years from 18 to 70 years of age in susceptible individuals (i.e., those with a family history of HCM) (Mann et al., 2015). Doppler echocardiography has been used for many years to detect HCM and blood flow alterations (Mann et al., 2015). More recently, the emergence of tissue Doppler imaging (TDI) has been useful in showing dysfunction of the myocardium despite preserved systolic function (Mann & Felker, 2016). Cardiovascular MRI has also become a more prevalent diagnostic tool given its high-resolution tomographic imaging capabilities and is often used in concert with traditional echocardiograms for diagnosis (Mann et al., 2015; Semsarian, Ingles, Maron, et al., 2015). Genetic testing may help identify those at risk before there are clinical manifestations of the disease (Mann & Felker, 2016; Semsarian et al., 2015).

In HCM, the heart muscle asymmetrically increases in size and mass, especially along the septum (see Fig. 28-8). HCM often affects nonadjacent areas of the ventricle. The increased thickness of the heart muscle reduces the size of the ventricular cavities and causes the ventricles to take a longer time to relax after systole. During the first part of diastole, it is more difficult for the ventricles to fill with blood. The atrial contraction at the end of diastole becomes critical for ventricular filling and systolic contraction.

Cardiac muscle cells normally lie parallel to and end to end with each other. The hypertrophied cardiac muscle cells are disorganized, oblique, and perpendicular to each other, decreasing the effectiveness of contractions and possibly increasing the risk of dysrhythmias such as ventricular tachycardia and ventricular fibrillation. In HCM, the coronary arteriole walls are thickened, which decrease the internal diameter of the arterioles. The narrow arterioles restrict the blood supply to the myocardium, causing numerous small areas of ischemia and necrosis. The necrotic areas of the myocardium ultimately fibrose and scar, further impeding ventricular contraction.

Arrhythmogenic Right Ventricular Cardiomyopathy/Dysplasia

ARVC/D occurs when the myocardium is progressively infiltrated and replaced by fibrous scar and adipose tissue. Initially, only localized areas of the right ventricle are affected, but as the disease progresses, the entire heart is affected. Eventually, the right ventricle dilates and develops poor contractility, right ventricular wall abnormalities, and dysrhythmias. ARVC/D is an uncommon form of inherited heart muscle disease and often is not recognized. Therefore, the prevalence is largely unknown, although it is estimated to affect about 1 in 5000 people (Rojas & Calkins, 2015; Fuster et al., 2011). Palpitations or syncope may develop between 15 and 40 years of age. ARVC/D should be considered in patients with ventricular tachycardia originating in the right ventricle (i.e., a left bundle branch block configuration on ECG) or sudden death, especially among young athletes (Mann et al., 2015). ARVC/D is genetic (i.e., autosomal dominant) (Corrado, Wichter, Link, et al., 2015; Fuster et al., 2011). First-degree blood relatives (e.g., parents, siblings, children) should be screened for the disease with a 12-lead ECG, Holter monitor, and echocardiography. Cardiac MRI is also more frequently used as a more conclusive diagnostic tool (Corrado et al., 2015; Mann & Felker, 2016). Some patients affected by dysrhythmias may benefit from having an implantable cardioverter defibrillator (ICD) placed (see Chapter 26).

Unclassified Cardiomyopathies

Unclassified cardiomyopathies are different from or have characteristics of more than one of the previously described types and are caused by fibroelastosis, noncompacted myocardium, systolic dysfunction with minimal dilation, and mitochondrial diseases (Mann et al., 2015). Examples of unclassified cardiomyopathies can include left ventricular noncompaction and stress-induced (Takotsubo) cardiomyopathy.

Clinical Manifestations

Patients with cardiomyopathy may remain stable and without symptoms for many years. As the disease progresses, so do the symptoms. Frequently, dilated or restrictive cardiomyopathy is first diagnosed when the patient presents with signs and symptoms of heart failure (e.g., DOE, fatigue). Patients with cardiomyopathy may also report PND, cough (especially with exertion), and orthopnea, which may lead to a misdiagnosis of bronchitis or pneumonia. Other symptoms include fluid retention, peripheral edema, and nausea, which are caused by poor perfusion of the gastrointestinal system. The patient also may experience chest pain, palpitations, dizziness, nausea, and syncope with exertion. However, with HCM, cardiac arrest (i.e., sudden cardiac death) may be the initial manifestation in young people, including athletes (Mann et al., 2015).

Regardless of type and cause, cardiomyopathy may lead to severe heart failure, lethal dysrhythmias, and death. The mortality rate is highest for African Americans and older adults (Mann et al., 2015).

Assessment and Diagnostic Findings

Physical examination at early stages may reveal tachycardia and extra heart sounds (e.g., S_3, S_4). Patients with DCM may have diastolic murmurs, and patients with DCM and HCM may have systolic murmurs. With disease progression, examination also reveals signs and symptoms of heart failure (e.g., crackles on pulmonary auscultation, jugular vein distention, pitting edema of dependent body parts, and enlarged liver).

Diagnosis is usually made from findings disclosed by the patient history and by ruling out other causes of heart failure such as myocardial infarction. The echocardiogram is one of the most helpful diagnostic tools because the structure and function of the ventricles can be observed easily. Cardiac MRI may also be used, particularly to assist with the diagnosis of HCM (Mann et al., 2015; Mann & Felker, 2016; Semsarian et al., 2015). ECG demonstrates dysrhythmias (atrial fibrillation, ventricular dysrhythmias) and changes consistent with left ventricular hypertrophy (left axis deviation, wide QRS, ST changes, inverted T waves). In ARVC/D, there often is a small deflection—an epsilon wave—at the end of the QRS. The chest x-ray reveals heart enlargement and possibly pulmonary congestion. Cardiac catheterization is sometimes used to rule out coronary artery disease as a causative factor. Endomyocardial biopsy may be performed to analyze myocardial cells.

Medical Management

Medical management is directed toward identifying and managing possible underlying or precipitating causes; correcting the heart failure with medications, a low-sodium diet, and an exercise/rest regimen (see Chapter 29); and controlling dysrhythmias with antiarrhythmic medications and possibly with an implanted electronic device, such as an ICD (see Chapter 26). Systemic anticoagulation to prevent thromboembolic events is usually recommended (Bennett, 2014). If the patient has signs and symptoms of congestion, fluid intake may be limited to 2 L each day. Patients with HCM should avoid dehydration and may need beta-blockers (atenolol [Tenormin], metoprolol [Lopressor], sotalol [Betapace], propranolol [Inderal]) to maintain cardiac output and minimize the risk of left ventricular outflow tract (LVOT) obstruction during systole. Patients with HCM or RCM may need to limit physical activity and avoid excessive weight gain to avoid a life-threatening dysrhythmia. To date, amiodarone (Cordarone) is the only drug shown to reduce the incidence of arrhythmogenic sudden cardiac death (Corrado et al., 2015; Mann & Felker, 2016; Marcus & Abidov, 2012).

A pacemaker may be implanted to alter the electrical stimulation of the muscle and prevent the forceful hyperdynamic contractions that occur with HCM. Atrial-ventricular and biventricular pacing have been used to decrease symptoms and obstruction of the LVOT. For some patients with DCM and HCM, biventricular pacing (also known as cardiac resynchronization therapy or CRT) increases the ejection fraction and reverses some of the structural changes in the myocardium.

Nonsurgical septal reduction therapy, also called *alcohol septal ablation*, has been used to treat obstructive HCM. This procedure is oftentimes indicated for patients with advanced age, patients with high operative risk or those with a preference to avoid surgery (Maron & Nishimura, 2014). In the cardiac catheterization laboratory, a percutaneous catheter is positioned in one or more of the septal coronary arteries. Once the position is verified, 1 to 3 mL of 95% to 98% ethanol (ethyl alcohol) is injected to destroy the myocardial cells (Mann et al., 2015; Maron & Nishimura, 2014). The procedure produces a septal myocardial infarction. The resulting scar is thinner than the living myocardium had been, so the obstruction is decreased. The patient may develop a left anterior hemibranch block or left bundle branch block (Elliott, Anastasakis, Borger, et al., 2014). Nitrates and morphine are not used because coronary artery dilation is contraindicated.

Surgical Management

When heart failure progresses and medical treatment is no longer effective, surgical intervention, including heart transplantation, is considered. However, because of the limited number of organ donors, many patients die waiting for transplantation. In some cases, a ventricular assist device (VAD) is implanted to support the failing heart until a suitable donor heart becomes available.

Left Ventricular Outflow Tract Surgery

When patients with HCM become symptomatic despite medical therapy and a difference in pressure of 50 mm Hg or more exists between the left ventricle and the aorta, surgery is considered (Elliott et al., 2014; Gersh et al., 2011; Mann et al., 2015). The most common procedure is a myectomy (sometimes referred to as a myotomy–myectomy or the Morrow procedure), in which some of the heart tissue is excised. Septal tissue approximately 1 cm wide and deep is cut from the enlarged septum below the aortic valve. The length of septum removed depends on the degree of obstruction caused by the hypertrophied muscle.

In about 11% to 20% of LVOT surgery cases, the surgeon may need to perform concomitant mitral valve surgery (Elliott et al., 2014; Maron & Nishimura, 2014). This procedure involves opening the LVOT to the aortic valve by mitral valvuloplasty involving the leaflets, chordae, or papillary muscles, or the patient's mitral valve may be replaced with a low-profile disc valve. The space taken up by the mitral valve is substantially reduced by the valvuloplasty or prosthetic valve, allowing blood to move around the enlarged septum to the aortic valve through the area the mitral valve once occupied. The primary complication of all procedures is

dysrhythmia. Additional complications include postoperative surgical complications such as pain, ineffective airway clearance, deep vein thrombosis, risk of infection, and delayed surgical recovery.

Heart Transplantation

Because of advances in surgical techniques and immunosuppressive therapies, heart transplantation is now a therapeutic option for patients with end-stage heart disease. Cyclosporine (Gengraf, Neoral, Sandimmune) and tacrolimus (Prograf, FK506) are some of the more common immunosuppressants that decrease the body's rejection of foreign proteins, such as transplanted organs. Unfortunately, these drugs also decrease the body's ability to resist infections and increase the risk of various cancers, and a satisfactory balance must be achieved between suppressing rejection and avoiding infection. In 2012, there were 4,196 adult and pediatric heart transplants performed worldwide. In the United States, approximately 2,400 heart transplants are performed annually, a number that has now plateaued over the previous years (Lund, Edwards, Kucheryavaya et al., 2014).

Cardiomyopathy, ischemic heart disease, valvular disease, rejection of previously transplanted hearts, and congenital heart disease are the most common indications for transplantation (Lund et al., 2014). Typical candidates have severe symptoms uncontrolled by medical therapy, no other surgical options, and a prognosis of less than 1 to 2 years to live. A multidisciplinary team screens the candidate before recommending the transplantation procedure. The person's age, pulmonary status, other chronic health conditions, psychosocial status, family support, infections, history of other transplantations, adherence to therapeutic regimens, and current health status are considered. The United Network for Organ Sharing (UNOS), a national organization that is regulated by the US government, is charged with maintaining organ transplant waiting lists and allocating donor organs. When a donor heart becomes available, UNOS generates a list of potential recipients on the basis of ABO blood group compatibility, the body sizes of the donor and the potential recipient, age, severity of illness, length of time on the waiting list, and the geographic locations of the donor and potential recipient. Distance is a factor because postoperative function depends on the heart being implanted within 4 hours of harvest from the donor (Costanzo, Dipchand, Starling, et al., 2010). Some patients are candidates for more than one organ transplant (e.g., heart–lung, heart–kidney, heart–liver).

Orthotopic transplantation is the most common surgical procedure for cardiac transplantation. Some surgeons prefer to remove the recipient's heart but leave a portion of the recipient's atria (with the vena cava and pulmonary veins) in place, which is known as the biatrial technique. However, this technique has been modified to a more common approach called the *bicaval technique*. This technique includes removal of the recipient's heart, and the implantation of the donor heart with intact atria at the vena cava and pulmonary veins (see Fig. 28-9) (Fuster et al., 2011; Mann & Felker, 2016). This newer approach is associated with decreased AV valve regurgitation, dysrhythmias, and conduction abnormalities.

Patients who have had heart transplantations are constantly balancing the risk of rejection with the risk of infection and diseases such as cancer. They must adhere to a

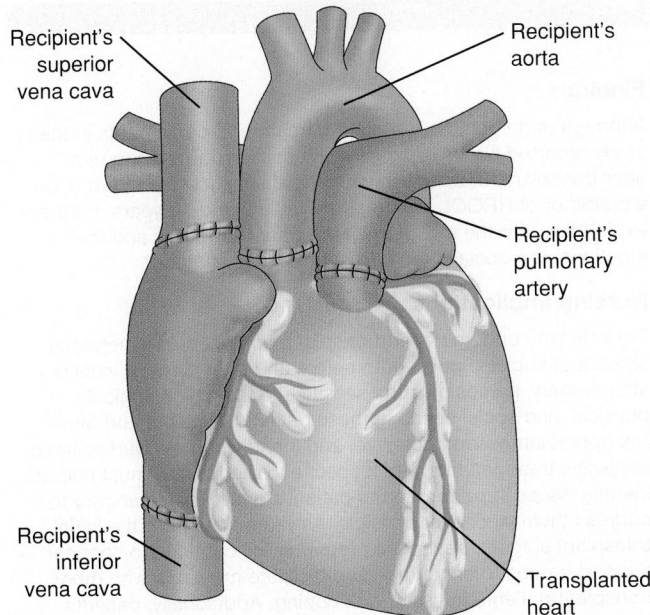

Recipient's superior vena cava

Recipient's aorta

Recipient's pulmonary artery

Recipient's inferior vena cava

Transplanted heart

Figure 28-9 • Orthotopic method of heart transplantation.

complex regimen of diet, medications, activity, follow-up laboratory studies, biopsies of the transplanted heart (to diagnose rejection), and clinic visits. There are three classes of medications that are prescribed for a transplant patient to help minimize rejection: corticosteroids (e.g., prednisone), calcineurin inhibitors (tacrolimus, cyclosporine), and antiproliferative agents (mycophenolate mofetil [CellCept], azathioprine [Imuran], or sirolimus [Rapamune]).

The transplanted heart has no nerve connections (i.e., denervated heart) to the recipient's body, so the sympathetic and vagus nerves do not affect the transplanted heart. The resting rate of the transplanted heart is approximately 90 to 110 bpm, but it increases gradually if catecholamines are in the circulation. Patients must gradually increase and decrease their exercise (i.e., extended warm-up and cool-down periods), because 20 to 30 minutes may be required to achieve the desired heart rate. Atropine does not increase the heart rate of transplanted hearts. Additionally, many heart transplant patients do not experience angina with ischemia and may present with congestive heart failure, silent myocardial infarction, or sudden death without a prior history of coronary artery disease (Fuster et al., 2011).

In addition to rejection and infection, complications may include accelerated atherosclerosis of the coronary arteries (i.e., cardiac allograft vasculopathy, accelerated graft atherosclerosis, transplant coronary artery disease). Both immunologic and nonimmunologic factors cause arterial injury and inflammation of the coronary arteries. The arterial smooth muscle proliferates, and there is hyperplasia of the coronary artery intima, accelerating atherosclerosis along the entire length of the coronary arteries (Mann et al., 2015; Mann & Felker, 2016). Hypertension may occur in patients taking cyclosporine or tacrolimus due to the effect these medications have on the kidneys. Osteoporosis is a frequent side effect of the antirejection medications as well as pretransplantation dietary insufficiency and medications. Patients with a long-term sedentary lifestyle are at greater risk for osteoporosis.

Posttransplantation lymphoproliferative disease and cancer of the skin and lips are the most common malignancies after transplantation, possibly caused by immunosuppression. Weight gain, obesity, diabetes, dyslipidemias (e.g., hypercholesterolemia), hypertension, and renal failure, as well as central nervous system, respiratory, and gastrointestinal disturbances, may be adverse effects of corticosteroids or other immunosuppressants. Toxicity from immunosuppressant medications may occur as well. The overall 1-year survival rate for patients with transplanted hearts is approximately 90% (Starling, 2013).

In the first year after transplantation, patients respond to the psychosocial stresses imposed by organ transplant in various ways. Most report a better quality of life after transplantation and are able to return to activities of daily living with little to no functional limitations (Fuster et al., 2011; Mann et al., 2015; Mann & Felker, 2016). Some experience guilt that someone had to die for them to be able to live, have anxiety about the new heart, experience depression or fear about rejection, or have difficulty with family role changes before and after transplantation (Fuster et al., 2011) (see Chart 28-1).

Mechanical Assist Devices and Total Artificial Hearts

The use of cardiopulmonary bypass in cardiovascular surgery and the possibility of performing heart transplantation in patients with end-stage cardiac disease, as well as the desire for a treatment option for patients with such disease who are not transplant candidates, have increased the need for mechanical assist devices. Patients who cannot be weaned from cardiopulmonary bypass and patients in cardiogenic shock may benefit from a period of mechanical heart assistance. The most commonly used device is the intra-aortic balloon pump (see Chapter 29). This pump decreases the work of the heart during contraction but does not perform the actual work of the heart.

Ventricular Assist Devices

More complex devices that perform some or all of the pumping function for the heart are being used. These more sophisticated **ventricular assist devices** (VADs) can circulate as much blood per minute as the heart, if not more (see Fig. 28-10). There are short- and long-term devices available, depending on the indication. Each VAD is used to support one ventricle, although in some instances, two VAD pumps may be used for biventricular support. Additionally, some VADs can be combined with an oxygenator; the combination is called *extracorporeal membrane oxygenation (ECMO)*. The oxygenator–VAD combination is used for the patient whose heart cannot pump adequate blood through the lungs or the body.

VADs may be used as (1) a "bridge to recovery" for patients who require temporary assistance for reversible ventricular failure, (2) a "bridge to transplant" for patients with end-stage heart failure until a donor organ becomes available for transplant (most common), and (3) "destination therapy" for patients with end-stage heart failure who are not candidates for or decline heart transplantation and have the VAD implanted for permanent use. As patients spend an increased length of time on the transplant list, and as more VADs are becoming approved for destination therapy, VAD patients are

Chart 28-1 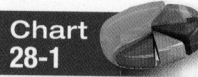 NURSING RESEARCH PROFILE
Quality of Life After Heart Transplant

White-Williams, C., Grady, K. L., Myers, S., et al. (2013). The relationships among satisfaction with social support, quality of life, and survival 5 to 10 years after heart transplantation. *Journal of Cardiovascular Nursing*, 28(5), 407–416.

Purpose

The purpose of this study was to explore the relationship between social support and patient outcomes after heart transplantation.

Design

This was a retrospective analysis of a larger prospective study of health-related quality of life (HRQOL). The sample consisted of 555 heart transplant patients over a 5-year period at 4 U.S. medical centers. Participants were 78% male, and 88% white, with a mean age of 53.8 years at the time of transplant. To generate data, five self-reported instruments were used: Social Support Index (SSI), Quality of Life Index, Heart Transplant Stressor Scale, Jalowiec Coping Scale, and Heart Transplant Symptoms Checklist. Medical record review was also utilized. Data were evaluated using a variety of statistical analyses, which included t-tests, correlations, Kaplan–Meier survival actuarials, and linear and multivariable regression.

Findings

Although undergoing a life-altering treatment, participants in the study reported high satisfaction with social support long term after transplant. Satisfaction with social support was found to be a predictor of HRQOL, but not survival at 5 and 10 years. Further exploration into the role of the heart transplant team and their functions as a social support resource is warranted.

Nursing Implications

Patients who undergo heart transplantation need a tremendous amount of social support both before and after surgery. Initially after surgery, nurses must be sensitive to the psychological, physical, and social needs of these patients. Patients and families appreciate warm, receptive, and friendly nurses. Nurses need to always treat patients with respect and dignity and must help to identify issues important to the patient's quality of life and try to address them whenever possible. As years pass from the initial transplant surgery, transplant programs will continue to sponsor support groups to encourage and facilitate meetings with other transplant patients to assist with coping. Additionally, patients appreciate spirituality, humor, peer support, and honesty to help them cope. These patients will rely heavily on support from the health care team, family, and friends.

---

being discharged from the hospital with the devices in place. Thus, the volume of patients with VADs in the community is rapidly expanding (Fuster et al., 2011; Mann & Felker, 2016). In some instances, the patient may request deactivation of the VAD, which may cause ethical controversy (see Chart 28-2).

Figure 28-10 • Left ventricular assist device. Reprinted with the permission from HeartWare, Inc.

VADs may be external, internal (i.e., implanted) with an external power source, or completely internal, and they may generate a pulsatile or continuous blood flow. There are four types of VADs: pneumatic, electric or electromagnetic, axial flow, and centrifugal. Pneumatic VADs are external or implanted pulsatile devices with a flexible reservoir housed in a rigid exterior. The reservoir usually fills with blood drained from the atrium or ventricle. The device then forces pressurized air into the rigid housing, compressing the reservoir and returning the blood to the circulation, usually into the aorta. Electric or electromagnetic VADs are similar to pneumatic VADs, but instead of using pressurized air to return the blood to the circulation, one or more flat metal plates are pushed against the reservoir. Generally, pneumatic and electric or electromagnetic VADs have been replaced by the newer generation of axial and centrifugal pumps; these earlier models were associated with higher rates of infections, thromboemboli, and mechanical failures (Lima, Mack, & Gonzalez-Stawinski, 2015). Axial flow VADs use a rotary mechanism (an impeller) to create nonpulsatile blood flow. The impeller spins rapidly within the VAD, creating a vacuum that pulls blood into the VAD and then pushes the blood out into the systemic circulation—the process is similar to a fan spinning in a tunnel, pulling air in one end of the tunnel and pushing it out the other. Centrifugal VADs are nonpulsatile devices that consist of a single moving impeller that is suspended in the pump housing by a combination of magnetic and hydrodynamic forces. The impeller rotates and pulls blood into the pump housing and ejects the blood out to the systemic circulation (Fuster et al., 2011).

Total Artificial Hearts

Total artificial hearts are designed to replace both ventricles. Some require the removal of the patient's heart to implant the total artificial heart, whereas others do not. Only one

Chart 28-2	**ETHICAL DILEMMA**

Should an Older Adult Be Allowed to Refuse Treatment When That Treatment Is Likely to Extend Life?

Case Scenario

The patient is an 88-year-old man with an extensive cardiac history who received a left ventricular assist device (LVAD). When the device was implanted, the patient knew the treatment was a destination therapy (i.e., a final treatment option) since he was not a candidate for a heart transplant. The goal was to improve his quality of life. Recently, he was hospitalized with sepsis from the device and reports significant pain at the site. He feels the quality of his life is poor and asks his physician to deactivate the device, which he realizes will lead to his death. The patient is mentally competent. His nurses, physician, and family are all stakeholders in this decision and have mixed feelings about his request.

Discussion

There are many ethical dilemmas inherent in this scenario. Although the LVAD is internally implanted, the control switch to deactivate the device is external. Some bioethicists argue that since the device has an external component, deactivating the device is similar to withdrawing treatment, which is ethical. Others argue that it becomes an integrated body part once it is implanted; therefore, to remove it is active euthanasia. There is an obligation to respect the patient's autonomy and self-determination, especially since he is deemed mentally competent. Yet, there is a "slippery slope" at play here in terms of the principle of nonmaleficence.

Analysis

- Identify the ethical principles that are in conflict in this case (see Chart 3-3 in Chapter 3).
- What arguments would you offer *in favor of* removal of the LVAD?
- What arguments would you offer *against* removal of the LVAD?
- Does removal of an LVAD constitute passive euthanasia? Does removal of an LVAD constitute active euthanasia?
- Assume that the patient is determined competent to make his own decisions and the deactivation is scheduled. Discuss the implications of this procedure on the stakeholders including the physician, nurse, and family. Does the physician or nurse have the right to refuse to participate in the procedure?

Resources

Kraemer, F. (2013). Ontology or phenomenology? How the LVAD challenges the euthanasia debate. *Bioethics, 27*(3), 140–150.
See Chapter 3, Chart 3-6 for ethics resources.

---

total artificial heart has been approved by the U.S. Food and Drug Administration (FDA) as a bridge to transplant. Although there has been some short-term success, the long-term results have been disappointing. Researchers hope to develop a device that can be permanently implanted and will eliminate the need for donated human heart transplantation for end-stage cardiac disease (Mann & Felker, 2016).

Complications of VADs and total artificial hearts include bleeding disorders, hemorrhage, thromboemboli, hemolysis, infection, kidney injury, right-sided heart failure, multisystem failure, and mechanical failure (Feldman, Pamboukian, Teuteberg, et al., 2013; Fuster et al., 2011; Mann et al., 2015; Starling, 2013). Nursing care of patients with these mechanical assist devices focuses on assessment for and minimization of these complications as well as providing emotional support and education about the device and the underlying cardiac disease. As the use of continuous flow devices increases and patients return to their community and to work, it is imperative that education regarding the potential inability to detect a pulse in these patients is disseminated to families and emergency personnel in the community.

NURSING PROCESS

The Patient With Cardiomyopathy

Assessment

Nursing assessment for the patient with cardiomyopathy begins with a detailed history of the presenting signs and symptoms. The nurse identifies possible etiologic factors, such as heavy alcohol intake, recent illness or pregnancy, or history of the disease in immediate family members. If the patient reports chest pain, a thorough review of the pain, including its precipitating factors, is warranted. The review of systems includes the presence of orthopnea, PND, and syncope or dyspnea with exertion. The number of pillows needed to sleep, usual weight, any weight change, and limitations on activities of daily living are assessed. The American College of Cardiology and American Heart Association Stages of Heart Failure classification is utilized to help identify disease progression, and the New York Heart Association Functional Classification for heart failure is determined based on the severity of the patient's symptoms (see Tables 29-1 and 29-2 in Chapter 29). The patient's usual diet is evaluated to determine the need to reduce sodium intake, optimize nutrition, or supplement with vitamins.

Because of the chronicity of cardiomyopathy, the nurse conducts a careful psychosocial history, exploring the impact of the disease on the patient's role within the family and community. Identification of perceived stressors helps the patient and the health care team to implement activities that relieve anxiety related to changes in health status. Very early on, the patient's support systems are identified, and members are encouraged to become involved in the patient's care and therapeutic regimen. The assessment addresses the effect the diagnosis has had on the patient and members of their support system and the patient's emotional status. Depression rates are two to three times higher in patients with heart failure (Rustad, Stern, Hebert, et al., 2013). Various screening tools are available to help assess symptoms associated with heart failure, including depression, though no one screening too has emerged as the generally accepted standard (Mann & Felker, 2016).

The physical assessment focuses on signs and symptoms of heart failure. The baseline assessment includes key components such as:

- Vital signs
- Calculation of pulse pressure and identification of pulsus paradoxus

- Current weight and any weight gain or loss
- Detection by palpation of the point of maximal impulse, often shifted to the left
- Cardiac auscultation for a systolic murmur and S₃ and S₄ heart sounds
- Pulmonary auscultation for crackles
- Measurement of jugular vein distention
- Assessment of edema and its severity

Diagnosis

NURSING DIAGNOSES

Based on the assessment data, major nursing diagnoses may include the following:

- Decreased cardiac output related to structural disorders caused by cardiomyopathy or to dysrhythmia from the disease process and medical treatments
- Risk for ineffective cardiac, cerebral, peripheral, and renal tissue perfusion related to decreased peripheral blood flow (resulting from decreased cardiac output)
- Impaired gas exchange related to pulmonary congestion caused by myocardial failure (resulting from decreased cardiac output)
- Activity intolerance related to decreased cardiac output or excessive fluid volume, or both
- Anxiety related to the change in health status and in role functioning
- Powerlessness related to disease process
- Nonadherence to medication and diet therapies

COLLABORATIVE PROBLEMS/POTENTIAL COMPLICATIONS

Potential complications may include the following:

- Heart failure
- Ventricular dysrhythmias
- Atrial dysrhythmias
- Cardiac conduction defects
- Pulmonary or cerebral embolism
- Valvular dysfunction

These complications are discussed earlier in this chapter and in Chapters 26 and 29.

Planning and Goals

The major goals for patients include improvement or maintenance of cardiac output, increased activity tolerance, reduction of anxiety, adherence to the self-care program, increased sense of power with decision-making, and absence of complications.

Nursing Interventions

IMPROVING CARDIAC OUTPUT AND PERIPHERAL BLOOD FLOW

During a symptomatic episode, rest is indicated. Many patients with DCM find that sitting up with their legs down is more comfortable than lying down in a bed. This position is helpful in pooling venous blood in the periphery and reducing preload. Assessing the patient's oxygen saturation at rest and during activity may assist with determining a need for supplemental oxygen. Oxygen usually is given through a nasal cannula when indicated.

Ensuring that medications are taken as prescribed is important to preserving adequate cardiac output. The nurse may assist the patient with planning a schedule for taking medications and identifying methods to remember to follow it, such

as associating the time to take a medication with an activity (e.g., eating a meal, brushing teeth). It is important to ensure that patients with DCM avoid verapamil, that patients with HCM avoid diuretics, and that patients with RCM avoid nifedipine to maintain contractility. In patients with HCM, the inotropic action of digoxin may create or worsen LVOT obstruction. Patients with RCM have increased sensitivity to digoxin, and the nurse must anticipate that low doses will be prescribed and assess for digoxin toxicity.

It is also important to ensure that the patient receives or chooses food selections that are appropriate for a low-sodium diet. One way to monitor a patient's response to treatment is to determine the patient's weight every day and identify any significant change. Another indication of the effect of treatment involves assessment of shortness of breath after activity and comparison to before treatment, as well as a change in the number of pillows needed to comfortably sleep. Patients with low cardiac output may need assistance keeping warm and frequently changing position to stimulate circulation and reduce the possibility of skin breakdown. Patients with HCM must be taught to avoid dehydration. One guideline that patients can use for self-assessment is to anticipate the urge to void at least every 4 hours while awake; if the urge to void is not present or the urine is a deep yellow color, more fluid intake is necessary.

INCREASING ACTIVITY TOLERANCE AND IMPROVING GAS EXCHANGE

The nurse plans the patient's activities so that they occur in cycles, alternating rest with activity periods. This benefits the patient's physiologic status, and it helps educate the patient about the need for planned cycles of rest and activity. For example, after taking a bath or shower, the patient should plan to sit and read a newspaper or engage in other relaxing activities. Suggesting that the patient sit while chopping vegetables, drying their hair, or shaving helps the patient learn to balance rest with activity. The nurse also makes sure that the patient recognizes the symptoms indicating the need for rest and actions to take when the symptoms occur. Patients with HCM or RCM must avoid strenuous activity, isometric exercises, and competitive sports.

REDUCING ANXIETY

Spiritual, psychological, and emotional support may be indicated for patients, families, and significant others. Interventions are directed toward eradicating or alleviating perceived stressors. Patients receive appropriate information about cardiomyopathy and self-management activities. It is important to provide an atmosphere in which patients feel free to verbalize concerns and receive assurance that their concerns are legitimate. If the patient is awaiting transplantation or facing death, it is necessary to allow time to discuss these issues. Providing the patient with realistic hope helps reduce anxiety while he or she awaits a donor heart. The nurse helps the patient, family, and significant others with anticipatory grieving.

DECREASING THE SENSE OF POWERLESSNESS

Patients often go through a grieving process when cardiomyopathy is diagnosed. The patient is assisted in identifying the things in life that he or she has lost (e.g., foods that the patient enjoyed eating but are high in sodium, the ability to engage in an active lifestyle, the ability to play sports, the ability to lift grandchildren) and their emotional responses to the loss (e.g., anger, feelings of sadness). The nurse assists the patient in identifying the amount of control that he or she still has over life, such as making food choices, managing medications, and working with the patient's primary provider to achieve the best possible outcomes. A diary in which the patient records food selections and weight may help with understanding the relationship between sodium intake and weight gain and give patients a sense of control over their disease. Some patients can manage a self-titrating diuretic regimen in which they adjust the dose of diuretic to their symptoms.

PROMOTING HOME, COMMUNITY-BASED, AND TRANSITIONAL CARE

Educating Patients About Self-Care. A key part of the plan of nursing care involves educating patients about the medication regimen, symptom monitoring, and symptom management. The nurse plays an integral role as the patient learns to balance lifestyle and work while accomplishing therapeutic activities. Helping patients cope with their disease status helps them adjust their lifestyles and implement a self-care program at home. Attainment of a goal, no matter how small, also promotes the patient's sense of well-being.

Continuing and Transitional Care. The nurse reinforces previous education and performs ongoing assessment of the patient's symptoms and progress. The nurse also assists the patient and family to adjust to lifestyle changes. Patients are taught to read nutrition labels, to maintain a record of daily weights and symptoms, and to organize daily activities to increase activity tolerance. In addition, the nurse assesses the patient's response to recommendations about diet and fluid intake and to the medication regimen and stresses the signs and symptoms that should be reported to the primary provider. Because of the risk of dysrhythmia, it may be necessary to educate the patient's family about cardiopulmonary resuscitation and the use of an automated external defibrillator (see Chapter 29). Women are often advised to avoid pregnancy, but each case is assessed individually. The nurse assesses the psychosocial needs of the patient and family on an ongoing basis. There may be concerns and fears about the prognosis, changes in lifestyle, effects of medications, and the possibility of others in the family having the same condition; these concerns often increase the patient's anxiety and interfere with effective coping strategies. Establishing trust is vital to the nurse's relationship with patients who are chronically ill and with these patients' families. This is particularly significant when the nurse is involved with a patient and family in discussions about end-of-life decisions. Patients who have significant symptoms of heart failure or other complications of cardiomyopathy may benefit from transitional or home care. Transitional Care Models have now emerged to assist the patient's transition from the hospital to home while dealing with a chronic illness (Naylor, Bowles, McCauley, et al., 2013).

Evaluation

Expected patient outcomes may include:
1. Maintains or improves cardiac function
   a. Exhibits heart and respiratory rates within normal limits
   b. Reports decreased dyspnea and increased comfort; maintains or improves gas exchange
   c. Reports no weight gain; appropriate weight for height
   d. Maintains or improves peripheral blood flow
2. Maintains or increases activity tolerance
   a. Carries out activities of daily living (e.g., brushes teeth, feeds self)
   b. Reports increased tolerance to activity
3. Is less anxious
   a. Discusses prognosis freely
   b. Verbalizes fears and concerns
   c. Participates in support groups if appropriate
   d. Demonstrates appropriate coping mechanisms
4. Decreases sense of powerlessness
   a. Identifies emotional response to diagnosis
   b. Discusses control that he or she has
5. Adheres to self-care program
   a. Takes medications according to prescribed schedule
   b. Modifies diet to accommodate sodium and fluid recommendations
   c. Modifies lifestyle to accommodate activity and rest behavior recommendations
   d. Identifies signs and symptoms to be reported to health care professionals

INFECTIOUS DISEASES OF THE HEART

Any of the heart's three layers may be affected by an infectious process. Infections are named for the layer of the heart most involved in the infectious process: infective endocarditis (endocardium), myocarditis (myocardium), and pericarditis (pericardium) (see Fig. 25-1). Rheumatic endocarditis is a unique infective endocarditis syndrome. Diagnosis of infection is made primarily on the basis of the patient's symptoms and echocardiography. Ideal management for all infectious diseases is prevention. IV antibiotics usually are necessary once an infection has developed in the heart.

Rheumatic Endocarditis

Acute rheumatic fever, which occurs most often in school-age children, may develop after an episode of group A beta-hemolytic streptococcal pharyngitis (see Chart 28-3). Patients with rheumatic fever may develop rheumatic heart disease as evidenced by a new heart murmur, cardiomegaly, pericarditis, and heart failure. Prompt and effective treatment of "strep" throat with antibiotics can prevent development of rheumatic fever. Streptococcus is spread by direct contact with oral or respiratory secretions. Although bacteria are the causative agents, malnutrition, overcrowding, poor hygiene, and lower socioeconomic status may predispose individuals to rheumatic fever. Incidence of rheumatic fever in the United States and other developed countries generally has decreased (Josephson, 2014); however, the exact incidence is difficult to determine because infection may go unrecognized and people may not seek treatment (Fuster et al., 2011). Further information about rheumatic fever and rheumatic endocarditis can be found in pediatric nursing books.

Infective Endocarditis

Infective endocarditis is a microbial infection of the endothelial surface of the heart. It usually develops in people with prosthetic heart valves, cardiac devices (e.g., pacemaker), or structural cardiac defects (e.g., valve disorders, HCM) (see Chart 28-4). It is more common in older adults (Josephson, 2014), who are more likely to have degenerative or calcific

valve lesions, reduced immunologic response to infection, and metabolic alterations associated with aging. Staphylococcal endocarditis infections of valves in the right side of the heart are common among IV drug abusers. Hospital-acquired infective endocarditis occurs most often in patients with debilitating disease or indwelling catheters and in patients who are receiving hemodialysis or prolonged IV fluid or antibiotic therapy. Patients taking immunosuppressive medications or corticosteroids are more susceptible to fungal endocarditis.

Invasive procedures, particularly those involving mucosal surfaces (e.g., those involving manipulation of gingival tissue or periapical regions of teeth), can cause a bacteremia, which rarely lasts more than 15 minutes. However, if a patient has any anatomic cardiac defects or implanted cardiac devices, bacteremia can cause bacterial endocarditis. Bacteremia also may be caused by IV drug abuse, body piercing (especially oral, nasal, and nipple), branding, and tattooing (Fuster et al., 2011; Josephson, 2014; Mann et al., 2015). Other patients who may be predisposed to infective endocarditis include those receiving therapeutic immunosuppression, or those with neutropenia, immunodeficiency, or malignancy (Grossman & Porth, 2014).

Pathophysiology

A deformity or injury of the endocardium leads to accumulation of fibrin and platelets (clot formation) on the endocardium. Infectious organisms, usually staphylococci or streptococci, invade the clot and endocardial lesion. Other causative microorganisms include fungi (e.g., *Candida*, *Aspergillus*) and *Rickettsiae*. Infection most frequently results in platelets, fibrin, blood cells, and microorganisms that cluster as vegetations on the endocardium. Vegetations may embolize to other tissues throughout the body. As the clot on the endocardium continues to expand, the infecting organism is covered by new clot and concealed from the body's normal defenses. Infection may erode through the endocardium into underlying structures (e.g., valve leaflets), causing tears or other deformities of valve leaflets, dehiscence of prosthetic valves, deformity of chordae tendineae, or mural abscesses.

Onset of infective endocarditis usually is insidious. Signs and symptoms develop from toxic effects of the infection, destruction of heart valves, and embolization of fragments of vegetative growths on the endocardium. Systemic emboli are more common with left-sided heart infective endocarditis when vegetations are larger than 10 mm in diameter (Josephson, 2014); pulmonary emboli may occur with right-sided heart infective endocarditis (Fuster et al., 2011).

Clinical Manifestations

Primary presenting symptoms of infective endocarditis are fever and a heart murmur. Fever may be intermittent or absent, especially in patients who are receiving antibiotics or corticosteroids, in older adults, and in those who have heart failure or kidney injury. A heart murmur may be absent initially but develops in almost all patients. Murmurs that worsen over time indicate progressive damage from vegetations or perforation of a valve or rupture of chordae tendineae.

In addition to fever and heart murmur, clusters of petechiae may be found on the body. Small, painful nodules (Osler nodes) may be present in pads of fingers or toes. Irregular, red or purple, painless flat macules (Janeway lesions) may be present on palms, fingers, hands, soles, and toes. Hemorrhages with pale centers (Roth spots) caused by emboli may be observed in fundi of the eyes. Splinter hemorrhages (i.e., reddish-brown lines and streaks) may be seen under the proximal half of fingernails and toenails. Petechiae may appear in conjunctiva and mucous membranes. Cardiomegaly, heart failure, tachycardia, or splenomegaly may occur.

Central nervous system manifestations of infective endocarditis include headache; temporary or transient cerebral ischemia; and strokes, which may be caused by emboli to cerebral arteries. Embolization may be a presenting symptom; it may occur at any time and may involve other organ systems. Embolic phenomena may occur, as discussed in the Rheumatic Endocarditis section.

Heart failure, which may result from perforation of a valve leaflet, rupture of chordae, blood flow obstruction due to vegetations, or intracardiac shunts from dehiscence of prosthetic valves, indicates a poor prognosis with medical therapy alone and a higher surgical risk. Valvular stenosis or regurgitation, myocardial damage, and mycotic (fungal) aneurysms are potential cardiac complications. First-, second-, and third-degree atrioventricular blocks may occur and are often a sign of a valve ring abscess. Emboli, immunologic responses, abscess of the spleen, mycotic aneurysms, cerebritis, and hemodynamic deterioration may cause complications in other organs.

Assessment and Diagnostic Findings

Although characteristics described previously may indicate infective endocarditis, signs and symptoms may indicate other diseases as well. Vague complaints of malaise, anorexia, weight loss, cough, and back and joint pain may be mistaken for influenza. Virulence of the causative organism usually correlates with the speed and degree of symptom development. A definitive diagnosis is made when a microorganism is found in two separate blood cultures, or in a vegetation or abscess. At least 2 sets of blood cultures (with each set including one aerobic and one anaerobic culture) drawn from different venipuncture sites over a 24-hour period (each set at least 12 hours apart), or every 30 minutes if the patient's condition is unstable, should be obtained before administration of any antimicrobial agents (Fuster et al., 2011; Mann et al., 2015; Nishimura et al., 2014). Negative blood cultures do not definitely rule out infective endocarditis. Patients may have elevated white blood cell (WBC) counts. In addition, patients may be anemic, have a positive rheumatoid factor, and an elevated erythrocyte sedimentation rate (ESR) or C-reactive protein.

Echocardiography may assist in diagnosis by demonstrating a mass on a valve, prosthetic valve, or supporting structures and by identifying vegetations, abscesses, new prosthetic valve dehiscence, or new regurgitation. An echocardiogram may reveal development of heart failure. TEE may provide additional data when transthoracic imaging is nondiagnostic; this method of echocardiography is superior in assessing vegetations and perivalvular complications (Fuster et al., 2011; Mann et al., 2015; Nishimura et al., 2014).

Prevention

Although rare, bacterial endocarditis may be life-threatening. A key strategy is primary prevention in high-risk patients (e.g., those with previous infective endocarditis, prosthetic heart valves, cardiac transplant patients with valve regurgitation, and some patients with congenital heart disease) (Grossman & Porth, 2014). Antibiotic prophylaxis is recommended for high-risk patients immediately before and sometimes after dental procedures that involve manipulation of gingival tissue or periapical area of teeth or perforation of oral mucosa (except routine anesthetic injections through noninfected tissue, placement of orthodontic brackets, loss of deciduous teeth, bleeding from trauma to lips or oral mucosa, dental x-rays, adjustment of orthodontic appliances, and placement of removable prosthodontic or orthodontic appliances). Updated guidelines no longer recommend antibiotic prophylaxis for patients undergoing nondental procedures (Nishimura et al., 2014).

The type of antibiotic used for prophylaxis varies with the type of procedure and degree of risk. Patients usually are instructed to take 2 g of amoxicillin (Amoxil) orally 1 hour before the procedure. If patients are allergic to penicillin, clindamycin (Cleocin), cephalexin (Keflex), cefazolin (Ancef, Kefzol), ceftriaxone (Rocephin), azithromycin (Zithromax), or clarithromycin (Biaxin) may be used (Fuster et al., 2011; Mann et al., 2015; Nishimura et al., 2014).

Equally important is ongoing good oral hygiene. Poor dental hygiene can lead to bacteremia, particularly in the setting of a dental procedure. Severity of oral inflammation and infection is a significant factor in the incidence and degree of bacteremia. Regular professional oral care combined with personal oral care may reduce the risk of bacteremia. Personal oral care includes using a soft toothbrush and toothpaste to brush teeth, gums, tongue, and oral mucosa at least twice a day, as well as rinsing the mouth with an antiseptic mouthwash for 30 seconds intermittently between tooth brushing. Patients must be advised to:

- Avoid using toothpicks or other sharp objects in the oral cavity
- Avoid nail biting
- Avoid body piercing, branding, tattooing
- Minimize outbreaks of acne, psoriasis

Female patients are advised not to use intrauterine devices (IUDs). Patients with substance abuse histories are referred to addiction treatment programs. Any fever of more than 7 days' duration is to be reported to a primary provider; patients should not self-medicate with antibiotics or stop taking them before the prescribed dosage has been completed.

Increased vigilance is also required in patients with IV catheters and during invasive procedures. To minimize the risk of infection, nurses must ensure meticulous hand hygiene, site preparation, and aseptic technique during insertion and maintenance procedures. All catheters, tubes, drains, and other devices are removed as soon as they are no longer needed or no longer function.

Medical Management

The objective of treatment is to eradicate invading organisms through adequate doses of an appropriate antimicrobial agent. Antibiotic therapy usually is given for 2 to 6 weeks every 4 hours or continuously by IV infusion. Parenteral therapy is given in doses that produce a high serum concentration for a significant period to ensure eradication of the dormant bacteria within dense vegetations. This therapy is often delivered in the patient's home and is monitored by a home care nurse. Serum levels of the antibiotic and blood cultures are monitored to gauge effectiveness of therapy. If there is insufficient bactericidal activity, increased dosages of the antibiotic are prescribed or a different antibiotic is used. Numerous antimicrobial regimens are in use, but penicillin usually is the medication of choice. In fungal endocarditis, an antifungal agent such as amphotericin B (Abelcet, Amphocin) is the usual treatment.

The patient's temperature is monitored at regular intervals because the course of fever is one indication of treatment effectiveness. However, febrile reactions also may occur as a result of medication. After adequate antimicrobial therapy is initiated, the infective organism is usually eliminated. The patient should begin to feel better, regain an appetite, and have less fatigue. During this time, patients require psychosocial support because although they feel well, they may find themselves confined to the hospital or home with restrictive IV therapy.

Surgical Management

Surgical intervention may be required if the infection does not respond to medications or the patient has prosthetic heart valve endocarditis, has a mobile vegetation, has heart failure, has heart block, or develops complications such as a septal perforation (Fuster et al., 2011; Josephson, 2014; Mann et al., 2015; Nishimura et al., 2014). Surgical interventions include valve débridement or excision, débridement of vegetations, débridement and closure of an abscess, and closure of a fistula. Aortic or mitral valve débridement, excision, or replacement is required in patients who:

- Develop congestive heart failure despite adequate medical treatment
- Have more than one serious systemic embolic episode
- Develop a valve obstruction
- Develop a periannular (heart valve), myocardial, or aortic abscess
- Have uncontrolled infection, persistent or recurrent infection, or fungal endocarditis

Surgical valve replacement greatly improves the prognosis for patients with severe symptoms from damaged heart valves. The aortic valve may best be treated with an autograft, as described previously. Most patients who have prosthetic valve endocarditis (i.e., infected valve replacements) require valve replacement.

Nursing Management

The nurse monitors the patient's temperature. The patient may have a fever for weeks. The nurse administers antibiotic, antifungal, or antiviral medication as prescribed or educates the patient to take them as prescribed. Patients need enough fluids to keep their urine light yellow. Fever often causes fatigue; rest periods should be planned and activities spaced to give to rest between activities. Good infection control and prevention practices include appropriate hand hygiene by both patients and caregivers. Nonsteroidal anti-inflammatory drugs (NSAIDs) may be prescribed as antipyretics or to decrease the discomfort of fever. Patients may be more comfortable with a light layer of linens and exposure of their skin

to air. They may be cooled with a fan, tepid water baths, or cloth compresses; if shivering or piloerection occurs, these interventions should be discontinued due to increased oxygen consumption and potential to further increase of body temperature.

Heart sounds are assessed. A new or worsening murmur may indicate dehiscence of a prosthetic valve, rupture of an abscess, or injury to valve leaflets or chordae tendineae. The nurse monitors for signs and symptoms of systemic embolization, or, for patients with right-sided heart endocarditis, for signs and symptoms of pulmonary infarction and infiltrates. In addition, the nurse assesses signs and symptoms of organ damage such as stroke (i.e., cerebrovascular disease or brain attack), meningitis, heart failure, myocardial infarction, glomerulonephritis, and splenomegaly.

Patient care is directed toward management of infection. Long-term IV antimicrobial therapy often is necessary; therefore, many patients have peripherally inserted central catheters or other long-term IV access. All invasive lines and wounds must be assessed daily for redness, tenderness, warmth, swelling, drainage, or other signs of infection. The patient and family are instructed about activity restrictions, medications, and signs and symptoms of infection. Patients with infective endocarditis are at high risk for another episode of infectious endocarditis. The nurse emphasizes the antibiotic prophylaxis described previously. If the patient has undergone surgical treatment, the nurse provides postoperative care and instructions (see Chapters 19 and 27).

As appropriate, the home care nurse supervises and monitors IV antibiotic therapy delivered in the home setting and educates the patient and family about prevention and health promotion. The nurse provides the patient and family with emotional support and facilitates coping strategies during the prolonged course of infection and antibiotic treatment.

Myocarditis

Myocarditis, an inflammatory process involving the myocardium, can cause heart dilation, thrombi on the heart wall (mural thrombi), infiltration of circulating blood cells around the coronary vessels and between the muscle fibers, and degeneration of the muscle fibers themselves. Mortality varies with the severity of symptoms. Most patients with mild symptoms recover completely; however, some patients develop cardiomyopathy and heart failure.

Pathophysiology

Myocarditis usually results from viral (e.g., coxsackievirus A and B, human immune deficiency virus, influenza A), bacterial, rickettsial, fungal, parasitic, metazoal, protozoal (e.g., Chagas disease), or spirochetal infection. It also may be immune related, occurring after acute systemic infections such as rheumatic fever. It may develop in patients receiving immunosuppressive therapy or in those with infective endocarditis, Crohn's disease, or systemic lupus erythematosus (Mann et al., 2015; Mann & Felker, 2016; Maron, Tobin, Thiene, et al., 2006).

Myocarditis may result from an inflammatory reaction to toxins such as pharmacologic agents used in the treatment of other diseases (e.g., anthracyclines for cancer therapy), ethanol, or radiation (especially to the left chest or upper back). It may begin in one small area of the myocardium and then spread throughout the myocardium. The degree of myocardial inflammation and necrosis determines the degree of interstitial collagen and elastin destruction. The greater the destruction, the greater is the hemodynamic effect and resulting signs and symptoms. It is thought that DCM and HCM are latent manifestations of myocarditis (Mann et al., 2015; Fuster et al., 2011).

 Concept Mastery Alert

> The most common pathogens involved in myocarditis tend to be viral, whereas in endocarditis they tend to be bacterial.

Clinical Manifestations

The symptoms of acute myocarditis depend on the type of infection, the degree of myocardial damage, and the capacity of the myocardium to recover. Patients may be asymptomatic, with an infection that resolves on its own. However, they may develop mild-to-moderate symptoms and seek medical attention, often reporting fatigue and dyspnea, syncope, palpitations, and occasional discomfort in the chest and upper abdomen. The most common symptoms are flulike. Patients may also sustain sudden cardiac death or quickly develop severe congestive heart failure.

Assessment and Diagnostic Findings

Assessment of the patient may reveal no detectable abnormalities; as a result, the illness can go undiagnosed. Patients may be tachycardic or may report chest pain. A cardiac catheterization demonstrates normal coronary arteries; however, cardiac MRI is being used more often as a diagnostic tool because of its noninvasive approach (Mann et al., 2015; Mann & Felker, 2016; Marx, 2014; Rapezzi, Arbustini, Caforio, et al., 2013). With contrast, cardiac MRI may be diagnostic and can guide clinicians to sites for endocardial biopsies, which may be diagnostic for an organism or its genome, an immune process, or a radiation reaction causing the myocarditis. Patients without any abnormal heart structure (at least initially) may suddenly develop dysrhythmias or ST–T-wave changes. If the patient has structural heart abnormalities (e.g., systolic dysfunction), a clinical assessment may disclose cardiac enlargement, faint heart sounds (especially S_1), pericardial friction rub, a gallop rhythm, or a systolic murmur. The WBC count, C-reactive protein, leukocyte count, and ESR may be elevated (Mann et al., 2015; Mann & Felker, 2016; Marx, 2014).

Prevention

Prevention of infectious diseases by means of appropriate immunizations (e.g., influenza, hepatitis) and early treatment appears to be important in decreasing the incidence of myocarditis (Mann et al., 2015).

Medical Management

Patients are given specific treatment for the underlying cause if it is known (e.g., penicillin for hemolytic streptococci) and are placed on bed rest to decrease cardiac workload. Bed rest also helps decrease myocardial damage and the complications of myocarditis. In young patients with myocarditis, activities, especially athletics, should be limited for a 6-month period or at least until heart size and function have returned to normal. Physical activity is increased slowly, and the patient is instructed to report any symptoms that occur with increasing activity, such as a rapidly beating heart. If heart failure or dysrhythmia develops, management is essentially the same as for all causes of heart failure and dysrhythmias (see Chapters 26 and 29). Although they are known for their anti-inflammatory effects, NSAIDs should not be used for pain control; they have been shown to be ineffective in relieving the inflammatory process in myocarditis and have been linked to worsening inflammation of the myocardium. This also can contribute to an increased mortality from increased virulence of the pathogen (Carforio, Pankuweit, Arbustini, et al., 2013).

Nursing Management

The nurse assesses for resolution of tachycardia, fever, and any other clinical manifestations. The cardiovascular assessment focuses on signs and symptoms of heart failure and dysrhythmias. Patients with dysrhythmias should have continuous cardiac monitoring with personnel and equipment readily available to treat life-threatening dysrhythmias.

 Quality and Safety Nursing Alert

> *Patients with myocarditis are sensitive to digitalis. Nurses must closely monitor these patients for digitalis toxicity, which is evidenced by a new onset of dysrhythmia, anorexia, nausea, vomiting, headache, and malaise. The primary provider should be notified immediately if this is suspected.*

Anti-embolism stockings and passive and active exercises should be used because embolization from venous thrombosis and mural thrombi can occur, especially in patients on bed rest. In some patients, pharmacologic prophylaxis may also be indicated (see Chapter 30) (Kahn, Comerota, Cushman, et al., 2014).

Pericarditis

Pericarditis refers to an inflammation of the pericardium, which is the membranous sac enveloping the heart. It may be a primary illness, or it may develop during various medical and surgical disorders. For example, pericarditis may occur after pericardiectomy (opening of the pericardium) following cardiac surgery. Pericarditis also may occur 10 days to 2 months after acute myocardial infarction (Dressler syndrome) (Curry, 2014; Mann et al., 2015). Pericarditis may be acute, chronic, or recurring. It is classified either as adhesive (constrictive), because the layers of the pericardium become attached to each other and restrict ventricular filling, or by what accumulates in the pericardial sac: serous (serum), purulent (pus), calcific (calcium deposits), fibrinous (clotting proteins), sanguinous (blood), or malignant (cancer). Pericarditis also may be described as exudative or noneffusive.

Pathophysiology

Causes underlying or associated with pericarditis are listed in Chart 28-5. The inflammatory process of pericarditis may lead to an accumulation of fluid in the pericardial sac (pericardial effusion) and increased pressure on the heart, leading to cardiac tamponade (see Chapter 29). Frequent or prolonged episodes of pericarditis also may lead to thickening and decreased elasticity of the pericardium, or scarring may fuse the visceral and parietal pericardium. These conditions restrict the heart's ability to fill with blood (constrictive pericarditis). The pericardium may become calcified, further restricting ventricular expansion during ventricular filling (diastole). With less filling, the ventricles pump less blood, leading to decreased cardiac output and signs and symptoms of heart failure. Restricted diastolic filling may result in increased systemic venous pressure, causing peripheral edema and hepatic failure.

Clinical Manifestations

Pericarditis may be asymptomatic. The most characteristic symptom of pericarditis is chest pain, although pain also may be located beneath the clavicle, in the neck, or in the left trapezius (scapula) region. Pain or discomfort usually remains fairly constant, but it may worsen with deep inspiration and when lying down or turning. The most characteristic clinical manifestation of pericarditis is a creaky or scratchy friction rub heard most clearly at the left lower sternal border. Other signs may include a mild fever, increased WBC count, anemia, and an elevated ESR or C-reactive protein level. Patients may have a nonproductive cough or hiccup. Dyspnea, as well as respiratory splinting because of pain upon inspiration, and other signs and symptoms of heart failure may occur as a result of pericardial compression due to

---

Chart 28-5 Causes of Pericarditis

- Idiopathic or nonspecific causes
- Infection: usually viral (e.g., human immune deficiency virus, coxsackievirus, influenza); rarely bacterial (e.g., staphylococci, streptococci, meningococci, gonococci, gram-negative rods, *Borrelia* [Lyme disease], tuberculosis); mycotic (fungal); and parasitic
- Disorders of connective tissue: systemic lupus erythematosus, rheumatic fever, rheumatoid arthritis, polyarteritis, and scleroderma
- Sarcoidosis
- Hypersensitivity states: immune reactions, medication reactions, and serum sickness
- Disorders of adjacent structures: myocardial infarction, dissecting aneurysm, pleural and pulmonary disease (pneumonia)
- Neoplastic disease: caused by metastasis from lung or breast cancer, leukemia, and primary (mesothelioma) neoplasms
- Radiation therapy of chest and upper torso (peak occurrence 5–9 months after treatment)
- Trauma: chest injury, cardiac surgery, cardiac catheterization, implantation of pacemaker, or implantable cardioverter defibrillator
- Kidney injury and uremia

Adapted from Fuster, V., Walsh, R. A., Harrington, R. A., et al. (Eds.). (2011). *Hurst's the heart* (13th ed.). New York: McGraw-Hill.

---

constrictive pericarditis or cardiac tamponade (Curry, 2014). The heart rate may increase to maintain cardiac output.

Assessment and Diagnostic Findings

The diagnosis most often is made on the basis of history, signs, and symptoms. An echocardiogram may detect inflammation, pericardial effusion or tamponade, and heart failure. It may help confirm the diagnosis and may be used to guide pericardiocentesis (needle or catheter drainage of the pericardium). TEE may be useful in diagnosis but may underestimate the extent of pericardial effusions. CT imaging may be the best diagnostic tool for determining size, shape, and location of pericardial effusions and may be used to guide pericardiocentesis. Cardiac MRI may assist with detection of inflammation and adhesions. Occasionally, a video-assisted pericardioscope-guided biopsy of the pericardium or epicardium is performed to obtain tissue samples for culture and microscopic examination. Because the pericardial sac surrounds the heart, a 12-lead ECG may show concave ST elevations in many, if not all, leads (with no reciprocal changes) and may show depressed PR segments or atrial dysrhythmias (Curry, 2014; Mann et al., 2015).

Medical Management

Objectives of pericarditis management are to determine the cause, administer therapy for treatment and symptom relief, and detect signs and symptoms of cardiac tamponade. When cardiac output is impaired, the patient is placed on bed rest until fever, chest pain, and friction rub have subsided.

Analgesic medications and NSAIDs such as aspirin or ibuprofen (Motrin) may be prescribed for pain relief during the acute phase. These agents also hasten reabsorption of fluid in patients with rheumatic pericarditis. Indomethacin (Indocin) is contraindicated because it may decrease coronary blood flow. Colchicine (Colcrys) or corticosteroids (e.g., prednisone) may be prescribed if the pericarditis is severe or if the patient does not respond to NSAIDs. Colchicine also may be used instead of NSAIDs during the acute phase (Curry, 2014; Imazio, Brucato, Cemin, et al., 2013; LeWinter, 2014; Mann et al., 2015; Marx, 2014).

Pericardiocentesis, a procedure in which some pericardial fluid is removed, rarely is necessary. It may be performed to assist in identification of the cause or relieve symptoms, especially if there are signs and symptoms of heart failure or tamponade. Pericardial fluid is cultured if bacterial, tubercular, or fungal disease is suspected; a sample is sent for cytology if neoplastic disease is suspected. A pericardial window, a small opening made in the pericardium, may be performed to allow continuous drainage into the chest cavity. Surgical removal of tough encasing pericardium (pericardiectomy) may be necessary to release both ventricles from constrictive and restrictive inflammation and scarring.

Nursing Management

Patients with acute pericarditis require pain management with analgesics, assistance with positioning, and psychological support. Patients with chest pain often benefit from education and reassurance that the pain is not due to a heart attack. Pain may be relieved with a forward-leaning or sitting position. To minimize complications, the nurse helps the patient with activity restrictions until pain and fever subside. As the patient's condition improves, the nurse encourages gradual increases of activity. However, if pain, fever, or friction rub recurs, activity restrictions must be resumed. The nurse educates the patient and family about a healthy lifestyle to enhance the patient's immune system.

Nurses caring for patients with pericarditis must be alert to cardiac tamponade (see Chapter 29). The nurse monitors the patient for heart failure. Patients with hemodynamic instability or pulmonary congestion are treated as if they had heart failure (see Chapter 29).

NURSING PROCESS
The Patient With Pericarditis

Assessment

The primary symptom of pericarditis is pain, which is assessed by evaluating the patient in various positions. The nurse tries to identify whether pain is influenced by respiratory movements, while holding an inhaled breath or holding an exhaled breath; by flexion, extension, or rotation of the spine, including the neck; by movements of shoulders and arms; by coughing; or by swallowing. Recognizing events that precipitate or intensify pain may help establish a diagnosis and differentiate pain of pericarditis from pain of myocardial infarction.

When pericardial surfaces lose their lubricating fluid because of inflammation, a pericardial friction rub occurs. The rub is audible on auscultation and is synchronous with the heartbeat. However, it may be elusive and difficult to detect.

⚑ Quality and Safety Nursing Alert

A pericardial friction rub is diagnostic of pericarditis. It is a creaky or scratchy sound and is louder at the end of exhalation. Nurses should monitor for pericardial friction rub by placing the diaphragm of the stethoscope tightly against the patient's thorax and auscultating the left sternal edge in the fourth intercostal space, which is the site where the pericardium comes into contact with the left chest wall. The rub may be heard best when a patient is sitting and leaning forward.

If there is difficulty in distinguishing a pericardial friction rub from a pleural friction rub, the patient is asked to hold their breath; a pericardial friction rub will continue to be heard.

The patient's temperature is monitored frequently. Pericarditis may cause an abrupt onset of fever in a patient who has been afebrile.

Diagnosis

NURSING DIAGNOSIS
Based on the assessment data, the major nursing diagnosis may be:
- Acute pain related to inflammation of the pericardium

COLLABORATIVE PROBLEMS/POTENTIAL COMPLICATIONS
Potential complications may include the following:
- Pericardial effusion
- Cardiac tamponade

Planning and Goals

The patient's major goals may include relief of pain and absence of complications.

Nursing Interventions

RELIEVING PAIN
Relief of pain is achieved by rest. Because sitting upright and leaning forward is the posture that tends to relieve pain, chair rest may be more comfortable. The nurse instructs the patient to restrict activity until pain subsides. As chest pain and friction rub abate, activities of daily living may be resumed gradually. If the patient is taking analgesics, antibiotics, or corticosteroids for pericarditis, their responses are monitored and recorded. Patients taking NSAIDs or colchicine are assessed for gastrointestinal adverse effects. If chest pain and friction rub recur, bed rest or chair rest is resumed.

MONITORING AND MANAGING POTENTIAL COMPLICATIONS
Pericardial Effusion. Abnormal accumulation of fluid between the pericardial linings (i.e., in the pericardial sac) is called *pericardial effusion* (see Chapter 29). Most patients have no effects or symptoms. However, enough fluid can accumulate to constrict the myocardium, impairing ventricular filling and the myocardium's ability to pump, a condition known as *cardiac tamponade* (discussed below) (Curry, 2014; Mann et al., 2015). Failure to identify and treat this problem can lead to death.

Cardiac Tamponade. Signs and symptoms of cardiac tamponade may begin with the patient reporting shortness of breath, chest tightness, or dizziness. The nurse may observe that the patient is becoming progressively more restless. Assessment of blood pressure may reveal a decrease of 10 mm Hg or more in systolic blood pressure during inspiration (pulsus paradoxus). Usually, the systolic pressure decreases and the diastolic pressure remains stable; hence, the pulse pressure narrows. The patient usually has tachycardia, and ECG voltage may be decreased or QRS complexes may alternate in height (electrical alternans). Heart sounds may progress from distant to imperceptible. Blood continues to return to the heart from the periphery but cannot flow into the heart to be pumped back into the circulation. The patient develops jugular vein distention and other signs of rising central venous pressure. Beck triad (hypotension, muffled heart sounds, and an elevated jugular venous pressure) is a useful diagnostic parameter of severe tamponade (Mann et al., 2015).

In such situations, the nurse notifies the primary provider immediately and prepares to assist with diagnostic echocardiography and pericardiocentesis (Mann et al., 2015) (see Chapter 29). The nurse stays with the patient and continues to assess and record signs and symptoms while intervening to decrease patient anxiety.

PROMOTING HOME, COMMUNITY-BASED, AND TRANSITIONAL CARE
Because patients, their family members, and health care providers tend to focus on the most obvious needs and issues related to pericarditis, the nurse reminds them about the importance of continuing health promotion and screening practices. The nurse educates patients who have not been involved in these practices in the past about their importance and refers them to appropriate health care providers.

Evaluation

Expected patient outcomes may include:
1. Freedom from pain
   a. Performs activities of daily living without pain, fatigue, or shortness of breath
   b. Temperature returns to normal range
   c. Exhibits no pericardial friction rub
2. Absence of complications
   a. Sustains blood pressure in normal range
   b. Heart sounds strong and can be auscultated
   c. Absence of jugular vein distention

CRITICAL THINKING EXERCISES

1 **ebp** A 19-year-old female college student presents to the student health clinic with recurrent tonsillitis. The physician on duty refers her to a surgeon for evaluation for tonsillectomy. Upon review of her medical history, the student reports an aortic valve replacement (prosthetic) as a child, but no other significant medical/surgical history. She remembers being told that she needs antibiotics before surgeries and asks if you agree. How would you respond to her questions? What complications are you focused on preventing? On what evidence do you base your response? What is the strength of your evidence?

2 Despite evidence-based medical management, a 57-year-old man with DCM continues to have significant functional limitations and is advised to consult with a cardiologist specializing in advanced heart failure therapy. The cardiologist recommends that the patient consider heart transplantation and begins the transplant workup. The patient expresses anxiety about what this entails and also fears about having "someone else's" heart. Based on what you know about transplant, how would you respond to these fears and anxiety?

3 **pq** A 47-year-old male presents to the emergency department complaining of malaise, fever, and painful nodules on the pads of his fingers. He admits to being an active IV drug abuser, while denying regular medical and dental care. Upon physical examination, the nurse notes a soft systolic murmur and small painful nodules on the pads of his fingers. Based upon these physical examination findings, the physician thinks that the patient may have infective endocarditis and prescribes antibiotics. What should the nurse ensure happens before the antibiotics are given? What are the care priorities for this patient?

4 A 39-year-old man presents to the cardiology clinic complaining of palpitations, fatigue, shortness of breath, and weakness over the last couple of weeks. On physical examination, you note a high-pitched systolic murmur and an irregular heartbeat. You suspect mitral regurgitation. What two diagnostic tests would be helpful in confirming your suspicion and directing treatment? What would you be concerned about for his future if this condition is not treated appropriately?

REFERENCES

*Asterisk indicates nursing research.
**Double asterisk indicates classic reference.

Books

Cohn, L. H. (2012). *Cardiac surgery in the adult* (4th ed.). New York: McGraw-Hill.

Fuster, V., Walsh, R. A., Harrington, R. A., et al. (Eds.). (2011). *Hurst's the heart* (13th ed.). New York: McGraw-Hill.

Grossman, S. C., & Porth, C. M. (2014). *Porth's pathophysiology* (9th ed.). Philadelphia, PA: Lippincott Williams & Wilkins.

Mann, D. L., & Felker, M. (2016). *Heart failure: A companion to Braunwald's heart disease* (3rd ed.). Philadelphia, PA: Elsevier Saunders.

Mann, D. L., Zipes, D. P., Bonow, R. O., et al. (Eds.). (2015). *Braunwald's heart disease: A textbook of cardiovascular medicine* (10th ed.). Philadelphia, PA: Saunders Elsevier.

Marx, J. A. (2014). *Rosen's emergency medicine: Concepts and clinical practice* (8th ed.). Philadelphia, PA: Elsevier Saunders.

Otto, C. M., & Bonow, R. O. (Eds.). (2013). *Valvular heart disease: A companion to Braunwald's heart disease* (4th ed.). Philadelphia, PA: Saunders Elsevier.

Runge, M. S., Stouffer, G. A., & Patterson, C. (Eds.). (2011). *Netter's cardiology* (2nd ed.). Philadelphia, PA: Saunders Elsevier.

Weber, J. R., & Kelley, J. H. (Eds.). (2014). *Health assessment in nursing* (5th ed.). Philadelphia, PA: Wolters Kluwer Health.

Journals and Electronic Documents

American Heart Association. (2015). *Physical changes to report.* Retrieved on 11/23/2015 at: www.heart.org/HEARTORG/Conditions/HeartFailure/PreventionTreatmentofHeartFailure/Physical-Changes-to-Report_UCM_306356_Article.jsp

American Society of Perianesthesia Nurses. (2014). *Perianesthesia nursing standards, practice recommendations and interpretive statements.* Retrieved on 3/2/2016 at:www.aspan.org/Clinical-Practice/FAQs#25

Badheka, A. O., Patel, N. J., Singh, V., et al. (2014). Percutaneous aortic balloon valvotomy in the United States: A 13-year perspective. *The American Journal of Medicine, 127*(8), 744–753.

Bennett, T., (2014). Treatment of dilated cardiomyopathy. *British Journal of Cardiac Nursing, 9*(6), 297–302.

Caforio, A. L., Pankuweit, S., Arbustini, E., et al. (2013). Current state of knowledge of etiology, diagnosis, management, and therapy of myocarditis: A position statement of the European Society of Cardiology Working Group on myocardial and pericardial diseases. *European Heart Journal, 34*, 2636–2648.

Centers for Disease Control and Prevention. (2015). *Is it strep throat?* Retrieved on 7/1/2016 at: www.cdc.gov/features/strepthroat

Corrado, D., Wichter, T., Link, M., et al. (2015). Treatment of arrhythmogenic right ventricular cardiomyopathy/dysplasia: An international task force consensus statement. *Circulation, 132*, 441–453.

**Costanzo, M. R., Dipchand, A., Starling, R., et al. (2010). The International Society of Heart and Lung Transplantation guidelines for the care of the heart transplant recipients. *Journal of Heart and Lung Transplantation, 29*(8), 914–956.

Curry, S., (2014). Acute pericarditis: An overview. *British Journal of Cardiac Nursing, 9*(3), 124–131.

Delling, F. N., & Vasan, R. S. (2014). Epidemiology and pathophysiology of mitral valve prolapse. *Circulation, 129*(21), 2158–2170.

Elliott, P. M., Anastasakis, A., Borger, M. A., et al. (2014). 2014 ESC guidelines on diagnosis and management of hypertrophic cardiomyopathy. *European Heart Journal, 35*, 2733–2779.

Feldman, D., Pamboukian, S., Teuteberg, J., et al. (2013). The International Society of Heart and Lung Transplantation guidelines for mechanical circulatory support: Executive Summary. *The Journal of Heart and Lung Transplantation, 32*(2), 157–187.

**Gersh, B. J., Maron, B. J., Bonow, R. O., et al. (2011). 2011 ACCF/AHA Guideline for the Diagnosis and Treatment of Hypertrophic Cardiomyopathy: Executive summary: A report of the American College of Cardiology Foundation/American Heart Association Task Force on Practice Guidelines developed in collaboration with the American Association for Thoracic Surgery, American Society of Echocardiography, American Society of Nuclear Cardiology,

Heart Failure Society of America, Heart Rhythm Society, Society for Cardiovascular Angiography and Interventions, and Society of Thoracic Surgeons. *Journal of American College of Cardiology, 58*(25), 2703–2738.

**Holmes, D. R., Mack, M. J., Kaul, S., et al. (2012). 2012 ACCF/AATS/SCAI/STS expert consensus document on transcatheter aortic valve replacement. *Annals of Thoracic Surgery, 93*(4), 1340–1395.

Hong, S., Hong, M., Ko, Y., et al. (2014). Multidisciplinary team approach for identifying potential candidate for transcatheter aortic valve implantation. *Yonsei Medical Journal, 55*(5), 1246–1252.

Imazio, M., Brucato, A., Cemin, R., et al. (2013). A randomized trial of colchicine for acute pericarditis. *New England Journal of Medicine, 369*(16), 1522–1528.

Josephson, L. (2014). Infective endocarditis: A review for nurses. *Dimensions of Critical Care Nursing, 33*(6), 327–240.

Kahn, S., Comerota, A., Cushman, M., et al. (2014). The postthrombotic syndrome: Evidence-based prevention, diagnosis, and treatment strategies. A scientific statement from the American Heart Association. *Circulation, 130*(13), 1636–1661.

Kaneko, R., & Davidson, M. J. (2014). Use of the hybrid operating room in cardiovascular medicine. *Circulation, 130*, 910–917.

Kapadia, S., Stewart, W. J., Anderson, W. N., et al. (2015). Outcomes of inoperable symptomatic aortic stenosis patients not undergoing aortic valve replacement: Insight into the impact of balloon aortic valvuloplasty from the PARTNER trial (Placement of AoRtic TraNscathER valve trial). *Journal of the American College of Cardiology: Cardiovascular Interventions, 8*(2), 324–333.

Kraemer, F. (2013). Ontology or phenomenology? How the LVAD challenges the euthanasia debate. *Bioethics, 27*(3), 140–150.

LeWinter, M. M. (2014). Acute pericarditis. *New England Journal of Medicine, 371*(25), 2410–2416.

Lima, B., Mack, M., & Gonzalez-Stawinski, G. (2015). Ventricular assist devices: The future is now. *Trends in Cardiovascular Medicine, 25*(4), 360–369.

Lund, L. H., Edwards, L. B., Kucheryavaya, A. Y., et al. (2014). The registry of the International Society for Heart and Lung Transplantation: Thirty-first official adult heart transplant report 0 2014; focus theme: Retransplantation. *Journal of Heart Lung Transplantation, 33*(10), 996–1008.

Marcus, F. I., & Abidov, A. (2012). Arrhythmogenic right ventricular cardiomyopathy 2012: Diagnostic challenges and treatment. *Journal of Cardiovascular Electrophysiology, 23*(10), 1149–1153.

Maron, B. J., & Nishimura, R. A. (2014). Surgical septal myectomy versus alcohol septal ablation assessing the status of the controversy in 2014. *Circulation, 130*, 1617–1624.

**Maron, B. J., Towbin, J. A., Thiene, G., et al. (2006). Contemporary definitions and classification of the cardiomyopathies: An American Heart Association scientific statement from the Council on Clinical Cardiology, Heart Failure and Transplantation Committee; Quality of Care and Outcomes Research and Functional Genomics and Translational Biology Interdisciplinary Working Groups; and Council on Epidemiology and Prevention. *Circulation, 113*(14), 1807–1816.

Munkholm-Larsen, S., Wan, B., Tian, D. H., et al. (2014). A systematic review on the safety and efficacy of percutaneous edge-to-edge mitral valve repair with the MitraClip System for high surgical risk candidates. *Heart, 100*(6), 473–478.

Naylor, M., Bowles, K., McCauley, K., et al. (2013). High-value transitional care: Translation of research into practice. *Journal of Evaluation in Clinic Practice, 19*(5), 727–733.

Nishimura, R. A., Otto, C. M., Bonow, R. O., et al. (2014). 2014 AHA/ACC guidelines for the management of patients with valvular heart disease. *Journal of the American College of Cardiology, 63*(22), e57–e185.

Pennell, D. J., Baksi, A. J., Kilner, P. J., et al. (2014). Review of The Journal of Cardiovascular Magnetic Resonance 2012. *Journal of Cardiovascular Magnetic Resonance, 16*(1), 100.

Rapezzi, C., Arbustini, E., Caforio, A., et al. (2013). Diagnostic work-up in cardiomyopathies: Bridging the gap between clinical phenotypes and final diagnosis. A position statement from the ESC Working Group on myocardial and pericardial diseases. *European Heart Journal, 34*, 1448–1458.

Rojas, L., & Calkins, H. (2015). Present understanding of the relationship between exercise and arrhythmogenic right ventricular dysplasia/cardiomyopathy. *Trends in Cardiovascular Medicine, 25*(3), 181–188.

Rustad, J., Stern, T., Hebert, K., et al. (2013). Diagnosis and treatment of depression in patients with congestive heart failure: A review of the literature. *The Primary Care Companion for CNS Disorders, 15*(4), PCC.13r01511.

Semsarian, C., Ingles, J., Maron, M., et al. (2015). New perspectives on the prevalence of hypertrophic cardiomyopathy. *Journal of the American College of Cardiology, 65*(12), 1249–1254.

Sheffle, N., & Bowden, T. (2014). Pre-participation screening for hypertrophic cardiomyopathy in young athletes. *British Journal of Cardiac Nursing, 9*(11), 551–559.

Starling, R. C. (2013). Advanced heart failure: Transplantation, LVADs, and beyond. *Cleveland Clinic Journal of Medicine, 80*(1), 33–40.

*White-Williams, C., Grady, K. L., Myers, S., et al. (2013). The relationships among satisfaction with social support, quality of life, and survival 5 to 10 years after heart transplantation. *Journal of Cardiovascular Nursing, 28*(5), 407–416.

Resources

American Heart Association, National Center, www.heart.org/HEARTORG/

Cardiomyopathy Association, www.cardiomyopathy.org

Heartmates, www.heartmates.us

National Heart, Lung, and Blood Institute, www.nhlbi.nih.gov

Management of Patients With Complications From Heart Disease

LEARNING OBJECTIVES

On completion of this chapter, the learner will be able to:

1 Identify the etiology, pathophysiology, and clinical manifestations of heart failure.
2 Describe management of patients with heart failure.
3 Use the nursing process as a framework for care of patients with heart failure.
4 Develop an education plan for patients with heart failure.
5 Identify the etiology, pathophysiology, and clinical manifestations of pulmonary edema.
6 Describe the medical and nursing management of patients with pulmonary edema.
7 Describe the medical and nursing management of patients with complications from heart disease.

GLOSSARY

acute decompensated heart failure: acute exacerbation of heart failure, with signs and symptoms of severe respiratory distress and poor systemic perfusion
anuria: urine output of less than 50 mL/24 h
ascites: an accumulation of serous fluid in the peritoneal cavity
cardiac resynchronization therapy (CRT): a treatment for heart failure in which a device paces both ventricles to synchronize contractions
congestive heart failure (CHF): a fluid overload condition (congestion) associated with heart failure
diastolic heart failure: the inability of the heart to pump sufficiently because of an alteration in the ability of the heart to fill; term used to describe a type of heart failure
ejection fraction (EF): percentage of blood volume in the ventricles at the end of diastole that is ejected during systole; a measurement of contractility
heart failure (HF): a clinical syndrome resulting from structural or functional cardiac disorders that impair the ability of a ventricle to fill or eject blood
left-sided heart failure (left ventricular failure): inability of the left ventricle to fill or eject sufficient blood into the systemic circulation

oliguria: diminished urine output; less than 0.5 mL/kg/h
orthopnea: shortness of breath when lying flat
paroxysmal nocturnal dyspnea (PND): shortness of breath that occurs suddenly during sleep
pericardiocentesis: procedure that involves aspiration of fluid from the pericardial sac
pericardiotomy: surgically created opening of the pericardium
pulmonary edema: abnormal accumulation of fluid in the interstitial spaces and alveoli of the lungs
pulseless electrical activity (PEA): condition in which electrical activity is present on an electrocardiogram, but there is not an adequate pulse or blood pressure
pulsus paradoxus: systolic blood pressure that is more than 10 mm Hg lower during inhalation than during exhalation; difference is normally less than 10 mm Hg
right-sided heart failure (right ventricular failure): inability of the right ventricle to fill or eject sufficient blood into the pulmonary circulation
systolic heart failure: inability of the heart to pump sufficiently because of an alteration in the ability of the heart to contract; term used to describe a type of heart failure

Today it is possible to help the patient with heart disease live longer and achieve a high quality of life. Advances in diagnostic procedures, treatments, technologies, and pharmacotherapies allow earlier and more accurate diagnoses and treatment that can begin well before significant debilitation occurs. However, heart disease remains a chronic and often progressive condition that is associated with serious complications. This chapter presents the complications most often associated with heart disorders and the collaborative treatment options for these complications.

HEART FAILURE

Heart failure (HF) is a clinical syndrome resulting from structural or functional cardiac disorders that impair the

ability of the ventricles to fill or eject blood (Yancy, Jessup, Bozkurt, et al., 2013). In the past, HF was often referred to as **congestive heart failure (CHF)**, because many patients experience pulmonary or peripheral congestion with edema. Currently, HF is recognized as a clinical syndrome characterized by signs and symptoms of fluid overload or inadequate tissue perfusion. Fluid overload and decreased tissue perfusion result when the heart cannot generate cardiac output (CO) sufficient to meet the body's demands for oxygen and nutrients. The term *heart failure* indicates myocardial disease in which impaired contraction of the heart (systolic dysfunction) or filling of the heart (diastolic dysfunction) may cause pulmonary or systemic congestion. Some cases of HF are reversible, depending on the cause. Most often, HF is a chronic, progressive condition that is managed with lifestyle changes and medications to prevent episodes of

acute decompensated heart failure. These episodes are characterized by increased symptoms, decreased CO, and low perfusion (Pinkerman, Sander, Breeding, et al., 2013). These episodes are also associated with increased hospitalizations, increased health care costs, and decreased quality of life.

Chronic Heart Failure

The incidence of HF increases with age. Approximately 6 million people in the United States have HF, and 870,000 new cases are diagnosed each year (American Heart Association [AHA], 2015). Although HF can affect people of all ages, it is most common in people older than 75 years. As the US population ages, HF has become an epidemic that challenges the country's health care resources. HF is the most common reason for hospitalization of people older than 65 years and is the second most common reason for visits to a physician's office. The rate of emergency department visits and hospital readmissions for this condition remains very high. Approximately 25% of patients discharged after treatment for HF are readmitted to the hospital within 30 days (Albert, Barnason, Deswal, et al., 2015). The estimated economic burden caused by HF in the United States is more than $30 billion annually in direct and indirect costs and is expected to increase (AHA, 2015).

The increased incidence of HF reflects not only the aging population but also improvements in treatment and survival rates of people with cardiac diagnoses such as myocardial infarction (MI). Many hospitalizations for HF can be prevented by appropriate outpatient care. Prevention and early intervention to arrest the progression of HF are major US health initiatives (AHA, 2015).

Two major types of HF are identified by assessment of left ventricular function, usually by echocardiogram. The most common type is an alteration in ventricular contraction called **systolic heart failure,** which is characterized by a weakened heart muscle. A second type is **diastolic heart failure,** which is characterized by a stiff and noncompliant heart muscle, making it difficult for the ventricle to fill. An assessment of the **ejection fraction (EF)** is performed by echocardiogram to assist in determining the type of HF. EF is calculated by subtracting the amount of blood present in the left ventricle at the end of systole from the amount present at the end of diastole and calculating the percentage of blood that is ejected. A normal EF is 55% to 65% of the ventricular volume; the ventricle does not completely empty between contractions. The EF is normal in diastolic HF; therefore, this condition is referred to as *heart failure with preserved EF.* Approximately one third of HF patients have systolic dysfunction, one third have diastolic dysfunction, and one third have both (Pinkerman et al., 2013).

Although a reduced EF is a hallmark of systolic HF, the severity of HF is frequently classified according to the patient's symptoms. The New York Heart Association (NYHA) classification of HF is described in Table 29-1. The American College of Cardiology and the American Heart Association (ACC/AHA) have developed another HF classification system (Yancy et al., 2013). This system, described in Table 29-2, takes into consideration the natural history and progressive nature of HF. Treatment guidelines have been developed for each stage, which are discussed later in this chapter.

TABLE 29-1 New York Heart Association Classification of Heart Failure

Classification	Signs and Symptoms
I	No limitation of physical activity Ordinary activity does not cause undue fatigue, palpitation, or dyspnea.
II	Slight limitation of physical activity Comfortable at rest, but ordinary physical activity causes fatigue, palpitation, or dyspnea.
III	Marked limitation of physical activity Comfortable at rest, but less than ordinary activity causes fatigue, palpitation, or dyspnea.
IV	Unable to carry out any physical activity without discomfort Symptoms of cardiac insufficiency at rest If any physical activity is undertaken, discomfort is increased.

Adapted from Yancy, C. W., Jessup, M., Bozkurt, B., et al. (2013). 2013 ACCF/AHA Guideline for the management of heart failure. A report of the American College of Cardiology Foundation/American Heart Association Task Force on Practice Guidelines. *Circulation, 128*(16), e240–e327.

Etiology

Myocardial dysfunction and HF can be caused by a number of conditions, including coronary artery disease, hypertension, cardiomyopathy, valvular disorders, and renal dysfunction with volume overload (McCance, Huether, Brashers, et al., 2014). Patients with diabetes are also at high risk for HF. Atherosclerosis of the coronary arteries is a primary cause of HF, and coronary artery disease is found in the majority of patients with HF. Ischemia causes myocardial dysfunction because it deprives heart cells of oxygen and causes cellular damage. MI causes focal heart muscle necrosis, the death of myocardial cells, and a loss of contractility; the extent of the infarction correlates with the severity of HF. Revascularization of the coronary artery by a percutaneous coronary intervention (PCI) or by coronary artery bypass surgery (coronary artery bypass graft [CABG]) may improve myocardial oxygenation and ventricular function and prevent more extensive myocardial necrosis that can lead to HF (see Chapter 27).

Systemic or pulmonary hypertension increases afterload (resistance to ejection), which increases cardiac workload and leads to hypertrophy of myocardial muscle fibers. This can be considered a compensatory mechanism because it initially increases contractility. However, sustained hypertension eventually leads to changes that impair the heart's ability to fill properly during diastole, and the hypertrophied ventricles may dilate and fail (Grossman & Porth, 2014).

Cardiomyopathy is a disease of the myocardium. The various types of cardiomyopathy lead to HF and dysrhythmias. Dilated cardiomyopathy, the most common type of cardiomyopathy, causes diffuse myocyte necrosis and fibrosis, and commonly leads to progressive HF (Grossman & Porth, 2014). Dilated cardiomyopathy can be idiopathic (unknown cause), or it can result from an inflammatory process, such as myocarditis, or from a cytotoxic agent, such as alcohol or certain antineoplastic drugs. Hypertrophic cardiomyopathy is an autosomal dominant disease which leads to severe

TABLE 29-2 American College of Cardiology and American Heart Association Classification of Heart Failure

Classification	Criteria	Patient Characteristics	Treatment Recommendations for Appropriate Patients
Stage A	Patients at high risk for developing left ventricular dysfunction but without structural heart disease or symptoms of HF	Hypertension Atherosclerotic disease Diabetes Metabolic syndrome	Heart healthy lifestyle Risk factor control of hypertension, lipids, diabetes, obesity
Stage B	Patients with left ventricular dysfunction or structural heart disease who have not developed symptoms of HF	History of myocardial infarction Left ventricular hypertrophy Low ejection fraction	Implement stage A recommendations, plus: • ACE inhibitor or ARB for low EF or history of MI • Beta blocker • Statin
Stage C	Patients with left ventricular dysfunction or structural heart disease with current or prior symptoms of heart disease	Shortness of breath Fatigue Decreased exercise tolerance	Implement stage A and B recommendations, plus: • Diuretics • Aldosterone antagonist • Sodium restriction • Implantable defibrillator • Cardiac resynchronization therapy
Stage D	Patients with refractory end-stage HF requiring specialized interventions	Symptoms despite maximal medical therapy Recurrent hospitalizations	Implement stage A, B, and C recommendations, plus: • Fluid restriction • End-of-life care • Extraordinary measures: • Inotropes • Cardiac transplantation • Mechanical support

ACE, angiotensin-converting enzyme; ARB, angiotensin receptor blocker; EF, ejection fraction; HF, heart failure; MI, myocardial infarction.
Adapted from Yancy, C. Jessup, M., Bozkurt, B., et al. (2013). 2013 ACCF/AHA guideline for the diagnosis and management of heart failure: A report of the American College of Cardiology Foundation/American Heart Association Task Force on Practice Guidelines. *Circulation, 128*(16), e240–e327.

ventricular hypertrophy and poor diastolic filling (diastolic failure). Usually, HF due to cardiomyopathy is chronic and progressive. However, cardiomyopathy and HF may resolve following removal of the causative agent (e.g., cessation of alcohol ingestion).

Valvular heart disease is also a cause of HF. The valves ensure that blood flows in one direction. With valvular dysfunction, it becomes increasingly difficult for blood to move forward, increasing pressure within the heart and increasing cardiac workload, leading to HF. See Chapter 28 for discussion of the effects of valvular heart disease.

Several systemic conditions, including progressive renal failure, contribute to the development and severity of HF. More than 40% of patients with chronic HF have impaired renal function. The term *cardiorenal syndrome* describes how dysfunction in one of these systems leads to dysfunction in the other, resulting in increased morbidity and mortality (Pinkerman et al., 2013). In addition, cardiac dysrhythmias such as atrial fibrillation may either cause or result from HF; in both instances, the altered electrical stimulation impairs myocardial contraction and decreases the overall efficiency of myocardial function. Other factors, such as hypoxia, acidosis, and electrolyte abnormalities, can worsen myocardial function.

Pathophysiology

Regardless of the etiology, the pathophysiology of HF results in similar changes and clinical manifestations. Significant myocardial dysfunction usually occurs before the patient experiences signs and symptoms of HF such as shortness of breath, edema, or fatigue.

As HF develops, the body activates neurohormonal compensatory mechanisms. These mechanisms represent the body's attempt to cope with the HF and are responsible for the signs and symptoms that develop (Grossman & Porth, 2014). Understanding these mechanisms is important because the treatment for HF is aimed at correcting them and relieving symptoms.

Systolic HF results in decreased blood ejected from the ventricle. The decreased blood flow is sensed by baroreceptors in the aortic and carotid bodies. The sympathetic nervous system is then stimulated to release epinephrine and norepinephrine (see Fig. 29-1). The purpose of this initial response is to increase heart rate and contractility and support the failing myocardium, but the continued response has multiple negative effects. Sympathetic stimulation causes vasoconstriction in the skin, gastrointestinal tract, and kidneys. A decrease in renal perfusion due to low CO and vasoconstriction then causes the release of renin by the kidneys. Renin converts the plasma protein angiotensinogen to angiotensin I, which then circulates to the lungs. Angiotensin-converting enzyme (ACE) in the lumen of pulmonary blood vessels converts angiotensin I to angiotensin II, a potent vasoconstrictor, which then increases the blood pressure and afterload. Angiotensin II also stimulates the release of aldosterone from the adrenal cortex, resulting in sodium and fluid retention by the renal tubules and an increase in blood

Physiology/Pathophysiology

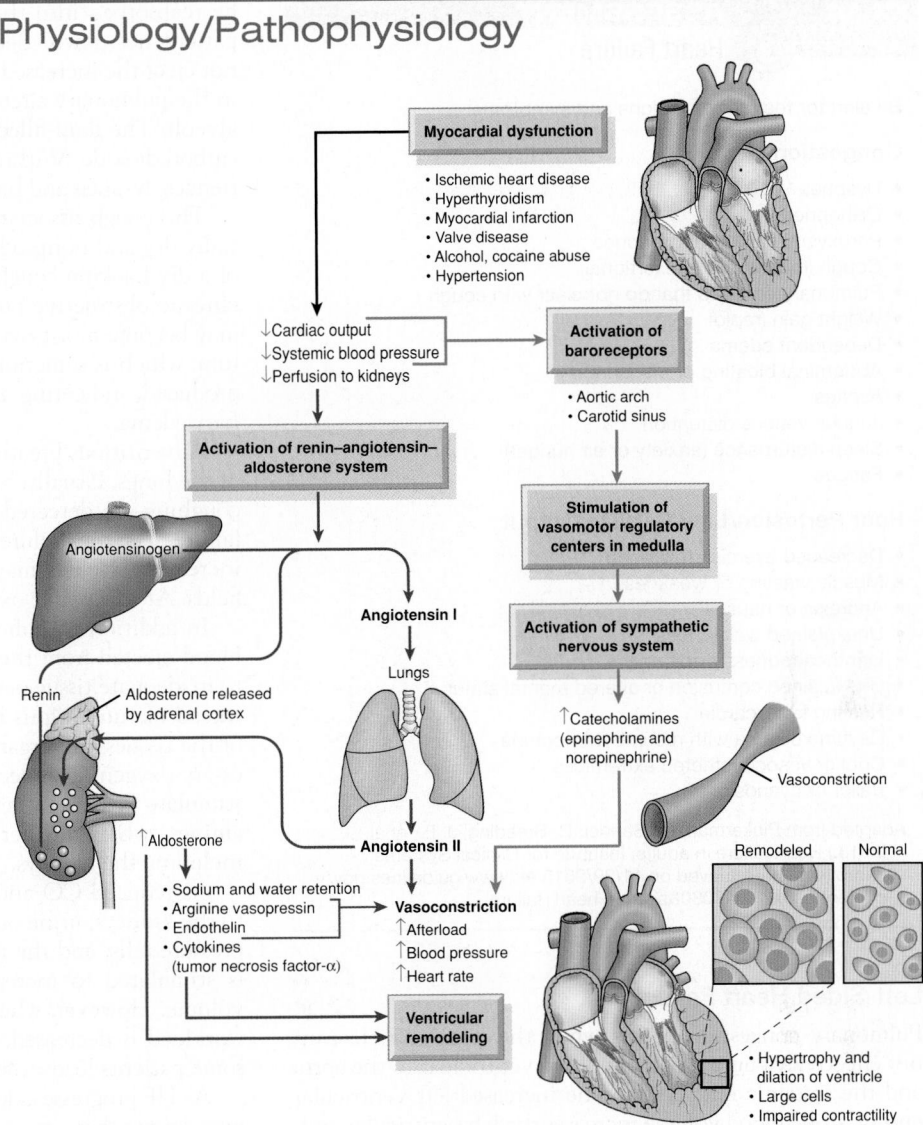

Myocardial dysfunction

- Ischemic heart disease
- Hyperthyroidism
- Myocardial infarction
- Valve disease
- Alcohol, cocaine abuse
- Hypertension

↓Cardiac output
↓Systemic blood pressure
↓Perfusion to kidneys

Activation of baroreceptors

- Aortic arch
- Carotid sinus

Activation of renin–angiotensin–aldosterone system

Angiotensinogen

Stimulation of vasomotor regulatory centers in medulla

Angiotensin I

Lungs

Activation of sympathetic nervous system

Renin   Aldosterone released by adrenal cortex

↑Catecholamines (epinephrine and norepinephrine)

Vasoconstriction

↑Aldosterone

Remodeled   Normal

Angiotensin II

- Sodium and water retention
- Arginine vasopressin
- Endothelin
- Cytokines (tumor necrosis factor-α)

Vasoconstriction
↑Afterload
↑Blood pressure
↑Heart rate

Ventricular remodeling

- Hypertrophy and dilation of ventricle
- Large cells
- Impaired contractility

Figure 29-1 • The pathophysiology of heart failure. A decrease in cardiac output activates multiple neurohormonal mechanisms that ultimately result in the signs and symptoms of heart failure.

volume. These mechanisms lead to the fluid volume overload commonly seen in HF. Angiotensin, aldosterone, and other neurohormones (e.g., endothelin) lead to an increase in preload and afterload, which increases stress on the ventricular wall, causing an increase in cardiac workload. A counter-regulatory mechanism is attempted through the release of natriuretic peptides. Atrial natriuretic peptide (ANP) and B-type natriuretic peptide (BNP; brain type) are released from the overdistended cardiac chambers. These substances promote vasodilation and diuresis. However, their effect is usually not strong enough to overcome the negative effects of the other mechanisms.

As the heart's workload increases, contractility of the myocardial muscle fibers decreases. Decreased contractility results in an increase in end-diastolic blood volume in the ventricle, stretching the myocardial muscle fibers and increasing the size of the ventricle (ventricular dilation). One way the heart compensates for the increased workload is to increase the thickness of the heart muscle (ventricular hypertrophy). However, hypertrophy results in abnormal changes in structure and function of myocardial cells, a process known as ventricular remodeling.

Under the influence of neurohormones (e.g., angiotensin II), enlarged myocardial cells become dysfunctional and die early (a process called *apoptosis*), leaving the other normal myocardial cells struggling to maintain CO.

As cardiac cells die and the heart muscle becomes fibrotic, diastolic HF can develop, leading to further dysfunction. A stiff ventricle resists filling, and less blood in the ventricles causes a further decrease in CO. All of these compensatory mechanisms of HF have been referred to as the "vicious cycle of HF" because low CO leads to multiple mechanisms that make the heart work harder, worsening the HF.

Clinical Manifestations

Many clinical manifestations are associated with HF (see Chart 29-1). These signs and symptoms are related to congestion and poor perfusion. The signs and symptoms of HF can also be related to the ventricle that is most affected. **Left-sided heart failure (left ventricular failure)** causes different manifestations than **right-sided heart failure (right ventricular failure).** In chronic HF, patients may have signs and symptoms of both left and right ventricular failure.

Chart 29-1 ASSESSMENT
Heart Failure

Be alert for the following signs and symptoms:

Congestion

- Dyspnea
- Orthopnea
- Paroxysmal nocturnal dyspnea
- Cough (recumbent or exertional)
- Pulmonary crackles that do not clear with cough
- Weight gain (rapid)
- Dependent edema
- Abdominal bloating or discomfort
- Ascites
- Jugular venous distention
- Sleep disturbance (anxiety or air hunger)
- Fatigue

Poor Perfusion/Low Cardiac Output

- Decreased exercise tolerance
- Muscle wasting or weakness
- Anorexia or nausea
- Unexplained weight loss
- Lightheadedness or dizziness
- Unexplained confusion or altered mental status
- Resting tachycardia
- Daytime oliguria with recumbent nocturia
- Cool or vasoconstricted extremities
- Pallor or cyanosis

Adapted from Pinkerman, C., Sander, P., Breeding, J. E., et al. (2013.) Heart failure in adults, Institute for Clinical Systems Improvement. Retrieved on 11/29/2015 at: www.guidelines.gov/content.aspx?id=47030&search=heart+failure

Left-Sided Heart Failure

Pulmonary congestion occurs when the left ventricle cannot effectively pump blood out of the ventricle into the aorta and the systemic circulation. The increased left ventricular end-diastolic blood volume increases the left ventricular end-diastolic pressure, which decreases blood flow from the left atrium into the left ventricle during diastole. The blood volume and pressure build up in the left atrium, decreasing flow through the pulmonary veins into the left atrium. Pulmonary venous blood volume and pressure increase in the lungs, forcing fluid from the pulmonary capillaries into the pulmonary tissues and alveoli, causing pulmonary interstitial edema and impaired gas exchange. The clinical manifestations of pulmonary congestion include dyspnea, cough, pulmonary crackles, and low oxygen saturation levels. An extra heart sound, the S_3, or "ventricular gallop," may be detected on auscultation. It is caused by abnormal ventricular filling (Pinkerman et al., 2013).

Dyspnea, or shortness of breath, may be precipitated by minimal to moderate activity (dyspnea on exertion [DOE]); dyspnea also can occur at rest. The patient may report **orthopnea**, difficulty breathing when lying flat. Patients with orthopnea may use pillows to prop themselves up in bed, or they may sit in a chair and even sleep sitting up. Some patients have sudden attacks of dyspnea at night, a condition known as **paroxysmal nocturnal dyspnea (PND).** Fluid that accumulates in the dependent extremities during the day may

be reabsorbed into the circulating blood volume when the patient lies down. Because the impaired left ventricle cannot eject the increased circulating blood volume, the pressure in the pulmonary circulation increases, shifting fluid into the alveoli. The fluid-filled alveoli cannot exchange oxygen and carbon dioxide. Without sufficient oxygen, the patient experiences dyspnea and has difficulty sleeping.

The cough associated with left ventricular failure is initially dry and nonproductive. Most often, patients complain of a dry hacking cough that may be mislabeled as asthma or chronic obstructive pulmonary disease (COPD). The cough may become moist over time. Large quantities of frothy sputum, which is sometimes pink or tan (blood tinged), may be produced, indicating acute decompensated HF with pulmonary edema.

Adventitious breath sounds may be heard in various areas of the lungs. Usually, bibasilar crackles that do not clear with coughing are detected in the early phase of left ventricular failure. As the failure worsens and pulmonary congestion increases, crackles may be auscultated throughout the lung fields. At this point, oxygen saturation may decrease.

In addition to pulmonary manifestations, the amount of blood ejected from the left ventricle decreases and can lead to inadequate tissue perfusion. The diminished CO has widespread manifestations because not enough blood reaches all of the tissues and organs (low perfusion) to provide the necessary oxygen. The decrease in stroke volume (SV) can also stimulate the sympathetic nervous system to release catecholamines, which further impedes perfusion to many organs, including the kidneys.

As reduced CO and catecholamines decrease blood flow to the kidneys, urine output drops (oliguria). Renal perfusion pressure falls, and the renin–angiotensin–aldosterone system is stimulated to increase blood pressure and intravascular volume. However, when the patient is sleeping, the cardiac workload is decreased, improving renal perfusion, which in some patients leads to frequent urination at night (nocturia).

As HF progresses, decreased output from the left ventricle may cause other symptoms. Decreased gastrointestinal perfusion causes altered digestion. Decreased brain perfusion causes dizziness, lightheadedness, confusion, restlessness, and anxiety due to decreased oxygenation and blood flow. As anxiety increases, so does dyspnea, increasing anxiety and creating a vicious cycle. Stimulation of the sympathetic system also causes the peripheral blood vessels to constrict, so the skin appears pale or ashen and feels cool and clammy.

A decrease in SV causes the sympathetic nervous system to increase the heart rate (tachycardia), often causing the patient to complain of palpitations. The peripheral pulses become weak. Without adequate CO, the body cannot respond to increased energy demands, and the patient becomes easily fatigued and has decreased activity tolerance. Fatigue also results from the increased energy expended in breathing and the insomnia that results from respiratory distress, coughing, and nocturia.

Right-Sided Heart Failure

When the right ventricle fails, congestion in the peripheral tissues and the viscera predominates. This occurs because the right side of the heart cannot eject blood effectively and cannot accommodate all of the blood that normally returns to it

Figure 29-2 • Example of pitting edema. **A.** The nurse applies pressure to an area near the ankle. **B.** When the pressure is released, an indentation remains in the edematous tissue. From Bickley, L. S. (2017). *Bates' guide to physical examination and history taking* (12th ed.). Philadelphia, PA: Lippincott Williams & Wilkins.

from the venous circulation. Increased venous pressure leads to jugular venous distention (JVD) and increased capillary hydrostatic pressure throughout the venous system. Systemic clinical manifestations include edema of the lower extremities (dependent edema), hepatomegaly (enlargement of the liver), **ascites** (accumulation of fluid in the peritoneal cavity), and weight gain due to retention of fluid.

Edema usually affects the feet and ankles and worsens when the patient stands or sits for a long period. The edema may decrease when the patient elevates the legs. Edema can gradually progress up the legs and thighs and eventually into the external genitalia and lower trunk. Ascites is evidenced by increased abdominal girth and may accompany lower body edema or may be the only edema present. Sacral edema is common in patients who are on bed rest, because the sacral area is dependent. Pitting edema, in which indentations in the skin remain after even slight compression with the fingertips (see Fig. 29-2), is generally obvious after retention of at least 4.5 kg (10 lb) of fluid (4.5 L).

Hepatomegaly and tenderness in the right upper quadrant of the abdomen result from venous engorgement of the liver. The increased pressure may interfere with the liver's ability to function (secondary liver dysfunction). As hepatic dysfunction progresses, increased pressure within the portal vessels may force fluid into the abdominal cavity, causing ascites. Ascites may increase pressure on the stomach and intestines and cause gastrointestinal distress. Hepatomegaly may also increase pressure on the diaphragm, causing respiratory distress.

Anorexia (loss of appetite), nausea, or abdominal pain may result from the venous engorgement and venous stasis within the abdominal organs. The generalized weakness that accompanies right-sided HF results from reduced CO and impaired circulation.

Assessment and Diagnostic Findings

HF may go undetected until the patient presents with signs and symptoms of pulmonary and peripheral edema. Some of the physical signs that suggest HF may also occur with other diseases, such as kidney injury and COPD; therefore, diagnostic testing is essential to confirm a diagnosis of HF.

Assessment of ventricular function is an essential part of the initial diagnostic workup. An echocardiogram is usually performed to determine the EF, identify anatomic features such as structural abnormalities and valve malfunction, and confirm the diagnosis of HF. This information may also be obtained noninvasively by radionuclide ventriculography or invasively by ventriculography as part of a cardiac catheterization procedure. Differential identification of systolic and diastolic HF is important, as treatment differs (Pinkerman et al., 2013).

A chest x-ray and a 12-lead electrocardiogram (ECG) are obtained to assist in the diagnosis. Laboratory studies usually performed during the initial workup include serum electrolytes, blood urea nitrogen (BUN), creatinine, liver function tests, thyroid-stimulating hormone, complete blood count (CBC), BNP, and routine urinalysis. The BNP level is a key diagnostic indicator of HF; high levels are a sign of high cardiac filling pressure and can aid in both the diagnosis and management of HF (Pinkerman et al., 2013). The results of these laboratory studies assist in determining the underlying cause and can also be used to establish a baseline to assess effects of treatment. Cardiac stress testing or cardiac catheterization may be performed to determine whether coronary artery disease and cardiac ischemia are causing the HF.

Medical Management

The goals of management of HF are to relieve patient symptoms, to improve functional status and quality of life, and to extend survival. The prognosis for HF patients has improved with the use of evidence-based protocols for patient management. Specific interventions are based on the stage of HF. The objectives of guideline-directed patient management include the following:

- Improvement of cardiac function with optimal pharmacologic management
- Reduction of symptoms and improvement of functional status
- Stabilization of patient condition and lowering of the risk of hospitalization
- Delay of the progression of HF and extension of life expectancy
- Promotion of a lifestyle conducive to cardiac health

Treatment options vary according to the severity of the patient's condition and may include oral and intravenous (IV) medications, major lifestyle changes, supplemental oxygen, and surgical interventions including implantation of cardiac devices and cardiac transplantation.

Managing the patient with HF begins with providing comprehensive education and counseling to the patient and family. The patient and family must understand the nature of HF and the importance of their participation in the treatment regimen. Lifestyle recommendations include restriction of dietary sodium; avoidance of smoking, including passive smoke; avoidance of excessive fluid and alcohol intake; weight reduction when indicated; and regular exercise. The patient must also know how to recognize signs and symptoms that need to be reported to the primary provider.

TABLE 29-3 Common Medications Used to Treat Heart Failure

Medication	Therapeutic Effects	Key Nursing Considerations
Angiotensin-Converting Enzyme Inhibitors		
Lisinopril (Prinivil) Enalapril (Vasotec)	↓ BP and ↓ afterload Relieves signs and symptoms of HF Prevents progression of HF	Observe for symptomatic hypotension, increased serum K⁺, cough, and worsening renal function.
Angiotensin Receptor Blockers		
Valsartan (Diovan) Losartan (Cozaar)	↓ BP and ↓ afterload Relieves signs and symptoms of HF Prevents progression of HF	Observe for symptomatic hypotension, increased serum K⁺, and worsening renal function.
Hydralazine and Isosorbide Dinitrate (Dilatrate)	Dilates blood vessels ↓ BP and ↓ afterload	Observe for symptomatic hypotension.
Beta-Adrenergic Blocking Agents (Beta-Blockers)		
Carvedilol (Coreg) Bisoprolol (Zebeta) Metoprolol (Lopressor; Toprol XL)	Dilates blood vessels and ↓ afterload ↓ Signs and symptoms of HF Improves exercise capacity	Observe for decreased heart rate, symptomatic hypotension, dizziness, and fatigue.
Diuretics		
Loop diuretic: Furosemide (Lasix) *Thiazide diuretics:* Metolazone (Zaroxolyn) Hydrochlorothiazide (HCTZ)	↓ Fluid volume overload ↓ Signs and symptoms of HF	Observe for electrolyte abnormalities, renal dysfunction, diuretic resistance, and decreased BP. Carefully monitor I&O and daily weight (see Chart 29-2).
Aldosterone antagonist: Spironolactone (Aldactone)	Improves HF symptoms in advanced HF	Observe for hyperkalemia, hyponatremia.
Digitalis		
Digoxin (Lanoxin)	Improves cardiac contractility ↓ Signs and symptoms of HF	Observe for bradycardia and digitalis toxicity.

↓, decreases; BP, blood pressure; HF, heart failure; K⁺, potassium; I&O, input and output.
Adapted from Birchum, J. R., & Rosenthal, L. D. (2014) *Lehne's pharmacology for nursing care* (9th ed.). St. Louis, MO: Elsevier.

Pharmacologic Therapy

Several medications are routinely prescribed for HF, including ACE inhibitors, beta-blockers, and diuretics (see Table 29-3). Many of these medications, particularly ACE inhibitors and beta-blockers, improve symptoms and extend survival. Others, such as diuretics, improve symptoms but may not affect survival. Target doses for these medications are identified in the ACC/AHA guidelines, and nurses and physicians work collaboratively toward achieving effective dosing of these medications (Yancy et al., 2013).

Angiotensin-Converting Enzyme Inhibitors

ACE inhibitors play a pivotal role in the management of systolic HF. They have been found to relieve the signs and symptoms of HF and significantly decrease mortality and morbidity, especially in patients with a left ventricular EF less than 35%. ACE inhibitors (e.g., lisinopril [Prinivil]) slow the progression of HF, improve exercise tolerance, and decrease the number of hospitalizations (Yancy et al., 2013). Available as oral and IV medications, ACE inhibitors promote vasodilation and diuresis, ultimately decreasing afterload and preload. Vasodilation reduces resistance to left ventricular ejection of blood, diminishing the heart's workload and improving ventricular emptying. ACE inhibitors decrease the secretion of aldosterone, a hormone that causes the kidneys to retain sodium and water. ACE inhibitors also promote renal excretion of sodium and fluid (while retaining potassium), thereby reducing left ventricular filling pressure and decreasing pulmonary congestion. ACE inhibitors may be the first medication prescribed for patients in mild failure—patients with fatigue or DOE but without signs of fluid overload and pulmonary congestion. These agents are also recommended for prevention of HF in patients at risk due to vascular disease and diabetes (Yancy et al., 2013).

ACE inhibitors are started at a low dose that is gradually increased until the optimal dose is achieved and the patient is hemodynamically stable. The final maintenance dose depends on the patient's blood pressure, fluid status, and renal status, as well as the severity of the HF.

Patients receiving ACE inhibitors are monitored for hypotension, hyperkalemia (increased potassium in the blood), and alterations in renal function, especially if they are also receiving diuretics. Because ACE inhibitors cause the kidneys to retain potassium, the patient who is also receiving a diuretic may not need to take oral potassium supplements. However, patients receiving potassium-sparing diuretics (which do not cause potassium loss with diuresis) must be carefully monitored for hyperkalemia. ACE inhibitors may be discontinued if the potassium level remains greater than 5.5 mEq/L or if the serum creatinine rises.

Other adverse effects of ACE inhibitors include a dry, persistent cough that may not respond to cough suppressants.

However, cough can also indicate a worsening of ventricular function and failure. Rarely, ACE inhibitors can cause an allergic reaction accompanied by angioedema. If angioedema affects the oropharyngeal area and impairs breathing, the ACE inhibitor must be stopped immediately and emergency care provided.

If the patient cannot continue taking an ACE inhibitor because of development of cough, an elevated creatinine level, or hyperkalemia, an angiotensin receptor blocker (ARB) or a combination of hydralazine and isosorbide dinitrate (Dilatrate) is prescribed (see Table 29-3).

Angiotensin Receptor Blockers

Although the action of ARBs is different from that of ACE inhibitors, they (e.g., valsartan [Diovan]) have similar hemodynamic effects and side effects (Pinkerman et al., 2013). Whereas ACE inhibitors block the conversion of angiotensin I to angiotensin II, ARBs block the vasoconstricting effects of angiotensin II at the angiotensin II receptors. ARBs are prescribed for HF patients as an alternative to ACE inhibitors (Yancy et al., 2013).

Hydralazine and Isosorbide Dinitrate

A combination of hydralazine and isosorbide dinitrate may be another alternative for patients who cannot take ACE inhibitors. Nitrates (e.g., isosorbide dinitrate) cause venous dilation, which reduces the amount of blood return to the heart and lowers preload. Hydralazine lowers systemic vascular resistance and left ventricular afterload. This combination of medications is also recommended in HF guidelines and may be more effective for African Americans who do not respond to ACE inhibitors (Yancy et al., 2013).

Beta-Blockers

Beta-blockers are also considered first-line therapy and are routinely prescribed in addition to ACE inhibitors. These agents block the adverse effects of the sympathetic nervous system. They relax blood vessels, lower blood pressure, decrease afterload, and decrease cardiac workload. Beta-blockers, such as carvedilol (Coreg), bisoprolol (Zebeta) and sustained-release metoprolol (Toprol XL), have been found to improve functional status and reduce mortality and morbidity in patients with HF (Burchum & Rosenthal, 2016). In addition, beta-blockers have been recommended for patients with asymptomatic systolic dysfunction, such as those with a decreased EF, to prevent the onset of symptoms of HF. The therapeutic effects of these drugs may not be seen for several weeks or even months.

Beta-blockers may produce a number of side effects, including dizziness, hypotension, bradycardia, fatigue, and depression. Side effects are most common in the initial few weeks of treatment. Because of the potential for side effects, beta-blockers are started at a low dose. The dose is titrated up slowly (every few weeks), with close monitoring after each dosage increase. Nurses educate patients about potential symptoms during the early phase of treatment and stress that adjustment to the drug may take several weeks. Nurses must also provide support to patients going through this symptom-provoking phase of treatment. Because beta-blockade can cause bronchiole constriction, these drugs are used with caution in patients with a history of bronchospastic diseases such as uncontrolled asthma.

Diuretics

Diuretics are prescribed to remove excess extracellular fluid by increasing the rate of urine produced in patients with signs and symptoms of fluid overload. HF guidelines advocate using the smallest dose of diuretic necessary to control fluid volume (Yancy et al., 2013). Loop, thiazide, and aldosterone blocking diuretics may be prescribed for patients with HF. These medications differ in their site of action in the kidney and their effects on renal electrolyte excretion and reabsorption.

Loop diuretics, such as furosemide (Lasix), inhibit sodium and chloride reabsorption mainly in the ascending loop of Henle. HF patients with severe volume overload are generally treated with a loop diuretic first (Burcham & Rosenthal, 2016). Thiazide diuretics, such as metolazone (Zaroxolyn), inhibit sodium and chloride reabsorption in the early distal tubules. Both of these classes of diuretics increase potassium excretion; therefore, patients treated with these medications must have their serum potassium levels closely monitored. Diuretics can also lead to orthostatic hypotension and kidney injury (Pinkerman et al., 2013). Both a loop and a thiazide diuretic may be used in patients with severe HF who are unresponsive to a single diuretic. The need for diuretics can be decreased if the patient avoids excessive fluid intake (e.g., more than 2 qt/day) and adheres to a low-sodium diet (e.g., no more than 2 g/day).

Aldosterone antagonists such as spironolactone (Aldactone) are potassium-sparing diuretics that block the effects of aldosterone in the distal tubule and collecting duct. They can effectively reduce mortality and morbidity in patients with moderate to severe HF (Pinkerman, et al., 2013). Serum creatinine and potassium levels are monitored frequently (e.g., within the first week and then every 4 weeks) when spironolactone is first given. These drugs are not prescribed for patients with an elevated serum creatinine.

The type and dose of diuretic prescribed depend on clinical signs and symptoms and renal function. Careful patient monitoring and dose adjustments are necessary to balance the effectiveness of these medications with the side effects (see Chart 29-2). Loop diuretics are administered IV for exacerbations of HF when rapid diuresis is necessary. Diuretics improve the patient's symptoms, provided that renal function is adequate. As HF progresses, cardiorenal syndrome may develop or worsen. Patients with this syndrome are resistant to diuretics and may require other interventions to deal with congestive signs and symptoms.

Digitalis

For many years, digitalis (digoxin) was considered an essential agent for the treatment of HF, but with the advent of new medications, it is not prescribed as often. Digoxin increases the force of myocardial contraction and slows conduction through the atrioventricular node. It improves contractility, increasing left ventricular output. Although the use of digoxin does not result in decreased mortality rates among patients with HF, it can be effective in decreasing the symptoms of systolic HF and may help prevent hospitalization (Pinkerman et al., 2013). Patients with renal dysfunction and older patients should receive smaller doses of digoxin, as it is excreted through the kidneys.

A key concern associated with digoxin therapy is digitalis toxicity. Clinical manifestations of toxicity include anorexia,

Chart 29-2 PHARMACOLOGY
Administering and Monitoring Diuretic Therapy

When nursing care involves diuretic therapy for conditions such as heart failure, the nurse needs to administer the medication and monitor the patient's response carefully, as follows:

- Prior to administration of the diuretic, check laboratory results for electrolyte depletion, especially potassium, sodium, and magnesium.
- Prior to administration of the diuretic, check for signs and symptoms of volume depletion, such as postural hypotension, lightheadedness, and dizziness.
- Administer the diuretic at a time conducive to the patient's lifestyle—for example, early in the day to avoid nocturia.
- Monitor urine output during the hours after administration, and analyze intake, output, and daily weights to assess response.
- Monitor blood pressure for orthostatic changes.
- Continue to monitor serum electrolytes for depletion. Replace potassium with increased oral intake of food rich in potassium or potassium supplements. Replace magnesium as needed.
- Monitor for hyperkalemia in patients receiving potassium-sparing diuretics.
- Continue to assess for signs of volume depletion.
- Monitor creatinine for increased levels indicative of diuretic-induced renal dysfunction.
- Monitor for elevated uric acid level and signs and symptoms of gout.
- Assess lungs sounds and edema to evaluate response to therapy.
- Monitor for adverse reactions such as dysrhythmias.
- Assist patients to manage urinary frequency and urgency associated with diuretic therapy.

nausea, visual disturbances, confusion, and bradycardia. The serum potassium level is monitored because the effect of digoxin is enhanced in the presence of hypokalemia and digoxin toxicity may occur. A serum digoxin level is obtained if the patient's renal function changes or there are symptoms of toxicity.

Intravenous Infusions

IV inotropes (milrinone [Primacor], dobutamine [Dobutrex]) increase the force of myocardial contraction; as such, they may be indicated for hospitalized patients with acute decompensated HF. These agents are used for patients who do not respond to routine pharmacologic therapy and are reserved for patients with severe ventricular dysfunction. They are used with caution, as some studies have associated their use with increased mortality (Ciuksza, Hebert, & Sokos, 2014). IV vasodilators such as nitroprusside (Nipride), nitroglycerin, or nesiritide (Natrecor) may also be used in patients with severe decompensated HF (Pinkerman et al., 2013). Patients usually require admission to the intensive care unit (ICU) and may also have hemodynamic monitoring with a pulmonary artery catheter or alternative technology (see Chapter 25). Hemodynamic data are used to assess cardiac function and volume status and to guide therapy with inotropes, vasodilators, and diuretics (Urden, Stacy, & Lough, 2014). Patients with end-stage HF who cannot be weaned from IV inotropes may be candidates for continuous therapy at home (Ciuksza et al., 2014).

Milrinone

Milrinone is a phosphodiesterase inhibitor that leads to an increase in intracellular calcium within myocardial cells, increasing their contractility (O'Donovan, 2013). This agent also promotes vasodilation, resulting in decreased preload and afterload and reduced cardiac workload. Milrinone is administered IV to patients with severe HF, including patients who are waiting for heart transplantation. Because the drug causes vasodilation, the patient's blood pressure is monitored prior to administration; if the patient is hypovolemic, the blood pressure could drop quickly. The major side effects are hypotension and increased ventricular dysrhythmias. Blood pressure and ECG are monitored closely during and following infusions of milrinone.

Dobutamine

Dobutamine is another IV medication given to patients with significant left ventricular dysfunction and hypoperfusion. A catecholamine, dobutamine stimulates the beta-1 adrenergic receptors. Its major action is to increase cardiac contractility and renal perfusion to enhance urine output. However, it also increases the heart rate and can precipitate ectopic beats and tachydysrhythmias (Burcham & Rosenthal, 2016).

Medications for Diastolic Dysfunction

Patients with predominant diastolic HF and preserved left ventricular EF are treated differently than patients with systolic HF. Contributing causes such as hypertension and ischemic heart disease are evaluated and treated. These patients do not tolerate tachycardia, because it does not allow time for ventricular filling. Beta-blockers may be used to control tachycardia from atrial fibrillation or other causes (Pinkerman et al., 2013).

Other Medications for Heart Failure

Anticoagulants may be prescribed, especially if the patient has a history of atrial fibrillation or a thromboembolic event. Antiarrhythmic drugs such as amiodarone (Cordarone) may be prescribed for patients with dysrhythmias, along with evaluation for device therapy with an implantable cardioverter defibrillator (ICD) (see Chapter 26). Medications that manage hyperlipidemia (e.g., statins) are also routinely prescribed. Nonsteroidal anti-inflammatory drugs (NSAIDs) such as ibuprofen (Motrin) should be avoided because they decrease renal perfusion, especially in older adults.

Nutritional Therapy

Following a low-sodium (no more than 2 g/day) diet and avoiding excessive fluid intake are usually recommended, although studies differ regarding the effectiveness of sodium restriction (Yancy et al., 2013). Decreasing dietary sodium reduces fluid retention and the symptoms of peripheral and pulmonary congestion. The purpose of sodium restriction is to decrease the amount of circulating blood volume, which decreases myocardial work. A balance needs to be achieved between the patient's ability to comply with the diet and the recommended dietary restriction. Any change in diet should consider good nutrition as well as the patient's likes, dislikes, and cultural food patterns. Patient adherence is important because dietary indiscretions may result in severe exacerbations

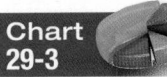

Chart 29-3

NURSING RESEARCH PROFILE

Helping Patients With Heart Failure Adhere to a Low-Sodium Diet.

Chung, M. L., Lennie, T. A., Mudd-Martin, G., et al. (2015). Adherence to a low-sodium diet in patients with heart failure is best when family members also follow the diet. *Journal of Cardiovascular Nursing, 30*(1), 44–50.

Purpose

Excess dietary sodium is associated with increased clinical manifestations of HF and an increased rate of hospitalization. Inadequate family support is one of the barriers to a patient's ability to follow a low-sodium diet (LSD). The purpose of this study was to evaluate the effect of family members' adherence to an LSD on the patient's ability to follow the diet.

Design

The study used data from 370 patients with HF. A 24-hour urinary sodium excretion was measured in each patient as an indicator of dietary sodium intake. A questionnaire on whether their family members followed the diet was also completed by the patients.

Findings

Patients whose family members followed the LSD had lower urine sodium levels, indicating adherence to the diet, when compared with patients whose family members did not. It did not make a difference whether the family member was a spouse or whether family members lived with the patient.

Nursing Implications

Strong support from family members can help patients effectively manage many aspects of their HF, including the important aspect of sodium restriction. Nursing interventions aimed at increasing adherence to an LSD should include encouraging family members to also follow the diet.

---

of HF requiring hospitalization (Chung, Lennie, Mudd-Martin, et al., 2015). However, behavioral changes in this area are difficult for many patients (see Chart 29-3).

Additional Therapy

Supplemental Oxygen

Oxygen therapy may become necessary as HF progresses. The need is based on the degree of pulmonary congestion and resulting hypoxia. Some patients require supplemental oxygen only during periods of activity.

Other Interventions

A number of procedures and surgical approaches may benefit patients with HF. If the patient has underlying coronary artery disease, coronary artery revascularization with PCI or coronary artery bypass surgery (see Chapter 27) may be considered. Ventricular function may improve in some patients when coronary flow is increased.

Patients with HF are at high risk for dysrhythmias, and sudden cardiac death is common among patients with advanced HF. In patients with severe left ventricular dysfunction and the possibility of life-threatening dysrhythmias, placement of an ICD can prevent sudden cardiac death and extend survival (see Chapter 26). Candidates for an ICD include those with an EF less than 35% and with NYHA functional class II or III, including those with and without a history of ventricular dysrhythmias (Yancy et al., 2013).

Patients with HF who do not improve with standard therapy may benefit from **cardiac resynchronization therapy (CRT)**. CRT involves the use of a biventricular pacemaker to treat electrical conduction defects. A prolonged QRS duration on ECG indicates left bundle branch block, which is a type of delayed conduction that is frequently seen in patients with HF. This problem results in dyssynchronous conduction and contraction of the right and left ventricles, which can further decrease EF (Yancy et al., 2013). (See Chapter 26 for discussion of dysrhythmias.) The use of a pacing device with leads placed in the right atrium, right ventricle, and left ventricular cardiac vein can synchronize the contractions of the right and left ventricles (see Fig. 29-3). This intervention improves CO, optimizes myocardial energy consumption, reduces mitral regurgitation, and slows the ventricular remodeling process. For selected patients, CRT results in fewer symptoms, increased functional status, fewer hospitalizations, and longer survival (Manne, Rickard, Varma, et al., 2013). Combination devices are available for patients who require CRT and an ICD. See Chapter 26 for further discussion of care of patients with pacemakers and ICDs.

Ultrafiltration is an alternative intervention for patients with severe fluid overload. It is reserved for patients with advanced HF who are resistant to diuretic therapy (Yancy et al., 2013). A dual-lumen central IV catheter is placed, and the patient's blood is circulated through a small bedside filtration machine.

Figure 29-3 • Cardiac resynchronization therapy. To pace both ventricles, pacemaker leads are placed in the right atrium and right ventricle; a third lead is threaded through the coronary sinus into a lateral vein on the wall of the left ventricle.

Liters of excess fluid and plasma are removed slowly from the patient's intravascular circulating volume over a number of hours. The patient's output of filtration fluid, blood pressure, and hemoglobin (analyzed for hemoconcentration) are monitored as indicators of volume status. Research continues regarding the effectiveness of ultrafiltration (Kazory & Ronco, 2013).

For some patients with end-stage HF, cardiac transplantation is one of the few options for long-term survival. Patients with ACC/AHA stage D HF who may be eligible are referred for consideration of transplantation. Some of these patients require mechanical circulatory assistance with an implanted ventricular assist device as a bridge therapy to cardiac transplantation (see Chapter 28). A left ventricular assist device may also be implanted as *destination therapy* (permanent therapy) for selected patients (Yancy et al., 2013).

Gerontologic Considerations

Several normal age-related changes increase the frequency of HF: increased systolic blood pressure, increased ventricular wall thickness, and increased myocardial fibrosis. There are a number of reasons that older adults are likely to be hospitalized with HF (Albert et al., 2015). Older adults may not always detect or accurately interpret common symptoms of HF such as shortness of breath, or they may have atypical symptoms such as weakness and somnolence. Decreased renal function can make the older patient resistant to diuretics and more sensitive to changes in volume. The administration of diuretics to older men requires nursing surveillance for bladder distention caused by urethral obstruction from an enlarged prostate gland. The bladder may be assessed with an ultrasound scanner or the suprapubic area palpated for an oval mass and percussed for dullness, indicative of bladder fullness. Urinary frequency and urgency may be particularly stressful to older patients, as many have arthritis and limited mobility.

NURSING PROCESS

The Patient With Heart Failure

Despite advances in treatment of HF, morbidity and mortality remain high. Nurses have a major impact on outcomes for patients with HF, especially in the areas of patient education and monitoring.

Assessment

Nursing assessment for the patient with HF focuses on observing for effectiveness of therapy and for the patient's ability to understand and implement self-management strategies. Signs and symptoms of increasing HF are analyzed and reported to the patient's provider so that therapy can be adjusted. The nurse also explores the patient's emotional response to the diagnosis of HF, because it is a chronic and often progressive condition that is commonly associated with depression and other psychosocial issues (Chapa, Akintade, Son, et al., 2014).

Health History

The health history focuses on the signs and symptoms of HF, such as dyspnea, fatigue, and edema. Sleep disturbances, particularly sleep suddenly interrupted by shortness of breath, may be reported. Patients are asked about the number of pillows needed for sleep, edema, abdominal symptoms, altered mental status, activities of daily living, and the activities that cause fatigue. Nurses need to be aware of the variety of clinical manifestations that may indicate worsening HF and assess the patient accordingly. While obtaining the patient's history, the nurse assesses the patient's understanding of HF, self-management strategies, and the patient's ability and willingness to adhere to those strategies.

Physical Examination

The patient is observed for restlessness and anxiety that might suggest hypoxia from pulmonary congestion. The patient's level of consciousness is also evaluated for any changes, as low CO can decrease the flow of oxygen to the brain.

The rate and depth of respirations are assessed along with the effort required for breathing. The lungs are auscultated to detect crackles and wheezes (Pinto & Kociol, 2015). Crackles are produced by the sudden opening of edematous small airways and alveoli. They may be heard at the end of inspiration and are not cleared with coughing. Wheezing may also be heard in some patients who have bronchospasm along with pulmonary congestion.

The blood pressure is carefully evaluated, because HF patients may present with hypotension or hypertension. Patients may be assessed for orthostatic hypotension, especially if they report lightheadedness, dizziness, or syncope. The heart is auscultated for an S_3 heart sound, which is an early sign that increased blood volume fills the ventricle with each beat. Heart rate and rhythm are also documented, and patients are often placed on continuous ECG monitoring in the hospital setting. When the heart rate is rapid or very slow, the CO decreases and potentially worsens the HF.

JVD is assessed with the patient sitting at a 45° angle; distention greater than 4 cm above the sternal angle is considered abnormal and indicative of right ventricular failure (Paul & Hice, 2014). This is an estimate, not a precise measurement, of high central venous pressure.

The nurse assesses peripheral pulses and rates their volume on a scale from 0 (not palpable) to 3+ (bounding). The skin is also assessed for color and temperature. With significant decreases in SV, there is a decrease in perfusion to the periphery, decreasing the volume of pulses and causing the skin to feel cool and appear pale or cyanotic. The feet and lower legs are examined for edema; if the patient is supine in bed, the sacrum and back are also assessed for edema. The upper extremities may also become edematous in some patients. Edema is typically rated on a scale from 0 (no edema) to 4+ (severe pitting edema).

The abdomen is examined for tenderness and hepatomegaly. The presence of firmness, distention, and possible ascites is noted. The liver may be assessed for hepatojugular reflux. The patient is asked to breathe normally while manual pressure is applied over the right upper quadrant of the abdomen for 30 to 60 seconds. If neck vein distention increases more than 1 cm, the finding is positive for increased venous pressure.

If the patient is hospitalized, the nurse measures urinary output and evaluates it in terms of diuretic use. Intake and output records are rigorously maintained and analyzed. It is important to track whether the patient has excreted excessive volume (i.e., negative fluid balance is generally the goal). The intake and output is then compared with changes in weight. Although diuresis is expected, the HF patient must also be monitored for **oliguria** (diminished urine output, less than 0.5 mL/kg/h) or **anuria** (urine output less than 50 mL/24 h) because of the risk of renal dysfunction.

The patient is weighed daily in the hospital or at home, at the same time of day, with the same type of clothing, and on the same scale. If there is a significant change in weight (i.e., 2- to 3-lb increase in a day or 5-lb increase in a week), the primary provider is notified and medications are adjusted (e.g., the diuretic dose is increased).

Diagnosis

Nursing Diagnoses

Based on the assessment data, major nursing diagnoses may include the following:

- Activity intolerance related to decreased CO
- Excess fluid volume related to the HF syndrome
- Anxiety related to clinical manifestations of HF
- Powerlessness related to chronic illness and hospitalizations
- Ineffective family health management

Collaborative Problems/Potential Complications

Potential complications may include the following:

- Hypotension, poor perfusion, and cardiogenic shock (see Chapter 14)
- Dysrhythmias (see Chapter 26)
- Thromboembolism (see Chapter 30)
- Pericardial effusion and cardiac tamponade

Planning and Goals

Major goals for the patient may include promoting activity and reducing fatigue, relieving fluid overload symptoms, decreasing anxiety or increasing the patient's ability to manage anxiety, encouraging the patient to verbalize their ability to make decisions and influence outcomes, and educating the patient and family about health management (Ackley & Ladwig, 2014).

Nursing Interventions

Promoting Activity Tolerance

Reduced physical activity caused by HF symptoms leads to physical deconditioning that worsens the patient's symptoms and exercise tolerance. Prolonged inactivity, which may be self-imposed, should be avoided because of its deconditioning effects and risks, such as pressure ulcers (especially in edematous patients) and venous thromboembolism. An acute illness that exacerbates HF symptoms or requires hospitalization may be an indication for temporary bed rest. Otherwise, some type of physical activity every day should be encouraged. Exercise training has many favorable effects for the HF patient, including increased functional capacity, decreased dyspnea, and improved quality of life (Georgantas, Dimopoulos, Tasoulis, et al., 2014). A typical program for a patient with HF might include a daily walking regimen, with the duration increased over a 6-week period. The primary provider, nurse, and patient collaborate to develop a schedule that promotes pacing and prioritization of activities. The schedule should alternate activities with periods of rest and avoid having two significant energy-consuming activities occur on the same

Chart 29-4	HEALTH PROMOTION

An Exercise Program for Patients With Heart Failure

Before undertaking physical activity, the patient should be given the following guidelines:

- Talk with your primary provider for specific exercise program recommendations.
- Begin with low-impact activities such as walking.
- Start with warm-up activity followed by sessions that gradually build up to about 30 minutes.
- Follow your exercise period with cool-down activities.
- Avoid performing physical activities outside in extreme hot, cold, or humid weather.
- Wait 2 hours after eating a meal before performing the physical activity.
- Ensure that you are able to talk during the physical activity; if you cannot do so, decrease the intensity of activity.
- Stop the activity if severe shortness of breath, pain, or dizziness develops.

Adapted from Piña, I. L. (2016) Cardiac rehabilitation in patients with heart failure. Retrieved on 3/17/16 at: www.uptodate.com/contents/cardiac-rehabilitation-in-patients-with-heart-failure

day or in immediate succession. Before undertaking physical activity, the patient should be given guidelines similar to those noted in Chart 29-4. Because some patients may be severely debilitated, they may need to limit physical activities to only 3 to 5 minutes at a time, one to four times per day. The patient should increase the duration of the activity, then the frequency, before increasing the intensity of the activity (Keteyian, Squires, Ades, et al., 2014).

Barriers to performing activities are identified, and methods of adjusting an activity are discussed. For example, vegetables can be chopped or peeled while sitting at the kitchen table rather than standing at the kitchen counter. Small, frequent meals decrease the amount of energy needed for digestion while providing adequate nutrition. The nurse helps the patient identify peak and low periods of energy, planning energy-consuming activities for peak periods. For example, the patient may prepare the meals for the entire day in the morning. Pacing and prioritizing activities help maintain the patient's energy to allow participation in regular physical activity.

The patient's response to activities needs to be monitored. If the patient is hospitalized, vital signs and oxygen saturation level are monitored before, during, and immediately after an activity to identify whether they are within the desired range. Heart rate should return to baseline within 3 minutes following the activity. If the patient is at home, the degree of fatigue felt after the activity can be used to assess the response. If the patient tolerates the activity, short- and long-term goals can be developed to gradually increase the intensity, duration, and frequency of activity.

Adherence to exercise training is essential if the patient is to benefit from it, but it may be difficult for patients with other conditions (e.g., arthritis) and longer duration of HF. Referral to a cardiac rehabilitation program may be indicated, especially for patients newly diagnosed with HF (Keteyian et al., 2014). A supervised program may also benefit those who need a structured environment, significant educational support, regular encouragement, and interpersonal contact.

MANAGING FLUID VOLUME

Patients with severe HF may receive IV diuretic therapy; however, patients with less severe symptoms are typically prescribed oral diuretics. Oral diuretics should be given early in the morning so that diuresis does not interfere with the patient's nighttime rest. Discussing the timing of medication administration is especially important for older patients who may have urinary urgency or incontinence. A single dose of a diuretic may cause the patient to excrete a large volume of fluid shortly after its administration.

The patient's fluid status is monitored closely by auscultating the lungs, monitoring daily body weight, and assisting the patient to adhere to a low-sodium diet by reading food labels and avoiding high-sodium foods such as canned, processed, and convenience foods (see Chart 29-5). Weight gain in a patient with HF almost always reflects fluid retention. If the diet includes fluid restriction, the nurse can assist the patient to plan fluid intake throughout the day while respecting the patient's dietary preferences. If the patient is receiving IV fluids and medications, the amount of fluid needs to be monitored closely, and the primary provider or pharmacist can be consulted about the possibility of maximizing the amount of medication in the same volume of IV fluid (e.g., double concentrating to decrease the fluid volume given).

The patient is positioned or taught how to assume a position that facilitates breathing. The number of pillows may be increased, the head of the bed may be elevated, or the patient may sit in a recliner. In these positions, the venous return to the heart (preload) is reduced, pulmonary congestion is reduced, and pressure on the diaphragm is minimized. The lower arms can be supported with pillows to eliminate the fatigue caused by the pull of the patient's weight on the shoulder muscles.

Because decreased circulation in edematous areas increases the risk of pressure ulcers, the nurse assesses for skin breakdown and institutes preventive measures. Positioning to avoid pressure and frequent changes of position help prevent pressure ulcers.

CONTROLLING ANXIETY

Patients with HF may exhibit signs and symptoms of anxiety. In addition to psychosocial sources of anxiety, the physiologic compensatory mechanisms include activation of neurohormones including catecholamines (Chapa et al., 2014). Complex medical interventions such as implantation of an ICD can provoke anxiety in patients and families. These sources of anxiety include living with the threat of shocks, role changes, and concerns about the patient's ability to carry out activities of daily living. The patient's anxiety may intensify at night and interfere with sleep. Emotional stress further stimulates the sympathetic nervous system, causing vasoconstriction, elevated arterial pressure, and increased heart rate. This sympathetic response increases cardiac workload.

When the patient exhibits anxiety, the nurse takes steps to promote physical comfort and provide psychological support. As mentioned previously, the patient may be more comfortable sitting in a recliner. Oxygen may be given during an acute event to diminish the work of breathing and increase the patient's comfort. In many cases, a family member's presence provides reassurance. Patients with HF rely on their families for many aspects of care; therefore, nurses should assess the needs of family caregivers and provide support to them (Pressler, Gradus-Pizlo, Chubinski, et al., 2013).

Chart 29-5 **HEALTH PROMOTION**

Facts About Dietary Sodium

Although the major source of sodium in the average American diet is salt, many types of natural foods contain varying amounts of sodium. Even if no salt is added in cooking and if salty foods are avoided, the daily diet will still contain about 2000 mg of sodium. Fresh fruits and vegetables are low in sodium and should be encouraged.

Additives in Food

In general, food prepared at home is lower in sodium than restaurant or processed foods. Added food substances (additives), such as sodium alginate, which improves food texture, sodium benzoate, which acts as a preservative, and disodium phosphate, which improves cooking quality in certain foods, increase the sodium intake when included in the daily diet. Therefore, patients on low-sodium diets should be advised to check labels carefully for words such as "salt" or "sodium," especially on canned foods. For example, without looking at the sodium content per serving found on the nutrition labels, when given a choice between a serving of potato chips and a cup of canned cream of mushroom soup, most would think that soup is lower in sodium. However, when the labels are examined, the lower-sodium choice is found to be the chips. Although potato chips are *not* recommended in a low-sodium diet, this example illustrates that it is important to read food labels to determine both sodium content and serving size.

Nonfood Sodium Sources

Sodium is contained in municipal water. Water softeners also increase the sodium content of drinking water. Patients on sodium-restricted diets should be cautioned against using nonprescription medications such as antacids, cough syrups, and laxatives. Salt substitutes may be allowed, but it is recognized that they are high in potassium. Over-the-counter medications should not be used without first consulting the patient's primary provider.

Promoting Dietary Adherence

If patients find food unpalatable because of the dietary sodium restrictions and/or the taste disturbances caused by the medications, they may refuse to eat or to adhere with the dietary regimen. For this reason, severe sodium restrictions should be avoided, and diuretic medication should be balanced with the patient's ability to restrict dietary sodium. A variety of flavorings, such as lemon juice, vinegar, and herbs, may be used to improve the taste of the food and facilitate acceptance of the diet. The patient's food preferences should be taken into account—diet counseling and educational handouts can be geared to individual and ethnic preferences—and the family should be involved in the dietary education.

Adapted from American Heart Association (2016b). *Shaking the salt habit.* Retrieved on 3/31/16 at: www.heart.org/HEARTORG/Conditions/High-BloodPressure/PreventionTreatmentofHighBloodPressure/Shaking-the-Salt-Habit_UCM_303241_Article.jsp#.Vzy9eNe3BK8

Along with reassurance, the nurse can begin educating the patient and family about techniques for controlling anxiety and avoiding anxiety-provoking situations. This includes how to identify factors that contribute to anxiety and how to use relaxation techniques to control anxious feelings. As the patient's anxiety decreases, cardiac function may improve and symptoms of HF may decrease, with overall feelings of relaxation.

> ### ◣ Quality and Safety Nursing Alert
>
> *When patients with HF are delirious, confused, or anxious, restraints should be avoided. Restraints are likely to be resisted, and resistance inevitably increases the cardiac workload.*

MINIMIZING POWERLESSNESS

Patients with HF may feel overwhelmed with their diagnosis and treatment regimen, leading to feelings of powerlessness. Contributing factors may include lack of knowledge and lack of opportunity to make decisions, particularly if health care providers or family members do not encourage the patient to participate in the treatment decision-making process.

Nurses should help patients recognize their choices, and that they can positively influence the outcomes of their diagnosis and treatment. Taking time to listen actively to patients encourages them to express their concerns and ask questions. Other strategies include providing the patient with decision-making opportunities, such as when activities are to occur, or encouraging food and fluid choices consistent with the dietary restrictions. Encouragement is provided, progress is identified, and the patient is assisted to differentiate between factors that can and cannot be controlled.

In addition to feelings of powerlessness, patients with HF have a high incidence of depressive symptoms, which are associated with increased morbidity and mortality (Chapa et al., 2014). Depression is related in part to physiologic changes associated with HF such as the presence of increased inflammatory mediators (Heo, Moser, Pressler, et al., 2014). Because these depressive symptoms are known to increase as the disease worsens, patients with HF need to be screened for depression so that it can be treated, hopefully maintaining the patient's functional status and quality of life.

ASSISTING PATIENTS AND FAMILY TO EFFECTIVELY MANAGE HEALTH

Therapeutic regimens for HF are complex and require the patient and family to make significant lifestyle changes. Inability to adhere to dietary and pharmacologic recommendations leads to episodes of acute decompensated HF and hospitalization. Nonadherence with prescribed diet and fluid restrictions and medications cause many hospital readmissions. Additionally, lack of coordination of care and clinical follow-up contribute to poor outcomes (Albert et al., 2015).

Nurses have a key role in managing episodes of acute decompensated HF and in developing a comprehensive teaching and discharge plan to prevent hospital readmissions and increase the patient's quality of life. Because of the high cost of hospitalization for HF, the Center for Medicare and Medicaid Services (CMS) initiated a program that reduces reimbursement to hospitals with a high 30-day readmission rate (U.S. Department of Health and Human Services, 2013).

Research continues to identify the most effective interventions that may decrease these rates (Bradley, Curry, Horwitz, et al., 2013).

A number of evidence-based components are known to increase the effectiveness of a discharge plan for patients with HF, including providing them with comprehensive, patient-centered instructions, scheduling follow-up visits with their primary providers within 7 days of discharge, and following up by telephone within 3 days of discharge (Albert et al., 2015; Yancy et al., 2013).

A number of programs and interventions are available to assist patients and families to effectively manage the HF regimen and to prevent hospitalizations and the associated increased costs and decreased quality of life. These options include home health care services, transitional care programs, HF clinics, and telehealth management programs. Nurses are an important part of the various types of outpatient management and transitional care programs led by advanced practice nurses can significantly reduce readmission rates for HF patients (Paul & Hice, 2014). See later discussion in the Continuing and Transitional Care section.

MONITORING AND MANAGING POTENTIAL COMPLICATIONS

Because HF is a complex and progressive condition, patients are at risk for many complications, including acute decompensated HF, pulmonary edema, kidney injury, and life-threatening dysrhythmias. Many potential problems associated with HF therapy relate to the use of diuretics. These problems require ongoing nursing assessment and collaborative intervention:

- Excessive and repeated diuresis can lead to hypokalemia (i.e., potassium depletion). Signs include ventricular dysrhythmias, hypotension, muscle weakness, and generalized weakness. In patients receiving digoxin, hypokalemia can lead to digitalis toxicity, which increases the likelihood of dangerous dysrhythmias. Patients with HF may also develop low levels of magnesium, which can add to the risk of dysrhythmias.
- Hyperkalemia may occur, especially with the use of ACE inhibitors, ARBs, or spironolactone. Hyperkalemia can also lead to profound bradycardia and other dysrhythmias.
- Prolonged diuretic therapy may produce hyponatremia (deficiency of sodium in the blood), which can result in disorientation, weakness, muscle cramps, and anorexia.
- Volume depletion from excessive fluid loss may lead to dehydration and hypotension. ACE inhibitors and beta-blockers may contribute to the hypotension.
- Other problems associated with diuretics include increased serum creatinine (indicative of renal dysfunction) and hyperuricemia (excessive uric acid in the blood), which leads to gout.

PROMOTING HOME, COMMUNITY-BASED, AND TRANSITIONAL CARE

Educating Patients About Self-Care. The nurse provides patient education and involves the patient and family in the therapeutic regimen to promote understanding and adherence to the plan. When the patient recognizes that the diagnosis of HF can be successfully managed with lifestyle changes and medications, recurrences of acute HF lessen, unnecessary hospitalizations decrease, and

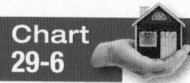

Chart 29-6   **HOME CARE CHECKLIST**
The Patient With Heart Failure

At the completion of education, the patient and/or caregiver will be able to:

- Identify heart failure as a chronic disease that can be managed with medications and specific self-management behaviors.
- State the impact of heart failure on physiologic functioning, ADLs, IADLs, roles, relationships, and spirituality.
- State the name, dose, side effects, frequency, and schedule for all medications.
- Take or administer medications daily, exactly as prescribed.
- Monitor effects of medication such as changes in breathing and edema.
- Know signs and symptoms of orthostatic hypotension and how to prevent it.
- Weigh self-daily at the same time with same clothes.
- Restrict sodium intake to no more than 2 g/day:
  - Adapt diet by examining nutrition labels to check sodium content per serving.
  - Avoid canned or processed foods, eating fresh or frozen foods.
  - Consult the written diet plan and the list of permitted and restricted foods.
  - Avoid salt use.
  - Avoid excesses in eating and drinking.
- Participate in prescribed activity program.
  - Participate in a daily exercise program.
  - Increase walking and other activities gradually, provided they do not cause unusual fatigue or dyspnea.
  - Conserve energy by balancing activity with rest periods.
  - Avoid activity in extremes of heat and cold, which increase the work of the heart.

- Recognize that air-conditioning may be essential in a hot, humid environment.
- Develop methods to manage and prevent stress.
  - Avoid tobacco.
  - Avoid alcohol.
  - Engage in social and diversional activities.
- Identify community resources for peer and caregiver/family support:
  - Identify sources of support (e.g., friends, relatives, faith community).
  - Identify phone numbers of support groups for people with heart failure and their caregivers/families.
  - State meeting locations and times.
- Report immediately to the primary provider or clinic any of the following:
  - Gain in weight of 2–3 lb (0.9–1.4 kg) in 1 day, or 5 lb (2.3 kg) in 1 week
  - Unusual shortness of breath with activity or at rest
  - Increased swelling of ankles, feet, or abdomen
  - Persistent cough
  - Loss of appetite
  - Development of restless sleep; increase in number of pillows needed to sleep
- Profound fatigue
- State how to reach primary provider with questions or complications
  - State time and date of follow-up appointments and diagnostic tests
- Identify the need for health promotion, disease prevention, and screening activities

ADL, activities of daily living; IADL, independent activities of daily living.

---

life expectancy increases. Nurses play a key role in instructing patients and their families about medication management, a low-sodium diet, moderate alcohol consumption, activity and exercise recommendations, smoking cessation, how to recognize the signs and symptoms of worsening HF, and when to contact the primary provider (Pinkerman et al., 2013). Use of the teach-back technique to assess the patient's comprehension of the instructions can increase teaching effectiveness and prevent rehospitalization (Peter, Robinson, Jordan, et al., 2015) (see Chapter 4 for further discussion of teach-back methods). Creation of an educational packet also facilitates effective patient teaching (Albert, 2013). A basic home education plan for the patient with HF is presented in Chart 29-6. The patient should receive a written copy of the instructions.

The patient's readiness to learn and potential barriers to learning are assessed. Patients with HF may have temporary or ongoing cognitive impairment due to their illness or other factors, increasing the need to rely on an identified caretaker (Peter et al., 2015). An effective treatment plan incorporates both the patient's goals and those of the health care providers. The nurse must consider cultural factors and adapt the education plan accordingly. Patients and families need to understand that effective HF management is influenced by choices made about treatment options and their ability to follow the treatment plan. They also need to be informed that

health care providers are available to assist them in reaching their health care goals.

Continuing and Transitional Care. Successful management of HF requires adherence to a complex medical regimen that includes multiple lifestyle changes for most patients. Assistance may be provided through a number of options that optimize evidence-based recommendations for effective management of HF. Depending on the patient's physical status and the availability of family assistance, a home care referral or another type of disease management program may be indicated for a patient who has been hospitalized. Transitional care programs (hospital to home) that include telephone contact along with home visits have been shown to decrease rehospitalizations and increase patient quality of life (Stamp, Machado, & Allen, 2014). Home visits by trained HF nurses provide assessment and management tailored to specific individualized patient needs. Older patients and those who have long-standing heart disease with compromised physical stamina often require assistance with the transition to home after hospitalization for an acute episode of HF. The home care nurse assesses the physical environment of the home and makes suggestions for adapting the home environment to meet the patient's activity limitations. If stairs are a concern, the patient can plan the day's activities so that stair-climbing is minimized; for some patients, a temporary bedroom may be set up on the main level of the home. The home care nurse works with the patient and family to maximize the benefits of these changes.

The home care nurse also reinforces and clarifies information about dietary changes and fluid restrictions, the need to monitor symptoms and daily body weight, and the importance of obtaining follow-up care with the primary provider's office or clinic. Assistance may be given in scheduling and keeping appointments as well. The patient is encouraged to gradually increase their self-care and responsibility for carrying out the therapeutic regimen.

Evidence-based HF guidelines also recommend patient referral to HF clinics, which provide intensive nursing management along with medical care in a collaborative model. Many of these clinics are managed by advanced practice nurses. Referral to an HF clinic gives the patient ready access to continuing education, professional nursing and medical staff, and timely adjustments to treatment regimens. HF clinics can also provide outpatient treatment (e.g., IV diuretics, laboratory monitoring) as an alternative to hospitalization. Because of the additional support and coordination of care, patients managed through HF clinics have fewer exacerbations of HF, fewer hospitalizations, decreased costs of medical care, and increased quality of life (Yancy, 2013).

Other disease management programs are carried out through telemonitoring, using telephones or computers to maintain contact with patients and to obtain patient data. This enables nurses and others to assess and manage patients on a frequent basis, without requiring patients to make frequent visits to health care providers. A variety of techniques ranging from simple telephone monitoring to sophisticated computer and video connections that monitor symptoms, daily weight, vital signs, heart sounds, and breath sounds may be used. Patient data may also include hemodynamics and other parameters transmitted from implantable devices. Studies have shown that telehealth management can decrease costs and hospitalizations for exacerbations of HF. More research is needed to determine which patients can benefit most from these interventions (Albert et al., 2015).

End-of-Life Considerations. Because HF is a chronic and often progressive condition, patients and families need to consider issues related to the end of life and when palliative or hospice care should be considered (Buonocore & Wallace, 2014). Although the prognosis in HF patients may be uncertain, issues often arise sooner or later related to the patient's thoughts and possible concerns about the use of complex treatment options (e.g., implantation of an ICD or a ventricular assist device [VAD]). VADs are an option for some patients with HF who have failed medical therapy and who are not candidates for cardiac transplantation. Elective, permanent implantation of a VAD (destination therapy) has been shown to extend survival and increase quality of life in some patients with end-stage HF (O'Neill & Kazer, 2014). Discussions concerning the use of technology, preferences for end-of-life care, and advance directives should take place while the patient is able to participate and express preferences. For example, with the expanded use of ICDs in the HF population, patients with ICDs, their families, and their primary providers should receive instructions for ICD inactivation at the end of life to prevent inappropriate discharges. See Chapter 16 for further discussion of end-of-life care.

Evaluation

Expected patient outcomes may include:

1. Demonstrates tolerance for desired activity
   a. Describes adaptive methods for usual activities
   b. Schedules activities to conserve energy and reduce fatigue and dyspnea
   c. Maintains heart rate, blood pressure, respiratory rate, and pulse oximetry within the targeted range
2. Maintains fluid balance
   a. Exhibits decreased peripheral edema
   b. Verbalizes understanding of fluid intake and diuretic use
3. Decreased anxiety
   a. Avoids situations that produce stress
   b. Sleeps comfortably at night
   c. Reports decreased stress and anxiety
   d. Denies symptoms of depression
4. Makes sound decisions regarding care and treatment
   a. Demonstrates ability to influence outcomes
5. Patients and family members adhere to healthy regimen
   a. Performs and records daily weights
   b. Limits dietary sodium intake to no more than 2 g/day
   c. Takes medications as prescribed
   d. Reports symptoms of worsening HF
   e. Makes and keeps appointments for follow-up care

 Concept Mastery Alert

For further review, visit thePoint to view an interactive tutorial on HF.

Pulmonary Edema

Pulmonary edema is the abnormal accumulation of fluid in the interstitial spaces and alveoli of the lungs. It is a diagnosis associated with acute decompensated HF that can lead to acute respiratory failure and death.

Pathophysiology

Pulmonary edema is an acute event that results from left ventricular failure. It can occur following acute MI or as an exacerbation of chronic HF. When the left ventricle begins to fail, blood backs up into the pulmonary circulation, causing pulmonary interstitial edema. This may occur quickly in some patients, a condition sometimes called *flash pulmonary edema.* Pulmonary edema can also develop slowly, especially when it is caused by noncardiac disorders such as kidney injury and other conditions that cause fluid overload. The pathophysiology is an extreme form of that seen in left-sided HF. The left ventricle cannot handle the volume overload, and blood volume and pressure build up in the left atrium. The rapid increase in atrial pressure results in an acute increase in pulmonary venous pressure, which produces an increase in hydrostatic pressure that forces fluid out of the pulmonary capillaries and into the interstitial spaces and alveoli (Grossman & Porth, 2014).

The fluid within the alveoli mixes with air, producing the classic sign of pulmonary edema—frothy pink (blood-tinged) sputum. The large amounts of alveolar fluid create a diffusion block that severely impairs gas exchange. The result is hypoxemia, which is often severe.

Clinical Manifestations

As a result of decreased cerebral oxygenation, the patient becomes increasingly restless and anxious. Along with a sudden onset of breathlessness and a sense of suffocation, the patient is tachypneic with noisy breathing and low oxygen saturation rates. The skin and mucous membranes may be pale to cyanotic, and the hands may be cool and moist. Tachycardia and JVD are common signs. Incessant coughing may occur, producing increasing quantities of foamy sputum. As pulmonary edema progresses, the patient's anxiety and restlessness increase. The patient may become confused and then stuporous. The patient, nearly suffocated by the blood-tinged, frothy fluid filling the alveoli, is literally drowning in secretions. The situation demands emergent action.

Assessment and Diagnostic Findings

The patient's airway and breathing are assessed to determine the severity of respiratory distress, along with vital signs. The patient is placed on a cardiac monitor, and IV access is confirmed or established for administration of drugs. Laboratory tests are obtained, including arterial blood gases, electrolytes, BUN, and creatinine (Pinto & Kociol, 2015). A chest x-ray is obtained to confirm the extent of pulmonary edema in the lung fields. Abrupt onset of signs of left-sided HF and pulmonary edema may occur without evidence of right-sided HF (e.g., no JVD, no dependent edema).

Prevention

Like many emergent conditions, pulmonary edema is easier to prevent than to treat. To recognize it early, the nurse assesses the degree of dyspnea, auscultates the lung fields and heart sounds, and assesses the degree of peripheral edema. A hacking cough, fatigue, weight gain, increased edema, and decreased activity tolerance may be early indicators of developing pulmonary edema.

In its early stage, pulmonary edema may be alleviated by increasing dosages of diuretics and by implementing other interventions to decrease preload. For instance, placing the patient in an upright position with the feet and legs dependent reduces left ventricular workload. The treatment regimen and the patient's understanding of and adherence to it are assessed. The long-range approach for preventing pulmonary edema must be directed at identifying and managing its precipitating factors.

 Medical Management

Clinical management of a patient with acute pulmonary edema due to left ventricular failure is directed toward reducing volume overload, improving ventricular function, and increasing oxygenation. These goals are accomplished through a combination of oxygen and ventilatory support, IV medication, and nursing assessment and interventions.

Oxygen Therapy

Oxygen is given in concentrations adequate to relieve hypoxemia and dyspnea. A nonrebreathing mask is used initially. If respiratory failure is severe or persists, noninvasive positive pressure ventilation is the preferred mode of assisted ventilation (Pinto & Kociol, 2015) (see Chapter 21 for further discussion). For some patients, endotracheal (ET) intubation and mechanical ventilation are required. The ventilator can provide positive end-expiratory pressure, which is effective in reducing venous return, decreasing fluid movement from the pulmonary capillaries to the alveoli, and improving oxygenation. Oxygenation is monitored by pulse oximetry and by measurement of arterial blood gases.

Diuretics

Diuretics promote the excretion of sodium and water by the kidneys. Furosemide or another loop diuretic is given by IV push or as a continuous infusion to produce a rapid diuretic effect. The blood pressure is closely monitored as the urine output increases, because it is possible for the patient to become hypotensive as intravascular volume decreases. The intake and output, daily weights, serum electrolytes, and creatinine are carefully monitored. As the clinical manifestations stabilize, the patient is transitioned to oral diuretics.

Vasodilators

Vasodilators such as IV nitroglycerin or nitroprusside may enhance symptom relief in pulmonary edema (Pinto & Kociol, 2015). Their use is contraindicated in patients who are hypotensive. Blood pressure is continually assessed in patients receiving IV vasodilator infusions.

 Nursing Management

Positioning the Patient to Promote Circulation

Proper positioning can help reduce venous return to the heart. The patient is positioned upright, preferably with the legs dangling over the side of the bed. This has the immediate effect of decreasing venous return, decreasing right ventricular SV, and decreasing lung congestion.

Providing Psychological Support

As the ability to breathe decreases, the patient's fear and anxiety rise proportionately, making the condition more severe. Reassuring the patient and providing skillful anticipatory nursing care are integral parts of the therapy. Because the patient is in an unstable condition, the nurse must remain with the patient. The nurse gives the patient simple, concise information in a reassuring voice about what is being done to treat the condition and the expected results.

Monitoring Medications

The patient receiving diuretic therapy may excrete a large volume of urine within minutes after a potent diuretic is given. A bedside commode may be used to decrease the energy required by the patient and to reduce the resultant increase in cardiac workload induced by getting on and off a bedpan. If necessary, in order to carefully monitor urine output, an indwelling urinary catheter may be inserted.

The patient receiving continuous IV infusions of diuretics and vasoactive medications requires continuous ECG monitoring and frequent measurement of vital signs. Patients who receive continuing therapy require management in an ICU.

OTHER COMPLICATIONS

Cardiogenic Shock

Cardiogenic shock occurs when decreased CO leads to inadequate tissue perfusion and initiation of the shock syndrome. Cardiogenic shock most commonly occurs following acute MI when a large area of myocardium becomes ischemic and hypokinetic. It also can occur as a result of end-stage HF, cardiac tamponade, pulmonary embolism (PE), cardiomyopathy, and dysrhythmias. Cardiogenic shock is a life-threatening condition with a high mortality rate. (See Chapter 14 for detailed information about the pathophysiology and management of cardiogenic shock.)

Medical Management

Goals in the treatment of cardiogenic shock include correcting the underlying problem when possible (e.g., opening the blocked coronary artery), reducing preload and afterload to decrease cardiac workload, improving oxygenation, and restoring tissue perfusion. In addition to standard critical care support with ventilatory and pharmacologic interventions, patients may require mechanical circulatory assistance.

Mechanical Circulatory Assistive Devices

Therapeutic modalities for cardiogenic shock include the use of circulatory assist devices, such as the intra-aortic balloon pump (IABP) (Hochman & Reyentovich, 2015). The IABP is a catheter with an inflatable balloon at the end. The catheter is usually inserted through the femoral artery and threaded toward the heart, and the balloon is positioned in the descending thoracic aorta (see Fig. 29-4). The IABP uses internal counterpulsation through the regular inflation and deflation of the balloon to augment the pumping action of the heart. It inflates during diastole, increasing the pressure in the aorta during diastole and therefore increasing blood flow through the coronary and peripheral arteries. It deflates just before systole, lessening the pressure within the aorta before left ventricular contraction, decreasing the amount of resistance the heart has to overcome to eject blood and therefore decreasing left ventricular workload. The device is connected to a console that synchronizes the inflation and deflation of the balloon with the ECG or the arterial pressure (as indicators for systole and diastole). Hemodynamic monitoring is often used to determine the patient's response to the IABP.

The IABP provides short-term (days) support for the failing myocardium. Other VADs for long-term support of the failing heart are described in Chapter 28.

Nursing Management

The patient in cardiogenic shock requires constant monitoring. Because of the frequency of nursing interventions and the technology required for safe and effective patient management, the patient is treated in an ICU. The critical care nurse must carefully assess the patient, observe the cardiac rhythm, monitor hemodynamic parameters, monitor fluid status, and adjust medications and therapies based on the assessment data. The patient is continuously evaluated for responses to the medical interventions and for the development of complications so that problems can be addressed immediately.

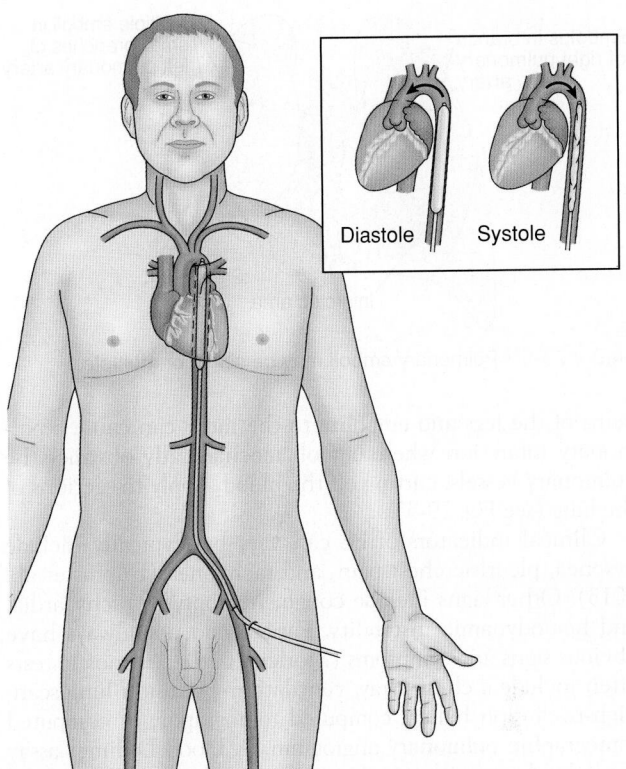

Figure 29-4 • The intra-aortic balloon pump inflates at the beginning of diastole, which results in increased perfusion of the coronary and peripheral arteries. It deflates just before systole, which results in a decrease in afterload (resistance to ejection) and in the left ventricular workload.

Thromboembolism

Patients with cardiovascular disorders are at risk for the development of arterial and venous thromboemboli. Intracardiac thrombi can form in patients with atrial fibrillation because the atria do not contract forcefully, resulting in slow and turbulent flow, and increasing the likelihood of thrombus formation. Mural thrombi can also form on ventricular walls when contractility is poor. Intracardiac thrombi can break off and travel through the circulation to other structures, including the brain, where they cause a stroke (i.e., cerebrovascular accident). Clots within the cardiac chambers can be detected by an echocardiogram and treated with anticoagulant agents, such as heparin and warfarin (Coumadin) (see Table 30-2 for further discussion of anticoagulants).

Decreased mobility and other factors in patients with cardiac disease also can lead to clot formation in the deep veins of the legs. Although signs and symptoms of deep vein thrombosis (DVT) can vary, patients may report leg pain and swelling and the leg may appear erythematous and feel warm. Diagnosis of DVT can be confirmed by duplex ultrasound of the lower extremities (Dupras, Bluhm, Felty, et al., 2013). These clots can break off and travel through the inferior vena cava and through the right side of the heart into the pulmonary artery, where they can cause a pulmonary embolus.

Pulmonary Embolism

PE is a potentially life-threatening disorder typically caused by blood clots in the lungs. Blood clots that form in the deep

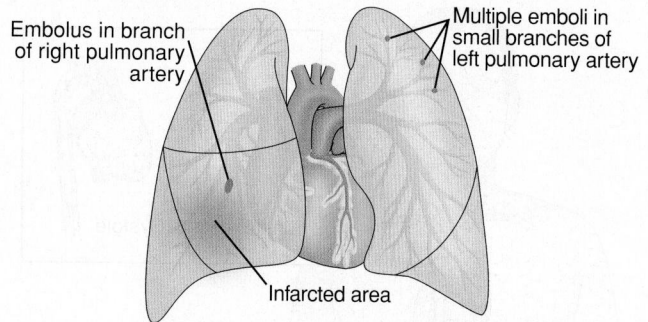

Embolus in branch
of right pulmonary
artery

Multiple emboli in
small branches of
left pulmonary artery

Infarcted area

Figure 29-5 • Pulmonary emboli may be single or multiple.

veins of the legs and embolize to the lungs can cause a pulmonary infarction where emboli mechanically obstruct the pulmonary vessels, cutting off the blood supply to sections of the lung (see Fig. 29-5).

Clinical indicators of PE can vary but typically include dyspnea, pleuritic chest pain, and tachypnea (Dupras et al., 2013). Other signs include cough, hemoptysis, tachycardia, and hemodynamic instability. Patients do not always have obvious signs and symptoms (Morici, 2014). Diagnostic tests often include a chest x-ray, ventilation–perfusion lung scan, high-resolution helical computed tomography, or computed tomographic pulmonary angiogram. A blood D-dimer assay is a helpful screening test that identifies whether clotting and fibrinolysis are taking place somewhere in the body.

Patient management begins with cardiopulmonary assessment and intervention. Emboli can cause hypoxic vasoconstriction and the release of inflammatory mediators in the pulmonary vessels, which can ultimately lead to right-sided HF and respiratory failure. Anticoagulant therapy with unfractionated heparin, low–molecular-weight heparin, fondaparinux (Arixtra) or rivaroxaban (Xarelto) is started when PE is suspected (Dobesh & Fanikos, 2014; Dupras et al., 2013). Thrombolytic (fibrinolytic) therapy may be used in patients with massive pulmonary emboli accompanied by hypotension and shock. Following initial therapy, patients are placed on oral anticoagulants for at least 3 to 6 months. Prevention of DVT and PE is an important aspect of patient management. Pharmacologic interventions are preferred, but mechanical devices (e.g., pneumatic compression devices) are acceptable for patients with contraindications to anticoagulation (e.g., bleeding ulcer). Care for patients with PE is further discussed in Chapter 23.

Pericardial Effusion and Cardiac Tamponade

Pathophysiology

Pericardial effusion (accumulation of fluid in the pericardial sac) may accompany advanced HF, pericarditis, metastatic carcinoma, cardiac surgery, or trauma. Normally, the pericardial sac contains about 20 mL of fluid, which is needed to decrease friction for the beating heart. An increase in pericardial fluid raises the pressure within the pericardial sac and compresses the heart. This has the following effects:

- Elevated pressure in all cardiac chambers
- Decreased venous return due to atrial compression
- Inability of the ventricles to distend and fill adequately

Pericardial fluid may build up slowly without causing noticeable symptoms until a large amount (1 to 2 L) accumulates (Hoit, 2015). However, a rapidly developing effusion (e.g., hemorrhage into the pericardial sac from chest trauma) can quickly stretch the pericardium to its maximum size and cause an acute problem. As pericardial fluid increases, pericardial pressure increases, reducing venous return to the heart and decreasing CO. This can result in cardiac tamponade, which causes low CO and obstructive shock.

Clinical Manifestations

The signs and symptoms of pericardial effusion can vary according to whether the problem develops quickly or slowly. In acute cardiac tamponade, the patient suddenly develops chest pain, tachypnea, and dyspnea. JVD results from poor right atrial filling and increased venous pressure. Hypotension occurs from low CO, and heart sounds are often muted. The subacute presentation of a pericardial effusion is less dramatic. The patient may report chest discomfort or a feeling of fullness. The feeling of pressure in the chest may result from stretching of the pericardial sac. These patients also develop dyspnea, JVD, and hypotension over time (Hoit, 2015). Patients with cardiac tamponade typically have tachycardia in response to low CO. In addition to hypotension, patients with cardiac tamponade may develop **pulsus paradoxus**, a systolic blood pressure that is markedly lower during inhalation. Also known as paradoxical pulse, this finding is characterized by an abnormal difference of at least 10 mm Hg in systolic pressure between the point that it is heard during exhalation and the point that it is heard during inhalation. This difference is caused by the variation in cardiac filling that occurs with changes in intrathoracic pressure during breathing. The cardinal signs of cardiac tamponade are illustrated in Figure 29-6.

Assessment and Diagnostic Findings

An echocardiogram is performed to confirm the diagnosis and quantify the amount of pericardial fluid. A chest x-ray may show an enlarged cardiac silhouette due to pericardial effusion. The ECG shows tachycardia and may also show low voltage (Hoit, 2015). See Chapter 27 for discussion of the significance of ECG abnormalities.

Medical Management

Pericardiocentesis

If cardiac function becomes seriously impaired, **pericardiocentesis** (puncture of the pericardial sac to aspirate pericardial fluid) is performed. During this procedure, the patient is monitored by continuous ECG and frequent vital signs. Catheter pericardiocentesis is performed using echocardiography to guide placement of the drainage catheter (Hoit, 2015).

A resulting decrease in central venous pressure and an associated increase in blood pressure after withdrawal of pericardial fluid indicate that the cardiac tamponade has been relieved. The patient almost always feels immediate relief. If there is a substantial amount of pericardial fluid aspirated, a small catheter may be left in place to drain recurrent accumulation of blood or fluid. Pericardial fluid is sent to the laboratory for examination for tumor cells, bacterial culture,

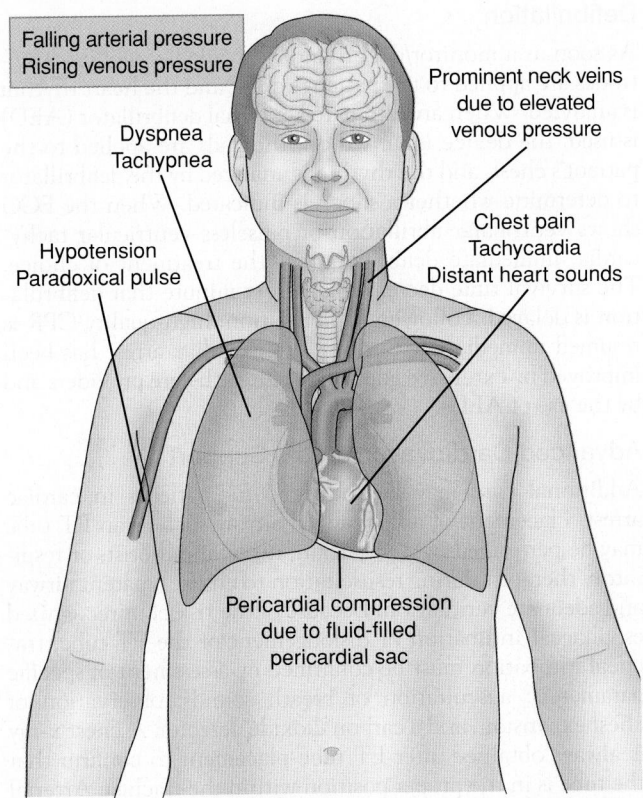

Falling arterial pressure
Rising venous pressure

Dyspnea
Tachypnea

Prominent neck veins
due to elevated
venous pressure

Hypotension
Paradoxical pulse

Chest pain
Tachycardia
Distant heart sounds

Pericardial compression
due to fluid-filled
pericardial sac

Figure 29-6 • Assessment findings in cardiac tamponade resulting from pericardial effusion include chest pain or fullness, dyspnea, tachypnea, jugular vein distention, hypotension, paradoxical pulse, tachycardia, and distant heart sounds.

chemical and serologic analysis, and differential blood cell count.

Complications of pericardiocentesis include coronary artery puncture, myocardial trauma, dysrhythmias, pleural laceration, and gastric puncture. After pericardiocentesis, the patient's heart rhythm, blood pressure, venous pressure, and heart sounds are monitored frequently to detect possible recurrence of cardiac tamponade. A follow-up echocardiogram is also performed. If the effusion recurs, repeat aspiration is necessary. Cardiac tamponade may require treatment by open surgical drainage (pericardiotomy) (Hoit, 2015).

Pericardiotomy

Recurrent pericardial effusions, usually associated with neoplastic disease, may be treated by a **pericardiotomy** (pericardial window). Under general anesthesia, a portion of the pericardium is excised to permit the exudative pericardial fluid to drain into the lymphatic system. The nursing care following the procedure includes routine postsurgical care (see Chapter 19) in addition to observation for recurrent tamponade.

Cardiac Arrest

In cardiac arrest, the heart is unable to pump and circulate blood to the body's organs and tissues. It is often caused by a dysrhythmia such as ventricular fibrillation, progressive bradycardia, or asystole (i.e., absence of cardiac electrical activity and heart muscle contraction). Cardiac arrest can also occur when electrical activity is present on the ECG but cardiac contractions are ineffective, a condition called **pulseless electrical activity (PEA).** PEA may be caused by a variety of problems such as profound hypovolemia (e.g., hemorrhage). Diagnoses that are associated with cardiac arrest include MI, massive pulmonary emboli, hyperkalemia, hypothermia, severe hypoxia, and medication overdose. Rapid identification of these problems and prompt intervention can restore circulation in some patients. Although survival after cardiac arrests that occur in the hospital is reported to be approximately 22%, survival is more likely when current AHA guidelines are followed (Anderson, Nichol, Dai, et al., 2016).

Clinical Manifestations

In cardiac arrest, consciousness, pulse, and blood pressure are lost immediately. Breathing usually ceases, but ineffective respiratory gasping may occur. The pupils of the eyes begin dilating in less than a minute, and seizures may occur. Pallor and cyanosis are seen in the skin and mucous membranes. The risk of organ damage, including irreversible brain damage, and of death increases with every minute that passes. A patient's age and overall health determine their vulnerability to irreversible damage. As soon as possible, the diagnosis of cardiac arrest must be made and action taken immediately to restore circulation.

Emergency Assessment and Management: Cardiopulmonary Resuscitation

Cardiopulmonary resuscitation (CPR) provides blood flow to vital organs until effective circulation can be reestablished. Following the recognition of unresponsiveness, a protocol for basic life support is initiated. The 2015 AHA Guidelines Update for Cardiopulmonary Resuscitation and Emergency Cardiovascular Care direct the current protocols (Neumar, Shuster, Callaway, et al., 2015). The resuscitation process begins with the immediate assessment of the patient and action to call for assistance, as CPR can be performed most effectively with the addition of more health care providers and equipment (e.g., defibrillator). The four basic steps in CPR are as follows:

1. *Recognition of sudden cardiac arrest.* The patient is checked for responsiveness and breathing.
2. *Activation of the Emergency Response System (ERS).* Within a medical facility, a call is made to alert the emergency response team, often called the "Code 4" or "Code Blue" team. Outside of a medical facility, 911 is called to activate the Emergency Medical Service (EMS).
3. *Performance of high-quality CPR.* If no carotid pulse is detected and no defibrillator is yet available, chest compressions are initiated. Rescue breathing may be added by a health care provider in a ratio of 30 compressions to 2 ventilations.
4. *Rapid cardiac rhythm analysis and defibrillation as soon as it is available.* Patients in ventricular fibrillation must be defibrillated as soon as possible.

Outcomes following CPR are improved by high-quality CPR (Meaney, Bobrow, Mancini, et al., 2013). Compressions are performed with the patient on a firm surface such as the

Figure 29-7 • Chest compressions in cardiopulmonary resuscitation are performed by placing the heel of one hand in the center of the chest over the sternum and the other hand on top of the first hand. Elbows are kept straight and body weight is used to apply forceful compressions to the lower sternum. The patient should be on a hard surface such as a cardiac board. From Field, J. M., Kudenchuk, P. J., O'Connor, R. E., et al., (2009). *The textbook of emergency cardiovascular care and CPR.* Philadelphia, PA: Lippincott Williams & Wilkins.

floor or a cardiac board. The provider, facing the patient's side, places one hand in the center of the chest on the lower half of the sternum and positions the other hand on top of the first hand (see Fig. 29-7). The chest is compressed 2 inches at a rate of 100 to 120 compressions per minute. Complete recoil of the chest is allowed between compressions. Interruptions in CPR to switch providers or check for a pulse are minimized. It is recommended that providers switch every 2 minutes due to the exertion of delivering effective compressions.

Maintaining Airway and Breathing

Rescue breathing is no longer recommended unless health care providers are present; if that is the case, it is then started after chest compressions. The airway is opened using a head-tilt/chin-lift maneuver, and any obvious material in the mouth or throat is removed. An oropharyngeal airway may be inserted if available to help maintain patency of the airway. Rescue ventilations are provided using a bag-valve mask or mouth-mask device. Oxygen is given at 100% during resuscitation to correct hypoxemia and improve tissue oxygenation. Excessive ventilation is avoided by the 30 to 2 ratio of compressions to ventilations (Meaney et al., 2013).

Defibrillation

As soon as a monitor/defibrillator is available, monitor electrodes are applied to the patient's chest and the heart rhythm is analyzed. When an automated external defibrillator (AED) is used, the device is turned on, the pads are applied to the patient's chest, and the rhythm is analyzed by the defibrillator to determine whether a shock is indicated. When the ECG shows ventricular fibrillation or pulseless ventricular tachycardia, immediate defibrillation is the treatment of choice. The survival time decreases for every minute that defibrillation is delayed. Following defibrillation, high-quality CPR is resumed immediately. Survival after cardiac arrest has been improved by extensive education of health care providers and by the use of AEDs.

Advanced Cardiovascular Life Support

Additional care may be indicated for patients in cardiac arrest. Placement of an advanced airway such as an ET tube may be performed by a physician, nurse anesthetist, or respiratory therapist during resuscitation to ensure a patent airway and adequate ventilation. Because of the risk of unrecognized esophageal intubation or dislodgement of the ET tube, tracheal intubation must be confirmed by assessment of specific parameters: auscultation of breath sounds, observation of chest expansion, and a carbon dioxide detector. A chest x-ray is always obtained after ET tube placement to confirm that the tube is in the proper position within the trachea. Arterial blood gases may also be obtained to assess ventilation and oxygenation.

Specific subsequent advanced support interventions depend on the assessment of the patient's condition and response to therapy. For example, if asystole is detected on the monitor, CPR is continued while IV epinephrine is given and an attempt is made to determine the cause of the arrest, such as severe hypovolemia or hypoxia. Additional medications (see Table 29-4) may be indicated for the patient during and after resuscitation.

CPR may be stopped when a pulse and blood pressure are detected, respirations are detected, and the patient responds. CPR efforts may also be stopped when rescuers are exhausted or at risk (e.g., a building is at risk of collapsing), or death is considered to be inevitable. If the patient does not respond to therapies given during the arrest, the resuscitation effort may be stopped by the physician or other provider in charge of the resuscitation. Many factors are considered in the decision, such as the initiating dysrhythmia, potential etiology, length of time for initiation of life support, and the patient's response to treatment.

 Follow-Up Monitoring and Care

The care provided to the patient following resuscitation is another determinant of survival (Williams, Calder, Cocchi, et al., 2013). The patient may be transferred to an ICU for close monitoring. Continuous ECG monitoring and frequent blood pressure assessments are essential until hemodynamic stability is established. Factors that precipitated the arrest such as dysrhythmias or electrolyte or metabolic imbalances are identified and treated.

Following resuscitation and return of spontaneous circulation, patients who are comatose may benefit from therapeutic

TABLE 29-4 Medications Used in Cardiopulmonary Resuscitation

Agent and Action	Indications	Nursing Considerations
Epinephrine—vasopressor used to optimize BP and cardiac output; improves perfusion and myocardial contractility	Given to patients in cardiac arrest caused by asystole, pulseless electrical activity, pulseless VT or VF	Administer 1 mg every 3–5 min by IV push or via IO route Follow peripheral IV administration with 20-mL flush and elevate extremity for 10–20 s
Vasopressin—increases systemic vascular resistance and BP	An alternative to epinephrine	Give 40 U IV one time only
Norepinephrine—vasopressor given to increase BP	Given for hypotension and shock	Give 0.1–0.5 mcg/kg/min as IV infusion, preferably through a central line
Dopamine—vasopressor given to increase BP and contractility	Given for hypotension and shock	Give 5–10 mcg/kg/min as IV infusion, preferably through a central line
Atropine—blocks parasympathetic action; increases SA node automaticity and AV conduction	Given to patients with symptomatic bradycardia (i.e., hemodynamically unstable with hypotension)	Give rapidly as 0.5-mg IV push; may repeat to dose of 3 mg
Amiodarone—acts on sodium–potassium and calcium channels to prolong action potential and refractory period	Used to treat pulseless VT and VF unresponsive to shock delivery	Give 300 mg IV; may give second dose of 150 mg in 3–5 min
Sodium bicarbonate (NaHCO₃)—corrects metabolic acidosis	Given to correct metabolic acidosis that is refractory to standard advanced cardiac life support interventions (cardiopulmonary resuscitation, intubation, and respiratory management)	Administer initial dose of 1 mEq/kg IV; then administer dose based on base deficit Recognize that to prevent development of rebound metabolic alkalosis, complete correction of acidosis is not indicated
Magnesium sulfate—promotes adequate functioning of cellular sodium—potassium pump	Given to patients with torsade de pointes, a type of VT	May give 1–2 g diluted in 10 mL D₅W over 5–20 min

BP, blood pressure; VT, ventricular tachycardia; VF, ventricular fibrillation; IV, intravenous; IO, intraosseous; SA, sinoatrial; AV, atrioventricular; D₅W, dextrose 5% in water.
Adapted from American Heart Association (2016a). Adult advanced cardiovascular life support. Retrieved on 3/31/16 at: cpr.heart.org/AHAECC/CPRAndECC/Training/HealthcareProfessional/AdvancedCardiovascularLifeSupportACLS/UCM_473186_Advanced-Cardiovascular-Life-Support-ACLS.jsp

hypothermia protocols. These induce a drop in core body temperature to 32° to 34°C (89.6° to 93.2°F) for 12 to 24 hours postresuscitation in order to decrease the cerebral metabolic rate and need for oxygen. Specific protocols have been developed to guide the use of both external cooling and catheter-based cooling methods and reduce associated complications such as shivering (Avery, O'Brien, Pierce, et al., 2015).

Advances in cardiac care, such as new techniques for effective resuscitation and postresuscitation hypothermia, have improved outcomes for patients with potentially lethal cardiac disorders, including those with cardiac arrest. Studies have demonstrated better neurologic recovery and overall survival for patients after cardiac arrest, and hope for even better outcomes in the future.

CRITICAL THINKING EXERCISES

1 A 76-year-old female is admitted to your unit with a diagnosis of acute decompensated HF. She complains of shortness of breath and swelling in her feet and lower legs. You administer furosemide and metolazone as prescribed. Identify your short-term expected outcomes of diuretic therapy. List three potential complications. Identify the physical assessment parameters and laboratory data you plan to monitor during the next 24 hours.

2 ebp As a member of your unit's practice council, you work on strategies to reduce the hospital's 30-day readmission rate for HF. Using your knowledge of evidence-based practice guidelines, list the most important topics to cover during discharge teaching. Compare and contrast the options for transitional care that are supported by the guidelines.

3 pq A 58-year-old male patient is recovering from an acute MI. He began coughing an hour ago, and now has a respiratory rate of 32 bpm and some pink-tinged sputum. The rapid response team arrives and the following are prescribed: chest x-ray, arterial blood gases and basic metabolic panel, furosemide 40 mg IV, and oxygen per nasal cannula. You know that you also need to explain what is happening to the patient and notify his wife. Identify which interventions you will do first and why.

REFERENCES

*Asterisk indicates nursing research.

Books

Ackley, B. J., & Ladwig, G. B. (2014). *Nursing diagnosis handbook* (10th ed.). Maryland Heights, MO: Elsevier.
Bickley, L. S. (2017). *Bates' guide to physical examination and history taking* (12th ed.). Philadelphia, PA: Lippincott Williams & Wilkins.

Burchum, J. R., & Rosenthal, L. D. (2016).*Lehne's pharmacology for nursing care* (9th ed.). St. Louis, MO: Elsevier.

Field, J. M., Kudenchuk, P. J., O'Connor, R. E., et al. (2009). *The textbook of emergency cardiovascular care and CPR*. Philadelphia, PA: Lippincott Williams & Wilkins.

Grossman, S. C., & Porth, C. M. (2014). *Porth's pathophysiology* (9th ed.). Philadelphia, PA: Lippincott Williams & Wilkins.

McCance, K. L., Huether, S. E., Brashers, V. L., et al. (2014). *Pathophysiology, The biologic basis for disease in adults and children* (7th ed.). St. Louis, MO: Elsevier.

Urden, L. D., Stacy, K. M., & Lough, M. E. (2014). *Critical care nursing* (7th ed.). St. Louis, MO: Elsevier.

Journals and Electronic Documents

Albert, N. M. (2013). Parallel paths to improve heart failure outcomes: Evidence matters. *American Journal of Critical Care, 22*(4), 289–297.

Albert, N. M., Barnason, S., Deswal, A., et al. (2015). Transitions of care in heart failure: A scientific statement from the American Heart Association. *Circulation & Heart Failure, 8*(2), 384–409.

American Heart Association. (2015). Heart disease and stroke statistics – 2015 Update. Retrieved on 9/24/2015 at: professional.heart.org/professional/ScienceNews/UCM_480113_Heart-Disease-and-Stroke-Statistics—2015-Update.jsp

American Heart Association (2016a). Adult advanced cardiovascular life support. Retrieved on 3/31/16 at: cpr.heart.org/AHAECC/CPRAndECC/Training/HealthcareProfessional/AdvancedCardiovascularLifeSupportACLS/UCM_473186_Advanced-Cardiovascular-Life-Support-ACLS.jsp

American Heart Association (2016b). *Shaking the salt habit*. Retrieved on 3/31/16 at: www.heart.org/HEARTORG/Conditions/HighBloodPressure/PreventionTreatmentofHighBloodPressure/Shaking-the-Salt-Habit_UCM_303241_Article.jsp#.Vzy9eNe3BK8

Anderson, M. L., Nichol, G., Dai, D., et al. (2016). Association between hospital process composite performance and patient outcomes after in-hospital cardiac arrest care. *JAMA Cardiology, 1*, 37–45. Retrieved on 3/1/2016 at: www.medscape.com/viewarticle/859491.

Avery, K. R., O'Brien, M., Pierce, C. D., et al. (2015). Use of a nursing checklist to facilitate implementation of therapeutic hypothermia after cardiac arrest. *Critical Care Nurse, 35*(1), 29–38.

Bradley, E. H., Curry, L., Horwitz, L. I., et al. (2013). Hospital strategies associated with 30-day readmission rates for patients with heart failure. *Circulation & Cardiovascular Quality Outcomes, 6*(4), 444–450.

Buonocore, D., & Wallace, E. (2014). Comprehensive guideline for care of patients with heart failure. *AACN Advanced Critical Care, 25*(2), 151–162.

Chapa, D. W., Akintade, B., Son, H., et al. (2014). Pathophysiological relationships between heart failure and depression and anxiety. *Critical Care Nurse, 34*(2), 14–25.

*Chung, M. L., Lennie, T. A., Mudd-Martin, G., et al. (2015). Adherence to a low-sodium diet in patients with heart failure is best when family members also follow the diet. *Journal of Cardiovascular Nursing, 30*(1), 44–50.

Ciuksza, M. S., Hebert, R., & Sokos, G. (2014). Use of home inotropes in patients near the end of life. *Journal of Palliative Medicine, 17*(10), 1178–1180.

Dobesh, P. P., & Fanikos, J. (2014). New oral anticoagulants for the treatment of venous thromboembolism: understanding differences and similarities. *Drugs, 74*(17), 2015–2032.

Dupras, D., Bluhm, J., Felty, C., et al. (2013). Venous thromboembolism diagnosis and treatment. Institute for Clinical Systems Improvement (ICSI). Retrieved on 9/21/15 at: www.guideline.gov/content.aspx?id=43864&search=pulmonary+embolism

Georgantas, A., Dimopoulos, S., Tasoulis, A., et al. (2014). Beneficial effects of combined exercise on early recovery cardiopulmonary exercise testing indices in patients with chronic heart failure. *Journal of Cardiopulmonary Rehabilitation and Prevention, 34*(6), 378–385.

*Heo, S., Moser, D. K., Pressler, S. J., et al. (2014). Depressive symptoms and the relationship of inflammation to physical signs and symptoms in heart failure patients. *American Journal of Critical Care, 23*(5), 404–413.

Hochman, J. S., & Reyentovoch, A. (2015). Prognosis and treatment of cardiogenic shock complicating myocardial infarction. Retrieved on 9/25/2015 at: www.uptodate.com/contents/prognosis-and-treatment-of-cardiogenic shock-complicating-acute myocardial infarction

Hoit, B. D. (2015). Diagnosis and treatment of pericardial effusion. Retrieved on 9/25/2015 at: www.uptodate.com/contents/diagnosis-and-treatment-of-pericardial-effusion

Kazory, A., & Ronco, C. (2013). Ultrafiltration therapy for acute decompensated heart failure: Lessons learned from 2 major trials. *American Heart Journal, 166*(5), 799–803.

Keteyian, S. J., Squires, R. W., Ades, P. A., et al. (2014). Incorporating patients with chronic heart failure into outpatient cardiac rehabilitation. *Journal of Cardiopulmonary Rehabilitation & Prevention, 34*(4), 223–232.

Manne, M., Rickard, J., Varma, N., et al. (2013). Normalization of left ventricular ejection fraction after cardiac resynchronization therapy also normalizes survival. *Pacing and Clinical Electrophysiology, 36*(8), 970–977.

Meaney, P. A., Bobrow, B. J., Mancini, M. E., et al. (2013). Cardiopulmonary resuscitation quality: Improving cardiac resuscitation outcomes both inside and outside the hospital. A consensus statement from the American Heart Association. *Circulation, 128*(4), 417–435.

Morici, B. (2014). Diagnosis and management of acute pulmonary embolism. *Journal of the American Academy of Physician Assistants, 27*(4), 18–22.

Neumar, R.W., Shuster, M., Callaway, C. W., et al. (2015). Part 1. Executive summary: 2015 American Heart Association guidelines update for cardiopulmonary resuscitation and emergency cardiovascular care. *Circulation, 132* (18), S315–S367.

O'Donovan, K. (2013). Milrinone therapy in adults with heart failure. *Nurse Prescribing, 11*(10), 493–498.

O'Neill, B. J., & Kazer, M. W. (2014). Destination to nowhere: A new look at aggressive treatment for heart failure – a case study. *Critical Care Nurse, 34*(2), 47–56.

Paul, S., & Hice, A. (2014). Role of the acute care nurse in managing patients with heart failure using evidence-based care. *Critical Care Nursing Quarterly, 37*(4), 357–376.

Peter, D., Robinson, P., Jordan, M., et al. (2015). Reducing readmissions using teach-back. *Journal of Nursing Administration, 45*(1), 35–42.

Piña, I. L. (2016). Cardiac rehabilitation in patients with heart failure. Retrieved on 3/17/16 at: www.uptodate.com/contents/cardiac-rehabilitation-in-patients-with-heart-failure

Pinkerman, C., Sander, P., Breeding, J. E., et al. (2013). Heart failure in adults. Institute for Clinical Systems Improvement (ICSI). Retrieved on 9/2/2015 at: www.guideline.gov/content.aspx?id=47030&search=heart failure

Pinto, D. S., & Kociol, R. D. (2015). Evaluation of acute decompensated heart failure. Retrieved 9/25/2015 at: www.uptodate.com/contents/evaluation-of-acute-decompensated-heart-failure

*Pressler, S. J., Gradus-Pizlo, I., Chubinski, S. D., et al. (2013). Family caregivers of patients with heart failure, a longitudinal study. *Journal of Cardiovascular Nursing, 28*(5), 417–428.

Stamp, K. D., Machado, M. A., & Allen, N. A. (2014). Transitional care programs improve outcomes for heart failure patients, an integrative review. *Journal of Cardiovascular Nursing, 29*(2), 140–154.

U.S. Department of Health and Human Services. (2013). Hospital quality overview. Retrieved on 9/6/2015 at: www.cms.gov/Medicare/Medicare-Fee-for-Service-Payment/AcuteInpatientPPS/Readmissions-Reduction-Program.html

Williams, D., Calder, S., Cocchi, M. N., et al. (2013). From door to recovery: A collaborative approach to the development of a post-cardiac arrest center. *Critical Care Nurse, 33*(5), 42–55.

Yancy, C. W., Jessup, M., Bozkurt, B., et al. (2013). 2013 ACCF/AHA Guideline for the management of heart failure. A report of the American College of Cardiology Foundation/American Heart Association Task Force on Practice Guidelines. *Circulation, 128*(16), e240–e327.

Resources

American Association of Heart Failure Nurses (AAHFN), aahfn.org
American College of Cardiology (ACC), www.acc.org
American Heart Association (AHA), www.heart.org/HEARTORG/
Heart Failure Society of America (HFSA), www.hfsa.org
National Heart, Lung, and Blood Institute, www.nhlbi.nih.gov

30

Assessment and Management of Patients With Vascular Disorders and Problems of Peripheral Circulation

LEARNING OBJECTIVES

On completion of this chapter, the learner will be able to:

1 Identify anatomic and physiologic factors that affect peripheral blood flow and tissue oxygenation.
2 Use assessment parameters appropriate for determining the status of peripheral circulation.
3 Apply the nursing process as a framework of care for patients with vascular insufficiency of the extremities.
4 Compare the various diseases of the arteries and their causes, pathophysiologic changes, clinical manifestations, management, and prevention.

5 Describe the prevention and management of venous thromboembolism (VTE).
6 Compare strategies to prevent and treat venous insufficiency, leg ulcers, and varicose veins.
7 Use the nursing process as a framework of care for patients with leg ulcers.
8 Describe the medical and nursing management of lymphatic disorders.

GLOSSARY

anastomosis: junction of two vessels
aneurysm: a localized sac or dilation of an artery formed at a weak point in the vessel wall
angioplasty: an invasive procedure that uses a balloon-tipped catheter to dilate a stenotic area of a blood vessel
ankle-brachial index (ABI): ratio of the ankle systolic pressure to the brachial systolic pressure; an objective measurement of arterial disease that provides quantification of the degree of stenosis
arteriosclerosis: diffuse process whereby the muscle fibers and the endothelial lining of the walls of small arteries and arterioles thicken
atherectomy: an invasive procedure that uses a cutting device or laser to remove or reduce plaque in an artery
atherosclerosis: inflammatory process involving the accumulation of lipids, calcium, blood components, carbohydrates, and fibrous tissue on the intimal layer of a large or medium-sized artery

bruit: sound produced by turbulent blood flow through an irregular, tortuous, stenotic, or dilated vessel
dissection: separation of the weakened elastic and fibromuscular elements in the medial layer of an artery
duplex ultrasonography: combines B-mode grayscale imaging of tissue, organs, and blood vessels with capabilities of estimating velocity changes by the use of a pulsed Doppler
intermittent claudication: a muscular, cramp-like pain or fatigue in the extremities consistently reproduced with the same degree of exercise or activity and relieved by rest
ischemia: deficient blood supply
rest pain: persistent pain in the foot or digits when the patient is resting, indicating a severe degree of arterial insufficiency
rubor: reddish-blue discoloration of the extremities; indicative of severe peripheral arterial damage in vessels that remain dilated and unable to constrict
stenosis: narrowing or constriction of a vessel

Conditions of the vascular system include arterial disorders, venous disorders, lymphatic disorders, and cellulitis. These disorders may be seen in patients in both the inpatient and the outpatient setting. Nursing management depends on an understanding of the vascular system.

Anatomic and Physiologic Overview

Adequate perfusion ensures oxygenation and nourishment of body tissues, and it depends in part on a properly functioning cardiovascular system. Adequate blood flow depends on the efficiency of the heart as a pump, the patency and responsiveness of the blood vessels, and the adequacy of circulating blood volume. Nervous system activity, blood viscosity, and

the metabolic needs of tissues influence the rate and adequacy of blood flow.

The vascular system consists of two interdependent systems. The right side of the heart pumps blood through the lungs to the pulmonary circulation, and the left side of the heart pumps blood to all other body tissues through the systemic circulation. The blood vessels in both systems channel the blood from the heart to the tissues and back to the heart (see Fig. 30-1). Contraction of the ventricles is the driving force that moves blood through the vascular system.

Arteries distribute oxygenated blood from the left side of the heart to the tissues, whereas the veins carry deoxygenated blood from the tissues to the right side of the heart. Capillary vessels located within the tissues connect the arterial and

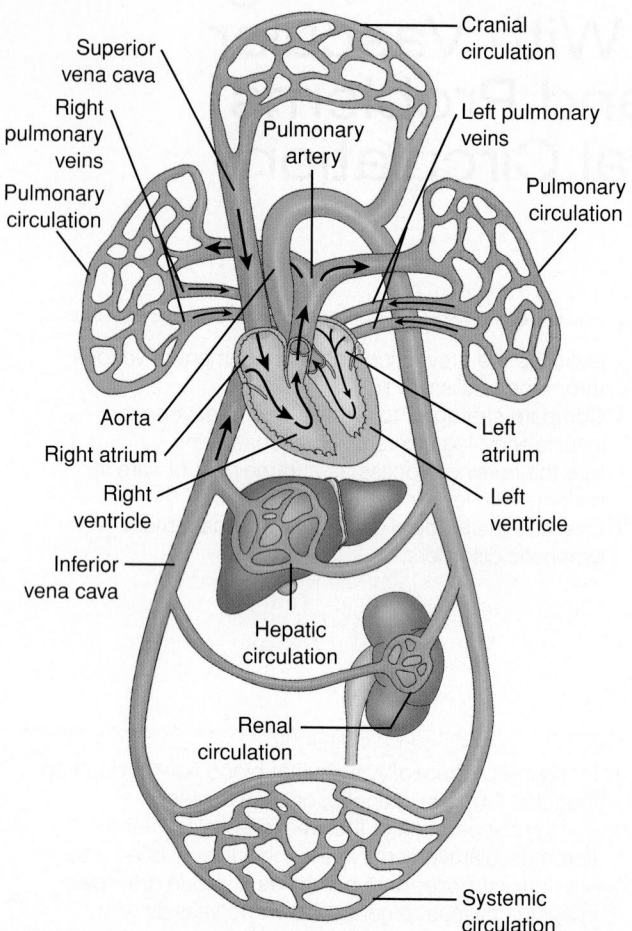

Figure 30-1 • Systemic and pulmonary circulation. Oxygen-rich blood from the pulmonary circulation is pumped from the left heart into the aorta and the systemic arteries to the capillaries, where the exchange of nutrients and waste products takes place. The deoxygenated blood returns to the right heart by way of the systemic veins and is pumped into the pulmonary circulation.

venous systems. These vessels permit the exchange of nutrients and metabolic wastes between the circulatory system and the tissues. Arterioles and venules immediately adjacent to the capillaries, together with the capillaries, make up the microcirculation.

The lymphatic system complements the function of the circulatory system. Lymphatic vessels transport lymph (a fluid similar to plasma) and tissue fluids (containing proteins, cells, and cellular debris) from the interstitial space to systemic veins.

Anatomy of the Vascular System

Arteries and Arterioles

Arteries are thick-walled structures that carry blood from the heart to the tissues. The aorta, which has a diameter of approximately 2.5 cm (1 in) in the average-sized adult, gives rise to numerous branches, which continue to divide into progressively smaller arteries that are 4 mm (0.16 in) in diameter. The vessels divide further, diminishing in size to approximately 30 mcm in diameter. These smallest arteries, called *arterioles*, are generally embedded within the tissues (Grossman & Porth, 2014).

The walls of the arteries and arterioles are composed of three layers: the intima, an inner endothelial cell layer; the media, a middle layer of smooth muscle and elastic tissue; and the adventitia, an outer layer of connective tissue. The intima, a very thin layer, provides a smooth surface for contact with the flowing blood. The media makes up most of the vessel wall in the aorta and other large arteries of the body. This layer is composed chiefly of elastic and connective tissue fibers that give the vessels considerable strength and allow them to constrict and dilate to accommodate the blood ejected from the heart during each cardiac cycle (stroke volume) and maintain an even, steady flow of blood. The adventitia is a layer of connective tissue that anchors the vessel to its surroundings. There is much less elastic tissue in the smaller arteries and arterioles, and the media in these vessels is composed primarily of smooth muscle (Grossman & Porth, 2014). Smooth muscle controls the diameter of the vessels by contracting and relaxing. Chemical, hormonal, and neuronal factors influence the activity of smooth muscle. Because arterioles offer resistance to blood flow by altering their diameter, they are often referred to as resistance vessels. Arterioles regulate the volume and pressure in the arterial system and the rate of blood flow to the capillaries. Because of the large amount of smooth muscle in the media, the walls of the arteries are relatively thick, accounting for approximately 25% of the total diameter of the artery.

The intima and the inner third of the smooth muscle layer of the media are in such close contact with the blood that the blood vessels receive their nourishment by direct diffusion. The adventitia and the outer media layers have a limited vascular system for nourishment and require their own blood supply to meet metabolic needs.

Capillaries

The walls of the capillaries, which lack smooth muscle and adventitia, are composed of a single layer of endothelial cells. This thin-walled structure permits rapid and efficient transport of nutrients to the cells and removal of metabolic wastes. The diameter of capillaries ranges from 5 to 10 mcm; this means that red blood cells must alter their shape to pass through these vessels. Changes in a capillary's diameter are passive and are influenced by contractile changes in the blood vessels that carry blood to and from a capillary. The capillary's diameter also changes in response to chemical stimuli. In some tissues, a cuff of smooth muscle, called the *precapillary sphincter*, is located at the arteriolar end of the capillary and is responsible, along with the arteriole, for controlling capillary blood flow (Grossman & Porth, 2014).

Some capillary beds, such as those in the fingertips, contain arteriovenous anastomoses, through which blood passes directly from the arterial to the venous system. These vessels are believed to regulate heat exchange between the body and the external environment.

The distribution of capillaries varies with the type of tissue. For example, skeletal tissue, which has high metabolic requirements, has a denser capillary network than cartilage, which has low metabolic needs.

Veins and Venules

Capillaries join to form larger vessels called *venules*, which join to form veins. The venous system is therefore structurally analogous to the arterial system; venules correspond to arterioles, veins to arteries, and the vena cava to the aorta. Analogous types of vessels in the arterial and venous systems have approximately the same diameters (see Fig. 30-1).

The walls of the veins, in contrast to those of the arteries, are thinner and considerably less muscular. In most veins, the wall makes up only 10% of the diameter, in contrast to 25% in most arteries. In veins, the walls are composed of three layers, like those of arteries; however, in veins, these layers are not as well defined.

The thin, less muscular structure of the vein wall allows these vessels to distend more than arteries. Greater distensibility and compliance permit large volumes of blood to remain in the veins under low pressure. For this reason, veins are referred to as capacitance vessels. Approximately 75% of total blood volume is contained in the veins. The sympathetic nervous system, which innervates the vein musculature, can stimulate the veins to constrict (venoconstriction), thereby reducing venous volume and increasing the volume of blood in the general circulation. Contraction of skeletal muscles in the extremities creates the primary pumping action to facilitate venous blood flow back to the heart (Grossman & Porth, 2014).

Some veins, unlike arteries, are equipped with valves. In general, veins that transport blood against the force of gravity, as in the lower extremities, have one-way bicuspid valves that prevent blood from seeping backward as it is propelled toward the heart. Valves are composed of endothelial leaflets, the competency of which depends on the integrity of the vein wall.

Lymphatic Vessels

The lymphatic vessels are a complex network of thin-walled vessels similar to the blood capillaries. This network collects lymphatic fluid from tissues and organs and transports the fluid to the venous circulation. The lymphatic vessels converge into two main structures: the thoracic duct and the right lymphatic duct. These ducts empty into the junction of the subclavian and the internal jugular veins. The right lymphatic duct conveys lymph primarily from the right side of the head, neck, thorax, and upper arms. The thoracic duct conveys lymph from the remainder of the body. Peripheral lymphatic vessels join larger lymph vessels and pass through regional lymph nodes before entering the venous circulation. The lymph nodes play an important role in filtering foreign particles.

The lymphatic vessels are permeable to large molecules and provide the only means by which interstitial proteins can return to the venous system. With muscular contraction, lymph vessels become distorted to create spaces between the endothelial cells, allowing protein and particles to enter. Muscular contraction of the lymphatic walls and surrounding tissues aids in propelling the lymph toward the venous drainage points (Zaleska, Olszewski, & Durlik, 2014).

Function of the Vascular System

Circulatory Needs of Tissues

The amount of blood flow needed by body tissues constantly changes. The percentage of blood flow received by individual organs or tissues is determined by the rate of tissue metabolism, the availability of oxygen, and the function of the tissues.

When metabolic requirements increase, blood vessels dilate to increase the flow of oxygen and nutrients to the tissues. When metabolic needs decrease, vessels constrict and blood flow to the tissues decreases. Metabolic demands of tissues increase with physical activity or exercise, local heat application, fever, and infection. Reduced metabolic requirements of tissues accompany rest or decreased physical activity, local cold application, and cooling of the body. If the blood vessels fail to dilate in response to the need for increased blood flow, tissue **ischemia** (deficient blood supply to a body part) results. The mechanism by which blood vessels dilate and constrict to adjust for metabolic changes ensures that normal arterial pressure is maintained (Grossman & Porth, 2014).

As blood passes through tissue capillaries, oxygen is removed and carbon dioxide is added. The amount of oxygen extracted by each tissue differs. For example, the myocardium tends to extract about 50% of the oxygen from arterial blood in one pass through its capillary bed, whereas the kidneys extract only about 7% of the oxygen from the blood that passes through them. The average amount of oxygen removed collectively by all of the body tissues is about 25%. This means that the blood in the vena cava contains about 25% less oxygen than aortic blood. This is known as the systemic arteriovenous oxygen difference (Grossman & Porth, 2014). This difference becomes greater when less oxygen is delivered to the tissues than they need.

Blood Flow

Blood flow through the cardiovascular system always proceeds in the same direction: left side of the heart to the aorta, arteries, arterioles, capillaries, venules, veins, vena cava, and right side of the heart. This unidirectional flow is caused by a pressure difference that exists between the arterial and venous systems. Because arterial pressure (approximately 100 mm Hg) is greater than venous pressure (approximately 40 mm Hg) and fluid always flows from an area of higher pressure to an area of lower pressure, blood flows from the arterial system to the venous system.

The pressure difference (ΔP) between the two ends of the vessel propels the blood. Impediments to blood flow offer the opposing force, which is known as resistance (R). The rate of blood flow is determined by dividing the pressure difference by the resistance:

$$\text{Flow rate} = \Delta P/R$$

This equation clearly shows that when resistance increases, a greater driving pressure is required to maintain the same degree of flow (Grossman & Porth, 2014). In the body, an increase in driving pressure is accomplished by an increase in the force of contraction of the heart. If arterial resistance is chronically elevated, the myocardium hypertrophies (enlarges) to sustain the greater contractile force.

In most long, smooth blood vessels, flow is laminar or streamlined, with blood in the center of the vessel moving slightly faster than the blood near the vessel walls. Laminar flow becomes turbulent when the blood flow rate increases, when blood viscosity increases, when the diameter of the vessel becomes greater than normal, or when segments of the vessel are narrowed or constricted (Krishna, Moxon, & Golledge, 2015). Turbulent blood flow creates an abnormal sound, called a **bruit**, which can be heard with a stethoscope.

Blood Pressure

Chapter 31 provides more information on the physiology and measurement of blood pressure.

Capillary Filtration and Reabsorption

Fluid exchange across the capillary wall is continuous. This fluid, which has the same composition as plasma without the proteins, forms the interstitial fluid. The equilibrium between hydrostatic and osmotic forces of the blood and interstitium, as well as capillary permeability, determines the amount and direction of fluid movement across the capillary. Hydrostatic force is a driving pressure that is generated by the blood pressure. Osmotic pressure is the pulling force created by plasma proteins. Normally, the hydrostatic pressure at the arterial end of the capillary is relatively high compared with that at the venous end. This high pressure at the arterial end of the capillaries tends to drive fluid out of the capillary and into the tissue space. Osmotic pressure tends to pull fluid back into the capillary from the tissue space, but this osmotic force cannot overcome the high hydrostatic pressure at the arterial end of the capillary. However, at the venous end of the capillary, the osmotic force predominates over the low hydrostatic pressure, and there is a net reabsorption of fluid from the tissue space back into the capillary (Grossman & Porth, 2014).

Except for a very small amount, fluid that is filtered out at the arterial end of the capillary bed is reabsorbed at the venous end. The excess filtered fluid enters the lymphatic circulation. These processes of filtration, reabsorption, and lymph formation aid in maintaining tissue fluid volume and removing tissue waste and debris. Under normal conditions, capillary permeability remains constant.

Under certain abnormal conditions, the fluid filtered out of the capillaries may greatly exceed the amounts reabsorbed and carried away by the lymphatic vessels. This imbalance can result from damage to capillary walls and subsequent increased permeability, obstruction of lymphatic drainage, elevation of venous pressure, or a decrease in plasma protein osmotic force. Accumulation of excess interstitial fluid that results from these processes is called *edema*.

Hemodynamic Resistance

The most important factor that determines resistance in the vascular system is the vessel radius. Small changes in vessel radius lead to large changes in resistance. The predominant sites of change in the caliber or width of blood vessels, and therefore in resistance, are the arterioles and the precapillary sphincter. Peripheral vascular resistance is the opposition to blood flow provided by the blood vessels. This resistance is proportional to the viscosity or thickness of the blood and the length of the vessel and is influenced by the diameter of the vessels. Under normal conditions, blood viscosity and vessel length do not change significantly, and these factors do not usually play an important role in blood flow. However, a large increase in hematocrit may increase blood viscosity and reduce capillary blood flow.

Peripheral Vascular Regulating Mechanisms

Even at rest, the metabolic needs of body tissues are continuously changing. Therefore, an integrated and coordinated regulatory system is necessary so that blood flow to individual tissues is maintained in proportion to the needs of those tissues. This regulatory mechanism is complex and consists of central nervous system influences, circulating hormones and chemicals, and independent activity of the arterial wall itself.

Sympathetic (adrenergic) nervous system activity, mediated by the hypothalamus, is the most important factor in regulating the caliber and therefore the blood flow of peripheral blood vessels. All vessels are innervated by the sympathetic nervous system except the capillary and precapillary sphincters. Stimulation of the sympathetic nervous system causes vasoconstriction. The neurotransmitter responsible for sympathetic vasoconstriction is norepinephrine (Grossman & Porth, 2014). Sympathetic activation occurs in response to physiologic and psychological stressors. Diminution of sympathetic activity by medications or sympathectomy results in vasodilation.

Other hormones affect peripheral vascular resistance. Epinephrine, released from the adrenal medulla, acts like norepinephrine in constricting peripheral blood vessels in most tissue beds. However, in low concentrations, epinephrine causes vasodilation in skeletal muscles, the heart, and the brain. Angiotensin I, which is formed from the interaction of renin (synthesized by the kidney) and angiotensinogen, a circulating serum protein, is then converted to angiotensin II by an enzyme secreted by the pulmonary vasculature, called *angiotensin-converting enzyme* (ACE). Angiotensin II is a potent vasoconstrictor, particularly of the arterioles. Although the amount of angiotensin II concentrated in the blood is usually small, its profound vasoconstrictive effects are important in certain abnormal states, such as heart failure and hypovolemia (Grossman & Porth, 2014).

Alterations in local blood flow are influenced by various circulating substances that have vasoactive properties. Potent vasodilators include nitric oxide, prostacyclin, histamine, bradykinin, prostaglandin, and certain muscle metabolites. A reduction in available oxygen and nutrients and changes in local pH also affect local blood flow. Proinflammatory cytokines are substances liberated from platelets that aggregate at the site of damaged vessels, causing arteriolar vasoconstriction and continued platelet aggregation at the site of injury (Favero, Paganelli, Buffoli, et al., 2014).

Pathophysiology of the Vascular System

Reduced blood flow through peripheral blood vessels characterizes all peripheral vascular diseases. The physiologic effects of altered blood flow depend on the extent to which tissue demands exceed the supply of oxygen and nutrients available. If tissue needs are high, even modestly reduced blood flow may be inadequate to maintain tissue integrity. Tissues then fall prey to ischemia, become malnourished, and ultimately die unless adequate blood flow is restored.

Pump Failure

Inadequate peripheral blood flow occurs when the heart's pumping action becomes inefficient. Left-sided heart failure (left ventricular failure) causes an accumulation of blood in the lungs and a reduction in forward flow or cardiac output, which results in inadequate arterial blood flow to the tissues. Right-sided heart failure (right ventricular failure) causes systemic venous congestion and a reduction in forward flow (see Chapter 29).

Alterations in Blood and Lymphatic Vessels

Intact, patent, and responsive blood vessels are necessary to deliver adequate amounts of oxygen to tissues and to remove metabolic wastes. Arteries can become damaged or obstructed as a result of atherosclerotic plaque, thromboemboli, chemical or mechanical trauma, infections or inflammatory processes, vasospastic disorders, and congenital malformations. A sudden arterial occlusion causes profound and often irreversible tissue ischemia and tissue death. When arterial occlusions develop gradually, there is less risk of sudden tissue death because collateral circulation may develop, giving that tissue the opportunity to adapt to gradually decreased blood flow.

Venous blood flow can be reduced by a thromboembolus obstructing the vein, by incompetent venous valves, or by a reduction in the effectiveness of the pumping action of surrounding muscles. Decreased venous blood flow results in increased venous pressure, a subsequent increase in capillary hydrostatic pressure, net filtration of fluid out of the capillaries into the interstitial space, and subsequent edema. Edematous tissues cannot receive adequate nutrition from the blood and consequently are more susceptible to breakdown, injury, and infection. Obstruction of lymphatic vessels also results in edema. Lymphatic vessels can become obstructed by a tumor or by damage from mechanical trauma or inflammatory processes.

Circulatory Insufficiency of the Extremities

Although many types of peripheral vascular diseases exist, most result in ischemia and produce some of the same symptoms: pain, skin changes, diminished pulse, and possible edema. The type and severity of symptoms depend in part on the type, stage, and extent of the disease process and on the speed with which the disorder develops. Table 30-1 highlights the distinguishing features of arterial and venous insufficiency. In this chapter, peripheral vascular disease is categorized as arterial, venous, or lymphatic.

 Gerontologic Considerations

Aging produces changes in the walls of the blood vessels that affect the transport of oxygen and nutrients to the tissues. The intima thickens as a result of cellular proliferation and fibrosis. Elastin fibers of the media become calcified, thin, and fragmented, and collagen accumulates in the intima and the media. These changes cause the vessels to stiffen, which results in increased peripheral resistance, impaired blood flow, and increased left ventricular workload causing hypertrophy, ischemia and failure of the left ventricle, and thrombosis and hemorrhage in microvessels in the brain and kidney (Favero et al., 2014).

Assessment of the Vascular System

Health History

The nurse obtains an in-depth description from the patient with peripheral vascular disease of any pain and its precipitating factors. A muscular, cramp-type pain, discomfort, or fatigue in the extremities consistently reproduced with the same degree of exercise or activity and relieved by rest is experienced by patients with peripheral arterial insufficiency. Referred to as **intermittent claudication**, this pain, discomfort, or fatigue is caused by the inability of the arterial system to provide adequate blood flow to the tissues in the face of increased demands for nutrients and oxygen during exercise. As the tissues are forced to complete the energy cycle without adequate nutrients and oxygen, muscle metabolites and lactic acid are produced. Pain is experienced as the metabolites aggravate the nerve endings of the surrounding tissue. Typically, about 50% of the arterial lumen or 75% of the cross-sectional area must be obstructed before intermittent claudication is experienced. When the patient rests and thereby decreases the metabolic needs of the muscles, the pain subsides. The progression of the arterial disease can be monitored by documenting the amount

TABLE 30-1 Characteristics of Arterial and Venous Insufficiency and Resulting Ulcers

Characteristic	Arterial	Venous
General Characteristics		
Pain	Intermittent claudication to sharp, unrelenting, constant	Aching, throbbing, cramping
Pulses	Diminished or absent	Present, but may be difficult to palpate through edema
Skin characteristics	Dependent rubor—elevation pallor of foot; dry, shiny skin; cool-to-cold temperature; loss of hair over toes and dorsum of foot; nails thickened and ridged	Pigmentation in gaiter area (area of medial and lateral malleolus), skin thickened and tough, may be reddish blue, frequently with associated dermatitis
Ulcer Characteristics		
Location	Tip of toes, toe webs, heel or other pressure areas if confined to bed	Medial malleolus, lateral malleolus, or anterior tibial area
Pain	Very painful	Minimal pain if superficial or may be very painful
Depth of ulcer	Deep, often involving joint space	Superficial
Shape	Circular	Irregular border
Ulcer base	Pale to black and dry gangrene	Granulation tissue—beefy red to yellow fibrinous in chronic long-term ulcer
Leg edema	Minimal unless extremity kept in dependent position constantly to relieve pain	Moderate to severe

of exercise or the distance the patient can walk before pain is produced. Persistent pain in the forefoot (i.e., the anterior portion of the foot) when the patient is resting indicates a severe degree of arterial insufficiency and a critical state of ischemia. Known as **rest pain**, this discomfort is often worse at night and may interfere with sleep. This pain frequently requires that the extremity be lowered to a dependent position to improve perfusion to the distal tissues.

The site of arterial disease can be deduced from the location of claudication, because pain occurs in muscle groups distal to the diseased vessel. Calf pain may accompany reduced blood flow through the superficial femoral or popliteal artery, whereas pain in the hip or buttock may result from reduced blood flow in the abdominal aorta or the common iliac or hypogastric (also known as internal iliac) arteries.

Physical Assessment

A thorough assessment of the patient's skin color and temperature and the character of the peripheral pulses is important in the diagnosis of arterial disorders.

Inspection of the Skin

Adequate blood flow warms the extremities and gives them a rosy coloring. Inadequate blood flow results in cool and pale extremities. Further reduction of blood flow to these tissues, which occurs when the extremity is elevated, for example, results in an even whiter or more blanched appearance (e.g.,

pallor). **Rubor**, a reddish-blue discoloration of the extremities, may be observed within 20 seconds to 2 minutes after the extremity is placed in the dependent position. Rubor suggests severe peripheral arterial damage in which vessels that cannot constrict remain dilated. Even with rubor, the extremity begins to turn pale with elevation. Cyanosis, a bluish tint of the skin, is manifested when the amount of oxygenated hemoglobin contained in the blood is reduced.

Additional changes resulting from a chronically reduced nutrient supply include loss of hair, brittle nails, dry or scaling skin, atrophy, and ulcerations. Edema may be apparent bilaterally or unilaterally and is related to the affected extremity's chronically dependent position because of severe rest pain. Gangrenous changes appear after prolonged, severe ischemia and represent tissue necrosis.

Palpation of Pulses

Determining the presence or absence, as well as the quality, of peripheral pulses is important in assessing the status of peripheral arterial circulation (see Fig. 30-2). Palpation of pulses is subjective, and the examiner may mistake their own pulse for that of the patient. To prevent this, the examiner should use light touch and avoid using only the index finger for palpation, because this finger has the strongest arterial pulsation of all the fingers. The thumb should not be used for the same reason. Absence of a pulse may indicate that the site of **stenosis** (narrowing or constriction) is proximal to that location. Occlusive arterial disease impairs blood flow and can reduce or

Figure 30-2 • Assessing peripheral pulses. **A.** Popliteal pulse. **B.** Dorsalis pedis pulse. **C.** Posterior tibial pulse. From Weber, J. R., & Kelley, J. H. (2014). *Health assessment in nursing* (5th ed.). Philadelphia, PA: Lippincott Williams & Wilkins.

obliterate palpable pulsations in the extremities. Pulses should be palpated bilaterally and simultaneously, comparing both sides for symmetry in rate, rhythm, and quality.

Diagnostic Evaluation

The nurse should educate the patient on the purpose of the studies, what to expect, and any possible side effects related to these examinations prior to diagnostic evaluation. The nurse should note trends in results because they provide information about disease progression as well as the patient's response to therapy. Various tests may be performed to identify and diagnose abnormalities that can affect the vascular structures (arteries, veins, and lymphatics).

Doppler Ultrasound Flow Studies

When pulses cannot be reliably palpated, a handheld continuous wave (CW) Doppler ultrasound device may be used to detect the blood flow in vessels. This handheld device emits a continuous signal through the patient's tissues. The signals are reflected by ("echo off") the moving blood cells and are received by the device. The filtered-output Doppler signal is then transmitted to a loudspeaker or headphones, where it can be heard for interpretation. Because CW Doppler emits a continuous signal, all vascular structures in the path of the sound beam are insonated, and differentiating arterial from venous flow and detecting the site of a stenosis may be difficult. The depth at which blood flow can be detected by Doppler is determined by the frequency (in megahertz [MHz]) it generates. The lower the frequency, the deeper the tissue penetration; a 5- to 10-MHz probe may be used to evaluate the peripheral arteries.

To evaluate the lower extremities, the patient is placed in the supine position with the head of the bed elevated 20 to 30 degrees; the legs are externally rotated, if possible, to permit adequate access to the medial malleolus. Acoustic gel is applied to the patient's skin to permit uniform transmission of the ultrasound wave. The tip of the Doppler transducer is positioned at a 45- to 60-degree angle over the expected location of the artery and angled slowly to identify arterial blood flow. Excessive pressure is avoided because severely diseased arteries can collapse with even minimal pressure.

Because the transducer can detect blood flow in advanced arterial disease states, especially if collateral circulation has developed, identifying a signal documents only the presence of blood flow. The patient's provider must be notified of the absence of a signal if one had been detected previously.

CW Doppler is more useful as a clinical tool when combined with ankle blood pressures, which are used to determine the **ankle-brachial index (ABI)** (see Fig. 30-3). The ABI is the ratio of the systolic blood pressure in the ankle to the systolic blood pressure in the arm. It is an objective indicator of arterial disease that allows the examiner to quantify the degree of stenosis. With increasing degrees of arterial narrowing, there is a progressive decrease in systolic pressure distal to the involved sites.

The first step in determining the ABI is to have the patient rest in a supine position (not seated) for approximately 5 minutes. An appropriate-sized blood pressure cuff (typically, a 10-cm cuff) is applied to the patient's ankle above the malleolus. After identifying an arterial signal at the posterior tibial and dorsalis pedis arteries, the systolic pressures,

Figure 30-3 • Continuous wave Doppler ultrasound detects blood flow in peripheral vessels. Combined with computation of ankle or arm pressures, this diagnostic technique helps health care providers characterize the nature of peripheral vascular disease. Photograph courtesy of Kim Cantwell-Gab.

are obtained in both ankles, while listening to the Doppler signal at each artery. Diastolic pressures in the ankles cannot be measured with Doppler. If pressure in these arteries cannot be measured, pressure can be measured in the peroneal artery, which can also be assessed at the ankle (see Fig. 30-4).

Doppler ultrasonography is used to measure brachial pressures in both arms. Both arms are evaluated because the patient may have an asymptomatic stenosis in the subclavian artery, causing brachial pressure on the affected side to be 20 mm Hg or more lower than systemic pressure. The abnormally low pressure should not be used for assessment.

To calculate ABI, the highest ankle systolic pressure for each foot is divided by the higher of the two brachial systolic pressures (see Chart 30-1). The ABI can be computed for a patient with the following systolic pressures:

Right brachial: 160 mm Hg
Left brachial: 120 mm Hg
Right posterior tibial: 80 mm Hg
Right dorsalis pedis: 60 mm Hg
Left posterior tibial: 100 mm Hg
Left dorsalis pedis: 120 mm Hg

Figure 30-4 • Location of peroneal artery; lateral malleolus.

Avoiding Common Errors in Calculating Ankle-Brachial Index

Take the following precautions to ensure an accurate ankle-brachial index (ABI) calculation:

- *Use correctly sized blood pressure (BP) cuffs.* To obtain accurate BP measurements, use a cuff with a bladder width at least 40% and length at least 80% of the limb circumference.
- *On the nursing plan of care, document the BP cuff sizes used* (e.g., "12-cm adult BP cuff used for brachial pressures; 10-cm pediatric BP cuff used for ankle pressures"). This minimizes the risk of shift-to-shift discrepancies in ABIs.
- *Use sufficient BP cuff inflation.* To ensure complete closure of the artery and the most accurate measurements, inflate cuffs 20–30 mm Hg beyond the point at which the last arterial signal is detected.
- *Do not deflate BP cuffs too rapidly.* Try to maintain a deflation rate of 2–4 mm Hg/s for patients without dysrhythmias and 2 mm Hg/s or slower for patients with dysrhythmias. Deflating the cuff more rapidly may miss the patient's highest pressure and result in recording an erroneous (low) BP measurement.
- *Suspect medial calcific sclerosis any time an ABI is 1.20 or greater or ankle pressure is more than 250 mm Hg.* Medial calcific sclerosis is associated with diabetes, chronic kidney disease, and hyperparathyroidism. It produces falsely elevated ankle pressures by hardening the media of the arteries, making the vessels noncompressible.
- *Be suspicious of arterial pressures recorded at less than 40 mm Hg.* This may mean the venous signal has been mistaken for the arterial signal. If the arterial pressure, which is normally 120 mm Hg, is measured at less than 40 mm Hg, ask a colleague to double-check the findings before recording this as an arterial pressure.

The highest systolic pressure for each ankle (80 mm Hg for the right, 120 mm Hg for the left) would be divided by the highest brachial pressure (160 mm Hg):

Right: 80/160 mm Hg = 0.50 ABI
Left: 120/160 mm Hg = 0.75 ABI

In general, systolic pressure in the ankle of a healthy person is the same or slightly higher than the brachial systolic pressure, resulting in an ABI of about 1.0 (no arterial insufficiency). Patients with claudication usually have an ABI of 0.90 to 0.50 (mild to moderate insufficiency); patients with ischemic rest pain have an ABI of less than 0.50; and patients with severe ischemia or tissue loss have an ABI of 0.40 or less (Zierler & Dawson, 2015).

Nursing Implications

Nurses should perform a baseline ABI on any patient with decreased pulses or any patient 70 years or older, especially patients with a history of diabetes or use of tobacco products (Conte, Pomposelli, Clair, et al., 2015). Patients who undergo an arterial interventional procedure or surgery should have ABIs performed per their institution's protocols. In addition, if there is a change in the clinical status of a patient, such as a sudden cold or painful limb, an ABI should be performed.

Prior to the procedure, nurses should educate patients about the indications for ABI and what to expect. Patients should be instructed to avoid use of tobacco products or drinking caffeinated beverages for at least 2 hours prior to testing

(if it is done on a nonurgent basis). There may be some discomfort involved when the cuffs are inflated.

Exercise Testing

Exercise testing is used to determine how long a patient can walk and to measure the ankle systolic blood pressure in response to walking. Typically, the patient walks on a treadmill at 1.5 mph with a 12% incline for a maximum of 5 minutes, or the test can be modified to walking a set distance in a hallway. Most patients can complete the test unless they have severe cardiac, pulmonary, or orthopedic problems or a physical disability. A normal response to the test is little or no drop in ankle systolic pressure after exercise. However, in a patient with true vascular claudication, the ankle pressure drops. Combining this hemodynamic information with the walking time helps the primary provider determine whether intervention is necessary. The nurse should reassure the patient that the treadmill test will not require running; rather, the test may require walking on a slight incline.

Duplex Ultrasonography

Duplex ultrasonography involves B-mode grayscale imaging of the tissue, organs, and blood vessels (arterial and venous) and permits estimation of velocity changes by use of a pulsed Doppler (see Fig. 30-5). Color flow techniques, which can identify vessels, may be used to shorten the examination time. Duplex ultrasound may be used to determine the level and extent of venous disease as well as chronicity of the disease. Using B mode and Doppler, it is possible to image and assess blood flow, evaluate flow of the distal vessels, locate the disease (stenosis versus occlusion), and determine anatomic morphology and the hemodynamic significance of plaque causing stenosis. Duplex ultrasound findings help in planning therapy and monitoring its outcomes. The test is noninvasive and usually requires no patient preparation. Patients who undergo abdominal vascular duplex ultrasound, however, should be advised to not eat or drink (i.e., NPO status) for at least 6 hours prior to the examination to decrease production of bowel gas that can interfere with the examination. The equipment is portable, making it useful anywhere for initial diagnosis, screening, or follow-up evaluations.

Figure 30-5 • Color flow duplex image of popliteal artery with normal triphasic Doppler flow.

Computed Tomography Scanning

Computed tomography (CT) scanning provides cross-sectional images of soft tissue and visualizes the area of volume changes to an extremity and the compartment where changes take place. CT of a lymphedematous arm or leg, for example, demonstrates a characteristic honeycomb pattern in the subcutaneous tissue. In multidetector-computed tomography (MDCT), a spiral CT scanner and rapid intravenous (IV) infusion of contrast agent are used to image very thin sections of the target area, and the results are configured in three dimensions so that the image can be rotated and viewed from multiple angles. The scan head moves circumferentially around the patient as the patient passes through the scanner, creating a series of overlapping images that are connected to one another in a continuous spiral. Scan times are short. However, the patient is exposed to x-rays, and a contrast agent is injected to visualize the blood vessels. The high volume of contrast agent injected into a peripheral vein may contraindicate the use of MDCT in children and patients with significantly impaired renal function (Conte et al., 2015).

Nursing Implications

Patients with impaired renal function scheduled for MDCT may require preprocedural treatment to prevent contrast-induced nephropathy. This may include oral or IV hydration 6 to 12 hours preprocedure or administration of sodium bicarbonate, which alkalinizes urine and protects against free radical damage. Meta-analysis of research studies that used oral and IV N-acetylcysteine do not support its use for protection against contrast-induced nephropathy (Sadat, 2013). The nurse should monitor the patient's urinary output post-procedurally, which should be at least 0.5 mL/kg/h. Contrast-induced acute kidney injury may occur within 48 to 96 hours postprocedure; therefore, the nurse should follow up with the patient's primary provider should this occur (see Chapter 54 for discussion of acute kidney injury). Patients who have known iodine or shellfish allergies may need premedication with steroids and histamine blockers.

Angiography

An arteriogram produced by angiography may be used to confirm the diagnosis of occlusive arterial disease when surgery or other interventions are considered. It involves injecting a radiopaque contrast agent directly into the arterial system to visualize the vessels. The location of a vascular obstruction or an **aneurysm** (abnormal dilation of a blood vessel) and the collateral circulation can be demonstrated. Typically, the patient experiences a temporary sensation of warmth as the contrast agent is injected, and local irritation may occur at the injection site. Infrequently, a patient may have an immediate or delayed allergic reaction to the iodine contained in the contrast agent. Manifestations include dyspnea, nausea and vomiting, sweating, tachycardia, and numbness of the extremities. Any such reaction must be reported to the interventionalist at once; treatment may include the administration of epinephrine, antihistamines, or corticosteroids. Additional risks include vessel injury, acute arterial occlusion, bleeding, or contrast nephropathy.

Magnetic Resonance Angiography

Magnetic resonance angiography (MRA) is performed with a standard magnetic resonance imaging (MRI) scanner and special software programmed to isolate the blood vessels. The resulting images can be rotated and viewed from multiple angles (Conte et al., 2015).

Nursing Implications

MRA is contraindicated in patients with any metal implants or devices such as pacemakers, including old tattoos, which may contain trace elements (newer materials used in tattoos such as nitinol and titanium are MRI compatible). The nurse should educate the patient regarding what to expect during and after the procedure. The patient should be prepared to lie on a cold, hard table that slides into an enclosed small tube. The nurse should instruct the patient that he or she will hear noises, including banging and popping sounds that will occur periodically. Patients with a history of claustrophobia may be prescribed a sedative prior to the procedure. Patients should be instructed to close their eyes before entering the tube, and to keep them closed, as this may decrease claustrophobic symptoms. Patients should be reassured that they will be provided with a panic button that they may press if they feel a need to stop the procedure. MRA procedures require the use of IV contrast dye; therefore, nursing implications following MRA are the same as those for MDCT (discussed in CT section).

Contrast Phlebography (Venography)

Also known as venography, contrast phlebography involves injecting a radiopaque contrast agent into the venous system. If a thrombus exists, the x-ray image reveals an unfilled segment of vein in an otherwise completely filled vein. Injection of the contrast agent may cause brief but painful inflammation of the vein. The test is generally performed if the patient is to undergo thrombolytic therapy; however, duplex ultrasonography is considered the standard for diagnosing lower extremity venous thrombosis (Zierler & Dawson, 2015). The nurse should instruct the patient anticipating a contrast venogram that he or she will receive contrast dye through a peripheral vein and will be monitored for 2 hours post venogram for access site oozing or hematoma. The guidelines for nursing care following venogram are the same as those for MDCT (see earlier discussion).

Lymphoscintigraphy

Lymphoscintigraphy involves injection of a radioactively labeled colloid subcutaneously in the second interdigital space. The extremity is then exercised to facilitate the uptake of the colloid by the lymphatic system, and serial images are obtained at preset intervals.

Nursing Implications

The nurse should educate the patient regarding what to expect. For instance, the blue dye typically used for this procedure may stain the injection site. If the patient has a lymphatic leak, as can occur with groin incisions, there may be blue drainage from the incision until the dye clears from the system, which may take several days.

ARTERIAL DISORDERS

Arterial disorders cause ischemia and tissue necrosis. These disorders may occur because of chronically progressive pathologic changes to the arterial vasculature (e.g., atherosclerotic changes) or due to an acute loss of blood flow to tissues (e.g., aneurysm rupture).

Arteriosclerosis and Atherosclerosis

Arteriosclerosis (hardening of the arteries) is the most common disease of the arteries. It is a diffuse process whereby the muscle fibers and the endothelial lining of the walls of small arteries and arterioles become thickened. **Atherosclerosis** involves a different process, affecting the intima of large and medium-sized arteries. These changes consist of the accumulation of lipids, calcium, blood components, carbohydrates, and fibrous tissue on the intimal layer of the artery. These accumulations are referred to as atheromas or plaques.

Although the pathologic processes of arteriosclerosis and atherosclerosis differ, rarely does one occur without the other, and the terms are often used interchangeably. Atherosclerosis is a generalized disease of the arteries, and when it is present in the extremities, it is usually present elsewhere in the body (Favero et al., 2014).

Pathophysiology

The most common direct results of atherosclerosis in arteries include narrowing (stenosis) of the lumen, obstruction by thrombosis, aneurysm, ulceration, and rupture. Its indirect results are malnutrition and the subsequent fibrosis of the organs that the sclerotic arteries supply with blood. All actively functioning tissue cells require an abundant supply of nutrients and oxygen and are sensitive to any reduction in the supply of these nutrients. If such reductions are severe and permanent, the cells undergo ischemic necrosis (death of cells due to deficient blood flow) and are replaced by fibrous tissue, which requires much less blood flow.

Atherosclerosis can develop at any point in the body, but certain sites are more vulnerable, such as regions where arteries bifurcate or branch into smaller vessels, with males having more below-the-knee pathology than females (Barochiner, Aparicio, & Waisman, 2014). In the proximal lower extremity, these include the distal abdominal aorta, the common iliac arteries, the orifice of the superficial femoral and profunda femoris arteries, and the superficial femoral artery in the adductor canal, which is particularly narrow. Distal to the knee, atherosclerosis can occur anywhere along the artery.

Although many theories exist about the development of atherosclerosis, no single theory explains the pathogenesis completely; however, tenets of several theories are incorporated into the reaction-to-injury theory. According to this theory, vascular endothelial cell injury results from prolonged hemodynamic forces, such as shearing stresses and turbulent flow, irradiation, chemical exposure, or chronic hyperlipidemia. Injury to the endothelium increases the aggregation of platelets and monocytes at the site of the injury. Smooth muscle cells migrate and proliferate, allowing a matrix of collagen and elastic fibers to form (Puranik, Dawson, & Peppas, 2013).

Atherosclerotic lesions are of two types: fatty streaks and fibrous plaque.

- Fatty streaks are yellow and smooth, protrude slightly into the lumen of the artery, and are composed of lipids and elongated smooth muscle cells. These lesions have been found in the arteries of people of all age groups, including infants. It is not clear whether fatty streaks predispose a person to the formation of fibrous plaques or whether they are reversible. They do not usually cause clinical symptoms.
- Fibrous plaques are composed of smooth muscle cells, collagen fibers, plasma components, and lipids. They are white to white-yellow and protrude in various degrees into the arterial lumen, sometimes completely obstructing it. These plaques are found predominantly in the abdominal aorta and the coronary, popliteal, and internal carotid arteries, and they are believed to be progressive lesions (see Fig. 30-6).

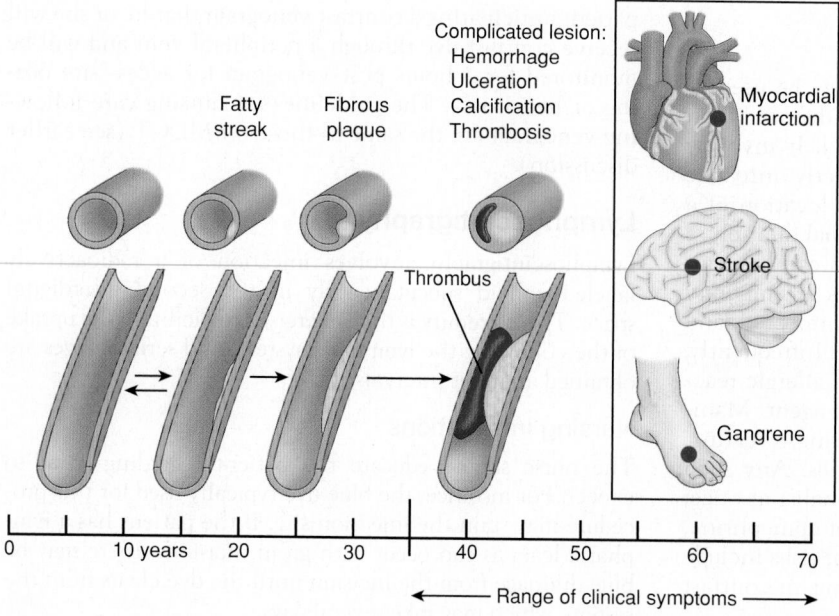

Figure 30-6 • Schematic concept of the progression of atherosclerosis. Fatty streaks constitute one of the earliest lesions of atherosclerosis. Many fatty streaks regress, whereas others progress to fibrous plaques and eventually to atheroma, which may be complicated by hemorrhage, ulceration, calcification, or thrombosis and may produce myocardial infarction, stroke, or gangrene.

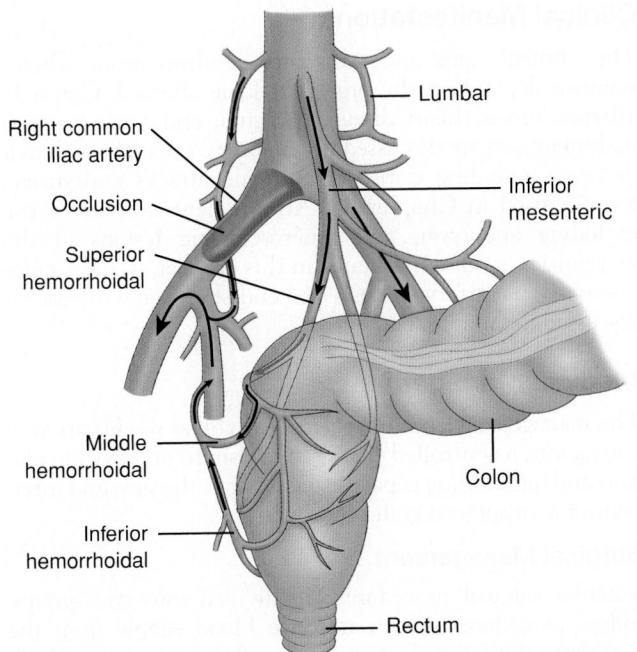

Right common iliac artery

Occlusion

Superior hemorrhoidal

Lumbar

Inferior mesenteric

Middle hemorrhoidal

Colon

Inferior hemorrhoidal

Rectum

Figure 30-7 • Development of channels for collateral blood flow in response to occlusion of the right common iliac artery and the terminal aortic bifurcation.

Gradual narrowing of the arterial lumen stimulates the development of collateral circulation (see Fig. 30-7). Collateral circulation arises from pre-existing vessels that enlarge to reroute blood flow around a hemodynamically significant stenosis or occlusion. Collateral flow allows continued perfusion to the tissues, but it is often inadequate to meet increased metabolic demand, and ischemia results.

Chart 30-2 ⚠️ RISK FACTORS
Atherosclerosis and Peripheral Arterial Disease

Modifiable Risk Factors

- Nicotine use (i.e., tobacco product such as cigarettes, e-cigarettes, or chewing tobacco)
- Diet (contributing to hyperlipidemia)
- Hypertension
- Diabetes (speeds the atherosclerotic process by thickening the basement membranes of both large and small vessels)
- Hyperlipidemia
- Stress
- Sedentary lifestyle
- Elevated C-reactive protein
- Hyperhomocysteinemia

Nonmodifiable Risk Factors

- Increasing age
- Female gender
- Familial predisposition/genetics

Adapted from Cronenwett, J. L., & Johnston, K. W. (2014). *Rutherford's vascular surgery* (8th ed., Vols. 1 and 2). Philadelphia, PA: W. B. Saunders.

Risk Factors

Many risk factors are associated with atherosclerosis (see Chart 30-2). Although it is not entirely clear whether modification of these risk factors prevents the development of cardiovascular disease, evidence indicates that it may slow the process. Recent studies have reported the prevalence of atherosclerosis in women is the same, if not higher, than in men, and that female gender is an independent risk factor for peripheral arterial disease (PAD) (Barochiner et al., 2014).

The use of tobacco products may be one of the most important risk factors in the development of atherosclerotic lesions. Nicotine in tobacco decreases blood flow to the extremities and increases heart rate and blood pressure by stimulating the sympathetic nervous system, causing vasoconstriction. It also increases the risk of clot formation by increasing the aggregation of platelets. Carbon monoxide, a toxin produced by burning tobacco, combines more readily with hemoglobin than oxygen, depriving the tissues of oxygen. There is evidence that smoking decreases high-density lipoprotein (HDL) levels and alters the ratios between HDL and low-density lipoprotein (LDL), HDL and triglycerides, and HDL and total cholesterol levels (see Chapter 27 for discussion of HDL and LDL and their association with atherosclerosis). The amount of tobacco used—inhaled in traditional or e-cigarette form, or chewed—is directly related to the extent of the disease, and cessation of any type of tobacco product use reduces the risks (Barochiner et al., 2014).

Diabetes increases the overall risk of PAD two- to four-fold, with amputation rates five to ten times higher than in patients without diabetes. Patients with diabetes show an earlier onset and more rapid progression of PAD than patients without diabetes; furthermore, they also exhibit a different anatomical distribution of pathology, with a greater severity of disease in the profunda femoris and in all segments below the knee (Conte et al., 2015). How diabetes affects the onset and progression of atherosclerosis is multifactorial and includes incitation of inflammatory processes, derangement of various cell types within vessel walls, promotion of coagulation, and inhibition of fibrinolysis (Thiruvoipati, Kielhorn, & Armstrong, 2015). Black race has been reported to increase the risk of developing PAD by over twofold and is also associated with higher rates of hypertension (Krishna et al., 2015). Many other factors, such as obesity, stress, and lack of exercise, have been identified as contributing to the disease process.

C-reactive protein (CRP) is a sensitive marker of cardiovascular inflammation, both systemically and locally. Slight increases in serum CRP levels are associated with an increased risk of damage in the vasculature, especially if these increases are accompanied by other risk factors, including increasing age, female gender, hypertension, hypercholesterolemia, obesity, elevated blood glucose levels, use of tobacco products, or a positive family history of cardiovascular disease (Krishna et al., 2015).

Hyperhomocysteinemia has been positively correlated with the risk of peripheral, cerebrovascular, and coronary artery disease as well as venous thromboembolism (VTE). Homocysteine is a protein that promotes coagulation by increasing factor V and factor XI activity while depressing protein C activation and increasing the binding of lipoprotein(a) in fibrin. These processes increase thrombin formation and the propensity for thrombosis. Folic acid and vitamin B_{12} have been reported to reduce serum homocysteine levels but there are no data demonstrating this therapy reduces adverse cardiovascular events (Conte et al., 2015).

Prevention

Intermittent claudication is a symptom of generalized atherosclerosis and may be a marker of occult coronary artery disease. Because it is suspected that a high-fat diet contributes to atherosclerosis, it is reasonable to measure serum cholesterol and to begin disease prevention efforts that include diet modification. The American Heart Association recommends reducing the amount of fat ingested in a healthy diet, substituting unsaturated fats for saturated fats, and decreasing cholesterol intake to reduce the risk of cardiovascular disease.

Certain medications that supplement dietary modification and exercise are used to reduce blood lipid levels. Current evidence-based guidelines established by the American College of Cardiology and the American Heart Association (ACC/AHA) recommend 3-hydroxy-3-methylglutaryl coenzyme A (HMG-CoA) reductase inhibitors (statins) for first-line use in patients with PAD for secondary prevention and cardiovascular risk reduction (Armstrong, Chen, Westin, et al., 2014). These statins may include medications such as atorvastatin (Lipitor), lovastatin (Mevacor), pitavastatin (Livalo), pravastatin (Pravachol), simvastatin (Zocor), fluvastatin (Lescol), and rosuvastatin (Crestor). Several other classes of medications used to reduce lipid levels include bile acid sequestrants (cholestyramine [Questran], colesevelam [WelChol], colestipol [Colestid]), nicotinic acid (niacin [Niacor, Niaspan]), fibric acid inhibitors (gemfibrozil [Lopid], fenofibrate [Tricor]), and cholesterol absorption inhibitors (ezetimibe [Zetia]). Patients receiving long-term therapy with these medications require close monitoring.

Hypertension, which may accelerate the rate at which atherosclerotic lesions form in high-pressure vessels, can lead to a stroke, ischemic renal disease, severe PAD, or coronary artery disease. Hypertension is a major risk factor for the development of PAD and may be a more significant risk factor for women than men based upon research findings from the classic Framingham Heart Study and a similar study performed in Europe (Barochiner et al., 2014). The majority of patients with hypertension require more than two antihypertensive agents to reach goal blood pressure, and at least one third require more than three antihypertensive agents to achieve effective blood pressure control (Cooper, Murphy, Cutlip, et al., 2014.). See Chapter 31 for further discussion of hypertension.

Although no single risk factor has been identified as the primary contributor to the development of atherosclerotic cardiovascular disease, it is clear that the greater the number of risk factors, the greater the risk of atherosclerosis. Elimination of all controllable risk factors, particularly the use of nicotine products, is strongly recommended.

Clinical Manifestations

The clinical signs and symptoms resulting from atherosclerosis depend on the organ or tissue affected. Coronary atherosclerosis (heart disease), angina, and acute myocardial infarction are discussed in Chapter 27. Cerebrovascular diseases, including transient ischemic attacks and stroke, are discussed in Chapter 67. Atherosclerosis of the aorta, including aneurysm, and atherosclerotic lesions of the extremities are discussed later in this chapter. Renovascular disease (renal artery stenosis and end-stage renal disease) is discussed in Chapter 54.

Medical Management

The management of atherosclerosis involves modification of risk factors, a controlled exercise program to improve circulation and functioning capacity, medication therapy, and interventional or surgical graft procedures.

Surgical Management

Vascular surgical procedures are divided into two groups: inflow procedures, which improve blood supply from the aorta into the femoral artery, and outflow procedures, which provide blood supply to vessels below the femoral artery. Inflow surgical procedures are described with diseases of the aorta and outflow procedures with peripheral arterial occlusive disease.

Radiologic Interventions

Several interventional radiologic techniques are important adjunctive therapies to surgical procedures. If an isolated lesion or lesions are identified during the arteriogram, **angioplasty**, also called *percutaneous transluminal angioplasty* (PTA), or an atherectomy, may be performed. After the patient receives a local anesthetic agent, a balloon-tipped catheter is maneuvered across the area of stenosis. Although some clinicians theorize that PTA improves blood flow by overstretching (and thereby dilating) the elastic fibers of the nondiseased arterial segment, most believe that the procedure widens the arterial lumen by "cracking" and flattening the plaque against the vessel wall (see Chapter 27). An **atherectomy** reduces the plaque build-up within an artery using a cutting device or laser. Complications from PTA and atherectomy include hematoma formation, embolus, **dissection** (separation of the intima) of the vessel, acute arterial occlusion, and bleeding. To decrease the risk of reocclusion, stents (small mesh tubes made of nitinol, titanium, or stainless steel) may be inserted to support the walls of blood vessels and prevent collapse immediately after balloon inflation (see Fig. 30-8). A variety of stents and stent grafts may be used for short-segment stenoses. Complications associated with stent or stent graft use include distal embolization, intimal damage (dissection), and dislodgment. The advantage of angioplasty, atherectomy, stents, and stent grafts is the decreased length of hospital stay required for the treatment; many of the procedures are performed on an outpatient basis.

Nursing Management

An overview of the care of a patient with peripheral arterial problems is provided in Chart 30-3.

Figure 30-8 • **A.** Flexible stent. © 2013 Medtronic, Inc. Used with permission. **B.** Representation of a common iliac artery with a wall stent.

Improving Peripheral Arterial Circulation

Arterial blood supply to a body part can be enhanced by positioning the part below the level of the heart. For the lower extremities, this is accomplished by elevating the head of the patient's bed or by having the patient use a reclining chair or sit with the feet resting on the floor.

 Concept Mastery Alert

For patients with PAD, blood flow to the lower extremities needs to be enhanced; therefore, the nurse encourages keeping the lower extremities in a neutral or dependent position. In contrast, for patients with venous insufficiency, blood return to the heart needs to be enhanced, so the lower extremities are elevated.

The nurse can assist the patient with walking or other moderate or graded isometric exercises that may be prescribed to promote blood flow and encourage the development of collateral circulation. The nurse instructs the patient to walk to the point of pain, rest until the pain subsides, and then resume walking so that endurance can be increased as collateral circulation develops. Pain can serve as a guide in determining the appropriate amount of exercise. The onset of pain indicates that the tissues are not receiving adequate oxygen, signaling the patient to rest before continuing activity. A regular exercise program can result in increased walking distance before the onset of claudication. The amount of exercise a patient can tolerate before the onset of pain is determined to provide a baseline for evaluation.

Not all patients with peripheral vascular disease should exercise. Before recommending any exercise program, the patient's primary provider should be consulted. Conditions that worsen with exercise include leg ulcers, cellulitis, gangrene, or acute thrombotic occlusions.

Promoting Vasodilation and Preventing Vascular Compression

Arterial dilation promotes increased blood flow to the extremities and is therefore a goal for patients with PAD. However, if the arteries are severely sclerosed, inelastic, or damaged,

dilation is not possible. For this reason, measures to promote vasodilation, such as medications, radiologic interventions or surgery, may be only minimally effective.

Nursing interventions may involve applications of warmth to promote arterial flow and instructions to the patient to avoid exposure to cold temperatures, which causes vasoconstriction. Adequate clothing and warm temperatures protect the patient from chilling. If chilling occurs, a warm bath or drink is helpful. A hot water bottle or heating pad may be applied to the patient's abdomen, causing vasodilation throughout the lower extremities.

 Quality and Safety Nursing Alert

Patients are instructed to test the temperature of bath water and to avoid using hot water bottles and heating pads on the extremities. It is safer to apply a hot water bottle or a heating pad to the abdomen; this can cause reflex vasodilation in the extremities.

In patients with vasospastic disorders (e.g., Raynaud disease), heat may be applied directly to ischemic extremities using a warmed or electric blanket; however, the temperature of the heat source must not exceed body temperature. Even at low temperatures, trauma to the tissues can occur in ischemic extremities.

Quality and Safety Nursing Alert

Excess heat may increase the metabolic rate of the extremities and the need for oxygen beyond that provided by the reduced arterial flow through the diseased artery. Heat must be used with great caution!

Nicotine from any tobacco product causes vasospasm and can thereby dramatically reduce circulation to the extremities. One study found that patients with PAD who smoked had shorter time to onset of claudication symptoms (Fritschi, Collins, O'Connell, et al., 2013). Tobacco smoke also impairs transport and cellular use of oxygen and increases blood viscosity. Patients with arterial insufficiency who smoke, chew tobacco, or use e-cigarettes must be fully informed of the

Chart 30-3 PLAN OF NURSING CARE

The Patient With Peripheral Vascular Problems

NURSING DIAGNOSIS: Ineffective peripheral tissue perfusion related to compromised circulation
GOAL: Increased arterial blood supply to extremities

Nursing Interventions	Rationale	Expected Outcomes
1. Lower the extremities below the level of the heart (if condition is arterial in nature). 2. Encourage moderate amount of walking or graded extremity exercises if no contraindications exist.	1. Dependency of lower extremities enhances arterial blood supply. 2. Muscular exercise promotes blood flow and the development of collateral circulation.	• Has extremities warm to touch • Has extremities with improved color • Experiences decreased muscle pain with exercise • Able to walk further distances

GOAL: Decrease in venous congestion

Nursing Interventions	Rationale	Expected Outcomes
1. Elevate extremities above heart level (if condition is venous in nature). 2. Discourage standing still or sitting for prolonged periods. 3. Encourage walking.	1. Elevation of extremities counteracts gravity, promotes venous return, and prevents venous stasis. 2. Prolonged standing still or sitting promotes venous stasis. 3. Walking promotes venous return by activating the "muscle pump."	• Elevates lower extremities as prescribed • Has decreased edema of extremities • Avoids prolonged standing still or sitting • Gradually increases walking time daily

GOAL: Promotion of vasodilation and prevention of vascular compression

Nursing Interventions	Rationale	Expected Outcomes
1. Maintain warm temperature and avoid chilling. 2. Discourage use of tobacco products. 3. Counsel in ways to avoid emotional upsets; stress management. 4. Encourage avoidance of constrictive clothing and accessories. 5. Encourage avoidance of crossing the legs. 6. Administer vasodilator medications and adrenergic blocking agents as prescribed, with appropriate nursing considerations.	1. Warmth promotes arterial flow by preventing the vasoconstriction effects of chilling. 2. Nicotine in all tobacco products causes vasospasm, which impedes peripheral circulation. 3. Emotional stress causes peripheral vasoconstriction by stimulating the sympathetic nervous system. 4. Constrictive clothing and accessories impede circulation and promote venous stasis. 5. Crossing the legs causes compression of vessels with subsequent impediment of circulation, resulting in venous stasis. 6. Vasodilators relax smooth muscle; adrenergic blocking agents block the response to sympathetic nerve impulses or circulating catecholamines.	• Protects extremities from exposure to cold • Avoids all tobacco products • Uses stress management program to minimize emotional upset • Avoids constricting clothing and accessories • Avoids crossing legs • Takes medication as prescribed

NURSING DIAGNOSIS: Chronic pain related to impaired ability of peripheral vessels to supply tissues with oxygen
GOAL: Relief of pain

Nursing Interventions	Rationale	Expected Outcomes
1. Promote increased circulation through exercise (e.g., walking program, upper extremity exercises, water aerobics, using stationary bicycle). 2. Administer analgesic agents as prescribed, with appropriate nursing considerations.	1. Enhancement of peripheral circulation increases the oxygen supplied to the muscle and decreases the accumulation of metabolites that cause muscle spasms. 2. Analgesic agents help reduce pain and allow the patient to participate in activities and exercises that promote circulation.	• Uses measures to increase arterial blood supply to extremities • Uses analgesic agents as prescribed

Chart 30-3

PLAN OF NURSING CARE (Continued)
The Patient With Peripheral Vascular Problems

NURSING DIAGNOSIS: Risk for impaired skin integrity related to compromised circulation
GOAL: Attainment/maintenance of tissue integrity

Nursing Interventions	Rationale	Expected Outcomes
1. Instruct in ways to avoid trauma to extremities.	1. Poorly nourished tissues are susceptible to trauma and bacterial invasion; healing of wounds is delayed or inhibited due to poor tissue perfusion.	• Inspects skin daily for evidence of injury or ulceration • Avoids trauma and irritation to skin • Wears protective shoes • Adheres to meticulous hygiene regimen • Eats a healthy diet that contains adequate protein and vitamins A and C
2. Encourage wearing protective shoes and padding for pressure areas; wear new shoes for short period of time and then inspect feet for signs of injury.	2. Protective shoes and padding prevent foot injuries and blisters.	
3. Encourage meticulous hygiene: bathing with neutral soaps, applying lotions, and carefully trimming nails.	3. Neutral soaps and lotions prevent drying and cracking of skin; avoid lotion between toes because the increased moisture can lead to maceration of tissue.	
4. Caution to avoid scratching or vigorous rubbing.	4. Scratching and rubbing can cause skin abrasions and bacterial invasion.	
5. Promote good nutrition; adequate intake of vitamins A and C, protein, and zinc; and weight reduction, if overweight or obese.	5. Good nutrition promotes healing and prevents tissue breakdown.	

NURSING DIAGNOSIS: Deficient knowledge regarding self-care activities
GOAL: Adherence to the self-care program

Nursing Interventions	Rationale	Expected Outcomes
1. Include family/significant others in education.	1. Adherence to the self-care program is enhanced when the patient receives support from family and from appropriate self-help groups and agencies.	• Practices frequent position changes as prescribed • Practices postural exercises as prescribed • Takes medications as prescribed • Avoids vasoconstrictors • Uses measures to prevent trauma • Uses stress management program • Accepts condition as chronic but amenable to therapies that will decrease symptoms
2. Provide written instructions about foot care, leg care, and exercise program.	2. Written instructions serve as reminder and reinforcement of information.	
3. Assist to obtain properly fitting clothing, shoes, and stockings.	3. Constrictive clothing and accessories impede circulation and promote venous stasis.	
4. Refer to self-help groups as indicated, such as smoking cessation clinics or stress management, weight management, and exercise programs.	4. Reducing risk factors may reduce symptoms or slow disease progression.	

effects of nicotine on circulation and encouraged to stop (see Chart 30-4).

Emotional upsets stimulate the sympathetic nervous system, resulting in peripheral vasoconstriction. Emotional stress can be minimized to some degree by avoiding stressful situations when possible or by consistently following a stress management program. Counseling services or alternative or complementary therapies (e.g., relaxation training, yoga, aromatherapy, mindfulness-based stress reduction) may be indicated for people who cannot cope effectively with situational stressors.

Constrictive clothing and accessories such as tight socks or shoelaces may impede circulation to the extremities and promote venous stasis and therefore should be avoided. Crossing the legs for more than 15 minutes at a time should be discouraged because it compresses vessels in the legs.

Relieving Pain

Frequently, the pain associated with peripheral arterial insufficiency is chronic, continuous, and disabling. It limits activities, affects work and responsibilities, disturbs sleep, and alters the patient's sense of well-being. Patients may be depressed, irritable, and unable to exert the energy necessary to execute prescribed therapies, making pain relief even more difficult. Analgesic agents such as hydrocodone plus acetaminophen (Vicodin, Norco, Lortab), oxycodone (Roxicodone), oxycodone plus acetylsalicylic acid (Percodan), or oxycodone plus acetaminophen (Percocet, Roxicet) may be helpful in reducing pain so that the patient can participate in therapies that can increase circulation and ultimately relieve pain more effectively.

Maintaining Tissue Integrity

Poorly perfused tissues are susceptible to damage and infection. When lesions develop, healing may be delayed or inhibited because of the poor blood supply to the area. Infected, nonhealing ulcerations of the extremities can be debilitating and may require prolonged and often expensive treatments. Amputation of an ischemic limb may eventually be necessary.

NURSING RESEARCH PROFILE

Chart 30-4

The Effects of Smoking on Walking and Quality-of-Life in Patients With Peripheral Arterial Disease

Fritschi, C., Collins, E. G., O'Connell, S., et al. (2013). The effects of smoking status on walking ability and health-related quality of life in patients with peripheral arterial disease. *Journal of Cardiovascular Nursing, 28*(4), 380–386.

Purpose

Peripheral arterial disease (PAD) is a common, chronic atherosclerotic vascular disease that affects up to 10% of the population, with an increase in prevalence from 15% to 20% among older adults, or among adults who have diabetes or smoke. The average risk of developing symptomatic PAD in smokers is reported to be over twice that of nonsmokers. Prior studies have shown that smoking is associated with poorer measures of exercise capacity during treadmill testing, including peak oxygen uptake, and earlier onset of claudication symptoms while walking among patients with PAD. There are limited data regarding the interrelationships between smoking status and health-related quality of life (HR-QoL) in patients with PAD, however. The aim of this study was to explore the differences in walking endurance and PAD-related factors (pain, calf muscle hemoglobin saturation, HR-QoL) between smokers and nonsmokers with PAD.

Design

This prospective cross-sectional, descriptive study solicited patients with PAD (N = 105) from a Midwestern Veterans Affairs and University Hospital, as well as through flyer distribution in urban communities. Participants had a diagnosis of PAD, an ankle-brachial index (ABI) less than 0.90 or had evidence of "stiff" vessels and a positive response from the Edinburgh Claudication Questionnaire, which evaluates lower extremity pain during walking and standing. Participants were all over age 55, 93% were men, with 36 of the 105 participants reporting that they were current smokers. Nearly half had diabetes, one third had some form of heart disease, and only nine reported never having smoked. Participants who were current smokers were instructed to refrain from smoking on the day of the study. Participants walked on a treadmill at a set speed and incline with the total distance in meters and distance walked at onset of claudication symptoms noted. Oxygen saturation of hemoglobin was measured in the gastrocnemius muscle during exercise testing using a tissue spectrometer probe attached to the muscle. A RAND Short Form-36 version 2 (SF-36 v2) was used to measure participants' perceived physical function and psychological well-being. Subjective walking ability was measured using the Walking Impairment Questionnaire (WIQ), and depression symptoms were measured with Center for Epidemiological Studies-Depression Scale (CES-D).

Findings

Walking endurance was poor among the 105 participants, but was similar in the smokers and nonsmokers. However, the time to onset of claudication symptoms was at a shorter distance among the smokers (142.6 vs. 247.7 m, $p = 0.01$). Moreover, current smokers had a steeper drop in calf muscle oxygenation from baseline to 2 minutes into the treadmill test than the nonsmokers (42.3% vs. 33%, $p < 0.05$). Covariate analyses including age as a factor did not change the relationship between smoking status and onset of claudication symptoms. There were no differences in other physiologic measures related to PAD, including ABI, nor any other measure of calf muscle tissue oxygenation. The composite score for mental health functioning from the SF-36 was lower in the smokers than the nonsmokers ($p < 0.0125$). The smokers had lower levels of self-reported physical functioning, lower levels of vitality, poorer social functioning, lower perceived emotional role functioning, and lower perceived mental health well-being. There were no differences identified in the self-perceived ability to walk a specified distance, walk fast, or climb stairs as measured by the WIQ.

Nursing Implications

Prior studies have reported reduced HR-QoL among patients with PAD; however, none have compared smokers to nonsmokers with PAD. The findings from this study suggest that smoking may have an additive detrimental effect on both mental and physical domains of HR-QoL in patients with PAD. While the mechanism by which smoking affects HR-QoL is unknown, a smoking cessation plan is an important adjunctive therapy to improve the quality of life in patients with PAD who smoke. In this study, the smokers were found to have an earlier onset of claudication symptoms during walking than the nonsmokers. Smoking cessation as part of a treatment plan for patients with PAD may enhance their walking ability. Promotion of disease self-management is a key principle to attaining positive outcomes. Nurses are at the forefront of patient care and play an essential role in the coordination of care, providing patient education and helping empower patients to take ownership of their health.

Measures to prevent these complications must be a high priority and vigorously implemented.

Trauma to the extremities must be avoided. Advising the patient to wear sturdy, well-fitting shoes or slippers to prevent foot injury and blisters may be helpful, and recommending neutral soaps and body lotions may prevent drying and cracking of skin. However, the nurse should instruct the patient not to apply lotion between the toes, because the increased moisture can lead to maceration of tissue. Scratching and vigorous rubbing can abrade skin and create sites for bacterial invasion; therefore, feet should be patted dry. Stockings should be clean and dry. Fingernails and toenails should be carefully trimmed straight across and sharp corners filed to follow the contour of the nail. If the nails cannot be trimmed safely, it is necessary to consult a podiatrist, who can also remove corns and calluses. Special shoe inserts may be needed to prevent calluses from recurring. All signs of blisters, ingrown toenails, infection, or other problems should be reported to health care professionals for treatment and follow-up. Patients with diminished vision and those with disabilities that limit mobility of the arms or legs may require assistance in periodically examining the lower extremities for trauma or evidence of inflammation or infection.

Good nutrition promotes healing and prevents tissue breakdown and is therefore included in the overall therapeutic program for patients with peripheral vascular disease. Eating a diet that contains adequate protein and vitamins is necessary for patients with arterial insufficiency. Key nutrients play specific roles in wound healing. However, a meta-analysis of randomized controlled trials found no evidence to support that supplementation with vitamins and antioxidants prevents vascular diseases (Myung, Ju, Cho, et al., 2013). Obesity strains the heart, increases venous congestion, and reduces circulation; therefore, a weight reduction plan may

Chart 30-5

HOME CARE CHECKLIST
Foot and Leg Care in Peripheral Vascular Disease

At the completion of education, the patient and/or caregiver will be able to:

- Describe the rationale for proper foot and leg care in managing peripheral vascular disease.
- Demonstrate daily foot bathing: Wash between toes with mild soap and lukewarm water, then rinse thoroughly and pat rather than rub dry.
- Recognize the dangers of thermal injury.
  - Wear clean, loose, soft cotton socks (they are comfortable, allow air to circulate, and absorb moisture)
  - In cold weather, wear extra socks in extra-large shoes.
  - Avoid heating pads, whirlpools, and hot tubs.
  - Avoid sunburn.
- Identify safety concerns.
  - Inspect feet daily with a mirror for redness, dryness, cuts, blisters, and so forth.
  - Always wear soft shoes or slippers when out of bed.
  - Trim nails straight across after showering.
  - Consult podiatrist to trim nails if vision is decreased and for care of corns, blisters, and ingrown nails.
  - Clear pathways in house to prevent injury.
  - Avoid wearing thong sandals.
  - Use lamb's wool between toes if they overlap or rub each other.
- Demonstrate the use of comfort measures.
  - Wear leather shoes with an extra-depth toe box. Synthetic shoes do not allow air to circulate.

- If feet become dry and scaly, use cream with lanolin. Never put cream between toes.
- Avoid scratching or vigorous rubbing which could cause abrasions.
- If feet perspire, especially between toes, use powder daily and/or lamb's wool between toes to promote drying.
- Demonstrate strategies to decrease risk of constricting blood vessels.
  - Avoid circular compression around feet or knees—e.g., by applying knee-high stockings or tight socks.
  - Do not cross legs at knees.
  - Stop using all tobacco products (i.e., smoking or chewing) because nicotine causes vasoconstriction and vasospasm.
  - Avoid applying tight, constricting bandages.
  - Participate in a regular walking exercise program to stimulate circulation.
- Recognize when to seek medical attention.
  - Contact health care provider at the onset of skin breakdown such as abrasions, blisters, fungus infection (athlete's foot), or pain.
  - Do not use any medication on feet or legs unless prescribed.
  - Avoid using iodine, alcohol, corn/wart-removing compound, or adhesive products before checking with primary provider.
- State understanding of community resources and referrals (if any).

---

be necessary for some patients. A diet low in lipids may be indicated for patients with atherosclerosis.

Gerontologic Considerations

In older adults, symptoms of PAD may be more pronounced than in younger people. In older patients who are inactive, limb ischemia or gangrene may be the first sign of disease (Walker, Bunch, Cavros, et al., 2015). These patients may have adjusted their lifestyle to accommodate the limitations imposed by the disease and may not walk far enough to develop symptoms of claudication due to other comorbid conditions such as chronic obstructive pulmonary disease (COPD) or congestive heart failure. Circulation is decreased, although this is not apparent to the patient until trauma occurs. At this point, gangrene develops when minimal arterial flow is impaired further by edema formation resulting from the traumatic event.

Intermittent claudication may occur after walking only one half to one block or after walking up a slight incline. Any prolonged pressure on the foot can cause pressure areas that become ulcerated, infected, and gangrenous. The outcomes of arterial insufficiency can include reduced mobility and activity as well as a loss of independence. Older adults with reduced mobility are less likely to remain in the community setting, have higher rates of hospitalizations, and experience a poorer quality of life (Walker et al., 2015).

Promoting Home, Community-Based, and Transitional Care

The self-care program is planned with the patient so that activities that promote arterial and venous circulation,

relieve pain, and promote tissue integrity are acceptable. The patient and family are helped to understand the reasons for each aspect of the program, the possible consequences of nonadherence, and the importance of keeping follow-up appointments. Long-term care of the feet and legs is of prime importance in the prevention of trauma, ulceration, and gangrene. Chart 30-5 provides detailed patient instructions for foot and leg care.

Peripheral Arterial Occlusive Disease

Arterial insufficiency of the extremities occurs most often in men and is a common cause of disability. The legs are most frequently affected; however, the upper extremities may be involved. The age of onset and the severity are influenced by the type and number of atherosclerotic risk factors (see Chart 30-2). In PAD, obstructive lesions are predominantly confined to segments of the arterial system extending from the aorta below the renal arteries to the popliteal artery (see Fig. 30-9). Distal occlusive disease is frequently seen in patients with diabetes and in older patients (Conte et al., 2015).

Clinical Manifestations

The hallmark symptom is intermittent claudication described as aching, cramping, or inducing fatigue or weakness that occurs with some degree of exercise or activity, which is relieved with rest. The pain commonly occurs in muscle groups distal to the area of stenosis or occlusion. As the disease progresses, the patient may have a decreased ability to walk the same distance as before or may notice increased pain with ambulation. When the arterial insufficiency becomes severe, the patient

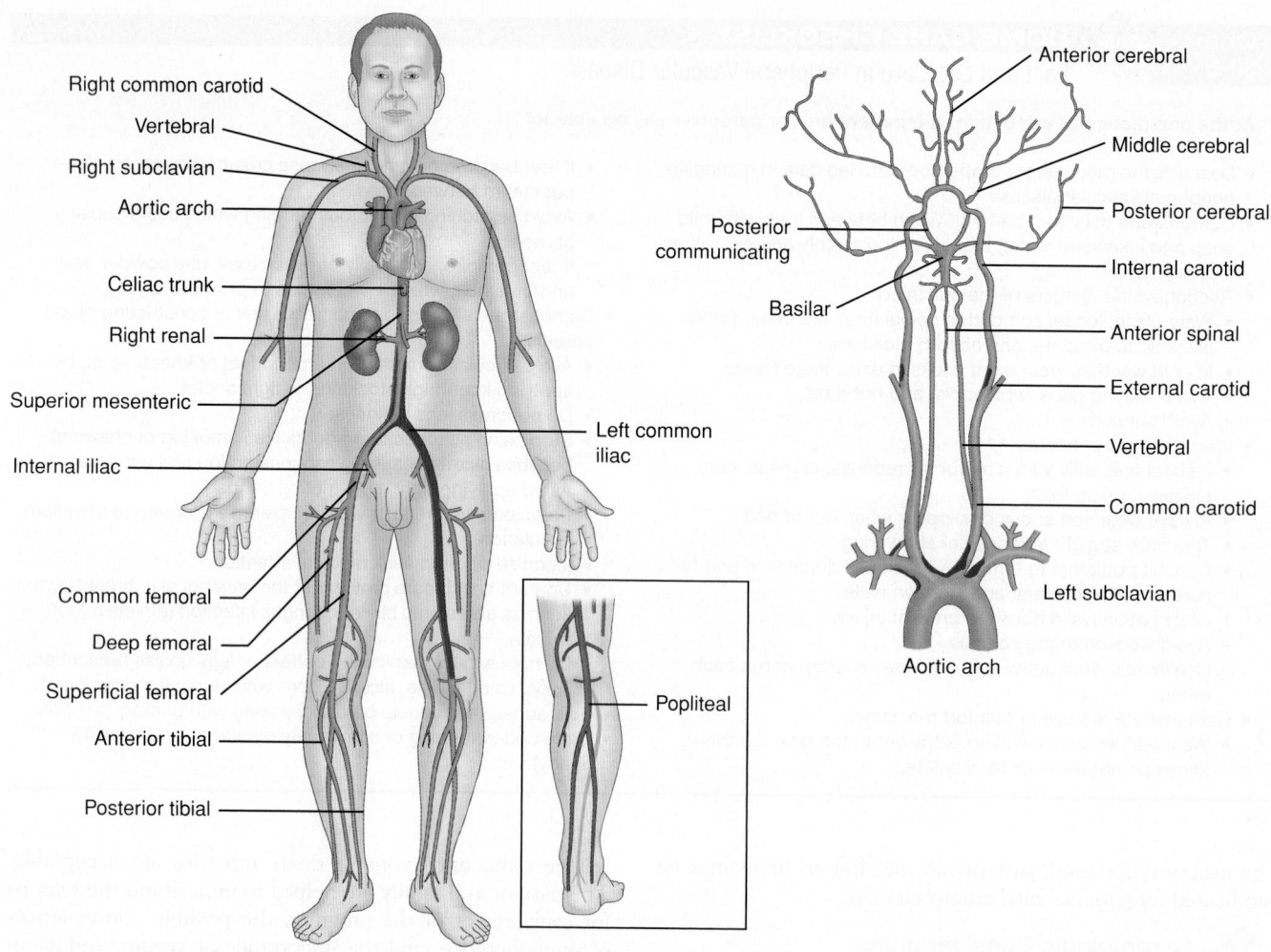

Figure 30-9 • Common sites of atherosclerotic obstruction in major arteries.

has rest pain. This pain is associated with critical ischemia of the distal extremity and is described as persistent, aching, or boring; it may be so excruciating that it is unrelieved by opioids and can be disabling. Ischemic rest pain is usually worse at night and often wakes the patient. Elevating the extremity or placing it in a horizontal position increases the pain, whereas placing the extremity in a dependent position reduces the pain. Some patients sleep with the affected leg hanging over the side of the bed. Some patients sleep in a reclining chair in an attempt to prevent or relieve the pain.

Assessment and Diagnostic Findings

A sensation of coldness or numbness in the extremities may accompany intermittent claudication and is a result of reduced arterial flow. The extremity is cool and pale when elevated or ruddy and cyanotic when placed in a dependent position. Skin and nail changes, ulcerations, gangrene, and muscle atrophy may be evident. Bruits may be auscultated with a stethoscope. Peripheral pulses may be diminished or absent.

Examination of the peripheral pulses is an important part of assessing arterial occlusive disease. Unequal pulses between extremities or the absence of a normally palpable pulse is a sign of PAD.

The presence, location, and extent of arterial occlusive disease are determined by a careful history of the symptoms and by physical examination. The color and temperature of the extremity are noted and the pulses palpated. The nails may be thickened and opaque, and the skin may be shiny, atrophic, and dry, with sparse hair growth. The assessment includes comparison of the right and left extremities.

The diagnosis of peripheral arterial occlusive disease may be made using CW Doppler and ABIs, treadmill testing for claudication, duplex ultrasonography, or other imaging studies described earlier in this chapter.

Medical Management

Generally, patients feel better and have fewer symptoms of claudication after they participate in an exercise program. Unsupervised walking exercise programs are attractive for many patients with PAD as they may not have access to a supervised exercise program, their insurance will not cover a supervised exercise program, or they like the independence that an unsupervised program gives them. Two recent trials of unsupervised walking exercise in patients with PAD found similar findings between the supervised and unsupervised groups, suggesting no greater therapeutic benefit for those who engage in supervised walking programs (McDermott, 2013).

These findings suggest that home-based programs may be a viable and efficacious option for patients unable to participate in a structured, on-site, supervised exercise program. If a walking program is combined with weight reduction and cessation of tobacco use, patients often can further improve their activity tolerance. Patients should not be promised that their symptoms will be relieved if they stop tobacco use, however, because claudication may persist, and they may lose their motivation to stop using tobacco. In addition to these interventions, arm-ergometer exercise training effectively improves physical fitness, central cardiorespiratory function, and walking capacity in patients with PAD claudication symptoms (McDermott, 2013).

Pharmacologic Therapy

Pentoxifylline (Trental) and cilostazol (Pletal) are approved by the U.S. Food and Drug Administration (FDA) for the treatment of symptomatic claudication. Pentoxifylline increases erythrocyte flexibility, lowers blood fibrinogen concentrations, and inhibits neutrophil adhesion and activation. Despite its physiologic effects, however, there has been no positive effect on ABIs at rest or postexercise in multiple trials; therefore, its usefulness is questionable in treatment of PAD (Conte et al., 2015). Cilostazol, a phosphodiesterase III inhibitor, is a direct vasodilator that inhibits platelet aggregation. Studies have shown it plays a role in decreasing intimal hyperplasia after angioplasty and stenting. Furthermore, patients prescribed cilostazol report improvement in maximal walking distance and pain-free walking distance within 4 to 6 weeks (Neel, Kruse, Drombrovskiy, et al., 2015). This agent is contraindicated in patients with a history of congestive heart failure or an ejection fraction less than 40%.

Antiplatelet agents such as aspirin or clopidogrel (Plavix) prevent the formation of thromboemboli, which can lead to myocardial infarction and stroke. Aspirin has been shown to reduce the risk of cardiovascular events (e.g., myocardial infarction, stroke, and cardiovascular death) in patients with vascular disease; however, adverse events associated with aspirin use include gastrointestinal upset or bleeding (Conte et al., 2015).

Statins improve endothelial function in patients with PAD. Studies suggest that statins improve symptoms of intermittent claudication and also increase walking distance to the onset of claudication (Barochiner et al., 2014). These medications have beneficial effects on vascular inflammation, plaque stabilization, endothelial dysfunction, and thrombosis, and have been linked to decreased rates of repeat peripheral interventions, amputations, and major adverse cardiovascular events up to 3 years postprocedure (Armstrong et al., 2014).

Endovascular Management

Radiologic interventional (endovascular) management can include a balloon angioplasty, stent, stent graft, or an atherectomy. These revascularization procedures are less invasive than conventional surgery; their objective is to establish adequate inflow to the distal vessels. A recent meta-analysis reported that the efficacy and safety of all of these endovascular procedures are comparable to surgical interventions. Some stents that may be selected are drug eluting. Although costly, these are particularly efficacious in patients who have recurrent disease. By releasing antiproliferative drugs such as paclitaxel, drug-eluting balloons and stents have been shown to reduce the risk of restenosis. Eligible candidates for drug-eluting stents must be able to take antiplatelet medications for 6 months post procedure (Di Minno, Spadarella, Cafaro, et al., 2014).

Surgical Management

Surgery is reserved for the treatment of severe and disabling claudication or when the limb is at risk for amputation because of tissue necrosis. The choice of the surgical procedure depends on the degree and location of the stenosis or occlusion. Other important considerations are the overall health of the patient and the length of the procedure that can be tolerated. For patients whose overall health is so compromised that they cannot tolerate an extensive vascular surgical procedure, it is sometimes necessary to provide the palliative therapy of primary amputation rather than arterial bypass. If endarterectomy is performed, an incision is made into the artery and the atheromatous obstruction is removed (see Fig. 30-10).

Bypass grafts are performed to reroute the blood flow around the stenosis or occlusion. Before bypass grafting, the surgeon determines where the distal **anastomosis** (site where the vessels are surgically joined) will be placed. The distal outflow vessel must be at least 50% patent for the graft to remain patent. If the atherosclerotic occlusion is below the inguinal ligament in the superficial femoral artery, the surgical procedure of choice is the femoral-to-popliteal graft. This procedure is further classified as above-knee and below-knee grafts, referring to the location of the distal anastomosis.

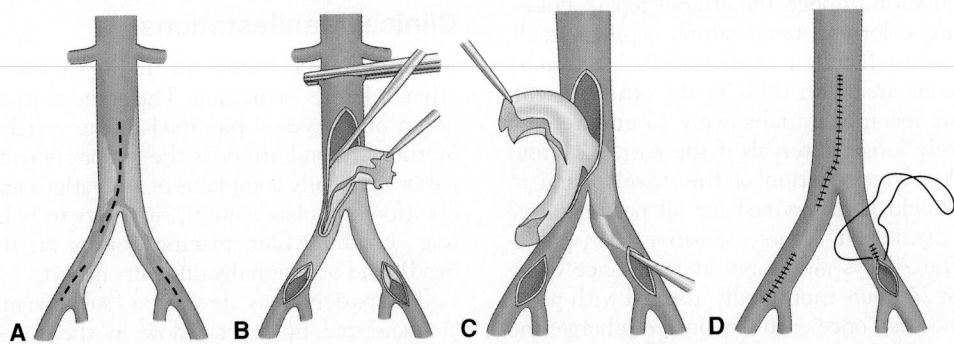

Figure 30-10 • In an aortoiliac endarterectomy, the vascular surgeon identifies the diseased area (**A**), clamps off the blood supply to the vessel (**B**), removes the plaque (**C**), and sutures the vessel shut (**D**), after which blood flow is restored. Adapted with permission from Cronenwett, J. L., & Johnston, K. W. (2014). *Rutherford's vascular surgery* (8th ed., *Vols. 1 and 2*). Philadelphia, PA: W. B. Saunders.

Lower leg or ankle vessels with occlusions may also require grafts. Occasionally, the popliteal artery is completely occluded and only collateral vessels maintain perfusion. The distal anastomosis may be made onto any of the tibial arteries (posterior tibial, anterior tibial, or peroneal arteries) or the dorsalis pedis or plantar artery. The distal anastomosis site is determined by the ease of exposure of the vessel in surgery and by which vessel provides the best flow to the distal limb. These grafts require the use of native vein (i.e., autologous—the patient's own vein) to ensure patency. The greater or lesser saphenous vein or a combination of one of the saphenous veins and an upper extremity vein such as the cephalic vein is used to provide the required length.

How long the graft remains patent is determined by several factors, including the size of the graft, graft location, and development of intimal hyperplasia at anastomosis sites (Conte et al., 2015). Bypass grafts may be synthetic or use autologous vein. Several synthetic materials are available for use as a peripheral bypass graft: woven or knitted Dacron or expanded polytetrafluoroethylene (PTFE, such as Gore-Tex or Impra). Cryopreserved saphenous veins and umbilical veins are also available. Infection can be a problem that threatens survival of the graft and almost always requires its removal.

If a vein graft is the surgical choice, care must be taken in the operating room not to damage the vein after harvesting (removing the vein from the patient's body). The vein is occluded at one end and inflated with a heparinized solution to check for leakage and competency. The graft is then placed in a heparinized solution to keep it from becoming dry and brittle.

Nursing Management

Nursing care for patients with peripheral vascular disease is reviewed in Chart 30-3. Nursing care for the patient who has had endovascular revascularization procedures mostly mirrors the care of patients who have had endovascular repair to aortic aneurysms (see later section). The patient who has had an endovascular procedure may be discharged home the day of the procedure, or by the following day.

Nursing Care of the Postoperative Patient

Maintaining Circulation

The primary objective in the postoperative period is to maintain adequate circulation through the arterial repair. Pulses, Doppler assessment, color and temperature, capillary refill, and sensory and motor function of the affected extremity are checked and compared with those of the other extremity; these values are recorded initially every 15 minutes and then at progressively longer intervals if the patient's status remains stable. Doppler evaluation of the vessels distal to the bypass graft should be performed for all postoperative vascular patients, because it is more sensitive than palpation for pulses. The ABI is monitored at least once every 8 hours for the first 24 hours (not usually assessed with pedal artery bypasses) and then once each day until discharge; the typical hospital length of stay is 3 to 5 days postoperatively. An adequate circulating blood volume should be established and maintained. Disappearance of a pulse that was present

may indicate thrombotic occlusion of the graft; the surgeon is immediately notified.

Monitoring and Managing Potential Complications

Continuous monitoring of urine output, central venous pressure, mental status, and pulse rate and volume permits early recognition and treatment of fluid imbalances. Bleeding can result from the heparin given during surgery or from an anastomotic leak. A hematoma may form as well.

Leg crossing and prolonged extremity dependency are avoided to prevent thrombosis. Edema is a normal postoperative finding; however, elevating the extremities and encouraging the patient to exercise the extremities while in bed reduces edema. Graduated compression or anti-embolism stockings may be prescribed for some patients, but care must be taken to avoid compressing distal vessel bypass grafts. Severe edema of the extremity, pain, and decreased sensation of toes or fingers can be an indication of compartment syndrome (see Chapter 42).

Promoting Home, Community-Based, and Transitional Care

Discharge planning includes assessing the patient's ability to manage activities of daily living (ADLs) independently. The nurse determines whether the patient has a network of family and friends to assist with ADLs. The patient is encouraged to make the lifestyle changes necessitated by the onset of a chronic disease, including pain management and modifications in diet, activity, and hygiene (skin care). The nurse ensures that the patient has the knowledge and ability to assess for any postoperative complications such as infection, occlusion of the artery or graft, and decreased blood flow. The nurse assists the patient in developing and implementing a plan to stop using tobacco products.

Upper Extremity Arterial Occlusive Disease

Arterial occlusions occur less frequently in the upper extremities (arms) than in the legs, and cause less severe symptoms because the collateral circulation is significantly better in the arms. The arms also have less muscle mass and are not subjected to the workload of the legs.

Clinical Manifestations

Stenosis and occlusions in the upper extremity result from atherosclerosis or trauma. The stenosis usually occurs at the origin of the vessel proximal to the vertebral artery, setting up the vertebral artery as the major contributor of flow. The patient typically complains of arm fatigue and pain with exercise (forearm claudication), inability to hold or grasp objects (e.g., combing hair, placing objects on shelves above the head), and occasionally difficulty driving.

The patient may develop a "subclavian steal" syndrome characterized by reverse flow in the vertebral and basilar arteries to provide blood flow to the arm. This syndrome may cause vertebrobasilar (cerebral) symptoms, including vertigo, ataxia, syncope, or bilateral visual changes.

Assessment and Diagnostic Findings

Assessment findings include coolness and pallor of the affected extremity, decreased capillary refill, and a difference in arm blood pressures of more than 20 mm Hg (Zierler & Dawson, 2015). Noninvasive studies performed to evaluate for upper extremity arterial occlusions include upper and forearm blood pressure determinations and duplex ultrasonography to identify the anatomic location of the lesion and to evaluate the hemodynamics of the blood flow. Transcranial Doppler evaluation is performed to evaluate the intracranial circulation and to detect any siphoning of blood flow from the posterior circulation to provide blood flow to the affected arm. If a surgical or interventional procedure is planned, a diagnostic arteriogram may be necessary.

Medical Management

If a short focal lesion is identified in an upper extremity artery, a PTA with possible stent or stent graft placement may be performed. If the lesion involves the subclavian artery with documented siphoning of blood flow from the intracranial circulation and an interventional radiologic (endovascular) procedure is not possible, a surgical bypass may be performed.

Nursing Management

Nursing assessment involves bilateral comparison of upper arm blood pressures (obtained by stethoscope and Doppler), radial, ulnar, and brachial pulses, motor and sensory function, temperature, color changes, and capillary refill every 2 hours. Disappearance of a pulse or Doppler flow that had been present may indicate an acute occlusion of the vessel, and the primary provider is notified immediately.

After surgery or endovascular procedure, the arm is kept at heart level or elevated, with the fingers at the highest level. Pulses are monitored with Doppler assessment of the arterial flow every hour for 2 hours and then every shift. Blood pressure (obtained by stethoscope and Doppler) is also assessed every hour for 4 hours and then every shift. Motor and sensory function, warmth, color, and capillary refill are monitored with each arterial flow (pulse) assessment.

> ◤ *Quality and Safety Nursing Alert*
>
> *Before surgery and for 24 hours after surgery, the patient's arm is kept at heart level and protected from cold, venipunctures or arterial sticks, tape, and constrictive dressings.*

Discharge planning is similar to that for the patient with peripheral arterial occlusive disease. Chart 30-3 describes nursing care for patients with peripheral vascular disease.

Aortoiliac Disease

If collateral circulation has developed, patients with a stenosis or occlusion of the aortoiliac segment may be asymptomatic, or they may complain of buttock or low back discomfort associated with walking. Men may experience impotence. These patients may have decreased or absent femoral pulses.

Medical Management

The treatment of aortoiliac disease is essentially the same as that for atherosclerotic peripheral arterial occlusive disease. An endovascular procedure, such as bilateral common iliac stents, may be attempted if the aorta has a less than 50% diameter reduction (Conte et al., 2015). If there is significant aortic disease, the surgical procedure of choice is the aortoiliac graft. If possible, the distal graft is anastomosed to the iliac artery, and the entire surgical procedure is performed within the abdomen. If the iliac vessels are occluded, the distal anastomosis is made to the femoral arteries (aortobifemoral graft). Bifurcated woven or knitted Dacron grafts are preferred for this surgical procedure.

Nursing Management

Preprocedural or preoperative assessment, in addition to the standard parameters (see Chapter 17), includes evaluating the brachial, radial, ulnar, femoral, posterior tibial, and dorsalis pedis pulses to establish a baseline for follow-up after arterial lines are placed and postoperatively. Patient education includes an overview of the procedure to be performed, the preparation for surgery, and the anticipated postoperative plan of care. Sights, sounds, and sensations that the patient may experience are discussed.

Postprocedural endovascular care mirrors the care described for the patient who has had endovascular repair of an aortic aneurysm (see later discussion). Postoperative care includes monitoring for signs of thrombosis in arteries distal to the surgical site. The nurse assesses color and temperature of the extremity, capillary refill time, sensory and motor function, and pulses by palpation and Doppler initially every 15 minutes and then at progressively longer intervals if the patient's status remains stable. Any dusky or bluish discoloration, coldness, decrease in sensory or motor function, or decrease in pulse quality is reported immediately to the primary provider.

Postoperative care also includes monitoring urine output and ensuring that output is at least 0.5 mL/kg/h. Renal function may be impaired as a result of hypoperfusion from hypotension, ischemia to the renal arteries during the surgical procedure, hypovolemia, or embolization of the renal artery or renal parenchyma. Vital signs, pain, and intake and output are monitored with the pulse and extremity assessments. Results of laboratory tests are monitored and reported to the primary provider. Abdominal assessment for bowel sounds and paralytic ileus is performed at least every 8 hours. Bowel sounds may not return before the third postoperative day. The absence of bowel sounds, absence of flatus, and abdominal distention are indications of paralytic ileus. Manual manipulation of the bowel during surgery may have caused bruising, resulting in decreased peristalsis. Nasogastric suction may be necessary to decompress the bowel until peristalsis returns. A liquid bowel movement before the third postoperative day may indicate bowel ischemia, which may occur when the mesenteric blood supply (celiac, superior mesenteric, or inferior mesenteric arteries) is occluded. Ischemic bowel usually causes increased pain and a markedly elevated white blood cell count (20,000 to 30,000 cells/mm^3).

Figure 30-11 • Characteristics of arterial aneurysm. **A.** Normal artery. **B.** False aneurysm—actually a pulsating hematoma. The clot and connective tissue are outside the arterial wall. **C.** True aneurysm. One, two, or all three layers of the artery may be involved. **D.** Fusiform aneurysm—symmetric, spindle-shaped expansion of entire circumference of involved vessel. **E.** Saccular aneurysm—a bulbous protrusion of one side of the arterial wall. **F.** Dissecting aneurysm—this usually is a hematoma that splits the layers of the arterial wall. Adapted with permission from Cronenwett, J. L., & Johnston, K. W. (2014). *Rutherford's vascular surgery* (8th ed., *Vols. 1 and 2*). Philadelphia, PA: W. B. Saunders.

Aneurysms

An aneurysm is a localized sac or dilation formed at a weak point in the wall of the artery (see Fig. 30-11). It may be classified by its shape or form. The most common forms of aneurysms are saccular and fusiform. A saccular aneurysm projects from only one side of the vessel. If an entire arterial segment becomes dilated, a fusiform aneurysm develops. Very small aneurysms due to localized infection are called *mycotic aneurysms*.

Historically, the cause of abdominal aortic aneurysm, the most common type of degenerative aneurysm, has been attributed to atherosclerotic changes in the aorta. Other causes of aneurysm formation are listed in Chart 30-6. Aneurysms are potentially serious; if they are located in large vessels that rupture, this can lead to hemorrhage and death.

Thoracic Aortic Aneurysm

Approximately 70% of all cases of thoracic aortic aneurysm are caused by atherosclerosis. They occur most frequently in men between the ages of 50 and 70 years, and are estimated to affect 10 of every 100,000 older adults. The thoracic area

---

Chart 30-6 · Etiologic Classification of Arterial Aneurysms

Congenital: Primary connective tissue disorders (Marfan syndrome, Ehlers–Danlos syndrome) and other diseases (focal medial agenesis, tuberous sclerosis, Turner syndrome, Menkes syndrome)

Mechanical (hemodynamic): Poststenotic and arteriovenous fistula and amputation related

Traumatic (pseudoaneurysms): Penetrating arterial injuries, blunt arterial injuries, pseudoaneurysms

Inflammatory (noninfectious): Associated with arteritis (Takayasu disease, giant cell arteritis, systemic lupus erythematosus, Behçet syndrome, Kawasaki disease) and periarterial inflammation (i.e., pancreatitis)

Infectious (mycotic): Bacterial, fungal, spirochetal infections

Pregnancy-related degenerative: Nonspecific, inflammatory variant

Anastomotic (postarteriotomy) and graft aneurysms: Infection, arterial wall failure, suture failure, graft failure

Adapted from Cronenwett, J. L., & Johnston, K. W. (2014). *Rutherford's vascular surgery* (8th ed., Vols. 1 and 2). Philadelphia, PA: W. B. Saunders.

---

is the most common site for a dissecting aneurysm. Thoracic aortic emergencies are associated with high morbidity and mortality rates, but with the emergence of endovascular aortic repair there is an improvement in the mortality rate; in particular, the mortality rate for patients treated at high-volume aortic centers can be as low as 4.8% (Patel, Williams, Drews, et al., 2014).

Clinical Manifestations

Symptoms vary and depend on how rapidly the aneurysm dilates and how the pulsating mass affects surrounding intrathoracic structures. Some patients are asymptomatic. In most cases, pain is the most prominent symptom. The pain is usually constant and boring but may occur only when the person is supine. Other conspicuous symptoms are dyspnea, the result of pressure of the aneurysm sac against the trachea, a main bronchus, or the lung itself; cough, frequently paroxysmal and with a brassy quality; hoarseness, stridor, or weakness or complete loss of the voice (aphonia), resulting from pressure against the laryngeal nerve; and dysphagia (difficulty in swallowing) due to impingement on the esophagus by the aneurysm.

Assessment and Diagnostic Findings

When large veins in the chest are compressed by the aneurysm, the superficial veins of the chest, neck, or arms become dilated, and edematous areas on the chest wall and cyanosis are often evident. Pressure against the cervical sympathetic chain can result in unequal pupils. Diagnosis of a thoracic aortic aneurysm is principally made by chest x-ray, computed tomography angiography (CTA), MRA, or transesophageal echocardiography (TEE). CTAs are typically performed because they are widely available, can be completed rapidly, and can remove cardiac motion artifacts, enhancing their accuracy (Rajiah, 2013).

Medical Management

Treatment is based on whether the aneurysm is symptomatic, is expanding in size, is caused by an iatrogenic injury, contains a dissection, and involves branch vessels. General measures such as controlling blood pressure and correcting risk factors are helpful. For decades, beta blockers (e.g., atenolol [Tenormin], metoprolol [Lopressor, Toprol XL], carvedilol [Coreg]), have been the mainstay of medical treatment for aortic aneurysms; however, angiotensin receptor blockers (ARBs) (e.g., losartan [Cozaar], valsartan [Diovan], irbesartan [Avapro]) may also retard aortic dilatation (Attenhofer Jost, Greutmann, Connolly, et al., 2014). It is also important to control blood pressure in patients with dissecting aneurysms. Preoperatively, the systolic pressure is maintained at approximately 90 to 120 mm Hg in order to maintain a mean arterial pressure at 65 to 75 mm Hg with a beta blocker such as esmolol (Brevibloc), or metoprolol. Occasionally, antihypertensive agents such as hydralazine (Apresoline) are used for this purpose. Sodium nitroprusside (Nipride) is the most established drug used for this purpose; it is given by continuous IV drip to emergently lower the blood pressure, as it has a rapid onset and short action of duration and is easily titrated (Suzuki, Eagle, Bossone, et al., 2014). The goal of surgery is to repair the aneurysm and restore vascular continuity with a vascular graft. Intensive monitoring is usually required after this type of surgery, and the patient is cared for in the critical care unit.

Repair of thoracic aneurysms using endovascular grafts placed percutaneously in an interventional suite (e.g., interventional radiology, cardiac catheterization laboratory) or combined interventional suite and operating room may decrease postoperative recovery time and decrease complications compared with traditional surgical techniques. Thoracic endografts are made of Gore-Tex or PTFE material reinforced with nitinol or titanium stents. These endovascular grafts are inserted into the thoracic aorta via various vascular access routes, usually the brachial or femoral artery. Because a large surgical incision is not necessary to gain vascular access, the overall patient recovery time tends to be shorter than with open surgical repair. Despite the absence of aortic cross-clamping, there is still a 2% to 15% chance of spinal cord ischemia as a potential complication (DeSart, Scali, Feezor, et al., 2013). To decrease the chances of spinal cord ischemia and paraplegia, lumbar spinal drains are usually placed in patients undergoing an endovascular repair of thoracic aortic aneurysms. Cerebrospinal fluid drainage is performed to decrease the arterial to cerebral spinal fluid gradient, thereby improving spinal perfusion. What appears to be most important in preventing neurologic deficit is to maintain the cerebrospinal fluid pressure less than or equal to 10 mm Hg (14 cm H_2O) and to keep the mean arterial pressure greater than 90 mm Hg for the first 36 to 48 hours postoperatively (DeSart et al., 2013).

Abdominal Aortic Aneurysm

The most common cause of abdominal aortic aneurysm is atherosclerosis. This condition affects men 2 to 6 times more often than women, is 2 to 3 times more common in Caucasian versus black men, and is most prevalent in patients older than 65 years of age (Kuivaniemi, Ryer, Elmore, et al., 2014). Most of these aneurysms occur below the renal arteries (infrarenal aneurysms). Untreated, the eventual outcome may be rupture and death.

Pathophysiology

All aneurysms involve a damaged media layer of the vessel. This may be caused by congenital weakness, trauma, or disease. After an aneurysm develops, it tends to enlarge. Risk factors include genetic predisposition, tobacco use, and

hypertension; more than half of patients with aneurysms have hypertension.

Clinical Manifestations

Only about 40% of patients with abdominal aortic aneurysms have symptoms. Some patients complain that they can feel their heart beating in their abdomen when lying down, or they may say that they feel an abdominal mass or abdominal throbbing. If the abdominal aortic aneurysm is associated with thrombus, a major vessel may be occluded or smaller distal occlusions may result from emboli. Small cholesterol, platelet, or fibrin emboli may lodge in the interosseous or digital arteries, causing cyanosis and mottling of the toes.

Signs of impending rupture include severe back or abdominal pain, which may be persistent or intermittent. Abdominal pain is often localized in the middle or lower abdomen to the left of the midline. Low back pain may be present because of pressure of the aneurysm on the lumbar nerves. Indications of a rupturing abdominal aortic aneurysm include constant, intense back pain; falling blood pressure; and decreasing hematocrit. Rupture into the peritoneal cavity is rapidly fatal. A retroperitoneal rupture of an aneurysm may result in hematomas in the scrotum, perineum, flank, or penis. Signs of heart failure or a loud bruit may suggest a rupture into the vena cava. If the aneurysm adheres to the adjacent vena cava, the vena cava may become damaged when rupture or leak of the aneurysm occurs. Rupture into the vena cava results in higher-pressure arterial blood entering the lower-pressure venous system and causing turbulence, which is heard as a bruit. The high blood pressure and increased blood volume returning to the right side of the heart from the vena cava may cause right-sided heart failure.

Assessment and Diagnostic Findings

The most important diagnostic indication of an abdominal aortic aneurysm is a pulsatile mass in the middle and upper abdomen. Most clinically significant aortic aneurysms are palpable during routine physical examination; however, the sensitivity depends upon the size of the aneurysm, abdominal girth of the patient (i.e., more difficult to find in the patient with obesity), and the skill of the examiner (Cronenwett & Johnston, 2014). A systolic bruit may be heard over the mass. Duplex ultrasonography or CTA is used to determine the size, length, and location of the aneurysm. When the aneurysm is small, ultrasonography is conducted at 6-month intervals until the aneurysm reaches a size so that surgery to prevent rupture is of more benefit than the possible complications of a surgical procedure. Some aneurysms remain stable over many years of monitoring.

 ## Gerontologic Considerations

Most abdominal aortic aneurysms occur in patients between 60 and 90 years of age. Rupture is likely with coexisting hypertension and with aneurysms more than 6 cm wide. In most cases at this point, the chances of rupture are greater than the chances of death during surgical repair. If the older patient is considered at risk for complications related to surgery or anesthesia, the aneurysm is not repaired until it is at least 5.5 cm (2 in) wide (DeMartino, Goodney, Nolan, et al., 2013).

Medical Management

Pharmacologic Therapy

If the aneurysm is stable in size based on serial duplex ultrasound scans, the blood pressure is closely monitored over time, because there is an association between increased blood pressure and aneurysm rupture (Kuivaniemi et al., 2014). Antihypertensive agents, including diuretics, beta blockers, ACE inhibitors, ARBs, and calcium channel blockers, are frequently prescribed to maintain the patient's blood pressure within acceptable limits (see Chapter 31).

Endovascular and Surgical Management

An expanding or enlarging abdominal aortic aneurysm is likely to rupture. When an abdominal aortic aneurysm measured at least 5.5 cm (2 in) wide or was enlarging, the standard treatment had been open surgical repair of the aneurysm by resecting the vessel and sewing a bypass graft in place. However, endovascular aortic repair has become a mainstay of therapy for treating an infrarenal abdominal aortic aneurysm and involves the transluminal placement and attachment of a sutureless aortic graft prosthesis across an aneurysm (see Fig. 30-12). This procedure can be performed under local or regional anesthesia. Endovascular grafting of abdominal aortic aneurysms may be performed if the patient's abdominal aorta and iliac arteries are not extremely tortuous, small, calcified, or filled with thrombi. Results from multiple, prospective studies suggest comparable mortality rates among patients with aneurysms treated by endovascular grafting and those treated with surgical repair, with similar 5-year survival rates (DeMartino et al., 2013). Potential complications include bleeding, hematoma, or wound infection at the arterial insertion site; distal ischemia or embolization; dissection or perforation of the aorta; graft thrombosis or infection; break of the attachment system; graft migration; proximal or distal graft leaks; delayed rupture; and bowel ischemia.

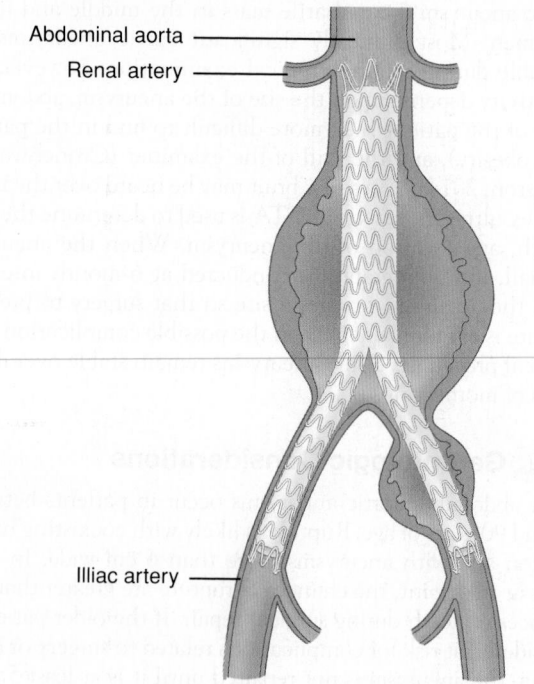

Abdominal aorta

Renal artery

Illiac artery

Figure 30-12 • Endograft repair of an abdominal aortic aneurysm.

Nursing Management

Before endovascular repair or surgery, nursing assessment is guided by anticipating a rupture and by recognizing that the patient may have cardiovascular, cerebral, pulmonary, and renal impairment from atherosclerosis. The functional capacity of all organ systems should be assessed. Medical therapies designed to stabilize physiologic function should be promptly implemented. Hemorrhage that leads to shock is a serious adverse consequence that must be treated decisively (see Chapter 14).

The patient who has had an endovascular repair must lie supine for 6 hours; the head of the bed may be elevated up to 45 degrees after 2 hours. The patient needs to use a bedpan or urinal while on bed rest. Vital signs and Doppler assessment of peripheral pulses are performed initially every 15 minutes and then at progressively longer intervals if the patient's status remains stable. The access site (usually the femoral artery) is assessed when vital signs and pulses are monitored. The nurse assesses for bleeding, pulsation, swelling, pain, and hematoma formation. Skin changes of the lower extremity, lumbar area, or buttocks that might indicate signs of embolization, such as extremely tender, irregularly shaped, cyanotic areas, as well as any changes in vital signs, pulse quality, bleeding, swelling, pain, or hematoma, are immediately reported to the primary provider.

The patient's temperature should be monitored every 4 hours, and any signs of postimplantation syndrome should be reported. Postimplantation syndrome typically begins within 24 hours of stent graft placement and consists of a spontaneously occurring fever, leukocytosis, and occasionally, transient thrombocytopenia. This condition has been attributed to complex immunologic changes that occur because of manipulations with sheaths and catheters with the aortic lumen, although the exact etiology is unknown. The symptoms are thought to be related to the activation of cytokines (Arnaoutoglou, Kouvelos, Koutsoumpelis, et al., 2015). They can be managed with a mild analgesic (e.g., acetaminophen [Tylenol]) or an anti-inflammatory agent (e.g., ibuprofen [Motrin]) and usually subside within a week.

Because of the increased risk of hemorrhage, the primary provider is also notified of persistent coughing, sneezing, vomiting, or systolic blood pressure greater than 180 mm Hg. Most patients can resume their preprocedure diet and are encouraged to drink fluids. An IV infusion may be continued until the patient can drink normally. Fluids are important to maintain blood flow through the arterial repair site and to assist the kidneys with excreting IV contrast agents and other medications used during the procedure. Six hours after the procedure, the patient may be able to roll from side to side and may be able to ambulate with assistance to the bathroom. Once the patient can take adequate fluids orally, the IV infusion may be discontinued.

Postoperative care requires frequent monitoring of pulmonary, cardiovascular, renal, and neurologic status. Possible complications of surgery include arterial occlusion, hemorrhage, infection, ischemic bowel, kidney injury, and impotence.

Other Aneurysms

Aneurysms may also arise in the peripheral vessels, most often as a result of atherosclerosis. These may involve such vessels as the subclavian artery, renal artery, femoral artery, or (most frequently) popliteal artery. Between 50% and 60% of popliteal aneurysms are bilateral; the true incidence is unknown but has been reported to be between 0.1% and 3% of the adult population and is associated with abdominal aortic aneurysms (Ronchey, Pecoraro, Alberti, et al., 2015).

The aneurysm produces a pulsating mass and disturbs peripheral circulation distal to it. Pain and swelling develop because of pressure on adjacent nerves and veins. Diagnosis is made by duplex ultrasonography or CTA to determine the size, length, and extent of the aneurysm. Arteriography may be performed to evaluate the level of proximal and distal involvement. The major complication associated with popliteal artery aneurysms is not rupture but distal embolization (Cronenwett & Johnston, 2014). Surgical repair is performed with replacement grafts. As an alternative, endovascular repair using a stent graft or wall graft, which is a Dacron or PTFE graft with external structures made from a variety of materials (e.g., nitinol, titanium, stainless steel) may be selected for additional support.

Dissecting Aorta

Occasionally, in an aorta diseased by arteriosclerosis, a tear develops in the intima or the media degenerates, resulting in a dissection (see Fig. 30-11). Arterial dissections are three times more common in men than in women, occur most commonly in the 50- to 70-year age group and are associated with hypertension (Bergmark, Sobieszczyk, Gravereaux, et al., 2013).

Pathophysiology

Arterial dissections (separations) are commonly associated with poorly controlled hypertension, blunt chest trauma, and cocaine use. The profound increase in sympathetic response caused by cocaine use creates an increase in the force of left ventricular contraction that causes heightened shear forces upon the aortic wall leading to disruption of the intima (Bergmark et al., 2013). Dissection is caused by rupture in the intimal layer. A rupture may occur through adventitia or into the lumen through the intima, allowing blood to reenter the main channel and resulting in chronic dissection (e.g., pseudoaneurysm) or occlusion of branches of the aorta.

As the separation progresses, the arteries branching from the involved area of the aorta shear and occlude. The tear occurs most commonly in the region of the aortic arch, with the highest mortality rate associated with ascending aortic dissection (Ziganshin, Dumfarth, & Elefteriades, 2014). The dissection of the aorta may progress backward in the direction of the heart, obstructing the openings to the coronary arteries or producing hemopericardium (effusion of blood into the pericardial sac) or aortic insufficiency, or it may extend in the opposite direction, causing occlusion of the arteries supplying the gastrointestinal tract, kidneys, spinal cord, and legs.

Clinical Manifestations

Onset of symptoms is usually sudden. Severe and persistent pain, described as tearing or ripping, may be reported. The pain is in the anterior chest or back and extends to the shoulders, epigastric area, or abdomen. Aortic dissection may be mistaken for an acute myocardial infarction, which confuses the clinical picture and initial treatment. Cardiovascular, neurologic, and gastrointestinal symptoms are responsible for other clinical manifestations, depending on the location and extent of the dissection. The patient may appear pale. Sweating and tachycardia may be detected. Blood pressure may be elevated or markedly different from one arm to the other if dissection involves the orifice of the subclavian artery on one side.

Assessment and Diagnostic Findings

Arteriography, multidetector-computed tomography angiography (MDCTA), TEE, duplex ultrasonography, and MRA, while limited in terms of expediency during an emergency situation, may aid in the diagnosis.

Medical Management

The medical or surgical treatment of a dissecting aorta depends on the type of dissection present and follows the general principles outlined for the treatment of thoracic aortic aneurysms.

Nursing Management

A patient with a dissecting aorta requires the same nursing care as a patient with an aortic aneurysm requiring intervention, as described earlier in this chapter. Nursing care as described in Chart 30-3 is also appropriate.

Arterial Embolism and Arterial Thrombosis

Acute vascular occlusion may be caused by an embolus or acute thrombosis. Acute arterial occlusions may result from iatrogenic injury, which can occur during insertion of invasive catheters such as those used for arteriography, PTA or stent placement, or an intra-aortic balloon pump, or it may occur as a result of IV drug abuse. Other causes include trauma from a fracture, crush injury, and penetrating wounds that disrupt the arterial intima. The accurate diagnosis of an arterial occlusion as embolic or thrombotic in origin is necessary to initiate appropriate treatment.

Pathophysiology

Arterial emboli arise most commonly from thrombi that develop in the chambers of the heart as a result of atrial fibrillation, myocardial infarction, infective endocarditis, or chronic heart failure. These thrombi become detached and are carried from the left side of the heart into the arterial system, where they lodge in and obstruct an artery that is smaller than the embolus. Emboli may also develop in advanced aortic atherosclerosis because the atheromatous plaques ulcerate or become rough. Acute thrombosis frequently occurs in patients with pre-existing ischemic symptoms.

Clinical Manifestations

Symptoms of arterial emboli depend primarily on the size of the embolus, organ involvement, and the state of collateral vessels. The immediate effect is cessation of distal blood flow. The blockage can progress distal and proximal to the site of the obstruction. Secondary vasospasm can contribute to the ischemia. The embolus can fragment or break apart, resulting in occlusion of distal vessels. Emboli tend to lodge at arterial bifurcations and areas narrowed by atherosclerosis. Cerebral, mesenteric, renal, and coronary arteries are often involved in addition to the large arteries of the extremities.

The symptoms of acute arterial embolism in extremities with poor collateral flow are acute, severe pain, and a gradual loss of sensory and motor function. The six Ps associated with acute arterial embolism are *p*ain, *p*allor, *p*ulselessness, *p*aresthesia, *p*oikilothermia (coldness), and *p*aralysis. Eventually, superficial veins may collapse because of decreased blood flow to the extremity. Because of ischemia, the part of the extremity distal to the occlusion is markedly colder and paler than the part proximal to the occlusion.

Arterial thrombosis can also acutely occlude an artery. A thrombosis is a slowly developing clot that usually occurs where the arterial wall has become damaged, generally as a result of atherosclerosis. Thrombi may also develop in an arterial aneurysm. The manifestations of an acute thrombotic arterial occlusion are similar to those described for embolic occlusion. However, treatment is more difficult with a thrombus because the arterial occlusion has occurred in a degenerated vessel and requires more extensive reconstructive surgery to restore flow than is required with an embolic event (Di Minno et al., 2014).

Assessment and Diagnostic Findings

An arterial embolus is usually diagnosed on the basis of the sudden nature of the onset of symptoms and an apparent source for the embolus. Two-dimensional transthoracic echocardiography or transthoracic echocardiogram (TTE), chest x-ray, and electrocardiography (ECG) may reveal underlying cardiac disease. Noninvasive duplex and Doppler ultrasonography can determine the presence and extent of underlying atherosclerosis, and arteriography may be performed.

Medical Management

Management of arterial thrombosis depends on its cause. Management of acute embolic occlusion usually requires surgery because time is of the essence. Because the onset of the event is acute, collateral circulation has not developed, and the patient quickly moves through the list of six Ps to paralysis, the most advanced stage. Heparin therapy is initiated immediately to prevent further development of emboli and to prevent the extension of existing thrombi. Typically, an initial IV bolus of 60 U/kg body weight is given, followed by a continuous infusion of 12 U/kg/h until the patient undergoes endovascular treatment or surgery.

Endovascular Management

Emergency embolectomy is the procedure of choice if the involved extremity is viable (see Fig. 30-13). Arterial emboli are usually treated by insertion of an embolectomy catheter. The catheter is passed through an incision into the affected artery and extended through the embolus that is causing the arterial occlusion. The catheter balloon is inflated with sterile saline solution, and the thrombus is extracted as the catheter is withdrawn. This procedure involves incising the vessel and removing the clot.

Figure 30-13 • Extraction of an embolus by a balloon-tipped embolectomy catheter. The deflated balloon-tipped catheter is advanced past the embolus, inflated, and then gently withdrawn, carrying the embolic material with it. Adapted with permission from Cronenwett, J. L. & Johnston, K. W. (2014). *Rutherford's vascular surgery* (8th ed., *Vols. 1 and 2*). Philadelphia, PA: W. B. Saunders.

Percutaneous mechanical thrombectomy devices may also be used for the treatment of an acute thrombosis. All endovascular devices necessitate obtaining access to the patient's arterial system and inserting a catheter into the patient's artery to obtain access to the thrombus. The approach is similar to that used for angiograms, in that it is made through the groin to the femoral artery. Some devices require that a small incision be made into the patient's artery. These devices may use (1) a jet of fluid to disrupt the thrombus and then aspirate the particles; (2) a rotating, sinusoidal-shaped wire that mixes a thrombolytic agent that simultaneously dissolves the clot; or (3) high-frequency, low-energy ultrasound to dissolve an occlusive thrombus. Complications arising from the use of any of the endovascular devices may include arterial dissection or distal artery embolization.

Pharmacologic Therapy

When the patient has adequate collateral circulation, treatment may include IV anticoagulation with heparin, which can prevent the thrombus from spreading and reduce muscle necrosis. Intra-arterial thrombolytic medications are used to dissolve the embolus. Fibrin-specific thrombolytic medications (e.g., tissue plasminogen activator [alteplase (Activase, t-PA)] and single-chain urokinase-type plasminogen activator [scu-PA, prourokinase]) do not deplete circulating fibrinogen and plasminogen, which prevents the development of systemic fibrinolysis. If t-PA is used for the treatment, heparin is usually given to prevent another thrombus from forming at the site of the lesion. The t-PA activates plasminogen on the thrombus, but it does not decrease the clotting factors as much as other thrombolytic therapies; therefore, patients receiving t-PA can make new thrombi more readily than if they receive other thrombolytics. Other thrombolytic medications are reteplase (r-PA, Retavase) and tenecteplase (TNKase) (Harter, Levine, & Henderson, 2015). Although these agents differ in their pharmacokinetics, they are given in a similar manner: A catheter is advanced under x-ray visualization to the clot, and the thrombolytic agent is infused.

Thrombolytic therapy should not be used when there are known contraindications to therapy or when the extremity cannot tolerate the several additional hours of ischemia that it takes for the agent to lyse (disintegrate) the clot. Contraindications to peripheral thrombolytic therapy include active internal bleeding, cerebrovascular hemorrhage, recent major surgery, uncontrolled hypertension, and pregnancy.

Nursing Management

Before an intervention or surgery, the patient remains on bed rest with the affected extremity level or slightly dependent (15 degrees). The affected part is kept at room temperature and protected from trauma. Heating and cooling pads are contraindicated because ischemic extremities are easily traumatized by alterations in temperature. If possible, tape and ECG electrodes should not be used on the extremity; sheepskin, protected padded boots, and foot cradles are used to protect an affected leg from mechanical trauma (Klein & Guha, 2014).

If the patient is treated with thrombolytic therapy, the dose is based on the patient's weight. The patient is admitted to a critical care unit for continuous monitoring. Vital signs are taken initially every 15 minutes and then at progressively longer intervals if the patient's status remains stable. The patient is closely monitored for bleeding. The nurse minimizes the number of punctures for inserting IV lines and obtaining blood samples, avoids intramuscular injections, prevents any possible tissue trauma, and applies pressure at least twice as long as usual after any puncture is performed.

During the recovery phase, the nurse collaborates with the primary provider about the patient's appropriate activity level based on the patient's condition. Generally, every effort is made to encourage the patient to move the extremity to stimulate circulation and prevent stasis. Anticoagulant therapy may be continued postendovascular intervention to prevent thrombosis of the affected artery and to diminish the development of subsequent thrombi at the initiating site. The nurse assesses for evidence of local and systemic hemorrhage, including mental status changes, which can occur when anticoagulants are given. Pulses, Doppler signals, ABI, and motor and sensory function are assessed every hour for the first 24 hours, because significant changes may indicate reocclusion. Metabolic abnormalities, kidney injury, and compartment syndrome may be complications after an acute arterial occlusion.

Raynaud Phenomenon and Other Acrosyndromes

Raynaud phenomenon is a form of intermittent arteriolar vasoconstriction that results in coldness, pain, and pallor of the fingertips or toes. There are two forms of this disorder. Primary or idiopathic Raynaud's (Raynaud disease) occurs in the absence of an underlying disease. Secondary Raynaud's (Raynaud syndrome) occurs in association with an underlying disease, usually a connective tissue disorder, such as systemic lupus erythematosus, rheumatoid arthritis, or scleroderma; trauma; or obstructive arterial lesions. Symptoms may result from a defect in basal heat production that eventually decreases the ability of cutaneous vessels to dilate. Episodes may be triggered by emotional factors or by unusual sensitivity to cold. Raynaud phenomenon is five times more common in women with the typical onset before age 30 (Ratchford & Evans, 2015). Acrocyanosis has been thought to be a variant of Raynaud phenomenon because both are aggravated by cold and emotional stress and both present with blue discoloration of the fingers and hyperhidrosis (excessive sweating).

The prognosis for patients with Raynaud phenomenon varies; some slowly improve, some become progressively worse, and others show no change. Raynaud symptoms may be mild so that treatment is not required. However, secondary Raynaud's is characterized by vasospasm and fixed blood vessel obstructions that may lead to ischemia, ulceration, and gangrene. Acrocyanosis is a poorly understood phenomenon that may be benign and require little or no treatment, or the patient may have chronic pain and ulcerations.

Clinical Manifestations

The classic clinical picture of Raynaud's reveals pallor brought on by sudden vasoconstriction. The skin then becomes bluish (cyanotic) because of pooling of deoxygenated blood during vasospasm. As a result of exaggerated reflow (hyperemia) due to vasodilation, a red color (rubor) is produced when oxygenated blood returns to the digits after the vasospasm stops. The characteristic sequence of color change of Raynaud phenomenon is described as white, blue, and red. Numbness, tingling, and burning pain occur as the color changes. The manifestations tend to be bilateral and symmetric and may involve toes and fingers.

Acrocyanosis is differentiated from Raynaud's by a relative persistence of skin color changes, symmetry, and an absence of the paroxysmal pallor that is found with Raynaud's. Almost all patients with acrocyanosis have marked clamminess and hyperhidrosis of their hands and feet, which tend to worsen in warmer temperatures while the color changes improve. Finger color normalizes when the hands are transferred from the dependent to horizontal position (Das & Maiti, 2013).

Medical Management

Avoiding the particular stimuli (e.g., cold, tobacco) that provoke vasoconstriction is a primary factor in controlling Raynaud phenomenon. Calcium channel blockers (nifedipine [Procardia], amlodipine [Norvasc]) may be effective in relieving symptoms. Sympathectomy (interrupting the sympathetic nerves by removing the sympathetic ganglia or dividing their branches) may help some patients.

Avoidance of exposure to cold and trauma and implementing measures to improve local circulation are the primary focus of treatment for acrocyanosis. Calcium channel blockers have not been effective in treating acrocyanosis (Das & Maiti, 2013).

Nursing Management

The nurse instructs the patient with Raynaud's or acrocyanosis to avoid situations that may be stressful or unsafe. Stress management classes may be helpful. Exposure to cold must be minimized, and in areas where the fall and winter months are cold, the patient should wear layers of clothing when outdoors. Hats and mittens or gloves should be worn at all times when outside. Fabrics specially designed for cold climates (e.g., Thinsulate) are recommended. Patients should warm up their vehicles before getting in so that they can avoid touching a cold steering wheel or door handle, which could elicit an attack. During summer, a sweater should be available when entering air-conditioned rooms.

Patients are often concerned about serious complications, such as gangrene and amputation; however, these complications are uncommon unless the patient has another underlying disease causing arterial occlusions. Patients should avoid all forms of nicotine; nicotine gum or patches used to help people quit smoking may induce attacks.

Patients should be cautioned to handle sharp objects carefully to avoid injuring their fingers. In addition, patients should be informed about the postural hypotension that may result from medications, such as calcium channel blockers, used to treat Raynaud's phenomenon.

VENOUS DISORDERS

Venous disorders cause reduction in venous blood flow, causing blood stasis. This may then cause a host of pathologic changes, including coagulation defects, edema formation and tissue breakdown, and an increased susceptibility to infections.

Venous Thromboembolism

Deep vein thrombosis (DVT) and pulmonary embolism (PE) collectively make up the condition called VTE. The annual incidence of VTE is estimated at 1 to 2 per 1000 population (Barnes, Kanthi, & Froehlich, 2015). The incidence of VTE is 10% to 20% in general medical patients and up to 80% in critically ill patients. Autopsy studies detected PE in 7% to 27% of critically ill patients; of these, only one third were clinically suspected (Minet, Potton, Bonadona, et al., 2015). VTE is frequently not diagnosed because DVT and PE are often clinically silent. It is estimated that as many as 30% of patients hospitalized with VTE develop long-term postthrombotic complications. The majority of symptomatic thromboembolic complications in surgical patients occur after hospital discharge due to short lengths of stay.

Pathophysiology

Superficial veins, such as the greater saphenous, short saphenous (also known as lesser saphenous), cephalic, basilic, and external jugular veins, are thick-walled muscular structures that lie just under the skin. Deep veins are thin walled and have less muscle in the media. They run parallel to arteries and bear the same names as the arteries. Deep and superficial veins have valves that permit unidirectional flow back to the heart. The valves lie at the base of a segment of the vein that is expanded into a sinus. This arrangement permits the valves to open without coming into contact with the wall of the vein, permitting rapid closure when the blood starts to flow backward. Other kinds of veins are known as perforating veins. These vessels have valves that allow one-way blood flow from the superficial system to the deep system.

Although the exact cause of VTE remains unclear, three factors, known as Virchow triad, are believed to play a significant role in its development: endothelial damage, venous

Chart 30-7

RISK FACTORS
Deep Vein Thrombosis and Pulmonary Embolism

Endothelial Damage

- Trauma
- Surgery
- Pacing wires
- Central venous catheters
- Dialysis access catheters
- Local vein damage
- Repetitive motion injury

Venous Stasis

- Bed rest or immobilization
- Obesity
- History of varicosities
- Spinal cord injury
- Age (>65 years)

Altered Coagulation

- Cancer
- Pregnancy
- Oral contraceptive use
- Protein C deficiency
- Protein S deficiency
- Antiphospholipid antibody syndrome
- Factor V Leiden defect
- Prothrombin G20210A defect
- Hyperhomocysteinemia
- Elevated factors II, VIII, IX, XI
- Antithrombin III deficiency
- Polycythemia
- Septicemia

Adapted from Heit, J. A. (2015). Epidemiology of venous thromboembolism. *Nature Reviews in Cardiology, 12*(8), 464–474.

stasis, and altered coagulation (see Chart 30-7). Damage to the intimal lining of blood vessels creates a site for clot formation. Direct trauma to the veins may occur with fractures or dislocation, diseases of the veins, and chemical irritation of the vein from IV medications or solutions. Venous stasis occurs when blood flow is reduced, as in heart failure or shock; when veins are dilated, as an effect of some medication therapies; and when skeletal muscle contraction is reduced, as in immobility, paralysis of the extremities, or anesthesia. Altered coagulation occurs most commonly in patients for whom anticoagulant medications have been abruptly withdrawn. Oral contraceptive use, elevated CRP levels (Piazza, 2015), and several blood dyscrasias (abnormalities) also can lead to hypercoagulability, with prevalence depending on the ethnicity of the patient. For example, factor V Leiden and prothrombin G20210A mutation is more prevalent in Caucasians, whereas antithrombin III deficiency, protein C deficiency, and protein S deficiency are found more commonly in patients of Southeast Asian descent (Lim & Moll, 2015). An increase in factor VIII concentrations is more common among African Americans (Zakai, McClure, Judd, et al., 2014). Pregnancy is also considered a hypercoagulable state, as it is accompanied by an increase in clotting factors that may not return to baseline until longer than 6 weeks postpartum, increasing the risk of thrombosis. In addition, there is a 50% decrease in venous outflow due to hormonally decreased venous capacitance and reduced venous outflow due to compression from the uterus (Lucania, Camiolo, Carmina, et al., 2014).

Formation of a thrombus frequently accompanies phlebitis, which is an inflammation of the vein walls. When a thrombus develops initially in the veins as a result of stasis or hypercoagulability but without inflammation, the process is referred to as phlebothrombosis. Venous thrombosis can occur in any vein, but it occurs more often in the veins of the lower extremities. The superficial and deep veins of the extremities may be affected.

Upper extremity venous thrombosis accounts for up to 2% of all cases of DVT, but its incidence may be as high as 65% in the presence of central venous cannulation or upper extremity compression (Cronenwett & Johnston, 2014). It typically involves more than one venous segment, with the subclavian vein the most frequently affected. In addition, upper extremity venous thrombosis is more common in patients with IV catheters or in patients with an underlying disease that causes hypercoagulability. Internal trauma to the vessels may result from pacemaker leads, chemotherapy ports, dialysis catheters, or parenteral nutrition lines (Joks, Czy , Popławski, et al., 2014). The lumen of the vein may be decreased as a result of the catheter or from external compression, such as by neoplasms or an extra cervical rib. Effort thrombosis, also known as Paget–Schroetter syndrome, of the upper extremity is caused by repetitive motion (e.g., in competitive swimmers, tennis players, baseball players, weight lifters, and construction workers) that irritates the vessel wall, causing inflammation and subsequent thrombosis and is a manifestation of venous thoracic outlet syndrome where the veins becomes distorted and narrowed (Shennib, Hickle, & Bowles, 2015).

Venous thrombi are aggregates of platelets attached to the vein wall that have a tail-like appendage containing fibrin, white blood cells, and many red blood cells. The "tail" can grow or can propagate in the direction of blood flow as successive layers of the thrombus form. A propagating venous thrombosis is dangerous because parts of the thrombus can break off and occlude the pulmonary blood vessels. Fragmentation of the thrombus can occur spontaneously as it dissolves naturally, or it can occur with an elevated venous pressure, as may occur after standing suddenly or engaging in muscular activity after prolonged inactivity. After an episode of acute DVT, recanalization (i.e., reestablishment of the lumen of the vessel) typically occurs. Lack of recanalization within the first 6 months after DVT appears to be an important predictor of postthrombotic syndrome, which is one complication of venous thrombosis (Kahn, Comerota, Cushman, et al., 2014) (see later discussion). Other complications of venous thrombosis are listed in Chart 30-8.

Clinical Manifestations

A major challenge in recognizing DVT is that the signs and symptoms are nonspecific. The exception is phlegmasia cerulea dolens (massive iliofemoral venous thrombosis), in which the entire extremity becomes massively swollen, tense, painful, and cool to the touch. The large DVT creates severe and sudden venous hypertension that leads to tissue ischemia with resultant translocation of fluid into the interstitial space. Venous gangrene occurs in 20% to 50% of cases

---

Chart 30-8 **Complications of Venous Thrombosis**

Chronic venous occlusion
Pulmonary emboli from dislodged thrombi
Valvular destruction:

- Chronic venous insufficiency
- Increased venous pressure
- Varicosities
- Venous ulcers

Venous obstruction:

- Increased distal pressure
- Fluid stasis
- Edema
- Venous gangrene

Adapted from Kahn, S. R., Comerota, A. J., Cushman, M., et al. American Heart Association Council on Peripheral Vascular Disease, Council on Clinical Cardiology, and Council on Cardiovascular and Stroke Nursing (2014). The postthrombotic syndrome: Evidence-based prevention, diagnosis, and treatment strategies. A scientific statement from the American Heart Association. *Circulation, 130,* 1636–1661.

---

and is associated with a poor prognosis for survival (Hu, Cai, Wang, et al., 2014).

Deep Veins

Clinical manifestations of obstruction of the deep veins include edema and swelling of the extremity because the outflow of venous blood is inhibited. The affected extremity may feel warmer than the unaffected extremity, and the superficial veins may appear more prominent. Tenderness, which usually occurs later, is produced by inflammation of the vein wall and can be detected by gently palpating the affected extremity. In some cases, signs and symptoms of a PE are the first indication of DVT.

Superficial Veins

Thrombosis of superficial veins produces pain or tenderness, redness, and warmth in the involved area. The risk of the superficial venous thrombi becoming dislodged or fragmenting into emboli is very low because most of them dissolve spontaneously. This condition can be treated at home with bed rest, elevation of the leg, analgesic agents, and possibly, anti-inflammatory medication.

Assessment and Diagnostic Findings

Careful assessment is invaluable in detecting early signs of venous disorders of the lower extremities. Patients with a history of varicose veins, hypercoagulation, neoplastic disease, cardiovascular disease, or recent major surgery or injury are at high risk. Other patients at high risk include those who are obese or older adults and women taking oral contraceptives (Heit, 2015).

When performing the nursing assessment, key concerns include limb pain, a feeling of heaviness, functional impairment, ankle engorement, and edema; increase in the surface temperature of the leg, particularly the calf or ankle; and areas of tenderness or superficial thrombosis (i.e., cord-like venous segment). The amount of swelling in the extremity can be determined by measuring the circumference of the affected extremity at various levels (i.e., thigh to ankle) with a tape measure and comparing one extremity with the other at the same level to determine size differences. If both extremities are swollen, a size difference may be difficult to detect. Homan sign (pain in the calf after the foot is sharply dorsiflexed) is *not* a reliable sign for DVT because it can be elicited in any painful condition of the calf and has no clinical value in assessment for DVT.

Prevention

Patients with a prior history of VTE are at increased risk of a new episode; the rate of recurrence can be as high as 17.5% at 2 years and 24.6% at 5 years (Barnes et al., 2015). VTE can be prevented, especially if patients who are considered at high risk are identified and preventive measures are instituted without delay. Preventive measures include the application of graduated compression stockings, the use of intermittent pneumatic compression devices, and encouragement of early ambulation and leg exercises. An additional method to prevent venous thrombosis in surgical patients is administration of subcutaneous unfractionated or low–molecular-weight heparin (LMWH). Patients should be advised to make lifestyle changes as appropriate, which may include weight loss, smoking cessation, and regular exercise.

Medical Management

The objectives of treatment for DVT are to prevent the thrombus from growing and fragmenting (thus risking PE), recurrent thromboemboli, and postthrombotic syndrome (discussed later in the chapter) (Barnes et al., 2015). Anticoagulant therapy (administration of a medication to delay the clotting time of blood, prevent the formation of a thrombus in postoperative patients, and forestall the extension of a thrombus after it has formed) can meet these objectives. However, anticoagulants cannot dissolve a thrombus that has already formed. Combining anticoagulation therapy with mechanical and ultrasonic-assisted thrombolytic therapy may eliminate venous obstruction, maintain venous patency, and prevent postthrombotic syndrome by early removal of the thrombus (Jenkins & Michael, 2014).

Pharmacologic Therapy

Medications for preventing or reducing blood clotting within the vascular system are indicated in patients with thrombophlebitis, recurrent embolus formation, and persistent leg edema from heart failure (see Table 30-2). They are also indicated in older patients with a hip fracture that may result in lengthy immobilization. Contraindications for anticoagulant therapy are noted in Chart 30-9.

Unfractionated Heparin

Unfractionated heparin is given subcutaneously to prevent development of DVT, or by intermittent or continuous IV infusion using weight-adjusted dosing guidelines along with a vitamin K antagonist (e.g., warfarin [Coumadin]) for 5 to 7 days to prevent the extension of a thrombus and the development of new thrombi (Jenkins & Michael, 2014). Medication dosage is regulated by monitoring the activated partial thromboplastin time (aPTT), the international normalized ratio (INR), and the platelet count.

TABLE 30-2 Summary of Anticoagulants and Thrombolytics Used to Treat Venous Thromboemboli

Medication	Major Indications
Unfractionated Heparin	
Heparin	Anticoagulation in patients with current VTE or VTE prophylaxis in patients at risk
Low–Molecular-Weight Heparin	
Dalteparin (Fragmin)	Prophylaxis in patients at risk for VTE or at risk for extension of current VTE
Enoxaparin (Lovenox)	Treatment of current VTE and prophylaxis in patients at risk for VTE or at risk for extension of current VTE
Oral Anticoagulant	
Warfarin (Coumadin)	Anticoagulation in patients with current VTE
Factor Xa Inhibitor	
Fondaparinux (Arixtra)	Prophylaxis in surgical patients at risk for VTE
Oral Factor Xa Inhibitor	
Rivaroxaban (Xarelto)	Fixed-dose regimen for treating acute deep vein thrombosis and for VTE prophylaxis
Apixaban (Eliquis)	Fixed-dose regimen for treating acute deep vein thrombosis and for VTE prophylaxis
Edoxaban (Savaysa)	Fixed-dose regimen for treating acute deep vein thrombosis and for VTE prophylaxis
Direct Thrombin Inhibitor	
Lepirudin (Refludan) Argatroban (Novastan)	Treatment for heparin-induced thrombocytopenia
Oral Direct Thrombin Inhibitor	
Dabigatran (Pradaxa)	Fixed-dose regimen for treating acute deep vein thrombosis and for VTE prophylaxis
Thrombolytic	
Alteplase (Activase, t-PA) Reteplase (Retavase) Tenecteplase (TNKase) Urokinase (Abbokinase)	Fibrinolysis/dissolution of existing VTE

VTE, venous thromboembolism.

Low–Molecular-Weight Heparin

Subcutaneous LMWHs that may include medications such as dalteparin and enoxaparin are effective treatments for some cases of DVT. These agents have longer half-lives than unfractionated heparin, so doses can be given in one or two subcutaneous injections each day. Doses are adjusted according to weight. LMWHs prevent the extension of a thrombus and development of new thrombi, and they are associated with fewer bleeding complications and lower risks of heparin-induced thrombocytopenia (HIT) than unfractionated heparin. Because there are several preparations, the dosing schedule must be based on the product used and the protocol at each institution. The cost of LMWH is higher than that of unfractionated heparin; however, LMWH may be used safely in pregnant women, and patients who take it may be more mobile and have an improved quality of life.

Oral Anticoagulants

Warfarin is a vitamin K antagonist that is indicated for extended anticoagulant therapy. Routine coagulation monitoring of the INR is essential to ensure that a therapeutic response is obtained and maintained over time. Interactions with a range of other medications can reduce or enhance the anticoagulant effects of warfarin, as can variable intake of foods containing vitamin K (see Chart 33-12). Warfarin has a narrow therapeutic window, and there is a slow onset of action. Treatment is initially supported with concomitant parenteral anticoagulation with heparin until the warfarin demonstrates anticoagulant effectiveness.

Factor Xa and Direct Thrombin Inhibitors

Fondaparinux (Arixtra) selectively inhibits factor Xa. This agent is given daily subcutaneously at a fixed dose, has a half-life of 17 hours, and is excreted unchanged via the kidneys (and therefore must be used with caution in patients with renal insufficiency). It has no effect on routine tests of coagulation, such as the aPTT or activated clotting time (ACT), so routine coagulation monitoring is unnecessary. Fondaparinux is approved for prophylaxis during major orthopedic surgery, such as hip or knee arthroplasties, and has been found to be effective for the treatment of VTE. Rivaroxaban (Xarelto) is an oral factor Xa inhibitor available for DVT prophylaxis and treatment that may be taken orally once daily; it is not indicated in patients with an estimated creatinine clearance less than 30 mL/min. Apixaban (Eliquis) is another oral factor Xa inhibitor available for DVT prophylaxis and treatment and is taken twice daily. Clinical trials have reported patients treated with apixaban had a lower risk of VTE recurrence without significantly increased risk of bleeding. Apixaban is not indicated in patients with an estimated creatinine clearance of less than 25 mL/min (Barnes et al., 2015). Dabigatran (Pradaxa), a direct thrombin inhibitor, which was FDA approved to reduce the risk of stroke and systemic embolism in patients with nonvalvular atrial fibrillation is also approved for acute and extended therapy for patients with VTE (Barnes et al., 2015). Dabigatran should be given twice daily but is not advised for patients with an estimated creatinine clearance of less than 30 mL/min. There is no need for routine coagulation laboratory monitoring or laboratory test–guided dosage adjustments; however, if measured, aPTT levels may be prolonged approximately 1.5 to 2 times (Skeik, Murphy, & Porten, 2014).

Thrombolytic Therapy

Catheter-directed thrombolytic therapy lyses and dissolves thrombi in at least 50% of patients. Thrombolytic therapy (e.g., alteplase) is given within the first 3 days after acute thrombosis. Therapy initiated beyond 14 days after the onset of symptoms is significantly less effective. The advantages of thrombolytic therapy include less long-term damage to the venous valves and a reduced incidence of postthrombotic syndrome and chronic venous insufficiency. Most of the reported complications associated with thrombolytic therapy are related to hemorrhage, but these happened less frequently if the lytic therapy was catheter-directed versus systemic (Jenkins & Michael, 2014).

Endovascular Management

Endovascular management is necessary for DVT when anticoagulant or thrombolytic therapy is contraindicated (see Chart 30-9), the danger of PE is extreme, or venous drainage is so severely compromised that permanent damage to the extremity is likely. A thrombectomy may be necessary. This mechanical method of clot removal may involve using intraluminal catheters with a balloon or other devices. Some of these spin to break the clot, and others use oscillation to break up the clot to facilitate removal. Ultrasound-assisted thrombolysis may be another option. This intervention uses bursts or continuous high-frequency ultrasound waves emanating from the catheters to cause cavitation of the thrombus, making it more permeable to the thrombolytic agent (Jenkins & Michael, 2014). A vena cava filter may be placed at the time of the thrombectomy or thrombolysis; this filter traps large emboli and prevents PE (see Chapter 23). Some retrievable caval filters can be left in place and then retrieved for up to 6 months. In patients with chronic iliac vein compression (e.g., as is seen in May–Thurner syndrome), balloon angioplasty with stent placement may successfully treat the patient's chronic leg symptoms (Birn &Vedantham, 2015).

Nursing Management

If the patient is receiving anticoagulant therapy, the nurse monitors the appropriate laboratory values. The aPTT, prothrombin time (PT), INR, ACT, hemoglobin and hematocrit values, platelet count, and fibrinogen levels are affected depending on the anticoagulant prescribed. Close observation is required to detect bleeding; if bleeding occurs, it must be reported immediately and anticoagulant therapy discontinued.

Assessing and Monitoring Anticoagulant Therapy

To prevent inadvertent infusion of large volumes of unfractionated heparin, which could cause hemorrhage, unfractionated heparin is always given by continuous IV infusion using an electronic infusion device. Dosage calculations are based on the patient's weight, and any possible bleeding tendencies are detected by a pretreatment-clotting profile. If renal insufficiency exists, lower doses of heparin are required. Periodic coagulation tests and hematocrit levels are obtained. Heparin is in the effective, or therapeutic, range when the aPTT is 1.5 times the control.

Oral anticoagulants, such as warfarin, are monitored by the PT or the INR. Because the full anticoagulant effect of warfarin is delayed for 3 to 5 days, it is usually given concurrently with heparin until desired anticoagulation has been achieved (i.e., when the PT is 1.5 to 2 times normal or the INR is 2.0 to 3.0) (Harter et al., 2015).

Monitoring and Managing Potential Complications

Bleeding

The principal complication of anticoagulant therapy is spontaneous bleeding. Bleeding from the kidneys is detected by microscopic examination of the urine and is often the first sign of excessive dosage. Bruises, nosebleeds, and bleeding gums are also early signs. To promptly reverse the effects of heparin, IV injections of protamine sulfate may be given. Risks of protamine administration include bradycardia and hypotension, which can be minimized by slow administration. Protamine sulfate can be used to reverse the effects of LMWH, but it is less effective with LMWH than with unfractionated heparin. Reversing the anticoagulation effects of warfarin is more difficult, but effective measures that may be prescribed include administration of vitamin K and/or infusion of fresh-frozen plasma or prothrombin complex concentrate (PCC). Oral and low-dose IV vitamin K significantly decreases the INR within 24 hours (Dobesh & Fanikos, 2014). Idarucizumab (Praxbind) is a humanized monoclonal antibody fragment that has been approved as a reversal agent for dabigatran (Pradaxa). It is administered IV at dosages of 5 g, provided as two separate infusions of 2.5 g/50 mL. At this time, there are no specific antidotes for the factor Xa inhibitors, although they are under development. The only option for reversal is by withholding the drugs, which have a relatively rapid rate of systemic clearance. It is recommended that activated charcoal be given within one to two hours following a dose. PCC may be used for patients with major bleeding, but its use carries the risk of disseminated intravascular coagulation (DIC) (Mohanty, Looser, Gokanapudy, et al., 2014).

Thrombocytopenia

HIT may be a complication of heparin therapy (see Chapter 33 for discussion).

Drug Interactions

Because oral anticoagulants, particularly warfarin, interact with many other medications and herbal and nutritional supplements, close evaluation of the patient's medications is necessary. Many medications and supplements potentiate or inhibit oral anticoagulants; it is always wise to check to see if any medications or supplements are contraindicated with warfarin (see Chart 33-12). Contraindications to anticoagulant therapy are summarized in Chart 30-9.

Providing Comfort

Elevation of the affected extremity, graduated compression stockings, and analgesic agents for pain relief are adjuncts to therapy. They help improve circulation and increase comfort. Warm, moist packs applied to the affected extremity reduce the discomfort associated with DVT. The patient is encouraged to walk once anticoagulation therapy has been initiated. The nurse should instruct the patient that walking is better than standing or sitting for long periods. Bed exercises, such as repetitive dorsiflexion of the foot, are also recommended.

Providing Compression Therapy

Stockings

Graduated compression stockings usually are prescribed for patients with venous disease. The amount of pressure gradient is determined by the amount and severity of venous disease. For example, a pressure gradient of 20 to 30 mm Hg is prescribed for patients with asymptomatic varicose veins, whereas at least a pressure gradient of 30 to 40 mm Hg is recommended for patients with venous stasis ulceration. These stockings should not be confused with antiembolism stockings (i.e., TED stockings) that provide less compression (12 to 20 mm Hg). Graduated compression stockings are designed to apply 100% of the prescribed pressure gradient at the ankle and then decrease along the length of the stocking, reducing the caliber of the superficial veins in the leg and increasing flow in the deep veins. These stockings may be knee high, thigh high, or pantyhose.

> ### Quality and Safety Nursing Alert
>
> *Any type of stocking can inadvertently become a tourniquet if applied incorrectly (i.e., rolled tightly at the top). In such instances, the stockings produce—rather than prevent—stasis. For ambulatory patients, graduated compression stockings are removed at night and reapplied before the legs are lowered from the bed to the floor in the morning.*

When the stockings are off, the skin is inspected for signs of irritation, and the calves are examined for tenderness. Any skin changes or signs of tenderness are reported. Stockings are contraindicated in patients with severe pitting edema, because they can produce severe pitting at the knee.

Gerontologic Considerations

Because of decreased strength and manual dexterity, older patients may be unable to apply graduated compression stockings properly. If this is the case, a family member or friend should be taught to assist the patient to apply the stockings so that they do not cause undue pressure on any part of the feet or legs. Frames have been designed to assist patients with applying stockings, and if there is any concern regarding patients' physical abilities, they should be referred to an occupational therapist who can provide examples of and training in the use of stocking assistance devices.

External Compression Devices and Wraps

Short stretch elastic wraps may be applied from the toes to the knee in a 50% spiral overlap. These wraps are available in a two-layer system, which includes an inner layer of soft padding. These wraps are rectangular and become squares on stretching, indicating the appropriate degree of stretch and reducing the possibility of wrapping a leg too loosely or too tightly. Three- and four-layer systems are also available (e.g., Profore, Dyna-Care), but these may be used only once compared with the two-layer system, which can be used multiple times.

Other types of compression are available. The Unna boot, which consists of a paste bandage impregnated with zinc oxide, glycerin, gelatin, and sometimes calamine, is applied without tension in a circular fashion from the base of the toes to the tibial tuberosity with a 50% spiral overlap. The foot must remain dorsiflexed at a 90-degree angle to the leg, thus avoiding excess pressure or trauma to the anterior ankle area. Once the bandage dries, it provides a constant and consistent compression of the venous system. This type of compression may remain in place for as long as 1 week, although it may be too heavy for debilitated patients to handle.

The CircAid, a nonelastic leg wrap with a series of over-lapping, interlocking Velcro straps, augments the effect of muscle while the patient is walking. The CircAid is usually worn during the day. Patients may find the CircAid easier to apply and wear than the Unna boot because it is lighter; they can remove it to shower, and it is adjustable. This readily adjustable feature may also be problematic; patients may be tempted to loosen the straps, and the compression achieved may not be adequate.

Intermittent Pneumatic Compression Devices

These devices can be used with elastic or graduated compression stockings to prevent DVT. They consist of an electric controller that is attached by air hoses to plastic knee-high or thigh-high sleeves. The leg sleeves are divided into compartments, which sequentially fill to apply pressure to the ankle, calf, and thigh at 30 to 70 mm Hg of pressure. These devices can increase blood velocity beyond that produced by the stockings. These devices are prescribed for patients who are unsuitable candidates for compression bandages, wraps, or stockings (Chi & Raffetto, 2015). Nursing measures in caring for patients who use these devices include ensuring that prescribed pressures are not exceeded, assessing for patient comfort, and ensuring compliance to therapy.

Positioning the Body and Encouraging Exercise

When the patient is on bed rest, the feet and lower legs should be elevated periodically above the level of the heart. This position allows the superficial and tibial veins to empty rapidly and to remain collapsed. Active and passive leg exercises, particularly those involving calf muscles, should be performed to increase venous flow. Early ambulation is most effective in preventing venous stasis. Deep breathing exercises are beneficial because they produce increased negative pressure in the thorax, which assists in emptying the large veins. Once ambulatory, the patient is instructed to avoid sitting for more than an hour at a time. The goal is to walk at least 10 minutes every 1 to 2 hours. The patient is also instructed to perform active and passive leg exercises as frequently as necessary when he or she cannot ambulate, such as during long car, bus, train, and plane trips.

Promoting Home, Community-Based, and Transitional Care

In addition to instructing the patient on how to apply graduated compression stockings and explaining the importance of

---

Chart 30-10

PATIENT EDUCATION
Taking Anticoagulant Medications

The nurse instructs the patient to:

- Take the anticoagulant medication at the same time each day, usually between 8:00 and 9:00 am.
- Wear or carry identification indicating the anticoagulant medication being taken.
- Keep all appointments for blood tests.
- Because other medications may affect the action of the anticoagulant medication, do not take any of the following medications or supplements without consulting with your primary provider: vitamins, cold medicines, antibiotics, aspirin, mineral oil, and anti-inflammatory agents, such as ibuprofen (Motrin) and similar medications or herbal or nutritional supplements. Your primary provider should be contacted before taking any over-the-counter drugs.
- Avoid alcohol if taking warfarin because it may change the body's response to an anticoagulant medication. There are no interactions with the oral factor Xa inhibitors (e.g., rivaroxaban [Xarelto], apixaban [Eliquis], edoxaban [Savaysa]) and alcohol.
- Avoid food fads, crash diets, or marked changes in eating habits if taking warfarin, dietary habits have no interactions with the oral factor Xa inhibitors.
- Do not take any anticoagulation therapy unless directed.
- Do not stop taking your anticoagulation therapy (when prescribed) unless directed.
- When seeking treatment from any health care provider, be sure to inform the caregiver that you are taking an anticoagulant medication.
- Contact your provider who manages your anticoagulation therapy before having dental work or elective surgery.
- If any of the following signs appear, report them immediately to your provider:
  Faintness, dizziness, or increased weakness
  Severe headaches or abdominal pain
  Reddish or brownish urine
  Any bleeding—e.g., cuts that do not stop bleeding
  Bruises that enlarge, nosebleeds, or unusual bleeding from any part of the body
  Red or black bowel movements
  Rash
- Avoid injury that can cause bleeding.
- *For women:* Notify your primary provider and obstetrical provider if you suspect pregnancy.

---

elevating the legs and exercising adequately, the nurse educates about the prescribed anticoagulant, its purpose, and the need to take the correct amount at the specific times, especially if warfarin is prescribed (see Chart 30-10). The patient should also be aware that if warfarin is prescribed, periodic blood tests are necessary to determine if a change in medication or dosage is required. If the patient fails to adhere to the therapeutic regimen, continuation of the medication therapy should be questioned. Caution should be used in a patient who refuses to discontinue the use of alcohol, because chronic alcohol use decreases the effectiveness of anticoagulation therapy. In patients with liver disease, the potential for bleeding may be exacerbated by anticoagulant therapy.

Chronic Venous Insufficiency/ Postthrombotic Syndrome

Venous insufficiency results from obstruction of the venous valves in the legs or a reflux of blood through the valves.

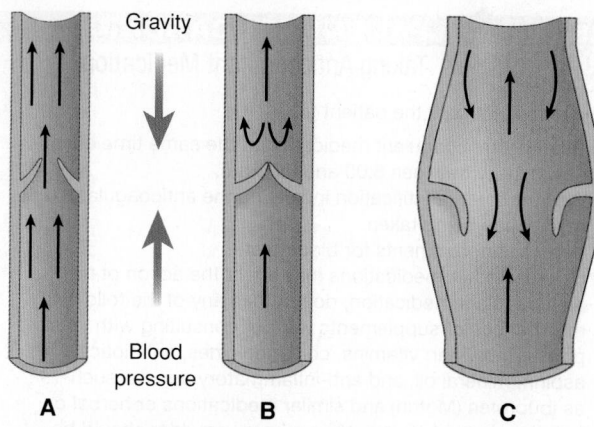

Figure 30-14 • Competent valves showing blood flow patterns when the valve is open (**A**) and closed (**B**), allowing blood to flow against gravity. **C.** With faulty or incompetent valves, the blood cannot move toward the heart.

Superficial and deep leg veins can be involved. Resultant venous hypertension can occur whenever there has been a prolonged increase in venous pressure, such as occurs with DVT. Because the walls of veins are thinner and more elastic than the walls of arteries, they distend readily when venous pressure is consistently elevated. In this state, leaflets of the venous valves are stretched and prevented from closing completely, causing a backflow or reflux of blood in the veins. Duplex ultrasonography confirms the obstruction and identifies the level of valvular incompetence. Twenty to 50% of patients who are post DVT that develop deep vein incompetence suffer from postthrombotic syndrome (Kahn et al., 2014) (see Fig. 30-14).

Clinical Manifestations

Postthrombotic syndrome is characterized by chronic venous stasis, resulting in edema, altered pigmentation, pain, and stasis dermatitis. The patient may notice the symptoms less in the morning and more in the evening. Obstruction or poor calf muscle pumping in addition to valvular reflux must be present for the development of severe postthrombotic syndrome and stasis ulcers. Superficial veins may be dilated. The disorder is long-standing, difficult to treat, and often disabling (Kahn et al., 2014).

Stasis ulcers develop as a result of the rupture of small skin veins and subsequent ulcerations. When these vessels rupture, red blood cells escape into surrounding tissues and then degenerate, leaving a brownish discoloration of the tissues, called *hemosiderin staining*. The pigmentation and ulcerations usually occur in the lower part of the extremity, in the area of the medial malleolus of the ankle. The skin becomes dry, cracks, and itches; subcutaneous tissues fibrose and atrophy. The risk of injury and infection of the extremities is increased.

Complications

Venous ulceration is the most serious complication of chronic venous insufficiency and can be associated with other conditions affecting the circulation of the lower extremities. Cellulitis or dermatitis may complicate the care of chronic venous insufficiency and venous ulcerations.

Medical and Nursing Management

Management of the patient with venous insufficiency is directed at reducing venous stasis and preventing ulcerations. Measures that increase venous blood flow are antigravity activities, such as elevating the leg, and compression of superficial veins with graduated compression stockings.

Elevating the legs decreases edema, promotes venous return, and provides symptomatic relief. The legs should be elevated frequently throughout the day (at least 15 to 20 minutes four times daily). At night, the patient should sleep with the foot of the bed elevated about 15 cm (6 in). Prolonged sitting or standing in one position is detrimental; walking should be encouraged. When sitting, the patient should avoid placing pressure on the popliteal spaces, as occurs when crossing the legs or sitting with the legs dangling over the side of the bed. Constricting garments, especially socks that are too tight at the top or that leave marks on the skin, should be avoided.

Compression of the legs with graduated compression stockings reduces the pooling of venous blood, enhances venous return to the heart, and is recommended for people with venous insufficiency. The American Heart Association recommends that compression stockings with at least 20 to 30 mm Hg pressure be used during the 6 months post DVT to decrease symptoms and development of postthrombotic syndrome, even though research-based evidence that supports this is weak at present (Kahn et al., 2014). Each stocking should fit so that pressure is greater at the foot and ankle and then gradually declines to a lesser pressure at the knee or groin. If the top of the stocking is too tight or becomes twisted, a tourniquet effect is created, which worsens venous pooling. Stockings should be applied after the legs have been elevated for a period, when the amount of blood in the leg veins is at its lowest.

Extremities with venous insufficiency must be carefully protected from trauma; the skin is kept clean, dry, and soft. Signs of ulceration are immediately reported to the primary provider for treatment and follow-up.

Leg Ulcers

A leg ulcer is an excavation of the skin surface that occurs when inflamed necrotic tissue sloughs off. In the United States the most common lower extremity ulcerations have a venous etiology (estimated between 45% and 90%), with PAD the second leading cause. The coexistence of both venous and arterial disease is estimated to be present in 26% of patients with leg ulcers (Hedayati, Carson, Chi, et al., 2015).

Pathophysiology

Inadequate exchange of oxygen and other nutrients in the tissue is the metabolic abnormality that underlies the development of leg ulcers. When cellular metabolism cannot maintain energy balance, cell death (necrosis) results. Alterations in blood vessels at the arterial, capillary, and venous levels may affect cellular processes and lead to the formation of ulcers.

Clinical Manifestations

The characteristics of leg ulcers are determined by the cause of the ulcer. Most ulcers, especially in older patients, have

Figure 30-15 • **A.** Ulcers resulting from arterial emboli. **B.** Gangrene of the toes resulting from severe arterial ischemia. **C.** Ulcer from venous stasis.

more than one cause. The symptoms depend on whether the problem is arterial or venous in origin (see Table 30-1). The severity of the symptoms depends on the extent and duration of the vascular insufficiency. The ulcer itself appears as an open, inflamed sore. The area may be draining or covered by eschar (dark, hard crust).

Arterial Ulcers

Chronic arterial disease is characterized by intermittent claudication, which is pain caused by activity and relieved after a few minutes of rest. The patient may also complain of digital or forefoot pain at rest. If the onset of arterial occlusion is acute, ischemic pain is unrelenting and rarely relieved even with opioids. Typically, arterial ulcers are small, circular, deep ulcerations on the tips of toes or in the webspaces between the toes. Ulcers often occur on the medial side of the hallux or lateral fifth toe and may be caused by a combination of ischemia and pressure (see Fig. 30-15).

Venous Ulcers

Chronic venous insufficiency is characterized by pain described as aching or heavy. The foot and ankle may be edematous. Ulcerations are in the area of the medial or lateral malleolus (gaiter area) and are typically large, superficial, and highly exudative. Venous hypertension causes extravasation of blood, which discolors the area

(see Fig. 30-15). Studies report the average venous ulcer requires as long as 6 to 12 months to heal completely and in patients who do not adhere to compression therapy, the recurrence rate is nearly 100% within 36 months (Chi & Raffetto, 2015). Patients with neuropathy (e.g., a common occurrence in patients with diabetes) frequently have ulcerations on the side of the foot over the metatarsal heads. These ulcers are painless and are described in further detail in Chapter 51.

Assessment and Diagnostic Findings

Because ulcers have many causes, the cause of each ulcer needs to be identified so that appropriate therapy can be prescribed. The history of the condition is important in determining venous or arterial insufficiency. The pulses of the lower extremities (femoral, popliteal, posterior tibial, and dorsalis pedis) are carefully examined. More conclusive diagnostic aids include Doppler and duplex ultrasound studies, arteriography, and venography. Cultures of the ulcer bed may be necessary to determine whether an infecting agent is the primary cause of the ulcer.

Medical Management

Patients with ulcers can be effectively managed by advanced practice nurses or wound-ostomy-continence nurses in collaboration with the patients' primary provider. All ulcers have the potential to become infected.

Pharmacologic Therapy

Antiseptic agents, such as povidone-iodine, cadexomer iodine, acetic acid, chlorhexidine, and silver wound products, inhibit growth and development of most skin organisms, are broad spectrum and generate relatively little antimicrobial resistance, and can be used for short periods of time. However, once a wound colonized with pathogens shows signs of infection (e.g., erythema, induration, exudate, edema, wound breakdown, foul odor), a systemic antibiotic is necessary. The specific antibiotic agent selected is based on culture and sensitivity test results. Oral antibiotics usually are prescribed because topical antibiotics have not proven to be effective for leg ulcers.

Compression Therapy

After the circulatory status of the patient is assessed and an absolute ankle pressure of greater than 60 mm Hg and an ABI that exceeds 0.50 are confirmed, compression therapy can be used up to 40 mm Hg without impeding arterial perfusion (Hedayati et al., 2015). Adequate compression therapy involves the application of external or counter pressure to the lower extremity to facilitate venous return to the heart. The pressure should be applied in a gradient or graduated fashion, with the pressure being somewhat higher at the ankle. Graduated compression stockings are one option; some of these are custom-made to the patient's anatomic specifications. The patient should be instructed to wear the stockings at all times except at night and to reapply the stockings in the morning before getting out of bed. Short stretch elastic wraps, Unna boots, and CircAids may be other effective options. See the discussion on compression therapy in the Venous Thromboembolism section.

Débridement

To promote healing, the wound is kept clean of drainage and necrotic tissue. The usual method is to flush the area with normal saline solution or clean it with a noncytotoxic wound-cleansing agent (Saf-Clens, Biolex, Restore). If this is unsuccessful, débridement may be necessary. Débridement is the removal of nonviable tissue from wounds. Removing the dead tissue is important, particularly in instances of infection. Débridement can be accomplished by several different methods:

- Surgical débridement is the fastest method and can be performed by a physician, skilled advanced practice nurse, or wound-ostomy-continence nurse in collaboration with the physician or advanced practice nurse.
- Nonselective débridement can be accomplished by applying isotonic saline dressings of fine mesh gauze to the ulcer. When the dressing dries, it is removed (dry), along with the debris adhering to the gauze. Pain management is usually necessary.
- Enzymatic débridement with the application of enzyme ointments may be prescribed to treat the ulcer. The ointment is applied to the lesion but not to normal surrounding skin. Most enzymatic ointments are covered with saline-soaked gauze that has been thoroughly wrung out. A dry gauze dressing and a loose bandage are then applied. The enzymatic ointment is discontinued when the necrotic tissue has been débrided, and an appropriate wound dressing is applied.
- Calcium alginate dressings (e.g., Kaltostat, Sorbsan, Aquacel Hydrofiber) may be used for débridement when absorption of exudate is needed. These dressings are changed when the exudate seeps through the cover dressing or at least every 7 days. The dressing can also be used on areas that are bleeding, because the material helps stop the bleeding. As the dry fibers absorb exudate, they become a gel that can be painlessly removed from the ulcer bed. Calcium alginate dressings should not be used on dry or nonexudative wounds.
- Foam dressings (e.g., Lyofoam, Allevyn, Cavi-Care) may be an option for exudative wounds because they absorb exudate into the foam, keeping the wound moist.

Arterial insufficiency may result in gangrene of the toe (digital gangrene), which usually is caused by trauma. The toe is stubbed and then turns black (see Fig. 30-15). Usually, patients with this problem are older people without adequate circulation to provide revascularization. Débridement is contraindicated in these instances. Although the toe is gangrenous, it is dry. Managing dry gangrene is preferable to débriding the toe and causing an open wound that will not heal because of insufficient circulation. If the toe were to be amputated, the lack of adequate circulation would prevent healing and might make further amputation necessary—a below-knee or an above-knee amputation. A higher-level amputation in an older adult could result in a loss of independence and possibly the need for institutional care. Dry gangrene of the toe in an older adult with poor circulation is usually left undisturbed. The nurse keeps the toe clean and dry until it separates (without creating an open wound).

Topical Therapy

A variety of topical agents can be used in conjunction with cleansing and débridement therapies to promote healing of leg ulcers. The goals of treatment are to remove devitalized tissue and to keep the ulcer clean and moist while healing takes place. The treatment should not destroy developing tissue. For topical treatments to be successful, adequate nutritional therapy must be maintained.

Wound Dressing

Semiocclusive or occlusive wound dressings prevent evaporative water loss from the wound and retain warmth; these factors favor healing. When determining the appropriate dressing to apply, the following should be considered: simplicity of application, frequency of required dressing changes, ability to absorb wound drainage, expense, and patient comfort. Available options that promote the growth of granulation tissue and reepithelialization include the hydrocolloids (e.g., Comfeel, DuoDERM CGF, Restore, Tegasorb). These materials also provide a barrier for protection because they adhere to the wound bed and surrounding tissue. Foam dressings (Allevyn, Mepilex, Biatain) are permeable to both gases and water vapor due to their hydrophilic properties and are indicated for wounds with moderate exudate, granulating or slough covered, and diabetic ulcerations. Semipermeable film dressings (e.g., Bioclusive, OpSite, Tegaderm) may be selected because they keep the wound moist and are impervious to bacteria while allowing some gas exchange. However, they may not be effective treatment for deep wounds and infected wounds (Sood, Granick, & Tomaselli, 2014).

Growth factor dressings (e.g., OASIS, becaplermin [Regranex], keratinocyte lysate, collagen matrix Promogran) may directly provide a growth factor, or they may stimulate important growth substances within the wound. Guidelines published by the Society of Vascular Surgery and American Venous Forum note no benefit in venous ulcer healing from using silver impregnated dressings (Chi & Raffetto, 2015). Calcium alginate, hydrofiber, and hydroconductive dressings are used for wounds with moderate to high amount of exudate. The hydroconductive dressings (Levafiber) provide a capillary action that lifts and moves exudate away from a wound into the core of the dressing from where it disperses into a second layer. These dressings can be left in place for up to 7 days (Sood et al., 2014).

Knowledge deficit, frustration, fear, and depression can decrease the patient's and family's compliance with the prescribed therapy; therefore, patient and family education is necessary before beginning and throughout the wound care program.

Stimulated Healing

Tissue-engineered human skin equivalent (e.g., Apligraf [Graftskin]) is a skin product cultured from human dermal fibroblasts and keratinocytes used in combination with therapeutic compression. When applied, it interacts with the patient's cells within the wound to stimulate the production of growth factors. Application is not difficult, no suturing is involved, and the procedure is painless. PriMatrix is a bioactive and regenerative extracellular matrix that binds with the patient's own cells and growth factors. PriMatrix has been used successfully for tunneling wounds, as well as wounds with exposed tendon and bone, in which Apligraf cannot be used. Dermagraft, which is a human fibroblast-derived dermal replacement, demonstrates efficacy similar to Apligraf (Chi & Raffetto, 2015).

Hyperbaric Oxygenation

Hyperbaric oxygenation (HBO) may be beneficial as an adjunct treatment in patients with diabetes with no signs of wound healing after 30 days of standard wound treatment. HBO is accomplished by placing the patient into a chamber that increases barometric pressure while the patient is breathing 100% oxygen. Treatment regimens vary from 90 to 120 minutes once daily for 30 to 90 sessions. The process by which HBO is thought to work involves several factors. The edema in the wound area is decreased because high oxygen tension facilitates vasoconstriction and enhances the ability of leukocytes to phagocytize and kill bacteria. In addition, HBO is thought to increase diffusion of oxygen to the hypoxic wound, thereby enhancing epithelial migration and improving collagen production. The two most common adverse effects of HBO are middle-ear barotrauma and confinement anxiety. The benefit from this therapy on wound healing in patients without diabetes is unclear (Gould, Abadir, Brem, et al., 2015).

Negative Pressure Wound Therapy

Research findings suggest that negative pressure wound therapy using vacuum-assisted closure (VAC) devices decreases time to healing in complex wounds that have not healed in a 3-week period. Groin incisions, common in vascular surgery, may be complicated by wound dehiscence, lymphatic fistula, or infections in 5% to 10% of patients. Wound VAC therapy has been found to be effective in treating patients who develop postoperative groin wound infections, decreasing hospital lengths of stay, rates of graft infection, and likelihood of limb loss (Ingargiola, Daniali, & Lee, 2013). Patients who are ambulatory may be given the small, portable VAC devices, giving patients the freedom to perform their ADLs. Research is underway to evaluate the bacterial load and changes in the bacterial spectrum in wounds while using a VAC device (Patmo, Krijnen, Tuinebreijer, et al., 2014).

NURSING PROCESS

The Patient With Leg Ulcers

Assessment

A careful nursing history and assessment are important. The extent and type of pain are carefully assessed, as are the appearance and temperature of the skin of both legs. The quality of all peripheral pulses is assessed, and the pulses in both legs are compared. The legs are checked for edema. If the extremity is edematous, the degree of edema is determined. Any limitation of mobility and activity that results from vascular insufficiency is identified. The patient's nutritional status is assessed, and a history of diabetes, collagen disease, or varicose veins is obtained.

Diagnosis

NURSING DIAGNOSES

Based on the assessment data, major nursing diagnoses may include:

- Impaired skin integrity related to vascular insufficiency
- Impaired physical mobility related to activity restrictions of the therapeutic regimen and pain

- Imbalanced nutrition: less than body requirements related to increased need for nutrients that promote wound healing

COLLABORATIVE PROBLEMS/POTENTIAL COMPLICATIONS

Potential complications may include the following:

- Infection
- Gangrene

Planning and Goals

The major goals for the patient may include restoration of skin integrity, improved physical mobility, adequate nutrition, and absence of complications.

Nursing Interventions

Caring for these patients can be challenging, whether the patient is in the hospital, in a long-term care facility, or at home. Leg ulcers are often long term and disabling causing a substantial drain on the patient's physical, emotional, and economic resources.

RESTORING SKIN INTEGRITY

To promote wound healing, measures are used to keep the area clean. Cleansing requires very gentle handling, a mild soap, and lukewarm water. Positioning of the legs depends on whether the ulcer is of arterial or venous origin. If there is arterial insufficiency, the patient should be referred for evaluation of vascular reconstruction. If there is venous insufficiency, dependent edema can be avoided by elevating the lower extremities. A decrease in edema promotes the exchange of cellular nutrients and waste products in the area of the ulcer, promoting healing.

Avoiding trauma to the lower extremities is imperative in promoting skin integrity. Protective boots may be used (e.g., Rooke vascular boots); they are soft and provide warmth and protection from injury and displace tissue pressure to prevent ulcer formation. If the patient is on bed rest, it is important to relieve pressure on the heels to prevent pressure ulcerations. When the patient is in bed, a bed cradle can be used to relieve pressure from bed linens and to prevent anything from touching the legs. When the patient is ambulatory, all obstacles are moved from the patient's path so that the patient's legs are not bumped. Heating pads, hot water bottles, or hot baths are avoided, because they increase the oxygen demands and thus the blood flow demands of the already compromised tissue. The patient with diabetes suffers from neuropathy with decreased sensation, and heating pads may produce injury before the patient is aware of being burned.

IMPROVING PHYSICAL MOBILITY

Generally, physical activity is initially restricted to promote healing. When infection resolves and healing begins, ambulation should resume gradually and progressively. Activity promotes arterial flow and venous return and is encouraged after the acute phase of the ulcer process. Until full activity is resumed, the patient is encouraged to move about when in bed, to turn from side to side frequently, and to exercise the upper extremities to maintain muscle tone and strength. Meanwhile, diversional activities are encouraged. Consultation with an occupational therapist and physical therapist may be helpful if prolonged immobility and inactivity are anticipated.

If pain limits the patient's activity, analgesic agents may be prescribed. The pain of peripheral vascular disease is typically chronic and often disabling. Analgesic agents may be taken before scheduled activities to help the patient participate more comfortably.

PROMOTING ADEQUATE NUTRITION

Nutritional deficiencies are common, requiring dietary alterations to remedy them. There is conflicting research and evidence that dietary supplementation aids in healing of ulcerations. Comorbidities that may contribute to ulceration may also cause ongoing inflammation, disuse atrophy, and other metabolic disturbances; these may have a greater effect on wound healing than nutritional intake. Further research is needed; however, eating a diet that is high in protein, vitamins C and A, iron, and zinc is encouraged to promote healing (Gould et al., 2015). Particular consideration should be given to iron intake, because many patients are older adults who are at risk for iron deficiency anemia. After a dietary plan has been developed that meets the patient's nutritional needs and promotes healing, diet instruction is provided to the patient and family.

PROMOTING HOME, COMMUNITY-BASED, AND TRANSITIONAL CARE

The self-care program is planned with the patient so that activities that promote arterial and venous circulation, relieve pain, and promote tissue integrity are encouraged. Reasons for each aspect of the program are explained to the patient and family. Leg ulcers are often chronic and difficult to heal; they frequently recur, even when the patient rigorously follows the plan of care. Long-term care of the feet and legs to promote healing of wounds and prevent recurrence of ulcerations is the primary goal. Leg ulcers increase the patient's risk of infection, may be painful, and may limit mobility, necessitating lifestyle changes. Participation of family members and home health care providers may be necessary for treatments such as dressing changes, reassessments, reinforcement of instruction, and evaluation of the effectiveness of the plan of care. Regular follow-up with a primary provider is necessary.

Evaluation

Expected patient outcomes may include:
1. Demonstrates restored skin integrity
   a. Exhibits absence of inflammation
   b. Exhibits absence of drainage; negative wound culture
   c. Avoids trauma to the legs
2. Increases physical mobility
   a. Progresses gradually to optimal level of activity
   b. Reports that pain does not impede activity
3. Attains adequate nutrition
   a. Selects foods high in protein, vitamins, iron, and zinc
   b. Discusses with family members dietary modifications that need to be made at home
   c. Plans, with the family, a diet that is nutritionally sound

Varicose Veins

Varicose veins (varicosities) are abnormally dilated, tortuous, superficial veins caused by incompetent venous valves (see Fig. 30-14). Most commonly, this condition occurs in the lower extremities, the saphenous veins, or the lower trunk, but it can occur elsewhere in the body, such as the esophagus (e.g., esophageal varices; see Chapter 49).

It is estimated that varicose veins occur in 23% of American adults, and if spider telangiectasias and reticular veins are included in these statistics, the prevalence increases to 80% of men and 85% of women (Piazza, 2014). The condition is most common in people whose occupations require prolonged standing, such as salespeople, hair stylists, teachers, nurses and ancillary medical personnel, and construction workers. A hereditary weakness of the vein wall may contribute to the development of varicosities, and it commonly occurs in several members of the same family. Varicose veins are rare before puberty. Pregnancy may cause varicosities because of hormonal effects related to decreased venous outflow, increased pressure by the gravid uterus, and increased blood volume (Costantine, 2014).

Pathophysiology

Varicose veins may be primary (without involvement of deep veins) or secondary (resulting from obstruction of deep veins). A reflux of venous blood results in venous stasis. If only the superficial veins are affected, the person may have no symptoms but may be troubled by their appearance.

Clinical Manifestations

Symptoms, if present, may include dull aches, muscle cramps, increased muscle fatigue in the lower legs, ankle edema, and a feeling of heaviness of the legs. Nocturnal cramps are common. When deep venous obstruction results in varicose veins, the patient may develop the signs and symptoms of chronic venous insufficiency: edema, pain, pigmentation, and ulcerations. Susceptibility to injury and infection is increased, thus increasing risk for ulcerations.

Assessment and Diagnostic Findings

Diagnostic tests for varicose veins include the duplex ultrasound scan, which documents the anatomic site of reflux and provides a quantitative measure of the severity of valvular reflux. These scans are typically performed in a reverse Trendelenburg position or with the patient standing. Venography is not routinely performed to evaluate for valvular reflux. However, when it is used, it involves injecting a radiopaque contrast agent into the leg veins so that the vein anatomy can be visualized by x-ray studies during various leg movements. CT venography can be helpful, especially if the pelvic venous structures are involved.

Prevention and Medical Management

The patient should avoid activities that cause venous stasis, such as wearing socks that are too tight at the top or that leave marks on the skin, crossing the legs at the thighs, and sitting or standing for long periods. Changing position frequently, elevating the legs 3 to 6 in higher than heart level when they are tired, and getting up to walk for several minutes of every hour promote circulation. The patient is encouraged to walk 30 minutes each day if there are no contraindications. Walking up the stairs rather than using the elevator or escalator is helpful, and swimming is good exercise.

Graduated compression stockings, especially knee-high stockings, are useful. The patient who is overweight should be encouraged to begin a weight reduction plan.

The most common treatment options for venous insufficiency and varicose veins are surgical ligation and stripping, micro (stab) phlebectomy, thermal ablation with radiofrequency and laser therapy, and foam sclerotherapy.

Ligation and Stripping

Surgery for symptomatic varicose veins requires that the deep veins be patent and functional. The saphenous vein is ligated high in the groin, where the saphenous vein meets the femoral vein. In addition, the vein may be removed (stripped). After the vein is ligated, an incision is made 2 to 3 cm below the knee, and a metal or plastic wire is passed the full length of the vein to the point of ligation. The wire is then withdrawn, pulling (removing, stripping) the vein as it is removed. Pressure and elevation minimize bleeding during surgery.

If there are superficial varicose veins that are close to the surface, a micro phlebectomy may be performed. This procedure involves removal of a superficial varicosity using anywhere from 1 to 20 small incisions. There can be extensive bruising and risk of infection with this procedure.

Thermal Ablation

Thermal ablation is a nonsurgical approach using thermal energy. Radiofrequency ablation uses an electrical contact inside the vein. As the device is withdrawn, the vein is sealed. Laser ablation uses a laser fiber tip that seals the vein (decompressed). Topical gel may be used first to numb the skin along the course of the saphenous vein. To protect the surrounding tissue, several small punctures are made along the vein, and 100 to 200 mL of dilute lidocaine is delivered to the perivenous space using ultrasound guidance. The goal of this tumescent anesthesia (i.e., anesthesia that causes localized swelling) is to provide analgesia, thermal protection (the cuff of fluid surrounds the veins and accompanying nerves), and extrinsic compression of the vein (Joh, Kim, Jung, et al., 2014). The saphenous vein is entered percutaneously near the knee using ultrasound guidance. A catheter is introduced into the saphenous vein and advanced to the saphenofemoral junction. The device is then activated and withdrawn, sealing the vein. Small bandages and graduated compression stockings are applied after the procedure. The patient is asked not to remove the stockings for at least 24 hours and then to rewrap the legs and wear the compression stockings while ambulatory for at least 1-week postprocedure. A simultaneous micro phlebectomy of branch varicosities may be performed at the same time; this is associated with a lower incidence of thrombophlebitis. This is also associated with quality of life improvements such as decreased leg swelling, pain, skin changes and healing of ulcerations, because all symptomatic veins may be treated at one time (Jarjous, Jarjous, & Nahhas, 2015). Patients are ambulatory prior to being discharged from the outpatient facility and have no activity restrictions, except that strenuous exercise, such as weight lifting, bicycle riding, or swimming is discouraged for 2 weeks. Nonsteroidal anti-inflammatory medications such as ibuprofen (Motrin) and cool compresses are used as needed for pain. The patient is informed that bruising may occur along the course of the saphenous vein and that he or she may experience leg cramps

for a few days and may find it difficult to straighten the knees for up to 1.5 weeks.

Cyanoacrylate embolization for varicose veins has recently been approved for the treatment of an incompetent greater saphenous vein. Cyanoacrylate adhesive has been used for the treatment of arteriovenous malformations and a modified cyanoacrylate adhesive was developed that has rapid polymerization on contact with blood and tissue, flexibility sufficient to tolerate dynamic movements in the legs without generation of symptoms or be perceptible by the patient, and has a high viscosity to decrease the risk of propagation or embolization into the deep veins (Morrison, Gibson, McEnroe, et al., 2015). During this procedure, a sheath is placed into the greater saphenous vein (guided by ultrasound). A catheter is advanced to the proximal saphenous vein and injections of cyanoacrylate are given, followed by local compression, and then repeated injections with repeated compression until the entire length of the target vein segment is treated. Cyanoacrylate embolization has been associated with less procedural ecchymosis because heat is not needed during this procedure.

Sclerotherapy

Sclerotherapy involves injection of an irritating chemical into a vein to produce localized phlebitis and fibrosis, thereby obliterating the lumen of the vein. This treatment may be performed alone for small varicosities or may follow vein ablation, ligation, or stripping. Sclerotherapy is typically performed in an examination or procedure room and does not require sedation. After the sclerosing agent is injected, graduated compression stockings are applied to the leg and are worn for approximately 7 days after the procedure. Ultrasound-guided foam sclerotherapy has been found to be more effective in achieving closure of the branch veins. It is also associated with decreased symptoms of leg aching, itching, and edema, less skin changes and ulcerations, and patient satisfaction in excess of 70% (Jarjous et al., 2015; Piazza, 2014). After sclerotherapy, walking activities are encouraged as prescribed to maintain blood flow in the leg.

Nursing Management

Ligation and stripping can be performed in an outpatient setting, or the patient may be admitted to the hospital on the day of surgery and discharged the next day if a bilateral procedure is to be performed and the patient is at high risk for postoperative complications. If the procedure is performed in an outpatient setting, nursing measures are the same as if the patient were hospitalized. Bed rest is discouraged, and the patient is encouraged to become ambulatory as soon as sedation has worn off. The patient is instructed to walk every hour for 5 to 10 minutes while awake for the first 24 hours if he or she can tolerate the discomfort, and then to increase walking and activity as tolerated. Graduated compression stockings are worn continuously for about 1 week after vein stripping. The nurse assists the patient to perform exercises and move the legs. The foot of the bed should be elevated. Standing and sitting are discouraged.

Promoting Comfort and Understanding

Analgesic agents are prescribed to help the patient move the affected extremities more comfortably. Dressings are inspected for bleeding, particularly at the groin, where the risk of bleeding is greatest. The nurse is alert for reported sensations of "pins and needles." Hypersensitivity to touch in the involved extremity may indicate a temporary or permanent nerve injury resulting from surgery, because the saphenous vein and nerve are close to each other in the leg. Any of these signs or symptoms should be reported to the primary provider.

Usually, the patient may shower after the first 24 hours. The patient is instructed to dry the incisions well with a clean towel using a patting technique rather than rubbing. Alternatively, the patient may be instructed to dry the area using a blow-dryer. Application of skin lotion is avoided until the incisions are completely healed to avoid infection. The patient is instructed to apply sunscreen or zinc oxide to the incisional area prior to sun exposure; otherwise, hyperpigmentation of the incision, scarring, or both may occur.

If the patient has undergone sclerotherapy, a burning sensation in the injected leg may be experienced for 1 or 2 days. The nurse may encourage the use of a mild analgesic medication as prescribed and walking to provide relief.

Promoting Home, Community-Based, and Transitional Care

Long-term venous compression is essential after discharge, and the patient needs to obtain adequate supplies of graduated compression stockings or elastic bandages. Exercise of the legs is necessary; the development of an individualized plan requires consultation with the patient and the health care team.

LYMPHATIC DISORDERS

The lymphatic system consists of a set of vessels that spread throughout most of the body, as described previously in this chapter. The fluid drained from the interstitial space by the lymphatic system is called *lymph*. The flow of lymph depends on the intrinsic contractions of the lymph vessels, the contraction of muscles, respiratory movements, and gravity. The lymphatic system of the abdominal cavity maintains a steady flow of digested fatty food (chyle) from the intestinal mucosa to the thoracic duct. In other parts of the body, the lymphatic system's function is regional; the lymphatic vessels of the head, for example, empty into clusters of lymph nodes located in the neck, and those of the extremities empty into nodes of the axillae and the groin.

Lymphangitis and Lymphadenitis

Lymphangitis is an acute inflammation of the lymphatic channels. It arises most commonly from a focus of infection in an extremity. Usually, the infectious organism is a hemolytic streptococcus. The characteristic red streaks that extend up the arm or the leg from an infected wound outline the course of the lymphatic vessels as they drain.

The lymph nodes located along the course of the lymphatic channels also become enlarged, red, and tender (acute lymphadenitis). They can also become necrotic and form an abscess (suppurative lymphadenitis). The nodes involved most often are those in the groin, axilla, or cervical region.

Because these infections are nearly always caused by organisms that are sensitive to antibiotics, it is unusual to see abscess formation. Recurrent episodes of lymphangitis are often associated with progressive lymphedema. After acute attacks, a graduated compression stocking should be worn on the affected extremity for several months to prevent long-term edema.

Lymphedema and Elephantiasis

Lymphedema may be primary (congenital malformations) or secondary (acquired obstructions). Tissue swelling occurs in the extremities because of an increased quantity of lymph that results from obstruction of lymphatic vessels. It is especially marked when the extremity is in a dependent position. Initially, the edema is soft and pitting. As the condition progresses, the edema becomes firm, nonpitting, and unresponsive to treatment. The most common type is congenital lymphedema (lymphedema praecox), which is caused by hypoplasia of the lymphatic system of the lower extremity. This disorder is usually seen in women and first appears before age 35 (Brouillard, Boon, & Vikkula, 2014).

The obstruction may be in the lymph nodes and the lymphatic vessels. Sometimes, it is seen in the arm after an axillary node dissection (e.g., for breast cancer) and in the leg in association with varicose veins or chronic thrombophlebitis. In the latter case, the lymphatic obstruction usually is caused by chronic lymphangitis. Lymphatic obstruction caused by a parasite (filaria) is most frequently seen in the tropics. When chronic swelling is present, there may be frequent bouts of acute infection characterized by high fever and chills and increased residual edema after the inflammation has resolved. These lead to chronic fibrosis, thickening of the subcutaneous tissues, and hypertrophy of the skin. This condition, in which chronic swelling of the extremity recedes only slightly with elevation, is referred to as elephantiasis. There are an estimated 120 million people in the world infected by lymph-dwelling filarial parasites; of these, 40 million have lymphedema and secondary infections, creating an enormous global burden (Mortimer & Rockson, 2014).

Medical Management

The goal of therapy is to reduce and control the edema and prevent infection. Active and passive exercises assist in moving lymphatic fluid into the bloodstream. External compression devices milk the fluid proximally from the foot to the hip or from the hand to the axilla. When the patient is ambulatory, custom-fitted graduated compression stockings or sleeves are worn; those with the highest compression strength (exceeding 40 mm Hg) are suggested; however, many patients cannot tolerate the pressure. When the leg is affected, continuous bed rest with the leg elevated may aid in mobilizing the fluids. Manual lymphatic drainage performed by specially trained therapists is a technique designed to direct or shift the congested lymph through functioning lymphatics that have preserved drainage. Manual lymphatic drainage is incorporated in a sequential treatment approach used in combination with multilayer compression bandages, exercises, skin care, pressure gradient sleeves, and pneumatic pumps, depending on the severity and stage of the lymphedema (Zaleska et al., 2014).

Pharmacologic Therapy

As initial therapy, the diuretic furosemide (Lasix) may be prescribed to prevent fluid overload due to mobilization of extracellular fluid. Diuretics have also been used along with elevation of the leg and the use of graduated compression stockings or sleeves. However, the use of diuretics alone has little benefit because their main action is to limit capillary filtration by decreasing the circulating blood volume. If lymphangitis or cellulitis is present, antibiotic therapy is initiated. Lymphedema carries a 71-fold enhancement of risk for cellulitis; therefore, the patient is taught to inspect the skin for evidence of infection (Mortimer & Rockson, 2014).

Surgical Management

Surgery is performed if the edema is severe and uncontrolled by medical therapy, if mobility is severely compromised, or if infection persists. One surgical approach involves the excision of the affected subcutaneous tissue and fascia, with skin grafting to cover the defect. Another procedure involves the surgical relocation of superficial lymphatic vessels into the deep lymphatic system, also known as lymph node transfer, by means of a buried dermal flap to provide a conduit for lymphatic drainage (Ciudad, Orfaniotis, Socas, et al., 2015). Lymphaticovenous bypasses also are performed with anastomosing the end of the lymphatic vessels to the side of veins to reduce lymphatic flow in the limbs (Qiu, Chen, & Cheng, 2014).

Nursing Management

After surgery, antibiotics may be prescribed for 3 to 7 days (Mortimer & Rockson, 2014). Constant elevation of the affected extremity and observation for complications are essential. Complications may include flap necrosis, hematoma or abscess under the flap, and cellulitis. The nurse instructs the patient or caregiver to inspect the dressing daily. Unusual drainage or any inflammation around the wound margin suggests infection and should be reported to the surgeon. The patient is informed that there may be a loss of sensation in the surgical area. The patient is also instructed to avoid the application of heating pads or exposure to sun to prevent burns or trauma to the area.

CELLULITIS

Cellulitis is the most common infectious cause of limb swelling. Cellulitis can occur as a single isolated event or a series of recurrent events. It is sometimes misdiagnosed as recurrent thrombophlebitis or chronic venous insufficiency.

Pathophysiology

Cellulitis occurs when an entry point through normal skin barriers allows bacteria to enter and release their toxins in the subcutaneous tissues. The etiologic pathogen of cellulitis is typically either *Streptococcus* species or *Staphylococcus aureus* (Horseman & Bowman, 2013).

Clinical Manifestations

The acute onset of swelling, localized redness, warmth, and pain is frequently associated with systemic signs of fever, chills, and sweating. The redness may not be uniform and often skips areas and eventually develops a pitting "orange peel" appearance. Regional lymph nodes may also be tender and enlarged (Horseman & Bowman, 2013).

 Concept Mastery Alert

Cellulitis needs to be differentiated from lymphangitis. With cellulitis, the swelling and redness is localized and anatomically nonspecific. With lymphangitis, characteristic red streaks appear denoting the outline of the lymphatic vessels that are affected.

Medical Management

Mild cases of cellulitis can be treated on an outpatient basis with oral antibiotic therapy. If the cellulitis is severe, the patient is treated with IV antibiotics. The key to preventing recurrent episodes of cellulitis lies in adequate antibiotic therapy for the initial event and in identifying the site of bacterial entry. Cracks and fissures that occur in the skin between the toes must be examined as potential sites of bacterial entry. Other locations include drug use injection sites, contusions, abrasions, ulceration, ingrown toenails, and hangnails.

Nursing Management

The patient is instructed to elevate the affected area 3 to 6 in above heart level and apply cool, moist packs to the site every 2 to 4 hours until the inflammation has resolved and then transition to warm moist packs. Patients with sensory and circulatory deficits, such as those caused by diabetes and paralysis, should use caution when applying warm packs because burns may occur; it is advisable to use a thermometer or have a caregiver ensure that the temperature is not more than lukewarm. Education should focus on preventing a recurrent episode. The patient with peripheral vascular disease or diabetes should receive education or reinforcement about skin and foot care.

CRITICAL THINKING EXERCISES

1 **pg** A 55-year-old female presents to the emergency department with 4- to 6-hour history of chest and back pain, hoarse voice, and difficulty swallowing. She is taking apixaban (Eliquis) for atrial fibrillation and has renal insufficiency (creatinine of 2.2 mg/dL) as a complication of poorly managed diabetes. Her blood glucose is 420 mg/dL and you note her blood pressure is 200/102 mm Hg. She admits to using methamphetamines today but insists she hasn't taken any other drugs. What additional assessment and vital signs need to be obtained? What are your priority assessments for this patient? Is the methamphetamine impacting the diagnosis and treatment? How would you triage and prioritize your nursing care for this patient?

2 **ebp** A 22-year-old female college student presents to campus health care with complaints of left upper extremity edema and a generalized ache of her shoulder and upper arm that is worse at the end of the day. She noted the onset of the symptoms 2 months ago after joining an intramural volleyball team. She is concerned as she has noted new veins across her left shoulder and upper chest wall. There is a positive maternal family history for DVT. What further diagnostic studies should be performed? Are there any labs that should be drawn? At the time of her clinic visit she mentions that she would like to begin taking birth control pills. What is the strength of the evidence that supports the best method of contraception for her, assuming she is at risk for thromboembolism? What additional information should you obtain? What risks should you discuss with this patient? Should she be given birth control pills at this visit?

3 A 54-year-old man presents to the community clinic. He needs a physical examination prior to beginning a job as a cashier at a local grocery store. The patient is found to have a history of diabetes that has not been consistently managed, and has a 38-year history of smoking a pack of cigarettes each day. Physical examination reveals blood pressure of 162/104 mm Hg, absent anterior tibial and posterior tibial artery pulses, bilateral varicose veins, and 1+ pitting ankle edema. What additional information is needed as part of the history and physical examination? What risk factor modifications would you want to address with this patient?

REFERENCES

*Asterisk indicates nursing research.

Books

Cronenwett, J. L., & Johnston, K. W. (2014). *Rutherford's vascular surgery* (8th ed., Vols. I and II). Philadelphia, PA: W. B. Saunders.

Grossman, S., & Porth, C.M. (2014). *Porth's pathophysiology: Concepts of altered health states* (9th ed.). Philadelphia, PA: Lippincott Williams & Wilkins.

Weber, J. R., & Kelley, J. H. (2014). *Health assessment in nursing* (5th ed.). Philadelphia, PA: Lippincott Williams & Wilkins.

Zierler, R. E., & Dawson, D. L. (2015). *Strandness's duplex scanning in vascular disorders* (5th ed.). Philadelphia, PA: Lippincott Williams & Wilkins.

Journals and Electronic Documents

Armstrong, E. J., Chen, D. C., Westin, G. G., et al. (2014). Adherence to guideline-recommended therapy is associated with decreased major adverse cardiovascular events and major adverse limb events among patients with peripheral arterial disease. *Journal of the American Heart Association, 3,* e000697.

Arnaoutoglou, E., Kouvelos, G., Koutsoumpelis, A., et al. (2015). An update on the inflammatory response after endovascular repair for abdominal aortic aneurysm. *Mediators of Inflammation,* Hindawi Publishing Corporation, Article ID 945035, 6 pages, dx.doi.org/10.1155/2015/945035.

Attenhofer Jost, C. H., Greutmann, M., Connolly, H. M., et al. (2014). Medical treatment of aortic aneurysms in Marfan syndrome and other heritable conditions. *Current Cardiology Reviews, 10*(2), 161–171.

Barnes, G. D., Kanthi, Y., & Froehlich, J. B. (2015). Venous thromboembolism: Predicting recurrence and the need for extended anticoagulation. *Vascular Medicine, 20*(2), 143–152.

Barochiner, J., Aparicio, L. S., & Waisman, G. D. (2014). Challenges associated with peripheral arterial disease in women. *Vascular Health and Risk Management, 10,* 115–128.

Bergmark, B. A., Sobieszczyk, P., Gravereaux, E. C., et al. (2013). Acute dissection of the descending aorta: A case report and review of the literature. *Cardiology Therapy, 2,* 199–213.

Birn, J., & Vedantham, S. (2015). May-Thurner syndrome and other obstructive iliac vein lesions: Meaning, myth, and mystery. *Vascular Medicine, 20*(1), 74–83.

Brouillard, P., Boon, L., & Vikkula, M. (2014). Genetics of lymphatic anomalies. *The Journal of Clinical Investigation, 124*(3), 898–904.

Chi, Y. W., & Raffetto, J. D. (2015). Venous leg ulceration pathophysiology and evidence based treatment. *Vascular Medicine, 20*(2), 168–181.

Ciudad, P., Orfaniotis, G., Socas, J., et al. (2015). Technical considerations to avoid microvascular complications during groin lymph node free flap transfer. *Archives of Plastic Surgery, 42*(5), 650–652.

Conte, M. S., Pomposelli, F. B., Clair, D. G., et al. (2015). Society for vascular surgery practice guidelines for atherosclerotic occlusive disease of the lower extremities: Management of asymptomatic disease and claudication. *Society for Vascular Surgery, 61*(3S), 2S–40S.

Cooper, C. J., Murphy, T. P., Cutlip, D. E., et al; CORAL Investigators (2014). Stenting and medical therapy for atherosclerotic renal-artery stenosis. *The New England Journal of Medicine, 370*(1), 13–22.

Costantine, M. M. (2014). Physiologic and pharmacokinetic changes in pregnancy. *Frontiers in Pharmacology, 5,* 65.

Das, S., & Maiti, A. (2013). Acrocyanosis: An overview. *Indian Journal of Dermatology, 58*(6), 417–420.

DeMartino, R. R., Goodney, P. P., Nolan, B. W., et al; Vascular Study Group of New England. (2013). Optimal selection of patients for elective abdominal aortic aneurysm repair based on life expectancy. *Journal of Vascular Surgery, 58*(3), 589–595.

DeSart, K., Scali, S. T., Feezor, R. J., et al. (2013). Fate of patients with spinal cord ischemia complicating thoracic endovascular aortic repair. *Journal of Vascular Surgery, 58*(3), 635–642.

Di Minno, G., Spadarella, G., Cafaro, G., et al. (2014). Systematic reviews and meta-analyses for more profitable strategies in peripheral artery disease. *Annals of Medicine, 46*(7), 475–489.

Dobesh, P. P., & Fanikos, J. (2014). New oral anticoagulants for the treatment of venous thromboembolism: Understanding differences and similarities. *Drugs, 74,* 2015–2032.

Favero, G., Paganelli, C., Buffoli, B., et al. (2014). Endothelium and its alterations in cardiovascular diseases: Life style intervention. *BioMed Research International,* 801896, 28 pages, http://dx.org/10.1155/2014/801896

*Fritschi, C., Collins, E. G., O'Connell, S., et al. (2013). The effects of smoking status on walking ability and health-related quality of life in patients with peripheral arterial disease. *Journal of Cardiovascular Nursing, 28*(4), 380–386.

Gould, L., Abadir, P., Brem, H., et al. (2015). Chronic wound repair and healing in older adults: Current status and future research. *Journal of the American Geriatrics Society, 63*(3), 427–438.

Harter, K., Levine M., & Henderson, S. O. (2015). Anticoagulation drug therapy: A review. *Western Journal of Emergency Medicine, 16*(1), 11–17.

Hedayati, N., Carson, J. G., Chi, Y. W., et al. (2015). Management of mixed arterial venous lower extremity ulceration: A review. *Vascular Medicine, 20*(5), 479–486.

Heit, J. A. (2015). Epidemiology of venous thromboembolism. *Nature Reviews in Cardiology, 12*(8), 464–474.

Horseman, M., & Bowman, J. D. (2013). Is community-acquired methicillin-resistant staphylococcus aureus coverage needed for cellulitis? *Infectious Disease Therapy, 2,* 175–185.

Hu, H., Cai, Y., Wang, C., et al. (2014). Successful treatment of post-traumatic phlegmasia cerulea dolens by reconstructing the external iliac vein: A case report. *Journal of Medical Case Reports, 8,* 149.

Ingargiola, M. J., Daniali, L. N., & Lee, E. S. (2013). Does the application of incisional negative pressure therapy to high-risk wounds prevent surgical site complications? A systematic review. *EPlasty, 13,* e49. Retrieved on 10/26/2015 at: www.eplasty.com

Jarjous, F., Jarjous, R., & Nahhas, G. (2015). One-step approach to treating venous insufficiency. *Journal of Clinical Medical Research, 7*(9), 681–684.

Jenkins, J. S., & Michael, P. (2014). Deep venous thrombosis: An interventionalist's approach. *The Ochsner Journal, 14,* 633–640.

Joh, J. H., Kim, W. S., Jung, I. M., et al; Consensus Working Group. (2014). Consensus for the treatment of varicose vein with radiofrequency ablation. *Vascular Specialist International, 30*(3), 105–112.

Joks, M., Czy , A., Popławski, D., et al. (2014). Incidence and risk factors for central venous catheter-related thrombosis in hematological patients. *Medical Oncology, 31,* 772.

Kahn, S. R., Comerota, A. J., Cushman, M., et al; American Heart Association Council on Peripheral Vascular Disease, Council on Clinical Cardiology, and Council on Cardiovascular and Stroke Nursing (2014). The postthrombotic syndrome: Evidence-based prevention, diagnosis, and treatment strategies: A scientific statement from the American Heart Association. *Circulation, 130,* 1636–1661.

Klein, K. C., & Guha, S. C. (2014). Cutaneous wound healing: Current concepts and advances in wound care. *Indian Journal of Plastic Surgery, 47*(3), 303–317.

Krishna, S. M., Moxon, J. V., & Golledge, J. (2015). A review of the pathophysiology and potential biomarkers for peripheral artery disease. *International Journal of Molecular Sciences, 16,* 11294–11322.

Kuivaniemi, H., Ryer, E. J., Elmore, J. R., et al. (2014). Update on abdominal aortic aneurysm research: From clinical to genetic studies. *Scientifica,* Article ID 564734, 14 pages, http://dx.doi.org/10.1155/2014/564734.

Lim, M. Y., & Moll, S. (2015). Thrombophilia. *Vascular Medicine, 20*(2), 193–196.

Lucania, G., Camiolo, E., Carmina, M. G., et al. (2014). Multidisciplinary approach in pregnancy-associated thrombotic thrombocytopenic purpura: A case report. *Blood Transfusion, 12*(Suppl 1), s137–s140.

McDermott, M. M. (2013). Functional impairment in peripheral artery disease and how to improve it in 2013. *Current Cardiology Reports, 15*(4), 347.

Minet, C., Potton, L., Bonadona, A., et al. (2015). Venous thromboembolism in the ICU: Main characteristics, diagnosis and thromboprophylaxis. *Critical Care, 19,* 287.

Mohanty, B. D., Looser, P. M., Gokanapudy, L. R., et al. (2014). Controversies regarding the new oral anticoagulants for stroke prevention in patients with atrial fibrillation. *Vascular Medicine, 19*(3), 190–204.

Morrison, N., Gibson, K., McEnroe, S., et al. (2015). Randomized trial comparing cyanoacrylate embolization and radiofrequency ablation for incompetent great saphenous veins (VeClose). *Journal of Vascular Surgery, 61*(4), 985–994.

Mortimer, P. S., & Rockson, S. G. (2014). New developments in clinical aspects of lymphatic disease. *The Journal of Clinical Investigation, 124*(3), 915–921.

Myung, S. K., Ju, W., Cho, B., et al. (2013). Efficacy of vitamin and antioxidant supplements in prevention of cardiovascular disease: Systematic review and meta-analysis of randomised controlled trials. *British Medical Journal, 346,* f10.

Neel, J. D., Kruse, R. L., Dombrovskiy, V. Y., et al. (2015). Cilostazol and freedom from amputation after lower extremity revascularization. *Journal of Vascular Surgery, 61*(4), 960–964.

Patel, H. J., Williams, D. M., Drews, J. D., et al. (2014). A 20-year experience with thoracic endovascular aortic repair. *Annals of Surgery, 260*(4), 691–696.

Patmo, A. S., Krijnen, P., Tuinebreijer, W. E., et al. (2014). The effect of vacuum-assisted closure on the bacterial load and type of bacteria: A systematic review. *Advances in Wound Care (New Rochelle), 3*(5), 383–389.

Piazza, G. (2014). Varicose veins. *Circulation, 130,* 582–587.

Piazza, G. (2015). Beyond Virchow's triad: Does cardiovascular inflammation explain the recurrent nature of venous thromoembolism? *Vascular Medicine, 20*(2), 102–104.

Puranik, A. S., Dawson, E. R., & Peppas, N. A. (2013). Recent advances in drug eluting stents. *International Journal of Pharmaceuticals, 441*(1–2), 665–679.

Qiu, S. S., Chen, H. Y., & Cheng, M. H. (2014). Vascularized lymph node flap transfer and lymphovenous anastomosis for klippel-trenaunay syndrome with congenital lymphedema. *Plastic Reconstructive Surgery Global Open, 2,* e167.

Rajiah, P. (2013). CT and MRI in the evaluation of thoracic aortic diseases. *Internal Journal of Vascular Medicine,* Article ID 797189, 16 pages, dx.doi.org/10.1155/2013/797189

Ratchford, E. V., & Evans, N. S. (2015). Raynaud's phenomenon. *Vascular Medicine, 20*(3), 269–271.

Ronchey, S., Pecoraro, F., Alberti, V., et al. (2015). Popliteal artery aneurysm repair in the endovascular era. Fourteen-years single center experience. *Medicine (Baltimore), 94*(30), e1130. Retrieved on 11/14/2015 at: www.md-journal.com

Sadat, U. (2013). Radiographic contrast-media-induced acute kidney injury: Pathophysiology and prophylactic strategies. *ISRN Radiology,* Article ID 496438, 21 pages, dx.doi.org/10.5402/2013/496438

Shennib, H., Hickle, K., & Bowles, B. (2015). Axillary vein thrombosis induced by an increasingly popular oscillating dumbbell exercise device: A case report. *Journal of Cardiothoracic Surgery, 10,* 73.

Skeik, N., Murphy, C. J., & Porten, B. R. (2014). The role of novel anticoagulants in the management of venous thromboembolism. *Vascular Medicine, 19*(3), 205–214.

Sood, A., Granick, M. S., & Tomaselli, N. L. (2014). Wound dressings and comparative effectiveness data. *Advances in Wound Care (New Rochelle), 3*(8), 511–529.

Suzuki, T., Eagle, K. A., Bossone, E., et al. (2014). Medical management in type B aortic dissection. *Annals of Cardiothoracic Surgery, 3*(4), 413–417.

Thiruvoipati, T., Kielhorn, C. E., & Armstrong, E. J. (2015). Peripheral artery disease in patients with diabetes: Epidemiology, mechanisms, and outcomes. *World Journal of Diabetes, 6*(7), 961–969.

Walker, C. M., Bunch, F. T., Cavros, N. G., et al. (2015). Multidisciplinary approach to the diagnosis and management of patients with peripheral arterial disease. *Clinical Interventions in Aging, 10,* 1147–1153.

Zakai, N. A., McClure, L. A., Judd, S. E., et al. (2014). Racial and regional differences in venous thromboembolism in the United States in 3 cohorts. *Circulation, 129*(14), 1502–1509.

Zaleska, M., Olszewski, W. L., & Durlik, M. (2014). The effectiveness of intermittent pneumatic compression in long-term therapy of lymphedema of lower limbs. *Lymphatic Research and Biology, 12*(2), 103–109.

Ziganshin, B. A., Dumfarth, J., & Elefteriades, J. A. (2014). Natural history of type B aortic dissection: Ten tips. *Annals of Cardiothoracic Surgery, 3*(3), 247–254.

Resources

American Venous Forum, www.veinforum.org
National Heart, Lung, and Blood Institute, www.nhlbi.nih.gov
Society for Vascular Nursing (SVN), www.svnnet.org
Society for Vascular Surgery (SVS), www.vascularweb.org
Society for Vascular Ultrasound (SVU), www.svunet.org
Society for Vascular Medicine (SVM), www.vascularmed.org
Vascular Disease Foundation, vasculardisease.org

31

Assessment and Management of Patients With Hypertension

LEARNING OBJECTIVES

On completion of this chapter, the learner will be able to:

1 Define normal blood pressure and categories of abnormal pressures.
2 Identify risk factors for hypertension.
3 Explain the differences between normal blood pressure and hypertension and discuss the significance of hypertension.

4 Describe treatment approaches for hypertension, including lifestyle modifications and medication therapy.
5 Use the nursing process as a framework for care of the patient with hypertension.
6 Describe hypertensive crises and their treatment.

GLOSSARY

dyslipidemia: abnormal blood lipid levels, including high total, low-density lipoprotein, and triglyceride levels as well as low high-density lipoprotein levels
hypertensive emergency: a situation in which blood pressure is severely elevated and there is evidence of actual or probable target organ damage
hypertensive urgency: a situation in which blood pressure is severely elevated but there is no evidence of impending or progressive target organ damage
isolated systolic hypertension: a condition most commonly seen in the older adult in which the systolic pressure is

greater than 140 mm Hg and the diastolic pressure is less than 80 mm Hg
monotherapy: medication therapy with a single agent
primary hypertension: denotes high blood pressure from an unidentified cause; also called essential hypertension
rebound hypertension: blood pressure that is controlled with medication and becomes uncontrolled (abnormally high) with the abrupt discontinuation of medication
secondary hypertension: high blood pressure from an identified cause, such as kidney disease

Hypertension is the most common chronic disease among adults in the United States and in the world (Weber, Schiffrin, White, et al., 2014). It is identified as the leading risk factor for premature death, disability, and overall disease burden worldwide because it may lead to myocardial infarction, heart failure, stroke, and chronic kidney disease when not appropriately treated (Mozaffarian, Benjamin, Go, et al., 2016). The overall risk of developing these cardiovascular and renal disorders is low among patients with blood pressures (BPs) that are consistently stable around 115/75 mm Hg; however, each increase of 20 mm Hg in the systolic BP or 10 mm Hg in the diastolic BP doubles the risk for having a cardiovascular event (e.g., heart attack or stroke) (Weber et al., 2014). And yet, most patients with hypertension may lower their blood pressure, thereby significantly modifying these risks, through lifestyle changes (e.g., diet, exercise, smoking cessation) and adhering to appropriate medication regimens. This chapter presents an overview of hypertension and how it is classified and managed so that nurses may appropriately assess, monitor, educate, and intervene with patients with hypertension.

Hypertension

Hypertension is defined by the *American Society of Hypertension (ASH)* and the *International Society of Hypertension*

(ISH) as a systolic blood pressure (SBP) of 140 mm Hg or higher or a diastolic blood pressure (DBP) of 90 mm Hg or higher, based on the average of two or more accurate blood pressure measurements taken 1 to 4 weeks apart by a health care provider (Weber et al., 2014). This mirrors the definition of hypertension published in the landmark *Seventh Report of the Joint National Committee on prevention, detection, evaluation, and treatment of high blood pressure* (JNC 7) (Chobanian, Bakris, Black, et al., 2003a); this definition was not revised in the more recent *Eighth Joint National Committee* (JNC 8) Report (James, Oparil, Carter, et al., 2014). Table 31-1 shows the classification of blood pressure established by JNC 7 and reinforced by ASH and ISH (Chobanian et al., 2003a; Weber et al., 2014). The blood pressure categories, from normal to stage 2 hypertension, emphasize the direct relationship between levels of systolic and diastolic BPs and the risks of morbidity, all-cause mortality, and, more specifically, cardiovascular disease mortality. Although increasing levels of either systolic or diastolic pressure are risky, treatment that controls blood pressure is so effective that mortality has been found to be no different between patients with hypertension who were appropriately treated and individuals without hypertension (Barengo, Antikainen, Kastarinen, et al., 2013).

The JNC 7 and ASH and ISH define a blood pressure of less than 120/80 mm Hg diastolic as normal, 120 to 139/80 to

TABLE 31-1 Classification of Blood Pressure for Adults Age 18 and Older[b]

BP Classification[a]	Systolic BP (mm Hg)		Diastolic BP (mm Hg)
Normal	<120	and	<80
Prehypertension	120–139	or	80–89
Stage 1 hypertension	140–159	or	90–99
Stage 2 hypertension	≥160	or	≥100

BP, blood pressure.

[a]Based on the average of two or more properly measured, seated readings taken on each of two or more office visits.

[b]A systolic blood pressure up to 150 mm Hg in adults older than 80 years of age is considered acceptable/does not require treatment.

Adapted from Chobanian, A. V., Bakris, G. L., Black, H. R., et al. (2003a). Seventh Report of the Joint National Committee on prevention, detection, evaluation, and treatment of high blood pressure: The JNC 7 Report. *JAMA*, 289(19), 2560–2572; Weber, M. A., Schiffrin, E. L., White, W. B., et al. (2014). Clinical practice guidelines for the management of hypertension in the community: A statement by the American Society of Hypertension and the International Society of Hypertension. *The Journal of Clinical Hypertension (Greenwich)*, 16(1), 14–26.

89 mm Hg as prehypertension, and 140/90 mm Hg or higher as hypertension (Chobanian et al., 2003a; Weber et al., 2014) (see Table 31-1). The term *stage* is used to define levels of hypertension; the classification system parallels what is used to describe cancer progression so that both the public and health care professionals will understand that consistently higher elevations in blood pressure from prehypertension to stage 1 or 2 are associated with greater health risks. The category of *prehypertension* is used to emphasize that people whose blood pressure begins to rise above 120/80 mm Hg are at risk to become hypertensive, and that even slight increases in pressure are associated with an adverse risk profile as well as increased risk of stroke, heart attack, heart failure, and cardiovascular death (Mozaffarian et al., 2016). To prevent or delay progression to hypertension and reduce risk, health care providers are encouraged to educate and inform patients with blood pressures in the prehypertension category to begin lifestyle modifications, which include weight loss, salt reduction, exercise, alcohol consumption reduction, and smoking cessation (Weber et al., 2014). Patients diagnosed with stage 1 hypertension are encouraged to adopt lifestyle changes while being treated with medications and seen by their primary provider every month until their blood pressure goal is reached and subsequently about every 3 to 6 months. People with stage 2 hypertension or with other complicating conditions need to be seen more frequently.

About 32.6% of the adults in the United States have hypertension, and the prevalence increases significantly as people get older or have other cardiovascular risk factors. Approximately 45.9% of persons with hypertension do not have their blood pressure under control (Mozaffarian et al., 2016). The prevalence of hypertension varies by ethnicity and gender, and is estimated at approximately 32.9% among Caucasian men, 30.1% among Caucasian women, 44.9% among African American men, 46.1% among African American women, 29.6% among Hispanic men, and 29.9% among Hispanic women. The prevalence of hypertension among African Americans is among the highest in the world. Moreover, African Americans tend to develop hypertension at younger ages than white Americans (Mozaffarian et al., 2016).

About 95% of patients with high blood pressure have **primary hypertension** (also called *essential hypertension*), which is defined as high blood pressure from an unidentified cause. The remaining small percentage, about 5%, have **secondary hypertension**, which occurs when a cause for the high blood pressure can be identified (Weber et al., 2014). These causes include chronic kidney disease, renal artery stenosis, hyperaldosteronism (mineralocorticoid hypertension), pheochromocytoma, and sleep apnea (Weber et al., 2014). High blood pressure can also occur with pregnancy; women who experience high blood pressure during pregnancy are at increased risk of ischemic heart disease, heart attacks, strokes, kidney disease, diabetes, and death from heart attack (Männistö, Mendola, Vääräsmäki, et al., 2013).

Hypertension is sometimes called the *silent killer* because people who have it are often symptom free. In the National Health and Nutrition Examination Survey (NHANES) conducted from 2009 to 2012, 18% of adults surveyed were unaware of their elevated blood pressure (Mozaffarian et al., 2016). Once identified, elevated blood pressure requires monitoring at regular intervals because hypertension is a lifelong condition.

High blood pressure can be viewed as a sign, as a risk factor for atherosclerotic cardiovascular disease, or as a disease. As a sign, blood pressure is used by nurses and other health care professionals to monitor a patient's clinical status. Elevated pressure may indicate an excessive dose of vasoconstrictive medication, stress, or other problems. As a risk factor, hypertension contributes to the rate at which atherosclerotic plaque accumulates within arterial walls. As a disease, hypertension is a major contributor to death related to cardiac, cerebrovascular, kidney, and peripheral vascular disease.

Hypertension often accompanies other risk factors for atherosclerotic heart disease, such as **dyslipidemia** (abnormal blood lipid levels, including high total, low-density lipoprotein [LDL], and triglyceride levels as well as low high-density lipoprotein [HDL] levels), obesity, diabetes, a family history of early cardiovascular events, metabolic syndrome, a sedentary lifestyle, and obstructive sleep apnea (Weber et al., 2014). The prevalence is also higher in patients who have other cardiovascular conditions, including heart failure, coronary artery disease, and a history of stroke. Cigarette smoking does not cause high blood pressure; however, if a patient with hypertension smokes, their risk of dying of a cardiovascular event increases significantly (Weber et al., 2014).

Prolonged blood pressure elevation gradually damages blood vessels throughout the body, particularly in target organs such as the heart, kidneys, brain, and eyes. The typical outcomes of prolonged, uncontrolled hypertension are myocardial infarction, heart failure, chronic kidney disease, strokes, and impaired vision. Hypertrophy (enlargement) of the left ventricle of the heart may occur as it works to pump blood against the elevated pressure. See Chapter 28 for discussion of ventricular hypertrophy.

Pathophysiology

Blood pressure is the product of cardiac output multiplied by peripheral resistance. Cardiac output is the product of the heart rate multiplied by the stroke volume. Each time the heart contracts, pressure is transferred from the contraction of the heart muscle to the blood and then pressure is exerted by the blood as it flows through the blood vessels. Hypertension can result from increases in cardiac output, increases in peripheral resistance (constriction of the blood vessels), or both. Increases in cardiac output are often related to an expansion in vascular volume. Although no precise cause can be identified for most cases of hypertension, it is understood that hypertension is a multifactorial condition. Because hypertension can be a sign, it is most likely to have many causes, just as fever has many causes.

For hypertension to occur there must be a change in one or more factors affecting peripheral resistance or cardiac output. In addition, there must also be a problem with the body's control systems that monitor or regulate pressure (see Fig. 31-1). More than 40 single-gene mutations associated with hypertension have been identified, but most types of hypertension are thought to be polygenic (i.e., mutations in more than one gene) (Ehret & Caulfield, 2013). The tendency to develop hypertension is inherited; however, genetic profiles alone cannot predict who will and will not develop hypertension. In fact, researchers estimate that genetics play a role in explaining blood pressure variation between individuals in 30% to 70% of cases (Ehret & Caulfield, 2013).

Many causes of hypertension have been suggested (Schiffrin, 2014):

- Increased sympathetic nervous system activity related to dysfunction of the autonomic nervous system
- Increased renal reabsorption of sodium, chloride, and water related to a genetic variation in the pathways by which the kidneys handle sodium
- Increased activity of the renin–angiotensin–aldosterone system, resulting in expansion of extracellular fluid volume and increased systemic vascular resistance
- Decreased vasodilation of the arterioles related to dysfunction of the vascular endothelium
- Resistance to insulin action, which may be a common factor linking hypertension, type 2 diabetes, hypertriglyceridemia, obesity, and glucose intolerance
- Activation of the innate and adaptive components of the immune response that may contribute to renal inflammation and dysfunction

Gerontologic Considerations

Structural and functional changes in the heart, blood vessels, and kidneys contribute to increases in blood pressure that occur with aging. These changes include accumulation of atherosclerotic plaque, fragmentation of arterial elastins, increased collagen deposits, impaired vasodilation, and renal

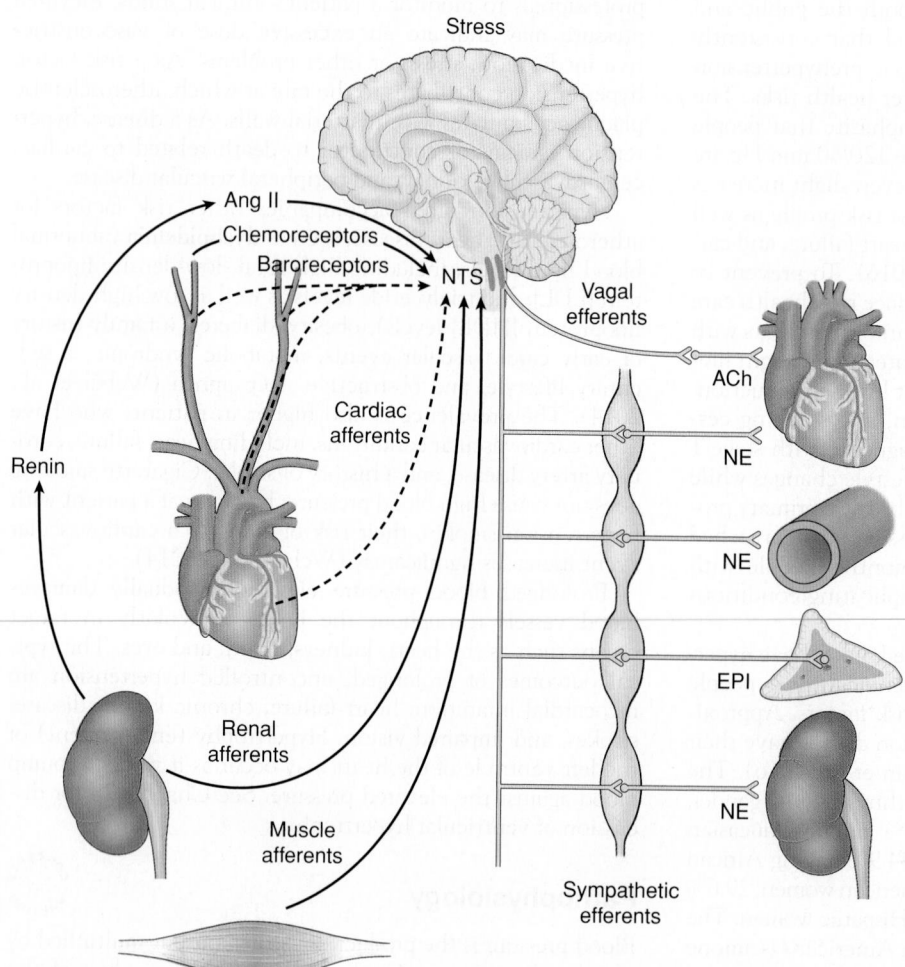

Figure 31-1 • Central and reflex mechanisms involved in the neural control of blood pressure. *Dotted arrows* represent inhibitory neural influences, and *solid arrows* represent excitatory neural influences on sympathetic outflow. EPI, epinephrine; NTS, nucleus tractus solitarius; NE, norepinephrine; ACh, acetylcholine; Ang II, angiotensin II. Adapted from Kaplan, N. M., & Victor, R. G. (2015). *Kaplan's clinical hypertension* (11th ed.). Philadelphia, PA: Lippincott Williams & Wilkins.

dysfunction. The result of these changes is decreased elasticity or stiffening of the major blood vessels, particularly the aorta, and volume expansion (Aronow, Fleg, Pepine, et al., 2011; Weber et al., 2014). Consequently, the aorta and large arteries are less able to accommodate the volume of blood pumped out by the heart (stroke volume), and the energy that would have stretched the vessels instead elevates the SBP, resulting in an elevated systolic pressure without a change in diastolic pressure. This condition, known as **isolated systolic hypertension** (see later discussion), is more common in older adults and is associated with significant cardiovascular and cerebrovascular morbidity and mortality (Weber et al., 2014).

Clinical Manifestations

Physical examination may reveal no abnormalities other than elevated blood pressure. Occasionally, retinal changes such as hemorrhages, exudates (fluid accumulation), arteriolar narrowing, and cotton-wool spots (small infarctions) occur. In severe hypertension, papilledema (swelling of the optic disc) may be seen. People with hypertension may be asymptomatic and remain so for many years. However, when specific signs and symptoms appear, they usually indicate vascular damage, with specific manifestations related to the organs served by the involved vessels. Coronary artery disease with angina and myocardial infarction are common consequences of hypertension. Left ventricular hypertrophy occurs in response to the increased workload placed on the ventricle as it contracts against higher systemic pressure. When heart damage is extensive, heart failure follows. Pathologic changes in the kidneys (indicated by increased blood urea nitrogen [BUN] and serum creatinine levels) may manifest as nocturia. Cerebrovascular involvement may lead to a transient ischemic attack (TIA) or stroke, manifested by alterations in vision or speech, dizziness, weakness, a sudden fall, or transient or permanent paralysis on one side (hemiplegia). Cerebral infarctions account for most of the strokes in patients with hypertension.

Assessment and Diagnostic Findings

A thorough health history and physical examination are necessary. The retinas are examined and laboratory studies are performed to assess possible target organ damage. Routine laboratory tests include urinalysis, blood chemistry (i.e., analysis of sodium, potassium, creatinine, fasting glucose, and total and HDL cholesterol levels), and a 12-lead electrocardiogram. Left ventricular hypertrophy can be assessed by echocardiography. Renal damage may be suggested by elevations in BUN and creatinine levels or by microalbuminuria or macroalbuminuria. Additional studies, such as creatinine clearance, renin level, urine tests, and 24-hour urine protein, may be performed (Weber et al., 2014).

A risk factor assessment is needed to classify and guide the treatment of those with hypertension who are at risk for cardiovascular damage. Risk factors for hypertension as well as cardiovascular problems related to hypertension are presented in Chart 31-1.

Medical Management

The goal of hypertension treatment is to prevent complications and death by achieving and maintaining the arterial blood pressure lower than 140/90 mm Hg. JNC 7 recommended more

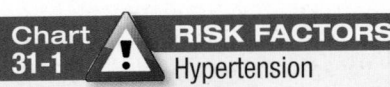

Chart 31-1 RISK FACTORS
Hypertension

Major Risk Factors

- Advancing adult age
- African American
- Drinking too much alcohol (i.e., more than two drinks per day for men and more than one drink per day for women)
- Family history
- Gender-related:
  - Men have greater risks until 45 years of age
  - Gender risks are approximately equal between 45 and 64 years of age
  - Women have greater risks at 65 years of age and later
- Overweight/obesity
- Poor diet habits, particularly if it includes too much salt
- Sedentary lifestyle

Possible Contributing Factors

- Use of tobacco products (e.g., cigarettes, e-cigarettes), and secondhand smoke
- Stress
- Sleep apnea

Risk of Target Organ Damage or Clinical Cardiovascular Disease Secondary to Hypertension

- Chronic kidney disease
- Heart disease (left ventricular hypertrophy, heart failure, angina, myocardial infarction)
- Peripheral arterial disease
- Retinopathy
- Stroke or transient ischemic attack (TIA)

Adapted from American Heart Association, Inc. (2016). *Know your risk factors for high blood pressure.* Retrieved on 10/29/2016 at: www.heart.org/HEARTORG/Conditions/HighBloodPressure/UnderstandYourRiskforHighBloodPressure/Understand-Your-Risk-for-High-Blood-Pressure_UCM_002052_Article.jsp#.WBUWC1u3BK9; Eckel, R. H., Jakicic, J. M., Ard, J. D., et al. (2014). 2013 AHA/ACC guideline on lifestyle management to reduce cardiovascular risk: A report of the American College of Cardiology/American Heart Association Task Force on Practice Guidelines. *Journal of the American College of Cardiology, 63*(25 Pt B), 2961–2984; Rosendorff, C., Lackland, D. T., Allison, M., et al. (2015). Treatment of hypertension in patients with coronary artery disease: A scientific statement from the American Heart Association, American College of Cardiology, and American Society of Hypertension. *Journal of the American Society of Hypertension, 9*(6), 453–498.

aggressive blood pressure management in patients with hypertension who also had chronic kidney disease or diabetes (Chobanian et al., 2003a). However, JNC 8 recommends treating patients with these concomitant conditions to the same blood pressure goals as patients with hypertension who do not also have either chronic kidney disease or diabetes (i.e., to lower than 140/90 mm Hg) (James et al., 2014). The experts diverge with regard to optimal blood pressure management of older adult patients with hypertension. JNC 8 recommends setting a goal of less than 150/90 mm Hg in patients older than 60 years of age (James et al., 2014); whereas, the ASH and ISH recommend setting a goal of less than 150/90 mm Hg in patients older than 80 years of age (Weber et al., 2014). Although these experts recommend different SBP management goals in patients between 61 and 79 years of age, JNC 8 and ASH and ISH are in agreement that treatment goals should not supplant

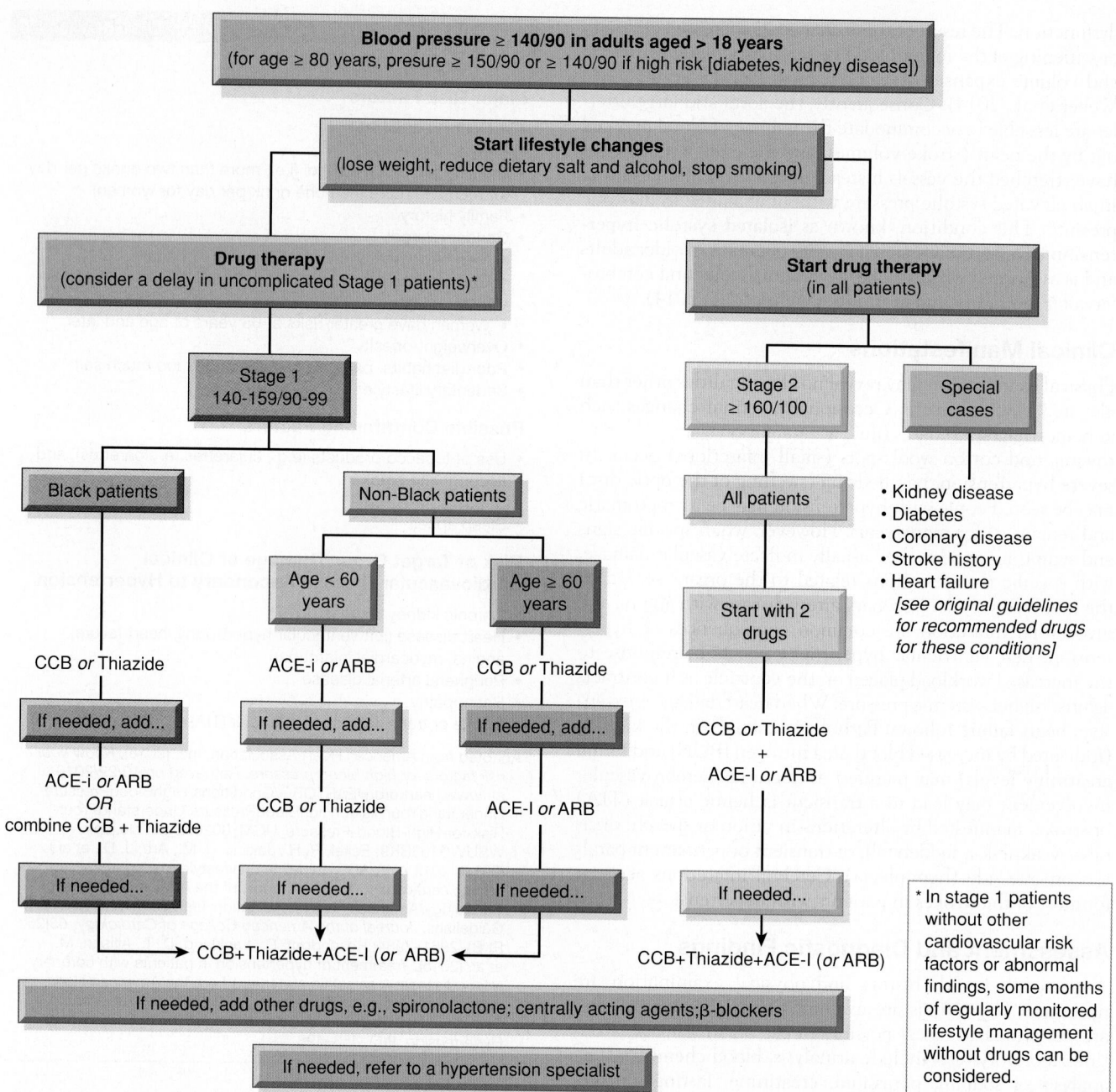

Figure 31-2 • Algorithm of hypertension treatment. Treatment begins with lifestyle modifications and continues with various medication regimens. ACE-I, angiotensin-converting enzyme inhibitor; ARB, angiotensin receptor blocker; CCB, calcium channel blocker; Thiazide, thiazide diuretic. From Weber, M. A., Schiffrin, E. L., White, W. B., et al. (2014). Clinical practice guidelines for the management of hypertension in the community: A statement by the American Society of Hypertension and the International Society of Hypertension. *The Journal of Clinical Hypertension (Greenwich), 16*(1), 14–26.

clinical judgment and individual patient considerations and preferences (James et al., 2014; Weber et al., 2014). The optimal management plan is one that is inexpensive, simple, and causes the least possible disruption in the patient's life.

The management options for hypertension are summarized in Figure 31-2; these include lifestyle modifications and pharmacologic therapy. Table 31-2 summarizes recommended lifestyle modifications. The clinician uses the algorithm with the risk factor assessment data and the patient's blood pressure category to choose the initial and subsequent treatment plans for the patient. Research findings demonstrate that

weight loss, reduced alcohol and sodium intake, and regular physical activity are effective lifestyle adaptations to reduce blood pressure (Appel, Champagne, Harsha, et al., 2003; Coxson, Cook, Joffres, et al., 2013; Eckel, Jakicic, Ard, et al., 2014; Knight, 2012; Weber et al., 2014). Studies suggest that diets high in fruits, vegetables, and low-fat dairy products can prevent the development of hypertension and lower elevated blood pressure (Appel, Sacks, Carey, et al., 2005). Table 31-3 shows the Dietary Approaches to Stop Hypertension (DASH) diet, which has been shown to lower blood pressure in people who follow it (Appel et al., 2003; Eckel et al., 2014).

TABLE 31-2 Lifestyle Modifications to Prevent and Manage Hypertension[a]

Modification	Recommendation	Goal of SBP Reduction (Range)[b]
Weight reduction	Maintain normal body weight (body mass index 18.5–24.9 kg/m²).	5–20 mm Hg/10 kg
Adopt DASH eating plan	Consume a diet rich in fruits, vegetables, and low-fat dairy products with a reduced content of saturated and total fat.	8–14 mm Hg
Dietary sodium reduction	Reduce dietary sodium intake to ≤2400 mg sodium daily. Further reduction to no more than 1500 mg sodium daily is better, as it is associated with an even greater reduction in blood pressure. Reduce overall sodium intake from baseline by at least 1000 mg daily, even if goal of ≤2400 mg is not achievable; that reduction from baseline is associated with blood pressure reduction.	2–8 mm Hg
Physical activity	Engage in regular aerobic physical activity such as brisk walking (≥30 min/day, most days of the week).	4–9 mm Hg
Moderation of alcohol consumption	Limit consumption to ≤2 drinks (e.g., 24 oz beer, 10 oz wine, or 3 oz 80-proof whiskey) per day in most men and to ≤1 drink per day in women and lighter-weight people.	2–4 mm Hg

SBP, systolic blood pressure; DASH, dietary approaches to stop hypertension.
[a]For overall cardiovascular risk reduction, stop smoking.
[b]The effects of implementing these modifications are dose and time dependent and could be greater for some individuals.
Adapted from Chobanian, A. V., Bakris, G. L., Black, H. R., et al. (2003b). Seventh Report of the Joint National Committee on prevention, detection, evaluation, and treatment of high blood pressure. *Hypertension*, 42(6), 1206–1252; Go, A. S., Bauman, M. A., Coleman, S. M., et al. (2014). An effective approach to high blood pressure control: A science advisory from the American Heart Association, the American College of Cardiology, and the Centers for Disease Control and Prevention. *Journal of the American College of Cardiology*, 63(12), 1230–1238.

Pharmacologic Therapy

The medications used for treating hypertension decrease peripheral resistance, blood volume, or the strength and rate of myocardial contraction. For African American patients and all patients 60 years of age and older with stage I hypertension, the recommended initial medications include a calcium channel blocker or a thiazide diuretic. Patients with stage I hypertension who are not African American and are less than 60 years of age are typically prescribed either an angiotensin-converting enzyme inhibitor (ACE-I) or an angiotensin receptor blocker (ARB). Patients are first given low doses of medication. If blood pressure does not fall to less than 140/90 mm Hg, the dose is increased gradually and additional medications are included as necessary to achieve control (see Fig. 31-2). Table 31-4 describes the various pharmacologic agents that are recommended for the treatment of hypertension.

TABLE 31-3 The DASH (Dietary Approaches to Stop Hypertension) Diet

Food Group	Number of Servings/Day
Grains and grain products	7 or 8
Vegetables	4 or 5
Fruits	4 or 5
Low-fat or fat-free dairy foods	2 or 3
Lean meat, fish, and poultry	≤2
Nuts, seeds, and dry beans	4 or 5 weekly

Note: The diet is based on 2000 calories/day.
Adapted from U.S. Department of Health and Human Services. (2003). *Your guide to lowering your blood pressure with DASH: DASH eating plan.* Retrieved on 11/27/2015 at: www.nhlbi.nih.gov/health/public/heart/hbp/dash/new_dash.pdf

When the blood pressure is less than 140/90 mm Hg for at least 1 year, gradual reduction of the types and doses of medication is indicated. To promote adherence to the regimen, clinicians try to prescribe the simplest treatment schedule possible, ideally one pill once each day. The pill may be a single agent or two or more agents combined into a single pill.

 ## Gerontologic Considerations

DBP tends to plateau in late middle age. However, age-related changes in the great vessels, related to an increase in collagen and decrease in elastin, cause them to stiffen. These age-related changes are associated with progressive increases in SBP, but do not have the same effects on the DBP (Aronow et al., 2011). Isolated systolic hypertension is the most common type of hypertension in adults older than 50 years of age (Busko, 2015). Isolated systolic hypertension is associated with increased risk of death, stroke, and heart failure, and treatment reduces this risk (Rosendorff, Lackland, Allison, et al., 2015). Like younger patients, older patients should begin treatment with lifestyle modifications.

Updated recommendations from the JNC 8 and from ASH and ISH suggest less rigid blood pressure control for patients older than 60 years of age, and for patients older than 80 years of age, respectively, to targets of less than 150/90 mm Hg, as noted previously (James et al., 2014; Weber et al., 2014). However, JNC 8 and ASH and ISH do not recommend changing the therapeutic regimen in older adult patients with hypertension who previously met the JNC 7 target goal of less than 140/90 mm Hg (James et al., 2014; Weber et al., 2014). Findings from the Atherosclerosis Risk in Communities (ARIC) cohort study revealed that among the over 6000 study participants, approximately 1 out of 6 were reclassified as meeting target blood pressure goals, using the new JNC 8 criteria, rather than the stricter JNC 7 criteria. However, (text continued on page 893)

TABLE 31-4 **Medication Therapy for Hypertension**

Medications	Major Action	Advantages and Contraindications	Effects and Nursing Considerations
Diuretics and Related Drugs			
Thiazide Diuretics			
chlorothiazide (Diuril) chlorthalidone (Hygroton) hydrochlorothiazide (Hydrodiuril) indapamide (Lozol) methyclothiazide (Enduron) metolazone (Zaroxolyn)	Decrease of blood volume, renal blood flow, and cardiac output Depletion of extracellular fluid Negative sodium balance (from natriuresis), mild hypokalemia Directly affect vascular smooth muscle	Relatively inexpensive Effective orally Effective during long-term administration Mild side effects Enhance other antihypertensive medications Counter sodium retention effects of other antihypertensive medications *Contraindications:* Gout, known sensitivity to sulfonamide-derived medications, severely impaired kidney function, and history of hyponatremia	Side effects include dry mouth, thirst, weakness, drowsiness, lethargy, muscle aches, muscular fatigue, tachycardia, GI disturbance Postural hypotension may be potentiated by alcohol, barbiturates, opioids, or hot weather Because thiazides cause loss of sodium, potassium, and magnesium, monitor for signs of electrolyte imbalance Encourage intake of potassium-rich foods (i.e., fruits) *Gerontologic considerations:* Risk of postural hypotension is significant because of volume depletion; measure blood pressure in 3 positions; caution patient to rise slowly
Loop Diuretics			
bumetanide (Bumex) ethacrynic acid (Edecrin) furosemide (Lasix) torsemide (Demadex)	Volume depletion Blocks reabsorption of sodium, chloride, and water in kidney	Action rapid Potent Used when thiazides fail or patient needs rapid diuresis *Contraindications:* Same as for thiazides	There is risk of volume and electrolyte depletion from the profound diuresis that can occur Fluid and electrolyte replacement may be required *Gerontologic considerations:* Same as for thiazides
Potassium-Sparing Diuretics			
amiloride (Midamor) triamterene (Dyrenium)	Blocks sodium reabsorption Acts on distal tubule independently of aldosterone	Causes potassium retention *Contraindications:* Kidney disease, azotemia, severe hepatic disease, hyperkalemia	Drowsiness, lethargy, headache Monitor for hyperkalemia if given with ACE inhibitor or angiotensin receptor blocker Diarrhea and other GI symptoms—administer medication after meals
Aldosterone Receptor Blockers			
eplerenone (Inspra) spironolactone (Aldactone)	Competitive inhibitors of aldosterone binding	Indicated for patients with a history of myocardial infarction or symptomatic ventricular dysfunction *Contraindications:* Hyperkalemia and impaired renal function Eplerenone is contraindicated in diabetes with microalbuminuria	Drowsiness, lethargy, headache Monitor for hyperkalemia if given with ACE inhibitor or angiotensin receptor blocker Diarrhea and other GI symptoms—administer medication after meals Avoid the use of potassium supplements or salt substitutes Educate patients, families, and caregivers about the signs and symptoms of hyperkalemia Spironolactone may cause gynecomastia
Central Alpha$_2$-Agonists and Other Centrally Acting Drugs			
clonidine (Catapres) clonidine patch (Catapres-TTS)	Exact mode of action is not understood, but acts through the central nervous system, apparently through centrally mediated alpha-adrenergic stimulation in the brain, producing blood pressure reduction	Little or no orthostatic effect; moderately potent, and sometimes is effective when other medications fail to lower blood pressure. *Contraindications:* Severe coronary artery disease, pregnancy	Dry mouth, drowsiness, sedation, and occasional headaches and fatigue. Anorexia, malaise, and vomiting with mild disturbance of liver function have been reported Rebound or withdrawal hypertension is relatively common; monitor blood pressure when stopping medication Common side effects include dry mouth, dizziness, sleepiness, fatigue, headache, constipation, and impotence
guanfacine (Tenex)	Stimulates central alpha$_2$-adrenergic receptors	Reduces heart rate and causes vasodilation. Serious adverse reactions are uncommon; use with caution in persons with diminished liver function, recent myocardial infarction, or known cardiovascular disease	If taking concurrent with another antihypertensive medication, administer at bedtime to avoid excessive sleepiness Do not administer extended release tablet formulation with high fat meal

TABLE 31-4 Medication Therapy for Hypertension (continued)

Medications	Major Action	Advantages and Contraindications	Effects and Nursing Considerations
methyldopa (Aldomet)	Dopa decarboxylase inhibitor; displaces norepinephrine from storage sites	Drug of choice for pregnant women with hypertension Useful in patients with chronic kidney disease or prostate disease Does not decrease cardiac output or renal blood flow Does not induce oliguria *Contraindications:* Liver disease	Drowsiness, dizziness Dry mouth; nasal congestion (troublesome at first but then tends to disappear) Use with caution with kidney disease *Gerontologic considerations:* May produce mental and behavioral changes in the older adult
Beta-Blockers			
atenolol (Tenormin) betaxolol (Kerlone) bisoprolol (Zebeta) metoprolol (Lopressor) metoprolol extended release (Toprol-XL) nadolol (Corgard) propranolol (Inderal) propranolol long acting (Inderal LA) timolol (Blocadren)	Block the sympathetic nervous system (beta-adrenergic receptors), especially the sympathetics to the heart, producing a slower heart rate and lowered blood pressure	Reduce pulse rate in patients with tachycardia and blood pressure elevation Indicated for patients who also have stable angina pectoris and silent ischemia *Contraindications:* Bronchial asthma, allergic rhinitis, right ventricular failure from pulmonary hypertension, heart failure, depression, diabetes, dyslipidemia, heart block, peripheral vascular disease, heart rate <60 bpm	Mental depression manifested by insomnia, lassitude, weakness, and fatigue Avoid sudden discontinuation. Lightheadedness and occasional nausea, vomiting, and epigastric distress Check heart rate before giving *Gerontologic considerations:* Risk of toxicity is increased for older adult patients with decreased renal and liver function. Take blood pressure in 3 positions, and observe for hypotension
Beta-Blockers With Intrinsic Sympathomimetic Activity			
acebutolol (Sectral) penbutolol (Levatol) pindolol (Visken)	Block both cardiac beta-1 and beta-2 receptors Also have antiarrhythmic activity by slowing atrioventricular conduction	Similar to beta-blockers *Contraindications:* Similar to beta-blockers	Avoid sudden discontinuation Withhold if bradycardia or heart block is present. Use with caution with COPD, diabetes Similar to beta-blockers
Beta-Blocker With Cardioselective and Vasodilatory Activity			
nebivolol (Bystolic)	Blocks beta-1 adrenergic receptors	Similar to other beta-blockers with additional capacity for vasodilation *Contraindications:* Similar to beta-blockers but with greater risk of severe bradycardia, heart block, cardiogenic shock, decompensated cardiac failure, sick sinus syndrome, severe hepatic impairment	Avoid sudden discontinuation. FDA warns that drug has not been shown to be more effective than any other beta-blocker
Alpha$_1$-Blockers			
doxazosin (Cardura) prazosin (Minipress) terazosin (Hytrin)	Peripheral vasodilator acting directly on the blood vessel; similar to hydralazine (see discussion of Vasodilators)	Act directly on the blood vessels and are effective agents in patients with adverse reactions to hydralazine *Contraindications:* Angina pectoris and coronary artery disease; induces tachycardia if not preceded by administration of propranolol and a diuretic	Occasional vomiting and diarrhea, urinary frequency, and cardiovascular collapse, especially if given in addition to hydralazine without lowering the dose of the latter. Patients occasionally experience drowsiness, lack of energy, and weakness
Combined Alpha- and Beta-Blockers			
carvedilol (Coreg) labetalol (Trandate)	Block alpha- and beta-adrenergic receptors; cause peripheral dilation and decrease peripheral vascular resistance	Fast acting No decrease in renal blood flow *Contraindications:* Asthma, cardiogenic shock, severe tachycardia, heart block	Orthostatic hypotension, tachycardia

(continued on page 892)

TABLE 31-4 Medication Therapy for Hypertension (continued)

Medications	Major Action	Advantages and Contraindications	Effects and Nursing Considerations
Vasodilators			
hydralazine (Apresoline)	Decreases peripheral resistance but concurrently elevates cardiac output Acts directly on smooth muscle of blood vessels	Not used as initial therapy; used in combination with other medications Used also in pregnancy-induced hypertension *Contraindications:* Angina or coronary disease, heart failure, hypersensitivity	Headache, tachycardia, flushing, and dyspnea may occur—can be prevented by pretreating with reserpine Peripheral edema may require diuretics May produce lupus erythematosus–like syndrome Tachycardia, angina pectoris, ECG changes, edema
minoxidil (Loniten)	Direct vasodilatory action on arteriolar vessels, causing decreased peripheral vascular resistance; reduces systolic and diastolic pressures	Hypotensive effect more pronounced than with hydralazine No effect on vasomotor reflexes, so does not cause postural hypotension *Contraindications:* Pheochromocytoma	Take blood pressure and apical pulse before administration Monitor intake and output and daily weights Causes hirsutism Dizziness, headache, nausea, edema, tachycardia, palpitations
nitroprusside (Nitropress) nitroglycerin	Peripheral vasodilation by relaxation of smooth muscle	Fast acting Used only in hypertensive emergencies *Contraindications:* Sepsis, azotemia, high intracranial pressure	Can cause thiocyanate and cyanide intoxication
ACE Inhibitors			
benazepril (Lotensin) captopril (Capoten) enalapril (Vasotec) enalaprilat (Vasotec IV) fosinopril (Monopril) lisinopril (Prinivil) moexipril (Univasc) perindopril (Aceon) quinapril (Accupril) ramipril (Altace) trandolapril (Mavik)	Inhibit conversion of angiotensin I to angiotensin II Lower total peripheral resistance	Fewer cardiovascular side effects Can be used with thiazide diuretic and digitalis Hypotension can be reversed by fluid replacement Angioedema is a rare but potentially life-threatening complication *Contraindications:* Renal impairment, pregnancy	*Gerontologic considerations:* Require reduced dosages and the addition of loop diuretics when there is renal dysfunction
Angiotensin II Receptor Blockers			
azilsartan (Edarbi) candesartan (Atacand) eprosartan (Teveten) irbesartan (Avapro) losartan (Cozaar) olmesartan (Benicar) telmisartan (Micardis) valsartan (Diovan)	Block the effects of angiotensin II at the receptor Reduce peripheral resistance	Minimal side effects *Contraindications:* Pregnancy, lactation, renovascular disease, hypersensitivity reaction to other ARBs	Monitor for hyperkalemia
Calcium Channel Blockers			
Nondihydropyridines			
diltiazem extended release (Cardizem CD, Dilacor XR, Tiazac) diltiazem long acting (Cardizem LA)	Inhibit calcium ion influx Reduce cardiac afterload	Inhibit coronary artery spasm not controlled by beta-blockers or nitrates *Contraindications:* Sick sinus syndrome, AV block, hypotension, heart failure	Do not discontinue suddenly Observe for hypotension Report irregular heartbeat, dizziness, edema Instruct on regular dental care because of potential gingivitis
verapamil immediate release (Calan, Isoptin) verapamil long acting (Calan SR, Isoptin SR) verapamil (Covera-HS, Verelan PM)	Inhibit calcium ion influx Slow velocity of conduction of cardiac impulse	Effective antiarrhythmic Rapid IV onset Block SA and AV node channels *Contraindications:* Sinus or AV node disease, severe heart failure, severe hypotension	Administer on empty stomach or before meal Do not discontinue suddenly Depression may subside when medication is discontinued To relieve headaches, reduce noise, monitor electrolytes Decrease dose for patients with liver or kidney disease

TABLE 31-4 Medication Therapy for Hypertension (continued)

Medications	Major Action	Advantages and Contraindications	Effects and Nursing Considerations
Dihydropyridines			
amlodipine (Norvasc) felodipine (Plendil) isradipine (Dynacirc CR) nicardipine (Cardene) nifedipine long acting (Procardia XL, Adalat CC) nisoldipine (Sular)	Inhibit calcium ion influx across membranes Vasodilatory effects on coronary arteries and peripheral arteriole Decrease cardiac work and energy consumption, increase delivery of oxygen to myocardium	Rapid action Effective by oral or sublingual route No tendency to slow SA nodal activity or prolong AV node conduction Isolated systolic hypertension *Contraindications:* None (except heart failure for nifedipine)	Administer on empty stomach Use with caution in patients with diabetes Small frequent meals if nausea Muscle cramps, joint stiffness, sexual difficulties may disappear when dose decreased Report irregular heartbeat, constipation, shortness of breath, edema May cause dizziness
clevidipine (Cleviprex)	Calcium channel antagonist causing rapid vasodilation	*Advantages:* Rapid acting with additional capacity for vasodilation; given IV *Contraindications:* Allergies to soybeans, soy products, eggs or egg products; impaired lipid metabolism as might be seen with pancreatitis and other hyperlipidemias; severe aortic stenosis	Monitor carefully for hypotension and tachycardia; there is risk of rebound hypertension, so careful monitoring after cessation of treatment is indicated
Direct Renin Inhibitors			
aliskiren (Tekturna)	Blocks the conversion of angiotensinogen to angiotensin I by inhibiting the activity of the enzyme renin	Given once daily for mild-to-moderate high blood pressure with minimal side effects Headaches, dizziness, and diarrhea are most frequent side effects Angioedema is a rare but potentially life-threatening complication Contraindicated in pregnancy; has not been studied in persons with diminished renal function	Monitor for hyperkalemia and hypotension

GI, gastrointestinal; ACE, angiotensin-converting enzyme; COPD, chronic obstructive pulmonary disease; FDA, U.S. Food and Drug Administration, IV, intravenous; ECG, electrocardiogram; ARBs, angiotensin receptor blockers; AV, atrioventricular; SA, sinoatrial.

Adapted from Karch, A. (2014). *2015 Lippincott's nursing drug guide.* Philadelphia, PA: Lippincott Williams & Wilkins; U.S. Food and Drug Administration (2016). Drug approvals and databases. Retrieved on 10/29/2016 at: www.fda.gov/Drugs/InformationOnDrugs/UCM079874

despite these changes, the blood pressure of over 1 in 5 participants still did not meet goals, suggesting that many community-dwelling older adults with hypertension are at risk for poor cardiovascular outcomes (Miedema, Lopez, Blaha, et al., 2015).

More than 75% of adults older than 75 years of age have hypertension, and yet, there has been less research on hypertension treatment and appropriate goals in this population than in younger adults. Furthermore, studies conducted to date have yielded contradictory results, with some showing a reduction in morbidity and mortality, whereas other studies have found either no benefit or increased risk associated with treatment. For instance, the Systolic Blood Pressure Intervention Trial (SPRINT) found that among 2,636 ambulatory participants (mean age of 79.9 years) with hypertension, those whose SBPs were treated to less than 120 mm Hg had significantly lower rates of death and cardiovascular morbidity than those whose SBPs were managed to less than 140 mm Hg (Williamson, Supiano, Applegate, 2016). However, another cohort-based study (Tinetti, Han, McAvay, et al., 2014) found that antihypertensive treatment, including high-intensity antihypertensive treatment, was associated with lower rates of death, but not cardiovascular morbidity, in a sample of 4,961 community-dwelling participants (mean age of 80.1 years). A parallel study in this same cohort found that antihypertensive treatment was associated with an increased risk of falls, particularly among those participants who had previously reported falls (Tinetti, Han, Lee, et al., 2014). One possible explanation for these discrepant results may be the health of the study participants. Odden, Peralta, Haan, et al. (2012) found that adults older than 65 years of age who were able to walk briskly (faster than 0.8 m/sec) benefited from hypertension treatment. Survey participants who walked more slowly or who could not complete a walk test of 20 ft actually benefited from having elevated blood pressures, and blood pressure treatment did not reduce mortality (Odden et al., 2012).

If medications are needed to achieve the blood pressure goal of less than 150/90 mm Hg in the older adult patient, the starting dose should be the lowest available and then gradually increased with a second medication from a different class added if control is difficult to achieve. As older adults often have other comorbid conditions, awareness of possible drug interactions is critical. In addition, older adults are at increased risk for the side effects of hyperkalemia and orthostatic hypotension, putting them at increased risk for falls and fractures (Tinetti et al., 2014).

NURSING PROCESS

The Patient With Hypertension

Assessment

When hypertension is initially detected, nursing assessment involves carefully monitoring the blood pressure at frequent intervals and then at routinely scheduled intervals. When the patient begins an antihypertensive treatment regimen, blood pressure assessments are needed to determine the effectiveness of medication therapy and to detect any changes in blood pressure that may indicate the need for a modification in the treatment plan.

The ASH and ISH have defined the standards for blood pressure measurement, including conditions required before measurements are made, equipment specifications, and techniques for measuring blood pressure to obtain accurate and reliable readings (Coogan, Marra, & Lomonaco, 2015; Weber et al., 2014) (see Chart 31-2).

A complete history is obtained to assess for other cardiovascular risk factors and for signs and symptoms that indicate target organ damage (i.e., whether specific tissues are damaged by the elevated blood pressure). Manifestations of target organ damage may include angina; shortness of breath; alterations in speech, vision, or balance; nosebleeds; headaches; dizziness; or nocturia. The patient's partner may be helpful in identifying whether the patient may be experiencing obstructive sleep apnea.

During the physical examination, the nurse must also pay specific attention to the rate, rhythm, and character of the apical and peripheral pulses to detect the effects of hypertension on the heart and blood vessels. A thorough assessment can yield valuable information about the extent to which the hypertension has affected the body and any other personal, social, or financial factors. For example, a patient's ability to adhere to an antihypertensive medication regimen may be influenced by the patient's financial resources to buy the medication and also by limited health insurance (Iuga & McGuire, 2014). Furthermore, patients' perceptions about the diagnosis of hypertension can affect whether they engage in key health behaviors, including exercising and modifying dietary habits (Stallings, 2016) (see Chart 31-3).

Diagnosis

NURSING DIAGNOSES

Based on the assessment data, nursing diagnoses may include the following:

- Deficient knowledge regarding the relation between the treatment regimen and control of the disease process
- Noncompliance with therapeutic regimen related to side effects of prescribed therapy

---

Chart 31-2 Measuring Blood Pressure

Equipment

For the Patient at Home

- Automatic or semiautomatic device with digital display of readings

For the Practitioner

- Preferably, a validated electronic device; if not available, a mercury sphygmomanometer, recently calibrated aneroid manometer
- Appropriately sized arm cuff

Instructions for the Patient

- Avoid smoking cigarettes or drinking caffeine for 30 minutes before blood pressure (BP) is measured.
- Empty bladder.
- Sit quietly for 5 minutes before the measurement.
- Sit comfortably, with back supported, with the forearm supported at heart level on a firm surface, with both feet on the ground; avoid talking while the measurement is being taken.

Instructions for the Practitioner

- Select the size of the cuff based on the size of the patient. (The cuff size should have a bladder width of at least 40% of limb circumference and length at least 80% of limb circumference.) The average adult cuff is 12–14 cm wide and 30 cm long. Using a cuff that is too small will give a higher BP measurement, and using a cuff that is too large results in a lower BP measurement compared to one taken with a properly sized cuff.

- Wrap the cuff firmly around the arm. Center the cuff bladder directly over the brachial artery.
- Position the patient's arm at the level of the heart.
- If a mercury sphygmomanometer is used, palpate the systolic pressure before auscultating. This technique helps to detect the presence of an auscultatory gap more readily.
- Ask the patient to sit quietly while the BP is measured, because the BP can increase when the patient is engaged in conversation.
- Initially, record BP results of both arms and take subsequent measurements from the arm with the higher BP. Normally, the BP should vary by no more than 5 mm Hg between arms.
- Take two readings 1–2 minutes apart and use the average of these measurements.
- Record the site where the BP was measured and the position of the patient (i.e., right arm).
- Inform the patient of their BP value and what it means. Emphasize the need for periodic reassessment, and encourage patients who measure BP at home to keep a written record of readings.

Interpretation

Assessment is based on the average of at least two readings. (If two readings differ by more than 5 mm Hg, additional readings are taken and an average reading is calculated from the results.)

Adapted from Coogan, N., Marra, A., & Lomonaco, E. A. (2015). Assessing accurate BP measurement: Size and technique matter! *Nursing, 45*(4), 16–18; Weber, M.A., Schiffrin, D. L., White, W. B., et al. (2014). Clinical practice guidelines for the management of hypertension in the community: A statement by the American Society of Hypertension and the International Society of Hypertension. *The Journal of Clinical Hypertension (Greenwich), 16*(1), 14–26.

Stallings, D. T. (2016). Illness perceptions and health behaviors of black women. *Journal of Cardiovascular Nursing, 31*(6), 492–499.

Chart 31-3 NURSING RESEARCH PROFILE
Perceptions of Hypertension and Health Behaviors Among African American Women

Purpose

African American women have the highest prevalence of hypertension in the world. Despite a plethora of research findings that indicate that health behaviors, including physical activity and diet, can influence hypertension and deter its morbid complications, many African American women who are at risk make poor diet choices and are physically inactive. The aim of this study was to analyze the relationships between perceptions of hypertension and self-reported health behaviors, specifically physical activity and fruit and vegetable consumption, among African American women with hypertension.

Design

This descriptive correlational study recruited African American women from five churches and a hair salon in Tennessee and Mississippi. Eligible participants were 18–65 years of age, able to read, write, and speak English, and self-reported that they had been diagnosed with hypertension. Participants ($n = 204$) completed a demographic form, the Illness Perception Questionnaire, a 7-day Physical Activity Recall, and the Fruit and Vegetable Quick Food Scan. In addition, they had their blood pressures and body mass indices measured by the investigators.

Findings

Most participants were married ($n = 108$; 52.9%), college-educated ($n = 102$; 50%) and were middle-aged (average age of 48.12 years

of age ±10.3 years). In this sample, the mean systolic blood pressure was 138.4 mm Hg (SD = 14.9 mm Hg), the mean diastolic blood pressure was 83.4 mm Hg (SD = 9.9 mm Hg), and the mean body mass index was 34.14 kg/m² (SD = 8.00 kg/m²). Hierarchical multiple regression analyses revealed that perceiving hypertension as chronic ($\beta = -0.149$; $P = 0.05$) and as caused by environmental factors ($\beta = -0.25$; $P = 0.05$) were both inversely associated with self-reported moderate-intensity physical activity. Emotional responses to hypertension, such as fear or anxiety, were positively correlated with moderate-intensity physical activity ($\beta = 0.32$; $P = 0.05$) and with fruit and vegetable consumption ($\beta = 0.28$; $P = 0.01$).

Nursing Implications

In this study, African American women with hypertension who saw hypertension as a chronic disease caused by environmental factors reported less moderate physical activity. This may imply that knowledge of the chronicity of hypertension may not be sufficient to motivate them to modify their health behaviors. However, fear and anxiety about hypertension seemed to motivate physical activity and fruit and vegetable consumption. Engaging in health coaching behaviors with African American women with hypertension that empowers them to cope and adapt to health challenges may assist them in self-managing hypertension. In particular, nurses who care for African American women with hypertension should assess their perceptions of hypertension, clarify any misperceptions, cultivate healthy coping skills, and motivate them to self-manage hypertension.

Collaborative Problems/Potential Complications

Potential complications may include the following:

- Left ventricular hypertrophy
- Myocardial infarction
- Heart failure
- TIA
- Cerebrovascular disease (stroke or brain attack)
- Renal insufficiency and chronic kidney disease
- Retinal hemorrhage

Planning and Goals

The major goals for the patient include understanding of the disease process and its treatment, participation in a self-care program, and absence of complications.

Nursing Interventions

The objective of nursing care for patients with hypertension focuses on lowering and controlling the blood pressure without adverse effects and without undue cost. To achieve these goals, the nurse's role is to support and educate the patient about the treatment regimen, including making lifestyle changes, taking medications as prescribed, and scheduling regular follow-up appointments with the patient's primary provider to monitor progress or identify and treat any complications of disease or therapy.

Increasing Knowledge

The patient needs to understand the disease process and how lifestyle changes and medications can control hypertension. The nurse needs to emphasize the concept of controlling hypertension rather than curing it. The nurse can encourage

the patient to consult a dietitian to help develop a plan for improving nutrient intake or for weight loss. The program usually consists of restricting sodium and fat intake, increasing intake of fruits and vegetables, and implementing regular physical activity. Explaining that it takes 2 to 3 months for the taste buds to adapt to changes in salt intake may help the patient adjust to reduced salt intake. The patient should be advised to limit alcohol intake (see Table 31-2 for specific recommendations), and tobacco should be avoided because anyone with high blood pressure is already at increased risk for heart disease, and smoking amplifies this risk.

Promoting Adherence to the Therapeutic Regimen

Deviation from the therapeutic program is a significant problem for people with hypertension and other chronic conditions requiring lifetime management. An estimated 50% of patients discontinue their medications within 1 year of beginning to take them. Blood pressure control is achieved by only 54% (Valderrama, Gillespie, King, et al., 2012). Adherence to the therapeutic regimen increases, however, when patients actively participate in self-care, including self-monitoring of blood pressure and diet, possibly because patients receive immediate feedback and have a greater sense of control. Nurse-led wellness programs that are tailored to take into account patients' behaviors and eating and exercise practices are more effective than generic programs. Patients with hypertension must make considerable effort to adhere to recommended lifestyle modifications (see Table 31-2) and to take regularly prescribed medications. The effort needed to follow the therapeutic plan may seem unreasonable to some, particularly when they have no symptoms without medications but do have side effects with medications. Continued education and encouragement are usually needed to enable patients to formulate an acceptable plan that helps them live with their hypertension and adhere to the treatment plan. Compromises may have to be made about some aspects of therapy to achieve higher-priority goals.

The nurse can assist with behavior change by supporting patients in making small changes with each visit that moves them toward their goals. Another important factor is following up at each visit to see how the patient has progressed with the plans made at the prior visit. If the patient has had difficulty with a particular aspect of the plan, the patient and nurse can work together to develop an alternative or modification to the plan that the patient believes will be more successful. Support groups for weight control, smoking cessation, and stress reduction may be beneficial for some patients; others can benefit from the support of family and friends. The nurse assists the patient to develop and adhere to an appropriate exercise regimen, because regular activity is a significant factor in weight reduction and a blood pressure–reducing intervention in the absence of any loss in weight (Weber et al., 2014).

PROMOTING HOME, COMMUNITY-BASED, AND TRANSITIONAL CARE

Blood pressure screenings with the sole purpose of case finding are not recommended by the National High Blood Pressure Education Program because approximately 83% of people with hypertension are already aware of their blood pressure levels (Mozaffarian et al., 2016). If asked to participate in a blood pressure screening program, the nurse should ensure that proper blood pressure measurement technique is being used (see Chart 31-2), that validated electronic devices are used or, if sphygmomanometers are used, that they are properly calibrated, and that provision has been made to provide follow-up for any person identified as having an elevated blood pressure level. Adequate time should also be allowed to educate each person screened about what the blood pressure numbers mean. Each person should be given a written record of their blood pressure at the screening.

Educating Patients About Self-Care. The therapeutic regimen is the responsibility of the patient in collaboration with the primary provider. The nurse can help the patient achieve blood pressure control through education about managing blood pressure (see earlier discussion), setting goal blood pressures, and providing assistance with social support. Involving family members in education programs enables them to support the patient's efforts to control hypertension. The American Heart Association and the National Heart, Lung, and Blood Institute both provide printed and electronic patient education materials.

Providing written information about the expected effects and side effects of medications is important. When side effects occur, patients need to understand the importance of reporting them and to whom they should be reported. Patients need to be informed that **rebound hypertension** (i.e., abnormally high blood pressure) can occur if antihypertensive medications are suddenly stopped. Thus, patients should be advised to have an adequate supply of medication, particularly when traveling and in case of emergencies such as natural disasters. If traveling by airplane, patients should pack the medication in their carry-on luggage. All patients should be informed that some medications, such as beta-blockers, might cause sexual dysfunction and that other medications are available if problems with sexual function or satisfaction occur. The nurse can encourage and educate patients to measure their blood pressure at home. This practice involves patients in their own care and emphasizes that failing to take medications may result in an identifiable rise in blood pressure. Patients need to know that blood pressure varies continuously and that the range within which their pressure varies should be monitored.

Gerontologic Considerations. Adherence to the therapeutic program may be more difficult for older adults. The medication regimen can be difficult to remember, and the expense can be a challenge. **Monotherapy** (treatment with a single agent), if appropriate, may simplify the medication regimen and make it less expensive. Special care must be taken to ensure that the older adult patient understands the regimen and can see and read instructions, open the medication container, and get the prescription refilled. The older adult's family or caregivers should be included in the educational program so that they understand the patient's needs, can encourage adherence to the treatment plan, and know when and whom to call if problems arise or information is needed.

Continuing and Transitional Care. Regular follow-up care is imperative so that the disease process can continue to be optimally assessed and treated, as shown in Table 31-5. A history and physical examination should be completed at each clinic visit. The history should include all data pertaining to any potential problem, specifically medication-related problems such as postural (orthostatic) hypotension (experienced as dizziness or lightheadedness on standing).

TABLE 31-5 Recommendations for Follow-Up Based on Initial Blood Pressure Measurements for Adults Without Acute End-Organ Damage

Initial BP (mm Hg)[a]	Follow-Up Recommended[b]
Normal	Recheck in 2 years
Prehypertension	Recheck in 1 year[c]
Stage 1 hypertension	Confirm within 1 month[c]
Stage 2 hypertension	Evaluate or refer to source of care within 1 month
	For those with higher pressures (e.g., >180/100 mm Hg), evaluate and treat immediately or within 1 week, depending on clinical situation and complications

BP, blood pressure.
[a]If systolic and diastolic values fall into different categories, follow recommendations for shorter follow-up (e.g., 160/86 mm Hg should be evaluated or referred to source of care within 1 month).
[b]Modify the scheduling of follow-up according to reliable information about past BP measurements, other cardiovascular risk factors, or target organ disease.
[c]Provide advice about lifestyle modifications.
Adapted from Weber, M. A., Schiffrin, D. L., White, W. B., et al. (2014). Clinical practice guidelines for the management of hypertension in the community: A statement by the American Society of Hypertension and the International Society of Hypertension. *The Journal of Clinical Hypertension (Greenwich), 16*(1), 14–26.

MONITORING AND MANAGING POTENTIAL COMPLICATIONS

Symptoms suggesting that hypertension is progressing to the extent that target organ damage is occurring must be detected early so that appropriate treatment can be initiated. When the patient returns for follow-up care, all body systems must be assessed to detect any evidence of vascular damage. An eye examination with an ophthalmoscope is particularly important because retinal blood vessel damage indicates similar damage elsewhere in the vascular system. The patient is questioned about blurred vision, spots in front of the eyes, and diminished visual acuity. The heart, nervous system, and kidneys are also carefully assessed. Any significant findings are promptly reported to determine whether additional diagnostic studies are required. Based on the findings, medications may be changed to improve blood pressure control.

Evaluation

Expected patient outcomes may include:

1. Reports knowledge of disease management sufficient to maintain adequate tissue perfusion
    a. Maintains blood pressure at less than 140/90 mm Hg (or less than 150/90 mm Hg for adults older than 60 years of age) with lifestyle modifications, medications, or both
    b. Demonstrates no symptoms of angina, palpitations, or vision changes
    c. Has stable BUN and serum creatinine levels
    d. Has palpable peripheral pulses
2. Adheres to the self-care program
    a. Adheres to the dietary regimen as prescribed: reduces calorie, sodium, and fat intake; increases fruit and vegetable intake
    b. Exercises regularly
    c. Takes medications as prescribed and reports any side effects
    d. Measures blood pressure routinely
    e. Abstains from tobacco and excessive alcohol intake
    f. Keeps follow-up appointments
3. Has no complications
    a. Reports no changes in vision
    b. Exhibits no retinal damage on vision testing
    c. Maintains pulse rate and rhythm and respiratory rate within normal ranges
    d. Reports no dyspnea or edema
    e. Maintains urine output consistent with intake
    f. Has renal function test results within normal range
    g. Demonstrates no motor, speech, or sensory deficits
    h. Reports no headaches, dizziness, weakness, changes in gait, or falls

Hypertensive Crises

Two classes of hypertensive crisis that require immediate intervention include hypertensive emergency and hypertensive urgency (pressures above 180 mm Hg systolic and/or above 120 mm Hg diastolic). Hypertensive emergencies and urgencies may occur in patients whose hypertension has been poorly controlled, whose hypertension has been undiagnosed, or in those who have abruptly discontinued their medications. Once the hypertensive crisis has been managed, a complete evaluation is performed to review the patient's ongoing treatment plan and strategies to minimize the occurrence of subsequent hypertensive crises are implemented (Hopkins, 2015).

A **hypertensive emergency** is a situation in which blood pressures are extremely elevated and must be lowered quickly (not necessarily to less than 140/90 mm Hg) to halt or prevent damage to the target organs (Monnet & Marik, 2015). Assessment will reveal actual or developing clinical dysfunction of the target organ. Conditions associated with a hypertensive emergency include hypertension of pregnancy, acute myocardial infarction, dissecting aortic aneurysm, and intracranial hemorrhage. Hypertensive emergencies are acute, life-threatening blood pressure elevations that require prompt treatment in an intensive care setting because of the serious target organ damage that may occur. The therapeutic goals are reduction of the mean blood pressure by 20% to 25% within the first hour of treatment, a further reduction to a goal pressure of about 160/100 mm Hg over a period of up to 6 hours, and then a more gradual reduction in pressure over a period of days. The exceptions to these goals are the treatment of ischemic stroke (in which there is no evidence of benefit from immediate pressure reduction) and treatment of aortic dissection (in which the goal is to lower systolic pressure to less than 100 mm Hg if the patient can tolerate the reduction) (Chobanian et al., 2003a).

The medications of choice in hypertensive emergencies are those that have an immediate effect. Intravenous vasodilators, including sodium nitroprusside (Nitropress), nicardipine (Cardene), clevidipine (Cleviprex), enalaprilat (Vasotec), and nitroglycerin have immediate actions that are short-lived (minutes to 4 hours), and they are therefore frequently used for initial treatment. Nicardipine and labetalol (Trandate) have demonstrated safety and effectiveness in treating hypertensive crises, with nicardipine demonstrating more predictability in controlling blood pressure (Monnet & Marik, 2015) (see Table 31-4.) Experts also recommend assessing the patient's fluid volume status. If there is volume depletion secondary to natriuresis caused by the elevated blood pressure, then volume replacement with normal saline can prevent large sudden drops in blood pressure when antihypertensive medications are given (Monnet & Marik, 2015).

Hypertensive urgency describes a situation in which blood pressure is very elevated but there is no evidence of impending or progressive target organ damage (Bisognano,

2015). Elevated blood pressures associated with severe headaches, nosebleeds, or anxiety are classified as urgencies. In these situations, oral agents can be given with the goal of normalizing blood pressure within 24 to 48 hours (Monnet & Marik, 2015). Oral doses of fast-acting agents such as beta-adrenergic blockers (i.e., labetalol [Trandate]), ACE inhibitors (i.e., captopril [Capoten]), or alpha₂-agonists (i.e., clonidine [Catapres]) are recommended for the treatment of hypertensive urgencies (see Table 31-4).

Extremely close hemodynamic monitoring of the patient's blood pressure and cardiovascular status is required during treatment of hypertensive emergencies and urgencies (see Chapter 25). The exact frequency of monitoring is a matter of clinical judgment and varies with the patient's condition. Taking vital signs every 5 minutes is appropriate if the blood pressure is changing rapidly; taking vital signs at 15- or 30-minute intervals in a more stable situation may be sufficient. A precipitous drop in blood pressure can occur that would require immediate action to restore blood pressure to an acceptable level.

CRITICAL THINKING EXERCISES

1 **pq** You are working as a nurse in a clinic that serves both an assisted living and skilled nursing facility. One of the patients is an 80-year-old woman who is a new resident of the facility. When you take her blood pressure, you note that it is 120/88 mm Hg. While talking with her, you find that she reports episodes of dizziness and has fallen twice in the past 2 weeks. She tells you that she takes her medications as prescribed and has had no other concerns. What additional assessment data do you plan to gather from this patient? What is your priority plan of action?

2 **ebp** You are employed as an occupational health nurse in a manufacturing facility. A 32-year-old man who operates a forklift presents to be treated after scraping his forearm on a piece of equipment. During your assessment, he tells you he takes a beta-blocker for his hypertension; you find that his blood pressure is 120/76 mm Hg. While dressing his wound, he tells you he is dedicated to staying healthy, by taking his meds and going to the gym, but he can't seem to get his heart rate up and feels tired all the time. What further follow-up would you recommend? Discuss the evidence that supports specific strategies aimed at treating hypertension.

3 **pq** You are working at the student health center at the local community college and a 28-year-old man comes into the office complaining of a headache and blurry vision. While obtaining assessment information, you discover his blood pressure to be 150/96 mm Hg. You continue to obtain assessment information and discover that he has been staying up late to get his assignments completed by drinking caffeinated energy drinks. What additional assessment data would you gather from this patient? What is your priority plan of action?

REFERENCES

*Asterisk indicates nursing research.
**Double asterisk indicates classic reference.

Books

Kaplan, N. M., & Victor, R. G. (2015). *Kaplan's clinical hypertension* (11th ed.). Philadelphia, PA: Lippincott Williams & Wilkins.
Karch, A. (2014). *2015 Lippincott's nursing drug guide*. Philadelphia, PA: Lippincott Williams & Wilkins.

Journals and Electronic Documents

American Heart Association, Inc. (2016). *Know your risk factors for high blood pressure*. Retrieved on 10/29/2016 at: www.heart.org/HEARTORG/Conditions/HighBloodPressure/UnderstandYourRiskforHighBloodPressure/Understand-Your-Risk-for-High-Blood-Pressure_UCM_002052_Article.jsp#.WBUWC1u3BK9
**Appel, L. J., Champagne, C. M., Harsha, D. W., et al; Writing Group of the PREMIER Collaborative Research Group. (2003). Effects of comprehensive lifestyle modification on blood pressure control: Main results of the PREMIER clinical trial. *JAMA, 289*(16), 2083–2093.
**Appel, L. J., Sacks, F. M., Carey, V. J., et al; OmniHeart Collaborative Research Group. (2005). Effects of protein, monounsaturated fat, and carbohydrate intake on blood pressure and serum lipids: Results of the OmniHeart randomized trial. *JAMA, 294*(19), 2455–2464.
**Aronow, W. S., Fleg, J. L., Pepine, C. J., et al; ACCF Task Force. (2011). ACCF/AHA 2011 expert consensus document on hypertension in the elderly: A report of the American College of Cardiology Foundation Task Force on Clinical Expert Consensus Documents. *Circulation, 123*(21), 2434–2506.
Barengo, N. C., Antikainen, R., Kastarinen, M., et al. (2013). The effects of control of systolic and diastolic hypertension on cardiovascular and all-cause mortality in a community-based population cohort. *Journal of Human Hypertension, 27*(11), 693–697.
Bisognano, J. D. (2015). *Malignant hypertension*. Medscape. Retrieved on 10/27/2016 at: emedicine.medscape.com/article/241640-overview
Busko, M. (2015). *Isolated systolic hypertension in young adults ups CVD risk*. Medscape. Retrieved on 10/27/2016 at: www.medscape.com/viewarticle/838941
**Chobanian, A. V., Bakris, G. L., Black, H. R., et al; National High Blood Pressure Education Program Coordinating Committee (2003a). Seventh Report of the Joint National Committee on prevention, detection, evaluation, and treatment of high blood pressure: The JNC 7 Report. *JAMA, 289*(19), 2560–2572.
**Chobanian, A. V., Bakris, G. L., Black, H. R., et al; National High Blood Pressure Education Program Coordinating Committee (2003b). Seventh Report of the Joint National Committee on prevention, detection, evaluation, and treatment of high blood pressure. *Hypertension, 42*(6), 1206–1252.
Coogan, N., Marra, A., & Lomonaco, E. A. (2015). Assessing accurate BP measurement: Size and technique matter! *Nursing, 45*(4), 16–18.
Coxson, P. G., Cook N. R., Joffres, M., et al. (2013). Mortality benefits from US population-wide reduction in sodium consumption: Projections from 3 modeling approaches. *Hypertension, 61*(3), 564–570.
Eckel, R. H., Jakicic, J. M., Ard, J. D., et al. (2014). 2013 AHA/ACC guideline on lifestyle management to reduce cardiovascular risk. A report of the American College of Cardiology/American Heart Association Task Force on Practice Guidelines. *Journal of the American College of Cardiology, 63*(25 Pt B), 2961–2984.
Ehret, G. B., & Caulfield, M. J. (2013). Genes for blood pressure: An opportunity to understand hypertension. *European Heart Journal, 34*(13), 951–961.
Go, A. S., Bauman, M. A., Coleman King, S. M., et al. (2014). An effective approach to high blood pressure control: A science advisory from the American Heart Association, the American College of Cardiology, and the Centers for Disease Control and Prevention. *Journal of the American College of Cardiology, 63*(12), 1230–1238.
Hopkins, C. (2015). *Hypertensive emergencies*. Medscape. Retrieved on 10/27/2016 at: emedicine.medscape.com/article/1952052-overview
Iuga, A. O., & McGuire, M. J. (2014). Adherence and health care costs. *Risk Management and Health Care Policy, 7*, 35–44.

James, P.A., Oparil, S., Carter, B.L, et al. (2014). 2014 evidence-based guideline for the management of high blood pressure in adults: Report from the panel members appointed to the Eighth Joint National Committee (JNC 8). *JAMA, 311*(5), 507–520.

Knight, J. A. (2012). Physical inactivity: Associated diseases and disorders. *Annals of Clinical & Laboratory Science, 42*(3), 320–337.

Männistö, T., Mendola, P., Vääräsmäki, M., et al. (2013). Elevated blood pressure in pregnancy and subsequent chronic disease risk. *Circulation, 127*(6), 681–690.

Miedema, M. D., Lopez, F. L., Blaha, S. S., et al. (2015). Implications of the Eighth Joint National Committee guidelines for the management of high blood pressure for aging adults: Atherosclerosis Risk in Communities Study. *Hypertension, 66*(3), 474–480.

Monnet, X., & Marik, P. E. (2015). What's new with hypertensive crises? *Intensive Care Medicine, 41*(1), 127–130.

Mozaffarian, D., Benjamin, E. J., Go, A. S., et al. (2016). Heart Disease and Stroke Statistics-2016 Update: A report from the American Heart Association. *Circulation, 133*(4), e38–e360.

Odden, M. C., Peralta, C. A., Haan, M. N., et al. (2012). Rethinking the association of high blood pressure with mortality in elderly adults: The impact of frailty. *Archives of Internal Medicine, 172*(15), 1162–1168.

Rosendorff, C., Lackland, D. T., Allison, M., et al. (2015). Treatment of hypertension in patients with coronary artery disease. A scientific statement from the American Heart Association, American College of Cardiology, and American Society of Hypertension. *Journal of the American Society of Hypertension, 9*(6), 453–498.

Schiffrin, E. L., (2014). Immune mechanisms in hypertension and vascular injury. *Clinical Science (London), 126*(4), 267–274.

*Stallings, D. T. (2016). Illness perceptions and health behaviors of black women. *Journal of Cardiovascular Nursing, 31*(6), 492–499.

Tinetti, M. E., Han, L., Lee, D. S., et al. (2014). Antihypertensive medications and serious fall injuries in a nationally representative sample of older adults. *JAMA Internal Medicine, 174*(4), 588–595.

Tinetti, M. E., Han, L., McAvay, G. J., et al. (2014). Anti-hypertensive medications and cardiovascular events in older adults with multiple chronic conditions. *PLoS One, 9*(3), e90733.

**U.S. Department of Health and Human Services. (2003). *Your guide to lowering your blood pressure with DASH: DASH eating plan*. Retrieved on 11/27/2015 at: www.nhlbi.nih.gov/health/public/heart/hbp/dash/new_dash.pdf

U.S. Food and Drug Administration. (2016). *Drug approvals and databases*. Retrieved on 10/29/2016 at: www.fda.gov/Drugs/InformationOnDrugs/UCM079874

Valderrama, A. L., Gillespie, C., King, S. C., et al. (2012). Vital signs: Awareness and treatment of uncontrolled hypertension among adults–United States, 2003-2010. *Morbidity and Mortality Weekly Report, 61*(35), 703–709.

Weber, M. A, Schiffrin, E. L., White, W. B., et al. (2014). Clinical practice guidelines for the management of hypertension in the community: A statement by the American Society of Hypertension and the International Society of Hypertension. *The Journal of Clinical Hypertension (Greenwich), 16*(1), 14–26.

Williamson, J. D., Supiano, M. A., Applegate, W. B., et al; SPRINT Research Group. (2016). Intensive versus standard blood pressure control and cardiovascular disease outcomes in adults aged ≥75 years: A randomized clinical trial. *JAMA, 315*(24), 2673–2682.

Resources

American Heart Association National Center, www.heart.org/HEARTORG/

American Society of Hypertension, www.ash-us.org/

Centers for Disease Control and Prevention (CDC), www.cdc.gov

Heart and Stroke Foundation of Canada, www.heartandstroke.com/site/c.ikIQLcMWJtE/b.3483933/

International Society of Hypertension, ish-world.com/index.htm

National Heart, Lung, and Blood Institute, www.nhlbi.nih.gov

World Health Association (WHO), Cardiovascular Disease Information, www.who.int/topics/cardiovascular_diseases/en

UNIT
7

Hematologic Function

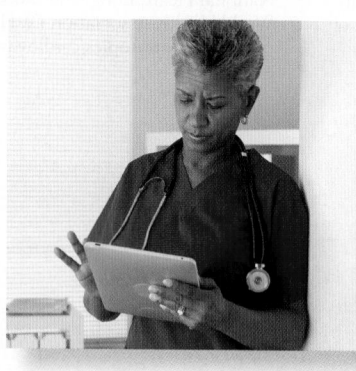

A 47-year-old patient is admitted to an inpatient oncology unit with a new diagnosis of acute myeloid leukemia (AML). She presented to the outpatient office of her primary provider with complaints of flu-like symptoms for the past four weeks, which have worsened over the past three days to now include weakness and dyspnea on exertion. Laboratory tests and a bone marrow biopsy confirmed the diagnosis of AML. The patient is scheduled to begin chemotherapy and a central venous catheter will be placed prior to treatment initiation. Prevention of infection is vital in patients with leukemia. Often patients with AML will not exhibit typical signs of infection such as elevated fever.

QSEN Competency Focus: Evidence-Based Practice (EBP)

The complexities inherent in today's health care system challenges nurses to demonstrate integration of specific interdisciplinary core competencies. These competencies are aimed at ensuring the delivery of safe, quality patient care (Institute of Medicine, 2003). The Quality and Safety Education for Nurses project (QSEN, 2017; Cronenwett, Sherwood, Barnsteiner, et al., 2007) provides a framework for the knowledge, skills, and attitudes (KSA) required for nurses to demonstrate competency in these key areas, which include **patient-centered care, interdisciplinary teamwork and collaboration, evidence-based practice, quality improvement, safety,** and **informatics.**

Evidence-Based Practice Definition: Integrate best current evidence with clinical expertise and patient/family preferences and values for delivery of optimal health care.

SELECTED PRE-LICENSURE KSAs	APPLICATION AND REFLECTION
Knowledge	
Explain the role of evidence in determining best clinical practice.	What is the strength of the evidence for strategies aimed at preventing infection in patients with AML? Identify the pathophysiologic relationships between the disease process in AML, the susceptibility to infection, and the atypical signs and symptoms of infection in patients with leukemias.
Skills	
Locate evidence reports related to clinical practice topics and guidelines.	What strategies would you use to search for and then identify appropriate evidence for decreasing rates of infection in patients with AML? What resources might you mobilize to provide education for this patient on the best strategies to prevent infection? What signs and symptoms should she monitor and report to her primary provider?
Attitudes	
Value the need for continuous improvement in clinical practice based on new knowledge.	Reflect on your attitudes toward patients with diseases susceptible to infection. Do you tend to think that infection is inevitable in patients with a cancer diagnosis?

Cronenwett, L., Sherwood, G., Barnsteiner, J., et al. (2007). Quality and safety education for nurses. *Nursing Outlook, 55*(3), 122–131.
Institute of Medicine. (2003). *Health professions education: A bridge to quality.* Washington, DC: National Academies Press.
QSEN Institute. (2017). *QSEN competencies: Definitions and pre-licensure KSAs.* Retrieved on 3/1/2017 at: www.qsen.org/competencies/pre-licensure-ksas

32

Assessment of Hematologic Function and Treatment Modalities

LEARNING OBJECTIVES

On completion of this chapter, the learner will be able to:

1 Describe hematopoiesis and the processes involved in maintaining hemostasis.
2 Discuss the significance of the health history to the assessment of hematologic health.
3 Specify the proper techniques utilized to perform a comprehensive physical assessment of hematologic function.
4 Explain the diagnostic tests and related nursing implications used to evaluate hematologic function.
5 Identify therapies for blood disorders, including nursing implications for the administration of blood components.

GLOSSARY

anemia: decreased red blood cell (RBC) count
band cell: slightly immature neutrophil
blast cell: primitive white blood cell (WBC)
cytokines: proteins produced by leukocytes that are vital to regulation of hematopoiesis, apoptosis, and immune responses
differentiation: development of functions and characteristics that are different from those of the parent stem cell
erythrocyte: a cellular component of blood involved in the transport of oxygen and carbon dioxide (*synonym:* red blood cell)
erythropoiesis: process of the formation of RBCs
erythropoietin: hormone produced primarily by the kidney; necessary for erythropoiesis
fibrin: filamentous protein; basis of thrombus and blood clot
fibrinogen: protein converted into fibrin to form thrombus and clot
fibrinolysis: process of breakdown of fibrin clot
granulocyte: granulated WBC (i.e., neutrophil, eosinophil, basophil); sometimes used synonymously with neutrophil
hematocrit: percentage of total blood volume consisting of RBCs
hematopoiesis: complex process of the formation and maturation of blood cells
hemoglobin: iron-containing protein of RBCs; delivers oxygen to tissues
hemostasis: intricate balance between clot formation and clot dissolution
histiocytes: cells present in all loose connective tissue, capable of phagocytosis
leukocyte: one of several cellular components of blood involved in defense of the body; subtypes include neutrophils, eosinophils, basophils, monocytes, and lymphocytes (*synonym:* white blood cell)
leukopenia: less-than-normal amount of WBCs in circulation
lymphocyte: form of WBC involved in immune functions
lymphoid: pertaining to lymphocytes
macrophage: reticuloendothelial cells capable of phagocytosis
monocyte: large WBC that becomes a macrophage when it leaves the circulation and moves into body tissues

myeloid: pertaining to nonlymphoid blood cells that differentiate into RBCs, platelets, macrophages, mast cells, and various WBCs
myelopoiesis: formation and maturation of cells derived from myeloid stem cell
natural killer (NK) cells: immune cells that accumulate in lymphoid tissue that are potent killers of virus-infected and cancer cells
neutrophil: fully mature WBC capable of phagocytosis; primary defense against bacterial infection
nucleated RBC: immature form of RBC; portion of nucleus remains within the RBC
oxyhemoglobin: combined form of oxygen and hemoglobin; found in arterial blood
phagocytosis: process of cellular ingestion and digestion of foreign bodies
plasma: liquid portion of blood
plasminogen: protein converted to plasmin to dissolve thrombi and clots
platelet: a cellular component of blood involved in blood coagulation (*synonym:* thrombocyte)
red blood cell (RBC): a cellular component of blood involved in the transport of oxygen and carbon dioxide (*synonym:* erythrocyte)
reticulocytes: slightly immature RBCs, usually only 1% of total circulating RBCs
reticuloendothelial system: complex system of cells throughout the body capable of phagocytosis
serum: portion of blood remaining after coagulation occurs
stem cell: primitive cell, capable of self-replication and differentiation into myeloid or lymphoid stem cell
stroma: component of the bone marrow not directly related to hematopoiesis but serves important supportive roles in this process
thrombocyte: a cellular component of blood involved in blood coagulation (*synonym:* platelet)
white blood cell (WBC): one of several cellular components of blood involved in defense of the body; subtypes include neutrophils, eosinophils, basophils, monocytes, and lymphocytes (*synonym:* leukocyte)

Unlike many other body systems, the hematologic system encompasses the entire human body. Patients with hematologic disorders often have significant abnormalities in blood tests but few or no symptoms. Therefore, the nurse must have a good understanding of the pathophysiology of the patient's condition and the ability to make a thorough assessment that relies heavily on the interpretation of laboratory tests. It is equally important for the nurse to anticipate potential patient needs and to target nursing interventions accordingly. Because it is so important to the understanding of most hematologic diseases, a basic appreciation of blood cells and bone marrow function is necessary.

Anatomic and Physiologic Overview

The hematologic system consists of the blood and the sites where blood is produced, including the bone marrow and the **reticuloendothelial system** (RES). Blood is a specialized organ that differs from other organs in that it exists in a fluid state. Blood is composed of plasma and various types of cells. **Plasma** is the fluid portion of blood; it contains various proteins, such as albumin, globulin, **fibrinogen**, and other factors necessary for clotting, as well as electrolytes, waste products, and nutrients. About 55% of blood volume is plasma (Mescher, 2013).

Structure and Function of the Hematologic System

Blood

The cellular component of blood consists of three primary cell types (see Table 32-1): **erythrocytes (red blood cells [RBCs], red cells), leukocytes (white blood cells [WBCs])**, and **thrombocytes (platelets)**. These cellular components of blood

TABLE 32-1 **Blood Cells**

Cell Type	Major Function
WBC (Leukocyte)	Fights infection
Neutrophil	Essential in preventing or limiting bacterial infection via phagocytosis
Monocyte	Enters tissue as macrophage; highly phagocytic, especially against fungus; immune surveillance
Eosinophil	Involved in allergic reactions (neutralizes histamine); digests foreign proteins
Basophil	Contains histamine; integral part of hypersensitivity reactions
Lymphocyte	Integral component of immune system
T lymphocyte	Responsible for cell-mediated immunity; recognizes material as "foreign" (surveillance system)
B lymphocyte	Responsible for humoral immunity; many mature into plasma cells to form antibodies
Plasma cell	Secretes immunoglobulin (antibody); most mature form of B lymphocyte
RBC (Erythrocyte)	Carries hemoglobin to provide oxygen to tissues; average lifespan is 120 days
Platelet (Thrombocyte)	Fragment of megakaryocyte; provides basis for coagulation to occur; maintains hemostasis; average lifespan is 10 days

WBC, white blood cell; RBC, red blood cell.

normally make up 40% to 45% of the blood volume. Because most blood cells have a short lifespan, the need for the body to replenish its supply of cells is continuous; this process is termed **hematopoiesis**. The primary site for hematopoiesis is the bone marrow. During embryonic development and in other conditions, the liver and spleen may also be involved.

Under normal conditions, the adult bone marrow produces about 175 billion erythrocytes, 70 billion **neutrophils** (a mature type of WBC), and 175 billion platelets each day. When the body needs more blood cells, as in infection (when neutrophils are needed to fight the invading pathogen) or in bleeding (when more RBCs are required), the marrow increases its production of the cells required. Thus, under normal conditions, the marrow responds to increased demand and releases adequate numbers of cells into the circulation.

Blood makes up approximately 7% to 10% of the normal body weight and amounts to 5 to 6 L of volume. Circulating through the vascular system and serving as a link between body organs, blood carries oxygen absorbed from the lungs and nutrients absorbed from the gastrointestinal (GI) tract to the body cells for cellular metabolism. Blood also carries hormones, antibodies, and other substances to their sites of action or use. In addition, blood carries waste products produced by cellular metabolism to the lungs, skin, liver, and kidneys, where they are transformed and eliminated from the body.

The danger that trauma can lead to excess blood loss always exists. To prevent this, an intricate clotting mechanism is activated when necessary to seal any leak in the blood vessels. Excessive clotting is equally dangerous, because it can obstruct blood flow to vital tissues. To prevent this, the body has a fibrinolytic mechanism that eventually dissolves clots (thrombi) formed within blood vessels. The balance between these two systems—clot (thrombus) formation and clot dissolution or **fibrinolysis**—is called **hemostasis**.

Bone Marrow

The bone marrow is the site of hematopoiesis, or blood cell formation. In adults, blood cell formation is usually limited to the pelvis, ribs, vertebrae, and sternum. Marrow is one of the largest organs of the body, making up 4% to 5% of total body weight. It consists of islands of cellular components (red marrow) separated by fat (yellow marrow). As people age, the proportion of active marrow is gradually replaced by fat; however, in healthy adults, the fat can again be replaced by active marrow when more blood cell production is required. In adults with disease that causes marrow destruction, fibrosis, or scarring, the liver and spleen can also resume production of blood cells by a process known as extramedullary hematopoiesis.

The marrow is highly vascular. Within it are primitive cells called **stem cells**. The stem cells have the ability to self-replicate, thereby ensuring a continuous supply of stem cells throughout the life cycle. When stimulated to do so, stem cells can begin a process of **differentiation** into either **myeloid** or **lymphoid** stem cells (see Fig. 32-1). These stem cells are committed to produce specific types of blood cells. Lymphoid stem cells produce either T or B **lymphocytes**. Myeloid stem cells differentiate into three broad cell types: erythrocytes, leukocytes, and platelets. Thus, with the exception of lymphocytes, all blood cells are derived from myeloid stem cells. A defect

Physiology/Pathophysiology

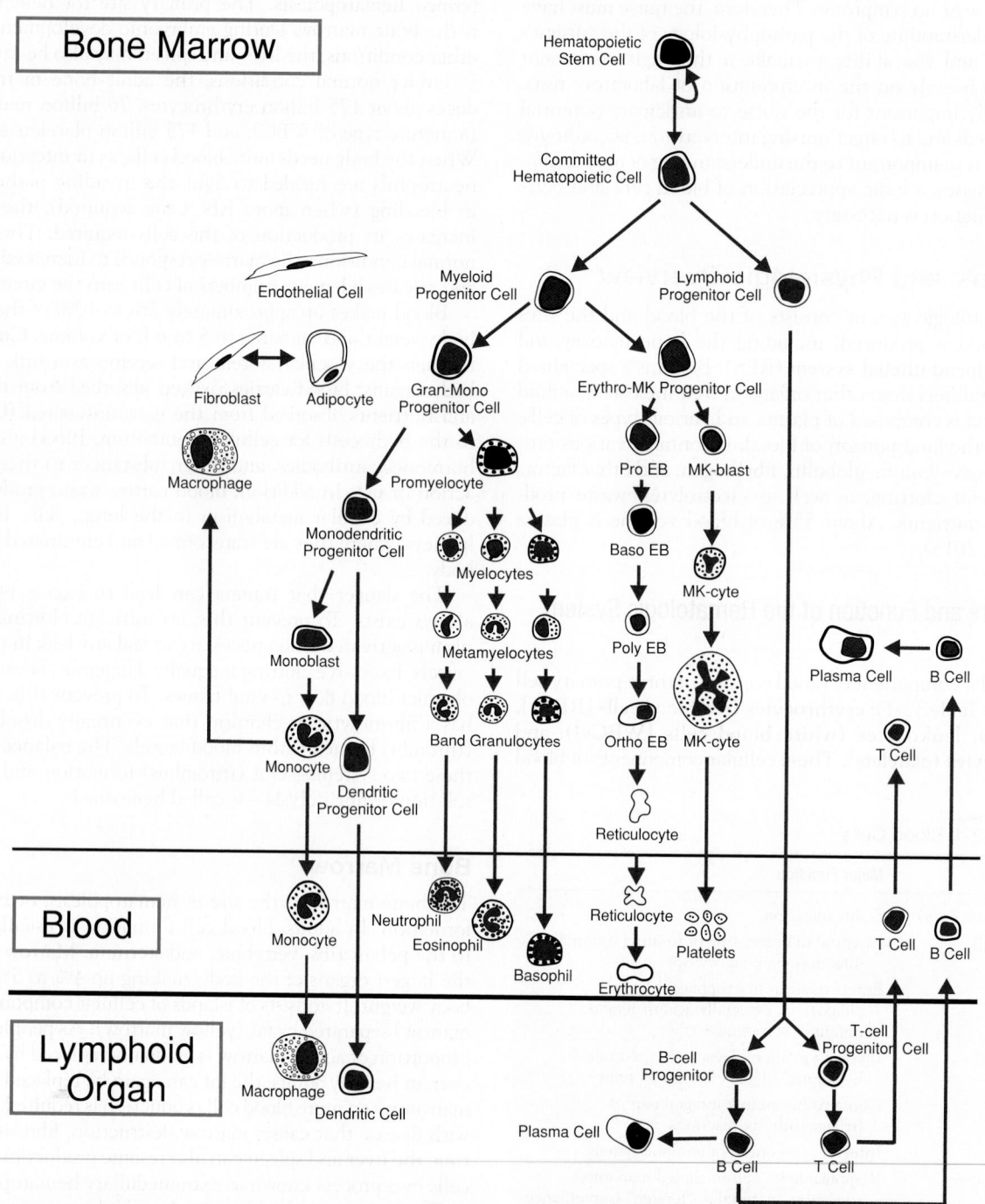

Figure 32-1 • Hematopoiesis and stromal stem cell differentiation. Uncommitted (pluripotent) stem cells can differentiate into myeloid or lymphoid stem cells. These stem cells then undergo a complex process of differentiation and maturation into normal cells that are released into the circulation. The myeloid stem cell is responsible not only for all nonlymphoid white blood cells but also for the production of red blood cells (RBCs) and platelets. Each step of the differentiation process depends in part on the presence of specific growth factors for each cell type. When the stem cells are dysfunctional, they may respond inadequately to the need for more cells, or they may respond excessively, and sometimes uncontrollably, as in leukemia. From Koury, M., Mahmud, N., & Rhodes, M. (2009). Origin and development of blood cells. In J. P. Greer, J. Foerster, G. M. Rodgers (Eds.). *Wintrobe's clinical hematology* (12th ed.). Philadelphia, PA: Lippincott Williams & Wilkins.

in a myeloid stem cell can cause problems with erythrocyte, leukocyte, and platelet production. In contrast, a defect in the lymphoid stem cell can cause problems with T or B lymphocytes, plasma cells (a more differentiated form of B lymphocyte), or natural killer (NK) cells. Over 100 billion cells are produced by the marrow each day (Davoren & Wang, 2013).

The **stroma** of the marrow refers to all tissue within the marrow that is not directly involved in hematopoiesis. However, the stroma is important in an indirect manner, in that it produces the colony-stimulating factors needed for hematopoiesis. The yellow marrow is the largest component of the stroma. Other cells comprising the stroma include fibroblasts (reticular connective tissue), osteoclasts, osteoblasts (both needed for remodeling of skeletal bone), and endothelial cells.

Blood Cells

Erythrocytes (Red Blood Cells)

The normal erythrocyte is a biconcave disc that resembles a soft ball compressed between two fingers (see Fig. 32-2). It has a diameter of about 8 mcm and is so flexible that it can pass easily through capillaries that may be as small as 2.8 mcm in diameter. The membrane of the red cell is very thin so that gases, such as oxygen and carbon dioxide, can easily diffuse across it; the disc shape provides a large surface area that facilitates the absorption and release of oxygen molecules.

Mature erythrocytes consist primarily of **hemoglobin**, which contains iron and makes up 95% of the cell mass.

Mature erythrocytes have no nuclei, and they have many fewer metabolic enzymes than do most other cells. The presence of a large amount of hemoglobin enables the red cell to perform its principal function, which is the transport of oxygen between the lungs and tissues. Occasionally, the marrow releases slightly immature forms of erythrocytes, called **reticulocytes**, into the circulation. This occurs as a normal response to an increased demand for erythrocytes (as in bleeding) or in some disease states.

The oxygen-carrying hemoglobin molecule is made up of four subunits, each containing a heme portion attached to a globin chain. Iron is present in the heme component of the molecule. An important property of heme is its ability to bind to oxygen loosely and reversibly. Oxygen readily binds to hemoglobin in the lungs and is carried as **oxyhemoglobin** in arterial blood. Oxyhemoglobin is a brighter red than hemoglobin that does not contain oxygen (reduced hemoglobin); thus, arterial blood is a brighter red than venous blood. The oxygen readily dissociates (detaches) from hemoglobin in the tissues, where the oxygen is needed for cellular metabolism. In venous blood, hemoglobin combines with hydrogen ions produced by cellular metabolism and thus buffers excessive acid. Whole blood normally contains about 15 g of hemoglobin per 100 mL of blood (Fischbach & Dunning, 2015).

Erythropoiesis

Erythroblasts arise from the primitive myeloid stem cells in bone marrow. The erythroblast is an immature nucleated cell that gradually loses its nucleus. At this stage, the cell is known

Blood smear

Platelet

Leukocyte

Erythrocytes

Erythrocytes

Platelets

Note the clump of platelets

Granulocytes

Nucleus

Neutrophil

Nucleus

Granules

Basophil

Granules

Nucleus

Eosinophil

Agranulocytes

Nucleus

Lymphocyte

Nucleus

Monocyte

Figure 32-2 • Normal types of blood cells. From Cohen, B. J. (2005). *Memmler's the human body in health and disease* (10th ed.). Philadelphia, PA: Lippincott Williams & Wilkins.

as a reticulocyte. Further maturation into an erythrocyte entails the loss of the dark-staining material within the cell and slight shrinkage. The mature erythrocyte is then released into the circulation. Under conditions of rapid **erythropoiesis** (i.e., erythrocyte production), reticulocytes and other immature cells (e.g., **nucleated RBCs**) may be released prematurely into the circulation. This is often seen when the liver or spleen takes over as the site of erythropoiesis and more nucleated red cells appear within the circulation.

Differentiation of the primitive myeloid stem cell into an erythroblast is stimulated by **erythropoietin**, a hormone produced primarily by the kidney. If the kidney detects low levels of oxygen, as occurs when fewer red cells are available to bind oxygen (i.e., **anemia**), or with people living at high altitudes with lower atmospheric oxygen concentrations, erythropoietin levels increase. The increased erythropoietin then stimulates the marrow to increase the production of erythrocytes. The entire process of erythropoiesis typically takes less than 5 days (Papayannopoulou & Migliaccio, 2013). For normal erythrocyte production, the bone marrow also requires iron, vitamin B$_{12}$, folate, pyridoxine (vitamin B$_6$), protein, and other factors. A deficiency of these factors during erythropoiesis can result in decreased red cell production and anemia.

Iron Stores and Metabolism

The average daily diet in the United States contains 10 to 15 mg of elemental iron, but only 1 to 2.5 mg of ingested iron is normally absorbed from the small intestine (Adamson, 2015). The rate of iron absorption is regulated by the amount of iron already stored in the body and by the rate of erythrocyte production. Additional amounts of iron, up to 2 mg daily, must be absorbed by women of childbearing age to replace that lost during menstruation. Total body iron content in the average adult is approximately 3 g, most of which is present in hemoglobin or in one of its breakdown products. Iron is stored as ferritin and when required, the iron is released into the plasma, binds to transferrin, and is transported into the membranes of the normoblasts (erythrocyte precursor cells) within the marrow, where it is incorporated into hemoglobin. Iron is lost in the feces, either in bile, blood, or mucosal cells from the intestine.

The concentration of iron in blood is normally about 50 to 150 μg/dL (Adamson & Longo, 2015). With iron deficiency, bone marrow iron stores are rapidly depleted; hemoglobin synthesis is depressed, and the erythrocytes produced by the marrow are small and low in hemoglobin. Iron deficiency in the adult generally indicates blood loss (e.g., from bleeding in the GI tract or heavy menstrual flow). Lack of dietary iron is rarely the sole cause of iron deficiency anemia in adults. The source of iron deficiency should be investigated promptly, because iron deficiency in an adult may be a sign of bleeding in the GI tract or colon cancer.

Vitamin B$_{12}$ and Folate Metabolism

Vitamin B$_{12}$ and folate are required for the synthesis of deoxyribonucleic acid (DNA) in RBCs. Both vitamin B$_{12}$ and folate are derived from the diet. Folate is absorbed in the proximal small intestine, but only small amounts are stored within the body. If the diet is deficient in folate, stores within the body quickly become depleted. Because vitamin B$_{12}$ is found only in foods of animal origin, strict vegetarians may ingest little

vitamin B$_{12}$. Vitamin B$_{12}$ combines with intrinsic factor produced in the stomach. The vitamin B$_{12}$–intrinsic factor complex is absorbed in the distal ileum. People who have had a partial or total gastrectomy may have limited amounts of intrinsic factor, and therefore the absorption of vitamin B$_{12}$ may be diminished. The effects of either decreased absorption or decreased intake of vitamin B$_{12}$ are not apparent for 2 to 4 years.

Vitamin B$_{12}$ and folate deficiencies are characterized by the production of abnormally large erythrocytes called *megaloblasts*. Because these cells are abnormal, many are sequestered (trapped) while still in the bone marrow, and their rate of release is decreased. Some of these cells actually die in the marrow before they can be released into the circulation. This results in megaloblastic anemia.

Red Blood Cell Destruction

The average lifespan of a normal circulating erythrocyte is 120 days. Aged erythrocytes lose their elasticity and become trapped in small blood vessels and the spleen. They are removed from the blood by the reticuloendothelial cells, particularly in the liver and the spleen. As the erythrocytes are destroyed, most of their hemoglobin is recycled. Some hemoglobin also breaks down to form bilirubin and is secreted in the bile. Most of the iron is recycled to form new hemoglobin molecules within the bone marrow; small amounts are lost daily in the feces and urine and monthly in menstrual flow.

Leukocytes (White Blood Cells)

Leukocytes are divided into two general categories: granulocytes and lymphocytes. In normal blood, the total leukocyte count is 4000 to 11,000 cells/mm³. Of these, approximately 60% to 80% are granulocytes and 20% to 40% are lymphocytes. Both of these types of leukocytes primarily protect the body against infection and tissue injury.

Granulocytes

Granulocytes are defined by the presence of granules in the cytoplasm of the cell. Granulocytes are divided into three main subgroups—eosinophils, basophils, and neutrophils—that are characterized by the staining properties of these granules (see Fig. 32-2). Eosinophils have bright-red granules in their cytoplasm, whereas the granules in basophils stain deep blue. The third and most numerous cell in this class is the neutrophil, with granules that stain a pink to violet hue. Neutrophils are also called *polymorphonuclear neutrophils* (PMNs, or polys) or *segmented neutrophils* (segs).

The nucleus of the mature neutrophil has multiple lobes (usually two to five) that are connected by thin filaments of nuclear material, or a "segmented" nucleus; it is usually two times the size of an erythrocyte. The somewhat less mature granulocyte has a single-lobed, elongated nucleus and is called a **band cell**. Ordinarily, band cells account for only a small percentage of circulating granulocytes, although their percentage can increase greatly under conditions in which neutrophil production increases, such as infection. The increased number of band cells is sometimes called a left shift or shift to the left. (Traditionally, the diagram of neutrophil maturation showed the myeloid stem cell on the left with progressive maturation stages toward the right, ending with a fully mature neutrophil on the far right side. A shift to the left indicates that more immature cells are present in the blood than normal.)

Fully mature neutrophils result from the gradual differentiation of myeloid stem cells, specifically myeloid **blast cells.** The process, called **myelopoiesis,** is highly complex and depends on many factors. These factors, including specific **cytokines** such as growth factors, are normally present within the marrow itself. As the blast cell matures, the cytoplasm of the cell changes in color (from blue to violet) and granules begin to form with the cytoplasm. The shape of the nucleus also changes. The entire process of maturation and differentiation takes about 10 days (see Fig. 32-1). Once the neutrophil is released into the circulation from the marrow, it stays there for only about 6 hours before it migrates into the body tissues to perform its function of **phagocytosis** (ingestion and digestion of bacteria and particles). Neutrophils die here within 1 to 2 days. The number of circulating granulocytes found in the healthy person is relatively constant; however, in infection, large numbers of these cells are rapidly released into the circulation.

Agranulocytes

Monocytes

Monocytes (also called *mononuclear leukocytes*) are leukocytes with a single-lobed nucleus and a granule-free cytoplasm—hence the term *agranulocyte* (see Fig. 32-2). In normal adult blood, monocytes account for approximately 5% of the total leukocytes. Monocytes are the largest of the leukocytes. Produced by the bone marrow, they remain in the circulation for a short time before entering the tissues and transforming into **macrophages.** Macrophages are particularly active in the spleen, liver, peritoneum, and alveoli; they remove debris from these areas and phagocytize bacteria within the tissues.

Lymphocytes

Mature lymphocytes are small cells with scanty cytoplasm (see Fig. 32-2). Immature lymphocytes are produced in the marrow from the lymphoid stem cells. A second major source of production is the thymus. Cells derived from the thymus are known as T lymphocytes (or T cells); those derived from the marrow can also be T cells but are more commonly B lymphocytes (or B cells). Lymphocytes complete their differentiation and maturation primarily in the lymph nodes and in the lymphoid tissue of the intestine and spleen after exposure to a specific antigen. Mature lymphocytes are the principal cells of the immune system, producing antibodies and identifying other cells and organisms as "foreign." **Natural killer (NK) cells** serve an important role in the body's immune defense system. Like other lymphocytes, NK cells accumulate in the lymphoid tissues (especially spleen, lymph nodes, and tonsils), where they mature. When activated, they serve as potent killers of virus-infected and cancer cells. They also secrete chemical messenger proteins, called *cytokines,* to mobilize the T and B cells into action.

Function of Leukocytes

Leukocytes protect the body from invasion by bacteria and other foreign entities. The major function of neutrophils is phagocytosis. Neutrophils arrive at a given site within 1 hour after the onset of an inflammatory reaction and initiate phagocytosis, but they are short-lived. An influx of monocytes follows; these cells continue their phagocytic activities for long periods as macrophages. This process constitutes a second line of defense for the body against inflammation and infection. Although neutrophils can often work adequately against bacteria without the help of macrophages, macrophages are particularly effective against fungi and viruses. Macrophages also digest senescent (aging or aged) blood cells, primarily within the spleen.

The primary function of lymphocytes is to attack foreign material. One group of lymphocytes (T lymphocytes) kills foreign cells directly or releases lymphokines, substances that enhance the activity of phagocytic cells. T lymphocytes are responsible for delayed allergic reactions, rejection of foreign tissue (e.g., transplanted organs), and destruction of tumor cells. This process is known as *cellular immunity.* The other group of lymphocytes (B lymphocytes) is capable of differentiating into plasma cells. Plasma cells, in turn, produce antibodies called *immunoglobulins* (Igs), which are protein molecules that destroy foreign material by several mechanisms. This process is known as humoral immunity.

Eosinophils and basophils function in hypersensitivity reactions. Eosinophils are important in the phagocytosis of parasites. The increase in eosinophil levels in allergic states indicates that these cells are involved in the hypersensitivity reaction; they neutralize histamine. Basophils produce and store histamine as well as other substances involved in hypersensitivity reactions. The release of these substances provokes allergic reactions. See Chapter 35 for further information on the immune response.

Platelets (Thrombocytes)

Platelets, or thrombocytes, are not technically cells; rather, they are granular fragments of giant cells in the bone marrow called *megakaryocytes* (see Fig. 32-2). Platelet production in the marrow is regulated in part by the hormone thrombopoietin, which stimulates the production and differentiation of megakaryocytes from the myeloid stem cell.

Platelets play an essential role in the control of bleeding. They circulate freely in the blood in an inactive state, where they nurture the endothelium of the blood vessels, maintaining the integrity of the vessel. When vascular injury occurs, platelets collect at the site and are activated. They adhere to the site of injury and to each other, forming a platelet plug that temporarily stops bleeding. Substances released from platelet granules activate coagulation factors in the blood plasma and initiate the formation of a stable clot composed of **fibrin,** a filamentous protein. Platelets have a normal lifespan of 7 to 10 days (Konkle, 2015).

Recently, researchers have discovered an additional role for platelets that is related to inflammatory function. Receptors on the surface of platelets permit them to interact with leukocytes, inflamed endothelium of the vessel, and pathogens (Weyrich, 2014). Through a complex process, activated platelets adhere to neutrophils and monocytes, amplifying the immune response. This process is beneficial in the context of exposure to various pathogens (e.g., bacteria). However, this process is also thought to contribute to the inflammatory injury that may be involved in the development of arthritis, cardiovascular and cerebrovascular diseases, cancer, and progression to sepsis.

Plasma and Plasma Proteins

After cellular elements are removed from blood, the remaining liquid portion is called *plasma*. More than 90% of plasma is water. The remainder consists primarily of plasma proteins; clotting factors (particularly fibrinogen); and small amounts of other substances, such as nutrients, enzymes, waste products, and gases. If plasma is allowed to clot, the remaining fluid is called **serum**. Serum has essentially the same composition as plasma, except that fibrinogen and several clotting factors have been removed during the clotting process.

Plasma proteins consist primarily of albumin and globulins. The globulins can be separated into three main fractions (alpha, beta, and gamma), each of which consists of distinct proteins that have different functions. Important proteins in the alpha and beta fractions are the transport globulins and the clotting factors that are made in the liver. The transport globulins carry various substances in bound form in the circulation. For example, thyroid-binding globulin carries thyroxin, and transferrin carries iron. The clotting factors, including fibrinogen, remain in an inactive form in the blood plasma until activated by the clotting cascade. The gamma-globulin fraction refers to the Igs, or antibodies. These proteins are produced by well-differentiated B lymphocytes and plasma cells. The actual fractionation of the globulins can be seen on a specific laboratory test (serum protein electrophoresis).

Albumin is particularly important for the maintenance of fluid balance within the vascular system. Capillary walls are impermeable to albumin, so its presence in the plasma creates an osmotic force that keeps fluid within the vascular space. Albumin, which is produced by the liver, has the capacity to bind to several substances that are transported in plasma (e.g., certain medications, bilirubin, and some hormones). People with impaired hepatic function may have low concentrations of albumin, with a resultant decrease in osmotic pressure and the development of edema.

Reticuloendothelial System (RES)

The RES is composed of special tissue macrophages. When released from the marrow, monocytes spend a short time in the circulation (about 24 hours) and then enter the body tissues. Within the tissues, the monocytes continue to differentiate into macrophages, which can survive for months or years. Macrophages have a variety of important functions. They defend the body against foreign invaders (i.e., bacteria and other pathogens) via phagocytosis. They remove old or damaged cells from the circulation. They stimulate the inflammatory process and present antigens to the immune system (see Chapter 35). Macrophages give rise to tissue **histiocytes**, including Kupffer cells of the liver, peritoneal macrophages, alveolar macrophages, and other components of the RES. Thus, the RES is a component of many other organs within the body, particularly the spleen, lymph nodes, lungs, and liver.

The spleen is the site of activity for most macrophages. Most of the spleen (75%) is made of red pulp; here, the blood enters the venous sinuses through capillaries that are surrounded by macrophages. Within the red pulp are tiny aggregates of white pulp, consisting of B and T lymphocytes. The spleen sequesters newly released reticulocytes from the marrow, removing nuclear fragments and other materials (e.g., denatured hemoglobin, iron) before the now fully mature

erythrocyte returns to the circulation. Although a minority of erythrocytes (less than 5%) pool in the spleen, a significant proportion of platelets (20% to 40%) pool here (Doherty, 2015). If the spleen is enlarged, a greater proportion of red cells and platelets can be sequestered. The spleen is a major source of hematopoiesis in fetal life. It can resume hematopoiesis later in adulthood if necessary, particularly when marrow function is compromised (e.g., in bone marrow fibrosis). The spleen has important immunologic functions as well. It forms substances called *opsonins* that promote the phagocytosis of neutrophils; it also forms the antibody immunoglobulin M (IgM) after exposure to an antigen.

Hemostasis

Hemostasis is the process of preventing blood loss from intact vessels and of stopping bleeding from a severed vessel, which requires adequate numbers of functional platelets. Platelets nurture the endothelium and thereby maintain the structural integrity of the vessel wall. Two processes are involved in arresting bleeding: primary and secondary hemostasis (see Fig. 32-3).

In primary hemostasis, the severed blood vessel constricts. Circulating platelets aggregate at the site and adhere to the vessel and to one another. An unstable hemostatic plug is formed. For the coagulation process to be correctly activated, circulating inactive coagulation factors must be converted to active forms. This process occurs on the surface of the aggregated platelets at the site of vessel injury.

The end result is the formation of fibrin, which reinforces the platelet plug and anchors it to the injury site. This process is referred to as secondary hemostasis. Blood coagulation is highly complex. It can be activated by the extrinsic pathway (also known as the tissue factor pathway) or the intrinsic pathway (also known as the contact activation pathway). Both pathways are needed for maintenance of normal hemostasis. Many factors are involved in the reaction cascade that forms fibrin. When tissue is injured, the extrinsic pathway is activated by the release of thromboplastin from the tissue. As the result of a series of reactions, prothrombin is converted to thrombin, which in turn catalyzes the conversion of fibrinogen to fibrin. Clotting by the intrinsic or contact activation pathway is activated when the collagen that lines blood vessels is exposed. Clotting factors are activated sequentially until, as with the extrinsic pathway, fibrin is ultimately formed (Camp, 2014). The intrinsic pathway is slower, and this sequence is less often responsible for clotting in response to tissue injury. However, it is important if a noninjured vessel wall comes into contact with lipoproteins (e.g., atherosclerosis) or with bacteria, resulting in a clot that is formed for purposes other than protection from trauma or bleeding.

As the injured vessel is repaired and again covered with endothelial cells, the fibrin clot is no longer needed. The fibrin is digested via two systems: the plasma fibrinolytic system and the cellular fibrinolytic system. The substance **plasminogen** is required to lyse (break down) the fibrin. Plasminogen, which is present in all body fluids, circulates with fibrinogen and is therefore incorporated into the fibrin clot as it forms. When the clot is no longer needed (e.g., after an injured blood vessel has healed), the plasminogen is activated to form plasmin. Plasmin digests the fibrinogen and fibrin. The breakdown particles of the clot, called *fibrin degradation products*, are released into the circulation. Through this system, clots are dissolved as tissue is repaired, and the vascular system returns to its normal baseline state.

Gerontologic Considerations

In older adults, the bone marrow's ability to respond to the body's need for blood cells (erythrocytes, leukocytes, and platelets) may be decreased, resulting in **leukopenia** (a decreased number of circulating leukocytes) or anemia. This decreased ability is a result of many factors, including diminished production of the growth factors necessary for hema-

topoiesis by stromal cells within the marrow or a diminished response to the growth factors (in the case of erythropoietin). Over time, stem cells within the marrow acquire damage to their DNA, which compromises their function. T and B cell development is also decreased (Snoeck, 2013). Therefore, the development of myeloid malignancies, such as acute myeloid leukemia (AML, see Chapter 34), is more common in older adults. In addition, in older patients, the bone marrow may be more susceptible to the myelosuppressive effects of medications. As a result of these factors, when an older adult needs more blood cells, the bone marrow may not be able to increase the production of these cells adequately.

Assessment

Health History

A careful health history and physical assessment can provide important information related to a patient's known or potential hematologic diagnosis. Because many hematologic disorders are more prevalent in certain ethnic groups, assessments of ethnicity and family history are useful (see Chart 32-1). Similarly, obtaining a nutritional history and assessing the use of prescription and over-the-counter medications, as well as herbal supplements, are important to note, because several conditions can result from nutritional deficiencies, or from the use of certain herbs or medications. Careful attention to the onset of a symptom or finding (e.g., rapid vs. gradual; persistent vs. intermittent), its severity, and any contributing factors can further differentiate potential causes. Of equal importance is assessing the impact of these findings on the patient's functional ability, manifestations of distress, and coping mechanisms.

Physical Assessment

The physical assessment should be comprehensive and include careful attention to the skin, oral cavity, lymph nodes, and spleen (see Fig. 32-4). Table 32-2 highlights a general approach to the physical assessment findings in hematologic disorders (more specific findings are presented in Chapters 33 and 34).

Diagnostic Evaluation

Most hematologic diseases reflect a defect in the hematopoietic, hemostatic, or RES. The defect can be quantitative (e.g., increased or decreased production of cells), qualitative (e.g., the cells that are produced are defective in their normal functional capacity), or both. Initially, many hematologic conditions cause few symptoms, and extensive laboratory tests are often required to establish a diagnosis. For most hematologic conditions, continued monitoring via specific blood tests is required because it is very important to assess for changes in test results over time. In general, it is important to assess trends in test results because these trends help the clinician decide whether the patient is responding appropriately to interventions.

Hematologic Studies

The most common tests used are the complete blood count (CBC) and the peripheral blood smear. The CBC identifies the total number of blood cells (leukocytes, erythrocytes, and platelets) as well as the hemoglobin, **hematocrit** (percentage of blood volume consisting of erythrocytes), and RBC

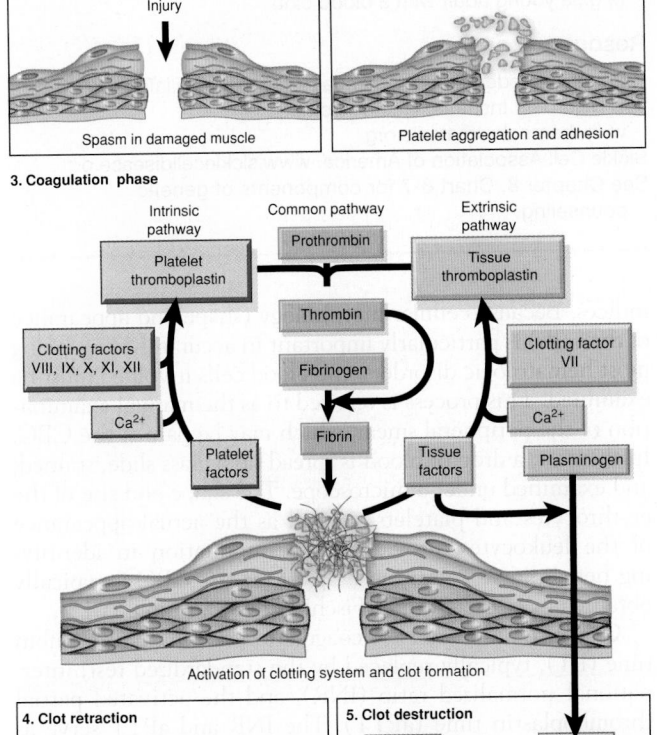

Figure 32-3 • Hemostasis. When the endothelial surface of a blood vessel is injured, several processes occur. In primary hemostasis, platelets within the circulation are attracted to the exposed layer of collagen at the site of injury. They adhere to the site of injury, releasing factors that stimulate other platelets to aggregate at the site, forming an unstable platelet plug. In secondary hemostasis, based on the type of stimulus, one of two clotting pathways is initiated—the intrinsic or extrinsic pathway—and the clotting factors within that pathway are activated. The end result from either pathway is the conversion of prothrombin to thrombin. Thrombin is necessary for fibrinogen to be converted into fibrin, the stabilizing protein that anchors the fragile platelet plug to the site of injury to prevent further bleeding and permit the injured vessel or site to heal. Modified from www.irvingcrowley.com/cls/clotting.gif

Chart 32-1 · GENETICS IN NURSING PRACTICE

Hematologic Disorders

Hematologic disorders are marked by aberrations in the structure or function of the blood cells or the blood clotting mechanism. Some examples of genetic hematologic disorders are:

Autosomal Dominant:
- Factor V Leiden
- Familial hypercholesterolemia
- Hereditary angioedema
- Hereditary spherocytosis
- Von Willebrand disease

Autosomal Recessive:
- Hemochromatosis
- Sickle cell disease
- Thalassemia

X Linked:
- Hemophilia

Nursing Assessments

Refer to Chart 5-2: Genetics in Nursing Practice: Genetic Aspects of Health Assessment

Family History Assessment Specific to Hematologic Disorders
- Collect family history information on maternal and paternal relatives from three generations of the family.

- Assess family history for other family members with histories of blood disorders or episodes of abnormal bleeding.
- If a family history or personal risk is suspected, the person should be carefully screened for bleeding disorders prior to surgical procedures.

Patient Assessment Specific to Hematologic Disorders
- Assess for specific symptoms of hematologic diseases:
  - Extreme fatigue (the most common symptom of hematologic disorders)
  - Delayed clotting of blood
  - Easy or deep bruising
  - Abnormal bleeding (e.g., frequent nosebleeds)
  - Abdominal pain (hemochromatosis) or joint pain (sickle cell disease)
- Review blood cell counts for abnormalities.
- Assess for presence of illness despite low risk for the illness (e.g., a young adult with a blood clot)

Resources

Hemophilia Federation of America, www.hemophiliafed.org
Iron Disorders Institute: Hemochromatosis, www.hemochromatosis.org
Sickle Cell Association of America, www.sicklecelldisease.org
See Chapter 8, Chart 8-7 for components of genetic counseling.

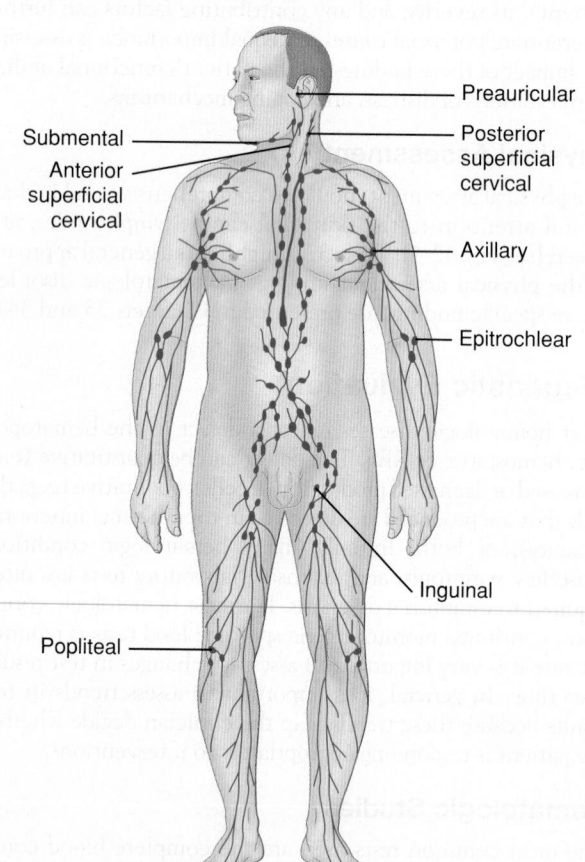

Figure 32-4 • Lymphatic system. *Arrows* indicate sites of lymph nodes accessible for palpation. Developed by Thomas, M., & Morrow, K. (2011). Veterans Administration Palo Alto Health Care System.

indices. Because cellular morphology (shape and appearance of the cells) is particularly important in accurately diagnosing most hematologic disorders, the blood cells involved must be examined. This process is referred to as the manual examination of the peripheral smear, which may be part of the CBC. In this test, a drop of blood is spread on a glass slide, stained, and examined under a microscope. The shape and size of the erythrocytes and platelets, as well as the actual appearance of the leukocytes, provide useful information in identifying hematologic conditions. Blood for the CBC is typically obtained by venipuncture (Fischbach & Dunning, 2015).

Other common tests of coagulation are the prothrombin time (PT), typically replaced by the standardized test, international normalized ratio (INR), and the activated partial thromboplastin time (aPTT). The INR and aPTT serve as useful screening tools for evaluating a patient's clotting ability and monitoring the therapeutic effectiveness of anticoagulant medications. In both tests, specific reagents are mixed into the plasma sample, and the time taken to form a clot is measured. For these tests to be accurate, the test tube must be filled with the correct amount of the patient's blood; either excess or inadequate blood volume within the tube can render the results inaccurate.

Bone Marrow Aspiration and Biopsy

Bone marrow aspiration and biopsy are crucial when additional information is needed to assess how a patient's blood cells are being formed and to assess the quantity and quality of each type of cell produced within the marrow. These tests are also used to document infection or tumor within the marrow. Other specialized tests can be performed on the marrow aspirate, such as cytogenetic analysis or immunophenotyping

TABLE 32-2 Health History and Physical Assessment in Hematologic Disorders[a]

	Findings	Potential Indications of Hematologic Disorder
Health History	Prior episodes of bleeding (epistaxis, tooth, gum, hematuria, menorrhagia, hematochezia, gastrointestinal bleeding and/or ulcers)	Thrombocytopenia, coagulopathy, anemia
	Prior blood clots, pulmonary emboli, miscarriages	Thrombotic disorder
	Fatigue and weakness	Anemia, infection, malignancy, clonal disorders
	Dyspnea, particularly dyspnea on exertion, orthopnea, shortness of breath	Anemia, infection
	Prior radiation therapy (especially pelvic irradiation)	Anemia, pancytopenia, myelodysplastic syndrome, leukemia
	Prior chemotherapy	Myelodysplastic syndrome, leukemia
	Hobbies/occupational/military exposure history (especially benzene, Agent Orange)	Myelodysplastic syndrome, leukemia, myeloma, lymphoma
	Diet history	Anemia (due to vitamin B_{12}, folate, iron deficiency)
	Alcohol consumption	Anemia (effect on hematopoiesis, nutritional deficiency)
	Use of herbal supplements	Platelet dysfunction
	Concurrent medications	Neutropenia, anemia, hemolysis, thrombocytopenia
	Family history/ethnicity	Some hematologic disorders have a higher prevalence in certain ethnic groups and families (see Chart 32-1)
Physical Assessment		
Skin	Gray-tan or bronze skin color (especially genitalia, scars, exposed areas)	Hemochromatosis (primary or secondary)
	Ruddy complexion (face, conjunctiva, hands, feet)	Polycythemia
	Ecchymoses (i.e., bruises)	Thrombocytopenia, coagulopathy
	Petechiae (i.e., pinpoint hemorrhagic lesions, usually more prominent on trunk or anterior aspects of lower extremities)	Severe thrombocytopenia
	Rash	Variable; if pruritic, may indicate polycythemia, other nonhematologic-related disorders (see Chapter 60)
	Bleeding (including around vascular lines, tubes)	Thrombocytopenia, coagulopathy
	Conjunctival hemorrhage	Severe thrombocytopenia, coagulopathy
	Pallor, especially in mucous membranes (including conjunctiva), nail beds	Anemia
	Jaundice in mucous membranes (including conjunctiva), nail beds, palate	Hemolysis
Oral cavity	Petechiae in the buccal mucosa, gingiva, hard palate	Severe thrombocytopenia
	Ulceration of oral mucosa	Infection, leukemia
	Tongue: Smooth	Pernicious anemia
	Beefy red	Vitamin B_{12}/folate deficiency
	Enlarged	Amyloidosis
	Angular cheilosis (ulceration at corners of mouth)	Anemia
	Enlarged gums: hyperplasia	Leukemia
Lymph nodes	Enlarged size, firm and fixed vs. mobile and tender	Leukemia, lymphoma
Respiratory	Increased rate and depth of respirations; adventitious breath sounds	Anemia; infection
Cardiovascular	Distended neck veins, edema, chest pain on exertion, murmurs, gallops	Severe anemia
	Hypotension (below baseline)	Polycythemia
	Hypertension (above baseline)	
Genitourinary	Hematuria	Hemolysis, thrombocytopenia
	Proteinuria	Myeloma
Musculoskeletal	Rib/sternal tenderness to palpation	Leukemia, myeloma
	Back pain; tenderness to palpation over spine, loss of height, kyphosis	Myeloma
	Pain/swelling in knees, wrists, hands	Hemophilia, sickle cell disease
Abdominal	Enlarged spleen	Leukemia, myelofibrosis
	Enlarged liver	Myelofibrosis
	Stool positive for occult blood	Anemia, thrombocytopenia
Central nervous system	Cranial nerve dysfunction	Vitamin B_{12} deficiency
	Peripheral nerve dysfunction (especially sensory)	Vitamin B_{12} deficiency, amyloidosis, myeloma
	Visual changes, headache, alteration in mental status	Severe thrombocytopenia
Gynecologic	Menorrhagia	Thrombocytopenia, coagulopathy
Constitutional	Fever, chills, sweats, asthenia	Leukemia, lymphoma; infection

[a]Common findings (obtained via health history and physical assessment) that occur in patients with hematologic disorders. Note that signs and symptoms are not disease specific but are useful in guiding the nurse to establishing an etiology for the findings noted.

(i.e., identifying specific proteins expressed by cells), which are useful in further identifying certain malignant conditions and, in some instances, establishing a prognosis.

Normal bone marrow is in a semifluid state and can be aspirated through a special large needle. In adults, bone marrow is usually aspirated from the iliac crest and occasionally from the sternum. The aspirate provides only a sample of cells. Aspirate alone may be adequate for evaluating certain conditions, such as anemia. However, when more information is required, a biopsy is also performed. Biopsy samples are taken from the posterior iliac crest; occasionally, an anterior approach is required. A marrow biopsy shows the architecture of the bone marrow as well as its degree of cellularity.

Patient preparation includes a careful explanation of the procedure, which may be done at the patient's bedside (for a hospitalized patient) or in the outpatient setting. Some patients may be anxious, thus an antianxiety agent may be prescribed. It is always important for the physician or nurse to describe and explain to the patient the procedure and the sensations that will be experienced. The risks, benefits, and alternatives are also discussed. A signed informed consent is needed before the procedure is performed.

Before aspiration, the skin is cleansed using aseptic technique. Then, a small area is anesthetized with a local anesthetic agent through the skin and subcutaneous tissue to the periosteum of the bone. It is not possible to anesthetize the bone itself. The bone marrow needle is introduced with a stylet in place. When the needle is felt to go through the outer cortex of bone and enter the marrow cavity, the stylet is removed, a syringe is attached, and a small volume (5 mL) of blood and marrow is aspirated. Patients typically feel a pressure sensation as the needle is advanced into position. The actual aspiration always causes sharp but brief pain, resulting from the suction exerted as the marrow is aspirated into the syringe; the patient should be warned about this. Taking deep breaths or using relaxation techniques often helps ease the discomfort (see Fig. 32-5).

If a bone marrow biopsy is necessary, it is best performed after the aspiration and in a slightly different location, because the marrow structure may be altered after aspiration (Ryan, 2015). A special biopsy needle is used. Because these needles are large, the skin may be punctured first with a surgical blade to make a 3- to 4-mm incision. The biopsy needle is advanced well into the marrow cavity. When the needle is properly positioned, a portion of marrow is cored out. The patient feels a pressure sensation but should not feel actual pain. The nurse should assist the patient in maintaining a comfortable position and encourage relaxation and deep breathing throughout the procedure. The patient should be instructed to inform the physician if pain occurs so that an additional anesthetic agent can be given.

Potential complications of either bone marrow aspiration or biopsy include bleeding and infection. The risk of bleeding is somewhat increased if the patient's platelet count is low or if the patient has been taking a medication (e.g., aspirin) that alters platelet function. After the marrow sample is obtained, pressure is applied to the site for several minutes. The site is then covered with a sterile dressing. Most patients have no discomfort after a bone marrow aspiration, but the site of a

Figure 32-5 • Bone marrow aspiration procedure. The posterior superior iliac crest is the preferred site for bone marrow aspiration and biopsy because no vital organs or vessels are nearby. The patient is placed either in the lateral position with one leg flexed or in the prone position. The anterior iliac crest or sternum may also be used. Note that the sternum cannot be used for a marrow biopsy. **A.** Bone marrow aspiration. **B.** Inserting a Jamshidi biopsy needle. **C.** Dispensing the bone marrow core. From Farhi, D. C. (2009). *Pathology of bone marrow and blood cells* (2nd ed.). Philadelphia, PA: Lippincott Williams & Wilkins.

biopsy may ache for 1 or 2 days. Warm tub baths and a mild analgesic agent (e.g., acetaminophen [Tylenol]) may be useful. Aspirin-containing analgesic agents should be avoided in the immediate postprocedure period because they can aggravate or potentiate bleeding.

Unfolding Patient Stories: Lloyd Bennett • Part 1

 Lloyd Bennett is a 76-year-old male who fell while working outdoors. He presents to the Emergency Department with a hip fracture. What physical assessment and laboratory data can assist the nurse in evaluation for possible internal blood loss from the fracture or indications that the patient is at higher risk of bleeding? (Lloyd Bennett's story continues in Chapter 53.)

Care for Lloyd and other patients in a realistic virtual environment: *vSim for Nursing* (**thepoint.lww.com/vSimMedicalSurgical**). Practice documenting these patients' care in DocuCare (**thepoint.lww.com/DocuCareEHR**).

Therapeutic Approaches to Hematologic Disorders

Splenectomy

The surgical removal of the spleen (splenectomy) is a possible treatment for some hematologic disorders. For example, an enlarged spleen may be the site of excessive destruction of blood cells. In addition, some patients with grossly enlarged spleens develop severe thrombocytopenia as a result of platelets being sequestered in the spleen. Splenectomy removes the "trap," and platelet counts may normalize over time.

Laparoscopic splenectomy is associated with decreased postoperative morbidity compared to open splenectomy. Postoperative complications include atelectasis, pneumonia, abdominal distention, and abscess formation. Although young children are at the highest risk after splenectomy, all age groups are vulnerable to acute lethal infections and should be vaccinated for pneumonia before undergoing splenectomy, if possible (Henry & Longo, 2015).

The patient is instructed to seek prompt medical attention for even minor symptoms of infection. Often, patients with high platelet counts have even higher counts after splenectomy (more than 1 million/mm^3), which can predispose them to serious thrombotic or hemorrhagic problems. However, this increase is usually transient and therefore often does not warrant additional treatment (Henry & Longo, 2015).

Therapeutic Apheresis

Apheresis is a Greek word meaning "separation." In therapeutic apheresis (or pheresis), blood is taken from the patient and passed through a centrifuge, where a specific component is separated from the blood and removed (Stowell & Hass, 2014) (see Table 32-3). The remaining blood is then returned to the patient. The entire system is closed, so the risk of bacterial contamination is low. When platelets or leukocytes are removed, the decrease in these cells within the circulation is temporary. However, the temporary decrease provides a window of time until suppressive medications (e.g., chemotherapy) can have therapeutic effects. Sometimes plasma is removed rather than blood cells—typically so that specific, abnormal proteins within the plasma are transiently lowered until a long-term therapy can be initiated.

Apheresis is also used to obtain larger amounts of platelets from a donor than can be provided from a single unit of whole blood. A unit of platelets obtained in this way is equivalent to 6 to 8 units of platelets obtained from six to eight separate donors via standard blood donation methods. Platelet donors can have their platelets apheresed as often as every 14 days. Leukocytes can be obtained similarly, typically after the donor has received growth factors (granulocyte colony-stimulating factor, granulocyte-macrophage colony-stimulating factor) to stimulate the formation of additional leukocytes and thereby increase the leukocyte count. The use of these growth factors also stimulates the

TABLE 32-3 Types of Apheresis[a]

Procedure	Purpose	Examples of Clinical Use
Plateletpheresis	Remove platelets	Extreme thrombocytosis, essential thrombocythemia (temporary measure); single-donor platelet transfusion
Leukapheresis	Remove WBCs (can be specific to neutrophils or lymphocytes)	Extreme leukocytosis (e.g., AML, CML) (very temporary measure); harvest WBCs for transfusion
Erythrocytapheresis (RBC exchange)	Remove RBCs	RBC dyscrasias (e.g., sickle cell disease); RBCs replaced via transfusion
Plasmapheresis (plasma exchange)	Remove plasma proteins	Hyperviscosity syndromes; treatment for some renal and neurologic diseases (e.g., Goodpasture syndrome, TTP, Guillain-Barré, myasthenia gravis)
Stem cell harvest	Remove circulating stem cells	Transplantation (donor harvest or autologous)

WBCs, white blood cells; AML, acute myeloid leukemia; CML, chronic myeloid leukemia; RBC, red blood cell; TTP, thrombotic thrombocytopenic purpura.
[a]Therapeutic apheresis can be used to treat a wide variety of conditions. When it is used to treat a disease that causes an increase in a specific cell type with a short life in circulation (i.e., WBCs, platelets), the reduction in those cells is temporary. However, this temporary reduction permits a margin of safety while waiting for a longer-lasting treatment modality (e.g., chemotherapy) to take effect. Apheresis can also be used to obtain stem cells for transplantation, either from a matched donor (allogeneic) or from the patient (autologous).
Adapted from Stowell, C. P., & Hass, J. J. (2014). Transfusion medicine. In M. Laposata (Ed.). *Laboratory medicine: The diagnosis of disease in the clinical laboratory*. New York: McGraw-Hill.

release of stem cells within the circulation. Apheresis is used to harvest these stem cells (typically over a period of several days) for use in peripheral blood stem cell transplant.

Hematopoietic Stem Cell Transplantation

Hematopoietic stem cell transplantation (HSCT) is a therapeutic modality that offers the possibility of cure for some patients with hematologic disorders such as severe aplastic anemia, some forms of leukemia, and thalassemia. It can also provide longer remission from disease even when cure is not possible, such as in multiple myeloma. Hematopoietic stem cells may be transplanted from either allogeneic or autologous donors. For most hematologic diseases, allogeneic transplant is more effective (Fakih, Shah, & Nieto, 2016); here, stem cells are obtained from a donor whose cells match those of the patient. In contrast, the patient's own stem cells are harvested and then used in autologous transplant. (See Chapter 15 for a detailed discussion of HSCT.)

Therapeutic Phlebotomy

Therapeutic phlebotomy is the removal of a certain amount of blood under controlled conditions. Patients with elevated hematocrits (e.g., those with polycythemia vera) or excessive iron absorption (e.g., hemochromatosis) can usually be managed by periodically removing 1 unit (about 500 mL) of whole blood. Over time, this process can produce iron deficiency, leaving the patient unable to produce as many erythrocytes. The actual procedure for therapeutic phlebotomy is similar to that for blood donation (see later discussion).

Blood Component Therapy

A single unit of whole blood contains 450 mL of blood and 50 mL of an anticoagulant, which can be processed and dispensed for administration. However, it is more appropriate, economical, and practical to separate that unit of whole blood into its primary components: erythrocytes, platelets, and plasma (leukocytes are rarely used; see later discussion). Because the plasma is removed, a unit of packed red blood cells (PRBCs) is very concentrated (hematocrit approximately 70%) (Butterworth, Mackey, & Wasnick, 2013).

Each component must be processed and stored differently to maximize the longevity of the viable cells and factors within it; thus, each individual blood component has a different storage life. PRBCs are stored at 4°C (39.2°F). With special preservatives, they can be stored safely for up to 42 days before they must be discarded (American Red Cross, 2015a).

In contrast, platelets must be stored at room temperature because they cannot withstand cold temperatures, and they last for only 5 days before they must be discarded. To prevent clumping, platelets are gently agitated while stored. Plasma is immediately frozen to maintain the activity of the clotting factors within; it lasts for 1 year if it remains frozen. Alternatively, plasma can be further pooled and processed into blood derivatives, such as albumin, immune globulin, factor VIII, and factor IX. Table 32-4 describes each blood component and how it is commonly used.

Special Preparations

Factor VIII concentrate (antihemophilic factor) is a lyophilized, freeze-dried concentrate of pooled fractionated human plasma. It is used in treating hemophilia A. Factor IX concentrate (prothrombin complex) is similarly prepared and contains factors II, VII, IX, and X. It is used primarily for the treatment of factor IX deficiency (hemophilia B). Factor IX concentrate is also useful in treating congenital factor VII and factor X deficiencies. Recombinant forms of factor VIII, such as Humate-P or Alphanate, are also useful. Because they contain von Willebrand factor, these agents are used in von Willebrand disease as well as in hemophilia A, particularly when patients develop factor VIII inhibitors.

Plasma albumin is a large protein molecule that usually stays within vessels and is a major contributor to plasma oncotic pressure. This protein is used to expand the blood volume of patients in hypovolemic shock and, rarely, to increase the concentration of circulating albumin in patients with hypoalbuminemia.

Immune globulin is a concentrated solution of the antibody immunoglobulin G (IgG), prepared from large pools of plasma. It contains very little immunoglobulin A (IgA) or IgM. Intravenous immunoglobulin (IVIG) is used in various clinical situations to replace inadequate amounts of IgG in patients who are at risk for recurrent bacterial infection (e.g., those with chronic lymphocytic leukemia, those receiving HSCT). It is also used in certain autoimmune disorders, such as idiopathic thrombocytopenic purpura (ITP). Albumin, antihemophilic factors, and IVIG, in contrast to all other fractions of human blood, cells, or plasma, can survive being subjected to heating at 60°C (140°F) for 10 hours to free them of the viral contaminants that may be present.

Procuring Blood and Blood Products

Blood Donation

To protect both the donor and the recipients, all prospective donors are examined and interviewed before they are allowed to donate their blood. The intent of the interview is to assess the general health status of the donor and to identify risk factors that might harm a recipient of the donor's blood. There is no upper age limit to donation. The American Red Cross (2015b) requires that donors be in good health and meet specific eligibility criteria related to medications and vaccinations, medical conditions and treatments, travel outside the United States, lifestyle and life events, and so on. Detailed information about these criteria is available on the American Red Cross Web site (see the Resources section). All donors are expected to meet the following minimal requirements (American Red Cross, 2015b):

- Body weight should be at least 50 kg (110 lb) for a standard 450-mL donation.
- People younger than 17 years require parental consent in some states.
- The oral temperature should not exceed 37.5°C (99.6°F).
- The systolic arterial blood pressure should be 80 to 180 mm Hg, and the diastolic pressure should be 50 to 100 mm Hg.
- The hemoglobin level should be at least 12.5 g/dL.

TABLE 32-4 Blood and Blood Components Commonly Used in Transfusion Therapy[a]

Component	Composition	Indications and Considerations
Whole blood	Cells and plasma, hematocrit about 40%	Volume replacement and oxygen-carrying capacity; usually used only in significant bleeding (>25% blood volume lost)
PRBCs	RBCs with little plasma (hematocrit about 75%); some platelets and WBCs remain	↑ RBC mass; symptomatic anemia: • Platelets within the unit are not functional • WBCs within the unit may cause reaction and are not functional
Platelets—random	Platelets (5.5×10^{10} platelets/unit), plasma; some RBCs, WBCs	Bleeding due to severe ↓ platelets Prevent bleeding when platelets <5,000–10,000/mm³ Survival ↓ in presence of fever, chills, infection Repeated treatment leads to ↓ survival due to alloimmunization.
Platelets—single donor	Platelets (3×10^{11} platelets/unit) 1 unit is equivalent to 6–8 units of random platelets.	Used for repeated treatment: • ↓ alloimmunization risk by limiting exposure to multiple donors
Plasma	Plasma; all coagulation factors Complement	Bleeding in patients with coagulation factor deficiencies; plasmapheresis
Granulocytes	Neutrophils (>1 $\times 10^{10}$/unit); some lymphocytes, RBCs, and platelets will remain within the unit.	Severe neutropenia in selected patients; controversial
Lymphocytes	Lymphocytes (number varies)	Stimulate graft-versus-host disease effect
Cryoprecipitate	Fibrinogen ≥150 mg/bag, AHF (VIII:C) 80–110 units/bag, von Willebrand factor; fibronectin	von Willebrand disease Hypofibrinogenemia Hemophilia A
AHF	Factor VIII	Hemophilia A
Factor IX concentrate	Factor IX	Hemophilia B (Christmas disease)
Factor IX complex	Factors II, VII, IX, X	Hereditary factor VII, IX, X deficiency; hemophilia A with factor VII inhibitors
Albumin	Albumin 5%, 25%	Hypoproteinemia; burns; volume expansion by 5% to ↑ blood volume; 25% leads to ↓ hematocrit
IV gamma-globulin	Immunoglobulin G antibodies	Hypogammaglobulinemia (in CLL, recurrent infections); ITP; primary immunodeficiency states
Antithrombin III concentrate (AT III)	AT III (trace amounts of other plasma proteins)	AT III deficiency with or at risk for thrombosis

PRBCs, packed red blood cells; RBCs, red blood cells; WBCs, white blood cells; ↑, increased; ↓, decreased; AHF, antihemophilic factor; IV, intravenous; CLL, chronic lymphocytic leukemia; ITP, idiopathic thrombocytopenic purpura.

[a]The composition of each type of blood component is described as well as the most common indications for using a given blood component. RBCs, platelets, and fresh-frozen plasma are the blood products most commonly used. When transfusing these blood products, it is important to realize that the individual product is always "contaminated" with very small amounts of other blood products (e.g., WBCs mixed in a unit of platelets). This contamination can cause some difficulties, particularly isosensitization, in certain patients.

Adapted from American Red Cross (2015a). Blood components.Retrieved on 9/14/2015 at: www.redcrossblood.org/learn-about-blood/blood components; Dzieczkowski, J. S., & Anderson, K. C. (2015).Transfusion biology and therapy. In D. Kasper, A. Fauci, S. Hauser, et al. (Eds.). *Harrison's principles of internal medicine*(19th ed.). Retrieved on 5/25/2016 at: accessmedicine.mhmedical.com.laneproxy.stanford.edu/content.aspx?bookid=1130&Sectionid=79732248

Directed Donation

At times, friends and family of a patient wish to donate blood for that person. These blood donations are referred to as directed donations. These donations are not any safer than those provided by random donors, because directed donors may not be as willing to identify themselves as having a history of any of the risk factors that disqualify a person from donating blood. Therefore, many blood centers no longer accept directed donations.

Standard Donation

Phlebotomy consists of venipuncture and blood withdrawal. Standard precautions are used. Donors are placed in a semi-recumbent position. The skin over the antecubital fossa is carefully cleansed with an antiseptic preparation, a tourniquet is applied, and venipuncture is performed. Withdrawal of 450 mL of blood usually takes less than 15 minutes. After the needle is removed, donors are asked to hold the involved arm straight up, and firm pressure is applied with sterile gauze for 2 to 3 minutes. A firm bandage is then applied. The donor remains recumbent until he or she feels able to sit up,

usually within a few minutes. Donors who experience weakness or faintness should rest for a longer period. The donor then receives food and fluids and is asked to remain another 15 minutes.

The donor is instructed to leave the dressing on and to avoid heavy lifting for several hours, to avoid smoking for 1 hour, to avoid drinking alcoholic beverages for 3 hours, to increase fluid intake for 2 days, and to eat healthy meals for at least 2 weeks. Specimens from the donated blood are tested to detect infections and to identify the specific blood type (see later discussion).

Autologous Donation

A patient's own blood may be collected for future transfusion; this method is useful for many elective surgeries where the potential need for transfusion is high (e.g., orthopedic surgery). Preoperative donations are ideally collected 4 to 6 weeks before surgery. Iron supplements are prescribed during this period to prevent depletion of iron stores. Typically, 1 unit of blood is drawn each week; the number of units obtained varies with the type of surgical procedure to be performed (i.e., the amount of blood anticipated to be transfused). Phlebotomies are not performed within 72 hours of surgery. Individual blood components can also be collected.

The primary advantage of autologous transfusions is the prevention of viral infections from another person's blood. Other advantages include safe transfusion for patients with a history of transfusion reactions, prevention of alloimmunization, and avoidance of complications in patients with alloantibodies. It is the policy of the American Red Cross that autologous blood is transfused only to the donor. If the blood is not required, it can be frozen until the donor needs it in the future (for up to 10 years). The blood is never returned to the general donor supply of blood products to be used by another person.

Needless autologous donation (i.e., performed when the likelihood of transfusion is small) is discouraged because it is expensive, takes time, and uses resources inappropriately. Moreover, in an emergency situation, the autologous units available may be inadequate, and the patient may still require additional units from the general donor supply. Furthermore, although autologous transfusion can eliminate the risk of viral contamination, the risk of bacterial contamination is the same as that in transfusion from random donors (Stowell & Hass, 2014).

Contraindications to donation of blood for autologous transfusion are acute infection, severely debilitating chronic disease, hemoglobin level less than 11 g/dL, unstable angina, and acute cardiovascular or cerebrovascular disease. A history of poorly controlled epilepsy may be considered a contraindication in some centers.

Intraoperative Blood Salvage

This transfusion method provides replacement for patients who cannot donate blood before surgery and for those undergoing vascular, orthopedic, or thoracic surgery. During a surgical procedure, blood lost into a sterile cavity (e.g., hip joint) is suctioned into a cell-saver machine. The whole blood or PRBCs are washed, often with saline solution; filtered; and then returned to the patient as an IV infusion. Salvaged blood cannot be stored, because bacteria cannot be completely removed from the blood and thus cannot be used when it is contaminated with bacteria. The use of intraoperative blood salvage has decreased the need for autologous blood donation but has not affected the need for allogeneic blood products (Vonk, Meesters, Garnier, et al., 2013).

Hemodilution

This transfusion method may be initiated before or after induction of anesthesia. About 1 to 2 units of blood are removed from the patient through a venous or arterial line and simultaneously replaced with a colloid or crystalloid solution. The blood obtained is then reinfused after surgery. The advantage of this method is that the patient loses fewer erythrocytes during surgery, because the added IV solutions dilute the concentration of erythrocytes and lower the hematocrit. However, patients who are at risk for myocardial injury should not be further stressed by hemodilution. Hemodilution has been associated with adverse outcomes in patients having cardiopulmonary bypass; it has also been linked to tissue ischemia, particularly in the kidneys (Mehta, Castelvecchio, Ballotta, et al., 2013).

Complications of Blood Donation

Excessive bleeding at the donor's venipuncture site is sometimes caused by a bleeding disorder but more often results from a technique error: laceration of the vein, excessive tourniquet pressure, or failure to apply enough pressure after the needle is withdrawn.

Fainting may occur after blood donation and may be related to emotional factors, a vasovagal reaction, or prolonged fasting before donation (McCullough, Refaai, & Cohn, 2015). Because of the loss of blood volume, hypotension and syncope may occur when the donor assumes an erect position. A donor who appears pale or complains of faintness should immediately lie down or sit with the head lowered below the knees. He or she should be observed for another 30 minutes.

Anginal chest pain may be precipitated in patients with unsuspected coronary artery disease. Seizures can occur in donors with epilepsy, although the incidence is very low. Both angina and seizures require further medical evaluation and treatment.

Blood Processing

Samples of the unit of blood are always taken immediately after donation so that the blood can be typed and tested. Each donation is tested for antibodies to human immune deficiency virus (HIV) types 1 and 2, hepatitis B core antibody (anti-HBc), hepatitis C virus (HCV), human T-cell lymphotropic virus type I (anti-HTLV-I/II), hepatitis B surface antigen (HbsAG), and syphilis. Negative reactions are required for the blood to be used, and each unit of blood is labeled to certify the results. Nucleic acid amplification testing has increased the ability to detect the presence of HCV, HIV, and West Nile virus infections, because it directly tests for genomic nucleic acids of the viruses rather than for the presence of antibodies to the viruses. This testing significantly shortens the "window" of inability to detect HIV and HCV from a donated unit, further ensuring the safety of the blood; the risk of transmission of HIV or HCV is now estimated at 1 in 2 million units and 1 in 1.6 million units of blood donated, respectively (American Cancer Society, 2013). Blood is also screened for cytomegalovirus (CMV). If it tests positive for CMV, it can still be used, except in recipients who are negative for CMV and who are severely immunocompromised; any components are labeled as CMV positive.

Equally important is accurate determination of the blood type. More than 200 antigens have been identified on the surface of RBC membranes. Of these, the most important for safe transfusion are the ABO and Rh systems. The ABO system identifies which sugars are present on the membrane of a person's erythrocytes: A, B, both A and B, or neither A nor B (type O). To prevent a significant reaction, the same type of PRBCs should be transfused. Previously, it was thought that in an emergency situation in which the patient's blood type was not known, type O blood could be safely transfused. This practice is no longer recommended.

The Rh antigen (also referred to as D) is present on the surface of erythrocytes in 85% of the population (Rh positive). Those who lack the D antigen are referred to as being Rh negative. PRBCs are routinely tested for the D antigen as well as ABO. Patients should receive PRBCs with a compatible Rh type.

The majority of transfusion reactions are due to clerical error where the patient is transfused an incompatible unit of blood product (McCullough et al., 2015). Reactions (other than those due to procedural error) are most frequently due to the presence of donor leukocytes within the blood component unit (PRBCs or platelets); the recipient may form antibodies to the antigens present on these leukocytes. PRBC components typically have 1 to 3×10^9 leukocytes remaining in each unit. Leukocytes from the blood product are frequently filtered to diminish the likelihood of developing reactions and refractoriness to transfusions, particularly in patients who have chronic transfusion needs. The process of leukocyte filtration renders the blood component "leukocyte poor" (i.e., leukopoor). Filtration can occur at the time the unit is collected from the donor and processed, which achieves better results but is more expensive, or at the time the blood component is transfused by attaching a leukocyte filter to the blood administration tubing. Many centers advocate routinely using leukopoor filtered blood components for people who have or are likely to develop chronic transfusion requirements.

When a patient is immunocompromised, as in the case following stem cell transplant, any donor lymphocytes must be removed from the blood components. In this situation, the blood component is exposed to low amounts of radiation (25 Gy) that kill any lymphocytes within the blood component. Irradiated blood products are highly effective in preventing transfusion-associated graft-versus-host disease, which is fatal in most cases. Irradiated blood products have a shorter shelf life.

Transfusion

Administration of blood and blood components requires knowledge of correct administration techniques and possible complications. It is very important to be familiar with the agency's policies and procedures for transfusion therapy. Methods for transfusing blood components are presented in Charts 32-2 and 32-3.

Chart 32-2 — Transfusion of Packed Red Blood Cells

Preprocedure

1. Confirm that the transfusion has been prescribed.
2. Check that patient's blood has been typed and cross-matched.
3. Verify that patient has signed a written consent form per institution or agency policy and agrees to procedure.
4. Explain procedure to patient. Instruct patient in signs and symptoms of transfusion reaction (itching, hives, swelling, shortness of breath, fever, chills).
5. Take patient's temperature, pulse, respiration, blood pressure and assess fluid volume status (e.g., auscultate lungs, assess for jugular venous distention) to serve as a baseline for comparison during transfusion.
6. Note if signs of increased fluid overload present (e.g., heart failure, see Chapter 29), contact primary provider to discuss potential need for a prescription for diuretic, as warranted.
7. Use hand hygiene and wear gloves in accordance with standard precautions.
8. Use appropriately sized needle for insertion in a peripheral vein.[a] Use special tubing that contains a blood filter to screen out fibrin clots and other particulate matter. Do not vent blood container.

Procedure

1. Obtain packed red blood cells (PRBCs) from the blood bank *after* the IV line is started. (Institution policy may limit release to only 1 unit at a time.)
2. Double-check labels with another nurse or physician to ensure that the ABO group and Rh type agree with the compatibility record. Check to see that number and type on donor blood label and on patient's medical record are correct. Confirm patient's identification by asking the patient's name and checking the identification wristband.
3. Check blood for gas bubbles and any unusual color or cloudiness. (Gas bubbles may indicate bacterial growth. Abnormal color or cloudiness may be a sign of hemolysis.)

4. Make sure that PRBC transfusion is initiated within 30 minutes after removal of PRBCs from blood bank refrigerator.
5. For the first 15 minutes, run the transfusion slowly—no faster than 5 mL/min. Observe patient carefully for adverse effects. If no adverse effects occur during the first 15 minutes, increase the flow rate unless patient is at high risk for circulatory overload.
6. Monitor closely for 15–30 minutes to detect signs of reaction. Monitor vital signs at regular intervals per institution or agency policy; compare results with baseline measurements. Increase frequency of measurements based on patient's condition. Observe patient frequently throughout the transfusion for any signs of adverse reaction, including restlessness, hives, nausea, vomiting, torso or back pain, shortness of breath, flushing, hematuria, fever, or chills. Should any adverse reaction occur, stop infusion immediately, notify primary provider, and follow the agency's transfusion reaction standard.
7. Note that administration time does not exceed 4 hours because of increased risk of bacterial proliferation.
8. Be alert for signs of adverse reactions: circulatory overload, sepsis, febrile reaction, allergic reaction, and acute hemolytic reaction.
9. Change blood tubing after every 2 units transfused to decrease chance of bacterial contamination.

Postprocedure

1. Obtain vital signs and breath sounds; compare with baseline measurements. If signs of increased fluid overload present (e.g., heart failure, see Chapter 29), consider obtaining prescription for diuretic as warranted.
2. Dispose of used materials properly.
3. Document procedure in patient's medical record, including patient assessment findings and tolerance to procedure.
4. Monitor patient for response to and effectiveness of procedure. If patient is at risk, monitor for at least 6 hours for signs of transfusion-associated circulatory overload (TACO); also monitor for signs of delayed hemolytic reaction.

Note: Never add medications to blood or blood products; if blood is too thick to run freely, normal saline may be added to the unit. If blood must be warmed, use an in-line blood warmer with a monitoring system.

[a]Most policies stipulate using an IV with a minimum of 20 gauge. A recent evidence-based synthesis did not find increased hemolysis when packed red cells are infused through a small-gauge needle (Stupnyckyj, Smolarek, Reeves, et al., 2014).

Adapted from Gorski, L., Hadaway, L., Hagle, M., et al. (2016). Infusion therapy: Standards of practice. *Journal of Infusion Nursing, 39*(1S), S135–S137; Stupnyckyj, C., Smolarek, S., Reeves, C., et al. (2014). Changing blood transfusion policy and practice. *The American Journal of Nursing, 114*(12), 50–59.

Chart 32-3 Transfusion of Platelets or Fresh-Frozen Plasma

Preprocedure

1. Confirm that the transfusion has been prescribed.
2. Verify that patient has signed a written consent form per institution or agency policy and agrees to procedure.
3. Explain procedure to patient. Instruct patient in signs and symptoms of transfusion reaction (itching, hives, swelling, shortness of breath, fever, chills).
4. Take patient's temperature, pulse, respiration, blood pressure, and assess fluid status, and auscultate breath sounds to establish a baseline for comparison during transfusion.
5. Note if signs of increased fluid overload present (e.g., heart failure, see Chapter 29), contact primary provider to discuss potential need for a prescription for diuretic, as warranted; this is particularly important when plasma is also infused.
6. Use hand hygiene and wear gloves in accordance with standard precautions.
7. Use a 22-gauge or larger needle for placement in a large vein, if possible. Use appropriate tubing per institution policy (platelets often require different tubing from that used for other blood products).

Procedure

1. Obtain platelets or fresh-frozen plasma (FFP) from the blood bank (only *after* the IV line is started.)
2. Double-check labels with another nurse or physician to ensure that the ABO group matches the compatibility record (not usually necessary for platelets; here only if compatible platelets are ordered). Check to see that the number and type on donor blood label and on patient's medical record are correct. Confirm patient's identification by asking the patient's name and checking the identification wristband.
3. Check blood product for any unusual color or clumps (excessive redness indicates contamination with larger amounts of red blood cells).

4. Make sure that platelets or FFP units are given immediately after they are obtained.
5. Infuse each unit of FFP over 30–60 minutes per patient tolerance; be prepared to infuse at a significantly lower rate in the context of fluid overload. Infuse each unit of platelets as fast as patient can tolerate to diminish platelet clumping during administration. Observe patient carefully for adverse effects, especially circulatory overload. Decrease rate of infusion if necessary.
6. Observe patient closely throughout transfusion for any signs of adverse reaction, including restlessness, hives, nausea, vomiting, torso or back pain, shortness of breath, flushing, hematuria, fever, or chills. Should any adverse reaction occur, stop infusion immediately, notify primary provider, and follow the agency's transfusion reaction standard.
7. Monitor vital signs at the end of transfusion per institution policy; compare results with baseline measurements.
8. Flush line with saline after transfusion to remove blood component from tubing.

Postprocedure

1. Obtain vital signs and auscultate breath sounds; compare with baseline measurements. If signs of increased fluid overload present, consider obtaining prescription for diuretic, as warranted.
2. Dispose of used materials properly.
3. Document procedure in patient's medical record, including patient assessment findings and tolerance to procedure.
4. Monitor patient for response to and effectiveness of procedure. A platelet count may be ordered 1 hour after platelet transfusion to facilitate this evaluation.
5. If patient is at risk for transfusion-associated circulatory overload (TACO), monitor closely for 6 hours after transfusion if possible.

Note: FFP requires ABO but not Rh compatibility. Platelets are not typically cross-matched for ABO compatibility. Never add medications to blood or blood products.

Setting

Most blood transfusions are performed in the acute care setting, and sometimes must be done emergently. However, the processes utilized to ensure safe transfusion of blood cannot be abridged for the sake of rapidity; all procedural details outlined in Chart 32-2 must be followed, including obtaining informed consent (see Chart 32-4).

Patients with chronic transfusion requirements often can receive transfusions in other settings. Freestanding infusion centers, ambulatory care clinics, physicians' offices, and even patients' homes may be appropriate settings for transfusion. Typically, patients who need chronic transfusions but are otherwise stable physically are appropriate candidates for outpatient therapy. Verification and administration of the blood product are performed as in a hospital setting. Although most blood products can be transfused in the outpatient setting, the home is typically limited to transfusions of PRBCs and factor components (e.g., factor VIII for patients with hemophilia).

Pretransfusion Assessment

Patient History

The patient history is an important component of the pretransfusion assessment to determine the history of previous transfusions as well as previous reactions to transfusion. The history should include the type of reaction, its manifestations, the interventions required, and whether any preventive interventions were used in subsequent transfusions. The nurse assesses the number of pregnancies a woman has had, because a high number can increase her risk of reaction due to antibodies developed from exposure to fetal circulation. Other concurrent health problems should be noted, with careful attention to cardiac, pulmonary, and vascular disease.

Physical Assessment

A systematic physical assessment and measurement of baseline vital signs and fluid status are important before transfusing any blood product. The respiratory system should be assessed, including careful auscultation of the lungs and the patient's use of accessory muscles. Cardiac system assessment should include careful inspection for any edema as well as other signs of heart failure (e.g., jugular venous distention; see Chapter 29). The skin should be observed for rashes, petechiae, and ecchymoses. The sclera should be examined for icterus. In the event of a transfusion reaction, a comparison of findings can help differentiate between types of reactions.

Concept Mastery Alert

The nurse should establish a baseline by taking vital signs before the transfusion. Also, written consent to perform the procedure is required.

 Patient Education

Reviewing the signs and symptoms of a transfusion reaction is crucial for patients who have not received a previous transfusion. Even for patients who have received prior transfusions, a brief review of the signs and symptoms of transfusion reactions is advised. Signs and symptoms of a reaction include fever, chills, respiratory distress, low back pain, nausea, pain at the IV site, or anything "unusual." Although a thorough review is very important, the nurse also reassures the patient that the blood is carefully tested against the patient's own blood (cross-matched) to diminish the likelihood of any untoward reaction. Similarly, the patient can be reassured about the very low possibility of contracting HIV from the transfusion; this fear persists among many people.

Complications

Any patient who receives a blood transfusion is at risk for developing complications from the transfusion. During patient education, the nurse explains the risks and benefits and what to expect during and after the transfusion. Patients must be informed that although it has been tested carefully, the supply of blood is not completely risk free. Nursing management is directed toward preventing complications, promptly recognizing complications if they develop, and promptly initiating measures to control complications. The following sections describe the most common or potentially severe transfusion-related complications.

Febrile Nonhemolytic Reaction

A febrile nonhemolytic reaction is caused by antibodies to donor leukocytes that remain in the unit of blood or blood component; it is the most common type of transfusion reaction (Dzieczkowski & Anderson, 2015). It occurs more frequently in patients who have had previous transfusions (exposure to multiple antigens from previous blood products) and in Rh-negative women who have borne Rh-positive children (exposure to an Rh-positive fetus raises antibody levels in the untreated mother).

The diagnosis of a febrile nonhemolytic reaction is made by excluding other potential causes, such as a hemolytic reaction or bacterial contamination of the blood product. The signs and symptoms of a febrile nonhemolytic transfusion reaction are chills (minimal to severe) followed by fever (more than 1°C elevation). The fever typically begins within 2 hours after the transfusion has begun. Although the reaction is not life-threatening, the fever, and particularly the chills and muscle stiffness, can be frightening to the patient.

This reaction can be diminished, even prevented, by further depleting the blood component of donor leukocytes; this is accomplished by a leukocyte reduction filter. Antipyretic agents can be given to prevent fever; however, routine premedication is not advised because it can mask the beginning of a more serious transfusion reaction.

Acute Hemolytic Reaction

The most dangerous, and potentially life-threatening, type of transfusion reaction occurs when the donor blood is incompatible with that of the recipient (i.e., type II hypersensitivity reaction). Antibodies already present in the recipient's plasma rapidly combine with antigens on donor erythrocytes, and the erythrocytes are destroyed in the circulation (i.e., intravascular hemolysis). The most rapid hemolysis occurs in ABO incompatibility. Rh incompatibility often causes a less severe reaction. This reaction can occur after transfusion of as little as 10 mL of PRBCs. Although the overall incidence of such reactions is not high (1:20,000 to 1:40,000 units transfused) (McCullough et al., 2015), they are largely preventable. The most common causes of acute hemolytic reaction are errors in blood component labeling and patient identification that result in the administration of an ABO-incompatible transfusion.

Symptoms consist of fever, chills, low back pain, nausea, chest tightness, dyspnea, and anxiety. As the erythrocytes are destroyed, the hemoglobin is released from the cells and excreted by the kidneys; therefore, hemoglobin appears in the urine (hemoglobinuria). Hypotension, bronchospasm, and vascular collapse may result. Diminished renal perfusion results in acute kidney injury, and disseminated intravascular coagulation may also occur. The reaction must be recognized promptly and the transfusion discontinued immediately (see the Nursing Management for Transfusion Reactions section).

Acute hemolytic transfusion reactions are preventable. Meticulous attention to detail in labeling blood samples and blood components and accurately identifying the recipient cannot be overemphasized. Bar coding methods can be useful safeguards in matching a patient's wristband with the label on the blood component; however, these methods are not fail proof and do not reduce the nurse's responsibility to ensure the correct blood component is transfused to the correct patient (Hurrell, 2014).

Allergic Reaction

Some patients develop urticaria (hives) or generalized itching during a transfusion; the cause is thought to be a sensitivity reaction to a plasma protein within the blood component being transfused. Symptoms of an allergic reaction are urticaria, itching, and flushing. The reactions are usually mild and respond to antihistamines. If the symptoms resolve after administration of an antihistamine (e.g., diphenhydramine [Benadryl]), the transfusion may be resumed. Rarely, the allergic reaction is severe, with bronchospasm, laryngeal edema, and shock. These reactions are managed with epinephrine, corticosteroids, and vasopressor support, if necessary.

Giving the patient antihistamines or corticosteroids before the transfusion may prevent future reactions. For severe reactions, future blood components are washed to remove any remaining plasma proteins. Leukocyte filters are not useful to prevent such reactions, because the offending plasma proteins can pass through the filter.

Transfusion-Associated Circulatory Overload (TACO)

If too much blood is infused too quickly, hypervolemia can occur. This condition can be aggravated in patients who already have increased circulatory volume (e.g., those with heart failure, renal dysfunction, advanced age, acute myocardial infarction) (Alam, Lin, Lima, et al., 2013). A careful assessment for signs of circulatory overload or positive fluid status prior to initiating the transfusion is required, particularly in those individuals at risk for developing transfusion-related acute lung injury (TRALI). PRBCs are safer to use than whole blood. If the administration rate is sufficiently slow, circulatory overload may be prevented.

For patients who are at risk for, or already in, circulatory overload, diuretics are given prior to the transfusion or between units of PRBCs. Patients receiving fresh-frozen plasma or even platelets may also develop circulatory overload. The infusion rate of these blood components must also be titrated to the patient's tolerance. Rates of transfusion may need to decrease to less than 100 to 120 mL/hr (Alam et al., 2013).

Signs of circulatory overload include dyspnea, orthopnea, tachycardia, an increase in blood pressure, and sudden anxiety. Jugular vein distention, crackles at the base of the lungs, and hypoxemia will also develop. Pulmonary edema can quickly develop, as manifested by severe dyspnea and coughing of pink, frothy sputum.

If fluid overload is mild, the transfusion can often be continued after slowing the rate of infusion and administering diuretics. However, if the overload is severe, the patient is placed upright with the feet in a dependent position, the transfusion is discontinued, and the primary provider is notified. The IV line is kept patent with a very slow infusion of normal saline solution or a saline lock device to maintain access to the vein in case IV medications are necessary. Oxygen and morphine may be needed to treat severe dyspnea (see Chapter 29).

TACO can develop as late as 6 hours after transfusion (Alam et al., 2013). Therefore, patients need close monitoring after the transfusion is completed, particularly those who are at higher risk for developing this complication (e.g., older adults, those with a positive fluid balance prior to transfusion, patients with renal dysfunction, patients with left ventricular dysfunction). Monitoring vital signs, auscultating breath sounds, and assessing for jugular venous distention should be included in patient monitoring.

Bacterial Contamination

The incidence of bacterial contamination of blood components is very low; however, administration of contaminated products puts the patient at great risk. Contamination can occur at any point during procurement or processing but often results from organisms on the donor's skin. Many bacteria cannot survive in the cold temperatures used to store PRBCs, but some organisms can do so. Platelets are at greater risk of contamination because they are stored at room temperature. In response to this, blood centers have developed rapid methods of culturing platelet units, thereby diminishing the risk of using a contaminated platelet unit for transfusion (Centers for Disease Control and Prevention, 2013).

Preventive measures include meticulous care in the procurement and processing of blood components. When PRBCs or whole blood is transfused, it should be given within a 4-hour period, because warm room temperatures promote bacterial growth. A contaminated unit of blood product may appear normal, or it may have an abnormal color.

The signs of bacterial contamination are fever, chills, and hypotension. These manifestations may not occur until the transfusion is complete, occasionally not until several hours after the transfusion. As soon as the reaction is recognized, any remaining transfusion is discontinued (see the Nursing Management for Transfusion Reactions section). If the condition is not treated immediately with fluids and broad-spectrum antibiotics, sepsis can occur. Sepsis is treated with IV fluids and antibiotics; corticosteroids and vasopressors are often also necessary (see Chapter 14).

Transfusion-Related Acute Lung Injury (TRALI)

TRALI is a potentially fatal, idiosyncratic reaction that is defined as the development of acute lung injury occurring within 6 hours after the blood transfusion. All blood components have been implicated in TRALI, including IVIG, cryoprecipitate, and stem cells. TRALI is the most common cause of transfusion-related death (Alam et al., 2013).

The underlying pathophysiologic mechanism for TRALI is unknown but is thought to involve specific human leukocyte antigen (HLA) or human neutrophil antigen (HNA) antibodies in the donor's plasma that react to the leukocytes in the recipient's blood. Occasionally, the reverse occurs, and antibodies present in the recipient's plasma agglutinate the antigens on the few remaining leukocytes in the blood component being transfused. Another theory suggests that an initial insult to the patient's vascular endothelium can predispose the neutrophils to aggregate at the injured endothelium. Various substances within the transfused blood component (lipids, cytokines) then activate these neutrophils. Each of these pathophysiologic mechanisms can contribute to the process. The end result of this process is interstitial and intra-alveolar edema, as well as extensive sequestration of WBCs within the pulmonary capillaries (Bockhold & Crumpler, 2015).

Onset is abrupt (usually within 6 hours of transfusion, often within 2 hours). Signs and symptoms include acute shortness of breath, hypoxia (arterial oxygen saturation [SaO_2] less than 90%; partial pressure of arterial oxygen [PaO_2] to fraction of inspired oxygen [FIO_2] ratio of less than 300), hypotension, fever, and eventual pulmonary edema. Diagnostic criteria include hypoxemia, bilateral pulmonary infiltrates (seen on chest x-ray), no evidence of cardiac cause for the pulmonary edema, and no other plausible alternative cause within 6 hours of completing transfusion. Aggressive supportive therapy (e.g., oxygen, intubation, fluid support) may prevent death. Immunological therapy (e.g., corticosteroids) has not been shown to be effective in this setting; diuretics can worsen the situation (Bockhold & Crumpler, 2015; Kenz & van der Linden, 2014).

Although TRALI can occur with the transfusion of any blood component, it is more likely to occur when plasma and, to a lesser extent, platelets are transfused. One commonly used preventive strategy involves limiting the frequency and amount of blood products transfused. Another entails obtaining plasma and possibly platelets only from men because women who have been pregnant may have developed offending antibodies. A third strategy involves screening donors for the presence of these antibodies and discarding any plasma-containing blood products from those donors who screen positive. The efficacy of these approaches in preventing TRALI remains unclear (Alam et al., 2013).

Delayed Hemolytic Reaction

Delayed hemolytic reactions usually occur within 14 days after transfusion, when the level of antibody has been increased to the extent that a reaction can occur. The hemolysis of the erythrocytes is extravascular via the RES and occurs gradually.

Signs and symptoms of a delayed hemolytic reaction are fever, anemia, increased bilirubin level, decreased or absent haptoglobin, and possibly jaundice. Rarely, there is hemoglobinuria. Generally, these reactions are not dangerous, but it is important to recognize them because subsequent transfusions with blood products containing these antibodies may cause a more severe hemolytic reaction. However, recognition is also difficult because the patient may not be in a health care setting to be tested for this reaction, and even if the patient is hospitalized, the reaction may be too mild to be recognized clinically. Because the amount of antibody present can be too low to detect, it is difficult to prevent delayed hemolytic reactions. Fortunately, the reaction is usually mild and requires no intervention.

Disease Acquisition

Despite advances in donor screening and blood testing, certain diseases can still be transmitted by transfusion of blood components (see Chart 32-5).

Complications of Long-Term Transfusion Therapy

The complications that have been described represent a real risk to any patient any time a blood component is given. However, patients with long-term transfusion requirements (e.g., those with myelodysplastic syndrome, thalassemia, aplastic anemia, sickle cell disease) are at greater risk for infection transmission and for becoming more sensitized to donor antigens, simply because they are exposed to more units of blood and, consequently, more donors. A summary of complications associated with long-term transfusion therapy is given in Table 32-5.

Iron overload is a complication unique to people who have had long-term PRBC transfusions. One unit of PRBCs contains 250 mg of iron. Patients with chronic transfusion requirements can quickly acquire more iron than they can use, leading to iron overload. Over time, the excess iron deposits in body tissues can cause organ damage, particularly in the liver, heart, testes, and pancreas. Promptly initiating a program of iron chelation therapy can prevent end-organ damage from iron toxicity (see Chapter 33, Hereditary Hemochromatosis, Nursing Management, and Chapter 34, Myelodysplastic Syndrome, Nursing Management).

Nursing Management for Transfusion Reactions

If a transfusion reaction is suspected, the transfusion must be stopped immediately and the primary provider notified. A thorough patient assessment is crucial, because many complications have similar signs and symptoms. The following steps are taken to determine the type and severity of the reaction:

- Stop the transfusion. Maintain the IV line with normal saline solution through new IV tubing, given at a slow rate.
- Assess the patient carefully. Compare the vital signs with baseline, including oxygen saturation. Assess the patient's respiratory status carefully. Note the presence of adventitious breath sounds; the use of accessory

Chart 32-5 Diseases Potentially Transmitted by Blood Transfusion

Hepatitis (Viral Hepatitis B, C)

- There is greater risk from pooled blood products and blood of paid donors than from volunteer donors.
- A screening test detects most hepatitis B and C.
- Transmittal risk for Hepatitis B is estimated at 1:350,000 donated units.

AIDS (HIV and HTLV)

- Donated blood is screened for antibodies to HIV.
- Transmittal risk is estimated at 1:1.5 million donated units.
- People with high-risk behaviors (multiple sex partners, anal sex, IV/injection drug use) and people with signs and symptoms that suggest AIDS should not donate blood.

Cytomegalovirus (CMV)

- Transmittal risk is greater for premature newborns with CMV antibody–negative mothers and for immunocompromised recipients who are CMV negative (e.g., those with acute leukemia, organ or tissue transplant recipients).
- Blood products rendered "leukocyte reduced" help reduce transmission of virus.

Graft-Versus-Host Disease (GVHD)

- GVHD occurs only in severely immunocompromised recipients (e.g., Hodgkin disease, bone marrow transplantation).
- Transfused lymphocytes engraft in recipient and attack host lymphocytes or body tissues; signs and symptoms are fever, diffuse reddened skin rash, nausea, vomiting, and diarrhea.
- Preventive measures include irradiating blood products to inactivate donor lymphocytes (no known radiation risks to transfusion recipient) and processing donor blood with leukocyte reduction filters.

Creutzfeldt-Jakob Disease (CJD)

- CJD is a rare, fatal disease that causes irreversible brain damage.
- There is no evidence of transmittal by transfusion.
- All blood donors must be screened for positive family history of CJD.
- Potential donors who spent a cumulative time of 5 years or more (January 1980 to present) in certain areas of Europe cannot donate blood; blood products from a donor who develops CJD are recalled.

AIDS, acquired immunodeficiency syndrome; HIV, human immunodeficiency virus; HTLV, human T-lymphotropic virus.
Adapted from Katz, L. M., & Dodd, R. Y. (2013). Transfusion-transmitted diseases. In B. A. Shaz, C. D. Hillyer, M. Roshal, et al. (Eds.), *Transfusion medicine and hemostasis: Clinical and laboratory aspects* (2nd ed.). Waltham, MA: Elsevier.

muscles; extent of dyspnea; and changes in mental status, including anxiety and confusion. Note any chills, diaphoresis, jugular vein distention, and reports of back pain or urticaria.

- Notify the primary provider of the assessment findings, and implement any treatments prescribed. Continue to monitor the patient's vital signs and respiratory, cardiovascular, and renal status.
- Notify the blood bank that a suspected transfusion reaction has occurred.
- Send the blood container and tubing to the blood bank for repeat typing and culture. The patient's identity and blood component identifying tags and numbers are verified.

If a hemolytic transfusion reaction or bacterial infection is suspected, the nurse does the following:

- Obtains appropriate blood specimens from the patient
- Collects a urine sample as soon as possible to detect hemoglobin in the urine
- Documents the reaction according to the institution's policy

Pharmacologic Alternatives to Blood Transfusions

Pharmacologic agents that stimulate the production of one or more types of blood cells by the marrow are commonly used (see Chart 32-6). Researchers continue to seek a blood

TABLE 32-5 Common Complications Resulting from Long-Term Packed Red Blood Cell Transfusion Therapy[a]

Complication	Manifestation	Management
Infection	Hepatitis (B, C)	May immunize against hepatitis B; treat hepatitis C; monitor hepatic function
	CMV	WBC filters to protect against CMV
Iron overload	Heart failure	Prevent by chelation therapy
	Endocrine failure (diabetes, hypothyroidism, hypoparathyroidism, hypogonadism)	
Transfusion reaction	Sensitization	Diminish by RBC phenotyping, using WBC-filtered products
	Febrile reactions	Diminish by using WBC-filtered products

CMV, cytomegalovirus; WBC, white blood cell; RBC, red blood cell.
[a]Patients with long-term transfusion therapy requirements are at risk not only for the transfusion reactions discussed in the text but also for the complications noted in the table. In many cases, the use of WBC-filtered (i.e., leukocyte-poor) blood products is standard for patients who receive long-term packed RBC transfusion therapy. An aggressive chelation program initiated early in the course of therapy can prevent problems with iron overload.
Adapted from McCullough, J., Refaai, M. A., & Cohn, C. S. (2015). Blood procurement and red cell transfusion. In K. Kaushansky, M. Lichtman, J. Prchal, et al. (Eds.). *Williams hematology* (9th ed.). New York: McGraw-Hill.

Chart 32-6 PHARMACOLOGY
Pharmacologic Alternatives to Blood Transfusions

Growth Factors

Recombinant technology has provided a means to produce hematopoietic growth factors necessary for the production of blood cells within the bone marrow. By increasing the body's production of blood cells, transfusions and complications resulting from diminished blood cells (e.g., infection from neutropenia) may be avoided. However, the successful use of growth factors requires functional bone marrow. Moreover, the safety of these products has been questioned, and the U.S. Food and Drug Administration is limiting their use in some patient populations.

Erythropoietin

Erythropoietin (epoetin alfa [Epogen, Procrit]; darbopoietin [Aranesp]) is an effective alternative treatment for patients with chronic anemia secondary to diminished levels of erythropoietin, as in chronic renal disease. This medication stimulates erythropoiesis. It also has been used for patients who are anemic from chemotherapy or zidovudine (AZT) therapy and for those who have diseases involving bone marrow suppression, such as myelodysplastic syndrome (MDS). The use of erythropoietin can also enable a patient to donate several units of blood for future use (e.g., preoperative autologous donation). The medication can be administered IV or subcutaneously, although plasma levels are better sustained with the subcutaneous route. Side effects are rare, but erythropoietin can cause or exacerbate hypertension. If the anemia is corrected too quickly or is overcorrected, the elevated hematocrit can cause headache and, potentially, seizures. Thrombosis has been noted in some patients whose hemoglobins were raised to a high level; thus, it is recommended that a target hemoglobin level of less than 12 g/dL be used. These adverse effects are rare except for patients with renal failure. Serial complete blood counts (CBCs) must be performed to evaluate the response to the medication. The dose and frequency of administration are titrated to the hemoglobin level.

Granulocyte Colony-Stimulating Factor (G-CSF)

G-CSF (filgrastim [Neupogen, Zarxio, Granix]) is a cytokine that stimulates the proliferation and differentiation of myeloid stem cells; a rapid increase in neutrophils is seen within the circulation. G-CSF is effective in improving transient but severe neutropenia after chemotherapy or in some forms of MDS. It is particularly useful in preventing bacterial infections that would be likely to occur with neutropenia. G-CSF is given subcutaneously on a daily basis. The primary side effect is bone pain; this probably reflects the increase in hematopoiesis within the marrow. Serial CBCs should be performed to evaluate the response to the medication and to ensure that the rise in white blood cells is not excessive. The effect of G-CSF on myelopoiesis is short; the neutrophil count drops once the medication is stopped.

Granulocyte-Macrophage Colony-Stimulating Factor (GM-CSF)

GM-CSF (sargramostim [Leukine]) is a cytokine that is naturally produced by a variety of cells, including monocytes and endothelial cells. It works either directly or synergistically with other growth factors to stimulate myelopoiesis. GM-CSF is not as specific to neutrophils as is G-CSF; thus, an increase in erythroid (red blood cell) and megakaryocytic (platelet) production may also be seen. GM-CSF serves the same purpose as G-CSF. However, it may have a greater effect on macrophage function and therefore may be more useful against fungal infections, whereas G-CSF may be better used to fight bacterial infections. GM-CSF is also given subcutaneously. Side effects include bone pain, fevers, and myalgias.

Thrombopoietin

Thrombopoietin (TPO) is a cytokine that is necessary for the proliferation of megakaryocytes and subsequent platelet formation. Nonimmunogenic second-generation thrombopoietic growth factors (romiplostim [Nplate]; eltrombopag [Promacta]) are used for the treatment of idiopathic thrombocytopenic purpura. Eltrombopag is also approved for use in certain situations for patients with aplastic anemia and in patients requiring hepatitis C treatment that can cause significant thrombocytopenia.

Adapted from Seeber, P., & Shander, A. (2012a). Anemia therapy I: Erythropoiesis-stimulating agents. In P. Seeber & A. Shander (Eds.). *Basics of blood management* (2nd ed.). Oxford, UK: Wiley-Blackwell; Seeber, P., & Shander, A. (2012b). Growth factors. In P. Seeber & A. Shander (Eds.). *Basics of blood management*(2nd ed.). Oxford, UK: Wiley-Blackwell.

---

substitute that is practical and safe. Manufacturing artificial blood is problematic, given the myriad functions of blood components. Currently, there are two types of products in development: hemoglobin-based oxygen carriers and perfluorocarbons (which have great ability to dissolve gases and thus carry oxygen indirectly) (Goodnough & Shander, 2013; van Veen & Hunt, 2015). None of these products are available for use in the United States (Tao & Ghoroghchian, 2014).

CRITICAL THINKING EXERCISES

1 **pq** You are caring for a 72-year-old male patient admitted to a medical unit with an exacerbation of chronic obstructive pulmonary disease. He is anemic, and you are transfusing him with 2 units of PRBCs. The second unit is almost completed when he complains of more shortness of breath and appears anxious. His pulse is 118 bpm, respirations 28 per minute, BP 104/60, and temperature 37.2° C (99° F). What might be the etiology of his respiratory distress? How will you distinguish between TACO, hemolytic transfusion reaction, and further exacerbation of his underlying pulmonary disease? What are the appropriate interventions to initiate? How will you prioritize your care for this patient?

2 **ebp** It is the beginning of "flu season" and you offer flu vaccinations to all patients in the surgery clinic where you work. You offer a flu vaccine to a 42-year-old woman who is seen for her initial postoperative visit after splenectomy. She tells you she doesn't need a "flu shot" because she received a "protective shot" prior to her splenectomy. How would you respond? What is the strength of the evidence supporting the role of vaccinations in this patient population?

REFERENCES

Books

Adamson, J. W. (2015). Iron deficiency and other hypoproliferative anemias. In D. Kasper, A. Fauci, S. Hauser, et al. (Eds.). *Harrison's principles of internal medicine* (19th ed.). Retrieved on 9/13/2015 at: accessmedicine.mhmedical.com.laneproxy.stanford.edu/content.aspx?bookid=1130&Sectionid=79731112.

Adamson, J. W., & Longo, D. L. (2015). Anemia and polycythemia. In D. Kasper, A. Fauci, S. Hauser, et al. (Eds.). *Harrison's principles of internal medicine* (19th ed.). Retrieved on 9/22/2015 at: accessmedicine.mhmedical.com.laneproxy.stanford.edu/content.aspx?bookid=1130&Sectionid=79727787.

Butterworth, J. F., Mackey, D. C., & Wasnick, J. D. (2013). Fluid management & blood component therapy. In J. F. IV. Butterworth, D. C. Mackey, & J. D. Wasnick (Eds.). *Morgan & Mikhail's clinical anesthesiology* (5th ed.). Retrieved on 9/15/2015 at: accessmedicine.mhmedical.com.laneproxy.stanford.edu/content.aspx?bookid=564&Sectionid=42800585

Davoren, J. B., & Wang, S. (2013). Blood disorders. In G. D. Hammer & S. J. McPhee (Eds.). *Pathophysiology of disease: An introduction to clinical medicine* (7th ed). Retrieved on 9/13/2015 at: accessmedicine.mhmedical.com.laneproxy.stanford.edu/content.aspx?bookid=961&Sectionid=53555687.

Doherty, G. M. (Ed.) (2015). Spleen. *Current diagnosis & treatment: Surgery* (14th ed.). Retrieved on 9/13/2015 at: accessmedicine.mhmedical.com.laneproxy.stanford.edu/content.aspx?bookid=1202&Sectionid=71521945.

Dzieczkowski, J. S., & Anderson, K.C.(2015). Transfusion biology and therapy. In D. Kasper, A. Fauci, S. Hauser, et al. (Eds.). *Harrison's principles of internal medicine* (19th ed.). Retrieved on 5/25/2016 at: accessmedicine.mhmedical.com.laneproxy.stanford.edu/content.aspx?bookid=1130&Sectionid=79732248

Fakih, R., Shah, N., & Nieto, Y. (2016). Autologous hematopoietic progenitor cell transplantation. In H. M. Kantarjian & R. A. Wolff (Eds.). *The MD Anderson manual of medical oncology* (3rd ed.). Retrieved on 05/25/2016 at: accessmedicine.mhmedical.com.laneproxy.stanford.edu/content.aspx?bookid=1772&Sectionid=121897865.

Fischbach, F., & Dunning, M. (2015). *A manual of laboratory and diagnostic tests.* (9th ed.). Philadelphia, PA: Lippincott, Williams & Wilkins.

Henry, P. H., & Longo, D. L. (2015). Enlargement of lymph nodes and spleen. In D. Kasper, A. Fauci, S. Hauser, et al. (Eds.). *Harrison's principles of internal medicine* (19th ed.) Retrieved on 5/25/2016 at: accessmedicine.mhmedical.com.laneproxy.stanford.edu/content.aspx?bookid=1130&Sectionid=7973242

Katz, L. M., & Dodd, R. Y. (2013). Transfusion-transmitted diseases. In B. A. Shaz, C. D. Hillyer, M. Roshal, et al. (Eds.), *Transfusion medicine and hemostasis: Clinical and laboratory aspects* (2nd ed.). Waltham, MA: Elsevier.

Konkle, B. A. (2015). Disorders of platelets and vessel wall. In D. Kasper, A. Fauci, S. Hauser, et al. (Eds.). *Harrison's principles of internal medicine* (19th ed.). Retrieved on 9/13/2015 at: accessmedicine.mhmedical.com.laneproxy.stanford.edu/content.aspx?bookid=1130&Sectionid=7973242

McCullough, J., Refaai, M. A., &Cohn, C. S. (2015). Blood procurement and red cell transfusion. In K. Kaushansky, M. Lichtman, J. Prchal, et al. (Eds.).*Williams hematology* (9th ed.). New York: McGraw-Hill.

Mescher, A. L. (2013). Blood. *Junqueira's basic histology: Text & atlas* (13th ed.). Retrieved on 9/13/2015 at: accessmedicine.mhmedical.com.laneproxy.stanford.edu/content.aspx?bookid=574&Sectionid=42524598.

Papayannopoulou, T., & Migliaccio, A. (2013). Biology of erythropoiesis, erythroid differentiation, and maturation. In R. Hoffman, L. Silberstein, et al. (Eds.).*Hematology: Basic principles and practice* (6th ed.). Waltham, MA: Elsevier.

Ryan, D. H. (2015). Examination of the marrow. In K. Kaushansky, M. Lichtman, J. Prchal, et al. (Eds.). *Williams hematology* (9th ed.). New York: McGraw-Hill.

Seeber, P., & Shander, A. (2012a). Anemia therapy I: Erythropoiesis-stimulating agents. In P. Seeber & A. Shander (Eds.). *Basics of blood management* (2nd ed.). Oxford, UK: Wiley-Blackwell.

Seeber, P., & Shander, A. (2012b). Growth factors. In P. Seeber & A. Shander (Eds.). *Basics of blood management* (2nd ed.). Oxford, UK: Wiley-Blackwell.

Stowell, C. P., & Hass, J. J. (2014). Transfusion medicine. In M. Laposata (Ed.). *Laboratory medicine: The diagnosis of disease in the clinical laboratory.* New York: McGraw-Hill.

Journals and Electronic Documents

Alam, A., Lin, Y., Lima, A., et al. (2013). The prevention of transfusion-associated circulatory overload. *Transfusion Medicine Reviews, 27*(2), 105–112.

American Cancer Society (2013). Possible risks of blood transfusions. Retrieved on 9/14/2015 at: www.cancer.org/treatment/treatmentsandsideeffects/treatmenttypes/bloodproductdonationandtransfusion/blood-product-donation-and-transfusion-possible-transfusion-risks.

American Red Cross (2015a). Blood components. Retrieved on 9/14/2015 at: www.redcrossblood.org/learn-about-blood/bloodcomponents.

American Red Cross (2015b). Eligibility requirements. Retrieved on 9/19/2015 at: www.redcrossblood.org/donating-blood/eligibility-requirements.

Bockhold, C., & Crumpler, S. (2015). Responding to pulmonary-related blood transfusion reactions. *Nursing, 45*(9), 36–41.

Camp, M. A. (2014). Hemostatic agents: A guide to safe practice for perioperative nurses. *AORN Journal, 100*(2), 131–147.

Centers for Disease Control and Prevention.(2013). Bacterial contamination of platelets.Retrieved on 9/20/2015 at: www.cdc.gov/bloodsafety/bbp/bacterial-contamination-of-platelets.html.

Goodnough, L. T., & Shander, A. (2013). Current status of pharmacologic therapies in patient blood management. *Anesthesia & Analgesia, 116*(1), 15–34.

Gorski, L., Hadaway, L., Hagle, M., et al. (2016). Infusion therapy: Standards of practice. *Journal of Infusion Nursing, 39*(1S), S135–S137.

Hurrell, K. (2014). Safe administration of blood components. *Nursing Times, 110*(38), 16–19.

Kenz, H. E., & Van der Linden, P. (2014). Transfusion-related acute lung injury. *The European Journal of Anaesthesiology, 31*(7), 345–350.

Mehta, R. H., Castelvecchio, S., Ballotta, A., et al. (2013). Association of gender and lowest hematocrit on cardiopulmonary bypass with acute kidney injury and operative mortality in patients undergoing cardiac surgery. *The Annals of Thoracic Surgery, 96*(1), 133–140.

Pavlish, C., Brown-Saltzman, K., Jakel, P., et al. (2014).The nature of ethical conflicts and the meaning of moral community in oncology practice. *Oncology Nursing Forum, 41*(2), 130–140.

Snoeck, H. W. (2013). Aging of the hematopoietic system. *Current Opinion In Hematology, 20*(4), 355–361.

Stupnyckyj, C., Smolarek, S., Reeves, C., et al. (2014). Changing blood transfusion policy and practice. *The American Journal of Nursing, 114*(12), 50–59.

Tao, Z.& Ghoroghchian, P. P. (2014). Microparticle, nanoparticle, and stem cell-based oxygen carriers as advanced blood substitutes. *Trends in Biotechnology, 32*(9), 466–473.

van Veen, T., & Hunt, J.A. (2015). Tissue engineering red blood cells: A therapeutic. *Journal of Tissue Engineering and Regenerative Medicine, 9*(7), 760–770.

Vonk, A. B., Meesters, M. I., Garnier, R. P., et al. (2013). Intraoperative cell salvage is associated with reduced postoperative blood loss and transfusion requirements in cardiac surgery: a cohort study. *Transfusion, 53*(11), 2782–2789.

Weyrich, A. S. (2014). Platelets: More than a sack of glue. *Hematology. American Society of Hematology. Education Program, 2014*(1), 400–403.

Resources

AABB (formerly known as the American Association of Blood Banks), www.aabb.org/Pages/default.aspx

American Cancer Society, www.cancer.org

American Red Cross, www.redcross.org

Blood and Marrow Transplant Information Network, www.bmtinfonet.org

Myelodysplastic Syndromes Foundation, www.mds-foundation.org

National Cancer Institute, www.cancer.gov

National Hemophilia Foundation, www.hemophilia.org

National Marrow Donor Program, https://bethematch.org

Oncology Nursing Society (ONS), www.ons.org

33

Management of Patients With Nonmalignant Hematologic Disorders

LEARNING OBJECTIVES

On completion of this chapter, the learner will be able to:

1 Differentiate between the hypoproliferative and the hemolytic anemias and compare and contrast the physiologic mechanisms, clinical manifestations, medical management, and nursing interventions for each.
2 Use the nursing process as a framework for care of patients with anemia.
3 Apply the nursing process as a framework for care of patients with sickle cell crises.

4 Discuss the diverse etiologies and management of secondary polycythemias.
5 Describe the processes involved in neutropenia and lymphopenia and the general principles of medical and nursing management of patients with these disorders.
6 Specify the medical and nursing management of patients with bleeding and thrombotic disorders.
7 Use the nursing process as a framework for care of patients with disseminated intravascular coagulation.

GLOSSARY

absolute neutrophil count (ANC): a calculation of the number of circulating neutrophils, derived from the total white blood cells (WBCs) and the percentage of neutrophils counted in a microscope's visual field
anemia: decreased red blood cell (RBC) count
aplasia: lack of cellular development (e.g., of cells within the bone marrow)
cytokines: proteins produced by leukocytes that are vital to regulation of hematopoiesis, apoptosis, and immune responses
erythrocyte: a cellular component of blood involved in the transport of oxygen and carbon dioxide; (synonym: RBC)
erythroid cells: any cell that is or will become a mature RBC
erythropoietin: hormone produced primarily by the kidney; necessary for erythropoiesis
haptoglobin: blood protein synthesized by liver; binds free hemoglobin released from erythrocytes, which is then removed by the reticuloendothelial system
hemolysis: destruction of RBCs; can occur within or outside of the vasculature
hemosiderin: iron-containing pigment derived from the breakdown of hemoglobin

hypochromia: pallor within the RBC caused by decreased hemoglobin content
leukemia: uncontrolled proliferation of WBCs, often immature
lymphopenia: a lymphocyte count less than 1500/mm³
megaloblastic anemia: a type of anemia characterized by the presence of abnormally large, nucleated RBCs
microcytosis: smaller-than-normal RBCs
neutropenia: lower-than-normal number of neutrophils
normochromic: normal RBC color, indicating normal amount of hemoglobin
normocytic: normal size of RBC
pancytopenia: abnormal decrease in WBCs, RBCs, and platelets
petechiae: tiny capillary hemorrhages
poikilocytosis: variation in shape of RBCs
polycythemia: excess RBCs
reticulocytes: slightly immature RBCs, usually only 1% of total circulating RBCs
spherocytes: small, spherically shaped erythrocytes
thrombocytopenia: lower-than-normal platelet count
thrombocytosis: higher-than-normal platelet count

The majority of hematologic disorders are considered benign (i.e., nonmalignant). Whereas many are relatively indolent, others have severe consequences and can be life-threatening. Most hematologic disorders are quite complex; a thorough understanding of the underlying processes associated with the disorders can assist nurses so that they may appropriately assess, monitor, educate, and intervene with patients with hematologic disorders.

ANEMIA

Anemia is a condition in which the hemoglobin concentration is lower than normal; it reflects the presence of fewer than the normal number of **erythrocytes** (i.e., red blood cells [RBCs]) within the circulation. As a result, the amount of oxygen delivered to body tissues is also diminished. Anemia is not a specific disease state but a sign of an underlying disorder. It is by far the most common hematologic condition.

Classification of Anemias

Anemia may be classified in several ways (see Table 33-1). A physiologic approach classifies anemia according to whether the deficiency in erythrocytes is caused by a defect in their production (i.e., hypoproliferative anemia), by their destruction (i.e., hemolytic anemia), or by their loss (i.e., bleeding).

TABLE 33-1 Classification of Anemias

Type of Anemia	Laboratory Findings	
	CBC	Other
Hypoproliferative (Resulting from Defective RBC Production)		
Iron deficiency	↓ MCV, ↓ reticulocytes	↓ Iron, % saturation, ferritin ↑ TIBC
Vitamin B$_{12}$ deficiency (megaloblastic)	↑ MCV	↓ Vitamin B$_{12}$
Folate deficiency (megaloblastic)	↑ MCV	↓ Folate
Decreased erythropoietin production (e.g., from renal dysfunction)	Normal MCV	↓ Erythropoietin level ↑ Creatinine
Cancer/inflammation	Normal MCV	↑ Ferritin, % saturation ↓ Iron, TIBC ↓ Erythropoietin level (usually)
Bleeding (Resulting from RBC Loss)		
Bleeding from gastrointestinal tract, epistaxis (nosebleed), trauma, bleeding from genitourinary tract (e.g., menorrhagia)	↓ Hgb and Hct (*Note:* Hgb and Hct may be normal if measured soon after bleeding starts) ↓ MCV (normal MCV initially) ↑ Reticulocytes	↓ Iron, % saturation, ferritin (later)
Hemolytic (Resulting from RBC Destruction)		
Altered erythropoiesis (sickle cell disease, thalassemia, other hemoglobinopathies)	↓ MCV ↑ Reticulocytes Fragmented RBCs (various shapes)	
Hypersplenism (hemolysis)	↑ MCV	
Drug-induced anemia	↑ Presence of spherocytes	
Autoimmune anemia	↑ Presence of spherocytes	
Mechanical heart valve–related anemia	Fragmented red cells	

CBC, complete blood count; RBC, red blood cell; ↓, decreased; MCV, mean corpuscular volume; %, percent; ↑, increased; TIBC, total iron-binding capacity; Hgb, hemoglobin; Hct, hematocrit.

Adapted from Prchal, J. T. (2016a). Clinical manifestations and classification of erythrocyte disorders. In K. Kaushansky, M. A. Lichtman, J. T. Prchal, et al. (Eds.). *Williams hematology* (9th ed.). New York: McGraw-Hill Medical.

In hypoproliferative anemias, the bone marrow does not produce adequate numbers of erythrocytes. Decreased erythrocyte production is reflected by a low or inappropriately normal reticulocyte count. Inadequate production of erythrocytes may result from marrow damage due to medications (e.g., chloramphenicol [Chloromycetin]), chemicals (e.g., benzene), or from a lack of factors (e.g., iron, vitamin B$_{12}$, folic acid, **erythropoietin**) necessary for erythrocyte formation.

In hemolytic anemias, premature destruction of erythrocytes results in the liberation of hemoglobin from the erythrocytes into the plasma; the released hemoglobin is converted in large part to bilirubin and, therefore, the bilirubin concentration rises. The increased erythrocyte destruction leads to tissue hypoxia, which in turn stimulates erythropoietin production. This increased production is reflected in an increased reticulocyte count as the bone marrow responds to the loss of erythrocytes. **Hemolysis** (destruction of red blood cells) can result from an abnormality within the erythrocyte itself (e.g., sickle cell disease [SCD], glucose-6-phosphate dehydrogenase [G-6-PD] deficiency), within the plasma (e.g., immune hemolytic anemias), or from direct injury to the erythrocyte within the circulation (e.g., hemolysis caused by a mechanical heart valve). Chart 33-1 identifies causes of hemolytic anemia.

It is usually possible to determine whether the presence of anemia in a given patient is caused by destruction or by inadequate production of erythrocytes on the basis of the following factors:

- The bone marrow's ability to respond to decreased erythrocytes (as evidenced by an increased reticulocyte count in the circulating blood)
- The degree to which young erythrocytes proliferate in the bone marrow and the manner in which they mature (as observed on bone marrow aspirate)
- The presence or absence of end products of erythrocyte destruction within the circulation (e.g., increased bilirubin level, decreased haptoglobin level)

Clinical Manifestations

Aside from the severity of the anemia itself, several factors influence the development of anemia-associated symptoms: the rapidity with which the anemia has developed, the duration of the anemia (i.e., its chronicity), the metabolic requirements of the patient, other concurrent disorders or disabilities (e.g., cardiac or pulmonary disease), and complications or concomitant features of the condition that produced the anemia.

In general, the more rapidly an anemia develops, the more severe its symptoms (Bunn, 2017). An otherwise healthy person can often tolerate as much as a 50% gradual reduction in hemoglobin (e.g., over months) without

Chart 33-1 Causes of Hemolytic Anemias

Inherited Hemolytic Anemia

Abnormal Hemoglobin

Sickle cell disease[a]
Thalassemia[a]

Red Blood Cell Membrane Abnormality

Acanthocytosis
Hereditary elliptocytosis
Hereditary spherocytosis
Stomatocytosis

Enzyme Deficiencies

Glucose-6-phosphate dehydrogenase deficiency[a]

Acquired Hemolytic Anemia

Antibody Related

Autoimmune hemolytic anemia[a]
Iso-antibody/transfusion reaction[b]
Cold agglutinin disease

Not Antibody Related

Disseminated intravascular coagulation[a]
Hypersplenism[a]
Infection
  Bacterial
  Parasitic
Liver disease
Mechanical heart valve
Microangiopathic hemolytic anemia
Paroxysmal nocturnal hemoglobinuria
Toxins
Trauma
Uremia

[a]Discussed in text.
[b]Discussed in Chapter 32.

pronounced symptoms or significant incapacity, whereas the rapid loss of as little as 30% (e.g., over minutes) may precipitate profound vascular collapse in the same person. A person who has become gradually anemic, with hemoglobin levels between 9 and 11 g/dL, usually has fewer or no symptoms other than slight tachycardia on exertion and possibly fatigue.

People who customarily are very active or who have significant demands on their lives (e.g., a single, working mother of small children) are more likely to have symptoms, and those symptoms are more likely to be pronounced than in more sedentary people. Patients with hypothyroidism with decreased oxygen needs may be completely asymptomatic, without tachycardia or increased cardiac output, at a hemoglobin level of 10 g/dL. Similarly, patients with coexistent cardiac, vascular, or pulmonary disease may develop more pronounced symptoms of anemia (e.g., dyspnea, chest pain, muscle pain or cramping) with a higher hemoglobin level than those without these concurrent health problems.

Finally, some anemias are complicated by various other abnormalities that do not result from the anemia but are inherently associated with these particular diseases. These abnormalities may give rise to symptoms that completely overshadow those of the anemia, as in the painful crises of SCD.

Assessment and Diagnostic Findings

A variety of hematologic studies are performed to determine the type and cause of the anemia. In an initial evaluation, the hemoglobin, hematocrit, reticulocyte count, and RBC indices, particularly the mean corpuscular volume (MCV) and red cell distribution width (RDW), are especially useful. Iron studies (serum iron level, total iron-binding capacity [TIBC], percent saturation, and ferritin), as well as serum vitamin B_{12} and folate levels, are also frequently obtained (Goroll & Mulley, 2014a). Other tests include haptoglobin and erythropoietin levels. The remaining complete blood count (CBC) values are useful in determining whether the anemia is an isolated problem or part of another hematologic condition, such as **leukemia** or myelodysplastic syndrome (MDS). Bone marrow aspiration may be performed. In addition, other diagnostic studies may be performed to determine the presence of underlying chronic illness, such as malignancy, or the source of any blood loss, such as polyps or ulcers within the gastrointestinal (GI) tract (see Chapter 32 for discussion of diagnostic tests).

Complications

Complications of severe anemia include heart failure, paresthesias, and delirium. Patients with underlying heart disease are far more likely to have angina or symptoms of heart failure than those without heart disease. Complications associated with specific types of anemia are included in the description of each type.

Medical Management

Management of anemia is directed toward correcting or controlling the cause of the anemia; if the anemia is severe, the erythrocytes that are lost or destroyed may be replaced with a transfusion of packed red blood cells (PRBCs). The management of the various types of anemia is covered in the discussions that follow.

 Gerontologic Considerations

Anemia is the most common hematologic condition affecting older patients, particularly those admitted to hospitals or in long-term care facilities. The overall prevalence of anemia increases with age, from 10% in persons 65 years of age to 50% in persons older than 85 years (Berliner, 2013). The impact of even mild anemia on function in older adults is significant and may include decreased physical performance, decreased mobility, increased frailty, increased rates of depression, increased risk for falling, and delirium (Goodnough & Schrier, 2014). Several studies found a significant association between anemia and declining cognitive function (Andro, Le Square, Estivan, et al., 2013; Hong, Falvey, Harris, et al., 2013). Older adults often cannot respond to anemia as well as younger individuals, in that heart rate and cardiac output do not increase as quickly; thus, fatigue, dyspnea, and confusion may be seen more readily in the older adult who is anemic. Those with pre-existing renal or cardiac disease or who have had recent surgery are also at increased risk for mortality when anemic.

NURSING PROCESS

The Patient With Anemia

Assessment

The health history and physical examination provide important data about the type of anemia involved, the extent and type of symptoms it produces, and the impact of those symptoms on the patient's life. Weakness, fatigue, and general malaise are common, as are pallor of the skin and mucous membranes (conjunctivae, oral mucosa) (see Fig. 33-1).

Jaundice; angular cheilosis (ulcerated corners of the mouth); and brittle, ridged, concave nails may be present in patients with **megaloblastic anemia** (characterized by the presence of abnormally large, nucleated RBCs) or hemolytic anemia. The tongue may be beefy red and sore in megaloblastic anemia, or smooth and red in iron deficiency anemia. Patients with iron deficiency anemia may infrequently crave ice, starch, or dirt; this craving is known as pica (Broadway-Duren & Klaassen, 2013). Restless leg syndrome is common in as many as 24% of

Figure 33-1 • Pallor seen in the patient with anemia. From Tkachuk, D. C., & Hirschman, J. V. (2007). *Wintrobe's atlas of clinical hematology* (Fig. 1.1, p. 9). Philadelphia, PA: Lippincott Williams & Wilkins.

those with iron deficiency anemia (Lopez, Cacoub, Macdougall, et al., 2015). The health history should include a medication history, because some medications can depress bone marrow activity, induce hemolysis, or interfere with folate metabolism. An accurate history of alcohol intake, including the amount and duration, should be obtained. Family history is important, because certain anemias are inherited. It is necessary to ask about athletic endeavors, because extreme exercise can decrease erythropoiesis and erythrocyte survival.

A nutritional assessment is important, because it may indicate deficiencies in essential nutrients such as iron, vitamin B_{12}, and folate. Strict vegetarians are at risk for megaloblastic anemias if they do not supplement their diet with vitamin B_{12}. Older adults also may have a diminished intake of vitamin B_{12} or folate.

Cardiac status should be carefully assessed. When the hemoglobin level is low, the heart attempts to compensate by pumping faster and harder in an effort to deliver more blood to hypoxic tissue. This increased cardiac workload can result in such symptoms as tachycardia, palpitations, dyspnea, dizziness, orthopnea, and exertional dyspnea. Heart failure may eventually develop, as evidenced by an enlarged heart (cardiomegaly) and liver (hepatomegaly) and by peripheral edema.

Assessment of the GI system may disclose complaints of nausea, vomiting (with specific questions about the appearance of any emesis [e.g., looks like "coffee grounds"]), melena (dark stools), diarrhea, anorexia, and glossitis (inflammation of the tongue). Stools should be tested for occult blood (see Chapter 32). Women should be questioned about their menstrual periods (e.g., excessive menstrual flow, other vaginal bleeding) and the use of iron supplements during pregnancy.

Neurologic examination is also important because pernicious anemia affects the central and peripheral nervous systems. Assessment should include the presence and extent of peripheral numbness and paresthesias, ataxia, poor coordination, and confusion. Delirium can sometimes result from other types of anemia, particularly in older adults. Finally, it is important to monitor relevant laboratory test results and to note any changes over time (see Chapter 32).

Diagnosis

NURSING DIAGNOSES

Based on the assessment data, major nursing diagnoses may include:

- Fatigue related to decreased hemoglobin and diminished oxygen-carrying capacity of the blood
- Imbalanced nutrition, less than body requirements, related to inadequate intake of essential nutrients
- Activity intolerance related to inadequate hemoglobin and hematocrit
- Noncompliance with prescribed therapy

Collaborative Problems/Potential Complications

Potential complications may include the following:

- Heart failure
- Angina
- Paresthesias
- Confusion
- Injury related to falls
- Depressed mood

Planning and Goals

The major goals for the patient may include decreased fatigue, attainment or maintenance of adequate nutrition, maintenance of adequate tissue perfusion, compliance with prescribed therapy, and absence of complications.

Nursing Interventions

MANAGING FATIGUE

The most common symptom and complication of anemia is fatigue. Fatigue is often the symptom that has the greatest negative impact on a patient's level of functioning and consequent quality of life. Therefore, it should not be minimized. Patients often describe the fatigue from anemia as oppressive. Fatigue can be significant, yet the anemia may not be severe enough to warrant transfusion. Fatigue can interfere with a person's ability to work and to participate in activities with family and friends. Patients often lose interest in hobbies and activities, including sexual activity. The distress from fatigue is often related to a person's responsibilities and life demands as well as the amount of assistance and support received from others.

Nursing interventions can focus on assisting the patient to prioritize activities and to establish a balance between activity and rest that is acceptable to the patient. Patients with chronic anemia need to maintain some physical activity and exercise to prevent the deconditioning that results from inactivity. It is also important to assess for other conditions that can exacerbate fatigue, such as pain, depression, and sleep disturbance.

MAINTAINING ADEQUATE NUTRITION

Inadequate intake of essential nutrients, such as iron, vitamin B_{12}, folic acid, and protein, can cause some anemias. The symptoms associated with anemia (e.g., fatigue, anorexia) can in turn interfere with maintaining adequate nutrition. A healthy diet should be encouraged. The nurse should inform the patient that alcohol interferes with the utilization of essential nutrients and advise moderation in the intake of alcoholic beverages (Cylwik, Naklick, Gruszewska, et al., 2013) (see Chapter 5). Dietary education sessions should be individualized, involve family members, and include cultural aspects related to food preferences and food preparation. Dietary supplements (e.g., vitamins, iron, folate, protein) may be prescribed.

Equally important, the patient and family must understand the role of nutritional supplements in the proper context, because many forms of anemia are not the result of a nutritional deficiency. In such cases, even an excessive intake of nutritional supplements will not improve the anemia. A potential problem in patients with chronic transfusion requirements occurs with the indiscriminate use of iron supplements. Unless an aggressive program of chelation therapy is implemented, these patients are at risk for iron overload from their transfusions (Jordan, Adams-Graves, Kanter-Wasko, et al., 2015). The addition of an iron supplement only exacerbates the situation.

ACTIVITY INTOLERANCE

Patients with acute blood loss or severe hemolysis may not tolerate typical activities because of decreased blood volume or reduced circulating erythrocytes (decreased hematocrit).

Lost volume is replaced with transfusions or intravenous (IV) fluids, based on symptoms and laboratory test results. Supplemental oxygen may be necessary, but it is rarely needed on a long-term basis unless there is underlying severe cardiac or pulmonary disease. The nurse monitors the patient's vital signs and pulse oximeter readings closely; other medications, such as antihypertensive agents, may need to be adjusted or withheld.

PROMOTING ADHERENCE WITH PRESCRIBED THERAPY

For patients with anemia, medications or nutritional supplements are often prescribed to treat the condition. These patients need to understand the purpose of the medication, how to take the medication and over what time period, and how to manage any side effects of therapy. To enhance adherence, the nurse assists the patient to develop ways to incorporate the therapeutic plan into everyday activities rather than merely giving the patient a list of instructions. For example, many patients have difficulty taking iron supplements because of related GI effects. Rather than seeking assistance from a health care provider in managing the problem, some patients simply stop taking the iron.

Abruptly stopping some medications can have serious consequences, as in the case of high-dose corticosteroids to manage hemolytic anemias. Some medications, such as growth factors, are extremely expensive. Patients receiving these medications may need assistance to obtain needed insurance coverage or to explore alternative ways to obtain these medications.

MONITORING AND MANAGING POTENTIAL COMPLICATIONS

A significant complication of anemia is heart failure from chronic diminished blood volume and the heart's compensatory effort to increase cardiac output. Patients with anemia should be assessed for signs and symptoms of heart failure (see Chapter 29).

In megaloblastic forms of anemia, the significant potential complications are neurologic. A neurologic assessment should be performed for patients with known or suspected megaloblastic anemia. Patients may initially complain of paresthesias in their lower extremities. These paresthesias are usually manifested as numbness and tingling on the bottom of the foot, and they gradually progress. As the anemia progresses, other signs become apparent. Position and vibration sense may be diminished. Difficulty maintaining balance is not uncommon, and some patients have gait disturbances as well. Initially mild confusion may develop; it may become severe (Stabler, 2013).

Evaluation

Expected patient outcomes may include:

1. Reports less fatigue
   a. Follows a progressive plan of rest, activity, and exercise
   b. Prioritizes activities
   c. Paces activities according to energy level
2. Attains and maintains adequate nutrition
   a. Eats a healthy diet
   b. Develops a meal plan that promotes optimal nutrition
   c. Maintains adequate amounts of iron, vitamins, and protein from diet or supplements

   d. Adheres to nutritional supplement therapy when prescribed

   e. Verbalizes understanding of rationale for using recommended nutritional supplements

   f. Verbalizes understanding of rationale for avoiding nonrecommended nutritional supplements

3. Maintains adequate activity level

   a. Has vital signs within baseline for patient

   b. Has pulse oximetry (arterial oxygenation) value within normal limits

4. Absence of complications

   a. Avoids or limits activities that trigger dyspnea, palpitations, dizziness, or tachycardia

   b. Uses rest and comfort measures to alleviate dyspnea

   c. Has vital signs within baseline for patient

   d. Has no signs of increasing fluid retention (e.g., peripheral edema, decreased urine output, neck vein distention)

   e. Remains oriented to time, place, and situation

   f. Remains engaged in social situations, exhibits no signs of depression

   g. Ambulates safely, using assistive devices as necessary

   h. Remains free of injury

   i. Verbalizes understanding of importance of serial CBC measurements

   j. Maintains safe home environment; obtains assistance as necessary

Hypoproliferative Anemias

Iron Deficiency Anemia

Iron deficiency anemia typically results when the intake of dietary iron is inadequate for hemoglobin synthesis. The body can store about one fourth to one third of its iron, and it is not until those stores are depleted that iron deficiency anemia actually begins to develop. Iron deficiency can also occur when total body iron stores are adequate, but the supply of iron to the bone marrow is inadequate; this type is referred to as functional iron deficiency (Lopez et al., 2015). Iron deficiency anemia is the most common type of anemia in all age groups, and it is the most common anemia in the world, affecting one in eight persons (Camaschella, 2015). It is particularly prevalent in developing countries, where inadequate iron stores can result from inadequate intake of iron (seen with vegetarian diets) or from blood loss (e.g., from intestinal hookworm). Iron deficiency is also common among adults in the United States, and the most common cause is blood loss. In fact, bleeding should be considered the cause of iron deficiency anemia until proven otherwise.

The most common cause of iron deficiency anemia in men and postmenopausal women is bleeding from ulcers, gastritis, inflammatory bowel disease, or GI tumors. The most common causes of iron deficiency anemia in premenopausal women are menorrhagia (i.e., excessive menstrual bleeding) and pregnancy with inadequate iron supplementation. Patients with chronic alcoholism or who take aspirin, steroids, or nonsteroidal anti-inflammatory drugs (NSAIDs) often have chronic blood loss from the GI tract, which causes iron loss and eventual anemia. Other causes include iron malabsorption, as is seen after gastrectomy, bariatric surgery, or with celiac or other inflammatory bowel disease; medications (proton pump inhibitors, H_2 blockers) can also decrease iron absorption (Camaschella, 2015; Nielson, Ainsworth, Coskun, et al., 2015).

Clinical Manifestations

Patients with iron deficiency primarily have symptoms of anemia. If the deficiency is severe or prolonged, they may also have a smooth, red tongue; brittle and ridged nails; and angular cheilosis. These signs subside after iron replacement therapy. The health history may be significant for multiple pregnancies, GI bleeding, and pica (Lopez et al., 2015).

Assessment and Diagnostic Findings

The definitive method of establishing the diagnosis of iron deficiency anemia is bone marrow aspiration (see Chapter 32 for further discussion of bone marrow aspiration.). The aspirate is stained to detect iron, which is at a low level or even absent. However, few patients with suspected iron deficiency anemia undergo bone marrow aspiration. In many patients, the diagnosis can be established with other tests, particularly in patients with a history of conditions that predispose them to this type of anemia.

A strong correlation exists between laboratory values that measure iron stores and hemoglobin levels. After iron stores are depleted (as reflected by low serum ferritin levels), the hemoglobin level falls. The diminished iron stores cause small erythrocytes to be produced by the marrow. Therefore, as the anemia progresses, the MCV, which measures the size of the erythrocytes, also decreases. Hematocrit and RBC levels are also low in relation to the hemoglobin level. Other laboratory tests that measure iron stores are useful but not as precise as ferritin levels. Typically, patients with iron deficiency anemia have a low serum iron level and an elevated TIBC, which measures the transport protein supplying the marrow with iron as needed (also referred to as transferrin) (Lopez et al., 2015). However, other disease states, such as infection and inflammatory conditions, can also cause a low serum iron level and TIBC, as well as an elevated ferritin level. If these are suspected, measuring the soluble transferring receptor can aid in differentiating the cause of anemia. This test result will be increased in the setting of iron deficiency, but not in chronic inflammation.

Medical Management

Except in the case of pregnancy, the cause of iron deficiency should be investigated. Anemia may be a sign of a curable GI cancer or of uterine fibroid tumors. Stool specimens should be tested for occult blood. People 50 years of age or older should have a colonoscopy, endoscopy, or x-ray examination of the GI tract to detect ulcerations, gastritis, polyps, or cancer (American Cancer Society, 2015). Individuals with celiac disease or who have had gastric surgery may not absorb iron adequately from their diet and therefore become iron deficient (Broadway-Duren & Klassen, 2013).

Oral iron supplementation is considered to be the primary mode of treating iron deficiency anemia. Several oral iron preparations—ferrous sulfate, ferrous gluconate, and ferrous fumarate—are available for treating iron deficiency anemia.

Chart 33-2 Parenteral Iron Formulations

- Older formulations of parenteral iron had a high molecular weight, and the risk of hypersensitivity reactions, including anaphylaxis, was significant. Newer formulations have a low molecular weight, and the risk of anaphylaxis is markedly reduced.
- Ferric gluconate (Ferrlecit): Each 5 mL contains 62.5 mg elemental iron; 125 mg is diluted in 100 mL normal saline and infused over 1 hour, or 5 mL undiluted is given as a slow IV push injection over 5 minutes. Although the likelihood of an allergic reaction is extremely low, a test dose is often given prior to the first infusion.
- Iron sucrose (Venofer): Each 5 mL contains 100 mg elemental iron; 100–200 mg can be given undiluted as a slow IV push injection over 2 to 5 minutes. This procedure can be repeated as often as every 3 days for a total cumulative dose of 1000 mg within a 2-week period.

Chart 33-3 PATIENT EDUCATION — Taking Oral Iron Supplements

The nurse instructs the patient to:

- Take iron on an empty stomach (1 hour before or 2 hours after a meal), preferably with orange juice or other forms of vitamin C. Iron absorption is reduced with food, especially dairy products.
- Prevent gastrointestinal distress by using the following schedule if more than one tablet a day is prescribed: Start with only one tablet per day for a few days, then increase to two tablets per day, then three tablets per day. This method permits the body to adjust gradually to the iron. If unable to tolerate oral iron supplements due to gastrointestinal distress and these interventions are inadequate, take at least one tablet daily rather than stop completely. However, reduced dosage will necessitate longer treatment duration to adequately replete iron stores.
- Increase the intake of vitamin C (citrus fruits and juices, strawberries, tomatoes, broccoli) to enhance iron absorption.
- Eat foods high in fiber to minimize problems with constipation; add stool softener if needed.
- Remember that stools will become dark in color.
- Prevent staining the teeth with a liquid preparation by using a straw or placing a spoon at the back of the mouth to take the supplement. Rinse the mouth thoroughly afterward.

The hemoglobin level may increase in only a few weeks, and the anemia can be corrected in a few months. Iron store replenishment takes much longer, so the patient must continue taking the iron for as long as 6 to 12 months.

In some cases, oral iron is poorly absorbed or poorly tolerated, or iron supplementation is needed in large amounts. In these situations, IV administration of iron may be needed. Several doses are required to replenish the patient's iron stores (see Chart 33-2).

Nursing Management

Preventive education is important, because iron deficiency anemia is common in menstruating and pregnant women. Food sources high in iron include organ meats (e.g., beef or calf's liver, chicken liver), other meats, beans (e.g., black, pinto, and garbanzo), leafy green vegetables, raisins, and molasses. Taking iron-rich foods with a source of vitamin C (e.g., orange juice) enhances the absorption of iron.

The nurse helps the patient select a healthy diet. Nutritional counseling can be provided for those whose usual diet is inadequate. Patients with a history of eating fad diets or strict vegetarian diets are counseled that such diets often contain inadequate amounts of absorbable iron. The nurse encourages the patient to continue iron therapy for as long as it is prescribed even though the patient may no longer feel fatigued.

Iron supplements are usually given in the oral form. Because iron is best absorbed on an empty stomach, the patient is instructed to take the supplement an hour before meals. Most patients can use the less expensive, more standard forms of ferrous sulfate. Many patients have difficulty tolerating iron supplements because of GI side effects (primarily constipation, but also cramping, nausea, and vomiting). Decreasing the frequency of taking iron supplements, or taking with food can mitigate the GI symptoms, but will diminish absorption of the iron; thus, it may take longer to replete the iron stores. While taking iron with vitamin C increases absorption of the iron, it also increases the frequency of side effects (Lopez et al., 2015). Some iron formulations are designed to limit GI side effects by the addition of a stool softener or the use of sustained-release formulations to limit nausea or gastritis. However, tablets with enteric coating may be poorly absorbed. Slow-release formulations should be avoided because the iron is released beyond the duodenum, the site of maximal iron absorption (Camaschella, 2015). Specific education aids (see Chart 33-3) can assist patients with the use of iron supplements.

If taking iron on an empty stomach causes gastric distress, the patient may need to take it with meals. However, doing so diminishes iron absorption by as much as 40%, thus prolonging the time required to replenish iron stores. Antacids or dairy products should not be taken with iron, because they greatly diminish its absorption. Polysaccharide iron complex forms are also available; they have less GI toxicity but are more expensive.

Liquid forms of iron that cause less GI distress are available. Iron replacement therapy should not cause a false-positive result on stool analyses for occult blood even though it may change the color of stool.

IV supplementation may be used when the patient's iron stores are completely depleted, the patient cannot tolerate oral forms of iron supplementation (see earlier Medical Management section), or both. The nurse needs to be aware of the type of parenteral formulation of iron ordered so that the risk of anaphylaxis may be determined. High molecular formulations are associated with a much higher incidence of anaphylaxis and therefore are now infrequently used. Administering a test dose of low-molecular formulations of iron dextran is still recommended by many manufacturers. The nurse needs to assist the patient in understanding the need for repeated dosing to replenish iron stores or to maintain iron stores in the setting of chronic blood loss, such as dialysis, or chronic GI bleeding.

Anemias in Renal Disease

The degree of anemia in patients with chronic kidney disease (CKD) varies greatly; however, in general, patients do not become significantly anemic until the glomerular filtration rate (GFR) is less than 30 mL/min/1.73² (Dmitrieva, de Lusignan, Macdougall, et al., 2013). The symptoms of anemia are often the most disturbing of the patient's symptoms. In patients with CKD, anemia contributes to increased cardiac output, reduced oxygen utilization, decreased concentration and cognitive function, reduced immune responsiveness, and reduced libido (National Clinical Guideline Centre [UK], 2015). Anemia in patients with CKD is discussed in Chapter 54.

Anemia of Inflammation

The term *anemia of inflammation* is a relatively new term that delineates the chronic diseases of inflammation, infection, and malignancy as causes for this type of anemia; this classification was previously referred to as anemia of chronic disease (Ganz, 2016b). Included in this term is the anemia of critical illness that develops within days after the onset of serious illness and also the anemia associated with aging. Many chronic inflammatory diseases are associated with a **normochromic, normocytic** anemia (i.e., the erythrocytes are normal in color and size). These disorders include rheumatoid arthritis; severe, chronic infections; and many cancers. It is therefore imperative that the "chronic disease" be diagnosed when this form of anemia is identified so that it can be appropriately managed.

The anemia is usually mild to moderate and nonprogressive. The hemoglobin level rarely falls below 9 g/dL, and the bone marrow has normal cellularity with increased stores of iron as the iron is diverted from the serum. Erythropoietin levels are low, perhaps because of decreased production, and iron use is blocked by **erythroid cells** (cells that are or will become mature erythrocytes). A moderate shortening of erythrocyte survival also occurs.

Most of these patients have fewer symptoms related to the anemia and do not require treatment. With successful treatment of the underlying disorder, the bone marrow iron is used to make erythrocytes and the hemoglobin level rises. These patients do not benefit from additional iron supplementation.

 Gerontologic Considerations

Increasing evidence suggests that inflammation may have a significant role in the development of anemia in older adults (Goodnough & Schrier, 2014). Higher-than-normal levels of inflammatory **cytokines** (proteins) are found in the older adult population, which may also be associated with anemia (Fairweather-Tait, Wawer, Gilings, et al., 2014). This proinflammatory state may predispose older adults to frailty, manifested by weight loss, decreased mobility, generalized weakness, and poor balance; frailty is strongly associated with the anemia of inflammation (Chang, Weis, Xue, et al., 2013). Erythropoietin levels may not rise appropriately in response to decreased hemoglobin.

Aplastic Anemia

Aplastic anemia is a rare disease caused by a decrease in or damage to marrow stem cells, damage to the microenvironment within the marrow, and replacement of the marrow with fat. Stem cell damage is caused by the body's T cells mediating an inappropriate attack against the bone marrow, resulting in bone marrow **aplasia** (i.e., markedly reduced hematopoiesis). Therefore, in addition to severe anemia, significant neutropenia and thrombocytopenia also occur.

Pathophysiology

Aplastic anemia can be acquired or, rarely, congenital, but most cases are idiopathic (i.e., without apparent cause) (Segel & Lichtman, 2016). Viral infections and pregnancy can trigger it, or it may be caused by certain medications, chemicals, or radiation damage. Agents that may produce marrow aplasia include benzene and benzene derivatives (e.g., airplane glue, paint remover, dry-cleaning solutions). Certain toxic materials, such as inorganic arsenic, glycol ethers, plutonium, and radon, have also been implicated as potential causes.

Clinical Manifestations

The manifestations of aplastic anemia are often insidious. Complications resulting from bone marrow failure may occur before the diagnosis is established. Typical complications are infection and the symptoms of anemia (e.g., fatigue, pallor, dyspnea). Purpura (bruising) may develop later and should trigger a CBC and hematologic evaluation if these were not performed initially. If the patient has had repeated throat infections, cervical lymphadenopathy may be seen. Other lymphadenopathies and splenomegaly sometimes occur. Retinal hemorrhages are common.

Assessment and Diagnostic Findings

In many situations, aplastic anemia occurs when a medication or chemical is ingested in toxic amounts. However, in a few people, it develops after a medication has been taken at the recommended dosage. This may be considered an idiosyncratic reaction in those who are highly susceptible, possibly caused by a genetic defect in the medication biotransformation or elimination process. A CBC reveals **pancytopenia** (a decrease in all myeloid stem cell–derived cells) with a neutrophil count less than 1500/μL, hemoglobin less than 10 g/dL, and platelets less than 50,000/μL (Segel & Lichtman, 2016). A bone marrow aspirate shows an extremely hypoplastic or even aplastic (very few to no cells) marrow replaced with fat.

Medical Management

It is presumed that the T lymphocytes of patients with aplastic anemia destroy the stem cells and consequently impair the production of erythrocytes, leukocytes, and platelets. Despite its severity, aplastic anemia can be successfully treated in most people. Those who are younger than 60 years, who are otherwise healthy, and who have a compatible donor can be cured of the disease with hematopoietic stem cell transplant (HSCT) (Maury & Aljurf, 2013). In others, the disease can be managed with immunosuppressive therapy, commonly using a combination of antithymocyte globulin (ATG) and cyclosporine or androgens (Marsh & Kulasekararaj, 2013). ATG, a purified gamma-globulin solution, is obtained from horses or rabbits immunized with human T lymphocytes. Side effects during the infusion are common and include fever and chills. The sudden onset of a rash or bronchospasm may herald anaphylaxis and requires prompt management (see Chapters 37 and 72). Serum sickness, as evidenced by fever, rash, arthralgias, and pruritus, may develop in some patients, but the incidence can be reduced by using corticosteroids concomitantly (Segel & Lichtman, 2016). If it does develop, serum sickness may take weeks to resolve.

Immunosuppressants prevent the patient's lymphocytes from destroying the stem cells. If relapse occurs (i.e., the patient becomes pancytopenic again), reinstitution of the same immunologic agents may induce another remission, although response rates are much lower (30% to 35%) (Marsh & Kulasekararaj, 2013). Corticosteroids are not very useful as immunosuppressive agents in the long term, because patients with aplastic anemia are particularly susceptible to the development of bone complications from corticosteroids (e.g., aseptic necrosis of the head of the femur).

Supportive therapy plays a major role in the management of aplastic anemia. Any offending agent is discontinued. The patient is supported with transfusions of PRBCs and platelets as necessary; infections are aggressively treated. Death usually is caused by infection, either bacterial or fungal (Marsh & Kulasekararaj, 2013).

Nursing Management

Patients with aplastic anemia are vulnerable to problems related to erythrocyte, leukocyte, and platelet insufficiencies. They should be assessed carefully for signs of infection and bleeding. (Specific interventions are delineated in the Neutropenia and Thrombocytopenia sections.) Nurses must also monitor for side effects of therapy, particularly for hypersensitivity reaction while administering ATG. If patients require long-term cyclosporine therapy, they should be monitored for long-term effects, including renal or liver dysfunction, hypertension, pruritus, visual impairment, tremor, and skin cancer. They should also be informed that the metabolism of ATG is altered by many other medications; thus, each new prescription needs careful assessment for drug–drug interactions. Patients also need to understand the importance of not abruptly stopping their immunosuppressive therapy.

Megaloblastic Anemias

In the anemias caused by deficiencies of vitamin B_{12} or folic acid, identical bone marrow and peripheral blood changes occur because both vitamins are essential for normal DNA synthesis. In either case, the erythrocytes that are produced are abnormally large and called *megaloblastic red cells*. Other cells derived from the myeloid stem cell (nonlymphoid leukocytes, platelets) are also abnormal. A bone marrow analysis reveals hyperplasia (an abnormal increase in the number of cells), and the precursor erythroid and myeloid cells are large and bizarre in appearance. However, many of these abnormal erythroid and myeloid cells are destroyed within the marrow, so the mature cells that do leave the marrow are actually fewer in number. Thus, pancytopenia can develop. Those cells that are released into the circulation are often abnormally shaped. The neutrophils are hypersegmented. The platelets may be abnormally large. The erythrocytes are abnormally shaped, and the shapes may vary widely (**poikilocytosis**). Because the erythrocytes are very large, the MCV is very high, usually exceeding 110 fl. Megaloblastic anemias develop slowly (e.g., over months) and thus the body can compensate well for a long time; symptoms of anemia may not develop until the anemia is very severe (Green, 2016). In Caucasians, the skin develops a lemon-yellow color resulting from simultaneous pallor and mild jaundice that results from a mild hemolysis of red cells.

Pathophysiology

Folic Acid Deficiency

Folic acid is stored as compounds referred to as folates. The folate stores in the body are much smaller than those of vitamin B_{12} and can become depleted within months when the dietary intake of folate is deficient (Green, 2016). Folate is found in green vegetables and liver. Thus, folate deficiency occurs in people who rarely eat uncooked vegetables. Alcohol increases folic acid requirements, and, at the same time, patients with alcoholism usually have a diet that is deficient in the vitamin. Folic acid requirements are also increased in patients with liver disease, chronic hemolytic anemias and in women who are pregnant, because the need for erythrocyte production is increased in these conditions. Some patients with malabsorptive diseases of the small bowel, such as celiac disease, may not absorb folic acid normally (Green, 2016).

Vitamin B_{12} Deficiency

A deficiency of vitamin B_{12} can occur in several ways. Inadequate dietary intake is rare but can develop in strict vegans who consume no meat or dairy products. Faulty absorption from the GI tract is more common, particularly in the older adult. Ten percent to 20% of older adults have low B_{12}; 5% to 10% have symptoms related to this deficiency (Broadway-Duren & Klaassen, 2013). Decreased B_{12} absorption also occurs in conditions such as Crohn's disease or after ileal resection, bariatric surgery, or gastrectomy. Chronic use of histamine blockers, antacids, or proton pump inhibitors to reduce gastric acid production can also inhibit B_{12} absorption, as can the use of the drug metformin (Glucophage) in managing diabetes (Goroll & Mulley, 2014b; Singh, Kumar, Karmakar, et al., 2013). Another cause is the absence of intrinsic factor; in this particular context, the resultant anemia is called *pernicious anemia*. Intrinsic factor is normally secreted by cells within the gastric mucosa; it binds with dietary vitamin B_{12} and travels with it to the ileum, where the vitamin is absorbed. Without intrinsic factor, orally consumed vitamin B_{12} cannot be adequately absorbed, and erythrocyte production is eventually diminished. Even if adequate vitamin B_{12} and intrinsic factor are present, a deficiency may occur if disease involving the ileum or pancreas impairs absorption. Pernicious anemia tends to run in families; it is primarily a disorder of adults, particularly older adults.

The body normally has large stores of vitamin B_{12}, so years may pass before the deficiency results in anemia. Because the body compensates so well, the anemia can be severe before the patient becomes symptomatic. Patients with pernicious anemia have a higher incidence of gastric cancer than the general population; these patients may benefit from having endoscopies at regular intervals to screen for early gastric cancer (Vannella, Lahner, Osborn, et al., 2013).

Clinical Manifestations

Symptoms of folic acid and vitamin B_{12} deficiencies are similar, and the two anemias may coexist. However, the neurologic manifestations of vitamin B_{12} deficiency do not occur with folic acid deficiency, and they persist if vitamin B_{12} is not replaced. Therefore, careful distinction between the two anemias must be made.

After the body stores of vitamin B_{12} are depleted, the patient may begin to show signs and symptoms of the anemia. However, because the onset and progression of the anemia are so gradual, the body can compensate well until the anemia is severe, so the typical manifestations of anemia (weakness, listlessness, fatigue) may not be apparent initially. The hematologic effects of vitamin B_{12} deficiency are accompanied by effects on other organ systems, particularly the GI tract and nervous system. Patients with pernicious anemia develop a smooth, sore, red tongue and mild diarrhea. They are extremely pale, particularly in the mucous membranes. They may become confused; more often, they have paresthesias in the extremities (particularly numbness and tingling in the feet and lower legs). They may have difficulty maintaining their balance because of damage to the spinal cord, and they also lose position sense (proprioception). These symptoms are progressive, although the course of illness may be marked by spontaneous partial remissions and exacerbations. Without treatment, patients can die after several years, usually from heart failure secondary to anemia.

Assessment and Diagnostic Findings

Serum levels of both vitamins can be measured. In the case of folic acid deficiency, even small amounts of folate increase the serum folate level, sometimes to normal. Measuring the amount of folate within the red cell itself (red cell folate) is therefore a more sensitive test in determining true folate deficiency, although not commonly performed.

The classic method of determining the cause of vitamin B_{12} deficiency was the Schilling test, but because of decreased availability of test components and cost, this test is rarely used. Other methods of establishing the diagnosis are now more commonly used. The vitamin B_{12} assay is typically the initial test used, but current methods render the test results to be either falsely positive (i.e., not indicative of a true deficiency) or falsely negative (Stabler, 2013). Although it is possible to measure methylmalonic acid and homocysteine levels in vitamin B_{12} deficiency, these levels also increase in the setting of renal insufficiency. Furthermore, it is expensive to measure these levels, which also limits the utility of the test. A more useful, easier test is the intrinsic factor antibody test. A positive test indicates the presence of antibodies that bind the vitamin B_{12}–intrinsic factor complex and prevent it from binding to receptors in the ileum, thus preventing its absorption. Although this test is not specific for pernicious anemia alone, it can aid in the diagnosis.

Medical Management

Folate deficiency is treated by increasing the amount of folic acid in the diet and administering 1 mg of folic acid daily. Folic acid is given intramuscularly only to people with malabsorption problems. Although many multivitamin preparations now contain folic acid, additional supplements may be necessary because the amount may be inadequate to fully replace deficient body stores. Patients who abuse alcohol should receive folic acid as long as they continue to consume alcohol.

Vitamin B_{12} deficiency is treated by vitamin B_{12} replacement. Vegans can prevent or treat deficiency with oral supplements with vitamins or fortified soy milk. When the deficiency is due to the more common defect in absorption or the absence of intrinsic factor, replacement is by monthly intramuscular injections of vitamin B_{12}. A small amount of an oral dose of vitamin B_{12} can be absorbed by passive diffusion, even in the absence of intrinsic factor; however, large doses are required if vitamin B_{12} is to be replaced orally (Shipton & Thachil, 2015).

As vitamin B_{12} is replaced, the reticulocyte count rises within 1 week, and in 4 to 8 weeks the blood counts return to normal (Green, 2016). The tongue feels better and appears less red in several days. However, the neurologic manifestations require more time for recovery; if there is severe neuropathy, the patient may never recover fully. To prevent recurrence of pernicious anemia, vitamin B_{12} therapy must be continued for life.

Nursing Management

Assessment of patients who have or are at risk for megaloblastic anemia includes inspection of the skin, mucous membranes, and tongue. Mild jaundice may be apparent and is best seen in the sclera without using fluorescent lights. Vitiligo (patchy loss of skin pigmentation) and premature graying of the hair are often seen in patients with pernicious anemia. Because of the neurologic complications associated with these anemias, a careful neurologic assessment is important, including tests of position, vibration sense, and cognitive function.

The nurse needs to pay particular attention to ambulation and should assess the patient's gait and stability, as well as the need for assistive devices (e.g., canes, walkers) and for assistance in managing daily activities. Of particular concern is ensuring safety when position sense, coordination, and gait are affected. Physical and occupational therapy referrals may be needed. If sensation is altered, the patient needs to be instructed to avoid excessive heat and cold.

Because mouth and tongue soreness may limit nutritional intake, the nurse advises the patient to eat small amounts of bland, soft foods frequently. The nurse also may explain that other nutritional deficiencies, such as alcohol-induced anemia, can induce neurologic problems.

Promoting Home, Community-Based, and Transitional Care

The patient must be taught about the chronicity of the disorder and the need for monthly vitamin B_{12} injections or daily oral vitamin B_{12} even in the absence of symptoms. If parenteral replacement is used, many patients can be taught to self-administer their injections. The gastric atrophy associated with pernicious anemia increases the risk for gastric carcinoma, so the patient needs to understand that ongoing medical follow-up and screening are important.

Hemolytic Anemias

In hemolytic anemias, the erythrocytes have a shortened lifespan; thus, their number in the circulation is reduced. Fewer erythrocytes result in decreased available oxygen, causing hypoxia, which in turn stimulates an increase in erythropoietin release from the kidney. Erythropoietin then stimulates the bone marrow to compensate by producing new erythrocytes and releasing some of them into the circulation somewhat prematurely as **reticulocytes**. If the red cell destruction persists, the hemoglobin is broken down excessively; the majority of the heme is converted to bilirubin, conjugated in the liver, and excreted in the bile (Packman, 2016). Five percent of all anemias are due to hemolysis (Broadway-Duren & Klaassen, 2013).

The mechanism of erythrocyte destruction varies, but all types of hemolytic anemia share certain laboratory features: the reticulocyte count is elevated, the fraction of indirect (unconjugated) bilirubin is increased, and the supply of **haptoglobin** (a binding protein for free hemoglobin) is depleted as more hemoglobin is released. As a result, the plasma haptoglobin level is low. If the marrow cannot compensate to replace the erythrocytes destroyed in the circulation, the anemia will progress.

Hemolytic anemia has various forms. Inherited forms include SCD, thalassemia and thalassemia major, G-6-PD deficiency, and hereditary spherocytosis. Acquired forms include autoimmune hemolytic anemia, non–immune-mediated paroxysmal nocturnal hemoglobinuria, microangiopathic hemolytic anemia, and heart valve hemolysis, as well as anemias associated with hypersplenism.

Sickle Cell Disease

SCD can cause a severe hemolytic anemia that results from inheritance of the sickle hemoglobin (HbS) gene, which causes the hemoglobin molecule to be defective. HbS acquires a crystal-like formation when exposed to low oxygen tension. The oxygen level in venous blood can be low enough to cause this change; consequently, the erythrocyte containing HbS loses its round, pliable, biconcave disc shape and becomes dehydrated, rigid, and sickle shaped (see Fig. 33-2). These long, rigid erythrocytes can adhere to the endothelium of small vessels; when they adhere to each other, blood flow to a region or an organ may be reduced. If ischemia or infarction results, the patient may have pain, swelling, and fever.

Figure 33-2 • A normal red blood cell (**upper left**) and a sickled red blood cell.

The sickling process takes time; if the erythrocyte is again exposed to adequate amounts of oxygen before the membrane becomes too rigid (e.g., when it travels through the pulmonary circulation), it can revert to a normal shape. For this reason, the "sickling crises" are intermittent. Cold can aggravate the sickling process, because vasoconstriction slows the blood flow. Oxygen delivery can also be impaired by an increased blood viscosity, with or without occlusion due to adhesion of sickled cells; in this situation, the effects are seen in larger vessels, such as arterioles.

The *HbS* gene is inherited in people of African descent and to a lesser extent in people from the Middle East, the Mediterranean area, and aboriginal tribes in India. Sickle cell anemia is the most severe form of SCD. This form of the disease is found in about 1 in 365 African American live births (National Heart, Lung, and Blood Institute, 2015). Less severe forms include sickle cell hemoglobin C (SC) disease, sickle cell hemoglobin D (SD) disease, and sickle cell beta-thalassemia. The clinical manifestations and management are the same as for sickle cell disease. The term *sickle cell trait* refers to the carrier state for SCD; it is the most benign type of SCD, in that less than 50% of the hemoglobin within an erythrocyte is HbS. One in 13 African Americans have sickle cell trait (National Heart, Lung, and Blood Institute, 2015). However, if two people with sickle cell trait have children, the children may inherit two abnormal genes and will have sickle cell disease (see Chapter 8 for additional discussion of genetic diseases).

Clinical Manifestations

Symptoms of SCD vary and are only somewhat based on the amount of HbS. Symptoms and complications result from chronic hemolysis or thrombosis. Sickled cells are rapidly hemolyzed and thus have a very short lifespan. Anemia is always present; usually, hemoglobin values range between 5 and 11 g/dL (Natrajan & Kutlar, 2016). Jaundice is characteristic and is usually obvious in the sclerae. The bone marrow expands in childhood in a compensatory effort to offset the anemia, sometimes leading to enlargement of the bones of the face and skull. The chronic anemia is associated with tachycardia, cardiac murmurs, and often an enlarged heart (cardiomegaly). Dysrhythmias and heart failure may occur in adults.

Virtually any organ may be affected by thrombosis, but the primary sites involve those areas with slower circulation, such as the spleen, lungs, and central nervous system. All tissues and organs are vulnerable to microcirculatory interruptions by the sickling process and therefore are susceptible to hypoxic damage or ischemic necrosis. Patients with SCD are unusually susceptible to infection, particularly pneumonia and osteomyelitis. Complications of sickle cell disease include infection, stroke, kidney injury, impotence, heart failure, and pulmonary hypertension (see Table 33-2).

Sickle Cell Crisis

There are three types of sickle cell crisis in the adult population. The most common is the very painful *acute vaso-occlusive crisis*, which results from entrapment of erythrocytes and leukocytes in the microcirculation, causing tissue hypoxia, inflammation, and necrosis due to inadequate blood flow to a specific region of tissue or organ. When perfusion is resumed,

TABLE 33-2 Complications in Sickle Cell Disease[a]

Organ Involved	Mechanisms[a]	Diagnostic Findings	Signs and Symptoms
Spleen	Primary site of sickling → infarctions → ↓ phagocytic function of macrophages	Autosplenectomy; ↑ infection (especially pneumonia, osteomyelitis)	Abdominal pain; fever, signs of infection
Lungs	Infection Infarction → ↑ pulmonary pressure → pulmonary hypertension	Pulmonary infiltrate ↑ sPLA$_2$[b]	Chest pain; dyspnea Chest pain; dyspnea
Central nervous system	Infarction	Stroke	Weakness (if severe); learning difficulties (if mild)
Kidney	Sickling → damage to renal medulla	Hematuria; inability to concentrate urine; kidney injury	Dehydration
Heart	Anemia	Tachycardia; cardiomegaly → heart failure	Weakness, fatigue, dyspnea
Bone	↑ Erythroid production Infarction of bone	Widening of medullary spaces and cortical thinning Osteosclerosis → avascular necrosis	Ache, arthralgias Bone pain, especially hips
Liver	Hemolysis	Jaundice and gallstone formation; hepatomegaly	Abdominal pain
Skin and peripheral vasculature	↑ Viscosity/stasis → infarction → skin ulcers	Skin ulcers; ↓ wound healing	Pain
Eye	Infarction	Scarring, hemorrhage, retinal detachment	↓ Vision; blindness
Penis	Sickling → vascular thrombosis	Priapism → impotence	Pain, impotence

→, leading to; ↓, decreased; ↑, increased; sPLA$_2$, secretory phospholipase A$_2$.
[a]Problems encountered in sickle cell disease vary and are the result of a variety of mechanisms, as depicted in this table. Common physical findings and symptoms are also variable.
[b]Elevated sPLA$_2$ levels can predict impending acute chest syndrome (see text).

substances are released (e.g., free radicals, free plasma hemoglobin) that cause oxidative damage to the vessel. In turn, the endothelium of the vessel becomes dysfunctional and vasculopathy develops (Ataga & Stocker, 2015). *Aplastic crisis* results from infection with the human parvovirus. The hemoglobin level falls rapidly and the marrow cannot compensate, as evidenced by an absence of reticulocytes (Natrajan & Kutlar, 2016). *Sequestration crisis* results when other organs pool the sickled cells. Although the spleen is the most common organ responsible for sequestration in children, most children with SCD have had a splenic infarction by 10 years of age, and the spleen is then no longer functional (autosplenectomy) (Natrajan & Kutlar, 2016). In adults, the common organs involved in sequestration are the liver and, more seriously, the lungs.

Acute Chest Syndrome

Acute chest syndrome is manifested by fever, respiratory distress (tachypnea, cough, wheezing), and new infiltrates seen on the chest x-ray; it is the main cause of death in young adults with SCD (de Prost, Sasanelli, Deux, et al., 2015). These signs often mimic infection, which is often the cause. However, the infectious etiology appears to be atypical bacteria such as *Chlamydia pneumoniae* and *Mycoplasma pneumoniae* as well as viruses such as respiratory syncytial virus and parvovirus. Other causes include pulmonary fat embolism, pulmonary infarction, pulmonary thromboembolism, and bone marrow embolism (Yawn, Buchanan, Afenyi-Annan, et al., 2014). Clinically, the patient's condition can deteriorate

rapidly, resulting in respiratory failure. Medical management includes red cell transfusion, antimicrobial therapy, bronchodilators, inhaled nitric oxide therapy, and when respiratory failure ensues, mechanical ventilation. Risk of acute chest syndrome can be reduced by the use of incentive spirometry during episodes of vaso-occlusive crisis and red cell transfusion preoperatively (Yawn et al., 2014). Although this syndrome can rapidly progress to acute respiratory distress syndrome and death, prompt and aggressive intervention can result in a favorable outcome.

Pulmonary Hypertension

Pulmonary hypertension is a common sequela of SCD, and is a common cause of death (Ataga & Klings, 2014). Diagnosing pulmonary hypertension is difficult because clinical symptoms rarely occur until damage is irreversible. Patients may complain of fatigue, dyspnea on exertion, dizziness, chest pain or syncope; however, pulse oximetry measurements are typically normal, and breath sounds are clear to auscultation until the disease has progressed to later stages. Pulmonary artery pressures are elevated above baseline but typically much lower than that seen in idiopathic or hereditary pulmonary hypertension. Screening patients with SCD with Doppler echocardiography may be useful in identifying those with elevated pulmonary artery pressures (Caughey, Poole, Ataga, et al., 2015). High levels of the amino-terminal form of brain natriuretic peptide can serve as a useful biomarker for pulmonary hypertension in this patient population and as an independent predictor of mortality (Natrajan & Kutlar,

2016). Although changes are not evident on chest x-ray, computed tomography (CT scan) of the chest often demonstrates microvascular pulmonary occlusion and diminished perfusion of the lung.

Stroke

Stroke is a devastating complication of SCD that affects 11% of patients under 20 years of age (Natrajan & Kutlar, 2016). While ischemic strokes are most common, particularly in young children and older adults, hemorrhagic stroke is more common in younger adults. The mechanisms are varied, but often result from decreased cerebral blood flow due to anemia, hemolysis, and increased hypoxic stress. Silent cerebral infarction is more common, with a prevalence of 40% (Quinn, 2014). Even without abnormal brain imaging, asymptomatic adults may have evidence of decline in neurocognitive function. These individuals are at risk for developing overt stroke (Quinn, 2014). Medical management of stroke includes red cell transfusions to reduce the level of hemoglobin S to less than 30%, thereby preventing cerebral edema (Chou, 2013).

Reproductive Problems

As patients live longer with SCD, the adverse impact on sexual function is now better appreciated. Almost 25% of men with SCD develop hypogonadism (Smith-Whitley, 2014). Low testosterone levels, low libido, erectile dysfunction, and infertility can occur. Frequent episodes of priapism (prolonged erection of the penis, typically without sexual stimulation) can also contribute to significant pain, decreased libido, and impotence. These problems can be a source of extreme embarrassment and depression. Menarche may be delayed in females, but menstrual patterns appear normal (Smith-Whitley, 2014). Pain episodes may be increased during menstruation. Fertility issues are not well assessed in women. Contraception is important when hydroxyurea (Hydrea) is used to treat SCD as it may be teratogenic. Concerns about infertility when using hydroxyurea may adversely influence adherence to this therapy among men (DeBaun, 2014). The nurse should initiate open discussions about sexual and reproductive concerns with patients prescribed this therapy.

Assessment and Diagnostic Findings

The patient with sickle cell trait usually has a normal hemoglobin level, a normal hematocrit, and a normal blood smear. In contrast, the patient with sickle cell disease has a low hematocrit and sickled cells on the smear. The white blood cell (WBC) and platelet counts are often higher than normal, attributed to a chronic inflammatory state (Natrajan & Kutlar, 2016). The diagnosis is confirmed by hemoglobin electrophoresis.

Prognosis

Patients with SCD are usually diagnosed in childhood because they become anemic in infancy and begin to have sickle cell crises at 1 or 2 years of age. Some children die in the first years of life, typically of infection, but antibiotic use and parent education strategies have greatly improved the outcomes for these children. Despite current management strategies, the average life expectancy is still suboptimal, rarely exceeding the sixth decade (Elmariah, Garrett, De Castro, et al., 2014).

Young adults often live with multiple, often severe, complications from their disease. In some patients, the symptoms and complications diminish by 30 years of age. Currently, there is no way to predict which patients will fall into this subgroup. Death is most commonly due to heart disease (32%), lung disease (28%), kidney disease (16%), infection (14%), and neurologic system disease (12%); less commonly, death results from GI tract or liver disease (9%) and cancer (<1%) (Hamideh & Alvarez, 2013).

Medical Management

Treatment for SCD is the focus of continued research. However, aside from the equally important aggressive management of symptoms and complications, there are few primary treatment modalities for SCD.

Hematopoietic Stem Cell Transplant

HSCT may cure SCD. However, this treatment modality is available to only a small subset of affected patients, either due to the lack of a compatible donor or due to severe organ damage (e.g., renal, liver, lung) that may be already present in the patient (see Chapter 15).

Pharmacologic Therapy

Hydroxyurea is a chemotherapy agent that is effective in increasing fetal hemoglobin (i.e., hemoglobin F) levels in patients with SCD, thereby decreasing the formation of sickled cells; it currently is the only FDA-approved drug for this disease (Ataga & Stocker, 2015). In a landmark study, patients who received hydroxyurea had fewer painful episodes of sickle cell crisis, a lower incidence of acute chest syndrome, and less need for transfusions (Charache, Terrin, Moore, et al., 1995); subsequent studies revealed a 40% decrease in mortality in those individuals who received the drug (Natrajan & Kutler, 2016). However, whether hydroxyurea can prevent or reverse actual organ damage remains unknown. Side effects of hydroxyurea include chronic suppression of leukocyte formation, teratogenesis, and potential for later development of a malignancy. Patient response to this agent varies significantly. The incidence and severity of side effects are also highly variable within a dose range. Adherence to taking this medication as prescribed is a common problem.

Patients with SCD may require daily folic acid replacements to maintain the supply required for increased erythropoiesis from hemolysis. Infections must be treated promptly with appropriate antibiotics; infection, particularly pneumococcal infection, is common in children. In adults, *Staphylococcus aureus* is more common, often developing within bones or joints (Natrajan & Kutlar, 2016). These patients should receive pneumococcal and annual influenza vaccinations.

Acute chest syndrome is managed by prompt initiation of antibiotic therapy. Incentive spirometry has been shown to decrease the incidence of pulmonary complications significantly (Yawn et al., 2014). In severe cases, bronchoscopy may be required to identify the source of pulmonary disease. Hydration is important but must be carefully monitored as fluid overload can develop quickly. Corticosteroids may also be useful. Transfusions reverse the hypoxia and decrease the level of secretory phospholipase A_2. Pulmonary function should be monitored regularly to detect pulmonary hypertension early, when therapy (hydroxyurea, arginine, transfusions, or HSCT) may have a positive impact.

Transfusion Therapy

RBC transfusions have been shown to be highly effective in several situations: in an acute exacerbation of anemia (e.g., aplastic crisis, severe vaso-occlusive crisis), in the prevention of severe complications from anesthesia and surgery, in improving the response to infection (when it results in exacerbated anemia), in the case of acute chest syndrome and multiorgan failure, and in thwarting the cerebral edema from a stroke. Transfusions are also effective in diminishing episodes of sickle cell crisis in pregnant women, although such transfusions do not improve fetal survival. Chronic transfusion therapy may be effective in preventing or managing complications from SCD by keeping the HbS level to less than 30% (Kim, 2014).

The risk of complications from transfusion is important to consider. These complications include poor venous access, which necessitates a vascular access device (and its attendant risk of infection or thrombosis); delayed hemolytic transfusion reactions, infections (particularly hepatitis); and iron overload, which necessitates chelation therapy (see Chapter 34, Myelodysplastic Syndromes, Nursing Management). Iron overload is likely, with the majority of iron deposition occurring within the liver; however, other organs can also develop iron deposition, notably the heart, pancreas, kidney, and pituitary. The rate of iron deposition in these organs appears to occur later than is seen in other diseases such as thalassemia major (Porter & Garbowski, 2013). In a longitudinal study of transfusions in young adults with SCD, those individuals who received chelation therapy had fewer complications; however, this reduction may have resulted from more frequent visits with health care providers than a direct effect from chelation therapy (Jordan et al., 2015). Another complication from transfusion is increased blood viscosity without reduction in the concentration of hemoglobin S. Exchange transfusion (in which the patient's own blood is removed and then replaced via transfusion) may be performed to diminish the risk of increasing the viscosity excessively; the objective is to reduce the patient's own blood volume with transfused (non-sickled) packed red cells to a target hemoglobin of 10 g/dL (Kim, 2014). Finally, it is important to consider the significant financial cost of an aggressive transfusion and chelation program. Because repeated blood transfusions are necessary, patients may develop multiple antibodies to other blood antigens, making cross-matching difficult; this process is known as alloimmunization (Yawn et al., 2014). In a study of 319 patients with SCD, 27% were alloimmunized; these patients had higher rates of avascular necrosis and end-organ damage, and shorter survival (Telen, Afenyi-Annan, Garrett, et al., 2015). Alloimmunization can develop from disparity in blood group antigens irrespective of ABO antigens between the donor (usually of European descent) and the recipient (usually of African descent). In this patient population, a hemolytic transfusion reaction (see Chapter 32) may mimic the signs and symptoms of a sickle cell crisis. The classic distinguishing factor is that with a hemolytic transfusion reaction, the patient becomes *more* anemic after being transfused. These patients need very close observation. Further transfusion is

Figure 33-3 • Chronic skin ulcers seen in a patient with sickle cell anemia. From Tkachuk, D. C., & Hirschman, J. V. (2007). *Wintrobe's atlas of clinical hematology* (Fig. 1.71, p. 36). Philadelphia, PA: Lippincott Williams & Wilkins.

avoided if possible until the hemolytic process abates, which can occur as late as 1 week after the transfusion. If possible, the patient is supported with corticosteroids (prednisone), and possibly intravenous immunoglobulin (IVIG) and erythropoietin (epoetin alfa [Epogen]).

Supportive Therapy

Supportive care is equally important. Pain management is a significant issue. Acute pain is typically caused by vaso-occlusive crisis, and is the most common reason for hospitalization or emergency department (ED) visits. Pain may also be neuropathic, resulting from damage or inflammation of peripheral nerves, as seen in avascular necrosis, or leg ulcers (see Fig. 33-3) (Darbari, Ballas, & Clauw, 2014). Chronic, non-neuropathic pain may result from central nervous system (CNS) dysfunction, increased CNS sensitivity to peripheral afferent pain signals, or differences in psychosocial aspects of pain perception (Darbari et al., 2014). The severity of the pain may not be enough to cause the patient to seek assistance from health care providers but severe enough to interfere with the ability to work and function within the family unit. The incidence of pain increases with age. In a landmark study of pain in individuals with SCD, children reported pain at home 9% of the time, but the rate increased to 55% in adults (McClish, Smith, Dahman, et al., 2009).

The use of medication to relieve acute pain is important and should be appropriate to the etiology of the pain. Aspirin is very useful in diminishing mild to moderate pain; it also diminishes inflammation and potential thrombosis (due to its ability to decrease platelet adhesion). NSAIDs are useful for moderate pain or in combination with opioid analgesics. Although no tolerance develops with NSAIDs, a "ceiling effect" does develop whereby an increase in dosage does not increase analgesia. NSAID use must be carefully monitored, because these medications can precipitate renal dysfunction. Acute pain should be treated promptly with parenteral opioids (Yawn et al., 2014). Patient-controlled analgesia is frequently used in the acute care setting (see Chapter 12 for a discussion of pain management). Neuropathic pain may be effectively managed with serotonin and norepinephrine reuptake inhibitors, tricyclic antidepressants, or gabapentinoids (Darbari et al., 2014). With chronic pain management, the principal goal is to maximize functioning; pain may not be completely eliminated without sacrificing function. This concept may be difficult for patients to accept; they may need repeated explanations and support from nonjudgmental health care providers. Nonpharmacologic approaches to pain management are crucial in this setting. Examples include physical and occupational therapy, physiotherapy (including the use of heat, massage, and exercise), cognitive and behavioral intervention (including distraction, relaxation, and motivational therapy), and support groups.

Adequate hydration is important during a painful sickling episode. Oral hydration is acceptable if the patient can maintain adequate fluid intake; IV hydration with dextrose 5% in water (D_5W) or dextrose 5% in 0.25 normal saline solution (3 $L/m^2/24$ h) may be required for a sickle crisis. Supplemental oxygen may also be needed.

Another significant problem for patients with SCD is fatigue; like pain, its cause is multifactorial. Fatigue is due to hypoxia, which in turn is due to low levels of normal hemoglobin and decreased oxygen affinity of sickled hemoglobin. The vascular endothelium becomes inflamed from the sickled red cells and resultant hypoxia. Inflammatory cytokines are increased in patients with SCD and are known to decrease muscle strength, decrease exercise capacity, increase resting energy expenditure, and decrease rapid eye movement stage of sleep—all exacerbating fatigue. Sleep disturbance and depression are common and exacerbate fatigue (Wallen, Minnitti, Krumlauf, et al., 2014). Fatigue is further increased in the setting of pain, stress, and anxiety. In a study of adolescents and young adults with SCD, fatigue was rated as moderate in intensity and interfered with school, work, exercise, and quality of life (Ameringer, Elswick, & Smith, 2014).

Working with patients who have multiple episodes of severe pain and fatigue can be challenging. Health care providers must realize that patients with SCD face a lifelong experience with severe, unpredictable pain and fatigue. These disrupt the patient's level of functioning, including social functioning, and may result in a feeling of helplessness. Patients with inadequate social support systems may have more difficulty coping with these problems.

NURSING PROCESS
The Patient With Sickle Cell Crisis

Assessment

The patient is asked to identify factors that precipitated previous crises and measures taken to prevent and manage crises. If a sickle cell crisis is suspected, the nurse needs to determine whether the pain currently experienced is the same as or different from the pain typically encountered in crisis. Pain levels should always be assessed (see Chapter 12). A similar assessment should be made of the patient's fatigue, including the impact of fatigue on current lifestyle, quality of life, and the extent that fatigue exacerbates pain and interferes with sleep.

Because the sickling process can interrupt circulation in any tissue or organ, with resultant hypoxia and ischemia, a careful assessment of all body systems is necessary. Particular emphasis is placed on pain, swelling, and fever. All joint areas are carefully examined for pain and swelling. The abdomen is assessed for pain and tenderness because of the possibility of splenic infarction.

The cardiopulmonary systems must be assessed carefully, including auscultation of breath sounds, measurement of oxygen saturation levels, and signs of cardiac failure, such as the presence and extent of dependent edema, an increased point of maximal impulse, and cardiomegaly (as seen on a chest x-ray). The patient is assessed for signs of dehydration by a history of fluid intake and careful examination of mucous membranes, skin turgor, urine output, and serum creatinine and blood urea nitrogen values.

A careful neurologic examination is important to elicit symptoms of cerebral hypoxia. However, ischemic findings on magnetic resonance imaging (MRI) or Doppler studies may precede findings on the physical examination. MRI and Doppler studies may be used for early diagnosis and may result in improved patient outcome because therapy can be initiated promptly. Cognitive dysfunction frequently occurs and may reflect inadequate oxygen delivery to the brain; it is a source of significant decline in quality of life (Quinn, 2014). Assessing for these problems is important as they develop prior to silent cerebral ischemic events or infarction.

Because patients with SCD are susceptible to infections, they are assessed for the presence of any infectious process. Particular attention is given to examination of the chest, long bones, and femoral head, because pneumonia and osteomyelitis are especially common. Leg ulcers, which may become infected and slow to heal, are common (see Fig. 33-3).

The extent of anemia and the ability of the marrow to replenish erythrocytes are assessed by the hemoglobin level, hematocrit, and reticulocyte counts; these are compared with the patient's baseline values. The patient's current and past history of medical management is also obtained, particularly chronic transfusion therapy, hydroxyurea use, and prior treatment for infection.

Diagnosis

NURSING DIAGNOSES
Based on the assessment data, major nursing diagnoses may include:

- Acute pain and fatigue related to tissue hypoxia due to agglutination of sickled cells within blood vessels
- Risk for infection
- Risk for powerlessness related to illness-induced helplessness
- Deficient knowledge regarding sickle crisis prevention

COLLABORATIVE PROBLEMS/POTENTIAL COMPLICATIONS
Potential complications may include the following:

- Hypoxia, ischemia, infection, and poor wound healing leading to skin breakdown and ulcers
- Dehydration
- Cerebrovascular disease (stroke)
- Anemia
- Acute kidney injury and chronic kidney failure
- Heart failure, pulmonary hypertension, and acute chest syndrome
- Impotence and impaired fertility
- Cognitive dysfunction
- Poor adherence to therapy
- Mutual conflict and distrust between patient and health care provider due to poorly managed acute and chronic pain

Planning and Goals

The major goals for the patient are relief of pain, decreased incidence of crisis, enhanced sense of self-esteem and power, and absence of complications.

Nursing Interventions

MANAGING PAIN

Acute pain during a sickle cell crisis can be severe and unpredictable. The patient's subjective description and rating of pain on a pain scale must guide the use of analgesic agents (see Chapter 12). Any joint that is acutely swollen should be supported and elevated until the swelling diminishes. Relaxation techniques, breathing exercises, and distraction are helpful for some patients. After the acute painful episode has diminished, aggressive measures should be implemented to preserve function. Physical therapy, whirlpool baths, and transcutaneous electrical nerve stimulation (TENS) are examples of such modalities.

MANAGING FATIGUE

The fatigue experienced can be acute or chronic in nature. Assisting the patient to find an appropriate balance between exercise and rest can be a useful strategy. Patients will need to develop strategies to cope with daily life demands in the setting of chronic fatigue. Maximizing nutrition, hydration, healthy sleep cycles, and diminishing tissue hypoxia can all serve to minimize fatigue. Research is needed to better understand fatigue in this patient population as well as to delineate the most effective ways to ameliorate it.

PREVENTING AND MANAGING INFECTION

Nursing care focuses on monitoring patients for signs and symptoms of infection. Prescribed antibiotics should be initiated promptly, and patients should be assessed for signs of dehydration. If patients are to take prescribed oral antibiotics at home, they must understand the importance of completing the entire course of antibiotic therapy.

PROMOTING COPING SKILLS

This illness can leave the patient feeling powerless and with decreased self-esteem because the acute exacerbations often result in chronic health problems. These feelings can be exacerbated by inadequate management of pain and fatigue, and enhancing management of pain and fatigue can be extremely useful in establishing a therapeutic relationship based on mutual trust. Nursing care that focuses on the patient's strengths rather than deficits can enhance effective coping skills. Providing the patient with opportunities to make decisions about daily care may increase the patient's feelings of control. The patient needs to understand the rationale for and importance of compliance with a therapeutic medication regimen.

MINIMIZING DEFICIENT KNOWLEDGE

Patients with SCD benefit from understanding what situations can precipitate a sickle cell crisis and the steps they can take to prevent or diminish such crises. Keeping warm and providing adequate hydration can be effective in diminishing the occurrence and severity of attacks.

If hydroxyurea is prescribed for a woman of childbearing age, she should be informed that the drug can cause congenital harm to unborn children and advised about pregnancy prevention.

MONITORING AND MANAGING POTENTIAL COMPLICATIONS

Management measures for many of the potential complications have been described in previous sections. Other measures follow.

Leg Ulcers. Leg ulcers require careful management and protection from trauma and contamination. Referral to a wound-ostomy-continence nurse may facilitate healing and assist with prevention. If leg ulcers fail to heal, skin grafting may be necessary. Scrupulous aseptic technique is warranted to prevent hospital-acquired infections.

Priapism Leading to Impotence. Male patients may develop sudden, painful episodes of priapism. The patient is taught to empty his bladder at the onset of the attack, exercise, and take a warm bath. If an episode persists longer than 3 hours, medical attention, which consists of IV hydration, administration of analgesic agents, and possible penile intracavernosal aspiration, is recommended. Repeated episodes may lead to extensive vascular thrombosis, resulting in impotence.

Chronic and Acute Pain. Many patients have considerable difficulty coping with chronic pain and repeated episodes of sickle cell crisis and may find it difficult to adhere to a prescribed treatment plan. Some patients with SCD develop problems with substance abuse, although the rate of abuse in this patient population is similar to populations of patients with other diseases (Natrajan & Kutler, 2016). This results from inadequate management of acute pain during episodes of crisis, which then promotes mistrust of the health care system and (from the patient's perspective) the need to seek care from other sources. In a qualitative study of health care system engagement and opioid pain use, patients with SCD who viewed themselves as "allies" and used interpersonal and symptom-specific strategies used the hospital setting less frequently for pain management than those who had a more defensive and reactive approach with their health care providers (Brown, Weisberg, Balf-Soran, et al., 2014). Receiving care from a single provider over time is much more beneficial than receiving care from rotating physicians and staff in an ED. Prior negative ED experiences often result in the patient delaying appropriate care during a subsequent painful episode (Jenerette, Brewer, & Ataga, 2014). When crises occur, the staff in the ED should be in contact with the patient's primary provider so that optimal management can be achieved. Frank, open discussion can be instrumental in promoting trust and improved outcomes. Health care providers' attitudes toward patients with SCD are also important if improved outcomes are to be achieved (Freiermuth, Haywood, Silva, et al., 2014) (see Chart 33-4).

PROMOTING HOME, COMMUNITY-BASED, AND TRANSITIONAL CARE

Educating Patients About Self-Care. Because patients with SCD are typically diagnosed as children, parents participate in the initial education. As the child ages, educational interventions prepare the child to assume more responsibility for self-care. Most families can learn about vascular access device management and chelation therapy. Nurses in outpatient facilities or home care nurses may need to provide follow-up care for patients with vascular access devices.

Continuing and Transitional Care. The illness trajectory of SCD is highly varied, with unpredictable episodes

Chart
33-4

NURSING RESEARCH PROFILE

Attitudes Toward Patients With Sickle Cell Disease in a Multicenter Sample of Emergency Department Providers

Freiermuth, C.E., Haywood, C., Silva, S., et al. (2014). Attitudes toward patients with sickle cell disease in a multicenter sample of emergency department providers. *Advanced Emergency Nursing Journal*, 36(4), 335–347.

Purpose

Pain management for vaso-occlusive crisis is a common reason patients with sickle cell disease (SCD) seek care in the emergency department (ED). An earlier systematic literature review noted strong evidence that negative attitudes from health care providers can be a barrier to adequate pain management in this patient population. Being able to accurately measure health care provider attitudes toward patients with SCD is important for assessing the efficacy of interventions to address these barriers. The purpose of this study was threefold: (1) to validate an assessment scale to assess attitudes of health care providers toward patients with SCD, (2) to measure the attitudes of health care providers working in the ED setting toward patients with SCD, and (3) to explore differences in attitudes between types of health care professionals working in the ED.

Design

A convenience sample of 214 providers (120 registered nurses [RNs], 50 resident physicians, 33 attending physicians, 11 nurse practitioners and physician assistants) from two Level 1 trauma centers in North Carolina consented to participate in this study by completing the General Perceptions about SCD Patients Scale and the Medical Condition Regard Scale (used to test the

validity of the General Perceptions scale). Demographic data from the participants were also gathered, including age, gender, ethnicity, years of experience in the role, and average number of patients with SCD cared for during an average week.

Findings

The majority of all providers were white; only 6.5% were black. When compared with physicians, nurses reported higher negative attitude scores and lower uneasiness scores; there was no significant difference in positive attitude scores between these two groups of professionals. Nurses also reported higher mean levels of frustration in caring for adults with SCD than the physicians. When compared with physicians, more nurses reported feeling that opioid addiction was prevalent in the general population of adults with SCD and in those with SCD treated in the ED. Scores related to beliefs about addiction were markedly higher in the RN group than the physician group. Given the small numbers of non-white participants, it was not possible to analyze difference in scores between ethnic groups.

Nursing Implications

Data from this study suggest that the General Perceptions about SCD Patients Scale is reliable and valid for use in health care professional staff. The data also support the need to improve attitudes of those health care professionals caring for individuals with SCD, particularly RNs, in the context of pain and pain management. Developing appropriate education, peer support, and multidisciplinary quality improvement team tracking can improve the ED care experience of patients with SCD.

---

of complications and crises. Care is often provided on an emergency basis, especially for some patients with pain management problems (see previous section). All health care providers who provide services to patients with SCD and their families need to communicate regularly with each other. Alternate methods of care delivery are being explored, such as day hospitals for acute pain management or patient-centered medical homes, where multidisciplinary care is emphasized (Raphael & Oyeku, 2013). Nurses are in an excellent position to serve as coordinators and facilitators between health care providers in a variety of settings so that the care of these patients is optimized. Patients need to learn which parameters are important for them to monitor and how to monitor them. Guidelines should also be given regarding when it is appropriate to seek urgent care.

Evaluation

Expected patient outcomes may include the following:

1. Control of pain and fatigue
   a. Uses analgesic agents to control acute pain
   b. Uses relaxation techniques, breathing exercises, and distraction to help relieve pain and fatigue
2. Absence of infection
   a. Has normal temperature
   b. Has leukocyte count within baseline range (normal: 4500/mm³ to 11,000/mm³)
   c. Identifies importance of continuing antibiotics at home (if applicable)

3. Expresses improved sense of control
   a. Participates in goal setting and in planning and implementing daily activities
   b. Participates in making decisions about care
   c. Adheres to prescribed therapy (hydroxyurea, transfusion, iron chelation)
4. Increases knowledge about disease process
   a. Identifies situations and factors that can precipitate sickle cell crisis
   b. Describes lifestyle changes needed to prevent crisis
   c. Describes the importance of warmth, adequate hydration, and prevention of infection in preventing crisis
5. Absence of complications

Thalassemias

The thalassemias are a group of hereditary anemias characterized by **hypochromia** (an abnormal decrease in the hemoglobin content of erythrocytes), extreme microcytosis (smaller-than-normal erythrocytes), hemolysis, and variable degrees of anemia. The thalassemias occur worldwide, but the highest prevalence is found in people of Mediterranean, African, and Southeast Asian ancestry (Weatherall, 2016).

Thalassemias are associated with defective synthesis of hemoglobin; the production of one or more globulin chains within the hemoglobin molecule is reduced. When this occurs, the imbalance in the configuration of the hemoglobin causes it to precipitate in the erythroid precursors or the erythrocytes themselves. This increases the rigidity of the erythrocytes and thus the premature destruction of these cells.

Thalassemias are classified into two major groups according to which hemoglobin chain is diminished: alpha or beta. The alpha-thalassemias occur mainly in people from Asia and the Middle East, and the beta-thalassemias are most prevalent in people from Mediterranean regions but also occur in those from the Middle East or Asia. However, because of extensive immigration, the prevalence of either type of thalassemia is no longer limited to geographic distribution (Weatherall, 2016). The alpha-thalassemias are milder than the beta forms and often occur without symptoms; the erythrocytes are extremely microcytic, but the anemia, if present, is mild. Alpha thalassemia seems to be very effective in protecting against severe malaria, but the mechanism of how this occurs is not well understood (Piel & Weatherall, 2014).

The severity of beta-thalassemia varies depending on the extent to which the hemoglobin chains are affected. Patients with mild forms have microcytosis and mild anemia. If left untreated, severe beta-thalassemia (i.e., thalassemia major or Cooley's anemia) can be fatal within the first few years of life. HSCT offers a chance of cure, but when this is not possible, the disease is usually treated with transfusion of PRBCs and iron chelation. Patient education during the reproductive years should include preconception counseling about the risk of thalassemia major in offspring (see Chapter 8 for discussion of genetic counseling and evaluation services).

Thalassemia major is characterized by severe anemia, marked hemolysis, and ineffective erythropoiesis. With early regular transfusion therapy, growth and development through childhood are facilitated. Organ dysfunction due to iron overload results from the excessive amounts of iron in multiple PRBC transfusions. Regular chelation therapy can reduce the complications of iron overload and prolong the life of these patients (see Myelodysplastic Syndromes section in Chapter 34). Long-term survivors of beta thalassemia may experience neurologic complications, such as cognitive dysfunction, peripheral neuropathy, and cerebrovascular disease (Nemtsas, Arnaoutoglou, Perifanis, et al., 2015). Death is often due to heart failure (Maggio, Vitrano, Calvaruso, et al., 2013).

Glucose-6-Phosphate Dehydrogenase Deficiency

The G-6-PD gene is the source of the abnormality in this disorder; this gene produces an enzyme within the erythrocyte that is essential for membrane stability. Some patients have inherited an enzyme that is so defective that they have a chronic hemolytic anemia; however, the most common type of defect results in hemolysis only when the erythrocytes are stressed by certain situations, such as fever or the use of certain medications. African Americans and people of Greek or Italian origin are those primarily affected by this disorder. In the United States, about 12% of African American males are affected (Broadway-Duren & Klaassen, 2013). The type of deficiency found in the Mediterranean population is more severe than that in the African American population, resulting in greater hemolysis and sometimes in life-threatening anemia. All types of G-6-PD deficiency are inherited as X-linked defects; however, women may also

develop the disease as one of the X chromosomes is inactivated in each cell of the female embryo. Thus, a female heterozygous for this deficiency would have half red cells normal for the enzyme and half deficient for it. Although those deficient cells are at risk for hemolysis, symptoms may be mild overall because the normal erythrocytes would not be subject to hemolysis.

Oxidant drugs have hemolytic effects for people with G-6-PD deficiency, particularly the antibacterial agents sulfadiazine, nitrofurantoin (Macrodantin) the antimalarial agents primaquine, and dapsone, as well as other medications, including phenazopyridine (Pyridium), rasburicase, (Elitek), methylthioninium chloride (methylene blue), and tolonium chloride (toluidine blue). Other medications that may be tried, but whose effectiveness is questionable, include other antimalarial agents such as chloroquine (Aralen), the sulfonamide trimethoprim–sulfamethoxazole (Bactrim, Septra), other antibacterial drugs such as moxifloxacin (Avelox) and chloramphenicol, as well as other medications that include tamsulosin (Flomax), glyburide (DiaBeta, Micronase), furosemide (Lasix), NSAIDs, and the street drug amyl nitrite ("poppers") (van Solinge & van Wijk, 2016; G6PD Deficiency Association, 2015). In affected people, a severe hemolytic episode can also result from ingestion of fava beans, menthol, tonic water, and some Chinese herbs.

Clinical Manifestations

Patients are asymptomatic and have normal hemoglobin levels and reticulocyte counts most of the time. However, several days after exposure to an offending medication or substance, they may develop pallor, jaundice, and hemoglobinuria (i.e., hemoglobin in the urine). The reticulocyte count increases, and symptoms of hemolysis develop. Special stains of the peripheral blood may then disclose Heinz bodies (degraded hemoglobin) within the erythrocytes. Hemolysis is often mild and self-limited. However, in the more severe Mediterranean type of G-6-PD deficiency, spontaneous recovery may not occur.

Assessment and Diagnostic Findings

The diagnosis is made by a screening test for the deficiency or by a quantitative assay of G-6-PD.

Medical Management

The treatment is to arrest the source and stop the offending medication. Transfusion is necessary only in the severe hemolytic state, which is more commonly seen in the Mediterranean variety of G-6-PD deficiency.

Nursing Management

Patients are educated about the disease and given a list of medications and substances to avoid. Individuals with G-6-PD deficiency should always seek advice before taking any new medication or supplement. An excellent source of this information is the G6PD Deficiency organization website (see Resources). If hemolysis develops, nursing interventions are the same as for hemolysis from other causes. Patients should be instructed to wear Medic-Alert bracelets that identify that they have G-6-PD deficiency. Genetic counseling may be indicated (see Chapter 8).

Immune Hemolytic Anemias

Hemolytic anemias can result from exposure of the erythrocyte to antibodies. Alloantibodies (i.e., antibodies against the host, or "self") result from the immunization of a person with foreign antigens (e.g., the immunization of an Rh-negative person with Rh-positive blood). Alloantibodies tend to be of the immunoglobulin G (IgG) type and cause immediate destruction of the sensitized erythrocytes, either within the blood vessel (intravascular hemolysis) or within the liver. An example of alloimmune hemolytic anemia in adults is anemia that results from a hemolytic transfusion reaction.

Autoantibodies may develop for many reasons. In many instances, the person's immune system is dysfunctional and falsely recognizes its own erythrocytes as foreign and produces antibodies against them. This mechanism is seen in people with chronic lymphocytic leukemia (CLL). Another mechanism is a deficiency in suppressor lymphocytes, which normally prevent antibody formation against a person's own antigens. The erythrocytes are sequestered in the spleen and destroyed by the macrophages outside the blood vessel (extravascular hemolysis).

Autoimmune hemolytic anemias can be classified based on the body temperature involved when the antibodies react with the RBC antigen. Warm-body antibodies are the most common (80%) and bind to erythrocytes most actively in warm conditions (37°C [98.6°F]); cold-body antibodies react in cold conditions (0°C [32°F]) (Packman, 2016). Autoimmune hemolytic anemia is associated with other disorders in most cases (e.g., medication exposure, lymphoma, CLL, other malignancy, collagen vascular disease, autoimmune disease, infection). In idiopathic autoimmune hemolytic states, the reason why the immune system produces the antibodies is not known. This primary form affects patients of all ages and both genders equally, whereas the incidence of secondary forms is greater in people older than 45 years and in females (Packman, 2016).

Clinical Manifestations

Clinical manifestations vary and usually reflect the degree of anemia. The hemolysis may range from very mild, in which the patient's marrow compensates adequately and the patient is asymptomatic, to so severe that the resultant anemia is life-threatening. Most patients complain of fatigue and dizziness. Splenomegaly is the most common physical finding; hepatomegaly, lymphadenopathy, and jaundice are also common.

Assessment and Diagnostic Findings

Laboratory tests show a low hemoglobin level and hematocrit, most often with an accompanying increase in the reticulocyte count. Erythrocytes appear abnormal; **spherocytes** (small, spherically shaped erythrocytes) are common. The serum bilirubin level is elevated, and if the hemolysis is severe, the haptoglobin level is low or absent. The Coombs test (also referred to as the direct antiglobulin test), which detects antibodies on the surface of erythrocytes, shows a positive result.

Medical Management

Any possible contributing medication should be immediately discontinued. The treatment consists of high doses of corticosteroids until hemolysis decreases; this is particularly effective in treating warm-antibody–induced hemolytic anemia (Packman, 2016). Corticosteroids decrease the macrophage's ability to clear the antibody-coated erythrocytes. If the hemoglobin level returns toward normal, usually after several weeks, the corticosteroid dose can be lowered or, in some cases, tapered and discontinued. However, corticosteroids rarely produce a lasting remission. In severe cases, blood transfusions may be required. Because the antibody may react with all possible donor cells, careful blood typing is necessary, and the transfusion should be given slowly and cautiously (Michel, 2014; Packman, 2016). Folic acid supplementation should be provided when the hemolysis is severe and the marrow is aggressively attempting to compensate by increasing erythropoietic activity (Michel, 2014).

Splenectomy (i.e., removal of the spleen) may be performed if corticosteroids do not produce a remission, because it removes the major site of erythrocyte destruction. If neither corticosteroid therapy nor splenectomy is successful, immunosuppressive agents may be given (Zanella & Barcellini, 2014). The two immunosuppressive agents most frequently used are cyclophosphamide (Cytoxan), which has a more rapid effect but more toxicity, and azathioprine (Imuran), which has a less rapid effect but less toxicity. The synthetic androgen danazol (Danocrine) can be useful in some patients, particularly in combination with corticosteroids. If corticosteroids or immunosuppressive agents are used, the taper must be very gradual over a period of several months to prevent a rebound "hyperimmune" response and exacerbation of the hemolysis. Monoclonal antibodies (e.g., rituximab [Rituxan]) can also be effective for some patients and the long-term efficacy is often years (Diericix, Kentos, & Delannoy, 2015), although this is a non–FDA-approved indication. Immunoglobulin administration is effective in about one third of patients, but the effect is transient and the medication is expensive. Transfusions may be necessary if the anemia is severe; it may be extremely difficult to cross-match samples of available units of PRBCs with that of the patient.

> ### Quality and Safety Nursing Alert
>
> *Cross-matching blood when antibodies are present can be difficult. If imperfectly cross-matched RBCs must be transfused, the nurse should begin the infusion very slowly (10 to 15 mL over 20 to 30 minutes) and monitor the patient very closely for signs and symptoms of a hemolytic transfusion reaction.*

For patients with cold-antibody hemolytic anemia, no treatment may be required other than to advise the patient to keep warm; relocation to a warm climate may be advisable. However, in other situations, the hemolysis may warrant more aggressive interventions as described previously.

Nursing Management

Patients may have great difficulty understanding the pathologic mechanisms underlying the disease and may need repeated explanations in terms they can understand. Patients who have had a splenectomy should receive the pneumonia vaccine and annual influenza vaccine and be informed that they are permanently at greater risk for infection. Patients receiving long-term corticosteroid therapy, particularly those with concurrent diabetes or hypertension, need careful monitoring. They must understand the need for the medication and the importance of never abruptly discontinuing it. A written explanation and a tapering schedule should be provided, and adjustments based on hemoglobin levels should be emphasized. Similar education should be provided when immunosuppressive agents are used. Corticosteroid therapy is not without significant risk, and patients need to be monitored closely for complications (see Table 52-5: Corticosteroid therapy and implications for nursing practice).

Hereditary Hemochromatosis

Hemochromatosis is a genetic condition in which excess iron is absorbed from the GI tract. Normally, the GI tract absorbs 1 to 2 mg of iron daily, but in those with hereditary hemochromatosis, this rate increases significantly. The excess iron is deposited in various organs, particularly the liver, skin, and pancreas; and less frequently, the heart, testes, and thyroid. Eventually, the affected organs become dysfunctional. Although hereditary hemochromatosis is diagnosed in 1% to 6% of the population in the United States (i.e., more than 1 million people), the actual prevalence is unknown because it is not always diagnosed (Reyes, Blanck, & Grossniklaus, 2015). The genetic defect associated with hemochromatosis is most commonly seen as a specific mutation (C282Y homozygosity) of the *HFE* gene. Despite the high prevalence of the genetic mutation, the actual expression of the disease is much lower; the reason for this discrepancy is unclear. The actual prevalence of hemochromatosis is lower among Asian Americans, African Americans, Latinos, and Pacific Islanders and higher in people of European descent (Adams, 2015). Women are less often affected than men because women lose iron through menses.

Clinical Manifestations

Often there is no evidence of tissue damage until middle age, because the accumulation of iron in body organs occurs gradually. Symptoms of weakness, lethargy, arthralgia, and weight loss are common and occur earlier in the illness trajectory. The skin may appear hyperpigmented from melanin deposits (and occasionally **hemosiderin**, an iron-containing pigment) or appear bronze in color. Cardiac dysrhythmias and cardiomyopathy can occur, with resulting dyspnea and edema. Endocrine dysfunction is manifested as hypothyroidism, diabetes, and hypogonadism (testicular atrophy, diminished libido, and impotence). Cirrhosis is common in later stages of the disease, shortens life expectancy, and is a risk factor for hepatocellular carcinoma (van Meer, de Man, Siersema, et al., 2013).

Assessment and Diagnostic Findings

Diagnostic laboratory findings include an elevated serum iron level and high transferrin saturation (more than 60% in men, more than 50% in women). CBC values are typically normal. The definitive diagnostic test for hemochromatosis was formerly the liver biopsy, but testing for the associated genetic mutation (i.e., C282Y homozygosity) is now more commonly used. While the prevalence of this genetic mutation is high

(1 in 200 to 300 in individuals of Northern European ancestry), the penetrance is low (13.5%) and therefore few individuals with the gene will actually develop sufficient iron overload to cause symptoms or organ dysfunction (Heeney, 2014; Kanwar & Kowdley, 2014).

Medical Management

Therapy involves the removal of excess iron via therapeutic phlebotomy (removal of whole blood from a vein). Each unit of blood removed results in a decrease of 200 to 250 mg of iron. To achieve this, frequent phlebotomy is required, initially one unit weekly. As the ferritin level decreases, the frequency of phlebotomy can be decreased as well. The goal is to maintain an iron saturation between 10% and 50% and a serum ferritin of less than 100 mcg/L (Ganz, 2016a). Evaluation of iron studies should be repeated regularly and phlebotomy resumed when the ferritin level rises. CBCs and iron panel tests should be performed regularly during a phlebotomy program to ensure the patient does not become significantly anemic. If anemia becomes moderate, a delay in phlebotomy is often adequate to correct the problem. Aggressive removal of excess iron can prevent end-organ dysfunction, particularly cardiac (e.g., cardiomyopathy, dysrhythmias), pancreas (e.g., increased insulin resistance and diabetes), skeletal (e.g., joint damage), and liver dysfunction (e.g., cirrhosis) and the complications from liver dysfunction (e.g., ascites, hemorrhage, hepatocellular carcinoma). Fatigue, skin pigmentation changes, and fibrosis may be partially reversed by achieving and maintaining normal ferritin levels (Kanwar & Kowdley, 2014).

Nursing Management

Patients with hemochromatosis often limit their dietary intake of iron, although this is not effective; however, they should be advised to refrain from taking any additional iron supplements. In addition, vitamin C intake should be limited because it enhances iron absorption. These patients must avoid any additional insults to the liver, such as alcohol abuse. Serial screening tests for hepatoma (e.g., through monitoring alpha-fetoprotein) is commonly done, despite the lack of sensitivity of the test. Other body systems should be monitored for signs of organ dysfunction, particularly the endocrine and cardiac systems, so that appropriate management can be implemented promptly. Children of patients who are homozygous for the *HFE* gene mutation should be screened for the mutation as well. Patients who are heterozygous for the *HFE* gene do not develop the disease but need to be advised that they can transmit the gene to their children.

POLYCYTHEMIA

Polycythemia refers to an increased volume of RBCs. The term is used when the hematocrit is elevated (more than 55% in males, more than 50% in females). Dehydration (decreased volume of plasma) can cause an elevated hematocrit but not typically to the level to be considered polycythemia. Polycythemia is classified as either primary or secondary. Primary polycythemia, also called *polycythemia vera,* is a proliferative disorder that is discussed in Chapter 34.

Secondary Polycythemia

Secondary polycythemia is caused by excessive production of erythropoietin. This may occur in response to a reduced amount of oxygen, which acts as a hypoxic stimulus, as in heavy cigarette smoking, obstructive sleep apnea (OSA), chronic obstructive pulmonary disease (COPD), or cyanotic heart disease, or with conditions such as living at a high altitude or exposure to low levels of carbon monoxide. It can also result from certain hemoglobinopathies (e.g., hemoglobin Chesapeake), in which the hemoglobin has an abnormally high affinity for oxygen or from genetic mutations that cause abnormally high erythropoietin levels and thus increased erythropoiesis (Prchal, 2016b). Secondary polycythemia can also occur from neoplasms (e.g., renal cell carcinoma) that stimulate erythropoietin production, excess erythropoietin-stimulating agent use, or androgen use.

Medical Management

When secondary polycythemia is mild, treatment may not be necessary; when treatment is necessary, it involves treating the primary condition. If the cause cannot be corrected (e.g., by treating the OSA or improving pulmonary function with smoking cessation), therapeutic phlebotomy may be necessary in symptomatic patients to reduce blood viscosity and volume as well as when the hematocrit is significantly elevated. However, therapeutic phlebotomy should not be used when the cause for an elevated RBC level is an appropriate, compensatory response to tissue hypoxia (Prchal, 2016b).

NEUTROPENIA

Neutropenia (a neutrophil count of less than 2000/mm³) results from decreased production of neutrophils or increased destruction of these cells (see Chart 33-5). Neutrophils are essential in preventing and limiting bacterial infection. A patient with neutropenia is at increased risk for infection from both exogenous and endogenous sources. (The GI tract and

---

Chart 33-5 Causes of Neutropenia

Decreased Production of Neutrophils

- Aplastic anemia, due to medications or toxins
- Chemotherapy
- Metastatic cancer, lymphoma, leukemia
- Myelodysplastic syndromes
- Radiation therapy

Ineffective Granulocytopoiesis

- Megaloblastic anemia

Increased Destruction of Neutrophils

- Bacterial infections
- Hypersplenism
- Immunologic disorders (e.g., systemic lupus erythematosus)
- Medication induced[a]
- Viral disease (e.g., infectious hepatitis, mononucleosis)

[a]Formation of antibody to medication, leading to a rapid decrease in neutrophils.

---

skin are common endogenous sources.) The risk of infection is based not only on the severity of the neutropenia but also on its duration. The actual number of neutrophils, known as the **absolute neutrophil count** (ANC), is determined by a simple mathematical calculation using data obtained from the CBC and differential (see Chapter 15). The risk of infection increases proportionately with the decrease in neutrophil count. The risk is low when the ANC is greater than 1000/mm³, is high when it is less than 500/mm³, and is almost certain when it is less than 100/mm³ (Dale & Welte, 2016). The duration of neutropenia is another risk factor for developing infection, as is the underlying etiology (see Chart 33-6).

Clinical Manifestations

There are no definite symptoms of neutropenia until the patient develops an infection. A routine CBC with differential, as obtained after chemotherapy treatment, can reveal neutropenia before the onset of infection.

> **Quality and Safety Nursing Alert**
>
> Patients with neutropenia often do not exhibit classic signs of infection. Fever is the most common indicator of infection, yet it is not always present, particularly if the patient is taking corticosteroids or is an older adult.

Medical Management

Treatment of the neutropenia varies depending on its cause. If the neutropenia is medication induced, the offending agent is stopped immediately, if possible. Treatment of an underlying neoplasm can temporarily make the neutropenia worse, but with bone marrow recovery, treatment may actually improve it. Corticosteroids may be used if the cause is an immunologic disorder. The use of growth factors such as granulocyte colony-stimulating factor or granulocyte-macrophage colony-stimulating factor can be effective in increasing neutrophil production when the cause of the neutropenia is decreased production. Withholding or reducing the dose of chemotherapy or radiation therapy may be required when the neutropenia is caused by these treatments; however, in the case of potentially curative therapy, administration of growth factor is considered to be preferable so that the maximum antitumor effect can be achieved by maintaining the chemotherapy regimen as originally planned (O'Brien, Dempsey, & Kennedy, 2014).

If the neutropenia is accompanied by fever, the patient is considered to have an infection and usually is admitted to the hospital. Cultures of blood, urine, and sputum, as well as a chest x-ray, are obtained. To ensure adequate therapy against the infectious organisms, broad-spectrum antibiotics are initiated as soon as the cultures are obtained, although the antibiotics may be changed after culture and sensitivity results are available.

Nursing Management

Nurses in all settings have a crucial role in assessing the severity of neutropenia and in preventing and managing complications, which most often include infections. Knowing risk factors for developing febrile neutropenia is an integral part of nursing practice, particularly for those who work with patients with cancer (O'Brien et al., 2014). Patient education is equally important, particularly at the time of

Chart 33-6 ⚠️ **RISK FACTORS**
Development of Infection and Bleeding in Patients With Hematologic Disorders

Risk of Infection

- *Severity of neutropenia:* Risk of infection is proportional to severity of neutropenia.
- *Duration of neutropenia:* Increased duration leads to increased risk of infection.
- *Nutritional status:* Decreased protein stores lead to decreased immune response and anergy.
- *Deconditioning:* Decreased mobility leads to decreased respiratory effort, leading to increased pooling of secretions.
- *Lymphocytopenia; disorders of lymphoid system (chronic lymphocytic leukemia, lymphoma, myeloma):* Decreased cell-mediated and humoral immunity.
- *Invasive procedures:* Break in skin integrity leads to increased opportunity for organisms to enter blood system.
- *Hypogammaglobulinemia:* Decreased antibody formation.
- *Poor hygiene:* Increased organisms on skin and mucous membranes, including perineum.
- *Poor dentition; mucositis:* Decreased endothelial integrity leads to increased opportunity for organisms to enter blood system.
- *Antibiotic therapy:* Increased risk for superinfection, often fungal.
- *Certain medications:* See text.

Risk of Bleeding

- *Severity of thrombocytopenia:* Risk increases when platelet count decreases; usually not a significant risk until platelet count is less than 10,000/mm^3, or less than 50,000/mm^3 when invasive procedure is performed.
- *Duration of thrombocytopenia:* Risk increases when duration increases (e.g., risk is less when duration is transient after chemotherapy than when duration is permanent with poor marrow production).
- *Sepsis:* Mechanism unknown; appears to cause increased platelet consumption.
- *Increased intracranial pressure:* Increased blood pressure leads to rupture of blood vessels.
- *Liver dysfunction:* Decreased synthesis of clotting factors.
- *Renal dysfunction:* Decreased platelet function.
- *Dysproteinemia:* Protein coats surface of platelet, leading to decreased platelet function; protein causes increased viscosity, which leads to increased stretching of capillaries and thus increased bleeding.
- *Alcohol abuse:* Suppressive effect on marrow leads to decreased platelet production and decreased ability to function; decreased liver function results in decreased production of clotting factors.
- *Splenomegaly:* Increased platelet destruction; spleen traps circulating platelets.
- *Concurrent medications:* See text.

---

hospital discharge or in the outpatient setting, so that the patient can implement appropriate self-care measures and know when and how to seek medical care (see Chart 33-7). Patients at risk for neutropenia should have blood drawn for a CBC with differential; the frequency is based on the suspected severity and duration of the neutropenia. To assess the severity of neutropenia and the risk of infection, nurses must assess patients' ANC (see Chapter 15 for formula). Nursing interventions related to neutropenia are delineated in Chapter 34.

LYMPHOPENIA

Lymphopenia (a lymphocyte count less than 1500/mm^3) can result from ionizing radiation, long-term use of corticosteroids, uremia, infections (particularly viral infections), some neoplasms (e.g., breast and lung cancers, advanced Hodgkin disease), and some protein-losing enteropathies (in which the lymphocytes within the intestines are lost) (Vasu & Caligiuri, 2016). When lymphopenia is mild, it is often without sequelae;

Chart 33-7 🏠 **HOME CARE CHECKLIST**
The Patient at Risk for Infection

At the completion of education, the patient and/or caregiver will be able to:

- State the impact of alterations in neutrophils, lymphocytes, immunoglobulins on physiologic functioning, ADLs, IADLs, roles, relationships, and spirituality.
- State changes in lifestyle (e.g., diet, activity) or home environment necessary to decrease risk for infection.
  - Maintain good hand hygiene technique, oral hygiene, total body hygiene, and skin integrity.
  - Avoid cleaning birdcages and litter boxes; consider avoiding garden work (soil) and fresh flowers in stagnant water.
  - Maintain a high-calorie, high-protein diet, with fluid intake of 3000 mL daily (unless fluids are restricted).
  - Avoid people with infections and crowds.
  - Perform deep breathing; use incentive spirometer every 4 hours while awake if mobility is restricted.

- Provide adequate lubrication with gentle vaginal manipulation during sexual intercourse; avoid anal intercourse.
- Identify signs and symptoms of infection to report to the primary provider, such as fever; chills; wet or dry cough; breathing problems; white patches in the mouth; swollen glands; nausea; vomiting; persistent abdominal pain; persistent diarrhea; problems with urination or changes in the character of the urine; red, swollen, or draining wounds; sores or lesions on the body; persistent vaginal discharge with or without itching; and severe fatigue.
- Demonstrate how to monitor for signs of infection.
- Describe to whom, how, and when to report signs of infection.
- Describe appropriate actions to take should infection occur.

ADL, activities of daily living; IADL, independent activities of daily living.

when severe, it can result in bacterial infections (due to low B lymphocytes) or in opportunistic infections (due to low T lymphocytes). T-cell lymphocyte depletion is most common, typically due to viral infection, such as the human immune deficiency virus (HIV). Excessive or prolonged abuse of alcohol can impair lymphocyte production; lymphocyte counts can improve when alcohol intake ceases (Vasu & Caligiuri, 2016).

BLEEDING DISORDERS

Failure of normal hemostatic mechanisms can result in bleeding, which may be severe. Bleeding is commonly provoked by trauma; however, in certain circumstances, it can occur spontaneously. When the cause is platelet or coagulation factor abnormalities, the site of bleeding can be anywhere in the body. When the source is vascular abnormalities, the site of bleeding may be more localized. Some patients have simultaneous defects in more than one hemostatic mechanism.

The bone marrow may be stimulated to increase platelet production (thrombopoiesis). This may be a reactive response, as in a compensatory response to significant bleeding, or a more general response to increased hematopoiesis, as in iron deficiency anemia. Sometimes, the increase in platelets does not result from increased production but from a loss in platelet pooling within the spleen. The spleen typically holds about one third of the circulating platelets at any time. If the spleen is absent (e.g., splenectomy), the platelet reservoir is also lost, and an abnormally high number of platelets enter the circulation. In time, the rate of thrombopoiesis slows to reestablish a more normal platelet level.

Clinical Manifestations

Signs and symptoms of bleeding disorders vary according to the type of defect. A careful history and physical examination can be useful in determining the source of the hemostatic defect. Abnormalities of the vascular system give rise to local bleeding, usually into the skin. Because platelets are primarily responsible for stopping bleeding from small vessels, patients with platelet defects develop **petechiae**, often in clusters; these are seen on the skin and mucous membranes and can occur throughout the body (see Fig. 33-4). Bleeding from platelet disorders can be

Figure 33-4 • Petechiae. From Wintrobe's Clinical Hematology 10th ed. (1999a). Color plate 62.4. Philadelphia, PA: Lippincott Williams & Wilkins.

severe. Unless the platelet disorder is severe, bleeding can often be stopped promptly when local pressure is applied; it does not typically recur when the pressure is released.

In contrast, coagulation factor defects do not tend to cause superficial bleeding, because the primary hemostatic mechanisms are still intact. Instead, bleeding occurs deeper within the body (e.g., subcutaneous or intramuscular hematomas, hemorrhage into joint spaces). External bleeding diminishes very slowly when local pressure is applied; it often recurs several hours after pressure is removed. For example, severe bleeding may start several hours after a tooth extraction. Risk factors for bleeding are listed in Chart 33-6.

Medical Management

Management varies based on the underlying cause of the bleeding disorder. If bleeding is significant, transfusions of blood products are indicated. The specific blood product used is determined by the underlying defect and the extent of the blood loss. If fibrinolysis is excessive, hemostatic agents such as aminocaproic acid (Amicar) can be used to inhibit this process. This agent must be used with caution, because excessive inhibition of fibrinolysis can result in thrombosis. A patient scheduled for an invasive procedure, including a dental extraction, may need a transfusion prior to the procedure to minimize the risk of excessive bleeding.

Nursing Management

Patients who have bleeding disorders or who have the potential for development of such disorders as a result of disease or therapeutic agents must be educated to observe themselves carefully and frequently for signs of bleeding (see Chart 33-8).

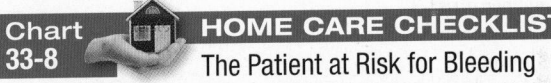

Chart 33-8 **HOME CARE CHECKLIST**
The Patient at Risk for Bleeding

At the completion of education, the patient and/or caregiver will be able to:

- Describe the source and function of platelets and clotting factors.
- State the impact of an alteration in platelets on physiologic functioning, ADLs, IADLs, roles, relationships, and spirituality.
- State changes in lifestyle (e.g., diet, activity) or home environment necessary to decrease risk of bleeding.
  - Avoid the use of suppositories, enemas, and tampons
  - Avoid constipation
  - Avoid vigorous sexual intercourse and anal sex
  - Avoid contact sports
  - Avoid or limit aggressive manual labor
  - Use an electric razor for shaving and a soft-bristled toothbrush for teeth brushing
  - Notify health care professional before having dental work or other invasive procedures
- Identify medications and other substances to avoid (e.g., aspirin-containing medications, alcohol).
- Identify signs and symptoms of bleeding.
- Demonstrate how to monitor for signs of bleeding.
- Describe to whom, how, and when to report signs of bleeding.
- Demonstrate appropriate actions to take should bleeding occur.

ADL, activities of daily living; IADL, independent activities of daily living.

They need to understand the importance of avoiding activities that increase the risk of bleeding, such as contact sports. It is necessary to examine the skin for petechiae and ecchymoses (bruises) and the nose and gums for bleeding. When bleeding disorders are severe, patients who are hospitalized are monitored for bleeding by testing all drainage and excreta (feces, urine, emesis, and gastric drainage) for occult blood as well as obvious blood.

Secondary Thrombocytosis

Increased platelet production is the primary mechanism of secondary, or reactive, **thrombocytosis**. The platelet count is above normal, but, in contrast to essential thrombocythemia (see Chapter 34), an increase of more than 1 million/mm³ is rare. Platelet function is normal; the platelet survival time is normal or decreased. Consequently, symptoms associated with hemorrhage or thrombosis are rare (Kaushansky, 2016). Many disorders or conditions can cause a reactive increase in platelets, including infection, iron deficiency, chronic inflammatory disorders, malignant disease, acute hemorrhage, and splenectomy. Treatment is aimed at the underlying disorder. With successful management, the platelet count usually returns to normal.

Thrombocytopenia

Thrombocytopenia (low platelet level) can result from various factors: decreased production of platelets within the bone marrow, increased destruction of platelets, or increased consumption of platelets (e.g., the use of platelets in clot formation). Causes and treatments are summarized in Table 33-3.

Clinical Manifestations

Bleeding and petechiae usually do not occur with platelet counts greater than 50,000/mm³, although excessive bleeding can follow surgery or other trauma. When the platelet count drops to less than 20,000/mm³, petechiae can appear, along with nasal and gingival bleeding, excessive menstrual bleeding, and excessive bleeding after surgery or dental extractions.

TABLE 33-3 Causes and Management of Thrombocytopenia

Cause	Management
Decreased Platelet Production	
Hematologic malignancy, especially acute leukemias	Treat leukemia; platelet transfusion
MDS	Treat MDS; platelet transfusion
Metastatic involvement of bone marrow from solid tumors	Treat solid tumor
Aplastic anemia	Treat underlying condition
Megaloblastic anemia	Treat underlying anemia
Toxins	Remove toxin
Medications (e.g., sulfa drugs, methotrexate)	Stop medication
Infection (especially septicemia, viral infection, tuberculosis, chronic hepatitis C)	Treat infection
Chronic alcohol abuse	Refrain from alcohol consumption
Chemotherapy	Delay or decrease dose; platelet transfusion
Chronic liver disease	Treat underlying disease
Radiation (e.g., pelvic irradiation)	Platelet transfusion
Delayed engraftment after stem cell transplantation	Platelet transfusion
Increased Platelet Destruction	
Due to antibodies:	Treat condition
ITP	
Lupus erythematosus	
Malignant lymphoma	
CLL	Treat CLL and/or treat as ITP
Medications	Stop medication
Due to infection:	Treat infection
Bacteremia/sepsis	
Postviral infection	
Sequestration of platelets in an enlarged spleen	If thrombocytopenia is severe, splenectomy may be needed
Increased Platelet Consumption	
DIC	Treat underlying condition triggering DIC; administer heparin, aminocaproic acid (Amicar), blood products
Major bleeding	Transfusion support, surgery if appropriate
Severe pulmonary embolism/severe thrombosis	Treat clot
Intravascular devices (intra-aortic balloon pump, cardiac assist devices)	Transfusion support as needed
Extracorporeal circulation (hemofiltration, extracorporeal lung assist)	Transfusion support as needed

MDS, myelodysplastic syndrome; ITP, idiopathic thrombocytopenic purpura; CLL, chronic lymphocytic leukemia; DIC, disseminated intravascular coagulation.

When the platelet count is less than 5000/mm³, spontaneous, potentially fatal central nervous system or GI hemorrhage can occur. If the platelets are dysfunctional as a result of disease (e.g., MDS) or medications (e.g., aspirin), the risk of bleeding may be much greater even when the actual platelet count is not significantly reduced, because the function of the platelets is altered.

Assessment and Diagnostic Findings

A platelet deficiency that results from decreased production (e.g., leukemia, MDS) can usually be diagnosed by examining the bone marrow via aspiration and biopsy. Numerous genetic causes of thrombocytopenia have been discovered, including autosomal dominant, autosomal recessive, and X-linked mutations. If platelet destruction is the cause of thrombocytopenia, the marrow shows increased megakaryocytes and normal or even increased platelet production as the body attempts to compensate for the decreased platelets in circulation. Hepatitis B or C can cause thrombocytopenia; thus, the patient should be screened for these diseases.

An important cause to exclude is pseudothrombocytopenia. Here, platelets aggregate and clump in the presence of ethylenediaminetetraacetic acid (EDTA), the anticoagulant present in the tube used for CBC collection. This clumping is seen in 0.8% to 1.25% of the population (Schuff-Werner, Steiner, Fenger, et al., 2013). A manual examination of the peripheral smear can easily determine platelet clumping as the cause of thrombocytopenia. Redrawing the blood in a tube anticoagulated with citrate rather than EDTA and rapidly analyzing the platelet count can provide a more accurate platelet count.

Medical Management

The management of secondary thrombocytopenia is usually treatment of the underlying disease. If platelet production is impaired, platelet transfusions may increase the platelet count and stop bleeding or prevent spontaneous hemorrhage. If excessive platelet destruction occurs, transfused platelets are also destroyed, and the platelet count does not increase. The most common cause of excessive platelet destruction is immune thrombocytopenic purpura (ITP) (see the following discussion). In some instances, splenectomy can be a useful therapeutic intervention, but often it is not an option. For example, in patients in whom the enlarged spleen is due to portal hypertension related to cirrhosis, splenectomy may cause more bleeding disorders.

Nursing Management

When selecting nursing interventions, the nurse considers the cause of the thrombocytopenia, the likely duration, and the overall condition of the patient. Education is important, as are interventions to promote patient safety, particularly fall prevention in the older adult or patient who is frail. The interventions for a patient with thrombocytopenia are the same as those for a patient with cancer who is at risk for bleeding (see Chapter 15).

Immune Thrombocytopenic Purpura

ITP is a disease that affects people of all ages, but it is more common among children and young women. Other names for the disorder are idiopathic thrombocytopenic purpura and immune thrombocytopenia. Primary ITP occurs in isolation; secondary ITP often results from autoimmune diseases (e.g., antiphospholipid antibody syndrome), viral infections (e.g., hepatitis C, HIV), and various drugs (e.g., sulfa drugs). Primary ITP is defined as a platelet count less than $100 \times 10^9/L$ with an inexplicable absence of a cause for thrombocytopenia (Neunert, 2013).

Pathophysiology

ITP is an autoimmune disorder characterized by a destruction of normal platelets by an unknown stimulus. Antiplatelet antibodies develop in the blood and bind to the patient's platelets. These antibody-bound platelets are then ingested and destroyed by the reticuloendothelial system (RES) or tissue macrophages. The body attempts to compensate for this destruction by increasing platelet production within the marrow. However, platelet production may also be impaired as the antibodies may also induce cell death (via apoptosis) of the megakaryocytes and thus inhibit platelet production within the bone marrow (Neunert, 2013).

Clinical Manifestations

Many patients have no symptoms, and the low platelet count is an incidental finding (often less than 30,000/mm³; less than 5000/mm³ is not uncommon). Common physical manifestations are easy bruising, heavy menses, and petechiae on the extremities or trunk (see Fig. 33-4). Patients with simple bruising or petechiae ("dry purpura") tend to have fewer complications from bleeding than those with bleeding from mucosal surfaces, such as the GI tract (including the mouth) and pulmonary system (e.g., hemoptysis), which is termed *wet purpura*. Patients with wet purpura have a greater risk of life-threatening bleeding than do those with dry purpura; aggressive treatment should be promptly initiated (Diz-Küçükkaya & López, 2016). Severe thrombocytopenia (platelet count less than 20,000/mm³), a history of prior minor bleeding episodes, and advanced age also are predictive of severe bleeding (Arnold, 2015). Despite low platelet counts, the platelets are young and very functional. They adhere to endothelial surfaces and to one another, so spontaneous bleeding does not always occur. Thus, treatment may not be initiated unless bleeding becomes severe or life-threatening, or the platelet count is extremely low (less than 30,000/mm³) (Diz-Küçükkaya & López, 2016).

Assessment and Diagnostic Findings

A careful history and physical assessment must be obtained to exclude causes of the thrombocytopenia and identify evidence of bleeding. Patients should be tested for hepatitis C and HIV, if not previously done to rule out these potential causes. If a bone marrow aspirate is performed, an increase in megakaryocytes may be seen. The severity of the thrombocytopenia is highly variable, but a platelet count that is less than 20,000/mm³ is a common finding.

Some patients are found to be infected with *Helicobacter pylori*, and eradicating the infection may improve platelet counts (Neunert, Lim, Crowther, et al., 2011). It is unclear why *H. pylori* and ITP are correlated, but possible causes are that *H. pylori* may trigger an autoimmune reaction or that it binds to von Willebrand factor (vWF), both of which may result in accelerated platelet demise.

Medical Management

The primary goal of treatment is a "safe" platelet count (i.e., platelets adequate to maintain hemostasis). Because the risk of bleeding typically does not increase until the platelet count is less than 30,000/mm^3, a patient whose count exceeds 30,000/mm^3 to 50,000/mm^3 may be carefully observed without additional intervention. However, if the count is less than 30,000/mm^3 or if bleeding occurs, the goal is to improve the patient's platelet count rather than to cure the disease. The decision to treat should not be made merely on the basis of the patient's platelet count but, more importantly, on the severity of bleeding (if any); likely treatment-related side effects; and the patient's lifestyle, activity level, concurrent use of medications, and overall preference. A person with a sedentary lifestyle can tolerate a low platelet count more safely than one with a more active lifestyle; however, increasing age is also associated with increased bleeding risk and mortality (Diz-Küçükkaya & López, 2016).

Treatment for ITP usually involves several approaches. If the patient is taking a medication known to be associated with ITP (e.g., quinine, sulfa-containing medications), then that medication must be stopped immediately. Transfusions tend to be ineffective because the patient's antiplatelet antibodies bind with the transfused platelets, causing them to be destroyed. Platelet counts can actually drop further after platelet transfusion. Thus, despite extremely low platelet counts, platelet transfusions are not indicated. Occasionally, transfusion of platelets may protect against catastrophic bleeding in patients with severe wet purpura. Aminocaproic acid—a fibrinolytic enzyme inhibitor that slows the dissolution of clots—may be useful for patients with significant mucosal bleeding refractory to other treatments.

The mainstay of short-term therapy is the use of immunosuppressive agents. These agents block the binding receptors on macrophages so that the platelets are not destroyed. The American Society of Hematology recommends administering the corticosteroid prednisone at a dose of 1 mg per kilogram of body weight for 21 days and then tapering the dose until the patient is off the medication (Neunert et al., 2011). Because of the associated side effects, patients cannot take high doses of corticosteroids indefinitely. Platelet counts typically begin to rise within a few days after institution of corticosteroid therapy. The platelet count tends to drop once the corticosteroid dose is tapered, but it often can remain at an adequate level.

IVIG is also commonly used to treat ITP. It is effective in binding the receptors on the macrophages; however, high doses are required, the drug is very expensive, and the effect is transient. Another approach to the management of chronic ITP involves the use of anti-D (WinRho) in patients who are Rh (D) positive. The actual mechanism of action is unknown. One theory is that the anti-D binds to the patient's erythrocytes, which are in turn destroyed by the body's macrophages. The receptors in the RES may become saturated with the sensitized erythrocytes, diminishing removal of antibody-coated platelets. Anti-D produces a transient decreased hematocrit

and increased platelet count in many, but not all, patients with ITP.

At some point, the platelet count will usually decline; at that time, additional therapy is required. Second-line therapy options should consider the patient's specific needs and potential treatment-related side effects.

Splenectomy is an alternative treatment and results in a sustained normal platelet count approximately 50% of the time, although many patients can maintain a "safe" platelet count of more than 30,000/mm^3 after the removal of the spleen (Rodeghiero & Ruggeri, 2015). Even those who do respond to splenectomy may have recurrences of severe thrombocytopenia months or years later. Patients who have undergone splenectomy are permanently at risk for sepsis and should receive pneumococcal, *Haemophilus influenzae* type B, and meningococcal vaccines, preferably 2 to 3 weeks before the splenectomy is performed (see Chapter 23 for information on pneumonia vaccine).

Other management options include certain monoclonal antibodies (e.g., rituximab). This agent may increase platelet counts for up to 1 year in 20% to 35% of those treated, but when that response is lost, the platelet count may not fall so low as to warrant additional therapy (Rodeghiero & Ruggeri, 2015).

In addition, two thrombopoietin receptor agonists have been approved for use in steroid-refractory ITP. Romiplostim (Nplate) is given weekly as a subcutaneous injection; eltrombopag (Promacta) is given orally. The timing of taking eltrombopag is somewhat complex, as the drug metabolism is altered with food and many medications. Side effects include headache, blistering of the oral mucosa, and ecchymoses. Platelet counts can fluctuate widely and treatment needs to be continued indefinitely (Rodeghiero & Ruggeri, 2015). However, in some situations, the platelet count can remain at a safe level after the drug is stopped.

Nursing Management

Nursing care includes an assessment of the patient's lifestyle to determine the risk of bleeding from activity. A careful medication history is also obtained, including use of over-the-counter (OTC) medications, herbs, and nutritional supplements. The nurse must be alert for sulfa-containing medications and others that alter platelet function (e.g., aspirin-based or other NSAIDs). The nurse assesses for any history of recent viral illness and reports of headache or visual disturbances, which could be initial symptoms of intracranial bleeding. Patients who are admitted to the hospital with wet purpura and low platelet counts should have a neurologic assessment incorporated into their routine vital sign measurements. All injections or rectal medications should be avoided, and rectal temperature measurements should not be performed, because they can stimulate bleeding.

Studies of patients with ITP have demonstrated a significant increase in fatigue compared to those without the disease that was not associated with the duration of the disease, corticosteroid use, bleeding episodes, and low platelet count (Diz-Küçükkaya & López, 2016). Nurses should explore the extent the patient experiences fatigue and offer strategies to ameliorate this problem.

Patient education addresses signs of exacerbation of disease (e.g., petechiae, ecchymoses), how to contact appropriate health care personnel, the name and type of medication inducing ITP (if appropriate), current medical treatment (medications, side effects, tapering schedule if relevant), and the frequency of monitoring the platelet count. The patient is instructed to avoid all agents that interfere with platelet function, including herbal therapies and OTC medications. The patient should avoid constipation, the Valsalva maneuver (e.g., straining at stool), and vigorous flossing of the teeth. Electric razors should be used for shaving, and soft-bristled toothbrushes should replace stiff-bristled ones. The patient may also be counseled to refrain from vigorous sexual intercourse when the platelet count is less than 10,000/mm³. Patients who are receiving corticosteroids long term are at risk for complications including osteoporosis, proximal muscle wasting, cataract formation, and dental caries (see Table 52-5). Bone mineral density should be monitored, and these patients may benefit from calcium and vitamin D supplementation and bisphosphonate therapy to prevent significant bone disease.

Platelet Defects

Quantitative platelet defects (i.e., thrombocytopenia, thrombocytosis) are relatively common; however, qualitative defects can also occur. With qualitative defects, the number of platelets may be normal but the platelets do not function normally. A platelet function analyzer is used to evaluate platelet function; this method is particularly valuable for rapid and simple screening. Examining the platelet morphology (via peripheral smear evaluation) can also be useful in assessing potential qualitative defects. The morphology of platelets is often hypogranular and pale, and may be larger than normal.

Aspirin may induce a platelet disorder. Even small amounts of aspirin reduce normal platelet aggregation, and the prolonged bleeding time lasts for several days after aspirin ingestion. Although this does not cause bleeding in most people, patients with a coagulation disorder (e.g., hemophilia) or thrombocytopenia can have significant bleeding after taking aspirin, particularly if invasive procedures or trauma have occurred.

NSAIDs can also inhibit platelet function, but the effect is not as prolonged as with aspirin (about 4 days vs. 7 to 10 days). Other causes of platelet dysfunction include end-stage renal disease, possibly from metabolic products affecting platelet function; MDS; multiple myeloma (due to abnormal protein interfering with platelet function); cardiopulmonary bypass; herbal therapy; and other medications (see Chart 33-9).

Clinical Manifestations

Bleeding may be mild or severe. Its extent is not necessarily correlated with the platelet count or with tests that measure coagulation (prothrombin time [PT], activated partial thromboplastin time [aPTT]). However, results from these tests may help determine the specific etiology of the bleeding disorder, if results from one are abnormal and the results from the other two are normal (Levi, Seligsohn, & Kaushansky, 2016). For example, an elevated PT in the setting of a normal aPTT and platelet count may suggest factor VII deficiency, whereas an elevated partial thromboplastin time (PTT) in the setting of a normal PT and platelet count may suggest hemophilia or von Willebrand disease (vWD). Ecchymoses are common,

particularly on the extremities. Patients with platelet dysfunction may be at risk for significant bleeding after trauma or invasive procedures (e.g., biopsy, dental extraction).

Medical Management

If the platelet dysfunction is caused by medication, its use should be stopped, if possible, particularly when bleeding occurs. If platelet dysfunction is marked, bleeding can often be prevented by transfusion of normal platelets before invasive procedures. Antifibrinolytic agents (e.g., aminocaproic acid) may be required to prevent significant bleeding after such procedures; desmopressin (DDAVP) can decrease the duration of bleeding in some situations and improve hemostasis (Levi et al., 2016).

Nursing Management

Patients with significant platelet dysfunction need to be instructed to avoid substances that can diminish platelet function, such as certain OTC medications, some herbal therapies, nutritional supplements, and alcohol. They also need to inform their health care providers (including dentists) of the underlying condition before any invasive procedure is performed so that appropriate steps can be initiated to diminish the risk of bleeding. Maintaining good oral hygiene is very important so that gingival bleeding can be minimized.

Hemophilia

Two inherited bleeding disorders—hemophilia A and hemophilia B—are clinically indistinguishable, although they can be distinguished by laboratory tests. Hemophilia A is caused by a genetic defect that results in deficient or defective factor VIII. Hemophilia B (also called *Christmas disease*) stems from a genetic defect that causes deficient or defective factor IX. Hemophilia is a relatively common disease; hemophilia A occurs in 1 of every 5000 to 7000 births and is five times more common than hemophilia B (Escobar & Key, 2016). Both types of hemophilia are inherited as X-linked traits, so most affected people are males; females can be carriers but are almost always asymptomatic. However, it is estimated that one third of cases result from spontaneous mutations, rather than through familial transmission (Dunn, 2015). The disease occurs in all ethnic groups (Escobar & Key, 2016).

The tendency for developing bleeding serves as the basis for hemophilia classification (Escobar & Key, 2016):

- Severe disease is defined as a plasma factor activity level of less than 1 IU/dL, or less than 1% normal factor VIII levels
- Moderate disease reflects a level of 1–5 IU/dL or factor VIII level between 1% and 5% of normal
- Mild disease reflects a level above 5 IU/dL or factor VIII level above 5%

Hemophilia is recognized in early childhood, usually in the toddler age group. However, patients with mild hemophilia may not be diagnosed until they experience severe trauma (e.g., a high school football injury) or surgery.

Clinical Manifestations

Hemophilia is manifested by hemorrhages into various parts of the body; these hemorrhages can be severe and can occur

Chart 33-9 PHARMACOLOGY
Medications and Substances That Impair Platelet Function

Anesthetic Agents

Halothane (Fluothane)
Local anesthetic agents

Antibiotics

Aminoglycosides
Beta-lactam antibiotics
  Penicillins
  Cephalosporins
Nitrofurantoin
Sulfonamides

Anticoagulation and Antiplatelet Agents

Abciximab (ReoPro)
Antithrombin agents
Clopidogrel (Plavix)
Dipyridamole (Persantine)
Fibrinolytic agents
Heparin
  Unfractionated heparin
  Low–molecular-weight heparins
Ticlopidine (Ticlid)
Tirofiban (Aggrastat)

Anti-Inflammatory Agents (Nonsteroidal)

Aspirin
Colchicine (Colcrys)
Ibuprofen (Advil, Motrin)
Indomethacin (Indocin)
Naproxen (Aleve)

Antineoplastic Agents

Carmustine (BCNU)
Daunorubicin (Cerubidine)
Mithramycin (Mithracin)
Vinblastine (Velban)
Vincristine (Oncovin)

Cardiovascular/Respiratory Drugs

Angiotensin-converting enzyme inhibitors
Angiotensin receptor blockers
Beta-blockers
Calcium channel blockers
Cilostazol (Pletal)
Clofibrate (Atromid-S)
Diuretics
  Ethacrynic acid (Edecrin)
  Furosemide (Lasix)
Hydralazine (Apresoline)
Methylxanthines
  Aminophylline
  Theophylline (Theo-Dur)

Nitrates
  Isosorbide (Isordil)
Phentolamine (Regitine)
Prasugel (Effient)
Prostacyclin
Quinidine

Food and Food Additives

Caffeine
Chinese black tree fungus
Clove
Cumin
Ethanol (i.e., alcohol)
Fish oils
Garlic
Ginger
Onion extract
Turmeric

Plasma Expanders

Dextrans
Hydroxyethyl starch (HES)

Psychotropic Agents

Phenothiazines
Serotonin Reuptake Inhibitors
  Fluoxetine (Prozac)
  Fluvoxamine (Luvox)
  Paroxetine (Plaxil)
  Sertraline (Zoloft)
Tricyclic antidepressants
  Doxepin (Sinequan)
  Imipramine (Tofranil)
Valproic acid (Dapacon)

Miscellaneous

Antihistamines
Contrast agents
Glyceryl guaiacolate (cough syrup base)
Hepatitis B vaccine
Heroin
Hydroxychloroquine (Plaquenil; Quineprox)
Phenytoin (Dilantin)
Vitamin E

Herbal Supplements

Feverfew
Gingko
Ginseng
Kava kava

even after minimal trauma. The frequency and severity of the bleeding depend on the degree of factor deficiency as well as the intensity of the precipitating trauma. For example, patients with a mild factor VIII deficiency rarely develop hemorrhage spontaneously; hemorrhage tends to occur secondary to trauma. In contrast, spontaneous hemorrhages, particularly hemarthroses and hematomas, can frequently occur in patients with severe factor VIII deficiency (Escobar & Key, 2016).

About 75% of all bleeding in patients with hemophilia occurs into joints. The most commonly affected joints are the knees, elbows, ankles, shoulders, wrists, and hips. Patients often note pain in a joint before they are aware of swelling and limitation of motion. Recurrent joint hemorrhages can result in damage so severe that chronic pain, ankylosis (fixation), or arthropathy of the joint occurs (see Fig. 33-5). Patients with severe factor deficiency can become disabled by the joint

Figure 33-5 • Hemophilic arthropathy: Sequelae of recurrent joint bleeding. From Wintrobe's Clinical Hematology 10th ed. (1999b). Color plate 68. Philadelphia, PA: Lippincott Williams & Wilkins.

damage before they become adults. Bleeding can be superficial as hematomas or as deep hemorrhages into muscle or subcutaneous tissue. With severe factor VIII deficiency, hematomas can occur without known trauma and progressively extend in all directions. When the hematomas occur within muscle, particularly in the extremities, peripheral nerves can be compressed. Over time, this compression results in decreased sensation, weakness, and atrophy of the area involved.

Bleeding is not limited to the joints and muscles. Bleeding is commonly associated with dental extraction. Spontaneous hematuria and GI bleeding can also occur. Bleeding is also common in other mucous membranes, such as the nasal passages, and in soft tissues. The most dangerous site of hemorrhage is in the head (intracranial or extracranial). Any head trauma requires prompt evaluation and treatment. Surgical procedures typically result in excessive bleeding at the surgical site. Because clot formation is poor, wound healing may also be poor.

Falls carry significant risk for morbidity in adults. A retrospective study of 74 adults over age 40 with severe or moderate hemophilia and independent in their mobility was evaluated for risk factors for falling (Sammels, Vandesande, Vlaeyen, et al., 2014). Falling was not uncommon in this sample; 32.4% fell in the previous year, and 42% of those who fell did so repeatedly (i.e., average 4 falls yearly). Most falls occurred outdoors and among those adults more physically active. This finding differs from other research that suggests physical activity decreased fall risk and may be due to higher confidence and thus less care when ambulating. Arthropathy and urinary incontinence were also associated with increased fall risk.

Medical Management

Recombinant forms of factor VIII and X concentrates are available and decrease the need for using factor concentrates, or, more infrequently, fresh-frozen plasma. Patients are given concentrates when they are actively bleeding; it is crucial to initiate treatment as soon as possible so that bleeding complications can be avoided. Prophylactic use of these factors as a preventive measure before traumatic procedures (e.g., lumbar puncture, dental extraction, surgery) is an important strategy

in preventing bleeding (Escobar & Key, 2016). Children typically receive factor administration prophylactically, three to four times each week; this approach has markedly reduced the incidence and severity of joint complications (Josephson, 2013). However, cost and adherence can limit the effectiveness of this approach. Studies suggest that initiating a prophylactic program later in life (adolescents or young adults) can still afford a positive outcome on joint complications, pain, physical function, and quality of life (Josephson, 2013).

Developing neutralizing antibodies (inhibitors) to factor concentrates is the most significant complication of factor replacement therapy. Between 13% and 33% of patients with hemophilia A and up to 3% of patients with hemophilia B develop antibodies (inhibitors) to factor concentrates (Kempton & Meeks, 2014). Although one third of such inhibitors are transient, their effects can be significant and induce partial or complete refractoriness to factor replacement, thus resulting in a markedly increased risk of bleeding. Treatment success is optimal when antibody titers remain low; thus, it is important to identify rising titers and act promptly. The mainstay of inhibitor management is inducing immune tolerance. Special formulations of factor replacement products are given on a daily basis. Some form of immunosuppression therapy (e.g., cyclophosphamide, IVIG, prednisone) may be used to facilitate eradicating the inhibitor. Patients with severe factor deficiency should be screened for antibodies, particularly before major surgery so that appropriate therapy can be initiated and major bleeding complications from surgery averted.

Other therapeutic options include administering recombinant factor VIIa (Novoseven, Novo Nordixk) or activated prothrombin complex concentrates (IaPCC, FEIBA) (Kempton & Meeks, 2014). An efficacy of 80% has been reported for both agents (Kempton & Meeks, 2014).

Aminocaproic acid inhibits fibrinolysis and therefore stabilizes the clot; it is very effective as an adjunctive measure after oral surgery and in treating mucosal bleeding. Another agent—desmopressin—induces a significant but transient rise in factor VIII levels; the mechanism for this response is unknown. In patients with mild forms of hemophilia A, desmopressin is extremely useful, significantly reducing the amount of blood products required. However, desmopressin is not effective in patients with severe factor VIII deficiency (Collins, Chalmers, Hart, et al., 2013).

Nursing Management

Most patients with hemophilia are diagnosed as children. They often require assistance in coping with the condition because it is chronic, places restrictions on their lives, and is an inherited disorder that can be passed to future generations. From childhood, patients are helped to cope with the disease and to identify the positive aspects of their lives. They are encouraged to be self-sufficient and to maintain independence by preventing unnecessary trauma that can cause acute bleeding episodes and temporarily interfere with normal activities. As they work through their feelings about the condition and progress to accepting it, they can assume more and more responsibility for maintaining optimal health.

Patients with mild factor deficiency may not be diagnosed until adulthood if they do not experience significant trauma or surgery as children. These patients need extensive education about activity restrictions and self-care measures to diminish the chance of hemorrhage and complications of bleeding. The nurse should emphasize safety at home and in the workplace.

Patients and family members are instructed how to administer the factor concentrate at home at the first sign of bleeding so that bleeding is minimized and complications avoided. The use of prophylactic factor replacement can be very effective in diminishing the morbidity associated with repeated bleeding. However, this method requires administration of these factors as often as two to three times each week. Adherence to prophylactic infusions can problematic. A recent study reported the adherence rate to be only 76%; those who had used prophylactic therapy for longer periods of time had higher adherence rates (Ho, Gue, McIntosh, et al., 2014). Nurses can assist patients to consider that the potential benefits of prophylactic therapy outweigh the disadvantages (i.e., time-consuming), particularly early in prophylaxis therapy. Patients with hemophilia are instructed to avoid agents that interfere with platelet aggregation, such as aspirin, NSAIDs, some herbal and nutritional supplements (e.g., chamomile, nettle, alfalfa), and alcohol. This restriction applies to OTC medications such as cold remedies. Oral hygiene is very important as a preventive measure because dental extractions are hazardous. Applying pressure to a minor wound may be sufficient to control bleeding if the factor deficiency is not severe. Nasal packing should be avoided, because bleeding frequently resumes when the packing is removed. Splints and other orthopedic devices may be useful in patients with joint or muscle hemorrhages. All injections should be avoided; invasive procedures (e.g., endoscopy, lumbar puncture) should be minimized or performed after administration of appropriate factor replacement. Patients with hemophilia should carry or wear medical identification (e.g., Medic-Alert bracelets). In addition, patients or families should have a written emergency plan that includes what to do in specific situations as well as names and phone numbers of emergency contacts.

During hemorrhagic episodes, the extent of bleeding must be assessed carefully. Patients who are at risk for significant compromise (e.g., bleeding into the respiratory tract or brain) warrant close observation and systematic assessment for emergent complications (e.g., respiratory distress, altered level of consciousness). If the patient has had recent surgery, the nurse frequently and carefully assesses the surgical site for bleeding. Frequent monitoring of vital signs is needed until the nurse is certain that there is no excessive postoperative bleeding.

Analgesic agents are commonly required to alleviate the pain associated with hematomas and hemorrhage into joints. Many patients report that warm baths promote relaxation, improve mobility, and lessen pain. However, during bleeding episodes, heat is avoided because it can accentuate bleeding; applications of cold are used instead.

Although the formulation of heat-solvent or detergent-treated factor concentrates has rendered factor VIII and IX preparations free of viruses such as HIV and hepatitis C, many patients treated prior to 1985 have already been exposed to these viruses through previous transfusions (Escobar & Key, 2016). These patients and their families may need assistance in coping with the diagnosis and the consequences of these infections.

Genetic testing and counseling should be provided to female carriers so that they can make informed decisions regarding having children and managing pregnancy (see Chapter 8).

Gerontologic Considerations

With improved therapy, the average lifespan of the patient with hemophilia continues to rise. Several unique challenges are seen in this patient population. The older adult patient with hemophilia was likely managed with blood component transfusion, at least early in life. Thus, hepatitis B and C infections are very common in this population, particularly hepatitis C (Canaro, Goranova-Marinova, & Berntorp, 2014); patients with HIV or hepatitis C are at increased risk for liver disease, which can be fatal. Intracranial hemorrhage is the third most common cause of death after HIV and hepatitis and may not result from trauma. The likelihood of acquiring inhibitors, especially hemophilia A inhibitors, also increases with age.

Although patients with hemophilia less commonly have concomitant cardiovascular disease, it is difficult to manage when it is present. Coronary bypass graft surgery is extremely high risk, as are stent placements. Antiplatelet therapy (including aspirin) can be challenging in those with severe hemophilia. Close coordination of care with a hematologist can improve outcomes.

Arthropathy is a major cause of morbidity in older patients with hemophilia and results in diminished range of motion, and chronic pain (Canaro et al., 2014). Pain management can be challenging as NSAID use is contraindicated due to the increased risk of bleeding.

Von Willebrand Disease (vWD)

Usually inherited as a dominant trait, vWD is a common bleeding disorder that affects males and females equally. The prevalence of this disease is estimated to be 1% to 2% of the population (National Hemophilia Foundation, 2014). The disease is caused by a deficiency of vWF, which is necessary for factor VIII activity. vWF is also necessary for platelet adhesion at the site of vascular injury. Although synthesis of factor VIII is normal, its half-life is shortened; therefore, factor VIII levels commonly are mildly low (15% to 50% of normal).

There are three types of vWD. Type 1, the most common, is characterized by decreases in structurally normal vWF. Type 2 shows variable qualitative defects based on the specific vWF subtype involved. Type 3 is very rare (less than 5% of cases) and is characterized by a severe vWF deficiency as well as significant deficiency of factor VIII. Figure 33-6 depicts the abnormal differences in clotting found in hemophilia and vWD.

Clinical Manifestations

Bleeding tends to be mucosal. Patients commonly have recurrent nosebleeds, easy bruising, heavy menses, prolonged bleeding from cuts, and postoperative bleeding. Massive soft tissue or joint hemorrhages are not often seen, unless the patient has severe type 3 vWD. As the laboratory values

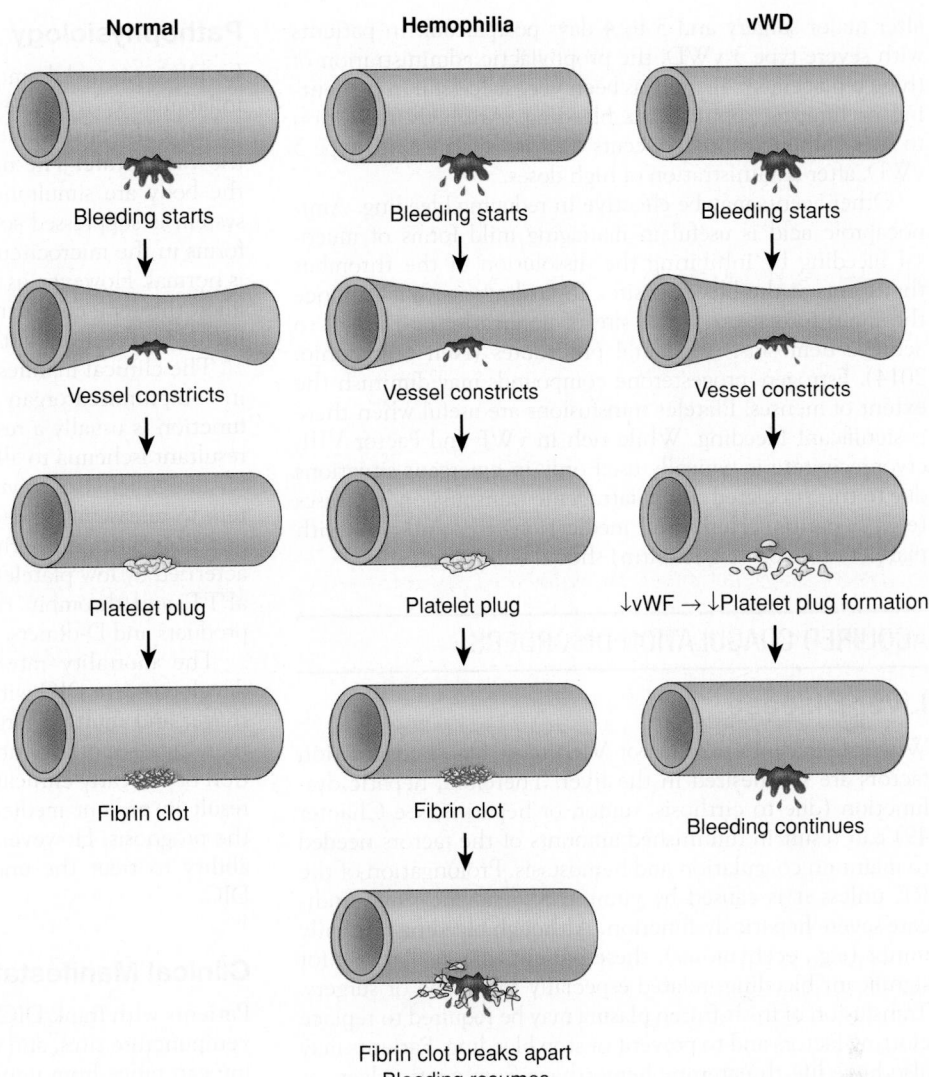

Normal	Hemophilia	vWD
Bleeding starts	Bleeding starts	Bleeding starts
Vessel constricts	Vessel constricts	Vessel constricts
Platelet plug	Platelet plug	↓vWF → ↓Platelet plug formation
Fibrin clot	Fibrin clot	Bleeding continues
		Fibrin clot breaks apart Bleeding resumes

Figure 33-6 • Differences in bleeding. Normal, hemophilia, and Von Willebrand disease (vWD). From Thomas, M., & Morrow, K. *Veterans Administration Palo Alto Health Care System*. Palo Alto: CA.

fluctuate (see the following Assessment and Diagnostic Findings section), so does the bleeding. For example, a careful history of prior bleeding may show little problem with postoperative bleeding on one occasion but significant bleeding from a dental extraction at another time.

Assessment and Diagnostic Findings

The diagnosis is established by the patient meeting all of these criteria: a history of bleeding since childhood, reduced vWF activity in plasma, and a history of bleeding within the family (Federici, 2014). Laboratory test results show a normal platelet count but a prolonged bleeding time and a slightly prolonged aPTT. These defects are not static, and laboratory test results can vary widely within the same patient over time. Thus, it is crucial to review these values over time rather than rely on a single measurement. More important tests include the ristocetin cofactor, or vWF collagen binding assay, which measures vWF activity. While these tests are specific for vWF abnormalities, they are not very sensitive. Thus, other tests are often needed to establish the diagnosis, such as the vWF antigen, factor VIII, and, for patients with suspected type 2 defects, vWF multimers, which measure specific subtypes of vWF.

Medical Management

The goal of treatment is to replace the deficient protein (e.g., vWF or factor VIII) at the time of spontaneous bleeding or prior to an invasive procedure to prevent subsequent bleeding. Desmopressin, a synthetic vasopressin analogue, can be used to prevent bleeding associated with dental or surgical procedures or to manage mild bleeding after surgery in those individuals with mild vWD, although it is often ineffective in treating those with type 3 vWD (Neff & Sidonio, 2014). Desmopressin provides a transient increase in factor VIII coagulant activity and may also correct the bleeding time. Desmopressin can be given as an IV infusion or intranasally. With major surgery or invasive procedures, IV administration is preferable. Side effects include headache, facial flushing, and tachycardia. With repeated doses, hyponatremia, and, rarely, seizures can occur; therefore, the drug is rarely given beyond 3 consecutive days.

Replacement products include Humate-P and Alphanate, which are commercial concentrates of vWF and factor VIII. The dosage and frequency of administration of these agents depend on the patient's factor VIII levels and the extent of bleeding. Treatment may be necessary for up to 7 to 10 days after major surgery and 3 to 4 days postpartum. In patients with severe type 3 vWD, the prophylactic administration of these replacement agents has been very successful in preventing or limiting spontaneous bleeding. Antibody formation to these products usually occurs only in patients with type 3 vWD, after administration of high doses.

Other agents may be effective in reducing bleeding. Aminocaproic acid is useful in managing mild forms of mucosal bleeding by inhibiting the dissolution of the thrombus that forms at the bleeding site. Topical agents that enhance thrombin formation at the site of application are useful to achieve hemostasis in dental procedures (Neff & Sidonio, 2014). Estrogen–progesterone compounds may diminish the extent of menses. Platelet transfusions are useful when there is significant bleeding. While rich in vWF and Factor VIII, cryoprecipitate is typically used only in emergent situations due to the associated risk of iatrogenic transmission of viruses (e.g., hepatitis). Herbs and medications that interfere with platelet function (e.g., aspirin) should be avoided.

ACQUIRED COAGULATION DISORDERS

Liver Disease

With the exception of factor VIII, most blood coagulation factors are synthesized in the liver. Therefore, hepatic dysfunction (due to cirrhosis, tumor, or hepatitis; see Chapter 49) can result in diminished amounts of the factors needed to maintain coagulation and hemostasis. Prolongation of the PT, unless it is caused by vitamin K deficiency, may indicate severe hepatic dysfunction. Although bleeding is usually minor (e.g., ecchymoses), these patients are also at risk for significant bleeding, related especially to trauma or surgery. Transfusion of fresh-frozen plasma may be required to replace clotting factors and to prevent or stop bleeding. Patients may also have life-threatening hemorrhage from peptic ulcers or esophageal varices. In these cases, replacement with fresh-frozen plasma, PRBCs, and platelets is usually required.

Vitamin K Deficiency

The synthesis of many coagulation factors depends on vitamin K. Vitamin K deficiency is common in malnourished patients. Prolonged use of some antibiotics decreases the intestinal flora that produces vitamin K, depleting vitamin K stores. Administration of vitamin K (phytonadione [Mephyton]), either orally or as a subcutaneous injection, can correct the deficiency quickly; adequate synthesis of coagulation factors is reflected by normalization of the PT.

Disseminated Intravascular Coagulation

Disseminated intravascular coagulation (DIC) is not an actual disease but a sign of an underlying condition. DIC may be triggered by sepsis, trauma, cancer, shock, abruptio placentae, toxins, allergic reactions, and other conditions; the vast majority (two thirds) of cases of DIC are initiated by an infection or a malignancy (Levi & Seligsohn, 2016). The severity of DIC is variable, but it is potentially life-threatening.

Pathophysiology

In DIC, normal hemostatic mechanisms are altered. The inflammatory response generated by the underlying disease initiates the process of inflammation and coagulation within the vasculature. The natural anticoagulant pathways within the body are simultaneously impaired, and the fibrinolytic system is suppressed so that a massive amount of tiny clots forms in the microcirculation. Initially, the coagulation time is normal. However, as the platelets and clotting factors form microthrombi, coagulation fails. Thus, the paradoxical result includes excessive clotting and bleeding (see Fig. 33-7).

The clinical manifestations of DIC are primarily reflected in compromised organ function or failure. Decline in organ function is usually a result of excessive clot formation (with resultant ischemia to all or part of the organ) or, less often, of bleeding. The excessive clotting triggers the fibrinolytic system to release fibrin degradation products, which are potent anticoagulants, furthering the bleeding. The bleeding is characterized by low platelet and fibrinogen levels; prolonged PT, aPTT, and thrombin time; and elevated fibrin degradation products and D-dimers.

The mortality rate can exceed 80% in patients who develop severe DIC with ischemic thrombosis, frank hemorrhage, and multiple organ dysfunction syndrome (MODS). Identification of patients who are at risk for DIC and recognition of the early clinical manifestations of this syndrome can result in prompt medical intervention, which may improve the prognosis. However, the primary prognostic factor is the ability to treat the underlying condition that precipitated DIC.

Clinical Manifestations

Patients with frank DIC may bleed from mucous membranes, venipuncture sites, and the GI and urinary tracts. The bleeding can range from minimal occult internal bleeding to profuse hemorrhage from all orifices. Patients typically develop MODS, and they may exhibit acute kidney injury as well as pulmonary and multifocal central nervous system infarctions as a result of microthromboses, macrothromboses, or hemorrhages.

During the initial process of DIC, the patient may have no new symptoms—the only manifestation being a progressive decrease in the platelet count. As the thrombosis becomes more extensive, the patient exhibits signs and symptoms of thrombosis in the organs involved. Then, as the clotting factors and platelets are consumed to form these thrombi, bleeding occurs. Initially, the bleeding is subtle, but it can develop into frank hemorrhage. Signs and symptoms depend on the organs involved and are listed in Chart 33-10.

Assessment and Diagnostic Findings

Clinically, the diagnosis of DIC is often established by laboratory tests that reflect consumption of platelets and clotting factors (i.e., drop in platelet count, an elevation in fibrin degradation products and D-dimer, an increase in PT and aPTT, and a low fibrinogen level) (see Table 33-4). Although each of these tests is useful in establishing the diagnosis of DIC, the specificity of each individual parameter is lacking, although D-dimer levels are more accurate than fibrin degradation

Physiology/Pathophysiology

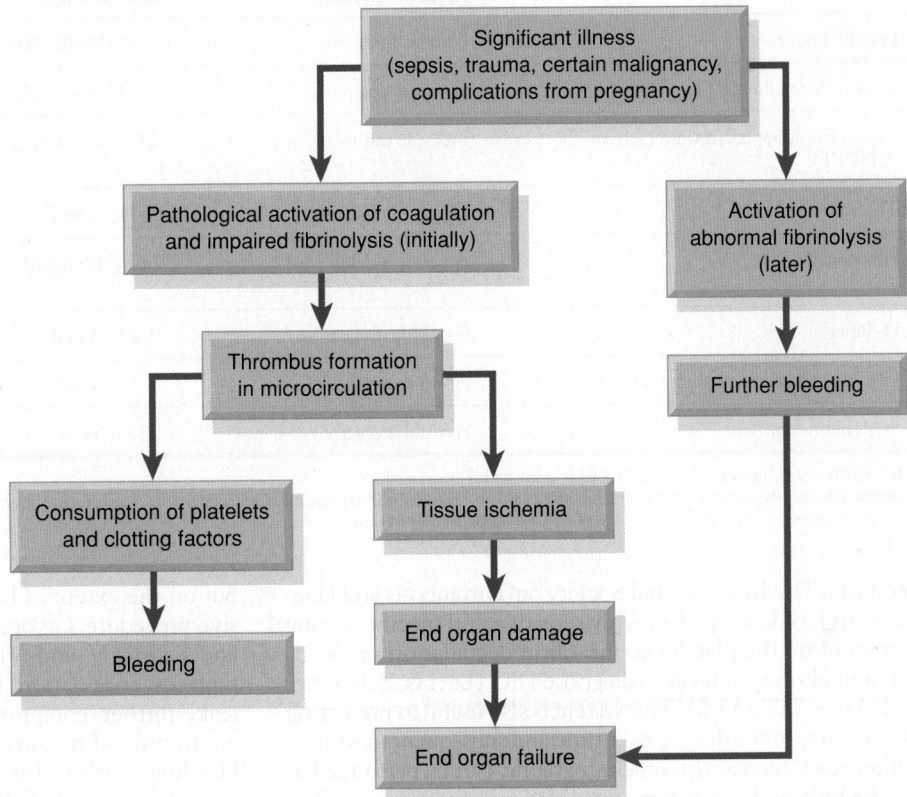

Figure 33-7 • Pathophysiology of disseminated intravascular coagulation.

Chart 33-10

ASSESSMENT

Assessing for Thrombosis and Bleeding in Disseminated Intravascular Coagulation

System	Signs and Symptoms of Microvascular Thrombosis	Signs and Symptoms of Microvascular and Frank Bleeding
Integumentary (skin)	↓ Temperature, sensation; ↑ pain; cyanosis in extremities, nose, earlobes; focal ischemia, superficial gangrene	Petechiae, including periorbital and oral mucosa; bleeding: gums, oozing from wounds, previous injection sites, around catheters (IVs, tracheostomies); epistaxis; diffuse ecchymoses; subcutaneous hemorrhage; joint pain
Circulatory	↓ Pulses; capillary filling time >3 seconds	Tachycardia
Respiratory	Hypoxia (secondary to clot in lung); dyspnea; chest pain with deep inspiration; ↓ breath sounds over areas of large embolism	High-pitched bronchial breath sounds; tachypnea; ↑ consolidation; signs and symptoms of acute respiratory distress syndrome
Gastrointestinal	Gastric pain; "heartburn"	Hematemesis (heme⊕ nasogastric output); melena (heme⊕ stools → tarry stools → bright-red blood from rectum); retroperitoneal bleeding (abdomen firm and tender to palpation; distended; ↑ abdominal girth)
Renal	↓ Urine output; ↑ creatinine, ↑ blood urea nitrogen	Hematuria
Neurologic	↓ Alertness and orientation; ↓ pupillary reaction; ↓ response to commands; ↓ strength and movement ability	Anxiety; restlessness; ↓ mentation, altered level of consciousness; headache; visual disturbances; conjunctival hemorrhage

↓, decreased; ↑, increased; IV, intravenous; heme⊕, positive for hemoglobin.
Note: Signs of microvascular thrombosis are the result of an inappropriate activation of the coagulation system, causing thrombotic occlusion of small vessels within all body organs. As the clotting factors and platelets are consumed, signs of microvascular bleeding appear. This bleeding can quickly extend into frank hemorrhage. Treatment must be aimed at the disorder underlying the disseminated intravascular coagulation; otherwise, the stimulus for the syndrome will persist.

TABLE 33-4 Laboratory Values Commonly Found in Disseminated Intravascular Coagulation[a]

Test	Function Evaluated	Normal Range	Changes in DIC
Platelet count	Platelet number	150,000–450,000/mm³	↓
Prothrombin time (PT)	Extrinsic pathway	11–12.5 seconds	↑
Partial thromboplastin time (activated) (aPTT)	Intrinsic pathway	23–35 seconds	↑
Thrombin time (TT)	Clot formation	8–11 seconds	↑
Fibrinogen	Amount available for coagulation	170–340 mg/dL	↓
D-dimer	Local fibrinolysis	0–250 ng/mL	↑
Fibrin degradation products (FDPs)	Fibrinolysis	0–5 mcg/mL	↑
Euglobulin clot lysis	Fibrinolytic activity	≥2 hours	≤1 hour

DIC, disseminated intravascular coagulation; ↓, decreased; ↑, increased.
[a]Because DIC is a dynamic condition, the laboratory values measured will change over time. Therefore, a progressive increase or decrease in a given laboratory value is likely to be more important than the actual value of a test at a single point in time.

products. The International Society on Thrombosis and Haemostasis has developed a highly sensitive and specific scoring system using the platelet count, fibrin degradation products, PT, and fibrinogen level to diagnose DIC (Levi & Seligsohn, 2016) (see Table 33-5). This system is also useful in predicting the severity of the disease over time and subsequent mortality. Other tests, such as thrombelastography, can be performed at the bedside and can better assess platelet function as well as fibrinolytic activity; studies suggest it is more useful to assess the status of the coagulation system in critically ill patients at the bedside than use more conventional laboratory tests (Haase, Ostrowski, Wettersley, et al., 2015; Mishra, Thekkudan, Sahajanadan, et al., 2015).

Medical Management

The most important factor in managing DIC is aggressively treating the underlying cause; until the cause is controlled, DIC will persist. Correcting the secondary effects of tissue ischemia by improving oxygenation, replacing fluids, correcting electrolyte imbalances, and administering vasopressor medications is also important. If serious hemorrhage occurs, the depleted coagulation factors and platelets may be replaced to reestablish the potential for normal hemostasis and thereby diminish bleeding. However, decisions to provide transfusion support should not be solely based on the laboratory results,

but on the extent of hemorrhage or need to initiate an invasive procedure. Cryoprecipitate is given to replace fibrinogen and factors V and VII. Administering fresh frozen plasma replaces coagulation factors, but can exacerbate capillary leak, further compromising pulmonary function. Platelets are transfused to correct severely low platelet levels, control bleeding (with factor replacement), or prior to an invasive procedure (Levi & Seligsohn, 2016).

A controversial treatment strategy is to interrupt the thrombosis process through the use of heparin infusion. Heparin may inhibit the formation of microthrombi and thus permit perfusion of the organs (skin, kidneys, or brain) to resume. Heparin use was traditionally reserved for patients in whom thrombotic manifestations predominated or in whom extensive blood component replacement failed to halt the hemorrhage or increased fibrinogen and other clotting levels. In the absence of bleeding, prophylactic doses of unfractionated heparin or low–molecular-weight heparin (LMWH) may be used to prevent venous thromboembolism (VTE), whereas therapeutic doses of unfractionated heparin may be used when severe thrombosis predominates. The effectiveness of heparin can be determined by observing for normalization of the plasma fibrinogen concentration and diminishing signs of bleeding. However, there is little evidence to suggest that heparin reverses organ dysfunction, whereas there is stronger

TABLE 33-5 Scoring System for Disseminated Intravascular Coagulation

Laboratory Test	0	1	2	3
Platelet count	>100,000/mm³	>50,000/mm³, <100,000/mm³	<50,000/mm³	
Fibrin degradation products	No increase		Moderate increase	Strong increase
Prothrombin time (upper limit of normal)	<3 seconds	>3 seconds, <6 seconds	>6 seconds	
Fibrinogen	>100 mg/dL	<100 mg/dL		

Note: 5 or more is compatible with overt disseminated intravascular coagulation.
Adapted from Taylor, F. B., Toh, C.-H., Hoots, W. K., et al. (2007). Towards a definition, clinical and laboratory criteria, and a scoring system for DIC. *Journal of Thrombosis and Haemostasis, 5*(3), 445–659.

evidence that LMWH may be associated with this benefit (Toh & Alhamdi, 2013). Fibrinolytic inhibitors, such as aminocaproic acid, are not routinely advised; they block the lysis of fibrin needed to preserve tissue perfusion. However, if the bleeding is profuse and there is evidence of excessive fibrinolysis, fibrinolytic inhibitors are used concomitantly with a continuous infusion of IV heparin (Levi & Seligsohn, 2016).

Recent studies suggest that recombinant forms of thrombomodulin can effectively bind to thrombin and inactivate thrombin's coagulant activity (Hoppensteadt, Tsuruta, Cunanan, et al., 2014; Matsushita, Watanabe, Honda, et al., 2014). This treatment may be a useful means to control profound bleeding associated with DIC. All management strategies must be individualized to the specific patient, underlying cause of DIC, and response to interventions.

Nursing Management

Nurses need to be aware of which patients are at risk for DIC (see previous discussion on "triggers"). Patients need to be assessed thoroughly and frequently for signs and symptoms of thrombi and bleeding and monitored for any progression of these signs (see Chart 33-10). Lab values must be monitored frequently, not only for the actual result but to note trends over time as well as the rate of change in values.

Chart 33-11 describes care of the patient with DIC. Assessment and interventions should target potential sites of end-organ damage. As organs become ischemic from microthrombi, organ function diminishes; the kidneys, lungs, brain, and skin are particularly vulnerable. Lack of renal perfusion may result in acute tubular necrosis and kidney injury, sometimes requiring dialysis. Placement of a large-bore dialysis catheter is extremely hazardous for this patient population and should be accompanied by adequate platelet and plasma transfusions. Hepatic dysfunction is also relatively common, reflected in altered liver function tests, depleted albumin stores, and diminished synthesis of clotting factors. Respiratory function warrants careful monitoring and aggressive measures to diminish alveolar compromise. Suctioning should be performed as gently as possible to diminish the risk of additional bleeding. Central nervous system involvement can be manifested as headache, visual changes, and alteration in level of consciousness.

Thrombotic Disorders

Several conditions can alter balance within the normal hemostasis process, causing excessive thrombosis that may be arterial (due to platelet aggregation) or venous (composed of platelets, red cells, and thrombin). Abnormalities that predispose a person to thrombotic events include decreased clotting inhibitors within the circulation (which enhances coagulation), altered hepatic function (which may decrease the production of clotting factors or clearance of activated coagulation factors), lack of fibrinolytic enzymes, and tortuous or atherosclerotic vessels (which promote platelet aggregation). Thrombosis may occur as an initial manifestation of an occult malignancy or as a complication from a pre-existing cancer. It can also be caused by more than one predisposing factor. Several inherited or acquired deficiency conditions, including hyperhomocysteinemia, antithrombin (AT) deficiency,

protein C deficiency, protein S deficiency, activated protein C (APC) resistance, and factor V Leiden deficiency, can predispose a patient to repeated episodes of thrombosis; they are referred to as hypercoagulable states or thrombophilia. Those disorders that are inherited should trigger the need for familial genetic testing for the disorder (see Chapter 8); acquired disorders do not warrant familial testing.

Conditions that may result from thrombosis include acute coronary syndrome (ACS) (see Chapter 27), ischemic stroke (see Chapter 67), and peripheral arterial occlusive disease (see Chapter 30). Anticoagulation therapy is necessary. The duration of therapy varies with the location and extent of the thrombosis, precipitating events (e.g., trauma, immobilization), and concurrent risk factors (e.g., the use of oral contraceptives or cigarettes, obesity, tortuous blood vessels, history of thrombotic events; see Table 33-6). A recent study found that taking aspirin after completing standard anticoagulation therapy for treating VTE reduced the risk of recurrent thrombosis (Simes, Becattini, Agnellis, et al., 2014). With some conditions, or with repeated thrombosis, lifelong anticoagulant therapy is necessary.

Hyperhomocysteinemia

Homocysteine can promote platelet aggregation. Increased plasma levels of homocysteine are a significant risk factor for VTE (e.g., deep vein thrombosis [DVT], pulmonary embolism [PE]), recurrent VTE, and arterial thrombosis (e.g., ischemic stroke, ACS) (Reitter-Pfoertner, Waldhoer, Mayerhofer, et al., 2013). Hyperhomocysteinemia can be hereditary, or it can result from a nutritional deficiency of folate and, to a lesser extent, of vitamins B_{12} and B_6, because these vitamins are cofactors in homocysteine metabolism. For unknown reasons, people who are older and those with kidney injury may also have elevated levels of homocysteine in the absence of nutritional deficiencies of these vitamins (Middeldorp & Coppens, 2016). Although a simple fasting measurement of plasma homocysteine can serve as a useful screening test, people with genetically inherited hyperhomocysteinemia and those who are vitamin B_6 deficient may have normal or minimally elevated levels. A more sensitive method involves obtaining a second measurement 4 hours after the patient consumes methionine; hyperhomocysteinemia is found twice as often when this method is used. In hyperhomocysteinemia, the endothelial lining of the vessel walls is denuded, which can precipitate thrombus formation. Research findings do not support that taking folic acid, vitamin B_6, and vitamin B_{12} supplements is effective in decreasing the risk of recurrent venous or arterial thromboembolism (Middeldorp & Coppens, 2016). Smoking causes low levels of vitamin B_6 and B_{12} and folate; thus, homocysteine levels rise. Patients need to be encouraged to refrain from smoking.

Antithrombin Deficiency

AT is a protein that inhibits thrombin and certain coagulation factors, and it may also play a role in diminishing inflammation within the endothelium of blood vessels. AT deficiency is most commonly a hereditary condition that can cause venous thrombosis, particularly when the AT level is less than 60% of normal. The most common sites for thrombosis are the

Chart 33-11

PLAN OF NURSING CARE

The Patient With Disseminated Intravascular Coagulation

NURSING DIAGNOSIS: Risk for deficient fluid volume related to bleeding
GOALS: Hemodynamic status maintained; urine output ≥0.5 mL/kg/h

Nursing Interventions	Rationale	Expected Outcomes
1. Avoid procedures/activities that can increase intracranial pressure (e.g., coughing, straining to have a bowel movement).	1. Prevents intracranial bleeding	• Level of consciousness (LOC) stable • Central venous pressure 5–12 cm H$_2$O, systolic blood pressure ≥70 mm Hg • Urine output ≥0.5mL/kg/h • Decreased bleeding • Decreased oozing • Decreased ecchymoses • Amenorrhea • Absence of oral and bronchial bleeding • Oral mucosa clean, moist, intact
2. Monitor vital signs closely, including neurologic checks: a. Monitor hemodynamics. b. Monitor abdominal girth. c. Monitor urine output.	2. Identifies signs of hemorrhage/shock quickly	
3. Avoid medications that interfere with platelet function if possible (e.g., aspirin, nonsteroidal anti-inflammatory drugs, beta-lactam antibiotics).	3. Decreases problems with platelet aggregation and adhesion	
4. Avoid rectal probes, rectal medications.	4. Decreases risk of rectal bleeding	
5. Avoid intramuscular injections.	5. Decreases risk of intramuscular bleeding	
6. Monitor amount of external bleeding carefully: a. Monitor number of dressings, percentage of dressing saturated; time to saturate a dressing is more objective than "dressing saturated a moderate amount." b. Assess suction output, all excreta for frank or occult blood. c. Monitor pad counts in women with vaginal bleeding. d. Females may receive progesterone to prevent menses.	6. a. Provides accurate, objective assessment of extent of bleeding b. Identifies presence of or quantifies extent of bleeding c. Quantifies extent of bleeding d. Decreases chance for gynecologic source of hemorrhage	
7. Use low pressure with any suctioning.	7. Prevents excessive trauma that could cause bleeding	
8. Administer oral hygiene carefully. a. Avoid lemon-glycerin swabs, hydrogen peroxide, commercial mouthwashes. b. Use sponge-tipped swabs, salt/baking soda (bicarbonate of soda) mouth rinses.	8. Prevents excessive trauma that could cause bleeding. Glycerin and alcohol (in commercial mouthwashes) will dry mucosa, increasing risk for bleeding.	
9. Avoid dislodging any clots, including those around IV sites and injection sites.	9. Prevents excessive bleeding at sites	

NURSING DIAGNOSIS: Risk for impaired skin integrity related to ischemia or bleeding
GOALS: Skin integrity remains intact; oral mucosa remains intact

Nursing Interventions	Rationale	Expected Outcomes
1. Assess skin, with particular attention to bony prominences, skin folds.	1. Prompt identification of any area at risk for skin breakdown or showing early signs of breakdown can facilitate prompt intervention and thus prevent complications.	• Skin integrity remains intact; skin is warm, and of normal color. • Oral mucosa is intact, pink, moist, without bleeding.
2. Reposition carefully; use pressure-reducing mattress.	2–4. Meticulous skin care and the use of measures to prevent pressure on bony prominences decrease the risk of skin trauma.	
3. Perform careful skin care every 2 hours, emphasizing dependent areas, all bony prominences, perineum.		
4. Use lamb's wool between digits, around ears, as needed.		
5. Use prolonged pressure after injection or procedure when such measures must be performed (at least 5 minutes).	5. Initial platelet plug is very unstable and easily dislodged, which can lead to increased bleeding.	
6. Perform oral hygiene carefully (see earlier discussion).	6. Meticulous care is needed to decrease trauma, bleeding, and risk of infection.	

Chart 33-11

PLAN OF NURSING CARE (Continued)
The Patient With Disseminated Intravascular Coagulation

NURSING DIAGNOSIS: Risk for imbalanced fluid volume related to excessive blood and/or factor component replacement
GOALS: Absence of edema; absence of crackles; intake not greater than output

Nursing Interventions	Rationale	Expected Outcomes
1. Auscultate breath sounds every 2–4 hours. 2. Monitor extent of edema. 3. Monitor volume of IVs, blood products; decrease volume of IV medications if indicated. 4. Administer diuretics as prescribed.	1. Crackles can develop quickly. 2. Fluid may extend beyond intravascular system. 3. Helps prevent fluid overload 4. Decreases fluid volume	• Breath sounds clear • Absence of edema • Intake does not exceed output • Weight stable

NURSING DIAGNOSIS: Risk for injury related to microthrombi
GOALS: Neurologic status remains intact; absence of hypoxemia; peripheral pulses remain intact; skin integrity remains intact; urine output remains ≥0.5 mL/kg/h

Nursing Interventions	Rationale	Expected Outcomes
1. Assess neurologic, pulmonary, integumentary systems. 2. Monitor response to heparin therapy. 3. Assess extent of bleeding. 4. Monitor fibrinogen levels. 5. Stop aminocaproic acid, if prescribed, if symptoms of thrombosis occur.	1. Initial signs of thrombosis can be subtle. 2. Assure anticoagulation effectiveness that may prevent formation of additional thromboses. 3. Objective measurements of all sites of bleeding are crucial to accurately assess extent of blood loss. 4. Response to heparin is most accurately reflected in fibrinogen level. 5. Aminocaproic acid should be used only in setting of extensive hemorrhage not responding to replacement therapy.	• Arterial blood gases, O$_2$ saturation, pulse oximetry, LOC within normal limits • Breath sounds clear • Absence of edema • Intake does not exceed output • Weight stable

NURSING DIAGNOSIS: Death anxiety related to uncertain prognosis or possible death
GOALS: Feelings verbalized/identified; realistic hope maintained

Nursing Interventions	Rationale	Expected Outcomes
1. Identify previous coping mechanisms, if possible; encourage patient to use them as appropriate. 2. Explain all procedures and their rationale in terms that patient and family can understand. 3. Assist family in supporting patient. 4. Use services from behavioral medicine, chaplain as needed.	1. Identifying previous stressful situations can aid in recall of successful coping mechanisms. 2. Decreased knowledge and uncertainty can increase anxiety. 3. Family can be useful in assisting patient to use coping strategies and to maintain hope. 4. Additional professional intervention may be necessary, particularly if previous coping mechanisms are maladaptive or ineffective. Spiritual dimension should be supported.	• Previously used coping strategies identified and tried, to extent patient is able to do so • Patient indicates understanding of procedures and situation as condition permits.

LOC, level of consciousness.

deep veins of the leg and the mesentery. Recurrent thrombosis often occurs, particularly as the patient ages. Patients tend to exhibit heparin resistance; thus, they may require greater amounts of heparin to achieve adequate anticoagulation. Patients with AT deficiency should be encouraged to have their family members tested for the deficiency.

AT deficiency can also be acquired by four mechanisms: accelerated consumption of AT (as in DIC), reduced synthesis of AT (as in hepatic dysfunction), increased excretion of AT (as in nephrotic syndrome), and medication induced (e.g., estrogens, L-asparaginase) (Truelove, Fielding, & Hunt, 2013).

Protein C Deficiency

Protein C is a vitamin K–dependent enzyme synthesized in the liver; when activated, it inhibits coagulation. When levels of protein C are deficient, the risk of thrombosis increases, and thrombosis can often occur spontaneously. People who are deficient in protein C are often without symptoms until their 20s; the risk of having a thrombotic event then increases. Individuals with Protein C deficiency are at higher risk for recurrent PE (Turan, Ündar, Güany, et al., 2013). A rare but significant complication of anticoagulation management in patients with protein C deficiency is warfarin-induced skin

TABLE 33-6 Risk Factors for Thrombosis

Acquired	Inherited	Mixed/Unknown
Advanced age	Antithrombin deficiency	Activated protein C resistance
Antiphospholipid antibody syndrome	Factor V Leiden	↑ Factor VII
Atrial fibrillation	Factor XII deficiency	↑ Factor VIII
Diabetes	Protein C deficiency	↑ Factor IX
Drugs (e.g., cocaine, ergot)	Protein S deficiency	↑ Factor XI
Estrogen use	Prothrombin 20210a	↓ Fibrinolytic activity
Hypertension		↑ Homocysteine
Inflammatory bowel disease		
Immobility		
Lupus anticoagulant		
Major surgery		
Myeloproliferative disease		
Nephrotic syndrome		
Obesity		
Paralysis		
Pregnancy/postpartum period		
Prior stroke		
Prior superficial vein thrombosis		
Smoking		
Trauma/fracture		
Vascular access catheters		

↑, increased; ↓, decreased.

Note: Risk factors for first, unprovoked venous thromboembolism. Note that the factor levels that are increased are procoagulant proteins.

Adapted from Heit J. A. (2015). Epidemiology of venous thromboembolism. *Nature Reviews. Cardiology*, 2015(8), 464–474; Kreidy, R. (2014). Influence of acquired and genetic risk factors on the prevention, management, and treatment of thromboembolic disease. *International Journal of Vascular Medicine*, 2014;2014: 859726.; Martinelli I., Passamonti, S. M., & Bucciarelli, P. (2014). Thrombophilic states. *Handbook of Clinical Neurology*, 120, 1061–1071.

necrosis. This complication appears to result from progressive thrombosis in the capillaries within the skin. The extent of the necrosis can be extreme. Prompt cessation of warfarin, treatment with vitamin K, and infusions of heparin and fresh-frozen plasma are crucial to arrest the pathophysiologic process and reverse the effects of the warfarin. Treatment with purified protein C concentrate is sometimes indicated.

Protein S Deficiency

Protein S is another natural anticoagulant normally produced by the liver. APC requires protein S to inactivate certain clotting factors. When the level of protein S is deficient, this inactivation process is diminished, and the risk of thrombosis can be increased. Like patients with protein C deficiency, those with protein S deficiency have a greater risk of recurrent venous thrombosis early in life, and also with recurrent PE (Turan et al., 2013).

Thromboses most commonly occur in the axillary, mesenteric, and cerebral veins. Warfarin-induced skin necrosis is possible. Acquired protein S deficiency can also occur. Pregnancy, DIC, liver disease, nephritic syndrome, HIV infection, and the use of L-asparaginase have all been associated with reduced protein S levels.

Activated Protein C Resistance and Factor V Leiden Mutation

APC resistance is a common condition that can occur with other hypercoagulable states. APC is an anticoagulant, and resistance to APC increases the risk of venous thrombosis.

A molecular defect in the factor V gene has been identified in most (90%) patients with APC resistance. This factor V Leiden mutation is the most common cause of inherited hypercoagulability in Caucasians, but its incidence appears to be much lower in other ethnic groups (Middeldorp & Coppens, 2016). Factor V Leiden mutation synergistically increases the risk of thrombosis in patients with other risk factors (e.g., the use of oral contraceptives, hyperhomocysteinemia, increased age). People who are homozygous for the factor V Leiden mutation are at extremely high risk of thrombosis (i.e., 80-fold increased risk) and therefore need anticoagulation for life. In contrast, those who are heterozygous for the mutation have a lower chance for developing a thrombus. The duration of anticoagulation is based upon the coexistence of other risk factors for thrombi formation (Donovan, Smith, & Ragni, 2013).

Acquired Thrombophilias

Acquired thrombophilias are types of clotting disorders that do not have inherited/genetic causes.

Etiology

Acquired thrombophilias result in inappropriate clot formation, typically caused by either an excess in antibodies that cause clotting or an increase in clotting factors.

Antiphospholipid Syndrome

Antibodies to phospholipids are common acquired causes of thrombophilia (i.e., hypercoagulable states); up to 5% of the general population may have this disorder. These antibodies reduce levels of annexin V, a protein that binds phospholipids and has anticoagulant activity (Chaturvedi & McCrae, 2015). The most common of these phospholipid antibodies are either lupus or anticardiolipin antibodies, or an antibody to B_2-glycoprotein (Rand & Wolgast, 2016). Antiphospholipid syndrome is classified as primary or secondary, with a reaction secondary to a pre-existing autoimmune disease—with systemic lupus erythematosus being the most common disease implicated. Primary antiphospholipid syndrome is associated with certain infections (hepatitis C, HIV, syphilis, malaria) or certain medications (e.g., antibiotics, quinine [Qualaquin], hydralazine [Apresoline], procainamide [Pronestyl]); a genetic predisposition to this syndrome has been postulated but not yet proven. Antiphospholipid antibodies are associated with repeated miscarriages and felt to be a significant cause of stroke. Most thrombotic events are venous, but arterial thrombosis can occur in up to one third of the cases. Recurrent thromboses tend to be of the same type—that is, venous thrombosis after an initial venous thrombosis, arterial thrombosis after an initial arterial thrombosis. Thrombi typically occur in large vessels. Therapy varies, based on the type of syndrome (e.g., secondary forms may be treated with immunosuppressive therapy), history of prior thrombosis, and location of thrombosis (venous versus arterial); arterial thrombosis often necessitates adding low-dose aspirin to some form of heparin (see later discussion).

Malignancy

Another common acquired cause of thrombophilia is cancer, particularly stomach, pancreatic, lung, and ovarian cancers. The type of thrombosis that results is unusual. Rather than DVT or PE, the thrombosis occurs in unusual sites, such as the portal, hepatic, or renal vein or the inferior vena cava. Migratory superficial thrombophlebitis or nonbacterial thrombotic endocarditis can also occur. In these patients, anticoagulation can be difficult to manage, and the thrombosis can progress despite standard doses of anticoagulants. LMWH appears to be a more effective anticoagulant than warfarin in treating this patient population (Connolly & Francis, 2013).

Medical Management

The primary method of treating thrombotic disorders is anticoagulation. However, in thrombophilic conditions, when to treat (prophylaxis or not) and how long to treat (lifelong or not) can be controversial. Anticoagulation therapy is not without risks; the most significant risk is bleeding. The most common anticoagulant medications are identified in the following section.

Pharmacologic Therapy

Anticoagulant agents are used in the treatment or prevention of thrombosis. These agents, particularly warfarin or unfractionated heparin (see later discussion), can cause bleeding, particularly if their use is not carefully monitored (see Chapter 32 for discussion of Hematologic Studies). Along with administering anticoagulant agents, any modifiable risk factors that predispose a patient to thrombosis should be identified and modified, as appropriate. When risk factors (e.g., immobility after surgery, pregnancy) are nonmodifiable, prophylactic anticoagulation may be necessary.

Heparin

Unfractionated Heparin

Heparin is a naturally occurring anticoagulant agent that enhances AT III and inhibits platelet function. To prevent thrombosis, heparin is typically given as a subcutaneous injection two or three times daily. A recent systematic review found that administering heparin slowly (over 30 seconds) resulted in less pain and smaller ecchymoses at the infection site than when the injection was given more rapidly (over 10 seconds) (Akbari, Janani, Mohammady, et al., 2014; Visvanathan, 2015).

To treat thrombosis, heparin is usually administered IV. The therapeutic effect of heparin is monitored by serial measurements of the aPTT; the dose is adjusted to maintain the range at 1.5 to 2.5 times the laboratory control. Protamine sulfate is rarely needed for heparin toxicity (to prevent or treat bleeding complications), because the half-life of heparin is very short (Sartori & Prandoni, 2015).

Low–Molecular-Weight Heparin

LMWHs (e.g., dalteparin [Fragmin], enoxaparin [Lovenox]) are special forms of heparin that have more selective effects on coagulation. Based on their biochemical properties, LMWHs have a longer half-life and a less variable anticoagulant response than unfractionated heparin. These differences permit LMWHs to be safely given only once or twice daily, without the need for laboratory monitoring for dose adjustments. The incidence of heparin-induced thrombocytopenia (HIT) (see later discussion) is much lower when an LMWH is used; however, LMWH is 100% cross-reactive with HIT antibodies and therefore contraindicated in HIT. In certain conditions, the use of an LMWH has allowed anticoagulation therapy to be moved entirely to the outpatient setting. Many cases of uncomplicated DVT are being managed outside the hospital. LMWHs are also used as "bridge therapy" when patients receiving anticoagulation therapy (warfarin) require a major invasive procedure such as surgery. In this situation, warfarin is stopped 2 to 3 days preoperatively, and an LMWH is used in its place until the procedure is performed. After the procedure, warfarin therapy is resumed. If the LMWH is resumed after the procedure, it is discontinued when a therapeutic level of warfarin is achieved.

Heparin-Induced Thrombocytopenia

HIT is a significant complication of heparin-based therapy. HIT involves the formation of antibodies against the heparin–platelet complex. HIT may occur in as many as 5% of patients receiving heparin (Lee & Arepally, 2013). The type of heparin used, duration of heparin therapy (beyond 4 days), and surgery (especially if it requires use of cardiopulmonary bypass) appear to be risk factors for developing HIT. Bovine preparations are more likely to lead to HIT than porcine preparations, and LMWH formulations carry a lower risk. Neither the dose nor the route of administration (IV vs. subcutaneous) is a risk. Women appear to be at a higher risk and young adults are at a very low risk for developing the disorder for reasons that are not clear. A decline in platelet count is a hallmark sign that typically occurs after 5 to 10 days of heparin therapy; therefore, the platelet count should be monitored in any patient beginning heparin therapy. The platelet count can drop significantly, usually by 50% of baseline over a period of 1 to 3 days (Greinacher, 2015). The antibodies typically disappear in 2 to 3 months.

Affected patients are at increased risk for thrombosis, either venous, arterial, or both, and the thrombosis can range from DVT to ACS or stroke, or to ischemic damage to an extremity, necessitating amputation. VTE is the most common, typically DVT or PE (Lee & Arepally, 2013).

Treatment for HIT includes prompt cessation of heparin (including any heparin-coated catheters) and initiation of an alternative means of anticoagulation. If the heparin is stopped without providing additional anticoagulation, the patient is at increased risk for developing new thrombi. Argatroban is an inhibitor of thrombin and an FDA-approved anticoagulant for the treatment of HIT. Oral anticoagulation with warfarin is contraindicated because it initially promotes thrombosis in the microvasculature by depleting protein C, which can lead to ischemia and gangrenous limbs (Greinacher, 2015). Once the platelet count has recovered, transitioning to treatment with warfarin is possible. Individuals who develop thrombosis in the setting of HIT should receive anticoagulation for 3 to 6 months; the duration of anticoagulation in the absence of thrombosis is shorter (Lee & Arepally, 2013). Patients need to be aware of their risk for reactivation of the disorder should they be exposed to any amount of heparin within 3 to 4 months after diagnosis. This time frame is thought to be sufficient to remove anti-heparin-platelet antibodies from the circulation by the RES.

Warfarin (Coumadin)

Warfarin (Coumadin) is a vitamin K antagonist; therefore, it interferes with the synthesis of vitamin K–dependent clotting factors. Warfarin binds to albumin, is metabolized in the liver, and has an extremely long half-life. Typically, a patient with VTE is initially treated with both heparin (either unfractionated or an LMWH) and warfarin. When the international normalized ratio (INR) reaches the desired therapeutic range, the heparin is stopped. The dosage required to maintain the therapeutic range (typically an INR of 2.0 to 3.0) varies widely among patients and even within the same patient, depending on the diagnosis and the rationale for anticoagulation. Frequent monitoring of the INR is extremely important so that the dosage of warfarin can be adjusted as needed.

Some patients can monitor their own INR testing and adjust their warfarin dosage based on pre-established algorithms (Michaels & Regan, 2013). Nurses play a critical role in evaluating which patients may be candidates for this self-management approach. Patient education is critical; eligible patients must demonstrate the ability to accurately calibrate and use the INR diagnostic machine, obtain a blood sample correctly, interpret the results, and adjust the warfarin dosage correctly.

Warfarin is affected by many medications; consultation with a pharmacist is important to assess the extent to which concurrently given medications, herbs, and nutritional supplements may interact with warfarin. It is also affected by many foods, so patients need dietary instruction and may benefit from consultation with a dietitian. In particular, foods with high vitamin K content antagonize the effects of warfarin. Some of these foods include spinach, broccoli, and lettuce. Patients need not avoid such foods but do need to maintain consistent intake; for example, eating a salad daily as opposed to weekly will diminish the antagonistic effect (although will likely necessitate a higher dose of warfarin). Chart 33-12 lists agents that interact with warfarin. A significant complication of

---

Chart 33-12 PHARMACOLOGY
Agents That Interact With Warfarin (Coumadin)

Although warfarin (Coumadin), an anticoagulant medication, is commonly used to treat and prevent thrombosis, many drug–drug and drug–food interactions are associated with its use. A careful medication history (including OTC medications, herbs, and other substances, such as vitamins and minerals) is important when oral anticoagulation therapy is prescribed. Consultation with a pharmacist is recommended to assess the extent to which concurrent medications may affect the anticoagulant and for appropriate dosage adjustments. The following list contains a few examples of agents that interact with warfarin.

Agents That Inhibit Warfarin Function

Azathioprine (Imuran)
Barbiturates
Carbamazepine (Tegretol)
Cholestyramine (Questran)
Corticosteroids
Cyclosporine (Sandimmune)
Dicloxacillin (Dynapen)
Digitalis
Estrogens
Ethanol (Alcohol)
Glutethimide (Doriden)
Griseofulvin (Grisovin)
Haloperidol (Haldol)
Herbal medicines: coenzyme Q, ginseng, St. John's wort, Cat's claw, green tea
Nafcillin
Oral contraceptives
Phenytoin (Dilantin) (long term)
Primidone (Mysoline)
Ribavirin (Copegus)
Rifampin (Rifadin)
Secobarbitol (Seconal)
Spironolactone (Aldactone)
Sucralfate (Carafate)
Trazodone (Desyrel)
Vitamin K

Agents That Potentiate Warfarin Function

Acetaminophen (Tylenol)
Allopurinol (Zyloprim)
Amiodarone
Anabolic steroids
Anti-inflammatory agents, including nonsteroidal anti-inflammatory drugs
Antimalarial agents
Argatroban

Aspirin
Broad-spectrum antibiotics
Chloral hydrate
Chloramphenicol
Cimetidine (Tagamet)
Colchicine (Colcrys)
Clofibrate (Atromid-S)
Chlorpromazine (Thorazine)
Danazol (Danocrine)
Diltiazem (Cardizem)
Disulfiram (Antabuse)
Erythromycin (E-Mycin)
Ethacrynic acid (Edecrin)
Feprazone (Prenazone)
Fluconazole (Diflucan)
Gemfibrozil (Lopid)
Herbal medicines: anise, danshen, devil's claw, dong quai, feverfew, fish oil, garlic, gingko, ginseng, green tea, licorice root, papain, turmeric, willow bark
Influenza vaccine
Isoniazid (INH)
Lovastatin (Mevacor)
Mefenamic acid (Ponstel)
Methotrexate (MTX)
Metronidazole (Flagyl)
Miconazole (Monistat)
Omeprazole (Prilosec)
Oral hypoglycemic agents
Oxyphenbutazone (Tandearil)
Phenytoin (Dilantin) (short term)
Piroxicam (Feldene)
Probenecid (Benemid)
Propranolol (Inderal)
Propylthiouracil (PTU)
Quinidine (Quinaglute)
Quinine (Qualiquin)
Salicylates
Simvastatin (Zocor)
Sulfinpyrazone (Anturane)
Sulfonamides (long acting)
Tamoxifen (Nolvadex)
Testosterone
Thyroxine
Triclofos
Tricyclic antidepressants
Vitamin C (in very large doses)
Vitamin E (in very large doses)
Voriconazole (Vfend)

warfarin therapy is bleeding; more than 60,000 people are treated for warfarin-associated hemorrhage in the ED annually (Levine & Goldstein, 2014). The antidote for warfarin is vitamin K, which will rapidly reverse its anti-coagulant effects (i.e., within 30 minutes when given IV) (Garcia, 2014). With significant bleeding, transfusions of fresh-frozen plasma are indicated to replace the vitamin K-dependent coagulation factors.

Thrombin and Factor Xa Inhibitors

Several oral anticoagulant agents have been approved for use that are not Vitamin K antagonists (such as warfarin). Dabigatran (Pradaxa) is a direct thrombin inhibitor, whereas rivaroxaban (Xarelto), apixiban (Eliquis), and edoxaban (Savaysa) are Factor Xa inhibitors. These drugs are indicated for prevention of DVT, PE, or stroke in patients with atrial fibrillation. With the exception of edoxaban, these drugs are also indicated as prophylaxis to prevent DVT in patients having knee or hip replacement surgery. These drugs appear to be as efficacious as warfarin but have the advantage of not requiring frequent INR monitoring and dose adjustment. All of these drugs are metabolized by the cytochrome P-450 pathway; therefore, it is important to assess for potential drug–drug interactions. Dabigatran is unique in that it must remain in its original packaging, because the potential for product breakdown and loss of potency is high if it becomes moist (Boehringer Ingelheim Pharmaceuticals, 2015). Therefore, this medication cannot be stored in a medication cassette (pillbox), which may limit its use in older adults or those with other issues limiting their ability to adhere to medication regimens.

Studies show that each of these new oral anticoagulant agents is associated with less risk of bleeding than warfarin. However, this benefit may not be seen in adults over 75 years of age; studies show similar rates of hemorrhage independent of oral anticoagulant used (Levine & Goldstein, 2014). Each of these agents still carries some risk of bleeding in all age groups. Dabigatran can be cleared if necessary via hemodialysis, and its absorption can be reduced with oral activated charcoal. Prothrombin complex concentrate, activated prothrombin concentrate, or recombinant factor VIIa can be used to reverse the effect of these oral anticoagulant agents; more specific antidotes are under development.

A challenge associated with the use of these oral agents is that it is not possible to easily measure their anticoagulant effect. Values obtained from standard tests of coagulation (e.g., PT, PTT) yield inconsistent results when measured during administration of these drugs. Measuring anti-Xa activity can be more reliable; however, this test is not available in many laboratories and the time required to obtain results limits its clinical utility (Garcia, 2014). Nevertheless, these drugs are rapidly cleared from the circulation, so long as the patient's renal function is normal. Therefore, their anticoagulant effect may be stopped simply by withdrawing drug administration.

When choosing an oral anticoagulant agent, bleeding risk (lower with thrombin or Factor Xa inhibitors) and ability to reverse the anticoagulant effect (easier to manage and control with warfarin) are important considerations. As noted previously, patients with poor renal function exhibit reduced drug clearance. Therefore, the risks of bleeding are higher when anticoagulant agents are prescribed for these patients and those risks need to be carefully weighed against the benefit of decreasing risk of thrombosis. There are additional factors that support the selection of warfarin over the newer agents. Concerns about adherence, the presence of a prosthetic heart valve, and extremes in body weight are factors that support the prescription of warfarin (Garcia, 2014). Drug cost is another important consideration; warfarin is inexpensive, the new drugs are not.

Aspirin

Patients with VTE (e.g., DVT, PE) remain at risk for recurrent thrombosis upon completion of anticoagulant therapy (10% risk within the first year, 5% risk with each subsequent year). An analysis of two large studies (1224 patients with VTE) revealed a 42% reduction in risk of recurrent VTE in patients who took 100 mg enteric-coated aspirin daily compared with those who took a placebo. Importantly, the risk of bleeding was not increased in those who took aspirin (Simes et al., 2014). The results of this study may increase the recommended use of aspirin after the conclusion of anticoagulation therapy in patients diagnosed with VTE.

Nursing Management

Patients with thrombotic disorders should avoid activities that lead to circulatory stasis (e.g., immobility, crossing the legs). Exercise, especially ambulation, should be performed frequently throughout the day, particularly during long trips by car or plane. Anti-embolism stockings are often prescribed, and patients usually need assistance in learning how to use them properly. Surgery further increases the risk of thrombosis. Medications that alter platelet aggregation, such as low-dose aspirin or clopidogrel (Plavix), may be prescribed. Some patients require lifelong therapy with anticoagulants such as warfarin. No evidence supports the use of bed rest as a therapeutic intervention in people with DVT or PE (Partsch, 2014; Pillai & Raval, 2015).

Patients with thrombotic disorders, particularly those with thrombophilia, should be assessed for concurrent risk factors for thrombosis and should avoid them if possible. For example, the use of tobacco and nicotine products should be avoided, blood pressure controlled, and alcohol consumption moderated (Levine & Goldstein, 2014). In many instances, younger patients with thrombophilia may not require prophylactic anticoagulation; however, with concomitant risk factors (e.g., pregnancy), increasing age, or subsequent thrombotic events, prophylactic or long-term anticoagulation therapy may be required. Being able to provide the health care provider with an accurate health history can be extremely useful and can help guide the selection of appropriate therapeutic interventions. Patients need to understand risk factors for thrombosis and what they can do to diminish or reduce them, such as avoiding smoking, using alternative forms of contraception, increasing mobility, and maintaining a healthy weight. Patients with hereditary disorders should encourage their siblings and children to be tested for the disorder.

When a patient with a thrombotic disorder is hospitalized, frequent assessments should be performed for signs and symptoms of beginning thrombus formation, particularly in the legs (DVT) and lungs (PE). Ambulation or range-of-motion exercises as well as the use of anti-embolism stockings should be initiated promptly to decrease stasis. Properly fitted graduated compression stockings may reduce pain and edema associated with the acute stage of DVT; however, studies evaluating their efficacy have yielded conflicting results and adherence to wearing them is often poor (Raskob, Hull, Buller, et al., 2016; Sachdeva, Dalton, Amaragiri, et al., 2014).

CRITICAL THINKING EXERCISES

1 `pq` A 23-year-old male presents to the emergency department (ED) with a chief complaint of unbearable pain in his chest. He is dyspneic, hypotensive, and tachycardic. From his medical record, you note he has sickle cell disease. How will you prioritize his care? Will it change if you note that he is febrile? What additional data do you need to elicit in your health history and physical assessment? What diagnostic tests and initial medical management interventions would you anticipate?

2 You are working in a pre-op clinic. A 47-year-old woman is evaluated prior to having a laparoscopic cholecystectomy. She informs you she has von Willebrand disease. How would you evaluate her risk for bleeding postoperatively? What information would you elicit in your health history? What lab values are of relevance for this situation? How will your education regarding postoperative management differ based on the information you elicit from her health history and lab data?

3 `ebp` You are working in home care. A 79-year-old man was admitted to your service after discharge from the hospital for a left lower extremity deep venous thrombosis (DVT) and you are making the initial visit to see him. He is in the middle of transitioning from a low–molecular-weight heparin (enoxaparin) to warfarin. He reports he dislikes the frequent blood tests required with this therapy and asks about "those new drugs" he hears about on the television. What is the evidence regarding efficacy of these novel oral anticoagulants (NOACs) as compared to warfarin for management of venous thromboemboli (VTE)? What physical, functional, and social assessments would be particularly important to include in your discussion regarding the advantages and disadvantages of one form of anticoagulation over another. How does this man's preference impact this discussion?

4 You are working on an orthopedic unit, and assigned to care for a 63-year-old woman who had a total knee replacement 2 days ago. You review her medical record and note that her platelet count today is 87,000/mm³. On further review, you note her pre-op complete blood count (CBC) was completely normal, including a platelet count of 205,000/mm³. What might be the cause of this decreased platelet count? Is your patient at an increased risk of bleeding? Of thrombosis? Why? What medication is important to look for? What additional information do you need to gather prior to contacting the patient's surgeon? What medical interventions would you anticipate being ordered? How does this finding alter your plan of care for this woman?

REFERENCES

*Asterisk indicates nursing research.
**Double asterisk indicates classic reference.

Books

Bunn, H. (2017). Overview of the anemias. In J. C. Aster, & H. Bunn (Eds.). *Pathophysiology of blood disorders* (2nd Ed.). New York: McGraw-Hill. Retrieved on 10/25/2016 at: accessmedicine.mhmedical.com.laneproxy. stanford.edu/content.aspx?bookid=1900&Sectionid=137394689.

Dale, D.C. , & Welte, K. (2016). Neutropenia and neutrophilia. In K. Kaushansky, M. A. Lichtman, J. T. Prchal, et al. (Eds.). *Williams hematology* (9th ed.). New York: McGraw-Hill Medical.

Diz-Küçükkaya, R., & López, J. (2016). Thrombocytopenia. In K. Kaushansky, M. A. Lichtman, J. T. Prchal, et al. (Eds.). *Williams hematology* (9th ed.). New York: McGraw-Hill Medical.

Escobar, M. A., & Key, N.S. (2016). Hemophilia A and hemophilia B. In K. Kaushansky, M. A. Lichtman, J. T. Prchal, et al. (Eds.). *Williams hematology* (9th ed.). New York: McGraw-Hill Medical.

Ganz, T. (2016a). Iron deficiency and overload. In K. Kaushansky, M. A. Lichtman, J. T. Prchal, et al. (Eds.). *Williams hematology* (9th ed.). New York: McGraw-Hill Medical.

Ganz, T. Ganz, Tomas(2016b). Anemia of chronic disease. In K. Kaushansky, M. A. Lichtman, J. T. Prchal, et al. (Eds.). *Williams hematology* (9th ed.). New York: McGraw-Hill Medical.

Goroll, A. H., & Mulley, A. G. (Eds.) (2014a). Evaluation of anemia. In: *Primary care medicine: Office evaluation and management of the adult patient*. Philadelphia, PA: Lippincott Williams & Wilkins.

Goroll, A.H., & Mulley, A.G. (Eds.). (2014b). Approach to the patient with heartburn and reflux (gastroesophageal disease). In *Primary care medicine: Office evaluation and management of the adult patient*. Philadelphia, PA: Lippincott Williams & Wilkins.

Green, R. (2016). Folate, cobalamin, and megaloblastic anemias. In K. Kaushansky, M. A. Lichtman, J. T. Prchal, et al. (Eds.). *Williams hematology* (9th ed.). New York: McGraw-Hill Medical.

Kaushansky, K. (2016). Reactive thrombocytosis. In K. Kaushansky, M. A. Lichtman, J. T. Prchal, et al. (Eds.). *Williams hematology* (9th ed.). New York: McGraw-Hill Medical.

Levi, M., & Seligsohn, U. (2016). Disseminated intravascular coagulation. In K. Kaushansky, M. A. Lichtman, J. T. Prchal, et al. (Eds.). *Williams hematology* (9th ed.). New York: McGraw-Hill Medical.

Levi, M., Seligsohn, U., & Kaushansky, K. (2016). Classification, clinical manifestations, and evaluation of disorders of hemostasis. In K. Kaushansky, M. A. Lichtman, J. T. Prchal, et al. (Eds.). *Williams hematology* (9th ed.). New York: McGraw-Hill Medical.

Middeldorp, S., & Coppens, M. (2016). Hereditary thrombophilia. In K. Kaushansky, M. A. Lichtman, J. T. Prchal, et al. (Eds.). *Williams hematology* (9th ed.). New York: McGraw-Hill Medical.

Natrajan, K., & Kutlar, A. (2016). Disorders of hemoglobin structure: Sickle cell anemia and related abnormalities. In K. Kaushansky, M. A. Lichtman, J. T. Prchal, et al. (Eds.). *Williams hematology* (9th ed.). New York: McGraw-Hill Medical.

Packman, C. H. (2016). Hemolytic anemia resulting from immune injury. In K. Kaushansky, M. A. Lichtman, J. T. Prchal, et al. (Eds.). *Williams hematology* (9th ed.). New York: McGraw-Hill Medical.

Prchal, J. T. (2016a). Clinical manifestations and classification of erythrocyte disorders. In K. Kaushansky, M. A. Lichtman, J. T. Prchal, et al. (Eds.). *Williams hematology* (9th ed.). New York: McGraw-Hill Medical.

Prchal, J. T. (2016b). Primary and secondary erythrocytoses. In K. Kaushansky, M. A. Lichtman, J. T. Prchal, et al. (Eds.). *Williams hematology* (9th ed.). New York: McGraw-Hill Medical.

Rand, J. H., & Wolgast, L. (2016). The antiphospholipid syndrome. In K. Kaushansky, M. A. Lichtman, J. T. Prchal, et al. (Eds.). *Williams hematology* (9th ed.). New York: McGraw-Hill Medical.

Raskob, G. E., Hull, R. D., Buller, H. R., et al. (2016). Venous thrombosis. In K. Kaushansky, M. A. Lichtman, J. T. Prchal, et al. (Eds.). *Williams hematology* (9th ed.). New York: McGraw-Hill Medical.

Segel, G. B., & Lichtman, M. A. Segel, George B. Marshall A. Lichtman.(2016). Aplastic anemia: Acquired and inherited. In K. Kaushansky, M. A. Lichtman, J. T. Prchal, et al. (Eds.). *Williams hematology* (9th ed.). New York: McGraw-Hill Medical.

Tkachuk, D. C., & Hirschman, J. V. (2007). *Wintrobe's atlas of clinical hematology* (Fig. 1.1, p. 9). Philadelphia, PA: Lippincott Williams & Wilkins.

van Solinge, W.W., & van Wijk, R. (2016). Erythrocyte enzyme disorders. In K. Kaushansky, M. A. Lichtman, J. T. Prchal, et al. (Eds.). *Williams hematology* (9th ed.). New York: McGraw-Hill Medical.

Vasu, S., & Caligiuri, M. A. (2016). Lymphocytosis and lymphocytopenia. In K. Kaushansky, M. A. Lichtman, J. T. Prchal, et al. (Eds.). *Williams hematology* (9th ed.). New York: McGraw-Hill Medical.

Weatherall, D. J. (2016). The thalassemias: Disorders of globin synthesis. In K. Kaushansky, M. A. Lichtman, J. T. Prchal, et al. (Eds.). *Williams hematology* (9th ed.). New York: McGraw-Hill Medical.

Journals and Electronic Documents

Adams, P.C. (2015). Epidemiology and diagnostic testing for hemochromatosis and iron overload. *International Journal of Laboratory Hematology, 37*(Suppl 1), 25–30.

Akbari, S., Janani, L., Mohammady, M., et al. (2014). Slow versus fast subcutaneous heparin injections for prevention of bruising and site-pain intensity. *The Cochrane Database of Systematic Reviews,* (7):CD008077.

American Cancer Society. (2015). *Colorectal cancer screening tests.* Retrieved on 10/31/2015 at: www.cancer.org/cancer/colonandrectumcancer/moreinformation/colonandrectumcancerearlydetection/colorectal-cancer-early-detection-screening-tests-used?gclid=CLfqt5mU7cgCFVGCfgodMG0E_Q

*Ameringer, S., Elswick, R. K., & Smith, W. (2014). Fatigue in adolescents and young adults with sickle cell disease: Biological and behavioral correlates and health-related quality of life. *Journal of Pediatric Oncology Nursing, 31*(1), 6–17.

Andro, M., Le Squere, P., Estivin, S., et al. (2013). Anaemia and cognitive performances in the elderly: A systematic review. *European Journal of Neurology, 20*(9), 1234–1240.

Arnold, D. M. (2015). Bleeding complications in immune thrombocytopenia. *Hematology American Society of Hematology Education Program, 2015*(1), 237–242.

Ataga, K. I., & Klings, E. S. (2014). Pulmonary hypertension in sickle cell disease: Diagnosis and management. *Hematology American Society of Hematology Education Program, 2014*(1), 425–431.

Ataga, K. I., & Stocker, J. (2015). The trials and hopes for drug development in sickle cell disease. *British Journal of Haematology, 170*(6), 768–780.

Berliner, N. (2013). Anemia in the elderly. *Transactions of the American Clinical and Climatological Association, 124,* 230–237.

Boehringer Ingelheim Pharmaceuticals. (2015). *Pradaxa product information.* Retrieved on 3/18/2016 at: http://docs.boehringer-ingelheim.com/Prescribing%20Information/PIs/Pradaxa/Pradaxa.pdf

Broadway-Duren, J. B., & Klaassen, H. (2013). Anemias. *Critical Care Nursing Clinics of North America, 25*(4), 411–426.

Brown, S. E., Weisberg, D. F., Balf-Soran, G., et al. (2014). Sickle cell disease patients with and without extremely high hospital use: Pain, opioids, and coping. *Journal of Pain and Symptom Management, 49*(3), 539–547.

Camaschella, C. (2015). Iron deficiency: New insights into diagnosis and treatment. *Hematology American Society of Hematology Education Program, 2015*(1), 8–13.

Canaro, M., Goranova-Marinova, V., & Berntorp, E. (2014). The ageing patient with haemophilia. *European Journal of Haematology, 94*(Suppl 77), 17–22.

Caughey, M. C., Poole, C., Ataga, K. I., et al. (2015). Estimated pulmonary artery systolic pressure and sickle cell disease: A meta-analysis and systematic review. *British Journal of Haematology, 170*(3), 416–424.

Chang, S., Weis, C., Xue, Q., et al. (2013). Association between inflammatory-related disease burden and frailty: Results from the Women's Health and Aging Studies (WHAS) I and II. *Archives of Gerontology and Geriatrics, 54*(1), 9–15.

**Charache, S., Terrin, M. L., Moore, R. D., et al. (1995). Effect of hydroxyurea on the frequency of painful crises in sickle cell anemia. Investigators of the Multicenter Study of Hydroxyurea in Sickle Cell Anemia. *New England Journal of Medicine, 332*(20), 1317–1322.

Chaturvedi, S., & McCrae, K. R. (2015). The antiphospholipid syndrome: Still an enigma. *Hematology American Society of Hematology Education Program, 2015*(1), 53–60.

Chou, S. T. (2013). Transfusion therapy for sickle cell disease: A balancing act. *Hematology. The American Society of Hematology Education Program, 2013*(1), 439–446.

Collins, W., Chalmers, E., Hart, D., et al. (2013). Diagnosis and management of acquired coagulation inhibitors: A guideline from UKHCDO. *British Journal of Haematology, 162*(6), 758–773.

Connolly, G. C., & Francis, C. W. (2013). Cancer-associated thrombosis. *Hematology American Society of Hematology, 2013* (1), 684–691.

Cylwik, B., Naklicki, N., Gruszewska, E., et al. (2013). The distribution of serum folate concentration and red blood cell indices in alcoholics. *Journal of Nutritional Science and Vitaminology, 59*(1), 1–8.

Darbari, D., Ballas, S. K., & Clauw, D. J. (2014). Thinking beyond sickling to better understand pain in sickle cell disease. *European Journal of Haematology, 93*(2), 89–95.

DeBaun, M. R. (2014). Hydroxyurea therapy contributes to infertility in adult men with sickle cell disease: A review. *Expert Review of Hematology, 7*(6), 767–773.

de Prost, N., Sasanelli, M., Deux, J. F., et al. (2015). Positron emission tomography with 18F-fluorodeoxyglucose in patients with sickle cell acute chest syndrome. *Medicine, 94*(18), e821.

Diericix, D., Kentos, A., & Delannoy, A. (2015). The role of rituximab in adults with warm antibody autoimmune hemolytic anemia. *Blood, 125*(21), 3223–3229.

Dmitrieva, O., de Lusignan, S., Macdougnall, I., et al. (2013). Association of anaemia in primary care patients with chronic kidney disease: Cross-sectional study of quality improvement in chronic kidney disease (QICKD) trial data. *BMC Nephrology, 14*(24).

Donovan, A. K., Smith, K.J., & Ragni, M. V. (2013). Anticoagulation duration in heterozygous factor V Leiden: A decision analysis. *Thrombosis Research, 132*(6), 724–728.

Dunn, A. (2015). The long and short of it: Using the new factor products. *Hematology American Society of Hematology Education Program, 2015*(1), 26–32.

Elmariah, H., Garrett, M. E., De Castro, L. M., et al. (2014). Factors associated with survival in a contemporary adult sickle cell disease cohort. *American Journal of Hematology, 89*(5), 530–535.

Fairweather-Tait, S., Wawer, A., Gilings, R., et al. (2014). Iron status in the elderly. *Mechanisms of Ageing and Development, 136–137*(100), 22–28.

Federici, A. B. (2014). Clinical and laboratory diagnosis of vWD. *Hematology American Society of Hematology, 2014*(1), 524–530.

*Freiermuth, C. E., Haywood, C., Silva, S., et al. (2014). Attitudes toward patients with sickle cell disease in a multicenter sample of emergency department providers. *Advanced Emergency Nursing Journal, 36*(4), 335–347.

G6PD Deficiency Association. (2015). *Drugs to avoid list.* Retrieved on 11/22/2015 at: g6pddeficiency.org/wp/living-with-g6pd-deficiency/drugs-to-avoid-list/#.VlfncHarRhE

Garcia, D. A. (2014). The target-specific oral anticoagulants: Practical considerations. *Hematology American Society of Hematology, 2014*(1), 510–513.

Goodnough, L. T., & Schrier, S. L. (2014). Evaluation and management of anemia in the elderly. *American Journal of Hematology, 89*(1), 88–96.

Greinacher, A. (2015). Heparin-induced thrombocytopenia. *New England Journal of Medicine, 373*(3), 252–261.

Haase, N., Ostrowski, S. R., Wettersley, J., et al. (2015). Thromboelastography in patients with severe sepsis: A prospective cohort study. *Intensive Care Medicine, 41*(1), 77–85.

Hamideh, D., & Alvarez, O. (2013). Sickle cell disease related mortality in the United States (1999–2009). *Pediatric Blood & Cancer, 60*(9), 1482–1486.

Heeney, M. M. (2014). Iron clad: Iron hemostasis and the diagnosis of hereditary iron overload. *Hematology American Society of Hematology, 2014*(1), 202–209.

Heit, J. A. (2015). Epidemiology of venous thromboembolism. *Nature Reviews. Cardiology, 2015*(8), 464–474.

Ho, S., Gue, D., McIntosh, K., et al. (2014). An objective method for assessing adherence to prophylaxis in adults with severe haemophilia. *Haemophilia, 20*(1), 39–43.

Hong, C. H., Falvey, C., Harris, T. B., et al. (2013). Anemia and risk of dementia in older adults: Findings from the Health ABC study. *Neurology, 81*(6), 528–533.

Hoppensteadt, D., Tsuruta, K., Cunanan, J., et al. (2014). Thrombin generation mediators and markers in sepsis-associated coagulopathy and their modulation by recombinant thrombomodulin. *Clinical and Applied Thrombosis/Hemostasis, 20*(2), 129–135.

*Jenerette, C. M., Brewer, C. A., & Ataga, K. I. (2014). Care seeking for pain in young adults with sickle cell disease. *Pain Management Nursing, 15*(1), 324–330.

Jordan, L., Adams-Graves, P., Kanter-Washko, J., et al. (2015). Multicenter COMPACT study of complications in patients with sickle cell disease and utilization of iron chelation therapy. *Current Medical Research and Opinion, 31*(3), 513–523.

Josephson, N. (2013). The hemophilias and their clinical management. *Hematology American Society of Hematology Education Program, 2013*(1), 261–267.

Kanwar, P., & Kowdley, K. D. (2014). Metal storage disorders. *Medical Clinics of North America, 98*(1), 87–102.

Kempton, C., & Meeks, S. L. (2014). Toward optimal therapy for inhibitors in hemophilia. *Hematology American Society of Hematology Education Program, 2014*(1), 364–371.

Kim, H. C. (2014). Red cell exchange: Special focus on sickle cell disease. *Hematology American Society of Hematology Education Program, 2014*(1), 450–456.

Kreidy, R. (2014). Influence of acquired and genetic risk factors on the prevention, management, and treatment of thromboembolic disease. *International Journal of Vascular Medicine, 2014:* 859726.

Lee, G. M., & Arepally, G. M. (2013). Heparin-induced thrombocytopenia. *Hematology American Society of Hematology, 2013*(1), 668–674.

Levine, M., & Goldstein, J. N. (2014). Bleeding complications of targeted oral anticoagulants: What is the risk? *Hematology American Society of Hematology, 2014*(1), 504–509.

Lopez, A., Cacoub, P., Macdougall, I., et al. (2015). Iron-deficiency anaemia. *Lancet, 387*(10021), 907–916.

Maggio, A., Vitrano, A., Calvaruso, G., et al. (2013). Serial echocardiographic left ventricular ejection fraction measurements: A tool for detecting thalassemia major patients at risk for cardiac death. *Blood Cells, Molecules, & Diseases, 50*(4), 241–246.

Marsh, J., & Kulasekararaj, A. (2013). Management of the refractory aplastic anemia patient: What are the options? *American Society of Hematology Educational Program, 2013*(1), 87–94.

Martinelli I., Passamonti, S. M., & Bucciarelli, P. (2014). Thrombophilic states. *Handbook of Clinical Neurology, 120,* 1061–1071.

Matsushita, T., Watanabe, J., Honda, G., et al. (2014). Thrombomodulin alpha treatment in patients with acute promyelocytic leukemia and disseminated intravascular coagulation: A retrospective analysis of an open-label, multicenter, post-marketing surveillance study cohort. *Thrombosis Research, 133*(5), 772–781.

Maury, S., & Aljurf, M. (2013). Management of adult patients older than 40 years refractory to at least one immunosuppressive course: HLA-identical sibling HSCT using fludarabine-based conditioning. *Bone Marrow Transplantation, 48*(2), 196–197.

**McClish, D. K., Smith, W. R., Dahman, B. A., et al. (2009). Pain site frequency and location in sickle cell disease: The PISCES project. *Pain, 145*(1–2), 246–251.

Michaels, K., & Regan, E. N. (2013). Teaching patients INR self-management. *Nursing, 43*(5), 67–69.

Michel, M. (2014). Warm autoimmune hemolytic anemia: Advances in pathophysiology and treatment. *Presse médicale, 43*(4 Pt 2), e97–e104.

Mishra, P. K., Thekkudan, J., Sahajanadan, R., et al. (2015). The role of point-of-care assessment of platelet function in predicting postoperative bleeding and transfusion requirements after coronary artery bypass grafting. *Annals of Cardiac Anaesthesia, 18*(1), 45–51.

National Clinical Guideline Centre (UK). (2015). *Anaemia management in chronic kidney disease: Partial update 2015 [Internet].* London: Royal College of Physicians (UK). Retrieved on 10/24/2016 at: ww-ncbi-nlm-nih-gov.laneproxy.stanford.edu/books/NBK299242/ PubMed PMID: 26065064.

National Heart, Lung, and Blood Institute. (2015). *Who is at risk for sickle cell anemia?* Retrieved on 3/14/2016 at: www.nhlbi.nih.gov/health/health-topics/topics/sca/atrisk.html.

National Hemophilia Foundation. (2014). *What is von Willebrand disease?* Retrieved on 11/19/2015 at: www.hemophilia.org

Neff, A. T., & Sidonio, R. F. (2014). Management of vWD. *Hematology American Society of Hematology, 2014*(1), 536–541.

Nemtsas, P., Arnaoutoglou, M., Perifanis, V., et al. (2015). Neurological complications of beta-thalassemia. *Annals of Hematology, 94*(8), 1261–1265.

Neunert, C. E. (2013). Current management of immunue thrombocytopenia. *Hematology American Society of Hematology Education Program, 2013*(1), 276–282.

**Neunert, C., Lim, W., Crowther, M., et al. (2011). The American Society of Hematology 2011 evidence-based practice guideline for immune thrombocytopenia. *Blood, 117*(16), 4190–4207.

Nielson, O., Ainsworth, M., Coskun, M., et al. (2015). Management of iron-deficiency anemia in inflammatory bowel disease: A systematic review. *Medicine, 94*(23), 1–14.

O'Brien, C., Dempsey, O., & Kennedy, M. J. (2014). Febrile neutropenia risk assessment tool: Improving clinical outcomes for oncology patients. *European Journal of Oncology Nursing, 18*(2), 167–174.

Partsch, H. (2014). The role of leg compression in the treatment of deep vein thrombosis. *Phlebology/Venous Forum of the Royal Society of Medicine, 29*(Suppl 1), 66–70.

Piel, F. B., & Weatherall, D. J. (2014). The α-Thalassemias. *The New England Journal of Medicine, 371*(20), 1908–1916.

Pillai, A. R., & Raval, J. S. (2015). Does early ambulation increase the risk of pulmonary embolism in deep vein thrombosis? A review of the literature. *Home Healthcare Nurse, 32*(6), 336–342.

Porter, J., & Garbowski, M. (2013). Consequences and management of iron overload in sickle cell disease. *Hematology American Society of Hematology Education Program, 2013*(1), 447–456.

Quinn, C. T. (2014). Breakthrough: New guidelines for silent cerebral ischemia and infarction in sickle cell disease. *Hematology American Society of Hematology Education Program, 2014*(1), 438–443.

Raphael, J. L., & Oyeku, S. O. (2013). Sickle cell disease pain management and the medical home. *Hematology American Society of Hematology Education Program, 2014*(1), 433–438.

Reitter- Pfoertner, S., Waldhoer, T., Mayerhofer, M., et al. (2013). The influence of thrombophilia on the long-term survival of patients with a history of venous thromboembolism. *Thrombosis and Haemostasis, 109*(1), 79–84.

Reyes, M., Blank, H. M., & Grossniklaus, D. (2015). *Hemochromatosis.* National Center on Birth Defects and Developmental Disabilities, Centers for Disease Control and Prevention. Retrieved on 11/26/2015 at: www.cdc.gov/ncbddd/hemochromatosis/training/epidemiology/prevalence.html

Rodeghiero, R., & Ruggeri, M. (2015). Treatment of immune thrombocytopenia in adults: The role of thrombopoietin-receptor agonists. *Seminars in Hematology, 52*(1), 16–24.

Sachdeva, A., Dalton, M., Amaragiri, S. V., et al. (2014). Graduated compression stockings for prevention of deep vein thrombosis. *The Cochrane Database of Systematic Reviews,* (12):CD001484.

Sammels, M., Vandesande, J., Vlaeyen, E., et al. (2014). Falling and fall risk factors in adults with haemophilia: An exploratory study. *Haemophilia, 20*(6), 836–845.

Sartori, M. T., & Prandoni, P. (2016). How to effectively manage the event of bleeding complications when using anticoagulants. *Expert Review of Hematology, 9*(1), 37–50.

Schuff-Werner, P., Steiner, M., Fenger, S., et al. (2013). Effective estimation of correct platelet counts in pseudothrombocytopenia using an alternative anticoagulant based on magnesium salt. *British Journal of Haematology, 162*(5), 684–692.

Shipton, M. J., & Thachil, J. (2015). Vitamin B_{12} deficiency: A 21st century perspective. *Clinical Medicine, 15*(2), 145–150.

Simes, J., Becattini, C., Agnellis, G., et al. (2014). Aspirin for the prevention of recurrent venous thromboembolism: The INSPIRE Collaboration. *Circulation, 130*(13), 1062–1071.

Singh, A. K., Kumar, A., Karmakar, D., et al. (2013). Association of B12 deficiency and clinical neuropathy with metformin use in type 2 diabetes patients. *Journal of Postgraduate Medicine, 60*(4), 253–257.

Smith-Whitley, K. (2014). Reproductive issues in sickle cell disease. *Hematology. American Society Hematology Education Program, 2014*(1), 418–424.

Stabler, S. (2013). Vitamin B12 deficiency. *The New England Journal of Medicine, 368*(2), 149–160.

**Taylor, F. B., Toh, C.-H., Hoots, W. K., et al. (2007). Towards a definition, clinical and laboratory criteria, and a scoring system for DIC. *Journal of Thrombosis and Haemostasis, 5*(3), 445–659.

Telen, M. J., Afenyi-Annan, A., Garrett, M. E., et al. (2015). Alloimmunization in sickle cell disease: Changing antibody specificities and association with chronic pain and decreased survival. *Transfusion, 55* (6 Pt 2), 1378–1387.

Toh, C. H., & Alhamdi, Y. (2013). Current consideration and management of disseminated intravascular coagulation. *Hematology American Society of Hematology Education Program, 2013*(1), 286–291.

Truelove, E., Fielding, A. K., & Hunt, B. J. (2013). The coagulopathy and thrombotic risk associated with L-asparaginase treatment in adults with acute lymphoblastic leukemia. *Leukemia, 27*(3), 553–559.

Turan, O., Ündar, B., Güany, T., et al. (2013). Investigation of inherited thrombophilias in patients with pulmonary embolism. *Blood Coagulation & Fibrinolysis, 24*(2), 140–149.

U.S. Food and Drug Administration. (2015). *Information on erythropoiesis-stimulating agents (ESA) epoetin alfa (marketed as Procrit, Epogen), darbepoetin alfa (marketed as Aranesp)*. Retrieved on 3/12/2016 at: www.fda.gov/drugs/drugsafety/postmarketdrugsafetyinformationforpatientsandproviders/ucm109375.htm

van Meer, S., de Man, R. A., Siersema, P. D., et al. (2013). Surveillance for hepatocellular carcinoma in chronic liver disease: Evidence and controversies. *World Journal of Gastroenterology, 19*(40), 6744–6756.

Vannella, L., Lahner, E., Osborn, J., et al. (2013). Systematic review: Gastric cancer incidence in pernicious anaemia. *Alimentary Pharmacology & Therapeutics, 37*(4), 375–382.

Visvanathan, V. (2015). Slow vs. fast subcutaneous heparin injections for prevention of pain and bruising. *American Journal of Nursing, 115*(12), 27.

Wallen, G. R., Minnitti, C.P., Krumlauf, M., et al. (2014). Sleep disturbance, depression and pain in adults with sickle cell disease. *BMC Psychiatry, 14*, 207.

Yawn, B. P., Buchanan, G .R., Afenyi-Annan, A. N., et al. (2014). Management of sickle cell disease: Summary of the 2014 evidence-based report by expert panel members. *Clinical Review & Education, 312*(10), 1033–1048.

Zanella A., & Barcellini, W. (2014). Treatment of autoimmune hemolytic anemias. *Haematologica, 99*(10), 1547–1554.

Resources

American Association of Blood Banks (AABB), www.aabb.org
Alternative Medicine Foundation, www.amfoundation.org
American Hemochromatosis Society, www.americanhs.org
American Pain Society (APS), ampainsoc.org
American Red Cross, www.redcross.org
American Society for Blood and Marrow Transplantation (ASBMT), asbmt.org
Aplastic Anemia and MDS International Foundation, www.aamds.org
APS Foundation of America (antiphospholipid antibody syndrome), www.apsfa.org
G6PD Deficiency, g6pddeficiency.org
ITP Support Association (immune thrombocytopenic purpura), www.itpsupport.org.uk/
MedlinePlus (information on drug–herb interaction), www.nlm.nih.gov/medlineplus/druginfo/herb_All.html
National Marrow Donor Program, bethematch.org
Platelet Disorder Support Association (PDSA), www.pdsa.org
Sickle Cell Disease Association of America (SCDAA), www.sicklecelldisease.org
National Heart, Lung, and Blood Institute, www.nhlbi.nih.gov

LEARNING OBJECTIVES

On completion of this chapter, the learner will be able to:

1 Distinguish between hematologic clonal disorders and frank malignancy.
2 Compare the leukemias in terms of their incidence, physiologic alterations, clinical manifestations, management, and prognosis.
3 Use the nursing process as a framework for care of patients with acute leukemia.
4 Compare the myeloproliferative disorders in terms of their incidence, clinical manifestations, management, complications, and prognosis.
5 Describe nursing management of patients with lymphoma or multiple myeloma.

GLOSSARY

absolute neutrophil count (ANC): a calculation of the number of circulating neutrophils, derived from the total white blood cells (WBCs) and the percentage of neutrophils counted in a microscope's visual field

angiogenesis: formation of new blood vessels

apoptosis: programmed cell death

blast cell: primitive leukocyte

clone: proliferation from same cell of origin so that descendent cells are identical to the cell of origin

cytokines: proteins produced by leukocytes that are vital to regulation of hematopoiesis, apoptosis, and immune responses

erythrocyte sedimentation rate (ESR): laboratory test that measures the rate of settling of red blood cells (RBCs); elevation is indicative of inflammation; also called the *sed rate*

granulocyte: granulated WBC (neutrophil, eosinophil, basophil); term sometimes used as synonymous with neutrophil

hematopoiesis: complex process of the formation and maturation of blood cells

indolent neoplasm: a slow-growing cancer that often remains localized or causes few symptoms

leukocyte: one of several cellular components of blood involved in defense of the body; subtypes include neutrophils, eosinophils, basophils, monocytes, and lymphocytes (*synonym:* white blood cell [WBC])

leukemia: uncontrolled proliferation of WBCs, often immature

leukopenia: less-than-normal amount of WBCs in circulation

lymphadenopathy: enlargement of a lymph node or lymph nodes

lymphocyte: type of WBC involved in immune functions

lymphoid: pertaining to lymphocytes

lysis: destruction of cells

monocyte: large WBC that becomes a macrophage when it leaves the circulation and moves into body tissues

myeloid: pertaining to nonlymphoid blood cells that differentiate into RBCs, platelets, macrophages, mast cells, and various WBCs

neutropenia: lower-than-normal number of neutrophils

neutrophil: fully mature WBC capable of phagocytosis; primary defense against bacterial infection

pancytopenia: abnormal decrease in WBCs, RBCs, and platelets

petechiae: tiny capillary hemorrhages

phagocytosis: process of cellular ingestion and digestion of foreign bodies

red blood cell (RBC): a cellular component of blood involved in the transport of oxygen and carbon dioxide (*synonym:* erythrocyte)

reticulocytes: slightly immature RBCs, usually only 1% of total circulating RBCs

splenomegaly: enlargement of the spleen

stem cell: primitive cell, capable of self-replication and differentiation into myeloid or lymphoid stem cell

thrombocytopenia: lower-than-normal platelet count

thrombocytosis: higher-than-normal platelet count

white blood cell (WBC): *synonym:* leukocyte

Hematopoiesis is characterized by a rapid, continuous turnover of blood cells. Normally, the production of specific blood cells from their **stem cell** precursors is carefully regulated according to the body's needs. If the mechanisms that control the production of these cells are disrupted, the cells can proliferate excessively, as seen in the development of hematologic neoplasms.

As is true with nonmalignant hematologic disorders, the pathophysiologic processes that undergird the development of hematologic neoplasms are complex. Understanding these processes and the rationale for treatments is important so that nurses may appropriately assess, monitor, educate, and intervene with patients with hematologic neoplasms.

Figure 34-1 • The development of myeloid neoplasms. Changes within the myeloid stem cell can cause the development of neoplasms that are either proliferative or, in the case of myelodysplastic syndrome, dysplastic. Although any indolent myeloid neoplasm can evolve into a malignant condition (e.g., acute myeloid leukemia [AML]), in most instances this will not occur. For example, the incidence of evolution from primary thrombocythemia is very low, yet it is much higher when from primary myelofibrosis. The actual incidence of evolution continues to change as therapy before more effective, as in the case of chronic myeloid leukemia. Note that AML can arise directly from the altered myeloid stem cell; it need not evolve from an existing indolent neoplasm. Similar events occur with lymphoid malignancy development.

Hematopoietic malignancies are often classified by the cells involved. **Leukemia** is a neoplastic proliferation of a particular cell type (granulocytes, **lymphocytes**, or infrequently erythrocytes or megakaryocytes). The defect originates in the hematopoietic stem cell, the myeloid, or the lymphoid stem cell. Lymphomas are neoplasms of lymphoid tissue, usually derived from B lymphocytes. Multiple myeloma is a malignancy of the most mature form of B lymphocyte—the plasma cell.

CLONAL STEM CELL DISORDERS

When some hematologic neoplasms develop, hematopoietic control mechanisms may be in place to continue to produce adequate numbers of normal blood cells. These are commonly referred to as **indolent neoplasms**, where the increased numbers of cells produced from a culprit clone all have the same genotype (see Chapter 8 for further discussion of genotypes). However, at some time, the control mechanisms may fail and the "indolent" **clone** may then evolve into a more aggressive clone.

Not all malignancies arise from an indolent neoplasm, however. Rather, they may evolve directly from changes in the stem cell. Similarly, not all indolent neoplasms will eventually evolve into a malignancy. Nonetheless, such evolution is possible for virtually any clonal disorder. Figure 34-1 illustrates this concept for myeloid stem cell disorders. Similar neoplastic conditions are derived from disorders within the lymphoid stem cell disorder (Shlush & Minden, 2015). Refer to later discussions about specific diseases noted in Figure 34-1.

LEUKEMIA

The term *leukocytosis* refers to an increased level of **leukocytes** (white blood cells [WBCs]) in the circulation. Typically, only one specific cell type is increased. Because the proportions of several types of leukocytes (e.g., eosinophils, basophils, monocytes) are small, an increase in other types can be great enough to elevate the total leukocyte count, particularly the neutrophil or lymphocyte. Although leukocytosis can be a normal response to increased need (e.g., in acute infection), the elevation in leukocytes should decrease as the physiologic need decreases. A prolonged or progressively increasing elevation in leukocytes is abnormal and should be evaluated. A significant cause of persistent leukocytosis is hematologic malignancy (i.e., **leukemia**).

The common feature of the leukemias is an unregulated proliferation of leukocytes in the bone marrow. In acute forms (or late stages of chronic forms), the proliferation of leukemic cells leaves little room for normal cell production. There can also be a proliferation of cells in the liver and spleen (extramedullary hematopoiesis). With acute forms, there can be infiltration of leukemic cells in other organs, such as the meninges, lymph nodes, gums, and skin. The cause of leukemia is not fully known, but exposure to radiation or chemicals, certain genetic disorders, and viral infections are known to be risk factors for certain types of leukemia. Bone marrow damage from pelvic radiation or certain types of chemotherapy drugs can cause acute leukemia, typically occurring years after treatment for another malignancy (Leukemia & Lymphoma Society, 2015a).

The leukemias are commonly classified according to the stem cell line involved, either **lymphoid** (referring to stem cells that produce lymphocytes) or **myeloid** (referring to stem cells that produce nonlymphoid blood cells). They are also classified as either acute or chronic, based on the time it takes for symptoms to evolve and the phase of cell development that is halted (i.e., with few leukocytes differentiating beyond that phase).

In acute leukemia, the onset of symptoms is abrupt, often occurring within a few weeks. Leukocyte development is halted at the blast phase, and thus most leukocytes are undifferentiated cells or blasts. Acute leukemia can progress rapidly, with death occurring within weeks to months without aggressive treatment.

In chronic leukemia, symptoms evolve over a period of months to years, and the majority of leukocytes produced are mature. Chronic leukemia progresses more slowly; the disease trajectory can extend for years.

Acute Myeloid Leukemia

Acute myeloid leukemia (AML) results from a defect in the hematopoietic stem cell that differentiates into all myeloid cells: **monocytes**, **granulocytes** (e.g., **neutrophils**, basophils, eosinophils), erythrocytes, and platelets. Any age group can be affected, although it infrequently occurs before age 45, and the incidence rises with age, with a peak incidence at age 67 (American Cancer Society [ACS], 2014a). AML is the most common non-lymphocytic leukemia.

The prognosis and survival rates are highly variable. Factors influencing a more positive outcome are younger age at diagnosis, more favorable cytogenetic alterations (which are strongly associated with younger age), and few concurrent (or mild) health problems. In contrast, individuals with significant comorbidities, of older age, with cytogenetic features deemed to be adverse, or who are frail, are more likely to have a poor prognosis. AML evolving from a preexisting clonal myeloid disease or from prior cytotoxic therapy for another malignancy or immune disease is also associated with a poorer prognosis (Liesveld & Lichtman, 2016).

Prior to the development of chemotherapy treatment for AML, the median survival rate was only 6 weeks. While platelet transfusion support and aggressive chemotherapy have markedly improved these statistics, survival rates remain suboptimal. Data from the Surveillance, Epidemiology, and End Results (SEER) Program of the National Cancer Institute established 5-year survival rates of 56% for those under age 45, 39% for those aged 45 to 54, 27% for those aged 55 to 64, 11% for those between 65 and 74 years old, and less than 2% for those over age 75 (Liesveld & Lichtman, 2016). Despite these poor statistics, cure is possible for some individuals, either with stem cell transplant or with chemotherapy. Death usually is due to infection or bleeding.

Clinical Manifestations

AML develops without warning, with symptoms typically occurring over a period of weeks. Signs and symptoms result from insufficient production of normal blood cells. Fever and infection result from **neutropenia** (low neutrophil count); weakness and fatigue, dyspnea on exertion, and pallor from anemia; and petechiae, ecchymoses, and bleeding tendencies from thrombocytopenia. The proliferation of leukemic cells within organs leads to a variety of additional symptoms: pain from an enlarged liver or spleen, hyperplasia of the gums, and bone pain from expansion of marrow (see Fig. 34-2). **Petechiae** (pinpoint red or purple hemorrhagic spots on the skin) or ecchymoses (bruises) are common on the skin (see Fig. 33-4 in Chapter 33); occasionally, leukemic infiltrates are also seen (see Fig. 34-3). Leukemic cells can also infiltrate the gingiva or synovial spaces of joints. **Lymphadenopathy** (enlargement of lymph nodes) or **splenomegaly** (enlargement of the spleen) is rare. Fevers may occur and are not always due to infection.

Assessment and Diagnostic Findings

The complete blood count (CBC) shows a decrease in both erythrocytes and platelets. Although the total leukocyte count can be low, normal, or high, the percentage of normal cells is usually vastly decreased. A bone marrow analysis shows an excess (more than 20%) of immature leukocytes, called **blast cells**; this is the hallmark of the diagnosis. AML

Figure 34-2 • Gingival infiltration of leukemic cells in a patient with acute myeloid leukemia. From Greer, J. P., Foerster, J., Rodgers, G. M., et al. (2009). *Wintrobe's clinical hematology* (12th ed., Fig. 72.8, p. 1680). Philadelphia, PA: Lippincott Williams & Wilkins.

Figure 34-3 • Leukemia cutis. Infiltration of leukemic cells in skin on extensor surface of forearms. Reproduced with permission from Stedman's Medical Dictionary. Copyright 2008 Lippincott Williams & Wilkins.

can be further classified into seven different subgroups, based on cytogenetics, histology, and morphology of the blasts. The actual prognosis varies somewhat between subgroups and with the extent of cytogenetic abnormalities and genetic mutations, yet the clinical course and treatment differ substantially with only one subtype. Patients with the specific AML subtype acute promyelocytic leukemia (APL, or AML-M3) have more potentially fatal bleeding episodes, because they have underlying coagulopathy and a higher incidence of disseminated intravascular coagulation (DIC); however, the potential to cure this form of AML is high (Coombs, Tavakkoli, & Tallman, 2015).

Medical Management

Despite advances in understanding of the biology of AML, substantive advances in treatment response rates and survival rates have not occurred for decades, with the exception of advances made in treating APL (see later discussion). Even for patients with AML subtypes that have not benefited from significant advances in treatment, cure is still possible. The overall objective of treatment is to achieve complete remission, in which there is no evidence of residual leukemia in the bone marrow. Attempts are made to achieve remission by the aggressive administration of chemotherapy, called *induction therapy*, which usually requires hospitalization for several weeks. Induction therapy typically involves high doses of cytarabine (Cytosar, Ara-C) and either daunorubicin (Cerubidine), idarubicin (Idamycin), or mitoxantrone (Novantrone); etoposide (VP-16, VePesid) is occasionally added to the regimen. The choice of agents is based on the patient's physical status and history of prior antineoplastic treatment. Older patients (especially those older than 70 years) tend to not tolerate standard therapy. Lower-intensity therapy (using hypomethylating agents, low doses of cytarabine, or hydroxyurea) may extend survival somewhat without a significant increase in toxicity beyond that of the underlying disease (Erba, 2015).

Treatment of APL revolves around induction therapy using the differentiating agent all-trans retinoic acid (ATRA), which induces the promyelocytic blast cells to differentiate, thereby deterring the blasts from proliferating at an immature stage. ATRA is typically combined with a formulation of arsenic (arsenic trioxide) and, in those deemed to be at high risk for relapse, a conventional anthracycline drug. This regimen yields a very high response rate, and cure is possible (Coombs et al., 2015).

In AML, the aim of induction therapy is to eradicate the leukemic cells; however, this is also accompanied by the eradication of normal types of myeloid cells. Thus, the patient becomes severely neutropenic; an **absolute neutrophil count** (**ANC**; a precise calculation of the number of circulating neutrophils) of 0 is not uncommon. Anemia, and severe thrombocytopenia (a platelet count of less than 5,000/mm^3), is also common. During this time, the patient is typically very ill, with bacterial, fungal, and occasionally viral infections; bleeding; and severe mucositis, which causes pain, diarrhea, and an inability to maintain adequate nutrition. Management consists of administering blood products (packed red blood cells and platelets) and promptly treating infections. The use of granulocytic growth factors, either granulocyte colony-stimulating factor (G-CSF; filgrastim [Neupogen]) or granulocyte-macrophage colony-stimulating factor (GM-CSF; sargramostim [Leukine]), can shorten the period of significant neutropenia by stimulating the bone marrow to produce leukocytes more quickly; these agents do not appear to increase the risk of producing more leukemic cells (Kam, Yiu, Loh, et al., 2015).

When the patient has recovered from the induction therapy (i.e., the neutrophil and platelet counts have returned to normal and any infection has resolved), consolidation therapy is given to eliminate any residual leukemia cells that are not clinically detectable and reduce the chance for recurrence. Multiple treatment cycles of various agents are used, usually containing some form of cytarabine. Frequently, the patient receives one cycle of treatment that is almost the same as, if not identical to, the induction treatment but at somewhat lower dosages. Because the amount of leukemia cells is dramatically reduced at this point, toxicity associated with therapy is less (Schiffer, 2014).

Another aggressive treatment option is hematopoietic stem cell transplantation (HSCT). When a suitable tissue match can be obtained, the patient embarks on an even more aggressive regimen of chemotherapy (sometimes in combination with radiation therapy), with the treatment goal of destroying the hematopoietic function of the patient's bone marrow. The patient is then "rescued" with the infusion of the donor stem cells to reinitiate blood cell production. Patients who undergo HSCT have a significant risk of infection and graft-versus-host disease (where the donor's lymphocytes [graft] recognize the patient's body as "foreign" and set up reactions to attack the "foreign" host, i.e., the patient). The most appropriate use and timing of HSCT remain unclear. Patients with a poorer prognosis may benefit from early HSCT; those with a good prognosis may not need transplant at all. See Chapter 15 for a discussion of nursing management in HSCT.

Another important option for the patient to consider is supportive care alone. In fact, supportive care may be the only option if the patient has significant comorbidity, such as extremely poor cardiac, pulmonary, renal, or hepatic function; is older and frail; or both. In such cases, aggressive antileukemia therapy is not used; occasionally, hydroxyurea (Hydrea) or hypomethylating agents such as azacitidine (Vidaza) may be used briefly to control the increase of blast cells. Patients are more commonly supported with antimicrobial therapy and transfusions as needed. This treatment approach provides the patient with some additional time outside the hospital; however, death frequently occurs within months, typically from infection or bleeding. Refer to Chapter 16 for a discussion of end-of-life care.

Complications

Complications of AML include bleeding and infection, which are the major causes of death. The risk of bleeding correlates with the level and duration of platelet deficiency (**thrombocytopenia**). The low platelet count can cause ecchymoses and petechiae. Major hemorrhages also may develop when the platelet count drops to less than 10,000/mm^3. The most common bleeding sources include gastrointestinal (GI), pulmonary, vaginal, and intracranial. For undetermined reasons, fever and infection also increase the likelihood of bleeding. DIC is common, particularly in patients with APL (Coombs et al., 2015). A very high WBC count (greater than $100,000 \times 10^9$/L) can cause stasis within the cerebral or pulmonary circulation.

Because of the lack of mature and normal granulocytes that help fight infection, patients with leukemia are prone to infection. The likelihood of infection increases with the degree and duration of neutropenia; neutrophil counts that persist at less than 100/mm^3 dramatically increase the risk of systemic infections. As the duration of severe neutropenia increases, the patient's risk of developing fungal infections also increases. Fungal infections remain difficult to treat despite the development of new antifungal agents, particularly if the patient has persistent neutropenia (Perfect, Hachem, & Wingard, 2014). However, improvement in reducing the incidence of fungal disease was noted in a study evaluating the efficacy of the drug posaconazole (Noxafil) as antifungal prophylaxis (Pagano, Verga, Busca, et al., 2014).

Massive leukemic cell destruction from chemotherapy results in the release of intracellular electrolytes and fluids into the systemic circulation. Increases in uric acid levels, potassium, and phosphate are seen; this process is referred to as tumor **lysis** (cell destruction) syndrome (see Chapter 15). The increased uric acid and phosphorus levels make the patient vulnerable to renal stone formation and renal colic, which can progress to acute kidney injury. Hyperkalemia and hypocalcemia can lead to cardiac dysrhythmias; hypotension; neuromuscular effects such as muscle cramps, weakness, and spasm/tetany; and confusion; and seizures may also develop. Patients require a high fluid intake, and prophylaxis with allopurinol (Zyloprim) to prevent crystallization of uric acid and subsequent stone formation. If necessary, uric acid degradation can be promoted by the administration of the enzyme rasburicase (Elitek) (Röllig & Ehninger, 2015).

GI problems may result from the infiltration of abnormal leukocytes into the abdominal organs and from the toxicity of the chemotherapeutic agents. Anorexia, nausea, vomiting, diarrhea, and severe mucositis are common. Because of the profound myelosuppressive effects of chemotherapy, significant neutropenia and thrombocytopenia typically result in serious infection and increased risk of bleeding.

Nursing Management

Nursing management of the patient with acute leukemia is presented at the end of the discussion of leukemia in this chapter.

Chronic Myeloid Leukemia

Chronic myeloid leukemia (CML) arises from a mutation in the myeloid stem cell. Normal myeloid cells continue to be produced, but there is a pathologic increase in the production of forms of blast cells. Therefore, a wide spectrum of cell types exists within the blood, from blast forms to mature neutrophils. Because there is an uncontrolled proliferation of cells, the marrow expands into the cavities of long bones, such as the femur, and cells are also formed in the liver and spleen (extramedullary hematopoiesis), resulting in enlargement of these organs that is sometimes painful. CML results from a chromosomal translocation, where a section of deoxyribonucleic acid (DNA) is shifted from chromosome 22 to chromosome 9. The specific location of these changes is on the *BCR* gene on chromosome 22 and the *ABL* gene on chromosome 9. When these two genes fuse (*BCR-ABL* gene), they produce an abnormal protein (a tyrosine kinase protein) that causes leukocytes to divide rapidly. This *BCR-ABL* gene is present in virtually all patients with this disease (ACS, 2015a).

CML accounts for 10% to 15% of all leukemias. The average age at diagnosis is 64; it rarely occurs in children (ACS, 2015b). Because of marked advances in treatment, patients diagnosed with CML in the chronic phase have an overall median life expectancy nearly equal to that of the general population (Thompson, Kantarjian, & Cortes, 2015).

Clinical Manifestations

The clinical picture of CML varies. Patients may be asymptomatic, and leukocytosis is detected by a CBC performed for some other reason. However, the leukocyte count may exceed 100,000/mm^3. Patients with extremely high leukocyte counts may be short of breath or slightly confused because of decreased perfusion to the lungs and brain from leukostasis (the excessive volume of leukocytes inhibits blood flow through the capillaries). The patient may have an enlarged, tender spleen, and occasionally the liver may also be enlarged and tender. Some patients have insidious symptoms, such as malaise, anorexia, and weight loss. Lymphadenopathy is uncommon. There are three stages in CML: chronic, transformation, and accelerated or blast crisis. During the chronic phase, patients have few symptoms and complications from the disease itself and problems with infections and bleeding are rare. However, if the disease transforms to the acute phase (blast crisis), the disease becomes more difficult to treat. Patients develop more symptoms and complications as the disease progresses.

Medical Management

Advances in understanding the pathology of CML at a molecular level have led to dramatic changes in treatment. An oral formulation of a tyrosine kinase inhibitor, imatinib mesylate (Gleevec), works by blocking signals within the leukemia cells that express the *BCR-ABL* protein, thus preventing a series of chemical reactions that cause the cell to grow and divide. Other tyrosine kinase inhibitors (dasatinib [Sprycel] or nilotinib [Tasigna]) are also approved for primary therapy; each has a slightly (but importantly) different toxicity profile. Tyrosine kinase inhibitor therapy can induce complete remission at the cellular and even molecular level. These drugs are metabolized by the cytochrome P450 pathway, which means that drug–drug interactions are common. In particular, antacids and grapefruit juice may limit drug absorption, and large doses of acetaminophen can cause hepatotoxicity. Despite the similarities, each drug has some unique side effects. Periorbital edema is common with long-term use of imatinib. Dasatinib is very myelosuppressive, and its use carries a significant risk for pleural effusion and for causing a prolonged QT interval; nilotinib has more cardiotoxic effects, including dysrhythmias and risk for sudden death (Hughes & White, 2013).

In those instances where imatinib taken at conventional doses does not elicit a molecular remission, or when that remission is not maintained, other treatment options may be considered. The dosage of imatinib can be increased (with potential increased toxicity), or another inhibitor of *BCR-ABL* (e.g., dasatinib or nilotinib) or HSCT can be used.

CML is a disease that can potentially be cured with HSCT in otherwise healthy patients who are younger than 65 years. However, with the development of tyrosine kinase inhibitors, the timing of transplant has come into question. Patients who receive such transplants while still in the chronic phase of the illness tend to have a greater chance for cure than those who receive them in the acute phase. The use of tyrosine kinase therapy has decreased the need for transplantation in CML. See Chapter 15 for more information on HSCT.

The transformation phase can be insidious or rapid; it marks the process of evolution (or transformation) to the acute form of leukemia (blast crisis). In the transformation phase, the patient may complain of bone pain and may report fevers (without any obvious sign of infection) and weight loss. Even with chemotherapy, the spleen may continue to enlarge. The patient may become more anemic and thrombocytopenic; an increased basophil level is detected by the CBC.

In the acute form of CML (blast crisis), treatment may resemble induction therapy for acute leukemia, using the same medications as for AML or acute lymphocytic leukemia (ALL). Patients whose disease evolves into a "lymphoid" blast crisis are more likely to be able to reenter a chronic phase after induction therapy. For those whose disease evolves into AML, therapy has been largely ineffective in achieving a second chronic phase. However, an increased dose of imatinib or dasatinib can be effective in the later stages of CML. Life-threatening infections and bleeding occur frequently in this phase.

Nursing Management

Advances in treatment of CML have changed the trajectory of the disease, from life-threatening and likely fatal to being a chronic illness. However, nurses must understand that the effectiveness of the drugs used to treat CML is based on the patient's ability to adhere to the prescribed medication regimen and on appropriate monitoring of the therapeutic response.

Drugs used to treat CML may cause side effects for the patient that may be difficult to manage. Fatigue, asthenia, pruritus, headache, skin rash, and oropharyngeal pain are common side effects that often can be effectively managed with nursing intervention (Coleman, 2014).

Blood testing, using a specific polymerase chain reaction (PCR) to detect the level of *BCR-ABL*, is performed at regular intervals to assess for a major molecular response. Major molecular response is the benchmark for determining the efficacy of therapy and the need to change to a different drug (Deninger, 2015). Yet studies have documented the lack of adherence to this assessment with rates of adherence from less than 40% (Goldberg, 2015) to only 21% within the initial 3 months of therapy (Di Bella, Bhowmik, Bhor, et al., 2015).

Patient adherence to therapy is critical for optimal outcomes to be achieved. Several studies have documented suboptimal adherence rates to taking tyrosine kinase inhibitors as prescribed. A large study conducted in Italy discovered a self-reported rate of complete adherence to be only 60% (Breccia, Efficace, Sica, et al., 2015). In that study, forgetting to take the drug was the most common reported reason for decreased adherence. A review of 34 studies was conducted to better determine adherence rates to therapy and issues related to poor adherence in patients receiving tyrosine kinase inhibitor therapy (Hall, Paul, Bryant, et al., 2016). In this review, 100% adherence rates ranged from 20% to 53%. The investigators explored factors associated with reduced adherence, many of which have significant relevance for nursing and are depicted in Table 34-1.

These data highlight the importance of nurses educating patients and assisting them to identify methods that help them remember to take their medication, to manage side effects, and to obtain prescription renewals on time. Furthermore, nurses must encourage patients to raise issues of concern that interfere with their adherence to their prescribed therapy. As adherence may decrease over time, it is important that nurses continue to assess patients for risk factors that may diminish adherence and proactively address them. To facilitate this process, acknowledging that the patient is ultimately responsible for their own care and targeting educational interventions to enhance the patient's ability to think critically are crucial (Coleman, 2014).

Acute Lymphocytic Leukemia

ALL results from an uncontrolled proliferation of immature cells (lymphoblasts) derived from the lymphoid stem cell. The cell of origin is the precursor to the B lymphocyte in approximately 75% of ALL cases; T-lymphocyte ALL occurs in approximately 25% of cases. The *BCR-ABL* translocation (see earlier CML discussion) is found in 20% of ALL blast cells. ALL is most common in young children, with boys affected more often than girls; the peak incidence is 4 years of age. After 15 years of age, it is relatively uncommon, until age 50 when the incidence again rises (Larson & Richard, 2016).

ALL is very responsive to treatment; complete remission or response rates are approximately 85% for adults (DeAngelo, 2015). Increasing age appears to be associated with diminished survival; the 5-year event-free survival rate is more than 85% for children, whereas the 3-year event-free survival rate drops to less than 45% for adults (DeAngelo, 2015). If relapse occurs, resumption of induction therapy can often achieve a second complete remission, but the duration of response is often brief. However, HSCT may be successful even after a second relapse, particularly in certain subsets of patients (e.g., those with Philadelphia chromosome–positive ALL [Ph+ ALL]).

Clinical Manifestations

Immature lymphocytes proliferate in the marrow and impede the development of normal myeloid cells. As a result, normal

TABLE 34-1 Risk Factors Associated With Lower Adherence to Oral Therapy for Chronic Myeloid Leukemia (CML)

Risk Factor Category	Risk Factor	Nursing Intervention
Patient Characteristics	Lower education level (below high school)	
	Higher self-report of functional status	
	Low self-efficacy regarding medication administration[a]	Explore with patient perceived barriers related to medication administration
	Taking medication independent of meals[a]	Develop medication administration schedule with patient; use timer/watch alarm to alert patient when to take medication
	Lack of knowledge regarding disease and treatment[a]	Provide relevant information in format understandable to patient
Social Characteristics	Living alone[a]	Evaluate need for phone follow-up, initiation of home care
	Low levels of social support	
	Low socioeconomic status	
Disease and Treatment Characteristics	Farther time from diagnosis	
	Higher rates of treatment-related side effects[a]	Monitor patient closely for side effects
	Higher number of cancer-related complications[a]	Monitor patient closely for complications
	Not participating in a clinical trial[a]	Provide patient with information on enrollment eligibility as advisable

[a]indicates risk factor amenable to nursing intervention

Adapted from Hall, A. E., Paul, C., Bryant, J., et al. (2016). To adhere or not to adhere: Rates and reasons of medication adherence in hematological cancer patients. *Critical Reviews in Oncology/Hematology, 97*(1), 247–262.

hematopoiesis is inhibited, resulting in reduced numbers of granulocytes, erythrocytes, and platelets. Leukocyte counts may be either low or high, but there is always a high proportion of immature cells. Manifestations of leukemic cell infiltration into other organs are more common with ALL than with other forms of leukemia and include pain from an enlarged liver or spleen and bone pain. The central nervous system (CNS) is frequently a site for leukemic cells; thus, patients may exhibit cranial nerve palsies or headache and vomiting because of meningeal involvement. Other extranodal sites include the testes and breasts.

Medical Management

The goal of treatment is to obtain remission without excess toxicity and with a rapid hematologic recovery so that additional therapy can be given if needed. Because of the heterogeneity of the disease, treatment plans are based on genetic markers of the disease as well as risk factors of the patient, primarily age. Because ALL frequently invades the CNS, preventive intrathecal chemotherapy or, less frequently, cranial irradiation is also a key part of the treatment plan.

Treatment protocols for ALL tend to be complex, using a wide variety of chemotherapeutic agents and complicated administration schedules. The expected outcome of treatment is complete remission. Lymphoid blast cells are typically very sensitive to corticosteroids and to vinca alkaloids; therefore, these medications are an integral part of the initial induction therapy. The corticosteroid dexamethasone is preferred to prednisone, as it is more toxic to lymphoid cells and has better CNS penetration. Typically, an anthracycline is included, sometimes with asparaginase (Elspar). Once a patient is in remission, special testing (immunophenotyping, immunoglobulin gene rearrangements, T-cell receptor genes, molecular testing) is done to look for residual leukemia cells; these tests can detect as fewer as 1 ALL cell among 10,000 to 100,000 normal cells. This minimal residual disease testing is useful as a prognostic indicator. Based on these results and the rapidity in which remission is achieved, a consolidation regimen ensues, using different combinations and dosages of the drugs used in induction therapy; the goal of consolidation is to improve outcomes in those patients at high risk for relapse. HSCT may be considered during initial remission if disease features and testing suggest the risk of relapse is high (Mathisen, Kantarjian, Thomas, et al., 2013). In the context of average-risk disease, HSCT may be postponed until the time of relapse, should it occur. The therapeutic goal at the time of relapse is to reinitiate treatment to obtain a remission and then move quickly to HSCT (Mathisen et al., 2013). HSCT can improve long-term disease-free survival; however, this potential benefit must be weighed with the risks associated with the procedure, including death and long-term morbid complications (see Chapter 15).

Despite its complexity, treatment can be provided in the outpatient setting in some circumstances until severe complications develop. Tyrosine kinase inhibitors (e.g., imatinib) appear effective in patients with Ph+ ALL; these drugs can be used alone or in combination with conventional chemotherapy (Chiaretti & Foà, 2015). Commercially available monoclonal antibodies (MoAbs), in which the antibody specific to the antigen expressed on the ALL blast cell is selected for treatment, are being utilized in the context of salvage therapy; new MoAbs are under investigation (DeAngelo, 2015).

Patients with ALL can experience some unique adverse effects from treatment. The use of corticosteroids to treat ALL increases the patient's susceptibility to infection; viral infections are common. Avascular necrosis can occur in patients treated with corticosteroid-based chemotherapy, as well as with transplantation. Patients treated with asparaginase are at increased risk for thrombosis. Hepatic toxicity is also common and may necessitate cessation of supportive drugs, such as proton pump inhibitors and certain antibacterial and antifungal drugs.

Nursing Management

Nursing management of the patient with acute leukemia is presented at the end of the leukemia section in this chapter.

Chronic Lymphocytic Leukemia

Chronic lymphocytic leukemia (CLL) is a common malignancy of older adults, and the most prevalent type of adult leukemia in the Western world (Randhawa & Ferrajoli, 2016). The average age at diagnosis is 72 years (Awan & Byrd, 2016). CLL is rarely seen in Native Americans and infrequently among persons of Asian descent. Unlike other forms of leukemia, a strong familial predisposition exists with CLL; the disease can occur in 10% of those with a first- or second-degree relative with the same diagnosis. Veterans of the Vietnam War who were exposed to Agent Orange may be at risk for developing this disease, but there is no definitive link to other pesticides or chemical exposure. While many patients will have a normal life expectancy, others will have a very short life expectancy due to the aggressive nature of the disease.

Pathophysiology

CLL is typically derived from a malignant clone of B lymphocytes. What was formerly called T-lymphocyte CLL is rare and is now reclassified as T-cell prolymphocytic leukemia (Hallek, 2015). In contrast to the acute forms of leukemia, most leukemia cells in CLL are fully mature. One possible mechanism that explains this oncogenesis is that these cells can escape **apoptosis** (programmed cell death), resulting in an excessive accumulation of the cells in the marrow and circulation. The disease is historically classified into three or four stages, based on the two classification systems that are used. In the early stage, an elevated lymphocyte count is seen; it can exceed 100,000/mm^3.

Because the lymphocytes are small, they can easily travel through the small capillaries within the circulation, and the pulmonary and cerebral complications of leukocytosis (as seen with myeloid leukemias) are not typically found in CLL. However, these cells often accumulate within the lymph nodes and spleen. When it takes less than 12 months for the absolute number of lymphocytes to double (lymphocyte doubling time), a more aggressive disease course may ensue.

Immunophenotyping of the circulating B cells is critical to establish the diagnosis by identifying the presence of a malignant clone of these cells; it is also used to gauge the prognosis (Hallek, 2015). Other special cytogenetic and molecular analyses (e.g., fluorescence in situ hybridization [FISH]) are also used to guide prognosis and therapy. Beta-2 microglobulin, a protein found on the surface of lymphocytes, can be measured in the serum; an elevated level correlates with more advanced clinical stage and poorer prognosis.

Autoimmune complications can occur at any stage, as either autoimmune hemolytic anemia or idiopathic thrombocytopenic purpura. In the autoimmune process, the reticuloendothelial system destroys the body's own erythrocytes or platelets. Patients with CLL also have a greater risk for developing other cancers; the risk is 2.2 times higher than the expected incidence per the SEER database (Randhawa & Ferrajoli, 2016). Second cancers typically involve the skin, colon, lung, breast, prostate, and kidney. Roughly 10% of patients will experience a gradual transformation of their disease to one that becomes refractory to chemotherapy (prolymphocytic leukemia transformation) (Awan & Byrd, 2016). Slightly fewer patients will experience a sudden transformation to a very aggressive lymphoma, known as Richter's transformation; this transformation results in markedly increased lymphadenopathy, splenomegaly, worsening B symptoms (see later discussion), and survival of only a few months despite treatment.

Clinical Manifestations

Many patients are asymptomatic and are diagnosed incidentally during routine physical examinations or during treatment for another disease. An increased lymphocyte count (lymphocytosis) is always present. The erythrocyte and platelet counts may be normal or, in later stages of the illness, decreased. Enlargement of lymph nodes (lymphadenopathy) is common; this can be severe and sometimes painful (see Fig. 34-4). The spleen can also be enlarged (splenomegaly).

Figure 34-4 • Massive lymphadenopathy in a patient with chronic lymphocytic leukemia. Note the enlarged liver and spleen as well. From Tkachuk, D. C., & Hirschman, J. V. (2007). *Wintrobe's atlas of clinical hematology* (Fig. 5.1, p. 154). Philadelphia, PA: Lippincott Williams & Wilkins.

Patients with CLL can develop "B symptoms," a constellation of symptoms including fevers, drenching sweats (especially at night), and unintentional weight loss. T-cell function is impaired and may be the cause of tumor progression and increased susceptibility to second malignancies and infections. Life-threatening infections are particularly common with advanced disease, and account for 50% to 60% of all deaths in this patient population (Randhawa & Ferrajoli, 2016). Viral infections, such as herpes zoster, can become widely disseminated. Defects in the complement system are also seen, which results in increased risk of developing infection with encapsulated organisms (e.g., *Haemophilus influenzae*). Patients should receive an annual comprehensive skin examination (as the incidence of skin cancer is higher in this group), and screening guidelines for other cancers should be followed, such as for breast, colorectal, lung, and prostate cancer (Randhawa & Ferrajoli, 2016).

Medical Management

For patients with no symptoms at the time of diagnosis, the traditional "watch and wait" approach is still used, even in the face of genetic markers associated with poor prognosis (Stilgenbauer, 2015). However, with the advent of newer treatment modalities and of more sensitive means of determining prognosis, achieving a complete remission and eradicating even minimal residual disease in patients in the early stages of CLL result in improved survival (Hallek, 2015). As a result, treatment may be initiated sooner in the illness trajectory; clinical trials are ongoing to assess for an advantage in survival with this approach. Various parameters are considered when treatment is selected, including the clinical stage of the disease, disease-associated symptoms, the functional status of the patient, genetic risk for poor prognosis, and the extent of any prior therapy and efficacy of that therapy (Hallek, 2015). Functional status is a complex consideration; in this context, it incorporates the individual's life expectancy independent of CLL (due to other health problems), the ability to tolerate aggressive therapy (where creatinine clearance is particularly important), and the ability to perform activities of daily living (Shanafelt, 2013). Individuals with good functional status can typically tolerate aggressive therapy and often achieve a lasting complete remission. Whereas, the objective of treatment in those with more impaired physical status focuses on controlling bothersome symptoms (e.g., drenching night sweats, painful lymphadenopathy).

The use of combination therapy, using an immunotherapeutic antibody against CD20 (e.g., rituximab [Rituxan], ofatumumab [Arzerra], or obinutuzumab [Gazyra]) with chemotherapy agents (e.g., fludarabine [Fludara], cyclophosphamide [Cytoxan], bendamustine [Treanda] and/or chlorambucil [Leukeran]) is typically given as initial therapy; the patient's functional status (as described above) guides the specific treatment selection. When the disease is accompanied by a deletion of the TP53 gene or a mutation of this gene, the combination of chemo-immunotherapy is largely ineffective. However, two kinase inhibitors, ibrutinib (Imbruvica) and idelalisib (Zydelig), are now available that are efficacious in this context (Hallek, 2015).

The effectiveness of conventional treatment must be balanced by the risk of toxicity. For example, the chemotherapy drugs fludarabine and cyclophosphamide are often given in combination with the MoAb rituximab. This regimen can result in remissions that last 5 years, but has a high associated rate of toxicity (76%) (Shanafelt, 2013). In contrast, chlorambucil has a remission time of 12 months, but the associated toxicity is negligible. These data emphasize the importance of determining the goals of treatment with the patient *a priori*.

The major side effect of fludarabine is prolonged bone marrow suppression, manifested by prolonged periods of neutropenia, lymphopenia, and thrombocytopenia, which puts patients at risk for such infections as *Pneumocystis jiroveci*, *Listeria*, mycobacteria, herpes viruses, and cytomegalovirus (CMV). The MoAb alemtuzumab (Campath) is often used in combination with other chemotherapeutic agents when the disease is refractory to fludarabine, the patient has very poor prognostic markers, or it is necessary to eradicate residual disease after initial treatment. Alemtuzumab targets the CD52 antigen commonly found on CLL cells, and it is effective in clearing the marrow and circulation of these cells without affecting the stem cells. Because CD52 is present on both B and T lymphocytes, patients receiving alemtuzumab are at significant risk for infection; prophylactic use of antiviral agents and antibiotics (e.g., trimethoprim–sulfamethoxazole [Bactrim, Septra]) is important and needs to continue for several months after treatment ends. CMV infection is also common with alemtuzumab and prophylaxis is important; among commonly prescribed antiviral agents, vancyclovir (Valacyclovir) is more effective than acyclovir (Zovirax) for treating CMV (Randhawa & Ferrajoli, 2016).

Virtually all patients with CLL have reduced levels of immunoglobulins, and bacterial infections are common, independent of treatment. Intravenous treatment with immunoglobulin (IVIG) may be given to selected patients with recurrent infection. While studies have not demonstrated improved survival, the rate of developing major infections is reduced (Randhawa & Ferrajoli, 2016). Patients with CLL should receive both pneumonia and flu vaccinations as indicated (see Chapter 23). Live vaccines should be avoided.

Because of the older age of most patients with CLL, transplantation may not be an option, particularly if significant comorbidities exist. Yet, allogeneic HSCT can be effective in patients with P53 deletions or mutations who otherwise have a poor prognosis. Morbidity and mortality rates remain high (20%); thus, this treatment modality may be reserved for those patients with high-risk disease, younger age, and high degree of match from the donor (Stilgenbauer, 2015).

NURSING PROCESS

The Patient With Acute Leukemia

Assessment

Although the clinical picture varies with the type of leukemia as well as with the treatment implemented, the health history may reveal a range of subtle symptoms reported by the patient before the problem is detectable on physical examination. If the patient is hospitalized, assessments should be performed daily, or more frequently as warranted. Because the physical findings may be subtle initially, a thorough, systematic assessment incorporating all body systems is essential. For example, a dry cough, mild dyspnea, and diminished breath sounds may indicate a pulmonary infection. However, the infection may

not be seen initially on the chest x-ray; the absence of neutrophils delays the inflammatory response against the pulmonary infection, thus delaying radiographic changes. When serial assessments are performed, current findings are compared with previous findings to evaluate improvement or worsening. Specific body system assessments are delineated in the neutropenic and bleeding precautions found in Chart 15-7 in Chapter 15.

The nurse also must closely monitor the results of laboratory studies, including tracking the leukocyte count, ANC, hematocrit, platelet, creatinine and electrolyte levels, and coagulation and hepatic function tests. Culture results need to be reported immediately so that appropriate antimicrobial therapy can begin or be modified.

Diagnosis

NURSING DIAGNOSES

Based on the assessment data, major nursing diagnoses may include:

- Risk for infection, bleeding, or both
- Impaired oral mucous membranes due to changes in epithelial lining of the GI tract from chemotherapy or prolonged use of antimicrobial medications
- Imbalanced nutrition: less than body requirements related to hypermetabolic state, anorexia, mucositis, pain, and nausea
- Acute pain and discomfort related to mucositis, leukocyte infiltration of systemic tissues, fever, and infection
- Fatigue and activity intolerance related to anemia, infection, inadequate nutrition, and deconditioning
- Risk for imbalanced fluid volume related to renal dysfunction, diarrhea, bleeding, infection, increased metabolic rate, hypoproteinemia, and need for multiple intravenous medications and blood products
- Self-care deficits (bathing, dressing, toileting) due to fatigue and malaise
- Anxiety and grieving due to uncertainty about future, anticipatory loss, and altered role functioning
- Risk for spiritual distress
- Deficient knowledge about disease process, treatment, complication management, and self-care measures

COLLABORATIVE PROBLEMS/POTENTIAL COMPLICATIONS

Potential complications may include the following (see Chapter 15 for further discussion):

- Infection
- Bleeding/DIC
- Renal dysfunction
- Tumor lysis syndrome

Planning and Goals

The major goals for the patient may include absence of complications and pain, attainment and maintenance of adequate nutrition, activity tolerance, ability to provide self-care and to cope with the diagnosis and prognosis, positive body image, and an understanding of the disease process and its treatment.

Nursing Interventions

PREVENTING OR MANAGING INFECTION AND BLEEDING

The nursing interventions related to diminishing the risk of infection and bleeding are delineated in Chart 15-7 in Chapter 15.

MANAGING MUCOSITIS

Although emphasis is placed on the oral mucosa, the entire GI mucosa can be altered, not only by the effects of chemotherapy but also from prolonged administration of antibiotics. See Chapter 15 for assessment and management of mucositis.

IMPROVING NUTRITIONAL INTAKE

The disease process can increase the patient's metabolic rate and nutritional requirements. Nutritional intake is often reduced because of pain and discomfort associated with stomatitis. Encouraging or providing mouth care before and after meals and administering analgesic agents before eating can help increase intake. If oral anesthetic agents are used, the patient must be warned to chew with extreme care to avoid inadvertently biting the tongue or buccal mucosa.

Nausea should not interfere with nutritional intake, because appropriate antiemetic therapy is highly effective. However, nausea can result from antimicrobial therapy, so some antiemetic therapy may still be required after the chemotherapy has been completed.

Small, frequent feedings of foods that are soft in texture and moderate in temperature may be better tolerated. Low-microbial diets may be prescribed (avoiding uncooked fruits or vegetables and those without a peelable skin), although there is little evidence to support this intervention (Foster, 2014). Nutritional supplements are frequently used. Daily body weight (as well as intake and output measurements) is useful in monitoring fluid status. Both calorie counts and more formal nutritional assessments are often useful. Parenteral nutrition may be required to maintain adequate nutrition.

EASING PAIN AND DISCOMFORT

Recurrent fevers are common in acute leukemia; at times, they are accompanied by shaking chills (rigors), which can be severe. Myalgias and arthralgias can result. Acetaminophen (Tylenol) is typically given to decrease fever, but it also increases diaphoresis. Sponging with cool water may be useful, but cold water or ice packs should be avoided because the heat cannot dissipate from constricted blood vessels. Bedclothes need frequent changing as well. Gentle back and shoulder massage may provide comfort.

Mucositis can also cause significant discomfort. In addition to oral hygiene practices, patient-controlled analgesia can be effective in controlling the pain (see Chapter 12). With the exception of severe mucositis, less pain is associated with acute leukemia than with many other forms of cancer. However, the amount of psychological suffering that the patient endures can be immense. Patients often benefit from active listening and possible referral for professional counseling.

DECREASING FATIGUE AND ACTIVITY INTOLERANCE

Fatigue is a common and oppressive symptom. Nursing interventions should focus on assisting the patient to establish a balance between activity and rest. Patients with acute leukemia need to maintain some physical activity and exercise to prevent the deconditioning that results from inactivity. The use of a high-efficiency particulate air (HEPA) filter mask can permit the patient to ambulate outside the room despite severe neutropenia. Stationary bicycles may also be set up in the room; however, many patients lack the motivation or stamina to use them. At a minimum, patients should be encouraged to sit up in a chair while awake rather than staying in bed; even

this simple activity can improve the patient's tidal volume and enhance circulation. Physical therapy can also be beneficial. Patients with acute leukemia may require hospitalization for extensive nursing care (either during induction or consolidation therapy or during resultant complications); sleep deprivation frequently results. Nurses need to implement creative strategies that permit uninterrupted sleep for at least a few hours while still administering necessary medications on schedule (see Chart 34-1: Nursing Research Profile: Sleep Disturbances Among Patients Post-HSCT).

MAINTAINING FLUID AND ELECTROLYTE BALANCE

Febrile episodes, bleeding, and inadequate or overly aggressive fluid replacement can alter the patient's fluid status. Similarly, persistent diarrhea, vomiting, and long-term use of certain antimicrobial agents can cause significant deficits in electrolytes. Intake and output need to be measured accurately, and daily weights should also be monitored. The patient should be assessed for signs of dehydration as well as fluid overload, with particular attention to pulmonary status and the development of dependent edema. Laboratory test results, particularly electrolytes, blood urea nitrogen, creatinine, and hematocrit, should be monitored and compared with previous results. Replacement of electrolytes, particularly potassium and magnesium, is commonly required. Patients receiving amphotericin or certain antibiotics are at increased risk for electrolyte depletion.

IMPROVING SELF-CARE: BATHING, DRESSING, AND TOILETING

Because hygiene measures are so important in this patient population, they must be performed by the nurse when the patient cannot do so. However, the patient should be encouraged to do as much as possible to preserve mobility and function as well as self-esteem. Patients may have negative feelings because they can no longer care for themselves. Empathetic listening is helpful, as is realistic reassurance that these deficits are temporary. As the patient recovers, the nurse assists him or her to resume more self-care. Patients are usually discharged from the hospital with a vascular access device (e.g., Hickman catheter, peripherally inserted central catheter [PICC]), and coordination with appropriate home care services is needed for catheter management.

MANAGING ANXIETY AND GRIEF

Being diagnosed with acute leukemia can be extremely frightening. In many instances, the need to begin treatment is emergent, and the patient has little time to process the fact that he or she has the illness before making decisions about therapy. Providing emotional support and discussing the uncertain future are crucial. The nurse also needs to assess how much information the patient wants to have regarding the illness, its treatment, and potential complications. This desire should be reassessed at intervals, because needs and interest in information change throughout the course of the disease and treatment. Priorities must be identified so that procedures, assessments, and self-care expectations are adequately explained even to those who do not wish extensive information.

Many patients exhibit depressive symptoms and begin to grieve for their losses, such as normal family functioning, professional roles and responsibilities, and social roles, as well as physical functioning. The nurse can assist the patient to identify the source of the grief and encourage him or her to allow time to adjust to the major life changes produced by the illness. Role restructuring, in both family and professional life, may be required. Again, when

Chart 34-1	**NURSING RESEARCH PROFILE**
	Sleep Disturbances Among Patients Post-HSCT

Hacker, E. D., Patel, P., & Stainthorpe, M. (2013). Sleep interrupted: Nocturnal care disturbances following hematopoietic stem cell transplantation. *Clinical Journal of Oncology Nursing, 17*(5), 517–523.

Purpose

Sleep is a physiologic process essential for health and well-being. Patients admitted to the hospital for hematopoietic stem cell transplantation (HCST) are at risk for sleep-wake disturbance due to the acuity of their illness, the need for continuous nursing care, environmental issues, and individual patient factors. The purpose of this exploratory retrospective study was to examine reports of sleep disturbance and nocturnal disturbances in patients receiving HSCT.

Design

Forty adults who were hospitalized for HSCT comprised the convenience sample for this study. Patients were receiving HSCT for a malignancy (not specified) on a single bone marrow transplantation unit in an academic medical center. Twenty-four of the participants were male, and 16 were female. Data were obtained from the patients' electronic medical records to complete the hourly nocturnal care interactions checklist, a standardized checklist designed to record interactions between the patient and all health care team members between the hours of 9 PM and 7 AM. Standardization of data abstraction was achieved by performing separate reviews of the record and identifying any inconsistencies in coding the data. The investigators also recorded any documentation of sleep disturbance within the progress notes of the medical record.

Results

Data were obtained from 160 unique nights; 1,642 care interactions were identified. The mean number of interactions over a

4-day time period was 41 per patient (range 20–58), approximately 10 interactions per patient per night. Five categories accounted for 88% of the nocturnal interactions: medication administration (40%), vital sign measurement (21%), obtaining blood samples (11%), intravenous catheter maintenance (10%), and patient assessment (6%). Nursing documentation of sleep disturbance was noted 145 times for 29 patients, and 17 times for 11 patients by physicians. Sleep aid medication was prescribed (*pro re nata* [PRN]) for 25 of the 40 patients. The peak time of nocturnal interaction occurred between 12 AM and 1 AM and between 4 AM and 5 AM, coinciding with obtaining routine vital sign measurements.

Nursing Implications

This study highlights that patients who have had HSCT have their sleep frequently interrupted while hospitalized. While the frequency is less than that reported in other studies documenting sleep interruption in the ICU setting, this study suggests that care (and thus sleep interruptions) is more clustered in the transplant unit setting. Nonetheless, clustering interventions is only partially responsible for disturbing sleep in that 50% of the interactions occur outside the two peak periods identified (i.e., 12 AM and 4 AM). Of note, toileting activities were not documented. As diarrhea is common in this patient population, the amount of sleep interruption may be greater than the data from this study suggest.

Given that a normal sleep cycle (REM sleep) is 90 to 120 minutes in length, most patients do not obtain the amount and quality of sleep needed to maximize—or regain—health. Nurses need to work collaboratively to cluster activities and interventions as much as possible. The timing of routine care practices may need to be modified so that the opportunity for patients to obtain needed sleep without interruption is realized.

---

possible, encouraging the patient to identify options and to take time making important decisions is helpful.

The patient's physical condition can deteriorate quickly and it is not often easy to discern if the patient may recover or will die from complications. Providing emotional support to both the patient and the family is critical and equally as important as is rendering expert physical care.

Discharge from the hospital can also provoke anxiety. Although most patients are eager to go home, they may lack confidence in their ability to manage potential complications and to resume their normal activity. Close communication between nurses across care settings can reassure patients that they will not be abandoned.

ENCOURAGING SPIRITUAL WELL-BEING

Because acute leukemia is a serious, potentially life-threatening illness, the nurse may offer support to enhance the patient's spiritual well-being. The patient's spiritual and religious practices should be assessed and pastoral services offered. Throughout the patient's illness, the nurse assists the patient to maintain hope. However, that hope should be realistic and will certainly change over the course of the illness. For example, the patient may initially hope to be cured, but with repeated relapses and a change to hospice or palliative care, the same patient may hope for a quiet, dignified death (see Chart 34-2: Ethical Dilemma: Can Comfort Care at End of Life Equate to Assisted Suicide or Active Euthanasia?). (Refer to Chapter 16 for a discussion of end-of-life care.)

PROMOTING HOME, COMMUNITY-BASED, AND TRANSITIONAL CARE

Educating Patients About Self-Care. Most patients cope better when they understand what is happening to them. Based on their health literacy level, and interest, educating the patient and family should begin with a focus on the disease (including some pathophysiology), its treatment, and certainly the resulting significant risk of infection and bleeding (see Charts 33-7 and 33-8 in Chapter 33).

Although management of a vascular access device can be taught to most patients or family members, this care is typically performed by a home care agency or outpatient clinic nursing staff. Patients and family members do need basic education regarding management of the vascular access device, particularly with regard to prevention of infections.

Continuing and Transitional Care. For patients who are clinically stable but require parenteral antibiotics or blood products, these procedures are most often performed in an outpatient setting. Nurses in these settings must communicate regularly. They need to inform the patient about parameters that are important to monitor, how to monitor them, and to give the patient specific instructions about when to seek care from the physician or other health care provider.

The patient and family need to have a clear understanding of the disease, the prognosis, and how to monitor for complications or recurrence. The nurse ensures that this information is provided. Should the patient no longer respond

Chart 34-2 ETHICAL DILEMMA
Can Comfort Care at End of Life Equate to Assisted Suicide or Active Euthanasia?

Case Scenario

A 34-year-old patient, wife and mother of two young children, has been on the oncology unit with a terminal diagnosis of acute myeloid leukemia (AML). She has recently decided to stop all treatments and begin palliative care. Over the course of the past few weeks, she has developed intractable bone pain, nausea, and episodes of severe bleeding. The patient, who is of sound mental capacity, discusses further treatment options with the oncologist and her family and wants to die peacefully. The patient is placed on a midazolam (Versed) and morphine intravenous drip that you titrate to achieve relief of symptoms. The patient dies peacefully within 72 hours of you starting this new medication regimen with her family at her bedside.

Discussion

There is a great deal of discomfort among both clinicians and laymen around what constitutes comfort care (i.e., palliative care) at end of life and what may constitute either assisted suicide or euthanasia. The premise is that palliative care should ameliorate pain and physical suffering in the patient who is terminally ill, but it should not significantly shorten the patient's life. There is never the intent to deliberately kill the patient. Although the American Nurses Association (ANA) clearly does not advocate that nurses participate in either assisted suicide or euthanasia, and avows that nurses should not participate in acts that intentionally cause patient death (ANA, 2015), the ANA does advocate that nurses provide competent palliative care at end of life that preserves each individual patient's dignity and autonomy (ANA, 2015).

Analysis

- Would you describe your role in this case as complicit in assisted suicide, active euthanasia, or providing palliation?

What distinction, if any, might there be among these three acts?

- Describe how the ethical principles of autonomy, beneficence, and nonmaleficence may intersect or be at odds with each other in this case (see Chart 3-3 in Chapter 3).
- Discuss how palliative sedation meets the moral justification of the four principles of the doctrine of double effect (see Chart 3-3 in Chapter 3).
- Note that the ANA (2015) Code of Ethics clearly states that nurses should not intentionally cause a patient's death. What were your "intentions" in this case? How might intentionality be instrumental in making this act of titrating medications that provided palliation morally defensible?

References

American Nurses Association (ANA). (2015). *Code of ethics for nurses with interpretive statements*. Washington, DC: Nursesbooks.org.

Broeckaert, B. (2011). Palliative sedation, physician assisted suicide, and euthanasia: "Same, same but different?" *American Journal of Bioethics, 11*(6), 62–64.

Carvalho, T. B., Radt, M. Y., Verheijde, J. L., et al. (2011). Continuous deep sedation in end-of-life care: disentangling palliation from physician-assisted death. *American Journal of Bioethics, 11*(6), 60–62.

Wilson, O., Avalos, G., & Dowling, M. (2016). Knowledge of palliative care and attitudes towards nursing the dying patient. *British Journal of Nursing, 25*(11), 600–605.

Resource

See Chapter 3, Chart 3-6 for ethics resources.

to therapy, it is important to respect the patient's choices about treatment and end-of-life care. Advance directives or other method should be used for patients to state their end-of-life preferences (see Chapter 16, Chart 16-4). In patients with acute leukemia, death typically occurs from infection or, less frequently, from bleeding. Family members need to have information about these complications and the measures to take should either occur. Many family members cannot cope with the care required when a patient begins to bleed actively. It is important to delineate alternatives to keeping the patient at home, such as inpatient hospice units.

Evaluation

Expected patient outcomes may include:
1. Shows no evidence of infection
2. Experiences no bleeding
3. Has intact oral mucous membranes
   a. Participates in oral hygiene regimen
   b. Reports no discomfort in mouth
4. Attains optimal level of nutrition
   a. Maintains weight with increased food and fluid intake
   b. Maintains adequate protein stores (e.g., albumin, prealbumin)
5. Reports satisfaction with pain and comfort levels
6. Has less fatigue and increased activity
7. Maintains fluid and electrolyte balance
8. Participates in self-care
9. Copes with anxiety and grief
   a. Discusses concerns and fears
   b. Uses stress management strategies appropriately
   c. Participates in decisions regarding end-of-life care
10. Reports sense of spiritual well-being
11. Absence of complications

MYELODYSPLASTIC SYNDROMES (MDS)

The MDS are a group of clonal disorders of the myeloid stem cell that cause dysplasia (abnormal development) in one or more types of cell lines. The most common feature of MDS—dysplasia of the erythrocytes—is manifested as a macrocytic anemia and is present in 80% to 90% of those with this disease (Pandita & Mukherjee, 2014). However, the leukocytes (myeloid forms, particularly neutrophils) and platelets can also be affected. Although the bone marrow is actually hypercellular, many of the cells within it die before being released into the circulation. Therefore, the actual number of cells in the circulation is typically lower than normal. In MDS, the affected cells do not function normally. The neutrophils have diminished ability to destroy bacteria by **phagocytosis**; platelets are less able to aggregate and are less adhesive than usual. The result of these defects is an increased risk of infection and bleeding, even when the actual number of circulating cells may not be excessively low.

Primary MDS tends to be a disease of older adults; the median age at diagnosis is 65 to 70 years (Adès, Itzykson, & Fenaux, 2014). Current data suggest the incidence is similar to that of AML and increases with increasing age (Troy, Atallah, Geyer, et al., 2014; Xie, Jiang, & Xie, 2015). Risk factors for developing this disease are unclear, although exposure to benzene and tobacco smoke (which also contains benzene) seem likely risks (Bowen, 2013). Thirty percent of cases evolve into AML, with the likelihood increasing based on severity of the underlying MDS (Troy et al., 2014). This type of AML tends to be resistant to standard therapy.

Secondary MDS can occur at any age and results from prior exposure to chemicals, including benzene, radiation, and chemotherapeutic medications (particularly alkylating agents and topoisomerase inhibitors). Secondary MDS is less common (10%), but has a poorer prognosis than does primary MDS, as it tends to be resistant to treatment, has more cytogenetic abnormalities associated with it, and evolves into AML more frequently (Adès et al., 2014; Bowen, 2013).

Clinical Manifestations

The manifestations of MDS can vary widely. Some patients are asymptomatic, with the illness being discovered incidentally when a CBC is performed for other purposes. Other patients have profound symptoms and complications from the illness. Because MDS tends to occur in older adults, other concurrent chronic health conditions may exacerbate symptoms associated with the disease. Fatigue is often present, with varying levels of intensity and frequency. Neutrophil dysfunction puts the person at risk for recurrent pneumonias and other infections. Because platelet function can also be altered, bleeding can occur. These problems may persist in a fairly steady state for months, even years. Over time, the marrow may fail to provide enough cells despite support with transfusion or growth factors; this is called *bone marrow failure*. MDS may also progress over time; as the dysplasia evolves into a leukemic state, the complications increase in severity. However, it is important to note that the majority of patients with MDS succumb to complications from the disease itself or from other comorbidities, and not to those from acute leukemia.

Assessment and Diagnostic Findings

The CBC typically reveals a macrocytic anemia; leukocyte and platelet counts may be diminished as well. Other potential causes for cytopenias (i.e., low blood cell counts), which may include vitamin deficiencies, viral infection, GI bleeding, autoimmune disease, splenomegaly, and liver dysfunction, should be excluded (Adès et al., 2014; Garcia-Manero, 2015). Serum erythropoietin levels may be variable and the **reticulocyte** count (immature RBCs) may be inappropriately low. If the disease evolves into AML, more immature blast cells are noted on the CBC.

The official diagnosis of MDS is based on the results of a bone marrow aspiration (to assess dysplasia) and biopsy (to assess characteristics of the affected cells). The clinical trajectory of these syndromes varies widely; thus, the nurse must understand the risk stratification category of each patient. Those patients with low-risk disease have a much longer survival (as much as 10 years) compared with untreated patients with high-risk disease (where survival is usually less than 9 months) (ACS, 2014b). Cytogenetic analysis of the bone marrow is important in determining the overall prog-

nosis, risk of evolution into AML, and method of treatment. See Chapter 32 for discussion of bone marrow biopsy.

Medical Management

Medical management strategies are based on the stage of disease and prognosis. The goal for treating patients with low-risk disease is to improve cytopenias, decrease blood transfusion requirements, and improve quality of life. The goal for treating patients with high-risk disease is to decrease the likelihood that the disease transforms into AML and to extend survival (Adès et al., 2014; Pandita & Mukherjee, 2014). HSCT is currently the only cure for MDS, but it is not often a viable option for most patients due to the presence of comorbidity or increased age.

Patients frequently need repeated transfusions (**red blood cells [RBCs]**, platelets, or both) throughout the illness trajectory to maintain adequate hemoglobin and platelet levels (termed *transfusion dependence*). Attempts to improve anemia and decrease RBC transfusion are often successful with the use of erythroid-stimulating agents (epoetin alfa [Procrit] or darbopoetin alfa [Aranesp]). Higher-than-normal doses may be required to achieve an adequate improvement in hemoglobin. Adding myeloid growth factors such as G-CSF (filgrastim [Neupogen]) or GM-CSF (sargramostim [Leukine]) can boost responsiveness to these agents (Pandita & Mukherjee, 2014). The median duration of response to this therapy is 2 years; transfusion requirements typically increase by this point.

Thrombocytopenia is a difficult challenge to manage in the MDS patient population. It develops in 40% to 80% of patients over the course of the disease (Santini & Fenaux, 2015) and is seen in 30% of those with lower-risk MDS (Pandita & Mukherjee, 2014). Severe thrombocytopenia is difficult to manage because patients can quickly develop refractoriness to platelet transfusions due to alloimmunization (Pandita & Mukherjee, 2014). Moreover, bleeding can develop even when the platelet level is not excessively low, due to poor platelet function. The cause of thrombocytopenia appears to be increased apoptosis (programmed cell death) and premature marrow destruction of the platelets prior to their release into the circulation (Santini & Fenaux, 2015). The recombinant thrombopoietin receptor agonists romiplostim (Nplate) and eltrombopag (Promacta) have been developed to stimulate the proliferation and differentiation of megakaryocytes into platelets within the bone marrow. These agents are now being evaluated for efficacy in the context of managing thrombocytopenia in MDS. Both drugs have demonstrated the ability to significantly raise platelet counts in this population, but their duration of action may not be long. Increased rates of marrow fibrosis and AML evolution seem to be ameliorated by discontinuing the drug, but additional study is needed.

Unique findings in subsets of MDS can be used to guide special approaches to therapy. Lenalidomide (Revlimid) is extremely effective in treating patients who have a specific cytogenetic/chromosomal abnormality, such as the deletion of 5q. Patients with hypocellular marrows may respond well to immunosuppressive therapy using antithymocyte globulin (Garcia-Manero, 2015).

Patients with intermediate-risk disease are typically treated with either of two available hypomethylating agents—

azacitidine or decitabine (Dacogen). These drugs work by inhibiting the abnormal genes regulating methylation, promoting tumor suppression genes, and permitting myeloid differentiation within the bone marrow. Neither drug has been shown to modify the natural trajectory of lower-risk MDS; therefore, hypomethylating agents are not typically used until erythroid-stimulating agents are no longer effective in controlling transfusion dependence (Garcia-Manero, 2015). Response to azacitidine can result in improved cytopenias, reduced transfusion requirements, reduced transformation to AML, and improved overall survival. A recent meta-analysis suggests a higher rate of partial and overall response and overall hematologic improvement with azacitidine compared with decitabine (Xie et al, 2015). Azacitidine also may be more effective when used in those of older age or who have higher-risk disease. However, as each drug has a slightly different mechanism of action, changing to the alternate drug may still be effective if the disease becomes resistant.

Traditionally, intensive chemotherapy has been used in patients with more aggressive forms of the illness. Results are disappointing, particularly in the context of unfavorable cytogenetic abnormalities (Adès et al., 2014). Secondary MDS and MDS that evolves into AML tend to be refractory to conventional therapy for leukemia.

Infection rates are high in the MDS population. In a retrospective review, infections were identified in 21% of MDS patients; infections requiring hospitalization occurred in 15% of these patients within the first year from the time of diagnosis (Sullivan, Sekeres, Shrestha, et al., 2013). In this study, rates of infection were similar between those patients with low-risk disease and those with high-risk disease. Severe neutropenia, coexisting chronic obstructive pulmonary disease (COPD) or autoimmune disease, and history of other malignancy were associated with higher risk for developing infection, whereas the extent of thrombocytopenia, age, MDS therapy, or diabetes were not. Pneumonia was the most common type of infection in this study; bacteria (gram negative and gram positive) were the predominant pathogens.

The administration of myeloid growth factors alone may be useful in some patients with infections and severe neutropenia, but they are not typically used to prevent infection. Studies have not found them useful in improving overall survival (Pandita & Mukherjee, 2014). Prophylactic antibiotics are not routinely used so that resistant organisms do not develop, but prompt initiation of antimicrobial therapy is crucial at the onset of infection to diminish the risk of increased mortality.

Iron overload is another significant problem for patients with MDS. Data suggest that ineffective erythropoiesis in MDS results in increased iron absorption from the intestinal tract, thereby resulting in elevated ferritin levels even in the absence of repeated red cell transfusions (Nolte, Angelucci, Breccia, et al., 2015; Steensma & Gatterman, 2013). However, red cell transfusion dependence is the primary cause for iron overload in this patient population. Here, surplus iron is deposited in cells within the reticuloendothelial system, and later in parenchymal organs (e.g., liver). While a true cause-and-effect has not yet been established, there is significant concern that patients with transfusion-dependent MDS are at high risk for developing cardiac events, particularly heart failure. Excess iron, and the resultant increased oxidative stress, is also associated with hepatic and pancreatic dysfunction, the development of diabetes, increased rates of infection, and decreased hematopoiesis. Studies are ongoing to further investigate if iron overload actually causes these complications.

In patients with MDS, iron overload is typically managed by chelation therapy. Iron is bound to the chelating agent and then excreted in the urine. Because chelation therapy removes only a small amount of iron with each treatment, patients with chronic iron overload from RBC transfusions need to continue chelation therapy as long as the iron overload exists. Oral iron chelation with deferasirox (Exjade) has replaced the need for long subcutaneous infusions of deferoxamine (Desferal). However, adherence remains a challenge, largely due to toxicity associated with the drug.

Nursing Management

Caring for patients with MDS can be challenging because the illness is unpredictable. As with other hematologic disorders, some patients (especially those with no symptoms) have difficulty perceiving that they have a serious illness that can place them at risk of life-threatening complications. At the other extreme, many patients have tremendous difficulty coping with the uncertain trajectory of the illness and fear that the illness will evolve into AML. Thus, it is important for patients to understand their unique risk of the disease transforming to AML and to recognize that, for most patients, MDS is a chronic illness. It is imperative that the nurse recognizes any concurrent health problems the patient may have. This knowledge will help the nurse better plan and manage the patient's care. For example, a patient with underlying heart failure or COPD may not tolerate anemia well, nor a more rapid rate of red cell transfusion.

Patients with MDS need extensive education about infection risk, measures to avoid it, signs and symptoms of developing infection, and appropriate actions to take should such symptoms occur. Instruction should also be given regarding the risk of bleeding. Patients need to be encouraged to serve as their own health advocate, by informing other health care providers, including dentists, that they have MDS, and their risks for infection and bleeding. Patients with MDS who are hospitalized may require neutropenic precautions.

Fatigue is often a debilitating symptom for the patient with MDS and significantly interferes with quality of life. It can impair the patient's ability to function in the work or home setting, to engage in meaningful activities, and overall cognitive function (Ryblom, Hast, Hellstrom-Lindberg, et al., 2015). Patients may benefit from anticipatory guidance in learning how to live with this symptom, and creative strategies may be required.

Laboratory values need to be monitored closely to anticipate the need for transfusion and to determine response to treatment with growth factors. Patients with chronic transfusion requirements often benefit from the insertion of a vascular access device for this purpose. Those patients receiving chemotherapy need extensive education regarding treatment side effects (and how to manage them) and treatment schedules. Patients receiving growth factors need instruction about these medications, administration schedules, and side effects.

Chelation therapy is a process that is used to remove excess iron acquired from chronic transfusions. Side effects from oral chelators commonly include diarrhea and abdominal cramping. Instructing the patient to take the medication in the evening prior to dinner and gradually increasing the dosage over time may diminish these side effects (Nolte et al., 2015; Steensma & Gatterman, 2013). Skin rash is usually mild and rarely warrants temporarily stopping the drug. Monitoring renal function is important as a rise in serum creatinine is common. The dosage should be reduced if the serum creatinine rises by more than one third of baseline. Patients with preexisting liver disease, including cirrhosis, should not receive oral iron chelators.

MYELOPROLIFERATIVE NEOPLASMS

Polycythemia Vera

Polycythemia vera (sometimes called *P vera* or primary polycythemia) is a proliferative disorder of the myeloid stem cells. The bone marrow is hypercellular, and the erythrocyte, leukocyte, and platelet counts in the peripheral blood are often elevated. However, erythrocyte elevation predominates; the hematocrit can exceed 60%. The median age at the onset is 65 years. Median survival is typically 14 years, but can be up to 24 years in patients who are diagnosed before age 60 (Tefferi & Barbui, 2015). Over time, the spleen may enlarge and resume its embryonic function of hematopoiesis. In some instances, the bone marrow may become fibrotic, with a resultant inability to produce as many cells; this process is referred to as the "burnt out" or "spent" phase of the disease. The disease may then evolve into myeloid metaplasia with myelofibrosis, or AML. This form of AML is usually refractory to standard treatment, and survival usually is less than a few months. Death from polycythemia vera typically results from thrombosis, hemorrhage, or, more rarely, evolution to AML (Prchal & Prchal, 2016).

The diagnosis is established by an elevated hemoglobin and the presence of an acquired mutation in the JAK2 gene resulting in an increased signaling of cell proliferation (Prchal & Prchal, 2016). Other mutations can also be seen. The serum erythropoietin level is lower than normal. Age at diagnosis, risk for thrombosis, and risk for transformation to AML vary based on the precise mutations involved. Survival is inferior when there are no mutations identified (Geyer & Mesa, 2014).

Clinical Manifestations

Patients typically have a ruddy complexion and splenomegaly. Symptoms result from increased blood volume and may include headache, dizziness, tinnitus, fatigue, paresthesias, and blurred vision. Symptoms also result from increased blood viscosity and may include angina, claudication, dyspnea, and thrombophlebitis, particularly if the patient has atherosclerotic blood vessels. For this reason, blood pressure is often elevated. Uric acid may be elevated as well, resulting in gout and renal stone formation. Another common problem is generalized pruritus, which may be caused by histamine release due to an increased number of basophils. Erythromelalgia, a burning sensation in the fingers and toes, may be reported and is only partially relieved by cooling.

Assessment and Diagnostic Findings

Diagnosis is based on an elevated hemoglobin or hematocrit and either the presence of a mutation of the JAK2 gene (which promotes cell proliferation and a hypersensitivity to erythropoietin) or a low serum erythropoietin level (Vannucchi, 2014). Causes of secondary erythrocytosis should not be present (see later discussion). Myeloid proliferation within the marrow can result in elevated white blood cells and platelets, as well.

Complications

Patients with polycythemia vera are at increased risk for thromboses that may be either venous or arterial. Thromboses can result in strokes or myocardial infarctions; thrombotic complications are the most common cause of death. Patients older than 60 years of age, those with a prior history of thrombosis, or those with an elevated platelet count (exceeding 1 million/mm³) are at greater risk for developing thrombotic complications (Tefferi & Barbui, 2015). Bleeding is also a complication, possibly because the platelets are often very large and somewhat dysfunctional. The bleeding can be significant and can occur in the form of nosebleeds, ulcers, frank GI bleeding, hematuria, and intracranial hemorrhage.

Medical Management

The objectives of management are to reduce the risk of thrombosis without increasing the risk of bleeding, reduce the risk of evolution to myelofibrosis or AML, and ameliorate symptoms associated with the disease (Geyer & Mesa, 2014; Vannucchi, 2014). Specific therapy is based on an established risk stratification where those less than age 60 and no prior history of thrombosis are considered "low risk;" age 60 or older, a history of thrombosis, or both are considered to be "high risk." Low-dose aspirin has been shown to reduce vascular thrombosis without increasing the risk of bleeding and is considered front-line therapy (Geyer & Mesa, 2014; Squizzato, Romualdi, Passamonti, et al., 2013).

Phlebotomy is an important part of therapy (see Fig. 34-5). It involves removing enough blood (initially 500 mL once or twice weekly) to reduce blood viscosity and to deplete the

Figure 34-5 • Phlebotomy can markedly reduce the plethora seen in polycythemia vera. This is evidenced here by a marked reduction in facial rubor in a patient with polycythemia vera. From Turgeon, M. L. (2012). *Clinical hematology: Theory & procedures* (5th ed., Fig. 21.10, p. 373). Philadelphia, PA: Lippincott Williams & Wilkins.

patient's iron stores, thereby rendering the patient iron deficient and consequently unable to continue to manufacture hemoglobin excessively. Many patients are well managed by routine phlebotomy on an intermittent basis, with the target of maintaining the hematocrit less than 45%.

The chemotherapeutic agent hydroxyurea can be used to suppress marrow function, thereby controlling blood counts. It has been reported to reduce thrombotic complications, and is often used in patients with high-risk disease (Tefferi & Barbui, 2015; Vannucchi, 2014).

Aggressive management of atherosclerosis, by treating hypertension and hyperlipidemia, is also important in diminishing the risk of thrombosis. Allopurinol (Zyloprim) is used to prevent gouty attacks in patients with elevated uric acid concentrations; such attacks are common in patients with polycythemia vera. Aspirin is useful in reducing the pain associated with erythromyalgia.

Anagrelide (Agrylin) inhibits platelet aggregation and has been used to control the **thrombocytosis** (abnormally high platelet count) associated with polycythemia vera. However, many patients have difficulty tolerating the medication; it can cause significant side effects, including headache, fluid retention, cardiac dysrhythmias, and heart failure. Furthermore, some studies suggest that anagrelide may be leukemogenic (i.e., may cause leukemia) and is associated with increased risk of arterial thromboses and bleeding. Thus, the use of anagrelide has declined significantly (Geyer & Mesa, 2014).

Interferon alfa-2b (Intron) is also very effective in controlling blood counts in this disorder. However, it may be difficult for patients to tolerate because of its frequent side effects (e.g., flu-like syndrome, depression) and high cost. Currently, it is more commonly used in younger patients or in those whose disease has become resistant to hydroxyurea.

Nursing Management

Patients with polycythemia vera can exhibit a variety of symptoms that have an adverse impact on quality of life (Abelsson, Andreasson, Samuelsson, et al., 2013; Stein, Moliterno, & Tiu, 2014). As symptoms vary and are not related to extent of disease (Scherber, Geyer, & Mesa, 2014), it is important to assess for symptoms carefully and regularly throughout the illness trajectory. Table 34-2 identifies common symptoms associated with polycythemia vera.

The nurse focuses on symptom management. Fatigue is the most common symptom, and can occur in 85% of patients (Radia & Geyer, 2015; Scherber, Kosiorek, Senyak, et al., 2016). Concurrent comorbidities (e.g., hypothyroidism, depression) and medications (e.g., antihypertensives, antihistamines) can exacerbate the fatigue (Scherber et al., 2016). Fatigue is not always correlated with the level of disease risk; patients with low-risk disease are as troubled with fatigue as are those with high-risk disease (Radia & Geyer, 2015).

Pruritus is also a common and frustrating symptom, occurring in up to 65% of patients with polycythemia vera (Radia & Geyer, 2015). It is described as strong itching, stinging, or burning. Pruritus is frequently triggered by contact with water (Siegel, Tauscher, & Petrides, 2013), alcohol consumption, diaphoresis, or change in body temperature. Antihistamines, including histamine-2 blockers, are not particularly effective in controlling itching, nor are emollient lotions. Interferon

TABLE 34-2 Common Symptoms Associated With Myeloproliferative Neoplasms

Symptoms vary between the three myeloproliferative neoplasms, both in frequency and severity. Nurses should assess these patients frequently for the presence of these symptoms and initiate appropriate measures to ameliorate them.

Symptom	P Vera	ET	Myelofibrosis
Fatigue	85%	84%	94%
Concentration	62%	58%	68%
Early satiety	60%	56%	74%
Night sweats	52%	47%	63%
Pruritus	62%	46%	52%
Abdominal discomfort	48%	48%	65%
Bone pain	48%	45%	53%
Weight loss	33%	28%	47%
Fever	19%	17%	24%

P vera, polycythemia vera; ET, essential thrombocythemia
Adapted from Geyer, H. L., & Mesa, R. A. (2014). Therapy for myeloproliferative neoplasms: When, which agent, and how? *Hematology American Society of Hematology Education Program, 2014*(1), 277–286.

alfa-2b, selective serotonin uptake inhibitors (e.g., paroxetine), and ultraviolet therapy have marginal effectiveness in diminishing the pruritus (Stein et al., 2014). As the efficacy of pharmacologic strategies may not be optimal, it is important to individualize therapy and monitor its effectiveness (Siegel et al., 2013). The nurse may recommend bathing in tepid or cool water and avoiding vigorous toweling off after bathing. Cocoa butter or oatmeal-based lotions and bath products or baking soda dissolved in bathwater may also be helpful.

Potentially life-threatening complications from the disease are thrombosis or hemorrhage. Risk factors for thrombotic complications, particularly a prior history of thrombosis, smoking, obesity, and poorly controlled hypertension and diabetes, should be assessed, and patients should be encouraged to modify the cardiovascular risk factors within their control (e.g., smoking, obesity). Adopting or maintaining a healthy lifestyle should be encouraged. Patients should be instructed about the signs and symptoms of thrombosis. To reduce the likelihood of deep vein thrombosis (DVT), sedentary behavior, crossing the legs, and wearing tight or restrictive clothing (particularly stockings) should be discouraged. Patients with a history of significant bleeding are usually advised to avoid high-dose aspirin and aspirin-containing medications, because these medications alter platelet function. Minimizing alcohol intake should also be emphasized to further diminish the risk of bleeding. Patients should be counseled about the signs of bleeding. The patient needs to be instructed to avoid iron supplements, including those in over-the-counter multivitamin supplements, because the iron can further stimulate RBC production.

Essential Thrombocythemia

Essential thrombocythemia (ET), also called *primary thrombocythemia*, is a stem cell disorder within the bone marrow. A mutation of the JAK2 gene promotes cell proliferation and resistance to cell death and a hypersensitivity to erythropoie-tin and thrombopoietin; it is found in 55% of patients with ET (Geyer & Mesa, 2014). A marked increase in platelet produc-tion occurs, with the platelet count consistently greater than 450,000/mm^3. The platelet count can exceed 1 to 2 million/mm^3. Occasionally, the increase in platelets (i.e., thrombocy-themia) is accompanied by an increase in erythrocytes, leu-kocytes, or both; however, these cells are not increased to the extent that they are in polycythemia vera, CML, or myelofi-brosis. Platelet size may be abnormal; these circulate through-out the vascular system in an activated state. Extremely high levels of platelets (exceeding 1 million/mm^3) are associ-ated with acquired von Willebrand disease; therefore, these patients are at higher risk for bleeding complications.

The exact cause of ET is unknown. This disease affects women twice as often as men and tends to occur later in life (median age at diagnosis is 65 to 70 years). Overall, survival does not differ from the general population. However, sur-vival rates vary based on the type of mutations seen in this disease. For example, 25% of patients with ET have a muta-tion in the calreticulin gene; the presence of this mutation appears to be associated with fewer thrombotic events and higher survival rates (Radia & Geyer, 2015). Patients without mutations may have a lower survival rate. The evolution to AML is very low (0.8%) (Birgegård, 2013). Death is typically due to thrombosis (arterial or venous) or hemorrhage.

Clinical Manifestations

Many patients with ET are asymptomatic; the illness is diag-nosed as the result of finding an elevated platelet count on a CBC. Symptoms occur most often when the platelet count exceeds 1 million/mm^3; however, they do not always correlate with the extent to which the platelet count is elevated. When symptoms do occur, they primarily result from vascular occlu-sion. This occlusion can occur in large arterial vessels (cere-brovascular, coronary, or peripheral arteries) and deep veins, as well as in the microcirculation. The interactive effects of platelet substances within the surface of the vascular endo-thelium can cause microthrombi in the arterioles and inflam-mation within the endothelium; these interactions result in erythromyalgia, the development of painful burning, warmth, and redness in a localized distal area of the extremities. More common forms of venous thromboembolism (VTE) include DVT and pulmonary embolism (PE).

Headaches are the most common neurologic manifesta-tions; other manifestations include transient ischemic attacks and diplopia. Tinnitus, paresthesias, or atypical chest pain may also occur (Tefferi & Barbui, 2015).

Because the platelets can be dysfunctional, minor or major hemorrhage may occur. Bleeding is commonly limited to recurrent skin manifestations (ecchymoses, hematomas, epi-staxis, gum bleeding), although significant GI bleeding and intracranial hemorrhage are both possible. Bleeding typically does not occur unless the platelet count exceeds 1.5 million/mm^3. It results from a deficiency in von Willebrand factor as the platelet count increases (Alvarez-Larrán & Besses, 2014; Tefferi & Barburi, 2015).

Assessment and Diagnostic Findings

The diagnosis of ET is made by ruling out other potential disorders—either other myeloproliferative disorders or underlying illnesses that cause a reactive or secondary throm-bocytosis (see later discussion). Iron deficiency should be excluded, because a reactive increase in the platelet count often accompanies this deficiency. Occult malignancy should be excluded. The CBC shows markedly large and abnormal platelets; the platelet count is persistently elevated (greater than 450,000/mm^3). An analysis of the JAK2 mutation or calreticulin is very useful, whereas an analysis of the bone marrow (by aspiration and biopsy) can aid in distinguishing between true ET and early myelofibrosis.

Complications

Complications include inappropriate formation of thrombi and hemorrhage. Patients with cardiovascular risk factors (such as poorly controlled hypertension, diabetes, obesity, hyperlipidemia, and smoking) are at higher risk for thrombotic complications (Barbui, Finazzi, & Falanga, 2013; Lekovic, Gotic, Sefer, et al., 2015). Patients older than 60 years and those with a history of prior thrombosis are also at higher risk for complications. Major bleeding tends to occur when the platelet count is very high (greater than 1.5 million/mm^3) and there is a prior history of major bleeding. In contrast, patients who are younger than 60 years, have no previous history of a thrombotic or hemorrhagic event, and have a normal WBC count and platelet counts less than 1 million/mm^3 are con-sidered to be at low risk for developing thrombotic or hemor-rhagic complications (Geyer & Mesa, 2014).

Medical Management

The management of ET is based on risk for developing throm-bosis or hemorrhage, and the presence of symptoms (see Table 34-2). A careful assessment of risk factors, history of periph-eral vascular disease, tobacco use, atherosclerosis, diabetes, and prior thrombotic or bleeding events are all considered in developing the treatment plan.

In younger patients with no risk factors, patients may receive no therapy and be closely observed. Low-dose aspirin therapy is commonly recommended as it is felt to be suffi-cient to prevent thrombotic complications (Alvarez-Larrán & Besses, 2014; Barbui et al., 2013; Tefferi & Barbui, 2015). However, the use of aspirin can increase the risk of hemor-rhagic complications, particularly when the platelet count exceeds 1 million/mm^3. Determining the presence of acquired von Willebrand disease is important prior to initiating aspi-rin therapy in these patients. Aspirin use in this context is associated with a much higher risk of hemorrhage. Aspirin therapy is also contraindicated in patients with a history of GI bleeding. Aspirin can relieve the neurologic symptoms (e.g., headache), erythromelalgias, and visual symptoms of ET, and is considered safe and effective in preventing complications during pregnancy (Tefferi & Barbui, 2015).

In older patients and in those with a history of prior throm-bosis, more aggressive measures are necessary to prevent thrombosis or bleeding. Hydroxyurea is effective in lowering the platelet count to a level below 400,000/mm^3 and is effec-tive in reducing the risk for developing arterial thrombosis and hemorrhage (Tefferi & Barbui, 2015). This agent is taken orally and causes minimal side effects other than dose-related **leukopenia**. With long-term use, some patients develop painful leg ulcers or actinic keratosis (Cozzani, Iurlo, Merlo, et al., 2015). Resistance develops in up to 25% of patients over time, necessitating changing pharmacologic management (Sever, Newberry, & Verstovsek, 2014).

Anagrelide is more specific in lowering the platelet count than hydroxyurea but has more side effects and may not be as effective. Severe headaches cause many patients to stop taking the medication. Tachycardia and chest pain may also occur, and anagrelide is contraindicated in patients with concurrent cardiac problems. Anagrelide is also associated with disease progression; for these reasons, it is infrequently used (Tefferi & Barbui, 2015).

Interferon alfa-2b has been shown to effectively lower platelet counts due to its antiproliferative effects on hematopoietic precursor cells and its ability to reduce the extent of molecular changes (Birgegård, 2013; Sever et al., 2014). Significant side effects such as fatigue, fever, depression, and flu-like symptoms are common. Subclinical depression may not be recognized until the drug is discontinued (Birgegård, 2013). A pegylated formulation of interferon alpha-2b is more commonly used, which may have improved tolerance and longer duration of use. Interferon is also safe for use in pregnancy.

Rarely, the occlusive symptoms require emergent reduction in the platelet count. When necessary, platelet apheresis (see Chapter 32) can reduce the amount of circulating platelets, but only transiently. The extent to which symptoms and complications (e.g., thromboses) are reduced by apheresis is unclear.

Patients who develop arterial or venous thrombosis may require additional therapy beyond reducing the platelet count (e.g., with hydroxyurea). Data suggest that those who develop cerebrovascular disease are more effectively managed with antiplatelet therapy (e.g., aspirin), whereas those who develop VTE may be more effectively managed with anticoagulation than antiplatelet therapy (Alvarez-Larrán & Besses, 2014).

Nursing Management

Symptoms associated with ET are now used as one criterion for initiating and selecting therapy (see Table 34-2). Because thrombosis and hemorrhage are the primary cause of morbidity or mortality, it is important to assess patients for a history of prior thrombotic or hemorrhagic events. Risk factors for thrombosis are assessed, such as obesity, hypertension, hyperlipidemia, diabetes, and smoking; measures to diminish these risk factors are strongly encouraged. Patients with ET need to be educated about the risks of hemorrhage and thrombosis. The patient is informed about signs and symptoms of thrombosis, particularly the neurologic manifestations, such as visual changes, numbness, tingling, and weakness. Patients taking aspirin should be informed about the importance of taking this medication as well as the increased risk of bleeding. Patients who are at risk for bleeding should be instructed about medications (e.g., aspirin, nonsteroidal anti-inflammatory agents [NSAIDs]) and other substances (e.g., alcohol, certain herbal therapies) that can alter platelet function. Patients taking interferon may be taught to self-administer the medication and how to manage side effects. Patients taking hydroxyurea should have CBCs monitored regularly; the dosage is adjusted based on the platelet and WBC count.

Primary Myelofibrosis

Primary myelofibrosis, also known as agnogenic myeloid metaplasia or myelofibrosis with myeloid metaplasia, is a chronic myeloproliferative disorder that arises from neoplastic transformation of an early hematopoietic stem cell. The disease is characterized by marrow fibrosis or scarring, extramedullary hematopoiesis (typically involving the spleen and the liver), leukocytosis, thrombocytosis, and anemia. Some patients have diminished leukocyte, platelet, and erythrocyte counts (i.e., **pancytopenia**). Patients with myelofibrosis have increased **angiogenesis** (formation of new blood vessels) within the marrow. Early forms of blood cells (including nucleated RBCs [immature RBCs] and megakaryocyte fragments) are frequently found in the circulation. The cause is unknown. Secondary myelofibrosis evolves from polycythemia vera or, much less frequently, from ET. As with ET and polycythemia vera, mutations of the JAK2 gene or calreticulin are frequently seen; prognosis is worse in those without genetic mutations (Lichtman & Prchal, 2016).

Myelofibrosis is the rarest of the classic myeloproliferative neoplasms that do not involve the BCR-ABL gene (i.e., CML). It is a disease of the older adult, with a median age at diagnosis of 65 to 70 years, and is more common in males. Symptoms may result from an often massively enlarged spleen, causing discomfort and early satiety. Other signs and symptoms include profound fatigue, pruritus, bone pain, weight loss, infection and bleeding (from pancytopenia), and cachexia (see Fig. 34-6). Arterial or venous thrombosis can

Figure 34-6 • Cachexia, severe wasting, and massively enlarged liver and spleen (hepatosplenomegaly) are seen in advanced myeloproliferative disorders, particularly myelofibrosis. (Note also the lack of adequate dressing over the patient's vascular access device.) From Tkachuk, D. C., & Hirschman, J. V. (2007). *Wintrobe's atlas of clinical hematology* (Fig. 4.1, p. 111). Philadelphia, PA: Lippincott Williams & Wilkins.

occur but is less frequent than that found in polycythemia vera or ET. Average survival ranges from 2 to 10 years based on the occurrence of such adverse prognostic indicators as increased age; anemia; leukocytosis; presence of blast cells in the circulation; and the presence of fever, diaphoresis, or weight loss at the time of diagnosis (Lichtman & Prchal, 2016). Common causes of death are heart or liver failure, complications of marrow failure (e.g., infection, bleeding), and transformation to AML. AML is especially difficult to treat successfully in these situations.

Medical Management

Goals of therapy are based on reducing the burden of the disease (by decreasing symptoms and splenomegaly) and improving blood counts (Geyer & Mesa, 2014). Risk is determined based on several factors, including age (over 65 years of age), elevated WBC count (above 25,000/mm^3), severe anemia (hemoglobin less than 10 g/dL), the presence of constitutional symptoms (e.g., weight loss), the presence of blast cells in the peripheral blood, RBC transfusion requirement, and unfavorable cytogenetic profile. Patients assessed to have low-risk disease may not require therapy initially, reserving it when more symptoms develop (see Table 34-2.)

Anemia is most commonly managed with RBC transfusions. Erythroid-stimulating agents may improve anemia to the extent that transfusion requirement is reduced but the effect is not durable (Manea, 2014). Androgens have been used in the past, but they are largely ineffective. Other pharmacologic agents are used to diminish splenomegaly and improve cytopenias. Hydroxyurea is often used to control high leukocyte and platelet counts and to reduce the size of the spleen. Thalidomide (Thalomid) or pomalidomide (Pomalyst) may be useful in improving anemia and reducing an enlarged spleen, but the effect is transient, lasting an average of 8 months (Odenike, 2013).

Ruxolitinib (Jakafi) is an inhibitor of the JAK2 kinase. It can be highly effective in decreasing splenomegaly, improves fatigue and weight gain, and decreases night sweats and pruritus and the need for RBC transfusions. Thrombocytopenia can be significant, as well as anemia. However, the anemia may improve after several months of therapy.

HSCT is a useful treatment modality in younger, otherwise healthy people, and is the only current therapy that can reverse the fibrosis within the marrow (Odenike, 2013). Patients with high risk of disease should be promptly evaluated to determine candidacy (Geyer & Mesa, 2014).

Splenectomy may be used to control the complications that result from a massively enlarged spleen. The mortality rate associated with this procedure is 10%, and the morbidity associated with the procedure (e.g., infection, bleeding, thrombosis) is 47% (Geyer & Mesa, 2014; Lichtman & Prchal, 2016). Furthermore, a reactive thrombocytosis and leukocytosis can develop because the cells are no longer sequestered out of the circulation. The decision to undergo splenectomy warrants careful consideration of the advantages and disadvantages.

Nursing Management

Splenomegaly can be profound in patients with myelofibrosis, with enlargement of the spleen that may extend to the pelvic rim. This condition is extremely uncomfortable and can severely limit nutritional intake. Analgesic agents are usually

TABLE 34-3 Fatigue in Patients With Myeloproliferative Neoplasms

Self-reported strategies used to ameliorate fatigue by patients with myeloproliferative neoplasms. Data obtained from online surveys ($N = 1,788$) gathered via myeloproliferative neoplasm web sites.

Strategy	% Patients Reported Use
Setting priorities	75%
Postponing nonessential activities	74%
Exercise	73%
Naps	70%
Walking	66%
Socializing	65%
Nutrition	64%
Reading	62%
Scheduling activity during peak energy periods	62%
Pacing activities	58%
Structured daily routine	54%
Delegation	52%

Adapted from Scherber, R. M., Kosiorek, H. E., Senyak, Z., et al. (2016). Comprehensively understanding fatigue in patients with myeloproliferative neoplasms. *Cancer*, 122(3), 477–485.

ineffective. Splenomegaly, coupled with a hypermetabolic state, results in significant weight loss and muscle wasting. Patients benefit from small, frequent meals of foods that are high in calories and protein. Weakness, fatigue, and altered body image are other significant problems. Energy conservation methods and active listening are important nursing interventions. The patient needs to be educated about signs and symptoms of infection, bleeding, and thrombosis, as well as appropriate interventions if these occur. Ensuring that the patient takes steps to decrease risks associated with developing thrombosis (e.g., smoking; obesity; poorly controlled hyperlipidemia, hypertension, or diabetes) is also important. Table 34-3 identifies useful strategies aimed at managing fatigue.

LYMPHOMA

The lymphomas are neoplasms of cells of lymphoid origin. These tumors usually start in lymph nodes but can involve lymphoid tissue in the spleen, GI tract (e.g., the wall of the stomach), liver, or bone marrow (see Fig. 35-1 in Chapter 35). They are often classified according to the degree of cell differentiation and the origin of the predominant malignant cell. Lymphomas can be broadly classified into two categories: Hodgkin lymphoma and non-Hodgkin lymphoma (NHL).

Hodgkin Lymphoma

Hodgkin lymphoma is a relatively rare malignancy that has a high cure rate. It is somewhat more common in men than in women and has two peaks of incidence: one from age 15 to 34 and the other after 60 years of age (Press, 2016). Disease occurrence has a familial pattern: First-degree relatives have a higher-than-normal frequency of disease, but the actual incidence of this pattern is low. No increased incidence for non-blood relatives (e.g., spouses) has been documented. The 5-year survival rate is 90% for more limited disease (stage I or II), and 65% for those with more extensive disease (stage IV) (ACS, 2015b).

Pathophysiology

Unlike other lymphomas, Hodgkin lymphoma is unicentric in origin in that it initiates in a single node. The disease spreads by contiguous extension along the lymphatic system. The malignant cell of Hodgkin lymphoma is the Reed-Sternberg cell, a gigantic tumor cell that is morphologically unique and thought to be of immature lymphoid origin (see Fig. 34-7). It is the pathologic hallmark and essential diagnostic criterion. However, the tumor is very heterogeneous and may actually contain few Reed-Sternberg cells. The remaining tumor volume is composed of benign, reactive, inflammatory cells that support the growth and survival of the Reed-Sternberg cell (Batlevi & Younes, 2013). Repeated biopsies may be required to establish the diagnosis.

The cause of Hodgkin lymphoma is unknown, but a viral etiology is suspected. Although fragments of the Epstein-Barr virus have been found in some Reed-Sternberg cells, the precise role of this virus in the development of Hodgkin lymphoma remains unknown. Other viruses may also be implicated, including human immune deficiency virus (HIV) and herpesvirus 8. Hodgkin lymphoma is seen more commonly in patients receiving chronic immunosuppressive therapy (e.g., for renal transplant) and also in veterans of the military who were exposed to the herbicide Agent Orange (Leukemia & Lymphoma Society, 2013).

Hodgkin lymphoma is customarily classified into five subgroups based on pathologic analyses that reflect the natural history of the malignancy and suggest the prognosis. For example, when lymphocytes predominate, with few Reed-Sternberg cells and minimal involvement of the lymph nodes,

the prognosis is much more favorable than when the lymphocyte count is low and the lymph nodes are virtually replaced by tumor cells of the most primitive type. Most patients with Hodgkin lymphoma have the types currently designated as "nodular sclerosis" or "mixed cellularity." The nodular sclerosis type tends to occur more often in young women, at an earlier stage, and is often cured by therapy. The mixed cellularity subgroup occurs more commonly in men and older individuals; it is associated with more constitutional symptoms, advanced stage disease, and immunodeficiency (Press, 2016).

Clinical Manifestations

Hodgkin lymphoma usually begins as an enlargement of one or more lymph nodes on one side of the neck. The individual nodes are painless and firm but not hard. The most common sites for lymphadenopathy are the cervical, supraclavicular, and mediastinal nodes; involvement of the iliac or inguinal nodes or spleen is much less common. A mediastinal mass may be seen on chest x-ray; occasionally, the mass is large enough to compress the trachea and cause dyspnea. Pruritus is common; it can be extremely distressing, and the cause is unknown. Some patients experience brief but severe pain after drinking alcohol, usually at the site of the tumor. The cause of this symptom is also unknown.

All organs are vulnerable to invasion by tumor cells. The symptoms result from compression of organs by the tumor, such as cough and pulmonary effusion (from pulmonary infiltrates), jaundice (from hepatic involvement or bile duct obstruction), abdominal pain (from splenomegaly or retroperitoneal adenopathy), or bone pain (from skeletal involvement). Herpes zoster infections are common. A cluster of constitutional symptoms has important prognostic implications. Referred to as B symptoms, they include fever (without chills), drenching sweats (particularly at night), and unintentional weight loss of more than 10% of body weight. B symptoms are found in 40% of patients, and are used in part in deciding appropriate treatment (Cheson, Fisher, Barrington, et al., 2014). A mild anemia is the most common hematologic finding. The leukocyte count may be elevated or decreased. The platelet count is typically normal, unless the tumor has invaded the bone marrow, suppressing hematopoiesis. The **erythrocyte sedimentation rate** (ESR) and the serum copper level are sometimes used to assess disease activity; elevations may reflect increases in disease activity. Patients with Hodgkin lymphoma have impaired cellular immunity, as evidenced by an absent or decreased reaction to skin sensitivity tests (e.g., *Candida*, mumps). Infections, including viral infections, are common (see Fig. 34-8).

Assessment and Diagnostic Findings

Because many manifestations are similar to those occurring with infection, diagnostic studies are performed to rule out an infectious origin of the disease. The diagnosis is made by means of an excisional lymph node biopsy and frequently, the finding of the Reed-Sternberg cell. Once the diagnosis is confirmed and the histologic type is established, it is necessary to assess the extent of the disease—a process referred to as staging.

During the health history, the patient is assessed for any B symptoms. Physical examination requires a careful, systematic

Figure 34-7 • Reed-Sternberg cell. Reed-Sternberg cells are large, abnormal lymphocytes that may contain more than one nucleus. These cells are found in Hodgkin lymphoma. Adapted with permission from Rubin, R., Strayer, D. S., & Rubin, E. (2011). *Rubin's pathology* (6th ed.).Philadelphia, PA: Lippincott Williams & Wilkins.

Figure 34-8 • Herpes zoster is a common complication in patients with lymphoproliferative disease, such as Hodgkin lymphoma here. Zoster infections are also common in patients on chronic steroid use for hematologic conditions and some chemotherapy regimens. From Tkachuk, D. C., & Hirschman, J. V. (2007). *Wintrobe's atlas of clinical hematology* (Fig. 5.152, p. 207). Philadelphia, PA: Lippincott Williams & Wilkins.

evaluation of all palpable lymph node chains (see Fig. 32–4 in Chapter 32), as well as the size of the spleen and liver. A chest x-ray and a computed tomography (CT) scan of the chest, abdomen, and pelvis are crucial to identify the extent of lymphadenopathy within these regions. A positron emission tomography (PET) scan may be the most sensitive imaging test in identifying residual disease and is being evaluated for its predictive value in this disease (Evens & Kostakoglu, 2014). Laboratory tests include CBC, platelet count, ESR, and liver and renal function studies. A bone marrow biopsy is not routinely performed (Cheson et al., 2014).

Medical Management

The goal in the treatment of Hodgkin lymphoma is cure. Cure rates are 85% to 90% for patients with early-stage disease and 65% to 85% for those with advanced-stage disease (Matasar, Ford, Riedel, et al., 2015). Treatment is determined primarily by the stage of the disease, not by the histologic type; however, extensive research is ongoing to target treatment regimens more to the histologic subtypes or prognostic features. Because of long-term survival and potential for cure from the disease, consideration must be made of potential long-term morbidity associated with treatment, particularly cardiac disease and second malignancies. Treatment choice must be balanced between using high-intensity therapy, where the likelihood of cure or long-lasting remission is high but has a risk of late toxicity and potential mortality, and less-intensive therapy that may have less toxicity but greater likelihood of relapsed disease. This dilemma is particularly relevant when treating young patients with early-stage disease (Johnson, 2013).

Treatment of limited-stage Hodgkin lymphoma commonly involves a short course (2 to 4 months) of chemotherapy followed by radiation therapy to the specific involved area. This strategy has reduced the radiation dosage, with subsequent decrease in long-term side effects (particularly second malignancies and late cardiovascular events) and without decreasing the likelihood of controlling the disease. However, with

the effectiveness of second-line therapies, even this amount of radiation is being questioned (Johnson, 2013). Combination chemotherapy with doxorubicin (Adriamycin), bleomycin (Blenoxane), vinblastine (Velban), and dacarbazine (DTIC), referred to as ABVD, is considered the standard treatment for more advanced disease (stages III and IV and all stages with B symptoms). Chemotherapy is often successful in obtaining remission even when relapse occurs. Other combinations of chemotherapy are used, which may have more toxicity. The MoAb brentuximab vedotin (Adcetris) has approval for use in refractory relapsed Hodgkin lymphoma. This drug targets a receptor that is expressed on the surface of activated T and B lymphocytes, but also on Reed-Sternberg cells. Current studies are ongoing to determine the best time to use this therapy: prior to transplant (HSCT), as maintenance therapy post-transplant, or when transplant is not an option (Graf & Gopal, 2014).

HSCT is used for advanced or refractory disease. Most patients diagnosed with Hodgkin lymphoma are either cured or experience prolonged remissions, and thus live for many years post diagnosis. As a result, much is now known about the long-term effects of chemotherapy and radiation therapy. Second malignancies are the leading cause of death in long-term survivors of Hodgkin lymphoma (Ng, 2014). There is a latency period of 5 years, after which time the risk progressively increases and remains greater than would be expected in the general population, at least 25 years after diagnosis (Ng, 2014). In a study of 465 adults previously treated for Hodgkin lymphoma, the risk of developing a nonfatal second malignancy was 3.41 times higher (Matasar et al., 2015). The most common to develop are breast, lung, GI, and skin cancers. Prior radiation therapy is more closely associated with the development of secondary cancers, but chemotherapy that used alkylator drugs is associated with lung and GI cancer development (Ng, 2014). Leukemia more commonly developed in patients who received the chemotherapy regimen MOPP (i.e., nitrogen mustard, vincristine, procarbazine, and prednisone).

Cardiovascular disease is also frequently seen in the Hodgkin lymphoma survivor population. The risk develops after a latency of 10 years after diagnosis and is directly related to doses of radiation to the anterior chest region. Coronary artery disease, dysrhythmias, valvular disease, and cardiomyopathy are noted after radiation; congestive heart failure, decreased systolic function, and dilated cardiomyopathy are more commonly associated with prior anthracycline therapy (Ng, 2014).

Other organ dysfunction is also well documented, including that of the endocrine system. A high incidence of anxiety and depression that also persist over time was reported in several studies (Matasar et al., 2015; Oerlemans, Mols, Nijziel, et al., 2014). Persistent fatigue is common in survivors and can be exacerbated by depression and other treatment-related comorbidities (Daniëls, Oerlemans, Krol, et al., 2013; Daniëls, Oerlemans, Krol, et al., 2014; Soares, Biasoli, Scheliga, et al., 2013). Chart 15-4 in Chapter 15 lists long-term potential complications associated with chemotherapy or radiation therapy.

Late effects of treatment can have an adverse effect on a survivor's quality of life (Oerlemans et al., 2014; Khimani, Chen, Mauch, et al., 2013). A study of 40 young adult survivors found improvements in quality of life as soon as 1 month after completing therapy, and this improvement was still noted 6 months after therapy (Roper, Cooley, McDermott, et al., 2013). These data need to be replicated in larger studies and for longer periods of time; it may be that early improvements in quality of life do not persist long term, particularly as late complications arise. Adequate social support and social network are associated with better quality of life (Soares et al., 2013).

Nursing Management

The potential development of a second malignancy should be addressed with the patient when initial treatment decisions are made. However, patients need to be informed that Hodgkin lymphoma is often curable. The nurse should encourage patients to reduce factors that increase the risk of developing second cancers, such as use of tobacco and alcohol and exposure to environmental carcinogens and excessive sunlight. Screening for late effects of treatment (see Chart 15-4, Chapter 15) is necessary. In addition, the nurse should provide education about relevant self-care strategies and disease management. See also the Nursing Management Section for Non-Hodgkin Lymphoma.

Non-Hodgkin Lymphomas

The NHLs are a heterogeneous group of cancers that originate from the neoplastic growth of lymphoid tissue. Similar to CLL, the neoplastic cells are thought to arise from a single clone of lymphocytes; however, in NHL, the cells may vary morphologically. Eighty-five percent of NHLs involve malignant B lymphocytes; the remaining 15% primarily involve T lymphocytes (ACS, 2015c). In contrast to Hodgkin lymphoma, the lymphoid tissues involved are largely infiltrated with malignant cells. The spread of these malignant lymphoid cells occurs unpredictably, and true localized disease is uncommon. Lymph nodes from multiple sites may be infiltrated, as may sites outside the lymphoid system (extranodal tissue; see Fig. 34-9).

NHL is the sixth most common type of cancer diagnosed in the United States; incidence rates have almost doubled in the past 35 years. The incidence increases with each decade of life; the median age at diagnosis is 66 years (Leukemia & Lymphoma Society, 2015b). Although no common etiologic factor has been identified, the incidence of NHL has increased in people with immunodeficiencies or autoimmune disorders; prior treatment for cancer; prior organ transplant; viral infections (including Epstein-Barr virus and HIV); and exposure to pesticides, solvents, dyes, or defoliating agents, including Agent Orange. The overall survival rate is 69% at 5 years, and 59% at 10 years (ACS, 2015d).

Clinical Manifestations

Symptoms are highly variable, reflecting the diverse nature of the NHLs. Lymphadenopathy is the most common; however, in indolent types of lymphomas, the lymphadenopathy can wax and wane. With early-stage disease, or with the types that are considered indolent, symptoms may be virtually absent or very minor, and the illness typically is not diagnosed until it progresses to a later stage, when the patient is symptomatic.

Figure 34-9 • Any extranodal location can be a site for diffuse B-cell lymphoma, such as the thyroid, as shown here. From Tkachuk, D. C., & Hirschman, J. V. (2007). *Wintrobe's atlas of clinical hematology* (Fig. 5.87, p. 183). Philadelphia, PA: Lippincott Williams & Wilkins.

At these stages (III or IV), lymphadenopathy is distinctly noticeable. One third of patients with NHLs have B symptoms (fever, drenching night sweats, and unintentional weight loss). Lymphomatous masses can compromise organ function. For example, a mass in the mediastinum can cause respiratory distress; abdominal masses can compromise the ureters, leading to renal dysfunction; and splenomegaly can cause abdominal discomfort, nausea, early satiety, anorexia, and weight loss.

Assessment and Diagnostic Findings

The actual diagnosis of NHL is categorized into a highly complex classification system based on histopathology, immunophenotyping, and cytogenetic analyses of the malignant cells (see Table 34-4). The specific histopathologic type of the disease has important prognostic implications. Treatment also varies and is based on these features. Indolent types tend to have small cells that are distributed in a circular or follicular pattern. Aggressive types tend to have large or immature cells distributed through the nodes in a diffuse pattern. Staging is typically based on data obtained from CT and PET scans, bone marrow biopsies, and occasionally cerebrospinal fluid analysis. The stage is based on the site of disease and its spread to other sites. For example, in stage I disease, only one area of involvement is detected; thus, stage I disease is highly localized and may respond well to localized therapy (e.g., radiation therapy). In contrast, in stage IV, disease in at least one extranodal site is detected.

TABLE 34-4 Types of Lymphomas[a]

Indolent	Aggressive	Highly Aggressive
Follicular	Diffuse large cell	Burkitt
Small lymphocytic	Mantle cell	Lymphoblastic

Marginal zone:
  MALT
  Splenic
  Nodal
		AIDS-related B cell

Lymphoplasmacytic:
  Waldenstrom's
    macroglobulinemia		

MALT, mucosa-associated lymphoidal tissue; AIDS, acquired immunodeficiency syndrome.
[a]Major types of lymphomas, many of which are indolent in nature. Table does not present an all-inclusive list.

Although the stage of disease is important, often it is not an accurate predictor of prognosis. Two prognostic classification systems have been developed that are particularly useful in the older patient population: the International Prognostic Index (IPI) and, for follicular lymphomas, the Follicular Lymphoma International Prognostic Index (FLIPI). Age, performance status, lactate dehydrogenase levels, stage of disease, and extranodal involvement are scored to determine risk of failure or death from disease. Based on the IPI, 5-year overall survival rates range from 75% (low risk) to 30% (high risk), and, based on the FLIPI, from 91% (low risk) to 53% (high risk) (ACS, 2015e).

Medical Management

Treatment is determined by the classification of disease, the stage of disease, prior treatment (if any), and the patient's ability to tolerate therapy. Tolerance to therapy is largely dictated by renal, hepatic, and cardiac function; the presence of concurrent diseases; functional status; and age. If the disease is not aggressive and is localized, radiation alone may be the treatment of choice. With aggressive types of NHL, aggressive combinations of chemotherapeutic agents are used; R-CHOP—the combination of the MoAb rituximab with conventional chemotherapy (cyclophosphamide, doxorubicin, vincristine, and prednisone)—is now considered standard treatment for common lymphomas (Martelli, Ferreria, Agostinelli, et al., 2013). CNS involvement is common with some aggressive forms of NHL; in this situation, cranial radiation or intrathecal chemotherapy is used in addition to systemic chemotherapy. Survival is very low when relapse occurs after being treated with rituximab-based regimens or with HSCT (Martelli et al., 2013).

More indolent lymphomas, such as follicular lymphoma, are not currently curable. However, the pace of the disease is slow and many patients have no or fewer symptoms at the time of diagnosis. "Watchful waiting," where therapy is delayed until symptoms develop, has often been used in those with indolent disease (Izutsu, 2014). More recently, immunotherapy (e.g., rituximab) is being used, often in combination with conventional chemotherapy, followed by rituximab as "maintenance therapy" (Hiddemann & Cheson, 2014; Izutsu,

2014). Patients with limited stage disease may be effectively treated with radiation therapy to the affected area.

Radiopharmaceutical agents (e.g., ibritumomab tiuxetan [Zevalin] or tositumomab/iodine-131 [Bexxar]) are also used, although they cause technical difficulties with administration due to the radioactivity of the agent. More aggressive treatment (often R-CHOP or rituximab plus bendamustine) may provide a longer duration of remission in which additional treatment is not needed. Unfortunately, in most situations, relapse is commonly seen in patients with low-grade lymphomas. Treatment after relapse is controversial; HSCT may be considered for patients younger than 60 years (see Chapter 15).

Nursing Management

Lymphoma is a highly complex constellation of diseases. When caring for patients with lymphoma, it is extremely important for the nurse to know the specific disease type, stage of disease, treatment history, and current treatment plan. Most of the care for patients with Hodgkin lymphoma or NHL takes place in the outpatient setting, unless complications occur (e.g., infection, respiratory compromise due to mediastinal mass). The most commonly used treatment methods are chemotherapy (often combined with an MoAb) and radiation therapy. Chemotherapy causes systemic side effects (e.g., myelosuppression, nausea, hair loss, risk of infection), whereas radiation therapy causes specific side effects that are limited to the area being irradiated. For example, patients receiving abdominal radiation therapy may experience nausea and diarrhea but not hair loss. Regardless of the type of treatment, all patients may experience fatigue (see Chart 15-7 in Chapter 15, Fatigue).

The risk of infection is significant for these patients, not only from treatment-related myelosuppression but also from the defective immune response that results from the disease itself. Patients need to be educated to minimize the risks of infection, to recognize signs of possible infection, and to contact their primary provider if such signs develop (see Chart 15-7 in Chapter 15, Infection).

Additional complications depend on the location of the lymphoma. Therefore, the nurse must know the tumor location so that assessments can be targeted appropriately. For example, patients with lymphomatous masses in the upper chest should be assessed for superior vena cava obstruction or airway obstruction, if the mass is near the bronchus or trachea.

Patient education is an integral component of nursing care. A longitudinal study of more than 1,000 patients with various types of lymphoma confirmed that informational needs vary over the course of the survival trajectory (Husson, Oerlemans, Mols, et al., 2014). Those patients diagnosed with lymphoma within the past 2 years voiced the need for disease and medical information; whereas, those diagnosed beyond 2 years voiced the need for information related to long-term effects of therapy. These results lend credence to the importance of tailoring information provided to the unique learning needs of the patient, as well as the coping styles that patient uses in living with lymphoma.

Many lymphomas can be cured with current treatments. However, as survival rates increase, the incidence of second malignancies, particularly AML or MDS, also increases.

Therefore, survivors should be screened regularly for the development of second malignancies. As is true with long-term survivors of Hodgkin lymphoma, survivors of NHL may be faced with managing persistent fatigue, depression, anxiety, cardiac, and pulmonary toxicity (Spector, Noonan, Mayer, et al., 2015). A study of quality of life among survivors of diffuse large B cell lymphoma found that younger-aged survivors (18 to 59 years of age) reported worse cognitive and social function and more financial problems and dyspnea compared to age-matched controls (van der Poel, Oerlemans, Schouten, et al., 2014). In contrast, the reported quality of life of older-aged survivors was similar to those of the control group, albeit lower than those of the younger-aged survivor group.

The American Cancer Society developed health behavior recommendations for cancer survivors, which include avoiding smoking, maintaining a normal body mass index (BMI), improving nutrition (i.e., consuming fruits and vegetables), and engaging in at least 150 minutes of aerobic physical activity per week. However, many survivors do not adhere to these recommendations. A study of more than 500 lymphoma survivors found that only 11% adhered to all four recommendations (Spector, et al., 2015). While most of these survivors reported they did not smoke (94%), 52% reported they did not adhere to the activity recommendations, 56% did not adhere to the dietary recommendations, and 64% were overweight or obese. Those individuals who did adhere to all four health behavior recommendations reported higher health-related quality of life (HRQOL) than those who did not. HRQOL scores were more strongly associated with non-smoking and exercise adherence. These data provide useful information for nurses in assisting patients to adapt and adhere to healthy lifestyles upon completing treatment for lymphoma.

MULTIPLE MYELOMA

Multiple myeloma is a malignant disease of the most mature form of B lymphocyte—the plasma cell. Plasma cells secrete immunoglobulins, which are proteins necessary for antibody production to fight infection. Myeloma is the second most common hematologic cancer in the United States. The incidence of multiple myeloma increases with age; the median age at diagnosis is 70 years (Wildes, Rosko, & Tuchman, 2014). The relative 5-year survival rate for newly diagnosed patients has steadily increased from 26.5% in 1975 to 46.6% in 2012 (National Cancer Institute, 2013).

Staging is based on four criteria: serum albumin (presumed to be a negative acute phase reactant), serum lactate dehydrogenase (an enzyme that, when elevated, is associated with a poorer prognosis), serum beta-2 microglobulin (presumed to be an indirect measure of tumor burden), and cytogenetic findings (where certain abnormalities are associated with a poor prognosis). Using this system, the 5-year overall survival rate for patients with early-stage disease (stage I) is 82%; the rate decreases to 40% in those with stage III disease (Palumbo, Avet-Loiseau, Oliva, et al., 2015). Methods to incorporate genetic information that may be useful in determining prognosis and even sensitivity to various drugs used in treating the disease are ongoing (Furukawa & Kikuchi,

2015). As with other B cell lymphoid malignancies, exposure to Agent Orange, used as a defoliating agent during the Vietnam War, is associated with the development of multiple myeloma (Chang, Boffetta, Adami, et al., 2015).

Pathophysiology

In multiple myeloma, the malignant plasma cells produce an increased amount of a specific immunoglobulin that is nonfunctional. Functional types of immunoglobulin are still produced by nonmalignant plasma cells, although in lower-than-normal quantity. The specific immunoglobulin secreted by the myeloma cells is detectable in the blood or urine and is referred to as the monoclonal protein, or M protein. This protein serves as a useful marker to monitor the extent of disease and the patient's response to therapy. It is commonly measured by serum or urine protein electrophoresis, or free light chain assay (see Fig. 34-10). The patient's total protein level is also typically elevated because of the production of M protein. Malignant plasma cells also secrete certain substances to stimulate angiogenesis to enhance the growth of these clusters of plasma cell. Occasionally, the plasma cells infiltrate other tissue, in which case they are referred to as plasmacytomas. Plasmacytomas can occur in the sinuses, spinal cord, and soft tissues.

Myeloma may evolve from a premalignant stage, known as monoclonal gammopathy of undetermined significance, or MGUS (Rajkumar, Dimopoulos, Palumbo, et al., 2014). At this point in the disease, there is no evidence of end-organ dysfunction that is seen in multiple myeloma: hypercalcemia, renal insufficiency, anemia, or bone lesions. This constellation of organ damage is referred to by the acronym CRAB (elevated *c*alcium, *r*enal insufficiency, *a*nemia, and/or *b*one

Figure 34-10 • Abnormal serum protein electrophoresis patterns contrasted with a normal pattern. Polyclonal peaks are characterized by a broad-based increase in immunoglobulin (Ig) by myriad reactive plasma cells and indicate a benign reactive process. In contrast, a narrow spike indicates homogeneity of the Ig secreted by a single clone of plasma cells. M spikes are seen in monoclonal gammopathies of undetermined significance or in plasma malignancies (myeloma, Waldenstrom's macroglobulinemia). From Turgeon, M. (2012). *Clinical hematology theory & procedures* (5th ed., Fig. 20.7, p. 347). Philadelphia, PA: Lippincott Williams & Wilkins.

lesions). In MGUS, while there is no evidence of CRAB features, there is a mild elevation in the M protein. The rate of progression from the MGUS state to multiple myeloma is 0.5% to 1% per year.

Clinical Manifestations

Clinical manifestations of the disease result not only from the malignant cells themselves, but also from the abnormal protein they produce (see Fig. 34-11). Bone disease is present in 80% of patients with multiple myeloma (Papamerkouriou, Kenanaidis, Gamie, et al., 2015). Bone pain is reported by the majority of patients with this disease; the classic presenting symptom of multiple myeloma is bone pain, usually in the back or ribs. Bone pain associated with myeloma increases with movement and decreases with rest; patients may report that they have less pain on awakening but more during the day. In myeloma, a substance secreted by the plasma cells, osteoclast activating factor, and other substances such as interleukin-6 (IL-6) are involved in stimulating osteoclasts. Both mechanisms appear to be involved in the process of bone breakdown. Thus, lytic lesions as well as osteoporosis may be seen on bone imaging, including combined PET-CT scan, CT scan, magnetic resonance imaging (MRI), and conventional x-ray; these lesions do not visualize on bone scans (Mihailovic & Goldsmith, 2015). The bone destruction can be severe enough to cause vertebral collapse and fractures, including spinal fractures, which can impinge on the spinal cord and result in spinal cord compression (see Fig. 34-12). When vertebral collapse occurs, the patient's height is reduced and kyphosis (an excessive curvature of the spine) is common.

If the bone destruction is extensive, excessive ionized calcium is lost from the bone and enters the serum; hypercalcemia may therefore develop and is frequently manifested by excessive thirst, dehydration, constipation, altered mental status, confusion, and perhaps coma. Kidney failure may also occur; the configuration of the circulating immunoglobulin molecule (particularly the shape of lambda light chains) can damage the renal tubules. Renal impairment occurs in 30% to 50% of patients at the time of diagnosis, can worsen when the disease

becomes refractory to treatment, and leads to dialysis in almost 10% of patients (O'Donnell, Cottini, Raje, et al., 2016).

> ### Quality and Safety Nursing Alert
>
> *Any older adult whose chief complaint is back pain and who has an elevated total protein level should be evaluated for possible myeloma.*

As more and more malignant plasma cells are produced, the marrow has less space for erythrocyte production, and anemia may develop. This anemia is also caused to a great extent by a diminished production of erythropoietin by the kidney. In the late stage of the disease, a reduced number of leukocytes and platelets may also be seen because the bone marrow is infiltrated by malignant plasma cells.

Infection is a concern and a frequent cause of morbidity and mortality. In contrast to other hematologic malignancies, the incidence of infection does not appear to be related to the extent of neutropenia in patients with multiple myeloma. Rather, the lack of adequate levels of normal immunoglobulin, as well as other alterations of the immune system, renders the patient at increased risk for developing infection, particularly due to *Streptococcus pneumoniae* or *H. influenzae*. Therapy for the disease also predisposes the patient for acquiring infections, particularly due to the high levels of corticosteroids used in treating the disease; herpes zoster and *Pneumocystis* are commonly causative organisms in this context (O'Donnell et al., 2016). Infection prophylaxis with antivirals and antibiotics (e.g., trimethoprim-sulfamethoxazole) is important to decrease infection risk.

Neurologic manifestations can also occur. Spinal cord compression is the most common, and other neurologic symptoms may be present, particularly peripheral nerve compression (see Chapter 15, Table 15-13: Oncologic Emergencies: Manifestations and Management). When the M protein is immunoglobulin M (IgM), peripheral neuropathy is more likely. Nerve root compression, the presence of intracranial neoplastic cells, and meningeal involvement are quite rare.

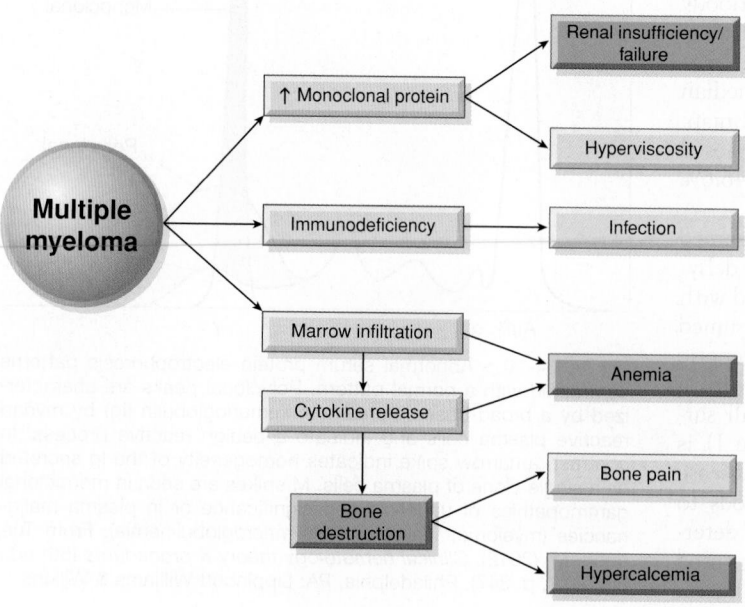

Figure 34-11 • Clinical manifestations of multiple myeloma and the mechanisms by which they develop. Those manifestations that are reflective of "end-organ damage" (i.e., CRAB features) are depicted in green. Adapted with permission from O'Donnell, E., Cottini, F., Raje, N., et al. (2016). Myeloma. In K. Kaushansky, M. A. Lichtman, J. T. Prchal, et al. (Eds.). *Williams hematology* (9th ed.). New York: McGraw-Hill.

Figure 34-12 • Lytic lesions seen in the humerus and skull in patients with multiple myeloma. These lesions typically occur in the long bones, vertebrae, and skull. Long bones are susceptible to fracture when the lesion occurs near the surface of the bone; vertebrae are susceptible to collapse, resulting in loss of height and potential for spinal cord compression. From (1999). *Wintrobe's clinical hematology* (10th ed., p. 2640). Philadelphia, PA: Lippincott Williams & Wilkins.

When plasma cells secrete excessive amounts of immunoglobulin, the serum viscosity can increase. Hyperviscosity may be manifested by bleeding from the nose or mouth, headache, blurred vision, paresthesias, or heart failure. Thromboembolic events (blood clots) may occur in patients with myeloma; the incidence is thought to be as high as 10% (Colson, 2015). The risk increases substantially when high doses of corticosteroids and immomodulatory drugs (e.g., thalidomide, lenalidomide, or pomalidomide) are used to treat the disease.

Assessment and Diagnostic Findings

An elevated monoclonal protein level in the serum (via serum protein electrophoresis), urine (via urine protein electrophoresis), or light chain ratio (via serum free light chain analysis) is a major criterion in the diagnosis of multiple myeloma. Evidence of end organ damage is typically necessary to establish the diagnosis, using the acronym CRAB, as noted previously. The diagnosis of myeloma is confirmed by bone marrow biopsy; the presence of more than 10% plasma cells is the hallmark diagnostic criterion.

Medical Management

There is no cure for multiple myeloma. Even autologous HSCT is considered to extend remission rather than provide a cure.

However, for many patients, it is possible to control the illness and maintain their level of functioning quite well for several years or longer. For those who are not candidates for HSCT, chemotherapy is the primary treatment. A significant improvement in response rates is largely due to the marked increase in new types of drugs used to treat this disease. The decision when to treat and with which regimen is highly complex. The time interval between treatment and relapse, development of drug resistance, adverse features of the disease (such as certain cytogenetic abnormalities), patient factors (especially comorbidities) and goals of treatment must all be considered.

Early Treatment Options

Because treatment has vastly improved, some experts advocate initiating therapy prior to the development of CRAB features, when the myeloma is considered "smoldering" (Rajkumar, Landgren, & Mateos, 2015). Corticosteroids, particularly dexamethasone, often form the backbone in myeloma therapy. They are typically combined with an immunomodulatory drug (lenalidomide, pomalidomide, or thalidomide) or a proteasome inhibitor (bortezomib [Velcade], carfilzomib [Kyprolis]). These drugs all target the disease via different mechanisms than do conventional chemotherapeutic agents. Combinations of two or three drugs are commonly used with the goal of reducing the tumor burden as much as possible.

Autologous Stem Cell Transplantation

Therapy has changed substantively for multiple myeloma, and has resulted in impressive increases in duration of survival. Importantly, patients not only live longer, the new treatment modalities provide the opportunity for enhanced quality of life. Therapeutic options are based on the determination of eligibility for receiving an autologous HSCT. Patient's age, functional status, and comorbidities are used to determine eligibility for transplant. For those deemed eligible, initial treatment is focused on reducing the amount of tumor burden (decrease the number of myeloma cells and reducing monoclonal protein) without damaging the patient's stem cells, which are harvested and then later used in the transplant process. Patients who are not eligible for autologous HSCT typically receive lower-intensity therapy with the objective of reducing tumor burden as much as possible. In both situations, maintenance therapy may be used to enhance the duration of remission. Therapeutic goals for patients who are frail when diagnosed focus on improving disease-associated symptoms and quality of life.

Pharmacologic Therapy

In the past decade, two new classes of drugs have been developed that have significant impact in treating multiple myeloma. Immunomodulatory drugs (IMiDs) have broad anti-myeloma effects by inhibiting angiogenesis and affecting specific **cytokines**, Il-6, tumor necrosis factor, both needed to support myeloma cell growth. Thalidomide, initially used as an antiemetic, was the first IMiD used in myeloma therapy. Fatigue, dizziness, constipation, rash, and peripheral neuropathy are commonly encountered in patients treated with thalidomide, whereas myelosuppression is not. There is also an increased incidence of DVT, particularly when the drug is used with corticosteroids; prophylactic anticoagulation should be used to prevent this complication. The thalidomide analogs lenalidomide and pomalidomide are also effective in treating myeloma. Side effects are quite different from those of thalidomide—myelosuppression, skin rash, and VTE are common, whereas sedation, neuropathy (including peripheral neuropathy), and constipation are not. Muscle cramps are more commonly associated with lenalidomide. These drugs are excreted by the kidneys, so careful monitoring of renal function is required, and dose reduction may be necessary. Because of teratogenic effects of all of these drugs, the female patient of child bearing age must be counseled and agree to use approved methods of birth control prior to taking any of them. While thalidomide is not used as frequently in treating multiple myeloma, the lack of associated myelosuppression makes it a viable option for select patients.

Proteasome inhibitors are a class of drugs that have significant anti-myeloma effects. Myeloma cells produce large amounts of immunoglobulin protein, and proteasomes are needed to process and clear the excess mis/unfolded protein that accumulates within the cell. Inhibiting this process causes an excess accumulation of these proteins that results in apoptosis of the myeloma cell (Merin & Kelly, 2015). Bortezomib (Velcade) was the first proteasome inhibitor used in treating multiple myeloma. A recent systematic review reported that the inclusion of bortezomib in various treatment regimens resulted in improved response to treatment and in some studies, in overall survival (Kouroukis, Baldassarre, Haynes, et al., 2014).

Side effects of bortezomib include transient thrombocytopenia, orthostatic hypotension, nausea and vomiting, skin rash, neuropathy, and asthenia (i.e., weakness, malaise, fatigue). Because neuropathy is potentially serious, the dosage needs to be decreased as soon as the neuropathy begins to interfere with function; however, administering the drug subcutaneously rather than intravenously markedly reduces this problem, as does changing the dosing schedule (weekly administration rather than twice weekly). Bortezomib is metabolized by the cytochrome P450 pathway, which means that a careful review of concurrent medications for drug–drug interaction is crucial. An oral formulation of the drug, ixazomib (Ninlaro) has been approved by the U.S. Food and Drug Administration (FDA, 2015).

Carfilzomib has greater proteasome selectivity than bortezomib and causes irreversible proteasome inhibition (Colson, 2015). It has a different side effect profile from bortezomib. Whereas peripheral neuropathy is not a side effect, pulmonary and cardiac toxicity are side effects, including dyspnea, which is more common early in treatment, as well as congestive heart failure, dysrhythmia formation, and ischemic heart disease (Wang & Cheng, 2013). Patients should be screened for cardiac disease prior to starting carfilzomib-based therapy, including obtaining baseline electrocardiograms (ECGs) and pulmonary function tests. Patients with preexisting heart disease should be carefully monitored throughout their treatment and hypertension well controlled.

Corticosteroids induce apoptosis in myeloma cells and markedly decrease bone pain (Colson, 2015). As a result, corticosteroids, particularly dexamethasone, have been used in combination with other myeloma therapy for decades. Reduced dosage (40 mg dexamethasone weekly as opposed to 160 mg weekly) has been associated with decreased adverse events, particularly VTE. Nonetheless, long-term use of corticosteroids can cause significant morbidity, including infection, VTE, proximal muscle weakness, osteoporosis, cataract formation, mood and behavior changes, and dental caries.

In additional to conventional chemotherapy, new drugs are now available for treating multiple myeloma (Lonial & Nooka, 2015). MoAbs have been targeted against specific antigens found on the surface of myeloma cells; daratumumab (Darzalex) is the first MoAb approved for myeloma therapy. Deacetylase inhibitors work to prevent the accumulation of mis/unfolded proteins that are not cleared by proteasomes; panobinostat (Farydak) is the first histone deacetylase inhibitor approved for use in multiple myeloma (Colson, 2015; Lonial & Nooka, 2015). Additional MoAbs, deacetylase inhibitors, and drugs with yet different mechanisms of action are under development. For all these new therapies, additional research is needed to guide clinicians and patients in determining how best—and when—to incorporate them in the multiple myeloma treatment armamentarium.

Managing Complications

Radiation therapy is useful in strengthening the bone at a specific lesion, particularly a bone at risk for fracture or spinal cord compression. It is also extremely useful in relieving bone pain and reducing the size of plasma cell tumors that occur outside the skeletal system as in plasmacytomas (Walker, Lawson, Buckle, et al., 2014). However, because it is a nonsystemic form of treatment, it does not diminish the source of the bone conditions (i.e., the production of malignant plasma cells). Therefore, radiation therapy is typically used in combination with systemic treatment such as chemotherapy.

When lytic lesions result in vertebral compression fractures, vertebroplasty may be performed (Jurczyszyn, Czepko, Banach, et al., 2015). This procedure may be enhanced by concomitant kyphoplasty (see Chapter 41 for further discussion of both vertebroplasty and kyphoplasty).

Some bisphosphonates, such as pamidronate (Aredia) and zoledronic acid (Zometa), have been shown to strengthen bone in multiple myeloma by diminishing survival of osteoclasts, thus controlling bone pain and potentially preventing bone fracture. These agents are also effective in managing and preventing hypercalcemia. Some evidence suggests that bisphosphonates may activate an antimyeloma immune response, inducing myeloma cell death, acting synergistically with antineoplastic drugs, and enhancing immune surveillance (van Acker, Anguille, Willemen, et al., 2015) (see Chapter 41 for further discussion of bisphosphonates).

When patients have significant signs and symptoms of hyperviscosity, plasmapheresis may be used to lower the immunoglobulin level. Symptoms may be more useful than serum viscosity levels in determining the need for this intervention.

 Gerontologic Considerations

Historically, aggressive myeloma therapy, particularly HSCT, was limited to patients younger than age 65, but recently this approach has been challenged. Patients older than age 65 who have excellent organ function (i.e., renal, hepatic, cardiopulmonary) and who have fewer comorbidities may tolerate more intense treatment, including reduced-dose autologous HSCT (Cerrato, Mina, & Palumbo, 2014). Determining an older adult patient's ability to tolerate therapy *a priori* is important. In addition to chronological age, organ function, and comorbidity, the ability to independently perform activities of daily living is another important factor. A comprehensive assessment of all these factors is useful to better determine the level of "fitness" in a given patient. Data suggest that patients categorized as frail develop more severe toxicity associated with therapy and consequently are more likely to discontinue that treatment (Wildes et al., 2014).

The older adult patient may have different goals of care from that of younger patients. Effective symptom control, preserving cognitive function, and maintaining independence are often viewed as higher priority than survival in the older adult (Wildes et al., 2014). Discussing these goals of care as well as the patient's physical and social needs can provide a more personalized approach to treating the older adult with multiple myeloma. Using lower doses and focusing on side effect management are important treatment strategies (Cerrato et al., 2014; Wildes et al., 2014). Side effects should be managed without additional medications to reduce the burden of "polypharmacy." Incorporating the expertise of a palliative care clinician may be extremely beneficial, not only in devising an appropriate treatment plan, but also in more effective symptom and side effect management.

Nursing Management

Pain management is very important in patients with multiple myeloma. NSAIDs can be very useful for mild pain or can be given in combination with opioid analgesics. Because NSAIDs can cause gastritis and renal dysfunction, renal function must be carefully monitored and patients assessed for gastritis; many patients are unable to use NSAIDs due to concurrent or newly developed renal insufficiency. Long-acting opioids are often prescribed to afford adequate pain relief.

Promoting Home, Community-Based, and Transitional Care

 Educating Patients About Self-Care

The patient needs to be educated about activity restrictions (e.g., lifting no more than 10 pounds, the use of proper body mechanics). Braces are occasionally needed to support the spinal column, but may be uncomfortable and hamper adherence. Bisphosphonate therapy has markedly reduced the severity and extent of bone pain. Patients need to understand the importance of comprehensive oral hygiene and good dental care to diminish the likelihood of developing osteonecrosis of the jaw that may arise from bisphosphonate therapy.

Renal function must be monitored closely. Kidney injury can become severe, and dialysis may be needed. Maintaining high urine output (3 L/day) can be very useful in preventing or limiting this complication, as is treating the underlying disease. The patient also needs to be instructed about the signs and symptoms of hypercalcemia. While hypercalcemia usually occurs at the onset of the disease, it can also develop at the time of disease progression or when multiple myeloma becomes refractory to therapy. Maintaining mobility and hydration are important to diminish exacerbations of this complication.

Because antibody production is impaired, infections, particularly bacterial infections, are common and can be life-threatening. The patient needs to be instructed in appropriate infection prevention measures and should be advised to contact the primary provider immediately if fever or other signs and symptoms of infection develop. The patient should receive pneumococcal and influenza vaccines. Prophylactic antibiotics, such as trimethoprim sulfamethoxazole, are often used, particularly when patients are treated with corticosteroid-containing regimens to prevent *Pneumocystis jirovecii* pneumonia (Raje, Yee, & Roodman, 2014). The antiviral agent acyclovir is recommended when patients are treated with bortezomib-based regimens to diminish the potential development of viral infection, such as herpes zoster.

Continuing and Transitional Care

Many newer medications, particularly the IMiDs, are associated with higher risks of thromboembolism formation, particularly when used concurrently with high doses of corticosteroids or erythropoietin (Raje et al., 2014). Other risk factors include decreased mobility, obesity, prior thromboembolic events, diabetes, cardiac or renal disease, and the presence of a vascular access device (e.g., PICC). It is important to maintain mobility and to use strategies that enhance venous return (e.g., anti-embolism stockings, avoid crossing the legs). For patients without additional risk factors, VTE can be prevented by taking low-dose aspirin. Those patients with additional risk factors for developing VTE should receive anticoagulation therapy.

TABLE 34-5 Peripheral Neuropathy

Type of Neuropathy	Manifestations	Nursing Intervention/Patient Education
Sensory	Hypoesthesia	Warn patient to avoid extreme temperatures (e.g., bathwater). Inspect feet for trauma, potential infection. Use loose-fitting stockings.
	Paresthesia (tingling)	Gentle massage Gentle ROM exercises
	Hyperalgesia (pain) Toes and fingers Soles of feet/palms	Gentle massage (cocoa butter or menthol-based cream/lotion) Apply lidocaine 5% patch to affected area every 12 hours. Consider gabapentin (Neurontin), tricyclic antidepressants (e.g., amitriptyline [Elavil]).
Motor	Muscle cramps Tremor ↓ Strength in distal muscles	Maximize hydration, ambulation. (Quinine is not recommended.)
	Gait disturbance ↓ Fine motor function (e.g., handwriting, buttoning clothes)	Encourage the use of appropriate footwear. Consider ambulatory aides (e.g., walker). Remove scatter rugs; perform a home safety evaluation. PT referral OT referral (if severe limitations)
Autonomic Nervous System	Orthostatic hypotension	Warn patient to avoid abrupt position change. Maximize hydration. Consider adjusting antihypertensive medications, diuretics.
	Bradycardia	Assess/warn patient for impact (fatigue, impairment in function). Consider adjusting drugs that cause bradycardia (e.g., calcium channel blockers, beta-blockers, alpha-/beta-adrenergic blockers, digoxin). Explore the use of activity to increase heart rate.
	Sexual dysfunction	Explore alternative means of sexual activity beyond intercourse. Consider the use of erectile dysfunction medication.
	Constipation	Maximize fluid intake, fiber. Use stool softeners, laxatives.

ROM, range of motion; ↓, decreased; PT, physical therapy; OT, occupational therapy.
Note: Peripheral neuropathy can be classified into three main categories. Within each category, specific manifestations are delineated as well as relevant nursing interventions. If the neuropathy is related to myeloma therapy, it is crucial to promptly stop the potentially offending medication. It is also important to reduce the impact from other predisposing factors. For example, diabetes should be well controlled and alcohol consumption reduced.

Peripheral neuropathy is a frequent issue for patients with multiple myeloma, affecting over 50% at the time of diagnosis (Koeppen, 2014). That incidence has increased with the use of thalidomide or bortezomib. The neuropathy is primarily sensory, but motor or autonomic nervous system neuropathy is also seen (Jongen, Broijl, & Sonneveld, 2015) (see Table 34-5). Painful neuropathy can be quite disabling and may interfere with the patient's ability to perform normal activities of daily living. The nurse needs to carefully assess for symptoms related to peripheral neuropathy and make assessments of the home for safety. Sensation (touch, temperature, pain, vibration, proprioception), ankle reflexes, distal muscle strength, and blood pressure should be evaluated. Other risk factors for peripheral neuropathy (e.g., diabetes, vitamin deficiencies, viral infection, or excessive alcohol consumption) should be aggressively managed. Patients should be educated to report any symptoms of peripheral neuropathy and to not minimize such symptoms, because prompt cessation of therapy or reducing the dose can prevent the neuropathy from progressing. Resuming treatment with a lower dosage and at a longer interval between dosing may diminish the worsening of peripheral nerve damage. Recovery can occur over time, although it may be incomplete. There is inadequate evidence to support the use of neuroprotective substances (e.g., l-carnitine) or additional nutritional supplements in treating this form of peripheral neuropathy (Jongen et al., 2015; Koeppen,

2014). Gabapentinoids (e.g., gabapentin [Neurontin], pregabalin [Lyrica]), tricyclic antidepressants (e.g., amitriptyline [Elavil], nortriptyline [Aventyl]), and selective serotonin reuptake inhibitors (e.g., duloxetine [Cymbalta]) can be used to diminish pain; opioids are fairly ineffective in this context.

As many drugs used in treating multiple myeloma are given orally, the nurse must ensure that the patient fully understands how to take the medication, manage side effects, and know what steps can be taken to diminish or mitigate toxicity. For example, cigarette smoking may decrease the efficacy of pomalidomide as it impacts its metabolism via the cytochrome P450 pathway. Therefore, patients need to be strongly encouraged to cease smoking and be provided assistance to do so.

CRITICAL THINKING EXERCISES

1 [pq] You are working in an emergency department. A 42-year-old man presents with a chief complaint of fever, fatigue, and a sore throat. His vital signs are notable for a temperature of 39°C (102.4°F), pulse of 112 bpm, BP 118/70, and respirations 28 per minutes. In your assessment, you note that he has mild crackles at the left lung base that clear with cough, and that he has petechiae on his back. He has multiple blood blisters on his buccal mucosa and beneath his tongue. His CBC shows a WBC of 42,000/mm³, hemoglobin of 7.2 g/dL, and platelet count of 8,000/mm³. What additional observations will you include in your assessment? What additional laboratory and radiologic data are important to consider? How will you prioritize your care of this patient?

2 **ebp** You are working in a woman's health clinic. A 26-year-old woman presents to the clinic; she remarks that she has completed treatment for Hodgkin lymphoma, and states she is anxious to "start to live again." She is worried about her prior radiation therapy and its long-term health consequences. What evidence is there for her developing subsequent health problems? What additional information do you need in order to assess her risk for late complications? What health behaviors are important for her to adopt? What evidence supports these behaviors? How will you respond to her statement regarding "starting to live again?"

3 **ebp** You are working on a med-surg unit and assigned to care for a 72-year-old male admitted for T8-9 vertebral fractures and pain control. He has multiple myeloma, receiving chemotherapy that includes long-term corticosteroids (dexamethasone 40 mg per week) and monthly bisphosphonate infusions. He has a PRN order for morphine 30 mg PO every 4 to 6 hours. Is this an appropriate pain regimen for this patient? What would you include in your assessment of the patient's pain and his prior pain management strategies? How might his health beliefs be a factor? What other medical interventions might be useful in this context? Would you advocate for including an NSAID? What evidence supports your decision? Why is pain a significant issue in the patient with multiple myeloma? What other complications from the underlying disease should be included in your assessment?

4 You are caring for a 57-year-old business executive who was recently diagnosed with polycythemia vera. He is very health conscious and is taking testosterone supplements to maintain his muscle mass. Does this behavior impact his risk for thrombosis? How? He reports he travels to Asia every 3 weeks. How does this impact his thrombosis risk? What other risk factors would you include in your assessment? What measures would you suggest to diminish his risk for developing a VTE?

REFERENCES

*Asterisk indicates nursing research.

Books

American Nurses Association (ANA). (2015). *Code of ethics for nurses with interpretive statements*. Washington, DC: Nursesbooks.org.

Awan, F. T., & Byrd, J. C. (2016). Chronic lymphocytic leukemia. In K. Kaushansky, M. A. Lichtman, J. T. Prchal, et al. (Eds.). *Williams hematology* (9th ed.). New York: McGraw-Hill.

Larson, R. A., & Richard, L. M. (2016). Acute lymphoblastic leukemia. In K.Kaushansky, M. A. Lichtman, J. T. Prchal, et al. (Eds.). *Williams hematology* (9th ed.). New York: McGraw-Hill.

Lichtman, M. A., & Prchal, J. T.(2016). Primary myelofibrosis. In K. Kaushansky, M. A. Lichtman, J. T. Prchal, et al. (Eds.). *Williams hematology* (9th ed.). New York: McGraw-Hill.

Liesveld, J. L., & Lichtman, M. A. (2016). Acute myelogenous leukemia. In K. Kaushansky, M. A. Lichtman, J. T. Prchal, et al. (Eds.). *Williams hematology* (9th ed.). New York: McGraw-Hill.

O'Donnell, E., Cottini, F., Raje, N., et al. (2016). Myeloma. In K. Kaushansky, M. A. Lichtman, J. T. Prchal, et al. (Eds.). *Williams hematology* (9th ed.). New York: McGraw-Hill.

Prchal, J. F., & Prchal, J. T. (2016). Polycythemia vera. In K. Kaushansky, M. A. Lichtman, J. T. Prchal, et al. (Eds.). *Williams hematology* (9th ed.). New York: McGraw-Hill.

Press, O. (2016). Hodgkin lymphoma. In K. Kaushansky, M. A. Lichtman, J. T. Prchal, et al. (Eds.). *Williams hematology* (9th ed.). New York: McGraw-Hill.

Journals and Electronic Documents

Abelsson, J., Andréasson, B., Samuelsson, J., et al. (2013). Patients with polycythemia have worst impairment of quality of life among patients with newly diagnosed acute myeloid leukemia. *Journal of Clinical Oncology*, 30(21), 2670–2677.

Adès, L., Itzykson, R., &Fenaux, P. (2014). Myelodysplastic syndromes. *Lancet*, 383(9936), 2239–2252.

Alvarez-Larrán, A., & Besses, C. (2014). Antiplatelet therapy in the management of myeloproliferative neoplasms. *Current Hematologic Malignancy Reports*, 9(4), 319–323.

American Cancer Society (ACS) (2014a). Leukemia—Acute myeloid (myelogenous). Last revised: 12/9/2014. Retrieved on 12/10/2015 at: www.cancer.org/cancer/leukemia-acutemyeloidaml/detailedguide/leukemia-acute-myeloid-myelogenous-key-statistics

American Cancer Society (ACS) (2014b). Survival rates for myelodysplastic syndrome. Retrieved on 12/20/2015 at: www.cancer.org/cancer/myelodysplasticsyndrome/overviewguide/myelodysplastic-syndromes-overview-survival

American Cancer Society (ACS) (2015a). Do we know what causes chronic myeloid leukemia? Retrieved on 12/16/2015 at: http://www.cancer.org/cancer/leukemia-chronicmyeloidcml/detailedguide/leukemia-chronic-myeloid-myelogenous-diagnosis

American Cancer Society (ACS) (2015b). Survival rates for Hodgkin disease by stage. Retrieved on 1/2/2016 at: www.cancer.org/cancer/hodgkindisease/detailedguide/hodgkin-disease-survival-rates

American Cancer Society (ACS) (2015c). Types of non-Hodgkin lymphoma. Retrieved on 1/10/2016 at: www.cancer.org/cancer/non-hodgkinlymphoma/detailedguide/non-hodgkin-lymphoma-types-of-non-hodgkin-lymphoma

American Cancer Society (ACS) (2015d). What are the key statistics about non-Hodgkin lymphoma? Retrieved on 1/10/2016 at: www.cancer.org/cancer/non-hodgkinlymphoma/detailedguide/non-hodgkin-lymphoma-key-statistics

American Cancer Society (ACS) (2015e). Survival rates and factors that affect prognosis (outlook) for non-Hodgkin lymphoma. Retrieved on 1/10/2016 at: www.cancer.org/cancer/non-hodgkinlymphoma/detailedguide/non-hodgkin-lymphoma-factors-prognosis

Barbui, T., Finazzi, G., & Falanga, A. (2013). Myeloproliferative neoplasms and thrombosis. *Blood*, 122(13), 2176–2184.

Batlevi, C. L., & Younes, A. (2013). Novel therapy for Hodgkin lymphomas. *Hematology American Society of Hematology Education Program*, 2013(1), 394–399.

Birgegård, G. (2013). Pharmacological management of essential thrombocythemia. *Expert Opinion on Pharmacotherapy*, 14(10), 1295–1306.

Bowen, D.T. (2013). Occupational and environmental etiology of MDS. *Best Practice and Research in Clinical Haematology*, 26(4), 319–326.

Breccia, M., Efficace, F., Sica, S., et al. (2015). Adherence and future discontinuation of tyrosine kinase inhibitors in chronic phase chronic myeloid leukemia. A patient-based survey on 1133 patients. *Leukemia Research*, 39(10), 1055–1059.

Broeckaert, B. (2011). Palliative sedation, physician assisted suicide, and euthanasia: "Same, same but different?" *American Journal of Bioethics*, 11(6), 62–64.

Carvalho, T. B., Radt, M. Y., Verheijde, J. L., et al. (2011). Continuous deep sedation in end-of-life care: disentangling palliation from physician-assisted death. *American Journal of Bioethics*,11(6), 60–62.

Cerrato, C., Mina, R., & Palumbo, A. (2014). Optimal management of elderly patients with myeloma. *Expert Review of Anticancer Therapy*, 14(2), 217–228.

Chang, E. T., Boffetta, P., Adami, H. O., et al. (2015). A critical review of the epidemiology of Agent Orange or 2,3,7,8-tetrachlorodibenzo-p-dioxin and lymphoid malignancies. *Annals of Epidemiology, 25*(4), 275–292.

Cheson, B. D., Fisher, R. I., Barrington, S. F., et al. (2014). Recommendations for initial evaluation, staging, and response assessment of Hodgkin and non-Hodgkin lymphoma: The Lugano classification. *Journal of Clinical Oncology, 32*(27), 3059–3067.

Chiaretti, S., &Foà, R. (2015). Management of adult Ph-positive acute lymphoblastic leukemia. *Hematology American Society of Hematology Education Program, 2015*(1), 406–413.

Coleman, M. (2014). Patient empowerment in the management of chronic myeloid leukemia. *Clinical Journal of Oncology Nursing, 18*(2), E12–E18.

Colson, K. (2015). Treatment-related symptom management in patients with multiple myeloma: A review. *Supportive Care in Cancer, 23*(5), 1431–1445.

Coombs, C. C., Tavakkoli, M., & Tallman, M. S. (2015). Acute promyelocytic leukemia: Where did we start, where are we not, and the future. *Blood Cancer Journal, 5*, e304.

Cozzani, E., Iurlo, A., Merlo, G., et al. (2015). Essential thrombocythemia: The dermatologic point of view. *Clinical Lymphoma Myeloma and Leukemia, 15*(12), 739–747.

Daniëls, L. A., Oerlemans, S., Krol, A. D., et al. (2013). Persisting fatigue in Hodgkin lymphoma survivors: A systematic review. *Annals of Hematology, 9*(8), 1023–1032.

Daniëls, L. A., Oerlemans, S., Krol, A. D., et al. (2014). Chronic fatigue in Hodgkin lymphoma survivors and associations with anxiety, depression and comorbidity. *British Journal of Cancer, 110*(4), 868–874.

DeAngelo, D. J. (2015). The use of novel monoclonal antibodies in the treatment of acute lymphoblastic leukemia. *Hematology American Society of Hematology Education Program, 2015*(1), 400–405.

Deninger, M. W. (2015). Molecular monitoring in CML and the prospects for treatment-free remissions. *Hematology American Society of Hematology Education Program, 2015*(1), 257–263.

Di Bella, N. J., Bhowmik, D., Bhor, M., et al. (2015). The effectiveness of tyrosine kinase inhibitors and molecular monitoring patterns in newly diagnosed patients with chronic myeloid leukemia in the community setting. *Clinical Lymphoma, Myeloma and Leukemia, 15*(10), 599–605.

Erba, H. P. (2015). Finding the optimal combination therapy for the treatment of newly diagnosed AML in older patients unfit for intensive therapy. *Leukemia Research, 39*(2), 183–191.

Evens, A. M., & Kostakoglu, L. (2014). The role of FDG-PET in defining prognosis of Hodgkin lymphoma for early stage disease. *Hematology. American Society of Hematology Education Program, 2014*(1), 135–143.

Food and Drug Administration (2015). Ixazomib. Retrieved on 1/13/2016 at: www.fda.gov/Drugs/InformationOnDrugs/ApprovedDrugs/ucm473804.htm

Foster, M. (2014). Reevaluating the neutropenic diet: Time to change. *Clinical Journal of Oncology Nursing, 18*(2), 239–241.

Furukawa, Y., & Kikuchi, J. (2015). Molecular pathogenesis of multiple myeloma. *International Journal of Clinical Oncology, 20*(3), 413–422.

Garcia-Manero, G. (2015). Myelodysplastic syndromes: 2015 update on diagnosis, risk-stratification and management. *American Journal of Hematology, 90*(9), 832–841.

Geyer, H. L.,& Mesa, R. A. (2014). Therapy for myeloproliferative neoplasms: When, which agent, and how? *Hematology American Society of Hematology Education Program, 2014*(1), 277–286.

Goldberg, S. L. (2015). Monitoring chronic myeloid leukemia in the real world: Gaps and opportunities. *Clinical Lymphoma Myeloma and Leukemia, 15*(12), 711–714.

Graf, S. A., &Gopal, A. K. (2014). Treatment of relapsed classical Hodgkin lymphoma in the brentuximab vedotin era. *Hematology American Society of Hematology Education Program, 2014*(1), 151–157.

*Hacker, E. D., Patel, P., & Stainthorpe, M. (2013). Sleep interrupted: Nocturnal care disturbances following hematopoietic stem cell transplantation. *Clinical Journal of Oncology Nursing, 17*(5), 517–523.

Hall, A. E., Paul, C., Bryant, J., et al. (2016). To adhere or not to adhere: Rates and reasons of medication adherence in hematological cancer patients. *Critical Reviews in Oncology/Hematology, 97*(1), 247–262.

Hallek, M. (2015). Chronic lymphocytic leukemia: 2015 update on diagnosis, risk stratification, and treatment. *American Journal of Hematology, 90*(5), 446–460.

Hiddemann, W., &Cheson, B. D. (2014). How we manage follicular lymphoma. *Leukemia, 28*(7), 1388–1395.

Hughes, T., & White, D. (2013). Which TKI? An embarrassment of riches for chronic myeloid leukemia patients. *Hematology American Society of Hematology Education Program, 2013*(1), 168–175.

Husson, O., Oerlemans, S., Mols, F., et al. (2014). Satisfaction with information provision is associated with baseline but not with follow-up quality of life among lymphoma patients: Results from the PROFILES registry. *Acta Ongologica, 53*(7), 917–926.

Izutsu, K. (2014). Treatment of follicular lymphoma. *Journal of Clinical and Experimental Hematopathology, 54*(1), 31–37.

Johnson, P. W. (2013). Management of early stage Hodgkin lymphoma: Is there still a role for radiation? *Hematology American Society of Hematology Education Program, 2013*(1), 400–405.

Jongen, J. L., Broijl, A., & Sonneveld, P. (2015). Chemotherapy-induced peripheral neuropathies in hematological malignancies. *Journal of Neuro-Oncology, 121*(2), 229–237.

Jurczyszyn, A., Czepko, R., Banach, M., et al. (2015). Percutaneous vertebroplasty for pathological vertebral compression fractures secondary to multiple myeloma—medium-term and long-term assessment of pain relief and quality of life. *Advances in Clinical and Experimental Medicine, 24*(4), 651–656.

Kam, G., Yiu, R., Loh, Y., et al. (2015). Impact of pegylated filgrastim in comparison to filgrastim for patients with acute myeloid leukaemia (AML) on high-dose cytarabine (HIDAC) consolidation therapy. *Supportive Care in Cancer, 23*(3), 643–649.

Khimani, N., Chen, Y. H., Mauch, P. M., et al. (2013). Influence of new late effects on quality of life over time in Hodgkin lymphoma survivors: A longitudinal study. *Annals of Oncology, 24*(1), 226–230.

Koeppen, S. (2014). Treatment of multiple myeloma: Thalidomide, bortezomib, and lenalidomide-induced peripheral neuropathy. *Oncology Research and Treatment, 37*(9), 506–513.

Kouroukis, T. C., Baldassarre, F. G., Haynes, A. E., et al. (2014). Bortezomib in multiple myeloma: Systematic review and clinical considerations. *Current Oncology, 21*(4), e573–e603.

Lekovic, D., Gotic, M., Sefer, D., et al. (2015). Predictors of survival and cause of death in patients with essential thrombocythemia. *European Journal of Haematology, 95*(5), 461–466.

Leukemia & Lymphoma Society. (2013). Hodgkin lymphoma. Retrieved on 6/2/2016 at: www.lls.org/sites/default/files/file_assets/PS57_Hogkin_Lymphoma%20FINAL_with%20insert%20May2016.pdf

Leukemia & Lymphoma Society. (2015a). Acute myeloid leukemia. Retrieved on 6/2/2015 at: www.lls.org/sites/default/files/file_assets/PS32_AML_Booklet_FINAL6.15.pdf

Leukemia & Lymphoma Society. (2015b). Somewhere is today. Facts 2014--2015.Retrieved on 12/10/2015 at: www.lls.org/sites/default/files/file_assets/facts.pdf

Lonial, S., & Nooka, A. K. (2015). Novel combination approaches for myeloma. *Hematology American Society of Hematology Education Program, 2015*(1), 286–293.

Manea, P. J. (2014). Optimizing the management of patients with myelofibrosis. *Clinical Journal of Oncology Nursing, 18*(3), 330–337.

Martelli, M., Ferreria, A., Agostinelli, C., et al. (2013). Diffuse B-cell lymphoma. *Critical Reviews in Oncology/Hematology, 87*(2), 146–171.

Matasar, M. J., Ford, J. S., Riedel, E. R., et al. (2015). Late morbidity and mortality in patients with Hodgkin's lymphoma treated during adulthood. *Journal of the National Cancer Institute, 107*(4), pii: djv018.

Mathisen, M. S., Kantarjian, H., Thomas, D., et al. (2013). Acute lymphoblastic leukemia in adults: Encouraging developments on the way to higher cure rates. *Leukemia & Lymphoma, 54*(12), 2592–2600.

Merin, N. M., & Kelly, K. R. (2015). Clinical use of proteosome inhibitors in treatment of multiple myeloma. *Pharmaceuticals, 8*(1), 1–20.

Mihailovic, J., &Goldsmith, S. J. (2015). Multiple myeloma: 18F-FDG-PET/CT and diagnostic imaging. *Seminars in Nuclear Medicine, 45*(1), 16–31.

National Cancer Institute. (2013). SEER Stat Fact Sheets: Myeloma. Retrieved on 1/13/2016 at: seer.cancer.gov/statfacts/html/mulmy.html

Ng, A. K. (2014). Current survivorship recommendations for patients with Hodgkin lymphoma: Focus on late effects. *Hematology American Society of Hematology Education Program, 2014*(1), 488–494.

Nolte, F, Angelucci, E., Breccia, M., et al. (2015). Updated recommendations on the management of gastrointestinal disturbances during iron chelation therapy with deferasirox in transfusion dependent patients with myelodysplastic syndrome: Emphasis on optimized dosing schedules and new formulations. *Leukemia Research, 39*(10), 1028–1033.

Odenike, O. (2013). Beyond JAK inhibitor therapy in myelofibrosis. *Hematology American Society of Hematology Education Program, 2015*(1), 545–552.

Oerlemans, S., Mols, F., Nijziel, M. R., et al. (2014). The course of anxiety and depression for patients with Hodgkin's lymphoma or diffuse large B cell lymphoma: A longitudinal study of the PROFILES registry. *Journal of Cancer Survivorship, 8*(4), 555–564.

Pagano, L., Verga, L., Busca, A., et al. (2014). Systemic antifungal treatment after posaconazole prophylaxis: Results from the SEIFEM 2010-C survey. *Journal of Antimicrobial Chemotherapy, 69*(11), 3142–3147.

Palumbo, A., Avet-Loiseau, H., Oliva, S., et al. (2015). Revised International Staging System for multiple myeloma: A report from International Myeloma Working Group. *Journal of Clinical Oncology, 33*(26), 2863–2869.

Pandita, A., & Mukherjee, S. (2014). Resuscitating a dying marrow: The role of hematopoietic growth factors. *Current Hematologic Malignancy Reports, 9*(4), 412–420.

Papamerkouriou, Y. M., Kenanaidis, E., Gamie, Z., et al. (2015). Treatment of multiple myeloma bone disease: Experimental and clinical data. *Expert Opinion on Biological Therapy, 15*(2), 213–230.

Perfect, J. R., Hachem, R., & Wingard, J. R. (2014). Update on epidemiology of and preventive strategies for invasive fungal infections in cancer patients. *Clinical Infectious Diseases, 59*(Suppl 5), S352–S355.

Radia, D., & Geyer, H. L. (2015). Management of symptoms in polycythemia vera and essential thrombocythemia patients. *Hematology American Society of Hematology Education Program, 2015*(1), 340–348.

Raje, N. S., Yee, A. J., & Roodman, G. D. (2014). Advances in supportive care for multiple myeloma. *Journal of the National Comprehensive Cancer Network, 12*(4), 502–511.

Rajkumar, S. V., Landgren, O., & Mateos, M. V. (2015). Smoldering multiple myeloma. *Blood, 125*(20), 3069–3075.

Rajkumar, S. V., Dimopoulos, M. A., Palumbo, A., et al. (2014). International Myeloma Working Group updated criteria for the diagnosis of multiple myeloma. *Lancet Oncology, 15*(12), e538–e548.

Randhawa, J. K., & Ferrajoli, A. (2016). A review of supportive care and recommendations to preventive approaches for patients with chronic lymphocytic leukemia. *Expert Review of Hematology, 9*(3), 235–244.

Röllig, C., & Ehninger, G. (2015). How I treat hyperleukocytosis in acute myeloid leukemia. *Blood, 125*(21), 3246–3252.

*Roper, K., Cooley, M. E., McDermott, K., et al. (2013). Health-related quality of life after treatment of Hodgkin lymphoma in young adults. *Oncology Nursing Forum, 40*(4), 349–360.

*Ryblom, H., Hast, R., Hellström-Lindberg, E., et al. (2015). Self-perception of symptoms of anemia and fatigue before and after blood transfusions in patients with myelodysplastic syndromes. *European Journal of Oncology Nursing, 19*(2), 99–106.

Santini, V., & Fenaux, P. (2015). Treatment of myelodysplastic syndrome with thrombomimetic drugs. *Seminars in Hematology, 52*(1), 38–45.

Scherber, R. M., Kosiorek, H. E., Senyak, Z., et al. (2016). Comprehensively understanding fatigue in patients with myeloproliferative neoplasms. *Cancer, 122*(3), 477–485.

Scherber, R. A., Geyer, H. L., & Mesa, R. A. (2014). Quality of life in MPN comes of age as a therapeutic target. *Current Hematologic Malignancy Reports, 9*(4), 324–330.

Schiffer, C. A. (2014). Optimal dose and schedule of consolidation in AML: Is there a standard? *Best Practice & Research. Clinical Haematology, 27*(3–4), 259–264.

Sever, M., Newberry, K. J., & Verstovsek, S. (2014). Therapeutic options for patients with polycythemia vera and essential thrombocythemia refractory/resistant to hydroxyurea. *Leukemia & Lymphoma, 55*(12), 2685–2690.

Shanafelt, T. (2013). Treatment of older patients with chronic lymphocytic leukemia: Key questions and current answers. *Hematology American Society of Hematology Education Program, 2013*(1), 158–167.

Shlush, L. I., & Minden, M. D. (2015). Preleukemia: The normal side of cancer. *Current Opinion in Hematology, 22*(2), 77–84.

Siegel, F. P., Tauscher, J., & Petrides, P. E. (2013). Aquagenic pruritus in polycythemia vera: Characteristics and influence on quality of life in 441 patients. *American Journal of Hematology, 88*(8), 665–669.

Soares, A., Biasoli, I., Scheliga, A., et al. (2013). Association of social network and social support with health-related quality of life and fatigue in long-term survivors of Hodgkin lymphoma. *Supportive Care in Cancer, 21*(8), 2153–2159.

*Spector, D. J., Noonan, D., Mayer, D. K., et al. (2015). Are lifestyle behavioral factors associated with health-related quality of life in long-term survivors of non-Hodgkin lymphoma? *Cancer, 121*(18), 3343–4451.

Squizzato, A., Romualdi, E., Passamonti, F., et al. (2013). Antiplatelet drugs for polycythemia vera and essential thrombocythemia. *Cochrane Database of Systematic Reviews, 4*:CD006503.

Steensma, D. P., & Gatterman, N. (2013). When is iron overload deleterious, and when and how should iron chelation therapy be administered in myelodysplastic syndromes? *Best Practice & Research. Clinical Hematology, 26*(4), 431–444.

Stein, B. L., Moliterno, A. R., & Tiu, R. V. (2014). Polycythemia vera disease burden: Contributing factors, impact on quality of life, and emerging treatment options. *Annals of Hematology, 93*(12), 1965–1976.

Stilgenbauer, S. (2015). Prognostic markers and standard management of chronic lymphocytic leukemia. *Hematology American Society of Hematology Education Program, 2015*(1), 368–377.

Sullivan, L. R., Sekeres M. A., Shrestha, N. K., et al. (2013). Epidemiology and risk factors for infections in myelodysplastic syndromes. *Transplant Infectious Disease, 15*(6), 652–657.

Tefferi, A., & Barbui, T. (2015). Polycythemia vera and essential thrombocythemia: 2015 update on diagnosis, risk-stratification and management. *American Journal of Hematology, 90*(2), 162–173.

Thompson, P. A., Kantarjian, H. M., & Cortes, J. E. (2015). Diagnosis and treatment of chronic myeloid leukemia in 2015. *Mayo Clinic Proceedings, 90*(10), 1440–1454.

Troy, J. D., Atallah, E., Geyer, J. T., et al. (2014). Myelodysplastic syndromes in the United States: An update for clinicians. *Annals of Medicine, 46*(5), 283–289.

van Acker, H. H., Anguille, S., Willemen, Y., et al. (2015). Bisphosphonates for cancer treatment: Mechanisms of action and lessons from clinical trials. *Pharmacology & Therapeutics, 158*(2016), 24–40.

van der Poel, M. W., Oerlemans, S., Schouten, H. C., et al. (2014). Quality of life more impaired in younger than in older diffuse large B cell lymphoma survivors compared to a normative population: A study from the population-based PROFILES registry. *Annals of Hematology, 93*(5), 811–819.

Vannucchi, A. M. (2014). How I treat polycythemia vera. *Blood, 124*(22), 3212–3220.

Walker, R. E., Lawson, M. A., Buckle, C. H., et al. (2014). Myeloma bone disease: Pathogenesis, current treatments and future targets. *British Medical Bulletin, 111*(1), 117–138.

Wang, M., & Cheng, J. (2013). Overview and management of cardiac and pulmonary adverse events in patients with relapsed and/or refractory multiple myeloma treated with single-agent carfilzomib. *Oncology, 27*(Suppl 3), 24–30.

Wildes, T. M., Rosko, A., & Tuchman, S. A. (2014). Multiple myeloma in the older adult: Better prospects, more challenges. *Journal of Clinical Oncology, 32*(24), 2531–2540.

Wilson, O., Avalos, G., & Dowling, M. (2016). Knowledge of palliative care and attitudes towards nursing the dying patient. *British Journal of Nursing, 25*(11), 600–605.

Xie, M., Jiang, Q., & Xie, Y. (2015). Comparison between decitabine and azacitidine for the treatment of myelodysplastic syndrome: A meta-analysis with 1392 participants. *Clinical Lymphoma, Myeloma & Leukemia, 15*(1), 22–28.

Resources

American Cancer Society, www.cancer.org

American College of Surgeons Commission on Cancer, www.facs.org/quality-programs/cancer/coc

American Pain Society, www.ampainsoc.org

American Society for Blood and Marrow Transplantation (ASBMT), www.asbmt.org

Aplastic Anemia & MDS International Foundation, www.aamds.org

Be The Match (Bone marrow transplantation network), bethematch.org

Blood and Marrow Transplant Information Network, www.bmtinfonet.org

International Myeloma Foundation, myeloma.org/Main.action

Leukemia and Lymphoma Society, www.lls.org

Lymphoma Research Foundation, www.lymphoma.org/site/pp.asp?c=bkLTKaOQLmK8E&b=6296735

Multinational Association of Supportive Care in Cancer, www.mascc.org

Myelodysplastic Syndromes Foundation (MDS Foundation), www.mds-foundation.org

National Cancer Institute, www.cancer.gov

National Comprehensive Cancer Network, www.nccn.org

National Heart, Lung, and Blood Institute, www.nhlbi.nih.gov

Oncology Nursing Society (ONS), www.ons.org

Immunologic Function

Case Study

SUPPORTING THE PATIENT WITH SYSTEMIC LUPUS ERYTHEMATOUS

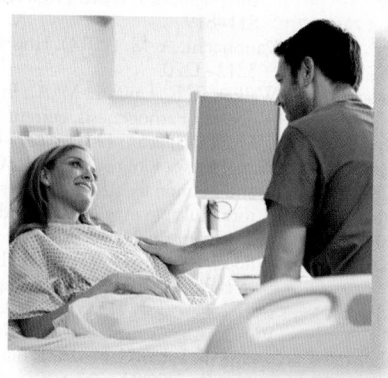

A 24-year-old female is hospitalized with an autoimmune disorder, systemic lupus erythematous (SLE). She has a toddler at home and reports that she and her husband wish to conceive another child. She has recently stopped taking her medications prescribed to treat SLE, which include hydroxychloroquine (Plaquenil) and prednisone. As a result of stopping her medications, she is experiencing a flare-up of SLE. She is currently experiencing fatigue, acute pain in her joints, and fever. She has a WBC of 2.1/mm^3 and Hgb 7.6 mg/dL. She is reluctant to resume medical treatment, including resuming her prescribed medications, as it may have teratogenic effects.

QSEN Competency Focus: Patient-Centered Care

The complexities inherent in today's health care system challenges nurses to demonstrate integration of specific inter-disciplinary core competencies. These competencies are aimed at ensuring the delivery of safe, quality patient care (Institute of Medicine, 2003). The Quality and Safety Education for Nurses project (QSEN, 2017; Cronenwett, Sherwood, Barnsteiner, et al., 2007) provides a framework for the knowledge, skills, and attitudes (KSA) required for nurses to demonstrate competency in these key areas, which include **patient-centered care, interdisciplinary teamwork and collaboration, evidence-based practice, quality improvement, safety,** and **informatics.**

Patient-Centered Care Definition: Recognize the patient or designee as the source of control and full partner in providing compassionate and coordinated care based on respect for patient's preferences, values, and needs.

SELECTED PRE-LICENSURE KSAs	APPLICATION AND REFLECTION
Knowledge	
Describe strategies to empower patients or families in all aspects of the health care process.	Describe strategies you would use to ensure that this patient is fully engaged in all aspects of her care. How might this empower her?
Skills	
Engage patients or designated surrogates in active partnerships that promote health, safety, well-being, and self-care management.	Discuss how you would assess the threats to this patient's active involvement in her health, safety, well-being, and self-care management. What measures might you take to mitigate these threats?
Attitudes	
Value active partnership with patients or designated surrogates in planning, implementation, and evaluation of care.	Reflect on your attitudes toward patients with chronic illness who stop taking their medication for personal reasons, such as wanting to conceive another child. What impact does this have on the plan of care?

Cronenwett, L., Sherwood, G., Barnsteiner, J., et al. (2007). Quality and safety education for nurses. *Nursing Outlook, 55*(3), 122–131.
Institute of Medicine. (2003). *Health professions education: A bridge to quality.* Washington, DC: National Academies Press.
QSEN Institute. (2017). *QSEN competencies: Definitions and pre-licensure KSAs.* Retrieved on 3/1/2017 at: www.qsen.org/competencies/pre-licensure-ksas

35 Assessment of Immune Function

LEARNING OBJECTIVES

On completion of this chapter, the learner will be able to:

1 Describe the body's general immune responses.
2 Discuss the stages of the immune response.
3 Differentiate between cellular and humoral immune responses.
4 Specify the effects of selected variables on function of the immune system.
5 Use assessment parameters for determining the status of patients' immune function.

GLOSSARY

agglutination: clumping effect occurring when an antibody acts as a cross-link between two antigens

antibody: a protein substance developed by the body in response to and interacting with a specific antigen

antigen: substance that induces the production of antibodies

antigenic determinant: the specific area of an antigen that binds with an antibody combining site and determines the specificity of the antigen–antibody reaction

apoptosis: programmed cell death that results from the digestion of deoxyribonucleic acid by end nucleases

B cells: cells that are important for producing a humoral immune response

cellular immune response: the immune system's third line of defense, involving the attack of pathogens by T cells

complement: series of enzymatic proteins in the serum that, when activated, destroy bacteria and other cells

cytokines: generic term for nonantibody proteins that act as intercellular mediators, as in the generation of immune response

cytotoxic T cells: lymphocytes that lyse cells infected with virus; also play a role in graft rejection

epitope: any component of an antigen molecule that functions as an antigenetic determinant by permitting the attachment of certain antibodies

genetic engineering: emerging technology designed to enable replacement of missing or defective genes

helper T cells: lymphocytes that attack foreign invaders (antigens) directly

humoral immune response: the immune system's second line of defense; often termed the *antibody response*

immune response: the coordinated response of the components of the immune system to a foreign agent or organism

immune system: the collection of organs, cells, tissues, and molecules that mediate the immune response

immunity: the body's specific protective response to a foreign agent or organism; resistance to disease, specifically infectious diseases

immunopathology: study of diseases resulting in dysfunctions within the immune system

immunoregulation: complex system of checks and balances that regulates or controls immune responses

immunosenescence: the gradual deterioration of the immune system brought on by the aging process

interferons: proteins formed when cells are exposed to viral or foreign agents; capable of activating other components of the immune system

lymphokines: substances released by sensitized lymphocytes when they come in contact with specific antigens

memory cells: cells that are responsible for recognizing antigens from previous exposure and mounting an immune response

natural killer (NK) cells: lymphocytes that defend against microorganisms and malignant cells

null lymphocytes: lymphocytes that destroy antigens already coated with the antibody

opsonization: the coating of antigen–antibody molecules with a sticky substance to facilitate phagocytosis

phagocytic cells: cells that engulf, ingest, and destroy foreign bodies or toxins

phagocytic immune response: the immune system's first line of defense, involving white blood cells that have the ability to ingest foreign particles

stem cells: precursors of all blood cells; reside primarily in bone marrow

suppressor T cells: lymphocytes that decrease B-cell activity to a level at which the immune system is compatible with life

T cells: cells that are important for producing a cellular immune response

Immunity is the body's specific protective response to a foreign agent or organism. The **immune system** functions as the body's defense mechanism against invasion and allows a rapid response to foreign substances in a specific manner. Genetic and cellular responses result. Any qualitative or quantitative change in the components of the immune system can produce profound effects on the integrity of the human organism. Immune function is affected by a variety of factors, such as central nervous system integrity; general physical and emotional status; medications; dietary patterns; and the stress of illness, trauma, or surgery. Dysfunctions involving the immune system occur across the lifespan. Many are genetically based; others are acquired. Immune memory is a property of the immune system that provides protection against harmful microbial agents despite the timing of re-exposure to the agent. Tolerance is the mechanism by which the immune system is programmed to eliminate foreign substances such as microbes, toxins, and cellular mutations but maintains the ability to accept self-antigens. Some credence is given to the concept of surveillance, in which the immune system is in a perpetual state of vigilance, screening and rejecting any invader that is recognized as foreign to the host. The term **immunopathology** refers to the study of diseases that result from dysfunctions within the immune system. Disorders of the immune system may stem from excesses or deficiencies of immunocompetent cells, alterations in the function of these cells, immunologic attack on self-antigens, or inappropriate or exaggerated responses to specific antigens (see Table 35-1).

Growing numbers of patients with primary immune deficiencies live to adulthood, and many others acquire immune disorders during their adult years. Thus, nurses in many practice settings need to understand how the immune system functions as well as immunopathologic processes. In addition, knowledge about assessment and care of people with immunologic disorders enables nurses to make appropriate management decisions.

Anatomic and Physiologic Overview

Anatomy of the Immune System

The immune system is composed of an integrated collection of various cell types, each with a designated function in defending against infection and invasion by other organisms. Supporting this system are molecules that are responsible for the interactions, modulations, and regulation of the system. These molecules and cells participate in specific interactions with immunogenic **epitopes** (antigenic determinants) present on foreign materials, initiating a series of actions in a host, including the inflammatory response, the lysis of microbial agents, and the disposal of foreign toxins. The major components of the immune system include central and peripheral organs, tissues, and cells (see Fig. 35-1).

Bone Marrow

The white blood cells (WBCs) involved in immunity are produced in the bone marrow (see Fig. 35-2). Like other blood cells, lymphocytes are generated from **stem cells** (undifferentiated cells). There are two types of lymphocytes—B lymphocytes (**B cells**) and T lymphocytes (**T cells**) (see Fig. 35-3).

Lymphoid Tissues

The spleen, composed of red and white pulp, acts somewhat like a filter. The red pulp is the site where old and injured red blood cells (RBCs) are destroyed. The white pulp contains concentrations of lymphocytes. The lymph nodes, which are connected by lymph channels and capillaries, are distributed throughout the body. They remove foreign material from the

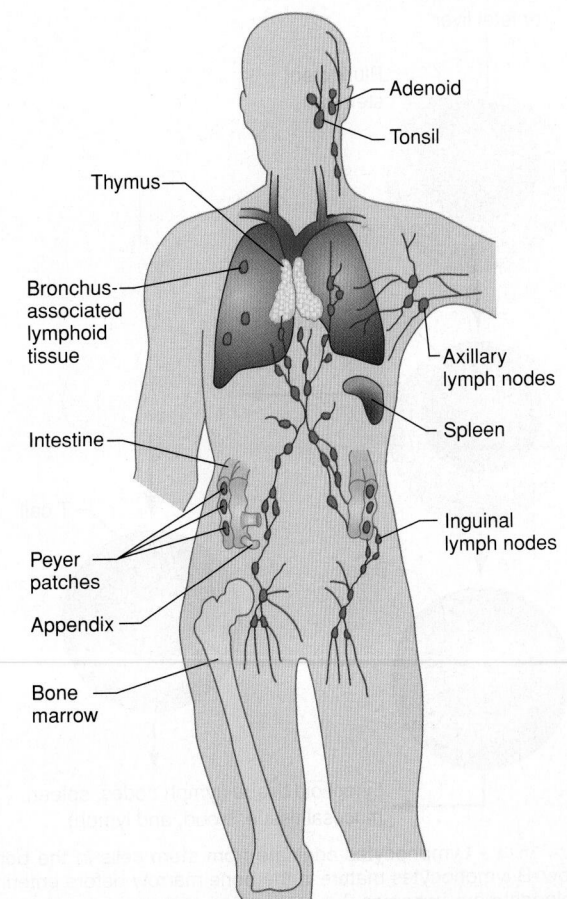

Figure 35-1 • Central and peripheral lymphoid organs, tissues, and cells. Reprinted with permission from Grossman, S. C., & Porth, C. M. (2014). *Porth's pathophysiology: Concepts of altered health states* (9th ed.). Philadelphia, PA: Lippincott Williams & Wilkins.

TABLE 35-1 Immune System Disorders

Disorder	Description
Autoimmunity	Normal protective immune response paradoxically turns against or attacks the body, leading to tissue damage
Hypersensitivity	Body produces inappropriate or exaggerated responses to specific antigens
Gammopathies	Overproduction of immunoglobulins
Immune deficiencies	
Primary	Deficiency results from improper development of immune cells or tissues; usually congenital or inherited
Secondary	Deficiency results from some interference with an already developed immune system; usually acquired later in life

Physiology/Pathophysiology

```
Bone marrow
     │
     ▼
Lymphoblasts
```

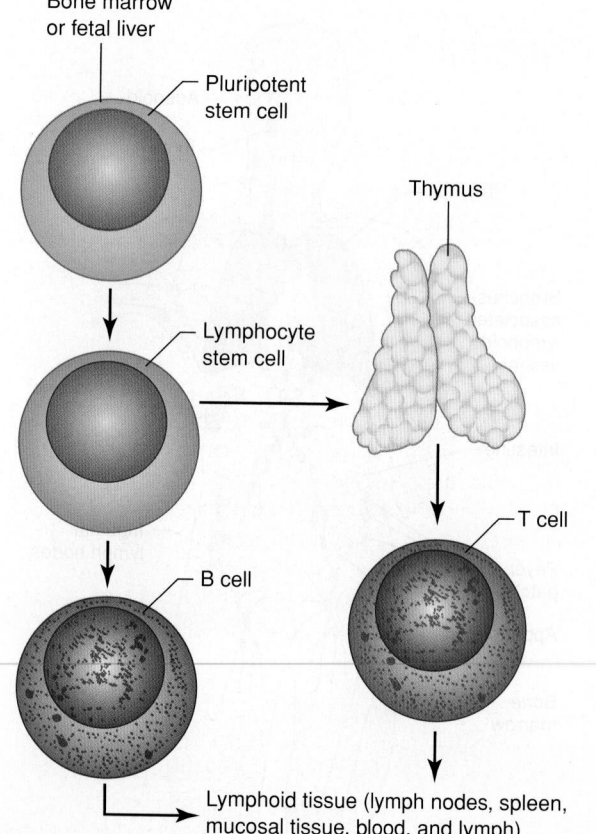

Figure 35-2 • Development of cells of the immune system.

Bone marrow
or fetal liver

Pluripotent
stem cell

Thymus

Lymphocyte
stem cell

T cell

B cell

Lymphoid tissue (lymph nodes, spleen,
mucosal tissue, blood, and lymph)

Figure 35-3 • Lymphocytes originate from stem cells in the bone marrow. B lymphocytes mature in the bone marrow before entering the bloodstream, whereas T lymphocytes mature in the thymus, where they also differentiate into cells with various functions. Reprinted with permission from Grossman, S. C., & Porth, C. M. (2014). *Porth's pathophysiology: Concepts of altered health states* (9th ed.). Philadelphia, PA: Lippincott Williams & Wilkins.

lymph system before it enters the bloodstream. The lymph nodes also serve as centers for immune cell proliferation. The remaining lymphoid tissues contain immune cells that defend the body's mucosal surfaces against microorganisms (McComb, Thiriot, Krishnan, et al., 2013).

Function of the Immune System

The basic function of the immune system is to remove foreign antigens such as viruses and bacteria to maintain homeostasis. There are two general types of immunity: natural (innate) and acquired (adaptive). Natural immunity or nonspecific immunity is present at birth. Acquired or specific immunity develops after birth. Each type of immunity has a distinct role in defending the body against harmful invaders, but the various components are usually interdependent (Levinson, 2014).

Natural Immunity

Natural immunity, which is nonspecific, provides a broad spectrum of defense against and resistance to infection. It is considered the first line of host defense following antigen exposure, because it protects the host without remembering prior contact with an infectious agent (Levinson, 2014). Responses to a foreign invader are very similar from one encounter to the next, regardless of the number of times the invader is encountered. Natural (innate) immunity co-coordinates the initial response to pathogens through the production of cytokines and other effector molecules, which either activate cells for control of the pathogen (by elimination) or promote the development of the acquired **immune response**. The cells involved in this response are monocytes, macrophages, dendritic cells, **natural killer (NK) cells**, basophils, eosinophils, and granulocytes. The early events in this process are critical in determining the nature of the adaptive immune response. Natural immune mechanisms can be divided into two stages: immediate (generally occurring within minutes) and delayed (occurring within several days after exposure) (Levinson, 2014).

White Blood Cell Action

The cellular response is the key to the effective initiation of the immune response. WBCs, or leukocytes, participate in both the natural and the acquired immune responses. Granular leukocytes, or granulocytes (so called because of granules in their cytoplasm), fight invasion by foreign bodies or toxins by releasing cell mediators, such as histamine, bradykinin, and prostaglandins, and by engulfing the foreign bodies or toxins. Granulocytes include neutrophils, eosinophils, and basophils.

Neutrophils (polymorphonuclear leukocytes) are the first cells to arrive at the site where inflammation occurs. Eosinophils and basophils, other types of granulocytes, increase in number during allergic reactions and stress responses. Nongranular leukocytes include monocytes or macrophages (referred to as histiocytes when they enter tissue spaces) and lymphocytes. Monocytes are the first to arrive on the scene and function as **phagocytic cells**, engulfing, ingesting, and destroying greater numbers and quantities of foreign bodies or toxins than granulocytes do. Lymphocytes, consisting of B cells and T cells, play major roles in humoral and cell-mediated immune responses. About 70% to 80% of lymphocytes in the blood are T cells, and about 10% to 15% are B cells (Haynes, Soderberg, & Fauci, 2015).

Inflammatory Response

The inflammatory response is a major function of the natural immune system that is elicited in response to tissue injury or invading organisms. Chemical mediators assist this response by minimizing blood loss, walling off the invading organism, activating phagocytes, and promoting formation of fibrous scar tissue and regeneration of injured tissue. The inflammatory response (discussed further in Chapter 6) is facilitated by physical and chemical barriers that are part of the human organism.

Physical and Chemical Barriers

Activation of the natural immunity response is enhanced by processes inherent in physical and chemical barriers. Physical surface barriers include intact skin, mucous membranes, and cilia of the respiratory tract, which prevent pathogens from gaining access to the body. The cilia of the respiratory tract, along with coughing and sneezing responses, filter and clear pathogens from the upper respiratory tract before they can invade the body further. Chemical barriers, such as mucus, acidic gastric secretions, enzymes in tears and saliva, and substances in sebaceous and sweat secretions, act in a nonspecific way to destroy invading bacteria and fungi. Viruses are countered by other means, such as interferon (see discussion later in chapter).

Immune Regulation

Regulation of the immune response involves balance and counterbalance. Dysfunction of the natural immune system can occur when the immune components are inactivated or when they remain active long after their effects are beneficial. A successful immune response eliminates the responsible antigen. If an immune response fails to develop and clear an antigen sufficiently, the host is considered to be immunocompromised or immunodeficient. If the response is overly robust or misdirected, allergies, asthma, or autoimmune disease results. The immune system's recognition of one's own cells or tissues as "foreign" rather than as self is the basis of many autoimmune disorders (Grossman & Porth, 2014). Despite the fact that the immune response is critical to the prevention of disease, it must be well controlled to curtail immunopathology. Most microbial infections induce an inflammatory response mediated by T cells and cytokines, which, in excess, can cause tissue damage (Haynes et al., 2015). Therefore, regulatory mechanisms must be in place to suppress or halt the immune response. This is mainly achieved by the production of cytokines and transformation of growth factor that inhibit macrophage activation. In some cases, T-cell activation is so acute that these mechanisms fail, and pathology develops. Ongoing research on **immunoregulation** holds the promise of preventing graft rejection and aiding the body in eliminating cancerous or infected cells (Kannan, Madden, & Andrews, 2013; Lo, Lee, & Powell, 2014).

Although natural immunity can often effectively combat infections, many pathogenic microbes have evolved that resist natural immunity. Acquired immunity is necessary to defend against these resistant agents.

Acquired Immunity

Acquired (adaptive) immunity usually develops as a result of prior exposure to an antigen through immunization (vaccination) or by contracting a disease, both of which generate a protective immune response. Weeks or months after exposure to the disease or vaccine, the body produces an immune response that is sufficient to defend against the disease on re-exposure. In contrast to the rapid but nonspecific natural immune response, this form of immunity relies on the recognition of specific foreign antigens. The acquired immune response is broadly divided into two mechanisms: (1) the cell-mediated response, involving T-cell activation, and (2) effector mechanisms, involving B-cell maturation and production of antibodies (Haynes et al., 2015).

The two types of acquired immunity are known as active and passive and are interrelated. Active acquired immunity refers to immunologic defenses developed by the person's own body. This immunity typically lasts many years or even a lifetime. Passive acquired immunity is temporary immunity transmitted from a source outside the body that has developed immunity through previous disease or immunization. Examples include immunity resulting from the transfer of antibodies from the mother to an infant in utero or through breast-feeding or receiving injections of immune globulin. Active and passive acquired immunity involve humoral and cellular (cell-mediated) immunologic responses (described later).

Response to Invasion

When the body is invaded or attacked by bacteria, viruses, or other pathogens, it has three means of defense:

- The phagocytic immune response
- The humoral or antibody immune response
- The cellular immune response

The first line of defense, the **phagocytic immune response**, primarily involves the WBCs (granulocytes and macrophages), which have the ability to ingest foreign particles and destroy the invading agent; eosinophils are only weakly phagocytic. Phagocytes also remove the body's own dying or dead cells. Cells in necrotic tissue that are dying release substances that trigger an inflammatory response. **Apoptosis**, or programmed cell death, is the body's way of destroying worn-out cells such as blood or skin cells or cells that need to be renewed (Grossman & Porth, 2014).

A second protective response, the **humoral immune response** (sometimes called the *antibody response*), begins with the B lymphocytes, which can transform themselves into plasma cells that manufacture antibodies. These antibodies are highly specific proteins that are transported in the bloodstream and attempt to disable invaders. The third mechanism of defense, the **cellular immune response**, also involves the T lymphocytes, which can turn into special cytotoxic (or killer) T cells that can attack the pathogens.

The structural part of the invading or attacking organism that is responsible for stimulating antibody production is called an **antigen** (or an immunogen). For example, an antigen can be a small patch of proteins on the outer surface of a microorganism. Not all antigens are naturally immunogenic; some must be coupled to other molecules to stimulate the immune response. A single bacterium or large molecule, such as a diphtheria or tetanus toxin, may have several antigens, or markers, on its surface, thus inducing the body to produce a number of different antibodies. Once produced, an antibody is released into the bloodstream and carried to the attacking organism. There, it combines with the antigen, binding with it like an interlocking piece of a jigsaw puzzle (see Fig. 35-4). There are four well-defined stages in an immune response: recognition, proliferation, response, and effector (see Fig. 35-5).

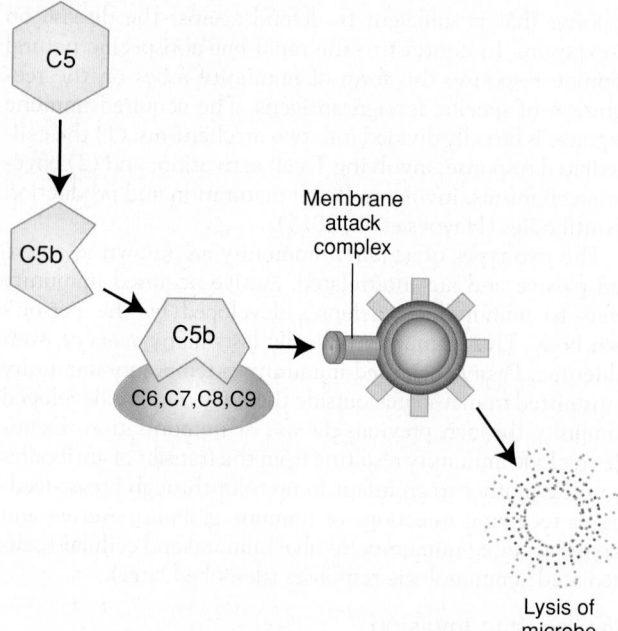

Figure 35-4 • Complement-mediated immune responses. Reprinted with permission from Grossman, S. C., & Porth, C. M. (2014). *Porth's pathophysiology: Concepts of altered health states* (9th ed.). Philadelphia, PA: Lippincott Williams & Wilkins.

Recognition Stage

Recognition of antigens as foreign, or non-self, by the immune system is the initiating event in any immune response. Recognition involves the use of lymph nodes and lymphocytes for surveillance. Lymph nodes are widely distributed internally throughout the body and in the circulating blood, as well as externally near the body's surfaces. They continuously discharge small lymphocytes into the bloodstream. These lymphocytes patrol the tissues and vessels that drain the areas served by that node. Lymphocytes recirculate from the blood to lymph nodes and from the lymph nodes back into the bloodstream in a continuous circuit. Lymphocytes and other cells have "microbial sensors" that identify molecules on microbes and other microorganisms. The interaction of these sensors with the offending agent sets off a cascade aimed at destroying the microbe (Paul, 2013). Invading organisms have pathogen-associated molecular patterns (PAMPs) contained in their cell membranes that are recognized by the immune system cells. Once the receptors on the immune cells come into contact with the PAMPs, the immune response is triggered (Grossman & Porth, 2014). Macrophages play an important role in helping the circulating lymphocytes process the antigens. Both macrophages and neutrophils have receptors for antibodies and complement; as a result, they coat microorganisms with antibodies, complement, or both, thereby enhancing phagocytosis.

In a streptococcal throat infection, for example, the streptococcal organism gains access to the mucous membranes of the throat. A circulating lymphocyte moving through the tissues of the throat comes in contact with the organism. The lymphocyte recognizes the antigens on the microbe as different (non-self) and the streptococcal organism as antigenic (foreign). This triggers the second stage of the immune response—proliferation.

Proliferation Stage

The circulating lymphocytes containing the antigenic message return to the nearest lymph node. Once in the node, these sensitized lymphocytes stimulate some of the resident T and B lymphocytes to enlarge, divide, and proliferate. T lymphocytes differentiate into cytotoxic (or killer) T cells, whereas B lymphocytes produce and release antibodies. Enlargement of the lymph nodes in the neck in conjunction with a sore throat is one example of the immune response.

Response Stage

In the response stage, the differentiated lymphocytes function in either a humoral or a cellular capacity. This stage begins with the production of antibodies by the B lymphocytes in response to a specific antigen. The cellular response stimulates the resident lymphocytes to become cells that attack microbes directly rather than through the action of antibodies. These transformed lymphocytes are known as cytotoxic (killer) T cells.

Viral rather than bacterial antigens induce a cellular response. This response is manifested by the increasing number of T lymphocytes (lymphocytosis) seen in the blood tests of people with viral illnesses such as infectious mononucleosis. (Cellular immunity is discussed in further detail later in this chapter.) Most immune responses to antigens involve both humoral and cellular responses, although one usually predominates. For example, during transplant rejection, the cellular response involving T cells predominates, whereas in the bacterial pneumonias and sepsis, the humoral response involving B cells plays the dominant protective role (see Chart 35-1).

Effector Stage

In the effector stage, either the antibody of the humoral response or the cytotoxic (killer) T cell of the cellular response reaches and connects with the antigen on the surface of the foreign invader. This initiates activities involving interplay of antibodies (humoral immunity), complement, and action by the cytotoxic T cells (cellular immunity).

Humoral Immune Response

The humoral response is characterized by the production of antibodies by B lymphocytes in response to a specific antigen. Whereas B lymphocytes are responsible for the production of antibodies, both the macrophages of natural immunity and the special T lymphocytes of cellular immunity are involved in recognition.

Antigen Recognition

Several theories explain the mechanisms by which B lymphocytes recognize the invading antigen and respond by producing antibodies. It is known that B lymphocytes recognize and respond to invading antigens in more than one way.

The B lymphocytes respond to some antigens by directly triggering antibody formation; however, in response to other antigens, they need the assistance of T cells to trigger antibody formation. With the help of macrophages, the T lymphocytes are believed to recognize the antigen of a foreign invader. The T lymphocyte picks up the antigenic message, or "blueprint," of the antigen and returns to the nearest lymph node with that message. B lymphocytes stored in the lymph nodes are subdivided into thousands of clones, which are stimulated to

Figure 35-5 • Stages of the immune response. **A.** In the *recognition stage,* antigens are recognized by circulating lymphocytes and macrophages. **B.** In the *proliferation stage,* the dormant lymphocytes proliferate and differentiate into cytotoxic (killer) T cells or B cells responsible for formation and release of antibodies. **C.** In the *response stage,* the cytotoxic T cells and the B cells perform cellular and humoral functions, respectively. **D.** In the *effector stage,* antigens are destroyed or neutralized through the action of antibodies, complement, macrophages, and cytotoxic T cells.

Chart 35-1 · Comparison of Cellular and Humoral Immune Responses

Humoral Responses (B Cells)

- Bacterial phagocytosis and lysis
- Anaphylaxis
- Allergic hay fever and asthma
- Immune complex disease
- Bacterial and some viral infections

Cellular Responses (T Cells)

- Transplant rejection
- Delayed hypersensitivity (tuberculin reaction)
- Graft-versus-host disease
- Tumor surveillance or destruction
- Intracellular infections
- Viral, fungal, and parasitic infections

enlarge, divide, proliferate, and differentiate into plasma cells capable of producing specific antibodies to the antigen. Other B lymphocytes differentiate into B-lymphocyte clones with a memory for the antigen. These memory cells are responsible for the more exaggerated and rapid immune response in a person who is repeatedly exposed to the same antigen.

Role of Antibodies

Antibodies are large proteins, called *immunoglobulins,* that consist of two subunits, each containing a light and a heavy peptide chain held together by a chemical link composed of disulfide bonds. Each subunit has one portion that serves as a binding site for a specific antigen and another portion that allows the antibody molecule to take part in the complement system.

Antibodies defend against foreign invaders in several ways, and the type of defense used depends on the structure and composition of both the antigen and the immunoglobulin.

Exact fit:
highly specific

No fit:
antigenic determinant
does not fit with antibody
binding site

Poor fit:
low specificity,
cross-reactivity

Figure 35-6 • Antigen–antibody binding. (**Left**) A highly specific antigen–antibody complex. (**Center**) No match and, therefore, no immune response. (**Right**) Poor fit or match with low specificity; antibody reacts to antigen with similar characteristics, producing cross-reactivity. LC, light chain; HC, heavy chain.

The antibody molecule has at least two combining sites, or Fab fragments (see Fig. 35-6). One antibody can act as a cross-link between two antigens, causing them to bind or clump together. This clumping effect, referred to as **agglutination**, helps clear the body of the invading organism by facilitating phagocytosis. Some antibodies assist in the removal of offending organisms through **opsonization**. In this process, the antigen–antibody molecule is coated with a sticky substance that also facilitates phagocytosis.

Antibodies also promote the release of vasoactive substances, such as histamine and slow-reacting substances, two of the chemical mediators of the inflammatory response. Antibodies do not function in isolation; rather, they mobilize other components of the immune system to defend against the invader.

The body can produce five different types of immunoglobulin (Ig). Each of the five types, or classes, is identified by a specific letter of the alphabet, IgA, IgD, IgE, IgG, and IgM. Classification is based on the chemical structure and biologic role of the individual immunoglobulin. Major characteristics of the immunoglobulins are summarized in Chart 35-2. The normal laboratory values for the three major Igs (IgA, IgG, and IgM) can be found in Table 38-1 in Chapter 38; see also Appendix A on at thepoint.lww.com/Brunner14e.

Antigen–Antibody Binding

The portion of the antigen involved in binding with the antibody is referred to as the **antigenic determinant**. The most efficient immunologic responses occur when the antibody and antigen fit like a lock and key. Poor fit can occur with an antibody that was produced in response to a different antigen. This phenomenon is known as cross-reactivity. For example, in acute rheumatic fever, the antibody produced against *Streptococcus pyogenes* in the upper respiratory tract may cross-react with the patient's heart tissue, leading to heart valve damage.

Cellular Immune Response

The T lymphocytes are primarily responsible for cellular immunity. Stem cells continuously migrate from the bone

Chart 35-2 Major Characteristics of the Immunoglobulins

IgG (75% of Total Immunoglobulin)

- Appears in serum and tissues (interstitial fluid)
- Assumes a major role in bloodborne and tissue infections
- Activates the complement system
- Enhances phagocytosis
- Crosses the placenta

IgA (15% of Total Immunoglobulin)

- Appears in body fluids (blood, saliva, tears, and breast milk, as well as pulmonary, gastrointestinal, prostatic, and vaginal secretions)
- Protects against respiratory, gastrointestinal, and genitourinary infections
- Prevents absorption of antigens from food
- Passes to neonate in breast milk for protection

IgM (10% of Total Immunoglobulin)

- Appears mostly in intravascular serum
- Appears as the first immunoglobulin produced in response to bacterial and viral infections
- Activates the complement system

IgD (0.2% of Total Immunoglobulin)

- Appears in small amounts in serum
- Possibly influences B-lymphocyte differentiation, but role is unclear

IgE (0.004% of Total Immunoglobulin)

- Appears in serum
- Takes part in allergic and some hypersensitivity reactions
- Combats parasitic infections

Ig immunoglobulin.
Adapted from Grossman, S. C., & Porth, C. M. (2014). *Porth's pathophysiology: Concepts of altered health states* (9th ed., p. 278). Philadelphia, PA: Lippincott Williams & Wilkins.

marrow to the thymus gland, where they develop into T cells. Despite the partial degeneration of the gland at puberty, T cells continue to develop in the thymus gland. Several types of T cells exist, each with designated roles in the defense against bacteria, viruses, fungi, parasites, and malignant cells. T cells attack foreign invaders directly rather than by producing antibodies.

Cellular reactions are initiated, with or without the assistance of macrophages, by the binding of an antigen to an antigen receptor located on the surface of a T cell. The T cells then carry the antigenic message, or blueprint, to the lymph nodes, where the production of other T cells is stimulated. Some T cells remain in the lymph nodes and retain a memory for the antigen. Other T cells migrate from the lymph nodes into the general circulatory system and ultimately to the tissues, where they remain until they either come in contact with their respective antigens or die (Grossman & Porth, 2014).

Types of T Lymphocytes

T cells include effector T cells, suppressor T cells, and memory T cells. The two major categories of effector T cells—helper T cells (also referred to as CD4+ cells) and cytotoxic T cells (also referred to as CD8+ cells)—participate in the destruction of foreign organisms. T cells interact closely with B cells, indicating that humoral and cellular immune responses are not separate, unrelated processes but rather are branches of the immune response that interact.

Helper T cells are activated on recognition of antigens and stimulate the rest of the immune system. When activated, helper T cells secrete **cytokines**, which attract and activate B cells, cytotoxic T cells, NK cells, macrophages, and other cells of the immune system. Cytokines are proteins produced by the cells of the immune system that determine the actions of the immune system cells. Separate subpopulations of helper T cells produce different types of cytokines and determine whether the immune response will be the production of antibodies or a cell-mediated immune response. Helper T cells also produce **lymphokines**, one category of cytokines (see Table 35-2).

Cytotoxic T cells (killer T cells) attack the antigen directly by altering the cell membrane, causing cell lysis

TABLE 35-2 Cytokines of Innate and Adaptive Immunity

Cytokines	Source	Biologic Activity
Interleukin 1 (IL-1)	Macrophages, endothelial cells, some epithelial cells	Wide variety of biologic effects; activates endothelium in inflammation; induces fever and acute-phase response; stimulates neutrophil production
Interleukin 2 (IL-2)	CD4$^+$, CD8$^+$ T cells	Growth factor for activated T cells; induces synthesis of other cytokines; activates cytotoxic T lymphocytes and NK cells
Interleukin 3 (IL-3)	CD4$^+$ T cells	Growth factor for progenitor hematopoietic cells
Interleukin 4 (IL-4)	CD4$^+$ T$_H$2 cells, mast cells	Promotes growth and survival o f T, B, and mast cells; causes T$_H$2 cell differentiation; activates B cells and eosinophils and induces IgE-type responses
Interleukin 5 (IL-5)	CD4$^+$ T$_H$2 cells	Induces eosinophil growth and development
Interleukin 6 (IL-6)	Macrophages, endothelial cells, T lymphocytes	Stimulates the liver to produce mediators of acute-phase inflammatory response; also induces proliferation of antibody-producing cells by the adaptive immune system
Interleukin 7 (IL-7)	Bone marrow stromal cells	Primary function in adaptive immunity; stimulates pre-B cells and thymocyte development and proliferation
Interleukin 8 (IL-8)	Macrophages, endothelial cells	Primary function in adaptive immunity; chemoattracts neutrophils and T lymphocytes; regulates lymphocyte homing and neutrophil infiltration
Interleukin 10 (IL-10)	Macrophages, some T-helper cells	Inhibitor of activated macrophages and dendritic cells; decreases inflammation by inhibiting T$_H$1 cells and release of interleukin 12 from macrophages
Interleukin 12 (IL-12)	Macrophages, dendritic cells	Enhances NK cell cytotoxicity in innate immunity; induces T$_H$1 cell differentiation in adaptive immunity
Type I interferons (IFN-α, IFN-β)	Macrophages, fibroblasts	Inhibit viral replication, activate NK cells, and increase expression of MHC-I molecules on virus-infected cells
Interferon-γ (IFN-γ)	NK cells, CD4$^+$ and CD8$^+$ T lymphocytes	Activates macrophages in both innate immune responses and adaptive cell-mediated immune responses; increases expression of MHC I and II and antigen processing and presentation
Tumor necrosis factor-α (TNF-α)	Macrophages, T cells	Induces inflammation, fever, and acute-phase response; activates neutrophils and endothelial cells; kills cells through apoptosis
Chemokines	Macrophages, endothelial cells, T lymphocytes	Large family of structurally similar cytokines that stimulate leukocyte movement and regulate the migration of leukocytes from the blood to the tissues
Granulocyte-monocyte CSF (GM-CSF)	T cells, macrophages, endothelial cells, fibroblasts	Promotes neutrophil, eosinophil, and monocyte maturation and growth; activates mature granulocytes
Granulocyte CSF (G-CSF)	Macrophages, fibroblasts, endothelial cells	Promotes growth and maturation of neutrophils consumed in inflammatory reactions
Monocyte CSF (M-CSF)	Macrophages, activated T cells, endothelial cells	Promotes growth and maturation of mononuclear phagocytes

NK, natural killer; T$_H$2, T-helper type 2; IgE, immunoglobulin E; T$_H$1, T-helper type 1; MHC, major histocompatibility complex; CSF, colony-stimulating factor.
Adapted from Grossman, S. C., & Porth, C. M. (2014). *Porth's pathophysiology: Concepts of altered health states* (9th ed.). Philadelphia, PA: Lippincott Williams & Wilkins.

TABLE 35-3 Lymphocytes Involved in Immune Responses

Type of Immune Response	Cell Type	Function
Humoral	B lymphocyte	Produces antibodies or immunoglobulins (IgA, IgD, IgE, IgG, IgM)
Cellular	T lymphocyte	
	Helper T	Attacks foreign invaders (antigens) directly
		Initiates and augments inflammatory response
	Helper T_1	Increases activated cytotoxic T cells
	Helper T_2	Increases B-cell (BG8) antibody production
	Suppressor T	Suppresses the immune response
	Memory T	Remembers contact with an antigen and on subsequent exposures mounts an immune response
	Cytotoxic T (killer T)	Lyses cells infected with virus; plays a role in graft rejection
Nonspecific	Non-T or non-B lymphocyte Null cell	Destroys antigens already coated with antibody
	Natural killer cell (granular lymphocyte)	Defends against microorganisms and some types of malignant cells; produces cytokines

(disintegration), and releasing cytolytic enzymes and cytokines. Lymphokines can recruit, activate, and regulate other lymphocytes and WBCs. These cells then assist in destroying the invading organism. Delayed-type hypersensitivity is an example of an immune reaction that protects the body from antigens through the production and release of lymphokines (see later discussion).

Suppressor T cells have the ability to decrease B-cell production, thereby keeping the immune response at a level that is compatible with health (e.g., sufficient to fight infection adequately without attacking the body's healthy tissues). **Memory cells** are responsible for recognizing antigens from previous exposure and mounting an immune response (see Table 35-3).

Null Lymphocytes and Natural Killer Cells

Null lymphocytes and NK cells are other lymphocytes that assist in combating organisms. These cells are distinct from B cells and T cells and lack the usual characteristics of those cells. **Null lymphocytes**, a subpopulation of lymphocytes, destroy antigens already coated with antibody. These cells have special receptor sites on their surface that allow them to connect with the end of antibodies; this is known as antibody-dependent, cell-mediated cytotoxicity.

NK cells are a class of lymphocytes that recognize infected and stressed cells and respond by killing these cells and by secreting macrophage-activating cytokine. The helper T cells contribute to the differentiation of null and NK cells.

Complement System

Circulating plasma proteins, known as **complement**, are made in the liver and activated when an antibody connects with its antigen. Complement plays an important role in the defense against microbes. Destruction of an invading or attacking organism or toxin is not achieved merely by the binding of the antibody and antigens; it also requires activation of complement, the arrival of killer T cells, or the attraction of macrophages. Complement has three major physiologic functions: defending the body against bacterial infection, bridging natural and acquired immunity, and disposing of immune complexes and the by-products associated with inflammation (Grossman & Porth, 2014).

The proteins that comprise complement interact sequentially with one another in a cascading effect. The complement cascade is important to modifying the effector arm of the immune system. Activation of complement allows important events, such as removal of infectious agents and initiation of the inflammatory response, to take place. These events involve active parts of the pathway that enhance chemotaxis of macrophages and granulocytes, alter blood vessel permeability, change blood vessel diameters, cause cells to lyse, alter blood clotting, and cause other points of modification. These macrophages and granulocytes continue the body's defense by devouring the antibody-coated microbes and by releasing bacterial products.

The complement cascade may be activated by any of three pathways: classic, lectin, and alternative. The classic pathway is triggered after antibodies bind to microbes or other antigens and is part of the humoral type of adaptive immunity. The lectin pathway is activated when a plasma protein (mannose-binding lectin) binds to terminal mannose residue on the surface glycoproteins of microbes. The alternative pathway is triggered when complement proteins are activated on microbial surfaces. This pathway is part of natural immunity.

Complement components, prostaglandins, leukotrienes, and other inflammatory mediators all contribute to the recruitment of inflammatory cells, as do chemokines, a group of cytokines. The activated neutrophils pass through the vessel walls to accumulate at the site of infection, where they phagocytize complement-coated microbes (Grossman & Porth, 2014). This response is usually therapeutic and can be lifesaving if the cell attacked by the complement system is a true foreign invader. However, if that cell is part of the human organism, the result can be devastating disease and even death. Many autoimmune diseases and disorders characterized by chronic infection are thought to be caused in part by continued or chronic activation of complement, which in turn results in chronic inflammation. The RBCs and platelets have complement receptors and, as a result, play an important role in the clearance of immune complexes that consist of antigen, antibody, and components of the complement system (Grossman & Porth, 2014).

Immunomodulators

Antimicrobial agents and vaccines have yielded considerable therapeutic success and the immune system usually works effectively; however, many infectious diseases remain difficult clinical challenges. Treatment success may be compromised by defects of the immune system; in this case, enhancement of the host immune response may be therapeutically beneficial. An immunomodulator (also known as a biologic response modifier) affects the host via direct or indirect effects on one or more components of the immunoregulatory network. Interferons, colony-stimulating factors, and monoclonal antibodies (MoAbs) are examples of agents used to help enhance the immune system (Page & Liles, 2015).

Interferons

Interferon, one type of biologic response modifier, is a nonspecific viricidal protein that is naturally produced by the body and is capable of activating other components of the immune system. Interferons continue to be investigated to determine their roles in the immune system and their potential therapeutic effects in disorders characterized by disturbed immune responses. These substances have antiviral and antitumor properties. In addition to responding to viral infection, interferons are produced by T lymphocytes, B lymphocytes, and macrophages in response to antigens. They are thought to modify the immune response by suppressing antibody production and cellular immunity. They also facilitate the cytolytic role of macrophages and NK cells. Interferons are used to treat immune-related disorders (e.g., multiple sclerosis) and chronic inflammatory conditions (e.g., chronic hepatitis). Research continues to evaluate the effectiveness of interferons in treating cancers (Booy, Hofland, & van Eijck, 2015) and acquired immunodeficiency syndrome.

Colony-Stimulating Factors

Colony-stimulating factors are a group of naturally occurring glycoprotein cytokines that regulate production, differentiation, survival, and activation of hematopoietic cells. Erythropoietin stimulates RBC production. Thrombopoietin plays a key regulatory role in the growth and differentiation of bone marrow cells. Interleukin 5 (IL-5) stimulates the growth and survival of eosinophils and basophils. Stem cell factor and IL-3 serve as stimuli for multiple hematopoietic cell lines. Granulocyte colony-stimulating factor, granulocyte-macrophage colony-stimulating factor, and macrophage colony-stimulating factor all serve as growth factors for specific cell lines. These cytokines have attracted considerable interest for their potential role in immunomodulation (Page & Liles, 2015).

Monoclonal Antibodies

MoAbs have become available through technologic advances, enabling investigators to grow and produce targeted antibodies for specific pathologic organisms. This type of specificity allows MoAbs to destroy pathologic organisms and spare normal cells. The specificity of MoAbs depends on identifying key antigen proteins that are present on the surface of tumors, but not on normal tissues. When the MoAb attaches to the cell surface antigen, it blocks an important signal transduction pathway for communication between the malignant cells and the extracellular environment. The results may include an inability to initiate apoptosis, reproduce, or invade surrounding tissues. To date, more than 1000 tumor antigens have been identified (Glassman & Balthasar, 2014). See Chapter 15 for a discussion on the use of MoAbs in cancer.

Advances in Immunology

Genetic Engineering

One of the more remarkable evolving technologies is **genetic engineering**, which uses recombinant deoxyribonucleic acid (DNA) technology. Two facets of this technology exist. The first permits scientists to combine genes from one type of organism with genes of a second organism. This type of technology allows cells and microorganisms to manufacture proteins, monokines, and lymphokines, which can alter and enhance immune system function. The second facet of recombinant DNA technology involves gene therapy. If a particular gene is abnormal or missing, experimental recombinant DNA technology may be capable of restoring normal gene function. For example, a recombinant gene is inserted onto a virus particle. When the virus particle splices its genes, the virus automatically inserts the missing gene and theoretically corrects the genetic anomaly. Extensive research into recombinant DNA technology and gene therapy is ongoing (Geering & Fussenegger, 2015).

Stem Cells

Stem cells are capable of self-renewal and differentiation; they continually replenish the body's entire supply of both RBCs and WBCs. Some stem cells, described as totipotent cells, have tremendous capacity to self-renew and differentiate. Embryonic stem cells, described as pluripotent, give rise to numerous cell types that are able to form tissues. Research has shown that stem cells can restore an immune system that has been destroyed (Kessler, 2015). Stem cell transplantation has been carried out in humans with certain types of immune dysfunction, such as severe combined immunodeficiency; clinical trials using stem cells are under way in patients with a variety of disorders having an autoimmune component, including systemic lupus erythematosus, rheumatoid arthritis, scleroderma, and multiple sclerosis. Research with embryonic stem cells has enabled investigators to make substantial gains in developmental biology, gene therapy, therapeutic tissue engineering, and the treatment of a variety of diseases (Kessler, 2015). However, along with these remarkable opportunities, many ethical challenges arise, which are largely based on concerns about safety, efficacy, resource allocation, and human cloning.

Cancer and Immunotherapy

It has long been understood that the immune system plays a role in fighting off malignancies. Recent advances in cancer treatment have sought to augment the body's natural antitumor activity and to shut down the pathways that allow malignancies to elude the immune system, which has led to the development of such treatments as MoAbs, cancer vaccines, immune adjuvants, immune checkpoint inhibitors, and cytokines (Kannan et al., 2013). These immunotherapeutic

Chart 35-3

ASSESSMENT

Assessing for Immune Dysfunction

Be alert for the following signs and symptoms:

Respiratory System

- Changes in respiratory rate
- Cough (dry or productive)
- Abnormal lung sounds (wheezing, crackles, rhonchi)
- Rhinitis
- Hyperventilation
- Bronchospasm

Cardiovascular System

- Hypotension
- Tachycardia
- Dysrhythmia
- Vasculitis
- Anemia

Gastrointestinal System

- Hepatosplenomegaly
- Colitis
- Vomiting
- Diarrhea

Genitourinary System

- Frequency and burning on urination
- Hematuria
- Discharge

Musculoskeletal System

- Joint mobility, edema, and pain

Skin

- Rashes
- Lesions
- Dermatitis
- Hematomas or purpura
- Edema or urticaria
- Inflammation
- Discharge

Neurosensory System

- Cognitive dysfunction
- Hearing loss
- Visual changes
- Headaches and migraines
- Ataxia
- Tetany

treatments are designed to stimulate the patient's immune system to mount its own defense against the cancer and have shown very promising results in a number of different cancer types. See Chapter 15 for a discussion on the use of immunotherapy in cancer.

Assessment of the Immune System

An assessment of immune function begins during the health history and physical examination. Areas to be assessed include nutritional status; infections and immunizations; allergies; disorders and disease states, such as autoimmune disorders, cancer, and chronic illnesses; surgeries; medications; and blood transfusions. In addition to inspection of general characteristics, palpation of the lymph nodes and examinations of the skin, mucous membranes, and respiratory, gastrointestinal, musculoskeletal, genitourinary, cardiovascular, and neurosensory systems are performed (see Chart 35-3).

Health History

The history should note the patient's age along with information about past and present conditions and events that may provide clues to the status of the patient's immune system.

Gender

There are differences in the immune system functions of men and women. For example, many autoimmune diseases have a higher incidence in females than in males, a phenomenon believed to be correlated with sex hormones. Sex hormones have long been recognized for their role in reproductive function; in the past two decades, research has revealed that these hormones are integral signaling modulators of the immune

system. Sex hormones play definitive roles in lymphocyte maturation, activation, and synthesis of antibodies and cytokines. In autoimmune disease, expression of sex hormones is altered, and this change contributes to immune dysregulation (Ngo, Steyn, & McCombe, 2014).

 Gerontologic Considerations

Immunosenescence is a complex route in which the aging process stimulates changes in the immune system (Shekarabi & Asgari, 2014). Some of the changes that occur in immunosenescence include, but are not limited to, bone marrow defects, dysfunction of the thymus gland, and impaired lymphocytes. Cellular changes occur as the result of aging and include impaired neutrophil function, decreased amount of circulating macrophages, impaired dendritic cell function, and reduced T-cell activation (Müller & Pawelec, 2014). As the immune system undergoes age-associated alterations, its response to infections progressively deteriorates. The capacity for self-renewal of hematopoietic stem cells diminishes. There is a notable decline in the total number of phagocytes, coupled with an intrinsic reduction in their activity. The cytotoxicity of NK cells decreases, contributing to a decline in humoral immunity (Müller & Pawelec, 2014). Acquired immunity may be negatively affected; the efficacy of vaccines is frequently decreased in older adults (Goronzy & Weyand, 2013). Inflammatory cytokines tend to increase with age.

Older adults have increased the incidence of infections, autoimmune diseases, metabolic diseases, osteoporosis, and neurologic disorders (Müller & Pawelec, 2014).The increased incidence of autoimmune diseases may be from a decreased ability of antibodies to differentiate between self and nonself. Failure of the surveillance system to recognize mutant or

TABLE 35-4 Age-Related Changes in Immunologic Function

Body System	Changes	Consequences
Immune	Impaired function of B and T lymphocytes Failure of lymphocytes to recognize mutant or abnormal cells Decreased antibody production Failure of immune system to differentiate "self" from "non-self" Suppressed phagocytic immune response	Suppressed responses to pathogenic organisms with increased risk for infection Increased incidence of cancers Anergy (lack of response to antigens applied to the skin [allergens]) Increased incidence of autoimmune diseases Absence of typical signs and symptoms of infection and inflammation Dissemination of organisms usually destroyed or suppressed by phagocytes (e.g., reactivation or spread of tuberculosis)
Gastrointestinal	Decreased gastric secretions and motility Decreased phagocytosis by the liver's Kupffer cells Altered nutritional intake with inadequate protein intake	Proliferation of intestinal organisms resulting in gastroenteritis and diarrhea Increased incidence and severity of hepatitis B; increased incidence of liver abscesses Suppressed immune response
Urinary	Decreased kidney function and changes in lower urinary tract function (enlargement of prostate gland, neurogenic bladder); altered genitourinary tract flora	Urinary stasis and increased incidence of urinary tract infections
Pulmonary	Impaired ciliary action due to exposure to smoke and environmental toxins	Impaired clearance of pulmonary secretions; increased incidence of respiratory infections
Integumentary	Thinning of skin with less elasticity; loss of adipose tissue	Increased risk of skin injury, breakdown, and infection
Circulatory	Impaired microcirculation	Stasis and pressure ulcers
Neurologic function	Decreased sensation and slowing of reflexes	Increased risk of injury, skin ulcers, abrasions, and burns

abnormal cells also may be responsible, in part, for the high incidence of cancer associated with increasing age.

Age-related changes in many body systems also contribute to impaired immunity (see Table 35-4). For example, postmenopausal females are at a greater risk for urinary tract infections due to residual urine, urinary incontinence, and estrogen deficiency (Mody & Juthani-Mehta, 2014). Secondary changes, including malnutrition and poor circulation, as well as the breakdown of natural mechanical barriers such as the skin, place the aging immune system at even greater disadvantage against infection (Carlsson, Haglin, Rosendahl, et al., 2013).

The effects of the aging process and psychological stress interact, with the potential to negatively influence immune integrity (Epel & Lithgow, 2014). Consequently, continual assessment of the physical and emotional status of older adults is imperative, because early recognition and management of factors influencing immune response may prevent or mitigate the high morbidity and mortality seen with illness in the older adult population (Müller & Pawelec, 2014).

Nutrition

The relationship of infection to nutritional status is a key determinant of health. Traditionally, this relationship focused on the effect of nutrients on host defenses and the effect of infection on nutritional needs. This has expanded in scope to encompass the role of specific nutrients in acquired immune function—the modulation of inflammatory processes and the virulence of the infectious agent itself. Iron and the immune system are linked in homeostasis and pathology, thus making it essential for max-

imum function (Cassat & Skaar, 2013). The list of nutrients affecting infection, immunity, inflammation, and cell injury has expanded from traditional proteins to several vitamins, multiple minerals, and, more recently, specific lipid components of the diet. One review looked at the role of Vitamins A, C, D, E, and K in treatment of pancreatic cancer but concluded that not enough evidence based on clinical trials is available to fully support the use of these vitamins as an intervention (Davis-Yadley & Malafa, 2015). The role of micronutrients and fatty acids on the response of cells and tissues to hypoxic and toxic damage has been recognized, suggesting that there is another dimension to the relationship. Deficiencies in micronutrients have been connected to impairment in various body functions, including immunity. Zinc deficiency in particular has been linked to the development of a number of diseases. Zinc plays an important role in homeostasis, immune function, and apoptosis, among other functions (Müller & Pawelec, 2014).

The effects exerted by polyunsaturated fatty acids on immune system functions are under investigation. Studies suggest that these elements play a role in diminishing the incidence and severity of inflammatory disorders. Recent studies suggest that diets high in olive oil are not as immunosuppressive as diets rich in fish oil. The contribution of immune modulation by lipids to the high risk of infectious complications associated with the use of parenteral nutrition is unclear; however, a recent meta-analysis revealed that the use of glutamine-supplemented parenteral nutrition decreased the incidence of infections postoperatively (Yue, Tian, Wang, et al., 2013).

Depletion of protein reserves results in atrophy of lymphoid tissues, depression of antibody response, reduction in the number of circulating T cells, and impaired phagocytic function. As a result, susceptibility to infection is greatly increased. During periods of infection or serious illness, nutritional requirements may be further altered, potentially contributing to depletion of protein, fatty acid, vitamin, and trace elements and causing even greater risk of impaired immune response and sepsis. Nutritional intake that supports a competent immune response plays an important role in reducing the incidence of infections; patients whose nutritional status is compromised have a delayed postoperative recovery and often experience more severe infections and delayed wound healing. The nurse must assess the patient's nutritional status, caloric intake, and quality of foods ingested. There is evidence that nutrition plays a role in the development of cancer and that diet and lifestyle can alter the risk of cancer development as well as other chronic diseases (Supic, Jagodic, & Magic, 2013). The nurse must assume a proactive role in ensuring the best possible nutritional intake for all patients as a vital step in preventing disease and poor outcomes (Slawson, Fitzgerald, & Morgan, 2013).

Immunization

The patient is asked about childhood and adult immunizations, including vaccinations to provide protection against influenza, pneumococcal disease (Pneumovax), pertussis, herpes simplex, and the usual childhood diseases (e.g., measles, mumps). Herpes simplex virus infections have a significant impact on health, causing a wide range of diseases (e.g., oral and genital herpes). Education about the importance of adhering to the recommended schedule for adult vaccines should be initiated. See Chapter 4, Table 4-3: Routine Health Promotion and Screening for Adults for more information about adult immunizations.

Infection

Known past or present exposure to tuberculosis is assessed, and the dates and results of any tuberculin tests (purified protein derivative [PPD] test) and chest x-rays are documented. Recent exposure to any infections and the exposure dates are elicited. The nurse must assess whether the patient has been exposed to any sexually transmitted infections (STIs) or bloodborne pathogens such as hepatitis B, C, and D viruses and human immune deficiency virus (HIV). A history of STIs such as gonorrhea, syphilis, human papillomavirus infection, and chlamydia can alert the nurse that the patient may have been exposed to HIV or hepatitis. Patients who have had an ischemic stroke or transient ischemic attack (TIA) are at risk for infection following the event (Ross, Lee, & Brewer, 2014). In an effort to fight infection, patients mount a peripheral immune response (PIR) consisting of neutrophilia, lymphocytopenia, and elevated monocytes (Ross et al., 2014). Researchers are investigating the time course, trajectory, and significance of the PIR following stroke or TIA (Ross et al., 2014; Ross & Lee, 2015) (see Chart 35-4).

A history of past and present infections and the dates and types of treatments, along with a history of any multiple persistent infections, fevers of unknown origin, lesions or sores, or any type of drainage, as well as the response to treatment, are obtained.

Allergy

The patient is asked about any allergies, including types of allergens (e.g., pollens, dust, plants, cosmetics, food, medications, vaccines, latex), the symptoms experienced, and seasonal variations in occurrence or severity in the symptoms. A history of testing and treatments, including prescribed and over-the-counter medications that the patient has taken or is currently taking for these allergies and the effectiveness of the treatments, is obtained. All medication and food allergies

---

Chart 35-4 — NURSING RESEARCH PROFILE
Peripheral Immune Response Trajectories

Ross, A.M., & Lee, C. (2015). Description and identification of the peripheral immune response trajectories over time in first-time and recurrent stroke/transient ischemic attack. *Journal of Neuroscience Nursing, 47*(5), 256–262.

Purpose

It is not known how the immune response changes over time in patients after a stroke or transient ischemic attack (TIA). The purpose of this study was to describe the peripheral immune response (PIR) trajectories over time following a first-time and recurrent stroke or transient ischemic attack. The two aims were first to compare changes in the PIR over time in patients with a first versus a recurrent stroke or TIA, and second to identify trajectories of change in the PIR in patients after a stroke or TIA.

Design

This was a secondary analysis of data collected during a retrospective cross-sectional study on the PIR in the acute phase of care after a stroke or TIA. Data for the parent study were collected using a detailed retrospective medical record review. Descriptive statistics and latent growth mixture modeling were used to investigate the changes in PIR over time.

Findings

Of the 192 adult men and women included in the study 84 (44%) had a first-time stroke or TIA and 108 (56%) had a recurrent event. Participants with recurrent stroke or TIA had a persistent elevation in lymphocyte percentage compared to a significant decline in lymphocyte percentage observed in patients with a first-time event. The first trajectory (80% of the sample) had persistently lower lymphocyte percentages and higher neutrophil percentages over time, while the second trajectory (20% of the sample) had higher lymphocyte percentages and lower neutrophil percentages over time.

Nursing Implications

Nurses monitoring laboratory values after stroke or TIA need to recognize that different trajectories of PIRs exist. This may have future implications for identification of patients who may benefit from novel immune therapies. Nurses caring for patients who have any signs of depressed immune function need to be more vigilant in their assessments, watching for possible signs and symptoms of infection.

Chart 35-5 GENETICS IN NURSING PRACTICE

Immunologic Disorders

An immunologic disorder is a disorder of an individual's immune system, which is a network of cells, tissues, and organs that work together to defend the body against attacks by foreign invaders such as bacteria, parasites, and fungi that can cause infection. A number of immunologic disorders have a known inheritance pattern, while others are noted to have a genetic abnormality that is influenced by environmental exposures. Therefore, the pattern of inheritance is unclear in some immunologic disorders. Examples of immunologic disorders caused by a genetic abnormality include:

- Adenosine deaminase deficiency (autosomal recessive)
- Alopecia areta
- Alopecia totalis
- Asthma
- Ataxia telangiectasia (autosomal recessive)
- Autoimmune polyglandular syndrome
- Bruton agammaglobulinemia (X linked)
- Burkitt lymphoma
- Crohn's disease
- Diabetes, type 1
- DiGeorge syndrome (Autosomal dominant)
- Familial Mediterranean fever
- Job syndrome (autosomal dominant and recessive)
- Purine nucleoside phosphorylase deficiency (autosomal dominant)
- Severe combined immunodeficiency (primarily X linked)
- Wiskott–Aldrich syndrome (X linked)

Nursing Assessments

Refer to Chapter 5, Chart 5-2: Genetics in Nursing Practice: Genetic Aspects of Health Assessment

Family History Assessment Specific to Immunologic Disorders

- Collect a family history for both maternal and paternal relatives for three generations.
- Assess family history for other family members with histories of immunologic disorders.

- Obtain information about family members with a history of recurrent infections or illness.
- Recognize ethnic risk (non-Ashkenazi Jewish, Armenian, Arab, and Turkish are at greater risk for Familial Mediterranean fever; Caucasians have a higher incidence of Crohn's disease)

Patient Assessment

- Assess for symptoms such as changes in respiratory status associated with asthma (e.g., wheezing, or airway hyperresponsiveness; mucosal edema; and mucus production).
- Gather information regarding immunizations and whether an altered response to any immunization has occurred.
- Assess for symptoms of immunodeficiency disorders, such as unexplained weight gain or loss, skin rashes, changes in hair texture or distribution, joint or muscle pain, intolerance to cold, irregular menstrual periods, abdominal discomfort, or the presence of diarrhea.
- Identify pattern of sickness with regard to frequency of colds, respiratory infections, or history of illness that tends to linger.
- Obtain history of childhood illnesses and details of the illness experience.
- Assess for medical history of frequent or recurrent infections.
- Learn about susceptibility to infections, assess for patterns (frequency, length of illness, severity of symptoms), and recognize infections that would be atypical for age.
- Inquire about environmental exposures (e.g., smoke, chloroform, metal or dust particles, paint).
- Ask about exposure to other viruses such as Epstein Barr or Influenza.

Resources

American Autoimmune Related Diseases Association, www.aarda.org

Genetic and Rare Diseases Information Center, rarediseases.info.nih.gov

See Chapter 8, Chart 8-7 for components of genetic counseling.

---

are listed on an allergy alert sticker and placed on the front of the patient's health or medical record to alert others. Continued assessment for potential allergic reactions in the patient is vital. See Chapter 37 for more information on allergies.

Disorders and Diseases

Autoimmune Disorders

Autoimmune disorders affect people of both genders of all ages, ethnicities, and social classes. Autoimmune disorders are a group of disorders that can affect almost any cell or tissue in the body (Grossman & Porth, 2014). As mentioned previously, they tend to be more common in women because estrogen tends to enhance immunity. Androgen, on the other hand, tends to be immunosuppressive. Autoimmune diseases are a leading cause of death by disease in females of reproductive age.

The patient is asked about any autoimmune disorders, such as lupus erythematosus, rheumatoid arthritis, multiple sclerosis, or psoriasis. The onset, severity, remissions and exacerbations, functional limitations, treatments that the patient has received or is currently receiving, and effectiveness of the treatments are described. The occurrence of different

autoimmune diseases within a family strongly suggests a genetic predisposition to more than one autoimmune disease (Brooks & Renaudineau, 2015) (see Chart 35-5).

Neoplastic Disease

If there is a history of cancer in the family, more information is obtained, including the type of cancer, age at onset, and relationship (maternal or paternal) of the patient to the affected family members. Dates and results of any cancer screening tests for the patient are documented.

A history of cancer in the patient is also obtained, along with the type of cancer, date of diagnosis, and treatment modalities used. Immunosuppression contributes to the development of cancers; however, cancer itself is immunosuppressive, as is the treatment for cancer. Large tumors can release antigens into the blood, and these antigens combine with circulating antibodies and prevent them from attacking the tumor cells. Furthermore, tumor cells may possess special blocking factors that coat tumor cells and prevent their destruction by killer T lymphocytes. During the early development of tumors, the body may fail to recognize the tumor antigens as foreign and subsequently fail to initiate destruction of the malignant cells. Hematologic cancers, such as leukemia and lymphoma, are associated with altered production and function of WBCs and lymphocytes.

All treatments that the patient has received or is currently receiving, such as radiation or chemotherapy, are recorded in the health history. In addition, the nurse should elicit information related to complementary or alternative modalities that have been used and the response to these efforts. Radiation destroys lymphocytes and decreases the ability to mount an effective immune response. The size and extent of the irradiated area determine the extent of immunosuppression. Whole-body irradiation may leave the patient totally immunosuppressed. Chemotherapy and other cancer treatments also affect bone marrow function, destroying cells that contribute to an effective immune response and resulting in immunosuppression (Morrison, 2014).

Chronic Illness and Surgery

The health assessment includes a history of chronic illness, such as diabetes, renal disease, chronic obstructive pulmonary disease (COPD), or fibromyalgia. The onset and severity of illnesses, as well as treatment that the patient is receiving for the illness, are obtained. Chronic illness may contribute to immune system impairments in various ways. Kidney injury is associated with a deficiency in circulating lymphocytes. In addition, immune defenses may be altered by acidosis and uremic toxins. In diabetes, an increased incidence of infection has been associated with vascular insufficiency, neuropathy, and poor control of serum glucose levels. Recurrent respiratory tract infections are associated with COPD as a result of altered inspiratory and expiratory function and ineffective airway clearance. In addition, a history of organ transplantation or surgical removal of the spleen, lymph nodes, or thymus is noted, because these conditions may place the patient at risk for impaired immune function (Bronte & Pittet, 2013).

Special Problems

Conditions such as burns and other forms of injury and infection may contribute to altered immune system function. Major burns cause impaired skin integrity and compromise the body's first line of defense. Loss of large amounts of serum occurs with burn injuries and depletes the body of essential proteins, including immunoglobulins. The physiologic and psychological stressors associated with surgery or injury stimulate cortisol release from the adrenal cortex; increased serum cortisol also contributes to suppression of normal immune responses (Eng, Kokolus, Reed, et al., 2014).

Medications and Blood Transfusions

A list of past and present medications is obtained. In large doses, antibiotics, corticosteroids, cytotoxic agents, salicylates, nonsteroidal anti-inflammatory drugs, and anesthetic agents can cause immune suppression (see Table 35-5).

A history of blood transfusions is obtained, because previous exposure to foreign antigens through transfusion may be associated with abnormal immune function. In addition, although the risk of HIV transmission through blood transfusion is extremely low in patients who received a transfusion after 1985 (when testing of blood for HIV was initiated in the United States), a small risk remains.

The patient is also asked about the use of herbal agents and over-the-counter medications. Because many of these products have not been subjected to rigorous testing, their effects have not been fully identified. It is important, therefore, to ask patients about their use of these substances, to document their use, and to educate patients about untoward effects that may alter immune responsiveness.

Lifestyle Factors

Like any other body system, the functions of the immune system are interrelated with other body systems. Poor nutritional status, smoking (Sheils, Katki, Freedman, et al., 2014), excessive consumption of alcohol, illicit drug use, STIs, and occupational or residential exposure to environmental radiation and pollutants have been associated with impaired immune function and are assessed in a detailed patient history. Although factors that are not consistent with a healthy lifestyle are predominately responsible for ineffective immune function, positive lifestyle factors can also negatively affect immune function and require assessment. For example, rigorous exercise or competitive exercise—usually considered a positive lifestyle factor—can be a physiologic stressor and cause negative effects on immune response (Jin, Paik, Kwak, et al., 2015). This outcome is compounded if the person also faces stressful environmental conditions while undergoing exercise. Given the cumulative impact of various environmental stressors on the immune system, every effort should be made to minimize the person's exposure to stressors other than the exercise performed (Jin et al., 2015).

Psychoneuroimmunologic Factors

Patient assessment must also address psychoneuroimmunologic factors. The bidirectional pathway between the brain and immune system is referred to as psychoneuroimmunology (Fagundes, Lindgren, & Kiecolt-Glaser, 2013). The immune response is regulated and modulated in part by neuroendocrine influences. Lymphocytes and macrophages have receptors that can respond to neurotransmitters and endocrine hormones. Lymphocytes can produce and secrete adrenocorticotropic hormone and endorphine-like compounds. Cells in the brain, especially in the hypothalamus, can recognize prostaglandins, interferons, and interleukins, as well as histamine and serotonin, all of which are released during the inflammatory process. Like all other biologic systems functioning to maintain homeostasis, the immune system is integrated with other psychophysiologic processes and is regulated and modulated by the brain. These relationships may have immunologic consequences.

Conversely, the immune processes can affect neural and endocrine function, including behavior. Growing evidence indicates that a measurable immune system response can be positively influenced by biobehavioral strategies such as relaxation and imagery techniques, biofeedback, humor, hypnosis, and conditioning (Bennett, Parsons, Ben-Moshe, et al., 2014; Palsson & van Tilburg, 2015). Therefore, the assessment should address the patient's general psychological status and the patient's use of and response to these strategies.

Physical Assessment

During the physical examination (see Chart 35-3), the skin and mucous membranes are assessed for lesions,

TABLE 35-5 Selected Medications and Effects on the Immune System

Drug Classification (and Examples)	Effects on the Immune System
Antibiotics (in large doses)	Bone Marrow Suppression
ceftriaxone (Rocephin)	Eosinophilia, hemolytic anemia, hypoprothrombinemia, neutropenia, thrombocytopenia
cefuroxime sodium (Ceftin)	Eosinophilia, hemolytic anemia, hypoprothrombinemia, neutropenia, thrombocytopenia
chloramphenicol (Chloromycetin)	Leukopenia, aplastic anemia
dactinomycin (Cosmegen)	Agranulocytosis, neutropenia
fluoroquinolones (ciprofloxacin [Cipro], levofloxacin [Levaquin])	Hemolytic anemia, methemoglobinemia, eosinophilia, leukopenia, pancytopenia
gentamicin sulfate (Garamycin)	Agranulocytosis, granulocytosis
macrolides (erythromycin, azithromycin [Zithromax], clarithromycin [Biaxin])	Neutropenia, leukopenia
Penicillins	Agranulocytosis
Streptomycin	Leukopenia, neutropenia, pancytopenia
vancomycin (Vancocin, Vancoled)	Transient leukopenia
Antithyroid Drugs	
propylthiouracil (PTU)	Agranulocytosis, leukopenia
Nonsteroidal Anti-Inflammatory Drugs (NSAIDs) (in large doses)	Inhibit Prostaglandin Synthesis or Release
Aspirin	Agranulocytosis
COX-2 inhibitors (celecoxib [Celebrex])	Anemia, allergy, no other major adverse effects
ibuprofen (Advil, Motrin)	Leukopenia, Neutropenia
indomethacin (Indocid, Indocin)	Agranulocytosis, leukopenia
Phenylbutazone	Pancytopenia, agranulocytosis, aplastic anemia
Adrenal Corticosteroids	Immunosuppression
Prednisone	
Antineoplastic Agents (cytotoxic agents)	Immunosuppression
cyclophosphamide (Cytoxan)	Leukopenia, neutropenia
mechlorethamine HCl (Mustargen)	Agranulocytosis, neutropenia
cyclosporine (Neoral)	Leukopenia, inhibits T-lymphocyte function
Antimetabolites	Immunosuppression
Pyrimidine antagonist (Fluorouracil [5-FU])	Leukopenia, eosinophilia
Folic acid antagonist (Methotrexate)	Leukopenia, aplastic bone marrow
Purine antagonist (Mercaptopurine[(6-MP])	Leukopenia, pancytopenia

COX, cyclo-oxygenase.
Adapted from Comerford, K. C. (2015). *Nursing 2015 drug handbook*. Philadelphia, PA: Wolters Kluwer.

dermatitis, purpura (subcutaneous bleeding), urticaria, inflammation, or any discharge. Any signs of infection are noted. The patient's temperature is recorded, and the patient is observed for chills and sweating. The anterior and posterior cervical, supraclavicular, axillary, and inguinal lymph nodes are palpated for enlargement; if palpable nodes are detected, their location, size, consistency, and reports of tenderness on palpation are noted. Joints are assessed for tenderness, swelling, increased warmth, and limited range of motion. The patient's respiratory, cardiovascular, genitourinary, gastrointestinal, and neurosensory systems are evaluated for signs and symptoms indicative of immune dysfunction. Any functional limitations or disabilities the patient may have are also assessed.

Diagnostic Evaluation

A series of blood tests and skin tests, as well as bone marrow biopsy, may be performed to evaluate the patient's immune competence. Specific laboratory and diagnostic tests are discussed in greater detail along with individual disease processes in subsequent chapters in this unit. Selected laboratory and diagnostic tests used to evaluate immune competence are summarized in Chart 35-6.

Nursing Management

The nurse needs to be aware that patients undergoing evaluation for possible immune system disorders experience not only physical pain and discomfort with certain types of diagnostic procedures but also many psychological reactions. It is the nurse's role to counsel, educate, and support patients throughout the diagnostic process. Many patients may be extremely anxious about the results of diagnostic tests and the possible implications of those results for their future health, employment, and personal relationships. This is an ideal time for the nurse to provide counseling and education, should these interventions be warranted.

Chart 35-6 Selected Tests for Evaluating Immunologic Status

Various laboratory tests may be performed to assess immune system activity or dysfunction. The studies assess leukocytes and lymphocytes, humoral immunity, cellular immunity, phagocytic cell function, complement activity, hypersensitivity reactions, specific antigen–antibodies, or human immunodeficiency virus infection.

Humoral (Antibody-Mediated) Immunity Tests

- B-cell quantification with monoclonal antibody
- In vivo immunoglobulin synthesis with T-cell subsets
- Specific antibody response
- Total serum globulins and individual immunoglobulins (electrophoresis, immunoelectrophoresis, single radial immunodiffusion, nephelometry, and isohemagglutinin techniques)

Cellular (Cell-Mediated) Immunity Tests

- Total lymphocyte count
- T-cell and T-cell-subset quantification with monoclonal antibody
- Delayed hypersensitivity skin test
- Cytokine production
- Lymphocyte response to mitogens, antigens, and allogenic cells
- Helper and suppressor T-cell functions

CRITICAL THINKING EXERCISES

1 An 80-year-old woman presents to her primary provider for evaluation of a recurrent urinary tract infection for which she has received several courses of antibiotics. What diagnostic tests would you expect to be prescribed? What is the rationale for these tests? What further assessment data would you want to obtain from this patient?

2 **ebp** A 40-year-old woman with systemic lupus erythematosus (SLE) is admitted to the hospital for a kidney transplant and is prescribed immunosuppressant medications. Describe how her altered immune system would affect the care you provide. Develop an evidence-based education plan for the patient and her family before hospital discharge. Discuss the criteria used to assess the strength of the evidence for your education plan.

3 **pq** A 35-year-old woman with rheumatoid arthritis presents with an acute flare-up of her symptoms and is prescribed corticosteroids. What are your priority nursing observations and assessments? Identify priorities for patient education appropriate for the new prescription of steroids.

REFERENCES

*Asterisk indicates nursing research.

Books

Comerford, K. C. (Ed.) (2015). *Nursing 2015 drug handbook.* Philadelphia, PA: Wolters Kluwer.

Fagundes, C. P., Lindgren, M . E., & Kiecolt-Glaser, J. K. (2013). Psychoneuroimmunology and cancer: Incidence, progression, and quality of life. In B. I. Carr, & J. Steel (Eds.). *Psychological aspects of cancer: A guide to emotional and psychological consequences of cancer, their causes and their management.* New York: Springer.

Grossman, S. C., & Porth, C. M. (2014). *Porth's pathophysiology: Concepts of altered health states* (9th ed.). Philadelphia, PA: Lippincott Williams & Wilkins.

Haynes, B. F., Soderberg, K. A., & Fauci, A. S. (2015). Introduction to the immune system. In D. L. Kasper, A. S. Fauci, S. L. Hauser, et al. (Eds.). *Harrison's principles of internal medicine* (19th ed.). New York: McGraw-Hill Education.

Kessler, J. A. (2015). Applications of stem cell biology in clinical medicine. In D. L. Kasper, A. S. Fauci, S. L. Hauser, et al. (Eds.). *Harrison's principles of internal medicine* (19th ed.). New York: McGraw-Hill Education.

Levinson, W. (2014). *Review of medical microbiology and immunology* (13th ed.). New York: McGraw-Hill Education.

McComb, S., Thiriot, A., Krishnan, L., et al. (2013). Introduction to the immune system. In K. M. Fulton, & S. M. Twine (Eds.). *Immunoproteomics: Methods and protocols.* Totowa: Humana Press.

Page, A. V., & Liles, W. C. (2015). Immunomodulators. In J. E. Bennett, R. Dolin, & M. J. Blaser (Eds.). *Principles and practices of infectious diseases* (8th ed.). Philadelphia, PA: Elsevier Saunders.

Paul, W. E. (Ed.) (2013). *Fundamental immunology* (7th ed.). Philadelphia, PA: Lippincott Williams & Wilkins.

Shekarabi, M., & Asgari, F. (2014). Aging immunity and infection. In A. N. Massoud, & N. Rezaei (Eds.). *Immunology of aging.* New York: Springer Heidelberg.

Journals and Electronic Documents

Bennett, P. N., Parsons, T., Ben-Moshe, R., et al. (2014). Laughter and humor therapy in dialysis. *Seminars in Dialysis, 27*(5), 488–493.

Bronte, V., & Pittet, M. J. (2013). The spleen in local and systemic regulation of immunity. *Immunity, 39*(5), 809–818.

Booy, S., Hofland, L., & van Eijck, C. (2015). Potentials of interferon therapy in the treatment of pancreatic cancer. *Journal of Interferon and Cytokine Research, 35*(5), 327–339.

Brooks, W. H., & Renaudineau, Y. (2015). Epigenetics and autoimmune diseases: The X chromosome-nucleolus nexus. *Frontiers in Genetics, 6*(22), 1–20.

Carlsson, M., Haglin, L., Rosendahl, E., et al. (2013). Poor functional status is associated with urinary tract infection among older people living in residential care facilities. *The Journal of Nutrition, Health & Aging, 17*(2), 186–191.

Cassat, J. E., & Skaar, E. P. (2013). Iron in infection and immunity. *Cell Host & Microbe, 13*(5), 509–519.

Davis-Yadley, A. H., & Malafa, M. P. (2015). Vitamins in pancreatic cancer: A review of underlying mechanisms and future applications. *Advances in Nutrition, 6,* 774–802.

Eng, J. W., Kokolus, K. M., Reed, C. B., et al. (2014). A nervous tumor microenvironment: The impact of adrenergic stress on cancer cells, immunosuppression, and immunotherapeutic response. *Cancer Immunology and Immunotherapy, 63*(11), 1115–1128.

Epel, E. S., & Lithgow, G. J. (2014). Stress biology and aging mechanisms: Toward understanding the deep connection between adaptation to stress and longevity. *The Journals of Gerontology Series A: Biological Sciences and Medical Sciences, 69*(Suppl 1), S10–S16.

Geering, B., & Fussenegger, M. (2015). Synthetic immunology: Modulating the human immune system. *Trends in Biotechnology, 33*(2), 65–79.

Glassman, P. M., & Balthasar, J. P. (2014). Mechanistic considerations for the use of monoclonal antibodies for cancer therapy. *Cancer Biology & Medicine, 11*(1), 20–33.

Goronzy, J. J., & Weyand, C. M. (2013). Understanding immunosenescence to improve responses to vaccines. *Nature Immunology, 14,* 428–436.

Jin, C.H., Paik, I.Y., Kwak, Y.S., et al. (2015). Exhaustive submaximal endurance and resistance exercises induce temporary immunosuppression via physical and oxidative stress. *Journal of Exercise and Rehabilitation, 11*(4), 198–203.

Kannan, R., Madden, K., & Andrews, S. (2013). Primer on immune-oncology and immune response. *Clinical Journal of Oncology Nursing, 18*(3), 311–317.

Lo, Y.C., Lee, C. F., & Powell, J. D. (2014). Insight into the role of mTOR and metabolism in T cells reveals new potential approaches to preventing graft rejection. *Current Opinion in Organ Transplantation*, *19*(4), 363–371.

Mody, L., & Juthani-Mehta, M. (2014). Urinary tract infections in older women: A clinical review. *JAMA*, *311*(8), 844–854.

Morrison, V. (2014). Immunosuppression associated with novel chemotherapy agents and monoclonal antibodies. *Clinical Infectious Diseases*, *59*(Suppl 5), S360–S364.

Müller, L., & Pawelec, G. (2014). Aging and immunity: Impact of behavioral intervention. *Brain, Behavior, and Immunity*, *39*, 8–22.

Ngo, S. T., Steyn, F. J., & McCombe, P. A. (2014). Gender differences in autoimmune disease. *Frontiers in Neuroendocrinology*, *35*(3), 347–369.

Palsson, O. S., & van Tilburg, M. (2015). Hypnosis and guided imagery treatment for gastrointestinal disorders: Experience with scripted protocols developed at the University of North Carolina. *American Journal of Clinical Hypnosis*, *58*(1), 5–21.

*Ross, A. M., & Lee, C. (2015). Description and identification of the peripheral immune response trajectories over time in first-time and recurrent stroke/transient ischemic attack. *Journal of Neuroscience Nursing*, *47*(5), 256–262.

*Ross, A. M., Lee, C. S., & Brewer, M. (2014). Peripheral immune response and infection in first-time and recurrent ischemic stroke or transient ischemic attack. *Journal of Neuroscience Nursing*, *46*(4), 199–206.

Sheils, M. S., Katki, H. A., Freedman, N. D., et al. (2014). Cigarette smoking and variations in systemic immune and inflammation markers. *Journal of the National Cancer Institute*, *106*(11), 1–8.

Slawson, D. L., Fitzgerald, N., & Morgan, K. T. (2013). Position of the academy of nutrition and dietetics: The role of nutrition in health promotion and chronic disease prevention. *Journal of the Academy of Nutrition and Dietetics*, *113*(7), 972–979.

Supic, C., Jagodic, M., & Magic, Z. (2013). Epigenetics: A new link between nutrition and cancer. *Nutrition and Cancer*, *65*(6), 781–792.

Yue, C., Tian, W., Wang, W., et al. (2013). The impact of perioperative glutamine-supplemented parenteral nutrition on outcomes of patients undergoing abdominal surgery: A meta-analysis of randomized clinical trials. *The American Surgeon*, *79*(5), 506–513.

Resources

Centers for Disease Control and Prevention, www.cdc.gov
National Institute of Allergy and Infectious Diseases, www.niaid.nih.gov/
National Institutes of Health, Health Information, www.nih.gov/health/infoline.htm
U.S. Department of Health and Human Services, www.hhs.gov
American Cancer Society, www.cancer.org

36

Management of Patients With Immune Deficiency Disorders

LEARNING OBJECTIVES

On completion of this chapter, the learner will be able to:

1 Identify the pathophysiology, clinical manifestations, and nursing management of patients with primary immune deficiency disorders (PIDD).
2 Describe the modes of transmission of human immune deficiency virus (HIV) infection and prevention strategies.

3 Explain the pathophysiology associated with the clinical manifestations of HIV and acquired immune deficiency syndrome (AIDS) and the purpose of antiretroviral therapy (ART).
4 Use the nursing process as a framework for care of the patient with HIV/AIDS.
5 Identify resources available to patient and family that promote self-management of immune deficiency disorders.

GLOSSARY

candidiasis: fungal infection, usually of skin or mucous membranes, caused by Candida species
enzyme immunoassay (EIA): a blood test that can determine the presence of antibodies to HIV in the blood or saliva; a variant of this test is called enzyme-linked immunosorbent assay (ELISA)
HIV-1: retrovirus isolated and recognized as the etiologic agent of HIV disease
HIV encephalopathy: clinical syndrome characterized by a progressive decline in cognitive, behavioral, and motor functions
immune reconstitution inflammatory syndrome (IRIS): a syndrome that results from rapid restoration of pathogen-specific immune responses to opportunistic infections
Kaposi sarcoma: malignancy that involves the epithelial layer of blood and lymphatic vessels
latent reservoir: the integrated HIV provirus within the CD4$^+$ T cell during the resting memory state; does not express viral proteins and is invisible to the immune system and antiviral medications
Mycobacterium avium **complex (MAC):** opportunistic infection caused by mycobacterial organisms that commonly causes a respiratory illness but can also infect other body systems
opportunistic infection: illness caused by various organisms, some of which usually do not cause disease in people with normal immune systems
peripheral neuropathy: disorder characterized by sensory loss, pain, muscle weakness, and wasting of muscles in the hands or legs and feet

Pneumocystis **pneumonia (PCP):** common opportunistic lung infection; pathogen implicated is most commonly a fungus
polymerase chain reaction: a sensitive laboratory technique that can detect and quantify HIV in a person's blood or lymph nodes
post-exposure prophylaxis (PEP): taking antiretroviral medicines as soon as possible, but no more than 72 hours (3 days) after possible HIV exposure; two to three drugs are usually prescribed which must be taken for 28 days.
pre-exposure prophylaxis (PrEP): prevention method for HIV-negative people who are at high risk of HIV infection; involves taking a specific combination of HIV medicines daily; use with condoms and other prevention tools.
progressive multifocal leukoencephalopathy: opportunistic infection that infects brain tissue and causes damage to the brain and spinal cord
retrovirus: a virus that carries genetic material in ribonucleic acid (RNA) instead of DNA and contains reverse transcriptase
reverse transcriptase: enzyme that transforms single-stranded RNA into a double-stranded DNA
viral load test: measures the quantity of HIV RNA or DNA in the blood
viral set point: amount of virus present in the blood after the initial burst of viremia and the immune response that follows
wasting syndrome: involuntary weight loss consisting of both lean and fat body mass

The human immune system is complex and multidimensional. It works to protect against invasion by foreign substances, protect against the proliferation of neoplastic cells, and plays a key role in inflammation and healing. Patients with primary or secondary immune system disorders require care from nurses who are knowledgeable about the pathophysiology, diagnostic procedures, and interventions that are used in the management of these disorders.

PRIMARY IMMUNE DEFICIENCIES

The majority of primary immune deficiency diseases (PIDDs) are diagnosed in infancy, with a male-to-female ratio of 5 to 1. However, some PIDDs are not diagnosed until adolescence or early adulthood, when the gender distribution equalizes. Diagnosis at this stage frequently is confounded by frequent use of antibiotics that mask symptoms. On occasion, adults present with clinical episodes of infectious diseases that are beyond the scope of normal immunocompetence. Examples include infections that are unusually persistent, recurrent, or resistant to treatment and those involving unexpected dissemination of disease or atypical pathogens.

Pathophysiology

There are more than 200 different forms of PIDDs affecting about 500,000 people in the United States. More than 270 different genes are associated with PIDDs that are recognized by the International Union of Immunological Societies (Hernandez-Trujillo, Orange, Roy, et al., 2015). These rare genetic diseases prevent the body from developing normal immune responses resulting in a complex group of disorders with a wide array of clinical presentations. Many present during the first year of life and may be chronic, debilitating, and costly (National Institute of Allergies and Infectious Diseases [NIAID], 2015).

Clinical Manifestations

Major signs and symptoms include multiple infections despite aggressive treatment, infections with unusual or opportunistic organisms, failure to thrive or poor growth, and a positive family history (Costa-Carvalho, Grumach, Franco, et al., 2014). Table 36-1 contains selected PIDDs along with some of their clinical manifestations.

Assessment and Diagnostic Findings

There is often a considerable delay between the onset of symptoms and time of diagnosis of PIDD (Lehman, Hernandez-Trujillo, & Ballow, 2015). Because of the genetic origins of PIDD, family history should be carefully assessed but epidemiologic data about specific infectious agents should be considered as well (Costa-Carvalho et al., 2014).

Laboratory tests are used to identify antibody deficiencies, cellular (T-cell) defects, neutrophil disorders and complement deficiencies (Blaese, Stiehm, Bonilla, et al., 2013). A complete blood cell count with manual differential should always be analyzed first. Lymphopenia may indicate an immunologic abnormality; serum Ig levels (IgG, IgM, and IgA) and antibody responses to vaccines should be assessed to detect a humoral immune defect. Age-matched normal ranges need to be used since antibody levels change as the person ages (Younger, Epland, Zampelli, et al., 2015).

Prevention

Live vaccines are contraindicated in patients with antibody deficiency disorders (Younger et al., 2015). The patient is incapable of generating antibodies and the live substance in the vaccine can cause disease. Family planning should be addressed in terms of future pregnancies; in some situations, prenatal in utero testing of a fetus can determine whether the infant will be affected (Blaese et al., 2013).

Medical Management

A pattern of unusually frequent, opportunistic, or severe infections generates the possibility of a PIDD and initial testing or referral to an immunologist (Younger et al., 2015). Patients with neutropenia are at increased risk for developing severe infections despite substantial advances in supportive care. Epidemiologic shifts occur periodically and must be detected early because they influence prophylactic, empiric, and specific strategies for medical management. Attention to infection control practices is important, especially with the emergence of multidrug-resistant organisms.

Hematopoietic stem cell transplantation (HSCT) is a curative modality. The stem cells may be from embryos or adults. Toxicity and reduced efficacy are frequent limitations of HSCT. See Chapter 15 for further discussion of HSCT.

Another therapy involves the use of cells as vehicles for the delivery of genes or gene products. Gene therapy has had many adverse effects; the first studies in human participants revealed numerous toxicities with this therapy. Knowledge of these toxicities is being used in planning further studies to increase tolerability (Blaese et al., 2013).

Pharmacologic Therapy

Pharmacologic treatment depends upon the type and severity of presenting infection and the particular PIDD diagnosis (see Table 36-1). Prophylactic drug treatment prevents some bacterial and fungal infections but it must be used with caution because it has been implicated in the emergence of resistant organisms. The choices for empiric therapy include combination regimens and monotherapy. Specific choices depend on local factors (epidemiology, susceptibility/resistance patterns, availability, cost). Patients with antibody deficiencies receive regular Ig replacement therapy including both IV immunoglobulin (IVIG) and subcutaneous immunoglobulin (SCIG) to provide functional antibodies (Cherin, Marie, Michallet, et al., 2016).

For the procedural guidelines for management of IVIG, go to **thepoint.lww.com/ Brunner14e.**

Nursing Management

Many patients with PIDDs have comorbid autoimmune disorders, such as thyroid disease, rheumatoid arthritis, cytopenias, and inflammatory bowel disease (Younger et al., 2015). Many patients require immunosuppression to ensure engraftment of depleted bone marrow during transplantation procedures. For this reason, nursing care must be meticulous. Appropriate hand hygiene and infection prevention precautions are essential. See Chapter 71, Chart 71-1 for hand hygiene methods and Chart 71-2 for a summary of infection prevention precautions. Institutional policies and procedures related to infection prevention care must be followed scrupulously until definitive evidence demonstrates that precautions are unnecessary. Continual monitoring of the patient's condition is critical, so early signs of impending infection may be detected and treated before they seriously compromise the patient's status.

Patients and caregivers in the home are taught how to administer medications, including regular Ig replacement therapy, if prescribed. Instruction is provided to the patient and family about how to administer the therapy at home (see Chart 36-1). Nurses provide ongoing education and support for the patient and family.

TABLE 36-1 Selected Primary Immune Deficiency Disorders (PIDDs)

Disorder	Characteristics
Autoimmune lymphoproliferative syndrome (ALPS)	Unusually high numbers of lymphocytes accumulate in the lymph nodes, liver, and spleen leading to enlargement of those organs. Causes numerous autoimmune problems including low levels of red blood cells, platelets, and neutrophils.
Autoimmune polyglandular syndrome type 1 (APS-1). (also called autoimmune polyendocrinopathy-candidiasis-ectodermal dystrophy [APECED])	Causes a diverse range of symptoms, including autoimmunity against different types of organs and candidiasis, a fungal infection caused by *Candida* yeast.
CARD9 Deficiency and other syndromes of susceptibility to candidiasis	Results in susceptibility to fungal infections such as candidiasis; fungi are usually present on the skin; does not cause severe problems in healthy people.
Chronic granulomatous disease (CGD)	May be caused by mutations in one of five different genes. Phagocytes are unable to kill certain bacteria and fungi resulting in increased susceptibility to infections.
Common variable immunodeficiency (CVID)	Caused by a variety of genetic abnormalities resulting in defective ability of immune cells to produce normal amounts of antibodies, resulting in frequent bacterial or viral infections of the upper airway, sinuses, and lungs.
Congenital neutropenia syndromes	Characterized by low levels of neutrophils from birth.
CTLA4 Deficiency	Autoimmunity, low levels of antibodies, and excessive numbers of lymphocytes which infiltrate the gut, lungs, bone marrow, central nervous system, kidneys resulting in recurrent infections.
DOCK8 Deficiency	Genetic defect named after mutated gene responsible for the disease which causes decreased numbers and defective function of immune cells and recurrent infections.
GATA2 Deficiency	Can manifest as five different syndromes with a wide variety of symptoms including severe infections, respiratory problems, hearing loss, leg swelling, and cancer. These symptoms can appear early in childhood but also later on in life.
Glycosylation disorders with immune deficiency	Defects in glycosylation, which refers to the attachment of sugars to proteins; can disrupt the immune system resulting in immune deficiency.
Hyper-immunoglobulin E syndrome (HIES). Also called Job syndrome	Results from mutations in a gene that encodes a signaling module called STAT3 resulting in recurrent bacterial infections of skin and lungs.
Hyper-immunoglobulin M (hyper-IgM) syndromes	Immune system fails to produce normal IgA, IgG, and IgE antibodies but can produce normal or elevated IgM. Infants usually develop severe respiratory infections.
Interferon gamma, interleukin 12, interleukin 23 deficiencies	Interferon gamma, interleukin 12, and interleukin 23 are key signals that raise alert against bacteria and other infectious microbes; deficiencies result in susceptibility to infections caused by bacteria and viruses.
Leukocyte adhesion deficiency (LAD)	Phagocytes are unable to move to the site of an infection resulting in an inability to fight pathogens resulting in recurrent, life-threatening infections and poor wound healing.
NF-κB Essential modifier (NEMO) mutations	Mutations in the NEMO gene cannot "turn on" other genes especially those involved in inflammation and the immune response and are, therefore, highly susceptible to infections with mycobacteria.
PI3 Kinase disease	Genetic mutations overactivate an important immune signaling pathway causing a change reaction that disrupts the infection-fighting B and T cells resulting in a weakened immune system and frequent bacterial and viral infections.
PLCG2-associated antibody deficiency and immune dysregulation (PLAID)	Rare disorder with allergic response to cold (cold urticaria) as the most distinct symptom.
Severe combined immune deficiency (SCID)	Group of rare, life-threatening disorders caused by mutations in different genes involved in development and function of T and B cells; infants appear healthy at birth but are highly susceptible to severe infections.
Warts, hypogammaglobulinemia, infections, and myelokathexis syndrome (WHIMS)	Low levels of white blood cells, especially neutrophils, which predispose to frequent infections and persistent warts.
Wiskott–Aldrich syndrome (WAS)	Problems with B and T cells and platelets resulting in prolonged episodes of bleeding, recurrent bacterial and fungal infections and increased risk of cancers and autoimmune diseases.

Adapted from National Institute of Allergies and Infectious Diseases (2015). Types of primary immune deficiency disorders. Retrieved on 5/10/1016 at: www.niaid.nih.gov/topics/immuneDeficiency/Pages/majorPIDDs.aspx.

Chart 36-1

HOME CARE CHECKLIST

Home Administration of Ig Replacement Therapy

At the completion of education, the patient and/or caregiver will be able to:

- State the impact of immune deficiency on physiologic functioning, ADLs, IADLs, roles, relationships, and spirituality.
- State what types of changes are needed (if any) to maintain a clean home environment and prevent infection.
- State how to contact the primary provider, the team of home care professionals overseeing care, and intravenous supply vendor.
- State how to obtain medical supplies and carry out dressing changes, IV access site care, and other prescribed regimens.
- Identify the benefits and expected outcome of regular Ig replacement therapy.
- State rationale for prophylactic use of acetaminophen (Tylenol) and diphenhydramine (Benadryl) before treatment begins.
- State the rationale for prehydration on the day before infusion.

- Demonstrate how to prepare regular Ig replacement therapy.
- Demonstrate how to administer regular Ig replacement therapy.
- Demonstrate how to clean and maintain IV equipment, as applicable.
- Identify side effects and adverse effects of regular Ig replacement therapy.
- Demonstrate how to monitor for adverse effects of regular Ig replacement therapy.
- Describe to whom, how, and when to report adverse effects of regular Ig replacement therapy.
- Describe appropriate actions to take for adverse effects.
- Verbalize understanding of emergency measures for anaphylactic shock.

ADL, activities of daily living; IADL, independent activities of daily living.

ACQUIRED IMMUNE DEFICIENCY

Immune deficiency can be acquired due to medical treatment such as chemotherapy (see Chapter 15) or infection from agents such as human immune deficiency virus (HIV). Advances have been made in treating HIV infection and acquired immune deficiency syndrome (AIDS); however, AIDS remains a critical public health issue in communities across the country and around the world. Prevention, early detection, and ongoing treatment remain important aspects of care for persons living with HIV infection or AIDS, sometimes referred to as PLWHA.

HIV Infection and AIDS

Since the disease now known as AIDS was first identified more than 35 years ago, remarkable progress has been made in improving the length and quality of life for people living with HIV disease. During the first decade, progress was associated with the recognition and treatment of opportunistic diseases and introduction of prophylaxis against **opportunistic infections** (illnesses caused by various organisms, some of which usually do not cause disease in people with normal immune systems). The second decade witnessed progress in the development of highly active antiretroviral drug therapies (HAART) as well as continuing progress in the treatment of opportunistic infections. The third decade has focused on issues of preventing new infections, adherence to antiretroviral therapy (ART), development of second-generation combination medications that affect different stages of the viral life cycle, and continued need for an effective vaccine. The HIV antibody test, an **enzyme immunoassay** (**EIA**; or a variant of this test called *enzyme-linked immunosorbent assay* [ELISA]), became available in 1984, allowing early diagnosis of the infection before the onset of symptoms. Since then, HIV infection has been best managed as a chronic disease, most appropriately in an outpatient care setting, whereas AIDS may involve acute conditions that require hospitalization.

Epidemiology

Since the first cases of AIDS were reported in the United States in 1981, surveillance case definitions for HIV infection and AIDS have undergone several revisions (in 1985, 1987, 1993, 2008, and 2014) in response to diagnostic advances. Criteria for a confirmed case of HIV infection can be met by either laboratory evidence or clinical evidence but laboratory evidence, usually obtained through blood tests, is preferred over clinical evidence (e.g., patient signs and symptoms). A case of HIV infection can be classified in one of five HIV infection stages (0, 1, 2, 3, or unknown). Stage 0 indicates early HIV infection, inferred from laboratory testing; stages 1, 2, and 3 are based on the CD4+ T-lymphocyte count; while cases with no information on CD4+ T-lymphocyte count or percentage are classified as stage unknown (Selik, Mokotoff, Branson, et al., 2014). See Table 36-2 for further explanation of stages.

In July 2015, the White House released the *National HIV/AIDS Strategy for the United States: Updated to 2020*. This document has four Strategic Goals, which include reducing new infections; increasing access to care and improving health outcomes for people living with HIV; reducing HIV-related health disparities and health inequities; and achieving a more coordinated national response to the HIV epidemic (White House, 2015).

About 1,218,400 persons aged 13 years and older are living with HIV infections in the United States, including 156,300 (12.8%) that are unaware that they are infected. HIV remains mainly an urban disease, with the majority of individuals diagnosed with HIV in 2013 residing in areas with 500,000 or more people (Centers for Disease Control and Prevention [CDC], 2015a). Due to a variety of factors, including stigma and lack of access to HIV testing, there are significant regional differences in the number of people who are unaware of their infection. The prevalence of HIV/AIDS cases has increased due to effective treatment and reduced mortality. In 2013, an estimated 47,352 people were diagnosed with HIV infection and an estimated 26,688 people were diagnosed with

TABLE 36-2 HIV Infection Stages 1, 2, and 3 Based on Age-Specific Laboratory Data

	Age on Date of CD4+ T-lymphocyte Test					
	<1 year		1–5 years		≥6 years	
Stage	Cells/μL	%	Cells/μL	%	Cells/μL	%
1	≥1,500	≥34	≥1,000	≥30	≥500	≥26
2	750–1,499	26–33	500–999	22–29	200–499	14–25
3	<750	<26	<500	<22	<200	<14

If a stage-3-defining opportunistic illness has been diagnosed, then the stage is 3 regardless of CD4+ T-lymphocyte test.

Stage-3-Defining Opportunistic Illnesses in HIV Infection
Bacterial infections, multiple or recurrent (only among children aged less than 6 years)
Candidiasis of bronchi, trachea, or lungs
Candidiasis of esophagus
Cervical cancer, invasive (only in persons aged 6 years or older)
Coccidioidomycosis, disseminated or extrapulmonary
Cryptococcosis, extrapulmonary
Cryptosporidiosis, chronic intestinal (>1 month's duration)
Cytomegalovirus disease (other than liver, spleen, or nodes), onset at age >1 month
Cytomegalovirus retinitis (with loss of vision)
Encephalopathy attributed to HIV
Herpes simplex: chronic ulcers (>1 month's duration) or bronchitis, pneumonitis, or esophagitis (onset at age >1 month)
Histoplasmosis, disseminated or extrapulmonary Isosporiasis, chronic intestinal (>1 month's duration)
Kaposi sarcoma
Lymphoma, Burkitt (or equivalent term)
Lymphoma, immunoblastic (or equivalent term)
Lymphoma, primary, of brain
Mycobacterium avium complex or *Mycobacterium kansasii*, disseminated or extrapulmonary
Mycobacterium tuberculosis of any site, pulmonary (only in persons aged 6 years or older) disseminated, or extrapulmonary
Mycobacterium, other species or unidentified species, disseminated or extrapulmonary
Pneumocystis jirovecii (previously known as "*Pneumocystis carinii*") pneumonia (PCP)
Pneumonia, recurrent (only in persons aged 6 years or older)
Progressive multifocal leukoencephalopathy
Salmonella septicemia (recurrent)
Toxoplasmosis of brain, onset at age >1 month
Wasting syndrome attributed to HIV

Adapted from Selik, R., Mokotoff, E., Branson, B., et al. (2014). Revised surveillance case definition for HIV infection—United States, 2014. *Morbidity and Mortality Weekly Report*, 63(RR03), 1–10.

AIDS. Gay, bisexual, and other men who have sex with men (MSM) of all races and ethnicities remain the population most profoundly affected by HIV. Although MSM represent about 4% of the male population, in 2010, MSM accounted for 78% of new HIV infections among males and 63% of all new infections. MSM accounted for 54% of all people living with HIV infection in 2011, the most recent year these data are available. In 2010, the greatest number of new HIV infections (4,800) among MSM occurred in young black/African American MSM aged 13 to 24. Young black MSM accounted for 45% of new HIV infections among black MSM and 55% of new HIV infections among young MSM overall (CDC, 2015b). Transgender individuals also experience a high prevalence of HIV (Wichinski, 2015).

In light of intensive efforts globally, the HIV pandemic has been addressed but the burden remains significant. According to the World Health Organization (WHO) (2015a), there were approximately 36.9 million people living with HIV at the end of 2014 with 2.0 million people becoming newly infected with HIV in 2014 globally. Sub-Saharan Africa is the most affected region, with 25.8 million people living with HIV in 2014 and almost 70% of the global total of new HIV infections. About 51% of people with HIV know that they are

infected; 40% of those needing ART are accessing treatment globally. Forty-seven percent of adults living with HIV/AIDS are female (17.4 million) (WHO, 2015b), many of whom are in their child-bearing years. The diagnosis and treatment of HIV infection remain highly dependent upon the geographic location of where the person is living.

HIV Transmission

Inflammation and breaks in the skin or mucosa result in the increased probability that an HIV exposure will lead to infection. Human immune deficiency virus type 1 (**HIV-1**) is transmitted in body fluids (blood, seminal fluid, vaginal secretions, amniotic fluid, and breast milk) that contain infected cells. Higher amounts of HIV and infected cells in the body fluid are associated with the probability that the exposure will result in infection. Mother-to-child transmission of HIV-1 may occur in utero, at the time of delivery, or through breast-feeding, but most perinatal infections are thought to occur after exposure during delivery. HIV is not transmitted through casual contact (see Chart 36-2).

Blood and blood products can transmit HIV to recipients. However, the risk associated with transfusions has been

Chart 36-2 — RISK FACTORS
Risks Associated With HIV Infection

- Sharing infected injection drug use equipment
- Having sexual relations with infected individuals (both male and female)
- Infants born to mothers with HIV infection and/or who are breast-fed by HIV-infected mothers
- People who received organ transplants, HIV-infected blood, or blood products (especially between 1978 and 1985)

virtually eliminated as a result of voluntary self-deferral, completion of a detailed health history, extensive testing, heat treatment of clotting factor concentrates, and more effective virus inactivation methods. Donated blood is tested for antibodies to HIV-1, human immunodeficiency virus type 2 ([retrovirus identified in 1986 in patients with AIDS in Western Africa]), and the p24 antigen; since 1999, additional testing has been performed.

Gerontologic Considerations

A growing number of adults aged 50 and older have HIV/AIDS (National Institute on Aging [NIA], 2015). Many were diagnosed with HIV in their younger years and are benefitting from effective treatment. However, thousands of older adults unknowingly become infected with HIV every year. Older adults are less likely than younger people to get tested. Signs of HIV/AIDS can be mistaken for the aches and pains of normal aging. Older adults might be coping with other diseases common to aging that can mask the signs of HIV/AIDS.

New York City has the oldest and largest HIV epidemic in the Western world and could serve as a future model for other locales. The proportion of New York City residents diagnosed with concurrent HIV/AIDS has increased with age—among the newly diagnosed, 14.9% of persons under 30 years of age were diagnosed concurrently, compared with 39.1% of persons 60 years and older, indicating that older persons are being tested for HIV after many years of living with the infection (Bureau of HIV/AIDS Prevention and Control, 2014).

Tillman and Mark (2015) examined published research on the frequency of HIV and sexually transmitted infection (STI) testing among older adults (aged 50 and older), factors related to HIV and STI testing among older adults, and the perspectives and practices of older adults and health care providers related to patient-provider communication regarding sexual health. They found that low rates of HIV and STI testing were influenced by low perceived risk of infection by older adults and their health care providers. Providers bring societal age and gender biases to their perceptions of patient sexuality, which influence their communication about sexual health with older adult patients. Providers' assumptions that discussions about sexual health will offend their patients, as well as their own discomfort with talking to older adults about sex, inhibit them from assessing risk factors that may indicate a need for HIV and STI testing. Older adults living with HIV/AIDS also experience the development of other comorbidities such as cardiovascular disease and diabetes occurring within that specific demographic population, and HIV/AIDS becomes a contributing, but not necessarily primary, cause of mortality.

Prevention of HIV Infection

Nurses need to help in efforts to prevent HIV infection by educating how to eliminate or reduce risks associated with HIV infection and AIDS. HIV is transmitted through the exchange of some infected body fluids (see Chart 36-2). While behavioral interventions such as encouraging the use of condoms are highly effective in reducing the transmission of HIV, the HIV-negative person must be motivated and have the freedom to choose to use the method. In some situations, however, that freedom is absent. For example, a lack of freedom exists in a discordant couple (those in which only one partner has HIV) if the husband refuses to use condoms and the wife's cultural and religious beliefs require intercourse with her husband. In this context, **pre-exposure prophylaxis (PrEP)** might be appropriate. PrEP involves taking one pill containing two HIV medications (tenofovir disoproxil fumarate 300 mg and emtricitabine 200 mg [Truvada]) daily in order to avoid the risk of sexual HIV acquisition in adults and adolescents age 12 and older (Comerford, 2015). HIV status should be checked every 3 months to be sure that the person has not become infected. The ultimate goal of PrEP is to reduce the acquisition of HIV infection with its resulting morbidity, mortality, and cost to individuals and society (US Public Health Service, 2014).

Preventive Education

Prevention of HIV infection is achieved through: (a) behavioral interventions have been effective in reducing the risk of acquiring or transmitting HIV by ensuring that people have the information, motivation, and skills necessary to reduce their risk; (b) HIV testing, because most people change behaviors to protect their partners if they know they are infected with HIV; and (c) linkage to treatment and care, which enables individuals with HIV to live longer, healthier lives and reduce their risk of transmitting HIV (CDC, 2015c). The CDC (2014a), through the HIV/AIDS Prevention Research Synthesis Project, provides information about evidence-based behavioral interventions that can be used in a number of settings with targeted populations. Strategies to protect against infection are outlined in Chart 36-3. Other than abstinence, consistent and correct use of condoms (see Chart 36-4) is the only effective method to decrease the risk of sexual transmission of HIV infection. When latex male condoms are used consistently and correctly during vaginal or anal intercourse, they are highly effective in preventing the sexual transmission of HIV (CDC, 2013). Nonlatex condoms made of natural materials such as lambskin are available for people with latex allergy but will not protect against HIV infection. A male condom should be used for oral contact with the penis, and a dental dam (a flat piece of latex used by dentists to isolate a tooth for treatment) or an altered condom can be used for oral contact with the vagina or rectum. Medical male circumcision, when safely provided by well-trained health professionals, reduces the risk of heterosexually acquired HIV infection in men by approximately 60%. This is a key intervention in generalized epidemic settings with high HIV prevalence and a low male circumcision rate (WHO, 2015 a).

The polyurethane female condom, which is an effective contraceptive, provides a physical barrier that

Chart 36-3 — HEALTH PROMOTION
Protecting Against HIV Infection

All patients should be advised to:

- Abstain from exchanging sexual fluids (semen and vaginal fluid).
- Reduce the number of sexual partners to one.
- Always use latex condoms. If the patient is allergic to latex, nonlatex condoms should be used; however, they will not protect against HIV infection.
- Not reuse condoms.
- Avoid using cervical caps or diaphragms without using a condom as well.
- Always use dental dams for oral–genital or anal stimulation.
- Avoid anal intercourse, because this practice may injure tissues; if not possible, use lubricant—there are water and silicone-based products designed for anal sex.
- Avoid manual–anal intercourse ("fisting").
- Avoid sharing needles, razors, toothbrushes, sex toys, or blood-contaminated articles.
- Consider PrEP if regularly engage in high-risk behaviors.

Patients who are HIV seropositive should also be advised to:

- Take ART regularly to achieve viral suppression.
- Inform previous, present, and prospective sexual and drug-using partners of their HIV-positive status. If the patient is concerned for their safety, advise the patient that many states have established mechanisms through the public health department in which professionals are available to notify exposed contacts.
- Avoid having unprotected sex with another HIV-seropositive person. Cross-infection with that person's HIV can increase the severity of infection.
- Not donate blood, plasma, body organs, or sperm.

ART, antiretroviral therapy; PrEP, pre-exposure prophylaxis.

Chart 36-4 — PATIENT EDUCATION
The Correct Way to Use a Male Condom

The nurse instructs the patient to:

1. Put on a new condom before any kind of sex.
2. Hold the condom by the tip to squeeze out the air.

3. Unroll the condom all the way over the erect penis.

4. Have sex.
5. Hold the condom so it cannot come off the penis.
6. Pull out.
7. Use a new condom if you want to have sex again or if you want to have sex in a different place (e.g., in the anus and then in the vagina).

Note: Keep condoms cool and dry. Never use skin lotions, baby oil, petroleum jelly, or cold cream as lubricants; the oil in these products will cause the latex condom to break. Products made with water (such as K-Y jelly or glycerin) are safer to use.

---

prevents exposure to genital secretions containing HIV, such as semen and vaginal fluid, and is inserted by the woman (see Chapter 56). Other safe and effective woman-controlled methods such as microbicides remain elusive although clinical trials continue globally. Microbicides are gels, films, or *suppositories* that can kill or neutralize viruses and bacteria; *vaginal* and *rectal* microbicides are being researched to see if they can prevent sexual transmission of HIV.

Total abstinence from addictive drugs might not be a realistic short-term goal. Using a harm reduction framework, the nurse works with people who inject drugs to assist them to increase their healthy behaviors. Harm reduction frameworks use practical strategies and ideas aimed at reducing negative consequences associated with drug use and a movement for social justice built on a belief in, and respect for, the rights of people who use drugs. Therefore, under this framework, needle exchange programs are usually free and do not promote increased drug use; on the contrary, they have been found to decrease the incidence of blood-borne infections in people who inject drugs. Nurses should refer clients to needle exchange programs in their neighborhood whenever available. If new needles and syringes are not available, cleaning used needles and syringes with bleach may reduce the risk of HIV (CDC, 2015d). Sharing of drug-use equipment is a high-risk behavior for a number of blood-borne infections and should be avoided.

Related Reproductive Education

Because HIV infection in women often occurs during the child-bearing years, family planning issues need to be addressed. Attempts to achieve pregnancy by couples in which only one partner has HIV (known as discordant couples) expose the unaffected partner to the virus. Efforts at artificial insemination using processed semen from an HIV-infected partner continue. Studies are needed, because HIV has been found in the spermatozoa of patients with HIV infection, and it is possible that HIV can replicate in the male germ cell. Women considering pregnancy need to have accurate information about the risks of transmitting HIV infection to themselves, their partner, and their future children, and about the benefits of taking ART to reduce perinatal HIV transmission. Women in resource-rich settings who are HIV positive should be instructed not to breast-feed their infants, because HIV is transmitted through breast milk.

An increased risk of HIV infection in women is associated with hormonal contraceptive use, but a cause-and-effect relationship has not been established (Sharma & Walmsley, 2015). Women who are HIV negative and who use hormonal contraceptives to prevent pregnancy should be encouraged to use methods to block HIV infection including PrEP; providers should explore drug–drug interactions between hormonal contraceptives and ART in women infected with HIV (Sharma & Walmsley, 2015).

Prevention in Lesbian, Gay, Bisexual, and Transgender

Many health care providers are insufficiently prepared to meet the unique health needs of those who identify as lesbian, gay, bisexual, and transgender (LGBT). LGBT youth, in particular, are at higher risk for contracting HIV (Bosse, Nesteby, & Randall, 2015; Johnson & Amella, 2013). At the same time, this population experiences significant challenges due to family rejection, lack of social support, stigma, isolation, minority stress, as well as abuse and harassment (Bosse, Nesteby, & Randall, 2015; Johnson & Amella, 2013). Nurses need to be nonjudgmental in order to be effective in educating this population about prevention methods.

Reducing the Risk of Transmission to Health Care Providers

Standard Precautions

Implementation of appropriate hand hygiene measures (see Chart 71-1 for further information on hand hygiene methods) remains the most effective measure to prevent transmission of organisms. To reduce the risk of exposure of health care workers to HIV, the CDC developed standard precautions (see Chart 36-5; also see Chapter 71, Chart 71-2) which are designed to reduce the risk of transmission of pathogens. Standard precautions are used when working with all patients in all health care settings, regardless of their diagnosis or presumed infectious status.

Post-Exposure Prophylaxis for Health Care Providers

Post-exposure prophylaxis (PEP) includes taking antiretroviral medicines as soon as possible, but no more than 72 hours (3 days) after possible HIV exposure; two to three drugs are usually prescribed which must be taken for 28 days.

Health care workers who are exposed to a needle stick involving HIV-infected blood in a health care setting have a 0.23% risk of becoming HIV infected; the risk of infection due to occupational exposure is very low. As of December 31, 2013, 58 confirmed occupational exposures to HIV and 150 possible transmissions had been reported in the United States and only one confirmed case has been reported since 1999. Occupational exposure is considered an urgent medical concern and should be managed immediately after possible exposure—the sooner the better; every hour counts (CDC, 2015e). The CDC is suggesting that these post-exposure guidelines be followed after occupational and other exposures

---

Chart 36-5 **Recommendations for Standard Precautions**

1. **Hand hygiene:** Use after touching blood, body fluids, secretions, excretions, or contaminated items; immediately after removing gloves; and between patient contacts.
2. **Personal protective equipment:**
   - *Gloves:* Use for touching blood, body fluids, secretions, excretions, and contaminated items, and for touching mucous membranes and nonintact skin.
   - *Gown:* Use during procedures and patient care activities when contact of clothing/exposed skin with blood or body fluids, secretions, and excretions is anticipated.
   - *Mask, eye protection (goggles), face shield[1]:* Use during procedures and patient care activities likely to generate splashes or sprays of blood, body fluids, and secretions, especially suctioning or endotracheal intubation.
3. **Soiled patient care equipment:** Handle in a manner that prevents transfer of microorganisms to others and to the environment; wear gloves if visibly contaminated; and perform hand hygiene.
4. **Environmental control:** Develop procedures for routine care, cleaning, and disinfection of environmental surfaces, especially frequently touched surfaces in patient care areas.
5. **Textiles and laundry:** Handle in a manner that prevents transfer of microorganisms to others and to the environment.
6. **Needles and other sharps:** Do not recap, bend, break, or hand manipulate used needles; if recapping is required, use a one-handed scoop technique only; use safety features when available; and place used sharps in a puncture-resistant container.
7. **Patient resuscitation:** Use mouthpiece, resuscitation bag, and other ventilation devices to prevent contact with mouth and oral secretions.
8. **Patient placement:** Prioritize for single-patient room if patient is at increased risk for transmission, is likely to contaminate the environment, does not maintain appropriate hygiene, or is at increased risk for acquiring infection or developing adverse outcome following infection.
9. **Respiratory hygiene/cough etiquette** (source containment of infectious respiratory secretions in symptomatic patients, beginning at initial point of encounter, such as triage and reception areas in emergency departments and physician offices): Instruct symptomatic people to cover mouth and nose when sneezing or coughing, use tissues and dispose in no-touch receptacle, observe hand hygiene after soiling of hands with respiratory secretions, and wear surgical mask if tolerated.

From Centers for Disease Control and Prevention (CDC). (2007). 2007 Guideline for Isolation Precautions: Preventing Transmission of Infectious Agents in Healthcare Settings. Retrieved on 5/13/2016 at: www.cdc.gov/hicpac/2007ip/2007ip_part1.html
[1]During aerosol-generating procedures on patients with suspected or proven infections transmitted by respiratory aerosols (e.g., severe acute respiratory syndrome), wear a fit-tested N95 or higher respirator in addition to gloves, gown, and face/eye protection.

---

such as sexual assault. Chart 36-6 provides the strategies and emphasizes the need for quick action. The phone number for the Health Resources and Service Administration (HRSA) Post-exposure Prophylaxis Hotline is listed in the Resources section at the end of this chapter; the hotline is answered by a health care provider.

Vaccination

In the face of a global pandemic, the search for an effective vaccine against the HIV remains an urgent priority (Fauci &

Post-HIV Exposure Prophylaxis for Health Care Providers

If you sustain an occupational exposure to HIV, take the following actions immediately:

- Alert your supervisor and initiate the occupational exposure reporting system used in the setting.
- Determine the HIV status of the exposure source (i.e., patient) when possible to guide appropriate use of HIV post-exposure prophylaxis (PEP). Use rapid-testing if the HIV status of the patient is unknown. Check laws in your state as you proceed to determine HIV status of the source patient.

Get counseling at the time of exposure and at follow-up appointments:

- Exposed health care providers (HCP) are advised to use precautions (e.g., use of barrier contraception and avoidance of blood or tissue donations, pregnancy, and, if possible, breast-feeding) to prevent secondary transmission, especially during the first 6–12 weeks after exposure.
- For exposures for which three drug PEP is prescribed, HCPs are informed regarding the following:
  - Possible drug toxicities (e.g., rash and hypersensitivity reactions that could imitate acute HIV seroconversion and the need for monitoring)
  - Possible drug interactions
  - The need for adherence to PEP regimens

Undergo early reevaluation after exposure:

- Regardless of whether an HCP is taking PEP, reevaluation of exposed HCP within 72 hours after exposure is strongly recommended, as additional information about the exposure or the source patient may be available.

Follow-up with HIV testing and appointments. At a minimum, this follow-up should include:

- HIV testing at baseline and at 6 weeks, 12 weeks, and 6 months after exposure; alternatively, if the HCP is certain that a fourth-generation combination HIV p24 antigen–HIV antibody test is being utilized, then HIV testing could be performed at baseline, 6 weeks after exposure, and 4 months after exposure
- Complete blood counts and renal and hepatic function tests (at baseline and 2 weeks after exposure; further testing may be indicated if abnormalities are detected)

Note: All HIV testing results should preferably be given to the exposed HCP during face-to-face appointments.
Adapted from Kuhar, D., Henderson, D., Struble, K., et al. (2013). Updated US Public Health Service guidelines for the management of occupational exposures to human immunodeficiency virus and recommendations for post-exposure prophylaxis. *Infection Control and Hospital Epidemiology, 34*(9), 875–892.

Marston, 2015). The first U.S. government-sponsored phase I trial of an HIV vaccine was launched in 1987 and intensive efforts worldwide using a variety of strategies continue.

Pathophysiology

Because HIV is an infectious disease, it is important to understand how HIV-1 integrates itself into a person's immune system and how the immune response plays a pivotal role in the course of HIV disease. This knowledge is also essential for understanding medication therapy and vaccine development. Viruses are intracellular parasites. HIV is in the subfamily of lentiviruses and is a **retrovirus** because it carries its genetic material in the form of ribonucleic acid (RNA)

Physiology/Pathophysiology

Figure 36-1 • A. Structure of HIV-1 virus. The virus surrounded by a lipid envelope. **B.** Life cycle of HIV-1. Reprinted with permission from Grossman, S., & Porth, C. M. (2014). *Porth's pathophysiology: Concepts of altered health states* (9th ed.). Philadelphia, PA: Lippincott Williams & Wilkins.

rather than deoxyribonucleic acid (DNA) (Grossman & Porth, 2014).

Two genetically different but closely related forms of HIV (HIV-1 and HIV-2) have been identified. The course of illness is slower when infection is caused by HIV-2, which seems to be more common in Western Africa compared to HIV-1, which is more common in other regions of the globe. Blood tests may be used to screen for both forms of HIV. As shown in Figure 36-1A, HIV consists of a viral core containing viral RNA, surrounded by an envelope consisting of protruding glycoproteins.

All viruses target specific cells. HIV targets cells with CD4+ receptors, which are expressed on the surface of T lymphocytes, monocytes, dendritic cells, and brain microglia. Mature T cells (T lymphocytes) are composed of two major subpopulations that are defined by cell surface receptors of CD4+ or CD8+. Approximately two thirds of peripheral blood T cells are CD4+, and approximately one third are CD8+. Most people have about 700 to 1,000 CD4+ cells/mm³, but a level as low as 500 cells/mm³ can be considered within normal limits. During stage 0, which is also known as acute/recent infection, most varieties of HIV-1 use the chemokine cell receptor molecule CCR5 (R5 virus) for entry to T cells in addition to the CD4+ receptor, which suggests that the R5 variant is preferred to a different variant (CXCR4) but the preferred coreceptor can shift over the course of infection.

The HIV life cycle is complex (see Fig. 36-1B) and consists of the following steps (Grossman & Porth, 2014):

1. *Attachment/Binding:* In this first step, the GP120 and GP41 glycoproteins of HIV bind with the host's uninfected CD4+ receptor and chemokine coreceptors, usually CCR5, which results in fusion of HIV with the CD4+ T-cell membrane.
2. *Uncoating/Fusion:* Only the contents of HIV's viral core (two single strands of viral RNA and three viral enzymes: **reverse transcriptase**, integrase, and protease) are emptied into the CD4+ T cell.

3. *DNA synthesis:* HIV changes its genetic material from RNA to DNA through action of reverse transcriptase, resulting in double-stranded DNA that carries instruction for viral replication.

4. *Integration:* New viral DNA enters the nucleus of the CD4+ T cell and through action of integrase is blended with the DNA of the CD4+ T cell, resulting in permanent, lifelong infection. Prior to this, the uninfected person has been only exposed to, not infected with, HIV. With this step, HIV infection is permanent.

5. *Transcription:* When the CD4+ T cell is activated, the double-stranded DNA forms single-stranded messenger RNA (mRNA), which builds new viruses.

6. *Translation:* The mRNA creates chains of new proteins and enzymes (polyproteins) that contain the components needed in the construction of new viruses.

7. *Cleavage:* The HIV protease enzyme cuts the polyprotein chain into the individual proteins that make up the new virus.

8. *Budding:* New proteins and viral RNA migrate to the membrane of the infected CD4+ T cell, exit from the cell, and start the process all over.

In resting (nondividing) CD4+ cells, HIV survives in a latent state as an integrated **provirus** that produces few or no viral particles. These resting CD4+ T cells can be stimulated to produce new particles if something activates them, such as another infection. When a resting T cell that harbors this integrated DNA (also known as provirus) becomes activated against HIV or other microbes, the cell begins to produce new copies of both RNA and viral proteins. Consequently, whenever the infected CD4+ cell is activated, HIV replication and budding occur, which can destroy the host cell. Newly formed HIV released into the blood can infect other CD4+ cells.

A mutation of CCR5 that is common in Caucasians, but not other ethnic groups, has been identified. About 1% of Caucasians lack functional CCR5 and are highly protected against HIV infection even if exposed (although protection is not absolute); about 18% are not markedly protected against infection but, if infected, demonstrate significantly slower rates of disease progression. CCR5 levels on T cells influence HIV acquisition, disease progression rates, viral load, and immune recovery during ART (Gornalusse, Mummidi, Gaitan, et al., 2015).

HIV-1 mutates quickly, at a relatively constant rate, with about 1% of the virus's genetic material changing annually. HIV-1 exhibits substantial genetic diversity, and several different genotypes of HIV-1 exist throughout the world. There is a major group (group M), which consists of subtypes A through L, and a more diverse collection of outliers, which has been referred to as groups N and O. Subtype B HIV-1 viruses predominate in the Western world; this genetic variation is one of the major reasons why effective vaccine development has been such a challenge.

Stages of HIV Infection

There are five stages of HIV infection based on clinical history, physical examination, laboratory evidence (Selik et al., 2014), signs and symptoms, and associated infections and malignancies. See Table 36-2.

The period from infection with HIV to the development of HIV-specific antibodies is known as **primary infection** or **acute HIV infection** (previously known as the window period) and is part of stage 0 (Selik et al., 2014). Acute HIV infection is the interval between the appearance of detectable HIV RNA and the first detection of antibodies. Its duration also depends on the design of the antibody immunoassay and the sensitivity of the immunoassay during seroconversion (CDC, 2014b). Initially, there is a period during which those who are HIV positive test negative on the HIV antibody blood test, although they are infected and highly infectious, because their viral loads are very high. About 40% to 80% of patients develop clinical symptoms of a nonspecific viral illness (e.g., fever, fatigue, or rash) lasting 1 to 2 weeks. After 2 to 3 weeks, antibodies to the glycoproteins of the HIV envelope can be detected in the sera of people infected with HIV, but most of these antibodies lack the ability to totally control the virus. By the time neutralizing antibodies can be detected (stage 1), HIV-1 is firmly established in the host.

Primary or acute infection is characterized by high levels of viral replication, widespread dissemination of HIV throughout the body, and destruction of CD4+ T cells, which leads to dramatic drops in CD4+ T-cell counts (normally 500 to 1,500 cells/mm³ of blood). The host responds to the HIV infection through a CD4+ T-cell response that causes other immune cells, such as CD8+ lymphocytes, to increase their killing of infected, virus-producing cells. The body produces antibody molecules in an effort to contain the free HIV particles (outside cells) and assist in their removal. During this stage, the virus is widely disseminated in lymphoid tissue, and a **latent reservoir** within resting memory CD4+ T cells is created.

The amount of virus in the body after the initial immune response subsides is referred to as the **viral set point**, which results in an equilibrium between HIV levels and the immune response that may be elicited. This can last for years and is inversely correlated with disease prognosis. The higher the viral set point, the poorer the prognosis. After the viral set point is reached, a chronic stage persists in which the immune system cannot eliminate the virus despite its best efforts. This set point varies greatly from patient to patient and dictates the subsequent rate of disease progression; on average, 8 to 10 years can pass before a major HIV-related complication develops. In this prolonged, chronic stage, patients feel well and have few, if any, symptoms. Apparent good health continues because CD4+ T-cell levels remain high enough to preserve immune defensive responses, but over time, the number of CD4+ T cells continues to decrease.

Stage 2 occurs when CD4+ T-lymphocyte cells are between 200 and 499, stage 3 when the count drops below 200 cells/mm³ of blood and at this point, the person is considered to have AIDS for surveillance purposes. HIV disease progression is classified from less to more severe; once a case is classified into a surveillance severity stage, it cannot be reclassified into a less severe stage even if the CD4+ T-lymphocytes increase, which often occurs when a person receives ART. A stage 3 diagnosis has implications for services (e.g., disability benefits, housing, and food stamps), because these programs are often linked to living with severe immune dysfunction.

Assessment and Diagnostic Findings in HIV Infection

During the first stage of HIV infection, the patient may be asymptomatic or may exhibit various signs and symptoms such as fatigue or skin rash. Patients who are in later stages of HIV infection may have a variety of symptoms related to their immunosuppressed state. The staging system requires laboratory evidence of HIV infection in order to diagnose HIV or AIDS (see Table 36-2).

HIV Tests

Several screening tests are used to diagnose HIV infection, and others are used to determine the stage and severity of the infection. A serologic testing algorithm for recent HIV sero-conversion (STARHS) analyzes HIV-positive blood samples to determine whether an HIV infection is recent or has been ongoing. In 2006, the CDC (2006) released recommendations for routine HIV testing in health care settings. Subsequently, the U.S. Preventive Services Task Force (Moyer, 2013) recommended routine screening of all persons aged 15 to 65 years, as well as screening for younger or older persons who are at risk. There are three types of HIV diagnostic tests: antibody tests, antigen/antibody tests, and nucleic acid (RNA) tests. Antibody tests detect antibodies, not HIV itself, while antigen and RNA tests directly detect HIV. The updated CDC recommendations (2014b) tests for HIV antigens and HIV nucleic acid because studies from populations at high risk for HIV demonstrated that antibody testing alone might miss a considerable percentage of HIV infections detectable by virologic tests, especially during stage 0.

Blood tests can detect HIV infection sooner after exposure than oral fluid tests because the level of antibody in blood is higher than it is in oral fluid. Likewise, antigen/antibody and RNA tests detect infection in blood before antibody tests. Some newer antigen/antibody laboratory tests can sometimes find HIV as soon as 3 weeks after exposure to the virus. No antigen/antibody or RNA tests are available for oral fluid.

Follow-up testing is performed if the initial test result is positive to ensure a correct diagnosis. These tests include (CDC, 2015f):

- antibody *differentiation tests*, which distinguishes HIV-1 from antibodies
- *HIV-1 nucleic acid tests*, which looks for the virus RNA directly

Table 36-3 identifies common blood tests used for screening.

Since negative perceptions and judgments associated with being HIV infected continue to persist, stigma remains one

TABLE 36-3 HIV Screening Blood Tests

Laboratory Test	Indications
HIV-1/HIV-2 immunoassay	Tests for both HIV-1 and antibodies
HIV/1-HIV-2 antigen/antibody combination immunoassay	Tests for both antibody and virus for both HIV-1 and HIV-2
HIV-1 differentiation assay	Differentiates HIV-1 from HIV-2
HIV-1 nucleic acid amplification test	Tests directly for virus
HIV-1 p24 antigen	Tests directly for virus

HIV, human immune deficiency virus.
Adapted from Centers for Disease Control and Prevention. (2014b). Laboratory Testing for the Diagnosis of HIV Infection: Updated Recommendations. Available at: stacks.cdc.gov/view/cdc/23447. Published June 27, 2014.

Chart 36-7 HIV Test Results: Implications for Patients

Interpretation of Positive Test Results

- Antibodies to HIV are present in the blood (the patient has been infected with the virus, and the body has produced antibodies).
- HIV is active in the body, and the patient can transmit the virus to others.
- Despite HIV infection, the patient does not necessarily have AIDS.
- The patient is not immune to HIV (the antibodies do not indicate immunity).

Interpretation of Negative Test Results

- Antibodies to HIV are not present in the blood at this time, which can mean that the patient has not been infected with HIV or, if infected, the body has not yet produced antibodies (stage 0).
- The patient should continue taking precautions. The test result does not mean that the patient is immune to the virus, nor does it mean the patient is not infected; it just means that the body may not have produced antibodies yet. If viral test used, a negative result is more consistent with the conclusion that the patient is uninfected.

HIV, human immune deficiency virus; AIDS, acquired immune deficiency syndrome.

---

of the biggest social challenges (Chambers, Rueda, Baker, et al., 2015). When the result of the HIV antibody test is received, it is carefully explained to the patient in private (see Chart 36-7). All test results are confidential. Education and counseling about the test result and about preventing transmission are essential. The patient's psychological response to a positive test result may include feelings of panic, depression, and hopelessness. The social and interpersonal consequences of a positive test result can be devastating. The patient may lose their sexual partner, housing, and their job because of disclosure. He or she may be subjected to physical abuse and, although illegal, experience discrimination in employment as well as social ostracism. For these reasons and others, patients who test positive may need ongoing counseling as well as referrals for social, financial, medical, and psychological support services. They must be connected to health care services to evaluate their stage of HIV infection and develop the treatment plan. Patients whose test results are seronegative may develop a false sense of security, possibly resulting in continued high-risk behaviors or feelings that they are immune to the virus. These patients may need ongoing counseling to help modify high-risk behaviors and to encourage returns for repeated testing. Other patients may experience anxiety regarding the uncertainty of their status. In addition to screening for HIV, patients should be screened for other blood-borne infections such as hepatitis; other STIs such as syphilis; and other infections associated with T-cell immunity such as tuberculosis (TB).

Staging

Two surrogate markers are used routinely to assess immune function and level of HIV viremia: CD4$^+$ T-cell count (CD4$^+$ count) and plasma HIV RNA (viral load). CD4$^+$ count should be measured in all patients at entry into care. **Viral**

load tests use target amplification methods to quantify HIV RNA or DNA levels in the plasma. Target amplification methods include reverse transcriptase–**polymerase chain reaction** (RT-PCR) and nucleic acid sequence–based amplification (NAT). A widely used viral load test measures plasma HIV RNA levels. Currently, these tests are used to track viral load and response to treatment of HIV infection. RT-PCR is also used to detect HIV in high-risk seronegative people before antibodies are measurable, to confirm a positive EIA result, and to screen neonates. HIV culture or quantitative plasma culture and plasma viremia are additional tests that measure viral burden, but they are used infrequently. Viral load is a better predictor of the risk of HIV disease progression than the CD4+ count. The lower the viral load, the longer the time to AIDS diagnosis and the longer the survival time. The key goal of ART is to achieve and maintain durable viral suppression.

Treatment of HIV Infection

The U.S. Department of Health and Human Services Panel on Antiretroviral Guidelines for Adults and Adolescents (Panel) (2016) is composed of HIV specialists from across the country who regularly meet to review the latest scientific evidence. The CD4+ count serves as the major laboratory indicator of immune function and prophylaxis for opportunistic infections, and is the strongest predictor of subsequent disease progression and survival (Panel, 2016). New drugs that offer new mechanisms of action, improvements in potency and activity even against multidrug-resistant viruses, dosing convenience, and tolerability have been approved. The overarching goal of ART is to suppress HIV replication to a level below which drug-resistant mutations do not emerge; related goals are to (1) reduce HIV-associated morbidity and prolong the duration and quality of survival, (2) restore and preserve immunologic function, (3) maximally and durably suppress plasma HIV viral load, and (4) prevent HIV transmission (Panel, 2016). In the United States, ART is now recommended for all HIV-infected patients regardless of their viral load or CD4+ count (Panel, 2016). Optimal viral suppression is defined generally as a viral load persistently below the level of detection (HIV RNA less than 20 to 75 copies/mL, depending on the assay used). Clinicians, in partnership with patients, make treatment decisions based on a number of factors, including whether the patient has already taken ART or is ART-naive and the willingness of the patient to adhere to the lifelong treatment regimen.

Achieving viral suppression requires the use of ART with at least two, and preferably three, active drugs from two or more drug classes and should occur within the first 12 to 24 weeks of therapy especially if the patient is new to ART (Panel, 2016). More than 25 antiretroviral (ARV) drugs (see Table 36-4) in 6 classes are Food and Drug Administration (FDA) approved for the treatment of HIV infection. The different drug classes of ART target some of the steps in the HIV/host cycle (see Fig. 36-1). These six classes include the nucleoside/nucleotide reverse transcriptase inhibitors (step 3), non-nucleoside reverse transcriptase inhibitors (step 3), protease inhibitors (step 6), a fusion inhibitor (step 1), a CCR5 antagonist (step 1), and integrase strand transfer inhibitors (step 4). In addition, two drugs (cobicistat and ritonavir) are used to improve the pharmacokinetic profiles of some of the other ART drugs. Some pharmaceutical companies have combined two to three agents into one tablet or capsule. The Panel (2016) provides clear directions regarding which medications should be prescribed for both ART-naive and experienced patients.

The CDC estimates that only 36% of the people living with HIV in the United States are prescribed ART and that among these individuals, only 76% have suppressed viral loads (Panel, 2016). Viral loads are often not suppressed because the patient is not adhering to the treatment plan. Psychosocial barriers such as depression and other mental illnesses, neurocognitive impairment, low health literacy, low levels of social support, stressful life events, high levels of alcohol consumption and active substance use, homelessness, poverty, nondisclosure of HIV serostatus, denial, stigma, and inconsistent access to medications affect adherence to ART. Failure to adopt practices that facilitate adherence, such as linking medication taking to daily activities or using a medication reminder system or a pill organizer, is also associated with treatment failure (Panel, 2016). Simplifying treatment regimens and decreasing the number of medications that must be taken each day increase patients' adherence to therapy. Although antiretroviral regimens have become less complex, side effects create barriers to adherence and inadequate dosing can lead to viral resistance. It is difficult to predict patients' adherence to medication regimens, but a positive relationship between the patient and health care provider is associated with better adherence. Individualized plans of care that consider housing and social support issues, in addition to health indicators including possible drug–drug interactions, are essential. Self-reported adherence measures can distinguish clinically meaningful patterns of medication-taking behaviors; therefore, nurses should assess if patients can describe how they are taking their ART.

Chart 36-8 summarizes strategies that health care providers can encourage to promote treatment regimen adherence. Every health care encounter should be used as an opportunity to briefly review the treatment regimen, identify any new issues, and reinforce successful behaviors.

Laboratory tests evaluate whether ART is effective for a specific patient. An adequate CD4+ response for most patients on ART is an increase in CD4+ count in the range of 50 to 150 mm^3 per year, generally with an accelerated response in the first 3 months (Panel, 2016). Viral load should be measured at baseline and on a regular basis thereafter because viral load is the most important indicator of response to ART.

Adverse effects associated with all HIV treatment regimens include hepatotoxicity, nephrotoxicity, and osteopenia, along with increased risk of cardiovascular disease and myocardial infarction (see Table 36-4). Many of the antiretroviral agents may cause fat redistribution syndrome and metabolic alterations such as dyslipidemia and insulin resistance, which put the patient at risk for early-onset heart disease and diabetes. The fat redistribution syndrome (lipodystrophy) consists of lipoatrophy (localized subcutaneous fat loss in the face, arms, legs, and buttocks) and lipohypertrophy (central visceral fat [lipomata] accumulation in the abdomen, although possibly in the breasts, dorsocervical region [buffalo hump], and within the muscle and liver). Facial wasting, characterized as a sinking of the cheeks, eyes, and temples caused by

(*text continued on page 1037*)

TABLE 36-4 Antiretroviral Agents[a]

Generic Name (Abbreviation) and Trade Names (Italic)	Food Interactions	Adverse Effects
Nucleoside Reverse Transcriptase Inhibitors (NRTIs)		
abacavir (ABC) *Ziagen* *Trizivir (ABC/ZDV/3TC)* *Epzicom (ABC/3TC)* *Triumeq (ABC/3TC/DTG)*	Take without regard to meals.	Hypersensitivity reaction, which can be fatal; symptoms may include fever, rash, nausea, vomiting, diarrhea, abdominal pain, malaise or fatigue, loss of appetite, and respiratory symptoms such as sore throat, cough, shortness of breath.
didanosine (ddI) *Videx* *Videx EC*	Take half hour before or 2 hours after meals.	Pancreatitis, peripheral neuropathy, retinal changes, nausea, diarrhea, lactic acidosis with fatty degeneration of the liver, insulin resistance/diabetes.
emtricitabine (FTC) *Emtriva* *Atripla (FTC/EFV/TDF)* *Complera (FTC/RPV/TDF)* *Stribild (FTC/EVG/c/TDF)* *Truvada (FTC/TDF)* lamivudine (3TC) *Epivir* *Combivir (3TC/ZDV)* Epzicom (3TC/ABC) *Trizivir (ABC/3TC/ZDV)* stavudine (d4 T) *Zerit*	Take without regard to meals. Take on empty stomach to reduce side effects. Take with a snack. Take with a snack. Take without regard to meals. Take without regard to meals.	Minimal toxicity, hyperpigmentation/skin discoloration. Severe acute exacerbation of hepatitis. Minimal toxicity, lactic acidosis with hepatic steatosis. Peripheral neuropathy, lipodystrophy, pancreatitis, lactic acidosis with hepatic steatosis (higher incidence with d4 T than with other NRTIs), hyperlipidemia, rapidly progressive ascending neuromuscular weakness (rare).
tenofovir disoproxil fumarate (TDF) *Viread*	Take without regard to meals.	Asthenia, headache, diarrhea, nausea, vomiting, and flatulence; kidney insufficiency; lactic acidosis with hepatic steatosis.
Zidovudine (AZT or ZDV) *Retrovir* *Combivir (3TC/AZT)* *Trizivir (ABC/3TC/AZT)*	Take without regard to meals.	Bone marrow suppression; macrocytic anemia or neutropenia; nail pigmentation, GI intolerance, headache, insomnia, asthenia; lactic acidosis with hepatic steatosis.
Non-Nucleoside Reverse Transcriptase Inhibitors		
efavirenz (EFV) *Sustiva* *Atripla (EFV/TDF/FTC)*	Take on empty stomach.	Rash (rare cases of Stevens–Johnson syndrome have been reported), central nervous system symptoms (dizziness, somnolence, insomnia, abnormal dreams, confusion, abnormal thinking, impaired concentration, amnesia, agitation, depersonalization, hallucinations, and euphoria), increased transaminase levels, false-positive cannabinoid test, teratogenic in monkeys and potentially teratogenic in humans during first trimester of pregnancy.
Etravirine (ETR) *Intelence*	Take following a meal.	Rash, including Stevens–Johnsons syndrome, hypersensitivity reaction, nausea.
nevirapine (NVP) *Viramune* *Viramune XR*	Take without regard to meals.	Rash including Stevens–Johnson syndrome, symptomatic hepatitis including fatal hepatic necrosis has been reported. Single dose has been used in developing countries to prevent vertical transmission.
Rilpivirine (RPV) *Edurant* *Complera (RPV/TDF/FTC)*	Take with a meal of between 400 and 600 calories.	Rash, depression, insomnia, headache, hepatotoxicity.
Protease Inhibitors		
atazanavir (ATV) *Reyataz* *Evotaz (ATV/c)*	Take with a snack.	Indirect hyperbilirubinemia; prolonged PR interval (some patients experience asymptomatic first-degree AV block); EKG changes; hyperglycemia; fat maldistribution; possible increased bleeding episodes in patients with hemophilia. Check creatinine clearance.
darunavir (DRV) *Prezista* *Prezcobix (DRV/c)*	Take with a snack.	Skin rash (10%), Stevens–Johnson syndrome, diarrhea, nausea, headache, cold-like symptoms (including runny nose or sore throat), inflammation of the liver, abnormal liver function tests, fever, and abnormally high cholesterol and triglyceride levels have been reported.

TABLE 36-4 Antiretroviral Agents (continued)

Generic Name (Abbreviation) and Trade Names (Italic)	Food Interactions	Adverse Effects
fosamprenavir (FPV) *Lexiva*	Tablets may be taken with or without food.	Skin rash (19%), diarrhea, nausea, vomiting, headache, hyperlipidemia, transaminase elevation, hyperglycemia, fat maldistribution, possible increased bleeding episodes in patients with hemophilia.
indinavir (IDV) *Crixivan*	For unboosted IDV: Should be taken 1 hour before or 2 hours after meals; may take with skim milk or low-fat meal. For RTV-boosted IDV: Can be taken with or without food.	Nephrolithiasis, GI intolerance, nausea, indirect hyperbilirubinemia, hyperlipidemia, headache, asthenia, blurred vision, dizziness, rash, metallic taste, thrombocytopenia, alopecia, hemolytic anemia, hyperglycemia, fat maldistribution, possible increased bleeding episodes in patients with hemophilia.
lopinavir + ritonavir (LPV/r) *Kaletra*	Liquid forms are taken with a snack; no restrictions for tablet.	GI intolerance, nausea, vomiting, diarrhea, asthenia, hyperlipidemia (especially hypertriglyceridemia), elevated serum transaminase, hyperglycemia, fat maldistribution, possible increased bleeding episodes in patients with hemophilia, EKG changes.
nelfinavir (NFV) *Viracept*	Take with a snack.	Diarrhea, hyperlipidemia, hyperglycemia, fat maldistribution, possible increased bleeding episodes in patients with hemophilia, serum transaminase elevation.
ritonavir (RTV) *Norvir*	Take with a snack.	GI intolerance, nausea, vomiting, diarrhea, paresthesias (circumoral and extremities), hyperlipidemia (especially hypertriglyceridemia), hepatitis, asthenia, taste perversion, hyperglycemia, fat maldistribution, possible increased bleeding in patients with hemophilia. Lower doses used as a booster.
saquinavir (SQV) *Invirase*	Take with meals or within 2 hours after meal.	GI intolerance, nausea, diarrhea, abdominal pain and dyspepsia, headache, hyperlipidemia, elevated transaminase enzymes, hyperglycemia, fat maldistribution, possible increased bleeding episodes in patients with hemophilia, EKG changes.
tipranavir (TPV) *Aptivus*	Take with a snack.	Serious liver problems, bleeding on the brain, skin rash (21%), increased cholesterol and triglyceride levels, and changes in body fat; women taking birth control pills that contain estrogen may be more likely to develop a rash. Individuals with hemophilia may have increased bleeding. Take with RTV, if prescribed.
Fusion Inhibitor		
enfuvirtide (T-20) *Fuzeon*	Injected subcutaneously, so meals are not an issue.	Local injection site reactions—almost 100% of patients (pain, erythema, induration, nodules and cysts, pruritus, ecchymosis); increased rate of bacterial pneumonia; hypersensitivity reaction—symptoms may include rash, fever, nausea, vomiting, chills, rigors, hypotension, or elevated serum transaminases.
Integrase Inhibitor (INSTIs)		
Dolutegravir (DTG) *Tivicay*	Take without regard to meals.	Hypersensitivity reaction including rash, constitutional symptoms, and organ dysfunction, insomnia, headache.
Elvitegravir (EVG) *Vitekta* *Stribild (EVG/c/FTC/TDF)*	Take with a snack. Take with a snack.	Nausea, diarrhea. Nausea, diarrhea, renal impairment, decrease in bone density, acute exacerbation of hepatitis, lactic acidosis.
raltegravir (RAL) *Isentress*	Take without regard to meals.	Rash including Stevens–Johnson syndrome, diarrhea, nausea, headache, fever, insomnia.
CCR5 Antagonist		
Maraviroc (MVC) *Selzentry*	Take without regard to meals; requires CCR5 tropism blood test before starting.	Cough, fever, dizziness, headache, orthostatic hypotension, nausea, bladder irritation; possible liver problems and cardiac events; an increased risk for some infections; a slight increase in cholesterol levels.

GI, gastrointestinal; AV, atrioventricular; EKG, electrocardiogram.
^aThis information changes often. Check the Panel and also the U.S. Food and Drug Administration website, http://www.fda.gov/forpatients/illness/hivaids/ucm118915.htm) for current information when using ART.
Adapted from Panel on Antiretroviral Guidelines for Adults and Adolescents (Panel). (2016). Guidelines for the use of antiretroviral agents in HIV-1-infected adults and adolescents. Department of Health and Human Services. Retrieved on 5/12/16 at: www.aidsinfo.nih.gov/ContentFiles/AdultandAdolescentGL.pdf. Appendix B, Tables 1 through 6.

Chart 36-8 Promoting Adherence to ART

Strategies	Examples
Use a multidisciplinary team approach. Provide an accessible, trustworthy health care team.	• Nonjudgmental providers, nurses, social workers, pharmacists, and medication managers.
Strengthen early linkage to care and retention in care.	• Encourage health care team participation in linkage to and retention in care.
Assess patient readiness to start ART.	
Evaluate patient's knowledge about HIV disease, prevention and treatment and, on the basis of the assessment, provide HIV-related information.	• Consider the patient's current knowledge base, provide information about HIV, including the natural history of the disease, HIV viral load and CD4$^+$ count and expected clinical outcomes according to these parameters, and therapeutic and prevention consequences of nonadherence.
Identify facilitators, potential barriers to adherence, and necessary medication management skills before starting ART medication.	• Assess patient's cognitive competence and any impairment. • Assess behavioral and psychosocial challenges including depression, mental illnesses, levels of social support, high levels of alcohol consumption and active substance use, nondisclosure of HIV serostatus and stigma. • Identify and address language and literacy barriers. • Assess beliefs, perceptions, and expectations about taking ART (e.g., impact on health, side effects, disclosure issues, consequences of nonadherence). • Ask about medication taking skills and foreseeable challenges with adherence (e.g., past difficulty keeping appointments, adverse effects from previous medications, issues managing other chronic medications, need for medication reminders and organizers). • Assess structural issues including unstable housing, lack of income, unpredictable daily schedule, lack of prescription drug coverage, lack of continuous access to medications.
Provide needed resources.	• Provide or refer for mental health and/or substance abuse treatment. • Provide resources to obtain prescription drug coverage, stable housing, social support, and income and food security.
Involve the patient in ARV regimen selection.	• Review regimen potency, potential side effects, dosing frequency, pill burden, storage requirements, food requirements, and consequences of nonadherence. • Assess daily activities and tailor regimen to predictable and routine daily events. • Consider use of fixed-dose combination formulation. • Assess if cost/co-payment for drugs can affect access to medications and adherence.
Assess adherence at every clinic visit.	• Monitor viral load as a strong biologic measure of adherence. • Use a simple behavioral rating scale. • Employ a structured format that normalizes or assumes less-than-perfect adherence and minimizes socially desirable or "white coat adherence" responses. • Ensure that other members of the health care team also assess adherence.
Use positive reinforcement to foster adherence success.	• Inform patients of low or nondetectable levels of HIV viral load and increases in CD4+ cell counts. • When needed, consider providing incentives and rewards for achieving high levels of adherence and treatment success.
Identify the type of and reasons for nonadherence.	• Failure to fill the prescription(s). • Failure to understand dosing instructions. • Complexity of regimen (e.g., pill burden, size, dosing schedule, food requirements). • Pill aversion. • Pill fatigue. • Adverse effects. • Inadequate understanding of drug resistance and its relationship to adherence. • Cost-related issues. • Depression, drug and alcohol use, homelessness, poverty. • Stigma. • Nondisclosure. • Other potential barriers.
Select from among available effective treatment adherence interventions.	• Use evidence-based interventions to promote adherence. • Use adherence-related tools to complement education and counseling interventions (e.g., pill boxes, dose planners, reminder devices). • Use community resources to support adherence (e.g., visiting nurses, community workers, family, peer advocates). • Use patient prescription assistance programs. • Use motivational interviews.
Systematically monitor retention in care.	• Record and follow-up on missed visits.
On the basis of any problems identified through systematic monitoring, consider options to enhance retention in care given resources available	• Provide outreach for those patients who drop out of care. • Use peer or paraprofessional treatment navigators. • Employ incentives to encourage clinic attendance or recognize positive clinical outcomes resulting from good adherence. • Arrange for directly observed therapy (if feasible).

Adapted from Panel on Antiretroviral Guidelines for Adults and Adolescents (Panel). (2016). Guidelines for the use of antiretroviral agents in HIV-1-infected adults and adolescents. Department of Health and Human Services. Retrieved on 5/12/16 at: www.aidsinfo.nih.gov/ContentFiles/AdultandAdolescentGL.pdf. Table 13. Strategies to Improve Adherence to Antiretroviral Therapy and Retention in Care.

Figure 36-2 • Facial lipoatrophy.

the loss of fat tissue under the skin, may be treated by inject-able fillers such as poly-l-lactic acid (Sculptra) (see Fig. 36-2). These changes can disturb the body image of people living with HIV/AIDS and may be a reason they decline or stop ART nurses could use an instrument such as the assessment of body change distress (ABCD) questionnaire that assesses subjective report of bodily changes and body dissatisfaction and the impact of bodily changes on psychosocial variables, quality of life, and HIV self-care behaviors (Blashill, Wilson, Baker, et al., 2014).

 Concept Mastery Alert

Nurses must recognize the differences among common laboratory tests used to diagnose and assess HIV infection and guide therapy. For example, the EIA is a diagnostic screening test that determines the presence of antibod-ies to HIV. The RT-PCR test, which measures viral load, is used along with the CD4+ count, which indicates the level of immune dysfunction, to assess the stage and severity of HIV infection. It is important to assess the extent of damage to the immune system before initiation of ART and/or pro-phylactic treatment for opportunistic infections.

Drug Resistance

Drug resistance is the ability of pathogens to withstand the effects of medications that should be toxic to them. There are two major components of ART resistance: (1) transmission of drug-resistant HIV at the time of initial infection and (2) selective drug resistance in patients who are receiving non-suppressive regimens. Genotypic and phenotypic resistance assays are used to assess viral strains and inform selection of treatment strategies. Genotypic assays detect drug-resistant mutations present in relevant viral genes while phenotypic assays measure the ability of a virus to grow in different con-centrations of ART drugs. Resistance testing in persons who are chronically infected is recommended at the time of entry into HIV care. Although no definitive prospective data exist

to support the choice of one type of resistance testing over another, genotypic testing is generally preferred because of lower cost, more rapid turnaround time, the assay's ability to detect mixtures of wild-type and resistant virus, and the relative ease of interpreting test results. If therapy is deferred, repeat testing soon before initiation of ART should be con-sidered because the patient may have acquired drug-resistant virus (i.e., superinfection) (Panel, 2016).

Immune Reconstitution Inflammatory Syndrome

Immune reconstitution inflammatory syndrome (IRIS) results from rapid restoration of organism-specific immune responses to infections that cause either the deterioration of a treated infection or new presentation of a subclinical infection. This syndrome typically occurs during the initial months after beginning ART and is associated with a wide spectrum of organisms, most commonly mycobacteria, herpes viruses, and deep fungal infections. IRIS is characterized by fever, respiratory and/or abdominal symptoms, and worsen-ing of the clinical manifestations of an opportunistic infec-tion or the appearance of new manifestations. IRIS is treated with anti-inflammatory medications such as cortisone. The nurse should be alert to the possibility of IRIS, especially in the 3-month period after treatment with ART is initiated, because this syndrome is associated with significant morbidity and patients often require hospital admission.

Paradoxical tuberculosis-associated immune reconstitution inflammatory syndrome (TB-IRIS) is a serious complication that arises during successful ART in patients with HIV-TB co-infection who are receiving TB treatment. In the majority of patients, TB-IRIS occurs within the first few weeks of ART but can occur much later. Patients with HIV-TB co-infection with low CD4+ counts who start ART are at high risk of develop-ing TB-IRIS. Although the immunopathogenesis of TB-IRIS is still not completely understood, the explosive restoration of T-cell function is believed to play a distinct role (Goovaerts, Jennes, Massinga-Loembé, et al., 2015).

Clinical Manifestations

Patients with HIV/AIDS experience a number of symptoms related to the disease, side effects of treatment, and other comorbidities, including pancreatitis, hepatitis, and cardio-metabolic abnormalities. The clinical manifestations of HIV/AIDS are widespread and may involve virtually any organ sys-tem. Patients in stage 3 or AIDS (see Table 36-2) are severely immune depressed and can develop opportunistic infections. Nurses need to understand the causes, signs and symptoms, and interventions, including self-management strategies that can enhance the quality of life for patients throughout the dif-ferent stages of the illness. Symptom assessment tools can be used to assess patients' symptom intensity and severity. People with HIV/AIDS use a variety of self-management strategies to minimize common symptoms (Schnall, Wantland, Velez, et al., 2014) (see Chart 36-9).

Respiratory Manifestations

Shortness of breath, dyspnea (labored breathing), cough, chest pain, and fever are associated with various opportunis-tic infections, such as those caused by *Pneumocystis jirovecii*, *Mycobacterium avium-intracellulare*, cytomegalovirus (CMV), and *Legionella* species.

| Chart 36-9 | **NURSING RESEARCH PROFILE** |
Symptom Self-Management Using Technology

Schnall, R., Wantland, D., Velez, O., et al. (2014). Feasibility testing of a web-based symptom self-management system for persons living with HIV. *Journal of the Association of Nurses in AIDS Care*. 25(4), 364–371.

Purpose

The purpose of this study was to explore the feasibility of using a web-based tool to provide tailored symptom management strategies for persons living with HIV. The web-based system provided tailored strategies for six symptoms: (a) depression, (b) anxiety, (c) fatigue, (d) diarrhea, (e) neuropathy, and (f) nausea. The hypothesis was that using the tool would decrease symptom intensity and frequency.

Design

This quantitative study used repeated-measures to test the components of the web-based system on symptom frequency and intensity, use of symptom management strategies, and engagement with health care providers over a 12-week period. Symptom intensity and frequency was measured by the items related to the six symptoms using the HIV Sign and Symptom Check List-Revised tool. Engagement with care was measured by the Engagement with Health Care Provider Scale.

Findings

The average age of participants was 50 years; the majority were male and most had completed high school ($N = 42$). At baseline, the most frequently reported symptom was fatigue, followed by anxiety. There was a trend toward a decrease in symptom frequency over time for all symptoms except diarrhea, and engagement with health care providers improved. One purpose of a feasibility study is to demonstrate the ability to recruit and retain study participants, which was achieved. Forty-two participants were recruited in 30 days, which demonstrates the interest of patients to use web-based tools to assist with symptom self-management. Almost 80% of the participants completed the 12-week longitudinal study.

Nursing Implications

Web-based tools have the potential to support patients to self-manage symptoms and are accessible to anyone who can access the internet. Patients are interested in and willing to use the web-based tool to manage HIV-related symptoms. Use of this tool decreased symptom intensity and increased engagement with health care providers. This sample was not particularly well educated and yet the intervention was effective. Use of multiple sources of health information should be encouraged by nurses in order to support patients in becoming more informed in self-management strategies.

Pneumocystis Pneumonia

Pneumocystis pneumonia (PCP) is caused by *P. jirovecii* (formerly *P. carinii*) (Panel on Opportunistic Infections in HIV-Infected Adults and Adolescents [OI-Panel], 2015) and the incidence has declined substantially with widespread use of PCP prophylaxis, which is used to prevent PCP, and ART. The most common manifestations of PCP are subacute onset of progressive dyspnea, fever, nonproductive cough, and chest discomfort that worsens within days to weeks. In mild cases, pulmonary examination usually is normal at rest. With exertion, tachypnea, tachycardia, and diffuse dry (cellophane) rales may be auscultated. Oral thrush is a common co-infection. Fever is apparent in most cases and may be the predominant symptom. Hypoxemia is the most characteristic laboratory abnormality, along with elevated lactate dehydrogenase levels. Because clinical presentation, blood tests, and chest radiographs are not pathognomonic for PCP, and because the organism cannot be cultivated routinely, histopathologic or cytopathologic demonstration of organisms in tissue, bronchoalveolar lavage fluid, or induced sputum samples is required for a definitive diagnosis (OI-Panel, 2015).

Mycobacterium avium Complex

Mycobacterium avium complex (MAC) disease is a common opportunistic infection that typically occurs in patients with CD4+ T-lymphocyte (CD4+) cell counts less than 50 cells/mm³. MAC is caused by infection with different types of mycobacterium: *Mycobacterium avium*, *Mycobacterium intracellulare*, or *Mycobacterium kansasii*. Early symptoms may be minimal and can precede detectable mycobacteremia by several weeks and include fever, night sweats, weight loss, fatigue, diarrhea, and abdominal pain. A confirmed diagnosis of disseminated MAC disease is based on compatible clinical signs and symptoms coupled with the isolation of MAC from cultures of blood, lymph node, bone marrow, or other normally sterile tissue or body fluids (OI-Panel, 2015).

Tuberculosis

The estimated annual risk of reactivation with TB among those with untreated HIV infection and latent TB infection is 3% to 16% and approximates the lifetime risk for individuals without HIV infection who have latent TB infection. TB disease can occur at any CD4+ T-lymphocyte (CD4+ cell) count, although the risk increases with progressive immune deficiency. Testing for latent TB at the time of HIV diagnosis should be routine, regardless of an individual's risk of TB exposure. Individuals with negative diagnostic tests for latent TB who have stage 3 HIV infection should be retested once their CD4+ count increases due to ART. Screening for symptoms (asking for cough of *any* duration) coupled with chest radiography is recommended to exclude TB disease in a patient with a positive skin test or interferon-gamma release assays. Latent TB in a person with HIV infection is treated with isoniazid (INH), supplemented with pyridoxine (Aminoxin) to prevent peripheral neuropathy, for 9 months since it has proven efficacy, good tolerability, and infrequent severe toxicity.

TB disease can develop in the lungs as well as in extrapulmonary sites such as the central nervous system (CNS), bone, pericardium, stomach, peritoneum, and scrotum and initial diagnostic testing is directed at the anatomic site of symptoms or signs, such as the lungs, lymph nodes, and cerebrospinal fluid. TB in individuals with advanced immune deficiency can be rapidly progressive and fatal if treatment is delayed and such patients often have smear-negative sputum specimens. Therefore, after collection of available specimens for culture and molecular diagnostic tests, empiric treatment for TB is warranted in patients with clinical and radiographic presentation suggestive of HIV-related TB. Treatment of suspected TB in individuals with HIV infection is the same as for those who are HIV uninfected and should include an initial four-drug combination of isoniazid, rifampin (Rifadin), pyrazinamide, and ethambutol (Etibi) (OI-Panel, 2015).

Gastrointestinal Manifestations

The gastrointestinal manifestations of HIV infection and AIDS include loss of appetite, nausea, vomiting, oral and esophageal candidiasis, and chronic diarrhea. Gastrointestinal symptoms may be related to the direct inflammatory effect of HIV on the cells lining the intestines. Some of the enteric pathogens that occur most frequently, identified by stool cultures or intestinal biopsy, are *Cryptosporidium muris*, *Salmonella* species, *Isospora belli*, *Giardia lamblia*, cytomegalovirus (CMV), *Clostridium difficile*, and *M. avium-intracellulare*. In patients with AIDS, the effects of diarrhea can be devastating in terms of profound weight loss (more than 10% of body weight), fluid and electrolyte imbalances, perianal skin excoriation, weakness, and inability to perform the usual activities of daily living.

Candidiasis

Oropharyngeal and esophageal **candidiasis** (fungal infections) are common in patients with HIV infection. Oropharyngeal candidiasis is characterized by painless, creamy white, plaque-like lesions that can occur on the buccal surface, hard or soft palate, oropharyngeal mucosa, or tongue surface. Lesions can be easily scraped off with a tongue depressor or other instrument which is in contrast to lesions associated with oral hairy leukoplakia. In women with early-stage HIV infection, *Candida* vulvovaginitis usually presents the same as in women without HIV infection, with white adherent vaginal discharge associated with mucosal burning and itching of mild-to-moderate severity and sporadic recurrences (OI-Panel, 2015).

HIV Wasting Syndrome

Wasting syndrome is defined as the involuntary loss of more than 10% of one's body weight while having experienced diarrhea or weakness and fever for more than 30 days. Wasting refers to the loss of muscle mass, although part of the weight loss may also be due to loss of fat.

Oncologic Manifestations

Those with HIV/AIDS are at greater risk of developing certain cancers. These include **Kaposi sarcoma** (KS), lymphoma, and invasive cervical cancer. KS and lymphomas are discussed next. Cervical carcinoma is described later in the Gynecologic Manifestations section.

Kaposi Sarcoma

KS is caused by human herpesvirus-8 (HHV-8); affects eight times more men than women; and may spread through sexual contact. It involves the epithelial layer of blood and lymphatic vessels. AIDS-related KS exhibits a variable and aggressive course, ranging from localized cutaneous lesions to disseminated disease involving multiple organ systems.

Figure 36-3 • Lesions of the AIDS-related Kaposi sarcoma. Whereas some patients may have lesions that remain flat, others experience extensively disseminated, raised lesions with edema. From DeVita, V. T., Jr., Hellman, S., & Rosenberg, S. (Eds.). (1993). *AIDS: Etiology, diagnosis, treatment, and prevention* (4th ed.). Philadelphia: Lippincott Williams & Wilkins.

Cutaneous signs may be the first manifestation of HIV; they can appear anywhere on the body and are usually brownish pink to deep purple. They may be flat or raised and surrounded by ecchymosis (hemorrhagic patches) and edema (see Fig. 36-3). Rapid development of lesions involving large areas of skin is associated with extensive disfigurement and significant body image issues. The location and size of some lesions can lead to venous stasis, lymphedema, and pain. Ulcerative lesions disrupt skin integrity and increase discomfort and susceptibility to infection. The most common sites of visceral involvement are the lymph nodes, gastrointestinal tract, and lungs. Involvement of internal organs may eventually lead to organ failure, hemorrhage, infection, and death.

Diagnosis of KS is confirmed by biopsy of suspected lesions. Prognosis depends on the extent of the tumor, the presence of other symptoms of HIV infection, and the CD4⁺ count. Death may result from tumor progression. More often, however, it results from other complications of HIV infection.

AIDS-Related Lymphomas

AIDS-related lymphomas include both Hodgkin lymphoma and non-Hodgkin lymphoma. Non-Hodgkin lymphoma is more common. AIDS-related lymphoma is usually aggressive; there are three main types: diffuse large B-cell; B-cell immunoblastic; and small noncleaved cell lymphoma. Symptoms include weight loss, night sweats, and fever. The complete blood count might be abnormal and a biopsy will confirm the diagnosis (National Cancer Institute [NCI], 2015).

Neurologic Manifestations

HIV-related brain changes have profound effects on cognition, including motor function, executive function, attention, visual memory, and visuospatial function. Neurologic dysfunction results from direct effects of HIV on nervous system tissue, opportunistic infections, primary or metastatic neoplasm, cerebrovascular changes, metabolic encephalopathies, or complications secondary to therapy. Immune system response to HIV infection in the CNS includes inflammation, atrophy, demyelination, degeneration, and necrosis.

Chart 36-10 Care of the Patient With HIV Encephalopathy

Chronic Confusion

- Assess mental status and neurologic functioning.
- Monitor for medication interactions, infections, electrolyte imbalance, and depression.
- Frequently orient the patient to time, place, person, reality, and the environment.
- Use simple explanations.
- Instruct the patient to perform tasks in incremental steps.
- Provide memory aids (clocks and calendars).
- Provide memory aids for medication administration.
- Post activity schedule.
- Give positive feedback for appropriate behavior.
- Educate caretakers about orienting patient to time, place, person, reality, and the environment.
- Encourage the patient to designate a responsible person to assume power of attorney.

Disturbed Sensation

- Assess sensory impairment.
- Decrease amount of stimuli in the patient's environment.
- Correct inaccurate perceptions.
- Provide reassurance and safety if the patient displays fear.
- Provide a secure and stable environment.
- Educate caregivers about recognizing inaccurate sensory perceptions.
- Provide caregivers techniques to correct inaccurate perceptions.
- Instruct the patient and caregivers to report any changes in the patient's vision to the patient's health care provider.

Risk for Injury

- Assess the patient's level of anxiety, confusion, or disorientation.
- Assess the patient for delusions or hallucinations.
- Remove potentially dangerous objects from the patient's environment.
- Structure the environment for safety (ensure adequate lighting, avoid clutter, provide bed rails if needed).
- Supervise smoking.
- Do not let the patient drive a car if confusion is present.
- Instruct the patient and caregiver in home safety.
- Provide assistance as needed for ambulation and in getting in and out of bed.
- Pad headboard and side rails if the patient has seizures.

Self-Care Deficits

- Encourage activities of daily living within the patient's level of ability.
- Encourage independence, but assist if the patient cannot perform an activity.
- Demonstrate any activity that the patient is having difficulty accomplishing.
- Monitor food and fluid intake.
- Weigh patient weekly.
- Encourage the patient to eat, and offer nutritious meals, snacks, and adequate fluids.
- If patient is incontinent, establish a routine toileting schedule.
- Educate caregivers about meeting the patient's self-care needs.

Peripheral Neuropathy

Peripheral neuropathy is the most common neurologic symptom at any stage of HIV infection. It may be a side effect of some ART drugs, and may occur in a variety of patterns, with distal sensory polyneuropathy or distal symmetric polyneuropathy the most frequently occurring type. It can lead to significant pain of feet and hands and functional impairment. Patients use a variety of physical and psychological self-management strategies to minimize this symptom (Nicholas, Corless, & Evans, 2014).

HIV Encephalopathy

HIV encephalopathy was formerly referred to as AIDS dementia complex (see Chart 36-10). It is a clinical syndrome that is characterized by a progressive decline in cognitive, behavioral, and motor functions as a direct result of HIV infection. HIV has been found in the brain and cerebrospinal fluid (CSF) of patients with HIV encephalopathy. The brain cells infected by HIV are predominantly the CD4+ cells of monocyte–macrophage lineage. HIV infection is thought to trigger the release of toxins or lymphokines that result in cellular dysfunction, inflammation, or interference with neurotransmitter function rather than cellular damage.

Signs and symptoms may be subtle and difficult to distinguish from fatigue, depression, or the adverse effects of treatment for infections and malignancies. Early manifestations include memory deficits, headache, difficulty concentrating, progressive confusion, psychomotor slowing, apathy, and ataxia. Later stages include global cognitive impairments, delay in verbal responses, a vacant stare, spastic paraparesis, hyperreflexia, psychosis, hallucinations, tremor, incontinence, seizures, mutism, and death.

Confirming the diagnosis of HIV encephalopathy can be difficult. Extensive neurologic evaluation includes a computed tomography scan, which may indicate diffuse cerebral atrophy and ventricular enlargement. Other tests that may detect abnormalities include magnetic resonance imaging, analysis of CSF through lumbar puncture, and brain biopsy.

Cryptococcus Neoformans

A fungal infection, *Cryptococcus neoformans* is another common opportunistic infection among patients with AIDS, and it causes neurologic disease. Cryptococcal meningitis is characterized by symptoms such as fever, headache, malaise, stiff neck, nausea, vomiting, mental status changes, and seizures. Diagnosis is confirmed by CSF analysis.

Progressive Multifocal Leukoencephalopathy

Progressive multifocal leukoencephalopathy (PML) is a demyelinating CNS disorder that affects the oligodendroglia. Clinical manifestations often begin with mental confusion and rapidly progress to include blindness, aphasia, muscle weakness, paresis (partial or complete paralysis), and death. ART has greatly reduced the threat of mortality associated with this disorder.

Other Neurologic Disorders

Other infections involving the nervous system include *Toxoplasma gondii*, CMV, and *Mycobacterium tuberculosis* infections.

Depressive Manifestations

Depression and apathy are neuropsychiatric complications of HIV infection. Estimates suggest that the prevalence of current depression is between 30% and 40% in persons with HIV/AIDS. Similarly, apathy, which refers to reduced, self-initiated, cognitive, emotional, and behavioral activity, is also commonly reported among those living with a diagnosis of HIV with rates as high as 65% (Bryant, Whitehead, Burrell, et al., 2015). Alcohol and cocaine use—both current and former—have been associated with depression and apathy in this population, and depression has been associated with less adherence with ART.

Integumentary Manifestations

Cutaneous manifestations are associated with HIV infection and the accompanying opportunistic infections and malignancies. KS (described earlier) and opportunistic infections such as herpes zoster and herpes simplex are associated with painful vesicles that disrupt skin integrity. Molluscum contagiosum is a viral infection characterized by deforming plaque formation. Seborrheic dermatitis is associated with an indurated, diffuse, scaly rash involving the scalp and face. Patients with AIDS may also exhibit a generalized folliculitis associated with dry, flaking skin or atopic dermatitis, such as eczema or psoriasis. Many patients treated with the antibacterial agent trimethoprim–sulfamethoxazole (TMP–SMZ) develop a drug-related rash that is pruritic with pinkish-red macules and papules (Comerford, 2015). Patients with any of these rashes experience discomfort, have body image changes, and are at increased risk for infection from disrupted skin integrity.

Gynecologic Manifestations

Persistent, recurrent vaginal candidiasis may be the first sign of HIV infection in women. Past or present genital ulcers are a risk factor for the transmission of HIV infection. Women with HIV infection are more susceptible to genital ulcers and venereal warts and have increased rates of incidence and recurrence of these conditions. Ulcerative STIs such as chancroid, syphilis, and herpes are more severe in women with HIV infection. Human papillomavirus (HPV) causes venereal warts and is a risk factor for cervical intraepithelial neoplasia, a cellular change that is frequently a precursor to cervical cancer. Women who are HIV seropositive and have cervical carcinoma present at a more advanced stage of disease and have more persistent and recurrent disease and a shorter interval to recurrence and death than women without HIV infection.

Women with HIV are at increased risk for pelvic inflammatory disease, a reportable infection, and the associated inflammation may increase HIV transmission to the uninfected sexual partner. Moreover, women with HIV infection appear to have a higher incidence of menstrual abnormalities, including amenorrhea or bleeding between periods, than do women without HIV infection.

Medical Management

Treatment of Opportunistic Infections

Guidelines for the treatment of opportunistic infections should be consulted for the most current recommendations (OI-Panel, 2015). Although ART is highly effective in keeping the CD4+ cell count high, opportunistic infections continue to cause considerable morbidity and mortality for three main reasons: (1) many patients are unaware of their HIV infection and present with an opportunistic infection as the initial indicator of their disease, (2) some patients are aware of their HIV infection but do not take antiretroviral agents because of psychosocial or economic factors, and (3) others receive prescriptions for antiretroviral medications but fail to attain adequate virologic and immunologic response as a result of issues related to adherence, pharmacokinetics, or unexplained biologic factors.

Pneumocystis Pneumonia

Persons in stage 3 HIV infection should receive chemoprophylaxis to prevent PCP with trimethoprim–sulfamethoxazole (TMP–SMX) if they have CD4+ counts less than 200 cells/mm^3 or a history of oropharyngeal candidiasis (OI-Panel, 2015). Once the CD4+ count improves, prophylaxis can be discontinued. When a person is diagnosed with PCP, TMP–SMX is the treatment of choice, lowering the dose if there is abnormal renal function. Adjunctive corticosteroids (Prednisone) are indicated as early as possible, preferentially within 72 hours after starting specific PCP therapy. Treatment duration is usually 21 days; rates of adverse reaction to TMP–SMX are high including rash (30% to 55%) (including Stevens–Johnson syndrome), fever (30% to 40%), leukopenia (30% to 40%), hepatitis (20%), thrombocytopenia (15%), azotemia (1% to 5%), and hyperkalemia. Because long-term survival is possible for patients in whom ART is effective, individuals with AIDS and severe PCP should be given the option to choose mechanical ventilation and critical care management if their functional status is such that it would be appropriate, just as with patients without HIV infection. Paradoxical IRIS has been reported following PCP and starting ART (OI-Panel, 2015).

Mycobacterium avium Complex

Initial treatment of MAC disease should consist of two or more antimycobacterial drugs to prevent or delay the emergence of resistance. Clarithromycin (Biaxin) is the preferred first agent; however, azithromycin (Zithromax) can be substituted for clarithromycin when drug interactions or intolerance to clarithromycin preclude its use. Ethambutol is the recommended second drug (OI-Panel, 2015).

Cryptococcal Meningitis

Cryptococcosis among patients with HIV infection most commonly occurs as a subacute meningitis or meningoencephalitis with fever, malaise, and headache. Treating cryptococcosis consists of three phases: induction, consolidation, and maintenance therapy. The preferred induction treatment for cryptococcal meningitis and other forms of extrapulmonary cryptococcosis is the IV lipid formulation of amphotericin B in combination with fluconazole (Diflucan). Serious potential adverse effects of amphotericin B include anaphylaxis, kidney and hepatic impairment, electrolyte imbalances, anemia, fever, and severe chills. After at least 2 weeks of successful induction therapy—defined as substantial clinical improvement and a negative CSF culture after repeat lumbar puncture—amphotericin B and flucytosine can be discontinued. Follow-up or consolidation therapy is then initiated with oral fluconazole daily which should continue for at least 8 weeks (OI-Panel, 2015).

Cytomegalovirus Retinitis

Retinitis caused by CMV is a leading cause of blindness in patients with AIDS. Oral valganciclovir (Valcyte), IV ganciclovir (Cytovene), IV ganciclovir followed by oral valganciclovir, IV foscarnet (Foscavir), IV cidofovir (Vistide), and a ganciclovir intraocular implant coupled with valganciclovir are all effective treatments for CMV retinitis (OI-Panel, 2015). All of these drugs have significant toxicities (bone marrow suppression, neutropenia, hepatitis, renal toxicity, seizures, etc.) and are used with caution (Comerford, 2015).

Antidiarrheal Therapy

Although many forms of diarrhea respond to treatment, it is not unusual for this condition to recur and become a chronic problem for the patient with HIV infection. Therapy with octreotide acetate (Sandostatin), a synthetic analog of somatostatin, has been shown to effectively manage chronic severe diarrhea. High concentrations of somatostatin receptors have been found in the gastrointestinal tract and in other tissues. Somatostatin inhibits many physiologic functions, including gastrointestinal motility and intestinal secretion of water and electrolytes.

Chemotherapy

Kaposi Sarcoma

KS can be treated with local therapy, radiation therapy, chemotherapy, and biologic therapy depending upon the location of the lesions.

Lymphoma

There is no standard treatment for AIDS-related peripheral or systemic lymphoma. The treatment plan is adjusted for each patient and usually includes one or more of combination chemotherapy, high-dose chemotherapy and stem cell transplant. There are many ongoing clinical trials (using monoclonal antibodies; different treatment combinations) that patients with AIDS-related lymphoma may be eligible to enter (NCI, 2015).

Antidepressant Therapy

Treatment for depression in people with HIV infection involves cognitive behavioral therapy integrated with pharmacotherapy. If depressive symptoms are severe and of sufficient duration, treatment with antidepressants may be initiated. Antidepressants such as imipramine (Tofranil), desipramine (Norpramin), and fluoxetine (Prozac) may be used, because these medications also alleviate the fatigue and lethargy that are associated with depression. A psychostimulant such as methylphenidate (Ritalin) may be used in low doses in patients with neuropsychiatric impairment. Electroconvulsive therapy may be an option for patients with severe depression who do not respond to pharmacologic interventions.

Nutrition Therapy

Alterations in lipid metabolism are associated with HIV infection and ART. Malnutrition increases the risk of infection and the incidence of opportunistic infections. Nutrition therapy should be part of the overall management plan and should be tailored to meet the nutritional needs of the patient, whether by oral diet, enteral tube feedings, or parenteral nutritional support, if needed. As with all patients, a healthy diet is essential for the patient with HIV infection. For all patients with AIDS who experience unexplained weight loss, calorie counts and weight monitoring should be obtained to evaluate nutritional status and initiate appropriate therapy. The goal is to maintain the ideal weight and, when necessary, to increase weight.

Appetite stimulants have been successfully used in patients with AIDS-related anorexia. Megestrol acetate (Megace), a synthetic oral progesterone preparation, promotes significant weight gain and inhibits cytokine IL-1 synthesis. In patients with HIV infection, it increases body weight primarily by increasing body fat stores. Dronabinol (Marinol), which is a synthetic tetrahydrocannabinol (THC), the active ingredient in marijuana, has been used to relieve nausea and vomiting associated with cancer chemotherapy. After beginning dronabinol therapy, almost all patients with HIV infection experience a modest weight gain. The effects on body composition are unknown.

Oral supplements may be used when the diet is deficient in calories and protein. Ideally, oral supplements should be lactose free (people with HIV infection may be intolerant to lactose), high in calories and easily digestible protein, low in fat with the fat easily digestible, palatable, inexpensive, and tolerated without causing diarrhea. Nutritional supplements have been developed specifically for people with HIV infection and AIDS. Parenteral nutrition is the final option because of its prohibitive cost and associated risks, including possible infection.

Complementary, Alternative, and Integrative Health Therapies

People with HIV infection, along with 20% of all Americans, report the use of complementary, alternative, and integrative therapies within the last year (National Center for Complementary and Integrative Health [NCCIH], 2015). Combined with traditional therapies, these may improve the patient's overall well-being. However, there can be adverse drug–drug interactions between certain therapies (e.g., St. John wort) and some ART.

Although there is insufficient research on the effects of complementary, alternative, and integrative therapies, a growing body of literature reports benefits for modalities involving nutrition, exercise, psychosocial treatment, and Chinese medicine (NCCIH, 2015). See Chapter 7 for further information on complementary, alternative, and integrative therapies.

Many patients who use these therapies do not report their use to their health care providers. To obtain a complete health history, the nurse should ask about the patient's use of complementary, alternative, and integrative therapies. Patients may need to be encouraged to report their use of these therapies to their primary provider. Problems may arise, for example, when patients are using complementary, alternative, and integrative therapies while participating in clinical drug trials; alternative therapies can have significant adverse side effects, making it difficult to assess the effects of the medications in the clinical trial. The nurse needs to become familiar with the potential adverse side effects of these therapies. The nurse who suspects that complementary, alternative, and integrative therapies is causing a side effect needs to discuss this with the patient, the alternative therapy provider, and the primary provider. The nurse needs to view complementary, alternative, and integrative therapies with an open mind and try to understand the importance of this treatment to the patient. This approach will improve communication with the patient and reduce conflict.

Supportive Care

Patients who are weak and debilitated as a result of chronic illness associated with HIV infection and AIDS typically require many kinds of supportive care. Nutritional support may be as simple as providing assistance in obtaining or preparing meals. For patients with more advanced nutritional impairment resulting from decreased intake, wasting syndrome, or gastrointestinal malabsorption associated with diarrhea, parenteral feedings may be required. Imbalances that result from nausea, vomiting, and profuse diarrhea often necessitate IV fluid and electrolyte replacement.

Management of skin breakdown associated with KS, perianal skin excoriation, or immobility entails thorough and meticulous skin care that involves regular turning, cleansing, and applications of medicated ointments and dressings. To combat pain associated with skin breakdown, abdominal cramping, peripheral neuropathy, or KS, the nurse administers analgesic agents at regular intervals around the clock. Patients with a history of drug abuse will need to have tailored approaches for pain management. Relaxation and guided imagery may help reduce pain and anxiety.

Pulmonary symptoms, such as dyspnea and shortness of breath, may be related to opportunistic infections, KS, or fatigue. For patients with these symptoms, oxygen therapy, relaxation training, and energy conservation techniques may be effective. Patients with severe respiratory dysfunction may require mechanical ventilation. Before mechanical ventilation is instituted, the procedure is explained to the patient and the caregiver.

As noted previously, with the advent of ART, there are generally more positive outcomes than could be achieved a few years ago, and a patient mechanically ventilated has a reasonable likelihood of survival. However, if the patient decides to forego mechanical ventilation, their wishes must be followed. Ideally, the patient has prepared an advance directive identifying preferences for treatments and end-of-life care, including hospice care. If the patient has not identified preferences in advance, treatment options are described so that the patient can make informed decisions and have those wishes respected.

Nurses should anticipate that patients as well as family and friends will need support and time to share concerns. In some family systems, more than one person might be living with HIV/AIDS.

NURSING PROCESS

The Patient With HIV/AIDS

The nursing care of patients with HIV/AIDS is challenging because of the potential for any organ system to be involved due to infections or cancer. In addition, this disease is complicated by many emotional, social, and ethical issues. The plan of care for the patient with AIDS (see Chart 36-11) is individualized to meet the needs of the patient. Care includes many of the interventions and concerns cited in the Supportive Care section.

Assessment

Nursing assessment includes identification of potential risk factors, including a history of risky sexual practices or IV/injection drug use. The patient's physical status and psychological status are assessed. All factors affecting immune system functioning are thoroughly explored. A number of instruments can be used to assess symptoms and self-management strategies (Fierz, Nicca, & Spirig, 2013).

NUTRITIONAL STATUS

Nutritional status is assessed by obtaining a dietary history and identifying factors that may interfere with oral intake, such as anorexia, nausea, vomiting, oral pain, or difficulty swallowing. In addition, the patient's ability to purchase, prepare, and store food safely is assessed. Weight history (i.e., changes over time), anthropometric measurements, and blood urea nitrogen (BUN), serum protein, albumin, and transferrin levels provide objective measurements of nutritional status.

SKIN INTEGRITY

The skin and mucous membranes are inspected daily for evidence of breakdown, ulceration, or infection. The oral cavity is monitored for redness, ulcerations, and the presence of creamy-white patches indicative of candidiasis. Assessment of the perianal area for excoriation and infection in patients with profuse diarrhea is important. Wounds are cultured to identify infectious organisms.

RESPIRATORY STATUS

Respiratory status is assessed by monitoring the patient for cough, sputum production (i.e., amount and color), shortness of breath, orthopnea, tachypnea, and chest pain. The presence and quality of breath sounds are investigated. Other measures of pulmonary function include chest x-ray results, arterial blood gas values, pulse oximetry, and pulmonary function test results.

NEUROLOGIC STATUS

Neurologic status is determined by assessing level of consciousness; orientation to person, place, and time; and memory lapses. Mental status is assessed as early as possible to provide a baseline. The patient is also assessed for sensory deficits (visual changes, headache, or numbness and tingling in the extremities), motor involvement (altered gait, paresis, or paralysis), and seizure activity.

FLUID AND ELECTROLYTE BALANCE

Fluid and electrolyte status is assessed by examining the skin and mucous membranes for turgor and dryness. Dehydration may be indicated by increased thirst, decreased urine output, postural hypotension, weak and rapid pulse, and urine-specific gravity of 1.025 or more. Electrolyte imbalances, such as decreased serum sodium, potassium, calcium, magnesium, and chloride, typically result from profuse diarrhea. The patient is assessed for signs and symptoms of electrolyte deficits, including decreased mental status, muscle twitching, muscle cramps, irregular pulse, nausea and vomiting, and shallow respirations.

(text continued on page 1048)

Chart 36-11

PLAN OF NURSING CARE

Care of the Patient With AIDS

NURSING DIAGNOSIS: Diarrhea related to enteric pathogens or HIV infection
GOAL: Resumption of usual bowel habits

Nursing Interventions	Rationale	Expected Outcomes
1. Assess patient's normal bowel habits.	1. Provides baseline for evaluation	• Exhibits return to normal bowel patterns
2. Assess for diarrhea: frequent, loose stools; abdominal pain or cramping, volume of liquid stools, and exacerbating and alleviating factors.	2. Detects changes in status, quantifies loss of fluid, and provides basis for nursing measures	• Reports decreasing episodes of diarrhea and abdominal cramping • Identifies and avoids foods that irritate the gastrointestinal tract
3. Obtain stool cultures, and administer antimicrobial therapy as prescribed.	3. Identifies pathogenic organism; therapy targets specific organism	• Takes appropriate therapy as prescribed
4. Initiate measures to reduce hyperactivity of bowel.	4. Promotes bowel rest, which may decrease acute episodes	• Exhibits normal stool cultures • Maintains adequate fluid intake
a. Maintain food and fluid restrictions as prescribed. Suggest BRAT diet (*bananas, rice, applesauce, tea,* and *toast*).	a. Reduces stimulation of bowel	• Maintains body weight and reports no additional weight loss • States rationale for avoiding smoking
b. Discourage smoking.	b. Eliminates nicotine, which acts as bowel stimulant	• Enrolls in program to stop smoking • Uses medication as prescribed
c. Avoid bowel irritants such as fatty or fried foods, raw vegetables, and nuts. Offer small, frequent meals.	c. Prevents stimulation of bowel and abdominal distention and promotes adequate nutrition	• Maintains adequate fluid status • Exhibits normal skin turgor, moist mucous membranes, adequate urine output, and absence of excessive thirst
5. Administer anticholinergic antispasmodics and opioids or other medications as prescribed.	5. Decreases intestinal spasms and motility	
6. Maintain fluid intake of at least 3 L/day unless contraindicated.	6. Prevents hypovolemia	

NURSING DIAGNOSIS: Risk for infection related to immune deficiency
GOAL: Absence of infection

Nursing Interventions	Rationale	Expected Outcomes
1. Monitor for infection: fever, chills, and diaphoresis; cough; shortness of breath; oral pain or painful swallowing; creamy-white patches in oral cavity; urinary frequency, urgency, or dysuria; redness, swelling, or drainage from wounds; vesicular lesions on face, lips, or perianal area.	1. Allows for early detection of infection, essential for prompt initiation of treatment. Repeated and prolonged infections contribute to patient's debilitation.	• Identifies reportable signs and symptoms of infection • Reports signs and symptoms of infection if present • Exhibits and reports absence of fever, chills, and diaphoresis
2. Educate patient or caregiver about need to report possible infection.	2. Allows early detection of infection	• Exhibits normal (clear) breath sounds without adventitious breath sounds • Maintains weight
3. Monitor white blood cell (WBC) count and differential.	3. Elevated WBC count possibly associated with infection	• Reports adequate energy level without excessive fatigue
4. Obtain cultures of wound drainage, skin lesions, urine, stool, sputum, mouth, and blood as prescribed. Administer antimicrobial therapy as prescribed.	4. Assists in determining offending organism to initiate appropriate treatment	• Reports absence of shortness of breath and cough • Exhibits pink, moist oral mucous membranes without fissures or lesions
5. Instruct patient in ways to prevent infection.	5. Minimizes exposure to infection and transmission of HIV infection to others	• Takes appropriate therapy as prescribed • Experiences no infection
a. Clean kitchen and bathroom surfaces with disinfectants.		• States rationale for strategies to avoid infection
b. Clean hands thoroughly after exposure to body fluids.		• Modifies activities to reduce exposure to infection or infectious persons
c. Avoid exposure to others' body fluids or sharing eating utensils.		• Practices "safer sex" • Avoids sharing eating utensils and toothbrush
d. Turn, cough, and deep breathe, especially when activity is decreased.		• Exhibits normal body temperature
e. Maintain cleanliness of perianal area.		• Uses recommended techniques to maintain cleanliness of skin, skin lesions, and perianal area
f. Avoid handling pet excreta or cleaning litter boxes, birdcages, or aquariums.		• Has others handle pet excreta and cleanup
g. Cook meat and eggs thoroughly.		• Uses recommended cooking techniques
6. Maintain aseptic technique when performing invasive procedures such as venipunctures, bladder catheterizations, and injections.	6. Prevents hospital-acquired infections	

Chart 36-11

PLAN OF NURSING CARE (Continued)
Care of the Patient With AIDS

NURSING DIAGNOSIS: Ineffective airway clearance related to *Pneumocystis* pneumonia, increased bronchial secretions, and decreased ability to cough related to weakness and fatigue

GOAL: Improved airway clearance

Nursing Interventions	Rationale	Expected Outcomes
1. Assess and report signs and symptoms of altered respiratory status, tachypnea, the use of accessory muscles, cough, color and amount of sputum, abnormal breath sounds, dusky or cyanotic skin color, restlessness, confusion, or somnolence.	1. Indicates abnormal respiratory function	• Maintains normal airway clearance: • Respiratory rate <20 breaths/min • Unlabored breathing without the use of accessory muscles and flaring nares (nostrils) • Skin color pink (without cyanosis) • Alert and aware of surroundings • Arterial blood gas values normal • Normal breath sounds without adventitious breath sounds
2. Obtain sputum sample for culture as prescribed. Administer antimicrobial therapy as prescribed.	2. Aids in identification of pathogenic organisms	• Begins appropriate therapy • Takes medication as prescribed • Reports improved breathing • Maintains clear airway
3. Provide pulmonary care (cough, deep breathing, postural drainage, and vibration) every 2–4 hours.	3. Prevents stasis of secretions and promotes airway clearance	• Coughs and takes deep breaths every 2–4 hours as recommended
4. Assist patient in attaining semi- or high Fowler position.	4. Facilitates breathing and airway clearance	
5. Encourage adequate rest periods.	5. Maximizes energy expenditure and prevents excessive fatigue	• Demonstrates appropriate positions and practices postural drainage every 2–4 hours

6. Initiate measures to decrease viscosity of secretions.
  a. Maintain fluid intake of at least 3 L/day unless contraindicated.
  b. Humidify inspired air as prescribed.
  c. Consult with primary provider concerning the use of mucolytic agents delivered through nebulizer or intermittent positive pressure breathing treatment.
	6. Facilitates expectoration of secretions; prevents stasis of secretions	• Reports reduced breathing difficulty when in semi- or high Fowler position
		• Practices energy-conserving strategies and alternates rest with activity
		• Demonstrates reduction in thickness (viscosity) of pulmonary secretions
		• Reports increased ease in coughing up sputum

7. Perform tracheal suctioning as needed.	7. Removes secretions if patient is unable to do so	• Uses humidified air or oxygen as prescribed and indicated
8. Administer oxygen therapy as prescribed.	8. Increases availability of oxygen	• Indicates need for assistance with removal of pulmonary secretions
9. Assist with endotracheal intubation; maintain ventilator settings as prescribed.	9. Maintains ventilation	• Understands need for and cooperates with endotracheal intubation and the use of a mechanical ventilator • Verbalizes concerns about respiratory difficulty, intubation, and mechanical ventilation

NURSING DIAGNOSIS: Imbalanced nutrition: less than body requirements related to decreased oral intake

GOAL: Intake of nutrients sufficient to meet metabolic needs

Nursing Interventions	Rationale	Expected Outcomes
1. Assess nutritional status with height, weight, age; blood urea nitrogen, serum protein, albumin, transferrin, hemoglobin, and hematocrit levels; and cutaneous anergy.	1. Provides objective measurement of nutritional status	• Identifies factors limiting oral intake, and uses resources to promote adequate dietary intake • Reports increased appetite
2. Obtain dietary history, including likes and dislikes and food intolerances.	2. Defines need for nutritional education; helps individualize interventions	• States understanding of nutritional needs
3. Assess factors that interfere with oral intake.	3. Provides basis and directions for interventions	• Identifies ways to reduce factors that limit oral intake • Rests before meals
4. Consult with dietitian to determine patient's nutritional needs.	4. Facilitates meal planning	• Eats in pleasant, odor-free environment

(continued on page 1046)

Chart 36-11

PLAN OF NURSING CARE (Continued)

Care of the Patient With AIDS

Nursing Interventions	Rationale	Expected Outcomes

5. Reduce factors limiting oral intake.
  a. Encourage patient to rest before meals.
  b. Plan meals so that they do not occur immediately after painful or unpleasant procedures.
  c. Encourage patient to eat meals with visitors or others when possible.
  d. Encourage patient to prepare simple meals or to obtain assistance with meal preparation if possible.
  e. Serve small, frequent meals: 6/day.
  f. Limit fluids 1 hour before meals and with meals.
6. Instruct patient in ways to supplement nutrition: consume protein-rich foods (meat, poultry, fish) and carbohydrates (pasta, fruit, breads).
7. Consult with primary provider and dietitian about alternative feeding (enteral or parenteral nutrition).
8. Consult with social worker or community liaison about financial assistance if patient cannot afford food.
	5. Addresses factors limiting intake.
	  a. Minimizes fatigue, which can decrease appetite
	  b. Decreases noxious stimuli
	
	  c. Limits social isolation
	
	  d. Limits energy expenditure
	
	  e. Prevents overwhelming patient
	  f. Reduces satiety
	6. Provides additional proteins and calories
	
	7. Provides nutritional support if patient is unable to take sufficient amounts by mouth
	8. Increases availability of resources and nutrition
		• Arranges meals to coincide with visitors' visits
		• Reports increased dietary intake
		• Uses oral hygiene before meals
		• Takes analgesic agents before meals as prescribed
		• Identifies ways to increase protein and caloric intake
		• Identifies foods high in protein and calories
		• Consumes foods high in protein and calories
		• Reports decreased rate of weight loss
		• Maintains adequate caloric intake
		• States rationale for enteral or parenteral nutrition if needed
		• Demonstrates skill in preparing alternate sources of nutrition

NURSING DIAGNOSIS: Deficient knowledge related to means of preventing HIV transmission
GOAL: Increased knowledge concerning means of preventing disease transmission

Nursing Interventions	Rationale	Expected Outcomes

1. Instruct patient, family, and friends about routes of transmission of HIV.
 	
2. Instruct patient, family, and friends about means of preventing transmission of HIV.
  a. Avoid sexual contact with multiple partners, and use precautions if sexual partner's HIV status is not certain.
  b. Use condoms during sexual intercourse (vaginal, anal, oral–genital); avoid mouth contact with the penis, vagina, or rectum; avoid sexual practices that can cause cuts or tears in the lining of the rectum, vagina, or penis.
  c. Avoid sex with sex workers and others at high risk.
 	
  d. Do not use IV/injection drugs; if addicted and unable or unwilling to change behavior, use clean needles and syringes.
 	
  e. Women who may have been exposed to HIV through sexual or drug practices should consult with a physician before becoming pregnant; consider the use of antiretroviral agents if pregnant.
  f. Consider using PrEP
	1. Knowledge about disease transmission can help prevent spread of disease; may also alleviate fears.
	2. Reduces transmission risk
	
	  a. The risk of infection increases with the number of sexual partners, male or female, and sexual contact with those who engage in high-risk behaviors.
	  b. Risk of HIV transmission is reduced.
	
	  c. Many sex workers are infected with HIV through sexual contact with multiple partners or IV/injection drug use.
	  d. Clean needles and syringes are the only way to prevent HIV transmission for those who continue to use drugs. Taking precautions is important for those who are antibody positive to prevent transmitting HIV.
	  e. HIV can be transmitted from mother to child in utero; the use of antiretroviral agents during pregnancy significantly reduces perinatal transmission of HIV.
	  f. Taking ART before engaging in high-risk activity seems to protect against infection.
		• Patient, family, and friends state means of transmission
		• Reports and demonstrates practices to reduce exposure of others to HIV
		• Demonstrates knowledge of safer sexual practices
		• Identifies means of preventing disease transmission
		• States that sexual partners are informed about patient's positive HIV status in blood
		• Avoids IV/injection drug use and sharing of drug equipment with others
		• Understands risks and benefits associated with PrEP

Chart 36-11

PLAN OF NURSING CARE (Continued)

Care of the Patient With AIDS

NURSING DIAGNOSIS: Social isolation related to stigma of the disease, withdrawal of support systems, isolation procedures, and fear of infecting others

GOAL: Decreased sense of social isolation

Nursing Interventions	Rationale	Expected Outcomes
1. Assess patient's usual patterns of social interaction. 2. Observe for behaviors indicative of social isolation, such as decreased interaction with others, hostility, noncompliance, sad affect, and stated feelings of rejection or loneliness. 3. Provide instruction concerning modes of transmission of HIV. 4. Assist patient to identify and explore resources for support and positive mechanisms for coping (e.g., contact with family, friends, AIDS task force). 5. Allow time to be with patient other than for medications and procedures. 6. Encourage participation in diversional activities such as reading, television, or handcrafts.	1. Establishes basis for individualized interventions 2. Promotes early detection of social isolation, which may be manifested in several ways 3. Provides accurate information, corrects misconceptions, and alleviates anxiety 4. Enables mobilization of resources and supports 5. Promotes feelings of self-worth and provides social interaction 6. Provides distraction	• Shares with others the need for valued social interaction • Demonstrates interest in events, activities, and communication • Verbalizes feelings and reactions to diagnosis, prognosis, and life changes • Identifies modes of transmission of HIV • States ways of preventing transmission of HIV to others while maintaining contact with valued friends and relatives • Reveals HIV/AIDS diagnosis to others when appropriate • Identifies resources (i.e., family, friends, and support groups) • Uses resources when appropriate • Accepts offers of assistance and support • Reports decreased sense of isolation • Maintains contacts with those of importance to him or her • Develops or continues hobbies that effectively serve as diversion or distraction

COLLABORATIVE PROBLEMS: Opportunistic infections; impaired breathing; wasting syndrome and fluid and electrolyte imbalances; adverse reaction to medications

GOAL: Absence of complications

Nursing Interventions	Rationale	Expected Outcomes
Opportunistic Infections 1. Monitor vital signs including temperature. 2. Obtain laboratory specimens, and monitor test results. 3. Instruct the patient and caregiver about signs and symptoms of infection and the need to report them early.	1. Changes in vital signs such as increases in pulse rate, respirations, blood pressure, and temperature may indicate infection. 2. Smears and cultures can identify causative agents such as bacteria, fungi, and protozoa, and sensitivity studies can identify antibiotics or other medications effective against the causative agent. 3. Early recognition of symptoms facilitates prompt treatment and avoids extra complications.	• Exhibits stable vital signs • Experiences control of infection • Identifies signs and symptoms correctly and experiences no complications • Identifies signs and symptoms that are reportable to the primary provider • Takes medications as prescribed
Impaired Breathing 1. Monitor respiratory rate and pattern. 2. Auscultate the chest for breath sounds and abnormal lung sounds. 3. Monitor pulse rate, blood pressure, and oxygen saturation levels.	1. Rapid shallow breathing, diminished breath sounds, and shortness of breath may indicate respiratory failure resulting in hypoxia. 2. Crackles and wheezes may indicate fluid in the lungs, which disrupts respiratory function and alters the blood's oxygen-carrying capacity. 3. Changes in pulse rate, blood pressure, and oxygen levels may indicate the development of respiratory or cardiac failure.	• Maintains stable respiratory rate and pattern within the normal limits • Exhibits no adventitious lung sounds; normal breath sounds • Has stable pulse rate and blood pressure within normal limits, and exhibits no evidence of hypoxia • Oxygen saturation levels within acceptable range

(continued on page 1048)

Chart 36-11

PLAN OF NURSING CARE (Continued)

Care of the Patient With AIDS

Nursing Interventions	Rationale	Expected Outcomes
Wasting Syndrome and Fluid and Electrolyte Disturbances		
1. Monitor weight and laboratory values for nutritional status.	1. Weight loss, malnutrition, and anemia are common in HIV infection and increase risk of superinfection.	• Maintains stable weight • Eats a nutritious diet • Attains and maintains hemoglobin, hematocrit, and ferritin levels within normal limits • Sustains fluid and electrolyte balance within normal limits • Exhibits no signs and symptoms of dehydration
2. Monitor intake and output and laboratory values for fluid and electrolyte imbalance (potassium, sodium, calcium, phosphorus, magnesium, and zinc).	2. Chronic diarrhea, inadequate oral intake, vomiting, and profuse sweating deplete electrolytes. Small intestine inflammation may impair the absorption of fluids and electrolytes.	
3. Monitor for and report signs and symptoms of dehydration.	3. Fluid loss results in decreased circulating volume leading to tachycardia, dry skin and mucous membranes, poor skin turgor, elevated urine specific gravity, and thirst. Early detection allows early treatment.	
Reactions to Medications		
1. Monitor for medication interactions.	1. People with HIV infection receive many medications for HIV and for disease complications. Early detection of medication interactions is necessary to prevent complications.	• Experiences no serious side effects or complications from medications • Correctly describes medication regimen and complies with therapy, including adaptations in eating routines and type of food used with prescribed medications
2. Monitor for and promptly report side effects from antiretroviral agents.	2. Side effects from antiretroviral agents can be life threatening. Serious side effects include anemia, pancreatitis, peripheral neuropathy, mental confusion, and persistent nausea and vomiting. Corrective measures need to be instituted.	
3. Instruct the patient and caregiver in the medication regimen.	3. Knowledge of the medication purpose, correct administration, side effects, and strategies to manage or prevent side effects promotes safety and greater compliance with treatment.	

KNOWLEDGE LEVEL

The patient's level of knowledge about the disease, modes of disease transmission, and adherence to ART are evaluated. In addition, the level of knowledge of family (biologic and family of choice) and friends is assessed. The patient's psychological reaction to the diagnosis of HIV infection or AIDS is important to explore. Reactions vary among patients and may include denial, anger, fear, shame, withdrawal from social interactions, and depressive symptoms. It is often helpful to gain an understanding of how the patient has dealt with illness and major life stresses in the past. The patient's resources for support are also identified.

Diagnosis

NURSING DIAGNOSES

The list of potential nursing diagnoses is extensive because of the complex nature of HIV/AIDS. However, based on the assessment data, major nursing diagnoses may include the following:

- Impaired skin integrity related to cutaneous manifestations of HIV infection, excoriation, and diarrhea
- Diarrhea related to enteric pathogens or HIV infection
- Risk for infection related to immune deficiency

- Activity intolerance related to weakness, fatigue, malnutrition, impaired fluid and electrolyte balance, and hypoxia associated with pulmonary infections
- Chronic confusion related to cognitive changes associated with HIV encephalopathy
- Ineffective airway clearance related to infection, increased bronchial secretions, and decreased ability to cough related to weakness and fatigue
- Acute and chronic pain related to impaired perianal skin integrity secondary to diarrhea, KS, and peripheral neuropathy
- Imbalanced nutrition: less than body requirements related to decreased oral intake
- Social isolation related to stigma of the disease, withdrawal of support systems, isolation procedures, and fear of infecting others
- Grieving related to changes in lifestyle and roles and unfavorable prognosis
- Deficient knowledge related to HIV infection, means of preventing HIV transmission, ART, and self-management strategies

COLLABORATIVE PROBLEMS/POTENTIAL COMPLICATIONS

Possible complications may include the following:

- Opportunistic infections
- Impaired breathing or respiratory failure

- Wasting syndrome and fluid and electrolyte imbalance
- Adverse effects of medications
- Body image changes

Planning and Goals

Goals for the patient may include achievement and maintenance of skin integrity, resumption of usual bowel patterns, absence of infection, improved activity tolerance, coherent thought processes, improved airway clearance, increased comfort, improved nutritional status, increased socialization, expression of grief, increased knowledge regarding disease prevention and self-care, and absence of complications.

Nursing Interventions

PROMOTING SKIN INTEGRITY

The skin and oral mucosa are assessed routinely for changes in appearance, location and size of lesions, and evidence of infection and breakdown. The patient is encouraged to maintain a balance between rest and mobility whenever possible. Patients who are immobile are assisted to change position at least every 2 hours and more often as needed. Devices such as alternating-pressure mattresses and low-air-loss beds are used to prevent skin breakdown. Patients are encouraged to avoid scratching, to use nonabrasive, nondrying soaps, and to apply nonperfumed skin moisturizers to dry skin. Regular oral care is also encouraged.

Medicated lotions, ointments, and dressings are applied to affected skin surfaces as prescribed. Adhesive tape is avoided. Skin surfaces are protected from friction and rubbing by keeping bed linens free of wrinkles and avoiding tight or restrictive clothing. Patients with foot lesions are advised to wear cotton socks and shoes that do not cause the feet to perspire. Antipruritic, antibiotic, and analgesic agents are given as prescribed.

The perianal region is assessed frequently for impairment of skin integrity and infection. The patient is instructed to keep the area as clean as possible. The perianal area is cleaned after each bowel movement with nonabrasive soap and water to prevent further excoriation and breakdown of the skin and infection. If the area is very painful, soft cloths or cotton sponges may be less irritating than washcloths. In addition, sitz baths or gentle irrigation may facilitate cleaning and promote comfort. The area is dried thoroughly after cleaning. Topical lotions or ointments may be prescribed to promote healing. Wounds are cultured if infection is suspected so that the appropriate antimicrobial treatment can be initiated. Debilitated patients may require assistance in maintaining hygienic practices.

PROMOTING USUAL BOWEL PATTERNS

Bowel patterns are assessed for diarrhea. The nurse monitors the frequency and consistency of stools and the patient's reports of abdominal pain or cramping associated with bowel movements. Factors that exacerbate frequent diarrhea are also assessed. The quantity and volume of liquid stools are measured to document fluid volume losses. Stool cultures are obtained to identify pathogenic organisms.

The patient is counseled about ways to decrease diarrhea. The primary provider may recommend restriction of oral intake to rest the bowel during periods of acute inflammation associated with severe enteric infections. As the patient's dietary intake is increased, foods that act as bowel irritants, such as raw fruits and vegetables, popcorn, carbonated beverages, spicy foods, and foods of extreme temperatures, should be avoided. Small, frequent meals help to prevent abdominal distention. Medications, such as anticholinergic agents, antispasmodic agents, or opioids, can be prescribed to decrease diarrhea by reducing intestinal spasms and motility. Administering antidiarrheal agents on a regular schedule may be more beneficial than administering them on an as-needed basis. Antibiotics and antifungal agents may also be prescribed to combat pathogens identified by stool cultures. Assessment of the patient's self-care strategies is essential.

PREVENTING INFECTION

The patient and caregivers are instructed to monitor for signs and symptoms of infection: fever; chills; night sweats; cough with or without sputum production; shortness of breath; difficulty breathing; oral pain or difficulty swallowing; creamy-white patches in the oral cavity; unexplained weight loss; swollen lymph nodes; nausea; vomiting; persistent diarrhea; frequency, urgency, or pain on urination; headache; visual changes or memory lapses; redness, swelling, or drainage from skin wounds; and vesicular lesions on the face, lips, or perianal area. The nurse also monitors laboratory test results that indicate infection, such as the white blood cell count and differential. Cultures of specimens from wound drainage, skin lesions, urine, stool, sputum, mouth, and blood are obtained to identify pathogenic organisms and the most appropriate antimicrobial therapy.

IMPROVING ACTIVITY TOLERANCE

Activity tolerance is assessed by monitoring the patient's ability to ambulate and perform activities of daily living. Patients may be unable to maintain their usual levels of activity because of weakness, fatigue, shortness of breath, dizziness, and neurologic involvement. Assistance in planning daily routines that maintain a balance between activity and rest may be necessary. In addition, patients benefit from instructions about energy conservation techniques, such as sitting while washing or preparing meals. Personal items that are frequently used should be kept within the patient's reach. Measures such as relaxation and guided imagery may be beneficial because they decrease anxiety, which contributes to weakness and fatigue.

Collaboration with other members of the health care team may uncover other factors associated with increasing fatigue and strategies to address them. For example, if fatigue is related to anemia, administering epoetin alfa (Epogen) as prescribed may relieve fatigue and increase activity tolerance.

MAINTAINING COHERENT THOUGHT PROCESSES

The patient is assessed for alterations in mental status that may be related to neurologic involvement, metabolic abnormalities, infection, side effects of treatment, and coping mechanisms. Manifestations of neurologic impairment may be difficult to distinguish from psychological reactions to HIV infection, such as anger and depression.

If the patient experiences altered mental or cognitive status, family and support network members are instructed to speak to the patient in simple, clear language and give the patient sufficient time to respond to questions. Reorientation to surroundings and location is conducted as needed. The patient's support network is encouraged to orient the patient to the daily routine by talking about what is taking place during daily activities and providing the patient with a regular daily schedule for medication administration, grooming, meal times, bedtimes, and awakening times. Posting the schedule in a prominent area (e.g., on the refrigerator), providing nightlights for the bedroom and bathroom, and planning safe leisure activities allow the patient to maintain a regular routine in a safe manner. Activities that the patient previously enjoyed are encouraged. These should be easy to accomplish and fairly short in duration. The nurse encourages the social support network to remain calm and not to argue with the patient while protecting the patient from injury. Around-the-clock supervision may be necessary, and strategies can be implemented to prevent the patient from engaging in potentially dangerous activities, such as driving, using the stove, or mowing the lawn. Strategies for improving or maintaining functional abilities and for providing a safe environment are used for patients with HIV encephalopathy and other cognitive impairments (see Chart 36-10).

IMPROVING AIRWAY CLEARANCE

Respiratory status, including rate, rhythm, the use of accessory muscles, and breath sounds, as well as mental status and skin color, must be assessed at least daily. Any cough and the quantity and characteristics of sputum are documented. Sputum specimens are analyzed for infectious organisms. Pulmonary therapy (coughing, deep breathing, postural drainage, percussion, and vibration) is provided as often as every 2 hours to prevent stasis of secretions and to promote airway clearance. Because of weakness and fatigue, many patients require assistance in attaining a position (such as a high Fowler position or semi-Fowler position) that facilitates breathing and airway clearance. Adequate rest is essential to minimize energy expenditure and prevent excessive fatigue. The fluid volume status is evaluated so that adequate hydration can be maintained. Unless contraindicated because of kidney or cardiac disease, daily intake of 3 L of fluid is encouraged. Humidified oxygen may be prescribed, and nasopharyngeal or tracheal suctioning, intubation, and mechanical ventilation may be necessary to maintain adequate ventilation.

RELIEVING PAIN AND DISCOMFORT

The patient is assessed for the quality and severity of pain associated with impaired perianal skin integrity, the lesions of KS, and peripheral neuropathy. In addition, the effects of pain on elimination, nutrition, sleep, affect, and communication are explored, along with exacerbating and relieving factors. Cleaning the perianal area, as described previously, can promote comfort. Topical anesthetic medications or ointments may be prescribed. The use of soft cushions or foam pads may increase comfort while sitting. The patient is instructed to avoid foods that act as bowel irritants. Antispasmodic and antidiarrheal medications may be prescribed to reduce the discomfort and frequency of bowel movements. If necessary, systemic analgesic agents may also be prescribed. Pain from KS is frequently described as a sharp, throbbing pressure, and heaviness, if lymphedema is present. Pain management may include the use of nonsteroidal anti-inflammatory drugs (NSAIDs) and opioids plus nonpharmacologic approaches such as relaxation techniques. When NSAIDs are given to

patients who are receiving ART, hepatic and hematologic status must be monitored (Comerford, 2015).

The patient with pain related to peripheral neuropathy frequently describes it as burning, numbness, and "pins and needles." Pain management approaches may include topical ointments, opioids, and tricyclic antidepressants. Tricyclic antidepressants can be helpful in controlling the symptoms of neuropathic pain (Comerford, 2015). They also potentiate the actions of opioids and can be used to relieve pain without increasing the dose of the opioid.

IMPROVING NUTRITIONAL STATUS

Nutritional status is assessed by monitoring weight; dietary intake; and serum albumin, BUN, protein, and transferrin levels. The patient is also assessed for factors that interfere with oral intake, such as anorexia, oral and esophageal candida infection, nausea, pain, weakness, fatigue, and lactose intolerance. Based on the results of assessment, the nurse can implement specific measures to facilitate oral intake. The dietitian is consulted to determine the patient's nutritional requirements.

Control of nausea and vomiting with antiemetic medications given on a regular basis may increase the patient's dietary intake. Inadequate food intake resulting from pain caused by oral lesions or a sore throat may be managed by administering prescribed opioids and viscous lidocaine (the patient is instructed to rinse the mouth and swallow). Additionally, the patient is encouraged to eat foods that are easy to swallow and to avoid spicy or sticky food items and foods that are excessively hot or cold. Oral hygiene before and after meals is encouraged. If fatigue and weakness interfere with intake, the nurse encourages the patient to rest before meals. If the patient is hospitalized, meals should be scheduled so that they do not occur immediately after painful or unpleasant procedures. The patient with diarrhea and abdominal cramping is encouraged to avoid foods that stimulate intestinal motility and abdominal distention, such as fiber-rich foods or lactose, if the patient is intolerant to lactose. The patient is instructed about ways to enhance the nutritional value of meals. Adding eggs, butter, or fortified milk (milk to which powdered skim milk has been added to increase the caloric content) to gravies, soups, or milkshakes can provide additional calories and protein. High-calorie, nutritional foods such as puddings, powders, milkshakes, and nutritional supplements may also be useful. Patients who cannot maintain their nutritional status through oral intake may require enteral feedings or parenteral nutrition.

DECREASING THE SENSE OF ISOLATION

People with AIDS are at risk for double stigmatization. They have what society refers to as a "dreaded disease," and they may have a lifestyle that differs from what is considered acceptable by many people. The diagnosis might prompt disclosure about hidden lifestyles or behaviors to family, friends, coworkers, and health care providers. As a result, people with HIV infection may be overwhelmed with emotions such as anxiety, guilt, shame, and fear. They also may be faced with multiple losses, such as loss of financial security, normal roles and functions, self-esteem, privacy, ability to control bodily functions, ability to interact meaningfully with the environment, and sexual functioning as well as rejection by sexual partners, family, and friends. Some patients may harbor feelings of guilt because of their lifestyle or because they may have infected others in current or previous relationships. Other patients may feel anger toward sexual partners who transmitted the virus to them. Infection control measures used in the hospital or at home may further contribute to the patient's emotional isolation. Any or all of these stressors may cause the patient with AIDS to withdraw both physically and emotionally from social contact.

Nurses are in a key position to provide an atmosphere of acceptance and understanding for people with AIDS and their social networks. The patient's usual level of social interaction is assessed as early as possible to provide a baseline for monitoring changes in behaviors that suggest social isolation (e.g., decreased interaction with staff or family, hostility, nonadherence). Patients are encouraged to express feelings of isolation and loneliness, with the assurance that these feelings are not unique or abnormal.

Providing information about how to protect themselves and others may help patients avoid social isolation. Patients, family, and friends must be reassured that HIV is not spread through casual contact. Education of ancillary personnel, nurses, and physicians helps reduce factors that might contribute to patients' feelings of isolation. Patient care conferences that address the psychosocial issues associated with HIV/AIDS may help sensitize the health care team to patients' needs.

COPING WITH GRIEF

The nurse can help the patient verbalize feelings and explore and identify resources for support and mechanisms for coping, especially when the patient is grieving anticipated losses. The patient is encouraged to maintain contact with family, friends, and coworkers and to use local or national AIDS support groups and hotlines. If possible, losses are identified and addressed. The patient is encouraged to continue usual activities whenever possible. Consultations with mental health counselors are useful for many patients and their families.

IMPROVING KNOWLEDGE OF HIV

The patient and family are educated about HIV infection, means of preventing HIV transmission, ART, and appropriate self-care measures. Information about the purpose of the medications, their correct administration, side effects, and strategies to manage or prevent side effects is provided. The patient is instructed to avoid others with active infections, such as upper respiratory infections.

MONITORING AND MANAGING POTENTIAL COMPLICATIONS

Opportunistic Infections. Patients who are severely immunosuppressed are at risk for opportunistic infections. Therefore, anti-infective agents may be prescribed and laboratory tests obtained to monitor their effect. Signs and symptoms of opportunistic infections, including fever, malaise, difficulty breathing, nausea or vomiting, diarrhea, difficulty swallowing, and any occurrences of swelling or discharge, should be reported as treated as indicated.

Respiratory Failure. Impaired breathing is a major complication that increases the patient's discomfort and anxiety and may lead to respiratory and cardiac failure. The respiratory rate and pattern are monitored, and the lungs are auscultated for abnormal breath sounds. The patient is instructed to report shortness of breath and increasing difficulty in carrying out usual activities. Pulse rate and rhythm, blood pressure, and oxygen saturation are monitored. Suctioning and oxygen therapy may be prescribed to ensure an adequate airway and to prevent hypoxia. Mechanical ventilation may be necessary for the patient who cannot maintain adequate ventilation as a result of pulmonary infection, fluid and electrolyte imbalance, or respiratory muscle weakness. Arterial blood gas values are used to guide ventilator settings. If the patient is intubated, methods must be established to allow communication with the nurse and others. The patient receiving mechanical ventilation will require support to cope with the stress associated with intubation and ventilator assistance. The use of mechanical ventilation should be consistent with the patient's decisions about end-of-life treatment. Further discussion of end-of-life care can be found in Chapter 16.

Wasting Syndrome. Wasting syndrome and fluid and electrolyte disturbances, including dehydration, are common complications of stage 3 of infection. The patient's nutritional and electrolyte status is evaluated by monitoring weight gains or losses, skin turgor, ferritin levels, hemoglobin and hematocrit values, and electrolyte levels. Fluid and electrolyte status is monitored on an ongoing basis; fluid intake and output and urine-specific gravity may be monitored daily if the patient is hospitalized with complications. The skin is assessed for dryness and adequate turgor. Vital signs are monitored for decreased systolic blood pressure or increased pulse rate on sitting or standing. Signs and symptoms of electrolyte disturbances, such as muscle cramping, weakness, irregular pulse, decreased mental status, nausea, and vomiting, are documented and reported to the primary provider. Serum electrolyte values are monitored, and abnormalities are reported.

The nurse helps the patient select foods that will replenish electrolytes, such as oranges and bananas (potassium) and cheese and soups (sodium). A fluid intake of 3 L or more per day, unless contraindicated, is encouraged to replace fluid lost with diarrhea, and measures to control diarrhea are initiated. If fluid and electrolyte imbalances persist, the nurse administers IV fluids and electrolytes as prescribed. Effects of parenteral therapy are monitored.

Side Effects of Medications. Adverse effects are of concern in patients who receive many medications to treat HIV infection or its complications. Many medications can cause severe toxic effects. Patients and their caregivers need to know which signs and symptoms of side effects should be reported immediately to their primary provider (see Table 36-4).

In addition to medications used to treat HIV infection, other medications that may be required include opioids, tricyclic antidepressants, and NSAIDs for pain relief; medications for treatment of opportunistic infections; antihistamines (diphenhydramine [Benadryl]) for relief of pruritus; acetaminophen (Tylenol) or aspirin for management of fever; and antiemetic agents for control of nausea and vomiting. Concurrent use of these medications can cause many drug interactions, resulting in hepatic and hematologic abnormalities. Therefore, careful monitoring of laboratory test results is essential.

During each contact with the patient, the nurse not only asks about side effects, but also about how well the patient is adhering to the medication regimen. To promote adherence, the nurse should assist the patient to organize and plan the medication schedule.

Body Image Changes. Body image changes often occur in patients with HIV and are an important collaborative problem. The nurse helps the patient verbalize feelings and explore and identify resources for support and mechanisms for coping with body image changes. Consultations with mental health counselors may be indicated for patients adjusting to body image changes.

PROMOTING, HOME, COMMUNITY-BASED, AND TRANSITIONAL CARE

Educating Patients About Self-Care. Patients, families, and friends are educated about the routes of transmission of HIV. As discussed earlier, the nurse discusses precautions the patient can use to avoid transmitting HIV sexually (see Charts 36-2 and 36-3) or through sharing of body fluids, especially blood. Patients and their families or caregivers must receive instructions about how to prevent disease transmission, including handwashing techniques and methods for safely handling and disposing of items soiled with body fluids. Clear guidelines about avoiding and controlling infection, keeping regular health care appointments, symptom management, nutrition, rest, and exercise are necessary (see Chart 36-12). The importance of personal and environmental hygiene is emphasized. Caregivers are taught hand hygiene and appropriate infection prevention precautions (see Chapter 71, Charts 71-1 and 71-2). Kitchen and bathroom surfaces should be cleaned regularly with disinfectants to prevent growth of fungi and bacteria. Patients with pets are encouraged to have another person clean areas soiled by animals, such as birdcages and litter boxes. If this is not possible, patients should use gloves to clean the area and then wash their hands afterward. Patients are advised to avoid exposure to others who are sick or who have been recently vaccinated, especially with live vaccine. The importance of avoiding smoking, excessive alcohol, and over-the-counter and street drugs is emphasized. Patients who are HIV positive or who inject drugs are instructed not to donate blood. IV/injection drug users who are unwilling to stop using drugs are advised to avoid sharing drug equipment with others.

Caregivers in the home are taught how to administer medications, including IV preparations. The medication regimens used for patients with HIV infection and AIDS are often complex and expensive. Patients receiving combination therapies for the treatment of HIV infection and its complications require careful education about the importance of taking medications as prescribed and explanations and assistance in fitting the medication regimen into their lives (see Chart 36-8). If the patient requires enteral or parenteral nutrition, instruction is provided to the patient and family about how to administer nutritional therapies at home. Nurses provide ongoing education and support for the patient and family.

Continuing and Transitional Care. Many people with HIV/AIDS remain in their community and continue their usual daily activities, whereas others can no longer work or maintain their independence. Families or caregivers may need assistance in providing supportive care. Many community-based organizations provide a variety of services for people living with HIV infection and AIDS; nurses can help identify these services.

Chart 36-12 — **HOME CARE CHECKLIST**

Infection Prevention for the Patient With Immune Deficiency

At the completion of education, the patient and/or caregiver will be able to:

- State the impact of immune deficiency on physiologic functioning, ADLs, IADLs, roles, relationships, and spirituality.
- State changes in lifestyle (e.g., hygiene, activity) necessary to decrease risk for infection.
  - Maintain good hand hygiene technique before eating, after using the bathroom, and before and after performing health care procedures.
  - Maintain total body hygiene and foot care to prevent bacterial and fungal diseases.
  - Maintain skin integrity, using cream and emollients to prevent or manage dry, chafed, or cracked skin.
  - Maintain good oral hygiene and dental checkups.
  - Avoid people with infections, recent vaccinations, and crowds.
  - Perform deep breathing; use incentive spirometer every 4 hours while awake if mobility is restricted.
  - Provide adequate lubrication with gentle vaginal manipulation during sexual intercourse; avoid anal intercourse.
- State changes in home environment necessary to decrease risk for infection.
  - Avoid cleaning birdcages and litter boxes; consider avoiding garden work (soil) and fresh flowers in stagnant water.
  - Identify the rationale for frequent cleaning of kitchen and bathroom surfaces with disinfectant.

- Verbalize understanding of ways to maintain a nutritious diet and adequate calories and necessary changes to decrease risk of infection.
  - State the reason for avoiding the eating of raw fruits and vegetables, cooking all foods thoroughly, and immediately refrigerating all leftover food.
- Identify rationale and benefits of avoiding alcohol, tobacco, and unprescribed medications.
- State the name, dose, side effects, frequency, and schedule for all medications.
- Verbalize ways to cope with stress successfully, plans for regular exercise, and rationale for obtaining adequate rest.
- Identify signs and symptoms of infection to report to the primary provider, such as fever; chills; wet or dry cough; breathing problems; white patches in the mouth; swollen glands; nausea; vomiting; persistent abdominal pain; persistent diarrhea; problems with urination or changes in the character of the urine; red, swollen, or draining wounds; sores or lesions on the body; persistent vaginal discharge with or without itching; and severe fatigue.
- Demonstrate how to monitor for signs of infection.
- Describe to whom, how, and when to report signs of infection.
- Describe appropriate actions to take should infection occur.

ADL, activities of daily living; IADL, independent activities of daily living.

Home, community-based, transitional, and hospice nurses are in an excellent position to provide the support and guidance that is so often needed in the home setting. Home care nurses are key to the safe and effective administration of parenteral antibiotics, chemotherapy, and nutrition in the home.

During home visits, the nurse assesses the patient's physical and emotional status and home environment. The patient's adherence to the therapeutic regimen is assessed, and strategies are suggested to assist with adherence. The patient is assessed for progression of disease and for adverse side effects of medications. Previous education is reinforced, and the importance of keeping follow-up appointments is stressed.

Complex wound care or respiratory care may be required in the home. Patients and families are often unable to meet these skilled care needs without assistance. Nurses may refer patients to community programs that offer a range of services for patients, friends, and families, including help with housekeeping, hygiene, and meals; transportation and shopping; individual and group therapy; support for caregivers; telephone networks for the homebound; and legal and financial assistance. These services are typically provided by both professionals and nonprofessional volunteers. A social worker may be consulted to identify sources of financial support, if needed.

Home care and hospice nurses are increasingly called on to provide physical and emotional support to patients and families as patients with AIDS enter the terminal stages of disease. This support takes on special meaning when people with AIDS lose friends and when family members fear the disease or feel anger concerning the patient's lifestyle. The nurse encourages the patient and family to discuss end-of-life decisions and to ensure that care is consistent with those decisions, all comfort measures are employed, and the patient is treated with dignity at all times.

Evaluation

Expected patient outcomes may include:

1. Maintains skin integrity
2. Resumes usual bowel habits
3. Experiences no infections
4. Maintains adequate level of activity tolerance
5. Maintains usual thought processes
6. Maintains effective airway clearance
7. Experiences increased sense of comfort and less pain
8. Maintains adequate nutritional status
9. Experiences decreased sense of social isolation
10. Progresses through grieving process
11. Reports increased understanding of AIDS, prevention of HIV transmission, and ART, and participates in self-management strategies as possible
12. Remains free of complications

Detailed outcomes are included in the plan of nursing care for a patient with AIDS (see Chart 36-11).

 Concept Mastery Alert

 For further review, visit thePoint. to view an interactive tutorial on HIV and AIDS.

Emotional and Ethical Concerns

Nurses in all settings are called on to provide care for patients with HIV infection. In doing so, they encounter not only the physical challenges of this epidemic but also emotional and ethical concerns. The concerns raised by health care professionals involve issues such as fear of infection, responsibility for giving care, values clarification, confidentiality, developmental stages of patients and caregivers, and poor prognostic outcomes.

Many patients with HIV infection have engaged in "stigmatized" behaviors. Because these behaviors challenge some traditional religious and moral values, nurses may feel reluctant to care for these patients. In addition, health care providers may still have fear and anxiety about disease transmission despite education concerning infection control and the low incidence of transmission to health care providers (see Chart 36-13). Nurses are encouraged to examine their personal beliefs and to use the process of values clarification to approach controversial issues (see Chapter 3, Chart 3-6). The American Nurses Association's Code of Ethics for Nurses (ANA, 2015) provides guidance including the first provision which states, "The nurse practices with compassion and respect for the inherent dignity, worth, and unique attributes of every person" (p.1).

Nurses are responsible for protecting the patient's right to privacy by safeguarding confidential information. Inadvertent disclosure of confidential patient information may result in personal, financial, and emotional hardships for the patient. The controversy surrounding confidentiality concerns the circumstances in which information may be disclosed to others. Health care team members need accurate patient information to conduct assessment, planning, implementation, and evaluation of patient care. Failure to disclose HIV status could compromise the quality of patient care. Sexual partners of patients infected with HIV should know about the potential for infection and the need to engage in safer sex practices, as well as the possible need for testing and health care. Nurses are advised to discuss concerns about confidentiality with nurse administrators and to consult professional nursing organizations such as the Association of Nurses in AIDS Care and legal experts in their state to identify the most appropriate course of action.

During the early years of the AIDS epidemic, the mortality rate was high. But medication advances have controlled the disease progression, resulting in what is called "functional cure" or HIV remission, which is characterized by viral loads at low or undetectable levels (Vanham, Buvé, Florence, et al., 2014). Many strategies have been used by nurses to cope with the stress associated with caring for patients with AIDS. Education and provision of up-to-date information help to alleviate apprehension and prepare nurses to deliver safe, high-quality patient care. Interdisciplinary meetings allow participants to support one another and provide comprehensive patient care. Staff support groups give nurses an opportunity to solve problems and explore values and feelings about caring for patients with AIDS and their families; they also provide a forum for grieving. Other sources of support include nursing administrators, peers, and spiritual advisors.

Chart 36-13 ETHICAL DILEMMA
Under What Circumstances May a Nurse Refuse to Care for a Patient?

Case Scenario

You are the charge nurse in the Intensive Care Unit (ICU). A 52-year-old male patient, who is married but is bisexual, is admitted with pneumocystic pneumonia. His bisexual status is unknown to his spouse. He appears malnourished and emaciated. His laboratory findings indicate he has HIV. His wife has been at his bedside daily but is unaware that he has HIV. The nurse assigned to care for him tells you, "I cannot believe what he has done to his wife! She is at his bedside and has no idea about his double lifestyle. I am a Christian and I want nothing to do with a man with no morals. I think someone needs to tell her the truth but it won't be me! I'm not going to take care of him—give me another assignment."

Discussion

Some health care providers may display a judgmental manner when providing care for patients with HIV/AIDS. The negative attitude often leads to a significant decrease in patient satisfaction regarding their health care. The American Nurses Association (ANA) clearly stipulates that nurses have an obligation to "provide fair and equal treatment to all patients" (ANA, 2016, p. 3) and also stipulates in its *Code of Ethics* that nurses must provide fair and equitable treatment to all individuals regardless of gender, socioeconomic status, religious, culture, or sexual orientation (ANA, 2015).

Analysis

- Does a nurse have the right to refuse treating a patient? What if a nurse refuses to care for a patient because he or she believes that by doing so the nurse may suffer harm or it may conflict with tenets of their religious beliefs?
- There are several statements that the staff nurse in this case makes with regard to this patient assignment. Analyze each of these in turn. Does the staff nurse demonstrate respect for the patient's autonomy? Is he or she adhering to the ethical principles of beneficence and nonmaleficence? Is the nurse's actions and statements in conflict with the ANA Code of Ethics? (see Chart 3-3)
- What might be the legal implications of the staff nurse refusing this assignment? As the charge nurse, how would you act to ensure that applicable hospital policies are adhered to, that you do not permit any type of negligent or other potentially criminal act to occur, and that the patient and his partner receive just and equitable health care?
- What responsibility does the health care team have to the patient's wife? Since her health may be at risk due to her husband's disease, does the health care provider have an obligation to disclose the patient's diagnosis? Does the health care team have any responsibility to inform the patient's sexual partners of his HIV status? What health agencies must be notified of this patient's newly diagnosed HIV status?

References

American Nurses Association. (2015). *Code of ethics for nurses with interpretive statements.* Washington, DC: American Nurses Publishing, American Nurses Foundation/American Nurses Association.

American Nurses Association. (2016). Position statement on the nurse's role in ethics and human rights: Protecting and promoting individual worth, dignity, and human rights in practice settings. Retrieved on 8/28/2016 at: www.nursingworld.org/MainMenuCategories/EthicsStandards/Ethics-Position-Statements/NursesRole-EthicsHumanRights-PositionStatement.pdf

Li, L., Comulada, W.S., Wu, Z., et al. (2011). Providers HIV avoidance and attitude and patient satisfaction. *Health Connection, 16,* 105–112.

Resource

See Chapter 3, Chart 3-6 for ethics resources.

CRITICAL THINKING EXERCISES

1 ebp A 43-year-old man who is an IV drug user and in a committed relationship wants to reduce the risk of HIV infection. What is the evidence base on strategies to reduce risk from use of IV/injection drugs? What is the evidence about the effectiveness of needle exchange programs? What is the evidence for the effectiveness of PrEP? How would you determine the strength of the evidence and how would you present information to him?

2 pq A 20-year-old female college student comes to the student health clinic stating she had unprotected sex with a partner she suspects is HIV positive. What further questions do you have for her? What is your priority focus for her physical examination? What diagnostic tests and treatments may you anticipate?

3 You are making a home visit to a patient with AIDS who lives alone and has become weak and debilitated. Describe the aspects of the home environment that you would assess to ensure safety and adequate care. Describe the nursing plan of care to promote adherence with ART and other medications since the patient is taking multiple different medications many times during the day. Identify the resources you could use to help support this patient to remain at home.

REFERENCES

*Asterisk indicates nursing research.
**Double asterisk indicates classic reference.

Books

American Nurses Association (ANA). (2015). *Code of ethics for nurses with interpretive statements.* Silver Spring, MD: Author.

American Nurses Association. (2016). Position statement on the nurse's role in ethics and human rights: Protecting and promoting individual worth, dignity, and human rights in practice settings. Retrieved on 8/28/2016 at: www.nursingworld.org/MainMenuCategories/EthicsStandards/Ethics-Position-Statements/NursesRole-EthicsHumanRights-PositionStatement.pdf

Blaese, R., Stiehm, E., Bonilla, F., et al. (2013). *Patient & family handbook for primary immunodeficiency diseases* (5th ed.). Towson, MD: Immune Deficiency Foundation.

Comerford, K. C. (2015). *Nursing 2015 drug handbook*. Philadelphia, PA: Wolters Kluwer.

Grossman, S. & Porth, C. (2014). *Porth's pathophysiology: Concepts of altered health states* (9th ed.). Philadelphia, PA: Lippincott Williams & Wilkins.

Journals and Electronic Documents

Blashill, A., Wilson, J. Baker, et al., (2014). Assessing appearance-related disturbances in HIV- infected men who have sex with men (MSM): Psychometrics of the body change and distress questionnaire—Short Form (ABCD-SF). *AIDS Behavior, 18*(6), 1075–1084.

Bosse, J. D., Nesteby, A., & Randall, C. E. (2015). Integrating sexual minority health issues into a health assessment class. *Journal of Professional Nursing, 31*(6) 498–507.

Bryant, V., Whitehead, N., Burrell, L., et al. (2015). Depression and apathy among people living with HIV: Implications for treatment of HIV. *Associated Neurocognitive Disorders. AIDS and Behavior, 19*(8), 1430–1437.

Bureau of HIV/AIDS Prevention and Control. (2014). Comprehensive jurisdictional plan for HIV prevention in New York City 2012–2016. Retrieved on 5/11/2016 at: www.nyc.gov/html/doh/downloads/pdf/ah/ jurisdictional-plan-cdc.pdf

**Centers for Disease Control and Prevention (CDC). (2006). Revised recommendations for HIV testing of adults, adolescents, and pregnant women in health-care settings. Retrieved on 5/31/6102 at: www.cdc. gov/mmwr/preview/mmwrhtml/rr5514a1.htm

**Centers for Disease Control and Prevention (CDC). (2007). 2007 Guideline for isolation precautions: Preventing transmission of infectious agents in healthcare settings. Retrieved on 5/13/2016 at: www. cdc.gov/hicpac/2007ip/2007ip_part1.html

Centers for Disease Control and Prevention (CDC). (2013). Condoms and STDs: Fact sheet for public health personnel. Retrieved on 5/13/2016 at: www.cdc.gov/condomeffectiveness/brief.html

Centers for Disease Control and Prevention (CDC). (2014a). Compendium of evidence-based interventions and best practices for HIV prevention. Retrieved on 5/13/2016 at: www.cdc.gov/hiv/prevention/ research/compendium/index.html

Centers for Disease Control and Prevention (CDC). (2014b). Laboratory testing for the diagnosis of HIV infection: Updated recommendations. Retrieved on 5/13/2016 at: stacks.cdc.gov/view/cdc/23447

Centers for Disease Control and Prevention (CDC). (2015a). Today's HIV/AIDS epidemic. Retrieved on 5/13/2016 at: www.cdc.gov/nchh-stp/newsroom/docs/HIVFactSheets/TodaysEpidemic-508.pdf

Centers for Disease Control and Prevention (CDC). (2015b). *HIV in the United States: At a glance.* Retrieved on 5/31/6102 :at www.cdc.gov/hiv/ statistics/basics/ataglance.html

Centers for Disease Control and Prevention (CDC). (2015c). *CDC's HIV prevention progress in the United States.* Retrieved on 5/13/2016 at: www. cdc.gov/hiv/dhap/progress/index.html

Centers for Disease Control and Prevention (CDC). (2015d). HIV and injection drug use in the United States. Retrieved on 5/31/6102: www. cdc.gov/hiv/riskbehaviors/idu.html

Centers for Disease Control and Prevention (CDC). (2015e). *Occupational HIV transmission and prevention among health care workers.* Retrieved on 5/13/2016 at: www.cdc.gov/hiv/workplace/occupational.html

Centers for Disease Control and Prevention (CDC). (2015f). HIV testing. Retrieved on 5/31/6102 at: www.cdc.gov/hiv/testing/index.html

Chambers, L., Rueda, S., Baker, N., et al. (2015). Stigma, HIV and health: A qualitative synthesis. *BMC Public Health, 15,* 848, 1–17.

Cherin, P., Marie, I., Michallet, M., et al. (2016). Management of adverse events in the treatment of patients with immunoglobulin therapy: A review of evidence. *Autoimmunity Reviews, 15,* 71–81.

Costa-Carvalho, B., Grumach, A., Franco, J., et al. (2014). Attending to warning signs of primary immunodeficiency diseases across the range of clinical practice. *Journal of Clinical Immunology, 34*(1), 10–22.

**DeVita, V. T., Jr., Hellman, S., & Rosenberg, S. (Eds.). (1993). *AIDS: Etiology, diagnosis, treatment, and prevention* (4th ed.). Philadelphia: Lippincott Williams & Wilkins.

Fauci, A., & Marston, H. (2015). Toward an HIV vaccine: A scientific journey. *Science, 349*(6246), 386–387.

Fierz, K., Nicca, D., & Spirig, R. (2013). Perceived HIV symptom manageability: Synthesis of a new use for a known concept. *Journal of Advanced Nursing, 69*(1), 229–241.

Goovaerts, O., Jennes, W., Massinga-Loembé, M., et al. (2015). Lower pre-treatment T cell activation in early- and late-onset tuberculosis-associated immune reconstitution inflammatory syndrome. *PLoS ONE, 10*(7), e0133924.

Gornalusse, G., Mummidi, S., Gaitan, A., et al. (2015). Epigenetic mechanisms, T-cell activation, and CCR5 genetics interact to regulate T-cell expression of CCR5, the major HIV-1 coreceptor. *Proceedings of the National Academy of Sciences of the United States of America, 112*(34), E4762-E4771.

Hernandez-Trujillo, H., Orange, J., Roy, J., et al. (2015). Validity of primary immunodeficiency disease diagnoses in United States Medicaid data. *Journal of Clinical Immunology, 35*(6), 566–572.

Johnson, M. J., & Amella, E. J. (2013). Isolation of lesbian, gay, bisexual and transgender youth: A dimensional concept analysis. *Journal of Advanced Nursing, 70*(3), 523–532.

Kuhar, D., Henderson, D., Struble, K. et al. (2013). Updated US Public Health Service guidelines for the management of occupational exposures to human immunodeficiency virus and recommendations for postexposure prophylaxis. *Infection Control and Hospital Epidemiology, 34*(9), 875–892.

Lehman, H., Hernandez-Trujillo, V., & Ballow, M. (2015). Brief review: Diagnosing primary immunodeficiency: A practical approach for the non-immunologist. *Current Medical Research & Opinion, 31*(4), 697–706.

Li, L., Comulada, W.S., Wu, Z., et al. (2011). Providers HIV avoidance and attitude and patient satisfaction. *Health Connection, 16,* 105–112.

Moyer, V. on behalf of the U.S. Preventive Services Task Force (2013). Screening for HIV: U.S. Preventive Services Task Force recommendation statement. *Annals of Internal Medicine, 159,* 51–60.

National Cancer Institute (NCI). (2015). AIDS-related lymphoma treatment. Retrieved on 5/31/2016 at: www.cancer.gov/types/lymphoma/ patient/aids-related-treatment-pdq

National Institute on Aging (NIA). (2015). HIV, AIDS, and older people. Retrieved on 5/11/2016: www.nia.nih.gov/health/publication/ hiv-aids-and-older-people

National Institute of Allergies and Infectious Diseases (NIAID). (2015). Types of primary immune deficiency disorders. Retrieved on 5/10/2016 at: www.niaid.nih.gov/topics/immuneDeficiency/Pages/majorPIDDs. aspx.

National Institutes of Health, National Center for Complementary and Integrative Health (NCCIH). (2015). Complementary, alternative, or integrative health: What's in a name? Retrieved on 10/10/2015 at: nccih.nih.gov/health/integrative-health

Nicholas, P., Corless, I., & Evans, L. (2014). Peripheral neuropathy in HIV: An analysis of evidence-based approaches. *Journal of the Association of Nurses in AIDS Care, 25*(4), 318–29.

Panel on Antiretroviral Guidelines for Adults and Adolescents (Panel). (2016). Guidelines for the use of antiretroviral agents in HIV-1-infected adults and adolescents. Department of Health and Human Services. Retrieved on 5/12/16 at: www.aidsinfo.nih.gov/ContentFiles/ AdultandAdolescentGL.pdf

Panel on Opportunistic Infections in HIV-Infected Adults and Adolescents (OI-Panel). (2015). Guidelines for the prevention and treatment of opportunistic infections in HIV-infected adults and adolescents: recommendations from the Centers for Disease Control and Prevention, the National Institutes of Health, and the HIV Medicine Association of the Infectious Diseases Society of America (OI-Panel). Retrieved on 5/12/16 at: aidsinfo.nih.gov/contentfiles/lvguidelines/adult_oi.pdf

*Schnall, R., Wantland, D., Velez, O., et al. (2014). Feasibility testing of a web-based symptom self-management system for persons living with HIV. *Journal of the Association of Nurses in AIDS Care, 25*(4), 364–371.

Selik, R., Mokotoff, E., Branson, B., et al. (2014). Revised surveillance case definition for HIV infection—United States, 2014. *Morbidity and Mortality Weekly Report, 63*(RR03),1–10.

Sharma, M., & Walmsley, S. (2015) Contraceptive options for HIV-positive women: Making evidence-based patient centered decisions. *HIV Medicine, 16*(6), 329–336.

*Tillman, J. L., & Mark, H. D. (2015). HIV and STI testing in older adults: An integrative review. *Journal of Clinical Nursing. 24*(15/16), 2074–2095.

US Public Health Service. (2014). Preexposure prophylaxis for the prevention of HIV infection in the United States: Clinical practice guideline. Retrieved on 5/11/2016 :www.cdc.gov/hiv/pdf/prepguidelines2014. pdf

Vanham, G., Buvé, A., Florence, E., et al. (2014). What is the significance of post treatment control of HIV infection vis-à-vis functional
cure? *AIDS, 28*(4), 603–605.

White House. (2015). National HIV/AIDS strategy for the United States:
Updated to 2020. Retrieved on 5/11/2016 at: www.aids.gov/federal-
resources/national-hiv-aids-strategy/nhas-update.pdf

Wichinski, K. (2015). Providing culturally proficient care for transgender.
Nursing, 45(2), 58–63.

World Health Organization (WHO). (2015a). HIV/AIDS: Fact sheet
N°360. Retrieved on 8/8/6102 at:www.who.int/mediacentre/factsheets/
fs360/en/

World Health Organization (WHO). (2015b). Global summary of the
AIDS epidemic/2014. Retrieved on 8/8/2016 at: www.who.int/hiv/data/
epi_core_july2015.png

Younger, E., Epland, K., Zampelli, A., et al. (2015). Primary immunodeficiency diseases: A primer for PCPs. *The Nurse Practitioner. 40*(2), 1–7.

Resources

AIDS Community Research Initiative of America (ACRIA), www.acria.org

AIDS Education and Training Centers (AETCs) Program (regional,
national, and international training opportunities), www.aidsetc.org

AIDSinfoglossary 8th edition. https://aidsinfo.nih.gov/contentfiles/
glossaryhivrelatedterms_english.pdf

AIDS vaccines, http://www.avac.org/prevention-option/aids-vaccines

American Red Cross, www.redcross.org

Antiretroviral medication information websites: www.AIDSmeds.com;
www.projectinform.org; www.sfaf.org; hivinsite.ucsf.edu/; www.amfAR.
org; www.natap.org; www.thebody.com

Centers for Disease Control and Prevention, HIV/AIDS Prevention
Research Synthesis Project, http://www.cdc.gov/hiv/dhap/prb/prs/

Gay Men's Health Crisis Network (GMHC), www.gmhc.org.

Harm Reduction Coalition, http://harmreduction.org/about-us/

Health Resources and Service Administration (HRSA), National Clinician's Postexposure Prophylaxis Hotline (health care providers only),
1-888-HIV-4911

Health Resources and Service Administration (HRSA), National HIV
Telephone Consultation Service, 1-800-933-3413

International AIDS Vaccine Initiative (AVI), www.iavi.org

International Partnership for Microbicides, www.ipmglobal.org

National Institutes of Health, HIV/AIDS Treatment, Prevention, and
Research, www.aidsinfo.nih.gov

National Pediatric and Family HIV Resource Center,
www.womenchildrenhiv.org

Office of Minority Health Resource Center, http://www.minorityhealth.
hhs.gov/omh/browse.aspx?lvl=4&lvlid=21

Pharmaceutical Research and Manufacturers of America (PhRMA),/www.
phrma.org/phrmapedia/search?search_api_views_fulltext=HIV

POZ, Health, Life, & HIV. Published by Smart+Strong, 500 Fifth Avenue,
Suite 320, New York, NY 10110, http://www.poz.com/

37

Assessment and Management of Patients With Allergic Disorders

LEARNING OBJECTIVES

On completion of this chapter, the learner will be able to:

1 Explain the physiologic events involved with allergic reactions.
2 Describe the types of hypersensitivity.
3 Use appropriate parameters for assessment of the status of patients with allergic disorders.
4 Describe the pathophysiologic changes, clinical manifestations, and management of patients with allergic disorders.
5 Specify measures to prevent and manage anaphylaxis.
6 Use the nursing process as a framework for care of the patient with allergic rhinitis.
7 Discuss the different allergic disorders according to type.

GLOSSARY

allergen: substance that causes manifestations of allergy

allergy: inappropriate and often harmful immune system response to substances that are normally harmless

anaphylaxis: rapid clinical response to an immediate immunologic reaction between a specific antigen and antibody

angioneurotic edema: condition characterized by urticaria and diffuse swelling of the deeper layers of the skin (i.e., angioedema)

antibody: protein substance developed by the body in response to and interacting with a specific antigen

antigen: substance that induces the production of antibodies

antihistamine: medication that opposes the action of histamine

atopic dermatitis: type I hypersensitivity involving inflammation of the skin evidenced by itching, redness, and a variety of skin lesions

atopy: term often used to describe immunoglobulin E–mediated diseases (i.e., atopic dermatitis, asthma, and allergic rhinitis) with a genetic component

B cells: lymphocyte cells that are important in producing circulating antibodies

bradykinin: a substance that stimulates nerve fibers and causes pain

eosinophil: granular leukocyte

erythema: diffuse redness of the skin

hapten: incomplete antigen

histamine: substance in the body that causes increased gastric secretion, dilation of capillaries, and constriction of the bronchial smooth muscle

hypersensitivity: abnormal heightened reaction to a stimulus of any kind

immunoglobulins: a family of closely related proteins capable of acting as antibodies

leukotrienes: a group of chemical mediators that initiate the inflammatory response

mast cells: connective tissue cells that contain heparin and histamine in their granules

prostaglandins: unsaturated fatty acids that have a wide assortment of biologic activity

serotonin: chemical mediator that acts as a potent vasoconstrictor and bronchoconstrictor

T cells: lymphocyte cells that can cause graft rejection, kill foreign cells, or suppress production of antibodies

urticaria: hives

The human body is bombarded by a host of potential invaders—allergens as well as microbial organisms—that constantly threaten its defenses. After penetrating those defenses, these allergens and organisms, if allowed to continue unimpeded, disrupt the body's enzyme systems and destroy its vital tissues. To protect against these agents, the body is equipped with an elaborate defense system.

The epithelial cells that coat the skin and make up the lining of the respiratory, gastrointestinal, and genitourinary tracts provide the first line of defense against microbial invaders. The structure and continuity of these surfaces and their resistance to penetration are initial deterrents to invaders.

One of the most effective defense mechanisms is the body's capacity to equip itself rapidly with antibodies individually designed to meet each new invader—namely, specific protein antigens. Antibodies react with antigens in a variety of ways: (1) by coating the antigens' surfaces if they are particular substances, (2) by neutralizing the antigens if they are toxins, and (3) by precipitating the antigens out of solution if they are dissolved. The antibodies prepare the antigens so that the phagocytic cells of the blood and the tissues can dispose of them. However, although this system is normally protective, in some cases the body produces inappropriate or exaggerated responses to specific antigens, and the result is an allergic or hypersensitivity disorder.

ALLERGIC ASSESSMENT

Physiologic Overview

An allergic reaction is a manifestation of tissue injury resulting from interaction between an antigen and an antibody. **Allergy** is an inappropriate and often harmful response of the immune system to normally harmless substances, called **allergens** (e.g., dust, weeds, pollen, dander). Chemical mediators released in allergic reactions may produce symptoms that range from mild to life-threatening.

In allergic reactions, the body encounters allergens that are types of **antigens**, usually proteins that the body's defenses recognize as foreign, and a series of events occurs in an attempt to render the invaders harmless, destroy them, and remove them from the body. When lymphocytes respond to the antigens, **antibodies** (protein substances that protect against antigens) are produced.

Antibodies combine with antigens in a special way, which has been likened to keys fitting into a lock. Antigens (the keys) fit only certain antibodies (the locks). Hence, the term *specificity* refers to the specific reaction of an antibody to an antigen. There are many variations and complexities in these patterns.

Function of Immunoglobulins

Antibodies that are formed by lymphocytes and plasma cells in response to an immunogenic stimulus constitute a group of serum proteins called **immunoglobulins**. Grouped into five classes (IgG, IgA, IgM, IgD, and IgE), immunoglobulins can be found in the lymph nodes, tonsils, appendix, and Peyer patches of the intestinal tract or circulating in the blood and lymph. These antibodies are capable of binding with a wide variety of antigens. Immunoglobulins of the IgE class are involved in allergic disorders and some parasitic infections. IgE-producing cells are located in the respiratory and intestinal mucosa. Two or more IgE molecules bind together to an allergen and trigger **mast cells** or basophils to release chemical mediators, such as histamine, serotonin, kinins, slow-reacting substances of anaphylaxis, and the neutrophil factor, which produces allergic skin reactions, asthma, and hay fever. **Atopy** refers to IgE-mediated diseases, such as allergic rhinitis, that have a genetic component. See Chapter 35 for more information on immunoglobulins.

Role of B Cells

B cells, or B lymphocytes, are programmed to produce one specific antibody. On encountering a specific antigen, B cells stimulate production of plasma cells, the site of antibody production. The result is the outpouring of antibodies for the purpose of destroying and removing the antigens.

Role of T Cells

T cells, or T lymphocytes, assist the B cells. T cells secrete substances that direct the flow of cell activity, destroy target cells, and stimulate the macrophages. The macrophages present the antigens to the T cells and initiate the immune response. They also digest antigens and assist in removing cells and other debris. Unlike a specific antibody, a T cell does not bind free antigens.

Function of Antigens

Antigens are divided into two groups: complete protein antigens and low–molecular-weight substances. Complete protein antigens, such as animal dander, pollen, and horse serum, stimulate a complete humoral response. See Chapter 35 for a discussion of humoral immunity. Low–molecular-weight substances, such as medications, function as **haptens** (incomplete antigens), binding to tissue or serum proteins to produce a carrier complex that initiates an antibody response. In an allergic reaction, the production of antibodies requires active communication between cells. When the allergen is absorbed through the respiratory tract, gastrointestinal tract, or skin, allergen sensitization occurs. Macrophages process the antigen and present it to the appropriate cells. These cells mature into allergen-specific secreting plasma cells that synthesize and secrete antigen-specific antibodies.

Function of Chemical Mediators

Mast cells, which are located in the skin and mucous membranes, play a major role in IgE-mediated immediate hypersensitivity. When mast cells are stimulated by antigens, powerful chemical mediators are released, causing a sequence of physiologic events that result in symptoms of immediate hypersensitivity (see Fig. 37-1). There are two types of chemical mediators: primary and secondary. Primary mediators are preformed and are found in mast cells or basophils. Secondary mediators are inactive precursors that are formed or released in response to primary mediators. Table 37-1 summarizes the actions of primary and secondary chemical mediators.

Primary Mediators

Histamine

Histamine, which is released by mast cells, plays an important role in the immune response. It is the first chemical

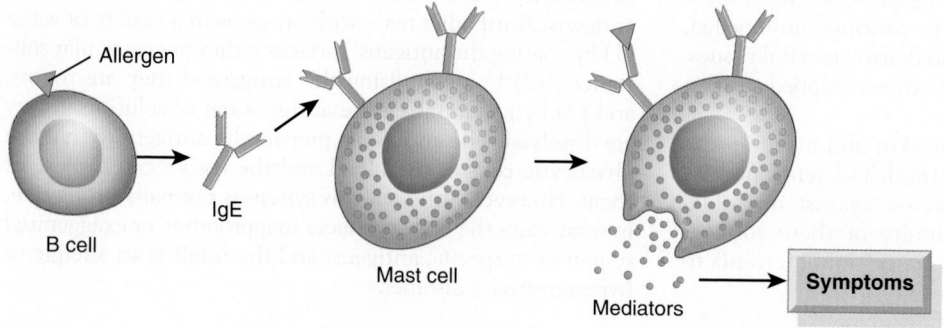

Figure 37-1 • Allergen triggers the B cell to make immunoglobulin E (IgE) antibody, which attaches to the mast cell. When that allergen reappears, it binds to the IgE and triggers the mast cell to release its chemicals. Courtesy of the U.S. Department of Health and Human Services, National Institutes of Health.

TABLE 37-1 Chemical Mediators of Hypersensitivity

Mediators	Action
Primary Mediators	
Preformed and Found in Mast Cells or Basophils	
Histamine (preformed in mast cells)	Vasodilation Smooth muscle contraction, increased vascular permeability, increased mucus secretions
Eosinophil chemotactic factor of anaphylaxis (preformed in mast cells)	Attracts eosinophils
Platelet-activating factor (requires synthesis by mast cells, neutrophils, and macrophages)	Smooth muscle contraction Incites platelets to aggregate and release serotonin and histamine
Prostaglandins (chemically derived from arachidonic acid; require synthesis by cells)	D and F series → bronchoconstriction E series → bronchodilation D, E, and F series → vasodilation
Basophil kallikrein (preformed in mast cells)	Frees bradykinin, which causes bronchoconstriction, vasodilation, and nerve stimulation
Secondary Mediators	
Inactive Precursors Formed or Released in Response to Primary Mediators	
Bradykinin (derived from precursor kininogen)	Smooth muscle contraction, increased vascular permeability, stimulates pain receptors, increased mucus production
Serotonin (preformed in platelets)	Smooth muscle contraction, increased vascular permeability
Heparin (preformed in mast cells)	Anticoagulant
Leukotrienes (derived from arachidonic acid and activated by mast cell degranulation) C, D, and E or slow-reacting substance of anaphylaxis	Smooth muscle contraction, increased vascular permeability

Adapted from Grossman, S. C., & Porth, C. M. (2014). *Porth's pathophysiology: Concepts of altered health states* (9th ed.). Philadelphia, PA: Lippincott Williams & Wilkins.

mediator to be released in immune and inflammatory responses. It is synthesized and stored in high concentrations in body tissues exposed to environmental substances (Frandsen & Pennington, 2014). Histamine's effects peak 5 to 10 minutes after antigen contact and include the following: erythema; localized edema in the form of wheals; pruritus; contraction of bronchial smooth muscle, resulting in wheezing and bronchospasm; dilation of small venules and constriction of larger vessels; and increased secretion of gastric and mucosal cells, resulting in diarrhea (Abbas, Lichtman, & Pillai, 2014; Fleisher, Shearer, Schroeder, et al., 2013). Histamine action results from stimulation of histamine-1 (H_1) and histamine-2 (H_2) receptors. H_1 receptors are found predominantly on bronchiolar and vascular smooth muscle cells; H_2 receptors are found on gastric parietal cells.

Certain medications are categorized by their action at these receptors. Diphenhydramine (Benadryl) is an example of an **antihistamine**, a medication that displays an affinity for H_1 receptors. Cimetidine (Tagamet) and ranitidine (Zantac) target H_2 receptors to inhibit gastric secretions in peptic ulcer disease.

Eosinophil Chemotactic Factor of Anaphylaxis

Eosinophil chemotactic factor of anaphylaxis affects the movement of **eosinophils** (granular leukocytes) to the site of allergens. It is preformed in the mast cells and is released from disrupted mast cells.

Platelet-Activating Factor

Platelet-activating factor is responsible for initiating platelet aggregation and leukocyte infiltration at sites of immediate hypersensitivity reactions. It also causes vasodilation, bronchoconstriction, and increased vascular permeability (Frandsen & Pennington, 2014).

Prostaglandins

Prostaglandins produce smooth muscle contraction as well as vasodilation and increased capillary permeability. They sensitize pain receptors and increase the pain associated with inflammation. In addition, prostaglandins induce inflammation and enhance the effects of mediators of inflammatory response. Local manifestations include erythema, heat, and edema (Frandsen & Pennington, 2014).

Secondary Mediators

Leukotrienes

Leukotrienes are chemical mediators that initiate the inflammatory response. Many manifestations of inflammation can be attributed in part to leukotrienes. In addition, leukotrienes cause smooth muscle contraction, bronchial constriction, mucus secretion in the airways, and the typical wheal-and-flare reactions of the skin. Compared with histamine, leukotrienes are 100 to 1000 times more potent in causing bronchospasm.

Bradykinin

Bradykinin is a substance that has the ability to cause increased vascular permeability, vasodilation, hypotension, and contraction of many types of smooth muscle, such as the bronchi. Increased permeability of the capillaries results in edema. Bradykinin stimulates nerve cell fibers and produces pain.

Serotonin

Serotonin acts as a potent vasoconstrictor and causes contraction of bronchial smooth muscle.

Hypersensitivity

Although the immune system defends the host against infections and foreign antigens, immune responses can themselves cause tissue injury and disease. **Hypersensitivity** is an excessive or aberrant immune response to any type of stimulus (Abbas et al., 2014). It usually does not occur with the first exposure to an allergen. Rather, the reaction follows a re-exposure after sensitization, or buildup of antibodies, in a predisposed person. Injurious or pathologic immune reactions are classed as hypersensitivity reactions. To promote understanding of the immunopathogenesis of disease, hypersensitivity reactions have been classified into four specific types of reactions (see Fig. 37-2). Most allergic reactions are either type I or type IV hypersensitivity reactions.

Type I

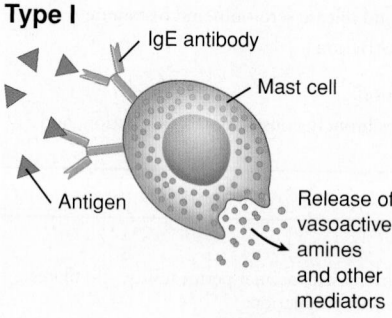

Type I. An anaphylactic reaction is characterized by vasodilation, increased capillary permeability, smooth muscle contraction, and eosinophilia. Systemic reactions may involve laryngeal stridor, angioedema, hypotension, and bronchial, GI, or uterine spasm; local reactions are characterized by hives. Examples of type I reactions include extrinsic asthma, allergic rhinitis, systemic anaphylaxis, and reactions to insect stings.

Type II

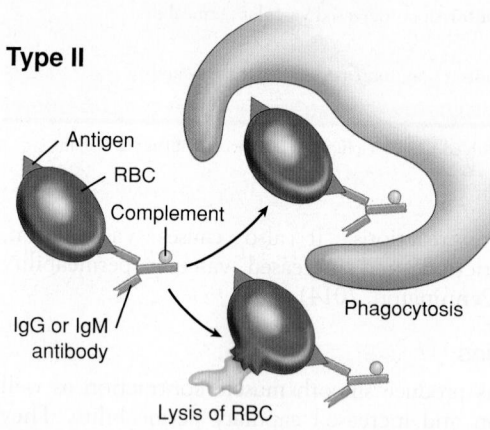

Type II. A cytotoxic reaction, which involves binding either the IgG or IgM antibody to a cell-bound antigen, may lead to eventual cell and tissue damage. The reaction is the result of mistaken identity when the system identifies a normal constituent of the body as foreign and activates the complement cascade. Examples of type II reactions are myasthenia gravis, Goodpasture syndrome, pernicious anemia, hemolytic disease of the newborn, transfusion reaction, and thrombocytopenia.

Type III

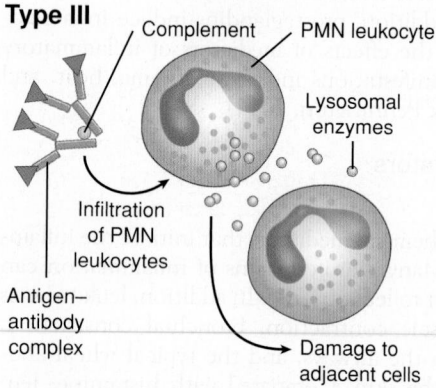

Type III. An immune complex reaction is marked by acute inflammation resulting from formation and deposition of immune complexes. The joints and kidneys are particularly susceptible to this kind of reaction, which is associated with systemic lupus erythematosus, serum sickness, nephritis, and rheumatoid arthritis. Some signs and symptoms include urticaria, joint pain, fever, rash, and adenopathy (swollen glands).

Type IV

Type IV. A delayed, or cellular, reaction occurs 1 to 3 days after exposure to an antigen. The reaction, which results in tissue damage, involves activity by lymphokines, macrophages, and lysozymes. Erythema and itching are common; a few examples include contact dermatitis, graft-versus-host disease, Hashimoto's thyroiditis, and sarcoidosis.

Figure 37-2 • Four types of hypersensitivity reactions. GI, gastrointestinal; Ig, immunoglobulin; PMN, polymorphonuclear; RBC, red blood cell.

Anaphylactic (Type I) Hypersensitivity

The most severe hypersensitivity reaction is **anaphylaxis**. An unanticipated severe allergic reaction that is rapid in onset, anaphylaxis is characterized by edema in many tissues, including the larynx, and is often accompanied by hypotension, bronchospasm, and cardiovascular collapse in severe cases. Type I or anaphylactic hypersensitivity is an immediate reaction beginning within minutes of exposure to an antigen. Primary chemical mediators are responsible for the symptoms of type I hypersensitivity because of their effects on the skin, lungs, and gastrointestinal tract. If chemical mediators continue to be released, a delayed reaction may occur and may last for up to 24 hours.

Clinical symptoms are determined by the amount of the allergen, the amount of mediator released, the sensitivity of the target organ, and the route of allergen entry. Type I hypersensitivity reactions may include both local and systemic anaphylaxis.

Cytotoxic (Type II) Hypersensitivity

Type II, or cytotoxic, hypersensitivity occurs when the system mistakenly identifies a normal constituent of the body as foreign. This reaction may be the result of a cross-reacting antibody, possibly leading to cell and tissue damage.

Type II hypersensitivity reactions are associated with several disorders. For example, in myasthenia gravis, the body mistakenly generates antibodies against normal nerve ending receptors. In Goodpasture syndrome, it generates antibodies against lung and renal tissue, producing lung damage and kidney injury (Grossman & Porth, 2014).

Immune Complex (Type III) Hypersensitivity

Type III, or immune complex, hypersensitivity involves immune complexes that are formed when antigens bind to antibodies. These complexes are cleared from the circulation by phagocytic action. If these type III complexes are deposited in tissues or vascular endothelium, two factors contribute to injury: the increased amount of circulating complexes and the presence of vasoactive amines. As a result, there is an increase in vascular permeability and tissue injury.

Delayed-Type (Type IV) Hypersensitivity

Type IV, or delayed-type, hypersensitivity (DTH), is an immune reaction in which T-cell–dependent macrophage activation and inflammation cause tissue injury. This type of reaction to the subcutaneous injection of antigen is often used as an assay for cell-mediated immunity (e.g., the purified protein derivative skin test for immunity to *Mycobacterium tuberculosis*) (Abbas et al., 2014).

Assessment

A comprehensive allergy history and a thorough physical examination provide useful data for the diagnosis and management of allergic disorders. An allergy assessment form is useful for obtaining and organizing pertinent information (see Chart 37-1).

The degree of difficulty and discomfort experienced by the patient because of allergic symptoms and the degree of improvement in those symptoms with and without treatment are assessed and documented. The relationship of symptoms to exposure to possible allergens is noted.

Diagnostic Evaluation

Diagnostic evaluation of the patient with allergic disorders commonly includes blood tests, smears of body secretions, skin tests, and the serum-specific IgE test (formerly known as radioallergosorbent test [RAST]). Results of laboratory blood studies provide supportive data for various diagnostic possibilities; however, they are not the major criteria for the diagnosis of allergic disease.

Complete Blood Count With Differential

The white blood cell (WBC) count is usually normal except with infection and inflammation (Pagana & Pagana, 2013). Eosinophils, which are granular leukocytes, normally make up 2% to 5% of the total number of WBCs. They can be found in blood, sputum, and nasal secretions. A level greater than 5% to 10% is considered abnormal and may be found in patients with allergic disorders (Fleisher et al., 2013).

Eosinophil Count

An actual count of eosinophils can be obtained from blood samples or smears of secretions. During symptomatic episodes, smears obtained from nasal secretions and sputum of patients with allergies usually reveal an increase in eosinophils, indicating an active allergic response (Fleisher et al., 2013).

Total Serum Immunoglobulin E Levels

High total serum IgE levels support the diagnosis of allergic disease. In the majority of cases, the antibody typically responsible for an allergic reaction belongs to the IgE isotype. Patients with this disorder are said to have an IgE-mediated allergic disease (Portnoy, 2015).

Skin Tests

Skin testing entails the intradermal injection or superficial application (epicutaneous) of solutions at several sites. Depending on the suspected cause of allergic signs and symptoms, many different solutions may be applied at separate sites. These solutions contain individual antigens representing an assortment of allergens most likely to be implicated in the patient's disease. Positive (wheal-and-flare) reactions are clinically significant when correlated with the history, physical findings, and results of other laboratory tests. Skin testing is considered the most accurate confirmation of allergy (Oppenheimer, Durham, Nelson, et al., 2014).

The results of skin tests complement the data obtained from the history. They indicate which of several antigens are most likely to provoke symptoms and indicate the intensity of the patient's sensitization. The dosage of the antigen (allergen) injected is also important. Most patients are hypersensitive to more than one allergen. Under testing conditions, they may not react (although they usually do) to the specific allergens that induce their attacks.

In cases of doubt about the validity of the skin tests, a serum-specific IgE test or a provocative challenge test may be performed. If a skin test is indicated, there is a reasonable suspicion that a

Chart 37-1 ASSESSMENT

Allergy Assessment Form

Name _____ Age _____ Sex _____ Date _____

I. Chief complaint: _____

II. Present illness: _____

III. Collateral allergic symptoms: _____

Eyes:	Pruritus _____	Burning _____	Lacrimation _____
	Swelling _____	Injection _____	Discharge _____
Ears:	Pruritus _____	Fullness _____	Popping _____
	Frequent infections _____		
Nose:	Sneezing _____	Rhinorrhea _____	Obstruction _____
	Pruritus _____	Mouth breathing _____	
	Purulent discharge _____		
Throat:	Soreness _____	Postnasal discharge _____	
	Palatal pruritus _____	Mucus in the morning _____	
Chest:	Cough _____	Pain _____	Wheezing _____
	Sputum _____	Dyspnea _____	
	Color _____	Rest _____	
	Amount _____	Exertion _____	
Skin:	Dermatitis _____	Eczema _____	Urticaria _____

IV. Family allergies: _____

V. Previous allergic treatment or testing: _____

Prior skin testing: _____

Medications:			
	Antihistamines	Improved _____	Unimproved _____
	Bronchodilators	Improved _____	Unimproved _____
	Nose drops	Improved _____	Unimproved _____
	Hyposensitization	Improved _____	Unimproved _____
	Duration _____		
	Antigens _____		
	Reactions _____		
	Antibiotics	Improved _____	Unimproved _____
	Corticosteroids	Improved _____	Unimproved _____

VI. Physical agents and habits: _____

Bothered by:

Tobacco for _____ years	Alcohol _____	Air-conditioning _____
Cigarettes _____ packs/day	Heat _____	Muggy weather _____
Cigars _____ per day	Cold _____	Weather changes _____
Pipes _____ per day	Perfumes _____	Chemicals _____
Never smoked _____	Paints _____	Hair spray _____
Bothered by smoke _____	Insecticides _____	Newspapers _____
	Cosmetics _____	Latex _____

VII. When symptoms occur: _____

Time and circumstances of 1st episode: _____

Prior health: _____

Course of illness over decades: progressing _____ regressing _____

Time of year: _____ Exact dates: _____

    Perennial _____

    Seasonal _____

    Seasonally exacerbated _____

Monthly variations (menses, occupation): _____

Time of week (weekends vs. weekdays): _____

Time of day or night: _____

After insect stings: _____

VIII. Where symptoms occur: _____

Living where at onset: _____

Living where since onset: _____

Effect of vacation or major geographic change: _____

Symptoms better indoors or outdoors: _____

Effect of school or work: _____

Effect of staying elsewhere nearby: _____

Effect of hospitalization: _____

Effect of specific environments: _____

Do symptoms occur around:

    old leaves _____ hay _____ lakeside _____ barns _____

    summer homes _____ damp basement _____ dry attic _____

    lawn mowing _____ animals _____ other _____

Chart 37-1 ASSESSMENT (Continued)

Allergy Assessment Form

Do symptoms occur after eating:

cheese _____ mushrooms _____ beer _____ melons _____
bananas _____ fish _____ nuts _____ citrus fruits _____
other foods (list) _____

Home: city _____ rural _____
        house _____ age _____
        apartment _____ basement _____ damp _____ dry _____
        heating system _____
        vacuum cleaner system _____ use of HEPA filter _____
        pets (how long) _____ dog _____ cat _____ other _____

Bedroom:	Type	Age	*Living room:*	Type	Age
Pillow	_____	_____	Rug	_____	_____
Mattress	_____	_____	Matting	_____	_____
Blankets	_____	_____	Furniture	_____	_____
Quilts	_____	_____			
Furniture	_____	_____			

Anywhere in home symptoms are worse: _____
IX. What does patient think makes symptoms worse? _____
X. Under what circumstances is patient free of symptoms? _____
XI. Summary and additional comments: _____

specific allergen is producing symptoms in a patient with allergies. However, several precautionary steps must be observed before skin testing with allergens is performed:

- Testing is not performed during periods of bronchospasm.
- Epicutaneous tests (scratch or prick tests) are performed before other testing methods, in an effort to minimize the risk of systemic reaction.
- Emergency equipment must be readily available to treat anaphylaxis.

Types of Skin Tests

The methods of skin testing include prick skin tests, scratch tests, and intradermal skin testing (see Fig. 37-3). After

Figure 37-3 • Intradermal testing. A 0.5- or 1-mL sterile syringe with a 26/27-gauge intradermal needle is used to inject 0.02 to 0.03 mL of intradermal allergen. The needle is inserted with the bevel facing upward and the syringe parallel to the skin. The skin is penetrated superficially, and a small amount of the allergen solution is injected to create a bleb (raised area) approximately 5 mm in diameter. A separate sterile syringe and needle are used for each injection. From Taylor, C., Lillis C., LeMone, P., & Lynn, P. (2011). *Fundamentals of nursing: The art and science of nursing care* (7th ed.). Philadelphia, PA Lippincott Williams & Wilkins.

negative prick or scratch tests, intradermal skin testing is performed with allergens that are suggested by the patient's history to be problematic. The back is the most suitable area of the body for skin testing because it permits the performance of many tests. A multitest applicator with multiple test heads is commercially available for simultaneous administration of antigens by multiple punctures at different sites. A negative response on a skin test cannot be interpreted as an absence of sensitivity to an allergen. Such a response may occur with insufficient sensitivity of the test or with the use of an inappropriate allergen in testing. Therefore, it is essential to observe the patient undergoing skin testing for an allergic reaction even if the previous response was negative.

Interpretation of Skin Test Results

Familiarity with and consistent use of a grading system are essential. The grading system used should be identified on a skin test record for later interpretation. A positive reaction, evidenced by the appearance of an urticarial wheal (round, reddened skin elevation) (see Fig. 37-4), localized **erythema** (diffuse redness) in the area of inoculation or contact, or pseudopodia (irregular projection at the end of a wheal) with associated erythema is considered indicative of sensitivity to the corresponding antigen. False-positive results may occur because of improper preparation or administration of allergen solutions.

▶ *Quality and Safety Nursing Alert*

Corticosteroids and antihistamines, including over-the-counter allergy medications, suppress skin test reactivity and should be stopped 48 to 96 hours before testing, depending on the duration of their activity. False-positive results may occur because of improper preparation or administration of allergen solutions.

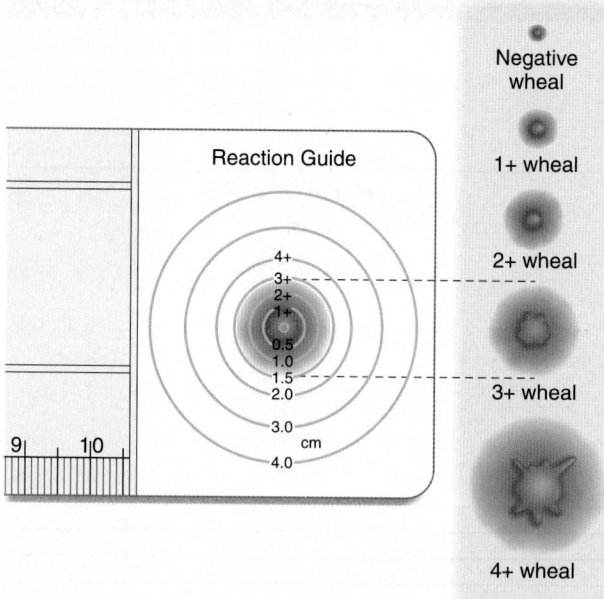

Negative
wheal

1+ wheal

2+ wheal

3+ wheal

4+ wheal

Figure 37-4 • Interpretation of reactions: Negative = wheal soft with minimal erythema; 1+ = wheal present (5 to 8 mm) with associated erythema; 2+ = wheal (7 to 10 mm) with associated erythema; 3+ = wheal (9 to 15 mm), slight pseudopodia possible with associated erythema; 4+ = wheal (12 mm+) with pseudopodia and diffuse erythema.

Positive or negative skin tests are interpreted in the context of a patient's history, clinical signs, and exposure to allergens (Australasian Society of Clinical Immunology and Allergy [ASCIA], 2015). The following guidelines are used for the interpretation of skin test results:

- Skin tests are used most frequently with the diagnosis of allergic rhinitis (Baran, Ozcan, Selcuk, et al., 2014).
- Negative test results are helpful in ruling out food allergy.
- Positive skin tests correlate highly with food allergy (ASCIA, 2015).

The use of skin tests to diagnose immediate hypersensitivity to medications is limited, because metabolites of medications, not the medications themselves, are usually responsible for causing hypersensitivity.

Provocative Testing

Provocative testing involves the direct administration of the suspected allergen to the sensitive tissue, such as the conjunctiva, nasal or bronchial mucosa, or gastrointestinal tract (by ingestion of the allergen), with observation of target organ response. This type of testing is helpful in identifying clinically significant allergens in patients who have a large number of positive tests. Major disadvantages of this type of testing are the limitation of one antigen per session and the risk of producing severe symptoms, particularly bronchospasm, in patients with asthma.

Serum-Specific IgE Test

The serum-specific IgE test, formerly known as RAST, is an automated test performed on blood samples by a pathology laboratory. As the name suggests, it detects free antigen-specific

IgE in serum as opposed to antigen-specific IgE bound to mast cells in the skin (ASCIA, 2015; Portnoy, 2015). The advantages of this test over other tests include decreased risk of systemic reaction, stability of antigens, and lack of dependence on skin reactivity modified by medications. The major disadvantages include limited allergen selection and reduced sensitivity compared with intradermal skin tests, lack of immediate results, and higher cost (ASCIA, 2015).

ALLERGIC DISORDERS

There are two types of IgE-mediated allergic reactions: atopic and nonatopic disorders. Although the underlying immunologic reactions of the two types of disorders are the same, the predisposing factors and manifestations are different. Atopy is defined as the genetic predisposition to mount an IgE response to inhaled or ingested innocuous proteins (Fleisher et al., 2013). Atopic diseases consist of asthma, allergic rhinitis, and atopic dermatitis. All share a common pathogenesis, mediated by IgE, and are frequently present together in the same individual and in families. The nonatopic disorders lack the genetic component and organ specificity of the atopic disorders (Fleisher et al., 2013). Latex allergy (see later discussion) can present as an IgE-mediated anaphylaxis, type I reaction, or a type IV hypersensitivity referred to as contact dermatitis (American Academy of Allergy, Asthma, & Immunology [AAAAI], 2015; Fleisher et al., 2013; Habif, 2016).

Unfolding Patient Stories: Jennifer Hoffman • Part 2

Recall from Chapter 24 Jennifer Hoffman, who came to the clinic with continued symptoms of asthma. The nurse confirmed that she was following the asthma action plan; however, Jennifer now returns to the clinic with worsening symptoms. What assessment findings would indicate to the nurse that Jennifer is having a hypersensitivity reaction to an allergen(s)? What questions can assist the nurse in identifying the causative agent(s)? What interventions should be implemented when allergen(s) are identified?

Care for Jennifer and other patients in a realistic virtual environment: *vSim for Nursing* (**thepoint.lww.com/vSimMedicalSurgical**). Practice documenting these patients' care in DocuCare (**thepoint.lww.com/DocuCareEHR**).

Anaphylaxis

Anaphylaxis is a clinical response to an immediate (type I hypersensitivity) immunologic reaction between a specific antigen and an antibody. The reaction results from a rapid release of IgE-mediated chemicals, which can induce a severe, life-threatening reaction (Abbas et al., 2014).

Pathophysiology

Anaphylaxis is a type I IgE allergic reaction to an antigen, a foreign substance that has entered the body (Frandsen & Pennington, 2014). It is caused by the cross-links of an allergen with allergen-specific IgE antibodies found on the surface membrane of mast cells and basophils, leading to cellular degranulation. The subsequent release of histamine and other bioactive mediators causes activation of platelets, eosinophils, and neutrophils. Histamine, prostaglandins, and inflammatory leukotrienes are potent vasoactive mediators that are implicated in the vascular permeability changes, flushing, urticaria, angioedema, hypotension, and broncho-constriction that characterize anaphylaxis. Smooth muscle spasm, bronchospasm, mucosal edema and inflammation, and increased capillary permeability result. Symptoms of anaphy-laxis are sudden in onset and progress in severity over minutes to hours (Campbell, Li, Nicklas, et al., 2014).

Closely resembling anaphylaxis is an anaphylactoid reac-tion, which is caused by the release of mast cell and basophil mediators triggered by non–immunoglobulin E (IgE)-medi-ated events. This nonallergenic anaphylaxis reaction may occur with medications, food, exercise, or cytotoxic anti-body transfusions. The reaction may be local or systemic. Local reactions usually involve urticaria and angioedema at the site of the antigen exposure. Although possibly severe, nonallergenic anaphylaxis reactions are rarely fatal. Systemic reactions occur within about 30 minutes after exposure and involve cardiovascular, respiratory, gastrointestinal, and integumentary organ systems. For the most part, the treat-ment of nonallergenic anaphylaxis reaction is identical to that of anaphylaxis.

Common causes of anaphylaxis are listed in Chart 37-2. Antibiotics and radiocontrast agents cause the most seri-ous anaphylactic reactions. Penicillin is the most common medication to cause anaphylaxis. In a study of an outpatient adult population, the prevalence of penicillin allergy was found to be 12% (Albin & Agarwal, 2014). However, only 6% of these patients were referred to an allergist for testing. Patients with reported penicillin allergy who were evaluated with skin testing experienced decreased use of broad spec-trum antibiotics and fewer anaphylactic reactions (Albin & Agarwal, 2014).

Chart 37-2 Common Causes of Anaphylaxis

Foods

Peanuts, tree nuts (e.g., walnuts, pecans, cashews, almonds), shellfish (e.g., shrimp, lobster, crab), fish, milk, eggs, soy, wheat

Medications

Antibiotics, especially penicillin and sulfa antibiotics, allopurinol, radiocontrast agents, anesthetic agents (lidocaine, procaine), vaccines, hormones (insulin, vasopressin, adrenocorticotropic hormone), aspirin, nonsteroidal anti-inflammatory drugs

Other Pharmaceutical/Biologic Agents

Animal serums (tetanus antitoxin, snake venom antitoxin, rabies antitoxin), antigens used in skin testing

Insect Stings

Bees, wasps, hornets, yellow jackets, ants (including fire ants)

Latex

Medical and nonmedical products containing latex

Clinical Manifestations

Anaphylactic reactions produce a clinical syndrome that affects multiple organ systems. Reactions may be categorized as mild, moderate, or severe. The time from the exposure to the antigen to the onset of symptoms is a good indicator of the severity of the reaction—the faster the onset, the more severe the reaction. The severity of previous reactions does not determine the severity of subsequent reactions, which could be the same or more or less severe. The severity depends on the degree of allergy and the dose of allergen exposure (Campbell et al., 2014).

Mild systemic reactions consist of peripheral tingling and a sensation of warmth, possibly accompanied by a sensation of fullness in the mouth and throat. Nasal congestion, perior-bital swelling, pruritus, sneezing, and tearing of the eyes can also be expected. The onset of symptoms begins within the first 2 hours after the exposure.

Moderate systemic reactions may include flushing, warmth, anxiety, and itching in addition to any of the milder symptoms. More serious reactions include bronchospasm and edema of the airways or larynx with dyspnea, cough, and wheezing. The onset of symptoms is the same as for a mild reaction.

Severe systemic reactions have an abrupt onset with the same signs and symptoms described previously. These symp-toms progress rapidly to bronchospasm, laryngeal edema, severe dyspnea, cyanosis, and hypotension. Dysphagia (dif-ficulty swallowing), abdominal cramping, vomiting, diarrhea, and seizures can also occur. Cardiac arrest and coma may follow. Severe reactions are also referred to as anaphylactic shock (see Chapter 14).

Prevention

Strict avoidance of potential allergens is an important pre-ventive measure for the patient at risk for anaphylaxis. Those at risk for anaphylaxis from insect stings should avoid areas populated by insects and should use appropriate clothing, insect repellent, and caution to avoid further stings.

If avoidance of exposure to allergens is impossible, an auto-injector system for epinephrine will be prescribed. The patient should be instructed to carry and administer epinephrine to prevent an anaphylactic reaction in the event of exposure to the allergen. People who are sensitive to insect bites and stings, those who have experienced food or medication reac-tions, and those who have experienced idiopathic or exer-cise-induced anaphylactic reactions should always carry an emergency kit that contains epinephrine. The EpiPen and Auvi-Q are auto-injection devices that are commercially available for first aid that deliver premeasured doses of epi-nephrine (Comerford, 2015; Frandsen & Pennington, 2014). The auto-injector system requires no preparation, and the self-administration technique is not complicated. The patient must be given an opportunity to demonstrate the correct technique for use; an EpiPen training device can be used for educating about the correct technique. Verbal and written information about the emergency kit, as well as strategies to avoid exposure to threatening allergens, must also be provided.

Screening for allergies before a medication is prescribed or first given is an important preventive measure. A care-ful history of any sensitivity to suspected antigens must be obtained before administering any medication, particularly in parenteral form, because this route is associated with the most severe anaphylaxis. Nurses caring for patients in any setting (hospital, home, outpatient diagnostic testing sites, long-term care facilities) must assess patients' risks for anaphylactic reactions. Patients are asked about previous exposure to contrast agents used for diagnostic tests and any allergic reactions, as well as reactions to any medications, foods, insect stings, and latex. People who are predisposed to anaphylaxis should wear medical identification such as a bracelet or necklace, which names allergies to medications, food, and other substances.

People who are allergic to insect venom may require venom immunotherapy, which is used as a control measure and not a cure. The most common serious allergic reactions to insect stings are from the Hymenoptera family, which includes bees, ants, wasps, and yellow jackets (Perez-Riverol, Justo-Jacomini, de Lima Zollner, et al., 2015). Venom is an effective treatment for people with systemic reactions to an insect sting. It reduces the systemic reaction, reduces the risk of future large local reactions, and improves quality of life (Ludman & Boyle, 2015).

Insulin-allergic patients with diabetes and those who are allergic to penicillin may require desensitization. Desensitization is based on controlled anaphylaxis, with a gradual release of mediators. Patients who undergo desensitization are cautioned to avoid lapses in therapy, because this may lead to the reappearance of the allergic reaction when the use of the medication is resumed.

Medical Management

Management depends on the severity of the reaction. Initially, respiratory and cardiovascular functions are evaluated. If the patient is in cardiac arrest, cardiopulmonary resuscitation (CPR) is instituted (Link, Berkow, Kudenchuk, et al., 2015). Supplemental oxygen is provided during CPR or if the patient is cyanotic, dyspneic, or wheezing. Epinephrine, in a 1:1000 dilution, is given subcutaneously in the upper extremity or thigh and may be followed by a continuous intravenous infusion. Most adverse events associated with administration of epinephrine (i.e., adrenaline) occur when the dose is excessive or is given intravenously. Patients at risk for adverse effects include older patients and those with hypertension, arteriopathies, or known ischemic heart disease.

Antihistamines and corticosteroids should not be given in place of epinephrine. However, they may also be given as adjunct therapy (Campbell et al., 2014).

Intravenous fluids (e.g., normal saline solution), volume expanders, and vasopressor agents are given to maintain blood pressure and normal hemodynamic status. In patients with episodes of bronchospasm or a history of bronchial asthma or chronic obstructive pulmonary disease, aminophylline and corticosteroids may also be given to improve airway patency and function. (See Chapter 14 for management of anaphylactic shock.)

Patients who have experienced anaphylactic reactions and received epinephrine should be transported to the local emergency department (ED) for observation and monitoring because of the risk for a "rebound" or delayed reaction 4 to 8 hours after the initial allergic reaction. However, the observation time should be individualized based on the severity of the anaphylaxis. Longer periods of observation should be considered for patients who ingested the allergen, required more than one dose of epinephrine, had hypotension or pharyngeal edema, or have a history of asthma (Campbell et al., 2014).

Nursing Management

If a patient is experiencing an allergic response, the nurse assesses the patient for signs and symptoms of anaphylaxis. Airway, breathing pattern, and vital signs are assessed. The patient is observed for signs of increasing edema and respiratory distress. Prompt notification of the rapid response team, the provider, or both is required. Rapid initiation of emergency measures (e.g., intubation, administration of emergency medications, insertion of intravenous lines, fluid administration, and oxygen administration) is important to reduce the severity of the reaction and to restore cardiovascular function. The nurse documents the interventions used and the patient's vital signs and response to treatment.

The patient who has recovered from anaphylaxis needs an explanation of what occurred, instruction about avoiding future exposure to antigens, and how to administer emergency medications to treat anaphylaxis. The patient must be instructed about antigens that should be avoided and about other strategies to prevent recurrence of anaphylaxis. All patients who have experienced an anaphylactic reaction should receive a prescription for auto-injectable epinephrine devices. The nurse instructs the patient and family in their use and has the patient and family demonstrate correct administration (see Chart 37-3).

Allergic Rhinitis

Allergic rhinitis (hay fever, seasonal allergic rhinitis) is the most common form of respiratory allergy, which is presumed to be mediated by an immediate (type I hypersensitivity) immunologic reaction. It is among the top 11% of all primary care visits and affects about 12% (1 in 8 adults) in the United States (Rosenfeld, Piccirillo, Chandrasekhar et al., 2015). Symptoms are similar to those of viral rhinitis (see Chapter 22) but are usually more persistent and demonstrate seasonal variation; rhinitis is considered to be the allergic form if the symptoms are caused by an allergen-specific IgE-mediated immunologic response. However, approximately one third of patients with rhinitis have associated conjunctivitis, sinusitis, and asthma (Baran et al, 2014; Lehrer, Mullol, Agredo, et al., 2014). The proportion of patients with the allergic form of rhinitis increases with age. It often occurs with other conditions, such as asthma, and cystic fibrosis (Rosenfeld et al., 2015). If symptoms are severe, allergic rhinitis may interfere with sleep, leisure, school, and overall quality of life (Sheikh, 2015). Chronic rhinitis accounts for an average of 1 to 2 missed work days per patient per year. These patients experience a 36% reduction in on-the-job effectiveness and 38% loss of productivity (Sheikh, 2015).

Early diagnosis and adequate treatment are essential to reduce complications and relieve symptoms.

Because allergic rhinitis is induced by airborne pollens or molds, it is characterized by the following seasonal occurrences (Sheikh, 2015):
- Early spring—tree pollen (oak, elm, poplar)
- Early summer—grass pollen (Timothy, Redtop)
- Early fall—weed pollen (ragweed)

Chart
37-3

PATIENT EDUCATION
Self-Administration of Epinephrine

The nurse instructs the patient to:

1. After removing the EpiPenautoinjector from its carrying tube, grasp the unit with the orange tip (injecting end) pointing downward. Form a fist around the unit with the orange tip down; with your other hand, remove the blue safety release cap.

2. Hold the black tip near outer thigh. Swing and **jab firmly** into the outer thigh until a click is heard with the device perpendicular (90-degree angle) to the thigh. Do NOT inject into buttocks.

3. Hold firmly against the thigh for approximately 10 seconds. Remove the unit from the thigh, and gently massage the injection area for 10 seconds. Call 911 and seek immediate medical attention. Carefully place the used autoinjector unit, needle-end first, into the device storage tube without bending the needle. Screw on the storage tube completely, and take it with you to the hospital emergency room.

~10 seconds

Each year, attacks begin and end at about the same time. Airborne mold spores require warm, damp weather. Although there is no rigid seasonal pattern, these spores appear in early spring, are rampant during the summer, then taper off and disappear by the first frost in areas that experience dramatic seasonal temperature variation. In temperate areas that do not experience freezing temperatures, these allergens, especially mold, can persist throughout the year.

Pathophysiology

Sensitization begins by ingestion or inhalation of an antigen. On re-exposure, the nasal mucosa reacts by the slowing of ciliary action, edema formation, and leukocyte (primarily eosinophil) infiltration. Histamine is the major mediator of allergic reactions in the nasal mucosa. Tissue edema results from vasodilation and increased capillary permeability.

Clinical Manifestations

The four major signs and symptoms of allergic rhinitis include copious amounts of serous nasal discharge, nasal congestion, sneezing, as well as nose and throat itching. Patients may experience post-nasal drip, itching, watery eyes, headache, and hyposomnia (Baran et al., 2014). Bronchial asthma is more persistent in patients with chronic rhinitis than in those with allergic rhinitis (Lehrer et al., 2014). The symptoms of this chronic condition depend on environmental exposure and intrinsic host responsiveness. Allergic rhinitis can affect quality of life by also producing sleep disturbance, impairment of daily activities, and missed school and work (Fleisher et al., 2013).

Assessment and Diagnostic Findings

Diagnosis of seasonal allergic rhinitis is based on history, physical examination, and diagnostic test results. Diagnostic tests include nasal smears, peripheral blood counts, total serum IgE, epicutaneous and intradermal testing, serum-specific IgE, and nasal provocation tests. Results indicative of allergy as the cause of rhinitis include increased IgE and eosinophil levels and positive reactions on allergen testing. False-positive and false-negative responses to these tests, particularly skin testing, may occur (Fleisher et al., 2013).

Medical Management

The goal of therapy is to provide relief from symptoms. Therapy may include one or all of the following interventions: avoidance therapy, pharmacologic therapy, and immunotherapy. Verbal instructions must be reinforced by written information. Knowledge of general concepts regarding assessment and therapy in allergic diseases is important so that the patient can learn to manage certain conditions as well as prevent severe reactions and illnesses.

Avoidance Therapy

In avoidance therapy, every attempt is made to remove the allergens that act as precipitating factors. Simple measures and environmental controls are often effective in decreasing symptoms. Examples include the use of air conditioners, air cleaners, humidifiers, and dehumidifiers; removal of dust-catching furnishings, carpets, and window coverings; removal of pets from the home or bedroom; the use of pillow and mattress covers that are impermeable to dust mites; and a smoke-free environment (Sheikh, 2015). Additional measures include changing clothing when coming in from outside, showering to wash allergens from hair and skin, and using an over-the-counter nasal irrigation device or saline nasal spray to reduce allergens in the nasal passages Because multiple allergens are often implicated, multiple measures to avoid exposure to allergens are often necessary (Bleier, 2015; Sheikh, 2015). High-efficiency particulate air (HEPA) purifiers and vacuum cleaner filters may also be used to reduce allergens in the environment. Research suggests that multiple avoidance strategies tailored to a person's risk factors can reduce the severity of symptoms, the number of work or school days missed because of symptoms, and the number of unscheduled health care visits for treatment (Sheikh, 2015). In many cases, it is impossible to avoid exposure to all environmental allergens, so pharmacologic therapy or immunotherapy is needed.

Pharmacologic Therapy

Antihistamines

Antihistamines, classified as H_1 receptor antagonists (or H_1 blockers), are used in the management of mild allergic disorders. H_1 blockers bind selectively to H_1 receptors, preventing the actions of histamines at these sites. They do not prevent the release of histamine from mast cells or basophils. The H_1 antagonists have no effect on H_2 receptors, but they do have the ability to bind to nonhistaminic receptors. The ability of certain antihistamines to bind to and block muscarinic receptors underlies several of the prominent anticholinergic side effects of these medications.

Oral antihistamines, which are readily absorbed, are most effective when given at the first occurrence of symptoms, because they prevent the development of new symptoms. The effectiveness of these medications is limited to certain patients with hay fever, vasomotor rhinitis, urticaria (hives), and mild asthma. They are rarely effective in other conditions or in any severe conditions (Frandsen & Pennington, 2014; Hodgson & Kizior, 2014).

Antihistamines are frequently prescribed for the symptomatic relief of allergic rhinitis. The major side effects are drowsiness and dry mouth (Hwang & Patel, 2015; Rosenfeld et al., 2015). Additional side effects include anxiety, agitation, urinary retention, blurred vision, anorexia, nausea, and vomiting (Frandsen & Pennington, 2014; Hodgson & Kizior, 2014).

Antihistamines are contraindicated during pregnancy, in nursing mothers and newborns, in children and older adults, and in patients with hypersensitivity to the drugs whose conditions may be aggravated by muscarinic blockade (e.g., asthma, urinary retention, open-angle glaucoma, hypertension, prostatic hyperplasia) (Frandsen & Pennington, 2014; Hodgson & Kizior, 2014; Katzung & Trevor, 2015).

Second-generation or nonsedating H_1 receptor antagonists are newer types of antihistamines. Unlike first-generation H_1 receptor antagonists, they do not readily enter the brain from the blood (Fleisher, et al., 2013; Frandsen & Pennington, 2014). They bind to peripheral rather than central nervous system H_1 receptors, causing less sedation. Examples of these medications are loratadine (Claritin), cetirizine (Zyrtec), and fexofenadine (Allegra). Selected H_1 antihistamines are shown in Table 37-2.

Antihistamines may also be combined with decongestants to reduce the nasal congestion associated with allergies. Most combination products are available as over-the-counter (nonprescription) medications; examples are loratadine/pseudoephedrine (Claritin-D) and cetirizine/pseudoephedrine (Zyrtec-D). Decongestants can cause an increase in blood pressure; therefore, patients with a history of hypertension should be cautioned about long-term use of any medication that contains decongestants (Bleier, 2015; Hodgson & Kizior, 2014).

Adrenergic Agents

Adrenergic agents, which are vasoconstrictors of mucosal vessels, are used topically in nasal (Afrin) and ophthalmic (Alphagan P) formulations in addition to the oral route (pseudoephedrine [Sudafed]) (Frandsen & Pennington, 2014; Hodgson & Kizior, 2014). The topical route (drops and sprays) causes fewer side effects than oral administration; however, the use of drops and sprays should be limited to a few days to avoid rebound congestion. Adrenergic nasal decongestants are applied topically to the nasal mucosa for the relief of nasal congestion. They activate the alpha-adrenergic receptor sites on the smooth muscle of the nasal mucosal blood vessels, reducing local blood flow, fluid exudation, and mucosal edema. Topical ophthalmic drops are used for symptomatic relief of eye irritations caused by allergies. Potential side effects include hypertension, dysrhythmias, palpitations, central nervous system stimulation, irritability, tremor, and tachyphylaxis (acceleration of hemodynamic status).

Mast Cell Stabilizers

Intranasal cromolyn sodium (NasalCrom) is a spray that acts by stabilizing the mast cell membrane, thus reducing the release of histamine and other mediators of the allergic response. In addition, it inhibits macrophages, eosinophils, monocytes, and platelets involved in the immune response (Arcangelo & Peterson, 2013). Cromolyn interrupts the physiologic response to nasal antigens, and it is used prophylactically (before the exposure to allergens) to prevent the onset of symptoms and to treat symptoms once they occur. It is also used therapeutically in chronic allergic rhinitis. This spray is as effective as antihistamines but is less effective than intranasal corticosteroids in the treatment of seasonal allergic rhinitis. The patient must be informed that the beneficial effects of the medication may take a week or so to manifest. The medication is of no benefit in the treatment of nonallergic rhinitis.

TABLE 37-2 Selected H₁ Antihistamines

H₁ Antihistamine	Contraindications	Major Side Effects	Nursing Implications and Patient Education
First-Generation H₁ Antihistamines (Sedating)			
Diphenhydramine (Benadryl)	Allergy to any antihistamines Third trimester of pregnancy Lactation Use cautiously with narrow-angle glaucoma, asthma, stenosing peptic ulcer, benign prostatic hyperplasia (BPH) or bladder neck obstruction, first and second trimester of pregnancy, older patients, hypertension.	Drowsiness, confusion, dizziness, dry mouth, nausea, vomiting, photosensitivity, urinary retention	Administer with food if gastrointestinal (GI) upset occurs. Caution patients to avoid alcohol, driving, or engaging in any hazardous activities until central nervous system (CNS) response to medication is stabilized. Suggest sucking on sugarless lozenges or ice chips for relief of dry mouth. Encourage the use of sunscreen and hat while outdoors. Assess for urinary retention; monitor urinary output.
Chlorpheniramine (Chlor-Trimeton)	Allergy to any antihistamines Third trimester of pregnancy Lactation Use cautiously with narrow-angle glaucoma, asthma, stenosing peptic ulcer, BPH or bladder neck obstruction, first and second trimester of pregnancy, older patients, hypertension.	Drowsiness, sedation, and dizziness, although less than other sedating agents; confusion, dry mouth, nausea, vomiting, urinary retention, epigastric distress, thickening of bronchial secretions	Caution patients to avoid alcohol, driving, or engaging in any hazardous activities until CNS response to medication is stabilized. Suggest sucking on sugarless lozenges or ice chips for relief of dry mouth. Recommend the use of a humidifier.
Hydroxyzine (Atarax)	Allergy to hydroxyzine or cetirizine (Zyrtec), pregnancy, lactation, hypertension	Drowsiness; dry mouth; involuntary motor activity, including tremor and seizures	Caution patients to avoid alcohol, driving, or engaging in any hazardous activities until CNS response to medication is stabilized. Suggest sucking on sugarless lozenges or ice chips for relief of dry mouth. Instruct patients to report tremors.
Second-Generation H₁ Antihistamines (Nonsedating)			
Cetirizine (Zyrtec)	Allergy to any antihistamines Narrow-angle glaucoma Asthma Stenosing peptic ulcer BPH or bladder neck obstruction Lactation Hypertension	Dry nasal mucosa, thickening of bronchial secretions	Can be taken without regard to meals. Instruct patients to use caution if driving or performing tasks that require alertness. Recommend the use of a humidifier.
Desloratadine (Clarinex)	Allergy to loratadine (Alavert, Claritin) Lactation Use cautiously with renal or hepatic impairment, pregnancy, hypertension.	Somnolence, nervousness, dizziness, fatigue, dry mouth	Can be taken without regard to meals. Suggest sucking on sugarless lozenges or ice chips for relief of dry mouth. Recommend the use of a humidifier.
Loratadine (Alavert, Claritin)	Allergy to any antihistamines Narrow-angle glaucoma Asthma Stenosing peptic ulcer BPH or bladder neck obstruction Hypertension	Headache, nervousness, dizziness, depression, edema, increased appetite	Instruct patients to take on empty stomach (1 hour before or 2 hours after meals or food). Instruct patients to avoid alcohol and to use caution if driving or performing tasks that require alertness. Suggest sucking on sugarless lozenges or ice chips for relief of dry mouth. Recommend the use of a humidifier.
Fexofenadine (Allegra)	Allergy to any antihistamines Pregnancy Lactation Use cautiously with hepatic or renal impairment, older patients, hypertension.	Fatigue, drowsiness, GI upset	Should not be given within 15 minutes of ingestion of antacids. Instruct patients to use caution if driving or performing tasks that require alertness. Recommend the use of a humidifier.
Levocetirizine (Xyzal)	Hypersensitivity to any antihistamines End-stage renal disease Hemodialysis Use cautiously with pregnancy, lactation, older patients.	Drowsiness, GI disturbance, headache	Can be taken without regard to meals. Instruct patients to use caution if driving or performing tasks that require alertness. Recommend the use of a humidifier.

Adapted from Comerford, K. C. (2015). *Nursing 2015 drug handbook.* Philadelphia, PA: Wolters Kluwer.

Adverse effects (e.g., sneezing, local stinging and burning sensations) are usually mild.

Corticosteroids

Intranasal corticosteroids are indicated in more severe cases of allergic and perennial rhinitis that cannot be controlled by more conventional medications, such as decongestants, antihistamines, and intranasal cromolyn. Examples of these medications include beclomethasone (Beconase, Qnasl), budesonide (Rhinocort), flunisolide (AeroSpan), and triamcinolone (Nasacort) (Comerford, 2015).

Because of their anti-inflammatory actions, corticosteroids are equally effective in preventing or suppressing the major symptoms of allergic rhinitis. These medications are given by metered-spray devices. If the nasal passages are blocked, a topical decongestant may be used to clear the passages before the administration of the intranasal corticosteroid. Patients must be aware that full benefit may not be achieved for several days to 2 weeks. Adverse effects of intranasal corticosteroids are mild and include drying of the nasal mucosa and burning and itching sensations caused by the vehicle used to administer the medication. Recommended use of this medication is limited to 30 days. Beclomethasone, budesonide, flunisolide, and triamcinolone are deactivated rapidly after absorption, so they do not achieve significant blood levels. Because corticosteroids suppress host defenses, they must be used with caution in patients with tuberculosis or untreated bacterial infections of the lungs. Patients taking corticosteroids are at risk for infection and suppression of typical manifestations of inflammation, because host defenses are compromised. Inhaled corticosteroids do not affect the immune system to the same degree as systemic corticosteroids (i.e., oral corticosteroids). Because corticosteroids are inhaled into the upper respiratory tract, tuberculosis or untreated bacterial infections of the lungs may become apparent and progress. Whenever possible, patients with tuberculosis or other bacterial infections of the lungs should avoid inhaled corticosteroids.

Oral and parenteral corticosteroids are used when conventional therapy has failed and symptoms are severe and of short duration (Frandsen & Pennington, 2014; Hodgson & Kizior, 2014). They can control symptoms of allergic reactions such as hay fever, medication-induced allergies, and allergic reactions to insect stings. Because the response to corticosteroids is delayed, these agents have little or no value in acute therapy for severe reactions such as anaphylaxis.

> ### ▶ Quality and Safety Nursing Alert
>
> *Patients who receive high-dose or long-term corticosteroid therapy must be cautioned not to stop taking the medication suddenly. Doses are tapered when discontinuing this medication to avoid adrenal insufficiency.*

The patient is also instructed about side effects, which include fluid retention, weight gain, hypertension, gastric irritation, glucose intolerance, and adrenal suppression.

Further discussion of corticosteroids is provided in Chapter 52, Table 52-4.

Leukotriene Modifiers

Leukotrienes have many effects on the inflammatory cycle. Leukotriene modifiers, such as zafirlukast (Accolate) and montelukast (Singulair), block the synthesis or action of leukotrienes and prevent the signs and symptoms associated with asthma (see Table 37-3).

Leukotriene modifiers are for long-term use, and patients should be advised to take their medication daily. Patients take appropriate "rescue" medications for symptom exacerbation but continue to take the leukotriene modifier on a daily basis. The National Asthma Education and Prevention Program (NAEPP) suggests using a leukotriene modifier in conjunction with an inhaled corticosteroid for mild persistent asthma (National Institute of Allergy and Infectious Disease [NIAID], 2013).

Immunotherapy

Allergen desensitization (allergen immunotherapy, hyposensitization) is primarily used to treat IgE-mediated diseases by injections of allergen extracts. Immunotherapy, also referred to as allergy vaccine therapy, involves the administration of gradually increasing quantities of specific allergens to the patient until a dose is reached that is effective in reducing disease severity from natural exposure. This is an effective treatment for 80% to 90% of certain allergens such as grass and pollen (ASCIA, 2015; Senti, von Moos, Graf, et al., 2015; Sheikh, 2015). This type of therapy provides an adjunct to symptomatic pharmacologic therapy and can be used when avoidance of allergens is not possible. Specific immunotherapy has been used in the treatment of allergic disorders for many years. Goals of immunotherapy include reducing the level of circulating IgE, increasing the level of blocking antibody IgG, and reducing mediator cell sensitivity. Immunotherapy has been most effective for ragweed pollen; however, treatment for grass, tree pollen, cat dander, and house dust mite allergens has also been effective. Indications and contraindications for immunotherapy are presented in Chart 37-4.

Correlation of a positive skin test with a positive allergy history is an indication for immunotherapy if the allergen cannot be avoided. The benefit of immunotherapy has been fairly well established in instances of allergic rhinitis and bronchial asthma that are clearly due to sensitivity to one of the common pollens, molds, or household dust. Unlike antiallergy medication, allergen immunotherapy has the potential to alter the allergic disease course after 3 to 5 years of therapy.

TABLE 37-3 Leukotriene Modifiers

Leukotriene Modifier	Available Formulations	Frequency of Dosing
Leukotriene-Receptor Antagonists		
Zafirlukast (Accolate)	Tablets: 10 mg; 20 mg	Taken twice a day
Montelukast (Singulair)	Tablets: 10 mg Chewable tablets: 4 mg; 5 mg Granules: 4 mg/packet	Taken once a day in pm
Leukotriene-Receptor Inhibitors		
Zileuton (Zyflo CR)	Tablets: 600 mg extended release	Taken twice a day within 1 hour after morning and evening meals

Chart 37-4 Immunotherapy: Indications and Contraindications

Indications

- Allergic rhinitis, conjunctivitis, or allergic asthma
- History of a systemic reaction to Hymenoptera and specific immunoglobulin E antibodies to Hymenoptera venom
- Desire to avoid the long-term use, potential adverse effects, or costs of medications
- Lack of control of symptoms by avoidance measures or the use of medications

Contraindications

- The use of beta-blocker or angiotensin-converting enzyme inhibitor therapy, which may mask early signs of anaphylaxis
- Presence of significant pulmonary or cardiac disease or organ failure
- Inability of the patient to recognize or report signs and symptoms of a systemic reaction
- Nonadherence of the patient to other therapeutic regimens and nonlikelihood that the patient will adhere to the immunization schedule (often weekly for an indefinite period)
- Inability to monitor the patient for at least 30 minutes after administration of immunotherapy
- Absence of equipment or adequate personnel to respond to allergic reaction if one occurs

Because it may prevent the progression or development of asthma or multiple or additional allergies, it is also considered to be a potential preventive measure (Sheikh, 2015). The patient must understand what to expect and the importance of continuing therapy for several years before immunotherapy is accomplished. When skin tests are performed, the results are correlated with symptoms; treatment is based on the patient's needs rather than on the results of skin tests.

There are three methods of immunotherapy: subcutaneous immunotherapy (SIT), sublingual immunotherapy (SLIT), and epicutaneous immunotherapy (EPIT).

Subcutaneous Immunotherapy

The most common method of treatment is SIT, which consists of the serial injection of one or more antigens that are selected in each particular case on the basis of skin testing. This method provides a simple and efficient technique for targeting IgE antibodies to specific antigens. Specific treatment consists of injecting extracts of the allergens that cause symptoms in a particular patient. Injections begin with very small amounts and are gradually increased, usually at weekly intervals, until a maximum tolerated dose is attained. Although severe systemic reactions are rare, the risk of systemic and potentially fatal anaphylaxis exists. It tends to occur most frequently at the induction or "up-dosing" phase. Therefore, the patient must be monitored after administration of immunotherapy. Because of the risk of anaphylaxis, injections should not be given by a lay person or by the patient. The patient must remain in the office or clinic for at least 30 minutes after the injection and is observed for possible systemic symptoms. If a large, local swelling develops at the injection site, the next dose should not be increased, because this may be a warning sign of a possible systemic reaction (ASCIA, 2015; Sheikh, 2015).

Maintenance booster injections are given at 2- to 4-week intervals, frequently for a period of several years, before the maximum benefit is achieved, although some patients will note early improvement in their symptoms. Long-term benefit seems to be related to the cumulative dose of vaccine given over time (ASCIA, 2015; Sheikh, 2015).

Quality and Safety Nursing Alert

Because the injection of an allergen may induce systemic reactions, such injections are given only in a setting where epinephrine is immediately available (i.e., primary provider's office, clinic).

Sublingual Immunotherapy.

In April 2014, the U.S. Food and Drug Administration (FDA) approved the use of a SLIT. SLIT has been reported to have a 30% to 40% reduction in reactions and rescue medication usage in seasonal allergic rhinitis. Administration of SLIT includes a buildup phase that is followed by a treatment plan of three times per week with a rapid dissolving tablet or liquid containing allergen extracts. Recent studies show comparable efficacy of SLIT with SIT (Senti et al., 2015). Systemic side effects are rare but have been reported in patients who also report systemic reactions with SIT. Side effects include irritation, minor swelling or itching inside the mouth, and stomach upset and nausea.

Epicutaneous Immunotherapy

EPIT represents an alternative allergen immunotherapy with delivery of the allergen to the epidermis. Because the epidermis is less vascular, there is reduced risk of systemic allergic side effects due to inadvertent intravascular allergen delivery. Reports from the completed trials of EPIT may find potential application in the management of IgE-mediated allergies, but more research is needed to define an optimal regimen that balances clinical efficacy and safety (Senti et al., 2015).

Immunotherapy should not be initiated during pregnancy; for patients who have been receiving immunotherapy before pregnancy, the dosage should not be increased during pregnancy.

Therapeutic failure is evident when a patient does not experience a decrease of symptoms within 12 to 24 months, fails to develop increased tolerance to known allergens, and cannot decrease the use of medications to reduce symptoms. Potential causes of treatment failure include misdiagnosis of allergies, inadequate doses of allergen, newly developed allergies, and inadequate environmental controls.

NURSING PROCESS

The Patient With Allergic Rhinitis

Assessment

The examination and history of the patient reveal sneezing, often in paroxysms; thin and watery nasal discharge; itching eyes and nose; lacrimation; and occasionally headache. The health history includes a personal or family history of allergy. The allergy assessment identifies the nature of antigens, seasonal changes in symptoms, and medication history. The nurse also obtains subjective data about how the patient feels just before symptoms become obvious, such as the occurrence of pruritus, breathing problems, and tingling sensations. In addition to these symptoms, hoarseness, wheezing, hives, rash, erythema, and edema are noted. Any relationship between emotional problems or stress and the triggering of allergy symptoms is assessed.

Diagnosis

NURSING DIAGNOSES
Based on the assessment data, major nursing diagnoses may include:
- Ineffective breathing pattern related to allergic reaction
- Deficient knowledge about allergy and the recommended modifications in lifestyle and self-care practices
- Ineffective coping with chronicity of condition and need for environmental modifications

COLLABORATIVE PROBLEMS/POTENTIAL COMPLICATIONS
Potential complications may include the following:
- Anaphylaxis
- Impaired breathing
- Nonadherence to the therapeutic regimen

Planning and Goals

The goals for the patient may include restoration of a breathing pattern that provides adequate ventilation, increased knowledge about the causes and control of allergic symptoms, improved coping with alterations and modifications, and absence of complications.

Nursing Interventions

IMPROVING BREATHING PATTERN
The patient is instructed and assisted to modify the environment to reduce the severity of allergic symptoms or to prevent their occurrence. The patient is also instructed to reduce exposure to people with upper respiratory tract infections. Adherence to medication schedules and other treatment regimens is encouraged and reinforced.

PROMOTING UNDERSTANDING OF
ALLERGY AND ALLERGY CONTROL
Instruction includes strategies to minimize exposure to allergens and explanation about desensitization procedures and correct use of medications. The nurse informs and reminds the patient of the importance of keeping appointments for desensitization procedures, because dosages are usually adjusted on a weekly basis, and missed appointments may interfere with the dosage adjustment.

Patients need to understand the difference between rescue medications for allergy exacerbation and seasonal flares (e.g., antihistamines) and medications used for allergy control throughout the year (e.g., inhaled corticosteroids, leukotriene modifiers). Patients also need to understand that medications for allergy exacerbation and seasonal flares should be used only when the allergy is apparent. Continued use of these medications when not required can result in tolerance; consequently, the medications will be ineffective when needed.

COPING WITH A CHRONIC DISORDER
Although allergic reactions are infrequently life-threatening, they require vigilance to avoid allergens and modification of the lifestyle or environment to prevent recurrence of symptoms. Allergic symptoms are often present year-round and create discomfort and inconvenience for the patient. Although patients may not feel ill during allergy seasons, they often do not feel well, either. The need to be alert for possible allergens in the environment may be tiresome, placing a burden on the patient's ability to lead a normal life. Stress related to these difficulties may in turn increase the frequency or severity of symptoms. To assist the patient in adjusting to these modifications, the nurse must have an appreciation of the difficulties encountered by the patient. The patient is encouraged to verbalize feelings and concerns in a supportive environment and to identify strategies to deal with them effectively.

MONITORING AND MANAGING POTENTIAL COMPLICATIONS
Anaphylaxis and Impaired Breathing. Respiratory and cardiovascular functioning can be significantly altered during allergic reactions by the reaction itself or by the medications used to treat reactions. The respiratory status is evaluated by monitoring the respiratory rate and pattern and by assessing for breathing difficulties or abnormal lung sounds. The pulse rate and rhythm and blood pressure are monitored to assess cardiovascular status regularly or any time the patient reports symptoms such as itching or difficulty breathing. In the event of signs and symptoms suggestive of anaphylaxis, emergency medications and equipment must be available for immediate use. See Chapter 14 for treatment of anaphylactic shock.

Nonadherence to the Therapeutic Regimen. Knowledge about the treatment regimen does not ensure adherence. Having the patient identify potential barriers and explore acceptable solutions for effective management of the condition (e.g., installing tile floors rather than carpet, not gardening in the spring) can increase adherence to the treatment regimen.

PROMOTING HOME, COMMUNITY-BASED,
AND TRANSITIONAL CARE
Educating Patients About Self-Care. The patient is instructed about strategies to minimize exposure to allergens, the actions and adverse effects of medications, and the correct use of medications. The patient should know the name, dose, frequency, actions, and side effects of all medications taken.

Instruction about strategies to control allergic symptoms is based on the needs of the patient as determined by the results of tests, the severity of symptoms, and the motivation of the patient and family to deal with the condition. Suggestions for patients who are sensitive to dust and mold in the home are given in Chart 37-5.

If the patient is to undergo SIT immunotherapy, the nurse reinforces the primary provider's explanation regarding the purpose and procedure. Instructions are given regarding the series of injections, which usually are given initially every week and then at 2- to 4-week intervals. These instructions include remaining in the primary provider's office or the clinic for at least 30 minutes after the injection, so that emergency treatment can be given if the patient has a reaction; avoiding rubbing or scratching the injection site; and continuing with the series for the period of time required. In addition, the patient and family are instructed about emergency treatment of severe allergic symptoms.

Because antihistamines may produce drowsiness, the patient is cautioned about this and other side effects applicable to the

Chart 37-5

HOME CARE CHECKLIST

Allergy Management

At the completion of education, the patient, caregiver, or both will be able to:

- State the impact of environmental allergens (e.g., dust, molds, perfumes, foods) on physiologic functioning, ADLs, IADLs, roles, relationships, and spirituality.
- State changes in home environment necessary to minimize exposure to allergens.
  - Removing drapes, curtains, and venetian blinds and replacing them with pull shades; covering the mattress with a hypoallergenic cover that can be zipped; and removing rugs and replacing them with wood flooring or linoleum.
  - Reducing dust in the house as a whole by using steam or hot water for heating and using high-efficiency particulate air (HEPA) purifiers or air-conditioning.
  - Washing the floor and dusting and vacuuming daily, using clean filters, wearing a mask whenever cleaning is being done.
  - Replacing stuffed furniture with wood pieces that can easily be dusted.
  - Avoiding the use of tufted bedspreads, stuffed toys, and feather pillows and replacing them with washable cotton material.
  - Avoiding the use of any clothing that causes itching.

- Verbalize ways to reduce exposure to pollens or molds by identifying seasons of the year when pollen counts are high; wearing a mask at times of increased exposure (windy days and when grass is being cut); and avoiding contact with weeds, dry leaves, and freshly cut grass.
- State rationale for seeking air-conditioned areas at the height of the allergy season.
- State rationale for avoiding sprays and perfumes.
- State rationale for the use of hypoallergenic cosmetics.
- State rationale for taking prescribed medications as ordered.
- Identify specific foods that may cause allergic symptoms and develop a list of foods to avoid (e.g., fish, nuts, eggs, chocolate).
- Verbalize ways to cope with stress successfully, plans for regular exercise, and rationale for obtaining adequate rest.
- State how to reach primary provider with questions or complications.
- State time and date of follow-up appointments, testing.
- Identify the need for health promotion, disease prevention, and screening activities.

ADLs, activities of daily living; IADLs, independent activities of daily living.

medication. Operating machinery, driving a car, and performing activities that require intense concentration should be postponed. The patient is also informed about the dangers of drinking alcohol when taking antihistamines, because they tend to exaggerate the effects of alcohol.

The patient must be aware of the effects caused by overuse of the sympathomimetic agents in nose drops or sprays, because a condition referred to as rhinitis medicamentosa may result. After topical application of the medication, a rebound period occurs in which the nasal mucous membranes become more edematous and congested than they were before the medication was used. Such a reaction encourages the use of more medication, and a cyclic pattern results. The topical agent must be discontinued immediately and completely to correct this problem.

Concept Mastery Alert

In rhinitis medicamentosa, the rebound reaction from the overuse of sympathomimetic nose drops or sprays worsens the congestion, causing the patient to use more of the medication and thus leads to more nasal congestion. This condition should not be confused with a patient developing tolerance to the drug.

Continuing and Transitional Care. Follow-up telephone calls to the patient are often reassuring to the patient and family and provide an opportunity for the nurse to answer any questions. The patient is reminded to keep follow-up appointments and informed about the importance of continuing with treatment. The importance of participating in health promotion activities and health screening is also emphasized.

Evaluation

Expected patient outcomes may include:
1. Exhibits a breathing pattern that provides adequate ventilation
   a. Demonstrates lungs clear on auscultation
   b. Exhibits absence of adventitious breath sounds (crackles, rhonchi, wheezing)
   c. Has a normal respiratory rate and pattern
   d. Reports no complaints of respiratory distress (shortness of breath, difficulty on inspiration or expiration)
2. Demonstrates knowledge about allergy and strategies to control symptoms
   a. Identifies causative allergens, if known
   b. States methods of avoiding allergens and controlling indoor and outdoor precipitating factors
   c. Removes from the environment items that retain dust
   d. Wears a dampened mask if dust or mold may be a problem
   e. Avoids smoke-filled rooms and dust-filled or freshly sprayed areas
   f. Uses air-conditioning for a major part of the day when allergens are high
   g. Takes antihistamines as prescribed; participates in hyposensitization program, if applicable
   h. Describes name, purpose, side effects, and method of administration of prescribed medications
   i. Identifies when to seek immediate medical attention for severe allergic responses
   j. Describes activities that are possible, including ways to participate in activities without activating the allergies

3. Adapts to the inconveniences of an allergy
   a. Relates the emotional aspects of the allergic response
   b. Demonstrates the use of measures to cope positively with allergy
4. Demonstrates absence of complications
   a. Exhibits vital signs within normal limits
   b. Reports no symptoms or episodes of anaphylaxis (urticaria, itching, peripheral tingling, fullness in the mouth and throat, flushing, difficulty swallowing, coughing, wheezing, or difficulty breathing)
   c. Demonstrates correct procedure to self-administer emergency medications to treat severe allergic reaction
   d. Correctly states medication names, dose and frequency of administration, and medication actions
   e. Correctly identifies side effects and untoward signs and symptoms to report to primary provider
   f. Discusses acceptable lifestyle changes and solutions for identified potential barriers to adherence to treatment and medication regimen

Contact Dermatitis

Contact dermatitis, a type IV delayed hypersensitivity reaction, is an acute or chronic skin condition caused by contact with an exogenous substance that elicits an allergic response. There are four basic types: allergic, irritant, phototoxic, and photo allergic (see Table 37-4). Eighty percent of cases are caused by excessive exposure to or additive effects of irritants (e.g., soaps, detergents, organic solvents). Skin sensitivity may develop after brief or prolonged periods of exposure, and the clinical picture may appear hours or weeks after the sensitized skin has been exposed.

Clinical Manifestations

Symptoms include itching, burning, erythema, skin lesions (vesicles and papules), and edema, followed by skin thickening, hardening, and scaling (Fonacier, Bernstein, Pancheco, et al., 2015). In severe responses, hemorrhagic bullae may develop. Repeated reactions may be accompanied by thickening of the skin and pigmentary changes. Secondary invasion by bacteria may develop in skin that is abraded by rubbing or scratching. Usually, there are no systemic symptoms unless the eruption is widespread (Habif, 2016).

Assessment and Diagnostic Findings

Determining allergens responsible requires a history, physical examination, and patch testing.

Assessment should include the date of onset, and any identifiable relationship to work environment and skin care products (Habif, 2016). The location of the lesions, distribution of the dermatitis, absence of other etiologies, and the history of exposure aid in determining the condition (Fonacier et al., 2015). Patch testing and environmental history of exposure to contact allergens are required to verify the diagnosis. Patch testing is indicated in cases in which inflammation persists despite avoidance therapy. The patch test most commonly used is the Thin-layer Rapid Use Epicutaneous (T.R.U.E.) test (Habif, 2016).

Atopic Dermatitis

Atopic dermatitis is a type I immediate hypersensitivity disorder characterized by inflammation and hyper reactivity of the skin. The term is used synonymously with atopic eczema (AAAAI, 2015). Other terms used to describe this kind of

TABLE 37-4 Types, Testing, and Treatment of Contact Dermatitis

Type	Etiology	Clinical Presentation	Diagnostic Testing	Treatment
Allergic	Results from contact of skin and allergenic substance; has a sensitization period of 10–14 days	Vasodilation and perivascular infiltrates on the dermis Intracellular edema Usually seen on dorsal aspects of hand	Patch testing (contraindicated in acute, widespread dermatitis)	Avoidance of offending material Aluminum acetate (Burow Solution, Domeboro Powder) or cool water compress Systemic corticosteroids (prednisone) for 7–10 days Topical corticosteroids for mild cases Oral antihistamines to relieve pruritus
Irritant	Results from contact with a substance that chemically or physically damages the skin on a nonimmunologic basis; occurs after first exposure to irritant or repeated exposures to milder irritants over an extended time	Dryness lasting days to months Vesiculation, fissures, cracks Hands and lower arms most common areas	Clinical picture Appropriate negative patch tests	Identification and removal of source of irritation Application of hydrophilic cream or petrolatum to soothe and protect Topical corticosteroids and compresses for weeping lesions Antibiotics for infection and oral antihistamines for pruritus
Phototoxic	Resembles the irritant type but requires sun and a chemical in combination to damage the epidermis	Similar to irritant dermatitis	Photo-patch test	Same as for allergic and irritant dermatitis
Photo allergic	Resembles allergic dermatitis but requires light exposure in addition to allergen contact to produce immunologic reactivity	Similar to allergic dermatitis	Photo-patch test	Same as for allergic and irritant dermatitis

Adapted from Comerford, K. C. (2015). *Nursing 2015 drug handbook*. Philadelphia, PA: Wolters Kluwer.

disorder include atopic eczema, atopic dermatitis, and atopic dermatitis/eczema syndrome (AEDS). In a revised classification system developed to clarify terminology, AEDS includes both allergic and nonallergic disorders (Habif, 2016). Currently, *atopic dermatitis* is the most commonly used term and will be used for the purpose of this discussion.

Atopic dermatitis is a chronic pruritis inflammatory skin disease. Increased serum IgE levels have been indicated in 80% of the patients with a family history of type 1 allergies, allergic rhinitis, and asthma. This disorder affects 15% to 30% of children and 2% to 10% of adults in developed countries (AAAAI, 2015). Most patients have significant elevations of serum IgE and peripheral eosinophilia. The eosinophil count may be increased depending on concomitant respiratory allergies (Habif, 2016).

Pruritus and hyperirritability of the skin are the most consistent features of atopic dermatitis and are related to large amounts of histamine in the skin. Excessive dryness of the skin with resultant itching is related to changes in lipid content, sebaceous gland activity, and sweating. In response to stroking of the skin, immediate redness appears on the skin. Pallor follows in 15 to 30 seconds and persists for 1 to 3 minutes. Patterns of inflammation result from scratching of erythematous papules. Lesions develop secondary to the trauma of scratching and appear in areas of increased sweating and hypervascularity. Atopic dermatitis is chronic, with remissions and exacerbations. This condition has a tendency to recur, with remission from adolescence to 20 years of age (Habif, 2016).

Nurses should be aware that atopic dermatitis is often linked in a process called the atopic march that often leads to asthma, allergic rhinitis, or food allergy (Fonacier et al., 2015). It is the result of interactions between susceptibility genes, the environment, defective function of the skin barrier, and immunologic responses.

Medical Management

Treatment of patients with atopic dermatitis must be individualized. Guidelines for treatment include identification and avoidance of contact with the offending agents; elimination of inflammatory disorders and infections; prescription of topical corticosteroids and non-steroidal anti-inflammatory agents; preservation and restoration of the stratum corneum layer; and prescription of antipuritic agents, oral antibiotics, and oral immunosuppressants for severely affected patients (Fonacier et al., 2015; Habif, 2016).

Itching can be decreased by wearing cotton fabrics; washing with a mild detergent; humidifying dry heat in winter; maintaining room temperature at 20°C to 22.2°C (68°F to 72°F); using antihistamines such as diphenhydramine; and avoiding animals, dust, sprays, and perfumes. Keeping the skin moisturized with daily baths to hydrate the skin and the use of topical skin moisturizers is encouraged. Topical corticosteroids are used to prevent inflammation, and any infection is treated with antibiotics to eliminate *Staphylococcus aureus* when indicated (Fonacier et al., 2015; Habif, 2016).

The use of immunosuppressive agents, such as cyclosporine (Neoral, Sandimmune), tacrolimus (Prograf, Protopic), and pimecrolimus (Elidel), may be effective in inhibiting T cells and mast cells involved in atopic dermatitis (Fonacier et al., 2015; Habif, 2016).

Research is needed to assess the effectiveness and the adverse side effects of medications used to treat atopic dermatitis.

Nursing Management

Patients who experience atopic dermatitis and their families require assistance and support from the nurse to cope with the disorder. The symptoms are often disturbing to the patient and disruptive to the family. The appearance of the skin may affect the patient's self-esteem and their willingness to interact with others. Instructions and counseling about strategies to incorporate preventive measures and treatments into the lifestyle of the family may be helpful.

The patient and family need to be aware of signs of secondary infection and of the need to seek treatment if infection occurs. The nurse also educates the patient and family about the side effects of medications used in treatment.

Dermatitis Medicamentosa (Drug Reactions)

Dermatitis medicamentosa, a type I hypersensitivity disorder, is the term applied to skin rashes associated with certain medications. Although people react differently to each medication, certain medications tend to induce eruptions of similar types. This disorder is the leading cause of fatal anaphylaxis, comprising 43% of deaths from anaphylaxis. All routes of administration are potentially fatal, but drugs given parenterally incur the greatest risk. Cutaneous rashes are among the most common adverse reactions to medications and occur in approximately 2% to 3% of hospitalized patients (Fleisher et al., 2013; Habif, 2016).

In general, drug reactions appear suddenly with characteristics that are more intense than the somewhat similar eruptions of infectious origin, and, with the exception of bromide and the iodide rashes, disappear rapidly after the medication is withdrawn (Comerford, 2015). Rashes may be accompanied by systemic or generalized symptoms. On discovery of a medication allergy, patients are warned that they have a hypersensitivity to a particular medication and are advised not to take it again. Penicillin, cephalosporin, and sulfonamide antibiotics are most commonly implicated (Habif, 2016). Patients should carry information identifying the hypersensitivity with them at all times.

Skin eruptions related to medication therapy suggest more serious hypersensitivities. Frequent assessment and prompt reporting of the appearance of any eruptions are important so that early treatment can be initiated. Some cutaneous drug reactions may indicate involvement of other organs and are known as complex drug reactions. Patients who suspect that a new rash may be caused by a drug allergy (newly prescribed medications, especially antibiotics such as penicillin or sulfa medications) should stop taking the medication immediately and contact their prescribing clinician, who will determine whether the medication and the rash are related.

Urticaria and Angioneurotic Edema

Urticaria (hives) is a type I hypersensitive allergic reaction of the skin that is characterized by the sudden appearance of edematous, pink or red wheals of variable size from 2 to 4 mm, and general pruritus. They may involve any part of the body, including the mucous membranes (especially those of the mouth), the larynx (occasionally with serious respiratory complications), and the gastrointestinal tract. This is a common condition with approximately 10% to 20% of people having one episode during their lifetime. Urticaria is most commonly instigated by infections, allergic reaction to food, insect stings, and medications (American Osteopathic College of Dermatology, 2015).

Each hive remains for a few minutes to several hours before disappearing. They usually fade within 24 to 48 hours, but new lesions may be developing simultaneously at other skin sites (Bernstein, Lang, Khan, et al., 2014). The condition usually resolves in 3 weeks. However, if this sequence continues for longer than 6 weeks, the condition is called *chronic urticaria*.

Management of the condition includes eliminating the causative drug or food; avoiding the use of nonsteroidal anti-inflammatory drugs (NSAIDs); minimizing potential aggravators, including heat, stress, alcohol, and tight clothes; administering antihistamines, and possibly a short course of corticosteroids (Prednisone) (AAAAI, 2015; American Osteopathic College of Dermatology, 2015; Fleisher et al., 2013; Habif, 2016).

Angioneurotic edema (i.e., angioedema) involves the deeper layers of the skin, resulting in more diffuse swelling rather than the discrete lesions characteristic of hives. It is manifested by non-pruritic, brawny, non-pitting edema with well-defined margins and erythema similar to urticaria (Bernstein et al., 2014). Urticaria and angioedema often occur together (Habif, 2016).

The regions most often involved in angioedema are the lips, eyelids, cheeks, hands, feet, genitalia, and tongue; the mucous membranes of the larynx, bronchi, and gastrointestinal canal may also be affected, particularly in the hereditary type (see discussion in the following section). On occasion, this reaction covers the entire back. Swellings may appear suddenly, in a few seconds or minutes, or slowly in 1 or 2 hours. In the latter case, their appearance is often preceded by itching or burning sensations. Seldom does more than a single swelling appear at one time, although one may develop while another is disappearing. Infrequently, swelling recurs in the same region. Individual lesions usually resolve in 24 hours (Fleisher et al., 2013; AAAAI, 2015). On rare occasions, swelling may recur with remarkable regularity at intervals of 3 to 4 weeks.

Several frequently prescribed medications, such as angiotensin-converting enzyme inhibitors (captopril [Capoten]) and penicillin, may cause angioedema. The nurse needs to be aware of all medications the patient is taking and be alert to the potential of angioedema as a side effect.

Hereditary Angioedema

Hereditary angioedema is a rare, potentially life-threatening, autosomal dominant disorder (Cicardi & Zuraw, 2015). Although not an immunologic disorder in the usual sense, this condition is included because of its resemblance to allergic angioedema and because of the potential seriousness of the condition. Symptoms are caused by edema of the skin, the respiratory tract, or the digestive tract. Attacks may be precipitated by trauma, or they may seem to occur spontaneously.

Clinical Manifestations

When skin is involved, the swelling usually is diffuse, does not itch, and usually is not accompanied by urticaria. Gastrointestinal edema may cause abdominal pain severe enough to be incapacitating. Typically, attacks last 2 to 4 days and resolve without intervention; however, attacks can occasionally affect the subcutaneous and submucosal tissues in the region of the upper airway and can be associated with respiratory obstruction and asphyxiation (Cicardi & Zuraw, 2015).

Medical Management

Attacks usually subside within 2 to 4 days, but during this time the patient should be observed carefully for signs of laryngeal obstruction, which may necessitate tracheostomy as a lifesaving measure. Epinephrine, antihistamines, and corticosteroids are usually used in treatment, although their success is limited. (Cicardi & Zuraw, 2015; Fleisher et al., 2013; Habif, 2016).

Cold Urticaria

Familial atypical cold urticaria (FACU) and acquired cold urticaria (ACU) are additional diseases within the spectrum of urticaria induced by temperature exposure. FACU is an autosomal dominant condition, inherited from one affected parent, and symptoms usually begin at birth within the first 6 months of life (Fleisher et al., 2013). ACU most frequently affects children and young adults (Fleisher et al., 2013; Habif, 2016).

Clinical Manifestations

Patients with FACU break out in hives (i.e., urticaria) when exposed to cold. The urticaria may be prompted by exposure to cold weather or cold water or after coming in contact with cold objects. Lesions occur within a few hours and usually subside in 2 days (Fleisher et al., 2013). Symptoms include fever, chills, conjunctiva infection, sweating, headache, and arthralgia. During the attack, the patient may develop leukocytosis, an increase in the erythrocyte sedimentation rate (ESR) and raised C-reactive protein levels (Ciccarelli, De Martinis, & Ginaldi, 2014).

Cold uticaria is diagnosed by physical testing. Ice cube provocation testing involves applying an ice cube to the skin of the forearm for 1 to 5 minutes. A positive test results in development of urticaria at the site in a patient with ACU. Clinical manifestations of FACU can be precipitated by the patient merely entering a 4°C (39°F) room.

Medical Management

Prevention involves avoidance of cold stimuli. Treatment involves bed rest, warmth, and corticosteroids to treat an acute attack (Ciccarelli et al., 2014).

All patients with any form of cold urticaria should carry an auto-injectable epinephrine device for emergency use because hives can progress to anaphylaxis.

Food Allergy

IgE-mediated food allergy, a type I hypersensitivity reaction, occurs in about 2% of the adult population; it is thought to occur in people who have a genetic predisposition combined with exposure to allergens early in life through the gastrointestinal or respiratory tract or nasal mucosa. More than 170 foods have been reported to cause IgE-mediated reactions (Sampson, Aceves, Brock, et al., 2014).

Almost any food can cause allergic symptoms. Any food can contain an allergen that results in anaphylaxis. The most common offenders are seafood (lobster, shrimp, crab, clams, fish), peanuts, tree nuts, berries, eggs, wheat, milk, and chocolate (Sampson et al., 2014). Peanut and tree nut (e.g., cashew, walnut) allergies are responsible for the most severe food allergy reactions. There is insufficient evidence that maternal diet during pregnancy or lactation affects the development of food allergies later in life (AAAAI, 2015; NIAID, 2013; Sampson et al., 2014).

One of the dangers of food allergens is that they may be hidden in other foods and not apparent to people who are susceptible to the allergen. For example, peanuts and peanut butter are often used in salad dressings and Asian, African, and Mexican cooking and may result in severe allergic reactions, including anaphylaxis. Previous contamination of equipment with allergens (e.g., peanuts) during preparation of another food product (e.g., chocolate cake) is enough to produce anaphylaxis in people with severe allergy (Fleischer, Sicherer, Greenhawt, et al., 2015).

Clinical Manifestations

Food allergy is the most common trigger for anaphylaxis. Symptoms occur in a few minutes to hours from exposure. The clinical symptoms are classic allergic symptoms (urticaria, dermatitis, wheezing, cough, laryngeal edema, angioedema) and gastrointestinal symptoms (itching; swelling of lips, tongue, and palate; abdominal pain; nausea; cramps; vomiting; and diarrhea) (NIAID, 2013; Sampson et al., 2015).

Assessment and Diagnostic Findings

A careful diagnostic workup is required in any patient with suspected food hypersensitivity. Included are a detailed allergy history, a physical examination, and pertinent diagnostic tests. Skin prick testing is used to identify the source of symptoms and assists in identifying specific foods as causative agents.

Medical Management

Therapy for food hypersensitivity includes elimination of the food responsible for the hypersensitivity (see Chart 37-6). Pharmacologic therapy is necessary for patients who cannot avoid exposure to offending foods and for patients with multiple food sensitivities not responsive to avoidance measures. Medication therapy involves the use of H_1 blockers, antihistamines, adrenergic agents, corticosteroids, and cromolyn sodium. All patients with food allergies, especially seafood and nuts, should have an auto-injectable epinephrine (e.g., EpiPen or Auvi-Q) device prescribed. Another essential aspect of management is educating patients and family members about how to recognize and manage the early stages of an acute anaphylactic reaction (AAAAI, 2015; Campbell et al., 2014). Many food allergies disappear with time, particularly in children.

Nursing Management

In addition to participating in management of the allergic reaction, the nurse focuses on preventing future exposure of the patient to the food allergen. If a severe allergic or anaphylactic reaction to food allergens has occurred, the nurse must instruct the patient and family about strategies to prevent its recurrence (see Chart 37-6). Patients' food allergies should be noted on their medical records, because there may be risk of allergic reactions not only to food but also to

---

Chart 37-6 **HOME CARE CHECKLIST**
Managing Food Allergies

At the completion of education, the patient, caregiver, or both will be able to:

- State the impact of food allergies on physiologic functioning, ADLs, IADLs, roles, relationships, and spirituality.
- Verbalize understanding of the need to maintain an allergen-free diet.
- Demonstrate reading of food labels to identify hidden allergens in food.
- Identify ways to manage an allergen-free diet when eating away from home.
- State the need to wear medical identification bracelet or necklace.
- List symptoms of food allergy.

- Demonstrate emergency administration of epinephrine.
- State the importance of replacing epinephrine when outdated.
- State the importance of prompt treatment of allergic reactions and health care follow-up.
- State how to reach primary provider with questions or complications.
- State time and date of follow-up appointments, testing.
- Verbalize ways to cope with stress successfully, plans for regular exercise, and rationale for obtaining adequate rest.
- Identify the need for health promotion, disease prevention, and screening activities.

ADLs, activities of daily living; IADLs, independent activities of daily living.

some medications containing similar substances (Sampson et al., 2014).

Latex Allergy

Latex allergy—the allergic reaction to natural rubber proteins—has been implicated in rhinitis, conjunctivitis, contact dermatitis, urticaria, asthma, and anaphylaxis. The prevalence has been steadily declining, possibly because of the use of nonpowdered latex and latex-free gloves (Mayo Foundation for Medical Education and Research, 2015).

Natural rubber latex is derived from the sap of the rubber tree (*Heveabrasiliensis*). The conversion of the liquid rubber latex into a finished product entails the addition of more than 200 chemicals. The proteins in the natural rubber latex (Hevea proteins) or the various chemicals that are used in the manufacturing process are thought to be the source of the allergic reactions. Not all objects composed of latex have the same ability to stimulate an allergic response. For example, the antigenicity of latex gloves can vary widely depending on the manufacturing method used (AAAAI, 2015; Mayo Foundation for Medical Education and Research, 2015).

Those at risk include 8% to 17% of health care workers, patients with atopic allergies or multiple surgeries, people working in factories that manufacture latex products, females, and 67% of patients with spina bifida (Fleisher et al., 2013). Because more food handlers, hairdressers, automobile mechanics, and police wear latex gloves, they are at risk for latex allergy. Patients are at risk for anaphylactic reactions as a result of contact with latex during medical treatments, especially surgical procedures. Food that has been handled by people wearing latex gloves may stimulate an allergic

TABLE 37-5 Selected Products Containing Natural Rubber Latex and Latex-Free Alternatives

Products Containing Latex	Examples of Latex-Safe Alternatives[a]
Hospital Environment	
Ace bandage (brown)	Ace bandage, white all cotton
Adhesive bandages, Band-Aid dressing, Telfa	Cotton pads and plastic or silk tape, Active Strips (3M), DuoDERM
Anesthesia equipment	Neoprene anesthesia kit (King)
Blood pressure cuff, tubing, and bladder	Clean Cuff, single-use nylon or vinyl blood pressure cuffs or wrap with stockinette or apply over clothing
Catheters	All-silicone or vinyl catheters
Catheter leg bag straps	Velcro straps
Crutch axillary pads and hand grips, tips	Cover with cloth, tape
ECG pads	Baxter, Red Dot 3M ECG pads
Elastic compression stockings	Kendall SCD stockings with stockinette
Gloves	Derma Prene, neoprene, polymer, or vinyl gloves
IV catheters	Jelco, Deseret IV catheters
IV rubber injection ports	Cover Y-sites and ports; do not puncture. Use three-way stopcocks on plastic tubing.
Levin tube	Salem sump tube
Medication vials	Remove rubber stopper.
Penrose drains	Jackson-Pratt, Zimmer Hemovac drains
Prepackaged enema kits	Therevac, Fleet Ready-to-Use
Pulse oximeters	Noninoximeters
Resuscitation bags	Laerdal, Puritan Bennett, *certain* Ambu
Stethoscope tubing	PVC tubing; cover with latex-free stockinette
Suction tubing	PVC (Davol, Laerdal)
Syringes—single use (Monoject, BD)	Terumo syringes, Abbott PCA Abboject
Tapes	Dermicel, Micropore
Theraband	New Thera-band Exercisers, plastic tubing
Thermometer probes	Diatek probe covers
Tourniquets	X-Tourn straps (Avcor)
Home Environment	
Balloons	Mylar balloons
Condoms, diaphragms	Polyurethane products, Durex Avanti and Reality products (female condom)
Diapers, incontinence pads	Huggies, Always, *some* Attends
Feminine hygiene pads	Kimberly-Clark products
Wheelchair cushions	ROHO cushions, Sof Care bed/chair cushions

ECG, electrocardiogram; IV, intravenous; PVC, polyvinyl chloride.
[a]Confirmation is essential to verify that all items are latex free before using, especially if risk of latex allergy is present.
Adapted from American Academy of Allergy, Asthma, and Immunology (AAAAI). (2015). Anaphylaxis overview. Retrieved on 11/15/ 2015 at: www.aaaai.org; Australasian Society of Clinical Immunology and Allergy (ASCIA). (2015). Immunotherapy for treatment of allergy. Retrieved on 11/15/ 2015 at: allergy.org.au; Campbell, R. L., Li, J., Nicklas, R. A., et al. (2014). Emergency department diagnosis and treatment of anaphylaxis: A practice parameter. *Annals of Allergy Asthma & Immunology*, 113, 599–608; Centers for Disease Control and Prevention (CDC)(2014). *Latex allergy: A prevention guide.* Retrieved on 11/20/2015 at: www.cdc.gov/niosh/docs/98-113/default.html; Mayo Foundation for Medical Education and Research. (2015). *Diseases and conditions: Latex allergy.* Retrieved on 11/20/2015 at: www.mayoclinic.org/diseases-conditions/latex-allergy/basics/definition/CON-20024233

response. Cross-reactions have been reported in people who are allergic to certain food products, such as kiwis, bananas, pineapples, mangoes, passion fruit, avocados, and chestnuts (AAAAI, 2015; Mayo Foundation for Medical Education and Research, 2015).

Routes of exposure to latex products can be cutaneous, percutaneous, mucosal, parenteral, or aerosol. Allergic reactions are more likely with parenteral or mucous membrane exposure but can also occur with cutaneous contact or inhalation. The most frequent source of exposure is cutaneous, which usually involves the wearing of natural latex gloves. The powder used to facilitate putting on latex gloves can become a carrier of latex proteins from the gloves; when the gloves are put on or removed, the particles become airborne and can be inhaled or settle on skin, mucous membranes, or clothing. Mucosal exposure can occur from the use of latex condoms, catheters, airways, and nipples. Parenteral exposure can occur from intravenous lines or hemodialysis equipment. In addition to latex-derived medical devices, many household items also contain latex. Examples of medical and household items containing latex and a list of alternative products are found in Table 37-5. It is estimated that more than 40,000 medical devices and nonmedical products contain latex. Chemical additives used in the manufacture of nonlatex gloves and other items have been associated with allergic symptoms, although these otherwise have a low potential to stimulate an allergic response (AAAAI, 2015; Mayo Foundation for Medical Education and Research, 2015).

Clinical Manifestations

Many different types of reactions to latex are possible (see Table 37-6). Irritant contact dermatitis, a nonimmunologic response, may be caused by mechanical skin irritation or an alkaline pH associated with latex gloves. Common symptoms of irritant dermatitis include erythema and pruritus. These symptoms can be eliminated by changing the brand of gloves or by using powder-free gloves. The use of hand lotion before donning latex gloves can worsen the symptoms, because lotions may leach latex proteins from the gloves, thus increasing skin exposure and the risk of developing true allergic reactions (Mayo Foundation for Medical Education and Research, 2015).

Delayed hypersensitivity to latex, a type IV reaction mediated by T cells in the immune system, is localized to the area of exposure and is characterized by symptoms of contact dermatitis, including vesicular skin lesions, papules, pruritus, edema, erythema, and crusting and thickening of the skin. These symptoms usually appear on the back of the hands. This reaction is thought to be caused by chemicals that are used in the manufacturing of latex products. It is the most common allergic reaction to latex. Although usually not life-threatening, delayed hypersensitivity reactions often require major changes in the patient's home and work environment to avoid further exposure. People who are sensitized to latex are at increased risk for development of type I allergic reactions (AAAAI, 2015; Mayo Foundation for Medical Education and Research, 2015).

Immediate hypersensitivity, a type I allergic reaction, is mediated by the IgE mast cell system (Abbas et al., 2014). Symptoms can include rhinitis, conjunctivitis, asthma, and anaphylaxis. Clinical manifestations have a rapid onset and can include urticaria, wheezing, dyspnea, laryngeal edema, bronchospasm, tachycardia, angioedema, hypotension, and cardiac arrest.

Localized itching, erythema, or local urticaria within minutes after exposure to latex is often the initial symptom. Symptoms of subsequent reactions can include generalized urticaria, angioedema, rhinitis, conjunctivitis, asthma, and anaphylactic shock minutes after dermal or mucosal exposure to latex. An increasing number of people who are allergic to latex experience severe reactions characterized by generalized urticaria, bronchospasm, and hypotension.

Assessment and Diagnostic Findings

The diagnosis of latex allergy is based on the history and diagnostic test results (Mayo Foundation for Medical Education and Research, 2015). Sensitization is detected by skin testing; serum-specific IgE, EIA, or ELISA; or the level of Hevea latex-specific IgE antibody in the serum. Testing for the chemicals found in the rubber production that makes latex is performed using the patch test. Skin patch testing is the preferred method for patients with contact allergies. The T.R.U.E. test and other skin tests should be performed only by clinicians who have expertise in their administration and interpretation and who have the necessary equipment available to treat local or systemic allergic reactions to the reagent (Habif, 2016).

Medical Management

The best treatment available for latex allergy is the avoidance of latex-based products, although avoidance is often difficult because of the widespread use of such products. Patients who have experienced an anaphylactic reaction to latex should be instructed to wear medical identification. Antihistamines and an emergency kit containing epinephrine should be provided to these patients, along with instructions about emergency management of latex allergy symptoms. Patients should be counseled to notify all health care workers, as well as local paramedic and ambulance companies, about their allergy. Warning labels can be attached to car windows to alert police and paramedics about the driver's or passenger's latex allergy in case of a motor vehicle crash. People with latex allergy should be provided with a list of alternative products and referred to local support groups; they are also urged to carry their own supply of nonlatex gloves.

People with type I latex sensitivity may be unable to continue to work if a latex-free work environment is not possible. This may occur with surgeons, dentists, operating room personnel, or intensive care nurses. Occupational implications for employees with type IV latex sensitivity are usually easier to manage by changing to nonlatex gloves and avoiding direct contact with latex-based medical equipment. Although latex-specific immunotherapy has been attempted, this method of treatment remains experimental.

Nursing Management

The nurse can assume a pivotal role in the management of latex allergies in both patients and staff. All patients should be asked about latex allergy, although special attention should be given

TABLE 37-6 Types of Reactions to Latex

Type of Reaction	Cause	Signs/Symptoms	Treatment
Irritant contact dermatitis	Damage to skin because of irritation and loss of epidermoid skin layer; not an allergic reaction. Can be caused by excessive use of soaps and cleansers, repeated handwashing, inadequate hand drying, mechanical irritation (e.g., sweating, rubbing inside powdered gloves), exposure to chemicals added during the manufacturing of gloves, and alkaline pH of powdered gloves. Reaction may occur with first exposure, is usually benign, and is not life-threatening.	*Acute:* Redness, edema, burning, discomfort, itching *Chronic:* Dry, thickened, cracked skin	Referral for diagnostic testing Avoidance of exposure to irritant Thorough washing and drying of hands Use of powder-free gloves with more frequent changes of gloves Changing glove types Use of water- or silicone-based moisturizing creams, lotions, or topical barrier agents Avoidance of oil- or petroleum-based skin agents with latex products, because they cause breakdown of the latex product
Allergic contact dermatitis	Delayed hypersensitivity (type IV) reaction. Usually affects only area in contact with latex; reaction is usually to chemical additives used in the manufacturing process rather than to latex itself. Cause of reaction is T-cell–mediated sensitization to additives of latex. Reaction is not life-threatening and is far more common than a type I reaction. Slow onset; occurs 18–24 hours after exposure. Resolves within 3–4 days after exposure. More severe reactions may occur with subsequent exposures.	Pruritus, erythema, swelling, crusty thickened skin, blisters, other skin lesions	Referral for diagnosis (patch tests) and treatment Thorough washing and drying of hands Use of water- or silicone-based moisturizing creams, lotions, or topical barrier agents Avoidance of oil- or petroleum-based products unless they are latex compatible Avoidance of identified causative agent, because continued exposure to latex products in presence of breaks in skin may contribute to latex protein sensitization
Latex allergy	Type I IgE-mediated immediate hypersensitivity to plant proteins in natural rubber latex. In sensitized people, antilatex IgE antibody stimulates mast cell proliferation and basophil histamine release. Exposure can be through contact with the skin, mucous membranes, or internal tissues, or through inhalation of traces of powder from latex gloves. Severe reactions usually occur shortly after parenteral or mucous membrane exposure. People with any type I reaction to latex are at high risk for anaphylaxis. Local swelling, redness, edema, itching, and systemic reactions, including anaphylaxis, occur within minutes after exposure.	Rhinitis, flushing, conjunctivitis, urticaria, laryngeal edema, bronchospasm, asthma, severe vasodilation angioedema, anaphylaxis, cardiovascular collapse, death	Immediate treatment of reaction with epinephrine, fluids, vasopressors, and corticosteroids, and airway and ventilator support, with close monitoring for recurrence for the next 12–14 hours Prompt referral for diagnostic evaluation Treatment and diagnostic evaluation in latex-free environment Assessment of all patients for symptoms of latex allergy Educating patients and family members about the disorder and the importance of preventing future reactions by avoiding latex (e.g., wearing medical identification, carrying EpiPen)

IgE, immunoglobulin E.

to those at particularly high risk (e.g., patients with spina bifida, patients who have undergone multiple surgical procedures). Every time an invasive procedure must be performed, the nurse should consider the possibility of latex allergies. Nurses working in operating rooms, intensive care units, short procedure units, and EDs need to pay particular attention to latex allergy. See Figure 17-1 in Chapter 17 for a latex allergy assessment form.

Although the type I reaction is the most significant of the reactions to latex, care must be taken in the presence of irritant contact dermatitis and delayed hypersensitivity reaction to avoid further exposure of the person to latex. Patients with latex allergy are advised to notify their health care providers and to wear medical identification. Patients must become knowledgeable about what products contain latex and what products are safe, nonlatex alternatives. They must also become knowledgeable about signs and symptoms of latex allergy and emergency treatment and self-injection of epinephrine in case of allergic reaction.

Nurses can be instrumental in establishing and participating in multidisciplinary committees to address latex allergy and to promote a latex-free environment. Latex allergy protocols and education of staff about latex allergy and precautions

are important strategies to reduce this growing problem and to ensure assessment and prompt treatment of those affected by allergy to latex.

CRITICAL THINKING EXERCISES

1 **pq** You are the nurse working in a preoperative holding area. A 38-year-old patient tells you that she has had a reaction to latex in the past. What are the immediate nursing priorities in providing care to this patient? What assessment data are needed to determine if this patient has a latex allergy?

2 **ebp** A 47-year-old mail carrier presents to the ED complaining of difficulty breathing after being stung by a bee. He states that this has happened two other times in his recent past and seems to be worse each time. What are the priority interventions? What medication is the drug of choice for severe allergic reactions, and how is it given? Describe the strength of the evidence and criteria used to assess its strength.

REFERENCES

*Asterisk indicates nursing research.

Books

Abbas, A., Lichtman, A., &Pillai, S. (2014). *Basic immunology functions and disorders of the immune system* (4th ed.). Philadelphia, PA: Elsevier Saunders.

Arcangelo, V. P., & Peterson, A. (Eds.). (2013). *Pharmacotherapeutics for advanced practice: A practical approach* (3rd ed.). Philadelphia, PA: Lippincott Williams & Wilkins.

Comerford, K. C. (2015). *Nursing 2015 drug handbook*. Philadelphia, PA: Wolters Kluwer.

Fleisher, T., Shearer, W., Schroeder, H., et al. (2013). *Clinical immunology* (4th ed.). St Louis, MO: Elsevier.

Frandsen, G., &Pennington, S. (2014). *Abrams's clinical drug therapy* (10th ed.). Philadelphia, PA: Wolters Kluwer Health/Lippencott Williams & Wilkens.

Grossman, S. C., & Porth, C. M. (2014). *Porth's pathophysiology: Concepts of altered health states* (9th ed.). Philadelphia, PA: Lippincott Williams & Wilkins.

Habif, T. (2016). *Clinical dermatology a color guide to diagnosis and therapy* (6th ed.). St Louis, MO: Elsevier.

Hodgson, B., & Kizior, R. (2014). *Saunders nursing drug book*. St Louis, MO: Elsevier.

Katzung, B., & Trevor, A. (2015). *Basic & clinical pharmacology* (13th ed.). New York: McGraw-Hill Education.

Pagana, K., &Pagana, T. (2013). *Mosby's diagnostic & laboratory test reference* (11th ed.). St Louis, MO: Elsevier

Turley, S. (2014). *Medical language* (3rd ed.). Saddle River, NJ: Pearson.

Journals & Electronic Documents

Albin, S., & Agarwal, S. (2014). Prevalence and characteristics of reported penicillin allergy in an urban outpatient population. *Allergy and Asthma Proceedings, 35*(6), 489–494.

American Academy of Allergy, Asthma, and Immunology (AAAAI). (2015). *Anaphylaxis overview*. Retrieved on 11/15/ 2015 at: www. aaaai.org

American Osteopathic College of Dermatology. (2015). *Urticaria*. Retrieved on 11/15/ 2015 at: www.aocd.org

Australasian Society of Clinical Immunology and Allergy (ASCIA). (2015). *Immunotherapy for treatment of allergy*. Retrieved on 11/15/ 2015 at: allergy.org.au

Baran, H., Ozcan, K., Selcuk, A., et al. (2014). Allergic rhinitis and its impact on asthma classification correlations. *The Journal of Laryngology & Otology,128*, 431–437.

Bernstein, J., Lang, D., Khan, D., et al. (2014). The diagnosis and management of acute and chronic urticaria: 2014 update. *Journal of Allergy and Clinical Immunology in Practice, 133*(5), 1270–1277.

Bleier, B. (2015). *Nasal/sinus irrigation*. Retrieved on 11/15/ 2015 at: care.american-rhinologic.org

Campbell, R. L., Li, J., Nicklas, R. A., et al. (2014). Emergency department diagnosis and treatment of anaphylaxis: A practice parameter. *Annals of Allergy Asthma & Immunology, 113*, 599–608.

Centers for Disease Control and Prevention (CDC). (2014). *Latex allergy: A prevention guide*. Retrieved on 11/20/2015 at: www.cdc. gov/niosh/docs/98-113/default.html

Cicardi, M., & Zuraw, B. (2015). *Hereditary andioedema: Treatment of acute attacks*. Retrieved on 11/15/ 2015 at: www.uptodate.com/ contents/hereditary-angioedema-treatment-of-acute-attacks

Ciccarelli, F., De Martinis, M., & Ginaldi, L. (2014). An update on autoinflammatory diseases. *Current Medical Chemistry, 21*(3),261–269.

Fleischer, D., Sicherer, S., Greenhawt, M., et al. (2015). Consensus communication on early peanut introduction and the prevention of peanut allergy in high risk infants. *Journal of Allergy and Immunology, 136*(2), 258–261.

Fonacier, L., Bernstein, D., Pacheco, K., et al. (2015). Contact dermatitis: A practice parameter-update 2015. *Journal of Allergy and Clinical Immunology in Practice, 3*, S1–S39.

Herro, E., & Jacob, S. (2014). An update on pediatric allergic contact dermatitis patch testing for common allergens. *Consultant for Pediatrics, 13*(8), 350–355.Retrieved on November 2015, from Consultant for Pediatrics at: www.pediatricsconsultant360.com

Hwang, P., & Patel, Z. (2015). Acute sinusitis and rhinosinusitis in adults: Treatment. *Retrieved* on November 2015 at: www.uptodate.co

Lehrer, E., Mullol, J., Agredo, F., et al (2014). Management of chronic rhinitis in asthma patients: Is there still a debate. *Current Allergy and Asthma Report, 14*(6), 1–6.

Link, M.S., Berkow, L.C., Kudenchuk, P.J., et al. (2015). Part 7: Adult advanced cardiovascular life support: 2015 American Heart Association Guidelines Update for Cardiopulmonary Resuscitation and Emergency Cardiovascular Care. *Circulation, 132*(Suppl 2), S444–S464

Ludman, S., & Boyle, R. (2015). Stinging insect allergy: Current perspectives on venom immunotherapy. *Journal of Allergy and Asthma, 2015*(8), 75–86.

Mayo Foundation for Medical Education and Research. (2015). *Diseases and conditions: Latex allergy*. Retrieved on 11/20/2015 at: www. mayoclinic.org/diseases-conditions/latex-allergy/basics/definition/ CON-20024233

National Institute of Allergy and Infectious Disease (NIAID). (2013). *The national asthma education and prevention program*.Retrieved on 11/20/2015 at: www.nhlbi.nih.gov/about/org/naepp/

Oppenheimer, J., Durham, S., Nelson, H., et al. (2014). *Allergy diagnostic testing*. Retrieved on 11/20/2015 at: www.worldallergy.org

Perez-Riverol, A., Justo-Jacomini, D., de Lima Zollner, R., et al. (2015). Facing hymenoptera venom allergy: From natural to recombinant allergens. *Toxins, 7*(7), 2551–2570.

Portnoy, J. (2015). *World allergy*. Retrieved on 11/20/2015 at: www. worldallergy.org

Rosenfeld, R., Piccirillo, J. F., Chandrasekhar, S., et al. (2015). Clinical practice guideline (Update): Adult sinusitis. *Otolaryngology-Head and Neck Surgery, 152*(2S), S1–S39.

Sampson, H., Aceves, S., Brock, S., et al. (2014). Food allergy: A practice parameter update-2014. *Journal of Allery and Clinical Immunology, 134*(5), 1025.e1–e43.

Senti, G., von Moos, S., Graf, N., et al. (2015). Determinants of efficacy and safety in epicutaneous allergen immunotherapy: Summary of three clinical trials. *European Journal of Allergy and Clinical Immunology, 70*(6), 707–710.

Sheikh, J. (2015). *Allergic rhinitis treatment and management*. Retrieved on 11/15/15 at: emedicine.medscape.com/ article/134825-treatment

Resources

American Academy of Allergy, Asthma, and Immunology (AAAAI), www.aaaai.org

American College of Allergy, Asthma, and Immunology (ACAAI), www.acaai.org

Asthma and Allergy Foundation of America (AAFA), www.aafa.org

Centers for Disease Control and Prevention (CDC), www.cdc.gov

Food Allergy Research Education (FARE), www.foodallergy.org

Mayo Foundation for Medical Education and Research, www.mayoclinic.org

MD Junction, Urticaria Support Group, www.mdjunction.com/urticaria

National Institute of Allergy and Infectious Diseases, www.niaid.nih.gov

Occupational Safety and Health Administration (OSHA), www.osha.gov

38 Assessment and Management of Patients With Rheumatic Disorders

LEARNING OBJECTIVES

On completion of this chapter, the learner will be able to:

1 Explain the pathophysiology of rheumatic diseases.
2 Describe the assessment and diagnostic findings seen in patients with rheumatic diseases or disorders.
3 Use the nursing process as a framework for the care of patients with rheumatic disorders.
4 Describe the systemic effects of a connective tissue disease.
5 Devise an education plan for the patient with newly diagnosed rheumatic disease.
6 Identify modifications in interventions to accommodate changes in patients' functional ability that may occur with disease progression.

GLOSSARY

ankylosis: fixation or immobility of a joint
arthritis: inflammation of a joint
arthroplasty: replacement of a joint
cytokines: proteins that can be produced by leukocytes that are vital to regulation of hematopoiesis, apoptosis, and immune responses
exacerbation: period when disease symptoms occur or increase
osteophyte: a bony outgrowth or protuberance; bone spur
pannus: proliferation of newly formed synovial tissue infiltrated with inflammatory cells

remission: period when disease symptoms are reduced or absent
rheumatic diseases: numerous disorders affecting skeletal muscles, bones, cartilage, ligaments, tendons, and joints
rheumatoid arthritis: a systemic autoimmune disease with symmetric arthritic manifestations and multiple extra-articular features
subchondral bone: bony plate that supports the articular cartilage
tophi: accumulation of crystalline deposits in articular surfaces, bones, soft tissue, and cartilage

---

The **rheumatic diseases** encompass autoimmune, degenerative, inflammatory, and systemic conditions that affect the joints, muscles, and soft tissues of the body. Rheumatic diseases most commonly manifest the clinical features of **arthritis** (inflammation of a joint) and pain. There are more than 100 types of rheumatic diseases. The problems caused by rheumatic diseases include limitations in mobility and activities of daily living, pain, fatigue, altered self-image, and sleep disturbances, as well as systemic effects that can lead to organ failure and death. An understanding of rheumatic diseases and their effects on a patient's function and well-being is essential to developing an appropriate plan of nursing care.

Rheumatic Diseases

An estimated 52.5 (22.7%) million adults in the United States have self-reported arthritis or other rheumatologic disease. Approximately 22.7 million (43.2% of those diagnosed with arthritis) have arthritis-attributable activity limitation. By 2030, an estimated 67 million (25%) adults will have arthritis or a rheumatologic condition, and an estimated 25 million adults (37%) will report arthritis-attributable activity limitations (Barbour, Helmick, Theis, et al., 2013).

Arthritis and other rheumatologic diseases and the physical limitations that occur with them are becoming more prominent and a larger public health issue, which can be attributed to the older adults in the United States.

Rheumatologic disease processes affect males and females of all ages and ethnic groups. Some disorders are more likely to occur at a particular time of life or to affect one gender more often than the other. In general, women are two to nine times more commonly affected by rheumatologic diseases than men (Barbour et al., 2013). The onset of these conditions may be acute or insidious, with a course possibly marked by periods of **remission** (a period when disease symptoms are reduced or absent) and **exacerbation** (a period when symptoms occur or increase). Treatment can be simple, aimed at localized relief, or it can be complex, directed toward relief of systemic effects. Permanent changes and disability may result from these disorders.

Nurses need to understand the classification of rheumatic diseases. One system is to classify disease as either monoarticular (affecting a single joint) or polyarticular (affecting multiple joints). Another system is to classify the disease as either inflammatory or noninflammatory. Conditions that may secondarily affect the musculoskeletal structure are also considered in disease classification.

Pathophysiology

Each of the rheumatologic diseases exhibits unique pathophysiologic features. Three distinct characteristics of pathophysiology include inflammation, autoimmunity, and degeneration.

Inflammation

Inflammation is a complex physiologic process mediated by the immune system that occurs in response to harmful stimuli like damaged cells or antigens, which may include pathogens (e.g., viruses, bacteria). Inflammation is meant to protect the body from insult by removing the triggering antigen or event. In response to a triggering episode, the antigen stimulus activates the body's immune system to form antibodies like monocytes and T lymphocytes (also referred to as T cells). Next, the immunoglobulin antibodies form immune complexes with antigens. Phagocytosis of the immune complexes is initiated, generating an inflammatory reaction (joint effusion, pain, and edema) (see Fig. 38-1). Phagocytosis produces chemicals such as leukotrienes and prostaglandins. Leukotrienes contribute to the inflammatory process by attracting other white blood cells to the area. Prostaglandins act as modifiers to inflammation. In some cases, they increase inflammation; in other cases, they decrease it. Leukotrienes and prostaglandins produce enzymes such as collagenase that break down collagen, which is a vital part of a normal joint. The release of these enzymes in the joint causes edema and proliferation of synovial membrane. In patients with chronic inflammation, the immune response can deviate from normal. Instead of resolution of swelling and joint pain once the triggering event has subsided, **pannus** (proliferation of newly formed synovial tissue infiltrated with inflammatory cells) formation occurs. Destruction of the joint's cartilage and erosion of bone soon follow.

The immunologic inflammatory process begins when antigens are presented to T lymphocytes, leading to a proliferation of T and B cells. B cells (also referred to as plasma cells) are a source of antibody-forming cells. In response to specific antigens, plasma cells produce and release antibodies. Antibodies combine with corresponding antigens to form pairs, or immune complexes. The immune complexes build up and are deposited in synovial tissue or other organs in the body, triggering the inflammatory reaction that can ultimately damage the involved tissue.

Autoimmunity

A hallmark of rheumatologic diseases is autoimmunity, where the body mistakenly recognizes its own tissue as a foreign antigen. Autoimmunity leads to destruction of tissue via the same inflammatory process as discussed earlier, along with chronic and long-standing pain. Although focused in the joints, inflammation and autoimmunity also involve other areas. The blood vessels (vasculitis and arteritis), lungs, heart, and kidneys may be affected by the autoimmunity and inflammation. See Chapter 35 for more information on autoimmune disease. A large group of genes, called *human leukocyte antigen* (HLA) genes, has been linked to the immune response and the development of multiple rheumatologic diseases (Di Lorenzo, 2015).

Degeneration

In degenerative rheumatic diseases, inflammation also occurs, but as a secondary process. Although the cause of degeneration of the articular cartilage is poorly understood, the process is known to be metabolically active and therefore is more accurately called *degradation*. One theory of degradation is that genetic or hormonal influences, mechanical factors, and prior joint damage cause cartilage failure. Degradation of

Figure 38-1 • Pathophysiology and associated physical signs of rheumatoid arthritis. ROM, range of motion.

cartilage ensues, and increased mechanical stress on bone ends causes stiffening of bone tissue. Another theory is that bone stiffening occurs and results in increased mechanical stress on cartilage, which in turn initiates the processes of degradation. See Chapter 39 for more information on the structure and function of the articular system.

Clinical Manifestations

The most common symptom in the rheumatic diseases is pain. Other common symptoms include joint swelling, limited movement, stiffness, weakness, and fatigue.

Assessment and Diagnostic Findings

Assessment begins with a general health history, which includes the onset of symptoms and how they evolved, family history, past health history, and any other contributing factors. Because many of the rheumatic diseases are chronic conditions, the health history should also include information about the patient's perception of the problem, previous treatments and their effectiveness, the patient's support systems, and the patient's current knowledge base and the source of that information. A complete health history is followed by a complete physical assessment (see Chapter 5).

Assessment for rheumatic diseases combines the physical examination with a functional assessment. Inspection of the patient's general appearance occurs during the initial contact. Gait, posture, and general musculoskeletal size and structure are observed. Gross deformities and abnormalities in movement are noted. The symmetry, size, and contour of other connective tissues, such as the skin and adipose tissue, are also noted and recorded. Chart 38-1 outlines the important areas for consideration during the physical assessment. The functional assessment is a combination of history (what the patient reports that he or she can and cannot do) and examination (observation of activities, in which the patient demonstrates what he or she can and cannot do, such as dressing and getting in and out of a chair). Observation also includes the adaptations and adjustments the patient may have made (sometimes without awareness)—for example, with shoulder or elbow involvement, the person may bend over to reach a fork rather than raising the fork to the mouth.

Laboratory Studies

In Table 38-1, some of the most common laboratory studies are listed with their corresponding normal ranges and significance. Many of the tests require special laboratory techniques and may not be performed in every health care facility. The primary provider determines which tests are necessary based on symptoms, stage of disease, cost, and likely benefit. In some instances, tests are used to monitor the course of the disease.

Other Diagnostic Studies

Imaging studies commonly used for patients with rheumatic diseases include x-ray studies, computed tomography (CT) scans, magnetic resonance imaging (MRI) scans, and arthrography. See Chapter 39 for further information about these and other diagnostic studies.

Medical Management

The chronic nature of rheumatic conditions requires cooperation between the patient and the provider. The patient needs to understand the disease process and to be active in making good decisions for their care. Patient education regarding the disease process and treatment options is imperative to enable the patient to make informed decisions regarding their care. Management of rheumatologic diseases is based on the patient's symptom self-assessment, quality of life, and objective assessment by the provider (Schur & Moreland, 2016). Table 38-2 outlines goals and strategies for care of the patient with rheumatic diseases.

Pharmacologic Therapy

Medications are used with the rheumatic diseases to manage symptoms, to control inflammation, and, in some instances, to modify the disease. Useful medications include the salicylates, nonsteroidal anti-inflammatory drugs (NSAIDs), and both biologic and nonbiologic disease-modifying antirheumatic drugs (DMARDs). As their name suggests, DMARDs have the ability to suppress the autoimmune response; alter disease progression; and stop or decrease further tissue damage on the joints, cartilage, and organs. DMARDs have been found to halt the progression of bone loss and destruction and can induce remission (Carter, Patty-Resk, Ruffing, et al., 2015). Nonbiologic DMARDs are thought to reduce proinflammatory **cytokines** (cell signaling proteins) and increase anti-inflammatory cytokines. Biologic DMARDs, in contrast, have been specifically engineered to target a certain cell or molecule within the immune system to treat the specific rheumatologic condition. Specific biologic DMARDs target tumor necrosis factor alpha (TNF-α), B cells, T cells, interleukin 1 (IL-1), and interleukin 6 (IL-6). Table 38-3 reviews commonly used medications.

Controlling the inflammation related to the disease process helps manage pain, but this is often a delayed response. Nonopioid medications are often used for pain management, especially early in the treatment program, until other measures can be instituted.

Nonpharmacologic Pain Management

Nonpharmacologic methods of pain management are important. Heat applications are helpful in relieving pain, stiffness, and muscle spasm. Superficial heat may be applied in the form of warm tub baths or showers and warm moist compresses. Paraffin baths (dips), which offer concentrated heat, are helpful to patients with wrist and small-joint involvement. Maximum benefit is achieved within 20 minutes after application. More frequent use for shorter lengths of time is most beneficial. Therapeutic exercises can be carried out more comfortably and effectively after heat has been applied.

Devices such as braces, splints, and assistive devices for ambulation (e.g., canes, crutches, walkers) ease pain by limiting movement or stress from putting weight on painful joints. Acutely inflamed joints can be rested by applying splints to limit motion. Splints also support the joint to relieve spasm. Canes and crutches can relieve stress from inflamed and painful weight-bearing joints while promoting safe ambulation. Cervical collars may be used to support the weight of the head and limit cervical motion. A metatarsal bar or special pads may be put into the patient's shoes if foot pain or deformity is

Chart 38-1	**ASSESSMENT**
	Assessing for Rheumatic Disorders

In addition to the head-to-toe assessment or systems review, the following are important areas of consideration to be noted when performing the complete physical assessment of a patient with a known or suspected rheumatic disorder.

Manifestation	Significance
Skin (inquire and inspect)	
Rash, lesions	Associated with systemic lupus erythematosus (SLE) vasculitis, adverse effect of medication
Increased bruising	Associated with several rheumatic diseases and adverse effect of medication
Erythema	Sign of inflammation
Thinning	Adverse effect of medication
Warmth	Sign of inflammation
Photosensitivity	Associated with SLE, dermatomyositis, adverse effect of medication
Hair (inquire and inspect)	
Alopecia or thinning	Associated with rheumatic diseases or adverse effect of medication
Eye (inquire and inspect)	
Dryness, grittiness	Associated with Sjögren's syndrome (commonly occurring with rheumatoid arthritis [RA] and SLE)
Decreased acuity or blindness	Associated with temporal arteritis, medication complications
Cataracts	Adverse effect of medication
Decreased peripheral vision	Adverse effect of medication
Conjunctivitis, uveitis	Associated with ankylosing spondylitis and Reiter's syndrome
Ear (inquire)	
Tinnitus	Adverse effect of medication
Decreased acuity	Adverse effect of medication
Mouth (inquire and inspect)	
Buccal, sublingual lesions	Associated with vasculitis, dermatomyositis, adverse effect of medication
Altered sense of taste	Adverse effect of medication
Dryness	Associated with Sjögren's syndrome
Dysphagia	Associated with myositis
Difficulty chewing	Associated with decreased range of motion of jaw
Chest (inspect and inquire)	
Pleuritic pain	Associated with RA and SLE
Decreased chest expansion	Associated with ankylosing spondylitis
Activity intolerance (dyspnea)	Associated with pulmonary hypertension in scleroderma
Cardiovascular system (inquire, inspect, palpate)	
Blanching of fingers on exposure to cold	Associated with Raynaud's phenomenon
Peripheral pulses	Deficit may indicate vascular involvement or edema associated with medication effect or rheumatic diseases, especially SLE or scleroderma
Abdomen (inquire and palpate)	
Altered bowel habits	Associated with scleroderma, spondylosis, ulcerative colitis, decreased physical mobility, medication effect
Nausea, vomiting, bloating, and pain	Adverse effect of medication
Weight change (measure)	Associated with RA (decreased), adverse effect of medication (increased or decreased)
Genitalia (inquire and inspect)	
Dryness, itching	Associated with Sjögren's syndrome
Abnormal menses	Adverse effect of medication
Altered sexual performance	Fear of pain (or of pain caused by partner) and limitation of motion may affect sexual mobility.
Hygiene	Poor hygiene may be related to limitations in activities of daily living.
Urethritis, dysuria	Associated with ankylosing spondylitis and Reiter's syndrome
Lesions	Associated with vasculitis
Neurologic (inquire and inspect)	
Paresthesias of extremities; abnormal reflex pattern	Nerve compressions (e.g., carpal tunnel syndrome, spinal stenosis)
Headaches	Associated with temporal arteritis, adverse effect of medication
Musculoskeletal (inspect and palpate)	
Joint redness, warmth, swelling, tenderness, deformity—location of first joint involved, pattern of progression, symmetry, acute vs. chronic nature	Signs of inflammation
Joint range of motion	Decreased range of motion may indicate severity or progression of disease.
Surrounding tissue findings	
Muscle atrophy, subcutaneous nodules, popliteal cyst	Extra-articular manifestations
Muscle strength (grip)	Muscle strength decreases with increased disease activity.

TABLE 38-1 Common Blood Studies for Rheumatic Diseases

Test	Normal Value	Significance
Serum		
Creatinine Metabolic waste excreted through the kidneys	0.7–1.4 mg/dL (62–124 mcmol/L)	Increase may indicate kidney damage in SLE, scleroderma, and polyarteritis.
Erythrocyte Count Measures circulating erythrocytes	*Men:* 4,600,000–6,200,000/mm³ (4.6–6.2 × 10¹²/L) *Women:* 4,200,000–5,400,000/mm³ (4.2–5.4 × 10¹²/L)	Decrease can be seen in RA, SLE.
Erythrocyte Sedimentation Rate (ESR) Measures the rate at which RBCs settle out of unclotted blood in 1 hour	Westergren: Men under 50 yrs: <15 mm/hr Men over 50 yrs: <20 mm/hr Women under 50 yrs: <25 mm/hr Women over 50 yrs: <30 mm/hr	Increase is usually seen in inflammatory connective tissue diseases. An increase indicates rising inflammation, resulting in clustering of RBCs, which makes them heavier than normal. The higher the ESR, the greater the inflammatory activity.
Hematocrit Measures the size, capacity, and number of cells present in blood	Men: 42%–52% Women: 35%–47%	Decrease can be seen in chronic inflammation (anemia of chronic disease); also, blood loss through GI bleed.
White Blood Cell Count Measures circulating leukocytes	4,500–11,000 cells/mm³	Decrease may be seen in SLE.
VDRL (Venereal Disease Research Laboratory) Measures antibody to syphilis	Nonreactive	False-positive results are sometimes found with SLE.
Uric Acid Measures level of uric acid in serum	2.5–8 mg/dL (0.15–0.5 mmol/L)	Increase is seen with gout. During acute flare, levels may be normal. After flare has subsided, levels will be elevated in gout.
Serum Immunology		
Antinuclear Antibody (ANA) Measures antibodies that react with a variety of nuclear antigens If antibodies are present, further testing determines the type of ANA circulating in the blood (anti-DNA, anti-RNP).	Negative Healthy adults may also have a positive ANA.	Positive test may be associated with SLE, RA, scleroderma, Raynaud's disease, Sjögren's syndrome, necrotizing arteritis. The higher the titer, the greater the inflammation. The pattern of immunofluorescence (speckled, homogeneous, or nucleolar) helps determine the diagnosis.
Anti-DNA, DNA Binding Titer measurement of antibody to double-stranded DNA	Negative	High titer is seen in SLE; increases in titer may indicate an increase in disease activity.
Complement Levels—C3, C4 Complement is a protein substance that binds with antigen–antibody complexes for the purpose of lysis. When the number of complexes increases markedly, complement is used for lysis, thus depleting the amount available in the blood.	C3: 80–170 mg/dL (0.8–1.7 g/L) C4: 18–51 mg/dL (180–510 mg/L)	Decrease may be seen in RA and SLE. Decrease indicates autoimmune and inflammatory activity.
C-Reactive Protein (CRP) Shows presence of abnormal glycoprotein due to inflammatory process	<1 mg/dL (<10 mg/L)	A positive reading indicates active inflammation.
Immunoglobulin Electrophoresis Measures the values of immunoglobulins	IgA: 80–400 mg/dL (0.8–4 g/L) IgG: 600–1,800 mg/dL (6–18 g/L) IgM: 55–250 mg/dL (0.55–2.5 g/L)	Increased levels are found in people who have autoimmune disorders.
Rheumatoid Factor (RF) Determines the presence of abnormal antibodies seen in connective tissue disease	Negative	Positive titer >1:80 Present in 80% of those with RA Positive RF may also suggest SLE, Sjögren's syndrome, or mixed connective tissue disease. The higher the titer (number at right of colon), the greater the inflammation.
Tissue Typing		
HLA-B27 Antigen Measures presence of HLA antigens, which are used for tissue recognition	Negative	Found in 80%–90% of those with ankylosing spondylitis and Reiter's syndrome

SLE, system lupus erythematosus; RBCs, red blood cells; GI, gastrointestinal; RA, rheumatoid arthritis; DNA, deoxyribonucleic acid; RNP, ribonucleoprotein; IgA, immunoglobulin A; IgG, immunoglobulin G; IgM, immunoglobulin M; HLA, human leukocyte antigen.
Adapted from Fischbach, F., & Dunning, M. B. (2015). *A manual of laboratory and diagnostic tests* (9th ed.). Philadelphia, PA: Lippincott Williams & Wilkins.

TABLE 38-2 Management Goals and Strategies for Rheumatic Diseases

Goals	Management Strategies
Suppress inflammation and the autoimmune response	Optimize pharmacologic therapy (anti-inflammatory and disease-modifying agents).
Control pain	Protect joints; ease pain with splints, thermal modalities, relaxation techniques.
Maintain or improve joint mobility	Implement exercise programs for joint motion, muscle strengthening, weight loss as appropriate, and overall health.
Maintain or improve functional status	Make use of adaptive devices and techniques.
Increase patient's knowledge of disease process	Provide and reinforce patient education.
Promote self-management by patient adherence with the therapeutic regimen	Emphasize compatibility of therapeutic regimen and lifestyle.

present. A combination of methods may be required, because different methods often work better at different times.

Exercise and Activity

The ongoing nature of most rheumatic diseases makes it important to maintain and, when possible, improve joint mobility and overall functional status. Appropriate programs of exercise have been shown to decrease pain and improve function (Miller, 2015). Changes in gait as well as joint limitations commonly require referral for rehabilitation therapy. An individualized exercise program is crucial to improve movement. Table 38-4 summarizes the exercises appropriate for patients with rheumatic diseases. Physical and occupational therapy programs and interventions are beneficial in improving physical activity and maintaining range of motion. Such interventions may include stretching exercises, muscle conditioning, aerobic exercise, massage, acupuncture, chiropractic and osteopathic manipulation. Other strategies for decreasing pain include muscle relaxation techniques, imagery, self-hypnosis, and distraction. The use of transcutaneous electrical nerve stimulation (TENS) unit has also been found to improve pain and enhance physical activity (Carter et al., 2015). A mild analgesic agent may be suggested before exercise to improve pain during exercise. A weight reduction program may be recommended to relieve stress on painful joints for some patients. Any patient who experiences acute or prolonged pain associated with exercise should report the symptoms to their primary provider for evaluation.

The major challenge for the patient and the health care provider is the need to adjust all aspects of treatment according to the activity of the disease. Especially for the patient with an active diffuse connective tissue disease, such as rheumatoid arthritis (RA) or systemic lupus erythematosus (SLE), activity levels may vary from day to day and even within a single day.

Sleep

Short-term use of low-dose antidepressant medications, such as amitriptyline (Elavil), may be prescribed to reestablish adequate sleep patterns and improve pain management (Papadakis, McPhee, & Rabow, 2015). Patients need restful sleep so that they can cope with pain, minimize physical fatigue, and deal with the changes related to having a chronic disease. In patients with acute disease, sleep time is frequently reduced and fragmented by prolonged awakenings. Stiffness, depression, and medications may also compromise the quality of sleep and increase daytime fatigue. A sleep-inducing routine, medication, and comfort measures may help improve the quality of sleep.

Education about sleep hygiene strategies may help promote restorative sleep. These strategies include establishing a set time to sleep and a regular wake-up time, creating a quiet sleep environment with a comfortable room temperature, avoiding factors that interfere with sleep (e.g., the use of alcohol and caffeine), using relaxation exercises, and getting out of bed and engaging in another activity (e.g., reading) if unable to sleep.

Nursing Management

Chart 38-2 details the nursing diagnoses, interventions, and expected outcomes for the patient with a rheumatic disorder.

 Gerontologic Considerations

The various rheumatologic disease conditions in the older adult pose unique challenges. These challenges relate to disability, cognitive changes, comorbid conditions, and diagnosis. Musculoskeletal problems are the most frequently reported conditions in older adults (Miller, 2015) and will be seen more frequently by health professionals in the coming years along with associated disability, especially among frail older adults.

Comorbid conditions pose a unique challenge in diagnosing rheumatologic disease in older adults because they have the potential to mask or alter presenting symptoms (Papadakis et al., 2015). The frequency, pattern of onset, clinical features, severity, and effects on function of the rheumatic disease in older patients may be different in very old patients. In addition, other medical conditions may take precedence over the rheumatic disease, which commonly becomes a secondary diagnosis and concern. Decreased vision and altered balance, often present in older adults, may be problematic if rheumatic disease in the lower extremities affects locomotion. The combination of decreased hearing and visual acuity, memory loss, and depression contributes to failure to follow the treatment regimen in older adult patients as well (Miller, 2015). Special techniques for promoting patient safety, self-management, and strategies such as memory aids for medications may be necessary.

Behavioral clues such as gait patterns, guarding, and joint flexion may aid the nurse in assessing the patient's pain when cognitive impairment is present. Older adults, especially men, may also neglect to communicate their pain unless elicited by the provider. Pain, in general, in this population that is not treated or undertreated may impact the quality of life for these patients, which can exacerbate all other medical conditions (Carter et al., 2015).

Older adults have an increased risk of osteoporosis. Pain, loss of mobility, diminished self-image, and increasing morbidity can result from progressive osteoporosis. Therefore, diagnosis and treatment of osteoporosis should not be overlooked in

TABLE 38-3 Selected Medications Used in Rheumatic Diseases

Medication	Action, Use, and Indication	Nursing Considerations
Salicylates		
Acetylated: aspirin *Nonacetylated:* choline trilisalicylate (Arthropan, Trilisate), salsalate (Disalcid), sodium salicylate	*Action:* Anti-inflammatory, analgesic, antipyretic Acetylated salicylates are platelet aggregation inhibitors Anti-inflammatory doses will produce blood salicylate levels of 20–30 mg/dL	Administer with meals to prevent gastric irritation. Assess for tinnitus, gastric intolerance, GI bleeding, and purpura. Monitor for possible confusion in the older adult.
Nonsteroidal Anti-inflammatory Drugs (NSAIDs)		
diclofenac (Voltaren), diflunisal (Dolobid), etodolac (Lodine), flurbiprofen (Ansaid), ibuprofen (Motrin), ketoprofen (Orudis, Oruvail), meclofenamate (Meclomen), meloxicam (Mobic), nabumetone (Relafen), naproxen (Naprosyn), oxaprozin (Daypro), piroxicam (Feldene), sulindac (Clinoril), tolmetin sodium (Tolectin) *COX-2 enzyme blockers:* celecoxib (Celebrex)	*Action:* Anti-inflammatory, analgesic, antipyretic, platelet aggregation inhibitor Anti-inflammatory effect occurs 2–4 weeks after initiation All NSAIDs are useful for short-term treatment of acute gout attack NSAIDs are an alternative to salicylates for first-line therapy in several rheumatic diseases *Action:* Inhibit only COX-2 enzymes, which are produced during inflammation, and spare COX-1 enzymes, which can be protective to the stomach	Administer NSAIDs with food. Monitor for GI, CNS, cardiovascular, renal, hematologic, and dermatologic adverse effects. Avoid salicylates; use acetaminophen for additional analgesia. Watch for possible confusion in older adults. Monitoring is the same as for other NSAIDs. Increased risk of cardiovascular events, including myocardial infarction and stroke Appropriate for older adults and patients who are at high risk for gastric ulcers
Disease-Modifying Antirheumatic Drugs (DMARDs)		
Antimalarials: hydroxychloroquine (Plaquenil), chloroquine (Aralen)	*Action:* Anti-inflammatory, inhibit lysosomal enzymes Slow acting; onset may take 2–4 months. May be used in conjunction with other DMARD therapy. Useful in RA and SLE	Administer concurrently with NSAIDs. Assess for visual changes, GI upset, skin rash, headaches, photosensitivity, bleaching of hair. Emphasize need for ophthalmologic examinations (every 6–12 months).
Janus Kinase (JAK) inhibitors (Xeljanz).	*Action:* Enters the cell and binds to the active JAK site, inhibits autophosphorylation and JAK activation that inhibits cytokine production. May be used in combination with methotrexate or other nonbiologic DMARDs. May also be used as monotherapy	Administer twice a day. Do not administer with biologic DMARDs or potent immunosuppressants. Monitor lipids 4–8 weeks following initiation of therapy. Monitor liver enzymes routinely.
sulfasalazine (Azulfidine)	*Action:* Anti-inflammatory, reduces lymphocyte response, inhibits angiogenesis Useful in RA, seronegative spondyloarthropathies	Administer concurrently with NSAIDs. Do not use in patients with allergy to sulfa medications or salicylates. Emphasize adequate fluid intake. Assess for GI upset, skin rash, headache, liver abnormalities, anemia.
Immunosuppressives: methotrexate (Rheumatrex), azathioprine (Imuran), cyclophosphamide (Cytoxan)	*Action:* Nonbiologic immune suppression, affect DNA synthesis and other cellular effects Have teratogenic potential; azathioprine and cyclophosphamide reserved for more aggressive or unresponsive disease Methotrexate is generally the first-line agent for RA treatment; also useful in SLE. Methotrexate may be given orally or by intramuscular or subcutaneous injection	Assess for bone marrow suppression, GI ulcerations, skin rashes, alopecia, bladder toxicity, increased infections. Monitor CBC, liver enzymes, creatinine at 6 weeks after initiation, then every 2–3 months or accordingly. Advise patient of contraceptive measures because of teratogenicity.
cyclosporine (Neoral)	*Action:* Nonbiologic immune suppression by inhibiting T lymphocytes Used for severe, progressive RA, unresponsive to other DMARDs Used in combination with methotrexate	Assess slow dose titration upward until response noted or toxicity occurs. Assess for toxic effects, such as bleeding gums, fluid retention, hair growth, tremors. Monitor blood pressure and renal function (creatinine) every 2 weeks until stable.
Immunomodulators		
Pyrimidine synthesis inhibitor: leflunomide (Arava)	*Action:* Nonbiologic with antiproliferative and anti-inflammatory effects; used in moderate to severe RA May be used alone or in combination with other DMARDs	Long half-life; requires loading dose followed by daily administration. Assess for diarrhea, hair loss, skin rash, mouth sores. Monitor liver function tests. Contraindicated in pregnancy and breast-feeding Given orally

TABLE 38-3 Selected Medications Used in Rheumatic Diseases (continued)

Medication	Action, Use, and Indication	Nursing Considerations
TNF blocking agents: adalimumab (Humira), certolizumabpegol (Cimzia), etanercept (Enbrel), infliximab (Remicade), golimumab (Simponi)	*Action:* Biologic response modifier that binds to TNF, a cytokine involved in inflammatory and immune responses. Used in moderate to severe RA. Can be used alone or with methotrexate or other nonbiologic DMARDs. Adalimumab is given by subcutaneous injection every 2 weeks, but may be used every week if efficacy not reached. Certolizumabpegol is given by subcutaneous injection every 2 weeks. Etanercept is given by subcutaneous injection weekly. Infliximab is given intravenously over 2 hours or more. Medication must be refrigerated Golimumab is given by subcutaneous injection once a month. Golimumab SQ is a second alternative that is administered intravenously every 8 weeks after initial 2 loading doses	Patient should be tested for tuberculosis before beginning this medication. Educate patient about subcutaneous self-injection. Monitor for injection site reactions. Educate patient about increased risk for infection and to withhold medication if fever occurs. Notify provider if any illness or infection occurs and medication is held.
T-cell costimulation modulator: abatacept (Orencia)	*Action:* Blocks one of the pathways needed to fully activate T cells, decreasing inflammatory and immunologic responses. Used in moderate to severe RA unresponsive to TNF inhibitors. Used with methotrexate or DMARDs other than TNF inhibitors or anakinra	Administered IV initially, then transitions to subcutaneous dosage once weekly. Educate patient about subcutaneous self-injections given daily. Monitor for injection site reactions. Educate patient about increased risk of infection and to withhold medication if fever occurs. IV infusions are given every 4 weeks over 30-minute infusion.
B-cell production blocker: rituximab (Rituxan)	*Action:* Binds to B-lymphocyte CD20 surface antigens. Used in refractory RA in patients with inadequate response to TNF antagonist. Given with methotrexate	Rituximab is given as two 1,000-mg doses via IV infusion separated by 2 weeks. Given on weeks 0 and 2, and then subsequent doses are infused 24 weeks later or based on clinical diagnosis (commonly given every 6 months). Premedicate with acetaminophen, antihistamine, and methylprednisolone (Solumedrol) 30 minutes prior to infusion of rituximab. Educate patient about increased risk of infection.
Human IL-1 receptor antagonist: anakinra (Kineret)	*Action:* Blocks IL-1 receptors, decreasing inflammatory and immunologic responses. Used in moderate to severe RA. Can be used alone or with methotrexate or DMARDs other than TNF-blocking agents	Given daily by subcutaneous injection. Educate patient about subcutaneous self-injections given daily. Medication must be refrigerated. Monitor for injection site reactions. Educate patient about increased risk of infection and to withhold medication if fever occurs.
Human IL-6 receptor antagonist: tocilizumab (Actemra)	*Action:* Binds to and inhibits IL-6 receptors, decreasing inflammatory and immunologic responses. Can be used alone or with methotrexate or in combination with other nonbiologic DMARDs	Administered IV every 4 weeks. Educate patient about increased risk of infection.
Corticosteroids prednisone, prednisolone, hydrocortisone	*Action:* Anti-inflammatory. Used for shortest duration and at lowest dose possible to minimize adverse effects. Useful for unremitting RA, SLE, polymyalgia rheumatica, myositis, arteritis Fast acting; onset in days Intra-articular injections useful for joints unresponsive to NSAIDs	Assess for toxicity: Cataracts, GI irritation, hyperglycemia, hypertension, fractures, avascular necrosis, hirsutism, psychosis. Joints most amenable to injections include ankles, knees, hips, shoulders, and hands. Repeated injections can cause joint damage. Use caution in patients diagnosed with diabetes, due to effects causing elevation in blood sugar.
Topical Analgesics capsaicin (Zostrix)	*Action:* Analgesic	Instruct patient to apply sparingly, avoid areas of open skin, and avoid contact with eyes and mucous membranes. Wash hands carefully after application. Assess for local skin irritation.

GI, gastrointestinal; CNS, central nervous system; COX, cyclo-oxygenase; RA, rheumatoid arthritis; SLE, systemic lupus erythematosus; IM, intramuscular; WBCs, white blood cells; CBC, complete blood count; TNF, tumor necrosis factor; IV, intravenous; IL-1, interleukin 1; IL-6, interleukin 6.
Adapted from Karch, A. (2014). *Lippincott's nursing drug guide.* Philadelphia, PA: Lippincott Williams & Wilkins.

TABLE 38-4 Exercise to Promote Mobility

Type of Exercise	Purpose	Recommended Performance	Precautions
Range of motion	Maintain flexibility and joint motion	Active or active/self-assisted at least daily	Reduce the number of repetitions when inflammation is present
Isometric exercise	Improve muscle tone, static endurance, and strength; prepare for dynamic and weight-bearing exercises	Perform at 70% of maximal voluntary contraction daily	Monitor blood pressure; isometric exercises may increase blood pressure and decrease blood flow to muscles
Dynamic exercise	Maintain or increase dynamic strength and endurance; increase muscle power; enhance synovial blood flow; promote strength of bone and cartilage	Start with repetitions against gravity and add progressive resistance; perform 2–3 days per week	May increase biomechanical stress on unstable or misaligned joints
Aerobic exercise	Improve cardiovascular fitness and endurance	Perform 3–5 days per week for 20–30 minutes of moderate-intensity exercise	Progress slowly as activity tolerance and fitness improve
Pool exercise	Water supports or resists movement; warm water may provide muscle relaxation	Provide buoyant medium for performance of dynamic or aerobic exercise	Heated swimming pool; deep water to minimize joint compression; nonslip footwear for safety and comfort. Receive appropriate instruction in a program designed for people with arthritis

Adapted from Carter S. C., Patty-Resk, C., Ruffing, V., et al. (2015). *Core curriculum for rheumatology nursing*(1st ed.). Greenville, SC: Lyons Den Solutions, LLC.

this population. Pharmacologic therapy (including analgesic agents), exercise, postural assistance, modification of activities of daily living, and psychological support are useful components of the treatment program for the older adult.

Identifying the effects of the rheumatic disease on the patient's lifestyle, independence, and psychological status is important and can improve the quality of life for older adults. Depressed mood is routinely found in those suffering from chronic joint disease. The body image and self-esteem of the older adult with rheumatic disease, combined with underlying depression, may interfere with the use of assistive devices such as canes. The use of adaptive equipment such as long-handled reachers or tongs may be viewed by the older adult as evidence of aging rather than as a means of increasing independence.

Because most rheumatologic diseases involve pain, especially with joints, some older adults may consider their symptoms as inevitable consequences of aging. In fact, many older adults expect and accept the immobility and self-care problems related to the rheumatic diseases and do not seek help, thinking that nothing can be done.

The older adult usually has a lifelong pattern of dealing with the stresses of daily life. Depending on the success of that pattern, the older adult can often maintain a positive attitude and self-esteem when faced with a rheumatic disease, especially if support is available. Previous stress management strategies are assessed. If these strategies have been effective, the patient is encouraged and supported in their use. If they were ineffective, the nurse assists the patient in identifying alternative strategies, encourages the use of new strategies, and assesses their effectiveness.

Pharmacologic treatment of rheumatic disease in older patients is more difficult than in younger patients. If therapeutic medications have an effect on the senses (hearing, cognition), this effect is intensified in the older adult. The cumulative effect of medications, in general, is accentuated because of the physiologic changes of aging. For example,

decreased renal function in the older adult alters the metabolism of certain medications, such as NSAIDs. Older adults are more prone to side effects associated with the use of multiple-drug therapy.

Partly because of the more frequent contact of older adults with health care providers for a variety of health issues, overtreatment or inappropriate treatment is possible. Complaints of pain may be met with a prescription for an opioid analgesic agent rather than instructions for rest, the use of an assistive device, and local comfort measures such as heat or cold. Acetaminophen (Tylenol) may be appropriate and worth trying before other medications that pose a greater chance of side effects. NSAIDs can be used; however, studies report that long-term use of NSAIDs can increase the risks of peptic ulcers, hemorrhage and cardiovascular toxicity. New guidelines recommend NSAIDs should be used in conjunction with a proton pump inhibitor (i.e., omeprazole [Prilosec]) to decrease the likelihood of gastric ulcers forming, hemorrhage and cardiovascular toxicity (Fujita, Kutsumi, Sanuki, et al., 2013).

Intra-articular corticosteroid injections, with their usually rapid relief of symptoms, may be requested by the patient who is unaware of the consequences of too-frequent use of this treatment. In addition, exercise programs may not be instituted or may be ineffective because the patient expects results to occur quickly or fails to appreciate the effectiveness of a program of exercise. In fact, strength training is encouraged in the older adult with chronic diseases.

Diffuse Connective Tissue Diseases

Diffuse connective tissue disease refers to a group of systemic disorders that are chronic in nature and are characterized by diffuse inflammation and degeneration in the connective tissues. These disorders share similar clinical features and may affect some of the same organs. The characteristic clinical
(*text continued on page 1093*)

Chart 38-2 · PLAN OF NURSING CARE

Care of the Patient With a Rheumatic Disorder

NURSING DIAGNOSIS: Acute and chronic pain related to inflammation and increased disease activity, tissue damage, fatigue, or lowered tolerance level

GOAL: Improvement in comfort level; incorporation of pain management techniques into daily life

Nursing Interventions	Rationale	Expected Outcomes
1. Provide variety of comfort measures: a. Application of heat or cold b. Massage, position changes, rest c. Foam mattress, supportive pillow, splints d. Relaxation techniques, diversional activities 2. Administer anti-inflammatory, analgesic, and slow-acting antirheumatic medications as prescribed. 3. Individualize medication schedule to meet patient's need for pain management. 4. Encourage verbalization of feelings about pain and chronicity of disease. 5. Assess for subjective changes in pain.	1. Pain may respond to nonpharmacologic interventions, such as exercise, relaxation, and thermal modalities. 2. Pain of rheumatic disease responds to individual or combination medication regimens. 3. Previous pain experiences and management strategies may be different from those needed for persistent pain. 4. Verbalization promotes coping. 5. The impact of pain on an individual's life often leads to misconceptions about pain and pain management techniques. 6. The individual's description of pain is a more reliable indicator than objective measurements such as change in vital signs, body movement, and facial expression.	• Identifies factors that exacerbate or influence pain response • Identifies and uses pain management strategies • Verbalizes decrease in pain • Reports signs and symptoms of side effects in timely manner to prevent additional problems • Verbalizes that pain is characteristic of rheumatic disease • Establishes realistic pain relief goals • Identifies changes in quality or intensity of pain

NURSING DIAGNOSIS: Fatigue related to increased disease activity, pain, inadequate sleep/rest, deconditioning, inadequate nutrition, and emotional stress/depression

GOAL: Incorporates as part of daily activities strategies necessary to modify fatigue

Nursing Interventions	Rationale	Expected Outcomes
1. Provide instruction about fatigue. a. Describe relationship of disease activity to fatigue. b. Describe comfort measures while providing them. c. Develop and encourage a sleep routine (warm bath and relaxation techniques that promote sleep). d. Explain importance of rest for relieving systematic, articular, and emotional stress. e. Explain how to use energy conservation techniques (pacing, delegating, setting priorities). f. Identify physical and emotional factors that can cause fatigue. 2. Facilitate development of appropriate activity/rest schedule. 3. Encourage adherence to the treatment program. 4. Refer to and encourage a conditioning program. 5. Encourage adequate nutrition, including source of iron from food and supplements.	1. The patient's understanding of fatigue will affect their actions. a. The amount of fatigue is directly related to the activity of the disease. b. Relief of discomfort can relieve fatigue. c. Effective bedtime routine promotes restorative sleep. d. Different kinds of rest are needed to relieve fatigue and are based on patient's need and response. e. A variety of measures can be used to conserve energy. f. Awareness of the various causes of fatigue provides the basis for measures to modify the fatigue. 2. Alternating rest and activity conserves energy while allowing most productivity. 3. Overall control of disease activity can decrease the amount of fatigue. 4. Deconditioning resulting from lack of mobility, understanding, and disease activity contributes to fatigue. 5. A nutritious diet can help counteract fatigue.	• Self-evaluates and monitors fatigue pattern • Verbalizes the relationship of fatigue to disease activity • Uses comfort measures as appropriate • Practices effective sleep hygiene and routine • Makes use of various assistive devices (splints, canes) and strategies (bed rest, relaxation techniques) to ease different kinds of fatigue • Incorporates time management strategies in daily activities • Uses appropriate measures to prevent physical and emotional fatigue • Has an established plan to ensure well-paced, therapeutic activity schedule • Adheres to therapeutic program • Follows a planned conditioning program • Consumes a nutritious diet consisting of the five major groups and recommended daily allowance of vitamins and minerals

(continued on page 1092)

Chart 38-2

PLAN OF NURSING CARE (Continued)
Care of the Patient With a Rheumatic Disorder

NURSING DIAGNOSIS: Impaired physical mobility related to decreased range of motion, muscle weakness, pain on movement, limited endurance, lack of or improper use of ambulatory devices
GOAL: Attains and maintains optimal functional mobility

Nursing Interventions	Rationale	Expected Outcomes
1. Encourage verbalization regarding limitations in mobility.	1. Mobility is not necessarily related to deformity. Pain, stiffness, and fatigue may temporarily limit mobility. The degree of mobility is not synonymous with the degree of independence. Decreased mobility may influence a person's self-concept and lead to social isolation.	• Identifies factors that interfere with mobility • Describes and uses measures to prevent loss of motion • Identifies environmental (home, school, work, community) barriers to optimal mobility • Uses appropriate techniques, assistive equipment, or both to aid mobility • Identifies community resources available to assist in managing decreased mobility

2. Assess need for occupational or physical therapy consultation.
  a. Emphasize range of motion of affected joints.
  b. Promote the use of assistive ambulatory devices.
  c. Explain the use of safe footwear.
  d. Use individual appropriate positioning/posture.
	2. Therapeutic exercises, proper footwear, and/or assistive equipment may improve mobility. Correct posture and positioning are necessary for maintaining optimal mobility.	

3. Assist to identify environmental barriers.	3. Furniture and architectural adaptations may enhance mobility.	

4. Encourage independence in mobility and assist as needed.
  a. Allow ample time for activity.
  b. Provide rest period after activity.
  c. Reinforce principles of pacing and work simplification.
	4. Changes in mobility may lead to a decrease in personal safety.	

5. Initiate referral to community health agency.	5. The degree of mobility may be slow to improve or may not improve with intervention.	

NURSING DIAGNOSIS: Readiness for enhanced self-care related to contractures, fatigue, or loss of motion
GOAL: Performs self-care activities independently or with the use of resources

Nursing Interventions	Rationale	Expected Outcomes
1. Assist patient to identify self-care deficits and factors that interfere with ability to perform self-care activities.	1. The ability to perform self-care activities is influenced by the disease activity and the accompanying pain, stiffness, fatigue, muscle weakness, loss of motion, and depression.	• Identifies factors that interfere with the ability to perform self-care activities • Identifies alternative methods for meeting self-care needs • Uses alternative methods for meeting self-care needs • Identifies and uses other health care resources for meeting self-care needs

2. Develop a plan based on the patient's perceptions and priorities on how to establish and achieve goals to meet self-care needs, incorporating energy conservation, and work simplification concepts.
  a. Provide appropriate assistive devices.
  b. Reinforce correct and safe use of assistive devices.
  c. Allow patient to control timing of self-care activities.
  d. Explore with the patient different ways to perform difficult tasks or ways to enlist the help of someone else.
	2. Assistive devices may enhance self-care abilities. Effective planning for changes must include the patient, who must accept and adopt the plan.	

3. Consult with community health care agencies when individuals have attained a maximum level of self-care yet still have some deficits, especially regarding safety.	3. Individuals differ in ability and willingness to perform self-care activities. Changes in ability to care for self may lead to a decrease in personal safety.	

Chart 38-2

PLAN OF NURSING CARE (Continued)

Care of the Patient With a Rheumatic Disorder

NURSING DIAGNOSIS: Disturbed body image related to physical and psychological changes and dependency imposed by chronic illness

GOAL: Adapts to physical and psychological changes imposed by the rheumatic disease

Nursing Interventions	Rationale	Expected Outcomes
1. Help patient identify elements of control over disease symptoms and treatment. 2. Encourage patient's verbalization of feelings, perceptions, and fears. a. Help to assess present situation and identify problems.	1. The individual's self-concept may be altered by the disease or its treatment. 2. The individual's coping strategies reflect the strength of their self-concept.	• Verbalizes an awareness that changes taking place in self-concept are normal responses to rheumatic disease and other chronic illnesses • Identifies strategies to cope with altered self-concept

NURSING DIAGNOSIS: Ineffective coping related to actual or perceived lifestyle or role changes

GOAL: Use of effective coping behaviors for dealing with actual or perceived limitations and role changes

Nursing Interventions	Rationale	Expected Outcomes

1. Identify areas of life affected by disease. Answer questions and dispel possible myths.
    a. Assist to identify past coping mechanisms.
    b. Assist to identify effective coping mechanisms.
2. Develop plan for managing symptoms and enlisting support of family and friends to promote daily function.
	1. The effects of disease may be more or less manageable once identified and explored reasonably.
	
	2. By taking action and involving others appropriately, patient develops or draws on coping skills and community support.
		• Names functions and roles affected and not affected by disease process
		• Describes therapeutic regimen and states actions to take to improve, change, or accept a particular situation, function, or role

COLLABORATIVE PROBLEMS: Complications secondary to effects of medications

GOAL: Absence or resolution of complications

Nursing Interventions	Rationale	Expected Outcomes
1. Perform periodic clinical assessment and laboratory evaluation. 2. Provide education about correct self-administration, potential side effects, and importance of monitoring. 3. Counsel regarding methods to reduce side effects and manage symptoms. 4. Administer medications in modified doses as prescribed if complications occur.	1. Skillful assessment helps detect early symptoms of side effects of medications. 2. The patient needs accurate information about medications and potential side effects to avoid or manage them. 3. Appropriate identification and early intervention may minimize complications. 4. Modifications may help minimize side effects or other complications.	• Adheres to monitoring procedures and experiences minimal side effects • Takes medication as prescribed and lists potential side effects • Identifies strategies to reduce or manage side effects • Reports that side effects or complications have subsided

course is one of exacerbations and remissions. Although diffuse connective tissue diseases have unknown causes, they are thought to be the result of immunologic abnormalities. They include RA, SLE, scleroderma, polymyositis, Sjögren's syndrome, polymyalgia rheumatica (PMR), and giant cell arteritis (GCA).

Rheumatoid Arthritis

RA is an autoimmune disease of unknown origin that affects 1% of the population worldwide, with females having a 2.5 times greater incidence than males. It may occur at any age but the onset commonly occurs between the third and sixth decade of life. The incidence of RA increases after the sixth decade of life (Carter et al., 2015). Risk factors for the development of RA include environmental factors such as

pollution and smoking, family history of first-degree relatives, and illnesses such as bacterial and viral illnesses. Cigarette smoking is one modifiable risk factor that has been shown to be highly related to RA (Carter et al., 2015).

Pathophysiology

The exact mechanism of action for the etiology of RA is unknown. Research has, however, identified that the autoimmune reaction (see Fig. 38-1) originates in the synovial tissue. It is hypothesized that both environmental factors, such as cigarette smoking, and genetic factors coalesce to produce inflammatory and destructive synovial fluid, starting in the more distal joints. This RA synovium breaks down collagen, causing edema, proliferation of the synovial membrane, and ultimately pannus formation. Pannus destroys cartilage and erodes the bone. The consequence is the loss of articular surfaces and joint motion. Muscle fibers undergo degenerative changes. Tendon and ligament elasticity and contractile power are lost.

The RA inflammatory process has also been implicated in other disease processes (i.e., arteriosclerosis). It is hypothesized that the RA disease process somehow interferes with the production of high-density lipoprotein cholesterol, which is the form of cholesterol responsible for decreasing cellular lipids and, therefore, is considered antiatherosclerotic.

The nervous system is also affected by the RA inflammatory process. The synovial inflammation can compress the adjacent nerve, causing neuropathies and paresthesias. Axonal degeneration and neuronal demyelination are also possible due to the infiltration of polymorphonuclear leukocytes, eosinophils, and mononuclear cells, causing necrotizing or occlusive vasculitis (Ramos-Remus, Duran-Barragan, & Castillo-Ortiz, 2012).

Clinical Manifestations

The American College of Rheumatology and the European League Against Rheumatism have collaborated and established new criteria for classifying RA. These criteria are based on a point system where a total score of 6 or greater is required for the diagnosis of RA. The scoring system is based on joint involvement (number of joints affected), serology (low positive or high positive rheumatoid factor [RF] or anti-citrullinated peptide antibody [ACPA]), abnormal results of the acute phase reactants (erythrocyte sedimentation rate [ESR] or C- reactive protein [CRP]), and duration of symptoms greater than 6 weeks. Patients diagnosed with RA who are excluded from these diagnostic criteria include: (1) patients who have one joint with synovitis that is not related to any other clinical disease and who also score at least 6 to 10 points on the scale, and (2) patients diagnosed with bony erosions on X-ray (Aletaha, Neogi, Silman, et al. 2010).

The initial clinical manifestations of RA include symmetric joint pain and morning joint stiffness lasting longer than 1 hour. Over the course of the disease, clinical manifestations of RA vary, usually reflecting the stage and severity of the disease. Symmetric joint pain, swelling, warmth, erythema, and lack of function are classic symptoms. Palpation of the joints reveals spongy or boggy tissue. Often, fluid can be aspirated from the inflamed joint. Characteristically, the pattern of joint involvement begins in the small joints of the hands, wrists, and feet (Klippel, Stone, Crofford, et al., 2008; Papadakis et al., 2015). As the disease progresses, the knees, shoulders, hips, elbows, ankles, cervical spine, and temporomandibular joints are affected. The onset of symptoms is usually acute. Symptoms are usually bilateral and symmetric.

In the early stages of disease, even before the presentation of bony changes, limitation in function can occur when there is active inflammation in the joints. Joints that are hot, swollen, and painful are not easily moved. The patient tends to guard or protect these joints by immobilizing them. Immobilization for extended periods can lead to contractures, creating soft tissue deformity.

Deformities of the hands (e.g., ulnar deviation and swan neck deformity) and feet are common in RA (see Fig. 39-6 in Chapter 39). The deformity may be caused by misalignment resulting from swelling, progressive joint destruction, or the subluxation (partial dislocation) that occurs when one bone slips over another and eliminates the joint space. Deformities of RA differ from those seen with osteoarthritis (OA), such as Heberden's and Bouchard's nodes.

RA is a systemic disease with multiple extra-articular features. Most common are fever, weight loss, fatigue, anemia, lymph node enlargement, and Raynaud's phenomenon (cold- and stress-induced vasospasm causing episodes of digital blanching or cyanosis). Rheumatoid nodules may be noted in patients with more advanced RA, and they develop at some time in the course of the disease in about 20% of patients (Papadakis et al., 2015). These nodules are usually nontender and movable in the subcutaneous tissue. They usually appear over bony prominences such as the elbow, are varied in size, and can disappear spontaneously. Nodules occur only in people who have rheumatoid factor. The nodules often are associated with rapidly progressive and destructive disease. Other extra-articular features include arteritis, neuropathy, pericarditis, splenomegaly, and Sjögren's syndrome (dry eyes and dry mucous membranes).

Assessment and Diagnostic Findings

Several assessment findings are associated with RA: rheumatoid nodules, joint inflammation detected on palpation, and laboratory findings. The history and physical examination focus on manifestations, such as bilateral and symmetric stiffness, tenderness, swelling, and temperature changes in the joints. The patient is also assessed for extra-articular changes; these often include weight loss, sensory changes, lymph node enlargement, and fatigue. Symptoms and examination findings are often recorded using a Disease Activity Score-28 (DAS28) form to evaluate disease activity and help guide treatment decisions.

RA inflammatory processes have also been implicated in arterial wall stiffness and endothelial dysfunction. It is now believed that cardiovascular risks are similar to the risks of patients with diabetes. Therefore, cardiovascular risk assessment should be included in the patient's physical assessment (Palmer & El Miedany, 2014).

Rheumatoid factor is present in about 70% to 80% of patients with RA, but its presence alone is not diagnostic of RA, and its absence does not rule out the diagnosis. Antibodies to cyclic citrullinated peptide (anti-CCP) have a specificity of approximately 95% at detecting RA (Papadakis et al., 2015). The ESR and CRP tend to be significantly elevated in the acute phases of RA and are therefore useful in monitoring active disease and disease progression. The complete blood count (CBC) should be assessed to establish a baseline count especially prior to starting medications. Patients may exhibit anemia, and platelets may be elevated due to the inflammatory process. A tuberculin (TB) skin test should be done prior to the initiation of certain medications to rule out tuberculosis. In the event the patient has latent TB and has never been treated, the infection can be reactivated. Hepatitis B and Hepatitis C should also be assessed for diagnosis, which could impact treatment strategies if positive. If the client tests positive for hepatitis, the infection should be treated prior to starting medication. Liver and kidney monitoring is recommended for most DMARD therapy because it can cause elevation of the liver enzymes and can also affect kidney function.

X-ray, ultrasound, or both of the hands, wrists, and feet can be useful in establishing a baseline for joint evaluation, and assessing the joints for erosions and synovitis. Joint damage may occur within the first 6 to 12 months of diagnosis and should be followed as indicated. MRI can also be useful to detect small erosions that may not be visible on x-ray or ultrasound.

Arthrocentesis may also be performed on any affected joint. Results of the arthrocentesis may show synovial fluid that is cloudy, milky, or dark yellow and may contain numerous inflammatory components. Recommended tests to perform on synovial fluid include WBC with differential, cultures, gram stain and crystals (Sholter & Russell, 2016).

Medical Management

The goal of treatment at all phases of the RA disease process is to decrease joint pain and swelling, achieve clinical remission, decrease the likelihood of joint deformity, and minimize disability. Initial treatment delays have been implicated in greater long-term joint deformity. Aggressive and early treatment regimens are warranted.

Early Rheumatoid Arthritis

Once the diagnosis of RA is made, treatment should begin with either a nonbiologic or biologic DMARD. The goal of using DMARD therapy is preventing inflammation and joint damage. Recommended treatment guidelines include beginning with the nonbiologic DMARDs (methotrexate [Rheumatrex], leflunomide [Arava], sulfasalazine [Azulfidine]), or hydroxychlorotquine (Plaquenil) within 3 months of disease onset. Care should be used with each of these medications, by performing routine blood testing for liver and kidney function, along with monitoring the CBC for anemia. Dosage may need to be modified for patients with renal impairment. Annual eye examinations are also recommended with the use of sulfasalazine and hydroxychloroquine (Carter et al., 2015).

After initiating treatment with a DMARD, patients generally report a beneficial effect within 6 weeks and tolerate the medication relatively well (Papadakis et al., 2015). However, some patients may take longer to see improvement. Research suggests that methotrexate combined with low-dose prednisone improves patient outcome compared to the use of methotrexate alone for early RA.

Another treatment approach for RA is the use of biologic DMARDs. These agents have been specifically engineered to target the most prominent proinflammatory mediators in RA—TNF-α, B cells, T cells, IL-1, and IL-6 (Klippel et al., 2008) (see Table 38-3). Biologic DMARDs are the first targeted therapy for RA. Clinical evidence suggests that biologic DMARDs work more quickly and show a greater delay in radiologic disease progression when compared to nonbiologic DMARDs (Klippel et al., 2008). The biologic DMARDs are more expensive and have fewer years of usage with the RA population. Therefore, they tend to be reserved for patients with persistent moderate-to-severe RA who have not responded adequately to synthetic DMARDs (Papadakis et al., 2015).

NSAIDs and specifically the cyclo-oxygenase 2 (COX-2) enzyme blockers are used for pain and inflammation relief. NSAIDs, such as ibuprofen (Motrin) and naproxen (Naprosyn), are commonly prescribed because of their low cost and analgesic properties. They must be used, however, with caution in long-term chronic diseases because of the possibility of gastric ulcers.

Several COX-2 enzyme blockers have been approved for treatment of RA. Cyclo-oxygenase is an enzyme that is involved in the inflammatory process. COX-2 medications block the enzyme involved in inflammation (COX-2) while leaving intact the enzyme involved in protecting the stomach lining (COX-1). As a result, COX-2 enzyme blockers are less likely to cause gastric irritation and ulceration than other NSAIDs; however, they are associated with increased risk of cardiovascular disease and must be used with caution (Karch, 2014). The nurse should be aware that no NSAIDs, not even the COX-2 inhibitors, prevent erosions or alter disease progression and, consequently, are medications useful only for symptom relief.

Additional analgesia may be prescribed for periods of extreme pain. Opioid analgesic agents are avoided because of the potential for continuing need for pain relief. Nonpharmacologic pain management techniques (e.g., relaxation techniques, heat and cold applications) are taught (Carter et al., 2015).

Moderate, Erosive Rheumatoid Arthritis

For moderate, erosive RA, a formal program with occupational and physical therapy is prescribed to educate the patient about principles of pacing activities, work simplification, range of motion, and muscle-strengthening exercises. The patient is encouraged to participate actively in the management program. The medication program is reevaluated periodically, and appropriate changes are made if indicated. Cyclosporine, an immunosuppressant, may be added to enhance the disease-modifying effect of methotrexate (Klippel et al., 2008). Combination therapy using one nonbiologic DMARD and one biologic DMARD is common.

Persistent, Erosive Rheumatoid Arthritis

For persistent, erosive RA, reconstructive surgery and corticosteroids are often used. Reconstructive surgery is indicated when pain cannot be relieved by conservative measures and the threat of loss of independence is eminent. Surgical procedures include synovectomy (excision of the synovial membrane), tenorrhaphy (suturing of a tendon), arthrodesis (surgical fusion of the joint), surgical repair, and replacement of the joint. Surgery is not performed during exacerbations.

Systemic corticosteroids are used when the patient has unremitting inflammation and pain or needs a "bridging" medication while waiting for the slower DMARDs (e.g., methotrexate) to begin taking effect. Low-dose corticosteroid therapy is prescribed for the shortest time necessary to minimize side effects (Papadakis et al., 2015). Single large joints that are severely inflamed and fail to respond promptly to the measures outlined previously may be treated by local injection of a corticosteroid.

Advanced, Unremitting Rheumatoid Arthritis

For advanced, unremitting RA, immunosuppressive agents are prescribed because of their ability to affect the production of antibodies at the cellular level. These include high-dose methotrexate, cyclophosphamide (Cytoxan), and azathioprine (Imuran). However, these medications are highly toxic and can produce bone marrow suppression, anemia, gastrointestinal disturbances, severe birth defects, and rashes (Karch, 2014).

For most patients with RA, the emotional and possible financial burden of the disease can lead to depressive symptoms and sleep deprivation. The patient may require the short-term use of low-dose antidepressant medications, such as amitriptyline (Elavil), paroxetine (Paxil), or sertraline (Zoloft), to reestablish an adequate sleep pattern and manage depressive symptoms. Patients may benefit from referrals for talk therapy or group support.

Nutrition Therapy

Patients with RA frequently experience anorexia, weight loss, and anemia. A dietary history identifies usual eating habits and food preferences. Two common problems seen in these patients are weight loss and rheumatoid cachexia (loss of skeletal muscle). Increased metabolism and decreased intake contribute to these losses. Increased and prolonged flares contribute to the increased expenditure as well. The dietician will counsel the patient about better food choices. Food selection should include the five major groups (grains, vegetables, fruits, dairy, and protein), with emphasis on foods high in vitamins, protein, and iron for tissue building and repair. For the patient who is extremely anorexic, small, frequent feedings with increased protein supplements may be prescribed. Supplemental vitamins and minerals may also be prescribed as needed. Boswellia, ginger, green tea, and turmeric have been studied for helping with inflammation and pain. However, the American College of Rheumatology does not recommend herbal supplements to treat RA as the U.S. Food and Drug Administration (FDA) does not regulate the safety and effectiveness of herbal supplements (Afshar, 2015).

Certain medications (i.e., oral corticosteroids) used in RA treatment stimulate the appetite and, when combined with decreased activity, may lead to weight gain. Therefore, patients may need to be counseled about eating a healthy, calorie-restricted diet.

Nursing Management

Nursing care of the patient with RA follows the basic plan of care presented earlier (see Chart 38-2). The most common issues for the patient with RA include pain, sleep disturbance, fatigue, altered mood, and limited mobility. The patient with newly diagnosed RA needs information about the disease to make daily self-management decisions and cope with having a chronic disease. Consultation with a dietician for assessment and assistance with appropriate food choices may be helpful.

Monitoring and Managing Potential Complications

Patients commonly have comorbid conditions such as cardiovascular disease that can lead to complications. It has been estimated that the primary cause of death for up to 40% of patients diagnosed with RA is cardiovascular disease. The cause of cardiovascular disease in these patients is thought to be due to elevated lipid values, chronic inflammation, dysfunction of the endothelium, and/or abnormal homocysteine levels (Palmer & El Miedany, 2014).

Medications used for treating RA may cause serious and adverse effects. The primary provider bases the prescribed medication regimen on clinical findings and past medical history, and then, with the help of the nurse, monitors for side effects using periodic clinical assessments and laboratory testing. The nurse, who can be available for consultation between visits with the primary provider, works to help the patient recognize and deal with these side effects (see Table 38-3). Medication may need to be stopped or the dose reduced. If the patient experiences an increase in symptoms while the complication is being resolved or a new medication is being initiated, the nurse's counseling regarding symptom management may relieve potential anxiety and distress.

Promoting Home, Community-Based, and Transitional Care

 Educating Patients About Self-Care

Patient education is an essential aspect in nursing care of the patient with RA to enable the patient to maintain as much independence as possible, to take medications accurately and safely, and to use adaptive devices correctly (Cottrell, Jonas, Bergsten, et al., 2013). Patient education focuses on the disorder itself, the possible changes related to the disorder, the therapeutic regimen prescribed to treat it, and the potential side effects of medications (see Nursing Research Profile in Chart 38-3). Patients undergoing

---

Chart 38-3 | NURSING RESEARCH PROFILE

Addressing Unmet Needs of Patients With Rheumatoid Arthritis

Cottrell, J. D., Jonas, M., Bergsten, U., et al. (2013). The nurse's role in addressing unmet treatment and management needs of patients with rheumatoid arthritis: Delphi-based recommendations. *International Journal of Nursing Knowledge, 24*(2), 66–76.

Purpose

Nurses spend a lot of time with patients with rheumatoid arthritis (RA). The purpose of this research was to evaluate the nurse's role in management of patients with RA.

Design

The modified Delphi methodology was the design for this study. Three rheumatology nurses developed a survey questionnaire. An additional group of 12 international rheumatology nurses, with extensive patient management experience, served as an expert panel. The survey was given to the panel of 12 rheumatology nurses in two online rounds and then in a third round during an in-person meeting.

Findings

The nurse has many roles in the management of patients with RA. In this study, the nurse's reported roles involved providing care, educating about treatment, performing a disease assessment, giving the patient treatment feedback, helping patients with unmet physical and emotional needs, and explaining complex treatments.

Nursing Implications

Rheumatology nurses are in a position to be able to expand the nursing role for patients diagnosed with RA. These nurses already perform the roles of caregiver and educator, and provide disease assessment. It is important for nurses to also address unmet patient needs, provide improved patient care, and perform additional functions for the patients to meet unmet physical and emotional needs.

Chart 38-4

HOME CARE CHECKLIST

The Patient With Rheumatoid Arthritis

At the completion of education, the patient, caregiver, or both will be able to:

- State the impact of rheumatoid arthritis on physiologic functioning, ADLs, IADLs, roles, relationships, and spirituality.
- State changes in lifestyle (e.g., diet, activity, rest) necessary to maintain health.
- State the name, dose, side effects, frequency, and schedule for all medications.
- Demonstrate accurate and safe self-administration of medications.
- Describe and demonstrate the use of pain management techniques.
- Demonstrate ability to perform ADLs independently or with assistive devices/adaptive equipment.
- Verbalize ways to cope with stress successfully, plans for regular, safe exercise, and rationale for obtaining adequate rest. Demonstrate a relaxation technique.

- Verbalize a dietary plan that includes increased vitamins, protein, and iron for tissue building and repair
- State how to reach primary provider with questions or complications
- State time and date of follow-up appointments, testing
- Identify the need for health promotion, disease prevention, and screening activities
- Identify community resources for peer and caregiver/family information and support:
- Identify sources of support (e.g., friends, relatives, faith community)
- Identify phone numbers of support groups for people with chronic illness/disabilities and their caregivers/families
- State meeting locations and times

ADLs, activities of daily living; IADLs, independent activities of daily living.

surgery need education as well. The nurse works with the patient and family on strategies to maintain independence, function, and safety in the home (see Chart 38-4).

The patient and family are encouraged to verbalize their concerns and ask questions. Because RA commonly affects young women, major concerns may be related to the effects of the disease on childbearing potential, caring for family, or work responsibilities. The patient with a chronic illness may seek a "cure" or have questions about alternative therapies. There is not enough evidence of the effectiveness of complementary, alternative, and integrative health therapies, and more rigorous research is needed (Marcus, 2015).

Pain, fatigue, and depressive symptoms can interfere with the patient's ability to learn and should be addressed before the instruction is initiated. Various educational strategies may then be used, depending on the patient's previous knowledge base, interest level, degree of comfort, social or cultural influences, and readiness to learn. The nurse educates the patient about basic disease management and necessary adaptations in lifestyle. Some types of aerobic exercise and strength training should be discussed. Because suppression of inflammation and autoimmune responses requires the use of anti-inflammatory, disease-modifying antirheumatic, and immunosuppressive agents, the patient is taught about prescribed medications, including type, dosage, rationale, potential side effects, self-administration, and required monitoring procedures. If hospitalized, the patient is encouraged to practice new self-management skills with support from caregivers and significant others. The nurse then reinforces disease management skills during each patient contact. Barriers are assessed, and measures are taken to promote adherence to medications and the treatment program.

Continuing and Transitional Care

Depending on the severity of the disease and the patient's resources and supports, referral for home care may be warranted. For example, the patient who is an older adult or frail, has RA

that limits function significantly, and lives alone may need referral for home care.

The impact of RA on everyday life is not always evident when the patient is seen in the hospital or in an ambulatory care setting. The increased frequency with which nurses see patients in the home provides opportunities for recognizing problems and implementing interventions aimed at improving the quality of life of patients with RA.

During home visits, the nurse has the opportunity to assess the home environment and its adequacy for patient safety and management of the disorder. Adherence to the treatment program can be more easily monitored in the home setting, where physical and social barriers to adherence are more readily identified. For example, a patient who also has diabetes and requires insulin may be unable to fill the syringe accurately or unable to administer the insulin because of impaired joint mobility. Appropriate adaptive equipment needed for increased independence is often identified more readily when the nurse sees how the patient functions in the home. Any barriers to adherence are identified, and appropriate referrals are made.

For patients at risk for impaired skin integrity, the home care nurse can closely monitor skin status and also educate, provide, or supervise the patient and family in preventive skin care measures. The nurse also assesses the patient's need for assistance in the home and supervises home health aides, who may meet many of the needs of the patient with RA. Referrals to physical and occupational therapists may be made as problems are identified and limitations increase. A home care nurse may visit the home to make sure that the patient can function as independently as possible despite mobility problems and can safely manage treatments, including pharmacotherapy. The patient and family should be informed about support services such as Meals on Wheels and local Arthritis Foundation chapters.

Because many of the medications used to suppress inflammation are injectable, the nurse may administer the medication to the patient or educate about self-injection. These frequent contacts allow the nurse to reinforce other disease management techniques.

The nurse also assesses the patient's physical and psychological status, adequacy of symptom management, and adherence to the management plan. Patients should know which type of rheumatic disease they have, not just that they have "arthritis" or "arthritis of the knee." The importance of attending follow-up appointments is emphasized to the patient and family, and they should be reminded about the importance of participating in other health promotion activities and health screening.

Systemic Lupus Erythematosus

SLE is an inflammatory, autoimmune disorder that affects nearly every organ in the body. The overall incidence of SLE is estimated to be 1.8 to 7.6 per 100,000 persons (Centers for Disease Control and Prevention [CDC], 2015a). It occurs 6 to 10 times more frequently in women than in men and occurs 3 times more in African American populations than among Caucasians (CDC, 2015a; Lim, Bayakly, Helmick, et al., 2014). In addition to SLE, many other forms of adult lupus exist, including discoid lupus erythematosus (which primarily affects the skin on the face), subacute cutaneous lupus erythematous (sun exposed areas affected with sores), and drug-induced lupus (rarely includes brain or kidney effects and is usually temporary).

Pathophysiology

SLE starts with the body's immune system inaccurately recognizing one or more components of the cell's nucleus as foreign, seeing it as an antigen. The immune system starts to develop antibodies to the nuclear antigen. In particular, B cells begin to overproduce antibodies with the help of multiple cytokines such as B-lymphocyte stimulator (BLyS), which is overexpressed in SLE. The antibodies and antigens form antigen–antibody complexes and have the propensity to get trapped in the capillaries of visceral structures. The antibodies also act to destroy host cells. It is thought that those two mechanisms are responsible for the majority of the clinical manifestations of this disease process. It is hypothesized that the immunoregulatory disturbance is brought about by some combination of four distinct factors: genetic, immunologic, hormonal, and environmental (Carter et al., 2015).

Research into the genetic origins of SLE has thus far revealed that multiple genes are likely implicated in the development of SLE. In support of this theory, research with homozygous twins has shown a higher incidence of SLE, especially considering that the prevalence of SLE was low in other family members (Bartels, 2015). The large majority of SLE cases, however, remain sporadic and unrelated to family medical history.

Given the acute number of women with SLE compared with men, it is hypothesized that female sex hormones (estrogen) play a role in the predisposition to SLE. Estrogen may contribute to the body's response of overreacting to the body's own tissues.

Although genetics and hormones likely play a role in the predisposition of SLE, it is hypothesized that an exogenous or environmental trigger is implicated in the onset of the disease

process. These triggers may include cigarette smoke, ultraviolet rays exposure from sunlight and fluorescent light bulbs, medications (sulfa drugs, penicillin, or antibiotic drugs), viral, infections, emotional stress, stress on the body (e.g., surgery, pregnancy), and silica dust exposure in the occupational setting (Carter et al., 2015).

Clinical Manifestations

SLE is an autoimmune, systemic disease that can affect any body system. The disease process involves chronic states where symptoms are minimal or absent and acute flares where symptoms and lab results are elevated. Systemic symptoms include fever, malaise, weight loss, and anorexia. The mucocutaneous, musculoskeletal, renal, nervous, cardiovascular, and respiratory systems are most commonly involved. Less commonly affected are the gastrointestinal tract and liver as well as the ocular system.

Some type of cutaneous system manifestation is experienced in 80% to 90% of patients with SLE (Bartels, 2015; Klippel et al., 2008). Four of the 11 criteria used for diagnosing SLE by the American College of Rheumatology involve the cutaneous system. The most familiar skin manifestation (occurring in less than 50% of patients with SLE) is an acute cutaneous lesion consisting of a butterfly-shaped erythematous rash across the bridge of the nose and cheeks (see Fig. 38-2). Several other skin manifestations may occur in patients with SLE, including subacute cutaneous lupus erythematosus, which involves papulosquamous or annular polycyclic lesions, and a discoid rash, which is a chronic rash with erythematous papules or plaques and scaling and can cause scarring and pigmentation changes. In some cases, the only skin involvement may be a discoid rash. In some patients with SLE, the initial skin involvement is the precursor to more systemic involvement. The lesions often worsen during **exacerbations** (flares)

Figure 38-2 • The characteristic butterfly rash of systemic lupus erythematosus.

of the systemic disease and possibly are provoked by sunlight or artificial ultraviolet light (Bartels, 2015; Klippel et al., 2008). Oral ulcers, which may accompany skin lesions, may involve the buccal mucosa or the hard palate, occur in crops, and are often associated with exacerbations. Other cutaneous manifestations include splinter hemorrhages, alopecia, and Raynaud's phenomenon.

Joint symptoms, with arthralgias, arthritis (synovitis), or both, occur in more than 90% of patients with SLE and are commonly the earliest manifestation of the disease process (Papadakis et al., 2015). Joint swelling, tenderness, and pain on movement are also common. Frequently, these are accompanied by morning stiffness.

The cardiac system is also commonly affected in SLE. Pericarditis is the most common cardiac manifestation (Bartels, 2015; Klippel et al., 2008). Patients may present with substernal chest pain that is aggravated by movement or inspiration. Symptoms can be acute and severe or last for weeks at a time. Other cardiac symptoms may involve myocarditis, hypertension, cardiac dysrhythmias, and valvular incompetence. Women who have SLE are also at risk for early-onset atherosclerosis, making them much more likely to suffer myocardial infarction or stroke. These events, which are believed to be secondary to the accelerated atherosclerosis, may contribute to higher rates of death for women with SLE. Inflammation is believed to be the key factor in the development and progression of atherosclerosis (Bartels, 2015).

Nephritis as a result of SLE, also referred to as lupus nephritis, occurs due to a buildup of antibodies and immune complexes that cause damage to the nephrons. Serum creatinine levels and urinalysis are used in screening for renal involvement. Early detection allows for prompt treatment so that renal damage can be prevented. Renal involvement may lead to hypertension, which also requires careful monitoring and management (see Chapter 31).

Central nervous system involvement is widespread, encompassing the entire range of neurologic disease. The varied and frequent neuropsychiatric presentations of SLE are now widely recognized and include psychosis, cognitive impairment, seizures, peripheral and cranial neuropathies, transverse myelitis, and strokes. These are generally demonstrated by subtle changes in behavior patterns or cognitive ability.

Assessment and Diagnostic Findings

Diagnosis of SLE is based on a complete history, physical examination, and blood tests. In addition to the general assessment performed for any patient with a rheumatic disease, assessment for known or suspected SLE has special features. The skin is inspected for erythematous rashes. Cutaneous erythematous plaques with an adherent scale may be observed on the scalp, face, or neck. Areas of hyperpigmentation or depigmentation may be noted, depending on the phase and type of disease. The patient should be questioned about skin changes (because these may be transitory) and specifically about sensitivity to sunlight or artificial ultraviolet light. The scalp should be inspected for alopecia and the mouth and throat for ulcerations reflecting gastrointestinal involvement.

Cardiovascular assessment includes auscultation for pericardial friction rub, possibly associated with myocarditis

and accompanying pleural effusions. The pleural effusions and infiltrations, which reflect respiratory insufficiency, are demonstrated by abnormal lung sounds. Papular, erythematous, and purpuric lesions developing on the fingertips, elbows, toes, and extensor surfaces of the forearms or lateral sides of the hand that may become necrotic suggest vascular involvement.

Joint swelling, tenderness, warmth, pain on movement, stiffness, and edema may be detected on physical examination. The joint involvement is often symmetric and similar to that found in RA.

The neurologic assessment is directed at identifying and describing any central nervous system changes. The patient and family members are asked about any behavioral changes, including manifestations of neurosis or psychosis. Signs of depression are noted, as are reports of seizures, chorea, or other central nervous system manifestations.

The American College of Rheumatology has established criteria for the classification of SLE involving 11 distinct elements (American College of Rheumatology, 1997) (see Chart 38-5). The diagnosis of SLE is generally made if 4 of the 11 criteria are present, either serially or simultaneously.

The ANA is positive in more than 95% of patients with SLE, indicating exceptional specificity. Other laboratory tests include anti-DNA (antibody that develops against the patient's own DNA), anti-ds DNA (antibody against DNA that is highly specific to SLE, which helps differentiate it from drug-induced lupus), and anti-Sm (antibody against Sm, which is a specific protein found in the nucleus). Other blood work includes the CBC, which may reveal anemia,

---

Chart 38-5

Criteria for Classifying Systemic Lupus Erythematosus

The American College of Rheumatology (ACR) established criteria for the classification of systemic lupus erythematosus (SLE) in 1982. These were updated in 1997, and include four cutaneous, four systemic, and three laboratory criteria. Diagnosis is determined by evaluating presenting signs and symptoms, laboratory results, and the patient's medical history and medical history of family members. The ACR-established criteria are as follows:

- Malar rash
- Discoid rash
- Photosensitivity
- Oral ulcers
- Nonerosive arthritis
- Pleuritis or pericarditis
- Kidney disease
- Neurologic disease
- Hematologic disorder
- Immunologic disorder
- Positive antinuclear antibody

Based on the 11 criteria above, a person is diagnosed with systemic lupus erythematosus if any 4 or more of the criteria are met at any time.

Reprinted with permission from Hochberg, C. (1997).Updating the American college of rheumatology revised criteria for the classification of systemic lupus erythematosus. *Arthritis and Rheumatism*, 40(9), 1725; Tan, E. M., Cohen, A. S., Fries, J. F., et al. (1982). The 1982 revised criteria for the classification of systemic lupus erythematosus. *Arthritis and Rheumatism*, 25(11), 1271–1277.

thrombocytopenia, leukocytosis, or leukopenia (Klippel et al., 2008).

Medical Management

SLE can be life-threatening, but advances in its treatment have led to improved survival and reduced morbidity. Acute disease requires interventions directed at controlling increased disease activity or exacerbations that can involve any organ system. Disease activity is a composite of clinical and laboratory features that reflect active inflammation secondary to SLE. Management of the more chronic condition involves periodic monitoring and recognition of meaningful clinical changes requiring adjustments in therapy.

The goals of treatment include preventing progressive loss of organ function, reducing the likelihood of acute disease, minimizing disease-related disabilities, and preventing complications from therapy. Management of SLE involves regular monitoring to assess disease activity and therapeutic effectiveness.

Pharmacologic Therapy

The mainstay of SLE treatment is based on pain management and nonspecific immunosuppression. Therapy includes monoclonal antibodies, corticosteroids, antimalarial agents, NSAIDs, and immunosuppressive agents. Each of these medications has potentially serious side effects, including organ damage.

Belimumab (Benlysta) is approved by the FDA for the treatment of SLE (Carter et al., 2015). Belimumab is a monoclonal antibody that specifically recognizes and binds to BLyS. BLyS acts to stimulate B cells to produce antibodies against the body's own nuclei, which is an integral part of the disease process in SLE. Belimumab acts to render BLyS inactive, preventing it from binding to B-cell surfaces and stimulating B-cell activity. This action then halts the production of unnecessary antibodies and decreases disease activity in SLE. Research suggests that belimumab reduces disease activity and flares in patients with SLE. Live vaccines are contraindicated while taking this medication, and caution should be used with all concurrent medications given the short duration that belimumab has been available.

Corticosteroids are another medication used topically for cutaneous manifestations, in low oral doses for minor disease activity, and in high doses for major disease activity. Intravenous (IV) administration of corticosteroids is an alternative to traditional high-dose oral administration. One of the most important risk factors associated with the use of corticosteroids in SLE is osteoporosis and fractures. In fact, osteopenia is reported in 25% to 74% and osteoporosis in 1.4% to 68% of patients with SLE (Bultink, 2012).

An antimalarial medication approved by the FDA, hydroxychloroquine, is effective for managing cutaneous, musculoskeletal, and mild systemic features of SLE. The NSAIDs used for minor clinical manifestations are often used in conjunction with corticosteroids in an effort to minimize corticosteroid requirements.

Immunosuppressive agents (alkylating agents and purine analogues) are used because of their effect on overall immune function. These medications are generally reserved for patients who have serious forms of SLE that have not responded to conservative therapies. Examples include cyclophosphamide, azathioprine, mycophenolic acid (Myfortic), and methotrexate, which are contraindicated in pregnancy and have been used most frequently in SLE nephritis (Carter et al., 2015).

Nursing Management

Nursing care of the patient with SLE is based on the fundamental plan presented earlier in the chapter (see Chart 38-2). The most common nursing diagnoses include fatigue, impaired skin integrity, body image disturbance, and deficient knowledge for self-management decisions. The disease or its treatment may produce dramatic changes in appearance and considerable distress for the patient. The changes and the unpredictable course of SLE necessitate expert assessment skills and nursing care with sensitivity to the psychological reactions of the patient. In particular, patients with SLE report feelings of depression and anxiety as well as difficulty coping with the disease and the financial strain associated with it (Fonseca, Bernardes, Terroso, et al., 2014). The patient may benefit from participation in support groups, which can provide disease information, daily management tips, and social support. Because sun and ultraviolet light exposure can increase disease activity or cause an exacerbation, patients should be instructed to avoid exposure or to protect themselves with sunscreen and clothing.

Because of the increased risk of involvement of multiple organ systems, patients should understand the need for routine periodic screenings as well as health promotion activities. A dietary consultation may be indicated to ensure that the patient is knowledgeable about dietary recommendations, given the increased risk of cardiovascular disease, including hypertension and atherosclerosis. Smoking tobacco accelerates complications in patients with SLE (Chasset, Frances, Barete, et al., 2015). In the healthy population, smoking increases the incidence of respiratory infections, lung cancer, risk of coronary artery disease; increases blood pressure, which can worsen kidney function; inhibits liver function (which can also inhibit treatment medications from working appropriately, such as hydroxychloroquine); increases the risk for skin diseases; and increases the risk for osteoporosis. Patients diagnosed with SLE are at even higher risk of developing lung cancer and other rare cancers. Therefore, smoking cessation programs should be offered to all patients who report smoking habits (Montes, Mocarzel, Lanzieri, et al, 2016).

The nurse educates the patient about the importance of continuing prescribed medications and addresses the changes and potential side effects that are likely to occur with their use. The patient is reminded of the importance of monitoring because of the increased risk of systemic involvement, including renal and cardiovascular effects.

Because of the immunosuppression associated with systemic corticosteroid usage, the nurse must watch for signs and symptoms of infection, especially with acutely ill patients.

The nurse should also screen the patient for osteoporosis, because long-term use of corticosteroids increases the incidence of osteoporosis. Patients should have a bone mineral density test performed at diagnosis and prior to beginning steroid use to determine a baseline status and then every 2 years thereafter. Educating the patient regarding calcium and Vitamin D supplementation daily is encouraged, along with the benefits of weight-bearing activities to support bone health (Cash & Glass, 2015).

Sjögren's Syndrome

Sjögren's syndrome is a systemic autoimmune disease that progressively affects the lacrimal and salivary glands of the body. More than 90% of patients affected are women, and the onset tends to begin between 35 and 50 years of age (Carter et al., 2015).

It is one of the most common autoimmune disorders, affecting approximately 1 out of 1000 people or 2 to 4 million people in the United States (Carter et al., 2015). Sjögren's syndrome very commonly manifests in conjunction with other autoimmune diseases such as RA or SLE.

Pathophysiology

B-cell–mediated antibodies infiltrate the exocrine glands, leading to gland dysfunction and gland destruction. This phenomenon seems to be somewhat regulated by genetics (HLA subtype). There also appears to be environmental triggers such as viruses. Given the clinical makeup and antibodies present, it may also be that Sjögren's disease is a subtype of SLE (Klippel et al., 2008).

Clinical Manifestations

The most common symptoms involve dry eyes (kerotoconjunctivitis sicca) and dry mouth (xerostomia). Some patients will complain that their eyes feel "gritty," as if there is sand present. The patient's eyes will exhibit increased redness and lack of tearing. These ocular symptoms can also lead to increased levels of anxiety and depression. The mouth will have dry and sticky mucous membranes. The reduced saliva production may lead to difficulty swallowing.

Sjögren's syndrome can also exhibit symptoms in many other organ systems. Vasculitis (5% to 10%) can manifest with palpable purpura on the skin (Quemeneur, Mouthon, Cacoub, et al., 2013). Lesions may ulcerate and can be painful. Optic neuritis, trigeminal neuralgia, and sensory neuropathy may be present, with symptoms such as burning pain in the extremities, numbness, vertigo, arthralgia, and/or myalgia. Raynaud's phenomenon, which involves blood vessel spasms leading to decreased circulation to the toes, fingers, nose and ears, is noted in 13% to 62% of patients (Klippel et al., 2008). Symptoms such as cough, dyspnea, and abdominal pain may also occur.

Assessment and Diagnostic Findings

The classification criteria for diagnosis of Sjögren's syndrome identify six distinct indices (Klippel et al., 2008):
- Ocular symptoms such as chronic dry eye (Kerotoconjunctivitis Sicca).
- Positive ocular tests (evaluating tear production, corneal, and conjunctival damage). Ocular testing may include Schemer tear test or Rose Bengal tests.
- Oral symptoms, dry mouth.
- Histopathology evaluation (of salivary glands). This will help differentiate the cause of dry mouth from other causes, such as infection, malignancy, stones, and sarcoidosis.
- Salivary gland involvement.

Laboratory tests include autoantibodies to ribonucleoprotein particles (Ro[SS-A] and/or La[SS-B]), which act as antigens in this disease process. Other laboratory indices are also useful in diagnosing Sjögren's syndrome. Rheumatoid factor is present in 50% to 70% of patients. ANA, circulating DNA (cDNA), anti-CCP, and anticentromere antibody (ACA) are all potentially present in Sjögren's syndrome and in some cases may act as markers for disease activity (Moerman, Bootsma, Kroese, et al., 2013).

For vasculitis manifestations, a skin biopsy can yield useful information such as leukocytoclasticvasculitis found on histologic examination. If neurologic symptoms are present, nerve conduction studies, MRI, electroencephalograms, and cerebrospinal fluid testing may be used to aid in diagnosis and treatment planning.

Medical Management

There is no cure for Sjögren's syndrome, and treatment is aimed at symptom management. Artificial tears, drops such as pilocarpine (Piloptic), and ocular ointments such as topical cyclosporine are used for dry eyes. Tears normally drain through the lacrimal puncta to the nose, which can render artificial tears ineffective. Therefore, punctum plugs have become very important management tools. For dry mouth, systemic cholinergic agents such as cevimeline (Evoxac) are used regularly (Klippel et al., 2008). Biotene oral rinse may also be useful for some patients. Additional suggestions include eating small frequent meals; omitting spicy, salty, and irritating food; and avoiding smoking, excessive alcohol use, and drugs with anticholinergic side effects. For severe cases, biologic DMARDs such as rituximab and belimumab and nonbiologic DMARDs such as hydroxychloroquine are sometimes used, but evidence regarding their effectiveness is limited (Carter et al., 2015).

Nursing Management

Nursing care is based on the fundamental plan of nursing care presented earlier (see Chart 38-2). The most frequent nursing diagnoses for the patient with Sjögren's syndrome are altered skin integrity, self-care deficit, and deficient knowledge of self-management techniques.

The nurse is in the unique position to reinforce the treatment regimen with the patient, especially involving the ocular treatments to avoid sequelae-like eye infections secondary to the dry eyes.

Scleroderma

Scleroderma is a compilation of autoimmune diseases affecting the connective tissue of the skin, blood vessel walls, and internal organs. There are two general types: localized (affecting only the cutaneous system) and systemic (routinely referred to as systemic sclerosis and affecting multiple organ systems). Scleroderma is a rare disease affecting 250 patients per million population (Klippel et al., 2008). Similar to other autoimmune diseases, women are affected three to five times more than men, and the onset occurs typically between the ages of 30 and 50 years. African American patients are affected much younger and have more diffuse symptoms with more severe lung disease. Scleroderma has a variable course with remissions and exacerbations (Varga, 2014).

Pathophysiology

The pathogenesis is poorly understood. Scleroderma commonly begins with skin involvement. Mononuclear cells cluster on the skin and stimulate lymphokines to stimulate procollagen. Insoluble collagen is formed and accumulates excessively in the tissues. Initially, the inflammatory response causes edema, with a resulting taut, smooth, and shiny skin appearance. The skin then undergoes fibrotic changes, leading to loss of elasticity and movement. Eventually, the tissue degenerates and becomes nonfunctional. This chain of events, from inflammation to degeneration, also occurs in blood vessels, major organs, and body systems (Varga, 2014). Both genetics and environmental factors can influence the disease process.

Clinical Manifestations

Scleroderma starts insidiously with Raynaud's phenomenon and swelling in the hands. Raynaud's phenomenon is observed in 90% of patients with scleroderma and can precede the official scleroderma diagnosis for years (Varga, 2014). The skin and subcutaneous tissues become increasingly hard and rigid and cannot be pinched up from the underlying structures. Wrinkles and lines are obliterated. The skin is dry because sweat secretion over the involved region is suppressed. The extremities stiffen and lose mobility. The condition spreads slowly; for years, these changes may remain localized in the hands and the feet. The face appears masklike, immobile, and expressionless, and the mouth becomes rigid (Jordan, Maurer, Toniolo, et al., 2015).

The changes within the body, although not visible directly, are vastly more important than the visible changes. Pulmonary hypertension is one problem that can result and is the leading cause of related death (Varga & Steen, 2015). The esophagus hardens, interfering with swallowing. The lungs become scarred, impeding respiration. Digestive disturbances occur because of hardening (sclerosing) of the intestinal mucosa. Progressive kidney failure may occur.

The patient may manifest a variety of symptoms referred to as the CREST syndrome. CREST stands for calcinosis (calcium deposits in the tissues), Raynaud's phenomenon, esophageal hardening and dysfunction, sclerodactyly (scleroderma of the digits), and telangiectasia (capillary dilation that forms a vascular lesion) (Papadakis et al., 2015).

Assessment and Diagnostic Findings

Assessment focuses on the sclerotic changes in the skin, contractures in the fingers, and color changes or lesions in the fingertips. Assessment of systemic involvement requires a systems review with special attention to gastrointestinal, pulmonary, renal, and cardiac symptoms. Limitations in mobility and self-care activities should be assessed, along with the impact the disease has had (or will have) on body image.

There is no one conclusive diagnostic test used to diagnose scleroderma. High-resolution CT is used to diagnose the presence of pulmonary hypertension. Pulmonary function tests and echocardiogram are recommended at diagnosis and yearly thereafter (Varga & Steen, 2015). Echocardiography identifies pericardial effusion (often present with cardiac involvement). Echocardiograms show some promise as well in detecting vascular changes in the early stages of the disease process. Esophageal studies demonstrate decreased motility in most patients with scleroderma. Blood tests may detect ANAs, indicating a connective tissue disorder and possibly distinguishing the subgroup (diffuse or limited) of scleroderma. A positive ANA test result is common in patients with scleroderma (Varga, 2014).

Medical Management

Treatment of scleroderma depends on the clinical manifestations. All patients require counseling, during which realistic individual goals may be determined. Support measures include strategies to decrease pain and limit disability. A moderate exercise program is encouraged to prevent joint contractures. Patients are advised to avoid extreme temperatures and to use lotion to minimize skin dryness.

Pharmacologic Therapy

No medication regimen is effective in modifying the disease process in scleroderma, but various medications are used to treat organ system involvement. Calcium channel blockers and other antihypertensive agents may provide improvement in symptoms of Raynaud's phenomenon. Anti-inflammatory medications can be used to control arthralgia, stiffness, and general musculoskeletal discomfort. Proton pump inhibitors are used for symptoms of gastric reflux. Aspirin and HMG-CoA (3-hydroxy-3-methylglutaryl coenzyme A) reductase inhibitors (statins) are used to help reduce cardiovascular risk factors. Given the propensity toward digital ulcers due to Raynaud's phenomenon and the potential for pulmonary hypertension, vasoactive medications such as epoprostenol (Flolan), bosentan (Tracleer), and sildenafil (Viagra) are used. Immunosuppressive agents such as cyclophosphamide and methotrexate have been used to improve skin and lung function. The antifibrotic agent imatinibmesylate is used to decrease fibrosis in various organs. Ultraviolet A irradiation is sometimes used to decrease the synthesis of collagen in dermal fibrosis and improve skin symptoms (Carter et al., 2015).

Nursing Management

Nursing care of the patient with scleroderma is based on the fundamental plan of nursing care presented earlier (see Chart 38-2). The most common nursing diagnoses are impaired skin integrity; self-care deficits; imbalanced nutrition: less than body requirements; and disturbed body image. The patient with advanced disease may also have impaired gas exchange, decreased cardiac output, impaired swallowing, and constipation.

Providing meticulous skin care and preventing the effects of Raynaud's phenomenon are major nursing challenges. See Chapter 30 for further discussion of Raynaud's phenomenon.

Polymyositis

Polymyositis is a group of diseases that are termed *idiopathic inflammatory myopathies* (Klippel et al., 2008). They are rare conditions, with an incidence estimated at 2 cases per 10,000 adults per year. Polymyositis is most commonly seen in women versus men (2:1) and usually seen between 40 and 50 years of age (Miller & Viegels, 2016).

Pathophysiology

Polymyositis is classified as autoimmune because autoantibodies are present. However, these antibodies do not cause damage to muscle cells, indicating only an indirect role in tissue damage. The pathogenesis is multifactorial, and a genetic predisposition is likely. Drug-induced disease is rare.

Clinical Manifestations

The onset may be very slow and insidious, with symptoms gradually worsening over weeks to months. Proximal muscle weakness is typically the first symptom. Muscle weakness is usually symmetric and diffuse. Common complaints include having difficulty rising from a chair, climbing steps, or holding up the head. Myalgia and muscle tenderness occur in 25% to 50% of patients. Dermatomyositis, a related condition, is most commonly identified by an erythematous smooth or scaly lesion found over the joint surface, which often occurs prior to symptoms of weakness in 50% to 60% of patients (Miller & Viegels, 2016).

Assessment and Diagnostic Findings

A complete history and physical examination help exclude other muscle-related disorders. As with other diffuse connective tissue disorders, no single test confirms polymyositis. An electromyogram is performed to rule out degenerative muscle disease. A muscle biopsy may reveal inflammatory infiltrate in the tissue. Serum studies indicate increased muscle enzyme activity.

Medical Management

Management involves high-dose corticosteroid therapy initially, followed by a gradual dosage reduction over several months as muscle enzyme activity decreases. Patients who do not respond to corticosteroids require the addition of an immunosuppressive agent, such as azathioprine, methotrexate, cyclosporine, or cyclophosphamide. The IV immune globulin given in combination with corticosteroids or another immunosuppressive agent has been noted to be beneficial (Carter et al., 2015). Plasmapheresis, lymphapheresis, and total-body irradiation have been used if there is no response to corticosteroids and immunosuppressive medications. The antimalarial agent hydroxychloroquine may be effective for skin rashes. Physical therapy is initiated slowly, with range-of-motion exercises to maintain joint mobility, followed by gradual strengthening exercises (Klippel et al., 2008).

Nursing Management

Nursing care is based on the fundamental plan of nursing care presented earlier (see Chart 38-2). The most frequent nursing diagnoses for the patient with polymyositis are impaired physical mobility, fatigue, self-care deficit, and deficient knowledge of self-management techniques.

Patients with polymyositis may have symptoms similar to those of other inflammatory diseases. However, proximal muscle weakness is characteristic, making activities such as combing the hair, reaching overhead, and using stairs difficult. Therefore, the use of assistive devices may be recommended, and referral to occupational or physical therapy may be warranted.

Polymyalgia Rheumatica and Giant Cell Arteritis

PMR involves stiffness of muscles and pain in the neck, shoulder, and pelvic girdle. GCA is a form of vasculitis affecting the medium-sized and large arteries of the body (Klippel et al., 2008). GCA is also sometimes referred to as temporal arteritis because the majority of arteries affected are extracranial branches of the carotid artery. It is widely agreed, however, that both PMR and GCA represent a spectrum of one disease (Papadakis et al., 2015). Both primarily affect individuals older than 50 years and are associated with the same HLA haplotype genetic markers. PMR and GCA occur predominately in Caucasians and often in first-degree relatives. PMR has an annual incidence rate of 52 cases per 100,000 people older than 50 years. GCA varies by geographic location and has the highest incidence in Scandinavian countries. PMR is two to three times more common than GCA (Klippel et al., 2008).

Pathophysiology

The underlying mechanism of action involved with PMR and GCA is unknown. It is clear, however, that the immune system is abnormally activated in both disease processes with increases in circulating monocytes that produce IL-1 and IL-6. These circulating monocytes make the endothelial linings of blood vessels more vulnerable to vasculitis (Klippel et al., 2008). Immunoglobulin deposits in the walls of inflamed temporal arteries suggest that an autoimmune process is at work.

Clinical Manifestations

PMR is characterized by severe proximal muscle discomfort with mild joint swelling. Severe aching in the neck, shoulder, and pelvic muscles is common. Stiffness is noticeable most often in the morning and after periods of inactivity. This stiffness can become so severe that patients struggle putting on a coat or combing their hair. Systemic features include low-grade fever, weight loss, malaise, anorexia, and depression. Because PMR usually occurs in people 50 years and older, it may be confused with, or dismissed as, an inevitable consequence of aging.

GCA may cause headaches, changes in vision, and jaw claudication. These symptoms should be evaluated immediately because of the potential for a sudden and permanent loss of vision if the condition is left untreated. PMR and GCA have a self-limited course, lasting several months to several years (Klippel et al., 2008).

Assessment and Diagnostic Findings

Assessment focuses on musculoskeletal tenderness, weakness, and decreased function. Careful attention should be directed toward assessing the head (for changes in vision, headaches, and jaw claudication). An MRI scan may be used in the assessment of extra-articular synovitis in patients with PMR, regardless of symptoms.

Often, diagnosis is difficult because of the lack of specificity of tests. A markedly high ESR is a screening test but is not definitive. The CRP level and platelet count also provide valuable data. In fact, simultaneous elevation in the ESR and CRP has a sensitivity of 98.6% and a specificity of 75.7% in making the diagnosis of GCA when coupled with clinical findings (Seetharaman, 2015). Diagnosis of both GCA and PMR is more likely to be made by eliminating other potential diagnoses. The dramatic and immediate response to treatment with corticosteroids is considered by some to be diagnostic.

In the case of GCA, biopsy of the temporal artery is the definitive diagnostic tool (Seetharaman, 2015). High-resolution MRI is an alternative or adjunct to the traditional temporal artery biopsy.

Medical Management

The treatment for patients with PMR (without GCA) is moderate doses of corticosteroids. Longer durations of corticosteroid treatment are required with patients who have higher baseline inflammatory markers. Gradual tapering of the corticosteroid treatment should be monitored. NSAIDs are sometimes given in mild disease. The treatment for patients with GCA is rapid initiation of and strict adherence to a regimen of corticosteroids. This is essential to avoid the complication of blindness. Aspirin is a useful adjunctive treatment that also helps reduce the risk of visual loss (Yurdakul, Bodur, Sivas, et al., 2015).

Nursing Management

Nursing care of the patient with PMR is based on the fundamental plan of nursing care presented earlier (see Chart 38-2). The most common nursing diagnoses are pain and deficient knowledge of medications.

A management concern is that the patient will take the prescribed medication, frequently corticosteroids, until symptoms improve and then discontinue the medication. The decision to discontinue the medication should be based on clinical and laboratory findings and the prescription. Nursing implications are related to helping the patient prevent and monitor adverse effects of medications (e.g., infections, diabetes, gastrointestinal problems, and depression) and adjust to those side effects that cannot be prevented (e.g., increased appetite and altered body image).

> ### ► Quality and Safety Nursing Alert
>
> *The nurse must emphasize to the patient the need for continued adherence to the prescribed medication regimen to avoid complications of GCA, such as blindness.*

The loss of bone mass with corticosteroid use increases the risk of osteoporosis in this already at-risk population. Interventions to promote bone health, such as adequate dietary calcium and vitamin D, measurement of bone mineral density, weight-bearing exercise, smoking cessation, and reduction of alcohol consumption if indicated, should be emphasized.

Osteoarthritis (Degenerative Joint Disease)

OA is a noninflammatory degenerative disorder of the joints. It is the most common form of joint disease and is routinely referred to as degenerative joint disease. OA is classified as either primary (idiopathic), with no prior event or disease

related to the OA, or secondary, resulting from previous joint injury or inflammatory disease, similar to RA (Papadakis et al., 2015). Unlike most of the disease processes discussed in this chapter, the pathophysiology of primary OA does not involve autoimmunity or inflammation. It can occur as an end result of an autoimmune disorder where joint destruction occurs. Another distinguishing characteristic of OA is that it is limited to the affected joints; there are no systemic symptoms associated with it.

OA often begins in the third decade of life and peaks between the fifth and sixth decades. By 40 years of age, 90% of the population has degenerative joint changes in their weight-bearing joints, even though clinical symptoms are usually absent (Papadakis et al., 2015). Women, especially those who are Hispanic or African American, are more commonly affected. The incidence of OA increases with age. It is estimated that over 85% of the general population over 65 years of age has radiographic changes indicating OA (Cash & Glass, 2015). Although OA is usually thought of as a disease of aging, it also affects younger patients and results in significant losses in work-related productivity and higher costs (CDC, 2015).

Pathophysiology

All joints consist of bone, particularly **subchondral bone** or the bony plate to which the articular cartilage is attached. This articular cartilage is a lubricated, smooth tissue that protects the bone from damage with physical activity. Between the articular cartilage of the bones forming the joint is a space (called the *joint space*) that allows for movement. To aid in fluidity, each joint contains synovial fluid to help lubricate and protect the joint's movement. With OA, the articular cartilage breaks down, leading to progressive damage to the underlying bone and eventual formation of **osteophytes** (bone spurs) that protrude into the joint space. The result is that the joint space is narrowed, leading to decreased joint movement and the potential for more damage. Consequently, the joint can progressively degenerate (see Fig. 38-3). Understanding of OA pathophysiology has been greatly expanded beyond what was previously thought of as simply "wear and tear" related to aging. The basic degenerative process in the joint exemplified in OA is presented in Figure 38-4. In addition to the degeneration, an infectious arteritis can occur. See Chapter 41 for discussion of septic (infectious) arthritis.

Figure 38-3 • Joint space narrowing and osteophytes (bone spurs) are characteristic of degenerative changes in joints.

Physiology/Pathophysiology

Figure 38-4 • Pathophysiology of osteoarthritis.

Risk factors for the disease and its progression include older age, female gender, and obesity. In addition, certain occupations (e.g., those requiring laborious tasks); engaging in sport activities; and a history of previous injuries, muscle weakness, genetic predisposition, and certain diseases can also place patients at risk for joint destruction. The most prominent modifiable risk factor for OA is obesity. In fact, both quality and quantity of life are reduced with OA, especially when obesity and OA are combined. A program of diet and exercise can help minimize symptoms of OA in patients who are obese (CDC, 2015).

Clinical Manifestations

The main clinical manifestations of OA are pain, stiffness, and functional impairment. The joint pain is usually aggravated by movement or exercise and relieved by rest. If morning stiffness is present, it is usually brief, lasting less than 30 minutes. The onset is routinely insidious, progressing over multiple years.

On physical examination, the affected joint may be enlarged with a decreased range of motion. Although OA occurs most often in weight-bearing joints (hips, knees, cervical and lumbar spine), the proximal interphalangeal (PIP) and distal interphalangeal (DIP) joints are also often involved causing bony enlargements of the DIP (Heberden's nodes) and PIP (Bouchard's nodes) joints. Crepitus may be palpated, especially over the knee. Joint effusion, a sign of inflammation, is usually mild. No systemic manifestations are found.

Assessment and Diagnostic Findings

Blood tests and examination of joint fluid are not useful in the diagnosis of OA but are occasionally indicated to rule out an autoimmune cause for the joint pain, such as RA. X-rays may show a narrowing of the joint space; osteophyte formation; and dense, thickened subchondral bone (Papadakis et al., 2015).

Medical Management

The goals of management are to decrease pain and stiffness and to maintain or, when possible, improve joint mobility. Exercise, especially in the form of cardiovascular aerobic exercise and lower extremity strength training, has been found to prevent OA progression and decrease symptoms of OA. Along with exercise, weight loss, which in turn decreases excess load on the joint, can also be extremely beneficial. Occupational and physical therapy can help the patient adopt self-management strategies (Kalunian, 2015a).

Wedged insoles, knee braces, and other modalities are being evaluated as possible therapies aimed at treating the abnormalities in biomechanics found in OA. The use of orthotic devices (e.g., splints, braces) and walking aids (e.g., canes) can improve pain and function by decreasing force on the affected joint (Kalunian, 2015a).

Patients with arthritis often use complementary, alternative, and integrative health therapies, such as massage, yoga, pulsed electromagnetic fields, TENS, and music therapy. These may also include herbal and dietary supplements, other special diets, acupuncture, acupressure, wearing copper bracelets or magnets, and participation in T'ai chi. Research is under way to determine the effectiveness of many of these treatments. To date, no definitive evidence has been found regarding their efficacy (Kalunian, 2015a).

Pharmacologic Therapy

Pharmacologic management of OA is directed toward symptom management and pain control. Selection of medication is based on the patient's needs, the stage of disease, and the risk of side effects. Medications are used in conjunction with nonpharmacologic strategies. In most patients with OA, the initial analgesic therapy is acetaminophen. Some patients respond to the nonselective NSAIDs, and patients who are at increased risk for gastrointestinal complications, especially gastrointestinal bleeding, have been managed effectively with COX-2 enzyme blockers. However, COX-2 enzyme blockers must be used with caution because of the associated risk of cardiovascular disease. Other medications that may be considered are the opioids and intra-articular corticosteroids. Topical analgesic agents such as capsaicin (Capsin, Zostrix) and methylsalicylate are also used (Carter et al., 2015). Topical diclofenac sodium gel (Voltaren gel) has been FDA approved for the use of osteoarthritic joint pain in the hands and knees.

Other therapeutic approaches include glucosamine and chondroitin. Although it has been suggested that these substances modify cartilage structure, studies have not shown them to be effective (Martin, Van Sell, & Danter, 2012). Viscosupplementation, the injection of gel-like substances (hyaluronates) into a joint (intra-articular), is thought to supplement the viscous properties of synovial fluid. These viscosupplements aim to prevent the loss of cartilage and repair chondral defects (Kalunian, 2015b).

Surgical Management

In moderate to severe OA, when pain is severe or because of loss of function, surgical intervention may be used. The procedures most commonly used are osteotomy (to alter the distribution of weight within the joint) and arthroplasty. In **arthroplasty**, diseased joint components are replaced (see Chapter 40). Rehabilitation with physical therapy that is initiated within the first 24 hours is associated with decreased hospital length of stay and improved balance and gait function (Martin, Thornhill, & Katz, 2015).

Nursing Management

Pain management and optimal functional ability are major goals of nursing intervention. With those goals in mind, nursing management of the patient with OA includes pharmacologic and nonpharmacologic approaches as well as education. The patient's understanding of the disease process and symptom pattern is critical to the plan of care. Because patients with OA usually are older, they may have other health problems. Commonly they are overweight, and they may have a sedentary lifestyle. Weight loss and exercise are important approaches to lessen pain and disability. Canes or other assistive devices for ambulation should be considered, and any stigma about the use of these devices should be explored. Exercises such as walking should be begun in moderation and increased gradually. Patients should plan their daily exercise for a time when the pain is least severe or plan to use an analgesic agent, if appropriate, before exercising. Adequate pain management is important for the success of an exercise program. Open discussion regarding the use of complementary, alternative, and integrative health therapies is important to maintain safe and effective practices for patients looking for relief.

Spondyloarthropathies

The spondyloarthropathies are another category of systemic inflammatory disorders of the skeleton. The spondyloarthropathies include ankylosing spondylitis (AS), reactive arthritis (formerly known as Reiter's syndrome), and psoriatic arthritis. Spondyloarthritis is also associated with inflammatory bowel diseases such as Crohn's disease (regional enteritis) and ulcerative colitis (Grossman & Porth, 2014).

These rheumatic diseases share several clinical features. The inflammation tends to occur peripherally at the sites of attachment—at tendons, joint capsules, and ligaments. Periosteal inflammation may be present. Many patients have arthritis of the sacroiliac joints. The onset tends to occur during young adulthood, with the disease affecting men more often than women. There is a strong tendency for these conditions to occur in families. Frequently, the HLA-B27 genetic marker is found. In addition, more than one of these conditions can be found simultaneously in the same person or another family member (Carter et al., 2015).

As with other inflammatory conditions, patients with spondyloarthropathies have an increased risk for cardiovascular disease. These findings may be related to a state of chronic systemic inflammation and an increase in traditional cardiac risk factors, such as lack of exercise due to increased pain (Carter et al., 2015).

Ankylosing Spondylitis

AS is a chronic and inflammatory disease of the spine. It is more prevalent in males than in females and is usually diagnosed in the second or third decade of life. The disease is also more severe in males, and significant systemic involvement is likely.

AS affects the cartilaginous joints of the spine and surrounding tissues, making them rigid, decreasing mobility, and leading to kyphosis (a stooped position). This kyphosis can, in turn, lead to decreased stability and balance. Back pain is the characteristic feature. The back pain can be so severe that it may mask symptoms of a cervical fracture, which can lead to neurologic problems if left untreated. Occasionally, the large synovial joints, such as the hips, knees, or shoulders, may be involved (Carter et al., 2015).

AS also exhibits systemic effects. Uveitis occurs in 20% to 25% of patients with AS and may be a presenting feature (Smith, 2013). Another potential complication of AS is the risk of osteoporosis, which appears to be related to the inflammatory process as well as bone turnover and low vitamin D levels. Other complications involve atrioventricular conduction defects, aortic insufficiency, and pulmonary fibrosis (Papadakis et al., 2015). As the disease progresses, ankylosis of the entire spine may occur, leading to respiratory compromise and further complications.

Reactive Arthritis (Reiter's Syndrome)

The disease process involved in reactive arthritis is called *reactive* because the arthritis occurs after an infection, primarily gastrointestinal or genitourinary (Carter et al., 2015). It mostly affects young adult males and is characterized primarily by urethritis, arthritis, and conjunctivitis. Dermatitis and ulcerations of the mouth and penis may also be present. Low back pain is common.

Psoriatic Arthritis

Psoriatic arthritis is an inflammatory arthritis associated with the skin disease psoriasis. In fact, research has suggested that between 10% and 20% of people with psoriasis will eventually develop psoriatic arthritis (Carter et al., 2015; Dewing, 2015). Psoriasis is the most common autoimmune disease in the United States, affecting 2% to 3% of the population. Psoriatic arthritis onset occurs between 30 and 50 years of age and affects equal numbers of men and women (Dewing, 2015).

Pathogenesis of the disease process is hypothesized to start in the skin with an exaggerated immune response to environmental factors and then spreads to the joints in genetically susceptible individuals. Genetics is found to be a strong predictor. Many men and women diagnosed with psoriatic arthritis usually have a first-degree relative with psoriasis. Research shows that the HLAs are also present in up to 50% of patients diagnosed with psoriatic arthritis testing positive for the HLA-B27 antigen (Dewing, 2015). Although these patients test negative for rheumatoid factor, levels of TNF-α and other cytokines are elevated (Dewing, 2015). The body is triggered to activate the T cells of the immune system, producing inflammatory cytokines and mediators that cause changes and inflammation in the body, which also may result in erosions and joint destruction. In addition to joint damage, this cascade may also damage the ligaments, tendons, skin, and nails. Nail psoriasis occurs in approximately 90% of patients (Dewing, 2015).

Psoriatic arthritis is characterized by synovitis, polyarthritis, and spondylitis. Inflammatory back pain is a common symptom, which is differentiated from other back pain by symptoms of back pain presenting at a young age, pain improving with activity, and pain occurring at night. Radiographic evidence of asymetricalsacroilitis or spondylitis may also assist with diagnosing psoriatic arthritis (Dewing, 2015). Other sites of pain commonly seen in these patients are the Achilles tendon, plantar fascia, or tibial tuberosity areas. Pain in these areas is common from the inflammation that occurs at the entheses, where tendons and ligaments attach to the bone.

In addition to pain, infections can also occur since this is a systemic disease. Uveitis occurs in approximately 1.5% to 25% of patients diagnosed with psoriatic arthritis. Uveitis should be quickly diagnosed and treated by the ophthalmologist to prevent vision loss (Dewing, 2015).

Medical Management

Medical management of spondyloarthropathies focuses on treating pain and maintaining mobility by suppressing inflammation. For the patient with AS, good body positioning and posture are essential so that if **ankylosis** (fixation) does occur, the patient is in the most functional position. Maintaining range of motion with regular exercise and a muscle-strengthening program is especially important and has been linked with higher quality of life for the patient (Carter et al., 2015).

Pharmacologic Management

The European League Against Rheumatism guidelines recommend NSAIDs as the first-line therapy for treating all spondylarthropathies. All chronic conditions (cardiac, renal, and gastrointestinal) should be taken into consideration when prescribing long-term NSAIDS. Methotrexate, sulfasalazine, and leflunomide may also be used; these drugs may help with skin and peripheral joint disease but may not prevent spinal changes. Corticosteroid injections may be used for periodic flares; however, oral and long-term use of steroids is not recommended due to the possibility of psoriatic skin flare when discontinuing use. More recently, anti-TNF therapy has been approved by the FDA for psoriatic arthritis. Anti-TNF medications that have been used effectively include etanercept (Enbrel), infliximab (Remicade), adalimumab (Humira), golimumab (Simponi), and certolizumabpegol (Cimzia). Two additional agents include apremilast (Otezla), which is a PDE4 inhibitor, and ustekinumab (Stelara), an anti-IL12/anti-IL23 agent (Carter et al., 2015; Dewing, 2015).

Surgical Management

With advanced AS and subsequent debilitating kyphosis, an osteotomy of the spine can be done. One study showed that an average correction of 45 degrees in the cervical spine was obtained and that quality of life also improved. Surgical management may also include total joint replacement (see Chapter 40) (Carter et al., 2015).

Nursing Management

Major nursing interventions in the spondyloarthropathies are related to symptom management and maintenance of optimal functioning. Affected patients are primarily young men. Their major concerns are often related to prognosis and job modification, especially among those who perform physical work. Patients may also express concerns about leisure and recreational activities. Focusing on physical activity and staying active and maintaining good posture will help to prevent chronic changes that may lead to deformities. It is important to address psychological changes, such as depression and emotional stress, that can occur with the diagnosis and chronicity of the disease (Carter et al., 2015). If symptoms are present, the primary provider should assess for emotional stress and treat as appropriate.

Metabolic and Endocrine Diseases Associated With Rheumatic Disorders

Metabolic and endocrine diseases may be associated with rheumatic disorders. These include biochemical abnormalities (amyloidosis and scurvy), endocrine diseases (diabetes and acromegaly), immune deficiency diseases (human immune deficiency virus infection, acquired immune deficiency syndrome), and some inherited disorders (hypermobility syndromes). However, the most common conditions are the crystal-induced arthropathies, in which crystals such as monosodium urate (gout) or calcium pyrophosphate (calcium pyrophosphate dihydrate disease or pseudogout) are deposited within joints and other tissues (Papadakis et al., 2015).

Gout

Gout is the most common form of inflammatory arthritis. More than 8.3 million Americans self-report the diagnosis of gout (CDC, 2015b). The prevalence is reported to be about 3.9% and appears to be on the rise. Men are three to four times more likely to be diagnosed with gout than women. The incidence of gout increases with age, body mass index, alcohol consumption, hypertension, and diuretic use (CDC, 2015b). Evidence links the consumption of fructose-rich beverages with the risk of gout for both men and women (CDC, 2015b). Patients with gout have an increased risk of cardiovascular disease. Comorbid conditions such as hypertension, dyslipidemia, diabetes, OA, and kidney disease may be present in patients with gout (Papadakis et al., 2015).

Given that the incidence of gout increases with age, its management can be complicated by other medical conditions, medications, and age-related changes (Carter et al., 2015).

Pathophysiology

Gout is caused by hyperuricemia (increased serum uric acid). Uric acid is a by-product of purine metabolism; purines are basic chemical compounds found in high concentrations in meat products. Urate levels are affected by diet, medications, overproduction in the body, and inadequate excretion by the kidneys. Hyperuricemia (serum concentration greater than 6.8 mg/dL) can, but does not always, cause urate crystal deposition. However, as uric acid levels increase, the risk becomes greater. The initial cause for the gout attack occurs when macrophages in the joint space phagocytize urate crystals. Through a series of immunologic steps, interleukin 1 beta is secreted, increasing the inflammation. This process is exacerbated by the presence of free fatty acids. Both alcohol and consumption of a large meal, especially with red meat, can lead to increases in free fatty acid concentrations; they also are implicated as triggers to acute gout attacks (Carter et al., 2015).

With repeated attacks, accumulations of sodium urate crystals, called tophi, are deposited in peripheral areas of the body, such as the great toe, the hands, and the ear. Renal uratelithiasis (kidney stones), with chronic kidney disease secondary to urate deposition, may develop.

Primary hyperuricemia may be caused by severe dieting or starvation, excessive intake of foods that are high in purines (shellfish, organ meats), or heredity. In secondary hyperuricemia, gout is a clinical feature secondary to any of a number of genetic or acquired processes, including conditions in which there is an increase in cell turnover (leukemia, multiple myeloma, some types of anemias, psoriasis) and an increase in cell breakdown. Altered renal tubular function, either as a major action or as an unintended side effect of certain pharmacologic agents (e.g., diuretics such as thiazides and furosemide), low-dose salicylates, or ethanol can contribute to uric acid underexcretion (Klippel et al., 2008). The finding of urate crystals in the synovial fluid of asymptomatic joints suggests that factors other than crystals may be related to the inflammatory reaction. Recovered monosodium urate crystals are coated with immunoglobulins that are mainly IgG. IgG enhances crystal phagocytosis, thereby demonstrating immunologic activity (Klippel et al., 2008).

Clinical Manifestations

Manifestations of the gout syndrome include acute gouty arthritis (recurrent attacks of severe articular and periarticular inflammation), **tophi** (crystalline deposits accumulating in articular tissue, osseous tissue, soft tissue, and cartilage), gouty nephropathy (renal impairment), and uric acid urinary calculi. Four stages of gout can be identified: asymptomatic hyperuricemia, acute gouty arthritis, intercritical gout, and chronic tophaceous gout (Neoai, Jansen, Dalbeth, et al., 2015). The subsequent development of gout is directly related to the duration and magnitude of the hyperuricemia. Therefore, the commitment to lifelong pharmacologic treatment of hyperuricemia is deferred until there is an initial attack of gout.

For hyperuricemic people who are going to develop gout, acute arthritis is the most common early clinical manifestation. The metatarsophalangeal joint of the big toe is a commonly affected joint. The tarsal area, ankle, or knee may also be affected. Less commonly, the wrists, fingers, and elbows may be affected. Trauma, alcohol ingestion, dieting, medications, surgical stress, or illness may trigger the acute attack. The abrupt onset often occurs at night, awakening the patient with severe pain, redness, swelling, and warmth of the affected joint. Early attacks tend to subside spontaneously over 3 to 10 days even without treatment. The attack is followed by a symptom-free period (the intercritical stage) until the next attack, which may not come for months or years.

However, with time, attacks tend to occur more frequently, involve more joints, and last longer (Becker, 2015).

Tophi (seen in chronic tophaceous gout) are generally associated with more frequent and severe inflammatory episodes. Higher serum concentrations of uric acid are also associated with more extensive tophus formation. Tophi most commonly occur in the synovium, olecranon bursa, subchondral bone, infrapatellar and Achilles tendons, and subcutaneous tissue on the extensor surface of the forearms and overlying joints. They have also been found in the aortic walls, heart valves, nasal and ear cartilage, eyelids, cornea, and sclera. Joint enlargement may cause a loss of joint motion. Uric acid deposits may cause renal stones and kidney damage.

Medical Management

A definitive diagnosis of gouty arthritis is established by polarized light microscopy of the synovial fluid of the involved joint. Uric acid crystals are seen within the polymorphonuclear leukocytes in the fluid.

Acute attacks are managed with colchicine (Colcrys) (oral or parenteral), an NSAID such as indomethacin (Indocin), or a corticosteroid. Management of hyperuricemia, tophi, joint destruction, and renal disorders is usually initiated after the acute inflammatory process has subsided. Once the acute attack has subsided, uric acid lowering therapy should be considered. Xanthine oxidase inhibitors, such as allopurinol (Zyloprim) and febuxostat (Uloric), are the agents of choice. Given the role of IL-1 in the pathogenesis of gout, some experts suggest that there may be a role for anakinra (Kineret), an IL-1 receptor antagonist in the management of acute gout (Papadakis et al., 2015).

Management between gout attacks needs to include lifestyle changes such as avoiding purine-rich foods, weight loss, decreasing alcohol consumption, and avoiding certain medications. Uricosuric agents, such as probenecid (Benemid), may be indicated in patients with frequent acute attacks. Uricosuric medications correct hyperuricemia and dissolve deposited urate. Corticosteroids may also be used in patients who have no response to other therapy. In patients with refractory chronic gout who are not controlled with the regimens mentioned earlier, pegloticase (Krystexxa), a newer agent, has been shown to be effective in lowering uric acid levels (Becker, 2016). Specific treatment is based on the serum uric acid level, 24-hour urinary uric acid excretion, and renal function (see Table 38-5) (Carter et al., 2015).

Nursing Management

Severe dietary restriction is not necessary; however, the nurse encourages the patient to restrict consumption of foods high in purines, especially organ meats, and to limit alcohol intake. Maintenance of normal body weight should be encouraged. In an acute episode of gouty arthritis, pain management with prescribed medications is essential, along with avoidance of factors that increase pain and inflammation, such as trauma, stress, and alcohol. Medication adherence is critical; therefore, counseling needs to be initiated by the nurse when appropriate. Between acute episodes, the patient feels well and may abandon preventive behaviors, which may result in an acute attack. Acute attacks are most effectively treated if therapy is begun early (Carter et al., 2015).

TABLE 38-5 Common Medications Used to Treat Gout

Medication	Actions and Use	Nursing Implications
colchicine (Colcrys)	Lowers the deposition of uric acid and interferes with leukocyte infiltration, thus reducing inflammation; does not alter serum or urine levels of uric acid; used in acute and chronic management	*Acute management:* Administer when attack begins; dosage increased until pain is relieved or diarrhea develops, then stop medication *Chronic management:* Causes gastrointestinal upset in most patients.
probenecid (Benemid)	Uricosuric agent; inhibits renal reabsorption of urates and increases the urinary excretion of uric acid; prevents tophi formation	Be alert for nausea and rash.
allopurinol (Zyloprim), febuxostat (Uloric)	Xanthine oxidase inhibitors; interrupt the breakdown of purines before uric acid is formed; inhibit xanthinoxidase because uric acid formation is blocked	Monitor for side effects, including bone marrow depression, vomiting, and abdominal pain. Avoid starting medication or increasing dose if active flare present.

Adapted from Karch, A. (2014). *Lippincott's nursing drug guide.* Philadelphia, PA: Lippincott Williams & Wilkins.

Fibromyalgia

Fibromyalgia is a chronic pain syndrome that involves chronic fatigue, generalized muscle aching, stiffness, sleep disturbances, and functional impairment. It is estimated to affect more than 5 million Americans, representing 2% to 5% of the general population, with women affected more than men. Between 25% and 65% of patients with fibromyalgia have other rheumatologic conditions such as RA, SLE, and AS (CDC, 2015c).

Pathophysiology

The amplified pain experienced by patients with fibromyalgia is neurogenic in origin (Carter et al., 2015). Specifically, the central nervous system's ascending and descending pathways (that regulate and moderate pain processing) function abnormally, causing amplification of pain signals. Some scientists describe this as if the "volume control setting" for pain were abnormally high (Carter et al., 2015). Therefore, stimulation that may not normally elicit pain, such as touch, may do so. In addition, there are a number of predisposing factors to pain, including anxiety, depression, physical trauma, emotional stress, sleep disorder, and viral infection (Carter et al., 2015).

Assessment and Diagnostic Findings

The American College of Rheumatology established preliminary diagnostic criteria and symptom severity indices for fibromyalgia (Carter et al., 2015). These criteria emphasize the regions of pain, rather than specific points, and take into account the fatigue, cognitive symptoms, and unrefreshed sleep that patients with fibromyalgia also tend to experience (Carter et al., 2015).

Medical Management

Treatment consists of attention to the specific symptoms reported by the patient. NSAIDs may be used to treat the diffuse muscle aching and stiffness. Tricyclic antidepressants such as amitriptyline (Elavil) and nortriptyline (Pamelor) as well as sleep hygiene measures are used to improve or restore normal sleep patterns (Cash & Glass, 2015). Muscle relaxants such as cyclobenzaprine (Amrix) may also be used to help with relaxation and pain. Cognitive behavioral therapy is also useful in improving sleep and attentional dysfunction. In addition, serotonin norepinephrine reuptake inhibitors, such as duloxetine (Cymbalta), venlafaxine (Effexor), and milnacipran (Savella); selective serotonin reuptake inhibitors, including fluoxetine (Prozac), paroxetine (Paxil), and sertraline (Zoloft); as well as anticonvulsants such as gabapentin (Neurontin) and pregabalin (Lyrica) have been reported to be effective (Carter et al., 2015). Individualized programs of exercise are used to decrease muscle weakness and discomfort and to improve the general deconditioning that occurs in affected patients. There has also been some promising research in complementary, alternative, and integrative health therapies, such as acupuncture, massage, homeopathy, hydrotherapy, craniosacral therapy, and myofascial therapy (Carter et al., 2015).

Nursing Management

Typically, patients with fibromyalgia have endured their symptoms for a long period of time. They may feel as if their symptoms have not been taken seriously. Nurses need to pay special attention to supporting these patients and providing encouragement as they begin their program of therapy. Patient support groups may be helpful. Careful listening to patients' descriptions of their concerns and symptoms is essential to help them make the changes that are necessary to improve their quality of life (Carter et al., 2015).

Miscellaneous Disorders

The last category in the classification of the rheumatic diseases is aptly labeled miscellaneous disorders because it contains a mix of disorders that are frequently associated with arthritis and other conditions. These include the direct consequences of trauma (including internal derangement and loose bodies of joints), pancreatic disease (related to avascular necrosis or osteonecrosis), sarcoidosis (a multisystem disorder particularly of the lymph nodes and lungs), and palindromic rheumatism (an uncommon variety of recurring and acute arthritis and periarthritis that in some may progress to RA but is characterized by symptom-free periods of days to months). Other conditions include villonodularsynovitis, chronic active hepatitis, and drug-related rheumatic syndromes. The nursing interventions related to these varied conditions are specific to the multisystemic problems experienced by the patient. However, the musculoskeletal components should not be neglected or overlooked. Further information about these rare disorders can be found in specialty references.

CRITICAL THINKING EXERCISES

1 A 62-year-old patient who was recently diagnosed with osteoarthritis (OA) comes in for her follow-up appointment. She wants to know why she is not being prescribed "stronger medications" for her arthritis like her friend is taking. Her friend has RA and her pain improved significantly after starting adalimumab injections. Describe your teaching plan to explain the physiologic differences between OA and RA, medications commonly used for OA and the difference between treatment regimens for OA and RA.

2 `pa` Your patient is a 52-year-old male patient with a history of hypertension, stage 3 kidney disease, diabetes, and hyperlipidemia. He smokes 1 pack of cigarettes a day and drinks alcohol on occasion. He is 6'2" and weighs 240 lbs. Today he presents with complaints of severe pain in his right great toe that started Sunday morning. He spent a long weekend with friends, drank a lot of alcohol, and ate a lot of rich food. He woke Sunday morning with pain in his foot that has progressively gotten worse. He has been diagnosed with gout. Identify the priorities, approach, and techniques you would use to provide nursing care to this patient. How would you prioritize the physical examination and techniques performed since his pain scale is 8/10? What lifestyle modifications are a priority for this patient?

3 `ebp` You are the nurse taking care of a woman with Sjögren's syndome. What is the evidence for symptom management for this patient? What criteria would you use to assess the strength of the evidence? What is the evidence for treatment options to improve her symptoms?

REFERENCES

*Asterisk indicates nursing research.
**Double asterisk indicates classic reference.

Books

Cash, J. C., &Glass, C. A. (2015). *Adult-gerontology practice guidelines.* New York: Springer Publishing Company.

Carter S. C., Patty-Resk, C., Ruffing, V., et al. (2015). *Core curriculum for rheumatology nursing* (1st ed.).Greenville, SC: Lyons Den Solutions, LLC.

Fischbach, F., & Dunning, M. B. (2015). *A manual of laboratory and diagnostic tests* (9th ed.). Philadelphia, PA: Lippincott Williams & Wilkins.

Grossman, S. C., &Porth, C. M. (2014). *Porth's pathophysiology: Concepts of altered health states* (9th ed.). Philadelphia, PA: Lippincott Williams & Wilkins.

Karch, A. (2014). *Lippincott's nursing drug guide.* Philadelphia, PA: Lippincott Williams & Wilkins.

**Klippel, J. H., Stone, J. H., Crofford, L. J., et al. (Eds.). (2008). *Primer on the rheumatic diseases* (13th ed.). New York: Springer.

Miller, C. A. (2015). *Nursing for wellness in older adults* (7th ed.). Philadelphia: Lippincott Williams & Wilkins.

Papadakis, M. A., McPhee, S. J., & Rabow, M. W. (2015). *Current medical diagnosis and treatment 2016* (55th ed.). New York: McGraw-Hill.

Journals and Electronic Documents

Afshar, B. (2015). *RA: Best and worse supplements and herbs.* Retrieved on 5/14/2016 at: www.webmd.com/rheumatoid-arthritis/guide/rheumatoid-arthritis-best-wrose-supplements-herbs.

American College of Rheumatology (1997). *ACR-endorsed criteria for Rheumatic diseases.* Retrieved on 1/13/2016 at: www.rheumatology.org/Portals/0/Files/1997%20Update%20of%201982%20Revised.pdf

**Aletaha, D., Neogi, T., Silman, A. J., et al. (2010). 2010 Rheumatoid arthritis classification criteria: An American College of Rheumatology/European League Against Rheumatism collaborative initiative. *Arthritis and Rheumatism,* 62(9), 2569–2581.

Barbour, K. E., Helmick, C. G., Theis, K. A., et al. (2013). Prevalence of doctor-diagnosed arthritis and arthritis-attributable activity limitation—United States, 2010–2012. *MMWR: Morbidity and Mortality Weekly Report,* 62(44), 869–873.

Bartels, C. (2015). *Systemic Lupus Erythematosus.* Retrieved on 5/14/2016 at: ww.emedicine.medscape.com/article/332244-overview.

Becker, M. A. (2015). Clinical manifestations and diagnosis of gout. Retrieved on 5/14/2016 at: www.uptodate.com/contents/search?search=Clinical+manifestations+and+diagnosis+of+gout&x=4&y=8

Becker, M.A. (2016). Prevention of recurrent gout: Pharmacologic urate-lowering therapy and treatment of tophi. Retrieved on 5/14/2016 at: www.uptodate.com/contents/search?search=Prevention+of+recurrent+gout%3A+Pharmacologic+urate-lowering+therapy+and+%09treatment+of+tophi&x=4&y=9

Bultink, I. E. (2012). Osteoporosis and fractures in systemic lupus erythematosus. *Arthritis Care and Research,* 64(1), 2–8.

Centers for Disease Control and Prevention (CDC). (2015). *Osteoarthritis (OA).* Retrieved on 5/14/2016 at: www.cdc.gov.

Centers for Disease Control and Prevention (CDC). (2015a). *Systemic lupus erythematous (SLE or lupus): Prevalence and incidence.* Retrieved on 5/14/2016 at: www.cdc.gov/arthritis/basics/lupus.htm

Centers for Disease Control and Prevention (CDC). (2015b). *Gout.* Retrieved on 5/14/2016 at: www.cdc.gov/arthritis/basics/gout.htm

Centers for Disease Control and Prevention (CDC). (2015c). *Fibromyalgia.* Retrieved on 5/14/2016 at: www.cdc.gov/arthritis/basics/fibromyalgia.htm

Chasset, F., Frances, C., Barete, S., et al. (2015). Influence of smoking on the efficacy of antimalarials in cutaneous lupus: A meta-analysis of the literature. *Journal of the American Academy of Dermatology,* 72(4), 634–639.

*Cottrell, J. D., Jonas, M., Bergsten, U., et al. (2013). The nurse's role in addressing unmet treatment and management needs of patients with rheumatoid arthritis: Delphi-based recommendations. *International Journal of Nursing Knowledge,* 24(2), 66–76.

Dewing, K. A. (2015). Management of patients with psoriatic arthritis. *The Nurse Practitioner,* 40(4), 40–46.

Di Lorenzo, A. L. (2015). *HLA-B27 syndromes.* Retrieved on 5/14/2016 at: www.emedicine.medscape.come/article/1201027-overview

Fonseca, R., Bernardes, M., Terroso, G., et al. (2014). *Silent burdens in disease: Fatigue and depression in SLE.* Autoimmune Diseases, 2014, 790724.

Fujita, T., Kutsumi, H., Sanuki, T., et al. (2013). Adherence to the preventive strategies for nonsteroidal anti-inflammatory drug-or low–dose aspirin-induced gastrointestinal injuries. *Journal of Gastroenterology,* 48(5), 559–573.

**Hochberg, C. (1997). Updating the American College of Rheumatology revised criteria for the classification of systemic lupus erythematosus. *Arthritis and Rheumatism,* 40(9), 1725.

Jordan, S., Maurer, B., Toniolo, M., et al. (2015). Performance of the new ACR/EULAR classification criteria for systemic sclerosis in clinical practice. *Rheumatology,* 54(8), 1454–1458.

Kalunian, K. C. (2015a). *Nonpharmacologic therapy of osteoarthritis.* Retrieved on 5/15/2016 at: www.uptodate.com/contents/search?search=Nonpharmacologic+therapy+of+osteoarthritis+&x=13&y=8

Kalunian, K. C. (2015b). Treatment of osteoarthritis resistant to initial pharmacologic therapy. Retrieved on 5/15/2016 at: www.uptodate.com/contents/search?search=Treatment+of+osteoarthritis+resistant+to+initial+pharmacologic+therapy&x=8&y=16

Lim, S., Bayakly, A. R., Helmick, C. G., et al. (2014). The incidence and prevalence of systemic lupus erythematosus, 2002–2004. *Arthritis & Rheumatology,* 66(2), 357–368.

Marcus, D. M. (2015). *Herbal remedies, supplements & acupuncture for arthritis.* The American College of Rheumatology. Retrieved on 5/14/2016 at: www.rheumatology.org/i-am-a/patient-caregiver/treatments/herbal-remedies-supplements-acupuncture-for-arthritis.

Martin, G., M., Thornhill, T. S., & Katz, J.M. (2015). Total knee arthroplasty. Retrieved on 5/14/2016 at: www.uptodate.com/contents/search?search=Total+knee+arthroplastypolimiosite&x=16&y=10

Martin, M. S., Van Sell, S., &Danter, J. (2012). Glucosamine and chondroitin: An appropriate adjunct treatment of symptomatic osteoarthritis of the knee. *Orthopaedic Nursing, 31*(3), 160–166.

Miller, M. L., & Viegels, R. A. (2016). *Clinical manifestations of dermatomyositis and polymyositis in adults.* Retrieved on 5/14/2016 at: www.uptodate.com/contents/clinical-manifestations-of-dermatomyositis-and-polymyositis-in-adults?source=machineLearning&search=polimiosite&selectedTitle=2%7E150&sectionRank=1&anchor=H17269403

Moerman, R., Bootsma, H., Kroese, R., et al. (2013). Sjogren's syndrome in older patients: Aetiology, diagnosis and management. *Drugs and Aging, 30*(3), 137–153.

Montes, R. A., Mocarzel, L.O., Lanzieri, P. G., et al. (2016). Smoking and its association with morbidity in systemic lupus erythematosus. *Arthritis and Rheumatology, 68*(2), 441–448.

Neoai, T., Jansen, T. A., Dalbeth, N., et al. (2015). 2105 Gout classification criteria: An American College of Rheumatology collaborative project. Retrieved on 8/25/2016 at: www.rheumatology.org/Practice-Quality/Clinical-Support/Criteria.

Palmer, D., & El Miedany, Y. (2014). Rheumatoid arthritis: Recommendations for treat to target. *British Journal of Nursing, 23*(6), 310–315.

Quemeneur, T., Mouthon, L., Cacoub, P., et al. (2013). Systemic vasculitis during the course of systemic sclerosis: Report of 12 cases and review of the literature. *Medicine, 92*(1), 1–9.

Ramos-Remus, C., Duran-Barragan, S., &Castillo-Ortiz, J. (2012). Beyond the joints: Neurological involvement in rheumatoid arthritis. *Clinical Rheumatology, 31*(1), 1–12.

Seetharaman, M. (2015). *Giant Cell Arteritis (Temporal Arteritis) workup.* Retrieved on 5/15/2016 at: emedicine.medscape.com/article/332483-workup

Sholter, D. E., & Russell, A. S. (2016). *Synovial fluid analysis.* Retrieved on 5/14/2016 at: www. uptodate.com/contents/ synovial-fluid-analysis.

Schur, P. H., & Moreland, L. W. (2016). *General principles of management of rheumatoid arthritis in adults.* Retrieved on 5/14/2016 at: www.uptodate.com/contents/general- principles-of-management-of-rheumatoid-arthritis-in-adults?source=search_result&search=rheumatoid+arthritis&selectedTitle=3~150

Smith, W. M. (2013). Gender and spondyloarthropathy-associated uveitis. *Journal of Opthalmology, 2013,* 928264.

Tan, E. M., Cohen, A. S., Fries, J. F., et al. (1982). The 1982 revised criteria for the classification of systemic lupus erythematosus. *Arthritis and Rheumatism, 25*(11), 1271–1277.

Varga, J. (2014). *Diagnosis and differential diagnosis of systemic sclerosis (scleroderma) in adults.* Retrieved on 5/14/2016 at:www.uptodate.com/contents/search?search=Diagnosis+and+differential+diagnosis+of+systemic+sclerosis+%28scleroderma%29+in+%09adults&x=14&y=9

Varga, J., & Steen, V. (2015). Pulmonary arterial hypertension in systemic sclerosis (scleroderma): Definition, classification, risk factors, screening and prognosis. Retrieved on 5/14/2016 at: www.uptodate.com/contents/table-of-contents/rheumatology/scleroderma.

Yurdakul, F. G., Bodur, H., Sivas, F., et al. (2015). Clinical features, treatment and monitoring in patients with olymyalgiarheumatica. *Archives of Rheumatology, 30*(1), 28–33.

Resources

American College of Rheumatology and Association of Rheumatology Health Professionals, www.rheumatology.org

American Fibromyalgia Syndrome Association (AFSA), www.afsafund.org

Arthritis Foundation, www.arthritis.org

Centers for Disease Control and Prevention, www.cdc.gov

Lupus Foundation of America, www.lupus.org

National Institute of Arthritis and Musculoskeletal and Skin Diseases, National Institutes of Health, www.niams.nih.gov

Scleroderma Foundation, www.scleroderma.org

Sjögren's Syndrome Foundation, www.sjogrens.org

Spondylitis Association of America, www.spondylitis.org

UNIT 9

Musculoskeletal Function

Case Study | DEVELOPING A TEAM APPROACH TO CARE IN THE HOME SETTING

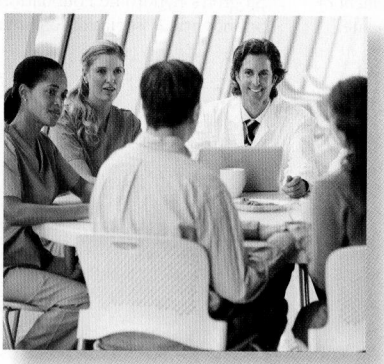

The nurse is participating in an interdisciplinary team meeting discussing patients in an inpatient acute rehabilitation unit. The team consists of a physician, nurse, pharmacist, social worker, occupational therapist, physical therapist, and registered dietician. The team is discussing the interdisciplinary management plan for a patient recently admitted for transitional care from the hospital, where he had an above the knee amputation of the right leg as a result of poorly controlled diabetes. The team has concerns for the patient because he lives alone and is unable to care for himself to achieve an optimal recovery. In addition, his last hemoglobin A1c was 9.8%, indicating that his diabetes is still not well controlled. The team must develop strategies necessary to help the patient recover from his recent surgery and develop a plan of care for controlling his diabetes before he can transition to an appropriate outpatient level of care.

QSEN Competency Focus: Teamwork and Collaboration

The complexities inherent in today's health care system challenges nurses to demonstrate integration of specific inter-disciplinary core competencies. These competencies are aimed at ensuring the delivery of safe, quality patient care (Institute of Medicine, 2003). The Quality and Safety Education for Nurses project (QSEN, 2017; Cronenwett, Sherwood, Barnsteiner, et al., 2007) provides a framework for the knowledge, skills and attitudes (KSA) required for nurses to demonstrate competency in these key areas, which include **patient-centered care, interdisciplinary teamwork and collaboration, evidence-based practice, quality improvement, safety,** and **informatics.**

Teamwork and Collaboration Definition: Function effectively within nursing and interprofessional teams, fostering open communication, mutual respect, and shared decision making to achieve quality patient care.

SELECTED PRE-LICENSURE KSAs	APPLICATION AND REFLECTION
Knowledge	
Recognize contributions of other individuals and groups in helping patient/family achieve health goals.	Collaborative problems require nursing interventions as well as those of other health care providers on the team. What are nursing interventions for managing diabetes? What contributions might the pharmacist and dietician have in regards to managing diabetes?
Skills	
Integrate the contributions of others who play a role in helping patient/family achieve goals.	Think of an example of a collaborative problem for this patient with both medical and nursing interventions. How does the nurse integrate the contributions of other team members into the nursing plan of care? What are some common goals that the team may share for this patient?
Attitudes	
Value the perspectives and expertise of all health team members. Value teamwork and the relationship upon which it is based.	Reflect on your experience with teamwork. What is the value of each team member's different area of expertise for this patient? How might perspectives differ between interdisciplinary team members? Considering these differences in perspectives, how might each individual member of this team foster a relationship for teamwork?

Cronenwett, L., Sherwood, G., Barnsteiner, J., et al. (2007). Quality and safety education for nurses. *Nursing Outlook, 55*(3), 122–131.

Institute of Medicine. (2003). *Health professions education: A bridge to quality.* Washington, DC: National Academies Press.

QSEN Institute. (2017). *QSEN Competencies: definitions and pre-licensure KSAs.* Retrieved on 3/1/2017 at: www.qsen.org/competencies/pre-licensure-ksas

39 Assessment of Musculoskeletal Function

LEARNING OBJECTIVES

On completion of this chapter, the learner will be able to:

1 Describe the basic structure and function of the musculoskeletal system.
2 Discuss the significance of the health history to the assessment of musculoskeletal health.

3 Recognize and evaluate the major manifestations of musculoskeletal dysfunction by applying concepts from the patient's health history and physical assessment findings.
4 Explain clinical indications, patient preparation, and other related nursing implications for common tests and procedures used to assess musculoskeletal function.

GLOSSARY

atonic: without tone; denervated muscle that atrophies

atrophy: decrease in the size of a muscle

bursa: fluid-filled sac found in connective tissue, usually in the area of joints

callus: cartilaginous/fibrous tissue at fracture site

cancellous bone: latticelike bone structure; trabecular bone

cartilage: tough, elastic, avascular tissue at ends of bone

clonus: rhythmic contractions of a muscle

contracture: abnormal shortening of muscle, joint, or both; fibrosis

cortical bone: compact bone

crepitus: grating or crackling sound or sensation; may occur with movement of ends of a broken bone or irregular joint surface

diaphysis: shaft of long bone

effusion: excess fluid in joint

endosteum: a thin, vascular membrane covering the marrow cavity of long bones and the spaces in cancellous bone

epiphysis: end of long bone

fascia (epimysium): fibrous tissue that covers, supports, and separates muscles

fasciculation: involuntary twitch of muscle fibers

flaccid: limp; without muscle tone

hypertrophy: enlargement; increase in the size of a muscle

isometric contraction: muscle tension is increased without changing its length; there is no associated joint motion

isotonic contraction: muscle is shortened without a change in its tension; a joint is moved as a result

joint: area where bone ends meet; provides for motion and flexibility

joint capsule: fibrous tissue that encloses bone ends and other joint surfaces

kyphosis: increase in the convex curvature of the thoracic spine

lamellae: mature compact bone structures that form concentric rings of bone matrix; lamellar bone

ligament: ropelike bundles of collagen fibrils connecting bones

lordosis: increase in concave curvature of the lumbar spine

ossification: process in which minerals (calcium) are deposited in bone matrix

osteoblast: bone-forming cell

osteoclast: bone resorption cell

osteocyte: mature bone cell

osteogenesis: bone formation

osteon: microscopic functional bone unit

osteopenic: refers to a reduction in bone mass to below normal levels

paresthesia: abnormal sensation (e.g., burning, tingling, numbness)

periosteum: fibrous connective tissue covering bone

remodeling: process that ensures bone maintenance through simultaneous bone resorption and formation

resorption: removal/destruction of tissue, such as bone

scoliosis: lateral curving of the spine

spastic: having greater-than-normal muscle tone

synovium: membrane in joint that secretes lubricating fluid

tendon: cord of fibrous tissue connecting muscle to bone

tone (tonus): normal tension (resistance to stretch) in resting muscle

trabeculae: latticelike bone structure; cancellous bone

The musculoskeletal system is composed of the bones, joints, muscles, tendons, ligaments, and bursae of the body. The major functions of this system are to support and protect the body and foster movement of the extremities. The components of this system are highly integrated; therefore, disease in or injury to one component adversely affects the others. For instance, an infection in a joint (e.g., septic arthritis) causes degeneration of the articular surfaces of the bones within the joint and local muscle atrophy.

Musculoskeletal disorders and injuries directly affect the quality of life of individuals and are the leading cause of disability in the United States. The economic impact of these collective conditions is estimated at more than 60 billion annually (Swartz, 2014). Of these musculoskeletal disorders, arthritis is the chief cause of musculoskeletal-related disability in the United States, with an estimated 52.5 million adults diagnosed with this disorder. Because the incidence of arthritis increases with age, the number of adults with arthritis is expected to increase to 67 million by 2030 (Centers for Disease Control and Prevention [CDC], 2015). Musculoskeletal disorders can significantly affect the overall productivity, independence, and quality of life in people of all ages (Swartz, 2014). Nurses in all practice areas may encounter patients with complaints about or impairment of the musculoskeletal system.

Anatomic and Physiologic Overview

The musculoskeletal system provides protection for vital organs, including the brain, heart, and lungs; serves as a framework to support body structures; and makes mobility possible. Muscles and tendons hold the bones together, and **joints** allow the body to move. They also move to produce heat that helps maintain body temperature. Movement facilitates the return of deoxygenated blood to the right side of the heart by massaging the venous vasculature. The musculoskeletal system serves as a reservoir for immature blood cells and essential minerals, including calcium, phosphorus, magnesium, and fluoride (Grossman & Porth, 2014). More than 98% of total body calcium is present in bone (International Osteoporosis Foundation [IOF], 2015).

Structure and Function of the Skeletal System

There are 206 bones in the human body, divided into four categories classified by their shape: long, short, flat, and irregular. The long bones are found in the upper and lower extremities (e.g., the femur). Long bones are shaped like rods or shafts with rounded ends (see Fig. 39-1). The shaft, known as the **diaphysis**, is primarily **cortical bone** (compact bone). The ends of the long bones, called **epiphyses**, are primarily **cancellous bone** (trabecular bone). During childhood and adolescence, there is a layer of cartilage known as the epiphyseal plate, or growth plate, that separates the epiphysis from the diaphysis. The epiphyseal plate nurtures and facilitates longitudinal growth. The epiphyseal plate is calcified in adults. The ends of long bones are covered at the joints by articular **cartilage**, which is tough, elastic, and avascular tissue (Grossman & Porth, 2014).

The short bones are the irregularly shaped bones located in the ankle and hand (e.g., metacarpals). The flat bones are located where extensive protection of underlying structures is needed (e.g., the sternum or skull). Finally, because of their shape, the irregular bones cannot be categorized in any other group and include bones such as the vertebrae and bones of the jaw.

The shape and construction of a specific bone are determined by its function and the forces exerted on it. Bones are constructed of cortical or cancellous bone tissue. Cortical bone exists in areas where support is needed, and cancellous bone is found where hematopoiesis and bone formation occur. For example, long bones are designed for weight bearing and movement and tend to be composed primarily of cortical bone, whereas flat bones, which are important sites of hematopoiesis and frequently protect vital organs, are made of cancellous bone layered between compact bone. Short bones consist of cancellous bone covered by a layer of cortical bone.

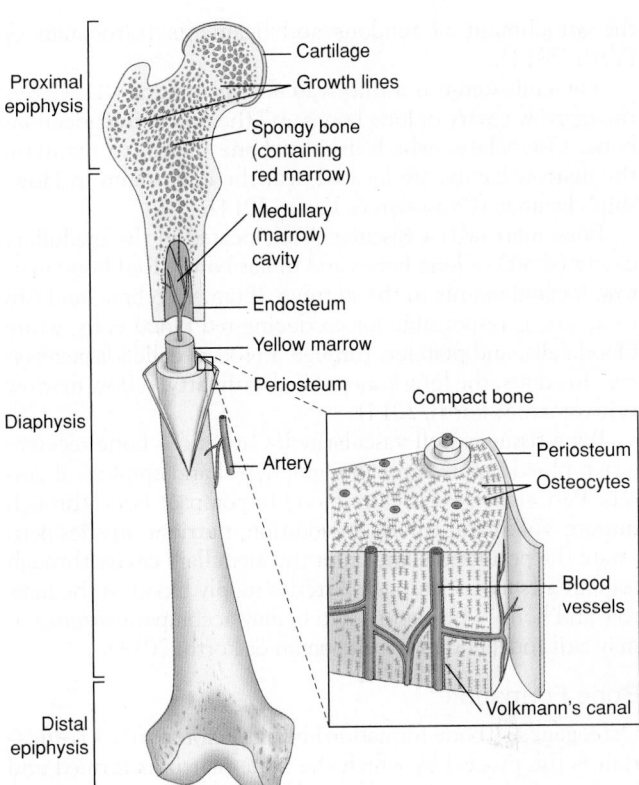

Figure 39-1 • Structure of a long bone; composition of compact bone.

Irregular bones have unique shapes related to their function. Generally, irregular bone structure is similar to that of flat bones (Grossman & Porth, 2014).

Bone is composed of cells, protein matrix, and mineral deposits. The cells are of three basic types—osteoblasts, osteocytes, and osteoclasts. **Osteoblasts** function in bone formation by secreting bone matrix. The matrix consists of collagen and ground substances (glycoproteins and proteoglycans) that provide a framework in which inorganic mineral salts are deposited. These minerals are primarily composed of calcium and phosphorus. **Osteocytes** are mature bone cells involved in bone maintenance; they are located in lacunae (bone matrix units). **Osteoclasts**, located in shallow Howship's lacunae (small pits in bones), are multinuclear cells involved in dissolving and resorbing bone. The microscopic functioning unit of mature cortical bone is the **osteon**, or Haversian system. The center of the osteon—the Haversian canal—contains a capillary. Around the capillary are circles of mineralized bone matrix called **lamellae**. Within the lamellae are lacunae that contain osteocytes. These are nourished through tiny structures called *canaliculi* (canals), which communicate with adjacent blood vessels within the Haversian system. Lacunae in cancellous bone are layered in an irregular lattice network known as **trabeculae**. Red bone marrow fills the lattice network. Capillaries nourish the osteocytes located in the lacunae (Grossman & Porth, 2014).

Covering the bone is a dense, fibrous membrane known as the **periosteum**. This membranous structure nourishes bone and facilitates its growth. The periosteum contains nerves, blood vessels, and lymphatics. It also provides for the attachment of tendons and ligaments (Grossman & Porth, 2014).

The **endosteum** is a thin, vascular membrane that covers the marrow cavity of long bones and the spaces in cancellous bone. Osteoclasts, which dissolve bone matrix to maintain the marrow cavity, are located near the endosteum in Howship's lacunae (Grossman & Porth, 2014).

Bone marrow is a vascular tissue located in the medullary cavity (shaft) of long bones and in flat bones. Red bone marrow, located mainly in the sternum, ilium, vertebrae, and ribs in adults, is responsible for producing red blood cells, white blood cells, and platelets through a process called *hematopoiesis*. In adults, the long bone is filled with fatty, yellow marrow (Grossman & Porth, 2014).

Bone tissue is well vascularized. Cancellous bone receives a rich blood supply through metaphyseal and epiphyseal vessels. Periosteal vessels carry blood to compact bone through minute Volkmann canals. In addition, nutrient arteries penetrate the periosteum and enter the medullary cavity through foramina (small openings). Arteries supply blood to the marrow and bone. The venous system may accompany arteries or may exit independently (Grossman & Porth, 2014).

Bone Formation

Osteogenesis (bone formation) begins before birth. **Ossification** is the process by which the bone matrix is formed and hard mineral crystals composed of calcium and phosphorus (e.g., hydroxyapatite) are bound to the collagen fibers. These mineral components give bone its characteristic strength, whereas the proteinaceous collagen gives bone its resilience (Grossman & Porth, 2014).

Bone Maintenance

Bone is a dynamic tissue in a constant state of turnover. Throughout the lifespan, a process known as bone **remodeling** occurs, in which old bone is removed and new bone is added to the skeleton (formation). During childhood and the teenage years, new bone is added faster than old bone is removed; therefore, bones become larger, heavier, and denser. This continues until peak bone mass is reached, typically by age 20 years. Remodeling maintains bone structure and function through simultaneous resorption and osteogenesis, and as a result, complete skeletal turnover occurs every 10 years (Grossman & Porth, 2014).

The balance between bone **resorption** (removal or destruction) and formation is influenced by the following factors: physical activity; dietary intake of certain nutrients, especially calcium; and several hormones, including calcitriol (i.e., activated vitamin D), parathyroid hormone (PTH), calcitonin, thyroid hormone, cortisol, growth hormone, and the sex hormones estrogen and testosterone (Florence, Allen, Benedict, et al., 2013).

Physical activity, particularly weight-bearing activity, acts to stimulate bone formation and remodeling. Bones subjected to continued weight bearing tend to be thick and strong. Conversely, people who are unable to engage in regular weight-bearing activities, such as those on prolonged bed rest or those with some physical disabilities, have increased bone resorption from calcium loss, and their bones become **osteopenic** (reduced in terms of mass) and weak. These weakened bones may fracture easily.

Concept Mastery Alert

Weight-bearing activity or exercise should not be confused with weight-resistance exercise. Weight-bearing activity, which supports bone maintenance, is any activity done while a person is on their feet that works a person's bones and muscles against gravity (e.g., walking, tennis). Weight-resistance exercise, on the other hand, uses weights or resistance to strengthen muscles.

Good dietary habits are integral to bone health. Daily intake of approximately 1000 to 1200 mg of calcium is essential to maintaining adult bone mass. Good sources of calcium include low-fat milk, yogurt, and cheese. Foods with added calcium such as orange juice, cereals, and bread are also beneficial (IOF, 2015). Vitamin D also plays a major role in calcium absorption and bone health. Young adults need a daily vitamin D intake of 600 IU, whereas adults 50 years and older require a daily intake of 800 to 1000 IU to ensure good bone health (Institute of Medicine [IOM], 2010). Dietary sources of vitamin D include vitamin D–fortified milk and cereals, egg yolks, saltwater fish, and liver.

Several hormones are vital in ensuring that calcium is properly absorbed and available for bone mineralization and matrix formation. Calcitriol functions to increase the amount of calcium in the blood by promoting absorption of calcium from the gastrointestinal tract. It also facilitates mineralization of osteoid tissue. A deficiency of vitamin D results in bone mineralization deficit, deformity, and fracture (IOF, 2015).

PTH and calcitonin are the major hormonal regulators of calcium homeostasis. PTH regulates the concentration of calcium in the blood, in part by promoting movement of calcium from the bone. In response to low calcium levels in the blood, increased levels of PTH prompt the mobilization of calcium, the demineralization of bone, and the formation of bone cysts. Calcitonin, secreted by the thyroid gland in response to elevated blood calcium levels, inhibits bone resorption and increases the deposit of calcium in bone (Grossman & Porth, 2014).

Both thyroid hormone and cortisol have multiple systemic effects with specific effects on bones. Excessive thyroid hormone production in adults (e.g., Graves' disease) can result in increased bone resorption and decreased bone formation. Increased levels of cortisol have these same effects. Patients receiving long-term synthetic cortisol or corticosteroids (e.g., prednisone) are at increased risk for steroid-induced osteopenia and fractures.

Growth hormone has direct and indirect effects on skeletal growth and remodeling. It stimulates the liver and, to a lesser degree, the bones to produce insulin-like growth factor 1 (IGF-I), which accelerates bone modeling in children and adolescents. Growth hormone also directly stimulates skeletal growth in children and adolescents. It is believed that the low levels of both growth hormone and IGF-I that occur with aging may be partly responsible for decreased bone formation and resultant osteopenia (Grossman & Porth, 2014).

The sex hormones testosterone and estrogen have important effects on bone remodeling. Estrogen stimulates osteoblasts and inhibits osteoclasts; therefore, bone formation is enhanced and resorption is inhibited. Testosterone has both direct and indirect effects on bone growth and formation. It directly causes skeletal growth in adolescence and has continued effects on skeletal muscle growth throughout the lifespan. Increased muscle mass results in greater weight-bearing stress on bones, resulting in increased bone formation. In addition, testosterone converts to estrogen in adipose tissue, providing an additional source of bone-preserving estrogen for aging men (U.S. Department of Health and Human Services [HHS], 2012).

During the process of bone remodeling, osteoblasts produce a receptor for activated nuclear factor-kappa B ligand (RANKL) that binds to the receptor for activated nuclear factor-kappa B (RANK) present on the cell membranes of osteoclast precursors, causing them to differentiate and mature into osteoclasts, which causes bone resorption. Conversely, osteoblasts may produce osteoprotegerin (OPG), which blocks the effects of RANKL, thereby turning off the process of bone resorption. T cells that may become activated as a result of the inflammatory process may also produce RANKL, overriding the effects of OPG and causing continued bone resorption during times of stress and injury, which can lead to loss of bone matrix and fractures (Khosla, 2013). Research focused on developing medications that block the effects of RANKL has resulted in U.S. Food and Drug Administration (FDA) approval of denosumab (Prolia) in treating postmenopausal women with osteoporosis (National Osteoporosis Foundation [NOF], 2014) (see Chapter 41).

Blood supply to the bone also affects bone formation. With diminished blood supply or hyperemia (congestion), osteogenesis and bone density decrease. Bone necrosis occurs when the bone is deprived of blood (Grossman & Porth, 2014).

Bone Healing

Most fractures heal through a combination of intramembranous and endochondral ossification processes. When a bone is fractured, the bone begins a healing process to reestablish continuity and strength. The bone fragments are not patched together with scar tissue; instead, the bone regenerates itself.

Fracture healing occurs in the bone marrow, where endothelial cells rapidly differentiate into osteoblasts; in the bone cortex, where new osteons are formed; in the periosteum, where a hard **callus** (fibrous tissue) is formed through intramembranous ossification peripheral to the fracture, and where cartilage is formed through endochondral ossification adjacent to the fracture site; and in adjacent soft tissue, where a bridging callus forms that provides stability to the fractured bones.

When a fracture occurs, the body's response is similar to that after injury elsewhere in the body. The repair of a simple fracture occurs in essentially four stages. These include the following (Grossman & Porth, 2014):

Stage I: Hematoma formation occurs during the first 1 to 2 days of the fracture. Bleeding into the injured tissue and local vasoconstriction occur, and a hematoma forms at the site of the fracture. Cytokines are released, initiating the fracture healing processes by causing replicating cells known as fibroblasts to proliferate, which in turn causes angiogenesis to occur (i.e., the growth of new blood vessels). Granulation tissue begins to form within the clot and becomes dense. At the same time, degranulated platelets and inflammatory cells release growth factor, which stimulates the generation of osteoclasts and osteoblasts.

Stage II: Fibrocartilaginous callus formation occurs with the formation of granulation tissue. Fibroblasts and osteoblasts migrate into the fractured site and begin the reconstruction of bone. The fibroblasts produce a fibrocartilaginous soft callus bridge that connects the bone fragments. Although tissue repair may reach maximum girth by the end of the second or third week, it is still not strong enough for weight bearing.

Stage III: Bony callus formation (ossification) usually begins during the third or fourth week of fracture healing and continues until a firm bony union is formed. During this stage, mature bone gradually replaces the fibrocartilaginous callus and the excess callus is gradually reabsorbed by the osteoclasts. During this stage, the fracture site feels immovable and appears aligned on x-ray. At this time, it is usually safe to remove a cast, if one is present.

Stage IV: Remodeling occurs as necrotic bone is removed by the osteoclasts. Compact bone replaces spongy bone around the periphery of the fracture. Although the final structure of the remodeled bone resembles the original unbroken bone, a thickened area on the surface of the bone may remain after healing. Remodeling may take months to years, depending on the extent of bone modification needed, the function of the bone, and the functional stresses on the bone.

Serial x-rays are used to monitor the progress of bone healing. The type of bone fractured, the adequacy of blood supply, the condition of the fracture fragments, the immobility of the fracture site, and the age and general health of the person influence the rate of fracture healing. Adequate immobilization is essential until there is x-ray evidence of bone formation with ossification.

When fractures are treated with internal or external fixation techniques, the bony fragments can be placed in direct contact. Primary bone healing occurs through cortical bone (Haversian) remodeling. Little or no cartilaginous callus develops. Immature bone develops from the endosteum. There is an intensive regeneration of new osteons, which develop in the fracture line by a process similar to normal bone maintenance. Fracture strength is obtained when the new osteons have become established.

Structure and Function of the Articular System

The junction of two or more bones is called a joint, or articulation. There are three basic kinds of joints: synarthrosis, amphiarthrosis, and diarthrosis joints. Synarthrosis joints, also referred to as fibrous joints, are immovable because of fibrous tissue banding (e.g., the skull sutures). Amphiarthrosis joints, also referred to as cartilaginous joints, allow limited motion (e.g., the vertebral joints and the symphysis pubis). Diarthrosis joints, also referred to as synovial joints, are freely movable joints (see Fig. 39-2).

There are several types of diarthrosis joints:

- *Ball-and-socket joints* (e.g., the hip and the shoulder) permit full freedom of movement.
- *Hinge joints* permit bending in only one direction, either flexion or extension (e.g., the elbow and the knee).
- *Saddle joints* allow movement in two planes at right angles to each other. The joint at the base of the thumb is a saddle, biaxial joint.

Femur

Articular cartilage

Medial meniscus

Tibia

Synovial (joint) cavity

Bursa

Patella

Synovial (joint) cavity

Fat pad

Infrapatellar bursa

Figure 39-2 • Hinge joint of the knee.

- *Pivot joints* allow one bone to move around a central axis without displacement. An example of a pivot joint is the articulation between the radius and the ulna. They permit rotation for such activities as turning a doorknob.
- *Gliding joints* allow for limited movement in all directions and are represented by the joints of the carpal bones in the wrist.

The ends of the articulating bones of a typical movable joint are covered with smooth hyaline cartilage. A tough, fibrous sheath called the **joint capsule** surrounds the articulating bones. The capsule is lined with a membrane, the **synovium**, which secretes the lubricating and shock-absorbing synovial fluid into the joint capsule. Therefore, the bone surfaces are not in direct contact. In some synovial joints (e.g., the knee), fibrocartilage discs (e.g., medial meniscus) are located between the articular cartilage surfaces. These discs provide shock absorption (Grossman & Porth, 2014).

Ligaments (ropelike bundles of collagen fibrils) bind the articulating bones together. **Tendons** are cords of fibrous tissue that connect muscle to bone. Ligaments and tendons, which pass over the joint, provide joint stability. In some joints, interosseous ligaments (e.g., the cruciate ligaments of the knee) are found within the capsule and add anterior and posterior stability to the joint. Ligaments are pliable enough to allow movement of the joints; however, they can tear rather than stretch if they are subjected to excess stress.

A **bursa** is a sac filled with synovial fluid that cushions the movement of tendons, ligaments, and bones over bones or other joint structures. Bursae can be found in the joints of the elbow, shoulder, hip, and knee. They may become inflamed, causing discomfort, swelling, and limited movement in that area.

Structure and Function of the Skeletal Muscle System

Muscles are attached by tendons to bones, connective tissue, other muscles, soft tissue, or skin. The muscles of the body are composed of parallel groups of muscle cells (fasciculi) encased in fibrous tissue called **fascia** (epimysium). The more fasciculi contained in a muscle, the more precise the movements.

Muscles vary in shape and size according to the activities for which they are responsible. Skeletal (striated) muscles are involved in body movement, posture, and heat-production functions. Muscles contract to bring the two points of attachment closer together, resulting in movement.

Skeletal Muscle Contraction

Each muscle cell (also referred to as a muscle fiber) contains myofibrils, which in turn are composed of a series of sarcomeres—the actual contractile units of skeletal muscle. Sarcomeres contain thick myosin and thin actin filaments.

Muscle cells contract in response to electrical stimulation delivered by an effector nerve cell at the motor end plate. When stimulated, the muscle cell depolarizes and generates an action potential in a manner similar to that described for nerve cells. These action potentials propagate along the muscle cell membrane and lead to the release of calcium ions that are stored in a specialized organelle called *sarcoplasmic reticulum*. When there is a local increase in calcium ion concentration, the myosin and actin filaments slide across one another. Shortly after the muscle cell membrane is depolarized, it recovers its resting membrane voltage. Calcium is rapidly removed from the sarcomeres by active reaccumulation in the sarcoplasmic reticulum. When the calcium concentration in the sarcomere decreases, the myosin and actin filaments cease to interact, and the sarcomere returns to its original resting length (relaxation). Actin and myosin do not interact in the absence of calcium (Grossman & Porth, 2014).

The contraction of muscle fibers can result in either isotonic or isometric contraction of the muscle. In **isometric contraction**, the length of the muscles remains constant but the force generated by the muscles is increased; an example of this is pushing against an immovable wall. **Isotonic contraction** is characterized by the shortening of the muscle without an increase in tension within the muscle; an example of this is flexing the forearm. In normal activities, many muscle movements are a combination of isometric and isotonic contraction. For example, during walking, isotonic contraction results in shortening of the leg, and isometric contraction causes the stiff leg to push against the floor.

Energy is consumed during muscle contraction and relaxation. The main source of energy for the muscle cells is adenosine triphosphate (ATP), which is generated through cellular oxidative metabolism. At low levels of activity (i.e., sedentary activity), the skeletal muscle synthesizes ATP from the oxidation of glucose to water and carbon dioxide. During periods of strenuous activity, when sufficient oxygen may not be available, glucose is metabolized primarily to lactic acid, an inefficient process compared with that of oxidative pathways. Stored muscle glycogen is used to supply glucose during periods of activity. Muscle fatigue is thought to be caused by depletion of glycogen and accumulation of lactic acid. As a result, the cycle of muscle contraction and relaxation cannot continue (Grossman & Porth, 2014).

During muscle contraction, the energy released from ATP is not completely used. The excess energy is dissipated in the form of heat. During isometric contraction, almost all of the energy is released in the form of heat; during isotonic contraction, some of the energy is expended in mechanical work. In some situations (i.e., shivering), the need to generate heat is the main stimulus for muscle contraction.

The speed of the muscle contraction is variable. Myoglobulin is a hemoglobin-like protein pigment present in striated muscle cells that transports oxygen. Muscles containing large quantities of myoglobulin (red muscles) have been observed to contract slowly and powerfully (e.g., respiratory and postural muscles). Muscles containing little myoglobulin (white muscles) contract quickly (e.g., extraocular eye muscles). Most muscles contain both red and white muscle fibers (Grossman & Porth, 2014).

Muscle Tone

Muscle **tone** (tonus) is produced by the maintenance of some of the muscle fibers in a contracted state. Muscle spindles, which are sense organs in the muscles, monitor muscle tone. Muscle tone is minimal during sleep and is increased when the person is anxious. A muscle that is limp and without tone is described as **flaccid**; a muscle with greater-than-normal tone is described as **spastic**. Typically, upper motor neuron lesions produce increased tone, whereas lower motor neuron lesions produce decreased tone. For example, in conditions characterized by upper motor neuron destruction (e.g., cerebral palsy), muscle becomes hypertonic and reflexes become hyperactive. In contrast, conditions characterized by lower motor neuron destruction (e.g., muscular dystrophy), denervated muscle becomes **atonic** (soft and flabby) and atrophies (Grossman & Porth, 2014). See Chapter 65 for assessment of upper and lower motor function.

Muscle Actions

Muscle contraction produces movement. The body is able to perform a wide variety of movements as a result of the coordination of muscle groups (see Fig. 39-3). The prime mover is the muscle that causes a particular motion. The muscles assisting the prime mover are known as synergists. The muscles causing movement opposite to that of the prime mover are known as antagonists. An antagonist must relax to allow the prime mover to contract, producing motion. For example, when contraction of the biceps causes flexion of the elbow joint, the biceps are the prime movers and the triceps are the antagonists. A person with muscle paralysis (a loss of movement, possibly from nerve damage) may be able to retrain functioning muscles within the synergistic group to produce the needed movement. Muscles of the synergistic group then become the prime movers.

Exercise, Disuse, and Repair

Muscles need exercise to maintain function and strength. When a muscle repeatedly develops maximum or close to maximum tension over a long time, as in regular exercise with weights, the cross-sectional area of the muscle increases. This enlargement, known as **hypertrophy**, results from an increase in the size of individual muscle fibers without an increase in their number. Hypertrophy persists only if the exercise is continued. The opposite phenomenon occurs with disuse of muscle over a long period of time. Age and disuse cause loss of muscular function as fibrotic tissue replaces the contractile muscle tissue. The decrease in the size of a muscle is called **atrophy**. Bed rest and immobility cause loss of muscle mass and strength. When immobility is the result of a treatment modality (e.g., casting, traction, or bed rest), the patient can decrease the effects of immobility by isometric exercise of the muscles of the immobilized part. Quadriceps contraction exercises (tightening the muscles of the thigh) and gluteal setting exercises (tightening of the muscles of the buttocks) help maintain the larger muscle groups that are important in ambulation. Active and weight-resistance exercises of uninjured parts of the body maintain muscle strength. When muscles are injured, they need rest and immobilization until tissue repair occurs. The healed muscle then needs progressive exercise to resume its preinjury strength and functional ability.

 ## Gerontologic Considerations

Multiple changes in the musculoskeletal system occur with aging (see Table 39-1) and bring complaints of pain and joint limitations. There is a loss of height due to osteoporosis (abnormal excessive bone loss), kyphosis (forward curvature of the thoracic spine), thinned intervertebral discs, compressed vertebral bodies, and flexion of the knees and hips. Numerous metabolic changes, including menopausal withdrawal of estrogen and decreased activity, contribute to osteoporosis (NOF, 2016a). Women lose more bone mass than men. In addition, bones change in shape and have reduced strength. Fractures are common. Collagen structures are less able to absorb energy. Increased inactivity, diminished neuron stimulation, and nutritional deficiencies contribute to the loss of muscle strength. In addition, remote musculoskeletal problems for which the patient has compensated may become new problems with age-related changes. For example, people who have had polio and who have been able to function normally by using synergistic muscle groups may discover increasing incapacity because of a reduced compensatory ability. Older adults may suffer from chronic musculoskeletal disorders that limit mobility and interfere with their ability to perform self-care. This may lead individuals to depend on others for completion of their activities of daily living (ADLs); in turn, they may grieve over the loss of independence. Despite these changes, the many effects of aging can be slowed if the body is kept healthy and active through positive lifestyle behaviors (Swartz, 2014).

Assessment

Health History

The nursing assessment of the patient with musculoskeletal dysfunction includes a health history and physical examination that evaluate the effects of the musculoskeletal disorder on the patient. The nurse is concerned with assisting patients who have musculoskeletal problems to maintain their general health and functional status, accomplish their ADLs, and manage their treatment programs. The nurse must promote a healthy lifestyle by discussing the importance of nutrition and nutritional supplements, regular exercise, and maintaining an appropriate weight. The nurse should also address problems associated with immobility and advocate for evidence-based periodic musculoskeletal health screenings. Through an individualized plan of nursing care, the nurse helps the patient achieve optimal health.

Common Symptoms

During the interview and physical assessment, the patient with a musculoskeletal disorder may report pain, tenderness,

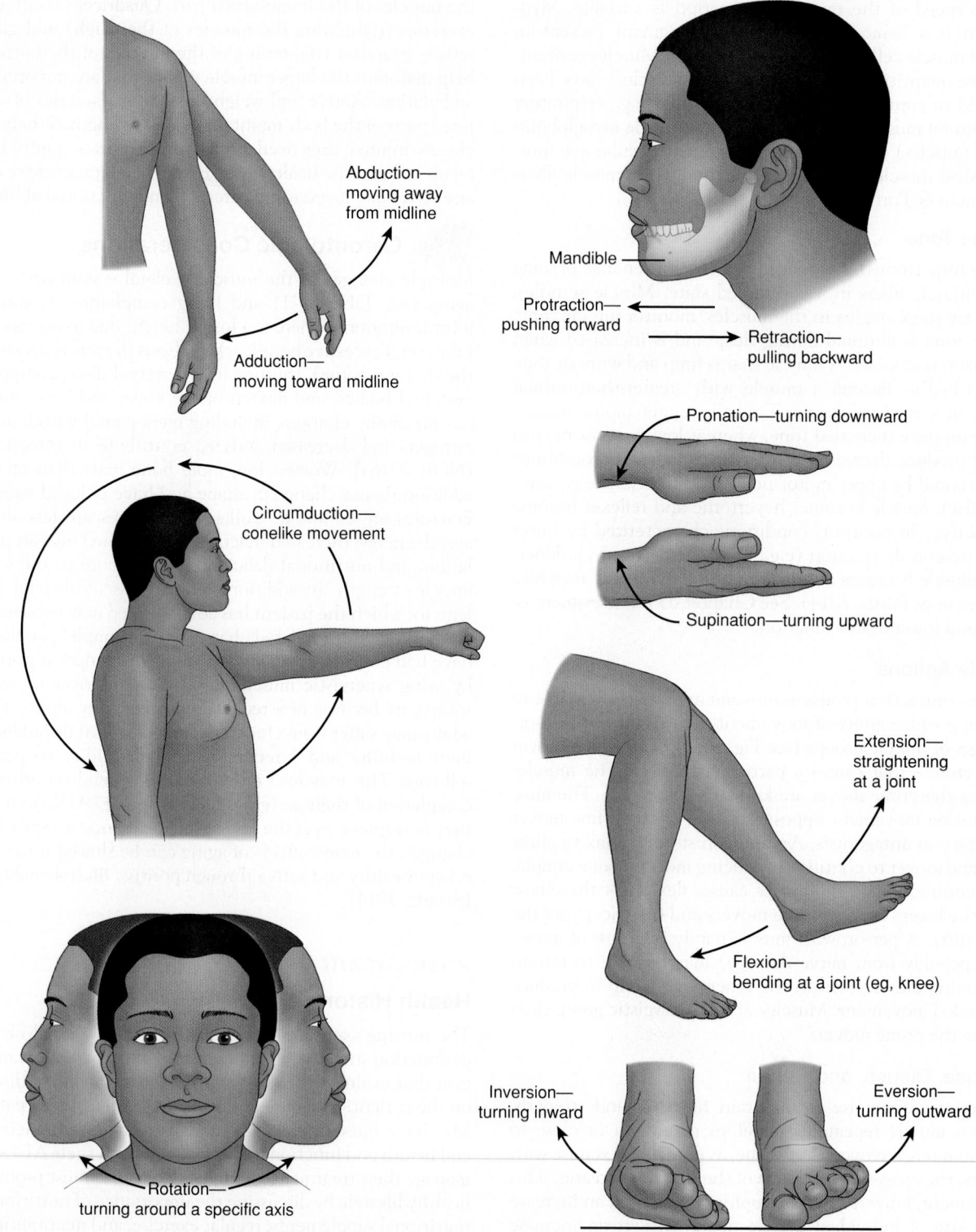

Figure 39-3 • Body movements produced by muscle contraction.

and altered sensations (Weber & Kelley, 2014). The nurse is responsible to assess and document this information.

Pain

Most patients with diseases and traumatic conditions or disorders of the muscles, bones, and joints experience pain. Bone pain is typically described as a dull, deep ache that is "boring" in nature. This pain is not typically related to movement and may interfere with sleep. Muscular pain is described as soreness or aching and is referred to as "muscle cramps." Fracture pain is sharp and piercing and is relieved by immobilization. Sharp pain may also result from bone infection with muscle

TABLE 39-1 Age-Related Changes of the Musculoskeletal System

Musculoskeletal System	Structural Changes	Functional Changes	History and Physical Findings
Bones	Gradual, progressive loss of bone mass after 30 years of age Vertebral collapse	Bones fragile and prone to fracture—vertebrae, hip, wrist	Loss of height Postural changes Kyphosis Loss of flexibility Flexion of hips and knees Back pain Osteoporosis Fracture
Muscles	Increase in collagen and resultant fibrosis Muscles diminish in size (atrophy); wasting Tendons less elastic	Loss of strength and flexibility Weakness Fatigue Stumbling Falls	Loss of strength Diminished agility Decreased endurance Prolonged response time (diminished reaction time) Diminished tone Broad base of support History of falls
Joints	Cartilage—progressive deterioration Thinning of intervertebral discs	Stiffness, reduced flexibility, and pain interfere with activities of daily living	Diminished range of motion Stiffness Loss of height
Ligaments	Lax ligaments (less-than-normal strength; weakness)	Postural joint abnormality Weakness	Joint pain on motion; resolves with rest Crepitus Joint swelling/enlargement Osteoarthritis (degenerative joint disease)

spasm or pressure on a sensory nerve. Joint pain is felt around or in the joint and typically worsens with movement (Swartz, 2014).

Rest relieves most musculoskeletal pain. Pain that increases with activity may indicate joint sprain, muscle strain, or compartment syndrome, whereas steadily increasing pain points to the progression of an infectious process (osteomyelitis), a malignant tumor, or neurovascular complications. Radiating pain occurs in conditions in which pressure is exerted on a nerve root.

The time of day that the pain occurs may be important to evaluate. Those experiencing pain with a rheumatic disorder experience pain that is worse in the morning, especially upon waking. Tendonitis worsens during the early morning and eases by midday, whereas osteoarthritis worsens as the day progresses (Swartz, 2014). Pain is variable, and its assessment and nursing management must be individualized.

The nurse assesses the patient's pain as described in Chapter 12. Specific assessments that the nurse should make regarding the pain include the following:
- Is the body in proper alignment?
- Are the joints symmetrical or are bony deformities present?
- Is there any inflammation or arthritis, swelling, warmth, tenderness, or redness?
- Is there pressure from traction, bed linens, a cast, or other appliances?
- Is there tension on the skin at a pin site?

The patient's pain and discomfort must be managed successfully. Not only is pain exhausting, but also, if prolonged, it can force the patient to become increasingly withdrawn and dependent on others as the musculoskeletal disorder continues.

Altered Sensations

Sensory disturbances are frequently associated with musculoskeletal problems. The patient may describe **paresthesias**, which are sensations of burning, tingling, or numbness. These sensations may be caused by pressure on nerves or by circulatory impairment. Soft tissue swelling or direct trauma to these structures can impair their function. The nurse assesses the neurovascular status of the involved musculoskeletal area.

Questions that the nurse should ask regarding altered sensations include the following:
- Is the patient experiencing abnormal sensations, such as burning, tingling, or numbness?
- If the abnormal sensation involves an extremity, how does this feeling compare to sensation in the unaffected extremity?
- When did the condition begin? Is it getting worse?
- Does the patient also have pain? (If the patient has pain, then the questions and assessments for pain discussed previously should be followed.)

Past Health, Social, and Family History

When assessing the musculoskeletal system, the nurse should gather pertinent data to include in the patient's health history, such as occupation (e.g., does the patient's work require physical activity or heavy lifting?), exercise patterns, alcohol consumption, tobacco use, and dietary intake (e.g., calcium and vitamin D). Concurrent health conditions (e.g., diabetes, heart disease, chronic obstructive pulmonary disease, infection, and preexisting disability) and related problems (e.g., familial or genetic abnormalities [see Chart 39-1]) need to be considered when developing and implementing the plan of care. Any previous history of trauma or injury to the musculoskeletal system or a history of falls should be included as well (Weber & Kelley, 2014).

Chart 39-1 · GENETICS IN NURSING PRACTICE

Musculoskeletal Disorders

Genetic musculoskeletal disorders vary in presentation and can tend to present at different points in time across the life span. Consideration must be given to other genetic disorders that will impact the musculoskeletal system. Some examples of inherited genetic musculoskeletal disorders include:

Autosomal Dominant:

- Achrondroplasia
- Nail-Patella syndrome
- Osteogenesisimperfecta
- Polydactyl
- Van der Woude syndrome

Autosomal Recessive:

- Tay Sachs

Forms of Muscular Dystrophy:

- Becker muscular dystrophy
- Congenital muscular dystrophy
- Distal muscular dystrophy
- Duchene muscular dystrophy (X-linked)
- Emery-Dreyfuss muscular dystrophy (X-linked)
- Facioscapulohumeral muscular dystrophy (autosomal dominant)
- Limb–girdle muscular dystrophy (autosomal dominant and autosomal recessive forms)

Other genetic disorders that impact the musculoskeletal system:

- Amyotrophic lateral sclerosis (neurologic disorder)
- Ehlers-Danlos syndrome (connective tissue disorder)
- Marfan syndrome (connective tissue disorder)
- Spina bifida (neurologic disorder)
- Stickler syndrome (connective tissue disorder)

Nursing Assessments

Refer to Chart 5-2: Genetics in Nursing Practice: Genetic Aspects of Health Assessment, in Chapter 5

DDH, developmental dysplasia of the hip(s)

Family History Assessment Related to Genetic Musculoskeletal Disorders

- Assess for other similarly affected family members in the past three generations.
- Assess for the presence of other related genetic conditions (e.g., hematologic, cardiac, integumentary conditions).
- Determine the age at onset (e.g., fractures present at birth such as osteogenesis imperfecta, hip dislocation present at birth in DDH, or early-onset osteoporosis).

Patient Assessment Specific to Genetic Musculoskeletal Disorders

- Assess stature for general screening purposes (unusually short stature may be related to achondroplasia; unusually tall stature may be related to Marfan syndrome).
- Assess for disease-specific skeletal findings (e.g., pectusexcavatum, scoliosis, long fingers [Marfan syndrome], osteoarthritis of the hip or waddling gait).
- Assessment findings that could indicate a genetic musculoskeletal disorder include:
  - Bone pain
  - Enlarged hands or feet
  - Excessive height, short stature, or decrease in height
  - Flat feet or highly arched feet
  - Frequency of bone-related injuries or unexplained fractures
  - Hypermobility of joints
  - Large or small head circumference
  - Protruding jaw or forehead
  - Unexplained changes in muscle tone (hypotonia)

Genetics Resources

The National Osteoporosis Foundation, www.nof.org
NIH Osteoporosis and Related Bone Diseases National Resource Center, www.niams.nih.gov/Health_Info/Bone
See Chapter 8, Chart 8-7 for components of genetic counseling.

The Fracture Risk Assessment Tool (FRAX®)

The Fracture Risk Assessment Tool (FRAX®) was developed in 2008 by a task force convened by the World Health Organization (WHO). It is a tool that predicts a patient's 10-year risk of fracturing a hip or other major bone, which includes the spine, forearm, or shoulder (NOF, 2016b). The tool may be accessed online, where it automatically calculates a patient's odds of fracture. Data entered are validated risks for fracture, and include:

- age (risk increases with increasing age)
- gender (risk is higher in females)
- body mass index (risk is higher with lower body mass indices)
- history of a previous fracture
- parental history of hip fracture
- current cigarette smoker
- current use of a corticosteroid (e.g., prednisone)
- history of rheumatoid arthritis
- alcohol intake of 3 or more drinks per day
- history of secondary causes/risks for osteoporosis, which include any of the following:
  - type I diabetes
  - osteogenesis imperfecta
  - untreated long-standing hyperthyroidism

- hypogonadism or premature menopause
- chronic malnutrition or malabsorption syndromes
- chronic liver disease

An additional validated risk factor that may be entered into the FRAX® is the patient's bone mineral density (BMD), based upon bone densitometry results, if those results are hip-based (see later discussion). However, while entering BMD results in the FRAX® provides a more accurate fracture risk calculation, it is not necessary (American College of Rheumatology, 2016). Thus, the FRAX® provides a good estimate of fracture risk in patients who may not have submitted to BMD testing. Patients who should be assessed for hip or major bone fracture risk include men and postmenopausal women over the age of 50, patients with known low BMD, and patients with known secondary causes/risks for osteoporosis See Chapter 41 for further discussion of osteoporosis.

Physical Assessment

An examination of the musculoskeletal system ranges from a basic assessment of functional capabilities to sophisticated physical examination maneuvers that facilitate diagnosis of specific bone, muscle, and joint disorders. The extent of assessment depends on the patient's physical complaints, health history, and physical clues that warrant further exploration. The nursing assessment is primarily a functional evaluation, focusing on the patient's ability to perform ADLs.

Techniques of inspection and palpation are used to evaluate the patient's posture, gait, bone integrity, joint function, and muscle strength and size. In addition, assessing the skin and neurovascular status is an important part of a complete musculoskeletal assessment. The nurse should also understand and be able to perform correct assessment techniques on patients with musculoskeletal trauma. When specific symptoms or physical findings of musculoskeletal dysfunction are apparent, the nurse carefully documents the examination findings and shares the information with the primary provider, who may decide that a more extensive examination and a diagnostic evaluation are necessary.

Posture

The normal curvature of the spine is convex through the thoracic portion and concave through the cervical and lumbar portions. Common deformities of the spine include **kyphosis**, which is an increased forward curvature of the thoracic spine that causes a bowing or rounding of the back, leading to a hunchback or slouching posture. The second deformity of the spine is referred to as **lordosis**, or swayback, an exaggerated curvature of the lumbar spine. A third deformity is **scoliosis**, which is a lateral curving deviation of the spine (see Fig. 39-4). Kyphosis can occur at any age and may be caused by degenerative diseases of the spine (e.g., arthritis or disc degeneration), fractures related to osteoporosis, and injury or trauma (Swartz, 2014). It may also be seen in patients with other neuromuscular disease. Lordosis can affect persons of any age. Common causes of lordosis include tight low back

muscles, excessive visceral fat, and pregnancy as the woman adjusts her posture in response to changes in her center of gravity. Scoliosis may be congenital, idiopathic (without an identifiable cause), or the result of damage to the paraspinal muscles (e.g., muscular dystrophy).

During inspection of the spine, the entire back, buttocks, and legs are exposed. The examiner inspects the spinal curves and trunk symmetry from posterior and lateral views. Standing behind the patient, the examiner notes any differences in the height of the shoulders or iliac crests. Shoulder and hip symmetry, as well as the line of the vertebral column, is inspected with the patient erect and with the patient bending forward (flexion). Scoliosis is evidenced by an abnormal lateral curve in the spine; shoulders that are not level; an asymmetric waistline; and a prominent scapula, which is accentuated by bending forward. The examiner should then instruct the patient to bend backward (extension) with the examiner supporting the patient by placing hands on the posterior iliac spine (Swartz, 2014). Older adults experience a loss in height due to the loss of vertebral cartilage and osteoporosis-related vertebral compression fractures. Therefore, an adult's height should be measured during each health screening.

Gait

Gait is assessed by having the patient walk away from the examiner for a short distance. The examiner observes the patient's gait for smoothness and rhythm. Any unsteadiness or irregular movements (frequently noted in older adult patients) are considered abnormal. A limping motion is most frequently caused by painful weight bearing. In such instances, the patient can usually pinpoint the area of discomfort, thus guiding further examination. If one extremity is shorter than

Figure 39-4 • A normal spine and three abnormalities. **A.** Kyphosis: an increased convexity or roundness of the spine's thoracic curve. **B.** Lordosis: swayback; exaggeration of the lumbar spine curve. **C.** Scoliosis: a lateral curvature of the spine.

another, a limp may also be observed as the patient's pelvis drops downward on the affected side with each step. The knee should be flexed during normal gait; therefore, limited joint motion may interrupt the smooth pattern of gait. Evaluation of the knee involves the joints, bones, ligaments, tendons, and cartilage, and may include tests for the anterior and collateral ligaments, medial and lateral ligaments, and medial meniscus (Swartz, 2014). In addition, a variety of neurologic conditions are associated with abnormal gait, such as a spastic hemiparesis gait (stroke), steppage gait (lower motor neuron disease), and shuffling gait (Parkinson's disease).

Bone Integrity

The bony skeleton is assessed for deformities and alignment. Symmetric parts of the body, such as extremities, are compared. Abnormal bony growths due to bone tumors may be observed. Shortened extremities, amputations, and body parts that are not in anatomic alignment are noted. Fracture findings may include abnormal angulation of long bones, motion at points other than joints, and **crepitus** (a grating or crackling sound or sensation) at the point of abnormal motion. Movement of fracture fragments must be minimized to avoid additional injury. The nurse should include the following observations (Weber & Kelley, 2014):

- If the affected part is an extremity, how does its overall appearance compare to the unaffected extremity?
- Can the patient move the affected part? If an extremity is involved, does each toe or finger have normal sensation and motion (flexion and extension), and is the skin warm or cool?
- What is the color of the part distal to the affected area? Is it pale? Dusky? Mottled? Cyanotic?
- Does rapid capillary refill occur? (The nurse can gently squeeze a nail until it blanches, then release the pressure. The amount of time for the color under the nail to return to normal is noted. Color normally returns within 3 seconds. The return of color is evidence of capillary refill.)
- Is a pulse distal to the affected area palpable? If the affected area is an extremity, how does the pulse compare to the pulse of the unaffected extremity?
- Is edema present?
- Is any constrictive device or clothing causing nerve or vascular compression?
- Does elevating the affected part or modifying its position affect the symptoms?

Joint Function

The articular system is evaluated by noting range of motion, deformity, stability, tenderness, and nodular formation. Range of motion is evaluated both actively (the joint is moved by the muscles surrounding the joint) and passively (the joint is moved by the examiner). The examiner is familiar with the normal range of motion of major joints. Precise measurement of range of motion can be made by a goniometer (a protractor designed for evaluating joint motion). Limited range of motion may be the result of skeletal deformity, joint pathology, or **contracture** (shortening of surrounding joint structures) of the surrounding muscles, tendons, and joint capsule. In older adult patients, limitations of range of motion associated with osteoarthritis may reduce their ability to perform ADLs.

If joint motion is compromised or the joint is painful, the joint is examined for **effusion** (excessive fluid within the capsule), swelling, and increased temperature that may reflect active inflammation. An effusion is suspected if the joint is swollen and the normal bony landmarks are obscured. The most common site for joint effusion is the knee. If large amounts of fluid are present in the joint spaces beneath the patella, it may be identified by assessing for the balloon sign and for ballottement of the knee (see Fig. 39-5). If inflammation or fluid is suspected in a joint, consultation with a specialist (e.g., orthopedic surgeon or rheumatologist) is indicated.

Joint deformity may be caused by contracture, dislocation (complete separation of joint surfaces), subluxation (partial separation of articular surfaces), or disruption of structures surrounding the joint. Weakness or disruption of joint-supporting structures may result in a weak joint that requires an external supporting appliance (e.g., brace).

Palpation of the joint while it is moved passively provides information about the integrity of the joint. Normally, the joint moves smoothly. A snap or crack may indicate that a ligament is slipping over a bony prominence. Slightly roughened surfaces, as in arthritic conditions, result in crepitus as the irregular joint surfaces move across one another.

The tissues surrounding joints are examined for nodule formation. Rheumatoid arthritis, gout, and osteoarthritis may produce characteristic nodules. The subcutaneous nodules of rheumatoid arthritis are soft and occur within and along tendons that provide extensor function to the joints. The nodules of gout are hard and lie within and immediately adjacent to the joint capsule itself. They may rupture, exuding white uric acid crystals onto the skin surface. Osteoarthritic nodules are hard and painless and represent bony overgrowth that has resulted from the destruction of the cartilaginous surface of bone within the joint capsule. They are frequently seen in older adults (Swartz, 2014).

Often, the size of the joint is exaggerated by atrophy of the muscles proximal and distal to that joint. This is seen in rheumatoid arthritis of the knees, in which the quadriceps muscle may atrophy dramatically. In rheumatoid arthritis, joint involvement assumes a symmetric pattern (see Fig. 39-6). See Chapter 38 for further information about rheumatoid arthritis.

Muscle Strength and Size

The muscular system is assessed by noting muscular strength and coordination, the size of individual muscles, and the patient's ability to change position. Weakness of a group of muscles may indicate a variety of conditions, such as polyneuropathy, electrolyte disturbances (particularly potassium and calcium), myasthenia gravis, poliomyelitis, and muscular dystrophy. By palpating the muscle while passively moving the relaxed extremity, the nurse can determine the muscle tone. The nurse assesses muscle strength by having the patient perform certain maneuvers with and without added resistance. For example, when the biceps are tested, the patient is asked to extend the arm fully and then to flex it against resistance applied by the nurse. A simple handshake may provide an indication of grasp strength.

The nurse may elicit muscle **clonus** (rhythmic contractions of a muscle) in the ankle or wrist by sudden, forceful, sustained dorsiflexion of the foot or extension of the wrist.

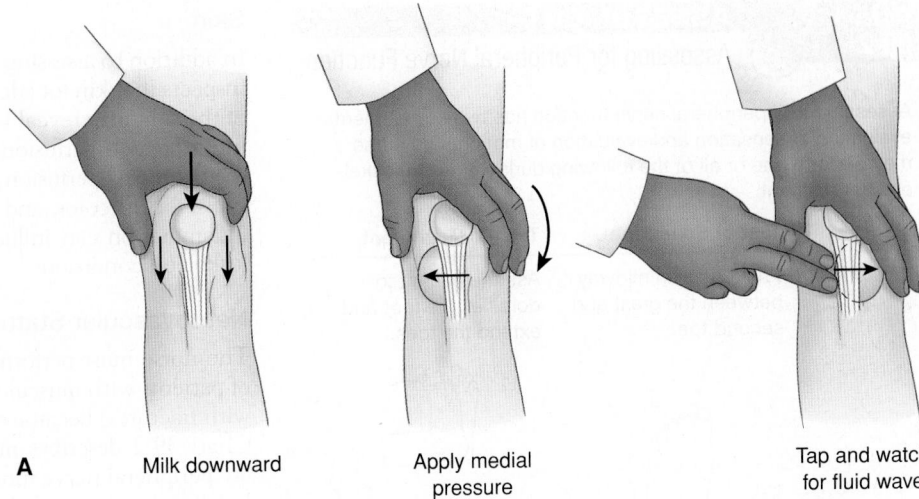

A   Milk downward   Apply medial   Tap and watch
                                   pressure   for fluid wave

Figure 39-5 • Tests for detecting fluid in the knee. **A.** Technique for balloon sign. The medial and lateral aspects of the extended knee are milked firmly in a downward motion, which displaces any fluid downward. The examiner feels for any fluid entering the space directly inferior to the patella. When larger amounts of fluid are present, the subpatellar region feels as if it is "ballooning," and the balloon sign test is positive. **B.** Technique for ballottement sign. The medial and lateral aspects of the extended knee are milked firmly in a downward motion. The examiner pushes the patella toward the femur and observes for fluid return to the region superior to the patella. When larger amounts of fluid are present, the patella elevates, there is visible return of fluid to the region directly superior to the patella, and the ballottement test is positive. Photograph used with permission from Bickley, L. S. (2017). *Bates' guide to physical examination and history taking* (12th ed.). Philadelphia, PA: Lippincott Williams & Wilkins.

B

Figure 39-6 • Rheumatoid arthritis joint deformity with ulnar deviation of fingers and "swan neck" deformity of fingers (i.e., hyperextension of proximal interphalangeal joints with flexion of distal interphalangeal joints).

Fasciculation (involuntary twitching of muscle fiber groups) may be observed.

The nurse measures the girth of an extremity to monitor increased size due to exercise, edema, or bleeding into the muscle. Girth may decrease due to muscle atrophy. The unaffected extremity is measured and used as the reference standard for the affected extremity. Measurements are taken at the maximum circumference of the extremity. It is important that the measurements be taken at the same location on the extremity, and with the extremity in the same position, with the muscle at rest. Distance from a specific anatomic landmark (e.g., 10 cm below the medial aspect of the knee for measurement of the calf muscle) should be indicated in the patient's record so that subsequent measurements can be made at the same point. For ease of serial assessment, the nurse may indicate the point of measurement by marking the skin. Variations in size greater than 1 cm are considered significant.

Chart 39-2 ASSESSMENT

Assessing for Peripheral Nerve Function

Assessment of peripheral nerve function has two key elements: evaluation of sensation and evaluation of motion. The nurse may perform one or all of the following during a musculoskeletal assessment.

Nerve	Test of Sensation	Test of Movement
Peroneal	Prick the skin midway between the great and second toe.	Ask the patient to dorsiflex the foot and extend the toes.
Tibial	Prick the medial and lateral surface of the sole.	Ask the patient to plantar flex toes and foot.
Radial	Prick the skin midway between the thumb and second finger.	Ask the patient to stretch out the thumb, then the wrist, and then the fingers at the metacarpal joints.
Ulnar	Prick the distal fat pad of the small finger.	Ask the patient to abduct all fingers.
Median	Prick the top or distal surface of the index finger.	Ask the patient to touch the thumb to the little finger. In addition, observe whether the patient can flex the wrist.

Skin

In addition to assessing the musculoskeletal system, the nurse inspects the skin for edema, temperature, and color. Palpation of the skin may reveal whether any areas are warmer, suggesting increased perfusion or inflammation, or cooler, suggesting decreased perfusion, and whether edema is present. Cuts, bruises, skin color, and evidence of decreased circulation or inflammation can influence nursing management of musculoskeletal conditions.

Neurovascular Status

The nurse must perform frequent neurovascular assessments of patients with musculoskeletal disorders (especially of those with fractures) because of the risk of tissue and nerve damage. Chart 39-2 describes methods the nurse may use to evaluate peripheral nerve function. The nurse needs to be particularly aware of signs and symptoms of compartment syndrome (which is described in detail later in this unit) when assessing the patient with a musculoskeletal injury. This neurovascular problem is caused by pressure within a muscle compartment that increases to such an extent that microcirculation diminishes, leading to nerve and muscle anoxia and necrosis. Function can be permanently lost if the anoxic situation continues for longer than 6 hours. Assessment of neurovascular status (see Chart 39-3) is frequently referred to as assessment of CMS (circulation, motion, and sensation).

Diagnostic Evaluation

X-Ray Studies

Bone x-rays determine bone density, texture, erosion, and changes in bone relationships. X-ray study of the cortex of the bone reveals any widening, narrowing, or signs of irregularity. Joint x-rays reveal fluid, irregularity, spur formation, narrowing, and changes in the joint structure. Multiple x-rays, with multiple views (e.g., anterior, posterior, lateral), are needed for full assessment of the structure being examined. Serial x-rays may be indicated to determine the status of the healing process.

Chart 39-3 Indicators of Peripheral Neurovascular Dysfunction

Circulation

Color: Pale, cyanotic, or mottled
Temperature: Cool
Capillary refill: More than 3 seconds

Motion

Weakness
Paralysis

Sensation

Paresthesia
Unrelenting pain
Pain on passive stretch
Absence of feeling

Computed Tomography

A computed tomography (CT) scan, which may be performed with or without the use of oral or intravenous (IV) contrast agents, shows a more detailed cross-sectional image of the body. It may be used to visualize and assess tumors; injury to the soft tissue, ligaments, or tendons; and severe trauma to the chest, abdomen, pelvis, head, or spinal cord. It is also used to identify the location and extent of fractures in areas that are difficult to evaluate (e.g., acetabulum) and not visible on x-ray (Van Leeuwen & Bladh, 2016).

Magnetic Resonance Imaging

Magnetic resonance imaging (MRI) is a noninvasive imaging technique that uses magnetic fields and radio waves to create high-resolution pictures of bones and soft tissues. It can be used to visualize and assess torn muscles, ligaments, and cartilage; herniated discs; and a variety of hip or pelvic conditions. The patient does not experience any pain during the procedure. The MRI scanner is noisy, and it may take 30 to 90 minutes to complete the test. Because an electromagnet is used, patients with any metal implants (i.e., cochlear implants), clips, or pacemakers are not candidates for MRI (Van Leeuwen & Bladh, 2016).

> ### ◤ Quality and Safety Nursing Alert
>
> *Jewelry, hair clips, hearing aids, credit cards with magnetic strips, and other metal-containing objects must be removed before the MRI is performed; otherwise, they can become dangerous projectile objects or cause burns. Credit cards with magnetic strips may be erased, and nonremovable cochlear devices can become inoperable; therefore, their presence is a contraindication for MRI. In addition, transdermal patches (e.g., nicotine patch [NicoDerm], nitroglycerin transdermal [Transderm-Nitro], scopolamine transdermal [TransdermScop], clonidine transdermal [Catapres-TTS]) that have a thin layer of aluminized backing must be removed before MRI because they can cause burns. The primary provider should be notified before the patches are removed.*

To enhance visualization of anatomic structures, an IV contrast agent may be used. Patients who experience claustrophobia may be unable to tolerate the confinement of closed MRI equipment without sedation. Open MRI systems are available, but they use lower-intensity magnetic fields, which produce lower-quality images. Advantages of open MRI include increased patient comfort, reduced problems with claustrophobic reactions, and reduced noise.

Arthrography

Arthrography is used to identify the cause of any unexplained joint pain and progression of joint disease. A radiopaque contrast agent or air is injected into the joint cavity to visualize the joint structures, such as the ligaments, cartilage, tendons, and joint capsule. The joint is put through its range of motion to distribute the contrast agent while a series of x-rays are obtained. If a tear is present, the contrast agent leaks out of the joint and is evident on the x-ray image (Van Leeuwen & Bladh, 2016).

Bone Densitometry

Bone densitometry is used to evaluate BMD. This can be performed through the use of x-rays or ultrasound. The most common modalities used include dual-energy x-ray absorptiometry (DXA or DEXA), quantitative computed tomography (QCT), and quantitative ultrasound (QUS). DXA measures BMD and predicts fracture risk through accurate monitoring of bone density changes in patients with osteoporosis who are undergoing treatment. The density of bones in the spine, hip, and wrist may be calculated, as well as the total body. Peripheral dual-energy x-ray absorptiometry (pDXA) may be an alternative test that measures BMD of the forearm, finger, or heel, although its ability to project hip or spine fracture risk is less accurate than DXA.

Bone density may vary among different skeletal areas; therefore, BMD results may be normal at one site but low at another. Because these tests only measure density at specific sites, they may miss abnormal findings in other skeletal areas. Thus, although the BMD of the heel can be used to diagnose and monitor osteoporosis, predicting bone fracture risk related to osteoporosis is best achieved through DXA of the hip and spine. Hence, DXA is the most commonly prescribed diagnostic test for determining BMD (NOF, 2014; Van Leeuwen & Bladh, 2016). See Chapter 42 for a further discussion of osteoporosis risks.

Nursing Interventions

Before the patient undergoes any of the imaging studies described previously (i.e., x-rays, CT scans, MRIs, arthrography, bone densitometry), the nurse prepares the patient. For these studies, the patient must lie still. During an MRI study, the patient may hear a knocking sound. In addition, the nurse assesses for conditions that may require special consideration during the study or that may be contraindications to the study (e.g., pregnancy; claustrophobia; inability to tolerate required positioning due to age, debility, or disability; metal implants). If contrast agents will be used for the CT scan, MRI, or arthrography, the patient is assessed for possible allergies (Van Leeuwen & Bladh, 2016).

The patient having an arthrogram may feel some discomfort or tingling during the procedure. After the arthrogram, a compression elastic bandage may be applied if prescribed, and the joint is usually rested for 12 hours. Strenuous activity should be avoided until approved by the primary provider. The nurse provides additional comfort measures (e.g., mild analgesia, ice) as appropriate and explains to the patient that it is normal to experience clicking or crackling in the joint for 24 to 48 hours after the procedure until the contrast agent or air is absorbed.

Bone Scan

A bone scan is performed to detect metastatic and primary bone tumors, osteomyelitis, some fractures, and aseptic necrosis, and to monitor the progression of degenerative bone diseases. A bone scan may accurately identify bone disease before it can be detected on x-ray; as such, it may diagnose a stress fracture in a patient who continues to experience pain after x-ray findings are negative (Van Leeuwen & Bladh, 2016). A bone scan requires the injection of a radioisotope through an IV line; the scan is performed 2 to 3 hours afterward. At this point, distribution and concentration of the isotope in the bone are measured. The degree of nuclide uptake is related to the metabolism of the bone; areas of abnormal bone formation will appear brighter. An increased uptake of the isotope is seen in primary skeletal disease (osteosarcoma), metastatic bone disease, inflammatory skeletal disease (osteomyelitis), and fractures that do not heal as expected.

Nursing Interventions

Prior to the bone scan, the nurse inquires about possible allergies to the radioisotope and assesses for any condition that would contraindicate performing the procedure (e.g., pregnancy, breast-feeding). The nurse should educate the patient about why the bone scan may be indicated and explain that it can assist in the identification of bone disease before it can be detected on an x-ray. The nurse should explain that the patient may experience moments of discomfort from the isotope (e.g., flushing, warmth) but provide reassurance that the radionuclide poses no radioactive hazard (Van Leeuwen & Bladh, 2016). In addition, the patient is encouraged to drink plenty of fluids to help distribute and eliminate the isotope. Before the scan, the nurse asks the patient to empty the bladder, because a full bladder interferes with accurate scanning of the pelvic bones.

Arthroscopy

Arthroscopy allows direct visualization of a joint through the use of a fiberoptic endoscope. Thus, it is a useful adjunct to diagnosing joint disorders. Biopsy and treatment of tears, defects, and disease processes may be performed through the arthroscope. The procedure takes place in the operating room under sterile conditions with either injection of a local anesthetic agent into the joint or general anesthesia. A large-bore needle is inserted, and the joint is distended with saline. The arthroscope is introduced, and joint structures, synovium, and articular surfaces are visualized. After the procedure, the puncture wound is closed with adhesive strips or sutures and covered with a sterile dressing. Complications are rare but may include infection, hemarthrosis, neurovascular compromise, thrombophlebitis, stiffness, effusion, adhesions, and delayed wound healing (Van Leeuwen & Bladh, 2016).

Nursing Interventions

After the arthroscopic procedure, the joint is wrapped with a compression dressing to control swelling. In addition, ice may be applied to control edema and enhance comfort. Frequently, the joint is kept extended and elevated to reduce swelling. The nurse monitors and documents the neurovascular status (see Chart 39-3). Analgesic agents are given as needed. The patient is instructed to avoid strenuous activity of the joint, and exercises must be approved by the primary provider. The patient and family are instructed to monitor for signs and symptoms of complications (e.g., fever, excessive bleeding, swelling, numbness, cool skin) and the importance of notifying the

primary provider should any of these occur (Van Leeuwen & Bladh, 2016).

Arthrocentesis

Arthrocentesis (joint aspiration) is carried out to obtain synovial fluid for purposes of examination or to relieve pain due to effusion. Examination of synovial fluid is helpful in the diagnosis of septic arthritis and other inflammatory arthropathies and reveals the presence of hemarthrosis (bleeding into the joint cavity), which suggests trauma or a bleeding disorder. Normally, synovial fluid is clear, pale, straw colored, and scanty in volume. Using aseptic technique, the physician inserts a needle into the joint and aspirates fluid. Anti-inflammatory medications may be injected into the joint. A sterile dressing is applied after aspiration. There is a risk of infection after this procedure.

Nursing Interventions

The nurse should review the procedure with the patient and its indications. Hair may need to be removed from the site before the procedure. Pain may be a concern; telling the patient that analgesics may be given to alleviate discomfort during the procedure may help decrease anxiety. Ice may be prescribed for the first 24 to 48 hours postprocedure; the patient should be educated about why ice may be indicated (i.e., to diminish edema formation and pain). If antibiotics are prescribed postprocedure, the patient must be educated about their use and reminded to take medications as prescribed. The patient and family are educated about the possible signs and symptoms of complications, particularly infection and bleeding (e.g., fever, excessive bleeding, swelling, numbness, cool skin) and the importance of promptly notifying the health care provider if any of these occur (Van Leeuwen & Bladh, 2016).

Electromyography

Electromyography (EMG) provides information about the electrical potential of the muscles and the nerves leading to them. The test is performed to evaluate muscle weakness, pain, and disability. The purpose of the procedure is to determine any abnormality of function and to differentiate muscle and nerve problems. An EMG can be used to identify the extent of damage if nerve function does not return within 4 months of an injury. Needle electrodes are inserted into selected muscles, and responses to electrical stimuli are recorded on an oscilloscope. Warm compresses may relieve residual discomfort after the study.

Nursing Interventions

Before the patient undergoes an EMG, the nurse inquires if the patient is taking any anticoagulant medications and assesses for any active skin infection. An EMG is usually contraindicated in patients receiving anticoagulant therapy (e.g., warfarin) because the needle electrodes may cause bleeding within the muscle. EMG also may be contraindicated in patients with extensive skin infections due to the risk of spreading infection from the skin to the muscle. The nurse instructs the patient to avoid using any lotions or creams on the day of the test (Van Leeuwen & Bladh, 2016). If the nurse finds that the patient is taking an anticoagulant or has a skin infection, the primary provider is notified.

Biopsy

Biopsy may be performed to determine the structure and composition of bone marrow, bone, muscle, or synovium to help diagnose specific diseases. It involves excising a sample of tissue that can be analyzed microscopically to determine cell morphology and tissue abnormalities.

Nursing Interventions

The nurse educates the patient about the procedure and assures the patient that analgesic agents will be provided. The nurse monitors the biopsy site for edema, bleeding, pain, hematoma formation, and infection. Ice is applied as prescribed to control bleeding and edema. In addition, antibiotics and analgesic agents are given as prescribed. The patient is instructed to report signs of redness, bleeding, or pain at the biopsy site as well as fever or chills to the primary provider (Van Leeuwen & Bladh, 2016).

Laboratory Studies

Examination of the patient's blood and urine is used to identify the presence and amount of chemicals and other substances. The results may indicate a primary musculoskeletal problem (e.g., Paget's disease of the bone), a developing complication (e.g., infection), the baseline for instituting therapy (e.g., anticoagulant therapy), or the response to therapy, as well as possible causes of bone loss. Before surgery, coagulation studies are performed to detect bleeding tendencies (because bone is vascular tissue).

Serum calcium levels are altered in patients with osteomalacia, parathyroid dysfunction, Paget's disease, metastatic bone tumors, or prolonged immobilization. Serum phosphorus levels are inversely related to calcium levels and are diminished in osteomalacia associated with malabsorption syndrome. Acid phosphatase is elevated in Paget's disease and metastatic cancer. Alkaline phosphatase is elevated during early fracture healing and in diseases with increased osteoblastic activity (e.g., metastatic bone tumors). Bone metabolism may be evaluated through thyroid studies and determination of calcitonin, PTH, and vitamin D levels. Serum enzyme levels of creatine kinase and aspartate aminotransferase become elevated with muscle damage. Serum osteocalcin indicates the rate of bone turnover. Urine calcium levels increase with bone destruction (e.g., parathyroid dysfunction, metastatic bone tumors, multiple myeloma) (Florence et al., 2013).

Specific urine and serum biochemical markers can be used to provide information about the speed of bone resorption or bone formation, as well as to document the effects of therapeutic interventions prescribed for patients diagnosed with musculoskeletal disorders. These include urinary N-telopeptide of type 1 collagen (N-Tx) and deoxypyridinoline (Dpd), both of which reflect increased osteoclast activity and increased bone resorption. Conversely, elevated serum levels of bone-specific alkaline phosphatase (ALP), osteocalcin, and intact N-terminal propeptide of type 1 collagen (P1NP) reflect increased activity of osteoblasts and enhanced bone remodeling activity (NOF, 2016a).

CRITICAL THINKING EXERCISES

1 **pq** You are a nurse working in a primary care office. You assess a 79-year-old man who complains of back pain for the past "month or so." The patient reports that the pain has been increasing and is no longer relieved with ibuprofen (Motrin). Vital signs are within normal limits. The patient weighs 118 pounds, and you note that he is 2 inches shorter than he was 5 years ago. What additional assessment information would you want to obtain from this patient? What appropriate diagnostic tests would you anticipate for this patient? What is your priority nursing diagnosis and plan of care for this patient? What musculoskeletal disorder is this patient at risk for?

2 **ebp** You are a nurse working in the Emergency Department (ED) and caring for a 75-year-old woman who arrived via ambulance after falling at home. She tells you she slipped on a rug and hurt her wrist trying to brace herself from the fall. You notice an obvious deformity of her right wrist. Her current weight is 90 pounds; she admits to smoking a half a pack of cigarettes a day for the past 45 years, and drinks 1 alcoholic drink a day. She has a medical history of chronic obstructive pulmonary disease (COPD) and hypertension. X-ray confirms a fractured right distal radius. What other health concerns should be evaluated for this patient? What is the evidence base that supports strategies for educating and planning care for this patient? In particular, what strategies can be implemented in order to educate this patient about fall prevention and maximize her musculoskeletal health? What is the strength of the evidence of the effectiveness of these strategies?

3 **ebp** You are a nurse working at an assisted living facility. You are developing an educational program regarding bone health and aging. What are the current evidence-based recommendations to maintain bone health? What is the level of evidence that supports each of the recommendations and strategies for reducing musculoskeletal risk for the aging adult?

REFERENCES

Books

Bickley, L. S. (2017). *Bates' guide to physical examination and history taking* (12th ed.). Philadelphia, PA: Lippincott Williams & Wilkins.
Grossman, S. C., & Porth, C. M. (2014). *Porth's pathophysiology: Concepts of altered health states* (9th ed.). Philadelphia, PA: Lippincott Williams & Wilkins.
National Osteoporosis Foundation (NOF). (2014). *Clinician's guide to prevention and treatment of osteoporosis.* Washington, DC: Author.
Swartz, M. (2014). *Textbook of physical diagnosis: History and examination* (7th ed.). Philadelphia, PA: Saunders.
Van Leeuwen, A., & Bladh, M. (2016). *Textbook of laboratory and diagnostic testing: Practical application of nursing process at the bedside.* Philadelphia, PA: F. A. Davis.
Weber, J., & Kelley, J. (2014). *Health assessment in nursing* (5th ed.). Philadelphia, PA: Lippincott Williams & Wilkins.

Journals and Electronic Documents

American College of Rheumatology. (2016). Fracture Risk Assessment Tool (FRAX). Retrieved on 05/05/16 at: www.rheumatology.

org/I-Am-A/Rheumatologist/Research/Clinician-Researchers/Fracture-Risk-Assessment-Tool-FRAX

Centers for Disease Control and Prevention (CDC). (2015). Arthritis: Addressing the nation's most common cause of disability. Retrieved on 03/03/2016 at: www.cdc.gov/chronicdisease/resources/publications/aag/arthritis.htm

Florence, R., Allen, S., Benedict, L., et al. (2013). Diagnosis and treatment of osteoporosis. Bloomington (MN): Institute for Clinical Systems Improvement (ICSI). Retrieved on 03/11/2016 at: www.icsi.org/_asset/vnw0c3/ Osteo.pdf

Institute of Medicine (IOM). (2010). Dietary reference intakes for calcium and vitamin D. Washington, DC: The National Academies Press. Retrieved on 03/09/2016 at: iom.nationalacademies.org/hmd/~/media/Files/Report%20Files/2010/Dietary-Reference-Intakes-for-Calcium-and-Vitamin-D/Vitamin%20D%20and%20Calcium%202010%20Report%20Brief.pdf

Khosla, S. (2013). Pathogenesis of age-related bone loss in humans. *Journals of Gerontology Series A: Biological Sciences & Medical Sciences*, 68, 1226–1235.

International Osteoporosis Foundation (IOF). (2015). Osteoporosis and musculoskeletal disorders. Retrieved on 03/09/2016 at: www.iofbone-health.org/osteoporosis-musculoskeletal-disorders

National Osteoporosis Foundation (NOF). (2016a). Bone basics. Washington, DC: Author. Retrieved on 04/3/2016 at: nof.org/learn/bonebasics

National Osteoporosis Foundation (NOF). (2016b). Making a diagnosis. Washington, DC: Author. Retrieved on 04/3/2016 at: nof.org/articles/8#lab

U.S. Department of Health and Human Services (HHS). (2012). The surgeon general's report on bone health and osteoporosis: What it means to you. Rockville, MD: Author. Retrieved on 03/01/2016 at: www.niams.nih.gov/Health_Info/Bone/SGR/surgeon_generals_report.asp

Resources

American College of Sports Medicine (ACSM), www.acsm.org

International Osteoporosis Foundation (IOF), www.iofbonehealth.org/

National Association of Orthopaedic Nurses (NAON), www.orthonurse.org

National Institute of Arthritis and Musculoskeletal and Skin Diseases, www.niams.nih.gov

National Osteoporosis Foundation, www.nof.org

World Health Organization (WHO) Collaborating Centre for Metabolic Bone Diseases: the fracture risk assessment tool (FRAX®), www.shef.ac.uk/FRAX/tool.aspx?country=9

40

Musculoskeletal Care Modalities

LEARNING OBJECTIVES

On completion of this chapter, the learner will be able to:

1 Identify the preventive and health education needs of the patient with a cast, splint, or brace.
2 Describe the nursing management of the patient with a cast, splint, or brace.
3 Compare the various types of traction and the principles of effective traction.
4 Describe the nursing management of the patient with an external fixator or in traction.
5 Compare the nursing needs of the patient undergoing total hip arthroplasty (THA) with those of the patient undergoing total knee arthroplasty (TKA).
6 Use the nursing process as a framework for care of the patient undergoing orthopedic surgery.

GLOSSARY

abduction: movement away from the center or median line of the body
adduction: movement toward the center or median line of the body
avascular necrosis: death of tissue due to insufficient blood supply
brace: externally applied device to support the body or a body part, control movement, and prevent injury
cast: rigid external immobilizing device molded to contours of body part
cast syndrome: psychological (claustrophobic reaction) or physiologic (superior mesenteric artery syndrome) responses to confinement in body cast
external fixator: external metal frame attached to bone fragments to stabilize them
fracture: a break in the continuity of the bone

heterotopic ossification: misplaced formation of bone
neurovascular status: neurologic (motor and sensory components) and circulatory functioning of a body part
osteolysis: lysis of bone from inflammatory reaction against polyethylene particulate debris
osteomyelitis: infection of the bone
osteotomy: surgical cutting of bone
paresthesia: an abnormal sensation of tingling or numbness or burning
sling: bandage used to support an arm
splint: device designed specifically to support and immobilize a body part in a desired position
traction: application of a pulling force to a part of the body
trapeze: overhead assistive device to promote patient mobility in bed

The management of musculoskeletal injuries and disorders frequently includes the use of casts, splints, braces, traction, surgery, or a combination of these. Because of the prevalence of musculoskeletal injuries and disorders, nurses practicing in many settings across the continuum of care, whether in the home, office, hospital, long-term care facility, or rehabilitation facility, must have an understanding of these modalities. Patient education is essential for optimal outcomes. The nurse prepares the patient for immobilization with casts or traction, and for surgery, when indicated. Nursing care is planned to maximize the effectiveness of these treatment modalities and to prevent potential complications associated with each of the interventions. The patient is instructed to manage care at home and how to safely resume activities.

The Patient in a Cast, Splint, or Brace

Casts

A **cast** is a rigid external immobilizing device that is molded to the contours of the body. The cast must fit the shape of the injured limb correctly to provide the best support possible (American Academy of Orthopaedic Surgeons [AAOS], 2015a). A cast is used to immobilize a reduced fracture, to correct or prevent a deformity (e.g., clubfoot, hip displacement), apply uniform pressure to underlying soft tissue, or support and stabilize weakened joints. Generally, casts permit mobilization of the patient while restricting movement of the affected body part.

Because of their ability to provide more complete immobilization, casting is the mainstay of treatment for many **fractures** (Alisangco, Asplund, & Benjamin, 2016), which are breaks in the continuity of the bones. The most common casting materials consist of fiberglass or plaster of Paris, as these are materials that can be molded. The choice of material depends on several factors, which include the condition being treated, availability, and costs. Generally, the joints proximal and distal to the area immobilized are included in the cast. However, with some fractures, cast construction and molding may allow movement of a joint while immobilizing a fracture (e.g., three-point fixation in a patellar tendon weight-bearing cast).

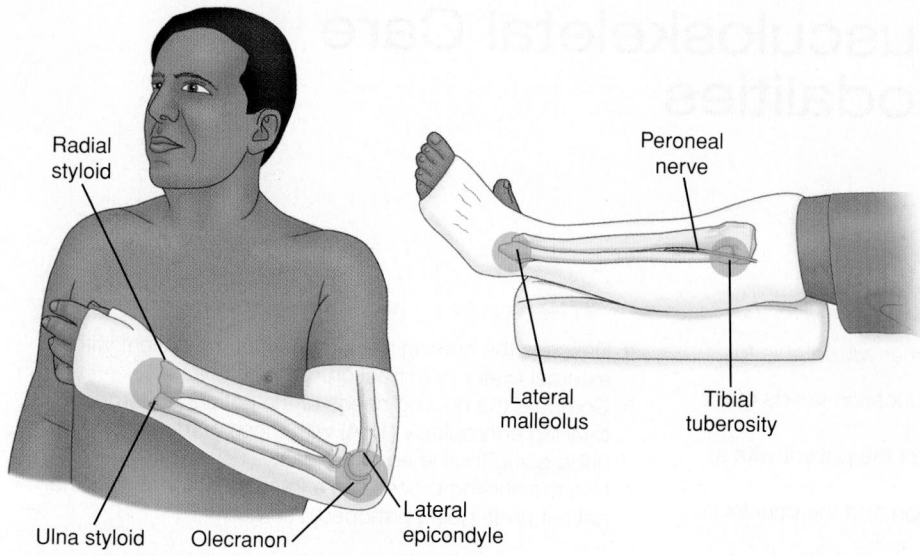

Radial styloid

Peroneal nerve

Lateral malleolus

Tibial tuberosity

Ulna styloid   Olecranon

Lateral epicondyle

Figure 40-1 • Pressure areas in common types of casts. **Left**. Long-arm cast. **Right**. Long-leg cast.

Generally, casts can be divided into three main groups: arm casts, leg casts, and body or spica casts:

Short-arm cast: Extends from below the elbow to the palmar crease, secured around the base of the thumb. If the thumb is included, it is known as a thumb spica or gauntlet cast.

Long-arm cast: Extends from the axillary fold to the proximal palmar crease. The elbow usually is immobilized at a right angle.

Short-leg cast: Extends from below the knee to the base of the toes. The foot is flexed at a right angle in a neutral position.

Long-leg cast: Extends from the junction of the upper and middle third of the thigh to the base of the toes. The knee may be slightly flexed.

Walking cast: A short- or long-leg cast reinforced for strength

Body cast: Encircles the trunk

Shoulder spica cast: A body jacket that encloses the trunk, shoulder, and elbow

Hip spica cast: Encloses the trunk and a lower extremity. A double hip spica cast includes both legs.

Figure 40-1 illustrates long-arm and long-leg casts and areas in which pressure problems commonly occur with these casts.

The application of a cast is a specialized skill, typically performed by orthopedic technologists. The skillset needed to apply and remove casts requires education, training, practice, and constant review of provider competence to ensure patients receive safe, high-quality care (Brubacher, Karg, Weinstock, et al., 2016; Newton-Triggs, Pugh, Rogers, et al., 2014).

Fiberglass Casts

Fiberglass casts are composed of polyurethane resins that have the versatility of plaster but are lighter in weight, stronger, water resistant, and more durable than plaster. In addition, fiberglass casts facilitate radiographic imaging better than plaster (AAOS, 2015a) and have the benefit of reaching full rigidity within 30 minutes of application. Because they tend to be more difficult to contour and mold, fiberglass casts are more commonly used for simple fractures of the upper and lower extremities. They consist of an open-weave, nonabsorbent fabric that requires tepid water for activation. Heat is given off (an exothermic reaction) while the cast is applied. The heat given off during this reaction can be uncomfortable, and the nurse should prepare the patient for the sensation of increasing warmth so that the patient does not become alarmed. Fiberglass casts can cause thermal injury like plaster casts, but the risk is less (Alisangco et al., 2016).

Some fiberglass casts use a waterproof lining (Gore-Tex), which permits the patient to shower, swim, or engage in hydrotherapy (the use of water for treatment). When the cast is wet, the patient is instructed to shake or drain water out of it; thorough drying is important to prevent skin breakdown, infection, or irritation. The best results are achieved with casts that can easily drain, such as short-arm casts. Heels and elbows encased in wet casts may become macerated from the trapped water and therefore are associated with more skin breakdown.

Plaster Casts

Casts made of plaster of Paris are less costly and achieve a better mold than fiberglass casts; however, they are heavy, not water resistant, and can take up to 24 to 72 hours to dry postapplication. The exothermic reaction during cast application has the potential to cause serious burns (Burghardt, Anderson, Reed, et al., 2014). Extra care should be taken when these types of casts are applied to older adults because their skin is more temperature sensitive than average adult skin (Burghardt et al., 2014). During the cast application process, clean, room temperature water should be used. Minimal layers of padding should be used. In addition, the cast should not be covered while it is drying because the heat generated by the chemical reaction cannot escape.

The time that it takes for a plaster cast to dry completely depends on its size, thickness, and location, as well as environmental drying conditions (Oron, Lindner, Bergman, et al., 2013). A freshly applied cast should be handled as little as possible to prevent denting and cracking (Alisangco et al., 2016). The wet plaster cast should be handled by only the palms so that indentations in the cast may be prevented; indentations can result in areas of pressure on the skin (Alisangco et al., 2016). The cast should be exposed to circulating air to dry and supported on a firm and smooth surface; it should not be placed on a metallic surface or one with sharp edges. If elevation is requested to reduce swelling, a cloth-covered pillow is preferred to one covered in plastic, which could retain heat and prevent drying. A wet plaster cast feels damp, appears dull and gray, sounds dull on percussion, and smells musty. The cast is dry when it feels hard and firm, has a white and shiny appearance, is resonant to percussion, and odorless.

On occasion, the plaster cast may have rough edges, which can crumble and cause skin irritation. Petaling, or smoothing the rough edges of the cast, resolves this problem if the underlying stockinette does not cover the edges of the cast. To prevent skin breakdown, moleskin can be used over any rough area of the cast that may rub against the patient's skin.

Splints and Braces

Many injuries that were treated previously with casts may now be treated with other immobilization devices such as splints and braces. Splinting is usually more practical and common and is the preferred method of fracture immobilization in the acute care setting and for the initial treatment of fractures that eventually require casting (Alisangco et al., 2016). Splints are often used for simple and stable fractures, sprains, tendon injuries, and other soft tissue injuries. They offer many advantages over casts in that they are faster and easier to apply. They are also noncircumferential and allow for natural swelling during the inflammatory phase of injury. Pressure-related complications (e.g., skin breakdown, necrosis, compartment syndrome [see later discussions]) are more prevalent when soft tissue swelling occurs within a contained space (e.g., a circumferential cast). Splints are easily removed, facilitating inspection of the injury site. In addition, splints can be indicated to provide initial stability for fractures that are unstable while awaiting definitive care.

Contoured **splints** of plaster or pliable thermoplastic materials may be used for conditions that do not require rigid immobilization, for those in which swelling may be anticipated, and for those that require special skin care. Splints made of thermoplastics are warmed and molded to custom-fit the affected body part (e.g., hand and thoracolumbosacral orthotics [TLSOs], clamshell-type back braces). The splint needs to immobilize and support the body part in a functional position, and it must be well padded to prevent pressure, skin abrasion, and skin breakdown. The splint is overwrapped with an elastic bandage applied in a spiral fashion and with pressure uniformly distributed so that circulation is not restricted.

Braces (i.e., orthoses) are used to provide support, control movement, and prevent additional injury. They are custom-fitted to various parts of the body; thus, they tend to be indicated for longer-term use than splints. The orthotist adjusts the brace for fit, positioning, and motion so that movement is enhanced, any deformities are corrected, and discomfort is minimized.

Many splints and braces are prefabricated and fastened with Velcro straps. They may be made of plastic and other materials such as cloth, leather, metal, and elastic. Knee immobilizers, ankle stirrups, and cock-up wrist splints are types of prefabricated splints and braces. Both splints and braces may be either custom-made or standard "off the shelf." Splints and braces are generally less compliant and permit more motion at the injury site than casts, which can be a serious disadvantage in that underlying injuries are not as well stabilized.

Nursing Management of a Patient in a Cast, Splint, or Brace

Before the cast, splint, or brace is applied, the nurse completes an assessment of the patient's general health, presenting signs and symptoms, emotional status, understanding of the need for the device, and condition of the body part to be immobilized. Physical assessment of the part to be immobilized must include a thorough assessment of the skin and **neurovascular status** (i.e., neurologic and circulatory functioning), including the degree and location of swelling, bruising, and skin abrasions.

To promote healing, any skin lacerations and abrasions that may have occurred as a result of the trauma that caused the fracture must be treated before the cast, brace, or splint is applied. The nurse thoroughly cleanses the skin and treats it as prescribed. The patient may require a tetanus booster if the wound is dirty and if the last known booster was given more than 5 years ago. Sterile dressings are used to cover the injured skin. If the skin wounds are extensive, an alternative method (e.g., external fixator) may be chosen to immobilize the body part.

The nurse gives the patient or family information about the underlying pathologic condition and the purpose and expectations of the prescribed treatment regimen. This knowledge promotes the patient's active participation in and adherence to the treatment program.

The nurse prepares the patient for the application of the cast, splint, or brace by describing the anticipated sights, sounds, and sensations (e.g., heat from the hardening reaction of the fiberglass or plaster) that he or she may experience. Asking the patient and family what they know about the application and care of the cast can help determine opportunities for education. The patient needs to know what to expect during application and the reason the body part must be immobilized.

For the procedural guidelines for applying a cast, go to **thepoint.lww.com/Brunner14e.**

The main concern following the application of an immobilization device is assessment and prevention of neurovascular dysfunction or compromise of the affected extremity. Assessments are performed at least every hour for the first 24 hours and every 1 to 4 hours thereafter to prevent neurovascular compromise related to edema and/or the device. Neurovascular assessment includes the assessment of peripheral circulation, motion, and sensation of the affected extremity, assessing the fingers or toes of the affected extremity, and comparing them with those of the opposite extremity. When assessing peripheral circulation, the nurse must check peripheral pulses as well as capillary refill response (within 3 seconds), edema, and the color and temperature of the skin. While assessing motion, the nurse should note any weakness or paralysis of the injured body part. While assessing sensation, the nurse monitors for **paresthesia** (numbness or tingling) or absence of feeling in the affected extremity, which could indicate nerve damage (Alisangco et al., 2016).

Nurses must be vigilant in assessing for subtle neurovascular changes in these patients (Turney, Noble, & Kim, 2013). The "6 Ps" indicative of symptoms of neurovascular compromise are *p*ain, *p*oikilothermia (i.e., takes on the ambient temperature), *p*allor, *p*ulselessness, *p*aresthesia, and *p*aralysis (Pechar & Lyons, 2016). Early recognition of diminished circulation and nerve function is essential to prevent loss of function. Swelling is a concern and can create excessive pressure under the cast (AAOS, 2015a). To augment the flow of fluid, the nurse elevates the extremity so that it is above the level of the heart during the first 24 to 48 hours postapplication to enhance arterial perfusion and control edema and notifies the primary provider at once if signs of compromised neurovascular status are present.

The nurse must carefully evaluate pain associated with the musculoskeletal condition, asking the patient to indicate the exact site and to describe the character and intensity of the pain using a pain rating scale (see Chapter 12). Pain associated with the underlying condition (e.g., fracture) is frequently controlled by immobilization. Pain due to edema that is associated with trauma, surgery, or bleeding into the tissues can frequently be controlled by elevation and, if prescribed, intermittent application of ice or cold packs (AAOS, 2015a). Ice bags (one third to one half full) or cold application devices are placed on each side of the cast, if prescribed, making sure not to indent or wet the cast. Unrelieved or pain out of proportion following cast application may indicate complications. Pain associated with compartment syndrome (see Chapter 42 and later in this chapter) is relentless and is not controlled by modalities such as elevation, application of ice or cold, and usual dosages of analgesic agents. Severe burning pain over bony prominences, especially the heels, anterior ankles, and elbows, warns of an impending pressure ulcer. This may also occur from too-tight elastic wraps used to hold splints in place.

> ### ▶ *Quality and Safety Nursing Alert*
>
> *The nurse must never ignore complaints of pain from the patient in a cast because of the possibility of problems, such as impaired tissue perfusion, compartment syndrome or pressure ulcer formation. A patient's unrelieved pain and increasing analgesic requirements must be reported immediately to the primary provider to avoid necrosis, neuromuscular damage, and possible paralysis.*

While the cast is on, the nurse observes the patient for systemic signs of infection, which include an unpleasant odor from the cast, splint, or brace, and purulent drainage staining the cast. Infection is more common from an open wound, but the moist, warm environment of a splint or cast can be an ideal conduit for infection. Foul-smelling casts should be removed to prevent skin and wound infections (Alisangco et al., 2016). If the infection progresses, a fever may develop. The nurse must notify the primary provider if any of these signs occur.

Finally, some degree of joint stiffness is an inevitable complication of immobilization. Every joint that is not immobilized should be exercised and moved through its range

of motion to maintain function. The nurse encourages the patient to move all fingers or toes hourly when awake to stimulate circulation.

Monitoring and Managing Potential Complications

It is important to assess for potential complications resulting from casts, splints, and braces that can be serious and life threatening, such as compartment syndrome, pressure ulcer formation, and disuse syndrome.

Compartment Syndrome

Compartment syndrome—the most serious complication of casting and splinting—occurs when increased pressure within a confined space (e.g., cast, muscle compartment) compromises blood flow and tissue perfusion (Alisangco et al., 2016). Ischemia and potentially irreversible damage to the soft tissues within that space can occur within a few hours if action is not taken (see Fig. 40-2). A tight or rigid cast/splint that constricts a swollen limb is associated with this complication.

Diagnosis of compartment syndrome is based on clinical suspicion, assessment of the 6 P's (pain, poikilothermia, pallor, paresthesia, pulselessness, and paralysis), and intracompartmental pressure (ICP) (Garner, Taylor, Gausden, et al., 2014). The earliest indicator of developing compartment syndrome is pain that seems out of proportion to the underlying injury and pain on passive stretch of other muscles in the immobilized limb (Ali, Santy-Tomlinson, & Watson, 2014). The patient may complain that the cast, brace, or splint is too tight. The primary provider must be notified immediately as a delay in diagnosis increases the risk of failed treatment, poor outcomes, additional operations, and the possibility of amputation. Pulselessness, paresthesia, and complete paralysis are found in the late stages of compartment syndrome (Donaldson, Haddad, & Khan, 2014).

If the complication is due to a cast or tight splint, the splint may be loosened or removed and the cast univalved or bivalved (cut in half longitudinally, on one side or two parallel sides of the cast, respectively) to release constriction and allow for inspection of the skin. The nurse assists in maintaining limb alignment, and the extremity must then be elevated no higher than heart level to maintain arterial perfusion. If pressure is not relieved and circulation is not restored, an emergent surgical fasciotomy may be necessary to relieve the pressure within the muscle compartment. The nurse closely monitors the patient's response to conservative and surgical management of compartment syndrome. The nurse records frequent neurovascular responses and promptly reports changes to the primary provider (see Chapter 42).

 For the procedural guidelines for univalving or bivalving a cast, go to **thepoint.lww.com/Brunner14e.**

Pressure Ulcers

Casts or splints can put pressure on soft tissues, particularly if they are inappropriately applied, causing tissue anoxia and pressure ulcers. Lower extremity sites most susceptible are the heel, malleoli, dorsum of the foot, head of the fibula, and anterior surface of the patella. The main pressure sites on the

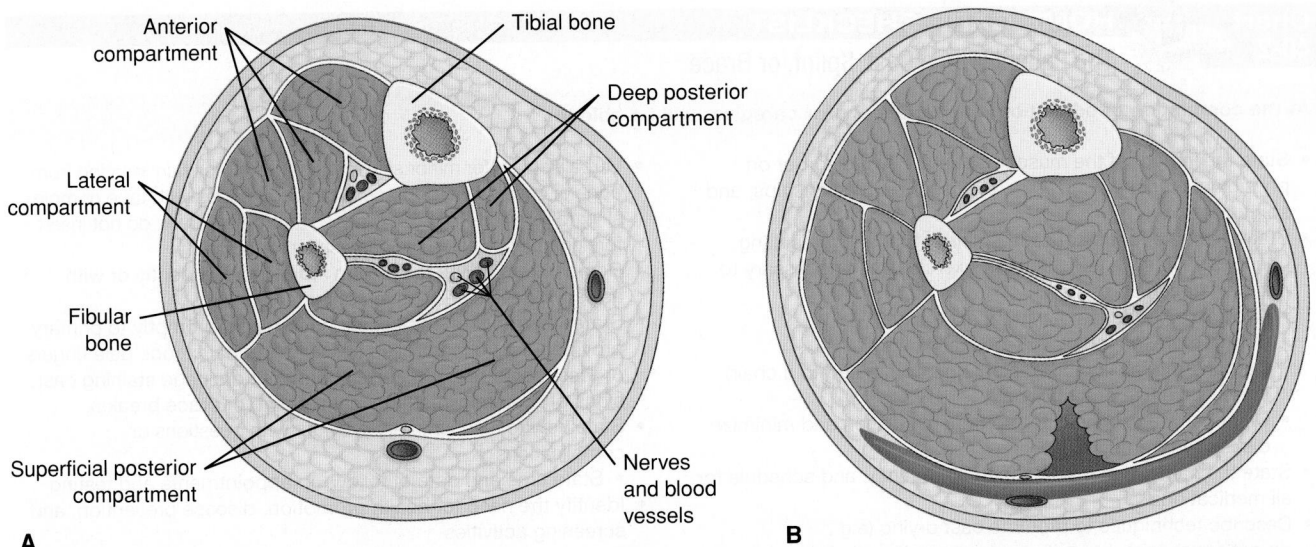

Figure 40-2 • **A.** Cross-section of normal lower leg with muscle compartments. **B.** Cross-section of lower leg with compartment syndrome. Swelling of muscles causes compression of nerves and blood vessels.

upper extremity are located at the medial epicondyle of the humerus and the ulnar styloid (see Fig. 40-1).

If pressure necrosis occurs, the patient typically reports a very painful "hot spot" and tightness under the cast. The cast may feel warmer in the affected area, suggesting underlying tissue erythema. Drainage may stain the cast or splint and emit an unpleasant odor. Even if discomfort does not occur, there may still be extensive loss of tissue with skin breakdown and tissue necrosis. To assess for pressure ulcer development, the primary provider may univalve, bivalve, or cut an opening (window) in the cast to allow for inspection, access, and possible treatment. A dressing may be applied over the exposed skin, and the cutout portion of the cast is replaced and held in place by an elastic compression dressing or tape. This prevents "window edema" from occurring, which is the swelling or bulging of the underlying soft tissue through the window opening.

Disuse Syndrome

Immobilization in a cast, splint, or brace can cause muscle atrophy and loss of strength, and can place patients at risk for disuse syndrome, which is the deterioration of body systems as a result of prescribed or unavoidable musculoskeletal inactivity (Herdman & Kamitsuru, 2014). To prevent this, the nurse instructs the patient to tense or contract muscles (e.g., isometric muscle contraction) without moving the underlying bone. Isometric exercises, such as instructing the patient with a leg or arm cast to splint or brace to "push down" the knee or to "make a fist," respectively, helps reduce muscle atrophy and maintain strength. Muscle setting exercises (e.g., quadriceps and gluteal setting exercises) are important in maintaining muscles essential for walking (see Chart 40-1). Isometric exercises should be performed hourly while the patient is awake.

Promoting Home, Community-Based, and Transitional Care

Educating the Patient About Self-Care

Self-care deficits occur when a portion of the body is immobilized. The nurse encourages the patient to participate actively in personal care and to use assistive devices safely. The nurse must assist the patient in identifying areas of self-care deficit and in developing strategies to achieve independence in activities of daily living (ADLs) (see Chart 40-2). Patient and family education is also described in Chart 40-2.

Continuing and Transitional Care

For the patient with a cast that is ready for removal, the nurse should prepare the patient by explaining what to expect. For instance, the patient should be instructed to never remove the cast themselves and that a cast saw will be used to remove the cast (AAOS, 2015a). The cast saw uses an oscillating blade that vibrates but does not spin; thus, it cuts through the outer cast layer but does not penetrate deeply enough to injure the patient's skin. The cast will be cut in several places,

---

Chart 40-1 **PATIENT EDUCATION**
Muscle Setting Exercises

The nurse instructs the patient to perform isometric contractions of the muscle to maintain muscle mass and strength and to prevent atrophy:

Quadriceps Setting Exercise

- Position patient supine with leg extended.
- Instruct patient to push knee back onto the mattress by contracting the anterior thigh muscles.
- Encourage patient to hold the position for 5 to 10 seconds.
- Let patient relax.
- Have patient repeat the exercise 10 times each hour when awake.

Gluteal Setting Exercise

- Position patient supine with legs extended, if possible.
- Instruct patient to contract the muscles of the buttocks.
- Encourage patient to hold the contraction for 5 to 10 seconds.
- Let the patient relax.
- Have patient repeat the exercise 10 times each hour when awake.

Chart 40-2 HOME CARE CHECKLIST

The Patient With a Cast, Splint, or Brace

At the completion of education, the patient and/or caregiver will be able to:

- State the impact of the musculoskeletal injury/disorder on physiologic functioning, ADLs, IADLs, roles, relationships, and spirituality.
- State rationale for use of cast, splint or brace and resulting changes in lifestyle (e.g., activity, exercise, rest) necessary to maintain health and safety.
  - Avoid excessive use of injured extremity.
  - Observe prescribed weight-bearing limits.
  - Demonstrate ability to transfer (e.g., from a bed to a chair) and/or safe use of mobility aid.
  - Demonstrate exercises to promote circulation and minimize disuse syndrome.
- State the name, dose, side effects, frequency, and schedule for all medications.
- Describe techniques to promote cast drying (e.g., do not cover cast; expose cast to circulating air; handle damp plaster cast with palms of hands; do not rest the cast on hard surfaces or sharp edges that can dent soft cast).
- Describe approaches to controlling swelling and pain (e.g., elevate immobilized extremity to heart level, apply ice bag intermittently if prescribed, take analgesic agents as prescribed).
- Report pain uncontrolled by elevating the immobilized limb and by analgesic agents (may be an indicator of impaired tissue perfusion—compartment syndrome or pressure ulcer).

- Verbalize care for minor skin irritations (e.g., for skin irritation from edge of cast, splint, or brace, pad rough edges with tape or moleskin; to relieve itching, blow cool air from hair dryer; do not insert foreign objects inside the cast, splint, or brace).
- Demonstrate ability to perform ADLs independently or with assistive devices/adaptive equipment.
- State indicators of complications to report promptly to primary provider (e.g., uncontrolled swelling and pain; cool, pale fingers or toes; paresthesia; paralysis; purulent drainage staining cast; signs of systemic infection; cast, splint, or brace breaks).
- State how to reach primary provider with questions or complications
  - State time and date of follow-up appointments and testing
- Identify the need for health promotion, disease prevention, and screening activities
- Describe care of extremity following cast, splint, or brace removal (e.g., skin care, gradual resumption of normal activities to protect limb from undue stresses, management of swelling).

Resources

See Chapter 10, Chart 10-8 for additional information related to durable medical equipment, adaptive equipment, mobility skills, skin, bowel, and bladder care.

ADL, activities of daily living; IADL, independent activities of daily living.

---

usually along both sides of the cast. The cast is then spread and opened and a special tool is used to lift it off. Scissors are used to cut through the protective padding and stockinette layers to ensure that the patient's skin will not be cut.

The formerly immobilized body part will be weak from disuse, stiff, and may appear atrophied. As the cast or splint is removed, the affected body part should be supported to prevent injury. The skin, which is usually dry and scaly from accumulated dead skin, is vulnerable to injury from scratching. The skin needs to be washed gently and lubricated with an emollient lotion. The patient should be instructed to avoid rubbing and scratching the skin, because doing so can cause damage to newly exposed skin.

The nurse and physical therapist educate the patient to resume activities gradually within the prescribed therapeutic regimen. Exercises prescribed to help the patient restore muscle strength, joint motion, and flexibility are explained and demonstrated. Because the muscles are weak from disuse, the body part that has been immobilized cannot withstand normal stresses immediately. In addition, the patient should be instructed to control swelling by elevating the formerly immobilized body part, no higher than the heart, until normal muscle tone and use are reestablished.

Nursing Management of the Patient With an Immobilized Upper Extremity

The patient whose arm is immobilized must readjust to many routine tasks. The unaffected arm will assume all upper extremity activities. The nurse, in consultation with an occupational therapist, suggests devices designed to aid one-handed activities. The patient may experience fatigue due to

modified activities and the weight of the cast, splint, or brace. Frequent rest periods are necessary.

To control swelling, the immobilized arm is elevated above heart level with a pillow. When the patient is lying down, the arm is elevated so that each joint is positioned higher than the preceding proximal joint (e.g., elbow higher than the shoulder, hand higher than the elbow).

A sling may be used when the patient ambulates. To prevent pressure on the cervical spinal nerves, the **sling** should distribute the supported weight over a large area of the shoulders and trunk, not just the back of the neck. The nurse encourages the patient to remove the arm from the sling and elevate it frequently.

Circulatory disturbances in the hand may become apparent with signs of cyanosis, swelling, and an inability to move the fingers. A missed compartment syndrome in the arm can result in a Volkmann's ischemic contracture, which may lead to devastating impairment of motor function and sensibility (Hovius & Nijhuis, 2015). Contracture of the fingers and wrist occurs as the result of obstructed arterial blood flow to the forearm and hand. The patient is unable to extend the fingers, describes abnormal sensation (e.g., unrelenting pain, pain on passive stretch), and exhibits signs of diminished circulation to the hand. Irreversible damage develops within a few hours if action is not taken (see Chapter 42). This serious complication can be prevented with nursing surveillance and proper care.

Nursing Management of the Patient With an Immobilized Lower Extremity

The application of a leg cast, splint, or brace imposes a degree of immobility on the patient. Casts may include short-leg casts, extending to the knees, or long-leg casts, extending to the groin. Hinged knee braces and immobilizers typically extend from ankle to groin.

The patient's leg must be supported on pillows to the level of the heart to control swelling. Cold therapy or ice packs should be applied as prescribed over the fracture site for 1 to 2 days. The patient is taught to elevate the immobilized leg when seated. The patient should also assume a recumbent position several times a day with the immobilized leg elevated to promote venous return and control swelling. Gentle toe and ankle exercises that allow for isometric contraction of muscles beneath the cast have also been shown to increase venous return and diminish edema (Hickey, Morgan, Pugh, et al., 2014).

The nurse assesses circulation by observing the color, temperature, and capillary refill of the exposed toes. Nerve function is assessed by observing the patient's ability to move the toes and by asking about the sensations in the foot. Numbness, tingling, and burning may indicate peroneal nerve injury resulting from pressure at the head of the fibula.

> ### ◄ Quality and Safety Nursing Alert
>
> *Injury to the peroneal nerve as a result of pressure is a cause of footdrop (the inability to maintain the foot in a normally flexed position). Consequently, the patient drags the foot when ambulating.*

The nurse and physical therapist instruct the patient how to transfer and ambulate safely with assistive devices (e.g., crutches, walker) (see Chapter 10). The gait to be used depends on whether the patient is permitted to bear weight. If weight bearing is allowed, the cast, splint, or brace is reinforced to withstand the body weight. A cast boot or shoe, which is worn over the casted foot, provides a broad, nonskid walking surface.

Nursing Management of the Patient With a Body or Spica Cast

Casts that encase the trunk of the body (body cast) and portions of one or two extremities (spica cast) require special nursing strategies. Body casts are used to immobilize the spine. Hip spica casts are utilized to treat various fractures of the hip or femur or to correct or maintain the correction of hip deformities after reduction or surgery. These casts typically remain in place for 4 to 6 weeks (Horn & Badowski, 2015). Shoulder spica casts are used for some humeral neck fractures.

Nursing responsibilities include preparing and positioning the patient, assisting with skin care and hygiene, and monitoring for cast syndrome (see later discussion). Explaining the casting procedure helps reduce the patient's apprehension about being encased in a large cast. The nurse reassures the patient that several people will provide care during the application, support for the injured area will be adequate, and care providers will be as gentle as possible. Patients immobilized in large casts may develop **cast syndrome**, which may include psychological or physiologic manifestations, and can occur weeks or months after the cast has been applied (Alisangco et al., 2016). The psychological component is similar to a claustrophobic reaction. The patient exhibits an acute anxiety reaction characterized by behavioral changes and autonomic responses (e.g., increased respiratory rate, diaphoresis, dilated pupils, increased heart rate, elevated blood pressure). The nurse needs to recognize the anxiety reaction and provide an environment in which the patient feels secure. The administration of pain and antianxiety medications prior to the procedure may help to reduce this reaction.

Superior mesenteric artery syndrome is the physiologic manifestation associated with immobilization from a body cast (Gebhart, 2015). With decreased physical activity, gastrointestinal motility decreases, and intestinal gases accumulate. The patient exhibits abdominal distention and discomfort, nausea, and vomiting, leading to food aversion, poor intake, and weight loss. This may eventually lead to increased abdominal pressure, and ileus. As with other instances of adynamic ileus, the patient is treated conservatively with decompression (nasogastric intubation connected to suction) and intravenous (IV) fluid therapy until gastrointestinal motility is restored. Rarely, the abdominal distention can place added pressure on the superior mesenteric artery, reducing the blood supply to the bowel, which can result in gangrenous bowel. The descending aorta may also sustain pressure, as it may be compressed between the spine and pressure of abdominal distention, which results in ischemia. Cutting a window in the abdominal portion of the cast or bivalving the cast may be sufficient to prevent or relieve pressure on the duodenum.

> ### ◄ Quality and Safety Nursing Alert
>
> *The nurse monitors the patient in a large body cast for potential physiologic cast syndrome, noting bowel sounds every 4 to 8 hours, and reports abdominal discomfort and distention, nausea, and vomiting to the primary provider.*

Caring for a patient with a body or spica cast at home can be very stressful for the caregiver(s); therefore, it is essential that nurses provide appropriate support and discharge education. To minimize complications after the cast is applied, the nurse should give the patient a comprehensive discharge package that supplements home care instructions with visual training instructions, as well as provide telephone counseling after discharge (Demir, Erden, Bulut, et al., 2015). Specifically, the nurse educates the family about how to care for the patient, which includes providing hygienic, cast and skin care, ensuring proper positioning, preventing complications, and recognizing symptoms that should be reported to the primary provider.

The Patient With an External Fixator

External fixators are used to manage fractures with soft tissue damage. Complicated fractures of the humerus, forearm, femur, tibia, and pelvis are managed with external skeletal fixators. They are also used to correct defects, treat nonunion, and lengthen limbs. Their use has increased in recent years with advances in orthopedic trauma care. The fixator provides skeletal stability for severe comminuted (crushed or splintered) fractures while permitting active treatment of extensive soft tissue damage (see Fig. 40-3).

External fixation involves the surgical insertion of pins through the skin and soft tissues into and through the bone.

Figure 40-3 • External fixation device. Pins are inserted into bone. The fracture is reduced and aligned and then stabilized by attaching the pins to a rigid portable frame. The device facilitates treatment of soft tissue damaged in complex fractures.

A metal external frame is attached to these pins and is designed to hold the fracture in proper alignment to enable healing to occur (Lethaby, Temple, & Santy-Tomlinson, 2013). Advantages of external fixation, compared to other modes of treatment, include immediate fracture stabilization, minimization of blood loss (in comparison to internal fixation), increased patient comfort, improved wound care, promotion of early mobilization and weight bearing on the affected limb, and active exercise of adjacent uninvolved joints (Lethaby et al., 2013). The disadvantages are an increased risk for pin site loosening and infection, which can lead to osteomyelitis (Jennison, McNally, & Pandit, 2014).

Nursing Management

Patients should be prepared psychologically for application of the external fixator, as they may be at risk for an altered body image related to the size and bulk of the apparatus. To promote acceptance of the device, patients should be given comprehensive information about the frame, reassurance that the discomfort associated with the device is minimal, and that early mobility is anticipated; however, among patients who have had significant trauma there may not be time to engage them in this type of preparation (Newton-Triggs et al., 2014). Clothing and other materials may need to be altered or used to cover the device.

After the external fixator is applied, the extremity is elevated to the level of the heart to reduce swelling, if appropriate. Any sharp points on the fixator or pins are covered with caps to prevent device-induced injuries. The nurse must be alert for potential problems caused by pressure from the device on the skin, nerves, or blood vessels and for the development of compartment syndrome (see Chapter 42). The nurse monitors the neurovascular status of the extremity every 2 to 4 hours and promptly reports changes to the primary provider (Pechar & Lyons, 2016). Because the pins are inserted externally, particular attention is focused on the pin sites for signs of inflammation and infection. The end goal is to avoid **osteomyelitis** (infection of the bone) (see Chapter 41 for a discussion of osteomyelitis). The nurse assesses each pin site at least every 8 to 12 hours for redness, swelling, pain around the pin sites, warmth, and purulent drainage, because these are the most common indicators of pin site infections. In the first 48 to 72 hours postinsertion, some serous drainage, skin warmth, and mild redness at the pin sites are expected (Lethaby et al., 2013); these are expected to subside after 72 hours.

Currently, there is no consensus or research-based evidence to direct the best method for cleansing and dressing percutaneous pin sites to minimize infection rates and complications (Jennison et al., 2014; Ktistakis, Gueradob, & Giannoudis, 2015; Lethaby et al., 2013; Newton-Triggs et al., 2014). In the absence of such research, aseptic technique during pin insertion (Ktistakis et al., 2015) is advised, along with general strategies such as cleansing each pin site separately to avoid cross contamination with nonshedding material (e.g., gauze, cotton-tip swab) and using chlorhexidine 2 mg/mL solution once weekly (Lethaby et al., 2013). Pin sites should be cleaned and dressed as prescribed unless there is copious drainage, the dressing becomes wet, or infection is suspected, in which case cleaning and dressing may be more frequent. If signs of infection are present or if the pins or clamps seem loose, the nurse notifies the primary provider.

 Quality and Safety Nursing Alert

The nurse never adjusts the clamps on the external fixator frame. It is the primary provider's responsibility to do so.

If activity is restricted, the nurse encourages isometric exercises as tolerated to prevent complications of mobility (e.g., thrombus formation). When the swelling subsides, the nurse helps the patient become mobile within the prescribed weight-bearing limits (non–weight bearing to full weight bearing). Adherence to weight-bearing instructions minimizes the chance of loosening of the pins when stress is applied to the bone–pin interface. The external fixator may be removed once the soft tissue heals and there are no signs of infection. The fracture may require additional stabilization by a cast, molded orthosis, or internal fixation while healing.

Ilizarov fixation is a specialized type of external fixator consisting of numerous wires that penetrate the limb and are attached to a circular metal frame. This device is used to correct angulation and rotational defects, to treat nonunion

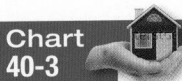

Chart 40-3 · HOME CARE CHECKLIST
The Patient With an External Fixator

At the completion of education, the patient and/or caregiver will be able to:

- State the impact of the musculoskeletal injury/disorder on physiologic functioning, ADLs, IADLs, roles, relationships, and spirituality.
- State rationale for use of external fixation and resulting changes in lifestyle (e.g., activity, exercise, rest) necessary to maintain health and safety.
  - Avoid excessive use of injured extremity.
  - Observe prescribed weight-bearing limits.
  - Demonstrate ability to transfer (e.g., from a bed to a chair) and/or safe use of mobility aid.
  - Demonstrate exercises to promote circulation and minimize disuse syndrome.
- State signs of pin site infection (e.g., redness, tenderness, increased or purulent pin site drainage) to be reported promptly.
- Describe approaches to controlling swelling and pain (e.g., elevate extremity to heart level, take analgesic agents as prescribed).
- Verbalize plan to report pain uncontrolled by elevation and analgesic agents (may be an indicator of impaired tissue perfusion, compartment syndrome, or pin tract infection).

- State indicators of complications to report promptly to primary provider (e.g., uncontrolled swelling and pain; cool, pale fingers or toes; paresthesia; paralysis; purulent drainage; signs of systemic infection; loose fixator pins or clamps).
- State how to reach primary provider with questions or complications
  - State time and date of follow-up appointments and testing
- State the name, dose, side effects, frequency, and schedule for all medications.
- Identify the need for health promotion, disease prevention, and screening activities
- Describe care of extremity after fixator removal (e.g., gradual resumption of normal activities to protect limb from undue stresses).

Resources

See Chapter 10, Chart 10-8 for additional information related to durable medical equipment, adaptive equipment, mobility skills, skin, bowel, and bladder care.

ADL, activities of daily living; IADL, independent activities of daily living.

(failure of bone fragments to heal), and to lengthen limbs. The device gently pulls apart the cortex of the bone and stimulates new growth through daily adjustment of the telescoping rods. The nurse must educate the patient about adjusting the telescoping rods and caring for the pin sites and apparatus, because this fixator can be in place for many months. When discharge is anticipated, the nurse educates the patient or caregiver about how to perform pin site care according to the prescribed protocol (clean technique can be used at home) and to promptly report any signs of pin site infection (Newton-Triggs et al., 2014). The nurse also instructs the patient or family to monitor neurovascular status and report any changes promptly. The patient or family members are instructed to check the integrity of the fixator frame daily and to report loose pins or clamps. A physical therapy referral is helpful in educating the patient how to transfer, use ambulatory aids safely, and adjust to weight-bearing limits and altered gait patterns (see Chart 40-3).

The Patient in Traction

Traction uses a pulling force to promote and maintain alignment to an injured part of the body. The goals of traction include decreasing muscle spasms and pain, realignment of bone fractures, and correcting or preventing deformities. The type of traction, amount of weight, and whether traction can be removed for nursing care must be determined to obtain its therapeutic effects.

At times, traction needs to be applied in more than one direction to achieve the desired line of pull. When this is done, one of the lines of pull counteracts the other. These lines of pull are known as the vectors of force. The actual resultant pulling force is somewhere between the two lines of pull (see Fig. 40-4). The effects of traction are evaluated with x-ray studies, and adjustments are made if necessary.

Traction is used primarily as a short-term intervention until other modalities, such as external or internal fixation,

are possible. These modalities reduce the risk of disuse syndrome and minimize hospital lengths of stay, often allowing the patient to be cared for in the home setting.

Principles of Effective Traction

Whenever traction is applied, countertraction must be used to achieve effective results. Countertraction is the force acting in the opposite direction. Usually, the patient's body weight and bed position adjustments supply the needed countertraction.

When caring for the patient in traction, the nurse should follow these additional principles:
- Traction must be continuous to be effective in reducing and immobilizing fractures.
- Skeletal traction is *never* interrupted.

Figure 40-4 • Traction may be applied in different directions to achieve the desired therapeutic line of pull. Adjustments in applied forces may be prescribed over the course of treatment.

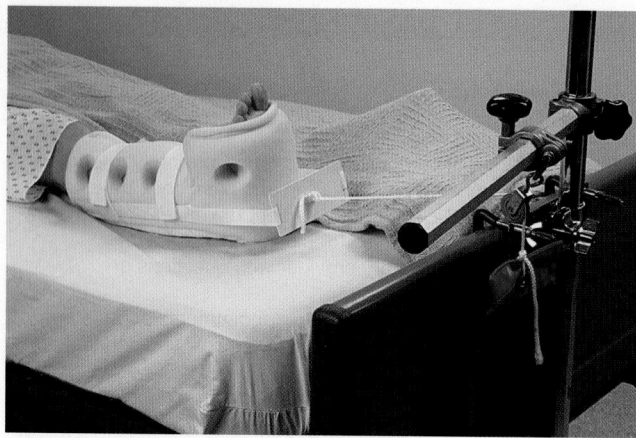

Figure 40-5 • Buck's extension traction. Lower extremity in unilateral Buck's extension traction is aligned in a foam boot and traction applied by the free-hanging weight. The Heelift® Traction Boot is shown here. Photo courtesy of DM Systems, Inc.

- Weights are not removed unless intermittent traction is prescribed.
- Any factor that might reduce the effective pull or alter its resultant line of pull must be eliminated.
- The patient must be in good body alignment in the center of the bed when traction is applied.
- Ropes must be unobstructed.
- Weights must hang freely and not rest on the bed or floor.
- Knots in the rope or the footplate must not touch the pulley or the foot of the bed.

Types of Traction

The use of traction has decreased significantly due to advances in the surgical reduction of fractures, shortened lengths of hospital stay, and research that queries the effectiveness of its use (Newton-Triggs et al., 2014). However, a basic working knowledge of the use of traction is necessary, because some orthopedic surgeons still prescribe traction for their patients (Hajbaghery & Moradi, 2013).

There are several types of traction. *Straight* or *running traction* applies the pulling force in a straight line with the body part resting on the bed. The countertraction is provided by the patient's body and movement can alter the traction provided. Buck's extension traction (discussed later; see Fig. 40-5) is an example of straight traction. *Balanced suspension traction* (see Fig. 40-6) supports the affected extremity off the bed and allows for some patient movement without disruption of the line of pull. With this traction, the countertraction is produced by devices such as slings or splints.

Traction may be applied to the skin (*skin traction*) or directly to the bony skeleton (*skeletal traction*). The mode of application is determined by the purpose of the traction. Traction can be applied with the hands (*manual traction*). This is temporary traction that may be used when applying a cast, giving skin care under a Buck's extension foam boot, or adjusting the traction apparatus.

Skin Traction

Skin traction is used less frequently than in years past; the AAOS (2014) recently reported that there was no reduction in pain or complications associated with its use compared with other standard interventions. Nonetheless, skin traction may be prescribed for short-term use to stabilize a fractured leg, control muscle spasms, and immobilize an area before surgery. The pulling force is applied by weights that are attached to the client with Velcro, tape, straps, boots, or cuffs. The amount of weight applied must not exceed the tolerance of the skin. No more than 2 to 3.5 kg (4.5 to 8 lb) of traction can be used on an extremity. Pelvic traction is usually limited to 4.5 to 9 kg (10 to 20 lb), depending on the weight of the patient.

Types of skin traction used for adults include Buck's extension traction (applied to the lower leg) (described next), the chin halter strap (occasionally used to treat chronic neck pain), and the pelvic belt (sometimes used to treat lower back pain).

Buck's Extension Traction

Buck's extension traction (unilateral or bilateral) is skin traction to the lower leg. The pull is exerted in one plane when partial or temporary immobilization is desired (see Fig. 40-5).

Figure 40-6 • Balanced suspension skeletal traction with Thomas leg splint. The patient can move vertically as long as the resultant line of pull is maintained. Note the use of overhead trapeze.

It is used as a temporary measure to overcome muscle spasms and promote immobilization of hip fractures in adult patients waiting for more definitive treatment such as surgery. However, current data show no direct benefit to using this traction with patients with hip fractures (AAOS, 2014).

Before the traction is applied, the nurse inspects the skin for abrasions and circulatory disturbances. The skin and circulation must be in healthy condition to tolerate the traction. The extremity should be clean and dry before the foam boot or traction tape is applied.

To apply Buck's traction, the extremity is elevated and supported under the patient's heel and knee while the foam boot is placed under the leg, with the patient's heel in the heel of the boot. Next, the Velcro straps are secured around the leg. Traction tape that is overwrapped with an elastic bandage in a spiral fashion may be used instead of the boot. Excessive pressure is avoided over the malleolus and proximal fibula during application to prevent pressure ulcers and nerve damage. The rope is then affixed to the spreader or footplate over a pulley fastened to the end of the bed and attaches the prescribed weight—usually 5 to 8 lb—to the rope. The weight should hang freely, not touching the bed or the floor as this compromises the efficiency of the traction system (Newton-Triggs et al., 2014).

Nursing Interventions

Ensuring Effective Skin Traction

To ensure effective skin traction, it is important to avoid wrinkling and slipping of the traction bandage and to maintain countertraction. Proper positioning must be maintained to keep the leg in a neutral position. To prevent bony fragments from moving against one another, the patient should not turn from side to side; however, the patient may shift position slightly with assistance.

Monitoring and Managing Potential Complications

Skin Breakdown

During the initial assessment, the nurse identifies sensitive, fragile skin (common in older adults). The nurse also inspects the skin area that is in contact with tape, foam, or shearing forces, at least every 8 hours, for signs of irritation or inflammation. The nurse performs the following procedures to monitor and prevent skin breakdown:

- Removes the foam boots to inspect the skin, the ankle, and the Achilles tendon three times a day. A second person is needed to support the extremity during the inspection and skin care.
- Palpates the area of the traction tapes daily to detect underlying tenderness.
- Provides frequent repositioning to alleviate pressure and discomfort, because the patient who must remain in a supine position is at increased risk for development of a pressure ulcer.
- Uses advanced static mattresses or overlays rather than standard hospital foam or alternating-air/low-air-loss mattresses to reduce the risk of pressure ulcer formation (Qaseem, Mir, Starkey, et al., 2015).

Nerve Damage

Skin traction can place pressure on peripheral nerves. Care must be taken to avoid pressure on the peroneal nerve at the point at which it passes around the neck of the fibula just below the knee when traction is applied to the lower extremity. Pressure at this point can cause footdrop. The nurse regularly questions the patient about sensation and asks the patient to move the toes and foot. The nurse should immediately investigate any complaint of a burning sensation under the traction bandage or boot. Dorsiflexion of the foot demonstrates function of the peroneal nerve. Weakness of dorsiflexion or foot movement and inversion of the foot might indicate pressure on the common peroneal nerve. Plantar flexion demonstrates function of the tibial nerve. In addition, the nurse should promptly report altered sensation or impaired motor function.

Circulatory Impairment

After skin traction is applied, the nurse assesses circulation of the foot within 15 to 30 minutes and then every 1 to 2 hours. Circulatory assessment consists of:

- Peripheral pulses, color, capillary refill, and temperature of the fingers or toes.
- Manifestations of deep vein thrombosis (DVT), which include unilateral calf tenderness, warmth, redness, and swelling.

The nurse also encourages the patient to perform active foot exercises every hour when awake.

Skeletal Traction

Skeletal traction is often used when continuous traction is desired to immobilize, position, and align a fracture of the femur, tibia, and cervical spine. It is used when traction is to be maintained for a significant amount of time, when skin traction is not possible, and when greater weight (11 to 18 kg [25 to 40 lb]) is needed to achieve the therapeutic effect. Skeletal traction involves passing a metal pin or wire (e.g., Steinmann pin, Kirschner wire) through the bone (e.g., proximal tibia or distal femur) under local anesthesia, avoiding nerves, blood vessels, muscles, tendons, and joints. Traction is then applied using ropes and weights attached to the end of the pin. Alternatively, skeletal traction may involve the application of tongs to the head that are fixed to the skull to immobilize cervical fractures (see Chapter 68).

The surgeon applies skeletal traction using surgical asepsis. The insertion site is prepared with a surgical scrub agent such as chlorhexidine solution. A local anesthetic agent is given at the insertion site and periosteum. The surgeon makes a small skin incision and drills the sterile pin or wire through the bone. The patient feels pressure during this procedure and possibly some pain when the periosteum is penetrated.

After insertion, the pin or wire is attached to the traction bow or caliper. The ends of the pin or wire are covered with caps to prevent injury to the patient or caregivers. The weights are attached to the pin or wire bow by a rope and pulley system that exerts the appropriate amount and direction of pull for effective traction. The weights applied initially must overcome the shortening spasms of the affected muscles. As the muscles relax, the traction weight is reduced to prevent fracture dislocation and to promote healing.

Often, skeletal traction is balanced traction, which supports the affected extremity, allows for some patient movement, and facilitates patient independence and nursing care while maintaining effective traction. The Thomas splint with a Pearson attachment is frequently used with skeletal traction for fractures of the femur (see Fig. 40-6). Because upward traction is required, an overbed frame is used.

When skeletal traction is discontinued, the extremity is gently supported while the weights are removed. The pin is cut close to the skin and removed by the surgeon. Internal fixation, casts, or splints are then used to immobilize and support the healing bone.

Nursing Interventions

Maintaining Effective Skeletal Traction

When skeletal traction is used, the nurse checks the traction apparatus to see that the ropes are in the wheel grooves of the pulleys, the ropes are not frayed, the weights hang freely, and the knots in the rope are tied securely. The nurse also evaluates the patient's position, because slipping down in bed results in ineffective traction (Zhang, 2015).

> **Quality and Safety Nursing Alert**
>
> *The nurse must never remove weights from skeletal traction unless a life-threatening situation occurs. Removal of the weights defeats their purpose and may result in injury to the patient.*

Maintaining Positioning

The nurse must maintain alignment of the patient's body in traction as prescribed to promote an effective line of pull (Zhang, 2015). The nurse positions the patient's foot to avoid footdrop (plantar flexion), inward rotation (inversion), and outward rotation (eversion). The patient's foot may be supported in a neutral position by orthopedic devices (e.g., foot supports).

If the patient reports severe pain from muscle spasm, the weights may be too heavy or the patient may need realignment. Pain must be reported to the primary provider if body alignment fails to reduce discomfort. Opioid and nonopioid analgesics may be used to control pain. Muscle relaxants may be prescribed to relieve muscles spasms as needed.

Preventing Skin Breakdown

The patient's elbows frequently become sore, and nerve injury may occur if the patient repositions by pushing on the elbows. In addition, patients frequently push on the heel of the unaffected leg when they raise themselves. This digging of the heel into the mattress may injure the tissues. It is important to instruct patients not to use their heels or elbows to push themselves up in bed (Levin & Morris, 2013). To encourage movement without using the elbows or heel, a **trapeze** can be suspended overhead within easy reach of the patient (see Fig. 40-6). The trapeze helps the patient move about in bed and move on and off the bedpan. Transparent film, hydrocolloid dressings, or skin sealants may also be applied to bony prominences (such as elbows) or critical areas to decrease the force of shearing and friction (Clark, Black, Alves, et al., 2014).

Specific pressure points are assessed for irritation and inflammation at least every 8 hours. Patients at high risk for skin breakdown (e.g., older adults, malnourished patients) may need to be assessed more frequently (Call, Pedersen, Bill, et al., 2015). Areas that are particularly vulnerable to pressure caused by a traction apparatus applied to the lower extremity include the ischial tuberosity, popliteal space, Achilles tendon, and heel. If the patient is not permitted to turn on one side or the other, the nurse must make a special effort to provide back care and to keep the bed dry and free of crumbs and wrinkles. The patient can assist by holding the overhead trapeze and raising the hips off the bed. If the patient cannot do this, the nurse can push down on the mattress with one hand to relieve pressure on the back and bony prominences and to provide for some shifting of weight. Advanced static mattresses or overlays should be used rather than foam or alternating-air/low-air-loss mattresses to reduce the risk of pressure ulcer formation (Qaseem et al., 2015). The patient's heel should be placed on a pillow or heel suspension device to keep the heel from the bed's surface (Baath, Engstrom, Gunningberg, et al., 2016).

For change of bed linens, the patient raises the torso while caregivers on both sides of the bed roll down and replace the upper mattress sheet. Then, as the patient raises the buttocks off the mattress, the sheets are slid under the buttocks. Finally, the lower section of the bed linens is replaced while the patient rests on the back. Sheets and blankets are placed over the patient in such a way that the traction is not disrupted.

Monitoring Neurovascular Status

The nurse evaluates the body part to be placed in traction and compares its neurovascular status (e.g., color, temperature, capillary refill, edema, pulses, ability to move, and sensations) to the unaffected extremity every hour for the first 24 hours after traction is applied and every 4 hours thereafter. The nurse instructs the patient to report any changes in sensation or movement immediately so that they can be promptly evaluated. Venous thromboembolus (VTE) formation is a significant risk for the immobilized patient. The nurse encourages the patient to do active flexion–extension ankle exercises and isometric contraction of the calf muscles (calf-pumping exercises) 10 times an hour while awake to decrease venous stasis. In addition, antiembolism stockings, compression devices, and anticoagulant therapy may be prescribed to help prevent thrombus formation.

> **Quality and Safety Nursing Alert**
>
> *The nurse must immediately investigate every report of discomfort expressed by the patient in traction. Prompt recognition of a developing neurovascular problem is essential so that corrective measures can be instituted quickly.*

Providing Pin Site Care

The wound at the pin insertion site requires attention, and it is important to follow the facility's specific policy pertaining to skeletal pin care. The goal is to avoid infection and development of osteomyelitis (see Chapter 41). For the first 48 hours after insertion, the site is covered with a sterile absorbent nonstick dressing and a rolled gauze or Ace-type bandage. After this time, a loose cover dressing or no dressing is recommended (a bandage is necessary if the patient is exposed to airborne dust). Evidence-based recommendations (Smith & Dahlen, 2013) for pin site care include the following:

- Pins located in areas with soft tissue are at greatest risk for infection.
- After the first 48 to 72 hours following skeletal pin placement, pin site care should be performed daily or weekly.

- Chlorhexidine 2 mg/mL solution is the most effective cleansing solution. If chlorhexidine is contraindicated (due to known sensitivity or skin reaction), saline solution should be used for cleansing.
- Strict handwashing before and after skeletal pin site care should always take place.

The nurse must inspect the pin sites every 8 hours for reaction (i.e., normal changes that occur at the pin site after insertion) and infection. Signs of reaction may include redness, warmth, and serosanguineous drainage at the site, which tend to subside after 72 hours. Signs of infection may mirror those of reaction but also include the presence of purulent drainage, pin loosening, tenting of skin at pin site, odor, and fever. Prophylactic broad-spectrum IV antibiotics may be given for 24 to 48 hours postinsertion to prevent infection; however, the evidence is confounding and there is no general consensus on the advisability of this practice (Smith & Dahlen, 2013). Minor infections may be readily treated with antibiotics, and infections that result in systemic manifestations may additionally warrant pin removal until the infection resolves.

> ### ◤ Quality and Safety Nursing Alert
> *The nurse must inspect the pin site at least every 8 hours for signs of inflammation and evidence of infection.*

Due to a lack of evidence-based research findings, controversy exists about skeletal pin care, showering, and the use of massage to release skin adherence to pins. Some evidence suggests that crusting at the pin site should be retained as long as the pin site remains uninfected as the retained crusts provides a natural barrier from bacterial contamination (Britten, Ghoz, Duffield, et al., 2013). The patient and family should be taught to perform any prescribed pin site care prior to discharge from the hospital and should be provided with written follow-up instructions that include the signs and symptoms of infection.

Promoting Exercise

Patient exercises, within the therapeutic limits of the traction, assist in maintaining muscle strength and tone, and in promoting circulation. Active exercises include pulling up on the trapeze, flexing and extending the feet, and range-of-motion and weight-resistance exercises for noninvolved joints. Isometric exercises of the immobilized extremity (quadriceps and gluteal setting exercises) are important for maintaining strength in major ambulatory muscles (see Chart 40-1). Without exercise, the patient will lose muscle mass and strength, and rehabilitation will be greatly prolonged.

Nursing Management

Assessing Anxiety

The nurse must consider the psychological and physiologic impact of the musculoskeletal problem, traction device, and immobility. Traction restricts mobility and independence. The equipment can look threatening, and its application can be frightening. Confusion, disorientation, and behavioral problems may develop in patients who are confined in a limited space for an extended time. Therefore, the nurse must assess and monitor the patient's anxiety level and psychological responses to traction.

Assisting With Self-Care

Initially, the patient may require assistance with self-care activities. The nurse helps the patient eat, bathe, dress, and toilet. Convenient arrangement of items such as the telephone, tissues, water, and assistive devices (e.g., reachers, overbed trapeze) may facilitate self-care. With resumption of self-care activities, the patient feels less dependent and less frustrated and experiences improved self-esteem. Because some assistance is required throughout the period of immobility, the nurse and the patient can creatively develop routines that maximize the patient's independence.

Monitoring and Managing Potential Complications

Immobility-related complications may include pressure ulcers (see Chapter 10), atelectasis, pneumonia, constipation, loss of appetite, urinary stasis, urinary tract infections, and VTE formation. Early identification of pre-existing or developing conditions facilitates prompt interventions to resolve them.

Atelectasis and Pneumonia

The nurse auscultates the patient's lungs every 4 to 8 hours to assess respiratory status and educates the patient about performing deep breathing and coughing exercises to aid in fully expanding the lungs and clearing pulmonary secretions. If the patient history and baseline assessment indicate that the patient is at risk for development of respiratory complications, specific therapies (e.g., the use of an incentive spirometer) may be indicated. If a respiratory complication develops, prompt institution of prescribed therapy is needed.

Constipation and Anorexia

Reduced gastrointestinal motility results in constipation and anorexia. A diet high in fiber and fluids may help stimulate gastric motility. If constipation develops, therapeutic measures may include stool softeners, laxatives, suppositories, and enemas. To improve the patient's appetite, the patient's food preferences are included, as appropriate, within the prescribed therapeutic diet.

Urinary Stasis and Infection

Incomplete emptying of the bladder related to positioning in bed can result in urinary stasis and infection. In addition, the patient may find the use of a bedpan uncomfortable and may limit fluids to minimize the frequency of urination. The nurse monitors the fluid intake and the character of the urine. Adequate hydration is important; therefore, the nurse instructs the patient to consume adequate amounts of fluid and to void every 3 to 4 hours. If the patient exhibits signs or symptoms of urinary tract infection (e.g., burning or pain on urination, hematuria), the nurse notifies the primary provider.

Venous Thromboembolism

Venous stasis that predisposes the patient to VTE occurs with immobility. The nurse educates the patient about how to perform ankle and foot exercises within the limits of the traction therapy every 1 to 2 hours when awake to prevent DVT. Involving family members in performing these exercises can increase adherence and promote the family's involvement with the patient's care (Miller & Walsh, 2015). The patient is encouraged to drink fluids to prevent dehydration and associated hemoconcentration, which contribute to stasis. The nurse monitors the patient for signs of DVT, including unilateral calf tenderness, warmth, redness, and swelling (increased calf circumference). The nurse promptly reports findings to the primary provider for evaluation and therapy.

During traction therapy, the nurse encourages the patient to exercise muscles and joints that are not in traction to prevent deterioration, deconditioning, and venous stasis. The physical therapist can design bed exercises that minimize loss of muscle strength. During the patient's exercise, the nurse ensures that traction forces are maintained and that the patient is properly positioned to prevent complications resulting from poor alignment.

The Patient Undergoing Orthopedic Surgery

Many patients with musculoskeletal dysfunction undergo surgery to correct the condition. Conditions that may be corrected by surgery include unstable fractures, deformity, joint disease, necrotic or infected tissue, and tumors. Frequent surgical procedures include open reduction with internal fixation (ORIF) and closed reduction with internal fixation (fracture fragments are not surgically exposed) for fractures; arthroplasty, meniscectomy, and joint replacement for joint conditions; amputation for severe extremity conditions (e.g., gangrene, massive trauma); bone graft for joint stabilization, defect filling, or stimulation of bone healing; and tendon transfer for improving motion. The goals include improving function by restoring motion and stability and relieving pain and disability. Chart 40-4 describes common orthopedic surgeries.

Chart 40-4 **Common Orthopedic Surgical Procedures**

Open reduction: Correction and alignment of the fracture after surgical dissection and exposure of the fracture

Internal fixation: Stabilization of the reduced fracture by the use of metal screws, plates, wires, nails, and pins

Arthroplasty: Repair of joint problems through the operating arthroscope (an instrument that allows the surgeon to operate within a joint without a large incision) or through open joint surgery

Hemiarthroplasty: Replacement of one of the articular surfaces (e.g., in a hip hemiarthroplasty, the femoral head and neck are replaced with a femoral prosthesis—the acetabulum is not replaced)

Joint arthroplasty or replacement: Replacement of joint surfaces with metal or synthetic materials

Total joint arthroplasty or replacement: Replacement of both articular surfaces within a joint with metal or synthetic materials

Meniscectomy: Excision of damaged joint fibrocartilage

Amputation: Removal of a body part

Bone graft: Placement of bone tissue (autologous or homologous grafts) to promote healing, to stabilize, or to replace diseased bone

Tendon transfer: Insertion of tendon to improve function

Fasciotomy: Incision and diversion of the muscle fascia to relieve muscle constriction, as in compartment syndrome, or to reduce fascia contracture

---

Indications for a surgical procedure are based on the patient's age, underlying orthopedic condition, and general physical health and the impact of disability on daily activities. Timing of these procedures is important to ensure maximum function. In general, surgery should be performed before surrounding muscles become contracted and atrophied and serious structural abnormalities occur.

Despite advances in surgical and anesthetic techniques as well as blood conservation strategies, orthopedic surgery is still associated with perioperative bleeding, and many patients require blood transfusions (Park, Rasouli, Mortazavi, et al., 2013). Acute postoperative anemia due to perioperative blood loss frequently occurs in patients undergoing total joint replacement and has been found to occur in up to 50% of patients who had routine total hip and knee arthroplasties (Rasouli, Maltenfort, Erkocak, et al., 2016). A blood loss of up to 1500 mL during the procedure may be anticipated; therefore, several units of typed and cross-matched blood (allogeneic blood) should be available. Because most orthopedic surgeries are elective procedures, many patients may donate their own blood (autologous blood) during the weeks preceding their surgery. Autologous blood donations are cost-effective and eliminate many of the risks of transfusion therapy (see Chapter 32); however, recent evidence suggests that autologous donations may lower preoperative hemoglobin levels and therefore increase the need for allogeneic blood transfusions (Hazel, Bern, Reilly, et al., 2015; Park et al., 2013).

A proactive approach to blood management in orthopedic surgery aims to reduce the need for allogeneic blood transfusions, which eliminates the associated complications of transfusion (Liu, 2015) (see Chapter 32). One approach to minimize blood loss during orthopedic limb surgery (e.g., total knee arthroplasty [TKA]) is the application of a pneumatic tourniquet (Unver, Karatosun, & Tuncalli, 2013). The tourniquet may be used intraoperatively to prevent bleeding and to maintain a clean surgical field. Although this technique may decrease the time needed for the operation and enables the surgeon to visualize the surgical field, the evidence is conflicting about how and when to use the tourniquet, whether bleeding is reduced, and whether its use has any effect on postoperative rehabilitation and recovery (Dennis, Kittleson, Yang, et al., 2016). Intraoperative red blood cell salvage with reinfusion is used when a large volume of blood loss is anticipated. A promising intervention to decrease total blood loss and reduce the need for allogeneic blood transfusions without an increase in surgical complications is the administration of intraoperative thrombolytics such as tranexamic acid (TXA) (Lee, 2016; Suggs & Holt, 2015; Zhou, Tao, Li, et al., 2013). Postoperative red blood cell salvage with intermittent autotransfusion also reduces the need for blood transfusions.

Joint Replacement

Patients with severe joint pain and disability may undergo joint replacement. Conditions contributing to joint degeneration include osteoarthritis, rheumatoid arthritis, trauma, and congenital deformity. Some fractures (e.g., femoral neck fracture) may cause disruption of the blood supply and subsequent **avascular necrosis** (death of tissue due to insufficient blood supply); management with joint replacement

Figure 40-7 • Examples of hip and knee replacement.

Acetabular (pelvic) component

Femoral (proximal) component

Femoral (distal) component

Tibial component

the femoral component is inserted without cement, and the tibial and patellar components are inserted with cement. Use of each of these materials and techniques have different benefits and risks. Current research evidence supports the use of either component fixation methods (cemented or cementless) because postoperative functional outcomes, rates of complications, and rates of reoperations are similar (AAOS, 2015b; Karachalios & Antoniou, 2015). Identifying patient-specific factors that may inform the decision to utilize a particular fixation technique is important. Considerations include gender, age, diagnosis, weight and activity level as well as the presence of healthy bone with adequate blood supply (Khan, Osman, Green, et al., 2016). Issues of cost and cost-effectiveness should also be considered (Mullaji & Shetty, 2015).

With joint replacement, patients may expect pain relief, return of joint motion, and improved functional status and quality of life. The scope of these improvements depends in part on patients' preoperative soft tissue condition and general muscle strength. Serious complications seldom occur, and recent innovations in total joint replacement surgery have made this a safer and more routinely performed surgery (AAOS, 2015b). In fact, minimally invasive surgical techniques, biomaterials, postoperative rehabilitation protocols, and multimodal analgesia strategies have led to earlier hospital discharge and quicker recovery (Lee, 2016). The American Joint Replacement Registry (AJRR) monitors the performance of devices and evaluates the cost-effectiveness of procedures. The data generated from the AJRR can provide orthopedic researchers and practitioners with the information necessary to improve the quality of health care among patients in need of knee and hip replacement procedures (Dy, Bumpass, Makhni, et al., 2016; Smith & Smith, 2012).

Nursing Interventions

Assessment of the patient and preoperative management are aimed at having the patient in optimal health at the time of surgery (see Chapter 17). If a patient is at risk for postoperative bleeding or is anemic, epoetin alfa (Epogen, Procrit) or iron supplements (e.g., ferrous sulfate) may be prescribed preoperatively to increase hemoglobin (Loftus, Spratling, Stone, et al., 2016).

Preventing Deep Vein Thrombosis

Patients having orthopedic surgery are particularly at risk for VTE, including DVT and pulmonary embolism (PE). Therefore, factors that compound or further increase this risk are assessed preoperatively. Increasing age (older than age 40), obesity, taking prescription hormonal medications, preoperative leg edema, previous history of any VTE, and varicose veins increase the risk for postoperative DVT and PE (Miller & Walsh, 2015). The use of medications that increase the risk of clotting, such as certain hormones and nonsteroidal anti-inflammatory drugs (NSAIDs), may be discontinued a week before surgery. Prophylactic low–molecular-weight heparin (LMWH) or another anticoagulant agent may be prescribed prior to or after surgery (Miller & Walsh, 2015). Intermittent pneumatic compression devices should be applied intraoperatively or immediately postoperatively (Lee, 2016).

may be elected over ORIF. Joints frequently replaced include the hip, knee (see Fig. 40-7), and finger joints. More complex joints (shoulder, elbow, wrist, ankle) are replaced less frequently.

Joint arthroplasty refers to the surgical removal of an unhealthy joint and replacement of joint surfaces with metal or synthetic materials. Total joint arthroplasty, also known as total joint replacement, involves the replacement of all components of an articulating joint. Most joint replacements consist of metal (e.g., stainless steel, cobalt-chromium, titanium) and high-density polyethylene components. In order to achieve fixation of components, the material can be cemented, cementless, or a hybrid of both of these materials. Cemented fixation uses a fast-curing bone cement (polymethylmethacrylate [PMMA]) to hold implants in place. Cementless fixation relies on new bone growing into the surface of the implant by using a press-fit, porous-coated prosthesis. There is also a hybrid fixation technique for TKA where

Assessing the neurovascular status of the extremity undergoing joint replacement is important, because postoperative assessment data are compared with preoperative assessment data to identify changes and any arterial impairment to the affected extremity. For example, an absent pulse postoperatively is of concern unless the pulse was also absent preoperatively. Nerve palsy could occur as a result of surgery.

Preventing Infection

Preoperative assessment of the patient for recent or active infections, including urinary tract infection, is necessary because of the risk for postoperative infection. Any infection presenting 2 to 4 weeks before planned surgery may result in postponement of surgery. Preoperative skin preparations, such as showers with antiseptic soap, are recommended the evening before and the morning of surgery (Smith & Dahlen, 2013). Scrubbing of the surgical site with a prescribed antiseptic soap the night before or on the morning of surgery decreases bacterial count on the skin and helps lower the chance of infection.

Research findings suggest that prophylactic broad-spectrum antibiotics given 60 minutes prior to skin incision and discontinued within 24 hours postoperatively are effective in preventing surgical site infections (Wu, Chen, Wang, et al., 2016). If antibiotics are given too early (60 or more minutes before surgery), the patient's risk for infection may increase. An important consideration in total knee replacements is that the antibiotic should ideally be infused 10 minutes prior to tourniquet inflation

(Smith & Dahlen, 2013). In addition to timely antibiotic prophylaxis, the use of antibiotic-loaded bone cement and preoperative nasal swabbing to screen for patients who are carriers of methicillin-resistant *Staphylococcus aureus* (MRSA) or methicillin-sensitive *Staphylococcus aureus* (MSSA) may help in further reducing postoperative infections; the effectiveness of these modalities is under research (Bosco, Bookman, Slover, et al., 2015; Smith & Dahlen, 2013).

Culture of the joint during surgery may be important in identifying and treating subsequent infections. If osteomyelitis develops, it is difficult to treat (see Chapter 41). Persistent infection at the site of the prosthesis usually requires removal of the implant and joint revision. It is not always possible to achieve a functional joint when the reconstruction procedure has to be repeated.

Managing Pain

Assessment of the patient's pain preoperatively and any cultural and personal preferences are important components related to the control of pain following joint surgery. Assessing the patient's level of understanding of the surgery and explaining what to expect in the postoperative period (e.g., incentive spirometry, pain control methods, activity limits) can improve outcomes. In particular, research findings suggest that patients who attend structured preoperative education classes report feeling better prepared for surgery and better able to control their pain after surgery (Louw, Diener, Butler, et al., 2013) (see Chart 40-5) (see Chapter 12).

Chart 40-5 | **NURSING RESEARCH PROFILE**

Guided Imagery for Pain Relief after Total Knee Replacement

Draucker, C., Jacobson, A. F., Umberger, W. A., et al. (2015). Acceptability of a guided imagery intervention for persons undergoing a total knee replacement *Orthopaedic Nursing, 34*(6), 356–364.

Purpose

Complementary health modalities with mind–body approaches can be valid and effective adjuncts used by the patient with orthopedic conditions. Guided imagery (GI), the generation of positive sensory and affective images to promote healing outcomes, has been shown to be an effective intervention for the reduction of pain and anxiety in patients having orthopedic surgery. Despite its popularity, little is known about the acceptability of the intervention. The purpose of this study was to describe the perceptions of patients undergoing total knee replacement (TKR) surgery regarding the acceptability of a customized GI intervention to promote TKR outcomes.

Design

This study was part of a larger mixed-methods study involving a randomized controlled trial (RCT) to evaluate a GI intervention for patients undergoing TKR. Eighty-two participants were randomly assigned to receive a GI (n = 42) or placebo (audiobook) (n = 40) intervention. Eligible participants were recruited from an orthopedic practice that performs a large volume of total joint replacements using a standardized approach. Participants who met the inclusion criteria (first-time TKR; no history of autoimmune disease or steroid use; no current use of GI; body mass index <40; no sensory or cognitive impairment) were randomly assigned to the treatment (GI) or control (audiobook) intervention. For this study, only narrative and interview data were analyzed to assess

the acceptability of the intervention from only the individuals that experienced the GI intervention.

Findings

Overall, most participants were generally satisfied and felt actively engaged with the GI intervention. Participants specifically liked the content of the GI messages and appreciated hearing that their pain before and after surgery was temporary. The majority of participants in the study described that the GI intervention improved relaxation, enhanced pain management, and improved outlook and mood during the pre-, intra-, and postoperative time periods. Many participants reported being engaged with the intervention and enjoyed it; very few individuals were nonadherent or dropped out of the study. A smaller subgroup of participants did not find the intervention to be acceptable and described their reasons for dissatisfaction and disengagement. One aspect of the intervention that the participants did not find satisfactory was that the CDs were too repetitious. These comments provide helpful information for refining the intervention in the future.

Nursing Implications

The results of this study suggest that the utilization of a GI intervention is an acceptable approach to promote positive outcomes for patients undergoing TKR. The qualitative findings enhanced the understanding of the participants' experience. The findings of this study may be useful as nurses can play a pivotal role in helping patients understand complementary therapies that can help them recover from orthopedic surgery. A tailored GI intervention to meet individual patient needs and preferences warrants further research.

Total Hip Arthroplasty

Total hip arthroplasty (THA) is the replacement of a severely damaged hip with an artificial joint. Indications for this surgery include osteoarthritis, rheumatoid arthritis, femoral neck fractures (i.e., hip fracture), failure of previous reconstructive surgeries, such as a failed prosthesis with **osteotomy** (surgical cutting of the bone), and conditions resulting from developmental dysplasia or Legg–Calvé–Perthes disease (avascular necrosis of the hip in childhood). A variety of total hip prostheses are available. Most consist of a metal femoral component topped by a spherical ball made of metal, ceramic, or plastic that is fitted into a plastic or metal acetabular socket (see Fig. 40-7).

The surgeon selects the prosthesis that is best suited to the individual patient, considering various factors including skeletal structure and activity level. The patient has irreversibly damaged hip joints, and the potential benefits, including improved quality of life, outweigh the surgical risks. With the advent of improved prosthetic materials and operative techniques, the life of the prosthesis has been extended, and today younger patients with severely damaged and painful hip joints are undergoing total hip replacement.

Nursing Interventions

The nurse must be aware of and monitor for specific potential complications associated with THA. Complications that may occur include dislocation of the hip prosthesis, excessive wound drainage, VTE, infection, and heel pressure ulcer (see Chart 40-6). The nurse also monitors for complications associated with immobility. Long-term complications include **heterotopic ossification** (formation of bone in the periprosthetic space), avascular necrosis, and loosening of the prosthesis.

Gerontologic Considerations

The older adult patient who has had THA merits special postoperative care considerations. Early THA surgery for hip fractures (within 24 to 36 hours) is recommended for most patients once a medical assessment has been made and the patient's condition has been stabilized appropriately. If there are no contraindications (e.g., history of a bleeding disorder), these patients should receive LMWH for DVT prophylaxis; mechanical devices should be used for patients in whom anticoagulants and antiplatelet agents are contraindicated. Providing an appropriate postoperative analgesic regimen for older adults can be challenging in the presence of impaired cognition, medical comorbidities, and possible drug interactions. Consulting with a pain management specialist to specifically tailor the analgesic type and dose may be helpful (see Chapter 12).

All older adult patients' post-THA should be placed on a higher-specification, foam pressure-relieving mattress rather than a standard hospital mattress (Qaseem et al., 2015). A major goal following surgery in this patient population is early mobilization, in an effort to prevent the complications associated with prolonged immobility and to return the patient to functional activity (Mohanty, Rosenthal, Russell, et al., 2016). Early assisted mobilization and ambulation on the day of surgery can decrease hospital length of stay, complications, and hospital costs and can prepare patients to care for themselves at home with a higher level of independent

functioning (Yager & Stichler, 2015). Patients who are assigned to restricted hip precautions have slower rehabilitation and return to usual ADLs (Barnsley, Barnsley, & Page, 2015).

Preventing Dislocation of the Hip Prosthesis

For patients undergoing a posterior or posterolateral approach for THA, maintenance of the femoral head component in the acetabular cup is essential. The risk for dislocation is more common with this approach and may occur when the hip is in full flexion, adducted (legs together), and internally rotated. Therefore, correct positioning is maintained at all times. The patient should be in a supine position with their head slightly elevated and the affected leg in a neutral position. The use of an abduction splint, a wedge pillow (see Fig. 40-8), or two or three pillows placed between the legs prevent adduction beyond the midline of the body. A cradle boot may be used to prevent leg rotation and to support the heel off the bed, preventing development of a pressure ulcer (Hanna-Bull, 2015). When the nurse turns the patient in bed to the unaffected side, it is important to keep the operative hip in **abduction** (movement away from the center or median line of the body). The patient should not be turned to the operative side, which could cause dislocation, unless specified by the surgeon.

The patient's hip is never flexed more than 90 degrees. When using a fracture bedpan, the nurse instructs the patient to flex the unaffected hip and to use the trapeze to lift the pelvis onto the pan. The patient is also reminded not to flex the affected hip.

Limited flexion is maintained during transfers and when sitting. When the patient is initially assisted out of bed, an abduction splint or pillows are kept between the legs. The nurse encourages the patient to keep the affected hip in extension, instructing the patient to pivot on the unaffected leg with assistance by the nurse, who protects the affected hip from **adduction** (movement toward the center or median line of the body), flexion, internal or external rotation, and excessive weight bearing.

High-seat (orthopedic) chairs with arm rests, semi-reclining chairs, and raised toilet seats are used to minimize hip joint flexion. When sitting, the patient's hips should be higher than the knees. The patient's affected leg should not be elevated when sitting. The patient may flex the knee.

The nurse educates the patient about protective positioning, which includes maintaining abduction and avoiding internal and external rotation, hyperextension, and acute flexion, as described previously. At no time should the patient cross their legs or bend at the waist past 90 degrees (e.g., to put on shoes and socks). Occupational therapists can provide the patient with devices to assist with dressing below the waist. Hip precautions for patients who had a posterior or posterolateral approach for THA should be enforced for 4 months or longer after surgery (see Chart 40-7). A patient who has had an anterior surgical approach may not need these precautions. Several studies have reported an anterolateral approach to THA results in a lower rate of dislocation than a posterior approach owing to its ease of access, superior visualization, and a predictable healing pattern. Using a less restrictive mobility protocol in these patients can lead to earlier and better resumption of ADL, earlier return to work, a *(text continued on page 1151)*

Chart 40-6

PLAN OF NURSING CARE

The Patient With a Total Hip Arthroplasty

NURSING DIAGNOSIS: Acute pain related to total hip arthroplasty
GOAL: Relief of pain

Nursing Interventions	Rationale	Expected Outcomes
1. Assess patient for pain using a standard pain intensity scale.	1. Pain is expected after a surgical procedure because of the surgical trauma and tissue response. Muscle spasms occur after total hip replacements. Immobility causes discomfort at pressure points.	• Describes discomfort • Expresses confidence in efforts to control pain • States pain is reduced; pain intensity scores are decreasing • Appears comfortable and relaxed • Uses physical, psychological, and pharmacologic measures to reduce pain and discomfort
2. Ask patient to describe discomfort.	2. Pain characteristics may help to determine the cause of discomfort. Pain may be due to complications (hematoma, infection, dislocation). Pain is an individual experience—it means different things to different people.	
3. Acknowledge existence of pain; inform patient of available analgesic agents or muscle relaxants.	3. The nurse can reduce the stress experienced by patient by communicating concern and availability of assistance to help the patient deal with the pain.	
a. Use pain-modifying techniques. Administer analgesic agents as prescribed.	a. Patient will require parenteral opioids during the first 24–48 hours and then will progress to oral analgesic agents.	
b. Change position within prescribed limits.	b. The use of pillows to provide adequate support and relief of pressure on bony prominences assists in minimizing pain.	
c. Modify environment.	c. Interactions with others, distractions, and sensory overload or deprivation may affect pain experience.	
d. Notify primary provider about persistent pain.	d. Surgical intervention may be necessary if pain is due to hematoma or excessive edema.	
4. Evaluate and record discomfort and effectiveness of pain-modifying techniques.	4. Effectiveness of action is based on experience; data provide a baseline about pain experiences, pain management, and pain relief.	

NURSING DIAGNOSIS: Impaired physical mobility related to positioning, weight bearing, and activity restrictions after total hip arthroplasty
GOAL: Achieves pain-free, functional, stable hip joint

Nursing Interventions	Rationale	Expected Outcomes
1. Maintain proper positioning of hip joint (abduction, neutral rotation, limited flexion).	1. Prevents dislocation of hip prosthesis.	• Maintains prescribed position • No heel pressure • Assists in position changes • Shows increased independence in transfers • Exercises hourly while awake • Participates in progressive ambulation program • Actively participates in exercise regimen • Uses ambulatory aids correctly and safely
2. Keep pressure off heel.	2. Prevents pressure ulcer on heel.	
3. Instruct and assist in position changes and transfers.	3. Encourages patient's active participation while preventing dislocation.	
4. Instruct and supervise isometric quadriceps and gluteal setting exercises.	4. Strengthens muscles needed for walking.	
5. In consultation with physical therapist, instruct and supervise progressive safe ambulation within limitations of weight-bearing prescription.	5. Amount of weight bearing depends on patient's condition and prosthesis; ambulatory aids are used to assist the patient with non–weight-bearing and partial weight-bearing ambulation.	
6. Offer encouragement and support exercise regimen.	6. Reconditioning exercises can be uncomfortable and fatiguing; encouragement helps patient comply with exercise program.	
7. Instruct and supervise safe use of ambulatory aids.	7. Prevents injury from unsafe use and prevents falls.	

Chart 40-6

PLAN OF NURSING CARE (Continued)
The Patient With a Total Hip Arthroplasty

COLLABORATIVE PROBLEMS: Hemorrhage; neurovascular compromise; dislocation of prosthesis; deep vein thrombosis; infection related to surgery
GOAL: Absence of complications

Nursing Interventions	Rationale	Expected Outcomes
Hemorrhage		
1. Monitor vital signs, observing for shock.	1. Changes in pulse, blood pressure, and respirations may indicate development of shock. Blood loss and stress of surgery may contribute to development of shock.	• Vital signs stabilize within normal limits • Amount of drainage decreases • No bright-red bloody drainage • Hematology values are within normal limits.
2. Note character and amount of drainage.	2. Within 48 hours, bloody drainage collected in portable suction device, if in use, should decrease to 25–30 mL per 8 hours. Excessive drainage (>250 mL in first 8 hours after surgery) and bright-red drainage may indicate active bleeding.	
3. Notify primary provider if patient develops shock or excessive bleeding, and prepare for administration of fluids, blood component therapy, and medications.	3. Corrective measures need to be instituted.	
4. Monitor hemoglobin and hematocrit values.	4. Anemia due to blood loss may develop. Blood replacement or iron supplementation may be needed.	
Neurovascular Dysfunction		
1. Assess affected extremity for color and temperature.	1. The skin becomes pale and feels cool with decreased tissue perfusion. Venous congestion may produce cyanosis.	• Color normal • Extremity warm • Normal capillary refill • Moderate edema and swelling; tissue not palpably tense • Pain controllable • No pain with passive dorsiflexion • Normal sensations • No paresthesia • Normal motor abilities • No paresis or paralysis • Pulses strong and equal
2. Assess toes for capillary refill response.	2. After compression of the nail, rapid return of pink color indicates good capillary perfusion.	
3. Assess extremity for edema and swelling. Report patient complaints of leg tightness.	3. The trauma of surgery will cause edema. Excessive swelling and hematoma formation can compromise circulation and function.	
4. Elevate lower extremity. Keep elevated extremity lower than hip when in chair.	4. Minimizes dependent edema. Hip is never flexed more than 90 degrees to prevent dislocation.	
5. Assess for deep, throbbing, unrelenting pain.	5. Surgical pain can be controlled; pain due to neurovascular compromise is not relieved by treatment.	
6. Assess for pain on passive flexion of foot.	6. With nerve ischemia, there will be pain on passive stretch. Additionally, pain or tenderness may indicate deep vein thrombosis.	
7. Assess for change in sensations and numbness.	7. Diminished pain and sensory function may indicate nerve damage. Sensation in web between great and second toe—peroneal nerve; sensation on sole of foot—tibial nerve.	
8. Assess ability to move foot and toes.	8. Dorsiflexion of ankle and extension of toes indicate function of peroneal nerve. Plantar flexion of ankle and flexion of toes indicate function of tibial nerve.	
9. Assess pedal pulses in both feet.	9. Indicator of extremity circulation	
10. Notify surgeon if altered neurovascular status is noted.	10. Function of extremity needs to be preserved.	

(continued on page 1150)

Chart 40-6

PLAN OF NURSING CARE (Continued)

The Patient With a Total Hip Arthroplasty

Interventions	Rationale	Expected Outcomes
Dislocation of Prosthesis 1. Position patient as prescribed. 2. Use abductor splint or pillows to maintain position and to support extremity. 3. Support leg and place pillows between legs when patient is turning and side-lying; turn to the unaffected side. 4. Avoid acute flexion of hip (head of bed ≤90 degrees). 5. Avoid crossing legs. 6. Assess for dislocation of prosthesis (extremity shortens, internally or externally rotated, severe hip pain, patient unable to move extremity). 7. Notify surgeon of possible dislocation.	1. Hip component positioning (femoral component in acetabular component) needs to be maintained. 2. Keeps hip in abduction and in a neutral rotation to prevent dislocation. 3. Prevent dislocation. 4. Findings may indicate dislocation of prosthesis. 5. Joint dislocations compromise neurovascular status and future function of extremity.	• Prosthesis not dislocated • Adheres to recommendations to prevent dislocation
Deep Vein Thrombosis 1. Use antiembolism stocking and sequential compression device as prescribed. 2. Remove stocking for 20 minutes twice a day and provide skin care. 3. Assess popliteal, dorsalis pedis, and posterior tibial pulses. 4. Assess skin temperature of legs. 5. Assess for unilateral calf pain or tenderness every 8 hours. 6. Avoid pressure on popliteal blood vessels from equipment (e.g., abductor splint straps, sequential compression stockings) or pillows. 7. Change position and increase activity as prescribed. 8. Supervise ankle exercises hourly. 9. Monitor body temperature. 10. Encourage fluids.	1. Aids in venous blood return and prevents stasis. 2. Skin care is necessary to avoid breakdown. Extended removal of stocking defeats purpose of stocking. 3. Pulses indicate arterial perfusion of extremity. 4. Local inflammation will increase local skin temperature. 5. Pain or tenderness may indicate deep vein thrombosis. 6. Compression of blood vessels diminishes blood flow. 7. Activity promotes circulation and diminishes venous stasis. 8. Muscle exercise promotes circulation. 9. Body temperature increases with inflammation. 10. Dehydration increases blood viscosity.	• Wears antiembolism stocking; uses compression device • No skin breakdown • Pulses equal and strong • Skin temperature normal • No calf pain or tenderness • Changes position with assistance and supervision • Participates in exercise regimen • Well hydrated • No chest pain; lungs clear to auscultation; no evidence of pulmonary emboli
Infection 1. Monitor vital signs. 2. Use aseptic technique for dressing changes and emptying of portable drainage. 3. Assess wound appearance and character of drainage. 4. Assess complaints of pain. 5. Administer prophylactic antibiotics if prescribed, and observe for side effects.	1. Temperature, pulse, and respirations increase in response to infection. (Magnitude of response may be minimal in older adults.) 2. Avoids introducing organisms. 3. Red, swollen, draining incision is indicative of infection. 4. Pain may be due to wound hematoma—a possible locus of infection—that needs to be surgically evacuated. 5. Infected prosthesis is avoided.	• Vital signs normal • Well-approximated incision without drainage or excessive inflammatory response • Minimal discomfort; no hematoma • Tolerates antibiotics

Figure 40-8 • An abduction pillow may be used after a total hip arthroplasty to prevent dislocation of the prosthesis.

shorter length of hospital stay, and improved patient satisfaction (van der Weegen, Kornuijt, & Das, 2016).

Dislocation may occur with positioning that exceeds the limits of the prosthesis. The nurse must monitor for signs and symptoms of dislocation of the prosthesis, which include:

- Increased pain at the surgical site, swelling, and immobilization
- Acute groin pain in the affected hip or increased discomfort
- Shortening of the affected extremity

- Abnormal external or internal rotation of the affected extremity
- Restricted ability or inability to move the leg
- Reported "popping" sensation in the hip

If any of these clinical manifestations occur, the nurse (or the patient, if at home) immediately notifies the surgeon, because the hip must be reduced and stabilized promptly so that the leg does not sustain circulatory and nerve damage. After closed reduction, the hip may be stabilized with Buck's traction or a brace to prevent recurrent dislocation. As the muscles and joint capsule heal, the chance of dislocation diminishes. Stresses to the new hip joint should be avoided for the first 8 to 12 weeks, when the risk of dislocation is greatest.

Promoting Ambulation

Patients begin ambulation with the assistance of a walker or crutches within a day after surgery. The nurse and the physical therapist assist the patient in achieving the goal of independent ambulation. At first, the patient may be able to stand for only a brief period because of orthostatic hypotension. Specific weight-bearing limits on the prosthesis are based on the patient's condition, the procedure, and the fixation method. Usually, patients with cemented prostheses can proceed to weight bearing as tolerated. If the patient has a press-fit, cementless, ingrowth prosthesis, weight bearing immediately after surgery may be limited to minimize micromotion of the prosthesis in the bone. As the patient is able to tolerate more activity, the nurse encourages transferring to

---

Chart 40-7 **PATIENT EDUCATION**

Avoiding Hip Dislocation After Arthroplasty With Posterior or Posterolateral Approach

The nurse instructs the patient to:

Until the hip prosthesis stabilizes after hip replacement surgery, it is necessary to follow instructions for proper positioning so that the prosthesis remains in place. Dislocation of the hip is a serious complication of surgery that causes pain and loss of function and necessitates reduction under anesthesia to correct the dislocation. Desirable positions include abduction, neutral rotation, and flexion of less than 90 degrees. When you are seated, the knees should be lower than the hip.

The nurse notes the following methods for avoiding displacement:

- Keep the knees apart at all times.
- Put a pillow between the legs when sleeping.
- Never cross the legs when seated.
- Avoid bending forward when seated in a chair.
- Avoid bending forward to pick up an object on the floor.
- Use a high-seated chair and a raised toilet seat.
- Do not flex the hip to put on clothing such as pants, stockings, socks, or shoes. Positions to avoid after total hip replacement are shown in the illustrations.

Affected leg should not cross the center of the body

Hip should not bend more than 90 degrees

Affected leg should not turn inward

a chair several times a day for short periods and walking for progressively greater distances.

Monitoring Wound Drainage

Fluid and blood accumulating at the surgical site, which could contribute to discomfort and provide a source for infection, may be drained with a closed suction portable suction device. However, the efficacy of using a wound drainage system is a controversial practice that is neither supported nor refuted in the research-based literature. Therefore, its use is most often based on the preference of the surgeon (AAOS, 2015b; Tsang, Cheng, Ho, et al., 2016). If a wound drainage system is used, drainage of 200 to 500 mL in the first 24 hours is expected; by 48 hours postoperatively, the total drainage in 8 hours usually decreases to 30 mL or less, and the suction device is then removed; drains that remain in place for longer than 24 hours are at an increased risk for contamination, and infection may occur (Tsang, 2015). The nurse promptly notifies the primary provider of excessive or foul-smelling drainage. If extensive blood loss is anticipated after total joint replacement surgery, an autotransfusion drainage system (in which the drained blood is filtered and reinfused into the patient during the immediate postoperative period) may be used to decrease the need for allogeneic blood transfusions.

Preventing Venous Thromboembolism (VTE)

In the absence of prophylactic therapy, which includes mechanical (e.g., intermittent compression devices) and pharmacologic prophylaxis (e.g., anticoagulant medications for at least 10 days), the risk of postoperative VTE is particularly high after orthopedic surgery (Budhiparama, Abdel, Ifran, et al., 2014; Lieberman & Pensak, 2013). Without prophylaxis, DVT formation can develop within 7 to 14 days following surgery and lead to PE, which can be fatal. Early identification of the patient's VTE risk, ensuring that the patient receives the appropriate prophylaxis, instituting preventive measures, and monitoring the patient closely for clinical signs of the development of DVT and PE are key nursing responsibilities (Miller & Walsh, 2015).

Physical signs of DVT include pain and tenderness at or below the area of the clot, swelling or tightness of the affected leg, possibly with pitting edema, with either warmth or cooling, and skin discoloration; PE symptoms may include acute onset of dyspnea, tachycardia, confusion, and pleuritic chest pain (Miller & Walsh, 2015).

Intermittent compression devices should be applied either intraoperatively or immediately postoperatively; these devices must remain on the legs at all times, even when the patient is out of bed. Patients should be instructed to dorsi- and plantar flex the ankles and the toes 10 to 20 times every half hour while awake. In addition, patients who are post-THA should be mobilized as soon as possible to assist with decreasing venous stasis; even patients with epidural catheters should stand and ambulate when they are physically able (Miller & Walsh, 2015).

Clinical practice guidelines support the use of anticoagulants as the primary effective DVT prophylaxis (Budhiparama et al., 2014). The decisions about which medications to use are based on patient risk for PE as well as risk for bleeding, and the dosage is based on patient weight. The use of aspirin, LMWH (e.g., enoxaparin [Lovenox], dalteparin [Fragmin]), and synthetic pentasaccharides (fondaparinux [Arixtra]) are recom-

mended as prophylaxis for VTE should continue for up to 35 days following surgery (Miller & Walsh, 2015). The duration of therapy can be variable and is based on surgeon preference and patient risk level.

Preventing Infection

Infection—a serious complication of THA—may necessitate removal of the prosthesis. Patients who are older, obese, poorly nourished, smoke cigarettes, or use corticosteroid medications (e.g., prednisone) and patients who have diabetes, rheumatoid arthritis, concurrent infections (e.g., urinary tract infection, dental abscess), carry MRSA, or have hematomas are at high risk for infection (Smith & Dahlen, 2013).

Over time, one in five patients with THA will undergo revision of the prosthesis, most commonly because of aseptic loosening, infection, instability, or a mechanical complication. Because these joint infections are difficult to treat, strategies for preventing infections should be implemented at various steps of the process of care. Strict hand hygiene and utilization of appropriate infection control practices can prevent transmission of infectious organisms. Proper preoperative patient skin cleansing reduces risk of bacteria entering sites caused by invasive devices or procedures. Appropriate antibiotic administration and discontinuation, as well as thorough patient education regarding subsequent antibiotic use is important. The presence of drains provides a means by which bacteria may enter the body and attach to prosthetic equipment (Smith & Dahlen, 2013; Tsang, 2015). Using a standard recording document to note and describe wound drainage may improve physician and nurse communication and promote decreased infection rates (Tsang et al., 2016). Moreover, caution should be exercised during the drain removal process to prevent the drain from breaking. After the drain is removed, the nurse should clean the drain tube site with an antiseptic solution and apply a small gauze dressing if there is any oozing at the site (Kneedler, Moss, Pfister, et al., 2015).

Acute infections may occur within 3 months after surgery and are associated with progressive superficial infections or hematomas. Delayed surgical infections may appear 4 to 24 months after surgery and may cause return of discomfort in the hip. Previously, prophylactic antibiotics were prescribed if the patient needed any future surgical or invasive procedures, such as tooth extraction or cystoscopic examination. However, the routine use of antibiotic prophylaxis prior to dental procedures for patients with total joint prostheses remains controversial and is not recommended (Sollecito, Abt, Lockhart, et al., 2015). Antibiotic prophylaxis can still be prescribed for some patients considered at higher risk of infection (e.g., patients who are immunosuppressed) (Jevsevar, Cummins, Azar, et al., 2015).

Infections occurring more than 2 years after surgery are attributed to the spread of infection through the bloodstream from another site in the body. If an infection occurs, antibiotics are prescribed. Severe infections may require surgical débridement or removal of the prosthesis.

Promoting Home, Community-Based, and Transitional Care

Educating the Patient About Self-Care

Before the patient leaves the acute care setting, the nurse provides thorough education to promote continuity of the therapeutic regimen and active participation

Chart 40-8 Providing Home Care After Total Hip Arthroplasty

Considerations

- Pain management
- Wound care
- Mobility
- Self-care (activities of daily living)
- Potential complications

Nursing Interventions

Discuss with patient the following methods to reduce pain:

- Periodic rest
- Distraction and relaxation techniques
- Medication therapy (e.g., nonsteroidal anti-inflammatory drugs, opioid analgesic agents): actions of medications, administration, schedule, side effects

Instruct patient in the following:

- Keeping incision clean and dry
- Cleansing incision daily with soap and water and changing the dressing
- Recognizing signs of wound infection (e.g., pain, increased redness, swelling, purulent drainage, fever)

Explain that sutures or staples will be removed 10 to 14 days after surgery.

Educate patient about the following:

- Safe use of assistive devices
- Weight-bearing limits
- How to change positions frequently
- Limitations on hip flexion and adduction (e.g., avoid acute flexion and crossing legs)

- How to stand without flexing hip acutely
- Avoidance of low-seated chairs
- Sleeping with pillow between legs to prevent adduction
- Gradual increase in activities and participation in prescribed exercise regimen
- Use of important medications such as warfarin (Coumadin) and aspirin

Assess home environment for physical barriers.

Instruct patient to use elevated toilet seat and to use reachers to aid in dressing.

Encourage patient to accept assistance with activities of daily living during early convalescence until mobility and strength improve.

Arrange services and accommodations to address the patient's disability or illness, as appropriate.

Assess patient for development of potential problems, and instruct patient to report signs of potential complications:

- Dislocation of prosthesis (e.g., increased pain, shortening of leg, inability to move leg, popping sensation in hip, abnormal rotation)
- Deep vein thrombosis (e.g., calf pain, swelling, redness)
- Wound infection (e.g., pain, increased redness, swelling, purulent drainage, fever)
- Pulmonary emboli (e.g., shortness of breath, tachypnea, pleuritic chest pain)

Discuss with patient the need to continue regular health care (routine physical examinations) and screenings.

---

in the rehabilitation process (see Chart 40-8). The patient may be discharged to their home, a rehabilitation unit, a transitional care unit, or a long-term care facility. The nurse advises the patient of the importance of a daily exercise program in maintaining the functional motion of the hip joint and strengthening the abductor muscles of the hip, and reminds the patient that it will take time to strengthen and retrain the muscles.

The patient will need physical therapy to regain mobility. Assistive devices (crutches, walker, or cane) may be used for a time. After sufficient muscle tone has developed to permit a normal gait without discomfort, these devices are not necessary. In general, by 3 months, the patient can resume routine ADLs. Stair climbing typically may resume within 3 to 6 weeks following surgery (AAOS, 2015b). Some discomfort with activity and at night is common for several weeks. Frequent walks, swimming, and the use of a high rocking chair are excellent for hip exercises.

Restrictions must be kept in mind when resuming sexual activity. Patients should be questioned about sexual concerns and counseled on physical and functional aspects of sexual activity. Sexual intercourse can be resumed based upon the surgeon's recommendation (typically 3 to 6 months postoperatively) and should be carried out with the patient in the supine position (flat on the back) to avoid excessive adduction and flexion of the new hip (Meiri, Rosenbaum, & Kalichman, 2014). Attention to positioning and comfort may enhance the intimacy of the experience.

At no time during the first 4 months should the patient cross the legs or flex the hip more than 90 degrees. Assistive devices should be used for dressing, such as long-handled shoehorns or dressing sticks for putting on shoes and socks. The patient should avoid low chairs and sitting for longer than 45 minutes at a time. These precautions minimize hip flexion and the risks of prosthetic dislocation, hip stiffness, and flexion contracture. Driving requires sufficient range of motion and muscle strength; most patients are given permission to drive 4 to 6 weeks postoperatively. Traveling long distances should be avoided unless frequent position changes are possible. Other activities to avoid include tub baths, jogging, lifting heavy loads, and excessive bending and twisting (e.g., lifting, shoveling snow, forceful turning). The primary provider may give the patient a card indicating that he or she has had a joint replacement; this card may be used to alert security personnel who use screening devices at airports or malls.

Continuing and Transitional Care

A nurse may assess the patient's home for potential problems and monitor wound healing (see Chart 40-9). The nurse, physical therapist, or occupational therapist assesses the home environment for physical barriers that may impede the patient's rehabilitation. In addition, the nurse or therapist may need to assist the patient in acquiring devices such as reachers and long-handled shoehorns or tongs to help with dressing or a toilet seat extender to elevate the toilet seat. After successful surgery and rehabilitation, the patient can

Chart 40-9

HOME CARE CHECKLIST
The Patient Who Has Had Orthopedic Surgery

At the completion of education, the patient and/or caregiver will be able to:

- Name the procedure that was performed and identify any permanent changes in anatomic structure or function as well as changes in ADLs, IADLs, roles, relationships, and spirituality.
- Identify modification of home environment, interventions, and strategies (e.g., durable medical equipment, adaptive equipment) used in safely adapting to changes in structure or function and promote effective recovery and rehabilitation.
- Describe ongoing postoperative therapeutic regimen, including diet and activities to perform (e.g., exercises) and to limit or avoid (e.g., lifting weights, driving a car, contact sports)
  - Consume a healthy diet to promote wound and bone healing.
  - Observe prescribed weight-bearing and activity limits.
  - Participate in prescribed exercise regimen to promote circulation and mobility
  - Demonstrate safe use of mobility aid.
- State the name, dose, side effects, frequency, and schedule for all prescribed therapeutic and prophylactic medications (e.g., antibiotics, anticoagulants, analgesic agents).
- State how to obtain medical supplies and carry out dressing changes, wound care, and other prescribed regimens.

- State indicators of wound infections (e.g., redness, swelling, tenderness, purulent drainage, fever).
- State indicators of complications to report promptly to primary provider (e.g., uncontrolled swelling and pain; cool, pale fingers or toes; paresthesia; paralysis; purulent drainage; signs of systemic infection; signs of deep vein thrombosis or pulmonary embolism).
- State time and date of follow-up appointments and testing.
- Relate how to reach primary provider with questions or complications.
- State understanding of community resources and referrals as appropriate.
- Identify the need for health promotion (e.g., weight reduction, smoking cessation, stress management), disease prevention, and screening activities

Resources

See Chapter 10, Chart 10-8 for additional information related to durable medical equipment, adaptive equipment, mobility skills, skin, bowel, and bladder care.

ADL, activities of daily living; IADL, independent activities of daily living.

expect a hip joint that is free or almost free of pain, has good motion, is stable, and permits normal or near-normal ambulation and function.

Total Knee Arthroplasty

A TKA is considered for patients whose joint pain cannot be managed by nonsurgical treatment and who have severe pain and functional disability related to destruction of joint surfaces by osteoarthritis, rheumatoid arthritis, or posttraumatic (osteonecrotic) arthritis. When activity and mobility severely prevent patients from participating in ADLs, TKA is a successful, cost-effective, low-risk therapy that offers significant pain relief and restores quality of life and function (Shan, Shan, Suzuki, et al., 2015). The femoral joint component can be metal or ceramic; the tibial component has a polyethylene surface that is either fixed to the metal tray attached to the tibia or slides freely (Lee, 2016). If the patient's ligaments have weakened, a fully constrained (hinged) or semiconstrained prosthesis may be used to provide joint stability. A nonconstrained (components are not linked) prosthesis depends on the patient's ligaments for joint stability.

Nursing Interventions

Postoperatively, the knee is dressed with a compression bandage. Ice or cold packs may be applied to reduce postoperative swelling and bleeding. The nurse assesses the neurovascular status (movement, sensation, color, pulse, capillary refill) of the surgical extremity and compares it with the contralateral extremity every 2 to 4 hours. It is important to encourage active flexion of the foot every hour when the patient is awake. Postoperative efforts are directed at preventing complications (VTE, peroneal nerve palsy, infection, bleeding, limited range of motion).

A wound suction drain may be present to remove fluid accumulating in the joint. If a drain is used, it is usually left

in place for only 24 to 48 hours to reduce the risk of infection (Tsang, 2015). Antibiotics are given prophylactically and continued for 24 hours postoperatively (Smith & Dahlen, 2013). If extensive bleeding is anticipated, an autotransfusion drainage system may be used during the immediate postoperative period. All blood must be transfused within 6 hours of collection (Tsang, 2015). The color, type, and amount of drainage are documented, and any excessive drainage or change in characteristics of the drainage is promptly reported to the primary provider.

A continuous passive motion (CPM) device may be prescribed to promote range of motion, circulation, and healing, and to prevent scar tissue from forming in the knee, which could decrease mobility and increase postoperative pain. The patient's leg is usually placed in this device immediately after surgery. The degree of flexion and extension of the joint and the cycle rate (the number of revolutions per minute) are prescribed by the surgeon, but it is often the responsibility of the nurse to maintain the device and monitor the patient's response to the therapy.

Recent research findings suggest that CPM has no influence on functional recovery, drainage, pain, or decreasing adverse outcomes in patients post-TKA; in fact, it necessitates that the patient spend more time in bed (Tabor, 2013). Additional considerations include the time it takes for staff to repeatedly place the patient in and out of the machine. Additionally, care and maintenance of the machine can be costly, time-consuming and burdensome.

The physical therapist supervises exercises for strength and range of motion and educates the patient about how to use assistive devices based on weight-bearing restrictions. To avoid flexion contractures, patients are instructed to limit positions of flexion. A knee gatch position (i.e., raising the hospital bed so that the knee is flexed) and pillows placed behind the knee are both avoided. If satisfactory flexion is not achieved, gentle manipulation of the knee joint under general anesthesia may be necessary about 2 weeks after surgery.

Patients who are postoperative for TKA should mobilize and ambulate by the first postoperative day (Yager & Stichler, 2015). The patient's weight-bearing status is determined by the primary provider. The knee is usually protected with a knee immobilizer and is elevated when the patient sits in a chair. The typical requirements for discharge to home may include evidence of wound stability (e.g., no erythema, discharge, or redness), appropriate anticoagulation status by laboratory results (i.e., international normalized ratio [INR] between 1.5 and 2), progress toward physical therapy goals (e.g., appropriate use of walker), and satisfactory pain control with oral medications (Newton-Triggs et al., 2014).

Acute rehabilitation usually takes about 1 to 2 weeks; length of time and discharge destination (e.g., home, acute rehabilitation unit) depend on the age and tolerance of the patient. If discharge is to home, the patient may continue to use the CPM device if prescribed and may undergo physical therapy on an outpatient basis. Total recovery takes 6 weeks or longer, especially for those older than 75 years. Late complications that may occur include polyethylene-induced breakdown infection (**osteolysis**), periprosthetic joint infections, and aseptic loosening of prosthetic components (Osmon, Berbari, Berendt, et al., 2013).

More than 95% of patients who have TKA will still have a functioning prosthesis 15 to 20 years after surgery (Lee, 2016). TKA is a viable option for improving both disease-specific and generic health-related quality of life, especially pain and function, leading to positive patient satisfaction (Shan et al., 2015). Patients usually can achieve a pain-free, functional joint and participate more fully in life activities than before the surgery.

NURSING PROCESS

Postoperative Care of the Patient Undergoing Orthopedic Surgery

Assessment

After orthopedic surgery, the nurse reassesses the patient's needs related to pain, neurovascular status, health promotion, mobility, and self-esteem. Skeletal trauma and surgery performed on bones, muscles, or joints can produce significant pain, especially during the first 1 or 2 postoperative days. Tissue perfusion must be monitored closely, because edema and bleeding into the tissues can compromise circulation and result in compartment syndrome. Inactivity contributes to venous stasis and the development of VTE that may include DVT or PE (see Chapters 19, 23, and 30).

VTE is one of the most common and dangerous of all complications occurring in the postoperative orthopedic patient. Advanced age, venous stasis, lower extremity orthopedic surgery, and immobilization are significant risk factors. The nurse assesses the patient daily for unilateral calf swelling, tenderness, warmth cooling of the extremity, and redness (Miller & Walsh, 2015). The nurse promptly reports abnormal findings to the primary provider.

In addition, fat embolism syndrome (FES) (see Chapter 42) may occur with orthopedic surgery. The nurse must be alert to any signs and symptoms that may suggest the development of FES. These major symptoms are referred to as the classic triad and include respiratory distress (dyspnea, tachypnea, and hypoxemia), onset of delirium or any acute change in level of consciousness and development of a petechial rash in the conjunctiva, oral membranes, axillae, neck, or anterior chest (Ruda, 2013).

Diagnosis

NURSING DIAGNOSES

Based on the assessment data, major nursing diagnoses after orthopedic surgery may include the following:

- Acute pain related to the surgical procedure, swelling, and immobilization
- Risk for ineffective peripheral tissue perfusion related to swelling, constricting devices, or impaired circulation
- Impaired physical mobility related to pain, edema, or the presence of an immobilizing device (e.g., splint, cast, or brace)

COLLABORATIVE PROBLEMS/POTENTIAL COMPLICATIONS

Potential complications may include any of those noted in Chapter 19, with particular attention to the following:

- Infection
- VTE, including DVT or PE

Planning and Goals

The major goals for the patient after orthopedic surgery mirror those for any patient having surgery (see Chapter 19). The specific major goals for the patient after orthopedic surgery may include relief of pain, adequate neurovascular function, improved mobility, and absence of complications.

Nursing Interventions

RELIEVING PAIN

Pain can be intense following orthopedic surgery. Maximizing pain management is paramount to obtaining the best patient outcomes, decreasing complications, and reducing costs of care (Vanderbeck, 2013). Edema, hematomas, and muscle spasms may contribute to the pain.

The nurse's role in ensuring effective pain management is to assess the patient's level of pain, evaluate the patient's response to therapeutic measures, and make every effort to relieve the pain and discomfort. Early recognition of acute pain and accurate pain assessments are critical to optimal pain management and will facilitate the patient's rehabilitation (Barker & Murray, 2013). A comprehensive pain assessment should occur prior to the initiation of treatment followed by reassessment throughout the duration of treatment. The nurse must accept the patient's report of pain as accurate (Vanderbeck, 2013).

Treatment of pain is multidisciplinary, multimodal (*epidural, intravenous, patient-controlled analgesia [PCA] or regional techniques*), and should be flexible according to the needs of the patient (Vanderbeck, 2013). Regional intraoperative techniques can provide prolonged pain relief in the initial postoperative phase and include spinal, epidural, regional nerve blocks, and local wound infiltration. Continuous femoral nerve block infusions (CFNBIs) have been found to both decrease patient postoperative pain and improve postoperative joint mobilization, both of which impact patient satisfaction, outcome, and length of stay (Thomas, Barrett, Tupper, et al., 2014). Regional blockade offers site-specific pain relief and has fewer adverse effects than systemic analgesia (Vanderbeck, 2013). Epidural/intrathecal routes are usually more effective than intravenous PCA for patients who have had hip or knee arthroplasty in certain surgical procedures and should be considered in eligible patients (see Chapter 12.)

In addition to pharmacologic approaches to controlling pain, elevation of the operative extremity and application of ice and cold packs, if prescribed, help control edema and pain. Surgical drains inserted in the wound decrease fluid accumulation and hematoma formation. The nurse may find that nonpharmacologic interventions such as biofeedback, relaxation, distraction, guided imagery acupressure, and acupuncture may help in reducing the patient's pain (Barker & Murray, 2013; Draucker, Jacobson, Umberger, et al., 2015). Patients who are critically ill, older, cognitively impaired, or have communication difficulties may require some of these additional interventions to ensure optimal pain management (Brown, Boshers, Chapman, et al., 2015).

The nurse should report increasing and uncontrollable pain to the primary provider for evaluation. Pain should diminish rapidly after the initial postoperative period. After 2 to 3 days, most patients require only occasional oral analgesia for residual muscle soreness and spasm.

MAINTAINING ADEQUATE PERIPHERAL TISSUE PERFUSION

The nurse monitors the neurovascular status of the involved body part and notifies the primary provider promptly of any indications of diminished tissue perfusion. The patient is reminded to perform muscle setting, ankle, and calf-pumping exercises hourly while awake to enhance circulation.

IMPROVING PHYSICAL MOBILITY

Patients are frequently reluctant to move after orthopedic surgery. Preoperative education about the planned postoperative treatment regimen promotes patient adherence to an optimal rehabilitation regimen (Yager & Stichler, 2015). Patients often increase their mobility once they have been reassured that movement within therapeutic limits is beneficial, the nurse will provide assistance, and discomfort can be controlled.

Metal pins, screws, rods, and plates used for internal fixation are designed to maintain the position of the bone until ossification occurs. They are not designed to support the body's weight, and they can bend, loosen, or break if stressed. The estimated strength of the bone, the stability of the fracture, reduction, and fixation, and the amount of bone healing are important considerations in determining weight-bearing limits. Although the incision may appear healed, the underlying bone requires more time to repair and regain normal strength. Some orthopedic procedures require weight-bearing restrictions. The primary provider will prescribe the weight-bearing limits and the use of protective devices (orthoses), if necessary, after surgery.

The rehabilitation program is tailored to each patient's needs. The goal is the patient's return to the highest level of function in the shortest time possible. Rehabilitation involves progressive increases in the patient's activities and exercises. Assistive devices (crutches, walker) may be used for postoperative mobility. Preoperative practice with assistive devices helps the patient use them appropriately postoperatively. The nurse makes sure that the patient uses these devices safely (see Chapter 10).

MONITORING AND MANAGING POTENTIAL COMPLICATIONS

The patient undergoing orthopedic surgery is at risk for many postoperative complications that include hypovolemic shock (see Chapter 14), atelectasis and pneumonia (see previous discussion in this chapter and in Chapter 23), and urinary retention and constipation (see Chapter 19), as well as infection and VTE formation.

Infection. Infection is a risk after any surgery, but it is of particular concern for the patient postorthopedic surgery because of the risk of osteomyelitis. Osteomyelitis often requires prolonged courses of IV antibiotics. At times, the infected bone and prosthesis or internal fixation device must be surgically removed. Therefore, prophylactic systemic antibiotics are usually prescribed during the perioperative and immediate postoperative periods. The nurse assesses the patient's response to these antibiotics. Routine care, such as aseptic dressing changes, safe injection practices, and cleaning of portable equipment ensure that organisms are not introduced into the patient's wound or body fluid through outside means (National Association of Orthopedic Nurses [NAON], 2014). The nurse monitors the patient's vital signs, incision, and any drainage for signs of infection in surgical sites and other known portals of entry. Prompt assessment of and timely interventions for treating infection are essential.

Venous Thromboembolism and Deep Vein Thrombosis. Prevention of DVT requires the use of ankle and calf-pumping exercises, antiembolism stockings, and intermittent compression devices applied to the patient's legs at all times, even when the patient is out of bed. Adequate hydration and early mobilization are equally important (Lieberman & Pensak, 2013). Aspirin and prophylactic fondaparinux, LMWH (e.g., enoxaparin, dalteparin), warfarin (Coumadin), or low-dose unfractionated heparin may be prescribed in the immediate postoperative period and up to 6 weeks postoperatively (Miller & Walsh, 2015). The nurse monitors the patient for signs of DVT as described previously and promptly reports findings to the primary provider for management. Patient education is an essential component in the management of patients who are discharged on anticoagulants. Appropriate education is important for the prevention of postoperative DVT after patients are discharged from the acute care setting (Wittig-Wells, Higgins, Davis, et al., 2015) (see Chapter 30, Chart 30-10).

PROMOTING HOME, COMMUNITY-BASED, AND TRANSITIONAL CARE

Educating the Patient About Self-Care. Because the hospital length of stay after orthopedic surgery is usually short, most convalescence and rehabilitation take place at home or in a nonacute care setting. The nurse educates the patient and family to recognize complications that must be reported promptly to the primary provider (Wilson, Watt-Watson, Hodnett, et al., 2016). The patient must understand the prescribed medication regimen. The nurse should demonstrate proper wound care. The patient gradually resumes physical activities and adheres to weight-bearing limits. The patient must be able to perform transfers and use mobility aids safely. If the patient has a cast or other immobilizing device, family members are educated about how to assist the patient in a way that is safe for the patient and for the family member (e.g., using proper body mechanics when assisting the patient). Specific exercises need to be taught and practiced before discharge. The nurse discusses recovery and health promotion, emphasizing a healthy lifestyle and diet (see Chart 40-9).

Continuing and Transitional Care. If special equipment or home modifications are needed for safe care at home, they must be in place before the patient is discharged home. Discharge planning begins before surgery. The nurse, physical therapist, and social worker can assist the patient and family in identifying their needs and getting ready to care for the patient at home.

Frequently, home health nursing and home physical therapy are part of the discharge plan of care. These referrals provide resources and help the patient and family cope with the demands of care during recovery and rehabilitation. The nurse assesses the patient's progress and monitors for possible complications. Regular medical follow-up care after discharge needs to be arranged. The nurse reminds the patient and family about the importance of continuing health promotion and screening practices.

Evaluation

Expected patient outcomes may include:
1. Reports decreased level of pain
   a. Uses multiple approaches to reduce pain
   b. Uses oral analgesic medication as needed to control discomfort
   c. Elevates extremity to control edema and discomfort
   d. Moves with greater comfort
2. Exhibits normal peripheral tissue perfusion
   a. Exhibits normal color and temperature of skin
   b. Has normal capillary refill response
   c. Demonstrates intact sensory and motor function
   d. Demonstrates reduced swelling
3. Maximizes mobility within the therapeutic limits
   a. Requests assistance when moving
   b. Elevates edematous extremity after transfer
   c. Uses immobilizing devices as prescribed
   d. Complies with prescribed weight-bearing limitation
4. Exhibits absence of complications
   a. Does not experience shock
   b. Maintains normal vital signs and blood pressure
   c. Has clear lung sounds
   d. Demonstrates wound healing without signs of infection
   e. Does not experience urinary retention
   f. Voids clear urine
   g. Exhibits no signs of DVT or PE
   h. Does not experience constipation

CRITICAL THINKING EXERCISES

1 A 70-year-old woman is 3 days postoperative after a left TKA. She is moderately overweight, has extensive varicose veins, and has a history of smoking. She has been reluctant to ambulate and complains that her intermittent compression devices are uncomfortable and she does not want to wear them. Her morning assessment reveals a red, swollen, and painful left calf. She is questioning what is going on and does not understand why she is at risk for VTE. How would you respond to her? Describe the physical assessment that should be conducted for this patient. What are her risk factors for this disease process?

2 **ebp** You are caring for a 64-year-old man who had a right THA following a femoral neck fracture. It is the second postoperative day and he still has a closed suction portable wound device. The drainage for the last 8 hours was 10 mL. You inform the orthopedic surgeon and he tells you that he wants to leave the wound device in for another 24 hours. What are your concerns about leaving the wound device in place? What is the strength of the evidence that supports the best way to care for wound drainage systems to promote the best patient outcomes?

3 **pq** You are an experienced orthopedic nurse. You are completing an assessment of a 45-year old man who had an external fixation device applied 6 hours ago for a fracture of the right tibia and fibula. You note that he has intense pain of the right foot when it is passively moved and his calf is becoming hard and swollen. He has had adequate pain control with oral analgesics but he now reports that his pain is unrelieved by the analgesic medication and he has burning and tingling in his foot. What additional assessments might you make at this time? What is your priority nursing diagnosis and plan of care?

REFERENCES

*Asterisk indicates nursing research.

Books

Alisangco, J., Asplund, C., & Benjamin, H. (2016). Splinting and casting. In R. B. Birrer, F. G. O'Connor., & S. F. Kane (Eds.). *Musculoskeletal and sports medicine for the primary care practitioner.* (4th ed.). Boca Raton, Florida: CRC Press.

Barker, D. M., & Murray, P. A. (2013). Orthopaedic pain. In L. Schoenly (Ed.), *Core curriculum for orthopaedic nursing* (7th ed.). Chicago, IL: National Association of Orthopaedic Nurses.

Herdman, T. H., & Kamitsuru, S. (2014). *NANDA International nursing diagnoses: Definitions and classification, 2015–17.* Oxford: Wiley-Blackwell.

Hovius, S. E., & Nijhuis, T. H. (2015) Compartment syndrome in the extremities. In R. D. Farhadieh, N. W. Bulstrode, & S. Cugno (Eds.). *Plastic and reconstructive surgery: Approaches and techniques.* Chichester, UK: John Wiley & Sons.

Karachalios, T., & Antoniou, I. (2015). Long term outcome of total knee arthroplasty. The effect of implant fixation (cementless). In T. Karachalios (Ed.), *Total knee arthroplasty.* London: Springer.

Newton-Triggs, L., Pugh, H., Rogers, J., et al. (2014). Key musculoskeletal interventions. In S. Clarke., & J. Santy-Tomlinson (Eds.). *Orthopedics and nursing trauma, an evidence-based approach to musculoskeletal care.* Oxford: WILEY Blackwell.

Journals and Electronic Documents

*Ali, P., Santy-Tomlinson, J. & Watson, R. (2014). Assessment and diagnosis of acute limb compartment syndrome: A literature review. *International Journal of Orthopaedic and Trauma Nursing, 18*(4), 180–190.

American Academy of Orthopaedic Surgeons (AAOS). (2014). Management of hip fractures in the elderly evidence- based clinical practice guideline. Retrieved on 2/24/2016 at: www.aaos.org/research/guidelines/HipFxGuideline.pdf

American Academy of Orthopaedic Surgeons (AAOS). (2015a). OrthoInfo. Care of casts and splints. Retrieved on 2/24/2016 at: orthoinfo.aaos.org/topic.cfm?topic=A00095

American Academy of Orthopaedic Surgeons (AAOS). (2015b). *Surgical management of osteoarthritis of the knee evidence-based clinical practice guideline.* Retrieved on 2/24/2016 at: www.aaos.org/uploadedFiles/PreProduction/Quality/Guidelines_and_Reviews/SMOAK%20CPG__12.4.15.pdf

*Baath, C., Engstrom, M., Gunningberg, L., et al. (2016). Prevention of heel pressure ulcers among older patients–from ambulance care to hospital discharge: A multi-centre randomized controlled trial. *Applied Nursing Research, 30,* 170–175.

Barnsley, L., Barnsley, L., & Page, R. (2015). Are hip precautions necessary post total hip arthroplasty? A systematic review. *Geriatric Orthopaedic Surgery & Rehabilitation, 6*(3), 230–235.

Bosco, J. A., Bookman, J., Slover, J., et al. (2015). Principles of antibiotic prophylaxis in total joint arthroplasty: Current concepts. *Journal of the American Academy of Orthopaedic Surgeons, 23*(8), e27–e35.

Britten, S., Ghoz, A., Duffield, B., et al. (2013). Ilizarov fixator pin site care: The role of crusts in the prevention of infection. *Injury, 44*(10), 1275–1278.

*Brown, A., Boshers, B., Chapman, L. F., et al. (2015). Do elderly patients use patient-controlled analgesia medication delivery systems correctly?. *Orthopaedic Nursing, 34*(4), 203–208.

Brubacher, J. W., Karg, J., Weinstock, P., et al. (2016). A novel cast removal training simulation to improve patient safety. *Journal of Surgical Education, 73*(1), 7–11.

Budhiparama, N. C., Abdel, M. P., Ifran, N. N., et al. (2014). Venous thromboembolism (VTE) prophylaxis for hip and knee arthroplasty: Changing trends. *Current Review of Musculoskeletal Medicine, 7*(2), 108–116.

Burghardt, R. D., Anderson, J. G., Reed, R. A., et al. (2014). Exothermic properties of plaster-synthetic composite casts. *Journal of Children's Orthopaedics, 8*(12), 193–201.

Call, E., Pedersen, J., Bill, B., et al. (2015), Enhancing pressure ulcer prevention using wound dressings: What are the modes of action? *International Wound Journal, 12*(4), 408–413.

Clark, M., Black, J., Alves, P., et al. (2014). Systematic review of the use of prophylactic dressings in the prevention of pressure ulcers. *International Wound Journal, 11*(5), 460–471.

*Demir, S. G. Erden, S. Bulut, H., et al. (2015). The problems experienced by parents providing postoperative home care following their child's surgery for developmental dysplasia of the hip. *Orthopaedic Nursing, 34*(5), 280–286.

Dennis, D. A, Kittleson, A. J., Yang, C. C., et al. (2016). Does tourniquet use in TKA affect recovery of lower extremity strength and function? A randomized trial. *Clinical Orthopaedics and Related Research, 474*(1), 69–77.

Donaldson, J., Haddad, B., & Khan, W. S. (2014). The pathophysiology, diagnosis and current management of acute compartment syndrome. *Open Orthopaedic Journal, 8,* 185–193.

*Draucker, C. B., Jacobson, A. F., Umberger, W. A., et al. (2015). Acceptability of a guided imagery intervention for persons undergoing a total knee replacement. *Orthopaedic Nursing, 34*(6), 356–364.

Dy, C. J., Bumpass, D. B., Makhni, E. C., et al. (2016). The evolving role of clinical registries: Existing practices and opportunities for orthopaedic surgeons. *The Journal of Bone & Joint Surgery, 98*(2), e7.

Garner, M. R., Taylor, S. A. Gausden, E., et al. (2014). Compartment syndrome: Diagnosis, management, and unique concerns in the twenty-first century. *HSSJ: The Musculoskeletal Journal of Hospital for Special Surgery, 10*(2), 143–152.

Gebhart, T. (2015). Superior mesenteric artery syndrome. *Gastroenterology Nursing, 38*(3), 189–193.

Hajbaghery, M. A., & Moradi, T. (2013). Quality of care for patients with traction in Shahid Beheshti Hospital in 2012. *Archives of Trauma Research, 2*(2), 85–90.

*Hanna-Bull, D. (2015). Preventing heel pressure ulcers: Sustained quality improvement initiative in a Canadian acute care facility. *Journal of Wound, Ostomy and Continence Nursing: Official Publication of The Wound, Ostomy and Continence Nurses Society/WOCN, 43*(2), 129–132.

Hazel, D., Bern, J., Reilly, D., et al. (2015). Effect of preoperative autologous blood donation coupled with fluid resuscitation on transfusion requirements following orthopedic surgery. *Journal of Hematology, 4*(2), 157–163.

Hickey, B. A., Morgan, A., Pugh, N., et al. (2014). The effect of lower limb cast immobilization on calf muscle pump function: A simple strategy of exercises can maintain flow. *Foot & Ankle International, 35*(5), 429–433.

*Horn, P. L., & Badowski, E. (2015). To improve nurses' knowledge base and increase their comfort level when caring for patients in a spica cast. *Orthopaedic Nursing, 34*(6), 334–337.

Jennison, T., McNally, M., & Pandit. H. (2014). Prevention of infection in external fixator pin sites. *Acta Biomaterialia, 10*(2), 595–603.

Jevsevar, D. S., Cummins, D. S., Azar, F. M., et al. (2015). One size does not fit all: Involve orthopaedic implant patients in deciding whether to use prophylactic antibiotics with dental procedures. *Journal of the American Academy of Orthopaedic Surgeons, 23*(3), 141–142.

Khan, M., Osman, K., Green, G., et al. (2016). The epidemiology of failure in total knee arthroplasty avoiding your next revision. *Bone & Joint Journal, 98*(1), 105–112.

Kneedler, J. A., Moss, R., Pfister, J. I., et al. (2015). Wound drainage systems in perioperative nursing. Retrieved on 5/9/2015 at: www.pfiedler.com/ce/1200/files/assets/common/downloads/Wound%20Drain%20Systems%20in%20Perioperative%20Nursing.pdf

Ktistakisa, J., Gueradob, E., & Giannoudis, P. V. (2015). Pin-site care: Can we reduce the incidence of infections? *Injury, 46*(3), S35–S39.

Lee, G. C. (2016). What's new in adult reconstructive knee surgery. *Journal of Bone & Joint Surgery American, 98*(2), 156–165.

Lethaby A., Temple J., & Santy-Tomlinson J. (2013). Pin site care for preventing infections associated with external bone fixators and pins. *Cochrane Database of Systematic Reviews,* (12). Art. No.: CD004551; doi: 10.1002/14651858.CD004551.pub3.

*Levin, B. & Morris, N. (2013). Practice points: Pressure ulcer. *National Association of Orthopaedic Nurses.* Retrieved on 5/24/2016 at: www.orthonurse.org/p/do/sd/sid=1140&type=0

Lieberman, J. R., & Pensak, M. J. (2013). Prevention of venous thromboembolic disease after total hip and knee arthroplasty. *Journal of Bone & Joint Surgery American, 95*(19), 1801–1811. http://dx.doi.org/10.2106/JBJS.L.01328

Liu, D. (2015). Blood conservation strategies in total hip and knee arthroplasty. *Reconstructive Review, 4*(4), 39–45.

Loftus, T. J., Spratling, L., Stone, B. A., et al. (2016). A patient blood management program in prosthetic joint arthroplasty decreases blood use and improves outcomes. *The Journal of Arthroplasty, 31*(1), 11–14.

Louw A., Diener I., Butler D. S., et al. (2013). Preoperative education addressing postoperative pain in total joint arthroplasty: Review of content and educational delivery methods. *Physiotherapy Theory and Practice, 29*(3), 175–194.

Meiri, R., Rosenbaum, T. Y., & Kalichman, L. (2014). Sexual function before and after total hip replacement: Narrative review. *Sexual Medicine, 2*(4), 159–167.

*Miller, A., & Walsh, C. (2015). Clinical practice guideline thromboembolic disease prevention. *National Association of Orthopaedic Nurses.* Retrieved on 5/24/2016 at: www.orthonurse.org/p/do/vi/sid=2254

Mohanty, S., Rosenthal, R. A., Russell, M. M., et al. (2016). Optimal perioperative management of the geriatric patient: A best practices guideline from the American College of Surgeons NSQIP and the American Geriatrics Society. *Journal of the American College of Surgeons, 222*(5), 930–947.

Mullaji, A., & Shetty, G. (2015). Cemented total knee arthroplasty remains the "gold standard." *Seminars in Arthroplasty, 26*(2), 62–64.

National Association of Orthopedic Nurses (NAON). (2014). NAON position statement: Preventing infection in the inpatient orthopaedic patient. Retrieved on 5/24/2016 at: www.orthonurse.org/p/do/sd/sid=1601&type=0

Oron, A., Lindner, D., Bergman, A., et al. (2013). Molding significantly affects the mechanical properties of plaster of Paris in orthopaedic use. *Current Orthopaedic Practice, 24*(6), 647–650.

Osmon, D. R., Berbari, E. F., Berendt, A. R., et al. (2013). Diagnosis and management of prosthetic joint infection: Clinical practice guidelines by the Infectious Diseases Society of America. *Clinical Infectious Diseases, 56*(1), e1–e25.

Park, J. H., Rasouli, M. R., Mortazavi, S. M., et al. (2013). Predictors of perioperative blood loss in total joint arthroplasty. *The Journal of Bone & Joint Surgery American, 95*(19), 1777–1783.

*Pechar, J., & Lyons, M. M. (2016) Acute compartment syndrome of the lower leg: A review. *The Journal for Nurse Practitioners. 12*(4), 265–270.

Qaseem, A., Mir, T.P., Starkey, M., et al. for the Clinical Guidelines Committee of the American College of Physicians. (2015). Risk assessment and prevention of pressure ulcers: A clinical practice guideline from the American College of Physicians. *Annals of Internal Medicine, 162,* 359–369.

Rasouli, M. R., Maltenfort, M. G., Erkocak, O. F., et al. (2016). Blood management after total joint arthroplasty in the United States: 19 year trend analysis. *Transfusion, 56*(5), 1112–1120.

Ruda, S. (2013). NAON practice points: Fat embolism syndrome. Retrieved on 5/24/2016 at: www.orthonurse.org/p/do/sd/sid=875&type=0

Shan, L., Shan, B., Suzuki, A., et al. (2015). Intermediate and long-term quality of life after total knee replacement. *Journal of Bone & Joint Surgery American, 97*(2), 156–168.

Smith, M. A., & Dahlen, N. R. (2013). Clinical practice guideline surgical site infection prevention. *Orthopaedic Nursing, 32*(5), 242–248.

Smith, M., & Smith, T. (2012). The American joint replacement registry. *Orthopaedic Nursing, 31*(5), 296–299.

Sollecito, T. P., Abt, E., Lockhart, P. B., et al. (2015). The use of prophylactic antibiotics prior to dental procedures in patients with prosthetic joints: Evidence-based clinical practice guideline for dental practitioners—a report of the American Dental Association Council on Scientific Affairs. *The Journal of the American Dental Association, 146*(1), 11–16.

Suggs, S., & Holt, K. (2015). The use of tranexamic acid in joint replacement surgery. *Orthopaedic Nursing, 34*(2), 89–92.

*Tabor, D. (2013). An empirical study using range of motion and pain score as determinants for continuous passive motion: Outcomes following total knee replacement surgery in an adult population. *Orthopaedic Nursing, 32*(5), 261–265.

*Thomas, K., Barrett, B., Tupper, R., et al. (2014). Pain management after total knee arthroplasty: A case–control study of continuous nerve block therapy. *Orthopaedic Nursing, 33*(5), 268–276.

*Tsang, L. F. (2015). Developing an evidence-based nursing protocol on wound drain management for total joint arthroplasty. *International Journal of Orthopaedic and Trauma Nursing, 19*(2), 61–73.

*Tsang, L. F., Cheng, H. C., Ho, H. S., et al. (2016). Translating evidence-based protocol of wound drain management for total joint arthroplasty into practice: A quasi-experimental study. *International Journal of Orthopaedic and Trauma Nursing, 21,* 49–61.

*Turney, J., Noble, D., & Kim, S. C. (2013). Orthopaedic nurses' knowledge and interrater reliability of neurovascular assessments with 2-point discrimination test. *Orthopaedic Nursing, 32*(3), 167–172.

Unver, B., Karatosun, V., & Tuncali, B. (2013). Effects of tourniquet pressure on rehabilitation outcomes in patients undergoing total knee arthroplasty. *Orthopaedic Nursing, 32*(4), 217–222.

Vanderbeck, K. (2013). NAON practice points: Acute pain management. Retrieved on 5/24/2016 at: www.orthonurse.org/p/do/sd/?type=0

van der Weegen, W., Kornuijt, A., & Das, D. (2016). Do lifestyle restrictions and precautions prevent dislocation after total hip arthroplasty? A systematic review and meta-analysis of the literature. *Clinical Rehabilitation, 30*(4), 329–339.

*Wilson, R. A., Watt-Watson, J., Hodnett, E., et al. (2016). A randomized controlled trial of an individualized preoperative education intervention for symptom management after total knee arthroplasty. *Orthopaedic Nursing, 35*(1), 20–29.

*Wittig-Wells, D., Higgins, M., Davis, E., et al. (2015). Impact of a focused approach for discharge teaching regarding the use of aspirin as anticoagulant after joint replacement surgery. *Orthopaedic Nursing, 34*(4), 211–220.

Wu, C. T., Chen, I. L., Wang, J. W., et al. (2016). Surgical site infection following total knee arthroplasty: Risk factors in patients with timely administration of systemic prophylactic antibiotics. *The Journal of Arthroplasty, 31*(7), 1568–1573.

*Yager, M., & Stichler, J. (2015). The effect of early ambulation on patient outcomes for total joint replacement. *Orthopaedic Nursing, 34*(4), 197–200.

*Zhang, Y. (2015). The perioperative nursing of treating the elderly patients of femoral intertrochanteric fracture with PFNA. *Journal of Nursing, 4*(1), 1–4.

Zhou, X., Tao, L., Li, J., et al. (2013). Do we really need tranexamic acid in total hip arthroplasty? A meta-analysis of nineteen randomized controlled trials. *Archives of Orthopaedic and Trauma Surgery, 133*(7), 1017–1027.

Resources

American Academy of Orthopaedic Surgeons/American Association of Orthopaedic Surgeons (AAOS), www.aaos.org

National Association of Orthopaedic Nurses (NAON), www.orthonurse.org

National Institute of Arthritis and Musculoskeletal and Skin Diseases, National Institutes of Health, www.niams.nih.gov

41

Management of Patients With Musculoskeletal Disorders

LEARNING OBJECTIVES

On completion of this chapter, the learner will be able to:

1 Describe the nursing management, rehabilitation, and health education needs of the patient with low back pain.
2 Discuss common musculoskeletal disorders of the hand, wrist, shoulder, and foot, and nursing care of the patient undergoing surgery to correct these disorders.
3 Explain the pathogenesis, prevention, and management of osteoporosis.

4 Use the nursing process as a framework for care of the patient with osteoporotic vertebral fracture.
5 Identify the causes and related management of patients with osteomalacia, Paget disease, and septic arthritis.
6 Apply the nursing process as a framework for care of the patient with osteomyelitis.
7 Recognize the causes and related management of the patient with a primary or metastatic bone tumor.

GLOSSARY

bursitis: inflammation of a fluid-filled sac in a joint
contracture: abnormal shortening of muscle or fibrosis of joint structures
involucrum: new bone growth around a sequestrum
osteopenia: low bone mineral density
osteoporosis: degenerative disease of the bone characterized by reduced mass, deterioration of matrix, and diminished architectural strength

radiculopathy: disease of a spinal nerve root, often resulting in pain and extreme sensitivity to touch.
sciatica: inflammation of the sciatic nerve, resulting in pain and tenderness along the nerve through the thigh and leg
sequestrum: dead bone in abscess cavity
tendonitis: inflammation of muscle tendons

Musculoskeletal disorders, particularly impairment of the back and spine, are leading health problems and causes of disability. The functional and psychological limitations for the patient may be severe. Nurses provide care in both inpatient and outpatient settings; because of this, nurses should be cognizant of these limitations and the effects these disorders may have on these patients. The economic costs in terms of loss of productivity, medical expenses, and other costs are among the highest for any medical diagnosis (Schaafsma, Anema, & van der Beek, 2015).

Low Back Pain

Most low back pain is caused by one of many musculoskeletal problems, including acute lumbosacral strain, unstable lumbosacral ligaments and weak muscles, intervertebral disc problems, and unequal leg length. Depression, smoking, alcohol abuse, obesity, and stress are frequent comorbidities (Shemory, Pfefferle, & Gradisar, 2015). Generally, back pain due to musculoskeletal disorders is aggravated by activity, whereas pain due to other conditions is not.

Older patients may experience back pain associated with osteoporotic vertebral fractures, osteoarthritis of the spine, and spinal stenosis. Higher numbers of areas of pain are associated with a higher level of disability (Buchman, Shah, Leurgans, et al., 2010). Other nonmusculoskeletal causes

of back pain beyond the scope of this chapter include kidney disorders, pelvic problems, retroperitoneal tumors, and abdominal aortic aneurysms.

Pathophysiology

The spinal column can be considered a rod constructed of rigid units (vertebrae) and flexible units (intervertebral discs) held together by complex facet joints, multiple ligaments, and paravertebral muscles. Its unique construction allows for flexibility while providing maximum protection for the spinal cord. The spinal curves absorb vertical shocks from running and jumping. The abdominal and thoracic muscles are important in lifting activities, working together to minimize stress on the spinal units. Disuse weakens these supporting muscular structures. Obesity, postural problems, structural problems, and overstretching of the spinal supports may result in back pain (Grossman & Porth, 2014).

The intervertebral discs change in character as a person ages. A young person's discs are mainly fibrocartilage with a gelatinous matrix. Over time, the fibrocartilage becomes dense and irregularly shaped. Disc degeneration is a common cause of back pain. The lower lumbar discs, L4–5 and L5–S1, are subject to the greatest mechanical stress and the greatest degenerative changes. Disc protrusion or facet joint changes can cause pressure on nerve roots as they leave the spinal canal, which results in pain that radiates along the nerve (Grossman & Porth, 2014). See Chapter 70 for discussion of the management of intervertebral disc disease.

Clinical Manifestations

The typical patient reports either acute back pain (lasting fewer than 3 months) or chronic back pain (3 months or longer without improvement) and fatigue. The patient may report pain radiating down the leg, which is known as **radiculopathy** (i.e., pain radiating from a diseased spinal nerve root) or **sciatica** (i.e., pain radiating from an inflamed sciatic nerve); presence of this symptom suggests nerve root involvement. The patient's gait, spinal mobility, reflexes, leg length, leg motor strength, and sensory perception may be affected. Physical examination may disclose paravertebral muscle spasm (greatly increased muscle tone of the back postural muscles) with a loss of the normal lumbar curve and possible spinal deformity.

 Concept Mastery Alert

With back pain, chronic pain is considered to last 3 months or longer without improvement.

Assessment and Diagnostic Findings

The initial evaluation of acute low back pain includes a focused history and physical examination, including observation of the patient, gait evaluation, and neurologic testing (described in Chapter 39). The findings suggest either nonspecific lumbar strain or potentially serious problems, such as a spinal fracture, cancer, infection, or rapidly progressing neurologic deficits. The presence of bruising, older age and prolonged use of glucocorticoid medications increases the risk of a fracture posttraumatic injury (Williams, Henschke, Maher, et al., 2013).

The diagnostic procedures described in Chart 41-1 may be indicated for the patient with potentially serious or prolonged low back pain. Red flags that trigger prescribing these studies include suspected spinal infection, severe neurologic weakness, urinary or fecal incontinence, and a new onset of back

pain in a patient with cancer (Henschke, Maher, Osteolo, et al., 2013). The nurse prepares the patient for these studies, provides the necessary support during the testing period, and monitors the patient for any adverse responses to the procedures.

Medical Management

Most back pain is self-limited and resolves within 4 to 6 weeks with analgesics, rest, and avoidance of strain. Based on initial assessment findings indicating nonspecific back symptoms, the patient is reassured that the pain is not due to a serious condition and x-rays or other imaging modalities are not necessary (American Board of Internal Medicine [ABIM], 2015). Management focuses on relief of discomfort, activity modification, and patient education. The presence of other medical problems complicates the picture and has higher cost, less favorable outcomes and more long-term disability (Schaafsma et al., 2015).

Nonprescription analgesics such as nonsteroidal anti-inflammatory drugs (NSAIDs) and short-term prescription muscle relaxants (e.g., cyclobenzaprine [Flexeril]) are effective in relieving acute low back pain, but no one medication is considered superior to another (Michigan Quality Improvement Consortium [MQIC], 2016a). Tricyclic antidepressants (e.g., amitriptyline [Elavil]) and the dual-action serotonin-norepinephrine reuptake inhibitors (e.g., duloxetine [Cymbalta]) (National Institute of Neurological Disorders [NINDS], 2014) or atypical anticonvulsant medications (e.g., gabapentin [Neurontin], which is prescribed for pain from radiculopathy) are used effectively in chronic low back pain. Opioid medications are indicated only short term for acute moderate to severe cases of low back pain, except in older adults, those with kidney disease, or those who must avoid chronic NSAID exposure because of its adverse gastric effects. Systemic corticosteroids and acetaminophen (Tylenol) are not effective in alleviating low back pain (Morgan, Dhruva, Wright, et al., 2015).

Effective nonpharmacologic interventions include thermal applications (hot or cold) and spinal manipulation (e.g., chiropractic therapy). Lumbar support belts are not recommended to treat acute low back pain but may be marginally effective devices for preventing low back pain in occupational health settings (MQIC, 2016a). Orthopedic shoe inserts are not recommended for prevention, but may help correct an underlying issue contributing to the problem (e.g., unequal leg length). Cognitive-behavioral therapy (e.g., biofeedback), exercise regimens, spinal manipulation, physical therapy, acupuncture, massage, and yoga are all effective nonpharmacologic interventions for treating chronic low back pain (Schaafsma et al., 2015).

Most patients need to alter their activity patterns to avoid aggravating the pain. They should avoid twisting, bending, lifting, and reaching—all of which stress the back. The patient is taught to change position frequently. Sitting should be limited to 20 to 50 minutes based on level of comfort. Absolute bed rest is no longer recommended; typical activities of daily living (ADLs) should be resumed as soon as possible. A quick return to normal activities and a program of low-stress aerobic exercise are recommended (MQIC, 2016a). Conditioning exercises for both back and trunk muscles are begun after about 2 weeks to help prevent recurrence of pain.

Chart 41-1	Diagnostic Procedures for Low Back Pain

X-ray of the spine: may demonstrate a fracture, dislocation, infection, osteoarthritis, or scoliosis

Bone scan and blood studies: may disclose infections, tumors, and bone marrow abnormalities

Computed tomography (CT) scan: useful in identifying underlying problems, such as obscure soft tissue lesions adjacent to the vertebral column and problems of vertebral discs

Magnetic resonance imaging (MRI) scan: permits visualization of the nature and location of spinal pathology

Electromyogram (EMG) and nerve conduction studies: used to evaluate spinal nerve root disorders (radiculopathies)

Myelogram: permits visualization of segments of the spinal cord that may have herniated or may be compressed (infrequently performed); indicated when MRI scan is contraindicated

Ultrasound: useful in detecting tears in ligaments, muscles, tendons, and soft tissues in the back

Nursing Assessment

The nurse asks the patient to describe the discomfort (e.g., location, severity, duration, characteristics, radiation, and weakness in the legs). Descriptions of how the pain occurred, such as with a specific action (e.g., opening a garage door) or with an activity in which weak muscles were overused (e.g., weekend gardening), and how the patient has dealt with the pain often suggest areas for intervention and patient education.

If back pain is a recurring problem, information about previous successful pain control methods helps in planning current management. Information about work and recreational activities helps identify areas for back health education. Because stress and anxiety can evoke muscle spasms and pain (de Heer, Gerrits, Beekman, et al., 2014), the nurse assesses environmental variables, work situations, and family relationships. In addition, the nurse assesses the effect of chronic pain on the emotional well-being of the patient. Referral to a mental health professional for assessment and management of stressors contributing to the low back pain and related depression may be appropriate.

During the interview, the nurse observes the patient's posture, position changes, and gait. Often, the patient's movements are guarded, with the back kept as still as possible. The patient should be directed to a chair of standard seat height with arms for support. The patient may sit and stand in an unusual position, leaning away from the most painful side, and may need assistance when undressing for the physical examination.

On physical examination, the nurse assesses the spinal curve, any leg length discrepancy, and pelvic crest and shoulder symmetry. The nurse palpates the paraspinal muscles and notes spasm and tenderness. When the patient is in a prone position, the paraspinal muscles relax and any deformity caused by spasm can subside. The nurse asks the patient to bend forward and then laterally, noting any discomfort or limitations in movement. It is important to determine the effect of these limitations on ADLs. The nurse evaluates nerve involvement by assessing deep tendon reflexes, sensations (e.g., paresthesia), and muscle strength. Back and leg pain on straight-leg raising (with the patient supine, the patient's leg is lifted upward with the knee extended) suggests nerve root involvement.

Nursing Management

The major nursing goals for the patient include relief of pain, improved physical mobility, the use of back-conserving techniques of body mechanics, improved self-esteem, and weight reduction (as necessary) (see Chart 41-2).

The nurse assesses the patient's response to analgesic agents. As the acute pain subsides, medication dosages are reduced. The nurse evaluates and notes the patient's response to various pain management modalities (see Chapter 12). The nurse cautions the patient with severe pain not to remain on bed rest because extended periods of inactivity are not effective and result in deconditioning. A medium to firm, nonsagging mattress (a bed board may be used) is recommended; there is no evidence to support the use of a firm mattress (Canadian Agency for Drugs and Technologies in Health, 2014). Lumbar flexion is increased by elevating the head and thorax 30 degrees by using pillows or a foam wedge and slightly flexing the knees supported on a pillow. Alternatively, the patient can assume a lateral position with knees and hips flexed (curled position) with a pillow between the knees and legs and a pillow supporting the head (see Fig. 41-1). A prone position should be avoided because it accentuates lordosis. The nurse instructs the patient to get out of bed by rolling to one side and placing the legs down while pushing the torso up, keeping the back straight (NINDS, 2014).

As the patient achieves comfort, an exercise program is gradually initiated with low-stress aerobic exercises, such as short walks or swimming. The physical therapist designs an exercise program for the patient to reduce lordosis, increase flexibility, and reduce strain on the back. It may include hyperextension exercises to strengthen the paravertebral muscles, flexion exercises to increase back movement and strength, and isometric flexion exercises to strengthen trunk muscles. Each 30-minute daily exercise period begins and ends with relaxation.

The nurse encourages the patient to adhere to the prescribed exercise program. Some patients may find it difficult to

---

Chart 41-2 | **HEALTH PROMOTION**
Strategies for Preventing Acute Low Back Pain

Prevention

- Weight reduction as needed: Modify diet to achieve ideal body weight
- Avoid high heels
- Walk daily and gradually increase the distance and pace of walking
- Avoid jumping and jarring activities
- Stretch to enhance flexibility. Do strengthening exercises

Body Mechanics

- Practice good posture
- Avoid twisting, lifting above waist level, and reaching up for any length of time
- Push objects rather than pull them
- Keep load close to your body when lifting
- Lift with the large leg muscles, not the back muscles

- Squat while keeping the back straight when it is necessary to pick something up off the floor
- Bend your knees and tighten abdominal muscles when lifting
- Avoid overreaching or a forward flexion position
- Use a wide base of support

Work Modifications

- Adjust height of chair using a footstool to position knees higher than hips
- Adjust height of work area to avoid stress on back
- Avoid bending, twisting, and lifting heavy objects
- Avoid prolonged standing and repetitive tasks
- Avoid work involving continuous vibrations
- Use lumbar support in straight back chair with arm rests
- When standing for any length of time, rest one foot on a small stool or box to relieve lumbar lordosis

Figure 41-1 • Positioning to promote lumbar flexion. Photo by B. Proud.

do so for a long period. In these instances, alternating activities may help facilitate adherence to the regimen (NINDS, 2014). Activities should not cause excessive lumbar strain or twisting, with avoidance of activities such as horseback riding and weight lifting.

Good body mechanics and posture are essential to avoid recurrence of back pain. The patient must be taught how to stand, sit, lie, and lift properly (see Fig. 41-2). Providing the patient with a list of suggestions helps in making these long-term changes (see Chart 41-2). The patient who wears high heels is encouraged to change to low heels with good arch support. The patient who is required to stand for long periods should shift weight frequently and rest one foot on a low stool, which decreases lumbar lordosis. Standing on a foot cushion made of foam or rubber can be helpful. The proper posture can be verified by looking in a mirror to see whether the chest is up, the abdomen is tucked in, and the shoulders are down and relaxed. Locking the knees when standing is avoided as well as bending forward for long periods.

When sitting, the knees and hips should be flexed, with the knees in level with the hips or higher to minimize lordosis. The feet should be flat on the floor or supported on a raised surface. Patients should avoid sitting on stools or chairs that do not provide firm back support.

The nurse instructs the patient in the safe and correct way to lift objects—using the strong quadriceps muscles of the thighs, with minimal use of weak back muscles (see Fig. 41-3). With feet placed hip-width apart to provide a wide base of support, the patient should bend the knees, tighten the abdominal muscles, and lift the object close to the body with a smooth motion, avoiding twisting and jarring motions. To prevent recurrence of acute low back pain, the patient should avoid lifting more than one third of their ideal weight without help.

Role-related responsibilities may have to be modified with the onset of low back pain (e.g., carrying children). As recovery progresses, the patient may resume them. However, if these activities contributed to the development of low back pain, resuming them may lead to the development of chronic low back pain, with associated disability. If the patient experiences secondary gains associated with low back disability (e.g., workers' compensation, easier lifestyle or workload, increased emotional support), there is a risk that the patient will not fully resume work and family roles. Earlier return to work and lifestyle, even at a reduced level, have better outcomes than

Figure 41-2 • Proper and improper standing postures. (*Left*) Abdominal muscles contracted, giving a feeling of upward pull, and gluteal muscles contracted, giving a downward pull. (*Right*) Slouch position, showing abdominal muscles relaxed and body out of proper alignment.

waiting for full recovery (Schaafsma et al., 2015). Antidepressants and counseling may be needed to assist the person in resuming a full, productive life. Specialized back clinics use

Figure 41-3 • Proper and improper lifting techniques. (*Left*) Correct position for lifting. This person is using the long and strong muscles of the arms and legs and holding the object so that the line of gravity falls within the base of support. (*Right*) Incorrect position for lifting. In this position, pull is exerted on the back muscles, and leaning causes the line of gravity to fall outside the base.

multidisciplinary approaches to help the patient with chronic pain resume role-related responsibilities.

Obesity contributes to back strain by overtaxing the relatively weak back muscles in the absence of abdominal muscle support. Exercises are less effective and more difficult to perform when the patient is overweight. Weight reduction through diet modification is imperative to prevent recurrence of back pain. A sound nutritional plan that includes a change in eating habits and low-impact activities is vital. Noting achievement of weight reduction and providing positive reinforcement facilitate adherence. Back problems may or may not resolve as optimal weight is achieved (MQCI, 2016a).

Common Upper Extremity Disorders

The structures in the upper extremities are frequently the sites of painful syndromes. This is especially true in occupational health settings, where many patient visits involve the shoulder, wrist, and hand.

Bursitis and Tendonitis

Bursitis and tendonitis are inflammatory conditions that commonly occur in the shoulder. Bursae are fluid-filled sacs that prevent friction between joint structures during joint activity and are painful when inflamed; **bursitis** is the consequence when these sacs become inflamed. Muscle tendon sheaths also become inflamed with repetitive stretching, causing **tendonitis.** The inflammation causes proliferation of synovial membrane and pannus formation, which restricts joint movement. Conservative treatment includes rest of the extremity, intermittent ice and heat to the joint, and NSAIDs to control the inflammation and pain. Newer therapies that include extracorporeal shock waves, pulsed magnetic fields, laser phototherapy, radiofrequency ablation and stem cell therapies (Rodriguez, 2014) may accelerate tendon healing, although further research is needed to determine their overall effectiveness. These modalities are expensive and are therefore not first line treatments. Arthroscopic synovectomy may be considered if shoulder pain and weakness persist. Corticosteroid injections remain more evidence based than most other interventions for short-term, rapid improvement in the shoulder, but are not always helpful in the long term (Dong, Goost, Lin, et al., 2015). Most tendon and bursal inflammatory problems are self-limiting; as they go away on their own with or without therapy. The treatments are primarily aimed at pain relief, not cure.

Loose Bodies

Loose bodies ("joint mice") may occur in a joint space as a result of articular cartilage wear and bone erosion. These fragments can interfere with joint movement ("locking the joint"). Loose bodies are removed by arthroscopic surgery if they cause pain or mobility issues.

Impingement Syndrome

Impingement syndrome is a general term that describes impaired movement of the rotator cuff of the shoulder. Impingement usually occurs from repetitive overhead movement of the arm or from acute trauma resulting in irritation and eventual inflammation of the rotator cuff tendons or the subacromial

---

> **Chart 41-3**
>
> **PATIENT EDUCATION**
>
> ### Measures to Promote Shoulder Healing of Impingement Syndrome
>
> The nurse instructs the patient to:
>
> - Rest the joint in a position that minimizes stress on the joint structures to prevent further damage and the development of adhesions.
> - Support the affected arm on pillows while sleeping to keep from turning onto the shoulder.
> - Gradually resume motion and use of the joint. Assistance with dressing and other activities of daily living may be needed.
> - Avoid working and lifting above shoulder level or pushing an object against a "locked" shoulder.
> - Perform the prescribed daily range-of-motion and strengthening exercises.

bursa as they grate against the coracoacromial arch. Early manifestations of this syndrome are characterized by edema from hemorrhage of these structures, pain, shoulder tenderness, limited movement, muscle spasm, and eventual disuse atrophy. The process may progress to a partial or complete rotator cuff tear (see Chapter 42).

Medications used to treat early impingement syndrome include oral NSAIDs or intra-articular injections of corticosteroids. Application of superficial cold or heat may subjectively improve patients' symptoms; however, a therapeutic exercise program (see Chapter 42) is required to improve outcomes, including reduction of pain and improved shoulder function (see Chart 41-3).

Carpal Tunnel Syndrome

Carpal tunnel syndrome is an entrapment neuropathy that occurs when the median nerve at the wrist is compressed by a thickened flexor tendon sheath, skeletal encroachment, edema, or a soft tissue mass. It frequently occurs in women between 30 and 60 years of age. Commonly caused by repetitive hand and wrist movements, it is also associated with rheumatoid arthritis, diabetes, acromegaly, hyperthyroidism, or trauma (Grossman & Porth, 2014).

The patient experiences pain, numbness, paresthesia, and, possibly, weakness along the median nerve distribution (thumb, index, and middle fingers). Night pain and/or fist clenching upon awakening is common. A positive Tinel sign helps identify patients requiring intervention (see Fig. 41-4).

Evidence-based treatment of acute carpal tunnel syndrome includes oral or intra-articular injections of corticosteroids, use of NSAIDs and acupuncture with and without electrical stimulation (attached to the needles). Application of wrist splints to prevent hyperextension and prolonged flexion of the wrist is also effective; however, yoga, laser therapy, and ultrasound therapy are ineffective therapies, as are prolotherapies, or the injection of substances (e.g., dextrose, lidocaine) purported to stimulate healing, diuretics, and vitamin B_6 (American College of Occupational and Environmental Medicine, 2011). The risks of inhibiting the synthesis of reparative substrates like collagen can potentiate an increased risk for tendon rupture; therefore, use of corticosteroids over the long term is not supported (Dong et al., 2015).

Figure 41-4 • Tinel sign may be elicited in patients with carpal tunnel syndrome by percussing lightly over the median nerve, located on the inner aspect of the wrist. If the patient reports tingling, numbness, and pain, the test for Tinel sign is considered positive. From Weber, J. W., & Kelley, J. (2014). *Health assessment in nursing* (5th ed.). Philadelphia, PA: Lippincott Williams & Wilkins. Photo by B. Proud.

Traditional open nerve release or endoscopic laser surgery are the two most common surgical management options when nonsurgical treatments fail. Both of these procedures are performed under local anesthesia and involve making incisions into the affected wrist and cutting the carpal ligament so that the carpal tunnel is widened. Smaller incisions are made with the endoscopic laser procedure, resulting in less scar formation and a shorter recovery time than with the open method. Following either procedure, the patient wears a hand splint and limits hand use during healing. The patient may need assistance with personal care. Full recovery of motor and sensory function after either type of nerve release surgery may take several weeks or months.

Ganglion

A ganglion—a collection of neurologic gelatinous material near the tendon sheaths and joints—appears as a round, firm, cystic swelling, usually on the dorsum of the wrist. It frequently occurs in women younger than 50 years (Grossman & Porth, 2014). The swelling is locally tender and may cause an aching pain. When a tendon sheath is involved, weakness of the finger occurs. Treatment may include aspiration, corticosteroid injection, or surgical excision. After treatment, a compression dressing and immobilization splint are used.

Dupuytren Disease

Dupuytren disease results in a slowly progressive **contracture** (i.e., an abnormal shortening) of the palmar fascia that causes flexion of the fourth, fifth, and, sometimes, middle finger, rendering these fingers more or less useless (see Fig. 41-5). It is linked to an inherited autosomal dominant trait and occurs most frequently in men of Scandinavian or Celtic heritage who are older than 50 years (Grossman & Porth, 2014). Dupuytren disease is also associated with arthritis, diabetes, gout, cigarette smoking, and alcoholism (Sood, Paik, & Lee, 2013). Starting as a nodule, it may or may not progress, producing a contracture of the fingers and palmar skin changes.

Figure 41-5 • Dupuytren contracture, a flexion deformity caused by an inherited trait, is a slowly progressive contracture of the palmar fascia, which severely impairs the function of the fourth, fifth, and, sometimes, middle finger.

The patient may experience dull and aching discomfort, morning numbness, and stiffness in the affected fingers. This condition starts in one hand, but eventually both are affected. Finger-stretching exercises or intra-nodular injections of corticosteroids may prevent contractures. With loss of movement, palmar and digital fasciotomies are performed to improve function.

Nursing Management of the Patient Undergoing Surgery of the Hand or Wrist

Surgery of the hand or wrist, unless related to major trauma, is generally an ambulatory procedure. Before surgery, the nurse assesses the patient's level and type of discomfort, as well as limitations in function, caused by the condition.

Hourly neurovascular assessment of the exposed fingers for the first 24 hours following surgery is essential for monitoring function of the nerves and perfusion. This is especially important if an intraoperative tourniquet technique was used, which is implicated in neurovascular deficits. The nurse compares the affected extremity with the unaffected extremity and the postoperative status with the documented preoperative status. The nurse asks the patient to describe sensations in the digits and has the patient demonstrate mobility, while enforcing limitations in movement prescribed by the patient's surgeon. With tendon repairs and nerve, vascular, or skin grafts, more extensive function is tested (see Chapter 39, Chart 39-2). Percutaneous pins may be used to hold bones in position. These pins serve as potential sites of infection. Patient instructions concerning aseptic wound and pin care may be necessary.

Dressings provide support but should be nonconstrictive. Intermittent use of ice packs to the surgical area during the first 24 to 48 hours may be prescribed to control edema. Unless contraindicated, active extension and flexion of the fingers to promote circulation are encouraged, even though movement is limited by the bulky dressing.

Generally, pain and discomfort can be controlled by the use of oral analgesic agents. Patient education concerning the risk of falls and impaired cognition is important. Pain out of proportion to what is expected, particularly if it is accompanied with compromised neurovascular functioning, needs to be evaluated as an indication of compartment syndrome (see Chapter 42). Pain may be related to surgery, edema, hematoma formation, or restrictive bandages. To control swelling that may increase the patient's discomfort, the nurse instructs the patient to elevate the hand to heart level with pillows. If the patient is ambulatory, the arm is supported in a conventional sling with the hand elevated at heart level (see Chapter 42, Fig. 42-10).

During the first few days after surgery, independent self-care is impaired. The patient may need to arrange for assistance with feeding, bathing, dressing, and toileting. Within a few days, the patient develops skills in one-handed ADLs and is usually able to function with minimal help and assistive devices. The nurse encourages the patient to use the involved hand, unless contraindicated, within the limits of discomfort. As rehabilitation progresses, the patient resumes use of the limb. Physical or occupational therapy–directed exercises may be prescribed.

Promoting Home, Community-Based, and Transitional Care

 Educating Patients about Self-Care

After the patient has undergone surgery, the nurse instructs the patient how to monitor neurovascular status and the signs of complications that need to be reported to the surgeon (e.g., paresthesia, paralysis, uncontrolled pain, coolness of fingers, extreme swelling, excessive bleeding, purulent drainage, foul odor, fever). The nurse discusses prescribed medications and their side effects with the patient. In addition, the nurse instructs the patient how to elevate the extremity and to apply ice (if prescribed) to control swelling. The use of assistive devices is demonstrated if such devices would be helpful in promoting accomplishment of ADLs. For bathing, the nurse instructs the patient to keep the dressing dry by covering it with a secured plastic bag. Generally, the wound is not redressed until the patient's follow-up visit with the surgeon (see Chart 41-4). The nurse identifies any perceived barriers to being able to attend to this plan (such as childcare needs). The patient is referred to community-based resources as appropriate.

Common Foot Problems

Disorders of the foot may be caused by poorly fitting shoes, which distort normal anatomy while inducing deformity and pain. Dermatologic problems commonly affect the feet in the form of fungal infections and plantar warts. Several systemic diseases affect the feet. Patients with diabetes are prone to develop corns and peripheral neuropathies with diminished sensation, leading to ulcers at pressure points of the foot. Patients with peripheral vascular disease and arteriosclerosis complain of burning and itching feet, resulting in scratching and skin breakdown. Foot deformities may occur with rheumatoid arthritis. Obesity can cause a host of foot anomalies, including adult-onset pes planus (i.e., "fallen arches") and plantar fasciitis.

The discomforts of foot strain are treated with rest, elevation, physiotherapy, supportive taping, and orthotic devices (American College of Foot and Ankle Surgeons [ACFAS], 2010; Shirzad, Kiesau, DeOrio, et al., 2011). The patient must inspect the foot and skin under pads and orthotic devices for pressure and skin breakdown daily. If a "window" is cut into shoes to relieve pressure over a bony deformity, the skin must be monitored daily for breakdown from pressure exerted at the window area. Active foot exercises promote circulation and help strengthen the feet. Walking in properly fitting shoes is considered the ideal exercise.

Callus

A callus is a thickened area of the skin that has been exposed to persistent pressure or friction. Faulty foot mechanics usually precede the formation of a callus. Treatment consists of eliminating the underlying causes and having a painful callus

---

Chart 41-4 **HOME CARE CHECKLIST**

Hand or Foot Surgery

At the completion of education, the patient and/or caregiver will be able to:

- Name the procedure that was performed and identify any permanent changes in anatomic structure or function as well as changes in ADLs, IADLs, roles, relationships, and spirituality.
- Identify modification of home environment, interventions, and strategies (e.g., durable medical equipment, adaptive equipment) used in safely adapting to changes in structure or function and promote effective recovery and rehabilitation.
- Describe ongoing postoperative therapeutic regimen, including diet and activities to perform (e.g., immobilization) and to limit or avoid (e.g., lifting weights, driving a car, contact sports).
  - Describe methods to prevent wound infection (e.g., keeping dressing clean and dry during activities of daily living).
  - Demonstrate how to assess neurovascular status.
  - Demonstrate control of edema by elevating extremity and applying ice intermittently if prescribed.
  - Observe prescribed weight-bearing, activity and exercise limits.
  - Demonstrate safe use of assistive devices, if appropriate.
  - Consume a healthy diet to promote healing.
- State the name, dose, side effects, frequency, and schedule for all prescribed therapeutic and prophylactic medications (e.g., antibiotics and analgesic agents).

- State indicators of wound infections (e.g., redness, swelling, tenderness, purulent drainage, fever, signs of systemic infection) to report promptly to primary provider.
- State indicators of other potential complications to report promptly to primary provider (e.g., uncontrolled swelling and pain; cool, pale fingers or toes; paresthesia; paralysis; purulent drainage; signs of deep vein thrombosis or pulmonary embolism).
- Relate how to reach primary provider with questions or complications.
- Verbalize the need to keep appointment with surgeon for initial dressing change.
  - State time and date of follow-up appointments and testing.
- Identify the need for health promotion (e.g., weight reduction, smoking cessation, stress management), disease prevention and screening activities.

Resources

See Chapter 10, Chart 10-8 for additional information related to durable medical equipment, adaptive equipment, mobility skills, skin, bowel, and bladder care.

ADL, activities of daily living; IADL, independent activities of daily living.

treated by a podiatrist. A keratolytic ointment may be applied and a thin plastic cup worn over the heel if the callus is on this area. Felt padding with an adhesive backing is also used to prevent and relieve pressure. Orthotic devices can be made to remove the pressure from bony protuberances, or the protuberance may be excised (American College of Foot and Ankle Surgeons [ACFAS], 2009; ACFAS, 2010).

Corn

A corn is an area of hyperkeratosis (overgrowth of a horny layer of epidermis) produced by internal pressure (the underlying bone is prominent because of a congenital or acquired abnormality, commonly arthritis) or external pressure (ill-fitting shoes). The fifth toe is most frequently involved, but any toe may be involved.

Corns are treated by a podiatrist by soaking and scraping off the horny layer, by application of a protective shield or pad, or by surgical modification of the underlying offending osseous structure. Injection of bleomycin (Blenoxane; a chemotherapy drug) is being evaluated as a solution for hard to treat corns that are surgically treated (Lee, Lee, Won, et al., 2014). Soft corns are located between the toes and are kept soft by moisture. Treatment consists of drying the affected spaces and separating the affected toes with lamb's wool or gauze. A wider shoe and toe box may be helpful (ACFAS, 2009).

Hallux Valgus

Hallux valgus (bunion) is a deformity in which the great toe deviates laterally (see Fig. 41-6A). There is a marked prominence of the medial aspect of the first metatarsophalangeal joint. There is also osseous enlargement (exostosis) of the medial side of the first metatarsal head, over which a bursa may form (secondary to pressure and inflammation). Acute bursitis symptoms include a reddened area, edema, and tenderness.

Factors contributing to bunion formation include heredity, ill-fitting shoes, osteoarthritis, and the gradual lengthening and widening of the foot associated with aging. Treatment depends on the patient's age, the degree of deformity, and the severity of symptoms. In uncomplicated cases, wearing a shoe that conforms to the shape of the foot, or that is molded to the foot to prevent pressure on the protruding portions, may be the only treatment needed. Corticosteroid injections control acute inflammation. In advanced cases, surgical removal of the exostosis and toe realignment may be required to improve function, appearance, and symptoms.

Hammer Toe

Hammer toe is a flexion deformity of the interphalangeal joint, which may involve several toes (see Fig. 41-6B). Tight socks or shoes may push an overlying toe back into the line of the other toes. The toes usually are pulled upward, forcing the metatarsal joints (ball of the foot) downward. Corns develop on top of the toes, and tender calluses develop under the metatarsal area. Treatment consists of conservative measures: wearing open-toed sandals or shoes that conform to the shape of the foot, carrying out manipulative exercises, and protecting the protruding joints with pads. Surgery (osteotomy) may be used to correct a resulting deformity. There

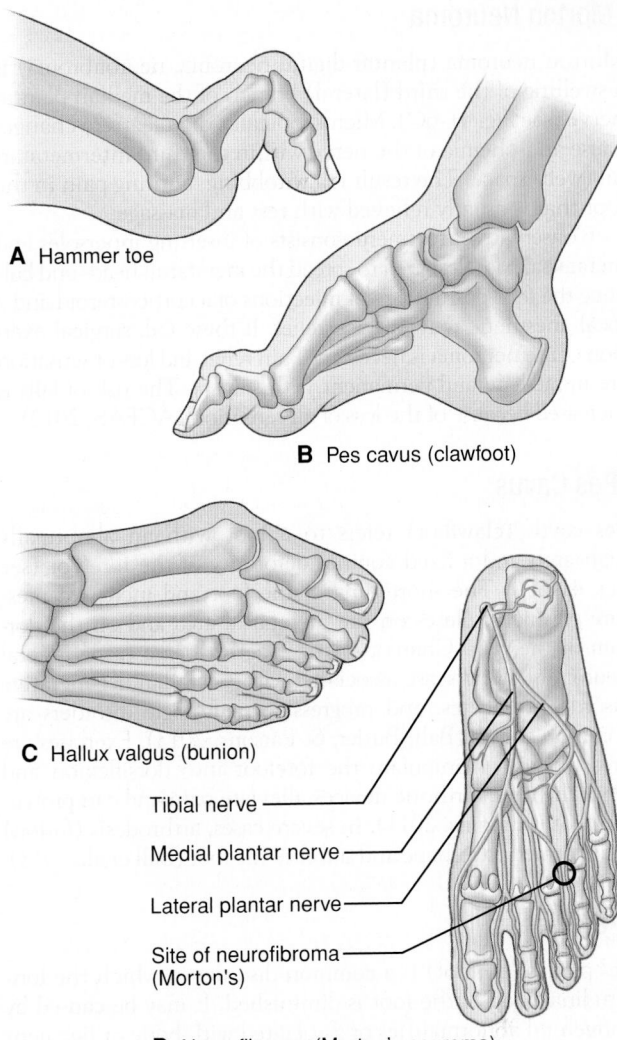

A Hammer toe

B Pes cavus (clawfoot)

C Hallux valgus (bunion)

Tibial nerve
Medial plantar nerve
Lateral plantar nerve
Site of neurofibroma (Morton's)

D Neurofibroma (Morton's neuroma)

Figure 41-6 • Common foot deformities.

is little evidence to support treatment of hammer toe when the patient does not report pain or other symptoms (ACFAS, 2009; Shirzad et al., 2011). Orthotics may help prevent them in persons with high arches.

Ingrown Toenail

An ingrown toenail (onychocryptosis) is a condition in which the free edge of a nail plate penetrates the surrounding skin. A secondary infection or granulation tissue may develop. This painful condition is caused by improper self-treatment, external pressure (tight shoes or stockings), internal pressure (deformed toes, growth under the nail), trauma, or infection. Trimming the nails properly (clipping them straight across and filing the corners consistent with the contour of the toe) can prevent this problem. Active treatment consists of washing the foot twice a day and relieving the pain by decreasing the pressure of the nail plate on the surrounding soft tissue (ACFAS, 2010). Warm, wet soaks help drain an infection. A toenail may need to be excised by the podiatrist or primary provider if there are recurrent infections.

Morton Neuroma

Morton neuroma (plantar digital neuroma, neurofibroma) is a swelling of the third (lateral) branch of the median plantar nerve (see Fig. 41-6C). Microscopically, digital artery changes cause an ischemia of the nerve within the third intermetatarsal (web) space. The result is a throbbing, burning pain in the foot that is usually relieved with rest and massage.

Conservative treatment consists of inserting innersoles and metatarsal pads designed to spread the metatarsal heads and balance the foot posture. Local injections of a corticosteroid and a local anesthetic may provide relief. If these fail, surgical excision of the neuroma is necessary. Pain relief and loss of sensation are immediate and permanent with surgery. The risk of falls is increased because of the loss of all sensation (ACFAS, 2010).

Pes Cavus

Pes cavus (clawfoot) refers to a foot with an abnormally high arch and a fixed equines deformity of the forefoot (see Fig. 41-6D). The shortening of the foot and increased pressure produce calluses on the metatarsal area and on the dorsum of the foot. Charcot–Marie–Tooth disease (a peripheral neuromuscular disease associated with a familial degenerative disorder), diabetes, and progressive neurologic disorders are common causes (Ball, Butler, & Parsons, 2013). Exercises are prescribed to manipulate the forefoot into dorsiflexion and relax the toes. Orthotic devices alleviate pain and can protect the foot (Huppins, 2011). In severe cases, arthrodesis (fusion) is performed to reshape and stabilize the foot (Ball et al., 2013).

Pes Planus

Pes planus (flatfoot) is a common disorder in which the longitudinal arch of the foot is diminished. It may be caused by congenital abnormalities or associated with bone or ligament injury, excessive weight, muscle fatigue, poorly fitting shoes, or arthritis. Signs and symptoms include a burning sensation, fatigue, clumsy gait, edema, and pain. Exercises to strengthen the muscles and to improve posture and walking habits are helpful. Foot orthoses can give the foot additional support (Banwell, Mackintosh, & Thewlis, 2014).

Plantar Fasciitis

Plantar fasciitis, an inflammation of the foot-supporting fascia, presents as an acute onset of heel pain experienced with the first steps in the morning. The pain is localized to the anterior medial aspect of the heel and diminishes with gentle stretching of the foot and Achilles tendon. Management includes stretching exercises, wearing shoes with support and cushioning to relieve pain, orthotic devices (e.g., heel cups, arch supports, night splints), and corticosteroid injections (Johnson, Haas, Lindow, et al., 2014). Unresolved plantar fasciitis may progress to fascial tears at the heel and eventual development of heel spurs.

Nursing Management of the Patient Undergoing Foot Surgery

Surgery of the foot may be necessary because of various conditions, including neuromas and foot deformities (bunion, hammer toe, clawfoot). Generally, foot surgery is performed on an outpatient basis. Before surgery, the nurse assesses the patient's gait and balance, as well as the neurovascular status of the foot. Additionally, the nurse considers the availability of assistance at home and the structural characteristics of the home in planning for care during the days after surgery.

Postoperative and home care follows the same principles as discussed earlier for hand surgery (see Chart 41-4). After surgery, neurovascular assessment of the exposed toes (every 1 to 2 hours for the first 24 hours) is essential to monitor the function of the nerves and the perfusion of the tissues. The nurse educates the patient and family about how to assess for edema and neurovascular status at home (circulation, motion, sensation). The affected foot is compared to the unaffected foot to determine differences in neurovascular function. Compromised neurovascular function can increase the patient's pain (see Chapter 39, Chart 39-3).

Pain experienced by patients who undergo foot surgery is related to inflammation and edema. Formation of a hematoma may contribute to the discomfort. To control the anticipated edema, the foot should be elevated on several pillows when the patient is sitting or lying. Support of the entire limb under the knee is preferable. Ice packs applied intermittently to the surgical area during the first 24 to 48 hours may be prescribed to control edema and provide some pain relief. As activity increases, the patient may find that dependent positioning of the foot is uncomfortable. Simply elevating the foot often relieves the discomfort. Oral analgesic agents may be used to control the pain. The nurse instructs the patient and family about appropriate use of these medications.

After surgery, the patient will have a bulky dressing on the foot, protected by a light cast or a special protective boot. Limits for weight bearing on the foot will be prescribed by the surgeon. Some patients are allowed to walk on the heel and progress to weight bearing as tolerated; other patients are restricted to non–weight-bearing activities. Assistive devices (e.g., crutches, walker) may be needed. The choice of the devices depends on the patient's general condition and balance and on the weight-bearing prescription. Safe use of the assistive devices must be ensured through adequate patient education and practice before discharge (see Chapter 10). Strategies to move around the house safely while using assistive devices are also discussed with the patient. As healing progresses, the patient gradually resumes ambulation within prescribed limits. The nurse emphasizes compliance with the therapeutic regimen.

The immobility of lower extremity surgery increases the risk of venous thromboembolism (VTE) development. See Chapter 30 for VTE risk assessment and treatment. Other postoperative complications may include limited range of motion, paresthesia, tendon injury, and recurrence of deformity (ACFAS, 2009). In addition, if percutaneous pins were used to hold bones in position, these pins may serve as potential sites of infection. Patient instructions concerning aseptic wound care and pin care may be necessary. See Chapter 40 for further discussion on pin care and infection prophylaxis. Care must be taken to protect the surgical wound from dirt and moisture. When bathing, the patient can secure a plastic bag over the dressing to prevent it from getting wet.

Metabolic Bone Disorders

Osteoporosis

Osteoporosis is the most prevalent bone disease in the world. More than 1.5 million osteoporotic fractures occur every year. Fractures requiring hospitalization have risen significantly over the past two decades (Cosman, de Beur, LeBoff, et al., 2014). More than 10 million Americans have osteoporosis, and an additional 33.6 million have **osteopenia** (i.e., low bone mineral density [BMD])—the precursor to osteoporosis. The consequence of osteoporosis is bone fracture. It is projected that one of every two Caucasian women and one of every five men will have an osteoporosis-related fracture at some point in their lives (Cosman et al., 2014).

Prevention

Peak adult bone mass is achieved between the ages of 18 and 25 years in both women and men and is affected by genetic factors, nutrition, physical activity, medications, endocrine status, and general health (Cosman et al., 2014).

Primary osteoporosis occurs in women after menopause (usually by age 51) and in men later in life, but it is not merely a consequence of aging. Failure to develop optimal peak bone mass and low vitamin D levels contribute to the development of osteopenia without associated bone loss. Early identification of at-risk teenagers and young adults, increased calcium and vitamin D intake, participation in regular weight-bearing exercise, and modification of lifestyle (e.g., reduced use of caffeine, tobacco products, carbonated soft drinks, and alcohol) are interventions that decrease the risk of fractures and associated disability later in life (Cosman et al., 2014).

Secondary osteoporosis is the result of medications or diseases that affect bone metabolism. Men are more likely than women to have secondary causes of osteoporosis, including the use of corticosteroids (especially if they receive doses in excess of 5 mg of prednisone daily for more than 3 months) and excessive alcohol intake. Specific disease states (e.g., celiac disease, hypogonadism) and medications such as anticonvulsants (phenytoin [Dilantin]), thyroid replacement agents (levothyroxine [Synthroid]), antiestrogens (medroxyprogesterone [Depo-Provera]), androgen inhibitors (leuprolide [Lupron]), and proton pump inhibitors (esomeprazole [Nexium]) that place patients at risk need to be identified and therapies instituted to reverse the development of osteoporosis (Cosman et al., 2014). The degree of bone loss is related to the duration of medication therapy. When the drugs are discontinued or the metabolic problem is corrected, the progression is halted but restoration of lost bone mass may not occur (see Chart 41-5).

Gerontologic Considerations

The prevalence of osteoporosis in women older than 80 years is 50%. The average 75-year-old woman has lost 25% of her cortical bone and 40% of her trabecular bone. Most residents of long-term care facilities have a low BMD and are at risk for bone fracture. One third of all hip fractures occur among men, and men have a higher mortality rate than women after sustaining a hip fracture (NPS Medicinewise, 2015). It is estimated that the number of hip fractures and their associated costs will at least double by the year 2040 because of the projected aging of the United States population (Cosman et al., 2014).

Routine vertebral fracture screenings are not recommended. However, 80% to 90% of these fractures can be seen incidentally on chest x-rays taken for other purposes. It is estimated that only one third of vertebral fractures are diagnosed. Vertebral fracture risk is five times higher among patients who have had prior fractures. Furthermore, 20% of women who are postmenopausal who have a vertebral fracture will have another one within one year (Wong & McGirt, 2013).

Older adults absorb dietary calcium less efficiently and excrete it more readily through their kidneys. Postmenopausal women and older adults need to consume approximately 1200 mg of daily calcium. Quantities larger than this may place patients at heightened risk of renal calculi or cardiovascular disease (United States Preventive Services Task Force [USPSTF], 2013).

Chart 41-5 **HEALTH PROMOTION** Strategies for Preventing Osteoporosis

Adolescents and Young Adults

- Educate so that they can:
  - Characterize risk factors for osteoporosis.
  - Consume diet with adequate calcium (1000–1300 mg/day) and vitamin D.
  - Engage in weight-bearing exercise daily.
  - Identify calcium- and vitamin D-rich foods.
  - Modify lifestyle choices—avoid smoking, alcohol, caffeine, and carbonated beverages.

Women Who Are Menopausal and Postmenopausal (in addition to above)

- Educate so that they can:
  - Assess home environment for hazards contributing to falls.
  - Demonstrate good body mechanics.
  - Describe appropriate calcium supplements and pharmacologic agents to maintain and enhance bone mass.

- Engage in exercise that improves balance to reduce risk of falls.
- Review concurrent medical conditions and medications with primary provider to identify factors that contribute to bone mass loss.

Men (in addition to above)

- Educate so that they can:
  - Characterize risk factors associated with osteoporosis in men, including medications (e.g., corticosteroids, anticonvulsants, aluminum-containing antacids), chronic diseases (e.g., kidney, lung, gastrointestinal), and undiagnosed low testosterone levels.
- Participate in screening for osteoporosis.
- Talk with primary provider about the use of medications (e.g., alendronate) to enhance bone mass or to correct testosterone deficiency.

Figure 41-7 • Progressive osteoporotic bone loss and compression fractures. From Rubin, E., Gorstein, F., Schwarting, R., et al. (2004). *Pathology* (4th ed.). Philadelphia, PA: Lippincott Williams & Wilkins.

| 10 yrs. postmenopause | 15 yrs. postmenopause height loss 1.5" | 25 yrs. postmenopause height loss 3.5" |

Figure 41-8 • Typical loss of height associated with osteoporosis and aging.

Pathophysiology

Osteoporosis is characterized by reduced bone mass, deterioration of bone matrix, and diminished bone architectural strength. Normal homeostatic bone turnover is altered; the rate of bone resorption that is maintained by osteoclasts is greater than the rate of bone formation that is maintained by osteoblasts, resulting in a reduced total bone mass. The bones become progressively porous, brittle, and fragile. They fracture easily under stresses that would not break normal bone. This occurs most commonly as compression fractures (see Fig. 41-7) of the thoracic and lumbar spine, hip fractures, and Colles fractures of the wrist. These fractures may be the first clinical manifestation of osteoporosis (Cosman et al., 2014).

The gradual collapse of a vertebra may be asymptomatic. With the development of kyphosis (i.e., Dowager hump), there is an associated loss of height (see Fig. 41-8). The postural changes result in relaxation of the abdominal muscles and a protruding abdomen. The deformity may also produce pulmonary insufficiency and increase the risk for falls related to balance issues.

Age-related loss begins soon after the peak bone mass is achieved (i.e., in the fourth decade). Calcitonin, which inhibits bone resorption and promotes bone formation, is decreased. Estrogen, which inhibits bone breakdown, also decreases with aging. On the other hand, parathyroid hormone (PTH) increases with aging, thus increasing bone turnover and resorption. The consequence of these changes is net loss of bone mass over time.

The withdrawal of estrogens at menopause or with oophorectomy causes an accelerated bone resorption within the first 5 years after cessation of menses. Most women lose 10% of their bone mass. More than half of all women older than 50 years show evidence of osteopenia (Cosman et al., 2014; MQIC, 2016b).

Risk Factors

Small-framed women are at greatest risk for osteoporosis. Men have a greater peak bone mass and do not experience a sudden midlife estrogen reduction. As a result, osteoporosis occurs about one decade later, but one in four men still sustain an osteopenic fracture (Cosman et al., 2014; Fasolino & Whitright, 2015). It is believed that both testosterone and estrogen are important in achieving and maintaining bone mass in men, although the risk profile for men is not as well established as it is for women (see Chart 41-6). Risk for osteoporosis rises with increasing age for both genders (Fasolino & Whitright, 2015; Wong & McGirt, 2013) (see Chart 41-7).

Nutritional factors contribute to the development of osteoporosis. A diet that includes adequate calories and nutrients needed to maintain bone, calcium, and vitamin D must be consumed. Patients who have had bariatric surgery are at increased risk for osteoporosis as the duodenum is bypassed, which is the primary site for absorption of calcium. Patients who have gastrointestinal diseases that cause malabsorption (e.g., celiac disease, alcoholism) may benefit from additional magnesium supplements (González-Reimers, Quintero-Platt, Rodríguez-Rodríguez, et al., 2015).

NURSING RESEARCH PROFILE

Chart 41-6

Osteoporosis Risks in Men

Fasolino, T. & Whitright, T. (2015). A pilot study to identify modifiable and non-modifiable variables associated with osteopenia and osteoporosis in men. *Orthopaedic Nursing 34*(5), 289–293.

Purpose

Modifiable and nonmodifiable risk factors for women with osteoporosis have been identified. However, one in four men over the age of 60 will have an osteoporotic fracture in their lifetime, scant evidence focuses on their risks, hampering the development of male specific osteoporosis screening and prevention programs. The purpose of this study was to identify risk factors that lead to osteoporosis in men.

Design

This was an exploratory pilot study conducted among patients affiliated with an internal medicine practice. Self-report surveys were completed by male participants between the ages of 65 and 75 years who had not previously been diagnosed with osteopenia or osteoporosis, were not taking bisphosphonate medications, and did not have a history of hyperthyroidism or parathyroid disease. Self-report measures on the survey included use of tobacco, alcohol consumption, exercise history, fracture history in adulthood, and family history of osteoporosis. Body mass indices (BMIs) were calculated based upon participants' height and weight. Bone Mineral Density (BMD) studies using DEXA imaging were completed on each participant.

Findings

Ninety-two of 101 participants (99% Caucasian; mean age 70.7 years) completed all portions of the study. Thirty-nine (38.6%) participants had normal BMDs, 43 (42.6%) participants had osteopenia, and 19 (18.8%) participants had previously undiagnosed osteoporosis. Among potential modifiable risk factors analyzed, only a lower BMI was significantly associated with lower BMD ($p = 0.02$). Tobacco use, alcohol consumption, and self-reported exercise levels were not statistically related to BMD results. None of the potential nonmodifiable risk factors, including age, history of fracture, and family history, correlated with BMD.

Nursing Implications

Over half of the men in this study had low BMDs, with 18.8% found to have osteoporosis that had not been previously diagnosed. These findings suggest that current recommendations set by the U.S. Preventive Services Task Force to not screen men for osteopenia and osteoporosis before the age of 70 should be reconsidered. However, results from this study do not clearly illuminate which osteoporosis risk factors are of significance to men. This research must be replicated with a larger sample and include men from more diverse ethnic backgrounds that better mirror the diversity among American men.

Bone formation is enhanced by the stress of weight and muscle activity. When immobilized by casts, general inactivity, paralysis, or other disability, the bone is resorbed faster than it is formed, and osteoporosis results (Grossman & Porth, 2014). Immobility contributes to the development of osteoporosis. Resistance and impact exercises are most beneficial in developing and maintaining bone mass (Fasolino & Whitwright, 2015).

Chart 41-7 ⚠ RISK FACTORS
Osteoporosis

- Alcohol intake of 3 or more drinks daily
- Current use of tobacco products
- Family history
- History of bone fracture during adulthood
- Inactive or sedentary lifestyle
- Inadequate calcium and vitamin D intake
- Low body mass index
- Malabsorption disorders (e.g., eating disorder, celiac disease, bariatric surgery)
- Men older than 60 years of age
- Women who are postmenopausal
- Prescribed corticosteroids (e.g., prednisone) for longer than 3 months

Adapted from Cosman, F., de Beur, S., J. LeBoff, M. S., et al. (2014). Clinician's guide to prevention and treatment of osteoporosis. *Osteoporosis International, 25*(10), 2359–2381; Fasolino, T. & Whitright, T. (2015). A pilot study to identify modifiable and non-modifiable variables associated with osteopenia and osteoporosis in men. *Orthopaedic Nursing 34*(5), 289–293; Smeltzer, S. C., & Qi, B. B. (2014). Practical implications for nurses caring for patients being treated for osteoporosis. *Nursing: Research and Reviews, 4*(4), 19–33.

Assessment and Diagnostic Findings

Osteoporosis may be undetectable on routine x-rays until there has been significant demineralization, resulting in radiolucency of the bones (Cosman et al., 2014). When the vertebrae collapse, causing compression fractures, the thoracic vertebrae become wedge shaped and the lumbar vertebrae become biconcave. Osteoporosis is diagnosed by dual-energy x-ray absorptiometry (DEXA), which provides information about BMD at the spine and hip (see Chapter 39). The DEXA scan data are analyzed and reported as T-scores (the number of standard deviations above or below the average BMD value for a 30-year-old healthy Caucasian woman). T-scores that are gender specific for men are not yet available.

Baseline DEXA testing is recommended for all women older than 65 years, for women who are postmenopausal older than 50 years with osteoporosis risk factors, and for all people who have had a fracture thought to occur as a consequence of osteoporosis (Cosman et al., 2014). BMD studies are also useful in assessing response to therapy and are recommended 3 months post any osteoporotic fracture. There is no evidence to support basic screening of men or for the optimal time interval to repeat studies following a normal baseline report.

Fracture risk can be estimated using the World Health Organization (WHO) Fracture Risk Assessment Tool (FRAX). Treatment is now reserved for those with a 10-year risk of more than 3% for hip fracture or 20% for other major fractures. The risks scores are based on BMD, personal and family history of fractures, body mass index, gender, age, and secondary factors such as medication use, smoking, and history of rheumatoid disease (Cosman et al., 2014).

Laboratory studies (e.g., serum calcium, serum phosphate, serum alkaline phosphatase [ALP], urine calcium excretion, urinary hydroxyproline excretion, hematocrit, erythrocyte sedimentation rate [ESR]), and x-ray studies are used to exclude other possible disorders (e.g., multiple myeloma, osteomalacia, hyperparathyroidism, malignancy) that contribute to bone loss. In men, low testosterone levels may be part of the cause (Cosman et al., 2014).

Medical Management

A diet rich in calcium and vitamin D throughout life, with an increased calcium intake during adolescence and the middle years, protects against skeletal demineralization. Such a diet includes three glasses of skimmed vitamin D–enriched milk or other foods high in calcium (e.g., cheese and other dairy products, steamed broccoli, canned salmon with bones) daily. A cup of milk or calcium-fortified orange juice contains about 300 mg of calcium. The recommended adequate intake level of calcium for men 50 to 70 years is 1000 mg daily, and for women aged 51 and older and men aged 71 and older is 1200 mg daily (Cosman et al., 2014). Some researchers are challenging these levels as too low for patients with low baseline values, while others express concern of administering higher dosages, noting that they are associated with adverse events (e.g., renal calculi) (Hansen, Johnson, Chambers, et al., 2015; Veugelers & Ekwaru, 2014). The recommended vitamin D intake for adults up to 70 years of age is 600 IU daily, and 800 IU daily for those over the age of 70 (Cosman et al., 2014).

Regular weight-bearing exercise promotes bone formation. Recommendations include 20 to 30 minutes of aerobic, bone-stressing exercise daily (e.g., not swimming). Weight training stimulates an increase in BMD. In addition, exercise improves balance, reducing the incidence of falls and fractures (Cosman et al., 2014). Women who are postmenopausal and men aged 50 and older should be advised to avoid excessive intake of alcohol. Those who use tobacco products should be advised to quit (Cosman, de Beur, LeBoff, et al., 2015).

Pharmacologic Therapy

To ensure adequate calcium intake, a calcium supplement (e.g., Caltrate, Citracal) with vitamin D may be prescribed and taken with meals or with a beverage high in vitamin C to promote absorption. The recommended daily dose should be split and not taken as a single dose. Common side effects of calcium supplements are abdominal distention and constipation. Calcium from foods is better absorbed, but calcium supplements may be necessary for patients who are lactose intolerant. Meta-analysis findings demonstrate that vitamin D taken alone is not effective in primary prevention of fractures. However, vitamin D plus calcium does reduce the risk of fractures (Avenell, Mak, & O'Connell, 2014). Calcium and vitamin D may be taken to prevent osteoporosis, or may be taken as supplements to drugs prescribed to prevent or treat osteoporosis. These types of drugs include bisphosphonates, estrogen agonist/antagonists, and receptor activator of nuclear factor kappa-B ligand (RANKL) inhibitors (see Table 41-1).

Fracture Management

Fractures of the hip that occur as a consequence of osteoporosis are managed surgically by joint replacement or by closed or open reduction with internal fixation (e.g., hip pinning) as described in Chapters 40 and 42, respectively. Management of Colles fractures is also described in Chapter 42.

Osteoporotic compression fractures of the vertebrae are managed conservatively. Patients with these findings should be referred to an osteoporosis specialist. Most patients who experience these fractures are asymptomatic and do not require acute care management; for those who experience pain, acute care management is indicated as outlined in the following Nursing Process section. Percutaneous vertebroplasty or kyphoplasty (injection of polymethylmethacrylate [PMMA] bone cement into the fractured vertebra, followed by inflation of a pressurized balloon to restore the shape of the affected vertebra) can provide rapid relief of acute pain and improve quality of life (Cosman et al., 2014). Patients who have not responded to first-line approaches to the treatment of vertebral compression fracture can be considered for these procedures. They are contraindicated in the presence of infection, multiple old fractures, and certain coagulopathies. The benefits of these expensive interventions are now questioned because of their association with increased rates of future fractures related to altered spinal mechanics (Song, Meng, Gan, et al., 2015).

NURSING PROCESS

The Patient With a Spontaneous Vertebral Fracture Related to Osteoporosis

Assessment

Recognition of risks and problems associated with osteoporosis form the basis for nursing assessment. The health history focuses on family history, previous fractures, dietary consumption of calcium, exercise patterns, onset of menopause, and the use of certain medications (e.g., corticosteroids), as well as alcohol, smoking, and caffeine intake. Any symptoms the patient is experiencing, such as back pain, constipation, or altered body image, are explored.

Physical examination may disclose localized pain, kyphosis of the thoracic spine, or shortened stature. Problems in mobility and breathing may exist as a result of changes in posture and weakened muscles.

Nursing Diagnoses

Based on the assessment data, major nursing diagnoses may include the following:
- Deficient knowledge about the osteoporotic process and treatment regimen
- Acute pain related to fracture and muscle spasm
- Risk for constipation related to immobility or development of ileus (intestinal obstruction)
- Risk for injury: additional fractures related to osteoporosis

Planning and Goals

The major goals for the patient may include knowledge about osteoporosis and the treatment regimen, relief of pain, improved bowel elimination, and absence of additional fractures.

TABLE 41-1 Selected Osteoporosis Medications

Medication	Therapeutic Effects and Indications	Key Nursing Considerations
Bisphosphonates	Inhibit osteoclasts, causing decreased bone loss and increased bone mass	Adequate calcium and vitamin D intake is needed to assure maximum effect; however, these supplements should not be taken at the same time as the bisphosphonates Side effects include gastrointestinal symptoms, including dyspepsia, nausea, flatulence, diarrhea, and constipation Adverse effects may include esophageal or gastric ulcers, osteonecrosis of the jaw, and atypical femur fractures; these effects may be mitigated by instituting a 1–2 year drug-free holiday in patients with mild osteoporosis after 4–5 years of treatment, and in patients with higher fracture risk after 10 years of treatment
Alendronate (Fosamax) Risedronate (Actonel)	• Prevention and treatment of osteoporosis in women who are postmenopausal • Treatment of osteoporosis in men, and in women and men taking corticosteroids	Administer PO, either daily or weekly Advise patient to take in AM on empty stomach with 250 mL of water while sitting upright and to remain upright for at least 30 minutes Effects of alendronate may be diminished in older adult patients who take proton pump inhibitors
Ibandronate (Boniva)	• Treatment of osteoporosis in women who are postmenopausal • IV dosing may be good option for patients either intolerant of PO bisphosphonates or nonadherent to prescribed therapy	May be given PO monthly or IV every 3 months
Zoledronic acid (Reclast)	• Prevention and treatment of osteoporosis in women who are postmenopausal • Treatment of osteoporosis in men and in both men and women taking corticosteroids for at least 12 months	Administer IV once yearly for osteoporosis treatment or once every 2 years for osteoporosis prevention This is the most potent bisphosphonate and is associated with acute kidney injury; therefore it is contraindicated in patients with creatinine clearances less than 35 mL/min or in patients with chronic kidney disease
Estrogen Agonist/ Antagonist (formerly called selective estrogen receptor modulator [SERM]) Raloxifene (Evista)	Promotes estrogenic effects on bone, preserving BMD, with concomitant antiestrogenic effects on the uterus and breasts • Prevention and treatment of osteoporosis in women who are postmenopausal, particularly those with breast cancer • May also reduce the risk of breast cancer in patients at risk	Administer PO once daily. May be given in tandem with calcium and vitamin D Side effects include hot flashes and leg cramps Adverse effects include VTE formation
RANKL Inhibitor Denosumab (Prolia)	Monoclonal antibody that increases BMD and reduces the porosity of cortical bone by inhibiting the effects of TNF on osteoclasts, inhibiting their activity • Treatment of osteoporosis in men and women who are postmenopausal at high risk of fracture; also indicated for women with osteoporosis and breast cancer receiving aromatase inhibitors and for men with osteoporosis and prostate cancer receiving gonadotropin-reducing hormones	Given once every 6 months SQ Side effects include skin rashes Adverse effects include hypocalcemia, cellulitis, osteonecrosis of the jaw, and atypical femur fracture Note: when treatment with denosumab is stopped, loss of BMD can be rapid; other drugs should be started to mitigate this response

BMD, bone mineral density; PO, orally; IV, intravenously; SQ, subcutaneous; TNF, tissue necrosis factor; VTE, venous thromboembolism.
Adapted from Cosman, F., de Beur, S., J. LeBoff, M. S., et al. (2014). Clinician's guide to prevention and treatment of osteoporosis. *Osteoporosis International, 25*(10), 2359–2381.

Nursing Interventions

PROMOTING UNDERSTANDING OF OSTEOPOROSIS AND THE TREATMENT REGIMEN

Patient education focuses on factors influencing the development of osteoporosis, interventions to arrest or slow the process, and measures to relieve symptoms. The nurse emphasizes that people of any age need sufficient calcium, vitamin D, and weight-bearing exercise to slow the progression of osteoporosis. Patient education related to medication therapy as described previously is important. Patients must understand that having one fracture increases the probability of sustaining another (Cosman et al., 2014).

RELIEVING PAIN

Relief of back pain resulting from compression fracture may be accomplished by short periods of resting in bed in a supine or side-lying position. The mattress should be supportive. Knee flexion increases comfort by relaxing back muscles. Intermittent local heat and backrubs promote muscle relaxation. The nurse instructs the patient to move the trunk as a unit and to avoid twisting. When the patient is assisted out of bed, a trunk orthosis (e.g., lumbosacral corset) may be worn for temporary support and immobilization, although such a device is frequently uncomfortable and is poorly tolerated by many older adults (Cosman et al., 2014). The patient gradually resumes activities as pain diminishes.

IMPROVING BOWEL ELIMINATION

Constipation is a problem related to immobility and medications. Early institution of a high-fiber diet, increased fluids, and the use of prescribed stool softeners help prevent or minimize constipation. If the vertebral collapse involves the T10–L2 vertebrae, the patient may develop a paralytic ileus. The nurse therefore monitors the patient's intake, bowel sounds, and bowel activity.

PREVENTING INJURY

Physical activity is essential to strengthen muscles, improve balance, prevent disuse atrophy, and retard progressive bone demineralization. Isometric exercises can strengthen trunk muscles. The nurse encourages walking, good body mechanics, and good posture. Daily weight-bearing activity, preferably outdoors in the sunshine to enhance the body's ability to produce vitamin D, is encouraged. Sudden bending, jarring, and strenuous lifting are avoided.

Gerontologic Considerations. Older adults fall frequently as a result of environmental hazards, diminished senses and cardiovascular responses, and responses to medications. The patient and family need to be included in planning for care and preventive management regimens. For example, the home environment should be assessed for elimination of potential hazards (e.g., scatter rugs, cluttered rooms and stairwells, toys on the floor, pets underfoot). A safe environment can then be created (e.g., well-lighted staircases with secure hand rails, grab bars in the bathroom, properly fitting footwear).

Evaluation

Expected patient outcomes may include:

1. Acquires knowledge about osteoporosis and the treatment regimen
   a. States relationship of calcium and vitamin D intake and exercise to bone mass
   b. Consumes adequate dietary calcium and vitamin D
   c. Takes prescribed medications, following instructions for administration
   d. Increases level of exercise
   e. Adheres to prescribed screening and monitoring procedures
2. Achieves pain relief
   a. Experiences pain relief at rest
   b. Experiences minimal discomfort during ADLs
   c. Demonstrates diminished tenderness at fracture site
3. Demonstrates usual pattern of bowel elimination
   a. Has active bowel sounds
   b. Reports regular pattern of bowel movements
4. Experiences no new fractures
   a. Maintains good posture
   b. Uses good body mechanics
   c. Engages in weight-bearing exercises (walks daily)
   d. Creates a safe home environment
   e. Accepts assistance and supervision as needed

Osteomalacia

Osteomalacia is a metabolic bone disease characterized by inadequate mineralization of bone. As a result, the skeleton softens and weakens, causing pain, tenderness to touch, bowing of the bones, and pathologic fractures. On physical examination, skeletal deformities (spinal kyphosis and bowed legs) give patients an unusual appearance and a waddling gait. These patients may be uncomfortable with their appearance and are at risk for falls and pathologic fractures, particularly of the distal radius and the proximal femur (Grossman & Porth, 2014).

Pathophysiology

The major defect in osteomalacia is a deficiency of activated vitamin D, which promotes calcium absorption from the gastrointestinal tract and facilitates mineralization of bone. The supply of calcium and phosphate in the extracellular fluid is low and does not move to calcification sites in bones.

Osteomalacia may result from failed calcium absorption or from excessive loss of calcium from the body (e.g., kidney failure). Gastrointestinal disorders (e.g., celiac disease, chronic biliary tract obstruction, chronic pancreatitis, small bowel resection) in which fats are inadequately absorbed are likely to produce osteomalacia through loss of vitamin D (along with other fat-soluble vitamins) and calcium, the latter being excreted in the feces with fatty acids. In addition, liver and kidney diseases can produce a lack of vitamin D because these are the organs that convert vitamin D to its active form.

Severe renal insufficiency results in acidosis. The body uses available calcium to combat the acidosis, and PTH stimulates the release of skeletal calcium in an attempt to reestablish a physiologic pH. During this continual drain of skeletal calcium, bony fibrosis occurs, and bony cysts form. Chronic glomerulonephritis, obstructive uropathies, and heavy metal poisoning result in a reduced serum phosphate level and demineralization of bone.

Hyperparathyroidism leads to skeletal decalcification and thus to osteomalacia by increasing phosphate excretion in the urine. Prolonged use of anticonvulsant medication (e.g., phenytoin [Dilantin], phenobarbital) poses a risk of osteomalacia, as does insufficient vitamin D (dietary, sunlight).

Osteomalacia that results from malnutrition (deficiency in vitamin D often associated with poor intake of calcium) is a result of poverty, poor dietary habits, and lack of knowledge about nutrition. It occurs most frequently in parts of the world where vitamin D is not added to food, where dietary deficiencies exist, and where sunlight is rare (Grossman & Porth, 2014).

Gerontologic Considerations

A nutritious diet is particularly important in older adults. Adequate intake of calcium and vitamin D is promoted. Because sunlight is necessary for synthesizing vitamin D, patients should be encouraged to spend some time in the sun, for at least 10 minutes and up to an hour daily (Vitamin D Council, 2016). Prevention, identification, and management of osteomalacia in older adults are essential to reduce the incidence of fractures. When osteomalacia is combined with osteoporosis, the risk of fracture increases.

Assessment and Diagnostic Findings

On x-ray studies, generalized demineralization of bone is evident. Studies of the vertebrae may show a compression fracture with indistinct vertebral end plates. Laboratory studies show low serum calcium and phosphorus levels and a moderately elevated ALP. Urine excretion of calcium and creatinine is low. Bone biopsy demonstrates an increased amount of osteoid, a demineralized, cartilaginous bone matrix that is sometimes referred to as prebone.

Medical Management

Physical, psychological, and pharmaceutical measures are used to reduce the patient's discomfort and pain. If the underlying cause of osteomalacia is corrected, the disorder may resolve. If kidney disease prevents activation of absorbed vitamin D, then supplementation requires the activated form (calcitriol). If osteomalacia is caused by malabsorption, increased doses of vitamin D, along with supplemental calcium, are usually prescribed. Exposure to sunlight may be recommended; ultraviolet radiation transforms a cholesterol substance (7-dehydrocholesterol) present in the skin into vitamin D (Singer, Bone, Hosking, et al., 2014).

If osteomalacia is dietary in origin, the interventions are akin to those discussed previously in the discussion on osteoporosis. Long-term monitoring of the patient is appropriate to ensure stabilization or reversal of osteomalacia. Some persistent orthopedic deformities may need to be treated with braces or surgery (e.g., osteotomy may be performed to correct long bone deformity).

Paget Disease of the Bone

Paget disease (osteitis deformans) is a disorder of localized rapid bone turnover, most commonly affecting the skull, femur, tibia, pelvic bones, and vertebrae. The disease occurs in about 2% to 3% of the population older than 50 years. The incidence is slightly greater in aging men than in women. A family history has been noted, with siblings often developing the disease. The cause of Paget disease is not known (Singer et al., 2014).

Pathophysiology

In Paget disease, a primary proliferation of osteoclasts occurs, which induces bone resorption. This is followed by a compensatory increase in osteoblastic activity that replaces the bone. As bone turnover continues, a classic mosaic (disorganized) pattern of bone develops. Because the diseased bone is highly vascularized and structurally weak, pathologic fractures occur. Structural bowing of the legs causes malalignment of the hip, knee, and ankle joints, which contributes to the development of arthritis and back and joint pain (Singer et al., 2014).

Clinical Manifestations

Paget disease is insidious. Some patients do not experience symptoms but only have skeletal deformity. The condition is most frequently identified on x-ray studies performed during a workup for another problem. Sclerotic changes and cortical thickening of the long bones occur.

In most patients, skeletal deformity involves the skull. The skull may thicken, and the patient may report that a hat no longer fits. In some cases, the cranium, but not the face, is enlarged. This gives the face a small, triangular appearance. Most patients with skull involvement have impaired hearing from cranial nerve compression and dysfunction. Other cranial nerves may also be similarly affected.

The femurs and tibiae tend to bow, producing a waddling gait. The spine is bent forward and is rigid; the chin rests on the chest. The thorax becomes immobile during respiration. The trunk is flexed on the legs to maintain balance and the arms are bent outward and forward, appearing long in relation to the shortened trunk (Grossman & Porth, 2014).

Tenderness and warmth over bones may be noted due to increased bone vascularity. Patients with large, highly vascular lesions may develop high-output cardiac failure due to the increased vascular bed and metabolic demands (Grossman & Porth, 2014). The pain is mild to moderate, deep, and aching. It increases with weight bearing. Pain and discomfort may precede skeletal deformities of Paget disease by years and are often wrongly attributed by the patient to old age or arthritis (Singer et al., 2014).

Assessment and Diagnostic Findings

Elevated serum ALP concentration and urinary hydroxyproline excretion reflect increased osteoblastic activity. Higher values suggest more active disease. Patients with Paget disease have normal blood calcium levels. X-rays confirm the diagnosis of Paget disease by revealing local areas of demineralization and bone overgrowth in the characteristic mosaic patterns. Bone scans demonstrate the extent of the disease. Bone biopsy may aid in the differential diagnosis with other bone diseases (Grossman & Porth, 2014).

Medical Management

Pain usually responds to NSAIDs. Gait problems from bowing of the legs are managed with walking aids, shoe lifts, and physical therapy. Weight is controlled to reduce stress on weakened bones and misaligned joints. Asymptomatic patients may be managed with diets adequate in calcium and vitamin D and periodic monitoring.

Fractures, arthritis, and hearing loss are complications of Paget disease. Fractures are managed according to location. Healing occurs if fracture reduction, immobilization, and stability are adequate. Severe degenerative arthritis may require total joint replacement; however, the afflicted "soft" bones do not make ideal surgical sites and are thus prone to complications. Loss of hearing is managed with hearing aids and communication techniques used with people who have hearing impairments (e.g., speech reading, body language) (see Chapter 64).

Pharmacologic Therapy

Patients with moderate to severe disease may benefit from specific antiosteoclastic therapy. These medications reduce bone turnover, reverse the course of the disease, relieve pain, and improve mobility.

Bisphosphonates are the cornerstone of Paget therapy in that they stabilize the rapid bone turnover. Their use may not suppress all Paget symptoms, but they reduce serum ALP and urinary hydroxyproline levels. See earlier discussion on bisphosphonates.

Plicamycin (Mithracin), a cytotoxic antibiotic, may be used to control the disease. This medication is reserved for severely affected patients with neurologic compromise and for those whose disease is resistant to other therapy. This medication has dramatic effects on pain reduction and on serum calcium, ALP, and urinary hydroxyproline levels; however, there are significant side effects. It is given by IV infusion; hepatic, kidney, and bone marrow function must be monitored during therapy. Clinical remissions may continue for months after the medication is discontinued.

 Gerontologic Considerations

Because Paget disease tends to affect older adults, patients and their families and caregivers should be educated about how to compensate for altered musculoskeletal functioning with an emphasis on the risk of falls. The home environment is assessed for safety to prevent falls and to reduce the risk of fracture. Strategies for coping with a chronic health problem and its effect on quality of life need to be developed. If age-related hearing loss is exacerbated by Paget disease, alternative communication devices (e.g., text telephone, telecommunication device for the deaf) and home safety alarms may be indicated.

Musculoskeletal Infections

Osteomyelitis

Osteomyelitis is an infection of the bone that results in inflammation, necrosis, and formation of new bone. Osteomyelitis is classified as:

- Hematogenous osteomyelitis (i.e., due to bloodborne spread of infection)
- Contiguous-focus osteomyelitis, from contamination from bone surgery, open fracture, or traumatic injury (e.g., gunshot wound)
- Osteomyelitis with vascular insufficiency, seen most commonly among patients with diabetes and peripheral vascular disease, most commonly affecting the feet (Grossman & Porth, 2014)

Patients who are at high risk for osteomyelitis include older adults and those who are poorly nourished or obese. Other patients at risk include those with impaired immune systems, those with chronic illnesses (e.g., diabetes, rheumatoid arthritis), those receiving long-term corticosteroid therapy or immunosuppressive agents, and those who use IV drugs (Lalani, 2016).

Postoperative surgical wound infections typically occur within 30 days after surgery. They are classified as incisional (superficial, located above the deep fascia layer) or deep (involving tissue beneath the deep fascia). If an implant has been used, deep postoperative infections may occur within a year. Osteomyelitis may become chronic and may affect the patient's quality of life.

Pathophysiology

More than 50% of bone infections are caused by *Staphylococcus aureus* and increasingly of the variety that is methicillin resistant (i.e., methicillin-resistant *Staphylococcus aureus* [MRSA]) (Kaplan, 2014). Surgical site ink markers have been linked to infections by cross contamination between preoperative patients who use their markers; therefore, these items are now considered one patient or one-time use items (Driessche, 2012). Other pathogens include the Gram-positive organisms *streptococci* and *enterococci*, followed by Gram-negative bacteria, including *pseudomonas* (Kaplan, 2014),

The initial response to infection is inflammation, increased vascularity, and edema. After 2 or 3 days, thrombosis of the local blood vessels occurs, resulting in ischemia with bone necrosis. The infection extends into the medullary cavity and under the periosteum and may spread into adjacent soft tissues and joints. Unless the infective process is treated promptly, a bone abscess forms. The resulting abscess cavity contains **sequestrum** (i.e., dead bone tissue), which does not easily liquefy and drain. Therefore, the cavity cannot collapse and heal, as it does in soft tissue abscesses. New bone growth, the **involucrum**, forms and surrounds the sequestrum. Although healing appears to take place, a chronically infected sequestrum remains and produces recurring abscesses throughout the patient's life. This is referred to as chronic osteomyelitis.

Clinical Manifestations

When the infection is bloodborne, the onset is usually sudden, occurring often with the clinical and laboratory manifestations of sepsis (e.g., chills, high fever, rapid pulse, general malaise). The systemic symptoms at first may overshadow the local signs. As the infection extends through the cortex of the bone, it involves the periosteum and the soft tissues. The infected area becomes painful, swollen, and extremely tender. The patient may describe a constant, pulsating pain that intensifies with movement as a result of the pressure of the collecting purulent material (i.e., pus). When osteomyelitis occurs from spread of adjacent infection or from direct contamination, there are no manifestations of sepsis. The surface area that lies over the infected bone is swollen, warm, painful, and tender to touch. The patient with chronic osteomyelitis presents with a nonhealing ulcer that overlies the infected bone with a connecting sinus that will intermittently and spontaneously drain pus (Bries, Kerr, & George, 2015).

Diabetic osteomyelitis can occur without any external wounds. Microvascular and macrovascular pathophysiologic changes, along with an impaired immune response by patients with diabetes who have poor glycemic control can exacerbate the spread of infection from other sources (Malhotra, Chan, & Nather, 2014).

Assessment and Diagnostic Findings

In acute osteomyelitis, early x-ray findings demonstrate soft tissue edema. In about 2 to 3 weeks, areas of periosteal elevation and bone necrosis are evident. Radioisotope bone scans, particularly the isotope-labeled white blood cell (WBC) scan, and MRI help with early definitive diagnosis. Blood studies reveal leukocytosis and an elevated ESR. Wound and blood culture studies are performed, although they are only positive in 50% of cases. Therefore, treatment with antibiotics may be prescribed without isolating the organism (Conterno & Turchi, 2013).

With chronic osteomyelitis, large, irregular cavities, raised periosteum, sequestra, or dense bone formations are seen on x-ray. Bone scans may be performed to identify areas of infection. The ESR and the WBC count are usually normal. Anemia, associated with chronic infection, may be evident. Cultures of blood specimens and drainage from the sinus tract are frequently unreliable for isolating the organisms involved. An open bone biopsy is indicated as percutaneous aspirations are not reliable for gathering cultures to identify the underlying pathogen (Bries et al., 2015).

Prevention

Prevention of osteomyelitis is the goal. Elective orthopedic surgery should be postponed if the patient has a current infection (e.g., urinary tract infection, sore throat). During surgery, careful attention is paid to the surgical environment. Prophylactic antibiotics, given to achieve adequate tissue levels at the time of surgery and for 24 hours after surgery, are helpful. Urinary catheters and drains are removed as soon as possible to decrease the incidence of hematogenous spread of infection.

Aseptic postoperative wound care reduces the incidence of superficial infections and osteomyelitis. Prompt management of soft tissue infections reduces extension of infection to the bone or hematogenous spread.

Medical Management

The initial goal of therapy is to control and halt the infective process. General supportive measures (e.g., hydration, diet high in vitamins and protein, correction of anemia) are instituted. The area affected with osteomyelitis is immobilized to decrease discomfort and to prevent pathologic fracture of the weakened bone.

Pharmacologic Therapy

Bone infections are more difficult to eradicate than soft tissue infections because bone is mostly avascular and less accessible to the body's natural immune response. Because there is decreased penetration by medications, antibiotic therapy is longer term than with other infections; typically it continues for 3 to 6 weeks. After the infection appears to be controlled, the antibiotic may be given orally. However, there is little evidence to support optimal length of therapy (Conterno & Turchi, 2013).

Surgical Management

If the infection is chronic and does not respond to antibiotic therapy, surgical débridement is indicated. The infected bone is surgically exposed, the purulent and necrotic material is removed, and the area is irrigated with sterile saline solution. A sequestrectomy (removal of enough involucrum to enable the surgeon to remove the sequestrum) is performed. In many cases, sufficient bone is removed to convert a deep cavity into a shallow saucer (saucerization). All dead, infected bone and cartilage must be removed before permanent healing can occur. A closed suction irrigation system may be used to remove debris. Wound irrigation using sterile physiologic saline solution may be performed for extended periods if the debris remains. Typically, irrigation does not need to extend beyond a week.

The wound is either closed tightly to obliterate the dead space or packed and closed later by granulation or possibly by grafting. The débrided cavity may be packed with cancellous bone graft to stimulate healing. With a large defect, the cavity may be filled with a vascularized bone transfer or muscle flap (in which a muscle is moved from an adjacent area with blood supply intact). These microsurgery techniques enhance the blood supply. The improved blood supply facilitates bone healing and eradication of the infection. These surgical procedures may be staged over time to ensure healing. Because surgical débridement weakens the bone, internal fixation or external supportive devices may be needed to stabilize or support the bone to prevent pathologic fracture (van Vugt, Geurts, & Arts, 2016).

NURSING PROCESS

The Patient With Osteomyelitis

Assessment

The patient reports an acute onset of signs and symptoms (e.g., localized pain, edema, erythema, fever) or recurrent drainage of an infected sinus with associated pain, edema, and low-grade fever. The nurse assesses the patient for risk factors (e.g., older age, diabetes, long-term corticosteroid therapy) and for a history of previous injury, infection, or orthopedic surgery. The gait may be altered as the patient avoids pressure and movement of the area. In acute hematogenous osteomyelitis, the patient exhibits generalized weakness due to the systemic reaction to the infection.

Physical examination reveals an inflamed, markedly edematous, warm area that is tender. Purulent drainage may be noted. The patient has an elevated temperature. With chronic osteomyelitis, the temperature elevation may be minimal, occurring in the afternoon or evening.

Nursing Diagnoses

Based on the assessment data, nursing diagnoses may include the following:

- Acute pain related to inflammation and edema
- Impaired physical mobility related to pain, use of immobilization devices, and weight-bearing limitations
- Risk for infection: bone abscess formation
- Deficient knowledge related to the treatment regimen

Planning and Goals

The patient's goals may include relief of pain, improved physical mobility within therapeutic limitations, control and eradication of infection, and knowledge of the treatment regimen.

Nursing Interventions

RELIEVING PAIN

The affected part may be immobilized with a splint to decrease pain and muscle spasm. The nurse monitors the skin and neurovascular status of the affected extremity. The wounds are frequently very painful, and the extremity must be handled with great care and gentleness. Elevation reduces swelling and associated discomfort. Pain is controlled with prescribed analgesic agents and other pain-reducing techniques.

IMPROVING PHYSICAL MOBILITY

Treatment regimens restrict weight-bearing activity. The bone is weakened by the infective process and must be protected by avoidance of stress on the bone. The patient must understand the rationale for the activity restrictions. The joints above and below the affected part should be gently moved through their range of motion. The nurse encourages full participation in ADLs within the prescribed physical limitations to promote general well-being.

CONTROLLING THE INFECTIOUS PROCESS

The nurse monitors the patient's response to antibiotic therapy and observes the IV access site for evidence of phlebitis, infection, or infiltration. With long-term, intensive antibiotic therapy, the nurse monitors the patient for signs of superinfection (e.g., oral or vaginal candidiasis, loose or foul-smelling stools). The nurse carefully monitors the patient for the development of additional sites that are painful or sudden increases in body temperature.

If surgery is necessary, the nurse takes measures to ensure adequate circulation to the affected area (wound suction to prevent fluid accumulation, elevation of the area to promote venous drainage, avoidance of pressure on the grafted area), to maintain needed immobility, and to ensure the patient's adherence to weight-bearing restrictions. The nurse changes dressings using aseptic technique to promote healing and to prevent cross contamination (Smith & Dahlen, 2013).

PROMOTING HOME, COMMUNITY-BASED, AND TRANSITIONAL CARE

Educating Patients About Self-Care. The patient and family are educated about the importance of strictly adhering to the therapeutic regimen of antibiotics. Patients and families often need to learn to maintain and manage the IV access and IV administration equipment in the home. Education includes the medication name, dosage, frequency, administration rate, safe storage and handling, adverse reactions, and necessary laboratory monitoring. In addition, the nurse provides instruction on aseptic dressing and warm compression techniques.

Continuing and Transitional Care. The patient must be medically stable and physically able and motivated to adhere strictly to the therapeutic regimen of antibiotic therapy. The transitional care environment needs to be conducive to the promotion of health and to the requirements of the therapeutic regimen.

If warranted, the nurse completes a home assessment to determine the patient's and family's abilities regarding continuation of the therapeutic regimen. If the patient's support system is questionable or if the patient lives alone, a home care nurse may be needed to assist with IV administration of the antibiotics, monitoring for response to the treatment and evaluation of signs and symptoms of superinfections, and adverse drug reactions. The nurse stresses the importance of follow-up health care appointments (see Chart 41-8).

Evaluation

Expected patient outcomes may include:

1. Experiences pain relief
   a. Reports decreased pain at rest
   b. Experiences no tenderness at site of previous infection
   c. Experiences minimal discomfort with movement
2. Increases in safe physical mobility
   a. Participates in self-care activities within restrictions
   b. Maintains full function of unimpaired extremities
   c. Demonstrates safe use of immobilizing and assistive devices
   d. Modifies environment to promote safety and to avoid falls
3. Shows absence of infection
   a. Takes antibiotic as prescribed
   b. Reports normal temperature
   c. Exhibits no edema
   d. Reports absence of drainage
   e. Laboratory results indicate normal WBC count and ESR
   f. Wound cultures are negative
4. Adheres to therapeutic plan
   a. Takes medications as prescribed
   b. Protects weakened bones
   c. Demonstrates proper wound care
   d. Reports signs and symptoms of complications promptly
   e. Consumes a healthy diet
   f. Keeps follow-up health care appointments

Septic (Infectious) Arthritis

Joints can become infected through spread of pathogens from other parts of the body (hematogenous spread) or directly through trauma or surgical instrumentation, causing septic arthritis. People at greatest risk include older adults, particularly those older than 80 years; people with comorbid conditions such as diabetes, rheumatoid arthritis, skin infection, or alcoholism; and people with a history of a joint replacement or other joint surgery or IV drug abuse. *S. aureus* is the most common cause of joint infections in all age groups, followed by other Gram-positive bacteria, including streptococci. Gonococcal infection may cause septic arthritis through hematogenous spread. When seen, it tends to afflict young adults (Goldenberg & Sexton, 2016).

Single knee or hip joints are most commonly infected in patients with septic arthritis, although up to 20% of cases involve more than one joint (i.e., polyarticular disease) (Kaplan, 2014). Prompt recognition and treatment of an infected joint are important because accumulating purulent material may result in chondrolysis (destruction of hyaline cartilage), and continued hematogenous spread may lead to sepsis and death. See Chapter 14 for further discussion of sepsis. The overall mortality rate is about 11% and approaches 50% in patients with polyarticular disease, which may be attributed to the fact that many patients with septic arthritis are older with a significant comorbidity and/or immunocompromised (Kaplan, 2014).

Clinical Manifestations

The patient with acute septic arthritis presents with a warm, painful, swollen joint with decreased range of motion. Systemic chills, fever, and leukocytosis are sometimes present (Kaplan, 2014). Although any joint may be infected, approximately half of all cases involve a knee (Goldenberg & Sexton, 2016).

Assessment and Diagnostic Findings

An assessment for the source and cause of infection is performed. Diagnostic studies include aspiration, examination,

HOME CARE CHECKLIST

Chart 41-8

The Patient With Osteomyelitis

At the completion of education, the patient and/or caregiver will be able to:

- State the impact of osteomyelitis on physiologic functioning, ADLs, IADLs, roles, relationships, and spirituality.
- Identify modification of home environment, interventions, and strategies (e.g., durable medical equipment, adaptive equipment) used in safely adapting to changes in structure or function and promote effective recovery and rehabilitation.
- State how to obtain medical supplies and carry out dressing changes, wound care, and other prescribed regimens.
- Describe ongoing postoperative therapeutic regimen, including diet and activities to perform (e.g., exercises) and to limit or avoid (e.g., lifting weights, driving a car, contact sports).
  - Consume a healthy diet to promote wound and bone healing.
  - Observe prescribed weight-bearing and activity limits.
  - Demonstrate proper wound care.
  - Demonstrate safe use of ambulatory aids and assistive devices.
- State the name, dose, side effects, frequency, and schedule for all medications.
- Demonstrate accurate and safe administration of medications.
- When indicated, identify the benefits and expected outcomes of intravenous antibiotic therapy and IV access management.

- Demonstrate how to prepare, infuse, maintain, and clean IV access and equipment.
- Identify adverse effects of antibiotic therapy and actions to take for adverse effects.
- Describe to whom, how, and when to report adverse effects.
- Relieve pain with pharmacologic and nonpharmacologic interventions.
- State indicators of wound infections (e.g., redness, swelling, tenderness, purulent drainage, fever) and systemic infection (e.g. fever, chills, rapid pulse, general malaise) to report promptly to primary provider.
- Relate how to reach primary provider with questions or complications.
- State time and date of follow-up appointments and testing.
- Identify the need for health promotion (e.g., weight reduction, smoking cessation, stress management), disease prevention and screening activities.

Resources

See Chapter 10, Chart 10-8 for additional information related to durable medical equipment, adaptive equipment, mobility skills, skin, bowel, and bladder care.

ADL, activities of daily living; IADL, independent activities of daily living; IV, intravenous.

---

and culture of the synovial fluid. Computed tomography (CT) and MRI scans may reveal damage to the joint lining. Radioisotope scanning may be useful in localizing the infectious process. There may not be any external wound or reported recent trauma.

Medical Management

Prompt treatment is essential and may save the prosthesis for patients who have had joint replacement surgery or prevent sepsis. Broad-spectrum IV antibiotics are started promptly and then changed to organism-specific antibiotics after culture results are available (Kaplan, 2014). The IV antibiotics are continued until symptoms resolve. The synovial fluid is aspirated and analyzed periodically for sterility and decrease in WBCs.

The primary provider may aspirate the joint with a needle to remove excessive joint fluid, exudate, and debris. This promotes comfort and decreases joint destruction caused by the action of proteolytic enzymes in the purulent fluid. Occasionally, arthrotomy or arthroscopy is used to drain the joint and remove dead tissue (Sharff, Richards, & Townes, 2013).

The inflamed joint is supported and immobilized in a functional position by a splint that increases the patient's comfort. Analgesic agents are prescribed to relieve pain. The patient's nutrition and fluid status is monitored. Progressive range-of-motion exercises are prescribed as soon as the patient can begin movement without exacerbating symptoms of acute pain. If septic joints are treated promptly, recovery of normal function is expected. If the articular cartilage was damaged during the inflammatory reaction, joint fibrosis and diminished function may result. The patient is assessed periodically for recurrence over the next year (Sharff et al., 2013).

Nursing Management

The nurse educates the patient and family about the septic arthritis physiologic process and explains the importance of supporting the affected joint, adhering to the prescribed antibiotic regimen, inspecting the skin under any splints that may be prescribed, and observing weight-bearing and activity restrictions. The patient is also educated that recurrence of infection in the near and far future is possible, and is educated about signs and symptoms to observe and report to the primary provider. The same interventions used for the patient with osteomyelitis are planned for the patient with septic arthritis. See previous discussion.

Bone Tumors

Neoplasms of the musculoskeletal system are of various types, including osteogenic, chondrogenic, fibrogenic, muscle (rhabdomyogenic), and marrow (reticulum) cell tumors as well as nerve, vascular and fatty cell tumors. They may be primary tumors or metastatic tumors from cancers elsewhere in the body (e.g., breast, lung, prostate, kidney).

Types

Benign Bone Tumors

Benign tumors of the bone and soft tissue are more common than malignant primary bone tumors. Benign bone tumors generally are slow growing, well circumscribed, and encapsulated; present few symptoms; and are not a cause of death. Benign masses include osteochondroma, enchondroma, bone cysts, osteoid osteoma, rhabdomyoma, and fibroma. Some benign tumors have the potential to become malignant.

Osteochondroma is the most common benign bone tumor. It usually occurs as a large projection of bone at the end of long bones (at the knee or shoulder), developing during growth. It then becomes a static bony mass. In fewer than 1% of patients, the cartilage cap of the osteochondroma may undergo malignant transformation after trauma, and a chondrosarcoma or osteosarcoma may develop (Czerniak, 2016).

Bone cysts are expanding lesions within the bone. Aneurysmal (widening) bone cysts are seen in young adults, who present with a painful, palpable mass of the long bones, vertebrae, or flat bone. Unicameral (single cavity) bone cysts occur more often in the first two decades of life and cause mild discomfort and possible pathologic fractures of the upper humerus and femur, which may heal spontaneously.

An osteoid osteoma is a painful tumor that occurs in children and young adults. The neoplastic tissue is surrounded by reactive bone formation that can be identified by x-ray. Enchondroma is a common tumor of the hyaline cartilage that develops in the hand, femur, tibia, or humerus. Usually, the only symptom is a mild ache. Pathologic fractures may occur in both types of tumors.

Giant cell tumors (osteoclastomas) are benign for long periods but may invade local tissue and cause destruction. They occur in young adults and are soft and hemorrhagic. Eventually, giant cell tumors may undergo malignant transformation and metastasize (Czerniak, 2016).

Malignant Bone Tumors

Primary malignant musculoskeletal tumors are relatively rare and arise from connective and supportive tissue cells (sarcomas) or bone marrow elements (multiple myeloma; see Chapter 34). Malignant primary musculoskeletal tumors include osteosarcoma, chondrosarcoma, Ewing sarcoma, and fibrosarcoma. Soft tissue sarcomas include liposarcoma, fibrosarcoma of soft tissue, and rhabdomyosarcoma. Bone tumor metastasis to the lungs is common (Davis, James, & Saifuddin, 2015).

Osteosarcoma is the most common and most often fatal primary malignant bone tumor. Prognosis depends on whether the tumor has metastasized to the lungs at the time the patient seeks health care. It appears most frequently in children, adolescents and young adults (in bones that grow rapidly), in older adults with Paget disease of the bone, and in persons with a prior history of radiation exposure. Clinical manifestations typically include localized bone pain that may be accompanied by a tender, palpable soft tissue mass. The primary lesion may involve any bone, but the most common sites are the distal femur, the proximal tibia, and the proximal humerus (Czerniak, 2016).

Malignant tumors of the hyaline cartilage are called *chondrosarcomas*. These tumors are the second most common primary malignant bone tumor. They may grow and metastasize slowly or very fast, depending on the characteristics of the tumor cells involved (i.e., grade). Patients with low-grade chondrosarcomas tend to have a much better prognosis than those with high-grade chondrosarcomas. See Chapter 15 for a discussion of tumor grades. The usual tumor sites include the pelvis, femur, humerus, spine, scapula, and tibia. Metastasis to the lungs occurs in fewer than half of patients. These tumors may recur after excision (Davis et al., 2015).

Metastatic Bone Disease

Metastatic bone disease (secondary bone tumor) is more common than primary bone tumors (Coleman, Body, Aapro, et al., 2014). Tumors arising from tissues elsewhere in the body may invade the bone and produce localized bone destruction (lytic lesions) or bone overgrowth (blastic lesions). The most common primary sites of tumors that metastasize to bone are the kidney, prostate, lung, breast, ovary, and thyroid (Coleman et al., 2014). Metastatic tumors are most frequently found in the skull, spine, pelvis, femur, and humerus and often involve more than one bone (polyostotic) (Grossman & Porth, 2014).

Pathophysiology

A tumor in the bone causes the normal bone tissue to react by osteolytic response (bone destruction) or osteoblastic response (bone formation). Adjacent normal bone responds to the tumor by altering its normal pattern of remodeling. The bone's surface changes and the contours enlarge in the tumor area.

Malignant bone tumors invade and destroy adjacent bone tissue (Coleman et al., 2014). Benign bone tumors, in contrast, have a symmetric, controlled growth pattern and place pressure on adjacent bone tissue. Malignant bone tumors invade and weaken the structure of the bone until it can no longer withstand the stress of ordinary use; pathologic fracture commonly results.

Clinical Manifestations

Patients with metastatic bone tumor may have a wide range of associated clinical manifestations. They may be symptom free or have pain that ranges from mild and occasional to constant and severe, varying degrees of disability, and, at times, obvious bone growth. Weight loss, malaise, and fever may be present. The tumor may be diagnosed only after pathologic fractures occur or as an incidental finding.

With spinal metastasis, spinal cord compression may occur. It can progress rapidly or slowly. Neurologic deficits (e.g., progressive pain, weakness, gait abnormality, paresthesia, paraplegia, urinary retention, loss of bowel or bladder control) must be identified early and treated with decompression laminectomy to prevent permanent spinal cord injury.

Assessment and Diagnostic Findings

The differential diagnosis is based on the history, physical examination, and diagnostic studies, including CT, bone scans, myelography, arteriography, MRI, biopsy, and biochemical assays of the blood and urine. A surgical biopsy is performed for histologic identification. Extreme care is taken during the biopsy to prevent seeding and resultant recurrence after excision of the tumor. Chest x-rays are performed to determine the presence of lung metastasis. Surgical staging of musculoskeletal tumors is based on tumor grade and site (intracompartmental or extracompartmental), as well as on metastasis. Staging is used for planning treatment (see Chapter 15).

Serum ALP levels are frequently elevated with osteogenic sarcoma or bone metastasis. Hypercalcemia is also present with bone metastases from breast, lung, or kidney cancer. Symptoms of hypercalcemia include muscle weakness, fatigue, anorexia, nausea, vomiting, polyuria, cardiac dysrhythmias, seizures, and coma. Hypercalcemia must be identified and treated promptly.

During the diagnostic period, the nurse explains the diagnostic tests and provides psychological and emotional support to the patient and family. The nurse assesses coping behaviors and encourages the use of support systems. Because the terminology associated with benign and malignant growths sound similar, the nurse can clarify the meaning of these in terms of treatment and prognosis and may allay fears.

Medical Management

Primary Bone Tumors

The goal of primary bone tumor treatment is to destroy or remove the tumor rapidly (Davis et al., 2015). This may be accomplished by surgical excision (ranging from local excision to amputation and disarticulation), radiation therapy if the tumor is radiosensitive, and chemotherapy (preoperative, intraoperative [neoadjuvant], postoperative, and adjunctive for possible micrometastases). Major gains are being made in the use of wide bloc excision with restorative grafting technique. Survival and quality of life are important considerations in procedures that attempt to save the involved extremity; however, surgical removal of the tumor may require amputation of the affected extremity, with the amputation extending well above the tumor to achieve local control of the primary lesion (see Chapter 42).

If possible, limb-sparing (salvage) procedures are used to remove the tumor and adjacent tissue. A customized prosthesis, total joint arthroplasty, or bone tissue from the patient (autograft) or from a cadaver donor (allograft) replaces the resected tissue. Soft tissue and blood vessels may need grafting because of the extent of the excision. Complications may include infection, loosening or dislocation of the prosthesis, allograft nonunion, fracture, devitalization of the skin and soft tissues, joint fibrosis, and recurrence of the tumor.

Because of the danger of metastasis with malignant bone tumors, chemotherapy is started before and continued after surgery in an effort to eradicate micrometastatic lesions. The goal of combined chemotherapy is greater therapeutic effect at a lower toxicity rate with reduced resistance to the medications. Soft tissue sarcomas are treated with radiation, limb-sparing excision, and adjuvant chemotherapy (see Chapter 15).

Secondary Bone Tumors

The treatment of advanced metastatic bone cancer is palliative. The therapeutic goal is to relieve the patient's pain and discomfort while promoting quality of life. If the bone is weakened, structural support and stabilization are needed to prevent pathologic fracture. Bones are strengthened by prophylactic internal fixation, arthroplasty, or PMMA (bone cement) reconstruction. Patients with metastatic disease are at higher risk than other patients for postoperative pulmonary congestion, hypoxemia, VTE, and hemorrhage.

Hematopoiesis is frequently disrupted by tumor invasion of the bone marrow or by treatment (chemotherapy, surgery, or radiation). Blood component therapy restores hematologic factors. Pain can result from multiple factors. Pain must be assessed accurately and managed with adequate interventions.

External-beam radiation to involved metastatic sites may be used. Patients with multiple bony metastases may achieve pain control with systemically given "bone-seeking" isotopes (e.g., strontium 89). See Chapter 12 for more information about pain management.

Additional therapies may be used to treat the original cancer. Radiation, chemotherapy, and hormonal therapy may also be effective in promoting healing of osteolytic lesions (see Chapter 15). Bisphosphonates are effective in stabilizing bone and may prevent cancer spread, as are the RANKL drugs (see Table 41-1).

Nursing Management

The nurse asks the patient about the onset and course of symptoms. During the interview, the nurse assesses the patient's understanding of the disease process, how the patient and the family have been coping, and how the patient has managed the pain. The nurse limits palpation of the mass to decrease any potential seeding process. The mass size and associated soft tissue swelling, pain, and tenderness are noted. Assessment of the neurovascular status and range of motion of the extremity provides baseline data for future comparisons. Evaluation of the patient's mobility and ability to perform ADLs is also documented.

The nursing care of a patient who has undergone excision of a bone tumor is similar in many respects to that of other patients who have had skeletal surgery. Explanation of diagnostic tests, treatments (e.g., wound care), and expected results (e.g., decreased range of motion, numbness, change of body contours) helps the patient deal with the procedures and changes and adhere to the therapeutic regimen. The nurse can most effectively reinforce and clarify information provided by the primary provider by being present during these discussions.

Accurate pain assessment and the use of pharmacologic and nonpharmacologic pain management techniques are used to relieve pain and increase the patient's comfort level. Oncology-associated bone pain is recognized as difficult to control. The nurse works with the patient in designing the most effective pain management regimen, thereby increasing the patient's self-efficacy.

Bone tumors weaken the bone to a point at which normal activities or even position changes can result in fracture. During nursing care, the affected extremities must be supported and handled gently. External supports (e.g., splints) may be used for additional protection. Surgery (e.g., open reduction with internal fixation, joint replacement) may be done in an attempt to prevent pathologic fracture. Prescribed weight-bearing restrictions must be followed. The nurse and physical therapist must educate the patient about using assistive devices safely and strengthening unaffected extremities.

The nurse encourages the patient and family to verbalize their fears, concerns, and feelings. They need to be supported as they deal with the impact of the malignant bone tumor. Details of nursing interventions for oncology patients covered in Chapter 15 are appropriate to initiate with these patients. Referral to a psychiatric advanced practice nurse, psychologist, counselor, or spiritual advisor may be indicated for specific psychological help and emotional support.

Monitoring and Managing Potential Complications

Delayed Wound Healing

Wound healing may be delayed because of tissue trauma from surgery, previous radiation therapy, inadequate nutrition, or infection. The nurse minimizes pressure on the wound site to promote circulation to the tissues. An aseptic, nontraumatic wound dressing promotes healing. Monitoring and reporting of laboratory findings facilitate initiation of interventions to promote homeostasis and wound healing.

Repositioning the patient at frequent intervals reduces the incidence of skin breakdown and pressure ulcers. Special therapeutic beds or mattresses may be needed to prevent skin breakdown and to promote wound healing after extensive surgical reconstruction and skin grafting.

Inadequate Nutrition

Because loss of appetite, nausea, and vomiting are frequent side effects of chemotherapy and radiation therapy, adequate nutrition must be provided for healing and health promotion. Antiemetic agents and relaxation techniques reduce the adverse gastrointestinal effects of chemotherapy. Stomatitis is controlled with anesthetic or antifungal mouthwash (see Chapter 15). Adequate hydration is essential. Nutritional supplements or parenteral nutrition may be prescribed to achieve adequate nutrition.

Osteomyelitis and Wound Infections

Prophylactic antibiotics and strict aseptic dressing techniques are used to diminish the occurrence of osteomyelitis and wound infections. During healing, other infections (e.g., upper respiratory infections) need to be prevented so that healing efforts are not divided between the cancer and the new, acute process. If the patient is receiving chemotherapy, the nurse monitors the WBC count and instructs the patient to avoid contact with people who have colds or other infections.

Hypercalcemia

Hypercalcemia is a dangerous complication of bone cancer or any process involved with breakdown of bone. Symptoms include muscular weakness, incoordination, anorexia, nausea and vomiting, constipation, electrocardiographic changes (e.g., shortened QT interval and ST segment, bradycardia, heart blocks), and altered mental states (e.g., confusion, lethargy, psychotic behavior). Treatment includes hydration with IV administration of normal saline solution, diuresis, mobilization, and medications such as IV bisphosphonates (e.g., zoledronic acid). Because inactivity leads to additional loss of bone mass and increased calcium in the blood, the nurse assists the patient to increase activity and ambulation. Denosumab may be prescribed if the calcium levels are not responsive to the IV bisphosphonates (Cicci, Buie, Bates, et al., 2014) (see Table 41-1). See Chapter 13 for further discussion of hypercalcemia and its management.

Promoting Home, Community-Based, and Transitional Care

 Educating Patients About Self-Care

Preparation for and coordination of continuing health care are begun early as a multidisciplinary effort. Patient education

---

Chart 41-9

HOME CARE CHECKLIST

The Patient With a Bone Tumor

At the completion of education, the patient and/or caregiver will be able to:

- State the impact of the bone tumor growth process and treatment on physiologic functioning, ADLs, IADLs, roles, relationships, and spirituality.
- Identify modification of home environment, interventions, and strategies (e.g., durable medical equipment, wound care/dressings, adaptive equipment, ADL assistance) used in safely adapting to changes in structure or function and promote effective recovery and rehabilitation.
- Describe ongoing therapeutic regimen, including diet and activities to perform (e.g., exercises) and to limit or avoid (e.g., lifting weights, driving a car, contact sports).
  - Consume a healthy diet to promote healing and health.
  - State weight-bearing and activity restrictions.
  - Support affected musculoskeletal area, position to decrease risk of skin breakdown.
  - Demonstrate safe use of ambulatory aids and assistive devices.
  - Engage in exercise that improves balance to reduce risk of falls.
- State the name, dose, side effects, frequency, and schedule for all prescribed therapeutic and prophylactic medications (e.g., antibiotics, analgesic agents).
- Control pain with pharmacologic and nonpharmacologic interventions.
- State indicators of complications to report promptly to primary provider such as:

  - Wound infection/delayed wound healing (e.g., redness, swelling, tenderness, purulent drainage, fever).
  - Osteomyelitis (e.g., localized pain, edema, erythema, fever).
  - Hypercalcemia (e.g., muscular weakness, anorexia, decreased coordination, nausea, vomiting, constipation).
- Relate how to reach primary provider with questions or complications.
- State time and date of follow-up appointments, therapy, and testing.
- Identify community resources for peer and caregiver/family support:
  - Identify sources of support (e.g., friends, relatives, faith community).
  - Identify phone numbers, meeting locations and times of support groups (e.g., cancer support groups, caregiver support groups).
- Identify the need for health promotion, disease prevention, and screening activities.

Resources

See Chapter 10, Chart 10-8 for additional information related to durable medical equipment, adaptive equipment, mobility skills, skin, bowel, and bladder care.

ADL, activities of daily living; IADL, independent activities of daily living.

addresses medication, dressing changes, treatment regimens, and the importance of physical and occupational therapy programs. The nurse educates the patient about weight-bearing limitations and special handling to prevent pathologic fractures. The patient and family must be educated about the signs and symptoms of possible complications as well as resources available for continuing care (see Chart 41-9).

Continuing and Transitional Care

Arrangements may be made for home, community-based, or transitional care. A home visit allows the nurse to assess the patient's and family's abilities to meet the patient's needs and determine whether other services are needed. The nurse advises the patient to have telephone numbers readily available so that providers can be contacted in case concerns arise.

The nurse emphasizes the need for long-term health monitoring to ensure cure or to detect tumor recurrence or metastasis and the need for recommended health screening. If the patient has metastatic disease, end-of-life issues may need to be explored. Referrals for hospice and palliative care are made if appropriate.

CRITICAL THINKING EXERCISES

1 `ebp` A 30-year-old nurse seeks treatment for acute low back pain in the hospital occupational health clinic after a lifting injury sustained from transferring a patient with obesity the previous evening. He tells you that his fellow nurses always ask him to help with heavy lifts. He wants to know if a lumbar brace will help to diminish his back pain. He also wonders if he should wear one all the time while at work. What is the strength of the evidence that supports or does not support the use of a lumbar brace for this patient, in either alleviating his pain or in preventing further lumbar strain?

2 `pg` A college student presents to the student health center after she jammed the first digit of her right foot on her dormitory room door. Describe the priority assessment process that you would follow when you examine her right foot. What is the expected care for a possible broken toe?

3 At the medical clinic where you work as a nurse, a 65-year-old man who is overweight presents with persistent low-grade pain along his lumbar spine. He believes it is related to moving around some boxes about a month ago. He has a history of heavy cigarette smoking, alcohol consumption and a personal history of prostatic cancer. What are the risk factors for problems other than muscle strain that must be considered, based on his medical history?

REFERENCES

*Asterisk indicates nursing research.

Books

Czerniak, B. (2016). *Dorfman and Czerniak's bone tumors* (2nd ed). Philadelphia, PA: WB Saunders.
Davis, A., James, S., & Saifuddin, A. (2015). Bone tumours (2): Malignant bone tumours. In A. Grainger & P. O'Connor (Eds).

Grainger and Allison's diagnostic radiology: The musculosketetal system. New York: Elsevier.
Grossman, S., & Porth, C. (2014). *Porth's pathophysiology: Concepts of altered health states* (9th ed.). Philadelphia, PA: Lippincott Williams and Wilkins.
Rubin, E., Gorstein, F., Schwarting, R., et al. (2004). *Pathology* (4th ed.). Philadelphia, PA: Lippincott Williams & Wilkins.
Weber, J. W., & Kelley, J. (2014). *Health assessment in nursing* (5th ed.). Philadelphia, PA: Lippincott Williams & Wilkins.

Journals and Electronic Documents

American Board of Internal Medicine (ABIM). (2015). *Choosing wisely campaign.* Retrieved on 2/13/2016 at: choosingwisely.org.
American College of Foot and Ankle Surgeons (ACFAS). (2009). Clinical practice guideline for the diagnosis and treatment of forefoot disorders. *Journal of Food and Ankle Surgery, 48*(2), 230–272.
American College of Foot and Ankle Surgeons (ACFAS). (2010). Diagnosis and treatment of heel pain. *Journal of Foot and Ankle Surgeons, 49*(3 Suppl.), S1–S19.
American College of Occupational and Environmental Medicine. (2011). *Carpal tunnel syndrome.* Retrieved on 2/13/2016 at: www.guideline.gov/content.aspx?id=34436&search=carpal+tunnel+syndrome.
Avenell, A., Mak, J. C., & O'Connell, D. (2014). Vitamin D and vitamin D analogues for preventing fractures in postmenopausal women and older men. *Cochrane Database of Systematic Reviews, 4,* CD000227.
Ball, T., Butler, M., & Parsons, S. (2013). Pes-cavis—Not just a clinical sign. Diagnosis, aetiology and management. *Advances in Clinical Neuroscience and Rehabilitation—Rehabilitation articles, 12*(6), 16–19.
Banwell, H., Mackintosh, S., & Thewlis, D. (2014). Foot orthoses for adults with flexible pes planus: a systematic review. *Journal of Foot & Ankle Research, 7*(1), 23. doi. 10.1186/1757–1146–7–23.
Bries, A., Kerr, B., & George, L. (2015). Osteomyelitis: an overview of imaging modalities. *Critical Care Nursing Quarterly, 38*(2), 154–164.
Buchman, A. S., Shah, R. C., Leurgans, S. E., et al. (2010). Musculoskeletal pain and incident disability in community-dwelling older adults. *Arthritis Care and Research, 62*(9), 1287–1293.
Canadian Agency for Drugs and Technologies in Health. (2014). *Mattresses for chronic back or neck pain: A review of the clinical effectiveness and guidelines.* Summary of Evidence. Retrieved on 11/29/2016 at: www.ncbi.nlm.nih.gov/books/NBK263383/.
Cicci, J., Buie, L., Bates, J., et al. (2014). Denosumab for the management of hyperglycemia of malignancy in patients with multiple myeloma and renal dysfunction. *Clinical Lymphoma, Myeloma & Leukemia, 14*(6), e207–e211.
Coleman, R., Body, J. J., Aapro, M., et al. (2014). Bone health in cancer patients: ESMO clinical practice guidelines. *Annals of Oncology, 25*(Suppl. 3), 124–137. doi: 10.1093/annonc/mdu103
Conterno, L. O., & Turchi, M. D. (2013). Antibiotics for treating chronic osteomyelitis in adults. *Cochrane Database of Systematic Reviews, 9,* CD004439.
Cosman, F., de Beur, S. J. LeBoff, M. S., et al. (2014). Clinician's guide to prevention and treatment of osteoporosis. *Osteoporosis International, 25*(10), 2359–2381.
Cosman, F., de Beur, S. J., LeBoff, M. S., et al. (2015). Erratum to: Clinician's guide to prevention and treatment of osteoporosis. *Osteoporosis International, 26*(7), 2045–2047.
de Heer, E., Gerrits, M., Beekman, A., et al. (2014). The association of depression and anxiety with pain: a study from NESDA. *PLoS ONE, 9*(10), e106907.
Dong, W., Goost, H., Lin, X. B., et al. (2015). Treatments for shoulder impingement syndrome: a PRISMA systematic review and network meta-analysis. *Medicine (Baltimore). 94*(10), e510.
*Driessche, A. M. (2012). Surgical site markers: Potential source of infection. *Orthopaedic Nursing, 31*(6), 344–347. doi: 10.1097/NOR.0b013e3182742609
*Fasolino, T. & Whitright, T. (2015). A pilot study to identify modifiable and nonmodifiable variables associated with osteopenia and osteoporosis in men. *Orthopaedic Nursing, 34*(5), 289–293.
Goldenberg, D. L., & Sexton, D. J. (2016). *Septic arthritis in adults.* Up To Date. Retrieved on 12/11/2016 at: www.uptodate.com/contents/septic-arthritis-in-adults.
González-Reimers, E., Quintero-Platt, G., Rodríguez-Rodríguez, E., et al. (2015). Bone changes in alcoholic liver disease. *World Journal of Hepatology, 7*(9), 1258–1264.

Hansen, K. E., Johnson, R. E., Chambers, K. R., et al. (2015). Treatment of vitamin D insufficiency in post menopausal women: a randomized clinical trial. *JAMA Internal Medicine*. *175*(10), 1612–1621.

Henschke, N., Maher, C. G., Osteolo, R. W., et al. (2013). Red flags to screen for malignancy in patients with low-back pain. *Cochrane Database of Systematic Reviews*, *2*, CD008686.

Huppins, L. (2011). Evidence-based medicine (EBM) and orthotic therapy. *Podiatry Management*, *4*(100), 97–102.

Johnson, R. E., Haas, K., Lindow, K., et al. (2014). Plantar fasciitis: what is the diagnosis and treatment? *Orthopaedic Nursing*, *33*(4), 198–204.

Kaplan, S. L. (2014). Recent lessons for the management of bone and joint infections. *Journal of Infection*, *68*(Suppl 1), S51–S56.

Lalani, T. (2016). *Overview of osteomyelitis in adults*. Up To Date. Retrieved on 4/4/2016 at: www.uptodate.com/contents/overview-of-osteomyelitis-in-adults.

Lee, W. J., Lee, S. M., Won, C. H, et al. (2014). Efficacy of intralesional bleomycin for the treatment of plantar hard corns. *International Journal of Dermatology*, *53*(12), e572–e577.

Malhotra, R., Chan, C., & Nather, A. (2014). Osteomyelitis in the diabetic foot. *Medical Clinics of North America*, *97*(5), 947–956.

Michigan Quality Improvement Consortium (MQIC). (2016a). *Management of acute low back pain in adults*. Retrieved on 11/29/2016 at: www.mqic.org/pdf/mqic_2016_lbp_guideline_update_alert.pdf.

Michigan Quality Improvement Consortium (MQIC). (2016b) *Management and prevention of osteoporosis*. Retrieved on 11/29/2016 at: www.guideline.gov/summaries/summary/47804/management-and-prevention-of-osteoporosis?q=Michigan+Quality+Improvement+Consortium.

Morgan, D. J., Dhruva, S. S., Wright, S. M., et al. (2015). Update on medical practices that should be questioned in 2015. *JAMA Internal Medicine*, *175*(12), 1960–1964.

National Institute of Neurological Disorders (NINDS). (2014). *Low back pain fact sheet*. Retrieved on 2/13/2016 at: www.ninds.nih.gov/disorders/backpain/detail_backpain.htm.

NPS Medicinewise. (2015). *Osteoporosis: not just a woman's disease*. Retrieved on 4/4/2016 at: www.nps.org.au/publications/health-professional/health-news-evidence/2015/osteoporosis

Rodriguez, J. A. (2014). Corticosteroid versus platelet-rich plasma injection in epicondylitis. *Orthopaedic Nursing*, *33*(5), 257–265.

Schaafsma, F. G., Anema, J. R., & van der Beek, A. J. (2015). Back pain: prevention and management in the workplace. *Best Practice & Research Clinical Rheumatology*, *29*(3), 483–494.

Sharff, K. A., Richards, E. P., & Townes, J. M. (2013). Clinical management of septic arthritis. *Current Rheumatology Reports*, *15*(6), 332.

Shemory, S. T., Pfefferle, K. J., & Gradisar, I. M. (2015). Modifiable risk factors in patients with low back pain. Paper presented at the 2015 Annual Meeting of the American Academy of Orthopedic Surgeons (AAOS), Las Vegas, NV.

Shirzad, K., Kiesau, C. D., DeOrio, J. K., et al. (2011). Lesser toe deformities. *Journal of the American Academy of Orthopaedic Surgeons*, *19*(8), 505–514.

Singer, F., Bone. H., Hosking, D., et al. (2014). Paget's disease of the bone: an endocrine society clinical practice guideline. *The Journal of Clinical Endocrinology & Metabolism*, *99*(12), 4408–4422.

Smeltzer, S. C., & Qi, B. B. (2014). Practical implications for nurses caring for patients being treated for osteoporosis. *Nursing: Research and Reviews*, *4*(4), 19–33.

Smith, M. A., & Dahlen, N. R. (2013). Clinical practice guideline: Surgical site infection prevention. *Orthopaedic Nursing*, *32*(5), 249–250.

Song, D., Meng, B., Gan, M., et al. (2015). The incidence of secondary vertebral fracture of vertebral augmentation techniques versus conservative treatment for painful osteoporotic vertebral fractures: a systematic review and meta-analysis, *Acta Radiologica*, *56*(8), 970–979.

Sood, A., Paik, A., & Lee, E. (2013). Dupuytren's contracture. *Eplasty*, *13*, ic1. Retrieved on 11/29/2016 at: www.ncbi.nlm.nih.gov/pmc/articles/PMC3552604/

United States Preventive Services Task Force (USPSTF). (2013). Menopausal hormone therapy for the primary prevention of chronic conditions. *Annals of Internal Medicine*, *158*(1), 47–54.

van Vugt, T. A., Geurts, J. & Arts, J. J. (2016). Clinical application of antimicrobial bone graft substitute in osteomyelitis treatment: a systematic review of different bone graft substitutes available in clinical treatment of osteomyelitis. *BioMed Research International*, doi:10.1155/2016/6984656.

Veugelers, P., & Ekwaru, J. (2014). A statistical error in the estimation of the recommended dietary allowance for vitamin D. *Nutrients*, *6*(10), 4472–4475. doi:10.3390/nu6104472

Vitamin D Council. (2016). *How do I get the vitamin D my body needs?* Retrieved on 12/11/2016 at: www.vitamindcouncil.org/about-vitamin-d/how-do-i-get-the-vitamin-d-my-body-needs/.

Williams, C., Henschke, N., Maher, C., et al. (2013). Red flags to screen for vertebral fracture in patients presenting with low-back pain. *Cochrane Database of Systematic Reviews*, *1*, CD008643.

Wong, C. C., & McGirt, M. J. (2013). Vertebral compression fractures: a review of current management and multimodal therapy. *Journal of Multidisciplinary Healthcare*, *6*, 205–214.

Resources

American Cancer Society, www.cancer.org

National Institute of Arthritis and Musculoskeletal and Skin Diseases, www.niams.nih.gov

National Bone Health Alliance, www.nbha.org

National Cancer Institute, www.cancer.gov

National Osteoporosis Foundation, www.nof.org

Paget Foundation, www.nbha.org/members/paget-foundation-pagets-disease-bone-and-related-disorders

Vitamin D Council, www.vitamindcouncil.org

42

Management of Patients With Musculoskeletal Trauma

LEARNING OBJECTIVES

On completion of this chapter, the learner will be able to:

1 Differentiate between contusions, strains, sprains, dislocations, and subluxations.
2 Identify the signs and symptoms of an acute fracture.
3 Describe common treatment modalities for fracture reduction, fracture immobilization, and management of open and intra-articular fractures.
4 Discuss the prevention and management of immediate and delayed complications of fractures.

5 Identify the rehabilitation needs of patients with fractures of the upper and lower extremities, pelvis, and hips.
6 Use the nursing process as a framework for care of the older adult patient with a fracture of the hip.
7 Recognize sports- and occupation-related musculoskeletal disorders and their signs, symptoms, and treatments.
8 Explain the rehabilitation and health education needs of the patient who has had an amputation.
9 Apply the nursing process as a framework for care of the patient with an amputation.

GLOSSARY

allograft: tissue harvested from a donor for use in another person
amputation: removal of a body part, usually a limb or part of a limb
arthroscope: surgical scope injected into the joint to examine or repair
autograft: tissue harvested from one area of the body and used for transplantation to another area of the same body
avascular necrosis (AVN): death of tissue secondary to a decrease or lack of perfusion; also called osteonecrosis
contusion: blunt force injury to soft tissue; bruise
crepitus: a grating sound or sensation made by rubbing bony fragments together
cryotherapy: application of cold compresses or packets
débridement: surgical removal of contaminated and devitalized tissues and foreign material

delayed union: prolongation of expected healing time for a fracture
disarticulation: amputation through a joint
dislocation: complete separation of joint surfaces
fracture: a break in the continuity of a bone
fracture reduction: restoration of fracture fragments into anatomic alignment
malunion: healing of a fractured bone in a malaligned position
nonunion: failure of fractured bones to heal together
phantom limb pain: pain perceived in an amputated section
PRICE: acronym for *protection, rest, ice, compression, elevation*
sprain: an injury to ligaments and muscles and other soft tissues at a joint
strain: a musculotendinous stress injury
subluxation: partial separation of joint surfaces

Unintentional injury is the fourth leading cause of death in the United States (National Center for Health Statistics [NCHS], 2015). Unintentional injuries are commonly called *accidents*; however, this term is considered inaccurate by trauma professionals. The term *accident* infers that there is no potential for prevention; yet, health care professionals understand that prevention plays a major role in decreasing the rate of unintentional injuries. The implementation of evidence-based primary prevention policies (e.g., mandatory use of seat belts for drivers and passengers in motor vehicles) may prevent many unintentional injuries from occurring.

Fracture injuries account for more than one million hospital discharges (NCHS, 2015). Therefore, nurses who work in emergency departments (EDs), critical care units, and inpatient medical-surgical units frequently encounter patients who have experienced musculoskeletal trauma. However, upon discharge from the hospital, many of these patients require extensive periods of rehabilitation and follow-up. Thus, nurses who work in rehabilitation centers, long-term care facilities, ambulatory surgery centers, occupational health settings, and primary care clinics may all care for patients with musculoskeletal injuries.

Contusions, Strains, and Sprains

A **contusion** is a soft tissue injury produced by blunt force, such as a blow, kick, or fall, causing small blood vessels to rupture and bleed into soft tissues (ecchymosis or bruising). A hematoma develops from bleeding at the site of impact, leaving a characteristic "black and blue" appearance. Contusions can be minor or severe, isolated or in conjunction with additional injuries (e.g., fracture). Local symptoms include pain, swelling, and discoloration. Contusions are managed with **PRICE**, an acronym that refers to **p**rotection, **r**est, **i**ce, **c**ompression, and **e**levation (American Academy of Orthopedic Surgeons [AAOS], 2014a). Most contusions resolve in 1 to 2 weeks.

Injury to a muscle or tendon from overuse, overstretching, or excessive stress may cause **strain** (National Association of Orthopaedic Nurses [NAON], 2013). Strains can be categorized as acute or chronic and are graded along a continuum based on postinjury symptoms and loss of function. Acute strains can result from a single injurious incident; whereas, chronic strains result from repetitive injuries. Chronic strains can result from improper management of acute strains. Three degrees of strains can be assessed (NAON, 2013):

- A first-degree strain is mild stretching of the muscle or tendon with no loss of range of motion (ROM). Signs and symptoms may include the gradual onset of palpation-induced tenderness and mild muscle spasm.
- A second-degree strain involves moderate stretching and/or partial tearing of the muscle or tendon. Signs and symptoms include acute pain during the precipitating event, followed by tenderness at the site with increased pain with passive ROM (PROM), edema, significant muscle spasm, and ecchymosis.
- A third-degree strain is severe muscle or tendon stretching with rupturing and tearing of the involved tissue. Signs and symptoms include immediate pain described as tearing, snapping, or burning, muscle spasm, ecchymosis, edema, and loss of function. An x-ray should be obtained to rule out bone injury, because an avulsion fracture (in which a bone fragment is pulled away from the bone by a tendon) may be associated with a third-degree strain. X-rays do not reveal injuries to soft tissue or muscles, tendons, or ligaments, but magnetic resonance imaging (MRI) and ultrasound can identify tendon injury.

A **sprain** is an injury to the ligaments and tendons that surround a joint. It is caused by a twisting motion or hyperextension (forcible) of a joint (NAON, 2013). Ligaments connect bone to bone, and tendons connect muscle to bone. The function of a ligament is to stabilize a joint while permitting mobility. An injured ligament causes joint instability. Sprains are graded in a manner similar to the grading system used for strains (NAON, 2013):

- A first-degree/mild grade sprain results from tears in some fibers of the ligament and mild, localized hematoma formation. Manifestations include mild pain, edema, and local tenderness.
- A second-degree/moderate grade sprain involves partial tearing of the ligament. Manifestations include increased edema, tenderness, pain with motion, joint instability, and partial loss of normal joint function.
- A third-degree/severe grade sprain occurs when a ligament is completely torn or ruptured. A third-degree sprain may also cause an avulsion of the bone. Symptoms include severe pain, increased edema, and abnormal joint motion.

Nursing Management

The treatment for contusions, strains, and sprains is guided by the severity of injury and consists of protecting from further injury, resting and elevating the affected part, applying cold, and using a compression bandage. (The acronym PRICE is helpful for remembering treatment interventions.) Protection from further injury is accomplished through support of the affected area (e.g., sling) and/or splinting. Rest prevents additional injury and promotes healing. Intermittent application of cold packs during the first 24 to 72 hours after injury produces vasoconstriction, which decreases bleeding, edema, and discomfort. Cold packs should not be in place for longer than 20 minutes at a time, and care must be taken to avoid skin and tissue damage from excessive cold (NAON, 2013). An elastic compression bandage controls bleeding, reduces edema, and provides support for the injured tissues. Elevation at or just above the level of the heart controls the swelling (NAON, 2013). If the sprain or strain is third degree, immobilization by a splint, brace, or cast may be necessary so that the joint will not lose its stability. Nonsteroidal anti-inflammatory drugs (NSAIDs) may be used for pain management (NAON, 2013). The neurovascular status (circulation, motion, sensation) of the injured extremity is monitored at frequent intervals (e.g., every 15 minutes for the first 1 to 2 hours after injury) and then at lesser intervals (e.g., every 30 minutes) until stable. Decreases in sensation or motion and increases in pain level should be documented and reported to the patient's primary provider immediately so that compartment syndrome can be prevented (see later discussion).

Joint Dislocations

A **dislocation** of a joint is a condition in which the articular surfaces of the distal and proximal bones that form the joint are no longer in anatomic alignment. A **subluxation** is a partial dislocation and does not cause as much deformity as a complete dislocation. In complete dislocation, the bones are literally "out of joint." Traumatic dislocations are orthopedic emergencies because the associated joint structures, blood supply, and nerves are displaced and may be entrapped with extensive pressure on them. If a dislocation or subluxation is not reduced immediately, **avascular necrosis (AVN)** may develop. AVN of bone is caused by ischemia, which leads to necrosis or death of the bone cells.

Signs and symptoms of a traumatic dislocation include acute pain, change in or awkward positioning of the joint, and decreased ROM. Bilateral assessment will make apparent the abnormality in the affected joint. X-rays confirm the diagnosis and reveal any associated fracture (NAON, 2013).

Medical Management

The affected joint needs to be immobilized at the scene and during transport to the hospital. The dislocation is promptly reduced, and displaced parts are placed back in proper anatomic position to preserve joint function. Analgesia, muscle relaxants, and possibly anesthesia are used to facilitate closed reduction. The joint is immobilized by splints, casts, or traction and is maintained in a stable position. Neurovascular status is assessed at a minimum of every 15 minutes until stable. After reduction, if the joint is stable, gentle, progressive, active and passive movement is begun to preserve ROM and restore strength. The joint is supported between exercise sessions.

Nursing Management

The focus of nursing care is on frequent assessment and evaluation of the injury, including complete neurovascular assessment with proper documentation and communication with the primary provider. The patient and family members are educated regarding proper exercises and activities as well as danger signs and symptoms to look for, such as increasing pain (even with analgesic agents), numbness or tingling, and increased edema in the extremity. These signs and symptoms may indicate compartment syndrome; if compartment syndrome is not identified and communicated to the primary provider, it may lead to disability or loss of the extremity (see later discussion).

Injuries to the Tendons, Ligaments, and Menisci

Rotator Cuff Tears

A rotator cuff tear is a rip in a tendon that connects one of the rotator muscles to the humeral head. The rotator cuff stabilizes the humeral head and is composed of four muscles and their tendons that include the supraspinatus, infraspinatus, teres minor, and subscapularis muscles (NAON, 2013).

Rotator cuff tears may result from acute or chronic stresses on the joint and from intrinsic (e.g., age-related factors) or extrinsic (e.g., overuse, fracture, etc.) factors. Physical examination should include bilateral evaluation of the joint. The patient complains of aching pain that is typically insidious in nature (unless related to an acute injury) and worsens with use. The patient will complain of tenderness to palpation and difficulty sleeping on affected side, and will exhibit decreased ROM and decreased strength. X-rays and MRIs aid in confirming diagnosis and extent of injury, but the most accurate diagnostic modality is arthroscopic (NAON, 2013).

Initial conservative management includes the use of physical therapy, NSAIDs, rest with modification of activities; and injection of a corticosteroid into the shoulder joint. If conservative methods fail, surgical management is warranted. Multiple surgical approaches (e.g., open, mini-open, and arthroscopic) can be employed. Selection of surgical modality is based upon the surgeon's preference, as there is no evidence based best practice guideline at present (NAON, 2013). Postoperatively, the shoulder is immobilized for several days to

4 weeks. Physical therapy with shoulder exercises is begun as prescribed, and the patient is instructed in how to perform the exercises at home. The course of rehabilitation is lengthy (i.e., 3 to 6 months); functionality post rehabilitation depends on the patient's dedication to the rehabilitation regimen (NAON, 2013).

Lateral and Medial Epicondylitis

Epicondylitis is a chronic, painful condition that is caused by excessive, repetitive extension, flexion, pronation, and supination motions of the forearm. These motions result in inflammation (tendonitis) and minor tears in the tendons at the origin of the muscles on the lateral or medial epicondyles. Lateral epicondylitis (i.e., tennis elbow) is frequently identified in someone who repeatedly extends the wrist with supination of the forearm. Pain develops over the lateral epicondyle and in the extensor muscles. Medial epicondylitis (i.e., golfer's elbow) is consistent with repetitive wrist flexion and pronation of the forearm. Extreme tenderness occurs at the medial epicondyle (NAON, 2013).

Rest, through cessation of aggravating actions, is the first-line treatment. Intermittent application of ice and administration of NSAIDs usually relieve the pain. In some instances, the arm is immobilized in a molded splint for support and pain relief. Local injection of corticosteroids may be used for symptom management, but because of its degenerative effects on tendons, this treatment is traditionally reserved for patients with severe pain who do not respond to first-line treatment methods. Rehabilitation exercises may also reduce pain and inflammation (NAON, 2013). Multiple electrophysical modalities, such as transcutaneous electrical nerve stimulation (TENS), ultrasound, extracorporeal shock wave therapy (ESWT), and laser therapy, may effectively manage epicondylitis; however, more research is necessary to validate their efficacy (Dingemanse, Randsdorp, Koes, et al., 2014). Surgical interventions are typically held as a last resort (NAON, 2013).

Lateral and Medial Collateral Ligament Injury

Lateral and medial collateral ligaments of the knee (see Fig. 42-1) provide stability to the knee. Injury to these ligaments occurs when the foot is firmly planted and the knee is struck—either medially, causing stretching and tearing injury

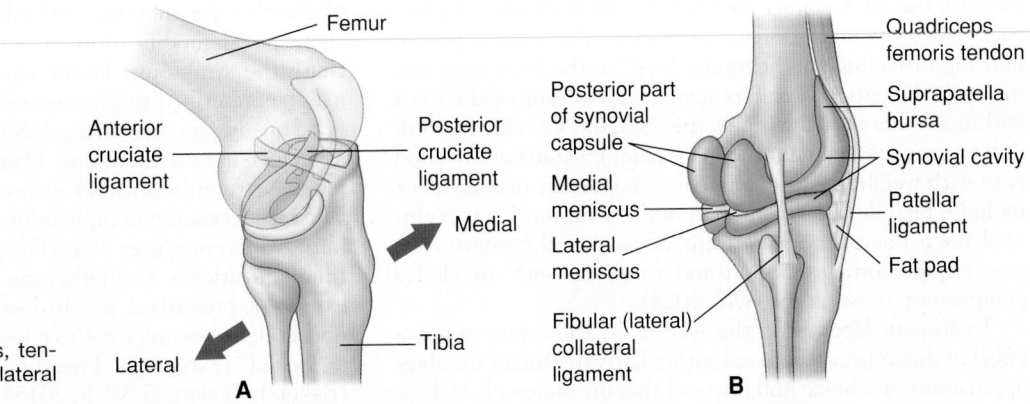

Figure 42-1 • Knee ligaments, tendons, and menisci. **A.** Anterolateral view. **B.** Posterolateral view.

to the lateral collateral ligament, or laterally, causing stretching and tearing injury to the medial collateral ligament. The patient experiences an acute onset of pain, point tenderness, joint instability, and inability to walk without assistance.

Medical Management

Early management includes PRICE. The joint is evaluated for fracture. Hemarthrosis (bleeding into the joint) may develop, contributing to the pain; should this occur, the joint fluid may be aspirated to relieve pressure.

Treatment depends on the severity of the injury. Conservative management includes PRICE, weight bearing as tolerated and the use of a hinged-brace for support. Crutches may be indicated to assist ambulation until weight bearing can be tolerated. Exercises to strengthen the supportive muscles to the knee without straining the ligaments are beneficial. Severe medial collateral ligament (MCL) injuries are initially treated with non–weight-bearing status with progression to weight bearing as tolerated (WBAT) in a hinged-brace for a lengthy timeframe; the healing process may take 8 to 12 weeks. Severe lateral collateral ligament (LCL) injuries usually require surgical intervention, followed by bracing and physical therapy (Agranoff, 2015). A progressive rehabilitation program helps restore the function and strength of the knee. Rehabilitation occurs over many months, and the patient may need to wear a derotational brace while engaging in sports to prevent reinjury.

Nursing Management

The nurse instructs the patient about proper use of ambulatory devices, the healing process, and activity limitation to promote healing. Education addresses pain management, the use of analgesic agents, the use of a brace, wound care, cold therapy, signs and symptoms of possible complications (e.g., altered neurovascular status, infection, skin breakdown, venous thromboembolism [VTE]), and self-care (NAON, 2013).

Cruciate Ligament Injury

The anterior cruciate ligament (ACL) and the posterior cruciate ligament (PCL) of the knee stabilize anterior and posterior motion of the tibia articulating with the femur (see Fig. 42-1A). These ligaments cross each other in the center of the knee. Injury occurs when the foot is firmly planted and the leg sustains direct force, either forward or backward. If the force is forward, the ACL suffers the impact from the force, whereas backward force places force on the PCL. The injured person may report feeling and hearing a "pop" in the knee with this injury. If the patient exhibits significant swelling of the joint within 2 hours after the injury, the ACL or PCL may be torn. A torn cruciate ligament produces pain, joint instability, and pain with weight bearing. Immediate postinjury management includes PRICE and stabilization of the joint until it is evaluated for a fracture. Severe joint effusion and hemarthrosis may require joint aspiration and wrapping with an elastic compression dressing (NAON, 2013).

Treatment depends on the severity of the injury and the effect of the injury on daily activities. Early treatment involves application of a brace and physical therapy. Surgical ACL or PCL reconstruction may be scheduled after near-normal joint ROM is achieved and includes tendon repair with grafting. This is typically performed as ambulatory arthroscopic surgery, a procedure in which the surgeon uses an **arthroscope** to visualize and repair the damage. The best surgical candidates include patients who are young and physically active. Older and less active patients, particularly with concomitant osteoarthritis, tend to benefit from nonsurgical therapy (NAON, 2013). After surgery, the patient is instructed to control pain with oral analgesic medications and **cryotherapy** (e.g., a cooling pad incorporated in a dressing). The patient and family are educated about monitoring the neurovascular status of the leg, wound care, and signs of complications (e.g., infection, VTE) that need to be reported promptly to the surgeon. Exercises (ankle pumps, quadriceps sets [see Chapter 40, Chart 40-1], and hamstring sets) are encouraged during the early postoperative period. The patient must protect the graft by complying with exercise restrictions. The physical therapist supervises progressive ROM and weight bearing (as permitted) (NAON, 2013).

Meniscal Injuries

Two crescent-shaped (semilunar) cartilages in the knee, called *menisci*, are located on the right and left side of the proximal tibia, between the tibia and the femur (see Fig. 42-1B). These structures act as shock absorbers in the knee. Normally, little twisting movement is permitted in the knee joint. Twisting of the knee or repetitive squatting and impact may result in either tearing or detachment of the cartilage from its attachment to the head of the tibia. The peripheral third of the menisci have a small amount of blood flow, which allows that portion to heal if torn.

These injuries leave loose cartilage in the knee joint that may slip between the femur and the tibia, preventing full extension of the leg. If this happens during walking or running, the patient often describes the leg as "giving way." The patient may hear or feel a click in the knee when walking, especially when extending the leg that is bearing weight. When the cartilage is attached to the front and back of the knee but torn loose laterally (bucket-handle tear), it may slide between the bones to lie between the condyles and prevent full flexion or extension. As a result, the knee "locks."

When a meniscus is torn, the synovial membrane secretes additional synovial fluid due to the irritation, and the knee becomes very edematous. Initial conservative treatment includes immobilization of the knee, cryotherapy, the use of crutches for support, anti-inflammatory agents, analgesic agents, and modification of activities to avoid those that cause the symptoms. Home exercises and physical therapy may be prescribed to increase strength in supporting muscles (e.g., quadriceps, hamstrings). MRI is the diagnostic tool used to detect a torn meniscus. Damaged cartilage is surgically removed (meniscectomy) arthroscopically (NAON, 2013). The most common complication is an effusion into the knee joint, which produces pain. The patient is instructed to continue quadriceps strengthening and ROM exercises. The extent of prescribed weight-bearing status can range from non–weight bearing for 4 to 6 weeks to full weight bearing in a "locked" (extension) knee brace. Full ROM is encouraged (Baker, Lubowitz, & Wolf, 2015).

Rupture of the Achilles Tendon

The Achilles tendon attaches the soleus and gastrocnemius muscles (i.e., calf muscles) to the os calcis (i.e., the heel). Traumatic rupture of the Achilles tendon occurs with the "pushing off" action of the gait (NAON, 2013). The patient experiences sudden posterior ankle pain with an audible "pop," difficulty in plantar flexion, and inability to fully bear weight on the affected leg (Cooper, 2015; NAON, 2013). Rupture of the Achilles tendon most commonly occurs in men with a mean age between 37 and 42 years (Cooper, 2015).

Clinical examination is paramount in diagnosis; the ability to plantar flex is decreased and to dorsiflex is improved. MRI or ultrasound is indicated to determine the extent of the injury (Cooper, 2015; NAON 2013). Nonoperative and operative treatment modalities are available for Achilles tendon rupture. Nonoperative modalities include casting (see Chapter 40 for further discussion of casts) while non–weight bearing. The cast is typically in place for 2 to 8 weeks; there is some controversy regarding optimal time. After immobilization with the cast, a boot and then a heel lift is worn with increasing weight-bearing status. Progressive physical therapy to promote ankle ROM and strength is implemented as well. Operative treatment has typically been reserved for young, healthy athletes, because surgery was associated with fewer cases of re-rupture; however, re-rupture rates are decreasing with nonoperative treatment when a holistic approach to physical therapy, called functional physical therapy, is instituted (Cooper, 2015). After surgery, a cast is used to immobilize the joint, as described previously (NAON, 2013).

Fractures

A **fracture** is a complete or incomplete disruption in the continuity of bone structure and is defined according to its type and extent. Fractures occur when the bone is subjected to stress greater than it can absorb (Porth, 2015). Fractures may be caused by direct blows, crushing forces, sudden twisting motions, and extreme muscle contractions. When the bone is broken, adjacent structures are also affected, which may result in soft tissue edema, hemorrhage into the muscles and joints, joint dislocations, ruptured tendons, severed nerves, and damaged blood vessels. Body organs may be injured by the force that caused the fracture or by fracture fragments.

Types of Fractures

Fractures types are classified by location (e.g., proximal, midshaft, distal) and type (Porth, 2015). Fractures are also described according to the degree of break (e.g., a *greenstick fracture* refers to a partial break) or the character of any fractured bone fragments (e.g., a *comminuted fracture* has more than two fragments). Select specific types of fractures are displayed in Figure 42-2.

A *closed fracture* (simple fracture) is one that does not cause a break in the skin. An *open fracture* (compound, or complex, fracture) is one in which the skin or mucous membrane wound extends to the fractured bone. Open fractures are graded according to the following criteria (Halawi & Morwood, 2015):

- Type I is a clean wound less than 1 cm long.

- Type II is a larger wound without extensive soft tissue damage or avulsions.
- Type III (A, B, C) is highly contaminated and has extensive soft tissue damage. It may be accompanied by traumatic amputation and is the most severe.

An *intra-articular fracture* extends into the joint surface of a bone. Because each end of a long bone is cartilaginous, if the fracture is nondisplaced, x-rays will not always reveal the fracture because cartilage is nonradiopaque. MRI or arthroscopy will identify the fracture and confirm the diagnosis. The joint is stabilized and immobilized with a splint or cast, and no weight bearing is allowed until the fracture has healed. Intra-articular fractures often lead to posttraumatic arthritis (Buckley & Page, 2016).

Clinical Manifestations

The clinical signs and symptoms of a fracture include acute pain, loss of function, deformity, shortening of the extremity, crepitus, and localized edema and ecchymosis (NAON, 2013). Not all of these are present in every fracture.

Pain

The pain is continuous and increases in severity until the bone fragments are immobilized. Immediately after a fracture, the injured area becomes numb and the surrounding muscles flaccid. The muscle spasms that accompany a fracture begin shortly thereafter, within a few to 30 minutes, and result in more intense pain than the patient reports at the time of injury. The muscle spasms can minimize further movement of the fracture fragments or can result in further bony fragmentation or malalignment (Porth, 2015).

Loss of Function

After a fracture, the extremity cannot function properly because normal function of the muscles depends on the integrity of the bones to which they are attached. Pain contributes to the loss of function. In addition, abnormal movement (false motion) may be present.

Deformity

Displacement, angulation, or rotation of the fragments in a fracture of the arm or leg causes a deformity that is detectable when the limb is compared with the uninjured extremity.

Shortening

In fractures of long bones, there is actual shortening of the extremity because of the compression of the fractured bone. Sometimes, muscle spasms can cause the distal and proximal site of the fracture to overlap, causing the extremity to shorten (Porth, 2015).

Crepitus

When the extremity is gently palpated, a crumbling sensation, called **crepitus,** can be felt or may be heard. It is caused by the rubbing of the bone fragments against each other.

Localized Edema and Ecchymosis

Localized edema and ecchymosis occur after a fracture as a result of trauma and bleeding into the tissues. These signs may not develop for several hours after the injury or may develop within an hour, depending on the severity of the fracture.

Avulsion
A fracture in which a fragment of bone has been pulled away by a tendon and its attachment

Comminuted
A fracture in which bone has splintered into several fragments

Compression
A fracture in which bone has been compressed (seen in vertebral fractures)

Depressed
A fracture in which fragments are driven inward (seen frequently in fractures of skull and facial bones)

Epiphyseal
A fracture through the epiphysis

Greenstick
A fracture in which one side of a bone is broken and the other side is bent

Impacted
A fracture in which a bone fragment is driven into another bone fragment

Oblique
A fracture occurring at an angle across the bone (less stable than a transverse fracture)

Open
A fracture in which damage also involves the skin or mucous membranes, also called a compound fracture

Pathologic
A fracture that occurs through an area of diseased bone (e.g., osteoporosis, bone cyst, Paget disease, bony metastasis, tumor); can occur without trauma or fall

Simple
A fracture that remains contained, with no disruption of the skin integrity

Spiral
A fracture that twists around the shaft of the bone

Stress
A fracture that results from repeated loading of bone and muscle

Transverse
A fracture that is straight across the bone shaft

Figure 42-2 • Specific types of fractures.

Emergency Management

Immediately after injury, if a fracture is suspected, the body part must be immobilized before the patient is moved. Adequate splinting is essential. Joints proximal and distal to the fracture also must be immobilized to prevent movement of fracture fragments. Immobilization of the long bones of the lower extremities may be accomplished by bandaging the legs together, with the unaffected extremity serving as a splint for the injured one. In an upper extremity injury, the arm may be bandaged to the chest, or an injured forearm may be placed in a sling. The neurovascular status distal to the injury should be assessed both before and after splinting to determine the adequacy of peripheral tissue perfusion and nerve function.

With an open fracture, the wound is covered with a sterile dressing to prevent contamination of deeper tissues. No attempt is made to reduce the fracture, even if one of the bone fragments is protruding through the wound. Splints are applied for immobilization (Schaller, 2016).

In the ED, the patient is evaluated completely. The clothes are gently removed, first from the uninjured side of the body and then from the injured side. The patient's clothing may be cut away. The fractured extremity is moved as little as possible to avoid more damage.

Medical Management

Reduction

Fracture reduction refers to restoration of the fracture fragments to anatomic alignment and positioning. Either closed reduction or open reduction may be used to reduce a fracture. The specific method selected depends on the nature of the fracture; however, the underlying principles are the same. Usually, the physician reduces a fracture as soon as possible to prevent loss of elasticity from the tissues through infiltration by edema or hemorrhage. In most cases, fracture reduction becomes more difficult as the injury begins to heal (Buckley & Page, 2016).

Before fracture reduction and immobilization, the patient is prepared for the procedure; consent for the procedure is obtained, and an analgesic agent is given as prescribed. Anesthesia may be given. The injured extremity must be handled gently to avoid additional damage.

Closed Reduction

In most instances, closed reduction is accomplished by bringing the bone fragments into anatomic alignment through manipulation and manual traction. The extremity is held in the aligned position while a cast, splint, or other device is applied. Reduction under anesthesia with percutaneous pinning may also be used. The immobilizing device maintains the reduction and stabilizes the extremity for bone healing. X-rays are obtained after reduction to verify that the bone fragments are correctly aligned (Buckley & Page, 2016).

Traction (skin or skeletal) may be used until the patient is physiologically stable to undergo surgical fixation. The use of traction and the nursing management of a patient in traction are discussed more fully in Chapter 40.

Open Reduction

Some fractures require open reduction. Through a surgical approach, the fracture fragments are anatomically aligned. Internal fixation devices (metallic pins, wires, screws, plates,

Figure 42-3 • Techniques of internal fixation. **A.** Plate and six screws for a transverse or short oblique fracture. **B.** Screws for a long oblique or spiral fracture. **C.** Screws for a long butterfly fragment. **D.** Plate and six screws for a short butterfly fragment. **E.** Medullary nail for a segmental fracture.

nails, or rods) may be used to hold the bone fragments in position until solid bone healing occurs. These devices may be attached to the sides of bone, or they may be inserted through the bony fragments or directly into the medullary cavity of the bone (see Fig. 42-3). Internal fixation devices ensure firm approximation and fixation of the bony fragments (Buckley & Page, 2016).

Immobilization

After the fracture has been reduced, the bone fragments must be immobilized and maintained in proper position and alignment until union occurs. Immobilization may be accomplished by external or internal fixation. Methods of external fixation include bandages, casts, splints, continuous traction, and external fixators.

Maintaining and Restoring Function

Reduction and immobilization are maintained as prescribed to promote bone and soft tissue healing. Edema is controlled by elevating the injured extremity and applying ice as prescribed. Neurovascular status (circulation, motion, and sensation) is monitored routinely, and the primary provider is notified immediately if signs of neurovascular compromise develop. Restlessness, anxiety, and discomfort are controlled with a variety of approaches, such as reassurance, position changes, and pain-relief strategies, including the use of analgesic medications. Isometric and muscle setting exercises are encouraged to minimize atrophy and to promote circulation. Participation in activities of daily living (ADLs) is encouraged to promote independent functioning and self-esteem. Gradual resumption of activities is promoted as prescribed. With internal fixation, the surgeon determines the amount of movement and weight-bearing stress the extremity can sustain and prescribes the level of activity (NAON, 2013). See Chapter 40 for more information about caring for patients who have a cast, are in traction, or are undergoing surgery.

Nursing Management

Patients With Closed Fractures

The patient with a closed fracture has no opening in the skin at the fracture site. The fractured bones may be nondisplaced or slightly displaced, but the skin is intact. The nurse educates the patient regarding the proper methods to control edema and pain (see Chart 42-1). It is important to educate about exercises to maintain the health of unaffected muscles and to increase the strength of muscles needed for transferring and for using assistive devices such as crutches, walkers, and special utensils. The patient is also educated to use assistive devices safely. Plans are made to help patients modify the home environment as needed and to ensure safety, such as removing floor rugs or anything that obstructs walking paths throughout the house. Patient education includes self-care, medication information, monitoring for potential complications, and the need for continuing health care supervision.

Fracture healing and restoration of strength and mobility may take an average of 6 to 8 weeks, depending on the quality of the patient's bone tissue (NAON, 2013).

Patients With Open Fractures

In an open fracture, there is a risk for osteomyelitis, tetanus, and gas gangrene. The objectives of management are to prevent infection of the wound, soft tissue, and bone, and to promote healing of bone and soft tissue. Intravenous (IV) antibiotics are given upon the patient's arrival in the hospital along with intramuscular (IM) tetanus toxoid if needed (Schaller, 2016).

Wound irrigation and **débridement** (removal of tissues and foreign material) are initiated in the operating room as soon as possible. The wound is cultured, and bone grafting may be performed to fill in areas of bone defects. The fracture is carefully reduced and stabilized by external fixation, and the wound is usually left open (see Chapter 40). If there is any damage to blood vessels, soft tissue, muscles, nerves, or tendons, appropriate treatment is implemented.

With open fractures, primary wound closure is usually delayed, particularly with higher-grade fractures. Heavily contaminated wounds are left unsutured and treated with vacuum-assisted closures (VAC) to facilitate wound drainage. Wound irrigation and débridement may be repeated, removing infected and devitalized tissue and increasing vascularity in the region (Schaller, 2016).

The extremity is elevated to minimize edema. Neurovascular status must be assessed frequently. Temperature is

---

Chart 42-1	**HOME CARE CHECKLIST**
	The Patient With a Closed Fracture

At the completion of education, the patient and/or caregiver will be able to:

- Name the procedure that was performed and identify any changes in anatomic structure or function as well as changes in ADLs, IADLs, roles, relationships, and spirituality.
- Identify modification of home environment, interventions, and strategies (e.g., durable medical equipment, adaptive equipment) used in safely promoting effective recovery and rehabilitation.
- Describe ongoing therapeutic regimen, including diet and activities to perform (e.g., exercises) and to limit or avoid (e.g., lifting weights, driving a car, contact sports).
  - Describe approaches to control swelling (e.g., elevate extremity to heart level).
  - Consume a healthy diet to promote bone healing.
  - Observe prescribed weight-bearing and activity limits.
  - Participate in prescribed exercise regimen to maintain the health of unaffected muscles and those muscles now needed for safe transfer, mobility, etc.
  - If indicated, demonstrate safe use of mobility aid, assistive device, immobilizing device and transfer technique.
- State the name, dose, side effects, frequency, and schedule for all prescribed therapeutic and prophylactic medications (e.g., antibiotics, analgesic agents).
- Control pain with pharmacologic and nonpharmacologic interventions.

- Report pain uncontrolled by elevation and analgesics (may be an indicator of impaired tissue perfusion or compartment syndrome).
- State indicators of complications to report promptly to primary provider (e.g., uncontrolled swelling and pain; cool, pale fingers or toes; paresthesia; paralysis; signs of local and systemic infection; signs of venous thromboembolism; problems with immobilization device).
- State possible complications of fractures (i.e., delayed union; nonunion; avascular necrosis; complex regional pain syndrome, formerly called *reflex sympathetic dystrophy syndrome;* heterotopic ossification).
- Describe gradual resumption of normal activities when medically cleared, and discuss how to protect fracture site from undue stresses.
- Relate how to reach primary provider with questions or complications.
- State time and date of follow-up appointments, therapy, and testing.
- Identify the need for health promotion, disease prevention, and screening activities.

Resources

See Chapter 10, Chart 10-8 for additional information related to durable medical equipment, adaptive equipment, mobility skills, skin, bowel, and bladder care.

ADL, activities of daily living; IADL, independent activities of daily living.

monitored at regular intervals, and the patient is monitored for signs of infection. Bone grafting may be necessary to bridge bone defects and to stimulate bone healing (Schaller, 2016).

Fracture Healing and Complications

Weeks to months are required for most fractures to heal. Many factors influence the time frame of the healing process (see Chart 42-2). With a comminuted fracture, fragments must be properly aligned to attain the best healing possible. It is essential for the fractured bone to have blood supply to the area to facilitate the healing process. In general, fractures of flat bones (pelvis, sternum, and scapula) heal rapidly. A complex, comminuted fracture may heal slowly. Fractures at the ends of long bones, where the bone is more vascular and cancellous, heal more quickly than do fractures in areas where the bone is dense and less vascular (midshaft). Fractures typically heal more quickly in younger patients (Porth, 2015).

If fracture healing is disrupted, bone union may be delayed or stopped completely. Factors that can impair fracture healing include inadequate fracture immobilization, inadequate

---

Chart 42-2   Factors That Inhibit Fracture Healing

- Age >40 years
- Avascular necrosis
- Bone loss
- Cigarette smoking
- Comorbidities (e.g., diabetes, rheumatoid arthritis)
- Corticosteroids, nonsteroidal anti-inflammatory drugs
- Extensive local trauma
- Inadequate immobilization
- Infection
- Local malignancy
- Malalignment of the fracture fragments
- Space or tissue between bone fragments
- Weight bearing prior to approval

Adapted from Buckley, R. & Page, J. L. (2016). *General principles of fracture care. Medscape.* Retrieved on 2/15/2016 at: emedicine. medscape.com/article/1270717-overview#showall; Porth, C.M., (2015). *Essentials of pathophysiology: Concepts of altered health states* (4th ed.). Philadelphia, PA: Lippincott Williams & Wilkins.

---

blood supply to the fracture site or adjacent tissue, multiple trauma, extensive bone loss, infection, poor adherence to prescribed restrictions, malignancy, certain medications (e.g., corticosteroids), older age, and some disease processes (e.g., rheumatoid arthritis) (Porth, 2015).

Complications of fractures may be either acute or chronic. Early complications include shock, fat embolism, compartment syndrome, and VTE (deep vein thrombosis [DVT], pulmonary embolism [PE]). Delayed complications include delayed union, malunion, nonunion, AVN of bone, complex regional pain syndrome (CRPS, formerly called *reflex sympathetic dystrophy*), and heterotopic ossification.

Early Complications

Shock

Hypovolemic shock resulting from hemorrhage is more frequently noted in trauma patients with pelvic fractures and in patients with a displaced or open femoral fracture in which the femoral artery is torn by bone fragments. Treatment for shock consists of stabilizing the fracture to prevent further hemorrhage, restoring blood volume and circulation, relieving the patient's pain, providing proper immobilization, and protecting the patient from further injury and other complications (NAON, 2013). See Chapter 14 for a discussion of shock.

 Fat Embolism Syndrome

Fat embolism syndrome (FES) describes the clinical manifestations that occur when fat emboli enter circulation following orthopedic trauma, especially long bone (e.g., femur) fractures. At the time of fracture, fat globules may diffuse from the marrow into the vascular compartment. The fat globules (i.e., emboli) may occlude the small blood vessels that supply the lungs, brain, kidneys, and other organs. The onset of symptoms is rapid, typically within 12 to 72 hours of injury (Kosova, Bergmark, & Piazza, 2015; Porth, 2015). FES occurs more frequently in males between the ages of 10 and 40 years after a traumatic injury. Although only a small percentage of patients who survive multitrauma have a diagnosis of FES by the time of hospital discharge (0.17% to 1.29%), fat emboli have been found in as many as 82% of trauma patient autopsies (Kosova et al., 2015).

Clinical Manifestations

The classic triad of clinical manifestations of FES include hypoxemia, neurologic compromise, and a petechial rash (Porth, 2015). The typical first manifestations are pulmonary and include hypoxia, tachypnea, and dyspnea accompanied by tachycardia, substernal chest pain, low-grade fever, crackles, and additional manifestations of respiratory failure. Chest x-ray may show evidence of acute respiratory distress syndrome (ARDS) or it may be normal. Petechial rash may develop 2 to 3 days after the onset of symptoms. This rash is secondary to dysfunction in the microcirculation and/or thrombocytopenia and is typically located in nondependent regions (e.g., chest, mucous membranes) of the body. There may be varying degrees of neurologic deficits that can include restlessness, agitation, seizures, focal deficits, and encephalopathy (Kosova et al., 2015; Porth, 2015). Diagnosis relies on clinical examination (Kosova et al., 2015).

> ### ⚑ Quality and Safety Nursing Alert
>
> *Subtle personality changes, restlessness, irritability, or confusion in a patient who has sustained a fracture are indications for immediate arterial blood gas studies.*

Prevention and Management

Immediate immobilization of fractures, including early surgical fixation, minimal fracture manipulation, and adequate support for fractured bones during turning and positioning, and maintenance of fluid and electrolyte balance are measures that may reduce the incidence of fat emboli. There is no specific treatment for FES; the treatment is supportive. Vasopressors, mechanical ventilation, and sometimes corticosteroids are used as supportive therapy (Kosova et al., 2015; Porth, 2015).

Compartment Syndrome

An anatomic compartment is an area of the body encased by bone or fascia (e.g., the fibrous membrane that covers and separates muscles) that contains muscles, nerves, and blood vessels. The human body has 46 anatomic compartments, and 36 of these are located in the extremities (see Fig. 43-4). Compartment syndrome is characterized by the elevation of pressure within an anatomic compartment that is above normal perfusion pressure. Compartment syndrome arises from an increase in compartment volume (e.g., from edema or bleeding), a decrease in compartment size (e.g., from a restrictive cast), or aspects of both. When the pressure within an affected compartment rises above normal, perfusion to the tissues is impaired, causing cell death, which may lead to tissue necrosis and permanent dysfunction (Porth, 2015). Compartment syndrome occurs more frequently in young adults, and although it may take up to 48 hours for symptoms to present, it typically develops quickly, within 6 to 8 hours after the initial injury or after fracture repair (NAON, 2013).

Assessment and Diagnostic Findings

The patient with acute compartment syndrome reports deep, throbbing, unrelenting pain, which is unrelieved by medications, seems disproportional to the injury, and intensifies with passive ROM. Frequent assessment of neurovascular function after a fracture is essential and focuses on the "five Ps": pain, pallor, pulselessness, paresthesias, and paralysis (von Keudell, Weaver, Appleton, 2015). Paresthesia (burning or tingling sensation) is an early sign of nerve involvement. With continued nerve ischemia and edema, the patient experiences diminished sensation followed by complete numbness. Motor weakness may occur as a late sign of nerve ischemia. Motion is evaluated by asking the patient to flex and extend the wrist or plantar flex and dorsiflex the foot. No movement (paralysis) indicates nerve damage (NAON, 2013).

Peripheral circulation is evaluated by assessing color, temperature, capillary refill time, edema, and pulses. Cyanotic nail beds suggest venous congestion. Pallor or dusky and cold digits, prolonged capillary refill time, and diminished pulses suggest impaired arterial perfusion. Edema may obscure the function of arterial pulsation, and Doppler ultrasonography may be used to verify a pulse. Pulselessness is a very late sign of compartment syndrome (NAON, 2013).

A patient may not exhibit all, or even more than just one of the "five Ps"; therefore, pain assessment is most crucial in early recognition of acute compartment syndrome (von Keudell et al., 2015). Palpation of the muscle, if possible, reveals it to be swollen and hard with the skin taut and shiny. The orthopedic surgeon may measure tissue pressure by inserting a tissue pressure-monitoring device, such as a handheld direct injection device (e.g., Stryker Intra-Compartmental Pressure Monitor), into the muscle compartment (normal pressure is 8 mmHg or less) (see Fig. 43-5). Nerve and muscle tissues deteriorate as compartment pressure increases. Prolonged pressure of more than 30 mmHg can result in permanent dysfunction (Porth, 2015).

Medical Management

Prompt management of acute compartment syndrome is essential. The surgeon needs to be notified immediately if neurovascular compromise is suspected. Delay in treatment may result in permanent nerve and muscle damage, necrosis, infection, rhabdomyolysis with acute kidney injury, and amputation (NAON, 2013; von Keudell et al., 2015).

If conservative measures do not restore tissue perfusion and relieve pain, a fasciotomy (surgical decompression with excision of the fascia) is indicated to relieve the constrictive muscle fascia (von Keudell et al., 2015). After fasciotomy, the wound is not sutured but is left open to allow the muscle tissues to expand; it is covered with moist, sterile saline dressings or with artificial skin. Alternatively, a vacuum dressing may be used to remove fluids and hasten wound closure. The affected arm or leg is splinted in a functional position and elevated to heart level, and prescribed intermittent passive ROM exercises are usually performed. In 2 to 3 days, when the swelling has resolved and tissue perfusion has been restored, the wound is débrided and closed (possibly with skin grafts) (NAON, 2013).

Nursing Management

The nurse should frequently assess pain and neurovascular status of the affected limb and report any negative changes that may suggest compartment syndrome immediately to the primary provider. The limb should be maintained in a functional position at the level of the heart to promote optimal blood flow.

> ### ⚑ Quality and Safety Nursing Alert
>
> *Compartment syndrome is managed by maintaining the extremity at the heart level (not above heart level), and opening and bivalving the cast (see Chapter 40) or opening the splint, if one or the other is present.*

Pain management is essential and is accomplished with opioid analgesia, as prescribed. Careful assessment of intake and output and urinalysis could alert the nurse to the development of rhabdomyolysis (see Chapter 54).

Education is necessary for those patients discharged to home-based or community settings with fractures and casts and should include recognition of the unique characteristics of acute compartment syndrome (increasing, refractory pain and neurovascular manifestations) and instructions when to contact the primary provider for emergent follow-up.

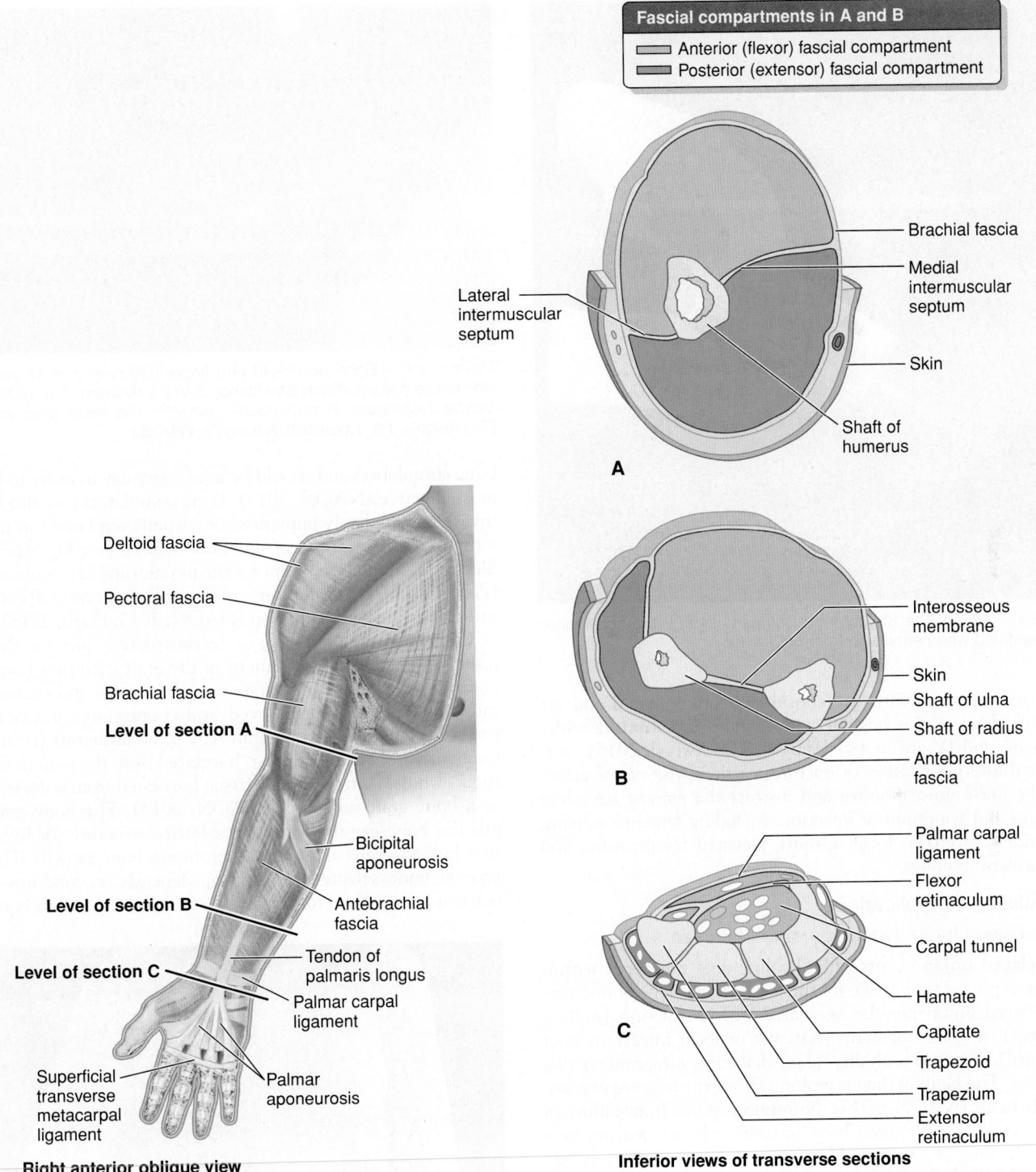

Figure 42-4 • Cross-sections of anatomic compartments. Compartments of the right forearm. From Moore, K. L., Agur, A. M. R., Dalley, A. F. II (2015). *Essential clinical anatomy* (5th ed.). Philadelphia, PA: Lippincott Williams & Wilkins.

Other Early Complications

VTE, including DVT and PE, are associated with reduced skeletal muscle contractions and bed rest. Patients with fractures of the lower extremities and pelvis are at high risk for VTE. PE may cause death several days to weeks after injury. See Chapter 23 for a discussion of PE and Chapter 30 for a discussion of DVT and VTE.

Disseminated intravascular coagulation (DIC) is a systemic disorder that results in widespread hemorrhage and microthrombosis with ischemia. Its causes are diverse and can include massive tissue trauma. Early manifestations of DIC include unexpected bleeding after surgery and bleeding from the mucous membranes, venipuncture sites, and gastrointestinal and urinary tracts. See Chapter 33 for discussion of treatment for DIC.

Figure 42-5 • The Stryker Intra-Compartmental Pressure Monitor. Reprinted with permission from Stryker Inc.

Figure 42-6 • Eight-month-old ring finger malunion in a 19-year-old female patient. (From Strickland, J. W., & Graham, T. J. (2005). *Master techniques in orthopaedic surgery: The hand* (2nd ed.). Philadelphia, PA: Lippincott Williams & Wilkins.)

All open fractures are considered contaminated and are treated as soon as possible with copious irrigation, débridement, and IV antibiotics (Halawi & Morwood, 2015). Surgical internal fixation of fractures carries a risk of infection. The nurse must monitor and instruct the patient regarding signs and symptoms of infection, including tenderness, pain, redness, swelling, local warmth, elevated temperature, and purulent drainage.

Delayed Complications

Delayed Union, Nonunion, and Malunion

Delayed union occurs when healing does not occur within the expected time frame for the location and type of fracture. Delayed union may be associated with distraction (pulling apart) of bone fragments, systemic or local infection, poor nutrition, or comorbidity (e.g., diabetes, autoimmune disease). The healing time is prolonged, but the fracture eventually heals (NAON, 2013). **Nonunion** results from failure of the ends of a fractured bone to unite, whereas **malunion** is the healing of a fractured bone in a malaligned position (see Fig. 42-6). In both of these instances, the patient complains of persistent discomfort and abnormal movement at the fracture site. Nonunion occurs most commonly in tibial fractures, whereas malunion occurs most commonly in fractures of the hand (or fingers) (Porth, 2015). Factors contributing to delayed union, nonunion, and malunion are those associated with impaired bone healing (see Chart 42-2).

Medical Management

Impaired bone healing can be treated with surgical interventions and nonsurgical interventions. Nonsurgical treatment modalities include ultrasound stimulation and electrical bone stimulation and should be used every day in order to be most effective (NAON, 2013). Bone stimulators can also be invasive: completely implanted or partially implanted in the form of pins to the site of impaired healing (see Fig. 42-7). Electrical stimulation promotes the functioning of osteoblasts (Porth, 2015). Surgical interventions include bone grafts and internal and external fixation (NAON, 2013; Porth, 2015).

Grafted bone undergoes a reconstructive process that results in a gradual replacement of the graft with new bone. During surgery, the bone fragments are débrided and aligned, infection (if present) is removed, and a bone graft is placed in the bony defect. The bone graft may be an **autograft** (tissue, frequently from the iliac crest, harvested from the patient for their own use), an **allograft** (tissue harvested from a donor), or a bone graft substitute (NAON, 2013). The bone graft fills the bone gap and provides a lattice structure for invasion by bone cells and actively promotes bone growth. The type of bone selected for grafting depends on function—cortical bone is used for structural strength, cancellous bone

Figure 42-7 • Bone healing stimulator applied to the arm. (Reprinted with permission from EBI Medical Systems, Parsippany, NJ.)

for osteogenesis, and corticocancellous bone for strength and rapid incorporation. Free vascularized bone autografts are grafted with their own blood supply, allowing for primary fracture healing.

After grafting, immobilization and non–weight-bearing exercises are required while the bone graft becomes incorporated and the fracture or defect heals. Depending on the type of bone grafted and the age of the patient, healing may take from 6 to 12 months or longer. Bone grafting complications include wound or graft infection, fracture of the graft, and nonunion. Specific problems associated with autografts include a limited quantity of bone available for harvest and harvest site pain that may persist for up to 2 years after harvest. Infrequent specific allograft complications include partial acceptance (lack of host and donor histocompatibility, which retards graft incorporation), graft rejection (rapid and complete resorption of the graft), and transmission of disease (rare) (Porth, 2015).

Nursing Management

The patient with a nonunion has experienced an extended time in fracture treatment and may become frustrated with prolonged therapy. The nurse provides emotional support and encouragement to the patient and encourages adherence to the treatment regimen. The orthopedic surgeon evaluates the progression of bone healing with periodic x-rays.

Nursing care for the patient with a bone graft includes pain management and monitoring the patient for possible complications. The nurse needs to reinforce educational information concerning the objectives of the bone graft, immobilization, non–weight-bearing exercises, wound care, monitoring for signs of infection, and the importance of follow-up care with the orthopedic surgeon (NAON, 2013).

Nursing care for the patient using bone stimulation devices focuses on patient education that addresses immobilization, weight-bearing restrictions, and correct daily use of the stimulator as prescribed (NAON, 2013).

Avascular Necrosis of Bone (AVN; Osteonecrosis)

AVN occurs when the bone loses its blood supply and dies. It may occur after a fracture with disruption of the blood supply to the distal area. It is also seen with prolonged high-dose corticosteroid therapy, radiation therapy, sickle cell disease, rheumatoid arthritis, and other diseases. The patient develops pain with movement that progresses to pain at rest. Diagnostics include history and physical examination with x-rays, CT scans, and bone scans. Medical management of AVN includes administration of NSAIDs, exercises, and limiting weight bearing of the affected region; however, total joint replacement is the definitive treatment when located in the hip or knee (Porth, 2015).

Complex Regional Pain Syndrome

CRPS is a rare condition characterized by chronic pain in a limb, typically after an injury. Dysfunctional peripheral and central nervous system responses that mount an excessive response to the precipitating event (e.g., fracture, surgery) are thought to be the cause of the pain. Women are affected more often than men, and the average age of diagnosis is 40 years (National Institute of Neurological Disorders and Stroke [NINDS], 2015). Two forms of CRPS exist: CRPS I

(formerly called *reflex sympathetic dystrophy*) and CRPS II, also called *causalgia*, which is characterized by nerve injury (Porth, 2015).

Clinical manifestations of CRPS include severe burning pain, local edema, hyperesthesia, stiffness, discoloration, vasomotor skin changes (i.e., fluctuating warm, red, dry and cold, sweaty, cyanotic), and trophic changes that may include glossy, shiny skin, and changes in hair and nail growth. This syndrome is frequently chronic, with extension of symptoms to adjacent areas of the body. Dysfunction of the affected limb may also be manifested in CRPS. The diagnosis is made through the history and physical examination and ruling out other organic causes (NINDS, 2015).

Nursing Management

Prevention may include early mobilization following an injury or after surgery (Porth, 2015). Early effective pain relief is the focus of management. Pain may be controlled with analgesic agents. NSAIDs, topical anesthetics (e.g., lidocaine patches), corticosteroids, and opioids. Anticonvulsants (e.g., gabapentin [Neurontin]) and antidepressants (e.g., amitriptyline [Elavil]) can be effective in treating neuropathic pain. Additional treatments may include sympathetic nerve blocks, neural stimulation, and delivering prescribed medications intrathecally. Novel treatments under investigation include infusions of immunoglobulin (IVIG) and ketamine and the use of hyperbaric oxygen. The nurse evaluates the effectiveness of these interventions and therapies (see Chapter 12) and helps the patient cope with CRPS manifestations through therapeutic listening, initiation of relaxation techniques and behavior modification, and referral for rehabilitation therapy. Rehabilitation initiated early can improve circulation to the affected area and maximize function. Depression and anxiety are often associated with severe pain disorders; therefore, the nurse should recommend a mental health referral as necessary (NINDS, 2015).

Quality and Safety Nursing Alert

The nurse avoids using the affected extremity for blood pressure measurements and venipuncture in the patient with CRPS.

Heterotopic Ossification

Heterotopic ossification refers to benign bone growth in an atypical location, such as in the soft tissue (Speed, 2015). Heterotopic ossification that is categorized as traumatic myositis ossificans usually develops in response to soft tissue trauma (e.g., contusion, sprain). It is characterized by pain and joint stiffness that causes decreased ROM. It typically occurs in young males after musculoskeletal sports injuries (Walczak, Johnson, & Howe, 2015). If significant ROM dysfunction persists, surgery may be indicated to remove the bone growth and restore function (NAON, 2013; Speed 2015).

Concept Mastery Alert

For further review of fractures, visit **thePoint** for an Interactive Tutorial.

Fractures of Specific Sites

Clavicle

Fracture of the clavicle (collar bone) is a common injury that can result from a fall or a direct blow to the shoulder. The clavicle helps maintain the shoulder in the upward, outward, and backward position from the thorax. Therefore, when the clavicle is fractured, the patient assumes a protective position, slumping the shoulders and immobilizing the arm to prevent shoulder movements. The treatment goal is to align the shoulder in its normal position by means of closed reduction and immobilization. Surgical intervention is not typical but may be indicated if the fracture is located in the distal third of the clavicle or is severely displaced, which may result in neurovascular compromise or pneumothorax (Kleinhenz, 2014; NAON, 2013).

Most of these fractures occur in the middle third of the clavicle and take 3 to 6 weeks to heal (NAON, 2013). A clavicular strap, also called a *figure-eight bandage* (see Fig. 42-8), may be used to pull the shoulders back, reducing and immobilizing the fracture. The nurse monitors the circulation and nerve function of the affected arm and compares it with the unaffected arm to determine variations, which may indicate disturbances in neurovascular status. A sling may be used to support the arm and relieve pain. The patient may be permitted to use the arm for light activities within the range of comfort (NAON, 2013).

Figure 42-9 • Exercises that promote shoulder range of motion include pendulum exercise (**A**) and wall climbing (**B**). The unaffected arm is used to assist with internal rotation (**C**), external rotation (**D**), and elevation (**E**). In **C**, **D**, and **E**, the unaffected arm is used for power.

Fracture of the distal third of the clavicle, without displacement and ligament disruption, is treated with a sling and restricted motion of the arm. When a fracture in the distal third is accompanied by a disruption of the coracoclavicular ligament that connects the coracoid process of the scapula and the inferior surface of the clavicle, the bony fragments are frequently displaced. This type of injury may be treated by open reduction with internal fixation (ORIF). See Chapter 40 for discussion of ORIF.

The nurse cautions the patient not to elevate the arm above shoulder level until the fracture has healed (about 3 to 6 weeks) but encourages the patient to exercise the elbow, wrist, and fingers as soon as possible. When prescribed, shoulder exercises are performed to obtain full shoulder motion (see Fig. 42-9). Vigorous activity is limited for approximately 3 months.

Complications of clavicular fractures include neurovascular injuries (brachial plexus, injury, subclavian vein or artery injury from a bony fragment), pneumothorax, and nonunion (Kleinhenz, 2014).

Humeral Neck

Fractures of the proximal humerus may occur through the neck of the humerus. Impacted fractures of the neck of the humerus are seen most frequently in older women after a fall on an outstretched arm. Active middle-aged patients who are injured in a fall may suffer severely displaced humeral neck fractures with associated rotator cuff damage (Emergency Nurses Association [ENA], 2013).

The patient presents with the affected arm hanging limp at the side or supported by the uninjured hand. Neurovascular assessment of the extremity is essential to evaluate the full

Figure 42-8 • Fracture of the clavicle. **A.** Anteroposterior view shows typical displacement in midclavicular fracture. **B.** Immobilization is accomplished with a clavicular strap.

Figure 42-10 • Immobilizers for proximal humeral fractures. **A.** Commercial sling with immobilizing strap permits easy removal for hygiene and is comfortable on the neck. **B.** Conventional sling and swathe. **C.** Stockinette Velpeau and swathe are used when there is an unstable surgical neck component. This position relaxes the pectoralis major.

extent of injury and the possible involvement of the nerves and blood vessels of the arm.

Many impacted fractures of the surgical neck of the humerus are not displaced and do not require reduction. The arm is supported and immobilized by a sling and swathe that secure the supported arm to the trunk (see Fig. 42-10). Limitation of motion and stiffness of the shoulder occur with disuse. Therefore, pendulum exercises begin as soon as tolerated by the patient. In pendulum or circumduction exercises, the physical therapist instructs the patient to lean forward and allow the affected arm to hang in abduction and rotate. These fractures require approximately 4 to 10 weeks to heal, and the patient should avoid vigorous arm activity for an additional 4 weeks. Residual stiffness, aching, and some limitation of ROM may persist for 6 months or longer (NAON, 2013).

When a humeral neck fracture is displaced, treatment consists of closed reduction with splinting, ORIF, or a hemiarthroplasty. Exercises are begun after an adequate period of immobilization (NAON, 2013).

Humeral Shaft

Fractures of the shaft of the humerus are most frequently caused by (1) direct trauma that results in a transverse, oblique, or comminuted fracture or (2) an indirect twisting force that results in a spiral fracture. The nerves and brachial blood vessels may be injured with these fractures, so neurovascular assessment is essential to monitor the status of the nerve or blood vessels. Damage to either requires immediate attention.

Well-padded splints are used to initially immobilize the upper arm and to support the arm in 90 degrees of flexion at the elbow. A sling or collar and cuff support the forearm. The weight of the hanging arm and splints put traction on the fracture site. External fixators are used to treat open fractures of the humeral shaft (see Chapter 40). ORIF of a fracture of the humerus is necessary with nerve palsy, blood vessel damage, comminuted fracture, or displaced fracture (ENA, 2013).

Functional bracing is another form of treatment used for these fractures. A contoured thermoplastic sleeve is secured in place with interlocking fabric (Velcro) closures around the upper arm, immobilizing the reduced fracture. As swelling

Figure 42-11 • Functional humeral brace with collar and cuff sling.

decreases, the sleeve is tightened, and uniform pressure and stability are applied to the fracture. The forearm is supported with a collar and cuff sling (see Fig. 42-11). Functional bracing allows active use of muscles, shoulder and elbow motion, and good approximation of fracture fragments. Pendulum shoulder exercises are performed as prescribed to provide active movement of the shoulder, thereby preventing a "frozen shoulder." Isometric exercises may be prescribed to prevent muscle atrophy. The callus that develops is substantial, and the sleeve can be discontinued in about 8 weeks. Complications that are seen with humeral shaft fractures include delayed union and nonunion because of decreased blood supply in that area.

Elbow

Fractures of the distal humerus result from motor vehicle crashes, falls on the elbow (in the extended or flexed position), or a direct blow. These fractures may result in injury to the median, radial, or ulnar nerves (NAON, 2013).

The patient is evaluated for paresthesia and signs of compromised circulation in the forearm and hand. The most serious complication of a supracondylar fracture of the humerus is Volkmann contracture (an acute compartment syndrome), which results from antecubital swelling or damage to the brachial artery and leads to a shortening (contracture) of the forearm muscles. This more commonly occurs in children than adults and will result in a "clawlike" appearance to the hand and wrist. The nurse needs to monitor the patient regularly for compromised neurovascular status and signs and symptoms of acute compartment syndrome. If Volkmann contracture develops, fasciotomy may be necessary with débridement of the muscle (Kare, 2015). Other potential complications are damage to the joint articular surfaces and hemarthrosis (i.e., blood in the joint), which may be treated by needle aspiration by the primary provider to relieve the pressure and pain.

The goal of therapy is prompt reduction and stabilization of the distal humeral fracture, followed by controlled active motion after swelling has subsided and healing has begun. If the fracture is not displaced, the arm is immobilized in a posterior long-arm splint for 2 to 3 weeks. At that point, ROM exercises can begin with the use of a hinged brace (NAON, 2013).

Usually, a displaced fracture is treated with ORIF. Excision of bone fragments may be necessary. Additional external support with a splint is then applied. Active finger exercises are encouraged. Gentle ROM exercise of the injured joint is begun early. Motion promotes healing of injured joints by producing movement of synovial fluid into the articular cartilage. Active exercise to prevent residual limitation of motion is performed as prescribed. Total elbow arthroplasty may be indicated in the presence of significant comminution (i.e., fragmentation of bone). Pain management is achieved through the use of NSAIDs or opioid medications (NAON, 2013).

Radial Head

Radial head fractures are fractures of the proximal radius. They are common and are usually produced by a fall on an outstretched hand with the elbow extended. If blood has collected in the elbow joint, it is aspirated to relieve pain and to allow early active elbow and forearm ROM exercises (NAON, 2013). Nondisplaced fractures are typically managed nonsurgically; recent studies demonstrate decreased joint stiffness with early mobilization (i.e., within 48 hours of injury), consisting of repeated extension and flexion exercises (Kodde, Kaas, Flipsen, et al., 2015; Paschos, Mitsionis, Vasiliadis, et al., 2013). If the fracture is displaced, surgery is typically indicated, with excision of or replacement of the radial head when necessary (Duckworth, McQueen, & Ring, 2013).

Radial and Ulnar Shafts

Fractures of the shaft of the bones of the forearm occur more frequently in children but can occur in adults. The radius or the ulna may be fractured at any level. Frequently, displacement occurs when both bones are broken. The forearm's unique functions of pronation and supination must be preserved with proper anatomic alignment (NAON, 2013).

If the fragments are not displaced, the fracture is treated by closed reduction with a long-arm cast applied from the upper arm to the proximal palmar crease. Circulation, motion, and sensation of the hand are assessed before and after the cast is applied. The arm is elevated to control edema. Frequent finger flexion and extension are encouraged to reduce edema. Active motion of the involved shoulder is essential. The reduction and alignment are monitored closely by x-rays to ensure proper alignment. The fracture is immobilized for about 12 weeks; during the last 6 weeks, the arm may be in a functional forearm brace that allows exercise of the wrist and elbow. Lifting and twisting are avoided.

Displaced fractures are managed by ORIF, using a compression plate with screws, intramedullary nails, or rods. The arm is usually immobilized in a plaster splint or cast. Open and displaced fractures may be managed with external fixation devices. The arm is elevated to control swelling. Neurovascular status is assessed and documented. Elbow, wrist, and hand exercises are begun when prescribed by the primary provider.

Chart 42-3 · PATIENT EDUCATION

Encouraging Exercise after Treatment for Wrist Fracture

The nurse encourages active motion of the fingers and shoulder. The patient is instructed to perform the following exercises to reduce swelling and prevent stiffness:

- Hold the hand at the level of the heart.
- Move the fingers from full extension to flexion. Hold and release. Repeat at least 10 times every hour when awake.
- Use the hand in functional activities.
- Actively exercise the shoulder and elbow, including complete range-of-motion exercises of both joints.

Wrist

Fractures of the distal radius (Colles fracture) are common and are usually the result of a fall on an open, dorsiflexed hand. This fracture is frequently seen in older adults with osteoporotic bones that do not dissipate the energy of the fall. The patient presents with a deformed wrist, pain, swelling, weakness, and limited finger ROM, and possibly reports of "tingling" in the affected hand. Tingling sensation may indicate injury to the median nerve (NAON, 2013).

Treatment usually consists of closed reduction and immobilization with a sugar-tong splint until swelling resides. A sugar-tong splint is a U-shaped splint (like tongs used for sugar cubes) that is placed so that it extends from the palm around the elbow to the back of the hand just below the fingers. Once the edema lessens a long or short-arm cast is applied. For fractures with extensive comminution, ORIF, plating, percutaneous pinning, or external fixation is used to achieve and maintain reduction. Pain medication is given as prescribed to aid in pain control (NAON, 2013).

Active motion of the fingers and shoulder should begin promptly to reduce swelling and prevent stiffness (see Chart 42-3).

The fingers may swell due to diminished venous and lymphatic return. The nurse assesses the sensory function of the median nerve by pricking the distal aspect of the index finger. The motor function is assessed by the patient's ability to touch the thumb to the little finger. Diminished circulation and nerve function must be treated promptly (see previous discussion of compartment syndrome).

Hand

Trauma to the hand is a frequent reason patients seek care in EDs (NAON, 2013). The most common type of metacarpal fracture in adults is referred to as boxer's fracture, which occurs when a closed fist bangs against a hard surface, fracturing the neck of the fifth finger. Falls and occupational injuries (e.g., machinery injuries, crushes) are the most common cause of phalangeal injury in adults (ENA, 2013). When any of the bones of the hand are fractured, the objectives of treatment are to regain maximum function of the hand and minimize cosmetic deformities. X-rays are the diagnostic studies of choice (NAON, 2013).

For a nondisplaced fracture of the phalanx (finger bone), the finger is splinted for 3 to 4 weeks to relieve pain and to protect the finger from further trauma. Splinting sometimes consists of "buddy taping" a fractured finger to an adjoining

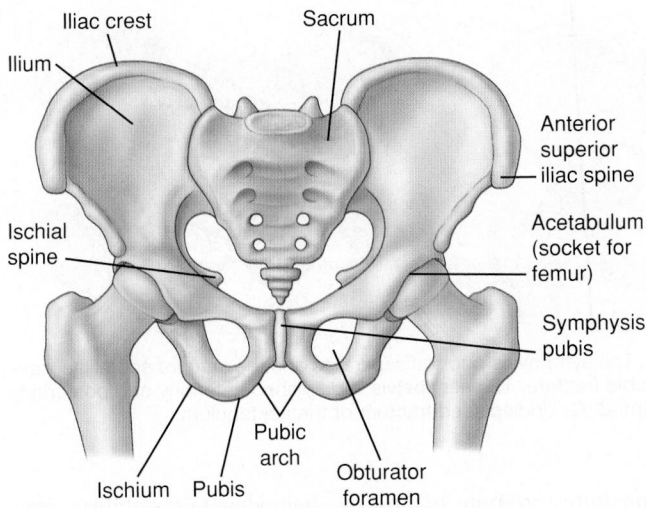

Figure 42-12 • Pelvic bones.

nonfractured finger. Serial x-rays may be done to monitor healing. Displaced fractures and open fractures may require ORIF, using wires or pins. If the fracture is open, or if a fingernail is avulsed, antibiotics may be prescribed (NAON, 2013).

The neurovascular status of the injured hand is evaluated and documented. Swelling is controlled by elevation of the hand. Functional use of the uninvolved portion of the hand is encouraged. Assistive devices might be recommended to aid the patient in performing ADLs until the hand has healed and functional status returns.

Pelvis

The sacrum, ilium, pubis, and ischium bones form the pelvis—a fused, stable, bony ring in adults (see Fig. 42-12). Falls from a great height, motor vehicle crashes, vehicle versus pedestrian, and crush injuries can cause pelvic fractures. There is a high mortality rate associated with unstable pelvic fractures, second only to head injuries among trauma-related deaths; this is primarily related to hemorrhage, although pulmonary complications, fat emboli, thromboembolic complications, and infection are also implicated (ENA, 2013; NAON, 2013). Management of severe, life-threatening pelvic fractures is coordinated with the trauma team (see Chapter 72).

Signs and symptoms of pelvic fracture may include ecchymosis; tenderness over the symphysis pubis, anterior iliac spines, iliac crest, sacrum, or coccyx; local edema; numbness or tingling of the pubis, genitals, and proximal thighs; inability to bear weight without discomfort; severe back pain (retroperitoneal bleed); alterations in neurovascular status of lower extremities (see later discussion of pedal pulse assessment); and clinical manifestations of shock (see Chapter 14). Computed tomography (CT) scanning of the pelvis helps determine the extent of injury by demonstrating sacroiliac joint disruption, soft tissue trauma, pelvic hematoma, and fractures. Neurovascular assessment of the lower extremities is completed to detect any injury to pelvic blood vessels and nerves. Assessment of underlying organs for injury is indicated especially in high-impact trauma (NAON, 2013). Trauma to the ureters, urethra, rectum, vagina; abdominal vascular trauma to veins (more common) and arteries; and neurologic trauma,

particularly spinal column and cord injury, should be assessed as potential concomitant injuries. (NAON, 2013; Russell & Jarrett, 2016). See chapter 72 for discussion of multi trauma and abdominal trauma.

Hemorrhage and shock are two of the most serious consequences that may occur. Bleeding arises mainly from the laceration of veins and arteries by bone fragments and possibly from a torn iliac artery. The peripheral pulses, especially the dorsalis pedis pulses of both lower extremities, are palpated; absence of a pulse may indicate a tear in the iliac artery or one of its branches. Abdominal CT may be performed to detect intra-abdominal hemorrhage. The patient is handled gently so that bony fragments are not displaced, which may exacerbate bleeding and shock. Exploratory laparotomy may be performed to further visualize the peritoneum (NAON, 2013).

Assessment of adjacent structures must be completed when pelvic injury is suspected.

Numerous classification systems have been used to describe pelvic fractures in relation to anatomy, stability, and mechanism of injury. Some fractures of the pelvis do not disrupt the pelvic ring; others disrupt the ring, which may be rotationally or vertically unstable. The severity of pelvic fractures varies. Long-term complications of pelvic fractures include malunion, nonunion, DVTs, residual gait disturbances, back pain from ligament injury, and dyspareunia and erectile dysfunction (Russell & Jarrett, 2016).

Stable Pelvic Fractures

Stable fractures of the pelvis (see Fig. 42-13) include fracture of a single pubic or ischial ramus, fracture of ipsilateral pubic and ischial rami, fracture of the pelvic wing of the ilium (Duverney's fracture), and fracture of the sacrum or coccyx. If injury results in only a slight widening of the pubic symphysis or the anterior sacroiliac joint and the pelvic ligaments are intact, the disrupted pubic symphysis is likely to heal spontaneously with conservative management. Most fractures of the pelvis heal rapidly because the pelvic bones are mostly cancellous bone, which has a rich blood supply.

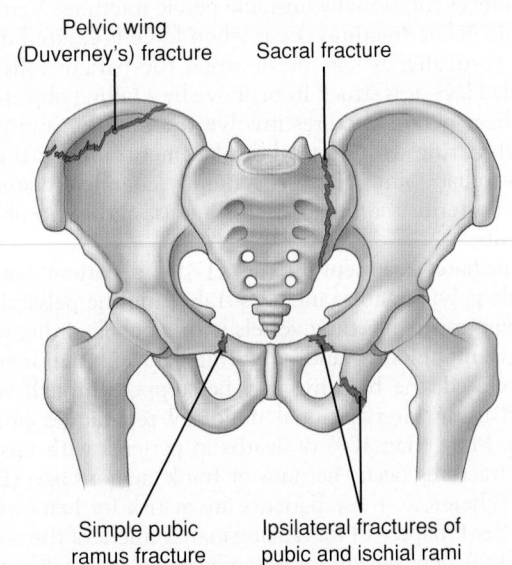

Figure 42-13 • Stable pelvic fractures.

Figure 42-14 • Unstable pelvic fracture. **A.** Rotationally unstable fracture. The symphysis pubis is separated and the anterior sacroiliac, sacrotuberous, and sacrospinous ligaments are disrupted. **B.** Vertically unstable fracture. The hemipelvis is displaced anteriorly and posteriorly through the symphysis pubis, and the sacroiliac joint ligaments are disrupted. **C.** Undisplaced fracture of the acetabulum.

Stable pelvic fractures are treated with a few days of bed rest and symptom management until discomfort is controlled. Fluids, dietary fiber, ankle and leg exercises, antiembolism stockings to aid venous return, logrolling, deep breathing, and skin care reduce the risk of complications and increase the patient's comfort. The patient with a fractured sacrum is at risk for paralytic ileus; therefore, bowel sounds should be monitored.

The patient with a fracture of the coccyx experiences pain when sitting and when defecating. Sitz baths may be prescribed to relieve pain, and stool softeners may be given to ease defecation. As pain resolves, activity is gradually resumed with the use of assistive mobility devices. Early mobilization reduces problems related to immobility (NAON, 2013). Rehabilitation focuses on the goal of full weight-bearing status by 3 months post injury (Russell & Jarrett, 2016).

Unstable Pelvic Fractures

Unstable fractures of the pelvis (see Fig. 42-14) may result in rotational instability (e.g., the "open book" type, in which a separation occurs at the symphysis pubis with sacroiliac ligament disruption), vertical instability, or a combination of both. Lateral or anteroposterior compression of the pelvis produces rotationally unstable pelvic fractures. Vertically unstable pelvic fractures occur when force is exerted on the pelvis vertically, as may occur when the patient falls onto extended legs or is struck from above by a falling object. Vertical shear pelvic fractures involve the anterior and posterior pelvic ring with vertical displacement, usually through the sacroiliac joint. There is generally complete disruption of the posterior sacroiliac, sacrospinous, and sacrotuberous ligaments.

Immediate treatment in the ED for a patient with an unstable pelvic fracture includes stabilizing the pelvic bones and compressing bleeding vessels with a pelvic girdle, which is an external binding and stabilizing device. If major vessels are lacerated, the bleeding may be stopped through embolization using interventional radiology techniques prior to surgery. More than 10% of deaths in patients with unstable pelvic fractures occur because of frank hemorrhage (ENA, 2013). Therefore, these patients are at risk for hemorrhagic shock. See Chapter 14 for nursing management of the patient in shock. When the patient is hemodynamically stable, treatment generally involves external fixation or ORIF. These measures promote hemostasis, hemodynamic stability, comfort, and early mobilization.

Acetabulum

Acetabular fractures are a type of intra-articular fracture. The typical mechanism of injury is that an external force drives the femoral shaft into the hip joint, fracturing the acetabulum. This may be caused by high-speed motor vehicle crashes (e.g., knees driven into dashboard, pedals forcibly driven upward into legs) or from falls from heights (Thacker, Tejwani, & Thakkar, 2014). Treatment depends on the pattern of fracture. Stable, nondisplaced fractures may be managed with traction and protective weight bearing so that the affected foot is placed on the floor only for balance. Displaced and unstable acetabular fractures are treated with open reduction, joint débridement, and internal fixation or arthroplasty. Internal fixation permits early non–weight-bearing ambulation and ROM exercise. Complications seen with acetabular fractures include malunion, nerve palsy, heterotopic ossification, and posttraumatic arthritis (Thacker et al., 2014).

Hip

Annually, more than 250,000 adults older than 65 years of age sustain a hip fracture requiring hospitalization (National Hospital Discharge Survey [NHDS], 2015). The 1-year mortality rate among these older adults is as high as 24% (NAON, 2013). Weak quadriceps muscles, slowed reflexes, decreased bone tensile strength, general frailty due to age, and conditions that produce decreased cerebral arterial perfusion (transient ischemic attacks, anemia, emboli, cardiovascular disease, effects of medications) contribute to the incidence of falls, which are the major cause of hip fracture.

There are three major types of hip fracture. *Extracapsular fractures* are fractures of the trochanteric region (between the base of the neck and the lesser trochanter of the femur) and of the subtrochanteric region. *Intracapsular fractures* are fractures of the neck of the femur. Fractures of the neck of the femur may damage the vascular system that supplies blood to the head and the neck of the femur, and the bone may become ischemic. For this reason, AVN is common in patients with femoral neck fractures (see Fig. 42-15). *Periprosthetic fractures* are fractures to the regions surrounding prosthetics joints (NAON, 2013).

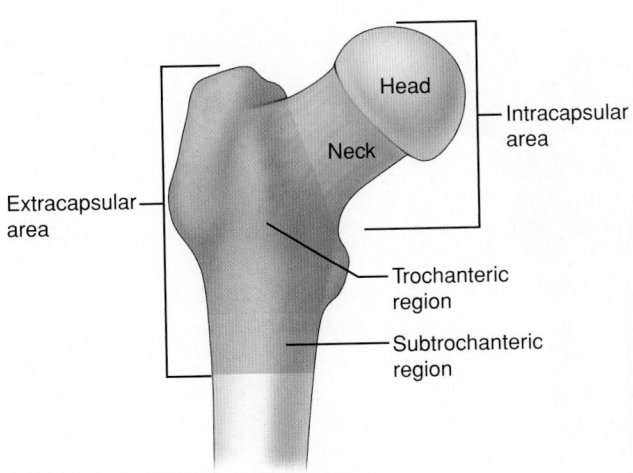

Figure 42-15 • Regions of the proximal femur.

Clinical Manifestations

With fractures of the femoral neck, the leg is shortened, adducted, and externally rotated. The patient reports pain in the hip and groin or in the medial side of the knee. With most fractures of the femoral neck, the patient cannot move the leg without a significant increase in pain. The patient is most comfortable with the leg slightly flexed in external rotation. Impacted intracapsular femoral neck fractures cause moderate discomfort (even with movement), may allow the patient to bear weight, and may not demonstrate obvious shortening or rotational changes. With extracapsular femoral fractures of the trochanteric or subtrochanteric regions, the extremity is significantly shortened, externally rotated to a greater degree than intracapsular fractures, exhibits muscle spasm that resists positioning of the extremity in a neutral position, and has an associated area of ecchymosis. The diagnosis is confirmed by x-ray (NAON, 2013).

Gerontologic Considerations

Older adults (particularly women) who have low bone density from osteoporosis and who tend to fall frequently have a high incidence of hip fracture. Stress and immobility related to the trauma predispose the older adult to atelectasis, pneumonia, sepsis, VTE, pressure ulcers, and reduced ability to cope with other health problems. Many older adults hospitalized with hip fractures exhibit delirium as a result of stress of the trauma, pain, unfamiliar surroundings, sleep deprivation, and medications. In addition, delirium that develops in some older adult patients may be caused by mild cerebral ischemia or mild hypoxemia. Other factors associated with delirium include responses to malnutrition, dehydration, infectious processes, mood disturbances, and blood loss (Holly, Rittenmyer, & Weeks, 2014). The same factors that may cause delirium may superimpose delirium on dementia in the older adult with a fractured hip, further complicating recovery.

To prevent complications, the nurse must assess the older patient for chronic conditions that require close monitoring. Examination of the legs may reveal edema due to heart failure or absence of peripheral pulses from peripheral vascular disease. Similarly, chronic respiratory problems may be present and may contribute to the possible development of atelectasis

or pneumonia. Coughing and deep-breathing exercises are encouraged. Frequently, older adults take cardiac, antihypertensive, or respiratory medications that need to be continued. The patient's responses to these medications should be monitored.

Dehydration and poor nutrition may be present. At times, older adults who live alone cannot call for help at the time of injury. A day or two may pass before assistance is provided, and as a result, dehydration occurs. Nutritional status may have been poor prior to admission, so the nurse should monitor for complications of dehydration and poor nutrition (e.g., pressure ulcers, etc.). Nutritional supplements are effective in improving outcomes in older adults and should be incorporated into the plan of care (AAOS, 2014b).

Muscle weakness may have initially contributed to the fall and fracture. Bed rest and immobility cause an additional loss of muscle strength unless the nurse encourages the patient to move all joints except the involved hip and knee. Patients are encouraged to use their arms and the overhead trapeze to reposition themselves. This strengthens the arms and shoulders, which facilitates walking with assistive devices.

Medical Management

Buck's extension traction, a type of temporary skin traction, was traditionally applied because it was believed to reduce muscle spasm, to immobilize the extremity, and to relieve pain. Its efficacy had never been established in clinical trials, however, so its routine prescription is not advocated (AAOS, 2014b). The goal of surgical treatment for hip fractures is to obtain a satisfactory fixation so that the patient can be mobilized quickly and avoid secondary medical complications. Surgical treatment consists of (1) open or closed reduction of the fracture and internal fixation, (2) replacement of the femoral head with a prosthesis (hemiarthroplasty), or (3) closed reduction with percutaneous stabilization for an intracapsular fracture. Surgical intervention is carried out as soon as possible after injury. The preoperative objective is to ensure that the patient is in as favorable a condition as possible for the surgery. Displaced femoral neck fractures are treated as emergencies, with reduction and internal fixation performed within 24 hours after fracture. The femoral head is often replaced with a prosthesis if there is complete disruption of blood flow to the femoral head, which may cause AVN (NAON, 2013).

After general or spinal anesthesia, the hip fracture is reduced under x-ray visualization. A stable fracture is usually fixed with nails, a nail and plate combination, multiple pins, or compression screw devices (see Fig. 42-16). The orthopedic surgeon determines the specific fixation device based on the fracture site or sites. Adequate reduction is important for fracture healing—the better the reduction, the better the healing.

Total hip arthroplasty (see Chapter 40) may be used in selected patients with intracapsular fractures (NAON, 2013).

Nursing Management

The immediate postoperative care for a patient with a hip fracture is similar to that for other patients undergoing major surgery (see Chapters 19 and 40). Attention is given to pain management, prevention of secondary medical problems, and

Cannulated screw fixation

Compression hip screw and side plate

Blade plate fixation

Figure 42-16 • Examples of internal fixation for hip fractures. Internal fixation is achieved through the use of screws and plates specifically designed for stability and fixation.

early mobilization of the patient so that independent functioning can be restored.

During the first 24 to 48 hours, relief of pain and prevention of complications are important, and continuous neurovascular assessment is essential. The nurse encourages deep breathing and dorsiflexion and plantar flexion exercises every 1 to 2 hours. Thigh-high antiembolism stockings or pneumatic compression devices are used, and anticoagulants are given as prescribed to prevent the formation of VTE. The nurse administers prescribed analgesic medications and monitors the patient's hydration, nutritional status, and urine output.

Repositioning the Patient

The most comfortable and safest way to turn the patient is to turn to the uninjured side. The standard method involves placing a pillow between the patient's legs to keep the affected leg in an abducted position. Proper alignment and supported abduction are maintained while turning (NAON, 2013).

Promoting Exercise

The patient is encouraged to exercise as much as possible by means of the overbed trapeze. This device helps strengthen the arms and shoulders in preparation for protected ambulation (e.g., toe touch, partial weight bearing). On the first postoperative day, the patient transfers to a chair with assistance and begins assisted ambulation. The amount of weight bearing that can be permitted depends on the stability of the fracture reduction. The primary provider prescribes the degree of weight bearing. In general, hip flexion and internal rotation restrictions apply only if the patient has had a hemiarthroplasty or total arthroplasty (NAON, 2013) (see Chapter 40). Physical therapists work with the patient on transfers, ambulation, and the safe use of assistive devices.

The patient can anticipate discharge to home or to an extended-care facility with the use of assistive devices (see Chapter 10). Some modifications in the home may be needed, such as installation of elevated toilet seats and grab bars.

Monitoring and Managing Potential Complications

Neurovascular complications may occur from direct injury or edema in the area that causes compression of nerves and blood vessels. With hip fracture, bleeding into the tissues and edema are expected. Monitoring and documenting the neurovascular status of the affected leg are vital.

To prevent VTE, the nurse encourages intake of fluids and ankle and foot exercises. Antiembolism stockings, pneumatic compression devices, and prophylactic anticoagulant therapy are indicated and should be prescribed (AAOS, 2014b). During hospitalization, the patient or the patient's caregiver should be educated regarding the signs, symptoms, and risks of VTE, and how to administer anticoagulant prophylaxis as prescribed (see Chart 42-4). Intermittent assessment of the patient's legs for signs of DVT, which may include unilateral calf tenderness, warmth, redness, and swelling, is indicated.

Pulmonary complications (e.g., atelectasis, pneumonia) are a threat to older patients undergoing hip surgery. Coughing and deep-breathing exercises, intermittent changes of position, and the use of an incentive spirometer may help prevent respiratory complications. Pain must be treated with analgesic agents, typically opioids; otherwise, the patient may not be able to cough, deep breathe, or engage in prescribed activities. The nurse assesses breath sounds to detect adventitious or diminished sounds.

Skin breakdown is often seen in older patients with hip fracture. Blisters caused by tape are related to the tension of soft tissue edema under a nonelastic tape. An elastic hip wrap dressing or elastic tape applied in a vertical fashion may reduce the incidence of tape blisters. In addition, patients with hip fractures tend to remain in one position and may develop pressure ulcers. Proper skin care, especially on the bony prominences, helps to relieve pressure. High-density foam mattress overlays may provide protection by distributing pressure evenly.

Loss of bladder control (incontinence or retention) may occur. In general, the routine use of an indwelling catheter is avoided because of the high risk of urinary tract infection.

NURSING RESEARCH PROFILE

Chart 42-4

Venous Thromboembolism Knowledge of Older Adults After Hip Fracture

Lee, J., Donaldson, J., Drake, D. et al. (2014). Venous thromboembolism knowledge among older post-hip fracture patients and their caregivers. *Geriatric Nursing*, 35(5), p. 374–380.

Purpose

Venous thromboembolism (VTE) is a serious complication following hip fracture injury in older adults. As VTE risk extends beyond the acute hospital phase, prevention of VTE should also be assured postdischarge. The purpose of this study was to assess older adults' knowledge of VTE prophylaxis after hip fracture and their satisfaction with VTE prophylaxis education provided during their hospitalization.

Design

The researchers used a survey to complete this descriptive cross-sectional study with adults older than 65 years of age following a hip fracture with surgical intervention. Patients ($n = 30$) or their caregivers ($n = 30$) consented to serve as participants and answered questions regarding VTE prophylaxis prior to discharge from the hospital.

Findings

Both patients and caregivers expressed the desire for more education on VTE prophylaxis, particularly information on medications used for VTE prevention and possible side effects and drug–drug interactions of these medications. The participants were also found to have insufficient knowledge of VTE risk factors, symptoms, and prevention measures.

Nursing Implications

Patients post hip fracture surgery or their caregivers may need to administer anticoagulant prophylaxis for several weeks postdischarge. Nurses administer medications to older adult patients post hip fracture surgery, and are in a prime position to educate patients about the indications, side effects, and risks involved with anticoagulant prophylaxis. These researchers assert that nurses should not only verbally instruct patients about anticoagulant prophylaxis, but also involve family members in education sessions and supplement verbal instruction with dissemination of written materials for future reference.

If a catheter is inserted at the time of surgery, it usually is removed on the first postoperative day followed by a trial to void (Street, Thompson, & Bailey, 2015). Because urinary retention is common after surgery, the nurse must assess the patient's voiding patterns. To ensure proper urinary tract function, the nurse encourages liberal fluid intake if the patient has no pre-existing cardiac disease.

Delayed complications of hip fractures include infection, nonunion, and AVN of the femoral head (particularly with femoral neck fractures) (NAON, 2013). Infection is suspected if the patient complains of constant pain in the hip and has an elevated erythrocyte sedimentation rate.

The nursing management of the older adult patient with a hip fracture is summarized in the Plan of Nursing Care (see Chart 42-5).

Promoting Home, Community-Based, and Transitional Care

Educating the Patient About Self-Care

Most patients are discharged from the hospital to an inpatient rehabilitation facility. The patient and family members or caregivers are assessed for their readiness to commence activities that promote healing and mobility. The nurse collaborates with other members of the multidisciplinary physiotherapy team (e.g., physical therapist, occupational therapist) to gather baseline data on the patient's anticipated long-term care environment post discharge, whether that is home or a long-term care facility, such as a skilled nursing facility. The patient begins a rehabilitation routine geared to meet the needs of this environment. For instance, if the patient is to be discharged home, and there are stairs in the home, then a goal of rehabilitation is that the patient will be able to get up and down stairs before discharge.

The patient engages in regular exercises to improve muscle tone and balance (see Chapter 10). The safe use of ambulatory aids, any specific activity restrictions (e.g., hip precautions if total hip arthroplasty was performed), and fall prevention measures (e.g., appropriate footwear, proper lighting, removal of throw rugs, getting rid of clutter) are also vitally important education topics that must be adequately addressed prior to discharge (Saccomano & Ferrara, 2015). The patient and caregiver are educated on the indications for any newly prescribed medications, wound care, and the importance of proper nutrition. Identification of any potential complications (e.g., reddened wound, fever) and when and how to contact the patient's primary provider are also important to understand.

Continuing and Transitional Care

Referral for home, community-based, or transitional care is important to enable assessment of the patient's home environment and the adequacy of resources and support of caregivers. Modifications may need to be made to ensure the patient's continuing care, safety, and mobility. During follow-up home health or outpatient clinic visits, the nurse reevaluates the patient's healing process and the continued adequacy of resources and support of caregivers. Modifications may need to be made based upon these findings. For instance, an older adult spouse may require assistance or respite care. Home health agencies, local area agencies on aging (for older adult patients), and faith community nursing organizations, may be tapped into to provide assistance within the home or with transporting the patient to follow-up outpatient appointments.

Osteoporosis screening of patients who have experienced hip fracture is important for prevention of future fractures. With dual-energy x-ray absorptiometry (DEXA) scan testing, the risk of additional fracture can be predicted. Specific patient education regarding dietary requirements, lifestyle changes, and weight-bearing exercise to promote bone health is needed. Vitamin D and calcium supplements are also recommended (AAOS, 2014b). Specific therapeutic interventions need to be initiated to slow bone loss and to build bone mineral density (see Chapter 41).

(text continued on page 1210)

Chart 42-5

PLAN OF NURSING CARE
Care of the Older Adult Patient With a Fractured Hip

NURSING DIAGNOSIS: Acute pain related to fracture, soft tissue damage, muscle spasm, and surgery
GOAL: Relief of pain

Nursing Interventions	Rationale	Expected Outcomes
1. Assess type and location of patient's pain whenever vital signs are obtained and as needed.	1. Pain is expected after fracture; soft tissue damage and muscle spasm contribute to discomfort; pain is subjective and is best evaluated on a pain scale of 0–10 and through description of characteristics and location, which are important for identifying cause of discomfort and for proposing interventions. Continuing pain may indicate development of neurovascular problems. Pain must be assessed periodically to gauge effectiveness of continuing analgesic therapy.	• Patient describes and rates pain on scale of 0–10. • Expresses confidence in efforts to control pain. • Expresses comfort with position changes. • Expresses comfort when leg is positioned and immobilized. • Minimizes movement of extremity before reduction and fixation. • Uses physical, psychological, and pharmacologic measures to reduce discomfort. • Describes acceptable pain level that does not interfere with ability to participate in rehabilitation activities within 24–48 hours after surgery. • Requests pain medications and uses pain-relief measures early in pain cycle. • States that positioning provides comfort. • Appears comfortable and relaxed. • Moves with increasing comfort as healing progresses.
2. Acknowledge existence of pain; inform patient of available analgesic agents and advocate for preemptive analgesia (e.g., prior to physical therapy); record patient's baseline discomfort.	2. Reduces stress experienced by the patient by communicating concern and availability of help in dealing with pain. Documentation provides baseline data.	
3. Handle the affected extremity gently, supporting it with hands or pillow.	3. Movement of bone fragments is painful; muscle spasms occur with movement; adequate support diminishes soft tissue tension.	
4. Apply Buck's traction if prescribed; advocate for its removal if pain worsens or is not improved; use trochanter roll.	4. Immobilizes fracture to decrease pain, muscle spasm, and external rotation of hip. Routine use of Buck's traction has not been proven to be effective.	
5. Use pain-modifying strategies. a. Modify the environment. b. Administer prescribed analgesic agents preemptively and as needed. c. Encourage patient to use pain-relief measures to relieve pain. d. Evaluate patient's response to medications and other pain reduction techniques. e. Consult with primary provider if relief of pain is not obtained.	5. Pain perception can be diminished by distraction and refocusing of attention. a. Interaction with others, distraction, and environmental stimuli may modify pain experiences. b. Analgesics reduce the pain; muscle relaxants may be prescribed to decrease discomfort associated with muscle spasm. c. Mild pain is easier to control than severe pain. d. Assessment of effectiveness of measures provides basis for future management interventions; early identification of adverse reactions is necessary for corrective measures and care plan modifications. e. Change in treatment plan may be necessary.	
6. Position for comfort and function.	6. Alignment of body facilitates comfort; positioning for function diminishes stress on musculoskeletal system.	
7. Assist with frequent changes in position.	7. Change of position relieves pressure and associated discomfort.	

NURSING DIAGNOSIS: Impaired physical mobility related to fractured hip
GOAL: Achieves pain-free, functional, stable hip

Nursing Interventions	Rationale	Expected Outcomes
1. Maintain neutral positioning of hip. 2. Use trochanter roll; roll to uninjured side. 3. Place pillow between legs when turning. 4. Instruct and assist in position changes and transfers.	1. Prevents stress at the site of fixation. 2. Minimizes external rotation. 3. Supports leg; prevents adduction. 4. Encourages patient's active participation while preventing stress on hip fixation.	• Patient engages in therapeutic positioning. • Uses pillow between legs when turning. • Assists in position changes; shows increased independence in transfers.

Chart 42-5

PLAN OF NURSING CARE (Continued)

Care of the Older Adult Patient With a Fractured Hip

Nursing Interventions	Rationale	Expected Outcomes
5. Instruct in and supervise isometric and quadriceps and gluteal setting exercises.	5. Strengthens muscles needed for walking.	• Exercises every 2 hours while awake.
6. Encourage the use of trapeze.	6. Strengthens shoulder and arm muscles necessary for use of ambulatory aids.	• Uses trapeze. • Participates in progressive ambulation program.
7. In consultation with physical therapist, instruct in and supervise progressive safe ambulation within limitations of weight-bearing prescription.	7. Amount of weight bearing depends on the patient's condition, fracture stability, and fixation device; ambulatory aids are used to assist the patient with non–weight-bearing and partial–weight-bearing ambulation.	• Actively participates in exercise regimen. • Uses ambulatory aids correctly and safely.
8. Offer encouragement and support exercise regimen.	8. Reconditioning exercises can be uncomfortable and fatiguing; encouragement helps patient comply with the program.	
9. Instruct in and supervise safe use of ambulatory aids.	9. Prevents injury from unsafe use.	

NURSING DIAGNOSIS: Risk for infection related to surgical incision
GOAL: Maintains asepsis

Nursing Interventions	Rationale	Expected Outcomes
1. Monitor vital signs.	1. Temperature, pulse, and respiration increase in response to infection. (Magnitude of response may be minimal in older adult patients.)	• Patient maintains vital signs within normal range. • Exhibits well-approximated incision without drainage or excessive inflammatory response.
2. Perform aseptic dressing changes.	2. Avoids introducing infectious organisms.	• Relates minimal discomfort; demonstrates no hematoma.
3. Assess wound appearance and character of drainage.	3. Red, swollen, draining incision is indicative of infection.	• Tolerates antibiotics if prescribed; exhibits no evidence of osteomyelitis.
4. Assess report of pain.	4. Pain may be due to wound hematoma, a possible locus of infection, which needs to be surgically evacuated.	
5. Administer preoperative antibiotic as prescribed and postoperative antibiotics if prescribed, and observe for side effects.	5. Administration of 1–3 doses of perioperative antibiotics improves outcomes and reduces the risk of wound infection.	

NURSING DIAGNOSIS: Readiness for enhanced urinary elimination related to immobility
GOAL: Maintains normal urinary elimination patterns

Nursing Interventions	Rationale	Expected Outcomes
1. Monitor intake and output.	1. Adequate fluid intake ensures hydration; adequate urinary output minimizes urinary stasis.	• Intake and output are adequate; patient exhibits normal voiding patterns. • Demonstrates no evidence of urinary tract infection.
2. Avoid or minimize use of indwelling catheter. 　a. Use bladder scanner if available to confirm urinary stasis; perform intermittent catheterization for urinary retention as prescribed.	2. Source of bladder infection. 3. Empties bladder; reduces urinary tract infections.	

NURSING DIAGNOSIS: Readiness for enhanced coping related to injury, anticipated surgery, and dependence
GOAL: Uses effective coping mechanisms to modify stress

Nursing Interventions	Rationale	Expected Outcomes
1. Encourage patient to express concerns and to discuss the possible impact of fractured hip.	1. Verbalization helps patient deal with problems and feelings. Clarification of thoughts and feelings promotes problem solving.	• Patient describes feelings concerning fractured hip and implications for lifestyle.
2. Support the use of coping mechanisms. Involve significant others and support services as needed.	2. Coping mechanisms modify disabling effects of stress; sharing concerns lessens the burden and facilitates necessary modification.	• Uses available resources and coping mechanisms; develops health promotion strategies. • Uses community resources as needed.
3. Contact social services, if needed.	3. Anxiety may be related to financial or social problems; facilitates management of problems associated with continuing care.	• Participates in development of health care plan.

(continued on page 1208)

Chart 42-5

PLAN OF NURSING CARE (Continued)
Care of the Older Adult Patient With a Fractured Hip

Nursing Interventions	Rationale	Expected Outcomes
4. Explain anticipated treatment regimen and routines to facilitate positive attitude in relation to rehabilitation.	4. Understanding of plan of care helps to diminish fears of the unknown.	
5. Encourage patient to participate in planning.	5. Participating in care provides for some control of self and environment.	

NURSING DIAGNOSIS: Risk for acute confusion related to age, stress of trauma, unfamiliar surroundings, and medication therapy
GOAL: Remains oriented and participates in decision making

Nursing Interventions	Rationale	Expected Outcomes
1. Assess orientation status.	1. Evaluate presenting orientation of patient; confusion may result from stress of fracture, unfamiliar surroundings, coexisting systemic disease, cerebral ischemia, hypoxemia, or other factors. Baseline data are important for determining change.	• Patient establishes effective communication. • Demonstrates orientation to time, place, and person. • Participates in self-care activities. • Remains mentally alert. • Does not exhibit episodes of confusion.
2. Interview family regarding patient's orientation and cognitive abilities before injury.	2. Provides data for evaluation of current findings.	
3. Assess patient for auditory and visual deficits.	3. Diminished vision and auditory acuity frequently occur with aging; glasses and hearing aid may increase patient's ability to interact with environment.	
a. Assist patient with the use of sensory aids (e.g., glasses, hearing aid)	a. Aids must be in good working order and available for use.	
b. Control environmental distractors.	b. Facilitates communication	
4. Orient to and stabilize environment.	4.	
a. Use orientation activities and aids (e.g., clock, calendar, pictures, introduction of self).	a. Short-term memory may be faulty in the older adult; frequent reorientation helps.	
b. Minimize number of staff working with patient.	b. Consistency of caregivers promotes trust.	
5. Give simple explanations of procedures and plan of care.	5. Promotes understanding and active participation.	
6. Encourage participation in hygiene and nutritional activities.	6. Participation in routine activities promotes orientation and increases awareness of self.	
7. Provide for safety.	7. Mechanism for securing assistance is available to patient; independent activities based on faulty judgment may result in injury.	
a. Keep light on at night.		
b. Have call bell available.		
c. Provide prompt response to requests for assistance.		
8. Assess mental responses to medications, especially sedative and analgesic agents.	8. Older adults tend to be more sensitive to medications; abnormal responses (e.g., hallucinations, depression) may occur.	

COLLABORATIVE PROBLEMS: Hemorrhage; pulmonary complications; peripheral neurovascular dysfunction; venous thromboemboli; pressure ulcers related to surgery and immobility
GOAL: Absence of complications

Nursing Interventions	Rationale	Expected Outcomes
Hemorrhage		
1. Monitor vital signs, observing for shock.	1. Changes in pulse, blood pressure, and respirations may indicate development of shock; blood loss and stress may contribute to development of shock.	• Vital signs are stabilized within normal limits. • Experiences no excessive or bright red drainage. • Exhibits stable postoperative hemoglobin and hematocrit values. • Patient has clear breath sounds. • Breath sounds are present in all fields. • Exhibits no shortness of breath, chest pain, or elevated temperature.
2. Consider preinjury blood pressure values and management of coexisting hypertension, if present.	2. Necessary for interpretation of current blood pressure determinations.	
3. Note character and amount of drainage.	3. Excessive drainage and bright red drainage may indicate active bleeding.	
4. Notify primary provider if patient develops shock or excessive bleeding.	4. Corrective measures need to be instituted.	

PLAN OF NURSING CARE (Continued)

Chart 42-5

Care of the Older Adult Patient With a Fractured Hip

Nursing Interventions	Rationale	Expected Outcomes
5. Note hemoglobin and hematocrit values, and report decreases in values.	5. Anemia due to blood loss may develop; bleeding into tissues after hip fracture may be extensive; blood replacement may be needed.	

Pulmonary Complications

Nursing Interventions	Rationale	Expected Outcomes
1. Assess respiratory status: respiratory rate, depth, and duration; breath sounds; sputum. Monitor temperature.	1. Anesthesia and bed rest diminish respiratory effort and cause pooling of respiratory secretions. Adventitious breath sounds, pain on respiration, shortness of breath, blood-tinged sputum, cough may indicate pulmonary dysfunction.	• Vital signs are stabilized within normal limits. • Patient has clear breath sounds. • Breath sounds are present in all fields. • Exhibits no shortness of breath, chest pain, or elevated temperature. • Arterial oxygen saturation (SaO_2) on room air is within normal limits. • Performs respiratory exercises; uses incentive spirometer as instructed. • Changes position frequently. • Consumes adequate fluids.
2. Report adventitious and diminished breath sounds and elevated temperature.	2. Elevated temperature in the early postoperative period may be due to atelectasis or pneumonia.	
3. Supervise deep-breathing and coughing exercises. Encourage the use of incentive spirometer if prescribed.	3. Deep-breathing and coughing exercises promote optimal ventilation. Coexisting respiratory conditions diminish lung expansion.	
4. Administer oxygen as prescribed.	4. Reduced ventilatory efforts may diminish SaO_2 when patient is breathing room air.	
5. Turn and reposition patient at least every 2 hours. Mobilize patient (assist patient out of bed) as soon as possible.	5. Promotes optimal ventilation; diminishes pooling of respiratory secretions.	
6. Ensure adequate hydration.	6. Liquefies respiratory secretions; facilitates expectoration.	

Peripheral Neurovascular Dysfunction

Nursing Interventions	Rationale	Expected Outcomes
1. Assess affected extremity for color and temperature.	1. The skin becomes pale and feels cool with decreased tissue perfusion. Venous congestion may cause cyanosis.	• Patient has normal color and the extremity is warm. • Demonstrates normal capillary refill response. • Exhibits moderate swelling; tissue not palpably tense. • States pain is tolerable. • Reports no pain with passive dorsiflexion. • Reports normal sensations and no paresthesia. • Demonstrates normal motor abilities and no paresis or paralysis. • Has strong and equal pulses.
2. Assess toes for capillary refill response.	2. After compression of the nail, rapid return of pink color indicates good capillary perfusion.	
3. Assess affected extremity for edema and swelling.	3. The trauma of surgery will cause swelling; excessive swelling and hematoma formation can compromise circulation and function; edema may be due to coexisting cardiovascular disease.	
4. Elevate affected extremity.	4. Minimizes dependent edema.	
5. Assess for deep, throbbing, unrelenting pain.	5. Surgical pain can be controlled; pain due to neurovascular compromise is refractory to treatment with analgesic medications.	
6. Assess for pain on passive flexion of foot.	6. With nerve ischemia, there will be pain on passive stretch.	
7. Assess for sensations and numbness.	7. Diminished pain and paresthesia may indicate nerve damage. Sensation in web between great and second toe—peroneal nerve; sensation on sole of foot—tibial nerve.	
8. Assess ability to move foot and toes.	8. Dorsiflexion of ankle and extension of toes indicate function of peroneal nerve. Plantar flexion of ankle and flexion of toes indicate functioning of tibial nerve.	
9. Assess pedal pulses in both feet.	9. Indicates circulatory status of extremities.	
10. Notify primary provider of changes in neurovascular status.	10. Function of extremity needs to be preserved.	

Venous Thromboemboli

Nursing Interventions	Rationale	Expected Outcomes
1. Apply thigh-high antiembolism stockings and/or sequential compression device as prescribed.	1. Compression aids venous blood return and prevents stasis.	• Wears thigh-high antiembolism stockings. • Uses sequential compression device. • Experiences no more warmth than usual in skin areas.

(continued on page 1210)

Chart 42-5 **PLAN OF NURSING CARE** (Continued)

Care of the Older Adult Patient With a Fractured Hip

Nursing Interventions	Rationale	Expected Outcomes
2. Remove stockings for 20 minutes twice a day, and provide skin care.	2. Skin care is necessary to avoid skin breakdown. Extended removal of stocking or device defeats purpose.	• Exhibits no increase in calf circumference.
3. Assess popliteal, dorsalis pedis, and posterior tibial pulses.	3. Pulses indicate arterial perfusion of extremity. With coexisting arteriosclerotic vascular disease, pulses may be diminished or absent.	• Demonstrates no evidence of calf tenderness, warmth, redness, or swelling. • Changes position with assistance and supervision.
4. Assess skin temperature of legs.	4. Local inflammation increases local skin temperature.	• Participates in exercise regimen. • Experiences no chest pain; has lungs clear to auscultation; presents no evidence of pulmonary emboli.
5. Assess calf intermittently for tenderness, warmth, redness, and swelling.	5. Unilateral calf tenderness, warmth, redness, and swelling may indicate deep vein thrombosis.	• Exhibits no signs of dehydration; has normal hematocrit.
6. Measure calf circumference daily.	6. Increased calf circumference indicates edema or altered perfusion.	• Maintains normal body temperature.
7. Avoid pressure on popliteal blood vessels from appliances or pillows.	7. Compression of blood vessels diminishes blood flow.	
8. Change patient's position and increase activity as prescribed.	8. Activity promotes circulation and diminishes venous stasis.	
9. Supervise ankle exercises hourly while patient is awake.	9. Muscle exercise promotes circulation.	
10. Ensure adequate hydration.	10. Older adults may become dehydrated because of low fluid intake, resulting in hemoconcentration.	
11. Monitor body temperature.	11. Body temperature increases with inflammation (magnitude of response minimal in older adults).	

Pressure Ulcers

Nursing Interventions	Rationale	Expected Outcomes
1. Monitor condition of skin at pressure points (e.g., heels, sacrum, shoulders); inspect heels at least twice a day.	1. Older adults are more prone to skin breakdown at points of pressure because of diminished subcutaneous tissue.	• Patient exhibits no signs of skin breakdown.
2. Reposition patient at least every 2 hours. Avoid skin shearing.	2. Avoids prolonged pressure and trauma to the skin.	• Skin remains intact.
3. Administer skin care, especially to pressure points.	3. Immobility causes pressure at bony prominences; position changes relieve pressure.	• Repositions self frequently. • Uses protective devices.
4. Use special care mattress and other protective devices (e.g., heel protectors); support heel off the mattress.	4. Devices minimize pressure on skin at bony prominences.	
5. Institute care according to protocol at first indication of potential skin breakdown.	5. Early interventions prevent tissue destruction and prolonged rehabilitation.	

Femoral Shaft

Considerable force is required to break the shaft of a femur in adults. Most femoral fractures occur in young adults who have been involved in motor vehicle crashes or who have fallen from heights. Frequently, these patients have associated multiple traumatic injuries (NAON, 2013).

The patient presents with an edematous, deformed, painful thigh and cannot move the hip or the knee. The fracture may be transverse, oblique, spiral, or comminuted. Frequently, the patient develops shock, because the loss of 1 to 2.5 L of blood into the tissues is common with these fractures (NAON, 2013). Types of femoral fractures are illustrated in Figure 42-17A.

Assessment and Diagnostic Findings

Assessment includes checking the neurovascular status of the extremity, especially circulatory perfusion of the lower leg and foot (popliteal, posterior tibial, and pedal pulses and toe capillary refill time), and comparing with the unaffected leg. A Doppler ultrasound may be indicated to assess blood flow. X-rays are used to confirm the diagnosis and determine the extent of injury (NAON, 2013). Dislocation of the hip and knee may accompany these fractures. Knee effusion suggests ligament damage and possible instability of the knee joint.

Medical Management

Continued neurovascular monitoring and documentation are important. The fracture is immobilized so that additional soft tissue damage does not occur. Generally, skeletal traction (see Fig. 42-17B,C) or splinting is used to immobilize fracture fragments until the patient is physiologically stable and ready for ORIF procedures. IV opioid analgesic agents (e.g., morphine) are typically given to treat pain (NAON, 2013).

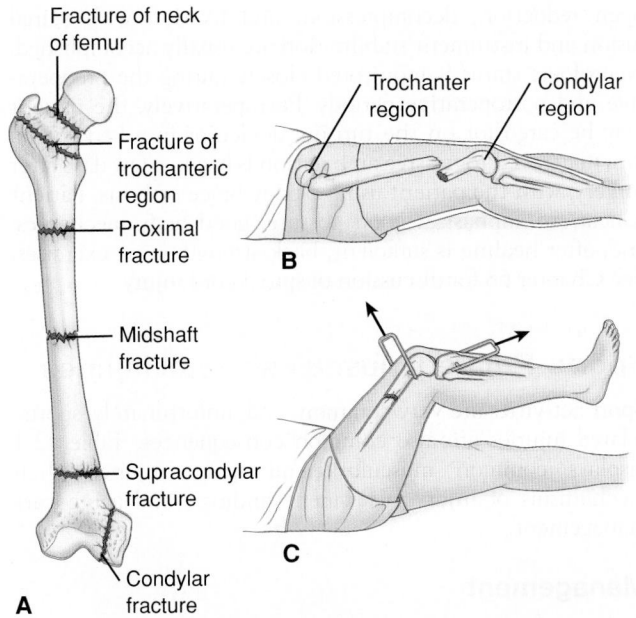

Figure 42-17 • **A.** Types of femoral fractures. **B.** Example of deformity on admission to hospital. **C.** Adequate reduction is achieved when additional wire is inserted in the lower femoral fragment and vertical lift is secured.

Internal fixation usually is carried out immediately. Intramedullary locking nail devices are typically used. Internal fixation permits early mobilization, which is associated with improved outcomes and recovery (Keany & McKeever, 2015). To preserve muscle strength, the patient is instructed to exercise the hip and the lower leg, foot, and toes on a regular basis. Active muscle movement enhances healing by increasing blood supply and electrical potentials at the fracture site. Prescribed weight-bearing limits are based on the type and location of the fracture and treatment approach. Physical therapy includes ROM and strengthening exercises, safe use of assistive devices, and gait training (NAON, 2013).

Traction may be used until surgery can be performed. Skeletal traction is a temporary intervention, however, until such time as the patient is stable and may tolerate surgical intervention (Keany & McKeever, 2015).

Open femoral fractures require immediate and extensive irrigation and débridement in the operating suite (see previous discussion of treatment for open fractures). Depending on needs for continued débridement, intramedullary nailing may be delayed (Keany & McKeever, 2015).

A common complication after fracture of the femoral shaft is restriction of knee motion. Active and passive knee exercises begin as soon as possible, depending on the stability of the fracture and knee ligaments. Other complications in the immediate postoperative period can include hemorrhage, compartment syndrome, and neurovascular compromise. Long-term complications may include malrotation, malunion, delayed union, and nonunion (Keany & McKeever, 2015).

Tibia and Fibula

Fractures of the tibia and fibula often occur in association with each other and tend to result from a direct blow, falls with the foot in a flexed position, or a violent twisting motion. Most of these fractures tend to be more distal than proximal; distal fractures may extend into the ankle joint (i.e., distal fractures of the tibia that extend into the joint are collectively referred to as pilon fractures). The patient presents with pain, deformity, obvious hematoma, and considerable edema (NAON, 2013).

Assessment and Diagnostic Findings

The peroneal nerve is assessed; if damaged, the patient cannot dorsiflex the great toe and has diminished sensation in the first web space. The tibial artery is assessed for damage by evaluating pulses, skin temperature, and color and by testing the capillary refill response. The affected leg and ankle are compared with the unaffected leg and ankle. X-rays are indicated to determine the location, type, and extent of the fracture (NAON, 2013).

Medical Management

Most closed, nondisplaced fractures that do not involve the ankle joint (i.e., extra-articular fractures) are treated with closed reduction and immobilization in a non–weight-bearing short-leg cast or brace. The leg is elevated to control edema. Weight-bearing status varies and depends on the type of fracture. Activity decreases edema and increases circulation. Fracture healing takes 6 to 10 weeks (NAON, 2013).

Displaced, open, or articular fractures may be treated with skeletal traction, internal fixation with intramedullary nails or plates and screws, or external fixation. External support may be used with internal fixation. Hip, foot, and knee exercises are encouraged within the limits of the immobilizing device. Partial weight bearing is begun when prescribed and is progressed as the fracture heals in 6 to 10 weeks (NAON, 2013).

As with any fracture, continued neurovascular evaluation is important. The development of acute compartment syndrome requires prompt recognition and communication to the primary provider. Other complications to monitor for include nonunion, delayed union, infection, and impaired wound edge healing (NAON, 2013).

Rib

Uncomplicated fractures of the lower ribs occur frequently in adults of all ages, typically from either motor vehicle crashes or falls, and usually result in no impairment of function. They are typically diagnosed based on clinical presentation and confirmed with x-rays or ultrasound scans (Melendez, 2015). Because these fractures cause pain with respiratory effort, the patient tends to decrease respiratory excursions and refrains from coughing. As a result, tracheobronchial secretions are not mobilized, aeration of the lung is diminished, and a predisposition to atelectasis and pneumonia results. To help the patient cough and take deep breaths and use an incentive spirometer (see Chapter 21), the nurse may splint the chest with their hands, or may educate the patient on using a pillow to temporarily splint the affected site. NSAIDs may be prescribed to provide analgesic relief. Occasionally, an anesthesia care provider administers intercostal nerve blocks or epidural analgesia to relieve pain and to improve respiratory function (Melendez, 2015).

Chest binders to immobilize the rib fracture are not used, because decreased chest expansion may result in atelectasis and pneumonia. Incentive spirometer use may aid in prevention of these complications. The fracture heals within 6 weeks. In addition to atelectasis and pneumonia, complications may include a flail chest, pneumothorax, and hemothorax (Melendez, 2015). The assessment and management of patients with these conditions are discussed in Chapter 23.

 Gerontologic Considerations

Older adults sustaining rib fractures are at an increased risk for complications. Even in the presence of isolated rib trauma, hospital admission is recommended for the older adult with multiple rib fractures or for the older adult who cannot effectively cough and mobilize sputum (Melendez, 2015). Careful monitoring of respiratory status and encouraging the patient to mobilize early, and, for the bedfast patient, encouraging turning, coughing, and deep breathing and use of an incentive spirometer, can prevent respiratory complications (see Chapter 21).

Thoracolumbar Spine

Fractures of the thoracolumbar spine may involve (1) the vertebral body, (2) the laminae and articulating processes, and (3) the spinous processes or transverse processes. The T12 to L2 area of the spine, called the *thoracolumbar junction,* is most vulnerable to fracture. Fractures generally result from indirect trauma caused by excessive loading, sudden muscle contraction, or excessive motion beyond physiologic limits. Osteoporosis contributes to vertebral body collapse (compression fracture) (NAON, 2013).

Stable spinal fractures are caused by flexion, extension, lateral bending, or vertical loading. The anterior structural column (vertebral bodies and discs) or the posterior structural column (neural arch, articular processes, ligaments) is disrupted. Unstable fractures occur with fracture dislocations and involve disruption of both anterior and posterior structural columns.

The patient with a spinal fracture presents with acute tenderness, swelling, paravertebral muscle spasm, and change in the normal curves or in the gap between spinous processes. Pain is greater with moving, coughing, or weight bearing. Immobilization is essential until initial assessments have determined if there is any spinal cord injury and whether the fracture is stable or unstable (see Chapter 68). X-rays are initially indicated to confirm the fracture(s), and CT scans or MRI studies are then indicated to precisely determine the extent of injury and spinal cord involvement (Vinas, 2015). If spinal cord injury with neurologic deficit does occur, it usually requires immediate surgery (laminectomy with spinal fusion) to decompress the spinal cord.

Stable spinal fractures are treated conservatively with limited bed rest. Analgesic medications are prescribed for pain relief. A spinal brace or plastic thoraco-lumbar-sacral orthosis (TLSO) is applied for support during progressive ambulation and resumption of activities. X-rays are taken to monitor the healing process at 6 weeks, 3 months, 6 months, and 1 year (NAON, 2013).

The patient with an unstable fracture is treated with bed rest, possibly with the use of a special turning device or bed to maintain spinal alignment. Within 24 hours after fracture,

open reduction, decompression, and fixation with spinal fusion and instrument stabilization are usually accomplished. Neurologic status is monitored closely during the preoperative and postoperative periods. Postoperatively, the patient may be cared for on the turning device or in a bed with a firm mattress. Progressive ambulation is begun a few days after surgery, with the patient using a body brace orthosis. Patient education emphasizes good posture, good body mechanics, and, after healing is sufficient, back-strengthening exercises. See Chapter 68 for discussion of spinal cord injury.

Sports-Related Musculoskeletal Injuries

Sport activities are very common, and, unfortunately, sports-related injuries are also common consequences. Table 42-1 displays common musculoskeletal sports injuries, their mechanisms of injury, assessment findings, and acute care management.

Management

Patients who have experienced sports-related musculoskeletal injuries are often highly motivated to return to their previous level of activity. Adherence to restriction of activities and gradual resumption of activities need to be reinforced. Injured athletes are at risk for reinjury and require follow-up and monitoring. With recurrence of symptoms, athletes need to diminish their level and intensity of activity to a comfortable level. The time required to recover from a sports-related injury can be as short as a few days or as long as 12 weeks, depending on the severity of the injury. The patient should be pain free with good ROM before returning to play (NAON, 2013).

Prevention

Sports-related musculoskeletal injuries can often be prevented by using proper equipment (e.g., running shoes for joggers, wrist guards for skaters) and by effectively training and conditioning the body. Specific training needs to be tailored to the person and the sport. Stretching, maintaining hydration, and proper nutrition aid in injury prevention (Porth, 2015).

Occupation-Related Musculoskeletal Disorders

According to the U.S. Department of Labor, occupation-related musculoskeletal disorders (MSDs) are injuries or illnesses of the muscles, nerves, tendons, joints, cartilage, and bones that occur because of exposure to work-related risks. In 2013, occupation-related MSDs, also called *ergonomic injuries,* accounted for 33% of all injury and illness cases with nursing assistants (highest) and registered nurses (fifth highest) making up 8.8% of total occupation-related MSDs (U.S. Department of Labor, Bureau of Labor Statistics, 2014).

The most frequent types of MSDs that occurred among workers in all occupations in 2013 and that required days away from work were sprains, strains, and tears (36.7%) and soreness and pain (17.45%), with smaller percentages of common MSDs including fractures, cuts, lacerations, and contusions and bruises (U.S. Department of Labor, Bureau of Labor Statistics, 2014).

TABLE 42-1 Common Musculoskeletal Sports Injuries

Anatomic Area	Mechanism of Injury	Assessment Findings	Sports Activity	Acute Management
Clavicle fracture	Fall on shoulder or outstretched arm Direct blow to the clavicle	Crepitus Holds arm closely to body Unable to raise affected arm above head Can feel movement of both ends of clavicle	Football Rugby Hockey Wrestling Gymnastics	Sling or shoulder immobilizer Ice NSAIDs
Dislocated shoulder	*Anterior:* Some combination of hyperextension, external rotation, and abduction Anterior blow to shoulder *Posterior:* Fall on flexed and adducted arm Direct axial load to humerus	Pain Lack of motion May feel empty shoulder socket Uneven posture in comparison to other shoulder Affected arm appears longer Abduction limited	Rugby Hockey Wrestling Skiing	Closed reduction Immobilizer Pendulum exercises
Dislocated elbow	Falling on a hand with a flexed elbow Elbow overextended	Intense pain Edema Limited motion Deformity Ecchymosis	Football Gymnastics Squash Wrestling Cycling Skiing	Immobilization Ice ROM exercises
Wrist sprain or fracture	Falling on an outstretched arm	Pain Edema Ecchymosis Deformity Limited motion	Skating Hockey Wrestling Skiing Soccer Handball Horseback riding	Ice Elevation Immobilization Gentle ROM for 4–6 weeks (for sprain only)
Knee sprain	Twisting injury that produces incomplete tear of ligaments and capsule around the joint	Pain Limited motion Edema Ecchymosis Tenderness over joint Joint appears stable	Basketball Football High jump	Ice Elevation Compression wrap Active ROM exercises Isometric exercises May immobilize
Knee strain	Sudden forced motion causing muscle to be stretched beyond normal capacity	Pain Limited motion Pain aggravated by activity	Soccer Swimming Skiing	Ice Elevation Rest Gradual return to activities
Meniscal tears of knee	Sharp, sudden pivot Direct blow to knee Forced internal rotation Wear from repetitive squatting or climbing Torsional weight-bearing force	Edema *Medial tear:* Pain occurs with hyperflexion, hyperextension, and turning in of knee with knee flexed. *Lateral tear:* Pain occurs with hyperflexion and hyperextension and internal rotation of foot with knee flexed. *Displaced fragment:* Inability to extend knee; "locked" Positive McMurray sign[a]	Hockey Basketball Football	*Conservative:* RICE Exercising of quadriceps and hamstrings Resistive exercising NSAIDs Physical therapy *Surgical:* Arthroscopy
Ankle sprain	Foot is twisted, causing stretching or tearing of ligaments.	Pain Edema Limited motion Ecchymosis	Tennis Basketball Football Skating	Immobilization in cast or brace Ice Elevation Rest
Ankle strain	Sudden forced motion, stretching muscles beyond normal capacity	*Acute:* Severe pain *Chronic:* Achy pain	Running All ball sports	Immobilization in cast or brace Ice Elevation Rest
Ankle fracture	Inward turning on sole of foot and front of foot Supination with internal rotation Pronation with external rotation	Pain Edema Deformity Inability to bear weight	Contact sports Tennis Basketball	Ice Elevation Cast (4–6 weeks) Surgery if fracture is displaced or unstable
Metatarsal stress fracture	Occurs with repeated loading of bone; often in an unconditioned extremity	Forefoot pain that progressively worsens with activity Minimal or no forefoot swelling	Running Dance Skating	Rest Stop sports-related activity for 6 weeks Ice Weight bearing as indicated

NSAIDs, nonsteroidal anti-inflammatory drugs; ROM, range of motion; RICE, rest, ice, compression, elevation.
[a]McMurray sign—manipulation of tibia while knee flexed produces audible "click."
Reprinted with permission from the National Association of Orthopedic Nurses (NAON). (2013).*Core curriculum for orthopaedic nursing* (7th ed.). Chicago: NAON.

Prevention of Occupation-Related Musculoskeletal Disorders in Nursing Personnel

Nursing is consistently ranked among the top 10 occupations that are most involved in occupation-related injuries and lost days of work (U.S. Department of Labor, Bureau of Labor Statistics, 2014). Most of these injuries result in MSDs and are linked to patient handling and movement activities. The American Nurses Association (ANA) (2017) recognizes the seriousness of MSDs among nurses, and advocates for the implementation of nonmanual methods for safe patient handling whenever feasible (see Resources).

Amputation

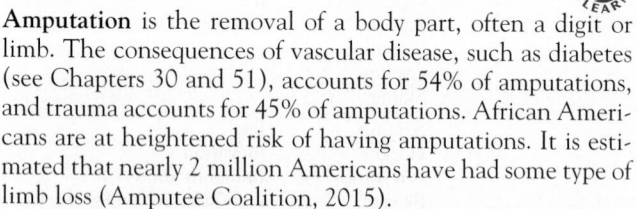

Amputation is the removal of a body part, often a digit or limb. The consequences of vascular disease, such as diabetes (see Chapters 30 and 51), accounts for 54% of amputations, and trauma accounts for 45% of amputations. African Americans are at heightened risk of having amputations. It is estimated that nearly 2 million Americans have had some type of limb loss (Amputee Coalition, 2015).

Amputation is used to relieve symptoms, to improve function, and to save or improve the patient's quality of life. If the health care team communicates a positive attitude, the patient adjusts to the amputation more readily and actively participates in the rehabilitative plan, learning how to modify activities and how to use assistive devices for ADLs and mobility (see Chart 42-6).

Levels of Amputation

Amputation is performed at the most distal point that will heal successfully. The site and extent of amputation is determined by circulation in the area (and whether or not necrosis is present) and functional usefulness (i.e., meets the requirements for the use of a prosthesis). If the cause for amputation is because of a tumor, then the extent of amputation is dictated by the requirement to fully excise the tumor (Morris, Potter, Athanasian, et al, 2015).

The circulatory status of the limb is evaluated through physical examination and diagnostic studies. Muscle and skin perfusion is important for healing. Doppler flow studies with duplex ultrasound, segmental blood pressure determinations, and transcutaneous partial pressure of arterial oxygen (PaO_2) of the limb are valuable diagnostic aids. Angiography is performed if revascularization is considered an option.

The objective of surgery is to conserve as much limb length as needed to preserve function and possibly to achieve a good prosthetic fit. Preservation of knee and elbow joints is desirable. Figure 42-18 shows the levels at which a limb may be amputated. Most amputations involving limbs eventually can be fitted with a prosthesis.

The amputation of toes and portions of the foot can cause changes in gait and balance. A Syme amputation (modified ankle disarticulation amputation) is performed most frequently for extensive foot trauma and aims to produce a durable residual limb that can withstand full weight bearing. Below-knee amputation (BKA) is preferred to above-knee amputation (AKA) because of the importance of the knee joint and the energy requirements for walking. A knee **disarticulation** (i.e., amputation through the joint) is most successful with a young, active patient who can develop precise control of the prosthesis. When AKAs are performed, all possible length is preserved, muscles are stabilized and shaped, and hip contractures are prevented to maximize ambulatory potential (NAON, 2013). Most people who have a hip disarticulation amputation must rely on a wheelchair for mobility.

Chart 42-6 — ETHICAL DILEMMA

Should a Health Care Agent Be Allowed to Refuse Treatment When That Treatment Is Likely to Extend Life?

Case Scenario

The patient is a 75-year-old man admitted to the emergency department following a motor vehicle crash. In addition to a significant head injury, he had crushing injuries of both legs. He has a history of poorly controlled type 2 diabetes and poor peripheral vascular circulation. He will require bilateral below the knee amputations (BKA). Despite his life-threatening injuries, he is not in a terminal state and the procedure could extend his life. His wife of 50 years states that he has often said he would never want to live if he "could not live his life plowing his fields." His wife refuses to sign the consent form for the surgery; however, his daughter is adamant that the surgery must be done. Within the past year, his wife was designated as his health care agent (i.e., authorized to make health care decisions by proxy for him should he become incapacitated).

Discussion

In order to address this ethical dilemma, a few considerations must be addressed. It is important to recognize that the patient is not in a terminal state, which means that the surgery could extend life albeit does not guarantee his quality of life. Since the patient does not have the mental capacity to consent to this procedure, the primary provider must determine if the patient has identified a proxy to make health care decisions for him. Each state specifies the types of decisions that may be made by the health care agent; it is important to know these specifications in the state where this patient is currently being treated. In all states, the document that designates a health care agent must be notarized.

Analysis

- Identify the ethical principles that are in conflict in this case (see Chapter 3, Chart 3-3).
- What arguments would you offer in favor of amputation of both legs?
- What arguments would you offer *against* amputation of both legs?
- What is the role of the health care agent in end-of-life decisions?
- Assume that the patient did not have a health care agent and permission for the surgery was required. How would the decision to consent to the surgery be made?

Resources

See Chapter 3, Chart 3-6 for ethics resources.

Paulson, S., Comfort, C. P., Lee, B. C., et al (2014), Prolonging life: Legal, ethical, and social dilemmas. *Annals of the New York Academy of Sciences*, 1330, 19–39.

Figure 42-18 • Levels of amputation are determined by circulatory adequacy, type of prosthesis, function of the part, and muscle balance. **A.** Levels of amputation of upper limb. **B.** Levels of amputation of lower limb.

Upper limb amputations are performed with the goal of preserving maximal functional length. The prosthesis is fitted early to ensure maximum function.

A "staged" amputation may be used when gangrene and infection exist. Initially, a guillotine amputation (e.g., nonclosed residual limb) is performed to remove the necrotic and infected tissue. The wound is débrided and allowed to drain. Sepsis is treated with systemic antibiotics. In a few days, after the infection has been controlled and the patient's condition has stabilized, a definitive amputation with skin closure is performed.

Complications

Complications that may occur with amputation include hemorrhage, infection, skin breakdown, phantom limb pain, and joint contracture. Because major blood vessels have been severed, hemorrhage may occur. Infection is a risk with all surgical procedures. The risk of infection increases with contaminated wounds after traumatic amputation. Skin irritation caused by the prosthesis may result in skin breakdown. **Phantom limb pain** (pain perceived in the amputated section) is caused by the severing of peripheral nerves. Joint contracture is caused by positioning and a protective flexion withdrawal pattern associated with pain and muscle imbalance (NAON, 2013).

Medical Management

The objective of treatment is to achieve healing of the amputation wound, the result being a nontender residual limb with healthy skin for prosthetic use. Healing is enhanced by gentle handling of the residual limb, control of residual limb edema through rigid or soft compression dressings, and the use of aseptic technique in wound care to avoid infection (Morris et al., 2015).

A rigid cast dressing, removable rigid dressing, or an elastic residual limb shrinker that covers the residual limb may be used to provide uniform compression, to support soft tissues, to control pain and edema, and to prevent joint contractures (Morris et al., 2015).

The rigid dressing is removed several days after surgery for wound inspection and is then replaced to control edema. However, edema is better controlled with semi-rigid dressings for certain types of amputations (e.g., transtibial) (Highsmith, Kahle, Miro, et al., 2016), and may facilitate earlier ambulation and improved readiness for prosthesis (Morris et al., 2015). The dressing facilitates residual limb shaping. A soft dressing with or without compression may be used if there is significant wound drainage and frequent inspection of the residual limb is required. An immobilizing splint may be incorporated in the dressing. Residual limb wound hematomas can be controlled with wound drainage devices (Morris et al., 2015).

Rehabilitation

The multidisciplinary rehabilitation team (patient, nurse, physician, social worker, physical therapist, occupational therapist, psychologist, prosthetist, vocational rehabilitation worker) helps the patient achieve the highest possible level of function and participation in life activities (see Fig. 42-19). Prosthetic clinics and support groups for people with amputations facilitate this rehabilitation process (Geertzen, van der Linde, Rosenbrand, et al., 2015).

Patients who undergo amputation need support as they grieve the loss and change in body image. Their reactions can include anger, bitterness, and hostility. Psychological issues (e.g., denial, anxiety, avoidance) may be influenced by the type of support the patient receives from the rehabilitation team, the effectiveness of pain management, and by how quickly ADLs and the use of the prosthesis are learned. Knowing the full options and capabilities available with the various prosthetic devices can give the patient a sense of control over the resulting disability (Geertzen et al., 2015).

Figure 42-19 • Many patients with amputations receive prostheses soon after surgery and begin learning how to use them with the help and support of the rehabilitation team, which includes nurses, physicians, physical therapists, and others.

Patients who require amputation because of severe trauma can be young and healthy. These patients heal rapidly and are physically able to participate in a vigorous rehabilitation program. Because the amputation is the result of an injury, the patient needs psychological support in accepting the sudden change in body image and in dealing with the stresses of hospitalization, long-term rehabilitation, and modification of lifestyle.

Within the past two decades, numerous U.S. soldiers have lost limbs because of ballistic injuries received while fighting in Iraq and Afghanistan, which has spurred advancements in amputation rehabilitation (Highsmith et al., 2016). In order to best meet the complex needs of these young, previously healthy men and women, the U.S. Army instituted both a specialized treatment center for patients with amputations and a database registry to facilitate their long-term treatment and management. Treatment for these injured soldiers addresses not only their physical rehabilitation needs but also their emotional needs. Behavioral health services are considered key components to their therapy (Department of Veterans Affairs & Department of Defense [VA/DoD], 2014).

NURSING PROCESS
The Patient Undergoing an Amputation

Assessment

Before surgery, the nurse must evaluate the neurovascular and functional status of the limb through history and physical assessment. If the patient has experienced a traumatic amputation, the nurse assesses the function and condition of the residual limb. The nurse also assesses the circulatory status and function of the unaffected limb. If infection or gangrene develops, the patient may have associated enlarged lymph nodes, fever, and purulent drainage. A culture and sensitivity test is obtained to determine the appropriate antibiotic therapy.

The nurse evaluates the patient's nutritional status and develops a plan for nutritional care in consultation with a dietitian or metabolic or nutrition support team, if indicated. A diet with adequate protein and vitamins is essential to promote wound healing.

Any concurrent health problems (e.g., dehydration, anemia, cardiac insufficiency, chronic respiratory problems, diabetes) need to be identified and treated so that the patient is in the best possible condition to withstand the surgical procedure. The use of corticosteroids, anticoagulants, vasoconstrictors, or vasodilators may influence management and prolong or delay wound healing.

The nurse assesses the patient's psychological status. Evaluation of the patient's emotional reaction to amputation is important. Grief responses to permanent alterations in body image, function, and mobility are likely. Professional counseling can help the patient cope in the aftermath of amputation surgery.

Diagnosis

Nursing Diagnoses

Based on the assessment data, major nursing diagnoses may include the following:
- Acute pain related to amputation
- Impaired skin integrity related to surgical amputation
- Disturbed body image related to amputation
- Grieving and/or risk for complicated grieving related to loss of body part and resulting disability
- Self-care deficit: bathing, dressing, feeding, or toileting, related to amputation
- Impaired physical mobility related to amputation

Collaborative Problems/Potential Complications

Potential complications may include the following:
- Hemorrhage
- Infection
- Skin breakdown

Planning and Goals

The major goals of the patient may include relief of pain, including phantom limb pain, wound healing, acceptance of altered body image, resolution of the grieving process, independence in self-care, restoration of physical mobility, and absence of complications.

Nursing Interventions

Relieving Pain

Pain may be incisional or may be caused by inflammation, infection, pressure on a bony prominence, hematoma, or phantom limb pain. Muscle spasms may add to the patient's discomfort. Surgical pain can be effectively controlled with opioid analgesics that may be accompanied with evacuation of a hematoma or accumulated fluid. Changing the patient's position or placing a light sandbag on the residual limb to counteract the muscle spasm may improve the patient's level of comfort. Evaluation of the patient's pain and responses to interventions is an important component of pain management.

Patients who have amputations may begin to experience phantom limb pain soon after surgery. It is estimated that 51% to 85% of these patients report persistent post amputation phantom limb pain (Kent, Hsia, Van de Ven, et al., 2016). The patient reports pain in the amputated limb as if it were still present. The pain is described as if the amputated limb feels crushed, cramped, or twisted in an abnormal position; this pain is sometimes accompanied by numbness, tingling, or burning sensations. Phantom pain occurs intermittently and unpredictably; episodes of pain may last seconds or hours. When a patient describes phantom pains or sensations, the nurse acknowledges these feelings as real and encourages the patient to verbalize when in pain so that effective treatment may be given. Phantom pain typically diminishes over time for most patients, with episodes gradually becoming less frequent and of lesser duration; however, some patients continue to experience phantom limb pain as long as 2 years after the amputation (Pirowska, Wloch, Nowobilski, et al., 2014).

The pathogenesis of the phantom limb pain phenomenon is believed to involve changes in both peripheral and central neuronal mechanisms. Disruption in neuronal pathways are thought to cause neuroplastic changes that in turn result in changes in cortical representation, or the proprioceptive, tactile, and visual image of body parts as perceived by the cerebral cortex (Pirowska et al., 2014). Perioperatively, the patient may be managed with acetaminophen, NSAIDs, gabapentinoids, opioids, and ketamine (infusion). Epidural and perineural catheter analgesia may be used during and immediately after the operation (Kent et al., 2016). Opioid analgesics may be effective in relieving postoperative pain. In addition, beta-blockers may relieve dull, burning discomfort; anticonvulsants control stabbing and cramping pain; and tricyclic antidepressants may not only alleviate phantom limb pain but may also be prescribed to improve mood and coping ability. Therapies that may be used as adjuncts to pharmacologic treatments include mirror therapy, massage, biofeedback, acupuncture, repositioning, TENS, guided imagery, and virtual reality (Amputee Coalition, 2015; Pirowska et al., 2014). The nurse monitors the effectiveness of these treatments and collaborates with the other members of the health care team to advocate for optimal pain control.

PROMOTING WOUND HEALING

The residual limb must be handled gently and should be measured once every 8 to 12 hours postoperatively to assess for edema formation. Neurovascular assessments are also performed at these intervals, to ensure that there is adequate blood supply. The dressing is changed as prescribed and whenever soiled, using aseptic technique to prevent infection and possible osteomyelitis (VA/DoD, 2014).

> ### Quality and Safety Nursing Alert
>
> *If the cast or elastic dressing inadvertently comes off, the nurse must immediately wrap the residual limb with an elastic compression bandage. If this is not done, excessive edema will develop in a short time, resulting in a delay in rehabilitation. The nurse notifies the surgeon if a cast dressing comes off so that another cast can be applied promptly.*

Application of consistent pressure to the residual limb reduces edema formation and helps to shape the residual limb so that it may fit a prosthetic. The wound should be assessed to ensure that it is healing and that there are no signs of infection (e.g., redness, purulent drainage), which can also hamper optimal prosthetic fit. After the incision is healed, the patient is instructed how to care for the residual limb (VA/DoD, 2014).

ENHANCING BODY IMAGE

Amputation is a procedure that alters the patient's body image. The nurse who has established a trusting relationship with the patient is better able to communicate acceptance of the patient who has experienced an amputation. The nurse encourages the patient to look at, feel, and care for the residual limb. It is important to identify the patient's strengths and resources to facilitate rehabilitation. The nurse helps the patient regain the previous level of independent functioning. The patient who is accepted as a whole person is more readily able to resume responsibility for self-care; self-concept improves, and body image changes are accepted. Even with highly motivated patients, this process may take months.

> ### Concept Mastery Alert
>
> The nurse can provide the following interventions to foster a positive self-image: encouraging the patient to care for the residual limb, allowing the expression of grief, and introducing the patient to local amputee support groups.

HELPING THE PATIENT TO RESOLVE GRIEVING

The loss of a limb (or part of one) may come as a shock even if the patient was prepared preoperatively. The patient's behavior (e.g., crying, withdrawal, apathy, anger) and expressed feelings (e.g., depression, fear, helplessness) reveal how the patient is coping with the loss and working through the grieving process.

The nurse creates an accepting and supportive atmosphere in which the patient and family are encouraged to express and share their feelings and work through the grief process. The support from family and friends promotes the patient's acceptance of the loss. The nurse helps the patient deal with immediate needs and become oriented to realistic rehabilitation goals and future independent functioning. Mental health and support group referrals and consulting with spiritual advisors (e.g., pastoral care) may be appropriate (Vincent, Horodyski, Vincent, et al., 2015).

PROMOTING INDEPENDENT SELF-CARE

Amputation affects the patient's ability to provide adequate self-care. The patient is encouraged to be an active participant in self-care. The patient needs time to accomplish these tasks and must not be rushed. Practicing an activity with consistent, supportive supervision in a relaxed environment enables the patient to learn self-care skills. The patient and the nurse need to maintain positive attitudes and minimize fatigue and frustration during the learning process.

Independence in dressing, toileting, and bathing depends on balance, transfer abilities, and physiologic tolerance of the activities. The nurse works with the physical therapist and occupational therapist to educate and supervise the patient in these self-care activities.

The patient with an upper limb amputation has self-care deficits in feeding, bathing, and dressing. Assistance is provided only as needed; the nurse encourages the patient to learn to do these tasks, using assistive feeding and dressing aids when needed. The nurse, therapists, and prosthetist work with the patient to achieve maximum independence.

HELPING THE PATIENT TO ACHIEVE PHYSICAL MOBILITY

Helping the Patient with a Lower Limb Amputation. Proper positioning prevents the development of hip or knee joint contracture in the patient with a lower limb amputation. Abduction, external rotation, and flexion of the lower limb are avoided. The patient with AKA may need to lie prone 20 to 30 minutes, three times per day to avoid contractures (Morris et al., 2015).

> ### Quality and Safety Nursing Alert
>
> *The residual limb should not be placed on a pillow because a flexion contracture of the hip may result.*

The nurse encourages the patient to turn from side to side and to assume a prone position, if possible, to stretch the flexor muscles and to prevent flexion contracture of the hip. The patient is encouraged not to sit for long periods of time to prevent flexion contracture. The legs should remain close together to prevent an abduction deformity. The nurse encourages the patient to use assistive devices to more readily perform self-care activities and to identify what home modifications, if any, should be made to perform these activities in the home environment.

Postoperative ROM exercises are started early because contracture deformities develop rapidly. ROM exercises include hip and knee exercises for patients with BKAs and hip exercises for patients with AKAs. It is important that the patient understands the importance of exercising the residual limb (Geertzen et al., 2015; Morris et al., 2015).

The upper limbs, trunk, and abdominal muscles are exercised and strengthened. The extensor muscles in the arm and the depressor muscles in the shoulder play an important part in crutch walking. The patient uses an overbed trapeze to change position and strengthen the biceps. The patient may flex and extend the arms while holding weights. Doing push-ups while seated strengthens the triceps muscles. Exercises (such as hyperextension of the residual limb), conducted under the supervision of the physical therapist, also aid in strengthening muscles as well as increasing circulation, reducing edema, and preventing atrophy.

Strength and endurance are assessed, and activities are increased gradually to prevent fatigue. As the patient progresses to independent use of the wheelchair, the use of ambulatory aids, or ambulation with a prosthesis, the nurse emphasizes safety considerations. Environmental barriers (e.g., steps, inclines, doors, throw rugs, wet surfaces) are identified, and methods of managing them are implemented. It is important to anticipate, identify, and manage problems associated with the use of the mobility aids. Proper instructions in using assistive devices will help prevent these problems.

Amputation of the leg changes the center of gravity; therefore, the patient may need to practice position changes (e.g., standing from sitting, standing on one foot). The patient is taught transfer techniques early and is reminded to maintain good posture when getting out of bed. A well-fitting shoe with a nonskid sole should be worn. During position changes, the patient should be guarded and stabilized with a transfer belt at the waist to prevent falling.

As soon as possible, the patient with a lower limb amputation is assisted to stand between parallel bars to allow extension of the temporary prosthesis to the floor with minimal weight bearing. How soon after surgery the patient is allowed to bear full body weight on the prosthesis depends on the patient's physical status and wound healing. As endurance increases and balance is achieved, ambulation is started with the use of parallel bars or crutches. The patient learns to use a normal gait, with the residual limb moving back and forth while walking with the crutches. To prevent a permanent flexion deformity from occurring, the residual limb should not be held up in a flexed position (Geertzen et al., 2015).

Helping the Patient with an Upper Limb Amputation. Because a patient who has had an upper limb amputated uses both shoulders to operate the prosthesis, the muscles of both shoulders are exercised. A patient with an above-elbow amputation or shoulder disarticulation is likely to develop a postural abnormality caused by loss of the weight of the amputated limb. Postural exercises are helpful.

The patient with an upper limb amputation is taught how to carry out ADLs with one arm. The patient is started on one-handed self-care activities as soon as possible. The use of a temporary prosthesis is encouraged. The patient who learns to use the prosthesis soon after the amputation is less dependent on one-handed self-care activities.

The patient with an upper limb amputation may wear a cotton T-shirt to prevent contact between the skin and shoulder harness and to promote absorption of perspiration.

The prosthetist advises about cleaning the washable portions of the harness. Periodically, the prosthesis is inspected for potential problems.

Preparing the Patient for a Prosthesis. The residual limb must be conditioned and shaped into a conical form to permit accurate fit, maximum comfort, and function of the prosthetic device. Elastic bandages, an elastic residual limb shrinker, or an air splint is used to condition and shape the residual limb. The nurse educates the patient or a member of the family about the correct method of bandaging.

Bandaging supports the soft tissue and minimizes the formation of edema while the residual limb is in a dependent position. The bandage is applied in such a manner that the remaining muscles required to operate the prosthesis are as firm as possible. An improperly applied elastic bandage contributes to circulatory problems and a poorly shaped residual limb.

Effective preprosthetic care is important to ensure proper fitting of the prosthesis. The major problems that can delay prosthetic fitting during this period are (1) flexion deformities, (2) nonshrinkage of the residual limb, and (3) abduction deformities of the hip.

The primary provider usually prescribes activities to condition or "toughen" the residual limb in preparation for a prosthesis. The patient begins by pushing the residual limb into a soft pillow, then into a firmer pillow, and finally against a hard surface. The patient is taught to massage the residual limb to mobilize the surgical incision site, decrease tenderness, and improve vascularity. Massage is usually started once healing has occurred and is first performed by the physical therapist. Skin inspection and preventive care are taught; mirrors may be used to visualize the skin on the residual limb (VA/DoD, 2014).

The prosthesis socket is custom-molded to the residual limb by the prosthetist. Prostheses are designed for specific activity levels and patient abilities. Types of prostheses include those that are hydraulic, pneumatic, biofeedback controlled, myoelectrically controlled, and synchronized. Adjustments of the prosthetic socket are made by the prosthetist to accommodate the residual limb changes that occur during the first 6 months to 1 year after surgery.

Helping the Patient Who Is Not a Candidate for a Prosthesis. Some patients are not candidates for a prosthesis (e.g., patients with amputations who are nonambulatory). If the use of a prosthesis is not possible, the patient is instructed in safe use of a wheelchair to achieve independence. A special wheelchair designed for patients who have had amputations is recommended. Because of the decreased weight in the front, a regular wheelchair may tip backward when the patient sits in it. In wheelchairs designed for patients who have had amputations, the rear axle is set back about 5 cm (2 inches) to compensate for the change in weight distribution.

MONITORING AND MANAGING POTENTIAL COMPLICATIONS

After any surgery, efforts are made to reestablish homeostasis and to prevent complications related to surgery, anesthesia, and immobility. The nurse assesses body systems (e.g., respiratory, hematologic, gastrointestinal, genitourinary, skin) for problems associated with immobility (e.g., atelectasis, pneumonia, DVT, PE, anorexia, constipation, urinary stasis, pressure ulcers).

Massive hemorrhage due to a loosened suture is a potentially life-threatening problem. The nurse monitors the patient for any signs or symptoms of bleeding and monitors the patient's vital signs and suction drainage.

> ### Quality and Safety Nursing Alert
>
> *Immediate postoperative bleeding may develop slowly or may take the form of massive hemorrhage resulting from a loosened suture. A large tourniquet should be in plain sight at the patient's bedside so that if severe bleeding occurs, it can be applied to the residual limb to control the hemorrhage. The nurse immediately notifies the surgeon in the event of excessive bleeding.*

Infection is a common complication of amputation. Patients who have undergone traumatic amputation have contaminated wounds. The nurse administers antibiotics as prescribed. The nurse must monitor the incision, dressing, and drainage for indications of infection (e.g., change in color, odor, or consistency of drainage; increasing discomfort). The nurse also assesses for systemic indicators of infection (e.g., elevated temperature, leukocytosis with an increase of more than 10% bands on the differential) and promptly reports indications of infection to the surgeon.

Skin breakdown may result from immobilization or pressure from various sources. The prosthesis may cause pressure areas to develop. The nurse and the patient assess for breaks in the skin. Careful skin hygiene is essential to prevent skin irritation, infection, and breakdown. The healed residual limb is washed and dried (gently) at least twice daily. The skin is inspected for persistent erythema, pressure areas, dermatitis, and blisters. If they are present, the prosthesis should not be worn until the complication is evaluated and treated in order to prevent further skin breakdown. Usually, a residual limb sock is worn to absorb perspiration and to prevent direct contact between the skin and the prosthetic socket. The sock is changed daily and must fit smoothly to prevent irritation caused by wrinkles. The socket of the prosthesis is washed with a mild detergent, rinsed, and dried thoroughly with a clean cloth. It must be thoroughly dry before the prosthesis is applied (VA/DoD, 2014).

PROMOTING HOME, COMMUNITY-BASED, AND TRANSITIONAL CARE

Educating the Patient About Self-Care. Before the patient is discharged to home or to a rehabilitation facility, the patient and family are encouraged to become active participants in care. They participate in care of the skin, residual limb, and prosthesis as appropriate. The patient receives ongoing education and practice sessions to learn to transfer and to use mobility aids and other assistive devices safely. The nurse explains the signs and symptoms of complications that must be reported to the primary provider (see Chart 42-7).

Continuing and Transitional Care. After the patient has achieved physiologic homeostasis and has demonstrated achievement of major health care goals, rehabilitation continues either in a rehabilitation facility or at home. Continued support and evaluation by the home, transitional or community-based nurse are essential.

HOME CARE CHECKLIST
Chart 42-7

The Patient With an Amputation

At the completion of education, the patient and/or caregiver will be able to:

- Name the procedure that was performed and identify any permanent changes in anatomic structure or function as well as changes in ADLs, IADLs, roles, relationships, and spirituality.
- Identify modification of home environment, interventions, and strategies (e.g., durable medical equipment, adaptive equipment, ADL assistance), used in safely adapting to changes in structure or function and promote effective recovery and rehabilitation.
  - Identify professionals and community agencies to help with transition to home.
- Describe ongoing postoperative therapeutic regimen, including diet and activities to perform (e.g., exercises) and to limit or avoid (e.g., lifting weights, driving a car, contact sports).
  - Describe care of residual limb and conditioning for prosthesis.
  - Consume a healthy diet to promote wound healing.
  - Participate in rehabilitation program to regain functional independence, promote circulation, maintain the health of unaffected muscles and those muscles now needed for safe transfer, mobility, etc.
  - If indicated, demonstrate safe use of mobility aid, assistive device, and transfer technique.
  - Observe prescribed weight-bearing and activity limits.
- State the name, dose, side effects, frequency, and schedule for all prescribed therapeutic and prophylactic medications (e.g., antibiotics, anticoagulants, analgesic agents).

- State how to obtain medical supplies and carry out dressing changes, wound care, and other prescribed regimens.
- Describe approaches to controlling pain (e.g., take analgesics as prescribed; use nonpharmacologic interventions).
- State indicators of complications to report promptly to primary provider (e.g., uncontrolled pain; signs of local or systemic infection; residual limb skin breakdown).
- Relate how to reach primary provider with questions or complications.
- State time and date of follow-up appointments, therapy, and testing.
- Identify community resources for peer and caregiver/family support:
  - Identify sources of support (e.g., friends, relatives, faith community).
  - Identify phone numbers, meeting locations and times of support groups (e.g., amputee support groups, caregiver support groups).
- Identify the need for health promotion, disease prevention, and screening activities.

Resources

See Chapter 10, Chart 10-8 for additional information related to durable medical equipment, adaptive equipment, mobility skills, skin, bowel, and bladder care.

ADL, activities of daily living; IADL, independent activities of daily living.

The patient's home environment should be assessed prior to discharge. Modifications are made to ensure the patient's continuing care, safety, and mobility. An overnight or weekend experience at home may be tried to identify problems that were not identified on the assessment visit. Physical therapy and occupational therapy may continue in the home or on an outpatient basis. Transportation to continuing health care appointments must be arranged. The social service department of the hospital or the home health agency may be of great assistance in securing personal assistance and transportation services.

During follow-up health visits, the nurse evaluates the patient's physical and psychosocial adjustment. Periodic preventive health assessments are necessary. An older adult spouse may not be able to provide the assistance required if needed at home. Modifications in the plan of care are made on the basis of such findings. Often, the patient and family find involvement in a postamputation support group to be of value; here, they can share problems, solutions, and resources. Talking with those who have successfully dealt with a similar problem may help the patient develop a satisfactory solution.

Because patients and their family members and health care providers tend to focus on the most obvious needs and issues, the nurse reminds the patient and family about the importance of continuing health promotion and screening practices, such as regular physical examinations and diagnostic screening tests. Accessible facilities for screening, health care, and exercise are identified. Patients are instructed about their importance and are referred to appropriate health care providers.

Evaluation

Expected patient outcomes may include:

1. Experiences no pain, including phantom limb pain
   a. Appears relaxed
   b. Verbalizes comfort
   c. Uses measures to increase comfort and mitigate pain
   d. Participates in self-care and rehabilitative activities
   e. Reports diminished phantom sensations
2. Achieves wound healing
   a. Controls residual limb edema
   b. Exhibits healed, nontender, nonadherent scar
   c. Demonstrates residual limb care
3. Demonstrates improved body image and effective coping
   a. Acknowledges change in body image
   b. Participates in self-care activities
   c. Demonstrates increasing independence
   d. Projects self as a whole person
   e. Resumes role-related responsibilities
   f. Reestablishes social contacts
   g. Demonstrates confidence in abilities
4. Exhibits resolution of grieving
   a. Expresses grief
   b. Works through feelings with family and friends
   c. Focuses on future functioning
   d. Participates in support group
5. Achieves independent self-care
   a. Asks for assistance when needed
   b. Uses aids and assistive devices to facilitate self-care
   c. Verbalizes satisfaction with abilities to perform ADLs

6. Achieves maximum independent mobility
   a. Avoids positions contributing to contracture development
   b. Demonstrates full active ROM
   c. Maintains balance when sitting and transferring
   d. Increases strength and endurance
   e. Demonstrates safe transferring technique
   f. Achieves functional use of prosthesis
   g. Overcomes environmental barriers to mobility
   h. Uses community services and resources as needed
7. Exhibits absence of complications of hemorrhage, infection, or skin breakdown
   a. Does not experience excessive bleeding
   b. Maintains normal blood values
   c. Is free of local or systemic signs of infection
   d. Repositions self frequently
   e. Is free of pressure-related problems
   f. Reports any skin discomfort and irritations promptly

CRITICAL THINKING EXERCISES

1 ebp You are a medical-surgical nurse working on a busy orthopedic unit caring for a 78-year-old female patient admitted one evening with a femoral neck fracture after a fall. The patient lives alone in her own home but remains very active within her community doing volunteer work. She is scheduled for surgery tomorrow. The patient tells you that she feels, "This is the beginning of the end for me." Identify this patient's unique nursing, medical, physical therapy, occupational therapy, social, and emotional needs. Devise a nursing plan of care that addresses these needs. What is the strength of the evidence that supports your plan of care for this patient?

2 A female college student athlete injures her knee during a soccer game the first week of the season. The trainer tells the student that she probably has an ACL injury and potentially also a meniscus injury. The student presents to the Student Health Center, where you work as a clinic nurse, unsure of the treatment plan for her injury. She expresses concern about how this injury will affect her chances at playing soccer for the remainder of the season. Describe the collaboration necessary to provide a comprehensive treatment plan for this patient. How will you, as the clinic nurse, support the student in this plan?

3 pg After a motorcycle crash, a 28-year-old male sustained a tibial fracture, which was surgically repaired yesterday afternoon. He was admitted to the inpatient orthopedic unit postoperatively, where you work as a staff nurse. During morning shift report, the night nurse reports to you, the oncoming day shift nurse, that the patient has been complaining of continuing pain all night that has not been alleviated despite administration of prescription opioid pain medication. The night shift nurse reports to you that she feels that the patient may have a high tolerance for pain medication due to his history of drug abuse. Describe your immediate assessments and interventions as your prioritize care for this patient.

REFERENCES

*Asterisk indicates nursing research.

Books

Emergency Nurses Association (ENA). (2013). *Sheehy's manual of emergency care*. St. Louis, MO: Mosby.

Moore, K. L., Agur, A. M. R., Dalley, A. F. II (2015). *Essential clinical anatomy* (5th ed.). Philadelphia, PA: Lippincott Williams & Wilkins

National Association of Orthopedic Nurses (NAON). (2013).*Core curriculum for orthopaedic nursing* (7th ed.). Boston, MA: Pearson.

Porth, C. M. (2015). *Essentials of pathophysiology: Concepts of altered health states*. (4th ed.). Philadelphia, PA: Lippincott Williams & Wilkins

Strickland, J. W., & Graham, T. J. (2005). *Master techniques in orthopaedic surgery: The hand* (2nd ed.). Philadelphia, PA: Lippincott Williams & Wilkins.

Journals and Electronic Documents

Agranoff, A. B. (2015). Medial collateral and lateral collateral ligament injury treatment and management. *Medscape*. Retrieved on 2/15/2016 at: emedicine.medscape.com/article/307959-treatment#d9

American Academy of Orthopaedic Surgeons (AAOS). (2014a). *Muscle contusion (bruise)*. Retrieved on 2/15/2016 at: orthoinfo.aaos.org/topic.cfm?topic=a00341

American Academy of Orthopaedic Surgeons (AAOS). (2014b). *Management of hip fractures in the elderly: Evidenced based clinical practice guidelines*. Retrieved on 2/15/2016 at: www.aaos.org/Research/guidelines/HipFxGuideline.pdf

Amputee Coalition. (2015). *Limb loss statistics*. Retrieved on 2/15/2016 at: www.amputee-coalition.org/resources/limb-loss-statistics/

American Nurses Association (ANA). (2017). *Safe patient handling and mobility*. Retrieved on 4/7/2017 at: nursingworld.org/Safe-Patient-Handling-and-Mobility

Baker, B., Lubowitz, J. H., & Wolf, B. T. (2015). Meniscus injuries treatment and management. *Medscape*. Retrieved on 2/15/2016 at: emedicine.medscape.com/article/90661-treatment#d11

Buckley, R. & Page, J. L. (2016). General principles of fracture care. *Medscape*. Retrieved on 2/14/2016 at: emedicine.medscape.com/article/1270717-overview#showall

Cooper, M. T. (2015). Acute Achilles tendon ruptures: Does surgery offer superior results (and other confusing issues)? *Clinical Sports Medicine, 34*(4), 595–606.

Department of Veterans Affairs & Department of Defense (VA/DoD). (2014). VA/DoD Clinical practice guideline for the management of upper extremity amputation rehabilitation. Retrieved on 12/17/2016 at: www.healthquality.va.gov/guidelines/rehab/uear/index.asp

Dingemanse, R., Randsdorp, M., Koes, B. et al. (2014). Evidence for the effectiveness of electrophysical modalities for treatment of medial and lateral epicondylitis: A systematic review. *The British Journal of Sports Medicine, 48*(12), 957–965.

Duckworth, A. D., McQueen, M. M., & Ring, D. (2013). Fractures of the radial head. *The Bone & Joint Journal, 95*-B(2), 151–159.

Geertzen, J., van der Linde, H., Rosenbrand, K., et al. (2015). Dutch evidence-based guidelines for amputation and prosthetics of the lower extremity: Rehabilitation process and prosthetics. Part 2. *Prosthetics and Orthotics International, 39*(5) 361–371.

Halawi, M. & Morwood, M. (2015). Acute management of open fractures: An evidence-based review. *Orthopedics, 38*(11), e1025–e1033.

Highsmith, M. J., Kahle, J. T., Miro, R. M., et al. (2016). Prosthetic interventions for people with transtibial amputation: Systematic review and meta-analysis of high-quality literature and systematic reviews. *Journal of Rehabilitation Research and Development, 53*(2), 157–184.

*Holly, C., Rittenmeyer, L., & Weeks, S. (2014). Evidenced-based clinical audit criteria for the prevention and management of delirium in the postoperative patient with hip fracture. *Orthopaedic Nursing, 33*(1), 27–34.

Kare, J. A. (2015). Volkmann contracture. *Medscape*. Retrieved on 2/15/2016 at: emedicine.medscape.com/article/1270462-overview

Keany, J. E. & McKeever, D. (2015). Femur fracture follow-up. *Medscape*. Retrieved on 2/15/2016 at: emedicine.medscape.com/article/824856-followup#e4

Kent, M., Hsia, H., Van de Ven, T., et al. (2016). Perioperative pain management strategies for amputation: A topical review. *Pain Medicine* (epublished July 8, 2016) doi: 10.1093/pm/pnw110

Kleinhenz, B. P. (2014). Clavicle fractures. *Medscape*. Retrieved on 2/15/2016 at: emedicine.medscape.com/article/92429-overview#a7

Kodde, I., Kaas, L., Flipsen, M., et al. (2015). Current concepts in the management of radial head fractures. *World Journal of Orthopedics, 6*(11), 954–960.

Kosova, E., Bergmark, B., & Piazza, G. (2015). Fat embolism syndrome. *Circulation, 131*(3), 317–320, doi: 10.1161/CIRCULATIONAHA.114.010835

*Lee, J., Donaldson, J., Drake, D. et al. (2014). Venous thromboembolism knowledge among older post-hip fracture patients and their caregivers. *Geriatric Nursing, 35*(5), 374–380.

Melendez, S. L. (2015). Rib fracture treatment and management. *Medscape*. Retrieved on 2/15/2016 at: emedicine.medscape.com/article/825981-overview

Morris, C., Potter, B., Athanasian, E., et al. (2015). Extremity amputations: Principles, techniques, and recent advancements. *Instructional Course Lectures, 64*, 105–117.

National Center for Health Statistics (NCHS). (2015). *Accidents or unintentional injuries*. Retrieved on 2/15/2016 at: www.cdc.gov/nchs/fastats/accidental-injury.htm

National Hospital Discharge Survey (NHDS). National Center for Health Statistics. (2015). Retrieved on 4/7/2017 at: www.cdc.gov/nchs/nhds/index.htm

National Institute of Neurological Disorders and Stroke (NINDS). (2015). *Complex regional rain syndrome factsheet*. Retrieved on 2/15/2016 at: www.ninds.nih.gov/disorders/reflex_sympathetic_dystrophy/detail_reflex_sympathetic_dystrophy.htm

Paschos, N., Mitsionis, G., Vasiliadis, H., et al. (2013). Comparison of early mobilization protocols in radial head fractures. *Journal of Orthopaedic Trauma, 27*(3), 134–139.

Paulson, S., Comfort, C. P., Lee, B. C., et al. (2014), Prolonging life: Legal, ethical, and social dilemmas. *Annals of the New York Academy of Sciences, 1330*, 19–39.

Pirowska, A., Wloch, T., Nowobilski, R., et al. (2014). Phantom phenomena and body scheme after amputation: A literature review. *Neurologia I Neurochirurgia Polska, 48*(1), 52–59.

Russell, G. V., & Jarrett, C. A. (2016). Pelvic fractures. *Medscape*. Retrieved on 2/15/2016 at: emedicine.medscape.com/article/1247913-overview#a10

*Saccomano, S., & Ferrara, L. (2015). Fall prevention in older adults. *Nurse Practitioner, 40*(6), 40–47.

Schaller, T. M. (2016). Open fractures. *Medscape*. Retrieved on 2/15/2016 at: emedicine.medscape.com/article/1269242-overview

Speed, J. (2015). Heterotopic ossification. *Medscape*. Retrieved on 2/15/2016 at: emedicine.medscape.com/article/327648-overview#showall

Street, P., Thompson, J., & Bailey, M. (2015). Management of urinary catheters following hip fracture. *Australasian Journal of Ageing, 34*(4), 241–246.

Thacker, M. M., Tejwani, N., & Thakkar, C. (2014). Acetabulum fractures. *Medscape*. Retrieved on 2/15/2016 at: emedicine.medscape.com/article/1246057-overview

U.S. Department of Labor, Bureau of Labor Statistics. (2014). *Nonfatal occupational injuries and illnesses requiring days away from work, 2013*. Retrieved on 2/15/2016 at: www.bls.gov/news.release/osh2.nr0.htm

Vinas, F. (2015). Lumbar spine fracture and dislocations. *Medscape*. Retrieved on 2/15/2016 at: emedicine.medscape.com/article/1264191-overview

Vincent, H., Horodyski, M., Vincent, K., et al. (2015). Psychological distress after orthopedic trauma: Prevalence in patients and implications for rehabilitation. *Physical Medicine and Rehabilitation, 7*(9), 978–989.

von Keudell, A. G., Weaver, M. J., Appleton, P. T. (2015). Diagnosis and treatment of acute extremity compartment syndrome. *The Lancet, 386*(1000), 1299–1310.

Walczak, B., Johnson, C., & Howe, B. M. (2015). Myositis ossificans. *Journal of the American Academy of Orthopaedic Surgeons, 23*(10), 612–622.

Resources

American College of Sports Medicine (ACSM), www.acsm.org

American Nurses Association (ANA), Safe Patient Handling and Mobility, nursingworld.org/Safe-Patient-Handling-and-Mobility

Amputee Coalition, www.amputee-coalition.org

Disabled American Veterans (DAV), www.dav.org

National Amputation Foundation (NAF), www.nationalamputation.org

National Association of Orthopaedic Nurses (NAON), www.orthonurse.org

National Institute for Occupational Safety and Health (NIOSH), www.cdc.gov/niosh/

National Institute of Arthritis and Musculoskeletal and Skin Diseases, www.niams.nih.gov

U.S. Department of Labor, Occupational Safety and Health Administration (OSHA), www.osha.gov

Wounded Warrior Project, www.woundedwarriorproject.org

UNIT 10

Digestive and Gastrointestinal Function

Case study

PROMOTING SELF-CARE IN THE PATIENT WITH A NEW OSTOMY

A 34-year-old woman with a long history of ulcerative colitis is admitted to a surgical unit following a total colectomy and an ileostomy. The patient had a preoperative evaluation with a wound–ostomy–continence (WOC) nurse, who had an educational session with the patient. The WOC nurse taught the patient basic principles of stoma care and recommended strategies for involvement in self-care in the postoperative period. It is now 4 days postoperative and the patient has had a good physical recovery without complications, but she refuses to participate in any ostomy care or even look at the stoma.

QSEN Competency Focus: Evidence-Based Practice (EBP)

The complexities inherent in today's health care system challenges nurses to demonstrate integration of specific interdisciplinary core competencies. These competencies are aimed at ensuring the delivery of safe, quality patient care (Institute of Medicine, 2003). The Quality and Safety Education for Nurses project (QSEN, 2017; Cronenwett, Sherwood, Barnsteiner, et al., 2007) provides a framework for the knowledge, skills, and attitudes (KSA) required for nurses to demonstrate competency in these key areas, which include *patient-centered care, interdisciplinary teamwork and collaboration, evidence-based practice, quality improvement, safety,* and *informatics.*

Evidence-Based Practice Definition: Integrate best current evidence with clinical expertise and patient/family preferences and values for delivery of optimal health care.

SELECTED PRE-LICENSURE KSAs	APPLICATION AND REFLECTION
Knowledge	
Discriminate between valid and invalid reasons for modifying evidence-based clinical practice based on clinical expertise or patient/family preferences.	What is the strength of the evidence that suggests that patients should be involved in their ostomy care? What do you think are this patient's reasons for not participating in her care? What is the psychological process patients go through after a disfiguring surgery?
Skills	
Consult with clinical experts before deciding to deviate from evidence-based protocols.	Identify members of the health care team you would consult with to help you craft the most appropriate, individualized plan of care for this patient.
Attitudes	
Acknowledge own limitations in knowledge and clinical expertise before determining when to deviate from evidence-based best practices.	Reflect on the complex interrelationships between the physical and psychological aspects of this patient's condition. Think about your own desire for this patient to accept her ostomy. How might your desire for her acceptance hamper the care you provide?

Cronenwett, L., Sherwood, G., Barnsteiner, J., et al. (2007). Quality and safety education for nurses. *Nursing Outlook, 55*(3), 122–131.
Institute of Medicine. (2003). *Health professions education: A bridge to quality.* Washington, DC: National Academies Press.
QSEN Institute. (2017). *QSEN Competencies: Definitions and pre-licensure KSAs.* Retrieved on 3/1/2017 at: www.qsen.org/competencies/pre-licensure-ksas

43 Assessment of Digestive and Gastrointestinal Function

LEARNING OBJECTIVES

On completion of this chapter, the learner will be able to:

1 Describe the structure and function of the organs of the gastrointestinal (GI) tract.
2 Explain the mechanical and chemical processes involved in digesting and absorbing nutrients and eliminating waste products.
3 Discriminate between normal and abnormal assessment findings identified by inspection, auscultation, percussion, and palpation of the gastrointestinal system.
4 Recognize and evaluate the major symptoms of gastrointestinal dysfunction by applying concepts from the patient's health history and physical assessment findings.
5 Identify the diagnostic tests used to evaluate GI tract function and related nursing implications.

GLOSSARY

absorption: phase of the digestive process that occurs when small molecules, vitamins, and minerals pass through the walls of the small and large intestine and into the bloodstream
amylase: an enzyme that aids in the digestion of starch
anus: last section of the gastrointestinal (GI) tract; outlet for waste products from the GI system
chyme: mixture of food with saliva, salivary enzymes, and gastric secretions that is produced as food passes through the mouth, esophagus, and stomach
digestion: phase of the digestive process that occurs when digestive enzymes and secretions mix with ingested food and when proteins, fats, and sugars are broken down into their component smaller molecules
dyspepsia: indigestion; upper abdominal discomfort associated with eating
elimination: phase of the digestive process that occurs after digestion and absorption, when waste products are evacuated from the body
esophagus: collapsible tube connecting the mouth to the stomach, through which food passes as it is ingested
hydrochloric acid: acid secreted by the glands in the stomach; mixes with chyme to break it down into absorbable molecules and to aid in the destruction of bacteria
ingestion: phase of the digestive process that occurs when food is taken into the GI tract via the mouth and esophagus
intrinsic factor: a gastric secretion that combines with vitamin B_{12} so that the vitamin can be absorbed
large intestine: the portion of the GI tract into which waste material from the small intestine passes as absorption continues and elimination begins; consists of several parts—ascending segment, transverse segment, descending segment, sigmoid colon, and rectum; also known as the colon
lipase: an enzyme that aids in the digestion of fats
pepsin: a gastric enzyme that is important in protein digestion
small intestine: longest portion of the GI tract, consisting of three parts—duodenum, jejunum, and ileum—through which food mixed with all secretions and enzymes passes as it continues to be digested and begins to be absorbed into the bloodstream
stomach: distensible pouch into which the food bolus passes to be digested by gastric enzymes
trypsin: enzyme that aids in the digestion of protein

Abnormalities of the gastrointestinal (GI) tract are numerous and represent every type of major pathology that can affect other organ systems, including bleeding, perforation, obstruction, inflammation, and cancer. Congenital, inflammatory, infectious, traumatic, and neoplastic lesions have been encountered in every portion and at every site along the length of the GI tract. As with all other organ systems, the GI tract is subject to circulatory disturbances, faulty nervous system control, and aging.

Apart from the many organic diseases to which the GI tract is susceptible, many extrinsic factors can interfere with its normal function and produce symptoms. Stress and anxiety, for example, often find their chief expression in indigestion, anorexia, or motor disturbances of the intestines, sometimes producing constipation or diarrhea. In addition, factors such as fatigue and an inadequate or abruptly changed dietary intake can markedly affect the GI tract. When assessing and instructing the patient, the nurse should consider the variety of mental and physical factors that affect the function of the GI tract.

Anatomic and Physiologic Overview

Anatomy of the Gastrointestinal System

The GI tract is a pathway 7 to 7.9 meters (23 to 26 feet) in length that extends from the mouth to the esophagus, stomach, small and large intestines, and rectum, to the

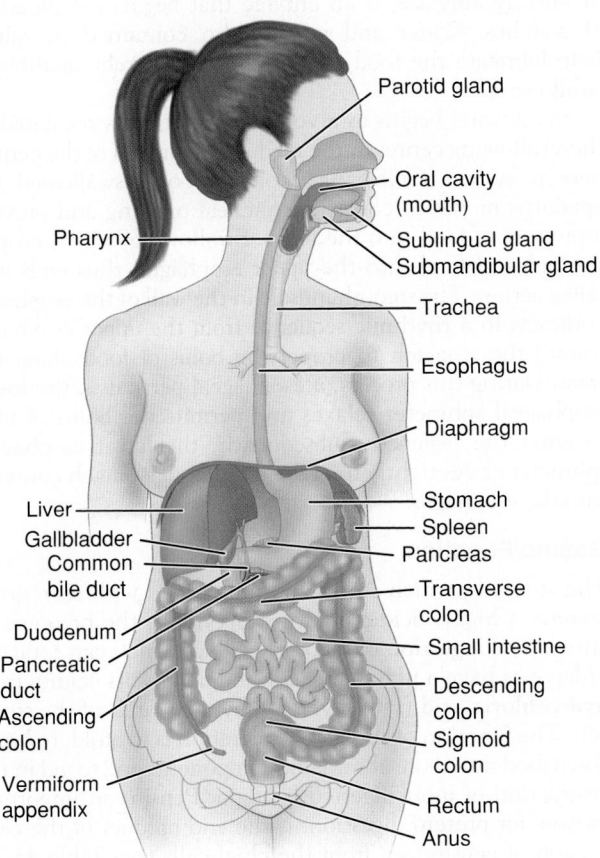

Figure 43-1 • Organs of the digestive system and associated structures.

terminal structure, the **anus** (see Fig. 43-1). The **esophagus** is located in the mediastinum, anterior to the spine and posterior to the trachea and heart. This hollow muscular tube, which is approximately 25 cm (10 inches) in length, passes through the diaphragm at an opening called the *diaphragmatic hiatus*.

The remaining portion of the GI tract is located within the peritoneal cavity. The **stomach** is situated in the left upper portion of the abdomen under the left lobe of the liver and the diaphragm, overlaying most of the pancreas (see Fig. 43-1). A hollow muscular organ with a capacity of approximately 1500 mL, the stomach stores food during eating, secretes digestive fluids, and propels the partially digested food, or chyme, into the small intestine. The gastroesophageal junction is the inlet to the stomach. The stomach has four anatomic regions: the cardia (entrance), fundus, body, and pylorus (outlet). Circular smooth muscle in the wall of the pylorus forms the pyloric sphincter and controls the opening between the stomach and the small intestine.

The **small intestine** is the longest segment of the GI tract, accounting for about two thirds of the total length. It folds back and forth on itself, providing approximately 70 m (230 ft) of surface area for secretion and **absorption,** the process by which nutrients enter the bloodstream through the intestinal walls. It has three sections: The most proximal section is the duodenum, the middle section is the jejunum, and the distal section is the ileum. The ileum terminates at the

ileocecal valve. This valve, or sphincter, controls the flow of digested material from the ileum into the cecal portion of the large intestine and prevents reflux of bacteria into the small intestine. Attached to the cecum is the vermiform appendix, an appendage that has little or no physiologic function. Emptying into the duodenum at the ampulla of Vater is the common bile duct, which allows for the passage of both bile and pancreatic secretions.

The **large intestine** consists of an ascending segment on the right side of the abdomen, a transverse segment that extends from right to left in the upper abdomen, and a descending segment on the left side of the abdomen. The sigmoid colon, the rectum, and the anus complete the terminal portion of the large intestine. A network of striated muscle that forms both the internal and the external anal sphincters regulates the anal outlet.

The GI tract receives blood from arteries that originate along the entire length of the thoracic and abdominal aorta and veins that return blood from the digestive organs and the spleen. This portal venous system is composed of five large veins: the superior mesenteric, inferior mesenteric, gastric, splenic, and cystic veins, which eventually form the vena portae that enters the liver. Once in the liver, the blood is distributed throughout and collected into the hepatic veins that then terminate in the inferior vena cava. Of particular importance are the gastric artery and the superior and inferior mesenteric arteries. Oxygen and nutrients are supplied to the stomach by the gastric artery and to the intestine by the mesenteric arteries (see Fig. 43-2). Venous blood is returned from the small intestine, cecum, and the ascending and transverse portions of the colon by the superior mesenteric vein, which corresponds with the distribution of the branches of the superior mesenteric artery. Blood flow to the GI tract is about 20% of the total cardiac output and increases significantly after eating.

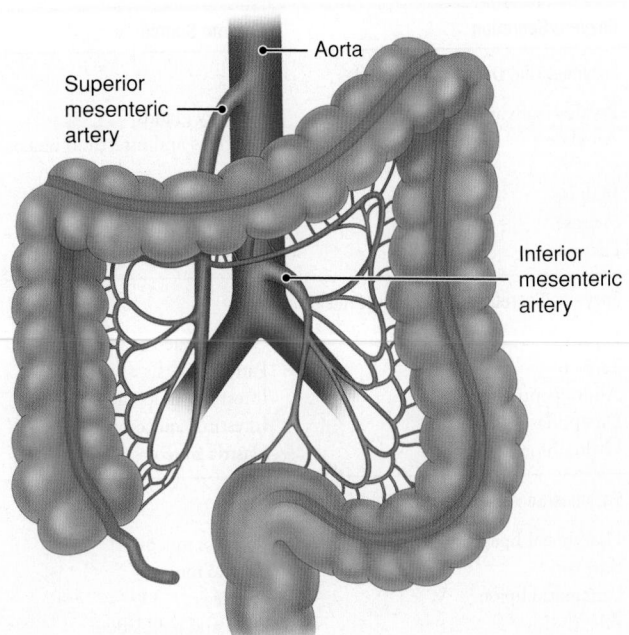

Figure 43-2 • Anatomy and blood supply of the large intestine.

Both the sympathetic and parasympathetic portions of the autonomic nervous system innervate the GI tract. In general, sympathetic nerves exert an inhibitory effect on the GI tract, decreasing gastric secretion and motility and causing the sphincters and blood vessels to constrict. Parasympathetic nerve stimulation causes peristalsis and increases secretory activities. The sphincters relax under the influence of parasympathetic stimulation, except for the sphincter of the upper esophagus and the external anal sphincter, which are under voluntary control (Grossman & Porth, 2014).

Function of the Digestive System

All cells of the body require nutrients. These nutrients are derived from the intake of food that contains proteins, fats, carbohydrates, vitamins, minerals, and cellulose fibers and other vegetable matter, some of which has no nutritional value. Major functions of the GI tract include:

- Breakdown of food particles into the molecular form for **digestion**
- Absorption into the bloodstream of small nutrient molecules produced by digestion
- **Elimination** of undigested unabsorbed foodstuffs and other waste products

After food is ingested, it is propelled through the GI tract, coming into contact with a wide variety of secretions that aid in its digestion, absorption, or elimination from the GI tract.

Chewing and Swallowing

The process of digestion begins with the act of chewing, in which food is broken down into small particles that can be swallowed and mixed with digestive enzymes. Eating—or even the sight, smell, or taste of food—can cause reflex salivation. Approximately 1.5 L of saliva is secreted daily from the parotid, the submaxillary, and the sublingual glands. Ptyalin,

or salivary **amylase**, is an enzyme that begins the digestion of starches. Water and mucus, also contained in saliva, help lubricate the food as it is chewed, thereby facilitating swallowing.

Swallowing begins as a voluntary act that is regulated by the swallowing center in the medulla oblongata of the central nervous system (CNS). As a bolus of food is swallowed, the epiglottis moves to cover the tracheal opening and prevent aspiration of food into the lungs. Swallowing, which propels the bolus of food into the upper esophagus, thus ends as a reflex action. The smooth muscle in the wall of the esophagus contracts in a rhythmic sequence from the upper esophagus toward the stomach to propel the bolus of food along the tract. During this process of esophageal peristalsis, the lower esophageal sphincter relaxes and permits the bolus of food to enter the stomach. Subsequently, the lower esophageal sphincter closes tightly to prevent reflux of stomach contents into the esophagus.

Gastric Function

The stomach, which stores and mixes food with secretions, secretes a highly acidic fluid in response to the presence or anticipated **ingestion** of food. This fluid, which can total 2.4 L/day, can have a pH as low as 1 and derives its acidity from **hydrochloric acid** (HCl) secreted by the glands of the stomach. The function of this gastric secretion is twofold: to break down food into more absorbable components and to aid in the destruction of most ingested bacteria. **Pepsin**, an important enzyme for protein digestion, is the end product of the conversion of pepsinogen from the chief cells (see Table 43-1). **Intrinsic factor**, also secreted by the gastric mucosa, combines with dietary vitamin B_{12} so that the vitamin can be absorbed in the ileum. In the absence of intrinsic factor, vitamin B_{12} cannot be absorbed, and pernicious anemia results (see Chapter 33).

TABLE 43-1 The Major Digestive Enzymes and Secretions

Enzyme/Secretion	Enzyme Source	Digestive Action
Enzymes That Digest Carbohydrates		
Ptyalin (salivary amylase)	Salivary glands	Starch→dextrin, maltose, glucose
Amylase	Pancreas and intestinal mucosa	Starch→dextrin, maltose, glucose
		Dextrin→maltose, glucose
Maltase	Intestinal mucosa	Maltose→glucose
Sucrase	Intestinal mucosa	Sucrose→glucose, fructose
Lactase	Intestinal mucosa	Lactose→glucose, galactose
Enzymes/Secretions That Digest Protein		
Pepsin	Gastric mucosa	Protein→polypeptides
Trypsin	Pancreas	Proteins and polypeptides→polypeptides, dipeptides, amino acids
Aminopeptidase	Intestinal mucosa	Polypeptides→dipeptides, amino acids
Dipeptidase	Intestinal mucosa	Dipeptides→amino acids
Hydrochloric acid	Gastric mucosa	Protein→polypeptides, amino acids
Enzymes/Secretions That Digest Fat (Triglyceride)		
Pharyngeal lipase	Pharynx mucosa	Triglycerides→fatty acids, diglycerides, monoglycerides
Steapsin	Gastric mucosa	Triglycerides→fatty acids, diglycerides, monoglycerides
Pancreatic lipase	Pancreas	Triglycerides→fatty acids, diglycerides, monoglycerides
Bile	Liver and gallbladder	Fat emulsification

→, converts to.

TABLE 43-2 The Major Gastrointestinal Regulatory Substances

Substance	Stimulus for Production	Target Tissue	Effect on Secretions	Effect on Motility
Neuroregulators				
Acetylcholine	Sight, smell, chewing food, stomach distention	Gastric glands, other secretory glands, gastric and intestinal muscle	↑gastric acid	Generally increased; decreased sphincter tone
Norepinephrine	Stress, other various stimuli	Secretory glands, gastric and intestinal muscle	Generally inhibitory	Generally decreased; increased sphincter tone
Hormonal Regulators				
Gastrin	Stomach distention with food	Gastric glands	↑ secretion of gastric juice, which is rich in HCl	Increased motility of stomach, decreased time required for gastric emptying Relaxation of ileocecal sphincter Excitation of colon Constriction of gastroesophageal sphincter
Cholecystokinin	Fat in duodenum	Gallbladder Pancreas Stomach	Release of bile into duodenum ↑production of enzyme-rich pancreatic secretions Inhibits gastric secretion somewhat	Slows gastric emptying
Secretin	pH of chyme in duodenum below 4–5	Stomach Pancreas	Inhibits gastric secretion somewhat ↑production of bicarbonate-rich pancreatic juice	Inhibits stomach contractions
Local Regulator				
Histamine	Unclear; substances in food	Gastric glands	↑gastric acid production	

HCl, hydrochloric acid, ↑ increased.

Peristaltic contractions in the stomach propel the stomach's contents toward the pylorus. Because large food particles cannot pass through the pyloric sphincter, they are churned back into the body of the stomach. In this way, food in the stomach is mechanically broken down into smaller particles. Food remains in the stomach for a variable length of time, from 30 minutes to several hours, depending on the volume, osmotic pressure, and chemical composition of the gastric contents. Peristalsis in the stomach and contractions of the pyloric sphincter allow the partially digested food to enter the small intestine at a rate that permits efficient absorption of nutrients. This partially digested food mixed with gastric secretions is called **chyme**. Hormones, neuroregulators, and local regulators found in the gastric secretions control the rate of gastric secretions and influence gastric motility (see Table 43-2).

Small Intestine Function

The digestive process continues in the duodenum. Duodenal secretions come from the accessory digestive organs—the pancreas, liver, and gallbladder—and the glands in the wall of the intestine itself. These secretions contain digestive enzymes: amylase, lipase, and bile. Pancreatic secretions have an alkaline pH due to their high concentration of bicarbonate. This alkalinity neutralizes the acid entering the duodenum from the stomach. Digestive enzymes secreted by the pancreas include **trypsin**, which aids in digesting protein; amylase, which aids in digesting starch; and **lipase**, which

aids in digesting fats. These secretions drain into the pancreatic duct, which empties into the common bile duct at the ampulla of Vater. Bile, secreted by the liver and stored in the gallbladder, aids in emulsifying ingested fats, making them easier to digest and absorb. The sphincter of Oddi, found at the confluence of the common bile duct and duodenum, controls the flow of bile. Hormones, neuroregulators, and local regulators found in these intestinal secretions control the rate of intestinal secretions and also influence GI motility. Intestinal secretions total approximately 1 L/day of pancreatic juice, 0.5 L/day of bile, and 3 L/day of secretions from the glands of the small intestine. Tables 43-1 and 43-2 give further information about the actions of digestive enzymes and GI regulatory substances.

Two types of contractions occur regularly in the small intestine: segmentation contractions and intestinal peristalsis. *Segmentation contractions* produce mixing waves that move the intestinal contents back and forth in a churning motion. *Intestinal peristalsis* propels the contents of the small intestine toward the colon. Both movements are stimulated by the presence of chyme.

Food, ingested as fats, proteins, and carbohydrates, is broken down into absorbable particles (constituent nutrients) by the process of digestion. Carbohydrates are broken down into disaccharides (e.g., sucrose, maltose, and galactose) and monosaccharides (e.g., glucose, fructose). Glucose is the major carbohydrate that tissue cells use as fuel. Proteins are a source of energy after they are broken down into amino acids and peptides. Ingested fats become monoglycerides and fatty acid through emulsification, which makes them smaller and easier to absorb. Chyme stays in the small intestine for 3 to 6 hours, allowing for continued breakdown and absorption of nutrients.

Small, fingerlike projections called *villi* line the entire intestine and function to produce digestive enzymes as well as to absorb nutrients. Absorption is the major function of the small intestine. Vitamins and minerals are absorbed essentially unchanged. Absorption begins in the jejunum and is accomplished by active transport and diffusion across the intestinal wall into the circulation. Nutrients are absorbed at specific locations in the small intestine and duodenum, whereas fats, proteins, carbohydrates, sodium, and chloride are absorbed in the jejunum. Vitamin B_{12} and bile salts are absorbed in the ileum. Magnesium, phosphate, and potassium are absorbed throughout the small intestine.

Colonic Function

Within 4 hours after eating, residual waste material passes into the terminal ileum and slowly into the proximal portion of the right colon through the ileocecal valve. With each peristaltic wave of the small intestine, the valve opens briefly and permits some of the contents to pass into the colon.

Bacteria, a major component of the contents of the large intestine, assist in completing the breakdown of waste material, especially of undigested or unabsorbed proteins and bile salts. Two types of colonic secretions are added to the residual material: an electrolyte solution and mucus. The electrolyte solution is chiefly a bicarbonate solution that acts to neutralize the end products formed by the colonic bacterial action, whereas the mucus protects the colonic mucosa from the interluminal contents and provides adherence for the fecal mass.

Slow, weak peristalsis moves the colonic contents along the tract. This slow transport allows for efficient reabsorption of water and electrolytes, which is the major function of the colon. Intermittent strong peristaltic waves propel the contents for considerable distances. This generally occurs after another meal is eaten, when intestine-stimulating hormones are released. The waste materials from a meal eventually reach and distend the rectum, usually in about 12 hours. As much as one fourth of the waste materials from a meal may still be in the rectum 3 days after the meal was ingested.

Waste Products of Digestion

Feces consist of undigested foodstuffs, inorganic materials, water, and bacteria. Fecal matter is about 75% fluid and 25% solid material (Grossman & Porth, 2014). The composition is relatively unaffected by alterations in diet because a large portion of the fecal mass is of nondietary origin, derived from the secretions of the GI tract. The brown color of the feces results from the breakdown of bile by the intestinal bacteria. Chemicals formed by intestinal bacteria are responsible in large part for the fecal odor. Gases formed contain methane, hydrogen sulfide, and ammonia, among others. The GI tract normally contains approximately 150 mL of these gases, which are either absorbed into the portal circulation and detoxified by the liver or expelled from the rectum as flatus.

Elimination of stool begins with distention of the rectum, which initiates reflex contractions of the rectal musculature and relaxes the normally closed internal anal sphincter. The internal sphincter is controlled by the autonomic nervous system; the external sphincter is under the conscious control of the cerebral cortex. During defecation, the external anal sphincter voluntarily relaxes to allow colonic contents to be expelled. Normally, the external anal sphincter is maintained in a state of tonic contraction. Thus, defecation is seen to be a spinal reflex (involving the parasympathetic nerve fibers) that can be inhibited voluntarily by keeping the external anal sphincter closed. Contracting the abdominal muscles (straining) facilitates emptying of the colon. The average frequency of defecation in humans is once daily, but this varies among people.

Gerontologic Considerations

Although an increased prevalence of several common GI disorders occurs in the older adult population, aging per se appears to have minimal direct effect on most GI functions, in large part because of the functional reserve of the GI tract. Normal physiologic changes of the GI system that occur with aging are identified in Table 43-3. Careful assessment and

TABLE 43-3 Age-Related Changes in the Gastrointestinal System

Structural Changes	Implications
Oral Cavity and Pharynx	
• Injury/loss or decay of teeth • Atrophy of taste buds • ↓ Saliva production • Reduced ptyalin and amylase in saliva	Difficulty chewing and swallowing
Esophagus	
• ↓ Motility and emptying • Weakened gag reflex • ↓ Resting pressure of lower esophageal sphincter	Reflux and heartburn
Stomach	
• Degeneration and atrophy of gastric mucosal surfaces with ↓ production of HCl • ↓ Secretion of gastric acids and most digestive enzymes • ↓ Gastric motility and emptying	Food intolerances, malabsorption, or ↓ vitamin B_{12} absorption
Small Intestine	
• Atrophy of muscle and mucosal surfaces • Thinning of villi and epithelial cells	↓ Motility and transit time, which lead to complaints of indigestion and constipation
Large Intestine	
• ↓ Mucus secretion • ↓ Elasticity of rectal wall • ↓ Tone of internal anal sphincter • Slower and duller nerve impulses in rectal area	↓ Motility and transit time, which lead to complaints of indigestion and constipation ↓ Absorption of nutrients (dextrose, fats, calcium, and iron) Fecal incontinence

↓, decreased; HCl, hydrochloric acid.
Adapted from Eliopoulos, C. (2018). *Gerontological nursing* (9th ed.). Philadelphia, PA: Lippincott Williams & Wilkins.

Schultz, H., Qvist, N., Morgensen, C. B., et al. (2013). Experiences of patients with acute abdominal pain in the ED or acute surgical ward–A qualitative comparative study. *International Emergency Nursing, 21*(2013), 228–235.

Purpose

The purpose of the study was to investigate the experience of patients with acute abdominal pain in an acute surgical ward (ASW) or in an emergency department (ED) observation unit.

Design

This was a comparative qualitative field study with participant observation and interviews that used the phenomenologic–hermeneutic approach. Data were interpreted through naïve reading, structural analysis, and critical interpretation and discussion. The study was conducted at two regional hospitals in Denmark. Both the ASW and ED were deemed comparable in terms of patient demographics.

Findings

Twenty four participants, 12 at each site, were observed during their stay. Twenty participants, 10 at each site were interviewed. The interviews were conducted at discharge or within 4 days of discharge. Five themes were identified after completion of data analysis. *Waiting* was identified in terms of waiting for admission, for an assessment by a surgeon, or for pain relief. *Waiting on the edge* entailed patient thoughts ranging from "nothing is wrong" to morbid thoughts anticipating death; these thoughts were affected by length of time with an unknown diagnosis. *Taking or not taking initiative* reflected that the patient rarely took initiative to change the situation. *Being the object of attention* reflected interactions with nurses while collecting vital signs and during interactions with the surgeons. While the object of attention, participants felt they were *being taken seriously,* the final theme. Importance was placed on the information relayed by the patients.

Nursing Implications

The findings of this study demonstrate the importance of communicating and interacting with patients. The findings shed light on the impact of the ebb and flow of provider–patient interactions. While nurses may recognize the importance of their interactions with patients, the time that they spend away from patients can be troubling for the patients. Nurses need to educate patients regarding communicating their needs to the healthcare team and also frequently assess the status and needs of the patient. Additionally, nurses should reaffirm the value placed on the patient and their stories.

---

monitoring of signs and symptoms related to these changes are imperative. Although irritable bowel symptoms decrease with aging, there seems to be an increase in many GI disorders of function and motility. Older adult patients frequently report dysphagia, anorexia, dyspepsia, and disorders of colonic function (Eliopoulos, 2018).

Assessment of the Gastrointestinal System

Health History

A focused GI assessment begins with a complete history. Information about abdominal pain, dyspepsia, gas, nausea and vomiting, diarrhea, constipation, fecal incontinence, jaundice, and previous GI disease is obtained (Weber & Kelley, 2014).

Common Symptoms

Pain

Pain can be a major symptom of GI disease; in particular, abdominal pain is a common presentation in the ambulatory setting (see Chart 43-1) (Cartwright & Knudson, 2015). The character, duration, pattern, frequency, location, distribution of referred abdominal pain (see Fig. 43-3), and time of the pain vary greatly depending on the underlying cause. Other factors such as meals, rest, activity, and defecation patterns may directly affect this pain (Weber & Kelley, 2014).

Dyspepsia

Dyspepsia—upper abdominal discomfort associated with eating (commonly called *indigestion*)—is the most common symptom of patients with GI dysfunction. Indigestion

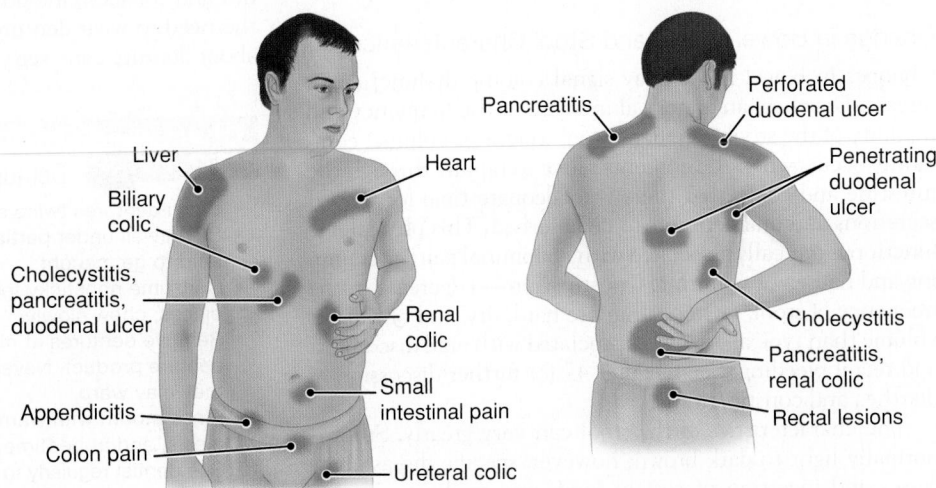

Figure 43-3 • Common sites of referred abdominal pain.

is an imprecise term that refers to a host of upper abdominal or epigastric symptoms such as pain, discomfort, fullness, bloating, early satiety, belching, heartburn, or regurgitation. Dyspepsia affects 25% to 40% of the population over a lifetime (Overland, 2014) while gastroesophageal reflux disease (GERD), which manifests with dyspepsia (most frequently with heartburn) affects approximately 20% of the U.S. population (Achem & DeVault, 2014; Grossman & Porth, 2014). Typically, fatty foods cause the most discomfort because they remain in the stomach for digestion longer than proteins or carbohydrates. Salads, coarse vegetables, and highly seasoned foods may also cause considerable GI distress.

Intestinal Gas

The accumulation of gas in the GI tract may result in belching (expulsion of gas from the stomach through the mouth) or flatulence (expulsion of gas from the rectum). Usually, gases in the small intestine pass into the colon and are released as flatus. Patients often complain of bloating, distention, or feeling "full of gas" with excessive flatulence as a symptom of food intolerance or gallbladder disease.

Nausea and Vomiting

Nausea is a vague, uncomfortable sensation of sickness or "queasiness" that may or may not be followed by vomiting. It can be triggered by odors, activity, medications, or food intake. The emesis, or vomitus, may vary in color and content and may contain undigested food particles, blood (hematemesis), or bilious material mixed with gastric juices.

The causes of nausea and vomiting are many; they may result from (1) visceral afferent stimulation (i.e., dysmotility, peritoneal irritation, infections, hepatobiliary or pancreatic disorders, mechanical obstruction); (2) CNS disorders (i.e., vestibular disorders, increased intracranial pressure, infections, psychogenic disorder); and/or (3) irritation of the chemoreceptor trigger zone from radiation therapy, systemic disorders, and endogenous and exogenous toxins, which may include specific classes of drugs (e.g., oncologic chemotherapy medications) (Grossman & Porth, 2014). Distention of the duodenum or upper intestinal tract is a common cause of nausea; it may also be an early warning sign of a pathologic process. Vomiting is a physiologic protective response that limits the effects of noxious agents by emptying the stomach contents and sections of the small intestine (Grossman & Porth, 2014).

Change in Bowel Habits and Stool Characteristics

Changes in bowel habits may signal colonic dysfunction or disease. Diarrhea, an abnormal increase in the frequency and liquidity of the stool or in daily stool weight or volume, commonly occurs when the contents move so rapidly through the intestine and colon that there is inadequate time for the GI secretions and oral contents to be absorbed. This physiologic function is typically associated with abdominal pain or cramping and nausea or vomiting. Constipation—a decrease in the frequency of stool, or stools that are hard, dry, and of smaller volume than typical—may be associated with anal discomfort and rectal bleeding. See Chapter 47 for further discussion of diarrhea and constipation.

The characteristics of the stool can vary greatly. Stool is normally light to dark brown; however, specific disease processes and ingestion of certain foods and medications may

TABLE 43-4 Foods and Medications That Alter Stool Color

Altering Substance	Color
Meat protein	Dark brown
Spinach	Green
Carrots, beets, red gelatin	Red
Cocoa	Dark red or brown
Senna	Yellow
Bismuth, iron, licorice, charcoal	Black
Barium	Milky white

change the appearance of stool (see Table 43-4). Blood in the stool can present in various ways and must be investigated. If blood is shed in sufficient quantities into the upper GI tract, it produces a tarry-black color (melena), whereas blood entering the lower portion of the GI tract or passing rapidly through it will appear bright or dark red. Lower rectal or anal bleeding is suspected if there is streaking of blood on the surface of the stool or if blood is noted on toilet tissue. Other common abnormalities in stool characteristics described by the patient may include:

- Bulky, greasy, foamy stools that are foul in odor and may or may not float
- Light-gray or clay-colored stool, caused by a decrease or absence of conjugated bilirubin
- Stool with mucus threads or pus that may be visible on gross inspection of the stool
- Small, dry, rock-hard masses occasionally streaked with blood
- Loose, watery stool that may or may not be streaked with blood

Past Health, Family, and Social History

The nurse asks about the patient's normal toothbrushing and flossing routine; frequency of dental visits; awareness of any lesions or irritated areas in the mouth, tongue, or throat; recent history of sore throat or bloody sputum; discomfort caused by certain foods; daily food intake; the use of alcohol and tobacco, including smokeless chewing tobacco; and the need to wear dentures or a partial plate. For information about denture care, see Chart 43-2.

Chart 43-2 **HEALTH PROMOTION**
Denture Care

- Brush dentures twice a day.
- Clean well under partial dentures, where food particles tend to get caught.
- Consume nonsticky foods that have been cut into small pieces; chew slowly.
- Remove dentures at night, and soak them in water or a denture product. Never put dentures in hot water, because they may warp.
- Rinse mouth with warm salt water in the morning, after meals, and at bedtime.
- See dentist regularly to assess and adjust fit.

Past and current medication use and any previous diagnostic studies, treatments, or surgery are noted. Current nutritional status is assessed via history; laboratory tests (complete metabolic panel including liver function studies, triglyceride, iron studies, and complete blood count [CBC]) are obtained. History of the use of tobacco and alcohol includes details about type, amount, length of use, and the date of discontinuation, if any. The nurse and patient discuss changes in appetite or eating patterns and any unexplained weight gain or loss over the past year. The nurse also asks questions about psychosocial, spiritual, or cultural factors that may be affecting the patient.

Physical Assessment

The physical examination includes assessment of the mouth, abdomen, and rectum and requires a good source of light, full exposure of the abdomen, warm hands with short fingernails, and a comfortable and relaxed patient with an empty bladder.

Oral Cavity Inspection and Palpation

Dentures should be removed to allow good visualization of the entire oral cavity.

Lips

The examination begins with inspection of the lips for moisture, hydration, color, texture, symmetry, and the presence of ulcerations or fissures. The lips should be moist, pink, smooth, and symmetric. The patient is instructed to open the mouth wide; a tongue blade is then inserted to expose the buccal mucosa for an assessment of color and lesions. Stensen duct of each parotid gland is visible as a small red dot in the buccal mucosa next to the upper molars.

Gums

The gums are inspected for inflammation, bleeding, retraction, and discoloration. The odor of the breath is also noted. The hard palate is examined for color and shape.

Tongue

The dorsum (back) of the tongue is inspected for texture, color, and lesions. A thin white coat and large, vallate papillae in a "V" formation on the distal portion of the dorsum of the tongue are normal findings. The patient is instructed to protrude the tongue and move it laterally. This provides the examiner with an opportunity to estimate the tongue's size as well as its symmetry and strength (to assess the integrity of the 12th cranial nerve [hypoglossal nerve]).

Further inspection of the ventral surface of the tongue and the floor of the mouth is accomplished by asking the patient to touch the roof of the mouth with the tip of the tongue. Any lesions of the mucosa or any abnormalities involving the frenulum or superficial veins on the undersurface of the tongue are assessed for location, size, color, and pain. This is a common area for oral cancer, which presents as a white or red plaque, lesions, ulcers, or nodules (Weber & Kelley, 2014).

A tongue blade is used to depress the tongue for adequate visualization of the pharynx. It is pressed firmly beyond the midpoint of the tongue; proper placement avoids a gagging response. The patient is told to tip the head back, open the mouth wide, take a deep breath, and say "ah." Often, this flattens the posterior tongue and briefly allows a full view of the tonsils, uvula, and posterior pharynx. These structures are inspected for color, symmetry, and evidence of exudate, ulceration, or enlargement. Normally, the uvula and soft palate rise symmetrically with a deep inspiration upon saying "ah"; this indicates an intact vagus nerve (10th cranial nerve).

A complete assessment of the oral cavity is essential because many disorders, such as cancer, diabetes, and immunosuppressive conditions resulting from medication therapy or acquired immunodeficiency syndrome, may be manifested by changes in the oral cavity, including stomatitis.

Abdominal Inspection, Auscultation, Percussion, and Palpation

The patient lies supine with knees flexed slightly for inspection, auscultation, percussion, and palpation of the abdomen. For the purposes of examination and documentation, the abdomen can be divided into either four quadrants or nine regions (see Fig. 43-4).

Consistent use of one of these mapping methods results in a thorough evaluation of the abdomen and appropriate documentation. The four-quadrant method involves the use of an imaginary line drawn vertically from the sternum to the pubis through the umbilicus and a horizontal line drawn across the abdomen through the umbilicus. Inspection is performed first, noting skin changes, nodules, lesions, scarring, discolorations, inflammation, bruising, or striae. Lesions are of particular importance, because GI diseases often produce skin changes. The contour and symmetry of the abdomen are noted, and any localized bulging, distention, or peristaltic waves are

Four quadrants
1 - right upper quadrant (RUQ)
2 - right lower quadrant (RLQ)
3 - left upper quadrant (LUQ)
4 - left lower quadrant (LLQ)

Nine regions
1 - epigastric region
2 - umbilical region
3 - hypogastric or suprapubic region
4 - right hypochondriac region
5 - left hypochondriac region
6 - right lumbar region
7 - left lumbar region
8 - right inguinal region
9 - left inguinal region

Figure 43-4 • Division of the abdomen into four quadrants or nine regions.

identified. Expected contours of the anterior abdominal wall can be described as flat, rounded, or scaphoid.

Auscultation always precedes percussion and palpation, because they may alter sounds. Auscultation is used to determine the character, location, and frequency of bowel sounds and to identify vascular sounds. Bowel sounds are assessed using the diaphragm of the stethoscope for soft clicks and gurgling sounds (Weber & Kelley, 2014). The frequency and character of the sounds are usually heard as clicks and gurgles that occur irregularly and range from 5 to 30 per minute. The terms *normal* (sounds heard about every 5 to 20 seconds), *hypoactive* (one or two sounds in 2 minutes), *hyperactive* (5 to 6 sounds heard in less than 30 seconds), or *absent* (no sounds in 3 to 5 minutes) are frequently used in documentation, but these assessments are highly subjective (Li, Wang, & Ma, 2012). Using the bell of the stethoscope, any bruits in the aortic, renal, iliac, and femoral arteries are noted. Friction rubs are high pitched and can be heard over the liver and spleen during respiration. Borborygmi ("stomach growling") is heard as a loud prolonged gurgle.

Percussion is used to assess the size and density of the abdominal organs and to detect the presence of air-filled, fluid-filled, or solid masses. Percussion is used either independently or concurrently with palpation because it can validate palpation findings. All quadrants are percussed for overall tympani and dullness. Tympani is the sound that results from the presence of air in the stomach and small intestines; dullness is heard over organs and solid masses. The use of light palpation is appropriate for identifying areas of tenderness or muscular resistance, and deep palpation is used to identify masses. Testing for rebound tenderness is not performed by many examiners because it can cause severe pain; light percussion is used instead to produce a mild localized response when peritoneal irritation is present.

Rectal Inspection and Palpation

The final part of the examination is evaluation of the terminal portions of the GI tract, the rectum, perianal region, and anus. The anal canal is approximately 2.5 to 4 cm (1 to 1.6 inches) in length and opens into the perineum. Concentric rings of muscle, the internal and external sphincters, normally keep the anal canal securely closed. Gloves, water-soluble lubrication, a penlight, and drapes are necessary tools for the evaluation. Although the rectal examination is generally uncomfortable and often embarrassing for the patient, it is a mandatory part of every thorough examination. For women, the rectal examination may be part of the gynecologic examination. Positions for the rectal examination include knee-chest, left lateral with hips and knees flexed, or standing with hips flexed and upper body supported by the examination table. Most patients are comfortable on the right side with knees brought up to the chest. External examination includes inspection for lumps, rashes, inflammation, excoriation, tears, scars, pilonidal dimpling, and tufts of hair at the pilonidal area. The discovery of tenderness, inflammation, or both should alert the examiner to the possibility of a pilonidal cyst, perianal abscess, or anorectal fistula or fissure. The patient's buttocks are carefully spread and visually inspected until the patient has relaxed the external sphincter control. The patient is asked to bear down, thus allowing the ready appearance of fistulas, fissures, rectal prolapse, polyps,

and internal hemorrhoids. Internal examination is performed with a gloved lubricated index finger inserted into the anal canal while the patient bears down. The tone of the sphincter is noted, as are any nodules or irregularities of the anal ring. Because this is an uncomfortable part of the examination for most patients, the patient is encouraged to focus on deep breathing and visualization of a pleasant setting during the brief examination.

Diagnostic Evaluation

GI diagnostic studies can confirm, rule out, stage, or diagnose various disease states, including cancer. After the diagnosis, time should be allotted for discussion with the patient, in addition to offering resource materials for information.

Many modalities are available for diagnostic assessment of the GI tract. The majority of these tests and procedures are performed on an outpatient basis in special settings designed for this purpose (e.g., endoscopy suite or GI laboratory). In the past, patients who required such tests typically were older adults; however, within the past 10 years, in part due to heightened media exposure and early diagnosis of colorectal cancer, the median age of patients evaluated for colorectal cancer has decreased significantly (American Cancer Society [ACS], 2015a). Preparation for many of these studies includes clear liquid diet, fasting, ingestion of a liquid bowel preparation, the use of laxatives or enemas, and ingestion or injection of a contrast agent or a radiopaque dye. These measures are poorly tolerated by some patients and are especially problematic in older adults or patients with comorbidities because bowel preparations can significantly alter the internal fluid and electrolyte balance. If further assessment or treatment is needed after any outpatient procedure, the patient may be admitted to the hospital.

Specific nursing interventions for each test are provided later in this chapter. General nursing interventions for the patient who is undergoing a GI diagnostic evaluation include:

- Establishing the nursing diagnosis
- Providing needed information about the test and the activities required of the patient
- Providing instructions about postprocedure care and activity restrictions
- Providing health information and procedural education to patients and significant others
- Helping the patient cope with discomfort and alleviating anxiety
- Informing the primary provider of known medical conditions or abnormal laboratory values that may affect the procedure
- Assessing for adequate hydration before, during, and immediately after the procedure, and providing education about maintenance of hydration

Serum Laboratory Studies

Initial diagnostic tests begin with serum laboratory studies, including but not limited to CBC, complete metabolic panel, prothrombin time/partial thromboplastin time, triglycerides, liver function tests, amylase, and lipase; possibly, more specific studies may be indicated, such as carcinoembryonic antigen (CEA), cancer antigen (CA) 19–9, and alpha-fetoprotein, which are sensitive and specific for colorectal and hepatocellular carcinomas, respectively. CEA is a protein that is normally not detected in the blood of a healthy person; therefore, when detected it indicates that cancer is present, although not what type of cancer is present. Primary providers can use CEA results to determine the stage and extent of the disease and the patient's prognosis for cancer, especially GI and, in particular, colorectal cancer (Standeven, Hiller, Mulder, et al., 2013). CA 19-9 is also a protein that exists on the surface of certain cells and is shed by tumor cells, making it useful as a tumor marker to follow the course of the cancer. CA 19-9 levels are elevated in most patients with advanced pancreatic cancer, but they may also be elevated in other conditions such as colorectal, stomach, and bile duct cancers; elevated levels may also be found in noncancer conditions (ACS, 2015b).

Stool Tests

Basic examination of the stool includes inspecting the specimen for consistency, color, and occult (not visible) blood. Additional studies, including fecal urobilinogen, fecal fat, nitrogen, *Clostridium difficile*, fecal leukocytes, calculation of stool osmolar gap, parasites, pathogens, food residues, and other substances, require laboratory evaluation.

Stool samples are usually collected on a random basis unless a quantitative study (e.g., fecal fat, urobilinogen) is to be performed. Random specimens should be sent promptly to the laboratory for analysis; however, the quantitative 24- to 72-hour collections must be kept refrigerated until transported to the laboratory. Some stool collections require the patient to follow a specific diet or refrain from taking certain medications before the collection; patient education is important.

Fecal occult blood testing (FOBT) is one of the most commonly performed stool tests. It can be useful in initial screening for several disorders, although it is used most frequently in early cancer detection programs. FOBT can be performed at the bedside, in the laboratory, or at home. Probably the most widely used in-office or at-home occult blood test is the Hemoccult II. It is inexpensive, noninvasive, and carries minimal risk to the patient. However, it should not be performed when there is hemorrhoidal bleeding. In the past, patients were advised to avoid ingesting red meats, aspirin, nonsteroidal anti-inflammatory drugs, turnips, and horseradish for 72 hours prior to the study because it was thought that these were associated with false-positive results; likewise, patients were advised to avoid ingesting vitamin C from supplements or foods as it was believed that this was associated with false-negative results. However, these restrictions are no longer advised as their actual effects on test results have not been established; plus, they unnecessarily restricted patient participation in screening (Garborg, 2015). A small amount of the specimen is applied to the guaiac-impregnated paper slide. If the test is performed at home, the patient mails the slide to the primary provider or the lab in an envelope provided for that purpose.

Fecal immunologic tests (FIT) use monoclonal or polyclonal antibodies to detect the globin protein in human hemoglobin. Dietary restrictions are not required prior to submission of the stool specimen (Wong, Ching, Chan, et al.,

2015). Since only one fecal stool sample is required, it is associated with improved screening participation (Garborg, 2015). Hematoporphyrin assays detect the broadest range of blood derivatives, but a strict dietary protocol is essential.

Stool DNA testing is a relatively new means to detect certain DNA related to colon cancer. More research is needed to determine how often the test needs to be performed. The stool DNA test does not require any dietary or medication restrictions and can detect neoplasia anywhere in the colon.

Breath Tests

The hydrogen breath test was developed to evaluate carbohydrate absorption, in addition to aiding in the diagnosis of bacterial overgrowth in the intestine and short bowel syndrome. This test determines the amount of hydrogen expelled in the breath after it has been produced in the colon (on contact of galactose with fermenting bacteria) and absorbed into the blood.

Urea breath tests detect the presence of *Helicobacter pylori*, the bacteria that can live in the mucosal lining of the stomach and cause peptic ulcer disease. After the patient ingests a capsule of carbon-labeled urea, a breath sample is obtained 10 to 20 minutes later. Because *H. pylori* metabolizes urea rapidly, the labeled carbon is absorbed quickly; it can then be measured as carbon dioxide in the expired breath to determine whether *H. pylori* is present. Prior to urea breath testing, the patient is instructed to avoid antibiotics or bismuth subsalicylate (Pepto-Bismol) for 1 month before the test; sucralfate (Carafate) and omeprazole (Prilosec) for 1 week before the test; and cimetidine (Tagamet), famotidine (Pepcid), and ranitidine (Zantac) for 24 hours before the test. *H. pylori* also can be detected by assessing serum antibody levels without requiring medication therapy adjustments (Overland, 2014).

Abdominal Ultrasonography

Ultrasonography is a noninvasive diagnostic technique in which high-frequency sound waves are passed into internal body structures, and the ultrasonic echoes are recorded on an oscilloscope as they strike tissues of different densities. It is particularly useful in the detection of an enlarged gallbladder or pancreas, the presence of gallstones, an enlarged ovary, an ectopic pregnancy, or appendicitis. Ultrasonography is an operator-dependent diagnostic technique; its diagnostic accuracy varies based on technologist skill and experience and patient body habitus (Cartwright & Knudson, 2015).

Advantages of abdominal ultrasonography include an absence of ionizing radiation, no noticeable side effects, relatively low cost, and almost immediate results. It cannot be used to examine structures that lie behind bony tissue, because bone prevents sound waves from traveling into deeper structures. Gas and fluid in the abdomen or air in the lungs also prevent transmission of ultrasound. An ultrasound produces no ill effects. However, some patients, typically pregnant women, have concerns regarding the energy emitted by the probe.

Endoscopic ultrasonography (EUS) is a specialized enteroscopic procedure that aids in the diagnosis of GI disorders by providing direct imaging of a target area. A small high-frequency ultrasonic transducer is mounted at the tip of the fiberoptic scope, which displays images that are of higher-quality resolution and definition than regular ultrasound imaging. Moderate sedation is typically indicated (Fischbach & Dunning, 2015) (see Chapter 18 for further discussion of moderate sedation). EUS may be used to evaluate submucosal lesions, specifically their location and depth of penetration. In addition, EUS may aid in the evaluation of Barrett esophagus, portal hypertension, chronic pancreatitis, suspected pancreatic neoplasm, biliary tract disease, and changes in the bowel wall due to ulcerative colitis. Intestinal gas, bone, and thick layers of adipose tissue that hamper conventional ultrasonography are not problems when EUS is used.

Nursing Interventions

The patient is instructed to fast for 8 to 12 hours before ultrasound testing to decrease the amount of gas in the bowel. If gallbladder studies are being performed, the patient should eat a fat-free meal the evening before the test. If barium studies are to be performed, they should be scheduled after ultrasonography; otherwise, the barium could interfere with the transmission of the sound waves. Patients who receive moderate sedation are observed for about 1 hour to assess for level of consciousness, orientation, and ability to ambulate. Patients treated on an outpatient basis are given instructions regarding diet, activity, and how to monitor for complications (American Society for Gastrointestinal Endoscopy [ASGE], 2013c).

Genetic Testing

Researchers have refined methods for genetics risk assessment, preclinical diagnosis, and prenatal diagnosis to identify people who are at risk for certain GI disorders (e.g., gastric cancer, lactose deficiency, inflammatory bowel disease, colon cancer) (see Chart 43-3). People who are identified as being at risk for certain GI disorders may choose to have genetic counseling to learn about the disease and options for preventing and treating the disease, and to receive support in coping with the situation. See Chapter 8 for further discussion of genetic counseling.

Imaging Studies

Numerous minimally invasive and noninvasive imaging studies, including x-ray and contrast studies, computed tomography (CT) scan, magnetic resonance imaging (MRI) scan, positron emission tomography (PET) scan, scintigraphy (radionuclide imaging), and virtual colonoscopy are available today.

Upper Gastrointestinal Tract Study

An upper GI fluoroscopy delineates the entire GI tract after the introduction of a contrast agent. A radiopaque liquid (e.g., barium sulfate) is commonly used; however, thin

---

Chart 43-3 · GENETICS IN NURSING PRACTICE
Digestive and Gastrointestinal Disorders

Several digestive and gastrointestinal disorders are associated with genetic abnormalities. Some examples include:

Autosomal dominant:

- Hereditary diffuse gastric cancer
- Hereditary nonpolyposis colorectal cancer (Lynch syndrome)
- Hirschsprung disease (aganglionic megacolon)

Autosomal recessive:

- Glucose galactose malabsorption
- Glycogen storage disease (von Gierke disease)
- Pompe disease
- Zellweger syndrome

Inheritance pattern includes autosomal dominant and autosomal recessive:

- Familial adenomatous polyposis

X-linked:

- Fabry disease

Inheritance pattern is not distinct; however, there is a genetic predisposition for the disease:

- Crohn's disease
- Type 1 diabetes
- Celiac disease
- Pancreatic cancer

Other genetic disorders that will impact the digestive and gastrointestinal system:

- Cleft lip and/or palate
- Cystic fibrosis

Nursing Assessments

Refer to Chart 5-2: Genetics in Nursing Practice: Genetic Aspects of Health Assessment

Family History Assessment Related to Digestive and Gastrointestinal Disorders

- Careful family history assessment for other family members with a similar condition (e.g., cleft lip/palate, pyloric stenosis).
- Assess for other family members in several generations with early-onset colorectal cancer.
- Inquire about other family members with inflammatory bowel disease.
- Assess family history for other cancers (e.g., endometrial, ovarian, kidney).

Patient Assessment Specific to Digestive and Gastrointestinal Disorders

- Ask about bowel pattern and color of stool.
- Assess if patient experiences episodes of abdominal cramping, diarrhea, or dehydration.
- Assess for unexplained weight loss.
- Identify intolerance to specific foods (e.g., gluten, high fat foods, lactose).
- Assess for prior history of liver disorders.

Assess for presence of other clinical conditions:

- With clefting—congenital heart defect, other birth defects suggestive of a genetic syndrome.
- With familial adenomatous polyposis—congenital hypertrophy of retinal pigment epithelium.

Genetics Resources

Celiac Support Association, www.csaceliacs.org
Crohn's & Colitis Foundation of America, www.ccfa.org
Cancer.Net, www.cancer.net
See Chapter 8, Chart 8-7 for components of genetic counseling.

barium, diatrizoate sodium (Hypaque), and at times water are used due to their low associated risks. The GI series enables the examiner to detect or exclude anatomic or functional disorders of the upper GI organs or sphincters. It also aids in the diagnosis of ulcers, varices, tumors, regional enteritis, and malabsorption syndromes. The procedure may be extended to examine the duodenum and small bowel (small bowel follow-through). As the barium descends into the stomach, the position, patency, and caliber of the esophagus are visualized, enabling the examiner to detect or exclude any anatomic or functional derangement of that organ. Fluoroscopic examination next extends to the stomach as its lumen fills with barium, allowing observation of stomach motility, thickness of the gastric wall, the mucosal pattern, patency of the pyloric valve, and the anatomy of the duodenum. Multiple x-ray images are obtained during the procedure, and additional images may be taken at intervals for up to 24 hours to evaluate the rate of gastric emptying. Small bowel x-rays taken while the barium is passing through that area allow for observation of the motility of the small bowel. Obstructions, ileitis, and diverticula can also be detected.

Variations of the upper GI study include double-contrast studies and enteroclysis. The double-contrast method of examining the upper GI tract involves administration of a thick barium suspension to outline the stomach and esophageal wall, after which tablets that release carbon dioxide in the presence of water are given. This technique has the advantage of showing the esophagus and stomach in finer detail, permitting signs of early superficial neoplasms to be noted.

Enteroclysis is a very detailed, double-contrast study of the entire small intestine that involves the continuous infusion (through a duodenal tube) of 500 to 1000 mL of a thin barium sulfate suspension; after this, methylcellulose is infused through the tube. The barium and methylcellulose fill the intestinal loops and are observed continuously by fluoroscopy and viewed at frequent intervals as they progress through the jejunum and the ileum. This process (even with normal motility) can take up to 6 hours and can be quite uncomfortable for the patient. The procedure aids in the diagnosis of partial small bowel obstructions or diverticula. After completion of the fluoroscopic component of the study, the patient undergoes a CT scan to check for lesions or adhesions (Bontrager & Lampignano, 2014).

Nursing Interventions

Instruction regarding dietary changes prior to the study should include a clear liquid diet, with nothing by mouth (NPO) from midnight the night before the study (ASGE, 2013c). In addition, the patient is advised to not smoke or chew gum during the NPO period because these can increase gastric secretions and salivation (Bontrager & Lampignano, 2014). Polyethylene glycol (PEG)-based solutions are considered the most effective bowel cleansing preparatory agent (Chen, Athilingam, Saloum, et al., 2015). Typically, oral medications are withheld on the morning of the study and resumed that evening, but each patient's medication regimen should be evaluated on an individual basis. When a patient with insulin-dependent diabetes is NPO, their insulin requirements will need to be adjusted accordingly (see Chapter 51).

Follow-up care is provided after the upper GI procedure to ensure that the patient has eliminated most of the ingested barium. Fluids may be increased to facilitate evacuation of stool and barium.

Lower Gastrointestinal Tract Study

Visualization of the lower GI tract is obtained after rectal installation of barium. The barium enema can be used to detect the presence of polyps, tumors, or other lesions of the large intestine and demonstrate any anatomic abnormalities or malfunctioning of the bowel. After proper preparation and evacuation of the entire colon, each portion of the colon may be readily observed. The procedure usually takes about 15 to 30 minutes, during which time x-ray images are obtained.

Other means for visualizing the colon include double-contrast studies and a water-soluble contrast study. These tests are still occasionally used because they are relatively inexpensive and simple. A double-contrast or air-contrast barium enema involves the instillation of a thicker barium solution, followed by the instillation of air. The patient may feel some cramping or discomfort during this process. This test provides a contrast between the air-filled lumen and the barium-coated mucosa, allowing easier detection of smaller lesions.

If active inflammatory disease, fistulas, or perforation of the colon is suspected, a water-soluble iodinated contrast agent (e.g., diatrizoic acid [Gastrografin]) can be used. The procedure is the same as for a barium enema, but the patient must first be assessed for allergy to iodine or contrast agent. The contrast agent is eliminated readily after the procedure, so there is no need for postprocedure laxatives. Some diarrhea may occur in some patients until the contrast agent has been totally eliminated.

Nursing Interventions

Preparation of the patient includes emptying and cleansing the lower bowel. This often necessitates a low-residue diet 1 to 2 days before the test, a clear liquid diet and a laxative the evening before, NPO after midnight, and cleansing enemas until returns are clear the following morning. The nurse makes sure that barium enemas are scheduled before any upper GI studies. If the patient has active inflammatory disease of the colon, enemas are contraindicated. Barium enemas also are contraindicated in patients with signs of perforation or obstruction; instead, a water-soluble contrast study may be performed. Active GI bleeding may prohibit the use of laxatives and enemas.

Postprocedural patient education includes information about increasing fluid intake, evaluating bowel movements for evacuation of barium, and noting increased number of bowel movements, because barium, due to its high osmolarity, may draw fluid into the bowel, thus increasing the intraluminal contents and resulting in greater output.

Computed Tomography

A CT scan provides cross-sectional images of abdominal organs and structures. Multiple x-ray images are taken from numerous angles, digitized in a computer, reconstructed, and then viewed on a computer monitor. As the sensitivity and specificity of CT scans have increased in recent years, so has its use. Volume CT scanners (i.e., helical or spiral scanning) provide more accurate reconstruction of patient data into alternate planes, require shorter scan times, and have less artifact when compared to single slice scanning (Bontrager & Lampignano, 2014). CT is a valuable tool for detecting and localizing many inflammatory conditions in the colon, such as appendicitis, diverticulitis, regional enteritis, and ulcerative colitis, as well as evaluating the abdomen for diseases of the liver, spleen, kidney, pancreas, and pelvic organs, and structural abnormalities of the abdominal wall. The CT procedure is completely painless, but radiation doses are considerable. A CT scan may be performed with or without oral or intravenous (IV) contrast, but the enhancement of the study is greater with the use of a contrast agent. For those patients who may be at risk for complications from use of contrast (see later discussion), the use of contrast should be contraindicated if the suspected pathology can be visualized from a non–contrast-enhanced study (Rawson & Pelletier, 2013).

Nursing Interventions

Common risks from IV contrast agents include allergic reactions and acute kidney injury; therefore, patients must be screened for these risks (Rawson & Pelletier, 2013). Any allergies to contrast agents, iodine, or shellfish, the patient's current serum creatinine level, and pregnancy status in females must be determined before administration of a contrast agent. Patients allergic to the contrast agent may be premedicated with a corticosteroid and antihistamine.

In addition, kidney protective measures include the administration of IV sodium bicarbonate 1 hour before and 6 hours after IV contrast and oral N-acetylcysteine (Mucomyst) before or after the study. N-acetylcysteine is thought to be a free radical scavenger that sequesters the contrast by-products that are destructive to kidney cells (Deek, Newton, Sheerin, et al., 2014). Research suggests the combination of these medications, hydration, and using less contrast agent may decrease the risk of acute kidney injury (Rawson & Pelletier, 2013).

Magnetic Resonance Imaging

MRI is used in gastroenterology to supplement ultrasonography and CT. This noninvasive technique uses magnetic fields and radio waves to produce images of the area being studied. The use of oral contrast agents to enhance the image has increased the application of this technique for the diagnosis of GI diseases. It is useful in evaluating abdominal soft tissues as well as blood vessels, abscesses, fistulas, neoplasms, and other sources of bleeding.

The physiologic artifacts of heartbeat, respiration, and peristalsis may create a less-than-clear image; however, newer, fast-imaging MRI techniques help eliminate these physiologic motion artifacts. MRI is not totally safe for all people; having the patient complete a preprocedure MRI tool that screens for contraindications to MRI is advocated by the American College of Radiology (Kanal, Barkovich, Bell, et al., 2013). Any ferromagnetic objects (metals that contain iron) can be attracted to the magnet and cause injury. Items that can be problematic or dangerous include jewelry, pacemakers, dental implants, paperclips, pens, keys, IV poles, clips on patient gowns, and oxygen tanks.

> ⚑ **Quality and Safety Nursing Alert**
>
> *MRI is contraindicated in patients with any device containing metal because the magnetic field could cause malfunction. MRI is also contraindicated for patients with internal metal devices (e.g., aneurysm clips), intraocular metallic fragments, or cochlear implants. Foil-backed skin patches (e.g., nicotine [NicoDerm], nitroglycerin [Transderm-Nitro], scopolamine [Transderm-Scop], clonidine [Catapres-TTS]) should be removed before an MRI because of the risk of burns; however, the patient's primary provider should be consulted before the patch is removed to determine whether an alternate form of the medication should be provided.*

Nursing Interventions

Before the study patient education includes NPO status 6 to 8 hours before the study and removal of all jewelry and other metals. The patient and family are informed that the study may take 60 to 90 minutes; during this time, the technician will instruct the patient to take deep breaths at specific intervals. The close-fitting scanners used in many MRI facilities may induce feelings of claustrophobia, and the machine will make a knocking sound during the procedure. Patients may choose to wear a headset and listen to music or wear a blindfold during the procedure. Open MRIs that are less close fitting eliminate the claustrophobia that many patients experience, although they produce lower-resolution images.

Positron Emission Tomography

PET scans produce images of the body by detecting the radiation emitted from radioactive substances. The radioactive substances are injected into the body IV and are usually tagged with radioactive isotopes of oxygen, nitrogen, carbon, or fluorine (Bontrager & Lampignano, 2014). These isotopes decay quickly, do not harm the body, have lower radiation levels than a typical x-ray or CT scan, and are eliminated in the urine or feces. The scanner essentially "captures" where the radioactive substances are in the body, transmits information to a scanner, and produces a scan with "hot spots" for evaluation by the radiologist or oncologist.

Scintigraphy

Scintigraphy (radionuclide testing) relies on the use of radioactive isotopes (i.e., technetium, iodine, and indium) to reveal displaced anatomic structures, changes in organ size, and the presence of neoplasms or other focal lesions such as cysts or abscesses. Scintigraphic scanning is also used to measure the uptake of tagged red blood cells and leukocytes. Tagging of red blood cells and leukocytes by injection of a radionuclide is performed to define areas of inflammation, abscess, blood loss, or neoplasm. A sample of blood is removed, mixed with a radioactive substance, and reinjected into the patient. Abnormal concentrations of blood cells are then detected at 24- and 48-hour intervals. Tagged red cell studies are useful in determining the source of internal bleeding when all other studies have returned a negative result.

Gastrointestinal Motility Studies

Radionuclide testing also is used to assess gastric emptying and colonic transit time. During gastric emptying studies, the liquid and solid components of a meal (typically scrambled eggs) are tagged with radionuclide markers. After ingestion of the meal, the patient is positioned under a scintiscanner, which measures the rate of passage of the radioactive substance from the stomach (Kar, Jones, Horowitz, et al., 2015). This is useful in diagnosing disorders of gastric motility, diabetic gastroparesis, and dumping syndrome.

Colonic transit studies are used to evaluate colonic motility and obstructive defecation syndromes. The patient is given a capsule containing 20 radionuclide markers and instructed to follow a regular diet and usual daily activities. Abdominal x-rays are taken every 24 hours until all markers are passed. This process usually takes 4 to 5 days; in the presence of severe constipation it may take as long as 10 days. Patients with chronic diarrhea may be evaluated at 8-hour intervals. The amount of time that it takes for the radioactive material to move through the colon indicates colonic motility.

Endoscopic Procedures

Endoscopic procedures used in GI tract assessment include fibroscopy/esophagogastroduodenoscopy (EGD), colonoscopy, anoscopy, proctoscopy, sigmoidoscopy, small bowel enteroscopy, and endoscopy through an ostomy.

Upper Gastrointestinal Fibroscopy/ Esophagogastroduodenoscopy

Fibroscopy of the upper GI tract allows direct visualization of the esophageal, gastric, and duodenal mucosa through a lighted endoscope (gastroscope) (see Fig. 43-5). EGD is valuable when esophageal, gastric, or duodenal disorders or inflammatory, neoplastic, or infectious processes are suspected. This procedure also can be used to evaluate esophageal and gastric motility and to collect secretions and tissue specimens for further analysis.

In EGD, the gastroenterologist views the GI tract through a viewing lens and can obtain images through the scope to document findings. Electronic video endoscopes also are available that attach directly to a video processor, converting the electronic signals into pictures that are projected on a screen. This allows larger and continuous viewing capabilities, as well as the simultaneous recording of the procedure.

Figure 43-5 • Patient undergoing gastroscopy.

PillCam ESO, or capsule endoscopy, requires that the patient swallows a capsule that travels by peristalsis through the small intestines. The capsule contains an oxide metal silicon chip video camera, which transmits digital images of the GI mucosa to a data recorder that is worn on the patient's waist. Transit time from the time the capsule is swallowed until it is passed is approximately 24 hours. This particular study provides superior visualization of the small intestines, and is particularly useful to detect occult areas of bleeding, inflammatory bowel disease, and celiac disease (Peralta & Contreras Pena, 2015).

Endoscopic retrograde cholangiopancreatography (ERCP) uses the endoscope in combination with x-rays to view the bile ducts, pancreatic ducts, and gallbladder (ASGE, 2013b). The side-viewing flexible scopes are used to visualize the common bile duct and the pancreatic and hepatic ducts through the ampulla of Vater in the duodenum. ERCP is helpful in evaluating jaundice, pancreatitis, pancreatic tumors, common bile duct stones, and biliary tract disease. However, ERCP is associated with postprocedure pancreatitis; therefore, alternative diagnostic studies such as magnetic resonance cholangiopancreatography or EUS are typically preferred for diagnosing obstructive biliary disease (Rustagi & Jamidar, 2015). ERCP is described further in Chapter 50.

Upper GI fibroscopy also can be a therapeutic procedure when combined with other procedures. Therapeutic endoscopy can be used to remove common bile duct stones, dilate strictures, and treat gastric bleeding and esophageal varices. Laser-compatible scopes can be used to provide laser therapy for upper GI neoplasms. Sclerosing solutions can be injected through the scope in an attempt to control upper GI bleeding.

After the patient is sedated, the endoscope is lubricated with a water-soluble lubricant and passed smoothly and slowly along the back of the mouth and down into the esophagus. The gastroenterologist views the gastric wall and the sphincters and then advances the endoscope into the duodenum for further examination. Biopsy forceps to obtain tissue specimens or cytology brushes to obtain cells for microscopic study can be passed through the scope. The procedure usually takes about 30 minutes.

The patient may experience nausea, gagging, or choking. The use of topical anesthetic agents and moderate sedation makes it important to monitor and maintain the patient's oral airway during and after the procedure. Finger or ear oximeters are used to monitor oxygen saturation, and supplemental oxygen may be given if needed. Precautions must be taken to protect the scope, because the fiberoptic bundles can be broken if the scope is bent at an acute angle. The patient wears a mouth guard to keep from biting the scope.

Nursing Interventions

The patient should be NPO for 8 hours prior to the examination. Before the introduction of the endoscope, the patient is given a local anesthetic gargle or spray. Midazolam (Versed), a sedative that provides moderate sedation with loss of the gag reflex and relieves anxiety during the procedure, is given. Atropine may be given to reduce secretions, and glucagon may be given to relax smooth muscle. The patient is positioned in the left lateral position to facilitate clearance of pulmonary secretions and provide smooth entry of the scope.

After gastroscopy, assessment includes level of consciousness, vital signs, oxygen saturation, pain level, and monitoring for signs of perforation (i.e., pain, bleeding, unusual difficulty swallowing, and rapidly elevated temperature). Temporary loss of the gag reflex is expected; after the patient's gag reflex has returned, lozenges, saline gargle, and oral analgesic agents may be offered to relieve minor throat discomfort. Patients who were sedated for the procedure must remain in bed until fully alert. After moderate sedation, the patient must be transported home with a family member or friend if the procedure was performed on an outpatient basis. Someone should stay with the patient until the morning after the procedure. Because of sedation, many patients will not remember postprocedure instructions. For this reason, discharge and follow-up verbal and written instructions are provided to the person accompanying the patient home, as well as to the patient. In addition, many endoscopy suites have a program in which a nurse telephones the patient the morning after the procedure to find out if the patient has any concerns or questions related to the procedure.

Fiberoptic Colonoscopy

Historically, direct visualization of the bowel was the only means to evaluate the colon, but virtual colonoscopy (also known as CT colonography) is now available. Virtual colonoscopy provides a computer-simulated view of the air-filled distended colon using conventional CT scanning (ACS, 2015c).

Direct visual inspection of the large intestine (anus, rectum, sigmoid, transcending and ascending colon) is possible by means of a flexible fiberoptic colonoscope (see Fig. 43-6). These scopes have the same capabilities as those used for EGD but are larger in diameter and longer. Still and video recordings can be used to document the procedure and findings.

This procedure is used commonly as a diagnostic aid and screening device. It is most frequently used for cancer screening and for surveillance in patients with previous colon cancer or polyps. See Chapter 15, Table 15-3 for details on the American Cancer Society's screening guidelines. In addition, tissue biopsies can be obtained as needed, and polyps can be removed and evaluated. Other uses of colonoscopy include the evaluation of patients with diarrhea of unknown cause,

occult bleeding, or anemia; further study of abnormalities detected on barium enema; and diagnosis, clarification, and determination of the extent of inflammatory or other bowel disease.

The procedure can be used to remove all visible polyps with a special snare and cautery through the colonoscope. Many colon cancers begin with adenomatous polyps of the colon; therefore, one goal of colonoscopic polypectomy is early detection and prevention of colorectal cancer. This procedure also can be used to treat areas of bleeding or stricture. The use of bipolar and unipolar coagulators and heater probes, as well as injections of sclerosing agents or vasoconstrictors, is possible during this procedure. Laser-compatible scopes provide laser therapy for bleeding lesions or colonic neoplasms. Bowel decompression (removal of intestinal contents to prevent gas and fluid from distending the coils of the intestine) can also be completed during the procedure.

Colonoscopy is performed while the patient is lying on the left side with the legs drawn up toward the chest. The patient's position may be changed during the test to facilitate advancement of the scope. Biopsy forceps or a cytology brush may be passed through the scope to obtain specimens for histology and cytology examinations. Complications during and after the procedure can include cardiac dysrhythmias and respiratory depression resulting from the medications given, vasovagal reactions, and circulatory overload or hypotension resulting from overhydration or underhydration during bowel preparation. The patient's cardiac and respiratory function and oxygen saturation are monitored continuously, with supplemental oxygen used as necessary. Typically, the procedure takes about 1 hour, and postprocedure discomfort results from instillation of air to expand the colon and insertion and movement of the scope during the procedure.

Capsule colonoscopy is another option for patients who cannot tolerate colonoscopy. This minimally invasive test consists of an ingestible capsule with a two-sided camera (similar to the PillCam ESO). This test requires that the patient completes the same type of extensive bowel preparation as for a colonoscopy. In addition, the patient must ingest a lot of fluids to ensure that the capsule transits through the colon (Garborg, 2015).

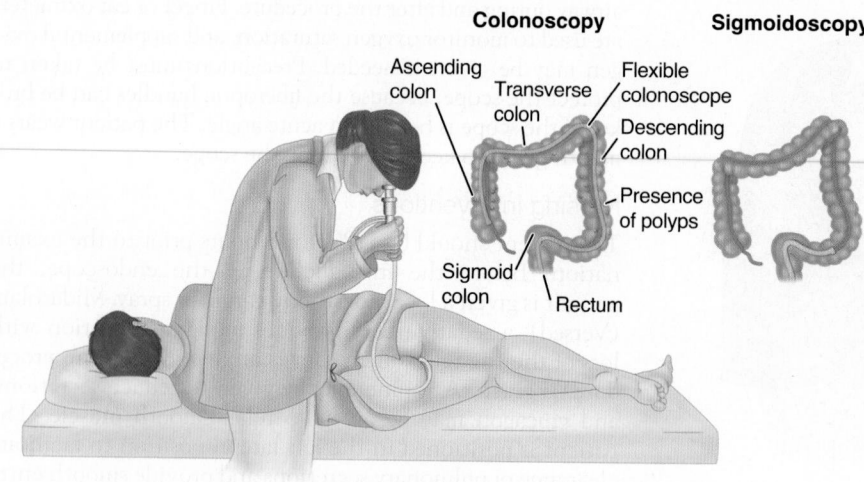

Colonoscopy

Ascending colon
Transverse colon
Sigmoid colon
Rectum

Sigmoidoscopy

Flexible colonoscope
Descending colon
Presence of polyps

Figure 43-6 • Colonoscopy and flexible fiberoptic sigmoidoscopy. For the colonoscopy, the flexible scope is passed through the rectum and sigmoid colon into the descending, transverse, and ascending colon. For the flexible fiberoptic sigmoidoscopy, the flexible scope is advanced past the proximal sigmoid and then into the descending colon.

Nursing Interventions

The success of colonoscopy depends on how well the colon is prepared (Chen et al., 2015). Adequate colon cleansing provides optimal visualization and decreases the time needed for the procedure. Cleansing of the colon can be accomplished in various ways. The primary provider may prescribe a laxative for two nights before the examination and a Fleet or saline enema until the return is clear the morning of the test. However, more commonly, PEG electrolyte lavage solutions (GoLYTELY, CoLyte, and NuLYTELY) are used as intestinal lavages for effective cleansing of the bowel. Current recommendations support use of 2-L PEG split-dose regimen in low or no risk patients, and 4-L split-dose with sodium picosulfate plus bisacodyl in patients with comorbidities such as diabetes, chronic constipation, or current history of opioid use, or with a history of problematic colonoscopies (Chen et al., 2015). The patient maintains a clear liquid diet starting at noon the day before the procedure. Then the patient ingests the lavage solution orally at intervals over 3 to 4 hours. If necessary, the nurse can give the solution through a feeding tube if the patient cannot swallow. Patients with a colostomy can receive this same bowel preparation. The use of lavage solutions is contraindicated in patients with intestinal obstruction or inflammatory bowel disease.

A sodium phosphate tablet (OsmoPrep, Visicol) can be used for colon cleansing prior to colonoscopy. Dosing consists of 32 tablets: 20 tablets (4 tablets every 15 minutes) with 8 oz of any clear liquid (water, any clear carbonated beverage, or juice) on the evening prior to the examination, and 12 tablets (taken in the same manner) on the morning of the examination.

With the use of lavage solutions, bowel cleansing is fast (rectal effluent is clear in about 4 hours) and is tolerated fairly well by most patients. Side effects of the electrolyte solutions include nausea, bloating, cramps or abdominal fullness, fluid and electrolyte imbalance, and hypothermia (patients are often told to drink the preparation as cold as possible to make it more palatable). The side effects are especially problematic for older adults, and sometimes they have difficulty ingesting the required volume of solution. Monitoring older patients after a bowel preparation is especially important because their physiologic ability to compensate for fluid loss is diminished. Many older adults take multiple medications each day; therefore, the nurse's knowledge of their daily medication regimen can prompt assessment for and prevention of potential problems and early detection of physiologic changes.

Additionally, the nurse advises the patient with diabetes to consult with their primary provider about medication adjustment to prevent hyperglycemia or hypoglycemia resulting from the dietary modifications required in preparing for the test. The nurse also instructs all patients, especially older adults, to maintain adequate fluid, electrolyte, and caloric intake while undergoing bowel cleansing.

Special precautions must be taken for some patients. Implantable defibrillators and pacemakers are at high risk for malfunction if electrosurgical procedures (i.e., polypectomy) are performed in conjunction with colonoscopy. A cardiologist should be consulted before the test is performed, and the defibrillator should be turned off. These patients require careful cardiac monitoring during the procedure.

Colonoscopy cannot be performed if there is a suspected or documented colon perforation, acute severe diverticulitis, or fulminant colitis. Patients with prosthetic heart valves or a history of endocarditis require prophylactic antibiotics before the procedure.

Informed consent is obtained by the practitioner before the patient is sedated. Before the examination, an opioid analgesic agent or sedative (e.g., midazolam) is given to provide moderate sedation and relieve anxiety during the procedure. Glucagon may be given, if needed, to relax the colonic musculature and to reduce spasm during the test. Older or debilitated patients may require a reduced dosage of the analgesic agent or sedative to decrease the risks of oversedation and cardiopulmonary complications.

During the procedure, the patient is monitored for changes in oxygen saturation, vital signs, color and temperature of the skin, level of consciousness, abdominal distention, vagal response, and pain intensity. After the procedure, patients are maintained on bed rest until fully alert. Some patients have abdominal cramps caused by increased peristalsis stimulated by the air insufflated into the bowel during the procedure.

Immediately after the test, the patient is monitored for signs and symptoms of bowel perforation (e.g., rectal bleeding, abdominal pain or distention, fever, focal peritoneal signs). Because of the amnesic effects of midazolam, the patient may be unable to recall verbal information and should receive written instructions. If the procedure is performed on an outpatient basis, someone must transport the patient home. After a therapeutic procedure, the nurse instructs the patient to report any bleeding to the primary provider.

Anoscopy, Proctoscopy, and Sigmoidoscopy

Endoscopic examination of the anus, rectum, and sigmoid and descending colon is used to evaluate chronic diarrhea, fecal incontinence, ischemic colitis, and lower GI hemorrhage and to observe for ulceration, fissures, abscesses, tumors, polyps, or other pathologic processes.

Flexible scopes have largely replaced the rigid scopes used in the past for routine examinations. The flexible fiberoptic sigmoidoscope (see Fig. 43-6) permits the colon to be examined up to 40 to 50 cm (16 to 20 inches) from the anus, much more than the 25 cm (10 inches) that can be visualized with the rigid sigmoidoscope. It has many of the same capabilities as the scopes used for the upper GI study, including the use of still or video images to document findings.

For flexible scope procedures, the patient assumes a comfortable position on the left side with the right leg bent and placed anteriorly. It is important to keep the patient informed throughout the examination and to explain the sensations associated with it. Biopsies and polypectomies can be performed during this procedure. Biopsy is performed with small biting forceps introduced through the endoscope; one or more small pieces of tissue may be removed. If polyps are present, they may be removed with a wire snare, which is used to grasp the pedicle, or stalk. An electrocoagulating current is then used to sever the polyp and prevent bleeding. It is extremely important that all excised tissue be placed immediately in moist gauze or in an appropriate receptacle, labeled correctly, and delivered without delay to the pathology laboratory for examination.

Nursing Interventions

These examinations require only limited bowel preparation, including a warm tap water or Fleet enema until returns are clear. Dietary restrictions usually are not necessary, and sedation usually is not required. During the procedure, the nurse monitors vital signs, skin color and temperature, pain tolerance, and vagal response. After the procedure, the nurse monitors the patient for rectal bleeding and signs of intestinal perforation (i.e., fever, rectal drainage, abdominal distention, and pain). On completion of the examination, the patient can resume their regular activities and diet.

Small Bowel Studies

Several methods are available for visualization of the small intestine, including capsule endoscopy and double-balloon enteroscopy. Capsule endoscopy allows the noninvasive visualization of the mucosa throughout the entire small intestine. It is particularly useful in the evaluation of obscure GI bleeding. The technique consists of the patient swallowing a capsule embedded with a wireless miniature camera, a light source, and an image transmission system. The capsule is the size of a large vitamin pill. It is propelled through the intestine by peristalsis. Images are transmitted from the end of the capsule to a recording device worn by the patient. Typically, the capsule passes from the rectum in 1 or 2 days. This procedure is limited because it is only diagnostic; it is not used to obtain specimens for biopsy or to treat conditions (ASGE, 2013a).

Double-balloon enteroscopy has made it possible to visualize the mucosa of the entire small bowel as well as carry out diagnostic and therapeutic interventions (ASGE, 2014). This endoscope is comprised of two balloons, one attached to the distal end of the scope and the other attached to the transparent overtube that slides over the endoscope. The endoscope is advanced alternately inflating and deflating the balloons; this causes telescoping of the small intestine onto the overtube. As a result of this telescoping, the endoscope can visualize much more of the small intestine than the length of the scope itself. The procedure takes between 1 and 3 hours and requires moderate sedation. Nursing interventions are similar to those for other endoscopic procedures.

Endoscopy Through an Ostomy

Endoscopy through an ostomy stoma is useful for visualizing a segment of the small or large intestine and may be indicated to evaluate the anastomosis for recurrent disease, or to visualize and treat bleeding in a segment of the bowel. Nursing interventions are similar to those for other endoscopic procedures.

Manometry and Electrophysiologic Studies

Manometry and electrophysiologic studies are methods for evaluating patients with GI motility disorders. The manometry test measures changes in intraluminal pressures and the coordination of muscle activity in the GI tract with the pressures transmitted to a computer analyzer.

Esophageal manometry is used to detect motility disorders of the esophagus and the upper and lower esophageal sphincter. Also known as esophageal motility studies, these studies are very helpful in the diagnosis of achalasia (i.e., absence of peristalsis), diffuse esophageal spasm, scleroderma, and other esophageal motor disorders. The patient must refrain from eating or drinking for 8 to 12 hours before the test. Medications that could have a direct effect on motility (e.g., calcium channel blockers, anticholinergic agents, sedatives) are withheld for 24 to 48 hours. A pressure-sensitive catheter is inserted through the nose and is connected to a transducer and a video recorder. The patient then swallows small amounts of water while the resultant pressure changes are recorded. Evaluation of a patient for gastroesophageal reflux disease typically includes esophageal manometry.

Gastroduodenal, small intestine, and colonic manometry procedures are used to evaluate delayed gastric emptying and gastric and intestinal motility disorders such as irritable bowel syndrome or atonic colon. This is often an ambulatory outpatient procedure lasting 24 to 72 hours. Anorectal manometry measures the resting tone of the internal anal sphincter and the contractibility of the external anal sphincter. It is helpful in evaluating patients with chronic constipation or fecal incontinence and is useful in biofeedback for the treatment of fecal incontinence. It can be performed in conjunction with rectal sensory functioning tests. Dibasic sodium (Phospho-soda) or a saline cleansing enema is given 1 hour before the test, and positioning for the test is either the prone or the lateral position.

Rectal sensory function studies are used to evaluate rectal sensory function and neuropathy. A catheter and balloon are passed into the rectum, with increasing balloon inflation until the patient feels distention. Then the tone and pressure of the rectum and anal sphincter are measured. The results are especially helpful in the evaluation of patients with chronic constipation, diarrhea, or incontinence.

Electrogastrography, an electrophysiologic study, also may be performed to assess gastric motility disturbances and can be useful in detecting motor or nerve dysfunction in the stomach. Electrodes are placed over the abdomen, and gastric electrical activity is recorded for up to 24 hours. Patients may exhibit rapid, slow, or irregular waveform activity.

Defecography measures anorectal function and is performed with very thick barium paste instilled into the rectum. Fluoroscopy is used to assess the function of the rectum and anal sphincter while the patient attempts to expel the barium. The test requires no preparation. The nurse educates the patient about what to expect during these procedures.

Gastric Analysis, Gastric Acid Stimulation Test, and pH Monitoring

Analysis of the gastric juice yields information about the secretory activity of the gastric mucosa and the presence or degree of gastric retention in patients thought to have pyloric or duodenal obstruction. It is also useful for diagnosing Zollinger–Ellison syndrome or atrophic gastritis.

The patient is NPO for 8 to 12 hours before the procedure. Any medications that affect gastric secretions are withheld for 24 to 48 hours before the test. Smoking is not allowed on the morning of the test because it increases gastric secretions. A small nasogastric tube with a catheter tip marked at various points is inserted through the nose. When the tube is at a point slightly less than 50 cm (21 inches), it should be within the stomach, lying along the greater curvature. Once in place, the tube is secured to the patient's cheek and the patient is placed in a semireclining position. The entire stomach contents are aspirated by gentle suction into a syringe, and gastric samples are collected every 15 minutes for the next hour.

Important diagnostic information to be gained from gastric analysis includes the ability of the mucosa to secrete HCl. This ability is altered in various disease states, including:

- *Pernicious anemia:* Patients with this disease secrete no acid under basal conditions or after stimulation.
- *Severe chronic atrophic gastritis or gastric cancer:* Patients with these diseases secrete little or no acid.
- *Gastric ulcer:* Patients with this disease secrete some acid.
- *Duodenal ulcers:* Patients with this disease usually secrete an excess amount of acid.

The gastric acid stimulation test usually is performed in conjunction with gastric analysis. Histamine or pentagastrin is given subcutaneously to stimulate gastric secretions. It is important to inform the patient that this injection may produce a flushed feeling. The nurse monitors the patient's blood pressure and pulse frequently to detect hypotension. Gastric specimens are collected after the injection every 15 minutes for 1 hour and are labeled to indicate the time of specimen collection after histamine injection. The volume and pH of the specimen are measured; in certain instances, cytologic study by the Papanicolaou technique may be used to determine the presence or absence of malignant cells.

Esophageal reflux of gastric acid may be diagnosed by ambulatory pH monitoring (Ang, Fock, Law, et al., 2015). The patient is NPO for 6 hours before the test, and all medications affecting gastric secretions are withheld for 24 to 36 hours before the test. A probe that measures pH is inserted through the nose and into position about 12.7 cm (5 inches) above the lower esophageal sphincter. It is connected to an external recording device and is worn for 24 hours while the patient continues usual daily activities. The result is a computer analysis and graphic display of the results.

The Bravo pH monitoring system offers the advantage of pH monitoring of the esophagus without the transnasal catheter. The clinician, by means of endoscopy, attaches a capsule (approximately the size of a gel cap) to the patient's esophageal wall. Data related to pH are transmitted from the capsule to a pager-sized receiver that the patient wears. Data are collected for up to 48 hours and then downloaded and analyzed. The capsule spontaneously detaches from the esophagus in 7 to 10 days and then is passed through the patient's digestive system. The accuracy of this method of pH testing is greater than methods in which a catheter is used because the patient can eat normally and continue typical activities during the testing. The patient is evaluated for both acid reflux and non-acid reflux events (Ang et al., 2015).

Laparoscopy (Peritoneoscopy)

With the tremendous advances in minimally invasive surgery, diagnostic laparoscopy is efficient, cost-effective, and useful in the diagnosis of GI disease. After a pneumoperitoneum (injecting carbon dioxide into the peritoneal cavity to separate the intestines from the pelvic organs) is created, a small incision is made lateral to the umbilicus, allowing for the insertion of the fiberoptic laparoscope. This permits direct visualization of the organs and structures within the abdomen, permitting visualization and identification of any growths, anomalies, and inflammatory processes. In addition, biopsy samples can be taken from the structures and organs as necessary. This procedure can be used to evaluate peritoneal disease, chronic abdominal pain, abdominal masses, and gallbladder and liver disease. However, laparoscopy has not become an important diagnostic modality in patients with acute abdominal pain, because less invasive tools (e.g., CT and MRI scans) are readily available. Laparoscopy usually requires general anesthesia and sometimes requires that the stomach and bowel be decompressed. Gas (usually carbon dioxide) is insufflated into the peritoneal cavity to create a working space for visualization. One of the benefits of this procedure is that after visualization of a problem, excision (e.g., removal of the gallbladder) can then be performed at the same time, if appropriate.

CRITICAL THINKING EXERCISES

1 **pg** You are caring for a 45-year-old man recently admitted to the emergency department (ED) with new onset of diffuse abdominal discomfort and nausea for the past 10 hours. He has a history of hypertension. Identify questions that should be asked when taking the patient's history. What are your priority assessments? What diagnostic tests would you expect? While in the ED, the patient reports that the pain has localized to the right lower quadrant. Given this new development, what questions will you now ask and what are your priority assessments?

2 **pg** You are working in a family practice clinic. A 45-year-old female comes into the office for a sick visit. She reports symptoms of abdominal pain, distention and bloating with episodes of constipation and diarrhea. The symptoms have been present for some time and seem to be worsening. Identify questions that should be asked when taking the patient's history. What assessment parameters would be addressed? What are your priority assessments? What diagnostic tests would you expect?

3 **ebp** You are working in a medical internist's office. A 56-year-old female patient comes into the office for a routine examination. She states that she has not been screened for colorectal cancer because no one in her family has colon cancer. However, she wants to discuss her options. The patient read on the internet that there are several diagnostic tests available for colorectal cancer screening. The patient asks you what test is recommended. How will you answer this question? What is the evidence base that supports your response? Discuss the strength of the evidence for this information. Identify the criteria used to evaluate the strength of the evidence.

REFERENCES

*Asterisk indicates nursing research

Books

Bontrager, K. L., & Lampignano, J. P. (2014). *Textbook of radiographic positioning and related anatomy* (8th ed.). St. Louis, MO: Elsevier.

Eliopoulos, C. (2018). *Gerontological nursing* (9th ed.). Philadelphia, PA: Lippincott Williams & Wilkins.

Fischbach, F., & Dunning, M. B. (2015). *A manual of laboratory and diagnostic tests* (9th ed.). Philadelphia, PA: Wolters Kluwer Health.

Grossman, S. C., & Porth, C. M. (2014). *Porth's pathophysiology. Concepts of altered health states* (9th ed.). Philadelphia, PA: Lippincott Williams & Wilkins.

Weber, J. R., & Kelley, J. H. (2014). *Health assessment in nursing.* (5th ed.). Philadelphia, PA: Lippincott Williams & Wilkins.

Journals and Electronic Documents

Achem, S. R., & DeVault, K. R. (2014). Gastroesophageal reflux disease and the elderly. *Gastroenterology Clinics of North America, 43*(1), 147–160.

American Cancer Society (ACS). (2015a). *Cancer facts & figures 2015.* Atlanta, GA: Author.

American Cancer Society (ACS). (2015b). *Cancer glossary.* Atlanta, GA: Author.

American Cancer Society (ACS). (2015c). *CT colonography (virtual colonoscopy).* Atlanta, GA: Author.

American Society for Gastrointestinal Endoscopy (ASGE). (2013a). *Understanding capsule endoscopy.* Retrieved on 5/31/2016 at: www.asge.org/publications/publications.aspx?id=390&terms=capsule%20endoscopy

American Society for Gastrointestinal Endoscopy (ASGE). (2013b). *Understanding ERCP.* Retrieved 5/31/2016 at: www.asge.org/publications/publications.aspx?id=386&terms=ercp

American Society for Gastrointestinal Endoscopy (ASGE). (2013c). *Understanding upper endoscopy.* Retrieved 5/31/2016 at: www.asge.org/publications/publications.aspx?id=378&terms=upper endoscopy

American Society for Gastrointestinal Endoscopy (ASGE). (2014). *Balloon assisted or "Deep" enteroscopy.* Retrieved on 5/31/2016 at: www.asge.org/press/press.aspx?id=8138

Ang, D., Fock, K. M., Law, N. M., et al. (2015). Current status of functional gastrointestinal evaluation in clinical practice. *Singapore Medical Journal, 56*(2), 69–80.

Cartwright, S. L., & Knudson, M. P. (2015). Diagnostic imaging of acute abdominal pain in adults. *American Family Physician, 91*(7), 452–459.

Chen, J., Athilingam, P., Saloum, Y., et al. (2015). Enhancing bowel preparation for screening colonoscopy: An evidence-based literature review. *The Journal for Nurse Practitioners, 11*(5), 519–525.

Deek, H., Newton, P., Sheerin, N., et al. (2014). Contrast media induced nephropathy: A literature review of the available evidence and recommendations for practice. *Australian Critical Care, 27*(4), 166–171.

Garborg, K. (2015). Colorectal cancer screening. *Surgical Clinics of North America, 95*(5), 979–989.

Kanal, E., Barkovich, A. J., Bell, C., et al. (2013). ACR guidance document on MR safe practices: 2013. *Journal of Magnetic Resonance Imaging, 37*(3), 501–530.

Kar, P., Jones, K. L., Horowitz, M., et al. (2015). Measurement of gastric emptying in the critically ill. *Clinical Nutrition, 34*(4), 557–564.

Li, B., Wang, J., & Ma, Y. (2012). Bowel sounds and monitoring gastrointestinal motility in critically ill patients. *Clinical Nurse Specialist, 26*(1), 29–34.

Overland, M. K. (2014). Dyspepsia. *Medical Clinics of North America, 98*(2014), 549–564.

Peralta, R., & Contreras Pena, F. A. (2015). Capsule endoscopy. MedScape. Retrieved on 12/18/2016 at: emedicine.medscape.com/article/197525-overview#a2

Rawson, J. V., & Pelletier, A. L. (2013). When to order contrast-enhanced CT. *American Family Physician, 88*(5), 312–316.

Rustagi, T., & Jamidar, P. A. (2015). Endoscopic retrograde cholangiopancreatography (ERCP)-related adverse events. *Gastrointestinal Endoscopy Clinics of North America, 25*(1), 107–121.

*Schultz, H., Qvist, N., Morgensen, C. B., et al. (2013). Experiences of patients with acute abdominal pain in the ED or acute surgical ward–A qualitative comparative study. *International Emergency Nursing, 21*(4), 228–235.

Standeven, L., Hiller, J. P., Mulder, K., et al. (2013). Impact of dedicated cancer center surveillance program on guideline adherence for patients with stage II and III colorectal cancer. *Clinical Colorectal Cancer, 12*(2), 103–112.

Wong, M. C., Ching, J. Y., Chan, V. C., et al. (2015). Factors associated with false-positive and false-negative fecal immunochemical test results for colorectal cancer screening. *Gastrointestinal Endoscopy, 81*(3), 596–607.

Resources

American Cancer Society, www.cancer.org
American Society for Gastrointestinal Endoscopy (ASGE), www.asge.org
Society of Gastroenterology Nurses and Associates (SGNA), www.sgna.org

44

Digestive and Gastrointestinal Treatment Modalities

GLOSSARY

aspiration: removal of substance by suction or the inhalation of fluids or foods into the trachea and bronchial tree

bolus feeding: a feeding given into the stomach in large amounts and at designated intervals

central venous access device (CVAD): a device designed and used for administration of sterile fluids, nutrition formulas, and medications into central veins

cyclic feeding: periodic infusion of feedings given over 8 to 18 hours

decompression (gastric/intestinal): removal of gastric or intestinal contents to prevent gas and fluid distention

dumping syndrome: physiologic response to rapid emptying of gastric contents into the small intestine, manifested by nausea, weakness, sweating, palpitations, syncope, and possibly diarrhea

duodenum: the first part of the small intestine, which arises from the pylorus of the stomach and extends to the jejunum

enteral nutrition: nutritional formula feedings infused through a tube directly into the gastrointestinal tract

enteric: of or relating to the intestines

gastroparesis: partial paralysis of the stomach that results in decreased gastric motility and emptying

gastrostomy: surgical creation of an opening into the stomach for the purpose of administering fluids, nutrition formulas, and medications or for decompression and drainage of stomach contents

intravenous fat emulsion (IVFE or lipid): an oil-in-water emulsion of oils, egg phospholipids, and glycerin; also referred to as intravenous lipid emulsion

intubation: the insertion or placement of a tube into a body structure or passageway

jejunostomy: surgical creation of an opening into the jejunum for the purpose of administering fluids, nutrition formulas, and medications

jejunum: second portion of the small intestine, which extends from the duodenum to the ileum

lavage: flushing of the stomach with water or other fluids with a gastric tube to clear it

lumen: the channel within a tube or catheter

nasoduodenal tube: tube inserted through the nose into the proximal portion of the small intestine (i.e., duodenum)

nasoenteric tube: tube inserted through the nose into the stomach and beyond the pylorus into the small intestine

nasogastric (NG) tube: tube inserted through the nose into the stomach

nasojejunal tube: tube inserted through the nose into the second portion of the small intestine (i.e., jejunum)

orogastric tube: tube inserted through the mouth into the stomach

osmolality: ionic concentration of fluid

parenteral nutrition (PN): method of supplying nutrients to the body by an intravenous route

percutaneous endoscopic gastrostomy (PEG): a feeding tube inserted endoscopically into the stomach

peripherally inserted central catheter (PICC): a device inserted into a peripheral vein and designed and used for administration of sterile fluids, nutrition formulas, and medications into central veins

peristalsis: wavelike movement that occurs involuntarily in the alimentary canal

radiopaque: can be easily localized on x-ray

stoma: artificially created opening between a body cavity (e.g., stomach or intestine) and the body surface

stylet: a stiff wire placed in a catheter or other tube that allows the tube to maintain its shape during insertion

total nutrient admixture (TNA): an admixture of lipid emulsions, proteins, carbohydrates, electrolytes, vitamins, trace minerals, and water

Nurses encounter patients using digestive and gastrointestinal treatment modalities across many practice settings. This chapter presents several topics related to gastrointestinal (GI) intubation, including managing the care of patients with gastric, enteric, gastrostomy and jejunostomy tubes and those with gastric drainage; providing enteral tube feedings; and educating patients about home care. In addition, parenteral nutrition (PN) is presented, including general indications for this nutritional modality and nursing care of patients receiving PN.

Gastrointestinal Intubation

GI **intubation** is the insertion of a flexible tube into the stomach, or beyond the pylorus into the **duodenum** (the first section of the small intestine) or the **jejunum** (the second section of the small intestine). The tube may be inserted through the mouth, the nose, or the abdominal wall. The tubes are of various diameters (French [Fr] size) and lengths, depending on their intended use. GI intubation may be performed in order to:

- Decompress the stomach and remove gas and fluid
- **Lavage** (flush with water or other fluids) the stomach and remove ingested toxins or other harmful materials
- Diagnose GI disorders
- Administer tube feedings, fluids, and medications
- Compress a bleeding site
- Aspirate GI contents for analysis

Tube Types

Gastric Tubes for Decompression, Drainage, Aspiration, and Lavage

A variety of tubes are used for decompression, drainage, **aspiration** (removal of substances by suction), and lavage of the stomach. Gastric tubes may also be labeled by their point of origin and end points. For instance, an **orogastric tube** is a large-bore tube inserted through the mouth into the stomach that contains a wide outlet for removal of gastric contents. Gastric tubes, commonly called **nasogastric (NG) tubes**, are introduced through the nose into the stomach, often before or during surgery or at the bedside, to remove fluid and gas from the upper GI tract by the process known as **decompression**

(gastric/intestinal). Other tubes, such as the Sengstaken–Blakemore and the Minnesota tube, are used to treat bleeding esophageal varices (see Chapter 49). Commonly used gastric tubes include the Levin and the Salem Sump tube (see Table 44-1).

Levin Tube

The Levin tube has a single **lumen** (channel within a tube or catheter) and is made of plastic or rubber. This tube is connected to low intermittent suction (30 to 40 mmHg) to avoid erosion or tearing of the stomach lining, which can result from adherence of the tube's lumen to the mucosa of the stomach. If this type of tube is removed inadvertently in a patient who has undergone esophageal or gastric surgery, it is usually replaced by the surgeon with care to avoid trauma to the suture line.

Salem Sump

The Salem Sump tube is a **radiopaque** (easily seen on x-ray), clear plastic, double-lumen gastric tube. The inner, smaller lumen (known as the blue port) vents the larger suction-drainage tube to the atmosphere by means of an opening at the distal end of the tube. The sump tube can protect fragile gastric mucosa by maintaining a low (25 mmHg) continuous force of suction at the drainage opening. The suction lumen may be irrigated to maintain patency.

The blue vent lumen should be kept above the patient's waist to prevent reflux of gastric contents through it; otherwise, it acts as a siphon. A one-way antireflux valve (prevents return or backward flow of fluid) seated in the blue pigtail can prevent the reflux of gastric contents out the vent lumen (see Fig. 44-1). The valve is removed for irrigation of the suction lumen. To reestablish a buffer of air between the gastric contents and the valve, 20 mL of air is injected through the blue vent with a catheter tip syringe and the valve is reinserted.

Nursing Management

The nurse explains the purpose of the tube to the patient prior to insertion to promote cooperation during the procedure. The general activities related to inserting the tube are then reviewed, including the fact that the procedure may cause gagging until the tube has passed beyond the throat. Periodically, the gastric tube's placement must be verified.

TABLE 44-1 Selected Gastric and Enteric Tubes

Tube Type	Length (cm)	Size (French)	Lumen	Other Characteristics
Gastric Tubes				
Levin (plastic or rubber)	125	14–18	Single	Circular markings at intervals along the tube serve as guidelines for insertion.
Salem Sump (plastic)	120	12–18	Double	Smaller lumen acts as a vent.
Moss	90	12–16	Triple	Contains both a gastric decompression lumen and a duodenal lumen for postoperative feedings.
Sengstaken–Blakemore (rubber)			Triple	Two lumens are used to inflate the gastric and esophageal balloons, and one tube is reserved for suction or drainage.
Enteric Feeding Tube				
Dobhoff or EnteraFlo (polyurethane or silicone rubber)	160–175	8–12	Single	Tungsten-weighted tip, radiopaque, stylet.

Figure 44-1 • Salem Sump tube equipped with a one-way valve that allows air to enter and can prevent reflux of gastric contents. The antireflux valve is designed with a pressure-activated air buffer (PAAB). The buffer is activated (1) and the valve closes (2) when pressure from gastric contents enters the tubing. ©2017 Medtronic. All rights reserved. Used with the permission of Medtronic.

For the procedural guidelines for inserting and confirming placement of a gastric tube, go to **thepoint.lww.com/Brunner14e.**

Gastric tubes used for decompression and drainage are connected to a wall mounted suction regulator and canister or to a suction machine. It is the nurse's responsibility to ensure that the suction is set at the prescribed pressure. Drainage should be assessed and noted as consistent with gastric drainage. Sterile saline or water can be used as irrigants, if prescribed and as needed, to keep the system patent. The nurse records the amount, color, and type of drainage. The nurse must ensure that oral and nasal hygiene are maintained to prevent discomfort, skin breakdown, and infection (see later discussion under feeding tubes: Providing Oral and Nasal Hygiene). When the gastric tube may be removed, the nurse explains the procedure to the patient and assesses for nausea and distention, delaying removal and notifying the primary provider if these are present.

For the procedural guidelines for gastric tube removal, go to **thepoint.lww.com/ Brunner14e.**

Gastric and Enteric Tubes for Administration of Tube Feedings, Fluids, and Medications

Some enteral tubes are manufactured to administer tube feedings, fluids, and medications. These tubes are made of various materials, including rubber, polyurethane, and silicone. They vary in length, diameter (Fr size), purpose, and placement in the GI tract. They are smaller bore (generally 5 to 12 Fr) than the tubes made for gastric decompression and drainage, which lessens patient discomfort and nasal irritation. An orally or nasally placed feeding tube is for short-term use and should stay in place for no more than 4 weeks before being replaced

with a new tube (Brantley & Mills, 2012) (see later discussion on stomal tubes). Any feeding solution given through a tube is regulated by a feeding infusion pump, poured through a syringe, or delivered by gravity drip.

Gastric or **enteric** (of or relating to the intestines) feeding tubes are used for patients who have the ability to receive and process nutrition, fluids, and medications adequately by the gastric route. For patients who have **gastroparesis** (reduced stomach motility), severe gastroesophageal reflux disease, impaired glottic closure, or undergone partial or total gastrectomy, or otherwise are at risk for **aspiration** (inhalation of substances into the airways), a **nasoenteric tube** (i.e., inserted through the nose into the stomach and beyond the pylorus into the small intestine) or oroenteric tube (i.e., inserted from the mouth to the small intestine) for feeding can be used.

Enteric tubes placed in the duodenum via the nares are called **nasoduodenal tubes**, whereas those placed in the jejunum (the portion of the small intestine distal to the duodenum) via the nares are called **nasojejunal tubes**. They can be inserted at the bedside, during surgery, fluoroscopically, or endoscopically. Due to the risk of complications associated with blind insertion of small bowel feeding tubes, some organizations only allow physicians or advanced practice clinicians (e.g., nurse practitioners, physician assistants) to insert these tubes (Hodin & Bordeianou, 2015). The nurse should demonstrate competency in and knowledge of small bowel feeding tube placement according to the Nurse Practice Act applicable in their state and should follow the rules and regulations, organizational policies and procedures, and practice guidelines of that state's board of nursing. Nasally inserted feeding tubes are soft and pliable; therefore, they may kink when a **stylet** (a stiff wire placed in a catheter or other tube that allows the tube to maintain its shape) is not used during insertion, particularly if the patient is unable to swallow. However, caution is required when inserting feeding tubes with a stylet because there is a risk of tissue puncture or placement error. Some enteric feeding tubes are weighted at the tip to facilitate movement into the duodenum; others are nonweighted.

Enteric tubes are never inserted in patients with basilar skull fractures, in those who have had maxillofacial surgery (including transsphenoidal approaches) or facial trauma, or in those with uncontrolled coagulation abnormalities (Hodin & Bordeianou, 2015). Nurses should also use caution when inserting these tubes in patients with esophageal varices due to the increased risk of bleeding.

During nasal insertion, the tip of the tube is initially directed toward the back of the nose, through the esophagus and into the stomach, and is further advanced through the pylorus into the small intestine if warranted. Fluoroscopic techniques may be used to visually direct feeding tubes into the stomach, duodenum, or jejunum. Several bedside techniques may be used to facilitate tube tip placements into the small intestine. These techniques include using air insufflation or manipulating the tube itself as it is being inserted (e.g., using a "corkscrew" technique). Research findings are inconclusive regarding the efficacy of prokinetic agents such as metoclopramide (Reglan) or erythromycin to facilitate movement of the feeding tube by **peristalsis** (involuntary wavelike movement) into the duodenum (Heuschkel & Duggan, 2015).

Some postpyloric feeding tubes, such as the Cortrak Enteral Access System or the Syncro BlueTube, have a magnetized tip and an external magnet device that is used with a bedside monitor to provide a visual guide during insertion. Use of these specific tubes precludes the need for postinsertion x-ray placement verification (Smithard, Barrett, Hargroves, et al., 2015). Although still widely used in practice, small bowel feeding tubes with tungsten-weighted tips do not always facilitate migration of the tube from the stomach into the intestine (Heuschkel & Duggan, 2015).

Clearing Tube Obstruction

If it is difficult to instill or withdraw contents from a feeding tube, several declogging steps can be taken, including warm water irrigation, milking the tube, infusing digestive enzymes, and employing mechanical declogging devices.

For the procedural guidelines for declogging a feeding tube, go to **thepoint.lww.com/ Brunner14e.**

A premanufactured declogging kit, such as the Clog Zapper, contains a syringe filled with enzymatic powder that is activated by pulling in water. An elongated hollow catheter is attached to this syringe so that the declogging solution gains close proximity to the clog. Inserting and twisting endoscopy or cytology brushes and commercial mechanical declogger devices into the feeding tube can only be used with larger-bore tubes and should be performed only by experienced providers. Of note, even though cola and cranberry juice are sometimes used to declog tubes, these fluids are not advocated because their acidic nature has been shown to worsen formula clogs by causing precipitation of proteins (Metheny, Eisenberg, & McSweeney, 1988; Nicalou & Davis, 1990; Wilson & Hayes-Johnson, 1987).

Quality and Safety Nursing Alert

Feeding tubes are more successfully declogged when intervention is initiated immediately after the obstruction is noted.

Monitoring the Patient and Maintaining Tube Function

Tubes used for **enteral nutrition** are attached to enteral delivery tubing or a syringe that contains the feeding formula. They can be connected continuously for pump feedings or intermittently (**bolus feeding**) so that the end of the tube may be capped between feedings. Malposition or dislodgement of the tube may be caused by tension on the tube with patient movement, coughing, suctioning, or airway intubation.

The nurse must keep an accurate record of all fluid intake, feedings, and irrigation volumes. To maintain patency, the tube is irrigated with water after every feeding and medication delivery and every 4 to 6 hours during continuous feedings, or if the tube is set to gravity drainage or suction. Sterile saline or water, or tap water can be used as irrigants, depending on the patient's electrolyte levels and ability to fight infection.

The nurse records the amount, color, and type of drainage. When double- or triple-lumen tubes are used, each lumen is labeled according to its intended use for drainage, medication delivery, or feeding.

Providing Oral and Nasal Hygiene

Regular, conscientious oral and nasal hygiene is a vital part of patient care because the tube may cause discomfort and pressure, and may be in place for an extended length of time. The nose is inspected daily for skin irritation, and the nasal tape is changed every 3 days and as needed. If the nasal and pharyngeal mucosae are excessively dry, steam or cool vapor inhalations may be beneficial. Throat lozenges, an ice collar, chewing gum, or sucking on hard candies (if permitted) and limiting talking also assist in relieving patient discomfort.

Monitoring and Managing Potential Complications

Patients with gastric or enteric intubation are susceptible to a variety of problems, including inadvertent misconnections and administrations, fluid volume deficit, pulmonary complications, and tube-related irritations. These potential complications require careful ongoing assessment.

The Institute for Safe Medication Practices (ISMP) has reported significant errors with inadvertent administration of liquid enteral medications into intravenous (IV) lines. To create a safer environment, a new industry-wide standard for enteral feeding connectors (which are incompatible with Luer lock or small-bore syringes) known as the ENFit is in the process of being fully implemented for use in all feeding tubes, feeding syringes, and feeding administration sets (ISMP, 2015; Joint Commission, 2014) (see Fig. 44-2).

The nurse should be vigilant for symptoms of fluid volume deficit in patients receiving enteral nutrition. These can include dry skin and mucous membranes, decreased urinary output, lethargy, lightheadedness, hypotension, and increased heart rate. Assessment involves maintaining an accurate record of intake and output (I&O). This includes measuring fluid intake from tube feeding and flushes, oral liquids, and intravenous (IV) fluids. Output of urine, emesis, gastric drainage, diarrhea, ostomies, fistulas, and drainage tubes should also be measured. The nurse assesses 24-hour fluid balance and reports negative fluid balance (output greater than intake, increased gastric tube output, interruption of IV therapy, or any other disturbance in fluid I&O). See Chapter 13 for further discussion of fluid volume deficit.

Pulmonary complications from gastric intubation can occur because coughing and clearing of the pharynx are impaired. Tubes may become malpositioned, retracting the distal end above the esophagogastric sphincter. Aspiration pneumonia occurs when regurgitated stomach contents or enteral feedings from an improperly positioned feeding tube are instilled into the pharynx or the trachea or when oral secretions are aspirated. Feeding patients through tubes placed beyond the pylorus or using prokinetic agents (e.g., erythromycin, metoclopramide) can decrease the frequency of feeding regurgitation and aspiration. In addition, feedings and medications should always be given with the patient in the semi-Fowler position, and the patient's head should be elevated at least 30 to 45 degrees to reduce the risk of reflux and pulmonary aspiration. This position is maintained at least 1 hour after completion of an intermittent tube feeding and is maintained

Figure 44-2 • **A.** ENFit connections on tubing. **B.** ENFit connection on syringe. **C.** ENFit connections on feeding bag. Reprinted with permission from Medline Industries.

whenever possible for patients receiving continuous tube feedings. A reverse Trendelenburg position can be considered when it is not possible or advisable to elevate the head of the patient's bed.

Patients at risk for aspiration pneumonia include those older than 70 years of age, unable to protect their airways, with altered mental status or other neurologic deficits, receiving mechanical ventilation, with gastric or enteral tubes, and in the supine position (McClave, Taylor, Martindale, et al., 2016). Although it has been thought that enteral feedings should be withheld when patients receiving mechanical ventilation are repositioned, research findings question the advisability of this practice (DiLebero, Lavieri, O'Donoghue, et al., 2015) (see Chart 44-1).

Signs and symptoms of pulmonary complications include coughing during the administration of foods or medications, difficulty clearing the airway, tachypnea, and fever. Assessment includes regular auscultation of lung sounds and monitoring of vital signs and laboratory values. The nurse also carefully confirms the proper placement of the tube with a

variety of methods before instilling any fluids or medications. If tube position is ever in question, radiographic confirmation is essential (Metheny, 2016).

Administering Tube Feedings

Tube feedings are given to meet nutritional requirements when oral intake is inadequate or not possible and the GI tract is functional. The feedings are delivered to the stomach, duodenum, or proximal jejunum and help preserve GI integrity by preserving normal intestinal and hepatic metabolism. Tube feedings have several advantages over parenteral nutrition (PN): they are lower in cost, safer, usually well tolerated by the patient, and easier to use in extended-care facilities and in the patient's home.

Nasoduodenal or nasojejunal feeding is indicated when the esophagus and stomach need to be bypassed or when the patient is at risk for aspiration. For tube feedings longer than 4 weeks, gastrostomy or jejunostomy tubes are preferred for administration of medications or nutrition. Indications for enteral nutrition are summarized in Table 44-2.

Chart 44-1 NURSING RESEARCH PROFILE
Enteral Feedings During Repositioning and the Incidence of Aspiration

DiLibero, J., Lavieri, M., O'Donoghue, S., et al. (2015). Withholding or continuing enteral feedings during repositioning and the incidence of aspiration. *American Journal of Critical Care*, 24(3), 258–261.

Purpose

The practice of continuing or withholding enteral feedings during repositioning of patients who are critically ill and mechanically ventilated varies among nurses, and is not necessarily research based. The purpose of this study was to see if there were differences in the incidence of aspiration between patients receiving mechanical ventilation and enteral feedings whose enteral feedings were either continued or stopped during repositioning.

Design

Twenty three adult patients who were intubated and mechanically ventilated in medical or surgical intensive care units and who were receiving enteral feedings at rates of at least 50 mL/hr comprised the study sample. Participants were required to tolerate backrest elevation of at least 30 degrees and maintain gastric residual volumes less than 200 mL. A crossover design was utilized, which allowed each patient to serve as their own control. Two samples of subglottal secretions were obtained on each participant, one during repositioning when feedings were withheld, and another during repositioning when feedings were continued ($N = 46$). The specimens were tested for presence of pepsin, which would indicate aspiration.

Findings

Of the 23 patients, 13 were admitted to medical intensive care units and 10 were admitted to surgical intensive care units. Patients were 31–91 years old (median, 64 years). Enteral feeding rates were 30 –75 mL/hr (mean; 52 mL/h; SD, 12.3 mL/hr). Feeding rates did not change between the time of collection of the first and second set of subglottal specimens.

There was no significant difference between the incidence of aspiration during repositioning when enteral feedings were withheld or when they were continued.

Nursing Implications

Results from this study suggest that precautionary withholding of enteral feedings during repositioning does not seem to reduce the incidence of aspiration in patients who are mechanically ventilated. However, further research is needed to provide definitive evidence for optimal enteral feeding practices.

Osmolality

The **osmolality** of normal body fluids (i.e., ionic concentration) is approximately 300 mOsm/kg. The body attempts to keep the osmolality of the contents of the stomach and intestines at this level. Osmolality is an important consideration for patients receiving tube feedings through the duodenum or jejunum because feeding formulas with a high osmolality may lead to undesirable effects. For example, when a concentrated solution of high osmolality entering the intestines is taken in quickly or in large amounts, water moves rapidly into the intestinal lumen from fluid surrounding the organs and the vascular compartment. The patient may have feelings of fullness, nausea, cramping, dizziness, diaphoresis, and osmotic diarrhea, collectively termed **dumping syndrome**. This can lead to dehydration, hypotension, and tachycardia. Patients fed by the small intestinal route vary in the degree to which they tolerate the effects of high osmolality; the nurse needs to be knowledgeable about the patient's formula and take steps to prevent this undesired effect. The small intestines may be able to adapt to a formula of high osmolality if it is initiated at a low hourly rate that is advanced slowly (Seres, 2016).

Formulas

The choice of formula to be delivered by tube feeding is influenced by the status of the GI tract and the nutritional needs of the patient. Formula characteristics that are considered include the chemical composition of the nutrient source (protein, carbohydrates, fat), caloric density, osmolality, fiber content, vitamins, minerals, electrolytes, and cost. Enteral formulas contain 70% to 85% free water and are not designed to meet total fluids needs (Seres, 2016). A wide variety of containers, delivery systems, and enteral pumps are available for use with tube feedings.

Various tube feeding formulas are available commercially. Polymeric formulas are the most common; are composed of protein, carbohydrates, and fats in a high–molecular-weight form, and require that the patient has normal digestive function. Chemically defined or "predigested" formulas contain easier-to-absorb nutrients. Modular products contain only one major nutrient, such as protein, and are used to enhance commercially prepared products. Disease-specific formulas

TABLE 44-2 Conditions that may Require Enteral Therapy

Condition or Need	Examples
Alcoholism, chronic depression, anorexia nervosa[a]	Chronic illness, psychiatric or neurologic disorder
Cancer therapy	Radiation, chemotherapy
Coma, semiconsciousness[a]	Stroke, head injury, neurologic disorder, neoplasm
Convalescent care	Surgery, injury, severe illness
Debilitation[a]	Disease or injury
Gastrointestinal problems	Fistula, short-bowel syndrome, mild pancreatitis, Crohn's disease, ulcerative colitis, nonspecific maldigestion or malabsorption
Hypermetabolic conditions	Burns, trauma, multiple fractures, sepsis, acquired immunodeficiency syndrome, organ transplantation
Maxillofacial or cervical surgery	Disease or injury
Oropharyngeal or esophageal paralysis[a]	Disease or injury, neoplasm, inflammation, trauma, respiratory failure
Preoperative bowel preparation	After administration of larger-volume cathartics

[a]Because some patients with these conditions are at risk for regurgitating or vomiting and aspirating administered formula, each condition must be considered individually.

are available as adjuncts to treat various conditions. Fiber, either premixed in or added to formulas, helps bulk the stool to decrease the occurrence of both diarrhea and constipation (McClave et al., 2016).

Some feedings are given as supplements, and others are given to meet the patient's total nutritional needs. Dietitians and certified nutrition support clinicians collaborate with primary providers and nurses to determine the best formula for each patient. The volume of formula delivered varies depending on the caloric density of the formula and the energy needs of the patient. The overall goal is to achieve positive nitrogen balance and weight maintenance or gain without producing discomfort or diarrhea.

Administration Methods

The tube feeding method chosen depends on the location of the tube in the GI tract, patient tolerance, convenience, and cost. Large-bore (larger than 12 Fr) gastric tubes can be uncomfortable and their usefulness for tube feedings is limited; however, they may be used for administration of feedings for several days (Brantley & Mills, 2012). Small-bore tubes manufactured for tube feedings are better tolerated; however, they require diligent monitoring and frequent flushing to remain patent.

Bolus and intermittent drip tube feeding methods are practical and inexpensive options for the patient receiving tube feedings who resides at home or in a long-term care facility; however, they may be poorly tolerated in patients who are acutely ill. Bolus feedings typically are divided into 3 to 4 feedings daily and can be given into the stomach through a large syringe with a plunger or by gravity (see Fig. 44-3). Bolus feedings can be delivered as quickly as the patient can tolerate them but are initiated slowly, increasing the rate as tolerated. With gravity feedings, raising or lowering the syringe above the abdominal wall regulates the rate of flow. The amount and flow rate is often determined by the patient's reaction. If the patient feels full, it may be desirable to slow the delivery time or give smaller volumes more frequently. The intermittent gravity drip feeding method requires administering feedings over 30 minutes or longer at designated intervals by a reservoir enteral bag and tubing,

Figure 44-3 • Bolus gastrostomy feeding by gravity. Syringe is raised perpendicular to the abdomen so that feeding can enter by gravity.

Figure 44-4 • Nasoenteric tube feeding by continuous controlled pump. The head of the bed should be elevated to prevent aspiration.

with the flow rate regulated by a roller clamp or automated pump.

Continuous feeding is the delivery of feedings incrementally by a slow infusion over long periods. Slow drip feedings may reduce aspiration rates, distention, nausea, vomiting, and diarrhea in patients with poor gastric emptying or who are receiving hypertonic feeding solutions, as well as patients with severe reflux or altered mental status (Blumenstein, Shastri, & Stein, 2014). This method may also be used to administer tube feedings into the small intestine. Enteral feeding pumps control the delivery rate of the formula (see Fig. 44-4). They allow for a constant flow rate and can infuse a viscous formula through a small-diameter feeding tube. However, they do not allow the patient as much flexibility as intermittent feedings. Portable lightweight enteral pumps are available for home use. In addition, feeding pumps have built-in alarms that signal when the bag is empty, the battery is low, or the tube is occluded. The patient and caregiver need to be aware of these alarms and know how to "troubleshoot" the pump.

An alternative to the continuous infusion method is **cyclic feeding,** in which the infused feeding is given by an enteral feeding pump over 8 to 18 hours. Feedings may be infused at night to avoid interrupting the patient's lifestyle. Cyclic infusions may be appropriate for patients who are being weaned from tube feedings to an oral diet, for patients who cannot eat enough and need supplements, and for patients at home who need daytime hours free from the pump.

Key assessment findings for patients receiving tube feedings are noted in Chart 44-2.

Maintaining Feeding Equipment and Nutritional Balance

The temperature and volume of the feeding, the flow rate, and the patient's total fluid intake are important factors to consider when tube feedings are given. The schedule of tube feedings, including the correct quantity and frequency, is maintained. The nurse must carefully monitor the drip rate and avoid administering fluids too rapidly.

For patients receiving tube feedings, measuring gastric residual volumes (GRVs) by removing gastric contents with

Chart 44-2

ASSESSMENT
Assessing Patients Receiving Tube Feedings

Be alert for the following assessment findings:

- Tube placement, patient's position (head of bed elevated 30–45 degrees), and formula flow rate
- Patient's ability to tolerate the formula; observe for fullness, bloating, distention, nausea, vomiting, and stool pattern
- Clinical responses, as noted in laboratory findings (blood urea nitrogen, serum protein, prealbumin, electrolytes, kidney function, hemoglobin, hematocrit)
- Signs of dehydration (dry mucous membranes, thirst, decreased urine output)
- Amount of formula actually taken in by the patient
- Elevated blood glucose level, decreased urinary output, sudden weight gain, and periorbital or dependent edema
- Infection control practices: Replace any formula given by an open system every 4–8 hours with fresh formula; change tube feeding container and tubing every 24 hours
- Check gastric residual volume before each feeding or, in the case of continuous feedings, every 4 hours; return the aspirate to the stomach
- Intake and output
- Weekly weights
- Recommendations made on dietitian consult

Adapted from McClave, S. A., Taylor, B. E., Martindale, R. G., et al. (2016). Guidelines for the provision and assessment of nutrition support therapy in the adult critically ill patient: Society of Critical Care Medicine (SCCM) and American Society for Parenteral and Enteral Nutrition (ASPEN). *Journal of Parenteral and Enteral Nutrition, 40*(2), 159–211.

a large syringe at routine intervals has been a commonly prescribed practice; however, the usefulness of measuring GRVs has not been validated by research (Reignier, Mercier, Le Gouge, et al., 2013; Williams, Leslie, Mills, et al., 2013). Previously, GRV in excess of 250 to 500 mL had been thought to indicate feeding intolerance. Other measures of feeding tolerance that the nurse may employ include physical assessment findings such as abdominal distention, patient reports of discomfort, vomiting, changes in passing flatus, and presence of diarrhea (McClave et al., 2016). The most recent guidelines for assessment and provision of nutrition in the patient who is critically ill, authored by the Society of Critical Care Medicine (SCCM) and the American Society for Parenteral and Enteral Nutrition (ASPEN), do not advocate using GRVs to monitor tolerance of enteral feedings (McClave et al., 2016). Recent research shows that GRVs between 250 and 500 mL did not increase the incidence of vomiting, aspiration, or pneumonia (McClave et al., 2016). Growing evidence supports moving away from routine assessment of GRVs (Seres, 2016).

Maintaining tube function is an ongoing responsibility of the nurse, patient, primary provider, and caregiver. To ensure patency and to decrease the chance of bacterial growth, sludge build-up, or occlusion of the tube, at least 30 mL of water is given in each of the following instances (Blumenstein et al., 2014).

- Before and after intermittent tube feeding and medication administration (with at least 5 mL of water in between each individual medication)
- After checking for gastric residuals and gastric pH

- Every 4 hours with continuous feedings
- When the tube feeding is discontinued or interrupted for any reason
- When the tube is not being used, where a minimum of once daily flushing is recommended

Water used to irrigate these tubes must be recorded as fluid intake. Sterile water or sterile saline should be used for patients who are immunocompromised or to flush postpyloric nasoduodenal and jejunostomy tubes (Blumenstein et al., 2014).

Potential complications of enteral therapy are noted in Table 44-3.

Providing Medications by Tube

When different types of medications are prescribed, a bolus method is used for administration that is compatible with the medication's preparation. The tube is flushed with 30 mL of water before and after medication administration, and this is recorded as intake. When small-bore feeding tubes for continuous infusion are irrigated after administration of medications, a 30-mL or larger syringe is used because the pressure generated by smaller syringes could rupture the tube.

 Quality and Safety Nursing Alert

Administering medications through postpyloric enteric tubes may adversely affect their absorption; therefore, this should be avoided if possible. In addition, to avoid nutrient and drug interactions, medications should not be mixed with the feeding formulas.

Maintaining Delivery Systems

Tube feeding formula is delivered to patients by either an open or a closed system. The open system is packaged as a liquid or a powder to be mixed with water that is either poured into a feeding container or given by a large syringe. The feeding container (which is hung on a pole) and the tubing used with the open system should be changed every 24 hours (Bankhead et al., 2009). The open system can be used for bolus feedings, intermittent feedings, or continuous drip feedings and can be delivered by push (with a syringe and plunger), gravity (syringe with plunger removed or gravity bag with roller clamp), or pump. To avoid bacterial contamination, the formula hang time in the bag at room temperature should never exceed what the formula manufacturer recommends, which is usually no more than 4 to 8 hours. Closed delivery systems use a prefilled, sterile container of about 1 L of formula that is spiked with enteral tubing and allows a hang time of 24 to 48 hours at room temperature. The closed delivery system must always use a pump to control formula rate in order to avoid dispensing a large formula volume in a short period of time.

Maintaining Normal Bowel Elimination Pattern

Patients receiving gastric or enteric tube feedings can experience diarrhea or constipation. Possible causes of diarrhea include:

- Malnutrition: A decrease in the intestinal absorptive area can cause diarrhea.

TABLE 44-3 Potential Complications of Enteral Therapy

Complications	Causes	Selected Nursing Interventions	
		Therapeutic	Preventive
Gastrointestinal			
Constipation	Lack of fiber Inadequate fluid intake/dehydration Opioid use	Check fiber and water content; report findings.	Administer adequate amount of hydration as flushes. Consider cathartic.
Diarrhea	Hyperosmolar feedings Rapid infusion/bolus feedings Cold formula Medications, especially antibiotic therapy	Assess fluid balance and electrolyte levels; report findings. Implement changes in tube feeding formula or rate. Review medications.	Appropriate rate of infusion and temperature of formula. Avoid multiple elixirs and prokinetic medications.
Gas/bloating/cramping	Air in tube Excess fiber	Notify primary provider if persistent.	Keep tubing free of air.
Nausea/vomiting	Change in formula or rate Inadequate gastric emptying	Review medications.	Check residuals; if ≥200 mL, reinstill and recheck; report if residual is consistently high.
Mechanical			
Aspiration pneumonia	Improper tube placement Vomiting with aspiration of tube feeding Flat in bed	Assess respiratory status and notify primary provider.	Implement reliable method for checking tube placement. Keep head of bed elevated 30 degrees.
Nasopharyngeal irritation	Tube position/improper taping Use of large tubes	Assess nasopharyngeal mucous membranes every 8 hours.	Tape tube to prevent pressure on nares. Reposition tape.
Tube displacement	Excessive coughing/vomitus Tension on the tube or unsecured tube Tracheal suctioning Airway intubation	Stop feeding, and notify primary provider.	Check tube placement before administering feeding.
Tube obstruction	Inadequate flushing/formula rate Inadequate crushing of medications and flushing after administration	Follow policy for declogging feeding tubes (see procedural guidelines on thePoint)	Obtain liquid medications when possible. Flush tube and crush medications adequately.
Metabolic			
Dehydration and azotemia (excessive urea in the blood)	Hyperosmolar feedings with insufficient fluid intake	Report signs and symptoms of dehydration. Implement changes in tube feeding formula, rate, or ratio to water.	Provide adequate hydration through flushes.
Hyperglycemia	Glucose intolerance High carbohydrate content of the feeding	Check blood glucose levels routinely. Dietary consult to reevaluate feeding regimen.	

Adapted from Blumenstein, I., Shastri, Y. H., & Stein, J. (2014). Gastroenteric tube feeding: Techniques, problems, and solutions. *World Journal of Gastroenterology, 20* (26), 8505–8524.

- Medication therapy:
  - Elixir-based medications—often contain sorbitol, which can act as a cathartic
  - Magnesium—acts as a cathartic
  - Antibiotics—thought to alter normal intestinal flora, allowing pathogenic bacteria to flourish
- *Clostridium difficile* (*C. difficile*) colitis: Can result after antibiotic use alters normal intestinal flora and promotes the abnormal growth of this potentially dangerous microbe. *C. difficile* colitis occurs most commonly in hospitalized older adult patients treated with antibiotics and causes significant, potentially lethal diarrhea (Gupta & Khanna, 2014).
- Zinc deficiency: Zinc is lost with diarrhea, and zinc deficiency can then cause continued diarrhea.
- Concomitant lactose intolerance

- Concomitant hyperthyroidism
- Dumping syndrome: Formula is infused into the small intestine quickly or formula bypasses the stomach too readily into the small intestine and causes expansion of the intestinal wall. This leads to bloating, cramping, diarrhea, dizziness, diaphoresis, and weakness. Measures for managing the GI symptoms associated with dumping syndrome are presented in Chart 44-3.
- Contamination of the formula and feeding equipment with diarrhea-causing pathogens

Possible causes of constipation include:
- Inadequate water intake: Tube feedings typically do not meet total fluid needs and additional water needs to be given.
- Administration of fiber-free tube feeding formulas
- Concomitant use of opioids

Chart 44-3 Preventing Dumping Syndrome

The following strategies may help prevent some of the uncomfortable signs and symptoms of dumping syndrome related to tube feeding:

- Slow the formula instillation rate to provide time for carbohydrates and electrolytes to be diluted.
- Administer feedings at room temperature, because temperature extremes stimulate peristalsis.
- Administer feeding by continuous drip (if tolerated) rather than by bolus, to prevent sudden distention of the intestine.
- Advise the patient to remain in semi-Fowler position for 1 hour after the feeding; this position prolongs intestinal transit time by decreasing the effect of gravity.
- Instill the minimal amount of water needed to flush the tubing before and after a feeding, because fluid given with a feeding increases intestinal transit time.

Maintaining Adequate Hydration

The nurse carefully monitors hydration because in many cases the patient cannot communicate the need for water. Water flushes are given every 4 hours and after feedings to prevent hypertonic dehydration. The feeding may be initially given as a continuous drip in order to help the patient develop tolerance, especially for hyperosmolar solutions. Key nursing interventions include observing for signs of dehydration (e.g., dry mucous membranes, thirst, decreased urine output); administering water routinely; and monitoring I&O, residual volume, and fluid balance.

Promoting Coping Ability

The psychosocial goal of nursing care is to support and encourage the patient to accept physical changes and to convey hope that daily progressive improvement is possible. If the patient is having difficulty adjusting to the treatment, the nurse intervenes by encouraging self-care within the parameters of the patient's activity level. In addition, the nurse reinforces an optimistic approach by identifying indicators of progress (daily weight trends, electrolyte balance, absence of nausea and diarrhea, improvement in plasma proteins).

Promoting Home, Community-Based, and Transitional Care

 Educating Patients about Self-Care

Patients who require long-term tube feedings may have had recent surgery, dysphagia due to a neuromuscular disease, radiation or other types of trauma to the throat, an obstruction of the upper GI tract, or decreased level of consciousness. For a patient to be considered for tube feeding at home, the patient should:

- Be medically stable and successfully tolerating at least 60% to 70% of the feeding regimen
- Be capable of self-care or have a caregiver willing to assume the responsibility
- Have access to supplies and interest in learning how to administer tube feedings at home

Preparation of the patient for home administration of enteral feedings begins while the patient is still hospital-ized. The nurse should educate the patient and caregiver while administering the feedings so that they can observe the mechanics and participate in the procedure, ask questions, and express any concerns. Before discharge, the nurse provides information about the equipment needed, formula purchase and storage, and administration of the feedings and water flushes (frequency, quantity, rate of instillation).

Family members who will be active in the patient's home care are encouraged to participate in education sessions. Available printed information about the equipment, the formula, and the procedure is reviewed. Arrangements are made to obtain the equipment and formula and have it ready for use before the patient's discharge.

Continuing and Transitional Care

Referral to home, community-based, or transitional care is important so that a nurse can supervise and provide support during the first tube feedings at home. Additional visits will depend on the skill and comfort of the patient or caregiver in administering the feedings. During all visits, the nurse monitors the patient's physical status (weight, hydration status, vital signs, activity level) and the ability of the patient and family to administer the tube feedings correctly and assess the enteral access device and site. Enteral access devices require periodic replacement, and the nurse should be sure that the patient and caregiver have the necessary information to set up these tube replacement appointments. In addition, the nurse assesses for any complications. The patient or caregiver is encouraged to record times and amounts of feedings and water flushes, bowel patterns, and any symptoms that occur. The nurse can review the record with the patient and caregiver during home visits.

Gastrostomy and Jejunostomy

A **gastrostomy** is a procedure in which an opening is created into the stomach either for the purpose of administering nutrition, fluids, and medications via a feeding tube, or for gastric decompression in patients with gastroparesis, gastroesophageal reflux disease, or intestinal obstruction. A gastrostomy is preferred over a nasally inserted tube to deliver enteral nutrition support longer than 4 weeks (Blumenstein et al., 2014). Gastrostomy is also preferred over nasogastric or orogastric feedings in the patient who is comatose because the gastroesophageal sphincter remains intact, making regurgitation and aspiration less likely.

Balloon and non-balloon gastrostomy tubes (G tubes) may be placed surgically, endoscopically, or fluoroscopically. Each technique requires an abdominal incision, and either a permanent gastric **stoma** (an artificially created opening) is created surgically that can be accessed with a feeding tube (Janeway gastrostomy), or a gastric stoma is established that remains open as long as it remains intubated (i.e., a tube remains in place). Insertion of a **percutaneous endoscopic gastrostomy (PEG)** requires the services of a provider skilled in endoscopy and utilizes moderate sedation. A lighted endoscope is inserted via the patient's mouth toward the stomach and then the stomach is inflated with air. The PEG tube is guided down the esophagus, into the stomach, and out through the abdominal incision. An internal fixation bolster is pulled snug against the stomach wall. An external

Figure 44-5 • **A.** A detail of the abdomen and the percutaneous endoscopic gastrostomy tube showing catheter fixation. **B.** A detail of the abdomen and the nonobturated low-profile gastrostomy device showing balloon fixation.

retention bolster (crossbar, circular, or star shaped) is threaded down the tube and positioned snug to the skin. The tension between the external and internal fixation bolsters keeps the tube in place (see Fig. 44-5A). G tubes can also be placed fluoroscopically by a skilled provider when an endoscope cannot be passed through a strictured or obstructed esophagus (DeLegge, 2015).

The initial G tube can be removed and replaced once the tract is well established, typically 6 weeks to 3 months after initial insertion. Routine replacement is indicated every 3 to 6 months for a balloon G tube and every 6 to 12 months for a non-balloon G tube. Replacement is also indicated for a tube that has clogged or fractured or has a ruptured balloon. The external G tube retention bolster should be fitted snugly to the stoma to prevent leakage of gastric secretions and is maintained in place through gentle traction between the internal and anchoring devices. The G tube site is cleaned daily and as needed with soap and water, or 2% chlorhexidine gluconate according to institution policy, and dried thoroughly. The site is assessed for tube deterioration, drainage, and signs and symptoms of possible infection, including redness, swelling and foul-smelling drainage. Abnormal findings are communicated to the primary provider. If there is excessive drainage, a gauze pad may be secured over the external anchor, taking caution to avoid excessive tension on the tube (Arora & Lukens, 2015; DeLegge, 2015).

An alternative to G tubes that are bulky (e.g., they are usually coiled under an elastic binder or secured to the abdomen with tape or some type of attachment device) are low-profile gastrostomy devices (LPGDs) (see Fig. 44-5B). Specific types of LPGDs include the MIC-KEY or the Bard Button. LPGDs may be inserted 6 weeks to 3 months after initial G tube placement or placed as the initial G tube. These devices are flush with the skin, eliminate the possibility of inward tube migration, have antireflux valves to prevent gastric leakage, and do not require tape or other securement devices. Patients requiring enteral nutrition support are able to conceal the feeding tube access site under their clothing. LPGDs require special connection tubing so they can be attached to the feeding container. Patients must be instructed to bring this connection tubing

with them when traveling, going to the emergency department or hospital, or undergoing diagnostic procedures that require access into the GI tract.

A **jejunostomy** is a surgically placed opening into the jejunum for the purpose of administering nutrition, fluids, and medications. A jejunostomy tube (J tube) is indicated when the gastric route is not accessible, or to decrease aspiration risk when the stomach is not functioning adequately to process and empty food and fluids (Gangadharan, 2015).

The small intestine can also be accessed by placing a jejunal extension tube through an existing G tube and manipulating it through the pylorus into the small intestine endoscopically, fluoroscopically, or during a surgical procedure. A transgastric J tube can be placed that contains both a gastric and jejunal port so that both the stomach and small intestine can be accessed. There are also low-profile jejunostomy devices (LPJDs) that are placed via a gastric stoma; the distal end is positioned in the small intestine via passage through the pylorus. These devices have the same advantages as the LPGDs described previously.

NURSING PROCESS

The Patient With a Gastrostomy or Jejunostomy

Assessment

The focus of the preoperative assessment is to determine the patient's ability to understand and cooperate with the procedure. The nurse assesses the ability of both patient and family to adjust to a change in body image and to participate in self-care. There are multiple medical and ethical issues that the patient, the caregivers, and the primary provider should discuss together (see Chart 44-4).

The purpose of the procedure and expected postoperative course should be explained. The patient needs to know that the feeding tube will bypass the mouth and esophagus so that liquid feedings can be given directly into the stomach or intestine. If the feeding tube is expected to be permanent,

Chart 44-4 ETHICAL DILEMMA
Is it Ethical to Withhold or Withdraw Nutrition and Hydration?

Case Scenario

You work as a staff nurse on a medical-surgical unit of a community hospital. An 85-year-old man was admitted to your unit several days ago after having a severe stroke. He has a history of moderate dementia and is not mentally competent. Prior to this hospitalization, he and his 82-year-old wife, who is cognitively intact, lived in separate units in a skilled nursing facility; the wife lived in an assisted living unit and the husband in the Alzheimer unit. Because the patient swallows poorly and is at risk for aspiration, enteral feedings have been recommended. The family has also been advised that given the patient's age and the severity of the stroke, the chance for a good outcome is not optimistic. The patient's wife wants the patient to begin enteral feedings, but an adult son who lives in the area says "This is ridiculous, Mom. Dad is not the man he used to be. We should not continue to prolong his end and make it worse than it already is. We both know he would not want this!" The patient's advanced directive identifies his wife as his health care representative; however, it does not include any information about the patient's consent for artificial nutrition.

Discussion

It is generally agreed that patients (or their designated decision makers) can refuse lifesaving treatment, particularly if the means of treatment are extraordinary (e.g., ventilators, dialysis machines, extracorporeal oxygenators). *Extraordinary means* include medications, treatments, and procedures that can be obtained only at excessive cost, pain, or inconvenience and offer no reasonable hope of benefit.

There has been much debate about medically given nutrition and hydration. *Ordinary means* are those medications, treatments, and procedures that offer a reasonable hope of benefit and can be obtained without excessive expense, pain, or inconvenience. Artificial nutrition and hydration therapy (ANH) are perceived as ordinary means by many health care professionals, and good nutrition improves outcomes in select cases. Withdrawing or withholding nutrition and hydration can in and of itself can hasten death; however, in patients who are terminally ill, hydration can prolong suffering. Some have argued that ANH should always be given. Yet, nurses and other health care professionals have mixed feelings on the ethical underpinnings of ANH. Since the patient's wife has been designated as the health care representative, she ultimately can consent or refuse nutrition for her husband. The American Nurses Association (2011) asserts that "the acceptance or refusal or food and fluids, whether delivered by normal or artificial means must be respected" (p. 1).

Analysis

- Describe the ethical principles that are in conflict in this case (see Chapter 3, Chart 3-3). Which principle should have preeminence as you proceed to work with this family?
- Is it possible to preserve this patient's autonomy? If so, what steps might you take to ensure that the patient's rights to "self-rule" are maintained?
- If a health care representative or a medical power of attorney had not been designated, how would this dilemma be addressed?
- Does withholding fluids and nutrition in the patient who is terminally ill violate the principle of non-maleficence? Does administering fluids and nutrition to the patient who is dying violate the principle of nonmaleficence?
- What resource might be available to you in your hospital to help you, the physician, and the patient and family determine what is in the patient's best interests?

References

American Nurses Association (ANA). (2011). Forgoing nutrition and hydration. Retrieved on 8/28/2016 at: www.nursingworld.org/MainMenuCategories/EthicsStandards/Ethics-Position-Statements/prtetnutr14451.pdf

Patterson, J. (2013). Providing artificial nutrition and hydration in palliative care. *Nursing Standard, 27*(20), 35–42.

Resources

See Chapter 3, Chart 3-6 for ethics resources.

---

the patient should be made aware of this. If the procedure is being performed to relieve discomfort, prolonged vomiting, debilitation, or an inability to eat, the patient may find it more acceptable.

In the postoperative period, the patient's fluid and nutritional needs are assessed to ensure proper intake and GI function. The nurse inspects the tube for proper maintenance and the incision for any drainage, skin breakdown, or signs of infection. As the nurse evaluates patients' responses to the change in body image and their understanding of the feeding methods, interventions are identified to help them cope with the tube and learn self-care measures.

Diagnosis

NURSING DIAGNOSES

Based on the assessment data, major nursing diagnoses may include the following:

- Imbalanced nutrition: less than body requirements
- Risk for infection related to presence of wound and tube
- Risk for impaired skin integrity at tube insertion site
- Disturbed body image related to presence of tube

COLLABORATIVE PROBLEMS/POTENTIAL COMPLICATIONS

Potential complications may include the following:

- Wound infection, cellulitis, and leakage
- GI bleeding
- Premature dislodgement of the tube

Planning and Goals

The major goals for the patient may include achieving nutritional requirements, preventing infection, maintaining skin integrity, adjusting to changes in body image, and preventing complications.

Nursing Interventions

MEETING NUTRITIONAL NEEDS

The first fluid nourishment is given soon after tube insertion and can consist of a sterile water or normal saline flush of at least 30 mL. Formula feeding can begin as prescribed, typically within 2 to 24 hours post tube insertion. The infusion rate or bolus amount given is gradually increased.

If the tube has been placed for gastric drainage, it can be connected to either low intermittent suction or to a gravity drainage bag. This drainage should be measured and recorded because it is a significant indicator of GI function. A decrease in the amount of drainage may indicate that the tube can be clamped for periods of time, allowing greater freedom of movement. High output can result in significant fluid and electrolyte losses.

PREVENTING INFECTION AND PROVIDING SKIN CARE

The skin surrounding a gastrostomy or jejunostomy requires special care because it may become irritated from the enzymatic action of gastric or intestinal juices that may leak around the tube. Left untreated, the skin becomes macerated and painful. The nurse washes the area around the tube under the bumper with soap and water or 2% chlorhexidine gluconate daily and as needed to remove any encrustation. If soap and water is used, the area is rinsed well with water and patted dry. If chlorhexidine is used, the area is allowed to air dry. A protective skin barrier may be applied. Skin at the exit site is evaluated daily for signs of breakdown, irritation, excoriation, and the presence of drainage, bleeding or hypertrophic tissue growth or scattered, raised red papules that could indicate a yeast or candidal infection. Candida may appear in warm moist areas of the body; the area beneath the G tube external retention bolster is a common location for it to develop and spread. The nurse encourages the patient and family members to participate in this evaluation and in hygiene activities.

A thin gauze or foam dressing is applied, if needed, under the external bumper. Dressings placed under the bumper may exert excessive tension on the tube tract (DeLegge, 2015). A tube stabilizer may also be used to anchor the G tube (Miller, McClave, Kiraly, et al., 2014).

It is normal to see scant serous drainage at the site for a few days post insertion. After this drainage ceases, the site may be left open to air. The nurse rotates the tube once daily to prevent skin breakdown and *buried bumper syndrome*. Buried bumper syndrome can occur when there is excessive traction on the G tube from the external retention bolster to the extent that the internal fixation bolster becomes embedded in the gastric mucosa. This causes pain during tube feedings and can lead to tube obstruction and peritonitis (DeLegge, 2015).

ENHANCING BODY IMAGE

Eating is a major physiologic and social function, and the patient with a gastrostomy has experienced a major change in body image. The patient is also aware that gastrostomy as a therapeutic intervention is performed only in the presence of a major, chronic, or perhaps terminal illness. It is necessary to evaluate the existing family support system, because adjustment takes time and is facilitated by family acceptance. G tubes, transgastric J tubes, and G tubes with jejunal extensions can be transitioned to LPGDs and LPJDs as described previously and may be indicated to minimize the bulkiness and visibility of these tubes.

MONITORING AND MANAGING POTENTIAL COMPLICATIONS

During the postoperative course, the most common complications are wound infection or cellulitis at the exit site, bleeding, leakage, excessive tightness of external retention bolster, and dislodgement. Because many patients who receive tube feedings are debilitated and have compromised nutritional status, any signs of infection are promptly reported to the primary provider so that appropriate therapy can be instituted.

Bleeding from the insertion site in the stomach can also occur and should be reported promptly. The nurse closely monitors the patient's vital signs and observes all operative site drainage, vomitus, and stool for evidence of bleeding. If an external retention bolster, tape, securement device, or sutures are present, they are evaluated for adequate tension and securement. Excessive tension of the external retention bolster can cause excruciating pain and will lead to skin breakdown and ulceration. The nurse should notify the primary provider if excessive pain occurs at the incision site post insertion. Dislodgement of a recently inserted tube requires immediate attention because the tract can close within 4 to 6 hours if the tube is not replaced promptly.

PROMOTING HOME, COMMUNITY-BASED, AND TRANSITIONAL CARE

Educating Patients About Self-Care. The patient with a G or J tube in the home setting must be capable of maintaining patency of the tube or have a caregiver who can do so. The nurse assesses the patient's level of knowledge and interest in learning about the tube, as well as an ability to understand how to flush, provide site care, and administer feedings or facilitate decompression and drainage. Education is similar to that described earlier. To facilitate self-care, the nurse encourages the patient to participate in flushing the tube, administering medications and tube feedings during hospitalization, and establishing as normal a routine as possible.

Adapters are available that can be secured to the end of the tube to create a "Y" site for ease of flushing, suction, or medication delivery. The flushing equipment is cleaned with warm, soapy water and rinsed after each use. The tube can be marked at skin level to provide the patient with a baseline for later comparison. The patient or caregiver should be advised to monitor the tube's length and to notify the primary provider or home care nurse if the segment of the tube outside the body becomes shorter or longer.

Continuing and Transitional Care. Referral to home, community-based, or transitional care is important to ensure initial supervision and support for the patient and caregiver. The nurse assesses the patient's status and progress and evaluates the care of the tube and healing status of the tube insertion site. Further instruction and supervision in the home setting may be required to help the patient and caregiver adapt to a physical environment and equipment that are different from the hospital setting (see Chart 44-5). The nurse also reviews with the patient and caregiver what complications to report and assists the patient and family in establishing as normal a routine as possible.

Evaluation

Expected patient outcomes may include:
1. Achieves nutrition goals
   a. Attains weight goal
   b. Tolerates tube feeding prescription without nausea, emesis, cramping, abdominal pain, or feelings of early satiety
   c. Has acceptable bowel movements without constipation or large-volume liquid stools
   d. Has normal plasma protein, glucose, vitamin, and mineral levels
   e. Has normal electrolyte values

Chart 44-5

HOME CARE CHECKLIST

The Patient Receiving Tube Feeding

At the completion of education, the patient and/or caregiver will be able to:

- Name the procedure that was performed and identify any permanent changes in anatomic structure or function as well as changes in ADLs, IADLs, roles, relationships, and spirituality.
- State what types of changes are needed (if any) to maintain a clean home environment and prevent infection.
- State how to contact the primary provider, the team of home care professionals overseeing care, and tube feeding supply vendor.
  - List emergency phone numbers.
- State how to obtain medical supplies and carry out dressing changes, site care, and other prescribed regimens.
- Demonstrate how to perform site care.
- Demonstrate how to prepare tube feeding.
- Demonstrate how to deliver tube feeding via prescribed method (e.g., bolus method, intermittent drip method, continuous feeding).
  - When indicated, demonstrate how to operate, disconnect, and clean the tube feeding pump.

- When indicated, demonstrate tube maintenance functions.
  - Flush before and after bolus and intermittent feeding and medication administration
  - Flush every 4 hours with continuous feeding
  - Flush once daily if tube is not being used
- Demonstrate how to record all fluid intake and output.
- Identify a plan for operation of tube feeding pump during a power outage or other emergency.
- State the name, dose, side effects, frequency, and schedule for all medications.
  - Demonstrate medication preparation and administration via bolus method, with flushing before, after and between medications.
- Identify possible tube feeding complications and interventions.
- Relate how to reach primary provider with questions or complications.
- State time and date of follow-up appointments and testing.
- State understanding of community resources and referrals (if any).
- Identify the need for health promotion (e.g., weight reduction, smoking cessation, stress management), disease prevention and screening activities.

ADL, activities of daily living; IADL, independent activities of daily living.

---

2. Is free of infection at enteral access site
   a. Is afebrile
   b. Has no induration, redness, pain, or purulent drainage
   c. Has no scattered papules indicative of a yeast infection
3. Has dry, intact skin surrounding enteral access site
   a. No evidence of excessive drainage or bleeding
   b. No skin breakdown or hypertrophic tissue growth
4. Adjusts to change in body image
   a. Is able to discuss expected changes
   b. Verbalizes concerns
5. Demonstrates skill in tube care
   a. Handles equipment competently
   b. Demonstrates how to maintain tube patency
   c. Keeps an accurate record of I&O
   d. Demonstrates how to gently wash tube site daily and keep clean and dry
6. Avoids other complications
   a. Exhibits adequate wound healing
   b. Tube remains intact and is routinely replaced for the duration of therapy

Parenteral Nutrition

Parenteral nutrition (PN) is a method of providing nutrients to the body by an IV route. The nutrients are a complex admixture containing proteins, carbohydrates, fats, electrolytes, vitamins, trace minerals, and sterile water in a single container. The goals of PN are similar to the goals of enteral feedings; namely, to improve nutritional status, establish a positive nitrogen balance, maintain muscle mass, promote weight maintenance or gain, and enhance the healing process (Seres, 2016).

Establishing Positive Nitrogen Balance

Most IV fluids do not provide sufficient calories or protein to meet the body's daily requirements. PN solutions can provide enough calories and nitrogen to meet the patient's daily nutritional needs. The patient with fever, trauma, burns, major surgery, or hypermetabolic disease requires additional daily calories (Gauglitz, 2014). When highly concentrated dextrose is given, caloric requirements are satisfied and the body uses amino acids for protein synthesis rather than for energy. Additionally, electrolytes such as calcium, phosphorus, magnesium, and sodium chloride are added to the solution to maintain proper electrolyte balance and to transport glucose and amino acids across cell membranes.

The volume of fluid necessary to provide these calories peripherally can surpass fluid tolerance. To provide the required calories in a smaller volume, it is necessary to increase the concentration of nutrients and use a route of administration that rapidly dilutes incoming nutrients to the proper levels of body tolerance. Typically, a large, high-flow vein such as the superior vena cava (at the right atriocaval junction) is the preferred site.

Clinical Indications

The indications for PN include an inability to ingest adequate oral food or fluids within a 7- to 10-day timeframe (McClave et al., 2016). Enteral nutrition should be considered before parenteral support because it assists in maintaining gut mucosal integrity and improved immune function and is typically associated with fewer complications. In both the home and hospital setting, PN is indicated in the situations listed in Table 44-4.

TABLE 44-4 Indications for Parenteral Nutrition

Condition or Need	Examples
Insufficient oral or enteral intake	Severe burns, malnutrition, short-bowel syndrome, acquired immune deficiency syndrome, sepsis, cancer
Impaired ability to ingest or absorb food orally or enterally	Paralytic ileus, Crohn's disease, short-bowel syndrome, postradiation enteritis, high-output enterocutaneous fistula
Patient unwilling or unable to ingest adequate nutrients orally or enterally	Major psychiatric illness (e.g., severe anorexia nervosa)
Prolonged preoperative and post-operative nutritional needs	Extensive bowel surgery, acute pancreatitis

Adapted from McClave, S. A., Taylor, B. E., Martindale, R. G., et al. (2016). Guidelines for the provision and assessment of nutrition support therapy in the adult critically ill patient: Society of Critical Care Medicine (SCCM) and American Society for Parenteral and Enteral Nutrition (ASPEN). *Journal of Parenteral and Enteral Nutrition, 40*(2), 159–211.

Formulas

A total of 1 to 3 L of solution is given over a 24-hour period. The label of the solution is verified with the prescription. **Intravenous fat emulsions (IVFEs or lipids)** may be infused simultaneously with PN through a Y connector close to the infusion site and should not be filtered. The PN solution is not to be piggybacked into the IVFE. Usually, 500 mL of a 10% IVFE or 250 mL of 20% IVFE is given over 6 to 12 hours, one to three times a week. IVFEs can provide up to 30% of the total daily calorie intake.

Quality and Safety Nursing Alert

Before PN infusion is given, the solution must be inspected for separation, oily appearance (also known as a "cracked solution"), or any precipitate (which appears as white crystals). If any of these are present, it is not used.

IVFEs can be mixed by the pharmacy staff with other components of PN to create a "three-in-one solution" commonly called a **total nutrient admixture (TNA)**. Whereas a filter is not used with IVFE, a special final filter (1.2 micron filter) is used with TNA to prevent the administration of a precipitate (i.e., calcium, phosphorus, incompatibilities) that cannot be seen due to the opacity of the solution. Advantages of TNA over PN are cost savings in preparation and equipment, decreased risk of catheter or nutrient contamination, decreased nursing time, and increased patient convenience and satisfaction (Gervasio, 2015). Ideally, the pharmacist, nutritionist, and primary provider should collaborate to determine the specific formula needed.

Initiating Therapy

PN solutions are initiated slowly and advanced gradually each day to the desired rate as the patient's fluid and dextrose tolerance permits. The patient's laboratory test results and response to PN therapy are monitored on an ongoing basis by the primary provider. Standing orders are initiated for weighing the patient; monitoring I&O and blood glucose; and baseline and periodic monitoring of complete blood count, platelet count, and chemistry panel, including serum carbon dioxide, magnesium, phosphorus, and triglycerides. A 24-hour urine nitrogen determination may be performed for analysis of nitrogen balance. In most hospitals, the PN solutions are prescribed on a daily standard PN order form. The formulation of the PN solutions is calculated carefully each day to meet the complete nutritional needs of the individual patient.

Administration Methods

Various vascular access devices are used to administer PN solutions in clinical practice. PN may be given through either peripheral or central IV lines, depending on the patient's condition and the anticipated length of therapy. An infusion pump is always used for administration of PN.

Peripheral Method

To supplement oral intake, peripheral parenteral nutrition (PPN) may be prescribed. PPN is given through a peripheral vein; this is possible because the solution is less hypertonic than a full-calorie PN solution. PPN formulas are not nutritionally complete because of their low dextrose content. Lipids are given simultaneously to buffer the PPN and to protect the peripheral vein from irritation. The usual length of therapy using PPN is 5 to 7 days.

Quality and Safety Nursing Alert

Formulations with dextrose concentrations of more than 10% should not be given through peripheral veins because they irritate the intima (innermost walls) of small veins, causing chemical phlebitis.

Central Method

Because central parenteral nutrition (CPN) solutions have five or six times the solute concentration of blood (and exert an osmotic pressure of about 2,000 mOsm/L), they are given into the vascular system through a catheter inserted into a high-flow, large blood vessel (e.g., ideally at the superior vena cava/right atriocaval junction). Concentrated solutions are then very rapidly diluted to isotonic levels by the blood in this vessel.

Several types of **central venous access devices (CVADs)** are available: percutaneous (or nontunneled), peripherally inserted central catheters (PICCs), surgically placed (or tunneled) catheters, and implanted vascular access ports.

Percutaneous (Nontunneled) Central Catheters

Percutaneous central catheters are used for short-term (less than 6 weeks) IV therapy in acute care settings. The subclavian vein is the most common vessel accessed because the subclavian area provides a stable insertion site to which the catheter can be anchored, is easily compressible (facilitating control of hemorrhage), allows the patient freedom of movement, and provides easy access to the dressing site. The subclavian access site should be avoided in patients with advanced kidney disease and those on hemodialysis to prevent subclavian vein stenosis. The second most common

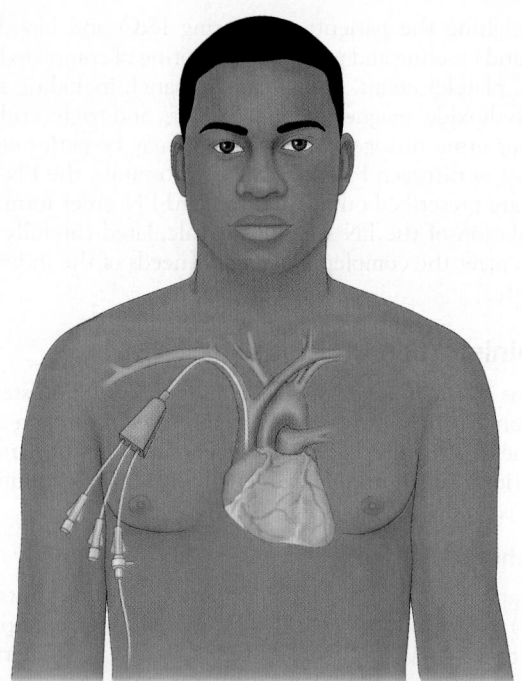

Figure 44-6 • Subclavian triple-lumen catheter used for parenteral nutrition and other adjunctive therapy. The catheter is threaded through the subclavian vein into the vena cava/right atriocaval junction. Each lumen is an avenue for solution administration. The lumens are secured with threaded needleless adapters or Luer lock–type caps when the device is not in use.

access sites include the basilic, brachial, or cephalic veins in the arm followed by the jugular vein. The femoral vein should be avoided for this purpose and should only be used as a last resort because of concerns about infection (Gorski, Hadaway, Hagle, et al., 2016). For a patient with limited IV access, a triple-lumen catheter can be used because it offers three ports for various uses (see Fig. 44-6). The use of a single-lumen catheter dedicated for the administration of PN is not typically feasible, because most patients require administration of medications and fluids in addition to PN, and the line used to administer PN cannot be used for other purposes.

When a patient requires IV access for PN, the insertion procedure is first explained so that the patient is aware of what to expect. The patient is placed supine in the Trendelenburg position to produce dilation of neck and shoulder vessels, which makes insertion easier and decreases the risk of air embolus. The skin is cleansed with 2% chlorhexidine to remove surface oils. To afford maximal accuracy in the placement of the catheter, the patient is instructed to turn their head away from the site of venipuncture and to remain motionless while the catheter is inserted and the wound is dressed. The nurse maintains the sterile field and supports the patient throughout the procedure. Maximal barrier precautions mandate that full-body sterile drapes are applied and sterile gloves, cap, gown, and masks are donned to reduce risk of central line-associated bloodstream infection (CLABSI) (Institute for Healthcare Improvement [IHI], 2012) (see Chapter 14, Chart 14-2). Lidocaine is injected to anesthetize the skin and underlying issues. A large-bore needle on a syringe is inserted and moved parallel to and beneath

the clavicle until it enters the vein. A radiopaque wire is inserted through the needle into the vein. The catheter is then advanced over the wire, the needle is withdrawn, and the hub of the catheter is attached to the IV tubing. Until the syringe is detached from the needle and the catheter is inserted, the patient may be asked to perform the Valsalva maneuver. The patient is instructed to take a deep breath, hold it, and bear down with the mouth closed to produce a positive phase in central venous pressure, thereby lessening the possibility of air being drawn into the circulatory system (air embolism). The catheter is sutured to the skin. A chlorhexidine-impregnated disc or gel with a semipermeable transparent dressing is applied using strict sterile technique (Marschall, Mermel, Fakih, et al., 2014).

The position of the tip of the catheter is verified with x-ray or fluoroscopy to confirm its location in the superior vena cava at the junction of the right atrium and to rule out a pneumothorax resulting from inadvertent puncture of the pleura. Once the catheter's position is confirmed, the prescribed CPN solution can be started. The initial rate of infusion is usually low, and the rate is gradually increased to the target rate.

An injection cap is attached to the end of each central catheter lumen, creating a closed system. IV infusion tubing is connected to the insertion cap of the central catheter with a threaded needleless adapter or Luer lock device. To ensure patency, all lumens are initially flushed according to institution policy with a 10-mL syringe. Smaller volume syringes are not to be used because the pressure from smaller syringes is potentially harmful to the catheter. Lumens are flushed with normal saline or diluted heparin (10 U/mL) after each intermittent infusion and after blood drawing; this flushing is necessary daily when the catheter is not in use. Force is never used to flush the catheter (Gorski et al., 2016). If resistance is met, aspiration may restore lumen patency; if this is not effective, the primary provider is notified. Low-dose tissue plasminogen activator may be prescribed to dissolve a clot or fibrin sheath. If attempts to clear the lumen are ineffective, the catheter should be changed.

Peripherally Inserted Central Catheters

Peripherally inserted central catheters (PICCs) are used for intermediate-term (several days to months) IV therapy in the hospital, long-term care, or home setting. These catheters may be inserted at the bedside or in the outpatient setting by a primary provider or specially trained nurse. The basilic, brachial, or cephalic vein is accessed above the antecubital space, and the catheter is threaded to the superior vena cava/right atriocaval junction (see Chapter 15, Fig. 15-6). Taking of blood pressure and blood specimens from the extremity with the PICC is avoided.

Surgically Placed (Tunneled) Central Catheters

Surgically placed central catheters are for long-term use and may remain in place for many years. These catheters are cuffed and can have single or double lumens; examples are the Power line (Power injectable), Hickman, Groshong, and Permacath. These catheters are inserted surgically. They are threaded (or tunneled) under the skin (reducing the risk of ascending infection) to the subclavian vein and advanced into the superior vena cava.

Implanted Vascular Access Ports

Implanted vascular access ports are also used for long-term IV therapy; examples include the Power injectable Port-A-Cath, Mediport, Hickman Port, and P.A.S. Port. Instead of exiting from the skin, the end of the catheter is attached to a small chamber that is placed in a subcutaneous pocket, either on the anterior chest wall or on the forearm. The port requires minimal care and allows the patient complete freedom of activity. Implanted ports are more expensive than the external catheters, and access requires passing a special noncoring needle (Huber tipped) through the skin into the chamber to initiate IV therapy (see Chapter 15, Fig. 15-5).

Discontinuing Parenteral Nutrition

The PN solution is discontinued gradually to allow the patient to adjust to decreased levels of glucose. If the PN solution is abruptly terminated, isotonic dextrose can be given at the same rate the PN solution was infusing for 1 to 2 hours to prevent rebound hypoglycemia. Symptoms of rebound hypoglycemia include weakness, faintness, sweating, shakiness, feeling cold, confusion, and increased heart rate. Once IV therapy is completed, the percutaneous central venous catheter or PICC is removed, pressure is held until hemostasis is achieved, and an occlusive dressing is applied to the exit site. Surgically placed central catheters and implanted vascular access ports are removed only by the primary provider.

NURSING PROCESS

The Patient Receiving Parenteral Nutrition

Assessment

The nurse assists in identifying patients unable to tolerate oral or enteral feedings who may be candidates for PN. Indicators include significant weight loss (10% or more of usual weight), a decrease in oral food intake for more than 1 week, muscle wasting, decreased tissue healing, abnormal urea nitrogen excretion, and persistent vomiting and diarrhea (McClave et al., 2016). The nurse carefully monitors the patient's hydration status, electrolyte levels, and calorie intake.

Diagnosis

NURSING DIAGNOSES

Based on the assessment data, major nursing diagnoses may include the following:

- Imbalanced nutrition: less than body requirements related to inadequate oral intake of nutrients
- Risk for infection related to contamination of the central catheter site or infusion line
- Risk for imbalanced fluid volume related to altered infusion rate
- Risk for activity intolerance related to restrictions because of the presence of IV access device

COLLABORATIVE PROBLEMS/POTENTIAL COMPLICATIONS

The most common complications are pneumothorax, air embolism, a clotted or displaced catheter, sepsis, hyperglycemia, fluid overload, and rebound hypoglycemia. These problems and the associated collaborative interventions are described in Table 44-5.

Planning and Goals

The major goals for the patient receiving PN may include optimal level of nutrition, absence of infection, adequate fluid volume, optimal level of activity (within individual limitations), knowledge of and skill in self-care, and absence of complications.

Nursing Interventions

MAINTAINING OPTIMAL NUTRITION

A continuous, uniform infusion of PN solution over a 24-hour period is desired. However, in some cases (e.g., home care patients), cyclic PN may be appropriate. Cyclic PN is infused during a set period of time. The time periods for infusion are sufficient to meet the patient's nutritional and pharmacologic needs. Ideally, cyclic PN is infused over a 10- to 15-hour period that continues through the night. The cyclic PN is titrated up during the beginning of the infusion cycle and down at the conclusion of the infusion to prevent hyperglycemia and hypoglycemia, respectively.

The patient is initially weighed daily (this may be decreased to 2 or 3 times per week once stable) at the same time of the day under the same conditions for accurate comparison. Under the PN regimen, satisfactory weight maintenance or gain can usually be achieved. It is important to keep accurate I&O records and calculations of fluid balance. A calorie count is kept of any oral nutrients. Trace elements (copper, zinc, chromium, manganese, and selenium) are included in PN solutions and are individualized for each patient.

PREVENTING INFECTION

The high dextrose and fat content of PN solutions makes them an ideal culture medium for bacterial and fungal growth, and CVADs provide a port of entry. Gram-positive cocci, Gram-negative bacilli, and Candida species are frequently isolated as causes of CLABSI. Common organisms include *Staphylococcus aureus*, *Staphylococcus epidermidis*, *Pseudomonas aeruginosa*, *Acinetobacter* species, and *Klebsiella pneumoniae*.

> ### Quality and Safety Nursing Alert
>
> *Meticulous aseptic technique is essential to prevent infection any time the IV line setup is manipulated.*

The skin and the catheter hub are the major sources for CLABSIs. The catheter site is covered with a chlorhexidine disc or gel and semipermeable transparent film dressing. The semipermeable transparent dressing allows frequent examination of the catheter site, adheres well to the skin, and is more comfortable for the patient. The transparent semipermeable membrane CVAD dressing is changed every 7 days unless the dressing is damp, bloody, loose, or soiled. Alternatively, an occlusive gauze dressing may be used and is changed every 48 hours or as needed (Gorski et al., 2016). During dressing changes, the nurse and patient wear masks to reduce the possibility of airborne contamination. Sterile technique is used (e.g., the nurse wears sterile gloves). The area is checked for leakage; bloody or purulent drainage; a kinked catheter; and skin reactions such as inflammation, redness, swelling, or tenderness. If chlorhexidine is used for skin asepsis, it is

TABLE 44-5 Potential Complications of Parental Nutrition

Complications	Cause	Nursing Actions and Collaborative Interventions	
		Treatment	Prevention
Pneumothorax	Improper catheter placement and inadvertent puncture of the pleura	Place patient in Fowler position. Offer reassurance. Monitor vital signs. Prepare for thoracentesis or chest tube insertion.	Assist patient to remain still in Trendelenburg position during catheter insertion.
Air embolism	Disconnected tubing Cap missing from port Blocked segment of vascular system	Replace tubing immediately and notify primary provider. Replace cap and notify primary provider. Turn patient on left side and place in the head-low position. Notify primary provider.	Examine all tubing connection sites for their security.
Clotted catheter line	Inadequate/infrequent saline/heparin flushes Disruption of infusion	At direction of primary provider, flush with thrombolytic medication as prescribed.	Flush lines per established protocols. Monitor infusion rate hourly and inspect integrity of the line.
Catheter displacement and contamination	Excessive movement, possibly with a nonsecured catheter Separation of tubing and contamination	Stop the infusion, and notify the primary provider.	Examine all tubing connection sites. Avoid interrupting the main line or piggybacking other lines.
Sepsis	Separation of dressings Contaminated solution Infection at insertion site of catheter	Reinforce or change dressing quickly using aseptic technique. Discard. Notify pharmacist. Notify primary provider. Monitor vital signs.	Maintain sterile technique when changing tubing, dressing, or PN bag. Scrub the hub for 15 seconds prior to accessing line for any reason; air-dry prior to use.
Hyperglycemia	Glucose intolerance	Notify primary provider; addition of insulin to PN solution may be prescribed.	Monitor glucose levels (blood and urine). Monitor urine output. Observe for stupor, confusion, or lethargy.
Fluid overload	Fluid infusing rapidly	Decrease infusion rate. Monitor vital signs. Notify primary provider. Treat respiratory distress by sitting patient upright and administering oxygen as needed, if prescribed.	Use infusion pump. Verify correct infusion rate ordered.
Rebound hypoglycemia	Feedings stopped too abruptly	Monitor for symptoms (weakness, tremors, diaphoresis, headache, hunger, and apprehension); notify primary provider.	Gradually wean patient from PN.

PN, parenteral nutrition.
Adapted from McClave, S. A., Taylor, B. E., Martindale, R. G., et al. (2016). Guidelines for the provision and assessment of nutrition support therapy in the adult critically ill patient: Society of Critical Care Medicine (SCCM) and American Society for Parenteral and Enteral Nutrition (ASPEN). *Journal of Parenteral and Enteral Nutrition, 40*(2), 159–211.

important to allow it to completely dry before applying the new dressing to avoid skin irritation.

The catheter is another major source of colonization and infection. The use of chlorhexidine/silver sulfadiazine- or minocycline/rifampin-impregnated catheters is recommended for a patient whose catheter is expected to remain in place for longer than 5 days if there is concern over a possibility of the patient acquiring a CLABSI (National Healthcare Safety Network, 2015).

MAINTAINING FLUID BALANCE

The ubiquitous use of infusion pumps ensures that an accurate rate of PN administration can be achieved. A designated rate is set in milliliters per hour (i.e., mL/hr), and the rate is routinely verified per institution policy, generally every 4 hours. The infusion rate should not be increased or decreased to compensate for fluids that have infused too quickly or too slowly. If the solution runs out, 10% dextrose and water is infused at the same rate to prevent hypoglycemia until the next PN solution is available for administration.

If the rate is too rapid, hyperosmolar diuresis can occur. Excess glucose is excreted by the renal tubules, pulling large volumes of water into the tubules via osmosis, resulting in higher-than-normal urine output and intravascular fluid volume deficit. If the flow rate is too slow, the patient does not receive the maximal benefit of calories and nitrogen. I&O is recorded every 8 hours so that fluid imbalance can be readily detected.

ENCOURAGING ACTIVITY

Activities and ambulation are encouraged when the patient is physically able. With a central catheter, the patient is free to move the extremities, and normal activity should be encour-

Chart 44-6 ASSESSMENT
Assessing for Home Nutrition Support

Be alert to the following assessment findings:

- Water: Water is necessary for hand hygiene and cleaning of work areas.
- Electricity: A reliable power source is needed to provide proper lighting and charging of pumps.
- Refrigeration: Refrigeration must be adequate for accommodation of several bags of parenteral nutrition solution.
- Telephone: A telephone is necessary for contacting home health personnel, arranging for prompt delivery of supplies, and for emergency purposes.
- Environment:
  - Should be free of rodents and insects
  - Should have storage that is not accessible to pets and small children
  - Should be assessed for stairs, carpets, and inaccessible areas, which can limit mobility with infusion pumps if the patient has a disability

Adapted from Durfee, S. M., Adams, S. C., Arthur, E., et al.; Home and Alternate Site Care Task Force and the American Society for Parenteral and Enteral Nutrition (ASPEN). (2014). ASPEN standards for nutrition support: Home and alternate site care. *Nutrition in Clinical Practice, 29*(4), 542–555.

aged to maintain good muscle tone. If applicable, the education and exercise program initiated by occupational and physical therapists is reinforced.

PROMOTING HOME, COMMUNITY-BASED, AND TRANSITIONAL CARE

Educating Patients About Self-Care. Successful home PN requires educating the patient and family in specialized skills using an intensive training program and follow-up supervision in the home. This is best accomplished through a team effort. Initiation of a home program facilitates the patient's discharge from the hospital.

Ideal candidates for home PN are patients who have a reasonable life expectancy after return home, have a limited number of illnesses other than the one that has resulted in the need for PN, and are highly motivated and fairly self-sufficient. Ethical dilemmas occur when the patient and family, as well as the caregiver, do not thoroughly understand what is involved in home PN. In addition, the ability to learn, availability of family interest and support, adequate finances, and physical plan of the home are factors that must be assessed when the decision about home PN is made (see Chart 44-6).

Many home health care agencies have developed education brochures and videos for home PN treatment. Topics include catheter and dressing care, the use of an infusion pump, administration of fat emulsions, and catheter maintenance. Education begins in the hospital and continues in the home or ambulatory infusion center.

Continuing and Transitional Care. The home, community-based, or transitional care nurse should be aware that the typical patient needs several instruction sessions for assessment of learning and reinforcement. More information about home patient education is presented in Chart 44-7. Special considerations for older adult patients who go home with nutrition support are presented in Chart 44-8.

Evaluation

Expected patient outcomes may include the following:

1. Attains or maintains nutritional balance
2. Is free of catheter-related infection
   a. Is afebrile
   b. Has no purulent drainage from the catheter insertion site
3. Is hydrated, as evidenced by good skin turgor
4. Achieves an optimal level of activity, within limitations
5. Demonstrates skill in managing PN regimen
6. Prevents complications
   a. Maintains proper catheter and equipment function
   b. Maintains metabolic balance within normal limits

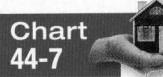

Chart 44-7 HOME CARE CHECKLIST
The Patient Receiving Parenteral Nutrition

At the completion of education, the patient and/or caregiver will be able to:

- State the goal and purpose of parenteral nutrition (PN) therapy and any impact on physiologic functioning, ADLs, IADLs, roles, relationships, and spirituality.
- State what types of changes are needed (if any) to support home PN therapy and maintain a clean home environment and prevent infection.
- State how to contact the primary provider, the team of home care professionals overseeing care, and parental nutrition supply vendor.
  - List emergency phone numbers
- State how to obtain medical supplies and carry out catheter and dressing care, and other prescribed regimens.
- Demonstrate how to perform catheter and dressing care.
- Discuss basic components of PN solution and intravenous fat emulsions.
- State the name, dose, side effects, frequency, and schedule for all medications.
- Demonstrate accurate and safe administration of medications.

- Demonstrate how to handle solutions and medications correctly.
- Demonstrate correct administration of PN
  - Operate infusion pump
  - Prime tubing and filter
  - Connect and disconnect PN infusion
  - Flush central line
  - Clean and maintain pump
  - Change tubing and filters as directed
- Discuss pump warning signals and how to address these signals.
- Identify possible PN complications and interventions.
- Relate how to reach primary provider with questions or complications.
- Identify a plan for refrigeration of PN solutions and operation of parental nutrition pump during a power outage or other emergency.
- State time and date of follow-up appointments and testing.
- Identify the need for health promotion, disease prevention and screening activities.

ADL, activities of daily living; IADL, independent activities of daily living.

Chart 44-8 — The Older Adult Patient and Home Parenteral and Enteral Nutrition

Age-related conditions that affect home nutrition support goals include the following:

- Arthritis—possible decreased hand dexterity and fine motor coordination
- Sensory impairment—inability to hear pump alarms; vision loss may affect ability to see pump menus or fill syringes
- Constipation—decreased overall bowel tone, which can cause intolerance of enteral feedings; water and fiber intake should be assessed
- Impaired thirst—may require close clinical management of fluid needs
- Obesity—decreased basal metabolic rate increases tendency toward weight gain; may require a kilocalorie reduction to compensate
- Diabetes—increased insulin resistance, which makes glucose control during PN infusion more challenging
- Depression/dementia—mood and memory disorders, which may present as low motivation to learn and adhere to the nutrition support regimen
- Multiple medications—conversion to an appropriate route or form required

Adapted from Durfee, S. M., Adams, S. C., Arthur, E., et al.; Home and Alternate Site Care Task Force and the American Society for Parenteral and Enteral Nutrition (ASPEN). (2014). ASPEN standards for nutrition support: Home and alternate site care. *Nutrition in Clinical Practice, 29*(4), 542–555.

CRITICAL THINKING EXERCISES

1 **ebp** A patient with a small bowel obstruction needs a central intravenous catheter for parenteral nutrition. Outline the steps you will take to assist the primary provider during insertion of the central line, including evidence-based infection prevention measures.

2 **ebp** You are caring for a patient with a small bowel feeding tube. As you prepare to administer medications through the tube, you observe that the tape that was securing the tube to the patient's cheek has come undone and the tube appears to be dislodged. Identify the evidence-based actions you will take to assess the tube location and the strength of the evidence for each method.

3 **pq** A 72-year-old patient with a G tube with continuous tube feedings is admitted to your unit from a skilled nursing facility for decreased level of consciousness. As you evaluate her tolerance of the tube feedings, you notice purulent drainage and red pustules around the insertion site of the G tube. The patient grimaces as you clean around the G tube. Is this an assessment finding that you should report to the primary provider? Describe your priority nursing interventions.

REFERENCES

*Asterisk indicates nursing research.
**Double asterisk indicates classic reference.

Books

American Nurses Association (ANA). (2011). *Forging nutrition and hydration.* Retrieved on 8/28/2016 at: www.nursingworld.org/MainMenuCategories/EthicsStandards/Ethics-Position-Statements/prtetnutr14451.pdf

Brantley, S. L., & Mills, M. E. (2012). Chapter 10: Overview of enteral nutrition. In C. M. Mueller (Ed.): *The ASPEN nutrition support core curriculum* (2nd ed.). Silver Springs, MD: American Society for Parenteral and Enteral Nutrition.

Gangadharan, S. P. (2015). Jejunal feeding tube complications. In T. M. Pawlick, S. K. Maithel, & N. B. Merchant (Eds.). *Gastrointestinal surgery.* New York: Springer.

Journals and Electronic Documents

Arora, G., & Lukens, F. J. (2015). Percutaneous endoscopic gastrostomy (PEG) tube placement. In D. A. Sherwinter (Ed.): *Medscape News and Perspective.* Retrieved on 06/24/2016 at: www.emedicine.medscape.com/article/149665-overview#a9.

**Bankhead, R., Boullata, J., Brantley, S., et al. (2009). ASPEN enteral nutrition practice recommendations. *Journal of Parenteral and Enteral Nutrition, 33*(2), 122–167. Retrieved on 5/30/2016 at: pen.sagepub.com/content/33/2/122

Blumenstein, I., Shastri, Y. H., & Stein, J. (2014). Gastroenteric tube feeding: Techniques, problems, and solutions. *World Journal of Gastroenterology, 20* (26), 8505–8524.

DeLegge, M. H. (2015). Gastrostomy tubes: Placement and routine care. In J. R. Saltzman, T. O. Lipman, & A. C. Travis (Eds.). *UpToDate.* Retrieved on 06/08/2016 at: www.uptodate-com.medjournal.hmc.psu.edu

*DiLibero, J., Lavieri, M., O'Donoghue, S., et al. (2015). Withholding or continuing enteral feedings during repositioning and the incidence of aspiration. *American Journal of Critical Care, 24*(3), 258–261.

Durfee, S. M., Adams, S. C., Arthur, E., et al.; Home and Alternate Site Care Task Force and the American Society for Parenteral and Enteral Nutrition (ASPEN). (2014). ASPEN standards for nutrition support: Home and alternate site care. *Nutrition in Clinical Practice, 29*(4), 542–555.

Gauglitz, G. G. (2014). Hypermetabolic response to severe burn injury: Recognition and treatment. In M. G. Jeschke (Ed.): *UpToDate.* Retrieved on 06/25/2016 at: www.uptodate.com/contents/hypermetabolic-response-to-severe-burn-injury-recognition-and-treatment

Gervasio, J. (2015). Total nutrient admixtures (3-in-1) pros vs cons for adults. *Nutrition in Clinical Practice, 30*(3). doi: 10.1177/0884533615578458.

Gorski, L., Hadaway, L., Hagle, M. E., et al. (2016). Infusion therapy standards of practice. *Journal of Infusion Nursing (Supplement), 39*(1S), S1–S159.

Gupta, A., & Khanna, S. (2014). Community-acquired Clostridium difficile infection: An increasing public health threat. *Infectious Drug Resistance Journal, 7,* 63–72. doi: 10.2147/IDR.S46780.

Heuschkel, R., & Duggan, C. (2015). Enteral feeding: Gastric versus post-pyloric. In T. Lipman & S. Grover (Eds.). *UpToDate.* Retrieved on 06/08/2016 at: www.uptodate-com.medjournal.hmc.psu.edu

Hodin, R. A., & Bordeianou, L. (2015). Nasogastric and nasoenteric tubes. In H. Sanfey & K. A. Collins (Eds.). *UpToDate.* Retrieved on 06/08/2016 at: www.uptodate-com.medjournal.hmc.psu.edu

Institute for Healthcare Improvement (IHI). (2012). *How-to Guide: Prevent Central Line-Associated Bloodstream Infection.* Retrieved on 11/28/2015 at: www.ihi.org/knowledge/Pages/Tools/HowtoGuidePreventCentralLineAssociatedBloodstreamInfection.aspx

Institute for Safe Medication Practices (ISMP). (2015). *Update on Implementation of the New ENFit Enteral Connectors.* Retrieved on 08/27/2015 at: www.ismp.org/newsletters/acutecare/showarticle.aspx?id=114

Joint Commission (2014). Managing risk during transition to new ISO tubing connector standards. *Joint Commission Sentinel Event Alert. Issue 53.* Retrieved on 06/20/2016 at www.jointcommission.org/assets/1/6/SEA_53_Connectors_8_19_14_final.pdf

Marschall, J., Mermel, L. A., Fakih, M., et al. (2014). Strategies to prevent central line-associated bloodstream in acute care hospitals: 2014 update. *Infection Control and Hospital Epidemiology, 35*(7), 753–771.

McClave, S. A., Taylor, B. E., Martindale, R. G., et al. (2016). Guidelines for the provision and assessment of nutrition support therapy in the adult critically ill patient: Society of Critical Care Medicine (SCCM) and American Society for Parenteral and Enteral Nutrition (ASPEN). *Journal of Parenteral and Enteral Nutrition, 40*(2), 159–211.

Metheny, N. (2016). AACN Practice Alert: Initial and ongoing verification of feeding tube placement in adults. *Critical Care Nurse, 36*(2), e8–e13.

**Metheny, N. Eisenberg, P., & McSweeney, M. (1988). Effect of feeding tube properties and three irrigants on clogging rates. *Nursing Research, 37,* 165–169.

Miller, K. R., McClave, S. A., Kiraly, L. N., et al. (2014). A tutorial on enteral access in adult patients in the hospitalized setting. *Journal of Parenteral and Enteral Nutrition, 38*(3), 282–295.

National Healthcare Safety Network. (2015). Adherence for central line insertion practices (CLIP) surveillance. Retrieved on 06/27/2016 at: www.cdc.gov/nhsn/acute-care-hospital/clip/imdex.html

**Nicalou, D. P., & Davis, S. K. (1990). Carbonated beverages as irrigants for feeding tubes. *Annals of Pharmacotherapy, 24,* 840.

Patterson, J. (2013). Providing artificial nutrition and hydration in palliative care. *Nursing Standard, 27*(20), 35–42.

Reignier, J., Mercier, E., Le Gouge, A., et al. (2013). Effect of not monitoring residual gastric volume on risk of ventilator-associated pneumonia in adults receiving mechanical ventilation and early enteral feeding: A randomized controlled study. *JAMA, 309*(3), 249–256.

Seres, D. (2016). Nutrition support in critically ill patients: Enteral nutrition. In P. E. Parsons & T. O. Lipman (Eds.). *UpToDate.* Retrieved on 06/20/2016 at www.uptodate-com.medjournal.hmc.psu.edu:2048

Smithard, D., Barrett, N. A., Hargroves, D., et al. (2015). Electromagnetic sensor-guided enteral access systems: A literature review. *Dysphagia.* doi: 10.1007/s00455-015-9607-4.

Williams, T. A., Leslie, G., Mills, L., et al. (2013). Frequency of aspirating gastric tubes for patients receiving enteral nutrition in the ICU: A randomized controlled trial. *Journal of Parenteral and Enteral Nutrition, 38*(7), 809–816.

**Wilson, M. F., & Hayes-Johnson, V. (1987). Cranberry juice or water? A comparison of feeding-tube irrigants. *Nutrition Support Service, 7*(7), 23–24.

Resources

American Cancer Society, www.cancer.org

American Society for Gastrointestinal Endoscopy (ASGE), www.asge.org

American Society for Nutrition (ASN), www.nutrition.org

American Society for Parenteral and Enteral Nutrition (A.S.P.E.N.), www.nutritioncare.org

Infusion Nurses Society (INS), www.ins1.org/i4a/pages/index.cfm?pageid=1

Oley Foundation, oley.org/?

Society of Gastroenterology Nurses and Associates (SGNA), www.sgna.org

45

Management of Patients With Oral and Esophageal Disorders

LEARNING OBJECTIVES

On completion of this chapter, the learner will be able to:

1 Define the relationship of dental hygiene and dental problems to nutrition and disease.
2 Describe the nursing management of patients with abnormalities of the oral cavity, jaw, and salivary glands.
3 Explain the nursing management of patients with cancer of the oral cavity.

4 Use the nursing process as a framework for care of patients undergoing neck dissection.
5 Apply the nursing process as a framework for care of patients with various conditions of the esophagus.
6 Identify various disorders of the esophagus and their clinical manifestations and management.

GLOSSARY

achalasia: absent or ineffective peristalsis (wavelike contraction) of the distal esophagus accompanied by failure of the esophageal sphincter to relax in response to swallowing

Boerhaave syndrome: spontaneous esophageal rupture due to forceful vomiting or straining

dysphagia: difficulty swallowing

dysplasia: abnormal change in cells

Frey syndrome: a rare syndrome characterized by undesirable sweating and flushing occurring on the cheek, temporal region, and behind the ears after eating certain foods; also called auriculotemporal syndrome

gastroesophageal reflux disease (GERD): disorder marked by backflow of gastric or duodenal contents into the esophagus that causes troublesome symptoms and/or mucosal injury to the esophagus

gingivitis: inflammation of the gums; change in color from pink to red, with associated swelling, bleeding, and sensitivity/tenderness

halitosis: foul odor from the oral cavity; in laymen's terms, "bad breath"

hernia: protrusion of an organ or part of an organ through the wall of the cavity that normally contains it

lithotripsy: the use of shock waves to break up or disintegrate stones

odynophagia: pain on swallowing

parotitis: inflammation of the parotid gland

periapical abscess: abscessed tooth

pyrosis: a burning sensation in the stomach and esophagus that moves up to the mouth; commonly called heartburn

sialadenitis: inflammation of the salivary glands

stomatitis: inflammation of the oral mucosa

temporomandibular disorders: a group of conditions that cause pain or dysfunction of the temporomandibular joint and surrounding structures

vagotomy syndrome: dumping syndrome; gastrointestinal symptoms, such as diarrhea and abdominal cramping, resulting from rapid gastric emptying

xerostomia: dry mouth

Because digestion normally begins in the mouth, adequate nutrition is related to good dental health and the general condition of the mouth. Any discomfort, abnormalities, or disease processes in the oral cavity can affect a person's nutritional status. Changes in the oral cavity can influence the type and amount of food ingested as well as the degree to which food particles are properly mixed with salivary enzymes. Disorders of the mouth or tongue can interfere with speech and thus affect communication and self-image. Esophageal problems related to swallowing can also adversely affect food and fluid intake, thereby jeopardizing general health and well-being. Given the close relationship between adequate nutritional intake and the structures of the upper gastrointestinal (GI) tract (lips, mouth, teeth, pharynx, esophagus), health education can help prevent disorders associated with these structures (see Fig. 45-1).

DISORDERS OF THE ORAL CAVITY

Oral health is a very important component of a person's physical and psychological sense of well-being. Periodontal disease, which encompasses both **gingivitis** (inflammation of the gums) and periodontitis (which involves the soft tissue and bone supporting the teeth), is the most common cause of tooth loss among adults (U.S. Department of Health and Human Services [HHS], 2000; HHS, 2014). Approximately 8.52% of adults between the ages of 20 and 64 years have periodontal disease, with 5.08% of adults having moderate to severe periodontal disease. In addition, 47.2% of adults aged 30 or older (64.7 million adults) have some form of periodontal disease, with 38.5% having either moderate or severe periodontal disease

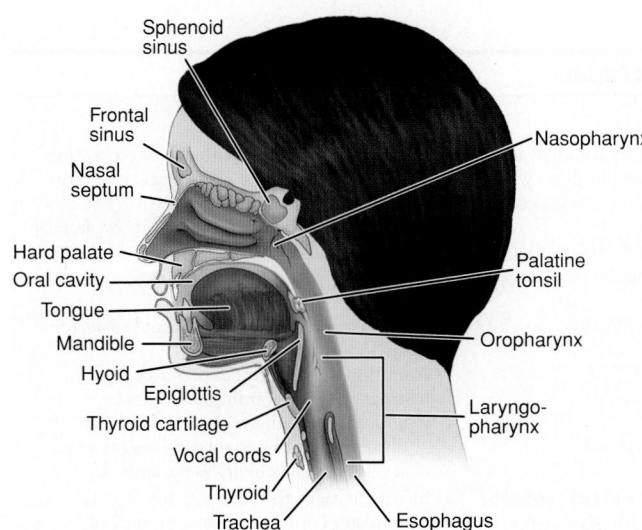

Figure 45-1 • Anatomy of the head and neck.

(Eke, Dye, Wei, et al., 2012). Individuals at risk for periodontal disease are older, black or Hispanic, current smokers, and have lower incomes and less education (Eke et al., 2012). Periodontal disease can be connected to a variety of other systemic diseases, such as cardiovascular disease, diabetes, and rheumatoid disease (American Academy of Periodontology [AAP], 2015). Table 45-1 reviews common abnormalities of the oral cavity, their possible causes, and nursing considerations. Figure 45-2 illustrates structures of the oral cavity.

Dental Plaque and Caries

Tooth decay is an erosive process that begins with the action of bacteria on fermentable carbohydrates in the mouth, which produces acids that dissolve tooth enamel. Despite the

fact tooth enamel is the hardest substance in the human body, caries and periodontal disease can occur for several reasons. Contributing factors include nutrition, soft drink consumption, and genetic predisposition. In addition, the extent of damage to the teeth may be related to the following:

- Presence of dental plaque, which is a gluey, gelatin-like substance that adheres to the teeth. The initial action that causes damage to a tooth occurs under dental plaque.
- Length of time acids are in contact with the teeth
- Strength of acids and the ability of the saliva to neutralize them
- Susceptibility of the teeth to decay

Dental decay begins with a small hole, usually in a fissure (a break in the tooth's enamel) or in an area that is hard to clean. Left unchecked, the decay extends into the dentin. Because dentin is not as hard as enamel, decay progresses more rapidly and in time reaches the pulp of the tooth.

Dentists can determine the extent of damage and the type of treatment needed using x-ray studies. Treatment for dental caries includes fillings, dental implants, or extraction, if necessary. In general, dental decay can occur in anyone. Older adults are subject to decay from drug-induced or age-related oral dryness (see Chart 45-1).

Prevention

Measures used to prevent and control primary dental caries include applying fluoride varnish/gel (Marinho, Worthington, Walsh, et al., 2015), using fluoride toothpaste, applying dental sealants (Twetman, 2015), and ensuring community water fluoridation (HHS, 2000; HHS, 2014). Other recommendations include implementing daily oral hygiene practices, seeking routine professional dental treatment, refraining from smoking and excessive alcohol use, making good dietary choices, and managing related systemic diseases (HHS, 2016).

Mouth Care

Healthy teeth must be cleaned on a daily basis. Brushing and flossing are particularly effective in mechanically breaking up the bacterial plaque that collects around teeth.

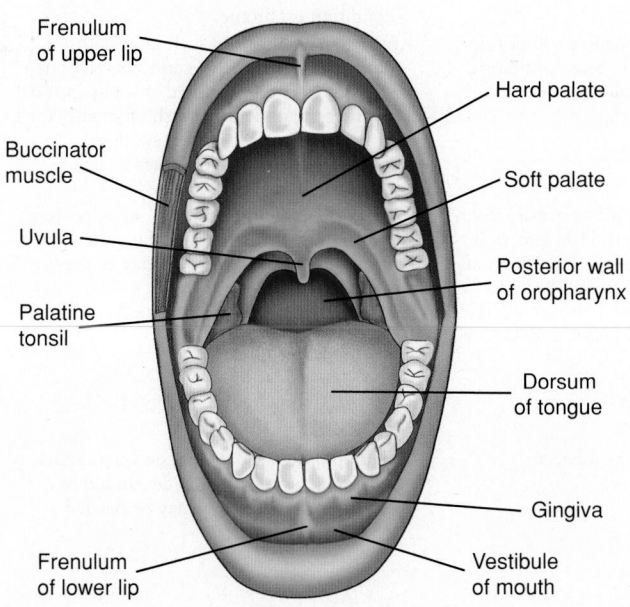

Figure 45-2 • Structures of the mouth, including the tongue and palate.

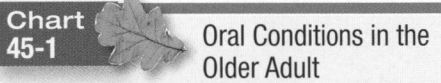

Chart 45-1 Oral Conditions in the Older Adult

Many medications taken by older adults cause dry mouth, which is uncomfortable, impairs communication, and increases the risk of oral infection. These medications include the following:

- Antidepressant medications
- Antihypertensive medications
- Anti-inflammatory agents
- Diuretic agents

Poor dentition can exacerbate problems of aging, such as:

- Decreased food intake
- Increased susceptibility to systemic infection (from periodontal disease)
- Loss of appetite
- Social isolation
- Trauma to the oral cavity secondary to thinner, less vascular oral mucous membranes

TABLE 45-1 Disorders of the Lips, Mouth, and Gums

Condition	Signs and Symptoms	Possible Causes and Sequelae	Nursing Considerations
Abnormalities of the Lips			
Actinic cheilitis	Irritation of lips associated with scaling, crusting, fissure; white overgrowth of horny layer of epidermis (hyperkeratosis) Considered a premalignant squamous cell skin cancer	Exposure to sun; more common in fair-skinned people and in those whose occupations involve sun exposure, such as farmers Chronic inflammatory lesion that may lead to squamous cell cancer of the lip	Educate patient on importance of protecting lips from the sun by using protective ointment such as sun block. Instruct patient to have a periodic checkup by primary provider.
Chancre	Reddened circumscribed lesion that ulcerates and becomes crusted	Primary lesion of syphilis	Use comfort measures such as cold soaks to lip, mouth care. Administer antibiotics as prescribed. Instruct patient regarding contagion. Use topical over-the-counter agents (e.g., Blistex, Carmex) or antiviral agents (e.g., acyclovir, penciclovir) as prescribed.
Contact dermatitis (i.e., allergic contact cheilitis)	Red area or rash; itching	Allergic reaction to lipstick, cosmetic ointments, or toothpaste	Instruct patient to avoid possible causes. Administer corticosteroids as prescribed.
Herpes simplex virus-1 (cold sore or fever blister)	Symptoms may be delayed up to 20 days after exposure; singular or clustered, irregular, painful vesicles throughout the oral cavity and lips that may rupture	An opportunistic infection; frequently seen in patients who are immunosuppressed May recur with menstruation, fever, or sun exposure	Use acyclovir ointment or systemic medications as prescribed. Administer analgesic agents as prescribed. Instruct patient to avoid irritating foods.
Abnormalities of the Mouth			
Leukoplakia	White patches; may be hyperkeratotic; usually in buccal mucosa; typically painless	Fewer than 2% are malignant, but may progress to cancer (premalignant) Common among tobacco users	Instruct patient to see the primary provider if leukoplakia persists >2 weeks. Eliminate risk factors, such as cigarettes, smokeless tobacco.
Oral hairy leukoplakia	White patches with rough hair-like projections; typically found on lateral border of the tongue	Possibly viral Related to smoking and the use of tobacco Associated with HIV infection	Instruct patient to see the primary provider if condition persists >2 weeks.
Lichen planus	Radiating white striations on the tongue and buccal mucosa; often association with painful ulcerations and erythema	Chronic inflammatory condition of unknown cause Recurrences are common May lead to a malignant process	Apply topical corticosteroids such as fluocinolone acetonide gel. Avoid foods that irritate. Administer corticosteroids systemically or intralesionally as prescribed. Instruct the patient of need for follow-up if condition is chronic.
Candidiasis (moniliasis/thrush)	Cheesy white plaque that looks like milk curds; when rubbed off, it leaves an erythematous and often bleeding base.	*Candida albicans* fungus; predisposing factors include diabetes, antibiotic therapy, and immunosuppression	Antifungal medications such as nystatin or clotrimazole may be prescribed as suspensions or troche; when used as a suspension, instruct the patient to swish vigorously for at least 1 minute and then swallow. If these treatments fail, oral agents such as fluconazole may be prescribed.
Aphthous stomatitis (canker sore) (Classified as *major* or *minor* depending upon size)	Shallow ulcer with a white or yellow center and typically a well-defined red border; seen on the inner side of the lip and cheek or on the tongue; it begins with a burning or tingling sensation and slight swelling; painful; usually lasts 7–10 days (*minor*) and heals without a scar.	Immune-mediated inflammatory disorder associated with HIV infection Associated with emotional or mental stress, fatigue, hormonal factors, minor trauma (e.g., biting), allergies, acidic foods and juices, and dietary deficiencies May recur	Instruct the patient in comfort measures (e.g., saline rinses) and a soft or bland diet. Antibiotics or corticosteroids may be prescribed. Use over-the-counter benzocaine as indicated.
Nicotine stomatitis (smoker's patch)	Two stages—begins as a red stomatitis; over time, the tongue and mouth become covered with a creamy, thick, white mucous membrane, which may slough, leaving a beefy red base.	Chronic irritation by tobacco	Cessation of tobacco use; if condition exists >2 weeks, a primary provider should be consulted and a biopsy may be needed.

TABLE 45-1 Disorders of the Lips, Mouth, and Gums (continued)

Condition	Signs and Symptoms	Possible Causes and Sequelae	Nursing Considerations
Erythroplakia	Red patch on the oral mucous membrane	Nonspecific inflammation; more frequently seen in older adults	
Kaposi sarcoma	Appears first on the oral mucosa as a red, purple, or blue lesion; may be singular or multiple; may be flat or raised Lesions can occur in other parts of the body: skin, lymph nodes, lungs, digestive tract	Cancer that develops from the cells that line the blood vessels and lymph system Associated with HIV infection (AIDS), men who are HIV negative and who have sex with men, organ transplantation, and geographic region (Mediterranean, Africa)	Instruct patient regarding side effects of planned treatment for HIV.
Stomatitis	Mild erythema and edema; severe forms include painful ulcerations, bleeding, and secondary infection.	Inflammation of the mucous lining of the mouth Associated with chemotherapy; radiation therapy; severe drug allergy; myelosuppression (bone marrow depression)	Prophylactic mouth care, including brushing, flossing, and rinsing, for any patient receiving chemotherapy or radiation therapy. Educate patient about proper oral hygiene, including the use of a soft-bristled toothbrush and nonabrasive toothpaste; for painful ulcers, oral swabs with spongelike applicators can be used in place of a toothbrush; avoid alcohol-based mouth rinses and hot or spicy foods. Apply topical anti-inflammatory, antibiotic, and anesthetic agents as prescribed.
Abnormalities of the Gums			
Gingivitis	Painful, inflamed, swollen gums; usually, the gums bleed in response to light contact	Reversible form of inflammation of the gingiva (i.e., mild form of periodontal disease) Associated with poor oral hygiene: food debris, bacterial plaque, and calculus (tartar) accumulate Gums may also swell in response to normal processes such as puberty and pregnancy, with certain medications (phenytoin [Dilantin], calcium channel blockers, cyclosporine [Neoral]), or with a deficiency in the immune system (i.e., AIDS) or nutritional status	Educate patient about proper oral hygiene; tooth-brushing, flossing, rinsing (i.e., chlorhexidine), dental appointments every 3–6 months. Remove causal agents as appropriate—medications, smoking, dental appliances.
Necrotizing gingivitis (trench mouth)	Gray-white pseudomembranous ulcerations affecting the edges of the gums, mucosa of the mouth, tonsils, and pharynx; halitosis; painful, bleeding gums; swallowing and talking are painful.	Progressive, painful bacterial infection Related to poor oral hygiene, lack of access to dental care, inadequate rest, overwork, emotional stress, smoking, and poor nutrition	Educate patient about proper oral hygiene; see Chart 45-2. Irrigate with 2–3% hydrogen peroxide or normal saline solution. Avoid irritants such as smoking and spicy foods.
Herpetic gingivostomatitis	Burning sensation with the appearance of small vesicles 24–48 hours later; vesicles may rupture, forming sore, shallow ulcers covered with a gray membrane.	Herpes simplex viral infection Occurs most frequently in people who are immunosuppressed; may occur in other infectious processes such as streptococcal pneumonia, meningococcal meningitis, and malaria	Apply topical anesthetics as prescribed; may need opioids if pain is severe. Saline or 2–3% hydrogen peroxide irrigations Antiviral agents such as acyclovir may be prescribed.
Periodontitis	Little discomfort at onset; may have bleeding, infection, gum recession, and loosening of teeth; later in the disease, tooth loss may occur.	Deep, chronic inflammation of the gingiva May result from untreated gingivitis Poor or inadequate dental hygiene and inadequate diet contribute to development	Instruct patient in proper oral hygiene, chlorhexidine rinses. Instruct patient to consult a dentist or periodontist for antibiotic prescription, deep root scaling.

AIDS, acquired immunodeficiency syndrome; HIV, human immunodeficiency virus.

Adapted from American Cancer Society (ACS). (2016). *Kaposi sarcoma*. Retrieved on 6/13/2016 at: www.cancer.org/cancer/kaposisarcoma/detailedguide/kaposi-sarcoma-what-is-kaposi-sarcoma; Anderson, W. D., Treister, N. S., Mayeaux, E. J., et al. (2015). Oral lesions you can't afford to miss. *Journal of Family Practice, 64*(7), 392–399; O'Gorman, S. M., & Torgerson, R. R. (2016). Contact allergy in cheilitis. *International Journal of Dermatology, 55*(7), 386–391; Silk, H. (2014). Disease of the mouth. *Primary Care: Clinics in Office Practice, 41*(1), 75–90.

Mastication (chewing) and the normal flow of saliva also aid greatly in keeping the teeth clean. Because many ill patients do not consume adequate nutrients, they produce less saliva, which in turn reduces this natural tooth-cleaning process. The nurse may need to assume the responsibility for brushing the patient's teeth. Merely wiping the patient's mouth and teeth with a swab is ineffective. The most effective method is mechanical cleansing (brushing). If brushing is not possible, it is better to wipe the teeth with a gauze pad and then have the patient swish an antiseptic mouthwash several times before expectorating into an emesis basin. A soft-bristled toothbrush is more effective than a sponge or foam stick. Flossing should be performed daily. To prevent drying, the lips may be coated with a water-soluble gel.

Diet

Dental caries may be prevented by decreasing the amount of sugar and starch in the diet. Patients who snack should be encouraged to choose less cariogenic alternatives, such as fruits, vegetables, nuts, cheeses, or plain yogurt. Brushing after meals is recommended.

Fluoridation

Fluoridation of public water supplies has been found to decrease dental caries. Some areas of the country have natural fluoridation; other communities have added fluoride to public water supplies. As of 2012, 67.1% of Americans receive fluoridated water (Centers for Disease Control and Prevention [CDC], 2013). Studies suggest that by instituting a community water fluoridation program, tooth decay is reduced by 25% in both children and adults (Weno, 2015).

Fluoridation may also be achieved by having a dentist apply a concentrated gel or solution to the teeth; adding fluoride to home water supplies; using fluoridated toothpaste or mouth rinse; or using sodium fluoride tablets, drops, or lozenges.

Pit and Fissure Sealants

The occlusal surfaces of the teeth have pits and fissures—areas that are prone to caries. Some dentists apply a coating to fill and seal these areas on the primary and permanent molars to protect them from potential exposure to cariogenic processes. These sealants can last at least 48 months and significantly prevent tooth decay (Ahovuo-Saloranta, Forss, Walsh, et al., 2013).

Dental Health and Disease

Studies are ongoing that show the link between oral health and chronic disease such as diabetes, heart disease, low birth weight, premature births, and stroke. As early as 1989, it was posited that bacteria, specifically gram-negative bacteria, were the culprits that link periodontal disease to other systemic diseases, specifically coronary artery disease, including myocardial infarction, and stroke. More recently, it was confirmed that these bacteria cause an inflammatory response that initiates an increase in inflammatory markers such as C-reactive protein, white blood cells, and fibrinogen. These markers are associated with an increased risk of cardiovascular disease. Although research has not proven periodontal disease to be a direct cause of cardiovascular disease, data from short-term studies suggest that if periodontal disease is treated, systemic inflammation and endothelial dysfunction are reduced (Papapanou, 2015).

The World Health Organization (WHO) Global Oral Health Programme (2015) espouses a global focus on oral health promotion and disease prevention, with an emphasis on policy and guideline development to support equitable implementation of evidence-based practices in global communities. The Programme supports an emphasis on addressing modifiable risk factors (e.g., diet, nutrition, tobacco, alcohol, and oral hygiene), water sanitation, and fluoride initiatives (WHO, 2015).

Periapical Abscess

A **periapical abscess**, more commonly referred to as an abscessed tooth, involves a collection of pus in the apical dental periosteum (fibrous membrane supporting the tooth structure) and the tissue surrounding the apex of the tooth (where it is suspended in the jaw bone). The abscess may be acute or chronic. An acute periapical abscess arises from an infection, usually secondary to dental caries. The infection of the dental pulp extends through the apical foramen of the tooth to form an abscess around the apex.

A chronic periodontal abscess occurs from a slowly progressive infectious process. In contrast to the acute form, a fully formed abscess may occur without the patient's knowledge. The infection eventually leads to a "blind dental abscess," which is actually a periapical granuloma. It may enlarge to as much as 1 cm in diameter. It is often discovered on x-ray images and is treated by extraction or root canal therapy, often with apicoectomy (excision of the apex of the tooth root).

Clinical Manifestations

The abscess produces a dull, gnawing, continuous pain, often with a surrounding cellulitis and edema of the adjacent facial structures, and mobility of the involved tooth. The gum opposite the apex of the tooth is usually swollen on the cheek side. Swelling and cellulitis of the facial structures may make it difficult for the patient to open the mouth. There may also be a systemic reaction, fever, and malaise.

Medical Management

In the early stages of an infection, a dentist or oral surgeon may perform a needle aspiration or drill an opening into the pulp chamber to relieve pressure and pain and to provide drainage. Drainage is provided by an incision through the gingiva down to the jawbone. Purulent material escapes under pressure. This procedure may be performed in a dentist's office, an outpatient surgery center, or a same-day surgery department. After the inflammatory reaction has subsided, the tooth may be extracted or root canal therapy performed. Antibiotics, in the presence of overt spreading infection, and analgesics may be prescribed (Robertson, Keys, Rautemaa-Richardon, et al., 2015).

Nursing Management

The patient is assessed for bleeding after treatment and is instructed to use a warm saline or warm water mouth rinse to keep the area clean. The patient is also instructed to take antibiotic and analgesic agents as prescribed, to advance from a liquid diet to a soft diet as tolerated, and to keep follow-up appointments.

DISORDERS OF THE JAW

Abnormal conditions affecting the mandible (jaw) and the temporomandibular joint (which connects the mandible to the temporal bone at the side of the head in front of the ear) include congenital malformation, fracture, chronic dislocation, cancer, and syndromes characterized by pain and limited motion. Temporomandibular disorders and jaw surgery, a treatment common in many structural abnormalities or cancer of the jaw, are presented in this section.

Temporomandibular Disorders

Temporomandibular disorders are categorized as follows (National Institute of Dental and Craniofacial Research [NIDCR], 2013b):

- Myofascial pain—a discomfort in the muscles controlling jaw function and in neck and shoulder muscles
- Internal derangement of the joint—a dislocated jaw, a displaced disc, or an injured condyle
- Degenerative joint disease—rheumatoid arthritis or osteoarthritis in the jaw joint

Diagnosis and treatment of temporomandibular disorders remain somewhat ambiguous, but the condition is thought to affect about 10 million people in the United States (NIDCR, 2013b). Misalignment of the joints in the jaw and other problems associated with the ligaments and muscles of mastication are thought to result in tissue damage and muscle tenderness. Suggested causes include arthritis of the jaw, head injury, trauma or injury to the jaw or joint, stress, and malocclusion, although research does not support malocclusion or associated orthodonture as a cause (NICDR, 2013b).

Clinical Manifestations

Patients have jaw pain ranging from a dull ache to throbbing, debilitating pain that can radiate to the ears, teeth, neck muscles, and facial sinuses. They often have restricted jaw motion and locking of the jaw. There also may be a sudden change in the way the upper and lower teeth fit together. The patient may hear clicking, popping, and grating sounds when the mouth is opened, and chewing and swallowing may be difficult. Symptoms such as headaches, earaches, dizziness, and hearing problems may sometimes be related to temporomandibular disorders (Gauer & Semidey, 2015; NIDCR, 2013b).

Assessment and Diagnostic Findings

Diagnosis is based on the patient's report of pain, limitations in range of motion, **dysphagia** (difficulty swallowing), difficulty chewing, difficulty with speech, or hearing difficulties. Magnetic resonance imaging and other imaging studies are generally only used for severe or chronic symptoms.

Medical Management

Signs and symptoms improve over time for the majority of patients with temporomandibular joint disorders, with or without treatment. Conservative treatment is recommended (Reid & Greene, 2013). Most patients improve with a combination of simple noninvasive therapies that may include patient education on self-care, cognitive behavioral therapy, physical therapy, exercise and manual therapy, analgesics (nonsteroidal anti-inflammatory drugs [NSAIDs] and muscle relaxants initially), and oral appliance therapy (Gauer & Semidey, 2015; Reid & Greene, 2013).

Jaw Disorders Requiring Surgical Management

Correction of mandibular structural abnormalities may require surgery involving repositioning or reconstruction of the jaw. Simple fractures of the mandible without displacement, resulting from a blow to the chin, and planned surgical interventions, as in the correction of long or short jaw syndrome, may require treatment by these means. Jaw reconstruction may be necessary in the aftermath of trauma from a severe injury or cancer, both of which can cause tissue and bone loss. New research supports screening for concussion (see Chapter 68) with mandibular fractures associated with high-force impacts (Sobin, Kopp, Walsh, et al., 2016).

Mandibular fractures are usually closed fractures. Rigid plate fixation (insertion of metal plates and screws or arch bars into the bone to approximate and stabilize the bone) is the current treatment of choice in many cases of mandibular fracture and in some mandibular reconstructive surgery procedures. Current research revolves around the use of various types of reconstruction plates and fixation devices, quality of life after specific instrumentation, and device choice (van den Bergh, de Mol van Otterloo, van der Ploeg, et al., 2015), and surgical advances such as the use of endoscopic-assisted positioning of the fixator and surgical reduction (Belli, Liberatore, Elidon, et al., 2015). Bone grafting may be performed to replace structural defects using bones from the patient's own ilium, ribs, or cranial sites.

Nursing Management

Depending on the fracture, surgical reduction, and extent of maxillomandibular fixation (referred to as "wiring the jaw shut"), patients may have various levels of diet restrictions (Haggerty, 2015). A liquid or soft diet may be recommended for up to 4 to 6 weeks; if this is the case, dietary counseling should be obtained to ensure optimal caloric and protein intake. Nutritional supplements may be recommended. The patient needs specific guidelines for mouth care and feeding. Any irritated areas in the mouth should be reported to the primary provider. The importance of keeping scheduled appointments to assess the stability of the fixation appliance is emphasized.

DISORDERS OF THE SALIVARY GLANDS

The salivary glands consist of: the parotid glands, one on each side of the face below the ear; the submandibular glands, located below the jawbone; the sublingual glands, in the floor of the mouth under the tongue; and the minor salivary glands in the lips, buccal mucosa, and the lining of the mouth and throat. About 1500 mL of saliva is produced daily and swallowed. The major functions of the salivary glands include lubrication, protection against harmful bacteria, and digestion.

Parotitis

Parotitis (inflammation of the parotid gland) is the most common inflammatory condition of the salivary glands. Inflammation of the parotid, may be due to mumps (epidemic parotitis), a communicable disease caused by viral infection and most commonly affecting unvaccinated children.

People who are older, acutely ill, or debilitated with decreased salivary flow from general dehydration or medications are at high risk for bacterial parotitis. The infecting organism, typically *Staphylococcus aureus*, travels from the mouth through the salivary duct. The onset of parotitis is sudden and associated with fever, chills, and other systemic signs of infection. The gland swells and becomes tense and tender. The patient feels pain in the ear, and swollen glands interfere with swallowing. The swelling increases rapidly, and the overlying skin soon becomes red and shiny.

Medical management includes maintaining adequate nutritional and fluid intake, good oral hygiene, and discontinuing medications (e.g., tranquilizers, diuretic agents) that can diminish salivation. Antibiotic therapy is necessary for bacterial parotitis, and analgesics may be prescribed to control pain. If antibiotic therapy is not effective, the gland may need to be drained by a surgical procedure known as parotidectomy. This procedure may be necessary to treat chronic parotitis. The patient is advised to have any necessary dental work performed prior to surgery.

Sialadenitis

Sialadenitis (inflammation of the salivary glands) may be caused by dehydration, radiation therapy, stress, malnutrition, salivary gland calculi (stones; sialolithiasis), or improper oral hygiene. The inflammation is commonly associated with infection by *S. aureus*. In hospitalized or institutionalized patients, the infecting organism may be methicillin-resistant *S. aureus* (MRSA). Symptoms include pain, swelling, and purulent discharge. Antibiotics are used to treat infections. Massage, hydration, warm compresses, and sialagogues (substances that trigger saliva flow like hard candy or lemon juice) frequently cure the problem. Chronic sialadenitis is typically due to decreased salivary flow. Surgical drainage or excision of the gland and its duct are considered in cases of sialadenitis that are recurrent or refractory to antibiotics.

Salivary Calculus (Sialolithiasis)

Sialolithiasis, or salivary calculi (stones), usually occur (in 80% to 90% of cases) in the submandibular gland (Sigismund, Zenk, Koch, et al., 2015). Salivary gland ultrasonography or sialography (x-ray studies imaged after the injection of a radiopaque substance into the duct) may be required to demonstrate obstruction of the duct. Salivary calculi are formed mainly from calcium phosphate. If located within the gland, the calculi are irregular and vary in diameter from 1 to 35 mm (Sigismund et al., 2015).

Calculi within the salivary gland itself may cause no symptoms unless infection arises; however, a calculus that obstructs the gland's duct causes swelling and sudden, local, and often colicky pain, which is abruptly relieved by a gush of saliva. This characteristic symptom is often disclosed in the patient's health history. On physical assessment, the gland is swollen and quite tender, the stone itself can be palpable, and its shadow may be seen on x-ray images.

The calculus can be extracted fairly easily from the duct in the mouth. Sometimes, enlargement of the ductal orifice permits the stone to pass spontaneously. Occasionally, **lithotripsy**, a procedure that uses shock waves to disintegrate the stone, may be used instead of surgical extraction for parotid stones and smaller submandibular stones. Lithotripsy requires no anesthesia, sedation, or analgesia. Side effects can include local hemorrhage and swelling. Surgery may be necessary to remove the gland if symptoms and calculi recur repeatedly.

Neoplasms

Although they are uncommon, neoplasms (tumors or growths) of almost any type may develop in the salivary gland; 50% of these are benign, with 70% to 80% of all salivary neoplasms beginning in the parotid gland. Neoplasm accounts for more than 0.5% of all malignancies and 3% to 5% of all head and neck cancers (National Cancer Institute [NCI], 2015b). Risk factors include prior exposure to radiation to the head and neck, older age, and specific carcinogens introduced in specific work environments (asbestos, plumbing, and woodworking). Most patients with a benign tumor present with painless swelling of the glands; patients with a malignancy tend to have neurologic symptoms (weakness or numbness) and persistent facial pain. Diagnosis is based on the health history, physical examination, and the results of fine-needle aspiration biopsy.

Early-stage salivary gland tumors are usually curable with surgery alone. Dissection is carefully performed to preserve the seventh cranial nerve (facial nerve), although it may not be possible to do so if the tumor is extensive. Complications from surgery may involve facial nerve dysfunction and Frey syndrome. **Frey syndrome,** also known as auriculotemporal syndrome, involves facial sweating and flushing in the general location of the (removed) parotid gland that occurs while eating. Frey syndrome may be successfully treated with botulinum toxin type A injections (Xie, Wang, Xu, et al., 2015). If the salivary gland tumor is malignant, radiation therapy may follow surgery. Radiation therapy alone may be a treatment choice for tumors thought to be localized or if there is risk of facial nerve damage from surgical intervention. Chemotherapy may be considered in late stages. Recurrent tumors usually are more aggressive than initial tumors (NCI, 2015b).

CANCER OF THE ORAL CAVITY AND PHARYNX

Cancers of the oral cavity and pharynx, which can occur in any part of the mouth or throat, are curable if discovered early. Risk factors for cancer of the oral cavity and pharynx include any use of any form of tobacco (cigarette, cigar, and pipe, and smokeless tobacco), excessive use of alcohol, infection with human papillomavirus (HPV), and a history of previous head and neck cancer (NCI, 2015a). Oral cancers are often associated with the combined use of alcohol and tobacco—these substances have a synergistic carcinogenic effect. People who smoke and drink have a 30-fold increased risk of developing oral cavity or oropharyngeal cancer (American Cancer Society [ACS], 2015). Patient education directed toward avoiding high-risk behaviors is critical to prevent oral cancers.

In the United States, approximately 45,780 new cases of oral cavity and oropharyngeal cancer occur annually, with an estimated 8650 deaths. Men are diagnosed with oral and oropharyngeal cancer twice as often as women, with only Caucasian men showing an increase (by 1.3%) in rates each year between 2007 and 2011. Regardless of stage, patients with cancer of the oral cavity and oropharynx have a 5-year survival rate of 66%, which is a statistically significant increase in survival rates (53%) since 1977 (ACS, 2015).

Pathophysiology

Malignancies of the oral cavity are usually squamous cell carcinomas (Steinau, Saraiya, Goodman, et al., 2014). Any area of the oropharynx can be a site of malignant growths, but the lips, the lateral aspects of the tongue, and the floor of the mouth are most commonly affected. HPV is known to be associated with the development of cervical and other forms of cancer. A recent study retrospectively examined tumor tissue samples from patients diagnosed with oropharyngeal cancer from 1995 to 2005 to determine the prevalence of HPV infection before the HPV vaccine became readily available. More than 72% of the sample had some type of the HPV virus, with 60.5% testing positive for HPV-16 (Steinau et al., 2014).

Clinical Manifestations

Many oral cancers produce few or no symptoms in the early stages. Later, the most frequent symptom is a painless sore or lesion that bleeds easily and does not heal. Oral cancer may also present as a red or white patch in the mouth or throat (ACS, 2015). A typical lesion in oral cancer is a painless indurated (hardened) ulcer with raised edges. As the cancer progresses, the patient may complain of tenderness, difficulty in chewing, swallowing, or speaking, coughing of blood-tinged sputum, or enlarged cervical lymph nodes.

Assessment and Diagnostic Findings

Diagnostic evaluation consists of an oral examination as well as an assessment of the cervical lymph nodes to detect possible metastases. Biopsies are performed on suspicious lesions (those that have not healed in 2 weeks). In people who use snuff or smoke cigars or pipes, high-risk areas include the buccal mucosa and gingiva. In those who smoke cigarettes and drink alcohol, high-risk areas include the floor of the mouth, the ventrolateral tongue, and the soft palate complex (soft palate, anterior and posterior tonsillar area, uvula, and the area behind the molar and tongue junction).

Human Papillomavirus Prevention

HPV vaccine is generally recommended for all children ages 11 or 12, up to the age of 26 years for women and 21 years for men. Men who have sex with men may receive the vaccine up to 26 years of age (CDC, 2015). These vaccines protect against HPV-16, which is associated with oropharyngeal cancer (Steinau et al., 2014).

Medical Management

In patients diagnosed with oropharyngeal cancer, management varies with the nature of the lesion, the preference of the physician, and patient choice. Surgical resection and radiation therapy are standard treatment. Chemotherapy may be useful for advanced disease (ACS, 2015).

In cancer of the lip, small lesions are usually excised liberally. Radiation therapy may be more appropriate for larger lesions involving more than one third of the lip because of superior cosmetic results. The choice depends on the extent of the lesion and what is necessary to cure the patient while preserving the best appearance. Tumors larger than 4 cm often recur.

In cancer of the tongue, treatment with radiation therapy and chemotherapy may preserve function and maintain quality of life. A combination of radioactive interstitial implants (surgical implantation of a radioactive source into the tissue adjacent to or at the tumor site) and external-beam radiation may be used. Surgical procedures include hemiglossectomy (surgical removal of half of the tongue) and total glossectomy (removal of the tongue). Glossectomy remains the principal treatment of advanced stage or cancers at the base of the tongue; long-term data on functional outcomes following these procedures are being studied (Lin, Yarlagadda, Sethi, et al., 2015).

Often, cancer of the oral cavity has metastasized through the extensive lymphatic channel in the neck region, requiring a neck dissection and reconstructive surgery of the oral cavity. Reconstructive techniques involve the use of a free (cut and removed) or pedicled (attached and tunneled) tissue flap (graft of tissue with its own blood supply) most commonly obtained from the pectoralis major, rectus abdominis, or radial forearm (Rihani, Lee, Lee, et al., 2013). Laryngeal preservation is associated with better speech and verbal communication (Lin et al., 2015).

Nursing Management

The nurse assesses the patient's nutritional status preoperatively, and a dietary consultation may be necessary. The patient may require enteral (through the GI tract) or parenteral (intravenous [IV]) feedings before and after surgery to maintain adequate nutrition (see Chapter 44). Continual assessment and reevaluation are necessary. If a radial graft is to be performed, an Allen test on the donor arm must be performed to ensure that the ulnar artery is patent and can provide blood flow to the hand after removal of the radial artery. The Allen test is performed by asking the patient to make a fist and then manually compressing the ulnar artery. The patient is then asked to open the hand into a relaxed, slightly flexed position. The palm becomes pale. Pressure on the ulnar artery is released. If the ulnar artery is patent, the palm flushes within about 3 to 5 seconds.

Verbal communication may be impaired by radical surgery for oral cancer, especially if the larynx is removed. It is therefore vital to assess the patient's ability to communicate in writing before surgery. Pen and paper are provided postoperatively to patients who can use them to communicate. A communication board with commonly used words or pictures is obtained preoperatively and given after surgery to patients who cannot write so that they may point to needed items. Electronic devices, such as tablets or smartphones, may also be options for facilitating communication. A speech therapist is also consulted postoperatively.

Postoperatively, the nurse assesses for a patent airway. The patient may be unable to manage oral secretions, making suctioning necessary. If grafting was part of the surgery, suctioning must be performed with care to prevent damage to the graft. The graft is assessed postoperatively for viability. Although color should be assessed (white may indicate arterial occlusion, and blue mottling may indicate venous congestion), it can be difficult to assess the graft by looking into the mouth. A Doppler ultrasound device may be used to locate the radial pulse at the graft site and to assess tissue perfusion. Depending on the extent of the surgery, the patient may require a temporary or permanent tracheostomy after surgery (see Chapter 21).

NURSING MANAGEMENT OF THE PATIENT WITH DISORDERS OF THE ORAL CAVITY

Promoting Mouth Care

The nurse educates the patient regarding the importance and techniques of preventive mouth care. If a patient cannot tolerate brushing or flossing, rinsing or irrigating with a solution of ½ to 1 teaspoon of baking soda (or ¼ teaspoon salt) in 8 oz of warm water is recommended (NIDCR, 2013a). The nurse reinforces the need to perform oral care and provides such care to patients who cannot provide it for themselves.

If a bacterial or fungal infection is present, the nurse administers the prescribed medications and instructs the patient how to administer the medications at home. The nurse monitors the patient's physical and psychological response to treatment.

Xerostomia (dryness of the mouth) is a frequent sequela of oral cancer, particularly when the salivary glands have been exposed to radiation or major surgery. It is also seen in patients who are receiving psychopharmacologic agents, patients who are taking multiple medications, patients who use drugs recreationally, patients with rheumatic diseases, patients with eating disorders (Villa, Nordio, & Gohel, 2015), patients with human immune deficiency virus (HIV) infection, and patients who cannot close the mouth and as a result, breathe through the mouth instead of the nose. To minimize this problem, the patient is advised to avoid dry, bulky, and irritating foods and fluids, as well as alcohol and tobacco. The patient is also encouraged to increase intake of fluids (when not contraindicated) and to use a humidifier while sleeping. The use of synthetic saliva, chewing gum (Miranda-Rius, Brunet-Llobet, Lahor-Soler, et al., 2015), or a saliva production stimulant such as pilocarpine may be helpful (Cheng, Xu, Liu, et al., 2016).

Stomatitis, a type of oral mucositis, which involves inflammation and breakdown of the oral mucosa, is often a side effect of chemotherapy or radiation therapy. Prophylactic mouth care is started when the patient begins receiving treatment;

however, mucositis may become so severe that a break in treatment is necessary. Current evidence suggests not using chlorhexidine with patients receiving head and neck radiation therapy, but instead recommends benzydamine mouthwash, a type of NSAID, be used to prevent oral mucositis (Lalla, Bowen, Barasch, et al., 2014). The nurse may also use what is informally referred to as *magic mouthwash* or *BMX*, a solution that contains equal parts diphenhydramine (Benadryl), aluminum-magnesium hydroxide (Maalox), and viscous lidocaine (Xylocaine) to both numb and protect the mouth (see Chapter 15).

Ensuring Adequate Food and Fluid Intake

The patient's weight, age, and level of activity are recorded to determine whether nutritional intake is adequate. A daily calorie count may be necessary to determine the exact quantity of food and fluid ingested. The frequency and pattern of eating are recorded to determine whether any psychosocial or physiologic factors are affecting ingestion. Based on the disorder and the patient's preferences, the nurse recommends changes in the consistency of foods and the frequency of eating. Intensive nutritional counseling with a dietitian may be indicated (Bossola, 2015). The goal is to help the patient attain and maintain desirable body weight and level of energy, as well as to promote the healing of tissue.

Supporting a Positive Self-Image

A patient who has a disfiguring oral condition or has undergone disfiguring surgery may experience an alteration in self-image. The patient is encouraged to verbalize the perceived and actual change in body appearance and to realistically discuss changes or losses. The nurse offers support while the patient verbalizes fears and negative feelings (withdrawal, depressed mood, anger). The nurse listens attentively and determines the patient's needs and individualizes the plan of care.

The nurse should determine the patient's concerns about relationships with others. Referral to support groups, a psychiatric liaison nurse, a social worker, or a spiritual advisor may be useful in helping the patient cope with anxieties and fears. The patient's progress toward development of positive self-esteem is documented. The nurse should be alert to signs of grieving and should document emotional changes. By providing acceptance and support, the nurse encourages the patient to verbalize feelings.

Minimizing Pain and Discomfort

Oral lesions can be painful. Strategies to reduce pain and discomfort include avoiding foods that are spicy, hot, or hard (e.g., pretzels, nuts). A soft or liquid diet may be preferred. The patient is instructed about mouth care. The use of a soft toothbrush may prevent secondary trauma. The patient may require an analgesic agent such as viscous lidocaine or opioids, as prescribed. The nurse can reduce the patient's fear of pain by providing information about pain control methods.

Preventing Infection

Leukopenia (a decrease in white blood cells) may result from radiation, chemotherapy, acquired immune deficiency syndrome, and some medications used to treat HIV infection.

Leukopenia reduces defense mechanisms, increasing the risk of infections. Malnutrition, which is also common among these patients, may further decrease resistance to infection. If the patient has diabetes, the risk of infection is further increased.

Laboratory results should be evaluated frequently and the patient's temperature checked every 4 to 8 hours for an elevation that may indicate infection. Visitors who might transmit microorganisms are prohibited if the patient's immunologic system is depressed. Sensitive skin tissues are protected from trauma to maintain skin integrity and prevent infection. Aseptic technique is necessary when changing dressings. Desquamation (shedding of the epidermis) is a reaction to radiation therapy that causes dryness and itching and can lead to a break in skin integrity and subsequent infection.

Signs of wound infection (redness, swelling, drainage, tenderness) are reported to the primary provider. Antibiotics may be prescribed prophylactically.

Promoting Home, Community-Based, and Transitional Care

 Educating Patients About Self-Care

The patient who is recovering from treatment of an oral disorder is instructed about mouth care, nutrition, prevention of infection, and signs and symptoms of complications (see Chart 45-2). Methods of preparing nutritious foods that are seasoned according to the patient's preference and at the preferred temperature are explained to the patient and family. For some patients, it may be more convenient (but also more expensive) to use commercial baby foods than to prepare liquid and soft diets. The patient who cannot take foods orally may receive enteral or parenteral nutrition; the administration of these feedings is explained and demonstrated to the patient and the caregiver.

For patients with oral cancer, instructions are provided in the use and care of any dentures. The importance of keeping dressings clean and the need for conscientious oral hygiene are emphasized.

Continuing and Transitional Care

The need for ongoing care in the home depends on the patient's condition. The patient, family members, and other health care team members responsible for home care (e.g., nurse, speech therapist, nutritionist, and psychologist) work together to prepare an individual plan of care.

If suctioning of the mouth or tracheostomy tube is required, the necessary equipment is obtained and the patient and caregivers are taught how to use it. Considerations include the control of odors and humidification of the home to keep secretions moist. The patient and caregivers are educated to assess for obstruction, hemorrhage, and infection, as well as what actions to take if they occur. The nurse may provide physical care, monitor for changes in the patient's physical status (e.g., skin integrity, nutritional status, respiratory function), and assess the adequacy of pain control measures. The nurse also assesses the patient's and family's ability to manage incisions, drains, and feeding tubes and the use of recommended strategies for communication. The ability of the patient and family to accept physical, psychological, and role changes is assessed and addressed.

Follow-up visits to the primary provider are important to monitor the patient's condition and to determine the need for modifications in treatment and general care. Because patients and their family members, as well as health care providers, tend to focus on the most obvious needs and issues, the nurse reminds the patient and family about the importance of continuing health promotion and screening practices and refers them to appropriate practitioners. The nurse also reinforces instructions in an effort to promote the patient's self-care and comfort.

 HOME CARE CHECKLIST

Chart 45-2 · The Patient With an Oral Disorder

At the completion of education, the patient and/or caregiver will be able to:

- State the impact of the oral disorder and treatment on communication and other physiologic functioning, ADLs, IADLs, body image, roles, relationships, and spirituality.
- Identify modification of home environment, interventions, and strategies (e.g., durable medical equipment, home health aide) used in safely adapting to changes in structure or function and promote effective recovery and rehabilitation.
- Describe ongoing therapeutic regimen, including diet and activities to perform (e.g., oral care, suctioning) and to limit or avoid (e.g., oral foods if NPO).
  - Identify foods or therapies necessary to meet caloric needs and dietary needs (e.g., change in consistency, seasoning limitations, supplements, enteral or parenteral therapy).
  - Participate in prescribed therapy (e.g., speech therapy) to promote recovery and rehabilitation.
  - Demonstrate the use of suction equipment if indicated.
  - Demonstrate use of humidification if indicated.
  - Demonstrate effective oral hygiene.
  - Demonstrate care of incision as appropriate.

- State the name, dose, side effects, frequency, and schedule for all medications.
  - Describe approaches to controlling pain (e.g., take analgesics as prescribed; use nonpharmacologic interventions).
- Identify possible complications and interventions.
- Relate how to reach primary provider with questions or complications.
- State time and date of follow-up medical/dental appointments, therapy, and testing.
- Identify sources of support (e.g., friends, relatives, faith community, cancer support, caregiver support).
- Identify the need for health promotion, disease prevention, and screening activities.

Resources

See Chapter 44 for Digestive and Gastrointestinal Treatment Modalities, Chart 44-5 and Chart 44-7 The Patient Receiving Parenteral Nutrition.

ADL, activities of daily living; IADL, independent activities of daily living; NPO, nothing by mouth.

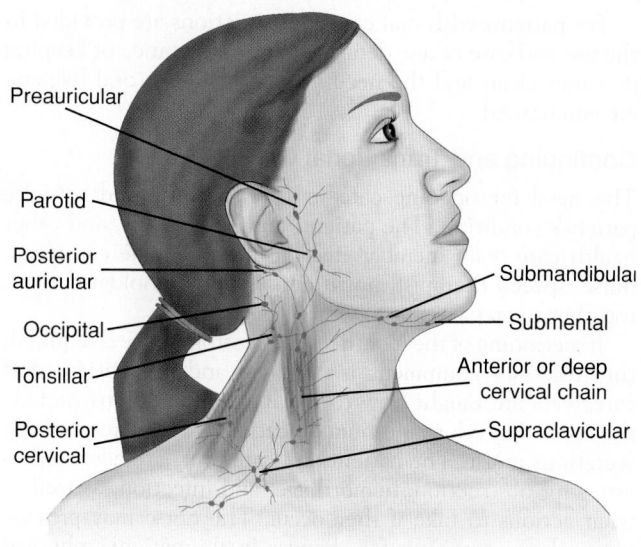

Figure 45-3 • Lymphatic drainage of the head and neck.

Labels: Preauricular, Parotid, Posterior auricular, Occipital, Tonsillar, Posterior cervical, Submandibular, Submental, Anterior or deep cervical chain, Supraclavicular

NECK DISSECTION

Deaths from malignancies of the head and neck are primarily attributable to local–regional metastasis to the cervical lymph nodes in the neck. This often occurs by way of the lymphatics before the primary lesion has been treated. This local–regional metastasis is not amenable to surgical resection and responds poorly to chemotherapy and radiation therapy. The cervical lymph nodes are classified as anterior or posterior and divided into regions for classification (Grègoire, Ang, Budach, et al., 2014; Robbins, Clayman, Levine, et al., 2002) (see Fig. 45-3).

A radical neck dissection involves removal of all cervical lymph nodes from the mandible to the clavicle and removal of the sternocleidomastoid muscle, internal jugular vein, and spinal accessory muscle on one side of the neck. The associated complications include shoulder drop and poor cosmesis (visible neck depression). Modified radical neck dissection, which preserves one or more of the nonlymphatic structures (internal jugular vein, sternocleidomastoid muscle, and the spinal accessory nerve) is used more often (Fonseca, Turvey, & Marciani, 2008). A selective neck dissection (in comparison to a radical or modified dissection) preserves one or more of the lymph node groups that are typically removed in a radical neck dissection. The selective neck dissection is the treatment usually used in oral cavity cancer (Robbins et al., 2002; see Fig. 45-4).

Reconstructive techniques may be performed with a variety of grafts. A cutaneous flap (skin and subcutaneous tissue), such as the deltopectoral flap, may be used. A myocutaneous flap (subcutaneous tissue, muscle, and skin) is a more frequently used graft; the pectoralis major muscle is usually used. For large grafts, a microvascular free flap may be used. This involves the transfer of muscle, skin, or bone with an artery and vein to the area of reconstruction, using microinstrumentation. Areas used for a free flap include the scapula, the radial area of the forearm, or the fibula. The fibula, which provides a larger bone area, may be used if mandibular reconstruction is involved (Fonseca et al., 2008).

NURSING PROCESS

The Patient Undergoing a Neck Dissection

Assessment

Preoperatively, the patient's physical and psychological preparation for major surgery is assessed, along with their knowledge of the preoperative and postoperative procedures. Postoperatively, the patient is assessed for complications such as altered respiratory status, wound infection, and hemorrhage. As healing occurs, neck range of motion is assessed to determine whether there has been a decrease in range of motion due to nerve or muscle damage.

Diagnosis

NURSING DIAGNOSES

Based on the assessment data, major nursing diagnoses may include the following:

- Deficient knowledge about preoperative and postoperative procedures

Label: Intact sternocleidomastoid muscle

Figure 45-4 • **A.** A classic radical neck dissection in which the sternocleidomastoid and smaller muscles are removed. All tissue is removed, from the ramus of the jaw to the clavicle. The jugular vein has also been removed. **B.** The modified neck dissection is similar, but preserves the sternocleidomastoid muscle, internal jugular vein, and/or spinal accessory nerve. **C.** The wound is closed, and portable suction drainage tubes are in place.

- Ineffective airway clearance related to obstruction by mucus, hemorrhage, or edema
- Acute pain related to surgical incision
- Impaired tissue integrity secondary to surgery and grafting
- Imbalanced nutrition: less than body requirements related to disease process or treatment
- Risk for situational low self-esteem related to diagnosis or prognosis
- Risk for caregiver role strain related to physical and emotional effects of disease and related surgical procedure
- Impaired verbal communication secondary to surgical resection
- Impaired physical mobility secondary to nerve injury

COLLABORATIVE PROBLEMS/POTENTIAL COMPLICATIONS

Potential complications include the following:

- Hemorrhage
- Chyle fistula
- Nerve injury

Planning and Goals

The major goals for the patient include increased knowledge of surgical procedure and treatment plan, maintenance of respiratory status, decreased pain, viability of the graft, maintenance of adequate intake of food and fluids, effective coping strategies (for patient and caregivers), effective communication, maintenance of shoulder and neck motion, and absence of complications.

Nursing Interventions

PROVIDING PREOPERATIVE PATIENT EDUCATION

Before surgery, the patient should be informed about the nature and extent of the surgery and what to expect in the postoperative period. The patient is encouraged to ask questions and to express concerns about the upcoming surgery and the expected results. During this exchange, the nurse has an opportunity to assess the patient's coping abilities, answer questions, and develop a plan for offering assistance. A sense of mutual understanding and rapport make the postoperative experience less traumatic for the patient. The patient's expressions of concern, anxieties, and fears guide the nurse in providing support postoperatively.

PROVIDING GENERAL POSTOPERATIVE CARE

The general postoperative nursing interventions are similar to those presented in Chapter 19 and are directed toward the identified nursing diagnoses and goals.

MAINTAINING AIRWAY CLEARANCE

After the endotracheal tube or airway has been removed and the effects of the anesthesia have worn off, the patient may be placed in the Fowler position to facilitate breathing and promote comfort. This position also increases lymphatic and venous drainage, facilitates swallowing, decreases venous pressure on the skin flaps, and prevents regurgitation and aspiration of stomach contents. If the patient has a tracheostomy, the nurse performs focused assessment and care of the stoma (see Chapter 21). Signs of respiratory distress, such as dyspnea, cyanosis, changes in mental status, and changes in vital signs, are assessed because they may suggest edema, hemorrhage, inadequate oxygenation, or inadequate drainage.

> **Quality and Safety Nursing Alert**
>
> *In the immediate postoperative period, the nurse assesses for stridor (coarse, high-pitched sound on inspiration) by listening frequently over the trachea with a stethoscope. This finding must be reported immediately because it indicates obstruction of the airway.*

Pneumonia may occur in the postoperative phase if pulmonary secretions are not removed. To aid in the removal of secretions, coughing and deep breathing are encouraged. With the nurse supporting the neck, the patient should assume a sitting position so that excessive secretions can be coughed up and expectorated. If this is ineffective, the patient's respiratory tract may have to be suctioned. Care is taken to protect the suture lines during suctioning. If a tracheostomy tube is in place, suctioning is performed through the tube. The patient may also be instructed on use of Yankauer suction (tonsil-tip suction) to remove oral secretions. Humidified air or oxygen is provided through the tracheostomy to keep secretions thin. Temperature should not be taken orally.

RELIEVING PAIN

Pain and the patient's fear of pain are assessed and managed. Patients with head and neck cancer often report less pain than patients with other types of cancer; however, the nurse needs to be aware that each person's pain experience is subjective. Pain management is monitored on a continual basis by the nursing staff and adjusted on an individual basis. Patient-controlled analgesia may be prescribed for postoperative pain management (see Chapter 12).

PROVIDING WOUND CARE

Wound drainage tubes are usually inserted during surgery to prevent the collection of fluid subcutaneously. The drainage tubes are connected to a portable suction device (e.g., Jackson-Pratt), and the container is emptied periodically. Between 80 and 120 mL of serosanguineous secretions may drain over the first 24 hours. Excessive drainage may be indicative of a chyle fistula or hemorrhage (see later discussion). Dressings are reinforced as needed and are observed for evidence of hemorrhage and constriction, which impair respiration and perfusion of the graft. A graft, if present, is assessed for color and temperature and for the presence of a pulse, if applicable, to determine viability. The graft should be pale pink and warm to the touch. The surgical incisions are also assessed for signs of infection (purulent, malodorous drainage), which are reported immediately. Prophylactic antibiotics may be prescribed in the early postoperative period. Aseptic technique is used when cleansing skin around the drains; dressings are changed as prescribed by the surgeon, usually on the second through the fifth postoperative days. Care should be taken to not apply excessive pressure to the surgical site in order to not impair flap perfusion and viability (Carr, 2016).

MAINTAINING ADEQUATE NUTRITION

Nutritional status is assessed preoperatively; early intervention to correct nutritional imbalances may decrease the risk of postoperative complications. Frequently, nutrition is less than optimal because of inadequate intake, and the patient often requires enteral or parenteral supplements preoperatively and postoperatively to attain and maintain a nutritional balance. Prophylactic nutritional support (before chemoradiation therapy or surgery) using a tube feeding is common and may prevent weight loss, reduce fluid imbalances, decrease hospitalizations, and prevent nonadherence to treatment (Bossola, 2015). Supplements that are nutritionally dense may help reestablish a positive nitrogen balance. They may be taken enterally by mouth, by a nasogastric (NG) feeding tube, or by a gastrostomy feeding tube (see Chapter 44).

The patient who can chew may take food by mouth; the patient's chewing ability determines whether some diet modification (e.g., soft, puréed, or liquid foods) is necessary. Food preferences should also be discussed with the patient. Oral care before eating may enhance the patient's appetite, and oral care after eating is important to prevent infection and dental caries.

SUPPORTING PATIENT SELF-ESTEEM AND THE NEEDS OF CAREGIVERS

Preoperatively, information about the planned surgery is given to the patient and family. Any questions are answered as accurately as possible. Postoperatively, psychological nursing interventions are aimed at supporting the patient who has had a change in body image or who has major concerns related to the prognosis. The patient may have difficulty communicating and may be concerned about their ability to breathe and swallow normally. The nurse supports the patient's family in encouraging and reassuring the patient that adjusting to the results of this surgery will take time. The nurse is also sensitive to the needs of family caregivers who are often responsible for both the physical and psychosocial care of the patient (Fronczek, 2015) (see Chart 45-3).

The person who has had extensive neck surgery often is sensitive about their appearance. This can occur when the operative area is covered by bulky dressings, when the incision line is visible, or later after healing has occurred and the appearance of the neck and possibly the lower face has been significantly altered. If the nurse accepts the patient's appearance and expresses a positive, optimistic attitude, the patient is more likely to be encouraged. The patient also needs an opportunity to express fears and concerns regarding the success of the surgery and the prognosis. The ACS may be a resource to provide a volunteer who meets with the patient either preoperatively or postoperatively and shares their own experience about the diagnosis, treatment, and recovery. The Look Good Feel Better programs of the ACS provide information about clothing and cosmetics that can be used to improve body image and self-esteem (see the Resources section at the end of this chapter).

People with cancer of the head and neck frequently have used alcohol or tobacco before surgery; postoperatively, they are encouraged to abstain from these substances. Alternative methods of coping need to be explored. A referral to Alcoholics Anonymous, a smoking cessation program, and family counseling may be appropriate.

PROMOTING EFFECTIVE COMMUNICATION

Communication plans begin preoperatively, when the patient and family determine which method of communication will be the best postoperatively. Useful communication methods for the patient who has undergone a laryngectomy include, dry-erase boards, writing materials, pictorial guides, computer aids, smart phones, tablets, and hand signals. During the postoperative period, the call bell must be readily accessible to the patient at all times.

The nurse obtains a consultation with a speech or language therapist. Alternative speech techniques, such as a voice prosthesis or esophageal speech, may be taught by a speech or language therapist (see Chapter 22).

MAINTAINING PHYSICAL MOBILITY

Excision of the sternocleidomastoid muscle and spinal accessory nerve results in weakness at the shoulder that can cause

---

Chart 45-3 · NURSING RESEARCH PROFILE
Family Caregivers of Patients with Head and Neck Cancers

Fronczek, A. E. (2015). A phenomenological study of family caregivers of patients with head and neck cancers. *Oncology Nursing Forum, 42*(6), 593–600.

Purpose

As patients transition from the acute care hospital environment to the home setting, family members often find themselves functioning as the patient's primary caregivers. These family caregivers must learn to manage the fairly complex physical, psychosocial, and economic challenges inherent in caring for patients diagnosed with head and neck cancers.

Design

This qualitative study explored the lived experience of family caregivers of patients with head and neck cancers, including cancer of the tonsil, larynx, nasopharynx, tongue, oral cavity, and lip. Nine family caregivers (eight female spouses and one adult son) participated in semi-structured interviews designed to elicit a description of their experience using van Manen's human science approach to phenomenology.

Findings

The analysis and associated reflection led to the identification of five major themes related to the lived experience of the caregivers in this study. Although the caregivers appreciated the need, most felt overwhelmed by the sheer amount of detailed information provided to them. They used such words as "absorb," "tremendous," and "huge" to describe the *information overload.* Caregivers recognized the need for *support from others,* both health care providers and personal contacts. Caregivers discovered they required adjustment to new routines and responsibilities, especially the sometimes *complicated procedures* associated with eating. Caregivers also had to adjust to their newly developed *vigilance and desire to protect their loved one from harm.* Due in large part to the experience of caregiving itself, these caregivers expressed *feelings of fear* (the most common emotion expressed), *sympathy, and guilt.*

Nursing Implications

Nurses need to support caregivers in their desire to provide care to their loved ones. Providing them the information and tools they need to be successful is important; however, nurses also need to involve the caregiver in the care early and assist the caregiver in identifying sources of ongoing social support. Recognizing the link between vigilance and fear provides a starting point for developing individualized interventions designed to address caregiver distress.

Exercise 1

Gently turn head to each side and look as far as possible. Gently tip right ear toward right shoulder as far as possible. Repeat on left side. Move chin to chest and then lift head up and back.

Exercise 2

Place hands in front with elbows at right angles away from body. Rotate shoulders back, bringing elbows to side. Then relax whole body.

Exercise 3: Using the hand on the unaffected side, lean or hold onto a low table or chair.

Bend body slightly at waist and swing shoulder and arm from left to right.

Swing shoulder and arm from front to back

Swing shoulder and arm in a wide circle, gradually bringing arm above head.

Figure 45-5 • Three rehabilitation exercises after head and neck surgery. The objective is to regain maximum shoulder function and neck motion after neck surgery. Adapted from Exercise for radical neck surgery patients. Head and Neck Service, Department of Surgery, Memorial Hospital, New York, NY.

shoulder drop, which is a forward curvature of the shoulder. Many problems can be avoided with a conscientious exercise program. These exercises are usually started after the drains have been removed and the neck incision is sufficiently healed. The purpose of the exercises depicted in Figure 45-5 is to promote maximal shoulder function and neck motion after surgery.

MONITORING AND MANAGING POTENTIAL COMPLICATIONS

Hemorrhage. Hemorrhage may occur from carotid artery rupture as a result of necrosis of the graft or damage to the artery itself from tumor or infection. The following measures are indicated:

- Vital signs are assessed frequently (every 1 to 2 hours or every 15 minutes if the patient is critical). Once the patient is stabilized, assessment is performed every 4 hours. Tachycardia, tachypnea, and hypotension may indicate hemorrhage and impending hypovolemic shock.
- The patient is instructed to avoid the Valsalva maneuver to prevent stress on the graft and carotid artery.

- Signs of impending rupture, such as high epigastric pain or discomfort, are reported.
- Dressings and wound drainage are observed for excessive bleeding.
- If hemorrhage occurs, assistance is summoned immediately.
- Hemorrhage requires the continuous firm application of pressure to the bleeding site or major associated vessel.
- The head of the patient's bed should be elevated at least 30 degrees to maintain airway patency and prevent aspiration.
- A controlled, calm manner allays the patient's anxiety.
- The surgeon is notified immediately, because a vascular or ligature tear requires surgical intervention.

Chyle Fistula. A chyle fistula (milk-like drainage from the thoracic duct into the thoracic cavity) may develop as a result of damage to the thoracic duct during surgery. Although not very common (1% to 2.5% of cases), this complication is serious and life-threatening (Swanson, Hudson, Bhandari, et al., 2015). The diagnosis is made if there is excess drainage present in the chest tube drainage that has a 3% fat content and a specific gravity of 1.012 or greater. Treatment of a small leak (500 mL or less) requires a diet of medium-chain fatty acids or parenteral nutrition (Tessier, 2015), although there is emerging support for the use of IV or subcutaneous administration of octreotide (Sandostatin) in conservative management (Swanson et al., 2015). Octreotide, a synthetic analog of the natural hormone somatostatin, works primarily by decreasing the absorption of triglycerides and inhibiting gastrointestinal circulation and motility, thereby reducing lymph flow and decreasing the chyle flow (Swanson et al., 2015). Surgical intervention may be needed to repair the damaged duct (Tessier, 2015).

Nerve Injury. Nerve injury can occur if the cervical plexus or spinal accessory nerves are severed during surgery. Because lower facial paralysis may occur as a result of injury to the facial nerve, this complication is observed for and reported. Likewise, if the superior laryngeal nerve is damaged, the patient may have difficulty swallowing liquids and food because of the partial lack of sensation of the glottis. Speech therapy may be indicated to assist with the problems related to nerve injury.

PROMOTING HOME, COMMUNITY-BASED, AND TRANSITIONAL CARE

Educating Patients About Self-Care. The patient and caregiver require instructions about management of the wound, the dressing, and any drains that remain in place. Patients who require oral suctioning or who have a tracheostomy may be very anxious about their care at home; the transition to home can be eased if the caregiver is given several opportunities to demonstrate the ability to meet the patient's needs (see Chart 45-4). The patient and caregiver are also instructed about possible complications, specifically bleeding and respiratory distress, and when to notify the primary provider.

If the patient cannot take food by mouth, detailed instructions and demonstration of enteral or parenteral feedings will be required. Education in techniques of effective oral hygiene is also important.

Continuing and Transitional Care. A referral for home, community-based, or transitional care may be necessary in the early period after discharge. The nurse assesses healing, ensures that feedings are being given properly, and monitors for any complications. The patient's adjustment to changes in physical appearance and status and ability to communicate and eat normally is also assessed.

Chart 45-4	HOME CARE CHECKLIST

The Patient Recovering From Neck Surgery

At the completion of education, the patient and/or caregiver will be able to:

- Name the procedure that was performed and identify any permanent changes in anatomic structure or function as well as changes in communication, ADLs, IADLs, roles, body image, relationships, and spirituality.
- Identify modification of home environment, interventions, and strategies (e.g., durable medical equipment, home health aide) used in safely adapting to changes in structure or function and promote effective recovery and rehabilitation.
- Describe ongoing therapeutic regimen, including diet and activities to perform (e.g., oral care, suctioning) and to limit or avoid (e.g., lifting weights, driving a car, contact sports).
  - Identify foods or therapies necessary to meet caloric needs and dietary needs (e.g., change in consistency, seasoning limitations, supplements, enteral or parenteral therapy).
  - Participate in prescribed therapy (e.g. speech therapy, PT, OT) to promote recovery and rehabilitation.
  - Demonstrate the use of tracheostomy care and suctioning if indicated.
  - Demonstrate use of humidification if indicated.
  - Demonstrate effective oral hygiene.
  - Demonstrate care of incision and drains.

- State the name, dose, side effects, frequency, and schedule for all medications.
- Describe approaches to controlling pain (e.g., take analgesics as prescribed; use nonpharmacologic interventions).
- Identify possible complications (e.g., bleeding, respiratory distress) and interventions.
- Relate how to reach primary provider with questions or complications.
- State time and date of follow-up medical/dental appointments, therapy, and testing.
- Identify sources of support (e.g., friends, relatives, faith community, cancer support, caregiver support).
- Identify the need for health promotion, disease prevention, and screening activities.

Resources

See Chapter 44, Chart 44-5 for additional information on The Patient Receiving Tube Feeding, and Chart 44-7 The Patient Receiving Parenteral Nutrition.

ADL, activities of daily living; IADL, independent activities of daily living; PT, physical therapy; OT, occupational therapy.

Physical and speech therapy also are likely to be continued at home.

The patient is given information regarding local support groups such as "I Can Cope" or "New Voice Club," if indicated. The local chapter of the ACS may be contacted for information and equipment needed for the patient (see the Resources section).

Evaluation

Expected patient outcomes may include:
1. Exhibits increased knowledge of course of treatment
2. Demonstrates adequate respiratory exchange
   a. Lungs are clear to auscultation
   b. Breathes easily with no shortness of breath
   c. Demonstrates ability to use suction effectively
3. Verbalizes comfort and relief of pain
4. Graft is pink and warm to touch
5. Maintains adequate intake of foods and fluids
   a. Accepts altered route of feeding
   b. Is well hydrated
   c. Maintains or gains weight
6. Demonstrates ability to cope (both patient and caregivers)
   a. Discusses emotional responses to the diagnosis
   b. Attends support group meetings
7. Communicates effectively with caregivers and family members
8. Attains maximal mobility
   a. Adheres to physical therapy exercises
   b. Attains maximal range of motion
9. Exhibits no complications
   a. Vital signs stable
   b. No excessive bleeding or discharge
   c. Able to move muscles of lower face and shoulders

DISORDERS OF THE ESOPHAGUS

The esophagus is a mucus-lined, muscular tube that carries food from the mouth to the stomach. It begins at the base of the pharynx and ends about 4 cm below the diaphragm. Its ability to transport food and fluid is facilitated by two sphincters. The upper esophageal sphincter, also called the *hypopharyngeal sphincter*, is located at the junction of the pharynx and the esophagus. The lower esophageal sphincter, also called the *gastroesophageal sphincter* or *cardiac sphincter*, is located at the junction of the esophagus and the stomach. An incompetent lower esophageal sphincter allows reflux (backward flow) of gastric contents. Because there is no serosal layer of the esophagus, if surgery is necessary, it is more difficult to perform suturing or anastomosis.

Disorders of the esophagus include motility disorders (achalasia, spasms), hiatal hernias, diverticula, perforation, foreign bodies, chemical burns, gastroesophageal reflux disease (GERD), Barrett esophagus (BE), benign tumors, and carcinoma. Dysphagia, the most common symptom of esophageal disease, may vary from an uncomfortable feeling that a bolus of food is caught in the upper esophagus to acute **odynophagia** (pain on swallowing). Obstruction of food (solid and soft) and even liquids may occur anywhere along the esophagus. Often, the patient can indicate that the problem is located in the upper, middle, or lower third of the esophagus.

Achalasia

Achalasia is absent or ineffective peristalsis of the distal esophagus accompanied by failure of the esophageal sphincter to relax in response to swallowing. Narrowing of the esophagus just above the stomach results in a gradually increasing dilation of the esophagus in the upper chest. Achalasia may progress slowly and occurs most often in people 40 years or older.

Clinical Manifestations

The main symptom is dysphagia (solids and liquids). The patient has a sensation of food sticking in the lower portion of the esophagus. As the condition progresses, food is commonly regurgitated either spontaneously or intentionally by the patient to relieve the discomfort produced by prolonged distention of the esophagus by food that will not pass into the stomach. The patient may also report non-cardiac chest or epigastric pain and **pyrosis** (heartburn) that may or may not be associated with eating. Secondary pulmonary complications may result from aspiration of gastric contents (Pandolfino & Gawron, 2015).

Assessment and Diagnostic Findings

X-ray studies show esophageal dilation above the narrowing at the gastroesophageal junction. Barium swallow, computed tomography (CT) scan of the chest, and endoscopy may be used for diagnosis; however, manometry, a process in which peristalsis, contraction amplitudes, and esophageal pressure is measured by a radiologist or gastroenterologist, confirms the diagnosis (Pandolfino & Gawron, 2015).

Management

The patient is instructed to eat slowly and to drink fluids with meals. As a temporary measure, oral calcium channel blockers and nitrates have been used to decrease esophageal pressure and improve swallowing. Injection of botulinum toxin (Botox) into quadrants of the esophagus via endoscopy has been helpful because it inhibits the contraction of smooth muscle (Pandolfino & Gawron, 2015).

Achalasia may be treated conservatively by pneumatic dilation to stretch the narrowed area of the esophagus (see Fig. 45-6). Pneumatic dilation has a high success rate. Although perforation is a potential complication, its incidence is low (see later discussion). The procedure can be painful; therefore, moderate sedation in the form of an analgesic or tranquilizer, or both, is given for the treatment (Pandolfino & Gawron, 2015).

Achalasia may be treated surgically by esophagomyotomy, which involves cutting the esophageal muscle fibers. The procedure is usually performed laparoscopically, either with a complete lower esophageal sphincter myotomy and an antireflux procedure or without an antireflux procedure. A new technique, an endoscopic myotomy (per-oral endoscopic myotomy [POEM]) may provide an alternative procedure (Pandolfino & Gawron, 2015).

Esophageal Spasm

The two types of esophageal spasm include diffuse esophageal spasm (DES) and hypertensive peristalsis, also known as

Catheter passed through narrowed end of esophagus

Fully inflated balloon

Figure 45-6 • Treatment of achalasia by pneumatic dilation. **A–C.** The dilator is passed, guided by a previously inserted guide wire. **D.** When the balloon is in proper position, it is distended by pressure sufficient to dilate the narrowed area of the esophagus.

nutcracker esophagus (NE). In DES, the spasms are normal in amplitude, but are uncoordinated, move quickly, or occur at various places in the esophagus at once. In NE, peristalsis is coordinated, but the amplitude is very high. Hypercontractile esophagus, also known as jackhammer esophagus, is an extreme form of NE in which the contractions involve the entire esophagus and occur over a prolonged period (Malas, 2015). NE is more common in women and usually manifests in middle age. The cause is unknown, but stress may be a factor. There may also be a relationship between NE and psychiatric disorders or psychotropic medications (Lufrano, Heckman, Diehl, et al., 2015).

Clinical Manifestations

Both DES and NE are characterized by dysphagia, odynophagia, and chest pain similar to that of coronary artery spasm. Dysphagia is more common in DES from the noncoordinated peristalsis.

Assessment and Diagnostic Findings

Esophageal manometry, which measures the motility and internal pressure of the esophagus, can test for irregular and high-amplitude spasms.

Management

Conservative, first-line therapy includes calcium channel blockers (nifedipine [Procardia], verapamil [Calan]) and nitrates (nitroglycerin). Smooth muscle relaxants (sildenafil [Viagra]), anticholinergics (botulinum toxin), antianxiety medications (tricyclic antidepressants), and proton-pump inhibitors (PPIs; omeprazole [Prilosec]) may also be indicated (Malas, 2015). Small, frequent feedings and a soft diet are usually recommended to decrease the esophageal pressure and irritation that lead to spasm. If conservative therapies do not provide relief, dilation or myotomy procedures may be performed. Since many patients also experience gastroesophageal

reflux disease (GERD), surgical procedures that also address GERD may be beneficial (see later discussion).

Hiatal Hernia

In the condition known as hiatal **hernia**, the opening in the diaphragm through which the esophagus passes becomes enlarged, and part of the upper stomach moves up into the lower portion of the thorax. Hiatal hernia occurs more often in women than in men. There are two main types of hiatal hernias: sliding and paraesophageal. Sliding, or type I, hiatal hernia occurs when the upper stomach and the gastroesophageal junction are displaced upward and slide in and out of the thorax (see Fig. 45-7A). About 95% of patients with esophageal hiatal hernia have a sliding hernia. A paraesophageal hernia occurs when all or part of the stomach pushes through the diaphragm beside the esophagus (see Fig. 45-7B). Paraesophageal hernias are further classified as types II, III, or IV, depending on the extent of herniation. Type IV has the greatest herniation, with other intra-abdominal viscera such as the colon, spleen, or small bowel evidencing displacement into the chest along with the stomach (Oleynikov & Jolley, 2015).

Clinical Manifestations

The patient with a sliding hernia may have pyrosis, regurgitation, and dysphagia, but many patients are asymptomatic. The patient may present with vague symptoms of intermittent epigastric pain or fullness after eating. Large hiatal hernias may lead to intolerance to food, nausea, and vomiting. Sliding hiatal hernias are commonly associated with GERD. Hemorrhage, obstruction, and strangulation can occur with any type of hernia (Oleynikov & Jolley, 2015).

Assessment and Diagnostic Findings

Diagnosis is typically confirmed by x-ray studies; barium swallow; esophagogastroduodenoscopy (EGD), which is the

Figure 45-7 • **A.** Sliding esophageal hernia. The upper stomach and gastroesophageal junction have moved upward and slide in and out of the thorax. **B.** Paraesophageal hernia. All or part of the stomach pushes through the diaphragm next to the gastroesophageal junction.

passage of a fiberoptic tube through the mouth and throat into the digestive tract for visualization of the esophagus, stomach, and small intestine; esophageal manometry; or chest CT scan (Kohn, Price, Demeester, et al., 2013).

Management

Management for a hiatal hernia includes frequent, small feedings that can pass easily through the esophagus. The patient is advised not to recline for 1 hour after eating, to prevent reflux or movement of the hernia, and to elevate the head of the bed on 4- to 8-inch (10- to 20-cm) blocks to prevent the hernia from sliding upward. Surgical hernia repair is indicated in patients who are symptomatic, although the primary reason for the surgery is typically to relieve GERD symptoms and not repair the hernia. Current guidelines recommend a laparoscopic approach, with an open transabdominal or transthoracic approach reserved for patients with complications such as bleeding, dense adhesions, or injury to the spleen.

Up to 50% of patients may experience early postoperative dysphagia; therefore, the nurse advances the diet slowly from liquids to solids, while managing nausea and vomiting, tracking nutritional intake, and monitoring weight. The nurse also monitors for postoperative belching, vomiting, gagging, abdominal distension, and epigastric chest pain, which may indicate the need for surgical revision; these should be reported immediately to the primary provider. Surgical repair is often reserved for patients with more extreme cases that involve gastric outlet obstruction or suspected gastric strangulation, which may result in ischemia, necrosis, or perforation of the stomach (Kohn et al., 2013).

Diverticulum

An esophageal diverticulum is an out-pouching of mucosa and submucosa that protrudes through a weak portion of the musculature of the esophagus. Diverticula may occur in one of the three areas of the esophagus—pharyngoesophageal (upper), midesophageal (middle), or epiphrenic (lower).

The most common type of diverticulum is Zenker diverticulum. Located in the pharyngoesophageal area, Zenker diverticula are caused by a dysfunctional sphincter that fails to open, which leads to increased pressure that forces the mucosa and submucosa to herniate through the esophageal musculature (called a pulsion diverticulum) (Smith, 2015) (see Fig. 45-8). It is usually seen in people older than 60 years of age.

Midesophageal diverticula are uncommon. Symptoms are less acute, and usually the condition does not require surgery. Epiphrenic diverticula are usually larger diverticula in the lower esophagus just above the diaphragm. They may be related to the improper functioning of the lower esophageal sphincter or to motor disorders of the esophagus. Intramural diverticulosis is the occurrence of numerous small diverticula associated with a stricture in the upper esophagus.

Clinical Manifestations

Symptoms experienced by the patient with a pharyngoesophageal pulsion diverticulum include dysphagia, fullness in the neck, belching, regurgitation of undigested food, and gurgling noises after eating. The diverticulum, or pouch, becomes filled with food or liquid. When the patient assumes a recumbent position, undigested food is regurgitated, and coughing may be caused by irritation of the trachea or aspiration. **Halitosis** (bad breath) and a sour taste in the mouth are also common because of the decomposition of food retained in the diverticulum. Although less acute, dysphagia is the primary symptom in the other types of diverticula (Smith, 2015).

Assessment and Diagnostic Findings

A barium swallow may determine the exact nature and location of a diverticulum. Manometric studies may be performed

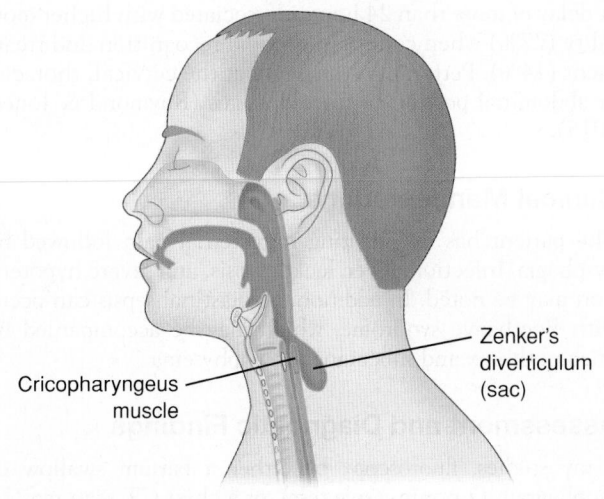

Figure 45-8 • Zenker diverticulum.

for patients with epiphrenic diverticula to rule out a motor disorder. Esophagoscopy usually is contraindicated because of the danger of perforation of the diverticulum, with resulting mediastinitis (inflammation of the organs and tissues that separate the lungs). Blind insertion of an NG tube should be avoided.

Management

Because Zenker diverticulum is progressive, the only means of cure is surgical removal of the diverticulum. During surgery, care is taken to avoid trauma to the common carotid artery and internal jugular veins. In addition to a diverticulectomy, a myotomy of the cricopharyngeal muscle is often performed to relieve spasticity of the musculature, which seems to contribute to a continuation of symptoms. An NG tube may be inserted at the time of surgery. Postoperatively, the nurse observes the incision for evidence of leakage from the esophagus and a developing fistula. Food and fluids are withheld until x-ray studies show no leakage at the surgical site. The diet begins with liquids and is progressed as tolerated. Advances in technology include the minimally invasive endoscopic stapler diverticulotomy, which expedites oral intake and discharge, reduces the risk of fistula formation, and does not require an NG tube. Patients who are not good candidates for this endoscopic procedure include those with a stiff or short neck, poor mouth opening, prominent teeth, large tongue, and with larger diverticula (Yuan, Zhao, Hu, et al., 2013).

Surgery is indicated for epiphrenic and midesophageal diverticula only if the symptoms are troublesome and becoming worse. Treatment consists of a diverticulectomy and long myotomy. Intramural diverticula usually regress after the esophageal stricture is dilated.

Perforation

Esophageal perforation is a surgical emergency. It may result from iatrogenic causes, such as endoscopy or intraoperative injury, or from spontaneous perforation associated with forceful vomiting or severe straining (**Boerhaave syndrome**), foreign-body ingestion, trauma, and malignancy. Immediate diagnosis and treatment are essential to minimize mortality. A delay of more than 24 hours is associated with higher mortality (27%) when compared to rapid recognition and treatment (14%). Perforation can occur at the cervical, thoracic, or abdominal portion of the esophagus (Raymond & Jones, 2015).

Clinical Manifestations

The patient has excruciating retrosternal pain followed by dysphagia. Infection, fever, leukocytosis, and severe hypotension may be noted. In addition, mediastinal sepsis can occur with Boerhaave syndrome, which may be accompanied by pneumothorax and subcutaneous emphysema.

Assessment and Diagnostic Findings

X-ray studies, fluoroscopy by either a barium swallow or esophagram (a noninvasive test), or a chest CT scan may be used to identify the site and scope of the injury.

Management

Esophageal perforation requires immediate treatment. Treatment includes having the patient remain NPO (nothing by mouth), beginning IV fluid therapy, administering broad-spectrum antibiotics (ampicillin-sulbactam [Unasyn], piperacillin-tazobactam [Zosyn], or a carbapenem [e.g., imipenem{Primaxin}]), considering the need for antifungal therapy (if the patient is immunosuppressed, has HIV infection, or shows no improvement with antibiotics), supportive monitoring and care (intensive care unit level-of-care often required), and evaluating and preparing the patient for surgery (Raymond & Jones, 2015). Surgical repair of the perforation site is performed in most cases, even if the diagnosis is made after 24 hours. If surgical repair of the perforation is not possible due to the clinical status of the patient, then drainage, diversion, stent placement, or an esophagostomy (removal of the esophagus) may be performed (Raymond & Jones, 2015).

Postoperative nutritional status is a major concern. The patient remains NPO for approximately 7 days, so enteral (e.g., jejunal feeding) or parenteral nutrition is started on postoperative day 2 or 3 (see Chapter 44). The nurse uses water to moisten the patient's mouth for comfort measures only. A repeat esophagram is obtained on postoperative day 7 to verify there is no leak or ileus before the NG tube is removed and oral intake is permitted. It is common for broad-spectrum antibiotics to continue for 7 to 10 days postoperatively (Raymond & Jones, 2015).

Foreign Bodies

Many swallowed foreign bodies pass through the GI tract without the need for medical intervention. However, some swallowed foreign bodies (e.g., dentures, fish bones, pins, small batteries, items containing mercury or lead) may injure the esophagus or obstruct its lumen and must be removed. Pain and dysphagia may be present, and dyspnea may occur as a result of pressure on the trachea. The foreign body may be identified by x-ray. Perforation may have occurred (see earlier discussion).

> ### ▶ Quality and Safety Nursing Alert
>
> The nurse performs an initial and ongoing respiratory (airway-focused) assessment of a patient with a foreign body in the esophagus. Intubation may be required to protect the airway.

Glucagon, because of its relaxing effect on the esophageal muscle, may be injected IV. A flexible endoscope and retrieval devices (e.g., forceps, graspers) may be used to remove the impacted food or object from the esophagus. Foreign bodies such as short-blunt objects, long objects, sharp-pointed objects, disc batteries, magnets, coins, or narcotic packets require special consideration (American Society for Gastrointestinal Endoscopy Standards of Practice Committee, 2011). For example, dilation techniques such as the bougienage procedure can be used to facilitate the passage of foreign objects (Allie, Blackshaw, Losek, et al., 2014). In bougienage, cylindrical rubber tubes of different sizes, called *bougies*, are advanced into the esophagus via the oral cavity; the dilator can manually advance the foreign object. The procedure usually is performed in the endoscopy suite or clinic by the gastroenterologist.

Chemical Burns

Chemical burns of the esophagus occur most often when a patient, either intentionally (67%; typically adults) or unintentionally (33%; typically children), swallows a strong acid or base, with alkaline agents being the most common (Byard, 2015). The patient is often emotionally distraught as well as in acute physical pain. Chemical burns of the esophagus may also be caused by undissolved medications in the esophagus, or they may also occur after swallowing of a battery, which may release a caustic alkaline. An acute chemical burn of the esophagus may be accompanied by severe burns of the lips, mouth, and pharynx, with pain on swallowing. Breathing difficulties due to either edema of the throat or a collection of mucus in the pharynx may occur.

The patient, who may be profoundly toxic, febrile, and in shock, is treated immediately for shock, pain, and respiratory distress. Esophagoscopy and barium swallow are performed as soon as possible to determine the extent and severity of damage. Vomiting and gastric lavage are avoided to prevent further exposure of the esophagus to the caustic agent. Emergent esophagectomy or gastrectomy may be required (Byard, 2015). The patient remains NPO and IV fluids are given. The use of corticosteroids to reduce inflammation and minimize subsequent scarring and stricture formation is of questionable value. Antibiotics are prescribed if there is documented infection.

After the acute phase has subsided, the patient may need nutritional support via enteral or parenteral feedings. The patient may require further treatment to prevent or manage strictures of the esophagus. Dilation by bougienage may be sufficient, but may need to be repeated periodically (see previous discussion). Progressively larger bougies are used to dilate the esophagus. Some strictures require rigid dilators, such as Savary dilators. These dilators are used in the same fashion as bougies but may be more successful for opening difficult strictures. For strictures that do not respond to either method of dilation, surgical management may be necessary. Reconstruction may be accomplished by esophagectomy and colon interposition to replace the portion of esophagus removed. This surgery is quite complex and should be considered only when other options have failed.

Gastroesophageal Reflux Disease

Gastroesophageal reflux disease (GERD) is a fairly common disorder marked by backflow of gastric or duodenal contents into the esophagus that causes troublesome symptoms and/or mucosal injury to the esophagus. Excessive reflux may occur because of an incompetent lower esophageal sphincter, pyloric stenosis, hiatal hernia, or a motility disorder. The incidence of GERD seems to increase with aging and is seen in patients with irritable bowel syndrome and obstructive airway disorders (asthma, COPD, cystic fibrosis) (Robinson & DiMango, 2014), BE (see later discussion), peptic ulcer disease, and angina. GERD is associated with tobacco use, coffee drinking, alcohol consumption, and gastric infection with *Helicobacter pylori*.

Clinical Manifestations

Symptoms may include pyrosis (heartburn, specifically more commonly described as a burning sensation in the esophagus),

dyspepsia (indigestion), regurgitation, dysphagia or odynophagia, hypersalivation, and esophagitis. The symptoms may mimic those of a heart attack. GERD can result in dental erosion, ulcerations in the pharynx and esophagus, laryngeal damage, esophageal strictures, adenocarcinoma, and pulmonary complications (Hart, 2013).

Assessment and Diagnostic Findings

The patient's history aids in obtaining an accurate diagnosis. Diagnostic testing may include an endoscopy or barium swallow to evaluate damage to the esophageal mucosa (Hart, 2013). Ambulatory 12- to 36-hour esophageal pH monitoring is used to evaluate the degree of acid reflux. Esophageal pH monitoring was historically an uncomfortable procedure, but the advent of wireless capsule pH monitoring is better tolerated and quite accurate (Singhal & Khaitan, 2015).

Management

Management begins with educating the patient to avoid situations that decrease lower esophageal sphincter pressure or cause esophageal irritation. The patient is instructed to eat a low-fat diet; avoid caffeine, tobacco, beer, milk, foods containing peppermint or spearmint, and carbonated beverages; avoid eating or drinking 2 hours before bedtime; maintain normal body weight; avoid tight-fitting clothes; and elevate the head of the bed by at least 30 degrees (Hart, 2013). See Table 45-2 for a list of medications commonly used to manage GERD.

If medical management is unsuccessful, surgical intervention may be necessary. Surgical management involves an open or laparoscopic Nissen fundoplication (wrapping of a portion of the gastric fundus around the sphincter area of the esophagus) (Garg & Gurusamy, 2015).

Barrett Esophagus

BE is a condition in which the lining of the esophageal mucosa is altered. It affects 5.6% of the population in the United States, occurs predominantly in white men aged 50 or older, and occurs in association with GERD (Sharma, Katzka, Gupta, et al., 2015). Reflux eventually causes changes in the cells lining the lower esophagus. The cells that are laid to cover the exposed area no longer form the normal, squamous mucosa, but instead form columnar-lined epithelium that resembles the intestines. BE is the only known precursor to esophageal adenocarcinoma (EAC).

Clinical Manifestations

The patient complains of symptoms of GERD, notably frequent heartburn. The patient may also complain of symptoms related to peptic ulcers or esophageal stricture, or both.

Assessment and Diagnostic Findings

An EGD is performed. This usually reveals an esophageal lining that is red rather than pink. Biopsies are performed, and high-grade **dysplasia** (HGD; abnormal changes in cells) is evidenced by the squamous mucosa of the esophagus replaced by columnar epithelium that resembles that of the stomach or intestines.

TABLE 45-2 Pharmacologic Management of GERD

Key Examples	Actions/Class	Key Nursing Considerations
Antacids/Acid neutralizing agents • Calcium carbonate (Tums) • Aluminum hydroxide, magnesium, hydroxide, and simethicone (Maalox)	**Neutralize acid** *Therapeutic and Pharmacologic class*—Antacid	• Potential risk of gastric acid suppression is the loss of protective flora and an increased risk of infection, especially *Clostridium difficile*
Histamine-2 (H₂) receptor antagonists • Famotidine (Pepcid) • Ranitidine (Zantac) • Cimetidine (Tagamet)	**Decrease gastric acid production** *Therapeutic class*—Antiulcer drugs *Pharmacologic class*—H₂-receptor antagonists	• Potential risk of gastric acid suppression is the loss of protective flora and an increased risk of infection, especially *Clostridium difficile* • For direct injection (IVP), dilute 2 mL (20 mg) with compatible solution to a total volume of either 5 or 10 mL; administer over at least 2 minutes • Monitor for QT-interval prolongation in patients with kidney injury
Prokinetic agents Metoclopramide (Reglan)	**Accelerate gastric emptying** *Therapeutic class*—GI stimulants *Pharmacologic class*—Dopamine antagonist	• May cause tardive dyskinesia • Typically used short term
Proton pump inhibitors (PPIs) • Pantoprazole (Protonix) • Omeprazole (Prilosec) • Esomeprazole (Nexium) • Lansoprazole (Prevacid) • Rabeprazole (AcipHex) • Dexlansoprazole (Dexilant)	**Decrease gastric acid production** *Therapeutic class*—Antiulcer drugs *Pharmacologic class*—Proton pump inhibitors	• Potential risk of gastric acid suppression is the loss of protective flora and an increased risk of infection, especially *Clostridium difficile* • For a 2-minute infusion (IVP), give the reconstituted vials (4 mg/mL) over at least 2 minutes • May increase the risk of hip fractures and interfere with some vitamin and mineral absorption (B12, iron, magnesium) • Interact with commonly prescribed medications such as diuretics and clopidogrel
Reflux inhibitors Bethanechol chloride (Urecholine)	**Stimulates parasympathetic** *Therapeutic and Pharmacologic class*—Cholinergic	• Primary use is for urinary retention • Do not use with possible GI obstruction or peptic ulcer
Surface Agents/Alginate-based barriers • Sucralfate	**Preserve mucosal barrier** *Therapeutic class*—Antiulcer drugs *Pharmacologic class*--GI protectants	• Give on an empty stomach hour before or 2 hours after meals • Separate from doses of antacid by 30 minutes

Adapted from Frandsen, G., & Pennington, S. S. (2014). *Abrams' clinical drug therapy: Rationales for nursing practice* (10th ed.). Philadelphia, PA: Wolters Kluwer Health/Lippincott Williams & Wilkins; Garg, S. K., & Gurusamy, K. S. (2015). Laparoscopic fundoplication surgery versus medical management for gastro-oesophageal reflux disease (GORD) in adults. *Cochrane Database Systematic Reviews*, 11: CD003243; Hart, A. M. (2013). Evidence-based recommendations for GERD treatment. *The Nurse Practitioner*, 38(8), 26–34.

Management

Monitoring varies depending on the extent of cell changes. Follow-up biopsies are recommended no sooner than 3 to 5 years after a biopsy shows no evidence of dysplasia (Sharma et al., 2015). Treatment is individualized for each patient. Recommendations include surveillance with biopsies, use of proton pump inhibitors (PPIs) (see Table 45-2) to control reflux symptoms, endoscopic resection, radiofrequency ablation (high-frequency heat energy that kills surrounding cells and tissues), and consideration of metal stents for severe dysphagia palliation (Sharma et al., 2015).

Benign Tumors of the Esophagus

Benign tumors are rare, but can arise anywhere along the esophagus. The most common lesion is a leiomyoma (tumor of the smooth muscle), which can occlude the lumen of the esophagus and cause dysphagia, pain, and pyrosis. Half of patients with benign tumors are asymptomatic and the other half present with multiple symptoms that have been present for a long period of time. The diagnosis may be made incidentally and is confirmed by endoscopy and needle biopsy. Due to the slow growth of most of these tumors, monitoring and minimally invasive techniques (endoscopic, thoracic, or laparoscopic resections) tend to be indicated rather than surgical resection (Ha, Regan, Cetindag, et al., 2015).

NURSING PROCESS

The Patient With a Noncancerous Condition of the Esophagus

Assessment

Emergency conditions of the esophagus (perforation, chemical burns) usually occur in the home or away from medical help and require emergency medical care. The patient is treated for shock and respiratory distress and transported as quickly as possible to a health care facility. Foreign bodies in the esophagus do not pose an immediate threat to life unless pressure is exerted on the trachea, resulting in dyspnea or interfering with respiration, or unless there is leakage of caustic alkali from a battery or exposure to another corrosive agent.

For nonemergency symptoms, a complete health history may reveal the nature of the esophageal disorder. The nurse asks about the patient's appetite. Has it remained the same, increased, or decreased? Is there any discomfort with swallowing? If so, does it occur only with certain foods? Is it associated with pain? Does a change in position affect the discomfort? The patient is asked to describe the pain. Does anything aggravate it? Are there any other symptoms that occur regularly, such as regurgitation, nocturnal regurgitation, eructation (belching), pyrosis, substernal pressure, a sensation that food is sticking in the throat, a feeling of fullness after eating a small amount of food, nausea, vomiting, or weight loss? Are the symptoms aggravated by emotional upset? If the patient reports any of these symptoms, the nurse asks about when they occur, their relationship to eating, and factors that relieve or aggravate them (e.g., position change, belching, antacids, vomiting) (Bickley, 2013).

This history also includes questions about past or present causative factors, such as infections and chemical, mechanical, or physical irritants; alcohol and tobacco use; and the amount of daily food intake. The nurse determines whether the patient appears emaciated and auscultates the patient's chest to assess for pulmonary complications (Bickley, 2013).

Nursing Diagnosis

Based on the assessment data, nursing diagnoses may include the following:

- Imbalanced nutrition: less than body requirements related to difficulty swallowing
- Risk for aspiration related to difficulty swallowing or tube feeding
- Acute pain related to difficulty swallowing, ingestion of an abrasive agent, tumor, or frequent episodes of gastric reflux
- Deficient knowledge about the esophageal disorder, diagnostic studies, medical management, surgical intervention, and rehabilitation

Planning and Goals

The major goals for the patient may include attainment of adequate nutritional intake, avoidance of respiratory compromise from aspiration, relief of pain, and increased knowledge level.

Nursing Interventions

ENCOURAGING ADEQUATE NUTRITIONAL INTAKE

The patient is encouraged to eat slowly and to chew all food thoroughly so that it can pass easily into the stomach. Small, frequent feedings of nonirritating foods are recommended to promote digestion and to prevent tissue irritation. Sometimes liquid swallowed with food helps the food pass through the esophagus, but usually liquids should be consumed between meals. Food should be prepared in an appealing manner to help stimulate the appetite. Irritants such as tobacco and alcohol should be avoided. A baseline weight is obtained, and daily weights are recorded. The patient's intake of nutrients is assessed.

DECREASING RISK OF ASPIRATION

The patient who has difficulty swallowing or difficulty handling secretions should be kept in at least a semi-Fowler position to decrease the risk of aspiration. The patient is instructed in the use of oral suction to decrease the risk of aspiration further.

RELIEVING PAIN

Small, frequent feedings (6 to 8 per day) are recommended because large quantities of food overload the stomach and promote gastric reflux. The patient is advised to avoid any activities that increase pain and to remain upright for 1 to 4 hours after each meal to prevent reflux. The head of the bed should be placed on 4- to 8-inch (10- to 20-cm) blocks. Eating before bedtime is discouraged.

The patient is advised that excessive use of over-the-counter antacids can cause rebound acidity. Antacid use should be directed by the primary provider, who can recommend the daily, safe dose needed to neutralize gastric juices and prevent esophageal irritation. H_2 antagonists or PPIs are given as prescribed to decrease gastric acid irritation.

PROVIDING PATIENT EDUCATION

The patient is prepared physically and psychologically for diagnostic tests, treatments, and possible surgery. Nursing interventions include reassuring the patient and explaining the procedures and their purposes. Some disorders of the esophagus evolve over time, whereas others are the result of trauma (e.g., chemical burns, perforation). In instances of trauma, the emotional and physical preparation for treatment is more difficult because of the short time available and the circumstances of the injury. Treatment interventions must be evaluated continually, and the patient is given sufficient information to participate in care and diagnostic tests. If endoscopic diagnostic methods are used, the patient is instructed regarding the moderate sedation that will be used during the procedure. If outpatient procedures are performed with the use of moderate sedation, someone must be available to drive the patient home after the procedure. If surgery is required, immediate and long-term evaluation is similar to that for a patient undergoing thoracic surgery.

PROMOTING HOME, COMMUNITY-BASED, AND TRANSITIONAL CARE

Educating Patients About Self-Care. The self-care required of the patient depends on the nature of the disorder and on the surgery or treatment measures used (e.g., diet, positioning, medications). If an ongoing condition exists, the nurse helps the patient plan for needed physical and psychological adjustments and for follow-up care (see Chart 45-5).

Special equipment, such as suction or enteral or parenteral feeding devices, may be required. The patient may need assistance in planning meals, using medications as prescribed, and resuming activities. Education about nutritional requirements and how to measure the adequacy of nutrition is important. Older adults and patients who are debilitated in particular often need assistance and education about ways they can adjust to their limitations and resume activities that are important to them.

Continuing and Transitional Care. Patients with chronic esophageal conditions require an individualized approach to their management at home. Foods may need to be prepared in a special way (blenderized foods, soft foods), and the patient may need to eat more frequently (e.g., 6 to 8 small servings per day). The medication schedule is adjusted to the patient's daily activities as much as possible. Analgesic medications

---

HOME CARE CHECKLIST

The Patient With an Esophageal Disorder

At the completion of education, the patient and/or caregiver will be able to:

- State the impact of the esophageal disorder and treatment on physiologic functioning, ADLs, IADLs, body image, roles, relationships, and spirituality.
- Identify modification of home environment, interventions, and strategies (e.g., durable medical equipment, home health aide) used in safely adapting to changes in structure or function and promote effective recovery and rehabilitation.
- Describe ongoing therapeutic regimen, including diet and activities to perform (e.g., suctioning) and to limit or avoid (e.g., oral foods if NPO).
  - Identify foods or therapies necessary to meet caloric needs and dietary needs (e.g., change in consistency, seasoning limitations, supplements, enteral or parenteral therapy).
  - Participate in prescribed therapy (e.g., speech therapy) to promote recovery and rehabilitation.
  - Demonstrate the use of suction equipment if indicated.
  - Demonstrate care of incision if indicated.
- State the name, dose, side effects, frequency, and schedule for all medications.

- Describe approaches to controlling pain (e.g., take analgesics as prescribed; use nonpharmacologic interventions).
- Identify possible complications (e.g., difficulty swallowing, pain, respiratory distress) and interventions.
- Relate how to reach primary provider with questions or complications.
- State time and date of follow-up medical appointments, therapy, and testing.
- Identify sources of support (e.g., friends, relatives, faith community, cancer support, caregiver support).
- Identify the need for health promotion, disease prevention, and screening activities.

Resources

See Chapter 44, Chart 44-5 for additional information on The Patient Receiving Tube Feeding, and Chart 44-7 The Patient Receiving Parenteral Nutrition.

ADL, activities of daily living; IADL, independent activities of daily living; NPO, nothing by mouth.

---

and antacids can usually be taken as needed every 3 to 4 hours.

Postoperative home health care focuses on nutritional support, management of pain, and respiratory function. Some patients are discharged from the hospital with enteral feeding by means of a gastrostomy or jejunostomy tube, or parenteral nutrition. The patient and caregiver need specific instructions regarding management of the equipment and treatments. Home care visits by a nurse may be necessary to assess the patient and the caregiver's ability to provide the necessary care (see Chapter 44). A multidisciplinary team that includes a dietitian, a social worker, and family members is helpful. Hospice care and consideration of end-of-life issues are appropriate for some patients.

Evaluation

Expected patient outcomes may include:
1. Achieves an adequate nutritional intake
   a. Eats small, frequent meals
   b. Drinks small sips of water with small servings of food
   c. Avoids irritants (alcohol, tobacco, very hot beverages)
   d. Maintains desired weight
2. Does not aspirate or develop pneumonia
   a. Maintains upright position during feeding
   b. Uses oral suction equipment effectively
3. Is free of pain or able to control pain within a tolerable level
   a. Avoids large meals and irritating foods
   b. Takes medications as prescribed and with adequate fluids (at least 4 oz), and remains upright for at least 10 minutes after taking medications
   c. Maintains an upright position after meals for 1 to 4 hours
   d. Reports that there is less eructation (belching) and chest pain

4. Increases knowledge level of esophageal condition, diagnostic tests, treatment, and prognosis
   a. States cause of condition
   b. Discusses rationale for medical or surgical management and diet or medication regimen
   c. Describes treatment program
   d. Practices preventive measures so that injuries are avoided

Cancer of the Esophagus

In the United States, there are about 16,980 newly diagnosed cases of carcinoma of the esophagus annually; of these, 13,570 are men and 3140 are women. Carcinoma of the esophagus is seen more frequently in African Americans than in Caucasians and usually occurs in the fifth or sixth decade of life (ACS, 2015).

Pathophysiology

Esophageal cancer can be of two cell types: adenocarcinoma and squamous cell carcinoma. The rate of adenocarcinoma is rapidly increasing in the United States as well as in other Western countries. It is found primarily in the distal esophagus and gastroesophageal junction (NCI, 2014).

Risk factors for esophageal cancer include chronic esophageal irritation or GERD. In the United States, cancer of the esophagus has been associated with ingestion of alcohol and the use of tobacco. There is an apparent association between GERD and adenocarcinoma of the esophagus. Patients with BE (which is caused by chronic irritation of the mucous membranes due to reflux of gastric and duodenal contents) have a higher incidence of esophageal cancer (Sharma et al., 2015). Risk factors for squamous cell carcinoma of the esophagus include chronic ingestion of hot liquids or foods, nutritional deficiencies, poor oral hygiene, exposure to nitrosamines in the environment or food, cigarette smoking or chronic alcohol exposure (especially in Western cultures), and some esophageal medical conditions such as caustic injury.

Early stages of esophageal cancer are limited to the mucosa or submucosa; these stages of cancer have a 5-year survival rate of about 90% (Levine & Rubesin, 2012). In later stages, tumor cells of adenocarcinoma and of squamous cell carcinoma may spread beneath the esophageal mucosa or directly into, through, and beyond the muscle layers into the lymphatics. Obstruction of the esophagus is noted, with possible perforation into the mediastinum and erosion into the great vessels (Levine & Rubesin, 2012). Five-year survival rates at this point drop to 20% (ACS, 2015).

Clinical Manifestations

Many patients have an advanced ulcerated lesion of the esophagus before symptoms are manifested. Symptoms include dysphagia, initially with solid foods and eventually with liquids; a sensation of a mass in the throat; painful swallowing; substernal pain or fullness; and, later, regurgitation of undigested food with halitosis and hiccups. The patient first becomes aware of intermittent and increasing difficulty in swallowing. As the tumor grows and the obstruction becomes nearly complete, even liquids cannot pass into the stomach. Regurgitation of food and saliva occurs, hemorrhage may take place, and progressive loss of weight and strength occurs from inadequate nutrition. Later symptoms include substernal pain, persistent hiccup, respiratory difficulty, and halitosis.

The delay between the onset of early symptoms and the patient seeking medical advice is often 12 to 18 months. Any person having swallowing difficulties should be encouraged to consult the primary provider immediately.

Assessment and Diagnostic Findings

Currently, diagnosis is confirmed most often by EGD with biopsy and brushings (95% to 100% sensitivity), although the double-contrast esophagography also has a sensitivity of more than 95% (Levine & Rubesin, 2012). The biopsy can be used to determine the presence of disease and cell differentiation. At presentation, most patients have moderately differentiated tumors.

Several imaging techniques may provide useful diagnostic information. A CT scan of the chest and abdomen is beneficial for detecting any anatomic evidence of metastatic disease, especially of the lungs, liver, and kidney. A positron emission tomography (PET) scan may also help detect metastasis. Endoscopic ultrasound is used to determine whether the cancer has spread to the lymph nodes and other mediastinal structures; it can also determine the size and invasiveness of the tumor. Exploratory laparoscopy is the best method for finding positive lymph nodes in patients with distal lesions.

Future diagnostic techniques that may serve as predictors for dysplastic progression in patients with BE involve molecular markers. Some data have shown that a small percentage of people may have a genetic predisposition to esophageal cancer. Researchers have identified at least four biomarkers with strong potential to predict outcomes in esophageal cancer (Chen, Huang, Zhu, et al., 2013). The usefulness of molecular markers in treating esophageal cancer continues to be researched.

Figure 45-9 • Esophageal reconstruction with free jejunal transfer. A portion of the jejunum is grafted between the esophagus and pharynx to replace the abnormal portion of the esophagus. The vascular structures are also anastomosed.

Medical Management

If esophageal cancer is detected at an early stage, treatment goals may be directed toward cure; however, it is often detected in late stages, making relief of symptoms the only reasonable goal of therapy. Treatment may include surgery, radiation, chemotherapy, or a combination of these modalities, depending on the type of cancer cell, the extent of the disease, and the patient's condition. A standard treatment plan for a patient who is newly diagnosed with esophageal cancer includes the following: preoperative combination chemotherapy and radiation therapy for 4 to 6 weeks, followed by a period of no medical intervention for 4 weeks, and, finally, surgical resection of the esophagus (NCI, 2014).

Although minimally invasive surgery may be possible in some cases, standard surgical management includes a total resection of the esophagus (esophagectomy) with removal of the tumor plus a wide tumor-free margin of the esophagus and the lymph nodes in the area (Cox, 1999; Kűper, Eisner, Kőnigsrainer, et al., 2014). The surgical approach may be through the thorax or the abdomen, depending on the location of the tumor. When tumors occur in the cervical or upper thoracic area, esophageal continuity may be maintained by a free jejunal graft transfer, in which the tumor is removed and the area is replaced with a portion of the jejunum (see Fig. 45-9). A segment of the colon may be used, or the stomach can be elevated into the chest and the proximal section of the esophagus anastomosed to the stomach (Cox, 1999).

Tumors of the lower thoracic esophagus are more amenable to surgery than are tumors located higher in the esophagus. GI tract integrity is maintained by anastomosing the lower esophagus to the stomach (see Fig. 45-10).

Surgical resection of the esophagus has a relatively high mortality rate because of infection, pulmonary complications, or leakage through the anastomosis. Postoperatively, the patient has an NG tube in place that should not be manipulated. The patient remains NPO until x-ray studies confirm

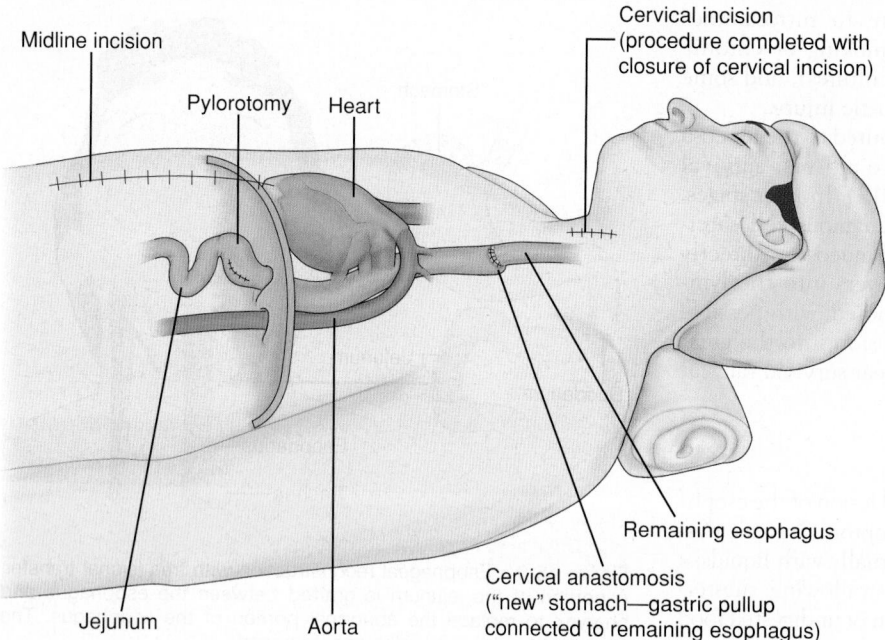

Midline incision

Pylorotomy   Heart

Cervical incision
(procedure completed with
closure of cervical incision)

Remaining esophagus

Cervical anastomosis
("new" stomach—gastric pullup
connected to remaining esophagus)

Jejunum   Aorta

Figure 45-10 • Transhiatal esophagectomy. Surgical removal of tumor of the lower esophagus with anastomosis of the remaining esophagus to the stomach. Redrawn with permission from Heitmiller, R. F. Closed chest esophageal resection. *Operative Techniques in Thoracic and Cardiovascular Surgery, 4*(3), 263 © 1999 Elsevier Inc.

that the anastomosis is free from an esophageal leak, there is no obstruction, and there is no evidence of pulmonary aspiration.

Palliative treatment may be necessary to keep the esophagus open, to assist with nutrition, and to control saliva. Palliation may be accomplished with dilation of the esophagus, laser therapy, placement of an endoprosthesis (stent) via EGD, radiation, or chemotherapy.

 Nursing Management

Preoperative nursing management is directed toward improving the patient's nutritional and physical status in preparation for surgery, radiation therapy, or chemotherapy. A program to promote weight gain based on a high-calorie and high-protein diet, in liquid or soft form, is provided if adequate food can be taken by mouth. If this is not possible, parenteral or enteral nutrition is initiated. Nutritional status is monitored throughout treatment. The patient is informed about the nature of the postoperative equipment that will be used, including that required for closed chest drainage, NG suction, parenteral fluid therapy, and gastric intubation.

Immediate postoperative care is similar to that provided for patients undergoing thoracic surgery. It is not uncommon for patients to have a tracheostomy and be placed in an intensive care unit or step-down unit. After recovering from the effects of anesthesia, the patient is placed in a low Fowler position, and later in a Fowler position, to help prevent reflux of gastric secretions. The patient is observed carefully for regurgitation and dyspnea. A common postoperative complication is aspiration pneumonia. Therefore, the patient is placed on a vigorous pulmonary plan of care that includes incentive spirometry, sitting up in a chair, and, if necessary, nebulizer treatments. Chest physiotherapy is avoided due to the risk of aspiration. The patient's temperature is monitored to detect any elevation that may indicate aspiration or seepage of fluid through the operative site into

the mediastinum, which would indicate an esophageal leak. Drainage from the cervical neck wound, usually saliva, is evidence of an early esophageal leak. Typically, no treatment other than maintaining NPO status and parenteral or enteral support is warranted.

Cardiac complications include atrial fibrillation, which occurs due to irritation of the vagus nerve at the time of surgery. Typical medical management includes digitalization or the use of beta-blockers, depending on the patient's response. Rarely, cardioversion may be used.

During surgery, an NG tube is inserted and taped in place. It is connected to low intermittent suction. The NG tube is not manipulated; if displacement occurs, it is not replaced because damage to the anastomosis may occur. The NG tube is typically removed 5 days after surgery; before the patient is allowed to eat, a barium swallow is performed to assess for any anastomotic leak.

Once feeding begins, the nurse encourages the patient to swallow small sips of water. Eventually, the diet is advanced as tolerated to a soft, mechanical diet. When the patient can increase their food and fluid intake to an adequate amount, parenteral fluids are discontinued. After each meal, the patient remains upright for at least 2 hours to allow the food to move through the GI tract. It is a challenge to encourage the patient to eat because the appetite is usually poor. Family involvement and home-cooked favorite foods may help the patient to eat. Antacids may help patients with gastric distress. Metoclopramide is useful in promoting gastric motility.

If chemotherapy and radiation are part of the therapy, the patient's appetite will be further depressed, and esophagitis may occur, causing pain when food is eaten. Liquid supplements may be more easily tolerated. However, supplements such as Boost and Ensure should be avoided because they promote **vagotomy syndrome** (dumping syndrome), which can occur with each meal or approximately 20 minutes to 2 hours after eating. The vagotomy syndrome occurs due to interruption of vagal nerve fibers, which in turn causes an alteration in the storage function of the stomach and the pyloric emptying mechanism. As a result, large amounts of solids and liquids rapidly "dump" into the duodenum. The patient experiences severe abdominal cramping, followed by a liquid bowel movement that may or may not be associated with diaphoresis, rapid heart rate or rapid respirations, or both. It can be quite disabling but typically resolves without incident, and the patient is left feeling extremely tired. The vagotomy syndrome is common following esophageal surgery, but as the patient's recovery progresses and the patient begins to eat soft foods and remains in an upright position for 2 hours after eating, the frequency and severity of episodes decrease.

Often, in either the preoperative or the postoperative period, an obstructed or nearly obstructed esophagus causes difficulty with excess saliva, and drooling becomes a problem. Oral suction may be used if the patient cannot handle oral secretions, or a wick-type gauze may be placed at the corner of the mouth to direct secretions to a dressing or emesis basin. The possibility that the patient may aspirate saliva into the tracheobronchial tree and develop pneumonia is a concern.

When the patient is ready to go home, the family is instructed about how to promote nutrition, what observations to make, what measures to take if complications occur, how to keep the patient comfortable, and how to obtain needed physical and emotional support.

CRITICAL THINKING EXERCISES

1 `ebp` A 52-year-old female patient presents to a primary care clinic with a mostly painless, but sometimes sore, hardened white patch in her oral cavity. What questions should the nurse ask her? What are the primary risk factors for oral cancer? If she is diagnosed with oral cancer, what treatment protocol would likely be recommended?

2 `pq` You are a nurse working on an inpatient oncology unit and have been assigned a postoperative patient who has had a modified radical neck resection due to cancer. What are the primary differences between a radical, modified, and selective neck dissection? You learn that the patient's internal jugular vein is intact, but that the sternocleidomastoid muscle and the spinal accessory nerve have both been impacted by the surgery. Based on this information, what are the key priority nursing interventions that will prevent long-term complications in this patient?

3 A patient diagnosed with esophageal cancer undergoes the standard treatment of chemoradiation prior to an esophagostomy. After the esophagostomy, the patient receives enteral nutrition through an NG tube. Although several days have passed, the patient remains disengaged from the staff and his family, making little eye contact, admitting to extreme pain only when asked, and refusing to engage in postoperative care. What are your two major nursing diagnoses for this patient? Identify three expected outcomes and interventions that address each of these diagnoses.

REFERENCES

*Asterisk indicates nursing research article.
**Double asterisk indicates classic reference.

Books

Bickley, L. S. (2013). *Bates' guide to physical examination and history taking* (11th ed.). Philadelphia, PA: Lippincott Williams & Wilkins.

Carr, E. (2016). Head and neck cancers. In J. K. Itano (Ed.): *Core curriculum for oncology nursing* (5th ed.). St. Louis, MO: Elsevier Inc.

**Cox, J. L. (1999). *Operative techniques in thoracic and cardiovascular surgery: A comparative atlas*. Philadelphia, PA: W. B. Saunders.

Fonseca, R. J., Turvey, T. A., Marciani, R. D. (Eds.). (2008). *Oral and maxillofacial surgery* (2nd ed.). Philadelphia, PA: W. B. Saunders.

Frandsen, G., & Pennington, S. S. (2014). *Abrams' clinical drug therapy: Rationales for nursing practice* (10th ed.). Philadelphia, PA: Wolters Kluwer Health/Lippincott Williams & Wilkins.

Haggerty, C. J. (2015). Mandibular fractures. In C. J. Haggerty & R. M. Laughlin (Eds.), *Atlas of operative oral and maxillofacial surgery*. Ames, Iowa: John Wiley & Sons, Inc.

Levine, M. S., & Rubesin, S. E. (2012). Radiology of the pharynx and esophagus. In D. O. Castell & J. E. Richter, (Eds.), (*The esophagus* (5th ed.). Philadelphia, PA: Lippincott Williams & Wilkins.

Journals and Electronic Documents

Ahovuo-Saloranta, A., Forss, H., Walsh, T., et al. (2013). Sealants for preventing dental decay in the permanent teeth. *Cochrane Database of Systematic Reviews, 3*, CD001830.

Allie, E. H., Blackshaw, A. M., Losek, J. D., et al. (2014). Clinical effectiveness of bougienage for esophageal coins in a pediatric ED. *American Journal of Emergency Medicine, 32*(10), 1263–1269.

American Academy of Periodontology. (2015). *Periodontal disease fact sheet*. Retrieved on 11/17/2015 at: www.perio.org/newsroom/periodontal-disease-fact-sheet

American Cancer Society (ACS). (2015). *Cancer facts and figures 2015*. Atlanta, GA: American Cancer Society. Retrieved on 11/17/2015 at: www.cancer.org/acs/groups/content/@editorial/documents/document/acspc-044552.pdf

American Cancer Society (ACS). (2016). *Kaposi sarcoma*. Retrieved on 6/13/2016 at: www.cancer.org/cancer/kaposisarcoma/detailedguide/kaposi-sarcoma-what-is-kaposi-sarcoma

American Society for Gastrointestinal Endoscopy Standards of Practice Committee. (2011). Guideline: Management of ingested foreign bodies and food impactions. *Gastrointestinal Endoscopy, 73*(6), 1085–1091.

Anderson, W. D., Treister, N. S., Mayeaux, E. J., et al. (2015). Oral lesions you can't afford to miss. *Journal of Family Practice, 64*(7), 392–399.

Belli, E., Liberatore, G., Elidon, M., et al. (2015). Surgical evolution in the treatment of mandibular condyle fractures. *BMC Surgery, 15*(16), 1–6.

Bossola, M. (2015). Nutritional interventions in head and neck cancer patients undergoing chemoradiotherapy: A narrative review. *Nutrients, 7*(1), 265–276.

Byard, R. W. (2015). Caustic ingestion: A forensic overview. *Journal of Forensic Science, 60*(3), 812–815.

Centers for Disease Control and Prevention (CDC). (2013). *2012 Water fluoridation statistics*. Retrieved on 11/17/2015 at: www.cdc.gov/fluoridation/statistics/2012stats.htm

Centers for Disease Control and Prevention (CDC). (2015). *Human papillomavirus (HPV): HPV vaccines: Vaccinating your preteen or teen*. Retrieved on 11/17/2015 at: www.cdc.gov/hpv/parents/vaccine.html

Chen, M., Huang, J., Zhu, Z., et al. (2013). Systematic review and meta-analysis of tumor biomarkers in predicting prognosis in esophageal cancer. *BMC Cancer, 13*, 539.

Cheng, C. Q., Xu, H., Liu, L., et al. (2016). Efficacy and safety of pilocarpine for radiation-induced xerostomia in patients with head and neck cancer: A systematic review and meta-analysis. *The Journal of the American Dental Association, 147*(4), 236–243.

Eke, P. I., Dye, B. A., Wei, L., et al. (2012). Prevalence of periodontitis in adults in the United States: 2009 and 2010. *Journal of Dental Research, 91*(10), 914–920.

*Fronczek, A. E., (2015). A phenomenological study of family caregivers of patients with head and neck cancers. *Oncology Nursing Forum, 42*(6), 593–600.

Garg, S. K., & Gurusamy, K. S. (2015). Laparoscopic fundoplication surgery versus medical management for gastro-oesophageal reflux disease (GORD) in adults. *Cochrane Database Systematic Reviews, 11*, CD003243.

Gauer, R. L., & Semidey, M. J. (2015). Diagnosis and treatment of temporomandibular disorders. *American Family Physician, 91*(6), 378–386.

Grègoire, V., Ang, K., Budach, W., et al. (2014). Delineation of the neck node levels for head and neck tumors: A 2013 update. DAHANCA, EORTC, HKNPCSG, NCIC CTG, NCRI, RTOG, TROG consensus guidelines. *Radiotherapy and Oncology, 110*(1), 172–181.

Ha, C., Regan, J., Cetindag, I. B., et al. (2015). Benign esophageal tumors. *Surgical Clinics of North America, 95*(3), 491–514.

Hart, A. M. (2013). Evidence-based recommendations for GERD treatment. *The Nurse Practitioner, 38*(8), 26–34.

**Heitmiller, R. F. (1999). Closed chest esophageal resection. *Operative Techniques in Thoracic and Cardiovascular Surgery, 4*(3), 252–265.

Kohn, G. P., Price, R. R., Demeester, S. R., et al. (2013). *Guidelines for the management of hiatal hernia.* Retrieved on 11/17/2015 from: www.sages.org/publications/guidelines/guidelines-for-the-management-of-hiatal-hernia/

Kűper, M. A., Eisner, F. Kőnigsrainer, A., et al. (2014). Laparoscopic surgery for benign and malign diseases of the digestive system: Indications, limitations, and evidence. *World Journal of Gastroenterology, 20*(17), 4883–4891.

Lalla, R. V., Bowen, J., Barasch, A., et al. (2014). MASCC/ISOO clinical practice guidelines for the management of mucositis secondary to cancer therapy. *Cancer, 120*, 1453–1461.

Lin, D. T., Yarlagadda, B. B., Sethi, R. K., et al. (2015). Long-term functional outcomes of total glossectomy with or without laryngectomy. *JAMA Otolaryngology – Head and Neck Surgery, 141*(9), 797–803.

Lufrano, R., Heckman, M. G., Diehl, N., et al. (2015). Nutcracker esophagus: Demographic, clinical features, and esophageal tests in 115 patients. *Diseases of the Esophagus, 28*(1), 11–18.

Malas, A. (2015). *Esophageal spasm.* Retrieved on 11/17/2015 at: emedicine.medscape.com/article/174975-overview

Marinho, V. C., Worthington, H. V., Walsh, T., et al. (2015). Fluoride gels for preventing dental caries in children and adolescents. *Cochrane Database of Systematic Reviews, 15*(6). doi: 10.1002/14651858.CD002280.pub2

Miranda-Rius, J., Brunet-Llobet, L., Lahor-Soler, E., et al. (2015). Salivary secretory disorders, inducing drugs, and clinical management. *International Journal of Medical Sciences, 12*(10), 811–824.

National Cancer Institute (NCI). (2014). *A snapshot of esophageal cancer.* Retrieved on 11/17/2015 at: www.cancer.gov/research/progress/snapshots/esophageal

National Cancer Institute (NCI). (2015a). *PDQ cancer information summaries [internet]: Oral cavity and oropharyngeal cancer prevention-health professional version (PDQ®).* Bethesda, MD: National Cancer Institute, PDQ Screening and Prevention Editorial Board. Retrieved on 11/17/2015 at: www.ncbi.nlm.nih.gov/books/NBK65979/#

National Cancer Institute (NCI). (2015b). *Salivary gland cancer treatment-for health professionals (PDQ®).* Retrieved on 11/17/2015 at: www.cancer.gov/types/head-and-neck/hp/salivary-gland-treatment-pdq

National Institute of Dental and Craniofacial Research (NIDCR). (2013a). *Chemotherapy and your mouth.* Retrieved on 11/17/2015 at: www.nidcr.nih.gov/oralhealth/Topics/CancerTreatment/ChemotherapyYourMouth.htm

National Institute of Dental and Craniofacial Research (NIDCR). (2013b). *TMJ (temporomandibular joint and muscle disorders).* Retrieved on 11/17/2015 at: www.nidcr.nih.gov/oralhealth/Topics/TMJ/TMJDisorders.htm

O'Gorman, S. M., & Torgerson, R. R. (2016). Contact allergy in cheilitis. *International Journal of Dermatology, 55*(7), 386–391.

Oleynikov, D., & Jolley, J. M. (2015). Paraesophageal hernia. *Surgical Clinics of North America, 95*(3), 555–565.

Pandolfino, J. E., & Gawron, A. J. (2015). Achalasia: A systematic review. *JAMA, 313*(18), 1841–1852. doi:10.1001/jama.2015.2996

Papapanou, P. N. (2015). Systemic effects of periodontitis: Lessons learned from research on atherosclerotic vascular disease and adverse pregnancy outcomes. *International Dental Journal, 65*(6), 283–291

Raymond, D. P., & Jones, C. (2015). Surgical management of esophageal perforation. *Up to Date.* Retrieved on 11/17/15 at: www.uptodate.com/contents/surgical-management-of-esophageal-perforation

Reid, K. I., & Greene, C. S. (2013). Diagnosis and treatment of temporomandibular disorders: An ethical analysis of current practices. *Journal of Oral Rehabilitation, 40*, 546–561.

Rihani, J., Lee, M. R., Lee, T., et al. (2013). Flap selection and functional outcomes in total glossectomy with laryngeal preservation. *JAMA Otolaryngology – Head and Neck Surgery, 149*(4), 547–553.

**Robbins, K. T., Clayman, G., Levine, P. A., et al. (2002). Neck dissection classification update: Revisions proposed by the American Head and Neck Society and the American Academy of Otolaryngology – Head and Neck Surgery. *Archives of Otolaryngology - Head and Neck Surgery, 128*(7), 751–758.

Robertson, D. P., Keys, W., Rautemaa-Richardson, R., et al. (2015). Management of severe acute dental infections. *British Dental Journal, 350*:h1300.

Robinson, N. B., & DiMango, E. (2014). Prevalence of gastroesophageal reflux in cystic fibrosis and implications for lung disease. *Annals of the American Thoracic Society, 11*(6), 964–968.

Sharma, P., Katzka, D. A., Gupta, N., et al. (2015). Consensus statement: Quality indicators for the management of Barrett's esophagus, dysplasia, and esophageal adenocarcinoma: International consensus recommendations from the American Gastroenterological Association symposium. *Gastroenterology, 149*(6), 1599–1606. doi: http://dx.doi.org/10.1053/j.gastro.2015.08.007

Sigismund, P. E., Zenk, J., Koch, M., et al. (2015). Nearly 3,000 salivary stones: Some clinical and epidemiologic aspects. *The Laryngoscope, 125*(8), 1879–1882. doi: 10.1002/lary.25377

Silk, H. (2014). Disease of the mouth. *Primary Care: Clinics in Office Practice, 41*(1), 75–90.

Singhal, V., & Khaitan, L. (2015). Preoperative evaluation of gastroesophageal reflux disease. *Surgical Clinics of North America, 95*(3), 615–627.

Smith, C. D. (2015). Esophageal strictures and diverticula. *Surgical Clinics of North America, 95*(3), 669–681.

Sobin, L., Kopp, R., Walsh, R., et al. (2016). Incidence of concussion in patients with isolated mandible fractures. *JAMA Facial Plastic Surgery, 18*(1), 15–18.

Steinau, M., Saraiya, M., Goodman, M. T., et al. (2014). Human papillomavirus prevalence in oropharyngeal cancer before vaccine introduction, United States. *Emerging Infectious Diseases, 20*(5), 822–828.

Swanson, M. S., Hudson, R. L., Bhandari, N., et al. (2015). Use of octreotide for the management of chyle fistula following neck dissection. *JAMA Otolaryngology – Head and Neck Surgery, 141*(8), 723–727.

Tessier, D. J. (2015). Chyle fistula. *Medscape.* Retrieved on 6/10/2016 at: emedicine.medscape.com/article/190025-overview

Twetman, S. (2015). The evidence base for professional and self-care prevention – caries, erosion and sensitivity. *BMC Oral Health, 15*(Suppl 1): S4. 10.1186/1472–6831–15-S1-S4

**U.S. Department of Health and Human Services (HHS). (2000). *Oral health in America: A report of the surgeon general. Executive summary.* Rockville, MD: US Department of Health and Human Services, National Institutes of Dental and Craniofacial Research, National Institutes of Health. Retrieved on 11/17/2015 at: silk.nih.gov/public/hck1ocv.@www.surgeon.fullrpt.pdf

U.S. Department of Health and Human Services (HHS). (2014). *A national call to action to promote oral health.* Rockville, MD: U.S. Department of Health and Human Services, Public Health Service, Centers for Disease Control and Prevention, National Institutes of Health, National Institute of Dental and Craniofacial Research. NIH Publication No. 03–5303. Retrieved on 6/12/2016 at: www.nidcr.nih.gov/DataStatistics/SurgeonGeneral/NationalCalltoAction/nationalcalltoaction.htm

U.S. Department of Health and Human Services (HHS), Office of Disease Prevention and Health Promotion. (2016). *Healthy People 2020: Oral health.* Retrieved on 6/11/2016 at: www.healthypeople.gov/2020/topics-objectives/topic/oral-health

van den Bergh, B., de Mol van Otterloo, J. J., van der Ploeg, T., et al. (2015). IMF-screws or arch bars as conservative treatment for mandibular condyle fractures: Quality of life aspects. *Journal of Cranio-Maxillo-Facial Surgery, 43*(7), 1004–1009.

Villa, A., Nordio, F., & Gohel, A. (2015). A risk prediction model for xerostomia: A retrospective cohort study. *Gerodontology 33*(4), 562–568.

Weno, K. (2015). *Statement on the evidence supporting the safety and effectiveness of community water fluoridation.* Atlanta, GA: Centers for Disease Control and Prevention. Retrieved on 11/17/2015 at: www.cdc.gov/fluoridation/pdf/statement-cwf-6–8–2015.pdf

World Health Organization (WHO). (2015). *Strategies for oral disease prevention and health promotion.* Retrieved on 11/17/2015 at www.who.int/oral_health/strategies/en/.

Xie, S., Wang, K., Xu, T., et al. (2015). Efficacy and safety of botulinum toxin type A for treatment of Frey's syndrome: Evidence from 22 published articles. *Cancer Medicine, 4*(11), 1639–1650

Yuan, Y., Zhao, Y. F., Hu, Y., et al. (2013). Surgical treatment of Zenker's diverticulum. *Digestive Surgery, 30*(3), 207–218.

Resources

Academy of General Dentistry (AGD), www.agd.org
American Cancer Society (ACS), www.cancer.org
American Dental Association (ADA), www.ada.org/en/
Healthy People 2020, www.healthypeople.gov
I Can Cope Online (ACS), www.cancer.org/treatment/supportprograms-services/onlinecommunities/participateinacancereducationclass/icancopeonline/index
Look Good Feel Better, www.lookgoodfeelbetter.org
National Institute of Dental and Craniofacial Research (NIDCR), National Institutes of Health, www.nidcr.nih.gov

LEARNING OBJECTIVES

On completion of this chapter, the learner will be able to:

1 Compare the etiology, clinical manifestations, and management of acute gastritis, chronic gastritis, and peptic ulcer.
2 Use the nursing process as a framework for care of patients with peptic ulcer.
3 Describe the pharmacologic, dietary, and surgical treatment of peptic ulcer.
4 Apply the nursing process as a framework for care of patients with gastric cancer.
5 Discuss the etiology, clinical manifestations, and management of tumors of the small intestine.

GLOSSARY

achlorhydria: lack of hydrochloric acid in digestive secretions of the stomach
antrectomy: removal of the pyloric (antrum) portion of the stomach with anastomosis (surgical connection) either to the duodenum (gastroduodenostomy or Billroth I) or to the jejunum (gastrojejunostomy or Billroth II)
duodenum: first portion of the small intestine, between the stomach and the jejunum
dumping syndrome: physiologic response to rapid emptying of gastric contents into the small intestines, manifested by nausea, weakness, sweating, palpitations, syncope, and diarrhea
dyspepsia: indigestion; upper abdominal discomfort associated with eating
gastric: refers to the stomach
gastric outlet obstruction: any condition that mechanically impedes normal gastric emptying; there is obstruction of the channel of the pylorus and duodenum through which the stomach empties; also called pyloric obstruction
gastritis: inflammation of the stomach
Helicobacter pylori (H. pylori): a spiral-shaped Gram-negative bacterium that colonizes the gastric mucosa; is involved in most cases of peptic ulcer disease

hematemesis: vomiting of blood
hematochezia: bright red, bloody stools
melena: tarry or black stools; indicative of occult blood in stools
omentum: fold of the peritoneum that surrounds the stomach and other organs of the abdomen
peritoneum: thin membrane that lines the inside of the wall of the abdomen and covers all of the abdominal organs
pyloroplasty: surgical procedure to increase the opening of the pyloric orifice
pylorus: opening between the stomach and the duodenum
pyrosis: a burning sensation in the stomach and esophagus that moves up to the mouth; commonly called heartburn
serosa: thin membrane that covers the outer surface of the stomach; visceral peritoneum covering the outer surface of the stomach
steatorrhea: fatty stool; typically malodorous with an oily appearance and floats in water
stenosis: narrowing or tightening of an opening or passage in the body

A person's nutritional status depends not only on the type and amount of intake, but also on the functioning of the gastric and intestinal portions of the gastrointestinal (GI) system. The scope of disorders that may affect a person's nutritional status is of particular note. According to the National Institute of Diabetes and Digestive and Kidney Diseases (NIDDK, 2013), as many as 70 million Americans are known to have at least one digestive disease. Given the high prevalence of Americans who have gastric and duodenal disorders, nurses will encounter adults and older adults with these disorders in virtually every inpatient and outpatient clinical setting. This chapter describes disorders of the stomach and small intestine, as well as their etiology, clinical manifestations, management, and related nursing care.

Gastritis

Gastritis (inflammation of the gastric or stomach mucosa) is a common GI problem, accounting for approximately 2 million visits to outpatient clinics annually in the United States (Wehbi, Yang, Sarver, et al., 2014). It affects women and men about equally and is more common in older adults. Gastritis may be acute, lasting several hours to a few days, or chronic, resulting from repeated exposure to irritating agents or recurring episodes of acute gastritis.

Acute gastritis may be classified as erosive or nonerosive, based upon pathologic manifestations present in the gastric mucosa (Wehbi et al., 2014). The erosive form of acute gastritis is most often caused by local irritants such as aspirin and other nonsteroidal anti-inflammatory drugs (NSAIDs) (e.g., ibuprofen [Motrin]); alcohol consumption; and gastric radiation therapy (Grossman & Porth, 2014; NIDDK, 2015; Wehbi et al., 2014). The nonerosive form of acute gastritis is most often caused by an infection with **Helicobacter pylori (H. pylori)** (Wehbi et al., 2014). It is estimated that 70% of individuals in developing countries and between 30% and 40% of individuals in the United States and other industrialized countries are infected with H. pylori (Centers for Disease Control and Prevention [CDC], 2016).

A more severe form of acute gastritis is caused by the ingestion of strong acid or alkali, which may cause the mucosa to become gangrenous or to perforate (see Chapter 72). Scarring can occur, resulting in pyloric **stenosis** (narrowing or tightening) or obstruction. Acute gastritis also may develop in acute illnesses, especially when the patient has had major traumatic injuries; burns; severe infection; hepatic, kidney, or respiratory failure; or major surgery. This type of acute gastritis is often referred to as *stress-related gastritis* (Clark, Gbadehan, Dim, et al., 2015; NIDDK, 2015).

Chronic gastritis is often classified according to the underlying causative mechanism, which most often includes an infection with H. pylori (Marcus & Greenwald, 2014). Chronic H. pylori gastritis is implicated in the development of peptic ulcers, gastric adenocarcinoma (cancer), and gastric mucosa-associated lymphoid tissue lymphoma (Ruggiero & Censini, 2014; Yazbek, Trindade, Chin, et al., 2015). Chronic gastritis may also be caused by a chemical gastric injury (gastropathy) as the result of long-term drug therapy (e.g., aspirin and other NSAIDs) or reflux of duodenal contents into the stomach, which most often occurs after gastric surgery (e.g., gastrojejunostomy and gastroduodenostomy). Autoimmune disorders such as Hashimoto thyroiditis, Addison disease, and Graves' disease are also associated with the development of chronic gastritis (see Chapter 52) (Grossman & Porth, 2014; Marcus & Greenwald, 2014).

Pathophysiology

Gastritis is characterized by a disruption of the mucosal barrier that normally protects the stomach tissue from digestive juices (e.g., hydrochloric acid [HCl] and pepsin). The impaired mucosal barrier allows corrosive HCL, pepsin, and other irritating agents (e.g., NSAIDs and H. pylori) to come in contact with the gastric mucosa, resulting in inflammation. In acute gastritis, this inflammation is usually transient and self-limiting in nature. Inflammation causes the gastric mucosa to become edematous and hyperemic (congested with fluid and blood) and to undergo superficial erosion (see Fig. 46-1). Superficial ulceration may occur as a result of erosive disease and may lead to hemorrhage. In chronic gastritis, persistent or repeated insults lead to chronic inflammatory changes, and eventually atrophy (or thinning) of the gastric tissue (Grossman & Porth, 2014).

Clinical Manifestations

The patient with acute gastritis may have a rapid onset of symptoms, such as epigastric pain or discomfort, **dyspepsia** (indigestion), anorexia, hiccups, or nausea and vomiting, which can last from a few hours to a few days. Erosive gastritis may cause bleeding, which may manifest as blood in vomit or as **melena** (black, tarry stools) or **hematochezia** (bright red, bloody stools) (NIDDK, 2015; Wehbi et al., 2014).

The patient with chronic gastritis may complain of fatigue, **pyrosis** (a burning sensation in the stomach and esophagus that moves up to the mouth; heartburn) after eating, belching, a sour taste in the mouth, early satiety, anorexia,

Cells secrete hydrochloric (HCl) acid or pepsinogen and intrinsic factor

Damaged mucosa

Mucosa (provides a barrier to protect stomach from HCl acid)

Submucosa

Muscularis

Serosa

Figure 46-1 • Endoscopic view of erosive gastritis (*left*). Damage from irritants (*right*) results in increased intracellular pH, impaired enzyme function, disrupted cellular structures, ischemia, vascular stasis, and tissue death. Image at left reproduced with permission from Strayer, D.S. & Rubin, E. (2015). Rubin's pathology: Clinicopathologic foundations of medicine (7th ed.). Philadelphia, PA: Lippincott Williams & Wilkins.

TABLE 46-1 Clinical Manifestations of Acute and Chronic Gastritis

	Acute Gastritis	Chronic Gastritis
Gastrointestinal Symptoms	• Anorexia • Epigastric pain (rapid onset) • Hematemesis • Hiccups • Melena or hematochezia • Nausea and vomiting	• Belching • Early satiety • Intolerance of spicy or fatty foods • Nausea and vomiting • Pyrosis • Sour taste in mouth • Vague epigastric discomfort relieved by eating
Systemic Symptoms	• Possible signs of shock	• Anemia • Fatigue

Adapted from Marcus, A. J., & Greenwald, D. (2014). Chronic gastritis. *Medscape*. Available at: emedicine.medscape.com/article/176156; Wehbi, M., Yang, V. W., Sarver, G., et al. (2014). Acute gastritis. *Medscape*. Retrieved on 5/5/2016 at: emedicine.medscape.com/article/175909

or nausea and vomiting. Some patients may have only mild epigastric discomfort or report intolerance to spicy or fatty foods or slight pain that is relieved by eating (Marcus & Greenwald, 2014; NIDDK, 2015). Patients with chronic gastritis may not be able to absorb vitamin B$_{12}$ because of diminished production of intrinsic factor by the stomach's parietal cells due to atrophy, which may lead to pernicious anemia (see Chapter 33) (Zayouna & Piper, 2014). Some patients with chronic gastritis have no symptoms (Marcus & Greenwald, 2014) (see Table 46-1).

Assessment and Diagnostic Findings

The definitive diagnosis of gastritis is determined by an endoscopy and histologic examination of a tissue specimen obtained by biopsy (Marcus & Greenwald, 2014; Wehbi et al., 2014). A complete blood count (CBC) may be drawn to assess for anemia as a result of hemorrhage or pernicious anemia. Diagnostic measures for detecting *H. pylori* infection may be used and are discussed later in this chapter in the Peptic Ulcer Disease section.

Medical Management

The gastric mucosa is capable of repairing itself after an episode of acute gastritis. As a rule, the patient recovers in about 1 day, although the patient's appetite may be diminished for an additional 2 or 3 days. Acute gastritis is also managed by instructing the patient to refrain from alcohol and food until symptoms subside. When the patient can take nourishment by mouth, a nonirritating diet is recommended. If the symptoms persist, intravenous (IV) fluids may need to be given. If bleeding is present, management is similar to the procedures used to control upper GI tract hemorrhage discussed later in this chapter.

Therapy is supportive and may include nasogastric (NG) intubation, antacids, histamine-2 receptor antagonists (H$_2$ blockers) (e.g., famotidine [Pepcid], ranitidine [Zantac]), proton pump inhibitors (e.g., omeprazole [Prilosec], lansoprazole [Prevacid]), and IV fluids (NIDDK, 2015; Wehbi et al., 2014). Fiberoptic endoscopy may be necessary. In extreme cases, emergency surgery may be required to remove gangrenous or perforated tissue. A gastric resection or a gastrojejunostomy (anastomosis of jejunum to stomach to detour around the **pylorus**) may be necessary to treat **gastric outlet obstruction**, also called *pyloric obstruction*, a narrowing of the pyloric orifice, which cannot be relieved by medical management.

Chronic gastritis is managed by modifying the patient's diet, promoting rest, reducing stress, recommending avoidance of alcohol and NSAIDs, and initiating medications that may include antacids, H$_2$ blockers, or proton pump inhibitors (NIDDK, 2015). *H. pylori* may be treated with selected drug combinations which typically include a proton pump inhibitor, antibiotics, and sometimes bismuth salts (see Table 46-2).

Nursing Management

Reducing Anxiety

If the patient has ingested acids or alkalis, emergency measures may be necessary (see Chapter 72). The nurse offers supportive therapy to the patient and family during treatment and after the ingested acid or alkali has been neutralized or diluted. In some cases, the nurse may need to prepare the patient for additional diagnostic studies (endoscopies) or surgery. The patient may be anxious because of pain and planned treatment modalities. The nurse uses a calm approach to assess the patient and to answer all questions as completely as possible.

Promoting Optimal Nutrition

For acute gastritis, the nurse provides physical and emotional support and helps the patient manage the symptoms, which may include nausea, vomiting, and pyrosis (heartburn). The patient should take no foods or fluids by mouth—possibly for a few days—until the acute symptoms subside, thus allowing the gastric mucosa to heal. If IV therapy is necessary, the nurse monitors fluid intake and output along with serum electrolyte values. After the symptoms subside, the nurse may offer the patient ice chips followed by clear liquids. Introducing solid food as soon as possible may provide adequate oral nutrition, decrease the need for IV therapy, and minimize irritation to the gastric mucosa. As food is introduced, the nurse evaluates and reports any symptoms that suggest a repeat episode of gastritis.

The nurse discourages the intake of caffeinated beverages, because caffeine is a central nervous system stimulant that increases gastric activity and pepsin secretion. The nurse also discourages alcohol use. Discouraging cigarette smoking is important because nicotine reduces the secretion of pancreatic bicarbonate, which inhibits the neutralization of gastric acid in the **duodenum** (the first part of the small intestine) (Hannah, 2014; Li, Chan, Lu, et al., 2014). When appropriate, the nurse initiates and refers the patient for alcohol counseling and smoking cessation programs.

Promoting Fluid Balance

Daily fluid intake and output are monitored to detect early signs of dehydration (minimal fluid intake of 1.5 L/day, minimal urine output of 0.5 mL/kg/h). If food and oral fluids are withheld, IV fluids (3 L/day) usually are prescribed and a record of fluid intake plus caloric value (1 L of 5% dextrose in water = 170 calories of carbohydrate) needs to be maintained. Electrolyte values (sodium, potassium, chloride) are assessed every 24 hours to detect any imbalance.

TABLE 46-2 Selected Pharmacotherapy for Peptic Ulcer Disease and Gastritis

Pharmacologic Agent	Major Action	Key Nursing Considerations
Antibiotics		
Amoxicillin (Amoxil)	A bactericidal antibiotic that assists with eradicating *H. pylori* bacteria in the gastric mucosa	• May cause diarrhea • Should not be used in patients allergic to penicillin
Clarithromycin (Biaxin)	Exerts bactericidal effects to eradicate *H. pylori* bacteria in the gastric mucosa	• May cause GI upset, headache, altered taste • Many drug–drug interactions (e.g., colchicine [Colcrys], lovastatin [Mevacor], warfarin [Coumadin])
Metronidazole (Flagyl)	A synthetic antibacterial and antiprotozoal agent that assists with eradicating *H. pylori* bacteria in the gastric mucosa when given with other antibiotics and proton pump inhibitors	• Should be given with meals to decrease GI upset; may cause anorexia and metallic taste • Patient should avoid alcohol; increases blood-thinning effects of warfarin
Tetracycline	Exerts bacteriostatic effects to eradicate *H. pylori* bacteria in the gastric mucosa	• May cause photosensitivity reaction; advise patient to use sunscreen • May cause GI upset • Must be used with caution in patients with renal or hepatic impairment • Milk or dairy products may reduce effectiveness
Antidiarrheal		
Bismuth subsalicylate (Pepto-Bismol)	Suppresses *H. pylori* bacteria in the gastric mucosa and assists with healing of mucosal ulcers	• Given concurrently with antibiotics to eradicate *H. pylori* infection • Should be taken on empty stomach
H₂ Receptor Antagonists		
Cimetidine (Tagamet)	Decreases amount of HCl produced by stomach by blocking action of histamine on histamine receptors of parietal cells in the stomach	• Least expensive of H₂ receptor antagonists • May cause confusion, agitation, or coma in older adults or those with renal or hepatic insufficiency • Long-term use may cause diarrhea, dizziness, and gynecomastia • Many drug–drug interactions (e.g., amiodarone [Cordarone], amitriptyline [Elavil], benzodiazepines, metoprolol [Lopressor], nifedipine [Procardia], phenytoin [Dilantin], warfarin)
Famotidine (Pepcid)	Same as for cimetidine	• Best choice for patient who is critically ill because it is known to have the least risk of drug–drug interactions; does not alter liver metabolism • Prolonged half-life in patients with renal insufficiency • Short-term relief for GERD
Nizatidine (Axid)	Same as for cimetidine	• Used for treatment of ulcers and GERD • Prolonged half-life in patients with renal insufficiency • May cause headache, dizziness, diarrhea, nausea/vomiting, GI upset, and urticaria
Ranitidine (Zantac)	Same as for cimetidine	• Prolonged half-life in patients with renal and hepatic insufficiency • Causes fewer side effects than cimetidine • May cause headache, dizziness, constipation, nausea and vomiting, or abdominal discomfort
Proton Pump Inhibitors of Gastric Acid		
Esomeprazole (Nexium)	Decreases gastric acid secretion by slowing the H⁺, K⁺-ATPase pump on the surface of the parietal cells of the stomach	• Used mainly for treatment of duodenal ulcer disease and *H. pylori* infection • A delayed-release capsule that is to be swallowed whole and taken before meals
Lansoprazole (Prevacid)	Decreases gastric acid secretion by slowing the H⁺, K⁺-ATPase pump on the surface of the parietal cells	• A delayed-release capsule that is to be swallowed whole and taken before meals
Omeprazole (Prilosec)	Same as for lansoprazole	• A delayed-release capsule that is to be swallowed whole and taken before meals • May cause diarrhea, nausea, constipation, abdominal pain, vomiting, headache, or dizziness
Pantoprazole (Protonix)	Same as for lansoprazole	• A delayed-release tablet that is to be swallowed whole and taken before meals • May cause diarrhea and hyperglycemia, headache, abdominal pain, and abnormal liver function tests
Rabeprazole (AcipHex)	Same as for lansoprazole	• A delayed-release tablet to be swallowed whole • May cause abdominal pain, diarrhea, nausea, and headache • Drug–drug interactions with digoxin, iron, and warfarin
Prostaglandin E₁ Analog		
Misoprostol (Cytotec)	Synthetic prostaglandin; protects the gastric mucosa from agents that cause ulcers; also increases mucus production and bicarbonate levels	• Used to prevent ulceration in patients using NSAIDs • Administer with food • May cause diarrhea and cramping (including uterine cramping) • Used mainly for the treatment of duodenal ulcers
Sucralfate (Carafate)	Creates a viscous substance in the presence of gastric acid that forms a protective barrier, binding to the surface of the ulcer, and prevents digestion by pepsin	• Should be taken without food but with water • Other medications should be taken 2 hours before or after this medication • May cause constipation or nausea

H. pylori, *Helicobacter pylori*; GI, gastrointestinal; H₂, histamine-2; HCl, hydrochloric acid; GERD, gastroesophageal reflux disease; H⁺, K⁺-ATPase, hydrogen-potassium adenosine triphosphatase; NSAIDs, nonsteroidal anti-inflammatory drugs; CNS, central nervous system.
Adapted from Karch, A. M. (2014). *Lippincott nursing drug guide.* Philadelphia, PA: Lippincott Williams & Wilkins.

The nurse must always be alert to any indicators of hemorrhagic gastritis, which include **hematemesis** (vomiting of blood), tachycardia, and hypotension. All stools should be examined for the presence of frank or occult bleeding. If these occur, the primary provider is notified and the patient's vital signs are monitored as the patient's condition warrants. Guidelines for managing upper GI tract bleeding are discussed later in this chapter.

Relieving Pain

Measures to help relieve pain include instructing the patient to avoid foods and beverages that may irritate the gastric mucosa as well as the correct use of medications to relieve chronic gastritis. The nurse must regularly assess the patient's level of pain and the extent of comfort achieved through the use of medications and avoidance of irritating substances.

Promoting Home, Community-Based, and Transitional Care

 Educating Patients About Self-Care

The nurse evaluates the patient's knowledge about gastritis and develops an individualized education plan that includes information about stress management, diet, and medications (see Table 46-2). Dietary instructions take into account the patient's daily caloric needs as well as cultural aspects of food preferences and patterns of eating. The nurse and patient review foods and other substances to be avoided (e.g., spicy, irritating, or highly seasoned foods; caffeine; nicotine; alcohol). Consultation with a dietitian may be recommended (see Chart 46-1).

Providing information about prescribed medications, which may include antacids, H₂ blockers, or proton pump inhibitors, may help the patient to better understand why these medications assist in recovery and prevent recurrence. The importance of completing the medication regimen as prescribed to eradicate *H. pylori* infection must be reinforced to the patient and caregiver (see later discussion).

Continuing and Transitional Care

The nurse reinforces previous instruction and conducts ongoing assessment of the patient's symptoms and progress. Patients with malabsorption of vitamin B₁₂ need information about lifelong vitamin B₁₂ injections; the nurse may instruct a family member or caregiver how to administer the injections or make arrangements for the patient to receive the injections from the primary provider. Finally, the nurse emphasizes the importance of keeping follow-up appointments with the primary provider.

Figure 46-2 • Deep peptic ulcer. Adapted from Strayer, D. S. & Rubin, E. (2015). Rubin's pathology: Clinicopathologic foundations of medicine (7th ed.). Philadelphia, PA: Lippincott Williams & Wilkins.

Peptic Ulcer Disease

Peptic ulcer disease affects approximately 4.5 million Americans annually, and it requires inpatient hospitalization for an estimated 30 out of every 100 patients (Anand, 2015). A peptic ulcer may be referred to as a gastric, duodenal, or esophageal ulcer, depending on its location. A peptic ulcer is an excavation (hollowed-out area) that forms in the mucosa of the stomach, in the pylorus (the opening between the stomach and duodenum), in the duodenum or in the esophagus. Erosion of a circumscribed area of mucosa is the cause (see Fig. 46-2). This erosion may extend as deeply as the muscle layers or through the muscle to the **peritoneum** (thin membrane that lines the inside of the wall of the abdomen) (Grossman & Porth, 2014; NIDDK, 2014).

Chart 46-1 **HOME CARE CHECKLIST**
The Patient With Gastritis

At the completion of education, the patient and/or caregiver will be able to:

- State the impact of gastritis on physiologic functioning, ADLs, IADLs, roles, relationships, and spirituality.
- State need for vitamin B₁₂ injections if patient has pernicious anemia.
- Explain the importance of and necessity for adherence with prescribed medication regimen.
- Demonstrate methods of keeping track of the medication regimen and storage of the prescribed medications, and use reminders such as beepers and/or pillboxes.
- State the name, dose, side effects, frequency, and schedule for all medications.

- Identify foods and other substances that may cause gastritis (e.g., spicy, highly seasoned foods, caffeine, nicotine, alcohol).
- Identify side effects and complications (e.g., increased or return of abdominal discomfort, inability to ingest adequate solids and liquids) that should be reported to primary provider.
- State how to reach primary provider with questions or complications.
- State time and date of follow-up appointments and testing.

ADL, activities of daily living; IADL, independent activities of daily living.

Peptic ulcers are more likely to occur in the duodenum than in the stomach. As a rule they occur alone, but they may occur in multiples. Chronic gastric ulcers tend to occur in the lesser curvature of the stomach, near the pylorus. Esophageal ulcers occur as a result of the backward flow of HCl from the stomach into the esophagus (gastroesophageal reflux disease [GERD]).

Women and men have about equivalent lifetime risk of developing peptic ulcers (Anand, 2015). The rates of peptic ulcer disease among middle-aged adults have diminished over the past several decades, whereas the rates among older adults have increased (Anand, 2015; Pilotto & Franceschi, 2014). Those who are 65 years and older present to both outpatient and inpatient settings for treatment of peptic ulcers more than any other age group. This trend may be explained, at least in part, by higher rates of NSAID use and *H. pylori* infections in older adult populations (Anand, 2015; Pilotto & Franceschi, 2014).

In the past, stress and anxiety were thought to be causes of peptic ulcers, but research has documented that most peptic ulcers result from infection with the gram-negative bacteria *H. pylori*, which may be acquired through ingestion of food and water. Person-to-person transmission of the bacteria also occurs through close contact and exposure to emesis. Although *H. pylori* infection is common in the United States, most infected people do not develop ulcers. It is not known why *H. pylori* infection does not cause ulcers in all people, but most likely the predisposition to ulcer formation depends on certain factors, such as the type of *H. pylori* and other as yet unknown factors (Anand, 2015; Ruggiero & Censini, 2014; Grossman & Porth, 2014).

The use of NSAIDs such as ibuprofen and aspirin is also a major risk factor for peptic ulcers. Furthermore, infection with *H. pylori* and concomitant use of NSAIDs are synergistic risks (Anand, 2015). It is believed that smoking and alcohol consumption may be risks, although the evidence is inconclusive. There is no evidence that the ingestion of milk, caffeinated beverages, and spicy foods are associated with the development of peptic ulcers (Anand, 2015; NIDDK, 2014).

Familial tendency also may be a significant predisposing factor. People with blood type O are more susceptible to the development of peptic ulcers than are those with blood type A, B, or AB. There also is an association between peptic ulcer disease and chronic obstructive pulmonary disease, cirrhosis of the liver, and chronic kidney disease (Anand, 2015).

Peptic ulcer disease is also associated with Zollinger–Ellison syndrome (ZES). ZES is a rare condition in which benign or malignant tumors form in the pancreas and duodenum that secrete excessive amounts of the hormone gastrin (Anand, 2015; NIDDK, 2014). The excessive amount of gastrin results in extreme gastric hyperacidity and severe peptic ulcer disease. While the exact cause of ZES is unknown, 25% of cases are linked to an inherited, genetic condition called multiple endocrine neoplasia, type 1 (MEN 1) (Epelboy & Mazeh, 2014).

Pathophysiology

Peptic ulcers occur mainly in the gastroduodenal mucosa because this tissue cannot withstand the digestive action of gastric acid (HCl) and pepsin. The erosion is caused by the increased concentration or activity of acid–pepsin or by decreased resistance of the normally protective mucosal barrier. A damaged mucosa cannot secrete enough mucus to act as a barrier against normal digestive juices. Exposure of the mucosa to gastric acid (HCl), pepsin, and other irritating agents (e.g., NSAIDs or *H. pylori*) leads to inflammation, injury, and subsequent erosion of the mucosa. Patients with duodenal ulcers secrete more acid than normal, whereas patients with gastric ulcers tend to secrete normal or decreased levels of acid. When the mucosal barrier is impaired, even normal or decreased levels of HCl may result in the formation of peptic ulcers.

The use of NSAIDs inhibits prostaglandin synthesis, which is associated with a disruption of the normally protective mucosal barrier. Damage to the mucosal barrier also results in decreased resistance to bacteria, and thus infection from *H. pylori* bacteria may occur (Anand, 2015; Grossman & Porth, 2014).

ZES is suspected when a patient has several peptic ulcers or an ulcer that is resistant to standard medical therapy. It is identified by the following: hypersecretion of gastrin, duodenal ulcers, and gastrinomas (islet cell tumors) in the pancreas or duodenum. More than 80% of gastrinomas are found in the "gastric triangle," which encompasses the cystic and common bile ducts, the second and third portions of the duodenum, and the junction of the head and body of the pancreas (Bonheur & Nachimuthu, 2014). Most gastrinomas tend to grow slowly; however, more than 50% of these tumors are malignant (Epelboym & Mazeh, 2014). The patient with ZES may experience epigastric pain, pyrosis diarrhea, and **steatorrhea** (fatty stools). Patients with ZES associated with MEN-1 syndrome may have coexisting pituitary or parathyroid tumors. Fifty percent of patients with ZES-associated MEN-1 syndrome are diagnosed with hyperparathyroidism and therefore may exhibit signs of hypercalcemia (Epelboym & Mazeh, 2014).

Stress ulcer is the term given to the acute mucosal ulceration of the duodenal or gastric area that occurs after physiologically stressful events, such as burns, shock, sepsis, and multiple organ dysfunction syndrome (Clark et al., 2015). Stress ulcers, which are clinically different from peptic ulcers, are most common in patients who are ventilator-dependent after trauma or surgery. Fiberoptic endoscopy within 24 hours of trauma or surgery reveals shallow erosions of the stomach wall; by 72 hours, multiple gastric erosions are observed. As the stressful condition continues, the ulcers spread. When the patient recovers, the lesions are reversed. This pattern is typical of stress ulceration.

Differences of opinion exist as to the actual cause of mucosal ulceration in stress ulcers. Usually, the ulceration results from a disruption of the normally protective mucosal barrier and decreased mucosal blood flow (ischemia). Mucosal ischemia results in the reflux of duodenal contents into the stomach, which increases exposure of the unprotected gastric mucosa to the digestive effects of gastric acid (HCl) and pepsin (Anand, 2015; Clark et al., 2015; Frandah, Colmer-Hamood, & Nugent, 2014; Grossman & Porth, 2014). The combination of mucosal ischemia and increased gastric acid and pepsin exposure creates an ideal climate for ulceration.

Specific types of ulcers that result from stressful conditions include Curling ulcers and Cushing ulcers. Curling ulcer is frequently observed about 72 hours after extensive burn injuries and often involves the antrum of the stomach or the duodenum (Anand, 2015). Cushing ulcer is common in patients with a traumatic head injury, stroke, brain tumor, or following intracranial surgery. Cushing ulcer is thought to be caused by increased intracranial pressure, which results in overstimulation of the vagal nerve and an increased secretion of gastric acid (HCl) (Grossman & Porth, 2014). Curling ulcers and Cushing ulcers may occur in the esophagus, stomach, or duodenum and are usually deeper and more penetrating than typical stress ulcers (Kemp, Bashir, Dababneh, et al., 2015).

Clinical Manifestations

Symptoms of peptic ulcer disease may last for a few days, weeks, or months and may disappear only to reappear, often without an identifiable cause. Many patients with peptic ulcers have no signs or symptoms. These *silent peptic ulcers* most commonly occur in older adults and those taking aspirin and other NSAIDs (Anand, 2015).

As a rule, the patient with an ulcer complains of dull, gnawing pain or a burning sensation in the midepigastrium or the back. There are few clinical manifestations that differentiate gastric ulcers from duodenal ulcers; however, classically, the pain associated with gastric ulcers most commonly occurs immediately after eating, whereas the pain associated with duodenal ulcers most commonly occurs 2 to 3 hours after meals. In addition, approximately 50% to 80% of patients with duodenal ulcers awake with pain during the night, whereas 30% to 40% of patients with gastric ulcers voice this type of complaint. Patients with duodenal ulcers are more likely to express relief of pain after eating or after taking an antacid than patients with gastric ulcers (Anand, 2015).

Other nonspecific symptoms of either gastric ulcers or duodenal ulcers may include pyrosis vomiting, constipation or diarrhea, and bleeding. These symptoms are often accompanied by sour eructation (burping), which is common when the patient's stomach is empty.

Although vomiting is rare in an uncomplicated peptic ulcer, it may be a symptom of a complication of an ulcer. It results from gastric outlet obstruction, caused by either muscular spasm of the pylorus or mechanical obstruction from scarring or acute swelling of the inflamed mucous membrane adjacent to the ulcer. Vomiting may or may not be preceded by nausea; usually, it follows a bout of severe pain and bloating, which is relieved by vomiting. Emesis may contain undigested food eaten many hours earlier. Constipation or diarrhea may occur, probably as a result of diet and medications.

The patient with bleeding peptic ulcers may present with evidence of GI bleeding, such as hematemesis (vomiting blood) or the passage of melena (black, tarry stools) (Anand, 2015). Between 30% and 50% patients with bleeding peptic ulcers do not experience abdominal pain at the time of diagnosis (Gururatsakul, Holloway, Bellon, et al., 2014). Peptic ulcer perforation results in the sudden onset of signs and symptoms. The patient often reports severe, sharp upper abdominal pain, which may be referred to the shoulder; extreme abdominal tenderness; and nausea or vomiting. Hypotension and tachycardia may occur, indicating the onset of shock (Anand, 2015; Dimou & Velanovich, 2015).

Assessment and Diagnostic Findings

A physical examination may reveal pain, epigastric tenderness, or abdominal distention. Upper endoscopy is the preferred diagnostic procedure because it allows direct visualization of inflammatory changes, ulcers, and lesions. Through endoscopy, a biopsy of the gastric mucosa and any suspicious lesions can be obtained. Endoscopy may reveal lesions that, because of their size or location, are not evident on x-ray studies. *H. pylori* infection may be determined by endoscopy and histologic examination of a tissue specimen obtained by biopsy, or a rapid urease test of the biopsy specimen. Other less invasive diagnostic measures for detecting *H. pylori* include serologic testing for antibodies against the *H. pylori* antigen, stool antigen test, and urea breath test (Anand, 2015).

The patient who has a bleeding peptic ulcer may require periodic CBCs to determine the extent of blood loss and whether or not blood transfusions are advisable (see Chapter 32). Stools may be tested periodically until they are negative for occult blood. Gastric secretory studies are of value in diagnosing ZES and **achlorhydria** (lack of hydrochloric acid [HCl], hypochlorhydria (low levels of HCl), or hyperchlorhydria (high levels of HCl).

Medical Management

Once the diagnosis is established, the patient is informed that the condition can be managed. Recurrence may develop; however, peptic ulcers treated with antibiotics to eradicate *H. pylori* have a lower recurrence rate than those not treated with antibiotics. The goals are to eradicate *H. pylori* as indicated and to manage gastric acidity. Methods used include medications, lifestyle changes, and surgical intervention.

Pharmacologic Therapy

Currently, the most commonly used therapy for peptic ulcers is a combination of antibiotics, proton pump inhibitors, and sometimes bismuth salts that suppress or eradicate *H. pylori*. Recommended combination drug therapy is typically prescribed for 10 to 14 days and may include triple therapy with two antibiotics (e.g., metronidazole [Flagyl] or amoxicillin [Amoxil] and clarithromycin [Biaxin]) plus a proton pump inhibitor (e.g., lansoprazole [Prevacid], omeprazole [Prilosec], or rabeprazole [AcipHex]), or quadruple therapy with two antibiotics (metronidazole and tetracycline) plus a proton pump inhibitor and bismuth salts (Pepto-Bismol) (Anand, 2015; Marcus & Greenwald, 2014). Research is currently being conducted to develop a vaccine against *H. pylori* (Ruggiero & Censini, 2014).

H_2 blockers and proton pump inhibitors that reduce gastric acid secretion are used to treat ulcers not associated with *H. pylori* infection. Table 46-3 provides information about the medication regimens for peptic ulcer disease.

The patient is advised to adhere to and complete the medication regimen to ensure complete healing of the ulcer. The patient is advised to avoid the use of aspirin and other NSAIDs. Because most patients become symptom free within a week, the nurse stresses to the patient the importance of following the prescribed regimen so that the healing process can continue uninterrupted and the return of chronic ulcer

TABLE 46-3 Drug Regimens for Peptic Ulcer Disease

Indications	Drug Regimen	Nursing Considerations
Ulcer healing	**H₂ receptor antagonists:** Ranitidine 150 mg bid or 300 mg at bedtime Cimetidine 400 mg bid or 800 mg at bedtime Famotidine 20 mg bid or 40 mg at bedtime Nizatidine 150 mg bid or 300 mg at bedtime	Should be used for 6–8 weeks for complete peptic ulcer healing; patients who are at high risk require a maintenance dose for 1 year
	PPIs: Omeprazole 20 mg daily Lansoprazole 30 mg daily Rabeprazole 20 mg daily Pantoprazole 40 mg daily Esomeprazole 40 mg daily	Should be used for 4–8 weeks for complete peptic ulcer healing; patients who are at high risk require a maintenance dose for 1 year
H. pylori infection	*Triple therapy* with a PPI bid, plus clarithromycin 500 mg bid, plus amoxicillin 1000 mg bid (or metronidazole 500 mg bid) for 10–14 days. *Quadruple therapy* with bismuth subsalicylate 525 mg qid, plus tetracycline 500 mg qid, plus metronidazole 250 mg qid, plus a PPI daily for 10–14 days	Efficacy of therapy is approximately 85% qid dosing may decrease adherence to the regimen
Prophylactic therapy for NSAID ulcers	Peptic ulcer healing doses of PPIs (above) Misoprostol 100–200 mcg qid	Prevents recurrent ulceration in approximately 80–90% of patients; qid dosing may decrease adherence to the regimen

H₂, histamine-2; bid, two times a day; PPIs, proton pump inhibitors; qid, four times a day; NSAID, nonsteroidal anti-inflammatory drug.
Adapted from Anand, B. S. (2015). Peptic ulcer disease. *Medscape*. Retrieved on 5/3/2016 at: emedicine.medscape.com/article/181753

symptoms can be prevented. Maintenance dosages of H₂ blockers are usually recommended for 1 year.

For patients with ZES, hypersecretion of gastrin stimulates the release of gastric acid (HCl), which may be controlled with high doses of H₂ blockers. These patients may require twice the normal dose, and dosages usually need to be increased with prolonged use (Epelboym & Mazeh, 2014). Octreotide (Sandostatin), a medication that suppresses gastrin levels, also may be prescribed.

Patients at high risk for stress ulcers (e.g., patients who are mechanically ventilated for more than 48 hours) may be treated prophylactically with either H₂ blockers or proton pump inhibitors, and cytoprotective agents (e.g., misoprostol, sucralfate) because of the increased risk of upper GI tract hemorrhage (Clarke et al., 2015; Plummer, Blaser, & Deane, 2014).

Smoking Cessation

Smoking decreases the secretion of bicarbonate from the pancreas into the duodenum, resulting in increased acidity of the duodenum. Continued smoking is also associated with delayed healing of peptic ulcers (Li et al., 2014). Therefore, the patient is encouraged to stop smoking. Refer to Chapter 27 for information on how the nurse may promote cessation of tobacco use.

Dietary Modification

The intent of dietary modification for patients with peptic ulcers is to avoid oversecretion of acid and hypermotility in the GI tract. These can be minimized by avoiding extremes of temperature in food and beverages and overstimulation from the consumption of alcohol, coffee (including decaffeinated coffee, which also stimulates acid secretion), and other caffeinated beverages. In addition, an effort is made to neutralize acid by eating three regular meals a day. Small, frequent feedings are not necessary as long as an antacid or an H₂ blocker is taken. Diet compatibility becomes an individual matter: The patient eats foods that are tolerated and avoids those that produce pain.

Surgical Management

The introduction of antibiotics to eradicate *H. pylori* and of H₂ blockers as treatment for ulcers has greatly reduced the need for surgical intervention (Epelboym & Mazeh, 2014; Soreide, Thorsen, & Soreide, 2014). However, surgery is usually recommended for patients with intractable ulcers (those failing to heal after 12 to 16 weeks of medical treatment), life-threatening hemorrhage, perforation, or obstruction and for those with ZES that is unresponsive to medications (Anand, 2015; Epelboym & Mazeh, 2014; Soreide et al., 2014). Surgical procedures include vagotomy, with or without **pyloroplasty** (transecting nerves that stimulate acid secretion and opening the pylorus), and **antrectomy**, which is removal of the pyloric (antrum) portion of the stomach with anastomosis (surgical connection) to either the duodenum (gastroduodenostomy or Billroth I) or jejunum (gastrojejunostomy or Billroth II) (see Table 46-4.)

Surgery may be performed using a traditional open abdominal approach (requiring a long abdominal incision) or through the use of laparoscopy (only requiring small abdominal incisions). Laparoscopy is a type of minimally invasive surgery that involves the indirect visualization of the abdominal cavity through the use of a laparoscope (a thin flexible tube) attached to a camera. The laparoscope is placed into the abdomen through small "keyhole" incisions (0.5 to 1.5 cm in length). Laparoscopy has been associated with decreased postoperative bleeding, pain, infection, and recovery time (American College of Gastroenterology, 2015). The choice of using an open abdominal approach or laparoscopy is determined by the surgeon's preference and expertise as well as clinical factors, such as the patient's current health status; the

TABLE 46-4 Surgical Procedures for Peptic Ulcer Disease

Operation	Description	Adverse Effects
Vagotomy Vagotomy	Severing of the vagus nerve. Decreases gastric acid by diminishing cholinergic stimulation to the parietal cells, making them less responsive to gastrin. May be performed via an open surgical approach or laparoscopy. May be performed to reduce gastric acid secretion. A drainage type of procedure (see pyloroplasty) is usually performed to assist with gastric emptying (because there is total denervation of the stomach).	Some patients experience problems with feeling of fullness, dumping syndrome, diarrhea, and gastritis.
Truncal vagotomy	Severs the right and left vagus nerves as they enter the stomach at the distal part of the esophagus; most commonly used to decrease acid secretions.	Some patients experience problems with feeling of fullness, dumping syndrome, diarrhea, or constipation.
Selective vagotomy	Severs vagal innervation to the stomach but maintains innervation to the rest of the abdominal organs.	Fewer associated adverse effects than with truncal vagotomy.
Proximal (parietal cell) gastric vagotomy without drainage	Denervates acid-secreting parietal cells but preserves vagal innervation to the gastric antrum and pylorus.	No associated dumping syndrome
Pyloroplasty Pylorus—note longitudinal incision Vertical suture	Longitudinal incision is made into the pylorus and transversely sutured closed to enlarge the outlet and relax the muscle; usually accompanies truncal and selective vagotomies.	See adverse effects associated with truncal and selective vagotomies, as appropriate.
Antrectomy Billroth I (gastroduodenostomy) Fundus, Body, Antrectomy, Duodenum, Duodenal anastomosis	Removal of the lower portion of the antrum of the stomach (which contains the cells that secrete gastrin) as well as a small portion of the duodenum and pylorus. The remaining segment is anastomosed to the duodenum. May be performed in conjunction with a truncal vagotomy.	Patients may have problems with feeling of fullness, dumping syndrome, and diarrhea.

TABLE 46-4 Surgical Procedures for Peptic Ulcer Disease (continued)

Operation	Description	Adverse Effects
Billroth II (gastrojejunostomy)	Removal of lower portion (antrum) of stomach with anastomosis to jejunum. Dotted lines show portion removed (antrectomy). A duodenal stump remains and is oversewn.	Patients frequently have associated dumping syndrome, anemia, weight loss, and malabsorption.

presence of coexisting medical conditions; and a history of previous abdominal surgery.

Follow-Up Care

Recurrence of peptic ulcer disease within 1 year may be prevented with the prophylactic use of H_2 blockers taken at a reduced dose. Not all patients require maintenance therapy; it may be prescribed only for those with two or three recurrences per year, those who have had a complication such as bleeding or gastric outlet obstruction, or those for whom gastric surgery poses too high a risk. The likelihood of recurrence is reduced if the patient avoids smoking, coffee (including decaffeinated coffee) and other caffeinated beverages, alcohol, and ulcerogenic medications (e.g., NSAIDs).

NURSING PROCESS

The Patient With Peptic Ulcer Disease

Assessment

The nurse asks the patient to describe the pain, its pattern and whether or not it occurs predictably (e.g., after meals, during the night), and strategies used to relieve it (e.g., food, antacids). If the patient reports a recent history of vomiting, the nurse determines how often emesis has occurred and notes important characteristics of the vomitus: Is it bright red, does it resemble coffee grounds, or is there undigested food from previous meals? Has the patient noted any bloody or tarry stools?

The nurse also asks the patient to list their usual food intake for a 72-hour period. Lifestyle and other habits are a concern as well. For example, do they smoke cigarettes? If yes, how many? Does the patient ingest alcohol? If yes, how much and how often? Are NSAIDs used? Is there a family history of ulcer disease?

The nurse assesses the patient's vital signs and reports tachycardia and hypotension, which may indicate anemia from GI bleeding. The stool is tested for occult blood, and

a physical examination, including palpation of the abdomen for localized tenderness, is performed.

Diagnosis

NURSING DIAGNOSES

Based on the assessment data, nursing diagnoses may include the following:

- Acute pain related to the effect of gastric acid secretion on damaged tissue
- Anxiety related to an acute illness
- Imbalanced nutrition: less than body requirements related to changes in diet

COLLABORATIVE PROBLEMS/POTENTIAL COMPLICATIONS

Potential complications may include the following:

- Hemorrhage
- Perforation
- Penetration
- Gastric outlet obstruction

Planning and Goals

The goals for the patient may include relief of pain, reduced anxiety, maintenance of nutritional requirements, and absence of complications.

Nursing Interventions

RELIEVING PAIN

Pain relief can be achieved with prescribed medications. The patient should avoid aspirin and other NSAIDs as well as alcohol. In addition, meals should be eaten at regularly paced intervals in a relaxed setting. Medications prescribed to treat the peptic ulcer should provide relief of ulcer-associated pain. Some patients benefit from learning relaxation techniques to help manage stress and pain.

REDUCING ANXIETY

The nurse assesses the patient's level of anxiety. Explaining diagnostic tests and administering medications as scheduled help reduce anxiety. The nurse interacts with the patient in a relaxed manner; helps identify stressors; and explains various coping techniques and relaxation methods, such as biofeedback, hypnosis, or behavior modification. The patient's family is also encouraged to participate in care and to provide emotional support.

MAINTAINING OPTIMAL NUTRITIONAL STATUS

The nurse assesses the patient for malnutrition and weight loss. After recovery from an acute phase of peptic ulcer disease, the patient is advised about the importance of adhering to the medication regimen and dietary restrictions.

MONITORING AND MANAGING POTENTIAL COMPLICATIONS

Hemorrhage. Gastritis and hemorrhage from peptic ulcer are the two most common causes of upper GI tract bleeding (which may also occur with esophageal varices, as discussed in Chapter 49). Hemorrhage in patients with peptic ulcers is associated with a 10% mortality rate (Wong & Sung, 2013). Bleeding peptic ulcers account for 36% of all upper GI bleeds and it may be manifested by hematemesis or melena (Anand, 2015; Wong & Sung, 2013). The vomited blood can be bright red, or it can have a dark coffee grounds appearance from the oxidation of hemoglobin to methemoglobin. When the hemorrhage is large (2000 to 3000 mL), most of the blood is vomited. Because large quantities of blood may be lost quickly, immediate correction of blood loss may be required to prevent hemorrhagic shock. When the hemorrhage is small, much or all of the blood is passed in the stools, which appear tarry black because of the digested hemoglobin. Management depends on the amount of blood lost and the rate of bleeding.

The nurse assesses the patient for faintness or dizziness and nausea, which may precede or accompany bleeding. The nurse must monitor vital signs frequently and evaluate the patient for tachycardia, hypotension, and tachypnea. Other nursing interventions include monitoring the hemoglobin and hematocrit, testing the stool for gross or occult blood, and recording hourly urinary output to detect anuria or oliguria (absence of or decreased urine production).

Many times, the bleeding from a peptic ulcer stops spontaneously; however, the incidence of recurrent bleeding is high. Because bleeding can be fatal, the cause and severity of the hemorrhage must be identified quickly and the blood loss treated to prevent hemorrhagic shock. The nurse monitors the patient carefully so that bleeding can be detected quickly. Patients suspected of having an ulcer who present with symptoms of GI bleeding should undergo evaluation with endoscopy within 24 hours to confirm the diagnosis and allow targeted endoscopic interventions (Lau, Barkun, Fan, et al., 2013; Wong & Sung, 2013). These endoscopic interventions may include injecting the bleeding site with epinephrine or alcohol, or cauterizing the site, or clipping the ulcer, all in efforts to stop the bleeding (Anand, 2015; Wong & Sung, 2013). Arteriography with embolization may be needed if there is persistent and severe bleeding (Lau et al., 2013; Loffroy, Favelier, Pottecher, et al., 2015; Wong & Sung, 2013). If bleeding cannot be managed by these methods, surgery may be indicated, in which the area of the ulcer is removed or the bleeding vessels are ligated. Many patients also undergo procedures (e.g., vagotomy and pyloroplasty, gastrectomy) aimed at controlling the underlying cause of the ulcers (see Table 46-4).

For patients who are not candidates for surgery or for those with persistent, severe bleeding despite medical and endoscopic treatment, arteriography with embolization may be indicated (Lau et al., 2013; Loffroy et al., 2015; Wong & Sung, 2013). Arteriography with embolization is more commonly referred to as Transcatheter Arterial Embolization (TAE). TAE is an interventional radiologic procedure in which a catheter is placed percutaneously (through the skin) into an artery (e.g., femoral or brachial artery) and is advanced under use of fluoroscopy to the site of the bleeding peptic ulcer. An embolic agent is then delivered via the catheter, which selectively occludes blood flow to the bleeding vessel(s), and thus stops bleeding of the peptic ulcer. Common embolic agents used include metallic coils (a small metal device), polyvinyl alcohol particles (tiny balls), and a gelfoam (an absorptive gelatin sponge) (Loffroy et al., 2015).

The patient with GI bleeding may require treatment for hemorrhagic shock. If that is the case, then the collaborative treatment guidelines described in Chapter 14 must be followed (e.g., hemodynamic monitoring, IV line insertion for fluid resuscitation and blood component therapy). In addition, other related nursing and collaborative interventions may include inserting an NG tube to distinguish fresh blood from "coffee grounds" material, to aid in the removal of clots and acid through administering a saline lavage, to prevent nausea and vomiting through suction decompression of gastric contents, and to provide a means of monitoring further bleeding.

Perforation and Penetration. Perforation is the erosion of the ulcer through the gastric serosa into the peritoneal cavity without warning. It is an abdominal emergency and requires immediate surgery. Perforation of a peptic ulcer is associated with a 10% to 25% mortality rate, making it the most lethal of all complications (Soreide et al., 2014). Penetration is erosion of the ulcer through the gastric serosa into adjacent structures such as the pancreas, biliary tract, or gastrohepatic omentum (membranous fold of the peritoneum). Symptoms of penetration include back and epigastric pain not relieved by medications that were effective in the past. Like perforation, penetration usually requires surgical intervention.

Signs and symptoms of perforation include the following:
- Sudden, severe upper abdominal pain (persisting and increasing in intensity); pain may be referred to the shoulders, especially the right shoulder, because of irritation of the phrenic nerve in the diaphragm
- Vomiting
- Collapse (fainting)
- Extremely tender and rigid (boardlike) abdomen
- Hypotension and tachycardia, indicating shock

Because chemical peritonitis develops within a few hours of perforation and is followed by bacterial peritonitis, the perforation must be closed as quickly as possible and the abdominal cavity lavaged of stomach or intestinal contents. In some patients, it may be safe and advisable to perform surgery to treat the ulcer disease in addition to suturing the perforation.

During surgery and postoperatively, the stomach contents are drained by means of an NG tube. The nurse monitors fluid and electrolyte balance and assesses the patient for localized infection or peritonitis (increased temperature, abdominal pain, paralytic ileus, increased or absent bowel sounds, abdominal distention). Antibiotic therapy is given as prescribed.

GASTRIC OUTLET OBSTRUCTION

Peptic ulcer disease is the leading benign (noncancerous) cause of gastric outlet obstruction (Castellanos & Podolsky, 2014). Gastric outlet obstruction occurs when the area distal to the pyloric sphincter becomes scarred and stenosed from spasm or edema or from scar tissue that forms when an ulcer alternately heals and breaks down. The patient may have nausea and vomiting, constipation, epigastric fullness, anorexia, and, later, weight loss.

In treating the patient with gastric outlet obstruction, the first consideration is to insert an NG tube to decompress the stomach. Confirmation that obstruction is the cause of the discomfort is accomplished by assessing the amount of fluid aspirated from the NG tube. A residual of more than 400 mL suggests obstruction. Usually, an upper GI study or endoscopy is performed to confirm gastric outlet obstruction. Decompression of the stomach and management of extracellular fluid volume and electrolyte balances may improve the patient's condition and avert the need for surgical intervention. Balloon dilation of the pylorus via endoscopy may be beneficial. If the obstruction is unrelieved by medical management, surgery (in the form of a vagotomy and antrectomy or gastrojejunostomy and vagotomy) may be required.

PROMOTING HOME, COMMUNITY-BASED, AND TRANSITIONAL CARE

Educating Patients About Self-Care. The nurse instructs the patient about the factors that relieve and those that aggravate the condition. The nurse reviews information about medications to be taken at home, including name, dosage, frequency, and possible side effects, stressing the importance of continuing to take medications even after signs and symptoms have decreased or subsided (see Chart 46-2). The patient is instructed to avoid medications and foods that exacerbate symptoms (e.g., NSAIDs, alcohol). If relevant, the nurse also informs the patient about the irritant effects of smoking on the ulcer and provides information about smoking cessation programs.

Continuing and Transitional Care. The nurse reinforces the importance of follow-up care; the need to report recurrence of symptoms; and the need for treating possible problems that occur after surgery, such as intolerance to specific foods. The nurse also reminds the patient and family of the importance of participating in health promotion activities and recommended health screening.

Evaluation

Expected patient outcomes may include:

1. Reports freedom from pain between meals and at night
2. Reports feeling less anxiety
3. Maintains weight
4. Demonstrates knowledge of self-care activities
   a. Avoids irritating foods and beverages (alcohol) and medications (NSAIDs)
   b. Takes medications as prescribed
5. No evidence of complications (e.g., hemorrhage, perforation or penetration, gastric outlet obstruction)

Gastric Cancer

More than 24,500 Americans are diagnosed with gastric (stomach) cancer each year (Siegel, Miller, & Jemal, 2015). Although the number of Americans diagnosed with gastric cancer has decreased over the past decade, the disease still accounts for more than 10,700 deaths annually. Gastric cancer is a more common diagnosis among older adults, with the mean age at diagnosis of 69 years (American Cancer Society [ACS], 2015a). Men have a higher incidence of gastric cancer than women. Hispanic Americans, African Americans, and Asian/Pacific Islanders are at higher risk of developing gastric cancer than Caucasian Americans.

Worldwide, gastric cancer is the fifth most common cancer diagnosis, with the highest incidence in Eastern Asia (e.g., Republic of Korea, Mongolia, and Japan) (Ferlay, Soerjomataram, Ervik, et al., 2014). Countries with high incidence of gastric cancer, such as Japan, have implemented mass screening programs, which resulted in earlier diagnosis (at a more curable stage of disease), and may have reduced the number of deaths from gastric cancer (ACS, 2015a).

Chart 46-2	HOME CARE CHECKLIST

The Patient With Peptic Ulcer Disease

At the completion of education, the patient and/or caregiver will be able to:

- State the impact of peptic ulcer disease on physiologic functioning, ADLs, IADLs, roles, relationships, and spirituality.
- Explain the importance of and necessity for adherence with prescribed medication regimen.
- Demonstrate methods of keeping track of the medication regimen and storage of the prescribed medications, and use reminders such as beepers and/or pillboxes.
- State the name, dose, side effects, frequency, and schedule for all medications.
- Identify foods and other substances to avoid (e.g., food and drinks with extreme temperatures, coffee and other caffeinated beverages, alcohol, foods that were not tolerated in the past).
- Identify side effects and complications that should be reported to primary provider:

- Hemorrhage—cool skin, confusion, increased heart rate, labored breathing, blood in stool (either bright red or tarry black)
- Penetration and perforation—severe abdominal pain, rigid and tender abdomen, vomiting, elevated temperature, increased heart rate
- Gastric outlet obstruction—nausea and vomiting, distended abdomen, abdominal pain
- State how to reach primary provider with questions or complications.
- State time and date of follow-up appointments and testing.
- Identify the need for health promotion (e.g., cessation of use of tobacco products, stress management), disease prevention and screening activities.

ADL, activities of daily living; IADL, independent activities of daily living.

Diet appears to be a significant risk factor for the development of gastric cancer. A diet high in smoked, salted, or pickled foods and low in fruits and vegetables may increase the risk of gastric cancer (ACS, 2015a). *H. pylori* infection is a major risk factor the development of gastric cancer. It is estimated that 60% of all gastric cancers worldwide are attributed to *H. pylori* infection (Fock, 2014). Other factors related to the incidence of gastric cancer include chronic inflammation of the stomach (gastritis), pernicious anemia, smoking, obesity, achlorhydria, gastric ulcers, previous partial gastrectomy (more than 20 years ago), and genetics.

The vast majority of gastric cancers are sporadic or occurring as a result of acquired, not inherited, gene mutations. However, it is estimated that 5% to 10% gastric cancers have a familial component (e.g., blood type A and those with and another first-degree relative [parent, sibling, or child] with gastric cancer) and another 3% to 5% are associated with inherited cancer predisposition syndromes (ACS, 2015a; National Comprehensive Cancer Network [NCCN], 2015). Inherited cancer predisposition syndromes associated with increased risk of developing gastric cancer include hereditary diffuse gastric cancer, Lynch syndrome (i.e., hereditary nonpolyposis colorectal cancer), juvenile polyposis syndrome, familial adenomatosis polyposis, and Peutz–Jeghers syndrome (ACS, 2015a; NCCN, 2015).

The prognosis for patients with gastric cancer is generally poor. The 5-year survival rate for all patients with gastric cancer is only about 29% (ACS, 2015a). One reason for the poor survival rate is that the diagnosis is usually made late because most patients are asymptomatic during the early stages of the disease. Most cases of gastric cancer are discovered only after the cancer has spread from the stomach to involve the lymph nodes or has metastasized to distant organs.

Pathophysiology

Ninety to 95% of gastric cancers are adenocarcinomas, which arise from the mucus-producing cells of the inner-most lining of the stomach (ACS, 2015a). They can occur anywhere, although up to 40% develop in the lower part, 40% in the middle part, and 15% in the upper part; 10% involve more than one of these parts of the stomach (Cabebe, 2015). Gastric cancer begins with a lesion involving cells on the top layer of the stomach mucosa. The lesion then penetrates cells in the deeper layers of the mucosa, submucosa, and stomach wall. Eventually the lesion infiltrates the stomach wall and extends to organs or structures adjacent to the stomach. Lymph node involvement and metastasis tend to occur early due to the abundant lymphatic and vascular networks of the stomach. Common sites of metastasis include the liver, peritoneum, lungs, and brain (ACS, 2015a).

Clinical Manifestations

Gastric cancer is associated with few if any symptoms in the early stages of the disease (ACS, 2015a). Symptoms of early-stage disease may include pain that is relieved by antacids, resembling those of benign ulcers, and are seldom definitive. Symptoms of advanced disease are similar to those of peptic ulcer disease, such as dyspepsia (indigestion), early satiety, weight loss, abdominal pain just above the umbilicus, loss or decrease in appetite, bloating after meals, and nausea or vomiting. Fatigue often occurs as a result of the cancer itself or blood loss from the lesion infiltrating the stomach or surrounding tissue.

Assessment and Diagnostic Findings

The physical examination is usually not helpful in detecting the cancer because most early gastric tumors are not palpable. Advanced gastric cancer may be palpable as a mass. Ascites and hepatomegaly (enlarged liver) may be apparent if the cancer cells have metastasized to the liver. Palpable nodules around the umbilicus, called *Sister Mary Joseph's nodules,* are a sign of a GI malignancy, usually a gastric cancer.

Esophagogastroduodenoscopy for biopsy and cytologic washings is the diagnostic study of choice, and a barium x-ray examination of the upper GI tract may also be performed (Cabebe, 2015; Pasechnikov, Chukov, Fredorov, et al., 2014). Endoscopic ultrasound is an important tool to assess tumor depth and any lymph node involvement. Computed tomography (CT) scanning completes the diagnostic studies, particularly to assess for surgical resectability of the tumor before surgery is scheduled. CT scans of the chest, abdomen, and pelvis are valuable in staging gastric cancer.

A CBC may be used to evaluate for the presence of anemia. Assessment of tumor markers (blood analysis for antigens indicative of cancer), such as carcinoembryonic antigen (CEA), carbohydrate antigen (CA 19-9), and CA 50 are monitored to determine the effectiveness of treatment(s). Tumor marker values are usually elevated in the presence of gastric cancer before treatment and decrease if the tumor is responding to the treatment (NCCN, 2015).

Medical Management

The treatment of gastric cancer is multimodal, often involving surgery, chemotherapy, targeted therapy, and radiation therapy. In general, the patient with a resectable tumor undergoes a surgical procedure to remove the tumor and appropriate lymph nodes. If the tumor can be removed while it is still localized to the stomach, the patient may be cured. In patients with a tumor that is not surgically resectable or those with advanced disease, cure is less likely. Treatment may include surgery to control the cancer growth or for the palliation of symptoms, chemotherapy, targeted therapy, and radiation therapy.

Surgical Management

A total gastrectomy may be performed for a resectable cancer in the midportion or body of the stomach. The entire stomach is removed along with the duodenum, the lower portion of the esophagus, supporting mesentery, and lymph nodes. Reconstruction of the GI tract is performed by anastomosing the end of the jejunum to the end of the esophagus, a procedure called an *esophagojejunostomy.* A radical partial (subtotal) gastrectomy is performed for a resectable tumor in the middle and distal portions of the stomach. A Billroth I or a Billroth II operation (see Table 46-4) is performed. The Billroth I involves a limited resection and offers a lower cure rate than the Billroth II. The Billroth II procedure is a wider resection that involves removing approximately 75% of the stomach and decreases the possibility of lymph node spread or metastatic recurrence. A proximal partial (subtotal) gastrectomy may be performed for a resectable tumor located in the proximal portion of the stomach or cardia. A total gastrectomy or an esophagogastrectomy is usually performed in place of this procedure to achieve a more extensive resection (Orditura, Galizia, Sforza, et al., 2014).

Surgery may be also required to treat common complications of advanced gastric cancer, which may include gastric outlet obstruction, bleeding, and severe pain. Gastric perforation is an emergency situation requiring surgical intervention. A gastric resection may be the most effective palliative procedure for advanced gastric cancer. Palliative procedures such as gastric or esophageal bypass, gastrostomy, or jejunostomy may temporarily alleviate symptoms such as nausea and vomiting. Palliative rather than radical surgery may be performed if there is metastasis to other vital organs, such as the liver, or to achieve a better quality of life.

Complications of Gastric Surgery

The patient undergoing gastric surgery may experience complications, including hemorrhage, dumping syndrome, bile reflux, and gastric outlet obstruction. Postoperative bleeding from the surgical site is a common complication of gastric surgery. Bleeding may be severe (hemorrhage) and manifest as vomiting large amounts of bright red blood, which may result in hemorrhagic shock (see Chapter 14). The medical management and nursing care of the patient experiencing hemorrhage is discussed in the peptic ulcer disease section of this chapter.

Dumping syndrome may occur as a result of any surgical procedure that involves the removal of a significant portion of the stomach or includes resection or removal of the pylorus (see Table 46-4). The rapid bolus of hypertonic food from the stomach to the small intestines draws extracellular fluid into the lumen of the intestines to dilute the high concentrations of electrolytes and sugars, which results in intestinal dilation, increased intestinal transit, hyperglycemia, and the rapid onset of GI and vasomotor symptoms (Kanth & Roy, 2014; NIDDK, 2013). It is estimated that 25% to 50% of all patients who have undergone gastric surgery experience at least some symptoms of dumping syndrome (Kanth & Roy, 2014). Early symptoms tend to occur within 10 to 30 minutes after a meal and often include early satiety, cramping abdominal pain, nausea, vomiting, and diarrhea. Vasomotor symptoms may manifest as a headache, flushing and feelings of warmth, diaphoresis, dizziness, palpations, drowsiness, faintness, or syncope. Early symptoms tend to resolve within 1 hour or with bowel evacuation (defecation) (NIDDK, 2013). Later, the rapid elevation in blood glucose is followed by the increased secretion of insulin, which results in hypoglycemia 2 to 3 hours after eating. Manifestations of hypoglycemia may include irritability, anxiety, shakiness, weakness, fatigue, diaphoresis, palpitations, and hunger. Dumping syndrome typically lasts for a few months after surgery, although in some patients symptoms may persist on a long-term basis.

Bile reflux may occur with any gastric surgery that involves manipulation or removal of the pylorus, which acts as a barrier to prevent reflex of duodenal contents back into the stomach (Roses & Fraker, 2015). Prolonged exposure of bile acid from the duodenum results in irritation and damage to the gastric mucosa, which may lead to gastritis, esophagitis, and possibly peptic ulcer formation. The patient with bile reflux may experience burning epigastric pain that may increase after meals. Vomiting usually does not provide relief from pain. Pharmacologic management of bile reflux includes the administration of sucralfate (Carafate) or cholestyramine (Questran), which may provide relief from symptoms. Cholestyramine binds with bile acids in the GI tract to prevent reabsorption and facilitate the elimination of bile acids in stool.

Gastric outlet obstruction may occur as a complication of gastric surgery. Postoperative gastric outlet obstruction may be caused by narrowing (stenosis) or scar tissue (stricture) formation at the surgical anastomosis site. Typical clinical manifestations and management of gastric outlet obstruction were previously discussed (see the peptic ulcer disease section of this chapter).

Chemotherapy and Targeted Therapy

In instances where the gastric tumor is not resectable, treatment with chemotherapy may offer further control of the disease or palliation. Chemotherapy may also be used in addition to surgery as adjuvant treatment of gastric cancer. Chemotherapeutic agents often include fluorouracil (5-FU), carboplatin (Paraplatin), capecitabine (Xeloda), cisplatin (Platinol), docetaxel (Taxotere), epirubicin (Ellence), irinotecan (campostar), oxaliplatin (Eloxatin), and paclitaxel (Taxol). For improved tumor response rates, it is more common to administer combination chemotherapy, primarily 5-FU–based therapy, with other agents (e.g., 5-FU plus cisplatin or oxaliplatin) (ACS, 2015a, NCCN, 2015).

Targeted therapies have become an important addition to the treatment of advanced gastric cancers (NCCN, 2015). Trastuzumab (a recombinant humanized anti–HER-2 monoclonal antibody) prescribed in combination with fluorouracil or capecitabine and cisplatin has shown an improvement in survival by nearly 3 months in patients with advanced gastric cancer who are HER-2 positive (Bang, Van Cutsem, Feyereislova, et al., 2010). Other targeted therapies are currently being investigated for the treatment of advanced gastric cancers. For example, the Food and Drug Administration (FDA) recently approved ramucirumab (a recombinant humanized monoclonal antibody that inhibits vascular endothelial growth receptor 2 [VEGFR2]), alone or along with paclitaxel, for the treatment of advanced gastric cancers in certain clinical situations. Ramucirumab works by blocking VEGFR2, which reduces the blood supply to the tumor to decrease tumor growth (NCCN, 2015).

Radiation Therapy

Radiation therapy is primarily used for advanced gastric cancers to slow the rate of tumor growth or for the palliation of symptoms related to obstruction, bleeding, and significant pain (ACS, 2015a). Radiation therapy may also be used alone or along with chemotherapy before surgery to decrease the size of the tumor or after surgery to destroy any remaining cancer cells and to delay or prevent reoccurrence of the cancer (ACS, 2015a, NCCN, 2015). Common approaches to radiation therapy for gastric cancer include traditional external beam radiation therapy or newer specialized approaches to external beam radiation therapy, such as 3-dimensional conformal radiation therapy (3D-CRT) and intensity-modulated radiation therapy (IMRT). These specialized approaches to external radiation therapy precisely direct the radiation beam to the site of the tumor, thus limiting damage to the healthy surrounding tissue (ACS, 2015a).

 Gerontologic Considerations

Gastric cancer mostly affects older adults. It is estimated that 6 of every 10 patients diagnosed with gastric cancer each year are 65 years old or older (ACS, 2015a). According to most recent Surveillance, Epidemiology, and End Results (SEER) data 66.4% of all deaths from gastric cancer occur in patients 65 years old or older (National Cancer Institute, 2015). Confusion, agitation, and restlessness may be the only symptoms seen in older adult patients, who may have no gastric symptoms until their tumors are well advanced. At this time, they present with reduced functional ability and other signs and symptoms of malignancy.

Surgery is more hazardous for the older adult, and the risk increases proportionally with increasing age. Nonetheless, gastric cancer should be treated with surgery in older patients. Patient education is important to prepare older patients with cancer for treatment, to help them manage adverse effects, and to face the challenges that cancer and aging present.

NURSING PROCESS

The Patient With Gastric Cancer

Assessment

The nurse obtains a dietary history from the patient, focusing on recent nutritional intake and status. Has the patient lost weight? If so, how much and over what period of time? Can the patient tolerate a full diet? If not, what foods can they eat? What other changes in eating habits have occurred? Does the patient have an appetite? Does the patient feel full after eating a small amount of food? Is the patient in pain? Do foods, antacids, or medications relieve the pain, make no difference, or worsen the pain? Is there a history of infection with *H. pylori*? Other health information to obtain includes the patient's smoking and alcohol history and family history (e.g., any first- or second-degree relatives with gastric or other cancer). A psychosocial assessment, including questions about social support, individual and family coping skills, and financial resources, helps the nurse plan for care in acute and community settings.

After the interview, the nurse performs a complete physical examination, carefully assesses the patient's abdomen for tenderness or masses, and palpates and percusses the abdomen to detect ascites.

Nursing Diagnosis

Based on the assessment data, major nursing diagnoses may include the following:

- Anxiety related to the disease and anticipated treatment
- Imbalanced nutrition: less than body requirements related to early satiety or anorexia
- Acute pain related to tumor mass
- Grieving related to the diagnosis of cancer
- Deficient knowledge regarding self-care activities

Planning and Goals

The major goals for the patient may include reduced anxiety, optimal nutrition, relief of pain, and adjustment to the diagnosis and anticipated lifestyle changes.

Nursing Interventions

REDUCING ANXIETY

A relaxed, nonthreatening atmosphere is provided so the patient can express fears, concerns, and possibly anger about the diagnosis and prognosis. The nurse encourages the family or significant other to support the patient, offering reassurance and supporting positive coping measures. The nurse educates the patient about any procedures and treatments so that the patient knows what to expect.

PROMOTING OPTIMAL NUTRITION

The nurse encourages the patient to eat small, frequent portions of nonirritating foods to decrease gastric irritation. Food supplements should be high in calories, as well as vitamins A and C and iron, to enhance tissue repair. Because the patient may develop dumping syndrome when enteral feeding resumes after gastric resection, the nurse explains ways to prevent and manage it and informs the patient that symptoms often resolve after several months. Management of dumping syndrome includes encouraging 6 small feedings daily that are low in carbohydrates and sugar and the consumption of fluids between meals rather than with meals. If a total gastrectomy is performed, injection of vitamin B_{12} will be required for life, because intrinsic factor, secreted by parietal cells in the stomach, binds to vitamin B_{12} so that it may be absorbed in the ileum. This deficiency in vitamin B_{12} metabolism can result in decreased production of red blood cells, or pernicious anemia. If the patient is unable to eat adequately prior to surgery to meet nutritional requirements, parenteral nutrition may be necessary. Weight loss is a common occurrence in the postoperative period following gastric surgery; research findings suggest that individualizing dietary interventions based upon patient preferences can improve outcomes (Kim, Suh, Lee, et al., 2014) (see Chart 46-3). The nurse monitors the IV therapy and nutritional status and records intake, output, and daily weights to ensure that the patient is maintaining or gaining weight. The nurse assesses for signs of dehydration (thirst, dry mucous membranes, poor skin turgor, tachycardia, decreased urine output) and reviews the results of daily laboratory studies to note any metabolic abnormalities (sodium, potassium, glucose, BUN). Antiemetic agents are given as prescribed.

RELIEVING PAIN

The nurse administers analgesic agents as prescribed. A continuous IV infusion of an opioid or a patient-controlled analgesia (PCA) pump set to infuse an opioid may be necessary to mitigate postoperative pain. The nurse routinely assesses the frequency, intensity, and duration of the pain to determine the effectiveness of the analgesic agent. The nurse works with the patient to help manage pain by suggesting nonpharmacologic methods for pain relief, such as position changes, imagery, distraction, relaxation exercises (using relaxation audiotapes), backrubs, massage, and periods of rest and relaxation. See Chapter 12 for further discussion of pain management.

Chart 46-3	NURSING RESEARCH PROFILE

The Effects of a Dietary Intervention on Patients With Gastrectomy

Kim, H., Suh, E. E., Lee, H. J., et al. (2014). The effects of patient participation-based dietary intervention on nutritional and functional status for patients with gastrectomy. *Cancer Nursing, 37*(2), E10–E20.

Purpose

Patients undergoing a gastrectomy for gastric cancer often have poor oral intake, which may lead to weight loss, malnutrition, and poor treatment outcomes. Previous researchers have not examined the effectiveness of a patient participation-based dietary intervention (PPDI) that was individualized based upon patient preferences and motivated patients in this population to monitor their own food tolerance and dietary intake. The purpose of this nursing research was to develop a PPDI and evaluate its effects on nutritional and functional status in patients following a partial or total gastrectomy for gastric cancer.

Design

This study used a true experimental design. Participants were recruited using convenience sampling techniques from one cancer center in South Korea. Participants were randomly assigned to either the control group or experimental group. The control group received standard care. The experimental group received the PPDI, which included two face-to-face and two telephone interventional sessions within 6 weeks of hospital discharge. Study data were collected from participants in both groups on the day before hospital discharge and again 12 weeks later.

The intervention (PPDI) included individualized nutritional assessments and interventions guided by the acronym CAN-CER (conversation, assessment, nutrition plan, complications, evaluation, and reassurance or removal). During PPDI sessions, participants worked with nurse researchers to develop a dietary plan that was tailored to their food preferences. All dietary plans were approved by a clinical dietician. Participants were also provided two educational booklets and encouraged to closely monitor and record their dietary plan, food intake, and any food tolerances/negative dietary symptoms.

Findings

Forty-eight participants, of the 56 participants recruited, completed the study. Participants were primarily middle-age, married adults, from a socioeconomically middle class with higher than a high school education. Participants in the intervention (PPDI) group demonstrated a statistically significant reduction in adverse dietary symptoms and statistically significant improvements in functional status, dietary intake, performance status, adherence to dietary guidelines, dietary knowledge, and satisfaction as compared with participants in the control group over time. The researchers concluded that PPDI is a promising approach to individualize and motivate patients to participate in a dietary intervention program. However, the researchers cautioned that additional research is needed to determine the effects of the PPDI in a more diverse population of patients with gastric cancer undergoing a gastrectomy.

Nursing Implications

This study highlights the value of using a patient-centered approach to enhance motivation and incorporate patient perspectives and opinions into dietary interventions following a gastrectomy for gastric cancer, which may contribute to improved patient outcomes and quality of nursing care.

PROVIDING PSYCHOSOCIAL SUPPORT

The nurse helps the patient express fears, concerns, and grief about the diagnosis. The nurse answers the patient's questions honestly and encourages the patient to participate in treatment decisions. Some patients mourn the loss of a body part and perceive their surgery as a type of mutilation. Some express disbelief and need time and support to accept the diagnosis.

The nurse offers emotional support and involves family members and significant others whenever possible. This includes recognizing mood swings and defense mechanisms (e.g., denial, rationalization, displacement, regression) and reassuring the patient, family members, and significant others that emotional responses are normal and expected. The services of clergy, psychiatric clinical nurse specialists, psychologists, social workers, and psychiatrists are made available, if needed. The nurse projects an empathetic attitude and spends time with the patient. Many patients may begin to participate in self-care activities after they have acknowledged their loss.

PROMOTING HOME, COMMUNITY-BASED, AND TRANSITIONAL CARE

Educating Patients About Self-Care. Self-care activities depend on the type of treatments used—surgery, chemotherapy, radiation, or palliative care. Patient and family education include information about diet and nutrition, treatment regimens, activity and lifestyle changes, pain management, and possible complications (see Chart 46-4). Consultation with a dietitian is essential to determine how the patient's nutritional needs can best be met at home. The nurse instructs the patient or caregiver about administration of enteral or parenteral nutrition. If chemotherapy or radiation is prescribed, the nurse provides explanations to the patient and family about what to expect, including the length of treatments, the expected side effects (e.g., nausea, vomiting, anorexia, fatigue, neutropenia), and the need for transportation to appointments for treatment. Psychological counseling may also be helpful (see Chapter 15).

Continuing and Transitional Care. The need for ongoing care in the home depends on the patient's condition and treatment. The nurse reinforces nutritional counseling and supervises the administration of any enteral or parenteral feedings; the patient or caregiver must become skillful in administering the feedings and in detecting and preventing untoward effects or complications related to the feedings (see Chapter 45). The nurse instructs the patient or caregiver to record the patient's daily intake, output, and weight and explains strategies to manage pain, nausea, vomiting, or other symptoms. The nurse also educates the patient or caregiver to recognize and report signs and symptoms of complications that require immediate attention, such as bleeding, obstruction, perforation, or any symptoms that become progressively worse. The nurse must explain the chemotherapy or radiation therapy regimen and ensure that the patient and family or significant other understand the care that will be needed during

---

Chart 46-4	HOME CARE CHECKLIST
	The Patient With Gastric Cancer

At the completion of education, the patient and/or caregiver will be able to:

- State the impact of cancer and treatment on physiologic functioning, ADLs, IADLs, roles, relationships, and spirituality.
- Identify modification of home environment, interventions, and strategies (e.g., durable medical equipment, home health aide) used in safely adapting to changes in structure or function and promote effective recovery and rehabilitation.
- Identify foods or therapies necessary to meet caloric needs and dietary needs (e.g., change in consistency, seasoning limitations or other dietary restrictions, supplements, enteral or parenteral therapy).
- Demonstrate safe management of enteral or parenteral feedings, if applicable.
- State the name, dose, side effects, frequency, and schedule for all medications.
- Describe approaches to controlling pain (e.g., take analgesics as prescribed; use nonpharmacologic interventions).
- When indicated, list possible side effects of chemotherapeutic agents and suggested management approaches.

ADL, activities of daily living; IADL, independent activities of daily living.

- When indicated, list possible side effects of radiation therapy and suggested management approaches.
- Identify possible complications (e.g., infection, bleeding, obstruction, perforation or worsening pain or other symptoms) and interventions.
- Relate how to reach primary provider with questions or complications.
- State time and date of follow-up medical appointments, therapy, and testing.
- Identify sources of support (e.g., friends, relatives, faith community, cancer support, caregiver support)
- Identify the need for health promotion, disease prevention, and screening activities.
- Make decisions about end-of-life care as appropriate.

Resources

See Chapter 44, Chart 44-5 for additional information on The Patient Receiving Tube Feeding, and Chart 44-7 The Patient Receiving Parental Nutrition.

---

and after treatments (see Chapter 15). Because the prognosis for gastric cancer is poor, the nurse may need to assist the patient, family, or significant other with decisions regarding end-of-life care and make referrals as warranted.

Evaluation

Expected patient outcomes may include the following:

1. Reports less anxiety
   a. Expresses fears and concerns about surgery
   b. Seeks emotional support
2. Attains optimal nutrition
   a. Eats small, frequent meals high in calories, iron, and vitamins A and C
   b. Adheres to enteral or parenteral nutrition as needed
3. Has decreased pain
4. Performs self-care activities and adjusts to lifestyle changes
   a. Resumes typical activities within 3 months
   b. Alternates periods of rest and activity
   c. Manages enteral feedings
5. Verbalizes knowledge of disease management
   a. Acknowledges disease process
   b. Reports control of symptoms
   c. Verbalizes fears and concerns about dying; involves family/caregiver in discussions
   d. Completes advance directives and other appropriate documents

Tumors of the Small Intestine

Benign or malignant tumors of the small intestine are rare. Approximately 64% of all tumors of the small intestines are malignant (Somasundar, Fisichella, & Espat, 2013).

Malignant tumors of the small intestine account for only about 2% of all GI cancers (Somasundar et al., 2013); annually, there are approximately 9400 new diagnoses of cancer of the small intestine in the United States (ACS, 2015b). Rates are higher among older adults (mean age at diagnosis of 60 years) and are also higher among African Americans and men (ACS, 2015b). Malignant tumors are often not discovered until they have metastasized to distant sites. Benign tumors may place patients at an increased risk for malignancy (Terry & Santora, 2015). The relative rarity of tumors of the small intestine, the diversity of tumor types (that may include adenocarcinomas, carcinoid tumors, lymphomas, or sarcomas), and the nonspecific nature of their manifestations complicate their diagnosis and treatment (Aparicio, Zaanan, Svrcek, et al., 2014; Somasundar et al., 2013).

Clinical Manifestations

Tumors of the small intestine often present insidiously with vague, nonspecific symptoms. Most benign tumors are discovered incidentally on an x-ray study, during surgery, or at autopsy. When the patient is symptomatic, benign tumors often present with intermittent pain. The next most common presentation is occult bleeding. Malignant tumors often result in symptoms that lead to their diagnosis, although these symptoms may reflect advanced disease. Most patients have sustained weight loss and may be malnourished at the time of diagnosis. Occult GI bleeding is less common than is found in patients with benign tumors, and complaints of pain are common. The patient also frequently presents with complaints of weakness, fatigue, nausea, vomiting, and intestinal obstruction (ACS, 2015b). Intestinal perforation is rare and associated with a poorer overall prognosis (ACS, 2015b; Somasundar et al., 2013). Clinical manifestations and management of the patient experiencing an intestinal obstruction and intestinal perforation are discussed in Chapter 47.

Assessment and Diagnostic Findings

A CBC may reveal a low hematocrit and hemoglobin level that is consistent with anemia if the patient has an occult source of GI bleeding. The bilirubin may also be elevated if tumor mass has caused biliary obstruction. CEA levels may also be elevated, consistent with a malignant mass.

An upper GI x-ray series with small bowel follow-through using oral water-insoluble contrast with frequent and detailed x-rays to follow the contrast through the small bowel is the traditional approach to diagnosis. A more sensitive examination is an enteroclysis, in which an NG tube is advanced into the small bowel to a position above the area in question; the area is then studied by single- and double-contrast techniques. Abdominal CT scan is used to determine the extent of disease (Somasundar et al., 2013).

Management

Benign tumors of the small intestine include adenomas, lipomas, hemangiomas, and hamartomas (a focal malformation that resembles a neoplasm, but unlike a neoplasm does not result in compression of adjacent tissue). These tumors may be treated endoscopically by excision/resection or electrocautery if the patient is symptomatic. Routine monitoring is recommended to assess for malignant transformation (Terry & Santora, 2015).

The most common primary malignant tumor of the small intestine is adenocarcinoma; the second and third portions of the duodenum are most often involved. These tumors may present with obstruction. If the tumor is located at the ampulla of Vater, obstructive jaundice is likely. Other rare malignant tumors of the small intestine include carcinoid tumors, lymphoma, and GI stromal tumors (Aparicio et al., 2014; Terry & Santora, 2015). Abdominal surgery may be required to remove these rare tumors. Chemotherapy and radiation therapy are commonly part of the treatment regimen.

The nursing process related to the care of the patient with a tumor of the small intestine is similar to that of the patient with gastric cancer. Each patient requires specialized care, astute assessment for complications, prompt interventions, and individualized education for self-care.

CRITICAL THINKING EXERCISES

1 `ebp` A 70-year-old woman is diagnosed with chronic *H. pylori* gastritis after experiencing fatigue, mild epigastric discomfort, anorexia, and occasional nausea for several months. She is started on treatment for *H. pylori* with triple therapy, including amoxicillin (Amoxil), clarithromycin (Biaxin), and omeprazole (Prilosec). The patient asks you if taking these medications will be successful in treating her infection. How would you respond to this patient? On what evidence do you base your response?

2 `pq` A 55-year-old female patient returns to your unit following a partial gastrectomy for the treatment of gastric cancer. Upon admission, she is awake, alert, and oriented. Her pain level is 2 (on a 0 to 10 numeric pain scale). She denies nausea. Her blood pressure is 128/78 mmHg, heart rate is 98 bpm, respiratory rate is 16 breaths/min and regular, and temperature is 36.7°C (98.1°F). Her nasogastric (NG) tube is patent and draining scant amounts of bloody secretions. Two hours later, you observe that her NG tube has drained 200 mL of bright red blood. What is your first nursing action? Describe the priorities of care for this patient.

3 `ebp` You are caring for a 67-year-old man with chronic lower back pain who was recently diagnosed with peptic ulcer disease. As you are providing discharge education, the patient asks if he can continue to take ibuprofen (Motrin) to manage his lower back pain. How would you respond to this patient? On what evidence do you base your response?

REFERENCES

*Asterisk indicates nursing research.
**Double asterisk indicates classic reference.

Books

Centers for Disease Control and Prevention (CDC). (2016). *CDC health information for international travel 2016*. New York: Oxford University Press.

Grossman, S. C., & Porth, C. M. (2014). *Porth's pathophysiology: Concepts of altered health states* (9th ed.). Philadelphia, PA: Lippincott Williams & Wilkins.

Karch, A. M. (2014). *Lippincott nursing drug guide*. Philadelphia, PA: Lippincott Williams & Wilkins.

National Institute of Diabetes and Digestive and Kidney Diseases (NIDDK). (2013). *Digestive diseases statistics for the United States*. NIH Publication No. 13–3873. Bethesda, MD: U.S. Department of Health and Human Services; National Institutes of Health.

National Institute of Diabetes and Digestive and Kidney Diseases (NIDDK). (2014). *H. Pylori and peptic ulcer disease*. NIH Publication No. 14–4225. Bethesda, MD: U.S. Department of Health and Human Services; National Institutes of Health.

Roses, R. E., & Fraker, D. L. (2015). Bile reflux and gastroparesis. In T. M. Pawlik, S. K. Maithel, & N. B. Merchant (Eds.). *Gastrointestinal surgery: Management of complex perioperative complications*. New York: Springer.

Strayer, D. S., & Rubin, E. (2015). *Rubin's pathology: Clinicopathologic foundations of medicine* (7th ed.). Philadelphia, PA: Lippincott Williams & Wilkins.

Journals and Electronic Documents

American Cancer Society (ACS). (2015a). Stomach cancer. Retrieved on 5/5/2016 at: www.cancer.org/cancer/stomachcancer/

American Cancer Society (ACS). (2015b). Small intestines cancer. Retrieved on 5/5/2016 at: www.cancer.org/cancer/smallintestinecancer/

American College of Gastroenterology. (2015). *Laparoscopic surgery*. Retrieved on 5/5/2016 at: patients.gi.org/topics/laparoscopic-surgery/

Anand, B. S. (2015). Peptic ulcer disease. *Medscape*. Retrieved on 5/3/2016 at: emedicine.medscape.com/article/181753

Aparicio, T., Zaanan, A., Svrcek, M., et al. (2014). Small bowel adenocarcinoma: Epidemiology, risk factors, diagnosis and treatment, *Digestive and Liver Disease*, 46(2), 97–104.

**Bang, Y. J., Van Cutsem, E., Feyereislova, A., et al. (2010). Trastuzumab in combination with chemotherapy versus chemotherapy alone for treatment of HER2-positive advanced gastric or gastro-oesophageal junction cancer (ToGA): a phase 3, open-label, randomised controlled trial. *Lancet, 376*(9742), 687–697.

Bonheur, J. L., & Nachimuthu, S. (2014). Gastrinoma. *Medscape.* Retrieved on 5/3/2016 at: emedicine.medscape.com/article/184332

Cabebe, E. W. (2015). Gastric cancer. *Medscape.* Retrieved on 5/5/2016 at: www.emedicine.medscape.com/article/278744-overview

Castellanos, A. E., & Podolsky, E. R. (2014) Gastric outlet obstruction. *Medscape* Retrieved on 5/5/2016 at: emedicine.medscape.com/article/190621

Clarke, R. C., Gbadehan, E., Dim, V. R., et al. (2015). Stress-induced gastritis. *Medscape.* Retrieved on 5/3/2016 at: emedicine.medscape.com/article/176319

Dimou, F., & Velanovich, V. (2015). Perforations of the esophagus and stomach: What should I do? *Journal of Gastrointestinal Surgery, 19*(2), 400.

Epelboym, I., & Mazeh, H. (2014). Zollinger- Ellison syndrome: Classical considerations and current controversies. *The Oncologist, 19*(1), 44–55.

Ferlay, J., Soerjomataram, I., Ervik, M., et al. (2014). Cancer incidence and mortality worldwide. *International Agency for Research on Cancer;* Retrieved on 5/5/2016 at: globocan.iarc.fr

Fock, K. M. (2014). The epidemiology and prevention of gastric cancer. *Alimentary Pharmacology & Therapeutics, 40*(3), 250–260.

Frandah, W., Colmer-Hamood, J., & Nugent, R. R. (2014). Patterns of use of prophylaxis for stress-related mucosal disease in patients admitted to the intensive care unit. *Journal of Intensive Care Medicine, 29*(2), 96–103.

Gururatsakul, M., Holloway, R. H., Bellon. M., et al. (2014). Complicated and uncomplicated peptic ulcer disease: Altered symptom response to a nutrient challenge linked to gastric motor dysfunction. *Digestion, 89*(3), 239–246.

Hannah, J. (2014). The noncancer effects of smoking on the gastrointestinal tract. *Gastroenterology Nursing, 37*(5), 366–367.

Kanth, R., & Roy, P. K. (2014). Dumping syndrome. *Medscape.* Retrieved on 5/5/2016 at: emedicine.medscape.com/article/173594

Kemp, W. J., Bashir, A., Dababneh, H., et al. (2015). Cushing's ulcer: Further reflections. *Asian Journal of Neurosurgery, 10*(2), 87–94.

*Kim, H., Suh, E. E., Lee, H. J., et al. (2014). The effects of patient participation-based dietary intervention on nutritional and functional status for patients with gastrectomy. *Cancer Nursing, 37*(2), E10–E20.

Lau, J. Y., Barkun, A., Fan, D. M., et al. (2013). Challenges in the management of acute peptic ulcer bleeding. *Lancet, 381*(9882), 2033–2043.

Li, L. F., Chan, R. L., Lu, L., et al. (2014). Cigarette smoking and gastrointestinal diseases: The causal relationship and underlying molecular mechanisms. *International Journal of Molecular Medicine, 34*(2), 372–380.

Loffroy, R., Favelier, S., Pottecher, P., et al. (2015). Transcatheter arterial embolization for acute nonvariceal upper gastrointestinal bleeding: Indications, techniques, and outcomes. *Diagnostic and Interventional Imaging, 96*(7-8), 731–744.

Marcus, A. J., & Greenwald, D. (2014). Chronic gastritis. *Medscape.* Retrieved on 5/5/2016 at: emedicine.medscape.com/article/176156

National Cancer Institute. (2015). *SEER cancer statistics factsheets: Stomach cancer.* National Cancer Institute Bethesda, MD: National Cancer Institute. Retrieved on 5/5/2016 at: seer.cancer.gov/statfacts/html/stomach.html

National Comprehensive Cancer Network (NCCN). (2015). *NCCN clinical guidelines version 3.2015 gastric cancer.* Retrieved on 6/7/2016 at: www.nccn.org/professionals/physician_gls/pdf/gastric.pdf

National Institute of Diabetes and Digestive and Kidney Diseases (NIDDK). (2013). *Dumping syndrome. National Digestive Diseases Information Clearinghouse.* Retrieved on 5/5/2016 at: www.niddk.nih.gov/health-information/health-topics/digestive-diseases/dumping-syndrome/Pages/facts.aspx

National Institute of Diabetes and Digestive and Kidney Diseases (NIDDK). (2015). *Gastritis. National Digestive Diseases Information Clearinghouse.* Retrieved on 5/5/2016 at: digestive.niddk.nih.gov/ddiseases/pubs/gastritis/index.aspx

Orditura, M., Galizia, G., Sforza, V., et al. (2014). Treatment of gastric cancer. *World Journal of Gastroenterology, 20*(7), 1635–1649.

Pasechnikov, V., Chukov, S. Fedorov, E., et al. (2014). Gastric cancer: Prevention, screening and early diagnosis. *World Journal of Gastroenterology, 20*(38), 13842–13862.

Pilotto, A., & Franceschi, M. (2014). Helicobacter pylori infection in older people. *World Journal of Gastroenterology, 20*(21), 6364–6373.

Plummer, M. P., Blaser, A. R., & Deane, A. M. (2014). Stress ulceration: Prevalence, pathology and association with adverse outcomes. *Critical Care, 18*(2), 213.

Ruggiero, P., & Censini, S. (2014). Helicobacter pylori: A brief history of a still lacking vaccine. *Digestion, 2*(2), 187–208.

Siegel, R. L., Miller, K. D., & Jemal, A. J. (2015). Cancer statistics, 2015. *CA: A Cancer Journal for Clinicians, 65*(1), 5-29.

Somasundar, P. S., Fisichella, P. M., & Espat, N. J. (2013). Malignant neoplasms of the small intestine. *Medscape.* Retrieved on 5/5/2016 at: emedicine.medscape.com/article/282684

Soreide, K., Thorsen, K., & Soreide, J. A. (2014) Strategies to improve the outcome of emergency surgery for perforated peptic ulcer. *British Journal of Surgery, 101*(1), E51–E64.

Terry, S. M., & Santora, T. (2015). Benign neoplasm of the small intestines. *Medscape.* Retrieved on 5/5/2016 at: emedicine.medscape.com/article/189390

Wehbi, M., Yang, V. W., Sarver, G., et al. (2014). Acute gastritis. *Medscape.* Retrieved on 5/5/2016 at: emedicine.medscape.com/article/175909

Wong, S. H., & Sung, J. Y. (2013). Management of GI emergencies: Peptic ulcer acute bleeding. *Best Practice & Research Clinical Gastroenterology, 27*(5), 639–646.

Yazbek, P. B., Trindade, A. B., Chin, C. M., et al. (2015). Challenges to the treatment and new perspectives for the eradication of Helicobacter pylori. *Digestive Diseases and Sciences, 60*(10), 2901-2912.

Zayouna, N., & Piper, M. H. (2014). Atrophic gastritis. *Medscape.* Retrieved on 5/5/2016 at: emedicine.medscape.com/article/176036

Resources

Agency for Healthcare Research and Quality (AHRQ), www.ahrq.gov
American Cancer Society, www.cancer.org
American Gastroenterological Association (AGA), www.gastro.org
Centers for Disease Control and Prevention (CDC), www.cdc.gov
Cochrane Library, www.cochranelibrary.com
Joanna Briggs Institute, www.joannabriggs.org
National Comprehensive Cancer Network (NCCN) Clinical Practice Guidelines, www.nccn.org
National Digestive Diseases Information Clearinghouse (NDDIC), digestive.niddk.nih.gov
Society of Gastroenterology Nurses and Associates, www.sgna.org

47 Management of Patients With Intestinal and Rectal Disorders

LEARNING OBJECTIVES

On completion of this chapter, the learner will be able to:

1. Describe the pathophysiology, clinical manifestations, and management of patients with constipation, diarrhea, fecal incontinence, and irritable bowel syndrome.
2. Identify celiac disease as a disorder of malabsorption; describe its pathophysiology, clinical manifestations, and management.
3. Discuss the nursing management of the patient with appendicitis, diverticular disease, and intestinal obstruction.
4. Compare Crohn's disease and ulcerative colitis with regard to their pathophysiology; clinical manifestations; diagnostic evaluation; and medical, surgical, and nursing management.
5. Use the nursing process as a framework for care of the patient with inflammatory bowel disease.
6. Identify the responsibilities of the nurse in meeting the needs of the patient with an intestinal diversion.
7. Apply the nursing process as a framework for care of the patient with colorectal cancer.
8. Explain the nursing management of the patient with an anorectal disorder.

GLOSSARY

abscess: localized collection of purulent material surrounded by inflamed tissues

colostomy: surgical opening into the colon by means of a stoma to allow drainage of bowel contents; one type of fecal diversion

constipation: fewer than three bowel movements weekly or bowel movements that are hard, dry, small, or difficult to pass

diarrhea: an increased frequency of bowel movements or an increased amount of stool with altered consistency (i.e., increased liquidity) of stool.

diverticulitis: inflammation of a diverticulum from obstruction by fecal matter resulting in abscess formation

diverticulosis: presence of several diverticula in the intestine

diverticulum: saclike out-pouching of the lining of the bowel protruding through the muscle of the intestinal wall

fecal incontinence: involuntary passage of feces

fissure: normal or abnormal fold, groove, or crack in body tissue

fistula: anatomically abnormal tract that arises between two internal organs or between an internal organ and the body surface

gastrocolic reflex: peristaltic movements of the large bowel occurring five to six times daily that are triggered by distention of the stomach

hemorrhoids: dilated portions of the anal veins

ileostomy: surgical opening into the ileum by means of a stoma to allow drainage of bowel contents; one type of fecal diversion

inflammatory bowel disease (IBD): group of chronic disorders (ulcerative colitis and Crohn's disease) that result in inflammation or ulceration (or both) of the bowel lining

irritable bowel syndrome (IBS): chronic functional disorder characterized by recurrent abdominal pain that affects frequency of defecation and consistency of stool; is associated with no specific structural or biochemical alterations

malabsorption: impaired transport across the mucosa

peritonitis: inflammation of the lining of the abdominal cavity

steatorrhea: excess of fatty wastes in the feces

tenesmus: ineffective and sometimes painful straining and urge to eliminate either feces or urine

Between 60 and 70 million people in the United States are diagnosed with some type of disease of the gastrointestinal (GI) tract. These diseases account for more than 48.3 million office visits to health care facilities and clinics and approximately 21.7 million hospital admissions annually. GI diseases cost the American public more than $141.8 billion and account for approximately 246,000 deaths each year (National Institute of Diabetes and Digestive and Kidney Diseases [NIDDK], 2014e). The types of diseases and disorders that affect the lower GI tract are many and varied; examples include constipation, diarrhea, diverticulitis, and inflammatory bowel disease (IBD).

In all age groups, a fast-paced lifestyle, high levels of stress, irregular eating habits, insufficient intake of fiber and water, and lack of daily exercise contribute to GI disorders. There is a growing understanding of the biopsychosocial implications of GI disease. The mind and emotions can have a profound impact on the GI system. Nurses can have an impact on these GI disorders by identifying behavior patterns that put patients at risk, by educating the public about prevention and management, and by helping those affected to improve their condition and prevent complications.

ABNORMALITIES OF FECAL ELIMINATION

Changes in patterns of fecal elimination are symptoms of functional disorders or diseases of the GI tract. The most common changes seen are constipation, diarrhea, and fecal incontinence.

Constipation

Constipation is defined as fewer than three bowel movements weekly or bowel movements that are hard, dry, small, or difficult to pass. Approximately 42 million Americans are constipated, making it a very common GI disorder. People more likely to become constipated are women, particularly pregnant women, patients who recently had surgery, older adults, non-Caucasians, and those of lower socioeconomic status (NIDDK, 2014c). Notably, constipation is a symptom and not a disease; however, constipation can indicate an underlying disease or motility disorder of the GI tract.

Constipation can be caused by certain medications, such as anticholinergic agents, antidepressants, anticonvulsants, antispasmodics (muscle relaxants), calcium channel antagonists, diuretic agents, opioids, aluminum- and calcium-based antacids, and iron preparations. Other causes of constipation may include weakness, immobility, debility, fatigue, and an inability to increase intra-abdominal pressure to facilitate the passage of stools, as may occur in patients with emphysema or spinal cord injury, for instance. Many people develop constipation because they do not take the time to defecate or ignore the urge to defecate. Constipation is also a result of dietary habits (i.e., low consumption of fiber and inadequate fluid intake), lack of regular exercise, and a stress-filled life (NIDDK, 2014c). Fiber is particularly important to bowel health because it increases the bulk of stool, generally easing the passage. More importantly, it also promotes optimal fermentation, providing good bowel wall health (McRorie, 2015).

Perceived constipation can also be an issue. This subjective problem occurs when a person's bowel elimination pattern is not consistent with what they consider normal. Chronic enema, laxative, and suppository abuse are defining characteristics of this problem (Herdman & Kamitsuru, 2014).

Pathophysiology

The pathophysiology of constipation is poorly understood, but it is thought to include interference with one of three major functions of the colon: mucosal transport (i.e., mucosal secretions facilitate the movement of colon contents), myoelectric activity (i.e., mixing of the rectal mass and propulsive actions), or the processes of defecation (e.g., pelvic floor dysfunction). There are three classes of constipation, based upon their underlying pathophysiologic mechanisms (Grossman & Porth, 2014):

- Functional constipation, which involves normal transit mechanisms of mucosal transport. This type of constipation is most common and can be successfully treated by increasing intake of fiber and fluids.

- Slow-transit constipation, which is caused by inherent disorders of the motor function of the colon (e.g., Hirschsprung disease), and is characterized by infrequent bowel movements.
- Defecatory disorders, which are caused by dysfunctional motor coordination between the pelvic floor and anal sphincter. This can cause not only constipation but also fecal incontinence (see later discussion).

The urge to defecate is stimulated normally by rectal distention that initiates a series of four actions: stimulation of the inhibitory rectoanal reflex, relaxation of the internal sphincter muscle, relaxation of the external sphincter muscle and muscles in the pelvic region, and increased intra-abdominal pressure. Interference with any of these processes can lead to constipation.

When the urge to defecate is ignored, the rectal mucous membrane and musculature become insensitive to the presence of fecal masses, and consequently a stronger stimulus is required to produce the necessary peristaltic rush for defecation. The initial effect of fecal retention is to produce irritability of the colon, which at this stage frequently goes into spasm, especially after meals, giving rise to colicky midabdominal or low abdominal pains. After several years of this process, the colon loses muscular tone and becomes essentially unresponsive to normal stimuli (similar to an overstretched balloon). Atony or decreased muscle tone occurs with aging. This may lead to constipation because the stool is retained for longer periods.

Clinical Manifestations

Clinical manifestations of constipation include fewer than three bowel movements per week; abdominal distention; pain and bloating; a sensation of incomplete evacuation; straining at stool; and the elimination of small-volume, lumpy, hard, dry stools. To make diagnosis more efficient, an international committee developed the Rome criteria (in the city of Rome, Italy) (see Chart 47-1) (Lacy, Mearin, Chang, et al., 2016).

Chart 47-1 **ASSESSMENT**
Rome IV Diagnostic Criteria for Functional Constipation

Reported signs and symptoms must be present for the past 3 months with onset at least 6 months prior to diagnosis; these must include 2 or more of the following:

- Straining during at least 25% of bowel movements
- Lumpy or hard stools from at least 25% of bowel movements
- Sensation of incomplete evacuation during at least 25% of bowel movements
- Sensation of anorectal obstruction or blockage during at least 25% of bowel movements
- Manual maneuvers (e.g., digital stimulation, support of pelvic floor) needed to facilitate at least 25% of bowel movements
- Less than three spontaneous bowel movements weekly

In addition to these, loose stools are rarely present without the use of laxatives, and there must be insufficient suspicion of irritable bowel syndrome.

Adapted from Lacy, B. E., Mearin, F., Chang, L., et al. (2016). Bowel disorders. *Gastroenterology, 150*(6), 1393–1407.

Assessment and Diagnostic Findings

Secondary causes of constipation should be excluded. In patients with severe, intractable constipation, further diagnostic testing is needed (Basson, 2015a). The diagnosis of constipation is based on the patient's history, physical examination, possibly the results of a barium enema or sigmoidoscopy, and stool testing for occult blood. These tests are used to determine whether this symptom results from spasm or narrowing of the bowel. Anorectal manometry (i.e., pressure studies such as a balloon expulsion test) may be performed to assess malfunction of the sphincter. Defecography and colonic transit studies can also assist in the diagnosis because they permit assessment of active anorectal function. Tests such as pelvic floor magnetic resonance imaging (MRI) may identify occult pelvic floor defects (Basson, 2015a).

Complications

Increased arterial pressure can occur with defecation. Straining at stool, which results in the Valsalva maneuver (i.e., forcibly exhaling with the glottis closed), has a striking effect on arterial blood pressure. During active straining, the flow of venous blood in the chest is temporarily impeded because of increased intrathoracic pressure. This pressure tends to collapse the large veins in the chest. The atria and the ventricles receive less blood, and consequently less blood is ejected by the left ventricle. Cardiac output is decreased, and there is a transient drop in arterial pressure, which may cause orthostasis, dizziness, or syncope (Grossman & Porth, 2014).

Additional complications of constipation include fecal impaction, which may lead to fecal incontinence, **hemorrhoids** (dilated portions of anal veins), **fissures** (normal or abnormal folds, grooves, or cracks in body tissue), rectal prolapse, and megacolon. Fecal impaction occurs when an accumulated mass of dry feces cannot be expelled. The mass may be palpable on digital examination, may produce pressure on the colonic mucosa that results in ulcer formation, and may cause fecal incontinence, with seepage of liquid stools. Treatment can be embarrassing and also painful, because impaction removal usually involves digital dislodgement and enema administration (NIDDK, 2014c).

Hemorrhoids develop as a result of perianal vascular congestion caused by straining. Anal fissures may result from the passage of the hard stool through the anus, tearing the lining of the anal canal. The rectum may prolapse through the anal canal, causing seepage of mucus (NIDDK, 2014c).

Megacolon is a dilated and atonic colon caused by a fecal mass that obstructs the passage of colon contents. Symptoms include constipation, liquid fecal incontinence, and abdominal distention. Megacolon can lead to perforation of the bowel (Grossman & Porth, 2014).

 ### Gerontologic Considerations

Visits to primary providers for treatment of constipation are common in people 65 years and older. The most common complaint they voice is the need to strain at stool. The aging process inevitably generates changes in the colon; but the extent and physiologic implications for defecation remain unclear. The clinical situation is made more complex by ubiquitous factors among the aged (Bailes & Reeve, 2013; Eliopoulos, 2018). For instance, older adults who have loose-fitting dentures or have lost their teeth have difficulty chewing and frequently choose soft, processed foods that are low in fiber. Older adults tend to have decreased food intake, reduced mobility, and weak abdominal and pelvic muscles, and they are more likely to have multiple chronic illnesses requiring multiple medications (polypharmacy) that often cause constipation. Low-fiber convenience foods are widely used by people who have lost interest in eating. Some older adults reduce their fluid intake if they are not eating regular meals. Depression, weakness, and prolonged bed rest also contribute to constipation by decreasing intestinal motility and anal sphincter tone. Nerve impulses are dulled, and there is a decreased urge to defecate. Many older adults overuse laxatives in an attempt to have a daily bowel movement and become dependent on them. Chronic constipation profoundly impairs quality of life comparable to other conditions such as diabetes, rheumatoid arthritis, and osteoarthritis (Bailes & Reeve, 2013; Eliopoulos, 2018).

Medical Management

Treatment targets the underlying cause of constipation and prevention of recurrence. It includes education, exercise, bowel habit training, increased fiber and fluid intake, and judicious use of laxatives. Management may also include discontinuing laxative use or replacing medications that could cause or exacerbate constipation with other nonconstipating medications (Lacy et al., 2016). Patients can be educated to sit on the toilet with legs supported and to utilize the **gastrocolic reflex** (peristaltic movements of the large bowel occurring five to six times daily that are triggered by distention of the stomach) by attempting to defecate following a meal and a warm drink. Routine exercise to strengthen abdominal muscles is encouraged. Biofeedback is a technique that can be used to help patients learn to relax the sphincter mechanism to expel stool. It is considered first-line therapy once anorectal structural lesions have been excluded as the cause for constipation (Collins, Hibberts, Lyons, et al., 2014). Daily dietary intake of 25 to 30 g/day of fiber (soluble and bulk forming) is recommended, especially for the treatment of constipation in the older adult. If laxative use is necessary, one of the following may be prescribed: bulk-forming agents (fiber laxatives), saline and osmotic agents, lubricants, stimulants, or fecal softeners. The physiologic action and patient education information related to these laxatives are presented in Table 47-1. Enemas and rectal suppositories are generally not recommended for treating constipation unless other medications have failed; then, glycerin suppositories may be tried (Bailes & Reeve, 2013).

Nursing Management

The nurse elicits information about the onset and duration of constipation, current and past elimination patterns, the patient's expectation of normal bowel elimination, and lifestyle information (e.g., exercise and activity level, occupation, food and fluid intake, and stress level) during the health history interview. Past medical and surgical history, current medications, and laxative and enema use are important, as is information about the sensation of rectal pressure or fullness, abdominal pain, excessive straining at defecation, and flatulence.

TABLE 47-1 Selected Laxative Medications

Classification/Medications	Action	Patient Education
Bulk Forming methylcellulose (Citrucel), psyllium (Metamucil), wheat dextrin (Benefiber)	Polysaccharides and cellulose and wheat derivatives mix with intestinal fluids, swell, and stimulate peristalsis.	Take with 8-oz water and follow with 8-oz water; do not take dry. Report abdominal distention or unusual amount of flatulence.
Saline Agent magnesium hydroxide (Milk of Magnesia)	Nonabsorbable magnesium ions alter stool consistency by drawing water into the intestines by osmosis; peristalsis is stimulated. Action occurs within 2 hours.	Be aware that the liquid preparation is more effective than the tablet form. Note that only short-term use is recommended because of toxicity (central nervous system or neuromuscular depression, electrolyte imbalance). Do not take magnesium laxatives with renal insufficiency.
Lubricant Mineral oil, glycerin suppository	Nonabsorbable hydrocarbons soften fecal matter by lubricating the intestinal mucosa; the passage of stool is facilitated. Action occurs within 6–8 hours for mineral oil and within 30 minutes for glycerin suppository.	Do not take mineral oil with meals, because it can impair the absorption of fat-soluble vitamins and delay gastric emptying. Swallow carefully, because drops of oil that gain access to the pharynx can produce a lipid pneumonia. Insert glycerin suppositories fully and retain.
Stimulant bisacodyl (Dulcolax), senna (Senokot)	Irritates the colonic epithelium by stimulating sensory nerve endings and increasing mucosal secretions and decreasing large intestinal water absorption. Action occurs within 6–8 hours.	Be aware that catharsis may cause fluid and electrolyte imbalance, especially in the older adult. Do not swallow, crush, or chew tablets. Avoid milk or antacids within 1 hour of taking medication, because the enteric coating may dissolve prematurely. Note that stimulant laxatives are *not* indicated for long-term use.
Fecal Softener docusate (Colace)	Hydrates the stool by its surfactant action on the colonic epithelium (increases the wetting efficiency of intestinal water); aqueous and fatty substances are mixed. Does *not* exert a laxative action.	Note that this can be used safely by patients who should avoid straining (cardiac patients, patients with anorectal disorders). Be aware that this will not evacuate hard stool because it is not a true laxative.
Osmotic Agent polyethylene glycol (PEG) and electrolytes (CoLyte, GoLYTELY)	Cleanses colon rapidly and induces diarrhea	Note that because this is a large-volume product, it takes time to consume it safely. Recognize that it can cause considerable nausea and bloating. Know that it has high level of research evidence support.
Chloride Channel Activator Lubiprostone (Amitiza)	Stimulates chloride channels in the colonic mucosa, causing passive passage of sodium and fluid into the colon.	Avoid pregnancy during treatment, keep in mind that it may cause increase flatulence and loose stools. Do not use for more than 4 weeks.

Adapted from Bailes, B. K. & Reeve, K. (2013). Constipation in older adults. *The Nurse Practitioner, 38*(8), 21–25.

Providing patient education is an important function of the nurse (see Chart 47-2). After the health history is obtained, the nurse sets specific goals for education. Goals for the patient include restoring or maintaining a regular pattern of elimination by responding to the urge to defecate, ensuring adequate intake of fluids and high-fiber foods, learning about methods to avoid constipation, relieving anxiety about bowel elimination patterns, and avoiding complications.

Diarrhea

Diarrhea is an increased frequency of bowel movements (more than 3 per day) with altered consistency (i.e., increased liquidity) of stool. It can be associated with urgency, perianal discomfort, incontinence, nausea, or a combination of these

factors (NIDDK, 2014d). Any condition that causes increased intestinal secretions, decreased mucosal absorption, or altered motility can produce diarrhea.

Diarrhea can be classified as acute, persistent, or chronic. Acute diarrhea is self-limiting, lasting 1 or 2 days; persistent diarrhea typically lasts between 2 and 4 weeks; and chronic diarrhea persists for more than 4 weeks and may return sporadically. Acute and persistent diarrheas are frequently caused by viral infections (e.g., Norwalk virus). In addition, some drugs can cause acute or persistent diarrhea, including some antibiotics (e.g., erythromycin) and magnesium-containing antacids (e.g., magnesium hydroxide [Milk of Magnesia]). Chronic diarrhea may be caused by adverse effects of chemotherapy, antiarrhythmic agents, antihypertensive agents, metabolic and endocrine disorders (e.g., diabetes, Addison

PATIENT EDUCATION
Preventing Constipation

The nurse instructs the patient to:

- Recognize the physiology of defecation and the importance of responding to the urge to defecate.
- Understand the normal variations in patterns of defecation.
- Establish a bowel routine, and be aware that having a regular time for defecation (e.g., best time is after a meal) may aid in initiating the reflex.
- Ensure proper dietary habits, such as eating high-residue, high-fiber foods (e.g., fruits, vegetables); adding bran daily (must be introduced gradually); and increasing fluid intake (unless contraindicated) to help prevent constipation.
- Increase muscle strength through an exercise regimen, increased ambulation, and abdominal muscle toning to help propel colon contents.
- Perform abdominal toning exercises, including contracting abdominal muscles 4 times daily and leg-to-chest lifts 10–20 times each day.
- Use the normal position (semisquatting) to maximize the use of abdominal muscles and force of gravity.
- Avoid overuse or long-term use of stimulant laxatives.

disease, thyrotoxicosis), malabsorptive disorders (e.g., lactose intolerance, celiac disease), anal sphincter defect, Zollinger–Ellison syndrome, acquired immune deficiency syndrome (AIDS), and by parasitic or *Clostridium difficile* infections (NIDDK, 2014d).

C. difficile is the most commonly identified agent in antibiotic-associated diarrhea in the hospital (Murray, 2016). Moreover, it is the most common health care–associated infection in the United States, infecting nearly half a million patients annually (100,000 of these in long-term care facilities), causing 15,000 deaths (Centers for Disease Control and Prevention [CDC], 2015b).

Pathophysiology

Acute and persistent diarrheas are classified as either noninflammatory (large-volume) or inflammatory (small-volume). Enteric pathogens that are noninvasive (e.g., S. aureus, Giardia) do not cause inflammation but secrete toxins that disrupt colonic fluid transport. They cause noninflammatory diarrhea, which is characterized by a large volume of loose, watery stools. Other pathogens that invade the intestinal mucosa and cause inflammatory changes typically result in smaller volumes of stool that is bloody (e.g., dysentery). Organisms implicated may include *Shigella, Salmonella,* and *Yersinia* species (Grossman & Porth, 2014).

Types of chronic diarrhea include secretory, osmotic, malabsorptive, infectious, and exudative. Secretory diarrhea is usually high-volume diarrhea. Often associated with bacterial toxins and chemotherapeutic agents used to treat neoplasms, it is caused by increased production and secretion of water and electrolytes by the intestinal mucosa into the intestinal lumen. Osmotic diarrhea occurs when water is pulled into the intestines by the osmotic pressure of unabsorbed particles, slowing the reabsorption of water. It can be caused by lactase deficiency, pancreatic dysfunction, or intestinal hemorrhage. Malabsorptive diarrhea combines mechanical and biochemical actions, inhibiting effective absorption of nutrients. Low serum albumin levels lead to intestinal mucosa swelling and

liquid stool. Infectious diarrhea results from infectious agents invading the intestinal mucosa. Exudative diarrhea is caused by changes in mucosal integrity, epithelial loss, or tissue destruction by radiation or chemotherapy. Diarrhea may also be caused by laxative misuse (Grossman & Porth, 2014).

Clinical Manifestations

In addition to the increased frequency and fluid content of stools, the patient usually has abdominal cramps, distention, borborygmus (i.e., a rumbling noise caused by the movement of gas through the intestines), anorexia, and thirst. Painful spasmodic contractions of the anus and **tenesmus** (i.e., ineffective, sometimes painful straining with a strong urge) may occur with defecation. Other symptoms depend on the cause and severity of the diarrhea but are related to dehydration and to fluid and electrolyte imbalances.

Voluminous, greasy stools suggest intestinal **malabsorption** (impaired transport across the mucosa), and the presence of blood, mucus, and pus in the stools suggests inflammatory enteritis or colitis. Oil droplets on the toilet water may be suggestive of pancreatic insufficiency. Nocturnal diarrhea may be a manifestation of diabetic neuropathy (NIDDK, 2014d; Weber & Kelley, 2014). The possibility of C. *difficile* infection should be considered in all patients with unexplained diarrhea who are taking or have recently taken antibiotics (Murray, 2016).

Assessment and Diagnostic Findings

When the cause of the diarrhea is not obvious, the following diagnostic tests may be performed: complete blood cell count (CBC); serum chemistries; urinalysis; routine stool examination; and stool examinations for infectious or parasitic organisms, bacterial toxins, blood, fat, electrolytes, and white blood cells. Endoscopy or barium enema may assist in identifying the cause (NIDDK, 2014d).

Complications

The most common complication of diarrhea is dehydration. Dehydration with electrolyte loss (especially loss of potassium) may cause cardiac dysrhythmias. Loss of bicarbonate with diarrhea can also lead to metabolic acidosis. Urinary output less than 0.5 mL/kg/h for 2 to 3 consecutive hours, muscle weakness, paresthesia, hypotension, anorexia, and drowsiness with a potassium level less than 3.5 mEq/L (3.5 mmol/L) must be reported. Chronic diarrhea can also result in skin care issues related to irritant dermatitis (NIDDK, 2014d). Cleansing with a wet wipe and applying barrier cream can prevent dermatitis.

 Gerontologic Considerations

Older patients can become dehydrated quickly and develop low potassium levels (i.e., hypokalemia) as a result of diarrhea. The nurse observes for clinical manifestations of muscle weakness, dysrhythmias, or decreased peristaltic motility that may lead to paralytic ileus. The older patient taking digitalis (e.g., digoxin [Lanoxin]) must be aware of how quickly dehydration and hypokalemia can occur with diarrhea. The nurse educates the patient to recognize the symptoms of hypokalemia, because low levels of potassium potentiate the action of digitalis, leading to digitalis toxicity (Eliopoulos, 2018).

The skin of an older person is more sensitive to excoriation due to decreased turgor and reduced subcutaneous fat layers. Gentle cleansing with a perineal cleansing solution (i.e., wet wiping method) and the use of a barrier cream or a liquid skin sealant will prevent and/or treat the excoriation (Eliopoulos, 2018).

Medical Management

Management is directed at controlling symptoms, preventing complications, and eliminating or treating the underlying disease. Until the definitive cause is discovered, infection control measures that restrict the transmission of infectious organisms (e.g., *C. difficile*–associated diarrhea) are warranted (Murray, 2016) (see Chapter 71 for further discussion of *C. difficile* prevention). Certain medications (e.g., antibiotics, anti-inflammatory agents) and antidiarrheal agents (e.g., loperamide [Imodium], diphenoxylate with atropine [Lomotil]) may be prescribed to reduce the severity of the diarrhea and treat the underlying disease. In most cases, loperamide is the medication of choice because it has fewer side effects than diphenoxylate with atropine. Some research supports the use of probiotics (live organisms given to a host) in some forms of diarrhea. These organisms consist of *Saccharomyces boulardii* (yeast) or lactic acid bacteria such as *Lactobacillus* species (Avadhani & Steefel, 2015).

Nursing Management

The nurse assesses and monitors the characteristics and pattern of diarrhea. A health history should address the patient's medication therapy, medical and surgical history, and dietary patterns and intake. Reports of recent acute illness or recent travel to another geographic area are important (Moore, 2015). Assessment includes abdominal auscultation and palpation for tenderness. Inspection of the abdomen, mucous membranes, and skin is important to determine hydration status. Stool samples are obtained for testing. The perianal area should also be assessed for skin excoriation.

During an episode of diarrhea, the patient is encouraged to increase intake of liquids and foods low in bulk until the symptoms subside. When the patient is able to tolerate food intake, the patient should avoid caffeine, alcoholic beverages, dairy products, and fatty foods for several days (NIDDK, 2014d). Antidiarrheal medications such as diphenoxylate with atropine or loperamide may be taken as prescribed. Intravenous (IV) fluid therapy may be necessary for rapid rehydration in some patients, especially in older adults and in patients with pre-existing GI conditions (e.g., IBD). It is important to monitor serum electrolyte levels closely. The nurse immediately reports evidence of dysrhythmias or a change in a patient's level of consciousness.

The perianal area may become excoriated because diarrheal stool contains digestive enzymes that can irritate the skin. The patient should follow a perianal skin care routine to decrease irritation and excoriation (see Chapter 61).

Fecal Incontinence

Fecal incontinence describes the recurrent involuntary passage of stool from the rectum for at least 3 months. Factors that influence this disorder include the ability of the rectum to sense and accommodate stool, the amount and consistency of stool, the integrity of the anal sphincters and musculature, and rectal motility. Fecal incontinence can have a substantially negative impact on quality of life (Rao, Bharucha, Chiarioni, et al., 2016; Wald, Bharucha, Cosman, et al., 2014).

Pathophysiology

Fecal incontinence has many causes and risk factors and may be a symptom of an underlying condition. In general, it results from conditions that interrupt or disrupt the structure or function of the anorectal unit. Common causes include anal sphincter weakness, both traumatic (e.g., after surgical procedures involving the rectum) and nontraumatic (e.g., scleroderma); neuropathies both peripheral (e.g., pudendal) and generalized (e.g., diabetes); disorders of the pelvic floor (e.g., rectal prolapse); inflammation (radiation proctitis, IBD); central nervous system disorders (e.g., dementia, stroke, spinal cord injury, multiple sclerosis); diarrhea; fecal impaction with overflow; and behavioral disorders. It is less commonly a long-term consequence of vaginal childbirth injuries than in years past, most likely because of improved delivery methods. It is more common with advancing age (i.e., weakness or loss of anal or rectal muscle tone) (Rao et al., 2016; Wald et al., 2014).

Clinical Manifestations

Patients may have minor soiling, occasional urgency and loss of control, or complete incontinence. Patients may also experience poor control of flatus, diarrhea, or constipation. Passive incontinence occurs without warning; whereas, patients with urge incontinence have the sensation of the urge to defecate but cannot reach the toilet in time (Rao et al., 2016).

Assessment and Diagnostic Findings

Assessing the patient's medical history is helpful in identifying the most likely etiology. Diagnostic studies are necessary because the treatment of fecal incontinence depends on the cause. A rectal examination and an endoscopic examination such as a flexible sigmoidoscopy are performed to rule out tumors, inflammation, fissures, or impaction. Anorectal manometry, anal endosonography, pelvic MRI scan, and transit studies may be helpful in identifying alterations in intestinal mucosa and muscle tone or in detecting other structural or functional problems (Rao et al., 2016; Wald et al., 2014).

Medical Management

Medical management of fecal incontinence is directed at correcting the underlying cause. If fecal incontinence is related to diarrhea, the incontinence may disappear when diarrhea is successfully treated. Fecal incontinence secondary to a fecal impaction may cease after the impaction is removed and the rectum is cleansed. If the fecal incontinence is related to the use of contributory drugs (e.g., laxatives, antacids containing magnesium), the incontinence may improve or cease when the drug regimen is altered. When fecal incontinence is related to other disorders, treatments targeted at correcting the underlying disorder are initiated. Some patients benefit from the addition of psyllium (Metamucil) as a fiber supplement. In addition, administering loperamide 30 minutes prior to meals can be an effective intervention in some patients.

Biofeedback therapy with pelvic floor muscle training can be of assistance if the problem is decreased sensory awareness or sphincter control. Bowel training programs can also be effective (Rao et al., 2016; Wald et al., 2014). Sacral nerve stimulation, provided by implanting a subcutaneous stimulator that delivers low amplitude electrical stimulation to the sacral nerve, may be an option for some patients refractory to other interventions (Yong, 2016). Surgical procedures include surgical reconstruction or repair of anal sphincter, artificial sphincter implantation, anal sphincter bulking by injection of synthetic agents, sacral nerve stimulation, or fecal diversion (Rao et al., 2016; Wald et al., 2014).

Nursing Management

The nurse obtains a thorough health history, including information about previous surgical procedures, chronic illnesses, dietary patterns, bowel habits and problems, and current medication regimen. Stool charts (e.g., Bristol Stool Form, see later discussion) may help with identifying frequency, volume, and consistency of the feces. The nurse also completes an examination of the rectal area. If a fecal impaction is noted, it must be removed before instituting any preventive therapies (Gump & Schmelzer, 2016).

The nurse initiates a bowel training program that involves setting a schedule to establish bowel regularity. The goal is to help the patient achieve fecal continence. If this is not possible, the goal should be to manage the problem so the patient can have predictable, planned elimination. Sometimes it is necessary to use suppositories to stimulate the anal reflex. After the patient has achieved a regular schedule, the suppository can be discontinued. Biofeedback in conjunction with pelvic floor exercises can be used to help the patient improve sphincter contractility and rectal sensitivity. Bowel regulation also involves the therapeutic use of diet and fiber. Foods that thicken stool (e.g., applesauce) and fiber supplements help improve continence (Gump & Schmelzer, 2016). In particular, participants enrolled in a randomized controlled trial who took psyllium supplements had less frequent stools and improved stool consistency than participants who took other fiber supplements, such as carboxymethylcellulose (MCM) or gum Arabic (GA) (Bliss, Savak, Jung, et al., 2014). Conversely, foods that loosen stool (e.g., rhubarb, figs, prunes, plums) should be avoided. Some patients with fecal incontinence may benefit from the use of antidiarrheal medications (Gump & Schmelzer, 2016). Loperamide and diphenoxylate with atropine can be used; loperamide is the preferred medication because it does not cause central nervous system adverse effects (Rao et al., 2016).

Fecal incontinence can disrupt perineal skin integrity. Maintaining skin integrity is a priority, especially in the debilitated or older adult patient. Incontinence briefs or adult diapers, although helpful in containing the fecal material, permit increased skin contact with feces and may cause skin excoriation. In general, incontinence briefs are to be used only for brief periods of time. The nurse encourages and instructs about meticulous skin hygiene and uses perineal skin cleansers and skin protection products to protect perineal skin. Some patients may benefit from occasional use of foam anal plugs. However, many people find them unacceptable (Gump & Schmelzer, 2016).

Continence sometimes cannot be achieved, and the nurse assists the patient and family to accept and cope with this chronic situation. Patients with dementia may benefit from toileting assistance, including prompted or timed voiding and habit training, which is the setting of a regular time to go to the bathroom (e.g., after breakfast to have a bowel movement) (Gump & Schmelzer, 2016). The patient can use fecal incontinence devices, which include external collection devices and internal drainage systems. External devices are special rectal pouches (called *fecal incontinence collectors*) that are drainable. They are attached to a synthetic adhesive skin barrier specially designed to conform to the buttocks. Designed for patients with chronic, debilitating illnesses (e.g., in long-term care facilities) or acute illnesses, fecal management systems (e.g., Flexi-Seal Fecal Management System) can be used to eliminate fecal skin contact and are especially useful when there is extensive excoriation or skin breakdown. These systems, which consist of a tube with a low-pressure balloon that conforms to the internal rectal area, may be used for short-term management of liquid stools (no more than 4 consecutive weeks) (see Fig. 47-1) (Girard & Ousey, 2015; Gump & Schmelzer, 2016).

Irritable Bowel Syndrome (IBS)

Irritable bowel syndrome (IBS) is a chronic functional disorder characterized by recurrent abdominal pain associated with disordered bowel movements, which may include diarrhea, constipation, or both (Lacy et al., 2016; Skrastins & Fletcher, 2016). Global prevalence of IBS is 11.2% (Lacy et al., 2016) and prevalence among American adults is 15% (NIDDK, 2015). Women are affected more often than men, with twice as many women diagnosed with IBS in the United States than men. IBS is typically diagnosed in adults younger than 45 years of age (NIDDK, 2015). A complex interplay of genetic, environmental, and psychosocial factors are thought to be associated with the onset of IBS. It

Figure 47-1 • Flexi-Seal Fecal Management System. Reprinted with permission from ConvaTec, Inc.

is believed that some triggers can either herald the initial onset of IBS or exacerbate symptoms in those with diagnosed IBS; these may include chronic stress, sleep deprivation, surgery, infections, diverticulitis, and some foods (e.g., milk, yeast products, eggs, wheat products, red meat) (Lacy et al., 2016; Zigich & Heuberger, 2013). The diagnosis of IBS is made after tests confirm the absence of structural or other disorders (Lacy et al., 2016).

Pathophysiology

IBS results from a functional disorder of intestinal motility. The change in motility may be related to neuroendocrine dysregulation, especially changes in serotonin signaling, infection, irritation, or a vascular or metabolic disturbance. The peristaltic waves are affected at specific segments of the intestine and in the intensity with which they propel the fecal matter forward. There is no evidence of inflammation or tissue changes in the intestinal mucosa (Grossman & Porth, 2014; Lacy et al., 2016).

Clinical Manifestations

Symptoms can vary widely, ranging in intensity and duration from mild and infrequent to severe and continuous. The main symptom is an alteration in bowel patterns: constipation (classified as IBS-C), diarrhea (classified as IBS-D), or a combination of both (classified as IBS-M for "mixed"). The few patients with IBS who do not fit any of these three categories of IBS-C, IBS-D, or IBS-M, are classified as IBS-U for "unknown." Pain, bloating, and abdominal distention often accompany changes in bowel pattern. The abdominal pain is sometimes precipitated by eating and is frequently relieved by defecation. IBS frequently occurs concomitant with other GI disorders, including gastroesophageal reflux disease (GERD) and with a variety of non-GI functional disorders, including chronic fatigue syndrome, chronic pelvic pain, fibromyalgia, interstitial cystitis, migraine headaches, anxiety, and depression (Lacy et al., 2016; NIDDK, 2015).

Assessment and Diagnostic Findings

The clinical manifestations of IBS must be present sometime during the last 3 months with onset for at least 6 months prior to diagnosis. These manifestations include recurrent abdominal pain for at least one day weekly that is associated with 2 or more of the following (Lacy et al., 2016):

- Abdominal pain related to defecation;
- Abdominal pain associated with a change in frequency of stool;
- Abdominal pain associated with a change in form/appearance of stool.

Recording the quality and quantity of bowel movements in a stool diary such as the Bristol Stool Form Scale can be useful in determining the category of IBS (Lacy et al., 2016) (see Fig. 47-2).

A definite diagnosis of IBS also necessitates testing to confirm the absence of structural or other disorders. Results from a CBC and C-reactive protein or fecal calprotectin can rule out IBD (see later discussion) for patients who may have IBS-D or IBS-M, as well as serologic tests for celiac disease (see later discussion). Stool studies and colonoscopy may be performed to rule out other colon diseases (e.g., colorectal cancer, colitis) (Lacy et al., 2016).

Medical Management

The goals of treatment are to relieve abdominal pain and control diarrhea or constipation. Lifestyle modification, including stress reduction, ensuring adequate sleep, and instituting an exercise regimen, can result in symptom improvement. The introduction of soluble fiber (e.g., psyllium) to the diet is important to IBS management (Lacy et al., 2016). Restriction and then gradual reintroduction of foods that are possibly irritating may help determine what types of food are acting as irritants (e.g., beans, caffeinated products, corn, wheat, dairy lactose, fried foods, alcohol, spicy foods, aspartame) (Zigich & Heuberger, 2013).

For patients with IBS-D, antidiarrheal agents (e.g., loperamide) may be given to control the diarrhea and fecal urgency. Women with severe IBS-D that persists for more than 6 months that does not respond to other therapies may be prescribed alosetron (Lotronex), a highly selective 5-HT3 antagonist that slows colonic motility (Lacy et al. 2016). Other newer drugs that can mitigate IBS-D symptoms include rifaximin (Xifaxan), a nonabsorbable oral antibiotic, and eluxadoline (Viberzi, Allergan), a mu-receptor agonist/delta-receptor antagonist that neuromodulates colonic motility (Lembo, Lacy, Zuckerman, et al., 2016). Lubiprostone (Amitiza), a chloride channel regulator in the gut, can be prescribed for patients with IBS-C (Lacy et al., 2016).

Patients with all types of IBS complain of abdominal pain. This symptom may be mitigated by prescribing smooth muscle antispasmodic agents (e.g., dicyclomine [Bentyl]). Antidepressants can assist in treating underlying anxiety and depression but also have secondary benefits. Antidepressants may affect serotonin levels, thus modulating intestinal transit time and improving abdominal comfort. Peppermint oil, a complementary medication, has proven effective in diminishing abdominal discomfort (Lacy et al., 2016). Other alternatives for IBS management include probiotics. Probiotics are bacteria that include *Lactobacillus* and *Bifidobacterium* that can be given to help decrease abdominal bloating and gas (Lacy et al., 2016).

Nursing Management

The nurse's role is to provide patient and family education and encourage self-care activities (Ghiyasvandian, Ghorbani, Zakerimoghadam, et al., 2016) (see Chart 47-3). The nurse may provide education on the appropriate use of a bowel habit diary, such as the Bristol Stool Form Scale (see Fig. 47-2A). The nurse emphasizes and reinforces good sleep habits and good dietary habits (e.g., avoidance of food triggers). A good way to identify problem foods is to keep a 1- to 2-week food diary. Patients are encouraged to eat at regular times and to avoid food triggers. They should understand that although adequate fluid intake is necessary, fluid should not be taken with meals because this results in abdominal distention. Alcohol use and cigarette smoking are discouraged. Stress management via relaxation techniques, cognitive-behavioral therapy, yoga, and exercise can be recommended (Ghiyasvandian et al., 2016; Skrastins & Fleccher, 2016).

DISORDERS OF MALABSORPTION

The inability of the digestive system to absorb one or more of the major vitamins (especially A and B_{12}), minerals (i.e., iron and calcium), and nutrients (i.e., carbohydrates, fats, and

Figure 47-2 • **A.** The Bristol Stool Form Scale (BSFS) is used to evaluate bowel movement (BM) habit. **B.** Characteristics of stools as recorded on the BSFS are then used to determine category of irritable bowel syndrome (IBS), where IBS-C (constipation), IBS-D (diarrhea), IBS-M (mixed), and IBS-U (uncategorized). Reprinted with permission from Lacy, B. E., Mearin, F., Chang, L., et al. (2016). Bowel disorders. *Gastroenterology, 150*(6), 1393–1407.

proteins) occurs in disorders of malabsorption. Interruptions in the complex digestive process may occur anywhere in the digestive system and cause decreased absorption (Goebel, 2014; Grossman & Porth, 2014). The conditions that cause malabsorption can be grouped into the following categories (Grossman & Porth, 2014):

- Mucosal (transport) disorders causing generalized malabsorption (e.g., celiac disease, Crohn's disease, radiation enteritis)
- Luminal disorders causing malabsorption (e.g., bile acid deficiency, Zollinger–Ellison syndrome, pancreatic insufficiency, small bowel bacterial overgrowth, or chronic pancreatitis)
- Lymphatic obstruction, interfering with transport of fat by products of digestion into the systemic circulation (e.g., neoplasms, surgical trauma).

Table 47-2 lists the clinical and pathologic aspects of selected malabsorptive disorders. Chart 47-4 provides an education plan for a patient with lactose intolerance, a common malabsorptive disorder caused by a deficiency in lactase.

Celiac Disease

Celiac disease is a disorder of malabsorption caused by an autoimmune response to consumption of products that contain the protein gluten. Gluten is most commonly found in wheat, barley, rye, and other grains, malt, dextrin, and brewer's yeast. Celiac disease has become more common in the past decade, with an estimated prevalence of 1% in the United States. Women are afflicted twice as often as men. This disease is more common among Caucasians, although the rates of celiac disease are on the rise among non-Caucasians. Celiac

NURSING RESEARCH PROFILE

The Efficacy of a Self-Care Program on Symptoms and Quality of Life of Patients With Irritable Bowel Syndrome

Ghiyasvandian, S., Ghorbani, M., Zakermoghadam, M., et al. (2016). The effects of a self-care program on the severity of symptoms and quality of life of patients with irritable bowel syndrome. *Gastroenterology Nursing, 39*(5), 359–365.

Purpose

Patients with irritable bowel syndrome (IBS) experience abdominal pain, bloating, flatulence, and disordered bowel movements that can include diarrhea, constipation, or a combination of both. These symptoms can lead to embarrassment, anxiety, and depression, and negatively affect overall quality of life. Nurses can educate patients in self-care activities, including treatment, diet, and stress management activities, which can mitigate the effects of IBS. The purpose of this study was to examine the effects of a nurse-led self-care management program on the severity of symptoms and quality of life (QOL) of patients with IBS.

Design

This study was a randomized controlled trial that enrolled patients diagnosed with mild to moderate IBS who were treated in gastroenterology clinics in Arak, Iran. Criteria for participation included being between 18 and 65 years of age, able to read the training booklet, and able to complete the questionnaire. Sixty participants were randomized into the experimental group, and 59 participants were randomized into the control group. All participants received usual treatment of IBS by a gastroenterologist. Participants in the experimental group were educated in the self-care program, which consisted of a series of individual

and group sessions that included education on the causes and treatment of IBS and the role of stress management, medications, and complementary medicine on alleviating IBS symptoms. Two follow-up phone calls were made to receive feedback on the effectiveness of the education. QOL was measured by having all participants complete the IBS-QOL questionnaire before and 2 months after the intervention. IBS symptom severity was measured by having all participants complete the IBS Symptom Severity Scale (IBS-SSS) during those same two intervals.

Findings

Independent t tests for the experimental and control groups pre-intervention showed no significant differences in either severity of symptoms or QOL. Paired t tests showed no difference in either severity of symptoms or QOL from pre-intervention to post-intervention in the control group. However, paired t tests in the experimental group demonstrated significant differences from pre-intervention to post-intervention in terms of both severity of symptoms ($p < 0.0001$) and QOL ($p < 0.0001$).

Nursing Implications

Findings from this study confirm that a nurse-led self-care intervention with patients with mild to moderate IBS can significantly improve symptom severity and overall QOL. Designing a specific training booklet, mixing individual and group education sessions, and scheduling follow-up phone calls appear to ensure successful delivery of this type of intervention. This self-care intervention can be modified and replicated for use in patients with other chronic disorders that adversely affect QOL.

---

disease also has a familial risk component, particularly among first-degree relatives. Others at heightened risk include those with type 1 diabetes, Down syndrome, and Turner syndrome. Celiac disease may manifest at any age in a person who is genetically predisposed (Ferrara & Saccamano, 2015; Heavey

PATIENT EDUCATION

Managing Lactose Intolerance

The nurse instructs the patient to:

- Recognize that deficiency of lactase, a digestive enzyme essential for the digestion and absorption of lactose ("milk sugar") from the intestines, results in an intolerance to milk.
- Prevent symptoms by eliminating milk and milk substances.
- Eliminate processed foods that have fillers, such as dried milk, added to them; recognizing this can help determine which foods may need to be eliminated.
- Reduce symptoms by pretreating foods with lactase preparations (e.g., Lactaid drops) before ingestion or by ingesting lactase enzyme tablets with the first bite of food.
- Understand that most people can tolerate 1–2 cups of milk or milk products daily without major problems; they are best tolerated if ingested in small amounts during the day.
- Be aware that lactase activity of yogurt with "active cultures" helps the digestion of lactose within the intestine better than lactase preparations.
- Recognize that milk and milk products are rich sources of calcium and vitamin D; elimination of milk from the diet may result in calcium and vitamin D deficiencies; decreased intake without supplements can lead to osteoporosis.

& Stoltman, 2016; NIDDK, 2016a; Robinson, Davis, Vess, et al., 2015; Roos, Hellstrom, Hallert, et al., 2013).

Pathophysiology

Nearly 30% of the population in the United States may be genetically predisposed to developing celiac disease. Individuals who are predisposed share a major histocompatibility complex (MHC) class II allele human leukocyte antigen (HLA), HLA-DQ2 or HLA-DQ8. Those who develop celiac disease exhibit an autoimmune response to gluten products that is both humoral and cell mediated. It is not known what trigger or triggers may incite this autoimmune response, although it cannot occur if gluten is not ingested. As a result of this response, the epithelial cells that line the small intestines become inflamed, particularly the proximal portion, where most absorption of nutrients occurs. Eventually, the mucosal villi of the small intestine become denuded and cannot function. This results in loss of ability to absorb both micronutrients and macronutrients, causing systemic nutritional deficits (Ferrara & Saccomano, 2015; Grossman & Porth, 2014).

Clinical Manifestations

The most common GI clinical manifestations of celiac disease include diarrhea, steatorrhea, abdominal pain, abdominal distention, flatulence, and weight loss. However, these manifestations are more common among children than adults. Adults can present with non-GI signs and symptoms of celiac disease, which are highly variable and can

TABLE 47-2 Selected Disorders of Malabsorption

Diseases/Disorders	Pathophysiology	Clinical Features
Gastric resection with gastrojejunostomy	Decreased pancreatic stimulation because of duodenal bypass; poor mixing of food, bile, pancreatic enzymes; decreased intrinsic factor	Weight loss, moderate steatorrhea, anemia (combination of iron deficiency, vitamin B_{12} malabsorption, folate deficiency)
Pancreatic insufficiency (chronic pancreatitis, pancreatic carcinoma, pancreatic resection, cystic fibrosis)	Reduced intraluminal pancreatic enzyme activity, with maldigestion of lipids and proteins	History of abdominal pain followed by weight loss; marked steatorrhea, azotorrhea (excess of nitrogenous matter in the feces or urine); also frequent glucose intolerance (70% in pancreatic insufficiency)
Ileal dysfunction (resection or disease)	Loss of ileal absorbing surface leads to reduced bile salt pool size and reduced vitamin B_{12} absorption; bile in colon inhibits fluid absorption	Diarrhea, weight loss with steatorrhea, especially when >100-cm resection, decreased vitamin B_{12} absorption
Stasis syndromes (surgical strictures, blind loops, enteric fistulas, multiple jejunal diverticula, scleroderma)	Overgrowth of intraluminal intestinal bacteria, especially anaerobic organisms, to >10^6/mL results in deconjugation of bile salts, leading to decreased effective bile salt pool size, also bacterial utilization of vitamin B_{12}	Weight loss, steatorrhea; low vitamin B_{12} absorption; may have low D-xylose absorption
Zollinger–Ellison syndrome	Hyperacidity in duodenum inactivates pancreatic enzymes	Ulcer diathesis, steatorrhea
Lactose intolerance	Deficiency of intestinal lactase results in high concentration of intraluminal lactose with osmotic diarrhea	Varied degrees of diarrhea and cramps after ingestion of lactose-containing foods; positive lactose intolerance test, decreased intestinal lactase
Celiac disease (gluten-sensitive enteropathy)	Toxic response to a gluten fraction gliadin by surface epithelium results in destruction of absorbing surface of intestine	Weight loss, diarrhea, bloating, anemia (low iron, folate), osteomalacia, steatorrhea, azotorrhea, low D-xylose absorption; folate and iron malabsorption
Tropical sprue	Unknown toxic factor results in mucosal inflammation, partial villous atrophy	Weight loss, diarrhea, anemia (low folate, vitamin B_{12}); steatorrhea; low D-xylose absorption, low vitamin B_{12} absorption
Whipple disease	Bacterial invasion of intestinal mucosa	Arthritis, hyperpigmentation, lymphadenopathy, serous effusions, fever, weight loss, steatorrhea, azotorrhea
Certain parasitic diseases (giardiasis, strongyloidiasis, coccidiosis, capillariasis)	Damage to or invasion of surface mucosa	Diarrhea, weight loss; steatorrhea; organism may be seen on jejunal biopsy or recovered in stool
Immunoglobulinopathy	Decreased local intestinal defenses, lymphoid hyperplasia, lymphopenia	Frequent association with *Giardia*: hypogammaglobulinemia or isolated immunoglobulin A deficiency

Adapted from Goebel, S. U. (2014). Malabsorption. *Medscape*. Retrieved on 12/27/2016 at: emedicine.medscape.com/article/180785-overview; Grossman, S. C., & Porth, C. M. (2014). *Porth's pathophysiology: Concepts of altered health states* (9th ed.). Philadelphia, PA: Wolters Kluwer.

include fatigue, general malaise, depression, hypothyroidism, migraine headaches, osteopenia, anemia, seizures, paresthesias in the hands and feet, and a red, shiny tongue. Some adults and children may evidence ridges in the enamel of their adult teeth, as well as discoloration or yellowing. Dermatitis herpetiformis is a rash that is frequently associated with celiac disease in adults; it manifests as clusters of erythematous macules that develop into itchy papules and vesicles on the forearms, elbows, knees, face, or buttocks (Heavy & Stoltman, 2016; NIDDK, 2016a).

Assessment and Diagnostic Findings

A comprehensive assessment of the patient's presenting signs and symptoms, as well as a family history and risk factor assessment, may provide the first clues that the patient may have celiac disease. The definitive diagnosis is based upon a series of serologic tests and endoscopic biopsy. It is important that the patient continues to consume gluten products during testing, or there could be a false negative serologic finding. The first serologic test is the immunoglobulin A (IgA)

anti-tissue transglutaminase (tTG), which is 90% sensitive and 95% specific to celiac disease. Findings are confirmed with upper endoscopy with biopsies of the proximal small intestine (Heavey & Stoltman, 2016; Robinson et al., 2015).

Medical Management

Celiac disease is a chronic, noncurable, lifelong disease. There are no drugs that induce remission; the treatment is to refrain from exposure to gluten in foods and other products (see later discussion). A consult with a dietician may be advisable. The patient should be advised that it will likely take time before bothersome signs and symptoms resolve; indeed, it will take a full year before the integrity of the intestinal villi can be restored. Other manifestations of celiac disease may require specific, targeted treatment. For instance, patients who present with anemia may require folate, cobalamin, or iron supplements (see Chapter 33). Patients with osteopenia may require treatment for osteoporosis (see Chapter 41) (Ferrera & Saccomano, 2015; Heavey & Stoltman, 2016; Robinson et al., 2015).

Nursing Management

The nurse provides patient and family education regarding adherence to a gluten-free diet (see Chart 47-5), and how to avoid other gluten products. For instance, oats are not contraindicated in gluten-free diets; however, many oat products are produced in facilities that are cross-contaminated with wheat or other contraindicated grains. Likewise, gluten-free foods prepared in restaurants or dining areas that share preparatory space can become gluten-contaminated. For instance, gluten-free toast prepared in a toaster that is also used for wheat-based toast can become gluten-contaminated. Patients must become vigilant in asking restaurant and dining hall staff about how gluten-free foods are prepared.

Products that are not foods can also contain gluten. Many generic and over-the-counter drugs can be prepared with gluten gels. Toothpastes, communion wafers, and some cosmetics (e.g., lipsticks) and art supplies (e.g., modeling clay) can also contain gluten. Patients must understand how to carefully read labels on both foods and nonfood products to determine if they contain gluten. Since 2013, the U.S. Food and Drug Administration (FDA) has regulated and monitored the appropriate application of gluten-free labels (Heavey & Stoltman, 2016; Robinson et al., 2015).

ACUTE ABDOMEN

An acute abdomen, sometimes called a *surgical abdomen* is characterized by an acute onset of abdominal pain that does not have a traumatic etiology and that most typically requires swift surgical intervention to prevent peritonitis, sepsis, and septic shock. Disorders of the lower GI tract that may cause similar initial presenting clinical manifestations, causing acute abdominal pain and an acute abdomen include appendicitis, severe diverticulitis, and intestinal obstruction, all of which may lead to **peritonitis**, which is an inflammation of the lining of the abdominal cavity (Ansari, 2014; Saccomano & Ferrara, 2013).

Peritonitis

Peritonitis is inflammation of the peritoneum, which is the serous membrane lining the abdominal cavity and covering the viscera. Usually, it is a result of bacterial infection but may occur secondary to a fungal or mycobacterial infection; the organisms come from diseases or disorders of the GI tract or, in women, from the internal reproductive organs (e.g., fallopian tube). The most common bacteria implicated are *Escherichia coli* and *Klebsiella, Proteus, Pseudomonas,* and *Streptococcus species.* Peritonitis can also result from external sources such as abdominal surgery or trauma (e.g., gunshot wound, stab wound) or an inflammation that extends from an organ outside the peritoneal area, such as the kidney, or from continuous ambulatory peritoneal dialysis (CAPD) (see Chapter 54) (Ansari, 2014; Daley, 2015). Peritonitis can be categorized as (Daley, 2015):

- Primary peritonitis, also called *spontaneous bacterial peritonitis (SBP)*, occurs as a spontaneous bacterial infection of ascitic fluid. This occurs most commonly in adult patients with liver failure (see Chapter 49).
- Secondary peritonitis occurs secondary to perforation of abdominal organs with spillage that infects the serous peritoneum. The most common causes include a perforated appendix (see later discussion), perforated peptic ulcer (see Chapter 46), perforated sigmoid colon caused by severe diverticulitis (see later discussion), volvulus of the colon (see later discussion), and strangulation of the small intestine (see later discussion). The major focus of this section is on secondary peritonitis.
- Tertiary peritonitis occurs as a result of a suprainfection in a patient who is immunocompromised. Tuberculous peritonitis in a patient with AIDS is an example of tertiary peritonitis; these are rare causes of peritonitis.

Pathophysiology

Secondary peritonitis is caused by leakage of contents from abdominal organs into the abdominal cavity, usually as a result of inflammation, infection, ischemia, trauma, or tumor perforation. Bacterial proliferation occurs. Edema of the tissues results, and exudation of fluid develops in a short time. Fluid in the peritoneal cavity becomes turbid with increasing amounts of protein, white blood cells, cellular debris, and blood. The immediate response of the intestinal tract is hypermotility, soon followed by paralytic ileus with an accumulation of air and fluid in the bowel (Daley, 2015; Grossman & Porth, 2014).

Clinical Manifestations

Symptoms depend on the location and extent of the inflammation. The early clinical manifestations of peritonitis frequently are the signs and symptoms of the disorder causing the condition (e.g., manifestations of infection). At first, pain is diffuse but then becomes constant, localized, and more intense over the site of the pathologic process (site of maximal peritoneal irritation). Movement usually aggravates it. The affected area of the abdomen becomes extremely tender and distended, and the muscles become rigid. Rebound tenderness may be present. Usually, anorexia, nausea, and vomiting occur and peristalsis is diminished, followed by paralytic ileus. An initial temperature of 37.8° to 38.3°C (100° to 101°F) can be expected, along with an increased pulse rate. With progression of the condition, patients may become hypotensive. Without swift and decisive intervention, clinical manifestations will mirror those of sepsis and septic shock (Ansari, 2014; Daley, 2015; Saccomano & Ferrera, 2013) (see Chapter 14).

Assessment and Diagnostic Findings

The white blood cell count is elevated and may demonstrate a relative increase in the immature neutrophils (i.e., bands), consistent with bacterial infection. The hemoglobin and hematocrit levels may be low if blood loss has occurred. Serum electrolyte studies may reveal altered levels of potassium, sodium, and chloride.

An abdominal x-ray may show air and fluid levels as well as distended bowel loops. Abdominal ultrasound may reveal **abscesses** (localized collection of purulent material surrounded by inflamed tissues) and fluid collections, and ultrasound-guided aspiration may assist in easier placement of drains. A computed tomography (CT) scan of the abdomen may show abscess formation. Peritoneal aspiration and culture and sensitivity studies of the aspirated fluid may reveal infection and identify the causative organisms. MRI may be used for diagnosis of intra-abdominal abscesses (Daley, 2015).

Medical Management

Fluid, colloid, and electrolyte replacement is the major focus of medical management. The administration of several liters of an isotonic solution is prescribed. Hypovolemia occurs because massive amounts of fluid and electrolytes move from the intestinal lumen into the peritoneal cavity and deplete the fluid in the vascular space.

Analgesic medications are prescribed for pain. Antiemetic agents are given as prescribed for nausea and vomiting. Intestinal intubation and suction assist in relieving abdominal distention and in promoting intestinal function. Fluid in the abdominal cavity can cause pressure that restricts expansion of the lungs and causes respiratory distress. Oxygen therapy by nasal cannula or mask generally promotes adequate oxygenation, but airway intubation and ventilatory assistance occasionally are required.

Antibiotic therapy is initiated early in the treatment of peritonitis. Large doses of a broad-spectrum antibiotic are given IV until the specific organism causing the infection is identified and appropriate antibiotic therapy can be initiated.

The main focus of treatment in secondary peritonitis is to identify the source of infection and eradicate it. Surgical treatment is directed toward excision (e.g., appendix), resection with or without anastomosis (e.g., intestine), repair (e.g., perforation), and drainage (e.g., abscess). With extensive sepsis, a fecal diversion may need to be created (see later dis-

cussions). In selected instances, ultrasound-guided and CT-guided peritoneal drainage of abdominal and extraperitoneal abscesses has allowed for avoidance or delay of surgical therapy until the acute septic process has subsided (Ansari, 2014; Daley, 2015; Saccomano & Ferrara, 2013). Antibiotics are continued postoperatively; a systematic review of antibiotic regimens noted that no one regimen of antibiotics is superior to another in terms of improving outcomes (Wong, Gilliam, Kumar, et al., 2012).

 ## Nursing Management

Intensive care is needed for the patient with septic shock (see Chapter 14). Signs indicating that peritonitis is subsiding include a decrease in temperature and pulse rate, softening of the abdomen, return of peristaltic sounds, passing of flatus, and bowel movements. The nurse increases fluid and food intake gradually and reduces parenteral fluids as prescribed. A worsening clinical condition may indicate a complication, and the nurse must prepare the patient for emergency surgery. The nursing management of a patient treated for secondary peritonitis is based upon the patient's primary diagnosis and treatment (see later discussions of Nursing Management of Patients with Appendicitis, Diverticular Disease, and Intestinal Obstruction).

Appendicitis

The appendix is a small, vermiform (i.e., wormlike) appendage about 8 to 10 cm (3 to 4 inches) long that is attached to the cecum just below the ileocecal valve. The appendix fills with by products of digestion and empties regularly into the cecum. Because it empties inefficiently and its lumen is small, the appendix is prone to obstruction and is particularly vulnerable to infection (i.e., appendicitis). Appendicitis, the most frequent cause of acute abdomen in the United States, is the most common reason for emergency abdominal surgery. Although it can occur at any age, it typically occurs between the ages of 10 and 30 years. Its incidence is slightly higher among males and there is a familial predisposition (Craig, 2015; NIDDK, 2014a).

Pathophysiology

The appendix becomes inflamed and edematous as a result of becoming kinked or occluded by a fecalith (i.e., hardened mass of stool), lymphoid hyperplasia (secondary to inflammation or infection), or rarely, foreign bodies (e.g., fruit seeds) or tumors. The inflammatory process increases intraluminal pressure, causing edema and obstruction of the orifice. Once obstructed, the appendix becomes ischemic, bacterial overgrowth occurs, and eventually gangrene or perforation occurs (Craig, 2015; Saccomano & Ferrara, 2013).

Clinical Manifestations

Vague periumbilical pain (i.e., visceral pain that is dull and poorly localized) with anorexia progresses to right lower quadrant pain (i.e., parietal pain that is sharp, discrete, and well localized) and nausea in approximately 50% of patients with appendicitis (Craig, 2015). A low-grade fever may be present. Local tenderness may be elicited at McBurney point when pressure is applied (see Fig. 47-3). Rebound tenderness

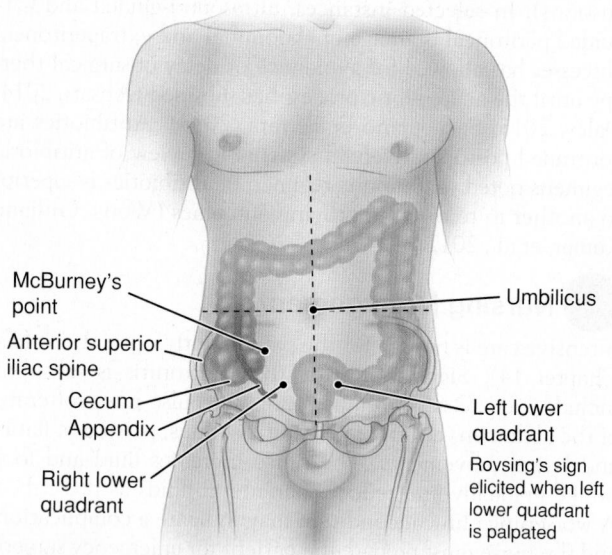

McBurney's point

Umbilicus

Anterior superior iliac spine

Cecum

Appendix

Left lower quadrant

Right lower quadrant

Rovsing's sign elicited when left lower quadrant is palpated

Figure 47-3 • When the appendix is inflamed, tenderness can be noted in the right lower quadrant at McBurney point, which is between the umbilicus and the anterior superior iliac spine. Rovsing sign is pain felt in the right lower quadrant after the left lower quadrant has been palpated.

(i.e., production or intensification of pain when pressure is released) may be present. Rovsing sign may be elicited by palpating the left lower quadrant; this paradoxically causes pain to be felt in the right lower quadrant (see Fig. 47-3). If the appendix has ruptured, the pain becomes consistent with peritonitis (see previous discussion); abdominal distention develops as a result of paralytic ileus, and the patient's condition worsens (Craig, 2015; Saccomano & Ferrara, 2013).

Constipation can also occur with appendicitis. Laxatives given in this instance may result in perforation of the inflamed appendix. In general, a laxative or cathartic should not be given when a person has fever, nausea, and abdominal pain.

Assessment and Diagnostic Findings

Diagnosis is based on the results of a complete history and physical examination and on laboratory findings and imaging studies. The CBC demonstrates an elevated white blood cell count with an elevation of the neutrophils. C-reactive protein levels are typically elevated. A CT scan may reveal a right lower quadrant density or localized distention of the bowel; enlargement of the appendix by at least 6 mm is suggestive of appendicitis (Saccomano & Ferrara, 2013). A pregnancy test may be ordered for women of childbearing age to rule out ectopic pregnancy and before radiologic studies are done. As an alternative, a transvaginal ultrasound may be used to confirm the diagnosis (Craig, 2015). A urinalysis is usually obtained to rule out urinary tract infection or renal calculi (Saccomano & Ferrara, 2013). A diagnostic laparoscopy may be used to rule out acute appendicitis in equivocal cases (Ansari, 2014).

Complications

The major complications of appendicitis are gangrene or perforation of the appendix, which can lead to peritonitis, abscess

formation, or portal pylephlebitis, which is septic thrombosis of the portal vein caused by vegetative emboli that arise from septic intestines. Perforation generally occurs within 6 to 24 hours after the onset of pain and leads to peritonitis (Craig, 2015; Saccomano & Ferrara, 2013).

 Gerontologic Considerations

Acute appendicitis is uncommon in older adults. When appendicitis does occur, classic signs and symptoms are altered and may vary greatly. Pain may be absent or minimal. Symptoms may be vague, suggesting bowel obstruction or another process. Fever and leukocytosis may not be present. As a result, diagnosis and prompt treatment may be delayed, causing complications and mortality. The patient may have no symptoms until the appendix becomes gangrenous or perforates. The incidence of complications is higher in older adults because many of these patients do not seek health care as quickly as younger patients (Craig, 2015; Eliopoulos, 2018).

Medical Management

Immediate surgery is typically indicated if appendicitis is diagnosed (Craig, 2015; Saccomano & Ferrara, 2013). However, conservative nonsurgical medical management for uncomplicated appendicitis (i.e., absence of gangrene or perforation of the appendix, empyema or abscess formation, or peritonitis) has been instituted in some instances with a reduced risk of complications and similar hospital length of stay as appendectomy (Salminen, Paajanen, Rautio, et al., 2015). To correct or prevent fluid and electrolyte imbalance, dehydration, and sepsis, antibiotics and IV fluids are given until surgery is performed. Appendectomy (i.e., surgical removal of the appendix) is performed as soon as possible to decrease the risk of perforation. It is typically performed using general anesthesia with either a low abdominal incision (laparotomy) or by laparoscopy. Both laparotomy and laparoscopy are safe and effective in the treatment of appendicitis with or without perforation. However, recovery after laparoscopic surgery is generally quicker (Andersson, 2014; Bozkurt, Unsal, Kapan, 2015). For complicated appendicitis (e.g., with gangrene or perforation), the patient is typically treated with a 3- to 5-day course of antibiotics postoperatively (van Rossem, Schreinemacher, Treskes, et al., 2014). Although it had been common practice for the surgeon to place a surgical drain, recent research findings suggest there is no improvement in outcomes but longer hospital lengths of stay when drains are used (Cheng, Zhou, Zhou, et al., 2015).

Some patients may have abscess formation that involves the cecum and/or terminal ileum. In these selected cases, appendectomy may be deferred until the mass is drained. Most commonly, these abscesses are drained percutaneously or surgically. The patient continues to receive treatment with antibiotics. After the abscess is drained and there is no further evidence of infection, an appendectomy is then performed (Ansari, 2014; Craig, 2015).

Nursing Management

Goals include relieving pain, preventing fluid volume deficit, reducing anxiety, preventing or treating surgical site infection, preventing atelectasis, maintaining skin integrity, and attaining optimal nutrition.

The nurse prepares the patient for surgery, which includes an IV infusion to replace fluid loss and promote adequate renal function, antibiotic therapy to prevent infection, and administration of analgesic agents for pain (Saccomano & Ferrera, 2013). An enema is not given because it can lead to perforation.

After surgery, the nurse places the patient in a high Fowler position. This position reduces the tension on the incision and abdominal organs, helping to reduce pain. It also promotes thoracic expansion, diminishing the work of breathing, and decreasing the likelihood of atelectasis. The patient is educated on the use of an incentive spirometer and encouraged to use it at least every 2 hours while awake. A parenteral opioid (e.g., morphine) is typically prescribed to relieve pain; this is switched to an oral agent when the patient is able to tolerate oral fluids and foods. Any patient who was dehydrated before surgery receives IV fluids. When tolerated, oral fluids are given. Food is provided as desired and tolerated on the day of surgery when bowel sounds are present. The nurse auscultates for the return of bowel sounds and queries the patient for passing of flatus. Urine output is monitored to ensure that the patient is not hampered by postoperative urinary retention and to ensure that hydration status is adequate. The patient is encouraged to ambulate the day of surgery to reduce risks of atelectasis and venous thromboemboli (VTE) formation.

The patient may be discharged on the day of surgery if the temperature is within normal limits, there is no undue discomfort in the operative area, and the appendectomy was performed laparoscopically. Discharge instruction for the patient and family is imperative. The nurse instructs the patient to make an appointment to have the surgeon remove any sutures and inspect the wound between 1 and 2 weeks after surgery (Evans & Curtin, 2014). Incision care and activity guidelines are discussed; heavy lifting is to be avoided postoperatively, although normal activity can usually be resumed within 2 to 4 weeks.

Patients with a gangrenous or perforated appendix are at greater risk for infection and peritonitis; therefore, they may be kept in the hospital for several days. Secondary abscesses may form in the pelvis, under the diaphragm, or in the liver, causing elevation of the temperature, pulse rate, and white blood cell count. When the patient is ready for discharge, the patient and family are educated about how to care for the incision and perform dressing changes and irrigations as prescribed. A home care nurse may be needed to assist with this care and to monitor the patient for complications and wound healing.

Diverticular Disease

A **diverticulum** is a saclike herniation of the lining of the bowel that extends through a defect in the muscle layer. Diverticula may occur anywhere in the GI tract, from the esophagus to the colon, but occur most commonly in the colon, particularly in the sigmoid colon (DiMarino, 2013; Shahedi, Dea, Chudasama, et al., 2016). However, Asian Americans may develop diverticula in the right colon, probably because of genetic differences (Shahedi et al., 2016).

Diverticulosis is defined by the presence of multiple diverticula without inflammation or symptoms. Diverticular disease of the colon is very common in developed countries, and its prevalence increases with increasing age; indeed, it is present in half of all adults over 65 years of age, and nearly all adults by 90 years of age (DiMarino, 2013). Diverticulosis is the most common pathologic incidental finding on colonoscopy. Approximately 80% of patients with diverticulosis never develop any complications or symptoms of disease. A low intake of dietary fiber is considered a risk factor, as well as obesity, a history of cigarette smoking, regular use of nonsteroidal anti-inflammatory drugs (NSAIDs) and acetaminophen (Tylenol), and a positive family history. Although there is an equal prevalence of diverticulosis between men and women, complications related to diverticulosis more commonly happen in men younger than 44 years of age, and in women older than 54 years of age (Razik & Nguyen, 2015).

Diverticulitis occurs when a diverticulum becomes inflamed, causing perforation, and potential complications such as obstruction, abscess, **fistula** (abnormal tract) formation, peritonitis, and hemorrhage (DiMarino, 2013).

Pathophysiology

Diverticula form when the mucosal and submucosal layers of the colon herniate through the muscular wall because of high intraluminal pressure, low volume in the colon (i.e., fiber-deficient contents), and decreased muscle strength in the colon wall (i.e., muscular hypertrophy from hardened fecal masses). Bowel contents can accumulate in the diverticulum and decompose, causing inflammation and infection. The diverticulum can also become obstructed and then inflamed if the obstruction continues. The inflammation of the weakened colonic wall of the diverticulum can cause it to perforate, giving rise to irritability and spasticity of the colon (i.e., diverticulitis). In addition, abscesses may develop and may eventually perforate, leading to peritonitis and erosion of the arterial blood vessels, resulting in bleeding. When a patient develops symptoms of diverticulitis, microperforation of the colon has occurred (DiMarino, 2013; Shahedi et al., 2016).

Clinical Manifestations

Chronic constipation sometimes precedes the development of diverticulosis by many years. Most commonly, no problematic symptoms occur with diverticulosis. Some patients may have mild signs and symptoms that include bowel irregularity with intervals of alternating constipation and diarrhea, with nausea, anorexia, and bloating or abdominal distention (Shahedi et al., 2016).

With diverticulitis, up to 70% of patients report an acute onset of mild to severe pain in the left lower quadrant. This may be accompanied by a change in bowel habits, most typically constipation, with nausea, fever, and leukocytosis. Acute complications of diverticulitis may include abscess formation, bleeding, and peritonitis. If an abscess develops, the associated findings are tenderness, a palpable mass, fever, and leukocytosis. Inflamed diverticula may erode areas adjacent to arterial branches, causing massive rectal bleeding. An inflamed diverticulum that perforates results in abdominal pain localized over the involved segment, usually the sigmoid;

local abscess or peritonitis follows (see previous discussion) (DiMarino, 2013; Shahedi et al., 2016).

Recurrent episodes of diverticulitis may cause chronic complications that include fistula formation, including colovesicular fistulas (i.e., between the colon and bladder) and, in women, colovaginal fistulas (i.e., between the colon and vagina). As a response to repeated inflammation, the colon may narrow with scar tissue and fibrotic strictures, leading to cramps, narrow stools, and increased constipation, or, at times, intestinal obstruction (DiMarino, 2013; Shahedi et al., 2016) (see later discussion).

Assessment and Diagnostic Findings

Diverticulosis is typically diagnosed by colonoscopy, which permits visualization of the extent of diverticular disease (DiMarino, 2013; Shahedi et al., 2016). Laboratory tests that assist in diagnosis of diverticulitis include a CBC, revealing an elevated white blood cell count; if the patient has frank blood in the stool, a hemoglobin level should also be analyzed. Urinalysis and urine cultures should be analyzed in patients with suspected colovesicular fistulas.

An abdominal CT scan with contrast agent is the diagnostic test of choice to confirm diverticulitis; it can also reveal perforation and abscesses. Abdominal x-rays may demonstrate free air under the diaphragm if a perforation has occurred from the diverticulitis. Results from these radiologic tests confirm whether or not the patient has uncomplicated diverticulitis or complicated diverticulitis that could require surgical intervention. The Hinchey classification is used as a guide to determine treatment (DiMarino, 2013; Shahedi et al., 2016) (see Table 47-3).

 Gerontologic Considerations

The incidence of diverticular disease increases with age because of degeneration and structural changes in the circular muscle layers of the colon and because of cellular hypertrophy. The symptoms are less pronounced in the older adult than in other adults. Older adults may not have abdominal pain until infection occurs. They may delay reporting symptoms because they fear surgery or are afraid that they may have cancer (Eliopoulos, 2018).

Medical Management

Medical management is guided by the presence of complications. Treatment for patients with uncomplicated diverticulitis or with Hinchey Stage I diverticulitis (see Table 47-3) is on an outpatient basis with diet and medication. This is the

typical treatment for 80% of patients with diagnosed diverticulitis (DiMarino, 2013). Rest, oral fluids, and analgesic medications are recommended. Initially, a clear liquid diet is consumed until the inflammation subsides; then a high-fiber, low-fat diet is recommended. This type of diet helps increase stool volume, decrease colonic transit time, and reduce intraluminal pressure. Although antibiotics are typically prescribed for 7 to 10 days, results from a systematic review did not find that the use of antibiotics improved outcomes (Shabanzadeh & Wille-Jorgensen, 2012).

In acute cases of diverticulitis with significant symptoms, hospitalization is required. Hospitalization is often indicated for those who are older, immunocompromised, or taking corticosteroids. Patients with Hinchey Stage 2 diverticulitis (see Table 47-3) can require hospitalization; those with higher stages require surgery and hospitalization (see later discussion). Withholding oral intake, administering IV fluids, and instituting nasogastric (NG) suctioning if vomiting or distention occurs are used to rest the bowel. Broad-spectrum antibiotics (e.g., ampicillin/sulbactam [Unasyn], ticarcillin/clavulanate [Timentin]) (Shahedi et al., 2016) are prescribed. An opioid (e.g., oxycodone) or other analgesic agents may be prescribed for pain relief. Oral intake is increased as symptoms subside. A low-fiber diet may be necessary until signs of infection decrease.

Surgical Management

Although acute diverticulitis usually subsides with medical management, immediate surgical intervention is necessary if complications (e.g., perforation, peritonitis, hemorrhage, obstruction) occur. In particular, patients with Hinchey Stage III or IV diverticulitis are considered surgical candidates (Shahedi, 2016). In cases of abscess formation without peritonitis, hemorrhage, or obstruction, CT-guided percutaneous drainage may be performed to drain the abscess, and IV antibiotics are given. After the abscess is drained and the acute

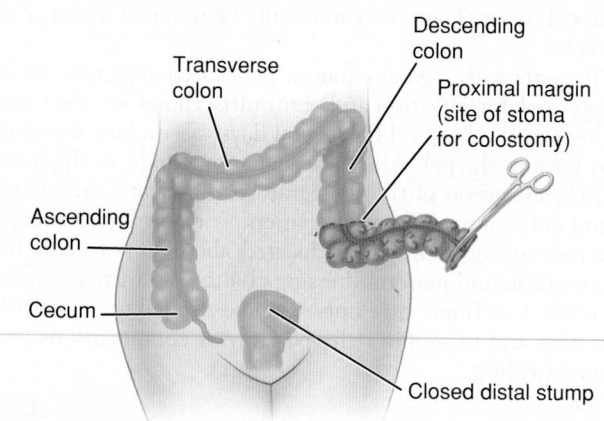

Figure 47-4 • Hartmann procedure for diverticulitis: primary resection for diverticulitis of the colon. The affected segment (*clamp attached*) has been divided at its distal end. In a primary anastomosis, the proximal margin (*dotted line*) is transected and the bowel attached end to end. In a two-stage procedure, a colostomy is constructed at the proximal margin with the distal stump oversewn (Hartmann procedure, as shown) and the stump is left in the pelvis. The distal stump may be brought to the surface as a mucous fistula if there is concern about blood supply. The second stage consists of colostomy takedown and anastomosis.

TABLE 47-3 Hinchey Classification: Staging of Acute, Complicated Diverticulitis

Hinchey Stage	Complication of Acute Diverticulitis
I	Localized pericolic or mesenteric abscess
II	Walled-off pelvic, intra-abdominal, or retroperitoneal abscess
III	Generalized purulent peritonitis
IV	Generalized fecal peritonitis

Adapted from Hinchey, E. J., Schaal, P. G., & Richards, G. K. (1978). Treatment of perforated diverticular disease of the colon. *Advances in Surgery, 12,* 85–109.

episode of inflammation has subsided (after approximately 6 weeks), surgery may be recommended to prevent repeated episodes. Two types of surgery are typically considered either to treat acute complications or prevent further episodes of inflammation:

- One-stage resection, in which the inflamed area is removed and a primary end-to-end anastomosis is completed
- Multiple-stage procedures for complications such as obstruction or perforation (see Fig. 47-4)

The type of surgery performed depends on the extent of complications found during the procedure. When possible, the area of diverticulitis is resected and the remaining bowel is joined end to end (i.e., primary resection and end-to-end anastomosis). This is performed using traditional surgical or laparoscopically assisted colectomy with lavage. A two-stage resection may be performed in patients with Hinchey Stage IV diverticulitis; the diseased colon is resected (as in a one-stage procedure) but no anastomosis is performed. In this procedure, one end of the bowel is brought out to the abdominal wall and the distal end is closed over and left in the abdomen (Hartmann procedure), or if the blood supply to the distal colon is questionable, both ends of the bowel are brought out to the abdominal wall (double-barrel) (Hupfeld, Burcharth, Pommergaard, et al., 2014). Both Hartmann procedures and double-barrel colostomies are usually reanastomosed at a later time.

Nursing Management

The nurse recommends a fluid intake of 2 L/day (within limits of the patient's cardiac and renal reserve) and suggests foods that are soft but have increased fiber, such as prepared cereals or soft-cooked vegetables, to increase the bulk of the stool and facilitate peristalsis, thereby promoting defecation. An individualized exercise program is encouraged to improve abdominal muscle tone. It is important to review the patient's daily routine to establish a schedule for meals and a set time for defecation and to assist in identifying habits that may have suppressed the urge to defecate. The nurse encourages daily intake of bulk laxatives such as psyllium, which helps propel feces through the colon. Some people with diverticulosis may have food triggers such as nuts and popcorn that bring on a diverticulitis attack, whereas others may not report food triggers. If triggers are identified, patients should be urged to avoid them.

For the patient who has had a colostomy placed, refer to the later section on Nursing Management of the Patient Requiring an Ostomy.

Intestinal Obstruction

Intestinal obstruction exists when blockage prevents the normal flow of intestinal contents through the intestinal tract. Two types of processes can impede this flow:

- *Mechanical obstruction:* An intraluminal obstruction or a mural obstruction from pressure on the intestinal wall occurs. Examples are intussusception, polypoid tumors and neoplasms, stenosis, strictures, adhesions, hernias, abscesses, and bezoars (i.e., foreign objects created by ingesting unusual substances) (Ansari, 2014).
- *Functional or paralytic obstruction:* The intestinal musculature cannot propel the contents along the bowel.

Examples are amyloidosis, muscular dystrophy, endocrine disorders such as diabetes, or neurologic disorders such as Parkinson disease. The blockage also can be temporary and the result of the manipulation of the bowel during surgery (i.e., ileus) (Grossman & Porth, 2014).

The obstruction can be partial or complete. Severity depends on the region of bowel affected, the degree to which the lumen is occluded, and especially the degree to which the vascular supply to the bowel wall is disturbed (Ansari, 2014).

Most bowel obstructions occur in the small intestine. Adhesions are the most common cause of small bowel obstruction, followed by tumors, Crohn's disease, and hernias (Ansari, 2014; Nobie, 2015). Other causes include intussusception, volvulus (i.e., twisting of the bowel), and paralytic ileus. Most obstructions in the large bowel occur in the sigmoid colon. The most common causes are carcinoma, diverticulitis, inflammatory bowel disorders, and fecal impaction (Ansari, 2014; Hopkins, 2016). Table 47-4 and Figure 47-5 list mechanical causes of obstruction and describe how they occur.

Small Bowel Obstruction

Pathophysiology

Intestinal contents, fluid, and gas accumulate proximal to the intestinal obstruction. The abdominal distention and retention of fluid reduce the absorption of fluids and stimulate more gastric secretion. With increasing distention, pressure within the intestinal lumen increases, causing a decrease in venous and arteriolar capillary pressure. This causes edema, congestion, necrosis, and eventual rupture or perforation of the intestinal wall, with resultant peritonitis (Ansari, 2014; Nobie, 2015; Saccomano & Ferrara, 2013).

Figure 47-5 • Three causes of intestinal obstruction. **A.** Intussusception; invagination or shortening of the colon caused by the movement of one segment of bowel into another. **B.** Volvulus of the sigmoid colon; the twist is counterclockwise in most cases. Note the edematous bowel. **C.** Hernia (inguinal). The sac of the hernia is a continuation of the peritoneum of the abdomen. The hernial contents are intestine, omentum, or other abdominal contents that pass through the hernial opening into the hernial sac.

TABLE 47-4 Mechanical Causes of Intestinal Obstruction

Cause	Course of Events	Result
Adhesions	Loops of intestine become adherent to areas that heal slowly or scar after abdominal surgery; occurs most commonly in small intestine	After surgery, adhesions produce a kinking of an intestinal loop.
Intussusception	One part of the intestine slips into another part located below it (like a telescope shortening); occurs more commonly in infants than adults	The intestinal lumen becomes narrowed, and blood supply becomes strangulated.
Volvulus	Bowel twists and turns on itself and occludes the blood supply	Intestinal lumen becomes obstructed. Gas and fluid accumulate in the trapped bowel.
Hernia	Protrusion of intestine through a weakened area in the abdominal muscle wall	Intestinal flow may be completely obstructed. Blood flow to the area may be obstructed as well.
Tumor	A tumor that exists within the wall of the intestine extends into the intestinal lumen, or a tumor outside the intestine causes pressure on the wall of the intestine. Most common type is colorectal adenocarcinoma	Intestinal lumen becomes partially obstructed; if the tumor is not removed, complete obstruction results.

Clinical Manifestations

The initial symptom is usually crampy pain that is wavelike and colicky due to persistent peristalsis both above and below the blockage. The patient may pass blood and mucus but no fecal matter and no flatus. Vomiting occurs. If the obstruction is complete, the peristaltic waves initially become extremely vigorous and eventually assume a reverse direction, with the intestinal contents propelled toward the mouth instead of toward the rectum. The signs of dehydration become evident: intense thirst, drowsiness, generalized malaise, aching, and a parched tongue and mucous membranes. The patient may continue to have flatus and stool early in the process due to distal peristalsis. The abdomen becomes distended. The lower the obstruction in the GI tract, the more marked the abdominal distention; this may cause reflux vomiting. Vomiting results in loss of hydrogen ions and potassium from the stomach, leading to reduction of chloride and potassium in the blood and to metabolic alkalosis. Dehydration and acidosis develop from loss of water and sodium. With acute fluid losses, hypovolemic shock may occur; septic shock may also occur (Ansari, 2014; Nobie, 2015; Saccomano & Ferrara, 2013) (see Chapter 14).

Assessment and Diagnostic Findings

Diagnosis is based on the symptoms described previously and on imaging studies. Abdominal x-ray and CT scan findings include abnormal quantities of gas, fluid, or both in the intestines and sometimes collapsed distal bowel. Laboratory studies (i.e., electrolyte studies and a CBC) reveal a picture of dehydration, loss of plasma volume, and possible infection. The approach to small bowel obstruction focuses on (1) confirming the diagnosis, (2) identifying the etiology, and (3) determining the likelihood of strangulation (Ansari, 2014; Nobie, 2015; Saccomano & Ferrara, 2013).

Medical Management

Decompression of the bowel through an NG tube (see Chapter 44) is necessary for all patients with small bowel obstruction; this may be tried for up to 3 days for patients with partial obstructions; resting the bowel in this manner can result in resolution of the obstruction (Nobie, 2015). When the bowel is completely obstructed, the possibility of strangulation and tissue necrosis (i.e., tissue death) warrants surgical intervention. Before surgery, IV fluids are necessary to replace the depleted water, sodium, chloride, and potassium.

Surgical Management

The surgical treatment of intestinal obstruction depends on the cause of the obstruction. For the most common causes of obstruction, such as hernia and adhesions, the surgical procedure involves repairing the hernia or dividing the adhesion to which the intestine is attached. In some instances, the portion of affected bowel may be removed and an anastomosis performed. The complexity of the surgical procedure depends on the duration of the intestinal obstruction and the condition of the intestine. Laparoscopy has become increasingly common because it can facilitate diagnosis and is easily converted to open laparotomy if warranted (Nobie, 2015).

Nursing Management

Nursing management of the patient with a small bowel obstruction who does not require surgery includes maintaining the function of the NG tube, assessing and measuring the NG output, assessing for fluid and electrolyte imbalance, monitoring nutritional status, and assessing for manifestations consistent with resolution (e.g., return of normal bowel sounds, decreased abdominal distention, subjective improvement in abdominal pain and tenderness, passage of flatus or stool).

> ▶ **Quality and Safety Nursing Alert**
>
> *Maintaining fluid and electrolyte balance is a priority area to monitor in the patient with a small bowel obstruction. The presence of the NG tube in conjunction with the patient's nothing-by-mouth (NPO) status place the patient at significant risk of fluid imbalance. Thus, measures to promote fluid balance are critically important.*

The nurse reports discrepancies in I&O, worsening of pain or abdominal distention, and increased NG output. If the patient's condition does not improve, the nurse prepares him or her for surgery. Nursing care of the patient after surgical repair of a small bowel obstruction is similar to that for other abdominal surgeries (see Chapter 19).

Large Bowel Obstruction

Pathophysiology

A large bowel obstruction results in an accumulation of intestinal contents, fluid, and gas proximal to the obstruction. It can lead to severe distention and perforation unless some gas and fluid can flow back through the ileocecal valve. Large bowel obstruction, even if complete, may be undramatic if the blood supply to the colon is not disturbed. However, if the blood supply is cut off, intestinal strangulation and necrosis occur; this condition is life threatening. In the large intestine, dehydration occurs more slowly than in the small intestine because the colon can absorb its fluid contents and can distend to a size considerably beyond its normal full capacity.

Adenocarcinoid tumors account for the majority of large bowel obstructions (Hopkins, 2016). Most tumors occur distal to the splenic flexure, making them accessible with a flexible sigmoidoscope.

Clinical Manifestations

Large bowel obstruction differs clinically from small bowel obstruction in that the symptoms develop and progress relatively slowly. In patients with obstruction in the sigmoid colon or the rectum, constipation may be the only symptom for weeks. The shape of the stool is altered as it passes the obstruction that is gradually increasing in size. Blood loss in the stool may result in iron deficiency anemia. The patient may experience weakness, weight loss, and anorexia. Eventually, the abdomen becomes markedly distended, loops of large bowel become visibly outlined through the abdominal wall, and the patient has crampy lower abdominal pain (Ansari, 2014; Hopkins, 2016).

Assessment and Diagnostic Findings

Diagnosis is based on symptoms and on imaging studies. Abdominal x-ray and abdominal CT or MRI findings reveal a distended colon and pinpoint the site of the obstruction (Hopkins, 2016).

Medical Management

Restoration of intravascular volume, correction of electrolyte abnormalities, and NG aspiration and decompression are instituted immediately. A colonoscopy may be performed to untwist and decompress the bowel. A cecostomy, in which a surgical opening is made into the cecum, may be performed in patients who are poor surgical risks and urgently need relief from the obstruction. The procedure provides an outlet for releasing gas and a small amount of drainage. A rectal tube may be used to decompress an area that is lower in the bowel. As an alternative, a metal colonic stent may be used as either a palliative intervention or as a bridge to definitive surgery. The colonic stent is placed endoscopically with the assistance of an image intensifier, which creates a fluoroscopic image (Hopkins, 2016). The usual treatment is surgical resection to remove the obstructing lesion. A temporary or permanent colostomy may be necessary. An ileoanal anastomosis may be performed if removal of the entire large bowel is necessary (Ansari, 2014; Hopkins, 2016).

Nursing Management

The nurse's role is to monitor the patient for symptoms indicating that the intestinal obstruction is worsening and to provide emotional support and comfort. The nurse administers IV fluids and electrolytes as prescribed. If the patient's condition does not respond to nonsurgical treatment, the nurse prepares the patient for surgery. This preparation includes preoperative education as the patient's condition indicates. After surgery, routine postoperative nursing care is provided, including abdominal wound care.

INFLAMMATORY BOWEL DISEASE

Inflammatory bowel disease (IBD) is a group of chronic disorders: Crohn's disease (i.e., regional enteritis) and ulcerative colitis that result in inflammation or ulceration (or both) of the bowel. Both disorders have striking similarities but also several differences. Table 47-5 compares Crohn's disease and ulcerative colitis.

The prevalence of IBD in the United States has increased in the past century; it is estimated that between 1 and 1.3 million Americans have an IBD (CDC, 2015a). Family history predisposes people to IBD, particularly if a first-degree relative has the disease (NIDDK, 2014f; NIDDK, 2016b). Other risk factors for IBD include being Caucasian, of Ashkenazi Jewish background, living in a northern climate, and living in an urban area (CDC, 2015a). Men are at a slightly higher risk for ulcerative colitis (NIDDK, 2014f); whereas, women are at greater risk for Crohn's disease (NIDDK, 2016b). People between the ages of 20 and 29 are at greatest risk for Crohn's disease (NIDDK, 2016b); whereas, people between the ages of 15 and 30 are at greatest risk and those older than 60 years of age are at slightly greater risk for ulcerative colitis (NIDDK, 2014f). Current smokers are at risk for Crohn's disease, but those who are ex-smokers or nonsmokers are at risk for ulcerative colitis (CDC, 2015a).

Despite extensive research, the cause of IBD is still unknown. Researchers theorize that environmental triggers (e.g., exposure to air pollutants), food, tobacco, and viral

TABLE 47-5 Comparison of Crohn's Disease and Ulcerative Colitis

	Crohn's Disease	Ulcerative Colitis
Course	Prolonged, variable	Exacerbations, remissions
Pathology		
Early	Transmural thickening	Mucosal ulceration
Late	Deep, penetrating granulomas	Minute, mucosal ulcerations
Clinical Manifestations		
Location	Ileum, ascending colon (usually)	Rectum, descending colon
Bleeding	Usually not, but if it occurs, it tends to be mild	Common—severe
Perianal involvement	Common	Rare—mild
Fistulas	Common	Rare
Diarrhea	Less severe	Severe
Abdominal mass	Common	Rare
Diagnostic Study Findings		
Barium studies	Regional, discontinuous skip lesions	Diffuse involvement
	Narrowing of colon	No narrowing of colon
	Thickening of bowel wall	No mucosal edema
	Mucosal edema	Stenosis rare
	Stenosis, fistulas	Shortening of colon
Sigmoidoscopy	May be unremarkable unless accompanied by perianal fistulas	Abnormal inflamed mucosa
Colonoscopy	Distinct ulcerations separated by relatively normal mucosa in ascending colon	Friable mucosa with pseudopolyps or ulcers in descending colon
Therapeutic Management	Corticosteroids, aminosalicylates (sulfasalazine [Azulfidine])	Corticosteroids, aminosalicylates (sulfasalazine) useful in preventing recurrence
	Immunomodulators (e.g., azathioprine [Imuran]) or monoclonal antibodies (e.g., infliximab [Remicade], adalimumab [Humira]) may be tried if refractory to corticosteroids and aminosalicylates	Immunomodulators (e.g., azathioprine [Imuran]) or monoclonal antibodies (e.g., infliximab [Remicade], adalimumab [Humira]) may be tried if refractory to corticosteroids and aminosalicylates
	Antibiotics	Bulk hydrophilic agents
	Parenteral nutrition	Antibiotics
	Partial or complete colectomy, with ileostomy or anastomosis	Proctocolectomy, with ileostomy
	Rectum can be preserved in some patients	Rectum can be preserved in only a few patients "cured" by colectomy
	Recurrence common	
Systemic Complications	Small bowel obstruction	Toxic megacolon
	Right-sided hydronephrosis	Perforation
	Nephrolithiasis	Hemorrhage
	Colon cancer	Colon cancer
	Cholelithiasis	Pyelonephritis
	Arthritis	Nephrolithiasis
	Uveitis	Cholangiocarcinoma
	Erythema nodosum	Arthritis
		Uveitis
		Erythema nodosum

Adapted from Walfish, A. E. (2016). Inflammatory bowel disease. *Merck Manual: Professional Version.* Retrieved on 12/29/2016 at: www.merckmanuals.com/professional/gastrointestinal-disorders/inflammatory-bowel-disease-ibd

illnesses in people genetically predisposed to developing an IBD can trigger the cell-mediated immune response that results in the inflammatory changes that characterize IBDs (Walfish, 2016).

Crohn's Disease (Regional Enteritis)

Crohn's disease is characterized by periods of remission and exacerbation. It is a subacute and chronic inflammation of the GI tract wall that extends through all layers (i.e., transmural lesion). Although its characteristic histopathologic changes can occur anywhere in the GI tract, it most commonly occurs in the distal ileum and the ascending colon. Approximately 35% of patients have only ileal involvement (ileitis), 45% of patients have diseased ileum and colon (ileocolitis), and 20% of patients have only colon involvement (granulomatous colitis) (Walfish, 2016).

Pathophysiology

The inflammatory process in Crohn's disease begins with crypt inflammation and abscesses, which develop into small, focal ulcers. These initial lesions then deepen into longitudinal and transverse ulcers, separated by edematous patches, creating a characteristic *cobblestone* appearance to the affected bowel. Fistulas, fissures, and abscesses form as the inflammation extends into the peritoneum. Granulomas can occur in lymph nodes, the peritoneum, and through the layers of the bowel in about half of patients. Diseased bowel segments are sharply demarcated by adjoining areas of normal bowel tissue. These are called *skip* lesions, from which the label *regional enteritis* is derived. As the disease advances, the bowel wall thickens and becomes fibrotic, and the intestinal lumen narrows. Diseased bowel loops sometimes adhere to other loops surrounding them (Smith & Harris, 2014; Walfish, 2016).

Clinical Manifestations

The onset of symptoms is usually insidious in Crohn's disease, with prominent right lower quadrant abdominal pain and diarrhea unrelieved by defecation. Scar tissue and the formation of granulomas interfere with the ability of the intestine to transport products of upper intestinal digestion through the constricted lumen, resulting in crampy abdominal pain. There is abdominal tenderness and spasm. Because eating stimulates intestinal peristalsis, the crampy pains occur after meals. To avoid these bouts of crampy pain, the patient tends to limit food intake, reducing the amounts and types of food to such a degree that normal nutritional requirements are often not met. As a result, weight loss, malnutrition, and secondary anemia occur (NIDDK, 2016b). Ulcers in the membranous lining of the intestine and other inflammatory changes result in a weeping, edematous intestine that continually empties an irritating discharge into the colon. Disrupted absorption causes chronic diarrhea and nutritional deficits. The result is a person who is thin and emaciated from inadequate food intake and constant fluid loss. In some patients, the inflamed intestine may perforate, leading to intra-abdominal and anal abscesses. Fever and leukocytosis occur. Chronic symptoms include diarrhea, abdominal pain, **steatorrhea** (i.e., excessive fat in the feces), anorexia, weight loss, and nutritional deficiencies.

Abscesses, fistulas, and fissures occur in approximately one third of patients (Smith & Harris, 2014). Manifestations may extend beyond the GI tract and can include joint disorders (e.g., arthritis), skin lesions (e.g., erythema nodosum), ocular disorders (e.g., uveitis), and oral ulcers. The clinical course and symptoms can vary; in some patients, periods of remission and exacerbation occur, but in others, the disease follows a fulminating course. When intestinal symptoms worsen, some extraintestinal manifestations can worsen, whereas the clinical course of some extraintestinal manifestations seems independent of the clinical course of the Crohn's disease (Walfish, 2016).

Assessment and Diagnostic Findings

The traditional conclusive diagnostic test for Crohn's disease was a barium study of the upper GI tract that showed a "string sign" on an x-ray image of the terminal ileum, indicating the constriction of a segment of intestine. However, this study has fallen out of favor with the introduction of improved CT scan and MRI techniques that can more accurately assess bowel and pelvic disease. CT scan can highlight bowel wall thickening and mesenteric edema, as well as obstructions, abscesses, and fistulae. Therefore, CT scan is considered more sensitive in diagnosing Crohn's disease than barium studies, and may help specify abscess formation and location, guiding percutaneous access and drainage. MRI is both highly sensitive and specific in terms of identifying pelvic and perianal abscesses and fistulae (Ghazi, 2016).

A CBC is performed to assess hematocrit and hemoglobin levels (which may be decreased) as well as the white blood cell count (may be elevated). The erythrocyte sedimentation rate (ESR) is usually elevated. Albumin and protein levels may be decreased, indicating malnutrition (Ghazi, 2016).

Complications

Complications of Crohn's disease include intestinal obstruction or stricture formation, perianal disease, fluid and electrolyte imbalances, malnutrition from malabsorption, and fistula and abscess formation. The most common type of small bowel fistula caused by Crohn's disease is the enterocutaneous fistula (i.e., an abnormal opening between the small bowel and the skin). Abscesses can be the result of an internal fistula that results in fluid accumulation and infection. Patients with colonic Crohn's disease are also at increased risk of colon cancer (NIDDK, 2016b; Walfish, 2016).

Ulcerative Colitis

Ulcerative colitis is a chronic ulcerative and inflammatory disease of the mucosal and submucosal layers of the colon and rectum that is characterized by unpredictable periods of remission and exacerbation with bouts of abdominal cramps and bloody or purulent diarrhea. The inflammatory changes typically begin in the rectum and progress proximally through the colon (Harris & Jelemensky, 2014; Walfish, 2016).

Pathophysiology

Ulcerative colitis affects the superficial mucosa of the colon and is characterized by multiple ulcerations, diffuse inflammations, and desquamation or shedding of the colonic epithelium. Bleeding occurs as a result of the ulcerations. The mucosa becomes edematous and inflamed. The lesions are contiguous, occurring one after the other. Eventually, the bowel narrows, shortens, and thickens because of muscular hypertrophy and fat deposits. Because the inflammatory process is not transmural (i.e., it affects the inner lining only), abscesses, fistulas, obstruction, and fissures are uncommon in ulcerative colitis (Harris & Jelemensky, 2014; Walfish, 2016).

Clinical Manifestations

The clinical course is usually one of exacerbations and remissions. The predominant symptoms of ulcerative colitis include diarrhea, with passage of mucus, pus, or blood; left lower quadrant abdominal pain; and intermittent tenesmus. The bleeding may be mild or severe, and pallor, anemia, and fatigue result. The patient may have anorexia, weight loss, fever, vomiting, and dehydration, as well as cramping, tenesmus, and the passage of six or more liquid stools each day. The disease is classified as mild, severe, or fulminant, depending on the severity of the symptoms. Hypoalbuminemia, electrolyte imbalances, and anemia frequently develop. Extraintestinal manifestations include skin lesions (e.g., erythema nodosum), eye lesions (e.g., uveitis), joint abnormalities (e.g., arthritis), and liver disease (Harris & Jelemensky, 2014; NIDDK, 2014f; Walfish, 2016).

Assessment and Diagnostic Findings

Abdominal x-ray studies are useful for determining the cause of symptoms. Free air in the peritoneum and bowel dilation or obstruction should be excluded as a source of the presenting symptoms. Colonoscopy is the definitive screening test that can distinguish ulcerative colitis from other diseases of the colon with similar symptoms. It may reveal friable, inflamed mucosa with exudate and ulcerations. Biopsies are typically taken to determine histologic characteristics of the colonic tissue and extent of disease. CT scanning, MRI, and ultrasound studies can identify abscesses and perirectal involvement (Basson, 2015b).

The stool is positive for blood, and laboratory test results reveal low hematocrit and hemoglobin levels in addition to an elevated white blood cell count, low albumin levels (indicating malabsorptive disorders), and an electrolyte imbalance. C-reactive protein levels are elevated. Elevated antineutrophil cytoplasmic antibody levels are common. Careful stool examination for parasites and other microbes is performed to rule out dysentery caused by common intestinal organisms, especially *Entamoeba histolytica*, *C. difficile* and *Campylobacter*, *Salmonella*, *Shigella*, and *Cryptospora species* (Basson, 2015b).

Complications

Complications of ulcerative colitis include toxic megacolon, perforation, and bleeding as a result of ulceration, vascular engorgement, and highly vascular granulation tissue. In toxic megacolon, the inflammatory process extends into the muscularis, inhibiting its ability to contract and resulting in colonic distention. Symptoms include fever, abdominal pain and distention, vomiting, and fatigue. If the patient with toxic megacolon does not respond within 72 hours to medical management with NG suction, IV fluids with electrolytes, corticosteroids, and antibiotics, surgery is required. A subtotal colectomy may be performed if bowel perforation has not occurred. Otherwise, colectomy is indicated; it is ultimately needed in up to one third of patients with severe ulcerative colitis (Walfish, 2016). For many patients, surgery becomes necessary to relieve the effects of the disease and to treat these serious complications; an ileostomy usually is performed. The surgical procedures involved and the care of patients with this type of fecal diversion are discussed later in this chapter.

Patients with ulcerative colitis also have a significantly increased risk of osteoporotic fractures due to decreased bone mineral density. Corticosteroid therapy may also contribute to the diminished bone density. Patients with ulcerative colitis area are also at increased risk for colon cancer. It is estimated that 20 years post diagnosis, approximately 7% to 10% of patients with extensive ulcerative colitis (i.e., not contained to the rectum) will have colon cancer (Walfish, 2016).

Medical Management of Chronic Inflammatory Bowel Disease

Medical treatment for both Crohn's disease and ulcerative colitis is aimed at reducing inflammation, suppressing inappropriate immune responses, providing rest for a diseased bowel so that healing may take place, improving quality of life, and preventing or minimizing complications. Most patients have long periods of well-being interspersed with short intervals of illness. Management depends on the disease location, severity, and complications (Harris & Jelemensky, 2014; Smith & Harris, 2014; Walfish, 2016).

Nutritional Therapy

Oral fluids and a low-residue, high-protein, high-calorie diet with supplemental vitamin therapy and iron replacement are prescribed to meet nutritional needs, reduce inflammation, and control pain and diarrhea. Fluid and electrolyte imbalances from dehydration caused by diarrhea are corrected by IV therapy as necessary if the patient is hospitalized or by oral fluids if the patient is managed at home. Any foods that exacerbate diarrhea are avoided. Milk may contribute to diarrhea in those with lactose intolerance. Cold foods and smoking are avoided because both increase intestinal motility. Parenteral nutrition may be indicated (see Chapter 44).

Pharmacologic Therapy

Sedatives and antidiarrheal and antiperistaltic medications are used to minimize peristalsis in order to rest the inflamed bowel. They are continued until the patient's stools approach normal frequency and consistency.

Aminosalicylates such as sulfasalazine (Azulfidine) are often effective for mild or moderate inflammation and are used to prevent or reduce recurrences in long-term maintenance regimens. Sulfa-free aminosalicylates (e.g., mesalamine [Asacol, Pentasa]) are effective in preventing and treating recurrence of inflammation. Antibiotics (e.g., metronidazole [Flagyl]) are used for complications such as abscesses or fistula formation (Walfish, 2016).

Corticosteroids are used to treat severe and fulminant disease and can be given orally (e.g., prednisone) in outpatient treatment or parenterally (e.g., hydrocortisone [Solu-Cortef]) in hospitalized patients. Topical (i.e., rectal administration) corticosteroids (e.g., budesonide [Entocort]) are also widely used in the treatment of distal colon disease. When the dosage of corticosteroids is reduced or stopped, the symptoms of disease may return. If corticosteroids are continued, numerous adverse sequelae may ensue; these are discussed in Chapter 52 and summarized in Table 52-5 (Walfish, 2016).

Immunomodulators (e.g., azathioprine [Imuran], mercaptopurine [6-MP], methotrexate [MTX], cyclosporine [Neoral]) have been used to alter the immune response. The exact mechanism of action of these medications in treating IBD is unknown. They are used in patients with severe disease who have not responded favorably to other therapies. These medications are useful in maintenance regimens to prevent relapses (Walfish, 2016). Newer biologic therapies incorporate monoclonal antibodies, including infliximab (Remicade), adalimumab (Humira), certolizumab pegol (Cimzia), and natalizumab (Tysabri) for treating Crohn's disease (Walfish, 2016) and infliximab and adalimumab for treating ulcerative colitis (Walfish, 2016). Clinical outcomes for the biologic therapies are promising, although adverse effects may seriously limit their usefulness. A major issue associated with appropriate pharmacologic treatment of IBD is nonadherence. Patients who are nonadherent may suffer a greater chance of disease relapse with severe associated symptoms.

Surgical Management

When nonsurgical measures fail to relieve severe symptoms of IBD, surgery may be necessary. Nearly one third of patients with severe ulcerative colitis and between 60% and 70% of patients with Crohn's disease require surgery (NIDDK, 2016b; Walfish, 2016). Common indications for surgery in patients with ulcerative colitis include the presence of colon cancer or colonic dysplasia/polyps (see later discussion); megacolon; severe, intractable bleeding; or perforation (NIDDK, 2014f; Walfish, 2016). Common indications for surgery in patients with Crohn's disease include recurrent partial intestinal obstructions; complete intestinal obstructions; intractable fistulas; or intractable abscesses (NIDDK, 2016b; Smith & Harris, 2014; Walfish, 2016). Furthermore, patients with either ulcerative colitis or Crohn's disease may require surgery to relieve strictures, or to correct underlying pathology in disease not responsive to long-term use of corticosteroids (NIDDK, 2014f; NIDDK, 2016b; Walfish, 2016). For the patient with ulcerative colitis, if the surgery is a proctocolectomy, which is removal of the rectum and colon, the surgery cures the disease (NIDDK, 2014f). Surgical cure is not possible with Crohn's disease, however; nearly 50% of patients with Crohn's disease who require surgical intervention will eventually require additional future surgery (Walfish, 2016).

A common procedure performed for strictures of the small intestines is laparoscope-guided strictureplasty, in which blocked or narrowed sections of the intestines are widened, leaving the intestines intact. In some cases, a small bowel resection is performed; diseased segments of the small intestines are resected, and the remaining portions of the intestines are anastomosed. Surgical removal of up to 50% of the small bowel usually can be tolerated.

A newer surgical procedure developed for patients with severe Crohn's disease is intestinal transplant. This technique is now available to children and to young and middle-aged adults who have lost intestinal function from disease. It may provide improvement in quality of life for some patients. The associated technical and immunologic problems remain formidable, and the costs and mortality rates continue to be high (Dunn, Greenstein, Prowse, et al., 2014).

Proctocolectomy with ileostomy (i.e., complete excision of colon, rectum, and anus) is recommended in patients with severe ulcerative colitis refractory to medical therapy with a severely diseased rectum. If the rectum can be preserved, restorative proctocolectomy with ileal pouch anal anastomosis (IPAA) is the procedure of choice for ulcerative colitis. Although complications following IPAA may occur, quality of life is generally good to excellent (Fazio, Kiran, Remzi, et al., 2013; Francone & Champagne, 2013).

Other types of surgical procedures, also known as fecal diversions, are discussed later in this chapter (see Colorectal Cancer: Surgical Management).

Total Colectomy With Ileostomy

An ileostomy is commonly performed after a total colectomy (i.e., excision of the entire colon) and is either temporary (see next section on restorative proctocolectomy with IPAA) or, less commonly, permanent. It allows for drainage of fecal matter (i.e., effluent) from the ileum to the outside of the body. The drainage is liquid to unformed and occurs at frequent intervals. Nursing management of the patient with an ileostomy is discussed later in this chapter.

Restorative Proctocolectomy With Ileal Pouch Anal Anastomosis

A restorative proctocolectomy with IPAA is the surgical procedure of choice in cases where the rectum can be preserved because it eliminates the need for a permanent ileostomy. It establishes an ileal reservoir that functions as a "new" rectum, and anal sphincter control of elimination is retained. The procedure involves connecting the ileum to the anal pouch (made from a small intestine segment), and the surgeon connects the pouch to the anus in conjunction with removing the colon and the rectal mucosa (i.e., total abdominal colectomy and mucosal proctectomy) (see Fig. 47-6). A temporary diverting loop ileostomy that promotes healing of the surgical

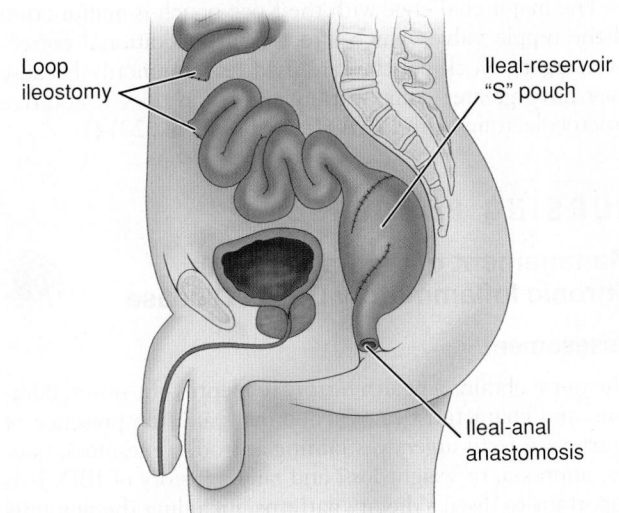

Figure 47-6 • A mucosal proctectomy precedes anastomosis of the ileal reservoir. A temporary loop ileostomy diverts effluent for several months to allow healing.

anastomoses is constructed at the time of surgery and closed about 3 months later (Francone & Champagne, 2013).

With IPAA or restorative proctocolectomy, the diseased colon and rectum are removed, voluntary defecation is maintained, and anal continence is preserved. The ileal reservoir decreases the number of bowel movements significantly. Nighttime elimination is gradually reduced to one bowel movement. Complications of ileoanal anastomosis include irritation of the perianal skin from leakage of fecal contents, stricture formation at the anastomosis site, small bowel obstruction, and "pouchitis" (inflammation of the ileoanal pouch due to altered microbial levels) (Francone & Champagne, 2013). For patients with IBD history, dietary intolerances may persist after the IPAA is formed. Increased stool output, flatulence, and perineal irritation are associated with consumption of nuts, corn, chocolate, spicy foods, onions, and citrus fruits. Consequently, some patients may need to alter their diet to avoid complications and perineal breakdown (Perrin, 2013) (see later discussion under Surgical Management in the Colorectal Cancer section).

Continent Ileostomy

A surgical procedure that is rarely performed involves the creation of a continent ileal reservoir (i.e., Kock pouch) by diverting a portion of the distal ileum to the abdominal wall and creating a stoma. This procedure eliminates the need for an external fecal collection bag. Approximately 30 cm (11 inches) of the distal ileum is reconstructed to form a reservoir with a nipple valve that is created by pulling a portion of the terminal ileal loop back into the ileum. GI effluent can accumulate in the pouch for several hours and then be removed by means of a catheter inserted through the nipple valve. In many patients, a total colectomy is also performed with the Kock pouch. Possible indications for a total colectomy with Kock pouch placement (rather than a restorative proctocolectomy with IPAA) include a badly diseased rectum, lack of rectal sphincter tone, or inability to achieve fecal continence post IPAA (Crawshaw, Williams, & Woodhouse, 2014).

The major challenge with the Kock pouch is malfunction of the nipple valve, which often requires additional corrective surgery. Kock pouches are used less commonly because they have greater complication rates than does restorative proctocolectomy with IPAA (Crawshaw et al., 2014).

NURSING PROCESS

Management of the Patient With Chronic Inflammatory Bowel Disease

Assessment

The nurse obtains a health history to identify the onset, duration, and characteristics of abdominal pain; the presence of diarrhea or fecal urgency, straining at stool (tenesmus), nausea, anorexia, or weight loss; and family history of IBD. It is important to discuss dietary patterns, including the amounts of alcohol, caffeine, and nicotine-containing products used daily and weekly. The nurse asks about patterns of bowel elimination, including character, frequency, and presence of blood, pus, fat, or mucus. Allergies and food intolerance, especially milk (lactose) intolerance, must be noted. The patient may identify sleep disturbances if diarrhea or pain occurs at night.

Diagnosis

NURSING DIAGNOSES

Based on the assessment data, nursing diagnoses may include the following:

- Diarrhea related to the inflammatory process
- Acute pain related to increased peristalsis and GI inflammation
- Deficient fluid volume related to anorexia, nausea, and diarrhea
- Imbalanced nutrition: less than body requirements related to dietary restrictions, nausea, and malabsorption
- Activity intolerance related to generalized weakness
- Anxiety related to impending surgery
- Ineffective coping related to repeated episodes of diarrhea
- Risk for impaired skin integrity related to malnutrition and diarrhea
- Deficient knowledge concerning the process and management of the disease

COLLABORATIVE PROBLEMS/POTENTIAL COMPLICATIONS

Potential complications may include the following:

- Electrolyte imbalance
- Cardiac dysrhythmias related to electrolyte imbalances
- GI bleeding with fluid volume loss
- Perforation of the bowel

Planning and Goals

The major goals for the patient include attainment of normal bowel elimination patterns, relief of abdominal pain and cramping, prevention of fluid volume deficit, maintenance of optimal nutrition and weight, avoidance of fatigue, reduction of anxiety, promotion of effective coping, absence of skin breakdown, increased knowledge about the disease process and self-health management, and avoidance of complications.

Nursing Interventions

MAINTAINING NORMAL ELIMINATION PATTERNS

The nurse assists the patient in determining if there is a relationship between diarrhea and certain foods, activities, or emotional stressors. Identifying precipitating factors, the frequency of bowel movements, and the character, consistency, and amount of stool passed is important. The nurse provides ready access to a bathroom, commode, or bedpan and keeps the environment clean and odor free. It is important to administer antidiarrheal medications as prescribed. Loperamide may be prescribed 30 minutes before meals (see previous discussion on interventions for diarrhea). The nurse should record the frequency and consistency of stools after therapy is initiated.

RELIEVING PAIN

The character of the pain is described as dull, burning, or crampy. It is important to ask about its onset. Does it occur before or after meals, during the night, or before elimination? Is the pattern constant or intermittent? Is it relieved with medications? The nurse administers analgesic agents as prescribed for pain. Position changes, local application of heat (as prescribed), diversional activities, and prevention of fatigue also are helpful for reducing pain.

MAINTAINING FLUID INTAKE

To detect fluid volume deficit, the nurse keeps an accurate record of I&O. The nurse monitors daily weights for fluid gains or losses and assesses the patient for signs of fluid volume deficit (i.e., dry skin and mucous membranes, decreased skin turgor, oliguria, fatigue, decreased temperature, increased hematocrit, elevated urine specific gravity, and hypotension). It is important to encourage oral intake of fluids and to monitor the flow rate of any IV fluids. The nurse initiates measures to decrease diarrhea (e.g., dietary restrictions, stress reduction, antidiarrheal agents).

MAINTAINING OPTIMAL NUTRITION

Parenteral nutrition is indicated in patients who have Crohn's disease with severe malnutrition and intolerance to enteral nutrition and who are expected to likely remain intolerant to enteral nutrition for more than 1 to 2 weeks (Smith & Harris, 2014). With parenteral nutrition, the nurse maintains an accurate record of fluid I&O as well as the daily weight. The patient should gain 0.5 kg (1.1 lb) daily during parenteral nutrition therapy. Because parenteral nutrition is very high in glucose and can cause hyperglycemia, blood glucose levels are monitored every 6 hours. Once the symptoms of any exacerbation have diminished and the patient has gained or stabilized weight, parenteral nutrition is stopped and the patient is advanced on oral elemental feedings. Elemental feedings are high in protein and low in fat and residue. They are digested primarily in the jejunum, do not stimulate intestinal secretions, and allow the bowel to continue to rest. The nurse notes intolerance if the patient exhibits nausea, vomiting, diarrhea, or abdominal distention. See Chapter 44 for further discussion of enteral and parenteral nutrition.

If oral foods are tolerated, small, frequent, low-residue feedings are given to avoid overdistending the stomach and stimulating peristalsis. The patient must restrict activity to conserve energy, reduce peristalsis, and reduce caloric requirements.

PROMOTING REST

The nurse recommends intermittent rest periods during the day and schedules or restricts activities to conserve energy and reduce the metabolic rate. It is important to encourage activity within the limits of the patient's capacity. The nurse suggests naps and periods of bed rest for a patient who is febrile, has frequent diarrheal stools, or is bleeding. However, the patient should perform active exercises to maintain muscle tone and prevent venous thromboembolic complications. If the patient cannot perform these active exercises, the nurse performs passive exercises and joint range of motion. Activity restrictions are modified as needed on a day-to-day basis.

REDUCING ANXIETY

Rapport can be established by being attentive and displaying a calm, confident manner. The nurse allows time for the patient to ask questions and express feelings. Careful listening and sensitivity to nonverbal indicators of anxiety (e.g., restlessness, tense facial expressions) are helpful. The patient may be emotionally labile because of the consequences of the disease and the uncertainty of exacerbations with complications. The nurse tailors information about possible impending surgery to the patient's level of understanding and desire for detail. If surgery is planned, pictures, illustrations, websites, and blogs help explain the surgical procedure and help the patient visualize what a stoma looks like.

ENHANCING COPING MEASURES

Because the patient may feel isolated, helpless, and out of control, understanding and emotional support are essential. The patient may respond to stress in a variety of ways that may alienate others (e.g., anger, denial, social self-isolation).

The nurse needs to recognize that the patient's behavior may be affected by a number of factors. Any patient suffering the discomforts of frequent bowel movements and rectal soreness is anxious, discouraged, and unhappy. It is important to develop a relationship with the patient that supports their attempts to cope with these stressors. It is also important to communicate that the patient's feelings are understood by encouraging the patient to talk and express their feelings and to discuss any concerns. Stress reduction measures that may be used include relaxation techniques, visualization, breathing exercises, and biofeedback. Professional counseling may be needed to help the patient and family manage issues associated with chronic illness and resulting disability.

PREVENTING SKIN BREAKDOWN

The nurse examines the patient's skin frequently, especially the perianal skin. Perianal care, including the use of a skin barrier (e.g., petroleum ointment [Vaseline]), is important after each bowel movement. The nurse gives immediate attention to reddened or irritated areas over bony prominences and uses pressure-relieving devices to prevent skin breakdown. Consultation with a wound-ostomy-continence (WOC) nurse (or WOCN; a nurse specially educated in the management of a variety of fecal and urinary diversions) is often helpful.

MONITORING AND MANAGING POTENTIAL COMPLICATIONS

Serum electrolyte levels are monitored daily, and electrolyte replacements are given as prescribed. Evidence of dysrhythmias or changes in level of consciousness must be reported immediately.

The nurse closely monitors rectal bleeding and administers blood component therapy and volume expanders as prescribed to prevent hypovolemia. It is important to monitor the blood pressure for hypotension and to obtain coagulation profiles and hemoglobin and hematocrit levels frequently. Vitamin K may be prescribed to increase clotting factors.

The nurse closely monitors the patient for indications of perforation (i.e., acute increase in abdominal pain, rigid abdomen, vomiting, or hypotension) and obstruction and toxic megacolon (i.e., abdominal distention, decreased or absent bowel sounds, change in mental status, fever, tachycardia, hypotension, dehydration, and electrolyte imbalances).

PROMOTING HOME, COMMUNITY-BASED, AND TRANSITIONAL CARE

Educating Patients About Self-Care. The nurse assesses the patient's understanding of the disease process and their need for additional information about medical management (e.g., medications, diet) and surgical interventions. The nurse provides information about nutritional management; a bland, low-residue, high-protein, high-calorie, and high-vitamin diet relieves symptoms and decreases diarrhea. It is important to explain the rationale for the use of corticosteroids and anti-inflammatory, antibacterial, and antidiarrheal medications. The nurse emphasizes the importance of taking medications as prescribed and not abruptly discontinuing them (especially corticosteroids) to avoid development of serious medical problems (see Chart 47-6). The nurse reviews ileostomy care as necessary (see Nursing Management of the Patient Requiring an Ostomy section). Patient education information can be obtained from the Crohn's and Colitis Foundation of America (CCFA) and from a patient skills education program developed by the American College of Surgeons (see Resources section).

Continuing and Transitional Care. Patients with chronic IBD are managed at home with follow-up care by their primary provider or through an outpatient clinic. Those whose nutritional status is compromised and who are receiving parenteral nutrition need the home care or transitional care nurse to consult and ensure that their nutritional requirements are being met and that they or their caregivers can follow through with the instructions for parenteral nutrition. Patients who are undergoing medical treatment need to understand that their disease can be controlled and that they can lead a healthy life between exacerbations. Control implies management based on an understanding of the disease and its treatment. Patients in the home or transitional setting need information about their medications (i.e., name, dose, side effects, and frequency of administration) and need to take medications on schedule. Medication reminders such as containers that separate pills according to day and time or daily checklists are helpful.

During a flare-up, the nurse encourages the patient to rest as needed and to modify activities according to their energy level. Patients should limit tasks that impose strain on the lower abdominal muscles. They should sleep in a room close to the bathroom because of the frequent diarrhea; quick access to a toilet helps alleviate worry about having an "accident." Room deodorizers help control odors.

Dietary modifications can control but do not cure the disease; the nurse recommends a low-residue, high-protein, high-calorie diet, especially during an acute phase. It is important to encourage the patient to keep a record of the foods that irritate the bowel and to avoid them and to drink at least eight glasses of water each day.

The prolonged nature of the disease has an impact on the patient and often strains their family life and financial resources. Family support is vital; however, some family members may be resentful or feel guilty, tired, or unable to cope with the emotional demands of the illness and the physical demands of providing care. Some patients with IBD do not socialize for fear of being embarrassed. Because they have lost control over elimination, they may fear losing control over other aspects of their lives. They need time to express their fears and frustrations. Individual and family counseling may be helpful.

Evaluation

Expected patient outcomes may include:

1. Reports a decrease in the frequency of diarrheal stools
   a. Adheres to dietary restrictions; maintains bed rest
   b. Takes medications as prescribed
2. Has reduced pain
3. Maintains fluid volume balance
   a. Drinks 1 to 2 L of oral fluids daily
   b. Has normal body temperature
   c. Displays adequate skin turgor and moist mucous membranes
4. Attains optimal nutrition; tolerates small, frequent feedings without diarrhea
5. Avoids fatigue
   a. Rests periodically during the day
   b. Adheres to activity restrictions
6. Is less anxious
   a. Seeks emotional support as appropriate
   b. Verbalizes fewer feelings of anxiety and concern
7. Copes successfully with diagnosis
   a. Verbalizes feelings freely
   b. Uses appropriate stress reduction behaviors
8. Maintains skin integrity
   a. Cleans perianal skin after defecation
   b. Uses appropriate skin barrier
9. Acquires an understanding of the disease process
   a. Modifies diet appropriately to decrease diarrhea
   b. Adheres to medication regimen as prescribed
10. Recovers without complications
    a. Electrolytes within normal ranges
    b. Normal sinus or baseline cardiac rhythm
    c. Maintains fluid balance
    d. Experiences no perforation or rectal bleeding

NURSING MANAGEMENT OF THE PATIENT REQUIRING AN OSTOMY

Nearly 100,000 patients have surgery to create fecal diversions in the United States annually. Common indications for these include not only IBD and diverticulitis, but also advanced colorectal cancer (see later discussion) (Hendren, Hammon, Glasgow, et al., 2015). Fecal diversions may be either ileostomies or colostomies, both of which may be permanent or temporary. An **ileostomy** is the surgical creation of an opening into the ileum or small intestine. A **colostomy** is the surgical opening into the colon by means of a stoma to allow drainage of contents of the colon. The Plan of Nursing Care summarizes care for the patient requiring an ostomy (see Chart 47-7).

Providing Preoperative Care

A period of preparation with replacement of fluid, blood, and protein is necessary prior to surgery. Antibiotics may be prescribed. If the patient has been taking corticosteroids (i.e., to treat IBD), they will be continued during the surgical phase to prevent steroid-induced adrenal insufficiency. Usually, the patient is given a low-residue diet, provided in frequent, small feedings. All other preoperative measures are similar to those for general abdominal surgery. The abdomen is marked for the proper placement of

---

Chart 47-6 | **HOME CARE CHECKLIST**
The Patient with Inflammatory Bowel Disease

At the completion of education, the patient and/or caregiver will be able to:

- State the impact of inflammatory bowel disease on physiologic functioning, ADLs, IADLs, roles, relationships, and spirituality.
- Discuss nutritional management: bland, low-residue, high-protein, high-vitamin diet; identify foods to include and foods to be avoided.
- Explain the importance of and necessity for adherence with prescribed medication regimen.
- Demonstrate methods of keeping track of the medication regimen, storing the prescribed medications, and using reminders such as beepers and/or pillboxes.
- State the name, dose, side effects, frequency, and schedule for all medications.
- Identify measures to be used to treat exacerbation of symptoms, to include rest, dietary modifications, and medications.
- Identify measures to be used to promote fluid and electrolyte balance during acute exacerbations.

- Demonstrate management of parenteral nutrition therapy, if applicable; identify possible complications and interventions.
- State how to reach primary provider with questions or complications.
- State time and date of follow-up appointments, testing.
- Verbalize ways to cope with stress successfully, plans for regular exercise, and rationale for obtaining adequate rest.
- Identify the need for health promotion (e.g., cessation of use of tobacco products, alcohol avoidance), disease prevention and screening activities.

Resources

See Chapter 44 for Digestive and Gastrointestinal Treatment Modalities and Chart 44-8 The Older Adult Patient and Home Parenteral and Enteral Nutrition.

ADL, activities of daily living; IADL, independent activities of daily living.

Chart 47-7 PLAN OF NURSING CARE
The Patient Undergoing Ostomy Surgery

NURSING DIAGNOSIS: Deficient knowledge about the surgical procedure and preoperative preparation
GOAL: Understands the surgical process and the necessary preoperative preparations

Nursing Interventions	Rationale	Expected Outcomes
Preoperative Care 1. Ascertain whether the patient has had a previous surgical experience, and ask for recollections of positive and negative impressions. 2. Determine what information the surgeon gave the patient and family and whether it was understood. Clarify and elaborate as necessary. Determine whether the stoma is permanent or temporary. Be aware of the patient's prognosis if carcinoma exists. 3. Use pictures, drawings, or websites to illustrate the location and appearance of the surgical wounds (abdominal, perineal) and the stoma if the patient is receptive. 4. Explain that oral/parenteral antimicrobial agents will be given to cleanse the bowel preoperatively. Mechanical cleansing may also be required. 5. Assist the patient during nasogastric/nasoenteric intubation, if indicated. Measure drainage from the tube.	1. Fear of a repeated negative experience increases anxiety. Talking about the experience with a nurse helps clarify misconceptions and helps the patient ventilate any repressed emotions. Positive experiences are reinforced. 2. Clarification prevents misunderstandings and alleviates anxiety. 3. Knowledge, for some, alleviates anxiety because fear of the unknown is decreased. Others choose not to know because it makes them more anxious. 4. Antimicrobial agents and mechanical cleansing (e.g., laxatives, enemas) reduce intestinal bacterial flora. 5. Nasoenteral intubation is used for decompression and drainage of GI contents before surgery.	• Expresses anxieties and fears about the surgical process • Projects a positive attitude toward the surgical procedure • Repeats in own words information given by the surgeon • Identifies normal anatomy and physiology of gastrointestinal (GI) tract and how it will be altered; can point to expected location of abdominal wound and stoma; describes stoma appearance and size • Adheres to "bowel prep" regimen of antimicrobial agents or mechanical cleansing • Tolerates the presence of nasogastric/nasoenteric tube, if present

NURSING DIAGNOSIS: Disturbed body image
GOAL: Attainment of a positive self-concept

Nursing Interventions	Rationale	Expected Outcomes
1. Encourage the patient to verbalize feelings about the stoma. Offer to be present when the stoma is first viewed and touched. 2. Suggest that the spouse or significant other view the stoma. 3. Offer counseling, if desired. 4. Arrange for a visit, phone call, or online chat with another patient with a stoma.	1. Free expression of feelings allows the patient the opportunity to verbalize and identify concerns. Expressed concerns can be therapeutically addressed by health care team members. 2. Helps patient to overcome fears about the response of significant other. 3. Provides opportunity for additional support. 4. People with stomas can offer support and share mutual feelings and experiences.	• Freely expresses concerns and fears • Accepts support • Seeks help as needed • States is willing to talk with another patient with a stoma or participate in support groups or blog sites

NURSING DIAGNOSIS: Anxiety related to the loss of bowel control
GOAL: Reduction of anxiety

Nursing Interventions	Rationale	Expected Outcomes
Postoperative Care 1. Provide information about expected bowel function: a. Characteristics of effluent b. Frequency of discharge	1. Emotional adjustment is facilitated if adequate information is provided at the level of the learner.	• Expresses interest in learning about altered bowel function • Handles equipment correctly • Changes the appliance unassisted • Irrigates colostomy successfully, if indicated • Progresses toward a regular schedule of elimination

(continued on page 1338)

Chart 47-7

PLAN OF NURSING CARE (Continued)

The Patient Undergoing Ostomy Surgery

Nursing Interventions	Rationale	Expected Outcomes

2. Explain how to prepare the appliance for an adequate fit.
  a. Choose the drainage appliance that will provide a secure fit around the stoma. Measure the stoma size with a measuring guide provided by the ostomy equipment manufacturer and compare with the opening on the pouch. The barrier opening should be sized to "hug" the stoma and cover the peristomal skin; wafer barriers can be pulled or molded to the size of the stoma.
  b. Remove any plastic covering that protects the appliance adhesive. *Note:* The pouch is applied by pressing the adhesive for 30 seconds to the skin barrier.
3. Demonstrate how to change the appliance or empty the pouch before leakage occurs. Be aware that the older adult may have diminished vision and difficulty handling equipment.
4. If appropriate, demonstrate how to irrigate the colostomy (usually on the 4th or 5th day). Recommend that irrigation be performed at a consistent time, depending on the type of colostomy.
	2. Adequate fit is necessary for successful use of the appliance.
	  a. The appliance opening should be larger than the stoma for an adequate fit. Available brands come in different sizes to fit the stoma. Adjustments are made as necessary.
	
	  b. The appliance is ready to apply directly to the skin or skin protector.
	
	3. Manipulation of the appliance is a learned motor skill that requires practice and positive reinforcement.
	
	4. Colostomy irrigation is used to regulate the passage of fecal material; alternatively, the bowel can be allowed to evacuate naturally. Irrigation is not routinely indicated.	

NURSING DIAGNOSIS: Risk for impaired skin integrity related to irritation of the peristomal skin by the effluent
GOAL: Maintenance of skin integrity

Nursing Interventions	Rationale	Expected Outcomes
1. Provide information about signs and symptoms of irritated or inflamed skin. Use pictures if possible. 2. Instruct patient how to cleanse the peristomal skin gently. 3. Demonstrate how to apply a skin barrier (e.g., wafer). 4. Demonstrate how to remove the pouch.	1. Peristomal skin should be slightly pink without abrasions and similar to that of the entire abdomen. 2. Mild friction with warm water and a gentle soap cleanses the skin and minimizes irritation and possible abrasions. After rinsing the soap, patting the skin dry prevents tissue trauma. 3. Skin barriers protect the peristomal skin from enzymes and bacteria. 4. Gently separate adhesive from the skin to avoid irritation. Never pull!	• Describes appearance of healthy skin • Correctly cleanses the skin • Successfully applies a skin barrier • Gently removes the drainage appliance without skin damage • Demonstrates intact skin around the stoma

NURSING DIAGNOSIS: Imbalanced nutrition: less than body requirements related to avoidance of foods that may cause GI discomfort
GOAL: Achievement of an optimal nutritional intake

Nursing Interventions	Rationale	Expected Outcomes
1. Conduct a complete nutritional assessment to identify any foods that may increase peristalsis by irritating the bowel. 2. Advise the patient to avoid food products with a cellulose or hemicellulose base (nuts, seeds). 3. Recommend moderation in intake of certain irritating fruits such as prunes, grapes, and bananas.	1. Patients react differently to certain foods because of individual sensitivity. 2. Cellulose food products are the nondigestible residue of plant foods. They hold water, provide bulk, and stimulate elimination. 3. These fruits tend to increase the quantity of effluent.	• Modifies diet to avoid offensive foods yet maintains adequate nutritional intake • Avoids cellulose-based foods, such as peanuts • Modifies intake of certain fruits

Chart 47-7

PLAN OF NURSING CARE (Continued)
The Patient Undergoing Ostomy Surgery

NURSING DIAGNOSIS: Sexual dysfunction related to altered body image
GOAL: Attainment of satisfactory sexual performance

Nursing Interventions	Rationale	Expected Outcomes
1. Encourage the patient to verbalize concerns and fears. The sexual partner is welcomed to participate in the discussion. 2. Recommend alternative sexual positions. 3. Seek assistance from a sexual therapist or wound-ostomy-continence nurse.	1. Expressed needs help to develop a plan of care. 2. Avoids patient embarrassment with the visual appearance of the stoma. Avoids peristomal skin irritation or stomal trauma secondary to friction. 3. Some patients may benefit from professional sexual counseling.	• Expresses fears and concerns • Discusses alternative sexual positions • Accepts services of a professional counselor

NURSING DIAGNOSIS: Risk for deficient fluid volume related to anorexia and vomiting and increased loss of fluids and electrolytes from GI tract
GOAL: Attainment of fluid balance

Nursing Interventions	Rationale	Expected Outcomes

1. Estimate fluid intake and output (I&O):
  a. Record I&O
 	
  b. Daily weights
 	
2. Assess serum and urinary values of sodium and potassium.
 	
3. Observe and record skin turgor and the appearance of the tongue.
	1. Provides indication of fluid balance
	  a. An early indicator of fluid imbalance is a daily, significant difference between I&O. The average person ingests (food, fluids) and loses (from urine, feces, lungs) about 2 L of fluid every 24 hours.
	  b. A gain/loss of 1 L of fluid is reflected in a body weight change of 1 kg (2.2 lb).
	2. Sodium is the major electrolyte regulating water balance. Vomiting results in decreased urinary and serum sodium levels. Urinary sodium values, in contrast to serum values, reflect early, sensitive changes in sodium balance. Sodium works in conjunction with potassium, which is also decreased with vomiting. A significant deficiency in potassium is associated with a decrease in intracellular potassium bicarbonate, which leads to acidosis and compensatory hyperventilation.
	3. Adequate hydration is reflected by the skin's ability to return to its normal shape after being grasped between the fingers. *Note:* In the older person, it is normal for the return to be delayed. Changes in the mucous membrane covering the tongue are accurate and early indicators of hydration status.
		• Maintains fluid balance
		• Maintains normal serum and urinary values for sodium and potassium
		• Normal skin turgor
		• Surface of tongue is pink, with a moist mucous membrane.

the stoma by the surgeon or the WOC nurse (Hendren et al., 2015). Care is taken to ensure that the stoma is conveniently placed—for instance, ileostomy stomas are usually placed in the right lower quadrant about 5 cm (2 inches) below the waist, in an area away from previous scars, bony prominences, skin folds, or fistulas. The stoma site must be visible to the patient.

The patient must have a thorough understanding of the surgery to be performed and what to expect after surgery.

Preoperative education ideally should be delivered by a WOC nurse and include information about the ostomy by means of written materials, models, websites, and discussion. Preoperative education should also include management of drainage from the stoma; the nature of drainage; an introduction to use of common stoma appliances; and the need for NG intubation, parenteral fluids, and possibly perineal packing (Hendren et al., 2015).

Providing Postoperative Care

General abdominal surgery care is required. As with other patients undergoing abdominal surgery, the nurse encourages those with an ostomy to engage in early ambulation. It is important to administer prescribed pain medications as required. The nurse observes the stoma for color and size. It should be pink to bright red and shiny. Typically, a temporary clear or transparent plastic bag (i.e., appliance or pouch) with an adhesive facing is placed over the ostomy in the operating room and firmly pressed onto the surrounding skin. The nurse monitors the ostomy for fecal drainage, which should begin about 24 to 48 hours after surgery for an ileostomy and within 3 to 6 days after surgery for a colostomy.

The drainage from an ileostomy is a continuous liquid from the small intestine because the stoma does not have a controlling sphincter. The contents drain into the pouch and are thus kept from coming into contact with the skin. They are collected, measured, and discarded when the pouch becomes full. If a continent ileal reservoir was created, as described for the Kock pouch, continuous drainage is provided by an indwelling reservoir catheter for 2 to 3 weeks after surgery. This allows the suture lines to heal. Stool drainage from transverse colostomies may be soft and unformed; whereas, stool from descending and sigmoid colostomies is more solid (see Fig. 47-7).

Because patients lose large fluid volumes in the early postoperative period, an accurate record of fluid I&O, including fecal discharge, is necessary to help gauge each patient's fluid needs. There may be 1,000 to 2,000 mL of fluid lost each day in addition to expected fluid loss through urine, perspiration, respiration, and other sources. With this loss, sodium and potassium are depleted. The nurse monitors laboratory values and administers electrolyte replacements as prescribed. Fluids are given IV for 4 to 5 days to replace lost fluids.

NG suction may be a part of the immediate postoperative care, with the tube requiring frequent irrigation, as prescribed. The purpose of NG suction is to prevent a buildup of gastric contents while the intestines are not functioning. After the tube is removed, the nurse offers sips of clear liquids and gradually progresses the diet. Nausea and abdominal distention, which may indicate intestinal obstruction, must be reported immediately.

If rectal packing has been used, it is removed by the end of the first week. Because this procedure may be uncomfortable, the nurse may administer an analgesic agent an hour before the removal. After the packing is removed, the perineum is irrigated two or three times daily until full healing takes place.

Providing Emotional Support

The patient may think that everyone is aware of the ostomy and may view the stoma as a mutilation compared with other abdominal incisions that heal and are hidden. Because there is loss of a body part and a major change in anatomy and function, the patient often goes through the phases of grief—denial, anger, bargaining, depression, and acceptance. Nursing support through these phases is important, and understanding of the patient's emotional state should determine the approach taken. For example, education may be ineffective until the patient is ready to learn. Concern about body image may lead to questions related to family relationships, sexual function,

Figure 47-7 • Placement of permanent colostomies. The nature of the discharge varies with the site. *Shaded areas* show sections of bowel removed. **A.** With a sigmoid colostomy, the feces are formed. **B.** With a descending colostomy, the feces are semiformed. **C.** With a transverse colostomy, the feces are unformed. **D.** With an ascending colostomy, the feces are fluid.

and, for women, the ability to become pregnant and deliver a baby normally (Watson, Nicol, Donaldson, et al., 2013). Patients need to know that someone understands and cares about them. A calm, nonjudgmental attitude exhibited by the nurse aids in gaining the patient's confidence. It is important to recognize that treatment of a possibly terminal illness (e.g., cancer) makes patients irritable, anxious, and unhappy. The nurse can coordinate patient care through meetings attended by consultants such as the physician, psychologist, psychiatrist, social worker, WOC nurse, and dietitian.

Conversely, a surgical procedure to create an ileostomy can produce dramatic positive changes in patients who have suffered from IBD for several years. After the discomfort of the disease has decreased and the patient learns how to take care of the ileostomy, he or she often develops a more positive outlook. Until the patient progresses to this phase, an empathetic and tolerant approach by the nurse plays an important part in recovery. The sooner the patient masters the physical care of the ostomy, the sooner he or she will psychologically accept it. Strong self-care skills are associated with better outcomes and adjustment for patients (Perrin, 2013).

Support from other people with ostomies is also helpful. The United Ostomy Associations of America (UOAA) is dedicated to the rehabilitation of people with ostomies. This organization gives patients useful information about living with an ostomy through an educational program of literature, lectures, and exhibits (see Resources section at the end of this chapter). Local associations offer visiting services by qualified members who provide hope and rehabilitation services to patients with new ostomies. Hospitals and other health care agencies may have a WOC nurse on staff who can serve as a valuable resource person for the patient with an ileostomy.

Managing Skin and Stoma Care

The patient with an ileostomy cannot establish regular bowel habits because the contents of the ileum are fluid and are discharged continuously. The patient must wear a pouch at all times. Stomal size and pouch size vary initially; the stoma should be rechecked 3 weeks after surgery, when the edema has subsided. The final size and type of appliance is selected in 3 months, after the patient's weight has stabilized and the stoma shrinks to a stable shape.

The incidence of complications related to a colostomy is usually less than that of an ileostomy. Postoperatively, the stoma is examined for swelling (slight edema from surgical manipulation is normal), color (a healthy stoma is pink or red), discharge (a small amount of oozing is normal), and bleeding (an abnormal sign if bright red or more than trace amounts) (Watson et al., 2013).

Skin excoriation around the stoma can be a persistent problem, particularly for ileostomies. Peristomal skin integrity may be compromised by several factors, such as an allergic reaction to the ostomy appliance, skin barrier, or paste; chemical irritation from the effluent; mechanical injury from the removal of the appliance; and infection. If irritation and yeast growth occur, nystatin powder (Mycostatin) is dusted lightly on the peristomal skin and a pouch with skin barrier is applied over the affected area (Watson et al., 2013).

Changing an Appliance

A regular schedule for changing the pouch before leakage occurs must be established for those with an ostomy. The patient should be educated to change the pouch.

For the procedural guidelines for changing an ostomy appliance, go to **thepoint.lww.com/ Brunner14e.**

The amount of time a person can keep the appliance sealed to the body surface depends on the location of the stoma and on body structure. The usual wearing time, which also depends on the type of skin barrier, is 5 to 10 days. The appliance is emptied every 4 to 6 hours, or at the same time the patient empties the bladder. An emptying spout at the bottom of the appliance is closed with a special clip or Velcro closure made for this purpose. If the patient wishes to bathe or shower before putting on a clean appliance, micropore tape applied to the sides of the pouch keeps it secure during bathing.

Most pouches are disposable and odor proof. Foods such as spinach and parsley act as deodorizers in the intestinal tract; foods that cause odors include asparagus, cabbage, onions, and fish. Bismuth subcarbonate tablets, which may be prescribed and taken orally three or four times each day, are effective in reducing odor. Oral diphenoxylate with atropine can be prescribed to diminish intestinal motility, thereby thickening the stool and assisting in odor control. Foods such as rice, mashed potatoes, and applesauce may also thicken stool.

Irrigating a Colostomy

The purpose of irrigating a colostomy is to empty the colon of gas, mucus, and feces so that the patient can go about social and business activities without fear of fecal drainage. A stoma does not have voluntary muscular control and may empty at irregular intervals. Regulating the passage of fecal material is achieved by irrigating the colostomy or allowing the bowel to evacuate naturally without irrigations. This choice depends on the person and the type of the colostomy (i.e., descending or sigmoid colostomies). By irrigating the stoma at a regular time, there is less gas and retention of the irrigant. The time for irrigating the colostomy should be consistent with the schedule that the person will follow after leaving the hospital.

For the procedural guidelines on irrigating a colostomy, **go to thepoint.lww.com/ Brunner14e.**

Colostomy irrigation is not recommended for persons with extensive pelvic irradiation because it carries a risk of perforation. Likewise, it is contraindicated in patients currently receiving chemotherapy, those with IBS, Crohn's disease, diverticulitis, and peristomal hernias (Bauer, Arnold-Long, & Kent, 2016).

As soon as the patient with a descending or sigmoid colostomy has established a routine for evacuation with irrigations, pouches may be dispensed with, and a closed ostomy appliance or a stoma cap is used to cover the stoma. Except for gas and a slight amount of mucus, nothing escapes from the colostomy opening between irrigations. New assistive devices and ostomy care algorithms are available to help nurses learn ostomy assessment and ostomy product selection (see Resources section at the end of this chapter).

Irrigating a Continent Ileostomy

For a continent ileostomy (i.e., Kock pouch), the nurse educates the patient how to drain the pouch.

For the procedural guidelines for draining a continent ileostomy (Kock pouch), **go to thepoint.lww.com/Brunner14e.**

Managing Dietary and Fluid Needs

A low-residue diet is followed for the first 6 to 8 weeks. Strained fruits and vegetables are ingested. These foods are important sources of vitamins A and C. Later, there are few dietary restrictions, except for avoiding foods that are high in fiber or hard-to-digest kernels, such as celery, popcorn, corn, poppy seeds, caraway seeds, and coconut, which may result in a stomal obstruction (food blockage) for the person with an ileostomy. Foods are reintroduced one at a time.

Getting enough fluids during the summer may be a challenge, when fluid lost through perspiration adds to the fluid loss through the ileostomy. Fluids such as sports drinks (Gatorade) are helpful in maintaining electrolyte balance. If the fecal discharge is too watery, fibrous foods (e.g., whole-grain cereals, fresh fruit skins, beans, corn, nuts) are restricted. If the effluent is excessively dry, salt intake is increased. Increased intake of water or fluid does not increase the effluent, because excess water is excreted in the urine.

Gerontologic Considerations

Some older adults may require an ostomy but have difficulty managing care due to decreased vision, impaired hearing, and difficulty with fine motor coordination. It may be helpful for patients to handle ostomy equipment and simulate cleaning the peristomal skin and irrigating the stoma before surgery. Skin care is a major concern in older patients with an ostomy because of the skin changes that occur with aging—the epithelial and subcutaneous fatty layers become thin, and the skin is irritated easily (Eliopoulos, 2018). To prevent skin breakdown, special attention is paid to skin cleansing and the proper fit of an appliance. Stoma skin barriers should be molded into shape around the stoma (e.g., ConvaTec; see Fig. 47-8). Arteriosclerosis may also be an issue; it causes decreased blood flow to the wound and stoma site, which may lead to delayed nutrient transport and prolonged healing time. Some patients have delayed elimination after irrigation because of decreased peristalsis and mucus production. Most patients require 6 months before they feel comfortable with their ostomy care.

Preventing Complications

Monitoring for complications is an ongoing activity for the patient with an ostomy. Peristomal skin irritation, which results from leakage of effluent, is the most common complication of an ileostomy. A drainable pouching system that does not fit well is often the cause. Components of the drainable pouching system include the pouch, a solid skin barrier, and adhesive. The WOC nurse typically recommends the appropriate drainable pouching system. The solid skin barrier is the component of this system that is most important in ensuring healthy peristomal skin. Solid skin barriers are typically shaped as rectangular or elliptical wafers and are composed of polymers and hydrocolloids. They protect the skin around the stoma from effluent from the stoma and provide a stable interface between the stoma and the pouch. It is critical that the barrier be sized appropriately to "hug" the stoma (up to the stoma but not touching) and not expose peristomal skin.

Other common complications include diarrhea, stomal stenosis, urinary calculi, and cholelithiasis. Even in the presence of a properly fitted drainable pouching system, diarrhea can be problematic. Diarrhea, manifested by very irritating effluent that rapidly fills the pouch (every hour or sooner), can quickly lead to dehydration and electrolyte losses. Supplemental water, sodium, and potassium are given to prevent hypovolemia and hypokalemia. Antidiarrheal agents are given. Stenosis is caused by circular scar tissue that forms at the stoma site. The scar tissue must be surgically released. Urinary calculi may occur in patients with ileostomies and are at least partly attributed to dehydration from decreased fluid intake. Crohn's disease is a risk factor for cholelithiasis (i.e., gallstones) due to altered absorption of bile acids (NIDDK, 2016b) (see Chapter 50).

Promoting Home, Community-Based, and Transitional Care

 Educating Patients About Self-Care

The spouse and family should be familiar with the adjustments that will be necessary when the patient returns home. They need to know why it is necessary for the patient to occupy the bathroom for 10 minutes or more at certain times of the day and why certain equipment is needed. Their understanding is necessary to reduce tension; a relaxed patient tends to have fewer problems. Visits from a home care, WOC, or transitional care nurse may be arranged to ensure that the patient is progressing as expected and to provide additional guidance and education as needed.

Continuing and Transitional Care

The patient needs to know the commercial name of the drainable pouching system to be used so that he or she can obtain a ready supply; the patient should also know how to obtain other supplies. The names and contact information of a local WOC nurse and local self-help groups are often helpful. Any restrictions on driving or working also need to be reviewed. The nurse instructs the patient about common postoperative complications and how to recognize and report them (see Chart 47-8).

 Concept Mastery Alert

Visit thePoint to view an Interactive Tutorial on IBD and related fundamental concepts.

COLORECTAL NEOPLASMS

The term *neoplasm* means new growth. Colorectal neoplasms encompass both cancerous and benign growths, including colorectal cancer and cancerous and benign colorectal polyps.

Figure 47-8 • Moldable stomal skin barrier. Reprinted with permission of ConvaTec, Inc.

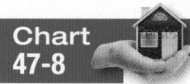

Chart 47-8

HOME CARE CHECKLIST

Managing Ostomy Care

At the completion of education, the patient and/or caregiver will be able to:

- Name the procedure that was performed and identify changes in anatomic structure or function as well as changes in ADLs, IADLs, roles, relationships, and spirituality.
  - Describe the frequency and character of effluent.
- Identify sources for obtaining ostomy care/appliance supplies.
- State the name, dose, side effects, frequency, and schedule for all medications.
- Demonstrate ostomy care, including wound cleansing, irrigation, and appliance changing.
- Describe the importance of assessing and maintaining peristomal skin integrity.
- Identify dietary restrictions (foods that can cause diarrhea and constipation), process for reintroduction of foods, as well as foods that may be encouraged.

- Identify measures to be used to promote fluid and electrolyte balance.
- Describe potential complications and necessary actions to be taken if complications occur.
- Relate how to reach primary provider with questions or complications.
  - Identify how to contact wound-ostomy-continence or home health nurse.
- State time and date of follow-up medical appointments, therapy, and testing.
- Identify sources of support (e.g., friends, relatives, faith community, ostomy support, caregiver support).
- Identify the need for health promotion, disease prevention, and screening activities.

ADL, activities of daily living; IADL, independent activities of daily living.

Colorectal Cancer

Tumors of the colon and rectum are relatively common; the colorectal area (the colon and rectum combined) is the third most common site of new cancer cases in the United States. In the United States, almost 145,000 new cases and 50,000 deaths from colorectal cancer occur annually (American Cancer Society [ACS], 2016; National Cancer Institute [NCI], 2016a). Colorectal cancer is the third leading cause of cancer death in men or women and the second leading cause of cancer death among all adults in the United States (ACS, 2016; NCI, 2016a).

The most significant risk factor for colorectal cancer is older age. It is most frequently diagnosed in adults between 65 and 74 years of age; the median age for patients who die from colorectal cancer is 68 years (Bibbins-Domingo, Grossman, Curry, et al., 2016). However, recent trends in epidemiologic data from the Surveillance, Epidemiology, and End Results registry (SEER) of the NCI found an increased incidence of colorectal cancer in adults younger than 50 years of age. The SEER data revealed that nearly one in seven new diagnoses of colorectal cancer were among younger adults; furthermore, these patients were more likely to have more advanced disease at the time of diagnosis but better long-term survival than among adults older than 50 years of age (Abdelsattar, Wong, Reggenbogen, et al., 2016; Pfeifer, 2016).

Approximately 20% of patients with colorectal cancer have a family history of the disease. The exact cause of colon and rectal cancer is still unknown, but risk factors have been identified (see Chart 47-9). A specific form of hereditary colorectal cancer is *Lynch syndrome,* or hereditary nonpolyposis colorectal cancer (HNPCC) (Bibbins-Domingo et al., 2016). HNPCC-defining cancers include those of the colorectum, uterus, stomach, ovaries, urinary epithelium, and small bowel. HNPCC is characterized by early age of onset. Another disorder with high risk of colorectal cancer is familial adenomatous polyposis (FAP), in which patients develop hundreds of colonic polyps that can become malignant (Bibbins-Domingo et al., 2016).

A drop in the numbers of Americans who smoke cigarettes and improved screening strategies have helped reduce the number of deaths from colon cancer (ACS, 2016; Greenwald, 2015a). The stage at presentation affects the prognosis in colon cancer. If the disease is detected and treated at an early stage before it spreads, the 5-year survival rate is 90%; however, only 39% of colorectal cancers are detected at an early stage (ACS, 2016). Survival rates after late diagnosis are very low. Most people are asymptomatic for long periods and seek health care only when they notice a change in bowel habits or rectal bleeding (ACS, 2016). Prevention and early screening are key to detection and reduction of mortality rates (Bibbins-Domingo et al., 2016).

Chart 47-9

RISK FACTORS

Colorectal Cancer

- Cigarette smoking
- Family history of colon cancer (Lynch syndrome) or polyps (familial adenomatous polyposis)
- High consumption of alcohol (i.e., >2 drinks daily in men, >1 drink daily in women)
- High-fat, high-protein (with high intake of beef), low-fiber diet
- History of genital cancer (e.g., endometrial cancer, ovarian cancer) or breast cancer (in women)
- History of inflammatory bowel disease
- History of type 2 diabetes
- Increasing age
- Male gender
- Overweight or obesity
- Previous colon cancer or adenomatous polyps
- Racial/ethnic background: African American or Ashkenazi Jewish

Adapted from American Cancer Society (ACS). (2016). *Cancer facts and figures 2016.* Atlanta, GA: American Cancer Society; Bibbins-Domingo, K., Grossman, D. C., Curry, S. J., et al. (2016). Screening for colorectal cancer: U.S. Preventive Services Task Force Recommendation Statement. *JAMA, 315*(23), 2564–2575. National Cancer Institute (NCI). (2016a). *Colorectal cancer prevention: Who is at risk?* Retrieved on 1/1/2017 at: www.cancer.gov/types/colorectal/hp/colorectal-prevention-pdq

Pathophysiology

Cancer of the colon and rectum is predominantly (95%) adenocarcinoma (i.e., arising from the epithelial lining of the intestine) (NCI, 2016b). It may start as a benign polyp but may become malignant, invade and destroy normal tissues, and extend into surrounding structures. Cancer cells may migrate away from the primary tumor and spread to other parts of the body (most often to the liver, peritoneum, and lungs) (NCI, 2016b).

Clinical Manifestations

The symptoms are determined by the location of the tumor, the stage of the disease, and the function of the affected intestinal segment. The most common presenting symptom is a change in bowel habits. The passage of blood in or on the stools is the second most common symptom. Symptoms may also include unexplained anemia, anorexia, weight loss, and fatigue (ACS, 2016).

The symptoms most commonly associated with right-sided lesions are dull abdominal pain and melena (i.e., black, tarry stools). The symptoms most commonly associated with left-sided lesions are those associated with obstruction (i.e., abdominal pain and cramping, narrowing stools, constipation, distention), as well as bright red blood in the stool. Symptoms associated with rectal lesions are tenesmus, rectal pain, the feeling of incomplete evacuation after a bowel movement, alternating constipation and diarrhea, and bloody stool (Livstone, 2014).

Assessment and Diagnostic Findings

The U.S. Preventive Services Task Force (USPSTF) (Bibbins-Domingo et al., 2016) notes that "Screening for colorectal cancer is a substantially underused preventive health strategy in the United States" (p. 2573) and that there is a high level of evidence that multiple screening tests are similarly effective in screening for early-stage colorectal cancer, when it can be most effectively treated. It is recommended that all adults should begin periodic screening for colorectal cancer at the age of 50 years (Bibbins-Domingo et al., 2016) (see Chapter 15, Table 15-3). Whether or not to continue screening adults after the age of 75 years should be made based upon each patient's preference and overall health status. Adults older than 85 years of age should not continue to be screened. While the USPSTF does not endorse any one screening practice as the most effective, it does note that "...the best screening test is the one that gets done" (p. 2573). It is estimated that one third of all adults older than 50 years of age do not participate in any type of colorectal cancer screening (Greenwald, 2015a).

Because colonoscopy is the only screening test that can also simultaneously remove precancerous polyps, thus preventing colorectal cancer, other experts recommend 10-year colonoscopies beginning at the age of 50 years as the major screening test for colorectal cancer, including the American College of Gastroenterology (ACG; Rex, Johnson, Anderson, et al., 2009) and the National Comprehensive Cancer Network (NCCN; Burt, Cannon, David, et al., 2013) (see Chapter 43 for discussion of colonoscopies). Most experts suggest commencing periodic screening at 40 years of age for those at higher risk of

colorectal cancer (e.g., family history of Lynch syndrome or FAP, first-degree relative with a history of colorectal cancer) (Abdelsattar et al., 2016).

Given the effectiveness of periodic colonoscopy in both screening for and preventing colorectal cancers, the ACS established the National Colorectal Roundtable, whose broad goal is to ensure that 80% of all Americans older than 50 years of age have screening colonoscopies done by 2018 (Greenwald, 2015a). The National Colorectal Roundtable is a major public health awareness initiative, which includes toolkits, educational webinars, blogs, and a variety of other resources that may be used by participating community members (see Resources section at the end of the chapter).

A patient who has a tumor found on screening colonoscopy should have the tumor biopsied and tattooed during the colonoscopy to facilitate further workup. For the patient whose tumor was found on a diagnostic test other than a colonoscopy (e.g., flexible sigmoidoscopy, FIT), a colonoscopy is indicated to biopsy and tattoo the tumor (Chang, Kaiser, Mills, et al., 2012).

The patient is referred to a colorectal surgeon. The preoperative workup consists of a focused history, to determine if there are any symptoms suggestive of colorectal cancer (see previous discussion in Clinical Manifestations). A family history is done to screen for a genetic predisposition (e.g., Lynch syndrome, FAP). Laboratory studies are done, including a CBC (may or may not reveal anemia), chemistry panel (to determine baseline status), and liver function tests (to screen for possible liver metastasis) (Chang et al., 2012). A baseline carcinoembryonic antigen (CEA) level is also obtained (Chang et al., 2012). CEA is a tumor marker that is recommended for assessing the presence of colorectal cancer, as well as its progression or recurrence, although it does yield both false-positives and false-negatives (NCI, 2016b). However, at present there is no other readily available tumor marker test. Therefore, CEA is not used as the sole predictor of tumor status, including progression or recurrence (ACS, 2016; Chang et al., 2012). Other tests indicated include contrast CT scans of the abdomen, pelvis, and chest, to screen for extent of the tumor and any metastases (Chang et al., 2012).

Complications

Tumor growth may cause partial or complete bowel obstruction or perforation. Extension of the tumor and ulceration into the surrounding blood vessels can result in hemorrhage. Each of these complications is treated surgically. Obstruction may be resected without anastomosis (e.g., Hartmann procedure) (see Fig. 47-4) or with anastomosis (e.g., colectomy or partial colectomy). Perforation typically carries a grim prognosis; it is typically treated with an ostomy. Acute hemorrhage is a rare complication; when it occurs, it is most effectively treated with surgical resection (Chang et al., 2012).

Gerontologic Considerations

Carcinomas of the colon and rectum are common malignancies in advanced age. In men, only the incidence of prostate cancer and lung cancer exceeds that of colorectal cancer. In women, only the incidence of breast cancer and lung cancer exceeds that of colorectal cancer (NCI, 2016a). Symptoms are often insidious. Patients with colorectal cancer usually report fatigue, which is caused primarily by iron deficiency anemia. In early stages, minor changes in bowel patterns and occasional bleeding may occur. The later symptoms most commonly reported by the older adult are abdominal pain, obstruction, tenesmus, and rectal bleeding.

Colon cancer in the older adult has been closely associated with dietary carcinogens. Lack of fiber is a major causative factor because the passage of feces through the intestinal tract is prolonged, which extends exposure to possible carcinogens. Excess dietary fat, high alcohol consumption, and smoking all increase the incidence of colorectal tumors. Physical activity and nonsteroidal anti-inflammatory drugs (NSAIDs) and aspirin have protective effects (ACS, 2016; NCI, 2016a).

Prevention

Several primary prevention strategies might thwart the onset of colorectal cancer. Use of tobacco products is implicated in one third of all cancers, including colorectal cancer (see Chapter 27 for discussion of smoking cessation programs). Physical activity, diet, and weight reduction strategies mirror those for other cancers (see previous discussion of Life Style Factors in Chapter 15) (Greenwald, 2015b). In addition to these strategies, the USPSTF recommends that adults between the ages of 50 and 59 who are also at risk for developing cardiovascular disease (see Chapter 25), and who have no contraindication to aspirin, take daily or alternate-day aspirin (dosage ≥75 mg) for 5 to 10 years, as an effective primary prevention strategy for both cardiovascular disease and colorectal cancer (Chubak, Kamineni, Buist, et al., 2015). In addition, some evidence shows that patients with a diagnosis of colorectal cancer may benefit from aspirin therapy; however, these benefits may be specific to the genetic subtype of the tumor (Chan, Ogino, & Fuchs, 2009; Liao, Lochhead, Nishihara, et al., 2012). To date, there is no expert consensus guideline that advocates routine prescription of aspirin postcolorectal cancer diagnosis.

Medical Management

Treatment for colorectal cancer depends on the stage of the disease (see Chart 47-10) and consists of surgery to remove the tumor, supportive therapy, and adjuvant therapy. Definitive staging can only be done after surgical excision (Chang et al., 2012; NCI, 2016b).

Chart 47-10	Staging of Colorectal Cancer: American Joint Committee on Cancer (AJCC) Stage Groupings

Note: This is based upon AJCC and National Cancer Institute (NCI) recommendations that at least 12 regional lymph nodes are examined in patients with colorectal cancer to confirm staging.

Stage	TNM	Description
Stage 0	Tis, N0, M0	Tis: carcinoma in situ; intraepithelial or invasion of lamina propria N0: no regional lymph node metastasis M0: no distant metastasis
Stage I	T1, N0, M0 T2, N0, M0	T1: Tumor invades submucosa T2: Tumor invades muscularis propria
Stage IIA	T3, N0, M0	T3: Tumor invades through the muscularis propria into pericolorectal tissues
Stage IIB	T4a, N0, M0	T4a: Tumor penetrates to the surface of the visceral peritoneum
Stage IIC	T4b, N0, M0	T4b: Tumor directly invades or is adherent to other organs or structures
Stage IIIA	T1–T2, N1–N1c, M0 T1, N2a, M0	N1: Metastases in 1–3 regional lymph nodes N1a: Metastasis in 1 regional lymph node N1b: Metastases in 2–3 regional lymph nodes N1c: Tumor deposit(s) in the subserosa, mesentery, or nonperitonealized pericolic or perirectal tissues without regional nodal metastasis N2: Metastases in ≥4 regional lymph nodes N2a: Metastases in 4–6 regional lymph nodes
Stage IIIB	T3–T4a, N1–N1c, M0 T2–T3, N2a, M0 T1–T2, N2b, M0	N2b: Metastases in ≥7 regional lymph nodes
Stage IIIC	T4a, N2a, M0 T3–T4a, N2b, M0 T4b, N1–N2, M0	
Stage IVA	Any T, Any N, M1a	M1a: Metastasis confined to 1 organ or site (e.g., liver, lung, ovary, nonregional node)
Stage IVB	Any T, Any N, M1b	M1b: Metastasis in >1 organ/site or the peritoneum

T, primary tumor; N, regional lymph nodes; M, distant metastasis.
Adapted from National Cancer Institute (NCI). (2016b). *Stage information for colon cancer.* Retrieved on 1/1/2017 at: www.cancer.gov/types/colorectal/hp/colon-treatment-pdq#link/_331

Surgical Management

Surgery is the mainstay of treatment for colorectal cancer. It may be curative or palliative. Advances in surgical techniques can enable the patient with rectal cancer to have sphincter-sparing devices that restore continuity of the GI tract. The type of surgery recommended depends on the location and size of the tumor; in up to 10% of patients with new diagnoses of colorectal cancer, there is more than one tumor, which is known as a synchronous tumor (Chang et al., 2012).

Patients who have Stage 0 tumors typically have endoscopic or laparoscopic excision of their tumors (NCI, 2016b). Laparoscopic surgery for Stage I, II, and III colorectal tumors achieves equivalent oncologic outcomes to surgery done by traditional open laparotomy (Chang et al., 2012). In addition, laparoscopic surgery is associated with shorter hospital lengths of stay, fewer postoperative complications, improved pain control, and earlier progression to a normal diet (Kapritsou, Korkolis, & Konstantinou, 2013).

Possible surgical procedures include the following (note that only segmental resections with anastomoses may be done by laparoscope):

- Segmental resection with anastomosis (i.e., removal of the tumor and portions of the bowel on either side of the growth, as well as the blood vessels and lymphatic nodes) (see Fig. 47-9)
- Abdominoperineal resection with permanent sigmoid colostomy (i.e., removal of the tumor and a portion of the sigmoid and all of the rectum and anal sphincter, also called *Miles resection*) (see Fig. 47-10)
- Temporary colostomy followed by segmental resection and anastomosis and subsequent reanastomosis of the colostomy, allowing initial bowel decompression and bowel preparation before resection
- Permanent colostomy or ileostomy for palliation of unresectable obstructing lesions
- Construction of a coloanal reservoir called a *colonic J-pouch*, which is performed in two steps. A temporary loop ileostomy is constructed to divert intestinal flow, and the newly constructed J-pouch (made from 6 to 10 cm of colon) is reattached to the anal stump. About 3 months after the initial stage, the ileostomy is reversed and intestinal continuity is restored. The anal sphincter and therefore continence are preserved.

The colostomy can be created as a temporary or permanent fecal diversion. It allows the drainage or evacuation of colon contents to the outside of the body. The consistency of the drainage is related to the placement of the colostomy, which is dictated by the location of the tumor and the extent of invasion into surrounding tissues (see Fig. 47-7).

Adjuvant Therapy and Ongoing Management

Patients diagnosed with colorectal cancer are referred to a medical oncologist for further management after they are discharged from the hospital after surgery. Patients at the lowest risk for recurrence (i.e., those with Stage 0 or I disease) do not require chemotherapy or radiation therapy. Those with Stage 0 disease do not require specific follow-up. Patients with Stage I colorectal cancer should have follow-up colonoscopies 1-year postoperatively, then again in another 3 years, and then every 5 years (Benson, Bekaii-Saab, Chen, et al., 2013).

Cecum and lower ascending colon

Descending colon and upper sigmoid

Low sigmoid and upper rectum

Rectal sigmoid resection

Figure 47-9 • Examples of areas where cancer can occur, the area that is removed, and how the anastomosis is performed (*small diagrams*).

Most patients with Stage II disease do not require any adjuvant chemotherapy. However, some patients with Stage II tumors have mutations in their DNA mismatch repair genes (MMR) that are classified as proficient (MMR-P). Patients in this subset have improved survival and less disease recurrence if they take the antimetabolite chemotherapeutic drug capecitabine (Xeloda) for 6 months. In order to screen for the MMR-P gene, the tumor should be analyzed by a multigene assay (i.e., genetic test). Patients with Stage II disease who may also benefit from capecitabine are those who had inadequately sampled lymph nodes, with T4-sized tumors, or with poorly differentiated tumors (Benson et al., 2013). Capecitabine is equivalent to the dual chemotherapeutic drugs 5-fluorouracil and leucovorin. It may be given either orally or intravenously. The most common adverse effects of capecitabine include anemia, neutropenia, fatigue, diarrhea, and palmar-plantar erythrodysesthesia (PPE; hand-foot syndrome), which manifests by reddening, pain, and swelling of the palms of the hands and soles of the feet (NCI, 2016b).

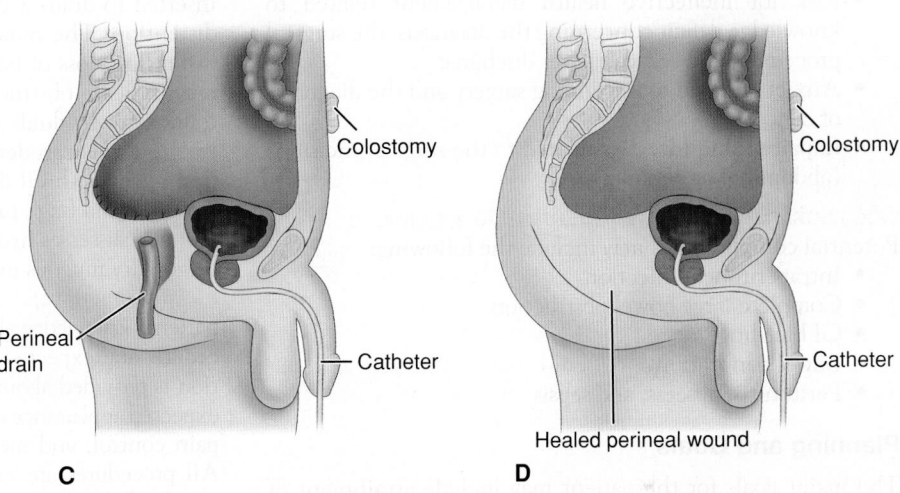

Figure 47-10 • Abdominoperineal resection for carcinoma of the rectum. **A.** Prior to surgery. Note tumor in rectum. **B.** During surgery, the sigmoid is removed and the colostomy is established. The distal bowel is dissected free to a point below the pelvic peritoneum, which is sutured over the closed end of the distal sigmoid and rectum. **C.** Perineal resection includes removal of the rectum and free portion of the sigmoid from below. A perineal drain is inserted. **D.** The final result after healing. Note the healed perineal wound and the permanent colostomy.

Patients with Stage III tumors are typically prescribed the combination chemotherapeutic drug of 5-fluorouracil, leucovorin, and oxaplatin, called FOLFOX. This combination chemotherapeutic drug must be administered IV in 2-week cycles over 6 months. The adverse effects mirrors that of capecitabine, plus patients frequently experience paresthesias of their hands and feet, which typically cease after the chemotherapy is completed (NCI, 2016b).

Patients with Stage II or Stage III tumors should have routine follow-ups and CEA testing every 3 to 6 months for 5 years. CT scans of the abdomen and chest should be done each year for 3 years. Colonoscopy should also be done 1-year postoperatively, and then every 5 years (Meyerhardt, Mangu, Flynn, et al., 2013).

Patients with Stage IV or recurrent colorectal tumors have metastases to distant organs. The treatment is highly variable and individualized, based upon the extent of the tumor mass(es), and the health status and wishes of the patient. Treatment might consist of targeted therapy aimed at possible cure, or palliative care (see Chapter 16). Chemotherapeutic drugs that might be tried include those previously described for treating Stage II or Stage III disease, as well as other categories of agents, including monoclonal antibodies (e.g., cetuximab, bevacizumab), and anti-vascular endothelial growth factor (anti-VEGF) agents (e.g., aflibercept), to

name a few. When metastasis occurs, the liver is implicated half the time. Therapy targeted to treat metastases to the liver can include surgical resection, radiofrequency ablation, and intra-arterial chemotherapy (NCI, 2016b). Surveillance for patients with Stage IV disease is also individualized, and is done on an ongoing basis (Steele, Chang, Hendren, et al., 2015).

NURSING PROCESS

The Patient With Colorectal Cancer

Assessment

The nurse obtains a health history about the presence of fatigue, abdominal or rectal pain (e.g., location, frequency, duration, association with eating or defecation), past and present elimination patterns, and characteristics of stool (e.g., color, odor, consistency, presence of blood or mucus). Additional information includes a history of IBD or colorectal polyps, a family history of colorectal disease, Lynch syndrome, or FAP, and current medication therapy. The nurse assesses dietary patterns, including fat and fiber intake, as well as amounts of alcohol consumed and history of smoking. The nurse describes and documents a history of weight loss and feelings of weakness and fatigue.

Assessment includes auscultation of the abdomen for bowel sounds and palpation of the abdomen for areas of tenderness, distention, and solid masses. Stool specimens are inspected for character and presence of blood.

Diagnosis

NURSING DIAGNOSES

Based on the assessment data, major nursing diagnoses may include the following:

- Imbalanced nutrition: less than body requirements related to nausea and anorexia
- Risk for infection related to surgery on bowel and disruption of colonic bacteria
- Risk for deficient fluid volume related to vomiting and dehydration
- Risk for ineffective health management related to knowledge deficit concerning the diagnosis, the surgical procedure, and self-care after discharge
- Anxiety related to impending surgery and the diagnosis of cancer
- Impaired skin integrity related to the surgical incisions (abdominal or perianal)

COLLABORATIVE PROBLEMS/POTENTIAL COMPLICATIONS

Potential complications may include the following:

- Intraperitoneal infection
- Complete large bowel obstruction
- GI bleeding
- Bowel perforation
- Peritonitis, abscess, and sepsis

Planning and Goals

The major goals for the patient may include attainment of optimal level of nutrition; prevention of infection; maintenance of fluid balance; reduction of anxiety; learning about the diagnosis, surgical procedure, and self-care after discharge; maintenance of optimal tissue healing; and avoidance of complications.

Nursing Interventions

The patient awaiting surgery for colorectal cancer has many concerns, needs, and fears. He or she may be physically debilitated and emotionally distraught with concerns about lifestyle changes after surgery, prognosis, ability to perform in established roles, and finances. Priorities for nursing care include preparing the patient physically for surgery; providing information about postoperative care; and supporting the patient and family emotionally.

PROVIDING PREOPERATIVE CARE

Maintaining Optimal Nutrition. Physical preparation for surgery involves building the patient's stamina in the days preceding surgery. If the patient's condition permits, the nurse recommends a diet high in calories, protein, and carbohydrates and low in residue for several days before surgery to provide adequate nutrition and minimize cramping by decreasing excessive peristalsis. A full or clear liquid diet may be prescribed for 24 to 48 hours before surgery to decrease bulk. If the patient is hospitalized in the days preceding surgery, parenteral nutrition may be required to replace depleted

nutrients, vitamins, and minerals. In some instances, parenteral nutrition is given at home before surgery.

Preventing Infection. The bowel is cleansed with laxatives, enemas, or colonic irrigations the evening before and the morning of surgery. Some surgeons prescribe antibiotics such as kanamycin (Kantrex), ciprofloxacin (Cipro), neomycin (Mycifradin), metronidazole, and cephalexin (Keflex) to be given orally the day before surgery to reduce intestinal bacteria. IV antibiotics such as cefazolin (Ancef) and metronidazole are given immediately before surgery (NCI, 2016b).

Maintaining Fluid Volume Balance. For the patient who is very ill and hospitalized, the nurse measures and records I&O, including vomitus, to provide an accurate record of fluid balance. The patient's intake of oral food and fluids may be restricted to prevent vomiting. The nurse administers antiemetic agents as prescribed. Full or clear liquids may be tolerated, or the patient may be NPO. An NG tube may be inserted to drain accumulated fluids and prevent abdominal distention. The nurse monitors the abdomen for increasing distention, loss of bowel sounds, and pain or rigidity, which may indicate obstruction or perforation. It also is important to monitor IV fluids and electrolytes. Monitoring serum electrolyte levels can detect the hypokalemia and hyponatremia that occur with GI fluid loss. The nurse observes for signs of hypovolemia (e.g., tachycardia, hypotension, decreased pulse volume); assesses hydration status; and reports decreased skin turgor, dry mucous membranes, and concentrated urine.

Providing Preoperative Education. The nurse assesses the patient's knowledge about the diagnosis, prognosis, surgical procedure, and expected level of functioning after surgery. Education is provided about the physical preparation for surgery, the expected appearance and care of the wound, dietary restrictions, pain control, and medication management (see Chart 47-5). All procedures are explained in language the patient understands. If the patient is going to have a colostomy, the nurse manages the plan of care as described previously (see Nursing Management of the Patient Requiring an Ostomy).

Providing Emotional Support. Patients anticipating bowel surgery for colorectal cancer may be very anxious. They may grieve about the diagnosis and the impending surgery. The nurse's role is to assess the patient's anxiety level and coping mechanisms and suggest methods for reducing anxiety, such as deep-breathing exercises and visualizing a successful recovery from surgery and cancer. The nurse can arrange a meeting with a spiritual advisor if the patient desires or with the physician if the patient wishes to discuss the treatment or prognosis. To promote patient comfort, the nurse projects a relaxed, professional, and empathetic attitude.

PROVIDING POSTOPERATIVE CARE

Postoperative nursing care for patients undergoing colon resection is similar to nursing care for any abdominal surgery patient (see Chapter 19), including pain management during the immediate postoperative period. The nurse also monitors the patient for complications. The nurse assesses the abdomen for returning peristalsis and assesses the initial stool characteristics. It is important to help patients out of bed on the first postoperative day to prevent atelectasis, VTE, and accelerate the return of peristalsis.

Maintaining Optimal Nutrition. The nurse educates all patients undergoing surgery for colorectal cancer about the health benefits to be derived from consuming a healthy diet. The diet is individualized as long as it is nutritionally sound and does not cause diarrhea or constipation. The return to normal diet is rapid.

Providing Wound Care. The nurse frequently examines the abdominal dressing during the first 24 hours after surgery to detect signs of hemorrhage. It is important to help the patient splint the abdominal incision during coughing and deep breathing to lessen tension on the edges of the incision. The nurse monitors temperature, pulse, and respiratory rate for elevations that may indicate an infectious process.

If the malignancy has been removed using the perineal route, the perineal wound is observed for signs of hemorrhage. This wound may contain a drain or packing that is removed gradually. Bits of tissue may slough off for a week. This process is hastened by mechanical irrigation of the wound or with sitz baths performed two or three times each day initially. The condition of the perineal wound and any bleeding, infection, or necrosis is documented.

Monitoring and Managing Potential Complications. The patient is observed for signs and symptoms of complications. It is important to frequently assess the abdomen, including bowel sounds and abdominal girth, to detect bowel obstruction. The nurse monitors vital signs for increased temperature, pulse, and respirations and for decreased blood pressure that may indicate an intra-abdominal infectious process. Rectal bleeding must be reported immediately because it indicates hemorrhage. The nurse monitors hemoglobin and hematocrit levels and administers blood component therapy as prescribed. Any abrupt change in abdominal pain is reported promptly. Elevated white blood cell counts and temperature or symptoms of shock are reported because they may indicate sepsis. The nurse administers antibiotics as prescribed. Table 47-6 lists additional potential postoperative complications.

Promoting Home, Community-Based, and Transitional Care

Educating Patients About Self-Care. Patient education and discharge planning require the combined efforts of the physician, nurse, social worker, and dietitian. Patients are given specific information about wound care and signs and symptoms of potential complications that is individualized to their needs. Dietary instructions are essential to help patients identify and eliminate irritating foods that can cause diarrhea or constipation. It is important to educate patients about their prescribed medications (i.e., action, purpose, and possible side and toxic effects).

Some patients who are older with multiple comorbid conditions may need referral to a home care agency and the telephone number of the local chapter of the ACS. The home care nurse provides further care and education and assesses the patient's and family's adjustment. The home environment is assessed for adequacy of resources that allow the patient to manage self-care activities. A family member may assume responsibility for purchasing the equipment and supplies needed at home.

Patients need very specific directions about when to call their primary provider. They need to know which complications require prompt attention (i.e., bleeding, abdominal distention and rigidity, diarrhea, fever, wound drainage, and disruption of suture line). If chemotherapy is planned, the possible side effects (i.e., diarrhea, fatigue, PPE) are reviewed.

Continuing and Transitional Care

Ongoing care of the patient with cancer often extends well beyond the initial hospital stay. Transitional care nurses who work in cancer care infusion centers manage follow-up care and coordinate adjuvant therapy and surveillance follow-ups. Some patients are interested in and can benefit from involvement in colorectal cancer support groups (see Resources section at the end of this chapter).

Evaluation

Expected patient outcomes may include:
1. Consumes a healthy diet
   a. Avoids foods and fluids that cause diarrhea, constipation, and obstruction
   b. Substitutes nonirritating foods and fluids for those that are restricted
2. Does not exhibit any signs or symptoms of infection
   a. Is afebrile
3. Maintains fluid balance
   a. Experiences no vomiting or diarrhea
   b. Experiences no signs or symptoms of dehydration
4. Acquires information about diagnosis, surgical procedure, preoperative preparation, and self-care after discharge
   a. Discusses the diagnosis, surgical procedure, and postoperative self-care
   b. Demonstrates techniques of ostomy care
5. Feels less anxious
   a. Expresses concerns and fears freely
   b. Uses coping measures to manage stress
6. Maintains clean wound(s)
7. Recovers without complications
   a. Regains normal bowel activity
   b. Exhibits no signs and symptoms of perforation or bleeding
   c. Identifies signs and symptoms that should be reported to the health care provider

Polyps of the Colon and Rectum

A polyp is a mass of tissue that protrudes into the lumen of the bowel. Polyps can occur anywhere in the intestinal tract and rectum. They can be classified as neoplastic (i.e., typically adenocarcinomas) or non-neoplastic (i.e., mucosal and hyperplastic). Non-neoplastic polyps, which are benign epithelial growths, are common in the Western world. They occur more commonly in the large intestine than in the small intestine. Because polyps might develop into malignant neoplasms, they should be removed when they are identified, typically during screening colonoscopy (Livstone, 2014). Adenomatous polyps are more common in men. The proportion of these polyps arising in the proximal part of the colon increases with age (after 50 years of age). Prevalence rates vary from 7% to 50%, depending on age.

Clinical manifestations depend on the size of the polyp and the amount of pressure it exerts on intestinal tissue. Most commonly, there are no symptoms. When there are clinical manifestations, the most common is rectal bleeding. Lower abdominal pain may also occur. If the polyp is large enough, symptoms of obstruction occur. The diagnosis is based on history and digital rectal examination, double-contrast barium

TABLE 47-6 Potential Complications and Nursing Interventions After Colorectal Surgery

Complication	Nursing Interventions
General Complications	
Paralytic ileus	Initiate or continue nasogastric intubation if prescribed (typically only indicated with vomiting or abdominal distention). Prepare patient for x-ray study or CT scan of abdomen. Ensure adequate fluid and electrolyte replacement; monitor serum electrolytes for abnormalities (e.g., hypokalemia, hyponatremia, hypomagnesemia). Prepare to institute or discontinue prescribed drugs or therapies that can increase motility (e.g., chewing gum increases motility, opioid analgesics can decrease motility).
Mechanical obstruction	Assess patient for intermittent colicky pain, nausea, and vomiting. Initiate or continue nasogastric intubation if prescribed. Prepare patient for x-ray study or CT scan of abdomen. Prepare patient for surgery.
Intra-abdominal Septic and Ischemic Conditions	
Peritonitis	Evaluate patient for nausea, hiccups, chills, spiking fever, tachycardia, boardlike abdomen. Administer antibiotics as prescribed. Prepare patient for drainage procedure. Administer parenteral fluid and electrolyte therapy as prescribed. Prepare patient for surgery if condition deteriorates.
Abscess formation	Administer antibiotics as prescribed. Apply warm compresses as prescribed. Prepare patient for surgical or percutaneous drainage.
Acute mesenteric ischemia	Assess patient for sudden onset of severe, colicky pain, abdominal distention, and sepsis. Prepare patient for x-ray study or CT scan of abdomen. Administer antibiotics as prescribed. Prepare patient for surgery.
Surgical Wound Complications	
Infection	Monitor temperature; report temperature elevation. Observe for redness, tenderness, hardening (induration), and pain around the surgical wound. Assist in establishing local drainage. Obtain specimen of drainage material for culture and sensitivity studies.
Wound dehiscence	Observe for sudden drainage of profuse serous fluid from wound. Cover wound area with sterile moist dressings.
Wound evisceration	Observe for wound dehiscence with protrusion of abdominal organs (e.g., intestines) through wound. Prepare patient immediately for surgery.
Abdominal wound infection	Monitor for evidence of constant or generalized abdominal pain, rapid pulse, and elevation of temperature. Prepare for tube decompression of bowel. Administer fluids and electrolytes by IV route as prescribed. Administer antibiotics as prescribed.
Anastomotic Complications	
Dehiscence of anastomosis	Prepare patient for surgery.
Fistulas	Prepare for tube decompression of bowel. Administer parenteral fluids as prescribed to correct fluid and electrolyte deficits.

Adapted from McCutcheon, T. (2013). The ileus and oddities after colorectal surgery. *Gastroenterology Nursing, 36*(5), 368–375.

enema studies, sigmoidoscopy, or colonoscopy (Livstone, 2014; NIDDK, 2014b).

After a polyp is identified, it should be removed. Several methods are used: colonoscopy with the use of special equipment (i.e., biopsy forceps and snares), laparoscopy, or colonoscopic excision with laparoscopic visualization. The latter technique enables immediate detection of potential problems and allows laparoscopic resection and repair of the major complications of perforation and bleeding that may occur with polypectomy. Microscopic examination of the polyp then identifies the type of polyp and indicates what further surgery is required, if any (Livstone, 2014; NIDDK, 2014b).

DISORDERS OF THE ANORECTUM

Anorectal disorders are common. Patients with anorectal disorders seek medical care primarily because of pain, rectal bleeding, or change in bowel habits. Other common complaints are protrusion of hemorrhoids, anal discharge, perianal itching, swelling, anal tenderness, stenosis, and ulceration. Constipation results from delaying defecation because of anorectal pain.

Proctitis

Proctitis refers to inflammation of the mucosa of the rectum, which may be secondary to infection, IBD, or radiation. Infectious diseases are the most frequent cause of proctitis; these etiologies may be either from enteric organism (e.g., *Shigella, Salmonella*) or from sexually transmitted infections (STIs; also called *sexually transmitted diseases,* or STDs).

Proctitis secondary to an STI may occur in any gender but is more prevalent among homosexual men who practice anorectal intercourse. It is commonly associated with recent anal-receptive intercourse with an infected partner. Symptoms include mucopurulent discharge or bleeding, rectal pain, and diarrhea. The pathogens most frequently involved are *Neisseria gonorrhoeae, Chlamydia trachomatis,* herpes simplex virus, and *Treponema pallidum.* These infections may progress into proctocolitis and enteritis. Proctocolitis involves the rectum and lowest portion of the descending colon. Symptoms are similar to proctitis but may also include watery or bloody diarrhea, cramps, pain, and bloating. Enteritis involves more of the descending colon, and symptoms include watery, bloody diarrhea; abdominal pain; and weight loss. The most common pathogens causing enteritis are *E. histolytica, Giardia lamblia, and Shigella,* and *Campylobacter* species (Irizarry & Yade, 2014).

Sigmoidoscopy is performed to identify portions of the anorectum involved. Samples are taken with rectal swabs, and cultures are obtained to identify the pathogens involved. Antibiotics (i.e., ceftriaxone [Rocephin] or cefixime [Suprax], doxycycline [Vibramycin], and penicillin G) are the treatment of choice for bacterial infections. Acyclovir [Zovirax] is given to patients with viral infections. Antiamebic therapy (i.e., metronidazole) is appropriate for infections with *E. histolytica* and *G. lamblia.* Ciprofloxacin (Cipro) is effective for *Shigella.* The antibiotics erythromycin and ciprofloxacin are the treatment of choice for *Campylobacter* infection (Ansari, 2014; Irizarry & Yade, 2014).

Anorectal Abscess

An anorectal abscess is caused by obstruction of an anal gland with dried debris, resulting in retrograde infection. People with Crohn's disease or immunosuppressive conditions such as AIDS are particularly susceptible to these infections. Many of these abscesses result in fistulas (Hebra, 2016).

An abscess may occur in a variety of spaces in and around the rectum, usually in the path of least resistance, where anatomic structures are in close proximity without hard or thick structures to separate them. Most patients with anorectal abscesses will complain of dull perianal discomfort and itching, and increased pain with defecation. Approximately half will present with perianal edema; only one quarter will report any abnormal fecal discharge, such as pus, mucous, or blood. Only 21% report fever or chills (Hebra, 2016).

Prompt surgical treatment to incise and drain the abscess is the treatment of choice, to prevent complications such as fistula formation, fecal incontinence, and sepsis. This may be done in the emergency department or in an outpatient clinic office setting. The wound may be packed with an absorptive dressing (e.g., calcium alginate or hydrofiber) and allowed to heal by granulation Hebra, 2016).

Anal Fistula

An anal fistula is a tiny, tubular, fibrous tract that extends into the anal canal from an opening located beside the anus in the perianal skin (see Fig. 47-11A). Fistulas usually result from an abscess. They may also develop from trauma, fissures, or Crohn's disease. Purulent drainage or stool may leak constantly from the cutaneous opening. Other symptoms may be the passage of flatus or feces from the vagina or bladder, depending on the location of the fistula tract. Untreated fistulas may cause systemic infection with related symptoms (Hebra, 2016).

Surgery is recommended because few fistulas heal spontaneously. A fistulectomy (i.e., excision of the fistulous tract) is the recommended surgical procedure. The lower bowel is evacuated thoroughly with several prescribed enemas. The fistula is dissected or laid open by an incision from its rectal opening to its outlet. The wound is packed with gauze. Postoperative medications include analgesics and antibiotics. Fistula recurrence occurs in up to half of patients (Hebra, 2016).

Anal Fissure

An anal fissure is a longitudinal tear or ulceration in the lining of the anal canal usually just distal to the dentate line (see Fig. 47-11B). Fissures are usually caused by the trauma of passing a large, firm stool or from persistent tightening of the anal canal because of stress and anxiety (leading to constipation). Other causes include childbirth, trauma, and or anal intercourse (Ansari, 2014).

Painful defecation, burning, and bleeding characterize fissures. Bright red blood may be seen on the toilet tissue after a bowel movement. Most of these fissures heal if treated by conservative measures that include dietary modification with addition of fiber supplements, stool softeners and bulk agents, an increase in water intake, and sitz baths (Wald et al., 2014). Anal dilation under anesthesia may be required. Therapies such as perianal or intra-anal application of nitroglycerin ointment, calcium channel blockers, minoxidil, or botulinum toxin (Botox) injections have increased the rate of healing and lowered pain levels in chronic anal fissures; these therapies should be tried before surgery. These agents work by increasing blood supply to the region and relaxing the anal sphincter (Wald et al., 2014).

If fissures do not respond to conservative treatment, surgery is indicated. The procedure of choice is the lateral internal sphincterotomy with excision of the fissure (Wald et al., 2014).

Hemorrhoids

Hemorrhoids are dilated portions of veins in the anal canal. They are very common, affecting approximately 38.9% of adults in the United States (Evans, Manley, & Rooney, 2016). Shearing of the mucosa during defecation results in the sliding of the structures in the wall of the anal canal, including the hemorrhoidal and vascular tissues. Increased pressure in the hemorrhoidal tissue due to pregnancy may initiate hemorrhoids or aggravate existing ones. Hemorrhoids are classified into two types: those above the internal sphincter are called

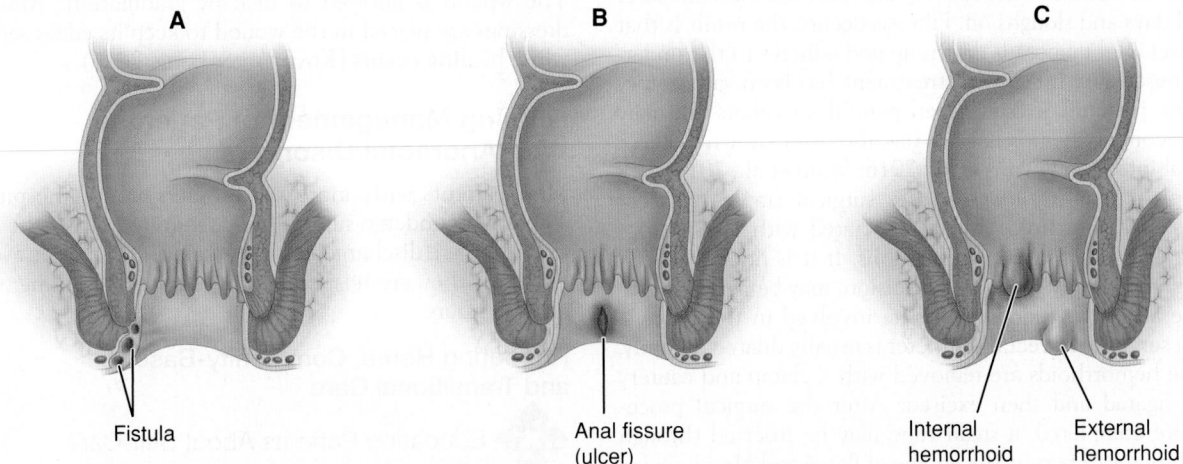

Fistula   Anal fissure (ulcer)   Internal hemorrhoid   External hemorrhoid

Figure 47-11 • Various types of anal lesions. **A.** Fistula. **B.** Fissure. **C.** External and internal hemorrhoids.

internal hemorrhoids, and those appearing outside the external sphincter are called *external hemorrhoids* (Ansari, 2014) (see Fig. 47-11C). Internal hemorrhoids are also classified by degree of prolapse (Thornton, Rosh, & Perry, 2015):

- First degree—do not prolapse and protrude into anal canal
- Second degree—prolapse outside the anal canal during defecation but reduce spontaneously
- Third degree—prolapsed to the extent that they require manual reduction
- Fourth degree—prolapsed to the extent that they may not be reduced

Hemorrhoids cause itching and pain and are the most common cause of bright red bleeding with defecation. External hemorrhoids are associated with severe pain from the inflammation and edema caused by thrombosis (i.e., clotting of blood within the hemorrhoid). This may lead to ischemia of the area and eventual necrosis. Internal hemorrhoids are not usually painful until they bleed or prolapse when they become enlarged.

Hemorrhoid symptoms and discomfort can be relieved by good personal hygiene and by avoiding excessive straining during defecation. A high-residue diet that contains fruit and bran along with an increased fluid intake may be all the treatment that is necessary to promote the passage of soft, bulky stools to prevent straining. If this treatment is not successful, the addition of hydrophilic bulk-forming agents such as psyllium may help. Warm compresses, sitz baths, analgesic ointments and suppositories, and astringents (e.g., witch hazel) reduce engorgement (Ansari, 2014; Wald et al., 2014).

There are several types of nonsurgical treatments for hemorrhoids. Infrared photocoagulation, bipolar diathermy, and laser therapy are used to affix the mucosa to the underlying muscle. Injection of sclerosing agents is also effective for small, bleeding hemorrhoids. Sclerotherapy involves injecting a sclerosing agent (5% phenol in saline) into the base of the hemorrhoid to cause blood vessel thrombosis. These procedures help prevent prolapse (Wald et al, 2014).

A conservative surgical treatment of internal hemorrhoids is the rubber band ligation procedure. The hemorrhoid is visualized through the anoscope, and its proximal portion above the mucocutaneous lines is grasped with an instrument. A small rubber band is then slipped over the hemorrhoid. Tissue distal to the rubber band becomes necrotic after several days and sloughs off. Fibrosis occurs; the result is that the lower anal mucosa is drawn up and adheres to the underlying muscle. Although this treatment has been satisfactory for some patients, it has proven painful for others and may cause secondary hemorrhage. It has also been known to cause perianal infection (Evans et al., 2016; Wald et al., 2014).

Stapled hemorrhoidopexy uses surgical staples to treat prolapsing hemorrhoids and is associated with less postoperative pain and fewer complications. If it is not successful, hemorrhoidectomy, or surgical excision, may be performed to remove all of the redundant tissue involved in the process. During surgery, the rectal sphincter is usually dilated digitally, and the hemorrhoids are removed with a clamp and cautery or are ligated and then excised. After the surgical procedures are completed, a small tube may be inserted through the sphincter to permit the escape of flatus and blood; pieces of absorbable gelatin sponge (Gelfoam) or oxidized cellulose

Figure 47-12 • (*Left*) Pilonidal sinus on lower sacrum about 5 cm (2 inches) above the anus in the intergluteal cleft. (*Right*) Hair particles emerge from the sinus tract, and localized indentations (pits) can appear on the skin near the sinus openings.

(Oxycel) gauze may be placed over the anal wounds (Wald et al., 2014).

Pilonidal Sinus or Cyst

A pilonidal sinus or cyst is found in the intergluteal cleft on the posterior surface of the lower sacrum (see Fig. 47-12). Current theories suggest that it results from local trauma, causing penetration of hairs into the epithelium and subcutaneous tissue. It may also be formed congenitally by an infolding of epithelial tissue beneath the skin, which may communicate with the skin surface through one or several small sinus openings. Hair frequently is seen protruding from these openings, and this gives the cyst its name, *pilonidal* (i.e., a nest of hair). The cysts rarely cause symptoms until adolescence or early adult life, when infection produces an irritating drainage or an abscess. Perspiration and friction easily irritate this area (Ansari, 2014; Koyfman & Long, 2016).

The abscess is incised and drained under local anesthesia. After the acute process resolves, further surgery might be indicated to excise the cyst and any secondary sinus tracts. The wound is allowed to heal by granulation. Absorptive dressings are placed in the wound to keep its edges separated while healing occurs (Koyfman & Long, 2016).

Nursing Management of Patients With Anorectal Disorders

Most patients with anorectal disorders are not hospitalized. Those who undergo surgical procedures to correct the condition often are discharged directly from the outpatient surgical center. If they are hospitalized, it is for a short time, usually only 24 hours.

Promoting Home, Community-Based, and Transitional Care

 Educating Patients About Self-Care

Patient education is essential to facilitate recovery at home.

The nurse instructs the patient to keep the perianal area as clean as possible by gently cleansing with warm water and then drying with absorbent cotton wipes. The patient should avoid rubbing the area with toilet tissue. Instructions are provided about how to take a sitz bath and how to test the temperature of the water.

During the first 24 hours after rectal surgery, painful spasms of the sphincter and perineal muscles may occur. The nurse instructs the patient that ice and analgesic ointments may decrease the pain. Warm compresses may promote circulation and soothe irritated tissues. Sitz baths taken 3 to 4 times each day can relieve soreness and pain by relaxing sphincter spasm. Twenty-four hours after surgery, topical anesthetic agents may be beneficial in relieving local irritation and soreness. Medications may include topical anesthetics (i.e., suppositories), astringents, antiseptics, tranquilizers, and antiemetic agents. Patients are more adherent and less apprehensive if they are free of pain.

Wet dressings saturated with equal parts of cold water and witch hazel help relieve edema. When wet compresses are being used continuously, petrolatum is applied around the anal area to prevent skin maceration. The patient is instructed to assume a prone position at intervals because this position reduces edema of the tissue.

Continuing and Transitional Care

Sitz baths may be given in the bathtub or plastic sitz bath unit 3 to 4 times each day. Sitz baths should follow each bowel movement for 1 to 2 weeks after surgery. The nurse encourages intake of at least 2 L of water daily to provide adequate hydration and recommends high-fiber foods to promote bulk in the stool and to make it easier to pass fecal matter through the rectum. Bulk laxatives such as psyllium may be recommended, and stool softeners (e.g., docusate) may be prescribed. The patient is advised to set aside a time for bowel movements and to heed the urge to defecate as promptly as possible, in order to prevent constipation. The diet is modified to increase fluids and fiber. Moderate exercise is encouraged, and the patient is taught about the prescribed diet, the significance of proper eating habits and exercise, and the laxatives that can be taken safely.

CRITICAL THINKING EXERCISES

1 You work in a family practice clinic. A 25-year-old female patient presents to the clinic with iron deficiency anemia. After a thorough workup, she is diagnosed with celiac disease. How might her anemia have been caused by her celiac disease? Describe the education plan you would devise for this patient. What foods and other products must she learn to avoid?

2 [pq] You work as a staff nurse in an emergency department. A 22-year-old woman presents to triage with a 2-day history of increasingly worse, colicky abdominal pain. She is holding her abdomen and is doubled-over as you take her vital signs. She is febrile, with a temperature of 38.9°C (102°F), her BP is 160/96 and HR is 112 bpm. She tells you she has not passed any stool or flatus in the past 3 days, though she feels that she needs to have a bowel movement. She tells you that she was diagnosed with Crohn's disease when she was 14 years of age. Describe your priorities of care for this patient. What are your assessment priorities? What other important health history information will you gather from her? What focused physical assessments will you perform?

3 [ebp] You work in an infusion center that is part of a comprehensive inpatient and outpatient cancer network. A 62-year-old male with Stage IIIA colorectal cancer is a new patient to the infusion center. Six weeks ago, he had a laparoscopic hemicolectomy to surgically resect his tumor. His oncologist now recommends that he begin chemotherapy with FOLFOX. As a self-employed electrician, the patient is worried that side effects of FOLFOX might compromise the hand dexterity required for his work. He wonders if he should consent to begin FOLFOX treatment. What is the strength of the evidence that supports his consent or refusal to begin FOLFOX? What are the potential adverse effects to commencing FOLFOX and how might these effects interfere with this patient's ability to continue working?

REFERENCES

*Asterisk indicates nursing research.
**Double asterisk indicates classic reference.

Books

American Cancer Society (ACS). (2016). *Cancer facts and figures 2016.* Atlanta, GA: American Cancer Society.

Chubak, J., Kamineni, A., Buist, D. S., et al. (2015). *Aspirin use for the prevention of colorectal cancer: An updated systematic evidence review for the U.S. Preventive Services Task Force.* Evidence Synthesis No. 133. AHRQ Publication No. 15–05228-EF-1. Rockville, MD: Agency for Healthcare Research and Quality.

Eliopoulos, C. (2018). *Gerontological nursing* (9th ed.). Philadelphia, PA: Wolters Kluwer.

Grossman, S. C., & Porth, C. M. (2014). *Porth's pathophysiology: Concepts of altered health states* (9th ed.). Philadelphia, PA: Wolters Kluwer.

Herdman, T. H., & Kamitsuru, S. (2014). *NANDA International nursing diagnoses: Definitions and classification 2015–2017.* Oxford: Wiley Blackwell.

Weber, J. R., & Kelley, J. H. (2014). *Health assessment in nursing* (5th ed.). Philadelphia, PA: Wolters Kluwer.

Journals and Electronic Documents

Abdelsattar, Z. M., Wong, S. L., Regenbogen, S. E., et al. (2016). Colorectal cancer outcomes and treatment patterns in patients too young for average-risk screening. *Cancer, 122*(6), 929–934.

Andersson, R. E. (2014). Short-term complications and long-term morbidity of laparoscopic and open appendicectomy in a national cohort. *British Journal of Surgery, 101*(9), 1135–1142.

Ansari, P. (2014). Acute abdomen and surgical gastroenterology. *Merck Manual: Professional Version.* Retrieved on 12/28/2016 at: www.merckmanuals.com/professional/gastrointestinal-disorders/acute-abdomen-and-surgical-gastroenterology/introduction-to-acute-abdomen-and-surgical-gastroenterology

Avadhani, A., & Steefel, L. (2015). Probiotics: A review for NPs. *The Nurse Practitioner, 40*(8), 50–54.

Bailes, B. K., & Reeve, K. (2013). Constipation in older adults. *The Nurse Practitioner, 38*(8), 21–25.

Basson, M. D. (2015a). Constipation treatment and management. *MedScape.* Retrieved on 12/25/2016 at: emedicine.medscape.com/article/184704-overview

Basson, M. D. (2015b). Ulcerative colitis workup. *MedScape*. Retrieved on 12/31/2016 at: emedicine.medscape.com/article/183084-workup#showall

Bauer, C., Arnold-Long, M., & Kent, D. J. (2016). Colostomy irrigation to maintain continence: An old method revived. *Nursing2016, 46*(8), 59–62.

Benson, A. B., Bekaii-Saab, T., Chan, E., et al. (2013). Localized colon cancer, version 3.2013: Featured updates to the NCCN Guidelines. *Journal of the National Comprehensive Cancer Network, 11*(5), 519–528.

Bibbins-Domingo, K., Grossman, D. C., Curry, S. J., et al. (2016). Screening for colorectal cancer: U.S. Preventive Services Task Force Recommendation Statement. *JAMA, 315*(23), 2564–2575.

*Bliss, D. Z., Savik, K. Jung, H-J. G., et al. (2014). Dietary fiber supplementation for fecal incontinence: A randomized clinical trial. *Research in Nursing and Health, 37*(5), 367–378.

Bozkurt, M. A., Unsal, M. G., Kapan, S., et al. (2015). Is laparoscopic appendectomy going to be standard procedure for acute appendicitis; a 5-year single center experience with 1,788 patients. *European Journal of Emergency Surgery, 41*(1), 87–89.

Burt, R. W., Cannon, J. A., David, D. S., et al. (2013). Colorectal cancer screening. *Journal of the National Comprehensive Cancer Network, 11*(12), 1538–1575.

Centers for Disease Control and Prevention (CDC). (2015a). *Epidemiology of the IBD*. Retrieved on 12/31/2016 at: www.cdc.gov/ibd/ibd-epidemiology.htm

Centers for Disease Control and Prevention (CDC). (2015b). *Nearly half a million Americans suffered from Clostridium difficile infections in a single year*. Retrieved on 1/1/2017 at: www.cdc.gov/media/releases/2015/p0225-clostridium-difficile.html

Chan, A. T., Ogino, S., & Fuchs, C. S. (2009). Aspirin use and survival after diagnosis of colorectal cancer. *JAMA, 302*(6), 649–658.

Chang, G. J., Kaiser, A. M., Mills, S., et al. (2012). Practice parameters for the management of colon cancer. *Diseases of the Colon & Rectum, 55*(8), 831–843.

Cheng, Y., Zhou, S., Zhou, R., et al. (2015). Abdominal drainage to prevent intra-peritoneal abscess for complicated appendicitis. *Cochrane Database of Systematic Reviews, 2*, CD010168.

Collins, E., Hibberts, F., Lyons, M., et al. (2014). Outcomes in non-surgical management for bowel dysfunction. *British Journal of Nursing, 23*(14), 776–780.

Craig, S. (2015). Appendicitis. *MedScape*. Retrieved on 12/28/2016 at: emedicine.medscape.com/article/773895-overview

Crawshaw, A., Williams, J., & Woodhouse, F. (2014). The Kock pouch reconsidered: An alternative surgical technique. *British Journal of Nursing, 23*(17), S26–S29.

Daley, B. J. (2015). Peritonitis and abdominal sepsis. *MedScape*. Retrieved on 12/30/2016 at: emedicine.medscape.com/article/180234-overview

DiMarino, M. C. (2013). Diverticular disease. *Merck Manual: Professional Version*. Retrieved on 12/28/2016 at: www.merckmanuals.com/professional/gastrointestinal-disorders/diverticular-disease/definition-of-diverticular-disease

Dunn, P., Greenstein, S. M., Prowse, O., et al. (2014). Intestinal transplant. *MedScape*. Retrieved on 1/1/2017 at: emedicine.medscape.com/article/1013245-overview

Evans, M. M., & Curtin, M. (2014). Acute appendicitis: A case study describing standards of care. *Medsurg Nursing, 23*(6), 3, 15.

Evans, L., Manley, K., & Rooney, L. (2016). A technical note regarding hemorrhoid banding. *The Nurse Practitioner, 41*(5), 18–21.

Fazio, V. W., Kiran, R. P., Remzi, F. H., et al. (2013). Ileal pouch anastomosis: Analysis of outcome and quality of life in 3707 patients. *Annals of Surgery, 257*(4), 679–785.

Ferrara, L. R., & Saccomano, S. J. (2015). Celiac disease: A case of unresolved anemia. *The Nurse Practitioner, 40*(3), 20–22.

Francone, T. D., & Champagne, B. (2013). Considerations and complications in patients undergoing ileal pouch anal anastomosis. *Surgical Clinics of North America, 93*(1), 107–143.

Ghazi, L. J. (2016). Crohn disease workup. *MedScape*. Retrieved on 12/31/2016 at: emedicine.medscape.com/article/172940-workup#showall

*Ghiyasvandian, S., Ghorbani, M., Zakermoghadam, M., et al. (2016). The effects of a self-care program on the severity of symptoms and quality of life of patients with irritable bowel syndrome. *Gastroenterology Nursing, 39*(5), 359–365.

Girard, N. J., & Ousey, K. (2015). An easily forgotten tube. *AORN Journal, 101*(6), 718–719.

Goebel, S. U. (2014). Malabsorption. *Medscape*. Retrieved on 12/27/2016 at: emedicine.medscape.com/article/180785-overview

Greenwald, B. (2015a). 80% by 2018: How are you and your team and community doing on this endeavor? *Gastroenterology Nursing, 38*(6), 481–482.

Greenwald, B. (2015b). Reducing the risk for colon cancer with healthy food choices and physical activity. *Gastroenterology Nursing, 38*(4), 307–319

Gump, K., & Schmelzer, M. (2016). Gaining control over fecal incontinence. *Medsurg Nursing, 25*(2), 97–103.

Harris, H., & Jelemensky, L. (2014). Managing the ups and downs of ulcerative colitis. *Nursing, 44*(8), 36–42.

Heavey, E., & Stoltman, J. (2016). Caring for hospitalized patients with celiac disease. *Nursing, 46*(11), 50–55.

Hebra, A. (2016). Anorectal abscess. *MedScape*. Retrieved on 12/30/2016 at: emedicine.medscape.com/article/191975-overview#showall

Hendren, S., Hammond, K., Glasgow, S. C., et al. (2015). Clinical practice guidelines for ostomy surgery. *Diseases of the Colon & Rectum, 58*(4), 375–387.

**Hinchey, E. J., Schaal, P. G., & Richards, G. K. (1978). Treatment of perforated diverticular disease of the colon. *Advances in Surgery, 12*, 85–109.

Hopkins, C. (2016). Large-bowel obstruction. *MedScape*. Retrieved on 12/29/2016 at: emedicine.medscape.com/article/774045-overview

Hupfeld, L., Burcharth, J., Pommergaard, H.-C., et al. (2014). The best choice of treatment for acute colonic diverticulitis with purulent peritonitis is uncertain. *BioMed Research International*, Article ID 380607, doi:10.1155/2014/380607.

Irizarry, L., & Yade, I. (2014). Acute proctitis. *MedScape*. Retrieved on 12/30/2016 at: emedicine.medscape.com/article/775952-overview

Kapritsou, M., Korkolis, D. P., & Konstantinou, E. A. (2013). Open or laparoscopic surgery for colorectal cancer: A retrospective comparative study. *Gastroenterology Nursing, 36*(1), 37–41.

Koyfman, A., & Long, B. J. (2016). Pilonidal cyst and sinus. *MedScape*. Retrieved on 12/30/2016 at: emedicine.medscape.com/article/788127-overview

Lacy, B. E., Mearin, F., Chang, L., et al. (2016). Bowel disorders. *Gastroenterology, 150*(6), 1393–1407.

Lembo, A. J., Lacy, B. E., Zuckerman, M. J., et al. (2016). Eluxadoline for irritable bowel syndrome with diarrhea. *The New England Journal of Medicine, 374*(3), 242–253.

Liao, X., Lochhead, P., Nichihara, R., et al. (2012). Aspirin use, tumor PIK3CA mutation, and colorectal-cancer survival. *New England Journal of Medicine, 367*(17), 1596–1606.

Livstone, E. M. (2014). Colorectal cancer. *Merck Manual: Professional Version*. Retrieved on 12/29/2016 at: www.merckmanuals.com/professional/gastrointestinal-disorders/tumors-of-the-gi-tract/colorectal-cancer

McCutcheon, T. (2013). The ileus and oddities after colorectal surgery. *Gastroenterology Nursing, 36*(5), 368–375.

McRorie, J. W. (2015). Evidence-based approach to fiber supplements and clinically meaningful health benefits, Part 2: What to look for and how to recommend an effective fiber therapy. *Nutrition Today, 50*(2), 90–97.

Meyerhardt, J. A., Mangu, P. B., Flynn, P. J., et al. (2013). Follow-up care, surveillance protocol, and secondary prevention measures for survivors of colorectal cancer: American Society of Clinical Oncology Clinical Practice Guideline Endorsement. *Journal of Clinical Oncology, 31*(35), 4465–4470.

Moore, K. S. (2015). Traveler's diarrhea: Risk reduction and management. *The Nurse Practitioner, 40*(11), 1–5.

Murray, K. (2016). Cracking down on C. diff. *Nursing Management, 47*(7), 56.

National Cancer Institute (NCI). (2016a). *Colorectal cancer prevention: Who is at risk?* Retrieved on 1/1/2017 at: www.cancer.gov/types/colorectal/hp/colorectal-prevention-pdq

National Cancer Institute (NCI). (2016b). *Stage information for colon cancer*. Retrieved on 1/1/2017 at: www.cancer.gov/types/colorectal/hp/colon-treatment-pdq#link/_331

National Institute of Diabetes and Digestive and Kidney Diseases (NIDDK). (2014a). *Appendicitis*. Retrieved on 12/28/2016 at: www.niddk.nih.gov/health-information/digestive-diseases/appendicitis

National Institute of Diabetes and Digestive and Kidney Diseases (NIDDK). (2014b). *Colon polyps.* Retrieved on 1/3/2017 at: www.niddk.nih.gov/health-information/digestive-diseases/colon-polyps/treatment

National Institute of Diabetes and Digestive and Kidney Diseases (NIDDK). (2014c). *Constipation.* Retrieved on 12/25/2016 at: www.niddk.nih.gov/health-information/digestive-diseases/constipation

National Institute of Diabetes and Digestive and Kidney Diseases (NIDDK). (2014d). *Diarrhea.* Retrieved on 12/26/2016 at: https://www.niddk.nih.gov/health-information/digestive-diseases/diarrhea

National Institute of Diabetes and Digestive and Kidney Diseases (NIDDK). (2014e). *Digestive diseases statistics for the United States.* Retrieved on 12/25/2016 at: www.niddk.nih.gov/health-information/health-statistics/Pages/digestive-diseases-statistics-for-the-united-states.aspx

National Institute of Diabetes and Digestive and Kidney Diseases (NIDDK). (2014f). *Ulcerative colitis.* Retrieved on 12/31/2016 at: www.niddk.nih.gov/health-information/digestive-diseases/ulcerative-colitis

National Institute of Diabetes and Digestive and Kidney Diseases (NIDDK). (2015). *Irritable bowel syndrome.* Retrieved on 12/27/2016 at: www.niddk.nih.gov/health-information/digestive-diseases/irritable-bowel-syndrome

National Institute of Diabetes and Digestive and Kidney Diseases (NIDDK). (2016a). *Celiac disease.* Retrieved on 12/28/2016 at: www.niddk.nih.gov/health-information/digestive-diseases/celiac-disease

National Institute of Diabetes and Digestive and Kidney Diseases (NIDDK). (2016b). *Crohn's disease.* Retrieved on 12/31/2016 at: www.niddk.nih.gov/health-information/digestive-diseases/crohns-disease

Nobie, B. A. (2015). Small-bowel obstruction. *MedScape.* Retrieved on 12/29/2016 at: emedicine.medscape.com/article/774140-overview

Perrin, A. (2013). Quality of life after ileo-anal pouch formation: Patient perceptions. *Gastrointestinal Nursing, 11*(3), 35–44.

Pfeifer, G. M. (2016). Increase in colorectal cancer occurring before age 50: Earlier screening is needed in certain younger patients. *American Journal of Nursing, 116*(5), 15.

Rao, S. S., Bharucha, A. E., Chiaroni, G. et al. (2016). Anorectal disorders. *Gastroenterology, 150*(6), 1430–1442.

Razik, R., & Nguyen, G. C. (2015). Diverticular disease: Changing epidemiology and management. *Drugs and Aging, 32*(5), 349–360.

Rex, D. K., Johnson, D. A., Anderson, J. C., et al. (2009). American College of Gastroenterology Guidelines for colorectal cancer screening. *American Journal of Gastroenterology, 104*(3), 739–750.

Robinson, B. L., Davis, S. C., Vess, J., et al. (2015). Primary care management of celiac disease. *The Nurse Practitioner, 40*(2), 28–34.

*Roos, S., Hellstrom, I., Hallert, C., et al. (2013). Everyday life for women with celiac disease. *Gastroenterology Nursing, 36*(4), 266–273.

Saccomano, S. J., & Ferrara, L. R. (2013). Evaluation of acute abdominal pain. *The Nurse Practitioner, 38*(11), 46–53.

Salminen, P., Paajanen, H., Rautio, T., et al. (2015). Antibiotic therapy vs appendectomy for treatment of uncomplicated acute appendicitis: The APPAC randomized clinical trial. *JAMA, 313*(23), 2340–2348.

Shabanzadeh, D. M., & Wille-Jorgensen, P. (2012). Antibiotics for uncomplicated diverticulitis. *Cochrane Database of Systematic Reviews, 11*, CD009092.

Shahedi, K., Dea, S. K., Chudasama, Y. N., et al. (2016). Diverticulitis. *MedScape.* Retrieved on 12/29/2016 at: emedicine.medscape.com/article/173388-overview

*Skrastins, O & Fletcher, P. C. (2016). "One flar at a time:" Adaptive and maladaptive behaviors of women coping with inflammatory bowel disease and irritable bowel syndrome. *Clinical Nurse Specialist, 30*(5), e1–e11.

Smith, C. J., & Harris, J. (2014). Crohn disease: Taking charge of a life-long disorder. *Nursing, 44*(12), 37–42.

Steele, S. R., Chang, G. J., Hendren, S., et al. (2015). Practice guideline for the surveillance of patients after curative treatment of colon and rectal cancer. *Diseases of the Colon & Rectum, 58*(8), 713–725.

Thornton, S. C., Rosh, A. J., & Perry, K. R. (2015). Hemorrhoids. *MedScape.* Retrieved on 12/30/2016 at: emedicine.medscape.com/article/775407-overview

van Rossem, C. C., Schreinemacher, M. H., Treskes, K., et al. (2014). Duration of antibiotic treatment after appendicectomy for acute complicated appendicitis. *British Journal of Surgery, 101*(6), 715–719.

Wald, A., Bharucha, A. E., Cosman, B. C., et al. (2014). ACG clinical guideline: Management of benign anorectal disorders. *The American Journal of Gastroenterology, 109*(8), 1141–1157.

Walfish, A. E. (2016). Inflammatory bowel disease. *Merck Manual: Professional Version.* Retrieved on 12/29/2016 at: www.merckmanuals.com/professional/gastrointestinal-disorders/inflammatory-bowel-disease-ibd

Watson, A. J., Nicol, L., Donaldson, S., et al. (2013). Complications of stomas: Their aetiology and management. *British Journal of Community Nursing, 18*(3), 111–112, 114–116.

Wong, P. F., Gilliam, A. D., Kumar, S., et al. (2012). Antibiotic regimens for secondary peritonitis of gastrointestinal origin in adults. *Cochrane Database of Systematic Reviews, 2*, CD004539.

Yong, J. (2016). What's new in neuromodulation for anorectal dysfunction. *Australian-New Zealand Continence Journal, 22*(4), 93–94.

Zigich, S., & Heuberger, R. (2013). The relationship of food intolerance and irritable bowel syndrome in adults. *Gastroenterology Nursing, 36*(4), 275–282.

Resources

American Cancer Society, www.cancer.org

American College of Surgeons, Ostomy Home Skills Program, www.facs.org/education/patient-education/skills-programs/ostomy-program

American Society of Colon and Rectal Surgeons (ASCRS), www.fascrs.org

Beyond Celiac Disease, www.beyondceliac.org

Celiac Support Association, www.csaceliacs.org

Colon Cancer Alliance, www.ccalliance.org

Crohn's and Colitis Foundation of America (CCFA), www.ccfa.org

Gluten Free Drugs, www.glutenfreedrugs.com

International Foundation for Functional Gastrointestinal Disorders (IFFGD), www.iffgd.org

J-Pouch Group (source for J-Pouch surgery support), www.j-pouch.org

Meet an OstoMate, www.meetanostomate.org

National Association for Continence, www.nafc.org

National Cancer Institute, National Institutes of Health, www.cancer.gov

National Colorectal Cancer Roundtable, nccrt.wpengine.com/

National Comprehensive Cancer Network Guidelines for Patients with Colon Cancer, www.nccn.org/patients/guidelines/colon/index.html#114

National Institute of Diabetes and Digestive and Kidney Diseases (NIDDK), www.niddk.nih.gov

The Colon Club, colonclub.org

The Rome Foundation, theromefoundation.org

United Ostomy Associations of America (UOAA), www.ostomy.org

Wound Ostomy and Continence Nurses Society, www.wocn.org

UNIT 11

Metabolic and Endocrine Function

ENSURING OPEN COMMUNICATION AND APPROPRIATE DELEGATION

Anurse has just started a 12-hour day shift on a medical unit. The assignment includes five patients; a 24-year-old male with a new diagnosis of type 1 diabetes; a 45-year-old female admitted last night with diabetic ketoacidosis; a 55-year-old male with cancer of the liver who is scheduled for chemotherapy today; a 65-year-old female patient with a diagnosis of hepatitis B; and a 66-year-old male with acute pancreatitis receiving total parenteral nutrition through a central line. The nurse requests a "huddle" with the unlicensed assistant assigned to the team for the day. How can the nurse foster open communication, mutual respect, and shared decision making with her team to achieve quality patient care for these five patients?

QSEN Competency Focus: Teamwork and Collaboration

The complexities inherent in today's health care system challenges nurses to demonstrate integration of specific inter-disciplinary core competencies. These competencies are aimed at ensuring the delivery of safe, quality patient care (Institute of Medicine, 2003). The Quality and Safety Education for Nurses project (QSEN, 2017; Cronenwett, Sherwood, Barnsteiner, et al., 2007) provides a framework for the knowledge, skills, and attitudes (KSA) required for nurses to demonstrate competency in these key areas, which include *patient-centered care, interdisciplinary teamwork and collaboration, evidence-based practice, quality improvement, safety,* and *informatics.*

Teamwork and Collaboration Definition: Function effectively within nursing and interprofessional teams, fostering open communication, mutual respect, and shared decision making to achieve quality patient care.

SELECTED PRE-LICENSURE KSAs	APPLICATION AND REFLECTION
Knowledge	
Examine strategies for improving systems to support team functioning.	Discuss what should happen during the beginning of the shift "huddle" in this busy medical unit. What tasks can the nurse delegate to the aide? Are there other resources within the hospital the nurse can draw on to help support these five patients?
Skills	
Participate in designing systems that support effective teamwork.	Give examples of checklists or other tools that may be used so that consistent processes are followed during a "huddle".
Attitudes	
Value the influence of system solutions in achieving effective team functioning.	How can a team approach to job completion assure best outcomes, generally speaking? Why is teamwork and collaboration of such great importance in assuring best patient outcomes?

Cronenwett, L., Sherwood, G., Barnsteiner, J., et al. (2007). Quality and safety education for nurses. *Nursing Outlook, 55*(3), 122–131.
Institute of Medicine. (2003). *Health professions education: A bridge to quality.* Washington, DC: National Academies Press.
QSEN Institute. (2017). *QSEN Competencies: Definitions and pre-licensure KSAs.* Retrieved on 3/1/2017 at: www.qsen.org/competencies/pre-licensure-ksas

48

Assessment and Management of Patients With Obesity

LEARNING OBJECTIVES

On completion of this chapter, the learner will be able to:

1 Describe the causes, classifications, and diseases and disorders associated with obesity.
2 Identify strategies aimed at preventing and treating obesity, including lifestyle modification, pharmacologic therapy, and nonsurgical interventions.
3 Explain nursing management considerations for the patient with obesity using nonsurgical interventions.
4 Compare and contrast surgical modalities indicated to treat patients with obesity in terms of preoperative, postoperative, and long-term management and complications.
5 Use the nursing process as a framework for care of patients who undergo bariatric surgical procedures.

GLOSSARY

adiposopathy: dysfunction of adipose tissue that causes chronic inflammation and disease
bariatric: relating to obesity; term derives from two Greek words meaning "weight" and "treatment"
body mass index (BMI): a weight-to-height ratio, calculated by dividing weight in kilograms by height in meters squared; the most common measure used to classify and diagnose obesity
dumping syndrome: physiologic response to rapid emptying of gastric contents into the jejunum, manifested by nausea, weakness, sweating, palpitations, syncope, and possibly diarrhea

dysphagia: difficulty swallowing
genome: the total complement of individual genes in an organism
microbiome: the collective genome of all microbes in a microbiota
microbiota: the complement of microbes in a given environment
obesity: a disease characterized by an abnormal or excessive accumulation of body fat that impairs health
obesogenic: a factor that promotes weight gain and obesity
orexigenic: a factor that stimulates appetite
satiety: feeling of having eaten sufficient quantities of food

The rates of obesity in the United States and globally have reached pandemic proportions. Given the high prevalence of obesity, nurses will encounter adults with obesity in every inpatient and outpatient clinical setting. This chapter describes the etiology, clinical manifestations, management, and related nursing care of the patient with obesity. The management of patients with obesity using both nonsurgical and surgical treatments is discussed.

 Obesity

Obesity is defined by the World Health Organization (WHO) as an "abnormal or excessive fat accumulation that may impair health" (WHO, 2016, p. 1). As a response to endorsements by multiple health care organizations and societies, including the American College of Cardiology, the Endocrine Society, and the American College of Surgeons, to name a few, the American Medical Association (AMA) House of Delegates in 2013 officially resolved that obesity should be diagnosed as a disease (AMA, 2013). This resolution was based upon the scientific observation that obesity followed criteria commonly used for defining a disease; namely, it can be said that obesity impairs normal bodily function, possesses characteristic signs and symptoms, and causes morbidity (AMA, 2013).

Epidemiology of Obesity

Worldwide, over 600 million adults have obesity, and another 1.4 billion are overweight (WHO, 2016). The prevalence of obesity has more than doubled since 1975. In particular, 3% of the world's men and 6% of the world's women had obesity in 1975, whereas 11% of the world's men and 15% of the world's women had obesity in 2014 (WHO, 2016). The burden of obesity is significant in both developed and developing nations. The WHO (2016) notes that many developing nations are now facing a "double-burden" effect from disorders linked to nutrition and metabolism; that is, these nations must simultaneously deal with the public health threats of both undernutrition and obesity. In developing nations, obesity has become particularly prevalent in urban settings (WHO, 2016).

The proportion of adults with obesity in the United States had risen every decade for over three decades until 2012, when those rates were reported to have plateaued. However, the prevalence of obesity and overweight in the United States remains among the highest in the world (Ogden, Carroll, Kit, et al., 2014). Among American adults, an estimated 36.5% have obesity (Ogden, Carroll, Fryar, et al., 2015); an estimated 68.5% have obesity or are overweight (Levi, Segal,

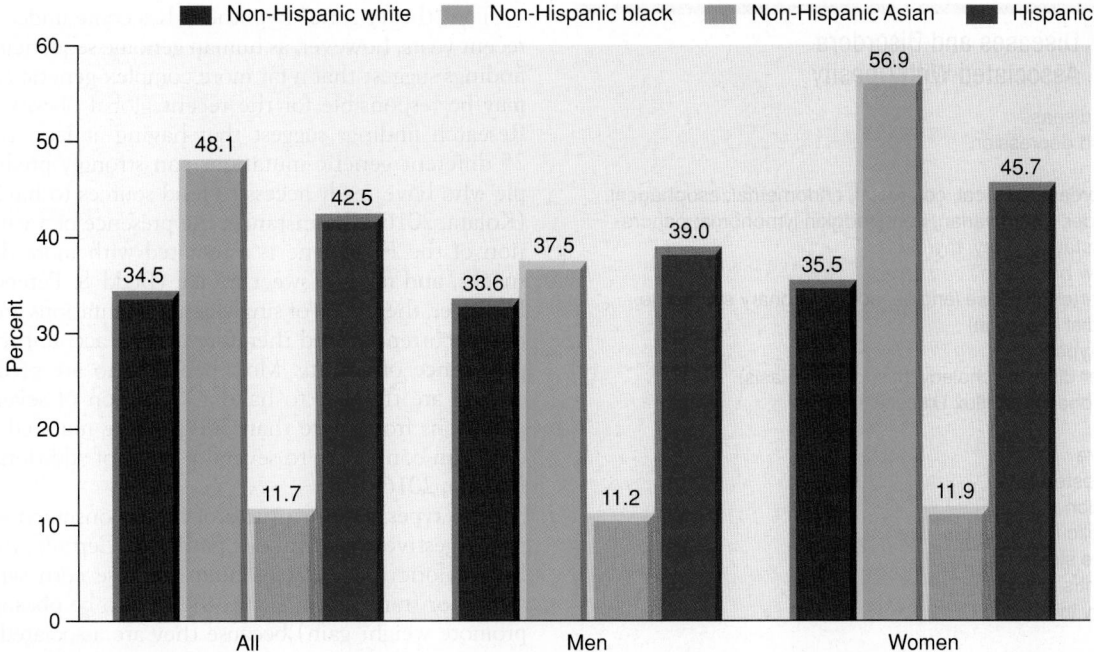

Figure 48-1 • Prevalence of obesity among adults aged 20 and older, by gender and race/ethnicity in the United States (2011–2014). Adapted from Ogden, C. L., Carroll, M. D., Fryar, C. D., et al. (2015). *Prevalence of obesity among adults and youth: United States, 2011–2014.* NCHS data brief, no 219. Hyattsville, MD: National Center for Health Statistics.

St. Laurent, et al., 2014). The prevalence of obesity is higher among American women than American men, and among African Americans and Hispanics than among Caucasians or Asian Americans (see Fig. 48-1). In general, those who are less educated and earn less income are more likely to have obesity, reflecting socioeconomic disparities in the disease burden of obesity (Segal, Rayburn, & Martin, 2016). Being overweight or obese is the primary reason why young American adults are excluded from military service (Segal et al., 2016).

The economic burden of obesity to American society extends beyond limiting young adults with obesity from pursuing military service commitments. It is estimated that annual health care costs tied to obesity are $147 billion, and that average annual health care expenditures for Americans with obesity are $1429 higher per person than for those Americans without obesity (Mozaffarian, Benjamin, Go, et al., 2016).

Obesity Risks

The causes of obesity are complex and multifactorial, and include behavioral, environmental, physiologic, and genetic factors. While there are certain demographic groups who seem to be at risk for obesity (see Fig. 48-1) and while there are notable familial patterns of obesity, identification of risk factors that specify odds of being diagnosed with obesity are not as clearly elucidated as those for other diseases (Centers for Disease Control and Prevention [CDC], 2016a), such as coronary artery disease (see Chapter 27) and cerebrovascular disease (see Chapter 67).

What is abundantly clear, however, is that obesity incurs a greater overall risk of mortality. Obesity is associated with a 6- to 20-year decrease in overall life expectancy (Moyer,

LeFevere, Siu, et al., 2012). Furthermore, obesity is associated with morbidity and mortality from numerous other diseases (see Fig. 48-2 and Chart 48-1). For instance, as body mass index (BMI) increases, so does the overall risk of cancer and risk for death from cancer; obesity is responsible for up to 90,000 deaths from cancer annually. Having obesity increases the likelihood of having type 2 diabetes by 10-fold and the likelihood of having either asthma or hypertension

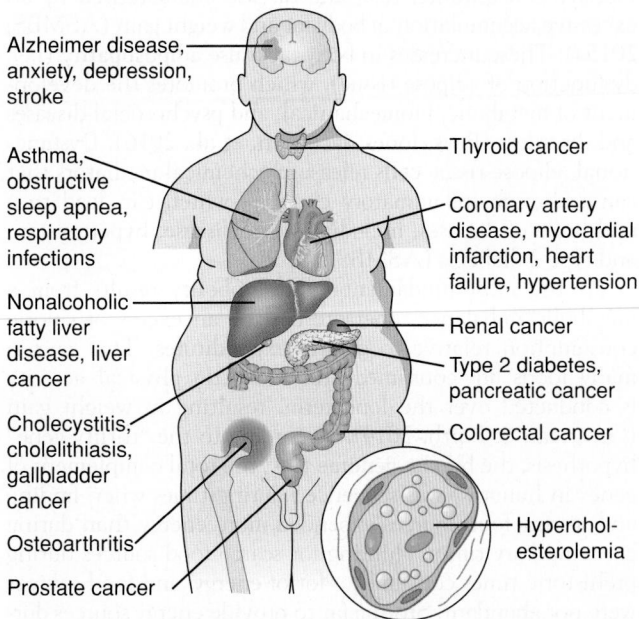

Figure 48-2 • Morbid diseases and disorders associated with obesity.

<table>
<tr><td>

Chart 48-1 Diseases and Disorders Associated With Obesity

Alzheimer disease
Anxiety and depression
Asthma
Cancers (breast, cervical, colorectal, endometrial, esophageal, gallbladder, liver, ovarian, non-Hodgkin lymphoma, pancreatic, prostate, kidney, thyroid)
Chronic low back pain
Coronary artery disease (angina, acute coronary syndrome, myocardial infarction)
Diabetes (type 2)
Gallbladder disease (cholecystitis, cholelithiasis)
Gastroesophageal Reflux Disease (GERD)
Gout
Heart failure
Hypercholesterolemia
Hypertension
Nonalcoholic fatty liver disease
Obstructive sleep apnea
Osteoarthritis
Respiratory infections
Stroke

Adapted from American Society for Metabolic and Bariatric Surgery (ASMBS). (2015b). *The impact of obesity on your body and health.* Retrieved on 11/19/2015 at: asmbs.org/patients/impact-of-obesity; Centers for Disease Control and Prevention (CDC). (2016a). Adult obesity causes & consequences. Retrieved on 1/8/2017 at: www.cdc.gov/obesity/adult/causes.html

</td></tr>
</table>

by nearly 4-fold (American Society for Metabolic and Bariatric Surgery [ASMBS], 2015b). Adults with obesity are twice as likely to eventually be diagnosed with Alzheimer disease than those adults who maintain a normal weight (Mozaffarian et al., 2016).

Pathophysiology

Obesity is a chronic, relapsing disease characterized by an excessive accumulation of body fat and weight gain (ASMBS, 2015a). These increases in body fat cause **adiposopathy** (i.e., dysfunction of adipose tissue), which promotes the development of metabolic, biomechanical, and psychosocial diseases and disorders (Bays, Jones, Jacobson, et al., 2016). Dysfunctional adipose tissue cells release biochemical mediators that cause chronic inflammatory changes, which can lead to a multitude of diseases, including heart disease, hypertension, and type 2 diabetes (ASMBS, 2013b).

At the most fundamental level, obesity results from a metabolic imbalance, characterized by an excess of caloric consumption relative to caloric expenditures. That is, too many foods are consumed and too little physical activity is conducted over the long term, resulting in weight gain (Grossman & Porth, 2014). According to the "thrifty gene" hypothesis, the human **genome** (i.e., the total complement of genes in humans) was sequenced during times when finding and storing food sources expended more energy than during contemporary times. Hunting for scarce food sources during prehistoric times consumed a lot of energy, and food sources were not abundant. Storing fat to provide energy sources during times of food scarcity was a physiologic adaptive response to these environmental challenges (Budd & Peterson, 2014).

The "thrifty gene" hypothesis has come under scrutiny in recent years, however, as human genome sequencing research findings suggest that a far more complex genetic explanation may be responsible for the recent global obesity pandemic. Research findings suggest that having at least one of over 25 different genetic mutations can strongly predispose people who have ready access to food sources to having obesity (Kolata, 2016). For instance, the presence of a variant mutation of the *FTO* gene is associated with more daily meals, snacks, and fat and sweet intake (Budd & Peterson, 2014). However, these type of single genetic mutations are relatively rare occurrences, and therefore cannot account for the high prevalence of obesity. Most people who are predisposed to obesity are thought to have a collection of several genetic mutations from more than 300 possible mutated genes that each can contribute to several pounds of additional body fat (Kolata, 2016).

The types and quantities of foods consumed affect complex digestive and metabolic pathways. Certain processed and high caloric foods that contain fructose corn syrup, simple sugars, or trans fats, are hypothesized to be **obesogenic** (i.e., promote weight gain) because they are associated with food cravings consonant with other type of addictive cravings (Budd & Peterson, 2014). Furthermore, the portions of foods served in restaurants and packaged on grocery shelves have increased over the past 20 years, subtly affecting consumers' feelings of **satiety** (i.e., feeling of having eaten sufficient amounts of food) (National Heart, Lung, and Blood Institute [NHLBI], 2016a). For instance, a typical bagel was 3 inches in diameter 20 years ago, but today is about 6 inches in diameter. Likewise, the average cheeseburger 20 years ago was 333 calories but today is larger and has 590 calories (NHLBI, 2016a).

Multiple hormones that control food cravings and feelings of fullness could be affected by individual genes. In response to periods of fasting, the hormone ghrelin is secreted by the stomach and the hormone neuropeptide Y (NPY) is secreted by the small intestines. These hormones are **orexigenic**, meaning that they stimulate appetite through central nervous system (CNS) pathways that lead to the hypothalamus, signaling higher neural pathways that lead to eating behaviors. Once eating occurs, multiple hormones are released throughout the gastrointestinal (GI) tract that promote satiety, including somatostatin, cholecystokinin (CCK), and insulin, to name a few. CCK also slows gastric motility and emptying, stimulates gallbladder contraction and release of bile into the duodenum, and stimulates the release of pancreatic digestive enzymes, all of which serve to enhance the digestive process. Somatostatin also slows gastric emptying but has other effects that are in opposition to CCK, such as decreasing the secretion of bile, depending on foods consumed and metabolic needs (Bays, Kothari, Azagury, et al., 2016).

Increases in fat stores, or adipose tissue, result in increases in the hormone leptin, which is secreted by fat cells. Leptin also has the effect of signaling satiety in the hypothalamus. Patients with obesity who lose weight are thought to also have drops in leptin levels that persist for the long term, creating persistent feelings of hunger, which may partially explain why many patients with obesity who lose weight tend to regain it (Budd & Peterson, 2014).

The GI tract **microbiota**, which is the complement of microbes within the gut, has been found to contain up to

100 trillion microbes, or 10 times the cells present in the human body (Davis, 2016). The collective genome of the microbiota, or the gut **microbiome**, has more than 100 times more genes than in the human genome (Davis, 2016). It has long been known that gut microbes perform numerous digestive, metabolic, and immunologic functions. The composition and diversity of these microbes may very well be tied in with obesity. For instance, patients with obesity tend to have less diverse microbiota than patients who are lean. In turn, these patients with obesity who have less diverse microbiota typically also have dyslipidemia, impaired glucose metabolism, and low-grade generalized inflammatory disorders. The effects of "Western-style diets," high in processed foods, fat, and sugars, and low in fiber, is thought to not only negatively affect the diversity of the gut microbiota, but also negatively affect the complement of *Bacteroidetes* species microbes, which are associated with a leaner type of microbiome (Davis, 2016). Whether or not it is possible to regulate the composition of the gut microbiota and prevent or treat obesity is the focus of ongoing research (Davis, 2016).

Assessment and Diagnostic Findings

Patient height and weight is measured to determine the **body mass index (BMI)**. The BMI is the definitive measure used to determine whether or not a patient is overweight or has

TABLE 48-1 Body Mass Index (BMI) Classification for Overweight and Obesity

Classification	BMI Range (kg/m²)
Overweight/Pre-obese	25–29.9
Class I Obesity	30–34.9
Class II Obesity	35–39.9
Class III (also called "extreme" or "severe") Obesity	≥40

Adapted from Centers for Disease Control and Prevention (CDC). (2016b). *Defining adult overweight and obesity.* Retrieved on 1/24/2017 at: www.cdc.gov/obesity/adult/defining.html

obesity; this is based upon a ratio of body weight in kilograms and height in meters (see Chapter 5, Table 5-1). Patients identified as overweight or pre-obese have a BMI of 25 to 29.9 kg/m² and those with obesity have a BMI that exceeds 30 kg/m². Those with a BMI exceeding 40 kg/m² are considered to have severe or extreme obesity (previously referred to as morbid obesity) (WHO, 2015) (see Fig. 48-3 and Table 48-1).

Patients with obesity may also have their waist circumferences assessed. Women with waist circumferences more than 35 inches and men with waist circumferences more than 40 inches have greater risks for obesity-related morbidity

Body Mass Index Table

	Normal						Overweight					Obese										Extreme Obesity														
BMI	19	20	21	22	23	24	25	26	27	28	29	30	31	32	33	34	35	36	37	38	39	40	41	42	43	44	45	46	47	48	49	50	51	52	53	54
Height (inches)																Body Weight (pounds)																				
58	91	96	100	105	110	115	119	124	129	134	138	143	148	153	158	162	167	172	177	181	186	191	196	201	205	210	215	220	224	229	234	239	244	248	253	258
59	94	99	104	109	114	119	124	128	133	138	143	148	153	158	163	168	173	178	183	188	193	198	203	208	212	217	222	227	232	237	242	247	252	257	262	267
60	97	102	107	112	118	123	128	133	138	143	148	153	158	163	168	174	179	184	189	194	199	204	209	215	220	225	230	235	240	245	250	255	261	266	271	276
61	100	106	111	116	122	127	132	137	143	148	153	158	164	169	174	180	185	190	195	201	206	211	217	222	227	232	238	243	248	254	259	264	269	275	280	285
62	104	109	115	120	126	131	136	142	147	153	158	164	169	175	180	186	191	196	202	207	213	218	224	229	235	240	246	251	256	262	267	273	278	284	289	295
63	107	113	118	124	130	135	141	146	152	158	163	169	175	180	186	191	197	203	208	214	220	225	231	237	242	248	254	259	265	270	278	282	287	293	299	304
64	110	116	122	128	134	140	145	151	157	163	169	174	180	186	192	197	204	209	215	221	227	232	238	244	250	256	262	267	273	279	285	291	296	302	308	314
65	114	120	126	132	138	144	150	156	162	168	174	180	186	192	198	204	210	216	222	228	234	240	246	252	258	264	270	276	282	288	294	300	306	312	318	324
66	118	124	130	136	142	148	155	161	167	173	179	186	192	198	204	210	216	223	229	235	241	247	253	260	266	272	278	284	291	297	303	309	315	322	328	334
67	121	127	134	140	146	153	159	166	172	178	185	191	198	204	211	217	223	230	236	242	249	255	261	268	274	280	287	293	299	306	312	319	325	331	338	344
68	125	131	138	144	151	158	164	171	177	184	190	197	203	210	216	223	230	236	243	249	256	262	269	276	282	289	295	302	308	315	322	328	335	341	348	354
69	128	135	142	149	155	162	169	176	182	189	196	203	209	216	223	230	236	243	250	257	263	270	277	284	291	297	304	311	318	324	331	338	345	351	358	365
70	132	139	146	153	160	167	174	181	188	195	202	209	216	222	229	236	243	250	257	264	271	278	285	292	299	306	313	320	327	334	341	348	355	362	369	376
71	136	143	150	157	165	172	179	186	193	200	208	215	222	229	236	243	250	257	265	272	279	286	293	301	308	315	322	329	338	343	351	358	365	372	379	386
72	140	147	154	162	169	177	184	191	199	206	213	221	228	235	242	250	258	265	272	279	287	294	302	309	316	324	331	338	346	353	361	368	375	383	390	397
73	144	151	159	166	174	182	189	197	204	212	219	227	235	242	250	257	265	272	280	288	295	302	310	318	325	333	340	348	355	363	371	378	386	393	401	408
74	148	155	163	171	179	186	194	202	210	218	225	233	241	249	256	264	272	280	287	295	303	311	319	326	334	342	350	358	365	373	381	389	396	404	412	420
75	152	160	168	176	184	192	200	208	216	224	232	240	248	256	264	272	279	287	295	303	311	319	327	335	343	351	359	367	375	383	391	399	407	415	423	431
76	156	164	172	180	189	197	205	213	221	230	238	246	254	263	271	279	287	295	304	312	320	328	336	344	353	361	369	377	385	394	402	410	418	426	435	443

Adapted from *Clinical Guidelines on the Identification, Evaluation, and Treatment of Overweight and Obesity in Adults: The Evidence Report.*

Figure 48-3 • Body mass index table. Adapted from National Heart, Lung, and Blood Institute (NHLBI) of the National Institutes of Health. (2016b). Aim for a healthy weight: Body mass index table. Retrieved on 3/2/2017 at: www.nhlbi.nih.gov/health/educational/lose_wt/BMI/bmi_tbl.pdf

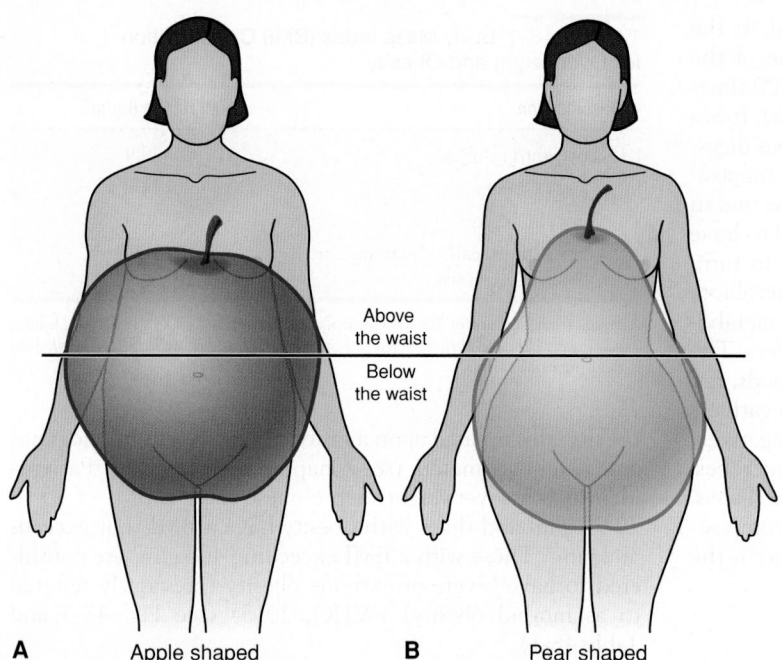

Above
the waist

Below
the waist

A Apple shaped

B Pear shaped

Figure 48-4 • **A.** Android obesity, with greater visceral/abdominal fat stores. **B.** Gynoid obesity. Reprinted with permission from Weber, J. R., & Kelley, J. H. (2014). *Health assessment in nursing* (5th ed.). Philadelphia, PA: Wolters Kluwer.

(see Chart 48-1) than those with smaller waistlines (Fitch, Everling, Fox, et al., 2013). The hip may also be measured and the waist-to-hip ratio assessed. Women with waist-to-hip ratios greater than 0.80 and men with waist-to-hip ratios greater than 0.90 are presumed to have proportionally more visceral (i.e., abdominal) fat stores. This morphological appearance is called android obesity, and is sometimes referenced as an "apple-shaped" appearance. Patients with android obesity have greater risk for developing hypertension, coronary artery disease, stroke, and type 2 diabetes, than patients who have gynoid obesity, also called the "pear-shaped" body (Weber & Kelley, 2014) (see Fig. 48-4).

Patients with obesity or who are overweight may have other diagnostic laboratory studies done to screen for cardiovascular diseases, such as cholesterol and triglycerides (see Chapter 27), for type 2 diabetes, such as fasting blood glucose and glycosylated hemoglobin (hemoglobin A1c) (see Chapter 51), or for nonalcoholic fatty liver disease, such as aspartate aminotransferase (AST) and alanine aminotransferase (ALT) (Orringer, Harrison, Nichani, et al., 2016) (see Chapter 49).

In some instances, obesity may be secondary to other diseases or disorders, such as hypothyroidism or Cushing syndrome (see Chapter 52). In those particular cases, the diagnostic workup follows that prescribed for the primary disease or disorder, and, when the therapeutic regimen is implemented, the patient may lose weight and the obesity may even resolve (Orringer et al., 2016). In addition, some patients who are overweight or have obesity may develop secondary diseases or disorders (see Chart 48-1) and may be prescribed medications aimed at treating those secondary diseases or disorders that can exacerbate weight gain (see Chart 48-2). Other patients may not have had a previous history of being overweight or having obesity, but may gain weight after being prescribed specific medications associated with weight gain. A history of weight gain that parallels the timeframe of commencing treatment with specific prescriptive medications may suggest that the medication has a key role in promoting weight gain. In some

instances, prescription medication dosages may be adjusted or another medication may be prescribed. For instance, patients with type 2 diabetes and obesity may reap the dual benefits of achieving better glycemic control and weight loss by taking the prescription drug metformin (Glucophage) (Apovian, Aronne, Bessesen, et al., 2015).

Medical Management

Treatment of obesity generally includes lifestyle modification, pharmacological management, and nonsurgical or surgical interventions.

Lifestyle Modification

The first approach used to treat obesity consists of lifestyle modification aimed at weight loss and then weight maintenance. The U.S. Preventive Services Task Force (USPSTF) recommends that all adults with BMIs in excess of 30 kg/m² be advised to engage in multicomponent behavioral interventions that include (Moyer et al., 2012):
- Setting weight-loss goals,
- Improving diet habits,
- Increasing physical activity,
- Addressing barriers to change, and,
- Self-monitoring and strategizing ongoing lifestyle changes aimed at a healthy weight.

The most effective behavioral interventions are those considered high intensity; that is, they consist of 12 to 26 sessions annually, which may include individual counseling sessions between the primary provider and patient, group nutrition education sessions, and physical activity sessions, to name a few (Moyer et al., 2012). The USPSTF notes that modest weight loss of 5% total body weight can be associated with significant clinical improvements and benefits to patients with obesity (Moyer et al., 2012).

A patient with obesity should be counseled to plan a caloric deficit of between 500 and 1000 calories daily from

Chart 48-2 — PHARMACOLOGY
Selected Medications That Affect Body Weight

Many medications prescribed to treat a variety of chronic diseases and disorders have the untoward side effect of weight gain, whereas others are associated with weight loss. The following list contains some examples of each of these.

Medications Associated with Weight Gain

Anticonvulsant Medications:
- carbamazepine (Tegretol)
- gabapentin (Neurontin)
- pregabalin (Lyrica)[a]
- valproate (Depakote)[a]

Antidepressant Medications:
- Selective Serotonin Reuptake Inhibitors (SSRIs) (*Note – these tend to be associated with early weight loss followed by gain within 6 months in some patients*):
  - citalopram (Celexa)
  - fluvoxamine (Luvox)
  - paroxetine (Paxil)
  - sertraline (Zoloft)
- Tricyclic Antidepressants:
  - amitriptyline (Elavil)
  - doxepin (Sinequan)
  - imipramine (Tofranil, Tofranil PM)
  - mirtazapine (Remeron)
  - nortriptyline (Aventyl)
  - trimipramine (Surmontil)

Antihistamines:
- cetirizine (Zyrtec)
- diphenhydramine (Benadryl)

Antihypertensive Medications:
- Beta Blockers:
  - atenolol (Tenormin)
  - metoprolol (Lopressor, Toprol)
  - propranolol (Inderal)
- Dihydropyridine Calcium Channel Blockers:
  - amlodipine (Norvasc)
  - felodipine (Plendil)
  - nifedipine (Procardia, Procardia XL)

Antipsychotic Medications:
- asenapine (Saphris)
- chlorpromazine (Thorazine)

- clozapine (Clozaril)[a]
- iloperidone (Fanapt)
- olanzapine (Zyprexa)[a]
- paliperidone (Invega)
- quetiapine (Seroquel)
- risperidone (Risperdal)

Diabetes Medications:
- Insulins:
  - insulin aspart (Novolog)
  - insulin glulisine (Apidra)
  - insulin lispro (Humalog)
- Meglitinides:
  - nateglinide (Starlix)
  - repaglinide (Prandin)
- Sulfonylureas:
  - chlorpropamide (Amaryl)
  - glimepiride (Glynase)
  - glipizide (Glucotrol, Glucotrol XL)
  - glyburide (Diabeta, Micronase)
  - tolbutamide (Diabinese)
- Thiazolidinediones:
  - Pioglitazone (Actos)

Hormones:
- Corticosteroids:
  - prednisone
  - budesonide (Pulmicort)
- Hormonal contraceptives:
  - Medroxyprogesterone (Depo-Provera)
- *Mood Stabilizers:*
  - lithium (Lithobid)
  - vigabatrin (Sabril)

Medications Associated with Weight Loss

Anticonvulsant Medications:
- lamotrigine (Lamictal)
- topiramate (Topamax)
- zonisamide (Zonegran)

Antidepressant Medications:
- bupropion (Wellbutrin, Zyban)

Diabetes Medications:
- metformin (Glucophage)

[a]Medications associated with significant weight gain.

Adapted from Bays, H. E., Seger, J. C., Primack, C., et al. (2016). *Obesity algorithm, presented by the Obesity Medicine Association.* Retrieved on 1/7/2017 at: www.obesityalgorithm.org; Budd, G. M., & Peterson, J. A. (2015). The obesity epidemic, part 2: Nursing assessment and intervention. *American Journal of Nursing*, 115(1), 38–46.; Kyle, T., & Kuehl, B. (2017). Prescription medications & weight gain – What you need to know. Retrieved on 1/7/2017 at: hwww.obesityaction.org/educational-resources/resource-articles-2/general-articles/prescription-medications-weight-gain

---

baseline, in order to achieve a 5% to 10% reduction in weight within about 6 months. This can be achieved through increasing physical activity and decreasing caloric dietary intake (Orringer et al., 2016).

Increasing physical activity through promotion of an exercise regimen is a key recommendation that can burn calories and result in weight loss. Physical activity recommendations for all adults (those with and without obesity) include at least 150 minutes of moderate-intensity aerobic exercise weekly or 75 minutes of vigorous-intensity aerobic exercise weekly. In addition, muscle strengthening exercises that engage all major muscle groups should be done at least twice weekly (Fitch et al., 2013; Orringer et al., 2016). Patients with obesity who were previously sedentary and deconditioned may

not be able to achieve this at the start; however, as little as 10 minutes of daily physical activity can result in weight loss and improved exercise tolerance (Fitch et al., 2013).

Patients with obesity should be counseled that reducing dietary caloric intake is a necessary component of weight loss therapy. This must also include a change in dietary habits in order for weight loss to be sustained over the long term. It is important to identify current dietary patterns and typical daily caloric intake in order to recommend an appropriate diet plan. Assessing food records or 24-hour recalls or conducting dietary interviews are all effective methods to gather baseline dietary information from patients (see Chapter 5: Dietary Data). There are a plethora of commercial diets that patients may select (see Chart 48-3). To date, there have not

Chart 48-3	Select Popular Commercial Diets

Atkins Diet, www.atkins.com
eDiets, www.ediets.com
Jenny Craig, www.jennycraig.com
Medifast, www.medifast1.com/index.jsp
Nutrisystem, www.nutrisystem.com/jsps_hmr/home/index.jsp
Optifast, www.optifast.com/Pages/index.aspx
South Beach Diet, www.southbeachdiet.com/home/index.jsp
The Biggest Loser Diet, www.biggestloserclub.com
Weight Watchers, www.weightwatchers.com/us/
Zone Diet, www.zonediet.com

been sufficiently rigorous longitudinal studies to determine which diet plans are superior to others in terms of achieving long-term weight loss (Katz & Meller, 2014).

Patients need not purchase commercial diet plans in order to achieve weight loss and embrace healthy diet habits. Most nutritionists advocate that healthy diets include few processed foods, sugars, and trans fats, and are heavy in plant-based foods (Katz & Meller, 2014). The Dietary Approaches to Stop Hypertension (DASH) diet is an example of a superior healthy noncommercial diet. Although initially promoted to manage hypertension, the DASH diet also provides a solid foundation for achieving and maintaining weight loss (Goldstein, Aoun, Gaar, et al., 2014) (see Chapter 31, Table 31-3: The DASH Diet). Other healthy diet plans that may form a basis for weight loss, though not specifically designed for this purpose, include the Mediterranean Diet and the Therapeutic Lifestyle Changes (TLC) Diet (see Chapter 27 for description of both diets, see Table 27-1: The TLC Diet). Patient education tips for managing ongoing healthy eating strategies are noted in Chart 48-4.

In addition to promoting healthy exercise and diet habits, ensuring healthy sleep habits is an additional lifestyle strategy that is associated with weight loss and maintenance of a healthy weight. It is posited that sleep deprivation can cause changes in cortisol levels that promote weight gain (Orringer et al., 2016). Advising patients with sleep disturbances to plan to be in bed with lights out at least 7 hours prior to wake-up time, to create a dark, relaxing bedroom environment, to avoid activities that can cause arousal around bedtime (e.g., texting), and to avoid beverages with caffeine after lunchtime can all be helpful strategies aimed at ensuring a restful night's sleep that is consonant with weight reduction (Orringer et al., 2016).

Pharmacologic Therapy

Patients who are not successful at meeting weight loss goals from lifestyle modification alone may be prescribed antiobesity medications. Some patients may exhibit initial success with lifestyle modifications, but be stymied with attempts to maintain a lower BMI over the long term. These patients may also benefit from antiobesity medications. Patients who are prescribed antiobesity medications should be counseled that these prescriptions are meant to supplement, not supplant diet modification and exercise (Yanovski & Yanovksi, 2014). Indications for antiobesity medications include a BMI >30 kg/m² or a BMI >27 kg/m² with concomitant morbidity that is related to being overweight (e.g., type 2 diabetes,

Chart 48-4	PATIENT EDUCATION
	Healthy Eating Strategies

The nurse instructs the patient about the healthy eating strategies outlined below.

Limit or eliminate the following:
- Processed foods with limited nutritional value (e.g., packaged cakes, cookies, chips)
- High caloric beverages (sugar-sweetened, juices, cream-enhanced)
- Fast foods
- Vending machine foods
- Foods high in sugars (e.g., candies) and saturated fats (e.g., fried foods, hot dogs)

Track the following:
- Daily food intake (food journals, diaries, smartphone, and tablet applications)
- Nutritional value and caloric content on food labels

Encourage the following:
- Reduce portions; use smaller plates and measure foods
- Schedule and plan meals and snacks in advance for each day; prepack lunches and snacks when you are out of the home (e.g., for work)
- Eat at home more often than you would eat outside the home; when eating out, avoid fried foods and choose lean meats and vegetables and salads with condiments on the side
- Eat breakfast
- Limit snacks
- Eat a variety of nutritious foods; monitoring quality of foods consumed is as important as the quantity of foods consumed
- Drink plenty of water
- Stay within your daily caloric intake plan; do not become discouraged if one day you do not adhere to your plan

Adapted from Fruh, S. M., Mulekar, M. S., & Dierking, J. (2013). Guiding patients to safe weight loss. *The Nurse Practitioner*, 38(10), 1–7; Orringer, K. A., Harrison, A. V., Nichani, S. S., et al. (2016). *University of Michigan Health System Clinical Alignment and Performance Excellence Guideline: Obesity prevention and management*. Retrieved on 1/25/2017 at: www.med.umich.edu/1info/FHP/practiceguides/obesity/obesity.pdf

hypertension) (Apovian et al., 2015; Bays, Seger, Primach, et al., 2016).

The U.S. Food and Drug Administration (FDA) has had a long history of approving antiobesity drugs and then rescinding those approvals. Thyroid hormone was approved in 1893 and then taken off the market for obesity treatment in 1949. Amphetamines were approved in 1937 and taken off the market in 1971 for cardiovascular toxic effects. More recently, fenfluramine was approved in 1973 and taken off the market in 1997, phenylpropanolamine was approved in 1960 and taken off the market in 2000, and sibutramine (Meridia) was approved in 1997 and taken off the market in 2010, all for life-threatening adverse effects (Bendich, 2013).

Today, there are five antiobesity medications that may be prescribed over the long term to assist in decreasing and then maintaining a lower BMI. Of these, only one, orlistat (Xenical), was FDA approved prior to 2012 (Bendich, 2013) (see Table 48-2). It is estimated that less than 3 million Americans take antiobesity medications, although many more may benefit from these prescriptions. It is thought that concerns about the safety of antiobesity medications coupled with the relatively recent FDA approval of safe and effective antiobesity

TABLE 48-2 Medications Prescribed to Treat Obesity

Medication	Adverse Effects	Nursing Considerations[a]
Gastrointestinal Lipase Inhibitor Mechanism of Action: Diminishes intestinal absorption and metabolism of fats, particularly triglycerides		
Orlistat (Xenical) *Note: Also available in lower dosages over-the-counter under the trade name of Alli*	Diarrhea Flatus Oily stools Fecal incontinence	Patients may have associated problems with malabsorption of nutrients; advise them to take a concomitant daily multivitamin. Caution in patients with known history of renal insufficiency, liver disease, or gallbladder disease as concomitant use is associated with renal calculi, liver failure, and cholelithiasis. Do not administer with cyclosporine (Neoral).
Selective Serotonergic 5-HT2C Receptor Agonist Mechanism of Action: Stimulates central 5-HT2C receptors, causing appetite suppression		
Lorcaserin (Belviq)	Fatigue Dizziness Nausea Headaches Cough Dry mouth Constipation	Can be associated with deficits in attention or memory; administer with caution in patients who drive or work with hazardous equipment when first prescribed until effects are realized. Can cause hypoglycemia in patients with diabetes Patients concomitantly taking antidepressants or migraine medications can have synergistic effects. Discontinue in patients who express suicidal ideation. Rarely, serotonin syndrome may develop—be alert for high fevers, brisk reflexes, agitation, and diarrhea; notify primary provider immediately and hold medication if these occur.
GLP-1 Receptor Agonists Mechanism of Action: Mimics the effects of incretins, resulting in delayed gastric emptying, thus curbing appetite		
Liraglutide (Saxenda) *Note: Also available in lower dosages under the trade name of Victoza to treat type 2 diabetes*	Nausea Diarrhea or constipation Headache Tachycardia	Must be given subcutaneously on a daily basis in the abdomen, thigh, or upper arm. Dosage increases weekly until week 5. Discontinue in patients who express suicide ideation. May be associated with pancreatitis; also associated with thyroid tumors in animal models.
Sympathomimetic Amines Mechanism of Action: Stimulate central noradrenergic receptors, causing appetite suppression		
Phentermine (Adipex-P, Fastin) Benzphetamine (Didrex) Diethylpropion (Tenuate) Phendimetrazine (Bontril)	Palpitations and tachycardia Tremors Hypertension Dizziness Insomnia Diarrhea or constipation Mouth dryness Restlessness Alterations in taste	These are only FDA-approved for short-term use (i.e., no more than 12 weeks). Contraindications include heart disease, uncontrolled hypertension, hyperthyroidism, and glaucoma. Caution patients to not drink alcohol while taking one of these medications.
Dual Agents Mechanism of Action: Each of these medications combines two medications with known anti-obesity effects; when taken together, the effects are synergistic.		
Phentermine/topiramate-ER (Qsymia) Mechanism of Action: combines the effectiveness of phentermine (see above) and topiramate, an anticonvulsant, which stimulates central GABA receptors & inhibits central glutamate receptors, suppressing appetite	Paresthesias Dizziness Insomnia Mouth dryness Alterations in taste Insomnia Constipation Tachycardia	Same contraindications apply as for phentermine (see above). May need to monitor electrolytes, as hypokalemia and metabolic acidosis are possible. Monitor creatinine and watch for manifestations of renal calculi.
Naltrexone/bupropion (Contrave) Mechanism of action: inhibits central opioid receptors and inhibits reuptake of dopamine and norepinephrine selectively, resulting in diminished appetite and cravings	Constipation or diarrhea Nausea Vomiting Insomnia Dizziness Mouth dryness Hypertension Tachycardia	Contraindications include uncontrolled hypertension, epilepsy, history of eating disorder such as anorexia nervosa or bulimia, and history of alcohol abuse of illicit drug abuse. Discontinue in patients who express suicidal ideation.

[a]All anti-obesity medications may be teratogenic; pregnancy is a contraindication to all of these agents.

FDA, U.S. Food and Drug Administration.

Adapted from Bays, H. E., Seger, J. C., Primack, C., et al. (2016). *Obesity algorithm, presented by the Obesity Medicine Association.* Retrieved on 1/7/2017 at: www.obesityalgorithm.org; National Institute of Diabetes and Digestive and Kidney Diseases (NIDDK). (2016). *Prescription medications to treat overweight and obesity.* Retrieved on 1/7/2017 at: www.niddk.nih.gov/health-information/health-topics/weight-control/prescription-medications-treat-overweight-obesity/Pages/facts.aspx; Yanovski, S. Z., & Yanovski, J. A. (2014). Long-term drug treatment for obesity: A systematic and clinical review. *JAMA, 311*(1), 74–86.

medications likely account for the relative dearth of these prescriptions (Yanovski & Yanovski, 2014).

Antiobesity medications work by either inhibiting gastrointestinal absorption of fats, or by altering central brain receptors to enhance satiety or reduce cravings (National Institute of Diabetes and Digestive and Kidney Diseases [NIDDK], 2016). Each of these medications has distinct side effects and contraindications; therefore, selection of these agents is very individualized. The patient is monitored while taking the selected medication; if the patient does not lose at least 5% body weight after 12 weeks, the prescription may need to be changed, or the patient may be referred for other weight-reduction therapy (e.g., bariatric surgery) (NIDDK, 2016).

The class of antiobesity medications known as the sympathomimetic amines have been FDA approved for many years. However, they are only supposed to be prescribed for short-term use (i.e., no longer than 12 weeks). They have many side effects (see Table 48-2), and patients do tend to regain weight once they are no longer taking these medications (NIDDK, 2016).

Nonsurgical Interventions

Adult patients with obesity that does not respond to lifestyle interventions or antiobesity medications and who have either Class III/severe/extreme obesity (i.e., BMI in excess of 40 kg/m^2) or Class II obesity (BMI 35–39.9 kg/m^2) with obesity-related diseases or disorders (e.g., obstructive sleep apnea, type 2 diabetes) may be candidates for bariatric surgical interventions (see later discussion). As an alternative, some patients may elect to pursue minimally invasive interventions that were approved by the FDA in 2015. These types of interventions include vagal blocking (i.e., neurometabolic modulation) or intragastric balloon therapy (Ali, Moustarah, Kim, et al., 2015; Papasavas, El Chaar, Kothari, et al., 2016).

Vagal blocking therapy involves placement of a pacemaker-like device (vBloc™) into the subcutaneous tissue in the lateral thoracic cavity with two leads that are laparoscopically implanted at the point where the vagus nerve truncates, at the gastroesophageal junction. A pre-programmed, pulsating signal is delivered for 12 hours daily. This signal causes intermittent "blocking" of the vagus nerve. Vagal blocking results in diminished gastric contraction and emptying, limited ghrelin secretion, and diminished pancreatic enzyme secretion; these cause increased satiety, decreased cravings, and diminished absorption of calories, all of which lead to weight loss (Papasavas et al., 2016). Results from a randomized controlled trial found greater initial and 18-month sustained weight loss with participants with obesity who received vagal blocking versus control sham device implantation (Ikramuddin, Blackstone, Bracatisano, et al., 2014; Shikora, Wolfe, Apovian, et al., 2015). There are few adverse effects noted with use of this device, which include GI symptoms (e.g., heartburn, belching). Patients must be educated to recharge the device twice weekly for about an hour with an external coil device.

Intragastric balloon therapy involves endoscopic placement of a saline-filled balloon (ORBERA™) or a saline-filled dual balloon (ReShape™) into the stomach. The mechanism by which these devices result in weight loss is poorly understood, but thought to be related to increased feelings of satiety and decreased gastric emptying. Post-insertion, the intragastric balloon(s) remain in place for 3 to 6 months, and are then deflated and removed. Studies suggest greater weight loss with these than with sham therapy or with lifestyle interventions alone (Ali et al., 2015). Early adverse effects include complaints of nausea and vomiting, which are generally transient and do not require balloon removal. Balloon rupture can occur over the long term, however, which may infrequently lead to intestinal obstruction. In order to monitor for this serious complication, it is recommended that the balloons be impregnated with methylene blue pre-insertion so that patients with silent ruptures can report the presence of green urine to their primary providers and receive timely interventions to remove the deflated balloons before they cause obstruction. Patients who seem unlikely to return for follow-up appointments should not be candidates for intragastric balloons. Balloons should be removed within 6 months of placement; longer placement periods are associated with increased likelihood of rupture and intestinal obstruction (Ali et al., 2015).

 Gerontologic Considerations

According to findings from the United States National Health and Nutrition Examination Survey (NHANES), the prevalence of obesity for adults over the age of 60 is 38.5%, slightly higher than the prevalence of obesity among all adults (Segal et al., 2016). Climbing rates of obesity among older adults mirrors the rate increases among all adults over the past few decades.

As adults age, lean skeletal mass decreases and adipose tissue increases. Adipose tissue does not burn calories as efficiently as lean skeletal mass; furthermore, basal metabolism drops by 2% for each additional decade of adult life. Therefore, older adults are more likely to gain weight unless they either increase activity levels or decrease their caloric intake (Eliopoulos, 2018).

Research suggests that older adults with obesity are at risk for complications that may negatively affect their quality of life. In particular, older adults with obesity may be at greater risk of falls (Joen, 2013) and mobility impairments (Murphy, Reinders, Register, et al., 2014). More older adults with obesity are admitted to nursing homes than normal weight older adults (Felix, Bradway, Chisholm, et al., 2015). One study found that older adults with obesity had lower resting hemoglobin–oxygen saturation levels (i.e., SpO$_2$ levels), which presumably could lead to hypoxemia, dyspnea, and ischemic complications (e.g., myocardial infarction) (Kapur, Wilsdon, Au, et al., 2013). Another study found that in one long-term care facility, more older adult residents who were overweight had indwelling urinary catheters than their counterparts who were leaner, which presumably could lead to urosepsis (Felix, Thostenson, Bursac, et al., 2013).

There is some evidence that older adults with an overweight body mass (i.e., between 25 and 29.9 kg/m^2) have reasonably good health outcomes; therefore, overweight older adults are not necessarily counseled to lose weight (Orringer et al., 2016). However, older adults with obesity (i.e., with BMIs in excess of 30 kg/m^2) should be encouraged to engage in lifestyle modifications, including diet and exercise, much as younger adults (Orringer et al., 2016). Along with decreasing dietary caloric intake, older adult patients should be counseled that the quality of calories consumed should be the focus of the daily diet (see Chapter 11, Fig. 11-2).

Fats should be limited to less than 30% of total calories, while proteins should comprise 10% to 20% of the daily diet. Intake of soluble fibers (e.g., oats, pectin) is particularly important since these can lower cholesterol levels and prevent cardiovascular diseases and cancers. Fewer than one third of older adults consume the recommended five servings of fruits and vegetables daily (Eliopoulos, 2018). Identifying barriers to consumption of these important sources of nutrients may help the older adult patient with obesity lose weight and adopt healthier eating habits. For instance, the older adult who has difficulty chewing raw fruits may enjoy fruit smoothies.

Whether or not older adult patients with obesity should be candidates for bariatric surgery (see later discussion) has been a point of contention. The Centers for Medicare and Medicaid Services (CMS), which provides insurance for most adults older than 65 years of age, had limited insurance coverage for bariatric surgery to only ASMBS Centers of Excellence (COEs). This policy was rescinded, however, after empirical research findings demonstrated no improvement in postoperative outcomes among patients who did and did not have their bariatric procedures done in COEs (Dimick, Nicholas, Ryan, et al., 2013). Other study findings suggest that many older adults with obesity benefit from bariatric surgery, although their weight loss tends to be less than that of younger adults who have bariatric surgery (Caceres, Moskowitz, & O'Connell, 2015). At present, there are no guidelines that identify the profile of which older adult patients with obesity can most benefit from bariatric surgery.

Nursing Management

Patients with obesity report feeling socially marginalized, judged, and unsupported by society at large. Many times, patients with obesity report that they suffer stigmatization by their health care providers, including nurses (Buxton & Snethen, 2013; Gilmartin, 2013; Puhl, Phelan, Nadglowski, et al., 2016). The bias that nurses may have against patients with obesity may not directly affect their nursing care; however, indirectly, the consequences of this stigmatization can lead to poor health outcomes. Patients with obesity who feel stigmatized by their health care providers report increased depression, low self-esteem, and avoidance of health care appointments and health maintenance activities (e.g., diet and exercise) (Budd & Peterson, 2015).

Nurses need to approach patients with obesity with the same respectful, courteous, and empathetic behavior that they extend to patients without obesity. Confronting their own attitudes and beliefs about patients with obesity may help to mitigate biases. For instance, using patient-first language for all patients with diagnosed diseases, including the disease of obesity, can be an effective way to dispel bias. By referencing *the patient with obesity*, the nurse is effectively noting that the patient, not the disease, is the central point of concern and that the disease is amenable to treatment. On the other hand, referencing *the obese patient* tends to define the person by having obesity, which can lead to subliminal impressions that the patient is somehow responsible for having obesity. Research studies report that many health care providers, including nurses, hold negative attitudes toward patients with obesity and believe that they are indulgent, lazy, and lack willpower (Puhl et al., 2016).

The patient with obesity who requires medical/surgical nursing care, whether it is because the patient is admitted to the hospital, needs home care, or is admitted to a transitional care setting, merits special considerations. Obesity can adversely affect the mechanics of ventilation and circulation, pharmacokinetics and pharmacodynamics, skin integrity, and body mechanics and mobility. These adverse effects are more common with higher BMIs; thus, the patient with Class III obesity (BMI in excess of 40 kg/m^2) is particularly vulnerable.

Obesity can result in anatomical remodeling, including compression of the oropharynx and increased neck circumference and chest diameter. These changes can predispose the patient with obesity to obstructive sleep apnea (OSA; see Chapter 22), respiratory failure (see Chapter 21), and obesity hypoventilation syndrome. Obesity hypoventilation syndrome is characterized by daytime hypoventilation with hypercapnea (i.e., PaCO$_2$ >45 mmHg) and hypoxemia (i.e., PaO$_2$ <80 mmHg), and sleep-disordered breathing. Potential adverse effects of obesity hypoventilation syndrome can be mitigated by maintaining the patient in the low Fowler position, which maximizes diaphragmatic chest expansion. Continuous pulse oximetry monitoring many be advisable, as well as supplemental oxygen therapy (see Chapter 21) and frequent respiratory assessments (at least every shift). For the patient with a known diagnosis of OSA, ensuring that the patient utilizes prescribed therapy (e.g., oral appliance, continuous positive airway pressure [CPAP]) if newly hospitalized or in a different transitional care environment is important in order to ensure breathing effectiveness and avert respiratory failure (Berrios, 2016; Dambaugh & Ecklund, 2016; Sturman-Floyd, 2013).

The patient with obesity may have central and peripheral circulatory compromise. Heart failure is more commonplace among patients with obesity (see Chapter 29). Hypertension is also more prevalent; the nurse must use appropriately sized blood pressure cuffs to obtain valid blood pressure readings (see Chapter 31). Peripheral blood flow can be compromised for the patient with obesity, resulting in stasis of blood flow, one of three components of Virchow triad, which are the broad categories of risk for venous thromboembolism (VTE) (see Chapter 30, Chart 30-7). Peripheral circulatory compromise not only can increase the risk for VTE formation (e.g., pulmonary embolism [PE] and deep vein thrombosis [DVT]), but it can also make finding venous access difficult when the patient with obesity requires intravenous (IV) therapy. Finding appropriate venous access can be exacerbated by the presence of increased adipose tissue in the extremities. Ultrasound guidance may be required in order to successfully gain IV access and place an IV cannula in the patient with obesity (Berrios, 2016; Dambaugh & Ecklund, 2016).

The patient with obesity may have differences in both pharmacokinetics (i.e., the movement of drug metabolites within the body) and pharmacodynamics (i.e., how drugs are metabolized and the effects of drugs) that can affect drug dosages, drug effectiveness, and patient safety. The effectiveness of many drugs is affected by the ratio of lean skeletal muscle mass to adipose tissue. The active metabolites of many drugs are protein bound in the plasma. In patients with greater adipose tissue, more of these active metabolites can be unbound in plasma, or free, and exert greater effects. Some drugs readily bind to adipose tissue, which may either inactivate them or prolong their effects. In addition, increased adiposity can have indirect effects on metabolic pathways within the liver, resulting in changes in drug metabolic pathways, which can result in either increased or decreased drug metabolism, depending upon the drug and the affected metabolic pathway. In other words, some drugs have enhanced effects while others have diminished effects with patients with obesity compared to patients of normal weight. For instance, one research study found that patients with obesity who were critically ill required proportionally lower dosages of IV drip norepinephrine, which is typically given based upon weight-based calculation, than patients with normal weight (Radosevich, Patanwal, & Erstad, 2016). On the other hand, patients with obesity who require opioid agents to treat pain many times require higher dosages of opioid agents to achieve pain relief, but are more likely to have serious adverse effects of sedation and respiratory depression (D'Arcy, 2015). The nurse should be cognizant that weight-based calculations of drug dosages for patients with obesity may need to be altered, depending upon the patient and the drug, and should consult with clinical pharmacologists and the patient's primary provider as needed to ensure optimal drug effectiveness and patient safety (Berrios, 2016).

Patients with obesity are particularly vulnerable to developing pressure ulcers. Increased adipose tissue can diminish the supply of blood, oxygen, and nutrients to peripheral tissue. The presence of more folds in the skin is associated with more skin moisture and increased skin friction, which are pressure ulcer risks. Moreover, skin folds may be present in uncommon areas, including under the breasts, under the lower abdomen, within gluteal folds, and at the nape of the neck (Berrios, 2016; Dambaugh & Ecklund, 2016; Sturman-Floyd, 2013). In addition, patients with obesity many times have more limitations in mobility than patients of normal weight. Immobility is another risk for pressure ulcer development (Hyun, Li, Vermillion, et al., 2014) (see Chart 48-5). Consultation with a wound-ostomy-continence (WOC) nurse may be advisable to ensure that pressure ulcer risks for the patient with obesity are minimized.

The nurse must ensure that the appropriate specialty equipment is utilized as needed so that the patient with obesity who is immobilized is turned and mobilized as indicated to prevent pressure ulcers. The typical nursing protocol is that the patient who is immobilized and bedfast should be turned every 2 hours to prevent pressure ulcers (Berrios, 2016). Nurses should be familiar with and comfortable using specialized durable medical bariatric equipment (e.g., lifts, transport equipment, commodes) so that the patient with obesity receives necessary care. It is also important to enforce and implement safe patient handling protocols so that the nurse does not incur musculoskeletal injury (Berrios, 2016).

Surgical Management

Bariatric surgery, or surgery for obesity, is typically performed after other nonsurgical attempts at weight control have failed. Insurance coverage for bariatric surgery varies widely, but most insurance companies will consider surgery as a treatment if the

---

Chart 48-5 | **NURSING RESEARCH PROFILE**

Pressure Ulcers Among Critically Ill Patients With Extreme Obesity

Hyun, S., Li, X., Vermillion, B., et al. (2014). Body mass index and pressure ulcers: Improved predictability of pressure ulcers in intensive care patients. *American Journal of Critical Care, 23*(6), 494–500.

Purpose

The Braden Scale is a validated tool used to assess pressure ulcer risk among multiple populations of patients at risk for pressure ulcers, and is commonly used in hospitals in the United States in a variety of settings. Patients who are admitted to intensive care units are at heightened risk for pressure ulcers. Those patients who are critically ill and who also have obesity are presumably at even higher risk for pressure ulcers, because they have heightened immobility problems as a consequence of their weight. This study sought to investigate whether or not body mass index (BMI) could serve as an additional predictor for pressure ulcer development that could complement Braden Scale Scores among patients who are critically ill who also had obesity.

Design

This retrospective study examined electronic health record data from adult patients admitted to the adult critical care units in one Midwest academic health center over a 3-year period. Patients were sorted into four groups; underweight, with a BMI less than 19 kg/m²; normal weight, with a BMI between 19 and 25 kg/m²; obese, with a BMI between 25 and 40 kg/m², and extremely obese, with a BMI greater than 40 kg/m². Patient demographics, the incidence of pressure ulcers, and Braden Scale Scores were compared and analyzed between groups.

Findings

Data gathering yielded information on 2632 patients admitted to both medical and surgical intensive care units. The incidence of pressure ulcers in the underweight cohort was 8.6%, in the normal weight cohort was 5.5%, in the obese cohort was 2.8%, and in the extremely obese cohort was 9.9%. Logistic regression analysis revealed that patients who were underweight or who had extreme obesity were more likely to develop pressure ulcers. The odds of pressure ulcer development, based upon BMI cohort groups was not more predictive than Braden Scale Scores, however.

Nursing Implications

Results from this study validated that the Braden Scale is a useful tool for predicting pressure ulcer risk among adults who are critically ill and who have obesity. BMI scores, although not more predictive of risk than Braden Scale Scores, may be roughly equivalent measures of ascertaining pressure ulcer risk. In particular, findings from this study suggest that patients who are critically ill and who have extreme obesity (i.e., with BMIs in excess of 40 kg/m²) are at high risk for developing pressure ulcers. This is particularly concerning, since 26% of this study sample of adults who were critically ill had extreme obesity. Additional nursing considerations for patients with extreme obesity who are critically ill are needed so that pressure ulcers may be prevented. These considerations may include the use of specialty lifts, turning devices, and other safe patient handling devices so that these patients may be appropriately mobilized to prevent pressure ulcers.

patient has Class III obesity or Class II obesity with a related medical condition (e.g., type 2 diabetes, OSA) (see Table 48-1) (Obesity Action Coalition [OAC], 2015a).

According to estimates by the ASMBS (2014), the number of bariatric surgeries performed in the United States grew by nearly 15% between 2011 and 2013. Bariatric surgical procedures work by restricting a patient's ability to eat (restrictive procedure), interfering with ingested nutrient absorption (malabsorptive procedures), or both. The different types of bariatric surgical procedures require unique lifestyle modifications. In order to optimize their success, patients should be well informed about the specific lifestyle changes, eating habits, and bowel habits that may result from each type of procedure.

Bariatric surgery typically results in a weight loss of 10% to 35% of total body weight within 2 to 3 years postoperatively (Colquitt, Pickett, Loveman, et al., 2014; OAC, 2015b), with the majority of weight loss occurring within the first year (Courcoulas, Christian, Belle, et al., 2013). Comorbid conditions such as type 2 diabetes, hypertension, and OSA may resolve; and dyslipidemia improves (ASMBS, 2013a; Courcoulas, Belle, Neiberg, et al., 2015). Bariatric surgery has been extended to carefully selected adolescents with severe obesity and comorbidity because of the positive results it has achieved in adults (Michalsky, Reichard, Inge, et al., 2012).

Patient selection is critical, and the preliminary process may necessitate months of counseling, education, and evaluation by a multidisciplinary team, including social workers, dietitians, a nurse counselor, a psychologist or psychiatrist, and a bariatric surgeon. The selection criteria for patients has changed considerably since the advent of bariatric surgery, with patients with BMIs as low as 30 kg/m² now considered candidates for surgical intervention if they have comorbid conditions that may demonstrably improve post weight loss (e.g., type 2 diabetes) (Mechanick, Youdim, Jones, et al., 2013) (see Chart 48-6).

Because bariatric surgery involves a drastic change in the functioning of the digestive system, patients need counseling before and after the surgery. Guidelines have been developed to assist in the care of patients having bariatric surgery (Broome, Ayala, Georgeson, et al., 2015; Mechanick et al., 2013).

Roux-en-Y gastric bypass (RYGB), gastric banding, sleeve gastrectomy, and biliopancreatic diversion with duodenal switch are the current bariatric procedures of choice. These procedures may be performed by laparoscopy or by an open surgical technique. The RYGB and the sleeve gastrectomy are the two most commonly used procedures (ASMBS, 2014); a systematic review found that outcomes were equally favorable between RYGB and sleeve gastrectomy, and generally better than outcomes with gastric banding (Colquitt et al., 2014). Biliopancreatic diversion with duodenal switch tends to result in the most postoperative weight loss, and is therefore more commonly indicated for patients with very high BMIs (Colquitt et al., 2014).

The RYGB is a combined restrictive and malabsorptive procedure. The gastric banding and sleeve gastrectomy are restrictive procedures, and the biliopancreatic diversion with duodenal switch combines gastric restriction with intestinal malabsorption. Figure 48-5A–D provides additional details about these procedures.

Chart 48-6 — Selection Criteria for Bariatric Surgery

BMI ≥40 kg/m² without excessive surgical risk

Patients with BMI ≥35 kg/m² and one or more severe obesity-associated comorbid conditions (e.g., hyperlipidemia, obstructive sleep apnea, obesity hypoventilation syndrome, nonalcoholic fatty liver disease, hypertension, asthma, debilitating arthritis, or considerably impaired quality of life)

Patients with *BMI* ≥30 kg/m² with type 2 diabetes or metabolic syndrome

Ability to perform activities of daily living and self-care

Presence of a support network of family and friends

Failure of previous nonsurgical attempts at weight loss, including nonprofessional programs

Expectation that patient will adhere to postoperative care, follow-up visits, and recommended medical management, including the use of dietary supplements

Exclusions

Reversible endocrine or other disorders that can cause obesity

Current drug or alcohol abuse

Uncontrolled, severe psychiatric illness

Lack of comprehension of risks, benefits, expected outcomes, alternatives, and lifestyle changes required with bariatric surgery

Adapted from Mechanick, J. I., Youdim, A., Jones, D. B., et al. (2013). Clinical practice guidelines for the perioperative nutritional, metabolic, and nonsurgical support of the bariatric surgery patient–2013 update: Cosponsored by the American Association of Clinical Endocrinologists, the Obesity Society, and American Society for Metabolic & Bariatric Surgery. *Surgery for Obesity and Related Diseases, 9*(2), 159–191.

NURSING PROCESS

The Patient Undergoing Bariatric Surgery

Assessment

Preoperatively, the nurse assesses for contraindications to major abdominal surgery. Previous attempts at losing weight are also assessed, including strategies such as nutritional counseling, dieting, or exercise programs. The nurse ensures the patient has received education and counseling regarding the possible risks and benefits of bariatric surgery including the complications, postsurgical outcomes, dietary changes, and the need for lifelong follow-up. The nurse also confirms that the patient has been screened for behavioral disorders that may interfere with postsurgical outcomes. Dietary counseling is initiated preoperatively to prepare for postoperative dietary changes (Mechanick et al., 2013; OAC, 2015b).

The nurse ensures that preoperative screening tests are obtained and scrutinizes the results. Typical laboratory tests include a complete blood cell count CBC, electrolytes, blood urea nitrogen (BUN), and creatinine. See Appendix A on thePoint for normal values for these laboratory tests. Patients with obesity may have OSA, gastroesophageal reflux disease (GERD), heart disease, nonalcoholic fatty liver disease, diabetes (or prediabetes), and vitamin and mineral deficiencies; thus, other screening tests that may be obtained include a sleep study, upper endoscopy, electrocardiogram (ECG), lipid panel, AST, ALT, glucose, and hemoglobin A1c, as well as iron, vitamin B₁₂, thiamine, folate, vitamin D, and calcium levels.

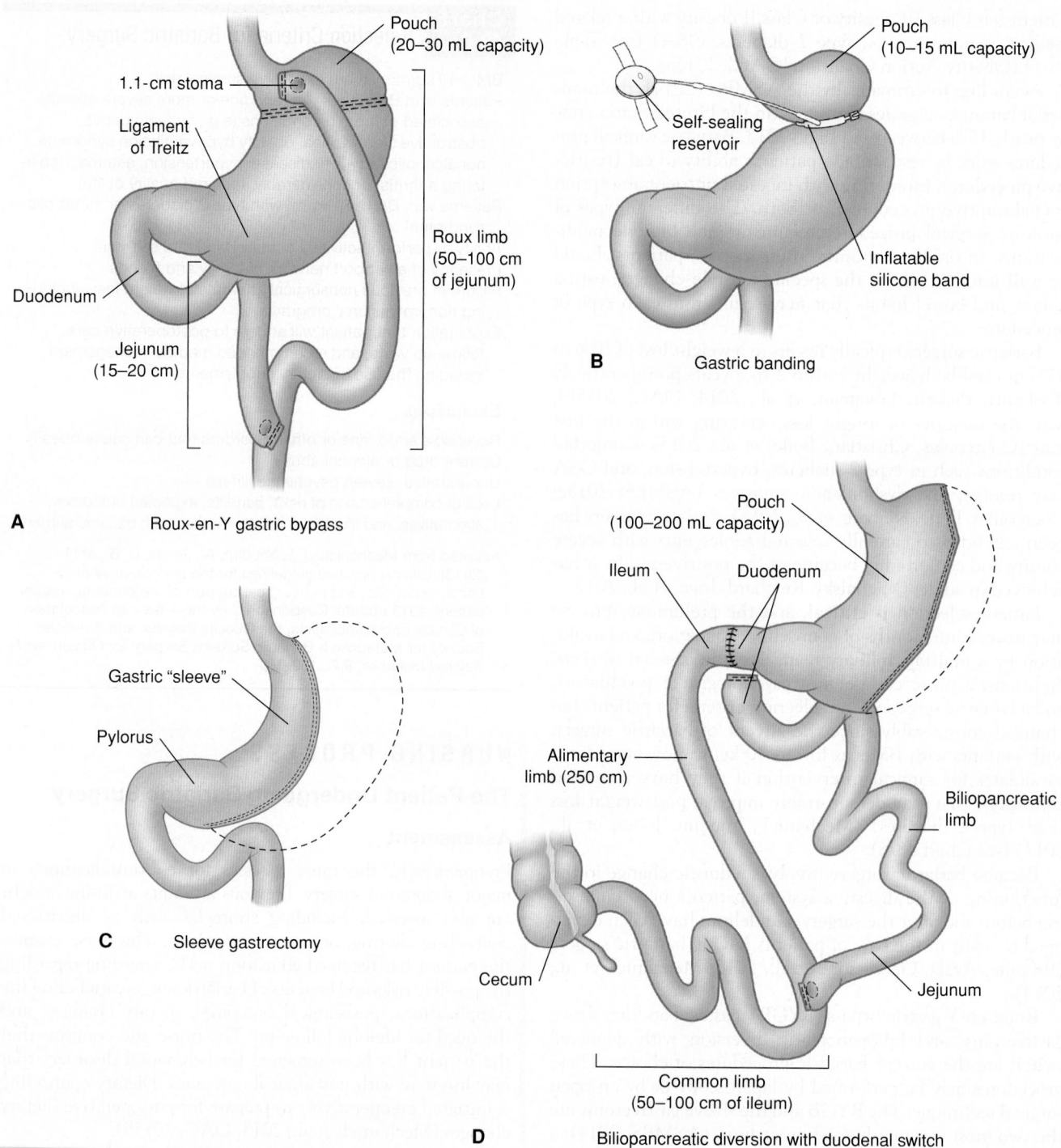

A Roux-en-Y gastric bypass

- Pouch (20–30 mL capacity)
- 1.1-cm stoma
- Ligament of Treitz
- Duodenum
- Jejunum (15–20 cm)
- Roux limb (50–100 cm of jejunum)

B Gastric banding

- Pouch (10–15 mL capacity)
- Self-sealing reservoir
- Inflatable silicone band

C Sleeve gastrectomy

- Gastric "sleeve"
- Pylorus

D Biliopancreatic diversion with duodenal switch

- Pouch (100–200 mL capacity)
- Ileum
- Duodenum
- Alimentary limb (250 cm)
- Biliopancreatic limb
- Cecum
- Jejunum
- Common limb (50–100 cm of ileum)

Figure 48-5 • Bariatric surgical procedures. **A.** Roux-en-Y gastric bypass. A horizontal row of staples across the fundus of the stomach creates a pouch with a capacity of 20 to 30 mL. The jejunum is divided distal to the ligament of Treitz, and the distal end is anastomosed to the new pouch. The proximal segment is anastomosed to the jejunum. **B.** Gastric banding. A prosthetic device is used to restrict oral intake by creating a small pouch of 10 to 15 mL that empties through the narrow outlet into the remainder of the stomach. **C.** Sleeve gastrectomy. The stomach is incised vertically and up to 85% of the stomach is surgically removed, leaving a "sleeve"-shaped tube that retains intact nervous innervation and does not obstruct or decrease the size of the gastric outlet. **D.** Biliopancreatic diversion with duodenal switch (also called *sleeve gastrectomy with duodenal switch*). Half of the stomach is removed, leaving a small area that holds about 60 mL. The entire jejunum is excluded from the rest of the gastrointestinal tract. The duodenum is disconnected and sealed off. The ileum is divided above the ileocecal junction, and the distal end of the jejunum is anastomosed to the first portion of the duodenum. The distal end of the biliopancreatic limb is anastomosed to the ileum.

Postoperatively, the nurse assesses the patient to ensure that goals for recovery are met and that the patient exhibits absence of complications secondary to the surgical intervention. See Chapter 19 for general assessment of the postoperative patient.

Diagnosis

NURSING DIAGNOSES

Based on the assessment data, major nursing diagnoses may include the following:

- Deficient knowledge about the dietary limitations during the immediate preoperative and postoperative phases
- Anxiety related to impending surgery
- Acute pain related to surgical procedure
- Risk for deficient fluid volume related to nausea, gastric irritation, and pain
- Risk for infection related to anastomotic leak
- Imbalanced nutrition: less than body requirements related to dietary restrictions
- Disturbed body image related to body changes from bariatric surgery
- Risk for constipation and/or diarrhea related to gastric irritation and surgical changes in anatomic structures from bariatric surgery

COLLABORATIVE PROBLEMS/POTENTIAL COMPLICATIONS

Potential complications may include the following:

- Hemorrhage
- Venous thromboembolism
- Bile reflux
- Dumping syndrome
- Dysphagia
- Bowel or gastric outlet obstruction

Planning and Goals

Preoperative goals include that the patient will become knowledgeable about the preoperative and postoperative dietary routine/restrictions and will have decreased anxiety about the surgery. Postoperative goals include relief of pain, maintenance of homeostatic fluid balance, prevention of infection, adherence to detailed diet instructions to include progression of food intake as well as fluid intake (to prevent dehydration), knowledge about vitamin supplements and the need for lifelong follow-up, achievement of a positive body image, and maintenance of normal bowel habits (ASMBS, 2013a; Mechanick et al., 2013).

Nursing Interventions

ENSURING DIETARY RESTRICTIONS

The nurse counsels the patient anticipating bariatric surgery to ingest nothing but clear liquids for a specified period of time preoperatively and postoperatively (typically about 24 to 48 hours before and after surgery). Nutritional support for patients scheduled for bariatric surgery is tailored to meet each patient's individual need to ensure optimal consumption of micronutrients. Bariatric diets usually follow a progression from clear liquids to full liquids to soft solids and eventually solid foods. This slow progression is necessary to maximize weight loss, and to prevent complications such as nausea, vomiting, bile reflux, and diarrhea.

The patient's diet will be limited upon discharge from the hospital; because of this, patients scheduled for bariatric surgery are given guidelines prior to surgery on which foods and liquids they may consume postoperatively so that they may stock up on these items at home before they are admitted to the hospital. These typically include sugar-free drinks, gelatins and puddings, flavored electrolyte drinks, fat-free milk, protein drinks, sugar-free applesauce, and low-fat soups (Cole, Beckman, & Earthman, 2014; Isom, Andromalos, Ariagno, et al., 2014; Mechanick et al., 2013).

REDUCING ANXIETY

The nurse provides the patient preparing for bariatric surgery anticipatory guidance as to what to expect during the surgery and postoperatively. In addition, the nurse may encourage the patient to join a bariatric surgery support group preoperatively, with the intent that the patient will continue to participate in this group postoperatively. Most bariatric surgery centers sponsor patient support groups that meet in person or online. These support groups provide a forum where patients contemplating bariatric surgery may talk with patients who have had the surgery and may provide them with guidance and tips that can help to lessen their anxiety (Mechanick et al., 2013).

RELIEVING PAIN

After surgery, analgesic agents may be given as prescribed to relieve pain and discomfort. Patients are usually prescribed opioid agents via patient-controlled analgesia (PCA) pumps; the nurse should educate the patient about its use and monitor its effectiveness. It is especially important to provide adequate pain relief so that the patient can perform pulmonary care activities (deep breathing and coughing) and leg exercises, turn from side to side, and ambulate. The nurse assesses the effectiveness of analgesic intervention and consults with other members of the health care team if pain is not adequately controlled (Patil & Melander, 2015) (see Chapter 12). Positioning the patient in a low Fowlers position promotes comfort and emptying of the stomach after any type of gastric surgery, including bariatric procedures.

ENSURING FLUID VOLUME BALANCE

Patients who have had bariatric surgery usually receive intravenous (IV) fluids for the first several hours postoperatively. Once they are awake and alert on the surgical unit, they are encouraged to begin intake of sugar-free oral fluids. Introducing small volumes of these liquids is believed to stimulate GI peristalsis and perfusion and thwart gastric reflux. Sugar-free fluids are preferred because they are not implicated in causing dumping syndrome (see later discussion). With a typical regimen, patients are encouraged to slowly sip 30 mL of these fluids every 15 minutes. Patients should stop ingesting fluids, however, if they feel nauseated or full. Antiemetic agents may be prescribed to relieve nausea and prevent vomiting, which could cause strain on the surgical site and cause either a hemorrhage or anastomotic leak (Mechanick et al., 2013).

PREVENTING INFECTION/ANASTOMOTIC LEAK

Disruption at the site of anastomosis (i.e., surgically resected site) may cause leakage of gastric contents into the peritoneal cavity, causing infection and possible sepsis. Patients at risk for this particular complication tend to be older, male, and with greater body mass. In addition, anastomotic leak is more commonly associated with open rather than laparoscopic procedures. Patients with anastomotic leaks typically exhibit nonspecific signs and symptoms that include fever, abdominal pain, tachycardia, and leukocytosis. This may progress to sepsis and possibly septic shock if not recognized and treated early (see Chapter 14). The nurse must be astute in recognizing these manifestations and alerting the patient's primary provider should they occur (Dunham, 2013; Patil & Melander, 2015).

A patient suspected of having an anastomotic leak may have an upper GI series that includes follow-up computed tomography (CT) scan with contrast dye, which may find leaking contrast dye, thus confirming the diagnosis. Treatment varies depending on the timing (early or late postoperatively) and severity of the leak. CT-guided drainage of the area may be appropriate for a less severe leak in the later postoperative phase of recovery, but an early or severe leak requires immediate open surgical intervention to repair the leak (Jacobsen, Nergard, Leifsson, et al., 2014).

ENSURING ADEQUATE NUTRITIONAL STATUS

After bowel sounds have returned and oral intake is resumed, six small feedings consisting of a total of 600 to 800 calories per day are provided, and consumption of fluids between meals is encouraged to prevent dehydration. The nurse instructs the patient to eat slowly and stop when feeling full. Eating too much or too fast or eating high-calorie liquids and soft foods can result in vomiting or painful esophageal distention. Gastric retention may be evidenced by abdominal distention, nausea, and vomiting. A nutritionist is typically consulted to assist with diet restrictions and diet progression (Mechanick et al., 2013) (see Chart 48-7).

Common dietary deficiencies in patients who have had bariatric surgery include malabsorption of organic iron, which may require supplementation with oral or parenteral iron, and a low serum level of vitamin B_{12}; the patient may be prescribed monthly vitamin B_{12} intramuscular injections to prevent pernicious anemia (Dunham, 2013; Isom et al., 2014) (see Chapter 33 for further discussion).

SUPPORTING BODY IMAGE CHANGES

Most patients post bariatric surgery report greatly improved perceptions of their body image, as well as improved quality of life. However, some patients report lingering dissatisfaction with their body images. In particular, some patients may report dissatisfaction related to loose skin folds and may eventually seek elective body-contouring surgical options (e.g., breast reductions, breast lifts, abdominoplasty). The nurse provides support to the patient who reports dissatisfaction with body image post weight loss by acknowledging the patient's feelings as real, sharing that these perceptions are not unusual, and providing links to live or online supports groups or counselors, as necessary (Gilmartin, 2013; Pfeil, 2014; Schauer, Woodruff, Hotz, & Kegler, 2014).

ENSURING MAINTENANCE OF BOWEL HABITS

Patients may complain of either diarrhea or constipation postoperatively. Diarrhea is more common an occurrence post bariatric surgery, particularly after malabsorptive procedures (Mechanick et al., 2013). Both may be prevented if the patient consumes a nutritious diet that is high in fiber. Steatorrhea also may occur as a result of rapid gastric emptying,

---

Chart 48-7	**PATIENT EDUCATION**

Dietary Guidelines for the Patient Who Has Had Bariatric Surgery

The nurse instructs the patient to:

- Eat smaller but more frequent meals that contain protein and fiber; each meal size should not exceed 1 cup.
- Eat only foods high in nutrients (e.g., peanut butter, cheese, chicken, fish, beans).
- Consume fat as tolerated.
- Ensure a low carbohydrate intake; in particular, avoid concentrated sources of carbohydrates (e.g., candy).
- Eat two protein snacks daily; animal protein may be poorly tolerated after Roux-en-Y gastric bypass, however.
- Eat slowly and chew thoroughly.
- Assume a low Fowler position during mealtime and then remain in that position for 20–30 minutes after mealtime—this delays stomach emptying and decreases the likelihood of dumping syndrome.
- Know that antispasmodic agents, as prescribed, also may aid in delaying the emptying of the stomach.
- Do not drink fluid with meals; instead, consume fluids up to 30 minutes before a meal and 30–60 minutes after mealtime.
- Do drink plenty of water; refrain from drinking liquid calories (e.g., alcoholic beverages, fruit drinks, nondiet sodas).
- Take prescribed dietary supplements of vitamins and medium-chain triglycerides.
- Follow up with primary provider for monthly injections of vitamin B_{12} and iron as prescribed.
- Walk for at least 30 minutes daily.

Adapted from Mechanick, J. I., Youdim, A., Jones, D. B., et al. (2013). Clinical practice guidelines for the perioperative nutritional, metabolic, and nonsurgical support of the bariatric surgery patient–2013 update: Cosponsored by the American Association of Clinical Endocrinologists, the Obesity Society, and American Society for Metabolic & Bariatric Surgery. *Surgery for Obesity and Related Diseases, 9*(2), 159–191.

---

which prevents adequate mixing with pancreatic and biliary secretions (Mechanick et al., 2013). In mild cases, reducing the intake of fat and administering an antimotility medication (e.g., loperamide [Imodium]) may control symptoms. Persistent diarrhea or steatorrhea may warrant further diagnostic testing, such as an upper endoscopy or colonoscopy with biopsies to rule out the presence of additional pathology, such as celiac diseases or *Clostridium difficile* infection (Mechanick et al., 2013) (see Chapter 47).

MONITORING AND MANAGING POTENTIAL COMPLICATIONS

After surgery, the nurse assesses the patient for complications from the bariatric surgery, such as hemorrhage, venous thromboembolism, bile reflux, dumping syndrome, dysphagia, and bowel or gastric outlet obstruction.

Hemorrhage. Postoperative hemorrhage may be a complication following bariatric surgery. Intra-abdominal hemorrhage may be evident by frank, bright red oral or rectal bleeding, tarry melena, bloody output from the wound or drains, if present, as well as typical clinical manifestations of severe bleeding and hemorrhagic shock (e.g., tachycardia, hypotension, syncope) (see Chapter 14). Bleeding within the first 72 hours postoperatively is most likely caused by disruption in a staple or suture. Bleeding 72 hours to 30 days postoperatively is most likely from formation of a gastric or duodenal ulcer (Patil & Melander, 2015) (see Chapter 46).

Venous Thromboembolism (VTE). Patients who have bariatric surgery are at moderate to high risk of VTE, including both PE and DVT. Patients who are older, have higher BMIs, and have a prior history of a VTE or coagulation defect are at higher risk (Brethauer, 2013). ASMBS guidelines for VTE prevention specify that in the immediate postoperative period, patients who have had bariatric surgery should be prescribed mechanical compression (e.g., intermittent pneumatic compression devices) and prophylactic anticoagulation with subcutaneous low molecular weight heparin (LMWH) agents (e.g., dalteparin [Fragmin], enoxaparin [Lovenox]). The duration of time that mechanical compression and anticoagulation should continue postoperatively are not described, however, and are left to the discretion of the patient and primary provider. In addition to implementing this prescribed therapy, nurses caring for patients post bariatric surgery should encourage them to begin early ambulation to further deter the advent of VTE (Brethauer, 2013) (see Chapter 30).

Bile Reflux. Bile reflux may occur with procedures that manipulate or remove the pylorus, which acts as a barrier to the reflux of duodenal contents. Reflux of bile can cause inflammation of the stomach (i.e., gastritis) or esophagus (i.e., esophagitis). Burning epigastric pain and vomiting of bilious material manifest this condition. Eating or vomiting does not relieve the symptoms. Bile reflux may be managed with proton pump inhibitors (e.g., omeprazole [Prilosec]) (Sifrim, 2013).

Dumping Syndrome. **Dumping syndrome** is an unpleasant set of vasomotor and GI symptoms that commonly occurs in patients who have had bariatric surgery. For many years, it had been theorized that the hypertonic gastric food boluses that quickly transit into the intestines drew extracellular fluid from the circulating blood volume into the small intestines to dilute the high concentration of electrolytes and sugars, resulting in symptoms. Now, it is thought that this rapid transit of the food bolus from the stomach into the small intestines instead causes a rapid and exuberant release of metabolic peptides that are responsible for the symptoms of dumping syndrome (Patil & Melander, 2015).

Symptoms of dumping syndrome typically occur 15 minutes to 2 hours after eating and include tachycardia, dizziness, sweating, nausea, vomiting, bloating, abdominal cramping, and diarrhea (Patil & Melander, 2015). These symptoms typically resolve once the intestine has been evacuated (i.e., with defecation). Later, blood glucose rises rapidly, followed by increased insulin secretion. This results in a reactive hypoglycemia, which also is unpleasant for the patient. Vasomotor symptoms that occur 10 to 90 minutes after eating are pallor, perspiration, palpitations, headache, and feelings of warmth, dizziness, and even drowsiness. Anorexia may also result from dumping syndrome, because the patient may be reluctant to eat (Patil & Melander, 2015).

 Concept Mastery Alert

> Dumping syndrome is a physiologic response to the rapid emptying of gastric contents into the jejunum. The rapid transit of the food bolus from the stomach into the small intestines causes a rapid and exuberant release of metabolic peptides that are responsible for the symptoms of dumping syndrome.

Dysphagia. **Dysphagia**, or difficulty swallowing, may occur in patients who have had any type of restrictive bariatric procedure. If it occurs, it tends to be most severe 4 to 6 weeks postoperatively and may persist for up to 6 months after surgery. Dysphagia may be prevented by educating patients to eat slowly, to chew food thoroughly, and to avoid eating tough foods such as steak or dry chicken or doughy bread. Patients with severe dysphagia who have had gastric banding may benefit from having their bands adjusted. Patients who have had other restrictive procedures may experience relief of symptoms after having stomal strictures relieved endoscopically (Mechanick et al., 2013).

Bowel and Gastric Outlet Obstruction. Bowel or gastric outlet obstruction may occur as a complication of bariatric surgery. The typical manifestations and treatments of gastric outlet obstruction are described in Chapter 46; however, there is a key difference in the treatment of a patient who has undergone bariatric surgery with a gastric outlet obstruction. It is contraindicated to insert a nasogastric (NG) tube in patients that have had bariatric surgery, even if they have a gastric outlet obstruction. Alternative treatment options may include endoscopic procedures aimed at relieving the obstruction, such as balloon dilation, or surgical revisions (Patil & Melander, 2015).

 Quality and Safety Nursing Alert

> *Insertion of NG tubes is contraindicated in the patient post bariatric surgery. This procedure may disrupt the surgical suture line and cause anastomotic leak or hemorrhage.*

PROMOTING HOME, COMMUNITY-BASED, AND TRANSITIONAL CARE

Patients are usually discharged from the hospital within 4 days postoperatively (this may be within 24 to 72 hours for patients who have had laparoscopic procedures) with detailed dietary instructions (see Chart 48-7) as well as instructions about how to either begin or resume an appropriate exercise regimen. Instructions on making follow-up appointments with the bariatric surgeon for routine postoperative visits or for complications are shared with the patient (Mechanick et al., 2013).

Educating Patients About Self-Care. The nurse provides education with the patient about nutrition, nutritional supplements, pain management, the importance of physical activity, and the symptoms of dumping syndrome and measures to prevent or minimize these symptoms. Patients who undergo laparoscopic or open RYGB procedures may have one or more Jackson–Pratt drains, which may remain in place after discharge. The nurse educates the patient or caregiver about how to empty, measure, and record the amount of drainage. Patients should be instructed to avoid taking nonsteroidal anti-inflammatory drugs (NSAIDs) (e.g., ibuprofen [Motrin]) postdischarge, as they have been implicated in development of stomach ulcers (Mechanick et al., 2013). The nurse must emphasize the continued need for follow-up (even after weight-loss goals are met) and continued support group participation (Wykowski & Krouse, 2013).

Continuing and Transitional Care. After bariatric surgery, all patients require lifelong monitoring of weight, comorbidities, metabolic and nutritional status, and dietary and activity behaviors because they are at risk for developing malnutrition or weight gain. Women of childbearing age who have bariatric surgery are advised to use contraceptives for at least 18 months after surgery to avoid pregnancy until their weight stabilizes. After weight loss, the patient may elect additional surgical interventions for body contouring. These may include breast reductions, lipoplasty to remove fat deposits, or a panniculectomy or abdominoplasty to remove excess abdominal skin folds (OAC, 2015b; Mechanick et al., 2013; Wykowski & Krouse, 2013).

Evaluation

Expected patient outcomes may include the following:
1. Relief of pain
   a. Reports relief of pain
   b. Engages in early mobilization activities as prescribed
2. Maintenance of fluid balance
   a. Able to tolerate progressive fluid intake without complaints of nausea or gastric reflux
   b. Voids 0.5 mL/kg/h
3. Maintenance of asepsis
   a. No evidence of infection (e.g., no fever, no leukocytosis, no complaints of abdominal pain)
4. Achievement of nutritional balance
   a. Able to consume small, frequent meals as prescribed
   b. Adheres to prescribed intake of vitamins and supplements
   c. Achieves and maintains weight reduction goals
5. Promotion of positive body image
   a. Verbalizes continued satisfaction with weight reduction plan and its effect on body image
6. Maintenance of usual bowel habits
   a. No evidence of diarrhea
   b. No evidence of constipation
7. Has no complications (e.g., no bleeding, VTE, bile reflux, dumping syndrome, dysphagia, or bowel or gastric outlet obstruction)

CRITICAL THINKING EXERCISES

1 **ebp** You work as a staff nurse in a women's health clinic. A 20-year-old woman presents to the clinic for her annual screening physical examination and is requesting a prescription refill for "birth control." You note that her height is 64 in and she weighs 163 lb. You note on her electronic health record that she weighed 152 lb last year. What is her BMI? She says to you "I would really like to lose some weight before I go on my vacation in 6 weeks. What diet do you think will help me to quickly lose the most weight?" Describe what other information you may gather from her that might help guide her to a healthier lifestyle. What is the strength of the evidence suggesting that any given commercial or other diet plan may offer her the healthiest weight loss outcomes?

2 **pq** A 51-year-old male patient is just over 24 hours post coronary artery bypass graft surgery and is a patient on your progressive care unit. You note on his electronic health record that his BMI is 42 kg/m^2. His BP is 124/72 mmHg, HR 112 bpm, RR 22 breaths/min, T 100.9°F and his SpO$_2$ is 90%. Describe your priority nursing assessments for this patient. What nursing interventions would you implement first?

3 **ebp** Your friend's mother is 9 months post bariatric surgery. She tells you that she is doing well and has been successful in reaching her weight loss goal. She says she does not feel the need to follow up with her nutritional counselor, primary provider, or support group, as she is "handling it on her own." What reasons would you give her for continuing with these follow-up appointments? On what evidence do you base your answer?

REFERENCES

*Asterisk indicates nursing research.

Books

Eliopoulos, C. (2018). *Gerontological nursing* (9th ed.). Philadelphia, PA: Lippincott Williams & Wilkins.

Grossman, S. C., & Porth, C. M. (2014). *Porth's pathophysiology: Concepts of altered health states* (9th ed.). Philadelphia, PA: Lippincott Williams & Wilkins.

Ogden, C. L., Carroll, M. D., Fryar, C. D., et al. (2015). *Prevalence of obesity among adults and youth: United States, 2011–2014.* NCHS data brief, no 219. Hyattsville, MD: National Center for Health Statistics.

Weber, J. R., & Kelley, J. H. (2014). *Health assessment in nursing* (5th ed.). Philadelphia, PA: Lippincott Williams & Wilkins.

Journals and Electronic Documents

Ali, M. R., Moustarah, F., Kim, J. J., et al. (2015). ASMBS position statement on intragastric balloon therapy endorsed by SAGES. Retrieved on 1/6/2017 at: asmbs.org/resources/position-statement-on-intragastric-balloon-therapy-endorsed-by-sages

American Medical Association (AMA) House of Delegates (2013). *Recognition of obesity as a disease.* Resolution: 420 (A-13); received 5/16/13. AMA: Author.

American Society for Metabolic and Bariatric Surgery (ASMBS). (2013a). *Medical and bariatric surgery: Medical outcomes of bariatric surgery.* Retrieved on 11/19/2015 at: asmbs.org/resources/metabolic-and-bariatric-surgery

American Society for Metabolic and Bariatric Surgery (ASMBS). (2013b). *Obesity in America: Fact sheet.* Retrieved on 1/22/2017 at: asmbs.org/wp/uploads/2014/06/Obesity-in-America-1.pdf

American Society for Metabolic and Bariatric Surgery (ASMBS). (2014). *New procedure estimates for bariatric surgery: What the numbers reveal.* Retrieved on 11/19/2015 at: connect.asmbs.org/may-2014-bariatric-surgery-growth.html

American Society for Metabolic and Bariatric Surgery (ASMBS). (2015a). *Disease of obesity.* Retrieved on 11/19/2015 at: asmbs.org/patients/disease-of-obesity (Accessed 11/19/15)

American Society for Metabolic and Bariatric Surgery (ASMBS). (2015b). *The impact of obesity on your body and health.* Retrieved on 11/19/2015 at: asmbs.org/patients/impact-of-obesity

Apovian, C. M., Aronne, L. J., Bessesen, D. H., et al. (2015). Pharmacological management of obesity: An Endocrine Society Clinical Practice Guideline. *Journal of Clinical Endocrinology and Metabolism,* 100(2), 342–362.

Bays, H. E., Jones, P. H., Jacobson, TA., et al. (2016). Lipids and bariatric procedures part 1 of 2: Scientific statement from the National Lipid Association, American Society for Metabolic and Bariatric Surgery, and Obesity Medicine Association: Executive summary. *Journal of Clinical Lipidology*, 10(1), 15–32.

Bays, H. E., Kothari, S. N., Azagury, D. E., et al. (2016). Lipids and bariatric procedures part 2 of 2: Scientific statement from the National Lipid Association, American Society for Metabolic and Bariatric Surgery, and Obesity Medicine Association. *Surgery for Obesity and Related Diseases*, 12(3), 468–495.

Bays, H. E., Seger, J. C., Primack, C., et al. (2016). Obesity algorithm, presented by the Obesity Medicine Association. Retrieved on 1/7/2017 at: www.obesityalgorithm.org.

Bendich, A. (2013). Prescription and over-the-counter options for weight loss. *Nutrition Today*, 48(2), 76–78.

Berrios, L. A. (2016). The ABCDs of managing morbidly obese patients in intensive care units. *Critical Care Nurse*, 36(5), 17–26.

Brethauer, S. A. (2013). ASMBS updated position statement on prophylactic measures to reduce the risk of venous thromboembolism in bariatric surgery patients. *Surgery for Obesity and Related Diseases*, 9(4), 493–497.

Broome, C. A., Ayala, E. M., Georgeson, K. A., et al. (2015). Nursing care of the super bariatric patient: Challenges and lessons learned. *Rehabilitation Nursing*, 40(2), 92–99.

Budd, G. M., & Peterson, J. A. (2014). The obesity epidemic, part 1: Understanding the origins. *American Journal of Nursing*, 114(12), 40–46.

Budd, G. M., & Peterson, J. A. (2015). The obesity epidemic, part 2: Nursing assessment and intervention. *American Journal of Nursing*, 115(1), 38–46.

*Buxton, B. K., & Snethen, J. (2013) Obese women's perceptions and experiences of healthcare and primary care providers: A phenomenological study. *Nursing Research*, 62(4), 252–259.

*Caceres, B. A., Moskowitz, D., & O'Connell, T. (2015). A review of the safety and efficacy of bariatric surgery in adults over the age of 60: 2002–2013. *Journal of the American Association of Nurse Practitioners*, 27(7), 403–410.

Centers for Disease Control and Prevention (CDC). (2016a). Adult obesity causes & consequences. Retrieved on 1/8/2017 at: www.cdc.gov/obesity/adult/causes.html

Centers for Disease Control and Prevention (CDC). (2016b). Defining adult overweight and obesity. Retrieved on 1/24/2017 at: www.cdc.gov/obesity/adult/defining.html

Cole, A. J., Beckman, L. M., & Earthman, C. P. (2014). Vitamin D status following bariatric surgery: Implications and Recommendations. *Nutrition in Clinical Practice*, 29(6), 751–758.

Colquitt, J. L., Pickett, K., Loveman, E., et al. (2014). Surgery for weight loss in adults. *Cochrane Database of Systematic Reviews*, 8, CD003641.

Courcoulas, A. P., Belle, S. H., Neiberg, R. H., et al. (2015). Three-year outcomes of bariatric surgery vs lifestyle intervention for type 2 diabetes mellitus treatment: A randomized controlled trial. *JAMA Surgery*, 150(10), 931–940.

Courcoulas, A. P., Christian, N. J., Belle, S. H., et al. (2013). Weight changes and health outcomes at three years after bariatric surgery among individuals with severe obesity. *JAMA*, 310(22), 2416–2425.

Dambaugh, L. A., & Ecklund, M. M. (2016). Progressive care of obese patients. *Critical Care Nurse*, 36(4), 58–63.

D'Arcy, Y. (2015). Managing pain in obese patients: Meeting weighty challenges. *Nursing*, 45(2), 42–49.

Davis, C. D. (2016). The gut microbiome and its role in obesity. *Nutrition Today*, 51(4), 167–174.

Dimick, J. B., Nicholas, L. H., Ryan, A. M., et al. (2013). Bariatric surgery complications before vs after implementation of a national policy restricting coverage to Centers of Excellence. *JAMA*, 309(8), 792–799.

Dunham, M. (2013). Caring for patients undergoing bariatric surgery. *American Journal of Nursing*, 43(10), 45–50.

*Felix, H. C., Bradway, C., Chisholm, L., et al. (2015). Prevalence of moderate to severe obesity among U. S. nursing home residents, 2000–2010. *Research in Gerontological Nursing*, 8(4), 173–178.

*Felix, H. C., Thostenson, J. D., Bursac, Z., et al. (2013). Effect of weight on indwelling catheter use among long-term care facility residents. *Urologic Nursing*, 33(4), 194–200.

Fitch, A., Everling, L., Fox, C., et al. (2013). *Prevention and management of obesity for adults*. Bloomington, MN: Institute for Clinical Systems Improvement. Retrieved on 1/25/2017 at: www.icsi.org/_asset/s935hy/ObesityAdults.pdf

Fruh, S. M., Mulekar, M. S., & Dierking, J. (2013). Guiding patients to safe weight loss. *The Nurse Practitioner*, 38(10), 1–7.

*Gilmartin, J. (2013). Body image concerns amongst massive weight loss patients. *Journal of Clinical Nursing*, 22(9–10), 1299–1309.

Goldstein, M., Aoun, A., Gaar, E., et al. (2014). *VA/DoD clinical practice guideline for screening and management of overweight and obesity*. Washington, DC: Department of Veterans Affairs. Retrieved on 1/25/2017 at: guideline.gov/summaries/summary/48461/vadod-clinical-practice-guideline-for-screening-and-management-of-overweight-and-obesity?q=obesity

*Hyun, S., Li, X., Vermillion, B., et al. (2014). Body mass index and pressure ulcers: Improved predictability of pressure ulcers in intensive care patients. *American Journal of Critical Care*, 23(6), 494–500.

Ikramuddin, S., Blackstone, R. P., Brancatisano, A, et al. (2014). Effect of reversible intermittent intra-abdominal vagal nerve blockade on morbid obesity: The ReCharge randomized clinical trial. *JAMA*, 312(9), 915–922.

Isom, K. A., Andromalos, L., Ariagno, M., et al. (2014). Nutrition and metabolic support recommendations for the bariatric patient. *Nutrition in Clinical Practice*, 29(6), 718–739.

Jacobsen, H. J., Nergard, B. J., Leifsson, B. G., et al. (2014). Management of suspected anastomotic leak after bariatric laparoscopic Roux-en-Y gastric bypass. *British Journal of Surgery*, 101(4), 417–423.

Joen, B.-Y. (2013). The effects of obesity on fall efficacy in elderly people. *Journal of Physical Therapy Science*, 25(11), 1485–1489.

Kapur, V. K., Wilsdon, A. G., Au, D., et al. (2013). Obesity is associated with lower resting oxygen saturation in the ambulatory elderly: Results from the cardiovascular health study. *Respiratory Care*, 58(5), 831–837.

Katz, D. L., & Meller, S. (2014). Can we say what diet is best for health? *Annual Reviews of Public Health*, 35, 83–103.

Kolata, G. (2016). One weight loss approach fits all? No, not even close. *New York Times, Health Section*, published on 12/12/2016. Retrieved on 1/22/2017 at: www.nytimes.com/2016/12/12/health/weight-loss-obesity.html

Kyle, T., & Kuehl, B. (2017). Prescription medications & weight gain – What you need to know. Retrieved on 1/7/2017 at: hwww.obesityaction.org/educational-resources/resource-articles-2/general-articles/prescription-medications-weight-gain

Levi, J., Segal, L. M., St. Laurent, R., et al. (2014). The state of obesity: 2014 – Better policies for a healthier America. Robert Wood Johnson Foundation. Retrieved on 1/6/2017 at: healthyamericans.org/assets/files/TFAH-2014-ObesityReport%20FINAL.pdf

Mechanick, J. I., Youdim, A., Jones, D. B., et al. (2013). Clinical practice guidelines for the perioperative nutritional, metabolic, and nonsurgical support of the bariatric surgery patient – 2013 update: Cosponsored by the American Association of Clinical Endocrinologists, the Obesity Society, and American Society for Metabolic & Bariatric Surgery. *Surgery for Obesity and Related Diseases*, 9(2), 159–191.

Michalsky, M., Reichard, K., Inge, T., et al. (2012). ASMBS pediatric committee best practice guidelines. *Surgery for Obesity and Related Diseases*, 8(1), 1–7.

Moyer, V. A., LeFevre, M. L., Siu, A. L., et al. (2012). Screening for and management of obesity in adults: U.S. Preventive Services Task Force recommendation statement. *Annals of Internal Medicine*, 157(5), 373–378.

Mozaffarian, D., Benjamin, E. J., Go, A. S., et al. (2016). Heart disease and stroke statistics–2016 update: A report from the American Heart Association. *Circulation*, 133(4), e38–3360.

Murphy, R. A., Reinders, I., Register, T. C., et al. (2014). Associations of BMI and adipose tissue area and density with incident mobility limitation and poor performance in older adults. *American Journal of Clinical Nutrition*, 99(5), 1059–1065.

National Heart, Lung, and Blood Institute (NHLBI) of the National Institutes of Health. (2016a). *Serving sizes and portions*. Retrieved on 1/22/2017 at: www.nhlbi.nih.gov/health/educational/wecan/eat-right/distortion.htm

National Heart, Lung, and Blood Institute (NHLBI) of the National Institutes of Health. (2016b). Aim for a healthy weight: Body mass index table. Retrieved on 3/2/2017 at: www.nhlbi.nih.gov/health/educational/lose_wt/BMI/bmi_tbl.pdf

National Institute of Diabetes and Digestive and Kidney Diseases (NIDDK). (2016). *Prescription medications to treat overweight and obesity*. Retrieved on 1/7/2017 at: www.niddk.nih.gov/health-information/

health-topics/weight-control/prescription-medications-treat-overweight-obesity/Pages/facts.aspx.

Obesity Action Coalition (OAC). (2015a). OAC insurance guide. Retrieved on 11/19/2015 at: www.obesityaction.org/educational-resources/brochures-and-guides/oac-insurance-guide/reviewing-your-insurance-policy-or-employer-sponsored-medical-benefits-plan

Obesity Action Coalition (OAC). (2015b). Obesity treatments: Bariatric surgery (severe obesity). Retrieved on 11/19/2015 at: www.obesityaction.org/obesity-treatments/bariatric-surgery

Ogden, C. L., Carroll, M. D., Kit, B. K., et al. (2014). Prevalence of childhood and adult obesity in the United States, 2011–2012. *JAMA, 311*(8), 806–814.

Orringer, K. A., Harrison, A. V., Nichani, S. S., et al. (2016). University of Michigan Health System Clinical Alignment and Performance Excellence Guideline: Obesity prevention and management. Retrieved on 1/25/2017 at: www.med.umich.edu/1info/FHP/practiceguides/obesity/obesity.pdf

Papasavas, P., El Chaar, M., Kothari, S. N., et al. (2016). American Society for Metabolic and Bariatric Surgery position statement on vagal blocking therapy for obesity. *Surgery for Obesity and Related Diseases, 12*(3), 460–461.

Patil, R., & Melander, S. (2015). Postoperative complications and emergency care for patients following bariatric surgery. *MEDSURG Nursing, 24*(4), 243–248.

*Pfeil, M. (2014). Patients' perception of the nursing contribution to gastric band surgery. *British Journal of Nursing, 23*(2), 95–99.

Puhl, R. M., Phelan, S. M., Nadglowski, J., et al. (2016). Overcoming weight bias in the management of patients with diabetes and obesity. *Clinical Diabetes Journals, 34*(1), 44–50.

Radosevich, J. J., Patanwala, A. E., & Erstad, B. L. (2016). Norepinephrine dosing in obese and nonobese patients with septic shock. *American Journal of Critical Care, 25*(1), 27–32.

Schauer, G. L., Woodruff, R. C., Hotz, J., & Kegler, M. C. (2014). A qualitative inquiry about weight counseling practices in community health centers. *Patient Education and Counseling, 97*(1), 82–87.

Segal, L. M., Rayburn, J., & Martin, A. (2016). The state of obesity: 2016 – Better policies for a healthier America. Robert Wood Johnson Foundation. Retrieved on 1/21/2017 at: stateofobesity.org/files/stateofobesity2016.pdf

Shikora, S. A., Wolfe, B. M., Apovian, D. M., et al. (2015). Sustained weight loss with vagal nerve blockade but not with sham: 18-month results of the ReCharge trial. *Journal of Obesity, 2015*:365604.

Sifrim, D. (2013). Management of bile reflux. *Gastroenterology and Hepatology, 9*(3), 179–180.

Sturman-Floyd, M. (2013). Moving and handling: Supporting bariatric residents. *Nursing and Residential Care, 15*(6), 432–437.

World Health Organization (WHO). (2015). *10 facts on obesity.* Retrieved on 11/19/2015 at: www.who.int/features/factfiles/obesity/facts/en/index1.html

World Health Organization (WHO). (2016). *Obesity and overweight: Fact sheet.* Retrieved on 1/21/2017 at: www.who.int/mediacentre/factsheets/fs311/en/

*Wykowski, K., & Krouse, H. J. (2013). Self-care predictors for success post-bariatric surgery. *Gastroenterology Nursing, 36*(2), 129–135.

Yanovski, S. Z., & Yanovski, J. A. (2014). Long-term drug treatment for obesity: A systematic and clinical review. *JAMA, 311*(1), 74–86.

Resources

American Society for Metabolic and Bariatric Surgery (ASMBS), www.asmbs.org

Centers for Disease Control and Prevention (CDC), www.cdc.gov/obesity/

DASH Diet for Healthy Eating, dashdiet.org

National Heart, Lung, and Blood Institute of the National Institutes of Health, Aim for a Healthy Weight, www.nhlbi.nih.gov/health/educational/lose_wt/index.htm

National Institute of Diabetes and Digestive and Kidney Diseases, Weight Management, www.niddk.nih.gov/health-information/weight-management

Obesity Action Coalition, www.obesityaction.org

Obesity Medicine Association, www.obesitymedicine.org

Obesity Society, www.obesity.org

Robert Wood Johnson Foundation The State of Obesity: Better Policies for a Healthier America, stateofobesity.org

Rudd Center for Food Policy and Obesity, www.uconnruddcenter.org

Therapeutic Lifestyle Changes (TLC) Diet, TLCdiet.org

LEARNING OBJECTIVES

On completion of this chapter, the learner will be able to:

1 Identify the metabolic functions of the liver and the alterations that occur with hepatic disorders.
2 Explain liver function tests and the clinical manifestations of liver dysfunction in relation to pathophysiologic alterations of the liver.
3 Relate jaundice, portal hypertension, ascites, varices, nutritional deficiencies, and hepatic encephalopathy and coma to pathophysiologic alterations of the liver.
4 Describe the medical, surgical, and nursing management of patients with esophageal varices.

5 Compare the various types of hepatitis and their causes, prevention, clinical manifestations, management, prognosis, and home health care needs.
6 Use the nursing process as a framework for care of the patient with cirrhosis of the liver.
7 Differentiate between the nonsurgical and surgical management of patients with cancer of the liver.
8 Specify the postoperative nursing care of the patient undergoing liver transplantation.

GLOSSARY

ascites: an albumin-rich fluid accumulation in the peritoneal cavity
asterixis: involuntary flapping movements of the hands
cirrhosis: a chronic liver disease characterized by fibrotic changes, the formation of dense connective tissue within the liver, subsequent degenerative changes, and loss of functioning cells
constructional apraxia: inability to draw figures in two or three dimensions
endoscopic variceal ligation (EVL): procedure that uses a modified endoscope loaded with an elastic rubber band passed through an overtube directly onto the varix (or varices) to be banded to ligate the area and stop bleeding
fetor hepaticus: sweet, slightly fecal odor to the breath, presumed to be of intestinal origin; prevalent with the extensive collateral portal circulation in chronic liver disease
fulminant hepatic failure: sudden, severe onset of acute liver failure that occurs within 8 weeks after the first symptoms of jaundice

hepatic encephalopathy: central nervous system dysfunction frequently associated with elevated ammonia levels that produce changes in mental status, altered level of consciousness, and coma
jaundice: condition where the body tissues, including the sclerae and the skin, become tinged yellow or greenish-yellow, due to high bilirubin levels
orthotopic liver transplantation (OLT): grafting of a donor liver into the normal anatomic location, with removal of the diseased native liver
portal hypertension: elevated pressure in the portal circulation resulting from obstruction of venous flow into and through the liver
sclerotherapy: the injection of substances into or around esophagogastric varices to cause constriction, thickening, and hardening of the vessel and stop bleeding
xenograft: transplantation of organs from one species to another

---

Liver function is complex, and hepatic dysfunction affects all body systems. For this reason, the nurse must understand how the liver functions and must have expert clinical assessment and management skills to care for patients undergoing diagnostic and treatment procedures. The nurse also must have an understanding of technologic advances in the management of hepatic disorders. Liver disorders are common and may result from a virus, obesity, and insulin resistance, or exposure to toxic substances, such as alcohol, or tumors.

ASSESSMENT OF THE LIVER

Anatomic and Physiologic Overview

The liver, the largest gland of the body and a major organ, can be considered a chemical factory that manufactures, stores, alters, and excretes a large number of substances involved in metabolism (Hall, 2015). The location of the liver is essential because it receives nutrient-rich blood directly from the gastrointestinal (GI) tract and then either stores or transforms

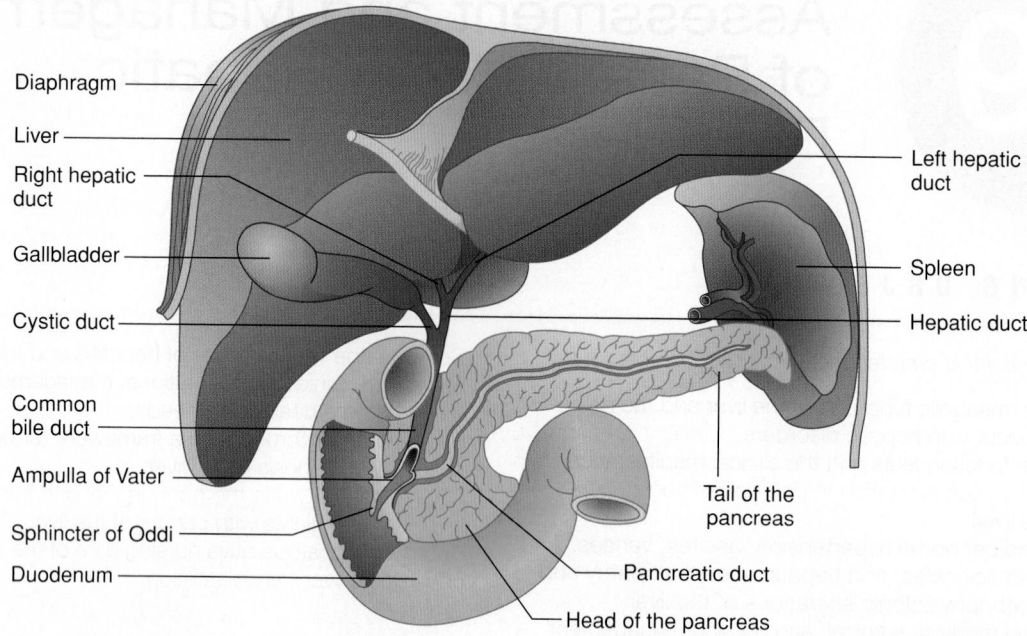

Figure 49-1 • The liver and biliary system, including the gallbladder and bile ducts. From Grossman, S. C., & Porth, C. M. (2014). *Pathophysiology: Concepts of altered health states* (9th ed.). Philadelphia, PA: Lippincott Williams & Wilkins.

these nutrients into chemicals that are used elsewhere in the body for metabolic needs. The liver is especially important in the regulation of glucose and protein metabolism. The liver manufactures and secretes bile, which has a major role in the digestion and absorption of fats in the GI tract. The liver removes waste products from the bloodstream and secretes them into the bile. The bile produced by the liver is stored temporarily in the gallbladder until it is needed for digestion, at which time the gallbladder empties and bile enters the intestine (see Fig. 49-1).

Anatomy of the Liver

The liver is a large, highly vascular organ located behind the ribs in the upper right portion of the abdominal cavity. It weighs between 1200 and 1500 g in the average adult and is divided into four lobes. A thin layer of connective tissue surrounds each lobe, extending into the lobe itself and dividing the liver mass into small, functional units called *lobules* (Hall, 2015).

The circulation of the blood into and out of the liver is of major importance to liver function. The blood that perfuses the liver comes from two sources. Approximately 80% of the blood supply comes from the portal vein, which drains the GI tract and is rich in nutrients but lacks oxygen. The remainder of the blood supply enters by way of the hepatic artery and is rich in oxygen. Terminal branches of these two blood vessels join to form common capillary beds, which constitute the sinusoids of the liver (see Fig. 49-2). Thus, a mixture of venous and arterial blood bathes the liver cells (hepatocytes). The sinusoids empty into venules that occupy the center of each liver lobule and are called the *central veins*. The central veins join to form the hepatic vein, which constitutes the venous drainage from the liver and empties into the inferior vena cava, close to the diaphragm (Hall, 2015).

In addition to hepatocytes, phagocytic cells belonging to the reticuloendothelial system are present in the liver. Other organs that contain reticuloendothelial cells are the spleen, bone marrow, lymph nodes, and lungs. In the liver, these cells are called *Kupffer cells* (Hall, 2015). As the most common phagocyte in the human body, their main function is to

Figure 49-2 • A section of liver lobule showing the location of hepatic veins, hepatic cells, liver sinusoids, and branches of the portal vein and hepatic artery.

engulf particulate matter (e.g., bacteria) that enters the liver through the portal blood.

The smallest bile ducts, called *canaliculi*, are located between the lobules of the liver. The canaliculi receive secretions from the hepatocytes and carry them to larger bile ducts, which eventually form the hepatic duct. The hepatic duct from the liver and the cystic duct from the gallbladder join to form the common bile duct, which empties into the small intestine. The sphincter of Oddi, located at the junction where the common bile duct enters the duodenum, controls the flow of bile into the intestine.

Functions of the Liver

Glucose Metabolism

The liver plays a major role in the metabolism of glucose and the regulation of blood glucose concentration. After a meal, glucose is taken up from the portal venous blood by the liver and converted into glycogen, which is stored in the hepatocytes. Subsequently, the glycogen is converted back to glucose (glycogenolysis) and released as needed into the bloodstream to maintain normal levels of blood glucose. However, this process provides a limited amount of glucose. Additional glucose can be synthesized by the liver through a process called *gluconeogenesis*. For this process, the liver uses amino acids from protein breakdown or lactate produced by exercising muscles. This process occurs in response to hypoglycemia (Hall, 2015).

Ammonia Conversion

The use of amino acids from protein for gluconeogenesis results in the formation of ammonia as a by-product. The liver converts this metabolically generated ammonia into urea. Ammonia produced by bacteria in the intestines is also removed from portal blood for urea synthesis. In this way, the liver converts ammonia, a potential toxin, into urea, a compound that is excreted in the urine (Hall, 2015; Lee & Moreau, 2015).

Protein Metabolism

The liver also plays an important role in protein metabolism. It synthesizes almost all of the plasma proteins (except gamma-globulin), including albumin, alpha-globulins and beta-globulins, blood clotting factors, specific transport proteins, and most of the plasma lipoproteins. Vitamin K is required by the liver for synthesis of prothrombin and some of the other clotting factors. Amino acids are used by the liver for protein synthesis (Hall, 2015; Lee & Moreau, 2015).

Fat Metabolism

The liver is also active in fat metabolism. Fatty acids can be broken down for the production of energy and ketone bodies (acetoacetic acid, beta-hydroxybutyric acid, and acetone). Ketone bodies are small compounds that can enter the bloodstream and provide a source of energy for muscles and other tissues. Breakdown of fatty acids into ketone bodies occurs primarily when the availability of glucose for metabolism is limited, as in starvation or in uncontrolled diabetes. Fatty acids and their metabolic products are also used for the synthesis of cholesterol, lecithin, lipoproteins, and other complex lipids (Hall, 2015).

Vitamin and Iron Storage

Vitamins A, B, and D and several of the B-complex vitamins are stored in large amounts in the liver. Certain substances, such as iron and copper, are also stored in the liver.

Bile Formation

Bile is continuously formed by the hepatocytes and collected in the canaliculi and bile ducts. It is composed mainly of water and electrolytes such as sodium, potassium, calcium, chloride, and bicarbonate, and it also contains significant amounts of lecithin, fatty acids, cholesterol, bilirubin, and bile salts. Bile is collected and stored in the gallbladder and is emptied into the intestine as needed for digestion. The functions of bile are excretory, as in the excretion of bilirubin; bile also serves as an aid to digestion through the emulsification of fats by bile salts.

Bile salts are synthesized by the hepatocytes from cholesterol. After conjugation or binding with amino acids (taurine and glycine), bile salts are excreted into the bile. The bile salts, together with cholesterol and lecithin, are required for emulsification of fats in the intestine, which is necessary for efficient digestion and absorption. Bile salts are then reabsorbed, primarily in the distal ileum, into portal blood for return to the liver and are again excreted into the bile. This pathway from hepatocytes to bile to intestine and back to the hepatocytes is called the *enterohepatic circulation*. Because of the enterohepatic circulation, only a small fraction of the bile salts that enter the intestine are excreted in the feces. This decreases the need for active synthesis of bile salts by the liver cells (Hall, 2015).

Bilirubin Excretion

Bilirubin is a pigment derived from the breakdown of hemoglobin by cells of the reticuloendothelial system, including the Kupffer cells of the liver. Hepatocytes remove bilirubin from the blood and chemically modify it through conjugation to glucuronic acid, which makes the bilirubin more soluble in aqueous solutions. The conjugated bilirubin is secreted by the hepatocytes into the adjacent bile canaliculi and is eventually carried in the bile into the duodenum.

In the small intestine, bilirubin is converted into urobilinogen, which is partially excreted in the feces and partially absorbed through the intestinal mucosa into the portal blood. Much of this reabsorbed urobilinogen is removed by the hepatocytes and secreted into the bile once again (enterohepatic circulation). Some of the urobilinogen enters the systemic circulation and is excreted by the kidneys in the urine. Elimination of bilirubin in the bile represents the major route of its excretion.

Drug Metabolism

The liver metabolizes many medications, such as barbiturates, opioids, sedatives, anesthetics, and amphetamines (Goldman & Schafer, 2015; Hall, 2015). Metabolism generally results in drug inactivation, although activation may also occur. One of the important pathways for medication metabolism involves conjugation (binding) of the medication with a variety of compounds, such as glucuronic acid or acetic acid, to form more soluble substances. These substances may be excreted in the feces or urine, similar to bilirubin excretion. Bioavailability is the fraction of the given medication that

Chart 49-1 Age-Related Changes of the Hepatobiliary System

- Atypical clinical presentation of biliary disease
- Decreases in the following:
  - Clearance of hepatitis B surface antigen
  - Drug metabolism and clearance capabilities
  - Intestinal and portal vein blood flow
  - Gallbladder contraction after a meal
  - Rate of replacement and or repair of liver cells after injury
  - Size and weight of the liver, particularly in women
- Increased prevalence of gallstones due to the increase in cholesterol secretion in bile
- More rapid progression of hepatitis C infection and lower response rate to therapy
- More severe complications of biliary tract disease

Adapted from Townsend, C. M., Beauchamp, R. D., Evers, B. M., et al. (2016). *Sabiston's textbook of surgery: The biological basis of modern surgical practice.* Philadelphia, PA: Elsevier.

actually reaches the systemic circulation. The bioavailability of an oral medication (absorbed from the GI tract) can be decreased if the medication is metabolized to a great extent by the liver before it reaches the systemic circulation; this is known as first-pass effect. Some medications have such a large first-pass effect that their use is essentially limited to the parenteral route, or oral doses must be substantially larger than parenteral doses to achieve the same effect.

 ## Gerontologic Considerations

Chart 49-1 summarizes age-related changes in the liver. In the older adult, the most common change in the liver is a decrease in size and weight, accompanied by a decrease in total hepatic blood flow. However, in general, these decreases are proportional to the decreases in body size and weight seen in normal aging. Results of liver function tests do not normally change with age; abnormal results in older patients indicate abnormal liver function and are not a result of the aging process itself.

Metabolism of medications by the liver decreases in the older adult, but such changes are usually accompanied by changes in intestinal absorption, renal excretion, and altered body distribution of some medications secondary to changes in fat deposition. These alterations necessitate careful medication administration and monitoring; if appropriate, reduced dosages may be needed to prevent medication toxicity.

Assessment

Health History

If liver function test results are abnormal, the patient is evaluated for liver disease. In such cases, the health history focuses on previous exposure of the patient to hepatotoxic substances or infectious agents. The patient's occupational, recreational, and travel history may assist in identifying exposure to hepatotoxins (e.g., industrial chemicals, other toxins). The patient's history of alcohol and drug use, including but not limited to the use of intravenous (IV) or injection drugs, provides additional information about exposure to toxins and infectious agents. Many medications (including acetaminophen [Tylenol],

ketoconazole [Nizoral], and valproic acid [Depakene]) are responsible for hepatic dysfunction and disease (Kathpalia & Ahn, 2015). A thorough medication history should address all current and past prescription medications, over-the-counter medications, herbal remedies, and dietary supplements.

Lifestyle behaviors that increase the risk of exposure to infectious agents are identified. IV or injection drug use, sexual practices, and foreign travel are all potential risk factors for liver disease. The amount and type of alcohol consumed are identified using screening tools (questionnaires) that have been developed for this purpose (see Chapter 5). The amount of alcohol required to produce chronic liver disease varies widely, but men who consume 60 to 80 g/day of alcohol (approximately four glasses of beer, wine, or mixed drinks) and women whose alcohol intake is 40 to 60 g/day are considered at high risk for **cirrhosis**. Cirrhosis is a chronic liver disorder characterized by fibrotic changes, the formation of dense connective tissue within the liver, subsequent degenerative changes, and loss of functional liver tissue (Lee & Moreau, 2015) (see later discussion).

The history also includes an evaluation of the patient's past medical history to identify risk factors for the development of liver disease. Current and past medical conditions, including those of a psychological or psychiatric nature, are identified. The family history includes questions about familial liver disorders that may have their origin in alcohol abuse or gallstone disease, as well as other familial or genetic disorders (see Chart 49-2).

The history also addresses symptoms that suggest liver disease. Symptoms that may have their origin in liver disease but are not specific to hepatic dysfunction include **jaundice**, malaise, weakness, fatigue, pruritus, abdominal pain, fever, anorexia, weight gain, edema, increasing abdominal girth, hematemesis, melena, hematochezia (passage of bloody stools), easy bruising, changes in mental acuity, personality changes, sleep disturbances, and decreased libido in men and secondary amenorrhea in women.

Physical Assessment

The nurse assesses the patient for physical signs that may occur with liver dysfunction, including the pallor often seen with chronic illness and jaundice. The skin, mucosa, and sclerae are inspected for jaundice, and the extremities are assessed for muscle atrophy, edema, and skin excoriation secondary to scratching. The nurse observes the skin for petechiae or ecchymotic areas (bruises), spider angiomas (see Fig. 49-3), and palmar erythema. The male patient is assessed for unilateral or bilateral gynecomastia and testicular atrophy due to hormonal changes. The patient's cognitive status (recall, memory, abstract thinking) and neurologic status are assessed. The nurse observes for general tremor, **asterixis** (involuntary flapping movements of the hands), weakness, and slurred speech. These symptoms are discussed later.

Nonalcoholic fatty liver disease (NAFLD) and nonalcoholic steatohepatitis (NASH) are two diseases within the spectrum of fatty liver to fibrosis and cirrhosis that are strongly associated with obesity (Lee & Moreau, 2015). Two preliminary studies further suggest that being overweight and drinking too much alcohol can cause severe harm to the liver (European Association for the Study of the Liver, 2013).

Chart 49-2 — GENETICS IN NURSING PRACTICE
Hepatic Disorders

A number of hepatic disorders have an underlying genetic cause. However, other genetic disorders associated with metabolic, gastrointestinal, or bleeding disorders will also impact the function of the liver. Some examples of hepatic disorders caused by genetic abnormalities include:

Autosomal Dominant:
- Alagille syndrome
- Hereditary coproporphyria
- Polycystic liver disease

Autosomal Recessive:
- Crigler–Najjar syndrome
- Dublin–Johnson syndrome
- Hemochromatosis
- Progressive familial intrahepatic cholestasis
- Thalassemia
- Wilson disease

Inheritance Pattern is not distinct; however, there is a genetic predisposition for the disorder:
- Biliary atresia
- Gilbert syndrome

Other genetic disorders that impact the hepatic system:
- Alpha-1 antitrypsin deficiency
- Cystic fibrosis
- Glycogen storage disease
- Lysosomal storage disease
- Polycystic kidney disease
- Zellweger syndrome

Nursing Assessments

Refer to Chapter 5, Chart 5-2: Genetics in Nursing Practice: Genetic Aspects of Health Assessment

Family History Assessment Related to Hepatic Disorders
- Collect family history for three generations of maternal and paternal relatives in the patient's family
- Assess family history for relatives with early-onset hepatic disease

Patient Assessment Related to Genetic Hepatic Disorders
- Assess for physical signs or history of the following:
  - Abdominal bloating, and constipation
  - Changes to skin color or yellow hue to sclera
  - Enlarged liver, spleen, or abdomen
  - Episodes of nausea and vomiting
  - Hemorrhoids, esophageal varices, or gallstones
  - Intolerance to fatty foods or alcohol
  - Pale-colored stools
  - Presence and frequency of indigestion or reflux
  - Unexplained weight loss
- Assess for associated nervous system disorders such as depression and mood changes especially anger and irritability (Wilson disease).
- Assess for associated blood sugar problems such as hypoglycemia
- Inquire about and assess for abnormal bleeding or bruising
- Obtain and review laboratory values: Liver function tests, ammonia, bilirubin, fat soluble vitamins (e.g., vitamins A, D, E, K)

Genetics Resources

American Liver Foundation www.liverfoundation.org
See Chapter 8, Chart 8-7 for components of genetic counseling.

One study found that overweight and obese women who were heavy drinkers had a significantly increased risk of developing and dying of chronic liver disease. The other study found an increased risk of liver cancer in people with alcoholic cirrhosis who also have fatty liver disease, type 2 diabetes, and are overweight or obese. In patients who are overweight, obese, or have high alcohol intake, the nurse observes for signs of associated liver dysfunction.

The nurse assesses for the presence of an abdominal fluid wave (discussed later). The abdomen is palpated to assess liver size and to detect any tenderness over the liver. The liver may be palpable in the right upper quadrant. A palpable liver presents as a firm, sharp ridge with a smooth surface (see Fig. 49-4). The nurse estimates the size of the liver by percussing its upper and lower borders. If the liver is not palpable but tenderness

Figure 49-3 • Spider angioma. This vascular (arterial) spider appears on the skin. Beneath the elevated center and radiating branches, the blood vessels are looped and tortuous.

Figure 49-4 • Technique for palpating the liver. The examiner places one hand under the right lower rib cage and presses downward during inspiration with light pressure with the other hand. From Bickley, L. S. (2017). *Bates' guide to physical examination and history taking* (12th ed.). Philadelphia, PA: Lippincott Williams & Wilkins.

is suspected, tapping the lower right thorax briskly may elicit tenderness. For comparison, the nurse then performs a similar maneuver on the left lower thorax (Lee & Moreau, 2015).

If the liver is palpable, the nurse notes and records its size, its consistency, any tenderness, and whether its outline is regular or irregular. If the liver is enlarged, the degree to which it descends below the right costal margin is recorded to provide some indication of its size. The nurse determines whether the liver's edge is sharp and smooth or blunt and whether the enlarged liver is nodular or smooth. The liver of a patient with cirrhosis is small and hard in late-stage cirrhosis, whereas the liver of a patient with acute hepatitis is soft and the hand easily moves the edge.

Tenderness of the liver indicates recent acute enlargement with consequent stretching of the liver capsule. The absence of tenderness may imply that the enlargement is of long-standing duration. The liver of a patient with viral hepatitis is tender, whereas that of a patient with alcoholic hepatitis is not. Enlargement of the liver is an abnormal finding that requires evaluation (Lee & Moreau, 2015).

Diagnostic Evaluation

A wide range of diagnostic studies may be performed in patients with hepatic disorders. The nurse should educate the patient about the purpose, what to expect, and any possible side effects related to these examinations prior to testing. The nurse should note trends in results because they provide information about disease progression as well as the patient's response to therapy.

Liver Function Tests

More than 70% of the parenchyma of the liver may be damaged before liver function test results become abnormal. Function is generally measured in terms of serum enzyme activity (i.e., serum aminotransferases, alkaline phosphatase, lactic dehydrogenase) and serum concentrations of proteins (albumin and globulins), bilirubin, ammonia, clotting factors, and lipids (Lee & Moreau, 2015; Woreta & Alqahtani, 2014). Several of these tests may be helpful for assessing patients with liver disease. However, the nature and extent of hepatic dysfunction cannot be determined by these tests alone, because other disorders can affect test results.

Serum aminotransferases are sensitive indicators of injury to the liver cells and are useful in detecting acute liver disease such as hepatitis. Alanine aminotransferase (ALT), aspartate aminotransferase (AST), and gamma-glutamyl transferase (GGT) (also called *gamma-glutamyl transpeptidase* [GGTP]) are the most frequently used tests of liver damage (Lee & Moreau, 2015; Woreta & Alqahtani, 2014). ALT levels increase primarily in liver disorders and may be used to monitor the course of hepatitis or cirrhosis or the effects of treatments that may be toxic to the liver. AST is present in tissues that have high metabolic activity; therefore, the level may be increased if there is damage to or death of tissues of organs such as the heart, liver, skeletal muscle, and kidney. Although not specific to liver disease, levels of AST may be increased in cirrhosis, hepatitis, and liver cancer. Increased GGT levels are associated with cholestasis but can also be due to alcoholic liver disease. Although the kidney has the highest level of the enzyme, the liver is considered the source of normal serum activity. The test determines liver cell dysfunction and is a sensitive indicator of cholestasis. Its main value in liver disease is confirming the hepatic origin of an elevated alkaline phosphatase level. Common liver function tests are summarized in Table 49-1, additional laboratory values can be found in Appendix A on thePoint.

Liver Biopsy

Liver biopsy is the removal of a small amount of liver tissue, usually through needle aspiration. It permits examination of liver cells. The most common indication is to evaluate diffuse disorders of the parenchyma and to diagnose space-occupying lesions. Liver biopsy is especially useful when clinical findings and laboratory tests are not diagnostic. Though rare due to the radiologic guidance now available, peritonitis caused by blood or bile after liver biopsy is the most common complication; therefore, coagulation studies are obtained, their values are noted, and abnormal results are treated before liver biopsy is performed (Feldman, Friedman, & Brandt, 2015). Other techniques for liver biopsy are preferred if **ascites** (an accumulation of albumin-rich fluid in the peritoneal cavity) or coagulation abnormalities exist. A liver biopsy can be performed percutaneously with ultrasound guidance or transvenously through the right internal jugular vein to right hepatic vein under fluoroscopic control. Liver biopsy can also be performed laparoscopically.

For the procedural guidelines for assisting with a percutaneous liver biopsy, go to **thePoint.lww.com/Brunner14e.**

Other Diagnostic Tests

Ultrasonography, computed tomography (CT) scans, and magnetic resonance imaging (MRI) are used to identify normal structures and abnormalities of the liver and biliary tree. A radioisotope liver scan may be performed to assess liver size, blood flow, and obstruction. Noninvasive liver stiffness measurements or elastography uses ultrasound-based vibration and scanning to identify liver fibrosis and determine its extent. Magnetic resonance elastography uses mechanical shear waves to identify stiff tissue (Bonder, Tapper, & Afdhal, 2015; Fabrellas, Alemany, Urquizu, et al., 2013) (see Chart 49-3). Liver fibrosis and other liver diseases can be identified, evaluated and monitored with a variety of other noninvasive studies. These studies may reduce the need for liver biopsy (Bonder et al. 2015).

Laparoscopy (insertion of a fiberoptic endoscope through a small abdominal incision) is used to examine the liver and other pelvic structures. It is also used to perform guided liver biopsy, to determine the cause of ascites, and to diagnose and stage tumors of the liver and other abdominal organs.

MANIFESTATIONS OF HEPATIC DYSFUNCTION

Hepatic dysfunction results from damage to the liver's parenchymal cells, directly from primary liver diseases, or indirectly from either obstruction of bile flow or derangements of hepatic circulation. Liver dysfunction may be acute or chronic; the latter is far more common.

TABLE 49-1 Common Laboratory Tests to Assess Liver Function

Test	Normal	Clinical Functions
Pigment Studies		
Serum bilirubin, direct	0.1–0.4 mg/dL (1.7–3.7 mcmol/L)	These studies measure the ability of the liver to conjugate and excrete bilirubin. Results are abnormal in liver and biliary tract disease and are associated with jaundice clinically.
Serum bilirubin, total	0.3–1 mg/dL (5–17 mcmol/L)	
Urine bilirubin	<0.25 mg/24 hr (<0.42 mcmol/24 hr)	
Urine urobilinogen	(Urine urobilinogen) 0.05–2.5 mg/24 hr (0.5–4 Ehrlich U/24 hr)	
Fecal urobilinogen (infrequently used)	(Fecal urobilinogen) 50–300 mg/24 hr (100–400 Ehrlich U/100 g)	
Protein Studies		
Total serum protein	7–7.5 g/dL (70–75 g/L)	Proteins are manufactured by the liver. Their levels may be affected in a variety of liver impairments: albumin is affected in cirrhosis, chronic hepatitis, edema; and ascites; globulins are affected in cirrhosis, liver disease, chronic obstructive jaundice, and viral hepatitis.
Serum albumin	3.5–5.5 g/dL (40–55 g/L)	
Serum globulin	2.3–3.5 g/dL (23–35 g/L)	
Serum protein electrophoresis		
Albumin	4–6 g/dL (40–60 g/L)	
α_1-Globulin	0.15–0.25 g/dL (1.5–2.5 g/L)	
α_2-Globulin	0.43–0.75 g/dL (4.3–7.5 g/L)	
β-Globulin	0.5–1 g/dL (5–10 g/L)	
γ-Globulin	0.6–1.3 g/dL (6–13 g/L)	
A/G ratio	A > G or 1.5:1–2.5:1	A/G ratio is reversed in chronic liver disease (decreased albumin and increased globulin).
Prothrombin Time	100% or 12–16 seconds	Prothrombin time may be prolonged in liver disease. It will not return to normal with vitamin K in severe liver cell damage.
Serum Alkaline Phosphatase	Varies with method: *Adults:* 30–120 U/L	Serum alkaline phosphatase is manufactured in bones, liver, kidneys, and intestine and excreted through biliary tract. In the absence of bone disease, it is a sensitive measure of biliary tract obstruction. Results may vary because this test is temperature and lab method dependent.
Serum Aminotransferase Studies		
AST	10–40 U/mL (0.34–0.68 U/L)	The studies are based on release of enzymes from damaged liver cells. These enzymes are elevated in liver cell damage. Normal values may differ in men and women.
ALT	8–40 U/mL (0.14–0.68 U/L)	
GGT, GGTP	0–30 U/L IU/L	Values are elevated in alcohol abuse and markers for biliary cholestasis.
LDH	100–200 units (100–225 U/L)	
Ammonia (plasma)	15–45 mcg/dL (11–32 mcmol/L)	Liver converts ammonia to urea. Ammonia level rises in liver failure.
Cholesterol		
Ester	60–70% of total cholesterol, fraction of total cholesterol 0.60–0.70	Cholesterol levels are elevated in biliary obstruction and decreased in parenchymal liver disease.
HDL	*Male:* 35–70 mg/dL; *Female:* 35–85 mg/dL	
LDL	<130 mcg/dL	

A/G, albumin/globulin; AST, aspartate aminotransferase; ALT, alanine aminotransferase; GGT, gamma-glutamyl transferase; GGTP, gamma-glutamyl transpeptidase; LDH, lactate dehydrogenase; HDL, high-density lipoprotein; LDL, low-density lipoprotein.
Adapted from Alldredge, B. K., Corelli, R. L., Ernst, M. E., et al., (Eds.). (2013). *Koda-Kimble & Young's applied therapeutics: The clinical use of drugs.* Philadelphia, PA: Lippincott Williams & Wilkins.

Chronic liver disease, including cirrhosis, is the 12th leading cause of death in the United States among young and middle-aged adults (James & Liou, 2015). At least 40% of those deaths are associated with alcohol use. The rate of chronic liver disease for men is twice that for women, and chronic liver disease is more common in Asian and African countries than it is in Europe and the United States. Compensated cirrhosis, in which the damaged liver is still able to perform normal functions, often goes undetected for extended periods, and as many as 1% of people may have subclinical or compensated cirrhosis (Bope & Kellerman, 2015). Approximately 80% of patients diagnosed with cirrhosis compensate and remain asymptomatic for the next 10 years (Fox, 2014; Nusrat, Khan, Fazili, et al., 2014).

Disease processes that lead to hepatocellular dysfunction may be caused by infectious agents such as bacteria and viruses and by anoxia, metabolic disorders, toxins and medications, nutritional deficiencies, and hypersensitivity states. The most common cause of parenchymal damage is malnutrition, especially that related to alcoholism (Fialla et al., 2015).

The parenchymal cells respond to most noxious agents by replacing glycogen with lipids, producing fatty infiltration with or without cell death or necrosis. This is commonly associated with inflammatory cell infiltration and growth of fibrous tissue. Cell regeneration can occur if the disease process is not too toxic to the cells. The result of chronic parenchymal disease is the shrunken, fibrotic liver seen in cirrhosis.

In some conditions, lipids may accumulate in the hepatocytes, resulting in the abnormal condition called *fatty liver disease*. If unrelated to alcohol, this disease is referred to as nonalcoholic fatty liver disease (NAFLD). A condition known as nonalcoholic steatohepatitis (NASH) represents a more serious condition within the broad spectrum of

Chart 49-3

NURSING RESEARCH PROFILE

Detecting Chronic Liver Diseases in a Primary Care Nurse Consultancy

Fabrellas, N., Alemany, M., Urquizu, M., et al. (2013). Using transient elastography to detect chronic liver diseases in a primary care nurse consultancy. *Nursing Research, 62*(6), 450–455.

Purpose

The purpose of this study was to assess the feasibility of performing screening for undiagnosed chronic liver diseases (CLD) in a primary care nurse consultancy program.

Design

Two experienced nurses in a primary care consultancy program were trained to perform transient elastography (TE). Patients were identified from a health registry and invited to participate in a feasibility pilot study. Participants were excluded if they had a history of liver disease. Nurses collected demographic and clinical data and performed the TE test to measure the degree of liver stiffness as an indicator of the presence of CLD with fibrosis.

Findings

Accurate measurements were obtained in 495 of 502 participants. Significant liver stiffness was observed in 28 of 495 participants (5.7%). Those with increased liver stiffness were older and were more likely to be male and to have metabolic syndrome. Upon further assessment of these participants nonalcoholic fatty liver disease was the most common cause of CLD.

Nursing Implications

Nurses who assess patients in primary care settings can be educated to perform additional noninvasive testing to identify liver stiffness. When identified this liver stiffness can indicate CLD and then can be further explored to achieve a definitive diagnosis. Patients will then be able to receive early interventions to treat, and in some cases, to ameliorate the disease process.

NAFLDs and may result in damage, fibrotic changes in the liver, and cirrhosis (Lee & Moreau, 2015).

The consequences of liver disease are numerous and varied. Their ultimate effects are often incapacitating or life threatening, and their presence is ominous. Among the most common and significant manifestations of liver disease are jaundice, portal hypertension, ascites and varices, nutritional deficiencies (resulting from the inability of damaged liver cells to metabolize certain vitamins), and **hepatic encephalopathy** or coma.

Jaundice

The bilirubin concentration in the blood may be increased in the presence of liver disease, if the flow of bile is impeded (e.g., by gallstones in the bile ducts), or if there is excessive destruction of red blood cells. With bile duct obstruction, bilirubin does not enter the intestine; as a consequence, urobilinogen is absent from the urine and decreased in the stool (Hall, 2015; Lee & Moreau, 2015).

When the bilirubin concentration in the blood is abnormally elevated, all of the body tissues, including the sclerae and the skin, become tinged yellow or greenish-yellow, a condition known as jaundice. Jaundice becomes clinically evident when the serum bilirubin level exceeds 2.0 mg/dL (34 mmol/L) (Lee & Moreau, 2015). Increased serum bilirubin levels and jaundice may result from impairment of hepatic uptake, conjugation of bilirubin, or excretion of bilirubin into the biliary system. There are several types of jaundice: hemolytic, hepatocellular, and obstructive jaundice, and jaundice due to hereditary hyperbilirubinemia. Hepatocellular and obstructive jaundice are the two types commonly associated with liver disease.

Hemolytic Jaundice

Hemolytic jaundice is the result of an increased destruction of the red blood cells; the effect is that the plasma is rapidly flooded with bilirubin so that the liver, although functioning normally, cannot excrete the bilirubin as quickly as it is formed. This type of jaundice is encountered in patients with hemolytic transfusion reactions and other hemolytic disorders.

In these patients, the bilirubin in the blood is predominantly unconjugated or free. Fecal and urine urobilinogen levels are increased, but the urine is free of bilirubin. Patients with this type of jaundice, unless their hyperbilirubinemia is extreme, do not experience symptoms or complications as a result of the jaundice per se. However, prolonged jaundice, even if mild, predisposes to the formation of pigment stones in the gallbladder, and extremely severe jaundice (levels of free bilirubin exceeding 20 to 25 mg/dL) poses a risk for central nervous system effects (Goldman & Schafer, 2015).

Hepatocellular Jaundice

Hepatocellular jaundice is caused by the inability of damaged liver cells to clear normal amounts of bilirubin from the blood. The cellular damage may be caused by hepatitis viruses, other viruses that affect the liver (e.g., yellow fever virus, Epstein–Barr virus), chemical toxins (e.g., carbon tetrachloride, phosphorus, arsenicals, certain medications), or alcohol. Cirrhosis of the liver is a form of hepatocellular disease that may produce jaundice. It is usually associated with excessive alcohol intake, but it may also be a late result of liver cell necrosis caused by viral infection. In prolonged obstructive jaundice, cell damage eventually develops, and both types of jaundice (i.e., obstructive and hepatocellular jaundice) appear together.

Patients with hepatocellular jaundice may be mildly or severely ill, with lack of appetite, nausea, malaise, fatigue, weakness, and possible weight loss. In some cases of hepatocellular disease, jaundice may not be obvious. The serum bilirubin concentration and the urine urobilinogen level may be elevated. In addition, AST and ALT levels may be increased, indicating cellular necrosis. The patient may report headache, chills, and fever if the cause is infectious. Depending on the cause and extent of the liver cell damage, hepatocellular jaundice may be completely reversible.

Obstructive Jaundice

Obstructive jaundice resulting from extrahepatic obstruction may be caused by occlusion of the bile duct from a gallstone, an inflammatory process, a tumor, or pressure from an enlarged organ (e.g., liver, gallbladder). The obstruction may also involve the small bile ducts within the liver (i.e., intrahepatic obstruction); this may be caused, for example, by pressure on these channels from inflammatory swelling of the liver or by an inflammatory exudate within the ducts themselves. Intrahepatic obstruction resulting from stasis and inspissation (thickening) of bile within the canaliculi may occur after the ingestion of certain medications, which are referred to as cholestatic agents. These include phenothiazines, antithyroid medications, sulfonylureas, tricyclic antidepressant agents, nitrofurantoin, androgens and estrogens, and some antibiotics.

Regardless of whether the obstruction is intrahepatic or extrahepatic, and regardless of its cause, bile cannot flow normally into the intestine and becomes backed up into the liver. It is then reabsorbed into the blood and carried throughout the entire body, staining the skin, mucous membranes, and sclerae. It is excreted in the urine, which becomes deep orange and foamy. Because of the decreased amount of bile in the intestinal tract, the stools become light or clay colored. The skin may itch intensely, requiring repeated soothing baths. Dyspepsia and intolerance to fatty foods may develop because of impaired fat digestion in the absence of intestinal bile. In general, AST, ALT, and GGT levels rise only moderately, but bilirubin and alkaline phosphatase levels are elevated.

Hereditary Hyperbilirubinemia

Increased serum bilirubin levels (hyperbilirubinemia), resulting from any of several inherited disorders, can also produce jaundice. Gilbert syndrome is a familial disorder characterized by an increased level of unconjugated bilirubin that causes jaundice. Although serum bilirubin levels are increased, liver histology and liver function test results are normal, and there is no hemolysis. This syndrome affects 3% to 8% of the population, predominantly males (Bope & Kellerman, 2015).

Other conditions that are probably caused by inborn errors of biliary metabolism include Dubin-Johnson syndrome (chronic idiopathic jaundice, with pigment in the liver) and Rotor syndrome (chronic familial conjugated hyperbilirubinemia, without pigment in the liver); the "benign" cholestatic jaundice of pregnancy, with retention of conjugated bilirubin, probably secondary to unusual sensitivity to the hormones of pregnancy; and benign recurrent intrahepatic cholestasis.

Portal Hypertension

Portal hypertension is the increased pressure throughout the portal venous system that results from obstruction of blood flow into and through the damaged liver. Commonly associated with hepatic cirrhosis, it can also occur with noncirrhotic liver disease. Although splenomegaly (enlarged spleen) with possible hypersplenism is a common manifestation of portal hypertension, the two major consequences of portal hypertension are ascites and varices.

Ascites

Pathophysiology

The mechanisms responsible for the development of ascites are not completely understood. Portal hypertension and

the resulting increase in capillary pressure and obstruction of venous blood flow through the damaged liver are contributing factors. The vasodilation that occurs in the splanchnic circulation (the arterial supply and venous drainage of the GI system from the distal esophagus to the midrectum, including the liver and spleen) is also a suspected causative factor. The failure of the liver to metabolize aldosterone increases sodium and water retention by the kidney. Sodium and water retention, increased intravascular fluid volume, increased lymphatic flow, and decreased synthesis of albumin by the damaged liver all contribute to the movement of fluid from the vascular system into the peritoneal space. The process becomes self-perpetuating; loss of fluid into the peritoneal space causes further sodium and water retention by the kidney in an effort to maintain the vascular fluid volume.

As a result of liver damage, large amounts of albumin-rich fluid, 20 L or more, may accumulate in the peritoneal cavity as ascites (Hall, 2015; Lee & Moreau, 2015). (Ascites may also occur with disorders such as cancer, kidney disease, and heart failure.) With the movement of albumin from the serum to the peritoneal cavity, the osmotic pressure of the serum decreases. This, combined with increased portal pressure, results in movement of fluid into the peritoneal cavity (see Fig. 49-5).

Physiology/Pathophysiology

Cirrhosis with portal hypertension

↓

Splanchnic arterial vasodilation

↓

Decrease in circulating arterial blood volume

↓

Activation of renin-angiotensin and sympathetic nervous systems and antidiuretic hormone

↓

Kidney retains sodium and water

↓

Hypervolemia

↓

Persistent activation of systems for retention of sodium and water; ascites and edema formation

↓

Continued arterial underfilling; cycle repeats

Figure 49-5 • Pathogenesis of ascites (arterial vasodilation theory).

Clinical Manifestations

Increased abdominal girth and rapid weight gain are common presenting symptoms of ascites. The patient may be short of breath and uncomfortable from the enlarged abdomen, and striae and distended veins may be visible over the abdominal wall. Umbilical hernias also occur frequently in those patients with cirrhosis. Fluid and electrolyte imbalances are common.

Assessment and Diagnostic Findings

The presence and extent of ascites are assessed by percussion of the abdomen. When fluid has accumulated in the peritoneal cavity, the flanks bulge when the patient assumes a supine position. The presence of fluid can be confirmed either by percussing for shifting dullness, by detecting a fluid wave (see Fig. 49-6), or by performing ballottement technique (see Fig. 49-7). A fluid wave is likely to be found only if a large amount of fluid is present (Lee & Moreau, 2015; Weber & Kelley, 2014). The ballottement technique is a palpation technique performed to identify a mass or enlarged organ within an abdomen with ascites (Weber & Kelley, 2009). Ballottement can be performed in two different ways: single handed or bimanually (see Fig. 49-7). Daily measurement and recording of abdominal girth and body weight are essential to assess the progression of ascites and its response to treatment.

Medical Management

The medical management of the patient with ascites includes dietary modifications, pharmacologic therapy, bed rest, paracentesis, the use of shunts, and other therapies.

Figure 49-6 • Assessing for abdominal fluid wave. The examiner places the hands along the sides of the patient's flanks, then strikes one flank sharply, detecting any fluid wave with the other hand. An assistant's hand is placed (ulnar side down) along the patient's midline to prevent the fluid wave from being transmitted through the tissues of the abdominal wall.

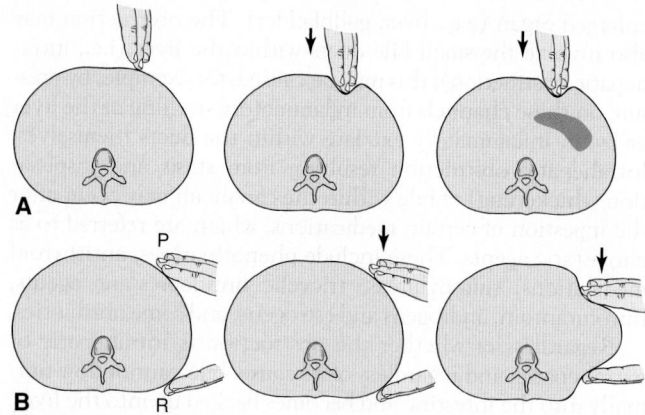

Figure 49-7 • Performing ballottement with one hand (**A**) and bimanually (**B**). From Weber, J., & Kelley, J. (2009). *Health assessment in nursing* (4th ed.). Philadelphia, PA: Lippincott Williams & Wilkins.

Nutritional Therapy

The goal of treatment for the patient with ascites is a negative sodium balance to reduce fluid retention. Table salt, salty foods, salted butter and margarine, and all canned and frozen foods that are not specifically prepared for low-sodium (2-g sodium) diets should be avoided (Lee & Moreau, 2015). It may take 2 to 3 months for the patient's taste buds to adjust to unsalted foods. In the meantime, the taste of unsalted foods can be improved by using salt substitutes such as lemon juice, oregano, and thyme. Commercial salt substitutes need to be approved by the patient's primary provider, because those that contain ammonia could precipitate hepatic encephalopathy and coma. Most salt substitutes contain potassium and should be avoided if the patient has impaired renal function. The patient should make liberal use of powdered, low-sodium milk and milk products. If fluid accumulation is not controlled with this regimen, the daily sodium allowance may be reduced further to 500 mg, and diuretic agents may be given. However, most patients will not accept such a severe sodium restriction as 500 mg, so clinicians often will not recommend it (Lee & Moreau, 2015).

Dietary control of ascites via strict sodium restriction is difficult to achieve at home. The likelihood that the patient will follow a 2-g sodium diet increases if the patient and the person preparing meals understand the rationale for the diet and receive periodic guidance about selecting and preparing appropriate foods. Approximately 10% of patients with ascites respond to these measures alone. Patients who do not respond and those who find sodium restriction difficult require diuretic therapy (Lee & Moreau, 2015).

Pharmacologic Therapy

The use of diuretic agents along with sodium restriction is successful in 90% of patients with ascites (Goldman & Schafer, 2015; Lee & Moreau, 2015). Spironolactone (Aldactone), an aldosterone-blocking agent, is most often the first-line therapy in patients with ascites from cirrhosis. When used with other diuretic agents, spironolactone helps prevent potassium loss. Oral diuretic agents such as furosemide (Lasix) may be added but should be used cautiously, because long-term use may induce severe sodium depletion (hyponatremia).

Ammonium chloride and acetazolamide (Diamox) are contraindicated because of the possibility of precipitating hepatic encephalopathy and coma. Daily weight loss should not exceed 1 kg (2.2 lb) in patients with ascites and peripheral edema or 0.5 to 0.75 kg (1.1 to 1.65 lb) in patients without edema (Bope & Kellerman, 2015; Feldman, et al., 2015; Lee & Moreau, 2015). Fluid restriction is not attempted unless the serum sodium concentration is very low.

Possible complications of diuretic therapy include fluid and electrolyte disturbances (including hypovolemia, hypokalemia, hyponatremia, and hypochloremic alkalosis) (see Chapter 13) and encephalopathy. Encephalopathy may be precipitated by dehydration and hypovolemia. In addition, when potassium stores are depleted, the amount of ammonia in the systemic circulation increases, which may cause impaired cerebral functioning and encephalopathy.

Bed Rest

In patients with ascites, an upright posture is associated with activation of the renin–angiotensin–aldosterone system and sympathetic nervous system (Lee & Moreau, 2015). This causes reduced renal glomerular filtration and sodium excretion and a decreased response to loop diuretics. Therefore, bed rest may be a useful therapy, especially for patients whose condition is refractory to diuretic agents.

Paracentesis

Paracentesis is the removal of fluid (ascites) from the peritoneal cavity through a puncture or a small surgical incision through the abdominal wall under sterile conditions (Goldman & Schafer, 2015). Ultrasound guidance may be indicated in some patients who are at high risk for bleeding because of an abnormal coagulation profile and in those who have had previous abdominal surgery and may have adhesions. Paracentesis was once considered a routine form of treatment for ascites. However, it is now performed primarily for diagnostic examination of ascitic fluid; in treatment for massive ascites that is resistant to nutritional and diuretic therapy and is causing severe problems to the patient; and as a prelude to diagnostic imaging studies, peritoneal dialysis, or surgery. A sample of the ascitic fluid may be sent to the laboratory for cell count, albumin and total protein levels, culture, and other tests.

Large-volume (5 to 6 L) paracentesis has been shown to be a safe method for treating patients with severe ascites. The use of this therapeutic intervention should not be restricted to patients in whom diuretic therapy has failed but should be considered the treatment of choice for all patients with large-volume ascites (Lee & Moreau, 2015). This technique, in combination with the IV infusion of salt-poor albumin or other colloid, has become a standard management strategy yielding an immediate effect. Refractive, massive ascites is unresponsive to multiple diuretic agents and sodium restriction for 2 weeks or more and can result in severe sequelae such as respiratory distress, which requires rapid intervention. Albumin infusions help to correct decreases in effective arterial blood volume that lead to sodium retention. The use of this colloid reduces the incidence of postparacentesis circulatory dysfunction with renal dysfunction, hyponatremia, and rapid reaccumulation of ascites associated with decreased effective arterial volume (Lee & Moreau, 2015). The beneficial effects of albumin adminis-

tration on hemodynamic stability and renal functional status may be related to an improvement in cardiac function as well as a decrease in the degree of arterial vasodilation. Although the patient with cirrhosis has a greatly increased extracellular blood volume, the kidney incorrectly senses that the intravascular volume has decreased. The renin–angiotensin–aldosterone axis is stimulated, and sodium is reabsorbed (Lee & Moreau, 2015; Nusrat et al. 2014). In addition, antidiuretic hormone secretion increases, which leads to increased retention of free water and sometimes to the development of dilutional hyponatremia. Therapeutic paracentesis provides only temporary removal of fluid; ascites rapidly recurs, necessitating repeated fluid removal.

For the procedural guidelines for assisting with a paracentesis, go to **thePoint.ww.com/ Brunner14e.**

Transjugular Intrahepatic Portosystemic Shunt

Transjugular intrahepatic portosystemic shunt (TIPS) is a method of treating ascites in which a cannula is threaded into the portal vein by the transjugular route (see Fig. 49-8). To reduce portal hypertension, an expandable stent is inserted to serve as an intrahepatic shunt between the portal circulation and the hepatic vein. This is extremely effective in decreasing sodium retention, improving the renal response to diuretic therapy, and preventing recurrence of fluid accumulation (Lee & Moreau, 2015; Nusrat et al. 2014). TIPS is an effective management strategy for refractive ascites. However, due to a higher risk of encephalopathy and higher cost of TIPS compared with large-volume paracentesis plus albumin, many consider TIPS a second-line therapy for refractive ascites that continues to occur despite medical management (Lee & Moreau, 2015; Nusrat et al. 2014).

Because the development of ascites in patients with cirrhosis is associated with a 50% mortality rate, patients considered candidates for liver transplantation may be referred for TIPS if paracentesis is contraindicated.

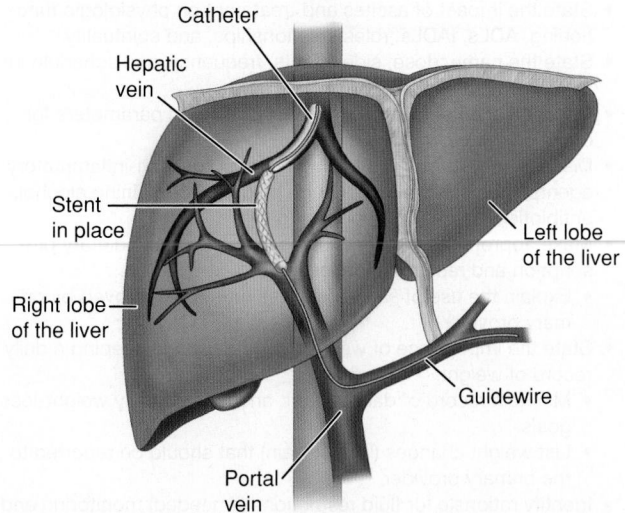

Figure 49-8 • Transjugular intrahepatic portosystemic shunt. A stent is inserted via catheter to the portal vein to divert blood flow and reduce portal hypertension.

Other Methods of Treatment

Ascites can also be treated by the insertion of a peritoneovenous shunt to redirect ascitic fluid from the peritoneal cavity into the systemic circulation via an abdominal and a thoracic catheter that drain into the superior vena cava through a one-way valve (Chen, Ge, Huang, et al., 2014; Lee & Moreau, 2015). However, this procedure is rarely used due to the availability of newer, more effective therapies such as TIPS.

Nursing Management

If a patient with ascites from liver dysfunction is hospitalized, nursing measures include assessment and documentation of intake and output (I&O), abdominal girth, and daily weight to assess fluid status. The nurse also closely monitors the respiratory status because large volumes of ascites can compress the thoracic cavity and inhibit adequate lung expansion. The nurse monitors serum ammonia, creatinine, and electrolyte levels to assess electrolyte balance, response to therapy, and indications of hepatic encephalopathy.

Promoting Home, Community-Based, and Transitional Care

Educating Patients About Self-Care

The patient treated for ascites is likely to be discharged with some ascites still present. Before hospital discharge, the nurse educates the patient and family about the treatment plan, including the need to avoid all alcohol intake, adhere to a low-sodium diet, take medications as prescribed, and check with the primary provider before taking any new medications. Additional home care education is summarized in Chart 49-4.

Continuing and Transitional Care

A referral for transitional, home, or community-based care may be warranted, especially if the patient lives alone or cannot provide self-care. The home visit enables the nurse to assess changes in the patient's condition and weight, abdominal girth, skin, and cognitive and emotional status. The nurse assesses the home environment and the availability of resources needed to adhere to the treatment plan (e.g., a scale to obtain daily weights, facilities to prepare and store appropriate foods, resources to purchase needed medications). The nurse also assesses the patient's adherence to the treatment plan and the ability to buy, prepare, and eat appropriate foods. The nurse reinforces previous education and emphasizes the need for regular follow-up and the importance of keeping scheduled health care appointments.

Esophageal Varices

Esophageal varices are present in 30% of patients with compensated cirrhosis and 60% of patients with decompensated cirrhosis at the time of diagnosis (Lee & Moreau, 2015; Satapathy & Sanyal, 2014) (see Clinical Manifestations in the Hepatic Cirrhosis section for further discussion). Varices are varicosities that develop from elevated pressure in the veins that drain into the portal system. They are prone to rupture and often are the source of massive hemorrhages from the upper GI tract and the rectum. In addition, abnormalities in blood clotting, often seen in patients with severe liver disease, increase the likelihood of bleeding with significant blood loss.

Once esophageal varices form, they increase in size over time and may eventually bleed (Lee & Moreau, 2015; Satapathy & Sanyal, 2014). In cirrhosis, varices are the most significant source of bleeding. The first bleeding episode has

---

Chart 49-4

HOME CARE CHECKLIST

Management of Ascites

At the completion of education, the patient and/or caregiver will be able to:

- State the impact of ascites and treatment on physiologic functioning, ADLs, IADLs, roles, relationships, and spirituality.
- State the name, dose, side effects, frequency, and schedule for all medications.
- Describe effects, side effects, and monitoring parameters for diuretic therapy.
- Discuss importance of avoiding nonsteroidal anti-inflammatory agents, medications (e.g., cough mixtures) containing alcohol, antibiotics, or antacids containing salt.
- Make appropriate dietary choices consistent with dietary prescription and recommendations.
  - Explain the use of salt substitutes must be approved by primary provider.
- State the importance of weighing self-daily and keeping a daily record of weight.
  - Maintain record of daily weight, and identify daily weight-loss goals.
  - List weight changes (loss or gain) that should be reported to the primary provider.
- Identify rationale for fluid restrictions (if needed) monitoring and keeping a daily record intake and output.

- Maintain a record of daily intake and output.
- Identify changes in output that should be reported to primary provider (e.g., decreasing urine output).
- Identify need to stop all alcohol intake as critical to well-being.
- Explain how to contact Alcoholics Anonymous or alcohol counselors in related organizations if indicated.
- Demonstrate how to inspect and care for skin, alleviate pressure over bony prominences by turning when in bed or chair, and decrease edema by position changes.
- Identify early signs and symptoms of complications (encephalopathy, spontaneous bacterial peritonitis, dehydration, electrolyte abnormalities, azotemia).
- Relate how to reach primary provider with questions or complications.
- State time and date of follow-up medical appointments, therapy, and testing.
- Identify sources of support (e.g., friends, relatives, faith community, support groups, caregiver support).
- Identify the need for health promotion, disease prevention, and screening activities.

ADL, activities of daily living; IADL, independent activities of daily living.

a mortality rate of 10% to 30% depending on the severity of the liver disease and is one of the major causes of death in patients with cirrhosis. Overall mortality associated with acute variceal bleeding ranges from 10% to 40%. The mortality rate is related to failure to control a bleeding episode and the occurrence of early rebleeding (Lee & Moreau, 2015; Satapathy & Sanyal, 2014). Patients surviving the first episode of variceal bleeding are at very high risk for recurrent bleeding (approximately 70%) and death (30% to 50%) (Lee & Moreau, 2015; Satapathy & Sanyal, 2014).

Pathophysiology

Esophageal varices are dilated, tortuous veins that are usually found in the submucosa of the lower esophagus but may develop higher in the esophagus or extend into the stomach. This condition is almost always caused by portal hypertension, which results from obstruction of the portal venous circulation within the damaged liver.

Because of increased obstruction of the portal vein, venous blood from the intestinal tract and spleen seeks an outlet through collateral circulation (new pathways for return of blood to the right atrium). The effect is increased pressure, particularly in the vessels in the submucosal layer of the lower esophagus and upper part of the stomach. These collateral vessels are not very elastic; rather, they are tortuous and fragile, and they bleed easily (see Fig. 49-9). Less common causes of varices are abnormalities of the circulation in the splenic vein or superior vena cava and hepatic venothrombosis.

Bleeding esophageal varices are life threatening and can result in hemorrhagic shock that produces decreased cerebral, hepatic, and renal perfusion. In turn, there is an increased nitrogen load from bleeding into the GI tract and an increased serum ammonia level, increasing the risk of encephalopathy. Usually, the dilated veins cause no symptoms. However, if the portal pressure increases sharply and the mucosa or supporting structures become thin, massive hemorrhaging occurs.

Factors that contribute to hemorrhage are muscular exertion from lifting heavy objects; straining at stool; sneezing, coughing, or vomiting; esophagitis; irritation of vessels by poorly chewed foods or irritating fluids; and reflux of stomach contents (especially alcohol). Salicylates and any medication that erodes the esophageal mucosa or interferes with cell replication also may contribute to bleeding.

Clinical Manifestations

The patient with bleeding esophageal varices may present with hematemesis, melena, or general deterioration in mental or physical status and often has a history of alcohol abuse. Signs and symptoms of shock (cool clammy skin, hypotension, tachycardia) may be present (see Chapter 14).

Assessment and Diagnostic Findings

Endoscopy is used to identify the bleeding site, along with ultrasonography, CT scanning, and angiography. Another diagnostic tool, the endoscopic video capsule, can detect esophageal varices but does not substitute for endoscopy unless this test cannot be performed. Standard endoscopy is superior to video capsule for the diagnosis of esophageal varices (Goldman & Schafer, 2015; Lee & Moreau, 2015). Because varices are present in 50% of patients with cirrhosis, it is recommended that patients who have been diagnosed with cirrhosis undergo screening endoscopy. If no varices are detected on initial endoscopy, the test should be repeated in 2 to 3 years in an effort to identify and treat large varices, which are the ones most likely to bleed. If small varices are identified on initial endoscopy, the test should be repeated in 1 to 2 years (Feldman et al., 2015; Lee & Moreau, 2015).

Endoscopy

Immediate endoscopy (see Chapter 43) is indicated to identify the cause and the site of bleeding; approximately 40% of patients with suspected bleeding from esophageal varices are actually bleeding from another source (gastritis, ulcer) (Lee & Moreau, 2015). Nursing support is essential during this often stressful experience. Careful monitoring can detect early signs of cardiac dysrhythmias, perforation, and hemorrhage.

After the examination, fluids are not given until the patient's gag reflex returns. Lozenges and gargles may be used to relieve throat discomfort if the patient's physical condition and mental status permit. If the patient is actively bleeding, oral intake will not be permitted, and the patient will be prepared for further diagnostic and therapeutic procedures.

Portal Hypertension Measurements

Portal hypertension may be suspected if dilated abdominal veins and hemorrhoids are detected. A palpable enlarged spleen (splenomegaly) and ascites may also be present. Portal venous pressure can be measured directly or indirectly. Indirect measurement of the hepatic vein pressure gradient is the most common procedure. The measurement requires insertion of a catheter with a balloon into the antecubital or femoral vein. The catheter is advanced under fluoroscopy to a hepatic

Physiology/Pathophysiology

Portal hypertension
(caused by resistance to portal flow
and increased portal venous inflow)

↓

Development of pressure gradient of 12 mmHg or greater
between portal vein and inferior vena cava
(portal pressure gradient)

↓

Venous collaterals develop from high portal system pressure to
systemic veins in esophageal plexus, hemorrhoidal plexus, and
retroperitoneal veins

↓

Abnormal varicoid vessels form in any of above locations

↓

Vessels may rupture causing life-threatening hemorrhage

Figure 49-9 • Pathogenesis of bleeding esophageal varices.

vein. Fluid is infused once the catheter is in position to inflate the balloon. A "wedged" pressure (similar to pulmonary artery wedge pressure) is obtained by occluding the blood flow in the blood vessel; pressure in the unoccluded vessel is also measured and the hepatic venous pressure gradient (HVPG) is obtained. An HVPG of over 10 mmHg is indicative of clinically significant portal hypertension (Abraldes, Sarlieve, & Tandon, 2014). Although the values obtained may underestimate portal pressure, this measurement may be taken several times to evaluate the results of therapy (Bloom, Kemp, & Lubel, 2015).

Direct measurement of portal vein pressure can be obtained by several methods. One direct measurement requires insertion of a catheter into the portal vein or one of its branches (Bloom et al., 2015). Endoscopic measurement of pressure within varices is used only in conjunction with endoscopic **sclerotherapy** (see later discussion).

Laboratory Tests

Laboratory studies may include various liver function tests, such as serum aminotransferases, bilirubin, alkaline phosphatase, and serum proteins. Splenoportography, which involves serial or segmental x-rays, is used to detect extensive collateral circulation in esophageal vessels, which would indicate varices. Other tests are hepatoportography and celiac angiography. These are usually performed in the operating room or x-ray department.

 ## Medical Management

Bleeding from esophageal varices is an emergency that can quickly lead to hemorrhagic shock. The patient is critically ill, requiring aggressive medical care and expert nursing care, and is usually transferred to the intensive care unit (ICU) for close monitoring and management. See Chapter 14 for a discussion of care of the patient in shock. The extent of bleeding is evaluated, and vital signs are monitored continuously if hematemesis and melena are present.

Because patients with bleeding esophageal varices have intravascular volume depletion and are subject to electrolyte imbalance, IV fluids, electrolytes, and volume expanders are provided to restore fluid volume and replace electrolytes. Transfusion of blood components also may be required.

Caution must be taken with volume resuscitation so that overhydration does not occur, because this would raise portal pressure and increase bleeding. An indwelling urinary catheter is usually inserted to permit frequent monitoring of urine output.

Although a variety of pharmacologic, endoscopic, and surgical approaches are used to treat bleeding esophageal varices, none is ideal, and most are associated with considerable risk to the patient. Nonsurgical treatment of bleeding esophageal varices is preferable because of the high mortality rate of emergency surgery to control bleeding esophageal varices and because of the poor physical condition that is typical of the patient with severe liver dysfunction.

Pharmacologic Therapy

In suspected variceal bleeding, vasoactive drugs need to be given as soon as possible and before endoscopy (Satapathy & Sanyal, 2014). In an actively bleeding patient, medications are given initially because they can be obtained and given more quickly than other therapies. Octreotide (Sandostatin),

a synthetic analog of the hormone somatostatin, is effective in decreasing bleeding from esophageal varices, and lacks the vasoconstrictive effects of vasopressin. Because of this safety and efficacy profile, octreotide is considered the preferred treatment regimen for immediate control of variceal bleeding. These medications cause selective splanchnic vasoconstriction by inhibiting glucagon release and are used mainly in the management of active hemorrhage. Adverse effects are rare with octreotide but mild hypoglycemia and abdominal cramping can occur (Satapathy & Sanyal, 2014).

Vasopressin (Pitressin) may be the initial mode of therapy in urgent situations because it produces constriction of the splanchnic arterial bed and decreases portal pressure. As described previously, splanchnic circulation comprises the arterial blood supply and venous drainage of the entire GI tract from the distal esophagus to the midrectum, including the liver and spleen. Vasopressin constricts distal esophageal and proximal gastric veins, thus reducing the inflow into the portal system and therefore the portal pressure. Vital signs and the presence or absence of blood in the gastric aspirate indicate the effectiveness of vasopressin. Monitoring of I&O and electrolyte levels is necessary because hyponatremia may develop, and vasopressin may have an antidiuretic effect.

Coronary artery disease is a contraindication to the use of vasopressin because coronary vasoconstriction is a side effect that may precipitate myocardial infarction. The combination of vasopressin with nitroglycerin (given by the IV, sublingual, or transdermal route) has been effective in reducing or preventing the side effects (constriction of coronary vessels and angina) caused by vasopressin alone. Side effects of vasopressin include myocardial and extremity ischemia as well as cardiac dysrhythmias; therefore, vasopressin is used only in urgent situations or when other agents such as octreotide are not available. Vasopressin must be given with close monitoring (Satapathy & Sanyal, 2014).

Beta-blocking agents such as propranolol or nadolol that decrease portal pressure are the most common medications used both to prevent a first bleeding episode in patients with known varices and to prevent rebleeding (James & Liou, 2015; Lee & Moreau, 2015; Liou, 2014; Tripathi & Hayes, 2014). Beta blockers have been shown to effectively reduce the risk of variceal bleeding and its associated mortality (Barrera, Zuniga, & Arrese, 2015). Beta-blockers should not be used in acute variceal hemorrhage, but they are effective prophylaxis against such an episode. Nitrates such as isosorbide (Isordil) lower portal pressure by venodilation and decreased cardiac output and may be used in combination with beta-blockers to reduce the risk of variceal bleeding (Bloom et al., 2015; Lee & Moreau, 2015).

 ## Balloon Tamponade

Although used infrequently today, balloon tamponade therapy may be used to temporarily control hemorrhage and to stabilize a patient with massive bleeding prior to other definitive management (Feldman et al., 2015; Liou, 2014; Satapathy & Sanyal, 2014).

When indicated, balloon tamponade can be successful; however, there are risks. Displacement of the tube and the inflated balloon into the oropharynx can cause life-threatening obstruction of the airway and asphyxiation. This may occur if the patient pulls on the tube because of confusion or discomfort. It may also result from rupture of the gastric balloon, which causes the esophageal balloon to move into the oropharynx. Sudden rupture of the balloon causes airway obstruction and aspiration of gastric contents into the lungs. Therefore, the tube must be tested before insertion to minimize this risk by ensuring that the balloons can attain and maintain inflation. Aspiration of blood and secretions into the lungs is frequently associated with balloon tamponade, especially in the stuporous or comatose patient. Endotracheal intubation before insertion of the tube protects the airway and minimizes the risk of aspiration. Ulceration and necrosis of the nose, the mucosa of the stomach, or the esophagus may occur if the tube is left in place too long, inflated too long, or inflated at too high a pressure. The therapy is used for as short a time as possible to control bleeding while emergency treatment is completed and definitive therapies are instituted (no longer than 12 hours, preferably less) (Liou, 2014; Satapathy & Sanyal, 2014).

> ### ◄ Quality and Safety Nursing Alert
>
> *The patient being treated with balloon tamponade must remain under close observation in the ICU and must be monitored continuously because of the risk of serious complications. Precautions must be taken to ensure that the patient does not pull on or inadvertently displace the tube.*

Nursing measures include frequent mouth and nasal care. For secretions that accumulate in the mouth, tissues should be within easy reach of the patient. Oral suction may be necessary to remove secretions.

Although balloon tamponade stops the bleeding in 90% of patients, bleeding recurs in 60% to 70%, necessitating other treatment modalities, such as endoscopic therapies (see later discussion) (Feldman et al., 2015; Satapathy & Sanyal, 2014). Once the tube is removed, the patient must be assessed frequently because of the high risk of recurrent bleeding.

Endoscopic Sclerotherapy

In endoscopic sclerotherapy (see Fig. 49-10), also referred to as injection sclerotherapy, a sclerosing agent (i.e., sodium morrhuate, ethanolamine oleate, sodium tetradecyl sulfate, or ethanol) is injected through a fiberoptic endoscope into or adjacent to the bleeding esophageal varices to promote thrombosis and eventual sclerosis (Lee & Moreau, 2015; Feldman et al., 2015; Liou, 2014). The process of sclerother-

apy causes inflammation of the involved vein with eventual thrombosis and loss of the lumen of the vessel. The procedure has been used successfully to treat acute GI hemorrhage but is not recommended for prevention of first and subsequent variceal bleeding episodes where **endoscopic variceal ligation (EVL)**, also known as esophageal banding therapy (discussed later), is the first-line treatment (Lee & Moreau 2015).

After treatment for acute hemorrhage, the patient must be observed for bleeding, perforation of the esophagus, aspiration pneumonia, and esophageal stricture. Antacids, histamine-2 (H₂) antagonists such as cimetidine (Tagamet), or proton pump inhibitors such as pantoprazole (Protonix) may be given after the procedure to counteract the chemical effects of the sclerosing agent on the esophagus and the acid reflux associated with the therapy.

Endoscopic Variceal Ligation (Esophageal Banding Therapy)

In variceal banding (see Fig. 49-11), also referred to as EVL, a modified endoscope loaded with an elastic rubber band is passed through an overtube directly onto the varix (or varices) to be banded. After the bleeding varix is suctioned into the tip of the endoscope, the rubber band is slipped over the tissue, causing necrosis, ulceration, and eventual sloughing of the varix.

Variceal banding is comparable to endoscopic sclerotherapy in its effectiveness in controlling acute bleeding. Compared with sclerotherapy, variceal banding also significantly reduces the rebleeding rate, mortality, procedure-related complications, and number of sessions needed to eradicate varices. Esophageal band ligation has replaced sclerotherapy

Figure 49-11 • Endoscopic variceal ligation. **A.** A rubber band–like ligature is slipped over an esophageal varix via an endoscope. **B.** Necrosis results, and the varix eventually sloughs off.

Figure 49-10 • Endoscopic or injection sclerotherapy. Injection of sclerosing agent into esophageal varices through an endoscope promotes thrombosis and eventual sclerosis, thereby obliterating the varices.

as the treatment of choice in the management of esophageal varices. Complications include superficial ulceration and dysphagia, transient chest discomfort, and, rarely, esophageal strictures. Band ligation in combination with pharmacologic therapy may be more effective than monotherapy (i.e., a single mode of therapy) in the treatment of acute hemorrhage. EVL is recommended for patients who have experienced variceal bleeding while receiving beta-blocker therapy and for those who cannot tolerate beta-blocking agents (Lee & Moreau, 2015; Liou, 2014).

Transjugular Intrahepatic Portosystemic Shunt

A TIPS procedure (see Fig. 49-8) is indicated for the treatment of an acute episode of uncontrolled variceal bleeding refractory to pharmacologic or endoscopic therapy. In 10% to 20% of patients for whom urgent band ligation or sclerotherapy and medications are not successful in eradicating bleeding, a TIPS procedure can effectively control acute variceal hemorrhage by rapidly lowering portal pressure. Polytetrafluoroethylene-covered TIPS placement should be considered in high-risk patients with cirrhosis and active bleeding at the time of endoscopy (Lee & Moreau, 2015). Potential complications of TIPS include bleeding, sepsis, heart failure, organ perforation, shunt thrombosis, and progressive liver failure.

Additional Therapies

The use of endoscopically placed tissue adhesives and fibrin glue has been successful in the treatment of gastric and esophageal varices. Coated expandable stents (placed via endoscope) have also been used effectively for the same purpose. These developing technologies require further study to determine their role in the management of bleeding esophageal varices (Lee & Moreau, 2015; Liou, 2014).

Surgical Management

Several surgical procedures have been developed to treat esophageal varices and to minimize rebleeding, but these procedures have significant risk. Procedures that may be used for esophageal varices are direct surgical ligation of varices; splenorenal, mesocaval, and portacaval venous shunts to relieve portal pressure; and esophageal transection with devascularization. The use of these procedures is controversial, and studies regarding their effectiveness and outcomes continue. What is known thus far is that these procedures are very effective in controlling variceal bleeding. They may be considered as second-line management (rescue therapy) in those patients for whom all other treatments have failed, those who are not candidates for liver transplantation, and those who require a bridge to transplantation. There is a high incidence of encephalopathy after the surgical shunting procedures, and morbidity and mortality statistics remain high (Lee & Moreau, 2015). The TIPS procedure has largely replaced the use of surgical decompression shunts and ligation procedures but these interventions may still be used in some cases to manage esophageal varices.

Surgical Bypass Procedures

Surgical decompression (shunt surgery) of the portal circulation may be used with the advent of a variceal bleeding episode. Although effective in eradicating bleeding, survival

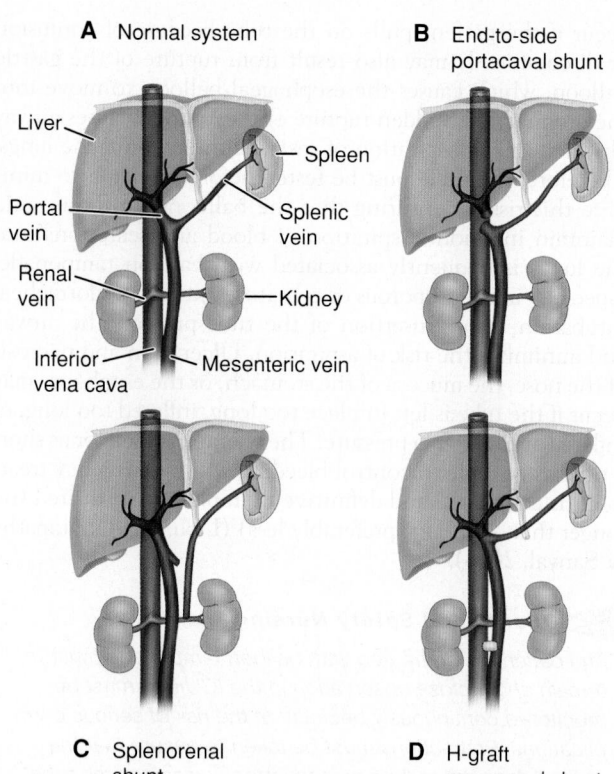

Figure 49-12 • Portosystemic shunts. **A.** Normal portal system. **B–D.** Examples of portal shunts to reduce portal pressure.

statistics and encephalopathy are worse than other preventative measures such as a TIPS procedure when this method is employed for prophylaxis, and shunt surgery for this purpose has largely been abandoned worldwide (Lee & Moreau, 2015; Nusrat et al. 2014).

One of the various surgical shunting procedures (see Fig. 49-12) is the distal splenorenal shunt, which is made between the splenic vein and the left renal vein after splenectomy. A mesocaval shunt is created by anastomosing the superior mesenteric vein to the proximal end of the vena cava or to the side of the vena cava using grafting material. The goal of distal splenorenal and mesocaval shunts is to decrease portal pressure by draining only a portion of venous blood from the portal bed; therefore, they are considered selective shunts. The liver continues to receive some portal flow, and the incidence of encephalopathy may be reduced. Portacaval shunts are considered nonselective shunts because they divert all portal flow to the vena cava via end-to-side or side-to-side approaches.

These procedures are extensive and are not always successful because of secondary thrombosis in the veins used for the shunt and because of complications (e.g., encephalopathy, accelerated liver failure). The effectiveness of these procedures has been studied extensively. All shunt procedures are equally effective in preventing recurrent variceal bleeding but may cause further impairment of liver function and encephalopathy. Partial portacaval shunts with interposition grafts are as effective as other shunts but are associated with a lower rate of encephalopathy (Doherty, 2015, Townsend, Beauchamp, Evers, et al., 2016). The severity of the disease (by a classification such as the Child–Pugh system, discussed later) and the potential for future liver transplantation guide the treatment decision. If the cause of portal hypertension is the rare Budd–Chiari syndrome (which is manifested by noncirrhotic portal hypertension caused by hepatic vein thrombosis) or other venous obstructive disease, a portacaval or a mesoatrial shunt may be performed (see Fig. 49-12). The mesoatrial shunt is required when the infrahepatic vena cava is thrombosed and must be bypassed.

Devascularization and Transection

Devascularization and staple-gun transection procedures to separate the bleeding site from the high-pressure portal system have been used in the emergency management of variceal bleeding. The lower end of the esophagus is reached through a small gastrostomy incision; a staple gun permits anastomosis of the transected ends of the esophagus. Rebleeding is a risk, and the outcomes of these procedures vary among patient populations.

> ### ▶ Quality and Safety Nursing Alert
>
> *The surgical procedures used to treat esophageal varices do not alter the course of the progressive liver disease, and bleeding may recur as new collateral vessels develop. The risk of complications (hypovolemic or hemorrhagic shock, hepatic encephalopathy, electrolyte imbalance, metabolic and respiratory alkalosis, alcohol withdrawal syndrome, and seizures) is high.*

Nursing Management

Nursing assessment includes monitoring the patient's physical condition and evaluating emotional responses and cognitive status. The nurse monitors and records vital signs and

assesses the patient's nutritional and neurologic status. This assessment assists in identifying hepatic encephalopathy (see later discussion).

If complete rest of the esophagus is indicated because of bleeding, parenteral nutrition is initiated. Gastric suction usually is initiated to keep the stomach as empty as possible and to prevent straining and vomiting. The patient often complains of severe thirst, which may be relieved by frequent oral hygiene and moist sponges to the lips. The nurse closely monitors the blood pressure. Vitamin K therapy and multiple blood transfusions often are indicated because of blood loss. A quiet environment and calm reassurance may help to relieve the patient's anxiety and reduce agitation.

Bleeding anywhere in the body is anxiety provoking, resulting in a crisis for the patient and family. If the patient has been a heavy user of alcohol, delirium secondary to alcohol withdrawal can complicate the situation. The nurse provides support and explanations about medical and nursing interventions to prepare both the patient and the family, because these procedures can be difficult to undergo and observe. Close monitoring of the patient helps in detecting and managing complications. Management modalities and nursing care of the patient with bleeding esophageal varices are summarized in Table 49-2.

Hepatic Encephalopathy and Coma

Hepatic encephalopathy, or portosystemic encephalopathy, is a life-threatening complication of liver disease that occurs with profound liver failure. Patients with this condition may have no overt signs of the illness but have abnormalities on neuropsychologic testing (Ellul, Gholkar, & Cross, 2015; Lee & Moreau, 2015; Nusrat et al. 2014). Hepatic encephalopathy is

TABLE 49-2 Select Modalities and Nursing Care for the Patient With Bleeding Esophageal Varices

Treatment Modality[a]	Nursing Interventions
Nonsurgical Modalities	
Pharmacologic agents	Observe response to therapy.
Propranolol (Inderal)/nadolol (Corgard) Vasopressin (Pitressin)	Monitor for side effects: *propranolol* and *nadolol*—decreased pulse pressure, impaired cardiovascular response to hemorrhage; *vasopressin*—angina (nitroglycerin may be prescribed to prevent or treat angina).
Octreotide (Sandostatin)	Support patient during treatment.
Injection sclerotherapy	Observe for aspiration, perforation of the esophagus, and recurrence of bleeding after treatment.
Endoscopic variceal ligation	Observe for recurrence of bleeding, esophageal perforation.
Transjugular intrahepatic portosystemic shunt	Observe for rebleeding and signs of infection.
Balloon tamponade	Explain procedure to patient briefly to obtain cooperation with insertion and maintenance of esophageal/gastric tamponade tube and reduce patient's fear of the procedure.
	Monitor closely to prevent inadvertent removal or displacement of tube, subsequent airway obstruction, and aspiration.
	Provide frequent oral hygiene.
Surgical Modalities	
Portal-systemic shunt	Observe for development of portal-systemic encephalopathy (altered mental status, neurologic dysfunction), hepatic failure, and rebleeding.
	Requires intensive, expert nursing care for prolonged period.
Surgical ligation of varices	Observe for rebleeding.
Esophageal transection and devascularization	Observe for rebleeding.
	Provide postthoracotomy care.

[a]Several modalities may be used concurrently or in sequence.

Adapted from Feldman, M., Friedman, L. S., & Brandt, L. J. (2015). *Sleisinger & Fordtran's gastrointestinal & liver disease* (10th ed.). Philadelphia, PA: Saunders Elsevier.

the neuropsychiatric manifestation of hepatic failure associated with portal hypertension and the shunting of blood from the portal venous system into the systemic circulation (Ellul et al., 2015; Lee & Moreau, 2015). This reversible metabolic form of encephalopathy can improve with recovery of liver function. The onset is often insidious and subtle, and initially the disease is termed *subclinical* or *minimal hepatic encephalopathy*.

Pathophysiology

Despite the frequency with which hepatic encephalopathy occurs, the precise pathophysiology is not fully understood (Ellul et al., 2015). Two major alterations underlie its development in acute and chronic liver disease. First, hepatic insufficiency may result in encephalopathy because of the inability of the liver to detoxify toxic by-products of metabolism. Second, portosystemic shunting, in which collateral vessels develop as a result of portal hypertension, allows elements of the portal blood (laden with potentially toxic substances usually extracted by the liver) to enter the systemic circulation (Ellul et al., 2015; Lee & Moreau, 2015). Ammonia is considered the major etiologic factor in the development of encephalopathy. Ammonia enters the brain and excites peripheral benzodiazepine-type receptors on astrocyte cells, increasing neurosteroid synthesis, and stimulating gamma-aminobutyric acid (GABA) neurotransmission. GABA causes depression of the central nervous system that inhibits neurotransmission and synaptic regulation (Ellul et al., 2015; Lee & Moreau, 2015), producing sleep and behavior patterns associated with hepatic encephalopathy.

Circumstances that increase serum ammonia levels tend to aggravate or precipitate hepatic encephalopathy. The largest source of ammonia is the enzymatic and bacterial digestion of dietary and blood proteins in the GI tract. Ammonia from these sources increases as a result of GI bleeding (i.e., bleeding esophageal varices, chronic GI bleeding), a high-protein diet, bacterial infection, or uremia. The ingestion of ammonium salts also increases the blood ammonia level. In the presence of alkalosis or hypokalemia, increased amounts of ammonia are absorbed from the GI tract and from the renal tubular fluid. Conversely, serum ammonia is decreased by elimination of protein from the diet and by the administration of antibiotics, such as neomycin sulfate (Mycifradin, Neo-Fradin), which reduce the number of intestinal bacteria capable of converting urea to ammonia (Ellul et al., 2015; Lee & Moreau, 2015).

Other factors unrelated to increased serum ammonia levels that can cause hepatic encephalopathy in susceptible patients include excessive diuresis, dehydration, infections, surgery, fever, and some medications (sedatives, tranquilizers, analgesics, and diuretics that cause potassium loss). Additional causes include elevated levels of serum manganese (Ellul et al., 2015; Romero-Gomez, Mantangnese, & Jalan, 2015), as well as changes in the types of circulating amino acids, mercaptans, and levels of dopamine and other neurotransmitters in the central nervous system (Feldman et al., 2015; Romero-Gomez et al., 2015). Mercaptans are toxic metabolites of sulfur-containing compounds that are excreted by the liver under normal conditions. Mercaptans and these other so-called "false" neurotransmitters may be generated from an intestinal source or from metabolism of protein by the liver and, with defective hepatic clearance, may precipitate encephalopathy.

Clinical Manifestations

The earliest symptoms of hepatic encephalopathy include mental status changes and motor disturbances. The patient appears confused and unkempt and has alterations in mood and sleep patterns. The patient tends to sleep during the day and has restlessness and insomnia at night. As hepatic encephalopathy progresses, the patient may become difficult to awaken and completely disoriented with respect to time and place. With further progression, the patient lapses into frank coma and may have seizures.

 Concept Mastery Alert

It is vital for the nurse to understand the four stages of hepatic encephalopathy and common signs and symptoms. These key points, as well as selected nursing diagnoses, are summarized in Table 49-3.

TABLE 49-3 Stages of Hepatic Encephalopathy and Applicable Nursing Diagnoses

Stage	Clinical Symptoms	Clinical Signs and EEG Changes	Selected Potential Nursing Diagnoses
1	Normal level of consciousness with periods of lethargy and euphoria; reversal of day–night sleep patterns	Impaired writing and ability to draw line figures. Normal EEG.	Activity intolerance Self-care deficit Disturbed sleep pattern
2	Increased drowsiness; disorientation; inappropriate behavior; mood swings; agitation	Asterixis; fetor hepaticus. Abnormal EEG with generalized slowing.	Impaired social interaction Ineffective role performance Risk for injury Confusion
3	Stuporous; difficult to rouse; sleeps most of time; marked confusion; incoherent speech	Asterixis; increased deep tendon reflexes; rigidity of extremities. EEG markedly abnormal.	Imbalanced nutrition Impaired mobility Impaired verbal communication
4	Comatose; may not respond to painful stimuli	Absence of asterixis; absence of deep tendon reflexes; flaccidity of extremities. EEG markedly abnormal.	Risk for aspiration Impaired gas exchange Impaired tissue integrity

EEG, electroencephalogram.
[a]Nursing diagnoses are likely to progress; thus, most nursing diagnoses present at earlier stages will occur during later stages as well.
Adapted from information in Feldman, M., Friedman, L. S., & Brandt, L. J. (2015). *Sleisinger & Fordtran's gastrointestinal & liver disease* (10th ed.). Philadelphia, PA: Saunders Elsevier.

Figure 49-13 • Asterixis ("liver flap") may occur in hepatic encephalopathy. The patient is asked to hold the arm out with the hand held upward (dorsiflexed). Within a few seconds, the hand falls forward involuntarily and then quickly returns to the dorsiflexed position.

Asterixis, an involuntary flapping of the hands, may be seen in stage II encephalopathy (see Fig. 49-13). Simple tasks, such as handwriting, become difficult. A handwriting or drawing sample (e.g., star figure), taken daily, may provide graphic evidence of progression or reversal of hepatic encephalopathy. Inability to reproduce a simple figure in two or three dimensions (see Fig. 49-14) is referred to as **constructional apraxia**. In the early stages of hepatic encephalopathy, the deep tendon reflexes are hyperactive; with worsening of the encephalopathy, these reflexes disappear and the extremities may become flaccid.

Occasionally, **fetor hepaticus**, a sweet, slightly fecal odor to the breath that is presumed to be of intestinal origin, may be noticed. The odor has also been described as similar to that of freshly mowed grass, acetone, or old wine. Fetor hepaticus is prevalent with extensive collateral portal circulation in chronic liver disease.

Figure 49-14 • Effects of constructional apraxia. Deterioration of handwriting and inability to draw a simple star figure occurs with progressive hepatic encephalopathy. With permission from Sherlock, S., & Dooley, J. (2002). *Diseases of the liver and biliary system* (11th ed.). Oxford, UK: Blackwell Scientific.

Assessment and Diagnostic Findings

Several diagnostic algorithms and a variety of psychometric tests are used in determining the presence and severity of hepatic encephalopathy. The electroencephalogram shows generalized slowing, an increase in the amplitude of brain waves, and characteristic triphasic waves. The survival rate after a first episode of overt hepatic encephalopathy in patients with cirrhosis is approximately 40% at 1 year. Eligible patients should be referred for liver transplantation after this initial episode (Ellul et al., 2015; Lee & Moreau, 2015; Romero-Gomez et al., 2015).

Medical Management

Medical management focuses on identifying and eliminating the precipitating cause, if possible, initiating ammonia-lowering therapy, minimizing potential medical complications of cirrhosis and depressed consciousness, and reversing the underlying liver disease, if possible. Correction of the possible reasons for the deterioration such as bleeding, electrolyte abnormalities, sedation, or azotemia is essential (Feldman et al., 2015; Lee & Moreau, 2015). Lactulose (Cephulac) is given to reduce serum ammonia levels. It acts by trapping and expelling the ammonia in the feces (Poordad, 2015; Romero-Gomez et al., 2015). Two or three soft stools per day are desirable; this indicates that lactulose is performing as intended.

> ### Quality and Safety Nursing Alert
>
> *The patient receiving lactulose is monitored closely for the development of watery diarrhea stools, because they indicate a medication overdose. Serum ammonia levels are closely monitored as well.*

Possible side effects of lactulose include intestinal bloating and cramps, which usually disappear within a week. To mask the sweet taste, which some patients dislike, it can be diluted with fruit juice. The patient is closely monitored for hypokalemia and dehydration. Other laxatives are not prescribed during lactulose administration because their effects disturb dosage regulation. Lactulose may be given by nasogastric tube or enema for patients who are comatose or for those in whom oral administration is contraindicated or not possible (Poordad, 2015; Romero-Gomez et al., 2015).

Other management strategies include IV administration of glucose to minimize protein breakdown, administration of vitamins to correct deficiencies, and correction of electrolyte imbalances (especially potassium). Antibiotics may also be added to the treatment regimen. Neomycin, metronidazole (Flagyl), and rifaximin (Xifaxan) have been used to reduce levels of ammonia-forming bacteria in the colon. However, no benefit has been shown for long-term treatment with these antibiotics (Poordad, 2015; Romero-Gomez et al., 2015). Additional principles of management of hepatic encephalopathy include the following:

- Neurologic status is assessed frequently.
- Mental status is monitored by keeping a daily record of handwriting and arithmetic performance.
- I&O and body weight are recorded each day.
- Vital signs are measured and recorded every 4 hours.

Chart 49-5	Nutritional Management of Hepatic Encephalopathy

- Minimize the formation and absorption of toxins, principally ammonia, from the intestine.
- Keep daily protein intake between 1.2 and 1.5 g/kg body weight per day.
- Avoid protein restriction if possible, even in those with encephalopathy.
- For patients who are truly protein intolerant, provide additional nitrogen in the form of an amino acid supplement. The use of branched-chain amino acids should be a consideration in patients with cirrhosis. It has improved outcomes in varied populations with the disease.
- Provide small, frequent meals and 3 small snacks per day in addition to a late-night snack before bed.

Adapted from Mueller, C. M. (2012). *The A.S.P.E.N. adult nutrition support core curriculum* (2nd ed.). Silver Spring, MD: American Society for Parenteral and Enteral Nutrition; Fialla, A. D., Israelsen, M., Hamberg, O., et al. (2015). Nutritional therapy in cirrhosis or alcoholic hepatitis: A systematic review and meta-analysis. *Liver International, 35*(9), 2072–2078.

- Potential sites of infection (peritoneum, lungs) are assessed frequently, and abnormal findings are reported promptly.
- Serum ammonia level is monitored daily.
- Dietary protein intake should not be restricted in hepatic encephalopathy as recommended in the past. Protein intake should be maintained at 1.2 to 1.5 g/kg per day (Ellul et al., 2015; Poordad, 2015) (see Chart 49-5). The danger of protein malnutrition far outweighs the risk of worsening hepatic encephalopathy caused by increased protein intake (James & Liou, 2015).
- Enteral feeding is provided for patients whose encephalopathic state persists.
- Reduction in the absorption of ammonia from the GI tract is accomplished by the use of gastric suction, enemas, or oral antibiotics.
- Electrolyte status is monitored and corrected if abnormal.
- Sedatives, tranquilizers, and analgesic medications are discontinued.
- Benzodiazepine antagonists such as flumazenil (Romazicon) may be administered IV to improve encephalopathy, whether or not the patient has previously taken benzodiazepines. This action may have short-term efficacy because patients with hepatic encephalopathy have an increased concentration of benzodiazepine receptors (Mastron, Siveen, Sethi, et al., 2015; Nusrat et al., 2014; Romero-Gomez et al., 2015; Siddiqui & Stravitz, 2014).

 Nursing Management

Table 49-3 presents the stages of hepatic encephalopathy, common signs and symptoms, and potential nursing diagnoses for each stage. The nurse is responsible for maintaining a safe environment to prevent injury, bleeding, and infection. The nurse administers the prescribed treatments and monitors the patient for the numerous potential complications. The potential for respiratory compromise is great given the patient's depressed neurologic status. The nurse encourages deep breathing and position changes to prevent the development of atelectasis, pneumonia, and other respiratory complications. Despite aggressive pulmonary care, patients may develop respiratory compromise. They may require intubation and mechanical ventilation to protect the airway, and they are frequently admitted to the ICU.

The nurse communicates with the patient's family to inform them about the patient's status and supports them by explaining the procedures and treatments that are part of the patient's care. If the patient recovers from hepatic encephalopathy and coma, rehabilitation is likely to be prolonged. Therefore, the patient and family will require assistance to understand the causes of this severe complication and to recognize that it may recur.

Promoting Home, Community-Based and Transitional Care

 ### Educating Patients About Self-Care

If the patient has recovered from hepatic encephalopathy and is to be discharged home, the nurse educates the family about subtle signs of recurrent encephalopathy. The goals for caloric intake and protein intake should be 35 to 40 kcal/kg body weight per day and 1.2 to 1.5 g/kg body weight per day (see Chart 49-5) (Ellul et al., 2015; Poordad, 2015). Protein intake should not be limited too severely, because doing so worsens nutritional status and increases mortality (Ellul et al., 2015; Poordad, 2015). Continued use of lactulose after discharge is not uncommon, and the patient and family should closely monitor its efficacy and side effects. They should also be cautioned that constipation can precipitate encephalopathy and should be prevented through the prescribed use of lactulose, which is crucial in preventing constipation.

Continuing and Transitional Care

Referral for transitional, home, or community-based care is warranted for the patient who returns home after recovery from hepatic encephalopathy. The nurse assesses the patient's physical and mental status and collaborates closely with the primary provider. The home visit provides an opportunity for the nurse to assess the home environment and the ability of the patient and family to monitor signs and symptoms and follow the treatment regimen. The nurse must evaluate the patient's fluid volume status and be alert for changes indicative of hypovolemia due to decreased intake and for decreased urine output associated with hepatorenal syndrome (see later discussion). Monitoring of laboratory values continues to be important, and the nurse must obtain prescriptions to correct abnormalities, especially electrolyte imbalances, which also can worsen encephalopathy.

The safety of the home environment is assessed closely to identify areas of risk for falls and other injuries. Home or transitional care visits are especially important if the patient lives alone because encephalopathy may affect the patient's ability to remember or follow the treatment regimen. The nurse reinforces previous education and reminds the patient and family about the importance of dietary restrictions, close monitoring, and follow-up. In addition, the nurse must observe the patient for subtle behavior changes of worsening hepatic encephalopathy. Patients with all types and stages of hepatic encephalopathy should have periodic neurologic evaluations to determine their cognitive function so that they do not engage in potentially harmful activities. Even subtle neuropsychiatric abnormalities may preclude patients from driving, operating machinery, or participating in other activities that require psychomotor coordination.

Patients and families may need additional support during those times that the patient exhibits mood disturbances and sleep disorders. Patients should be as active as possible during the day and develop a normal sleep–wake pattern. Sedating medications should be avoided because they may precipitate encephalopathy. Patients and families may require assistance in developing plans to cope with changes in mood and mental status changes. This plan should identify support persons to attend to the patient in the home situation if needed. Social workers and case managers may make appropriate referrals for assistance with physical and psychosocial support and care. Referrals to psychologists, psychiatric liaison nurses, case managers, social workers, or therapists may assist family members with coping. Spiritual advisors may also provide another outlet for communication and guidance. If alcohol played a role in the development of the liver disease and encephalopathy, referral to Alcoholics Anonymous or Al-Anon may provide needed support and education.

Other Manifestations of Hepatic Dysfunction

Edema and Bleeding

Many patients with liver dysfunction develop generalized edema caused by hypoalbuminemia due to decreased hepatic production of albumin. The production of blood clotting factors by the liver is also reduced, leading to an increased incidence of bruising, epistaxis, bleeding from wounds, and, as described previously, GI bleeding. Abnormalities in the number and effectiveness of platelets also contribute to the bleeding in liver dysfunction. Congestion of the spleen secondary to portal hypertension causes increased pooling of platelets in the organ (hypersplenism). The resultant thrombocytopenia generally correlates with spleen size. In patients who are alcoholics, suppression of bone marrow by the acute toxic effects of alcohol or folate deficiency may contribute to the thrombocytopenia (Goldman & Schafer, 2015). These factors predispose patients to easy bruising, petechiae formation, and bleeding from a variety of sources such as the GI or genitourinary tract (Goldman & Shafer, 2015).

Vitamin Deficiency

Decreased production of several clotting factors may be partially due to deficient absorption of vitamin K from the GI tract. This probably is caused by the inability of liver cells to use vitamin K to make prothrombin (Hall, 2015). Absorption of the other fat-soluble vitamins (vitamins A, D, and E) as well as dietary fats may also be impaired because of decreased secretion of bile salts into the intestine.

Another group of problems common to patients with severe chronic liver dysfunction results from inadequate intake of sufficient vitamins. These include the following:

- Vitamin A deficiency, resulting in night blindness and eye and skin changes

- Thiamine deficiency, leading to beriberi, polyneuritis, and Wernicke–Korsakoff psychosis
- Riboflavin deficiency, resulting in characteristic skin and mucous membrane lesions
- Pyridoxine deficiency, resulting in skin and mucous membrane lesions and neurologic changes
- Vitamin C deficiency, resulting in the hemorrhagic lesions of scurvy
- Vitamin K deficiency, resulting in hypoprothrombinemia, characterized by spontaneous bleeding and ecchymoses
- Folic acid deficiency, resulting in macrocytic anemia

Because of these potential vitamin deficiencies, the diet of every patient with chronic liver disease (especially if alcohol related) is supplemented with vitamins A, B complex, C, K, and folic acid (Fialla et al., 2015; O'Shea, Dasarathy, McCullough, et al., 2010).

Metabolic Abnormalities

Abnormalities of glucose metabolism also occur; the blood glucose level may be abnormally high shortly after a meal (similar to that when diabetes is present), but hypoglycemia may occur during fasting because of decreased hepatic glycogen reserves and decreased gluconeogenesis. Medications must be used cautiously and in reduced dosages because the ability to metabolize medications is decreased in the patient with liver failure.

Many endocrine abnormalities also occur with liver dysfunction because the liver cannot properly metabolize hormones, including androgens and sex hormones. Failure of the damaged liver to inactivate estrogens normally can cause gynecomastia, amenorrhea, testicular atrophy, loss of pubic hair in the male, menstrual irregularities in the female, and other disturbances of sexual function and sex characteristics.

Pruritus and Other Skin Changes

Patients with liver dysfunction resulting from biliary obstruction commonly develop severe pruritus due to retention of bile salts. Patients may develop vascular (or arterial) spider angiomas on the skin (see Fig. 49-3), usually above the waistline. These are numerous small vessels resembling a spider's legs. They are most often associated with cirrhosis, especially in alcoholic liver disease. Patients may also develop reddened palms ("liver palms" or palmar erythema).

VIRAL HEPATITIS

Viral hepatitis is a systemic, viral infection in which necrosis and inflammation of liver cells produce a characteristic cluster of clinical, biochemical, and cellular changes. To date, five definitive types of viral hepatitis that cause liver disease have been identified: hepatitis A, B, C, D, and E. Hepatitis A and E are similar in mode of transmission (fecal–oral route), whereas hepatitis B, C, and D share many other characteristics.

Hepatitis is easily transmitted and causes high morbidity and prolonged loss of time from school or employment. Acute viral hepatitis affects 0.5% to 1% of people in the United States each year. Hepatitis A virus (HAV) was responsible for 1,781 cases in the United States in

2013, with an overall incidence of 0.6 cases per 100,000 cases. During the same year, the hepatitis B virus (HBV) was the offending agent in a total of 3050 cases of acute viral hepatitis nationwide, with an incidence of 1.0 cases per 100,000 population. The occurrence rate of viral hepatitis C (HCV) in 2013 was 2138 cases, with an incidence rate of 0.7 cases per 100,000 population, which represents an increase of approximately 20% since 2012 (Centers for Disease Control and Prevention [CDC], 2013). The occurrence rate for HAV and HBV has been decreasing steadily since 1990, largely because of the use of hepatitis A and B vaccines, the introduction of universal precautions and blood supply safety measures as well as public health education regarding high-risk behaviors (Dan, Moses-Eisenstein, & Valdiserri, 2015; Goldman & Schafer, 2015). Conversely, the incidence of HCV infection has been on the rise. It is estimated that 60% to 90% of viral hepatitis cases go unreported (CDC, 2013). The occurrence of subclinical cases, failure to recognize mild cases, and misdiagnosis are thought to contribute to the underreporting. Table 49-4 compares the major forms of viral hepatitis.

Hepatitis A Virus

The HAV accounts for 20% to 25% of cases of clinical hepatitis in the United States (CDC, 2013). Hepatitis A, formerly called *infectious hepatitis*, is caused by an RNA virus of the enterovirus family. In the United States, the disease is seen mainly in the adult population. HAV is transmitted primarily through the fecal–oral route, by the ingestion of food or liquids infected with the virus. It is more prevalent in countries with overcrowding and poor sanitation. The virus has

been found in the stool of infected patients before the onset of symptoms and during the first few days of illness.

Typically, a child or a young adult acquires the infection at school through poor hygiene, hand-to-mouth contact, or other close contact. The virus is carried home, where haphazard sanitary habits spread it through the family. An infected food handler can spread the disease, and people can contract it by consuming water or shellfish from sewage-contaminated waters. Outbreaks have occurred in day care centers and institutions as a result of poor hygiene among people with developmental disabilities. Hepatitis A can be transmitted during sexual activity; this is more likely with oral–anal contact or anal intercourse and with multiple sex partners (Dan et al., 2015; Goldman & Schafer, 2015). Hepatitis A is not transmitted by blood transfusions.

The incubation period is estimated to be between 2 and 6 weeks, with a mean of approximately 4 weeks (CDC, 2013). The illness may be prolonged, lasting 4 to 8 weeks. It usually lasts longer and is more severe in those older than 40 years. Most patients recover from hepatitis A; it rarely progresses to acute liver necrosis or **fulminant hepatic failure** resulting in cirrhosis of the liver or death. The mortality rate of hepatitis A is approximately 0.5% for those younger than 40 years and 1% to 2% for older adults. In patients with underlying chronic liver disease, morbidity and mortality are increased in the presence of an acute hepatitis A infection. No carrier state exists, and no chronic hepatitis is associated with the HAV. The virus is present only briefly in the serum; by the time jaundice occurs, the patient is likely to be noninfectious. Although hepatitis A confers immunity against itself, the person may contract other forms of hepatitis.

TABLE 49-4 Comparison of Major Forms of Viral Hepatitis

	Hepatitis A	Hepatitis B	Hepatitis C	Hepatitis D	Hepatitis E
Previous names	Infectious hepatitis	Serum hepatitis	Non-A, non-B hepatitis		
Epidemiology					
Cause	Hepatitis A virus (HAV)	Hepatitis B virus (HBV)	Hepatitis C virus (HCV)	Hepatitis D virus (HDV)	Hepatitis E virus (HEV)
Immunity	*Average:* 30 days Homologous	*Average:* 70–80 days Homologous	*Average:* 50 days Second attack may indicate weak immunity or infection with another agent.	*Average:* 35 days Homologous	*Average:* 31 days Unknown
Nature of Illness					
Signs and symptoms	May occur with or without symptoms; flu-like illness *Preicteric phase:* Headache, malaise, fatigue, anorexia, fever *Icteric phase:* Dark urine, jaundice of sclera and skin, tender liver	May occur without symptoms May develop arthralgias, rash	Similar to HBV; less severe and anicteric	Similar to HBV	Similar to HAV; very severe in pregnant women
Outcome	Usually mild with recovery. No carrier state or increased risk of chronic hepatitis, cirrhosis, or hepatic cancer.	May be severe. Carrier state possible. Increased risk of chronic hepatitis, cirrhosis, and hepatic cancer.	Frequent occurrence of chronic carrier state and chronic liver disease. Increased risk of hepatic cancer.	Similar to HBV but greater likelihood of carrier state, chronic active hepatitis, and cirrhosis	Similar to HAV except very severe in pregnant women

Adapted from Kumar, V., Abbas, A. K., Fausto, N., et al. (2014). *Robbins and Cotran pathologic basis of disease* (9th ed.). Philadelphia, PA: Saunders Elsevier.

Clinical Manifestations

Many patients are anicteric (without jaundice) and symptomless. When symptoms appear, they resemble those of a mild, flu-like upper respiratory tract infection, with low-grade fever. Anorexia, an early symptom, is often severe. It is thought to result from release of a toxin by the damaged liver or from failure of the damaged liver cells to detoxify an abnormal product. Later, jaundice and dark urine may become apparent. Indigestion is present in varying degrees, marked by vague epigastric distress, nausea, heartburn, and flatulence. The patient may also develop a strong aversion to the taste of cigarettes or the presence of cigarette smoke and other strong odors (Papadakis & McPhee, 2016). These symptoms tend to clear as soon as the jaundice reaches its peak, perhaps 10 days after its initial appearance. Symptoms may be mild in children; in adults, they may be more severe and the course of the disease prolonged.

Assessment and Diagnostic Findings

The liver and spleen are often moderately enlarged for a few days after onset; other than jaundice, there are few other physical signs. An HAV antigen may be found in the stool 7 to 10 days before illness and for 2 to 3 weeks after symptoms appear. HAV antibodies are detectable in the serum, although usually not until symptoms appear. Analysis of subclasses of immunoglobulins can help determine whether the antibody represents acute or past infection.

Prevention

A number of strategies exist to prevent transmission of HAV. Patients and their families are encouraged to follow general precautions that can prevent transmission of the virus. Scrupulous hand hygiene, safe water supplies, and proper control of sewage disposal are just a few of these prevention strategies.

Effective (95% to 100% after two to three doses) and safe HAV vaccines include Havrix and Vaqta (Mandell, Bennett, & Dolin, 2014). It is recommended that the two-dose vaccine be given to adults 18 years of age or older, with the second dose given 6 to 12 months after the first. Protection against HAV develops within several weeks after the first dose of the vaccine. Children and adolescents 1 to 18 years of age receive three doses; the second dose is given 1 month after the first, and the third dose is given 6 to 12 months later. HAV routine immunization of young children has proved to be effective in reducing disease incidence and maintaining very low incidence levels among vaccine recipients and across all age groups in many settings (Goldman & Schafer, 2015). As a result of its effectiveness in decreasing HAV, the hepatitis A vaccination recommendations have been expanded to include all children at 1 year of age. Hepatitis A vaccine is also recommended for people traveling to locations where sanitation and hygiene are unsatisfactory. Vaccination is also recommended for those from high-risk groups, such as men who have sex with men, people who use IV or injection drugs, staff of day care centers, health care personnel and those who work with the virus in research or animal care settings (Dan et al., 2015; Mandell et al., 2014). The vaccine has also been used to interrupt community-wide outbreaks. A combined HAV and HBV vaccine (Twinrix) is available for vaccination of people 18 years of age or older with indications for both HAV and HBV vaccination. Vaccination consists of three doses, given on the same schedule as that used for single-antigen HBV vaccine.

For people who have not been previously vaccinated, HAV can be prevented by intramuscular administration of globulin during the incubation period, if given within 2 weeks of exposure. This bolsters the person's antibody production and provides 6 to 8 weeks of passive immunity. Immune globulin may suppress overt symptoms of the disease; the resulting subclinical case of HAV would produce immunity to subsequent episodes of the virus.

Immune globulin is also recommended for household members and sexual contacts of people with HAV. Susceptible people in the same household as the patient are usually also infected by the time the diagnosis is made and should receive immune globulin. Institutional contacts of patients with HAV should also receive post-exposure prophylaxis with immune globulin. Prophylaxis is not necessary for casual contacts of an infected person, such as classmates, coworkers, or hospital employees (Mandell et al., 2014). Although rare, systemic reactions to immune globulin do occur. Caution is required when anyone who has previously had angioedema, hives, or other allergic reactions is treated with any human immune globulin. Epinephrine should be available in case of systemic, anaphylactic reaction.

Pre-exposure prophylaxis is recommended for those traveling to developing countries or settings with poor or uncertain sanitation conditions who do not have sufficient time to acquire protection by administration of hepatitis A vaccine (Mandell et al., 2014). Prevention strategies for HAV are outlined in Chart 49-6.

Medical Management

Bed rest during the acute stage and a nutritious diet are important aspects of treatment. During the period of anorexia, the patient should receive frequent small feedings, supplemented if necessary by IV fluids with glucose. Because the patient often has an aversion to food, gentle persistence, and creativity may be required to stimulate appetite. Optimal food and fluid levels are necessary to counteract weight loss and to speed recovery. Even before the icteric phase, however, many patients recover their appetites (see Chart 49-7).

The patient's sense of well-being and laboratory test results are generally appropriate guides to bed rest and restriction of physical activity. Gradual but progressive ambulation hastens recovery, provided the patient rests after activity and does not participate in activities to the point of fatigue (Wu, Wu, Lien, et al., 2012).

Nursing Management

Management usually occurs in the home unless symptoms are severe. Therefore, the nurse assists the patient and family in coping with the temporary disability and fatigue that are common with HAV and educates them to seek additional health care if the symptoms persist or worsen. The patient and family also need specific guidelines about diet, rest, follow-up blood work, and the importance of avoiding alcohol, as well as sanitation and hygiene measures (particularly hand hygiene) to prevent spread of the disease to other family members.

Specific education for patients and families about reducing the risk of contracting HAV includes good personal hygiene,

Chart 49-6 HEALTH PROMOTION
Prevention of Hepatitis

Hepatitis A

- Educate patients regarding safe practices for preparing and dispensing food.
- Encourage conscientious individual hygiene.
- Encourage proper community and home sanitation.
- Facilitate mandatory reporting of viral hepatitis to local health departments.
- Promote community health education programs.
- Promote vaccination to interrupt community-wide outbreaks.
- Recommend pre-exposure vaccination for all children 12–23 months of age. Continue existing immunization programs for children 1–18 years of age.
- Recommend vaccination for travelers to developing countries, illegal drug users (injection and noninjection drug users), men who have sex with men, people with chronic liver disease, people who work with HAV-infected animals or work with HAV in research facilities and recipients (e.g., hemophiliacs) of pooled plasma products for clotting factor disorders.
- Support effective health supervision of schools, dormitories, extended care facilities, barracks, and camps.

Hepatitis B

- Advise avoidance of high-risk behaviors.
- Avoid multidose vials in patient care settings.

- Monitor cleaning, disinfection, and sterilization of reusable devices in patient care settings.
- Recommend vaccination for international travelers to regions with high or intermediate levels of endemic hepatitis B virus infection and for persons with chronic liver disease or with human immune deficiency virus infection.
- Recommend vaccination for persons at risk for infection by sexual exposure, by percutaneous or mucosal exposure to blood.
- Recommend vaccination of all infants in the United States regardless of the mother's hepatitis B.
- Use barrier precautions in situations of contact with blood or body fluids.
- Use needleless IV and injection systems in health care.
- Use standard precautions in clinical care.

Hepatitis C

- Advise avoidance of high-risk behaviors such as IV drug use.
- Avoid multidose vials in patient care settings.
- Monitor cleaning, disinfection, and sterilization of reusable devices in patient care settings.
- Use barrier precautions in situations of contact with blood or body fluids.
- Use needleless IV and injection systems in health care.
- Use standard precautions in clinical care.

Adapted from Ferri, F. F. (Ed.). (2014). *Practical guide to the care of the medical patient* (9th ed.). Philadelphia, PA: Mosby Elsevier.

---

stressing careful hand hygiene (after bowel movements and before eating) and environmental sanitation (safe food and water supply, effective sewage disposal).

Hepatitis B Virus

Unlike HAV, the HBV is transmitted primarily through blood (percutaneous and permucosal routes). HBV can be found in blood, saliva, semen, and vaginal secretions and can be transmitted through mucous membranes and breaks in the skin.

HBV is also transferred from carrier mothers to their infants, especially in areas with a high incidence (e.g., Southeast Asia). The infection usually is not transmitted via the umbilical vein but from the mother at the time of birth and during close contact afterward.

HBV has a long incubation period. It replicates in the liver and remains in the serum for relatively long periods, allowing transmission of the virus. Risk factors for HBV infection are summarized in Chart 49-8. Screening of blood

Chart 49-7 Dietary Management of Hepatitis

- Advise patient to avoid substances (medications, herbs, illicit drugs, and toxins) that may affect liver function, such as St. John wort in patients taking hepatitis C virus protease inhibitors.
- Be aware that that enteral feedings may be necessary if anorexia, nausea, and vomiting persist.
- Carefully monitor fluid balance.
- Instruct patient to abstain from alcohol during acute illness and for at least 6 months after recovery.
- Provide intake of 25–30 kcal/day.
- Provide protein intake of 1.2–1.5 g/kg/day.
- Recommend small, frequent meals; minimize periods without food intake.

Adapted from Mueller, C. M. (2012). *The A.S.P.E.N. adult nutrition support core curriculum* (2nd ed.). Silver Spring, MD: American Society for Parenteral and Enteral Nutrition; Fialla, A.D., Israelsen, M., Hamberg, et al. (2015). Nutritional therapy in cirrhosis or alcoholic hepatitis: A systematic review and meta-analysis. *Liver International, 35*(9), 2072–2078.

Chart 49-8 RISK FACTORS
Hepatitis B

- Close contact with carrier of hepatitis B virus
- Frequent exposure to blood, blood products, or other body fluids
- Health care workers: hemodialysis staff, oncology and chemotherapy nurses, personnel at risk for needlesticks, operating room staff, respiratory therapists, surgeons, dentists
- Hemodialysis
- IV/injection drug use
- Male homosexual and bisexual activity
- Mother-to-child transmission
- Multiple sexual partners
- Receipt of blood or blood products (e.g., clotting factor concentrate)
- Recent history of sexually transmitted infection
- Tattooing
- Travel to or residence in area with uncertain sanitary conditions

Adapted from Bope, E. T., & Kellerman, R. D. (Eds.). (2015). *Conn's current therapy*. Philadelphia, PA: Saunders.

donors has greatly reduced the occurrence of HBV after blood transfusion.

Most people (more than 90%) who contract HBV infection develop antibodies and recover spontaneously in 6 months. The mortality rate from acute HBV has been reported to be as high as 1%. Another 10% of patients who have HBV progress to a carrier state or develop chronic hepatitis with persistent HBV infection and hepatocellular injury and inflammation. It remains a major worldwide cause of cirrhosis and hepatocellular carcinoma (HCC) with higher mortality rates (Dan et al., 2015; Papadakis & McPhee, 2016). In fact, approximately 15% of those who develop chronic hepatitis B during adulthood die of cirrhosis or liver cancer. Mortality rates are even higher (25%) for those whose chronic infection occurs during childhood (McMahon, 2014). An estimated 730,000 adult residents of the United States are afflicted with chronic hepatitis B infection; however, there has been a small but significant decrease in the prevalence among U.S.-born adults who are 20 to 49 years of age (Dan et al., 2015; McMahon, 2014).

 ### Gerontologic Considerations

The immune system is altered in the aged. A less responsive immune system may be responsible for the increased incidence and severity of HBV among older adults and the increased incidence of liver abscesses secondary to decreased phagocytosis by the Kupffer cells. The older patient with HBV has a serious risk of severe liver cell necrosis or fulminant hepatic failure, particularly if other illnesses are present. With the advent of an HBV vaccine as the standard for prevention, the incidence of hepatic diseases may decrease in the future.

Clinical Manifestations

Clinically, HBV closely resembles HAV, but the incubation period is much longer (1 to 6 months). Signs and symptoms of HBV may be insidious and variable. Fever and respiratory symptoms are rare; some patients have arthralgias and rashes. The patient may have loss of appetite, dyspepsia, abdominal pain, generalized aching, malaise, and weakness. Jaundice may or may not be evident. If jaundice occurs, light-colored stools and dark urine accompany it. The liver may be tender and enlarged to 12 to 14 cm vertically. The spleen is enlarged and palpable in a few patients; the posterior cervical lymph nodes may also be enlarged. Subclinical episodes also occur frequently.

Assessment and Diagnostic Findings

HBV is a deoxyribonucleic acid (DNA) virus composed of the following antigenic particles:

- HBcAg—hepatitis B core antigen (antigenic material in an inner core)
- HBsAg—hepatitis B surface antigen (antigenic material on the viral surface, a marker of active replication and infection)
- HBeAg—an independent protein circulating in the blood
- HBxAg—gene product of X gene of HBV DNA

Each antigen elicits its specific antibody and is a marker for different stages of the disease process:

- anti-HBc—antibody to core antigen of HBV; persists during the acute phase of illness; may indicate continuing HBV in the liver
- anti-HBs—antibody to surface determinants on HBV; detected during late convalescence; usually indicates recovery and development of immunity
- anti-HBe—antibody to hepatitis B e-antigen; usually signifies reduced infectivity
- anti-HBxAg—antibody to the hepatitis B x-antigen; may indicate ongoing replication of HBV

HBsAg appears in the circulation in 80% to 90% of infected patients 1 to 10 weeks after exposure to HBV and 2 to 8 weeks before the onset of symptoms or an increase in transferase levels. Patients with HBsAg that persists for 6 months or longer after acute infection are considered to be HBsAg carriers (McMahon, 2014). HBeAg is the next antigen of HBV to appear in the serum. It usually appears within 1 week of the appearance of HBsAg but before changes in aminotransferase levels; it disappears from the serum within 2 weeks. HBV DNA, detected by polymerase chain reaction testing, appears in the serum at about the same time as HBeAg. HBcAg is not always detected in the serum in HBV infection.

In the United States, the number of cases of chronic HBV is estimated to be 0.8 to 1.4 million persons. However, an accurate estimate is difficult to obtain because there is no national chronic-hepatitis surveillance program (Cameron, 2015). In 2013, males who died with HBV had a mortality rate that was nearly three times the mortality rate of females who died with HBV (0.8 deaths/100,000 population compared to 0.3 deaths/100,000 population). From 2009 to 2013, HBV-related mortality remained relatively stable for males and females (CDC, 2013).

Prevention

Prevention of hepatitis B transmission requires a multifaceted approach, including public health interventions and education as well as programs to foster immunization against this virulent virus in an effort to reduce the disease burden.

Preventing Transmission

Continued screening of blood donors for the presence of hepatitis B antigen (HBAg) further decreases the risk of transmission by blood transfusion. The use of disposable syringes, needles, and lancets and the introduction of needleless IV administration systems have reduced the risk of spreading this infection from one patient to another or to health care personnel during the collection of blood samples or the administration of parenteral therapy. In the clinical laboratory and the hemodialysis unit, work areas are disinfected daily. Gloves are worn when handling all blood and body fluids, as well as HBAg–positive specimens, or when there is potential exposure to blood (e.g., blood drawing) or to patients' secretions. Eating is prohibited in the laboratory and in other areas exposed to secretions, blood, or blood products. Patient education regarding the nature of the disease, its infectiousness, and prognosis is a critical factor in preventing transmission and protecting contacts (see Chart 49-6).

Active Immunization: HBV

Active immunization is recommended for people who are at high risk for HBV (e.g., health care personnel, patients undergoing hemodialysis). In addition, people with HCV and other chronic liver diseases should receive the vaccine. A yeast-recombinant hepatitis B vaccine (Recombivax HB) is used to provide active immunity and has shown rates of protection greater than 90% in healthy people (Chan, Wong, Qin, et al., 2016; Dan et al., 2015; Mandell et al., 2014). Although antibody levels may become low or undetectable, immunologic memory may remain intact for at least 5 to 10 years. Measurable levels of antibodies may not be essential for protection. In general, in those with normal immune systems, booster doses are not required, and no data support the use of booster doses of hepatitis B vaccine among immunocompetent people who have responded to the vaccination series. However, booster doses are recommended for people who are immunocompromised (Chan et al., 2016; Mandell et al., 2014). Additional information is required to determine if booster injections are needed for adults 15 years or more after initial vaccination as well as those at high risk for HBV infection.

A hepatitis B vaccine prepared from plasma of humans chronically infected with HBV is used only rarely in patients who are immunodeficient or allergic to recombinant yeast-derived vaccines.

Both forms of the hepatitis B vaccine are given intramuscularly in three doses; the second and third doses are given 1 and 6 months, respectively, after the first dose. The third dose is very important in producing prolonged immunity. Hepatitis B vaccination should be given to adults in the deltoid muscle. Antibody response may be measured by anti-HBs levels 1 to 3 months after completion of the basic course of vaccine, but this testing is not routine and is not currently recommended. People who do not respond may benefit from one to three additional doses (Mandell et al., 2014).

People at high risk, including nurses and other health care personnel exposed to blood or blood products, should receive active immunization. Health care workers who have had frequent contact with blood are screened for anti-HBs to determine whether immunity is already present from previous exposure. The vaccine produces active immunity to HBV in 90% to 95% of healthy people (Dan et al., 2015). It does not provide protection to those already exposed to HBV nor does it provide protection against other types of viral hepatitis.

Because HBV infection is frequently transmitted sexually, hepatitis B vaccination is recommended for all people who are unvaccinated and are being evaluated for a sexually transmitted infection (STI). It is also recommended for those with a history of an STI, people with multiple sex partners, people who have sex with IV or injection drug users, and sexually active men who have sex with other men (Dan et al., 2015; Feldman et al., 2015; Mandell et al., 2014).

Universal childhood vaccination for hepatitis B prevention has been instituted in the United States, and universal vaccination of all infants is encouraged. Catch-up vaccination is recommended for all children and prepubertal adolescents up to the age of 19 years who have not been previously immunized (Feldman et al., 2015). Development of chronic carrier states has not been reported in adult responders to the vaccine.

Passive Immunity: Hepatitis B Immune Globulin

Hepatitis B immune globulin (HBIG) provides passive immunity to HBV and is indicated for people exposed to HBV who have never had hepatitis B and have never received hepatitis B vaccine. Specific indications for postexposure vaccine with HBIG include (1) inadvertent exposure to HBAg-positive blood through percutaneous (needlestick) or transmucosal (splashes in contact with mucous membrane) routes, (2) sexual contact with people positive for HBAg, and (3) perinatal exposure (infants born to HBV-infected mothers should receive HBIG within 12 hours after delivery). HBIG is prepared from plasma selected for high titers of anti-HBs. Prompt immunization with HBIG (within hours to a few days after exposure to hepatitis B) increases the likelihood of protection. Both active and passive immunization are recommended for people who have been exposed to HBV through sexual contact or through the percutaneous or transmucosal routes. If HBIG and hepatitis B vaccine are given at the same time, separate sites and separate syringes should be used. HBIG is considered very safe, and there has been no evidence that infectious diseases have been transmitted due its administration (Chan et al., 2016).

Medical Management

Goals are to minimize infectivity and liver inflammation and decrease symptoms. Of all the agents that have been used to treat chronic type B viral hepatitis, alpha-interferon is the single modality of therapy that offers the most promise. A regimen of 5 million U daily or 10 million U three times weekly for 16 to 24 weeks results in remission of disease in approximately one third of patients (Chan et al., 2016; Ferri, 2014; Ghaziani, Sendi, Shahraz, et al., 2014). A prolonged course of treatment may also have additional benefits and is under study. Interferon must be given by injection and has significant side effects, including fever, chills, anorexia, nausea, myalgias, and fatigue. Delayed side effects are more serious and may necessitate dosage reduction or discontinuation. These include bone marrow suppression, thyroid dysfunction, alopecia, and bacterial infections. Several recombinant forms of alpha-interferon are also available, including the pegylated form (peginterferon alfa-2a [Pegasys]), with once-weekly dosing. Pegylated interferon, also referred to as peginterferon, has largely replaced standard interferon due to its dosing schedule (Ferri, 2014).

Two antiviral agents, entecavir (ETV) and tenofovir (TDF), which are oral nucleoside analogs, have been approved for use in chronic hepatitis B in the United States. They are the currently recommended agents for patients with HBV-related decompensated cirrhosis. Either of these agents may be indicated for use in combination with peginterferon (Cholongitas, Tziomalos, & Pipili, 2015; Govan, Wu, Xin, et al., 2015). Studies have revealed improved seroconversion rates and loss of detectable virus, improved liver function, and reduced progression to cirrhosis with ETV and TDF. These agents can also be used for patients with decompensated cirrhosis who are awaiting liver transplantation (Chan et al., 2016; Cholongitas et al., 2015; Ferri, 2014). Patients with decompensated cirrhosis have such severely damaged liver parenchyma that normal liver function severely deteriorates, resulting in life-threatening ascites, encephalopathy, or variceal hemorrhage (Chan et al., 2016; Feldman et al., 2015).

Bed rest may be recommended until the symptoms of hepatitis have subsided. Activities are restricted until the hepatic enlargement and levels of serum bilirubin and liver enzymes have decreased. Gradually, increased activity is then allowed.

Adequate nutrition should be maintained. Proteins are not restricted. Protein intake should be 1.2 to 1.5 g/kg/day. Measures to control the dyspeptic symptoms and general malaise include the use of antacids and antiemetic agents, but all medications should be avoided if vomiting occurs. If vomiting persists, the patient may require hospitalization and fluid therapy. Because of the mode of transmission, the patient is evaluated for other bloodborne diseases (e.g., human immune deficiency virus infection).

Nursing Management

Convalescence may be prolonged, with complete symptomatic recovery sometimes requiring 3 to 4 months or longer (Papadakis & McPhee, 2016). During this stage, gradual resumption of physical activity is encouraged after the jaundice has resolved.

The nurse identifies psychosocial issues and concerns, particularly the effects of separation from family and friends if the patient is hospitalized during the acute and infective stages. Even if not hospitalized, the patient will be unable to work and must avoid sexual contact. Planning is required to minimize social isolation. Planning that includes the family helps to reduce their fears and anxieties about the spread of the disease.

Promoting Home, Community-Based and Transitional Care

 Educating Patients About Self-Care

Because of the prolonged period of convalescence, the patient and family must be prepared for care in the home. Provision for adequate rest and nutrition must be ensured. The nurse educates family members and friends who have had intimate contact with the patient about the risks of contracting HBV and makes arrangements for them to receive hepatitis B vaccine or HBIG as prescribed. Those at risk must be made aware of the early signs of HBV and of ways to reduce risk by avoiding all modes of transmission. Patients with all forms of hepatitis should avoid drinking alcohol (Chan et al., 2016; Dan et al., 2015; Feldman et al., 2015).

Continuing and Transitional Care

Follow-up visits by a transitional or home care nurse may be needed to assess the patient's progress and answer family members' questions about disease transmission. During a home visit, the nurse assesses the patient's physical and psychological status and confirms that the patient and family understand the importance of adequate rest and nutrition. The nurse also reinforces previous education. Because of the risk of transmission through sexual intercourse, strategies to prevent exchange of body fluids are recommended, such as abstinence or the use of condoms. The nurse emphasizes the importance of keeping follow-up appointments and participating in other health promotion activities and recommended health screenings.

Hepatitis C Virus

Blood transfusions and sexual contact once accounted for most cases of HCV in the United States, but other parenteral means, such as sharing of contaminated needles by those who use IV or injection drugs and unintentional needlesticks and other injuries in health care workers now account for a significant number of cases. Approximately 35,000 new cases of HCV are reported in the United States each year. About 4 million people (1.8% of the U.S. population) have been infected with the HCV, making it the most common chronic bloodborne infection nationally, though many of those infected are unaware of the disease (Dan et al., 2015). Between the years 2010 and 2013, there was an approximate 2.5-fold increase in the number of reported acute HCV cases from 850 to 2138 cases (CDC, 2013). The highest prevalence of HCV is in adults 40 to 59 years of age; in this age group, its prevalence is highest among African Americans. There are 10,000 to 12,000 deaths each year in the United States due to HCV, and it has been suggested that deaths from this cause are underestimated. HCV is the underlying cause of about one third of cases of HCC, and it is the most common reason for liver transplantation (Rude & Crippen, 2015; Salgia & Singal, 2014).

People who are at particular risk for HCV include those who use IV or injection drugs, people who are sexually active with multiple partners, patients receiving frequent transfusions, those who require large volumes of blood, and health care personnel (see Chart 49-9). The incubation period is variable and may range from 15 to 160 days. The clinical course of acute HCV is similar to that of HBV; symptoms are usually mild or absent. However, a chronic carrier state occurs frequently, and there is an increased risk of chronic liver disease, including cirrhosis or liver cancer, after HCV. It is for this reason that those in high- and moderate-risk groups as well as those known to have high prevalence rates (e.g., those born in certain countries or regions) be screened for HCV as well as for HBV (LeFevre, 2014; Moyer, 2013). Small amounts of alcohol taken regularly appear to cause progression of the disease. Therefore, alcohol and medications that may affect the liver should be avoided.

There is no benefit from rest, diet, or vitamin supplements. A combination of two antiviral agents, peginterferon and ribavirin (Rebetol), was effective in producing improvement in patients with hepatitis C and in treating relapses (Papadakis & McPhee, 2016). In the United States, this combination therapy was the standard treatment beginning in 2001. However, this treatment regimen is no longer employed in the United States for most genotypes of HCV since new antivirals agents are now recommended. Simeprevir (Olysio) plus sofosbuvir

---

Chart 49-9 ⚠️ **RISK FACTORS**
Hepatitis C

- Children born to women infected with hepatitis C virus
- Health care and public safety workers after needlestick injuries or mucosal exposure to blood
- Multiple contacts with a hepatitis C virus–infected person
- Multiple sex partners, history of sexually transmitted infection, unprotected sex
- Past/current illicit IV/injection drug use
- Recipient of blood products or organ transplant before 1992 or clotting factor concentrates before 1987

Adapted from Kumar, V., Abbas, A.K., Fausto, N., et al. (2014). *Robbins and Cotran pathologic basis of disease* (9th ed.). Philadelphia, PA: Saunders Elsevier.

(Sovaldi), ledipasvir-sofosbuvir (Harvoni) and ombitasvir-paritaprevir-ritonavir packaged with dasabuvir (Viekira Pak) have fewer side effects, shorter treatment durations and higher cure rates than the previously recommended antiviral agents (Chan et al., 2016; Dan et al., 2015). Peginterferon (Pegasys) and ribavirin are now used only for genotype 5 HCV and in countries which have not approved the newest antiviral drugs (American Association for the Study of Liver Diseases [AASLD], 2014; Dan et al., 2015). There are HCV treatments in development that are expected to be more effective in curing the disease and better tolerated with fewer adverse effects and contraindications (Dan et al., 2015). As a result of the rapidly changing landscape for treatment of viral infections, it is important to monitor related websites for the most up-to-date recommendations (AASLD, 2014).

Screening of blood has reduced the incidence of HCV associated with blood transfusion, and public health programs are helping to reduce the number of cases associated with shared needles in IV or injection drug use (see Chart 49-6).

Hepatitis D Virus

Hepatitis D virus (delta agent) infection occurs in some cases of hepatitis B. Because the virus requires HBsAg for its replication, only people with hepatitis B are at risk for hepatitis D. Anti-delta antibodies in the presence of HBAg on testing confirm the diagnosis. Hepatitis D is common among those who use IV or injection drugs, patients undergoing hemodialysis, and recipients of multiple blood transfusions. Sexual contact with those who have hepatitis B is considered to be an important mode of transmission of hepatitis B and D. The incubation period varies between 30 and 150 days (Feldman et al., 2015).

The symptoms of hepatitis D are similar to those of hepatitis B, except that patients are more likely to develop fulminant hepatic failure and to progress to chronic active hepatitis and cirrhosis. Treatment is similar to that of other forms of hepatitis. Currently, interferon alfa is the only licensed drug available in the treatment for HDV infection. The rate of recurrence is high, and the efficacy of interferon is related to the dose and duration of treatment. High-dose, long-duration therapy for at least a year is recommended (Greenberger, Blumberg, & Burakoff, 2015).

Hepatitis E Virus

It is believed that HEV is transmitted by the fecal–oral route, principally through contaminated water in areas with poor sanitation. The incubation period is variable, estimated to range between 15 and 65 days. In general, hepatitis E resembles hepatitis A. It has a self-limited course with an abrupt onset. Jaundice is almost always present. Chronic forms do not develop.

Avoiding contact with the virus through good hygiene, including handwashing, is the major method of prevention of hepatitis E. The effectiveness of immune globulin in protecting against HEV is uncertain.

Hepatitis G Virus and GB Virus-C

It has long been believed that there is another non-A–E agent causing hepatitis in humans. The incubation period for posttransfusion hepatitis is 14 to 145 days—too long for hepatitis B or C. In the United States, about 5% of chronic liver disease remains cryptogenic (i.e., does not appear to be autoimmune or viral in origin), and 50% of these patients have received blood transfusions before developing disease. Therefore, another form of hepatitis, referred to as hepatitis G virus (HGV) or GB virus-C (GBV-C), has been described; these are thought to be two different isolates of the same virus, which are percutaneously transmitted. Autoantibodies are absent.

The clinical significance of this virus remains uncertain. Risk factors are similar to those for hepatitis C. There is no clear relationship between HGV/GBV-C infection and progressive liver disease. Persistent infection does occur but does not affect the clinical course (Papadakis & McPhee, 2016).

NONVIRAL HEPATITIS

Certain chemicals have toxic effects on the liver and produce acute liver cell necrosis or toxic hepatitis when inhaled, injected parenterally, or taken by mouth. Some chemicals commonly implicated in this disease include carbon tetrachloride and phosphorus. These substances are true hepatotoxins. Many medications can induce hepatitis but are only sensitizing rather than toxic. Drug-induced hepatitis is similar to acute viral hepatitis, but parenchymal destruction tends to be more extensive. Medications that can lead to hepatitis include isoniazid (Nydrazid); halothane (Fluothane); acetaminophen; methyldopa (Aldomet); and certain antibiotics, antimetabolites, and anesthetic agents.

Toxic Hepatitis

At the onset of disease, toxic hepatitis resembles viral hepatitis. Obtaining a history of exposure to hepatotoxic chemicals, medications, botanical agents, or other toxic agents assists in early treatment and removal of the causative agent. Anorexia, nausea, and vomiting are the usual symptoms; jaundice and hepatomegaly are noted on physical assessment. Symptoms are more intense for the more severely toxic patient.

Recovery from acute toxic hepatitis is rapid if the hepatotoxin is identified early and removed or if exposure to the agent has been limited. Recovery is unlikely if there is a prolonged period between exposure and onset of symptoms. There are no effective antidotes. The fever rises; the patient becomes toxic and prostrated. Vomiting may be persistent, with the emesis containing blood. Clotting abnormalities may be severe, and hemorrhages may appear under the skin. The severe GI symptoms may lead to vascular collapse. Delirium, coma, and seizures develop, and within a few days the patient may die of fulminant hepatic failure (discussed later) unless they receive a liver transplant.

Short of liver transplantation, few treatment options are available. Therapy is directed toward restoring and maintaining fluid and electrolyte balance, blood replacement, and comfort and supportive measures. A few patients recover from acute toxic hepatitis only to develop chronic liver disease. If the liver heals, there may be scarring, followed by postnecrotic cirrhosis.

Drug-Induced Hepatitis

Drug-induced liver disease is the most common cause of acute liver failure, accounting for more than 50% of all cases in the United States (Lancaster, Hiatt, & Zarrinpar, 2015; Singanayagam & Bernal, 2015). Manifestations of sensitivity to a medication may occur on the first day of its use or not until several months later. Usually, the onset is abrupt, with chills, fever, rash, pruritus, arthralgia, anorexia, and nausea. Later, there may be jaundice, dark urine, and an enlarged and tender liver. After the offending medication is withdrawn, symptoms may gradually subside. However, reactions can be severe, or even fatal, even if the medication is stopped. If fever, rash, or pruritus occurs from any medication, its use should be stopped immediately.

Although any medication can affect liver function, the use of acetaminophen (found in many over-the-counter medications used to treat fever and pain) has been identified as the leading cause of acute liver failure (Lancaster et al., 2015; Singanayagam & Bernal, 2015). Other causes commonly associated with liver injury include many anesthetic agents, medications used to treat rheumatic and musculoskeletal disease, antidepressants, psychotropic medications, anticonvulsants, and antituberculosis agents (Whitehouse & Wendon, 2013).

A short course of high-dose corticosteroids may be used in patients with severe hypersensitivity reactions, although its efficacy is uncertain. Liver transplantation is an option for drug-induced hepatitis, but outcomes may not be as successful as with other causes of liver failure.

FULMINANT HEPATIC FAILURE

Fulminant hepatic failure is the clinical syndrome of sudden and severely impaired liver function in a previously healthy person. The generally accepted definition is that fulminant hepatic failure develops within 8 weeks after the first symptoms of jaundice (Feldman et al., 2015; Singanayagam & Bernal, 2015).

Patterns of the progression from jaundice to encephalopathy have been identified and have led to proposals of time-based classifications. However, no agreement about these classifications has been reached. Three categories are frequently cited: hyperacute, acute, and subacute liver failure. In hyperacute liver failure, the duration of jaundice before the onset of encephalopathy is 0 to 7 days; in acute liver failure, it is 8 to 28 days; and in subacute liver failure, it is 28 to 72 days. The prognosis for fulminant hepatic failure is much worse than for chronic liver failure. However, in fulminant failure, the hepatic lesion is potentially reversible, and survival rates are approximately 20% to 50%, depending greatly on the cause. Those who do not survive die of massive hepatocellular injury and necrosis (Feldman et al., 2015; Siddiqui & Stravitz, 2014; Singanayagam & Bernal, 2015).

Viral hepatitis is a common cause of fulminant hepatic failure; other causes include toxic medications (e.g., acetaminophen) and chemicals (e.g., carbon tetrachloride), metabolic disturbances (e.g., Wilson disease, a hereditary syndrome with deposition of copper in the liver), and structural changes (e.g., Budd–Chiari syndrome, an obstruction to outflow in major hepatic veins) (Whitehouse & Wendon, 2013).

Jaundice and profound anorexia may be the initial reasons the patient seeks health care. Fulminant hepatic failure is often accompanied by coagulation defects, kidney disease and electrolyte disturbances, cardiovascular abnormalities, infection, hypoglycemia, encephalopathy, and cerebral edema (Whitehouse & Wendon, 2013).

The key to optimized treatment is rapid recognition of acute liver failure and intensive intervention. Supporting the patient in the ICU and assessing the indications for and feasibility of liver transplantation are hallmarks of management. The use of antidotes for certain conditions may be indicated such as N-acetylcysteine for acetaminophen toxicity and penicillin for mushroom poisoning. Treatment modalities may include plasma exchanges (plasmapheresis) to correct coagulopathy, to reduce serum ammonia levels, and to stabilize the patient awaiting liver transplantation, and prostaglandin therapy to enhance hepatic blood flow. Although these treatment modalities may be implemented, no evidence exists indicating any clinical improvement with their use (Feldman et al., 2015; Siddiqui & Stravitz, 2014; Singanayagam & Bernal, 2015). Hepatocytes within synthetic fiber columns have been tested as liver support systems (liver assist devices) to provide a bridge to transplantation.

Research into interventions for acute liver failure has begun to focus on techniques that combine the efficacy of a whole liver with the convenience and biocompatibility of hemodialysis. The acronyms ELAD (extracorporeal *liver assist devices*) and BAL (*bioartificial liver*) have been used to describe these hybrid devices. These short-term devices, which remain experimental, may help patients survive until transplantation is possible (Whitehouse & Wendon, 2013). The BAL device exposes separated plasma to a cartridge containing porcine liver cells after the plasma has flowed through a charcoal column that removes substances toxic to hepatocytes. The ELAD exposes whole blood to cartridges containing human hepatoblastoma cells, resulting in removal of toxic substances. In the near future, similar extracorporeal circuits using **xenografts** (transplantation of organs from one species to another) may be studied as a bridge to liver transplantation. These approaches appear promising and have had success in animal studies. In human clinical application, the use of various BAL systems has resulted in improved neurologic and biochemical parameters. Adding albumin to extracorporeal dialysis in a process known as molecular adsorbent recirculating system (MARS) has been used to remove protein-bound toxins and is potentially useful in unstable patients with fulminant hepatic failure (Banares, Catalina, & Vaquero, 2014; Papadakis & McPhee, 2016; Romero-Gomez et al., 2015; Singanayagam & Bernal, 2015).

In patients who have fulminant hepatic failure with stage 4 encephalopathy (see Table 49-3), there is a high risk of cerebral edema, a life-threatening complication. The cause is not fully understood, although disruption of the blood–brain barrier and plasma leakage into the cerebrospinal fluid may be one cause. An increase in the intracellular osmolarity within cerebral astrocyte cells, possibly related to increased sodium and glutamine in these cells, may be another (Singanayagam & Bernal, 2015). These patients require intracranial pressure monitoring. Measures to promote adequate cerebral perfusion include careful fluid balance and hemodynamic assessments, a quiet environment, and diuresis with mannitol (Osmitrol), an osmotic diuretic.

The use of pharmacologic neuromuscular blockade (NMB) and sedation is indicated to prevent surges in intracranial pressure related to agitation. Other support measures include monitoring for and treating hypoglycemia, coagulopathies, and infection. Despite these treatment modalities, the mortality rate remains high. Consequently, liver transplantation (discussed later) is the treatment of choice for fulminant hepatic failure.

HEPATIC CIRRHOSIS

Cirrhosis is a chronic disease characterized by replacement of normal liver tissue with diffuse fibrosis that disrupts the structure and function of the liver. There are three types of cirrhosis or scarring of the liver:

* Alcoholic cirrhosis, in which the scar tissue characteristically surrounds the portal areas. This is most frequently caused by chronic alcoholism and is the most common type of cirrhosis.
* Postnecrotic cirrhosis, in which there are broad bands of scar tissue. This is a late result of a previous bout of acute viral hepatitis.
* Biliary cirrhosis, in which scarring occurs in the liver around the bile ducts. This type of cirrhosis usually results from chronic biliary obstruction and infection (cholangitis); it is much less common.

The portion of the liver chiefly involved in cirrhosis consists of the portal and the periportal spaces, where the bile canaliculi of each lobule communicate to form the liver bile ducts. These areas become the sites of inflammation, and the bile ducts become occluded with inspissated (thickened) bile and pus. The liver attempts to form new bile channels; hence, there is an overgrowth of tissue made up largely of disconnected, newly formed bile ducts and surrounded by scar tissue.

Pathophysiology

Several factors have been implicated in the etiology of cirrhosis. Nutritional deficiency with reduced protein intake contributes to liver destruction in cirrhosis, but excessive alcohol intake is the major causative factor in fatty liver and its consequences. However, cirrhosis can occur in people who do not consume alcohol and in those who consume a normal diet and have a high alcohol intake.

Some people appear to be more susceptible than others to this disease, whether or not they have alcoholism or are malnourished. Other factors may play a role, including exposure to certain chemicals (carbon tetrachloride, chlorinated naphthalene, arsenic, or phosphorus) or infectious schistosomiasis. Twice as many men as women are affected, although, for unknown reasons, women are at greater risk for development of alcohol-induced liver disease. Most patients are between 40 and 60 years of age. Each year, more than 31,000 people die of chronic liver diseases and cirrhosis in the United States (Poordad, 2015).

Alcoholic cirrhosis is characterized by episodes of necrosis involving the liver cells, which sometimes occur repeatedly throughout the course of the disease. The destroyed liver cells are gradually replaced by scar tissue. Eventually, the amount of scar tissue exceeds that of the functioning liver tissue. Islands of residual normal tissue and regenerating liver tissue

TABLE 49-5 Modified Child–Pugh Classification of the Severity of Liver Disease

Parameter	Points Assigned		
	1	2	3
Ascites	Absent	Slight	Moderate
Bilirubin (mg/dL)	≤2	2–3	>3
Albumin (g/dL)	>3.5	2.8–3.5	<2.8
Prothrombin time (seconds over control)	1–3	4–6	>6
Encephalopathy	None	Grade 1–2	Grade 3–4

Total score of 5–6, grade A; 7–9, grade B; 10–15, grade C.
Adapted from information in Feldman, M., Friedman, L. S., & Brandt, L. J. (2015). *Sleisinger & Fordtran's gastrointestinal & liver disease* (10th ed.). Philadelphia, PA: Saunders Elsevier.

may project from the constricted areas, giving the cirrhotic liver its characteristic hobnail appearance. The disease usually has an insidious onset and a protracted course, occasionally proceeding over a period of 30 or more years.

The prognoses for different forms of cirrhosis caused by various liver diseases have been investigated in several studies. Of the many prognostic indicators, the Child–Pugh classification seems most useful in predicting the outcome of patients with liver disease (see Table 49-5). It is also used in choosing management approaches.

Clinical Manifestations

Signs and symptoms of cirrhosis increase in severity as the disease progresses, and severity is used to categorize the disorder as compensated or decompensated cirrhosis (see Chart 49-10). Compensated cirrhosis, with its less severe, often vague symptoms, may be discovered secondarily at a routine physical examination. The hallmarks of decompensated cirrhosis result from failure of the liver to synthesize proteins, clotting factors, and other substances and manifestations of portal hypertension (see earlier sections of this chapter for clinical manifestations and management of portal hypertension, ascites, varices, and hepatic encephalopathy).

Liver Enlargement

Early in the course of cirrhosis, the liver tends to be large, and the cells are loaded with fat. The liver is firm and has a sharp edge that is noticeable on palpation. Abdominal pain may be present because of recent, rapid enlargement of the liver, which produces tension on the fibrous covering of the liver (Glisson capsule). Later in the disease, the liver decreases in size as scar tissue contracts the liver tissue. The liver edge, if palpable, is nodular.

Portal Obstruction and Ascites

Portal obstruction and ascites—late manifestations of cirrhosis—are caused partly by chronic failure of liver function and partly by obstruction of the portal circulation. Almost all of the blood from the digestive organs is collected in the portal veins and carried to the liver. Because a cirrhotic liver does not allow free blood passage, blood backs up into the spleen and the GI tract, and these organs become the seat of chronic passive congestion—that is, they are stagnant with blood and therefore cannot function properly. Indigestion and altered bowel function result. Fluid rich in protein may accumulate in the peritoneal cavity, producing ascites. This can be detected through percussion for shifting dullness or a fluid wave (see Fig. 49-5).

Infection and Peritonitis

Bacterial peritonitis may develop in patients with cirrhosis and ascites in the absence of an intra-abdominal source of infection or an abscess. This condition is referred to as spontaneous bacterial peritonitis (SBP). Bacteremia due to translocation of intestinal flora is believed to be the most likely route of infection. Clinical signs may be absent, necessitating paracentesis for diagnosis. Antibiotic therapy is effective in the treatment and prevention of recurrent episodes of SBP. The development of SBP is a precipitating factor to the onset of hepatorenal syndrome, a form of acute kidney injury unresponsive to administration of fluid or diuretic agents (Karvellas, Durand, & Nadim, 2015). This type of kidney disease is characterized by a lack of pathologic changes in the kidney; there is no evidence of dehydration or obstruction of the urinary tract or any other renal disorder.

Gastrointestinal Varices

The obstruction to blood flow through the liver caused by fibrotic changes also results in the formation of collateral blood vessels in the GI system and shunting of blood from the portal vessels into blood vessels with lower pressures. As a result, the patient with cirrhosis often has prominent, distended abdominal blood vessels, which are visible on abdominal inspection (caput medusae) and distended blood vessels throughout the GI tract. The esophagus, stomach, and lower rectum are common sites of collateral blood vessels. These distended blood vessels form varices or hemorrhoids, depending on their location.

Because these vessels were not intended to carry the high pressure and volume of blood imposed by cirrhosis, they may rupture and bleed. Therefore, assessment must include observation for occult and frank bleeding from the GI tract.

Edema

Another late symptom of cirrhosis is edema, which is attributed to chronic liver failure. A reduced plasma albumin concentration predisposes the patient to the formation of edema. Although edema is generalized, it often affects the lower extremities, the upper extremities, and the presacral area. Facial edema is not typical. Overproduction of aldosterone occurs, causing sodium and water retention and potassium excretion.

Vitamin Deficiency and Anemia

Because of inadequate formation, use, and storage of certain vitamins (notably vitamins A, C, and K), signs of deficiency are common, particularly hemorrhagic phenomena associated with vitamin K deficiency. Chronic gastritis and impaired GI function, together with inadequate dietary intake and impaired liver function, account for the anemia that is often associated with cirrhosis. The patient's anemia, poor nutritional status, and poor state of health result in severe fatigue, which interferes with the ability to carry out routine activities of daily living.

Mental Deterioration

Additional clinical manifestations include deterioration of mental and cognitive function with impending hepatic encephalopathy and hepatic coma, as described previously. Serial neurologic assessment is indicated, including assessment of the patient's general behavior, cognitive abilities, orientation to time and place, and speech patterns.

Assessment and Diagnostic Findings

The extent of liver disease and the type of treatment are determined after review of the laboratory findings. The functions of the liver are complex, and many diagnostic tests provide information about liver function (see Table 49-1). The patient needs to know why these tests are being performed and how to cooperate.

In severe parenchymal liver dysfunction, the serum albumin level tends to decrease, and the serum globulin level rises. Enzyme tests indicate liver cell damage: serum alkaline phosphatase, AST, ALT, and GGT levels increase, and the serum cholinesterase level may decrease. Bilirubin tests are performed to measure bile excretion or retention; increased levels of bilirubin can occur with cirrhosis and other liver disorders. Prothrombin time is prolonged. Normal values for laboratory data are listed in Appendix A on thePoint.

Ultrasound scanning is used to measure the difference in density of parenchymal cells and scar tissue. CT, MRI, radioisotope liver scans, and elastography studies give information about liver size, hepatic blood flow and obstruction and the presence of liver fibrosis. Diagnosis is confirmed by liver biopsy. Arterial blood gas analysis may reveal a ventilation–perfusion imbalance and hypoxia.

Medical Management

Management of the patient with cirrhosis is usually based on the presenting symptoms. For example, antacids or H_2 antagonists are prescribed to decrease gastric distress and minimize the possibility of GI bleeding. Vitamins and nutritional supplements promote healing of damaged liver cells and improve the patient's general nutritional status. Potassium-sparing diuretic agents such as spironolactone or triamterene (Dyrenium) may be indicated to decrease ascites, if present; these diuretics are preferred because they minimize the fluid and electrolyte changes commonly seen with other agents. An adequate diet and avoidance of alcohol are essential. Although the fibrosis of the cirrhotic liver cannot be reversed, its progression may be halted or slowed by such measures.

Many medications have been shown to possess antifibrotic activity for the treatment of cirrhosis. Some of these medications include colchicine, angiotensin system inhibitors, statins, diuretics including spironolactone (Aldactone), immunosuppressants, and glitazones such as pioglitazone (Acto) or rosiglitazone (Avandia). These medications have reasonable safety profiles, but their long-term safety and efficacy in patients with cirrhosis has yet to be demonstrated (Lee & Moreau, 2015; Poordad, 2015).

Many patients who have end-stage liver disease (ESLD) with cirrhosis use the herb milk thistle (*Silybum marianum*) to treat jaundice and other symptoms. This herb has been used for centuries because of its healing and regenerative properties for liver disease. Silymarin from milk thistle has anti-inflammatory and antioxidant properties that may have beneficial effects, especially in hepatitis, alcohol-induced liver injury and hepatocellular carcinoma (Lee & Moreau, 2015; Madrigal-Santillan, Madrigal-Bujaidair, Alvarez-Gonzalez, et al., 2014; Mastron et al., 2015). The natural compound SAM-e (S-adenosylmethionine) may improve outcomes in liver disease by improving liver function, possibly through enhancing antioxidant function. Primary biliary cirrhosis has been treated with ursodeoxycholic acid (Actigall, Urso) to improve liver function.

Nursing Management

Nursing management for the patient with cirrhosis of the liver is described in detail in Chart 49-11. Nursing interventions are directed toward promoting patient's rest, improving nutritional status, providing skin care, reducing risk of injury, and monitoring and managing potential complications.

Promoting Rest

The patient with cirrhosis requires rest and other supportive measures to permit the liver to reestablish its functional ability. If the patient is hospitalized, weight and I&O are measured and recorded daily. The nurse adjusts the patient's position in bed for maximal respiratory efficiency, which is especially important if ascites is marked, because it interferes with adequate thoracic excursion. Oxygen therapy may be required in liver failure to oxygenate the damaged cells and prevent further cell destruction.

Rest reduces the demands on the liver and increases the liver's blood supply. Because the patient is susceptible to the hazards of immobility, efforts to prevent respiratory, circulatory, and vascular disturbances are initiated. These measures may help prevent such problems as atelectasis, pneumonia, venous thromboemboli formation, and pressure ulcers. After nutritional status improves and strength increases, the nurse encourages the patient to increase activity gradually. Activity and mild exercise, as well as rest, are planned.

Improving Nutritional Status

The patient with cirrhosis without ascites, edema, or signs of impending hepatic coma should receive a nutritious, high-protein diet, if tolerated, supplemented by vitamins of the B complex, as well as A, C, and K. The nurse encourages the patient to eat. If ascites is present, small, frequent meals may be better tolerated than three large meals because of the abdominal pressure exerted by ascites.

The use of probiotics for the management of hepatic encephalopathy is currently the topic of ongoing research. Imbalance of the intestinal flora is not uncommon. Some research suggests that the oral ingestion of 1 cup of probiotic yogurt three times a day reduces intestinal flora imbalance by decreasing *Escherichia coli* counts and promoting the growth of non–urease-producing bacteria. This strategy is thought to then reduce ammonia levels and improve mental status (Nusrat et al., 2014).

Patients with fatty stools (steatorrhea) should receive water-soluble forms of fat-soluble vitamins A, D, and E (Aquasol A, D, and E). Folic acid and iron are prescribed to prevent anemia. Sodium restriction is also indicated to prevent ascites. Patients with prolonged or severe anorexia and those who are vomiting or eating poorly for any reason may receive nutrients by the enteral or parenteral route.

Providing Skin Care

Providing careful skin care is important because of subcutaneous edema, the patient's immobility, jaundice, and increased susceptibility to skin breakdown and infection. Frequent changes in position are necessary to prevent pressure ulcers. Irritating soaps and the use of adhesive tape are avoided to prevent trauma to the skin. Lotion may be soothing to irritated skin; the nurse takes measures to minimize scratching by the patient.

Reducing Risk of Injury

The nurse protects the patient with cirrhosis from falls and other injuries. The side rails should be in place and pads used in case the patient becomes agitated or restless. To minimize agitation, the nurse orients the patient to time and place and explains all procedures. The nurse instructs the patient to ask for assistance to get out of bed. The nurse carefully evaluates any injury because of the possibility of internal bleeding.

Because of the risk for bleeding from abnormal clotting, the patient should use an electric razor rather than a safety razor. A soft-bristled toothbrush helps minimize bleeding gums, and pressure applied to all venipuncture sites helps minimize bleeding.

(*text continued on page 1416*)

PLAN OF NURSING CARE
The Patient With Impaired Liver Function

NURSING DIAGNOSIS: Activity intolerance related to fatigue, lethargy, and malaise
GOAL: Patient reports decrease in fatigue and reports increased ability to participate in activities

Nursing Interventions	Rationale	Expected Outcomes
1. Assess level of activity tolerance and degree of fatigue, lethargy, and malaise when performing routine activities of daily living.	1. Provides baseline for further assessment and criteria for assessment of effectiveness of interventions.	• Exhibits increased interest in activities and events
2. Assist with activities and hygiene when fatigued.	2. Promotes exercise and hygiene within patient's level of tolerance.	• Participates in activities and gradually increases exercise within physical limits
3. Encourage rest when fatigued or when abdominal pain or discomfort occurs.	3. Conserves energy and protects the liver.	• Reports increased strength and well-being
4. Assist with selection and pacing of desired activities and exercise.	4. Stimulates patient's interest in selected activities.	• Reports absence of abdominal pain and discomfort
5. Provide diet high in carbohydrates with protein intake of 1.2–1.5 g/kg/day.	5. Provides calories for energy and protein for healing.	• Plans activities to allow ample periods of rest
6. Administer supplemental vitamins (A, B complex, C, and K).	6. Provides additional nutrients.	• Takes vitamins as prescribed

NURSING DIAGNOSIS: Imbalanced nutrition: less than body requirements related to abdominal distention and discomfort and anorexia
GOAL: Positive nitrogen balance, no further loss of muscle mass; meets nutritional requirements

Nursing Interventions	Rationale	Expected Outcomes
1. Assess dietary intake and nutritional status through diet history and diary, daily weight measurements, and laboratory data.	1. Identifies deficits in nutritional intake and adequacy of nutritional state.	• Exhibits improved nutritional status by increased weight (without fluid retention) and improved laboratory data
2. Provide diet high in carbohydrates with protein intake of 1.2–1.5 g/kg/day.	2. Provides calories for energy and protein for healing.	• States rationale for dietary modifications
3. Assist patient in identifying low-sodium foods.	3. Reduces edema and ascites formation.	• Identifies foods high in carbohydrates and protein
4. Elevate the head of the bed during meals.	4. Reduces discomfort from abdominal distention and decreases sense of fullness produced by pressure of abdominal contents and ascites on the stomach.	• Reports improved appetite
		• Participates in oral hygiene measures
5. Provide oral hygiene before meals and pleasant environment for meals at mealtime.	5. Promotes positive environment and increased appetite; reduces unpleasant taste.	• Reports increased appetite; identifies rationale for smaller, frequent meals
6. Offer smaller, more frequent meals (6/day).	6. Decreases feeling of fullness, bloating.	• Demonstrates intake of high-calorie diet; adheres to protein intake recommendations
7. Encourage patient to eat meals and supplementary feedings.	7. Encouragement is essential for the patient with anorexia and gastrointestinal discomfort.	• Identifies foods and fluids that are nutritious and permitted on diet
8. Provide attractive meals and an aesthetically pleasing setting at mealtime.	8. Promotes appetite and sense of well-being.	• Gains weight without increased edema or ascites formation
9. Eliminate alcohol.	9. Eliminates "empty calories" and further damage from alcohol.	• Reports increased appetite and well-being
		• Excludes alcohol from diet
10. Administer medications prescribed for nausea, vomiting, diarrhea, or constipation.	10. Reduces gastrointestinal symptoms and discomforts that decrease the appetite and interest in food.	• Takes medications for gastrointestinal disorders as prescribed
11. Encourage increased fluid intake and exercise if the patient reports constipation.	11. Promotes normal bowel pattern and reduces abdominal discomfort and distention.	• Reports normal gastrointestinal function with regular bowel function

NURSING DIAGNOSIS: Impaired skin integrity related to pruritus from jaundice and edema
GOAL: Decrease potential for pressure ulcer development; breaks in skin integrity

Nursing Interventions	Rationale	Expected Outcomes
1. Assess degree of discomfort related to pruritus and edema.	1. Assists in determining appropriate interventions.	• Exhibits intact skin without redness, excoriation, or breakdown

(continued on page 1410)

Chart
49-11

PLAN OF NURSING CARE (Continued)
The Patient With Impaired Liver Function

Nursing Interventions	Rationale	Expected Outcomes
2. Note and record degree of jaundice and extent of edema.	2. Provides baseline for detecting changes and evaluating effectiveness of interventions.	• Reports relief from pruritus • Exhibits no skin excoriation from scratching
3. Keep patient's fingernails short and smooth.	3. Prevents skin excoriation and infection from scratching.	• Uses nondrying soaps and lotions; states rationale for the use of nondrying soaps and lotions
4. Provide frequent skin care; avoid the use of soaps and alcohol-based lotions.	4. Removes waste products from skin while preventing dryness of skin.	• Turns self periodically; exhibits reduced edema of dependent parts of the body
5. Massage every 2 hours with emollients; turn every 2 hours.	5. Promotes mobilization of edema.	• Exhibits no areas of skin breakdown • Exhibits decreased edema; normal skin turgor
6. Initiate use of alternating-pressure mattress or low air loss bed.	6. Minimizes prolonged pressure on bony prominences susceptible to breakdown.	
7. Recommend avoiding the use of harsh detergents.	7. May decrease skin irritation and need for scratching.	
8. Assess skin integrity every 4–8 hours. Instruct patient and family in this activity.	8. Edematous skin and tissue have compromised nutrient supply and are vulnerable to pressure and trauma.	
9. Restrict sodium as prescribed.	9. Minimizes edema formation.	
10. Perform range-of-motion exercises every 4 hours; elevate edematous extremities whenever possible.	10. Promotes mobilization of edema.	

NURSING DIAGNOSIS: Risk for injury related to altered clotting mechanisms and altered level of consciousness
GOAL: Reduced risk of injury

Nursing Interventions	Rationale	Expected Outcomes
1. Assess level of consciousness and cognitive level.	1. Assists in determining patient's ability to protect self and comply with required self-protective actions; may detect deterioration of hepatic function.	• Is oriented to time, place, and person • Exhibits no hallucinations and demonstrates no efforts to get up unassisted or to leave hospital
2. Provide safe environment (pad side rails, remove obstacles in room, prevent falls).	2. Minimizes falls and injury if falls occur.	• Exhibits no ecchymoses (bruises), cuts, or hematoma
3. Provide frequent surveillance to orient patient, and avoid the use of restraints.	3. Protects patient from harm while stimulating and orienting patient; the use of restraints may disturb patient further.	• Uses electric razor rather than sharp-edged razor • Exhibits absence of frank bleeding from gastrointestinal tract
4. Replace sharp objects (razors) with safer items.	4. Avoids cuts and bleeding.	• Exhibits absence of restlessness, epigastric fullness, and other indicators of hemorrhage and shock
5. Observe each stool for color, consistency, and amount.	5. Permits detection of bleeding in gastrointestinal tract.	• Exhibits negative results of test for occult gastrointestinal bleeding
6. Be alert to symptoms of anxiety, epigastric fullness, weakness, and restlessness.	6. May indicate early signs of bleeding and shock.	• Is free of ecchymotic areas or hematoma formation
7. Test each stool and emesis for occult blood.	7. Detects early evidence of bleeding.	• Exhibits normal vital signs • Maintains rest and remains quiet if active bleeding occurs
8. Observe for hemorrhagic manifestations: ecchymosis, epistaxis, petechiae, and bleeding gums.	8. Indicates altered clotting mechanisms.	• Identifies rationale for blood transfusions and measures to treat bleeding
9. Record vital signs at frequent intervals, depending on patient acuity (every 1–4 hours).	9. Provides baseline and evidence of hypovolemia and hemorrhagic shock.	• Uses measures to prevent trauma (e.g., uses soft toothbrush, blows nose gently, avoids bumps and falls, avoids straining during defecation)
10. Keep patient quiet, and limit activity.	10. Minimizes risk of bleeding and straining.	• Experiences no side effects of medications
11. Assist physician in passage of tube for esophageal balloon tamponade, if its insertion is indicated.	11. Promotes nontraumatic insertion of tube in anxious and combative patient for immediate treatment of bleeding.	• Takes all medications as prescribed • Identifies rationale for precautions with the use of all medications
12. Observe during blood transfusions.	12. Permits detection of transfusion reactions (risk increased with multiple blood transfusions needed for active bleeding from esophageal varices).	• Adheres to prescribed treatment modalities
13. Measure and record nature, time, and amount of vomitus.	13. Assists in evaluating extent of bleeding and blood loss.	

Chart 49-11

PLAN OF NURSING CARE (Continued)

The Patient With Impaired Liver Function

Nursing Interventions	Rationale	Expected Outcomes
14. Maintain patient in fasting state, if indicated.	14. Reduces risk of aspiration of gastric contents and minimizes risk of further trauma to esophagus and stomach by preventing vomiting.	
15. Administer vitamin K as prescribed.	15. Promotes clotting by providing fat-soluble vitamin necessary for clotting.	
16. Remain with patient during episodes of bleeding.	16. Reassures anxious patient and permits monitoring and detection of further needs of the patient.	
17. Offer cold liquids by mouth when bleeding stops (if prescribed).	17. Minimizes risk of further bleeding by promoting vasoconstriction of esophageal and gastric blood vessels.	
18. Institute measures to prevent trauma. a. Maintain safe environment.	18. Promotes safety of patient. a. Minimizes risk of trauma and bleeding by avoiding falls and cuts, etc.	
b. Encourage *gentle* blowing of nose.	b. Reduces risk of nosebleed (epistaxis) secondary to trauma and decreased clotting.	
c. Provide soft toothbrush, and avoid the use of toothpicks.	c. Prevents trauma to oral mucosa while promoting good oral hygiene.	
d. Encourage intake of foods with high content of vitamin C.	d. Promotes healing.	
e. Apply cold compresses where indicated.	e. Minimizes bleeding into tissues by promoting local vasoconstriction.	
f. Record location of bleeding sites.	f. Permits detection of new bleeding sites and monitoring of previous sites of bleeding.	
g. Use small-gauge needles for injections.	g. Minimizes oozing and blood loss from repeated injections.	
19. Administer medications carefully; monitor for side effects.	19. Reduces risk of side effects secondary to damaged liver's inability to detoxify (metabolize) medications normally.	

NURSING DIAGNOSIS: Disturbed body image related to changes in appearance, sexual dysfunction, and role function
GOAL: Patient verbalizes feelings consistent with improvement of body image and self-esteem

Nursing Interventions	Rationale	Expected Outcomes
1. Assess changes in appearance and the meaning these changes have for patient and family.	1. Provides information for assessing impact of changes in appearance, sexual function, and role on the patient and family.	• Verbalizes concerns related to changes in appearance, life, and lifestyle • Shares concerns with significant others • Identifies past coping strategies that have been effective
2. Encourage patient to verbalize reactions and feelings about these changes.	2. Enables patient to identify and express concerns; encourages patient and significant others to share these concerns.	• Uses past effective coping strategies to deal with changes in appearance, life, and lifestyle
3. Assess patient's and family's previous coping strategies.	3. Permits encouragement of those coping strategies that are familiar to patient and have been effective in the past.	• Maintains good grooming and hygiene • Identifies short-term goals and strategies to achieve them
4. Assist and encourage patient to maximize appearance (such as strategies to limit the appearance of jaundice and ascites through careful selection of colors and type of clothing) and explore alternatives to previous sexual and role functions.	4. Encourages patient to continue safe roles and functions while encouraging exploration of alternatives.	• Takes an active role in decision making about self and care • Identifies resources that are not harmful • Verbalizes that some of previous lifestyle practices have been harmful • Uses healthy expressions of frustration, anger, anxiety
5. Assist patient in identifying short-term goals.	5. Accomplishing these goals serves as positive reinforcement and increases self-esteem.	
6. Encourage and assist patient in decision making about care.	6. Promotes patient's control of life and improves sense of well-being and self-esteem.	

(continued on page 1412)

Chart 49-11

PLAN OF NURSING CARE (Continued)

The Patient With Impaired Liver Function

Nursing Interventions	Rationale	Expected Outcomes
7. Identify with patient resources to provide additional support (counselor, spiritual advisor).	7. Assists patient in identifying resources and accepting assistance from others when indicated.	
8. Assist patient in identifying previous practices that may have been harmful to self (alcohol and drug abuse). Involve patient in goal setting, and provide positive feedback for accomplishments.	8. Recognition and acknowledgment of the harmful effects of these practices are necessary for identifying a healthier lifestyle.	

NURSING DIAGNOSIS: Readiness for enhanced comfort related to enlarged tender liver and ascites
GOAL: Increased level of comfort

Nursing Interventions	Rationale	Expected Outcomes
1. Maintain bed rest when patient experiences abdominal discomfort.	1. Reduces metabolic demands and protects the liver.	• Reports pain and discomfort if present
2. Administer antispasmodic and analgesic agents as prescribed.	2. Reduces irritability of the gastrointestinal tract and decreases abdominal pain and discomfort.	• Maintains bed rest and decreases activity in presence of pain
3. Observe, record, and report presence and character of pain and discomfort.	3. Provides baseline to detect further deterioration of status and to evaluate interventions.	• Takes antispasmodic and analgesic agents as indicated and as prescribed
4. Reduce sodium and fluid intake if prescribed.	4. Minimizes further formation of ascites.	• Reports decreased pain and abdominal discomfort
5. Prepare patient and assist with procedures for management of ascites such as paracentesis or TIPS procedure, if indicated.	5. Removal of ascites fluid may decrease abdominal discomfort.	• Reduces sodium and fluid intake to prescribed levels if indicated to treat ascites
		• Exhibits decreased abdominal girth and appropriate weight changes
6. Encourage the use of distracting activities such as music, reading, or meditation.	6. Distraction may limit the perception of pain.	• Reports decreased discomfort after paracentesis or other procedure to manage ascites such as TIPS procedure

NURSING DIAGNOSIS: Excess fluid volume related to ascites and edema formation
GOAL: Restoration of normal fluid volume

Nursing Interventions	Rationale	Expected Outcomes
1. Restrict sodium and fluid intake if prescribed.	1. Minimizes formation of ascites and edema.	• Consumes diet low in sodium and within prescribed fluid restriction
2. Administer diuretic agents, potassium, and protein supplements as prescribed.	2. Promotes excretion of fluid through the kidneys and maintenance of normal fluid and electrolyte balance.	• Takes diuretic agents, potassium, and protein supplements as indicated without experiencing side effects
3. Record intake and output every 1–8 hours depending on response to interventions and on patient acuity.	3. Indicates effectiveness of treatment and adequacy of fluid intake.	• Exhibits increased urine output
4. Measure and record abdominal girth and weight daily.	4. Monitors changes in ascites formation and fluid accumulation.	• Exhibits decreasing abdominal girth
5. Explain rationale for sodium and fluid restriction.	5. Promotes patient's understanding of restriction and cooperation with it.	• Exhibits no rapid increase in weight
		• Identifies rationale for sodium and fluid restriction
6. Prepare patient and assist with paracentesis or TIPS procedure, if indicated.	6. Paracentesis will temporarily decrease amount of ascites present and a TIPS procedure will lower portal pressure and thus limit the accumulation of ascitic fluid.	• Shows a decrease in ascites with decreased weight

NURSING DIAGNOSIS: Confusion related to abnormal liver function and increased serum ammonia level
GOAL: Improved mental status; safety maintained; ability to cope with cognitive and behavioral changes

Nursing Interventions	Rationale	Expected Outcomes
1. Give frequent, small feedings of carbohydrates and protein.	1. Promotes consumption of adequate carbohydrates for energy requirements and protein for healing.	• Demonstrates an interest in events and activities in environment
2. Protect from infection.	2. Minimizes risk of further increase in metabolic requirements.	• Demonstrates normal attention span
		• Follows and participates in conversation appropriately

Chart
49-11
PLAN OF NURSING CARE (Continued)
The Patient With Impaired Liver Function

Nursing Interventions	Rationale	Expected Outcomes
3. Keep environment warm and draft free.	3. Minimizes shivering, which would increase metabolic requirements.	• Is oriented to person, place, and time
4. Pad the side rails of the bed.	4. Provides protection for the patient should hepatic coma and seizure activity occur.	• Remains in bed when indicated • Experiences no seizures • No neurologic or respiratory depression
5. Limit visitors.	5. Minimizes patient's activity and metabolic requirements.	• Patient develops no cognitive impairments, but if they develop, they are quickly identified and treated, enhancing the potential of recovery
6. Provide careful nursing surveillance to ensure patient's safety.	6. Provides close monitoring of new symptoms and minimizes trauma to the confused patient.	• Patient and family describe adequate feelings of coping and lowered anxiety. They demonstrate ability to listen and to make decisions as able
7. Avoid opioids and barbiturates.	7. Prevents masking of symptoms of hepatic coma and prevents drug overdose secondary to reduced ability of the damaged liver to metabolize opioids and barbiturates; prevents respiratory depression.	• Patient and family communicate their feelings and their needs in a secure and caring environment
8. Awaken at intervals (every 2–4 hours during daytime hours for the stable patient) to assess cognitive status.	8. Provides stimulation to the patient and opportunity for observing patient's level of consciousness.	
9. Identify subtle changes in behavior or sleep–wake pattern (consistent staff caring for the patient enhances this assessment as they become familiar with patient's baseline).	9. These changes may herald worsening of encephalopathy, which requires rapid intervention, including medication.	
10. Assess handwriting or drawing skill daily as indication of cognitive ability.	10. These changes may herald worsening of encephalopathy, which requires rapid intervention, including medication.	
11. Encourage patient and family to participate in therapeutic strategies to enhance coping with episodes of mental deterioration.	11. Promoting activities such as listening to music, relaxation techniques, or preillness coping strategies can reduce anxiety.	
12. Encourage patient and family to discuss feeling of fear, powerlessness, or emotional distress related to patient's mental deterioration.	12. Actively listening demonstrates caring and concern.	

NURSING DIAGNOSIS: Risk for imbalanced body temperature: failure to maintain normal body temperature due to inflammatory process of cirrhosis or hepatitis

GOAL: Maintenance of normal body temperature, free from infection

Nursing Interventions	Rationale	Expected Outcomes
1. Record temperature regularly (every 4 hours).	1. Provides baseline to detect fever and to evaluate interventions.	• Exhibits normal temperature and reports absence of chills or sweating
2. Encourage fluid intake.	2. Corrects fluid loss from perspiration and fever and increases patient's level of comfort.	• Demonstrates adequate intake of fluids
3. Apply cool sponges or ice bag for elevated temperature.	3. Promotes reduction of fever and increases patient's comfort.	• Exhibits no evidence of local or systemic infection
4. Administer antibiotics as prescribed.	4. Ensures appropriate serum concentration of antibiotics to treat infection.	• Develops no nosocomial infections related to invasive procedures/lines
5. Avoid exposure to infections by frequent handwashing and limiting use of central lines and urinary catheters to the shortest period of time, only when they are necessary.	5. Minimizes risk of further infection and further increases in body temperature and metabolic rate.	
6. Keep patient at rest while temperature is elevated.	6. Reduces metabolic rate.	
7. Assess for abdominal pain, tenderness.	7. May occur with bacterial peritonitis.	
8. Use sterile technique for all invasive procedures.	8. Many evidence-based practice guidelines (e.g., central venous catheter care) recommend the use of sterile technique to prevent nosocomial infections.	

(continued on page 1414)

Chart 49-11

PLAN OF NURSING CARE (Continued)

The Patient With Impaired Liver Function

NURSING DIAGNOSIS: Ineffective breathing pattern related restriction of thoracic excursion secondary to ascites, abdominal distention, and fluid in the thoracic cavity
GOAL: Improved respiratory status

Nursing Interventions	Rationale	Expected Outcomes
1. Elevate head of bed to at least 30 degrees.	1. Reduces abdominal pressure on the diaphragm and permits fuller thoracic excursion and lung expansion.	• Experiences improved respiratory status • Reports decreased shortness of breath • Reports increased strength and sense of well-being
2. Conserve patient's strength by providing rest periods and assisting with activities.	2. Reduces metabolic and oxygen requirements.	• Exhibits normal respiratory rate (12–18 breaths/min) with no adventitious sounds
3. Change position every 2 hours.	3. Promotes expansion and oxygenation of all areas of the lungs.	• Exhibits full thoracic excursion without shallow respirations
4. Assist with paracentesis, TIPS or thoracentesis, if indicated.	4. Paracentesis, TIPS, and thoracentesis (performed to remove fluid from the abdominal and thoracic cavities, respectively) may be frightening to the patient.	• Exhibits normal arterial blood gases • Exhibits adequate oxygen saturation by pulse oximetry • Experiences absence of confusion or cyanosis
a. Explain procedure and its purpose to patient.	a. Helps obtain patient's cooperation with procedures.	
b. Have patient void before paracentesis.	b. Prevents inadvertent bladder injury.	
c. Support and maintain position during procedure.	c. Prevents inadvertent organ or tissue injury.	
d. Record both the amount and the character of fluid aspirated.	d. Provides record of fluid removed and indication of severity of limitation of lung expansion by fluid.	
e. Observe for evidence of coughing, increasing dyspnea, or pulse rate.	e. Indicates irritation of the pleural space and evidence of pneumothorax or hemothorax.	

COLLABORATIVE PROBLEM: Gastrointestinal bleeding and hemorrhage
GOAL: Absence of episodes of gastrointestinal bleeding and hemorrhage

Nursing Interventions	Rationale	Expected Outcomes

1. Assess patient for evidence of gastrointestinal bleeding or hemorrhage. If bleeding does occur:
  a. Monitor vital signs (blood pressure, pulse, respiratory rate) every 4 hours or more frequently, depending on acuity.
  b. Assess skin temperature, level of consciousness every 4 hours or more frequently, depending on acuity.
  c. Monitor gastrointestinal secretions and output (emesis, stool for occult or obvious bleeding). Test emesis for blood once per shift and with any color change. Hematest each stool.
  d. Monitor hematocrit and hemoglobin for trends and changes.
	1. Allows early detection of signs and symptoms of bleeding and hemorrhage.	• Experiences no episodes of bleeding and hemorrhage
		• Vital signs are within acceptable range for patient
		• No evidence of bleeding from gastrointestinal tract
		• Hematocrit and hemoglobin levels within acceptable limits
		• Turns and moves without straining and increasing intra-abdominal pressure
		• No straining with bowel movements
		• No further bleeding episodes if aggressive treatment of bleeding and hemorrhage was needed

2. Avoid activities that increase intra-abdominal pressure (straining, turning).
  a. Avoid coughing/sneezing.
  b. Assist patient to turn.
  c. Keep all needed items within easy reach.
  d. Use measures to prevent constipation such as adequate fluid intake, stool softeners.
  e. Ensure small meals.
	2. Minimizes increases in intra-abdominal pressure that could lead to rupture and bleeding of esophageal or gastric varices.	• Patient and family state rationale for treatments
		• Patient and family identify supports available to them
		• Patient and family describe signs and symptoms of a recurrent bleeding episode and identify needed action

PLAN OF NURSING CARE (Continued)

Chart 49-11

The Patient With Impaired Liver Function

Nursing Interventions	Rationale	Expected Outcomes
3. Have equipment (Sengstaken–Blakemore tube™, medications, IV fluids) available if indicated.	3. Equipment, medications, and supplies will be readily available if patient experiences bleeding from ruptured esophageal or gastric varices.	
4. Assist with procedures and therapy needed to treat gastrointestinal bleeding and hemorrhage.	4. Gastrointestinal bleeding and hemorrhage require emergency measures (e.g., insertion of Sengstaken–Blakemore tube™, administration of fluids and medications).	
5. Monitor respiratory status every hour, and minimize risk of respiratory complications if balloon tamponade is needed.	5. The patient is at high risk for respiratory complications, including asphyxiation if gastric balloon of tamponade tube ruptures or migrates upward.	
6. Prepare patient physically and psychologically for other treatment modalities if needed.	6. The patient who experiences hemorrhage is very anxious and fearful; minimizing anxiety assists in control of hemorrhage.	
7. Monitor patient for recurrence of bleeding and hemorrhage.	7. Risk of rebleeding is high with all treatment modalities used to halt gastrointestinal bleeding.	
8. Keep family informed of patient's status.	8. Family members are likely to be anxious about the patient's status; providing information will reduce their anxiety level and promote more effective coping.	
9. Once recovered from bleeding episode, provide patient and family with information regarding signs and symptoms of gastrointestinal bleeding.	9. Risk of rebleeding is high. Subtle signs may be more quickly identified.	

COLLABORATIVE PROBLEM: Hepatic encephalopathy
GOAL: Absence of changes in cognitive status and of injury

Nursing Interventions	Rationale	Expected Outcomes
1. Assess cognitive status every 4–8 hours. a. Assess patient's orientation to person, place, and time. b. Monitor patient's level of activity, restlessness, and agitation. Assess for presence of asterixis (flapping hand tremors). c. Obtain and record daily sample of patient's handwriting or ability to construct a simple figure (e.g., star). d. Assess neurologic signs (deep tendon reflexes, ability to follow instructions).	1. Data will provide baseline of patient's cognitive status and enable detection of changes.	• Remains awake, alert, and aware of surroundings • Is oriented to time, place, and person • Deep tendon reflexes remain within normal limits • Exhibits no restlessness or agitation • Record of handwriting demonstrates no deterioration in cognitive function • States rationale for treatment used to prevent or treat hepatic encephalopathy • Demonstrates stable serum ammonia level within acceptable limits • Takes medications as prescribed • Breath sounds normal without adventitious sounds • Skin and tissue intact without evidence of pressure or breaks in integrity • Verbalizes understanding of need for treatments and procedures to promote recovery
2. Monitor medications to prevent administration of those that may precipitate hepatic encephalopathy (sedative, hypnotic, analgesic agents).	2. Medications are a common precipitating factor in development of hepatic encephalopathy in patients at risk.	
3. Monitor laboratory data, especially serum ammonia level.	3. Increases in serum ammonia level are associated with hepatic encephalopathy and coma.	
4. Notify physician of even subtle changes in patient's neurologic assessment, cognitive function, sleep pattern, or mood.	4. Allows early initiation of treatment of hepatic encephalopathy and prevention of hepatic coma.	

(continued on page 1416)

Chart 49-11

PLAN OF NURSING CARE (Continued)

The Patient With Impaired Liver Function

Nursing Interventions	Rationale	Expected Outcomes
5. Limit sources of protein from diet if indicated.	5. Reduces breakdown and conversion of protein to ammonia.	
6. Administer medications prescribed to reduce serum ammonia level (e.g., lactulose, antibiotics, glucose, benzodiazepine antagonist [flumazenil] if indicated).	6. Reduces serum ammonia level.	
7. Assess respiratory status, and initiate measures to prevent complications.	7. The patient who develops hepatic coma is at risk for respiratory complications (i.e., pneumonia, atelectasis, infection).	
8. Protect patient's skin and tissue from pressure and breakdown.	8. The patient in coma is at risk for skin breakdown and pressure ulcer formation.	
9. Provide support and active listening for patient and family as patient's mental status deteriorates.	9. The patient with hepatic encephalopathy can experience episodes of mental deterioration due to liver failure. This can produce feelings of fear and anxiety.	

Monitoring and Managing Potential Complications

A major role of the nurse is monitoring of the patient with cirrhosis for complications.

Bleeding and Hemorrhage

The patient is at increased risk for bleeding and hemorrhage because of decreased production of prothrombin and decreased ability of the diseased liver to synthesize the necessary substances for blood coagulation (see the Esophageal Varices section).

 ### Hepatic Encephalopathy

Hepatic encephalopathy and coma, which are complications of cirrhosis, may manifest as deteriorating mental status (delirium) or as physical signs such as abnormal voluntary and involuntary movements. Hepatic encephalopathy was discussed earlier in the chapter in detail.

Monitoring is essential to identify early deterioration in mental status. The nurse monitors the patient's mental status closely and reports changes so that treatment for encephalopathy can be initiated promptly. An extensive baseline and ongoing neurologic evaluation is key to identify progression through the four stages of encephalopathy (see Table 49-3).

Each advancing stage demands more intensive nursing interventions aimed at providing for patient safety and prevention and early identification of life-threatening complications such as respiratory failure and cerebral edema, which would necessitate interventions in an ICU. Because electrolyte disturbances can contribute to encephalopathy, serum electrolyte levels are carefully monitored and corrected if abnormal. Oxygen is given if oxygen desaturation occurs. The nurse monitors for fever or abdominal pain, which may signal the onset of bacterial peritonitis or other infection (see earlier discussion of hepatic encephalopathy).

Fluid Volume Excess

Patients with advanced chronic liver disease develop cardiovascular abnormalities. These occur due to an increased cardiac output and decreased peripheral vascular resistance, possibly resulting from the release of vasodilators. A hyperdynamic circulatory state develops in patients with cirrhosis, and plasma volume increases. This increase in circulating plasma volume is probably multifactorial, but some studies have implicated excess production of nitrous oxide, such as that seen in sepsis, as one causative factor (Nusrat et al., 2014). The greater the degree of hepatic decompensation, the more severe the hyperdynamic state. Close assessment of cardiovascular and respiratory status is of key importance for the care of patients with this disorder. Pulmonary compromise is always a potential complication of ESLD because of plasma volume excess; consequently, the nurse has an important role in preventing pulmonary complications. Administering diuretic agents, implementing fluid restrictions, and enhancing patient positioning can optimize pulmonary function. Fluid retention may be noted in the development of ascites, lower extremity swelling, and dyspnea. Monitoring of I&O, daily weight changes, changes in abdominal girth, and edema formation is part of nursing assessment in the hospital or in the home setting. Patients are also monitored for nocturia and, later, for oliguria, because these states indicate increasing severity of liver dysfunction (Nusrat et al., 2014).

Promoting Home, Community-Based and Transitional Care

 ### Educating Patients About Self-Care

During the hospital stay, the nurse and other health care providers prepare the patient with cirrhosis for discharge, focusing on dietary education. Of greatest importance is the exclusion of alcohol from the diet. The patient may benefit from referral to Alcoholics Anonymous, psychiatric care, or counseling or support from a spiritual advisor. The patient should avoid the consumption of raw shellfish.

Sodium restriction will continue for a considerable time, if not permanently. The patient will require written education, reinforcement, and support from the staff as well as family members.

Successful treatment depends on convincing the patient of the need to adhere completely to the therapeutic plan. This includes rest, lifestyle changes, adequate dietary intake, and the elimination of alcohol. The nurse also instructs the patient and family about symptoms of impending encephalopathy, possible bleeding tendencies, and susceptibility to infection.

Recovery is neither rapid nor easy; there are frequent setbacks and apparent lack of improvement. Many patients find it difficult to refrain from using alcohol for comfort or escape. The nurse has a significant role in offering support and encouragement to the patient and in providing positive feedback when the patient experiences success.

Continuing and Transitional Care

Referral for transitional or home care may assist the patient in dealing with the transition from hospital to home. The use of alcohol may have been an important part of normal home and social life in the past. The nurse assesses the patient's progress at home and the manner in which the patient and family are coping with the elimination of alcohol and the dietary restrictions. The nurse also reinforces previous education and answers questions that may not have occurred to the patient or family until the patient is back home and trying to establish new patterns of eating, drinking, and lifestyle.

CANCER OF THE LIVER

Hepatic tumors may be malignant or benign. Benign liver tumors were uncommon until oral contraceptives were in widespread use. Now, benign liver tumors such as hepatic adenomas occur most frequently in women in their reproductive years who are taking oral contraceptives (Greenberger et al., 2015).

Primary Liver Tumors

Few cancers originate in the liver. Primary liver tumors usually are associated with chronic liver disease, hepatitis B and C infections, and cirrhosis. HCC is the most common type of primary liver cancer, responsible for 75% of all liver cancers, with more than half a million cases diagnosed each year on a worldwide basis. HCC is the third leading cause of cancer-related mortality worldwide. It is rare in the United States and northern Europe, accounting for fewer than 6 cases per 100,000 inhabitants (James & Liou, 2015; Nusrat et al., 2014). Other types of primary liver cancer include fibrolamellar carcinoma, angiosarcoma, hepatoblastoma, cholangiocellular carcinoma, and combined hepatocellular and cholangiocellular carcinoma. HCC is usually nonresectable because of rapid growth and metastasis. If found early, resection of primary liver cancer may be possible; however, early detection is not common.

Cirrhosis, chronic infection with HBV and HCV, and exposure to certain chemical toxins (e.g., vinyl chloride, arsenic) have been implicated as causes of HCC. Cigarette smoking has also been identified as a risk factor, especially when combined with alcohol use. Some evidence suggests that aflatoxin, a metabolite of the fungus *Aspergillus flavus*, may be a risk factor for HCC. This is especially true in areas where HCC is endemic (i.e., Asia and Africa). Aflatoxin and other similar toxic molds can contaminate food such as ground nuts and grains and may act as co-carcinogens with hepatitis B (Greenberger et al., 2015; Salgia & Singal, 2014). The risk of contamination is greatest when these foods are stored unrefrigerated in tropical or subtropical climates.

Liver Metastases

Metastases from other primary sites, particularly the digestive system, breast, and lung, are found in the liver 2.5 times more frequently than tumors due to primary liver cancers (Goldman & Schafer, 2015; Salgia & Singal, 2014). Malignant tumors are likely to reach the liver eventually, by way of the portal system or lymphatic channels, or by direct extension from an abdominal tumor. Moreover, the liver apparently is an ideal place for these malignant cells to thrive. Often, the first evidence of cancer in an abdominal organ is the appearance of liver metastases; unless exploratory surgery or an autopsy is performed, the primary tumor may never be identified.

Clinical Manifestations

The early manifestations of malignancy of the liver include pain—a continuous dull ache in the right upper quadrant, epigastrium, or back. Weight loss, loss of strength, anorexia, and anemia may also occur. The liver may be enlarged and irregular on palpation. Jaundice is present only if the larger bile ducts are occluded by the pressure of malignant nodules in the hilum of the liver. Ascites develops if such nodules obstruct the portal veins or if tumor tissue is seeded in the peritoneal cavity.

Assessment and Diagnostic Findings

The diagnosis of liver cancer is based on clinical signs and symptoms, the history and physical examination, and the results of laboratory and x-ray studies. Increased serum levels of bilirubin, alkaline phosphatase, AST, GGT, and lactic dehydrogenase may occur. Leukocytosis (increased white blood cells), erythrocytosis (increased red blood cells), hypercalcemia, hypoglycemia, and hypocholesterolemia may also be seen on laboratory assessment.

The serum level of alpha-fetoprotein, which serves as a tumor marker, is elevated in 30% to 40% of patients with primary liver cancer, commonly to levels greater than 200 ng/mL (Feldman et al., 2015; Salgia & Singal, 2014). The level of carcinoembryonic antigen, a marker of advanced cancer of the digestive tract, may be elevated. These two markers together are useful to distinguish between metastatic liver disease and primary liver cancer.

Many patients have metastases from the primary liver tumor to other sites by the time the diagnosis is made; metastases occur primarily to the lung but may also occur to regional lymph nodes, adrenals, bone, kidneys, heart, pancreas, or stomach.

X-rays, liver scans, CT scans, ultrasound studies, MRI, arteriography, and laparoscopy may be part of the diagnostic workup and may be performed to determine the extent of the cancer. Positron emission tomography (PET) scans are used to evaluate a wide range of metastatic tumors of the liver.

Confirmation of a tumor's histology can be made by biopsy under imaging guidance (CT scan or ultrasound) or laparoscopically. Local or systemic dissemination of the tumor by needle biopsy or fine-needle biopsy can occur. Because of the small but real risks of tumor seeding (0.5% to 2%), hemorrhage, and false-negative results from biopsy, many transplant centers avoid biopsy, particularly in patients who may be candidates for liver resection or liver transplantation. Assessment of the imaging characteristics for the diagnosis of HCC is preferred in these instances, and a confirmed diagnosis of HCC is made by frozen section at the time of surgery (Goldman & Schafer, 2015; Nusrat et al., 2014).

Medical Management

Although surgical resection of the liver tumor is possible in some patients, the underlying cirrhosis is so prevalent in cancer of the liver that it increases the risks associated with surgery. Radiation therapy and chemotherapy have been used to treat cancer of the liver with varying degrees of success. Although these therapies may prolong survival and improve quality of life by reducing pain and discomfort, their major effect is palliative.

Radiation Therapy

The use of external-beam radiation for the treatment of liver tumors has been limited by the radiosensitivity of normal hepatocytes and the risk of destruction of normal liver parenchyma. More effective methods of delivering radiation to tumors of the liver include (1) IV or transarterial injection of antibodies tagged with radioactive isotopes (also known as TARE-transarterial chemoembolization) that specifically attack tumor-associated antigens and (2) percutaneous placement of a high-intensity source for interstitial radiation therapy (delivery of radiation directly to the tumor cells). Internal radiotherapy can result in reduction in tumor size, but its effect on survival is yet to be determined (Salgia & Singal, 2014).

Chemotherapy

Typically, studies of patients with advanced cases of liver cancer have shown that the use of systemic chemotherapeutic agents leads to poor outcomes. For patients with stable hepatic function (Child class A), a targeted molecular therapy, sorafenib (Nexavar), has been developed and approved for use and has shown some degree of improvement in treating patients with HCC (Nusrat et al., 2014). Systemic chemotherapy may be used to treat metastatic liver lesions. Embolization of tumor vessels with chemotherapy (a process known as transarterial chemoembolization or TACE) produces anoxic necrosis with high concentrations of trapped chemotherapeutic agents. This therapy has begun to show some promising results. An implantable pump has been used to deliver a high concentration of chemotherapy by constant infusion to the liver through the hepatic artery in cases of metastatic disease. This method has shown a moderate response rate (Feldman et al., 2015).

Percutaneous Biliary Drainage

Percutaneous biliary or transhepatic drainage is used to bypass biliary ducts obstructed by liver, pancreatic, or bile duct tumors in patients who have inoperable tumors or are considered poor surgical risks. Under fluoroscopy, a catheter is inserted through the abdominal wall and past the obstruction into the duodenum. Such procedures are used to reestablish biliary drainage, relieve pressure and pain from the buildup of bile behind the obstruction, and decrease pruritus and jaundice. As a result, the patient is made more comfortable, and quality of life and survival are improved.

For several days after its insertion, the catheter is opened to external drainage. The bile is observed closely for amount, color, and presence of blood and debris. Complications of percutaneous biliary drainage include sepsis, leakage of bile, hemorrhage, and reobstruction of the biliary system by debris in the catheter or by encroaching tumor. Therefore, the patient is observed for fever and chills, bile drainage around the catheter, changes in vital signs, and evidence of biliary obstruction, including increased pain or pressure, pruritus, and recurrence of jaundice.

Other Nonsurgical Treatments

Laser hyperthermia has been used to treat hepatic metastases. Heat has been directed to tumors through several methods to cause necrosis of the tumor cells while sparing normal tissue. In radiofrequency thermal ablation, a needle electrode is inserted into the liver tumor under imaging guidance. Radiofrequency energy passes through to the noninsulated needle tip, causing heat and tumor cell death from coagulation necrosis.

Immunotherapy is another treatment modality under investigation. In this therapy, lymphocytes with antitumor reactivity are given to the patient with hepatic cancer. Tumor regression has been demonstrated in patients with metastatic cancer for whom standard treatment has failed.

Transcatheter arterial embolization interrupts the arterial blood flow to small tumors by injecting small particulate embolic or chemotherapeutic agents (as described previously) into the artery supplying the tumor. As a result, ischemia and necrosis of the tumor occur.

For multiple small lesions, ultrasound-guided injection of alcohol promotes dehydration of tumor cells and tumor necrosis (Feldman et al., 2015; Salgia & Singal, 2014).

Surgical Management

Surgical resection is the treatment of choice when HCC is confined to one lobe of the liver and the function of the remaining liver is considered adequate for postoperative recovery. In the case of metastasis, hepatic resection can be performed if the primary site can be completely excised and the metastasis is limited. However, metastases to the liver are rarely limited or solitary. Capitalizing on the regenerative capacity of the liver cells, some surgeons have successfully removed 90% of the liver. However, the presence of cirrhosis limits the ability of the liver to regenerate. Laparoscopic liver resection for malignant tumors has also been described. Staging of liver tumors aids in predicting the likelihood of surgical cure (Doherty, 2015; Feldman et al., 2015; Townsend et al., 2016).

In preparation for surgery, the patient's nutritional, fluid, and general physical status are assessed, and efforts are undertaken to ensure the best physical condition possible. Extensive diagnostic studies may be performed. Specific studies may include liver scan, liver biopsy, cholangiography, selective hepatic angiography, percutaneous needle biopsy, peritoneoscopy, laparoscopy, ultrasound, CT scan, PET scan, MRI, and blood tests, particularly determinations of serum alkaline phosphatase, AST, and GGT and its isoenzymes.

Lobectomy

Removal of a lobe of the liver is the most common surgical procedure for excising a liver tumor. If it is necessary to restrict blood flow from the hepatic artery and portal vein for longer than 15 minutes, it is likely that hypothermia will be used. For a right-liver lobectomy or an extended right lobectomy (including the medial left lobe), a thoracoabdominal incision is used. An extensive abdominal incision is made for a left lobectomy.

Local Ablation

In patients who are not candidates for resection or transplantation, ablation of HCC may be accomplished by chemicals such as ethanol or by physical means such as radiofrequency ablation (most frequently used local ablative therapy) or microwave coagulation. These techniques may be performed under ultrasound or CT guidance laparoscopically or percutaneously. Radiofrequency ablation is becoming a standard mode of treatment; a tumor up to 5 cm in size can be destroyed in one session. The most common complications following ablation are local pain or bleeding. Serious complications are rare (Feldman et al., 2015; Salgia & Singal, 2014).

Immunotherapy with interferon may be used after surgical resection for HCC to prevent recurrence of the lesion in those patients who have developed the lesion related to hepatitis B or C.

Liver Transplantation

Liver transplantation offers good patient outcomes. Candidates with liver cancer meet stringent selection criteria, including having small, early-stage lesions (Nusrat et al., 2014). The Milan criteria have been developed to limit transplantation to patients who are most likely to have better outcomes. The Milan criteria include that the patient must have a single tumor measuring less than 5 cm, or have three or fewer lesions with none over 3 cm in size (Nusrat et al., 2014). This treatment involves removing the liver and replacing it with a healthy donor organ. Studies report decreased recurrence rates of the primary liver malignancy after transplantation, with improvement in 4-year survival rates to approximately 85% (Nusrat et al., 2014). Metastasis and recurrence may be enhanced by the immunosuppressive therapy that is needed to prevent rejection of the transplanted liver. In patients with small (less than 5 cm), single lesions, liver transplantation has been shown to be beneficial, but its use is limited by organ shortages. The increasing use of living donor transplantation may improve this situation and decrease the waiting time and tumor proliferation that is characteristic of patients with liver cancer (see later discussion).

Nursing Management

For patients with liver cancer anticipating surgery, support, education, and encouragement are provided to help them prepare psychologically for the surgery. After surgery, potential problems related to cardiopulmonary involvement may include vascular complications and respiratory and liver dysfunction. Metabolic abnormalities require careful attention. Because extensive blood loss may occur as well, the patient receives infusions of blood and IV fluids. The patient requires constant, close monitoring and care for the first 2 or 3 days, similar to postsurgical abdominal and thoracic nursing care.

If the patient is to receive chemotherapy or radiation therapy in an effort to relieve symptoms, they may be discharged home while still receiving one or both of these therapies. The patient may also go home with a biliary drainage system or hepatic artery catheter in place. In most cases, the hepatic artery catheter has been inserted surgically and has a prefilled infusion pump implanted subcutaneously that delivers a continuous chemotherapeutic dose until completed (Yarbro, Wujcik, & Gobel, 2011). A hepatic artery port may also be inserted to provide access for intermittent chemotherapy infusion. This port dwells under the skin, but because it provides direct arterial access, it is not used for continuous infusion therapy in the home environment; the access line is discontinued once the chemotherapeutic agent has infused. The patient and family require education about care of the biliary catheter and the effects and side effects of hepatic artery chemotherapy. This education is necessary because of participation of the patient and family in patient care in the home setting.

Promoting Home, Community-Based and Transitional Care

Educating Patients About Self-Care

The nurse educates the patient to recognize and report the potential complications and side effects of the chemotherapy and the desirable and undesirable effects of the specific chemotherapy regimen. The nurse also emphasizes the importance of follow-up visits to assess the response to chemotherapy and radiation therapy. In addition, if the patient is receiving chemotherapy on an outpatient basis, the nurse explains the patient's and family's role in managing the chemotherapy infusion and in assessing the infusion or insertion site. The nurse encourages the patient to resume routine activities as soon as possible while cautioning about falls and activities that may damage the infusion pump or site.

Patients at home with a biliary drainage system in place typically fear that the catheter will become dislodged; this fear is often shared by the patient's family. Reassurance and instruction can help reduce their fear that the catheter will fall out easily. The patient and family also require education on catheter care, including instruction on how to keep the catheter site clean and dry and how to assess the catheter and its insertion site. Irrigation of the catheter with sterile normal saline solution or water may be prescribed to keep the catheter patent and free of debris. The patient and caregivers are taught proper technique to avoid introducing bacteria into the biliary system or catheter during irrigation. They are instructed not to aspirate or draw back on the syringe during irrigation in order to prevent entry of irritating duodenal contents into the biliary tree or catheter. The patient and caregivers are also instructed about the signs of complications and are encouraged to notify the nurse or primary provider if problems or questions arise.

Patients with implantable ports are instructed about the chemotherapy regimen, types of medications, effects and side effects that may occur, and appropriate management strategies if problems occur. If a hepatic artery port is inserted for intermittent chemotherapy, patients and their families are provided the same educational content. Such a port has an internal one-way valve; therefore, it is not aspirated for a blood return before the infusion is initiated. The patient is instructed to assess the port site between infusions and to note and report any sign of infection or inflammation.

Continuing and Transitional Care

In many cases, referral for transitional or home care enables the patient with liver cancer to be at home in a familiar environment with family and friends. Because of the poor prognosis associated with liver cancer, the nurse serves a vital role in assisting the patient and family to cope with the symptoms that may occur and the prognosis. The patient's physical and psychological status are assessed as well as adequacy of pain relief, nutritional status, and presence of symptoms indicating complications of treatment or progression of disease. During home visits, the nurse assesses the function of the chemotherapy pump, the infusion site, and the biliary drainage system, if indicated. The nurse collaborates with the other members of the health care team, the patient, and the family to ensure effective pain management and to manage potential problems, which include weakness, pruritus, inadequate dietary intake, jaundice, and symptoms associated with metastasis to other sites. The nurse also assists the patient and family in making decisions about hospice care and assists with initiation of referrals. The patient is encouraged to discuss preferences for end-of-life care with family members and health care providers (see Chapter 16).

LIVER TRANSPLANTATION

Liver transplantation is used to treat life-threatening ESLD for which no other form of treatment is available. The transplantation procedure involves total removal of the diseased liver and replacement with a healthy liver from a cadaver donor or with the right lobe from a live donor in the same anatomic location (**orthotopic liver transplantation [OLT]**). Removal of the liver creates a space for the new liver and permits anatomic reconstruction of the hepatic vasculature and biliary tract as close to normal as possible.

The success of liver transplantation depends on successful immunosuppression. Immunosuppressant agents currently used include cyclosporine (Neoral), tacrolimus (Prograf), corticosteroids, azathioprine (Imuran), mycophenolate mofetil (CellCept), sirolimus (formerly known as rapamycin [Rapamune]), everolimus [Afinitor], antithymocyte globulin (Thymoglobulin), basiliximab (Simulect), and daclizumab (Zenapax). There is no one, accepted, optimal immunosuppressive regimen. Most transplant centers have developed their own therapeutic practices, largely based on experience. Multiple immunosuppressive strategies can be used to prevent transplanted organ rejection. Most strategies involve the use of more than one agent but current recommendations advise the minimization of immunosuppression in order to avoid toxicity (Gotthardt, Bruns, Weiss, et al., 2014). Using multiple

immunosuppressive agents has the effect of blocking multiple targets in the immune response cascade. This allows the use of lower doses of each drug, thus avoiding toxicity associated with high doses of these powerful drugs. Some patients are treated with "triple therapy" using corticosteroids, a calcineurin inhibitor such as tacrolimus or cyclosporine, and either an antiproliferative agent (mycophenolate mofetil) or a TOR (target of rapamycin) inhibitor such as sirolimus and everolimus (Doherty, 2015; Gotthardt et al., 2014). Some transplant centers also prescribe steroid-free immunosuppressant regimens after liver transplantation. This regimen has been found to be a safe alternative. Still other transplant centers advocate monotherapy with a calcineurin inhibitor alone to provide long-term immunosuppression (Doherty, 2015; Gotthardt et al., 2014; Townsend, et al., 2016). In order to prevent acute rejection in the early, high-risk months after liver transplantation, some centers employ induction therapy, which is the use of prophylactic, perioperative course of immunosuppressant drugs that suppress the body's response to the foreign, transplanted tissue and may improve graft survival by reducing the risk of acute cellular rejection (Gotthardt et al., 2014). Medications used for induction include basiliximab and a lymphocyte immune globulin (Atgam). Over time, withdrawal of all immunosuppressants is possible but rare; randomized, prospective studies are needed before this clinical practice is accepted (Gotthardt et al., 2014).

Despite the success of immunosuppression in reducing the incidence of rejection of transplanted organs, liver transplantation is not routine and may be accompanied by complications related to the lengthy surgical procedure, immunosuppressive therapy, infection, and technical difficulties encountered in reconstructing the blood vessels and biliary tract. Long-standing systemic problems resulting from the primary liver disease may complicate the pre- and postoperative course. Previous surgery of the abdomen, including procedures to treat complications of advanced liver disease (i.e., shunt procedures used to treat portal hypertension and esophageal varices) increase the complexity of the transplantation procedure.

General indications for liver transplantation include irreversible advanced chronic liver disease, fulminant hepatic failure, metabolic liver diseases, and some hepatic malignancies. Examples of disorders that are indications for liver transplantation include hepatocellular liver diseases (e.g., viral hepatitis, drug- or alcohol-induced liver disease, Wilson disease) and cholestatic diseases (primary biliary cirrhosis, sclerosing cholangitis, NASH, and biliary atresia).

The patient being considered for liver transplantation frequently has many systemic problems that influence pre- and postoperative care. Because transplantation is more difficult if the patient has developed severe GI bleeding and hepatic coma, efforts are made to perform the procedure before the disease progresses to this stage. The patient must undergo a thorough evaluation of hepatic reserve and general health. Part of this evaluation includes classification of the degree of medical need, an objective determination known as the Model for End-Stage Liver Disease (MELD) classification, which stratifies the level of illness of those awaiting a liver transplant. The MELD score is derived from a complex formula incorporating bilirubin levels, prothrombin time (reported as international normalized ratio), creatinine, and the cause of the liver disease (i.e., cholestatic, alcoholic, or other). This system has replaced the Child–Pugh and Child Turcotte–Pugh (CTP) classifications and other related scoring systems for prioritizing patients on the liver transplantation list (Fox, 2014). Although the Child–Pugh score classifies the severity of liver disease and stratifies patients into levels for varied treatment regimens, the MELD score is an indicator of short-term mortality for those with ESLD. Organs are allocated using the MELD score in an effort to provide transplants to the most severely ill patients. The CTP score classification can be used to predict short-term prognosis in patients awaiting liver transplantation (Liou, 2014).

Liver transplantation is an established therapeutic modality, and the number of liver transplant centers is increasing. Patients requiring transplantation are often referred from distant hospitals to these centers. To prepare the patient and family for liver transplantation, nurses in all settings must understand the processes and procedures of liver transplantation.

Many ethical issues arise concerning liver transplantation, particularly concerning the allocation of organs. The way in which some persons contracted liver disease (e.g., alcohol use, hepatitis) leads others to question allocation of organs to them, and some believe that preference should be given to people who need liver transplants but do not have a history of socially unacceptable behavior. More issues arise when a patient requires a second transplant operation because of a return to alcohol or drug use or failure to follow immunosuppressive regimens (see Chart 49-12). Transplant recipients must go through a rigorous selection and preparation process that includes counseling and education to aid them in making critical choices for their improved health. Nurses and other health care providers need to be aware of and confront their own biases and work toward improved understanding and acceptance.

Surgical Procedure

During the procedure, the donor liver is freed from other structures, the bile is flushed from the gallbladder to prevent damage to the walls of the biliary tract, and the liver is perfused with a preservative and cooled. Before the donor liver is placed in the recipient, it is flushed with cold lactated Ringer solution to remove potassium and air bubbles. The presence of portal hypertension increases the difficulty of the procedure. To minimize this problem, many centers use venovenous bypass, which decompresses the venous system below the diaphragm by temporarily shunting blood to the superior vena cava via the axillary vein (Townsend et al., 2016).

Anastomoses (connections) of the blood vessels and bile duct are performed between the donor liver and the recipient liver. There are two types of biliary anastomoses. Biliary reconstruction is performed with an end-to-end anastomosis of the donor and recipient common bile ducts; a stented T-tube may be inserted for external drainage of bile. In patients with biliary disease such as primary sclerosing cholangitis or if the recipient's bile duct is not suitable for anastomosis for other reasons, a biliary-enteric end-to-side anastomosis with a 40- to 50-cm Roux-en-Y loop of jejunum is created for biliary drainage (known as a Roux-en-Y procedure) (see Fig. 49-15A); in this case, bile drainage is internal, and a T-tube is not inserted (Townsend et al., 2016). Figure 49-15B and C illustrates the final appearance of the grafted liver and final closure and drain placement.

Chart 49-12 **ETHICAL DILEMMA**

What Ethical Principles Apply When a Candidate for a Second Liver Transplantation Abuses Alcohol?

Case Scenario

You are a staff nurse working in a university health science center critical care unit that has a reputable organ transplant unit. A 60-year-old man is emergently admitted to the unit with hepatic failure and hemorrhagic shock from bleeding esophageal varices. He has a 30-year history of alcohol and substance abuse. Although he has been in rehabilitation for substance abuse, he recently relapsed following the death of his wife. He continues to be self-employed and is able to function well at work. Although he is at the top of the waiting list for a liver transplant, the transplant team has offered him a split liver segment. They inform him that there are increased complications with this type of procedure as compared to those associated with whole organ transplants which include longer hospitalization. He states, "I have been paying high insurance premiums for all of my life and cannot afford to miss any more work than I have to miss! I think I am entitled to receive a whole organ instead of a split organ!"

Discussion

A number of ethical concerns are inherent within the transplant community because there are a limited number of organs available for transplant. In order to provide the "greatest good" for the most people in need of this scarce resource, whole cadaver livers are split into two for transplant. Since there are complications unique to this procedure, the potential recipient must be informed of these factors prior to consent. Potential liver recipients have the right to refuse the split liver procedure in order to wait for a whole organ to be available. Refusal to receive a split liver should not compromise their decision to wait for a whole organ.

Analysis

- Describe the ethical principles that are in conflict in this case (see Chapter 3, Chart 3-3). Which principle has preeminence when making decisions about allocation of scarce resources, such as organs? How does the principle of distributive justice factor into the allocation of organs?
- Do you believe that this patient should have the right to deny transplant of a split liver? Should his past medical history of alcohol and substance abuse influence the decision to offer him a liver transplant since this is a scare resource?
- What resources or referrals should be made based on this clinical scenario?

Reference

Organ Procurement and Transplant Network (OPTN): U.S. Department of Health and Human Services (HHS) (2016). *Split versus whole liver transplantation*. Retrieved on 12/3/2016 at: optn.transplant.hrsa.gov/resources/ethics/split-versus-whole-liver-transplantation/

Resources

See Chapter 3, Chart 3-6 for ethics resources.

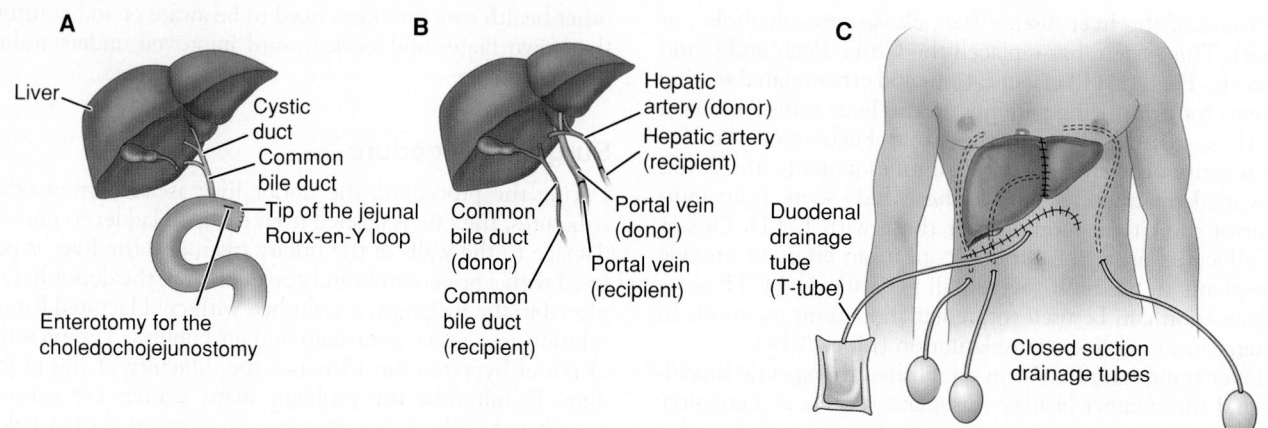

Figure 49-15 • **A.** Some transplant recipients have diseases or conditions that cause their bile ducts to be unusable for anastomosis to the donor liver bile duct. In this case, a loop of jejunum is used as a bridge from the donor liver bile duct to the recipient's small bowel for biliary continuity and drainage. This procedure is termed *Roux-en-Y hepaticojejunostomy*. **B.** Final appearance of implanted liver graft with an end-to-end biliary anastomosis. **C.** Final closure and drain placement after liver transplantation with an end-to-end biliary anastomosis and T-tube placement.

Several additional techniques have been developed to expand the donor pool for liver transplantation. In a split-liver transplant, a single organ is used to provide grafts for two individuals with ESLD, with the smaller patient receiving the smaller left lobe. This procedure has resulted in a higher complication rate and lower survival rate than traditional liver transplantation. Living donor transplantation is being increasingly performed from adult to adult using full right lobes, although it is controversial because it is a major surgical procedure for the donor, and some donor deaths have occurred.

Living donor liver transplantation (LDLT) is considered for patients who have a high potential for mortality while awaiting a cadaveric liver donor, such as those patients with HCC or those with severe complications of cirrhosis including GI bleeding or hepatic encephalopathy (Townsend et al., 2016). The results thus far have indicated that this procedure is most successful when donor and recipient are appropriately selected using careful screening criteria (Townsend et al., 2016). The option of LDLT decreases the waiting list mortality and produces positive recipient outcomes with a low risk of morbidity and mortality for the donor. The LDLT procedure involves transplantation of the right hepatic lobe from an adult donor to the recipient. Potential donors are evaluated by a donor advocate team. Donors must be completely healthy and have hepatic size and anatomy compatible with right lobe transplantation (Townsend et al., 2016). There is an extensive informed consent process for live liver donors. The donor advocate ensures that the concern for donor safety is paramount, especially in the intra- and postoperative period when complications can occur. The clear separation of donor and recipient teams ensures that the donor is treated without ulterior motives, which might occur if the same team cared for both the donor and recipient (Townsend et al., 2016).

In the LDLT procedure, the surgeon performs a formal right hepatic lobectomy. The right lobe is then flushed with preservative solution and vascular reconstruction is completed to prepare for implantation. The recipient operation involves an inferior vena cava–sparing hepatectomy with anastomosis of the donor right-sided vascular and biliary structures to the corresponding recipient structures (Townsend et al., 2016).

Liver transplantation is a long surgical procedure, partly because the patient with liver failure often has portal hypertension, requiring ligation of many venous collateral vessels. Blood loss during the surgical procedure may be extensive. If the patient has adhesions from previous abdominal surgery, lysis of adhesions is often necessary. If a shunt procedure was performed previously, it must be surgically reversed to permit adequate portal venous blood supply to the new liver. During the lengthy surgery, it is important to provide regular updates to the family about the progress of the operation and the patient's status.

Complications

The postoperative complication rate is high, primarily because of technical complications or infection. Immediate postoperative complications may include bleeding, infection, and rejection. Disruption, infection, obstruction of the biliary anastomosis, and impaired biliary drainage may occur. Vascular thrombosis and stenosis are other potential complications. These complications occur in patients receiving either a cadaver or live donor organ. Despite the development of some complications, the 1-year patient survival rate approaches 90% and the 5-year patient survival rate is approximately 80% (Townsend et al., 2016; Wong & Pagalilauan, 2015).

Bleeding

Bleeding is common in the postoperative period and may result from coagulopathy, portal hypertension, and fibrinolysis caused by ischemic injury to the donor liver. Hemodynamic instability and transient hypotension may occur in this phase, secondary to blood loss, loss of vasomotor tone, and vasodilatation due to rewarming the hypothermic patient or due to preexisting cardiac conditions such as cardiomyopathy (Goldman & Schafer, 2015; Wong & Pagalilauan, 2015). Administration of platelets, fresh-frozen plasma, or other blood products may be necessary. Hypertension may co-occur postoperatively but is more common later in the postoperative phase, although its cause is uncertain. Currently available hypertension guidelines do not have specific recommendations for management in the liver transplant population. However, calcium channel blockers such as nifedipine or amlodipine are frequently used for their vasodilatory effects. These drugs also are preferable due to their low interaction level with the cytochrome P450 enzyme system with resultant minimal risk of disruption of immunosuppressant levels. Angiotensin-converting enzyme inhibitors and angiotensin receptor blockers are not first-line drugs for the treatment of hypertension during the first year after transplant due to low levels of renin during this time period. Thiazide diuretics are reserved for patients requiring more than one medication for blood pressure control (Wong & Pagalilauan, 2015). Blood pressure elevation that is significant or sustained is also managed with lifestyle modifications, a low-sodium diet, and an exercise regimen.

 Infection

Infection is the leading cause of death after liver transplantation. Pulmonary and fungal infections are common; susceptibility to infection is increased by the immunosuppressive therapy that is needed to prevent rejection (Wong & Pagalilauan, 2015). Therefore, precautions must be taken to prevent health care–associated infections. The nurse uses strict asepsis when manipulating central venous catheters, arterial lines, and urine, bile, and other drainage systems; obtaining specimens; and changing dressings. Meticulous hand hygiene is crucial. In the ICU, the nurse vigilantly monitors for early clinical manifestations of sepsis (see Chapter 14, Charts 14-5 and 14-6) and uses evidence-based practice guidelines (or bundles) developed by the Institute for Healthcare Improvement (IHI) in the care of the postoperative liver transplant patient. Some of these care guidelines include prevention of sepsis through prevention of central line–associated bloodstream infections and its rapid treatment (see Chart 14-2) and prevention of ventilator-associated pneumonia (VAP) (see Chapter 21, Chart 21-11).

Rejection

Rejection is a major concern. A transplanted liver is perceived by the immune system as a foreign antigen. This triggers an immune response, leading to the activation of T lymphocytes that attack and destroy the transplanted liver. Immunosuppressive agents are used as long-term therapy to prevent this response and rejection of the transplanted liver. These agents inhibit the activation of immunocompetent T lymphocytes to prevent the production of effector T cells.

Although the 1- and 5-year survival rates have increased dramatically with the use of new immunosuppressive therapies, these advances are not without major side effects. A major side effect of cyclosporine, which has been widely used in transplantation, is nephrotoxicity; this problem seems to be dose related. Cyclosporine-related side effects have caused many transplant centers to use tacrolimus instead as first-line therapy because of its efficacy and lower side-effect profile.

Corticosteroids, azathioprine, mycophenolate mofetil, sirolimus, antithymocyte globulin, basiliximab, and daclizumab are also used in various regimens of immunosuppression. These agents may be used as the initial therapy to prevent rejection or used later to treat rejection. Liver biopsy and ultrasound may be required to evaluate suspected episodes of rejection.

Retransplantation is usually attempted if the transplanted liver fails, but the success rate of retransplantation does not approach that of initial transplantation. The greater rates of organ dysfunction and loss after a second or third liver transplant is related to technical intraoperative difficulties and higher bleeding risk (Townsend et al., 2016).

Complications of the LDLT Donor

Improved surgical techniques have made the LDLT procedure an increasingly safe one; however, complications do occur for donors as well. The most frequently occurring complications include pulmonary emboli, portal vein thrombosis, bile duct injury, and liver insufficiency secondary to a resection that is too extensive (Townsend et al., 2016).

Nursing Management

The patient considering transplantation, together with the family, must make difficult choices about treatment, the use of financial resources, and relocation to another area to be closer to the medical center. They must also be aware of the risks and benefits of the procedure and its consequences. In addition, they must also cope with the patient's long-standing health problems and any social and family problems associated with behaviors that may have caused the patient's liver failure. As a result, considerable emotional stress occurs while the patient and family consider liver transplantation and wait for an available liver. The nurse must be aware of these issues and attuned to the emotional and psychological status of the patient and family. Referral to a psychiatric liaison nurse, psychologist, psychiatrist, or spiritual advisor may help them cope with the stressors associated with ESLD and liver transplantation.

If the patient and family are considering undergoing an LDLT, they are subject to additional stressors. Both the patient and the potential donor must undergo a thorough and exhaustive physical and psychological workup to ensure that all involved parties are physically and emotionally prepared. Often, but not always, the donor is a close family member. Coercion must be excluded as influencing the decision to donate a portion of one's liver to another. The potential donor must be aware of the risks associated with the procedure.

If the patient and family believe that liver transplantation may be appropriate, the nurse, surgeon, hepatologist, and other health care team members provide the patient and family with full explanations about the procedure, the chances of success, and the risks (for the donor—bleeding and venous thromboembolism), including the side effects of long-term immunosuppression and postoperative complications in the recipient as well as bleeding and biliary abnormalities (Townsend et al., 2016). The need for close follow-up and lifelong adherence to the therapeutic regimen, including immunosuppression, is emphasized to the patient and family.

Preoperative Nursing Interventions

Once the patient has been accepted as a candidate, they are placed on a waiting list at the transplant center, and patient information is entered into the United Network for Organ Sharing (UNOS) computer system. The UNOS system uses the MELD score to determine organ allocation priorities so that the patient with the highest MELD score will receive the first available organ. Candidates may be matched with appropriate organs as they become available. MELD scores provide the necessary information regarding medical need.

Except in the case of LDLT, a liver becomes available for transplantation only with the death of another person, usually someone who had been healthy except for severe brain injury and brain death. Therefore, the patient and family undergo a stressful waiting period, and the nurse is often their major source of support. The patient must be accessible at all times in case an appropriate liver becomes available. During this time, liver function may deteriorate further, and the patient may experience complications from the progressing disease. Because of the shortage of donor organs, many patients die awaiting transplantation.

Malnutrition, massive ascites, and fluid and electrolyte disturbances are treated before surgery to increase the likelihood of a successful outcome. If the patient's liver dysfunction has a very rapid onset, as in fulminant hepatic failure, there is little time or opportunity for the patient to consider and weigh options and their consequences; the patient may be in a coma and the decision to proceed with transplantation made by the family.

The nurse coordinator is an integral member of the transplant team and plays an important role in preparing the patient for liver transplantation. The nurse serves as an advocate for the patient and family and assumes the important role of liaison between the patient and the other members of the transplant team. The nurse also serves as a resource to other nurses and health care team members involved in evaluating and caring for the patient.

 ## Postoperative Nursing Interventions

The organ recipient is maintained in an environment as free from bacteria, viruses, and fungi as possible, because immunosuppressive medications reduce the body's natural defenses. In the immediate postoperative period, cardiovascular, pulmonary, renal, neurologic, and metabolic functions are monitored continuously. Mean arterial and pulmonary artery pressures are also monitored continuously. Cardiac output, central venous pressure, pulmonary capillary wedge pressure, arterial and mixed venous blood gases, oxygen saturation, oxygen demand and delivery, urine output, heart rate, and blood pressure are used to evaluate the patient's hemodynamic status and intravascular fluid volume. Liver function tests, electrolyte levels, the coagulation profile, chest x-ray, electrocardiogram, and fluid output (including urine, bile from the T-tube, and drainage from Jackson–Pratt tubes) are monitored closely. Because the liver is responsible for the storage of glycogen and the synthesis of protein and clotting factors, these substances need to be monitored and replaced in the immediate postoperative period.

There is a high risk of atelectasis and an altered ventilation–perfusion ratio caused by insult to the diaphragm during the surgical procedure, prolonged anesthesia, immobility, and postoperative pain. The patient will have an endotracheal tube in place and will require mechanical ventilation during the initial postoperative period. Suctioning is performed as required, and sterile humidification is provided. Evidence-based practice guidelines are implemented to prevent the development of pneumonia in the postoperative liver transplant recipient (see Chapter 21, Chart 21-11).

As the patient's condition stabilizes, efforts are made to promote recovery from the trauma of this complex surgery. After removal of the endotracheal tube, the nurse encourages the patient to use an incentive spirometer to decrease the risk of atelectasis. Following extubation, the patient is assisted to get out of bed, to ambulate as tolerated, and to participate in self-care to prevent the complications associated with immobility. Close monitoring for signs and symptoms of liver dysfunction and rejection continue throughout the hospital stay. Plans are made for close follow-up after discharge as well. Education is initiated during the preoperative period and continues after surgery.

The live donor is frequently admitted to an ICU setting along with the recipient. The donor also requires close monitoring for cardiovascular, hemodynamic, and pulmonary stability. The nurse closely assesses the donor for signs of hemorrhage, biliary complication, respiratory decompensation, and infection. The donor is mobilized early in the postoperative phase to prevent the development of complications such as pulmonary embolism. Studies suggest that the donor may experience more pain than the recipient, possibly requiring more analgesia for pain control (Lee, 2015). Patient education focuses on prevention and recognition of complications as well as activity progression and pain management.

Promoting Home, Community-Based and Transitional Care

 ### Educating Patients About Self-Care

Educating the patient, family, and caregivers about long-term measures to promote health is crucial for the success of transplantation and is an important role of the nurse. The patient and family must understand why they need to adhere closely to the therapeutic regimen, with special emphasis on the methods of administration, rationale, and side effects of the prescribed immunosuppressive agents. The nurse provides written and verbal education about how and when to take the medications. To avoid running out of medication or skipping a dose, the patient must make sure that an adequate supply of medication is available. Education is provided about the signs and symptoms that indicate problems necessitating consultation with the transplant team. The patient with a T-tube in place must be educated about how to manage the tube, drainage, and skin care.

Continuing and Transitional Care

The nurse emphasizes the importance of follow-up laboratory tests and appointments with the transplant team. Trough blood levels of immunosuppressive agents are obtained, along with other blood tests that assess the function of the liver and kidneys. During the first months, the patient is likely to require blood tests two or three times a week. As the patient's condition stabilizes, laboratory studies and visits to the transplant team are less frequent. The importance of routine ophthalmologic examinations is emphasized because of the increased incidence of cataracts and glaucoma associated with the long-term corticosteroid therapy used with transplantation. Regular oral hygiene and follow-up dental care, with administration of prophylactic antibiotics before dental examinations and treatments, are recommended because of the immunosuppression.

The nurse reminds the patient that preventing rejection and infection is essential and increases the chances for survival and a more normal life than before transplantation. Many patients live successful and productive lives after receiving a liver transplant. In fact, pregnancy can be considered one to two years after transplantation (Wong & Pagalilauan, 2015). Although successful outcomes have been reported, these pregnancies are considered high risk for both mother and infant and referral should be made to a high risk pregnancy center well before conception. Transplant recipients should be advised about birth control. The waiting period allows time to establish good health, stable liver function, and lower maintenance levels of immunosuppressive therapy (Feldman et al., 2015; Wong & Pagalilauan, 2015).

LIVER ABSCESSES

Two categories of liver abscess have been identified: amebic and pyogenic. Amebic liver abscesses are most commonly caused by *Entamoeba histolytica*. Most amebic liver abscesses occur in the developing countries of the tropics and subtropics because of poor sanitation and hygiene. Pyogenic liver abscesses are much less common, but they are more common in developed countries than the amebic type (Townsend et al., 2016).

Pathophysiology

Whenever an infection develops anywhere along the biliary or GI tract, infecting organisms may reach the liver through the biliary system, portal venous system, or hepatic arterial or lymphatic system. Most bacteria are destroyed promptly, but occasionally some gain a foothold. The bacterial toxins destroy the neighboring liver cells, and the resulting necrotic tissue serves as a protective wall for the organisms.

Meanwhile, leukocytes migrate into the infected area. The result is an abscess cavity full of a liquid containing living and dead leukocytes, liquefied liver cells, and bacteria. Pyogenic abscesses of this type may be either single or multiple and small. Examples of causes of pyogenic liver abscess include cholangitis (usually related to benign or malignant obstruction of the biliary tree) and abdominal trauma.

Clinical Manifestations

The clinical picture is one of sepsis with few or no localizing signs. Fever with chills and diaphoresis, malaise, anorexia, nausea, vomiting, and weight loss may occur. The patient may complain of dull abdominal pain and tenderness in the right upper quadrant of the abdomen. Hepatomegaly, jaundice, anemia, and pleural effusion may develop. Sepsis and shock may be severe and life threatening. In the past, the mortality rate was 100% because of the vague clinical symptoms, inadequate diagnostic tools, and inadequate surgical drainage of the abscess. With the aid of ultrasound, CT, MRI, and liver scans, early diagnosis and surgical drainage of abscesses have greatly reduced the mortality rate.

Assessment and Diagnostic Findings

Although blood cultures are obtained, the organism may not be identified. Aspiration of the liver abscess, guided by ultra-sound, CT, or MRI, may be performed to assist in diagnosis and to obtain cultures of the organism. Percutaneous drainage of pyogenic abscesses is carried out to evacuate the abscess material and promote healing. A catheter may be left in place for continuous drainage; the patient must be instructed about its management.

Medical Management

Treatment includes IV antibiotic therapy; the specific antibiotic used in treatment depends on the organism identified. Continuous supportive care is indicated because of the serious condition of the patient. Open surgical drainage may be required if antibiotic therapy and percutaneous drainage are ineffective (Lardiere-Deguelte, Ragot, Amroun, et al., 2015).

Nursing Management

Although the manifestations of liver abscess vary with the type of abscess, most patients appear acutely ill. Others appear to be chronically ill and debilitated. The nursing management depends on the patient's physical status and the medical management that is indicated. For patients who undergo evacuation and drainage of an abscess, monitoring the drainage and providing skin care are imperative. Strategies must be implemented to contain the drainage and to protect the patient from other sources of infection. Vital signs are monitored to detect changes in the patient's physical status. Deterioration in vital signs or the onset of new symptoms such as increasing pain, which may indicate rupture or extension of the abscess, is reported promptly. The nurse administers IV antibiotic therapy as prescribed. The white blood cell count and other laboratory test results are monitored closely for changes consistent with worsening infection. The nurse prepares the patient for discharge by providing instruction about symptom management, signs and symptoms that should be reported to the primary provider, management of drainage, and the importance of taking antibiotics as prescribed.

CRITICAL THINKING EXERCISES

1 **pq** A 56-year-old woman is at high risk for hepatitis B and C due to a history of IV drug abuse. What laboratory testing is likely to be done first for this patient? If laboratory testing is positive for either or both diseases, what invasive and noninvasive testing is warranted next? Describe the education a nurse working with this patient should provide about these tests.

2 **ebp** A 68-year-old man is admitted to the hospital with a diagnosis of ESLD with hepatic encephalopathy. What is the evidence base for meeting the nutritional needs of this patient? What are the most appropriate caloric and protein intake recommendations? Identify the criteria used to evaluate the strength of the evidence for the treatment practices you have identified.

3 A 66-year-old man underwent an orthotopic liver transplant for decompensated cirrhosis. He is placed on an immunosuppressant regimen including corticosteroids, mycophenolate mofetil, and tacrolimus. On day 10 postoperatively, he develops an acute change in mental status with confusion and severe extremity tremors. As this patient's nurse, you are in attendance when the patient appears to have a generalized clonic seizure. Identify the priorities, approach, and techniques you would use to provide immediate interventions for this patient. What are your concerns regarding the potential causes of these neurologic abnormalities? What testing would you anticipate? Could his medication regimen have a role in the symptomatology? What laboratory testing would be important in identifying a cause for the seizure?

4 ebp A 44-year-old woman with obesity is diagnosed with NAFLD and is symptomatic with jaundice and fatigue. What are the best risk reduction tactics for this patient? How should the nurse prepare and educate the patient to achieve specific evidence-based management goals and potentially control the disease?

REFERENCES

*Asterisk indicates nursing research.

Books

Alldredge, B. K., Corelli, R. L., Ernst, M. E., et al., (Eds.). (2013). *Koda-Kimble & Young's applied therapeutics: The clinical use of drugs.* Philadelphia, PA: Lippincott Williams & Wilkins

Bickley, L. S. (2017). *Bates' guide to physical examination and history taking* (12th ed.). Philadelphia, PA: Lippincott Williams & Wilkins.

Bope, E. T., & Kellerman, R. D. (Eds.). (2015). *Conn's current therapy.* Philadelphia, PA: Saunders.

Doherty, G. (2015). *Current diagnosis and treatment: Surgery* (14th ed.). New York: McGraw-Hill.

Feldman, M., Friedman, L. S., & Brandt, L. J. (2015). *Sleisinger & Fordtran's gastrointestinal & liver disease* (10th ed.). Philadelphia, PA: Saunders Elsevier.

Ferri, F. F. (Ed.). (2014). *Practical guide to the care of the medical patient* (9th ed.). Philadelphia, PA: Mosby Elsevier.

Goldman, L., & Schafer, A. I. (2015). *Goldman's Cecil medicine* (25th ed.). Philadelphia, PA: Saunders Elsevier.

Greenberger, N. J., Blumberg, R. S., & Burakoff, R. (Eds.). (2015). *Current diagnosis and treatment: Gastroenterology, hepatology & endoscopy.* New York: McGraw-Hill.

Grossman, S. C., & Porth, C. M. (2014). *Pathophysiology: Concepts of altered health states* (9th ed.). Philadelphia, PA: Lippincott Williams & Wilkins.

Hall, J. E. (2015). *Guyton & Hall textbook of medical physiology* (13th ed.). Philadelphia, PA: Saunders Elsevier.

Kumar, V., Abbas, A. K., Fausto, N., et al. (2014). *Robbins and Cotran pathologic basis of disease* (9th ed.). Philadelphia, PA: Saunders Elsevier.

Lee, S. S., & Moreau, R. (2015). *Cirrhosis: A practical guide to management* (1st ed.). Hoboken, NJ: John Wiley & Sons, Ltd.

Mandell, G. L., Bennett, J. E., & Dolin, R. (2014). *Mandell, Douglas and Bennett's principles and practice of infectious diseases* (8th ed.). Philadelphia, PA: Elsevier.

Mueller, C. M. (2012). *The A.S.P.E.N. adult nutrition support core curriculum* (2nd ed.). Silver Spring, MD: American Society for Parenteral and Enteral Nutrition.

Papadakis, M. A., & McPhee, S. J. (Eds.). (2016). *Current medical diagnosis and treatment* (55th ed.). New York: McGraw-Hill.

Sherlock, S., & Dooley, J. (2002). *Diseases of the liver and biliary system* (11th ed.). Oxford, UK: Blackwell Scientific.

Townsend, C. M., Beauchamp, R. D., Evers, B. M., et al. (2016). *Sabiston's textbook of surgery: The biological basis of modern surgical practice.* Philadelphia, PA: Elsevier.

Weber, J., & Kelley, J. (2009). *Health assessment in nursing* (4th ed.). Philadelphia, PA: Lippincott, Williams & Wilkins.

Weber, J., & Kelley, J. (2014). *Health assessment in nursing* (5th ed.). Philadelphia, PA: Lippincott, Williams & Wilkins.

Yarbro, C. H., Wujcik, D., & Gobel, B. H. (2011). *Cancer nursing: Principles & practice* (7th ed.). Burlington, MA: Jones & Bartlett.

Journals and Electronic Documents

Abraldes, J. G., Sarlieve, P., & Tandon, P. Measurement of portal pressure. (2014). *Clinics in Liver Disease, 18*(4), 779–792.

American Association for the Study of Liver Diseases Society of America, International Antiviral Society-USA. (2014). Recommendations for testing, managing and treating hepatitis C. Alexandria, VA. Retrieved on 12/1/2015 at: www.hcvguidelines.org.

Banares, R., Catalina, M. V., & Vaquero, J. (2014). Molecular adsorbent recirculating system and bioartificial devices for liver failure. *Clinics in Liver Disease, 18*(2014), 945–956.

Barrera, F., Zuniga, P., & Arrese, M. (2015). Prediction of esophageal variceal bleeding in liver cirrhosis: Is there a role for hemostatic factors? *Seminars in Thrombosis and Hemostasis, 41*(05), 481–487.

Bloom, S., Kemp, W., & Lubel, J. (2015). Portal hypertension: Pathophysiology, diagnosis and management. *Internal Medicine Journal, 45*(1), 16–26.

Bonder, A., Tapper, E. B., & Afdhal, N. H. (2015). Contemporary assessment of hepatic fibrosis. *Clinics in Liver Disease, 19*(2015), 123–134.

Cameron, A. M. (2015). Screening for viral hepatitis and hepatocellular carcinoma. *Surgical Clinics of North America, 95*(5), 1013–1021.

Centers for Disease Control and Prevention (CDC), Division of Viral Hepatitis. (2013). *Viral hepatitis surveillance—United States, 2013.* Retrieved on 12/1/2015 at: www.cdc.gov/hepatitis/Statistics/2010 Surveillance/index.htm

Chan, S. L., Wong, V. W. S., Qin, S., et al. (2016). Infection and cancer: The case of hepatitis B. *Journal of Clinical Oncology, 34*(1), 83–91.

Chen, R. P., Ge, X. J. Z., Huang, Z. M., et al. (2014). Prophylactic use of transjugular intrahepatic portosystemic shunt aids in treatment of refractory ascites. *Journal of Clinical Gastroenterology, 48*(3), 290–299.

Cholongitas, E., Tziomalos, K., & Pipili, C. (2015). Management of patients with hepatitis B in special populations. *World Journal of Gastroenterology, 21*(6), 1738–1748.

Dan, C., Moses-Eisenstein, M., & Valdiserri, R. O. (2015). Viral hepatitis: New U.S screening recommendations, assessment tools, and treatments. *American Journal of Nursing, 115*(7), 26–36.

Ellul, M. A., Gholkar, S. A., & Cross, T. J. (2015). Hepatic encephalopathy due to liver cirrhosis. *British Medical Journal, 351*, 26–30.

European Association for the Study of the Liver. (2013). Too much drinking, weight may harm liver. *News release*, April 25, 2013. Retrieved on 11/28/2015 at: www.easl.eu

*Fabrellas, N., Alemany, M., Urquizu, M., et al. (2013). Using transient elastography to detect chronic liver diseases in a primary care nurse consultancy. *Nursing Research, 62*(6), 450–455.

Fialla, A. D., Israelsen, M., Hamberg, O., Kraq, A., & Gluud, L. L. (2015). Nutritional therapy in cirrhosis or alcoholic hepatitis: A systematic review and meta-analysis. *Liver International, 35*(9), 2072–2078.

Fox, R. K. (2014). When to consider liver transplantation during the management of chronic liver disease. *Medical Clinics of North America, 98*(2014), 153–168.

Ghaziani, T., Sendi, H., Shahraz, S., et al. (2014). Hepatitis B and liver transplantation: Molecular and clinical features that influence recurrence and outcome. *World Journal of Gastroenterology, 20*(39), 14142–14155.

Gotthardt, D. N., Bruns, H., Weiss, K. H. et al., (2014). Current strategies for immunosuppression following liver transplantation. *Langenbeck's Archives of Surgery, 399*(8), 981–988.

Govan, L., Wu, O., Xin, Y., et al. (2015). Comparative effectiveness of antiviral treatment for hepatitis B: A systematic review and Bayesian network meta-analysis. *European Journal of Gastroenterology and Hepatology, 27*(8), 882–894.

James, J., & Liou, I. W. (2015). Comprehensive care of patients with chronic liver disease. *Medical Clinics of North America, 99*(2015), 913–933.

Karvellas, C. J., Durand, F., & Nadim, M. K. (2015). Acute kidney injury in cirrhosis. *Critical Care Clinics, 31*(4) 737–750.

Kathpalia, P., & Ahn, J. (2015). Assessment of jaundice in the hospitalized patient. *Clinics in Liver Disease, 19*(1), 155–170.

Lancaster, E. M., Hiatt, J. R., & Zarrinpar, A. (2015). Acetaminophen hepatotoxicity: An updated review. *Archives of Toxicology, 89*(2), 193–199.

Lardiere-Deguelte, S., Ragot, E., Amroun, K., et al. (2015). Hepatic abscess: Diagnosis and management. *Journal of Visceral Surgery, 152*(4), 231–243.

Lee, S. G. (2015). A complete treatment of adult living donor liver transplantation: A review of surgical technique and current challenges to expand indication of patients. *American Journal of Transplantation, 15*(1), 17–38.

LeFevre, M. L., U.S. Preventive Services Task Force. (2014). Screening for hepatitis B virus infection in nonpregnant adolescents and adults: U.S. Preventive Services Task Force recommendation statement. *Annals of Internal Medicine, 16*(1), 58–66.

Liou, I. W. (2014). Management of end-stage liver disease. *Medical Clinics of North America, 98*(2014), 119–152.

Madrigal-Santillan, E., Madrigal-Bujaidair, E., Alvarez-Gonzalez, I., et al. (2014). Review of natural products with hepatoprotective effects. *World Journal of Gastroenterology, 20*(40), 14787–14804.

Mastron, J. K., Siveen, K. S., Sethi, G., et al. (2015). Silymarin and hepatocellular carcinoma: A systematic, comprehensive and critical review. *Anti-Cancer Drugs, 26*(5), 475–486.

McMahon, B. J. (2014). Chronic hepatitis B virus infection. *Medical Clinics of North America, 98*(2014), 39–54.

Moyer, V. A., U.S. Preventive Services Task Force. (2013). Screening for hepatitis C virus infection in adults: U.S. Preventive Services Task Force recommendation statement. *Annals of Internal Medicine, 159*(5), 349–357.

Nusrat, S., Khan, M. S., Fazili, J., & Madhoun, M. T. (2014). Cirrhosis and its complications: Evidence-based treatment. *World Journal of Gastroenterology, 20*(18), 5442–5460.

Organ Procurement and Transplant Network (OPTN): U.S. Department of Health and Human Services (HHS). (2016). *Split versus whole liver transplantation.* Retrieved on 12/3/2016 at: optn.transplant.hrsa.gov/resources/ethics/split-versus-whole-liver-transplantation

O'Shea, R. S., Dasarathy, S., McCullough, A. J., & the Practice Guideline Committee of the American Association for the Study of Liver Diseases and the Practice Parameters Committee of the American College of Gastroenterology. (2010). Alcoholic liver disease. *Hepatology, 51*(1), 307–328.

Poordad, F. F. (2015). Presentation and complications associated with cirrhosis of the liver. *Current Medical Research & Opinion, 31*(5), 925–937.

Romero-Gomez, M., Mantagnese, S., & Jalan, R. (2015). Hepatic encephalopathy in patients with acute decompensation of cirrhosis and acute-on-chronic liver failure. *Journal of Hepatology, 62*(2), 437–667.

Rude, M. K., & Crippen, J. S. (2015). Liver transplantation for hepatocellular carcinoma. *Current Gastroenterology Reports, 17*(3), 11–15.

Salgia, R., & Singal, A. G. (2014). Hepatocellular carcinoma and other liver lesions. *Medical Clinics of North America, 98*(2014), 103–118.

Satapathy, S. K., & Sanyal, A. J. (2014). Nonendoscopic management strategies for acute esophagogastric variceal bleeding. *Gastroenterology Clinics of North America, 43*(4), 819–833.

Siddiqui, M. S., & Stravitz, R. T. (2014). Intensive care unit management of patients with liver failure. *Clinics in Liver Disease, 18*(2014), 957–978.

Singanayagam, A., & Bernal, W. (2015). Update on acute liver failure. *Current Opinion in Critical Care, 21*(2), 134–141.

Tripathi, D., & Hayes, P. C. (2014). Beta-blockers in portal hypertension: New developments and controversies. *Liver International, 34*(5), 655–667.

Whitehouse, T., & Wendon, J. (2013). Acute liver failure. *Best Practice & Research in Clinical Gastroenterology, 27*(5), 757–769.

Wong, C. J., & Pagalilauan, G. (2015). Primary care of the solid organ transplant recipient. *Medical Clinics of North America, 99*(2015), 1075–1103.

Woreta, T. A., & Alqahtani, S. A. (2014). Evaluation of abnormal liver tests. *Medical Clinics of North America, 98*(1), 1–16.

*Wu, L. J., Wu, M. S., Lien, G. S., et al. (2012). Fatigue and physical activity levels in patients with liver cirrhosis. *Journal of Clinical Nursing, 21*(1), 129–138.

Resources

Al-Anon Family Groups Headquarters, www.al-anon.alateen.org

Alcoholics Anonymous World Services (AAWS), www.aa.org

American Association for the Study of Liver Diseases (AASLD), www.aasld.org

American College of Gastroenterology (ACG), www.acg.gi.org

American Liver Foundation (ALF), www.liverfoundation.org

Hepatitis Foundation International (HFI), www.hepfi.org

National Council on Alcoholism and Drug Dependence (NCADD), www.ncadd.org

National Digestive Diseases Information Clearinghouse (NDDIC), www.digestive.niddk.nih.gov

National Institute on Alcohol Abuse and Alcoholism (NIAAA), www.niaaa.nih.gov

United Network for Organ Sharing (UNOS), www.unos.org

50

Assessment and Management of Patients With Biliary Disorders

LEARNING OBJECTIVES

On completion of this chapter, the learner will be able to:

1 Identify the structure and function of the biliary tract and pancreas.
2 Describe the pathophysiology, clinical manifestations, and medical management of cholelithiasis.
3 Use the nursing process as a framework for care of patients with cholelithiasis and those undergoing laparoscopic or open cholecystectomy.

4 Differentiate between acute and chronic pancreatitis.
5 Apply the nursing process as a framework for care of patients with acute pancreatitis.
6 Explain the nutritional and metabolic effects of surgical treatment of tumors of the pancreas.

GLOSSARY

amylase: pancreatic enzyme; aids in the digestion of carbohydrates
cholecystectomy: removal of the gallbladder
cholecystitis: inflammation of the gallbladder which can be acute or chronic
cholecystojejunostomy: anastomosis of the jejunum to the gallbladder to divert bile flow
cholecystokinin (CCK): hormone; major stimulus for digestive enzyme secretion; stimulates contraction of the gallbladder
cholecystostomy: surgical opening and drainage of the gallbladder
choledocholithiasis: stones in the common bile duct
choledochostomy: opening into the common bile duct
cholelithiasis: calculi in the gallbladder
dissolution therapy: the use of medications to break up/dissolve gallstones
endocrine: secreting internally; hormonal secretion of a ductless gland

endoscopic retrograde cholangiopancreatography (ERCP): procedure using fiberoptic technology to visualize the biliary system
exocrine: secreting externally; hormonal secretion from excretory ducts
lipase: pancreatic enzyme; aids in the digestion of fats
lithotripsy: disintegration of gallstones by shock waves
pancreatitis: inflammation of the pancreas; may be acute or chronic
secretin: hormone responsible for stimulating bicarbonate secretion from the pancreas; also used as an aid in diagnosing pancreatic exocrine disease
steatorrhea: frothy, foul-smelling stools with a high fat content; results from impaired digestion of proteins and fats due to a lack of pancreatic juice in the intestine
trypsin: pancreatic enzyme; aids in the digestion of proteins
Zollinger–Ellison syndrome: hypersecretion of gastric acid that produces peptic ulcers as a result of a non–beta-cell tumor of the pancreatic islets

Disorders of the biliary tract and pancreas are common and include gallbladder stones and pancreatic dysfunction. An understanding of the structure and function of the biliary tract and pancreas is essential, along with an understanding of how biliary tract disorders are closely linked with liver disease. Patients with acute or chronic biliary tract or pancreatic disease require care from nurses who are knowledgeable about the diagnostic procedures and interventions that are used in the management of gallbladder and pancreatic disorders.

ANATOMIC AND PHYSIOLOGIC OVERVIEW

The Gallbladder

The gallbladder, a pear-shaped, hollow, saclike organ that is 7.5 to 10 cm (3 to 4 inches) long, lies in a shallow depression

on the inferior surface of the liver, to which it is attached by loose connective tissue. The capacity of the gallbladder is 30 to 50 mL of bile. Its wall is composed largely of smooth muscle. The gallbladder is connected to the common bile duct by the cystic duct (see Fig. 50-1).

The gallbladder functions as a storage depot for bile. Between meals, when the sphincter of Oddi is closed, bile produced by the hepatocytes enters the gallbladder. During storage, a large portion of the water in bile is absorbed through the walls of the gallbladder; thus, bile in the gallbladder is 5 to 10 times more concentrated than that originally secreted by the liver. When food enters the duodenum, the gallbladder contracts and the sphincter of Oddi (located at the junction of the common bile duct with the duodenum) relaxes. Relaxation of this sphincter allows the bile to enter the intestine. This response is mediated by secretion of the hormone **cholecystokinin (CCK)** from the intestinal wall

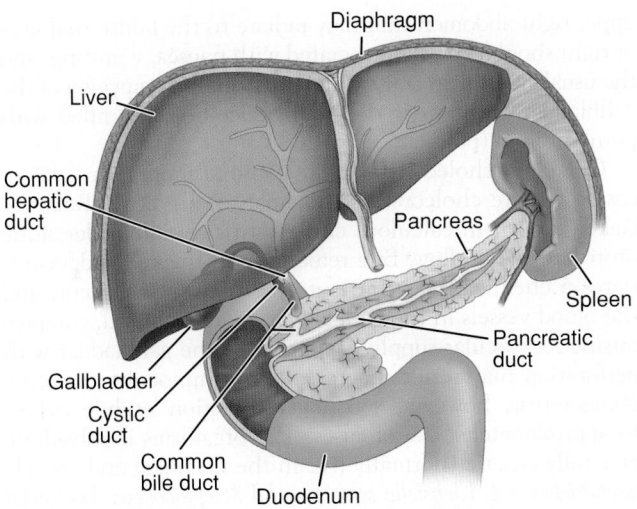

Figure 50-1 • The liver, biliary system, and pancreas.

(Ferri, 2014; Marx, Hockberger, & Walls, 2013). CCK is the major stimulus for digestive enzyme secretion and acts by stimulating the gallbladder to contract.

Bile is composed of water and electrolytes (sodium, potassium, calcium, chloride, and bicarbonate) along with significant amounts of lecithin, fatty acids, cholesterol, bilirubin, and bile salts. The bile salts, together with cholesterol, assist in emulsification of fats in the distal ileum. They are then reabsorbed into the portal blood for return to the liver, after which they are once again excreted into the bile. This pathway from hepatocytes to bile to intestine and back to the hepatocytes is called the *enterohepatic circulation*. Because of this circulation, only a small fraction of the bile salts that enter the intestine are excreted in the feces. This decreases the need for active synthesis of bile salts by the liver cells.

Approximately half of the bilirubin (a pigment derived from the breakdown of red blood cells) is a component of bile. It is converted by the intestinal flora into urobilinogen, which is a highly soluble substance. Urobilinogen is either excreted in the feces or returned to the portal circulation, where it is re-excreted into the bile. About 5% is normally absorbed into the general circulation and then excreted by the kidneys (Feldman, Friedman, & Brandt, 2015; Goldman & Schafer, 2015).

If the flow of bile is impeded (e.g., by gallstones in the bile ducts), bilirubin does not enter the intestine. As a result, blood levels of bilirubin increase. This causes increased renal excretion of urobilinogen, which results from conversion of bilirubin in the small intestine, and decreased excretion in the stool. These changes produce many of the signs and symptoms seen in gallbladder disorders.

The Pancreas

The pancreas is located in the upper abdomen (see Fig. 50-1). It has both **exocrine** (secreting externally; hormonal secretion from excretory ducts) and **endocrine** (secreting internally; hormonal secretion of a ductless gland) functions. The exocrine functions include secretion of pancreatic enzymes into the gastrointestinal (GI) tract through the pancreatic duct. The endocrine functions include secretion of insulin, glucagon, and somatostatin directly into the bloodstream.

The Exocrine Pancreas

The secretions of the exocrine portion of the pancreas are collected in the pancreatic duct, which joins the common bile duct and enters the duodenum at the ampulla of Vater. Surrounding the ampulla is the sphincter of Oddi, which partially controls the rate at which secretions from the pancreas and the gallbladder enter the duodenum.

The secretions of the exocrine pancreas are digestive enzymes high in protein content and an electrolyte-rich fluid. The secretions, which are very alkaline because of their high concentration of sodium bicarbonate, are capable of neutralizing the highly acid gastric juice that enters the duodenum. Pancreatic enzymes include **amylase**, which aids in the digestion of carbohydrates; **trypsin**, which aids in the digestion of proteins; and **lipase**, which aids in the digestion of fats. Other enzymes that promote the breakdown of more complex foodstuffs are also secreted.

Hormones originating in the GI tract stimulate the secretion of these exocrine pancreatic juices. The hormone **secretin** is the major stimulus for increased bicarbonate secretion from the pancreas, and the major stimulus for digestive enzyme secretion is the hormone CCK. The vagus nerve also influences exocrine pancreatic secretion.

The Endocrine Pancreas

The islets of Langerhans, the endocrine part of the pancreas, are collections of cells embedded in the pancreatic tissue. They are composed of alpha, beta, and delta cells. The hormone produced by the beta cells is called *insulin*, the alpha cells secrete glucagon, and the delta cells secrete somatostatin.

Insulin

A major action of insulin is to lower blood glucose by permitting entry of glucose into the cells of the liver, muscle, and other tissues, where it is either stored as glycogen or used for energy. Insulin also promotes the storage of fat in adipose tissue and the synthesis of proteins in various body tissues. In the absence of insulin, glucose cannot enter the cells and is excreted in the urine. This condition, called *diabetes*, can be diagnosed by high levels of glucose in the blood. In diabetes, stored fats and protein are used for energy instead of glucose, causing loss of body mass. Diabetes is discussed in detail in Chapter 51. The level of glucose in the blood normally regulates the rate of insulin secretion from the pancreas (Feldman et al., 2015; Goldman & Schafer, 2014).

Glucagon

The effect of glucagon (opposite to that of insulin) is chiefly to raise the blood glucose by converting glycogen to glucose in the liver. Glucagon is secreted by the pancreas in response to a decrease in the level of blood glucose.

Somatostatin

Somatostatin exerts a hypoglycemic effect by interfering with release of growth hormone from the pituitary and glucagon from the pancreas, both of which tend to raise blood glucose levels.

Endocrine Control of Carbohydrate Metabolism

Glucose required for energy is derived by metabolism of ingested carbohydrates and also from proteins by the process of gluconeogenesis. Glucose can be stored temporarily in the form of glycogen in the liver, muscles, and other tissues. The endocrine system controls the level of blood glucose by regulating the rate at which glucose is synthesized, stored, and moved to and from the bloodstream. Through the action of hormones, blood glucose is normally maintained at less than 100 mg/dL (5.6 mmol/L) (Papadakis & McPhee, 2016). Insulin is the primary hormone that lowers the blood glucose level. Hormones that raise the blood glucose level are glucagon, epinephrine, adrenocorticosteroids, growth hormone, and thyroid hormone.

The endocrine and exocrine functions of the pancreas are interrelated. The major exocrine function is to facilitate digestion through secretion of enzymes into the proximal duodenum. Secretin and CCK are hormones from the GI tract that aid in the digestion of food substances by controlling the secretions of the pancreas. Neural factors also influence pancreatic enzyme secretion. Considerable dysfunction of the pancreas must occur before enzyme secretion decreases and protein and fat digestion becomes impaired. Pancreatic enzyme secretion is normally 1500 to 3000 mL/day (Doherty, 2015; Papadakis & McPhee, 2016).

 ### Gerontologic Considerations

There is little change in the size of the pancreas with age. However, there is an increase in fibrous material and some fatty deposition in the normal pancreas in people older than 70 years. Some localized arteriosclerotic changes occur with age. There is also a decreased rate of pancreatic enzyme secretion (i.e., amylase, lipase, and trypsin) and decreased bicarbonate output in older adults. Some impairment of normal fat absorption occurs with increasing age, possibly because of delayed gastric emptying and pancreatic insufficiency (Eliopoulos, 2018; Papadakis & McPhee, 2016). Decreased calcium absorption may also occur. These changes require care in interpreting diagnostic test results in the normal older patient and in providing dietary counseling.

DISORDERS OF THE GALLBLADDER

Several disorders affect the biliary system and interfere with normal drainage of bile into the duodenum. These disorders include inflammation of the biliary system and carcinoma that obstructs the biliary tree. Gallbladder disease with stones is the most common disorder of the biliary system. Not all occurrences of cholecystitis are related to stones (calculi) in the gallbladder (**cholelithiasis**) or stones in the common bile duct (**choledocholithiasis**). However, most of the 15 million Americans with gallstones have no pain and are unaware of the presence of stones (Bope & Kellerman, 2015).

Cholecystitis

Cholecystitis (inflammation of the gallbladder which can be acute or chronic) causes pain, tenderness, and rigidity of the upper right abdomen that may radiate to the midsternal area or right shoulder and is associated with nausea, vomiting, and the usual signs of an acute inflammation. An empyema of the gallbladder develops if the gallbladder becomes filled with purulent fluid (pus).

Calculous cholecystitis is the cause of more than 90% of cases of acute cholecystitis (Feldman et al., 2015; Rakel & Rakel, 2015). In calculous cholecystitis, a gallbladder stone obstructs bile outflow. Bile remaining in the gallbladder initiates a chemical reaction; autolysis and edema occur; and the blood vessels in the gallbladder are compressed, compromising its vascular supply. Gangrene of the gallbladder with perforation may result. Bacteria play a minor role in acute cholecystitis; however, secondary infection of bile occurs in approximately 50% of cases. The organisms involved are generally enteric (normally live in the GI tract) and include *Escherichia coli*, *Klebsiella* species, and *Streptococcus*. Bacterial contamination is not believed to stimulate the actual onset of acute cholecystitis (Feldman et al., 2015).

Acalculous cholecystitis describes acute gallbladder inflammation in the absence of obstruction by gallstones. Acalculous cholecystitis occurs after major surgical procedures, orthopedic procedures, severe trauma, or burns. Other factors associated with this type of cholecystitis include torsion, cystic duct obstruction, primary bacterial infections of the gallbladder, and multiple blood transfusions. It is speculated that acalculous cholecystitis is caused by alterations in fluids and electrolytes and alterations in regional blood flow in the visceral circulation. Bile stasis (lack of gallbladder contraction) and increased viscosity of the bile are also thought to play a role. The occurrence of acalculous cholecystitis with major surgical procedures or trauma makes its diagnosis difficult (Doherty, 2015).

Cholelithiasis

Calculi, or gallstones, usually form in the gallbladder from the solid constituents of bile; they vary greatly in size, shape, and composition (see Fig. 50-2). They are uncommon in children and young adults but become more prevalent with increasing age. It is estimated that the prevalence of gallstones ranges from 5% to 20% in women between the ages of 20 and 55 years and from 25% to 30% in women older than 50 years. Cholelithiasis affects approximately 50% of women by the age of 70 years.

Pathophysiology

There are two major types of gallstones: those composed predominantly of pigment and those composed primarily of cholesterol. Pigment stones probably form when unconjugated pigments in the bile precipitate to form stones; these stones account for about 10% to 25% of cases in the United States (Feldman et al., 2015; Kumar, Abbas, Fausto, et al., 2014). The risk of developing such stones is increased in patients with cirrhosis, hemolysis, and infections of the biliary tract. Pigment stones cannot be dissolved and must be removed surgically.

Cholesterol stones account for most of the remaining 75% of cases of gallbladder disease in the United States. Cholesterol, which is a normal constituent of bile, is insoluble in

Figure 50-2 • Examples of cholesterol gallstones (*left*) made up of a coalescence of multiple small stones and pigment gallstones (*right*) composed of calcium bilirubinate. From Strayer, D. S., & Rubin, E. (2015). *Rubin's pathology: Clinicopathologic foundations of medicine* (7th ed.). Philadelphia, PA: Lippincott Williams & Wilkins.

water. Its solubility depends on bile acids and lecithin (phospholipids) in bile (Hall, 2015). In gallstone-prone patients, there is decreased bile acid synthesis and increased cholesterol synthesis in the liver, resulting in bile supersaturated with cholesterol, which precipitates out of the bile to form stones (Hall, 2015; Kumar et al., 2014). The cholesterol-saturated bile predisposes to the formation of gallstones and acts as an irritant that produces inflammatory changes in the mucosa of the gallbladder (Feldman et al., 2015; Lee, Keane, & Pereira, 2015).

Two to three times more women than men develop cholesterol stones and gallbladder disease; affected women are usually older than 40 years, multiparous, and obese (Feldman et al., 2015; Goldman & Schafer, 2015; Greenberger, Blumberg, & Burakoff, 2015; Lee et al., 2015). Stone formation is more frequent in people who use oral contraceptives, estrogens, or clofibrate (Atromid-S); these medications are known to increase biliary cholesterol saturation (Feldman et al., 2015; Kumar et al., 2014). The incidence of stone formation increases with age as a result of increased hepatic secretion of cholesterol and decreased bile acid synthesis (Greenberger et al., 2015; Kumar et al., 2014). In addition, there is an increased risk because of malabsorption of bile salts in patients with GI disease or T-tube fistula and in those who have undergone ileal resection or bypass. The incidence is also greater in people with diabetes (see Chart 50-1).

Clinical Manifestations

Gallstones may be silent, producing no pain and only mild GI symptoms. Such stones may be detected incidentally during surgery or evaluation for unrelated problems (Doherty, 2015; Greenberger et al., 2015; Lee et al., 2015).

The patient with gallbladder disease resulting from gallstones may develop two types of symptoms: those due to disease of the gallbladder itself and those due to obstruction of the bile passages by a gallstone. The symptoms may be acute or chronic. Epigastric distress, such as fullness, abdominal distention, and vague pain in the right upper quadrant of the abdomen, may occur. This distress may follow a meal rich in fried or fatty foods (Feldman et al., 2015; Greenberger et al., 2015; Lee et al., 2015).

Pain and Biliary Colic

If a gallstone obstructs the cystic duct, the gallbladder becomes distended, inflamed, and eventually infected

---

Chart 50-1 ⚠ **RISK FACTORS**
Cholelithiasis

- Cystic fibrosis
- Diabetes
- Frequent changes in weight
- Ileal resection or disease
- Low-dose estrogen therapy—carries a small increase in the risk of gallstones
- Obesity
- Rapid weight loss (leads to rapid development of gallstones and high risk of symptomatic disease)
- Treatment with high-dose estrogen (e.g., in prostate cancer)
- Women, especially those who have had multiple pregnancies or who are of Native American or U.S. southwestern Hispanic ethnicity

Adapted from Lee, J. Y. J., Keane, M. G., & Pereira, S. (2015). Diagnosis and treatment of gallstone disease. *Practitioner, 259*(1783), 15–19; Greenberger, N. J., Blumberg, R. S., & Burakoff, R. (Eds.). (2015). *Current diagnosis and treatment: Gastroenterology, hepatology & endoscopy.* New York: McGraw-Hill.

(acute cholecystitis). The patient develops a fever and may have a palpable abdominal mass. The patient may have biliary colic with excruciating upper right abdominal pain that radiates to the back or right shoulder. Biliary colic is usually associated with nausea and vomiting, and it is noticeable several hours after a heavy meal. The patient moves about restlessly, unable to find a comfortable position. In some patients, the pain is constant rather than colicky (Greenberger et al., 2015; Lee et al., 2015; Townsend, Beauchamp, Evers, et al., 2016).

Such a bout of biliary colic is caused by contraction of the gallbladder, which cannot release bile because of obstruction by the stone. When distended, the fundus of the gallbladder comes in contact with the abdominal wall in the region of the right 9th and 10th costal cartilages. This produces marked tenderness in the right upper quadrant on deep inspiration and prevents full inspiratory excursion.

The pain of acute cholecystitis may be so severe that analgesic medications are required. The use of morphine has traditionally been avoided because of concern that it could cause spasm of the sphincter of Oddi, and meperidine (Demerol) has been used instead. This is controversial, because morphine is the preferred analgesic agent for management of acute pain, and some metabolites of meperidine are toxic to the central nervous system (CNS). Furthermore, all opioids stimulate the sphincter of Oddi to some degree (Emmanuel & Lee, 2014; Papadakis & McPhee, 2016).

If the gallstone is dislodged and no longer obstructs the cystic duct, the gallbladder drains and the inflammatory process subsides after a relatively short time. If the gallstone continues to obstruct the duct, abscess, necrosis, and perforation with generalized peritonitis may result.

Jaundice

Jaundice occurs in a few patients with gallbladder disease, usually with obstruction of the common bile duct. The bile, which is no longer carried to the duodenum, is absorbed by the blood and gives the skin and mucous membranes a yellow color. This is frequently accompanied by marked pruritus (itching) of the skin.

Changes in Urine and Stool Color

The excretion of the bile pigments by the kidneys gives the urine a very dark color. The feces, no longer colored with bile pigments, are grayish (like putty) or clay colored.

Vitamin Deficiency

Obstruction of bile flow interferes with absorption of the fat-soluble vitamins A, D, E, and K. Patients may exhibit deficiencies of these vitamins if biliary obstruction has been prolonged. For example, a patient may have bleeding caused by vitamin K deficiency (vitamin K is necessary for normal blood clotting).

Assessment and Diagnostic Findings

A wide range of diagnostic studies may be performed in patients with biliary disorders. Table 50-1 identifies various procedures and their diagnostic uses. The nurse should educate the patient about the purpose, what to expect, and any possible side effects related to these examinations prior to testing. The nurse should note trends in results because they

TABLE 50-1 Studies Used in the Diagnosis of Biliary Tract and Pancreatic Disease

Studies	Diagnostic Uses
Magnetic resonance cholangiopancreatography (MRCP)	Visualizes the biliary tree and capable of detecting biliary tract obstruction
Cholecystogram, cholangiogram	Visualize gallbladder and bile duct
Celiac axis arteriography	Visualize liver and pancreas
Laparoscopy	Visualize anterior surface of liver, gallbladder, and mesentery through a trocar
Ultrasonography	Show size of abdominal organs and presence of masses
Helical computed tomography and magnetic resonance imaging	Detect neoplasms; diagnose cysts, pseudocysts, abscess, and hematomas; determine severity of pancreatitis based on the presence of necrosis and/or peripancreatic fluid collections
Endoscopic retrograde cholangiopancreatography	Visualize biliary structures and pancreas via endoscopy
Endoscopic ultrasound	Identify small tumors and facilitate fine-needle aspiration biopsy of tumors or lymph nodes for diagnosis
Serum alkaline phosphatase	In absence of bone disease, to measure biliary tract obstruction
Gamma-glutamyl, gamma-glutamyl transpeptidase, lactate dehydrogenase	Markers for biliary stasis; also elevated in alcohol abuse
Cholesterol levels	Elevated in biliary obstruction; decreased in parenchymal liver disease

provide information about disease progression as well as the patient's response to therapy.

Abdominal X-Ray

If gallbladder disease is suspected, an abdominal x-ray may be obtained to exclude other causes of symptoms. However, only 10% to 15% of gallstones are calcified sufficiently to be visible on such x-ray studies (Rakel & Rakel, 2015; Townsend et al., 2016).

Ultrasonography

Ultrasonography is the diagnostic procedure of choice because it is rapid and accurate and can be used in patients with liver dysfunction and jaundice. It does not expose patients to ionizing radiation. The procedure is most accurate if the patient fasts overnight so that the gallbladder is distended. Ultrasonography can detect calculi in the gallbladder or a dilated common bile duct with 90% accuracy (Rakel & Rakel, 2015; Townsend et al., 2016).

Radionuclide Imaging or Cholescintigraphy

Cholescintigraphy is used successfully in the diagnosis of acute cholecystitis or blockage of a bile duct (Goldman & Schafer, 2015; Greenberger et al., 2015; Lee et al., 2015; Rakel & Rakel, 2015). During this procedure, a radioactive agent is administered intravenously (IV) which is taken up by the hepatocytes and excreted rapidly through the biliary tract.

The biliary tract is then scanned, and images of the gallbladder and biliary tract are obtained. This test is more expensive than ultrasonography, takes longer to perform, and exposes the patient to radiation. It is often used when ultrasonography is not conclusive, such as in acalculous cholecystitis (Feldman et al., 2015; Goldman & Schafer, 2015; Greenberger et al., 2015; Lee et al., 2015).

Oral Cholecystography

Oral cholecystography is used if ultrasound equipment is not available or if the ultrasound results are inconclusive. This study may be performed to detect gallstones and to assess the ability of the gallbladder to fill, concentrate its contents, contract, and empty. If the patient is not allergic to iodine or seafood, an iodide-containing contrast agent that is excreted by the liver and concentrated in the gallbladder is given 10 to 12 hours before the x-ray study (Feldman et al., 2015; Marx et al., 2013). The normal gallbladder fills with this radiopaque substance. If gallstones are present, they appear as shadows on the x-ray image.

Oral cholecystography may be used as part of the evaluation of patients who have been treated with gallstone **dissolution therapy** (the use of medications to break up/dissolve gallstones) or **lithotripsy** (disintegration of gallstones by shock waves).

Endoscopic Retrograde Cholangiopancreatography

Endoscopic retrograde cholangiopancreatography (ERCP) permits direct visualization of structures that previously could be seen only during laparotomy. This procedure examines the hepatobiliary system via a side-viewing flexible fiberoptic endoscope inserted through the esophagus to the descending duodenum (see Fig. 50-3). Multiple position changes are required to pass the endoscope during the procedure, beginning in the left semiprone position.

Fluoroscopy and multiple x-rays are used during ERCP to evaluate the presence and location of ductal stones. Careful insertion of a catheter through the endoscope into the common bile duct is the most important step in sphincterotomy (division of the muscles of the biliary sphincter) for gallstone extraction via this technique (see later discussion). ERCP is not recommended for the evaluation of suspected common bile duct stones but can be used to treat confirmed choledocholithiasis before or during laparoscopic cholecystectomy (Lee et al., 2015).

Nursing Implications

An ERCP requires a cooperative patient to permit insertion of the endoscope without damage to the GI tract structures, including the biliary tree. Before the procedure, the patient is educated about the procedure and their role in it. The patient takes nothing by mouth for several hours before the procedure. Moderate sedation is used, and the sedated patient must be monitored closely. It may be necessary to administer medications, such as glucagon or anticholinergic agents, to make cannulation easier by decreasing duodenal peristalsis. The nurse observes closely for signs of respiratory and CNS depression, hypotension, oversedation, and vomiting (if glucagon is given). During ERCP, the nurse monitors IV fluids, administers medications, and positions the patient. After the procedure,

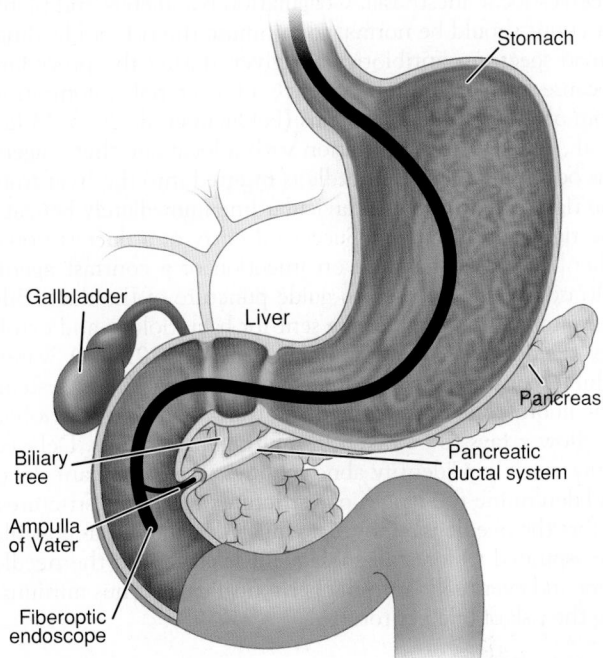

Figure 50-3 • Endoscopic retrograde cholangiopancreatography. A fiberoptic duodenoscope, with side-viewing apparatus, is inserted into the duodenum. The ampulla of Vater is catheterized, and the biliary tree is injected with contrast agent. The pancreatic ductal system is also assessed, if indicated. This procedure is of special value in visualizing neoplasms of the ampulla area and extracting a biopsy specimen.

the nurse monitors the patient's condition, observing vital signs and assessing for signs of perforation or infection. The nurse also monitors the patient for side effects of any medications received during the procedure and for return of the gag and cough reflexes after the use of local anesthetic agents.

Percutaneous Transhepatic Cholangiography

Percutaneous transhepatic cholangiography (PTC) is rarely used for diagnostic purposes alone due to the multitude of other less invasive and reliable imaging studies. PTC is reserved for those patients in whom an ERCP may be unsafe due to previous surgery involving the biliary tract (Doherty, 2015; Feldman et al., 2015). The use of PTC has mainly been replaced by ERCP and magnetic resonance cholangiopancreatography (MRCP). PTC involves the injection of dye directly into the biliary tract. Because of the relatively large concentration of dye that is introduced into the biliary system, including the hepatic ducts within the liver, the entire length of the common bile duct, the cystic duct, and the gallbladder is outlined clearly.

This procedure can be carried out even in the presence of liver dysfunction and jaundice. It is useful for (1) distinguishing jaundice caused by liver disease (hepatocellular jaundice) from that caused by biliary obstruction, (2) investigating the GI symptoms of a patient whose gallbladder has been removed, (3) locating stones within the bile ducts, and (4) diagnosing cancer involving the biliary system (Miller, Eriksson, Fleisher, et al., 2014).

This sterile procedure is performed under moderate sedation on a patient who has been fasting; the patient also receives local anesthesia. Coagulation parameters and plate-let count should be normal to minimize the risk of bleeding. Broad-spectrum antibiotics are given during the procedure because of the high prevalence of bacterial colonization from obstructed biliary systems (Feldman et al., 2015; Miller et al., 2014). After infiltration with a local anesthetic agent has occurred, a flexible needle is inserted into the liver from the right side in the midclavicular line immediately beneath the right costal margin. Successful entry of a duct is noted when bile is aspirated or on injection of a contrast agent. Ultrasound can be used to guide puncture of the duct. Bile is aspirated, and samples are sent for bacteriology and cytol-ogy (Feldman et al., 2015; Rakel & Rakel, 2015). A water-soluble contrast agent is injected to fill the biliary system. The fluoroscopy table is tilted and the patient is repositioned to allow x-rays to be taken in multiple projections. Delayed x-ray views can identify abnormalities of more distant ducts and determine the length of a stricture or multiple strictures. Before the needle is removed, as much dye and bile as possible are aspirated to forestall subsequent leakage into the needle tract and eventually into the peritoneal cavity, thus minimiz-ing the risk of bile peritonitis.

Nursing Implications

Although the complication rate after this procedure is low, the nurse must closely observe the patient for symptoms of bleed-ing, peritonitis, and sepsis. The nurse assesses the patient for pain and indications of these complications and reports them promptly to the primary provider, takes measures to reassure the patient, and ensures patient comfort. Antibiotic agents are often prescribed to minimize the risk of sepsis and septic shock.

Medical Management

The major objectives of medical therapy are to reduce the incidence of acute episodes of gallbladder pain and chole-cystitis by supportive and dietary management and, if pos-sible, to remove the cause of cholecystitis by pharmacologic therapy, endoscopic procedures, or surgical intervention. Although nonsurgical procedures eliminate risks associated with surgery, these approaches are associated with persistent symptoms or recurrent stone formation. Most of the non-surgical approaches, including lithotripsy and dissolution of gallstones, provide only temporary solutions to gallstone problems and are infrequently used in the United States. In some instances, other treatment approaches may be indi-cated; these are described later.

Removal of the gallbladder (**cholecystectomy**) through traditional surgical approaches has largely been replaced by laparoscopic cholecystectomy (removal of the gallbladder through a small incision through the umbilicus). As a result, surgical risks have decreased, along with the length of hospi-tal stay and the long recovery period required after standard surgical cholecystectomy. In relatively rare instances, a stan-dard surgical procedure may be necessary.

Nutritional and Supportive Therapy

Approximately 80% of the patients with acute gallbladder inflammation achieve remission with rest, IV fluids, naso-gastric suction, analgesia, and antibiotic agents. Unless the patient's condition deteriorates, surgical intervention is delayed just until the acute symptoms subside (usually within a few days). At this time, the patient undergoes a laparoscopic cholecystectomy (Goldman & Schafer, 2015; Michetti, Griffen, Tran, et al., 2015).

The diet immediately after an episode is usually low-fat liquids. These can include powdered supplements high in protein and carbohydrate stirred into skim milk. Cooked fruits, rice or tapioca, lean meats, mashed potatoes, non–gas-forming vegetables, bread, coffee, or tea may be added as tolerated. The patient should avoid eggs, cream, pork, fried foods, cheese, rich dressings, gas-forming vegetables, and alcohol. It is important to remind the patient that fatty foods may induce an episode of cholecystitis. Dietary management may be the major mode of therapy in patients who have had only dietary intolerance to fatty foods and vague GI symp-toms (Rakel & Rakel, 2015).

Pharmacologic Therapy

Ursodeoxycholic acid (UDCA [Urso, Actigall]) and che-nodeoxycholic acid (chenodiol or CDCA [Chenix]) have been used to dissolve small, radiolucent gallstones com-posed primarily of cholesterol (Comerford, 2015). UDCA has fewer side effects than chenodiol and can be given in smaller doses to achieve the same effect. It acts by inhib-iting the synthesis and secretion of cholesterol, thereby desaturating bile. Treatment with UDCA can reduce the size of existing stones, dissolve small stones, and prevent new stones from forming. Six to 12 months of therapy is required in many patients to dissolve stones, and monitor-ing of the patient for recurrence of symptoms or the occur-rence of side effects (e.g., GI symptoms, pruritus, headache) is required during this time. The effective dose of medica-tion depends on body weight. This method of treatment is generally indicated for patients who refuse surgery or for whom surgery is contraindicated. The success rate of this therapy is low as the recurrence following it is high (Lee et al., 2015).

Patients with significant, frequent symptoms, cystic duct occlusion, or pigment stones are not candidates for pharma-cologic therapy. Laparoscopic or open cholecystectomy is more appropriate for symptomatic patients with acceptable operative risk (Lee et al., 2015).

Nonsurgical Removal of Gallstones
Dissolving Gallstones

Several methods have been used to dissolve gallstones by infusion of a solvent (mono-octanoin or methyl tertiary butyl ether [MTBE]) into the gallbladder. The solvent can be infused through the following routes: through a tube or catheter inserted percutaneously directly into the gallbladder, through a tube or drain inserted through a T-tube tract to dissolve stones not removed at the time of surgery, endoscopi-cally with ERCP; or via a transnasal biliary catheter (a rarely used procedure due to its lack of success, potential side effects, and rates of recurrence rate of up to 50% (Lee et al., 2015; Townsend et al., 2016).

Laparoscopic cholecystectomy is the standard for man-agement. Dissolution therapies are used for those patients who may not be candidates for the procedure due to safety concerns regarding general anesthesia (Lee et al., 2015; Townsend et al., 2016).

A T-tube tract to remove stone

B Removal of stone with basket to catheter threaded through T-tube tract

C ERCP endoscope inserted into duodenum

D Papillotome inserted into common bile duct

E Enlarging opening of sphincter of Oddi

F Retrieval and removal of stone with basket inserted through endoscope

Figure 50-4 • A–F. Nonsurgical techniques for removing gallstones.

Stone Removal by Instrumentation

Several nonsurgical methods are used to remove stones that were not removed at the time of cholecystectomy or have become lodged in the common bile duct (see Fig. 50-4A,B). A catheter and instrument with a basket attached are threaded through the T-tube tract or fistula formed at the time of T-tube insertion; the basket is used to retrieve and remove the stones lodged in the common bile duct.

A second procedure involves the use of the ERCP endoscope (see Fig. 50-4C). After the endoscope is inserted, a cutting instrument is passed through the endoscope into the ampulla of Vater of the common bile duct. It may be used to cut the submucosal fibers, or papilla, of the sphincter of Oddi, enlarging the opening, which may allow the lodged stones to pass spontaneously into the duodenum. Another instrument with a small basket or balloon at its tip may be inserted through the endoscope to retrieve the stones (see Fig. 50-4D–F). The patient is observed closely for bleeding, perforation, and the development of pancreatitis (see later discussion) or sepsis.

The ERCP procedure is particularly useful in diagnosis and treatment of patients who have symptoms after biliary tract surgery, patients with intact gallbladders, and patients for whom surgery is particularly hazardous.

Intracorporeal Lithotripsy

Stones in the gallbladder or common bile duct may be fragmented by means of laser pulse technology. A laser pulse is directed under fluoroscopic guidance with the use of devices that can distinguish between stones and tissue. The laser pulse produces rapid expansion and disintegration of plasma on the stone surface, resulting in a mechanical shock wave. Electrohydraulic lithotripsy uses a probe with two electrodes that deliver electric sparks in rapid pulses, creating expansion of the liquid environment surrounding the gallstones. This results in pressure waves that cause stones to fragment. This technique can be used percutaneously with a basket or balloon catheter system or by direct visualization through an endoscope. Repeated procedures may be necessary because of stone size, local anatomy, bleeding, or technical difficulty. A nasobiliary tube can be inserted to allow for biliary decompression and to prevent stone impaction in the common bile duct. This approach allows time for improvement in the patient's clinical condition until gallstones are cleared endoscopically, percutaneously, or surgically.

Extracorporeal Shock Wave Lithotripsy

Extracorporeal shock wave therapy (lithotripsy or ESWL) has been used for nonsurgical fragmentation of gallstones. Lithotripsy, which is a noninvasive procedure, uses repeated shock waves directed at the gallstones in the gallbladder or common bile duct to fragment the stones. The waves are transmitted to the body through a fluid-filled bag or by immersing the patient in a water bath. After the stones are gradually broken up, the stone fragments can be spontaneously passed from the gallbladder or common bile duct, removed by endoscopy, or dissolved with oral bile acid or solvents. Because the procedure requires no incision and no hospitalization, patients are usually treated as outpatients, but usually several sessions are necessary. This procedure has largely been replaced by laparoscopic cholecystectomy. ESWL is used in some centers for a small percentage of suitable patients (those with common bile duct stones who may not be surgical candidates), sometimes in combination with dissolution therapy (Feldman et al., 2015; Lee et al., 2015; Rakel & Rakel, 2015).

Surgical Management

Surgical treatment of gallbladder disease and gallstones is carried out to relieve persistent symptoms, to remove the cause of biliary colic, and to treat acute cholecystitis. Surgery may be delayed until the patient's symptoms have subsided, or it may be performed as an emergency procedure, if necessitated by the patient's condition.

Preoperative Measures

Chest x-ray, electrocardiogram, and liver function tests may be performed in addition to imaging studies of the gallbladder. Vitamin K may be given if the prothrombin level is low. Nutritional requirements are considered, and, if the nutritional status is suboptimal, it may be necessary to provide IV glucose with protein supplements to aid wound healing and help prevent liver damage.

Patient education for gallbladder surgery is similar to that for any upper abdominal laparotomy or laparoscopy. Instructions and explanations are given before surgery about turning and deep breathing. Postoperative pneumonia and atelectasis can be avoided by deep-breathing exercises, frequent turning, and early ambulation. The patient should be informed that drainage tubes and a nasogastric tube and suction might be required during the immediate postoperative period if an open cholecystectomy is performed.

Laparoscopic Cholecystectomy

Laparoscopic cholecystectomy (see Fig. 50-5) is the standard of therapy for symptomatic gallstones. Approximately 700,000 patients in the United States require surgery each year for removal of the gallbladder, and 80% to 90% of them are candidates for laparoscopic cholecystectomy (Doherty,

2015; Feldman et al., 2015). If the common bile duct is thought to be obstructed by a gallstone, an ERCP with sphincterotomy may be performed to explore the duct before laparoscopy (Goldman & Schafer, 2015; Lee et al., 2015).

Before the procedure, the patient is educated that an open abdominal procedure may be necessary, and general anesthesia is given. Laparoscopic cholecystectomy is performed through a small incision or puncture made through the abdominal wall at the umbilicus. The abdominal cavity is insufflated with carbon dioxide (pneumoperitoneum) to assist in inserting the laparoscope and to aid in visualizing the abdominal structures. The fiberoptic scope is inserted through the small umbilical incision. Several additional punctures or small incisions are made in the abdominal wall to introduce other surgical instruments into the operative field. A camera attached to the laparoscope permits the surgeon to view the intra-abdominal field and biliary system on a television monitor. After the cystic duct is dissected, the common bile duct can be visualized by ultrasound or cholangiography to evaluate the anatomy and identify stones. The cystic artery is dissected free and clipped. The gallbladder is separated from the hepatic bed and removed from the abdominal cavity after bile and small stones are aspirated. Stone forceps also can be used to remove or crush larger stones.

With the laparoscopic procedure, the patient does not experience the paralytic ileus that occurs with open abdominal surgery and has less postoperative abdominal pain. The patient is often discharged from the hospital on the same day of surgery or within 1 or 2 days and resumes full activity and employment within 1 week after the procedure.

Conversion to a traditional abdominal surgical procedure occurs in 2.2% of cases in the United States and 3.6% to

Figure 50-5 • In laparoscopic cholecystectomy (**A**), the surgeon makes four small incisions (less than one half inch each) in the abdomen and inserts a laparoscope with a miniature camera through the umbilical incision (**B**). The camera apparatus displays the gallbladder and adjacent tissues on a screen, allowing the surgeon to visualize the sections of the organ for removal.

8.2% of cases internationally. Conversion to an open procedure occurs if there is inflammation in and around the gallbladder, making safe dissection of the porta hepatis difficult (Feldman et al., 2015). (The porta hepatis is the fissure of the liver where the portal vein and the hepatic artery enter and the hepatic ducts exit the liver.) Careful screening of patients and identification of those at low risk for complications limit the frequency of conversion to an open abdominal procedure. However, with increasing use of laparoscopic procedures, the number of such conversions may increase.

The most serious complication after laparoscopic cholecystectomy is a bile duct injury, which may be identified and corrected at the time of the procedure. Patients with a postoperative bile leak may not develop symptoms until several days after the procedure, and some have an even more prolonged period before injury to the bile duct becomes apparent (Doherty, 2015; Michetti et al., 2015). A bile leak may result in fluid collections, which can usually be managed by endoscopic stent placement. Bile peritonitis, a rare complication, may result in serious illness or death.

Because of the short length of hospital stay with uncomplicated laparoscopic cholecystectomies, it is important to provide patient education about managing postoperative pain and reporting signs and symptoms of intra-abdominal complications, including loss of appetite, vomiting, pain, distention of the abdomen, and temperature elevation. Although recovery from laparoscopic cholecystectomy is rapid, patients are drowsy afterward. The patient must have assistance at home during the first 24 to 48 hours. If pain occurs in the right shoulder or scapular area (from migration of the carbon dioxide used to insufflate the abdominal cavity during the procedure), the nurse may recommend a heating pad for 15 to 20 minutes hourly.

Cholecystectomy

In cholecystectomy, the gallbladder is removed through an abdominal incision (usually right subcostal) after the cystic duct and artery are ligated. The procedure is performed for acute and chronic cholecystitis. In some patients, a drain is placed close to the gallbladder bed and brought out through a puncture wound if there is a bile leak. The drain type is chosen based on the surgeon's preference. A small leak should close spontaneously in a few days, with the drain preventing accumulation of bile. Usually, only a small amount of serosanguineous fluid drains in the initial 24 hours after surgery; afterward, the drain is removed. The drain is typically maintained if there is excess oozing or bile leakage. Insertion of a T-tube into the common bile duct during the open procedure is now uncommon; it is used only in the setting of a complication (i.e., retained common bile duct stone). Bile duct injury is a serious complication of cholecystectomy, but it occurs less frequently than with the laparoscopic approach, which has largely replaced traditional surgical cholecystectomy.

Small-Incision Cholecystectomy

Small-incision cholecystectomy is a surgical procedure in which the gallbladder is removed through a small abdominal incision, as the name implies. If needed, the surgical incision is extended to remove larger gallbladder stones. Drains may or may not be used. The short length hospital stay has been identified as a major advantage of this type of procedure

(Doherty, 2015; Goldman & Schafer, 2015). The procedure is controversial because it limits exposure to all involved biliary structures.

Choledochostomy

Choledochostomy is reserved for the patient with acute cholecystitis who may be too ill to undergo a surgical procedure. This procedure involves making an incision in the common duct, usually for removal of stones. After the stones have been evacuated, a tube is usually inserted into the duct for drainage of bile until edema subsides. This tube is connected to gravity drainage tubing; the patient is monitored closely, and a laparoscopic cholecystectomy is planned for a future date after acute inflammation has resolved.

Surgical Cholecystostomy

Cholecystostomy is performed when the patient's condition precludes more extensive surgery or when an acute inflammatory reaction is severe. The gallbladder is surgically opened, stones and the bile or the purulent drainage are removed, and a drainage tube is secured with a purse-string suture. The drainage tube is connected to a drainage system to prevent bile from leaking around the tube or escaping into the peritoneal cavity. After recovery from the acute episode, the patient may return for subsequent laparoscopic cholecystectomy. Despite its lower risk, surgical cholecystostomy has a high mortality rate (reported to be as high as 10% to 30%) because of the underlying infectious disease process (Feldman et al., 2015; Goldman & Schafer, 2015).

Percutaneous Cholecystostomy

Percutaneous cholecystostomy has been used in the treatment and diagnosis of acute cholecystitis in patients who are poor risks for any surgical procedure or for general anesthesia. This at risk population may include patients with sepsis or severe cardiac, renal, pulmonary, or liver failure (Doherty, 2015; Gurusamy, Rossi & Davidson, 2013; Nikfarjam, Shen, Fink, et al., 2013). Under local anesthesia, a fine needle is inserted through the abdominal wall and liver edge into the gallbladder under the guidance of ultrasound or computed tomography (CT). Bile is aspirated to ensure adequate placement of the needle, and a catheter is inserted into the gallbladder to decompress the biliary tract. Almost immediate relief of pain and resolution of signs and symptoms of sepsis and cholecystitis have been reported with this procedure. Antibiotic agents are given before, during, and after the procedure.

 Gerontologic Considerations

Surgical intervention for disease of the biliary tract is the most common operative procedure performed in the older adult. Cholesterol saturation of bile increases with age because of increased hepatic secretion of cholesterol and decreased bile acid synthesis.

Although the incidence of gallstones increases with age, the older patient may not exhibit the typical symptoms of fever, pain, chills, and jaundice. Symptoms of biliary tract disease in the older adult may be accompanied or preceded by those of septic shock, which include oliguria, hypotension, changes in mental status, tachycardia, and tachypnea.

Although surgery in the older adult presents a risk because of pre-existing associated diseases, the mortality rate from serious complications of biliary tract disease itself is also high. The risk of death and complications is increased in the older patient who undergoes emergency surgery for life-threatening disease of the biliary tract. Despite the presence of chronic illness in many older patients, elective cholecystectomy is usually well tolerated and can be carried out with low risk if expert assessment and care are provided before, during, and after the surgical procedure (Doherty, 2015; Rao, Polanco, Qiu, et al., 2013).

Because of changes in reimbursement for health care expenses, there are fewer elective surgical procedures performed, including cholecystectomies. As a result, patients requiring the procedure are seen in later stages of disease. At the same time, patients undergoing surgery are increasingly older than 60 years and may have complicated acute cholecystitis (de Mestral, Rotstein, Laupacis, et al., 2014). The higher risk of complications and shorter length of hospital stay make it essential that older patients and their family members receive specific information about signs and symptoms of complications and measures to prevent them.

NURSING PROCESS

The Patient Undergoing Surgery for Gallbladder Disease

Assessment

The patient undergoing surgical treatment of gallbladder disease is often admitted to the hospital or same-day surgery unit on the morning of surgery. Preadmission testing is often completed a week or longer before admission. At that time, the nurse educates the patient about the need to avoid smoking, to enhance pulmonary recovery postoperatively, and to avoid respiratory complications. The need to avoid aspirin, nonsteroidal medications, and other agents (over-the-counter medications and herbal remedies) that can alter coagulation and other biochemical processes is also emphasized.

Assessment should focus on the patient's respiratory status. If a traditional surgical approach is planned, the high abdominal incision required during surgery may interfere with full respiratory excursion. The nurse notes a history of smoking, previous respiratory problems, shallow respirations, a persistent or ineffective cough, and the presence of adventitious breath sounds. Nutritional status is evaluated through a dietary history and a general examination performed at the time of preadmission testing. The nurse also reviews previously obtained laboratory results to obtain information about the patient's nutritional status.

Diagnosis

NURSING DIAGNOSES

Based on the assessment data, major postoperative nursing diagnoses may include the following:

- Acute pain and discomfort related to surgical incision
- Impaired gas exchange related to the high abdominal surgical incision (if traditional surgical cholecystectomy was performed)
- Impaired skin integrity related to altered biliary drainage after surgical intervention (if a T-tube was inserted because of retained stones in the common bile duct or another drainage device was employed)

- Imbalanced nutrition: less than body requirements related to inadequate bile secretion
- Deficient knowledge about self-care activities related to incision care, dietary modifications (if needed), medications, and reportable signs or symptoms (e.g., fever, bleeding, vomiting)

COLLABORATIVE PROBLEMS/POTENTIAL COMPLICATIONS

Potential complications may include the following:

- Bleeding
- GI symptoms (may be related to biliary leak or injury to the bowel)

Planning and Goals

The goals for the patient include relief of pain, adequate ventilation, intact skin and improved biliary drainage, optimal nutritional intake, absence of complications, and understanding of self-care routines.

Nursing Interventions

After recovery from anesthesia, the patient is placed in the low Fowler position. Fluids may be administered IV, and nasogastric suction (a nasogastric tube was probably inserted immediately before surgery for a nonlaparoscopic procedure) may be instituted to relieve abdominal distention. Water and other fluids are given within hours after laparoscopic procedures. A soft diet is started after bowel sounds return, which is usually the next day if the laparoscopic approach is used.

RELIEVING PAIN

The location of the subcostal incision in nonlaparoscopic gallbladder surgery often causes the patient to avoid turning and moving, to splint the affected site, and to take shallow breaths to prevent pain. Because full expansion of the lungs and gradually increased activity are necessary to prevent postoperative complications, the nurse administers analgesic agents as prescribed to relieve the pain and to help the patient turn, cough, breathe deeply, and ambulate as indicated. The use of a pillow or binder over the incision may reduce pain during these maneuvers.

IMPROVING RESPIRATORY STATUS

Patients undergoing biliary tract surgery are especially prone to pulmonary complications, as are all patients with upper abdominal incisions. Therefore, the nurse reminds the patient to take deep breaths and cough every hour to expand the lungs fully and prevent atelectasis. The early and consistent use of incentive spirometry also helps improve respiratory function. Early ambulation prevents pulmonary complications as well as other complications, such as venous thromboembolism (VTE) formation. Pulmonary complications are more likely to occur in patients who are older, those who are obese, and those with pre-existing pulmonary disease.

MAINTAINING SKIN INTEGRITY AND PROMOTING BILIARY DRAINAGE

In patients who have undergone a cholecystostomy or choledochostomy, the drainage tube must be connected immediately to a drainage receptacle. The nurse should fasten the tubing to the dressings or to the patient's gown, with enough leeway for the patient to move without dislodging or kinking the tube. Because a drainage system remains attached when the patient is ambulating, the drainage bag may be placed in a bathrobe pocket or fastened so that it is below the waist or common duct level. If a Penrose drain is used, the nurse changes the dressings as required.

After these surgical procedures, the patient is observed for indications of infection, leakage of bile into the peritoneal cavity, and obstruction of bile drainage. If bile is not draining properly, an obstruction is probably causing bile to be forced back into the liver and bloodstream. Because jaundice may result, the nurse should assess the color of the sclerae. The nurse should note and report right upper quadrant abdominal pain, nausea and vomiting, bile drainage around any drainage tube, clay-colored stools, and a change in vital signs.

Bile may continue to drain from the drainage tract in considerable quantities for some time, necessitating frequent changes of the outer dressings and protection of the skin from irritation (bile is corrosive to the skin).

To prevent total loss of bile, the surgeon may want the drainage tube (T-tube) or collection receptacle elevated above the level of the abdomen so that the bile drains externally only if pressure develops in the duct system. Every 24 hours, the nurse measures the bile collected and records the amount, color, and character of the drainage. After several days of drainage, the T-tube may be clamped for 1 hour before and after each meal to deliver bile to the duodenum to aid in digestion (Townsend et al., 2016). Within 7 days to 3 weeks, the drainage tube is removed (Townsend et al., 2016). The patient who goes home with a drainage tube in place requires instruction and reassurance about the function and care of the T-tube (Townsend et al., 2016).

In all patients with biliary drainage, the nurse (or the patient, if at home) observes the color of stools daily. Urine and stool specimens may be sent to the laboratory for examination for bile pigments. In this way, it is possible to determine whether the bile pigment is disappearing from the blood and is draining again into the duodenum. Maintaining a careful record of fluid intake and output is important.

IMPROVING NUTRITIONAL STATUS

The nurse encourages the patient to eat a diet that is low in fats and high in carbohydrates and proteins immediately after surgery. At the time of hospital discharge, there are usually no special dietary instructions other than to maintain a healthy diet and avoid excessive fats. Fat restriction usually is lifted in 4 to 6 weeks, when the biliary ducts dilate to accommodate the volume of bile once held by the gallbladder and when the ampulla of Vater again functions effectively. After this time, when the patient eats fat, adequate bile will be released into the GI tract to emulsify the fats and allow their digestion. This is in contrast to the condition before surgery, when fats may not have been digested completely or adequately and flatulence may have occurred. One purpose of gallbladder surgery is to allow a normal diet.

MONITORING AND MANAGING POTENTIAL COMPLICATIONS

Bleeding may occur as a result of inadvertent puncture or injury to a major blood vessel. Postoperatively, the nurse closely monitors vital signs and inspects the surgical incisions and any drains for bleeding. The nurse also assesses the patient for increased tenderness and rigidity of the abdomen. If these signs and symptoms occur, they are reported to the surgeon. The nurse instructs the patient and family to report any change in the color of stools, because this may indicate complications. GI symptoms, although not common, may occur with manipulation of the intestines during surgery.

After laparoscopic cholecystectomy, the nurse assesses the patient for anorexia, vomiting, pain, abdominal distension, and temperature elevation. These may indicate infection or disruption of the GI tract and should be reported to the surgeon promptly. Because the patient is discharged soon after laparoscopic surgery, the patient and family are instructed verbally and in writing about the importance of reporting these symptoms promptly.

PROMOTING HOME, COMMUNITY-BASED CARE, AND TRANSITIONAL CARE

Educating Patients About Self-Care. The nurse educates the patient about the medications that are prescribed (vitamins, anticholinergic and antispasmodic agents) and their actions. The nurse also informs the patient and family about symptoms that should be reported to the primary provider, including jaundice, dark urine, pale-colored stools, pruritus, and signs of inflammation and infection such as pain or fever.

Some patients report one to three bowel movements a day, which is a result of a continual trickle of bile through the choledochoduodenal junction after cholecystectomy. Usually, such frequency diminishes over a period of a few weeks to several months.

If a patient is discharged from the hospital with a drainage tube still in place, the patient and family need education about its management. The nurse educates them in proper care of the drainage tube and the importance of reporting promptly any changes in the amount or characteristics of drainage. Assistance in securing the appropriate dressings reduces the patient's anxiety about going home with the drain or tube still in place. Chart 50-2 provides additional details about self-care after laparoscopic cholecystectomy.

Continuing and Transitional Care. With sufficient support at home, most patients recover quickly from a cholecystectomy. However, older or frail patients and those who live alone may require a referral for transitional or home care. The hospital nurse can help ease the unpredictability of the postoperative and postdischarge experience for patients by providing relevant patient education, prompt pain relief, and an attentive approach to the nursing care (Lindseth & Denny, 2014). During home visits, the nurse assesses the patient's physical status, especially wound healing, and progress toward recovery. Assessing the patient for adequacy of pain relief and pulmonary exercises is also important. If the patient has a drainage system in place, the nurse assesses it for patency and appropriate management by the patient and family. Assessing for signs of infection and educating the patient about the signs and symptoms of infection are also important nursing interventions. The patient's understanding of the therapeutic regimen (medications, gradual return to normal activities) is assessed, and previous education is reinforced. The nurse emphasizes the importance of keeping follow-up appointments and reminds the patient and family of the importance of participating in health promotion activities and recommended health screening.

Chart 50-2

PATIENT EDUCATION

Managing Self-Care After Laparoscopic Cholecystectomy

The nurse instructs the patient about pain management, activity and exercise, wound care, nutrition, and follow-up care as described below.

Managing Pain

- You may experience pain or discomfort from the gas used to inflate your abdominal area during surgery. Sitting upright in bed or a chair, walking, or using a heating pad may ease the discomfort.
- Take analgesic medications as needed and as prescribed. Report to your surgeon if pain is unrelieved even with analgesic use.

Resuming Activity

- Begin light exercise (walking) immediately.
- Take a shower or bath after 1 or 2 days.
- Drive a car after 3 or 4 days.
- Avoid lifting objects exceeding 5 pounds after surgery, usually for 1 week.
- Resume sexual activity when desired.

Caring for the Wound

- Check puncture site daily for signs of infection.
- Wash puncture site with mild soap and water.
- Allow special adhesive strips on the puncture site to fall off. Do not pull them off.

Resuming Eating

- Resume your normal diet.
- If you had fat intolerance before surgery, gradually add fat back into your diet in small increments.

Managing Follow-Up Care

- Make an appointment with your surgeon for 7–10 days after discharge.
- Call your surgeon if you experience any signs or symptoms of infection at or around the puncture site: redness, tenderness, swelling, heat, or drainage.
- Call your surgeon if you experience a fever of 37.7°C (100°F) or more for 2 consecutive days.
- Call your surgeon if you develop nausea, vomiting, or abdominal pain.

Evaluation

Expected patient outcomes may include:

1. Reports decrease in pain
   a. Splints abdominal incision to decrease pain
   b. Avoids foods that cause pain
   c. Uses postoperative analgesia as prescribed
2. Demonstrates appropriate respiratory function
   a. Achieves full respiratory excursion, with deep inspiration and expiration
   b. Coughs effectively, using pillow to splint abdominal incision
   c. Uses postoperative analgesia as prescribed
   d. Exercises as prescribed (e.g., turns, ambulates)
3. Exhibits normal skin integrity around biliary drainage site (if applicable)
   a. Is free of fever; abdominal pain; change in vital signs; and presence of bile, foul-smelling drainage, or pus around drainage tube
   b. Demonstrates correct management of drainage tube (if applicable)
   c. Identifies signs and symptoms of biliary obstruction to be noted and reported
   d. Has serum bilirubin level within normal range
4. Obtains relief from dietary intolerance
   a. Maintains adequate dietary intake and avoids foods that cause GI symptoms
   b. Reports decreased or absent nausea, vomiting, diarrhea, flatulence, and abdominal discomfort
5. Absence of complications
   a. Has normal vital signs (blood pressure, pulse, respiratory rate and pattern, and temperature)
   b. Reports absence of bleeding from GI tract and from biliary drainage tube or catheter (if present) and no evidence of bleeding in stool
   c. Reports return of appetite and no evidence of vomiting, abdominal distention, or pain
   d. Lists symptoms that should be reported to surgeon promptly and demonstrates an understanding of self-care, including wound care

DISORDERS OF THE PANCREAS

Pancreatitis (inflammation of the pancreas) is a serious disorder. The most basic classification system used to describe or categorize the various stages and forms of pancreatitis divides the disorder into acute and chronic forms. Acute pancreatitis can be a medical emergency associated with a high risk of life-threatening complications and mortality, whereas chronic pancreatitis often goes undetected because classic clinical and diagnostic findings are not always present in the early stages of the disease (Feldman et al., 2015; Papadakis & McPhee, 2016). By the time symptoms occur in chronic pancreatitis, approximately 90% of normal acinar cell function (exocrine function) has been lost (Feldman et al., 2015; Papadakis & McPhee, 2016). Acute pancreatitis does not usually lead to chronic pancreatitis unless complications develop. However, chronic pancreatitis can be characterized by acute episodes.

Although the mechanisms causing pancreatic inflammation are unknown, pancreatitis is commonly described as autodigestion of the pancreas. It is believed that the pancreatic duct becomes temporarily obstructed, accompanied by hypersecretion of the exocrine enzymes of the pancreas. These enzymes enter the bile duct, where they are activated and, together with bile, back up (reflux) into the pancreatic duct, causing pancreatitis.

Acute Pancreatitis

Approximately 200,000 cases of acute pancreatitis occur in the United States each year, of which 80% are the result of cholelithiasis or sustained alcohol abuse (Feldman et al., 2015; Fagenholz & de Moya, 2014). Acute pancreatitis ranges from a mild, self-limited disorder to a severe, rapidly fatal disease that does not respond to any treatment. These two main types of acute pancreatitis (mild and severe) are classified as interstitial edematous pancreatitis and necrotizing pancreatitis, respectively. Interstitial pancreatitis affects the majority of patients. It is characterized by a lack of pancreatic or peripancreatic parenchymal necrosis with diffuse enlargement of the gland due to inflammatory edema (Wu & Banks, 2013). The edema and inflammation in interstitial pancreatitis is confined to the pancreas itself. Minimal organ dysfunction is present, and return to normal function usually occurs within 6 months. Although this is considered the milder form of pancreatitis, the patient is acutely ill and at risk for hypovolemic shock, fluid and electrolyte disturbances, and sepsis.

In the more severe form, necrotizing pancreatitis, there is presence of tissue necrosis in either the pancreatic parenchyma or in the tissue surrounding the gland. This type can be sterile or infected; if the parenchyma is involved this is a marker for more severe disease (Lankisch, Apte, & Banks, 2015; Wu & Banks, 2013). A more widespread and complete enzymatic digestion of the gland characterizes necrotizing pancreatitis. Enzymes damage the local blood vessels, and bleeding and thrombosis can occur. The tissue may become necrotic, with damage extending into the retroperitoneal tissues. Local complications include pancreatic cysts or abscesses and acute fluid collections in or near the pancreas. Patients who develop systemic complications with organ failure, such as pulmonary insufficiency with hypoxia, shock, kidney disease, and GI bleeding, are also characterized as having severe acute pancreatitis.

 ### Gerontologic Considerations

Acute pancreatitis affects people of all ages, but the mortality rate associated with acute pancreatitis increases with advancing age (Wu & Banks, 2013). In addition, the pattern of complications changes with age. Younger patients tend to develop local complications; the incidence of multiple organ dysfunction syndrome (MODS) increases with age, possibly as a result of progressive decreases in physiologic function of major organs with increasing age. Close monitoring of major organ function (i.e., lungs, kidneys) is essential, and aggressive treatment is necessary to reduce mortality from acute pancreatitis in the older adult patient.

Pathophysiology

Self-digestion of the pancreas by its own proteolytic enzymes, principally trypsin, causes acute pancreatitis. These patients usually have had undiagnosed chronic pancreatitis before their first episode of acute pancreatitis. Gallstones enter the common bile duct and lodge at the ampulla of Vater, obstructing the flow of pancreatic juice or causing a reflux of bile from the common bile duct into the pancreatic duct, thus activating the powerful enzymes within the pancreas. Normally, these remain in an inactive form until the pancreatic secretions reach the lumen of the duodenum (Hall, 2015). Activation of the enzymes can lead to vasodilation, increased vascular permeability, necrosis, erosion, and hemorrhage (Fagenholz & de Moya, 2014; Townsend et al., 2016).

Other less common causes of pancreatitis include bacterial or viral infection, with pancreatitis occasionally developing as a complication of mumps viral infection. Spasm and edema of the ampulla of Vater, caused by duodenitis, can probably produce pancreatitis. Blunt abdominal trauma, peptic ulcer disease, ischemic vascular disease, hyperlipidemia, hypercalcemia, and the use of corticosteroids, thiazide diuretics, oral contraceptives, and other medications have also been associated with an increased incidence of pancreatitis. Acute pancreatitis may develop after surgery on or near the pancreas or after instrumentation of the pancreatic duct. In addition to alcohol consumption, use of tobacco products is a risk factor for the development of acute and chronic pancreatitis (Alsamarrai, Das, Windsor, et al., 2014). Acute idiopathic pancreatitis accounts for up to 10% of the cases of acute pancreatitis. Some postulate that these cases may be related to occult microlithiasis (small stones in the bile) (De Waele, 2014; Fagenholz & de Moya, 2014; Townsend et al., 2016). In addition, there is a small incidence of hereditary pancreatitis.

The mortality rate of patients with acute pancreatitis is 2% to 10% because of shock, anoxia, hypotension, or fluid and electrolyte imbalances. This mortality rate may also be related to the 10% to 30% of patients with severe acute disease characterized by pancreatic and peripancreatic necrosis (De Waele, 2014; Townsend et al., 2016). Pancreatitis may result in complete recovery, may recur without permanent damage, or may progress to chronic pancreatitis. The patient who is admitted to the hospital with a diagnosis of pancreatitis is acutely ill and needs expert nursing and medical care.

The severity of acute pancreatitis and its outcomes can be predicted based on clinical and laboratory data (see Chart 50-3).

Clinical Manifestations

Severe abdominal pain is the major symptom of pancreatitis that causes the patient to seek medical care. Abdominal pain and tenderness and back pain result from irritation and edema of the inflamed pancreas. Increased tension on the pancreatic capsule and obstruction of the pancreatic ducts also contribute to the pain. Typically, the pain occurs in the midepigastrium. Pain is frequently acute in onset, occurring 24 to 48 hours

---

Chart 50-3   Criteria for Predicting Severity of Pancreatitis

Criteria on Admission to Hospital

Age >55 years
White blood cells (WBCs) >16,000 mm³
Serum glucose >200 mg/dL (>11.1 mmol/L)
Serum lactose dehydrogenase (LDH) >350 IU/L (>350 U/L)
AST >250 IU/L

Criteria Within 48 Hours of Hospital Admission

Fall in hematocrit >10% (>0.10)
Blood urea nitrogen (BUN) increase >5 mg/dL (>1.7 mmol/L)
Serum calcium <8 mg/dL (<2 mmol/L)
Base deficit >4 mEq/L (>4 mmol/L)
Fluid retention or sequestration >6 L
Partial pressure of oxygen (PO₂) <60 mmHg

Two or fewer signs, 1% mortality; 3 or 4 signs, 15% mortality; 5 or 6 signs, 40% mortality; >6 signs, 100% mortality.
Note: The more risk factors a patient has, the greater the severity and likelihood of complications or death.
Adapted from Ranson, J. H., Rifkind, K. M., Roses, D. F., et al. (1974). Prognostic signs and the role of operative management in acute pancreatitis. *Surgery, Gynecology & Obstetrics, 139*(1), 69–81.

after a very heavy meal or alcohol ingestion, and it may be diffuse and difficult to localize. It is generally more severe after meals and is unrelieved by antacids. Pain may be accompanied by abdominal distention; a poorly defined, palpable abdominal mass; decreased peristalsis; and vomiting that fails to relieve the pain or nausea.

The patient appears acutely ill. Abdominal guarding is present. A rigid or boardlike abdomen may develop and is generally an ominous sign, usually indicating peritonitis (Fagenholz & de Moya, 2014). Ecchymosis (bruising) in the flank or around the umbilicus may indicate severe pancreatitis. Nausea and vomiting are common in acute pancreatitis. The emesis is usually gastric in origin but may also be bile stained. Fever, jaundice, mental confusion, and agitation may also occur.

Hypotension is typical and reflects hypovolemia and shock caused by the loss of large amounts of protein-rich fluid into the tissues and peritoneal cavity. In addition to hypotension, the patient may develop tachycardia; cyanosis; and cold, clammy skin. Acute kidney injury is common.

Respiratory distress and hypoxia are common, and the patient may develop diffuse pulmonary infiltrates, dyspnea, tachypnea, and abnormal blood gas values. Myocardial depression, hypocalcemia, hyperglycemia, and disseminated intravascular coagulation may also occur with acute pancreatitis.

Assessment and Diagnostic Findings

The diagnosis of acute pancreatitis is based on a history of abdominal pain, the presence of known risk factors, physical examination findings, and diagnostic findings. Serum amylase and lipase levels are used in making the diagnosis of acute pancreatitis, although their elevation can be attributed to many other causes (Fagenholz & de Moya, 2014; Feldman et al., 2015; Wu & Banks, 2013). In most cases, serum amylase and lipase levels are elevated within 24 hours of the onset of the symptoms. Serum amylase usually returns to normal within 48 to 72 hours, but serum lipase levels may remain elevated for a longer period, often days longer than amylase. Urinary amylase levels also become elevated and remain elevated longer than serum amylase levels. The white blood cell count is usually elevated; hypocalcemia is present in many patients and correlates well with the severity of pancreatitis. Transient hyperglycemia and glucosuria and elevated serum bilirubin levels occur in some patients with acute pancreatitis.

X-ray studies of the abdomen and chest may be obtained to differentiate pancreatitis from other disorders that can cause similar symptoms and to detect pleural effusions. Ultrasound studies, contrast-enhanced CT scans, and magnetic resonance imaging (MRI) scans are used to identify an increase in the diameter of the pancreas and to detect pancreatic cysts, abscesses, or pseudocysts.

Hematocrit and hemoglobin levels are used to monitor the patient for bleeding. Peritoneal fluid, obtained through paracentesis or peritoneal lavage, may contain increased levels of pancreatic enzymes. ERCP is rarely used in the diagnostic evaluation of acute pancreatitis, because the patient is acutely ill; however, it may be valuable in the treatment of gallstone pancreatitis.

Medical Management

Management of acute pancreatitis is directed toward relieving symptoms and preventing or treating complications. All oral intake is withheld to inhibit stimulation of the pancreas and its secretion of enzymes. Ongoing research has shown positive outcomes with the use of enteral feedings. The current recommendation is that, whenever possible, the enteral route should be used to meet nutritional needs in patients with pancreatitis. This strategy also has been found to prevent infectious complications safely and cost-effectively (McClave, 2013; Townsend et al., 2016; Zerem, 2014). Enteral feedings should be started early in the course of acute pancreatitis (McClave, 2013; Zerem, 2014). Parenteral nutrition has a role in the nutritional support of patients with severe acute pancreatitis, particularly in those who are unable to tolerate enteral nutrition (Fagenholz & de Moya, 2014; Schepers, Besselink, van Santvoort, et al., 2013; Zerem, 2014). Nasogastric suction may be used to relieve nausea and vomiting and to decrease painful abdominal distention and paralytic ileus (Zerem, 2014). Research data do not support the routine use of nasogastric tubes to remove gastric secretions in an effort to limit pancreatic secretion. Though current literature discourages the use of acid-suppressive therapy, this practice is common for hospitalized patients. Histamine-2 (H$_2$) antagonists such as cimetidine (Tagamet) and ranitidine (Zantac) may be prescribed to decrease pancreatic activity by inhibiting secretion of gastric acid. Proton pump inhibitors such as pantoprazole (Protonix) may be used for patients who do not tolerate H$_2$ antagonists or for whom this therapy is ineffective (Hong, Monye, & Seifert, 2015).

Pain Management

Adequate administration of analgesia is essential during the course of acute pancreatitis to provide sufficient pain relief and to minimize restlessness, which may stimulate pancreatic secretion further. Pain relief may require parenteral opioids such as morphine, fentanyl (Sublimaze), or hydromorphone (Dilaudid) (Rakel & Rakel, 2015). There is no clinical evidence to support the use of meperidine for pain relief in pancreatitis; in fact, accumulation of its metabolites can cause CNS irritability and possibly seizures. The current recommendation for pain management is the use of opioids, with assessment for their effectiveness and altering therapy if pain is not controlled or increased (Marx et al., 2013). More research is needed to identify the best option for pain management in the patient with acute pancreatitis (Marx et al., 2013). Until evidence-based recommendations are developed, guidelines for acute pain management in the perioperative setting should be followed (Lankisch et al., 2015). Antiemetic agents may be prescribed to prevent vomiting.

 Intensive Care

Correction of fluid and blood loss and low albumin levels is necessary to maintain fluid volume and prevent acute kidney injury. The patient is usually acutely ill and is monitored in the intensive care unit, where hemodynamic monitoring and arterial blood gas monitoring are initiated. Antibiotic agents may be prescribed if infection is present. Prophylactic antibiotics are not recommended for patients with acute pancreatitis (Lankisch et al., 2015; Zerem, 2014). Insulin may be required if hyperglycemia occurs. Intensive insulin therapy (continuous infusion) in the critically ill patient has undergone much study and has shown promise in terms of positive patient outcomes when compared with intermittent insulin dosing. Glycemic control with near-normal blood glucose levels improves patient outcomes, most notably in critically ill surgical patients (McMahon, Nystrom, Braunschweig, et al., 2013).

Respiratory Care

Aggressive respiratory care is indicated because of the high risk of elevation of the diaphragm, pulmonary infiltrates and effusion, and atelectasis. Hypoxemia occurs in a significant number of patients with acute pancreatitis, even with normal x-ray findings. Respiratory care may range from close monitoring of arterial blood gases to the use of humidified oxygen to intubation and mechanical ventilation (see Chapter 21 for further discussion).

Biliary Drainage

Placement of biliary drains (for external drainage) and stents (indwelling tubes) in the pancreatic duct through endoscopy has been performed to reestablish drainage of the pancreas. This has resulted in decreased pain.

Surgical Intervention

Although the acutely ill patient is at high risk for surgical complications, surgery may be performed to assist in the diagnosis of pancreatitis (diagnostic laparotomy); to establish pancreatic drainage; or to resect or débride an infected, necrotic pancreas. The patient who undergoes pancreatic surgery may have multiple drains in place postoperatively, as well as a surgical incision that is left open for irrigation and repacking every 2 to 3 days to remove necrotic debris (see Fig. 50-6).

Postacute Management

Oral feedings that are low in fat and protein are initiated gradually. Caffeine and alcohol are eliminated from the diet.

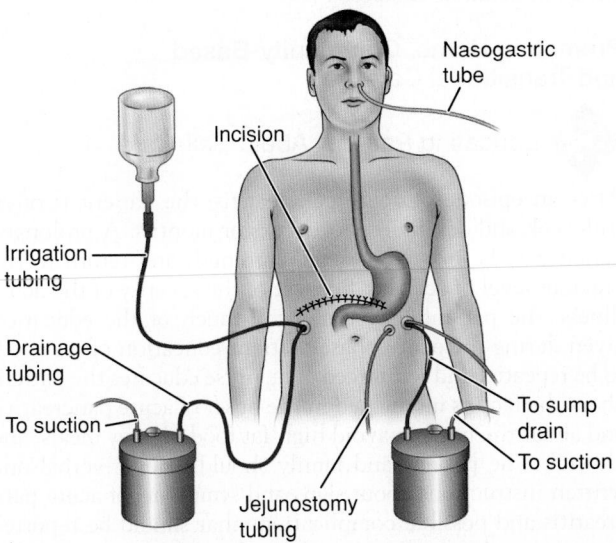

Figure 50-6 • Multiple sump tubes are used after pancreatic surgery. Triple-lumen tubes consist of ports that provide tubing for irrigation, air venting, and drainage.

If the episode of pancreatitis occurred during treatment with thiazide diuretics, corticosteroids, or oral contraceptives, these medications are discontinued. Follow-up may include ultrasound, x-ray studies, or ERCP to determine whether the pancreatitis is resolving and to assess for abscesses and pseudocysts. ERCP may also be used to identify the cause of acute pancreatitis if it is in question and for endoscopic sphincterotomy and removal of gallstones from the common bile duct.

Nursing Management

Relieving Pain and Discomfort

Because the pathologic process responsible for pain is autodigestion of the pancreas, the objectives of therapy are to relieve pain and decrease secretion of pancreatic enzymes. The pain of acute pancreatitis is often very severe, necessitating the liberal use of analgesic agents. The current recommendation for pain management in this population is parenteral opioids, including morphine, hydromorphone, or fentanyl via patient-controlled analgesia or bolus (Marx et al., 2013). In critically ill patients, a continuous infusion may be needed. Because most opioids stimulate spasm of the sphincter of Oddi to some degree, consensus has not been reached on the most effective agent. Ensuring patient comfort, regardless of the opioid prescribed, is the most essential aspect of care. The nurse frequently assesses the pain and the effectiveness of the pharmacologic (and nonpharmacologic) interventions. Changes may be needed in the regimen for pain management based on the achievement of pain control. Pain assessment tools (see Chapter 12) are available for the nurse to ensure an accurate rating of pain. Nonpharmacologic interventions such as proper positioning, music, distraction, and imagery may be effective in reducing pain when used along with medications.

In addition, oral feedings are withheld to decrease the secretion of secretin. Parenteral fluids and electrolytes are prescribed to restore and maintain fluid balance. Nasogastric suction may be used to relieve nausea and vomiting or to treat abdominal distention and paralytic ileus. The nurse provides frequent oral hygiene and care to decrease discomfort from the nasogastric tube and relieve dryness of the mouth.

The acutely ill patient is maintained on bed rest to decrease the metabolic rate and reduce the secretion of pancreatic and gastric enzymes. If the patient experiences increasing severity of pain, the nurse reports this to the primary provider because the patient may be experiencing hemorrhage of the pancreas or the dose of analgesic medication may be inadequate.

The patient with acute pancreatitis is often confused or delirious because of severe pain, fluid and electrolyte disturbances, and hypoxia. Therefore, the nurse provides frequent and repeated but simple explanations about the need for withholding fluids, maintenance of gastric suction, and bed rest.

Improving Breathing Pattern

The nurse maintains the patient in a semi-Fowler position to decrease pressure on the diaphragm by a distended abdomen and to increase respiratory expansion. Frequent changes of position are necessary to prevent atelectasis and pooling of respiratory secretions. Pulmonary assessment, including monitoring of pulse oximetry or arterial blood gases, is essential to detect changes in respiratory status so that early treatment can be initiated. The nurse instructs the patient in techniques of coughing and deep breathing and in the use of incentive spirometry to improve respiratory function and assists the patient to perform these activities every hour.

Improving Nutritional Status

The nurse assesses the patient's nutritional status and notes factors that alter the patient's nutritional requirements (e.g., temperature elevation, surgery, drainage). Laboratory test results and daily weights are useful to monitor the nutritional status.

Enteral or parenteral nutrition may be prescribed. In addition to administering enteral or parenteral nutrition, the nurse monitors serum glucose levels every 4 to 6 hours. As the acute symptoms subside, oral feedings are gradually reintroduced. Between acute attacks, the patient receives a diet that is high in protein and low in fat (Dudek, 2013). The patient should avoid heavy meals and alcoholic beverages.

Maintaining Skin Integrity

The patient is at risk for skin breakdown because of poor nutritional status, enforced bed rest, and restlessness, which may result in pressure ulcers and breaks in tissue integrity. In addition, the patient who has undergone surgery may have multiple drains or an open surgical incision and is at risk for skin breakdown and infection. The nurse carefully assesses the wound, drainage sites, and skin for signs of infection, inflammation, and breakdown. The nurse carries out wound care as prescribed and takes precautions to protect intact skin from contact with drainage. Consultation with a wound-ostomy-continence (WOC) nurse, a nurse specially educated in appropriate skin, wound, ostomy, and continence care is often helpful in identifying appropriate skin care devices and protocols. The patient must be turned every 2 hours; the use of specialty beds may be indicated to prevent skin breakdown.

 ### Monitoring and Managing Potential Complications

Fluid and electrolyte disturbances are common complications because of nausea, vomiting, movement of fluid from the vascular compartment to the peritoneal cavity, diaphoresis, fever, and the use of gastric suction. The nurse assesses the patient's fluid and electrolyte status by noting skin turgor and moistness of mucous membranes. The nurse weighs the patient daily and carefully measures fluid intake and output, including urine output, nasogastric secretions, and diarrhea. In addition, it is important to assess for other factors that may affect fluid and electrolyte status, including increased body temperature and wound drainage. The nurse assesses the patient for ascites and measures abdominal girth daily if ascites is suspected.

Fluids are administered IV and may be accompanied by infusion of blood or blood products to maintain the blood volume and to prevent or treat hypovolemic shock. Emergency medications must be readily available because of the risk of circulatory collapse and shock. The nurse promptly reports decreased blood pressure and reduced urine output, which indicate hypovolemia and shock or acute kidney injury. Low serum calcium and magnesium levels may occur and require prompt treatment.

Pancreatic necrosis is a major cause of morbidity and mortality in patients with acute pancreatitis because of resulting hemorrhage, septic shock, and MODS. The patient may

undergo diagnostic procedures for confirmation of pancreatic necrosis. If the patient is found to have pancreatic necrosis with infection, this may require surgical, percutaneous or endoscopic débridement and/or insertion of multiple drains. Percutaneous or endoscopic catheter drainage is the first step of what is known as the "Step-Up Approach." Here, catheters are placed via the left or right retroperitoneal approach to drain the infection. This intervention, coupled with appropriate, targeted antibiotic therapy may be the only necessary treatment for some patients (da Costa, Boerma, van Santvoort, et al., 2014; Lankisch et al., 2015; Martin & Hein, 2013). These procedures are considered first-line approaches with surgery reserved for patients for whom these interventions do not work. Prophylactic antibiotics are not indicated (Lankisch et al., 2015; Zerem, 2014). The patient with pancreatic necrosis with or without infection is usually critically ill and requires expert medical and nursing management, including hemodynamic monitoring in the intensive care unit.

In addition to carefully monitoring vital signs and other signs and symptoms, the nurse is responsible for administering prescribed fluids, medications, and blood products; assisting with supportive management, such as the use of a ventilator; preventing additional complications; and providing physical and psychological care.

Shock and MODS may occur with acute pancreatitis. Hypovolemic shock may occur as a result of hypovolemia and sequestering of fluid in the peritoneal cavity. Hemorrhagic shock may occur with hemorrhagic pancreatitis. Septic shock may occur with bacterial infection of the pancreas. Cardiac dysfunction may occur as a result of fluid and electrolyte disturbances, acid–base imbalances, and release of toxic substances into the circulation.

The nurse closely monitors the patient for early signs of neurologic, cardiovascular, renal, and respiratory dysfunction. The nurse must be prepared to respond quickly to rapid changes in the patient's status, treatments, and therapies. In addition, it is important to inform the family about the status and progress of the patient and to allow them to spend time with the patient. Management of shock and MODS is discussed in detail in Chapter 14.

Promoting Home, Community-Based and Transitional Care

 ### Educating Patients About Self-Care

After an episode of acute pancreatitis, the patient is often still weak and debilitated for weeks or months. A prolonged period may be needed to regain strength and return to the previous level of activity. Because of the severity of the acute illness, the patient may not recall much of the education given during the acute phase. Patient education often needs to be repeated and reinforced. The nurse educates the patient about the factors implicated in the onset of acute pancreatitis and about the need to avoid high-fat foods, heavy meals, and alcohol. The patient and family should receive verbal and written instructions about signs and symptoms of acute pancreatitis and possible complications that should be reported promptly to the primary provider.

If acute pancreatitis is a result of biliary tract disease, such as gallstones and gallbladder disease, additional explanations are needed about required dietary modifications. If the pancreatitis is a result of alcohol abuse, the nurse reinforces the need to avoid all alcohol.

Continuing and Transitional Care

A referral for home, community-based or transitional care is often indicated. This enables the nurse to assess the patient's physical and psychological status and adherence to the therapeutic regimen. The nurse also assesses the home situation and reinforces instructions about fluid and nutrition intake and avoidance of alcohol. After the acute attack has subsided, some patients may be inclined to return to their previous drinking habits. The nurse provides specific information about resources and support groups that may be of assistance in avoiding alcohol in the future. Referral to Alcoholics Anonymous as appropriate or other support groups is essential. See the accompanying plan of nursing care in Chart 50-4 for the patient with acute pancreatitis.

Chronic Pancreatitis

Chronic pancreatitis is an inflammatory disorder characterized by progressive destruction of the pancreas. As cells are replaced by fibrous tissue with repeated attacks of pancreatitis, pressure within the pancreas increases. The result is obstruction of the pancreatic and common bile ducts and the duodenum. In addition, there is atrophy of the epithelium of the ducts, inflammation, and destruction of the secreting cells of the pancreas.

Alcohol consumption in Western societies and malnutrition worldwide are the major causes of chronic pancreatitis. The median age of patients diagnosed with chronic pancreatitis has been reported to be 62 years (Muniraj, Aslanian, Farrell, et al., 2014). Frequently, at that age, patients already report a long history of alcohol abuse. Excessive and prolonged consumption of alcohol accounts for approximately 70% to 80% of all cases of chronic pancreatitis (Gupte & Forsmark, 2014; Muniraj et al., 2014; Townsend et al., 2016). The incidence of pancreatitis is 50 times greater in people with alcoholism than in those who do not abuse alcohol. Long-term alcohol consumption causes hypersecretion of protein in pancreatic secretions, resulting in protein plugs and calculi within the pancreatic ducts. Alcohol also has a direct toxic effect on the cells of the pancreas. Damage to these cells is more likely to occur and to be more severe in patients whose diets are poor in protein content and either very high or very low in fat.

Smoking is another factor in the development of chronic pancreatitis. Because they are often associated, it is difficult to separate the effects of the alcohol abuse and smoking (Muniraj et al., 2014; Townsend et al., 2016).

Clinical Manifestations

Chronic pancreatitis is characterized by recurring attacks of severe upper abdominal and back pain, accompanied by vomiting. Attacks are often so painful that opioids, even in large doses, do not provide relief. The risk of opioid dependence is increased in pancreatitis because of the chronic nature and severity of the pain. As the disease progresses, recurring attacks of pain are more severe, more frequent, and of longer duration. Some patients experience continuous severe pain, and others have dull, nagging constant pain. Periods of well-being sometimes follow the episodes of pain (Muniraj et al., 2014). In some patients, chronic pancreatitis is painless. The natural history of abdominal pain (character, timing, severity) is variable, and many studies have documented a decrease in pain ("burnout") over time in a majority of patients (Muniraj et al., 2014).

Weight loss is a major problem in chronic pancreatitis. More than 80% of patients experience significant weight loss, which is usually caused by decreased dietary intake secondary to anorexia or fear that eating will precipitate another attack (Bope & Kellerman, 2015). Malabsorption occurs late in the disease, when as little as 10% of pancreatic function remains (Bope & Kellerman, 2015). As a result, digestion, especially of proteins and fats, is impaired. The stools become frequent, frothy, and foul smelling because of impaired fat digestion, which results in stools with a high fat content referred to as **steatorrhea**. As the disease progresses, calcification of the gland may occur, and calcium stones may form within the ducts.

Assessment and Diagnostic Findings

ERCP is the most useful study in the diagnosis of chronic pancreatitis. It provides details about the anatomy of the pancreas and the pancreatic and biliary ducts. It is also helpful in obtaining tissue for analysis and differentiating pancreatitis from other conditions, such as carcinoma (Muniraj, Aslanian, Farrell, et al., 2015). Various imaging procedures, including MRI, CT scans, and ultrasound, are used in the diagnostic evaluation of patients with suspected pancreatic disorders. A CT scan or ultrasound study is also helpful to detect pancreatic cysts (Muniraj et al., 2015).

A glucose tolerance test evaluates pancreatic islet cell function and provides necessary information for making decisions about surgical resection of the pancreas. An abnormal glucose tolerance test may indicate the presence of diabetes associated with pancreatitis. Acute exacerbations of chronic pancreatitis may result in increased serum amylase levels. Steatorrhea is best confirmed by laboratory analysis of fecal fat content (Bope & Kellerman, 2015).

Medical Management

The management of chronic pancreatitis depends on its probable cause in each patient. Treatment is directed toward preventing and managing acute attacks, relieving pain and discomfort, and managing exocrine and endocrine insufficiency of pancreatitis (Muniraj et al., 2015).

Nonsurgical Management

Nonsurgical approaches may be indicated for the patient who refuses surgery, is a poor surgical risk, or when the disease and symptoms do not warrant surgical intervention. Endoscopy to remove pancreatic duct stones, correct strictures with stenting, and drain cysts may be effective in selected patients to manage pain and relieve obstruction via ERCP (Gupte & Forsmark, 2014; Muniraj et al., 2015; Talukdar & Nageshwar, 2014).

Management of abdominal pain and discomfort is similar to that of acute pancreatitis; however, the focus is usually on the use of nonopioid methods to manage pain and

(*text continued on page 1448*)

Chart 50-4

PLAN OF NURSING CARE
Care of the Patient With Acute Pancreatitis

NURSING DIAGNOSIS: Acute pain and discomfort related to edema, distention of the pancreas, peritoneal irritation, and excess stimulation of pancreatic secretions
GOAL: Relief of pain and discomfort

Nursing Interventions	Rationale	Expected Outcomes
1. Using a pain scale, assess pain level at baseline, before and after administration of analgesic medications.	1. Baseline assessment and control of pain are important because restlessness increases the body's metabolism, which stimulates the secretion of pancreatic and gastric enzymes.	• Patient rates pain using pain scale • Reports relief of pain, discomfort, and abdominal cramping • Moves and turns without increasing pain and discomfort • Rests comfortably and sleeps for increasing periods • Reports increased feelings of well-being and security with the health care team
2. Administer morphine, fentanyl, or hydromorphone frequently, as prescribed, to achieve level of pain acceptable to patient.	2. Morphine, fentanyl, and hydromorphone act by depressing the central nervous system and thereby increasing the patient's pain threshold. Meperidine (Demerol) is avoided because it has failed acute pain studies and possesses toxic metabolites.	
3. Maintain the patient NPO (nothing by mouth) as prescribed.	3. Pancreatic secretion is increased by food and fluid intake.	
4. Maintain the patient on bed rest.	4. Bed rest decreases body metabolism and thus reduces pancreatic and gastric secretions.	

5. Maintain continuous nasogastric drainage if paralytic ileus or nausea and vomiting, abdominal distention are present.
  a. Measure gastric secretions at specified intervals.
  b. Observe and record color and viscosity of gastric secretions.
  c. Ensure that the nasogastric tube is patent to permit free drainage.
	5. Nasogastric suction relieves nausea, vomiting, and abdominal distention. Decompression of the intestines (if intestinal intubation is used) also assists in relieving respiratory distress.	

6. Report unrelieved pain or increasing intensity of pain.	6. Pain may increase pancreatic enzymes and may also indicate pancreatic hemorrhage.	
7. Assist patient to assume positions of comfort; turn and reposition every 2 hours.	7. Frequent turning relieves pressure and assists in preventing pulmonary and vascular complications.	
8. Use nonpharmacologic interventions for relieving pain (e.g., relaxation, focused breathing, diversion).	8. The use of nonpharmacologic methods will enhance the effects of analgesic medications.	
9. Listen to patient's expression of pain experience.	9. Demonstration of caring can help to decrease anxiety.	

NURSING DIAGNOSIS: Impaired comfort related to nasogastric tube
GOAL: Relief of discomfort associated with nasogastric intubation used to treat ileus, vomiting, distention

Nursing Interventions	Rationale	Expected Outcomes
1. Use water-soluble lubricant around external nares.	1. Prevents irritation of nares.	• Exhibits intact skin and tissue of nares at site of nasogastric tube insertion • Reports no pain or irritation of nares or oropharynx • Exhibits moist, clean mucous membranes of mouth and nasopharynx • States that thirst is relieved by oral hygiene • Identifies rationale for nasogastric tube and suction
2. Turn patient at intervals; avoid pressure or tension on nasogastric tube.	2. Relieves pressure of tube on esophageal and gastric mucosa.	
3. Provide oral hygiene and gargling solutions without alcohol.	3. Relieves dryness and irritation of oropharynx.	
4. Explain rationale for the use of nasogastric drainage.	4. Assists patient to cooperate with the drainage, nasogastric tube, and suction.	

Chart 50-4

PLAN OF NURSING CARE (Continued)
Care of the Patient With Acute Pancreatitis

NURSING DIAGNOSIS: Imbalanced nutrition: less than body requirements related to inadequate dietary intake, impaired pancreatic secretions, increased nutritional needs secondary to acute illness, and increased body temperature

GOAL: Improvement in nutritional status

Nursing Interventions	Rationale	Expected Outcomes
1. Assess current nutritional status and increased metabolic requirements.	1. Alteration in pancreatic secretions interferes with normal digestive processes. Acute illness, infection, and fever increase metabolic needs.	• Maintains normal body weight • Demonstrates no additional weight loss • Maintains normal serum glucose levels • Reports decreasing episodes of vomiting and diarrhea
2. Monitor serum glucose levels and administer insulin as prescribed.	2. Impairment of endocrine function of the pancreas leads to increased serum glucose levels.	• Reports return of normal stool characteristics and bowel pattern • Consumes foods high in carbohydrates, low in fat and protein
3. Administer IV fluid and electrolytes, enteral or parenteral nutrition as prescribed.	3. Parenteral administration of fluids and electrolytes, and enteral or parenteral nutrients are essential to provide fluids, calories, electrolytes, and nutrients when oral intake is prohibited.	• Explains rationale for high-carbohydrate, low-fat, low-protein diet • Eliminates alcohol from diet • Explains rationale for limiting coffee intake and avoiding spicy foods
4. Provide high-carbohydrate, low-protein, low-fat diet when tolerated.	4. These foods increase caloric intake without stimulating pancreatic secretions beyond the ability of the pancreas to respond.	• Participates in Alcoholics Anonymous as appropriate or other counseling approach • Returns to and maintains desirable weight
5. Instruct patient to eliminate alcohol, and refer to Alcoholics Anonymous, if indicated.	5. Alcohol intake produces further damage to pancreas and precipitates attacks of acute pancreatitis.	
6. Counsel patient to avoid excessive use of coffee and spicy foods.	6. Coffee and spicy foods increase pancreatic and gastric secretions.	
7. Monitor daily weights.	7. This provides a baseline and a means to measure weight gain or weight loss.	

NURSING DIAGNOSIS: Ineffective breathing pattern related to splinting from severe pain, pulmonary infiltrates, pleural effusion, and atelectasis

GOAL: Improvement in respiratory function

Nursing Interventions	Rationale	Expected Outcomes
1. Assess respiratory status (rate, pattern, breath sounds), pulse oximetry, and arterial blood gases.	1. Acute pancreatitis produces retroperitoneal edema, elevation of the diaphragm, pleural effusion, and inadequate lung ventilation. Intra-abdominal infection and labored breathing increase the body's metabolic demands, which further decreases pulmonary reserve and leads to respiratory failure.	• Demonstrates normal respiratory rate and pattern and full lung expansion • Demonstrates normal breath sounds and absence of adventitious breath sounds • Demonstrates normal arterial blood gases and pulse oximetry • Maintains semi-Fowler position when in bed
2. Maintain semi-Fowler position.	2. Decreases pressure on diaphragm and allows greater lung expansion.	• Changes position in bed frequently • Coughs and takes deep breaths at least every hour
3. Instruct and encourage patient to take deep breaths and to cough every hour.	3. Taking deep breaths and coughing will clear the airways and reduce atelectasis.	• Demonstrates normal body temperature • Exhibits no signs or symptoms of respiratory infection or impairment
4. Assist patient to turn and change position every 2 hours.	4. Changing position frequently assists aeration and drainage of all lobes of the lungs.	• Is alert and responsive to environment

5. Reduce the excessive metabolism of the body.
  a. Administer antibiotics as prescribed.
  b. Place patient in an air-conditioned room.
  c. Administer nasal oxygen as required for hypoxia.
  d. Use a hypothermia blanket if necessary.
	5. Pancreatitis produces a severe peritoneal and retroperitoneal reaction that causes fever, tachycardia, and accelerated respirations. Placing the patient in an air-conditioned room and supporting the patient with oxygen therapy decrease the workload of the respiratory system and the tissue utilization of oxygen. Reduction of fever and pulse rate decreases the metabolic demands on the body.	

(continued on page 1448)

Chart 50-4

PLAN OF NURSING CARE (Continued)

Care of the Patient With Acute Pancreatitis

COLLABORATIVE PROBLEM: Fluid and electrolyte disturbances, hypovolemia, shock
GOAL: Improvement in fluid and electrolyte status, prevention of hypovolemia and shock

Nursing Interventions	Rationale	Expected Outcomes
1. Assess fluid and electrolyte status (skin turgor, mucous membranes, urine output, vital signs, hemodynamic parameters).	1. The amount and type of fluid and electrolyte replacement are determined by the status of the blood pressure, the laboratory evaluations of serum electrolyte and blood urea nitrogen levels, the urinary volume, and the assessment of the patient's condition.	• Exhibits moist mucous membranes and normal skin turgor • Exhibits normal blood pressure without evidence of postural (orthostatic) hypotension • Excretes adequate urine volume • Exhibits normal, not excessive, thirst • Maintains normal pulse and respiratory rate
2. Assess sources of fluid and electrolyte loss (vomiting, diarrhea, nasogastric drainage, excessive diaphoresis).	2. Electrolyte losses occur from nasogastric suctioning, severe diaphoresis, and emesis, and as a result of the patient being in a fasting state.	• Remains alert and responsive • Exhibits normal arterial pressures and blood gases • Exhibits normal electrolyte levels • Exhibits no signs or symptoms of calcium deficit (e.g., tetany, carpopedal spasm)

3. Combat shock if present.
  a. Administer corticosteroids as prescribed if patient does not respond to conventional treatment.
  b. Evaluate the amount of urinary output. Attempt to maintain this at ≥0.5 mL/kg/hr.
	3. Extensive acute pancreatitis may cause peripheral vascular collapse and shock. Blood and plasma may be lost into the abdominal cavity; therefore, there is a decreased blood and plasma volume. The toxins from the bacteria of a necrotic pancreas may cause shock.	• Exhibits no additional losses of fluids and electrolytes through vomiting, diarrhea, or diaphoresis
		• Reports stabilization of weight
		• Demonstrates no increase in abdominal girth

4. Administer blood products, fluids, and electrolytes (sodium, potassium, chloride) as prescribed.	4. Patients with hemorrhagic pancreatitis lose large amounts of blood and plasma, which decreases effective circulation and blood volume.	• Demonstrates no fluid wave on palpation of the abdomen • Demonstrates stable organ function without manifestations of failure
5. Administer plasma and blood products as prescribed.	5. Replacement with blood, plasma, or albumin assists in ensuring effective circulating blood volume.	
6. Keep a supply of IV calcium gluconate or calcium chloride readily available.	6. Calcium may be prescribed to prevent or treat tetany, which may result from calcium losses into retroperitoneal (peripancreatic) exudate.	

7. Assess abdomen for ascites formation.
  a. Measure abdominal girth daily.
  b. Weigh patient daily.
  c. Assess abdomen for ascites (see Figs. 49-6 and 49-7).
	7. During acute pancreatitis, plasma may be lost into the abdominal cavity, which diminishes the blood volume.	

8. Monitor for manifestations of multiple organ dysfunction syndrome: neurologic, cardiovascular, renal, and respiratory dysfunction.	8. All body systems may fail if pancreatitis is severe and treatment is ineffective.	

the implementation of the World Health Organization's (WHO) three-step ladder for the treatment of chronic pain. This involves initiating monotherapy and, if ineffective, instituting combination therapy with peripherally acting and centrally acting medications. Pain management in the early stages may respond to nonopioid analgesics, but if the pain becomes more constant or debilitating, introduction of opioid analgesics is appropriate. The abuse of opioids is possible in these patients, and may be more likely in patients with depression, higher pain intensity, and alcohol use (Gupte & Forsmark, 2014). Adjunct means of pain modulation, such as use of antioxidants, antidepressants, and nonnarcotic agents as well as avoidance of smoking and alcohol, are recommended before starting opioids for pain control (Gupte & Forsmark, 2014). Antioxidants have shown effect in the relief of pain and in improving quality of life and are often given to patients with chronic pancreatitis (Gupte & Forsmark,

2014). An endoscopic ultrasound (EUS)–guided placement of a celiac nerve block is a potential option for chronic, unrelieved pain of this disease (D'Haese, Ceyhan, Demir, et al., 2014). Yoga and other mindfulness-based therapies may be effective nonpharmacologic methods for pain reduction and for relief of other coexisting symptoms of chronic pancreatitis (Schulenburg, 2015). Persistent, unrelieved pain is often the most difficult aspect of management (Gupte & Forsmark, 2014; Muniraj et al., 2015). The primary provider, nurse, and dietitian emphasize to the patient and family the importance of avoiding alcohol and foods that have produced abdominal pain and discomfort in the past. The health care team stresses to the patient that no other treatment is likely to relieve pain if the patient continues to consume alcohol.

Diabetes resulting from dysfunction of the pancreatic islet cells is treated with diet, insulin, or oral antidiabetic agents. The hazard of severe hypoglycemia with alcohol consumption is stressed to the patient and family. Pancreatic enzyme replacement is indicated for the patient with malabsorption and steatorrhea.

Surgical Management

Chronic pancreatitis is not often managed by surgery. However, surgery may be indicated to relieve persistent abdominal pain and discomfort, restore drainage of pancreatic secretions, and reduce the frequency of acute attacks of pancreatitis and hospitalization (D'Haese et al., 2014; Gupte & Forsmark, 2014; Muniraj et al., 2015). The type of surgery performed depends on the anatomic and functional abnormalities of the pancreas, including the location of disease within the pancreas, the presence of diabetes, exocrine insufficiency, biliary stenosis, and pseudocysts of the pancreas. Other considerations for surgery selection include the patient's likelihood for continued use of alcohol and the likelihood that the patient will be able to manage the endocrine or exocrine changes that are expected after surgery.

Pancreaticojejunostomy (also referred to as Roux-en-Y), with a side-to-side anastomosis or joining of the pancreatic duct to the jejunum, allows drainage of the pancreatic secretions into the jejunum. Pain relief occurs within 6 months in more than 85% of the patients who undergo this procedure, but pain returns in a substantial number of patients as the disease progresses (D'Haese et al., 2014; Doherty, 2015; Gupte & Forsmark, 2014).

Other surgical procedures may be performed for different degrees and types of underlying disorders. These procedures include revision of the sphincter of the ampulla of Vater, internal drainage of a pancreatic cyst into the stomach (see later discussion), insertion of a stent, and wide resection or removal of the pancreas. A Whipple resection (pancreaticoduodenectomy) can be carried out to relieve the pain of chronic pancreatitis (see later discussion under Tumors of the Head of the Pancreas). In an effort to provide permanent pain relief and avoid endocrine and exocrine insufficiency that ensue with major resections of the pancreas, surgeons have designed new procedures that combine limited resection of the head of the pancreas with a pancreaticojejunostomy. These procedures, known as the Beger or Frey operations, remove most of the head of the pancreas except for a shell of pancreatic tissue posteriorly (D'Haese et al., 2014; Doherty, 2015; Gupte & Forsmark, 2014).

When chronic pancreatitis develops as a result of gallbladder disease, surgery is performed to explore the common duct and remove the stones; usually, the gallbladder is removed at the same time. In addition, an attempt is made to improve the drainage of the common bile duct and the pancreatic duct by dividing the sphincter of Oddi, a muscle that is located at the ampulla of Vater (this surgical procedure is known as a sphincterotomy). A T-tube usually is placed in the common bile duct, requiring a drainage system to collect the bile postoperatively. Nursing care after such surgery is similar to that indicated after other biliary tract surgery.

Approximately two thirds of all patients with chronic pancreatitis can be managed with endoscopic or laparoscopic intervention (D'Haese et al., 2014; Gupte & Forsmark, 2014; Muniraj et al., 2015). Endoscopic and laparoscopic procedures such as distal pancreatectomy, longitudinal decompression of the pancreatic duct, nerve denervation, and stenting

have been performed in patients with jaundice or recurrent inflammation and are being refined. Minimally invasive procedures to treat chronic pancreatitis may prove to be successful adjuncts in the management of this complex disorder (D'Haese et al., 2014; Gupte & Forsmark, 2014).

Patients who undergo surgery for chronic pancreatitis may experience weight gain and improved nutritional status; this may result from reduction in pain associated with eating rather than from correction of malabsorption. However, morbidity and mortality after these surgical procedures are high because of the poor physical condition of the patient before surgery and the concomitant presence of cirrhosis. Even after undergoing these surgical procedures, the patient is likely to continue to have pain and impaired digestion secondary to pancreatitis.

 Concept Mastery Alert

Visit thePoint to view an interactive Tutorial on pancreatitis and related fundamentals concepts.

Pancreatic Cysts

As a result of the local necrosis that occurs because of acute pancreatitis, collections of fluid may form close to the pancreas. These fluid collections become walled off by fibrous tissue and are called *pancreatic pseudocysts*. Pseudocysts are amylase-rich fluid collections contained within a wall of fibrous granulation tissue that occur within 4 to 6 weeks after an episode of acute pancreatitis. They are a result of pancreatic necrosis, which produces a pancreatic ductal leak *into* pancreatic tissue weakened by extravasating enzymes (Feldman et al., 2015; Goldman & Schafer, 2015). Pseudocysts are distinguished from true cysts by the characteristics of the lining of the walls of these anomalies. The lining of pseudocysts consists of fibrous granulation tissue, whereas true cysts have epithelium-lined walls (Feldman et al., 2015; Goldman & Schafer, 2015; Papadakis & McPhee, 2016). Pseudocysts are the most common type of pancreatic "cyst." Less common cysts occur as a result of congenital anomalies or secondary to chronic pancreatitis or trauma to the pancreas.

Diagnosis of pancreatic cysts and pseudocysts is made by ultrasound, CT scan, and ERCP. ERCP may be used to define the anatomy of the pancreas and evaluate the patency of pancreatic drainage. Pancreatic pseudocysts may be of considerable size. When pancreatic pseudocysts enlarge, they impinge on and displace the adjacent stomach or the colon because of the location of pseudocysts behind the posterior peritoneum. Eventually, through pressure or secondary infection, they produce symptoms and require drainage.

Drainage into the GI tract or through the skin and abdominal wall may be established. In the latter instance, the drainage is likely to be profuse and destructive to tissue because of the enzyme contents. Hence, steps (including application of skin ointment) must be taken to protect the skin near the drainage site from excoriation. A suction apparatus may be used to continuously aspirate digestive secretions from the drainage tract so that skin contact with the digestive enzymes is avoided. Expert nursing attention is required to ensure that the suction tube does not become dislodged and suction is not interrupted. Consultation with a WOC nurse is indicated to identify appropriate strategies for maintaining drainage and protecting the skin.

Cancer of the Pancreas

Pancreatic cancer is the fourth leading cause of cancer death in men in the United States and the fifth leading cause of cancer death in women. It is very rare before the age of 45 years, and the majority of patients present in or beyond the sixth decade of life (Feldman et al., 2015; Papadakis & McPhee, 2016; Yeo, 2015). The incidence of pancreatic cancer increases with age, peaking in the seventh and eighth decades for both men and women (American Cancer Society [ACS], 2015). The frequency of pancreatic cancer has decreased slightly over the past 25 years among non-Caucasian men. There is a slight male preponderance, and in the United States, incidence is highest in African American males (ACS, 2015; Feldman et al., 2015). Cigarette smoking, exposure to industrial chemicals or toxins in the environment, and a diet high in fat, meat, or both are associated risk factors (ACS, 2015; Alsamarrai et al., 2014; Feldman et al., 2015; Papadakis & McPhee, 2016).

The risk of pancreatic cancer is greater in those with a history of increased pack years of cigarette smoking. Diabetes, chronic pancreatitis, and hereditary pancreatitis are also associated with pancreatic cancer (Alsamarrai et al., 2014; Yeo, 2015). The pancreas can also be the site of metastasis from other tumors.

Cancer may develop in the head, body, or tail of the pancreas; clinical manifestations vary depending on the site and whether functioning insulin-secreting pancreatic islet cells are involved. Approximately 70% of pancreatic cancers originate in the head of the pancreas and give rise to a distinctive clinical picture (Feldman et al., 2015). Functioning islet cell tumors, whether benign (adenoma) or malignant (adenocarcinoma), are responsible for the syndrome of hyperinsulinism. The symptoms are typically nonspecific, and patients usually do not seek medical attention until late in the disease. Only about 7% of cases are diagnosed in early stages; 80% to 85% of patients have advanced, unresectable tumor when first detected. As a result, pancreatic carcinoma has only a 7% survival rate at 5 years regardless of the stage of disease at diagnosis or treatment (ACS, 2015; Yeo, 2015).

Clinical Manifestations

Pain, jaundice, or both are present in more than 80% of patients and, along with weight loss, are considered classic signs of pancreatic carcinoma (Feldman et al., 2015). However, they often do not appear until the disease is far advanced. Other signs include rapid, profound, and progressive weight loss as well as vague upper or midabdominal pain or discomfort that is unrelated to any GI function and is often difficult to describe. Such discomfort radiates as a boring pain in the midback and is unrelated to posture or activity. It is often progressive and severe, requiring the use of opioids. It is often more severe at night and is accentuated when lying supine. Relief may be obtained by sitting up and leaning forward.

Malignant cells from pancreatic cancer are often shed into the peritoneal cavity, increasing the likelihood of metastasis.

The formation of ascites is common. An important sign, if present, is the onset of symptoms of insulin deficiency: glucosuria, hyperglycemia, and abnormal glucose tolerance. Therefore, diabetes may be an early sign of carcinoma of the pancreas. Meals often aggravate epigastric pain, which usually occurs before the appearance of jaundice and pruritus.

Assessment and Diagnostic Findings

Spiral (helical) CT is more than 85% to 90% accurate in the diagnosis and staging of pancreatic cancer and currently is the most useful preoperative imaging technique. MRI may also be used. ERCP is also used in the diagnosis of pancreatic carcinoma. EUS is useful in identifying small tumors and in performing fine-needle aspiration biopsy of the primary tumor or lymph nodes (Goldman & Schafer, 2015; Papadakis & McPhee, 2016). Cells obtained during ERCP are sent to the laboratory for analysis. GI x-ray findings may demonstrate deformities in adjacent organs caused by the impinging pancreatic mass.

A histologic diagnosis is not usually required in patients who are candidates for surgery. The tissue diagnosis is made at the time of the surgical procedure. Percutaneous fine-needle aspiration biopsy of the pancreas, which is used to diagnose pancreatic tumors, is also used to confirm the diagnosis in patients whose tumors are not resectable so that a palliative plan of care can be determined. This may eliminate the stress and postoperative pain of ineffective surgery. In this procedure, a needle is inserted through the anterior abdominal wall into the pancreatic mass, guided by CT, ultrasound, ERCP, or other imaging techniques. The aspirated material is examined for malignant cells. Although percutaneous biopsy is a valuable diagnostic tool, it has some potential drawbacks: a false-negative result if small tumors are missed and the risk of seeding of cancer cells along the needle track. Low-dose radiation to the site may be used before the biopsy to reduce this risk.

PTC is another procedure that may be performed to identify obstructions of the biliary tract by a pancreatic tumor. Several tumor markers (e.g., cancer antigen 19-9, carcinoembryonic antigen, DU-PAN-2) may be used in the diagnostic workup, but they are nonspecific for pancreatic carcinoma. These tumor markers are useful as indicators of disease progression.

Angiography, CT scans, and laparoscopy may be performed to determine whether the tumor can be removed surgically. Intraoperative ultrasonography has been used to determine whether there is metastatic disease to other organs.

Medical Management

If the tumor is resectable and localized (typically tumors in the head of the pancreas), the surgical procedure to remove it is usually extensive (see later discussion). However, total excision of the lesion often is not possible for two reasons: (1) extensive growth of tumor before diagnosis and (2) probable widespread metastases (especially to the liver, lungs, and bones). More often, treatment is limited to palliative measures.

Although pancreatic tumors may be resistant to standard radiation therapy, the patient may be treated with radiation and chemotherapy (5-fluorouracil [5-FU, Adrucil], leucovorin

[Wellcovorin], and gemcitabine [Gemzar]). Currently, gemcitabine is the standard of care for patients with metastatic pancreatic cancer and has been found to lengthen survival (ACS, 2015; Feldman et al., 2015). The targeted anticancer drug erlotinib (Tarceva) has demonstrated a slight improvement in advanced pancreatic cancer survival when used in combination with gemcitabine (ACS, 2015). Clinical trials with new agents such as S-1 (an oral fluoropyrimidine), Folfirinox, or the use of nanoparticle albumin-bound paclitaxel (nab-paclitaxel) with gemcitabine therapy, combined with radiation and/or surgery may also result in improved survival (ACS, 2015; Kamisawa, Wood, Itoi, et al., 2016). If the patient undergoes surgery, intraoperative radiation therapy may be used to deliver a high dose of radiation to the tumor with minimal injury to other tissues; this may also be helpful in relief of pain. Interstitial implantation of radioactive sources has also been used, although the rate of complications is high. A large biliary stent inserted percutaneously or by endoscopy may be used to relieve jaundice (Alemi, Alseidi, Helton, et al., 2015; Li, Wang, Li, et al., 2015).

Nursing Management

Pain management and attention to nutritional requirements are important nursing measures that improve the level of patient comfort. Skin care and nursing measures are directed toward relief of pain and discomfort associated with jaundice, anorexia, and profound weight loss. Specialty mattresses are beneficial and protect bony prominences from pressure. Pain associated with pancreatic cancer may be severe and may require liberal use of opioids; patient-controlled analgesia should be considered for the patient with severe, escalating pain.

Because of the poor prognosis and likelihood of short survival, end-of-life preferences are discussed and honored. If appropriate, the nurse refers the patient to hospice care. See Chapters 15 and 16 for care of the patient with cancer and end-of-life care, respectively.

Promoting Home, Community-Based and Transitional Care

 Educating Patients About Self-Care

Specific education for the patient and family varies with the stage of disease and the treatment choices made by the patient. If the patient elects to receive chemotherapy, the nurse focuses on prevention of side effects and complications of the agents used. If surgery is performed to relieve obstruction and establish biliary drainage, education addresses management of the drainage system and monitoring for complications. The nurse educates the family about changes in the patient's status that should be reported to the primary provider.

Continuing and Transitional Care

A referral for home, community-based, or transitional care is indicated to help the patient and family deal with the physical problems and discomforts associated with pancreatic cancer and the psychological impact of the disease. The nurse assesses the patient's physical status, fluid and nutritional status, skin integrity, and the adequacy of pain management. The nurse educates the patient and family on strategies to prevent skin breakdown and relieve pain, pruritus, and anorexia. It is important to discuss and arrange palliative care (hospice services) as indicated in an effort to relieve patient discomfort, assist with care, and comply with the patient's end-of-life decisions and wishes (see Chart 50-5).

Tumors of the Head of the Pancreas

Tumors of the head of the pancreas comprise 60% to 80% of all pancreatic tumors (Goldman & Schafer, 2015; Muniraj et al., 2014; Yeo, 2015). Tumors in this region of the pancreas obstruct the common bile duct where the duct passes through the head of the pancreas to join the pancreatic duct and empty at the ampulla of Vater into the duodenum. The tumors producing the obstruction may arise from the pancreas, the common bile duct, or the ampulla of Vater (Alemi et al., 2015; Li et al., 2015).

Chart 50-5 **NURSING RESEARCH PROFILE**

Patients With Advanced Pancreatic Cancer and the Psychological Health of Their Family Caregivers

Sherman, D. W., & McMillan, S. C. (2015). The physical health of patients with advanced pancreatic cancer and the psychological health of their family caregivers when newly enrolled in hospice. *Journal of Hospice & Palliative Nursing, 17*(3), 235–241.

Purpose

The purpose of this study was to describe commonly occurring symptoms and level of associated patient distress as well as to explore the perceived social support, perceived health, and depressive symptoms of caregivers of hospice patients with advanced pancreatic cancer.

Design

The study used a descriptive design and enrolled a sample of 64 patients with advanced pancreatic cancer and their family caregivers who were newly enrolled in a hospice program. Self-report by participants and caregivers was used to determine patient symptoms and perceived levels of social support, perceived health, and depressive symptoms in caregivers.

Findings

More than 50% of participants reported symptoms of fatigue, lack of appetite, dry mouth, pain, feeling drowsy, and feeling sad. The symptoms causing the most distress were fatigue, pain, and lack of appetite. When perceived social support was measured, family caregivers reported satisfaction with emotional support and rated their perceived health as fair to good with relatively low depressive symptoms.

Nursing Implications

Nurses can be instrumental in aiding patients and families through the often painful and distressing experience of pancreatic cancer. This research reinforces the need for nurses to develop individualized plans of care for patients with this diagnosis and their families. More research is needed on how to best palliate symptoms and improve end-of-life care for these patients and their family caregivers.

Clinical Manifestations

The obstructed flow of bile produces jaundice, clay-colored stools, and dark urine. Malabsorption of nutrients and fat-soluble vitamins may result if the tumor obstructs the entry of bile to the GI tract. Abdominal discomfort or pain and pruritus may be noted, along with anorexia, weight loss, and malaise. If these signs and symptoms are present, cancer of the head of the pancreas is suspected.

The jaundice of this disease must be differentiated from that due to a biliary obstruction caused by a gallstone in the common duct. Jaundice caused by a gallstone is usually intermittent and occurs more commonly in women and in people who are obese and who have had previous symptoms of gallbladder disease.

Assessment and Diagnostic Findings

Diagnostic studies may include duodenography, angiography by hepatic or celiac artery catheterization, pancreatic scanning, PTC, ERCP, and percutaneous needle biopsy of the pancreas. Results of a biopsy of the pancreas may aid in the diagnosis.

Medical Management

Before extensive surgery can be performed, a period of preparation is necessary because the patient's nutritional status and physical condition are often quite compromised. Various liver and pancreatic function studies are performed. A diet high in protein along with pancreatic enzymes is often prescribed. Preoperative preparation includes adequate hydration, correction of prothrombin deficiency with vitamin K, and treatment of anemia to minimize postoperative complications. Enteral or parenteral nutrition and blood component therapy are frequently required.

A biliary drainage procedure may be performed, usually with a catheter via percutaneous access, to relieve the jaundice and, perhaps, to provide time for a thorough diagnostic evaluation. Total pancreatectomy (removal of the pancreas) may be performed if there is no evidence of direct extension of the tumor to adjacent tissues or regional lymph nodes. A pancreaticoduodenectomy (Whipple procedure or resection) is used for potentially resectable cancer of the head of the pancreas (see Fig. 50-7) (Alemi et al., 2015; Li et al., 2015). This procedure involves removal of the gallbladder, a portion of the stomach, duodenum, proximal jejunum, head of the pancreas, and distal common bile duct. Reconstruction involves anastomosis of the remaining pancreas and stomach to the jejunum (Townsend et al., 2016). A pylorus-preserving pancreaticojejunostomy (PPPD) may also be performed for tumors of the head of the pancreas and may reduce postgastrectomy symptoms and improve overall GI function (Feldman et al., 2015). The result of these procedures is removal of the tumor, allowing flow of bile into the jejunum. If the tumor cannot be excised, the jaundice may be relieved by diverting the bile flow into the jejunum by anastomosing the jejunum to the gallbladder, a procedure known as **cholecystojejunostomy** (Alemi et al., 2015; Li et al., 2015).

The postoperative management of patients who have undergone a pancreatectomy or a pancreaticoduodenectomy is similar to the management of patients after extensive GI or

Figure 50-7 • Pancreatoduodenectomy (Whipple procedure or resection). End result of resection of carcinoma of the head of the pancreas or the ampulla of Vater. The common duct is sutured to the side of the jejunum (choledochojejunostomy), and the remaining portion of the pancreas and the end of the stomach are sutured to the side of the jejunum.

biliary surgery. The patient's physical status is often suboptimal, increasing the risk of postoperative complications. Hemorrhage, vascular collapse, and hepatorenal failure remain the major postoperative complications. The mortality rate associated with these procedures has decreased because of advances in nutritional support and improved surgical techniques. A nasogastric tube with suction and parenteral nutrition allow the GI tract to rest while promoting adequate nutrition.

Nursing Management

Preoperatively and postoperatively, nursing care is directed toward promoting patient comfort, preventing complications, and assisting the patient to return to and maintain as normal and comfortable a life as possible. The nurse closely monitors the patient in the intensive care unit after surgery; in the immediate postoperative period, multiple IV and arterial lines are used for fluid and blood replacement and hemodynamic monitoring, and a mechanical ventilator may be used. It is important to note and report changes in vital signs, arterial blood gases and pressures, pulse oximetry, laboratory values, and urine output. The nurse must also consider the patient's compromised nutritional status and risk of bleeding. Depending on the type of surgical procedure performed, malabsorption syndrome and diabetes are likely; the nurse must address these issues during acute and long-term patient care.

Although the patient's physiologic status is the focus of the health care team in the immediate postoperative period, the patient's psychological and emotional states must be considered, along with those of the family. The patient has undergone a major high-risk surgery and is critically ill; anxiety and depression may affect recovery. The immediate and long-term outcomes of this extensive surgical resection are uncertain, and the patient and family require emotional support and understanding in the critical and stressful preoperative and postoperative periods.

Promoting Home, Community-Based and Transitional Care

 Educating Patients About Self-Care

The patient who has undergone this extensive surgery requires careful and thorough preparation for self-care at home. The nurse educates the patient and family about strategies to relieve pain and discomfort, along with strategies to manage drains, if present, and to care for the surgical incision. The patient and family members may require education about the use of appropriate analgesic medications, parenteral nutrition, wound care, skin care, and management of drainage.

The nurse may need to educate the patient and family about the need for modifications in the diet because of malabsorption and hyperglycemia resulting from the surgery. It is important to educate the patient and family about the continuing need for pancreatic enzyme replacement, a low-fat diet, and vitamin supplementation. The nurse describes—verbally and in writing—the signs and symptoms of complications and educates the patient and family about indicators of complications that should be reported promptly.

Discharge of the patient to a long-term care or rehabilitation facility may be warranted after surgery as extensive as pancreatectomy or pancreaticoduodenectomy, particularly if the patient's preoperative status was not optimal. Information about the education that has been provided is shared with the long-term care staff so that instructions can be clarified and reinforced. During the recovery or long-term phase of care, the patient and family receive further education about self-care in the home.

Continuing and Transitional Care

A referral for home, community-based, or transitional care may be indicated when the patient returns home. The nurse assesses the patient's physical and psychological status and the ability of the patient and family to manage needed care. The nurse provides needed physical care and monitors the adequacy of pain management. In addition, it is important to assess the patient's nutritional status and monitor the use of enteral or parenteral nutrition, if used. The nurse discusses the use of hospice services with the patient and family and makes a referral if indicated.

Pancreatic Islet Tumors

At least two types of tumors of the pancreatic islet cells are known: those that secrete insulin (insulinoma) and those in which insulin secretion is not increased (nonfunctioning

islet cell cancer). All of these types of tumors combined are termed *neuroendocrine tumors* (NETs). Insulinomas produce hypersecretion of insulin and cause an excessive rate of glucose metabolism. The resulting hypoglycemia may produce symptoms of weakness, mental confusion, and seizures. These symptoms may be relieved almost immediately by oral or IV administration of glucose. The 5-hour glucose tolerance test is helpful to diagnose insulinoma and to distinguish a diagnosis of NET from other causes of hypoglycemia.

Surgical Management

If a tumor of the islet cells (a type of NET) has been diagnosed, surgical treatment with removal of the tumor is usually recommended (Greenberger et al., 2015). The tumors may be benign adenomas, or they may be malignant. Complete removal usually results in almost immediate relief of symptoms. In some patients, symptoms may be produced by simple hypertrophy of this tissue rather than a tumor of the islet cells. In such cases, a partial pancreatectomy (removal of the tail and part of the body of the pancreas) is performed.

Nursing Management

In preparing the patient for surgery, the nurse must be alert for symptoms of hypoglycemia and be ready to administer glucose as prescribed if symptoms occur. Postoperatively, the nursing management is the same as after other upper abdominal surgical procedures, with special emphasis on monitoring serum glucose levels. Patient education is determined by the extent of surgery and alterations in pancreatic function.

Hyperinsulinism

Hyperinsulinism is caused by overproduction of insulin by the pancreatic islets. Symptoms resemble those of excessive doses of insulin and are attributable to the same mechanism: an abnormal reduction in blood glucose levels. Clinically, it is characterized by episodes during which the patient experiences unusual hunger, nervousness, sweating, headache, and faintness; in severe cases, seizures and episodes of unconsciousness may occur. The findings at the time of surgery or at autopsy may indicate hyperplasia (overgrowth) of the islets of Langerhans or a benign or malignant tumor involving the islets that is capable of producing large amounts of insulin (see preceding discussion). Occasionally, tumors of nonpancreatic origin produce an insulinlike material that can cause severe hypoglycemia and may be responsible for seizures coinciding with blood glucose levels that are too low to sustain normal brain function (i.e., lower than 30 mg/dL [1.6 mmol/L]) (Bope & Kellerman, 2015; Goldman & Schafer, 2015).

All of the symptoms that accompany spontaneous hypoglycemia are relieved by the oral or parenteral administration of glucose. Surgical removal of the hyperplastic or neoplastic tissue from the pancreas is the only successful method of treatment. About 15% of patients with spontaneous or functional hypoglycemia eventually develop diabetes.

Ulcerogenic Tumors

Some tumors of the islets of Langerhans are associated with hypersecretion of gastric acid that produces ulcers in the stomach, duodenum, and jejunum. This is referred to as **Zollinger–Ellison syndrome**. The hypersecretion is so excessive that even after partial gastric resection, enough acid is produced to cause further ulceration. If a marked tendency to develop gastric and duodenal ulcers is noted, an ulcerogenic tumor of the islets of Langerhans is considered (Dacha, Razvi, Massaad, et al., 2015).

These tumors, which may be benign or malignant, are treated by excision, if possible. Frequently, however, removal is not possible because of extension beyond the pancreas. In many patients, a total gastrectomy may be necessary to reduce the secretion of gastric acid sufficiently to prevent further ulceration. This procedure is also indicated to treat gastric carcinoid tumors that may arise from the effect of prolonged hypersecretion of gastric acids (Dacha et al., 2015; Doi, 2015).

The many disorders of the biliary and pancreatic systems result in a host of clinical and biochemical abnormalities presented in detail in this chapter. The recognition and management of these illnesses pose a challenge to nurses. There is now much evidence about the prevention, diagnosis, and treatment of these disorders. However, there is still much to learn as the medical and nursing communities strive to provide optimum care to patients afflicted with biliary and pancreatic disorders.

CRITICAL THINKING EXERCISES

1 `pq` A 77-year-old man underwent a right total hip replacement. His clinical course was initially stable but on day 4 postoperatively he became nauseated and began vomiting. He also complained of right upper quadrant pain and was hypotensive and tachycardic. His urine output has decreased to 10 mL/hr. What are the initial priorities of care for this patient? An abdominal ultrasound and abdominal CT scan were performed and revealed marked thickening of the gallbladder wall and pericholecystic effusion but no gallstones were identified. He was determined to have acalculous cholecystitis. What would be the initial treatment the nurse would expect to implement? If the patient continued to deteriorate with worsening pain and signs of systemic inflammation and hypovolemia, what additional interventions should the nurse be prepared to implement?

2 `ebp` A 58-year-old man presents to the emergency department with complaints of severe midepigastric pain. He is also nauseated and vomiting. His vital signs reveal hypotension and tachycardia and he is febrile. His history is significant for alcohol abuse and hypertension. What laboratory and imaging studies do you expect to be performed? His CT scan revealed pancreatic necrosis and multiple fluid collections. An evidence-based approach for managing infected pancreatic necrosis was implemented. What first-line intervention would you expect to be implemented in this case? What classification of pancreatitis is this patient experiencing?

3 A 55-year-old woman has been experiencing upper abdominal pain for several weeks. She believes that she has gallbladder disease but is concerned because her mother died from pancreatic cancer. She visits her physician who prescribes a CT scan and initial laboratory screening studies. Which laboratory tests would you expect to be assessed? The CT scan revealed no masses but did show dilatation of the pancreatic duct. The woman grew more concerned due to her family history even though her initial laboratory tests were normal. Her physician shared her concern and prescribed an MRI, which revealed a small mass at the head of the pancreas. The woman was referred to a surgeon who began an assessment to determine if the patient was a candidate for potentially curative resection. What testing is needed to assess if the mass was cancerous and if it may have metastasized? The patient is determined to be a candidate for surgery. List two postoperative nursing interventions that can be effective in preventing complications. What education will the nurse provide the patient to enhance comfort, nutrition and quality of life after discharge?

REFERENCES

*Asterisk indicates nursing research.
**Double asterisk indicates classic reference.

Books

Bope, E. T., & Kellerman, R. D. (Eds.). (2015). *Conn's current therapy.* Philadelphia, PA: Saunders.

Comerford, K. C. (2015). *Nursing 2015 drug handbook.* Philadelphia, PA: Wolters Kluwer.

Doherty, G. (2015). *Current diagnosis and treatment: Surgery* (14th ed.). New York: McGraw-Hill.

Dudek, S. G. (2013). *Nutrition essentials for nursing practice* (7th ed.). Philadelphia, PA: Lippincott Williams & Wilkins.

Eliopoulos, C. (2018). *Gerontological nursing* (9th ed.). Philadelphia, PA: Lippincott Williams & Wilkins.

Feldman, M., Friedman, L. S., & Brandt, L. J. (2015). *Sleisenger & Fordtran's gastrointestinal & liver disease* (10th ed.). Philadelphia, PA: Saunders Elsevier.

Ferri, F. F. (Ed.). (2014). *Practical guide to the care of the medical patient* (9th ed.). Philadelphia, PA: Mosby Elsevier.

Goldman, L., & Schafer, A. I. (2015). *Goldman's cecil medicine* (25th ed.). Philadelphia, PA: Saunders Elsevier.

Greenberger, N. J., Blumberg, R. S., & Burakoff, R. (Eds.). (2015). *Current diagnosis and treatment: Gastroenterology, hepatology & endoscopy.* New York: McGraw-Hill.

Hall, J. E. (2015). *Guyton & Hall textbook of medical physiology* (13th ed.). Philadelphia, PA: Saunders Elsevier.

Kumar, V., Abbas, A. K., Fausto, N., et al. (2014). *Robbins and Cotran pathologic basis of disease* (9th ed.). Philadelphia, PA: Saunders Elsevier.

Marx, J., Hockberger, R. & Walls, R. (Eds.). (2013). *Rosen's emergency medicine: Concepts and clinical practice.* Philadelphia, PA: Mosby Elsevier.

Miller, R. D., Eriksson, L. I., Fleisher, L. E., et al. (2014). *Miller's anesthesia* (8th ed.). Edinburgh, UK: Churchill Livingstone.

Papadakis, M. A., & McPhee, S. J. (Eds.). (2016). *Current medical diagnosis and treatment* (55th ed.). New York: McGraw-Hill.

Rakel, R. E., & Rakel, D. P. (Eds.). (2015). *Textbook of family medicine* (9th ed.). Philadelphia, PA: Saunders Elsevier.

Strayer, D. S., & Rubin, E. (2015). *Rubin's pathology: Clinicopathologic foundations of medicine* (7th ed.). Philadelphia, PA: Lippincott Williams & Wilkins.

Townsend, C. M., Beauchamp, R. D., Evers, B. M., et al. (2016). *Sabiston's textbook of surgery: The biological basis of modern surgical practice.* Philadelphia, PA: Elsevier.

Journals and Electronic Documents

Alemi, F., Alseidi, A., Helton, H. W., et al. (2015). Multidisciplinary management of locally advanced pancreatic ductal adenocarcinoma. *Current Problems in Surgery, 52*(9), 362–398.

Alsamarrai, A., Das, S. L. M., Windsor, J. A., et al. (2014). Factors that affect risk for pancreatic disease in the general population: A systematic review and meta-analysis of prospective cohort studies. *Clinical Gastroenterology and Hepatology, 12*(10), 1635–1644; quiz e103.

American Cancer Society (ACS). (2015). *Cancer Facts & Figures 2015*. Retrieved on 12/12/2015 at: www.cancer.org/Research/CancerFactsFigures.

Dacha, S., Razvi, M., Massaad, J., et al. (2015). Hypergastrinemia. *Gastroenterology Report. 3*(3), 201–208.

da Costa, D. W., Boerma, D., van Santvoort, H. C., et al. (2014). Staged multidisciplinary step-up management for necrotizing pancreatitis. *British Journal of Surgery, 10*(1), e65–e79.

de Mestral, C., Rotstein, O. D., Laupacis, A., et al. (2014). Comparative operative outcomes of early and delayed cholecystectomy for acute cholecystitis: A population-based propensity score analysis. *Annals of Surgery, 259*(1), 10–15.

De Waele, J. J. (2014). Acute pancreatitis. *Current Opinion in Critical Care, 20*(2), 189–195.

D'Haese, J. G., Ceyhan, G. O., Demir, I. E., et al. (2014). Treatment options in painful chronic pancreatitis: A systematic review. *HPB, 16*(6), 512–521.

Doi, R. (2015). Determinants of surgical resection for pancreatic neuroendocrine tumors. *Journal of Hepato-biliary-Pancreatic Sciences. 22*(8), 610–617.

Emmanuel, N., & Lee, P. (2014). Acute pain management. *International Journal of Nursing Education, 6*(2), 93–97.

Fagenholz, P. J., & de Moya, M. A. (2014). Acute inflammatory surgical disease. *Surgical Clinics of North America, 24*(2014), 1–30.

Gupte, A. R., & Forsmark, C. E. (2014). Chronic pancreatitis. *Current Opinion in Gastroenterology, 30*(5), 500–505.

Gurusamy, K. S., Rossi, M., & Davidson, B. R. (2013). Percutaneous cholecystostomy for high-risk surgical patients with acute calculous cholecystitis. *Cochrane Database of Systematic Reviews*, (8), CD007088.

Hong, M. T., Monye, L. C., & Seifert, C. F. (2015). Acid suppressive therapy for stress ulcer prophylaxis in noncritically ill patients. *Annals of Pharmacotherapy, 49*(9), 1004–1008.

Kamisawa, T., Wood, L. D., Itoi, T., et al. (2016). Pancreatic cancer. *The Lancet, 388*(10039), 73–85.

Lankisch, P. G., Apte, M. & Banks, P. A. (2015). Acute pancreatitis. *The Lancet, 386*(9988), 85–96.

Lee, J. Y., Keane, M. G., & Pereira, S. (2015). Diagnosis and treatment of gallstone disease. *Practitioner, 259*(1783), 15–19.

Li, C. C., Wang, Y. Q., Li, Y. P., et al. (2015). Critical appraisal of clinical practice guidelines for treating pancreatic cancer based on the global disease burden. *Journal of Evidence-Based Practice, 8*(1), 11–21.

*Lindseth, G. N., & Denny, D. L. (2014). Patients' experiences with cholecystitis and a choecystectomy. *Gastroenterology Nursing, 37*(6), 407–414.

Martin, R. F., & Hein, A. R. (2013). Operative management of acute pancreatitis. *Surgical Clinics of North America, 93*(3), 595–610.

McClave, S. A. (2013). Nutrition in pancreatitis. *World Review of Nutrition & Dietetics, 105*, 160–168.

McMahon, M., Nystrom, E., Braunschweig, C., et al. (2013). ASPEN guidelines: Nutrition support of adult patients with hyperglycemia. *Journal of Parenteral and Enteral Nutrition, 37*(1), 23–36.

Michetti, C. P., Griffen, M., Tran, H. T., et al. (2015). Laparoscopic cholecystectomy performed by acute care surgeons and general surgeons. *American Surgeon, 81*(5), E220–E221.

Muniraj, T., Aslanian, H. R., Farrell, J., et al. (2014). Chronic pancreatitis, a comprehensive review and update. Part I: Epidemiology, etiology, risk factors, genetics, pathophysiology, and clinical features. *Disease-A-Month, 60*(12), 530–550.

Muniraj, T., Aslanian, H. R., Farrell, J., et al. (2015). Chronic pancreatitis, a comprehensive review and update. Part II: Diagnosis, complications, and management, *Disease-A-Month, 61*(1), 5–37.

Nikfarjam, M., Shen, L., Fink, M. A., et al. (2013). Percutaneous cholecystostomy for treatment of acute cholecystitis in the era of early laparoscopic cholecystectomy. *Surgical Laparoscopy, Endoscopy & Percutaneous Techniques, 23*(5), 474–480.

**Ranson, J. H., Rifkind, K. M., Roses, D. F., et al. (1974). Prognostic signs and the role of operative management in acute pancreatitis. *Surgery, Gynecology & Obstetrics, 139*(1), 69–81.

Rao, A., Polanco, A., Qiu, S., et al. (2013). Safety of outpatient laparoscopic cholecystectomy in the elderly: Analysis of 15,248 patients using the NSQIP database. *Journal of the American College of Surgeons, 217*(6), 1038–1043.

Schepers, N. J., Besselink, M. G., van Santvoort, H. C., et al; Dutch Pancreatitis Study Group. (2013). Early management of acute pancreatitis. *Best practice & research Clinical gastroenterology, 27*(5), 727–743.

Schulenburg, J. (2015). Considerations for complementary and alternative interventions for pain. *AORN Journal, 101*(3), 319–326.

Sherman, D. W., & McMillan, S. C. (2015). The physical health of patients with advanced pancreatic cancer and the psychological health of their family caregivers when newly enrolled in hospice. *Journal of Hospice & Palliative Nursing, 17*(3), 235–241.

Talukdar, R., & Nageshwar, R. D. (2014). Endoscopic therapy for chronic pancreatitis. *Current Opinion in Gastroenterology, 30*(5), 484–489.

Wu, B., & Banks, P. A. (2013). Clinical management of patients with acute pancreatitis. *Gastroenterology, 144*(6), 1272–1281.

Yeo, T. P. (2015). Demographics, epidemiology, and inheritance of pancreatic ductal adenocarcinoma. *Seminars in Oncology, 42*(1), 8–18.

Zerem, E. (2014). Treatment of severe acute pancreatitis and its complications. *World Journal of Gastroenterology, 20*(38), 13879–13892.

Resources

American Gastroenterological Association (AGA), www.gastro.org

Endocrine Society, www.endo-society.org

National Digestive Diseases Information Clearinghouse (NDDIC), www.digestive.niddk.nih.gov

National Pancreas Foundation (NPF), www.pancreasfoundation.org

51

Assessment and Management of Patients With Diabetes

LEARNING OBJECTIVES

On completion of this chapter, the learner will be able to:

1 Differentiate between the types of diabetes.
2 Describe etiologic factors associated with diabetes.
3 Relate the clinical manifestations of diabetes to the associated pathophysiologic alterations.
4 Identify the diagnostic and clinical significance of blood glucose test results.
5 Explain the dietary modifications used for management of people with diabetes.
6 Describe the relationships among diet, exercise, and medication (i.e., insulin or oral antidiabetic agents) for people with diabetes.
7 Develop an education plan for insulin self-management.
8 Identify the role of oral antidiabetic agents in therapy for patients with diabetes.
9 Use the nursing process as a framework for care of patients who have hyperglycemia with diabetic ketoacidosis or hyperglycemic hyperosmolar syndrome.
10 Describe management strategies for a person with diabetes to use during "sick days."
11 Outline the major complications of diabetes and the self-care behaviors that are important in their prevention.
12 Identify the programs and community support groups available for people with diabetes.

GLOSSARY

diabetes: a group of metabolic diseases characterized by hyperglycemia resulting from defects in insulin secretion, insulin action, or both

diabetic ketoacidosis (DKA): a metabolic derangement in type 1 diabetes that results from a deficiency of insulin; highly acidic ketone bodies are formed, resulting in acidosis

fasting plasma glucose (FPG): blood glucose determination obtained in the laboratory after fasting for at least 8 hours

gestational diabetes: any degree of glucose intolerance with its onset during pregnancy

glycated hemoglobin (glycosylated hemoglobin, HgbA₁c, or A1C): a measure of glucose control that is a result of glucose molecule attaching to hemoglobin for the life of the red blood cell (120 days)

glycemic index: the amount a given food increases the blood glucose level compared with an equivalent amount of glucose

hyperglycemia: elevated blood glucose level

hyperglycemic hyperosmolar syndrome (HHS): a metabolic disorder of type 2 diabetes resulting from a relative insulin deficiency initiated by an illness that raises the demand for insulin

hypoglycemia: low blood glucose level

impaired fasting glucose (IFG) or impaired glucose tolerance (IGT): a metabolic stage intermediate between normal glucose homeostasis and diabetes; referred to as prediabetes

insulin: a hormone secreted by the beta cells of the islets of Langerhans of the pancreas that is necessary for the metabolism of carbohydrates, proteins, and fats; a deficiency of insulin results in diabetes

insulin pump: a continuous subcutaneous insulin infusion device that delivers insulin on a 24-hour basis

ketone: a highly acidic substance formed when the liver breaks down free fatty acids in the absence of insulin

latent autoimmune diabetes of adults (LADA): a subtype of diabetes

medical nutrition therapy (MNT): nutritional therapy prescribed for management of diabetes that usually is given by a registered dietician

nephropathy: a long-term complication of diabetes in which the kidney cells are damaged; characterized by microalbuminuria in early stages and progressing to end-stage kidney disease

neuropathy: a long-term complication of diabetes resulting from damage to the nerve cell

prediabetes: impaired glucose metabolism in which blood glucose concentrations fall between normal levels and those considered diagnostic for diabetes; includes impaired fasting glucose and impaired glucose tolerance, not clinical entities in their own right but risk factors for future diabetes and cardiovascular disease

retinopathy: a complication of diabetes in which the small blood vessels that nourish the retina in the eye are damaged

self-monitoring of blood glucose (SMBG): a method of capillary blood glucose testing

type 1 diabetes: a metabolic disorder characterized by an absence of insulin production and secretion from autoimmune destruction of the beta cells of the islets of Langerhans in the pancreas; formerly called *insulin-dependent diabetes, or juvenile diabetes*

type 2 diabetes: a metabolic disorder characterized by the relative deficiency of insulin production and a decreased insulin action and increased insulin resistance; formerly called *non–insulin-dependent diabetes, or adult-onset diabetes*

Diabetes is a group of metabolic diseases characterized by increased levels of glucose in the blood (**hyperglycemia**) resulting from defects in insulin secretion, insulin action, or both (American Diabetes Association [ADA], 2016a). Care of the patient with diabetes, formerly known as diabetes mellitus but now more commonly referred to as diabetes, requires an understanding of the epidemiology, pathophysiology, diagnostic testing, medical and nursing care, and rehabilitation of patients with diabetes. Nurses care for patients with diabetes in all settings. This chapter focuses on the nursing management of patients with diabetes.

DIABETES

Epidemiology

It is estimated that more than 29.1 million people in the United States have diabetes, although almost one third of these cases are undiagnosed. The number of people older than 20 years newly diagnosed with diabetes increases by 1.7 million per year (Centers for Disease Control and Prevention [CDC], 2014). If this trend continues, one in every three adults in the United States could have diabetes by 2050. In 2014, the worldwide estimate of the prevalence of diabetes was 422 million people, and by 2040, this is expected to increase to more than 642 million (World Health Organization [WHO], 2015a).

Minority populations are disproportionately affected by diabetes. The age-adjusted prevalence of diabetes is increasing among all gender and racial groups, but compared with Caucasians, African Americans and members of other racial and ethnic groups (Native Americans and persons of Hispanic origin) are more likely to develop diabetes, are at greater risk for many of the complications, and have higher death rates due to diabetes (CDC, 2014). Chart 51-1 summarizes risk factors for diabetes.

Diabetes can have far-reaching and devastating physical, social, and economic consequences, including the following (CDC, 2014):

- In the United States, diabetes is the leading cause of nontraumatic amputations, blindness in working-age adults, and end-stage kidney disease (ESKD).

> ## Chart 51-1 ⚠️ RISK FACTORS
> ### Diabetes
>
> - Family history of diabetes (e.g., parents or siblings with diabetes)
> - Obesity (i.e., ≥20% over desired body weight or body mass index ≥30 kg/m²)
> - Race/ethnicity (e.g., African Americans, Hispanic Americans, Native Americans, Asian Americans, Pacific Islanders)
> - Age equal to or greater than 45 years
> - Previously identified impaired fasting glucose or impaired glucose tolerance
> - Hypertension (≥140/90 mm Hg)
> - High-density lipoprotein (HDL) cholesterol level ≤35 mg/dL (0.90 mmol/L) and/or triglyceride level ≥250 mg/dL (2.8 mmol/L)
> - History of gestational diabetes or delivery of a baby over 9 lb
>
> Adapted from American Diabetes Association (ADA). (2016b). Standards of medical care in diabetes—2016. Classification and diagnosis of diabetes. *Diabetes Care, 39*(Suppl 1), S13–S24.

- Diabetes is a leading cause of death from disease, primarily because of the high rate of cardiovascular disease (myocardial infarction [MI], stroke, and peripheral vascular disease) among people with diabetes.
- Hospitalization rates for people with diabetes are 2.4 times greater for adults and 5.3 times greater for children than for the general population.

The economic cost of diabetes continues to increase because of increasing health care costs and an aging population. The U.S. Department of Health and Human Services (HHS) has identified diabetes as an important topic area. Nationwide efforts are needed to decrease its occurrence and to increase the quality of life of those people who have the disease (HHS, 2014).

Classification

The major classifications of diabetes are type 1 diabetes, type 2 diabetes, gestational diabetes, latent autoimmune diabetes of adults (LADA), and diabetes associated with other conditions or syndromes (ADA, 2016b). The different types of diabetes vary in cause, clinical course, and treatment (see Table 51-1). The classification system is dynamic in two ways. First, research findings suggest many differences among individuals within each category. Second, except for people with type 1 diabetes, patients may move from one category to another. For example, a woman with gestational diabetes may, after delivery, move into type 2 diabetes. **Prediabetes** is classified as **impaired glucose tolerance (IGT)** or **impaired fasting glucose (IFG)** and refers to a condition in which blood glucose concentrations fall between normal levels and those considered diagnostic for diabetes (CDC, 2014).

Pathophysiology

Insulin is a hormone secreted by beta cells, which are one of four types of cells in the islets of Langerhans in the pancreas (Grossman & Porth, 2014). Insulin is an anabolic, or storage, hormone. When a person eats a meal, insulin secretion increases and moves glucose from the blood into muscle, liver, and fat cells. In those cells, insulin has the following actions:

- Transports and metabolizes glucose for energy
- Stimulates storage of glucose in the liver and muscle (in the form of glycogen)
- Signals the liver to stop the release of glucose
- Enhances storage of dietary fat in adipose tissue
- Accelerates transport of amino acids (derived from dietary protein) into cells
- Inhibits the breakdown of stored glucose, protein, and fat

During fasting periods (between meals and overnight), the pancreas continuously releases a small amount of insulin (basal insulin); another pancreatic hormone called *glucagon* (secreted by the alpha cells of the islets of Langerhans) is released when blood glucose levels decrease, which stimulates the liver to release stored glucose. The insulin and the glucagon together maintain a constant level of glucose in the blood by stimulating the release of glucose from the liver.

Initially, the liver produces glucose through the breakdown of glycogen (glycogenolysis). After 8 to 12 hours without food, the liver forms glucose from the breakdown of noncarbohydrate substances, including amino acids (gluconeogenesis).

TABLE 51-1 Classification of Diabetes and Related Glucose Intolerances

Current Classification	Clinical Characteristics and Clinical Implications
Type 1 (5% of all diabetes; previously classified as juvenile diabetes, juvenile-onset diabetes, ketosis-prone diabetes, brittle diabetes, and insulin-dependent diabetes mellitus [IDDM])	Onset any age, but usually young (<30 years) Usually thin at diagnosis; recent weight loss Etiology includes genetic, immunologic, and environmental factors (e.g., virus) Often have islet cell antibodies Often have antibodies to insulin even before insulin treatment Little or no endogenous insulin Need exogenous insulin to preserve life Ketosis prone when insulin absent Acute complication of hyperglycemia: diabetic ketoacidosis
Type 2 (95% of all diabetes: obese—80% of type 2, nonobese—20% of type 2; previously classified as adult-onset diabetes, maturity-onset diabetes, ketosis-resistant diabetes, stable diabetes, and non–insulin-dependent diabetes mellitus [NIDDM])	Onset any age, usually >30 years Usually obese at diagnosis Causes include obesity, heredity, and environmental factors No islet cell antibodies Decrease in endogenous insulin, or increased with insulin resistance Most patients can control blood glucose through weight loss if obese Oral antidiabetic agents may improve blood glucose levels if dietary modification and exercise are unsuccessful May need insulin on a short- or long-term basis to prevent hyperglycemia Ketosis uncommon, except in stress or infection Acute complication: hyperglycemic hyperosmolar syndrome
Diabetes associated with other conditions or syndromes (previously classified as secondary diabetes)	Accompanied by conditions known or suspected to cause the disease: pancreatic diseases, hormonal abnormalities, medications such as corticosteroids and estrogen-containing preparations Depending on the ability of the pancreas to produce insulin, the patient may require treatment with oral antidiabetic agents or insulin.
Gestational diabetes	Onset during pregnancy, usually in the second or third trimester Because of hormones secreted by the placenta, which inhibit the action of insulin Above-normal risk for perinatal complications, especially macrosomia (abnormally large babies) Treated with diet and, if needed, insulin to strictly maintain normal blood glucose levels Occurs in about 18% of pregnancies Glucose intolerance transitory but may recur: • In subsequent pregnancies • 35–60% will develop diabetes (usually type 2) within 10 to 20 years, especially if obese Risk factors include obesity, age >30 years, family history of diabetes, previous large babies (>9 lb) Screening tests (glucose challenge test) should be performed on all pregnant women between 24 and 28 weeks of gestation Should be screened for diabetes periodically
Prediabetes (previously classified as previous abnormality of glucose tolerance)	Previous history of hyperglycemia (e.g., during pregnancy or illness) Current normal glucose metabolism Impaired glucose tolerance or impaired fasting glucose screening after age 40 years if there is a family history of diabetes or if symptomatic Encourage ideal body weight, because loss of 10–15 lb may improve glycemic control

Adapted from American Diabetes Association (ADA). (2016b). Standards of medical care in diabetes—2016. Classification and diagnosis of diabetes. *Diabetes Care, 39*(Suppl 1), S13–S24; American Diabetes Association (ADA). (2016c). Standards of medical care in diabetes—2016; Management of diabetes in pregnancy. *Diabetes Care, 39*(Suppl 1), S94–S98.

Type 1 Diabetes

Type 1 diabetes affects approximately 5% of adults with the disease (CDC, 2014). It is characterized by the destruction of the pancreatic beta cells (Grossman & Porth, 2014). Combined genetic, immunologic, and possibly environmental (e.g., viral) factors are thought to contribute to beta-cell destruction. Although the events that lead to beta-cell destruction are not fully understood, it is generally accepted that a genetic susceptibility is a common underlying factor in the development of type 1 diabetes. People do not inherit type 1 diabetes itself but rather a genetic predisposition, or tendency, toward the development of type 1 diabetes. This genetic tendency has been found in people with certain human leukocyte antigen types. There is also evidence of an autoimmune response in type 1 diabetes. This is an abnormal response in which antibodies are directed against normal tissues of the body, responding to these tissues as if they were foreign. Autoantibodies against islet cells and against endogenous (internal) insulin have been detected in people at the time of diagnosis and even several years before the development of clinical signs of type 1 diabetes. In addition to genetic and immunologic components, environmental factors such as viruses or toxins that may initiate destruction of the beta cell continue to be investigated.

Regardless of the specific cause, the destruction of the beta cells results in decreased insulin production, increased glucose production by the liver, and fasting hyperglycemia. In addition, glucose derived from food cannot be stored in the liver but instead remains in the bloodstream and contributes to postprandial (after meals) hyperglycemia. If the concentration of glucose in the blood exceeds the renal threshold for glucose, usually 180 to 200 mg/dL (9.9 to 11.1 mmol/L), the kidneys may not reabsorb all of the filtered glucose; the glucose then appears in the urine (glycosuria). When excess glucose is excreted in the urine, it is accompanied by excessive loss of fluids and electrolytes. This is called *osmotic diuresis*.

Because insulin normally inhibits glycogenolysis (breakdown of stored glucose) and gluconeogenesis (production of new glucose from amino acids and other substrates), these processes occur in an unrestrained fashion in people with insulin deficiency and contribute further to hyperglycemia. In addition, fat breakdown occurs, resulting in an increased production of **ketone** bodies, a highly acidic substance formed when the liver breaks down free fatty acids in the absence of insulin.

Diabetic ketoacidosis (DKA) is a metabolic derangement that occurs most commonly in persons with type 1 diabetes and results from a deficiency of insulin; highly acidic ketone bodies are formed, and metabolic acidosis occurs. The three major metabolic derangements are hyperglycemia, ketosis, and metabolic acidosis (Grossman & Porth, 2014). DKA is commonly preceded by a day or more of polyuria, polydipsia, nausea, vomiting, and fatigue with eventual stupor and coma if not treated. The breath has a characteristic fruity odor due to the presence of ketoacids.

 Type 2 Diabetes

Type 2 diabetes affects approximately 95% of adults with the disease (CDC, 2014). It occurs more commonly among people who are older than 30 years and obese, although its incidence is rapidly increasing in younger people because of the growing epidemic of obesity in children, adolescents, and young adults (CDC, 2014).

The two main problems related to insulin in type 2 diabetes are insulin resistance and impaired insulin secretion. Insulin resistance refers to a decreased tissue sensitivity to insulin. Normally, insulin binds to special receptors on cell surfaces and initiates a series of reactions involved in glucose metabolism. In type 2 diabetes, these intracellular reactions are diminished, making insulin less effective at stimulating glucose uptake by the tissues and at regulating glucose release by the liver (see Fig. 51-1). The exact mechanisms that lead to insulin resistance and impaired insulin secretion in type 2 diabetes are unknown, although genetic factors are thought to play a role.

To overcome insulin resistance and to prevent the buildup of glucose in the blood, increased amounts of insulin must be secreted to maintain the glucose level at a normal or slightly elevated level. If the beta cells cannot keep up with the increased demand for insulin, the glucose level rises and type 2 diabetes develops. Insulin resistance may also lead to metabolic syndrome, which is a constellation of symptoms, including hypertension, hypercholesterolemia, abdominal obesity, and other abnormities (Grossman & Porth, 2014).

Despite the impaired insulin secretion that is characteristic of type 2 diabetes, there is enough insulin present to prevent the breakdown of fat and the accompanying production of ketone bodies. Therefore, DKA does not typically occur in type 2 diabetes. However, uncontrolled type 2 diabetes may lead to another acute problem—**hyperglycemic hyperosmolar syndrome (HHS)** (see discussion later in chapter).

Physiology/Pathophysiology

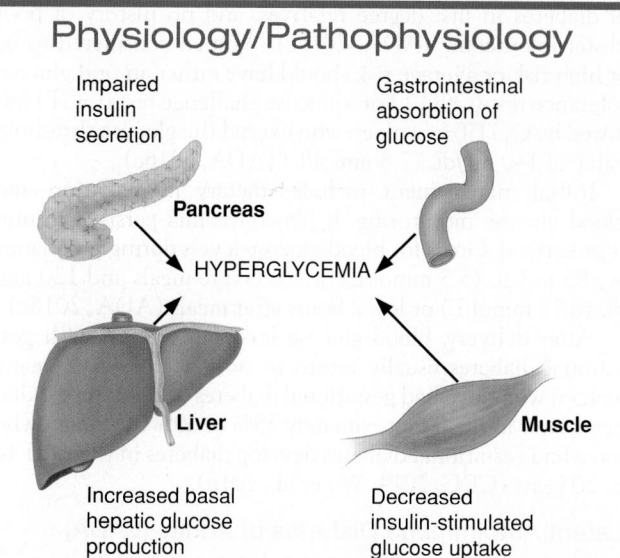

Figure 51-1 • Pathogenesis of type 2 diabetes.

Because type 2 diabetes is associated with a slow, progressive glucose intolerance, its onset may go undetected for many years. If the patient experiences symptoms, they are frequently mild and may include fatigue, irritability, polyuria, polydipsia, poorly healing skin wounds, vaginal infections, or blurred vision (if glucose levels are very high).

For most patients (approximately 75%), type 2 diabetes is detected incidentally (e.g., when routine laboratory tests or ophthalmoscopic examinations are performed). One consequence of undetected diabetes is that long-term diabetes complications (e.g., eye disease, peripheral neuropathy, peripheral vascular disease) may have developed before the actual diagnosis of diabetes is made (ADA, 2016b), signifying that the blood glucose has been elevated for a time before diagnosis.

Gestational Diabetes

Gestational diabetes is any degree of glucose intolerance with its onset during pregnancy. Hyperglycemia develops during pregnancy because of the secretion of placental hormones, which causes insulin resistance. Gestational diabetes occurs in as many as 18% of pregnant women and increases their risk for hypertensive disorders during pregnancy (CDC, 2014; Wu, Nien, Kuo, et al., 2016).

Women who are considered to be at high risk for gestational diabetes and should be screened by blood glucose testing at their first prenatal visit are those with marked obesity, a personal history of gestational diabetes, glycosuria, or a strong family history of diabetes. High-risk ethnic groups include Hispanic Americans, Native Americans, Asian Americans, African Americans, and Pacific Islanders. If these high-risk women do not have gestational diabetes at initial screening, they should be retested between 24 and 28 weeks of gestation. All women of average risk should be tested at 24 to 28 weeks of gestation. Testing is not specifically recommended for women identified as being at low risk. Low-risk women are those who meet all of the following criteria: age younger than 25 years, normal weight before pregnancy, member of an ethnic group with low prevalence of gestational diabetes, no history of abnormal glucose tolerance, no known history of diabetes in first-degree relatives, and no history of poor obstetric outcome (ADA, 2016c). Women considered to be at high risk or average risk should have either an oral glucose tolerance test (OGTT) or a glucose challenge test (GCT) followed by OGTT in women who exceed the glucose threshold value of 140 mg/dL (7.8 mmol/L) (ADA, 2016c).

Initial management includes dietary modification and blood glucose monitoring. If hyperglycemia persists, insulin is prescribed. Goals for blood glucose levels during pregnancy are 95 mg/dL (5.3 mmol/L) or less before meals and 120 mg/dL (6.72 mmol/L) or less 2 hours after meals (ADA, 2016c).

After delivery, blood glucose levels in women with gestational diabetes usually return to normal. However, many women who have had gestational diabetes develop type 2 diabetes later in life. Approximately 35% to 60% of women who have had gestational diabetes develop diabetes in the next 10 to 20 years (CDC, 2014; Wu et al., 2016).

Latent Autoimmune Diabetes of Adults (LADA)

In adults, LADA is a subtype of diabetes in which the progression of autoimmune beta cell destruction in the pancreas is slower than in types 1 and 2 diabetes (Deng, Xiang, Tan, et al., 2016). Patients with LADA are not insulin-dependent in the initial 6 months of disease onset. Clinical manifestation of LADA shares the features of types 1 and 2 diabetes (Deng et al., 2016). The emergence of this subtype has led some to propose the diabetes classification scheme should be revised to reflect changes in the beta cells in the pancreas (Schwartz, Epstein, Corkey, et al. 2016).

Prevention

The Diabetes Prevention Program Research Group (2002) reported that type 2 diabetes can be prevented with appropriate changes in lifestyle. Persons at high risk for type 2 diabetes (body mass index [BMI] greater than 24, fasting and postprandial plasma glucose levels elevated but not to levels diagnostic of diabetes) received standard lifestyle recommendations plus metformin (Glucophage), an oral antidiabetic agent, standard lifestyle recommendations plus placebo, or an intensive program of lifestyle modifications. The 16-lesson curriculum of the intensive program of lifestyle modifications focused on weight reduction of greater than 7% of initial body weight and physical activity of moderate intensity. It also included behavior modification strategies designed to help patients achieve the goals of weight reduction and participation in exercise. Compared to the placebo group, the lifestyle intervention group had a 58% lower incidence of diabetes and the metformin group had a 31% lower incidence of diabetes. These findings were found in both genders and all racial and ethnic groups. These findings demonstrate that type 2 diabetes can be prevented or delayed in persons at high risk for the disease (Diabetes Prevention Program Research Group, 2002). The Diabetes Prevention Program Outcomes Study followed these individuals for 15 years and demonstrated that those who participated in the program continued to develop type 2 diabetes at a lower rate compared to controls (Diabetes Prevention Program Research Group, 2015).

Clinical Manifestations

Clinical manifestations depend on the patient's level of hyperglycemia. Classic clinical manifestations of diabetes include the "three Ps": polyuria, polydipsia, and polyphagia. Polyuria (increased urination) and polydipsia (increased thirst) occur as a result of the excess loss of fluid associated with osmotic diuresis. Patients also experience polyphagia (increased appetite) that results from the catabolic state induced by insulin deficiency and the breakdown of proteins and fats (Grossman & Porth, 2014). Other symptoms include fatigue and weakness, sudden vision changes, tingling or numbness in hands or feet, dry skin, skin lesions or wounds that are slow to heal, and recurrent infections. The onset of type 1 diabetes may also be associated with sudden weight loss or nausea, vomiting, or abdominal pains, if DKA has developed.

Assessment and Diagnostic Findings

An abnormally high blood glucose level is the basic criterion for the diagnosis of diabetes. **Fasting plasma glucose (FPG)** (blood glucose determination obtained in the laboratory after fasting for at least 8 hours), random plasma glucose, and glucose level 2 hours after receiving glucose (2-hour postload) may be used (Fischbach & Dunning, 2015). The OGTT and the intravenous (IV) glucose tolerance test are no longer recommended for routine clinical use. See Chart 51-2 for the ADA's diagnostic criteria for diabetes (ADA, 2016a).

In addition to the assessment and diagnostic evaluation performed to diagnose diabetes, ongoing specialized assessment of patients with known diabetes and evaluation for complications in patients with newly diagnosed diabetes are important components of care. Parameters that should be regularly assessed are discussed in Chart 51-3.

 Gerontologic Considerations

Diabetes is particularly prevalent in older adults. In fact, type 2 diabetes is the seventh leading cause of death and affects approximately 20% of older adults (Eliopoulos, 2018). There

---

> **Chart 51-2** Criteria for the Diagnosis of Diabetes
>
> 1. Symptoms of diabetes plus casual plasma glucose concentration equal to or greater than 200 mg/dL (11.1 mmol/L). Casual is defined as any time of day without regard to time since last meal. The classic symptoms of diabetes include polyuria, polydipsia, and unexplained weight loss.
>
> Or
>
> 2. Fasting plasma glucose greater than or equal to 126 mg/dL (7.0 mmol/L). Fasting is defined as no caloric intake for at least 8 hours.
>
> Or
>
> 3. Two-hour postload glucose equal to or greater than 200 mg/dL (11.1 mmol/L) during an oral glucose tolerance test. The test should be performed as described by the World Health Organization, using a glucose load containing the equivalent of 75 g anhydrous glucose dissolved in water.
>
> Or
>
> 4. A1C ≥6.5% (48 mmol/mol).
>
> In the absence of unequivocal hyperglycemia with acute metabolic decompensation, these criteria should be confirmed by repeat testing on a different day. The third measure is not recommended for routine clinical use.
>
> Adapted from American Diabetes Association (ADA). (2016b). Standards of medical care in diabetes—2016. Classification and diagnosis of diabetes. *Diabetes Care, 39*(Suppl 1), S13–S24.

Chart 51-3 — ASSESSMENT
Assessing the Patient With Diabetes

History

- Symptoms related to the diagnosis of diabetes:
  Symptoms of hyperglycemia
  Symptoms of hypoglycemia
    Frequency, timing, severity, and resolution
- Results of blood glucose monitoring
- Status, symptoms, and management of chronic complications of diabetes:
  Eye; kidney; nerve; genitourinary and sexual, bladder, and gastrointestinal
  Cardiac; peripheral vascular; foot complications associated with diabetes
- Adherence to/ability to follow prescribed dietary management plan
- Adherence to prescribed exercise regimen
- Adherence to/ability to follow prescribed pharmacologic treatment (insulin or oral antidiabetic agents)
- Use of tobacco, alcohol, and prescribed and over-the-counter medications/drugs
- Lifestyle, cultural, psychosocial, and economic factors that may affect diabetes treatment
- Effects of diabetes or its complications on functional status (e.g., mobility, vision)

Physical Examination

- Blood pressure (sitting and standing to detect orthostatic changes)
- Body mass index (height and weight)
- Funduscopic examination and visual acuity
- Foot examination (lesions, signs of infection, pulses)
- Skin examination (lesions and insulin injection sites)
- Neurologic examination
  Vibratory and sensory examination using monofilament
  Deep tendon reflexes
- Oral examination

Laboratory Examination

- HgbA$_{1C}$ (A1C)
- Fasting lipid profile
- Test for microalbuminuria
- Serum creatinine level
- Urinalysis
- Electrocardiogram

Need for Referrals

- Ophthalmologist
- Podiatrist
- Dietitian
- Diabetes educator
- Others if indicated

is a high prevalence among African Americans and those who are 65 to 74 years of age (Eliopoulos, 2018).

Early detection is important but may be challenging because symptoms may be absent or nonspecific. A glucose tolerance test is more effective in diagnosis than urine testing for glucose in older patients due to the higher renal threshold for glucose (Eliopoulos, 2018).

Medical Management

The main goal of diabetes treatment is to normalize insulin activity and blood glucose levels to reduce the development of complications. The Diabetes Control and Complications Trial Research Group (DCCT), a 10-year prospective clinical trial conducted from 1983 to 1993, demonstrated the importance of achieving blood glucose control in the normal, nondiabetic range. This landmark trial demonstrated that intensive glucose control dramatically reduced the development and progression of complications such as **retinopathy** (damage to small blood vessels that nourish the retina), **nephropathy** (damage to kidney cells), and neuropathy (damage to nerve cells). Intensive treatment is defined as 3 or 4 insulin injections per day or an **insulin pump** (i.e., a continuous subcutaneous insulin infusion) plus frequent blood glucose monitoring and weekly contacts with diabetes educators (DCCT, 1993). The ADA now recommends that all patients with diabetes strive for glucose control (HgbA1c less than 7%) to reduce their risk of complications (ADA, 2016a).

Intensive therapy must be initiated with caution and must be accompanied by thorough education of the patient and family and by responsible behavior of the patient. Careful screening of patients for capability and responsibility is a key step in initiating intensive therapy.

The therapeutic goal for diabetes management is to achieve normal blood glucose levels (euglycemia) without **hypoglycemia** while maintaining a high quality of life. Diabetes management has five components: nutritional therapy, exercise, monitoring, pharmacologic therapy, and education. Diabetes management involves constant assessment and modification of the treatment plan by health professionals and daily adjustments in therapy by the patient. Although the health care team directs the treatment, it is the individual patient who must manage the complex therapeutic regimen. For this reason, patient and family education is an essential component of diabetes treatment and is as important as all other components of the regimen.

Nutritional Therapy

Nutrition, meal planning, weight control, and increased activity are the foundation of diabetes management (ADA, 2016d). The most important objectives in the dietary and nutritional management of diabetes are control of total caloric intake to attain or maintain a reasonable body weight, control of blood glucose levels, and normalization of lipids and blood pressure to prevent heart disease. Success in this area alone is often associated with reversal of hyperglycemia in type 2 diabetes. However, achieving these goals is not always easy. Because **medical nutrition therapy (MNT)**—nutritional therapy prescribed for management of diabetes usually given by a registered dietician—is complex, a registered dietitian who understands the therapy has the major responsibility for designing and educating about this aspect of the therapeutic plan. Nurses and all other members of the health care team must be knowledgeable about nutritional therapy and supportive of patients who need to implement nutritional and lifestyle changes. Nutritional management of diabetes includes the following goals:

1. To achieve and maintain:
   a. Blood glucose levels in the normal range or as close to normal as is safely possible
   b. A lipid and lipoprotein profile that reduces the risk for vascular disease
   c. Blood pressure levels in the normal range or as close to normal as is safely possible

2. To prevent, or at least slow, the rate of development of the chronic complications of diabetes by modifying nutrient intake and lifestyle
3. To address individual nutrition needs, taking into account personal and cultural preferences and willingness to change
4. To maintain the pleasure of eating by only limiting food choices when indicated by scientific evidence

For patients who are obese and have diabetes (especially those with type 2 diabetes), weight loss is the key to treatment. (It is also a major factor in preventing diabetes.) In general, overweight is considered to be a BMI of 25 to 29; obesity is defined as 20% above ideal body weight or a BMI equal to or greater than 30 (ADA, 2016d; WHO, 2015b). Calculation of BMI is discussed in Chapter 5. Patients who are obese, have type 2 diabetes, and require insulin or oral agents to control blood glucose levels may be able to reduce or eliminate the need for medication through weight loss. A weight loss as small as 5% to 10% of total weight may significantly improve blood glucose levels. For patients who are obese, have diabetes, and do not take insulin or sulfonylureas (a class of oral antidiabetic medication for treating type 2 diabetes that stimulates insulin secretion and insulin action), consistent meal content or timing is important but not as critical. Rather, decreasing the overall caloric intake is of greater importance. Meals should not be skipped. Pacing food intake throughout the day decreases demands on the pancreas.

A new class of medication that lowers glucose levels in persons with type 2 diabetes has also been associated with weight loss. This class of drugs, incretins, mimic hormones thus reducing appetite (Triplitt & Solis-Herrera, 2015).

Consistently following a meal plan is one of the most challenging aspects of diabetes management. It may be more realistic to restrict calories only moderately. For patients who have lost weight incorporating new dietary habits into their lifestyles, diet education, behavioral therapy, group support, and ongoing nutrition counseling are encouraged to maintain weight loss.

Meal Planning and Related Education

The meal plan must consider the patient's food preferences, lifestyle, usual eating times, and ethnic and cultural background. For patients who require insulin to help control blood glucose levels, maintaining as much consistency as possible in the amount of calories and carbohydrates ingested at each meal is essential. In addition, consistency in the approximate time intervals between meals, with the addition of snacks if necessary, helps prevent hypoglycemic reactions and maintain overall blood glucose control. For patients who can master the insulin-to-carbohydrate calculations, lifestyle can be more flexible and diabetes control more predictable. For those using intensive insulin therapy, there may be greater flexibility in the timing and content of meals by allowing adjustments in insulin dosage for changes in eating and exercise habits. Advances in insulin management (new insulin analogues, insulin algorithms, insulin pumps) permit greater flexibility of schedules than was previously possible. This contrasts with the concept of maintaining a constant dose of insulin, requiring strict scheduling of meals to match the onset and duration of the insulin.

The first step in preparing a meal plan is a thorough review of the patient's diet history to identify eating habits and lifestyle and cultural eating patterns (ADA, 2016d; Evert, Boucher, Cypress, et al., 2013). This includes a thorough assessment of the patient's need for weight loss, gain, or maintenance. In most instances, people with type 2 diabetes require weight reduction.

In educating about meal planning, clinical dietitians use various tools, materials, and approaches. Initial education addresses the importance of consistent eating habits, the relationship of food and insulin, and the provision of an individualized meal plan. In-depth follow-up education then focuses on management skills, such as eating at restaurants; reading food labels; and adjusting the meal plan for exercise, illness, and special occasions. The nurse plays an important role in communicating pertinent information to the dietitian and reinforcing the patient's understanding. Communication between the team is important.

Certain aspects of meal planning, such as the food exchange system, may be difficult to learn. This may be related to limitations in the patient's intellectual level or to emotional issues, such as difficulty accepting the diagnosis of diabetes or feelings of deprivation and undue restriction in eating. In any case, it helps to emphasize that using the exchange system (or any food classification system) provides a new way of thinking about food rather than a new way of eating. It is also important to simplify information as much as possible and to provide opportunities for the patient to practice and repeat activities and information.

Caloric Requirements

Calorie-controlled diets are planned by first calculating a person's energy needs and caloric requirements based on age, gender, height, and weight. An activity element is then factored in to provide the actual number of calories required for weight maintenance. To promote a 1- to 2-lb weight loss per week, 500 to 1000 calories are subtracted from the daily total. The calories are distributed into carbohydrates, proteins, and fats, and a meal plan is then developed, taking into account the patient's lifestyle and food preferences.

Patients may be underweight at the onset of type 1 diabetes because of rapid weight loss from severe hyperglycemia. The goal initially may be to provide a higher-calorie diet to regain lost weight and blood glucose control.

Caloric Distribution

A meal plan for diabetes focuses on the percentages of calories that come from carbohydrates, proteins, and fats.

Carbohydrates. The caloric distribution currently recommended is higher in carbohydrates than in fat and protein. In general, carbohydrate foods have the greatest effect on blood glucose levels because they are more quickly digested than other foods and are converted into glucose rapidly. However, research into the appropriateness of a higher-carbohydrate diet in patients with decreased glucose tolerance is ongoing, and recommendations may change accordingly. Currently, the ADA and the Academy of Nutrition and Dietetics (formerly the American Dietetic Association) recommend that for all levels of caloric intake, 50% to 60% of calories should be derived from carbohydrates, 20% to 30% from fat, and the remaining 10% to 20% from protein (Dudek, 2014; Evert et al., 2013). The majority of the selections for carbohydrates should come from whole grains. These recommendations are also consistent with those of the American Heart Association and American Cancer Society.

Carbohydrates consist of sugars (e.g., sucrose) and starches (e.g., rice, pasta, bread). Low **glycemic index** diets (described later) may reduce postprandial glucose levels. Therefore, the nutrition guidelines recommend that all carbohydrates should be eaten in moderation to avoid high postprandial blood glucose levels (Dudek, 2014; Evert et al., 2013).

Foods high in carbohydrates, such as sucrose (concentrated sweets), are not totally eliminated from the diet but should be eaten in moderation (up to 10% of total calories), because they are typically high in fat and lack vitamins, minerals, and fiber.

Fats. The recommendations regarding fat content of the diabetic diet include both reducing the total percentage of calories from fat sources to less than 30% of total calories and limiting the amount of saturated fats to 10% of total calories. Additional recommendations include limiting the total intake of dietary cholesterol to less than 300 mg/day. This approach may help reduce risk factors such as increased serum cholesterol levels, which are associated with the development of coronary artery disease—the leading cause of death and disability among people with diabetes (ADA, 2016d; Evert et al., 2013).

Protein. The meal plan may include the use of some non-animal sources of protein (e.g., legumes, whole grains) to help reduce saturated fat and cholesterol intake. In addition, the amount of protein intake may be reduced in patients with early signs of kidney disease.

Fiber. Increased fiber in the diet may improve blood glucose levels, decrease the need for exogenous insulin, and lower total cholesterol and low-density lipoprotein levels in the blood (ADA, 2016d; Evert et al., 2013).

There are two types of dietary fibers: soluble and insoluble. Soluble fiber—in foods such as legumes, oats, and some fruits—plays more of a role in lowering blood glucose and lipid levels than does insoluble fiber, although the clinical significance of this effect is probably small (ADA, 2016d; Evert et al., 2013). Soluble fiber slows stomach emptying and the movement of food through the upper digestive tract. The potential glucose-lowering effect of fiber may be caused by the slower rate of glucose absorption from foods that contain soluble fiber. Insoluble fiber is found in whole-grain breads and cereals and in some vegetables. This type of fiber along with soluble fiber increases satiety, which is helpful for weight loss. At least 25 g of fiber should be ingested daily.

One risk involved in suddenly increasing fiber intake is that it may require adjusting the dosage of insulin or oral agents to prevent hypoglycemia. Other problems may include abdominal fullness, nausea, diarrhea, increased flatulence, and constipation if fluid intake is inadequate. If fiber is added to or increased in the meal plan, it should be done gradually and in consultation with a dietitian. Exchange lists (ADA, 2016d) serve as an excellent guide for increasing fiber intake. Fiber-rich food choices within the vegetable, fruit, and starch/bread exchanges are highlighted in the lists.

Food Classification Systems

To educate about diet principles and help in meal planning, several systems have been developed in which foods are organized into groups with common characteristics, such as number of calories, composition of foods (i.e., amount of protein, fat, or carbohydrate in the food), or effect on blood glucose levels. Several of these are listed next.

Exchange Lists. A commonly used tool for nutritional management is the exchange lists for meal planning (ADA, 2016d). There are six main exchange lists: bread/starch, vegetable, milk, meat, fruit, and fat. Foods within one group (in the portion amounts specified) contain equal numbers of calories and are approximately equal in grams of protein, fat, and carbohydrate. Meal plans can be based on a recommended number of choices from each exchange list. Foods on one list may be interchanged with one another, allowing for variety while maintaining as much consistency as possible in the nutrient content of foods eaten. Table 51-2 presents three sample lunch menus that are interchangeable in terms of carbohydrate, protein, and fat content.

Exchange list information on combination foods such as pizza, chili, and casseroles, as well as convenience foods, desserts, snack foods, and fast foods, is available from the ADA (see the Resources section). Some food manufacturers and restaurants publish exchange lists that describe their products.

Nutrition Labels. Food manufacturers are required to have the nutrition content of foods listed on their packaging, and reading food labels is an important skill for patients to learn

TABLE 51-2 Selected Sample Menus From Exchange Lists

Exchanges	Sample Lunch #1	Sample Lunch #2	Sample Lunch #3
2 starch	2 slices bread	Hamburger bun	1 cup cooked pasta
3 meat	2 oz sliced turkey and 1 oz low-fat cheese	3 oz lean beef patty	3 oz boiled shrimp
1 vegetable	Lettuce, tomato, onion	Green salad	½ cup plum tomatoes
1 fat	1 tsp mayonnaise	1 tbsp salad dressing	1 tsp olive oil
1 fruit	1 medium apple	1¼ cup watermelon	1¼ cup fresh strawberries
"Free" items (optional)	Unsweetened iced tea Mustard, pickle, hot pepper	Diet soda 1 tbsp catsup, pickle, onions	Ice water with lemon Garlic, basil

and use when food shopping. The label includes information about how many grams of carbohydrate are in a serving of food. This information can be used to determine how much medication is needed. For example, a patient who takes pre-meal insulin may use the algorithm of 1 unit of insulin for 15 g of carbohydrate. Patients can also be educated to have a "carbohydrate budget" per meal (e.g., 45 to 60 g).

Carbohydrate counting is a nutritional tool used for blood glucose management because carbohydrates are the main nutrients in food that influence blood glucose levels. This method provides flexibility in food choices, can be less complicated to understand than the diabetic food exchange list, and allows more accurate management with multiple daily injections (insulin before each meal). However, if carbohydrate counting is not used with other meal-planning techniques, weight gain can result. A variety of methods are used to count carbohydrates. When developing a diabetic meal plan using carbohydrate counting, all food sources should be considered.

Once digested, 100% of carbohydrates are converted to glucose. Approximately 50% of protein foods (meat, fish, and poultry) are also converted to glucose, and this has minimal effect on blood glucose levels.

While carbohydrate counting is commonly used for blood glucose management with type 1 and type 2 diabetes, it is not a perfect system. All carbohydrates affect the blood glucose level to different degrees, regardless of equivalent serving size (i.e., the glycemic index—see later discussion). When carbohydrate counting is used, reading labels on food items is the key to success. Knowing what the "carbohydrate budget" for the meal is and knowing how many grams of carbohydrate are in a serving of a food, the patient can calculate the amount in one serving.

Healthy Food Choices. An alternative to counting grams of carbohydrate is measuring servings or choices. This method is used more often by people with type 2 diabetes. It is similar to the food exchange list and emphasizes portion control of total servings of carbohydrate at meals and snacks. One carbohydrate serving is equivalent to 15 g of carbohydrate. Examples of one serving are an apple 2 in in diameter and one slice of bread. Vegetables and meat are counted as one third of a carbohydrate serving. This system works well for those who have difficulty with more complicated systems.

MyPlate Food Guide. The Food Guide (i.e., MyPlate) is another tool used to develop meal plans. It is commonly used for patients with type 2 diabetes who have a difficult time following a calorie-controlled diet. Foods are categorized into five major groups (grains, vegetables, fruits, dairy, and protein), plus fats and oils (see Chapter 5). Foods (grains, fruits, and vegetables) that are lowest in calories and fat and highest in fiber should make up the basis of the diet. For those with diabetes, as well as for the general population, 50% to 60% of the daily caloric intake should be from these three groups. Foods higher in fat (particularly saturated fat) should account for a smaller percentage of the daily caloric intake. Fats, oils, and sweets should be used sparingly to obtain weight and blood glucose control and to reduce the risk for cardiovascular disease. Reliance on MyPlate may result in fluctuations in blood glucose levels, however, because high-carbohydrate foods may be grouped with low-carbohydrate foods. The guide is appropriately used only as a first-step educational tool for patients who are learning how to control food portions

and how to identify which foods contain carbohydrate, protein, and fat.

Glycemic Index. One of the main goals of diet therapy in diabetes is to avoid sharp, rapid increases in blood glucose levels after food is eaten. The term *glycemic index* is used to describe how much a given food increases the blood glucose level compared with an equivalent amount of glucose. The effects of the use of the glycemic index on blood glucose levels and on long-term patient outcomes are unclear, but it may be beneficial (ADA, 2016e). Although more research is necessary, the following guidelines may be helpful when making dietary recommendations:

- Combining starchy foods with protein- and fat-containing foods tends to slow their absorption and lower the glycemic index.
- In general, eating foods that are raw and whole results in a lower glycemic index than eating chopped, puréed, or cooked foods (except meat).
- Eating whole fruit instead of drinking juice decreases the glycemic index, because fiber in the fruit slows absorption.
- Adding foods with sugars to the diet may result in a lower glycemic index if these foods are eaten with foods that are more slowly absorbed.

Patients can create their own glycemic index by monitoring their blood glucose level after ingestion of a particular food. This can help improve blood glucose control through individualized manipulation of the diet. Many patients who use frequent monitoring of blood glucose levels can use this information to adjust their insulin doses in accordance with variations in food intake.

Other Dietary Concerns

Alcohol Consumption

Patients with diabetes do not need to give up alcoholic beverages entirely, but patients and primary providers must be aware of the potential adverse effects of alcohol specific to diabetes. Alcohol is absorbed before other nutrients and does not require insulin for absorption. Large amounts can be converted to fats, increasing the risk for DKA. In general, the same precautions regarding the use of alcohol by people without diabetes should be applied to patients with diabetes. Moderation is recommended. A major danger of alcohol consumption by the patient with diabetes is hypoglycemia, especially for patients who take insulin or insulin secretagogues (medications that increase the secretion of insulin by the pancreas). Alcohol may decrease the normal physiologic reactions in the body that produce glucose (gluconeogenesis). Therefore, if a patient with diabetes consumes alcohol on an empty stomach, there is an increased likelihood of hypoglycemia. In addition, excessive alcohol intake may impair the patient's ability to recognize and treat hypoglycemia or to follow a prescribed meal plan to prevent hypoglycemia. To reduce the risk of hypoglycemia, the patient should be cautioned to consume food along with the alcohol; however, carbohydrate consumed with alcohol may raise blood glucose.

Alcohol consumption may lead to excessive weight gain (from the high caloric content of alcohol), hyperlipidemia, and elevated glucose levels (especially with mixed drinks and liqueurs). Patient education regarding alcohol intake must emphasize moderation in the amount of alcohol consumed. Moderate intake is considered to be one alcoholic beverage per day for women and two per day for men. Lower-calorie or less-sweet drinks (e.g., light beer, dry wine) and food intake along with alcohol consumption are advised (ADA, 2016e). Patients with type 2 diabetes who wish to control their weight should incorporate the calories from alcohol into the overall meal plan.

Sweeteners

The use of artificial sweeteners is acceptable, especially if it assists in overall dietary adherence. Moderation in the amount of sweetener used is encouraged to avoid potential adverse effects. There are two main types of sweeteners: nutritive and nonnutritive. The nutritive sweeteners contain calories, and the nonnutritive sweeteners have few or no calories in the amounts normally used.

Nutritive sweeteners include fructose (fruit sugar), sorbitol, and xylitol, all of which provide calories in amounts similar to those in sucrose (table sugar). They cause less elevation in blood sugar levels than sucrose does and are often used in sugar-free foods. Sweeteners containing sorbitol may have a laxative effect.

Nonnutritive sweeteners have minimal or no calories. They are used in food products and are also available for table use. They produce minimal or no elevation in blood glucose levels, and the U.S. Food and Drug Administration (FDA) lists them as safe for people with diabetes.

Misleading Food Labels

Foods labeled "sugarless" or "sugar-free" may still provide calories equal to those of the equivalent sugar-containing products if they are made with nutritive sweeteners. Therefore, these foods should not be considered "free" foods to be eaten in unlimited quantity, because they can elevate blood glucose levels. Foods labeled "dietetic" are not necessarily reduced-calorie foods. Patients are advised that foods labeled dietetic may still contain significant amounts of sugar or fat.

Patients must read the labels of "health foods"—especially snacks—because they often contain carbohydrates (e.g., honey, brown sugar, corn syrup, flour) and saturated vegetable fats (e.g., coconut or palm oil), hydrogenated vegetable fats, or animal fats, which may be contraindicated in people with elevated blood lipid levels.

Exercise

Exercise is extremely important in diabetes management because of its effects on lowering blood glucose and reducing cardiovascular risk factors (ADA, 2016b). Exercise lowers blood glucose levels by increasing the uptake of glucose by body muscles and by improving insulin utilization. It also improves circulation and muscle tone. Resistance (strength) training, such as weight lifting, can increase lean muscle mass, thereby increasing the resting metabolic rate. These effects are useful in diabetes in relation to losing weight, easing stress, and maintaining a feeling of well-being. Exercise also alters blood lipid concentrations, increasing levels of high-density lipoproteins and decreasing total cholesterol and triglyceride levels. This is especially important for people with diabetes because of their increased risk of cardiovascular disease.

Chart 51-4 **PATIENT EDUCATION**

General Considerations for Exercise in People With Diabetes

The nurse instructs the patient to:

- Exercise three times each week with no more than 2 consecutive days without exercise.
- Perform resistance training twice a week if you have type 2 diabetes.
- Exercise at the same time of day (preferably when blood glucose levels are at their peak) and for the same duration each session.
- Use proper footwear and, if appropriate, other protective equipment (i.e., helmets for cycling).
- Avoid trauma to the lower extremities, especially if you have numbness due to peripheral neuropathy.
- Inspect feet daily after exercise.
- Avoid exercise in extreme heat or cold.
- Avoid exercise during periods of poor metabolic control.
- Stretch for 10 to 15 minutes before exercising.

Adapted from American Diabetes Association (ADA). (2016b). Standards of medical care in diabetes—2016. Classification and diagnosis of diabetes. *Diabetes Care, 39*(Suppl 1), S13–S24.

Exercise Recommendations

Ideally, a person with diabetes should engage in regular exercise. General considerations for exercise in patients with diabetes are presented in Chart 51-4. Exercise recommendations must be altered as necessary for patients with diabetic complications, such as retinopathy, autonomic neuropathy, sensorimotor neuropathy, and cardiovascular disease (ADA, 2016b). Increased blood pressure associated with exercise may aggravate diabetic retinopathy and increase the risk of a hemorrhage into the vitreous or retina.

In general, a slow, gradual increase in the exercise period is encouraged. For many patients, walking is a safe and beneficial form of exercise that requires no special equipment (except for proper shoes) and can be performed anywhere. People with diabetes should discuss an exercise program with their primary provider and undergo a careful medical evaluation with appropriate diagnostic studies before beginning a program (ADA, 2016f).

For patients who are older than 30 years and who have two or more risk factors for heart disease, an exercise stress test is recommended prior to starting an exercise program (ADA, 2016f). Risk factors for heart disease include hypertension, obesity, high cholesterol levels, abnormal resting electrocardiogram (ECG), sedentary lifestyle, smoking, male gender, and a family history of heart disease. An abnormal stress test may indicate cardiac ischemia. Typically, an abnormal stress test is followed by a cardiac catheterization and, in some cases, with an intervention such as angioplasty, stent placement, or cardiac surgery.

Exercise Precautions

Patients who have blood glucose levels exceeding 250 mg/dL (14 mmol/L) and who have ketones in their urine should not begin exercising until the urine test results are negative for ketones and the blood glucose level is closer to normal. Exercising with elevated blood glucose levels increases the secretion of glucagon, growth hormone, and catecholamines. The liver then releases more glucose, and the result is an increase in the blood glucose level (ADA, 2016b).

The physiologic decrease in circulating insulin that normally occurs with exercise cannot occur in patients treated with insulin. Initially, patients who require insulin should be taught to eat a 15-g carbohydrate snack (a fruit exchange) or a snack of complex carbohydrates with a protein before engaging in moderate exercise to prevent unexpected hypoglycemia. The exact amount of food needed varies from person to person and should be determined by blood glucose monitoring.

Another concern for patients who take insulin is hypoglycemia that occurs many hours after exercise. To avoid postexercise hypoglycemia, especially after strenuous or prolonged exercise, the patient may need to eat a snack at the end of the exercise session and at bedtime and monitor the blood glucose level more frequently. Patients who are capable, knowledgeable, and responsible can learn to adjust their own insulin doses by working closely with a diabetes educator. Others need specific instructions on what to do when they exercise.

Patients taking insulin and participating in extended periods of exercise should test their blood glucose levels before, during, and after the exercise period, and they should snack on carbohydrates as needed to maintain blood glucose levels. Other participants or observers should be aware that the person exercising has diabetes, and they should know what assistance to give if severe hypoglycemia occurs.

In people with type 2 diabetes who are overweight or obese, exercise in addition to dietary management both improves glucose metabolism and enhances loss of body fat. Exercise coupled with weight loss improves insulin sensitivity and may decrease the need for insulin or oral antidiabetic agents (ADA, 2016b). Eventually, the patient's glucose tolerance may return to normal. Patients with type 2 diabetes who are not taking insulin or an oral agent may not need extra food before exercise.

Gerontologic Considerations

Physical activity that is consistent and realistic is beneficial to older adults with diabetes. Physical fitness in the older adult population with diabetes may lead to improved glycemic control, decreased risk for chronic vascular disease, and an improved quality of life (Eliopoulos, 2018; Weinger, Beverly, & Smaldone, 2014). Advantages of exercise in this population include a decrease in hyperglycemia, a general sense of well-being, and better use of ingested calories, resulting in weight reduction. Because there is an increased incidence of cardiovascular problems in older adults, a physical examination and exercise stress test may be warranted before an exercise program is initiated. A pattern of gradual, consistent exercise, including a combination of stretching, aerobic exercise, and resistance training, should be planned that does not exceed the patient's physical capacity. Physical impairment because of other chronic diseases must also be considered. In some cases, a physical therapy evaluation may be indicated, with the goal of determining exercises specific to the patient's needs and abilities. Tools such as the *Armchair Fitness* video or the Go4Life senior fitness booklet may be helpful (see resource section at end of chapter).

Monitoring Glucose Levels and Ketones

Blood glucose monitoring is a cornerstone of diabetes management, and **self-monitoring of blood glucose (SMBG)** levels has dramatically altered diabetes care. SMBG is a method of capillary blood glucose testing in which the patient pricks their finger and applies a drop of blood to a test strip that is read by a meter. It is recommended that SMBG occurs when circumstances call for it (e.g., before meals, snacks, and exercise) for patients prescribed frequent insulin injections or an insulin pump (ADA, 2016e).

Self-Monitoring of Blood Glucose

Using SMBG and learning how to respond to the results enable people with diabetes to individualize their treatment regimen to obtain optimal blood glucose control. This allows for detection and prevention of hypoglycemia and hyperglycemia and plays a crucial role in normalizing blood glucose levels, which in turn may reduce the risk of long-term diabetic complications.

Various methods for SMBG are available. Most involve obtaining a drop of blood from the fingertip, applying the blood to a special reagent strip, and allowing the blood to stay on the strip for the amount of time specified by the manufacturer (usually 5 to 30 seconds). The meter gives a digital readout of the blood glucose value. The meters available for SMBG offer various features and benefits such as monthly averages, tracking of events such as exercise and food consumption, and downloading capacity. Most meters are biosensors that can use blood obtained from alternative test sites, such as the forearm. They have a special lancing device that is useful for patients who have painful fingertips or experience pain with fingersticks.

Because laboratory methods measure plasma glucose, most blood glucose monitors approved for patient use in the home and some test strips calibrate blood glucose readings to plasma values. Plasma glucose values are 10% to 15% higher than whole blood glucose values, and it is crucial for patients with diabetes to know whether their monitor and strips provide whole blood or plasma results.

Methods for SMBG must match the skill level and physical capabilities of patients. Factors affecting SMBG performance include visual acuity, fine motor coordination, cognitive ability, comfort with technology and willingness to use it, and cost (American Association of Diabetes Educators [AADE], 2014; Eliopoulos, 2018). Some meters can be used by patients with visual impairments; these meters have audio components to assist in performing the test and obtaining the result. In addition, meters are available to check both blood glucose and blood ketone levels by those who are particularly susceptible to DKA. Most insurance companies, and programs such as Medicare and Medicaid, cover some or all of the costs of meters and strips.

All methods of SMBG carry the risk that patients may obtain and report erroneous blood glucose values as a result of incorrect techniques. Some common sources of error include improper application of blood (e.g., drop too small), damage to the reagent strips caused by heat or humidity, the use of outdated strips, and improper meter cleaning and maintenance.

Nurses play an important role in providing initial education about SMBG techniques. Equally important is evaluating the techniques of patients who are experienced in self-monitoring. Every 6 to 12 months, patients should conduct a comparison of their meter result with a simultaneous laboratory-measured blood glucose level in their provider's office and have their technique observed (AADE, 2014; Unger, 2013). The accuracy of the meter and strips can also be assessed with control solutions specific to that meter whenever a new vial of strips is used and whenever the validity of the reading is in doubt.

Candidates for Self-Monitoring of Blood Glucose

SMBG is a useful tool for managing self-care for everyone with diabetes. It is a key component of treatment for any intensive insulin therapy regimen (i.e., 2 to 4 injections per day or the use of an insulin pump) and for diabetes management during pregnancy. It is also recommended for patients with the following conditions:

- Unstable diabetes (severe swings from very high to very low blood glucose levels within a 24-hour day)
- A tendency to develop severe ketosis or hypoglycemia
- Hypoglycemia without warning symptoms

For patients not taking insulin, SMBG is helpful for monitoring the effectiveness of exercise, diet, and oral antidiabetic agents. For patients with type 2 diabetes, SMBG is recommended during periods of suspected hyperglycemia (e.g., illness) or hypoglycemia (e.g., unusual increased activity levels) and when the medication or dosage of medication is modified (AADE, 2014; ADA, 2016d).

Frequency of Self-Monitoring of Blood Glucose

For most patients who require insulin, SMBG is recommended two to four times daily (usually before meals and at bedtime). For patients who take insulin before each meal, SMBG is required at least three times daily before meals to determine each dose (AADE, 2014; ADA, 2016d). Those not receiving insulin may be instructed to assess their blood glucose levels at least two or three times per week, including a 2-hour postprandial test. For all patients, testing is recommended whenever hypoglycemia or hyperglycemia is suspected; with changes in medications, activity, or diet; and with stress or illness.

Responding to Self-Monitoring of Blood Glucose Results

Patients are asked to keep a record or logbook of blood glucose levels so that they can detect patterns. Testing is done at the peak action time of the medication to evaluate the need for dosage adjustments. To evaluate basal insulin and determine bolus insulin doses, testing is performed before meals. To determine the need for bolus doses of regular or rapid-acting insulin (lispro [Humalog], aspart [NovoLog], or glulisine [Apidra]), testing is done 2 hours after meals. Patients with type 2 diabetes are encouraged to test daily before and 2 hours after the largest meal of the day until individualized blood glucose levels are reached. Thereafter, testing should be done periodically before and after meals. Patients who take insulin at bedtime or who use an insulin infusion pump should also test at 3 AM once a week to document that the blood glucose level is not decreasing during the night. If the patient is unwilling or cannot afford to test frequently, then once or twice a day may be sufficient if the time of testing is varied (e.g., before breakfast one day and before lunch the next day).

Patients are more likely to discontinue SMBG if they are not instructed how to use the results to alter the treatment regimen, if they receive no positive reinforcement, and if testing costs increase. At the very least, the patient should be given parameters for contacting the primary provider. Patients using intensive insulin therapy regimens may be instructed in the use of algorithms (rules or decision trees) for changing the insulin doses based on patterns of values greater or less than the target range and the amount of carbohydrate to be consumed. Baseline patterns should be established by SMBG for 1 to 2 weeks.

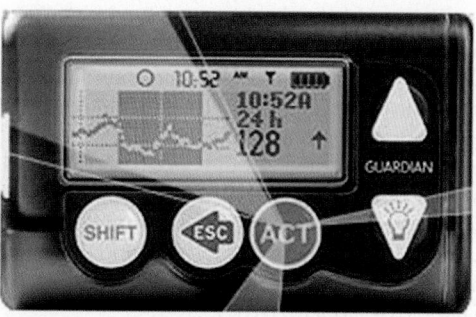

Figure 51-2 • MiniMed Guardian® REAL-Time CGM System. Manufactured by the diabetes division of Medtronic, Inc. Used with permission.

Using a Continuous Glucose Monitoring System

A continuous glucose monitoring system (CGMS) can be used to monitor blood glucose levels (see Fig. 51-2). A sensor attached to an infusion set, which is similar to an insulin pump infusion set, is inserted subcutaneously in the abdomen and connected to the device worn on the patient's clothing or placed in a pocket. After 120 to 168 hours, the data from the device are downloaded, and blood glucose readings are analyzed. Although the CGMS cannot be used for making decisions about specific insulin doses, it can be used to determine whether treatment is adequate over a 24-hour period. This device is most useful in patients with type 1 diabetes (ADA, 2016d).

Testing for Glycated Hemoglobin

Glycated hemoglobin (also referred to as glycosylated hemoglobin, $HgbA_{1C}$, or A1C) is a measure of glucose control for the past 3 months (ADA, 2016e). When blood glucose levels are elevated, glucose molecules attach to hemoglobin in red blood cells. The longer the amount of glucose in the blood remains above normal, the more glucose binds to hemoglobin and the higher the glycated hemoglobin level becomes. This complex (hemoglobin attached to the glucose) is permanent and lasts for the life of an individual red blood cell, approximately 120 days. If near-normal blood glucose levels are maintained, with only occasional increases, the overall value will not be greatly elevated. However, if the blood glucose values are consistently high, then the test result is also elevated. If the patient reports mostly normal SMBG results but the glycated hemoglobin is high, there may be errors in the methods used for glucose monitoring, errors in recording results, or frequent elevations in glucose levels at times during the day when the patient is not usually monitoring blood sugar levels. Normal values typically range from 4% to 6% and indicate consistently near-normal blood glucose concentrations. The target range for people with diabetes is less than 7% (ADA, 2016e).

Testing for Ketones

Ketones (or ketone bodies) are by-products of fat breakdown, and they accumulate in the blood and urine. Ketones in the urine signal that there is a deficiency of insulin and control of type 1 diabetes is deteriorating. When there is almost no effective insulin available, the body starts to break down stored fat for energy.

The patient may use a urine dipstick (Ketostix or Chemstrip uK) to detect ketonuria. The reagent pad on the strip turns purple when ketones are present. (One of the ketone bodies is called *acetone*, and this term is frequently used interchangeably with the term *ketones*.) Other strips are available for measuring both urine glucose and ketones (Keto-Diastix or Chemstrip uGK). Large amounts of ketones may depress the color response of the glucose test area, meters that text the blood for ketones are available.

Urine ketone testing should be performed whenever patients with type 1 diabetes have glycosuria or persistently elevated blood glucose levels (more than 240 mg/dL or 13.2 mmol/L for two testing periods in a row) and during illness, in pregnancy with preexisting diabetes, and in gestational diabetes (AADE, 2014; ADA, 2016e).

Pharmacologic Therapy

Insulin is secreted by the beta cells of the islets of Langerhans and lowers the blood glucose level after meals by facilitating the uptake and utilization of glucose by muscle, fat, and liver cells. In the absence of adequate insulin, pharmacologic therapy is essential.

Insulin Therapy

In type 1 diabetes, exogenous insulin must be given for life because the body loses the ability to produce insulin. In type 2 diabetes, insulin may be necessary on a long-term basis to control glucose levels if meal planning and oral agents are ineffective or when insulin deficiency occurs. In addition, some patients in whom type 2 diabetes is usually controlled by meal planning alone or by meal planning and an oral antidiabetic agent may require insulin temporarily during illness, infection, pregnancy, surgery, or some other stressful event. In many cases, insulin injections are given two or more times daily to control the blood glucose level. Because the insulin dose required by the individual patient is determined by the level of glucose in the blood, accurate monitoring of blood glucose levels is essential; thus, SMBG is a cornerstone of insulin therapy.

Preparations

A number of insulin preparations are available. They vary according to three main characteristics: time course of action, species (source), and manufacturer (Comer-

ford, 2015). Human insulins are produced by recombinant deoxyribonucleic acid (DNA) technology and are the only type of insulin available in the United States.

Time Course of Action. Insulins may be grouped into several categories based on the onset, peak, and duration of action (see Table 51-3).

Rapid-acting insulins produce a more rapid effect that is of shorter duration than regular insulin. Because of their rapid onset, the patient should be instructed to eat no more than 5 to 15 minutes after injection. Because of the short duration of action of these insulin analogues, patients with type 1 diabetes and some patients with type 2 or gestational diabetes also require a long-acting insulin (basal insulin) to maintain glucose control. Basal insulin is necessary to maintain blood glucose levels irrespective of meals. A constant level of insulin is required at all times. Intermediate-acting insulins function as basal insulins but may have to be split into 2 injections to achieve 24-hour coverage.

Short-acting insulins are called *regular insulin* (marked R on the bottle). Regular insulin is a clear solution and is usually given 15 minutes before a meal, either alone or in combination with a longer-acting insulin. Regular insulin can be administered IV (Comerford, 2015).

Intermediate-acting insulins are called *NPH insulin* (neutral protamine Hagedorn) or *Lente insulin*. Intermediate-acting insulins, which are similar in their time course of action, appear white and cloudy. If NPH or Lente insulin is taken alone, it is not crucial that it be taken before a meal but patients should eat some food around the time of the onset and peak of these insulins.

"Peakless" basal or very long-acting insulins are approved by the FDA for use as a basal insulin—that is, the insulin is absorbed very slowly over 24 hours and can be given once a day. Because the insulin is in a suspension with a pH of 4, it cannot be mixed with other insulins because this would cause precipitation. It was originally approved to be given once a day at bedtime; however, it has now been approved to be given once a day at any time of the day but must be given at

TABLE 51-3 Selected Categories of Insulin

Time Course	Agent	Onset	Peak	Duration	Indications
Rapid acting	lispro (Humalog)	10–15 minutes	1 hours	2–4 hours	Used for rapid reduction of glucose level, to treat postprandial hyperglycemia, and/or to prevent nocturnal hypoglycemia
	aspart (NovoLog)	5–15 minutes	40–50 minutes	2–4 hours	
	glulisine (Apidra)	5–15 minutes	30–60 minutes	2 hours	
Short acting	regular (Humulin R, Novolin R, Iletin II Regular)	30–60 minutes	2–3 hours	4–6 hours	Usually given 20–30 minutes before a meal; may be taken alone or in combination with longer-acting insulin
Intermediate acting	NPH (neutral protamine Hagedorn)	2–4 hours	4–12 hours	16–20 hours	Usually taken after food
	(Humulin N, Iletin II Lente, Iletin II NPH, Novolin N [NPH])	3–4 hours	4–12 hours	16–20 hours	
Very long acting	glargine (Lantus)	1 hours	Continuous (no peak)	24 hours	Used for basal dose
	detemir (Levemir)	6 hours		24–36 hours	
	glargine (Toujeo)				
Rapid-acting inhaled insulin	Afrezza	<15 minutes	~50 minutes	2–3 hours	Used as rapid-acting insulin

the same time each day to prevent overlap of action. Many patients fall asleep, forgetting to take their bedtime insulin, or may be wary of taking insulin before going to sleep. Having these patients take their insulin in the morning ensures that the dose is taken.

> ### ◤ Quality and Safety Nursing Alert
>
> *When administering insulin, it is very important to read the label carefully and to be sure that the correct type of insulin is given. It is also important to avoid mistaking Lantus insulin for Lente insulin and vice versa.*

The nurse should emphasize which meals—and snacks—are being "covered" by which insulin doses. In general, the rapid- and short-acting insulins are expected to cover the increase in glucose levels after meals, immediately after the injection; the intermediate-acting insulins are expected to cover subsequent meals; and the long-acting insulins provide a relatively constant level of insulin and act as a basal insulin.

Insulin Regimens

Insulin regimens vary from 1 to 4 injections per day. Usually, there is a combination of a short-acting insulin and a longer-acting insulin. The normally functioning pancreas continuously secretes small amounts of insulin during the day and night. In addition, whenever blood glucose increases after ingestion of food, there is a rapid burst of insulin secretion in proportion to the glucose-raising effect of the food. The goal of all but the simplest, 1-injection insulin regimens is to mimic this normal pattern of insulin secretion in response to food intake and activity patterns. Table 51-4 describes several insulin regimens and the advantages and disadvantages of each.

There are two general approaches to insulin therapy: conventional and intensive (described in detail later). The patient can learn to use SMBG results and carbohydrate counting to vary the insulin doses. This allows more flexibility in timing and content of meals and exercise periods. However, complex insulin regimens require a strong level of commitment, intensive education, and close follow-up by the health care team.

The patient should be very involved in the decision regarding which insulin regimen to use. The patient should compare the potential benefits of different regimens with the potential costs (e.g., time involved, number of injections or fingersticks for glucose testing, amount of record keeping). There are no set guidelines as to which insulin regimen should be used for which patient. Members of the health care team should not assume that older patients should automatically be given a simplified regimen, or that all people want to be involved in a complex treatment regimen. The nurse plays an important role in educating the patient about the various approaches to insulin therapy. The nurse should refer the patient to a diabetes specialist, certified diabetes educator (CDE), or a diabetes education center, if available, for further training and education in the insulin treatment regimens.

Conventional Regimen. One approach is to simplify the insulin regimen as much as possible, with the aim of avoiding the acute complications of diabetes (hypoglycemia and symptomatic hyperglycemia). With this type of simplified regimen (e.g., one or more injections of a mixture of short- and intermediate-acting insulins per day), the patient should not vary meal patterns and activity levels. The simplified regimen would be appropriate for the terminally ill, the older adult who is frail and has limited self-care abilities, or patients who are completely unwilling or unable to engage in the self-management activities that are part of a more complex insulin regimen.

Intensive Regimen. The second approach is to use a more complex insulin regimen to achieve as much control over blood glucose levels as is safe and practical. A more complex insulin regimen allows the patient more flexibility to change the insulin doses from day to day in accordance with changes in eating and activity patterns, with stress and illness, and as needed for variations in the prevailing glucose level.

While intensive treatment (3 or 4 injections of insulin per day) reduces the risk of complications, not all people with diabetes are candidates for very tight control of blood glucose. The risk of severe hypoglycemia increases threefold in patients receiving intensive treatment (ADA, 2016d). Patients who have received a kidney transplant because of nephropathy and chronic kidney failure should follow an intensive insulin regimen to preserve function of the new kidney.

Those who are not candidates include those with:

- Nervous system disorders rendering them unaware of hypoglycemic episodes (e.g., those with autonomic neuropathy)
- Recurring severe hypoglycemia
- Irreversible diabetic complications, such as blindness or ESKD
- Severe cerebrovascular or cardiovascular disease
- Ineffective self-care skills

Complications of Insulin Therapy

Local Allergic Reactions. A local allergic reaction (redness, swelling, tenderness, and induration or a 2- to 4-cm wheal) may appear at the injection site 1 to 2 hours after the administration of insulin. Reactions usually resolve in a few hours or days. If they do not resolve, another type of insulin can be prescribed (Comerford, 2015).

Systemic Allergic Reactions. Systemic allergic reactions to insulin are rare. When they do occur, there is an immediate local skin reaction that gradually spreads into generalized urticaria (hives). These rare reactions are occasionally associated with generalized edema or anaphylaxis. The treatment is desensitization, with small doses of insulin given in gradually increasing amounts using a desensitization kit.

Insulin Lipodystrophy. Lipodystrophy refers to a localized reaction, in the form of either lipoatrophy or lipohypertrophy, occurring at the site of insulin injections. Lipoatrophy is the loss of subcutaneous fat; it appears as slight dimpling or more serious pitting of subcutaneous fat. The use of human insulin has almost eliminated this disfiguring complication.

Lipohypertrophy, the development of fibrofatty masses at the injection site, is caused by the repeated use of an injection site. If insulin is injected into scarred areas, absorption may be delayed. This is one reason that rotation of injection sites is so important. Patients should avoid injecting insulin into these areas until the hypertrophy disappears.

Resistance to Injected Insulin. Patients may develop insulin resistance and require large insulin doses to control symptoms of diabetes (Comerford, 2015). In most patients with diabetes who take insulin, immune antibodies develop and bind the insulin, thereby decreasing the insulin available for use. All insulins cause some antibody production in humans.

TABLE 51-4 Insulin Regimens

Schematic Representation	Description	Advantages	Disadvantages
Normal pancreas 100 µU/mL 0 BR LU DI SN BR	Insulin release increases when blood glucose levels rise and continues at a low steady rate between meals		
1 injection per day Insulin effect Rapid-acting insulin NPH ↑BR LU DI SN BR	Before breakfast: • NPH or • NPH with rapid-acting insulin	Simple regimen	Difficult to control fasting blood glucose if effects of NPH do not last Afternoon hypoglycemia may result from attempts to control fasting glucose level by increasing NPH dose
2 injections per day–mixed Insulin effect Rapid-acting insulin NPH Rapid-acting insulin NPH ↑BR LU ↑DI SN BR	Before breakfast and dinner: • NPH or • NPH with rapid-acting insulin or • Premixed (rapid-acting insulin) insulin	Simplest regimen that attempts to mimic normal pancreas	Need relatively fixed schedule of meals and exercise Cannot independently adjust NPH or regular if premixed insulin is used
3 or 4 injections per day Insulin effect Rapid-acting insulin Rapid-acting insulin Rapid-acting insulin NPH ↑BR ↑LU ↑DI SN BR	Rapid-acting insulin before each meal with: • NPH at dinner or • NPH at bedtime or • Long-acting insulin one or two times a day	More closely mimics normal pancreas than 3-injection regimen Each premeal dose of regular insulin decided independently More flexibility with meals and exercise	Requires more injections than other regimens Requires multiple blood glucose tests on a daily basis Requires intensive education and follow-up
Insulin effect Rapid-acting insulin Rapid-acting insulin Rapid-acting insulin Long-acting insulin ↑BR ↑LU ↑DI SN BR			
Insulin pump BOLUS Insulin effect Rapid-acting insulin Rapid-acting insulin Rapid-acting insulin BASAL RATE Rapid-acting insulin BR LU DI SN BR	Uses ONLY rapid-acting insulin infused at continuous, low rate called *basal rate* (commonly 0.5–1.5 units/hr) and premeal *bolus doses* activated by pump wearer	Most closely mimics normal pancreas Decreases unpredictable peaks of intermediate- and long-acting insulins Increases meal and exercise flexibility	Requires intensive training and frequent follow-up Potential for mechanical problems Requires multiple blood glucose tests on a daily basis Potential increase in expenses (depending on insurance coverage)

Note: Rapid-acting insulin—lispro, aspart, or glulisine (Apidra).
BR, breakfast; LU, lunch; DI, dinner; SN, snack; NPH, neutral protamine Hagedorn; regular; ↑, insulin injections.
Adapted from Comerford, K. C. (2015). *Nursing 2015 drug handbook*. Philadelphia, PA: Wolters Kluwer; U.S. Food and Drug Administration (FDA). (2014). FDA approves Afrezza to treat diabetes. Retrieved on 6/21/16 at: www.fda.gov/newsevents/newsroom/pressannouncements/ucm403122.htm

Very few patients who are resistant develop high levels of antibodies. Many of these patients have a history of insulin therapy interrupted for several months or longer. Treatment consists of administering a more concentrated insulin preparation, such as U-500, which is available by special order (Comerford, 2015). Never store U-500 insulin with other insulin preparations due to the risk of overdose if accidentally given to the wrong patient (Comerford, 2015). Occasionally, prednisone is needed to block the production of antibodies. This may be followed by a gradual reduction in the insulin requirement. Therefore, patients must monitor their blood for hypoglycemia.

Morning Hyperglycemia. An elevated blood glucose level on arising in the morning is caused by an insufficient level of insulin, which may be caused by several factors: the dawn phenomenon, the Somogyi effect, or insulin waning. The dawn phenomenon is characterized by a relatively normal blood glucose level until approximately 3 AM, when blood glucose levels begin to rise. The phenomenon is thought to result from nocturnal surges in growth hormone secretion, which creates a greater need for insulin in the early morning hours in patients with type 1 diabetes. It must be distinguished from insulin waning (the progressive increase in blood glucose from bedtime to morning) and from the Somogyi effect (nocturnal hypoglycemia followed by rebound hyperglycemia). Insulin waning is frequently seen if the evening NPH dose is given before dinner; it is prevented by moving the evening dose of NPH insulin to bedtime.

It may be difficult to tell from a patient's history what the cause is for morning hyperglycemia. To determine the cause, the patient must be awakened once or twice during the night to test blood glucose levels. Testing at bedtime, at 3 AM, and on awakening provides information that can be used to make adjustments in insulin to avoid morning hyperglycemia.

Table 51-5 summarizes the differences among insulin waning, the dawn phenomenon, and the Somogyi effect.

Methods of Insulin Delivery

Methods of insulin delivery include traditional subcutaneous injections, insulin pens, jet injectors, and insulin pumps. (See Nursing Management later in this section for discussion of traditional subcutaneous injections.)

Insulin Pens. Insulin pens use small (150- to 300-unit) prefilled insulin cartridges that are loaded into a penlike holder. A disposable needle is attached to the device for insulin injection. Insulin is delivered by dialing in a dose or pushing a button for every 1- or 2-unit increment given. People using these devices still need to insert the needle for each injection (see Fig. 51-3); however, they do not need to carry insulin bottles or draw up insulin before each injection. These devices are most useful for patients who need to inject only one type of insulin at a time (e.g., premeal rapid-acting insulin three times a day and bedtime NPH insulin) or who can use the premixed insulins. These pens are convenient for those who administer insulin before dinner if eating out or traveling. They are also useful for patients with impaired manual dexterity, vision, or cognitive function, which makes the use of traditional syringes difficult.

Jet Injectors. As an alternative to needle injections, jet injection devices deliver insulin through the skin under pressure in an extremely fine stream. These devices are more expensive and require thorough training and supervision when first used. In addition, patients should be cautioned that absorption rates, peak insulin activity, and insulin levels may be different when changing to a jet injector. (Insulin given by jet injector is usually absorbed faster.) The use of jet injectors has been associated with bruising in some patients.

Figure 51-3 • Prefilled insulin syringe.

TABLE 51-5 Causes of Morning Hyperglycemia

Characteristic	Treatment
Insulin Waning	
Progressive rise in blood glucose from bedtime to morning	Increase evening (predinner or bedtime) dose of intermediate- or long-acting insulin, or institute a dose of insulin before the evening meal if one is not already part of the treatment regimen.
Dawn Phenomenon	
Relatively normal blood glucose until about 3 AM, when the level begins to rise	Change time of injection of evening intermediate-acting insulin from dinnertime to bedtime.
Somogyi Effect	
Normal or elevated blood glucose at bedtime, a decrease at 2–3 AM to hypoglycemic levels, and a subsequent increase caused by the production of counter-regulatory hormones	Decrease evening (predinner or bedtime) dose of intermediate-acting insulin, or increase bedtime snack.

Figure 51-4 • A. MiniMed Paradigm® REAL-Time Revel™ Insulin Pump. **B.** Patient using this insulin pump for self-management of blood glucose and insulin doses. Manufactured by the diabetes division of Medtronic, Inc. Used with permission.

Insulin Pumps. Continuous subcutaneous insulin infusion involves the use of small, externally worn devices (insulin pumps) that closely mimic the functioning of the normal pancreas (ADA, 2016f). Insulin pumps contain a 3-mL syringe attached to a long (24- to 42-in), thin, narrow-lumen tube with a needle or Teflon catheter attached to the end (see Fig. 51-4). The patient inserts the needle or catheter into subcutaneous tissue (usually on the abdomen) and secures it with tape or a transparent dressing. The needle or catheter is changed at least every 3 days. The pump is then worn either on the patient's clothing or in a pocket. Some women keep the pump tucked into the front or side of the bra.

When an insulin pump is used, insulin is delivered by subcutaneous infusion at a basal rate (e.g., 0.0.25 to 2 units per hour). When a meal is consumed, the patient calculates a dose of insulin to metabolize the meal by counting the total amount of carbohydrate for the meal using a predetermined insulin-to-carbohydrate ratio; for example, a ratio of 1 unit of insulin for every 15 g of carbohydrate would require 3 units for a meal with 45 g of carbohydrate. This allows flexibility of meal timing and content.

Possible disadvantages of insulin pumps are unexpected disruptions in the flow of insulin from the pump that may occur if the tubing or needle becomes occluded, if the supply of insulin runs out, or if the battery is depleted, increasing the risk of DKA. Effective education to produce knowledgeable patients minimizes this risk. There is the potential for infection at needle insertion sites. Hypoglycemia may occur with insulin pump therapy; however, this is usually related to the lowered blood glucose levels that many patients achieve rather than to a specific problem with the pump itself. The tight diabetes control associated with the use of an insulin pump may increase the incidence of hypoglycemia unawareness because of the very gradual decline in serum glucose level, from more than 70 mg/dL (3.9 mmol/L) to less than 60 mg/dL (3.3 mmol/L).

Some patients find that wearing the pump for 24 hours each day is inconvenient. However, the pump can easily be disconnected, per patient preference, for limited periods, such as for showering, exercise, swimming or sexual activity.

Candidates for the insulin pump must be willing to assess their blood glucose level several times daily. In addition, they must be psychologically stable and comfortable about having diabetes, because the insulin pump is often a visible sign to others and a constant reminder to patients that they have diabetes. Most important, patients using insulin pumps must have extensive education in the use of the pump and in self-management of blood glucose and insulin doses. They must work closely with a team of health care professionals who are experienced in insulin pump therapy—specifically, a diabetologist/endocrinologist, a dietitian, and a certified diabetes educator.

The most common risk of insulin pump therapy is ketoacidosis, which can occur if there is an occlusion in the infusion set or tubing. Because only rapid-acting insulin is used in the pump, any interruption in the flow of insulin may rapidly cause the patient to be without insulin. The patient should be taught to administer insulin by manual injection if an insulin interruption is suspected (e.g., no response in blood glucose level after a meal bolus).

Many insurance companies cover the cost of pump therapy. If not, the extra expense of the pump and associated supplies may be a deterrent for some patients. Medicare covers insulin pump therapy for patients with type 1 diabetes.

Insulin pumps have been used in patients with type 2 diabetes whose beta-cell function has diminished and who require insulin. Patients with a hectic lifestyle often do well with an insulin pump. There is no risk of DKA when there is an interruption of the flow of insulin in people with type 2 diabetes wearing an insulin pump.

Future Insulin Delivery. Research into mechanical delivery of insulin has involved implantable insulin pumps that can be externally programmed according to blood glucose test results. Clinical trials with these devices are continuing. In addition, there is research into the development of implantable devices that both measure the blood glucose level and deliver insulin as needed. Methods of administering insulin by the oral route (oral spray or capsule) and skin patch are undergoing intensive study. The FDA has conditionally approved an inhaled form of insulin to treat patients who require mealtime insulin administration (FDA, 2014). Afrezza is a fast-acting, powdered form of human insulin to treat type 1 or type 2 diabetes; however, because of the serious risk of acute bronchospasm, Afrezza will only be available once postmarketing studies and communication plans required by the FDA have been conducted (FDA, 2014).

Transplantation of Pancreatic Cells. Transplantation of the whole pancreas or a segment of the pancreas is being performed on a limited population (mostly patients with diabetes who are receiving a kidney transplantation simultaneously). Patients must weigh the risks of antirejection medications against the advantages of pancreas transplantation. Implantation of insulin-producing pancreatic islet cells is another approach. This latter approach involves a less extensive surgical procedure and a potentially lower incidence of immunogenic problems. However, thus far, independence from exogenous insulin has been limited to 2 years after transplantation of islet cells. Results of studies of patients with islet cell transplants using less toxic antirejection drugs have shown some promise. These procedures are not widely available due to a critical shortage of organs for transplantation (National Institute of Diabetes and Digestive and Kidney Diseases [NIDDK], 2013a).

Oral Antidiabetic Agents

Oral antidiabetic agents may be effective for patients who have type 2 diabetes that cannot be treated effectively with MNT and exercise alone. In the United States, oral antidiabetic agents include first- and second-generation sulfonylureas, biguanides, alpha-glucosidase inhibitors, non-sulfonylurea insulin secretogogues (meglitinides and phenylalanine derivatives), thiazolidinediones (glitazones), dipeptide peptidase-4 (DPP-4) inhibitors, glucagon-like peptide-1 receptor agonists (GLP-1), and sodium-glucose cotransporter 2 (SGL2) inhibitors (see Table 51-6). The thiazolidinediones are a class of oral antidiabetic medications that reduce insulin resistance in target tissues, enhancing insulin action without directly stimulating insulin secretion. Sulfonylureas and meglitinides are considered insulin secretagogues because their action increases the secretion of insulin by the pancreatic beta cells (Hinnen, 2015; Triplitt & Solis-Herrera, 2015; Vivian, 2015).

Patients must understand that oral agents are prescribed as an addition to (not as a substitute for) other treatment modalities, such as MNT and exercise. The use of oral antidiabetic medications may need to be halted temporarily and insulin prescribed if hyperglycemia develops that is attributable to infection, trauma, or surgery. See later section on glycemic control in the hospitalized patient.

Because mechanisms of action vary (see Fig. 51-5), effects may be enhanced with the use of a multidose, or more than one medication (ADA, 2016e). A combination of oral agents with insulin, usually glargine (Lantus) at bedtime, has also been used as a treatment for some patients with type 2 diabetes. Insulin therapy may be used from the onset for newly diagnosed patients with type 2 diabetes who are symptomatic and have high blood glucose and A1C levels (ADA, 2016e).

Other Pharmacologic Therapy

Additional medications are available for use in the pharmacologic management of diabetes. These are adjunct therapies, not a substitute for insulin if insulin is required to control diabetes.

Pramlintide (Symlin), a synthetic analogue of human amylin, a hormone that is secreted by the beta cells of the pancreas, is approved for treatment of both type 1 and type 2 diabetes (Comerford, 2015). It is used to control hyperglycemia in adults who have not achieved acceptable levels of glucose control despite the use of insulin at mealtimes. It is used with insulin, not in place of insulin. It acts to slow the rate at which food leaves the stomach and reduces appetite (Comerford, 2015). The goal of therapy is to minimize fluctuations in daily glucose levels and provide better glucose control. Pramlintide must be injected subcutaneously 2 in from an insulin injection site (Comerford, 2015). Patients are instructed to monitor their blood glucose levels closely during the initial period of use of pramlintide.

Exenatide (Byetta, Byduron) is used as an adjunct therapy or monotherapy for patient with type 2 diabetes (Comerford, 2015; ADA, 2016e). It is derived from a hormone that is produced in the small intestine and has been found to be deficient in type 2 diabetes. It is normally released after food is ingested to delay gastric emptying and enhance insulin secretion, resulting in dampening of the rise in blood glucose levels after meals and a feeling of satiety. The return of the blood glucose level to normal results in decreased production of the hormone. Hypoglycemia is not a side effect of exenatide if adjustments are made in the sulfonylurea dose. Exenatide is associated with appetite suppression and weight loss. Exenatide must be injected twice a day within 1 hour before breakfast and dinner (Comerford, 2015). There is also a once-a-week injection (Byduron) available. These medications are not substitutes for insulin in patients who require insulin to control their diabetes.

Nursing Management

Nursing management of patients with diabetes can involve treatment of a wide variety of physiologic disorders, depending on the patient's health status and whether the patient is newly diagnosed or seeking care for an unrelated health problem. Glucose control in patients diagnosed with diabetes as well as those who have not been diagnosed is an important consideration in the hospital setting. Nursing management of patients with DKA and HHS and of those with diabetes as a secondary diagnosis is discussed in subsequent sections of this chapter.

Because all patients with diabetes must master the concepts and skills necessary for long-term management and avoidance of potential complications of diabetes, a solid educational foundation is necessary for competent self-care and is an ongoing focus of nursing care.

Managing Glucose Control in the Hospital Setting

Hyperglycemia can prolong lengths of stay and increase infection rates and mortality; thus, nurses need to address glucose management in all hospital patients (Seggelke & Everhart, 2013). Hyperglycemia occurs most often in patients with known diabetes (i.e., type 1, type 2, gestational) and in those newly diagnosed with diabetes or stress hyperglycemia. Nursing management of hyperglycemia in the hospital uses the following principles (ADA, 2016g):

- Blood glucose targets are 140 to 180 mg/dL.
- Insulin (subcutaneous or IV) is preferred to oral antidiabetic agents to manage hyperglycemia.
- Hospital insulin protocols or order sets should minimize complexity, ensure adequate staff training, include

TABLE 51-6 Selected Oral Antidiabetic Agents

Generic (Trade) Name	Action/Indications	Side Effects	Implications
Second-Generation Sulfonylureas			
glipizide (Glucotrol, Glucotrol XL) glyburide (Micronase, Glynase, DiaBeta) glimepiride (Amaryl)	Stimulate beta cells of the pancreas to secrete insulin; may improve binding between insulin and insulin receptors or increase the number of insulin receptors Used in type 2 diabetes to control blood glucose levels Have more potent effects than first-generation sulfonylureas May be used in combination with metformin or insulin to improve glucose control	Hypoglycemia Mild GI symptoms Weight gain Drug–drug interactions (NSAIDs, warfarin, sulfonamides)	Monitor patient for hypoglycemia. Monitor blood glucose and urine ketone levels to assess effectiveness of therapy. Patients at high risk for hypoglycemia: advanced age, renal insufficiency. When taken with beta-adrenergic blocking agents, may mask usual warning signs and symptoms of hypoglycemia. Instruct patients to avoid the use of alcohol. Contraindicated with sulfa allergy.
Biguanides			
metformin (Glucophage, Glucophage XL, Fortamet) metformin with glyburide (Glucovance)	Inhibit production of glucose by the liver Increase body tissue sensitivity to insulin Decrease hepatic synthesis of cholesterol Used in type 2 diabetes to control blood glucose levels	Lactic acidosis Hypoglycemia if metformin is used in combination with insulin or other antidiabetic agents Drug–drug interaction GI disturbances Contraindicated in patients with impaired kidney or liver function, respiratory insufficiency, severe infection, or alcohol abuse	Monitor for lactic acidosis and hypoglycemia. Monitor kidney function. Patients taking metformin are at increased risk for acute kidney injury and lactic acidosis with the use of iodinated contrast material for diagnostic studies; metformin should be stopped 48 hours prior to and for 48 hours after the use of contrast agent or until kidney function is evaluated and normal. Check for interactions with other medications.
Alpha-Glucosidase Inhibitors			
acarbose (Precose) miglitol (Glyset)	Delay absorption of complex carbohydrates in the intestine and slow entry of glucose into systemic circulation Do not increase insulin secretion Used in type 2 diabetes to control blood glucose levels Can be used alone or in combination with sulfonylureas, metformin, or insulin to improve glucose control	Hypoglycemia (risk increased if used with insulin or other antidiabetic agents) GI side effects (abdominal discomfort or distention, diarrhea, flatulence) Drug–drug interactions	Must be taken with first bite of food to be effective Monitor for GI side effects (diarrhea, abdominal distention). Monitor for blood glucose levels to assess effectiveness of therapy. Monitor liver function studies every 3 months for 1 year, then periodically. Contraindicated in patients with GI or kidney dysfunction, or cirrhosis *Alert:* Hypoglycemia must be treated with glucose, not sucrose.
Non-Sulfonylurea Insulin Secretagogues			
repaglinide (Prandin) categorized as a meglitinide nateglinide (Starlix) categorized as a D-phenylalanine derivative	Stimulate pancreas to secrete insulin Used in type 2 diabetes to control blood glucose levels Can be used alone or in combination with metformin or thiazolidinediones to improve glucose control	Hypoglycemia/weight gain less likely than sulfonylureas Drug–drug interactions (with ketoconazole [Nizoral], fluconazole [Diflucan], erythromycin [E-Mycin], rifampin [Rifadin], isoniazid [INH])	Monitor blood glucose levels to assess effectiveness of therapy. Has rapid action and short half-life Should be taken only if able to eat a meal immediately Educate patients about symptoms of hypoglycemia. Monitor patients with impaired liver function and renal impairment. Has no effect on plasma lipids Is taken before each meal Check for interactions with other medications.

TABLE 51-6 Oral Antidiabetic Agents (continued)

Generic (Trade) Name	Action/Indications	Side Effects	Implications
Thiazolidinediones (or Glitazones)			
pioglitazone (Actos) rosiglitazone (Avandia)	Sensitize body tissue to insulin; stimulate insulin receptor sites to lower blood glucose and improve action of insulin May be used alone or in combination with sulfonylurea, metformin, or insulin	Hypoglycemia (risk increased with the use of insulin or other antidiabetic agents) Anemia Weight gain, edema Decrease effectiveness of oral contraceptives Possible liver dysfunction Drug–drug interactions Hyperlipidemia (has variable effect on lipids; pioglitazone may be preferred choice in patients with lipid abnormalities) Impaired platelet function	Monitor blood glucose levels to assess effectiveness of therapy. Monitor liver function tests. Arrange dietary education to establish weight control program. Instruct patient taking oral contraceptives about increased risk of pregnancy.
Dipeptidyl Peptidase-4 (DPP-4) Inhibitors			
sitagliptin (Januvia) vildagliptin (Galvus) saxagliptin (Onglyza) linaglipitin (Tradjenta) alogliptin (Nesina)	Increase and prolong the action of incretin, a hormone that increases insulin release and decreases glucagon levels, with the result of improved glucose control	Upper respiratory infection Stuffy or runny nose and sore throat Headache Stomach discomfort and diarrhea Hypoglycemia, if used with sulfonylurea	Usually given once a day Used alone or with other oral antidiabetic agents Instruct patient about signs and symptoms of hypoglycemia and other adverse effects to report. Monitor kidney function.
Glucagon-like peptide-1 agonist (GLP-1)			
liraglutide (Victoza) dulaglutide (Trulicity)	Enhances glucose-dependent insulin secretion and exhibit other antihyperglycemic actions following their release into the circulation from the gastrointestinal tract.	Pancreatitis, weight loss, diarrhea, nausea, vomiting, reaction at injection site, cough	Given once a day by subcutaneous injection. For patients with type 2 diabetes (not indicated for type 1 diabetes)
Sodium-glucose co-transporter 2 (SGL-2) Inhibitors			
dapagliflozin (Forxiga) anagliflozin (Invokana) empagliflozin (Jardiance)	For type 2 diabetes only. Prevents the kidneys from reabsorbing glucose back into the blood, therefore lowering glucose by releasing glucose into the urine	Urinary tract infections Hypoglycemia May increase LDL and HDL cholesterol	Improves glycemic control in patients with type 2 diabetes.

GI, gastrointestinal; NSAIDs, nonsteroidal anti-inflammatory drugs.
Adapted from Comerford, K. C. (2015). *Nursing 2015 Drug Handbook*. Philadelphia, PA: Wolters Kluwer.

standardized hypoglycemic treatment, and make guidelines available for glycemic goals and insulin dosing.
- Appropriate timing of blood glucose checks, meal consumption, and insulin dose are all crucial for glucose control and to avoid hypoglycemia.

 Providing Patient Education

Diabetes is a chronic illness that requires a lifetime of special self-management behaviors (ADA, 2016a). Because MNT, physical activity, medication, and physical and emotional stress affect diabetic control, patients must learn to balance a multitude of factors.

Developing a Diabetes Education Plan

Patients with new-onset type 1 diabetes are hospitalized for short periods or may be managed completely on an outpatient basis. Patients with new-onset type 2 diabetes are rarely hospitalized for initial care. Outpatient diabetes education

and training programs have proliferated with the availability of third-party reimbursement. All encounters with patients with diabetes are opportunities for reinforcement of self-management skills, regardless of the setting.

Many health systems employ nurses who specialize in diabetes education and management and who are certified by the National Certification Board for Diabetes Educators as certified diabetes educators. However, because of the large number of patients with diabetes all nurses play a vital role in identifying patients with diabetes, assessing self-care skills, providing basic education, reinforcing the education provided by the specialist, and referring patients for follow-up care. Diabetes patient education programs that have been peer-reviewed by the ADA as meeting National Standards for Diabetes Self-Management Education can be reimbursed for education.

Organizing Information

There are various strategies for organizing and prioritizing the vast amount of information that must be taught to patients

Figure 51-5 • Action sites of hypoglycemic agents and mechanisms of lowering blood glucose in type 2 diabetes. The incretins are the dipeptidyl peptidase-4 inhibitors and glucagonlike peptide-1 agonists.

Unfolding Patient Stories: Skyler Hansen • Part 2

Recall from Chapter 6 Skyler Hansen, a high school student recently diagnosed with type 1 diabetes. Outline a diabetes education plan for Skyler and his parents. What are important patient education topics, resources, and methods for the nurse to consider? How would the nurse evaluate whether the patient and his family understand the education provided?

Care for Skyler and other patients in a realistic virtual environment: *vSim for Nursing* (**thepoint.lww.com/vSimMedicalSurgical**). Practice documenting these patients' care in DocuCare (**thepoint.lww.com/DocuCareEHR**).

with diabetes. In addition, many hospitals and outpatient diabetes centers have devised written guidelines, care plans, and documentation forms (often based on ADA guidelines) that may be used to document and evaluate education. One approach is to organize education using the seven tips for managing diabetes identified and developed by the American Association of Diabetes Educators (AADE, 2011; AADE, 2014): healthy eating, being active, monitoring, taking medication, problem solving, healthy coping, and reducing risks. The AADE can be contacted for additional information about assessment and documentation of outcomes of this approach to education (see Resources at end of chapter).

Another general approach is to organize information and skills into two main categories: basic, initial and in-depth (advanced) or continuing education.

Educating Patients About Basic Skills. Basic skills must be learned by all patients with newly diagnosed type 1 or type 2 diabetes and all patients receiving insulin for the first time. Basic information that patients must know is included in Chart 51-5.

For patients with newly diagnosed type 2 diabetes, emphasis is initially placed on meal planning and exercise. Those who are starting to take oral antidiabetic agents need

Chart 51-5 — PATIENT EDUCATION
Basic Skills for People With Diabetes

The nurse includes the following basic information in education:

1. Pathophysiology
   a. Basic definition of diabetes (having a high blood glucose level)
   b. Normal blood glucose ranges and target blood glucose levels
   c. Effect of insulin and exercise (decrease glucose)
   d. Effect of food and stress, including illness and infections (increase glucose)
   e. Basic treatment approaches
2. Treatment modalities
   a. Administration of insulin and oral antidiabetes medications
   b. Meal planning (food groups, timing of meals)
   c. Monitoring of blood glucose and urine ketones
3. Recognition, treatment, and prevention of acute complications
   a. Hypoglycemia
   b. Hyperglycemia
4. Pragmatic information
   a. Where to buy and store insulin, syringes, and glucose monitoring supplies
   b. When and how to contact the primary provider

to know about detecting, preventing, and treating hypoglycemia. If diabetes has gone undetected for many years, the patient may already be experiencing some chronic complications from diabetes. Therefore, for some patients with newly diagnosed type 2 diabetes, basic diabetes education must include information on preventive skills, such as foot care (Fisher, 2016) and eye care (e.g., planning yearly or more frequent complete [dilated eye] examinations by an ophthalmologist, understanding that retinopathy is largely asymptomatic until advanced stages).

Patients also need to realize that once they master the basic skills and information, diabetes education is a life-long process. Acquiring in-depth and advanced diabetes knowledge occurs both formally through programs of continuing education and informally through experience and sharing of information with other people with diabetes.

Planning In-Depth and Continuing Education. This education involves more details related to basic skills (e.g., learning to vary food choices [carbohydrate counting] and insulin, preparing for travel) as well as learning preventive measures for avoiding long-term complications from diabetes. Preventive measures include foot care, eye care, general hygiene (e.g., skin care and oral hygiene), and risk factor management (e.g., blood pressure control and blood glucose normalization and cholesterol/lipid control) (AADE, 2014).

More advanced continuing education may include alternative methods for insulin delivery, such as the insulin pump, and algorithms or rules for evaluating and adjusting insulin doses. The degree of advanced diabetes education to be provided depends on the patient's interest and ability. However, learning preventive measures (especially foot and eye care) is mandatory for early detection and treatment to reduce the occurrence of amputations and blindness in patients with diabetes.

Assessing Readiness to Learn

Before initiating diabetes education, the nurse assesses the patient's (and family's) readiness to learn. When patients are first diagnosed with diabetes (or first told of their need for insulin), they often go through stages of the grieving process. These stages may include shock and denial, anger, depression, negotiation, and acceptance. The amount of time it takes for the patient and family members to work through the grieving process varies from patient to patient. They may experience helplessness, guilt, altered body image, loss of self-esteem, and concern about the future. The nurse must assess the patient's coping strategies and reassure the patient and family that feelings of depression and shock are normal.

Asking the patient and family about their major concerns or fears is an important way to learn about any misinformation that may be contributing to anxiety. Simple, direct information should be provided to dispel misconceptions. Once the patient masters basic skills, more information is provided.

Patients who are in the hospital rarely have the luxury of waiting until they feel ready to learn; short lengths of hospital stay necessitate initiation of basic skill education as early as possible. This gives the patient the opportunity to practice skills with supervision by the nurse before discharge. Follow-up in the home is often necessary for reinforcement of skills.

The nurse evaluates the patient's social situation for factors that may influence the diabetes treatment and education plan, such as:

- Low literacy level (may be evaluated while assessing for visual deficits by having the patient read from educational materials)
- Limited financial resources or lack of health insurance
- Presence or absence of family support
- Typical daily schedule (the patient is asked about the timing and number of usual daily meals, work and exercise schedule, plans for travel)
- Neurologic deficits caused by stroke, other neurologic disorders, or other disabling conditions, obtained from the patient's health history and physical assessment (the patient is assessed for aphasia or decreased ability to follow simple commands)

Cultural beliefs may also impact adherence to a regimen.

Educating Experienced Patients

Nurses need to continue to assess the skills and self-care behaviors of patients who have had diabetes for many years. Assessment of these patients must include direct observation of skills, not just the patient's self-report of self-care behaviors. In addition, these patients must be fully aware of preventive measures related to foot care, eye care, and risk factor management. Those experiencing long-term complications from diabetes for the first time may go through the grieving process again. Some patients may have a renewed interest in diabetes self-care in the hope of delaying further complications. Others may have guilt and depression. The patient is encouraged to discuss feelings and fears related to complications. Meanwhile, the nurse provides appropriate information regarding complications from diabetes.

Determining Education Methods

Maintaining flexibility with regard to education approaches is important. Providing education on skills and information in a logical sequence is not always the most helpful method for patients. For example, many patients fear self-injection. Before they learn how to prepare, purchase, store, and mix insulins, they should be taught to insert the needle and inject insulin (or practice with saline solution).

Various tools can be used to complement education. Many of the companies that manufacture products for diabetes self-care also provide booklets, videotapes, DVDs or on-line materials to assist in patient education. Educational materials are also available from the AADE, ADA, and CDC (see the Resources section). It is important to use a variety of written handouts that match the patient's learning needs (including different languages, low-literacy information, and large print) and reading level and to ensure that these materials are technically accurate. Patients can continue learning about diabetes care by participating in community based educational programs (Gaillard, Amponsah, & Osei, 2015) (see Chart 51-6).

Educating Patients to Self-Administer Insulin

Insulin injections are self-administered into the subcutaneous tissue with the use of special insulin syringes. Basic information includes explanations of the equipment, insulins, and syringes and how to mix insulin, if necessary.

Chart 51-6

NURSING RESEARCH PROFILE

Impact of Community Diabetes Education

Gaillard, T., Amponsah, G., & Osei K. (2015). Patient-centered community diabetes education program improves glycemic control in African American patients with poorly controlled type 2 diabetes: Importance of point of care metabolic measurements. *Journal of the National Black Nurses Association, 26*(1), 51–58.

Purpose

The purpose of this study was to evaluate the benefits of a 6-month patient-centered, intensive lifestyle and diabetes self-management education support (DSMES) program on improving glycemic control as assessed by point-of-care (POC) A1C testing, body weight, blood pressure, and lipids and lipoprotein levels in African Americans with poorly controlled type 2 diabetes compared to standard diabetes cares.

Design

This was a single center randomized clinical trial of participants with poorly controlled type 2 diabetes (A1C > 7.0%) residing in the inner city. Participants were randomized to DSMES (*n* = 58) or to standard diabetes care (*n* = 38). Participants in the DSMES group received intensive lifestyle and behavioral program that included didactic lectures provided by the Diabetes Care Team at 1 to 2 week intervals for 6 months. A community health worker, trained in diabetes self-management, provided support in the form of weekly phone calls and information about community resources. At the end of each didactic session, goals from the prior week, barriers, and challenges were discussed. The group then discussed alternate strategies

for goal attainment. Participants were provided with quarterly POC testing (A1C, blood pressure, cholesterol, weight) and were reminded of targets. Emphasis was placed on how lifestyle changes could assist in meeting targets/goals. Participants in the standard care group attended the initial orientation, but did not attend the didactic nor intensive self-management lectures. General diabetes topics were discussed to increase group participation. POC testing was done in both groups at baseline, 3 and 6 months.

Findings

At 6 months, the DSMES group had significant reduction in A1C ($8.2 \pm 1.4\%$ vs. $7.5 \pm 1.5\%$, $p = 0.02$) and random glucose (190.4 ± 77.6 vs. 160.6 ± 59.8 mg/dl, $p = 0.03$) when compared with the standard care group. However, there were no changes in body weight, blood pressure, or lipids/lipoprotein levels. In addition, participants in the DSMES verbalized enjoying meeting with the group to discuss strategies and challenges faced with controlling type 2 diabetes.

Nursing Implications

Nurses need to encourage patients with diabetes and prediabetes to attend diabetes self-management, education, and support groups. In addition, these programs should be culturally sensitive, located in the community, and offered at times that are convenient to participants. Finally, the addition of POC testing allows individuals to reconcile their results with goals of therapy and provides immediate feedback and suggestions for change.

Storing Insulin

Whether insulin is the short- or the long-acting preparation, vials not in use, including spare vials or pens, should be refrigerated. Extremes of temperature should be avoided; insulin should not be allowed to freeze and should not be kept in direct sunlight or in a hot car. The insulin vial in use should be kept at room temperature to reduce local irritation at the injection site, which may occur if cold insulin is injected. If a vial of insulin will be used up within 1 month, it may be kept at room temperature. The patient should be instructed to always have a spare vial of the type or types of insulin that he or she uses (ADA, 2016a). Cloudy insulins should be thoroughly mixed by gently inverting the vial or rolling it between the hands before drawing the solution into a syringe or a pen (Comerford, 2015). The patient needs to be educated to pay attention to the expiration date on any type of insulin.

Bottles of intermediate-acting insulin should also be inspected for flocculation, which is a frosted, whitish coating inside the bottle. This occurs most commonly with insulins that are exposed to extremes of temperature. If a frosted, adherent coating is present, some of the insulin is bound, inactive, and should not be used.

Selecting Syringes

Syringes must be matched with the insulin concentration (e.g., U-100). Currently, three sizes of U-100 insulin syringes are available:

- 1-mL syringe, 100-unit capacity
- 0.5-mL syringe, 50-unit capacity
- 0.3-mL syringe, 30-unit capacity

The concentration of insulin used in the United States is U-100; that is, there are 100 units per milliliter (or cubic

centimeter). Small syringes allow patients who require small amounts of insulin to measure and draw up the amount of insulin accurately. There is a U-500 (500 units/mL) concentration of insulin available by special order for patients who have severe insulin resistance and require massive doses of insulin.

Most insulin syringes have a disposable 27- to 29-gauge needle that is approximately 0.5 in long. The smaller syringes are marked in 1-unit increments and may be easier to use for patients with visual deficits and those taking very small doses of insulin. The 1-mL syringes are marked in 1- and 2-unit increments. A small disposable insulin needle (31 gauge, 8 mm long) is available for very thin patients and children.

Mixing Insulins

When rapid- or short-acting insulins are to be given simultaneously with longer-acting insulins, they are usually mixed together in the same syringe; the longer-acting insulins must be mixed thoroughly before drawing into the syringe. It is important that patients prepare their insulin injections consistently from day to day.

There are varying opinions regarding which type of insulin (short-acting or longer-acting) should be drawn up into the syringe first when they are going to be mixed, but the ADA recommends that the regular insulin be drawn up first. The most important issues are (1) that patients are consistent in technique, so as not to draw up the wrong dose in error or the wrong type of insulin, and (2) that patients not inject one type of insulin into the bottle containing a different type of insulin. Injecting cloudy insulin into a vial of clear insulin contaminates the entire vial of clear insulin and alters its action.

For patients who have difficulty mixing insulins, several options are available. They may use a premixed insulin, they may have prefilled syringes prepared (see Fig. 51-3), or they may take 2 injections. Premixed insulins are available in many different ratios of NPH insulin to regular insulin (Comerford, 2015). The ratio of 70/30 (70% NPH and 30% regular insulin in one bottle) is most common; this combination is available as Novolin 70/30 (Novo Nordisk) and Humulin 70/30 (Lilly). Combinations with a ratio of 75% NPL (neutral protamine lispro) and 25% insulin lispro are also available. NPL is used only in the mix with Humalog; its action is the same as NPH. The appropriate initial dosage of premixed insulin must be calculated so that the ratio of NPH to regular insulin most closely approximates the separate doses needed.

For patients who can inject insulin but who have difficulty drawing up a single or mixed dose, syringes may be prefilled with the help of home care nurses or family and friends. A 3-week supply of insulin syringes may be prepared and kept in the refrigerator but warmed to room temperature before administration. The prefilled syringes should be stored with the needle in an upright position to avoid clogging of the needle; they should be mixed thoroughly by inverting syringe several times before the insulin is injected.

Withdrawing Insulin

Most (if not all) of the printed materials available on insulin dose preparation instruct patients to inject air into the bottle of insulin equivalent to the number of units of insulin to be withdrawn. The rationale for this is to prevent the formation of a vacuum inside the bottle, which would make it difficult to withdraw the proper amount of insulin.

Selecting and Rotating the Injection Site

The four main areas for injection are the abdomen, upper arms (posterior surface), thighs (anterior surface), and hips (see Fig. 51-6). Insulin is absorbed faster in some areas of the body than others. The speed of absorption is greatest in the abdomen and decreases progressively in the arm, thigh, and hip, respectively.

Systematic rotation of injection sites within an anatomic area is recommended to prevent localized changes in fatty tissue (lipodystrophy). In addition, to promote consistency in insulin absorption, the patient should be encouraged to use all

available injection sites within one area rather than randomly rotating sites from area to area. For example, some patients almost exclusively use the abdominal area, administering each injection 0.5 to 1 in away from the previous injection. Another approach to rotation is always to use the same area at the same time of day. For example, patients may inject morning doses into the abdomen and evening doses into the arms or legs.

A few general principles apply to all rotation patterns. First, the patient should try not to use the exact same site more than once in 2 to 3 weeks. In addition, if the patient is planning to exercise, insulin should not be injected into the limb that will be exercised because this will cause the drug to be absorbed faster, which may result in hypoglycemia.

Preparing the Skin

The use of alcohol to cleanse the skin is not necessary, but patients who have learned this technique often continue to use it. They should be cautioned to allow the skin to dry after cleansing with alcohol. If the skin is not allowed to dry before the injection, the alcohol may be carried into the tissues, resulting in a localized reddened area and a burning sensation.

Inserting the Needle

There are varying approaches to inserting the needle for insulin injections. The correct technique is based on the need for the insulin to be injected into the subcutaneous tissue (see Chart 51-7). Injection that is too deep (e.g., intramuscular) or too shallow (intradermal) may affect the rate of absorption of the insulin. For a normal or overweight person, a 90-degree angle is the best insertion angle. Aspiration (inserting the needle and then pulling back on the plunger to assess for blood being drawn into the syringe and needle in vein) is not necessary. Many patients who have been using insulin for an extended period have eliminated this step from their insulin injection routine with no apparent adverse effects. Chart 51-8 details how to evaluate the effectiveness of self-injection of insulin education.

Disposing of Syringes and Needles

Insulin syringes and pens, needles, and lancets should be disposed of according to local regulations. If community disposal programs are unavailable, used sharps should be placed in a puncture-resistant container. The patient should contact local trash authorities for instructions about proper disposal of filled containers, which should not be mixed with containers to be recycled.

Promoting Home, Community-Based, and Transitional Care

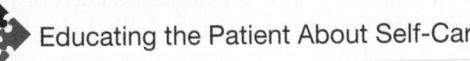 Educating the Patient About Self-Care

If poor glucose control or preventable complications occur, the nurse needs to assess the reasons for the patient's ineffective management of the treatment regimen. It should not be assumed that problems with diabetes management are related to the patient's decision to ignore self-management. The patient may have forgotten or may have never learned certain information, or there may be cultural or religious beliefs that interfere with adherence. The problem may be correctable simply through providing complete information and ensuring that the patient understands the information. The focus of diabetes education should be patient empowerment. Patient education must address behavior change, self-efficacy, and health beliefs.

Figure 51-6 • Suggested areas for insulin injection.

Chart 51-7 PATIENT EDUCATION
Self-Injection of Insulin

The nurse instructs the patient to:

1. With one hand, stabilize the skin by spreading it or pinching up a large area.

Pinching the skin

2. Pick up syringe with the other hand, and hold it as you would a pencil. Insert needle straight into the skin.[a]

Inserting the needle into the skin

3. To inject the insulin, push the plunger all the way in.

Injecting the insulin

4. Pull needle straight out of skin. Press cotton ball over injection site for several seconds.

Removing the needle and holding cotton ball over site

5. Use disposable syringe *only once* and discard into hard plastic container (with a tight-fitting top) such as an empty bleach or detergent container.[b] Follow state regulations for disposal of syringes and needles.

Disposing of syringe

[a]Some patients may be taught to insert the needle at a 45-degree angle.
[b]Although some studies suggest that reusing disposable syringes may be safe, it is recommended that this be done only in the absence of poor personal hygiene, an acute concurrent illness, open wounds on the hands, or decreased resistance to infection.

If knowledge deficit is not the issue, physical or emotional factors may be impairing the patient's ability to perform self-care skills. For example, decreased visual acuity may impair the patient's ability to administer insulin accurately, measure the blood glucose level, or inspect the skin and feet. In addition, decreased joint mobility (especially in older adults) or preexisting disability may impair the patient's ability to inspect the bottom of the feet. Denial of the diagnosis or depression may impair the patient's ability to carry out multiple daily self-care measures. The patient whose family, personal, or work problems may be of higher priority may benefit from assistance in establishing priorities. The nurse must also assess the patient for infection or emotional stress, which may lead to elevated blood glucose levels despite adherence to the treatment regimen.

The following approaches are helpful for promoting self-care management skills:

- Address any underlying factors (e.g., knowledge deficit, self-care deficit, illness) that may affect control of diabetes.
- Simplify the treatment regimen if it is too difficult for the patient to follow.

- Adjust the treatment regimen to meet patient requests (e.g., adjust diet or insulin schedule to allow increased flexibility in meal content or timing).
- Establish a specific plan or contract with each patient with simple, measurable goals.
- Provide positive reinforcement of self-care behaviors performed instead of focusing on behaviors that were neglected (e.g., positively reinforce blood glucose tests that were performed instead of focusing on the number of missed tests).
- Help the patient identify personal motivating factors rather than focusing on wanting to please primary providers.
- Encourage the patient to pursue life goals and interests, and discourage an undue focus on diabetes.

Continuing and Transitional Care

The degree to which patients interact with primary providers to obtain ongoing care depends on many factors. Age, socioeconomic level, existing complications, type of diabetes, and

Chart 51-8 — Criteria for Determining Effectiveness of Self-Injection of Insulin Education

Equipment

Insulin

1. Identifies information on label of insulin bottle:
   - Type (e.g., NPH, regular, 70/30)
   - Manufacturer (Lilly, Novo Nordisk)
   - Concentration (e.g., U-100)
   - Expiration date
2. Checks appearance of insulin:
   - Clear or milky white
   - Checks for flocculation (clumping, frosted appearance)
   - Identifies where to purchase and store insulin:
   - Indicates approximately how long bottle will last (1000 units per bottle U-100 insulin)
   - Indicates how long opened bottles can be used

Syringes

1. Identifies concentration (U-100) marking on syringe
2. Identifies size of syringe (e.g., 100 units, 50 units, 30 units)
3. Describes appropriate disposal of used syringe

Preparation and Administration of Insulin Injection

1. Draws up correct amount and type of insulin
2. Properly mixes 2 insulins if necessary
3. Inserts needle and injects insulin
4. Describes site rotation:
   - Demonstrates injection with all anatomic areas to be used
   - Describes pattern for rotation, such as using abdomen only or using certain areas at the same time of day
   - Describes system for remembering site locations, such as horizontal pattern across the abdomen as if drawing a dotted line

Knowledge of Insulin Action

1. Lists prescription:
   - Type and dosage of insulin
   - Timing of insulin injections
2. Describes approximate time course of insulin action:
   - Identifies long- and short-acting insulins by name
   - States approximate time delay until the onset of insulin action
   - Identifies need to delay food until 5 to 15 minutes after injection of rapid-acting insulin (lispro, aspart, glulisine [Apidra])
   - Knows that longer time delays are safe when blood glucose level is high and that time delays may need to be shortened when blood glucose level is low

Incorporation of Insulin Injections Into Daily Schedule

1. Recites proper order of premeal diabetes activities:
   - May use mnemonic device such as the word "tie," which helps the patient remember the order of activities ("t" = test [blood glucose], "i" = insulin injection, "e" = eat)
   - Describes daily schedule, such as test, insulin, eat before breakfast and dinner; test and eat, before lunch and bedtime
2. Describes information regarding hypoglycemia:
   - Symptoms: shakiness, sweating, nervousness, hunger, weakness
   - Causes: too much insulin, too much exercise, not enough food
   - Treatment: 15 g concentrated carbohydrate, such as 2 or 3 glucose tablets, 1 tube glucose gel, 0.5 cup juice
   - After initial treatment, follow with snack including starch and protein, such as cheese and crackers, milk and crackers, half sandwich.
3. Describes information regarding prevention of hypoglycemia:
   - Avoids delays in meal timing
   - Eats a meal or snack approximately every 4 to 5 hours (while awake)
   - Does not skip meals
   - Increases food intake before exercise if blood glucose level is less than 100 mg/dL
   - Checks blood glucose regularly
   - Identifies safe modification of insulin doses consistent with management plan
   - Carries a form of fast-acting sugar at all times
   - Wears a medical identification bracelet
   - Educates family, friends, and coworkers about signs and treatment of hypoglycemia
   - Has family, roommates, and traveling companions learn to use injectable glucagon for severe hypoglycemic reactions
4. Maintains regular follow-up for evaluation of diabetes control:
   - Keeps written record of blood glucose, insulin doses, hypoglycemic reactions, variations in diet
   - Keeps all appointments with health professionals
   - Sees primary provider regularly (usually two to four times per year)
   - States how to contact primary provider in case of emergency
   - States when to call primary provider to report variations in blood glucose levels

comorbid conditions may dictate the frequency of follow-up visits. Many patients with diabetes are seen by home health, community-based, or transitional care nurses for diabetes education, wound care, insulin preparation, or assistance with glucose monitoring. Even patients who achieve excellent glucose control and have no complications can expect to see their primary provider at least twice a year for ongoing evaluation and should receive routine nutrition updates. In addition, the nurse should remind the patient to participate in recommended health promotion activities (e.g., immunizations) and age-appropriate health screenings (e.g., pelvic examinations, mammograms).

Participation in support groups is encouraged for patients who have had diabetes for many years as well as for those who are newly diagnosed (Gaillard et al., 2015). Such participation may help the patient and family cope with changes in lifestyle that occur with the onset of diabetes and its complications. People who participate in support groups often share valuable information and experiences and learn from others. Support groups provide an opportunity for discussion of strategies to deal with diabetes and its management and to clarify and verify information with nurses or other health care professionals. Participation in support groups may also promote healthy activities.

ACUTE COMPLICATIONS OF DIABETES

There are three major acute complications of diabetes related to short-term imbalances in blood glucose levels: hypoglycemia, DKA, and HHS (Umpeirrez & Korytkowski, 2016).

Hypoglycemia (Insulin Reactions)

Hypoglycemia means low (hypo) sugar in the blood (glycemia) and occurs when the blood glucose falls to less than 70 mg/dL (3.7 mmol/L). Severe hypoglycemia is when glucose levels are less the 40 mg/dL (2.5 mmol/L) (Seggelke & Everhart, 2013). It can occur when there is too much insulin or oral hypoglycemic agents, too little food, or excessive physical activity. Hypoglycemia may occur at any time of the day or night. It often occurs before meals, especially if meals are delayed or snacks are omitted. For example, midmorning hypoglycemia may occur when the morning insulin is peaking, whereas hypoglycemia that occurs in the late afternoon coincides with the peak of the morning NPH insulin. Middle-of-the-night hypoglycemia may occur because of peaking evening or predinner NPH insulins, especially in patients who have not eaten a bedtime snack.

 Gerontologic Considerations

In older patients with diabetes, hypoglycemia is a particular concern for many reasons:

- Older adults frequently live alone and may not recognize the symptoms of hypoglycemia.
- With decreasing kidney function, it takes longer for oral hypoglycemic agents to be excreted by the kidneys.
- Skipping meals may occur because of decreased appetite or financial limitations.
- Decreased visual acuity may lead to errors in insulin administration.

Clinical Manifestations

The clinical manifestations of hypoglycemia may be grouped into two categories: adrenergic symptoms and central nervous system (CNS) symptoms.

In mild hypoglycemia, as the blood glucose level falls, the sympathetic nervous system is stimulated, resulting in a surge of epinephrine and norepinephrine. This causes symptoms such as sweating, tremor, tachycardia, palpitation, nervousness, and hunger.

In moderate hypoglycemia, the drop in blood glucose level deprives the brain cells of needed fuel for functioning. Signs of impaired function of the CNS may include inability to concentrate, headache, lightheadedness, confusion, memory lapses, numbness of the lips and tongue, slurred speech, impaired coordination, emotional changes, irrational or combative behavior, double vision, and drowsiness. Any combination of these symptoms (in addition to adrenergic symptoms) may occur with moderate hypoglycemia.

In severe hypoglycemia, CNS function is so impaired that the patient needs the assistance of another person for treatment of hypoglycemia. Symptoms may include disoriented behavior, seizures, difficulty arousing from sleep, or loss of consciousness.

 Concept Mastery Alert

It is important to check the patient's blood glucose level and correlate it with the patient's symptoms. If the patient's blood glucose level is low, but he or she is not exhibiting any symptoms, the nurse should double-check the glucose level to ensure that it is correct.

Assessment and Diagnostic Findings

Symptoms of hypoglycemia may occur suddenly and vary considerably from person to person. Decreased hormonal (adrenergic) response to hypoglycemia may contribute to lack of symptoms of hypoglycemia. This occurs in some patients who have had diabetes for many years. It may be related to autonomic neuropathy, which is a chronic diabetic complication (see later discussion). As the blood glucose level falls, the normal surge in adrenalin does not occur, and the usual adrenergic symptoms, such as sweating and shakiness, do not take place. The hypoglycemia may not be detected until moderate or severe CNS impairment occurs. Affected patients must perform SMBG on a frequent regular basis, especially before driving or engaging in other potentially dangerous activities.

Management

Treating With Carbohydrates

Immediate treatment must be given when hypoglycemia occurs (Seggelke & Everhart, 2013). The usual recommendation is for 15 g of a fast-acting concentrated source of carbohydrate (see Chart 51-8). It is not necessary to add sugar to juice, even if it is labeled as unsweetened juice, because the fruit sugar in juice contains enough carbohydrate to raise the blood glucose level. Adding table sugar to juice may cause a sharp increase in the blood glucose level, and patients may experience hyperglycemia for hours after treatment.

Initiating Emergency Measures

In emergency situations, for adults who are unconscious and cannot swallow, an injection of glucagon 1 mg can be given either subcutaneously or intramuscularly (Seggelke & Everhart, 2013). Glucagon is a hormone produced by the alpha cells of the pancreas that stimulates the liver to breakdown glycogen, the stored glucose. Injectable glucagon is packaged as a powder in 1-mg vials and must be mixed with a diluent immediately before being injected. After injection of glucagon, the patient may take as long as 20 minutes to regain consciousness. A concentrated source of carbohydrate followed by a snack should be given to the patient on awakening to prevent recurrence of hypoglycemia (because the duration of the action of 1 mg of glucagon is brief—its onset is 8 to 10 minutes, and its action lasts 12 to 27 minutes) and to replenish liver stores of glucose. Some patients experience nausea after the administration of glucagon. If this occurs, the patient should be turned to the side to prevent aspiration in case the patient vomits.

Glucagon is sold by prescription only and should be part of the emergency supplies available to patients with diabetes who require insulin. Family members, friends, neighbors, and coworkers should be instructed in the use of glucagon, especially for patients who have little or no warning of hypoglycemic episodes. Patients should be instructed to notify their primary provider after severe hypoglycemia has occurred and been treated. Close monitoring for 24 hours following a hypoglycemic episode is indicated because the patient is at increased risk of another episode (Seggelke & Everhart, 2013).

In hospitals and emergency departments, for patients who are unconscious or cannot swallow, 25 to 50 mL of dextrose 50% in water ($D_{50}W$) may be administered IV. The effect is usually seen within minutes. The patient may complain of a headache and of pain at the injection site. Ensuring patency of the IV line used for injection of 50% dextrose is essential because hypertonic solutions such as 50% dextrose are very irritating to veins.

 Providing Patient Education

Hypoglycemia is prevented by a consistent pattern of eating, administering insulin, and exercising. Between-meal and bedtime snacks may be needed to counteract the maximum insulin effect. In general, the patient should cover the time of peak activity of insulin by eating a snack and by taking additional food when physical activity is increased. Routine blood glucose tests are performed so that changing insulin requirements may be anticipated and the dosage adjusted. Because unexpected hypoglycemia can occur, all patients treated with insulin should wear an identification bracelet or tag stating that they have diabetes.

Patients, family members, and coworkers must be instructed to recognize the symptoms of hypoglycemia. Family members in particular must be made aware that any subtle (but unusual) change in behavior may be an indication of hypoglycemia. They should be taught to encourage and even insist that the person with diabetes assess blood glucose levels if hypoglycemia is suspected. Some patients become very resistant to testing or eating and become angry with family members who are trying to treat the hypoglycemia. Family members must be taught to persevere and to understand that the hypoglycemia can cause irrational behavior, due to low supply of glucose to the brain.

Autonomic neuropathy or beta-blockers such as propranolol (Inderal) to treat hypertension or cardiac dysrhythmias may mask the typical symptoms of hypoglycemia. It is very important that patients taking these medications perform blood glucose tests on a frequent and regular basis. Patients who have type 2 diabetes and who take oral sulfonylurea agents may also develop hypoglycemia, which can be prolonged and severe; this is a particular risk for older adult patients.

It is important that patients with diabetes, especially those receiving insulin, learn to carry some form of simple sugar with them at all times (ADA, 2016e). There are commercially prepared glucose tablets and gels that the patient may find convenient to carry. If the patient has a hypoglycemic reaction and does not have any of the recommended emergency foods available, he or she should eat any available food (preferably a carbohydrate food).

Patients are advised to refrain from eating high-calorie, high-fat dessert foods (e.g., cookies, cakes, doughnuts, ice cream) to treat hypoglycemia because their high fat content may slow the absorption of the glucose and resolution of the hypoglycemic symptoms. The patient may subsequently eat more of the foods when symptoms do not resolve rapidly, which may cause very high blood glucose levels for several hours and may contribute to weight gain.

Patients who feel unduly restricted by their meal plan may view hypoglycemic episodes as a time to reward themselves with desserts. Instructing these patients to incorporate occasional desserts into the meal plan may be more effective, because this may make it easier for them to limit their treatment of hypoglycemic episodes to simple (low-calorie)

carbohydrates such as juice or glucose tablets. Patients should be instructed to report all severe hypoglycemic episodes in addition to any increase in the incidence, frequency, and severity to the primary provider.

Diabetic Ketoacidosis

DKA is caused by an absence or markedly inadequate amount of insulin. This deficit in available insulin results in disorders in the metabolism of carbohydrate, protein, and fat. The three main clinical features of DKA are as follows:
- Hyperglycemia
- Dehydration and electrolyte loss
- Acidosis

Pathophysiology

Without insulin, the amount of glucose entering the cells is reduced, and the production and release of glucose by the liver (gluconeogenesis) are increased, leading to hyperglycemia (see Fig. 51-7). In an attempt to rid the body of the excess glucose, the kidneys excrete the glucose along with water and electrolytes (e.g., sodium, potassium). This osmotic diuresis, which is characterized by excessive urination (polyuria), leads to dehydration and marked electrolyte loss (Grossman & Porth, 2014). Patients with severe DKA may lose up to 6.5 L of water and up to 400 to 500 mEq each of sodium, potassium, and chloride over a 24-hour period.

Another effect of insulin deficiency or deficit is the breakdown of fat (lipolysis) into free fatty acids and glycerol. The free fatty acids are converted into ketone bodies by the liver. Ketone bodies are acids; their accumulation in the circulation due to lack of insulin leads to metabolic acidosis.

Three main causes of DKA are decreased or missed dose of insulin, illness or infection, and undiagnosed and untreated

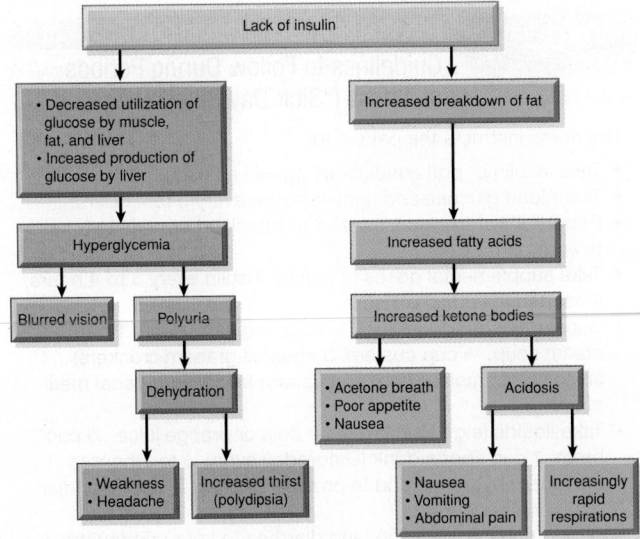

Figure 51-7 • Abnormal metabolism that causes signs and symptoms of diabetic ketoacidosis. Redrawn from Pearce, M. A., Rosenberg, C. S., & Davidson, M. D. (2003). Patient education. In Davidson, M. B. (Ed.). *Diabetes mellitus: Diagnosis and treatment.* New York: Churchill Livingstone.

diabetes (DKA may be the initial manifestation of type 1 diabetes). An insulin deficiency may result from an insufficient dosage of insulin prescribed or from insufficient insulin being given by the patient. Errors in insulin dosage may be made by patients who are ill and who assume that if they are eating less or if they are vomiting, they must decrease their insulin doses. (Because illness, especially infections, can cause increased blood glucose levels, the patient does not need to decrease the insulin dose to compensate for decreased food intake when ill and may even need to increase the insulin dose.)

Other potential causes of decreased insulin include patient error in drawing up or injecting insulin (especially in patients with visual impairments), intentional skipping of insulin doses (especially in adolescents with diabetes who are having difficulty coping with diabetes or other aspects of their lives), or equipment problems (e.g., occlusion of insulin pump tubing). Illness and infections are associated with insulin resistance. In response to physical (and emotional) stressors, there is an increase in the level of "stress" hormones—glucagon, epinephrine, norepinephrine, cortisol, and growth hormone. These hormones promote glucose production by the liver and interfere with glucose utilization by muscle and fat tissue, counteracting the effect of insulin. If insulin levels are not increased during times of illness and infection, hyperglycemia may progress to DKA (ADA, 2016e).

Prevention

For prevention of DKA related to illness, "sick day rules" for managing diabetes when ill (see Chart 51-9) should be reviewed with patients. The most important concept in this is to never eliminate insulin doses when nausea and vomiting occur. Instead, the patient should take the usual insulin dose (or previously prescribed special sick day doses) and then attempt to consume frequent small portions of carbohydrates

---

Chart 51-9

PATIENT EDUCATION

Guidelines to Follow During Periods of Illness ("Sick Day Rules")

The nurse instructs the patient to:

- Take insulin or oral antidiabetic agents as usual.
- Test blood glucose and urine ketones every 3 to 4 hours.
- Report elevated glucose levels as specified or urine ketones to your primary provider.
- Take supplemental doses of regular insulin every 3 to 4 hours, if needed, if you take insulin.
- Substitute soft foods (e.g., 1/3 cup regular gelatin, 1 cup cream soup, ½ cup custard, 3 squares graham crackers) six to eight times a day if you cannot follow your usual meal plan.
- Take liquids (e.g., ½ cup regular cola or orange juice, ½ cup broth, 1 cup sports drink [Gatorade]) every ½ to 1 hour to prevent dehydration and to provide calories, if vomiting, diarrhea, or fever persists.
- Report nausea, vomiting, and diarrhea to your primary provider, because extreme fluid loss may be dangerous.
- Be aware that if you are unable to retain oral fluids, you may require hospitalization to avoid diabetic ketoacidosis and possibly coma.

(including foods usually avoided, such as juices, regular sodas, and gelatin). Drinking fluids every hour is important to prevent dehydration. Blood glucose and urine ketones must be assessed every 3 to 4 hours.

If the patient cannot take fluids without vomiting, or if elevated glucose or ketone levels persist, the provider must be contacted. Patients are taught to have foods available for use on sick days. In addition, a supply of urine test strips (for ketone testing) and blood glucose test strips should be available. The patient must know how to contact their primary provider 24 hours a day. These materials should be assembled in a "sick day" kit.

After the acute phase of DKA has resolved, the nurse should assess for underlying causes. If there are psychological reasons for the patient missing insulin doses, the patient and family may be referred for evaluation and counseling or therapy.

Clinical Manifestations

The hyperglycemia of DKA leads to polyuria, polydipsia (increased thirst), and marked fatigue. In addition, the patient may experience blurred vision, weakness, and headache. Patients with marked intravascular volume depletion may have orthostatic hypotension (drop in systolic blood pressure of 20 mm Hg or more on changing from a reclining to a standing position). Volume depletion may also lead to frank hypotension with a weak, rapid pulse.

The ketosis and acidosis of DKA lead to gastrointestinal symptoms, such as anorexia, nausea, vomiting, and abdominal pain. The patient may have acetone breath (a fruity odor), which occurs with elevated ketone levels. In addition, hyperventilation (with very deep, but not labored, respirations) may occur. These Kussmaul respirations represent the body's attempt to decrease the acidosis, counteracting the effect of the ketone buildup (Grossman & Porth, 2014). In addition, mental status in DKA varies widely. The patient may be alert, lethargic, or comatose.

Assessment and Diagnostic Findings

Blood glucose levels may vary between 300 and 800 mg/dL (16.6 and 44.4 mmol/L). Some patients have lower glucose values, and others have values of 1000 mg/dL (55.5 mmol/L) or higher (usually depending on the degree of dehydration). The severity of DKA is not necessarily related to the blood glucose level. Evidence of ketoacidosis is reflected in low serum bicarbonate (0 to 15 mEq/L) and low pH (6.8 to 7.3) values. A low partial pressure of carbon dioxide (PCO_2 10 to 30 mm Hg) reflects respiratory compensation (Kussmaul respirations) for the metabolic acidosis. Accumulation of ketone bodies (which precipitates the acidosis) is reflected in blood and urine ketone measurements.

Sodium and potassium concentrations may be low, normal, or high, depending on the amount of water loss (dehydration). Despite the plasma concentration, there has been a marked total body depletion of these (and other) electrolytes, and they will need to be replaced.

Increased levels of creatinine, blood urea nitrogen (BUN), and hematocrit may also be seen with dehydration. After rehydration, continued elevation in the serum creatinine and BUN levels suggests underlying renal insufficiency.

Management

In addition to treating hyperglycemia, management of DKA is aimed at correcting dehydration, electrolyte loss, and acidosis before correcting the hyperglycemia with insulin.

Rehydration

In dehydrated patients, rehydration is important for maintaining tissue perfusion. In addition, fluid replacement enhances the excretion of excessive glucose by the kidneys. The patient may need as much as 6 to 10 L of IV fluid to replace fluid losses caused by polyuria, hyperventilation, diarrhea, and vomiting.

Initially, 0.9% sodium chloride (normal saline [NS]) solution is given at a rapid rate, usually 0.5 to 1 L per hour for 2 to 3 hours. Half-strength NS (0.45%) solution (also known as hypotonic saline solution) may be used for patients with hypertension or hypernatremia and those at risk for heart failure. After the first few hours, half-strength NS solution is the fluid of choice for continued rehydration, provided the blood pressure is stable and the sodium level is not low. Moderate to high rates of infusion (200 to 500 mL per hour) may be needed for several more hours. When the blood glucose level reaches 300 mg/dL (16.6 mmol/L) or less, the IV solution may be changed to dextrose 5% in water (D$_5$W) to prevent a precipitous decline in the blood glucose level (Umpeirrez & Korytkowski, 2016).

Monitoring of fluid volume status involves frequent measurements of vital signs (including monitoring for orthostatic changes in blood pressure and heart rate), lung assessment, and monitoring of intake and output. Initial urine output lags behind IV fluid intake as dehydration is corrected. Plasma expanders may be necessary to correct severe hypotension that does not respond to IV fluid treatment. Monitoring for signs of fluid overload is especially important for patients who are older, have renal impairment, or are at risk for heart failure.

Restoring Electrolytes

The major electrolyte of concern during treatment of DKA is potassium. The initial plasma concentration of potassium may be low, normal, or high, but more often than not, tends to be high (hyperkalemia) from disruption of the cellular sodium-potassium pump (in the face of acidosis). Therefore, the serum potassium level must be monitored frequently. Some of the factors related to treating DKA that affect potassium concentration include rehydration, which leads to increased plasma volume and subsequent decreases in the concentration of serum potassium. Rehydration also leads to increased urinary excretion of potassium. Insulin administration enhances the movement of potassium from the extracellular fluid into the cells.

Cautious but timely potassium replacement is vital to avoid dysrhythmias that may occur with hypokalemia. As much as 40 mEq per hour may be needed for several hours. Because extracellular potassium levels decrease during DKA treatment, potassium must be infused even if the plasma potassium level is normal.

Frequent (every 2 to 4 hours initially) ECGs and laboratory measurements of potassium are necessary during the first 8 hours of treatment. Potassium replacement is withheld only if hyperkalemia is present or if the patient is not urinating.

> **Quality and Safety Nursing Alert**
>
> *Because a patient's serum potassium level may drop quickly as a result of rehydration and insulin treatment, potassium replacement must begin once potassium levels drop to normal in the patient with DKA.*

Reversing Acidosis

Ketone bodies (acids) accumulate as a result of fat breakdown. The acidosis that occurs in DKA is reversed with insulin, which inhibits fat breakdown, thereby ending ketone production and acid buildup. Insulin is usually infused IV at a slow, continuous rate (e.g., 5 units per hour). Hourly blood glucose values must be measured. IV fluid solutions with higher concentrations of glucose, such as NS solution (e.g., D$_5$NS, D$_5$.45NS), are given when blood glucose levels reach 250 to 300 mg/dL (13.8 to 16.6 mmol/L) to avoid too rapid a drop in the blood glucose level (i.e., hypoglycemia) during treatment.

Regular insulin, the only type of insulin approved for IV use, may be added to IV solutions. The nurse must convert hourly rates of insulin infusion (frequently prescribed as units per hour) to IV drip rates. For example, if 100 units of regular insulin are mixed into 500 mL of 0.9% NS, then 1 unit of insulin equals 5 mL; therefore, an initial insulin infusion rate of 5 units per hour would equal 25 mL per hour. The insulin is often infused separately from the rehydration solutions to allow frequent changes in the rate and content of the latter.

Insulin must be infused continuously until subcutaneous administration of insulin can be resumed. Any interruption in administration may result in the reaccumulation of ketone bodies and worsening acidosis. Even if blood glucose levels are decreasing and returning to normal, the insulin drip must not be stopped until subcutaneous insulin therapy has been started. Rather, the rate or concentration of the dextrose infusion may be increased to prevent hypoglycemia. Blood glucose levels are usually corrected before the acidosis is corrected. Therefore, IV insulin may be continued for 12 to 24 hours, until the serum bicarbonate level increases (to at least 15 to 18 mEq/L) and until the patient can eat. In general, bicarbonate infusion to correct severe acidosis is avoided during treatment of DKA because it precipitates further, sudden (and potentially fatal) decreases in serum potassium levels. Continuous insulin infusion is usually sufficient for reversal of DKA (Noble-Bell & Cox, 2014; Umpeirrez & Korytkowski, 2016).

> **Quality and Safety Nursing Alert**
>
> *When hanging the insulin drip, the nurse must flush the insulin solution through the entire IV infusion set and discard the first 50 mL of fluid. Insulin molecules adhere to the inner surface of plastic IV infusion sets; therefore, the initial fluid may contain a decreased concentration of insulin.*

Hyperglycemic Hyperosmolar Syndrome

HHS is a metabolic disorder of type 2 diabetes resulting from a relative insulin deficiency initiated by an illness that raises the demand for insulin. This is a serious condition in which

TABLE 51-7 Comparison of Diabetic Ketoacidosis and Hyperglycemic Hyperosmolar Syndrome

Characteristics	DKA	HHS
Patients most commonly affected	Can occur in type 1 or type 2 diabetes; more common in type 1 diabetes	Can occur in type 1 or type 2 diabetes; more common in type 2 diabetes, especially older patients with type 2 diabetes
Precipitating event	Omission of insulin; physiologic stress (infection, surgery, stroke, MI)	Physiologic stress (infection, surgery, stroke, MI)
Onset	Rapid (<24 hours)	Slower (over several days)
Blood glucose levels	Usually >250 mg/dL (>13.9 mmol/L)	Usually >600 mg/dL (>33.3 mmol/L)
Arterial pH level	<7.3	Normal
Serum and urine ketones	Present	Absent
Serum osmolality	300–350 mOsm/L	>350 mOsm/L
Plasma bicarbonate level	<15 mEq/L	Normal
BUN and creatinine levels	Elevated	Elevated
Mortality rate	1%–5%	10%–20%

DKA, diabetic ketoacidosis; HHS, hyperglycemic hyperosmolar syndrome; MI, myocardial infarction; BUN, blood urea nitrogen.
Adapted from Umpeirrez, G., & Korytkowski, M. (2016). Diabetic emergencies—ketoacidosis, hyperglycaemic hyperosmolar state and hyperglycemia. *Nature Reviews. Endocrinology, 12,* 222–232.

hyperosmolarity and hyperglycemia predominate, with alterations of the sensorium (sense of awareness). At the same time, ketosis is usually minimal or absent. The basic biochemical defect is the lack of effective insulin (i.e., insulin resistance). Persistent hyperglycemia causes osmotic diuresis, which results in losses of water and electrolytes. To maintain osmotic equilibrium, water shifts from the intracellular fluid space to the extracellular fluid space. With glycosuria and dehydration, hypernatremia and increased osmolarity occur. Table 51-7 compares DKA and HHS.

HHS occurs most often in older adults (50 to 70 years of age) who have no known history of diabetes or who have type 2 diabetes (Umpeirrez & Korytkowski, 2016). HHS often can be traced to an infection or a precipitating event such as an acute illness (e.g., stroke), medications that exacerbate hyperglycemia (e.g., thiazides), or treatments such as dialysis. The history includes days to weeks of polyuria with adequate fluid intake. What distinguishes HHS from DKA is that ketosis and acidosis generally do not occur in HHS, partly because of differences in insulin levels. In DKA, no insulin is present, and this promotes the breakdown of stored glucose, protein, and fat, which leads to the production of ketone bodies and ketoacidosis. In HHS, the insulin level is too low to prevent hyperglycemia (and subsequent osmotic diuresis), but it is high enough to prevent fat breakdown. Patients with HHS do not have the ketosis-related gastrointestinal symptoms that lead them to seek medical attention. Instead, they may tolerate polyuria and polydipsia until neurologic changes or an underlying illness (or family members or others) prompts them to seek treatment.

Clinical Manifestations

The clinical picture of HHS is one of hypotension, profound dehydration (dry mucous membranes, poor skin turgor), tachycardia, and variable neurologic signs (e.g., alteration of consciousness, seizures, hemiparesis) (see Table 51-7).

Assessment and Diagnostic Findings

Diagnostic assessment includes a range of laboratory tests, including blood glucose, electrolytes, BUN, complete blood count, serum osmolality, and arterial blood gas analysis. The blood glucose level is usually 600 to 1200 mg/dL, and the osmolality exceeds 320 mOsm/kg (Umpeirrez & Korytkowski, 2016). Electrolyte and BUN levels are consistent with the clinical picture of severe dehydration (see Chapter 14). Mental status changes, focal neurologic deficits, and hallucinations are common secondary to the cerebral dehydration that results from extreme hyperosmolality. Postural hypotension accompanies the dehydration.

Management

The overall approach to the treatment of HHS is similar to that of DKA: fluid replacement, correction of electrolyte imbalances, and insulin administration. Because patients with HHS are typically older, close monitoring of volume and electrolyte status is important for prevention of fluid overload, heart failure, and cardiac dysrhythmias. Fluid treatment is started with 0.9% or 0.45% NS, depending on the patient's sodium level and the severity of volume depletion. Central venous or hemodynamic pressure monitoring guides fluid replacement. Potassium is added to IV fluids when urinary output is adequate and is guided by continuous ECG monitoring and frequent laboratory determinations of potassium (Noble-Bell & Cox, 2014; Umpeirrez & Korytkowski, 2016).

Extremely elevated blood glucose concentrations decrease as the patient is rehydrated. Insulin plays a less important role in the treatment of HHS because it is not needed for reversal of acidosis, as in DKA. Nevertheless, insulin is usually given at a continuous low rate to treat hyperglycemia, and replacement IV fluids with dextrose are given (as in DKA) after the glucose level has decreased to the range of 250 to 300 mg/dL (13.8 to 16.6 mmol/L) (Noble-Bell & Cox, 2014; Umpeirrez & Korytkowski, 2016).

Other therapeutic modalities are determined by the underlying illness and the results of continuing clinical and laboratory evaluation. It may take 3 to 5 days for neurologic symptoms to clear, and treatment of HHS usually continues well after metabolic abnormalities have resolved. After recovery from HHS, many patients can control their diabetes with MNT alone or with MNT and oral antidiabetic medications. Insulin may not be needed once the acute hyperglycemic complication is resolved. Frequent SBGM is important in prevention of recurrence of HHS.

NURSING PROCESS

The Patient With Diabetic Ketoacidosis or Hyperglycemic Hyperosmolar Syndrome

Assessment

For the patient with DKA, the nurse monitors the ECG for dysrhythmias indicating abnormal potassium levels. Vital signs (especially blood pressure and pulse), arterial blood gases, breath sounds, and mental status are assessed every hour and recorded on a flow sheet. Neurologic status checks are included as part of the hourly assessment because cerebral edema can be a severe and sometimes fatal outcome. Blood glucoses are checked every hour (Noble-Bell & Cox, 2014; Umpeirrez & Korytkowski, 2016).

For the patient with HHS, the nurse assesses vital signs, fluid status, and laboratory values. Fluid status and urine output are closely monitored because of the high risk of kidney failure secondary to severe dehydration. Because HHS tends to occur in older patients, the physiologic changes that occur with aging should be considered. Careful assessment of cardiovascular, pulmonary, and kidney function throughout the acute and recovery phases of HHS is important (Noble-Bell & Cox, 2014; Umpeirrez & Korytkowski, 2016).

Diagnosis

NURSING DIAGNOSES

Based on the assessment data, major nursing diagnoses may include the following:

- Risk for deficient fluid volume related to polyuria and dehydration
- Risk for electrolyte imbalance related to fluid loss or shifts
- Deficient knowledge about diabetes self-care skills or information
- Anxiety related to loss of control, fear of inability to manage diabetes, misinformation related to diabetes, fear of diabetes complications

COLLABORATIVE PROBLEMS/POTENTIAL COMPLICATIONS

Potential complications may include the following:

- Fluid overload, pulmonary edema, and heart failure
- Hypokalemia
- Hyperglycemia and ketoacidosis

- Hypoglycemia
- Cerebral edema

Planning and Goals

The major goals for the patient may include maintenance of fluid and electrolyte balance, increased knowledge about diabetes basic skills and self-care, decreased anxiety, and absence of complications.

Nursing Interventions

MAINTAINING FLUID AND ELECTROLYTE BALANCE

Intake and output are measured. IV fluids and electrolytes are given as prescribed, and oral fluid intake is encouraged when it is permitted. Laboratory values of serum electrolytes (especially sodium and potassium) are monitored. Vital signs are monitored hourly for signs of dehydration (tachycardia, orthostatic hypotension) along with assessment of breath sounds, level of consciousness, presence of edema, and cardiac status (ECG rhythm strips).

INCREASING KNOWLEDGE ABOUT DIABETES MANAGEMENT

The development of DKA or HHS suggests the need for the nurse to carefully assess the patient's understanding of and adherence to the diabetes management plan. Furthermore, factors that may have led to the development of DKA or HHS are explored with the patient and family. If the patient's blood glucose monitoring, dietary intake, use of antidiabetes (insulin or oral agents) medications, and exercise patterns differ from those identified in the diabetes management plan, their relationship to the development of DKA or HHS is discussed, along with early manifestations of DKA or HHS. If other factors, such as trauma, illness, surgery, or stress, are implicated, appropriate strategies to respond to these and similar situations in the future are described so that the patient can respond in the future without developing life-threatening complications. The nurse may need to provide education about basic skills again to patients who may not be able to recall the instructions. If the patient has omitted insulin or oral antidiabetes agents that have been prescribed, the nurse explores the reasons for doing so and addresses those issues to prevent future recurrence and readmissions for treatment of these complications.

If the patient has not previously been diagnosed with diabetes, the opportunity is used to educate the patient about the need for maintaining blood glucose at a normal level and learning about diabetes management and basic skills.

DECREASING ANXIETY

Educating the patient about cognitive strategies may be useful for relieving tension, overcoming anxiety, decreasing fear, and achieving relaxation (see Chapter 4). Examples include:

- *Imagery:* The patient concentrates on a pleasant experience or restful scene.
- *Distraction:* The patient thinks of an enjoyable story or recites a favorite poem or song.
- *Optimistic self-recitation:* The patient recites optimistic thoughts ("I know all will go well").
- *Music:* The patient listens to soothing music (an easy-to-administer, inexpensive, noninvasive intervention).

MONITORING AND MANAGING POTENTIAL COMPLICATIONS

Fluid Overload. Fluid overload can occur because of the administration of a large volume of fluid at a rapid rate, which is often required to treat patients with DKA or HHS. This risk is increased in older patients and in those with preexisting cardiac or kidney disease. To avoid fluid overload and resulting heart failure and pulmonary edema, the nurse monitors the patient closely during treatment by measuring vital signs and intake and output at frequent intervals. Central venous pressure monitoring and hemodynamic monitoring may be initiated to provide additional measures of fluid status. Physical examination focuses on assessment of cardiac rate and rhythm, breath sounds, venous distention, skin turgor, and urine output. The nurse monitors fluid intake and keeps careful records of IV and other fluid intake, along with urine output measurements.

Hypokalemia. Hypokalemia is a potential complication during the treatment of DKA. Low serum potassium levels may result from rehydration, increased urinary excretion of potassium, movement of potassium from the extracellular fluid into the cells with insulin administration, and restoration of the cellular sodium–potassium pump. Prevention of hypokalemia includes cautious replacement of potassium; however, before its administration, it is important to ensure that a patient's kidneys are functioning. Because of the adverse effects of hypokalemia on cardiac function, monitoring of the cardiac rate, cardiac rhythm, ECG, and serum potassium levels is essential.

Cerebral Edema. Although the exact cause of cerebral edema is unknown, rapid correction of hyperglycemia, resulting in fluid shifts, is thought to be the cause. Cerebral edema, which occurs more often in children than in adults, can be prevented by a gradual reduction in the blood glucose level. An hourly flow sheet is used to enable close monitoring of the blood glucose level, serum electrolyte levels, fluid intake, urine output, mental status, and neurologic signs. Precautions are taken to minimize activities that could increase intracranial pressure.

EDUCATING PATIENTS ABOUT SELF-CARE

The patient is educated about basic skills, including treatment modalities (diet, insulin administration, monitoring of blood glucose, and, for type 1 diabetes, monitoring of urine ketones); the patient is also educated about recognition, treatment, and prevention of DKA and HHS (Noble-Bell & Cox, 2014). Education addresses those factors leading to DKA or HHS. Follow-up education is arranged with a home care nurse and dietitian or an outpatient diabetes education center. This is particularly important for patients who have experienced DKA or HHS because of the need to address factors that led to its occurrence (i.e., dehydration). For patients who have had HHS, avoiding dehydration and paying attention to increased urination or thirst are even more important than insulin administration. The importance of self-monitoring and of monitoring and follow-up by primary providers is reinforced, and the patient is reminded about the importance of keeping follow-up appointments.

Evaluation

Expected patient outcomes may include:

1. Achieves fluid and electrolyte balance
   a. Demonstrates intake and output balance
   b. Exhibits electrolyte values within normal limits
   c. Exhibits vital signs that remain stable, with resolution of orthostatic hypotension and tachycardia

2. Demonstrates knowledge about DKA and HHS
   a. Identifies factors leading to DKA and HHS
   b. Describes signs and symptoms of DKA and HHS
   c. Describes short- and long-term consequences of DKA and HHS
   d. Identifies strategies to prevent the development of DKA and HHS
   e. States when contact with primary provider is needed to treat early signs of DKA and HHS
3. Decreased anxiety
   a. Identifies strategies to decrease anxiety and fear
4. Absence of complications
   a. Exhibits normal cardiac rate and rhythm and normal breath sounds
   b. Exhibits no jugular venous distention
   c. Exhibits blood glucose and urine ketone levels within target range
   d. Exhibits no manifestations of hypoglycemia or hyperglycemia
   e. Shows improved mental status without signs of cerebral edema

LONG-TERM COMPLICATIONS OF DIABETES

The number of deaths attributable to ketoacidosis and infection in patients with diabetes has steadily declined, but diabetes related complications have increased. Long-term complications are becoming more common as more people live longer with diabetes; these complications can affect almost every organ system of the body and are a major cause of disability. The general categories of long-term diabetic complications are macrovascular disease, microvascular disease, and neuropathy.

The causes and pathogenesis of each type of complication are still being investigated. However, it appears that increased levels of blood glucose play a role in neuropathic disease, microvascular complications, and risk factors contributing to macrovascular complications. Hypertension may also be a major contributing factor, especially in macrovascular and microvascular diseases (ADA, 2016b).

Long-term complications are seen in both type 1 and type 2 diabetes but usually do not occur within the first 5 to 10 years after diagnosis. However, evidence of these complications may be present at the time of diagnosis of type 2 diabetes, because patients may have had undiagnosed diabetes for many years. Kidney (microvascular) disease is more prevalent in patients with type 1 diabetes, and cardiovascular (macrovascular) complications are more prevalent in older patients with type 2 diabetes.

Macrovascular Complications

Diabetic macrovascular complications result from changes in the medium to large blood vessels. Blood vessel walls thicken, sclerose, and become occluded by plaque that adheres to the vessel walls. Eventually, blood flow is blocked. These atherosclerotic changes tend to occur more often and at an earlier age in patients with diabetes. Coronary artery disease, cerebrovascular disease, and peripheral vascular disease are the three main types of macrovascular complications that occur frequently in patients with diabetes.

MI is twice as common in men with diabetes and three times as common in women with diabetes, compared with people without diabetes. There is also an increased risk of complications resulting from MI and an increased likelihood of a second MI. Coronary artery disease accounts for an increased incidence of death among patients with diabetes. The typical ischemic symptoms may be absent in patients with diabetes. Therefore, the patient may not experience the early warning signs of decreased coronary blood flow and may have "silent" MIs, which may be discovered only as changes on the ECG. In some cases, ECG changes may not be apparent. This lack of ischemic symptoms may be secondary to autonomic neuropathy (see later discussion). See Chapter 27 for a detailed discussion of coronary vascular disorders.

Cerebral blood vessels are similarly affected by accelerated atherosclerosis. Occlusive changes or the formation of an embolus elsewhere in the vasculature that lodges in a cerebral blood vessel can lead to transient ischemic attacks and strokes. People with diabetes have twice the risk of developing cerebrovascular disease and an increased risk of death from stroke (Bader, Littlejohns, & Olson, 2016). In addition, recovery from a stroke may be impaired in patients who have elevated blood glucose levels at the time of and immediately after a stroke. Because symptoms of a stroke may be similar to symptoms of acute diabetic complications (HHS or hypoglycemia), it is very important to assess the blood glucose level (and treat abnormal levels) rapidly in patients with these symptoms so that testing and treatment of a stroke can be initiated promptly if indicated.

Atherosclerotic changes in the large blood vessels of the lower extremities are responsible for the increased incidence (two to three times higher than in nondiabetic people) of occlusive peripheral arterial disease in patients with diabetes (ADA, 2016b). Signs and symptoms of peripheral vascular disease include diminished peripheral pulses and intermittent claudication (pain in the buttock, thigh, or calf during walking). The severe form of arterial occlusive disease in the lower extremities is largely responsible for the increased incidence of gangrene and subsequent amputation in patients with diabetes. Neuropathy and impairments in wound healing also play a role in diabetic foot disease (see later discussion).

Role of Diabetes in Macrovascular Diseases

Researchers continue to investigate the relationship between diabetes and macrovascular diseases. The main feature unique to diabetes is elevated blood glucose; however, a direct link has not been found between hyperglycemia and atherosclerosis. Although it may be tempting to attribute the increased prevalence of macrovascular diseases to the increased prevalence of certain risk factors (e.g., obesity, increased triglyceride levels, hypertension) in patients with diabetes, there is a higher-than-expected rate of macrovascular diseases among patients with diabetes compared with patients without diabetes who have the same risk factors (ADA, 2016d). Therefore, diabetes itself is seen as an independent risk factor for accelerated atherosclerosis. Other potential factors that may play a role in diabetes-related atherosclerosis include platelet

and clotting factor abnormalities, decreased flexibility of red blood cells, decreased oxygen release, changes in the arterial wall related to hyperglycemia, and possibly hyperinsulinemia.

Management

The focus of management is an aggressive modification and reduction of risk factors. This involves prevention and treatment of the commonly accepted risk factors for atherosclerosis. MNT and exercise are important in managing obesity, hypertension, and hyperlipidemia. In addition, the use of medications to control hypertension and hyperlipidemia is indicated. Smoking cessation is essential. Control of blood glucose levels may reduce triglyceride concentrations and can significantly reduce the incidence of complications (ADA, 2016d; Evert et al., 2013).

Microvascular Complications

Diabetic microvascular disease (or microangiopathy) is characterized by capillary basement membrane thickening. The basement membrane surrounds the endothelial cells of the capillary. Researchers believe that increased blood glucose levels react through a series of biochemical responses to thicken the basement membrane to several times its normal thickness. Two areas affected by these changes are the retina and the kidneys (Grossman & Porth, 2014).

Diabetic Retinopathy

Diabetic retinopathy is the leading cause of blindness among people between 20 and 74 years of age in the United States; it occurs in both type 1 and type 2 diabetes (ADA, 2016b).

People with diabetes are subject to many visual complications (see Table 51-8). The pathology referred to as diabetic retinopathy is caused by changes in the small blood vessels in the retina, which is the area of the eye that receives images and sends information about the images to the brain (see Fig. 51-8). The retina is richly supplied with blood vessels of all kinds: small arteries and veins, arterioles, venules, and capillaries. Retinopathy has three main stages: nonproliferative (background), preproliferative, and proliferative.

Almost all patients with type 1 diabetes and the majority of patients with type 2 diabetes have some degree of retinopathy after 20 years (ADA, 2016b). Changes in the microvasculature include microaneurysms, intraretinal hemorrhage, hard exudates, and focal capillary closure. Although most patients do not develop visual impairment, it can be devastating if it occurs. A complication of nonproliferative retinopathy—macular edema—occurs in approximately 10% of people with type 1 or type 2 diabetes and may lead to visual distortion and loss of central vision (ADA, 2016b).

An advanced form of background retinopathy—preproliferative retinopathy—is considered to be a precursor to the more serious proliferative retinopathy. In preproliferative retinopathy, there are more widespread vascular changes and loss of nerve fibers. Epidemiologic evidence suggests that 10% to 50% of patients with preproliferative retinopathy will develop proliferative retinopathy within a short time (possibly as little as 1 year). As with background retinopathy, if visual changes occur during the preproliferative stage, they are usually caused by macular edema.

TABLE 51-8 Ocular Complications of Diabetes

Eye Disorder	Characteristics
Retinopathy	Damage to the small blood vessels that nourish the retina.
Background	Early-stage, asymptomatic retinopathy. Blood vessels within the retina develop microaneurysms that leak fluid, causing swelling and forming deposits (exudates). In some cases, macular edema causes distorted vision.
Preproliferative	Represents increased destruction of retinal blood vessels.
Proliferative	Abnormal growth of new blood vessels on the retina. New vessels rupture, bleeding into the vitreous and blocking light. Ruptured blood vessels in the vitreous form scar tissue, which can pull on and detach the retina.
Cataracts	Opacity of the lens of the eye; cataracts occur at an earlier age in patients with diabetes.
Lens Changes	The lens of the eye can swell when blood glucose levels are elevated. For some patients, visual changes related to lens swelling may be the first symptoms of diabetes. It may take up to 2 months of improved blood glucose control before hyperglycemic swelling subsides and vision stabilizes. Therefore, patients are advised not to change eyeglass prescriptions during the 2 months after discovery of hyperglycemia.
Extraocular Muscle Palsy	This may occur as a result of diabetic neuropathy. The involvement of various cranial nerves responsible for ocular movements may lead to double vision. This usually resolves spontaneously.
Glaucoma	Results from occlusion of the outflow channels by new blood vessels. Glaucoma may occur with slightly higher frequency in the diabetic population.

Proliferative retinopathy represents the greatest threat to vision and is characterized by the proliferation of new blood vessels growing from the retina into the vitreous. These new vessels are prone to bleeding. The visual loss associated with proliferative retinopathy is caused by this vitreous hemorrhage, retinal detachment, or both. The vitreous is normally clear, allowing light to be transmitted to the retina. When there is a hemorrhage, the vitreous becomes clouded and cannot transmit light, resulting in loss of vision. Another consequence of vitreous hemorrhage is that resorption of the blood in the vitreous leads to the formation of fibrous scar tissue. This scar tissue may place traction on the retina, resulting in retinal detachment and subsequent visual loss.

Clinical Manifestations

Retinopathy is a painless process. In nonproliferative and preproliferative retinopathy, blurry vision secondary to macular edema occurs in some patients, although many patients are asymptomatic. Even patients with a significant degree of proliferative retinopathy and some hemorrhaging may not experience major visual changes. However, symptoms indicative of hemorrhaging include floaters or cobwebs in the visual field, sudden visual changes including spotty or hazy vision, or complete loss of vision.

Assessment and Diagnostic Findings

Diagnosis is by direct visualization of the retina through dilated pupils with an ophthalmoscope or with a technique known as fluorescein angiography. Fluorescein angiography can document the type and activity of the retinopathy. Dye is injected into an arm vein and is carried to various parts of the body through the blood, but especially through the vessels of the retina of the eye. This technique allows an ophthalmologist, using special instruments, to see the retinal vessels in bright detail and gives useful information that cannot be obtained with just an ophthalmoscope.

Side effects of this diagnostic procedure may include nausea during the dye injection; yellowish, fluorescent discoloration of the skin and urine lasting 12 to 24 hours; and occasionally allergic reactions, usually manifested by hives or itching. However, the diagnostic procedure is generally safe.

Medical Management

The first focus of management of retinopathy is on primary and secondary prevention. The DCCT study (1993) demonstrated that in patients without preexisting retinopathy, maintenance of blood glucose to a normal or near-normal level in type 1 diabetes through intensive insulin therapy and patient education decreased the risk of retinopathy by 76%, compared with conventional therapy. The progression of retinopathy was decreased by 54% in patients with very mild to

Figure 51-8 • Diabetic retinopathy. **A.** In the fundus photograph of a normal eye, the light circular area over which a number of blood vessels converge is the optic disc, where the optic nerve meets the back of the eye. **B.** The fundus photograph of a patient with diabetic retinopathy shows characteristic waxy-looking retinal lesions, microaneurysms of the vessels, and hemorrhages. Courtesy of American Optometric Association.

moderate nonproliferative retinopathy at the time of initiation of treatment. Better control of blood glucose levels in patients with type 2 diabetes reduces the risk of retinopathy as well.

Other strategies that may slow the progression of diabetic retinopathy include control of hypertension, control of blood glucose, and cessation of smoking.

For advanced cases of diabetic retinopathy, the main treatment is argon laser photocoagulation. The laser treatment destroys leaking blood vessels and areas of neovascularization. For patients who are at increased risk for hemorrhage, panretinal photocoagulation may significantly reduce the rate of progression to blindness. Panretinal photocoagulation involves the systematic application of multiple (more than 1000) laser burns throughout the retina (except in the macular region). This stops the widespread growth of new vessels and hemorrhaging of damaged vessels. The role of "mild" panretinal photocoagulation (with only one third to one half as many laser burns) in the early stages of proliferative retinopathy or in patients with preproliferative changes is being investigated. For patients with macular edema, focal photocoagulation is used to apply smaller laser burns to specific areas of microaneurysms in the macular region. This may reduce the rate of visual loss from macular edema (ADA, 2016b).

Photocoagulation treatments are usually performed on an outpatient basis, and most patients can return to their usual activities by the next day. Limitations may be placed on activities involving weight bearing or bearing down. In most cases, the treatment does not cause intense pain, although patients may report varying degrees of discomfort such as a headache. Usually, an anesthetic eye drop is all that is needed during the treatment. A few patients may experience slight visual loss, loss of peripheral vision, or impairments in adaptation to the dark. However, the risk of slight visual changes from the laser treatment itself is much less than the potential for loss of vision from progression of retinopathy.

A major hemorrhage into the vitreous may occur, with the vitreous fluid becoming mixed with blood, preventing light from passing through the eye; this can cause blindness. A vitrectomy is a surgical procedure in which vitreous humor filled with blood or fibrous tissue is removed with a special drill-like instrument and replaced with saline or another liquid. A vitrectomy is performed for patients who already have visual loss and in whom the vitreous hemorrhage has not cleared on its own after 6 months. The purpose is to restore useful vision; recovery to near-normal vision is not usually expected.

Nursing Management

Nursing management of patients with diabetic retinopathy or other eye disorders involves implementing the individual plan of care and providing patient education. Education focuses on prevention through regular ophthalmologic examinations, blood glucose control, and self-management of eye care regimens. The effectiveness of early diagnosis and prompt treatment is emphasized in educating the patient and family.

If vision loss occurs, nursing care must also address the patient's adjustment to impaired vision and the use of adaptive devices for diabetes self-care as well as activities of daily living. See Chapter 63 for discussion of nursing care for patients with low vision and blindness.

Promoting Home, Community-Based, and Transitional Care

 Educating Patients About Self-Care

Because the course of the retinopathy may be long and stressful, patient education is essential. In educating and counseling patients, it is important to stress the following:

- Retinopathy may appear after many years of diabetes, and its appearance does not necessarily mean that the diabetes is on a downhill course.
- The odds for maintaining vision are in the patient's favor, especially with adequate control of glucose levels and blood pressure.
- Frequent eye examinations allow for the detection and prompt treatment of retinopathy.

A patient's response to vision loss depends on personality, self-concept, and coping mechanisms. Acceptance of blindness occurs in stages; some patients may learn to accept blindness in a rather short period, and others may never do so. An important issue in educating patients is that several complications of diabetes may occur simultaneously. For example, a patient who is blind due to diabetic retinopathy may also have peripheral neuropathy and may experience impairment of manual dexterity and tactile sensation, or kidney failure. This can be devastating to the patient and family. Psychological counseling may be warranted. To prevent further losses, glycemic control remains a priority.

Continuing and Transitional Care

The importance of careful diabetes management is emphasized as one means of slowing the progression of visual changes. The patient is reminded of the need to see an ophthalmologist regularly. If eye changes are progressive and unrelenting, the patient should be prepared for inevitable blindness. Therefore, consideration is given to making referrals for educating the patient in Braille and for training him or her with guide (i.e., service) dogs. Referral to state agencies should be made to ensure that the patient receives services for the blind. Family members are also taught how to assist the patient to remain as independent as possible despite decreasing visual acuity.

Referral for home care may be indicated for some patients, particularly those who live alone, those who are not coping well, and those who have other health problems or complications of diabetes that may interfere with their ability to perform self-care. During home visits, the nurse can assess the patient's home environment and their ability to manage diabetes despite visual impairments. See Chapter 63 for a detailed discussion of medical management and nursing care for patients with visual disturbances.

Nephropathy

Nephropathy, or kidney disease secondary to diabetic microvascular changes in the kidney, is a common complication of diabetes (ADA, 2016b). In the United States each year, people with diabetes account for almost 50% of new cases of ESKD, and about 25% of those require dialysis or transplantation. About 20% to 30% of people with type 1 or types 2 diabetes develop nephropathy, but fewer of those with type 2 diabetes progress to ESKD. Native American, Latino, African

American, Asian American, and Pacific Island people with type 2 diabetes are at greater risk for ESKD than non-Latino whites (ADA, 2016b).

Patients with type 1 diabetes frequently show initial signs of kidney disease after 10 to 15 years, while patients with type 2 diabetes tend to develop kidney disease within 10 years after the diagnosis of diabetes. Many patients with type 2 diabetes have had diabetes for many years before the diabetes is diagnosed and treated. Therefore, they may have evidence of nephropathy at the time of diagnosis (ADA, 2016b). If blood glucose levels are elevated consistently for a significant period of time, the kidney's filtration mechanism is stressed, allowing blood proteins to leak into the urine. As a result, the pressure in the blood vessels of the kidney increases. It is thought that this elevated pressure serves as the stimulus for the development of nephropathy. Various medications and diets are being tested to prevent these complications.

The DCCT (1993) results showed that intensive treatment for type 1 diabetes with a goal of achieving a glycolated hemoglobin level as close to the nondiabetic range as possible reduced the occurrence of early signs of nephropathy. Similarly, the United Kingdom Prospective Diabetes Study Group (UKPDS, 1998) demonstrated a reduced incidence of overt nephropathy in patients with type 2 diabetes who controlled their blood glucose levels.

Clinical Manifestations

Most of the signs and symptoms of kidney dysfunction in patients with diabetes are similar to those seen in patients without diabetes (see Chapter 54). In addition, as kidney failure progresses, the catabolism (breakdown) of both exogenous and endogenous insulin decreases, and frequent hypoglycemic episodes may result. Insulin needs change as a result of changes in the catabolism of insulin, changes in diet related to the treatment of nephropathy, and changes in insulin clearance that occur with decreased kidney function.

Assessment and Diagnostic Findings

Albumin is one of the most important blood proteins that leak into the urine. Although small amounts may leak undetected for years, its leakage into the urine is among the earliest signs that can be detected. Clinical nephropathy eventually develops in more than 85% of people with microalbuminuria but in fewer than 5% of people without microalbuminuria. The urine should be checked annually for the presence of microalbumin. If the microalbuminuria exceeds 30 mg/24 hours on two consecutive random urine tests, a 24-hour urine sample should be obtained and tested. If results are positive, treatment is indicated (see later discussion).

In addition, tests for serum creatinine and BUN levels should be conducted annually. Diagnostic testing for cardiac or other systemic disorders may also be required with progression of other complications, and caution is indicated if contrast agents are used with these tests. Contrast agents and dyes used for some diagnostic tests may not be easily cleared by the damaged kidney, and the potential benefits of these diagnostic tests must be weighed against their potential risks.

Hypertension often develops in patients (with and without diabetes) who are in the early stages of kidney disease. However, hypertension is the most common complication in all people with diabetes (ADA, 2016g). Therefore, this symptom may or may not be due to kidney disease; other diagnostic criteria must also be present.

Management

In addition to achieving and maintaining near-normal blood glucose levels, management for all patients with diabetes should include careful attention to the following:

- Control of hypertension (the use of angiotensin-converting enzyme [ACE] inhibitors, such as captopril [Capoten]), because control of hypertension may also decrease or delay the onset of early proteinuria
- Prevention or vigorous treatment of urinary tract infections
- Avoidance of nephrotoxic medications and contrast dye
- Adjustment of medications as kidney function changes
- Low-sodium diet
- Low-protein diet

If the patient has already developed microalbuminuria with levels that exceed 30 mg/24 hours on two consecutive tests, an ACE inhibitor should be prescribed. ACE inhibitors lower blood pressure and reduce microalbuminuria, thereby protecting the kidney. Alternatively, angiotensin receptor blocking agents may be prescribed. This preventive strategy should be part of the standard of care for all people with diabetes (ADA, 2016a). Carefully designed low-protein diets also appear to reverse early leakage of small amounts of protein from the kidney.

In chronic or ESKD, two types of treatment are available: dialysis (hemodialysis or peritoneal dialysis) and transplantation from a relative or a cadaver. Hemodialysis for patients with diabetes is similar to that for patients without the disease (see Chapter 54). Because hemodialysis creates additional stress on patients with cardiovascular disease, it may not be appropriate for some patients.

Continuous ambulatory peritoneal dialysis is being used by patients with diabetes, mainly because of the independence it allows. In addition, insulin can be mixed into the dialysate, which may result in better blood glucose control and end the need for insulin injections. In some cases, patients may require higher doses of insulin because the dialysate contains glucose. Major risks of peritoneal dialysis are infection and peritonitis. The mortality rate for patients with diabetes undergoing dialysis is higher than that for patients without diabetes undergoing dialysis and is closely related to the severity of cardiovascular problems.

Kidney disease is frequently accompanied by advancing retinopathy that may require laser treatments and surgery. Severe hypertension also worsens eye disease because of the additional stress it places on the blood vessels. Patients being treated with hemodialysis who require eye surgery may be changed to peritoneal dialysis and have their hypertension aggressively controlled for several weeks before surgery to prevent bleeding and damage to the retina. The rationale for this change is that hemodialysis requires anticoagulant agents that can increase the risk of bleeding after the surgery, and peritoneal dialysis minimizes pressure changes in the eyes.

In medical centers performing large numbers of transplantations, the chances are 75% to 80% that the transplanted kidney will continue to function in patients with diabetes for at least 5 years. Like the original kidneys, transplanted kidneys can eventually be damaged if blood glucose levels are consistently high after the transplantation. Therefore, monitoring blood glucose levels frequently and adjusting insulin levels in patients with diabetes are essential for long-term success of kidney transplantation.

Diabetic Neuropathies

Diabetic neuropathy refers to a group of diseases that affect all types of nerves, including peripheral (sensorimotor), autonomic, and spinal nerves. The disorders appear to be clinically diverse and depend on the location of the affected nerve cells. The prevalence increases with the age of the patient and the duration of the disease (NIDDK, 2013b).

The etiology of neuropathy may involve elevated blood glucose levels over a period of years. Control of blood glucose levels to normal or near-normal levels decreases the incidence of neuropathy. The pathogenesis of neuropathy may be attributed to either a vascular or metabolic mechanism or both. Capillary basement membrane thickening and capillary closure may be present. In addition, there may be demyelinization of the nerves, which is thought to be related to hyperglycemia. Nerve conduction is disrupted when there are aberrations of the myelin sheaths.

The two most common types of diabetic neuropathy are sensorimotor polyneuropathy and autonomic neuropathy. Sensorimotor polyneuropathy is also called *peripheral neuropathy*. Cranial mononeuropathies—those affecting the oculomotor nerve—also occur in diabetes, especially in older adults.

Peripheral Neuropathy

Peripheral neuropathy most commonly affects the distal portions of the nerves, especially the nerves of the lower extremities; it affects both sides of the body symmetrically and may spread in a proximal direction.

Clinical Manifestations

Although approximately half of patients with diabetic neuropathy do not have symptoms, initial symptoms may include paresthesias (prickling, tingling, or heightened sensation) and burning sensations (especially at night). As the neuropathy progresses, the feet become numb. In addition, a decrease in proprioception (awareness of posture and movement of the body and of position and weight of objects in relation to the body) and a decreased sensation of light touch may lead to an unsteady gait. Decreased sensations of pain and temperature place patients with neuropathy at increased risk for injury and undetected foot infections. Deformities of the foot may also occur; neuropathy-related joint changes are sometimes referred to as Charcot joints. These joint deformities result from the abnormal weight distribution on joints resulting from lack of proprioception.

On physical examination, a decrease in deep tendon reflexes and vibratory sensation is found. For patients who have fewer or no symptoms of neuropathy, these physical findings may be the only indication of neuropathic changes. For patients with signs or symptoms of neuropathy, it is important to rule out other possible causes, including alcohol-induced and vitamin-deficiency neuropathies.

Management

Intensive insulin therapy and control of blood glucose levels delay the onset and slow the progression of neuropathy. Pain, particularly of the lower extremities, is a disturbing symptom in some people with neuropathy secondary to diabetes. In some cases, neuropathic pain spontaneously resolves within 6 months; for others, pain persists for many years. Various approaches to pain management can be tried. These include analgesic agents (preferably nonopioid); tricyclic antidepressants and other antidepressant medications (duloxetine [Cymbalta]); anticonvulsant medications (pregabalin [Lyrica], carbamazepine [Tegretol], or gabapentin [Neurontin]); mexiletine (Mexitil, an antiarrhythmic agent); and transcutaneous electrical nerve stimulation.

Duloxetine and pregabalin are approved specifically for treating painful diabetic peripheral neuropathy (NIDDK, 2013b).

Autonomic Neuropathies

Neuropathy of the autonomic nervous system results in a broad range of dysfunctions affecting almost every organ system of the body (NIDDK, 2013b).

Clinical Manifestations

Three manifestations of autonomic neuropathy are related to the cardiac, gastrointestinal, and renal systems. Cardiovascular symptoms range from a fixed, slightly tachycardic heart rate and orthostatic hypotension to silent, or painless, myocardial ischemia and infarction. Delayed gastric emptying may occur with the typical gastrointestinal symptoms of early satiety, bloating, nausea, and vomiting. "Diabetic" constipation or diarrhea (especially nocturnal diarrhea) may occur as a result. In addition, there may be unexplained wide swings in blood glucose levels related to inconsistent absorption of the glucose from ingested foods secondary to the inconsistent gastric emptying.

Urinary retention, a decreased sensation of bladder fullness, and other urinary symptoms of neurogenic bladder result from autonomic neuropathy. The patient with a neurogenic bladder is predisposed to development of urinary tract infections because of the inability to empty the bladder completely. This is especially true of patients with poorly controlled diabetes because hyperglycemia impairs resistance to infection.

Hypoglycemic Unawareness

Autonomic neuropathy affecting the adrenal medulla is responsible for diminished or absent adrenergic symptoms of hypoglycemia. Patients may report that they no longer feel the typical shakiness, sweating, nervousness, and palpitations associated with hypoglycemia. Frequent blood glucose monitoring is recommended for these patients. The inability to detect and treat these warning signs of hypoglycemia puts patients at risk for development of dangerously low blood glucose levels. Therefore, goals for blood glucose levels may need to be adjusted to reduce the risk for hypoglycemia. Patients and families need to be taught to recognize subtle and atypical symptoms of hypoglycemia, such as numbness around the mouth and impaired ability to concentrate.

Sudomotor Neuropathy

The neuropathic condition called *sudomotor neuropathy* refers to a decrease or absence of sweating (anhidrosis) of the extremities, with a compensatory increase in upper body sweating. Dryness of the feet increases the risk for the development of foot ulcers.

Sexual Dysfunction

Sexual dysfunction, especially erectile dysfunction in men, is a complication of diabetes. The effects of autonomic neuropathy on female sexual functioning are not well documented. Reduced vaginal lubrication has been mentioned as a possible neuropathic effect. Other possible changes in sexual function in women with diabetes include decreased libido and lack of orgasm. Vaginal infection, which increases in the incidence in women with diabetes, may be associated with decreased lubrication and vaginal pruritus (itching) and tenderness. Urinary tract infections and vaginitis may also affect sexual function.

Erectile dysfunction occurs with greater frequency in men with diabetes than in other men of the same age. Some men with autonomic neuropathy have normal erectile function and can experience orgasm but do not ejaculate normally. Retrograde ejaculation occurs; seminal fluid is propelled backward through the posterior urethra and into the urinary bladder. Examination of the urine confirms the diagnosis because of the large number of active sperm present. Fertility counseling may be necessary for couples attempting conception.

Diabetic neuropathy is not the only cause of impotence in men with diabetes. Medications such as antihypertensive agents, psychological factors, and other medical conditions (e.g., vascular insufficiency) that may affect other men also play a role in erectile dysfunction in men with diabetes (see Chapter 59).

Management

Management strategies for autonomic neuropathy focus on alleviating symptoms and on modification and management of risk factors. Detection of painless cardiac ischemia is important so that education about avoiding strenuous exercise can be provided. Orthostatic hypotension may respond to a diet high in sodium, discontinuation of medications that impede autonomic nervous system responses, the use of sympathomimetic and other agents (e.g., caffeine) that stimulate an autonomic response, mineralocorticoid therapy, and the use of lower-body elastic garments that maximize venous return and prevent pooling of blood in the extremities.

Treatment of delayed gastric emptying includes a low-fat diet, frequent small meals, frequent blood glucose monitoring, and the use of agents that increase gastric motility (e.g., metoclopramide [Reglan], bethanechol [Myotonachol]). Treatment of diabetic diarrhea may include bulk-forming laxatives or antidiarrheal agents. Constipation is treated with a high-fiber diet and adequate hydration; medications, laxatives, and enemas may be necessary if constipation is severe. Management of sexual dysfunction in women and men is discussed in Chapters 57 and 59, respectively. Intermittent straight catheterization may be necessary to prevent urinary tract infections in patients with neurogenic bladders.

Treatment of sudomotor dysfunction focuses on education about skin care and heat intolerance.

Foot and Leg Problems

Between 50% and 75% of lower extremity amputations are performed on people with diabetes. More than 50% of these amputations are thought to be preventable, provided patients are taught foot care measures and practice them on a daily basis (ADA, 2016b). Complications of diabetes that contribute to the increased risk of foot problems and infections include the following:

- *Neuropathy:* Sensory neuropathy leads to loss of pain and pressure sensation, and autonomic neuropathy leads to increased dryness and fissuring of the skin (secondary to decreased sweating). Motor neuropathy results in muscular atrophy, which may lead to changes in the shape of the foot.
- *Peripheral vascular disease:* Poor circulation of the lower extremities contributes to poor wound healing and the development of gangrene.
- *Immunocompromise:* Hyperglycemia impairs the ability of specialized leukocytes to destroy bacteria. Therefore, in poorly controlled diabetes, there is a lowered resistance to certain infections.

The typical sequence of events in the development of a diabetic foot ulcer begins with a soft tissue injury of the foot, formation of a fissure between the toes or in an area of dry skin, or formation of a callus (see Fig. 51-9). Patients with an insensitive foot do not feel injuries, which may be thermal (e.g., from using heating pads, walking barefoot on hot concrete, testing bathwater with the foot), chemical (e.g., burning the foot while using caustic agents on calluses, corns, or bunions), or traumatic (e.g., injuring skin while cutting nails, walking with an undetected foreign object in the shoe, or wearing ill-fitting shoes and socks).

If the patient is not in the habit of thoroughly inspecting both feet on a daily basis, the injury or fissure may go unnoticed until a serious infection has developed. Drainage, swelling, redness of the leg (from cellulitis), or gangrene may be the first sign of foot problems that the patient notices. Treatment of foot ulcers involves bed rest, antibiotics, and débridement. In addition, controlling glucose levels, which tend to increase when infections occur, is important for promoting

Figure 51-9 • Neuropathic ulcers occur on pressure points in areas with diminished sensation in diabetic polyneuropathy. Because pain is absent, the ulcer may go unnoticed.

wound healing. When peripheral vascular disease is present, foot ulcers may not heal because of the decreased ability of oxygen, nutrients, and antibiotics to reach the injured tissue. Amputation (see Chapter 42) may be necessary to prevent the spread of infection, particularly if it involves the bone (osteomyelitis) (see Chapter 41).

Foot assessment and foot care instructions are most important when caring for patients who are at high risk for foot infections. Some of the high-risk characteristics include:

- Duration of diabetes more than 10 years
- Age greater than 40 years
- Current smoker and history of smoking
- Decreased peripheral pulses
- Decreased sensation
- Anatomic deformities or pressure areas (e.g., bunions, calluses, hammer toes)
- History of previous foot ulcers or amputation

Management

Educating patients about proper foot care is a nursing intervention that can prevent costly and painful complications that result in disability (see Chart 51-10).

In addition to the daily visual and manual inspection of the feet, the feet should be examined during every health care visit or at least once per year (more often if there is an increase in risk) by a podiatrist, physician, or nurse (ADA, 2016a; NIDDK, 2013b). All patients should be assessed for neuropathy and undergo evaluation of neurologic status by an experienced examiner using a monofilament device (ADA, 2016b) (see Fig. 51-10). Pressure areas, such as calluses, or

thick toenails should be treated by a podiatrist in addition to routine trimming of nails.

Additional aspects of preventive foot care include the following:

- Properly bathing, drying, and lubricating the feet, taking care not to allow moisture (water or lotion) to accumulate between the toes.
- Wearing closed-toed shoes that fit well. A podiatrist can provide the patient with inserts (orthotics) to remove pressure from pressure points on the foot. New shoes should be broken in slowly (i.e., worn for 1 to 2 hours initially, with gradual increases in the length of time worn) to avoid blister formation. Patients with bony deformities may need custom-made shoes with extra width or depth. High-risk behaviors, such as walking barefoot, using heating pads on the feet, wearing open-toed shoes, soaking the feet, and shaving calluses, should be avoided.
- Trimming toenails straight across and filing sharp corners to follow the contour of the toe. If the patient has visual deficits, is unable to reach the feet because of disability, or has thickened toenails, a podiatrist should cut the nails.
- Reducing risk factors, such as smoking and elevated blood lipids, that contribute to peripheral vascular disease.
- Avoiding home remedies, over-the-counter agents, and self-medicating to treat foot problems.

Blood glucose control is important for avoiding decreased resistance to infections and for preventing diabetic neuropathy.

Chart 51-10

PATIENT EDUCATION

Foot Care Tips

The nurse instructs the patient to:

1. Take care of your diabetes.
   - Work with your health care team to keep your blood glucose level within a normal range.
2. Inspect your feet every day.
   - Look at your bare feet every day for cuts, blisters, red spots, and swelling.
   - Use a mirror to check the bottoms of your feet, or ask a family member for help if you have trouble seeing.
   - Check for changes in temperature.
3. Wash your feet every day.
   - Wash your feet in warm, not hot, water.
   - Dry your feet well. Be sure to dry between the toes.
   - Do not soak your feet.
   - Do not check water temperature with your feet; use a thermometer or elbow.
4. Keep the skin soft and smooth.
   - Rub a thin coat of skin lotion over the tops and bottoms of your feet, but not between your toes.
5. Smooth corns and calluses gently.
   - Use a pumice stone to smooth corns and calluses.
6. Trim your toenails each week or when needed.
   - Trim your toenails straight across, and file the edges with an emery board or nail file.

7. Wear shoes and socks at all times.
   - Never walk barefoot.
   - Wear comfortable shoes that fit well and protect your feet.
   - Feel inside your shoes before putting them on each time to make sure that the lining is smooth and there are no objects inside.
8. Protect your feet from hot and cold.
   - Wear shoes at the beach or on hot pavement.
   - Wear socks at night if your feet get cold.
9. Keep the blood flowing to your feet.
   - Put your feet up when sitting.
   - Wiggle your toes and move your ankles up and down for 5 minutes, two or three times a day.
   - Do not cross your legs for long periods of time.
   - Do not smoke.
10. Check with your primary provider.
    - Have your primary provider check your bare feet and find out whether you are likely to have serious foot problems. Remember that you may not feel the pain of an injury.
    - Call your primary provider right away if a cut, sore, blister, or bruise on your foot does not begin to heal after 1 day.
    - Follow your primary provider's advice about foot care.
    - Do not self-medicate or use home remedies or over-the-counter agents to treat foot problems.

Adapted from National Institute of Diabetes and Digestive and Kidney Diseases (NIDDK). (2013b). *Diabetic neuropathies: The nerve damage of diabetes.* Retrieved on 6/21/16 at: www.niddk.nih.gov/health-information/health-topics/Diabetes/diabetic-neuropathies-nerve-damage-diabetes/Pages/diabetic-neuropathies-nerve-damage.aspx; Fisher T. (2016). Your annual comprehensive foot exam. Diabetes Self Management. AACE/ACE Consensus Statement. *Endocrine Practice, 22*(1), 84–102.

Figure 51-10 • The monofilament test is used to assess the sensory threshold in patients with diabetes. The test instrument—a monofilament—is gently applied to about five pressure points on the foot (as shown in image on *left*). **A.** Example of a monofilament used for advanced quantitative assessment. **B.** Semmes-Weinstein monofilament used by clinicians. **C.** Disposable monofilament used by patients. The examiner applies the monofilament to the test area to determine whether the patient feels the device. Adapted with permission from Cameron, B. L. (2002). Making diabetes management routine. *American Journal of Nursing, 102*(2), 26–32.

SPECIAL ISSUES IN DIABETES CARE

Patients With Diabetes Who Are Undergoing Surgery

During periods of physiologic stress, such as surgery, blood glucose levels tend to increase, because levels of stress hormones (epinephrine, norepinephrine, glucagon, cortisol, and growth hormone) increase. If hyperglycemia is not controlled during surgery, the resulting osmotic diuresis may lead to excessive loss of fluids and electrolytes. Patients with type 1 diabetes also risk developing ketoacidosis during periods of stress.

Hypoglycemia is also a concern in patients with diabetes who are undergoing surgery. This is a special concern during the preoperative period if surgery is delayed beyond the morning in a patient who received a morning injection of intermediate-acting insulin.

There are various approaches to managing glucose control during the perioperative period. Frequent blood glucose monitoring is essential throughout the pre- and postoperative periods, regardless of the method used for glucose control. Examples of these approaches are described in Chart 51-11. The use of IV insulin and dextrose has become widespread with the increased availability of meters for intraoperative glucose monitoring.

During the postoperative period, patients with diabetes must also be closely monitored for cardiovascular complications because of the increased prevalence of atherosclerosis, wound infections, and skin breakdown (especially in patients with decreased sensation in the extremities due to neuropathy). Maintaining adequate nutrition and blood glucose control promote wound healing.

Management of Hospitalized Patients With Diabetes

At any one time, as many as 25% of hospitalized general medical-surgical patients have diabetes (ADA, 2016g). Often, diabetes is not the primary medical diagnosis, yet problems with control of diabetes frequently result from changes in the patient's normal routine or from surgery or illness. Patients who are hospitalized and have a diagnosis of diabetes should have this clearly indicated on their medical record, and glucose monitoring needs to be prescribed (ADA, 2016g). During the course of treatment, blood glucose control may worsen. Control of blood glucose levels is important because hyperglycemia in patients who are hospitalized can increase the length of hospital stay, the risk of infection, and mortality (ADA, 2016g).

In addition, this is an opportunity for patients with diabetes to update their knowledge about diabetes self-care and prevention of complications. Nurses caring for patients with diabetes should focus attention on the diabetes as well as the primary health issue.

Self-Care Issues

For patients who are actively involved in diabetes self-management (especially insulin dose adjustment), relinquishing control over meal timing, insulin timing, and insulin dosage can be particularly difficult and anxiety provoking. The patient may fear hypoglycemia and express much concern over possible delays in receiving attention from the nurse if hypoglycemic symptoms occur or may disagree with a planned dose of insulin.

The nurse acknowledges the patient's concerns and involves the patient in the plan of care as much as possible. If the patient disagrees with certain aspects of the care related to diabetes, the nurse must communicate this to other members of the health care team. Nurses and other health care providers must pay particular attention to patients who are successful in managing self-care; they should assess these patients' self-care management skills and encourage them to continue if their performance is correct and effective.

Hospitalization of a patient with diabetes should be considered an opportunity to evaluate the patient's self-care skills and to reinforce and/or deliver education that might be needed. The nurse observes the patient preparing and injecting the insulin, monitoring blood glucose, and performing foot care. (Simply questioning the patient about these

Chart 51-11 Approaches to Management of Glucose Control During the Perioperative Period for Those With a Diagnosis of Diabetes

- Monitor blood glucose levels frequently (every 1 to 2 hours).
- For patients taking insulin:
  1. The morning of surgery, all subcutaneous insulin doses are withheld, unless the blood glucose level is elevated (e.g., >200 mg/dL [11.1 mmol/L]), in which case a small dose of subcutaneous regular insulin may be prescribed. The blood glucose level is controlled during surgery with the IV infusion of regular insulin, which is balanced by an infusion of dextrose. The insulin and dextrose infusion rates are adjusted according to frequent (hourly) capillary glucose determinations. After surgery, the insulin infusion may be continued until the patient can eat. If IV insulin is discontinued, subcutaneous regular insulin may be given at set intervals (every 4 to 6 hours), or intermediate-acting insulin may be given every 12 hours with supplemental regular insulin as necessary until the patient is eating and the usual pattern of insulin dosing is resumed.
     - Carefully monitor the insulin infusion rate and blood glucose levels in a patient with diabetes who is receiving IV insulin. IV insulin has a much shorter duration of action than subcutaneous insulin. If the infusion is interrupted or discontinued, hyperglycemia will develop rapidly (within 1 hour in type 1 diabetes and within a few hours in type 2 diabetes).
     - Ensure that subcutaneous insulin is given 30 minutes before the IV insulin infusion is discontinued.

  2. One half to two thirds of the patient's usual morning dose of insulin (either intermediate-acting insulin alone or both short- and intermediate-acting insulins) is given subcutaneously in the morning before surgery. The remainder is then given after surgery.
  3. The patient's usual daily dose of subcutaneous insulin is divided into 4 equal doses of regular insulin. These are then given at 6-hour intervals. The last 2 approaches do not provide the control achieved by IV administration of insulin and dextrose.
     - Patients with type 2 diabetes who do not usually take insulin may require insulin during the perioperative period to control blood glucose elevations. Patients who are taking metformin may be instructed to discontinue the oral agent 24 to 48 hours before surgery, if possible. Some of these patients may resume their usual regimen of diet and oral agent during the recovery period. Other patients (whose diabetes is probably not well controlled with diet and an oral antidiabetic agent before surgery) need to continue with insulin injections after discharge.
     - For patients with type 2 diabetes who are undergoing minor surgery but who do not normally take insulin, glucose levels may remain stable provided no dextrose is infused during the surgery. After surgery, these patients may require small doses of regular insulin until the usual diet and oral agent are resumed.

Adapted from Comerford, K. C. (2015). *Nursing 2015 drug handbook.* Philadelphia, PA: Wolters Kluwer.

---

skills without actually observing performance of the skills is not sufficient.) The patient's knowledge about diet can be assessed with the help of a dietitian through direct questioning and review of the patient's menu choices. The patient's understanding about signs and symptoms, treatment, and prevention of hypoglycemia and hyperglycemia is assessed, along with knowledge of risk factors for macrovascular disease, including hypertension, increased lipids, and smoking. In addition, the patient is asked the date of their last eye examination (including dilation of the pupils). Education about these issues is critical.

Hyperglycemia During Hospitalization

Hyperglycemia may occur in patients who are hospitalized as a result of the original illness that led to the need for hospitalization. A number of other factors may contribute to hyperglycemia; examples include:

- Changes in the usual treatment regimen (e.g., increased food, decreased insulin, decreased activity)
- Medications (e.g., corticosteroids such as prednisone, which are used in the treatment of a variety of inflammatory disorders)
- IV dextrose, which may be part of the maintenance fluids or may be used for the administration of antibiotics and other medications, without adequate insulin therapy
- Overly vigorous treatment of hypoglycemia
- Inappropriate withholding of insulin or inappropriate use of "sliding scales"
- Mismatched timing of meals and insulin (e.g., postmeal hyperglycemia may occur if short-acting insulin is given immediately before or even after a meal)

Nursing actions to correct some of these factors are important for avoiding hyperglycemia. Assessment of the patient's usual home routine is important. The nurse should try to approximate as much as possible the home schedule of insulin, meals, and activities. Monitoring blood glucose levels has been identified by the ADA as an additional "vital sign" essential in assessment of patients (ADA, 2016g). The results of blood glucose monitoring provide information needed to obtain orders for extra doses of insulin (at times when insulin is usually taken), which is an important nursing function. Insulin doses must not be withheld when blood glucose levels are normal. It is very important to test blood glucose before a meal and administer insulin at that time, not on a rigid set time schedule as other medications are given. Insulin should be given when the meal is served to prevent hypoglycemia and elicit a physiologic response.

Short-acting insulin is usually needed to avoid postprandial hyperglycemia (even in patients with normal premeal glucose levels), and NPH insulin does not peak until many hours after the dose is given. IV antibiotics should be mixed in NS (if possible) to avoid excess infusion of dextrose (especially in patients who are eating). It is important to avoid overly vigorous treatment of hypoglycemia, which may lead to hyperglycemia.

Hypoglycemia During Hospitalization

Hypoglycemia in patients who are hospitalized is usually the result of too much insulin or delays in eating. Specific examples include:

- Overuse of sliding-scale regular insulin, particularly as a supplement to regularly scheduled, twice-daily short- and intermediate-acting insulins

- Lack of change in insulin dosage when dietary intake is changed (e.g., in the patient taking nothing by mouth [NPO])
- Overly vigorous treatment of hyperglycemia (e.g., giving too-frequent successive doses of regular insulin before the time of peak insulin activity is reached), resulting in a cumulative effect
- Delayed meal after administration of lispro, aspart, or glulisine (Apidra) insulin (patient should eat within 5 to 15 minutes after insulin administration)

Treatment of hypoglycemia should be based on the established hospital protocol (ADA, 2016g). If the initial treatment does not increase the glucose level adequately, the same treatment may be repeated after 15 minutes. The nurse must assess the pattern of glucose values and avoid giving doses of insulin that repeatedly lead to hypoglycemia. Successive doses of subcutaneous regular insulin should be given no more frequently than every 3 to 4 hours. For patients receiving intermediate insulin before breakfast and dinner, the nurse must use caution in administering supplemental doses of regular insulin at lunch and bedtime. Hypoglycemia may occur when two insulins peak at similar times (e.g., morning NPH peaks with lunchtime regular insulin and may lead to late-afternoon hypoglycemia; dinnertime NPH peaks with bedtime regular insulin and may lead to nocturnal hypoglycemia). To avoid hypoglycemic reactions caused by delayed food intake, the nurse should arrange for snacks to be given to the patient if meals are going to be delayed because of procedures, physical therapy, or other activities.

Common Alterations in Diet

Dietary modifications commonly prescribed during hospitalization require special consideration for patients who have diabetes (ADA, 2016d; Evert et al., 2013).

Nothing by Mouth

For patients who must be NPO in preparation for diagnostic or surgical procedures, the nurse must ensure that the usual insulin dosage has been changed. These changes may include eliminating the rapid-acting insulin and giving a decreased amount (e.g., half the usual dose) of intermediate-acting insulin. Another approach is to use frequent (every 3 to 4 hours) dosing of rapid-acting insulin only. IV dextrose may be given to provide calories and to avoid hypoglycemia.

Even without food, glucose levels may increase as a result of hepatic glucose production, especially in patients with type 1 diabetes and lean patients with type 2 diabetes. Furthermore, in type 1 diabetes, elimination of the insulin dose may lead to the development of DKA. Administration of basal insulin to patients with type 1 diabetes who are NPO is an important nursing action.

For patients with type 2 diabetes who are taking insulin, DKA does not usually develop when insulin doses are eliminated because the patient's pancreas produces some insulin. Therefore, skipping the insulin dose altogether (when the patient is receiving IV dextrose) may be safe; however, close monitoring of blood glucose levels is essential.

For patients who are NPO for extended periods (24 hours), glucose testing and insulin administration should be performed at regular intervals, usually four times per day. Insulin regimens for the patient who is NPO for an extended period may include NPH insulin every 12 hours, rapid-acting insulin only every 4 to 6 hours, or an IV insulin drip. These patients should receive dextrose infusions to provide some calories and limit ketosis.

To prevent the problems that result from the need to withhold food, diagnostic tests and procedures and surgery should be scheduled early in the morning when possible.

Clear Liquid Diet

When the diet is advanced to include clear liquids, patients with diabetes receive more simple carbohydrate foods, such as juice and gelatin desserts, than are usually included in the diabetic diet. Because patients who are hospitalized should maintain their nutritional status as much as possible to promote healing, the use of reduced-calorie substitutes such as diet soda or diet gelatin desserts would not be appropriate when the only source of calories is clear liquids. Simple carbohydrates, if eaten alone, cause a rapid rise in blood glucose levels; therefore, it is important to try to match peak times of insulin effect with peaks in the blood glucose concentration. If the patient receives insulin at regular intervals while NPO, the scheduled times for glucose tests and insulin injections should match mealtimes.

Enteral Tube Feedings

Tube feeding formulas contain more simple carbohydrates and less protein and fat than the typical meal plan for diabetes. This results in increased levels of glucose in patients with diabetes who are receiving tube feedings. Insulin doses must be given at regular intervals (e.g., NPH every 12 hours or regular insulin every 4 to 6 hours) when continuous tube feedings are given. If insulin is administered at routine (prebreakfast and predinner) times, hypoglycemia during the day may result (because the patient receives more insulin without more calories); hyperglycemia may occur during the night if feedings continue but insulin action decreases.

A common cause of hypoglycemia in patients receiving both continuous tube feedings and insulin is inadvertent or purposeful discontinuation of the feeding. The nurse must discuss with the medical team any plans for temporarily discontinuing the tube feeding (e.g., when the patient is away from the unit). Planning ahead may allow for alterations to be made in the insulin dose or for administration of IV dextrose. In addition, if problems with the tube feeding develop unexpectedly (e.g., the patient pulls out the tube, the tube clogs, the feeding is discontinued when residual gastric contents are found), the nurse must notify the primary provider, assess blood glucose levels more frequently, and administer IV dextrose if indicated.

Parenteral Nutrition

Patients receiving parenteral nutrition may receive both IV insulin (added to the parenteral nutrition container) and subcutaneous intermediate- or short-acting insulins. If the patient is receiving continuous parenteral nutrition, the blood glucose level should be monitored and insulin given at regular intervals. If the parenteral nutrition is infused over a limited number of hours, subcutaneous insulin should be given so that peak times of insulin action coincide with times of parenteral nutrition infusion.

Hygiene

Nurses caring for hospitalized patients with diabetes must focus attention on oral hygiene and skin care. Because these patients are at increased risk for periodontal disease, the nurse assists with daily dental care. The patient may also require assistance in keeping the skin clean and dry, especially in areas of contact between two skin surfaces (e.g., groin, axilla, under the breasts), where chafing and fungal infections tend to occur.

Careful assessments of the oral cavity and the skin are important. The skin is assessed for dryness, cracks, breakdown, and redness, especially at pressure points and on the lower extremities. The patient is asked about symptoms of neuropathy, such as tingling and pain or numbness of the feet. Deep tendon reflexes are assessed.

As with any patient confined to bed, nursing care must emphasize the prevention of skin breakdown at pressure points. The heels are particularly susceptible to breakdown because of loss of sensation of pain and pressure associated with sensory neuropathy.

Feet should be cleaned, dried, lubricated with lotion (but not between the toes), and inspected frequently. If the patient is in the supine position, pressure on the heels can be alleviated by elevating the lower legs on a pillow, with the heels positioned over the edge of the pillow. When the patient is seated in a chair, the feet should be positioned so that pressure is not placed on the heels. If the patient has an ulcer on one foot, the nurse provides preventive care to the unaffected foot as well as special care of the affected foot.

As always, every opportunity should be taken to educate the patient about diabetes self-management, including daily oral, skin, and foot care. Female patients should also be instructed about measures for the avoidance of vaginal infections, which occur more frequently when blood glucose levels are elevated. Patients often take their cues from nurses and realize the importance of daily personal hygiene if this is emphasized during their hospitalization.

Stress

Physiologic stress, such as infections and surgery, contributes to hyperglycemia and may precipitate DKA or HHS. Emotional stress related to hospitalization for any reason can also have a negative impact on diabetic control. An increase in stress hormones leads to an increase in glucose levels, especially if intake of food and insulin remains unchanged. In addition, during periods of emotional stress, people with diabetes may alter their usual pattern of meals, exercise, and medication. This can contribute to hyperglycemia or even hypoglycemia (e.g., in the patient taking insulin or oral antidiabetic agents who stops eating in response to stress).

People with diabetes must be made aware of the potential deterioration in diabetic control that can accompany emotional stress. They must be encouraged to follow the diabetes treatment plan as much as possible during times of stress. In addition, learning strategies for minimizing stress and coping with stress when it does occur are important aspects of diabetes education. Healthy coping is one of the seven steps to managing diabetes identified by the AADE (AADE, 2014).

 ## Gerontologic Considerations

Because people with diabetes are living longer, both type 1 and type 2 diabetes are being seen more frequently in older patients hospitalized for various reasons. Regardless of the type or duration of diabetes, the goals of diabetes treatment may need to be altered when caring for older adults who are hospitalized. The focus is on quality-of-life issues, such as maintaining independent functioning and promoting general well-being.

Some of the barriers to learning and self-care during hospital stays and in preparing patients for discharge include decreased vision, hearing loss, memory deficits, decreased mobility and fine motor coordination, increased tremors, depression and isolation, decreased financial resources, and limitations related to disabilities and other medical disorders. Assessing these barriers is important in planning diabetes treatment and educational activities. Presenting brief, simplified instructions with ample opportunity for practice of skills is important. The use of special devices such as a magnifier for the insulin syringe, an insulin pen, or a mirror for foot inspection is helpful. Frequent evaluation of self-care skills (insulin administration, blood glucose monitoring, foot care, diet planning) is essential, especially in patients with deteriorating vision and memory. Providing written instructions with handouts to take home also assists with management in the home setting.

If appropriate, family members may be called on to assist with diabetes basic skills, and referral to community resources may be made. It is preferable to educate the patient or family members to test blood glucose at home; the choice of meter should be tailored to the patient's visual and cognitive status and dexterity.

> ### ⚑ Quality and Safety Nursing Alert
>
> *Careful monitoring for diabetes complications must not be neglected in older adults. Hypoglycemia is especially dangerous, because it may go undetected and result in falls. Dehydration is a concern in patients who have chronically elevated blood glucose levels. Assessment for long-term complications, especially eye and foot problems, is important. Avoiding blindness and amputation through early detection and treatment of retinopathy and foot ulcers may mean the difference between placement in a long-term care facility and continued independent living for the older adult with diabetes.*

Nursing Management

Monitoring and Managing Potential Complications

Assessment for hypoglycemia and hyperglycemia involves frequent blood glucose monitoring (usually prescribed before meals and at bedtime) and monitoring for signs and symptoms of hypoglycemia or prolonged hyperglycemia (including DKA or HHS), as described previously. Inadequate control of blood glucose levels may hinder recovery from the primary health problem. Blood glucose levels are monitored, and insulin is given as prescribed. The nurse must ensure that prescribed insulin dosage is modified as needed to compensate for changes in the patient's schedule or eating pattern. Treatment is given for hypoglycemia (with oral glucose) or hyperglycemia (with supplemental regular insulin no more often than every 3 to 4 hours). Blood glucose records are assessed for patterns of hypoglycemia and hyperglycemia at the same time of day, and findings are reported to the primary provider for modification in insulin orders. In the patient with prolonged elevations in blood glucose, laboratory values and the patient's physical condition are monitored for signs and symptoms of DKA or HHS.

Promoting Home, Community-Based, and Transitional Care

 ### Educating Patients About Self-Care

Even if patients have had diabetes for many years, their knowledge and adherence to the plan of care must be assessed. A new plan of care may need to be devised using updated evidence. The nurse also reminds the patient and family about the importance of health promotion activities and recommended health screening.

Continuing and Transitional Care

A patient who is hospitalized may require referral for home, community based or transitional care. The nurse can use this opportunity to assess the patient's knowledge about diabetes management and the patient's and family's ability to carry out that management. The nurse reinforces the education provided in the hospital, clinic, office, or diabetes education center and assesses the home care environment to determine its adequacy for self-care and safety.

CRITICAL THINKING EXERCISES

1 `ebp` A 25-year-old patient is newly diagnosed with type 1 diabetes. What is the evidence base for self glucose management? Identify the criteria used to evaluate the strength of the evidence for the practices you have identified.

2 A 45-year-old patient has had type 2 diabetes for 5 years. His current diet consists of high-fat and high-carbohydrate foods, high sodium intake, and minimal vegetable consumption. He does not exercise and has smoked one pack of cigarettes a day since his early 20s. Generate an education plan for this patient. Identify immediate and long-term goals of management for his diabetes. Identify community resources that may be useful to this patient.

3 `pq` An 85-year-old patient who lives alone was found at home unresponsive and is admitted to the emergency department with possible DKA. Identify the pathophysiology and signs and symptoms of DKA. What are your priorities for the assessment, medical management, and nursing care for this patient with DKA? What are your priorities for discharge planning given this patient lives alone?

REFERENCES

*Asterisk indicates nursing research.
**Double asterisk indicates classic reference.

Books

Bader, M. K, Littlejohns, L. R., & Olson, D. M (2016). *AANN core curriculum for neuroscience nursing* (6th ed.). Chicago, IL: American Association of Neuroscience Nurses.

Comerford, K. C. (2015). *Nursing 2015 drug handbook.* Philadelphia, PA: Wolters Kluwer.

Dudek, S. G. (2014). *Nutrition essentials for nursing practice* (7th ed.). Philadelphia: Lippincott Williams & Wilkins.

Eliopoulos, C. (2018). *Gerontological nursing* (9th ed.). Philadelphia, PA: Lippincott Williams & Wilkins.

Fischbach, F. T., & Dunning, M. B. (2015). *A manual of laboratory and diagnostic tests* (9th ed.). Philadelphia, PA: Lippincott Williams & Wilkins.

Grossman, S. C., & Porth, C. M. (2014). *Pathophysiology: Concepts of altered health states* (9th ed.). Philadelphia, PA: Lippincott Williams & Wilkins.

Journals and Electronic Documents

American Association of Diabetes Educators (AADE). (2011). The scope of practice, standards of practice, and standards of professional performance for diabetes educators. Retrieved on 6/20/16 at: www.diabeteseducator.org/docs

American Association of Diabetes Educators (AADE). (2014). AADE7 self-care behaviors. Retrieved on 6/20/16 at: www.diabeteseducator.org/patient-resources/aade7-self-care-behaviors

American Diabetes Association (ADA). (2016a). Standards of medical care in diabetes—2016. *Diabetes Care, 39*(Suppl 1), S1–S2.

American Diabetes Association (ADA). (2016b). Standards of medical care in diabetes—2016. Classification and diagnosis of diabetes. *Diabetes Care, 39*(Suppl 1), S13–S24.

American Diabetes Association (ADA). (2016c). Standards of medical care in diabetes—2016. Management of diabetes in pregnancy. *Diabetes Care, 39*(Suppl 1), S94–S98.

American Diabetes Association (ADA). (2016d). Standards of medical care in diabetes—2016. Foundations of care and comprehensive medical evaluation. *Diabetes Care, 39*(Suppl 1), S23–S35.

American Diabetes Association (ADA). (2016e). Standards of medical care in diabetes—2016. Glycemic targets. *Diabetes Care, 39*(Suppl 1), S39–S47.

American Diabetes Association. (2016f). Standards of medical care in diabetes—2016. Cardiovascular disease and risk management. *Diabetes Care, 39*(Suppl 1), S60–S71.

American Diabetes Association. (2016g). Standards of medical care in diabetes—2016. Diabetes care in the hospital. *Diabetes Care, 39*(Suppl 1), S99–S104.

**Cameron, B. L. (2002). Making diabetes management routine. *American Journal of Nursing, 102*(2), 26–32.

Centers for Disease Control and Prevention (CDC). (2014). Diabetes report card. Retrieved on 6/17/16 at: www.cdc.gov/diabetes/pdfs/library/diabetesreportcard2014.pdf

Deng, C., Xiang, Y., Tan, T., et al. (2016). Altered peripheral b-lymphocyte subsets in type 1 diabetes and latent autoimmune diabetes in adults. *Diabetes Care, 39*(3), 434–440.

**Diabetes Control and Complications Trial Research Group (DCCT). (1993). The effect of intensive treatment of diabetes on the development and progression of long-term complications in insulin-dependent diabetes mellitus. *New England Journal of Medicine, 329*(14), 977–986.

**Diabetes Prevention Program Research Group. (2002). Reduction in the incidence of type 2 diabetes with lifestyle intervention or metformin. *New England Journal of Medicine, 346*(6), 393–403.

Diabetes Prevention Program Research Group. (2015). Long-term effects of lifestyle intervention or metformin on diabetes development and microvascular complications over 15-year follow-up: The Diabetes Prevention Program Outcomes Study. *Lancet, Diabetes and Endocrinology, 3*(11), 866–875.

Evert, A. B., Boucher, J. L., Cypress, M., et al. (2013). Nutrition therapy recommendation for the management of adults with diabetes. *Diabetes Care, 36*(11), 3821–3842.

Food and Drug Administration (FDA). (2014). FDA approves Afrezza to treat diabetes. Retrieved on 6/21/16 at: www.fda.gov/newsevents/newsroom/pressannouncements/ucm403122.htm

Fisher, T. (2016) Your annual comprehensive foot exam. Diabetes self management. AACE/ACE Consensus Statement. *Endocrine Practice*, 22(1), 84–102.

*Gaillard, T., Amponsah, G., & Osei, K. (2015). Patient-centered community diabetes education program improves glycemic control in African American patients with poorly controlled type 2 diabetes: Importance of point of care metabolic measurements. *Journal of the National Black Nurses Association*, 26(1), 51–58.

Hinnen, D. (2015). Dipeptidyl peptidase-4 inhibitors in diverse patient populations with type 2 diabetes. *The Diabetes Educator*, 41(1), 19S–31S.

National Institute of Diabetes and Digestive and Kidney Diseases (NIDDK). (2013a). Pancreatic islet transplantation. Retrieved on 6/21/16 at: www.niddk.nih.gov/health-information/health-topics/Diabetes/pancreatic-islet-transplantation/Pages/index.aspx

National Institute of Diabetes and Digestive and Kidney Diseases (NIDDK). (2013b). Diabetic neuropathies: The nerve damage of diabetes. Retrieved on 6/21/16 at: www.niddk.nih.gov/health-information/health-topics/Diabetes/diabetic-neuropathies-nerve-damage-diabetes/Pages/diabetic-neuropathies-nerve-damage.aspx

Noble-Bell, G., & Cox, A. (2014). Management of diabetic ketoacidosis in adults. *Nursing Times, 110*(10), 14–17.

Pearce, M. A., Rosenberg, C. S., & Davidson, M. D. (2003). Patient education. In M. B. Davidson, (Ed.). *Diabetes mellitus: Diagnosis and treatment*. New York: Churchill Livingstone.

Schwartz, S. S., Epstein, S., Corkey, B. E., et al. (2016). The time is right for a new classification system for diabetes: Rationale and implications of the β-cell-centric classification schema. *Diabetes Care*, 39(2), 179–186.

Seggelke, S., & Everhart, B. (2013). Management of type 2 diabetes. *Nurse Practioner*, 38(6), 13–16.

Triplitt, C., & Solis-Herrera, C. (2015). GLP-1 receptor agonists. Practical considerations for clinical practice. *The Diabetes Educator*, 41(1), 32S–46S.

Umpeirrez, G., & Korytkowski, M. (2016). Diabetic emergencies—ketoacidosis, hyperglycaemic hyperosmolar state and hyperglycemia. *Nature Reviews. Endocrinology, 12*, 222–232.

Unger, J. (2013). Educating patients about hypoglycemia prevention and self-management. *Clinical Diabetes, 31*(4), 179–188.

**United Kingdom Prospective Diabetes Study Group. (1998). Intensive blood glucose control with sulfonylureas or insulin compared with conventional treatment and risk of complications with type 2 diabetes. *Lancet, 352*(9131), 837–853.

U.S. Department of Health and Human Services. (2014). Healthy people 2020. Retrieved on 6/17/16 at: https://www.healthypeople.gov/2020/topics-objectives/topic/diabetes

Vivian, E. (2015). Sodium-Glucose cotransporter 2 inhibitors in the treatment of type 2 diabetes mellitus. *The Diabetes Educator, 41*(1), 5S–18S.

Weinger, K., Beverly, E. A., & Smaldone, A. (2014). Diabetes self-care and the older adult. *Western Journal of Nursing Research, 36*(9), 1272–1298.

World Health Organization (WHO). (2015a). *Diabetes*. Fact Sheet No. 312. Retrieved on 6/17/16 at: www.who.int/mediacentre/factsheets/fs312/en/

World Health Organization (WHO). (2015b). *Obesity and overweight*. Retrieved on 6/17/16 at: www.who.int/mediacentre/factsheets/fs311/en/

Wu, E. T., Nien, F. J., Kuo, C. H., et al. (2016). Diagnosis of more gestational diabetes lead to better pregnancy outcomes: Comparing the International Association of the Diabetes and Pregnancy Study Group criteria, and the Carpenter and Coustan criteria. *Journal of Diabetes Investigation, 7*(1), 121–126.

Resources

Academy of Nutrition and Dietetics (formerly the American Dietetic Association), www.eatright.org

American Association of Diabetes Educators (AADE), www.diabeteseducator.org

American Diabetes Association, www.diabetes.org

American Foundation for the Blind (AFB), www.afb.org

Centers for Disease Control and Prevention (CDC), www.cdc.gov/diabetes/home/index.html

Go4Life. Physical Activity of Older adults, go4life.nia.nih.gov/

JDRF (formerly the Juvenile Diabetes Research Foundation), www.jdrf.org

MedicAlert Foundation, www.medicalert.org

National Diabetes Information Clearinghouse, www.niddk.nih.gov

National Library Services for the Blind and Physically Handicapped (NLS), www.loc.gov/nls/

52

Assessment and Management of Patients With Endocrine Disorders

LEARNING OBJECTIVES

On completion of this chapter, the learner will be able to:

1. Describe the functions of each of the endocrine glands and their hormones.
2. Identify the diagnostic tests used to determine alterations in function of each of the endocrine glands.
3. Use the nursing process as a framework for care of patients with hyperthyroidism.
4. Develop a plan of nursing care for the patient undergoing thyroidectomy.
5. Compare hyperparathyroidism and hypoparathyroidism in terms of their causes, clinical manifestations, management, and nursing interventions.
6. Compare Addison disease with Cushing syndrome: their causes, clinical manifestations, management, and nursing interventions.
7. Explain nursing management of patients with adrenal insufficiency.
8. Apply the nursing process as a framework for care of patients with Cushing syndrome.
9. Identify the education needs of patients requiring corticosteroid therapy.

GLOSSARY

acromegaly: progressive enlargement of peripheral body parts resulting from excessive secretion of growth hormone

Addison disease: chronic adrenocortical insufficiency due to inadequate adrenal cortex function

addisonian crisis: acute adrenocortical insufficiency; characterized by hypotension, cyanosis, fever, nausea/vomiting, and signs of shock

adrenalectomy: surgical removal of one or both adrenal glands

adrenocorticotropic hormone (ACTH): hormone secreted by the anterior pituitary, essential for growth and development

adrenogenital syndrome: masculinization in women, feminization in men, or premature sexual development in children; result of abnormal secretion of adrenocortical hormones, especially androgens

androgens: male sex hormones

basal metabolic rate: chemical reactions occurring when the body is at rest

calcitonin: hormone secreted by the thyroid gland; participates in calcium regulation

Chvostek sign: spasm of the facial muscles produced by sharply tapping over the facial nerve in front of the parotid gland and anterior to the ear; suggestive of latent tetany in patients with hypocalcemia

corticosteroids: hormones produced by the adrenal cortex or their synthetic equivalents; also referred to as adrenalcortical hormone and adrenocorticosteroid; consist of glucocorticoids, mineralocorticoids, and androgens

Cushing syndrome: group of symptoms produced by an oversecretion of adrenocorticotropic hormone; characterized by truncal obesity, "moon face," acne, abdominal striae, and hypertension

diabetes insipidus: condition in which abnormally large volumes of dilute urine are excreted as a result of deficient production of vasopressin

dwarfism: generalized limited growth resulting from insufficient secretion of growth hormone during childhood

endocrine: secreting internally; hormonal secretion of a ductless gland

euthyroid: state of normal thyroid hormone production

exocrine: secreting externally; hormonal secretion from excretory ducts

exophthalmos: abnormal protrusion of one or both eyeballs

glucocorticoids: steroid hormones secreted by the adrenal cortex in response to adrenocorticotropic hormone; produce a rise of liver glycogen and blood glucose

goiter: enlargement of the thyroid gland

Graves disease: a form of hyperthyroidism; characterized by a diffuse goiter and exophthalmos

hormones: chemical transmitter substances produced in one organ or part of the body and carried by the bloodstream to other cells or organs on which they have a specific regulatory effect; produced mainly by endocrine glands

hypophysectomy: removal or destruction of all or part of the pituitary gland

mineralocorticoids: steroid hormones secreted by the adrenal cortex

myxedema: severe hypothyroidism; can be with or without coma

negative feedback: regulating mechanism in which an increase or decrease in the level of a substance decreases or increases the function of the organ producing the substance

pheochromocytoma: adrenal medulla tumor

syndrome of inappropriate antidiuretic hormone (SIADH) secretion: excessive secretion of antidiuretic hormone from the pituitary gland despite low serum osmolality level

thyroidectomy: surgical removal of all or part of the thyroid gland

thyroiditis: inflammation of the thyroid gland; may lead to chronic hypothyroidism or may resolve spontaneously

thyroid-stimulating hormone (TSH): released from the pituitary gland; causes stimulation of the thyroid, resulting in release of T_3 and T_4

thyroid storm: severe life-threatening hyperthyroidism precipitated by stress; characterized by high fever, extreme tachycardia, and altered mental state

thyrotoxicosis: condition produced by excessive endogenous or exogenous thyroid hormone

thyroxine (T_4): thyroid hormone; active iodine compound formed and stored in the thyroid; deiodinated in peripheral tissues to form triiodothyronine; maintains body metabolism in a steady state

triiodothyronine (T_3): thyroid hormone; formed and stored in the thyroid; released in smaller quantities, biologically more active, and with faster onset of action than T_4; widespread effect on cellular metabolism

Trousseau sign: carpopedal spasm induced when blood flow to the arm is occluded using a blood pressure cuff or tourniquet, causing ischemia to the distal nerves; suggestive sign for latent tetany in hypocalcemia

vasopressin: antidiuretic hormone secreted by the posterior pituitary

---

The **endocrine** system plays a vital role in orchestrating cellular interactions, metabolism, growth, reproduction, aging, and response to adverse conditions (Porth, 2015). This interconnected network of glands is closely linked with the nervous and immune systems, regulating the functions of multiple body organs. Disorders of the endocrine system are common and are manifested as hyperfunction and hypofunction.

Nursing interventions are essential in the management of patients with endocrine disorders. This chapter focuses on the anatomy and physiology of the endocrine system; the most common endocrine disorders of the pituitary, thyroid, parathyroid, and adrenal glands; clinical manifestations; diagnostic studies; medical management; and nursing interventions. The unique endocrine and **exocrine** functions of the pancreas, pancreatic function, and associated pancreatic disorders are discussed in Chapters 50 and 51; reproductive structures, including the ovaries and testes, are discussed in Chapters 56 and 59, respectively.

ASSESSMENT OF THE ENDOCRINE SYSTEM

Anatomic and Physiologic Overview

The endocrine system involves the release of chemical transmitter substances known as **hormones**. These substances regulate and integrate body functions by acting on local or distant target sites. Hormones are generally produced by the endocrine glands but may also be produced by specialized tissues such as those found in the gastrointestinal (GI) system, the kidney, and white blood cells. The GI mucosa produces hormones (e.g., gastrin, enterogastrone, secretin, cholecystokinin) that are important in the digestive process; the kidneys produce erythropoietin, a hormone that stimulates the bone marrow to produce red blood cells; and the white blood cells produce cytokines (hormonelike proteins) that actively participate in inflammatory and immune responses.

The endocrine system has a unique relationship with the immune and the nervous systems. Chemicals such as neurotransmitters (e.g., epinephrine) released by the nervous system can also function as hormones when needed. The immune system responds to the introduction of foreign agents by means of chemical messengers (cytokines), and is also subject to regulation by adrenal corticosteroid hormones (Porth, 2015).

Glands of the Endocrine System

The endocrine system is composed of the pituitary gland, thyroid gland, parathyroid glands, adrenal glands, pancreatic islets, ovaries, and testes (see Fig. 52-1). Most hormones secreted from endocrine glands are released directly into the bloodstream. However, exocrine glands, such as sweat glands, secrete their products through ducts onto epithelial surfaces or into the GI tract.

Function and Regulation of Hormones

Hormones help regulate organ function in concert with the nervous system. The rapid action by the nervous system is balanced by slower hormonal action. This dual regulatory system permits precise control of organ functions in response to changes within and outside the body. Table 52-1 lists the major hormones, their target tissues, and some of their properties.

The endocrine glands are composed of secretory cells arranged in minute clusters known as acini. A rich blood supply provides a vehicle for the hormones produced by the endocrine glands to enter the bloodstream rapidly. The amount of circulating hormones depends on their unique function and the body's needs. In the healthy physiologic state, hormone concentration in the bloodstream is maintained at a relatively constant level. To prevent accumulation, these hormones must be inactivated continuously by a **negative feedback** system so that when the hormone concentration increases, further production of that hormone is inhibited. Conversely, when the hormone concentration decreases, the rate of production of that hormone increases.

Classification and Action of Hormones

Hormones are classified into four categories according to their structure: (1) amines and amino acids (e.g., epinephrine, norepinephrine, and thyroid hormones); (2) peptides, polypeptides, proteins, and glycoproteins (e.g., thyrotropin-releasing hormone [TRH], follicle-stimulating hormone [FSH], and growth hormone [GH]); (3) steroids (e.g., **corticosteroids,**

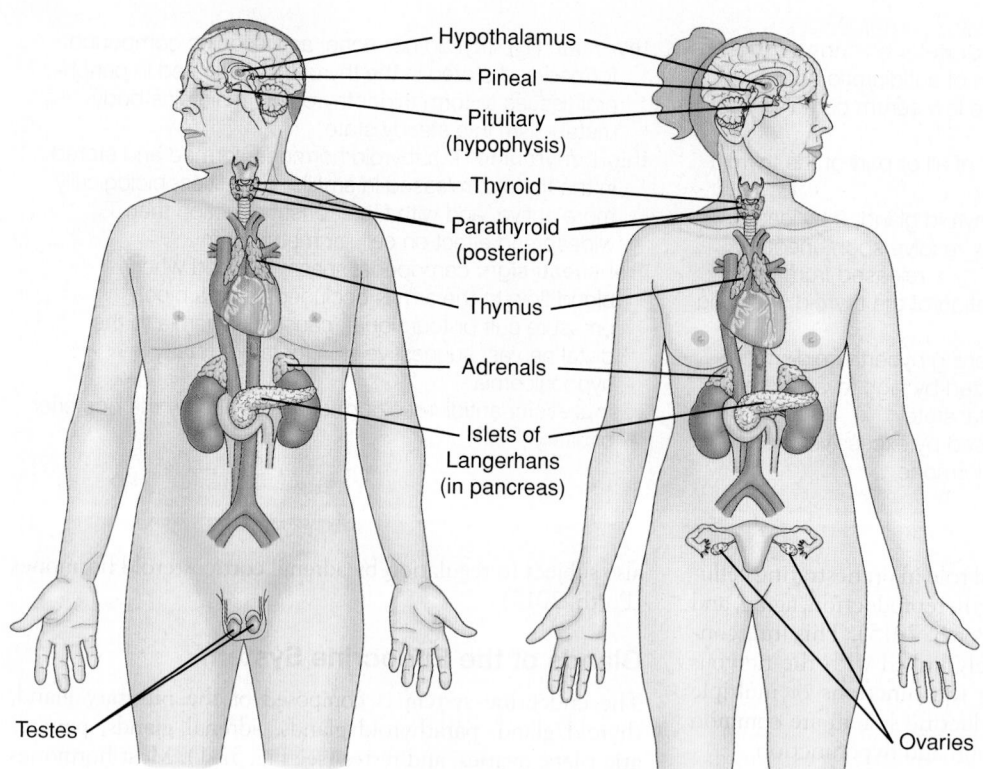

Figure 52-1 • Major hormone-secreting glands of the endocrine system.

Labels: Hypothalamus, Pineal, Pituitary (hypophysis), Thyroid, Parathyroid (posterior), Thymus, Adrenals, Islets of Langerhans (in pancreas), Testes, Ovaries

which are hormones produced by the adrenal cortex or their synthetic equivalents); and (4) fatty acid derivatives (e.g., eicosanoid, retinoids) (Porth, 2015). Although most hormones released by endocrine glands can be transported to distant target sites for action, some hormones never enter the bloodstream. Some hormones act locally in the area where they are released; this is called *paracrine action* (e.g., the effect of sex hormones on the ovaries). Others may act on the actual cells from which they were released; this is called *autocrine action* (e.g., the effect of insulin from pancreatic beta cells on those cells) (Lazar & Birnbaum, 2016).

Hormones can alter the function of the target tissue by interacting with chemical receptors located either on the cell membrane or in the interior of the cell. For example, *peptide* and *protein hormones* interact with receptor sites on the cell surface, resulting in stimulation of the intracellular enzyme adenyl cyclase. This causes increased production of cyclic 3′,5′-adenosine monophosphate (AMP). The cyclic AMP inside the cell alters enzyme activity. Thus, cyclic AMP is the "second messenger" that links the peptide hormone at the cell surface to a change in the intracellular environment. Some protein and peptide hormones also act by changing membrane permeability and act within seconds or minutes. The mechanism of action for *amine hormones* is similar to that for peptide hormones (Porth, 2015).

Steroid hormones, because of their smaller size and higher lipid solubility, penetrate cell membranes and interact with intracellular receptors. The steroid–receptor complex modifies cell metabolism and the formation of messenger ribonucleic acid (mRNA) from deoxyribonucleic acid (DNA). The mRNA then stimulates protein synthesis within the cell. Steroid hormones require several hours to exert their effects, because they exert their action by the modification of protein synthesis.

Assessment

Health History

Although specific endocrine disorders are often accompanied by specific clinical symptoms, more general manifestations may also occur. A thorough health history and review of systems are necessary for diagnosis and management of these disorders. Patients should be asked if they have experienced changes in energy level, tolerance to heat or cold, weight, thirst, frequency of urination, fat and fluid distribution, secondary sexual characteristics such as loss or growth of hair, menstrual cycle, memory, concentration, sleep patterns, and mood, as well as vision changes, joint pain, and sexual dysfunction. It is important to document (1) the severity of these changes, (2) the length of time the patient has experienced these changes, (3) the way in which these changes have affected the patient's ability to carry out activities of daily living, (4) the effect of the changes on the patient's self-perception, and (5) family history.

Physical Assessment

The physical examination should include vital signs; head-to-toe inspection; and palpation of skin, hair, and thyroid. Findings should be compared with previous findings, if available. Physical, psychological, and behavioral changes should be noted. Examples of changes in physical characteristics on examination may include appearance of facial hair in women, "moon face," "buffalo hump," **exophthalmos** (abnormal protrusion of one or both eyeballs), vision changes, edema, thinning of the skin, obesity of the trunk, thinness of the extremities, increased size of the feet and hands, edema, and hypo- or hyperreflexia. The patient may also exhibit changes

TABLE 52-1 Major Action and Source of Selected Hormones

Source	Hormone	Major Action
Hypothalamus	Releasing and inhibiting hormones CRH TRH GHRH GnRH Somatostatin Dopamine	Controls the release of pituitary hormones Inhibits GH and TSH Inhibits prolactin release from the pituitary Inhibits FSH and LH
Anterior pituitary	GH ACTH TSH FSH LH Prolactin	Stimulates growth of bone and muscle, promotes protein synthesis and fat metabolism, decreases carbohydrate metabolism Stimulates synthesis and secretion of adrenal cortical hormones Stimulates synthesis and secretion of thyroid hormone Female: stimulates growth of ovarian follicle, ovulation Male: stimulates sperm production Female: stimulates development of corpus luteum, release of oocyte, production of estrogen and progesterone Male: stimulates secretion of testosterone, development of interstitial tissue of testes Prepares female breast for breast-feeding
Posterior pituitary	ADH (Arginine Vasopressin [AVP]) Oxytocin	Increases water reabsorption by kidney Stimulates contraction of pregnant uterus, milk ejection from breasts after childbirth
Adrenal cortex	Mineralocorticosteroids, mainly aldosterone Glucocorticoids, mainly cortisol Adrenal androgens, mainly dehydroepian-drosterone (DHEA) and androstenedione	Increases sodium absorption, potassium loss by kidney Affects metabolism of all nutrients; regulates blood glucose levels, affects growth, has anti-inflammatory action, and decreases effects of stress Have minimal intrinsic androgenic activity; they are converted to testosterone and dihydrotestosterone (DHT) in the periphery
Adrenal medulla	Epinephrine Norepinephrine	Serve as neurotransmitters for the sympathetic nervous system
Thyroid (follicular cells)	Thyroid hormones: triiodothyronine (T_3), thyroxine (T_4) Calcitonin	Increase the metabolic rate; increase protein and bone turnover; increase responsiveness to catecholamines; necessary for fetal and infant growth and development Lowers blood calcium and phosphate levels
Parathyroid glands	Parathyroid hormone (PTH)	Regulates serum calcium
Pancreatic islet cells	Insulin Glucagon Somatostatin	Lowers blood glucose by facilitating glucose transport across cell membranes of muscle, liver, and adipose tissue Increases blood glucose concentration by stimulation of glycogenolysis and glyconeogenesis Delays intestinal absorption of glucose
Kidney	1,25-Dihydroxyvitamin D	Stimulates calcium absorption from the intestine
Ovaries	Estrogen Progesterone	Affects development of female sex organs and secondary sex characteristics Influences menstrual cycle; stimulates growth of uterine wall; maintains pregnancy
Testes	Androgens, mainly testosterone	Affect development of male sex organs and secondary sex characteristics; aid in sperm production

CRH, corticotropin-releasing hormone; TRH, thyrotropin-releasing hormone; GHRH, growth hormone–releasing hormone; GnRH, gonadotropin-releasing hormone; GH, growth hormone; ACTH, adrenocorticotropic hormone; TSH, thyroid-stimulating hormone; FSH, follicle-stimulating hormone; LH, luteinizing hormone; ADH, antidiuretic hormone.
Reprinted with permission from Grossman, S. C., & Porth, C. M. (2014). *Pathophysiology: Concepts of altered health states* (9th ed.). Philadelphia, PA: Lippincott Williams & Wilkins.

in mood and behavior such as nervousness, lethargy, and fatigue (Weber & Kelley, 2014).

Diagnostic Evaluation

A variety of diagnostic studies are used to evaluate the endocrine system. The nurse educates the patient about the purpose of the prescribed studies, what to expect, and any possible side effects related to these examinations prior to testing. The nurse notes trends in results that provide information about disease progression as well as the patient's response to therapy.

Blood Tests

Blood tests determine the levels of circulating hormones, the presence of autoantibodies, and the effect of a specific hormone on other substances (e.g., the effect of insulin on blood glucose levels). The serum levels of a specific hormone may provide information to determine the presence of hypofunction or hyperfunction of the endocrine system and the site of dysfunction. Radioimmunoassays are radioisotope-labeled antigen tests that are commonly indicated blood tests used to measure the levels of hormones or other substances (Sluss & Hayes, 2016).

Urine Tests

Urine tests are used to measure the amount of hormones or the end products of hormones excreted by the kidneys. One-time specimens or, in some disorders, 24-hour urine specimens are collected to measure hormones or their metabolites. For example, urinary levels of free catecholamines (norepinephrine, epinephrine, and dopamine) may be measured in patients with suspected tumors of the adrenal medulla (**pheochromocytoma**). Several disadvantages related to urine tests that must be considered are that patients may be unable to urinate at scheduled intervals and that some medications or disease states may affect the test results (Porth, 2015).

Additional Diagnostic Studies

Stimulation tests are used to confirm hypofunction of an endocrine organ. The tests determine how an endocrine gland responds to the administration of stimulating hormones that are normally produced or released by the hypothalamus or pituitary gland. If the endocrine gland responds to this stimulation, the specific disorder may be in the hypothalamus or pituitary. Failure of the endocrine gland to respond to this stimulation helps identify the problem as being in the endocrine gland itself.

Suppression tests are used to detect hyperfunction of an endocrine organ. They determine if the organ is not responding to the negative feedback mechanisms that normally control secretion of hormones from the hypothalamus or pituitary gland. Suppression tests measure the effect of an given exogenous dose of the hormone on the endogenous secretion of the hormone or on the secretion of stimulation hormones from the hypothalamus or pituitary gland.

Imaging studies include radioactive scanning, magnetic resonance imaging (MRI), computed tomography (CT), ultrasonography, positron emission tomography (PET), and dual-energy x-ray absorptiometry (DEXA) (Porth, 2015).

Genetic screening is increasingly becoming more routine in the assessment of endocrine disorders (see Chart 52-1). DNA testing can be used for the identification of specific genes associated with endocrine disorders, selective targeting for drug development, and increased understanding of the function of the endocrine system. Genetic screening is used to determine the presence of a gene mutation that may predispose an individual to a certain condition. The implications of genetic screening must be considered carefully by the primary provider and patient (Majithia, Altshuler, & Hirschhorn, 2016; Rosenthal, 2014).

THE PITUITARY GLAND

Anatomic and Physiologic Overview

The pituitary gland, or hypophysis, is commonly referred to as the master gland because of the influence it has on secretion of hormones by other endocrine glands (Porth, 2015)

Chart 52-1

GENETICS IN NURSING PRACTICE
Metabolic and Endocrine Disorders

Metabolic and endocrine disorders that are influenced by genetic factors are complex and typically impact multiple body systems. Some examples of genetic metabolic and endocrine disorders include:

- Diabetes
- Disorders in amino acids (e.g., phenylketonuria, homocystinuria, maple syrup urine disease)
- Disorders of carbohydrate metabolism (e.g., galactosemia)
- Disorders of fatty acid oxidation (e.g., medium-chain acyl-CoA dehydrogenase deficiency)
- Disorders of glycogen storage (e.g., Pompe disease, Von Gierke disease, Danon disease, Cori disease, Anderson disease, McArdle disease)
- Disorders of lysosomal storage disease (e.g., Tay Sachs, Gaucher, Niemann-Pick, Fabry disease)
- Disorders of mucopolysaccharides (e.g., Hurler syndrome, Hunter disease, Morquio syndrome)
- Disorders in urea cycle (e.g., ornithine transcarbamylase deficiency)
- Hemochromatosis
- McCune–Albright syndrome
- Multiple endocrine neoplasia type I and type II

Nursing Assessments

Refer to Chapter 5, Chart 5-2: Genetics in Nursing Practice: Genetic Aspects of Health Assessment

Family History Assessment

- Assess family history for relatives with early-onset hepatic, pancreatic, or endocrine disease.
- Inquire about family members with diabetes and their ages at onset.
- Assess family history of other related genetic conditions such as cystic fibrosis, alpha₁-antitrypsin deficiency, and hemochromatosis.

Patient Assessment

- Assess for physical symptoms such as mucosal neuromas, hypertrophied lips, skeletal abnormalities, and marfanoid appearance.
- Assess for signs of arthritis and bronze pigmentation of the skin (hemochromatosis).
- Assess for history of seizures, sweet smell to urine, jaundice, lethargy, vomiting, dehydration, acidosis, neutropenia, hepatomegaly, high ammonia levels

Genetics Resources

Society for Inherited Metabolic Disorders, www.simd.org
Association for Glycogen Storage Disease, www.agsdus.org.
See Chapter 8, Chart 8-7 for components of genetic counseling.

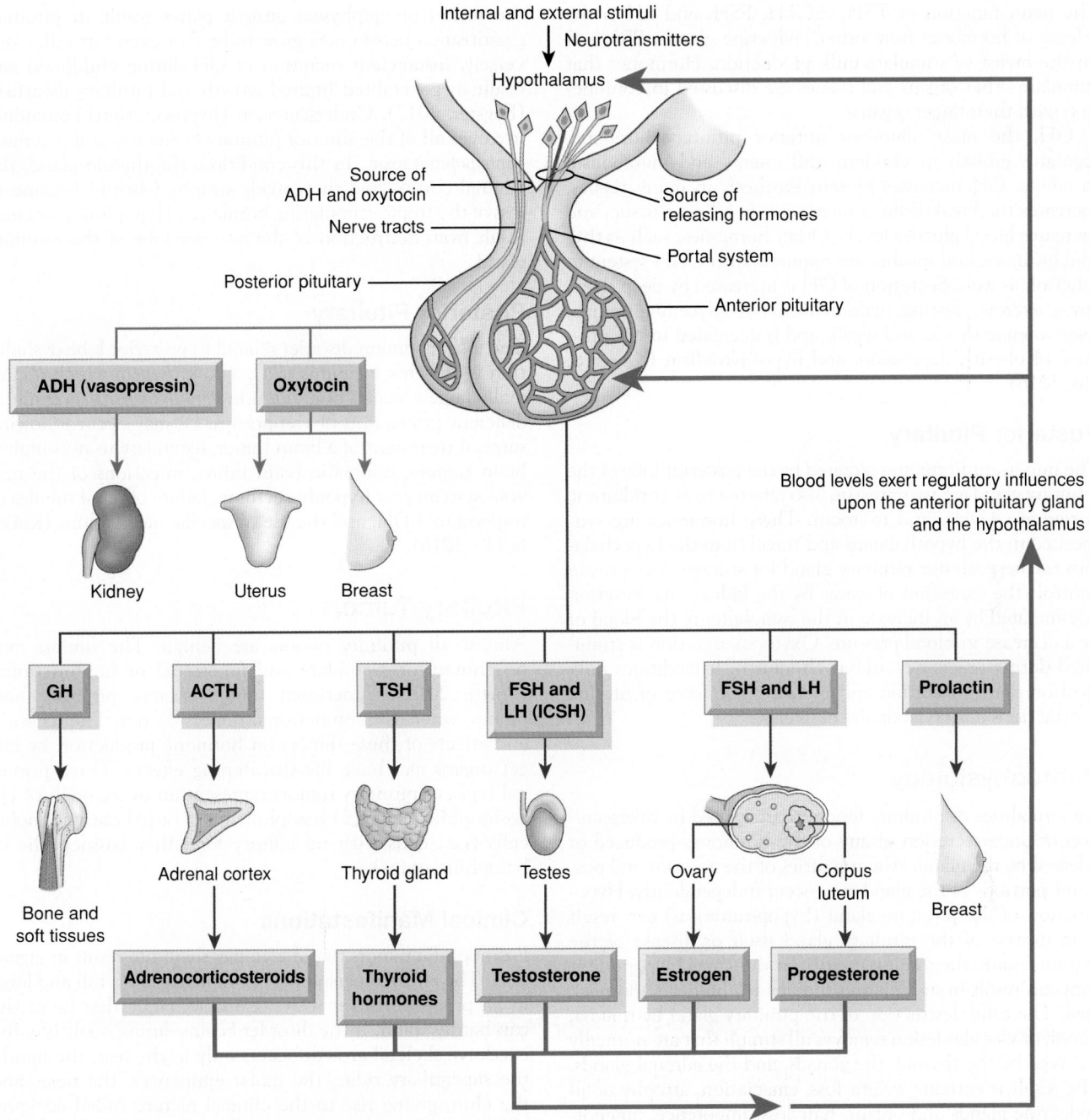

Figure 52-2 • The pituitary gland, the relationship of the brain to pituitary action, and the hormones secreted by the anterior and posterior pituitary lobes. ADH, antidiuretic hormone; GH, growth hormone; ACTH, adrenocorticotropic hormone; TSH, thyroid-stimulating hormone; FSH, follicle-stimulating hormone; LH, luteinizing hormone; ICSH, interstitial cell-stimulating hormone.

(see Fig. 52-2). The round structure, about 1.27 cm (1/2 in) in diameter, is located on the inferior aspect of the brain and is divided into anterior and posterior lobes. It is controlled by the hypothalamus, which is an adjacent area of the brain that is connected to the pituitary by the pituitary stalk.

Anterior Pituitary

The major hormones of the anterior pituitary gland are FSH, luteinizing hormone (LH), prolactin (PRL), **adrenocorticotropic hormone (ACTH)**, **thyroid-stimulating hormone (TSH)**, and GH (also referred to as somatotropin). The secretion of these major hormones is controlled by releasing factors secreted by the hypothalamus. These releasing factors reach the anterior pituitary by way of the bloodstream in a special circulation called the *pituitary portal blood system*. Other hormones include melanocyte-stimulating hormone and beta-lipotropin; the function of lipotropin is poorly understood.

The hormones released by the anterior pituitary enter the general circulation and are transported to their target organs.

The main function of TSH, ACTH, FSH, and LH is the release of hormones from other endocrine glands. PRL acts on the breast to stimulate milk production. Hormones that stimulate other organs and tissues are discussed in conjunction with their target organs.

GH, the most abundant anterior pituitary hormone, regulates growth in children and energy and metabolism in adults. GH increases protein synthesis in many tissues, increases the breakdown of fatty acids in adipose tissue, and increases blood glucose levels. Other hormones, such as thyroid hormone and insulin, are required for the GH system to function as well. Secretion of GH is increased by deep sleep, stress, exercise, fasting, malnutrition, hypoglycemia, trauma, hypovolemic shock, and sepsis, and is decreased in the presence of obesity, depression, and hypothyroidism (Kaiser & Ho, 2016).

Posterior Pituitary

The important hormones secreted by the posterior lobe of the pituitary gland are **vasopressin**, also referred to as antidiuretic hormone (ADH), and oxytocin. These hormones are synthesized in the hypothalamus and travel from the hypothalamus to the posterior pituitary gland for storage. Vasopressin controls the excretion of water by the kidney; its secretion is stimulated by an increase in the osmolality of the blood or by a decrease in blood pressure. Oxytocin secretion is stimulated during pregnancy and at childbirth. It facilitates milk ejection during lactation and increases the force of uterine contractions during labor and delivery.

Pathophysiology

Abnormalities of pituitary function are caused by oversecretion or undersecretion of any of the hormones produced or released by the gland. Abnormalities of the anterior and posterior portions of the gland may occur independently. Hypofunction of the pituitary gland (hypopituitarism) can result from disease of the pituitary gland itself or disease of the hypothalamus; the result is essentially the same. Hypopituitarism can result from radiation therapy to the head and neck area. The total destruction of the pituitary gland by trauma, tumor, or vascular lesion removes all stimuli that are normally received by the thyroid, the gonads, and the adrenal glands. The result is extreme weight loss, emaciation, atrophy of all endocrine glands and organs, hair loss, impotence, amenorrhea, hypometabolism, and hypoglycemia. Coma and death occur if the missing hormones are not replaced.

Anterior Pituitary

Oversecretion (hypersecretion) of the anterior pituitary gland most commonly involves ACTH or GH and results in **Cushing syndrome** (group of symptoms produced by an oversecretion of ACTH) or acromegaly, respectively. **Acromegaly**, a disorder caused by an excess of GH in adults, results in enlargement of peripheral body parts and soft tissue, after the fusion of the epiphyseal plates has occurred, without an increase in height (Woodworth, Lakhani, Aleryani, et al., 2014). It occurs in approximately four cases per 1 million people per year (Katznelson, Laws, Melmed, et al., 2014). Although rare, oversecretion of GH in children before

the fusion of epiphyseal growth plates result in pituitary gigantism; a person may grow to be 7 or even 8 ft tall. Conversely, insufficient secretion of GH during childhood can result in generalized limited growth and pituitary **dwarfism** (Eugster, 2017). Undersecretion (hyposecretion) commonly involves all of the anterior pituitary hormones and is termed *panhypopituitarism*. In this condition, the thyroid gland, the adrenal cortex, and the gonads atrophy (shrink) because of loss of the tropic-stimulating hormones. Hypopituitarism may result from destruction of the anterior lobe of the pituitary gland.

Posterior Pituitary

The most common disorder related to posterior lobe dysfunction is **diabetes insipidus** (DI), a condition in which abnormally large volumes of dilute urine are excreted as a result of deficient production of vasopressin. DI may occur following surgical treatment of a brain tumor, secondary to nonsurgical brain tumors, traumatic brain injury, infections of the nervous system, post **hypophysectomy**, failure of renal tubules to respond to ADH, and the use of specific medications (Kaiser & Ho, 2016).

Pituitary Tumors

Almost all pituitary tumors are benign. The tumors may be primary or secondary and functional or nonfunctional (Porth, 2015). Functional tumors secrete pituitary hormones, whereas nonfunctional tumors do not. The location and effects of these tumors on hormone production by target organs can have life-threatening effects. Three principal types of pituitary tumors represent an overgrowth of (1) eosinophilic cells, (2) basophilic cells, or (3) chromophobic cells (i.e., cells with no affinity for either eosinophilic or basophilic stains).

Clinical Manifestations

Eosinophilic tumors that develop early in life result in gigantism. The affected person may be more than 7 ft tall and large in all proportions, yet so weak and lethargic that he or she can hardly stand. If the disorder begins during adult life, the excessive skeletal growth occurs only in the feet, the hands, the superciliary ridge, the molar eminences, the nose, and the chin, giving rise to the clinical picture called *acromegaly*. However, enlargement involves all tissues and organs of the body (Porth, 2015). Many of these patients suffer from severe headaches and visual disturbances because the tumors exert pressure on the optic nerves (Porth, 2015). Assessment of central vision and visual fields may reveal loss of color discrimination, diplopia (double vision), or blindness in a portion of a field of vision. Decalcification of the skeleton, muscular weakness, and endocrine disturbances, similar to those occurring in patients with hyperthyroidism, also are associated with this type of tumor.

Basophilic tumors give rise to Cushing syndrome with features largely attributable to hyperadrenalism, including masculinization and amenorrhea in females, truncal obesity, hypertension, osteoporosis, and polycythemia.

Chromophobic tumors represent 90% of pituitary tumors. These tumors usually produce no hormones but destroy the rest of the pituitary gland, causing hypopituitarism. People with this disease are often obese and somnolent and exhibit fine, scanty hair; dry, soft skin; a pasty complexion; and small bones. They also experience headaches, loss of libido, and visual defects progressing to blindness. Other signs and symptoms include polyuria, polyphagia, a lowering of the **basal metabolic rate** (chemical reactions occurring when the body is at rest), and a subnormal body temperature.

Assessment and Diagnostic Findings

Diagnostic evaluation requires a careful history and physical examination, including assessment of visual acuity and visual fields. CT and MRI scans are used to diagnose the presence and extent of pituitary tumors. Serum levels of pituitary hormones may be obtained along with measurements of hormones of target organs (e.g., thyroid, adrenal) to assist in diagnosis.

Medical Management

Surgical removal of the pituitary gland (hypophysectomy) through a transsphenoidal approach is the usual treatment. Stereotactic radiation therapy, which requires the use of a neurosurgery-type stereotactic frame, may be used to deliver external-beam radiation therapy precisely to the pituitary tumor with minimal effect on normal tissue (see Chapter 15). Other treatments include conventional radiation therapy, bromocriptine (Parlodel, a dopamine antagonist), and octreotide (Sandostatin, a synthetic analog of GH). These medications inhibit the production or release of GH and may bring about marked improvement of symptoms (Mercado, 2016). Octreotide and lanreotide (Somatuline Depot, a somatostatin analog) may also be used preoperatively to improve the patient's clinical condition and to shrink the tumor (Comerford, 2015).

Surgical Management

Hypophysectomy is the treatment of choice in patients with Cushing syndrome resulting from excessive production of ACTH by a pituitary tumor. Hypophysectomy may also be performed on occasion as a palliative measure to relieve bone pain secondary to metastasis of malignant lesions of the breast and prostate.

Several approaches are used to remove or destroy the pituitary gland, including surgical removal by transfrontal, subcranial, or oronasal–transsphenoidal approaches; irradiation; and cryosurgery. The transsphenoidal approach and the nursing management of a patient undergoing cranial surgery are discussed in Chapter 66. Features or symptoms of acromegaly are unaffected by surgical removal of the tumor.

The absence of the pituitary gland alters the function of many body systems. Menstruation ceases and infertility occurs after total or near-total ablation of the pituitary gland. Replacement therapy with corticosteroids and thyroid hormone is necessary.

Diabetes Insipidus

DI is the most common disorder of the posterior lobe of the pituitary gland and is characterized by a deficiency of ADH (vasopressin). Excessive thirst (polydipsia) and large volumes of dilute urine are manifestations of the disorder. It may occur secondary to head trauma, brain tumor, or surgical ablation

or irradiation of the pituitary gland (Kaiser & Ho, 2016). It may also occur with infections of the central nervous system (meningitis, encephalitis, tuberculosis) or with tumors (e.g., metastatic disease, lymphoma of the breast or lung). Another cause of DI is failure of the renal tubules to respond to ADH; this nephrogenic form may be related to hypokalemia, hypercalcemia, and a variety of medications (e.g., lithium, demeclocycline [Declomycin]).

 Concept Mastery Alert

It is important to distinguish between DI, a disorder of insufficient output of pituitary ADH, and diabetes, a metabolic disorder characterized by hyperglycemia caused by deficient insulin secretion or action (or both).

Clinical Manifestations

Without the action of ADH on the distal nephron of the kidney, an enormous daily output (greater than 250 mL per hour) of very dilute urine with a specific gravity of 1.001 to 1.005 occurs (John & Day, 2012). The urine contains no abnormal substances such as glucose or albumin. Because of the intense thirst, the patient tends to drink 2 to 20 L of fluid daily and craves cold water. In adults, the onset of DI may be insidious or abrupt.

The disease cannot be controlled by limiting fluid intake, because the high-volume loss of urine continues even without fluid replacement. Attempts to restrict fluids cause the patient to experience an insatiable craving for fluid and to develop hypernatremia and severe dehydration.

Assessment and Diagnostic Findings

The fluid deprivation test is carried out by withholding fluids for 8 to 12 hours or until 3% to 5% of the body weight is lost. The patient is weighed frequently during the test. Plasma and urine osmolality studies are performed at the beginning and end of the test. The inability to increase the specific gravity and osmolality of the urine is characteristic of DI. The patient continues to excrete large volumes of urine with low specific gravity and experiences weight loss, increasing serum osmolality, and elevated serum sodium levels. The patient's condition needs to be monitored frequently during the test, and the test is terminated if tachycardia, excessive weight loss, or hypotension develops.

Other diagnostic procedures include concurrent measurements of plasma levels of ADH and plasma and urine osmolality as well as a trial of desmopressin (synthetic vasopressin) therapy and intravenous (IV) infusion of hypertonic saline solution. If the diagnosis is confirmed and the cause (e.g., head injury) is not obvious, the patient is carefully assessed for tumors that may be causing the disorder.

Medical Management

The objectives of therapy are (1) to replace ADH (which is usually a long-term therapeutic program), (2) to ensure adequate fluid replacement, and (3) to identify and correct the underlying intracranial pathology. Nephrogenic causes require different management approaches (John & Day, 2012).

Pharmacologic Therapy

Desmopressin (DDAVP), a synthetic vasopressin without the vascular effects of natural ADH, is particularly valuable because it has a longer duration of action and fewer adverse effects than other preparations previously used to treat the disease. It is given intranasally; the patient sprays the solution into the nose through a flexible calibrated plastic tube. One or two administrations daily (i.e., every 12 to 24 hours) usually control the symptoms (McPhee, Rabow, & Papadakis, 2016). Vasopressin causes vasoconstriction; thus, it must be used cautiously in patients with coronary artery disease.

Chlorpropamide (Diabinese) and thiazide diuretics are also used in mild forms of the disease because they potentiate the action of vasopressin (Comerford, 2015). Hyperglycemia is possible.

If the DI is renal in origin, the previously described treatments are ineffective. Thiazide diuretics, mild salt depletion, and prostaglandin inhibitors (ibuprofen [Advil, Motrin], indomethacin [Indocin], and aspirin) are used to treat the nephrogenic form of DI.

Nursing Management

Physical assessment and patient education are the pillars of skilled nursing management of the patient with a diagnosis of DI. Initially, the nurse reviews the patient history and physical assessment. The nurse is responsible to educate the patient, family, and other caregivers about follow-up care, prevention of complications, and emergency measures. Specific verbal and written instructions should include the dose, actions, side effects, and administration of all medications and the signs and symptoms of hyponatremia. The nurse should demonstrate and observe a return demonstration of medication administration to ensure that the patient received the prescribed dosage. The patient should be advised to wear a medical identification bracelet and carry required medication and information about DI at all times.

Syndrome of Inappropriate Antidiuretic Hormone Secretion

The **syndrome of inappropriate antidiuretic hormone (SIADH) secretion** includes excessive ADH secretion from the pituitary gland even in the face of subnormal serum osmolality. Patients with SIADH cannot excrete a dilute urine, retain fluids, and develop a sodium deficiency known as dilutional hyponatremia. SIADH is often of nonendocrine origin; for instance, the syndrome may occur in patients with bronchogenic carcinoma in which malignant lung cells synthesize and release ADH. SIADH has also occurred in patients with severe pneumonia, pneumothorax, and other disorders of the lungs, as well as malignant tumors that affect other organs (Kaiser & Ho, 2016; Porth, 2015).

Disorders of the central nervous system, such as head injury, brain surgery or tumor, and infection, are thought to produce SIADH by direct stimulation of the pituitary gland (Kaiser & Ho, 2016). Some medications (e.g., vincristine [Oncovin], phenothiazines, tricyclic antidepressants, thiazide diuretics) and nicotine have been implicated in SIADH; they either directly stimulate the pituitary gland or increase the sensitivity of renal tubules to circulating ADH.

Medical Management

Interventions include eliminating the underlying cause, if possible, and restricting fluid intake (John & Day, 2012). Because retained water is excreted slowly through the kidneys, the extracellular fluid volume contracts and the serum sodium concentration gradually increases toward normal. Diuretic agents such as furosemide (Lasix) may be used along with fluid restriction if severe hyponatremia is present.

Nursing Management

Close monitoring of fluid intake and output, daily weight, urine and blood chemistries, and neurologic status is indicated for the patient at risk for SIADH. Supportive measures and explanations of procedures and treatments assist the patient in managing this disorder.

THE THYROID GLAND

The thyroid gland—the largest endocrine gland—is a butterfly-shaped organ located in the lower neck, anterior to the trachea (Fig. 52-3). It consists of two lateral lobes connected by an isthmus. The gland is about 5 cm long and 3 cm wide and weighs about 30 g. The blood flow to the thyroid is very high (about 5 mL/min per gram of thyroid tissue), approximately five times the blood flow to the liver. The thyroid gland produces three hormones: **thyroxine (T_4)**, **triiodothyronine (T_3)**, and **calcitonin**.

Anatomic and Physiologic Overview

Various hormones and chemicals are responsible for normal thyroid function. Key among them are thyroid hormone, calcitonin, and iodine.

Thyroid Hormone

Thyroid hormone is comprised of T_4 and T_3, two separate hormones produced by the thyroid gland. Both are amino acids that contain iodine molecules bound to the amino acid structure; T_4 contains four iodine atoms in each molecule, and T_3 contains three. These hormones are synthesized and stored bound to proteins in the cells of the thyroid gland

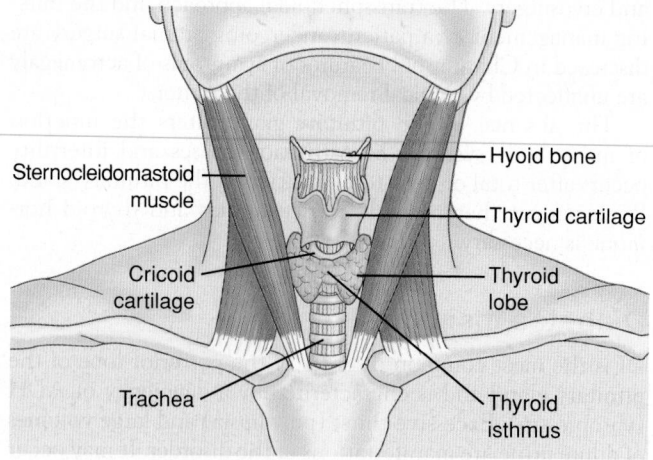

Figure 52-3 • The thyroid gland and surrounding structures.

Sternocleidomastoid muscle

Cricoid cartilage

Trachea

Hyoid bone

Thyroid cartilage

Thyroid lobe

Thyroid isthmus

until needed for release into the bloodstream. Three thyroid-binding hormones—thyroxine-binding globulin (TBG), transthyretin (formerly known as thyroid-binding prealbumin), and albumin—bind and transport T_3 and T_4 (Porth 2015).

Synthesis of Thyroid Hormone

Iodine is essential to the thyroid gland for synthesis of its hormones. The major use of iodine in the body is by the thyroid, and the major derangement in iodine deficiency is alteration of thyroid function. Iodide is ingested in the diet and absorbed into the blood in the GI tract. The thyroid gland is extremely efficient at taking up iodide from the blood and concentrating it within the cells, where iodide ions are converted to iodine molecules, which react with tyrosine (an amino acid) to form the thyroid hormones (Salvatore, Davies, Sclumberger, et al., 2016).

Regulation of Thyroid Hormone

The secretion of T_3 and T_4 by the thyroid gland is controlled by TSH (also called *thyrotropin*) from the anterior pituitary gland. TSH controls the rate of thyroid hormone release through a negative feedback mechanism. In turn, the level of thyroid hormone in the blood determines the release of TSH. If the thyroid hormone concentration in the blood decreases, the release of TSH increases, which causes increased output of T_3 and T_4. The term **euthyroid** refers to thyroid hormone production that is normal.

TRH, secreted by the hypothalamus, exerts a modulating influence on the release of TSH from the pituitary. Environmental factors, such as a decrease in temperature, may lead to increased secretion of TRH, resulting in elevated secretion of thyroid hormones. Figure 52-4 shows the hypothalamic–pituitary–thyroid axis, which regulates thyroid hormone production.

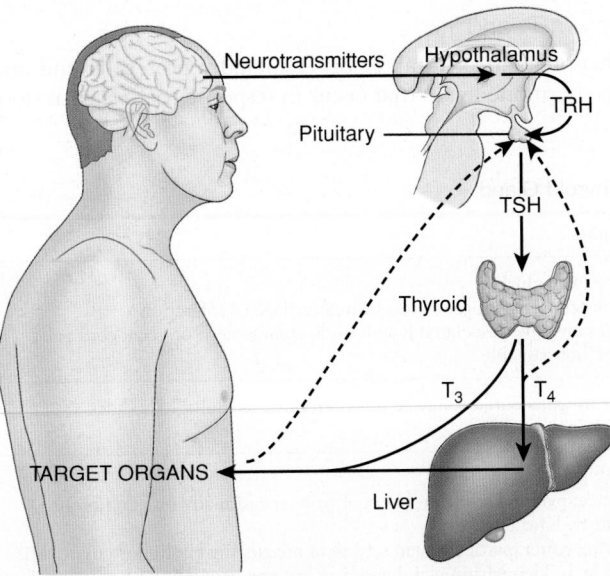

Figure 52-4 • The hypothalamic–pituitary–thyroid axis. Thyroid-releasing hormone (TRH) from the hypothalamus stimulates the pituitary gland to secrete thyroid-stimulating hormone (TSH). TSH stimulates the thyroid to produce thyroid hormone (triiodothyronine $[T_3]$ and thyroxine $[T_4]$). High circulating levels of T_3 and T_4 inhibit further TSH secretion and thyroid hormone production through a negative feedback mechanism (*dashed lines*).

Function of Thyroid Hormone

The main function of thyroid hormone is to control cellular metabolic activity. T_4, a relatively weak hormone, maintains body metabolism in a steady state. T_3 is about five times as potent as T_4 and has a more rapid metabolic action. These hormones accelerate metabolic processes by increasing the level of specific enzymes that contribute to oxygen consumption and altering the responsiveness of tissues to other hormones. The thyroid hormones influence cell replication and are important in brain development. Thyroid hormone is also necessary for normal growth. Thyroid hormones affect virtually every major organ system and tissue function, including the basal metabolic rate, tissue thermogenesis, serum cholesterol levels, and vascular resistance (Porth, 2015).

Calcitonin

Calcitonin, or thyrocalcitonin, is another important hormone secreted by the thyroid gland. It is secreted in response to high plasma levels of calcium, and it reduces the plasma level of calcium by increasing its deposition in bone.

Pathophysiology

Inadequate secretion of thyroid hormone during fetal and neonatal development results in intellectual disability and stunted physical growth (congenital hypothyroidism) because of general depression of metabolic activity (LaFranchi, 2016). In adults, hypothyroidism manifests as lethargy, slow mentation, weight gain, constipation, cold intolerance, and generalized slowing of body functions (Surks, 2016a).

Oversecretion of thyroid hormones (hyperthyroidism) is manifested by a greatly increased metabolic rate. Many of the other characteristics of hyperthyroidism result from the increased response to circulating catecholamines (epinephrine and norepinephrine). Oversecretion of thyroid hormones is usually associated with an enlarged thyroid gland known as a **goiter**. Goiter also commonly occurs with iodine deficiency. In this latter condition, lack of iodine results in low levels of circulating thyroid hormones, which causes increased release of TSH; the elevated TSH causes overproduction of thyroglobulin (a precursor of T_3 and T_4) and hypertrophy of the thyroid gland.

Assessment

Physical Examination

The thyroid gland is inspected and palpated routinely in all patients. Inspection begins with identification of landmarks. The lower neck region between the sternocleidomastoid muscles is inspected for swelling or asymmetry. The patient is instructed to extend the neck slightly and swallow. Thyroid tissue rises normally with swallowing. The thyroid is then palpated for size, shape, consistency, symmetry, and the presence of tenderness (Weber & Kelley, 2014).

The clinician may examine the thyroid from an anterior or a posterior position. In the posterior position, both hands encircle the patient's neck. The thumbs rest on the nape of the neck, while the index and middle fingers palpate for the thyroid isthmus and the anterior surfaces of the lateral lobes.

When palpable, the isthmus is perceived as firm and of a rubber-band consistency.

The left lobe is examined by positioning the patient so that the neck flexes slightly forward and to the left. The thyroid cartilage is then displaced to the left with the fingers of the right hand. This maneuver displaces the left lobe deep into the sternocleidomastoid muscle, where it can be more easily palpated. The left lobe is then palpated by placing the left thumb deep into the posterior area of the sternocleidomastoid muscle, while the index and middle fingers exert opposite pressure in the anterior portion of the muscle. Having the patient swallow during the maneuver may assist the examiner to locate the thyroid as it ascends in the neck. The procedure is reversed to examine the right lobe. The isthmus is the only portion of the thyroid that is normally palpable. If a patient has a very thin neck, two thin, smooth, nontender lobes may also be palpable.

If palpation discloses an enlarged thyroid gland, both lobes are auscultated using the diaphragm of the stethoscope. Auscultation identifies the localized audible vibration of a bruit. This is indicative of increased blood flow through the thyroid gland associated with hyperthyroidism and necessitates referral to a primary provider. Other abnormal findings that require referral for further evaluation may include a soft texture (**Graves disease**), firmness (Hashimoto **thyroiditis** or malignancy), and tenderness (thyroiditis) (see Table 52-2) (Weber & Kelley, 2014).

Diagnostic Evaluation

Assessment measures in addition to palpation and auscultation include thyroid function tests, such as laboratory measurement of thyroid hormones, thyroid scanning, biopsy, and ultrasonography. The most widely used tests are serum immunoassay for TSH and free T_4 (U.S. Preventive Services Task Force [USPSTF], 2015). Free T_4 levels correlate with metabolic status; they are elevated in hyperthyroidism and decreased in hypothyroidism. Ultrasound, CT, and MRI may be used to clarify or confirm the results of other diagnostic studies.

Thyroid Tests

Serum Thyroid-Stimulating Hormone

Measurement of the serum TSH concentration is the primary screening test of thyroid function (USPSTF, 2015). Measurement of TSH has a high sensitivity of about 98% and specificity of about 92% when used to confirm clinically suspected thyroid disease in persons referred to an endocrinologist (USPSTF, 2015). The ability to detect minute changes in serum TSH makes it possible to distinguish subclinical thyroid disease from euthyroid states in patients with low or high normal values. Measurement of TSH is also used for monitoring thyroid hormone replacement therapy and for differentiating between disorders of the thyroid gland itself and disorders of the pituitary or hypothalamus.

There are differing opinions among professional organizations regarding who should be screened for thyroid disease and when. The USPSTF (2015) does not recommend universal screening of asymptomatic nonpregnant adults. The American Academy of Family Physicians (AFP) supports this recommendation. The American Association of Clinical Endocrinologists (AACE) recommends screening for hypothyroidism in patients older than 60 years and aggressive case finding in persons at risk for hypothyroidism and in women who are planning pregnancy. The American Thyroid Association (ATA) recommends TSH screening for all adults beginning at 35 years of age and every 5 years thereafter (Garber, Cobin, Gharib, et al., 2012).

Serum Free T_4

Serum free T_4 is a direct measurement of free (unbound) thyroxine, the only metabolically active fraction of T_4. The range of free T_4 in serum is normally 0.9 to 1.7 ng/dL (11.5 to 21.8 pmol/L). When measured by the dialysis method, free T_4 is not affected by variations in protein binding and is the procedure of choice for monitoring the changes in T_4 secretion during treatment for hyperthyroidism.

Serum T_3 and T_4

Measurement of total T_3 or T_4 includes protein-bound and free hormone levels that occur in response to TSH secretion.

TABLE 52-2 Summary of Findings on Physical Examination of the Thyroid Gland

Physical Finding	Differential Diagnosis	Special Features
Single nodule	Autonomously functioning adenoma	Opposite lobe not palpable
	Adenoma or adenomatous nodule	Rubbery, firm; tenderness suggests recent hemorrhage or infarction
	Cancer	Usually hard; may have associated lymph node enlargement or vocal cord palsy
	Hyperplasia secondary to unilobar agenesis	Opposite lobe not palpable
Multiple nodules	Multinodular goiter	Firm lobes or irregular surface may be misinterpreted as multiple nodules
	Hashimoto thyroiditis	
Diffuse goiter	Graves disease	Bruit or thrill; pyramidal lobe
	Hashimoto thyroiditis	Irregular surface; pyramidal lobe; rubbery or firm; occasionally tender; fibrous variant may be hard
	Thyroid lymphoma	Rapidly growing goiter, particularly in setting of preexisting Hashimoto thyroiditis
	Multinodular goiter	Nodules may be hidden within gland and may become apparent with thyroid hormone suppression
Tenderness	Subacute thyroiditis	Unilateral or bilateral; tenderness often severe
	Hemorrhagic or infarcted adenoma	Discrete nodule with tenderness
	Hashimoto thyroiditis	Mild tenderness
	Cancer	Irregular, firm thyroid nodule with chronic tenderness

T_4 is 70% bound to TBG; T_3 is bound less firmly. Only 0.03% of T_4 and 0.3% of T_3 are unbound. Serious systemic illnesses, medications (e.g., oral contraceptives, corticosteroids, carbamazepine [Tegretol], salicylates), and protein wasting as a result of nephrosis or the use of androgens may interfere with accurate test results (Fischbach & Dunning, 2015). Normal range for T_4 is 5.4 to 11.5 µg/dL (57 to 148 nmol/L) (Fischbach & Dunning, 2015). Although serum T_3 and T_4 levels generally increase or decrease together, the T_3 level appears to be a more accurate indicator of hyperthyroidism or severity of the disorder, as T_4 levels are often within normal range. The normal range for serum T_3 is 80 to 200 ng/dL (1.2 to 3.1 nmol/L) (Fischbach & Dunning, 2015).

T_3 Resin Uptake Test

The T_3 resin uptake test is an indirect measure of unsaturated TBG. Its purpose is to determine the amount of thyroid hormone bound to TBG and the number of available binding sites. This provides an index of the amount of thyroid hormone already present in the circulation. Normally, TBG is not fully saturated with thyroid hormone, and additional binding sites are available to combine with radioiodine-labeled T_3 added to the blood specimen. The normal T_3 uptake value is 25% to 35% (relative uptake fraction, 0.25 to 0.35), which indicates that about one third of the available sites of TBG are occupied by thyroid hormone (Fischbach & Dunning, 2015). If the number of free or unoccupied binding sites is low, as in hyperthyroidism, the T_3 uptake is greater than 35% (0.35). If the number of available sites is high, as occurs in hypothyroidism, the test result is less than 25% (0.25).

T_3 uptake is useful in evaluating thyroid hormone levels in patients who have received diagnostic or therapeutic doses of iodine. The test results may be altered by the use of estrogens, androgens, salicylates, phenytoin, anticoagulants, or corticosteroids.

Thyroid Antibodies

Autoimmune thyroid diseases include both hypothyroid and hyperthyroid conditions. Results of testing by immunoassay techniques for antithyroid antibodies are positive in chronic autoimmune thyroid disease (90%), Hashimoto thyroiditis (100%), Graves disease (80%), and other organ-specific autoimmune diseases, such as systemic lupus erythematosus (SLE) and rheumatoid arthritis. Antithyroid antibody titers are normally present in 5% to 10% of the population and increase with age.

Radioactive Iodine Uptake

The radioactive iodine uptake test measures the rate of iodine uptake by the thyroid gland. The patient is given a tracer dose of iodine 123 (^{123}I) or another radionuclide, and a count is made over the thyroid gland with a scintillation counter, which detects and counts the gamma rays released from the breakdown of ^{123}I in the thyroid. It measures the proportion of the given dose that is present in the thyroid gland at a specific time after its administration. It is a simple test and provides reliable results. It is affected by the patient's intake of iodide or thyroid hormone; therefore, a careful preliminary clinical history is essential in evaluating results. Normal values vary from one geographic region to another and with the intake of iodine. Patients with hyperthyroidism

exhibit a high uptake of the ^{123}I (in some patients, as high as 90%), whereas patients with hypothyroidism exhibit a very low uptake.

Fine-Needle Aspiration Biopsy

The use of a small-gauge needle to sample the thyroid tissue for biopsy is a safe and accurate method of detecting malignancy. It is often the initial test for evaluation of thyroid masses. Results are reported as (1) negative (benign), (2) positive (malignant), (3) indeterminate (suspicious), and (4) inadequate (nondiagnostic) (Dhyani, Faquin, Lubitz, et al., 2013).

Thyroid Scan, Radioscan, or Scintiscan

In a thyroid scan, a scintillation detector or gamma camera moves back and forth across the area to be studied in a series of parallel tracks, and a visual image is made of the distribution of radioactivity in the area being scanned. The most commonly used isotopes of iodine are ^{123}I and iodine 131 (^{131}I) (Fischbach & Dunning, 2015).

Scans are helpful in determining the location, size, shape, and anatomic function of the thyroid gland, particularly when thyroid tissue is substernal or large (Fischbach & Dunning, 2015). Identifying areas of increased function ("hot" areas) or decreased function ("cold" areas) can assist in diagnosis. Although most areas of decreased function do not represent malignancies, lack of function increases the likelihood of malignancy, particularly if only one nonfunctioning area is present. Scanning of the entire body, to obtain the total body profile, may be carried out in a search for a functioning thyroid metastasis (i.e., a lesion that produces thyroid hormones).

Serum Thyroglobulin

Thyroglobulin (Tg) can be measured reliably in the serum by radioimmunoassay. Clinically, it is used to detect persistence or recurrence of thyroid carcinoma.

Nursing Implications

When thyroid tests are scheduled, it is necessary to determine if the patient is allergic to iodine (shellfish) and whether the patient has taken medications or agents that contain iodine, because these may alter the test results (Fischbach & Dunning, 2015). Obvious sources of iodine-containing medications include contrast agents and those used to treat thyroid disorders such as radioactive iodine. Less obvious sources of iodine are topical antiseptics; multivitamin preparations; food supplements that may contain kelp and seaweed (frequently found in health food stores); and amiodarone (Cordarone), an antiarrhythmic agent (Surks, 2016b). Other medications that may affect test results are estrogens, salicylates, amphetamines, chemotherapeutic agents, antibiotics, corticosteroids, and diuretics. This information should be documented in the patient's medical record and the laboratory requisition. Chart 52-2 gives a list of selected medications that may interfere with accurate testing of thyroid gland function.

Hypothyroidism

Hypothyroidism results from suboptimal levels of thyroid hormone. Thyroid deficiency can affect all body functions and

Chart 52-2

PHARMACOLOGY

Selected Medications That May Alter Thyroid Test Results

amiodarone (Cordarone)
aspirin
cimetidine (Tagamet)
diazepam (Valium)
furosemide (Lasix)
heparin
lithium (Lithotabs)
phenytoin (Dilantin) and other anticonvulsants
propranolol (Inderal)

Adapted from Fischbach, F., & Dunning, M. B. (2015). *A manual of laboratory and diagnostic tests* (9th ed.). Philadelphia, PA: Lippincott Williams & Wilkins.

can range from mild, subclinical forms to **myxedema** (severe deficiency discussed later), an advanced life-threatening form (Ross, 2016a). The most common cause of hypothyroidism in adults is autoimmune thyroiditis (Hashimoto disease), in which the immune system attacks the thyroid gland. Symptoms of hyperthyroidism may later be followed by those of hypothyroidism and myxedema. Hypothyroidism also commonly occurs in patients with previous hyperthyroidism that has been treated with radioiodine or antithyroid medications or **thyroidectomy** (surgical removal of all or part of the thyroid gland). In addition, there is an increased incidence of thyroid cancer in men who have undergone radiation therapy for head and neck cancer. Therefore, testing of thyroid function is recommended for all patients who receive such treatment. Other causes of hypothyroidism are presented in Chart 52-3.

More than 95% of patients with hypothyroidism have primary or thyroidal hypothyroidism, which refers to dysfunction of the thyroid gland itself. If the cause of the thyroid dysfunction is failure of the pituitary gland, the hypothalamus, or both, the hypothyroidism is known as central hypothyroidism. If the cause is entirely a pituitary disorder, it may be referred to as pituitary or secondary hypothyroidism. If the cause is a disorder of the hypothalamus resulting in inadequate secretion of TSH due to decreased stimulation of TRH, it is referred to as hypothalamic or tertiary hypothyroidism. If thyroid deficiency is present at birth, it is referred to as neonatal hypothyroidism. In such instances, the mother may also have thyroid deficiency. The term *myxedema* refers to the accumulation of mucopolysaccharides in subcutaneous and other interstitial tissues. Although myxedema occurs in long-standing hypothyroidism, the term is used appropriately only to describe the extreme symptoms of severe hypothyroidism (Ross, 2016a).

Clinical Manifestations

Extreme fatigue makes it difficult for the person to complete a full day's work or participate in usual activities. Reports of hair loss, brittle nails, and dry skin are common, and numbness and tingling of the fingers may occur. On occasion, the voice may become husky, and the patient may complain of hoarseness. Hypothyroidism affects women five to eight times more frequently than men and occurs most often between 40 and 70 years of age (Visser, Visser, & Peeters, 2013). Menstrual disturbances such as menorrhagia or amenorrhea occur, in addition to loss of libido. The prevalence of the disease increases with increasing age; however, experts question if the standard reference range for serum TSH levels (0.4-4.5 mU/L) should be used for diagnosis in the older adult. Women and older adults may exhibit different symptoms (Dunn & Turner, 2016; Harman, 2016; Visser et al., 2013).

Severe hypothyroidism results in a subnormal body temperature and pulse rate. The patient usually begins to gain weight even without an increase in food intake, although he or she may be cachectic. The skin becomes thickened because of an accumulation of mucopolysaccharides in the subcutaneous tissues. The hair thins and falls out, and the face becomes expressionless and masklike. The patient often complains of being cold even in a warm environment.

At first, the patient may be irritable and may complain of fatigue, but as the condition progresses, the emotional responses are subdued. The mental processes become dulled, and the patient appears apathetic. Speech is slow, the tongue enlarges, the hands and feet increase in size, and deafness may occur. The patient frequently reports constipation.

Advanced hypothyroidism may produce personality and cognitive changes characteristic of dementia. Inadequate ventilation and sleep apnea can occur with severe hypothyroidism (Morgan & Tsai, 2015). Pleural effusion, pericardial effusion, and respiratory muscle weakness may also occur.

Severe hypothyroidism is associated with an elevated serum cholesterol level, atherosclerosis, coronary artery disease, and poor left ventricular function. The patient with advanced hypothyroidism is hypothermic and abnormally sensitive to sedative, opioid, and anesthetic agents, which must be given with extreme caution.

Patients with unrecognized hypothyroidism who are undergoing surgery are at increased risk for intraoperative hypotension, postoperative heart failure, and altered mental status.

Myxedema coma is a rare life-threatening condition. It is the decompensated state of severe hypothyroidism in which the patient is hypothermic and unconscious (Ross, 2016a). This condition may develop with undiagnosed hypothyroidism and may be precipitated by infection or other systemic

Chart 52-3 Causes of Hypothyroidism

Autoimmune disease (Hashimoto thyroiditis, post-Graves disease)
Atrophy of thyroid gland with aging
Therapy for hyperthyroidism
   Radioactive iodine (^{131}I)
   Thyroidectomy
Medications
   Lithium
   Iodine compounds
   Antithyroid medications
Radiation to head and neck in treatment for head and neck cancers, lymphoma
Infiltrative diseases of the thyroid (amyloidosis, scleroderma, lymphoma)
Iodine deficiency and iodine excess

disease or by use of sedatives or opioid analgesic agents. Patients may also experience myxedema coma if they forget to take their thyroid replacement medication. The condition occurs most often among older women in the winter months and appears to be precipitated by cold. However, the disorder can affect any age group.

In myxedema coma, the patient may initially show signs of depression, diminished cognitive status, lethargy, and somnolence (Ross, 2016a). Increasing lethargy may progress to stupor. The patient's respiratory drive is depressed, resulting in alveolar hypoventilation, progressive carbon dioxide retention, narcosis, and coma. In addition, patients with myxedema coma can also exhibit hyponatremia, hypoglycemia, hypoventilation, hypotension, bradycardia, and hypothermia. These symptoms, along with cardiovascular collapse and shock, require aggressive and intensive supportive and hemodynamic therapy if the patient is to survive. Although there has been a decline in mortality rates over the past two decades due to early intervention and improved therapies, the mortality rate remains high at 30% to 40%. Patients at greatest risk are older adults, individuals with cardiac complications, reduced consciousness, persistent hypothermia, and sepsis (Ross, 2016a).

Medical Management

The objectives in the management of hypothyroidism are to restore a normal metabolic state by replacing the missing hormone, as well as prevention of disease progression and complications.

Pharmacologic Therapy

Synthetic levothyroxine (Synthroid or Levothroid) is commonly prescribed for treating hypothyroidism and suppressing nontoxic goiters (Jonklaas, Bianco, Bauer, et al., 2014). The dosage is based on the patient's serum TSH concentration. If replacement therapy is adequate, the symptoms of myxedema disappear and normal metabolic activity is resumed. Although rare, if the disease progresses to myxedema coma, IV administration of T_4 and T_3 are recommended rather than T_4 alone. T_4 is administered IV until the patient is able to safely take T_4 in oral form. T_3 is administered IV until the patient is stable (Ross, 2016a).

Administration of high-dose **glucocorticoids** (hydrocortisone) every 8 to 12 hours for 24 hours followed by low-dose therapy is recommended until coexisting adrenal insufficiency is ruled out (Ross, 2016a). Serum levels of T_4, TSH, and cortisol should be obtained before and after administration of ACTH and before administration of glucocorticoid and thyroid hormone therapies. Associated conditions such as infection, GI bleeding, hyponatremia, hypotension, bradycardia, hypoglycemia, and hypothermia will also require appropriate pharmacologic management (Ross, 2016a).

Prevention of Cardiac Dysfunction

Any patient who has had hypothyroidism for a long period usually has associated elevated serum cholesterol, atherosclerosis, and coronary artery disease. As long as metabolism is subnormal and the tissues (including the myocardium) require relatively little oxygen, a reduction in blood supply is tolerated without overt symptoms of coronary artery disease. When thyroid hormone is given, the oxygen demand increases, but oxygen delivery cannot be increased unless, or until, the atherosclerosis improves. This occurs very slowly, if at all. The occurrence of angina and acute coronary syndrome (see Chapter 27) is the signal that the oxygen needs of the myocardium exceed its blood supply. Angina or dysrhythmias can occur when thyroid replacement is initiated because thyroid hormones enhance the cardiovascular effects of catecholamines.

> ### ▶ Quality and Safety Nursing Alert
>
> *The nurse must monitor for signs and symptoms of ACS, which can occur in response to therapy in patients with severe, long-standing hypothyroidism or myxedema coma, especially during the early phase of treatment. ACS must be aggressively treated at once to avoid morbid complications (e.g., myocardial infarction).*

Obviously, if angina or dysrhythmias occur, thyroid hormone administration must be discontinued immediately. Later, when it can be resumed safely, it should be prescribed cautiously at a lower dosage and with close monitoring by the primary provider and the nurse.

Prevention of Medication Interactions

Oral thyroid hormones interact with many other medications. There is a decrease in thyroid hormone absorption when patients are also taking magnesium-containing antacids. Thyroid hormones may also decrease the pharmacologic effects of digitalis glycosides. Doses of anticoagulant agents need to be decreased when beginning thyroid replacement because of the increased risk of bleeding (Comerford, 2015).

Even in small IV doses, hypnotic and sedative agents may induce profound somnolence, lasting far longer than anticipated and leading to narcosis (stuporlike condition). Furthermore, they are likely to cause respiratory depression, which can easily be fatal because of decreased respiratory reserve and alveolar hypoventilation. The dose of these medications should be one half or one third of that typically prescribed for patients of similar age and weight with normal thyroid function.

Supportive Therapy

Severe hypothyroidism and myxedema coma require prompt, aggressive management to maintain vital functions. Arterial blood gases may be measured to determine carbon dioxide retention and to guide the use of assisted ventilation to combat hypoventilation. Oxygen saturation levels should be monitored using pulse oximetry. Fluids are given cautiously because of the danger of water intoxication. Passive rewarming with a blanket is recommended versus active rewarming such as application of external heat (e.g., heating pads) (Ross, 2016a). The latter should be avoided to prevent increased oxygen demands and hypotension. If myxedema has progressed to myxedema coma, refer to the current recommendations stated in the previous Pharmacologic Therapy section.

Nursing Management

Nursing care of the patient with hypothyroidism and myxedema is summarized in the plan of nursing care in Chart 52-4. In patients with hypothyroidism, the effects of

(*text continued on page 1518*)

PLAN OF NURSING CARE

Chart 52-4

Care of the Patient With Hypothyroidism

NURSING DIAGNOSIS: Activity intolerance related to insufficient physiologic or psychological energy
GOAL: Increased participation in activities and increased independence

Nursing Interventions	Rationale	Expected Outcomes

1. Promote independence in self-care activities.
  a. Space activities to promote rest and exercise as tolerated.
  b. Assist with self-care activities when patient is fatigued.
  c. Provide stimulation through conversation and nonstressful activities.
  d. Monitor patient's response to increasing activities.
	1. Encouragement needed in patients with decreased energy
	  a. Encourages activities while allowing time for adequate rest
	  b. Permits patient to participate to the extent possible in self-care activities
	  c. Promotes interest without stressing the patient
	  d. Guards against over- and underexertion by the patient
		• Participates in self-care activities
		• Reports increased level of energy
		• Displays interest and awareness in environment
		• Participates in activities and events in environment
		• Participates in family events and activities
		• Reports no chest pain, increased fatigue, or breathlessness with increased level of activity

NURSING DIAGNOSIS: Risk for imbalanced body temperature
GOAL: Maintenance of normal body temperature

Nursing Interventions	Rationale	Expected Outcomes
1. Provide extra layer of clothing or extra blanket. 2. Avoid and discourage the use of external heat source (e.g., heating pads, electric or warming blankets). 3. Monitor patient's body temperature and report decreases from patient's baseline value. 4. Protect from exposure to cold and drafts.	1. Minimizes heat loss 2. Reduces risk of peripheral vasodilation and vascular collapse 3. Detects decreased body temperature and onset of myxedema coma 4. Increases patient's level of comfort and decreases further heat loss	• Experiences relief of discomfort and cold intolerance • Maintains baseline body temperature • Reports adequate feeling of warmth and lack of chilling • Uses extra layer of clothing or extra blanket • Explains rationale for avoiding external heat source

NURSING DIAGNOSIS: Constipation related to diminished gastrointestinal peristalsis
GOAL: Return of normal bowel function

Nursing Interventions	Rationale	Expected Outcomes
1. Encourage increased fluid intake within limits of fluid restriction. 2. Provide foods high in fiber. 3. Instruct patient about foods with high water content. 4. Monitor bowel function. 5. Encourage increased mobility within patient's exercise tolerance. 6. Encourage patient to use laxatives and enemas sparingly.	1. Promotes passage of soft stools 2. Increases bulk of stools and more frequent bowel movements 3. Provides rationale for patient to increase fluid intake 4. Permits detection of constipation and return to normal bowel pattern 5. Promotes evacuation of the bowel 6. Minimizes patient's dependence on laxatives and enemas and encourages normal pattern of bowel evacuation	• Reports normal bowel function • Identifies and consumes foods high in fiber • Drinks recommended amount of fluid each day • Participates in gradually increasing exercises • Uses laxatives as prescribed and avoids excessive dependence on laxatives and enemas

NURSING DIAGNOSIS: Deficient knowledge about the therapeutic regimen for lifelong thyroid replacement therapy
GOAL: Knowledge and acceptance of the prescribed therapeutic regimen

Nursing Interventions	Rationale	Expected Outcomes
1. Explain rationale for thyroid hormone replacement. 2. Describe desired effects of medication to patient. 3. Assist patient to develop schedule and checklist to ensure self-administration of thyroid replacement.	1. Provides rationale for patient to use thyroid hormone replacement as prescribed 2. Provides encouragement to patient by identifying improved physical status and well-being that will occur with thyroid hormone therapy and return to a euthyroid state 3. Increases chances that medication will be taken as prescribed	• Describes therapeutic regimen correctly • Explains rationale for thyroid hormone replacement • Identifies positive outcomes of thyroid hormone replacement • Administers medication to self as prescribed • Identifies adverse side effects that should be reported promptly to primary provider: recurrence of symptoms of hypothyroidism and occurrence of symptoms of hyperthyroidism

Chart 52-4

PLAN OF NURSING CARE (Continued)
Care of the Patient With Hypothyroidism

Nursing Interventions	Rationale	Expected Outcomes
4. Describe signs and symptoms of over- and underdose of medication. 5. Explain the necessity for long-term follow-up to patient and family.	4. Serves as check for patient to determine if therapeutic goals are met 5. Increases likelihood that hypo- or hyperthyroidism will be detected and treated	• Restates need for periodic/long-term follow-up visits to primary provider

NURSING DIAGNOSIS: Ineffective breathing pattern related to depressed ventilation
GOAL: Improved respiratory status and maintenance of normal breathing pattern

Nursing Interventions	Rationale	Expected Outcomes
1. Monitor respiratory rate, depth, pattern, pulse oximetry, and arterial blood gases. 2. Encourage deep breathing, coughing, and the use of incentive spirometry. 3. Administer medications (hypnotics and sedatives) with caution. 4. Maintain patent airway through suction and ventilatory support if indicated (see Chapter 21 for care of patients requiring mechanical ventilation).	1. Identifies patient's baseline to monitor further changes and evaluate effectiveness of interventions 2. Prevents atelectasis and promotes adequate ventilation 3. Patients with hypothyroidism are very susceptible to respiratory depression with the use of hypnotics and sedatives 4. The use of an artificial airway and ventilatory support may be necessary with respiratory depression	• Shows improved respiratory status and maintenance of normal breathing pattern • Demonstrates normal respiratory rate, depth, and pattern • Takes deep breaths, coughs, and uses incentive spirometry when encouraged • Demonstrates normal breath sounds without adventitious sounds on auscultation • Explains rationale for cautious use of medications • Cooperates with suction procedure and ventilator support when necessary

NURSING DIAGNOSIS: Acute confusion related to depressed metabolism and altered cardiovascular and respiratory status
GOAL: Improved thought processes

Nursing Interventions	Rationale	Expected Outcomes
1. Orient patient to time, place, date, and events around him or her. 2. Provide stimulation through conversation and nonthreatening activities. 3. Explain to patient and family that change in cognitive and mental functioning is a result of disease process. 4. Monitor cognitive and mental processes and response of these to medication and other therapy.	1. Provides reality orientation to patient 2. Provides stimulation within patient's level of tolerance for stress 3. Reassures patient and family about the cause of the cognitive changes and that a positive outcome is possible with appropriate treatment 4. Permits evaluation of the effectiveness of treatment	• Shows improved cognitive functioning • Identifies time, place, date, and events correctly • Responds appropriately when stimulated • Responds spontaneously as treatment becomes effective • Interacts spontaneously with family and environment • Explains that change in mental and cognitive processes is a result of disease processes • Takes medications as prescribed to prevent decrease in cognitive processes

COLLABORATIVE PROBLEM: Myxedema and myxedema coma
GOAL: Evidence of progression to pre-coma baseline without incurring additional complications

Nursing Interventions	Rationale	Expected Outcomes

1. Monitor patient for increasing severity of signs and symptoms of hypothyroidism:
   a. Decreased level of consciousness
   b. Decreased vital signs (blood pressure, respiratory rate, temperature, pulse rate)
   c. Increasing difficulty in awakening or arousing patient
 2. Assist in ventilatory support if respiratory depression and failure occur.
 	
 3. Administer prescribed medications (e.g., thyroxine) with extreme caution.
 	
 4. Turn and reposition patient at intervals.
 5. Avoid the use of hypnotic, sedative, and analgesic agents.
	1. Extreme hypothyroidism may lead to myxedema, myxedema coma, and slowing of all body systems if untreated
	
	 2. Ventilatory support is necessary to maintain adequate oxygenation and maintenance of airway
	 3. The slow metabolism and atherosclerosis of myxedema may result in angina with administration of thyroxine
	 4. Minimizes risks associated with immobility
	 5. Altered metabolism of these agents greatly increases the risks of their use in myxedema
		• Exhibits reversal of myxedema and myxedema coma
		 • Responds appropriately to questions and surroundings
		 • Vital signs return to normal or near-normal ranges
		 • Respiratory status improves with adequate spontaneous ventilatory effort
		 • Reports no episodes of angina or other indicators of cardiac insufficiency
		 • Experiences minimal or no complications caused by immobility

analgesic, sedative, and anesthetic agents are prolonged. The nurse should carefully monitor patients who are prescribed these agents for adverse effects. Older patients are at increased risk because of age-related changes in liver and renal function.

> ### Quality and Safety Nursing Alert
>
> *Medications are given to the patient with hypothyroidism with extreme caution because of the potential for altered metabolism and excretion, as well as depressed metabolic rate and respiratory status.*

Promoting Home, Community-Based, and Transitional Care

Educating Patients About Self-Care

The patient and family require education and support to manage this complex disorder at home. Oral and written instructions should be provided regarding the following:

- Desired actions and side effects of medications
- Correct medication administration ("Take first thing in the morning with a full glass of water.")
- Importance of continuing to take the medications as prescribed even after symptoms improve
- When to seek medical attention
- Importance of nutrition and diet to promote weight loss and normal bowel patterns
- Importance of periodic follow-up testing

The patient and family should be educated that the symptoms observed during the course of the disorder will disappear with effective treatment (see Chart 52-5).

Continuing and Transitional Care

If indicated, a referral is made for home, community-based or transitional care. The nurse monitors the patient's recovery and ability to cope with the recent changes, and assesses the patient's physical and cognitive status and the patient's and family's understanding of previous education. The nurse documents and reports to the patient's primary provider subtle signs and symptoms that may indicate either inadequate or excessive thyroid hormone.

Gerontologic Considerations

The prevalence of hypothyroidism increases with age, most often among women (Visser et al., 2013). The higher prevalence of hypothyroidism among older adults may be related to age-related alterations in immune function and complicated by multiple comorbidities.

Most patients with primary hypothyroidism present with long-standing mild to moderate hypothyroidism. Subclinical disease is common among older women and can be asymptomatic or mistaken for other medical conditions. Subtle symptoms of hypothyroidism, such as fatigue, muscle aches, and mental confusion, may be attributed to the normal aging process by patients, families, and health care providers; therefore, these symptoms require close attention (Visser et al., 2013). In addition, signs and symptoms of hypothyroidism in older adults are often atypical, and manifestations of hypothyroidism and hyperthyroidism may blur. Patients may have few or no symptoms until dysfunction is severe. Depression, apathy, and decreased mobility or activity may be the major initial symptoms and may be accompanied by significant weight loss. Constipation affects one fourth of older patients.

In older patients, treatment is recommended for those who have a TSH in excess of 10 mU/L (Visser et al., 2013). In those with mild to moderate hypothyroidism, thyroid hormone replacement is individually tailored and must be started with low dosages and increased gradually to prevent serious cardiovascular side effects (Visser et al., 2013). Angina, for example, may occur with rapid thyroid replacement in the presence of coronary artery disease secondary to the hypothyroid state. Heart failure and tachydysrhythmias may worsen during the transition from the hypothyroid state to the normal metabolic state. Dementia may become more apparent during early thyroid hormone replacement in older patients with concomitant dementia.

Older patients with severe hypothyroidism and atherosclerosis may become confused and agitated if their metabolic rate is increased too quickly. Marked clinical improvement follows the administration of hormone replacement; such medication must be continued for life, even though signs of hypothyroidism disappear within 3 to 12 weeks.

Myxedema and myxedema coma usually occur exclusively in patients older than 50 years (Ross, 2016a). The

---

> ### Chart 52-5   HOME CARE CHECKLIST
> ### The Patient With Hypothyroidism (Myxedema)
>
> **At the completion of education, the patient and/or caregiver will be able to:**
>
> - State the impact of hypothyroidism and treatment on physiologic functioning, ADLs, IADLs, roles, relationships, and spirituality.
>   - State the need to avoid extreme cold temperature until condition is stable.
> - State precipitating factors and interventions for complications (hyperthyroidism, myxedema coma).
> - State the continuing potential effects of hypothyroidism on the body.
>   - State the potential for menstrual irregularities and potential for pregnancy in women.
>
> - State the importance of avoiding infection.
> - Relate how to reach primary provider with questions or complications.
> - State time and date of follow-up medical appointments, therapy, and testing.
> - Identify sources of support (e.g., friends, relatives, faith community, support groups, caregiver support).
> - Identify the need for health promotion, disease prevention, and screening activities
>
> ADL, activities of daily living; IADL, independent activities of daily living.

high mortality rate of myxedema coma mandates immediate IV administration of thyroid hormone and supportive management of other clinical manifestations such as hyponatremia, hypoglycemia, hypothermia, hypoventilation, and hypotension.

Older patients require periodic follow-up monitoring of serum TSH levels, because poor adherence with therapy may occur or the patient may take the medications erratically. A careful history can identify the need for further education about the importance of the medication.

Hyperthyroidism

Hyperthyroidism, a common endocrine disorder, is a form of **thyrotoxicosis** resulting from an excessive synthesis and secretion of endogenous or exogenous thyroid hormones by the thyroid (Bahn, Burch, Cooper, et al., 2011). The most common causes are Graves disease, toxic multinodular goiter, and toxic adenoma. Other causes include thyroiditis (inflammation of the thyroid gland) and excessive ingestion of thyroid hormone.

Graves disease, the most common cause of hyperthyroidism, is an autoimmune disorder that results from an excessive output of thyroid hormones caused by abnormal stimulation of the thyroid gland by circulating immunoglobulins (Bahn et al., 2011; Muldoon, Mai, & Burch, 2014). This disease affects women eight times more frequently than men, with onset usually between the second and fourth decades. The disorder may appear after an emotional shock, stress, or an infection, but the exact significance of these relationships is not understood.

Clinical Manifestations

Patients with hyperthyroidism exhibit a characteristic group of signs and symptoms. The presenting symptom is often nervousness. These patients are often emotionally hyperexcitable, irritable, and apprehensive; they cannot sit quietly; they suffer from palpitations; and their pulse is abnormally rapid at rest as well as on exertion. They tolerate heat poorly and perspire unusually freely. The skin is flushed continuously, with a characteristic salmon color in Caucasians, and is likely to be warm, soft, and moist. However, patients may report dry skin and diffuse pruritus. A fine tremor of the hands may be observed. Patients may exhibit ophthalmopathy, such as exophthalmos (abnormal protrusion of one or both eyeballs), which produces a startled facial expression. Despite treatment, these ocular changes are not always reversible (Weber & Kelley, 2014).

Other manifestations include an increased appetite and dietary intake, weight loss, fatigability and weakness (difficulty in climbing stairs and rising from a chair), amenorrhea, and changes in bowel function. Atrial fibrillation occurs in 15% of older adult patients with new-onset hyperthyroidism (Muldoon et al., 2014).

Cardiac effects may include sinus tachycardia or dysrhythmias, increased pulse pressure, and palpitations; these changes may be related to increased sensitivity to catecholamines or to changes in neurotransmitter turnover. Myocardial hypertrophy and heart failure may occur if the hyperthyroidism is severe and untreated.

The course of the disease may be mild, characterized by remissions and exacerbations, and terminate with spontaneous recovery in a few months or years. Conversely, it may progress relentlessly, with the untreated person becoming emaciated, intensely nervous, delirious, and even disoriented; eventually, the heart fails.

Symptoms of hyperthyroidism may occur with the release of excessive amounts of thyroid hormone as a result of inflammation after irradiation of the thyroid or destruction of thyroid tissue by tumor. Such symptoms may also occur with excessive administration of thyroid hormone for the treatment of hypothyroidism. Long-standing use of thyroid hormone in the absence of close monitoring may be a cause of symptoms of hyperthyroidism. It is also likely to result in premature osteoporosis, particularly in women.

Assessment and Diagnostic Findings

The thyroid gland is enlarged to some extent. It is soft and may pulsate; a thrill often can be palpated, and a bruit is heard over the thyroid arteries (Weber & Kelley, 2014). These are signs of greatly increased blood flow through the thyroid gland. In advanced cases, the diagnosis is made on the basis of the symptoms, a decrease in serum TSH, increased free T_4, and an increase in radioactive iodine uptake.

Medical Management

Appropriate treatment of hyperthyroidism depends on the underlying cause and often consists of a combination of therapies, including antithyroid agents, radioactive iodine, and surgery. Treatment of hyperthyroidism is directed toward reducing thyroid hyperactivity to relieve symptoms and preventing complications. The use of radioactive iodine is the most common form of treatment for Graves disease in North America. Beta-adrenergic blocking agents (e.g., propranolol [Inderal], atenolol [Tenormin], metoprolol [Lopressor]) are used as adjunctive therapy for symptomatic relief, particularly in transient thyroiditis (Ross, 2016c). The three treatments (radioactive iodine therapy, antithyroid medications [e.g., thionamides], and surgery) share the same complications: relapse or recurrent hyperthyroidism and permanent hypothyroidism. The rate of relapse increases in patients who have had very severe disease, a long history of dysfunction, ocular and cardiac symptoms, large goiter, or relapse after previous treatment.

Pharmacologic Therapy

Two forms of pharmacotherapy are available for treating hyperthyroidism and controlling excessive thyroid activity: (1) the use of irradiation by administration of the radioisotope ^{131}I for destructive effects on the thyroid gland and (2) antithyroid medications that interfere with the synthesis of thyroid hormones and other agents that control manifestations of hyperthyroidism.

Radioactive Iodine Therapy

Radioactive iodine has been used to treat toxic adenomas, toxic multinodular goiter, and most varieties of thyrotoxicosis. Radioactive iodine is contraindicated during pregnancy because it crosses the placenta. Women of childbearing age should be given a pregnancy test 48 hours before administration of radioactive iodine. They should also be instructed to not conceive for at least 6 months following treatment. To ensure that radioactivity is no longer actively concentrated in breast tissue, radioactive iodine should not be given until at least 6 weeks after lactation stops (Bahn et al., 2011).

The goal of radioactive iodine therapy (^{131}I) is to eliminate the hyperthyroid state with the administration of sufficient radiation in a single dose (Bahn et al., 2011). Almost all of the iodine that enters and is retained in the body becomes concentrated in the thyroid gland. Therefore, the radioactive isotope of iodine is concentrated in the thyroid gland, where it destroys thyroid cells without jeopardizing other radiosensitive tissues. Over a period of several weeks, thyroid cells exposed to the radioactive iodine are destroyed, resulting in reduction of the hyperthyroid state and inevitably hypothyroidism.

Some patients at high risk for complications of hyperthyroidism (e.g., older adults, patients with cardiovascular disease) may need pretreatment with antithyroid medications. Methimazole (MMI) is given 4 to 6 weeks prior to administration of radioactive iodine. The antithyroid medications are stopped 3 days before and restarted 3 days after administering radioactive iodine and then tapered over 4 to 6 weeks (Ross, 2016g).

The use of an ablative dose of radioactive iodine initially causes an acute release of thyroid hormone from the thyroid gland and may cause increased symptoms. The patient is observed for signs of **thyroid storm** (see Chart 52-6), a life-threatening condition manifested by cardiac dysrhythmias, fever, and neurologic impairment (Davies, Laurberg, & Bahn, 2016; Ross, 2016b). Beta-blockers are used to control these symptoms.

Thyroid hormone replacement is started 4 to 18 weeks after the antithyroid medications have been stopped based on the results of thyroid function tests. TSH measurements can be misleading in the early months following treatment with radioactive iodine. Therefore, serum free T_4 is the principal test (Bahn et al., 2011; Ross, 2016e) measured at 3 to 6 weeks following administration of radioactive iodine and then every 1 to 2 months until normal thyroid function is established. If TSH and free T_4 are both persistently low, the total T_3 then must be measured to differentiate between persistent hyperthyroidism (T_3 elevated) or transient hypothyroidism (T_3 normal or low) (Ross, 2016e). Once a normal thyroid state has been established, TSH should be measured every 6 to 12 months for life (Ross, 2016e).

A major advantage of treatment with radioactive iodine is that it avoids many of the side effects associated with antithyroid medications. However, some patients may elect to be treated with antithyroid medications rather than radioactive iodine for a variety of reasons, including fear of radiation.

Patients who receive radioactive iodine should be informed that they can contaminate their household and other persons through saliva, urine, or radiation emitting from their body. They should avoid sexual contact, sleeping in the same bed with other persons, having close contact with children and pregnant women, and sharing utensils and cups. The patient should follow the instructions provided by the primary provider regarding the time restrictions for these cautions because they are dose related (Ross, 2016e).

Chart 52-6   Thyroid Storm (Thyrotoxic Crisis, Thyrotoxicosis)

Thyroid storm (thyrotoxic crisis) is a form of severe hyperthyroidism, usually of abrupt onset. Untreated, it is almost always fatal, but with proper treatment the mortality rate is reduced substantially. The patient with thyroid storm or crisis is critically ill and requires astute observation and aggressive and supportive nursing care during and after the acute stage of illness.

Clinical Manifestations

Thyroid storm is characterized by:

- High fever (hyperpyrexia), >38.5°C (>101.3°F)
- Extreme tachycardia (>130 bpm)
- Exaggerated symptoms of hyperthyroidism with disturbances of a major system—for example, gastrointestinal (weight loss, diarrhea, abdominal pain) or cardiovascular (edema, chest pain, dyspnea, palpitations)
- Altered neurologic or mental state, which frequently appears as delirium psychosis, somnolence, or coma

Life-threatening thyroid storm is usually precipitated by stress, such as injury, infection, thyroid and nonthyroid surgery, tooth extraction, insulin reaction, diabetic ketoacidosis, pregnancy, digitalis intoxication, abrupt withdrawal of antithyroid medications, extreme emotional stress, or vigorous palpation of the thyroid. These factors can precipitate thyroid storm in the partially controlled or completely untreated patient with hyperthyroidism. Current methods of diagnosis and treatment for hyperthyroidism have greatly decreased the incidence of thyroid storm, making it uncommon today.

Management

Immediate objectives are reduction of body temperature and heart rate and prevention of vascular collapse. Measures to accomplish these objectives include:

- A hypothermia mattress or blanket, ice packs, a cool environment, hydrocortisone, and acetaminophen (Tylenol). Salicylates (e.g., aspirin) are not used because they displace thyroid hormone from binding proteins and worsen the hypermetabolism.
- Humidified oxygen is given to improve tissue oxygenation and meet the high metabolic demands. Arterial blood gas levels or pulse oximetry may be used to monitor respiratory status.
- IV fluids containing dextrose are given to replace liver glycogen stores that have been decreased in the patient who is hyperthyroid.
- Propylthiouracil (PTU) or methimazole is given to impede formation of thyroid hormone and block conversion of T_4 to T_3, the more active form of thyroid hormone.
- Hydrocortisone is prescribed to treat shock or adrenal insufficiency.
- Iodine is given to decrease output of T_4 from the thyroid gland. For cardiac problems such as atrial fibrillation, dysrhythmias, and heart failure, sympatholytic agents may be given. Propranolol, combined with digitalis, has been effective in reducing severe cardiac symptoms.

T_4, thyroxine; T_3, triiodothyronine.

Adapted from Davies, T. F., Laurberg, P., & Bahn, R. S. (2016). Thyroid disorders. In S. Melmed, K. Polonsky, Larsen, P., et al. (Eds.). *Williams textbook of endocrinology*. Philadelphia, PA: Elsevier.

TABLE 52-3 Pharmacologic Agents Used to Treat Hyperthyroidism

Agent	Action	Nursing Considerations
Propylthiouracil (PTU)	Blocks synthesis of hormones (conversion of T_4 to T_3)	Monitor cardiac parameters. Observe for conversion to hypothyroidism. Must be given by mouth. Watch for rash, nausea, vomiting, agranulocytosis, SLE.
Methimazole (Tapazole)	Inhibits synthesis of thyroid hormone	More toxic than PTU. Watch for rash and other symptoms as for PTU.
Sodium iodide	Suppresses release of thyroid hormone	Given 1 h after PTU or methimazole. Watch for edema, hemorrhage, gastrointestinal upset.
Potassium iodide	Suppresses release of thyroid hormone	Discontinue for rash. Watch for signs of toxic iodinism.
Saturated solution of potassium iodide (SSKI)	Suppresses release of thyroid hormone	Mix with juice or milk. Given by straw to prevent staining of teeth.
Beta-blocker (e.g., propranolol [Inderal])	Beta-adrenergic blocking agent	Monitor cardiac status. Hold for bradycardia or decreased cardiac output. Use with caution in patients with heart failure.

T_4, thyroxine; T_3, triiodothyronine; SLE, systemic lupus erythematosus.
Adapted from Morton, P. G., & Fontaine, D. K. (2013). *Critical care nursing: A holistic approach*. Philadelphia, PA: Lippincott Williams & Wilkins.

Antithyroid Medications

Antithyroid medications (thionamides) are summarized in Table 52-3. The objective of pharmacotherapy is to inhibit one or more stages in thyroid hormone synthesis or hormone release. Antithyroid agents block the utilization of iodine by interfering with the iodination of tyrosine and the coupling of iodotyrosines in the synthesis of thyroid hormones. This prevents the synthesis of thyroid hormone. The most commonly used antithyroid drugs in the United States are methimazole (MMI, Tapazole) or propylthiouracil (PTU). The medications are used until the patient is euthyroid (i.e., neither hyperthyroid nor hypothyroid). These medications block extrathyroidal conversion of T_4 to T_3 (Bahn et al., 2011).

Prior to initiating therapy with these drugs, baseline blood tests are performed, including complete blood count (white blood cell [WBC] count with differential) and liver profile (transaminases and bilirubin) (Bahn et al., 2011; Ross, 2016d). The therapeutic dose is determined on the basis of clinical criteria, including changes in pulse rate, pulse pressure, body weight, size of the goiter, and results of laboratory studies. The patient should be instructed to take the medication in the morning on an empty stomach 30 minutes before eating to avoid decrease in absorption associated with some foods such as walnuts, soybean flour, cottonseed meal, and dietary fiber. Because antithyroid medications do not interfere with release or activity of previously formed thyroid hormones, it may take several weeks until symptom relief occurs. At that time, the maintenance dose is established, and the medication is gradually tapered over several months.

Toxic complications of antithyroid medications are relatively uncommon; nevertheless, the importance of periodic follow-up is emphasized, because medication sensitization, fever, rash, urticaria, or even agranulocytosis and thrombocytopenia (decrease in granulocytes and platelets) may develop (Bahn et al., 2011). With any sign of infection, especially pharyngitis and fever or the occurrence of mouth ulcers, the patient is advised to stop the medication, notify the primary provider immediately, and undergo hematologic studies (Bahn et al., 2011). PTU is recommended during the first trimester of pregnancy rather than MMI due to the teratogenic effects of MMI (Ross, 2016f). Due to risk of hepatotoxicity, PTU should be discontinued after the first trimester and the patient should be switched to MMI for the remainder of the pregnancy and when breast feeding (Ross, 2016b).

Discontinuation of antithyroid medications before therapy is complete usually results in relapse within 6 months. It is important that the possibility of relapse be discussed so that a treatment strategy will be in place if relapse occurs.

Adjunctive Therapy

Iodine or iodide is necessary for thyroid function, and deficiency or excess can lead to thyroid dysfunction. Iodine or iodide solutions were once the only therapy available for patients with hyperthyroidism but are no longer the sole method of treatment. Antithyroid medications (MMI and PTU) and radioactive iodine are not the mainstays of pharmacologic treatment for hyperthyroidism. In the short term, iodine solutions are considered effective. When treating patients with thyroid storm and those requiring surgical intervention for hyperthyroidism, iodine solutions are considered highly effective. Iodine solutions inhibit the release of T_4 and T_3 within hours of administration and inhibit thyroid hormone synthesis. The maximum inhibitory effect on serum thyroid hormone production is only 10 days (Ross, 2016g). Solutions such as potassium iodide (KI), Lugol's solution, and saturated solution of potassium iodide (SSKI) may be used in combination with antithyroid agents or beta-adrenergic blockers to prepare the patient with hyperthyroidism for surgery. Solutions of iodine and iodide compounds are more palatable in milk or fruit juice and are administered through a straw to prevent staining of the teeth. The nurse should be aware that there have been reported cases of local esophageal or duodenal mucosal injury and hemorrhage as a result of administration of Lugol's solution (960 mg/day) to manage thyroid storm (Bahn et al., 2011).

Beta-adrenergic blocking agents (e.g., propranolol, atenolol, metoprolol) are important in decreasing heart rate, systolic blood pressure, muscle weakness, nervousness, tremor, anxiety, and heat intolerance. The patient continues taking the beta-blocker until the free T_4 is within the normal range and the TSH level approaches normal.

Surgical Management

Surgery to remove thyroid tissue is reserved for special circumstances—for example, in pregnant women who are allergic to antithyroid medications, in patients with large goiters, or in patients who are unable to take antithyroid agents. Surgery for treatment of hyperthyroidism is performed soon after the thyroid function has returned to normal (4 to 6 weeks).

The surgical removal of about five sixths of the thyroid tissue (subtotal thyroidectomy) reliably results in a prolonged remission in most patients with exophthalmic goiter. Its use today is reserved for patients with obstructive symptoms, for pregnant women in the second trimester, and for patients with a need for rapid normalization of thyroid function. Before surgery, an antithyroid medication is given until signs of hyperthyroidism have disappeared. A beta-adrenergic blocking agent (e.g., propranolol) may be used to reduce the heart rate and other signs and symptoms of hyperthyroidism. Medications that may prolong clotting (e.g., aspirin) are stopped several weeks before surgery to reduce the risk of postoperative bleeding. Patients receiving iodine medication must be monitored for evidence of iodine toxicity (iodinism), which requires immediate withdrawal of the medication. Symptoms of iodinism include swelling of the buccal mucosa, excessive salivation, cold symptoms, and skin eruptions. The incidence of relapse with a total thyroidectomy is nearly 0%, whereas recurrence following a subtotal thyroidectomy is 8% at 5 years (Bahn et al., 2011).

 Gerontologic Considerations

Although hyperthyroidism is much less common in older adults than hypothyroidism, patients 65 years and older need careful assessment to avoid missing subtle signs and symptoms. Subclinical hyperthyroidism has been reported in approximately 8% of this age group (Harman, 2016; Visser et al., 2013). This age group may present with atypical vague and nonspecific signs and symptoms of thyroid disease such as anorexia and weight loss with absence of ocular signs, or isolated atrial fibrillation. New or worsening heart failure or angina is more likely to occur in older patients rather than in younger patients. Symptoms such as tachycardia, fatigue, mental confusion, weight loss, change in bowel habits, and depression can be attributed to age and other illnesses that are common in older adults. The older patient may complain of difficulty climbing stairs or rising from a chair because of muscle weakness (Visser et al., 2013). Evaluation for thyroid disease with a serum TSH measurement is indicated in older patients who have unexplained physical or mental deterioration (Bahn et al., 2011). Free T_4 and T_3 should be included in the initial screening when hyperthyroidism is highly suspected. Once thyrotoxicosis is confirmed, additional tests such as radioactive iodine uptake and thyroid scan are prescribed to differentiate between causes such as Graves disease, toxic nodular goiter, acute thyroiditis, and other disorders. Toxic nodular goiter is the most common cause of thyrotoxicosis in older patients.

Patients have the option of treatment using antithyroid medications, radioactive iodine, and surgery. Radioactive iodine is generally recommended for treatment of thyrotoxicosis caused by toxic nodular goiter in older patients unless an enlarged thyroid gland is pressing on the airway. Prior to administration of radioactive iodine (Bahn et al., 2011) in this at-risk group, pretreatment with beta-blockade is indicated if the patient's resting heart rate is 90 bpm or if the patient has coexistent cardiovascular disease and symptomatic hyperthyroidism. MMI should be given prior to treatment with radioactive iodine to prevent complications due to worsening of hyperthyroidism. Patients who elect to have surgery to treat toxic nodular goiter must be pretreated with an antithyroid medication (methimazole) to achieve a euthyroid state. However, preoperative iodine should not be used to prevent exacerbating the hyperthyroidism (Bahn et al., 2011). Long-term use of certain antithyroid medications such as PTU is not recommended for treatment of toxic nodular goiter in older patients due to risk of side effects. Although rare, there is evidence that PTU can result in agranulocytosis and hepatic injury. However, the use of antithyroid medications versus radioactive iodine or surgery may be the patient's preferred choice or the option for some older patients and other ill persons with "limited longevity" who can be monitored at least every 3 months (Bahn et al., 2011).

The use of beta-adrenergic blocking agents (e.g., propranolol and atenolol) may be indicated to decrease the cardiovascular and neurologic signs and symptoms of thyrotoxicosis. These agents must be used with extreme caution in older patients to minimize adverse effects on cardiac function that may produce heart failure. The dosage of other medications used to treat other chronic illnesses in older patients may also need to be modified because of the altered rate of metabolism associated with hyperthyroidism.

NURSING PROCESS

The Patient With Hyperthyroidism

Assessment

The health history and examination focus on symptoms related to accelerated or exaggerated metabolism. These include the patient's and family's reports of irritability and increased emotional reaction and the impact that these changes have had on the patient's interactions with family, friends, and coworkers. The history includes other stressors and the patient's ability to cope with stress.

The nurse initially and periodically assesses the patient's nutritional status and the presence of symptoms related to the hypermetabolic state. This hypermetabolic state may affect the cardiovascular system including heart rate and rhythm, blood pressure, heart sounds, and peripheral pulses. Other specific changes may also include alteration in vision and appearance of the external eye. Because emotional changes are associated with hyperthyroidism, the patient's emotional state and psychological status are evaluated, as well as such symptoms as irritability, anxiety, sleep disturbances, apathy, and lethargy, all of which may occur with hyperthyroidism (Morgan & Tsai, 2015). The family may also provide information about recent changes in the patient's emotional status.

Diagnosis

NURSING DIAGNOSES

Based on the assessment data, major nursing diagnoses may include the following:

- Imbalanced nutrition: less than body requirements related to exaggerated metabolic rate, excessive appetite, and increased GI activity
- Ineffective coping related to irritability, hyperexcitability, apprehension, and emotional instability
- Situational low self-esteem related to changes in appearance, excessive appetite, and weight loss
- Risk for imbalanced body temperature

COLLABORATIVE PROBLEMS/POTENTIAL COMPLICATIONS

Potential complications may include the following:

- Thyrotoxicosis or thyroid storm
- Hypothyroidism

Planning and Goals

The goals for the patient may be improved nutritional status, improved coping ability, improved self-esteem, maintenance of normal body temperature, and absence of complications.

Nursing Interventions

IMPROVING NUTRITIONAL STATUS

Hyperthyroidism affects all body systems, including the GI system. The appetite is increased but may be satisfied by several well-balanced meals of small size, even up to six meals a day. Foods and fluids are selected to replace fluid lost through diarrhea and diaphoresis and to control the diarrhea that results from increased peristalsis. Rapid movement of food through the GI tract may result in nutritional imbalance and further weight loss. To reduce diarrhea, highly seasoned foods and stimulants such as coffee, tea, cola, and alcohol are discouraged. High-calorie, high-protein foods are encouraged. A quiet atmosphere during mealtime may aid digestion. Weight and dietary intake are recorded to monitor nutritional status.

ENHANCING COPING MEASURES

The patient with hyperthyroidism needs reassurance that the emotional reactions being experienced are a result of the disorder and that with effective treatment those symptoms will be controlled. Because of the negative effect that these symptoms can have on family and friends, they too need reassurance that the symptoms are expected to disappear with treatment.

It is important to use a calm, unhurried approach with the patient. Stressful experiences should be minimized and a quiet, uncluttered environment should be maintained. It is important to balance periods of activity with rest.

If thyroidectomy is planned, the patient needs to know that pharmacologic therapy is necessary to prepare the thyroid gland for surgical treatment. The nurse provides education and reminds the patient to take the medications as prescribed. Because of hyperexcitability and shortened attention span, the patient may require repetition of this education and written instructions.

IMPROVING SELF-ESTEEM

The patient with hyperthyroidism is likely to experience changes in appearance, appetite, and weight. These factors, along with the patient's inability to cope well with family and

the illness, may result in loss of self-esteem. The nurse conveys an understanding of the patient's concern about these problems and promotes the use of effective coping strategies. The patient and family should be reassured that these changes are a result of the thyroid dysfunction and are, in fact, out of the patient's control. The nurse refers the patient to professional counseling as necessary.

If the patient experiences ocular changes secondary to hyperthyroidism, eye care and protection may be necessary. The nurse educates the patient about instillation of eye drops or ointment prescribed to soothe the eyes and protect the exposed cornea. Smoking should be highly discouraged, and smoking cessation strategies are recommended. The patient may be embarrassed by the need to eat large meals. Caregivers and family should avoid commenting on the patient's large dietary intake while making sure that the patient receives sufficient nutritious food.

MAINTAINING NORMAL BODY TEMPERATURE

The patient with hyperthyroidism frequently finds a normal room temperature too warm because of an exaggerated metabolic rate and increased heat production. If the patient is hospitalized, the environment should be maintained at a cool, comfortable temperature, and the bedding and clothing should be changed as needed. Cool baths and cool or cold fluids may also provide relief.

MONITORING AND MANAGING POTENTIAL COMPLICATIONS

The nurse closely monitors the patient with hyperthyroidism for signs and symptoms that may be indicative of thyroid storm. Cardiac and respiratory functions are assessed by measuring vital signs and cardiac output, electrocardiographic (ECG) monitoring, arterial blood gases, and pulse oximetry. Assessment continues after treatment is initiated because of the potential effects of treatment on cardiac function. Oxygen is given to prevent hypoxia, to improve tissue oxygenation, and to meet the high metabolic demands. IV fluids may be necessary to maintain blood glucose levels and to replace lost fluids. Antithyroid medications (MMI or PTU) may be prescribed to reduce thyroid hormone levels. In addition, beta-blockers and digitalis may be prescribed to treat cardiac symptoms. If shock develops, treatment strategies must be implemented (see Chapter 14).

Hypothyroidism is likely to occur with any of the treatments used for hyperthyroidism. Therefore, the nurse periodically monitors the patient. Most patients report a greatly improved sense of well-being after treatment of hyperthyroidism, and some fail to continue to take prescribed thyroid replacement therapy. Therefore, part of patient and family education is instruction about the importance of continuing therapy indefinitely after discharge and a discussion of the consequences of failing to take medication.

PROMOTING HOME, COMMUNITY-BASED, AND TRANSITIONAL CARE

Educating Patients About Self-Care. The nurse educates the patient with hyperthyroidism about how and when to take prescribed medication and provides instruction about the essential role of the medication in the broader therapeutic plan. Because of the hyperexcitability and decreased attention span associated with hyperthyroidism, the nurse provides a written plan for the patient to take home and

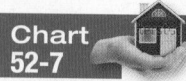

Chart 52-7

HOME CARE CHECKLIST
The Patient With Hyperthyroidism

At the completion of education, the patient and/or caregiver will be able to:

- State the impact of hyperthyroidism, treatment on physiologic functioning, ADLs, IADLs, roles, relationships, and spirituality.
- State that emotional lability is part of disease process.
- Identify the potential for menstrual irregularities and pregnancy, and increased risk of osteoporosis in women.
- State that long-term treatment and follow-up is necessary.
- Describe the potential benefits and risks of surgical intervention or radioactive iodine therapy.
- State the name, dose, side effects, frequency, and schedule for all medications.
- Explain the purpose, dose, route, schedule, side effects, and precautions of treatment of hyperthyroidism (antithyroid medications, radioactive iodine).
- State the need to contact primary provider before taking over-the-counter medications.
- State changes in lifestyle (e.g., diet, activity) necessary to maintain health.

- Identify the need for increased dietary intake until weight stabilizes.
- Identify foods to be avoided.
- Identify the need for planned rest periods and methods to improve sleep patterns.
- Identify areas of stress and management techniques.
- Identify rationale for smoking cessation and steps to stop use of any tobacco product.
- State precipitating factors and interventions for complications (hypothyroidism, thyroid storm).
- Relate how to reach primary provider with questions or complications.
- State time and date of follow-up medical appointments, therapy, and testing.
- Identify sources of support (e.g., friends, relatives, faith community, support groups, caregiver support).
- Identify the need for health promotion, disease prevention, and screening activities.

ADL, activities of daily living; IADL, independent activities of daily living.

---

use. The type and amount of information given depend on the patient's stress and anxiety levels. The patient and family members receive verbal and written education about the actions and possible side effects of the medications as well as adverse effects that should be reported if they occur (see Chart 52-7).

If a total or subtotal thyroidectomy is anticipated, the patient needs to be educated about what to expect. Information is repeated as the time of surgery approaches. The nurse also advises the patient to avoid stressful situations that may precipitate thyroid storm.

Continuing and Transitional Care. Referral for home, community-based or transitional care, if indicated, allows the nurse to assess the home and family environment, as well as the patient's and family's understanding of the importance of adhering to the therapeutic regimen and the recommended follow-up monitoring. The nurse reinforces to the patient and family the importance of long-term follow-up because of the risk of hypothyroidism after thyroidectomy or treatment with antithyroid medications or radioactive iodine. The nurse also assesses the patient for changes indicating return to normal thyroid function and signs and symptoms of hyperthyroidism and hypothyroidism. Furthermore, the nurse reminds the patient and family about the importance of health promotion activities and recommended health screening.

Evaluation

Expected patient outcomes may include:
1. Improves nutritional status
   a. Reports adequate dietary intake and decreased hunger
   b. Identifies high-calorie, high-protein foods; identifies foods to be avoided
   c. Avoids the use of alcohol and other stimulants
   d. Stops smoking
   e. Reports decreased episodes of diarrhea

2. Demonstrates effective coping methods in dealing with family, friends, and coworkers
   a. Explains reasons for irritability and emotional instability
   b. Avoids stressful situations, events, and people
   c. Participates in relaxing, nonstressful activities
3. Achieves increased self-esteem
   a. Verbalizes feelings about self and illness
   b. Describes feelings of frustration and loss of control
   c. Describes reasons for increased appetite
4. Maintains normal body temperature
5. Absence of complications
   a. Serum thyroid hormone and TSH levels within normal limits
   b. Identifies signs and symptoms of thyroid storm and hypothyroidism
   c. Vital signs and results of ECG, arterial blood gases, and pulse oximetry within normal limits
   d. States importance of regular follow-up and lifelong maintenance of prescribed therapy

Thyroid Tumors

Tumors of the thyroid gland are classified on the basis of being benign or malignant, the presence or absence of associated thyrotoxicosis, and the diffuse or irregular quality of the glandular enlargement. If the enlargement is sufficient to cause a visible swelling in the neck, the tumor is referred to as a goiter.

All grades of goiter are encountered, from those that are barely visible to those producing disfigurement. Some are symmetric and diffuse; others are nodular. Some are accompanied by hyperthyroidism, in which case they are described as toxic; others are associated with a euthyroid state and are referred to as nontoxic goiters.

Endemic (Iodine-Deficient) Goiter

The most common type of goiter that occurs when iodine intake is deficient is the simple or colloid goiter. In addition to being caused by an iodine deficiency, simple goiter may be caused by an intake of large quantities of goitrogenic substances in patients with unusually susceptible glands. These substances include excessive amounts of iodine. Lithium prescribed for the treatment of bipolar disorder has also been found to also have antithyroid actions (Janicak, 2016; Shine, McKnight, Leaver, et al., 2016; Surks, 2016c).

Simple goiter is a compensatory hypertrophy of the thyroid gland, caused by stimulation by the pituitary gland. The pituitary gland produces thyrotropin or TSH, a hormone that controls the release of thyroid hormone from the thyroid gland. Its production increases if there is subnormal thyroid activity, as when insufficient iodine is available for production of the thyroid hormone. Such goiters usually cause no symptoms, except for the swelling in the neck, which may result in tracheal compression when excessive swelling is present.

Many goiters of this type recede after the iodine imbalance is corrected. Supplementary iodine, such as SSKI, is prescribed to suppress the pituitary's thyroid-stimulating activity. When surgery is indicated, the risk of postoperative complications is minimized by ensuring a preoperative euthyroid state through treatment with antithyroid medications and iodide to reduce the size and vascularity of the goiter. The introduction of iodized salt has been the single most effective means of preventing goiter in at-risk populations.

Nodular Goiter

Some thyroid glands are nodular because of areas of hyperplasia (overgrowth). No symptoms may arise as a result of this condition, but not uncommonly these nodules slowly increase in size, with some descending into the thorax, where they cause local pressure symptoms. Some nodules become malignant, and some are associated with a hyperthyroid state. Therefore, the patient with many thyroid nodules may eventually require surgery.

Thyroid Cancer

Cancer of the thyroid is much less prevalent than other forms of cancer, but the incidence has been increasing steadily since the 1990s. It accounts for 90% of endocrine malignancies. Although it accounts for the fastest-growing cancer rate among both men and women, three of four cases occur in women. Unlike other cancers, two of three new cases are in patients under the age of 55 years (American Cancer Society [ACS], 2017a).

External radiation of the head, neck, or chest in infancy and childhood increases the risk of thyroid carcinoma. The incidence of thyroid cancer appears to increase 5 to 40 years after irradiation. Consequently, people who underwent radiation treatment or were otherwise exposed to radiation as children should consult their primary provider, request an isotope thyroid scan as part of the evaluation, follow recommended treatment of abnormalities of the gland, and continue with annual checkups.

Assessment and Diagnostic Findings

Lesions that are single, hard, and fixed on palpation or associated with cervical lymphadenopathy suggest malignancy. Thyroid function tests may be helpful in evaluating thyroid nodules and masses; however, results are rarely conclusive. Needle biopsy of the thyroid gland is used as an outpatient procedure to make a diagnosis of thyroid cancer, to differentiate cancerous thyroid nodules from noncancerous nodules, and to stage the cancer if detected. The procedure is safe and usually requires only a local anesthetic agent. However, patients who undergo the procedure are monitored closely, because cancerous tissues may be missed during the procedure. A second type of aspiration or biopsy uses a large-bore needle rather than the fine needle used in standard biopsy; it may be used when the results of the standard biopsy are inconclusive or with rapidly growing tumors. Additional diagnostic studies include ultrasound, MRI, CT, thyroid scans, radioactive iodine uptake studies, and thyroid suppression tests.

Medical Management

The treatment of choice for thyroid carcinoma is surgical removal. Total or near-total thyroidectomy is performed if possible (ACS, 2017b). Modified neck dissection or more extensive radical neck dissection is performed if there is lymph node involvement.

Efforts are made to spare parathyroid tissue to reduce the risk of postoperative hypocalcemia and tetany. After surgery, ablation procedures are carried out with radioactive iodine to eradicate residual microscopic disease (ACS, 2017c). Radioactive iodine is also used for thyroid cancers with metastasis (ACS, 2017c). The use of radioactive iodine therapy has been crucial in making thyroid one of the most curable types of cancer (Dagan & Amdur, 2013).

After surgery, thyroid hormone is given to lower the levels of TSH to a euthyroid state (Bahn et al., 2011). If the remaining thyroid tissue is inadequate to produce sufficient thyroid hormone, thyroxine is required permanently.

Several routes are available for administering radiation to the thyroid or tissues of the neck, including oral administration of radioactive iodine (Bahn et al., 2011) and external administration of radiation therapy. Short-term side effects of radioactive iodine treatment may include neck soreness, nausea, and upset stomach; salivary glands being tender and swollen; dry mouth; changes in taste; and, rarely, pain (Bahn et al., 2011). The patient who receives external sources of radiation therapy is at risk for mucositis, dryness of the mouth, dysphagia, redness of the skin, anorexia, and fatigue (see Chapter 15). Chemotherapy is infrequently used to treat thyroid cancer.

Patients whose thyroid cancer is detected early and who are appropriately treated have a good prognosis. Patients who have had papillary cancer—the most common and least aggressive tumor—have the best prognosis of all thyroid cancers (Dagan & Amdur, 2013). Long-term survival is also common in follicular cancer, which is a more aggressive form of thyroid cancer (Dagan & Amdur, 2013). However, continued thyroid hormone therapy and periodic follow-up and diagnostic testing are important to ensure the patient's well-being.

Later follow-up includes clinical assessment for recurrence of nodules or masses in the neck and signs of hoarseness, dysphagia, or dyspnea. The recommendations for long-term follow-up of patients with differentiated thyroid cancer are based on the stage of cancer and results of the follow-up examination 1 year following the initial treatment. The first year evaluation includes clinical examination, TSH and free thyroxine, and measurement of serum thyroglobulin within 6 months following the initial treatment, and a routine neck ultrasound with the first 6 to 12 months following initial treatment. Tests used to confirm sites of metastasis if there is clinical evidence of recurrence include radioiodine imaging, CT, MRI, skeletal x-rays, and skeletal radionucleotide imaging. Fluorodeoxyglucose (FGDA) PET is useful to establish prognosis if there is evidence of distant metastases (Tuttle, 2016). Free T_4, TSH, and serum calcium and phosphorus levels are monitored to determine whether the thyroid hormone supplementation is adequate and to note whether calcium balance is maintained.

Although local and systemic reactions to radiation may occur and may include neutropenia or thrombocytopenia, these complications are rare when radioactive iodine is used. Patients who undergo surgery that is combined with radioactive iodine have a higher survival rate than those who undergo surgery alone. Patient education emphasizes the importance of taking prescribed medications and following recommendations for follow-up monitoring. The patient who is undergoing radiation therapy is also instructed in how to assess and manage side effects of treatment (see Chapter 15).

Nursing Management

Important preoperative goals are to prepare the patient for surgery and reduce anxiety. Often, the patient's home life has become tense because of their restlessness, irritability, and nervousness secondary to hyperthyroidism. Efforts are necessary to protect the patient from tension and stress to avoid precipitating thyroid storm. Suggestions are made to limit stressful situations. Quiet and relaxing activities are encouraged.

Providing Preoperative Care

The nurse instructs the patient about the importance of eating a diet high in carbohydrates and proteins. A high daily caloric intake is necessary because of the increased metabolic activity and rapid depletion of glycogen reserves. Supplementary vitamins, particularly thiamine and ascorbic acid, may be prescribed. The patient is reminded to avoid tea, coffee, cola, and other stimulants.

The nurse also informs the patient about the purpose of preoperative tests, if they are to be performed, and explains what preoperative preparations to expect. This information should help to reduce the patient's anxiety about the surgery. In addition, special efforts are made to ensure a good night's rest before surgery.

Preoperative education includes demonstrating to the patient how to support the neck with the hands after surgery to prevent stress on the incision. This involves raising the elbows and placing the hands behind the neck to provide support and reduce strain and tension on the neck muscles and the surgical incision.

Providing Postoperative Care

The nurse periodically assesses the surgical dressings and reinforces as necessary. When the patient is in a recumbent position, the nurse observes the sides and the back of the neck as well as the anterior dressing for bleeding. In addition to monitoring the pulse and blood pressure for any indication of internal bleeding, the nurse must be alert for complaints of a sensation of pressure or fullness at the incision site. Such symptoms may indicate subcutaneous hemorrhage and hematoma formation and should be reported.

Difficulty in respiration can occur as a result of edema of the glottis, hematoma formation, or injury to the recurrent laryngeal nerve. This complication requires that an airway be inserted. Therefore, a tracheostomy set is kept at the bedside at all times, and the surgeon is summoned at the first indication of respiratory distress. If the respiratory distress is caused by hematoma, surgical evacuation is required.

The intensity of pain is assessed, and analgesic agents are given as prescribed for pain. The nurse should anticipate apprehension in the patient and should inform the patient that oxygen will assist breathing. When moving and turning the patient, the nurse carefully supports the patient's head and avoids tension on the sutures. The most comfortable position is the semi-Fowler position, with the head elevated and supported by pillows.

IV fluids are given during the immediate postoperative period. Water may be given by mouth as soon as nausea subsides and bowel sounds are present. Usually, there is a little difficulty in swallowing; initially, cold fluids and ice may be taken better than other fluids. Often, patients prefer a soft diet to a liquid diet in the immediate postoperative period.

The patient is advised to talk as little as possible to reduce edema to the vocal cords; however, when the patient does speak, any voice changes are noted, indicating possible injury to the recurrent laryngeal nerve, which lies just behind the thyroid next to the trachea. An overbed table is provided for access to frequently used items so that the patient avoids turning their head. The table can also be used to support a humidifier when vapor-mist inhalations are prescribed for the relief of excessive mucous accumulation.

The patient is encouraged to be out of bed as soon as possible and to eat foods that are easily swallowed. A high-calorie diet may be prescribed to promote weight gain. The incision may be closed using absorbable sutures, nonabsorbable sutures, and adhesive strips. Absorbable sutures dissolve within the body. If nonabsorbable sutures are used, the timeline for removal may vary; however, these types of sutures are usually removed 5 to 7 days following surgery. Adhesives will peel off spontaneously. The patient is usually discharged from the hospital on the day of surgery or soon afterward if the postoperative course is uncomplicated.

Monitoring and Managing Potential Complications

Hemorrhage, hematoma formation, edema of the glottis, and injury to the laryngeal nerve are complications reviewed previously in this chapter. Occasionally in thyroid surgery, the parathyroid glands are injured or removed, producing a disturbance in calcium metabolism. As the blood calcium level falls, hyperirritability of the nerves occurs, with spasms of the hands and feet and muscle twitching (see Chapter 13). This group of symptoms is termed *tetany*, and the nurse must immediately report its appearance because laryngospasm, although rare, may occur and obstruct the airway. Tetany of this type is usually treated with IV calcium gluconate. This calcium abnormality is usually temporary after thyroidectomy unless all parathyroid tissues were removed.

> ### ◢ Quality and Safety Nursing Alert
>
> *Following thyroid surgery, the patient should be monitored closely for signs of tetany, including hyperirritability of the nerves, with spasms of the hands and feet and muscle twitching. Laryngospasm, although rare, may occur and obstruct the airway.*

Promoting Home, Community-Based, and Transitional Care

Predischarge education is essential because the patient is usually discharged within 1 or 2 days. The patient, family, and caregivers need to be knowledgeable about the signs and symptoms that should be reported. Discharge education includes strategies for managing postoperative pain at home and for increasing humidification. The nurse explains to the patient and family the need for rest, relaxation, and adequate nutrition and to avoid putting strain on the incision and sutures. The patient is permitted to resume their former activities and responsibilities completely once recovered from surgery.

Family responsibilities and factors relating to the home environment that produce emotional tension have often been implicated as precipitating causes of thyrotoxicosis. A home visit provides an opportunity to evaluate these factors and to suggest ways to improve the home and family environment. If indicated, a referral to home, community-based or transitional care is made. The nurse reviews the history; performs a physical assessment; assesses the surgical incision; develops a plan of care with the patient and family; and educates the patient, family, and caregivers about wound care, signs and symptoms to report, stress reduction, and the importance of keeping appointments with the primary provider.

THE PARATHYROID GLANDS

Anatomic and Physiologic Overview

The parathyroid glands (normally four) are situated in the neck and embedded in the posterior aspect of the thyroid gland (see Fig. 52-5). Parathormone (parathyroid hormone)—the protein hormone produced by the parathyroid glands—regulates calcium and phosphorus metabolism. Increased secretion of parathormone results in increased calcium absorption from the kidney, intestine, and bones, which raises the serum calcium level (Grossman & Porth, 2014). Some actions of this hormone are increased by the presence of vitamin D. Parathormone also tends to lower the blood phosphorus level. The serum level of ionized calcium regulates the output of parathormone. Increased serum calcium results in decreased parathormone secretion, creating a negative feedback system.

Pathophysiology

Excess parathormone can result in markedly increased levels of serum calcium, which is a potentially life-threatening

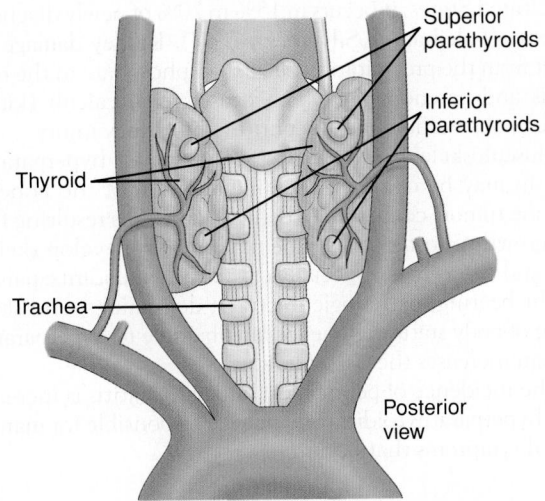

Figure 52-5 • The parathyroid glands are located behind the thyroid gland. The parathyroids may be embedded in the thyroid tissue.

situation. When the product of serum calcium and serum phosphorus (calcium × phosphorus) rises, calcium phosphate may precipitate in various organs of the body (e.g., the kidneys) and cause tissue calcification.

Hyperparathyroidism

Hyperparathyroidism is caused by overproduction of parathormone by the parathyroid glands and is characterized by bone decalcification and the development of renal calculi (kidney stones) containing calcium.

Primary hyperparathyroidism occurs two to four times more often in women than in men and is most common in people between 60 and 70 years of age. Its incidence is approximately 25 cases per 100,000 people. The disorder is rare in children younger than 15 years, but its incidence increases 10-fold between the ages of 15 and 65 years. Half of the people diagnosed with hyperparathyroidism do not have symptoms (Fuleihan & Silverberg, 2017).

Secondary hyperparathyroidism, with manifestations similar to those of primary hyperparathyroidism, occurs in patients who have chronic kidney failure and so-called renal rickets as a result of phosphorus retention, increased stimulation of the parathyroid glands, and increased parathormone secretion.

Clinical Manifestations

The patient may have no symptoms or may experience signs and symptoms resulting from involvement of several body systems. Apathy, fatigue, muscle weakness, nausea, vomiting, constipation, hypertension, and cardiac dysrhythmias may occur. All of these signs and symptoms are attributable to the increased concentration of calcium in the blood. Psychological effects may vary from irritability and neurosis to psychoses caused by the direct action of calcium on the brain and nervous system. An increase in calcium produces a decrease in the excitation potential of nerve and muscle tissue.

The formation of stones in one or both kidneys (nephrolithiasis), related to the increased urinary excretion of calcium and phosphorus, is one of the major complications of hyperparathyroidism. Although the incidence is on the decline in the United States, it occurs in 15% to 20% of newly diagnosed patients (Fuleihan & Silverberg, 2017). Kidney damage can result from the precipitation of calcium phosphate in the renal pelvis and parenchyma, which causes renal calculi (kidney stones), obstruction, pyelonephritis, and kidney injury.

Musculoskeletal symptoms accompanying hyperparathyroidism may be caused by demineralization of the bones or by bone tumors composed of benign giant cells resulting from overgrowth of osteoclasts. The patient may develop skeletal pain and tenderness, especially of the back and joints; pain on weight bearing; pathologic fractures; deformities; and shortening of body stature. Bone loss attributable to hyperparathyroidism increases the risk of fracture.

The incidence of peptic ulcer and pancreatitis is increased with hyperparathyroidism and may be responsible for many of the GI symptoms that occur.

Assessment and Diagnostic Findings

Primary hyperparathyroidism is diagnosed by persistent elevation of serum calcium levels and an elevated concentration of parathormone. Radioimmunoassays for parathormone are sensitive and differentiate primary hyperparathyroidism from other causes of hypercalcemia in more than 80% of patients with elevated serum calcium levels (Fuleihan & Silverberg, 2017). An elevated serum calcium level alone is a nonspecific finding, because serum levels may be altered by diet, medications, and kidney and bone changes. Bone changes may be detected on x-ray or bone scans in advanced disease. The double-antibody parathyroid hormone test is used to distinguish between primary hyperparathyroidism and malignancy as a cause of hypercalcemia. Ultrasound, MRI, thallium scan, and fine-needle biopsy have been used to evaluate the function of the parathyroids and to localize parathyroid cysts, adenomas, or hyperplasia.

Medical Management

Surgical Management

The recommended treatment for primary hyperparathyroidism is the surgical removal of abnormal parathyroid tissue (parathyroidectomy) (Fuleihan & Silverberg, 2017). In the past, the standard parathyroidectomy involved a bilateral neck exploration under general anesthesia. Today, minimally invasive parathyroidectomy techniques allow for unilateral neck exploration using local anesthesia; these are performed on an outpatient basis. In some cases, only the removal of a single diseased gland is necessary, reducing morbidity rates associated with surgery. For asymptomatic patients who have only mildly elevated serum calcium concentrations and normal kidney function, surgery may be delayed and the patient monitored closely for worsening of hypercalcemia, bone deterioration, renal impairment, or the development of kidney stones.

Surgery is recommended for asymptomatic patients who meet one or more of the following criteria: (1) younger than 50 years, (2) any patient unable or unlikely to participate in follow up care, (3) serum calcium level more than 1 mg/dL (0.25 mmol/L) above normal reference range, (3) GFR < 60 mL/min, (4) urinary calcium level greater than 400 mg/day (10 mmol/day), (5) bone density at hip, lumbar spine, or distal radius with T score < −2.5 or previous fracture fragility at any site, (6) nephrolethiasis or nephrocalcinosis (Fuleihan, & Silverberg, 2017).

Hydration Therapy

Patients with hyperparathyroidism are at risk for renal calculi. Therefore, a daily fluid intake of 2,000 mL or more is encouraged to help prevent calculus formation. The patient is instructed to report other manifestations of renal calculi, such as abdominal pain and hematuria. Thiazide diuretics are avoided, because they decrease the renal excretion of calcium and further elevate serum calcium levels. Because of the risk of hypercalcemic crisis (see later discussion), the patient is instructed to avoid dehydration and to seek immediate health care if conditions that commonly produce dehydration (e.g., vomiting, diarrhea) occur.

Mobility

The nurse encourages the patient to be mobile. The patient with limited mobility is encouraged to walk. Bones subjected to the normal stress of walking give up less calcium. Bed rest increases calcium excretion and the risk of renal calculi. Oral phosphates lower the serum calcium level in some patients; long-term use is not recommended because of the risk of ectopic calcium phosphate deposition in soft tissues.

Diet and Medications

Nutritional needs are met, but the patient is advised to avoid a diet with restricted or excess calcium. If the patient has a coexisting peptic ulcer, prescribed antacids and protein feedings are necessary. Because anorexia is common, efforts are made to improve the appetite. Prune juice, stool softeners, and physical activity, along with increased fluid intake, help offset constipation, which is common postoperatively.

Nursing Management

The insidious onset and chronic nature of hyperparathyroidism along with its diverse and commonly vague symptoms may result in depression and frustration. The family may have considered the patient's illness to be psychosomatic. An awareness of the course of the disorder and an understanding approach by the nurse may help the patient and family deal with their reactions and feelings.

The nursing management of the patient undergoing parathyroidectomy is essentially the same as that of a patient undergoing thyroidectomy. However, the previously described precautions about airway patency, dehydration, immobility, and diet are particularly important in the patient who is awaiting or recovering from parathyroidectomy. Although not all parathyroid tissue is removed during surgery in an effort to control the calcium–phosphorus balance, the nurse closely monitors the patient to detect symptoms of tetany (which may be an early postoperative complication). Most patients quickly regain function of the remaining parathyroid tissue and experience only mild, transient postoperative hypocalcemia. In patients with significant bone disease or bone changes, a more prolonged period of hypocalcemia should be anticipated. The nurse educates the patient and family about the importance of follow-up laboratory testing to ensure return of serum calcium levels to normal (see Chart 52-8).

Chart 52-8 HOME CARE CHECKLIST
The Patient With Hyperparathyroidism

At the completion of education, the patient and/or caregiver will be able to:

- State the impact of hyperparathyroidism and treatment on physiologic functioning, ADLs, IADLs, roles, relationships, and spirituality.
- Describe potential benefits and risks of parathyroidectomy.
- State the name, dose, side effects, frequency, and schedule for all medications.
- Explain the purpose, dose, route, schedule, side effects, and precautions of pharmacologic treatment (loop diuretics, phosphates, and calcitonin) of hyperparathyroidism.
- State the need to contact primary provider before taking over-the-counter medication containing calcium.
- State changes in lifestyle (e.g., diet, activity) necessary to maintain health, including:
  - Recommended intake of dietary calcium.

- Maintenance of regular bowel habits and management of constipation (e.g., prune juice, stool softeners, increased physical activity and fluids).
- Monitoring of fluid intake as indicated, generally 2,000 mL daily.
- Managing pain (medication and nonpharmacologic interventions).
- Increasing mobility as indicated
- Relate how to reach primary provider with questions or complications.
- State time and date of follow-up medical appointments, therapy, and testing.
- Identify sources of support (e.g., friends, relatives, faith community, support groups, caregiver support).
- Identify the need for health promotion, disease prevention, and screening activities

ADL, activities of daily living; IADL, independent activities of daily living.

Complications: Hypercalcemic Crisis

Acute hypercalcemic crisis can occur with extreme elevation of serum calcium levels. Serum calcium levels greater than 13 mg/dL (3.25 mmol/L) result in neurologic, cardiovascular, and kidney symptoms that can be life threatening (Fischbach & Dunning, 2015). Rapid rehydration with large volumes of IV isotonic saline fluids to maintain urine output of 100 to 150 mL per hour is combined with administration of calcitonin (Shane & Berenson, 2016). Calcitonin promotes renal excretion of excess calcium and reduces bone resorption. The saline infusion should be stopped and a loop diuretic may be needed if the patient develops edema. Dosage and rates of infusion depend on the patient profile. The patient should be monitored carefully for fluid overload. Loop diuretics are not recommended as initial therapy in the absence of heart failure and kidney insufficiency. Bisphosphonates are added to promote a sustained decrease in serum calcium levels by promoting calcium deposition in bone and reducing the GI absorption of calcium. Cytotoxic agents (e.g., mithramycin), calcitonin, and dialysis may be used in emergency situations to decrease serum calcium levels quickly.

> **Quality and Safety Nursing Alert**
>
> *The patient in acute hypercalcemic crisis requires close monitoring for life-threatening complications (e.g., airway obstruction) and prompt treatment to reduce serum calcium levels.*

A combination of calcitonin and corticosteroids is given in emergencies to reduce the serum calcium level by increasing calcium deposition in bone. Other agents that may be given to decrease serum calcium levels include bisphosphonates (e.g., etidronate [Didronel], pamidronate [Aredia]) (Shane & Berenson, 2016).

Expert assessment and care are required to minimize complications and reverse the life-threatening hypercalcemia. Medications are given with care, and attention is given to

fluid balance to promote return of normal fluid and electrolyte balance. Supportive measures are necessary for the patient and family. See Chapters 13 and 15 for further discussion of hypercalcemic crisis.

Hypoparathyroidism

Hypoparathyroidism is caused by abnormal parathyroid development, destruction of the parathyroid glands (surgical removal or autoimmune response), and vitamin D deficiency. The most common cause is the near-total removal of the thyroid gland. The result is inadequate secretion of parathormone (Goltzman, 2016).

Deficiency of parathormone results in increased blood phosphate (hyperphosphatemia) and decreased blood calcium (hypocalcemia) levels. In the absence of parathormone, there is decreased intestinal absorption of dietary calcium and decreased resorption of calcium from bone and through the renal tubules. Decreased renal excretion of phosphate causes hypophosphaturia, and low serum calcium levels result in hypocalciuria.

Clinical Manifestations

Hypocalcemia causes irritability of the neuromuscular system and contributes to the chief symptom of hypoparathyroidism—tetany. Tetany is general muscle hypertonia, with tremor and spasmodic or uncoordinated contractions occurring with or without efforts to make voluntary movements. Symptoms of latent tetany are numbness, tingling, and cramps in the extremities, and the patient complains of stiffness in the hands and feet. In overt tetany, the signs include bronchospasm, laryngeal spasm, carpopedal spasm (flexion of the elbows and wrists and extension of the carpophalangeal joints and dorsiflexion of the feet), dysphagia, photophobia, cardiac dysrhythmias, and seizures. Other symptoms include anxiety, irritability, depression, and even delirium. ECG changes and hypotension also may occur.

Assessment and Diagnostic Findings

A positive Chvostek sign or a positive Trousseau sign suggests latent tetany. **Chvostek sign** is positive when a sharp tapping over the facial nerve just in front of the parotid gland and anterior to the ear causes spasm or twitching of the mouth, nose, and eye (see Fig. 13-6A). **Trousseau sign** is positive when carpopedal spasm is induced by occluding the blood flow to the arm for 3 minutes with a blood pressure cuff (see Fig. 13-6B). The diagnosis of hypoparathyroidism often is difficult because of the vague symptoms, such as aches and pains. Therefore, laboratory studies are especially helpful. Tetany develops at very low serum calcium levels. Serum phosphate levels are increased, and x-rays of bone show increased density. Calcification is detected on x-rays of the subcutaneous or paraspinal basal ganglia of the brain.

Medical Management

The goal of therapy is to increase the serum calcium level to 9 to 10 mg/dL (2.2 to 2.5 mmol/L) and to eliminate the symptoms of hypoparathyroidism and hypocalcemia. Management is determined by the underlying cause and patient profile. Treatment may include combinations of calcitriol, calcium, magnesium, and vitamin D_2 (ergocalciferol) or vitamin D_3 (calcitriol), the latter being preferred. A thiazide diuretic (e.g., hydrochlorothiazide [HydroDIURIL]) may be given to help decrease urinary calcium excretion (Goltzman, 2016; Rosen, 2016). Recombinant parathyroid hormone has been approved for the treatment of osteoporosis but not for hypoparathyroidism at this time (Goltzman, 2016; Rosen, 2016).

When hypocalcemia and tetany occur after a thyroidectomy, the immediate treatment is administration of IV calcium gluconate. If this does not decrease neuromuscular irritability and seizure activity immediately, sedative agents such as pentobarbital may be given.

Because of neuromuscular irritability, the patient with hypocalcemia and tetany requires an environment that is free of noise, drafts, bright lights, or sudden movement. Tracheostomy or mechanical ventilation may become necessary, along with bronchodilating medications, if the patient develops respiratory distress.

Therapy for chronic hypoparathyroidism is determined after serum calcium levels are obtained. A diet high in calcium and low in phosphorus is prescribed. Although milk, milk products, and egg yolk are high in calcium, they are restricted because they also contain high levels of phosphorus. Spinach also is avoided because it contains oxalate, which would form insoluble calcium substances. Oral tablets of calcium salts, such as calcium gluconate, may be used to supplement the diet. Aluminum hydroxide gel or aluminum carbonate (Gelusil, Amphojel) also is given after meals to bind phosphate and promote its excretion through the GI tract.

Nursing Management

Nursing management of the patient with possible acute hypoparathyroidism includes the following:

- Care of postoperative patients who have undergone thyroidectomy, parathyroidectomy, or radical neck dissection is directed toward detecting early signs of hypocalcemia and anticipating signs of tetany, seizures, and respiratory difficulties.
- Calcium gluconate should be available for emergency IV administration. If the patient requiring administration of calcium gluconate has a cardiac disorder, is subject to dysrhythmias, or is receiving digitalis, the calcium gluconate is given slowly and cautiously.
- Calcium and digitalis increase systolic contraction and also potentiate each other; this can produce potentially fatal dysrhythmias. Consequently, the cardiac patient requires continuous cardiac monitoring and careful assessment.

An important aspect of nursing care is patient education about medications and diet therapy. The patient needs to know the reason for high calcium and low phosphate intake and the symptoms of hypocalcemia and hypercalcemia; he or she should know to contact the primary provider immediately if these symptoms occur (see Chart 52-9).

Chart 52-9

HOME CARE CHECKLIST

The Patient With Hypoparathyroidism

At the completion of education, the patient and/or caregiver will be able to:

- State the impact of hypoparathyroidism and treatment on physiologic functioning, ADLs, IADLs, roles, relationships, and spirituality.
- State purpose, dose, route, schedule, side effects, and precautions of prescribed medications (calcium, phosphate binders).
- State changes in lifestyle (e.g., diet, activity) necessary to maintain health, including:
  - Ensuring a diet high in calcium and vitamin D, low in phosphorous.
  - Alternating activity and rest periods.

- State precipitating factors and interventions for complications (seizure, cardiac dysrhythmias, cardiac arrest).
- State necessary actions for seizure activity.
- Relate how to reach primary provider with questions or complications.
- State time and date of follow-up medical appointments, therapy, and testing.
- Identify sources of support (e.g., friends, relatives, faith community, support groups, caregiver support).
- Identify the need for health promotion, disease prevention, and screening activities

ADL, activities of daily living; IADL, independent activities of daily living.

THE ADRENAL GLANDS

Anatomic and Physiologic Overview

Each person has two adrenal glands, one attached to the upper portion of each kidney (Porth, 2015). Each adrenal gland is, in reality, two endocrine glands with separate, independent functions. The adrenal medulla at the center of the gland secretes catecholamines, and the outer portion of the gland, the adrenal cortex, secretes steroid hormones (see Fig. 52-6). The secretion of hormones from the adrenal cortex is regulated by the hypothalamic–pituitary–adrenal axis. The hypothalamus secretes corticotropin-releasing hormone (CRH), which stimulates the pituitary gland to secrete ACTH, which in turn stimulates the adrenal cortex to secrete glucocorticoid hormone (cortisol). Increased levels of the adrenal hormone then inhibit the production or secretion of CRH and ACTH. This system is an example of a negative feedback mechanism.

Adrenal Medulla

The adrenal medulla functions as part of the autonomic nervous system. Stimulation of preganglionic sympathetic nerve fibers, which travel directly to the cells of the adrenal medulla, causes release of the catecholamine hormones epinephrine and norepinephrine. About 90% of the secretion of the human adrenal medulla is epinephrine (also called *adrenaline*). Catecholamines regulate metabolic pathways to promote catabolism of stored fuels to meet caloric needs from endogenous sources. The major effects of epinephrine release are to prepare to meet a challenge (fight-or-flight response). Secretion of epinephrine causes decreased blood flow to tissues that are not needed in emergency situations, such as the GI tract, and increased blood flow to tissues that are important for effective fight or flight, such as cardiac and skeletal muscle. Catecholamines also induce the release of free fatty acids, increase the basal metabolic rate, and elevate the blood glucose level.

Adrenal Cortex

A functioning adrenal cortex is necessary for life; adrenocortical secretions make it possible for the body to adapt to stress of all kinds. The three types of steroid hormones produced by the adrenal cortex are glucocorticoids, mainly cortisol; **mineralocorticoids**, mainly aldosterone; and sex hormones, mainly **androgens** (male sex hormones) (Porth, 2015). Without the adrenal cortex, severe stress would cause peripheral circulatory failure, circulatory shock, and prostration. Survival in the absence of a functioning adrenal cortex is possible only with nutritional, electrolyte, and fluid replacement and appropriate replacement with exogenous adrenocortical hormones.

Glucocorticoids

The glucocorticoids are so named because they have an important influence on glucose metabolism: Increased cortisol secretion results in elevated blood glucose levels. However, the glucocorticoids have major effects on the metabolism of almost all organs of the body. Glucocorticoids are secreted from the adrenal cortex in response to the release of ACTH from the anterior lobe of the pituitary gland. This system represents an example of negative feedback. The presence of glucocorticoids in the blood inhibits the release of CRH from the hypothalamus and also inhibits ACTH secretion from the pituitary. The resultant decrease in ACTH secretion causes diminished release of glucocorticoids from the adrenal cortex.

Corticosteroids are the classification of drugs that include glucocorticoids. These drugs are given to inhibit the inflammatory response to tissue injury and to suppress allergic manifestations. Their side effects include the development of diabetes, osteoporosis, peptic ulcer, increased protein breakdown resulting in muscle wasting and poor wound healing, and redistribution of body fat. When large doses of exogenous glucocorticoids are given, the release of ACTH and endogenous glucocorticoids are inhibited. This can cause the adrenal cortex to atrophy. If exogenous glucocorticoid administration is discontinued suddenly, adrenal insufficiency results because of the inability of the atrophied cortex to respond adequately.

Mineralocorticoids

Mineralocorticoids exert their major effects on electrolyte metabolism. They act principally on the renal tubular and GI epithelium to cause increased sodium ion absorption in exchange for excretion of potassium or hydrogen ions. ACTH only minimally influences aldosterone secretion. It is primarily secreted in response to the presence of angiotensin II in the bloodstream. Angiotensin II is a substance that elevates the blood pressure by constricting arterioles.

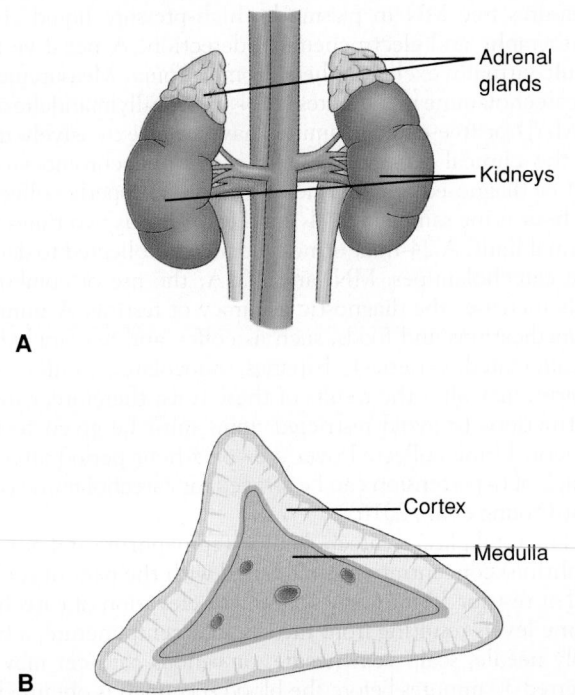

Figure 52-6 • A. The adrenal glands sit on top of the kidneys. **B.** Each gland is composed of an outer cortex and an inner medulla. Each area secretes specific hormones. The adrenal medulla secretes catecholamines—epinephrine and norepinephrine; the adrenal cortex secretes glucocorticoids, mineralocorticoids, and sex hormones. Adapted from Porth, C. (2006). *Essentials of pathophysiology: Concepts of altered health states* (2nd ed.). Philadelphia, PA: Wolters Kluwer.

Its concentration is increased when renin is released from the kidney in response to decreased perfusion pressure. The resultant increased aldosterone levels promote sodium reabsorption by the kidney and the GI tract, which tends to restore blood pressure to normal. The release of aldosterone is also increased by hyperkalemia. Aldosterone is the main hormone for the long-term regulation of sodium balance.

Adrenal Sex Hormones (Androgens)

Androgens, the third major type of steroid hormones produced by the adrenal cortex, exert effects similar to those of male sex hormones. The adrenal gland may also secrete small amounts of some estrogens, or female sex hormones. ACTH controls the secretion of adrenal androgens. When secreted in normal amounts, the adrenal androgens have little effect, but when secreted in excess, they produce masculinization in women, feminization in men, or premature sexual development in children. This is called the **adrenogenital syndrome**.

Pheochromocytoma

Pheochromocytoma is a tumor that is usually benign and originates from the chromaffin cells of the adrenal medulla. This tumor is the cause of high blood pressure in 0.1% of patients with hypertension and is usually fatal if undetected and untreated. Although uncommon, it is one form of hypertension that is usually cured by surgery. In 90% of patients (Porth, 2015), the tumor arises in the medulla; in the remaining patients, it occurs in the extra-adrenal chromaffin tissue located in or near the aorta, ovaries, spleen, or other organs. Pheochromocytoma may occur at any age, but its peak incidence is between 40 and 50 years of age and affects men and women equally (Young & Kaplan, 2016). Ten percent of the tumors are bilateral, and 10% are malignant. Because of the high incidence of pheochromocytoma in family members of affected people, the patient's family members should be alerted and screened for this tumor. Pheochromocytoma may occur in the familial form as part of multiple endocrine neoplasia type 2; therefore, it should be considered a possibility in patients who have medullary thyroid carcinoma and parathyroid hyperplasia or tumor.

Clinical Manifestations

The nature and severity of symptoms of functioning tumors of the adrenal medulla depend on the relative proportions of epinephrine and norepinephrine secretion. The typical triad of symptoms is headache, diaphoresis, and palpitations in the patient with hypertension. The tumor is discovered incidentally in approximately 10% of patients (Young, Kaplan, & Kebebew, 2016). Hypertension and other cardiovascular disturbances are common. The hypertension may be intermittent or persistent. If the hypertension is sustained, it may be difficult to distinguish from other causes of hypertension. Other symptoms may include tremor, headache, flushing, and anxiety. Hyperglycemia may result from conversion of liver and muscle glycogen to glucose due to epinephrine secretion; insulin may be required to maintain normal blood glucose levels.

The clinical picture in the paroxysmal form of pheochromocytoma is usually characterized by acute, unpredictable attacks lasting seconds or several hours. Symptoms usually begin abruptly and subside slowly. During these attacks, the patient is extremely anxious, tremulous, and weak. The patient may experience headache, vertigo, blurring of vision, tinnitus, air hunger, and dyspnea. Other symptoms include polyuria, nausea, vomiting, diarrhea, abdominal pain, and a feeling of impending doom. Palpitations and tachycardia are common (Porth, 2015). Blood pressures exceeding 250/150 mm Hg have been recorded. Such blood pressure elevations are life threatening and can cause severe complications, such as cardiac dysrhythmias, dissecting aneurysm, stroke, and acute kidney failure. Postural hypotension (decrease in systolic blood pressure, lightheadedness, dizziness on standing) occurs in 70% of patients with untreated pheochromocytoma.

Assessment and Diagnostic Findings

Pheochromocytoma is suspected if signs of sympathetic nervous system overactivity occur in association with marked elevation of blood pressure. These signs can be associated with the "five Hs": *h*ypertension, *h*eadache, *h*yperhidrosis (excessive sweating), *h*ypermetabolism, and *h*yperglycemia. The presence of these signs is highly predictive of pheochromocytoma. Paroxysmal symptoms of pheochromocytoma commonly develop in the fifth decade of life.

Measurements of urine and plasma levels of catecholamines and metanephrine (MN), a catecholamine metabolite, are the most direct and conclusive tests for overactivity of the adrenal medulla. A test for detecting pheochromocytoma measures free MN in plasma by high-pressure liquid chromatography and electrochemical detection. A negative test result virtually excludes pheochromocytoma. Measurements of catecholamine metabolites (MN and vanillylmandelic acid [VMA]) or free catecholamines have been extensively used in the clinical setting. In most cases, pheochromocytoma can be diagnosed or confirmed based on a properly collected 24-hour urine sample. Levels can be as high as two times the normal limit. A 24-hour urine specimen is collected to detect free catecholamines, MN, and VMA; the use of combined tests increases the diagnostic accuracy of testing. A number of medications and foods, such as coffee and tea (including decaffeinated varieties), bananas, chocolate, vanilla, and aspirin, may alter the results of these tests; therefore, careful instructions to avoid restricted items must be given to the patient. Urine collected over a 2- or 3-hour period after an attack of hypertension can be assayed for catecholamine content (Young et al., 2016).

The total plasma catecholamine (epinephrine and norepinephrine) concentration is measured with the patient supine and at rest for 30 minutes. To prevent elevation of catecholamine levels resulting from the stress of venipuncture, a butterfly needle, scalp vein needle, or venous catheter may be inserted 30 minutes before the blood specimen is obtained.

Factors that may elevate catecholamine concentrations must be controlled to obtain valid results; these factors include consumption of coffee or tea (including decaffeinated varieties), the use of tobacco, emotional and physical stress, and the use of many prescription and over-the-counter medications (e.g., amphetamines, nose drops or sprays, decongestant agents, bronchodilators).

Normal plasma values of epinephrine are 100 pg/mL (590 pmol/L); normal values of norepinephrine are generally less than 100 to 550 pg/mL (590 to 3,240 pmol/L). Values of epinephrine greater than 400 pg/mL (2,180 pmol/L) or norepinephrine values greater than 2,000 pg/mL (11,800 pmol/L) are considered diagnostic of pheochromocytoma. Values that fall between normal levels and those diagnostic of pheochromocytoma indicate the need for further testing.

A clonidine suppression test may be performed if the results of plasma and urine tests of catecholamines are inconclusive. Clonidine (Catapres) is a centrally acting antiadrenergic medication that suppresses the release of neurogenically mediated catecholamines. The suppression test is based on the principle that catecholamine levels are normally increased through the activity of the sympathetic nervous system. In pheochromocytoma, increased catecholamine levels result from the diffusion of excess catecholamines into the circulation, bypassing normal storage and release mechanisms. Therefore, in patients with pheochromocytoma, clonidine does not suppress the release of catecholamines (Young & Kaplan, 2016).

Imaging studies, such as CT, MRI, and ultrasonography, may also be carried out to localize the pheochromocytoma and to determine whether more than one tumor is present. The use of ^{131}I-metaiodobenzylguanidine (MIBG) scintigraphy may be required to determine the location of the pheochromocytoma and to detect metastatic sites outside the adrenal gland. MIBG is a specific isotope for catecholamine-producing tissue. It has been helpful in identifying tumors not detected by other tests or procedures. MIBG scintigraphy is a noninvasive, safe procedure that has increased the accuracy of diagnosis of adrenal tumors (Fischbach & Dunning, 2015).

Other diagnostic studies may focus on evaluating the function of other endocrine glands because of the association of pheochromocytoma in some patients with other endocrine tumors.

Medical Management

During an episode or attack of hypertension, tachycardia, anxiety, and the other symptoms of pheochromocytoma, bed rest with the head of the bed elevated is prescribed to promote an orthostatic decrease in blood pressure.

Pharmacologic Therapy

The patient may be treated preoperatively on an inpatient or outpatient basis. Regardless of the setting, monitoring of blood pressure and cardiac function is essential. The goals are to control hypertension before and during surgery and volume expansion. Although there are no randomized controlled studies that have compared the efficacy of different treatments, the use of an alpha-adrenergic blocker, sometimes in tandem with a beta-adrenergic blocker, has led to positive outcomes. In some instances, calcium channel blockers and metyrosine have been also been used successfully.

Preoperatively, the patient may begin treatment with a low dose of an alpha-adrenergic blocker (phenoxybenzamine [Dibenzyline]) 10 to 14 days or longer prior to surgery (Young et al., 2016). The patient should be informed about the potential for adverse effects of these medications, which include orthostasis, nasal stuffiness, increased fatigue, and retrograde ejaculation in men. The dosage is increased every 2 to 3 days as needed to control blood pressure, with the final dose usually ranging between 20 to 100 mg daily (Young et al., 2016). Some practitioners may prefer the use of a selective alpha$_1$-adrenergic blocker with fewer side effects, such as prazosin (Minipress), terazosin (Hytrin), or doxazosin (Cardura), when long-term therapy is indicated. Unless contraindicated, patients are encouraged to begin a high-sodium diet on the second or third day after the introduction of alpha-adrenergic blockade.

After administration of the alpha-blockers, the blood pressure should be monitored closely. In an outpatient setting, the blood pressure should be taken twice daily in a sitting and standing position. The targets are 120/80 mm Hg (seated) with a standing systolic pressure greater than 90 mm Hg. Age and comorbid disease should be taken into consideration when establishing and evaluating targets. Cautious low-dose beta-adrenergic blockade (e.g., propranolol) is only initiated once adequate alpha-adrenergic control has been achieved (Young et al., 2016). The dosage is adjusted according to the patient response and ability to tolerate the drug. The dosage may be initiated in daily divided doses and on day 2 adjusted to a single long-acting dose. On subsequent days, the dose may be increased to control tachycardia as needed with a target heart rate of 60 to 80 bpm.

Calcium channel blockers such as nifedipine (Procardia) are sometimes used as an alternative or supplement to preoperative alpha- and beta-blockers, when blood pressure control is inadequate or the patient is unable to tolerate the side effects. Nifedipine and nicardipine (Cardene) may be used safely without causing undue hypotension. For episodes of severe hypertension, nifedipine is a fast and effective treatment, because the capsules can be pierced and chewed. The patient needs to be well hydrated before, during, and after surgery to prevent hypotension. Additional medications that may be used preoperatively include catecholamine synthesis inhibitors, such as alpha-methyl-p-tyrosine (metyrosine [Demser]). These are occasionally used if adrenergic blocking agents (i.e., alpha- and beta-blockers) are not effective. Long-term use of metyrosine may result in many adverse effects, including sedation, depression, diarrhea, anxiety, nightmares, dysuria, impotence, elevated aspartate aminotransferase, anemia, thrombocytopenia, crystalluria, galactorrhea (breast discharge), and extrapyramidal signs (e.g., drooling, speech impairment, tremors).

Surgical Management

The definitive treatment of pheochromocytoma is surgical removal of the tumor, usually with **adrenalectomy** (removal of one or both adrenal glands). Surgery may be performed using a laparoscopic approach or an open operation. The laparoscopic approach is the preferred method for patients with solitary intra-adrenal pheochromocytomas less than 8 cm in diameter without malignancy (Young et al., 2016). Bilateral adrenalectomy may be necessary if tumors are present in both adrenal glands. Patient preparation includes control of blood pressure and blood volumes; usually, this is carried out over 10 to 14 days, as described previously. A calcium channel blocker (nicardipine [Cardene]) can be given intraoperatively exclusively or in combination with the alpha- and beta-blockers to control blood pressure.

A hypertensive crisis, however, can still arise as a result of manipulation of the tumor during surgical excision, causing a release of stored epinephrine and norepinephrine, with marked increases in blood pressure and changes in heart rate. In response to this crisis, sodium nitroprusside (Nitropress), phentolamine (OraVerse), or nicardipine can be given. Lidocaine (Xylocaine) or esmolol (Brevibloc) is used to control cardiac arrhythmias (Young et al., 2016). Exploration of other possible tumor sites is frequently undertaken to ensure removal of all tumor tissue. As a result, the patient is subject to the stress and effects of a long surgical procedure, which may increase the risk of hypertension postoperatively.

Corticosteroid replacement is required if bilateral adrenalectomy has been necessary. Corticosteroids may also be required for the first few days or weeks after removal of a single adrenal gland. IV administration of corticosteroids (methylprednisolone [Solu-Medrol]) may begin on the evening before surgery and continue during the early postoperative period to prevent adrenal insufficiency. Oral preparations of corticosteroids (prednisone) are prescribed after the acute stress of surgery diminishes.

Hypotension and hypoglycemia may occur in the postoperative period because of the sudden withdrawal of excessive amounts of catecholamines. Therefore, careful attention is directed toward monitoring and treating these changes. Hypertension may continue if not all pheochromocytoma tissue was removed, if pheochromocytoma recurs, or if the blood vessels were damaged by severe and prolonged hypertension. Several days after surgery, urine and plasma levels of catecholamines and their metabolites are measured to determine whether the surgery was successful.

Nursing Management

The patient who has undergone surgery to treat pheochromocytoma has experienced a stressful preoperative and postoperative course and may remain fearful of repeated attacks. Although it is usually expected that all pheochromocytoma tissue has been removed, there is a possibility that other sites were undetected and that attacks may recur. The patient is monitored until stable with special attention given to ECG changes, arterial pressures, fluid and electrolyte balance, and blood glucose levels. IV access will be required for administration of fluids and medications.

Promoting Home, Community-Based, and Transitional Care

 Educating Patients About Self-Care

During the pre- and postoperative phases of care, the nurse educates the patient about the importance of follow-up monitoring to ensure that pheochromocytoma does not recur undetected. After adrenalectomy, the use of corticosteroids may be needed. Therefore, the nurse educates the patient about their purpose, the medication schedule, and the risks of skipping doses or stopping their administration abruptly.

The nurse educates the patient and family about how to measure the patient's blood pressure and when to notify the primary provider about changes in blood pressure. In addition, the nurse provides verbal and written instructions about

the procedure for collecting 24-hour urine specimens to monitor urine catecholamine levels.

Continuing and Transitional Care

A follow-up visit from a home, community-based or transitional care nurse may be indicated to assess the patient's postoperative recovery, surgical incision, knowledge regarding medication, and adherence to the medication schedule. This may help reinforce previous education about management and monitoring. The nurse also obtains blood pressure measurements and assists the patient in preventing or dealing with problems that may result from long-term use of corticosteroids.

Because of the risk of recurrence of hypertension, periodic checkups are required, especially in young patients and in those whose families have a history of pheochromocytoma. The patient is scheduled for periodic follow-up appointments to observe for return of normal blood pressure and plasma and urine levels of catecholamines.

Adrenocortical Insufficiency (Addison Disease)

Addison disease, primary adrenal insufficiency (PAI), occurs when the adrenal glands are damaged and cannot produce sufficient amounts of cortical hormones (Bornstein, Allolio, Arlt, et al., 2016). Autoimmune or idiopathic atrophy of the adrenal glands is responsible for 80% to 90% of all cases. Other causes include surgical removal of both adrenal glands and infection of the adrenal glands. Tuberculosis and histoplasmosis are the most common infections that destroy adrenal gland tissue. The use of multiple pharmacologic therapies such as anticoagulants (resulting in adrenal hemorrhage), anticonvulsants (e.g., phenytoin [Dilantin] and phenobarbital), and antibiotics (e.g., rifampicin) for chronic and severe illnesses has also resulted in manifestations of PAI (Bornstein et al., 2016). Tuberculosis should be considered in the diagnostic workup. Inadequate secretion of ACTH from the pituitary gland is a secondary cause of adrenocortical insufficiency as a result of decreased stimulation of the adrenal cortex (Bornstein et al., 2016).

Therapeutic use of corticosteroids is the most common cause of adrenocortical insufficiency (Porth, 2015). Symptoms of adrenocortical insufficiency may result from the sudden cessation of exogenous adrenocortical hormonal therapy, which suppresses the body's normal response to stress and interferes with normal feedback mechanisms. Treatment with daily administration of corticosteroids for 2 to 4 weeks may suppress function of the adrenal cortex; therefore, adrenal insufficiency should be considered in any patient who has been treated with corticosteroids.

Clinical Manifestations

Addison disease is characterized by muscle weakness; anorexia; GI symptoms; fatigue; emaciation; dark pigmentation of the mucous membranes and the skin, especially of the knuckles, knees, and elbows; hypotension; and low blood glucose, low serum sodium, and high serum potassium levels. Depression, emotional lability, apathy, and confusion are present in 20% to 40% of patients (Nieman, 2016a). In severe cases, the disturbance of sodium and potassium metabolism may be marked by depletion of sodium and water and severe, chronic dehydration.

With disease progression, **addisonian crisis** (i.e., hypotension, cyanosis, fever, nausea, vomiting, and signs of shock) develops. In addition, the patient may have pallor; complain of headache, abdominal pain, and diarrhea; and may show signs of confusion and restlessness. Even slight overexertion, exposure to cold, acute infection, or a decrease in salt intake may lead to circulatory collapse, shock, and death, if untreated. The stress of surgery or dehydration resulting from preparation for diagnostic tests or surgery may precipitate an addisonian or hypotensive crisis.

Assessment and Diagnostic Findings

Although the clinical manifestations presented appear specific, the onset of Addison disease usually occurs with nonspecific symptoms. The diagnosis is confirmed by laboratory test results. Combined measurements of early-morning serum cortisol and plasma ACTH are performed to differentiate primary adrenal insufficiency from secondary adrenal insufficiency and from normal adrenal function. Patients with primary insufficiency have a greatly increased plasma ACTH level and a serum cortisol concentration lower than the normal range or in the low-normal range (Nieman, 2016b). Other laboratory findings include decreased levels of blood glucose (hypoglycemia) and sodium (hyponatremia), an increased serum potassium concentration (hyperkalemia), and an increased white blood cell count (leukocytosis).

Medical Management

Immediate treatment is directed toward combating circulatory shock: restoring blood circulation, administering fluids and corticosteroids, monitoring vital signs, and placing the patient in a recumbent position with the legs elevated. Hydrocortisone (Solu-Cortef) is administered by IV, followed by 5% dextrose in normal saline. Vasopressors may be required if hypotension persists.

Antibiotics may be given if infection has precipitated adrenal crisis in a patient with chronic adrenal insufficiency. In addition, the patient is assessed closely to identify other factors, stressors, or illnesses that led to the acute episode.

Oral intake may be initiated as soon as tolerated. IV fluids are gradually decreased after oral fluid intake is adequate to prevent hypovolemia. If the adrenal gland does not regain function, the patient needs lifelong replacement of corticosteroids and mineralocorticoids to prevent recurrence of adrenal insufficiency (Young & Kaplan, 2016). During stressful procedures or significant illnesses, additional supplementary therapy with glucocorticoids is required to prevent addisonian crisis. In addition, the patient may need to supplement dietary intake with salt during GI losses of fluids through vomiting and diarrhea.

Nursing Management

Assessing the Patient

The health history and examination focus on the presence of symptoms of fluid imbalance and the patient's level of stress. The nurse should monitor the blood pressure and pulse rate as the patient moves from a lying, sitting, and standing position to assess for inadequate fluid volume. A decrease in systolic pressure (20 mm Hg or more) may indicate depletion of fluid volume, especially if accompanied by symptoms. The skin should be assessed for changes in color and turgor, which could indicate chronic adrenal insufficiency and hypovolemia. The patient is assessed for change in weight, muscle weakness, fatigue, and any illness or stress that may have precipitated the acute crisis.

Monitoring and Managing Addisonian Crisis

The patient at risk is monitored for signs and symptoms indicative of addisonian crisis, which can include shock; hypotension; rapid, weak pulse; rapid respiratory rate; pallor; and extreme weakness (see Chapter 14). Physical and psychological stressors such as cold exposure, overexertion, infection, and emotional distress should be avoided.

The patient with addisonian crisis requires immediate treatment with IV administration of fluid, glucose, and electrolytes, especially sodium; replacement of missing steroid hormones; and vasopressors. The nurse anticipates and meets the patient's needs to promote return to a precrisis state.

Restoring Fluid Balance

The nurse encourages the patient to consume foods and fluids that assist in restoring and maintaining fluid and electrolyte balance. Along with the dietitian, the nurse helps the patient select foods high in sodium during GI disturbances and in very hot weather.

The nurse educates the patient and family to administer hormone replacement as prescribed and to modify the dosage during illness and other stressful situations. Written and verbal instructions are provided about the administration of corticosteroids (hydrocortisone, cortisone, and prednisone) and mineralocorticoids (fludrocortisone [Florinef]) as prescribed.

Improving Activity Tolerance

Until the patient's condition is stabilized, the nurse takes precautions to avoid unnecessary activity and stress that could precipitate another hypotensive episode. Efforts are made to detect signs of infection or the presence of other stressors. Explaining the rationale for minimizing stress during the acute crisis assists the patient to increase activity gradually.

Promoting Home, Community-Based, and Transitional Care

 Educating Patients About Self-Care

Because of the need for lifelong replacement of adrenal cortex hormones to prevent addisonian crises, the patient and family members receive explicit education about the rationale for replacement therapy and proper dosage. In addition, the patient, family, and caregivers are educated about the signs of excessive or insufficient hormone replacement. The patient should have an emergency kit in the form of corticosteroid in prefilled syringes, 100-mg vials of hydrocortisone or 4 mg of dexamethasone and 0.9% sterile saline to reconstitute the corticosteroid and syringes (Nieman, 2016c). Specific verbal and written instructions about how and when to use the injection are also provided to the patient and family

Chart 52-10

HOME CARE CHECKLIST
The Patient With Adrenal Insufficiency (Addison Disease)

At the completion of education, the patient and/or caregiver will be able to:

- State the impact of adrenal insufficiency and treatment on physiologic functioning, ADLs, IADLs, roles, relationships, and spirituality.
- State the purpose, dose, route, schedule, side effects, and precautions of prescribed medications (corticosteroid replacement).
- State that compliance with medical regimen is lifelong.
- Recognize the need for dosage adjustment during times of stress.
- State changes in lifestyle (e.g., diet, activity) necessary to maintain health, including:
  - Wearing medical alert identification, and carrying medical information card.
  - Avoiding strenuous activity in hot, humid weather.
  - Identifying strategies for dealing with stress and avoiding adrenal crisis.
  - Notifying primary providers about disease before treatment or procedure.

- Increasing fluid intake and salt with excessive perspiration.
- Ensuring high-carbohydrate, high-protein diet with adequate sodium intake.
- State warning signs of adrenal crisis and the need for emergency care.
- Explain components of an emergency kit and indications for their use; demonstrate how to use them.
- Relate how to reach primary provider with questions or complications.
- State time and date of follow-up medical appointments, therapy, and testing.
- Identify sources of support (e.g., friends, relatives, faith community, support groups, caregiver support).
- Identify the need for health promotion, disease prevention, and screening activities

ADL, activities of daily living; IADL, independent activities of daily living.

---

or caregivers. The entire dose of 100-mg hydrocortisone or 4 mg of dexamethasone should be given and medical attention sought immediately after administering the drug. Chart 52-10 summarizes education for patients with Addison disease and their caregivers.

Continuing and Transitional Care

Although most patients can return to their job and family responsibilities soon after hospital discharge, others cannot do so because of concurrent illnesses or incomplete recovery from the episode of adrenal insufficiency. In these circumstances, a referral for home, community-based or transitional care enables the nurse to assess the patient's recovery, monitor hormone replacement, and evaluate stress in the home. The nurse assesses the patient's and family's knowledge about medication therapy and dietary modifications and provides education as needed. The home care nurse educates the patient and family on the importance of keeping follow-up visits with the primary provider and participating in health promotion activities and health screening.

Cushing Syndrome

Cushing syndrome results from excessive, rather than deficient, adrenocortical activity (Porth, 2015). Cushing syndrome is commonly caused by the use of corticosteroid medications and is infrequently the result of excessive corticosteroid production secondary to hyperplasia of the adrenal cortex. However, overproduction of endogenous corticosteroids may be caused by several mechanisms, including a tumor of the pituitary gland that produces ACTH and stimulates the adrenal cortex to increase its hormone secretion despite production of adequate amounts. Primary hyperplasia of the adrenal glands in the absence of a pituitary tumor is less common. Another less common cause of Cushing syndrome is the ectopic production of ACTH by malignancies; bronchogenic carcinoma is the most common type. Regardless of the cause, the normal feedback mechanisms that control the function of the adrenal cortex become ineffective, and the usual diurnal pattern of cortisol is lost. The signs and symptoms of Cushing syndrome are primarily a result of oversecretion of glucocorticoids and androgens, although mineralocorticoid secretion may be affected as well (Porth, 2015).

 Concept Mastery Alert

Nurses must recognize that imbalanced adrenocortical hormone secretion characterizes both Addison disease (hypoproduction) and Cushing syndrome (hyperproduction).

Clinical Manifestations

When overproduction of the adrenocortical hormone occurs, arrest of growth, obesity, and musculoskeletal changes occur along with glucose intolerance. The classic picture of Cushing syndrome in the adult is that of central-type obesity, with a fatty "buffalo hump" in the neck and supraclavicular areas, a heavy trunk, and relatively thin extremities. The skin is thin, fragile, and easily traumatized; ecchymoses (bruises) and striae develop. The patient complains of weakness and lassitude. Sleep is disturbed because of altered diurnal secretion of cortisol.

Excessive protein catabolism occurs, producing muscle wasting and osteoporosis. Kyphosis, backache, and compression fractures of the vertebrae may result. Retention of sodium and water occurs as a result of increased mineralocorticoid activity, producing hypertension and heart failure.

The patient develops a "moon-faced" appearance and may experience increased oiliness of the skin and acne. Hyperglycemia or overt diabetes may develop. The patient may also report weight gain, slow healing of minor cuts, and bruises.

Women between the ages of 20 and 40 years are five times more likely than men to develop Cushing syndrome. In females of all ages, virilization may occur as a result of excess androgens. Virilization is characterized by the appearance of masculine traits and the recession of feminine traits. There is an excessive growth of hair on the face (hirsutism), the breasts atrophy, menses cease, the clitoris enlarges, and the voice deepens. Libido is lost in men and women. Distress and depression are common and are increased by the severity of the physical changes that occur with this syndrome. If Cushing syndrome is a consequence of pituitary tumor, visual disturbances may occur because of pressure of the growing tumor on the optic chiasm. Chart 52-11 summarizes the clinical manifestations of Cushing syndrome.

Assessment and Diagnostic Findings

The three tests used to diagnose Cushing syndrome are serum cortisol, urinary cortisol, and low-dose dexamethasone (Decadron) suppression tests (Nieman, 2016d). Two of these three tests need to be unequivocally abnormal to diagnose Cushing syndrome. If the results of all three tests are normal, the patient likely does not have Cushing syndrome (but may have a mild case, or the manifestations may be cyclic). For these patients, further testing is not recommended unless symptoms progress. If test results are either slightly abnormal or discordant, further testing is recommended.

Serum cortisol levels are usually higher in the early morning (6 to 8 AM) and lower in the evening (4 to 6 PM). This variation is lost in patients with Cushing syndrome (Fischbach & Dunning, 2015).

A urinary cortisol test requires a 24-hour urine collection. The nurse instructs the patient how to collect and store the specimen. If the results of the urinary cortisol test are three times the upper limit of the normal range and one other test is abnormal, Cushing syndrome can be assumed.

An overnight dexamethasone suppression test is used to diagnosis pituitary and adrenal causes of Cushing syndrome. It can be performed on an outpatient basis. Dexamethasone (1 mg or 8 mg) is given orally late in the evening or at bedtime, and a plasma cortisol level is obtained at 8 AM the next morning. Suppression of cortisol to less than 5 mg/dL indicates that the hypothalamic–pituitary–adrenal axis is functioning properly (Fischbach & Dunning, 2015). Stress, obesity, depression, and medications such as anticonvulsant agents, estrogen (during pregnancy or as oral medications), and rifampin (Rifadin) can falsely elevate cortisol levels.

Indicators of Cushing syndrome include an increase in serum sodium and blood glucose levels and a decrease in serum potassium, a reduction in the number of blood eosinophils, and disappearance of lymphoid tissue. Measurements of plasma and urinary cortisol levels are obtained. Several blood samples may be collected to determine whether the normal diurnal variation in plasma levels is present; this variation is frequently absent in adrenal dysfunction. If several blood samples are required, they must be collected at the times specified, and the time of collection must be noted on the requisition slip.

Chart 52-11	Clinical Manifestations of Cushing Syndrome

Ophthalmic
Cataracts
Glaucoma

Cardiovascular
Hypertension
Heart failure

Endocrine/Metabolic
Altered calcium metabolism
Adrenal suppression
Buffalo hump
Hyperglycemia
Hypokalemia
Impotence
Menstrual irregularities
Metabolic alkalosis
Moon face
Negative nitrogen balance
Sodium retention
Truncal obesity

Immune Function
Decreased inflammatory responses
Impaired wound healing
Increased susceptibility to infections

Skeletal
Aseptic necrosis of femur
Osteoporosis
Spontaneous fractures
Vertebral compression fractures

Gastrointestinal
Peptic ulcer
Pancreatitis

Muscular
Myopathy
Muscle weakness

Dermatologic
Acne
Ecchymoses
Petechiae
Striae
Thinning of skin

Psychiatric
Mood alterations
Psychoses

This woman with Cushing syndrome has several classic signs, including facial hair, buffalo hump, and moon face. From Rubin, R., Strayer, D. S., & Rubin, E. (2012). *Rubin's pathology* (6th ed.). Philadelphia, PA: Lippincott Williams & Wilkins.

Medical Management

If Cushing syndrome is caused by pituitary tumors rather than tumors of the adrenal cortex, treatment is directed at the pituitary gland. Surgical removal of the tumor by transsphenoidal hypophysectomy (see Chapter 66) is the treatment of choice and has an 80% success rate. Radiation of the pituitary gland also has been successful, although it may take several months for control of symptoms. Adrenalectomy is the treatment of choice in patients with unilateral primary adrenal hypertrophy. Medical management is recommended for bilateral adrenal dysplasia.

Postoperatively, symptoms of adrenal insufficiency may begin to appear 12 to 48 hours after surgery because of reduction of the high levels of circulating adrenal hormones. Temporary replacement therapy with hydrocortisone may be necessary for several months, until the adrenal glands begin to respond normally to the body's needs.

Adrenal enzyme inhibitors (e.g., metyrapone [Metopirone], aminoglutethimide [Cytadren], mitotane [Lysodren], and ketoconazole [Nizoral]) may be used to reduce hyperadrenalism if the syndrome is caused by ectopic ACTH secretion by a tumor that cannot be eradicated. Close monitoring is necessary, because symptoms of inadequate adrenal function may result and side effects of the medications may occur.

If Cushing syndrome is a result of the administration of corticosteroids, an attempt is made to reduce or taper the medication to the minimum dosage needed to treat the underlying disease process (e.g., autoimmune or allergic disease, rejection of a transplanted organ). Frequently, alternate-day therapy decreases the symptoms of Cushing syndrome and allows recovery of the adrenal glands' responsiveness to ACTH.

NURSING PROCESS

The Patient With Cushing Syndrome

Assessment

The health history and examination focus on the effects on the body of high concentrations of adrenal cortex hormones and on the inability of the adrenal cortex to respond to changes in cortisol and aldosterone levels. The history includes information about the patient's level of activity and ability to carry out routine and self-care activities. The skin is observed and assessed for trauma, infection, breakdown, bruising, and edema. Changes in physical appearance are noted, and the patient's responses to these changes are elicited. The nurse assesses the patient's mental function, including mood, responses to questions, awareness of environment, and level of depression. The family is often a good source of information about gradual changes in the patient's physical appearance as well as emotional status.

Diagnosis

NURSING DIAGNOSES

Based on the assessment data, major nursing diagnoses include the following:

- Risk for injury related to weakness
- Risk for infection related to altered protein metabolism and inflammatory response
- Risk for activity intolerance
- Impaired skin integrity related to edema, impaired healing, and thin and fragile skin
- Disturbed body image related to altered physical appearance, impaired sexual functioning, and decreased activity level
- Ineffective coping related to mood swings, irritability, and depression

COLLABORATIVE PROBLEMS/POTENTIAL COMPLICATIONS

Potential complications may include the following:

- Addisonian crisis
- Adverse effects of adrenocortical activity

Planning and Goals

The major goals for the patient include decreased risk of injury, decreased risk of infection, decreased risk of inactivity, improved skin integrity, improved body image, improved mental function, and absence of complications.

Nursing Interventions

DECREASING RISK OF INJURY

Establishing a protective environment helps prevent falls, fractures, and other injuries to bones and soft tissues. The patient who is very weak may require assistance from the nurse in ambulating to avoid falling or bumping into sharp corners of furniture. Foods high in protein, calcium, and vitamin D are recommended to minimize muscle wasting and osteoporosis. Referral to a dietitian may assist the patient in selecting appropriate foods that are also low in sodium and calories.

DECREASING RISK OF INFECTION

The patient should avoid unnecessary exposure to others with infections. The nurse frequently assesses the patient for subtle signs of infection, because the anti-inflammatory effects of corticosteroids may mask the common signs of inflammation and infection.

PREPARING THE PATIENT FOR SURGERY

The patient is prepared for adrenalectomy, if indicated, and the postoperative course (see later discussion). If Cushing syndrome is a result of a pituitary tumor, a transsphenoidal hypophysectomy may be performed (see Chapter 66). Diabetes and peptic ulcer are common in patients with Cushing syndrome. Therefore, insulin therapy and medication to prevent or treat peptic ulcer are initiated if needed. Before, during, and after surgery, blood glucose monitoring and assessment of stools for blood are carried out to monitor for these complications. If the patient has other symptoms of Cushing syndrome, these are considered in the preoperative preparation. For example, if the patient has experienced weight gain, special instruction is given about postoperative breathing exercises.

ENCOURAGING REST AND ACTIVITY

Although the patient with Cushing syndrome experiences insomnia, weakness, fatigue, and muscle wasting, the nurse should encourage moderate activity to prevent complications of immobility and promote increased self-esteem. It is important to help the patient plan and space rest periods throughout the day and promote a relaxing, quiet environment for rest and sleep.

PROMOTING SKIN INTEGRITY

Meticulous skin care is necessary to avoid traumatizing the patient's fragile skin. The use of adhesive tape is avoided, because it can irritate the skin and tear the fragile tissue when the tape is removed. The nurse frequently assesses the skin and bony prominences and encourages and assists the patient to change positions frequently to prevent skin breakdown.

IMPROVING BODY IMAGE

If treated successfully, the major physical changes associated with Cushing syndrome disappear in time. The patient may benefit from discussion of the effect the changes have had on their self-concept and relationships with others. Weight gain and edema may be modified by a low-carbohydrate, low-sodium diet, and a high-protein intake may reduce some of the other bothersome symptoms.

IMPROVING COPING

Explanations to the patient and family members about the cause of emotional instability are important in helping them cope with the mood swings, irritability, and depression that may occur. Psychotic behavior may occur in a few patients and should be reported. The nurse encourages the patient and family members to verbalize their feelings and concerns.

MONITORING AND MANAGING POTENTIAL COMPLICATIONS

Addisonian Crisis. The patient with Cushing syndrome whose symptoms are treated by withdrawal of corticosteroids, by adrenalectomy, or by removal of a pituitary tumor is at risk for adrenal hypofunction and addisonian crisis. If high levels of circulating adrenal hormones have suppressed the function of the adrenal cortex, atrophy of the adrenal cortex is likely. If the circulating hormone level is decreased rapidly because of surgery or abrupt cessation of corticosteroid agents, manifestations of adrenal hypofunction and addisonian crisis may develop. Therefore, the patient with Cushing syndrome should be assessed for signs and symptoms of addisonian crisis as discussed previously. If addisonian crisis occurs, the patient is treated for circulatory collapse and shock (see Chapter 14).

Adverse Effects of Adrenocortical Activity. The nurse assesses fluid and electrolyte status by monitoring laboratory values and daily weights. Because of the increased risk of glucose intolerance and hyperglycemia, blood glucose monitoring is initiated. The nurse reports elevated blood glucose levels to the primary provider so that treatment can be prescribed if indicated.

PROMOTING HOME, COMMUNITY-BASED, AND TRANSITIONAL CARE

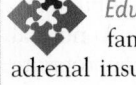

Educating Patients About Self-Care. The patient, family, and caregivers should be educated that acute adrenal insufficiency and underlying symptoms will recur if medication is stopped abruptly without medical supervision. The nurse stresses the need for dietary modifications to ensure adequate calcium intake without increasing the risks for hypertension, hyperglycemia, and weight gain. The nurse educates the patient and family about how to monitor blood pressure, blood glucose levels, and weight. Patients should be advised to wear a medical alert bracelet and to notify other health care providers (e.g., dentist) about their condition (see Chart 52-12).

Continuing and Transitional Care. The need for follow-up depends on the origin and duration of the disease and its management. The patient who has been treated by adrenalectomy or removal of a pituitary tumor requires close monitoring to ensure that adrenal function has returned to normal and adequacy of circulating adrenal hormones. Home care referral may be indicated to ensure a safe environment that minimizes stress and risk of falls and other side effects. The home care nurse assesses the patient's physical and psychological status and reports changes to the primary provider. The nurse also assesses the patient's understanding of the medication regimen and their compliance with the regimen and reinforces previous education about the medications and the importance of taking them as prescribed. The nurse emphasizes the importance of regular medical follow-up, the side effects and toxic effects of medications, and the need to wear medical identification with Addison and Cushing diseases. In addition, the nurse reminds the patient and family about the importance of health promotion activities and recommended health screening, including bone mineral density testing.

Evaluation

Expected patient outcomes may include:
1. Decreases risk of injury
   a. Is free of fractures or soft tissue injuries
   b. Is free of ecchymotic areas

Chart 52-12 | HOME CARE CHECKLIST
The Patient With Cushing Syndrome

At the completion of education, the patient and/or caregiver will be able to:

- State the impact of Cushing syndrome and treatment on physiologic functioning, ADLs, IADLs, roles, relationships, and spirituality.
  - State the relationship between adrenal hormones, emotional state, and stress.
- State the purpose, dose, route, schedule, side effects, and precautions for prescribed medications (adrenocortical inhibitors).
- State importance of compliance with medical regimen.
- State the need to contact primary provider before taking over-the-counter medications.
- State changes in lifestyle (e.g., diet, activity) necessary to maintain health, including:
  - Wearing medical alert identification, and carrying medical information card.
  - Identifying methods for managing labile emotions.
  - Describing protective skin care measures and the use of protective devices and practices to decrease injury/fracture.

- Identifying foods high in potassium and low in sodium, calories, and carbohydrates.
- Describing measures to decrease risk of infection.
- Balancing rest and activity.
- Monitoring blood pressure, blood glucose levels, and weight.
- Identify signs and symptoms of excessive and insufficient adrenal hormone.
- Relate how to reach primary provider with questions or complications.
- State time and date of follow-up medical appointments, therapy, and testing.
- Identify sources of support (e.g., friends, relatives, faith community, support groups, caregiver support).
- Identify the need for health promotion, disease prevention, and screening activities.

ADL, activities of daily living; IADL, independent activities of daily living.

2. Decreases risk of infection
   a. Experiences no temperature elevation, redness, pain, or other signs of infection or inflammation
   b. Avoids contact with others who have infections
3. Increases participation in self-care activities
   a. Plans activities and exercises to allow alternating periods of rest and activity
   b. Reports improved well-being
   c. Is free of complications of immobility
4. Attains/maintains skin integrity
   a. Has intact skin, without evidence of breakdown or infection
   b. Exhibits decreased edema in extremities and trunk
   c. Changes position frequently and inspects bony prominences daily
5. Achieves improved body image
   a. Verbalizes feelings about changes in appearance, sexual function, and activity level
   b. States that physical changes are a result of excessive corticosteroids
6. Exhibits improved thought processes
7. Exhibits absence of complications
   a. Exhibits normal vital signs and weight and is free of symptoms of addisonian crisis
   b. Identifies signs and symptoms of adrenocortical hypofunction that should be reported and measures to take in case of severe illness and stress
   c. Identifies strategies to minimize complications of Cushing syndrome
   d. Complies with recommendations for follow-up appointments and health screening

Primary Aldosteronism

The principal action of aldosterone is to conserve body sodium. Under the influence of this hormone, the kidneys excrete less sodium and more potassium and hydrogen. Excessive production of aldosterone, which occurs in some patients with functioning tumors of the adrenal gland, causes a distinctive pattern of biochemical changes and a corresponding set of clinical manifestations that are diagnostic of this condition.

Clinical Manifestations

Hypertension is the most prominent and almost universal sign of primary aldosteronism. Patients with uncomplicated, complicated, and treatment resistant hypertension and hypertension with hypokalemia should be considered at risk for this disorder. However, hypokalemia should no longer be considered a requisite for this diagnosis. It is now recognized that hypokalemia is not always present in primary aldosteronism. In some patients, hypokalemia only becomes evident after the introduction of a potassium-sparing diuretic (e.g., hydrochlorothiazide, furosemide) (Young, 2016; Young & Kaplan, 2016). If hypokalemia is present, it may be responsible for the variable muscle weakness or paralysis, cramping, and fatigue in patients with aldosteronism, as well as the kidneys' inability to acidify or concentrate the urine. Accordingly, the urine

volume is excessive, leading to polyuria. Serum, by contrast, becomes abnormally concentrated, contributing to excessive thirst (polydipsia) and arterial hypertension. A secondary increase in blood volume and possible direct effects of aldosterone on nerve receptors, such as the carotid sinus, are other factors that result in hypertension.

Hypokalemic alkalosis may decrease the ionized serum calcium level and predispose the patient to tetany and paresthesias. Chvostek and Trousseau signs may be used to assess neuromuscular irritability before overt paresthesia and tetany occur. Glucose intolerance may occur, because hypokalemia interferes with insulin secretion from the pancreas.

Assessment and Diagnostic Findings

Withholding antihypertensive medication before testing is not required (Young, 2016). A blood test to measure the ratio of PAC (plasma aldosterone concentration) to PRA (plasma renin activity) can be performed even while the patient is taking an antihypertensive. This should be followed by aldosterone suppression confirmatory tests and sub-type evaluation tests.

Medical Management

The recommended treatment of unilateral primary aldosteronism is total surgical removal of the adrenal tumor through laparoscopic adrenalectomy rather than open surgery. Open adrenalectomy is performed through an incision in the flank or the abdomen. In general, the postoperative care for open surgery resembles that for other abdominal surgery. However, the patient is susceptible to fluctuations in adrenocortical hormones and requires administration of corticosteroids, fluids, and other agents to maintain blood pressure and prevent acute complications. If the adrenalectomy is bilateral, replacement of corticosteroids will be lifelong. A normal serum glucose level is maintained with insulin, appropriate IV fluids, and dietary modifications.

Laparoscopic surgery is recommended over open surgery to reduce complications and hospital length of stay (Young & Kaplan, 2016). Hypokalemia should be treated with spironolactone (Aldactone) preoperatively. Hypokalemia typically resolves for all patients after surgery and hypertension is resolved in 35% to 60%. Postoperatively, spironolactone and potassium supplements should be discontinued and antihypertensives should be decreased. Potassium levels should be checked once a week for 4 weeks postoperatively (Young & Kaplan, 2016).

Medical treatment rather than surgery is recommended for patients with bilateral adrenal involvement due to poor blood pressure control and other risks.

Pharmacologic Therapy

Pharmacologic management is required for patients with bilateral adrenal hyperplasia or unilateral aldosterone hypersecretion who do not undergo surgery. Spironolactone is recommended as the first-line drug to control hypertension. Eplerenone (Inspra) a newer, more expensive drug is recommended as a second-line drug if the patient cannot tolerate side effects of spironolactone (Young & Kaplan, 2016). Serum potassium and creatinine should be monitored frequently during the first 4 to 6 weeks of taking spironolactone. Ongoing monitoring will be determined by the clinical course. The half-life of digoxin may be increased when taken with spironolactone, and its dosage may need to be adjusted. The effectiveness of spironolactone in controlling blood pressure may be affected if taken with salicylates or nonsteroidal anti-inflammatory drugs (Young & Kaplan, 2016).

Nursing Management

Nursing management in the postoperative period includes frequent assessment of vital signs to detect early signs and symptoms of adrenal insufficiency and crisis or hemorrhage. Explaining all treatments and procedures, providing comfort measures, and providing rest periods can reduce the patient's stress and anxiety level.

Corticosteroid Therapy

Corticosteroids are used extensively for adrenal insufficiency and are also widely used in suppressing inflammation and autoimmune reactions, controlling allergic reactions, and reducing the rejection process in transplantation. Commonly used corticosteroid preparations are listed in Table 52-4. Their anti-inflammatory and antiallergy actions make corticosteroids effective in treating rheumatic or connective tissue diseases, such as rheumatoid arthritis and SLE. They are also frequently used in the treatment of asthma, multiple sclerosis, and other autoimmune disorders.

High doses appear to allow patients to tolerate high degrees of stress. Such antistress action may be caused by the ability of corticosteroids to aid circulating vasopressor substances in keeping the blood pressure elevated; other effects, such as maintenance of the serum glucose level, also may keep blood pressure elevated.

TABLE 52-4 Commonly Used Corticosteroid Preparations

Generic Names	Trade Names
beclomethasone	Beconase, Beclovent, Vanceril, Vancenase, Propaderm
betamethasone	Celestone, Betameth, Betnesol, Betnelan
cortisone	Cortone, Cortate, Cortogen
dexamethasone	Dexamethasone Intensol, DexPak
hydrocortisone	Cortisol, Cortef, Hydrocortone, Solu-Cortef
methylprednisolone	Medrol, Solu-Medrol, Meprolone
prednisone	Meticorten, Deltasone, Orasone, Panasol, Novo-prednisone
prednisolone	Prelone
triamcinolone	Kenalog, Triderm

Adapted from Comerford, K. C. (2015). *Nursing 2015 drug handbook*. Philadelphia, PA: Wolters Kluwer.

Side Effects

Although the synthetic corticosteroids are safer for some patients because of relative freedom from mineralocorticoid activity, most natural and synthetic corticosteroids produce similar kinds of side effects. The dose required for anti-inflammatory and antiallergy effects also produces metabolic effects, pituitary and adrenal gland suppression, and changes in the function of the central nervous system. Therefore, although corticosteroids are highly effective therapeutically, they may also be very dangerous. Dosages of these medications are frequently altered to allow high concentrations when necessary and then tapered in an attempt to avoid undesirable effects. This requires that patients be observed closely for side effects and that the dose be reduced when high doses are no longer required. Suppression of the adrenal cortex may persist up to 1 year after a course of corticosteroids.

Therapeutic Uses of Corticosteroids

The dosage of corticosteroids is determined by the nature and chronicity of the illness as well as the patient's other medical conditions. Rheumatoid arthritis, bronchial asthma, and multiple sclerosis are chronic disorders that corticosteroids do not cure; however, these medications may be useful when other measures do not provide adequate control of symptoms. In addition, corticosteroids may be used to treat acute exacerbations of these disorders.

In such situations, the adverse effects of corticosteroids are weighed against the patient's current condition. These medications may be used for a period but then are gradually reduced or tapered as the symptoms subside. The nurse plays an important role in providing encouragement and understanding during times when the patient is experiencing (or is apprehensive about experiencing) recurrence of symptoms while taking smaller doses.

Treatment of Acute Conditions

Acute flare-ups and crises are treated with large doses of corticosteroids. Examples include emergency treatment for bronchial obstruction in status asthmaticus and for septic shock from septicemia caused by gram-negative bacteria. Other measures, such as anti-infective agents or medications, are also used with corticosteroids to treat shock and other major symptoms. At times, corticosteroids are continued past the acute flare-up stage to prevent serious complications.

Ophthalmologic Treatment

Outer eye infections can be treated by topical application of corticosteroid eye drops, because the agents do not cause systemic toxicity. However, long-term application can cause an increase in intraocular pressure, which leads to glaucoma in some patients. In addition, prolonged use of corticosteroids can sometimes lead to cataract formation.

Dermatologic Disorders

Topical administration of corticosteroids in the form of creams, ointments, lotions, and aerosols is especially effective in many dermatologic disorders. It may be more effective in some conditions to use occlusive dressings around the affected part to achieve maximum absorption of the medication. Penetration and absorption are also increased if the medication is applied when the skin is hydrated or moist (e.g., immediately after bathing).

Absorption of topical agents varies with body location. For example, absorption is greater through the layers of skin on the scalp, face, and genital area than on the forearm; as a result, the use of topical agents on these sites increases the risk of side effects. The availability of over-the-counter topical corticosteroids increases the risk of side effects in patients who are unaware of their potential risks. Excessive use of these agents, especially on large surface areas of inflamed skin, can lead to decreased therapeutic effects and increased side effects.

Dosage

Attempts have been made to determine the best time to administer pharmacologic doses of steroids. If symptoms have been controlled on a 6- or 8-hour program, a once-daily or every-other-day schedule may be implemented. In keeping with the natural secretion of cortisol, the best time of day

TABLE 52-5 Corticosteroid Therapy and Implications for Nursing Practice

Side Effects	Nursing Interventions
Cardiovascular Effects	
Hypertension	Monitor for elevated blood pressure.
Thrombophlebitis	Assess for signs and symptoms of deep venous thrombosis: redness, warmth, tenderness, and edema of an extremity.
Thromboembolism	Remind patient to avoid positions and situations that restrict blood flow (e.g., crossing legs, prolonged sitting in same position).
Accelerated atherosclerosis	Encourage foot and leg exercises when recumbent.
	Encourage low-sodium diet.
	Encourage limited intake of fat.
Immunologic Effects	
Increased risk of infection and masking of signs of infection	Assess for subtle signs of infection and inflammation.
	Encourage patient to avoid exposure to others with upper respiratory infection.
	Monitor patient for fungal infections.
	Encourage handwashing.
Ophthalmologic Changes	
Glaucoma	Encourage yearly eye examinations.
Corneal lesions	Refer patient to ophthalmologist if changes in visual acuity are detected.
Musculoskeletal Effects	
Muscle wasting	Encourage high-protein intake.
Poor wound healing	Encourage high-protein intake and vitamin C supplementation.
Osteoporosis with vertebral compression fractures, pathologic fractures of long bones, aseptic necrosis of head of the femur	Encourage diet high in calcium and vitamin D or calcium and vitamin D supplementation if indicated.
	Take measures to avoid falls and other trauma.
	Use caution in moving and turning patient.
	Encourage postmenopausal women on corticosteroids to consider bone mineral density testing and treatment, if indicated.
	Instruct patient to rise slowly from bed or chair to avoid falling due to postural hypotension.
Metabolic Effects	
Alterations in glucose metabolism	Monitor blood glucose levels at periodic intervals.
Steroid withdrawal syndrome	Instruct patient about medications, diet, and exercise prescribed to control blood glucose level.
	Report signs of adrenal insufficiency.
	Administer corticosteroids and mineralocorticoids as prescribed.
	Instruct patient about importance of taking corticosteroids as prescribed without abruptly stopping therapy.
	Encourage patient to obtain and wear a medical identification bracelet.
	Advise patient to notify all health care providers (e.g., dentist) about the need for corticosteroid therapy.
Changes in Appearance	
Moon face	Encourage low-calorie, low-sodium diet.
Weight gain	Assure patient that most changes in appearance are temporary and will disappear if and when corticosteroid therapy is no longer necessary.
Acne	
Fluid and Electrolyte Imbalances	Monitor intake and output and electrolytes.
	Administer fluids and electrolytes as prescribed.

for the total corticosteroid dose is in the early morning, between 7 and 8 AM. Large-dose therapy at 8 AM, when the adrenal gland is most active, produces maximal suppression of the gland. A large 8 AM dose is more physiologic because it allows the body to escape effects of the steroids from 4 PM to 6 AM, when serum levels are normally low, hence minimizing cushingoid effects. If symptoms of the disorder being treated are suppressed, alternate-day therapy is helpful in reducing pituitary–adrenal suppression in patients requiring prolonged therapy. Some patients report discomfort associated with symptoms of their primary illness on the second day; therefore, the nurse must explain to patients that this regimen is necessary to minimize side effects and suppression of adrenal function.

Tapering

Corticosteroid dosages are reduced gradually (tapered) to allow normal adrenal function to return and to prevent steroid-induced adrenal insufficiency. Up to 1 year or longer after the use of corticosteroids, the patient is still at risk for adrenal insufficiency in times of stress. For example, if surgery for any reason is necessary, the patient is likely to require IV corticosteroids during and after surgery to reduce the risk of acute adrenal crisis.

Nursing Management

Nursing management of corticosteroid therapy includes many important interventions. Table 52-5 provides an overview of the effects of corticosteroid therapy and the nursing implications.

Promoting Home, Community-Based, and Transitional Care

Educating Patients About Self-Care

The nurse educates the patient, family, and caregivers that acute adrenal insufficiency and underlying symptoms will recur if corticosteroid therapy is stopped abruptly without medical supervision. The patient should be instructed to always have an adequate supply of the corticosteroid medication to avoid running out.

Continuing and Transitional Care

The patient who requires continued corticosteroid therapy is monitored to ensure understanding of the medications and the need for a dosage that treats the underlying disorder while minimizing the side effects. Home care referral may be indicated to ensure a safe environment that minimizes stress, risk of falls, and other side effects. The nurse assesses the patient's physical and psychological status and reports changes to the primary provider. The nurse also assesses the patient's understanding of the medication regimen and their compliance with the regimen and reinforces previous education about the medications and the importance of taking them as prescribed. The nurse emphasizes the importance of regular medical follow-up, the side effects, and effects of abruptly discontinuing corticosteroids. In addition, the nurse reminds the patient and family about the importance of health promotion activities and recommended health screening, including bone mineral density testing.

CRITICAL THINKING EXERCISES

1 `ebp` A 42-year-old man has been recently diagnosed with hypothyroidism. What resources would you use to identify evidence-based practices for appropriate interventions and prevention of complications for this patient? Identify the evidence, as well as the criteria used to evaluate the strength of the evidence, for the practices identified.

2 `pq` Identify the priorities, approach, and techniques you would use to perform a comprehensive assessment on a 60-year-old patient newly diagnosed with Cushing syndrome. How will your priorities, approach, and techniques differ if the patient has a visual impairment or is hard of hearing? If the patient is from a culture with very different values from your own?

3 A 75-year-old patient has a new prescription for corticosteroid therapy. Describe the assessment techniques appropriate to evaluate the patient and the use of the medication. What instructions should you provide regarding precautions to take related to corticosteroid therapy? How will your assessment and instructions differ if the patient is disoriented?

REFERENCES

Books

Comerford, K. C. (2015). *Nursing 2015 drug handbook*. Philadelphia, PA: Wolters Kluwer.

Dagan, R., & Amdur, R. J. (2013). Thyroid cancer. In E. C. Halperin, D. E. Wazer, C. A. Perez, et al. (Eds.). *Perez and Brady's principles and practice of radiation oncology* (6th ed.). Philadelphia, PA: Lippincott Williams and Wilkins.

Davies, T. F., Laurberg, P., & Bahn, R. S. (2016). Thyroid disorders. In S. Melmed, K. Polonsky, P. Larsen, et al. (Eds.). *Williams textbook of endocrinology*. Philadelphia, PA: Elsevier.

Fischbach, F., & Dunning, M. B. (2015). *A manual of laboratory and diagnostic tests* (9th ed.). Philadelphia, PA: Lippincott Williams & Wilkins.

Grossman, S. C., & Porth, C. M. (2014). *Pathophysiology: Concepts of altered health states* (9th ed.). Philadelphia, PA: Lippincott Williams & Wilkins.

Kaiser, U., & Ho, K.K.Y. (2016). Pituitary physiology and diagnostic evaluation. In S. Melmed, K. Polonsky, P. Larsen, et al. (Eds.). *Williams textbook of endocrinology*. Philadelphia, PA: Elsevier.

Lazar, M. A., & Birnbaum, M. J. (2016). Principles of hormone action. In S. Melmed, K. Polonsky, P. Larsen, et al. (Eds.). *Williams textbook of endocrinology*. Philadelphia, PA: Elsevier.

Majithia, A., Altshuler, R. D., & Hirschhorn, J. N. (2016). Genetics of endocrinology. In S. Melmed, K. Polonsky, P. Larsen, et al. (Eds.). *Williams textbook of endocrinology*. Philadelphia, PA: Elsevier.

Mercado, M. (2016). Endocrine and metabolic disorders. In E. T. Bope & R. D. Kellerman (Eds.). *Conn's current therapy*. Philadelphia, PA: Elsevier.

McPhee, S. J, Rabow, M. W., & Papadakis, M. (Eds.). (2016). *Current medical diagnosis and treatment*. New York: Lange Medical Books/McGraw-Hill.

Morton, P. G., & Fontaine, D. K. (2013). *Critical care nursing: A holistic approach*. Philadelphia, PA: Lippincott Williams & Wilkins.

Porth, C. (2006). Essentials of pathophysiology: Concepts of altered health states (2nd ed.). Philadelphia, PA: Wolters Kluwer.

Porth, C. M. (2015). Essentials of pathophysiology: Concepts for altered health states (4th ed.). Philadelphia, PA: Wolters Kluwer.

Rubin, R., Strayer, D. S., & Rubin, E. (2012). *Rubin's pathology* (6th ed.). Philadelphia, PA: Lippincott Williams & Wilkins.

Salvatore, D., Davies, T. F., Sclumberger, M. J., et al. (2016). Thyroid physiology and diagnostic evaluation of patients with thyroid disorders. In S. Melmed, K. Polonsky, P. Larsen., et al. (Eds.). *Williams textbook of endocrinology.* Philadelphia, PA: Elsevier.

Sluss, P. M., & Hayes, F. J. (2016). *Laboratory techniques for recognition of endocrine disorders.* In S. Melmed, K. Polonsky, P. Larsen, et al. (Eds.). *Williams textbook of endocrinology.* Philadelphia, PA: Elsevier.

Weber, J. R., & Kelley, J. H. (2014). *Health assessment in nursing* (5th ed.). Philadelphia, PA: Lippincott Williams & Wilkins.

Woodworth, A, Lakhani, V., Aleryani, S. L., et al. (2014). The endocrine system. In M. Laposata (Ed.). *Laboratory medicine: The diagnosis of disease in the clinical laboratory.* New York: McGraw-Hill.

Young, W. F. (2016). Endocrine hypertension. In S. Melmed, K. Polonsky, P. Larsen, et al. (Eds.). *Williams textbook of endocrinology.* Philadelphia, PA: Elsevier.

Journals and Electronic Documents

American Cancer Society (2017a). Estimated new cases 2017. Atlanta, GA: Author. Retrieved on 3/29/17 at: www.cancerstatisticscenter.cancer.org/#/data-analysis/module/BmVYeqHT?type=barGraph

American Cancer Society (2017b). What are key statistics about thyroid cancer? Atlanta, GA: Author. Retrieved on 3/29/17 at: www.cancer.org/cancer/thyroid-cancer/about/key-statistics.html

American Cancer Society (2017c). Radioactive iodine treatment for thyroid cancer. Atlanta, GA: Author. Retrieved on 3/29/17 at: www.cancer.org/cancer/thyroid-cancer/treating/radioactive-iodine.html

Bahn, R. S., Burch, H. B., Cooper, D. S., et al. (2011). Hyperthyroidism and other causes of thyrotoxicosis: Management guidelines of the American Thyroid Association and American Association of Clinical Endocrinologists. *Thyroid, 21*(6), 593–646.

Bornstein, S. R., Allolio, B., Arlt, W., et al. (2016). Diagnosis and treatment of primary adrenal insufficiency: An Endocrine Society clinical practice guideline. *Journal of Clinical Endocrinology Metabolism, 101*(2), 364–389.

Dhyani, M., Faquin, W., Lubitz, C. C., et al. (2013). How to interpret thyroid fine-needle aspiration biopsy reports: A guide for the busy radiologist in the era of the Bethesda Classification System. *American Journal of Roentgenology, 201*(6), 1335–1339.

Dunn, D., & Turner, C. (2016). Hypothyroidism in women. *Nursing for Women's Health, 20*(1), 93–98.

Eugster, E. A. (2017). Pituitary gigantism. *UpToDate.* Retrieved on 3/31/17 at: www.uptodate.com/contents/pituitary-gigantism

Fuleihan, G. E., & Silverberg, S. S. (2017). Primary hyperparathyroidism: Diagnosis, differential diagnosis, and evaluation. *UpToDate.* Retrieved on 3/31/17 at: www.uptodate.com/contents/primary-hyperparathyroidism-diagnosis-differential-diagnosis-and-evaluation?source=search_result&search=primary +hyperparathyroidism&selectedTitle=1%7E98

Garber, J. R., Cobin, R. H., Gharib, H., et al. (2012). Clinical practice guidelines for hypothyroidism in adults. *Endocrine Practice18*(6), 988–1028.

Goltzman, D. (2016). Hypoparathyroidism. *UpToDate.* Retrieved on 6/29/16 at: www.uptodate.com/contents/hypoparathyroidism

Harman, S. M. (2016). Endocrine changes with aging. *UpToDate.* Retrieved on 6/22/16 at: http://www.uptodate.com/contents/endocrine-changes-with-aging

Janicak, P. (2016). Bipolar disorder in adults and lithium: Pharmacology, administration and side effects. *UpToDate.* Retrieved on 6/29/16 at: www.uptodate.com/contents/bipolar-disorder-in-adults-and-lithium-pharmacology-administration-and-side-effects/contributor-disclosure

John, C. A., & Day, M. W. (2012). Central neurogenic diabetes insipidus, syndrome of inappropriate secretion of antidiuretic hormone, and cerebral salt-wasting syndrome in traumatic brain injury. *Critical Care Nurse, 32*(2), e1–e7.

Jonklaas, J., Bianco, A. C., Bauer, A. J., et al. (2014). Guidelines for the treatment of hypothyroidism. *Thyroid, 24*(12), 1670–1751.

Katznelson, L., Laws, E. R., Melmed, S., et al. (2014). Acromegaly: An Endocrine Society clinical practice guideline. *Journal of Clinical Endocrinology Metabolism, 99*(11), 3933–3951.

LaFranchi, S. (2016). Congenital hypothyroidism. Retrieved on 6/21/16 at: www.uptodate.com/contents/clinical-features-and-detection-of-congenital-hypothyroidism

Morgan, D., & Tsai, S. C. (2015). Sleep and the endocrine system. *Critical Care Clinics, 31*(3), 403–418.

Muldoon, B. T., Mai, V. Q., & Burch, H. B. (2014). Management of Graves' disease. An overview and comparison of clinical practice guidelines with actual practice trends. *Endocrinology & Metabolism Clinics of North America, 43,* 495–516.

Nieman, L. K. (2016a). Clinical manifestations of adrenal insufficiency in adults. *UpToDate.* Retrieved on 6/29/16 at: www.uptodate.com/contents/clinical-manifestations-of-adrenal-insufficiency-in-aduMorganlts

Nieman, L. K. (2016b). Diagnosis of adrenal insufficiency in adults. *UpToDate.* Retrieved on 6/29/16 at: www.uptodate.com/contents/diagnosis-of-adrenal-insufficiency-in-adults

Nieman, L. K. (2016c). Treatment of adrenal insufficiency in adults. *UpToDate.* Retrieved on 6/29/16 at: www.uptodate.com/contents/diagnosis-of-adrenal-insufficiency-in-adults

Nieman, L. K. (2016d). Establishing the diagnosis of Cushing's syndrome. *UpToDate.* Retrieved on 6/29/16 at: www.uptodate.com/contents/establishing-the-diagnosis-of-cushings-syndrome

Rosen, C. J. (2016). Parathyroid hormone therapy for osteoporosis. *UpToDate.* Retrieved on 6/29/16 at: www.uptodate.com/contents/parathyroid-hormone-therapy-for-osteoporosis

Rosenthal, M. S. (2014). Ethical issues and management of thyroid disease. *Endocrinology & Metabolism Clinics of North America, 43*(2), 545–564.

Ross, D. S. (2016a). Myxedema coma. *UpToDate.* Retrieved on 6/22/16 at: www.uptodate.com/contents/myxedema-coma

Ross, D. S. (2016b). Thyroid storm. *UpToDate.* Retrieved on 6/22/16 at: www.uptodate.com/contents/thyroid-storm

Ross, D. S. (2016c). Beta blockers in the treatment of hyperthyroidism. *UpToDate.* Retrieved on 6/22/16 at: www.uptodate.com/contents/beta-blockers-in-the-treatment-of-hyperthyroidism

Ross, D. S. (2016d). Thionamides in the treatment of Graves' disease. *UpToDate.* Retrieved on 6/22/16 at: www.uptodate.com/contents/thionamides-in-the-treatment-of-graves-disease

Ross, D. S. (2016e). Radioiodine in the treatment of hyperthyroidism. *UpToDate.* Retrieved on 6/29/16 at: www.uptodate.com/contents/radioiodine-in-the-treatment-of-hyperthyroidism

Ross, D. S. (2016f). Pharmacology and toxicity of thionamides. *UpToDate.* Retrieved on 6/29/16 at: www.uptodate.com/contents/pharmacology-and-toxicity-of-thionamides

Ross, D. S. (2016g). Iodine in the treatment of hyperthyroidism. *UpToDate.* Retrieved on 6/29/16 at: www.uptodate.com/contents/iodine-in-the-treatment-of-hyperthyroidism?title=Hyperthyroidism

Shane, E., & Berenson, J. R. (2016). Treatment of hypercalcemia. *UpToDate.* Retrieved on 6/29/16 at: www.uptodate.com/contents/treatment-of-hypercalcemia

Shine, B., McKnight, R. F., Leaver, L. et al. (2015). Long-term effects of lithium on renal, thyroid, and parathyroid function: A retrospective analysis of laboratory data. *Lancet, 386,* 461–468.

Surks, M. I. (2016a). Manifestations of hypothyroidism. *UpToDate.* Retrieved on 6/21/16 at: www.uptodate.com/contents/hypothyroidism-underactive-thyroid-beyond-the-basics

Surks, M. I. (2016b). Iodine-induced thyroid dysfunction. *UpToDate.* Retrieved on 6/21/16 at: www.uptodate.com/contents/iodine-induced-thyroid-dysfunction

Surks, M. I. (2016c). Lithium and the thyroid. *UpToDate.* Retrieved on 6/21/16 at: www.uptodate.com/contents/lithium-and-the-thyroid

Tuttle, R. M. (2016). Surgical treatment of differentiated thyroid cancer. *UpToDate.* Retrieved on 6/29/16 at: www.uptodate.com/contents/differentiated-thyroid-cancer-surgical-treatment

U.S. Preventive Services Task Force (USPSTF). (2015). *Final Update Summary: Thyroid dysfunction: screening.* Retrieved on 6/21/16 at: www.uspreventiveservicestaskforce.org/Page/Document/UpdateSummaryFinal/thyroid-dysfunction-screening

Visser, W. E., Visser, T. J., & Peeters R. P. (2013). Thyroid disorders in older adults. *Endocrinology & Metabolism Clinics of North America, 42,* 287–303.

Young, F., & Kaplan, N. M. (2016). Clinical presentation and diagnosis of pheochromocytoma. *UpToDate.* Retrieved on 6/29/16 at: www.uptodate.com/contents/pathogenesis-of-behcets-disease/abstract/130

Young, F., Kaplan, N. M., & Kebebew, E. (2016). Treatment of pheochromocytoma in adults. *UpToDate*. Retrieved on 6/29/16 at: www.uptodate.com/contents/treatment-of-pheochromocytoma-in-adults

Resources

American Association of Clinical Endocrinologists (AACE), www.aace.com

American Thyroid Association, www.thyroid.org

Cushing's Support and Research Foundation (CSRF), www.csrf.net

Endocrine Society, www.endocrine.org

EndocrineWeb, www.endocrineweb

Hormone Health Network, www.hormone.org

National Adrenal Diseases Foundation (NADF), www.nadf.us

National Cancer Institute, Cancer Net for Health Professionals, www.cancer.gov

National Institute of Diabetes and Digestive and Kidney Disease, www.niddk.nih.gov

UNIT 12

Kidney and Urinary Tract Function

DECREASING CENTRAL LINE–ASSOCIATED BLOODSTREAM INFECTIONS (CLABSI)

A nurse working in an intermediate medical unit notes a high incidence of patients with CLABSI. After accessing data about hospital admissions for CLABSI, the nurse verifies these observations. The nurse determines that many of the patients with CLABSI are receiving hemodialysis or have new kidney transplants and thus have central line access sites. The nurse sees the need for a plan that includes a unit-wide response to this problem. The plan involves arranging education programs about strategies to prevent CLABSI, including a review of hand hygiene, standard precautions, and central line care.

QSEN Competency Focus: Quality Improvement (QI)

The complexities inherent in today's health care system challenges nurses to demonstrate integration of specific interdisciplinary core competencies. These competencies are aimed at ensuring the delivery of safe, quality patient care (Institute of Medicine, 2003). The Quality and Safety Education for Nurses project (QSEN, 2017; Cronenwett, Sherwood, Barnsteiner, et al., 2007) provides a framework for the knowledge, skills, and attitudes (KSA) required for nurses to demonstrate competency in these key areas, which include *patient-centered care, interdisciplinary teamwork and collaboration, evidence-based practice, quality improvement, safety,* and *informatics.*

Quality Improvement Definition: Use data to monitor the outcomes of care processes and use improvement methods to design and test changes to continuously improve the quality and safety of health care systems.

SELECTED PRE-LICENSURE KSAs	APPLICATION AND REFLECTION
Knowledge	
Describe approaches for changing processes of care.	Describe how the nurse's observation of CLABSI rates in a specific population was then linked to data-derived measures that verified a need to plan a quality improvement initiative.
Skills	
Design a small test of change in daily work (using an experiential learning method such as Plan-Do-Study-Act). Practice aligning the aims, measures, and changes involved in improving care. Use measures to evaluate the effect of change.	What tools might the nurse use to gain buy-in from key constituents in her or his unit? What benchmarks of quality might he or she wish to use with these constituents?
Attitudes	
Value local change (in individual practice or team practice on a unit) and its role in creating joy in work. Appreciate the value of what individuals and teams can to do to improve care.	Reflect on what you learned from this case study. Do you appreciate that variations may occur in specific populations (e.g., in this case, patients on hemodialysis and with new transplants)? If you practiced within the same setting, do you think you could have made the same observations and analyses?

Cronenwett, L., Sherwood, G., Barnsteiner, J., et al. (2007). Quality and safety education for nurses. *Nursing Outlook, 55*(3), 122–131.

Institute of Medicine. (2003). *Health professions education: A bridge to quality*. Washington, DC: National Academies Press.

QSEN Institute, (2017). *QSEN Competencies: Definitions and pre-licensure KSAs*. Retrieved on 3/1/2017 at: www.qsen.org/competencies/pre-licensure-ksas

53

Assessment of Kidney and Urinary Function

LEARNING OBJECTIVES

On completion of this chapter, the learner will be able to:

1 Describe the structure and function of the renal and urinary systems.
2 Explain the role of the kidneys in regulating fluid and electrolyte balance, acid–base balance, and blood pressure.

3 Identify the diagnostic studies used to determine upper and lower urinary tract function and related nursing implications.
4 Discriminate between normal and abnormal assessment findings of upper and lower urinary tract function.
5 Initiate education and preparation for patients undergoing assessment of the urinary system.

GLOSSARY

aldosterone: hormone synthesized and released by the adrenal cortex; causes the kidneys to reabsorb sodium
antidiuretic hormone (ADH): hormone secreted by the posterior pituitary gland; causes the kidneys to reabsorb more water; also called *vasopressin*
anuria: decreased urine output of less than 50 mL in 24 hours
bacteriuria: bacteria in the urine
creatinine: endogenous waste product of muscle energy metabolism
diuresis: increased urine volume
dysuria: painful or difficult urination
frequency: voiding more frequently than every 3 hours
glomerular filtration rate (GFR): amount of plasma filtered through the glomeruli per unit of time

glomerulus: tuft of capillaries forming part of the nephron through which filtration occurs
hematuria: red blood cells in the urine
micturition: urination or voiding
nephron: structural and functional unit of the kidney responsible for urine formation
nocturia: awakening at night to urinate
oliguria: urine output less than 0.5 mL/kg/hr
proteinuria: protein in the urine
pyuria: white blood cells in the urine
renal clearance: ability of the kidneys to clear solutes from the plasma
renal glycosuria: excretion of glucose in the urine
specific gravity: expression of the degree of concentration of the urine
urea nitrogen: end product of protein metabolism

Function of the renal and urinary systems is essential to life. The primary purpose of the renal and urinary systems is to maintain the body's state of homeostasis by carefully regulating fluid and electrolytes, removing wastes, and providing other functions (see Chart 53-1). Dysfunction of the kidneys and lower urinary tract is common and may occur at any age and with varying degrees of severity. Assessment of upper and lower urinary tract function is part of every health examination and requires that the nurse have an understanding of the anatomy and physiology of the urinary system as well as the effects of changes in the system on other physiologic functions.

Anatomic and Physiologic Overview

Anatomy of the Kidney and Urinary Systems

The kidney and urinary systems include the kidneys, ureters, bladder, and urethra. Urine is formed by the kidney and flows through the other structures to be eliminated from the body.

Kidneys

The kidneys are a pair of bean-shaped, brownish-red structures located retroperitoneally (behind and outside the peritoneal cavity) on the posterior wall of the abdomen—from the 12th thoracic vertebra to the 3rd lumbar vertebra in the adult (see Fig. 53-1A). The rounded outer convex surface of each kidney is called the hilum. Each hilum is penetrated with blood vessels, nerves, and the ureter (Eaton & Pooler, 2013). The average adult kidney weighs approximately 113 to 170 g (about 4.5 oz) and is 10 to 12 cm long, 6 cm wide, and 2.5 cm thick (Eaton & Pooler, 2013; Grossman & Porth, 2014). The right kidney is slightly lower than the left due to the location of the liver.

Externally, the kidneys are well protected by the ribs and by the muscles of the abdomen and back. Internally, fat deposits surround each kidney, providing protection against jarring. The kidneys and surrounding fat are suspended from the abdominal wall by renal fascia made of connective tissue which holds the kidney in place (Skorecki, Chertow,

Chart 53-1	Functions of the Kidney

- Urine formation
- Excretion of waste products
- Regulation of electrolytes
- Regulation of acid–base balance
- Control of water balance
- Control of blood pressure
- Renal clearance
- Regulation of red blood cell production
- Synthesis of vitamin D to active form
- Secretion of prostaglandins

Marsden, 2015). The fibrous connective tissue, blood vessels, and lymphatics surrounding each kidney are known as the renal capsule. An adrenal gland lies on top of each kidney. The kidneys and adrenals are independent in function, blood supply, and innervation.

The renal parenchyma is divided into two parts: the cortex and the medulla (see Fig. 53-1B). The medulla, which is approximately 5 cm wide, is the inner portion of the kidney. It contains the loops of Henle, the vasa recta, and the collecting ducts of the juxtamedullary nephrons. The collecting ducts from both the juxtamedullary and the cortical nephrons connect to the renal pyramids, which are triangular and are situated with the base facing the concave surface of the kidney and the point (papilla) facing the hilum, or pelvis. Each kidney contains approximately 8 to 18 pyramids. The pyramids drain into minor calyces, which drain into major calyces that open directly into the renal pelvis. The tip of each pyramid is called a papilla and projects into the minor calyx (Eaton & Pooler, 2013). The renal pelvis is the beginning of the collecting system and is composed of structures that are designed to collect and transport urine. Once the urine leaves the renal pelvis, the composition or amount of urine does not change.

The cortex, which is approximately 1 cm wide, is located farthest from the center of the kidney and around the outermost edges. It contains the **nephrons** (the structural and

functional units of the kidney responsible for urine formation), which are discussed later.

Blood Supply to the Kidneys

The hilum is the concave portion of the kidney through which the renal artery enters and the ureters and renal vein exit. The kidneys receive 20% to 25% of the total cardiac output, which means that all of the body's blood circulates through the kidneys approximately 12 times per hour (Grossman & Porth, 2014). The renal artery (arising from the abdominal aorta) divides into smaller and smaller vessels, eventually forming the afferent arterioles. Each afferent arteriole branches to form a **glomerulus**, which is the tuft of capillaries forming part of the nephron through which filtration occurs. Blood leaves the glomerulus through the efferent arteriole and flows back to the inferior vena cava through a network of capillaries and veins.

Nephrons

Each kidney has 1 million nephrons that are located within the renal parenchyma and are responsible for the formation of filtrate that will become urine (Eaton & Pooler, 2013). The large number of nephrons allows for adequate renal function even if the opposite kidney is damaged or becomes nonfunctional. If the total number of functioning nephrons is less than 20% of normal, renal replacement therapy needs to be considered.

There are two types of nephrons. The cortical nephrons (80% to 85%) are located in the outermost part of the cortex, and the juxtamedullary nephrons (15% to 20%) are located deeper in the cortex (Grossman & Porth, 2014). The juxtamedullary nephrons are distinguished by long loops of Henle and are surrounded by long capillary loops called *vasa recta* that dip into the medulla of the kidney. The length of the tubular component of the nephron is directly related to its ability to concentrate urine.

Nephrons are made up of two basic components: a filtering element composed of an enclosed capillary network (the glomerulus) and the attached tubule (see Fig. 53-2). The glomerulus is a unique network of capillaries suspended between the afferent and efferent blood vessels, which are

Figure 53-1 • A. Kidneys, ureters, and bladder. **B.** Internal structure of the kidney. Redrawn with permission from Porth, C. M., & Matfin, G. (2009). *Pathophysiology: Concepts of altered health states* (8th ed.). Philadelphia, PA: Lippincott Williams & Wilkins.

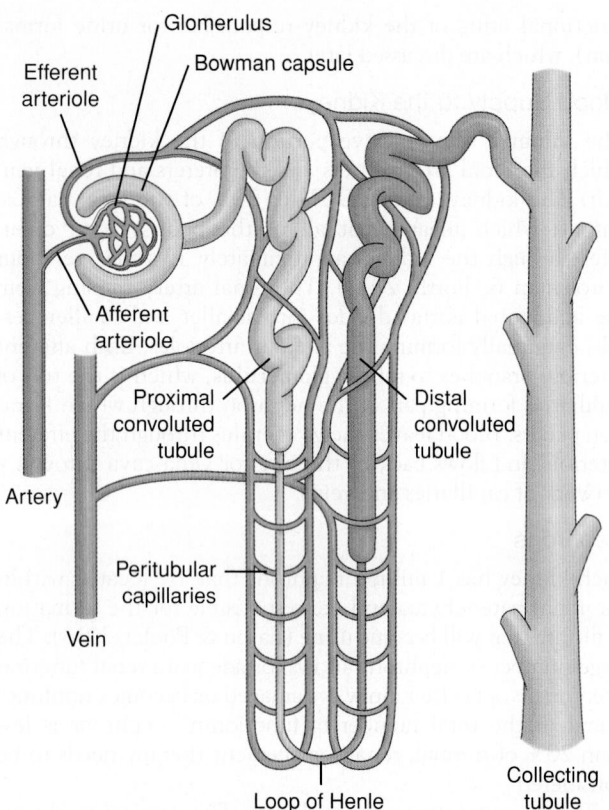

Figure 53-2 • Representation of a nephron. Each kidney has about 1 million nephrons of two types: cortical and juxtamedullary. Cortical nephrons are located in the cortex of the kidney; juxtamedullary nephrons are adjacent to the medulla.

enclosed in an epithelial structure called the *Bowman capsule*. The glomerular membrane is composed of three filtering layers: the capillary endothelium, the basement membrane, and the epithelium. This membrane normally allows filtration of fluid and small molecules yet limits passage of larger molecules, such as blood cells and albumin. Pressure changes and the permeability of the glomerular membrane of the Bowman capsule facilitate the passage of fluids and various substances from the blood vessels, filling the space within the Bowman capsule with this filtered solution.

The tubular component of the nephron begins in the Bowman capsule. The filtrate created in the Bowman capsule travels first into the proximal tubule, which is made up of epithelial cells resting on the basement membrane, then the loop of Henle, the distal tubule, and either the cortical or medullary collecting ducts (Eaton & Pooler, 2013). The structural arrangement of the tubule allows the distal tubule to lie in close proximity to where the afferent and efferent arterioles, respectively, enter and leave the glomerulus. The distal tubular cells located in this area, known as the macula densa, function with the adjacent afferent arteriole and create what is known as the juxtaglomerular apparatus. This is the site of renin production. Renin is a hormone directly involved in the control of arterial blood pressure; it is essential for proper functioning of the glomerulus (see later discussion).

The tubular component consists of the Bowman capsule, the proximal tubule, the descending and ascending limbs of the loop of Henle, and the cortical and medullary collecting

ducts. This portion of the nephron is responsible for making adjustments in the filtrate based on the body's needs. Changes are continually made as the filtrate travels through the tubules until it enters the collecting system and is expelled from the body (see Fig. 53-2).

Ureters, Bladder, and Urethra

The urine formed in the nephrons flows through the renal calyces and then into the ureters, which are long fibromuscular tubes that connect each kidney to the bladder (Hall, 2016). These narrow tubes, each 24 to 30 cm long, originate at the lower portion of the renal pelvis and terminate in the trigone (tissue between the opening of the ureters and urethra) of the bladder wall.

The lining of the ureters is made up of transitional cell epithelium called *urothelium*. The urothelium prevents reabsorption of urine. The movement of urine from each renal pelvis through the ureter into the bladder is facilitated by peristaltic contraction of the smooth muscles in the ureter wall. Each ureter has three narrow areas that are prone to obstruction by renal calculi (kidney stones) or stricture. These three areas include the ureteropelvic junction, the ureteral segment near the sacroiliac junction, and the ureterovesical junction. Obstruction of the ureteropelvic junction is the most serious because of its close proximity to the kidney and the risk of associated kidney dysfunction.

The urinary bladder is a distensible muscular sac located just behind the pubic bone (Weber & Kelley, 2014). The usual capacity of the adult bladder is 400 to 500 mL, but it can distend to hold a larger volume. The bladder is characterized by its central, hollow area, called the *vesicle*, which has two inlets (the ureters) and one outlet (the urethra). The area surrounding the bladder neck is called the *urethrovesical junction*. The angling of the ureterovesical junction is the primary means of providing antegrade, or downward, movement of urine, also referred to as efflux of urine. This angling prevents vesicoureteral reflux (retrograde, or backward, movement of urine) from the bladder, up the ureter, toward the kidney.

The wall of the bladder contains four layers. The outermost layer is the adventitia, which is made up of connective tissue. Immediately beneath the adventitia is a smooth muscle layer known as the detrusor. Beneath the detrusor is a submucosal layer of loose connective tissue that serves as an interface between the detrusor and the innermost layer, a mucosal lining. The inner layer contains specialized transitional cell epithelium, a membrane that is impermeable to water and prevents reabsorption of urine stored in the bladder. The bladder neck contains bundles of involuntary smooth muscle that form a portion of the urethral sphincter known as the internal sphincter. An important portion of the sphincter mechanism that helps maintain continence is the external urinary sphincter at the anterior urethra, which is the segment most distal from the bladder (Grossman & Porth, 2014). During **micturition** (voiding or urination), increased intravesical pressure keeps the ureterovesical junction closed and urine within the ureters. As soon as micturition is completed, intravesical pressure returns to its normal low baseline value, allowing efflux of urine to resume. Therefore, the only time that the bladder is completely empty is in the last seconds of micturition, before efflux of urine resumes.

The urethra arises from the base of the bladder: In the male, it passes through the penis; in the female, it opens just anterior to the vagina. In the male, the prostate gland, which lies just below the bladder neck, surrounds the urethra posteriorly and laterally.

Function of the Kidney and Urinary Systems

Urine Formation

The healthy human body is composed of approximately 60% water. Water balance is regulated by the kidneys and results in the formation of urine. Urine is formed in the nephrons through a complex three-step process: glomerular filtration, tubular reabsorption, and tubular secretion (see Fig. 53-3). Each nephron functions independently from other nephrons because each has its own blood supply (Eaton & Pooler, 2013). The various substances normally filtered by the glomerulus, reabsorbed by the tubules, and excreted in the urine include sodium, chloride, bicarbonate, potassium, glucose, urea, **creatinine,** and uric acid. Within the tubule, some of these substances are selectively reabsorbed into the blood. Others are secreted from the blood into the filtrate as it travels down the tubule.

Amino acids and glucose are usually filtered at the level of the glomerulus and reabsorbed so that neither is excreted in the urine. Normally, glucose does not appear in the urine. However, **renal glycosuria** (excretion of glucose in the urine) occurs if the amount of glucose in the blood and glomerular filtrate exceeds the amount that the tubules are able to reabsorb. Renal glycosuria can occur on its own as a benign condition (Hall, 2016). It also occurs in poorly controlled diabetes—the most common condition that causes the blood glucose level to exceed the kidney's reabsorption capacity.

Protein molecules also are not usually found in the urine; however, low–molecular-weight proteins (globulins and albumin) may periodically be excreted in small amounts. Protein in the urine is referred to as **proteinuria** (Eaton & Pooler, 2013).

Glomerular Filtration

The normal blood flow through the kidneys is between 1000 and 1300 mL/min (Grossman & Porth, 2014). As blood flows into the glomerulus from an afferent arteriole, filtration occurs. The filtered fluid, also known as filtrate or ultrafiltrate, then enters the renal tubules. Under normal conditions, about 20% of the blood passing through the glomeruli is filtered into the nephron, amounting to about 180 L/day of filtrate (Eaton & Pooler, 2013). The filtrate normally consists of water, electrolytes, and other small molecules, because water and small molecules are allowed to pass, whereas larger molecules stay in the bloodstream. As blood enters the glomerulus from the afferent arteriole, filtration depends on adequate blood flow that maintains a consistent pressure through the glomerulus called hydrostatic pressure. Many factors can alter this blood flow and pressure, including hypotension, decreased oncotic pressure in the blood, and increased pressure in the renal tubules from an obstruction (Eaton & Pooler, 2013; Grossman & Porth, 2014).

Tubular Reabsorption and Tubular Secretion

The second and third steps of urine formation occur in the renal tubules. In tubular reabsorption, a substance moves from the filtrate back into the peritubular capillaries or vasa recta. In tubular secretion, a substance moves from the peritubular capillaries or vasa recta into tubular filtrate. Of the 180 L (45 gallons) of filtrate that the kidneys produce each day, 99% is reabsorbed into the bloodstream, resulting in the formation of 1 to 2 L of urine each day. Although most reabsorption occurs in the proximal tubule, reabsorption occurs along the entire tubule. Reabsorption and secretion in the tubule frequently involve passive and active transport and may require the use of energy. Tubular secretion occurs when substances move from the peritubular capillary blood plasma (blood) into the tubular lumen (filtrate). Tubular secretion helps with the elimination of potassium, hydrogen ions, ammonia, uric acid, some drugs, and other waste products (Headly, 2015). Filtrate becomes concentrated in the distal tubule and collecting ducts under hormonal influence and becomes urine, which then enters the renal pelvis. In the absence of tubular reabsorption, volume depletion would rapidly occur (Headly, 2015).

Antidiuretic Hormone

Antidiuretic hormone (ADH), also known as vasopressin, is a hormone that is secreted by the posterior portion of the pituitary gland in response to changes in osmolality of the blood. With decreased water intake, blood osmolality tends to increase, stimulating ADH release. ADH then acts on the kidney, increasing reabsorption of water and thereby returning the osmolality of the blood to normal. With excess water intake, the secretion of ADH by the pituitary is suppressed; therefore, less water is reabsorbed by the kidney tubule, leading to **diuresis** (increased urine volume).

A dilute urine with a fixed **specific gravity** (about 1.010) or fixed osmolality (about 300 mOsm/L) indicates an inability

Physiology/Pathophysiology

① Filtration at glomerulus	
Water	180 L
Sodium	540.0 g
Chloride	630.0 g
Bicarbonate	300.0 g
Potassium	28.0 g
Glucose	140.0 g
Urea	53.0 g
Creatinine	1.4 g
Uric acid	8.5 g

② Absorption into peritubular capillaries	
Water	178.5 L
Sodium	536.5 g
Chloride	624.05 g
Bicarbonate	295.5 g
Potassium	24.0 g
Glucose	140.0 g
Urea	28.0 g
Creatinine	0.0 g
Uric acid	7.7 g

③ Reabsorption into tubule for excretion in urine	
Water	1.5 L
Sodium	3.5 g
Chloride	5.5 g
Bicarbonate	0.5 g
Potassium	4.0 g
Glucose	0.0 g
Urea	25.0 g
Creatinine	1.4 g
Uric acid	0.8 g

Figure 53-3 • Urine is formed in the nephrons in a three-step process: filtration, reabsorption, and secretion. Water, electrolytes, and other substances, such as glucose and creatinine, are filtered by the glomerulus; varying amounts of these substances are reabsorbed in the renal tubule or excreted in the urine. Approximate normal volumes of these substances during the steps of urine formation are shown at the top. Wide variations may occur in these values depending on diet.

to concentrate and dilute the urine, which is a common early sign of kidney disease (Skorecki et al., 2015).

Osmolarity and Osmolality

Osmolarity refers to the ratio of solute to water. The regulation of salt and water is paramount for control of the extracellular volume and both serum and urine osmolarity. Controlling either the amount of water or the amount of solute can change osmolarity. Osmolarity and ionic composition are maintained by the body within very narrow limits. As little as a 1% to 2% change in the serum osmolarity can cause a conscious desire to drink and conservation of water by the kidneys (Skorecki et al., 2015).

The degree of dilution or concentration of the urine is also measured in terms of osmolality (the number of osmoles [the standard unit of osmotic pressure] dissolved per kilogram of solution). The filtrate in the glomerular capillary normally has the same osmolality as the blood—280 to 300 mOsm/kg. Serum and urine osmolality and osmolarity are discussed in more detail in Chapter 13.

Regulation of Water Excretion

Regulation of the amount of water excreted is an important function of the kidney. With high fluid intake, a large volume of dilute urine is excreted. Conversely, with a low fluid intake, a small volume of concentrated urine is excreted. A person normally ingests about 1300 mL of oral liquids and 1000 mL of water in food per day. Of the fluid ingested, approximately 900 mL is lost through the skin and lungs (called *insensible loss*), 50 mL through sweat, and 200 mL through feces. It is important to consider all fluid gained and lost when evaluating total fluid status. Daily weight measurements are a reliable means of determining overall fluid status. One pound (1 lb) equals approximately 500 mL, so a weight change of as little as 1 lb could suggest an overall fluid gain or loss of 500 mL (Grossman & Porth, 2014).

Regulation of Electrolyte Excretion

When the kidneys are functioning normally, the volume of electrolytes excreted per day is equal to the amount ingested. For example, the average American daily diet contains 6 to 8 g each of sodium chloride (salt) and potassium chloride, and approximately the same amounts are excreted in the urine.

The regulation of sodium volume excreted depends on **aldosterone**, a hormone synthesized and released by the adrenal cortex. With increased aldosterone in the blood, less sodium is excreted in the urine, because aldosterone fosters renal reabsorption of sodium. Release of aldosterone from the adrenal cortex is largely under the control of angiotensin II. Angiotensin II levels are in turn controlled by renin, an enzyme that is released from specialized cells in the kidneys (see Fig. 53-4). This complex system is activated when pressure in the renal arterioles falls below normal levels, as occurs with shock, dehydration, or decreased sodium chloride delivery to the tubules. Activation of this system increases the retention of water and expansion of the intravascular fluid volume, thereby maintaining enough pressure within the glomerulus to ensure adequate filtration.

The regulation of serum sodium and potassium are discussed in detail in Chapter 13.

Physiology/Pathophysiology

Figure 53-4 • The renin–angiotensin system. GFR, glomerular filtration rate; ADH, antidiuretic hormone.

Regulation of Acid–Base Balance

The normal serum pH is about 7.35 to 7.45 and must be maintained within this narrow range for optimal physiologic function (Grossman & Porth, 2014). The kidney performs major functions to assist in this balance. One function is to reabsorb and return to the body's circulation any bicarbonate from the urinary filtrate; other functions are to excrete or reabsorb acid, synthesize ammonia, and excrete ammonium chloride (Headly, 2015). Because bicarbonate is a small ion, it is freely filtered at the glomerulus. The renal tubules actively reabsorb most of the bicarbonate in the urinary filtrate. To replace any lost bicarbonate, the renal tubular cells generate new bicarbonate through a variety of chemical reactions. This newly generated bicarbonate is then reabsorbed by the tubules and returned to the body.

The body's acid production is the result of catabolism, or breakdown, of proteins, which produces acid compounds, particularly phosphoric and sulfuric acids. The normal daily diet also includes a certain amount of acid materials. Unlike carbon dioxide (CO_2), phosphoric and sulfuric acids cannot be eliminated by the lungs. Because accumulation of these acids in the blood lowers pH (making the blood more acidic) and inhibits cell function, they must be excreted in the urine. However, if the hydrogen ions are low, they will be reabsorbed. A person with normal kidney function excretes about 70 mEq of acid each day. The kidney is able to excrete some of this acid directly into the urine until the urine pH reaches 4.5, which is 1000 times more acidic than blood (Grossman & Porth, 2014).

However, more acid usually needs to be eliminated from the body than can be secreted directly as free acid in the urine. These excess acids are bound to chemical buffers so that they can be excreted in the urine. Two important chemical buffers are phosphate ions and ammonia (NH_3). When buffered with acid, ammonia becomes ammonium (NH_4). Phosphate is present in the glomerular filtrate, and ammonia is produced by the cells of the renal tubules and secreted into the tubular fluid. Through the buffering process, the kidney is able to excrete large quantities of acid in a bound form without further lowering the pH of the urine.

Autoregulation of Blood Pressure

Regulation of blood pressure is an important function of the kidney. Specialized vessels of the kidney, called the *vasa recta*, constantly monitor blood pressure as blood begins its passage into the kidney. When the vasa recta detect a decrease in blood pressure, specialized juxtaglomerular cells near the afferent arteriole, distal tubule, and efferent arteriole, secrete the hormone renin. Renin converts angiotensinogen to angiotensin I, which is then converted to angiotensin II—the most powerful vasoconstrictor known; angiotensin II causes the blood pressure to increase (Hall, 2016). The adrenal cortex secretes aldosterone in response to stimulation by the pituitary gland, which occurs in response to poor perfusion or increasing serum osmolality. The result is an increase in blood pressure. When the vasa recta recognize the increase in blood pressure, renin secretion stops. Failure of this feedback mechanism is one of the primary causes of hypertension (see Fig. 53-4).

Renal Clearance

Renal clearance refers to the ability of the kidneys to clear solutes from the plasma. A 24-hour collection of urine is the primary test of renal clearance used to evaluate how well the kidney performs this important excretory function. Renal clearance depends on several factors: how quickly the substance is filtered across the glomerulus, how much of the substance is reabsorbed along the tubules, and how much of the substance is secreted into the tubules. It is possible to measure the renal clearance of any substance, but the one measure that is particularly useful is the creatinine clearance.

Creatinine is an endogenous waste product of skeletal muscle that is filtered at the glomerulus, passed through the tubules with minimal change, and excreted in the urine. Hence, creatinine clearance is a good measure of the **glomerular filtration rate (GFR)**, the amount of plasma filtered through the glomeruli per unit of time. To calculate creatinine clearance, a 24-hour urine specimen is collected. Midway through the collection, the serum creatinine level is measured. The following formula is then used to calculate the creatinine clearance:

$$\frac{(\text{Volume of urine [mL/min]} \times \text{Urine creatinine [mL/dL]})}{\text{Serum creatinine (mg/dL)}}$$

The adult GFR can vary from a normal of approximately 125 mL/min (1.67 to 2 mL/sec) to a high of 200 mL/min (Grossman & Porth, 2014). Creatinine clearance is the best approximation of renal function. As renal function declines, both creatinine clearance and renal clearance (the ability to excrete solutes) decrease.

Regulation of Red Blood Cell Production

When the kidneys detect a decrease in the oxygen tension in renal blood flow, because of anemia, arterial hypoxia, or inadequate blood flow, they release erythropoietin. Erythropoietin is a glycoprotein from the kidney that stimulates the bone marrow to produce red blood cells (RBCs), which carry oxygen throughout the body (Eaton & Pooler, 2013).

Vitamin D Synthesis

The kidneys are also responsible for the final conversion of inactive vitamin D to its active form, 1,25-dihydroxycholecalciferol. Vitamin D is necessary for maintaining normal calcium balance in the body.

Secretion of Prostaglandins and other Substances

The kidneys also produce prostaglandin E and prostacyclin, thromboxanes and leukotrienes, which have vasoactive effects. These substances help the afferent and efferent arterioles maintain renal blood flow by causing selective vasodilation or vasoconstriction (Headly, 2015).

Excretion of Waste Products

The kidneys eliminate the body's metabolic waste products. The major waste product of protein metabolism is urea, of which about 25 to 30 g are produced and excreted daily (Grossman & Porth, 2014). All of this urea must be excreted in the urine; otherwise, it accumulates in body tissues. Other waste products of metabolism that must be excreted are creatinine, phosphates, and sulfates. Uric acid, formed as a waste product of purine metabolism, is also eliminated in the urine. The kidneys serve as the primary mechanism for excreting drug metabolites.

Urine Storage

The bladder is the reservoir for urine. Both filling and emptying of the bladder are mediated by coordinated sympathetic and parasympathetic nervous system control mechanisms involving the detrusor muscle and the bladder outlet. Conscious awareness of bladder filling occurs as a result of sympathetic neuronal pathways that travel via the spinal cord to the level of T10 through T12, where peripheral, hypogastric nerve innervation allows for continued bladder filling. As bladder filling continues, stretch receptors in the bladder wall are activated, coupled with the desire to void. This information from the detrusor muscle is relayed back to the cerebral cortex via the parasympathetic pelvic nerves at the level of S1 through S4 (Grossman & Porth, 2014). Overall bladder pressure remains low due to the bladder's compliance (ability to expand or collapse) as urine volume changes.

Bladder compliance is due in part to the smooth muscle lining of the bladder and collagen deposits within the wall of the bladder, as well as to neuronal mechanisms that inhibit the detrusor muscle from contracting (specifically, adrenergic receptors that mediate relaxation). To maintain adequate kidney filtration rates, bladder pressure during filling must remain lower than 40 cm water (H_2O). This low pressure allows the urine to freely leave the renal pelvis and enter the ureters. The sensation of bladder fullness is transmitted to the central nervous system when the bladder has reached about 150 to 200 mL in adults, and an initial desire to void occurs (Hall, 2016). A marked sense of fullness and discomfort with a strong desire to void usually occurs when the bladder reaches its functional capacity of 400 to 500 mL of urine. Neurologic changes to the bladder at the level of the supraspinal nerves, the spinal nerves, or the bladder wall itself can cause abnormally high volumes (up to 2000 mL) of urine to be stored due to a decreased or absent urge to void.

Under normal circumstances with average fluid intake of approximately 1 to 2 L/day, the bladder should be able to store urine for periods of 2 to 4 hours at a time during the day (Hall, 2016). At night, the release of vasopressin in response to decreased fluid intake causes a decrease in the production of urine and makes it more concentrated. This phenomenon usually allows the bladder to continue filling for periods of 6 to 8 hours in adolescents and adults, making them able to sleep for longer periods before needing to void. In older adults, decreasing bladder compliance and decreased vasopressin levels often cause **nocturia** (awakening during the night to urinate).

Bladder Emptying

Micturition normally occurs approximately eight times in a 24-hour period. It is activated via the micturition reflex arc within the sympathetic and parasympathetic nervous systems, which causes a coordinated sequence of events. Initiation of voiding occurs when the efferent pelvic nerve, which originates in the S1 to S4 area, stimulates the bladder to contract, resulting in complete relaxation of the striated urethral sphincter. This is followed by a decrease in urethral pressure, contraction of the detrusor muscle, opening of the vesicle neck and proximal urethra, and flow of urine. This coordinated effort by the parasympathetic system is mediated by muscarinic and, to a lesser extent, cholinergic receptors within the detrusor muscle. The pressure generated in the bladder during micturition is about 20 to 40 cm H_2O in females. It is somewhat higher and more variable in males 45 years and older due to the normal hyperplasia of the cells of the middle lobes of the prostate gland, which surround the proximal urethra. Any obstruction of the bladder outlet, such as in advanced benign prostatic hyperplasia (BPH), results in a high voiding pressure. High voiding pressures make it more difficult to start urine flow and maintain it.

If the spinal pathways from the brain to the urinary system are destroyed (e.g., after a spinal cord injury), reflex contraction of the bladder is maintained, but voluntary control over the process is lost. In both situations, the detrusor muscle can contract and expel urine, but the contractions are generally insufficient to empty the bladder completely, so residual urine (urine left in the bladder after voiding) remains. Normally, residual urine amounts to no more than 50 mL in the middle-aged adult and less than 50 to 100 mL in the older adult (Weber & Kelley, 2014).

 ### Gerontologic Considerations

Upper and lower urinary tract function changes with age. The GFR decreases, starting between 35 and 40 years of age, and a yearly decline of about 1 mL/min continues thereafter. Older adults are more susceptible to acute and chronic kidney injury due to the structural and functional changes in the kidney. Examples include sclerosis of the glomerulus and renal vasculature, decreased blood flow, decreased GFR, altered tubular function, and acid–base

imbalance. Although renal function usually remains adequate, renal reserve is decreased and may reduce the kidneys' ability to respond effectively to drastic or sudden physiologic changes. This steady decrease in glomerular filtration, combined with the use of multiple medications in which metabolites are cleared by the kidneys, puts the older person at higher risk for adverse drug effects and drug–drug interactions (Eliopoulos, 2018).

Older adults are more prone to develop hypernatremia and fluid volume deficit, because increasing age is also associated with diminished osmotic stimulation of thirst. Thirst is defined as one's awareness of the desire to drink. The sense of thirst is so protective that hypernatremia almost never occurs in adults younger than 60 years.

Structural or functional abnormalities that occur with aging may also prevent complete emptying of the bladder. This may be due to decreased bladder wall contractility; secondary to myogenic or neurogenic factors; or related to bladder outlet obstruction, such as in BPH or after prostatectomy. Vaginal and urethral tissues atrophy (become thinner) in aging women due to decreased estrogen levels. This causes decreased blood supply to the urogenital tissues, resulting in urethral and vaginal irritation and urinary incontinence.

Urinary incontinence is present in 15% to 30% of community-dwelling older adults, 50% of older adults who are institutionalized, and 30% of older adults who are hospitalized (Eliopoulos, 2018). Many older adults and their families are unaware that urinary incontinence stems from many causes. The nurse needs to inform the patient and family that with appropriate evaluation, urinary incontinence can often be managed at home, and in many cases it can be eliminated. Many treatments are available for urinary incontinence in older adults, including noninvasive, behavioral interventions that the patient or caregiver can carry out. Treatment modalities for urinary incontinence are described in further detail in Chapter 55.

Preparation of the older adult patient for diagnostic tests must be managed carefully to prevent dehydration, which might precipitate kidney disease in a patient with marginal renal function. Limitations in mobility may affect an older patient's ability to void adequately or to consume an adequate volume of fluids. The patient may limit fluid intake to minimize the frequency of voiding or the risk of incontinence.

 Concept Mastery Alert

Providing education about the dangers of an inadequate fluid intake is an important role of the nurse caring for the older patient. The nurse emphasizes the need to drink throughout the day even if the patient does not feel thirsty, because the thirst stimulation is decreased.

Older women often have incomplete emptying of the bladder and urinary stasis, which may result in urinary tract infection or increasing bladder pressure, leading to overflow incontinence, hydronephrosis, pyelonephritis, or chronic kidney disease (Eliopoulos, 2018). Urologic symptoms can mimic disorders such as appendicitis, peptic ulcer disease, and cholecystitis, which can make diagnosis difficult in older adults due to decreased neurologic innervation (Eliopoulos, 2018).

Assessment of the Kidney and Urinary Systems

Health History

Obtaining a urologic health history requires excellent communication skills, because many patients are embarrassed or uncomfortable discussing genitourinary function or symptoms (Weber & Kelley, 2014). It is important to use language the patient can understand and to avoid medical jargon. It is also important to review risk factors, particularly for those patients who are at high risk. For example, the nurse needs to be aware that multiparous women delivering their children vaginally have a high risk for stress urinary incontinence, which, if severe enough, can also lead to urge incontinence. People with neurologic disorders such as diabetic neuropathy, multiple sclerosis, or Parkinson disease often have incomplete emptying of the bladder and urinary stasis, which may result in urinary tract infection or increasing bladder pressure, leading to overflow incontinence, hydronephrosis, pyelonephritis, or chronic kidney disease (Eliopoulos, 2018). Risk factors for specific disorders and kidney and lower urinary tract dysfunction are summarized in Table 53-1 and discussed in Chapters 54 and 55.

When obtaining the health history, the nurse should inquire about the following:

- The patient's chief concern or reason for seeking health care, the onset of the problem, and its effect on the patient's quality of life
- The location, character, and duration of pain, if present, and its relationship to voiding; factors that precipitate pain, and those that relieve it
- History of urinary tract infections, including past treatment or hospitalization for urinary tract infection
- Fever or chills
- Previous renal or urinary diagnostic tests, surgeries or procedures; or the use of indwelling urinary catheters

- **Dysuria** (painful or difficult urination), as well as during voiding (i.e., at initiation or at termination of voiding) this occurs
- Hesitancy, straining, or pain during or after urination
- Urinary incontinence (stress incontinence, urge incontinence, overflow incontinence, or functional incontinence)
- **Hematuria** (RBCs in the urine) or change in color or volume of urine
- Nocturia and its date of onset
- Renal calculi (kidney stones), passage of stones or gravel in urine
- In female patients, the number and type (vaginal or cesarean) of deliveries; the use of forceps; vaginal infection, discharge, or irritation; contraceptive practices
- History of **anuria** (decreased urine production of less than 50 mL in 24 hours) or other kidney problem
- Presence or history of genital lesions or sexually transmitted infections
- The use of tobacco, alcohol, or recreational drugs
- Any prescription and over-the-counter medications (including those prescribed for renal or urinary problems)

Common Symptoms

Dysfunction of the kidney can produce a complex array of symptoms throughout the body. Pain, changes in voiding, and gastrointestinal symptoms are particularly suggestive of urinary tract disease.

Pain

Genitourinary pain is usually caused by distention of some portion of the urinary tract as a result of obstructed urine flow or inflammation and swelling of tissues. Severity of pain is related to the sudden onset, rather than the extent of distention.

 TABLE 53-1 Risk Factors for Selected Renal or Urologic Disorders

Risk Factor	Possible Renal or Urologic Disorder
Advanced age	Incomplete emptying of bladder, leading to urinary tract infection and urosepsis
Benign prostatic hyperplasia	Obstruction to urine flow, leading to frequency, oliguria, anuria
Diabetes	Chronic kidney disease, neurogenic bladder
Gout, hyperparathyroidism, Crohn's disease, ileostomy	Kidney stone formation
Hypertension	Renal insufficiency, chronic kidney failure
Instrumentation of urinary tract, cystoscopy, catheterization	Urinary tract infection, incontinence
Immobilization	Kidney stone formation
Multiple sclerosis	Incontinence, neurogenic bladder, and other complications
Occupational, recreational, or environmental exposure to chemicals (plastics, pitch, tar, rubber)	Acute kidney failure
Obstetric injury, tumors	Incontinence
Parkinson disease	Incontinence and other complications
Pregnancy	Proteinuria, frequent voiding
Radiation therapy to pelvis	Cystitis, fibrosis of ureter, or fistula in urinary tract
Recent pelvic surgery	Inadvertent trauma to ureters or bladder
Sickle cell disease, multiple myeloma	Chronic kidney disease
Spinal cord injury	Neurogenic bladder, urinary tract infection, incontinence
Strep throat, impetigo, nephrotic syndrome	Chronic kidney disease
Systemic lupus erythematosus	Nephritis, chronic kidney disease

TABLE 53-2 Identifying Characteristics of Genitourinary Pain

Type	Location	Characteristics	Associated Signs and Symptoms	Possible Etiology
Kidney	Costovertebral angle, may extend to umbilicus	Dull constant ache; if sudden distention of capsule, pain is severe, sharp, stabbing, and colicky in nature	Nausea and vomiting, diaphoresis, pallor, signs of shock	Acute obstruction, kidney stone, blood clot, acute pyelonephritis, trauma
Bladder	Suprapubic area	Dull, continuous pain that may be intense with voiding; may be severe if bladder full	Urgency, pain at end of voiding, painful straining	Overdistended bladder, infection, interstitial cystitis; tumor
Ureteral	Costovertebral angle, flank, lower abdominal area, testis, or labium	Severe, sharp, stabbing pain, colicky in nature	Nausea and vomiting, paralytic ileus	Ureteral stone, edema or stricture, blood clot
Prostatic	Perineum and rectum	Vague discomfort, feeling of fullness in perineum, vague back pain	Suprapubic tenderness, obstruction to urine flow; frequency, urgency, dysuria, nocturia	Prostatic cancer, acute or chronic prostatitis
Urethral	*Male:* Along penis to meatus *Female:* Urethra to meatus	Pain variable, most severe during and immediately after voiding	Frequency, urgency, dysuria, nocturia, urethral discharge	Irritation of bladder neck, infection of urethra, trauma, foreign body in lower urinary tract

Table 53-2 lists the various types of genitourinary pain, characteristics of the pain, associated signs and symptoms, and possible causes. However, kidney disease does not always involve pain. It tends to be diagnosed because of other symptoms that cause a patient to seek health care, such as pedal edema, shortness of breath, and changes in urine elimination (Weber & Kelley, 2014).

Changes in Voiding

Micturition is normally a painless function that occurs approximately eight times in a 24-hour period. The average person voids 1 to 2 L of urine in 24 hours, although this amount varies depending on fluid intake, sweating, environmental temperature, vomiting, or diarrhea. Common problems associated with voiding include **frequency** (voiding more frequently than every 3 hours), urgency, dysuria, hesitancy, incontinence, enuresis, polyuria, **oliguria**, and hematuria. These problems and others are described in Table 53-3. Increased urinary urgency and frequency, coupled with decreasing urine volumes strongly suggest urine retention. Depending on the acuity of the onset of these symptoms, immediate bladder emptying via cath-

TABLE 53-3 Problems Associated With Changes in Voiding

Problem	Definition	Possible Etiology
Anuria	Urine output <50 mL/day	Acute or chronic kidney injury (see Chapter 54), complete obstruction
Bacteriuria	Bacterial count >100,000 colonies/mL in the urine	Infection
Dysuria	Painful or difficult voiding	Lower urinary tract infection, inflammation of bladder or urethra, acute prostatitis, stones, foreign bodies, tumors in bladder
Enuresis	Involuntary voiding during sleep	Delay in functional maturation of central nervous system (bladder control usually achieved by 5 years of age), obstructive disease of lower urinary tract, genetic factors, failure to concentrate urine, urinary tract infection, psychological stress
Frequency	Frequent voiding—more than every 3 hours	Infection, obstruction of lower urinary tract leading to residual urine and overflow, anxiety, diuretic agents, benign prostatic hyperplasia, urethral stricture, diabetic neuropathy
Hematuria	Red blood cells in the urine	Cancer of genitourinary tract, acute glomerulonephritis, renal stones, renal tuberculosis, blood dyscrasia, trauma, extreme exercise, rheumatic fever, hemophilia, leukemia, sickle cell trait or disease
Hesitancy	Delay, difficulty in initiating voiding	Benign prostatic hyperplasia, compression of urethra, outlet obstruction, neurogenic bladder
Incontinence	Involuntary loss of urine	External urinary sphincter injury, obstetric injury, lesions of bladder neck, detrusor dysfunction, infection, neurogenic bladder, medications, neurologic abnormalities
Nocturia	Awakening during the night to urinate	Decreased renal concentrating ability, heart failure, diabetes, incomplete bladder emptying, excessive fluid intake at bedtime, nephrotic syndrome, cirrhosis with ascites
Oliguria	Urine output <0.5 mL/kg/hr	Acute or chronic kidney failure (see Chapter 54), inadequate fluid intake
Polyuria	Increased volume of urine voided	Diabetes, diabetes insipidus, the use of diuretics, excess fluid intake, lithium toxicity, some forms of kidney disease (hypercalcemic and hypokalemic nephropathy)
Proteinuria	Protein in the urine	Acute and chronic kidney disease, nephrotic syndrome, vigorous exercise, heat stroke, severe heart failure, diabetic nephropathy, multiple myeloma
Urgency	Strong desire to void	Infection, chronic prostatitis, urethritis, obstruction of lower urinary tract leading to residual urine and overflow, anxiety, diuretic agents, benign prostatic hyperplasia, urethral stricture, diabetic neuropathy

GENETICS IN NURSING PRACTICE
Kidney and Urinary Disorders

Chart 53-2

Various conditions that affect the renal system and urinary tract function are influenced by genetic factors. Some examples of these genetic disorders are:

Autosomal Dominant:
- Familial Wilms tumor
- Polycystic kidney disease
- Renal cystic disease in tuberous sclerosis complex

X-Linked Recessive:
- Alport syndrome (primarily X-linked but autosomal dominant and recessive forms exist)

Congenital Kidney Disorders:
- Congenital absence of the vas deferens (caused by *CFTR* gene mutation for cystic fibrosis)
- Horseshoe kidney
- Multicystic dysplastic kidneys

Other Genetic Disorders that Impact the Renal System:
- Alpha-1 antitrypsin deficiency
- Anderson–Fabry disease
- Diabetes
- Coronary artery disease
- Pulmonary hypertension
- Von Hippel–Lindau syndrome

Nursing Assessments

Refer to Chapter 5, Chart 5-2: Genetics in Nursing Practice: Genetic Aspects of Health Assessment

Family History Specific to Kidney and Urinary Disorders
- Inquire about other family members with a history of renal and/or urinary tract malformations, kidney disease, or end-stage kidney disease and age of onset.

- Determine if other family members have diabetic kidney disease (clustering of this within the family could indicate genetic susceptibility).
- Identify family history of male infertility and cystic fibrosis (congenital absence of vas deferens).
- Be alert to family members with history of early-onset renal (Wilms tumor) or other cancers.

Physical Assessment Specific to Genetic Kidney and Urinary Disorders
- Be alert to signs and symptoms of kidney disease at an early age.
- Ascertain for presence and frequency of kidney stones or urinary tract infections.
- Assess for the presence and frequency of:
  - Abdominal pain or presence of an abdominal mass
  - Hematuria
  - Hypertension
  - Peripheral or orbital edema
  - Proteinuria
- Assess for clinical findings suggesting that kidney disease is a component of a genetic syndrome (e.g., seizures, intellectual disability, skin involvement).
- Assess for bleeding tendencies, abnormal clotting, or history of anemia.

Genetics Resources

Alport Syndrome Foundation, www.alportsyndrome.org
The American Kidney Fund, www.kidneyfund.org
See Chapter 8, Chart 8-7 for components of genetic counseling resources.

---

eterization and evaluation may be necessary to prevent kidney dysfunction.

Gastrointestinal Symptoms

Gastrointestinal signs and symptoms are often associated with urologic conditions because of shared autonomic and sensory innervation and renointestinal reflexes (see Table 53-3). The proximity of the right kidney to the colon, duodenum, head of the pancreas, common bile duct, liver, and gallbladder may cause gastrointestinal disturbances. The proximity of the left kidney to the colon (splenic flexure), stomach, pancreas, and spleen may also result in intestinal symptoms. The most common signs and symptoms are nausea, vomiting, diarrhea, abdominal discomfort, and abdominal distention.

Unexplained Anemia

Gradual kidney dysfunction can be insidious in its presentation, although fatigue is a common symptom. Fatigue, shortness of breath, and exercise intolerance all result from the condition known as "anemia of chronic disease."

Past Health, Family, and Social History

Data collection about previous health problems or diseases provides the health care team with useful information for evaluating the patient's current urinary status. People with diabetes who have hypertension are at risk for renal dysfunction. Older men are at risk for prostatic enlargement, which

causes urethral obstruction and can result in urinary tract infections and kidney disease. People with a family history of urinary tract problems are at increased risk for renal disorders. Genetics may also influence renal conditions (see Chart 53-2).

It is also important to assess the patient's psychosocial status, level of anxiety, perceived threats to body image, available support systems, and sociocultural patterns.

Physical Assessment

Several body systems can affect upper and lower urinary tract dysfunction, and conversely that dysfunction can affect several end organs; therefore, a head-to-toe assessment is indicated. Areas of emphasis include the abdomen, suprapubic region, genitalia, lower back, and lower extremities.

The kidneys are not usually palpable. However, palpation of the kidneys may detect an enlargement that could prove to be very important (Weber & Kelley, 2014). The correct technique for palpation is illustrated in Figure 53-5. It may be possible to palpate the smooth, rounded lower pole of the kidney between the hands. The right kidney is easier to detect, because it is somewhat lower than the left one. In patients who are obese, palpation of the kidneys is more difficult.

Renal dysfunction may produce tenderness over the costovertebral angle, which is the angle formed by the lower border of the 12th, or bottom, rib and the spine (see Fig. 53-6). The

Figure 53-5 • The left kidney is palpated by reaching over to the patient's left side and placing the right hand beneath the patient's lower left rib. Push the hand on top forward as the patient inhales deeply. Reprinted with permission from Weber, J. R., & Kelley, J. H. (2014). *Health assessment in nursing* (5th ed.). Philadelphia, PA: Lippincott Williams & Wilkins.

abdomen (just slightly to the right and left of the midline in both upper quadrants) is auscultated to assess for bruits (low-pitched murmurs that indicate renal artery stenosis or an aortic aneurysm). The abdomen is also assessed for the presence of ascites (accumulation of fluid in the peritoneal cavity), which may occur with kidney as well as liver dysfunction.

To check for residual urine, the bladder should be percussed after the patient voids. Percussion of the bladder begins at the midline just above the umbilicus and proceeds downward. The sound changes from tympanic to dull when percussing over the bladder. The bladder, which can be palpated only if it is moderately distended, feels like a smooth, firm, round mass rising out of the abdomen, usually at midline (see Fig. 53-7). Dullness to percussion of the bladder after voiding indicates incomplete bladder emptying (Weber & Kelley, 2014). Portable bladder ultrasonography is another

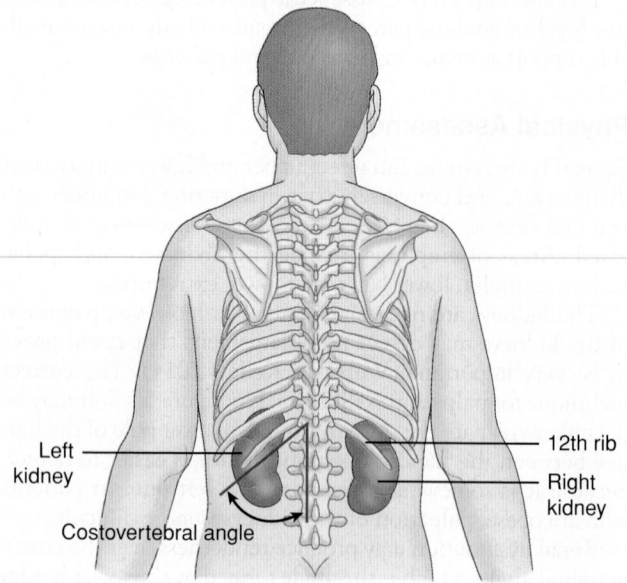

Figure 53-6 • Location of the costovertebral angle.

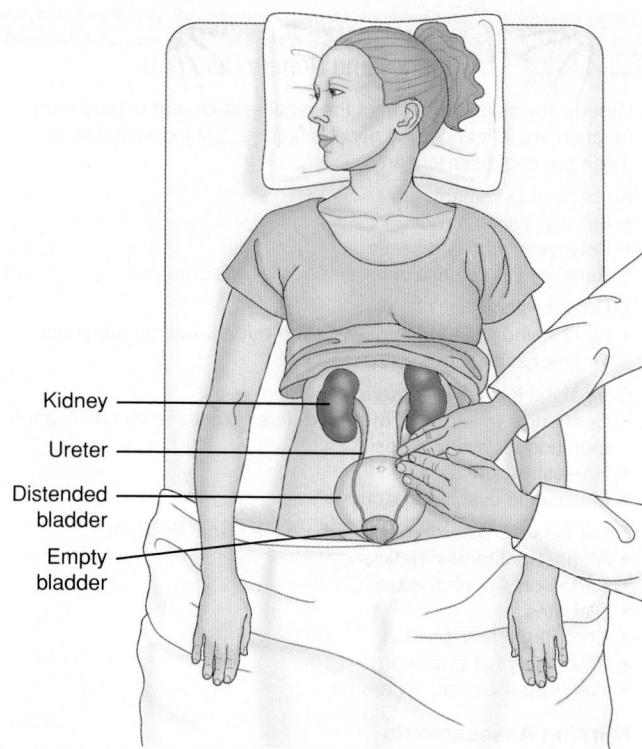

Figure 53-7 • Palpation of the bladder.

method of detecting urinary retention. These devices provide a three-dimensional image of the bladder and should be used 10 minutes after voiding to detect urine retention (Davis, Chrisman, & Walden, 2012). See later discussion in bladder ultrasonography section.

In older men, BPH or prostatitis can cause difficulty with urination. Because the signs and symptoms of prostate cancer can mimic those of BPH, the prostate gland is palpated by digital rectal examination (DRE) as part of the yearly physical examination in men 40 years and older (see Chapter 59). In addition, a blood specimen is obtained to test the prostate-specific antigen (PSA) level annually; the results of the DRE and PSA are then correlated. Blood is drawn for PSA before the DRE, because manipulation of the prostate can cause the PSA level to increase temporarily. The inguinal area is examined for enlarged nodes, an inguinal or femoral hernia, and varicocele (varicose veins of the spermatic cord).

In women, the vulva, urethral meatus, and vagina are examined (Weber & Kelley, 2014). The urethra is palpated for diverticula, and the vagina is assessed for adequate estrogen effect and any of five types of herniation: urethrocele, cystocele, pelvic prolapse, enterocele, and rectocele. Urethrocele is the bulging of the anterior vaginal wall into the urethra. Cystocele is the herniation of the bladder wall into the vaginal vault. Pelvic prolapse is bulging of the cervix into the vaginal vault. Enterocele is herniation of the bowel into the posterior vaginal wall. Rectocele is herniation of the rectum into the vaginal wall. These prolapses are graded depending on the degree of herniation. See Chapter 57 for more information.

The woman is asked to cough and perform a Valsalva maneuver to assess the urethra's system of muscular and ligament support. If urine leakage occurs, the index and middle fingers of the examiner's gloved hand are used to support either side of the urethra as the woman is asked to repeat the Valsalva maneuver; this is called the *Marshall–Bonney maneuver*. If this produces urinary leakage, referral is suggested.

The patient is assessed for edema and changes in body weight. Edema may be observed, particularly in the face and dependent parts of the body, such as the ankles and sacral areas, and suggests fluid retention. An increase in body weight commonly accompanies edema. A 1 kg weight gain equals approximately 1000 mL of fluid (1 lb is approximately 500 mL) (Hall, 2016).

The deep tendon reflexes of the knee are examined for quality and symmetry. This is an important part of testing for neurologic causes of bladder dysfunction, because the sacral area, which innervates the lower extremities, is the same peripheral nerve area responsible for urinary continence. The gait pattern of the person with bladder dysfunction is also noted, as well as the patient's ability to walk toe to heel. These tests evaluate possible supraspinal causes for urinary incontinence.

Unfolding Patient Stories: Lloyd Bennett • Part 2

Recall from Chapter 32 Lloyd Bennett, who presented to the emergency department with a hip fracture. What effect can significant blood loss from surgery to repair the fracture have on renal function? What clinical findings would indicate to the nurse that kidney function is impaired? What clinical assessment findings would alert the nurse of potential trauma to the urinary tract resulting from the hip fracture? What diagnostic tests may be used to identify a urinary tract complication that the nurse would consider for preparatory patient education?

Care for Lloyd and other patients in a realistic virtual environment: **vSim** *for Nursing* (**thepoint.lww. com/vSimMedicalSurgical**). Practice documenting these patients' care in DocuCare (**thepoint.lww.com/ DocuCareEHR**).

Diagnostic Evaluation

A wide range of diagnostic studies may be performed in patients with urinary conditions. A comprehensive health history is used to determine the appropriate laboratory and diagnostic tests. The following sections review some of the specific tests that might be used.

The nurse educates the patient about the purpose, what to expect, and any possible side effects related to these examinations prior to testing. The nurse should also note trends in results, because they provide information about disease progression as well as the patient's response to therapy.

Most patients undergoing urologic testing or imaging studies are apprehensive, even those who have had these tests in the past. Patients frequently feel discomfort and embarrassment about such a private and personal function as voiding. Voiding in the presence of others can frequently cause guarding, a natural reflex that inhibits voiding due to situational anxiety. Because the outcomes of these studies

---

Chart 53-3 • PATIENT EDUCATION
Before and After Urodynamic Testing

The nurse instructs the patient on what to expect before, during, and after the procedure:

Preprocedure

- A physician or nurse will conduct an in-depth interview. Questions related to your urologic symptoms and voiding habits will be asked.

During the Procedure

- You will be asked to describe sensations felt.
- You might be asked to change positions (e.g., from supine to sitting or standing).
- You may be asked to cough or perform the Valsalva maneuver (bear down).
- You will probably need to have one or two urethral catheters inserted so that bladder pressure and bladder filling can be measured. Another catheter may be placed in the rectum or vagina to measure abdominal pressure.
- You may also have electrodes (surface, wire, or needle) placed in the perianal area for electromyography. This may be uncomfortable initially during insertion and later during position changes.
- Your bladder will be filled through the urethral catheter one or more times.

After the Procedure

- You may experience urinary frequency, urgency, or dysuria from the urethral catheters. Avoid caffeinated, carbonated, and alcoholic beverages because they can further irritate the bladder. These symptoms usually decrease or subside by the day after the procedure.
- You might notice slight hematuria (blood-tinged urine) right after the procedure (especially in men with benign prostatic hyperplasia). Drinking fluids will help to clear the hematuria.
- If the urinary meatus is irritated, a warm sitz bath may be helpful.
- Be alert to signs of a urinary tract infection. Contact your primary provider if you experience fever, chills, lower back pain, or continued dysuria and hematuria.
- If you receive an antibiotic medication before the procedure, you should continue taking the complete course of medication after the procedure. This is a measure to prevent infection.

---

determine the plan of care, the nurse must help the patient relax by providing as much privacy and explanation about the procedure as possible (see Chart 53-3). In addition, Chart 53-4 provides a plan of care for patients undergoing diagnostic testing.

Urinalysis and Urine Culture

The urinalysis provides important clinical information about kidney function and helps diagnose other diseases, such as diabetes. The urine culture determines whether bacteria are present in the urine, as well as their strains and concentration. Urine culture and sensitivity also identify the antimicrobial therapy that is best suited for the particular strains identified, taking into consideration the antibiotic agents that have the best rate of resolution in that particular geographic region. Appropriate evaluation of any abnormality can assist in detecting serious underlying diseases.

Chart 53-4 PLAN OF NURSING CARE

Care of the Patient Undergoing Diagnostic Testing of the Renal–Urologic System

NURSING DIAGNOSIS: Deficient knowledge about procedures and diagnostic tests
GOAL: Patient demonstrates increased understanding of the procedure and tests and expected behaviors

Nursing Interventions	Rationale	Expected Outcomes
1. Assess patient's level of understanding of planned diagnostic tests 2. Provide a description of tests in language the patient can understand 3. Assess patient's understanding of test results after their completion 4. Reinforce information provided to patient about test results and implications for follow-up care	1. Provides basis for education and gives indication of patient's perception of tests 2. Understanding what is expected enhances patient adherence and cooperation 3. Apprehension may interfere with patient's ability to understand information and results provided by health care team 4. Provides opportunity for patient to clarify information and anticipate follow-up care	• States rationale for planned diagnostic tests and what tasks and behaviors are expected during the procedure • Adheres to prescribed urine collection, fluid modifications, or other procedures required for diagnostic evaluation • Restates in own words results of diagnostic tests • Asks for clarification of terms and procedures • Explains rationale for follow-up care • Participates in follow-up care

NURSING DIAGNOSIS: Acute pain related to infection, edema, obstruction, or bleeding along urinary tract or related to invasive diagnostic tests
GOAL: Patient reports decrease in pain and absence of discomfort

Nursing Interventions	Rationale	Expected Outcomes
1. Assess level of pain: dysuria, burning on urination, abdominal or flank pain, bladder spasm 2. Encourage fluid intake (unless contraindicated) 3. Encourage warm sitz baths 4. Report increased pain to primary provider 5. Administer analgesic and antispasmodic agents for pain and spasm as prescribed 6. Assess voiding patterns and hygiene practices and provide instructions about recommended voiding patterns and hygienic practices	1. Provides baseline for evaluation of pain-relief strategies and progression of dysfunction 2. Promotes dilute urine and flushing of the lower urinary tract 3. Relieves local discomfort and promotes relaxation 4. May indicate progression or recurrence of dysfunction, or untoward signs (e.g., bleeding, calculi) 5. Prescribed to relieve pain or spasm 6. Delayed emptying of the bladder and poor hygiene may contribute to pain secondary to renal or urinary tract dysfunction	• Reports decreasing levels of pain • Reports absence of local symptoms • States ability to start and stop urinary stream without discomfort • Consumes increased fluid intake if indicated • Uses sitz bath as indicated • Identifies signs and symptoms to be reported to the primary provider • Takes medications as prescribed • Does not delay in emptying bladder • Uses appropriate hygienic measures, avoids bubble baths, uses appropriate hygiene after bowel movements

NURSING DIAGNOSIS: Fear related to potential alteration in renal function and embarrassment secondary to discussion of urinary function and invasion of genitalia
GOAL: Patient appears relaxed and reports decreased fear and anxiety

Nursing Interventions	Rationale	Expected Outcomes
1. Assess patient's level of fear and apprehension 2. Explain all procedures and tests to patient 3. Provide privacy and respect patient's modesty by closing doors and keeping patient covered. Keep urinal and bedpan covered and out of sight 4. Use correct terminology in a factual manner when questioning patient about urinary tract dysfunction 5. Assess patient's fears about perceived changes associated with tests and other procedures 6. Instruct patient in relaxation techniques	1. A high level of fear or apprehension can interfere with learning and cooperation 2. Knowledge about what is expected helps reduce fear and apprehension 3. Communicates that you are aware of and accept patient's need for privacy and modesty 4. Conveys that you are comfortable discussing patient's urinary dysfunction and symptoms with patient 5. May uncover fears and misconceptions of the patient that can be alleviated by correct understanding 6. Promotes relaxation and assists patient in coping with uncertainty about outcomes	• Appears relaxed with a low level of fear or apprehension • States rationale for tests and procedures in a calm, relaxed manner • Maintains usual privacy and modesty • Discusses own urinary tract dysfunction using correct terminology without overt indications of embarrassment or discomfort • Relates fears and concerns • Demonstrates correct understanding of procedures and possible outcomes • Appears relaxed with low level of fear and apprehension

TABLE 53-4 Changes in Urine Color and Possible Causes

Urine Color	Possible Cause
Colorless to pale yellow	Dilute urine due to diuretic agents, alcohol consumption, diabetes insipidus, glycosuria, excess fluid intake, kidney disease
Yellow to milky white	Pyuria, infection, vaginal cream
Bright yellow	Multiple vitamin preparations
Pink to red	Hemoglobin breakdown, red blood cells, gross blood, menses, bladder or prostate surgery, beets, blackberries, medications (phenytoin [Dilantin], rifampin [Rifadin], thioridazine [Mellaril], cascara sagrada, senna products)
Blue, blue green	Dyes, methylene blue, *Pseudomonas* species organisms, medications (amitriptyline HCl [Amitriptyline], triamterene [Dyrenium])
Orange to amber	Concentrated urine due to dehydration, fever, bile, excess bilirubin or carotene, medications (phenazopyridine hydrochloride [Pyridium], nitrofurantoin [Furadantin])
Brown to black	Old red blood cells, urobilinogen, bilirubin, melanin, porphyrin, extremely concentrated urine due to dehydration, medications (cascara sagrada, metronidazole [Flagyl], iron preparations, quinine sulfate [Qualaquin], senna products, methyldopa [Aldomet], nitrofurantoin)

Components

Urine examination includes the following:
- Urine color (see Table 53-4)
- Urine clarity and odor
- Urine pH and specific gravity
- Tests to detect protein, glucose, and ketone bodies in the urine (proteinuria, renal glycosuria, and ketonuria, respectively)
- Microscopic examination of the urine sediment after centrifugation to detect RBCs (hematuria), white blood cells (**pyuria**), casts (cylindruria), crystals (crystalluria), and bacteria (**bacteriuria**) (see Table 53-3)

Researchers are working on additional noninvasive tests that can be performed on urine to detect conditions such as bladder cancer. For example, urine telomerase activity levels have been found to be sensitive and specific to detect bladder cancer in men (Lamarca & Barriuso, 2012).

Significance of Findings

Several abnormalities, such as hematuria and proteinuria, produce no symptoms but may be detected during a routine urinalysis using a dipstick. Normally, about 1 million RBCs pass into the urine daily, which is equivalent to one to three RBCs per high-power field. Hematuria (more than three RBCs per high-power field) can develop from an abnormality anywhere along the genitourinary tract and is more common in women than in men. Common causes include acute infection (cystitis, urethritis, or prostatitis), renal calculi, and neoplasm. Other causes include systemic disorders, such as bleeding disorders; malignant lesions; and medications, such as warfarin (Coumadin) and heparin. Although hematuria may initially be detected using a dipstick test, further evaluation is necessary with a 24-hour collection (Fischbach & Dunning, 2015).

Proteinuria may be a benign finding, or it may signify serious disease. Occasional loss of up to 150 mg/day of protein in the urine, primarily albumin and Tamm–Horsfall protein (also known as uromodulin), is considered normal and usually does not require further evaluation. A dipstick examination, which can detect from 30 to 1000 mg/dL of protein, should be used as a screening test only, because urine concentration, pH, hematuria, and radiocontrast materials all affect the results. Because dipstick analysis does not detect protein concentrations of less than 30 mg/dL, the test cannot be used for early detection of diabetic nephropathy. Microalbuminuria (excretion of 20 to 200 mg/dL of protein in the urine) is an early sign of diabetic nephropathy. Common benign causes of transient proteinuria are fever, strenuous exercise, and prolonged standing.

Causes of persistent proteinuria include glomerular diseases, malignancies, collagen diseases, diabetes, preeclampsia, hypothyroidism, heart failure, exposure to heavy metals, and the use of medications, such as nonsteroidal anti-inflammatory drugs and angiotensin-converting enzyme inhibitors (Comerford, 2015).

Specific Gravity

Specific gravity is an expression of the degree of concentration of the urine that measures the density of a solution compared to the density of water, which is 1.000. Specific gravity is altered by the presence of blood, protein, and casts in the urine. The normal range of urine-specific gravity is 1.010 to 1.025 (Grossman & Porth, 2014).

Methods for determination of specific gravity include the following:
- Multiple-test dipstick (most common method), with a specific reagent area for specific gravity
- Urinometer (least accurate method), in which urine is placed in a small cylinder and the urinometer is floated in the urine; a specific gravity reading is obtained at the meniscus level of the urine
- Refractometer, an instrument used in a laboratory setting, which measures differences in the speed of light passing through air and the urine sample; this is the most accurate test

Urine-specific gravity depends largely on hydration status. When fluid intake decreases, specific gravity normally increases. With high fluid intake, specific gravity decreases. In patients with kidney disease, urine-specific gravity does not vary with fluid intake, and the patient's urine is said to have a fixed specific gravity. Disorders or conditions that cause decreased urine-specific gravity include diabetes insipidus, glomerulonephritis, and severe renal damage. Those that can cause increased specific gravity include diabetes, nephritis, and fluid deficit.

Osmolality

Osmolality is the most accurate measurement of the kidney's ability to dilute and concentrate urine. It measures the number of solute particles in a kilogram of water. Serum and urine osmolality are measured simultaneously to assess the body's fluid status. In healthy adults, serum osmolality is 280 to 300 mOsm/kg, and normal urine osmolality is 200 to 800 mOsm/kg. For a 24-hour urine sample, the normal value is 300 to 900 mOsm/kg (Fischbach & Dunning, 2015).

Renal Function Tests

Renal function tests are used to evaluate the severity of kidney disease and to assess the status of the patient's kidney function. These tests also provide information about the effectiveness of the kidney in carrying out its excretory function. Renal function test results may be within normal limits until the GFR is reduced to less than 50% of normal. Renal function can be assessed most accurately if several tests are performed and their results are analyzed together. Common tests of renal function include renal concentration tests, creatinine clearance, and serum creatinine and blood **urea nitrogen** (end product of protein metabolism) levels (see Table 53-5).

Other tests for evaluating renal function that may be helpful include serum electrolyte levels as well as urinary biomarkers to detect acute kidney injury (Fallone & Cotton, 2015) (see Chapter 13).

Diagnostic Imaging

Kidney, Ureter, and Bladder Studies

An x-ray study of the abdomen or kidneys, ureters, and bladder (KUB) may be performed to delineate the size, shape, and position of the kidneys and to reveal urinary system abnormalities (Fischbach & Dunning, 2015).

General Ultrasonography

Ultrasonography is a noninvasive procedure that uses sound waves passed into the body through a transducer to detect abnormalities of internal tissues and organs. Abnormalities such as fluid accumulation, masses, congenital malformations, changes in organ size, and obstructions can be identified. During the test, the lower abdomen and genitalia may need to be exposed. Ultrasonography requires a full bladder; therefore, fluid intake is encouraged before the procedure.

Bladder Ultrasonography

Bladder ultrasonography is a noninvasive method of measuring urine volume in the bladder. It may be indicated for urinary frequency, inability to void after removal of an indwelling urinary catheter, measurement of postvoiding residual urine volume, inability to void postoperatively, or assessment of the need for catheterization during the initial stages of an intermittent catheterization training program. Portable, battery-operated devices are available for bedside use. The scan head is placed on the patient's abdomen and directed toward the bladder (see Fig. 53-8). The device automatically calculates and displays urine volume.

Computed Tomography and Magnetic Resonance Imaging

Computed tomography (CT) and magnetic resonance imaging (MRI) are noninvasive techniques that provide excellent cross-sectional views of the anatomy of the kidney and urinary tract. They are used to evaluate genitourinary masses, nephrolithiasis, chronic renal infections, renal or urinary tract trauma, metastatic disease, and soft tissue abnormalities. Occasionally, an oral or intravenous (IV) radiopaque contrast agent is used in CT scanning to enhance visualization.

Nursing Interventions

Preparation includes educating the patient about relaxation techniques and explaining that they will be able to communicate

---

TABLE 53-5 Renal Function Tests

Test	Purpose	Normal Values		
Renal Concentration				
Specific gravity	A measure of the degree of concentration of the urine.	1.010–1.025		
Urine osmolality	Concentrating ability is lost early in kidney disease; hence, these test findings may disclose early defects in renal function.	250–900 mOsm/kg/24 hr, 50–1200 mOsm/kg random sample		
24-Hour Urine				
Creatinine clearance	Detects and evaluates progression of kidney disease. Test measures volume of blood cleared of endogenous creatinine in 1 minute, which provides an approximation of the glomerular filtration rate. Sensitive indicator of kidney disease used to follow progression of kidney disease.	Measured in mL/min/1.73 m²		
		Age (Years)	**Male**	**Female**
		<30	88–146	81–134
		30–40	82–140	75–128
		40–50	75–133	69–122
		50–60	68–126	64–116
		60–70	61–120	58–110
		70–80	55–113	52–105
Serum				
Creatinine level	Measures effectiveness of renal function. Creatinine is the end product of muscle energy metabolism. In normal function, the level of creatinine, which is regulated and excreted by the kidneys, remains fairly constant in the body.	0.6–1.2 mg/dL (50–110 mmol/L)		
BUN	Serves as index of renal function. Urea is the nitrogenous end product of protein metabolism. Test values are affected by protein intake, tissue breakdown, and fluid volume changes.	7–18 mg/dL; patients >60 years: 8–20 mg/dL		
BUN-to-creatinine ratio	Evaluates hydration status. An elevated ratio is seen in hypovolemia; a normal ratio with an elevated BUN and creatinine is seen with intrinsic kidney disease.	About 10:1		

BUN, blood urea nitrogen.
Adapted from Fischbach, F., & Dunning, M. B. (2015). A manual of laboratory and diagnostic tests (9th ed.). Philadelphia, PA: Lippincott Williams & Wilkins.

Figure 53-8 • Bladder ultrasonography. **A.** The nurse puts on gloves and cleans the rounded end of the scan head with an alcohol pad. **B.** After locating the symphysis pubis, the nurse places the scan head about 2.5 cm (1 inch) superior to the symphysis pubis. Reprinted with permission from Springhouse. (2008). *Lippincott's visual encyclopedia of clinical skills.* Philadelphia, PA: Lippincott Williams & Wilkins.

with the staff by means of a microphone located inside the scanner. Many MRI suites provide headphones so that patients can listen to the music of their choice during the procedure. Nursing care guidelines for patient preparation and precautions for any imaging procedure that requires a contrast agent (contrast medium) are explained in Chart 53-5.

Before the patient enters the room where the MRI is to be performed, all metal objects and credit cards (the magnetic field can erase them) are removed. This includes medication patches (e.g., nicotine and nitroglycerin) that have a metal backing, which can cause burns if they are not removed. No metal objects (e.g., oxygen tanks, ventilators, stethoscopes) may be brought into the MRI room. The magnetic field is so strong that any metal-containing items will be pulled toward the magnet, causing severe injury and possible death. A patient history is obtained to determine the presence of any metal objects (e.g., aneurysm clips, orthopedic hardware, pacemakers, artificial heart valves, intrauterine devices). These objects could malfunction, be dislodged, or heat up as they absorb energy. Cochlear implants are inactivated by MRI; therefore, other imaging procedures are considered. A sedative agent may be prescribed, because claustrophobia is a problem for some patients.

Chart 53-5

Patient Care During Urologic Testing With Contrast Agents

For some patients, contrast agents are nephrotoxic and allergenic. Emergency equipment and medications should be available in case of an anaphylactic reaction to the contrast agent. Emergency supplies include epinephrine, corticosteroids, vasopressors, oxygen, and airway and suction equipment.

The following guidelines can help the nurse respond quickly in the event of a problem.

Nursing Actions for Patient Preparation

- Obtain the patient's allergy history with emphasis on allergy to iodine, shellfish, and other seafood, because many contrast agents contain iodine.
- Notify primary provider and radiologist if the patient is allergic or suspected to be allergic to iodine.
- Obtain health history. Contrast agents should be used with great caution in older patients and in patients who have multiple myeloma, renal impairment, or volume depletion.
- Obtain medication history. Nephrotoxic medications such as vancomycin, amphotericin B, metformin, and nonsteroidal anti-inflammatory drugs should be discontinued before contrast media administration.
- The use of both nonionic low-osmolar contrast media (LOCM, e.g., iohexol) and ionic high-osmolar contrast media (HOCM, e.g., diatrizoate), is indicated in patients with renal impairment and other risk factors to prevent contrast-induced nephropathy.
- Check kidney function in at-risk patients. Patients should receive IV hydration prior to the procedure.
- Inform the patient that they may experience a temporary feeling of warmth, flushing of the face, and an unusual flavor (similar to that of seafood) in the mouth when the contrast agent is infused.

Nursing Actions During and Post Procedure

- Monitor patient closely for allergic reaction, and monitor urine output.
- Maintain hydration status.

Adapted from Andreucci, M., Solomon, R., & Tasanarong, A. (2014). Side effects of radiographic contrast media: Pathogenesis, risk factors, and prevention. Retrieved on 4/17/2016 at: www.hindawi.com/journals/bmri/2014/741018/; Rank, W. (2013). Preventing contrast media–induced nephrotoxicity. *Nursing, 43*(4), 48–51.

Prior to MRI of the urinary system, the patient needs to be informed to avoid alcohol, caffeine-containing beverages, and smoking for at least 2 hours and food for at least 1 hour prior to the scan. Patients should continue taking their usual medication, except for iron supplements, which can interfere with the imaging (Fischbach & Dunning, 2015).

Nuclear Scans

Nuclear scans require injection of a radioisotope (a technetium 99m–labeled compound or iodine 123 [^{123}I] hippurate) into the circulatory system; the isotope is then monitored as it moves through the blood vessels of the kidneys. A scintillation camera is placed behind the kidney with the patient in a supine, prone, or seated position. Hypersensitivity to the radioisotope is rare. The technetium scan provides information about kidney perfusion. The ^{123}I-hippurate renal scan provides information about kidney function, such as GFR.

Nuclear scans are used to evaluate acute and chronic kidney injury, renal masses, and blood flow before and after kidney transplantation. The radioisotope is injected at a specified time to achieve the proper concentration in the kidneys. After the procedure is completed, the patient is encouraged to drink fluids to promote excretion of the radioisotope by the kidneys.

Intravenous Urography

IV urography includes various tests such as excretory urography, intravenous pyelography (IVP), and infusion drip pyelography. A radiopaque contrast agent is given IV. An IVP shows the kidneys, ureter, and bladder via x-ray imaging as the dye moves through the upper and then the lower urinary system. A nephrotomogram may be carried out as part of the study to visualize different layers of the kidney and the diffuse structures within each layer and to differentiate solid masses or lesions from cysts in the kidneys or urinary tract.

IV urography may be used as the initial assessment of many suspected urologic conditions, especially lesions in the kidneys and ureters. It also provides an approximate estimate of renal function. After the contrast agent (sodium diatrizoate or meglumine diatrizoate) is given IV, multiple x-rays are obtained to visualize drainage structures in the upper and lower urinary systems.

Infusion drip pyelography requires IV infusion of a large volume of a dilute contrast agent to opacify the renal parenchyma and fills the urinary tract. This examination method is useful when prolonged opacification of the drainage structures is desired so that tomograms (body-section radiography) can be made. Images are obtained at specified intervals after the start of the infusion. These images show the filled and distended collecting system. The patient preparation is the same as for excretory urography, except fluids are not restricted.

Retrograde Pyelography

In retrograde pyelography, catheters are advanced through the ureters into the renal pelvis by means of cystoscopy. A contrast agent is then injected. Retrograde pyelography is usually performed if IV urography provides inadequate visualization of the collecting systems. It may also be used before extracorporeal shock wave lithotripsy and in patients with urologic cancer who need follow-up and have an allergy to IV contrast agents. Possible complications include infection, hematuria, and perforation of the ureter. Retrograde pyelography is used infrequently because of improved techniques in excretory urography.

Cystography

Cystography aids in evaluating vesicoureteral reflux (backflow of urine from the bladder into one or both ureters) and in assessing for bladder injury. A catheter is inserted into the bladder, and a contrast agent is instilled to outline the bladder wall. The contrast agent may leak through a small bladder perforation stemming from bladder injury, but such leakage is usually harmless. Cystography can also be performed with simultaneous pressure recordings inside the bladder.

Voiding Cystourethrography

Voiding cystourethrography uses fluoroscopy to visualize the lower urinary tract and assess urine storage in the bladder. It is commonly used as a diagnostic tool to identify vesicoureteral reflux. A urethral catheter is inserted, and a contrast agent is instilled into the bladder. When the bladder is full and the patient feels the urge to void, the catheter is removed, and the patient voids.

Renal Angiography

A renal angiogram, or renal arteriogram, provides an image of the renal arteries. The femoral (or axillary) artery is pierced with a needle, and a catheter is threaded up through the femoral and iliac arteries into the aorta or renal artery. A contrast agent is injected to opacify the renal arterial supply. Angiography is used to evaluate renal blood flow in suspected renal trauma, to differentiate renal cysts from tumors, and to evaluate hypertension. It is used preoperatively for renal transplantation.

Nursing Interventions

Before the procedure, a laxative may be prescribed to evacuate the colon so that unobstructed x-rays can be obtained. Injection sites (groin for femoral approach or axilla for axillary approach) may be shaved. The peripheral pulse sites (radial, femoral, and dorsalis pedis) are marked for easy access during postprocedural assessment (Rank, 2013). See Chart 53-5 for considerations for the patient receiving a contrast agent.

After the procedure, vital signs are monitored until stable. If the axillary artery was the injection site, blood pressure measurements are taken on the opposite arm. The injection site is examined for swelling and hematoma. Peripheral pulses are palpated, and the color and temperature of the involved extremity are noted and compared with those of the uninvolved extremity. Cold compresses may be applied to the injection site to decrease edema and pain. Possible complications include hematoma formation, arterial thrombosis or dissection, false aneurysm formation, and altered renal function.

MAG3 Renogram

This scan is used to further evaluate kidney function in some centers by permitting visualization of renal clearance (Fischbach & Dunning, 2015). The patient is given an injection containing a small amount of radioactive material, which will show how the kidneys are functioning. The patient needs to lie still for about 35 minutes while special cameras take images (Fischbach & Dunning, 2015).

Urologic Endoscopic Procedures

Endourology, or urologic endoscopic procedures, can be performed in one of two ways: using a cystoscope inserted into the urethra, or percutaneously, through a small incision.

The cystoscopic examination is used to directly visualize the urethra and bladder. The cystoscope, which is inserted through the urethra into the bladder, has an optical lens system that provides a magnified, illuminated view of the bladder (see Fig. 53-9). The use of high-intensity light and interchangeable lenses allows excellent visualization and permits still and motion pictures to be taken. The cystoscope is manipulated to allow complete visualization of the urethra and bladder as well as the ureteral orifices and prostatic urethra. Small ureteral catheters can be passed through

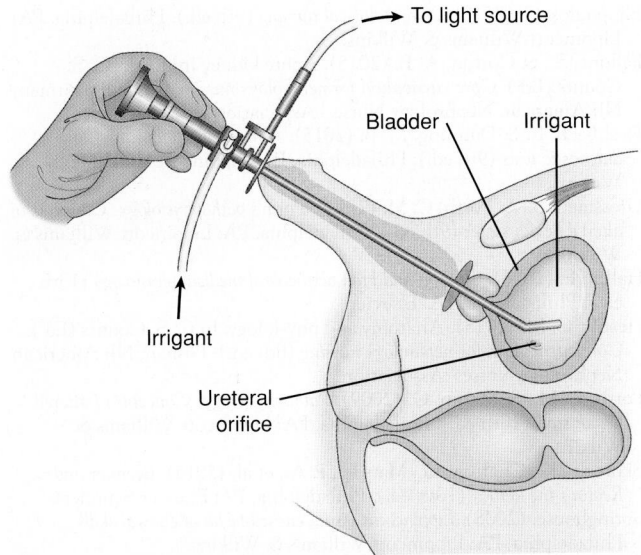

To light source

Bladder

Irrigant

Irrigant

Ureteral orifice

Figure 53-9 • Cystoscopic examination. A rigid or semirigid cystoscope is introduced into the bladder. The upper cord is an electric line for the light at the distal end of the cystoscope. The lower tubing leads from a reservoir of sterile irrigant that is used to inflate the bladder.

the cystoscope for assessment of the ureters and the pelvis of each kidney.

The cystoscope also allows the urologist to obtain a urine specimen from each kidney to evaluate its function. Cup forceps can be inserted through the cystoscope for biopsy. Calculi may be removed from the urethra, bladder, and ureter using cystoscopy. If a lower tract cystoscopy is performed, the patient is usually conscious, and the procedure is usually no more uncomfortable than a catheterization. To minimize posttest urethral discomfort, viscous lidocaine is given several minutes before the study. If the cystoscopy includes examination of the upper tracts, a sedative agent may be given before the procedure. General anesthesia is usually given to ensure that there are no involuntary muscle spasms when the scope is being passed through the ureters or kidneys.

Nursing Interventions

The nurse describes the procedure to the patient and family to prepare them and to allay their fears. If an upper cystoscopy is to be performed, the patient is usually restricted to nothing by mouth (NPO) for several hours beforehand.

Postprocedural management is directed at relieving any discomfort resulting from the examination. Some burning on voiding, blood-tinged urine, and urinary frequency from trauma to the mucous membranes can be expected. Moist heat to the lower abdomen and warm sitz baths are helpful in relieving pain and relaxing the muscles.

After a cystoscopic examination, the patient with obstructive pathology may experience urine retention if the instruments used during the examination caused edema. The nurse carefully monitors the patient with prostatic hyperplasia for urine retention. Warm sitz baths and antispasmodic medication, such as flavoxate (Urispas), may be prescribed to relieve temporary urine retention caused by poor relaxation of the urinary sphincter; however, intermittent catheterization may be necessary for a few hours after the examination. The nurse

monitors the patient for signs and symptoms of urinary tract infection. Because edema of the urethra secondary to local trauma may obstruct urine flow, the patient is also monitored for signs and symptoms of obstruction.

Biopsy

Renal and Ureteral Brush Biopsy

Brush biopsy techniques provide specific information when abnormal x-ray findings of the ureter or renal pelvis raise questions about whether a defect is a tumor, a stone, a blood clot, or an artifact. First, a cystoscopic examination is conducted. Then, a ureteral catheter is introduced, followed by a biopsy brush that is passed through the catheter. The suspected lesion is brushed back and forth to obtain cells and surface tissue fragments for histologic analysis.

Kidney Biopsy

Biopsy of the kidney is used to help diagnose and evaluate the extent of kidney disease. Indications for biopsy include unexplained acute kidney injury, persistent proteinuria or hematuria, transplant rejection, and glomerulopathies. A small section of renal cortex is obtained either percutaneously (needle biopsy) or by open biopsy through a small flank incision. Before the biopsy is carried out, coagulation studies are conducted to identify any risk of post biopsy bleeding. Contraindications to kidney biopsy include bleeding tendencies, uncontrolled hypertension, sepsis, a solitary kidney, large polycystic kidneys, kidney neoplasm, urinary tract infection, and morbid obesity (Doss-McQuitty, 2015).

The patient may be prescribed a fasting regimen 6 to 8 hours before the test. An IV line is established. A urine specimen is obtained and saved for comparison with the post biopsy specimen.

If a needle biopsy is to be performed, the patient is instructed to breathe in and hold that breath (to prevent the kidney from moving) while the needle is being inserted. The sedated patient is placed in a prone position with a sandbag under the abdomen. The skin at the biopsy site is infiltrated with a local anesthetic agent. The biopsy needle is introduced just inside the renal capsule of the outer quadrant of the kidney. The location of the needle may be confirmed by fluoroscopy or by ultrasound, in which case a special probe is used.

With open biopsy, a small incision is made over the kidney, allowing direct visualization. Preparation for an open biopsy is similar to that for any major abdominal surgery.

Nursing Interventions

After a biopsy procedure, nursing care includes monitoring vital signs for the first 24 hours to detect signs and symptoms of bleeding or infection. The nurse should assess for other signs and symptoms of internal bleeding such as pallor, dizziness, and flank or back pain. IV fluids may be given to help clear the kidneys and prevent clot formation. Urine may contain blood (usually clearing in 24 to 48 hours) from oozing at the site. Bed rest should be maintained and pressure dressings applied for prescribed periods of time to control bleeding. Puncture sites should be examined for signs and symptoms of infection. Analgesic agents should be given as prescribed and needed for pain (Doss-McQuitty, 2015).

CRITICAL THINKING EXERCISES

1 A patient you are caring for complains of urinary incontinence. Describe the assessment techniques appropriate to evaluate the patient. Review the possible causes and describe the actions you would take and the rationale for each action. Describe any differences in your assessments and possible action that are dependent on the gender of the patient.

2 `pq` A 30-year-old male is admitted to the emergency department for evaluation of urinary dysfunction and is scheduled for a renal angiography. The patient is now highly anxious. Describe your priorities for educating this patient about a kidney biopsy. What are your priority interventions for decreasing the patient's anxiety?

3 `ebp` You make a home visit to a 70-year-old female who had a urologic examination with contrast. She complains of flu-like symptoms and reports that she thinks she notices swelling in her lower extremities. She has a history of renal impairment. Identify assessments and possible interventions that you would use to evaluate and manage the patient's symptoms. Identify the evidence for the assessments and nursing interventions you chose and the strength of that evidence.

REFERENCES

Books

Comerford, K. C. (2015). *Nursing 2015 drug handbook.* Philadelphia, PA: Wolters Kluwer.

Doss-McQuitty, S. J. (2015). Assessment of kidney structure and function. In C. S. Counts (Ed.): *Core curriculum for nephrology nursing* (6th ed.). Pitman, NJ: American Nephrology Nurses' Association.

Eaton, D. C., & Pooler, J. P. (2013). *Vander's renal physiology* (8th ed.). New York: McGraw-Hill Education.

Eliopoulos, C. (2018). *Gerontological nursing* (9th ed.). Philadelphia, PA: Lippincott Williams & Wilkins.

Fallone, S., & Cotton, A. B. (2015). Acute kidney injury. In C. S. Counts (Ed.): *Core curriculum for nephrology nursing* (6th ed.). Pitman, NJ: American Nephrology Nurses' Association.

Fischbach, F., & Dunning, M. B. (2015). *A manual of laboratory and diagnostic tests* (9th ed.). Philadelphia, PA: Lippincott Williams & Wilkins.

Grossman, S., & Porth, C. M. (2014). *Porth's pathophysiology: Concepts of altered health states* (9th ed.). Philadelphia, PA: Lippincott Williams & Wilkins.

Hall, J. E. (2016). *Guyton and Hall textbook of medical physiology* (13th ed.). Philadelphia, PA: Elsevier.

Headly, C. M. (2015). Anatomy and physiology. In C. S. Counts (Ed.): *Core curriculum for nephrology nursing* (6th ed.). Pitman, NJ: American Nephrology Nurses' Association.

Porth, C. M., & Matfin, G. (2009). *Pathophysiology: Concepts of altered health states* (8th ed.). Philadelphia, PA: Lippincott Williams & Wilkins.

Skorecki, K., Chertow, G., Marsden P. A., et al. (2015). *Brenner and Rector's the kidney* (10th ed.). Philadelphia, PA: Elsevier Saunders.

Springhouse. (2008). *Lippincott's visual encyclopedia of clinical skills.* Philadelphia, PA: Lippincott Williams & Wilkins.

Weber, J. R., & Kelley, J. H. (2014). *Health assessment in nursing* (5th ed.). Philadelphia, PA: Lippincott Williams & Wilkins.

Journals and Electronic Documents

Andreucci, M., Solomon, R., & Tasanarong, A. (2014). Side effects of radiographic contrast media: pathogenesis, risk factors, and prevention. *BioMed Research International.* Retrieved on 4/17/2016 at: www.hindawi.com/journals/bmri/2014/741018/

Davis, C., Chrisman, J., & Walden, P. (2012). To scan or not to scan? Detecting urinary retention. *Nursing Made Incredibly Easy, 10*(4), 53–54.

Lamarca, A., & Barriuso, J. (2012). Urine telomerase for diagnosis and surveillance of bladder cancer. *Advances in Urology.* Retrieved on 12/29/15 at: www.hindawi.com/journals/au/2012/693631

Rank, W. (2013). Preventing contrast media–induced nephrotoxicity. *Nursing, 43*(4), 48–51.

Resources

American Association of Kidney Patients (AAKP), www.aakp.orgNational Kidney Foundation, www.kidney.org

National Institute of Diabetes and Digestive and Kidney Diseases, National Institutes of Health, www.niddk.nih.gov

54

Management of Patients With Kidney Disorders

LEARNING OBJECTIVES

On completion of this chapter, the learner will be able to:

1 Describe the key factors associated with the development of kidney disorders.
2 Differentiate between the causes of chronic kidney disease (CKD) and acute kidney injury (AKI).
3 Explain the pathophysiology, clinical manifestations, medical management, and nursing management for patients with kidney disorders.

4 Understand the nursing management of patients with chronic kidney disease and acute kidney injury.
5 Compare and contrast the renal replacement therapies, including hemodialysis, peritoneal dialysis, continuous renal replacement therapies, and kidney transplantation.
6 Identify the nursing management of the patient on dialysis who is hospitalized.
7 Develop a postoperative plan of nursing care for the patient undergoing kidney surgery and transplantation.

GLOSSARY

acute kidney injury (AKI): rapid loss of renal function due to damage to the kidneys; formerly called acute kidney injury

acute nephritic syndrome: type of kidney disease with glomerular inflammation

acute tubular necrosis (ATN): type of acute kidney injury in which there is damage to the kidney tubules

anuria: total urine output less than 50 mL in 24 hours

arteriovenous fistula: type of vascular access for dialysis; created by surgically connecting an artery to a vein

arteriovenous graft: type of surgically created vascular access for dialysis by which a piece of biologic, semibiologic, or synthetic graft material connects the patient's artery to a vein

azotemia: abnormal concentration of nitrogenous waste products in the blood

chronic kidney disease: kidney damage or a decrease in the glomerular filtration rate lasting for 3 or more months

continuous ambulatory peritoneal dialysis (CAPD): method of peritoneal dialysis whereby a patient manually performs exchanges or cycles throughout the day

continuous cyclic peritoneal dialysis (CCPD): method of peritoneal dialysis in which a peritoneal dialysis machine (cycler) automatically performs exchanges, usually while the patient sleeps

continuous renal replacement therapy (CRRT): method used to replace normal kidney function in patients who are hemodynamically unstable by circulating the patient's blood through a hemofilter and returning it to the patient

dialysate: the electrolyte solution that circulates through the dialyzer in hemodialysis and through the peritoneal membrane in peritoneal dialysis

dialyzer: artificial kidney; contains a semipermeable membrane through which particles of a certain size can pass

diffusion: movement of solutes (waste products) from an area of higher concentration to an area of lower concentration

effluent: term used to describe the drained fluid from a peritoneal dialysis exchange

end-stage kidney disease (ESKD): final stage of chronic kidney disease that results in retention of uremic waste products and the need for renal replacement therapies

exchange: denotes a complete cycle including fill, dwell, and drain phases of peritoneal dialysis

glomerular filtration rate (GFR): amount of plasma filtered through the glomeruli per unit of time

glomerulonephritis: inflammation of the glomerular capillaries

hemodialysis: procedure during which a patient's blood is circulated through a dialyzer to remove waste products and excess fluid

interstitial nephritis: inflammation within the renal tissue

nephrosclerosis: hardening of the renal arteries

nephrotic syndrome: type of kidney disease with increased glomerular permeability and massive proteinuria

nephrotoxic: any substance, medication, or action that destroys kidney tissue

oliguria: urine output less than 0.5 mL/kg/hr

osmosis: movement of water through a semipermeable membrane from an area of lower solute concentration to an area of higher solute concentration

peritoneal dialysis: procedure that uses the lining of the patient's peritoneal cavity as the semipermeable membrane for exchange of fluid and solutes

peritonitis: inflammation of the peritoneal membrane (lining of the peritoneal cavity)

polyuria: excessive urine production

ultrafiltration: process whereby water is removed from the blood by means of a pressure gradient between the patient's blood and the dialysate

uremia: an excess of urea and other nitrogenous wastes in the blood

urinary casts: proteins secreted by damaged kidney tubules

The kidneys and urinary system help regulate the body's internal environment and are essential for the maintenance of life. Nurses working in any clinical setting may encounter patients with various kidney injuries and diseases, and thus need to be knowledgeable about these disorders. This chapter provides an overview of electrolyte imbalances and systemic manifestations that are common in patients with kidney disorders. The main causes are discussed, together with management strategies to prevent damage and preserve renal function. Chronic kidney disease (CKD) and acute kidney injury (AKI) are discussed, as is the care of patients with other renal conditions requiring dialysis, continuous renal replacement therapies (CRRTs), transplantation, and kidney surgery.

FLUID AND ELECTROLYTE IMBALANCES IN KIDNEY DISORDERS

Patients with kidney disorders commonly experience fluid and electrolyte imbalances and require careful assessment and close monitoring for signs of potential problems. The patient whose fluid intake exceeds the ability of the kidneys to excrete fluid is said to have fluid overload. If fluid intake is inadequate, the patient is said to be volume depleted and may show signs and symptoms of fluid volume deficit. The intake and output (I&O) record, a key monitoring tool, is used to document important fluid parameters, including the amount of fluid taken in (orally or parenterally), the volume of urine excreted, and other fluid losses (diarrhea, vomiting, diaphoresis). Patient weight is also important, and documenting trends in weight is a key assessment strategy essential for determining the daily fluid allowance and indicating signs of fluid volume excess or deficit.

 Quality and Safety Nursing Alert

The most accurate indicator of fluid loss or gain in patients who are acutely ill is weight. An accurate daily weight must be obtained and recorded. A 1-kg weight gain is equal to 1000 mL of retained fluid.

Clinical Manifestations

The signs and symptoms of common fluid and electrolyte disturbances that can occur in patients with kidney disorders and general management strategies are listed in Table 54-1.

TABLE 54-1 Common Fluid and Electrolyte Disturbances in Kidney Disorders

Disturbance	Manifestations	General Management Strategies
Fluid volume deficit	Acute weight loss ≥5%, decreased skin turgor, dry mucous membranes, oliguria or anuria, increased hematocrit, BUN level increased out of proportion to creatinine level, hypothermia	Fluid challenge, fluid replacement orally or parenterally
Fluid volume excess	Acute weight gain ≥5%, edema, crackles, shortness of breath, decreased BUN, decreased hematocrit, distended neck veins	Fluid and sodium restriction, diuretic agents, dialysis
Sodium deficit	Nausea, malaise, lethargy, headache, abdominal cramps, apprehension, seizures	Diet, normal saline or hypertonic saline solutions
Sodium excess	Dry, sticky mucous membranes, thirst, rough dry tongue, fever, restlessness, weakness, disorientation	Fluids, diuretic agents, dietary restriction
Potassium deficit	Anorexia, abdominal distention, paralytic ileus, muscle weakness, ECG changes, dysrhythmias	Diet, oral or parenteral potassium replacement therapy
Potassium excess	Diarrhea, colic, nausea, irritability, muscle weakness, ECG changes	Dietary restriction, diuretics, IV glucose, insulin and sodium bicarbonate, cation-exchange resin, calcium gluconate, dialysis
Calcium deficit	Abdominal and muscle cramps, stridor, carpopedal spasm, hyperactive reflexes, tetany, positive Chvostek or Trousseau sign, tingling of fingers and around mouth, ECG changes	Diet, oral or parenteral calcium salt replacement
Calcium excess	Deep bone pain, flank pain, muscle weakness, depressed deep tendon reflexes, constipation, nausea and vomiting, confusion, impaired memory, polyuria, polydipsia, ECG changes	Fluid replacement, etidronate, pamidronate, mithramycin, calcitonin, glucocorticoids, phosphate salts
Bicarbonate deficit	Headache, confusion, drowsiness, increased respiratory rate and depth, nausea and vomiting, warm flushed skin	Bicarbonate replacement, dialysis
Bicarbonate excess	Depressed respirations, muscle hypertonicity, dizziness, tingling of fingers and toes	Fluid replacement if volume depleted; ensure adequate chloride
Protein deficit	Chronic weight loss, emotional depression, pallor, fatigue, soft flabby muscles	Diet, dietary supplements, hyperalimentation, albumin
Magnesium deficit	Dysphagia, muscle cramps, hyperactive reflexes, tetany, positive Chvostek or Trousseau sign, tingling of fingers, dysrhythmias, vertigo	Diet, oral or parenteral magnesium replacement therapy
Magnesium excess	Facial flushing, nausea and vomiting, sensation of warmth, drowsiness, depressed deep tendon reflexes, muscle weakness, respiratory depression, cardiac arrest	Calcium gluconate, mechanical ventilation, dialysis
Phosphorus deficit	Deep bone pain, flank pain, muscle weakness and pain, paresthesia, apprehension, confusion, seizures	Diet, oral or parenteral phosphorus supplementation therapy

BUN, blood urea nitrogen; ECG, electrocardiographic; IV, intravenous.

The nurse continually assesses, monitors, and informs appropriate members of the health care team if the patient exhibits any of these signs. Management strategies for fluid and electrolyte disturbances in kidney disease are discussed in greater depth later in this chapter (see Chapter 13).

 ### Gerontologic Considerations

With aging, the kidney is less able to respond to acute fluid and electrolyte changes. Older adult patients may develop atypical and nonspecific signs and symptoms of altered renal function and fluid and electrolyte imbalances. A fluid balance deficit in older adults can lead to constipation, falls, medication toxicity, urinary tract and respiratory tract infections, delirium, seizures, electrolyte imbalances, hyperthermia, and delayed wound healing. Recognition of acute changes in fluid and electrolytes is further hampered by their association with pre-existing disorders and the misconception that they are normal changes of aging.

KIDNEY DISORDERS

Chronic Kidney Disease

Chronic kidney disease is an umbrella term that describes kidney damage or a decrease in the glomerular filtration rate (GFR) lasting for 3 or more months. CKD is associated with decreased quality of life, increased health care expenditures, and premature death. Untreated CKD can result in **end-stage kidney disease (ESKD)**, which is the final stage of CKD. ESKD results in retention of uremic waste products and the need for renal replacement therapies, dialysis, or kidney transplantation. Risk factors include cardiovascular disease, diabetes, hypertension, and obesity. Recent research reported that 10% of the U.S. population aged 20 years and older has CKD (Centers for Disease Control and Prevention [CDC], 2014).

Diabetes is the primary cause of CKD. More than 35% of the U.S. population aged 20 years and older with diabetes have CKD (CDC, 2014). Diabetes is the leading cause of kidney disease in patients starting renal replacement therapy. The second leading cause is hypertension, followed by glomerulonephritis and pyelonephritis; polycystic, hereditary, or congenital disorders; and renal cancers (U.S. Renal Data System [USRDS], 2015). More than 20% of the U.S. population aged 20 years and older with hypertension have CKD (CDC, 2014).

Pathophysiology

In the early stages of CKD, there can be significant damage to the kidneys without signs or symptoms. The pathophysiology of CKD is not yet clearly understood, but the damage to the kidneys is thought to be caused by prolonged acute inflammation that is not organ specific and thus has subtle systemic manifestations.

Stages of Chronic Kidney Disease

CKD has been classified into five stages by the National Kidney Foundation (NKF) (see Chart 54-1). Stage 5 results when the kidneys cannot remove the body's metabolic wastes or perform their regulatory functions; thus, renal replacement therapies are required to sustain life. Screening and early

---

Chart 54-1

Stages of Chronic Kidney Disease

Stages are based on the GFR. The normal GFR is 125 mL/min/1.73 m².

Stage 1

GFR ≥90 mL/min/1.73 m²
Kidney damage with normal or increased GFR

Stage 2

GFR = 60–89 mL/min/1.73 m²
Mild decrease in GFR

Stage 3

GFR = 30–59 mL/min/1.73 m²
Moderate decrease in GFR

Stage 4

GFR = 15–29 mL/min/1.73 m²
Severe decrease in GFR

Stage 5

GFR <15 mL/min/1.73 m²
End-stage kidney disease or chronic kidney disease

GFR, glomerular filtration rate.
Adapted from Grossman, S. C., & Porth, C. M. (2014). *Pathophysiology: Concepts of altered health states* (9th ed.). Philadelphia, PA: Lippincott Williams & Wilkins.

---

intervention are important, because not all patients progress to stage 5 CKD. Patients with CKD are at increased risk for cardiovascular disease, which is the leading cause of morbidity and mortality (Kane-Gill, Sileanu, Murugan, et al., 2015). Treatment of hypertension, anemia, and hyperglycemia and detection of proteinuria all help to slow disease progression and improve patient outcomes (Lewis, 2013).

Clinical Manifestations

Elevated serum creatinine levels indicate underlying kidney disease; as the creatinine level increases, symptoms of CKD begin. Anemia, due to decreased erythropoietin production by the kidney, metabolic acidosis, and abnormalities in calcium and phosphorus herald the development of CKD (Taal, 2013). Fluid retention, evidenced by both edema and congestive heart failure, develops. As the disease progresses, abnormalities in electrolytes occur, heart failure worsens, and hypertension becomes more difficult to control.

Assessment and Diagnostic Findings

The **glomerular filtration rate (GFR)** is the amount of plasma filtered through the glomeruli per unit of time. Creatinine clearance is a measure of the amount of creatinine the kidneys are able to clear in a 24-hour period. Normal values differ in men and women. Calculation of GFR, an important assessment parameter in CKD, is discussed in Chapter 53.

Medical Management

The management of patients with CKD includes treatment of the underlying causes. Regular clinical and laboratory assessment is important to keep the blood pressure below 130/80 mmHg

(Klein-Kauric, 2015). Medical management also includes early referral for initiation of renal replacement therapies as indicated by the patient's renal status. Prevention of complications is accomplished by controlling cardiovascular risk factors; treating hyperglycemia; managing anemia; smoking cessation, weight loss, and exercise programs as needed; and reduction in salt and alcohol intake.

Gerontologic Considerations

Changes in kidney function with normal aging increase the susceptibility of older patients to kidney dysfunction and kidney disease (Kane-Gill et al., 2015). In addition, the incidence of systemic diseases, such as atherosclerosis, hypertension, heart failure, diabetes, and cancer, increases with advancing age, predisposing older adults to kidney disease associated with these disorders. Therefore, acute problems need to be prevented if possible or recognized and treated quickly to avoid kidney damage. Thus, nurses in all settings need to be alert to signs and symptoms of kidney dysfunction in older patients.

Older patients frequently take multiple prescription and over-the-counter medications. Because alterations in renal blood flow, glomerular filtration, and renal clearance increase the risk of medication-associated changes in renal function, precautions are indicated with all medications. When older patients undergo extensive diagnostic tests or when new medications (e.g., diuretic agents) are added, precautions must be taken to prevent dehydration, which can compromise marginal renal function and lead to kidney disease (Kane-Gill et al., 2015).

Nephrosclerosis

Nephrosclerosis (hardening of the renal arteries) is most often due to prolonged hypertension and diabetes. Nephrosclerosis is a major cause of CKD and ESKD secondary to many disorders.

Pathophysiology

There are two forms of nephrosclerosis: malignant (accelerated) and benign. Malignant nephrosclerosis is often associated with significant hypertension (diastolic blood pressure higher than 130 mmHg). It usually occurs in young adults and twice as often in men compared to women (Klein-Kauric, 2015). Damage is caused by decreased blood flow to the kidney resulting in patchy necrosis of the renal parenchyma. Over time, fibrosis occurs and glomeruli are destroyed.

The disease process progresses rapidly. Without dialysis, more than half of patients die of **uremia** (an excess of urea and other nitrogenous waste products in the blood) in a few years. Benign nephrosclerosis can be found in older adults, associated with atherosclerosis and hypertension.

Assessment and Diagnostic Findings

Symptoms are rare early in the disease, even though the urine usually contains protein and occasional casts. Renal insufficiency and associated signs and symptoms occur late in the disease.

Medical Management

Treatment of nephrosclerosis is aggressive antihypertensive therapy. An angiotensin-converting enzyme (ACE) inhibitor,

---

alone or in combination with other antihypertensive medications, significantly reduces its incidence. See Chapter 31 for additional information on hypertension.

Primary Glomerular Diseases

Diseases that destroy the glomerulus of the kidney are the third most common cause of stage 5 CKD. In these disorders, the glomerular capillaries are primarily involved. Antigen–antibody complexes form in the blood and become trapped in the glomerular capillaries (the filtering portion of the kidney), inducing an inflammatory response. Immunoglobulin G (IgG)—the major immunoglobulin (antibody) found in the blood—can be detected in the glomerular capillary walls. The major clinical manifestations of glomerular injury include proteinuria, hematuria, decreased GFR, decreased excretion of sodium, edema, and hypertension (see Chart 54-2).

Acute Nephritic Syndrome

Acute nephritic syndrome is a type of kidney disease with glomerular inflammation (Grossman & Porth, 2014). **Glomerulonephritis** is an inflammation of the glomerular capillaries that can occur in acute and chronic forms.

Pathophysiology

Primary glomerular diseases include postinfectious glomerulonephritis, rapidly progressive glomerulonephritis, membrane proliferative glomerulonephritis, and membranous glomerulonephritis. Postinfectious causes are group A beta-hemolytic streptococcal infection of the throat that precedes the onset of glomerulonephritis by 2 to 3 weeks (see Fig. 54-1). It may also follow impetigo (infection of the skin) and acute viral infections (upper respiratory tract infections, mumps, varicella zoster virus, Epstein–Barr virus, hepatitis B, and human immune deficiency virus [HIV] infection). In some patients, antigens outside the body (e.g., medications, foreign serum) initiate the process, resulting in antigen–antibody complexes being deposited in the glomeruli. In other patients, the kidney tissue itself serves as the inciting antigen.

Clinical Manifestations

The primary presenting features of an acute glomerular inflammation are hematuria, edema, **azotemia** (an abnormal

Physiology/Pathophysiology

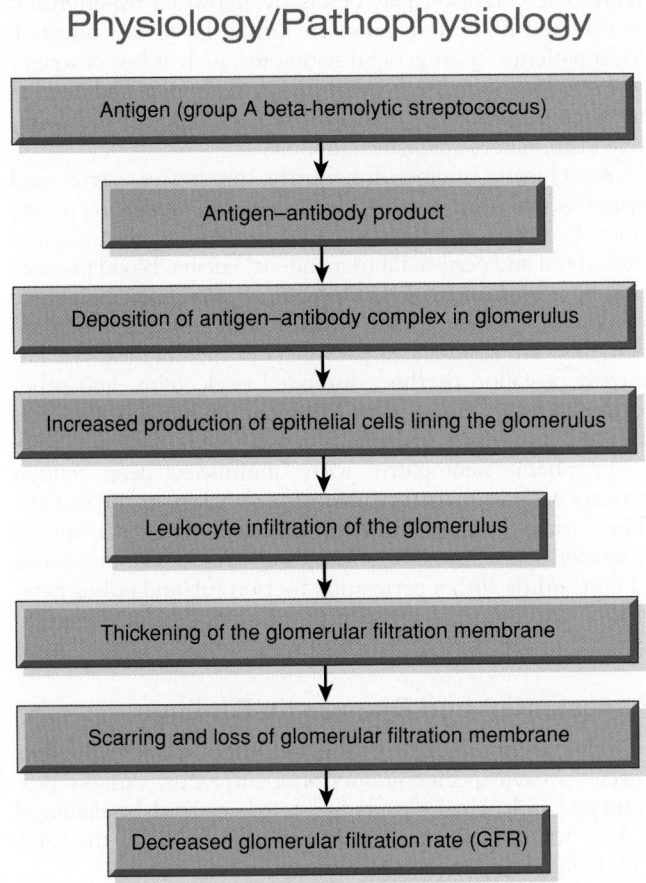

Figure 54-1 • Sequence of events in acute nephritic syndrome.

concentration of nitrogenous wastes in the blood), and **proteinuria** (excess protein in the urine) (Grossman & Porth, 2014). The hematuria may be microscopic (identifiable only through microscopic examination) or macroscopic (visible to the eye). The urine may appear cola colored because of red blood cells (RBCs) and protein plugs or casts; RBC casts indicate glomerular injury. Glomerulonephritis may be mild and the hematuria discovered incidentally through a routine urinalysis, or the disease may be severe, with AKI and oliguria.

Some degree of edema and hypertension is present in most patients. Marked proteinuria due to the increased permeability of the glomerular membrane may also occur, with associated pitting edema, hypoalbuminemia, hyperlipidemia, and fatty casts in the urine. Blood urea nitrogen (BUN) and serum creatinine levels may increase as urine output decreases. In addition, anemia may be present.

In the more severe form of the disease, patients also complain of headache, malaise, and flank pain. Older patients may experience circulatory overload with dyspnea, engorged neck veins, cardiomegaly, and pulmonary edema. Atypical symptoms include confusion, somnolence, and seizures, which are often confused with the symptoms of a primary neurologic disorder.

Assessment and Diagnostic Findings

In acute nephritic syndrome, the kidneys become large, edematous, and congested. All renal tissues, including the glomeruli, tubules, and blood vessels, are affected to varying degrees. Patients with an immunoglobulin A (IgA) nephropathy have an elevated serum IgA and low to normal complement levels. Electron microscopy and immunofluorescent analysis help identify the nature of the lesion; however, a kidney biopsy may be needed for definitive diagnosis. See Chapter 53 for discussion of kidney biopsy.

If the patient improves, the amount of urine increases and the urinary protein and sediment diminish. The percentage of adults who recover is unknown. Some patients develop severe **uremia** (an excess of urea and other nitrogenous wastes in the blood) within weeks and require dialysis for survival. Others, after a period of apparent recovery, insidiously develop chronic glomerulonephritis.

Complications

Complications of acute glomerulonephritis include hypertensive encephalopathy, heart failure, and pulmonary edema. Hypertensive encephalopathy is a medical emergency, and therapy is directed toward reducing the blood pressure without impairing renal function. This can occur in acute nephritic syndrome or preeclampsia with chronic hypertension of greater than 140/90 mmHg. Rapidly progressive glomerulonephritis is characterized by a rapid decline in renal function. Without treatment, ESKD develops in a matter of weeks or months. Signs and symptoms are similar to those of acute glomerulonephritis (hematuria and proteinuria), but the course of the disease is more severe and rapid. Crescent-shaped cells accumulate in Bowman space, disrupting the filtering surface. Plasma exchange (plasmapheresis) and treatment with high-dose corticosteroids and cytotoxic agents have been used to reduce the inflammatory response. Dialysis is initiated in acute glomerulonephritis if signs and symptoms of uremia are severe. The prognosis for patients with acute nephritic syndrome is excellent and rarely causes CKD (Grossman & Porth 2014).

Medical Management

Management consists primarily of treating symptoms, attempting to preserve kidney function, and treating complications promptly. Treatment may include prescribing corticosteroids, managing hypertension, and controlling proteinuria. Pharmacologic therapy depends on the cause of acute glomerulonephritis. If residual streptococcal infection is suspected, penicillin is the agent of choice; however, other antibiotic agents may be prescribed. Dietary protein is restricted when renal insufficiency and nitrogen retention (elevated BUN) develop. Sodium is restricted when the patient has hypertension, edema, and heart failure.

Nursing Management

Although most patients with acute uncomplicated glomerulonephritis are cared for as outpatients, nursing care is important in every setting.

Providing Care in the Hospital

In a hospital setting, carbohydrates are given liberally to provide energy and reduce the catabolism of protein. I&O is carefully measured and recorded. Fluids are given based on the patient's fluid losses and daily body weight. Insensible fluid loss through the lungs (300 mL) and skin (500 mL) is considered when estimating fluid loss (see Chapter 13; Table 13-2). If treatment is effective, diuresis will begin, resulting in decreased edema and blood pressure. Proteinuria and microscopic hematuria may persist for many months; in fact, 20% of patients have some degree of persistent protein-uria or decreased GFR 1 year after presentation (Grossman & Porth, 2014). Other nursing interventions focus on patient education about the disease process, explanations of labora-tory and other diagnostic tests, and preparation for safe and effective self-care at home.

Promoting Home, Community-Based, and Transitional Care

 Educating Patients About Self-Care

Patient education is directed toward managing symptoms and monitoring for complications. Fluid and diet restrictions must be reviewed with the patient to avoid worsening of edema and hypertension. The patient is instructed verbally and in writing to notify the primary provider if symptoms of kidney disease occur (e.g., fatigue, nausea, vomiting, diminishing urine output) or at the first sign of any infection.

Continuing and Transitional Care

The importance of follow-up evaluations of blood pressure, urinalysis for protein, and BUN and serum creatinine levels to determine if the disease has progressed is stressed to the patient. A referral for transitional, home, or community-based care may be indicated. A home visit from a nurse pro-vides an opportunity for careful assessment of the patient's progress and detection of early signs and symptoms of renal insufficiency. If corticosteroids, immunosuppressant agents, or antibiotic medications are prescribed, the nurse uses the opportunity to review the dosage, desired actions, and adverse effects of medications and the precautions to be taken.

Chronic Glomerulonephritis

Chronic glomerulonephritis may be due to repeated episodes of acute nephritic syndrome, hypertensive nephrosclerosis, hyperlipidemia, chronic tubulointerstitial injury, or hemody-namically mediated glomerular sclerosis. Secondary glomeru-lar diseases that can have systemic effects include systemic lupus erythematosus, Goodpasture syndrome (caused by antibodies to the glomerular basement membrane), diabetic glomerulosclerosis, and amyloidosis.

Pathophysiology

The kidneys are reduced to as little as one fifth their nor-mal size (consisting largely of fibrous tissue). The cortex layer shrinks to 1 to 2 mm in thickness or less. Bands of scar tissue distort the remaining cortex, making the surface of the kidney rough and irregular. Numerous glomeruli and their tubules become scarred, and the branches of the renal artery are thickened. The resulting severe glomerular damage can prog-ress to stage 5 CKD and require a renal replacement therapy.

Clinical Manifestations

The symptoms of chronic glomerulonephritis vary. Some patients with severe disease have no symptoms at all for many years. The condition may be discovered when hypertension or elevated BUN and serum creatinine levels are detected. Most patients report general symptoms, such as loss of weight and strength, increasing irritability, and an increased need to urinate at night (nocturia). Headaches, dizziness, and diges-tive disturbances are also common.

As chronic glomerulonephritis progresses, signs and symptoms of CKD may develop. The patient appears poorly nourished, with a yellow-gray pigmentation of the skin and periorbital and peripheral (dependent) edema. Blood pressure may be normal or severely elevated. Retinal findings include hemorrhage, exudate, narrowed tortuous arterioles, and pap-illedema. Anemia causes pale mucous membranes. Cardio-megaly, a gallop rhythm, distended neck veins, and other signs and symptoms of heart failure may be present. Crackles can be heard in the bases of the lungs.

Peripheral neuropathy with diminished deep tendon reflexes and neurosensory changes occur late in the disease. The patient becomes confused and demonstrates a limited attention span. An additional late finding includes evidence of pericarditis with a pericardial friction rub and pulsus para-doxus (difference in blood pressure during inspiration and expiration of greater than 10 mmHg).

Assessment and Diagnostic Findings

A number of laboratory abnormalities occur. Urinalysis reveals a fixed specific gravity of about 1.010, variable pro-teinuria, and **urinary casts** (proteins secreted by damaged kidney tubules). As kidney disease progresses and the GFR falls below 50 mL/min, the following changes occur:

- Hyperkalemia due to decreased potassium excretion, acidosis, catabolism, and excessive potassium intake from food and medications
- Metabolic acidosis from decreased acid secretion by the kidney and inability to regenerate bicarbonate
- Anemia secondary to decreased erythropoiesis (produc-tion of RBCs)
- Hypoalbuminemia with edema secondary to protein loss through the damaged glomerular membrane
- Increased serum phosphorus level due to decreased renal excretion of phosphorus
- Decreased serum calcium level (calcium binds to phos-phorus to compensate for elevated serum phosphorus levels)
- Mental status changes
- Impaired nerve conduction due to electrolyte abnor-malities and uremia

Chest x-rays may show cardiac enlargement and pulmo-nary edema. The electrocardiogram (ECG) may be normal or may indicate left ventricular hypertrophy associated with hypertension and signs of electrolyte disturbances, such as tall, tented (or peaked) T waves associated with hyperkale-mia. Computed tomography (CT) and magnetic resonance imaging (MRI) scans show a decrease in the size of the renal cortex.

Medical Management

Management of symptoms guides the treatment. If the patient has hypertension, efforts are made to reduce the blood pres-sure with sodium and water restriction, antihypertensive agents, or both. Weight is monitored daily, and diuretic medications are prescribed to treat fluid overload. Proteins of high biologic value (dairy products, eggs, meats) are provided to promote good nutritional status. Adequate calories are provided to spare protein for tissue growth and repair. Urinary tract infections (UTIs) must be treated promptly to prevent further kidney damage.

Dialysis is initiated early in the course of the disease to keep the patient in optimal physical condition, prevent fluid and electrolyte imbalances, and minimize the risk of complications of kidney disease. The course of dialysis is smoother if treatment begins before the patient develops complications.

Nursing Management

Whether the patient is hospitalized or cared for in the home, the nurse observes the patient for common fluid and electrolyte disturbances in kidney disease (see Table 54-1). Changes in fluid and electrolyte status and in cardiac and neurologic status are reported promptly to the primary provider. Throughout the course of the disease and treatment, the nurse gives emotional support by providing opportunities for the patient and family to verbalize their concerns, have their questions answered, and explore their options (Ahmad & Al Nazly, 2015).

Promoting Home, Community-Based, and Transitional Care

 Educating Patients About Self-Care

The nurse has a major role in educating the patient and family about the prescribed treatment plan and the risks associated with noncompliance. Instructions to the patient include explanations and scheduling for follow-up evaluations: blood pressure, urinalysis for protein and casts, and laboratory studies of BUN and serum creatinine levels. If long-term dialysis is needed, the nurse educates the patient and family about the procedure, how to care for the access site, dietary restrictions, and other necessary lifestyle modifications. These topics are discussed later in this chapter.

Periodic hospitalization, visits to the outpatient clinic or office, and home care referrals provide the nurse in each setting with the opportunity for careful assessment of the patient's progress and continued education about changes to report to the primary provider (worsening signs and symptoms of kidney disease, such as nausea, vomiting, and diminished urine output). Specific education may include explanations about recommended diet and fluid modifications and medications (purpose, desired effects, adverse effects, dosage, and administration schedule).

Continuing and Transitional Care

Periodic laboratory evaluations of creatinine clearance and BUN and serum creatinine levels are carried out to assess residual renal function and the need for dialysis or transplantation. If dialysis is initiated, the patient and family require considerable assistance and support in dealing with therapy and its long-term implications. The patient and family are reminded of the importance of participation in health promotion activities, including health screening. The patient is instructed to inform all health care providers about the diagnosis of glomerulonephritis so that all medical management,

including pharmacologic therapy, is based on altered renal function.

Nephrotic Syndrome

Nephrotic syndrome is a type of kidney disease characterized by increased glomerular permeability and is manifested by massive proteinuria (Grossman & Porth, 2014). Clinical findings include a marked increase in protein (particularly albumin) in the urine (proteinuria), a decrease in albumin in the blood (hypoalbuminemia), diffuse edema, high serum cholesterol, and low-density lipoproteins (hyperlipidemia).

The syndrome is apparent in any condition that seriously damages the glomerular capillary membrane and results in increased glomerular permeability to plasma proteins. Although the liver is capable of increasing the production of albumin, it cannot keep up with the daily loss of albumin through the kidneys. Thus, hypoalbuminemia results (see Fig. 54-2).

Pathophysiology

Nephrotic syndrome occurs with many intrinsic kidney diseases and systemic diseases that cause glomerular damage. It is not a specific glomerular disease but a constellation of clinical findings that result from the glomerular damage.

Clinical Manifestations

The major manifestation of nephrotic syndrome is edema. It is usually soft and pitting and commonly occurs around

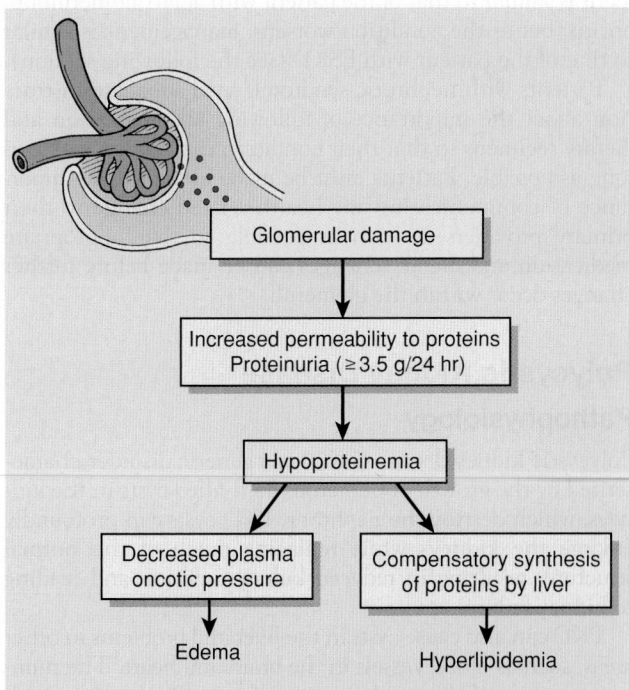

Physiology/Pathophysiology

Glomerular damage

↓

Increased permeability to proteins
Proteinuria (≥3.5 g/24 hr)

↓

Hypoproteinemia

Decreased plasma oncotic pressure → Edema

Compensatory synthesis of proteins by liver → Hyperlipidemia

Figure 54-2 • Sequence of events in nephrotic syndrome. Reprinted with permission from Grossman, S. C., & Porth, C. M. (2014). *Pathophysiology: Concepts of altered health states* (9th ed.). Philadelphia, PA: Lippincott Williams & Wilkins.

the eyes (periorbital), in dependent areas (sacrum, ankles, and hands), and in the abdomen (ascites). Patients may also exhibit irritability, headache, and malaise.

Assessment and Diagnostic Findings

Proteinuria (predominately albumin) exceeding 3.5 g/day is the hallmark of the diagnosis of nephrotic syndrome. Protein electrophoresis and immunoelectrophoresis may be performed on the urine to categorize the type of proteinuria. The urine may also contain increased white blood cells (WBCs) as well as granular and epithelial casts. A needle biopsy of the kidney may be performed for histologic examination of renal tissue to confirm the diagnosis.

Complications

Complications of nephrotic syndrome include infection (due to a deficient immune response), thromboembolism (especially of the renal vein), pulmonary embolism, AKI (due to hypovolemia), and accelerated atherosclerosis (due to hyperlipidemia).

Medical Management

Treatment is focused on addressing the underlying disease state causing proteinuria, slowing progression of CKD, and relieving symptoms. Typical treatment includes diuretic agents for edema, ACE inhibitors to reduce proteinuria, and lipid-lowering agents for hyperlipidemia.

Nursing Management

In the early stages of nephrotic syndrome, nursing management is similar to that of the patient with acute glomerulonephritis, but as the condition worsens, management is similar to that of the patient with ESKD (see the following section).

Patients with nephrotic syndrome need adequate instruction about the importance of following all medication and dietary regimens so that their condition can remain stable as long as possible. Patients must be made aware of the importance of communicating any health-related change to their primary providers as soon as possible so that appropriate medication and dietary changes can be made before further changes occur within the glomeruli.

Polycystic Kidney Disease

Pathophysiology

Polycystic kidney disease (PKD) is a genetic disorder characterized by the growth of numerous fluid-filled cysts in the kidneys, which destroy the nephrons. PKD cysts can profoundly enlarge the kidneys while replacing much of the normal structure, resulting in reduced kidney function and leading to kidney failure.

PKD can also cause cysts in the liver and problems in other areas, such as blood vessels in the brain and heart. The number of cysts and the resulting complications help distinguish PKD from the usually harmless cysts that can form in the kidneys in later years of life. In the United States, PKD and cystic diseases are a leading cause of kidney failure. Two major inherited forms of PKD exist:

- Autosomal dominant PKD is the most common inherited form. Symptoms usually develop between 30 and 40 years of age, but they can begin earlier, even in childhood. About 90% of all PKD cases are autosomal dominant PKD.
- Autosomal recessive PKD is a rare inherited form. Symptoms of autosomal recessive PKD begin in the earliest months of life or in utero.

When autosomal dominant PKD causes kidneys to fail, which usually happens after many years, the patient requires dialysis or kidney transplantation. Approximately one half of individuals with autosomal dominant PKD progress to stage 5 CKD, requiring renal replacement therapy.

Clinical Manifestations

Signs and symptoms of PKD result from loss of renal function and the increasing size of the kidneys as the cysts grow. Kidney damage can result in hematuria, **polyuria** (excessive urine production), hypertension, development of renal calculi and associated UTIs, and proteinuria. The growing cysts are noted with reports of abdominal fullness and flank pain (back and lower sides).

Assessment and Diagnostic Findings

PKD is a genetic disease; therefore, careful evaluation of family history is necessary. Palpation of the abdomen will often reveal enlarged cystic kidneys. Ultrasound imaging of the kidneys is the preferred technique for diagnosis (Grossman & Porth, 2014).

Medical Management

PKD has no cure, and treatment is largely supportive and includes blood pressure control, pain control, and antibiotic agents to resolve infections. Once the kidneys fail, renal replacement therapy is indicated (see later discussion in chapter). Genetic linkage studies and counseling may be indicated, particularly when screening family members for potential kidney donation (Grossman & Porth, 2014).

RENAL CANCER

Renal cancer accounts for about 5% of all cancers in the United States (American Cancer Society [ACS], 2015), where the incidence of renal cancer at all stages has increased in the past two decades. The incidence of renal cell carcinoma is higher in both men and women with an increased body mass index. Tobacco use continues to be a significant risk factor (see Chart 54-3). American Indians and Alaskans have a higher mortality rate from renal carcinoma compared to other races and population groups.

The most common type of renal carcinoma arises from the renal epithelium and accounts for more than 85% of all kidney tumors (ACS, 2015). These tumors may metastasize early to the lungs, bone, liver, brain, and contralateral kidney. One quarter of patients have metastatic disease at the time of diagnosis. Although enhanced imaging techniques account for improved detection of early-stage kidney cancer, it is unknown why the rate of late-stage kidney cancers is high.

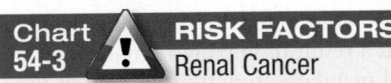

Clinical Manifestations

Many renal tumors produce no symptoms and are discovered on a routine physical examination as a palpable abdominal mass. Signs and symptoms, which occur in only 10% of patients, include hematuria, pain, and a mass in the flank. The usual sign that first calls attention to the tumor is painless hematuria, which may be either intermittent and microscopic or continuous and gross. There may be a dull pain in the back from the pressure produced by compression of the ureter, extension of the tumor into the perirenal area, or hemorrhage into the kidney tissue. Colicky pains occur if a clot or mass of tumor cells passes down the ureter. Symptoms from metastasis may be the first manifestations of renal tumor and may include unexplained weight loss, increasing weakness, and anemia.

Assessment and Diagnostic Findings

The diagnosis of a renal tumor may require intravenous (IV) urography, cystoscopic examination, renal angiograms, ultrasonography, or a CT scan (see Chapter 53). These tests may be exhausting for patients already debilitated by the systemic effects of a tumor as well as for older patients and those who are anxious about the diagnosis and outcome. The nurse assists the patient to prepare physically and psychologically for these procedures and monitors carefully for signs and symptoms of dehydration and exhaustion.

Medical Management

The goal of medical management is to detect the tumor early and to eradicate slow-growing tumors before metastasis occurs. Treatment most often includes a combination of surgery and pharmacologic management. Radiation therapy may be used for palliation in patients who are not candidates for surgery or other treatments.

Surgical Management

Nephrectomy

A radical nephrectomy is the preferred treatment if the tumor can be removed. This includes removal of the kidney (and tumor), adrenal gland, surrounding perinephric fat and Gerota fascia, and lymph nodes. Laparoscopic nephrectomy can be performed for removal of the kidney with a small tumor. This procedure incurs less morbidity and a shorter recovery time. Radiation therapy, hormonal therapy, or chemotherapy may

be used along with surgery. Immunotherapy may also be helpful. For patients with bilateral tumors or cancer of a functional single kidney, nephron-sparing surgery (partial nephrectomy) may be considered. Favorable results have been achieved in patients with small local tumors and a normal contralateral kidney.

Nephron-sparing surgery is increasingly being used to treat patients with solid renal lesions. The technical success rate of nephron-sparing surgery is excellent, and operative morbidity and mortality are low.

Patients with upper tract transitional cell carcinoma may benefit from laparoscopic nephroureterectomy. Although it is a lengthier surgical procedure, it has the same efficacy and is better tolerated by patients than open nephroureterectomy.

Renal Artery Embolization

In patients with metastatic renal carcinoma, the renal artery may be occluded to impede the blood supply to the tumor and thus kill the tumor cells. After angiographic studies are completed, a catheter is advanced into the renal artery, and embolizing materials (e.g., Gelfoam, autologous blood clot, steel coils) are injected into the artery and carried with the arterial blood flow to occlude the tumor vessels mechanically. This decreases the local blood supply, making removal of the kidney (nephrectomy) easier. It also stimulates an immune response because infarction of the renal cell carcinoma releases tumor-associated antigens that enhance the patient's response to metastatic lesions. The procedure may also reduce the number of tumor cells entering the venous circulation during surgical manipulation.

After renal artery embolization and tumor infarction, a characteristic symptom complex called postinfarction syndrome occurs, lasting 2 to 3 days. The patient has pain localized to the flank and abdomen, elevated temperature, and gastrointestinal (GI) symptoms. Pain is treated with parenteral analgesic agents, and acetaminophen (Tylenol) is given to control fever. Antiemetic medications, restriction of oral intake, and IV fluids are used to treat the GI symptoms.

Pharmacologic Therapy

Depending on the stage of the tumor, percutaneous partial or radical nephrectomy may be followed by treatment with chemotherapeutic agents. Treatment with biologic response modifiers such as interleukin 2 (IL-2) is effective. IL-2, a protein that regulates cell growth, is used alone or in combination with lymphokine-activated killer cells (WBCs that have been stimulated by IL-2 to increase their ability to kill cancer cells). Interferon, another biologic response modifier, appears to have a direct antiproliferative effect on renal tumors.

Another promising experimental approach to renal cell carcinoma is a vaccination to stimulate immune response, with autologous tumor cells with IL-2–, granulocyte-macrophage stimulating factor–, and dendritic cell–type vaccines. If patients with renal cancer do not respond to immunotherapy, allogeneic stem cell transplantation may be indicated (see Chapter 15).

Nursing Management

The patient with a renal tumor usually undergoes extensive diagnostic and therapeutic procedures. Treatment includes surgery, radiation therapy, and medications. After surgery, the patient usually has catheters and drains in place to maintain a patent urinary tract, to remove drainage, and to permit accurate measurement of urine output. Because of the location of the surgical incision, the patient's position during surgery, and the nature of the surgical procedure, pain and muscle soreness are common. Pharmacologic management often includes immunosuppressant agents; therefore, patients are monitored for infection.

The patient requires frequent analgesia during the postoperative period and assistance with turning, coughing, the use of incentive spirometry, and deep breathing to prevent atelectasis and other pulmonary complications. The patient and family require assistance and support to cope with the diagnosis and uncertain prognosis. See discussion later in this chapter of postoperative care of the patient undergoing kidney surgery and Chapter 15 for discussion of care of the patient with cancer.

Promoting Home, Community-Based, and Transitional Care

 Educating Patients About Self-Care

The nurse educates the patient about how to inspect and care for the incision and to perform other general postoperative care including activity and lifting restrictions, driving, and pain management. Instructions are provided about when to notify the primary provider about problems (e.g., fever, respiratory difficulty, wound drainage, blood in the urine, pain or swelling of the legs).

The nurse encourages the patient to eat a healthy diet and to drink adequate liquids to avoid constipation and to maintain an adequate urine volume. Education and emotional support are provided related to the diagnosis, treatment, and continuing care because many patients are concerned about the loss of the other kidney, the possible need for dialysis, or the recurrence of cancer.

Continuing and Transitional Care

Follow-up care is essential to detect signs of metastases and to reassure the patient and family about the patient's status and well-being. The patient who has had surgery for renal carcinoma should have a yearly physical examination and chest x-ray, because late metastases are not uncommon. All subsequent symptoms should be evaluated with possible metastases in mind.

If follow-up chemotherapy is necessary, the patient and family are informed about the treatment plan or chemotherapy protocol, what to expect with each visit, and when to notify the primary provider. Evaluation of remaining renal function (creatinine clearance, BUN, and serum creatinine levels) may also be carried out periodically. A home care nurse may monitor the patient's physical status and psychological well-being and coordinate other indicated services and resources.

KIDNEY DISEASE

Kidney disease results when the kidneys cannot remove the body's metabolic wastes or perform their regulatory functions.

The substances normally eliminated in the urine accumulate in the body fluids as a result of impaired renal excretion, affecting endocrine and metabolic functions as well as fluid, electrolyte, and acid–base disturbances. Kidney disease is a systemic disease and a final common pathway of many different kidney and urinary tract diseases. Each year, the number of deaths from irreversible kidney disease increases (USRDS, 2015).

Acute Kidney Injury

Acute kidney injury (AKI) is a rapid loss of renal function due to damage to the kidneys. Depending on the duration and severity of AKI, a wide range of potentially life-threatening metabolic complications can occur, including metabolic acidosis as well as fluid and electrolyte imbalances (Vritis, 2013). Treatment is aimed at replacing renal function temporarily to minimize potentially lethal complications and reduce potential causes of increased kidney injury with the goal of minimizing long-term loss of renal function. AKI is a problem seen in patients who are hospitalized and those in outpatient settings. A widely accepted criterion for AKI is a 50% or greater increase in serum creatinine above baseline (normal creatinine is less than 1 mg/dL) (Vritis, 2013). Urine volume may be normal, or changes may occur. Possible changes include nonoliguria (greater than 800 mL/day), **oliguria** (less than 0.5 mL/kg/hr), or **anuria** (less than 50 mL/day) (Vritis, 2013).

Pathophysiology

Although the pathogenesis of AKI and oliguria is not always known, many times there is a specific underlying cause. Some of the factors may be reversible if identified and treated promptly, before kidney function is impaired. This is true of the following conditions that reduce blood flow to the kidney and impair kidney function: (1) hypovolemia; (2) hypotension; (3) reduced cardiac output and heart failure; (4) obstruction of the kidney or lower urinary tract by tumor, blood clot, or kidney stone; and (5) bilateral obstruction of the renal arteries or veins. If these conditions are treated and corrected before the kidneys are permanently damaged, the increased BUN and creatinine levels, oliguria, and other signs may be reversed.

Although renal stones are not a common cause of AKI, some types may increase the risk of AKI. Some hereditary stone diseases (see Chapter 55), primary struvite stones, and infection-related urolithiasis associated with anatomic and functional urinary tract anomalies and spinal cord injury may cause recurrent bouts of obstruction as well as crystal-specific damage to tubular epithelial cells and interstitial renal cells.

Classifications of Acute Kidney Injury

The term acute kidney injury has replaced the term acute renal failure because it better describes this syndrome in patients, not only simply those who require renal replacement therapies but also those patients who experience minor changes in renal function. Classification criteria for AKI include assessment of three grades of severity and two outcome-level classifications. This 5-point system is known as the RIFLE classification system (Davies & Leslie, 2012). RIFLE stands for risk, injury, failure, loss, and ESKD (Vrtis, 2013). Risk, injury, and failure are

TABLE 54-2 The RIFLE Classification for Acute Kidney Injury

Class	GFR Criteria	Urinary Output Criteria
R (Risk)	Increased serum creatinine 1.5 × baseline OR GFR decreased ≥25%	0.5 mL/kg/hr for 6 hours
I (Injury)	Increased serum creatinine 2 × baseline OR GFR decreased ≥50%	0.5 mL/kg/hr for 12 hours
F (Failure)	Increased serum creatinine 3 × baseline OR GFR decreased ≥75% OR Serum creatinine ≥354 mmol/L with an acute rise of at least 44 mmol/L	<0.3 mL/kg/hr for 24 hours OR Anuria for 12 hours
L (Loss)	Persistent acute kidney injury = complete loss of kidney function >4 weeks	
E (ESKD)	ESKD >3 months	

GFR, glomerular filtration rate; ESKD, end-stage kidney disease.
Adapted from Davies, H., & Leslie, G. (2012). Acute kidney injury and the critically ill patient. *Dimensions of Critical Care Nursing, 31*(3), 135–152.

considered grades of AKI severity, whereas loss and ESKD are considered outcomes of loss that require some form of renal replacement therapy, at least temporarily (Dring & Hipkiss, 2015). Table 54-2 lists the classification criteria for the RIFLE system for AKI (Vritis, 2013). This classification system is used by health care professionals to identify kidney injury and improve patient outcomes.

Categories of Acute Kidney Injury

The major categories of AKI are prerenal (hypoperfusion of kidney), intrarenal (actual damage to kidney tissue), and postrenal (obstruction to urine flow). Prerenal AKI, which occurs in 60% to 70% of cases, is the result of impaired blood flow that leads to hypoperfusion of the kidney commonly caused by volume depletion (burns, hemorrhage, GI losses), hypotension (sepsis, shock), and renal artery stenosis, ultimately leading to a decrease in the GFR (Vritis, 2013). Intrarenal AKI is the result of actual parenchymal damage to the glomeruli or kidney tubules. **Acute tubular necrosis (ATN)**, or AKI in which there is damage to the kidney tubules, is the most common type of intrinsic AKI. Characteristics of ATN are intratubular obstruction, tubular back leak (abnormal reabsorption of filtrate and decreased urine flow through the tubule), vasoconstriction, and changes in glomerular permeability. These processes result in a decrease of GFR, progressive azotemia, and fluid and electrolyte imbalances. CKD, diabetes, heart failure, hypertension, and cirrhosis can lead to ATN. Postrenal AKI usually results from obstruction distal to the kidney by conditions such as renal calculi, strictures, blood clots, benign prostatic hypertrophy, malignancies, and pregnancy. Pressure rises in the kidney tubules, and eventually the GFR decreases. Common causes of each type of AKI are further summarized in Chart 54-4.

Chart 54-4 Causes of Acute Kidney Injury

Prerenal Failure

- Volume depletion resulting from:
  - Gastrointestinal losses (vomiting, diarrhea, nasogastric suction)
  - Hemorrhage
  - Renal losses (diuretic agents, osmotic diuresis)
- Impaired cardiac efficiency resulting from:
  - Cardiogenic shock
  - Dysrhythmias
  - Heart failure
  - Myocardial infarction
- Vasodilation resulting from:
  - Anaphylaxis
  - Antihypertensive medications or other medications that cause vasodilation
  - Sepsis

Intrarenal Failure

- Prolonged renal ischemia resulting from:
  - Hemoglobinuria (transfusion reaction, hemolytic anemia)
  - Rhabdomyolysis/myoglobinuria (trauma, crush injuries, burns)
  - Pigment nephropathy (associated with the breakdown of blood cells containing pigments that in turn occlude kidney structures)
- Nephrotoxic agents such as:
  - Aminoglycoside antibiotics (gentamicin, tobramycin)
  - Angiotensin-converting enzyme inhibitors
  - Heavy metals (lead, mercury)
  - Nonsteroidal anti-inflammatory drugs
  - Radiopaque contrast agents
  - Solvents and chemicals (ethylene glycol, carbon tetrachloride, arsenic)
- Infectious processes such as:
  - Acute glomerulonephritis
  - Acute pyelonephritis

Postrenal Failure

- Urinary tract obstruction, including:
  - Benign prostatic hyperplasia
  - Blood clots
  - Calculi (stones)
  - Strictures
  - Tumors

Phases of Acute Kidney Injury

There are four phases of AKI: initiation, oliguria, diuresis, and recovery.

- The initiation period begins with the initial insult and ends when oliguria develops.
- The oliguria period is accompanied by an increase in the serum concentration of substances usually excreted by the kidneys (urea, creatinine, uric acid, organic acids, and the intracellular cations [potassium and magnesium]). The minimum amount of urine needed to rid the body of normal metabolic waste products is 400 mL in 24 hours or 0.5 mL/kg/hr. In this phase, uremic symptoms first appear and life-threatening conditions such as hyperkalemia develop.
- The diuresis period is marked by a gradual increase in urine output, which signals that glomerular filtration has started to recover. Laboratory values stabilize and

eventually decrease. Although the volume of urinary output may reach normal or elevated levels, renal function may still be markedly abnormal. Because uremic symptoms may still be present, the need for expert medical and nursing management continues. The patient must be observed closely for dehydration during this phase; if dehydration occurs, the uremic symptoms are likely to increase.

- The recovery period signals the improvement of renal function and may take 3 to 12 months. Laboratory values return to the patient's normal level. Although a permanent 1% to 3% reduction in the GFR may occur, it is not clinically significant.

Some patients have decreased renal function with increasing nitrogen retention but actually excrete normal amounts of urine (1 to 2 L/day). This is the nonoliguric form of kidney injury and occurs predominantly after exposure of the patient to **nephrotoxic** agents (any substance, medication, or action that destroys kidney tissue), burns, traumatic injury, and the use of halogenated anesthetic agents.

Clinical Manifestations

Almost every system of the body is affected with failure of the normal renal regulatory mechanisms. The patient may appear critically ill and lethargic. The skin and mucous membranes are dry from dehydration. Central nervous system signs and symptoms include drowsiness, headache, muscle twitching, and seizures. Table 54-3 summarizes common clinical characteristics in all three categories of AKI.

Assessment and Diagnostic Findings

Assessment of the patient with AKI includes evaluation for changes in the urine, diagnostic tests that evaluate the kidney contour, and a variety of laboratory values. See Chapter 53 for information about the normal characteristics of urine, diagnostic findings, and laboratory values in the renal system.

In AKI, urine output varies from scanty to a normal volume, hematuria may be present, and the urine has a low specific gravity (compared with a normal value of 1.010 to 1.025). One of the earliest manifestations of tubular damage is the inability to concentrate the urine (Vritis, 2013). Patients with prerenal azotemia have a decreased amount of sodium in the urine (less than 20 mEq/L) and normal urinary sediment. Patients with intrarenal azotemia usually have urinary sodium levels greater than 40 mEq/L with **urinary casts** and other cellular debris.

Ultrasonography is a critical component of the evaluation of patients with kidney disease. A renal sonogram or a CT or MRI scan may show evidence of anatomic changes.

The BUN level increases steadily at a rate that depends on the degree of catabolism (breakdown of protein), renal perfusion, and protein intake. Serum creatinine levels are useful in monitoring kidney function and disease progression and increase with glomerular damage.

With a decline in the GFR, oliguria, and anuria, patients are at high risk for hyperkalemia. Protein catabolism results in the release of cellular potassium into the body fluids, causing severe hyperkalemia (high serum potassium levels). Hyperkalemia may lead to dysrhythmias, such as ventricular tachycardia and cardiac arrest. Sources of potassium include normal tissue catabolism, dietary intake, blood in the GI tract, or blood transfusion and other sources (e.g., IV infusions, potassium penicillin, and extracellular shift in response to metabolic acidosis).

Progressive metabolic acidosis occurs in kidney disease because patients cannot eliminate the daily metabolic load of acid-type substances produced by the normal metabolic processes. In addition, normal renal buffering mechanisms fail. This is reflected by decreased serum carbon dioxide (CO_2) and pH levels.

Blood phosphate concentrations may increase; calcium levels may be low due to decreased absorption of calcium from the intestine and as a compensatory mechanism for the elevated blood phosphate levels. Anemia is another common laboratory finding in AKI, as a result of reduced erythropoietin production, uremic GI lesions, reduced RBC lifespan, and blood loss from the GI tract.

TABLE 54-3 Comparing Clinical Characteristics of Acute Kidney Injury

Characteristics	Categories		
	Prerenal	Intrarenal	Postrenal
Etiology	Hypoperfusion	Parenchymal damage	Obstruction
Blood urea nitrogen value	↑ (out of normal 20:1 proportion to creatinine)	↑	↑
Creatinine	↑	↑	↑
Urine output	↓	Varies, often ↓	Varies, may be ↓, or sudden anuria
Urine sodium	↓ to <20 mEq/L	↑ to >40 mEq/L	Varies, often ↓ to ≤20 mEq/L
Urinary sediment	Normal, few hyaline casts	Abnormal casts and debris	Usually normal
Urine osmolality	↑ to 500 mOsm	~350 mOsm, similar to serum	Varies, ↑ or equal to serum
Urine specific gravity	↑	Low normal	Varies

↑, increased; ↓, decreased.

<table>
<tr><td>Chart 54-5</td><td>Preventing Acute Kidney Injury</td></tr>
</table>

- Continually assess renal function (urine output, laboratory values) when appropriate.
- Monitor central venous and arterial pressures and hourly urine output of critically ill patients to detect the onset of kidney disease as early as possible.
- Pay special attention to wounds, burns, and other precursors of sepsis.
- Prevent and treat infections promptly. Infections can produce progressive kidney damage.
- Prevent and treat shock promptly with blood and fluid replacement.
- Provide adequate hydration to patients at risk for dehydration, including:
  - Before, during, and after surgery
  - Patients undergoing intensive diagnostic studies requiring fluid restriction and contrast agents (e.g., barium enema, IV pyelograms), especially older patients who may have marginal renal reserve
  - Patients with neoplastic disorders or disorders of metabolism (e.g., gout) and those receiving chemotherapy
  - Patients with skeletal muscle injuries (e.g., crush injuries, compartment syndrome)
  - Patients with heat-induced illnesses (e.g., heat stroke, heat exhaustion)
- Take precautions to ensure that the appropriate blood is given to the correct patient in order to avoid severe transfusion reactions, which can precipitate kidney disease.
- To prevent infections from ascending in the urinary tract, give meticulous care to patients with indwelling catheters. Remove catheters as soon as possible.
- To prevent toxic drug effects, closely monitor dosage, duration of use, and blood levels of all medications metabolized or excreted by the kidneys.
- Treat hypotension promptly.

Prevention

AKI has a high mortality rate that ranges from 40% to 90%. Factors that influence mortality include increased age, comorbid conditions, and pre-existing kidney and vascular diseases and respiratory failure (Vritis, 2013). Therefore, prevention of AKI is essential (see Chart 54-5).

A careful history is obtained to identify exposure to nephrotoxic agents or environmental toxins. The kidneys are susceptible to the adverse effects of medications because the metabolic by-products of most medications are excreted by the kidneys. Patients taking nephrotoxic medications (e.g., aminoglycosides, gentamicin [Garamycin], tobramycin, colistimethate [Coly-Mycin], polymyxin B, amphotericin B, vancomycin, amikacin [Amikin], cyclosporine [Neoral]) should be monitored closely for changes in renal function. Kidney function needs to be monitored prior to initiation of these medications and during therapy (Prentice, 2013).

Any agent that reduces renal blood flow (e.g., long-term analgesic use) may cause renal insufficiency. Chronic use of analgesic agents, particularly nonsteroidal anti-inflammatory drugs (NSAIDs), may cause **interstitial nephritis** (inflammation within the renal tissue) and papillary necrosis. Patients with heart failure or cirrhosis with ascites are at particular risk for NSAID-induced kidney disease. Increased age, pre-existing kidney disease, and the simultaneous administration of several nephrotoxic agents increase the risk of kidney damage.

Radiocontrast-induced nephropathy (CIN) is a major cause of hospital-acquired AKI. Patients undergo more than 1 million radiocontrast studies in the United States annually; of these, approximately 150,000 patients will experience CIN, and at least 1% of them will require dialysis and experience a prolonged length of hospital stay (Kane-Gill et al., 2015). This is a potentially preventable condition. Baseline levels of creatinine greater than 2 mg/dL identify patients at high risk. Limiting the patient's exposure to contrast agents and nephrotoxic medications will reduce the risk of CIN (Rank, 2013). Administration of N-acetylcysteine and sodium bicarbonate before and during procedures reduces risk, but prehydration with saline is considered the most effective method to prevent CIN (Rank, 2013).

 ## Gerontologic Considerations

About half of all patients who develop AKI during hospitalization are older than 60 years. The etiology of AKI in older adults includes prerenal causes such as dehydration, intrarenal causes such as nephrotoxic agents (e.g., medications, contrast agents), and complications of major surgery (Elliott, 2012). Suppression of thirst, enforced bed rest, lack of access to drinking water, and confusion all contribute to the older patient's failure to consume adequate fluids and may lead to dehydration, further compromising already decreased renal function.

AKI in older adults is also often seen in the community setting. Nurses in the ambulatory setting need to be aware of the risk. All medications need to be monitored for potential side effects that could result in damage to the kidney either through reduced circulation or nephrotoxicity. Outpatient procedures that require fasting or a bowel preparation may cause dehydration and therefore require careful monitoring.

Medical Management

The kidneys have a remarkable ability to recover from insult. The objectives of treatment for AKI are to restore normal chemical balance and prevent complications until repair of renal tissue and restoration of renal function can occur. Management includes eliminating the underlying cause; maintaining fluid balance; avoiding fluid excesses; and, when indicated, providing renal replacement therapy. Prerenal azotemia is treated by optimizing renal perfusion, whereas postrenal failure is treated by relieving the obstruction. Intrarenal azotemia is treated with supportive therapy, with removal of causative agents, aggressive management of prerenal and postrenal failure, and avoidance of associated risk factors. Shock and infection, if present, are treated promptly (see Chapter 14). The presence of myoglobin in the urine (i.e., myoglobinuria) in the patient who has had a crush injury, compartment syndrome, or heat-induced illness is treated for rhabdomyolysis (see Chapter 72).

Maintenance of fluid balance is based on daily body weight, serial measurements of central venous pressure, serum and urine concentrations, fluid losses, blood pressure, and the clinical status of the patient. The parenteral and oral intake and the output of urine, gastric drainage, stools, wound drainage, and perspiration are calculated and are used as the basis for fluid replacement. The insensible fluid produced through the normal metabolic processes and lost through the skin and lungs is also considered in fluid management.

Fluid excesses can be detected by the clinical findings of dyspnea, tachycardia, and distended neck veins. The patient's lungs are auscultated for moist crackles. Because pulmonary edema may be caused by excessive administration of parenteral fluids, extreme caution must be used to prevent fluid overload. The development of generalized edema is assessed by examining the presacral and pretibial areas several times daily. Mannitol (Osmitrol), furosemide (Lasix), or ethacrynic acid (Edecrin) may be prescribed to initiate diuresis (Walton, 2015).

Adequate renal blood flow in patients with prerenal causes of AKI may be restored by IV fluids or transfusions of blood products. If AKI is caused by hypovolemia secondary to hypoproteinemia, an infusion of albumin may be prescribed. Dialysis may be initiated to prevent complications of AKI, such as hyperkalemia, metabolic acidosis, pericarditis, and pulmonary edema. Dialysis corrects many biochemical abnormalities; allows for liberalization of fluid, protein, and sodium intake; diminishes bleeding tendencies; and promotes wound healing. **Hemodialysis** (a procedure that circulates the patient's blood through an artificial kidney [dialyzer] to remove waste products and excess fluid), **peritoneal dialysis** (PD; a procedure that uses the patient's peritoneal membrane [the lining of the peritoneal cavity] as the semipermeable membrane to exchange fluid and solutes), or a variety of **continuous renal replacement therapies (CRRTs)** (methods used to replace normal kidney function by circulating the patient's blood through a hemofilter) may be performed (Dirkes, 2014). These and other treatment modalities for patients with renal dysfunction are discussed later in this chapter.

Pharmacologic Therapy

Hyperkalemia is the most life threatening of the fluid and electrolyte changes that occur in patients with kidney disorders. Therefore, the patient is monitored for hyperkalemia through serial serum electrolyte levels (potassium value greater than 5.0 mEq/L [5 mmol/L]), ECG changes (tall, tented, or peaked T waves), and changes in clinical status (see Chapter 13). Other symptoms of hyperkalemia include irritability, abdominal cramping, diarrhea, paresthesia, and generalized muscle weakness. Muscle weakness may present as slurred speech, difficulty breathing, paresthesia, and paralysis. As the potassium level increases, both cardiac and other muscular function declines, making this a medical emergency.

The elevated potassium levels may be reduced by administering cation-exchange resins (sodium polystyrene sulfonate [Kayexalate]) orally or by retention enema. Kayexalate works by exchanging sodium ions for potassium ions in the intestinal tract. Sorbitol may be given in combination with Kayexalate to induce a diarrhea-type effect (it induces water loss in the GI tract). If a Kayexalate retention enema is given (the colon is the major site of potassium exchange), a rectal catheter with a balloon may be used to facilitate retention if necessary. The patient should retain the Kayexalate for at least 30 to 60 minutes (preferable 6 to 10 hours) to promote potassium removal (Comerford, 2015). Afterward, a cleansing enema may be prescribed to remove remaining medication as a precaution against fecal impaction.

If the patient is hemodynamically unstable (low blood pressure, changes in mental status, dysrhythmia), IV dextrose 50%, insulin, and calcium replacement may be given to shift potassium back into the cells. The shift of potassium into the intracellular space is temporary, so arrangements for dialysis need to be made on an emergent basis.

Many medications are eliminated through the kidneys; therefore, dosages must be reduced when a patient has AKI.

Examples of commonly used agents that require adjustment are antibiotic medications (especially aminoglycosides), digoxin (Lanoxin), phenytoin (Dilantin), ACE inhibitors, and magnesium-containing agents.

In addition, many medications have been used in patients with AKI in an attempt to improve patient outcomes. Diuretic agents are often used to control fluid volume, but they have not been shown to improve recovery from AKI (Prentice, 2013).

In patients with severe acidosis, the arterial blood gases and serum bicarbonate levels (CO_2) must be monitored because the patient may require sodium bicarbonate therapy or dialysis. If respiratory problems develop, appropriate ventilatory measures must be instituted. The elevated serum phosphate level may be controlled with phosphate-binding agents (e.g., calcium or lanthanum carbonate) that help prevent a continuing rise in serum phosphate levels by decreasing the absorption of phosphate from the intestinal tract.

Nutritional Therapy

AKI causes severe nutritional imbalances (because nausea and vomiting contribute to inadequate dietary intake), impaired glucose use and protein synthesis, and increased tissue catabolism. The patient is weighed daily and loses 0.2 to 0.5 kg (0.5 to 1 lb) daily if the nitrogen balance is negative (i.e., caloric intake falls below caloric requirements). If the patient gains or does not lose weight or develops hypertension, fluid retention should be suspected.

Nutritional support is based on the underlying cause of AKI, the catabolic response, the type and frequency of renal replacement therapy, comorbidities, and nutritional status. Replacement of dietary proteins is individualized to provide the maximum benefit and minimize uremic symptoms. Caloric requirements are met with high-carbohydrate meals, because carbohydrates have a protein-sparing effect (i.e., in a high-carbohydrate diet, protein is not used for meeting energy requirements but is "spared" for growth and tissue healing). Foods and fluids containing potassium or phosphorus (e.g., bananas, citrus fruits and juices, coffee) are restricted.

The oliguric phase of AKI may last 10 to 14 days and is followed by the diuretic phase, at which time urine output begins to increase, signaling the patient is in the recovery phase (Prentice, 2013). Results of blood chemistry tests are used to determine the amounts of sodium, potassium, and water needed for replacement, along with assessment for over- or underhydration. Following the diuretic phase, the patient is placed on a high-protein, high-calorie diet and is encouraged to resume activities gradually.

Nursing Management

The nurse has an important role in caring for the patient with AKI. The nurse monitors for complications, participates in emergency treatment of fluid and electrolyte imbalances, assesses the patient's progress and response to treatment, and provides physical and emotional support. In addition, the nurse keeps family members informed about the patient's condition, helps them understand the treatments, and provides psychological support. Although the development of AKI may be the most serious problem, the nurse continues to provide nursing care indicated for the primary disorder (e.g., burns, shock, trauma, obstruction of the urinary tract).

Monitoring Fluid and Electrolyte Balance

Because of the serious fluid and electrolyte imbalances that can occur with AKI, the nurse monitors the patient's serum electrolyte levels and physical indicators of these complications during all phases of the disorder. IV solutions must be carefully selected based on the patient's fluid and electrolyte status. The patient's cardiac function and musculoskeletal status are monitored closely for signs of hyperkalemia.

> ### ▶ Quality and Safety Nursing Alert
>
> *Hyperkalemia is the most immediate life-threatening imbalance seen in AKI. Parenteral fluids, all oral intake, and all medications are screened carefully to ensure that sources of potassium are not inadvertently given or consumed.*

The nurse monitors fluid status by paying careful attention to fluid intake (IV medications should be given in the smallest volume possible), urine output, apparent edema, distention of the jugular veins, alterations in heart sounds and breath sounds, and increasing difficulty in breathing. Accurate daily weights, as well as I&O records, are essential. Indicators of deteriorating fluid and electrolyte status are reported immediately to the primary provider, and preparation is made for emergency treatment. Severe fluid and electrolyte disturbances may be treated with hemodialysis, PD, or CRRT.

Reducing Metabolic Rate

The nurse takes steps to reduce the patient's metabolic rate. Bed rest may be indicated to reduce exertion and the metabolic rate during the most acute stage of the disorder. Fever and infection, both of which increase the metabolic rate and catabolism, are prevented or treated promptly.

Promoting Pulmonary Function

Attention is given to pulmonary function, and the patient is assisted to turn, cough, and take deep breaths frequently to prevent atelectasis and respiratory tract infection. Drowsiness and lethargy may prevent the patient from moving and turning without encouragement and assistance.

Preventing Infection

Asepsis is essential with invasive lines and catheters to minimize the risk of infection and increased metabolism. An indwelling urinary catheter is avoided whenever possible due to the high risk of UTI associated with its use but may be required to provide ongoing data required to accurately monitor fluid I&O.

Providing Skin Care

The skin may be dry or susceptible to breakdown as a result of edema; therefore, meticulous skin care is important. In addition, excoriation and itching of the skin may result from the deposit of irritating toxins in the patient's tissues. Bathing the patient with cool water, frequent turning, and keeping the skin clean and well moisturized and the fingernails trimmed to avoid excoriation are often comforting and prevent skin breakdown.

Providing Psychosocial Support

The patient with AKI may require treatment with hemodialysis, PD, or CRRT. The length of time that these treatments are necessary varies with the cause and extent of damage to the kidneys. The patient and family need assistance, explanation, and support during this period. The purpose of the treatment is explained to the patient and family by the primary provider. However, high levels of anxiety and fear may necessitate repeated explanation and clarification by the nurse. The family members may initially be afraid to touch and talk to the patient during these procedures but should be encouraged and assisted to do so.

In an intensive care setting, many of the nurse's functions are devoted to the technical aspects of patient care; however, it is essential that the psychological needs and other concerns of the patient and family be addressed. Continued assessment of the patient for complications of AKI and precipitating causes is essential (Davies & Leslie, 2012).

End-Stage Kidney Disease or Chronic Kidney Disease

When a patient has sustained enough kidney damage to require renal replacement therapy on a permanent basis, the patient has moved into the fifth or final stage of CKD, also referred to as ESKD.

Pathophysiology

As renal function declines, the end products of protein metabolism (normally excreted in urine) accumulate in the blood. Uremia develops and adversely affects every system in the body. The greater the buildup of waste products, the more pronounced the symptoms.

The rate of decline in renal function and progression of ESKD is related to the underlying disorder, the urinary excretion of protein, and the presence of hypertension. The disease tends to progress more rapidly in patients who excrete significant amounts of protein or have elevated blood pressure than in those without these conditions.

Clinical Manifestations

Because virtually every body system is affected in ESKD, patients exhibit a number of signs and symptoms. The severity of these signs and symptoms depends in part on the degree of renal impairment, other underlying conditions, and the patient's age. Cardiovascular disease is the predominant cause of death in patients with ESKD (Walton, 2015). Peripheral neuropathy, a disorder of the peripheral nervous system, is present in some patients. Patients complain of severe pain and discomfort. Restless leg syndrome and burning feet can occur in the early stage of uremic peripheral neuropathy. The precise mechanisms for many of these systemic signs and symptoms have not been identified. However, it is generally thought that the accumulation of uremic waste products is the probable cause. Chart 54-6 summarizes the systemic signs and symptoms.

Assessment and Diagnostic Findings

Glomerular Filtration Rate

As the GFR decreases (due to nonfunctioning glomeruli), the creatinine clearance decreases, whereas the serum creatinine and BUN levels increase. Serum creatinine is a more

Chart
54-6

ASSESSMENT

Assessing for End-Stage Kidney Disease

Be alert to the following signs and symptoms:

Neurologic

- Asterixis
- Behavior changes
- Burning of soles of feet
- Confusion
- Disorientation
- Inability to concentrate
- Restlessness of legs
- Seizures
- Tremors
- Weakness and fatigue

Integumentary

- Coarse, thinning hair
- Dry, flaky skin
- Ecchymosis
- Gray-bronze skin color
- Pruritus
- Purpura
- Thin, brittle nails

Cardiovascular

- Engorged neck veins
- Hyperkalemia
- Hyperlipidemia
- Hypertension
- Pericardial effusion
- Pericardial friction rub
- Pericardial tamponade
- Pericarditis
- Periorbital edema
- Pitting edema (feet, hands, sacrum)

Pulmonary

- Crackles
- Depressed cough reflex
- Kussmaul-type respirations
- Pleuritic pain
- Shortness of breath
- Tachypnea
- Thick, tenacious sputum
- Uremic pneumonitis

Gastrointestinal

- Ammonia odor to breath ("uremic fetor")
- Anorexia, nausea, and vomiting
- Bleeding from gastrointestinal tract
- Constipation or diarrhea
- Hiccups
- Metallic taste
- Mouth ulcerations and bleeding

Hematologic

- Anemia
- Thrombocytopenia

Reproductive

- Amenorrhea
- Decreased libido
- Infertility
- Testicular atrophy

Musculoskeletal

- Bone fractures
- Bone pain
- Footdrop
- Loss of muscle strength
- Muscle cramps
- Renal osteodystrophy

---

sensitive indicator of renal function than BUN. The BUN is affected not only by kidney disease but also by protein intake in the diet, catabolism (tissue and RBC breakdown), parenteral nutrition, and medications such as corticosteroids.

Sodium and Water Retention

The kidney cannot concentrate or dilute the urine normally in ESKD. Appropriate responses by the kidney to changes in the daily intake of water and electrolytes, therefore, do not occur. Some patients retain sodium and water, increasing the risk for edema, heart failure, and hypertension. Hypertension may also result from activation of the renin–angiotensin–aldosterone axis and the concomitant increased aldosterone secretion. Other patients have a tendency to lose sodium and run the risk of developing hypotension and hypovolemia. Vomiting and diarrhea may cause sodium and water depletion, which worsens the uremic state.

Acidosis

Metabolic acidosis occurs in ESKD because the kidneys are unable to excrete increased loads of acid. Decreased acid secretion results from the inability of the kidney tubules to excrete ammonia (NH_3-) and to reabsorb sodium bicarbonate (HCO_3-). There is also decreased excretion of phosphates and other organic acids.

Anemia

Anemia develops as a result of inadequate erythropoietin production, the shortened lifespan of RBCs, nutritional deficiencies, and the patient's tendency to bleed, particularly from the GI tract. Erythropoietin, a substance normally produced by the kidneys, stimulates bone marrow to produce RBCs. In ESKD, erythropoietin production decreases and profound anemia results, producing fatigue, angina, and shortness of breath.

Calcium and Phosphorus Imbalance

Another abnormality seen in ESKD is a disorder in calcium and phosphorus metabolism. Serum calcium and phosphate levels have a reciprocal relationship in the body: As one increases, the other decreases. With a decrease in filtration through the glomerulus of the kidney, there is an increase in the serum phosphate level and a reciprocal or corresponding decrease in the serum calcium level. The decreased serum calcium level causes increased secretion of parathormone from the parathyroid glands. However, in kidney disease, the body does not respond normally to the increased secretion of parathormone; as a result, calcium leaves the bone, often producing bone changes and bone disease as well as calcification of major blood vessels in the body. In addition, the active metabolite of vitamin D (1,25-dihydroxycholecalciferol) normally manufactured by the kidney decreases as kidney disease progresses (Counts, 2015). Uremic bone disease, often called renal osteodystrophy, develops from the complex changes in calcium, phosphate, and parathormone balance. There is also evidence of calcification of blood vessels.

Complications

There are a number of potential complications of ESKD that necessitate a collaborative approach to care. These include the following:

- Anemia due to decreased erythropoietin production, decreased RBC lifespan, bleeding in the GI tract from irritating toxins and ulcer formation, and blood loss during hemodialysis
- Bone disease and metastatic and vascular calcifications due to retention of phosphorus, low serum calcium levels, abnormal vitamin D metabolism, and elevated aluminum levels
- Hyperkalemia due to decreased excretion, metabolic acidosis, catabolism, and excessive intake (diet, medications, fluids)
- Hypertension due to sodium and water retention and malfunction of the renin–angiotensin–aldosterone system
- Pericarditis, pericardial effusion, and pericardial tamponade due to retention of uremic waste products and inadequate dialysis

Medical Management

The goal of management is to maintain kidney function and homeostasis for as long as possible. All factors that contribute to ESKD and all factors that are reversible (e.g., obstruction) are identified and treated. Management is accomplished primarily with medications and diet therapy, although dialysis may also be needed to decrease the level of uremic waste products in the blood and to control electrolyte balance.

Pharmacologic Therapy

Complications can be prevented or delayed by administering prescribed phosphate-binding agents, calcium supplements, antihypertensive and cardiac medications, anticonvulsant medications, and recombinant human erythropoietin (epoetin alfa [Epogen]).

Calcium and Phosphorus Binders

Hyperphosphatemia and hypocalcemia are treated with medications that bind dietary phosphorus in the GI tract. Binders such as calcium carbonate (Os-Cal) or calcium acetate (PhosLo) are prescribed, but there is a risk of hypercalcemia. If calcium is high or the calcium–phosphorus product exceeds 55 mg/dL, a polymeric phosphate binder such as sevelamer hydrochloride (Renagel) may be prescribed (Walton, 2015). This medication binds dietary phosphorus in the intestinal tract; one to four tablets are given with food to be effective.

Magnesium-based antacid agents are avoided to prevent magnesium toxicity.

Antihypertensive and Cardiovascular Agents

Hypertension is managed by intravascular volume control and a variety of antihypertensive agents (Weiner, Brunelli, Hunt, et al., 2014). Heart failure and pulmonary edema may also require treatment with fluid restriction, low-sodium diets, diuretic agents, inotropic agents such as digoxin or dobutamine (Dobutrex), and dialysis. The metabolic acidosis of ESKD usually produces no symptoms and requires no treatment; however, sodium bicarbonate supplements or dialysis may be needed to correct the acidosis if it causes symptoms.

Anticonvulsant Agents

Neurologic abnormalities may occur, so the patient must be observed for early evidence of slight twitching, headache, delirium, or seizure activity. If seizures occur, the onset of the seizure is recorded along with the type, duration, and general effect on the patient. The primary provider is notified immediately. IV diazepam (Valium) or phenytoin is usually given to control seizures. The side rails of the bed should be raised and padded to protect the patient. See Chapter 66 for discussion of nursing management for the patient with seizures.

Erythropoietin

Anemia associated with ESKD is treated with erythrocyte-stimulating agents (recombinant human erythropoietin). Patients with anemia (hematocrit less than 30%) present with nonspecific symptoms, such as malaise, general fatigability, and decreased activity tolerance. Erythrocyte stimulation therapy is initiated to achieve a hematocrit of 33% to 38% and a target hemoglobin of 12 g/dL, which generally alleviates the symptoms of anemia.

Epoetin alfa is administered IV or subcutaneously three times a week in ESKD. It may take 2 to 6 weeks for the hematocrit to increase; therefore, the medication is not indicated for patients who need immediate correction of severe anemia. Adverse effects seen with erythropoietin therapy include hypertension (especially during early stages of treatment), increased clotting of vascular access sites, seizures, and depletion of body iron stores (Arslanian, 2015).

Management involves adjustment of heparin to prevent clotting of the lines during hemodialysis treatments, frequent monitoring of hemoglobin and hematocrit, and periodic assessment of serum iron and transferrin levels. Because adequate stores of iron are necessary for an adequate response to epoetin alfa, supplementary iron may be prescribed. Common iron supplements include iron sucrose (Venofer), iron dextran (INFeD or Dexferrum), and ferric gluconate (Ferrlecit). In addition, the patient's blood pressure and serum potassium level are monitored to detect hypertension and increasing serum potassium levels, which may occur with therapy and the increasing RBC mass. The occurrence of hypertension requires initiation or adjustment of the patient's antihypertensive therapy. Hypertension that cannot be controlled is a contraindication to recombinant erythropoietin therapy.

Patients who have received erythropoietin therapy have reported decreased levels of fatigue, increased feelings of well-being, better tolerance of dialysis, higher-energy levels, and improved exercise tolerance. In addition, this therapy has decreased the need for transfusion and its associated risks, including bloodborne infectious disease, antibody formation, and iron overload.

Nutritional Therapy

Dietary intervention is necessary with deterioration of renal function and includes careful regulation of protein intake, fluid intake to balance fluid losses, sodium intake to balance sodium losses, and some restriction of potassium. At the same time, adequate caloric intake and vitamin supplementation must be ensured. Protein is restricted because urea, uric acid, and organic acids—the breakdown products of dietary and tissue proteins—accumulate rapidly in the blood when there is impaired renal clearance. The allowed protein must be of high biologic value (dairy products, eggs, meats). High–biologic-value proteins are those that are complete proteins and supply the essential amino acids necessary for growth and cell repair.

Usually, the fluid allowance per day is 500 to 600 mL more than the previous day's 24-hour urine output. Calories are supplied by carbohydrates and fat to prevent wasting. Vitamin supplementation is necessary because a protein-restricted diet does not provide the necessary complement of vitamins. In addition, the patient on dialysis may lose water-soluble vitamins during the dialysis treatment.

Hyperkalemia is usually prevented by ensuring adequate dialysis treatments with potassium removal and careful monitoring of diet, medications, and fluids for their potassium content. Sodium polystyrene sulfonate (Kayexalate), a cation-exchange resin, may be needed for acute hyperkalemia.

Dialysis

The patient with increasing symptoms of kidney disease is referred to a dialysis and transplantation center early in the course of progressive kidney disease. Dialysis is usually initiated when the patient cannot maintain a reasonable lifestyle with conservative treatment.

Nursing Management

The patient with ESKD requires astute nursing care to avoid the complications of reduced renal function and the stresses and anxieties of dealing with a life-threatening illness.

Nursing care is directed toward assessing fluid status and identifying potential sources of imbalance, implementing a dietary program to ensure proper nutritional intake within the limits of the treatment regimen, and promoting positive feelings by encouraging increased self-care and greater independence. It is extremely important to provide explanations and information to the patient and family concerning ESKD, treatment options, and potential complications. A great deal of emotional support is needed by the patient and family because of the numerous changes experienced. Specific interventions, along with rationale and evaluation criteria, are presented in more detail in the plan of nursing care for the patient with ESKD (see Chart 54-7).

Promoting Home, Community-Based, and Transitional Care

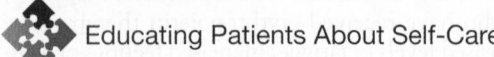 Educating Patients About Self-Care

The nurse plays an important role in educating the patient with ESKD. Because of the extensive education needed, the home care nurse, dialysis nurse, and nurses in the hospital and outpatient settings all provide ongoing education and reinforcement while monitoring the patient's progress and compliance with the treatment regimen.

A referral to a nutritionist is made because of the dietary changes required. The patient is instructed to check the vascular access device for patency and to use appropriate precautions, such as avoiding venipuncture and blood pressure measurements on the arm with the access device.

In addition, the patient and family need to know what problems to report to the primary provider. These include the following:

- Worsening signs and symptoms of kidney disease (nausea, vomiting, change in usual urine output [if any], ammonia odor on breath)
- Signs and symptoms of hyperkalemia (muscle weakness, diarrhea, abdominal cramps)
- Signs and symptoms of access problems (clotted fistula or graft, infection)

These signs and symptoms of decreasing renal function, in addition to increasing BUN and serum creatinine levels, may indicate a need to alter the dialysis prescription. The dialysis nurses also provide ongoing education and support at each treatment visit.

Continuing and Transitional Care

The importance of follow-up examinations and treatment is stressed with the patient and family because of changing physical status, renal function, and dialysis requirements. Referral for home care provides the home care nurse with the opportunity to assess the patient's environment, emotional status, and the coping strategies used by the patient and family to deal with the changes in family roles often associated with chronic illness.

The home care nurse also assesses the patient for further deterioration of renal function and signs and symptoms of complications resulting from the primary kidney disorder, the resulting kidney disease, and effects of treatment strategies (e.g., dialysis, medications, dietary restrictions) (Hain, 2015). Patients need education and reinforcement of the dietary restrictions required, including fluid, sodium, potassium, and protein restriction. Reminders about the need for health promotion activities and health screening are an important part of nursing care for the patient with kidney disease.

Gerontologic Considerations

Diabetes, hypertension, chronic glomerulonephritis, interstitial nephritis, and urinary tract obstruction are among the causes for ESKD in older adults. The signs and symptoms of kidney disease in older adults are often nonspecific. The occurrence of symptoms of other disorders (heart failure, dementia) can mask the symptoms of kidney disease and delay or prevent diagnosis and treatment.

Hemodialysis and PD are used effectively in treating older patients with ESKD. Initiation of dialysis among older patients has dramatically increased in the past decade. Implementation of palliative care has also increased among patients who choose not to start dialysis or who decide to stop dialysis. Although there is no specific age limitation for (*text continued on page 1589*)

Chart 54-7

PLAN OF NURSING CARE

The Patient With End-Stage Kidney Disease

NURSING DIAGNOSIS: Excess fluid volume related to decreased urine output, dietary excesses, and retention of sodium and water
GOAL: Maintenance of ideal body weight without excess fluid

Nursing Interventions	Rationale	Expected Outcomes

1. Assess fluid status:
  a. Daily weight
  b. Intake and output balance
  c. Skin turgor and presence of edema
  d. Distention of neck veins
  e. Blood pressure, pulse rate, and rhythm
  f. Respiratory rate and effort
2. Limit fluid intake to prescribed volume.
 	
3. Identify potential sources of fluid:
  a. Medications and fluids used to take or administer medications: oral and IV
  b. Foods
4. Explain to patient and family the rationale for fluid restriction.
5. Assist patient to cope with the discomforts resulting from fluid restriction.
6. Provide or encourage frequent oral hygiene.
	1. Assessment provides baseline and ongoing database for monitoring changes and evaluating interventions.
	
	2. Fluid restriction will be determined on basis of weight, urine output, and response to therapy.
	3. Unrecognized sources of excess fluids may be identified.
	
	4. Understanding promotes patient and family cooperation with fluid restriction.
	5. Increasing patient comfort promotes compliance with dietary restrictions.
	6. Oral hygiene minimizes dryness of oral mucous membranes.
		• Demonstrates no rapid weight changes
		• Maintains dietary and fluid restrictions
		• Exhibits normal skin turgor without edema
		• Exhibits normal vital signs
		• Exhibits no neck vein distention
		• Reports no difficulty breathing or shortness of breath
		• Performs oral hygiene frequently
		• Reports decreased thirst
		• Reports decreased dryness of oral mucous membranes

NURSING DIAGNOSIS: Imbalanced nutrition: less than body requirements related to anorexia, nausea, vomiting, dietary restrictions, and altered oral mucous membranes
GOAL: Maintenance of adequate nutritional intake

Nursing Interventions	Rationale	Expected Outcomes

1. Assess nutritional status:
  a. Weight changes
  b. Laboratory values (serum electrolyte, blood urea nitrogen [BUN], creatinine, protein, transferrin, and iron levels)
   (see Appendix A on thePoint)
2. Assess patient's nutritional dietary patterns:
  a. Diet history
  b. Food preferences
  c. Calorie counts
3. Assess for factors contributing to altered nutritional intake:
  a. Anorexia, nausea, or vomiting
  b. Diet unpalatable to patient
  c. Depression
  d. Lack of understanding of dietary restrictions
  e. Stomatitis
4. Provide patient's food preferences within dietary restrictions.
5. Promote intake of high–biologic-value protein foods: eggs, dairy products, meats.
 	
6. Encourage high-calorie, low-protein, low-sodium, and low-potassium snacks between meals.
 	
7. Alter schedule of medications so that they are not given immediately before meals.
	1. Baseline data allow for monitoring of changes and evaluating effectiveness of interventions.
	
	2. Past and present dietary patterns are considered in planning meals.
	
	3. Information about other factors that may be altered or eliminated to promote adequate dietary intake is provided.
	
	4. Increased dietary intake is encouraged.
	
	5. Complete proteins are provided for positive nitrogen balance needed for growth and healing.
	6. Reduces source of restricted foods and proteins and provides calories for energy, sparing protein for tissue growth and healing.
	7. Ingestion of medications just before meals may produce anorexia and feeling of fullness.
		• Consumes protein of high biologic value
		• Chooses foods within dietary restrictions that are appealing
		• Consumes high-calorie foods within dietary restrictions
		• Explains in own words rationale for dietary restrictions and relationship to urea and creatinine levels
		• Takes medications on schedule that does not produce anorexia or feeling of fullness
		• Consults written lists of acceptable foods
		• Reports increased appetite at meals
		• Exhibits no rapid increases or decreases in weight
		• Demonstrates normal skin turgor without edema; wound healing and acceptable plasma albumin levels

(continued on page 1586)

Chart 54-7

PLAN OF NURSING CARE (Continued)

The Patient With End-Stage Kidney Disease

Nursing Interventions	Rationale	Expected Outcomes
8. Explain rationale for dietary restrictions and relationship to kidney disease and increased urea and serum creatinine levels.	8. Promotes patient understanding of relationships between diet and urea and creatinine levels to kidney disease.	
9. Provide written lists of foods allowed and suggestions for improving their taste without the use of sodium or potassium.	9. Lists provide a positive approach to dietary restrictions and a reference for patient and family to use when at home.	
10. Provide pleasant surroundings at mealtimes.	10. Unpleasant factors that contribute to patient's anorexia are eliminated.	
11. Weigh patient daily.	11. Allows monitoring of fluid and nutritional status.	
12. Assess for evidence of inadequate protein intake: a. Edema formation b. Delayed wound healing c. Decreased serum albumin levels	12. Inadequate protein intake can lead to decreased albumin and other proteins, edema formation, and delay in wound healing.	

NURSING DIAGNOSIS: Deficient knowledge regarding condition and treatment
GOAL: Increased knowledge about condition and related treatment

Nursing Interventions	Rationale	Expected Outcomes
1. Assess understanding of cause of kidney disease, consequences of kidney disease, and its treatment: a. Cause of patient's kidney disease b. Meaning of kidney disease c. Understanding of renal function d. Relationship of fluid and dietary restrictions to kidney disease e. Rationale for treatment (hemodialysis, peritoneal dialysis, transplantation)	1. Provides baseline for further explanations and education.	• Verbalizes relationship of cause of kidney disease to consequences • Explains fluid and dietary restrictions as they relate to failure of kidney's regulatory functions • States in own words relationship of kidney disease and need for treatment
2. Provide explanation of renal function and consequences of kidney disease at patient's level of understanding and guided by patient's readiness to learn.	2. Patient can learn about kidney disease and treatment as they become ready to understand and accept the diagnosis and consequences.	• Asks questions about treatment options, indicating readiness to learn • Verbalizes plans to continue as normal a life as possible
3. Assist patient to identify ways to incorporate changes related to illness and its treatment into lifestyle.	3. Patient can see that their life does not have to revolve around the disease.	• Uses written information and instructions to clarify questions and seek additional information
4. Provide oral and written information as appropriate about: a. Renal function and failure b. Fluid and dietary restrictions c. Medications d. Reportable problems, signs, and symptoms e. Follow-up schedule f. Community resources g. Treatment options	4. Provides patient with information that can be used for further clarification at home.	

NURSING DIAGNOSIS: Activity intolerance related to fatigue, anemia, retention of waste products, and dialysis procedure
GOAL: Participation in activity within tolerance

Nursing Interventions	Rationale	Expected Outcomes
1. Assess factors contributing to activity intolerance: a. Fatigue b. Anemia c. Fluid and electrolyte imbalances d. Retention of waste products e. Depression	1. Indicates factors contributing to severity of fatigue.	• Participates in increasing levels of activity and exercise • Reports increased sense of well-being • Alternates rest and activity • Participates in selected self-care activities

Chart 54-7 | **PLAN OF NURSING CARE** (Continued)

The Patient With End-Stage Kidney Disease

Nursing Interventions	Rationale	Expected Outcomes
2. Promote independence in self-care activities as tolerated; assist if fatigued.	2. Promotes improved self-esteem.	
3. Encourage alternating activity with rest.	3. Promotes activity and exercise within limits and adequate rest.	
4. Encourage patient to rest after dialysis treatments.	4. Adequate rest is encouraged after dialysis treatments, which are exhausting to many patients.	

NURSING DIAGNOSIS: Risk for situational low self-esteem related to dependency, role changes, change in body image, and change in sexual function
GOAL: Improved self-esteem

Nursing Interventions	Rationale	Expected Outcomes
1. Assess patient's and family's responses and reactions to illness and treatment.	1. Provides data about problems encountered by patient and family in coping with changes in life.	• Identifies previously used coping styles that have been effective and those no longer possible due to disease and treatment (alcohol or drug use; extreme physical exertion)
2. Assess relationship of patient and significant family members.	2. Identifies strengths and supports of patient and family.	
3. Assess usual coping patterns of patient and family members.	3. Coping patterns that may have been effective in past may be harmful in view of restrictions imposed by disease and treatment.	• Patient and family identify and verbalize feelings and reactions to disease and necessary changes in their lives
4. Encourage open discussion of concerns about changes produced by disease and treatment: a. Role changes b. Changes in lifestyle c. Changes in occupation d. Sexual changes e. Dependence on health care team	4. Encourages patient to identify concerns and steps necessary to deal with them.	• Seeks professional counseling, if necessary, to cope with changes resulting from kidney disease
5. Explore alternate ways of sexual expression other than sexual intercourse.	5. Alternative forms of sexual expression may be acceptable.	• Reports satisfaction with method of sexual expression
6. Discuss role of giving and receiving love, warmth, and affection.	6. Sexuality means different things to different people, depending on stage of maturity.	

COLLABORATIVE PROBLEMS: Hyperkalemia; pericarditis, pericardial effusion, and pericardial tamponade; hypertension; anemia; bone disease and metastatic calcifications
GOAL: Absence of complications

Nursing Interventions	Rationale	Expected Outcomes
Hyperkalemia		
1. Monitor serum potassium levels. Notify primary provider if level is at or approaching >5.5 mEq/L, and prepare to treat hyperkalemia.	1. Hyperkalemia causes potentially life-threatening changes in the body.	• Has normal potassium level
2. Assess patient for muscle weakness, diarrhea, electrocardiographic (ECG) changes (tall-tented T waves and widened QRS).	2. Cardiovascular signs and symptoms are characteristic of hyperkalemia.	• Experiences no muscle weakness or diarrhea • Exhibits normal ECG pattern • Vital signs are within normal limits
Pericarditis, Pericardial Effusion, and Pericardial Tamponade		
1. Assess patient for fever, chest pain, and a pericardial friction rub (signs of pericarditis); if present, notify primary provider.	1. About 30–50% of patients with chronic kidney disease develop pericarditis due to uremia; fever, chest pain, and a pericardial friction rub are classic signs.	• Has strong and equal peripheral pulses • Absence of a paradoxical pulse • Absence of pericardial effusion or tamponade on cardiac ultrasound • Has normal heart sounds

(continued on page 1588)

Chart 54-7

PLAN OF NURSING CARE (Continued)

The Patient With End-Stage Kidney Disease

Nursing Interventions	Rationale	Expected Outcomes

2. If patient has pericarditis, assess for the following every 4 hours:
  a. Paradoxical pulse, >10 mmHg
  b. Extreme hypotension
  c. Weak or absent peripheral pulses
  d. Altered level of consciousness
  e. Jugular venous distention
	2. Pericardial effusion is a common fatal sequela of pericarditis. Signs of an effusion include a paradoxical pulse (>10 mmHg drop in blood pressure during inspiration) and signs of shock due to compression of the heart by a large effusion. Cardiac tamponade exists when the patient is severely compromised hemodynamically.	

3. Prepare patient for echocardiogram to aid in diagnosis of pericardial effusion and cardiac tamponade.	3. Echocardiogram is useful in visualizing pericardial effusions and cardiac tamponade.	
4. If cardiac tamponade develops, prepare patient for emergency pericardiocentesis.	4. Cardiac tamponade is a life-threatening condition, with a high mortality rate. Immediate aspiration of fluid from the pericardial space is essential.	

Hypertension

Nursing Interventions	Rationale	Expected Outcomes
1. Monitor and record blood pressure as indicated.	1. Provides objective data for monitoring. Elevated levels may indicate nonadherence to the treatment regimen.	• Blood pressure within normal limits • Reports no headaches, visual problems, or seizures • Edema is absent • Demonstrates adherence to dietary and fluid restrictions
2. Administer antihypertensive medications as prescribed.	2. Antihypertensive medications play a key role in treatment of hypertension associated with chronic kidney disease.	
3. Encourage adherence to dietary and fluid restriction therapy.	3. Adherence to diet and fluid restrictions and dialysis schedule prevents excess fluid and sodium accumulation.	
4. Instruct patient to report signs of fluid overload, vision changes, headaches, edema, or seizures.	4. These are indications of inadequate control of hypertension and the need to alter therapy.	

Anemia

Nursing Interventions	Rationale	Expected Outcomes
1. Monitor red blood cell (RBC) count and hemoglobin and hematocrit levels as indicated.	1. Provides assessment of degree of anemia.	• Patient has a normal skin color without pallor • Exhibits hemoglobin levels within acceptable limits • Experiences no bleeding from any site
2. Administer medications as prescribed, including iron and folic acid supplements, an erythrocyte stimulating agent, and multivitamins.	2. RBCs need iron, folic acid, and vitamins to be produced. An erythrocyte-stimulating agent stimulates the bone marrow to produce RBCs.	
3. Avoid drawing unnecessary blood specimens.	3. Anemia is worsened by drawing numerous specimens.	
4. Educate patient to prevent bleeding: Avoid vigorous nose blowing and contact sports, and use a soft toothbrush.	4. Bleeding from anywhere in the body worsens anemia.	
5. Administer blood component therapy as indicated.	5. Blood component therapy may be needed if the patient has symptoms.	

Bone Disease and Metastatic Calcifications

Nursing Interventions	Rationale	Expected Outcomes
1. Administer the following medications as prescribed: phosphate binders, calcium supplements, vitamin D supplements.	1. Chronic kidney disease causes numerous physiologic changes affecting calcium, phosphorus, and vitamin D metabolism.	• Exhibits serum calcium, phosphorus, and aluminum levels within acceptable ranges • Exhibits no symptoms of hypocalcemia • Has no bone demineralization on bone scan • Discusses importance of maintaining activity level and exercise program
2. Monitor serum laboratory values as indicated (calcium, phosphorus, aluminum levels), and report abnormal findings to primary provider.	2. Hyperphosphatemia, hypocalcemia, and excess aluminum accumulation are common in chronic kidney disease.	
3. Assist patient with an exercise program.	3. Bone demineralization increases with immobility.	

kidney transplantation, concomitant disorders (e.g., coronary artery disease, peripheral vascular disease) have made it a less common treatment for older adults. However, the outcome is comparable to that in younger patients. Some older patients elect not to undergo dialysis or transplantation. Conservative management and palliative care, including nutritional therapy, fluid control, and medications such as phosphate binders, may be considered in patients who are not suitable for or elect not to have dialysis or transplantation (Prentice, 2013). Palliative care for the patient with ESKD focuses on relieving suffering, promoting health-related quality of life, and facilitating dignity at the end of life (see Chapter 16).

 Concept Mastery Alert

Visit thePoint to view an Interactive Tutorial on kidney disease and associated fundamental concepts.

RENAL REPLACEMENT THERAPIES

The use of renal replacement therapies becomes necessary when the kidneys can no longer remove wastes, maintain electrolytes, and regulate fluid balance. This can occur rapidly or over a long period of time, and the need for replacement therapy can be acute (short term) or chronic (long term). The main renal replacement therapies include the various types of dialysis and kidney transplantation.

Dialysis

Types of dialysis include hemodialysis, CRRT, and PD. Acute or urgent dialysis is indicated when there is a high and increasing level of serum potassium, fluid overload, or impending pulmonary edema; increasing acidosis; pericarditis; and advanced uremia (Grossman & Porth, 2014). It may also be used to remove medications or toxins (poisoning or medication overdose) from the blood or for edema that does not respond to other treatment, hepatic coma, hyperkalemia, hypercalcemia, hypertension, and uremia.

Chronic or maintenance dialysis is indicated in advanced CKD and ESKD in the following instances: the presence of uremic signs and symptoms affecting all body systems (nausea and vomiting, severe anorexia, increasing lethargy, mental confusion), hyperkalemia, fluid overload not responsive to diuretics and fluid restriction, and a general lack of well-being. An urgent indication for dialysis in patients with kidney disease is pericardial friction rub, which is indicative of uremic pericarditis.

The decision to initiate dialysis should be reached only after thoughtful discussion among the patient, family, primary provider, and other health care team members. The nurse can assist the patient and family by answering their questions, clarifying the information provided, and supporting their decision.

Successful kidney transplantation eliminates the need for dialysis. Not only is the quality of life much improved in patients with ESKD who undergo transplantation, but physiologic function is improved as well. Patients who undergo kidney transplantation from living donors before dialysis is initiated generally have longer survival of the transplanted kidney than patients who receive transplantation after dialysis treatment is initiated (Trevitt, Dunsmore, Murphy, et al., 2012).

Hemodialysis

Hemodialysis is used for patients who are acutely ill and require short-term dialysis for days to weeks until kidney function resumes and for patients with advanced CKD and ESKD who require long-term or permanent renal replacement therapy. Hemodialysis prevents death but does not cure kidney disease and does not compensate for the loss of endocrine or metabolic activities of the kidneys. More than 90% of patients requiring long-term renal replacement therapy are on chronic hemodialysis (USRDS, 2015). Most patients receive intermittent hemodialysis that involves treatments three times a week with an average treatment duration of 3 to 5 hours in an outpatient setting. Hemodialysis can also be performed at home by the patient and a caregiver. With home dialysis, treatment time and frequency can be adjusted to meet optimal patient needs.

The objectives of hemodialysis are to extract toxic nitrogenous substances from the blood and to remove excess fluid. A **dialyzer** (also referred to as an artificial kidney) is a synthetic semipermeable membrane through which blood is filtered to remove uremic toxins and a desired amount of fluid. In hemodialysis, the blood, laden with toxins and nitrogenous wastes, is diverted from the patient to a machine via the use of a blood pump to the dialyzer, where toxins are filtered from the blood and the blood is returned to the patient.

Diffusion, osmosis, and **ultrafiltration** are the principles on which hemodialysis is based (see Chapter 13). The toxins and wastes in the blood are removed by **diffusion**—that is, they move from an area of higher concentration in the blood to an area of lower concentration in the dialysate. The **dialysate** is a solution that circulates through the dialyzer, made up of all the electrolytes in their ideal extracellular concentrations. The electrolyte level in the patient's blood can be brought under control by properly adjusting the electrolytes in the dialysate solution. The semipermeable membrane impedes the diffusion of large molecules, such as RBCs and proteins.

Excess fluid is removed from the blood by **osmosis**, in which water moves from an area of low concentration potential (the blood) to an area of high concentration potential (the dialysate bath). In **ultrafiltration**, fluid moves under high pressure to an area of lower pressure. This process is much more efficient than osmosis for fluid removal and is accomplished by applying negative pressure or a suctioning force to the dialysis membrane. Because patients with disease requiring dialysis usually cannot excrete water, this force is necessary to remove fluid to achieve fluid balance.

The body's buffer system is maintained using a dialysate bath made up of bicarbonate (most common) or acetate, which is metabolized to form bicarbonate. The anticoagulant heparin is given to keep blood from clotting in the extracorporeal dialysis circuit. Cleansed blood is returned to the body with the goal of removing fluid, balancing electrolytes, and managing acidosis.

Dialyzers

Dialyzers are hollow-fiber devices containing thousands of tiny capillary tubes that carry the blood through the artificial kidney. The tubes are porous and act as a semipermeable membrane, allowing toxins, fluid, and electrolytes to pass across the membrane. The constant flow of the solution maintains the

Figure 54-3 • Hemodialysis system. Blood from an artery is pumped (**A**) into a dialyzer, where it flows through the synthetic capillary tubes (**B**), which act as the semipermeable membrane (*inset*). The dialysate, which has a particular chemical composition, flows into the dialyzer around the capillary tubes that the blood flows through. The waste products in the blood diffuse across the semipermeable membrane into the dialysate solution.

concentration gradient to facilitate the exchange of wastes from the blood across the semipermeable membrane into the dialysate solution, where they are removed and discarded (see Fig. 54-3).

Dialyzers have undergone many technologic changes in performance and biocompatibility. High-flux dialysis uses highly permeable membranes to increase the clearance of low- and mid–molecular-weight molecules. These special membranes are used with higher than traditional rates of flow for the blood entering and exiting the dialyzer (500 to 550 mL/min). High-flux dialysis increases the efficiency of treatments while shortening their duration and reducing the need for heparin.

Vascular Access

Access to the patient's vascular system must be established to allow blood to be removed, cleansed, and returned to the patient's vascular system at the rapid rates of 300 and 800 mL/min. Several types of access can be surgically created or placed during procedures performed in interventional radiology suites or at the bedside.

Vascular Access Devices

Immediate access to the patient's circulation for acute hemodialysis is achieved by inserting a double-lumen, noncuffed, large-bore catheter into the subclavian, internal jugular, or femoral vein by the physician (see Fig. 54-4). This method of vascular access involves some risk (e.g., hematoma, pneumothorax, infection, thrombosis of the subclavian vein, inadequate flow). The catheter is removed when no longer needed (e.g., because the patient's condition has improved or another type of permanent access has been established). Double-lumen, cuffed catheters may also be inserted, usually by either a surgeon or interventional radiologist, into the internal jugular vein of the patient. Because these catheters have cuffs under the skin, the insertion site heals, sealing the wound and reducing the risk for ascending infection. This feature makes these catheters safe for longer-term use. However, infection rates remain high, and sepsis continues to be a common cause for hospital admission (Figueiredo, 2014).

Arteriovenous Fistula

The preferred method of permanent vascular access for dialysis is an **arteriovenous fistula** (AVF) that is created surgically (usually in the forearm) by joining (anastomosing) an artery to a vein, either side to side or end to side (see Fig. 54-5A). Needles are inserted into the vessel to obtain blood flow adequate to pass through the dialyzer. The arterial segment of the fistula is used for arterial flow to the dialyzer and the venous segment for reinfusion of the dialyzed blood. This access will exercises to increase the size of these vessels (i.e., squeezing a rubber ball for forearm fistulas) to accommodate the large-bore needles. Once established, this access has the longest useful life and thus is the best option for vascular access for the patient requiring ongoing hemodialysis (MacRae, Ahmed, & Hemmelgam, 2014).

Arteriovenous Graft

An **arteriovenous graft** can be created by subcutaneously interposing a biologic, semibiologic, or synthetic graft material between an artery and vein (see Fig. 54-5B). Usually, a graft is created when the patient's vessels are not suitable for creation of an AVF. Patients with compromised vascular systems (e.g., from diabetes) often require a graft because their native vessels may not be suitable for creation of an AVF. Grafts are usually placed in the arm but may be placed in the thigh or chest wall. Stenosis, infection, and thrombosis are the most common complications of this access. It is not at all uncommon to see a dialysis patient with numerous "old" or "nonfunctioning" accesses present on their arms. The patient is asked to identify the current access in use, and it is checked carefully for the presence of a bruit and thrill.

See the Special Considerations: Nursing Management of the Patient on Dialysis Who Is Hospitalized section later in this chapter for nursing interventions and care of the patient with an arteriovenous graft or fistula.

> ⚑ **Quality and Safety Nursing Alert**
>
> *Failure of the permanent dialysis access (fistula or graft) accounts for most hospital admissions of patients undergoing chronic hemodialysis. Thus, protection of the access is of high priority.*

Complications

Although hemodialysis can prolong life, it does not alter the natural course of the underlying CKD, nor does it completely replace kidney function. The CKD complications previously discussed will continue to worsen and require treatment. With the initiation of dialysis, disturbances of lipid metabolism (hypertriglyceridemia) are accentuated and contribute to cardiovascular complications. Heart failure, coronary artery disease, angina, stroke, and peripheral vascular disease may occur and can incapacitate the patient. Cardiovascular disease remains the leading cause of death in patients receiving dialysis (Deng & Forbes, 2015; Ludvigsen, Hermansen, & Lindberg, 2014).

Anemia is compounded by blood lost during hemodialysis. Gastric ulcers may result from the physiologic stress of chronic illness, medication, and pre-existing medical conditions (e.g., diabetes). Patients with uremia report a metallic taste and nausea when they require dialysis. Vomiting may occur during the hemodialysis treatment when rapid fluid shifts and hypotension occur. These contribute to the malnutrition seen in patients on dialysis. Poor calcium metabolism and renal osteodystrophy can result in bone pain and fractures, interfering with mobility. As time on dialysis continues, calcification of major blood vessels has been reported and linked to hypertension and other vascular complications. Phosphorus deposits in the skin can occur and cause itching.

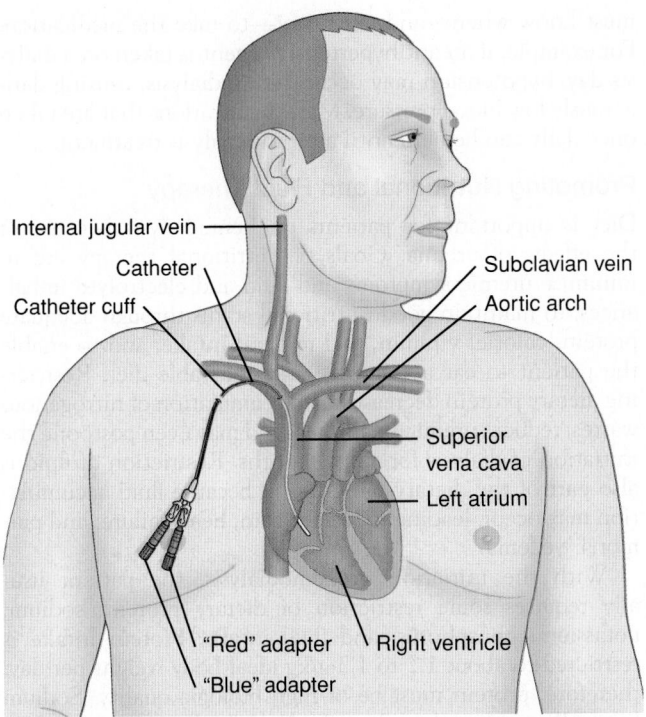

Figure 54-4 • Double-lumen, cuffed hemodialysis catheter used in acute hemodialysis. The red lumen is attached to a blood line through which blood is pumped from the patient to the dialyzer. After the blood passes through the dialyzer (artificial kidney), it returns to the patient through the blue lumen of the catheter.

need time (2 to 3 months) to "mature" before it can be used. As the AVF matures, the venous segment dilates due to the increased blood flow coming directly from the artery. Once sufficiently dilated, it will then accommodate two large-bore (14-, 15-, or 16-gauge) needles that are inserted for each dialysis treatment. The patient is encouraged to perform hand

Figure 54-5 • **A.** Arteriovenous fistulas are created by anastomosing a patient's vein to an artery. This illustrates a side-to-side anastomosis. **B.** Arteriovenous grafts are established by connecting the artery and vein using synthetic tubing.

Many people undergoing hemodialysis experience major sleep problems that further complicate their overall health status. Early-morning or late-afternoon dialysis may be a risk factor for developing sleep disturbances.

Other complications of dialysis treatment may include the following:

- Episodes of shortness of breath often occur as fluid accumulates between dialysis treatments.
- Hypotension may occur during the treatment as fluid is removed. Nausea and vomiting, diaphoresis, tachycardia, and dizziness are common signs of hypotension.
- Painful muscle cramping may occur, usually late in dialysis as fluid and electrolytes rapidly leave the extracellular space.
- Exsanguination may occur if blood lines separate or dialysis needles become dislodged.
- Dysrhythmias may result from electrolyte and pH changes or from removal of antiarrhythmic medications during dialysis.
- Air embolism is rare but can occur if air enters the vascular system.
- Chest pain may occur in patients with anemia or arteriosclerotic heart disease.
- Dialysis disequilibrium results from cerebral fluid shifts. Signs and symptoms include headache, nausea and vomiting, restlessness, decreased level of consciousness, and seizures. It is rare and more likely to occur in AKI or when BUN levels are very high (exceeding 150 mg/dL).

Nursing Management

The nurse in the dialysis unit has an important role in monitoring, supporting, assessing, and educating the patient. During dialysis, the patient, the dialyzer, and the dialysate bath require constant monitoring because numerous complications are possible, including clotting of the dialysis tubing or dialyzer, air embolism, inadequate or excessive fluid removal, hypotension, cramping, vomiting, blood leaks, contamination, and access complications. Nursing care of the patient and maintenance of the vascular access device are especially important and are discussed in the Special Considerations: Nursing Management of the Patient on Dialysis Who Is Hospitalized section.

Promoting Pharmacologic Therapy

Many medications are removed from the blood during hemodialysis; therefore, dosage or timing of the medication administration may require adjustment. Medications that are water soluble are readily removed during hemodialysis treatment, and those that are fat soluble or adhere to other substances (like albumin) are not dialyzed out very well. This is the reason some drug overdoses are treated with emergency hemodialysis and others are not.

Patients undergoing hemodialysis who require medications (e.g., cardiac glycosides, antibiotic agents, antiarrhythmic medications, antihypertensive agents) are monitored closely to ensure that blood and tissue levels of these medications are maintained without toxic accumulation. Antihypertensive therapy, often part of the regimen of patients on dialysis, is one example when communication, education, and evaluation can make a difference in patient outcomes. The patient must know when—and when not—to take the medication. For example, if an antihypertensive agent is taken on a dialysis day, hypotension may occur during dialysis, causing dangerously low blood pressure. Many medications that are taken once daily can be held until after the dialysis treatment.

Promoting Nutritional and Fluid Therapy

Diet is important for patients on hemodialysis because of the effects of uremia. Goals of nutritional therapy are to minimize uremic symptoms and fluid and electrolyte imbalances; to maintain good nutritional status through adequate protein, calorie, vitamin, and mineral intake; and to enable the patient to eat a palatable and enjoyable diet. Restricting dietary protein decreases the accumulation of nitrogenous wastes, reduces uremic symptoms, and may even postpone the initiation of dialysis for a few months. Restriction of fluid is also part of the dietary prescription because fluid accumulation may occur, leading to weight gain, heart failure, and pulmonary edema.

With the initiation of hemodialysis, the patient usually requires some restriction of dietary protein, sodium, potassium, phosphorus, and fluid intake. Protein intake is restricted to about 1.2 to 1.3 g/kg ideal body weight per day; therefore, protein must be of high biologic quality. Sodium is usually restricted to 2 to 3 g/day; fluids are restricted to an amount equal to the daily urine output plus 500 mL/day. The goal for patients on hemodialysis is to keep their interdialytic (between dialysis treatments) weight gain under 1.5 kg. Potassium restriction depends on the amount of residual renal function and the frequency of dialysis. Dietary restriction is an unwelcome change in lifestyle for many patients with ESKD. Patients can feel stigmatized in social situations because there may be few food choices available for their diet. If the restrictions are ignored, life-threatening complications, such as hyperkalemia and pulmonary edema, may result. Thus, the patient may feel punished for responding to basic human drives to eat and drink. The nurse who cares for a patient with symptoms or complications resulting from dietary indiscretion must avoid harsh, judgmental, or punitive tones when communicating with him or her. Regular education with reinforcement is needed to achieve these difficult changes in lifestyle.

Meeting Psychosocial Needs

Patients requiring long-term hemodialysis are often concerned about the unpredictability of the illness and the quality of their lives (Wright & Wilson, 2015). They often have financial problems, difficulty holding a job, waning sexual desire and impotence, clinical depression, and fear of dying. Younger patients worry about marriage, having children, and the burden that they bring to their families. The regimented lifestyle that frequent dialysis treatments and restrictions in food and fluid intake impose can be demoralizing to the patient and family. Researchers have studied the quality of life and self-efficacy in patient undergoing dialysis (see Chart 54-8).

Dialysis alters the lifestyle of the patient and family. The amount of time required for dialysis and primary provider visits and being chronically ill can create conflict, frustration, guilt, and depression. It may be difficult for the patient, spouse, and family to express anger and negative feelings.

Chart 54-8 NURSING RESEARCH PROFILE
Quality of life in Patients Receiving Dialysis

Wright, L. S. & Wilson, L. (2015). Quality of life and self-efficacy in three dialysis modalities: Incenter hemodialysis, home hemodialysis, and home peritoneal dialysis. *Nephrology Nursing Journal, 42*(5), 463–476.

Purpose

Previous research has focused almost exclusively on the quality of life among patients receiving incenter hemodialysis (HD). The purpose of this study was to describe the quality of life and self-efficacy of patients receiving incenter HD compared to those receiving a home HD (HD or peritoneal dialysis [PD]).

Design

This study utilized a correlational cross-sectional design and quota sampling to achieve equal group size. Patients were recruited from outpatient dialysis facilities and included 77 community dwelling adult patients who had been on dialysis for at least 6 months. Quality of life was measured using the Kidney Disease Quality of Life (QOL) Instrument, and self-efficacy was measured using the Strategies Used by People to Promote Health instrument.

Findings

The sample included 29 participants receiving incenter HD treatments, 22 on home HD, and 26 on home PD. There were no significant differences in demographic characteristics. Participants on PD scored the highest in 6 of the 11 CKD-specific to QOL measures. Patients on PD also scored highest in 8 of the 9 generic QOL measures. The results of this study suggest a possible benefit for patients on PD with regard to QOL and self-efficacy.

Nursing Implications

This information helps nurses to understand patient needs, both medical and social, and to recognize their key role in educating patients about treatment options and other care-related issues. By knowing the differences in reported self-efficacy and QOL across dialysis modalities, nurses can help empower patients to make decisions about which mode of dialysis treatment will meet their individual needs.

The nurse needs to give the patient and family the opportunity to express feelings of anger and concern about the limitations that the disease and treatment impose, possible financial problems, and job insecurity. If anger is not expressed, it may be directed inward and lead to depression, despair, and attempts at suicide (suicide is more prevalent in patients on dialysis); however, if anger is projected outward to other people, it may damage family relationships.

Although these feelings are normal in this situation, they are often profound. Counseling and psychotherapy may be useful. Depression may require treatment with antidepressant agents. Referring the patient and family to a mental health provider with expertise in the care of patients receiving dialysis may also be helpful. Clinical nurse specialists, psychologists, and social workers may be helpful in assisting the patient and family to cope with the changes brought about by kidney disease and its treatment.

The sense of loss that the patient experiences cannot be underestimated because every aspect of a "normal life" is disrupted. Some patients use denial to deal with the array of medical problems (e.g., infections, hypertension, anemia, neuropathy). Staff who are tempted to label the patient as noncompliant must consider the impact of kidney disease and its treatment on the patient and family and the coping strategies that they may use.

Palliative care principles that focus on symptom control are becoming increasingly important as greater attention is focused on quality-of-life issues (Hain, 2015). Patients and their families are encouraged to discuss end-of-life options and to develop advanced directives or living wills.

Promoting Home, Community-Based, and Transitional Care

Educating Patients About Self-Care

Preparing a patient for hemodialysis is essential. Assessment helps identify the learning needs of the patient and family members. In many cases, the patient is discharged home

before learning needs and readiness to learn can be thoroughly evaluated; therefore, hospital-based nurses, dialysis staff, and home care nurses must work together to provide appropriate education that meets the patient's and family's changing needs and readiness to learn (see Chart 54-9).

The diagnosis of ESKD and the need for dialysis can be devastating for the patient and family. In addition, many patients with ESKD have clinical depression, a shortened attention span, a decreased level of concentration, and altered perception. Therefore, education must occur in brief, 10- to 15-minute sessions, with time added for clarification, repetition, reinforcement, and questions from the patient and family. The nurse needs to convey a nonjudgmental attitude to enable the patient and family to discuss options and their feelings about those options. Team conferences are helpful for sharing information and providing every team member the opportunity to discuss the needs of the patient and family.

Home Hemodialysis

Most patients who undergo hemodialysis do so in an outpatient setting, but home hemodialysis is an option for some. Home hemodialysis requires a highly motivated patient who is willing to take responsibility for the procedure and is able to adjust each treatment to meet the body's changing needs. It also requires the commitment and cooperation of a caregiver to assist the patient. However, many patients are not comfortable imposing on others this way and do not wish to subject family members to the feeling that their home is being turned into a clinic. The health care team never forces a patient to use home hemodialysis, because this treatment requires changes in the home and family. Home hemodialysis must be the patient's and family's decision (Wright & Wilson, 2015).

The patient undergoing home hemodialysis and the caregiver assisting that patient must be trained to prepare, operate, and disassemble the dialysis machine; maintain and clean the equipment; administer medications (e.g., heparin) into the machine lines; and handle emergency problems (hemodialysis dialyzer rupture, electrical or mechanical problems,

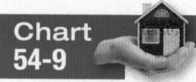

Chart 54-9	**HOME CARE CHECKLIST**

The Patient Undergoing Hemodialysis

At the completion of education, the patient and/or caregiver will be able to:

- Discuss kidney disease and its effects on the body.
- State the goal and purpose of hemodialysis and its impact on physiologic functioning, ADLs, IADLs, roles, relationships, and spirituality.
- Discuss common problems that may occur during hemodialysis and their prevention and management.
- State the name, dose, side effects, frequency, and schedule for all medications on dialysis and nondialysis days.
- Describe commonly measured laboratory values, results, and implications.
- State changes in lifestyle (e.g., diet, activity) necessary to maintain health.
  - Acknowledge dietary and fluid restrictions, rationale, and consequences of nonadherence.
  - State dietary restrictions and changes required to provide adequate protein, calorie, vitamin, and mineral intake.
- List guidelines for prevention and detection of fluid overload, meaning of "dry" weight, and how to weigh self.

- Demonstrate vascular access care, how to check patency, signs and symptoms of infection, and prevention of complications.
- Develop strategies to manage or reduce anxiety and maintain independence.
- Discuss strategies for detection, management, and relief of pruritus, neuropathy, and other potential complications of kidney disease.
- Relate how to reach primary provider with questions or complications.
- State time and date of follow-up medical appointments, therapy, and testing.
- Coordinate financial arrangements for hemodialysis and strategies to identify and obtain resources.
- Identify sources of support (e.g., friends, relatives, faith community, support groups, caregiver support).
- Identify the need for health promotion, disease prevention, and screening activities.

ADL, activities of daily living; IADL, independent activities of daily living.

---

hypotension, shock, and seizures) (Tennankore, d'Gama, Faratro, et al., 2015). Because home hemodialysis places primary responsibility for the treatment on the patient and the family member, they must understand and be capable of performing all aspects of the hemodialysis procedure.

Before home hemodialysis is initiated, the home environment, household and community resources, and ability and willingness of the patient and family to carry out this treatment are assessed. The home is surveyed to see if electrical outlets, plumbing facilities, and storage space are adequate. Modifications may be needed to enable the patient and assistant to perform dialysis safely and to deal with emergencies.

Once home hemodialysis is initiated, the home care nurse must visit periodically to evaluate compliance with the recommended techniques, to assess the patient for complications, to reinforce previous instruction, and to provide reassurance.

Continuing and Transitional Care

The health care team's goal in treating patients with CKD is to maximize their vocational potential, functional status, and quality of life (Wright & Wilson, 2015). To facilitate renal rehabilitation, appropriate follow-up and monitoring by members of the health care team (physicians, dialysis nurses, social worker, psychologist, home care nurses, and others as appropriate) are essential to identify and resolve problems early on. Many patients with chronic kidney disease can resume relatively normal lives, doing the things that are important to them: traveling, exercising, working, or actively participating in family activities. If appropriate interventions are available early in the course of dialysis, the potential for better health improves, and the patient can remain active in family and community life. Outcome goals for renal rehabilitation include employment for those able to work, improved physical functioning of all patients, improved understanding about adaptation and options for living well, increased

control over the effects of kidney disease and dialysis, and resumption of activities enjoyed before dialysis.

 Continuous Renal Replacement Therapies

Continuous renal replacement therapies (CRRTs) may be indicated for patients with acute or chronic kidney disease who are too clinically unstable for traditional hemodialysis, for patients with fluid overload secondary to oliguric (low urine output) kidney disease, and for patients whose kidneys cannot handle their acutely high metabolic or nutritional needs. Some forms of CRRT may not require dialysis machines or dialysis personnel to carry out the procedures and can be initiated quickly. Several types of CRRT are available and widely used in critical care units (see Fig. 54-6). The methods are similar, as they require access to the circulation and blood to pass through an artificial filter. A hemofilter (an extremely porous blood filter containing a semipermeable membrane) is used in all types.

 Continuous Venovenous Hemofiltration

Continuous venovenous hemofiltration (CVVH) is often used to manage AKI. Blood from a double-lumen venous catheter is pumped (using a small blood pump) through a hemofilter and then returned to the patient through the same catheter (Richardson & Whatmore, 2015). CVVH provides continuous slow fluid removal (**ultrafiltration**); therefore, hemodynamic effects are mild and better tolerated by patients with unstable conditions. CVVH requires a dual-lumen venous catheter and critical care nurses trained in management of the therapy who can set up, initiate, maintain, and terminate the system. Many hospitals have developed a collaborative approach to managing the CVVH therapy between the critical care and nephrology nursing staff.

A **B** **C**

Figure 54-6 • Devices for administering continuous renal replacement therapy (CRRT) offer an integrated fluid warmer for the heating of infusion and dialysate fluids, a weighing system to reduce the possibility of error in assessing fluid balance, and a battery backup that allows treatments to continue when the patient is moved. **A.** Diapact CRRT System, B-Braun Medical, Inc., Bethlehem, PA. **B.** PRISMA, Gambro Corporation, Lakewood, CO. **C.** System One, NxStage Medical Inc., Lawrence, MA.

 Continuous Venovenous Hemodialysis

Continuous venovenous hemodialysis (CVVHD) is similar to CVVH. Blood is pumped from a double-lumen venous catheter through a hemofilter and returned to the patient through the same catheter. In addition to the benefits of **ultrafiltration**, CVVHD uses a concentration gradient to facilitate the removal of uremic toxins and fluid by adding a dialysate solution into the circuit. A dual-lumen venous catheter is required; hemodynamic effects are usually mild; and critical care nurses can set up, initiate, maintain, and terminate the system with the support of the nephrology nursing staff.

Peritoneal Dialysis

The goals of PD are to remove toxic substances and metabolic wastes and to reestablish normal fluid and electrolyte balance. PD may be the treatment of choice for patients with kidney disease who are unable or unwilling to undergo hemodialysis or kidney transplantation. Patients who are susceptible to the rapid fluid, electrolyte, and metabolic changes that occur during hemodialysis experience fewer of these problems with the slower rate of PD. Therefore, patients with diabetes or cardiovascular disease, many older patients, and those who may be at risk for adverse effects of systemic heparin are likely candidates for PD. In addition, severe hypertension, heart failure, and pulmonary edema not responsive to usual treatment regimens have been successfully treated with PD. Fewer than 8% of patients with ESKD receive PD as their treatment modality (USRDS, 2015).

In PD, the peritoneal membrane that covers the abdominal organs and lines the abdominal wall serves as the semipermeable membrane. A sterile dextrose dialysate fluid is introduced into the peritoneal cavity through an abdominal catheter at established intervals (see Fig. 54-7). Once the

Figure 54-7 • In peritoneal dialysis and in acute intermittent peritoneal dialysis, dialysate is infused into the peritoneal cavity by gravity, after which the clamp on the infusion line is closed. After a dwell time (when the dialysate is in the peritoneal cavity), the drainage tube is unclamped and the fluid drains from the peritoneal cavity, again by gravity. A new container of dialysate is infused as soon as drainage is complete. The duration of the dwell time depends on the type of peritoneal dialysis.

sterile solution is in the peritoneal cavity, uremic toxins such as urea and creatinine begin to be cleared from the blood. Diffusion and osmosis occur as waste products move from an area of higher concentration (the bloodstream) to an area of lesser concentration (the dialysate fluid) through a semipermeable membrane (the peritoneum). This movement of solute from the blood into the dialysate fluid is called clearance. Because substances cross the peritoneal membrane at different rates, adjustments in solution dwell time in the peritoneal cavity and amount of fluid used are made to facilitate the process. **Ultrafiltration** (water removal) occurs in PD through an osmotic gradient created by using a dialysate fluid with a higher glucose concentration than the blood.

Procedure

As with other forms of treatment, the decision to begin PD is made by the patient and family in consultation with the primary provider. The patient may be acutely ill, thus requiring short-term treatment to correct severe disturbances in fluid and electrolyte status, or may have ESKD and need to receive ongoing treatments.

Preparing the Patient

The nurse's preparation of the patient and family for PD depends on the patient's physical and psychological status, level of alertness, previous experience with dialysis, and understanding of and familiarity with the procedure.

The nurse explains the procedure to the patient and assists in obtaining signed consent for insertion of the catheter. Baseline vital signs, weight, and serum electrolyte levels are recorded. Evaluation of the abdomen for placement of the catheter is done to facilitate self-care. Typically, the catheter is placed on the nondominant side to allow the patient easier access to the catheter connection site when exchanges are done. The patient is encouraged to empty the bladder and bowel to reduce the risk of puncture of internal organs during the insertion procedure. Broad-spectrum antibiotic agents may be given to prevent infection. The peritoneal catheter can be inserted in interventional radiology, in the operating room, or at the bedside. Depending on the situation, this will need to be explained to the patient and family.

Preparing the Equipment

In addition to assembling the equipment for PD, the nurse consults with the physician to determine the concentration of dialysate to be used and the medications to be added. Heparin may be added to prevent fibrin formation and resultant occlusion of the peritoneal catheter. Potassium chloride may be prescribed to prevent hypokalemia. Antibiotic agents may be added to treat **peritonitis** (inflammation of the peritoneal membrane) caused by infection. Regular insulin may be added for patients with diabetes due to the high dextrose concentration of the PD solution. Aseptic technique is imperative whenever medications are added to the PD solution.

Before medications are added, the dialysate is warmed to body temperature to prevent patient discomfort and abdominal pain and to dilate the vessels of the peritoneum to increase urea clearance. Solutions that are too cold cause pain, cramping, and vasoconstriction and reduce clearance. Dry heating (heating cabinet, incubator, or heating pad) is recommended.

Methods not recommended include soaking the bags of solution in warm water (can introduce bacteria to the exterior of the bags of solution and increase the chance of peritonitis) and the use of a microwave oven to heat the fluid (increases the danger of burning the peritoneum).

Immediately before initiating dialysis, using aseptic technique, the nurse assembles the administration set and tubing. The tubing is filled with the prepared dialysate to reduce the amount of air entering the catheter and peritoneal cavity, which could increase abdominal discomfort and interfere with instillation and drainage of the fluid.

Inserting the Catheter

Ideally, the peritoneal catheter is inserted in the operating room or radiology suite to maintain surgical asepsis and minimize the risk of contamination. Catheters for long-term use are usually soft and flexible and made of silicone with a radiopaque strip to permit visualization on x-ray. These catheters have three sections: (1) an intraperitoneal section, with numerous openings and an open tip to allow dialysate to flow freely; (2) a subcutaneous section that passes from the peritoneal membrane and tunnels through muscle and subcutaneous fat to the skin; and (3) an external section for connection to the dialysate and tubing system. Most of these catheters have 2 cuffs made of Dacron polyester. The cuffs stabilize the catheter, limit movement, prevent leaks, and provide a barrier against microorganisms. One cuff is placed just distal to the peritoneum, and the other cuff is placed subcutaneously. The subcutaneous tunnel (5 to 10 cm long) further protects against bacterial infection (see Fig. 54-8).

Performing the Exchange

PD involves a series of exchanges or cycles. An **exchange** is the entire cycle including the infusion (fill), dwell, and drainage of the dialysate. This cycle is repeated throughout the course of the dialysis. The dialysate is infused by gravity into the peritoneal cavity. A period of about 5 to 10 minutes is usually required to infuse 2 to 3 L of fluid. The prescribed dwell, or equilibration, time allows diffusion and osmosis to occur. At the end of the dwell time, the drainage portion of the exchange begins. The tube is unclamped, and the solution drains from the peritoneal cavity by gravity through a closed system. Drainage is usually completed in 10 to 20 minutes. The drainage fluid is normally colorless or straw colored and should not be cloudy. Bloody drainage may be seen in the first few exchanges after insertion of a new catheter but should not occur after that time. The number of cycles or exchanges and their frequency are prescribed based on monthly laboratory values and the presence of uremic symptoms. The exchanges can be performed manually during the waking hours by the patient (continuous ambulatory peritoneal dialysis [CAPD]) or via the use of a PD machine (cycler) that automatically performs exchanges, usually while the patient is sleeping at night (continuous cycling peritoneal dialysis [CCPD]).

The removal of excess water during PD occurs because dialysate has a high dextrose concentration, making it hypertonic. An osmotic gradient is created between the blood and the dialysate solution. Dextrose solutions of 1.5%, 2.5%, and 4.25% are available in several volumes, from 1000 to 3000 mL. The higher the dextrose concentration, the greater the osmotic gradient and the more water will be

Figure 54-8 • Continuous ambulatory peritoneal dialysis. **A.** The peritoneal catheter is implanted through the abdominal wall. **B.** Dacron cuffs and a subcutaneous tunnel provide protection against bacterial infection. **C.** Dialysate flows by gravity through the peritoneal catheter into the peritoneal cavity. After a prescribed period of time, the fluid is drained by gravity and discarded. New solution is then infused into the peritoneal cavity until the next drainage period. Dialysis thus continues on a 24-hour-a-day basis, during which the patient is free to move around and engage in their usual activities.

removed. Selection of the appropriate solution is based on the patient's fluid status.

Complications

Most complications of PD are often minor; however, several, if unattended, can have serious consequences.

Acute Complications

Peritonitis

Peritonitis is the most common and serious complication of PD. The first sign of peritonitis is cloudy dialysate drainage fluid. Diffuse abdominal pain and rebound tenderness occur much later. Hypotension and other signs of shock may also occur with advancing infection. The patient with peritonitis may be treated as an inpatient or outpatient (most common), depending on the severity of the infection and the patient's clinical status. Drainage fluid is examined for cell count; Gram stain and culture are used to identify the organism and guide treatment. Antibiotic agents (aminoglycosides or cephalosporins) are usually added to subsequent exchanges until Gram stain or culture results are available for appropriate antibiotic determination. Intraperitoneal administration of antibiotic agents is as effective as IV administration and therefore most often used. Antibiotic therapy continues for 10 to 14 days (Figueiredo, 2014). Careful selection and calculation of the antibiotic dosage are needed to prevent nephrotoxicity and further compromise of residual renal function.

Regardless of the organism causing peritonitis, the patient loses large amounts of protein through the peritoneum. Acute malnutrition and delayed healing may result. Therefore, attention must be given to detecting and promptly treating peritonitis.

Leakage

Leakage of dialysate through the catheter site may occur immediately after the catheter is inserted. Usually, the leak stops spontaneously if dialysis is withheld for several days, giving the tissue surrounding the cuffs located on the abdominal catheter a chance to infiltrate the Dacron and seal the insertion tunnel. It also allows the exit site time to heal. During this time, it is important to reduce factors that might delay healing, such as undue abdominal muscle activity and straining during bowel movement. In many cases, leakage can be avoided by using small volumes (500 mL) of dialysate, gradually increasing the volume up to 2000 to 3000 mL.

Bleeding

A bloody **effluent** (drainage) may be observed occasionally, especially in young, menstruating women. (The hypertonic fluid pulls blood from the uterus, through the opening in the fallopian tubes, and into the peritoneal cavity.) Bleeding is also common during the first few exchanges after a new catheter insertion because some blood enters the abdominal cavity following insertion. In many cases, no cause can be found for the bleeding, although catheter displacement from the pelvis has occasionally been associated with bleeding. Some patients have had bloody effluent after an enema or from minor trauma. Most often, bleeding stops in 1 to 2 days and requires no specific intervention. More frequent exchanges and the addition of heparin to the dialysate during this time may be necessary to prevent blood clots from obstructing the catheter.

Long-Term Complications

Hypertriglyceridemia is common in patients undergoing long-term PD, suggesting that the therapy may accelerate atherogenesis. Cardiovascular disease is the leading cause of morbidity and mortality in patients with kidney failure, and many patients have suboptimal blood pressure control. Beta-blockers and ACE inhibitors should be used to control hypertension or protect the heart, and the use of aspirin and statins should be considered (James, Oparil, Carter, et al., 2014).

Other complications that may occur with long-term PD include abdominal hernias (incisional, inguinal, diaphragmatic, and umbilical), probably resulting from continuously increased intra-abdominal pressure. The persistently elevated intra-abdominal pressure also aggravates symptoms of hiatal hernia and hemorrhoids. Low back pain and anorexia from fluid in the abdomen and a constant sweet taste related to glucose absorption may also occur.

Mechanical problems occasionally occur and may interfere with instillation or drainage of the dialysate. Formation of clots in the peritoneal catheter and constipation are factors that may contribute to these problems.

Approaches

PD can be performed using several different approaches: acute intermittent peritoneal dialysis, CAPD, and CCPD.

Acute Intermittent Peritoneal Dialysis

Indications for acute intermittent PD, a variation of PD, include uremic signs and symptoms (nausea, vomiting, fatigue, altered mental status), fluid overload, acidosis, and hyperkalemia. Although PD is not as efficient as hemodialysis in removing solute and fluid, it permits a more gradual change in the patient's fluid volume status and in waste product removal. Therefore, it may be the treatment of choice for the hemodynamically unstable patient. It can be carried out manually (the nurse warms, spikes, and hangs each container of dialysate) or by a cycler machine. Exchange times range from 30 minutes to 2 hours. One routine is hourly exchanges consisting of a 10-minute infusion, a 30-minute dwell time, and a 20-minute drain time (Figueiredo, 2014).

Maintaining the PD cycle is a nursing responsibility. Aseptic technique is maintained when changing solution containers and emptying drainage containers. Vital signs, weight, I&O, laboratory values, and patient status are frequently monitored. The nurse uses a flow sheet or the electronic medical record to document each exchange and records vital signs, dialysate concentration, medications added, exchange volume, dwell time, dialysate fluid balance for each exchange (fluid lost or gained), and cumulative fluid balance. The nurse also carefully assesses skin turgor and mucous membranes to evaluate fluid status and monitor the patient for edema.

> ### ▶ Quality and Safety Nursing Alert
>
> *If the peritoneal fluid does not drain properly, the nurse can facilitate drainage by turning the patient from side to side or raising the head of the bed. The catheter should never be pushed further into the peritoneal cavity.*

Other measures to promote drainage include checking the patency of the catheter by inspecting for kinks, closed clamps, or an air lock. The nurse monitors for complications, including peritonitis, bleeding, respiratory difficulty, and leakage of peritoneal fluid. Abdominal girth may be measured periodically to determine if the patient is retaining large amounts of dialysis solution. In addition, the nurse must ensure that the PD catheter remains secure and that the dressing remains dry. Physical comfort measures, frequent turning, and skin care are provided. The patient and family are educated about the procedure and are kept informed about progress (fluid loss, weight loss, laboratory values). Emotional support and encouragement are given to the patient and family during this stressful and uncertain time.

Continuous Ambulatory Peritoneal Dialysis

Continuous Ambulatory Peritoneal Dialysis (CAPD) is the second most common form of dialysis for patients with ESKD (USRDS, 2015). CAPD is performed at home by the patient or a trained caregiver who is usually a family member. The procedure allows the patient reasonable freedom and control of daily activities but requires a serious commitment to be successful. Chart 54-10 discusses suitability for CAPD.

CAPD works on the same principles as other forms of PD: diffusion and osmosis. Less extreme fluctuations in the patient's laboratory values occur with CAPD than with intermittent PD or hemodialysis because the dialysis is constantly in progress. The serum electrolyte levels usually remain in the normal range.

Procedure

The patient performs exchanges 4 or 5 times a day, 24 hours a day, 7 days a week, at intervals scheduled throughout the day. Different manufacturers supply different equipment. A Y-shaped system is most commonly used, in which a bag containing dialysate solution comes connected to one branch of the "Y" and a sterile empty bag is connected to the second branch. This leaves the third part of the "Y" open and available for connection to the transfer set on the PD catheter. To perform an exchange, the patient (or person doing the exchange) washes their hands, dons a mask, and then removes the cap from the transfer set while maintaining sterility. The open end of the "Y" set is connected to the end of the transfer set and the dialysate infused where it will dwell. After the dialysate is infused, the patient clamps off the transfer set and the tubing set, disconnects the tubing set, and applies a new cap to the transfer set, making it a closed system. The patient drains the fluid (effluent) from the peritoneal cavity through the catheter (over about 20 to 30 minutes) into an empty bag. Once the effluent has been fully drained, fresh fluid is instilled into the peritoneal cavity.

The longer the dwell time, the better the clearance of uremic toxins. If dwell time is excessive, the patient will absorb some of the effluent back into the body simply because the osmotic gradient is lost. Once equilibrium is reached, the movement of fluid and toxins stops.

Complications

To reduce the risk of peritonitis, the patient (and all caregivers) must use meticulous care to avoid contaminating the catheter, fluid, or tubing and to avoid accidentally disconnecting the catheter from the tubing. Whenever a connection or disconnection is made, hand hygiene must be used and a mask worn by anyone within 6 ft of the area to avoid contamination with airborne bacteria. Excess manipulation

| Chart 54-10 | Considerations in Continuous Ambulatory Peritoneal Dialysis |

Although continuous ambulatory peritoneal dialysis (CAPD) is not suitable for all patients with end-stage kidney disease (ESKD), it is a viable therapy for those who can perform self-care and fluid exchanges and fit therapy into their own routines. Often, patients report having more energy and feeling healthier once they begin CAPD. Nurses can be instrumental in helping patients with ESKD find the dialysis therapy that best suits their lifestyle. Those considering CAPD need to understand the advantages and disadvantages along with the indications and contraindications for this form of therapy.

Advantages

- Freedom from a hemodialysis machine
- Control over daily activities
- Opportunities to eat a more liberal diet than allowed with hemodialysis, increase fluid intake, raise serum hematocrit values, improve blood pressure control, avoid venipuncture, and gain a sense of well-being

Disadvantages

- Continuous dialysis 24 hours a day, 7 days a week
- Dietary alterations related to protein and potassium losses. Patients may be encouraged to increase the intake of protein and potassium in the diet due to these losses with peritoneal dialysis fluid exchanges

Indications

- Patient's willingness, motivation, and ability to perform dialysis at home
- Strong family or community support system (essential for success), particularly if the patient is an older adult
- Special problems with long-term hemodialysis, such as dysfunctional or failing vascular access devices, excessive thirst, severe hypertension, postdialysis headaches, and severe anemia requiring frequent transfusion
- Interim therapy while awaiting kidney transplantation
- ESKD secondary to diabetes because hypertension, uremia, and hyperglycemia are easier to manage with CAPD than with hemodialysis

Contraindications

- Adhesions from previous surgery (adhesions reduce clearance of solutes) or systemic inflammatory disease
- Chronic backache and pre-existing disc disease, which could be aggravated by the continuous pressure of dialysis fluid in the abdomen
- Severe arthritis or poor hand strength necessitating assistance in performing the exchange. However, patients who are blind or partially blind and those with other physical limitations can learn to perform CAPD

should be avoided, and meticulous care of the catheter entry site is provided using a standardized protocol.

Continuous Cyclic Peritoneal Dialysis

Continuous cyclic peritoneal dialysis (CCPD) uses a machine called a cycler to provide the fluid exchanges. It is programmed to deliver an established amount of PD solution that will dwell in the peritoneal cavity for a programmed period of time before it drains from the peritoneal cavity via gravity. The cycler is also set to deliver a specific number of fluid changes in a designated period of time. Because it is programmed, it also keeps track of the total amounts removed and will sound an alarm if limits are not met. It requires that a person set up and break down the system for use, which typically takes about 15 minutes.

CCPD combines overnight intermittent PD with a prolonged dwell time during the day. The peritoneal catheter is connected to a cycler machine every evening, usually just before the patient goes to sleep for the night. Because the machine is very quiet, the patient can sleep, and the extra-long tubing allows the patient to move and turn normally during sleep.

In the morning, the patient disconnects from the cycler. Sometimes, dialysate is left in the abdominal cavity for a longer day dwell cycle. This day exchange is drained during the day either by using a "Y" set or reattaching to the cycler. This process is done every day to achieve the effects of dialysis required.

CCPD has a lower infection rate than other forms of PD because there are fewer opportunities for contamination with bag changes and tubing disconnections (Hain & Chan, 2013). It also allows the patient to be free from exchanges throughout the day, making it possible to engage in work and activities of daily living more freely.

Nursing Management

Meeting Psychosocial Needs

In addition to the complications of PD described previously, patients who elect to do PD may experience altered body image because of the presence of the abdominal catheter, bag, tubing, and cycler. Waist size increases from 1 to 2 inches (or more) with fluid in the abdomen. This affects clothing selection and may make the patient feel "fat." Body image may be threatened if patients do not want to look at or care for the catheter. The nurse may arrange for the patient to talk with other patients who have adapted well to PD. Although some patients have no psychological problems with the catheter—they think of it as their lifeline and as a life-sustaining device—other patients feel they are doing exchanges all day long and have no free time, particularly in the beginning. They may experience depression because they feel crushed with the responsibility of self-care.

Patients undergoing PD may also experience altered sexuality patterns and sexual dysfunction. The patient and partner may be reluctant to engage in sexual activities, partly because of the catheter being psychologically "in the way" of sexual performance. The peritoneal catheter, drainage bag, and about 2 L of dialysate may interfere with the patient's sexual function and body image as well. In patients on CCPD, the presence of the dialysis cycler in the bedroom and the continual connection during the sleeping hours can also cause interference with intimacy. Although these problems may resolve with time, some problems may warrant special counseling. Questions by the nurse about concerns related to sexuality and sexual function often provide the patient with a welcome opportunity to discuss these issues and a first step toward their resolution.

Chart 54-11

HOME CARE CHECKLIST

Peritoneal Dialysis, Continuous Ambulatory Peritoneal Dialysis, or Continuous Cycling Peritoneal Dialysis

At the completion of education, the patient and/or caregiver will be able to:

- Discuss kidney disease and its effects on the body.
- State the goal and purpose of dialysis and its impact on physiologic functioning, ADLs, IADLs, roles, relationships, and spirituality.
- Describe the basic principles of peritoneal dialysis (PD) and exchange options such as continuous ambulatory peritoneal dialysis (CAPD), or continuous cycling peritoneal dialysis (CCPD).
- State what types of changes are needed (if any) to support home PD therapy and maintain a clean home environment and prevent infection.
- State how to contact the primary provider, the team of home care professionals overseeing care, and supply vendor.
  - Discuss ordering, storage, and inventory of dialysis supplies.
  - List emergency phone numbers.
- State the name, dose, side effects, frequency, and schedule for all medications.
  - Demonstrate procedure for adding medications to the dialysis solution.
- Demonstrate catheter and exit site care.
- Demonstrate measurement of vital signs and weight measurement.
- Discuss monitoring and management of fluid balance.
- Discuss basic principles of aseptic technique.

- Demonstrate the CAPD or CCPD exchange procedure using aseptic technique (patients receiving CCPD should also demonstrate exchange procedure in case of failure or unavailability of cycling machine) and discuss cycling machine warning signals and how to address these signals.
- Demonstrate maintenance of home dialysis records.
- Demonstrate procedure for obtaining sterile peritoneal dialysis fluid samples.
- Discuss routine laboratory tests needed and implications of results.
- Discuss high protein diet and diet to avoid constipation, any other dietary restrictions as indicated.
- Discuss complications of peritoneal dialysis; prevention, recognition, and management of complications.
- Describe actions in case of emergency.
- Relate how to reach primary provider with questions or complications.
- State time and date of follow-up medical appointments, therapy, and testing.
- Coordinate financial arrangements for peritoneal dialysis and strategies to identify and obtain resources.
- Identify sources of support (e.g., friends, relatives, faith community, support groups, caregiver support).
- Identify the need for health promotion, disease prevention, and screening activities.

ADL, activities of daily living; IADL, independent activities of daily living.

Promoting Home, Community-Based, and Transitional Care

Educating Patients About Self-Care

Patients are educated as inpatients or outpatients to perform PD once their condition is medically stable. Education usually takes 5 days to 2 weeks. Patients are taught according to their own learning ability and knowledge level and only as much at one time as they can handle without feeling uncomfortable or becoming saturated. Education topics for the patient and family who will be performing PD at home are described in Chart 54-11. The use of an adult learning theory–based curriculum may decrease peritonitis and exit site infection rates (Hain & Chan, 2013).

Because of protein loss with continuous PD, the patient is instructed to eat a high-protein, nutritious diet. The patient is also encouraged to increase their daily fiber intake to help prevent constipation, which can impede the flow of dialysate into or out of the peritoneal cavity. Many patients gain 3 to 5 lb within a month of initiating PD, so they may be asked to limit their carbohydrate intake to avoid excessive weight gain. Potassium, sodium, and fluid restrictions are not usually needed. Patients commonly lose about 2 to 3 L of fluid over and above the volume of dialysate infused into the abdomen during a 24-hour period, permitting a normal fluid intake even in a patient who is anephric (a patient without kidneys).

Continuing and Transitional Care

Follow-up care through phone calls, visits to the dialysis clinic, outpatient department, and continuing home care assists patients in the transition to home and promotes their active participation in their own health care. Patients often check with the nurse to see if they are making the correct choices about dialysate or control of blood pressure, or simply to discuss a problem.

Patients may be seen by the PD team as outpatients once a month or more often if needed. The exchange procedure is evaluated at that time to see that strict aseptic technique is being used. Blood chemistry values are followed closely to make certain the therapy is adequate for the patient.

If a referral is made for home care, the home care nurse assesses the home environment and suggests modifications to accommodate the equipment and facilities needed to carry out PD. In addition, the nurse assesses the patient's and family's understanding of PD and evaluates their technique in performing PD. Assessments include checking for changes related to kidney disease; complications such as peritonitis; and treatment-related problems such as heart failure, inadequate drainage, and weight gain or loss. The nurse continues to reinforce and clarify education about PD and ESKD and assesses the patient's and family's progress in coping with the procedure. This is also an opportunity to remind patients about the need to participate in appropriate health promotion activities and health screening (e.g., gynecologic examinations, colonoscopy).

Special Considerations: Nursing Management of the Patient on Dialysis Who Is Hospitalized

Whether undergoing hemodialysis or PD, the patient may be hospitalized for treatment of complications related to the dialysis treatment, the underlying kidney disorder, or health problems not related to renal dysfunction or its treatment.

Protecting Vascular Access

When the patient undergoing hemodialysis is hospitalized for any reason, care must be taken to protect the vascular access. The nurse assesses the vascular access for patency and takes precautions to ensure that the extremity with the vascular access is not used for measuring blood pressure or for obtaining blood specimens; tight dressings, restraints, or jewelry over the vascular access must be avoided as well (Arslanian, 2015).

The bruit, or "thrill," over the venous access site must be evaluated at least every shift. Absence of a palpable thrill or audible bruit may indicate blockage or clotting in the vascular access. Clotting can occur if the patient has an infection anywhere in the body (serum viscosity increases) or if the blood pressure has dropped. When blood flow is reduced through the access for any reason (hypotension, application of blood pressure cuff or tourniquet), the access can clot. If a patient has a hemodialysis catheter or implanted hemodialysis access device, the nurse must observe for signs and symptoms of infection such as redness, swelling, drainage from the exit site, fever, and chills. The nurse must assess the integrity of the dressing and change it as needed. Patients with kidney disease are more prone to infection; therefore, appropriate infection control measures must be used for all procedures. The patient's vascular access device should not be used for any purpose other than dialysis, unless it is an emergency situation and no other access is available. In this situation, a dialysis nurse or physician should cannulate the vascular access.

Taking Precautions During Intravenous Therapy

When the patient needs IV therapy, the rate of administration must be as slow as possible. Accurate I&O records are essential.

Quality and Safety Nursing Alert

Because patients on dialysis cannot excrete water, rapid administration of IV fluid can result in pulmonary edema.

Monitoring Symptoms of Uremia

As metabolic end products accumulate, symptoms of uremia worsen. Patients whose metabolic rate accelerates (those receiving corticosteroid medications or parenteral nutrition, those with infections or bleeding disorders, those undergoing surgery) accumulate waste products more quickly and may require daily dialysis. These same patients are more likely than other patients receiving dialysis to experience complications.

Detecting Cardiac and Respiratory Complications

Cardiac and respiratory assessment must be conducted frequently. As fluid builds up, fluid overload, heart failure, and pulmonary edema develop. Crackles in the bases of the lungs may indicate pulmonary edema.

Pericarditis may result from the accumulation of uremic toxins. If not detected and treated promptly, this serious complication may progress to pericardial effusion and cardiac tamponade. Pericarditis is detected by the patient's report of substernal chest pain (if the patient can communicate), low-grade fever, and pericardial friction rub. A pulsus paradoxus (a decrease in blood pressure of more than 10 mmHg during inspiration) is often present. When pericarditis progresses to effusion, the friction rub disappears, heart sounds become distant and muffled, ECG waves show very low voltage, and the pulsus paradoxus worsens (Yamamoto, Shoji, Yamakawa, et al., 2015).

The effusion may progress to life-threatening cardiac tamponade, noted by narrowing of the pulse pressure in addition to muffled or inaudible heart sounds, crushing chest pain, dyspnea, and hypotension.

Quality and Safety Nursing Alert

Although pericarditis, pericardial effusion, and cardiac tamponade can be detected by chest x-ray, they should also be detected through astute nursing assessment. Because of their clinical significance, assessment of the patient for these complications is a priority.

Controlling Electrolyte Levels and Diet

Electrolyte alterations are common, and potassium changes can be life threatening. All IV solutions and medications to be given are evaluated for their electrolyte content. Serum laboratory values are assessed daily. If blood transfusions are required, they may be given during hemodialysis, if possible, so that excess potassium can be removed and hypervolemia is avoided. Dietary intake must also be monitored. The patient's frustrations related to dietary restrictions typically increase if the food is unappetizing. The nurse needs to recognize that this may lead to dietary indiscretion and hyperkalemia.

Hypoalbuminemia is an indicator of malnutrition in patients undergoing long-term or maintenance dialysis. Although some patients can be treated with adequate nutrition alone, some patients remain hypoalbuminemic for reasons that are poorly understood.

Managing Discomfort and Pain

Complications such as pruritus and pain secondary to neuropathy must be managed. Antihistamine agents, such as diphenhydramine (Benadryl), are commonly used, and analgesic medications may be prescribed. However, because elimination of the metabolites of medications occurs through dialysis rather than through renal excretion, medication dosages may need to be adjusted. Keeping the skin clean and well moisturized using bath oils, superfatted soap, and creams or lotions helps promote comfort and reduce itching. Instructing the patient to keep the nails trimmed to avoid scratching and excoriation also promotes comfort.

Monitoring Blood Pressure

Hypertension in kidney disease is common. It is usually the result of fluid overload and, in part, oversecretion of renin. Many patients undergoing dialysis receive some form of antihypertensive therapy. Patients require detailed education and reinforcement of information regarding their antihypertensive regimen, because it is not uncommon for patients to need more than one antihypertensive agent. Rapid fluid fluctuations in patients receiving dialysis also create challenges to maintaining blood pressure control. Antihypertensive agents must be withheld before dialysis to avoid hypotension due to the combined effect of fluid removal with the dialysis treatment and the medication (Doss-McQuitty, 2014).

Typically, these patients require single or multiple antihypertensive agents to achieve normal blood pressure, thus adding to the total number of medications needed on an ongoing basis (James et al., 2014).

Preventing Infection

Patients with ESKD commonly have low WBC counts (and decreased phagocytic ability), low RBC counts (anemia), and impaired platelet function. Together, these pose a high risk of infection and potential for bleeding after even minor trauma. Preventing and controlling infection are essential because the incidence of infection is high. Infection of the vascular access site and pneumonia are common.

Caring for the Catheter Site

Patients receiving CAPD usually know how to care for the catheter site; however, the hospital stay is an opportunity to assess catheter care technique and correct misperceptions or deviations from recommended technique. Recommended daily or 3 or 4 times-weekly routine catheter site care is typically performed during showering or bathing (Hain & Chan, 2013). The exit site should not be submerged in bathwater. The most common cleaning method is soap and water; liquid soap is recommended. During care, the nurse and patient need to make sure that the catheter remains secure to avoid tension and trauma. The patient may wear a gauze or semitransparent dressing over the exit site.

Administering Medications

All medications and the dosage prescribed for any patient on dialysis must be closely monitored to avoid those that are toxic to the kidneys and may threaten remaining renal function. Medications are also scrutinized for potassium and magnesium content; those medications that contain them are avoided. Care must be taken to evaluate all problems and symptoms that the patient reports without automatically attributing them to kidney disease or to dialysis therapy.

Providing Psychological Support

Patients undergoing dialysis for a while may begin to reevaluate their status, the treatment modality, their satisfaction with life, and the impact of these factors on their families and support systems. Nurses must provide opportunities for these patients to express their feelings and reactions and to explore options. The decision to begin dialysis does not require that dialysis be continued indefinitely, and it is not uncommon for patients to consider discontinuing treatment. These feelings and reactions must be taken seriously, and the patient should have the opportunity to discuss them with the dialysis team as well as with a psychologist, psychiatrist, psychiatric nurse, trusted friend, or spiritual advisor. The patient's informed decision about discontinuing treatment, after thoughtful deliberation, should be respected.

KIDNEY SURGERY

A patient may undergo surgery to remove obstructions that affect the kidney (tumors or calculi), to insert a tube for draining the kidney (nephrostomy, ureterostomy), or to remove the kidney involved in unilateral kidney disease, renal carcinoma, or kidney transplantation.

Management of Patients Undergoing Kidney Surgery

Preoperative Considerations

Surgery is performed only after a thorough evaluation of renal function. Patient preparation to ensure that optimal renal function is maintained is essential. Fluids are encouraged to promote increased excretion of waste products before surgery unless contraindicated because of pre-existing renal or cardiac dysfunction. If kidney infection is present preoperatively, broad-spectrum antimicrobial agents may be prescribed to prevent bacteremia. Antibiotic agents must be given with extreme care because many are toxic to the kidneys. Coagulation studies (prothrombin time, partial thromboplastin time, platelet count) may be indicated if the patient has a history of bruising and bleeding. The preoperative preparation is similar to that described in Chapter 17.

Because many patients facing kidney surgery are apprehensive, the nurse encourages the patient to recognize and verbalize concerns. Confidence is reinforced by establishing a relationship of trust and by providing expert care. Patients faced with the prospect of losing a kidney may think that they will have to depend on dialysis for the rest of their lives. The nurse reassures the patient and family that normal function may be maintained by a single healthy kidney.

Perioperative Concerns

Kidney surgery requires various patient positions to expose the surgical site adequately. Three surgical approaches are common: flank, lumbar, and thoracoabdominal (see Fig. 54-9). During surgery, plans are carried out for managing altered urinary drainage. These may include inserting a nephrostomy or other drainage tube.

Postoperative Management

Because the kidney is a highly vascular organ, hemorrhage and shock are the chief potential complications of kidney surgery. Fluid and blood component replacement is frequently necessary in the immediate postoperative period to treat intraoperative blood loss.

Abdominal distention and paralytic ileus are fairly common after renal and ureteral surgery and are thought to be due to a reflex paralysis of intestinal peristalsis and manipulation of

Figure 54-9 • Patient positioning and incisional approaches—flank (**A**), lumbar (**B**), thoracoabdominal (**C**)—for kidney surgery are associated with significant postoperative discomfort.

A Flank approach   **B** Lumbar approach   **C** Thoracoabdominal approach

the colon or duodenum during surgery. Abdominal distention is relieved by decompression through a nasogastric tube. See Chapter 48 for treatment of paralytic ileus. Oral fluids are permitted when the passage of flatus is noted.

If infection occurs, antibiotics are prescribed after a culture reveals the causative organism. The toxic effects that antibiotic agents have on the kidneys (nephrotoxicity) must be kept in mind when assessing the patient. Low-dose heparin therapy may be initiated postoperatively to prevent thromboembolism in patients who have had any type of urologic surgery.

Nursing Management

In addition to those interventions listed in this section, Chart 54-12 provides a plan of nursing care for the patient undergoing kidney surgery.

(*text continued on page 1606*)

Chart 54-12

PLAN OF NURSING CARE

Care of the Patient Undergoing Kidney Surgery

NURSING DIAGNOSIS: Ineffective airway clearance related to pain of high abdominal or flank incision, abdominal discomfort, and immobility; risk for ineffective breathing pattern related to high abdominal incision

GOAL: Improved airway clearance

Nursing Interventions	Rationale	Expected Outcomes

1. Assess respiratory status:
   a. Rate
   b. Breath sounds
	1. Baseline data allow for monitoring of changes and evaluating effectiveness of interventions.	• Exhibits respiratory rate of 12–18 breaths/min and normal breath sounds without adventitious sounds

2. Administer analgesic agent as prescribed.	2. Adequate pain relief enables patient to take deep breaths and cough.	• Takes deep breaths and coughs adequately when encouraged and assisted sounds
3. Splint incision with hands or pillow to assist patient in coughing.	3. Splints incision and promotes adequate cough and prevention of atelectasis.	• Exhibits full thoracic excursion without shallow respirations
4. Assist patient to change positions frequently.	4. Promotes drainage and inflation of all lobes of the lungs.	• Uses incentive spirometer with encouragement
5. Encourage the use of incentive spirometer if indicated or prescribed.	5. Encourages adequate deep breaths.	• Splints incision while taking deep breaths and coughing
6. Assist with and encourage early ambulation.	6. Mobilizes pulmonary secretions.	• Reports progressively less pain and discomfort with coughing and deep breaths

NURSING DIAGNOSIS: Acute pain and discomfort related to surgical incision, positioning, and stretching of muscles during kidney surgery

GOAL: Relief of pain and discomfort

Nursing Interventions	Rationale	Expected Outcomes
1. Assess level of pain.	1. Provides baseline for later evaluation of pain relief strategies.	• Reports relief of severe pain and discomfort
2. Administer analgesic agents as prescribed.	2. Promotes pain relief.	• Takes analgesia as prescribed

(*continued on page 1604*)

Chart 54-12 **PLAN OF NURSING CARE** (Continued)

Care of the Patient Undergoing Kidney Surgery

Nursing Interventions	Rationale	Expected Outcomes
3. Splint incision with hands or pillow during movement or deep breathing and coughing exercises.	3. Minimizes sensation of pulling or tension on incision and provides sense of support to the patient.	• Exercises aching muscles within recommendations
4. Assist and encourage early ambulation.	4. Promotes resumption of muscle activity exercise.	• Uses distraction, relaxation exercises, and imagery to relieve pain
5. Offer and educate patient how to use appropriate nonpharmacologic interventions.	5. Many nonpharmacologic interventions, such as distraction, relaxation exercises, and imagery assist patients to decrease their pain.	• Exhibits no behavioral manifestations of pain and discomfort (e.g., restlessness, perspiration, verbal expressions of pain)
		• Participates in deep-breathing and coughing exercises
		• Gradually increases physical activity and exercise

NURSING DIAGNOSIS: Fear and anxiety related to diagnosis, outcome of surgery, and alteration in urinary function
GOAL: Reduction of fear and anxiety

Nursing Interventions	Rationale	Expected Outcomes
1. Assess patient's anxiety and fear before surgery if possible.	1. Provides a baseline for postoperative assessment.	• Verbalizes reactions and feelings to staff
2. Assess patient's knowledge about procedure and expected surgical outcome preoperatively.	2. Provides a basis for further education.	• Shares reactions and feelings with family or partner
3. Evaluate the meaning of alterations resulting from surgical procedure for the patient and family or partner.	3. Enables understanding of patient's reactions and responses to expected and unexpected results of surgery.	• Grieves appropriately for self and for changes in role and function
		• Identifies information needed to promote own adaptation and coping
4. Encourage patient to verbalize reactions, feelings, and fears.	4. Affirms patient's understanding of and ultimate resolution of feelings and fears.	• Participates in activities and events in immediate environment
5. Encourage patient to share feelings with spouse or partner.	5. Enables patient and partner to receive mutual support and reduces sense of isolation from each other.	• Accepts visit from support group if indicated
6. Offer and arrange for visit from member of support group (e.g., ostomy group, transplant group, if indicated).	6. Provides support from another person who has encountered the same or a similar surgical procedure and an example of how others have coped with the alteration.	• Identifies support person or support group

NURSING DIAGNOSIS: Impaired urinary elimination related to urinary drainage; risk for infection related to altered urinary drainage
GOAL: Maintenance of urinary elimination; infection-free urinary tract

Nursing Interventions	Rationale	Expected Outcomes
1. Assess urinary drainage system immediately.	1. Provides basis for further assessment and action.	• Exhibits adequate urinary output and patent drainage system
2. Assess adequacy of urinary output and patency of drainage system.	2. Provides baseline.	• Exhibits urinary output consistent with fluid intake
3. Assess pertinent laboratory values (see Table 53-5).	3. Provides basis for further assessment and action.	• Demonstrates normal laboratory values: blood urea nitrogen, serum creatinine levels, urine specific gravity, and osmolality
4. Use asepsis and hand hygiene when providing care and manipulating drainage system.	4. Prevents or reduces risk of contamination of urinary drainage system.	• Exhibits sterile urine on urine culture
5. Maintain closed urinary drainage system.	5. Reduces risk of bacterial contamination and infection.	• Exhibits clear, dilute urine without debris or encrustation in the drainage system
6. If irrigation of the drainage system is necessary, use sterile gloves and sterile irrigating solution and a closed drainage and irrigation system.	6. Permits irrigation when necessary while maintaining closed drainage system, minimizing risk of infection.	• States rationale for avoiding manipulation of catheter, drainage, or irrigation system
7. If irrigation is necessary and prescribed, perform it gently with sterile saline and the prescribed amount of irrigating fluid.	7. Maintains patency of the catheter or drainage system and prevents sudden increases in pressure in the urinary tract that may cause trauma, pressure on sutures or urinary tract structures, and pain.	• Exhibits normal placement of urinary stent or ureteral catheters until removed by physician
		• Maintains closed urinary drainage system

PLAN OF NURSING CARE (Continued)

Care of the Patient Undergoing Kidney Surgery

Chart 54-12

Nursing Interventions	Rationale	Expected Outcomes
8. Assist patient in turning and moving in bed and when ambulating to prevent displacement or inadvertent removal of urinary stent or ureteral catheters if in place.	8. Prevents trauma from accidental displacement of urinary stent or ureteral catheter necessitating repeated instrumentation of the urinary tract (e.g., cystoscopy) to replace them.	• Exhibits normal body temperature without signs or symptoms of urinary tract infection • Cleans catheter with soap and water • Consumes adequate fluid intake (6–8 glasses of water or more per day, unless contraindicated)
9. Observe urine color, volume, odor, and components.	9. Provides information about adequacy of urine output, condition and patency of drainage system, and debris in urine.	• Urinary drainage system remains in place until physician removes or discontinues it • Maintains urinary drainage system without infection or obstruction
10. Minimize trauma and manipulation of catheter, drainage system, and urethra.	10. Reduces risk of contamination of drainage system and eliminates site of bacterial invasion.	• Maintains urinary diversion as instructed • Maintains self-care so that environment is odor free
11. Clean catheter gently with soap during bathing, avoiding any to-and-fro movement of catheter.	11. Removes debris and encrustations without causing trauma to or contamination of urethra.	
12. Anchor drainage tube.	12. Prevents movement or slipping of drainage tube, minimizing trauma to and contamination of urethra or catheter.	
13. Maintain adequate fluid intake.	13. Promotes adequate urine output and prevents urinary stasis.	
14. Assist with and encourage early ambulation while ensuring placement of urinary drainage system.	14. Minimizes cardiovascular and pulmonary complications while preventing loss, dislodging, or disruption of drainage system.	
15. If patient is to be discharged with urinary drainage system (catheter) in place or a urinary diversion, instruct patient and family member in care.	15. Knowledge and understanding of the drainage system or urinary diversion are essential to prevent infection and other complications.	

NURSING DIAGNOSIS: Risk for imbalanced fluid volume related to surgical fluid loss, altered urinary output, parenteral fluid administration

GOAL: Normal fluid balance will be maintained

Nursing Interventions	Rationale	Expected Outcomes
1. Weigh patient daily.	1. Daily weight is the most sensitive indicator of fluid loss or gain.	• Patient's weight will be within 2–3 lb of patient's baseline.
2. Take accurate intake and output measurements.	2. Detects fluid retention due to poor cardiac or renal output.	• Intake that exceeds output will be detected early.
3. Place all parenteral therapy on an infusion pump.	3. Ensures that the patient does not receive excess or insufficient IV fluids.	• The exact amount of solution is infused with no adverse effects resulting from over- or underinfusion.
4. Monitor amount and characteristics of urine.	4. Assists in early detection of possible complications of surgery or tube insertion.	• Urine is clear and absent of blood, pus, or any foreign substances.
5. Monitor vital signs: temperature, pulse, respirations, and blood pressure.	5. When fluid volume or cardiac output is altered, vital signs are affected.	• Temperature, pulse, respiration, and blood pressure are normal. • Normal heart and lung sounds are present.
6. Auscultate heart and lungs every shift.	6. When fluid volume is increased because of poor cardiac or renal output, fluid accumulates in the lungs. In addition, heart sounds change as heart failure develops; frequent auscultation ensures early detection.	

Providing Immediate Postoperative Care

Immediate postoperative care of the patient who has undergone surgery of the kidney includes assessment of all body systems. Respiratory and circulatory status, pain level, fluid and electrolyte status, and patency and adequacy of urinary drainage systems are assessed.

Respiratory Status

As with any surgery, the use of anesthesia increases the risk of respiratory complications. Noting the location of the surgical incision assists the nurse in anticipating respiratory problems and pain. Respiratory status is assessed by monitoring the rate, depth, and pattern of respirations. The location of the incision frequently causes pain on inspiration and coughing; therefore, the patient tends to splint the chest wall and take shallow respirations. Auscultation is performed to assess normal and adventitious breath sounds.

Circulatory Status and Blood Loss

The patient's vital signs and arterial or central venous pressure are monitored. Skin color and temperature and urine output provide information about circulatory status. The surgical incision and drainage tubes are observed frequently to help detect unexpected blood loss and hemorrhage.

Pain

Postoperative pain is a major problem for the patient because of the location of the surgical incision and patient's position on the operating table to permit access to the kidney. The location and severity of pain are assessed before and after analgesic medications are given. Abdominal distention, which increases discomfort, is also noted.

Urinary Drainage

Urine output and drainage from tubes inserted during surgery are monitored for amount, color, and type or characteristics. Decreased or absent drainage is promptly reported to the primary provider because it may indicate obstruction that could cause pain, infection, and disruption of the suture lines.

Monitoring and Managing Potential Complications

Bleeding is a major complication of kidney surgery. If undetected and untreated, it can result in hypovolemia and hemorrhagic shock. The nurse's role is to observe for these complications, to report their signs and symptoms, and to administer prescribed parenteral fluids and blood and blood components. Monitoring of vital signs, skin condition, the urinary drainage system, the surgical incision, and the level of consciousness is necessary to detect evidence of bleeding, decreased circulating blood, and fluid volume and cardiac output. Frequent monitoring of vital signs (initially monitored at least at hourly intervals) and urinary output is necessary for early detection of these complications.

If bleeding goes undetected or is not detected promptly, the patient may lose significant amounts of blood and may experience hypoxemia. In addition to hypovolemic shock due to hemorrhage, this type of blood loss may precipitate a myocardial infarction or transient ischemic attack. Bleeding may be suspected when the patient experiences fatigue and when urine output is less than 0.5 mL/kg/hr. As bleeding persists,

late signs of hypovolemia occur, such as cool skin, flat neck veins, and change in level of consciousness or responsiveness. Transfusions of blood components are indicated, along with surgical repair of the bleeding vessel.

Pneumonia may be prevented through the use of an incentive spirometer, adequate pain control, and early ambulation. Early signs of pneumonia include fever, increased heart and respiratory rates, and adventitious breath sounds.

Preventing infection involves using asepsis when changing dressings and handling and preparing catheters, other drainage tubes, central venous catheters, and IV catheters for administration of fluids. Insertion sites are monitored closely for signs and symptoms of inflammation: redness, drainage, heat, and pain. Special care must be taken to prevent UTI, which is associated with the use of indwelling urinary catheters. Catheters and other invasive tubes are removed as soon as they are no longer needed.

Antibiotics are commonly given postoperatively to prevent infection. If antibiotic agents are prescribed, serum creatinine and BUN values must be monitored closely because many antibiotic agents are toxic to the kidney or can accumulate to toxic levels if renal function is decreased.

Preventing fluid imbalance is critical when caring for a patient undergoing kidney surgery, because both fluid loss and fluid excess are possible adverse effects of the surgery. Fluid loss may occur during surgery as a result of excessive urinary drainage when the obstruction is removed, or it may occur if diuretic agents are used. Such loss may also occur with GI losses, with diarrhea resulting from antibiotic use, or with nasogastric drainage. When postoperative IV therapy is inadequate to match the output or fluids lost, a fluid deficit results. Fluid excess, or overload, may result from cardiac effects of anesthesia, administration of excessive amounts of fluids, or the patient's inability to excrete fluid because of changes in renal function. Decreased urine output may be an indication of fluid excess.

Astute assessment skills are needed to detect early signs of fluid excess (such as weight gain, pedal edema, urine output below 0.5 mL/kg/hr, and slightly elevated pulmonary artery wedge pressure if available) before they become severe (appearance of adventitious breath sounds, shortness of breath).

Fluid excess may be treated with fluid restriction and administration of furosemide (Lasix) or other diuretic agents. If renal insufficiency is present, these medications may prove ineffective; therefore, dialysis may be necessary to prevent heart failure and pulmonary edema.

Deep vein thrombosis (DVT) may occur postoperatively because of surgical manipulation of the iliac vessels during surgery or prolonged immobility. Antiembolism stockings are applied, and the patient is monitored closely for signs and symptoms of thrombosis and encouraged to exercise the legs. Heparin may be given postoperatively to reduce the risk of thrombosis.

Promoting Home, Community-Based, and Transitional Care

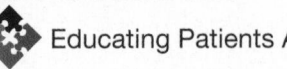 Educating Patients About Self-Care

If the patient has a drainage system in place, measures are taken to ensure that both the patient and family understand the importance of maintaining the system correctly at home and preventing infection. Verbal and written instructions and guidelines are provided to the patient and family at the time of hospital discharge. The patient may be asked to demonstrate management of the drainage system to ensure understanding. The importance of strategies to prevent postoperative complications (urinary tract obstruction and infection, DVT, atelectasis, and pneumonia) is stressed to the patient and family. The nurse reviews the signs, symptoms, problems, and questions that should be referred to the physician or other primary provider with the patient and family.

Continuing and Transitional Care

The need for postoperative assessment and care after kidney surgery continues regardless of the setting: the home, subacute care unit, outpatient clinic or office, or rehabilitation facility. Referral for home care is indicated for the patient going home with a urinary drainage system in place. During the home visit, the home care nurse reviews the instructions and guidelines given to the patient at hospital discharge. The nurse assesses the patient's ability to carry out the instructions in the home and answers questions that the patient or family has about management of the drainage system and the surgical incision.

In addition, the home care nurse obtains vital signs and assesses the patient for signs and symptoms of urinary tract obstruction and infection. The nurse also ensures that pain is adequately controlled and that the patient is complying with recommendations. The home care nurse encourages adequate fluid intake and increased levels of activity. Together, the nurse, patient, and family review the signs, symptoms, problems, and questions that should be referred to the primary provider. If the patient has a drainage tube in place, the nurse assesses the site and the patency of the system and monitors the patient for complications, such as DVT, bleeding, or pneumonia.

Because it is easy for the patient, family, and health care team to focus on the patient's immediate disorder to the exclusion of other health issues, the nurse reminds the patient and family about the importance of participating in health promotion activities, including appropriate health screenings.

Kidney Transplantation

Kidney transplantation has become the treatment of choice for most patients with ESKD. In the United States and globally, there are many more patients on the waiting list for kidney transplantation than there are organ donors. More than 99,000 Americans are on the waiting list to receive a kidney (Organ Procurement and Transplantation Network [OPTN], 2016). Patients choose kidney transplantation for various reasons, such as the desire to avoid dialysis or to improve their sense of well-being and the wish to lead a more normal life. In addition, the cost of maintaining a successful transplantation is one third the cost of dialysis treatment (Trevitt et al., 2012). Kidney transplantation is an elective procedure, not an emergency lifesaving procedure. Therefore, patients should be in the best possible condition prior to transplantation.

Kidney transplantation involves transplanting a kidney from a living or deceased donor to a recipient who no longer has renal function (see Chart 54-13). A living donor is a

---

> ### Chart 54-13 Kidney Donation
>
> An inadequate number of available kidneys remain the greatest limitation to treating patients with end-stage kidney disease successfully. For those interested in donating a kidney, the National Kidney Foundation provides written information describing the organ donation program and a card specifying the organs to be donated in the event of death.
>
> The organ donation card is signed by the donor and two witnesses and should be carried by the donor at all times. Procurement of an adequate number of kidneys for potential recipients is still a major problem, despite national legislation that requires relatives of deceased patients or patients declared brain dead to be asked if they would consider organ donation.
>
> In some states in the United States, drivers can indicate their desire to be organ donors on their driver's license application or renewal; however, this decision should be discussed with the family because the organ procurement agency will approach the family to discuss this option.

---

person who is alive at the time of donation and may or may not be related to the recipient. A deceased or cadaveric transplant comes from someone who has died and donated their organs. Transplantation from well-matched living donors who are related to the patient (those with compatible ABO and human leukocyte antigens) is slightly more successful than from cadaver donors (Gaber, Knight, & Patel, 2013). A contemporary development in kidney transplantation is paired donor exchange. In paired donor exchange, recipients essentially swap willing donors (Gaber et al., 2013). Although medically eligible to donate a kidney, a willing donor may be incompatible with the intended recipient due to blood type or antigens. The donor then agrees to donate the kidney to a compatible and unknown recipient, with the intention that the donor's originally intended organ recipient will be part of the donation chain and be the recipient of a donated kidney through organized donor and recipient matches.

Prior to either receiving or donating an organ, an extensive medical evaluation is performed. Not everyone is suitable for kidney transplantation. Contraindications include recent malignancy, active or chronic infection, severe irreversible extrarenal disease (e.g., inoperable cardiac disease, chronic lung disease, severe peripheral vascular disease), active infection (e.g., HIV, hepatitis B and C), Class II obesity (body mass index greater than 35 kg/m^2), current substance abuse, inability to give informed consent, and history of nonadherence to treatment regimens (Dring & Hipkiss 2015). Donors may be rejected for the same reasons or any condition that is determined to have an impact on the remaining kidney. Examples include hypertension and diabetes because both are known causes of kidney disease. It is imperative when donors are evaluated that serious consideration be given to the overall long-term health of the donor. Every precaution must be taken to ensure that the remaining kidney in the donor will remain healthy. If these conditions are met, the donor should remain healthy after donation and have a normal lifespan. Because one kidney can easily handle the body's needs, no long-term adjustments will need to be made.

The recipient's native kidneys are not usually removed. The transplanted kidney is placed in the patient's iliac fossa anterior to the iliac crest because it allows for easier access to

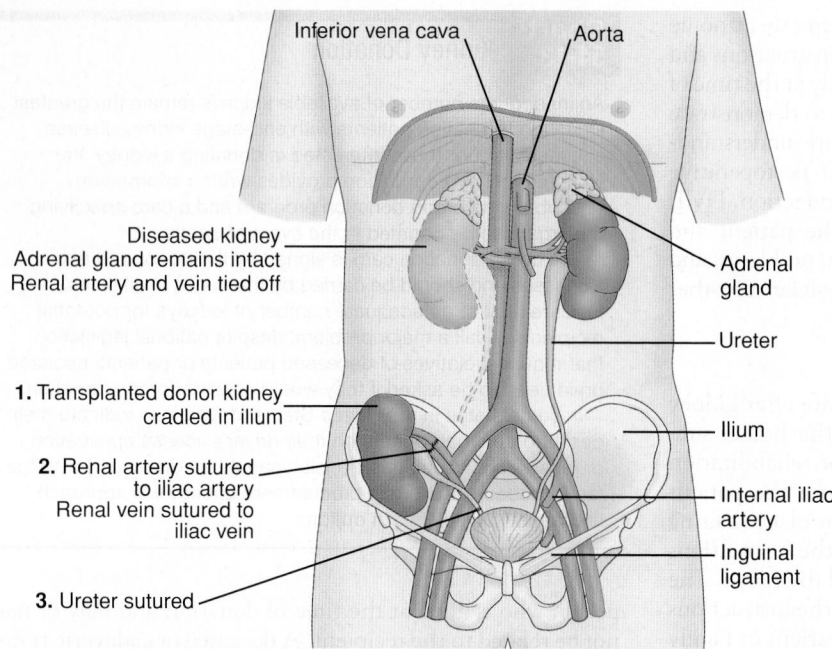

Figure 54-10 • Kidney transplantation. **1.** The transplanted kidney is placed in the iliac fossa. **2.** The renal artery of the donated kidney is sutured to the iliac artery, and the renal vein is sutured to the iliac vein. **3.** The ureter of the donated kidney is sutured to the bladder or to the patient's ureter.

the blood supply needed to perfuse the kidney. The ureter of the newly transplanted kidney is transplanted into the bladder or anastomosed to the ureter of the recipient (see Fig. 54-10). Once the blood supply has been reestablished to the transplanted kidney in the operating room, urine should begin to flow. The production of urine at this stage is an important indicator of the overall success of the procedure and ultimate long-term outcome.

Preoperative Management

Preoperative management goals include bringing the patient's metabolic state to a level as close to normal as possible through diet, possibly dialysis and medical management, making sure that the patient is free of infection, and preparing the patient for surgery and the postoperative course.

Medical Management

A complete physical examination is performed on the donor and the recipient to detect and treat any conditions that could cause complications after the donor and transplantation procedure. Tissue typing, blood typing, and antibody screening are performed to determine compatibility of the tissues and cells of the donor and recipient. Other diagnostic tests must be completed to identify conditions requiring treatment before transplantation for either individual. The lower urinary tract is studied to assess bladder neck function and to detect ureteral reflux.

Both patients must be free of infection at the time of kidney transplantation. After surgery, medications to prevent transplant rejection will be prescribed to the transplant recipient. These medications suppress the immune response, leaving the patient immunosuppressed and at risk for infection. Therefore, both the donor and recipient are evaluated and treated for any infections, including gingival (gum) disease and dental caries.

A psychosocial evaluation is conducted to assess the organ recipient's ability to adjust to the transplant, coping styles, social history, social support available, and financial resources. A history of psychiatric illness is important to obtain because psychiatric conditions are often aggravated by the corticosteroids needed for immunosuppression after transplantation (Colaneri, 2014). A psychosocial evaluation is also conducted to assess the organ donor's motive for giving the organ. The donor should not be coerced to donate this organ; it should be an altruistic act (Choudhury, Jotterand, Casenave, et al., 2014; Robbins, 2014) (see Chart 54-14). If a dialysis routine has been established, hemodialysis is often performed the day before the scheduled transplantation procedure to optimize the physical status of the patient receiving the transplant.

Nursing Management

The nursing aspects of preoperative care for the patient undergoing kidney transplant and donation are similar to those for patients undergoing other types of kidney or elective abdominal surgery. Preoperative education can be conducted in a variety of settings, including the outpatient preadmission area, the hospital, or the transplantation clinic during the preliminary workup phase. Patient education directed at the kidney transplant donor and recipient addresses postoperative pulmonary hygiene, pain management options, dietary restrictions, IV and arterial lines, tubes (indwelling catheter and possibly a nasogastric tube), and early ambulation. Most patients have been on dialysis for months or years before transplantation. Many have waited months to years for a kidney transplant and are anxious about the surgery, possible rejection, and the need to return to or begin dialysis. Helping the patient to deal with these concerns is part of the nurse's role in preoperative management, as is educating the patient about what to expect after surgery.

The patient who receives a kidney from a living related donor is often concerned about the donor and how the donor will tolerate the surgical procedure. If the patient is receiving a cadaveric donor transplant, the recipient may express sadness and grief over the loss of the donor's life. The nurse must

Chart 54-14 ETHICAL DILEMMA
The Gift of Life for Whom? Whose Life Is It?

Case Scenario

You are a nurse working in a solid organ transplant clinic that is affiliated with a university health science center. A 52-year-old man with a history of type 2 diabetes and end-stage kidney disease and each of his three biologic siblings, none of whom have diabetes, have been worked up to see if one may be a match for a living transplant. The youngest sibling, who is the only sister in the family, is a perfect donor match. The patient assumes that his sister will donate a kidney, which will improve his quality of life. However, the sister confides in you when other family members are not present, "You know, his need for a kidney is because he never managed his diabetes and everyone is pressuring me into donating. I'm not really certain I want to do this. What if I need this kidney one day?"

Discussion

Living donor transplants offer the best possibility for successful organ engraftment. Biologic siblings are the best candidates for finding good organ matches; there is a greater likelihood that siblings will share all human leukocyte antigens. Patient advocacy and informed consent are imperative as a potential living donor contemplates donating an organ. In 2007, the United Network for Organ Sharing mandated that all transplant centers provide any potential donor with an unbiased advocate. The goal is to ensure that the donor is mentally competent, adequately educated about the risks of the procedure, and capable of autonomous decision making.

Analysis

- Describe the ethical principles that are in conflict in this case (see Chapter 3, Chart 3-3). Which principle should have preeminence as you proceed to work with the potential living donor?
- There are two patients in this case—one is the brother with end-stage kidney disease who is hoping to receive a donated kidney from a sibling, and the other is the sister with healthy kidneys who is reluctant to donate one to her brother. Should the autonomous right of one patient have preeminence over the autonomous right of the other? How would you respond to the sister when she confides in you?
- For whom is there an obligation to advocate for in this situation—the brother, the sister, or the extended family? What resources might you mobilize to help them reconcile their differences?
- Is it morally ethical to donate an organ to a patient whose noncompliance in the management of their disease may have directly caused the organ to fail?

Resources

Choudhury, D., Jotterand, F., Casenave, G., et al. (2014). Independent donor ethical assessment: Aiming to standardize donor advocacy. *Progress in transplantation*, *24*(2), 163–168.

Robbins, K. C. (2014). The independent living donor advocate: An essential role for living kidney donation. *Nephrology Nursing Journal*, *41*(6), 569–586.

See Chapter 3, Chart 3-6 for ethics resources.

---

maintain open communication with the recipient of the organ and allow the patient to express these concerns.

The nurse working in an intensive care setting may provide care to the organ donor who is brain dead prior to organ removal. The overall goal is to preserve the function of the organs through maintaining hemodynamic stability, decreasing the risk for infection, and monitoring laboratory values while providing dignified care to the donor and family members (Derkowski, 2014). Continuing care for the donor can be complex and last several hours. Care is often provided in collaboration with the organ procurement coordinator and transplant coordinator.

Postoperative Management

The goal of postoperative care is to maintain homeostasis until the transplanted kidney is functioning well. The patient whose kidney functions immediately has a more favorable prognosis than the patient whose kidney does not.

Often, the organ donor will be on the same unit as the transplant recipient. The donor will require the same level of care provided to the recipient, including follow-up after the procedure and lifelong. The organ donor may experience more pain than the recipient, possibly requiring more analgesia for pain control. Fluid, electrolyte, and hemodynamic status will also be closely monitored in the organ donor.

Medical Management

After a kidney transplantation, rejection and failure can occur within 24 hours (hyperacute), within 3 to 14 days (acute),

or after many years. A hyperacute rejection is caused by an immediate antibody-mediated reaction that leads to generalized glomerular capillary thrombosis and necrosis. An acute rejection typically occurs within a few days to weeks of the transplant surgery, and the patient experiences tenderness at the transplant site, a decrease in serum creatinine values, fever, malaise, and oliguria (Colaneri, 2014). An acute rejection requires early recognition and treatment with immunosuppressant therapy, whereas a hyperacute reaction requires immediate removal of the transplanted organ (Colaneri, 2014). The long-term survival of a transplanted kidney depends on how well it matches the recipient and how well the body's immune response is controlled. The body's immune system views the transplanted kidney as "foreign"; therefore, it continually works to reject it. To overcome or minimize the body's defense mechanisms, immunosuppressive agents are given. Optimally, medications modify the immune system enough to prevent rejection, although not enough to allow infections or malignancies to occur (see Table 54-4).

Combinations of corticosteroids and medications specifically developed to affect the action of lymphocytes are used to minimize the body's reaction to the transplanted organ. Treatment with combinations of new agents has dramatically improved survival rates, and now 90% to 95% of transplanted kidneys still function after 1 year (Colaneri, 2014). Doses of immunosuppressive agents are often adjusted depending on the patient's immunologic response to the transplant. However, the patient will be required to take some form of immunosuppressive therapy for the entire time that they have the transplanted kidney.

TABLE 54-4 Immunosuppressant Agents Used Following Organ Transplant

Agent	Action	Nursing Implications
azathioprine (Azasan, Imuran)	Antagonizes purine metabolism and appears to inhibit DNA, RNA, and normal protein synthesis in rapidly growing cells; suppresses T-cell effects	Give oral drug in divided doses with food. Monitor leukocyte and platelet counts and bleeding.
belatacept (Nulojix)	Inhibition of T-lymphocyte proliferation and cytokine production	Contraindicated in patients with EBV seronegativity or unknown EBV serostatus, liver transplantation, breast-feeding. Monitor for symptoms of infection, hypertension, progressive multifocal leukoencephalopathy. Administer IV.
cyclosporine (Gengraf, Neoral, Sandimmune)	Selective and reversible inhibition of first phase of T-cell activation with T lymphocytes	Do not dilute oral solution with grapefruit juice (use orange juice, regular or chocolate milk, or apple juice and administer immediately after mixing). Observe for adverse reactions for 30 minutes after initiation of the IV infusion. Be aware that nephrotoxicity is reported in up to 1/3 of transplant recipients. Give medication with food to reduce gastrointestinal upset. Administer medication at the same time each day.
everolimus (Afinitor, Zortess)	Protein–tyrosine kinase inhibitor	Monitor for hypersensitivity reaction. Watch for changes in pulmonary status and cough. Avoid administration of live vaccines. Administer at the same time each day with food; do not crush or allow patient to chew tablet.
mycophenolate mofetil (CellCept) mycophenolic acid (Myfortic)	Inhibition of T- and B-lymphocyte responses, thus inhibiting antibody formation and generation of cytotoxic T cells	Administer on an empty stomach. Do not crush or open capsules. Avoid contact with powder in capsules; wash thoroughly with soap and water if contact occurs. Obtain baseline complete blood count with differential prior to initiating therapy. Instruct the patient to avoid over-the-counter antacids.
prednisone (Apo-Prednisone, Deltasone, Orasone, Panasol, Winpred)	Immediate-acting synthetic analog of hydrocortisone that has anti-inflammatory and immunosuppressant properties	Give with meals or a snack. Crush tablet and give with fluid if patient is unable to swallow it whole. Note that the drug should not be stopped abruptly; the dosage is reduced gradually. Monitor weight, blood pressure, blood glucose levels, and sleep patterns. Monitor for hypocalcemia. Instruct patient to avoid or minimize alcohol intake.
sirolimus (Rapamune)	Inhibits the response of helper T and B lymphocytes	Administer 4 hours after oral cyclosporine. Instruct patient to swallow tablets whole and to avoid chewing or crushing tablets. Refrigerate drug and protect from light. Instruct patient to avoid grapefruit juice within 2 hours of taking drug and to mix the drug only with orange juice or water. Instruct the patient to limit exposure to sunlight.
tacrolimus (Prograf)	Inhibits helper T lymphocytes	Monitor for neurotoxicity (tremors and changes in mental status). Assess for hypertension. Monitor tacrolimus levels.

DNA, deoxyribonucleic acid; RNA, ribonucleic acid; EBV, Epstein–Barr virus; IV, intravenous.
Adapted from Comerford, K. C. (2015). *Nursing 2015 drug handbook*. Philadelphia, PA: Wolters Kluwer.

The risks associated with taking these medications include nephrotoxicity, hypertension, hyperlipidemia, hirsutism, tremors, blood dyscrasias, cataracts, gingival hyperplasia, and several types of cancer (Colaneri, 2014).

Nursing Management

Assessing the Patient for Transplant Rejection

After kidney transplantation, the nurse assesses the patient for signs and symptoms of transplant rejection: oliguria, edema, fever, increasing blood pressure, weight gain, and swelling or tenderness over the transplanted kidney or graft. Patients receiving cyclosporine (Neoral) may not exhibit the usual signs and symptoms of acute rejection. In these patients, the only sign may be an asymptomatic rise in the serum creatinine level (more than a 20% rise is considered acute rejection) (Colaneri, 2014).

Preventing Infection

The results of blood chemistry tests and leukocyte and platelet counts are monitored closely because immunosuppression depresses the formation of leukocytes and platelets. The patient is closely monitored for infection because of susceptibility to impaired healing and infection related to immunosuppressive therapy and complications of kidney disease. Clinical manifestations of infection include shaking chills,

Chart
54-15 **Kidney Transplant Rejection and Infection**

Renal graft rejection and failure may occur within 24 hours (hyperacute), within 3–14 days (most commonly acute), or after many years (most commonly chronic). It is not uncommon for rejection to occur during the first year after transplantation.

Detecting Rejection

Ultrasonography may be used to detect enlargement of the kidney; percutaneous renal biopsy (most reliable) and x-ray techniques are used to evaluate transplant rejection. If the body rejects the transplanted kidney, the patient needs to commence dialysis. The rejected kidney may or may not be removed, depending on when the rejection occurs (acute vs. chronic) and the risk for infection if the kidney is left in place.

Potential Infection

About 75% of kidney transplant recipients have at least one episode of infection in the first year after transplantation because of immunosuppressant therapy. Immunosuppressants of the past made the transplant recipient more vulnerable to opportunistic infections (candidiasis, cytomegalovirus, Pneumocystis pneumonia) and infection with other relatively nonpathogenic viruses, fungi, and protozoa, which can be a major hazard. Immunosuppressive therapy, such as cyclosporine (Neoral) has reduced the incidence of opportunistic infections because it selectively exerts its effect, sparing T cells that protect the patient from life-threatening infections. In addition, combination immunosuppressant therapy and improved clinical care have produced 1-year patient survival rates approaching 100% and graft survival exceeding 90%. Infections, however, remain a major cause of death at all points in time for kidney transplant recipients.

Adapted from Colaneri, J. (2014). An overview of transplant immunosuppression—History, principles, and current practices in kidney transplantation. *Nephrology Nursing Journal, 41*(6), 549–560.

fever, rapid heartbeat (tachycardia), and respirations (tachypnea), as well as either an increase or a decrease in WBCs (leukocytosis or leukopenia).

Infection may be introduced through many sources. Urine cultures are performed frequently because of the high incidence of bacteriuria during early and late stages of transplantation. Any type of wound drainage should be viewed as a potential source of infection because drainage is an excellent culture medium for bacteria. Catheter and drain tips may be cultured when removed by cutting off the tip of the catheter or drain (using aseptic technique) and placing the tip in a sterile container to be taken to the laboratory for culture (see Chart 54-15).

The nurse ensures that the patient is protected from exposure to infection by hospital staff, visitors, and other patients with active infections. Attention to hand hygiene by all who come in contact with the patient is imperative.

Monitoring Urinary Function

A kidney from a living donor who is related to the patient usually begins to function immediately after surgery and may produce large quantities of dilute urine. A kidney from a cadaver donor may undergo ATN and therefore may not function for 2 or 3 weeks, during which time anuria, oliguria, or polyuria may be present. During this stage, the patient may experience

significant changes in fluid and electrolyte status. Therefore, careful monitoring is indicated. The output from the urinary catheter (connected to a closed drainage system) is measured every hour. IV fluids are given on the basis of urine volume and serum electrolyte levels and as prescribed by the primary provider. Hemodialysis may be necessary postoperatively to maintain homeostasis until the transplanted kidney is functioning well. It also may be required if fluid overload and hyperkalemia occur. After successful kidney transplantation, the vascular access device may clot, possibly from improved coagulation with the return of renal function. The vascular access for hemodialysis is monitored to ensure patency and to evaluate for evidence of infection.

Addressing Psychological Concerns

The rejection of a transplanted kidney is of great concern to the patient, the family, and the health care team for many months. The fear of kidney rejection and the complications of immunosuppressive therapy (Cushing syndrome, diabetes, capillary fragility, osteoporosis, glaucoma, cataracts, acne, nephrotoxicity) place tremendous psychological stress on the patient. If the organ donor was a family member there may be added feelings of guilt and anger that need to be addressed. Anxiety and uncertainty about the future and difficult posttransplantation adjustment are often sources of stress for the patient and family.

An important nursing function is the assessment of the patient's stress and coping. The nurse uses each visit with the patient to determine if the patient and family are coping effectively and the patient is adhering to the prescribed medication regimen. If indicated or requested, the nurse refers the patient for counseling.

Monitoring and Managing Potential Complications

The patient undergoing kidney transplantation is at risk for the postoperative complications that are associated with any surgical procedure. In addition, the patient's physical condition may be compromised because of the effects of long-standing kidney disease and its treatment. Therefore, careful assessment of the complications related to kidney disease and those associated with a major surgery are important aspects of nursing care. Breathing exercises, early ambulation, and care of the surgical incision are important aspects of postoperative care.

GI ulceration and corticosteroid-induced bleeding may occur. Fungal colonization of the GI tract (especially the mouth) and urinary bladder may occur secondary to corticosteroid and antibiotic therapy. Closely monitoring the patient and notifying the primary provider about the occurrence of these complications are important nursing interventions. In addition, the patient is monitored closely for signs and symptoms of adrenal insufficiency if the treatment has included the use of corticosteroids.

Promoting Home, Community-Based, and Transitional Care

 Educating Patients About Self-Care

The nurse works closely with the patient and family to be sure that they understand the need for continuing immunosuppressive therapy as prescribed. In addition, the patient and family are instructed to assess for and report signs and symptoms of transplant rejection, infection, or significant adverse effects of the immunosuppressive regimen. These include decreased urine output; weight gain; malaise; fever; respiratory distress; tenderness over the transplanted kidney; anxiety; depression; changes in eating, drinking, or other habits; and changes in blood pressure. The patient is instructed to inform other health care providers (e.g., dentist) about the kidney transplant and the use of immunosuppressive agents.

Continuing and Transitional Care

The patient needs to know that follow-up care after transplantation is a lifelong necessity. Individual verbal and written instructions are provided concerning diet, medication, fluids, daily weight, daily measurement of urine, management of I&O, prevention of infection and chronic rejection, resumption of activity, and avoidance of contact sports in which the transplanted kidney may be injured. Because of the risk of other potential complications, the patient is followed closely by a health care team that includes the nephrologist, transplant surgeon, transplant coordinator or nurse, social worker, and dietician. Medications are often obtained at one pharmacy or through the pharmacy at the hospital where the transplant surgery was performed for the purpose of quality control. Follow-up with providers from the transplant team will initially occur once a week upon discharge from the hospital and taper with time. Laboratory studies will also be obtained and followed on an ongoing basis to monitor the function of the kidney.

Cardiovascular disease is the major cause of morbidity and mortality after transplantation, due in part to the increasing age of patients with transplants. An additional problem is possible malignancy; patients receiving long-term immunosuppressive therapy are at higher risk for cancers than the general population. The nurse reminds the patient of the importance of health promotion and health screening and provides information on local transplantation support groups at the transplant hospital or through the procurement organization.

The American Association of Kidney Patients and the NKF (listed in the Resources section of this chapter) are nonprofit organizations that serve the needs of those with kidney disease. These groups can provide many helpful suggestions for patients and family members learning to cope with dialysis and transplantation.

RENAL TRAUMA

The kidneys are protected by the rib cage and musculature of the back posteriorly and by a cushion of abdominal wall and viscera anteriorly. They are highly mobile and are fixed only at the renal pedicle (stem of renal blood vessels and the ureter). With traumatic injury, the kidneys can be thrust against the lower ribs, resulting in contusion and rupture. Rib fractures or fractures of the transverse process of the upper lumbar vertebrae may be associated with renal contusion or laceration. Failure to wear seat belts contributes to the incidence of renal trauma in motor vehicle crashes. Up to 80% of patients with renal trauma have associated injuries of other internal organs.

Injuries may be blunt (automobile and motorcycle crashes, falls, athletic injuries, assaults) or penetrating (gunshot

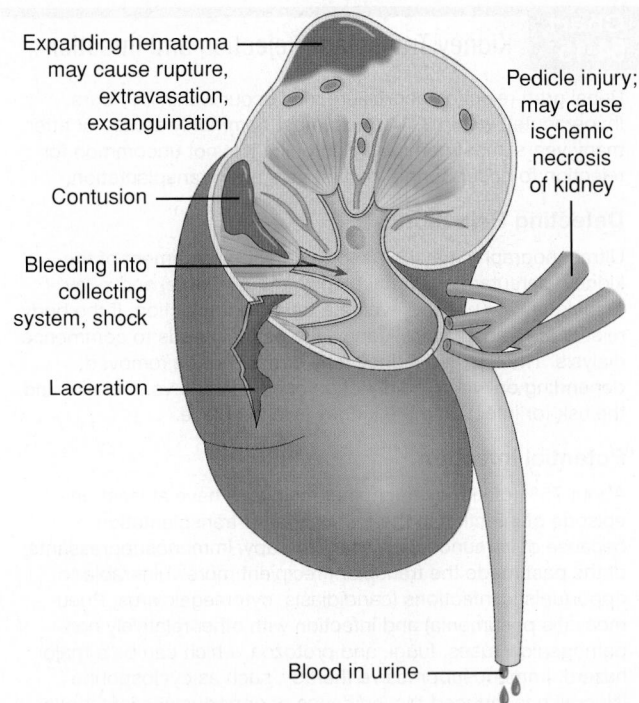

Figure 54-11 • Types and pathophysiologic effects of kidney injuries: contusions, lacerations, rupture, and pedicle injury.

wounds, stabbings). Blunt renal trauma accounts for 80% to 90% of all renal injuries; penetrating renal trauma accounts for the remaining 10% to 20% (Counts, 2015; USRDS, 2015).

Blunt renal trauma is classified into one of four groups, as follows:

- Contusion: Bruises or hemorrhages under the renal capsule; capsule and collecting system intact
- Minor laceration: Superficial disruption of the cortex; renal medulla and collecting system are not involved
- Major laceration: Parenchymal disruption extending into cortex and medulla, possibly involving the collecting system
- Vascular injury: Tears of renal artery or vein

The most common renal injuries are contusions, lacerations, ruptures, and renal pedicle injuries or small internal lacerations of the kidney (see Fig. 54-11). The kidneys receive half of the blood flow from the abdominal aorta; therefore, even a fairly small renal laceration can produce massive bleeding. The majority of patients are in shock when admitted to the hospitals. In some cases, there is an isolated renal artery thrombosis.

Clinical manifestations include pain, renal colic (due to blood clots or fragments obstructing the collecting system), hematuria, mass or swelling in the flank, ecchymoses, and lacerations or wounds of the lateral abdomen and flank. Hematuria is the most common manifestation of renal trauma; its presence after trauma suggests kidney injury. There is no relationship between the degree of hematuria and the degree of injury. Hematuria may not occur, or it may be detectable only on microscopic examination. Signs and symptoms of hypovolemia and shock (see Chapter 14) are likely with significant hemorrhage.

Medical Management

The goals of management in patients with renal trauma are to control hemorrhage, pain, and infection as well as to preserve and restore renal function. All urine is saved and sent to the laboratory for analysis to detect RBCs and to evaluate the course of bleeding. Hematocrit and hemoglobin levels are monitored closely; decreasing values indicate hemorrhage.

The patient is monitored for oliguria and signs of hemorrhagic shock, because a pedicle injury or shattered kidney can lead to rapid exsanguination (lethal blood loss). An expanding hematoma may cause rupture of the kidney capsule. To detect hematoma, the area around the lower ribs, upper lumbar vertebrae, flank, and abdomen is palpated for tenderness. A palpable flank or abdominal mass with local tenderness, swelling, and ecchymosis suggests renal hemorrhage. The area of the original mass can be outlined with a marking pen so that the examiner can evaluate the area for change.

Renal trauma is often associated with other injuries to the abdominal organs (liver, colon, small intestines); therefore, the patient is assessed for skin abrasions, lacerations, and entry and exit wounds of the upper abdomen and lower thorax, because these may be associated with kidney injury.

With a contusion of the kidney, healing may take place with conservative measures. If the patient has microscopic hematuria and a normal IV urogram, outpatient management is possible. If gross hematuria or a minor laceration is present, the patient is hospitalized and kept on bed rest until the hematuria clears. Antimicrobial medications may be prescribed to prevent infection from perirenal hematoma or urinoma (a cyst containing urine). Patients with retroperitoneal hematomas may develop low-grade fever as absorption of the clot takes place.

Surgical Management

In renal trauma, any sudden change in the patient's condition suggests hemorrhage and requires rapid surgical intervention. Depending on the patient's condition and the nature of the injury, major lacerations may be treated through surgical intervention or conservatively (bed rest, no surgery). Vascular injuries require immediate exploratory surgery because of the high incidence of involvement of other organ systems and the serious complications that may result if these injuries are untreated. The patient is often in shock and requires aggressive fluid resuscitation. The damaged kidney may have to be removed (nephrectomy).

Early postoperative complications (within 6 months) include rebleeding, perinephritic abscess formation, sepsis, urine extravasation, and fistula formation. Other complications include stone formation, infection, cysts, vascular aneurysms, and loss of renal function. Hypertension can be a complication of any surgery but usually is a late complication of kidney injury.

Nursing Management

The patient with renal trauma must be assessed frequently during the first few days after injury to detect flank and abdominal pain, muscle spasm, and swelling over the flank. During this time, the patient who has undergone surgery is educated about care of the incision and the importance of an adequate fluid intake. In addition, instructions about changes that should be reported to the physician, such as fever, hematuria, flank pain, or any signs and symptoms of decreasing kidney function, are provided. Guidelines for gradually increasing activity, lifting, and driving are also provided in accordance with the physician's prescription.

Follow-up nursing care includes monitoring the blood pressure to detect hypertension and advising the patient to restrict activities for about 1 month after trauma to minimize the incidence of delayed or secondary bleeding. The patient should be advised to schedule periodic follow-up assessments of renal function (creatinine clearance, BUN, and serum creatinine analyses). If a nephrectomy was necessary, the patient is advised to wear medical identification.

CRITICAL THINKING EXERCISES

1 **pq** You are a staff nurse in an outpatient dialysis facility. A 40-year-old man with ESKD is seen in the clinic for the first time and states that he wants to begin home hemodialysis. The patient lives alone and is employed full-time. What should be the priorities for educating this patient about the options for dialysis? How should the priorities change if the patient decides on PD?

2 **ebp** You are caring for a 75-year-old patient who has been recently diagnosed with renal cancer. What is the evidence base for her treatment options? Identify the criteria used to evaluate the strength of the evidence.

3 A 23-year-old man is admitted to the surgical intensive care unit after a motor vehicle crash. The patient sustained multiple abdominal injuries that resulted in intra-abdominal hemorrhage requiring emergent surgery. The patient's blood pressure was 58/42 upon arrival to the emergency department, and the patient was not responsive. Due to broken ribs and a pneumothorax, the patient is also being mechanically ventilated. The nurse notes that the patient's urine output is less than 0.5 mL/kg/hr and that the patient remains hypotensive. Based on the assessment information, what type of AKI is this patient most likely experiencing? Describe the nursing plan of care for this patient.

REFERENCES

*Asterisk indicates nursing research.

Books

Comerford, K. C. (2015). *Nursing 2015 drug handbook*. Philadelphia, PA: Wolters Kluwer.

Counts, C. S. (2015). *ANNA core curriculum for nephrology nursing* (6th ed.). Pitman, NJ: American Nephrology Nurses Association.

Grossman, S. C., & Porth, C. M. (2014). *Pathophysiology: Concepts of altered health states* (9th ed.). Philadelphia, PA: Lippincott Williams & Wilkins.

U.S. Renal Data System (USRDS). (2015). *Annual data report: Atlas of chronic kidney disease and end-stage renal disease in the United States*. Bethesda, MD: National Institutes of Health, National Institute of Diabetes and Digestive and Kidney Diseases.

Journals and Electronic Documents

Ahmad, M. M., & Al Nazly, E. K. (2015). Hemodialysis: Stressors and coping strategies. *Psychology Health and Medicine*, 20(4), 477–487.

American Cancer Society. (2015). *Kidney cancer.* Retrieved on 1/10/2015 at: www.cancer.org/cancer/kidneycancer/detailedguide/kidney-cancer-adult-key-statistics

Arslanian, J. (2015). Monitoring and surveillance of the hemodialysis vascular access. *Nephrology News and Issues*, 29(3), 38–42.

Centers for Disease Control and Prevention (CDC). (2014). *National chronic kidney disease fact sheet 2014.* Retrieved 7/4/2016 at: www.cdc.gov/diabetes/pubs/pdf/kidney_Factsheet.pdf

Choudhury, D., Jotterand, F., Casenave, G., et al. (2014). Independent donor ethical assessment: Aiming to standardize donor advocacy. *Progress in transplantation*, 24(2), 163–168.

Colaneri, J. (2014). An overview of transplant immunosuppression—History, principles, and current practices in kidney transplantation. *Nephrology Nursing Journal*, 41(6), 549–560.

Davies, H., & Leslie, G. (2012). Acute kidney injury and the critically ill patient. *Dimensions of Critical Care Nursing*, 31(3), 135–152.

Deng, D., & Forbes, A. (2015). Cardiovascular risk factors in patients on dialysis. *Nephrology Nursing Journal*, 42(1), 45–50.

Derkowski, D. (2014). Understanding the changes to the national deceased donor allocation system. *Nephrology Nursing Journal*, 41(6), 589–591, 608.

Dirkes, S. M. (2014). Continuous renal replacement therapy: Dialysis for critically ill patients. *American Nurse Today*, 9(5), 8–11.

Doss-McQuitty, S. (2014). Strategies for removing fluids during hemodialysis. *Nephrology Nursing Journal*, 41(3), 257–263.

Dring, B., & Hipkiss, V. (2015). Managing and treating chronic kidney disease. *Nursing Times*, 111(7), 16–19.

Elliott, R. W. (2012). Demographics of the older adult and chronic kidney disease: A literature review. *Nephrology Nursing Journal*, 39(6), 491–496.

Figueiredo, A. E. (2014). The challenges in preventing infection in peritoneal dialysis: A nurse's viewpoint. *Renal Society of Australasia Journal*, 10(3), 120–125.

Gaber, L. W., Knight, R. J., & Patel, S. J. (2013). A surgeons' guide to renal transplant immunopathology, immunology, and immunosuppression. *Surgical Clinics of North America*, 93(6), 1293–1307.

Hain, D. J. (2015). Where's the evidence? Care coordination for adults with chronic kidney disease. *Nephrology Nursing Journal*, 42(1), 77–83.

Hain, D. J., & Chan, J. (2013). Best available evidence for peritoneal dialysis catheter exit-site care. *Nephrology Nursing Journal*, 40(1), 63–69.

James, P. A., Oparil, S., Carter, B. L, et al. (2014). 2014 Evidence-based guidelines for the management of high blood pressure in adults: Report from the panel members appointed to the Eighth Joint National Committee (JNC 8). *JAMA*, 311(5), 507–520.

*Kane-Gill, S. L., Sileanu, F. E., Murugan, R., et al. (2015). Risk factors for acute kidney injury in older adults with critical illness: A retrospective cohort study. *American Journal of Kidney Diseases*, 65(6), 860–869.

Klein-Kauric, Z. (2015). Understanding hypertension in patients on hemodialysis. *Nephrology Nursing Journal*, 42(1), 69–75.

Lewis, R. (2013). An overview of chronic kidney disease in older people. *Nursing Older People*, 25(10), 31–38.

Ludvigsen, M. S., Hermansen, H. M., & Lindberg, M. (2014). The quality of nursing care during intradialytic fluid removal in hemodialysis: Time to change practice? *Journal of Clinical Nursing*, 24(11–12), 1733–1736.

*MacRae, J. M., Ahmed, S. B., & Hemmelgam, B. R. (2014). Arteriovenous fistula survival and needling technique: Long-term results from a randomized buttonhole trial. *American Journal of Kidney Disease*, 63(4), 636–642.

Organ Procurement and Transplantation Network (OPTN). (2016). Waiting list candidates as of today. Retrieved 7/5/2016 at: optn.transplant.hrsa.gov/data/

Prentice, M. (2013). Conservative care in advanced kidney disease. *British Journal of Primary Care Nursing*, 10(2), 83–86.

Rank, W. (2013). Preventing contrast media-induced nephrotoxicity. *Nursing 2013*, 43(4), 48–51.

Richardson, A., & Whatmore, J. (2015). Nursing essential principles: Continuous renal replacement therapy. *Nursing in Critical Care*, 20(1), 8–15.

Robbins, K. C. (2014). The independent living donor advocate: An essential role for living kidney donation. *Nephrology Nursing Journal*, 41(6), 569–586.

Taal, M. W. (2013). Chronic kidney disease in general populations and primary care: Diagnostic and therapeutic considerations. *Current Opinion in Nephrology and Hypertension*, 22(6), 593–598.

Tennankore, K. K., d'Gama, C., Faratro, R., et al. (2015). Adverse technical events in home hemodialysis. *American Journal of Kidney Diseases*, 65(1), 116–121.

Trevitt, R., Dunsmore, V., Murphy, F., et al. (2012). Pre- and post- transplant care: Nursing management of the renal transplant recipient: Part 2. *Journal of Renal Care*, 38(2), 107–114.

Vritis, M. C. (2013). Preventing and responding to acute kidney injury. *The American Journal of Nursing*, 113(4), 38–47.

Walton, B. (2015). Chronic kidney disease. *Ohio Nurse*, 8(3), 5–6.

*Weiner, D. E., Brunelli, S. M., Hunt, A., et al. (2014). Improving clinical outcomes among hemodialysis patients: A proposal for a "volume first" approach from the chief medical officers of US dialysis providers. *American Journal of Kidney Diseases*, 64(5), 685–695.

*Wright, L. S., & Wilson, L. (2015). Quality of life and self-efficacy in three dialysis modalities: Incenter hemodialysis, home hemodialysis, and home peritoneal dialysis. *Nephrology Nursing Journal*, 42(5), 463–476.

*Yamamoto, T., Shoji, S., Yamakawa, T., et al. (2015). Predialysis and postdialysis pH and bicarbonate and risk of all-cause and cardiovascular mortality in long-term hemodialysis patients. *American Journal of Kidney Disease*, 66(3), 469–478.

Resources

American Association of Kidney Patients (AAKP), www.aakp.org

American Kidney Fund, www.kidneyfund.org

American Nephrology Nurses' Association (ANNA), www.annanurse.org

American Urological Association (AUA), www.auanet.org

Arteriovenous Fistula First, www.fistulafirst.org

National Institute of Diabetes and Digestive and Kidney Diseases (NIDDK), www.niddk.nih.gov

National Kidney and Urologic Diseases Information Clearinghouse (NKUDIC), digestive.niddk.nih.gov

National Kidney Foundation (NKF), www.kidney.org

United Network for Organ Sharing (UNOS), www.unos.org

United States Renal Data System (USRDS, www.usrds.org

55

Management of Patients With Urinary Disorders

LEARNING OBJECTIVES

On completion of this chapter, the learner will be able to:

1 Explain the factors contributing to upper and lower urinary tract infections (UTIs).
2 Use the nursing process as a framework for care of the patient with a lower UTI.
3 Differentiate between the various adult dysfunctional voiding patterns.
4 Develop an education plan for a patient who has mixed (stress and urge) urinary incontinence.

5 Identify potential causes of an obstruction of the urinary tract along with the medical and surgical management of the patient with this condition.
6 Apply the nursing process as a framework for care of the patient with kidney stones.
7 Describe the pathophysiology, clinical manifestations, medical management, and nursing management for patients with genitourinary trauma and urinary tract cancers.
8 Use the nursing process as a framework for care of the patient undergoing urinary diversion surgery.

GLOSSARY

bacteriuria: bacteria in the urine
cystectomy: surgical removal of the urinary bladder
cystitis: inflammation of the urinary bladder
ileal conduit: transplantation of the ureters to an isolated section of the terminal ileum, with one end of the ureters brought to the abdominal wall
interstitial cystitis: inflammation of the bladder wall that eventually causes disintegration of the lining and loss of bladder elasticity
micturition: voiding or urination
neurogenic bladder: bladder dysfunction that results from a disorder or dysfunction of the nervous system and leads to urinary incontinence
nocturia: awakening at night to urinate
overflow incontinence: involuntary urine loss associated with overdistention of the bladder
prostatitis: inflammation of the prostate gland
pyelonephritis: inflammation of the renal pelvis

pyuria: white blood cells in the urine
residual urine: urine that remains in the bladder after voiding
suprapubic catheter: a urinary catheter that is inserted through a suprapubic incision into the bladder
ureterosigmoidostomy: transplantation of the ureters into the sigmoid colon, allowing urine to flow through the colon and out the rectum
ureterovesical or vesicoureteral reflux: backward flow of urine from the bladder into one or both ureters
urethritis: inflammation of the urethra
urethrovesical reflux: An obstruction to free-flowing urine leading to the reflux of urine from the urethra into the bladder
urinary frequency: voiding more often than every 3 hours
urinary incontinence: involuntary or uncontrolled loss of urine from the bladder
urosepsis: spread of infection from the urinary tract to the bloodstream that results in a systemic infection

The urinary system is responsible for providing the route for drainage of urine formed by the kidneys. Care of the patient with disorders of the urinary tract requires an understanding of the anatomy, physiology, diagnostic testing, medical, and nursing care, as well as rehabilitation of patients with the multiple processes that affect the urinary system. Nurses care for patients with urologic disorders in all settings. This chapter focuses on the nursing management of patients with common urinary dysfunctions, including infections, dysfunctional voiding patterns, urolithiasis, genitourinary trauma, cancer of the urinary tract, and urinary diversions.

INFECTIONS OF THE URINARY TRACT

Urinary tract infections (UTIs) are caused by pathogenic microorganisms in the urinary tract (the normal urinary tract is sterile above the urethra). UTIs are generally classified as infections involving the upper or lower urinary tract and further classified as uncomplicated or complicated, depending on other patient-related conditions (see Chart 55-1).

Lower UTIs include bacterial **cystitis** (inflammation of the urinary bladder), bacterial **prostatitis** (inflammation of the prostate gland), and bacterial **urethritis** (inflammation of the urethra). Acute or chronic nonbacterial causes of inflammation in any of these areas can be misdiagnosed as bacterial infections. Upper UTIs are much less common and include acute or chronic **pyelonephritis** (inflammation of the renal pelvis), interstitial nephritis (inflammation of the kidney), and kidney abscesses. Upper and lower UTIs are further classified as uncomplicated or complicated, depending on whether the UTI is recurrent and the duration of the infection. Most uncomplicated UTIs are community acquired (Hopkins,

Urinary tract infections (UTIs) are classified by location: the lower urinary tract (which includes the bladder and structures below the bladder) or the upper urinary tract (which includes the kidneys and ureters). They can also be classified as uncomplicated or complicated UTIs.

Lower UTIs

Cystitis, prostatitis, urethritis

Upper UTIs

Acute pyelonephritis, chronic pyelonephritis, renal abscess, interstitial nephritis, perirenal abscess

Uncomplicated Lower or Upper UTIs

Community-acquired infection; common in young women and not usually recurrent

Complicated Lower or Upper UTIs

Often acquired in the hospital and related to catheterization; occur in patients with urologic abnormalities, pregnancy, immunosuppression, diabetes, and obstructions and are often recurrent

- Contributing conditions such as:
  - Female gender
  - Diabetes
  - Pregnancy
  - Neurologic disorders
  - Gout
  - Altered states caused by incomplete emptying of the bladder and urinary stasis
- Decreased natural host defenses or immunosuppression
- Inability or failure to empty the bladder completely
- Inflammation or abrasion of the urethral mucosa
- Instrumentation of the urinary tract (e.g., catheterization, cystoscopic procedures)
- Obstructed urinary flow caused by:
  - Congenital abnormalities
  - Urethral strictures
  - Contracture of the bladder neck
  - Bladder tumors
  - Calculi (stones) in the ureters or kidneys
  - Compression of the ureters

Adapted from Hagerty, T., Kertesz, L., Schmidt, J. M., et al. (2015). Risk factors for catheter associated urinary tract infections in critically ill patients with subarachnoid hemorrhage. *Journal of Neuroscience Nursing, 47*(1), 51–54; Hopkins, L., McCroskey, D., Reeves, G., et al. (2014). Implementing a urinary tract infection clinical practice guideline in an ambulatory urgent care practice. *The Nurse Practitioner, 39*(4), 50–54.

McCroskey, Reeves, et al., 2014). Complicated UTIs usually occur in people with urologic abnormalities or recent catheterization and are often acquired during hospitalization.

A UTI is the second most common infection in the body. Most cases occur in women; one out of every five women in the United States will develop a UTI during her lifetime. The urinary tract is the most common site of nosocomial infection, accounting for greater than 40% of the total number reported by hospitals and affecting about 600,000 patients each year. In most of these hospital-acquired UTIs, instrumentation of the urinary tract or catheterization is the precipitating cause. More than 250,000 cases of acute pyelonephritis occur in the United States each year, with 100,000 patients requiring hospitalization. Approximately 8.1 million women are diagnosed with uncomplicated UTIs in the United States annually (Hopkins et al., 2014).

Lower Urinary Tract Infections

Several mechanisms maintain the sterility of the bladder: the physical barrier of the urethra, urine flow, ureterovesical junction competence, various antibacterial enzymes and antibodies, and antiadherent effects mediated by the mucosal cells of the bladder. Abnormalities or dysfunctions of these mechanisms are contributing risk factors for lower UTIs (see Chart 55-2).

Pathophysiology

For infection to occur, bacteria must gain access to the bladder, attach to and colonize the epithelium of the urinary tract to avoid being washed out with voiding, evade host defense mechanisms, and initiate inflammation. Many UTIs result from fecal organisms ascending from the perineum to the urethra and the bladder and then adhering to the mucosal surfaces.

Bacterial Invasion of the Urinary Tract

By increasing the normal slow shedding of bladder epithelial cells (resulting in bacteria removal), the bladder can clear large numbers of bacteria. Glycosaminoglycan (GAG), a hydrophilic protein, normally exerts a nonadherent protective effect against various bacteria. The GAG molecule attracts water molecules, forming a water barrier that serves as a defensive layer between the bladder and the urine. GAG may be impaired by certain agents (cyclamate, saccharin, aspartame, and tryptophan metabolites). The normal bacterial flora of the vagina and urethral area also interfere with adherence of *Escherichia coli*. Urinary immunoglobulin A (IgA) in the urethra may also provide a barrier to bacteria.

Reflux

An obstruction to free-flowing urine is a condition known as **urethrovesical reflux**, which is the reflux (backward flow) of urine from the urethra into the bladder (see Fig. 55-1). With coughing, sneezing, or straining, the bladder pressure increases, which may force urine from the bladder into the urethra. When the pressure returns to normal, the urine flows back into the bladder, bringing into the bladder bacteria from the anterior portions of the urethra. Urethrovesical reflux is also caused by dysfunction of the bladder neck or urethra. The urethrovesical angle and urethral closure pressure may be altered with menopause, increasing the incidence of infection in postmenopausal women. Reflux is most often noted in young children, and treatment is based on its severity.

Ureterovesical or vesicoureteral reflux refers to the backward flow of urine from the bladder into one or both ureters (see Fig. 55-1). Normally, the ureterovesical junction

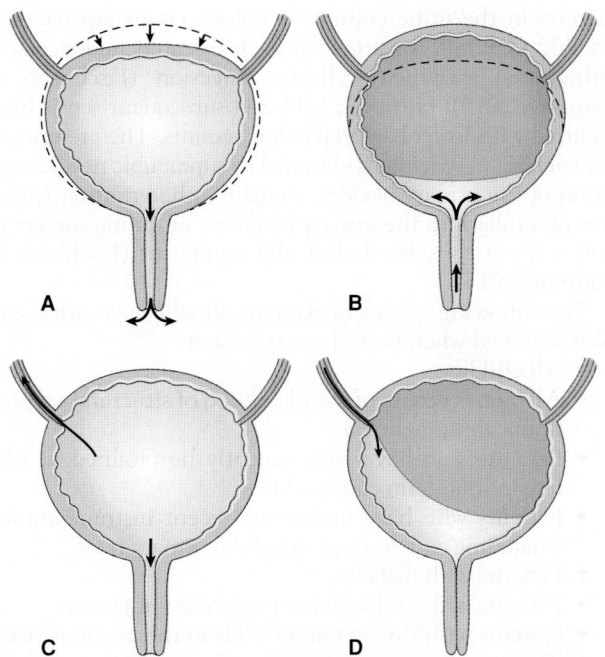

Figure 55-1 • Mechanisms of urethrovesical and ureterovesical reflux may cause urinary tract infection. *Urethrovesical reflux:* With coughing and straining, bladder pressure rises, which may force urine from the bladder into the urethra. **A.** When bladder pressure returns to normal, the urine flows back to the bladder (**B**), which introduces bacteria from the urethra to the bladder. *Ureterovesical reflux:* With failure of the ureterovesical valve, urine moves up the ureters during voiding (**C**) and flows into the bladder when voiding stops (**D**). This prevents complete emptying of the bladder. It also leads to urinary stasis and contamination of the ureters with bacteria-laden urine.

prevents urine from traveling back into the ureter. The ureters tunnel into the bladder wall so that the bladder musculature compresses a small portion of the ureter during normal voiding. When the ureterovesical valve is impaired by congenital causes or ureteral abnormalities, the bacteria may reach the kidneys and eventually destroy them.

Uropathogenic Bacteria

Bacteriuria is the term used to describe the presence of bacteria in the urine. Because urine samples (especially in women) can be easily contaminated by the bacteria normally present in the urethral area, a clean-catch midstream urine specimen is the measure used to establish bacteriuria. In men, contamination of the collected urine sample occurs less frequently. Bacteriuria is defined as 100,000 colony-forming units (CFU)/mL urine (Fischbach & Dunning, 2015; Grossman & Porth, 2014). Community-acquired UTIs are among the most common bacterial infections in women (Hopkins, et al., 2014). The organisms most frequently responsible for UTIs are those normally found in the lower gastrointestinal (GI) tract, usually *Escherichia coli* (Grossman & Porth, 2014).

Routes of Infection

Bacteria enter the urinary tract in three ways: by the transurethral route (ascending infection), through the bloodstream (hematogenous spread), or by means of a fistula from the intestine (direct extension).

The most common route of infection is transurethral, in which bacteria (often from fecal contamination) colonize the periurethral area and subsequently enter the bladder by means of the urethra (Grossman & Porth, 2014). In women, the short urethra offers little resistance to the movement of uropathogenic bacteria. Sexual intercourse forces the bacteria from the urethra into the bladder. This accounts for the increased incidence of UTIs in sexually active women. Bacteria may also enter the urinary tract by means of the blood from a distant site of infection or through direct extension by way of a fistula from the intestinal tract.

Clinical Manifestations

Signs and symptoms of UTI depend on whether the infection involves the lower (bladder) or upper (kidney) urinary tract and whether the infection is acute or chronic. Signs and symptoms of an uncomplicated lower UTI include burning on urination, **urinary frequency** (voiding more than every 3 hours), urgency, **nocturia** (awakening at night to urinate), incontinence, and suprapubic or pelvic pain. Hematuria and back pain may also be present. In older adults, these symptoms are less common (see Gerontologic Considerations section).

In patients with complicated UTIs, manifestations can range from asymptomatic bacteriuria to gram-negative sepsis with shock. Complicated UTIs often are caused by a broader spectrum of organisms, have a lower response rate to treatment, and tend to recur. Many patients with catheter-associated UTIs are asymptomatic; however, any patient with a catheter who suddenly develops signs and symptoms of septic shock should be evaluated for **urosepsis** (the spread of infection from the urinary tract to the bloodstream that results in a systemic infection).

 Gerontologic Considerations

The incidence of bacteriuria in older adults differs from that in younger adults. Bacteriuria increases with age and disability, and women are affected more frequently than men. UTI is the most common infection of older adults and increases in prevalence with age. UTIs occur more frequently in women than in men at younger ages but the gap between the sexes narrows in later life, which is due to reduced sexual intercourse in women and a higher incidence of bladder outlet obstruction secondary to benign prostatic hyperplasia in men (Eliopoulos, 2018).

In older adults, structural abnormalities secondary to decreased bladder tone, **neurogenic bladder** (dysfunctional bladder) secondary to stroke, or autonomic neuropathy of diabetes may prevent complete emptying of the bladder and increase the risk of UTI (Eliopoulos, 2018). When indwelling catheters are used, the risk of UTI increases dramatically (Hagerty, Kertesz, Schmidt, et al., 2015). Older women often have incomplete emptying of the bladder and urinary stasis. In the absence of estrogen, postmenopausal women are susceptible to colonization and increased adherence of bacteria to the vagina and urethra. Oral or topical estrogen has been used to restore the glycogen content of vaginal epithelial cells and an acidic pH for some postmenopausal women with recurrent cystitis.

The antibacterial activity of prostatic secretions that protect men from bacterial colonization of the urethra and

Chart 55-3 Factors That Contribute to Urinary Tract Infection in Older Adults

- Cognitive impairment
- Frequent use of antimicrobial agents
- High incidence of multiple chronic medical conditions
- Immunocompromise
- Immobility and incomplete emptying of bladder
- Obstructed flow of urine (e.g., urethral strictures, neoplasms, or a clogged indwelling catheter)

Adapted from Eliopoulos, C. (2018). *Gerontological nursing* (9th ed.). Philadelphia, PA: Lippincott Williams & Wilkins.

bladder decreases with aging. The use of catheterization or cystoscopy in evaluation or treatment for prostatic hyperplasia or carcinoma, strictures of the urethra, and neuropathic bladder may contribute to the higher incidence of UTIs in men. The incidence of bacteriuria also increases in men with confusion, dementia, or bowel or bladder incontinence. The most common cause of recurrent UTIs in older males is chronic bacterial prostatitis. Resection of the prostate gland may help reduce its incidence (see Chapter 59).

Chart 55-3 lists other factors that may contribute to UTI in older patients. Diligent hand hygiene, careful perineal care, and frequent toileting may decrease the incidence of UTIs.

The organisms responsible for UTIs in the institutionalized older adult may differ from those found in patients residing in the community; this is thought to result in part from the frequent use of antibiotic agents by patients in long-term care facilities. *E. coli* is the most common organism seen in older patients in the community or hospital. However, patients with indwelling catheters are more likely to be infected with organisms such as *Proteus, Klebsiella, Pseudomonas,* or *Staphylococcus.* Patients who have been previously treated with antibiotics may be infected with *Enterococcus* species. Frequent reinfections are common in older adults.

Early symptoms of UTI in older adults include burning, urgency, and fever (Eliopoulos, 2018). Some patients develop incontinence and delirium with the onset of a UTI.

Antibiotics are prescribed when bacteriuria is present (Eliopoulos, 2018). Treatment regimens are generally the same as those for younger adults, although age-related changes in the intestinal absorption of medications and decreased kidney function and hepatic flow may necessitate alterations in the antimicrobial regimen. Kidney function must be monitored, and medication dosages should be altered accordingly. The nurse carefully monitors fluid intake and output. Increasing fluid intake is advisable, provided that the patient's cardiac status does not contraindicate this action (Eliopoulos, 2018).

Assessment and Diagnostic Findings

Results of various tests, such as bacterial colony counts, cellular studies, and urine cultures, help confirm the diagnosis of UTI. In an uncomplicated UTI, the strain of bacteria determines the antibiotic of choice (Grossman & Porth, 2014).

Urine Cultures

Urine cultures are useful for documenting a UTI and identifying the specific organism present. UTI is diagnosed by

bacteria in the urine culture. A colony count greater than 100,000 CFU/mL. of urine on a clean-catch midstream or catheterized specimen indicates infection (Fischbach & Dunning, 2015). However, UTI and subsequent sepsis have occurred with lower bacterial colony counts. The presence of any bacteria in specimens obtained by suprapubic needle aspiration of the urinary bladder, straight catheterization (insertion of a tube into the urinary bladder), or during surgery or cystoscopy is considered clinically significant (Fischbach & Dunning, 2015).

The following groups of patients should have urine cultures obtained when bacteriuria is present:

- All children
- All men (because of the likelihood of structural or functional abnormalities)
- Patients who have been recently hospitalized or who live in long-term care facilities
- Patients who have undergone recent instrumentation (including catheterization) of the urinary tract
- Patients with diabetes
- Patients with prolonged or persistent symptoms
- Patients with three or more UTIs in the previous year
- Women who are postmenopausal
- Women who are pregnant
- Women who are sexually active
- Women who have new sexual partners
- Women with a history of compromised immune function or renal problems

Cellular Studies

Microscopic hematuria is present in about half of patients with an acute UTI (see Chapter 53). **Pyuria** (white blood cells [WBCs] in the urine) occurs in all patients with UTI; however, it is not specific for bacterial infection. Pyuria can also be seen with kidney stones, interstitial nephritis, and renal tuberculosis.

Other Studies

A multiple-test dipstick often includes testing for WBCs, known as the leukocyte esterase test, and nitrite testing (Grossman & Porth, 2014). Tests for sexually transmitted infections may be performed because acute urethritis caused by sexually transmitted organisms (i.e., *Chlamydia trachomatis, Neisseria gonorrhoeae,* herpes simplex) or acute vaginitis infections (caused by *Trichomonas* or *Candida* species) may be responsible for symptoms similar to those of UTIs.

X-ray images, computed tomography (CT) scan, ultrasonography, and kidney scans are useful diagnostic tools. A CT scan may detect pyelonephritis or abscesses. Ultrasonography and kidney scans are extremely sensitive for detecting obstruction, abscesses, tumors, and cysts (Grossman & Porth, 2014).

Medical Management

Management of UTIs typically involves pharmacologic therapy and patient education. Various prescribed medication regimens are used to treat UTI.

Acute Pharmacologic Therapy

The ideal medication for treatment of UTI is an antibacterial agent that eradicates bacteria from the urinary tract with

TABLE 55-1 Examples of Medications Used to Treat Urinary Tract Infections and Pyelonephritis

Drug Classes	Generic (Brand) Name	Major Indications
Anti-infective, urinary tract Bactericidal	nitrofurantoin (Macrodantin, Furadantin) cephalexin (Keflex)	UTI Genitourinary infection
Cephalosporin	cefadroxil (Duricef, Ultracef)	UTI
Fluoroquinolone	ciprofloxacin (Cipro) ofloxacin (Floxin) norfloxacin (Noroxin) gatifloxacin (Zymar)	UTI Pyelonephritis
Fluoroquinolone	levofloxacin (Levaquin)	Uncomplicated UTI
Penicillin	ampicillin (Principen, Omnipen) amoxicillin (Amoxil)	UTI—not commonly used alone due to *Escherichia coli* resistance Pyelonephritis UTI—not commonly used alone due to *E. coli* resistance
Trimethoprim–sulfamethoxazole combination	Co-trimoxazole (Bactrim, Septra)	UTI Pyelonephritis
Urinary analgesic agent	Phenazopyridine (Pyridium)	For relief of burning, pain, and other symptoms associated with UTI

UTI, urinary tract infection.
Adapted from Comerford, K. C. (2015). *Nursing 2015 drug handbook.* Philadelphia, PA: Wolters Kluwer; Hopkins, L., McCroskey, D., Reeves, G., et al. (2014). Implementing a urinary tract infection clinical practice guideline in an ambulatory urgent care practice. *The Nurse Practitioner, 39*(4), 50–54.

minimal effects on fecal and vaginal flora, thereby minimizing the incidence of vaginal yeast infections. The antibacterial agent should be affordable and should have few adverse effects and low resistance. Because the organism in initial, uncomplicated UTIs in women is most likely *E. coli* or other fecal flora, the agent should be effective against these organisms. Various treatment regimens have been successful in treating uncomplicated lower UTIs in women: single-dose administration, short-course (3-day) regimens, or 7-day regimens (Hopkins et al., 2014). The trend is toward a shortened course of antibiotic therapy for uncomplicated UTIs, because most cases are cured after 3 days of treatment. Medications commonly used to treat UTIs are listed in Table 55-1. Regardless of the regimen prescribed, the patient is instructed to take all doses prescribed, even if relief of symptoms occurs promptly. Longer medication courses are indicated for men, pregnant women, and women with pyelonephritis and other types of complicated UTIs. Hospitalization and intravenous (IV) antibiotics are occasionally necessary (Hopkins et al., 2014).

Long-Term Pharmacologic Therapy

Although brief pharmacologic treatment of UTIs for 3 days is usually adequate in women, infection recurs in about 20% of women treated for uncomplicated UTIs. Infections that recur within 2 weeks of therapy do so because organisms of the original offending strain remain. Relapses suggest that the source of bacteriuria may be the upper urinary tract or that initial treatment was inadequate or given for too short a time. Recurrent infections in men are usually caused by persistence of the same organism; further evaluation and treatment are indicated (Hopkins et al., 2014).

If infection recurs after completing antimicrobial therapy, another short course (3 to 4 days) of full-dose antimicrobial therapy followed by a regular bedtime dose of an antimicrobial agent may be prescribed. If there is no recurrence, medication is taken every other night for 6 to 7 months. Long-term use of antimicrobial agents decreases the risk of reinfection and may be indicated in patients with recurrent infections.

If recurrence is caused by persistent bacteria from preceding infections, the cause (i.e., kidney stone, abscess), if known, must be treated. After treatment and sterilization of the urine, low-dose prophylactic therapy (trimethoprim with or without sulfamethoxazole) each night at bedtime may be prescribed (Hopkins et al., 2014).

Daily intake of cranberry juice can help prevent and control symptoms of UTI (Bass-Ware, Weed, Johnson, et al., 2014; Hopkins et al., 2014). One group of researchers reported that daily consumption of cranberry juice over an 8-week period decreased symptoms (i.e., urgency, frequency, nocturia, dysuria, and pain) in women diagnosed with a UTI in an ambulatory setting (Bass-Ware, et al., 2014).

NURSING PROCESS

The Patient With a Lower Urinary Tract Infection

Nursing care of the patient with a lower UTI focuses on treating the underlying infection and preventing its recurrence.

Assessment

A history of pertinent signs and symptoms is obtained from the patient with a suspected UTI. The presence of pain, frequency, urgency, hesitancy, and changes in urine are assessed, documented, and reported. The patient's usual pattern of voiding is assessed to detect factors that may predispose him or her to UTI. Infrequent emptying of the bladder, the association of symptoms of UTI with sexual intercourse, contraceptive practices, and personal hygiene are assessed. The patient's knowledge about prescribed antimicrobial medications and preventive health care measures is also assessed. In addition, the urine is assessed for volume, color, concentration, cloudiness, and odor—all of which are altered by bacteria in the urinary tract. Patients need to be asked specifically about the use of complementary and alternative therapies. Researchers in one study reported that women with interstitial cystitis (inflammation of the bladder wall) used both complementary and conventional therapies. The most common complementary therapies reported included diet, biofeedback, dietary supplements, meditation, yoga, and massage (Anderson & Zinkgraf, 2013).

Diagnosis

Nursing Diagnoses

Based on the assessment data, nursing diagnoses may include the following:

- Acute pain related to infection within the urinary tract
- Deficient knowledge about factors predisposing the patient to infection and recurrence, detection and prevention of recurrence, and pharmacologic therapy

Collaborative Problems/Potential Complications

Potential complications may include the following:

- Sepsis (urosepsis)
- Acute kidney injury and/or chronic kidney disease may occur as the long-term result of either an extensive infective or inflammatory process

Planning and Goals

Major goals for the patient may include relief of pain and discomfort, increased knowledge of preventive measures and treatment modalities, and absence of complications.

Nursing Interventions

Relieving Pain

The pain associated with a UTI is quickly relieved once effective antimicrobial therapy is initiated. Antispasmodic agents may also be useful in relieving bladder irritability and pain. Analgesic agents and the application of heat to the perineum help relieve pain and spasm. The patient is encouraged to drink liberal amounts of fluids (water is the best choice) to promote renal blood flow and to flush the bacteria from the urinary tract. Urinary tract irritants (e.g., coffee, tea, citrus, spices, colas, alcohol) should be avoided. Frequent voiding (every 2 to 3 hours) is encouraged to empty the bladder completely, because doing so can lower urine bacterial counts, reduce urinary stasis, and prevent reinfection (Bass-Ware, et al., 2014; Hopkins et al., 2014).

Monitoring and Managing Potential Complications

Early recognition of UTI and prompt treatment are essential to prevent recurrent infection and the possibility of complications, such as kidney disease, sepsis (urosepsis), strictures, and obstructions. The goal of treatment is to prevent infection from progressing and causing permanent kidney damage and injury. Thus, the patient must be educated to recognize early signs and symptoms, to test for bacteriuria, and to initiate treatment as prescribed. Appropriate antimicrobial therapy, liberal fluid intake, frequent voiding, and hygienic measures are commonly prescribed for managing UTIs. The patient is instructed to notify the primary provider if fatigue, nausea, vomiting, fever, or pruritus occurs. Periodic monitoring of renal function and evaluation for strictures, obstructions, or stones may be indicated for patients with recurrent UTIs.

Patients with UTIs are at increased risk for gram-negative sepsis. For each day a urinary catheter is in place, the risk of developing catheter-associated urinary tract infection (CAUTI) increases. The risk of sepsis in patients with a urinary catheter is about 15% (Booker, 2015). CAUTIs should be avoided as they result in unpleasant symptoms, additional pharmacologic therapy, serious complications, and delayed discharge (Booker, 2015; Carter, Reitmeier, & Goodloe, 2014).

If an indwelling catheter is necessary, the following specific nursing interventions are initiated to prevent infection and urosepsis:

- Using strict aseptic technique during insertion of the smallest catheter possible
- Securing the catheter to prevent movement
- Frequently inspecting urine color, odor, and consistency
- Performing meticulous daily perineal care with soap and water
- Maintaining a closed system
- Following the manufacturer's instructions when using the catheter port to obtain urine specimens

Careful assessment of vital signs and level of consciousness may alert the nurse to kidney involvement or impending sepsis. Positive blood cultures and elevated WBC counts must be reported immediately. At the same time, appropriate antibiotic therapy and increased fluid intake are prescribed (IV antibiotic therapy and fluids may be required). Aggressive early treatment is the key to reducing the mortality rate associated with CAUTI especially in older patients, those with anemia, and those with elevated blood sugar levels (Hagerty et al., 2015). See Chart 55-4 for more information on risk factors for CAUTIs.

Promoting Home, Community-Based, and Transitional Care

Educating Patients About Self-Care. In helping patients learn about and prevent or manage a recurrent UTI, the nurse implements education that meets the patient's needs. Health-related behaviors that help prevent recurrent UTIs include practicing careful personal hygiene, increasing fluid intake to promote voiding and dilution of urine, urinating regularly and more frequently, and adhering to the therapeutic regimen. For a detailed discussion of patient education, see Chart 55-5.

Evaluation

Expected patient outcomes may include:

1. Experiences relief of pain
   a. Reports absence of pain, urgency, frequency, nocturia, or hesitancy on voiding
   b. Takes analgesic, antispasmodic, and antibiotic agents as prescribed
2. Explains UTIs and their treatment
   a. Demonstrates knowledge of preventive measures and prescribed treatments
   b. Drinks 8 to 10 glasses of fluids daily

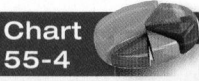

NURSING RESEARCH PROFILE

Chart 55-4

Risk Factors for Catheter-Associated Urinary Tract Infections

Hagerty, T., Kertesz, L., Schmidt, J. M., et al. (2015). Risk factors for catheter associated urinary tract infections in critically ill patients with subarachnoid hemorrhage. *Journal of Neuroscience Nursing, 47*(1), 51–54.

Purpose

The use of indwelling urinary catheters can lead to complications, most importantly catheter-associated urinary tract infections (CAUTI). These infections are the most common health care–associated infection in the United States. The purpose of this study was to assess the prevalence of and risk factors for CAUTIs among patients with subarachnoid hemorrhage (SAH) in one neurologic intensive care unit.

Design

This quantitative study used a retrospective design and included 242 patients with SAH admitted between 2005 and 2012 for whom data had been included in an existing data set. Logistic regression was used to identify predictors of CAUTI.

Findings

Catheterized adult patients (n = 242) with SAH over the 8-year period were included in the analysis. The rate of CAUTIs was 21%, or 6 times higher than the reported national average. Variables statistically significantly associated with CAUTI were older age (odds ratio [OR] = 1.06, 95% confidence interval [CI] [1.01, 1.11]), increased blood sugar levels (OR = 13.0, 95% CI [1.28, 107.4]), and anemia requiring transfusion (OR = 3.78, 95% CI [0.977, 14.67]).

Nursing Implications

Nurses should know that the high rates of CAUTI in this study were likely associated with prolonged catheterization. These findings indicate that nurses should carefully assess the need for catheterization and have increased vigilance regarding urinary catheter care in patients admitted with an SAH. Particular attention should be paid to patients who are older, those with anemia requiring transfusion, and those with elevated blood glucose levels due to their increased risk of CAUTI.

---

    c. Voids every 2 to 3 hours
    d. Produces urine that is clear and odorless
  3. Experiences no complications
    a. Reports no symptoms of infection (fever, frequency)
    b. Has normal kidney function, negative urine and blood cultures
    c. Exhibits normal vital signs and temperature; no signs or symptoms of sepsis (urosepsis)
    d. Maintains adequate urine output more than 0.5 mL/kg/hr

Upper Urinary Tract Infections

Pyelonephritis is a bacterial infection of the renal pelvis, tubules, and interstitial tissue of one or both kidneys. Causes involve either the upward spread of bacteria from the bladder or spread from systemic sources reaching the kidney via the bloodstream. Pathogenic bacteria from a bladder infection can ascend into the kidney, resulting in pyelonephritis. An incompetent ureterovesical valve or obstruction occurring in the urinary tract increases the susceptibility of the kidneys to infection (see Fig. 55-1), because static urine provides a good

---

PATIENT EDUCATION

Chart 55-5

Preventing Recurrent Urinary Tract Infections

The nurse instructs the patient on the following basic information:

Hygiene

- Shower rather than bathe in the tub because bacteria in the bathwater may enter the urethra.
- Clean the perineum and urethral meatus from front to back after each bowel movement. This will help reduce concentrations of pathogens at the urethral opening and, in women, the vaginal opening.

Fluid Intake

- Drink liberal amounts of fluids daily to flush out bacteria. It may be helpful to include at least one glass of cranberry juice per day.
- Avoid coffee, tea, colas, alcohol, and other fluids that are urinary tract irritants.

Voiding Habits

Void every 2–3 hours during the day, and completely empty the bladder. This prevents overdistention of the bladder and

compromised blood supply to the bladder wall. Both predispose the patient to urinary tract infection. Precautions expressly for women include voiding immediately after sexual intercourse.

Interventions

- Take medication *exactly* as prescribed. Special timing of administration may be required.
- Keep in mind that if bacteria continue to appear in the urine, long-term antimicrobial therapy may be required to prevent colonization of the periurethral area and recurrence of infection.
- For recurrent infection, consider acidification of the urine through ascorbic acid (vitamin C), 1000 mg daily, or daily consumption of cranberry juice.
- To decrease recurrences, consider *Lactobacillus* probiotics use in oral or vaginal form.
- If prescribed, test urine for presence of bacteria following manufacturer's and health care provider's instructions.
- Notify the primary provider if fever occurs or if signs and symptoms persist.
- Consult the primary provider regularly for follow-up.

Adapted from Bass-Ware, A., Weed, D., Johnson. T., et al. (2014). Evaluation of the effect of cranberry juice on symptoms associated with a urinary tract infection. *Urologic Nursing, 34*(3), 121–127; Chisholm, A. H. (2015). Probiotics in preventing recurrent urinary tract infections in women: A literature review. *Urologic Nursing, 35*(1), 18–21, 29.

medium for bacterial growth. Bladder or prostate tumors, strictures, benign prostatic hyperplasia, and urinary stones are some potential causes of obstruction that can lead to infections. Systemic infections (such as tuberculosis) can spread to the kidneys and result in abscesses.

Pyelonephritis may be acute or chronic. Acute pyelonephritis usually leads to enlargement of the kidneys with interstitial infiltrations of inflammatory cells (Grossman & Porth, 2014). Abscesses may be noted on or within the renal capsule and at the corticomedullary junction. Eventually, atrophy and destruction of tubules and the glomeruli may result. When pyelonephritis becomes chronic, the kidneys become scarred, contracted, and nonfunctioning. Chronic pyelonephritis is a cause of chronic kidney disease that can result in the need for renal replacement therapies such as transplantation or dialysis.

Acute Pyelonephritis

Clinical Manifestations

The patient with acute pyelonephritis has chills, fever, leukocytosis, bacteriuria, and pyuria. Low back pain, flank pain, nausea and vomiting, headache, malaise, and painful urination are common findings. Physical examination reveals pain and tenderness in the area of the costovertebral angle (see Fig. 53-6 in Chapter 53). In addition, symptoms of lower urinary tract involvement, such as urgency and frequency, are common.

Assessment and Diagnostic Findings

An ultrasound study or a CT scan may be performed to locate an obstruction in the urinary tract. Relief of obstruction is essential to prevent complications and eventual kidney damage. An IV pyelogram may be indicated with pyelonephritis if functional and structural renal abnormalities are suspected (Fischbach & Dunning, 2015). Radionuclide imaging with gallium citrate and indium-111 (^{111}In)–labeled WBCs may be useful to identify sites of infection that may not be visualized on CT scan or ultrasound. Urine culture and sensitivity tests are performed to determine the causative organism so that appropriate antimicrobial agents can be prescribed (Fischbach & Dunning, 2015).

Medical Management

Patients with acute uncomplicated pyelonephritis are most often treated on an outpatient basis if they are not exhibiting acute symptoms of sepsis, dehydration, nausea, or vomiting. In addition, they must be responsible and reliable to ensure that all medications will be taken as prescribed. For outpatients, a 2-week course of antibiotic agents is recommended because renal parenchymal disease is more difficult to eradicate than mucosal bladder infections. Commonly prescribed agents include many of the same medications prescribed for the treatment of UTIs (see Table 55-1).

Following acute pyelonephritis treatment, the patient may develop a chronic or recurring symptomless infection persisting for months or years. After the initial antibiotic regimen, the patient may need antibiotic therapy for up to 6 weeks if a relapse occurs. A follow-up urine culture is obtained 2 weeks after completion of antibiotic therapy to document clearing of the infection.

Hydration with oral or parenteral fluids is essential in all patients with UTIs when there is adequate kidney function. Hydration helps facilitate "flushing" of the urinary tract and reduces pain and discomfort.

Chronic Pyelonephritis

Repeated bouts of acute pyelonephritis may lead to chronic pyelonephritis.

Clinical Manifestations

The patient with chronic pyelonephritis usually has no symptoms of infection unless an acute exacerbation occurs. Noticeable signs and symptoms may include fatigue, headache, poor appetite, polyuria, excessive thirst, and weight loss. Persistent and recurring infection may produce progressive scarring of the kidney, resulting in chronic kidney disease (see Chapter 54).

Assessment and Diagnostic Findings

The extent of the disease is assessed by an IV urogram and measurements of creatinine clearance, blood urea nitrogen, and creatinine levels (Fischbach & Dunning, 2015).

Complications

Complications of chronic pyelonephritis include end-stage kidney disease (from progressive loss of nephrons secondary to chronic inflammation and scarring), hypertension, and formation of kidney stones (from chronic infection with urea-splitting organisms).

Medical Management

Bacteria, if detected in the urine, are eradicated if possible. Long-term use of prophylactic antimicrobial therapy may help limit recurrence of infections and kidney scarring. Impaired kidney function alters the excretion of antimicrobial agents and necessitates careful monitoring of kidney function, especially if the medications are potentially toxic to the kidneys.

Nursing Management

The patient may require hospitalization or may be treated as an outpatient. When the patient requires hospitalization, fluid intake and output are carefully measured and recorded. Unless contraindicated, 3 to 4 L of fluids per day is encouraged to dilute the urine, decrease burning on urination, and prevent dehydration. The nurse assesses the patient's temperature every 4 hours and administers antipyretic and antibiotic agents as prescribed.

Patient education focuses on prevention of further infection by consuming adequate fluids, emptying the bladder regularly, and performing recommended perineal hygiene. The importance of taking antimicrobial medications exactly as prescribed is stressed, as is the need for keeping follow-up appointments.

ADULT VOIDING DYSFUNCTION

Both neurogenic and nonneurogenic disorders can cause adult voiding dysfunction (see Table 55-2). The **micturition**

TABLE 55-2 Conditions Causing Adult Voiding Dysfunction

Condition	Voiding Dysfunction	Treatment
Neurogenic Disorders		
Cerebellar ataxia	Incontinence or dyssynergia	Timed voiding; anticholinergic agents
Stroke	Retention or incontinence	Anticholinergic agents; bladder retraining
Dementia	Incontinence	Prompted voiding; anticholinergic agents
Diabetes	Incontinence and/or incomplete bladder emptying	Timed voiding; EMG/biofeedback; pelvic floor nerve stimulation; anticholinergic/antispasmodic agents; well-controlled blood glucose levels
Multiple sclerosis	Incontinence or incomplete bladder emptying	Timed voiding; EMG/biofeedback to learn pelvic muscle exercises and urge inhibition; pelvic floor nerve stimulation; antispasmodic agents
Parkinson disease	Incontinence	Anticholinergic/antispasmodic agents
Spinal Cord Dysfunction		
Acute injury	Urinary retention	Indwelling catheter
Degenerative disease	Incontinence and/or incomplete bladder emptying	EMG/biofeedback; pelvic floor nerve stimulation; anticholinergic agents
Nonneurogenic Disorder		
"Bashful bladder"	Inability to initiate voiding in public bathrooms	Relaxation therapy; EMG/biofeedback
Overactive bladder	Urgency, frequency, and/or urge incontinence	EMG/biofeedback; pelvic floor nerve stimulation; bladder drill (see Chart 55-8); anticholinergic agents
Post general surgery	Acute urine retention	Catheterization
Post prostatectomy	Incontinence	*Mild:* Biofeedback; bladder drill (see Chart 55-8); pelvic floor nerve stimulation *Moderate/severe:* Surgery—artificial sphincter
Stress incontinence	Incontinence with cough, laugh, sneeze, position change	*Mild:* Biofeedback; bladder drill (see Chart 55-8); periurethral bulking with collagen *Moderate/severe:* Surgery

EMG, electromyogram.

Adapted from Bader, M. K., Littlejohns, L. R., & Olson, D. M. (2016). *AANN core curriculum for neuroscience nursing* (6th ed.). Chicago, IL: American Association of Neuroscience Nurses.

(voiding or urination) process involves several highly coordinated neurologic responses that mediate bladder function. A functional urinary system allows for appropriate bladder filling and complete bladder emptying (see Chapter 53). If voiding dysfunction goes undetected and untreated, the upper urinary system may be compromised. Chronic incomplete bladder emptying from poor detrusor pressure results in recurrent bladder infection. Incomplete bladder emptying due to bladder outlet obstruction (such as benign prostatic hyperplasia), causing high-pressure detrusor contractions, can result in hydronephrosis from the high detrusor pressure that radiates up the ureters to the renal pelvis.

Urinary Incontinence

More than 25 million adults in the United States are estimated to have **urinary incontinence** (involuntary or uncontrolled loss of urine from the bladder), with most of them experiencing overactive bladder syndrome, making this disorder more prevalent than diabetes or ulcer disease (Miller, 2015). Despite widespread media coverage, urinary incontinence remains underdiagnosed and underreported. Patients may be too embarrassed to seek help, causing them to ignore or conceal symptoms. Many patients use absorbent pads or other devices without having their condition properly diagnosed and treated (Day, Leahy-Warren, Loughran, et al., 2014). Health care providers must be alert to subtle cues of urinary incontinence and stay informed about current management strategies.

The costs of care for patients with urinary incontinence include the expenses of absorbent products, medications, and surgical or nonsurgical treatment modalities, as well as psychosocial costs (i.e., embarrassment, loss of self-esteem, and social isolation) (Day et al., 2014; McCooty & Latthe, 2014).

Although urinary incontinence is commonly regarded as a condition that occurs in older multiparous women, it can occur in young nulliparous women, especially during vigorous high-impact activity. Age, gender, and number of vaginal deliveries are established risk factors that explain, in part, the increased incidence in women (see Chart 55-6). Men can have urinary incontinence, especially those with certain comorbid conditions. One group of researchers, for example, reported that 40% of men with Parkinson disease reported urinary incontinence (Robinson, Bradway, Bunting-Perry, et al., 2013). Urinary incontinence is a symptom of many possible disorders.

Types of Urinary Incontinence

There are many types of urinary incontinence, including the following:

Stress incontinence is the involuntary loss of urine through an intact urethra as a result of sneezing, coughing, or changing position (Miller, 2015; Weber & Kelley, 2014). It predominantly affects women who have had vaginal deliveries and is thought to be the result of decreasing ligament and pelvic floor support

Chart 55-6 RISK FACTORS
Urinary Incontinence

- Age-related changes in the urinary tract
- Caregiver or toilet unavailable
- Cognitive disturbances—dementia, Parkinson disease
- Diabetes
- Genitourinary surgery
- High-impact exercise
- Immobility
- Incompetent urethra due to trauma or sphincter relaxation
- Medications—diuretic, sedative, hypnotic, and opioid agents
- Menopause
- Morbid obesity
- Pelvic muscle weakness
- Pregnancy—vaginal delivery, episiotomy
- Stroke

Adapted from Robinson, J. P., Bradway. C. W., Bunting-Perry, L., et al. (2013). Lower urinary tract symptoms in men with Parkinson's disease. *Journal of Neuroscience Nursing, 45*(6). 382–392.

of the urethra and decreasing or absent estrogen levels within the urethral walls and bladder base. In men, stress incontinence is often experienced after a radical prostatectomy for prostate cancer because of the loss of urethral compression that the prostate had supplied before the surgery, and possibly bladder wall irritability.

Urge incontinence is the involuntary loss of urine associated with a strong urge to void that cannot be suppressed (Miller, 2015; Weber & Kelley, 2014). The patient is aware of the need to void but is unable to reach a toilet in time. An uninhibited detrusor contraction is the precipitating factor. This can occur in a patient with neurologic dysfunction that impairs inhibition of bladder contraction or in a patient without overt neurologic dysfunction.

Functional incontinence refers to those instances in which lower urinary tract function is intact but other factors, such as severe cognitive impairment (e.g., Alzheimer dementia), make it difficult for the patient to identify the need to void or physical impairments make it difficult or impossible for the patient to reach the toilet in time for voiding (Miller, 2015).

Iatrogenic incontinence refers to the involuntary loss of urine due to extrinsic medical factors, predominantly medications. One such example is the use of alpha-adrenergic agents to decrease blood pressure. In some people with an intact urinary system, these agents adversely affect the alpha receptors responsible for bladder neck closing pressure; the bladder neck relaxes to the point of incontinence with a minimal increase in intra-abdominal pressure, thus mimicking stress incontinence. As soon as the medication is discontinued, the apparent incontinence resolves.

Mixed urinary incontinence, which encompasses several types of urinary incontinence, is involuntary leakage associated with urgency and also with exertion, effort, sneezing, or coughing (Miller, 2015).

Only with appropriate recognition of the problem, assessment, and referral for diagnostic evaluation and treatment can the outcome of incontinence be determined. All people with incontinence should be considered for evaluation and treatment.

Gerontologic Considerations

Although urinary incontinence is not a normal consequence of aging, age-related changes in the urinary tract do predispose the older person to incontinence. However, if nurses and other health care providers accept incontinence as an inevitable part of illness or aging or consider it irreversible and untreatable, it cannot be treated successfully. Collaborative, interdisciplinary efforts are essential in assessing and effectively treating urinary incontinence. Urinary incontinence can decrease an older person's ability to maintain an independent lifestyle, which increases dependence on caregivers and may lead to institutionalization. Between 25% and 45% of older women have urinary incontinence (Day et al., 2014).

Many older adults experience transient episodes of incontinence that tend to be abrupt in onset. When this occurs, the nurse should question the patient, as well as the family if possible, about the onset of symptoms and any signs or symptoms of a change in other organ systems. Acute UTI, infection elsewhere in the body, constipation, decreased fluid intake, and a change in a chronic disease pattern, such as elevated blood glucose levels in patients with diabetes or decreased estrogen levels in menopausal women, can provoke the onset of urinary incontinence. If the cause is identified and modified or eliminated early at the onset of incontinence, the incontinence itself may be eliminated. Although the bladder of the older person is more vulnerable to altered detrusor activity, age alone is not a risk factor for urinary incontinence (Miller, 2015).

Decreased bladder muscle tone is a normal age-related change found in older adults. This leads to decreased bladder capacity, increased **residual urine** (urine remaining in the bladder after voiding), and an increase in urgency.

Many medications affect urinary continence in addition to causing other unwanted or unexpected effects (Miller, 2015). All medications need to be assessed for potential interactions.

Assessment and Diagnostic Findings

Once incontinence is recognized, a thorough history is necessary. This includes a detailed description of the problem and a history of medication use. The patient's voiding history, a diary of fluid intake and output, and bedside tests (e.g., residual urine, stress maneuvers) may be used to help determine the type of urinary incontinence involved. Extensive urodynamic tests may be performed (see Chapter 53). Urinalysis and urine culture are performed to identify infection.

Urinary incontinence may be transient or reversible if the underlying cause is successfully treated and the voiding pattern reverts to normal. Chart 55-7 provides causes of transient incontinence.

Medical Management

Management depends on the type of urinary incontinence and its causes. Management of urinary incontinence may be behavioral, pharmacologic, or surgical.

Behavioral Therapy

Behavioral therapies are the first choice to decrease or eliminate urinary incontinence (see Chart 55-8). In using these techniques, health care professionals help patients avoid potential adverse effects of pharmacologic or surgical

Chart 55-7

Causes of Transient Incontinence

- Atrophic vaginitis, urethritis, prostatitis
- Delirium or confusion
- Excessive urine production (increased intake, diabetes, diabetic ketoacidosis)
- Limited or restricted activity

- Pharmacologic agents (anticholinergic agents, sedatives, alcohol, analgesic agents, diuretics, muscle relaxants, adrenergic agents)
- Psychological factors (depression, regression)
- Stool impaction or constipation
- Urinary tract infections (UTI)

Chart 55-8

HEALTH PROMOTION
Interventions for Urinary Incontinence

Behavioral strategies are largely carried out, coordinated, and monitored by the nurse. These interventions may or may not be augmented by the use of medications.

Fluid Management

An adequate daily fluid intake of approximately 50–60 oz (1500–1600 mL), taken as small increments between breakfast and the evening meal, helps to reduce urinary urgency related to concentrated urine production, decreases the risk of urinary tract infection, and maintains bowel functioning. (Constipation, resulting from inadequate daily fluid intake, can increase urinary urgency and urine retention.) The best fluid is water, although some suggest it may be helpful to include at least one glass of cranberry juice per day. Fluids containing caffeine, carbonation, alcohol, or artificial sweetener should be avoided because they irritate the bladder wall, thus resulting in urinary urgency. Some patients who have heart failure or end-stage kidney disease need to discuss their daily fluid limit with their primary provider.

Standardized Voiding Frequency

After establishing a patient's natural voiding and urinary continence tendencies, voiding on a schedule can be very effective in those with and without cognitive impairment, although patients with cognitive impairment may require assistance with this technique from nursing personnel or family members. The object is to purposely empty the bladder before the bladder reaches the critical volume that would cause an urge or stress incontinence episode. This approach involves the following:

- **Timed voiding** involves establishing a set voiding frequency (such as every 2 hours if incontinent episodes tend to occur 2 or more hours after voiding). The individual chooses to "void by the clock" at the given interval while awake rather than wait until a voiding urge occurs.
- **Prompted voiding** is timed voiding that is carried out by staff or family members when the individual has cognitive difficulties that make it difficult to remember to void at set intervals. The caregiver checks the patient to assess if he or she has remained dry and, if so, assists the patient to use the bathroom while providing positive reinforcement for remaining dry.
- **Habit retraining** is timed voiding at an interval that is more frequent than the individual would usually choose. This technique helps to restore the sensation of the need to void in individuals who are experiencing diminished sensation of bladder filling due to various medical conditions such as a stroke.
- **Bladder retraining**, also known as "bladder drill," incorporates a timed voiding schedule and urinary urge inhibition exercises to inhibit voiding, or leaking urine, in an attempt to remain dry for a set time. When the first timing interval is easily reached on a consistent basis without urinary urgency or incontinence, a new

voiding interval, usually 10–15 minutes beyond the last, is established. Again, the individual practices urge inhibition exercises to delay voiding or avoid incontinence until the next preset interval arrives. When an acceptable voiding interval is reached, the patient continues that timed voiding sequence throughout the day.

Pelvic Muscle Exercise

Also known as Kegel exercises, pelvic muscle exercise (PME) aims to strengthen the voluntary muscles that assist in bladder and bowel continence in both men and women. Research shows that written or verbal instruction alone is usually inadequate to educate an individual about how to identify and strengthen the pelvic floor for sufficient bladder and bowel control. Biofeedback-assisted PME uses either electromyography or manometry to help the individual identify the pelvic muscles as they attempt to learn which muscle group is involved when performing PME. The biofeedback method also allows assessment of the strength of this muscle area.

PME involves gently tightening the same muscles used to stop flatus or the stream of urine for 5–10-second increments, followed by 10-second resting phases. To be effective, these exercises need to be performed 2 or 3 times a day for at least 6 weeks. Depending on the strength of the pelvic musculature when initially evaluated, anywhere from 10–30 repetitions of PME are prescribed at each session. Older patients may need to exercise for an even longer time to strengthen the pelvic floor muscles. Pelvic muscle exercises are helpful for women with stress, urge, or mixed incontinence and for men who have undergone prostate surgery.

Vaginal Cone Retention Exercises

Vaginal cone retention exercises are an adjunct to the Kegel exercises. Vaginal cones of varying weight are inserted intravaginally twice a day. The patient tries to retain the cone for 15 minutes by contracting the pelvic muscles.

Transvaginal or Transrectal Electrical Stimulation

Commonly used to treat urinary incontinence, electrical stimulation is known to elicit a passive contraction of the pelvic floor musculature, thus re-educating these muscles to provide enhanced levels of continence. This modality is often used with biofeedback-assisted pelvic muscle exercise training and voiding schedules. At high frequencies, it is effective for stress incontinence. At low frequencies, electrical stimulation can also relieve symptoms of urinary urgency, frequency, and urge incontinence. Intermediate ranges are used for mixed incontinence.

Neuromodulation

Neuromodulation via transvaginal or transrectal nerve stimulation of the pelvic floor inhibits detrusor overactivity and hypersensory bladder signals and strengthens weak sphincter muscles.

Adapted from Bader, M. K., Littlejohns, L. R., & Olson, D. M. (2016). *AANN core curriculum for neuroscience nursing* (6th ed.). Chicago, IL: American Association of Neuroscience Nurses; Bass-Ware, A., Weed, D., Johnson. T., et al. (2014). Evaluation of the effect of cranberry juice on symptoms associated with a urinary tract infection. *Urologic Nursing, 34*(3), 121–127; Chisholm, A. H. (2015). Probiotics in preventing recurrent urinary tract infections in women: A literature review. *Urologic Nursing, 35*(1), 18–21, 29.

interventions. Pelvic floor muscle exercises (sometimes referred to as Kegel exercises) represent the cornerstone of behavioral intervention for addressing symptoms of stress, urge, and mixed incontinence (Miller, 2015; Weber & Kelley, 2014). Other behavioral treatments include the use of a voiding diary, biofeedback, verbal instruction (prompted voiding), and physical therapy (Day et al., 2014; McCooty & Latthe, 2014).

Pharmacologic Therapy

Pharmacologic therapy works best when used as an adjunct to behavioral interventions. Anticholinergic agents inhibit bladder contraction and are considered first-line medications for urge incontinence. A tricyclic antidepressant medication (e.g., amitriptyline [Elavil]) can also decrease bladder contractions as well as increase bladder neck resistance (Comerford, 2015). Pseudoephedrine sulfate (Sudafed), which acts on alpha-adrenergic receptors, causing urinary retention, may be used to treat stress incontinence; it needs to be used with caution in men with prostatic hyperplasia and patients with hypertension.

Surgical Management

Surgical correction may be indicated in patients who have not achieved continence using behavioral and pharmacologic therapy. Surgical options vary according to the underlying anatomy and the physiologic problem. Most procedures involve lifting and stabilizing the bladder or urethra to restore the normal urethrovesical angle or to lengthen the urethra.

Women with stress incontinence may undergo an anterior vaginal repair, retropubic suspension, or needle suspension to reposition the urethra. Procedures to compress the urethra and increase resistance to urine flow include sling procedures and placement of periurethral bulking agents such as artificial collagen.

Periurethral bulking is a semipermanent procedure in which small amounts of artificial collagen are placed within the walls of the urethra to enhance the closing pressure of the urethra (Matsuoka, Locali, Pacetta, et al., 2016). This procedure takes only 10 to 20 minutes and may be performed under local anesthesia or moderate sedation. A cystoscope is inserted into the urethra. An instrument is inserted through the cystoscope to deliver a small amount of collagen into the urethral wall at locations selected by the urologist. The patient is usually discharged home after voiding. There are no restrictions following the procedure, although occasionally more than one collagen bulking session may be necessary if the initial procedure did not halt stress incontinence. Collagen placement anywhere in the body is considered semipermanent because its durability averages between 12 and 24 months, until the body absorbs the material. Periurethral bulking with collagen is a relatively safe alternative to surgery (Matsuoka et al., 2016). It is also an option for people who are seeking help with stress incontinence who prefer to avoid surgery and who do not have access to behavioral therapies.

An artificial urinary sphincter can be used to close the urethra and promote continence. Two types of artificial sphincters are a periurethral cuff and a cuff inflation pump.

Men with overflow and stress incontinence may undergo a transurethral resection to relieve symptoms of prostatic enlargement. An artificial sphincter can be used after

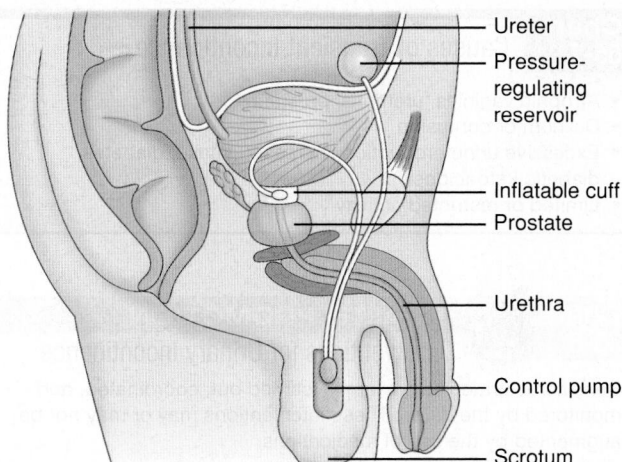

Figure 55-2 • Male artificial urinary sphincter. An inflatable cuff is inserted surgically around the urethra or neck of the bladder. To empty the bladder, the cuff is deflated by squeezing the control pump located in the scrotum.

prostatic surgery for sphincter incompetence (see Fig. 55-2). After surgery, periurethral bulking agents can be injected into the periurethral area to increase compression of the urethra (Matsuoka et al., 2016).

Nursing Management

Nursing management is based on the premise that incontinence is not inevitable with illness or aging and that it is often reversible and treatable. The nursing interventions are determined in part by the type of treatment that is undertaken. For behavioral therapy to be effective, the nurse must provide support and encouragement, because it is easy for the patient to become discouraged if therapy does not quickly improve the level of continence. Patient education is important and should be provided verbally and in writing (see Chart 55-9). The patient should be educated to develop and use a log or

PATIENT EDUCATION

Chart 55-9

Strategies for Promoting Urinary Continence

The nurse instructs the patient to:

- Avoid bladder irritants, such as caffeine, alcohol, and aspartame (NutraSweet).
- Avoid taking diuretic agents after 4 pm.
- Increase awareness of the amount and timing of all fluid intake.
- Perform all pelvic floor muscle exercises as prescribed, every day.
- Stop smoking (smokers usually cough frequently, which increases incontinence).
- Take steps to avoid constipation: Drink adequate fluids, eat a well-balanced diet high in fiber, exercise regularly, and take stool softeners if recommended.
- Void regularly, 5–8 times a day (about every 2–3 hours):
  - First thing in the morning
  - Before each meal
  - Before retiring to bed
  - Once during the night if necessary

diary to record timing of pelvic floor muscle exercises, frequency of voiding, any changes in bladder function, and any episodes of incontinence (Miller, 2015).

If pharmacologic treatment is used, the patient and family are educated about its purpose. Patients with mixed incontinence must be informed that anticholinergic and antispasmodic agents can help decrease urinary urgency and frequency and urge incontinence but do not decrease the urinary incontinence related to stress incontinence. If surgical correction is undertaken, the procedure and its desired outcomes are described to the patient and family. Follow-up contact with the patient enables the nurse to answer the patient's questions and to provide reinforcement and encouragement.

Urinary Retention

Urinary retention is the inability to empty the bladder completely during attempts to void. Chronic urine retention often leads to **overflow incontinence** (involuntary urine loss associated with overdistention of the bladder). Residual urine is urine that remains in the bladder after voiding. In a healthy adult younger than 60 years, complete bladder emptying should occur with each voiding. In adults older than 60 years, 50 to 100 mL of residual urine may remain after each voiding because of the decreased contractility of the detrusor muscle.

Urinary retention can occur postoperatively in any patient, particularly if the surgery affected the perineal or anal regions and resulted in reflex spasm of the sphincters. General anesthesia reduces bladder muscle innervation and suppresses the urge to void, impeding bladder emptying.

Pathophysiology

Urinary retention may result from diabetes, prostatic enlargement, urethral pathology (infection, tumor, calculus), trauma (pelvic injuries), pregnancy, or neurologic disorders (e.g., stroke, spinal cord injury, multiple sclerosis, or Parkinson disease). Some medications cause urinary retention either by inhibiting bladder contractility or by increasing bladder outlet resistance (Comerford, 2015).

Assessment and Diagnostic Findings

The assessment of a patient for urinary retention is multifaceted because the signs and symptoms are challenging to detect. The following questions serve as a guide in assessment:

- What was the time of the last voiding, and how much urine was voided?
- Is the patient voiding small amounts of urine frequently?
- Is the patient dribbling urine?
- Does the patient complain of pain or discomfort in the lower abdomen? (Discomfort may be relatively mild if the bladder distends slowly.)
- Is the pelvic area rounded and swollen (could indicate urine retention and a distended bladder)?
- Does percussion of the suprapubic region elicit dullness (possibly indicating urine retention and a distended bladder)?
- Are other indicators of urinary retention present, such as restlessness and agitation?
- Does a postvoid bladder ultrasound test reveal residual urine?

The patient may verbalize an awareness of bladder fullness and a sensation of incomplete bladder emptying. Signs and symptoms of UTI (hematuria, urgency, frequency, and nocturia) may be present. A series of urodynamic studies (described in Chapter 53) may be performed to identify the type of bladder dysfunction and to aid in determining appropriate treatment. A voiding diary can be used to provide a written record of the amount of urine voided and the frequency of voiding. Postvoid residual urine may be assessed by using either straight catheterization or an ultrasound bladder scanner and is considered diagnostic of urinary retention. Normally, residual urine amounts to no more than 50 mL in the middle-aged adult and less than 50 to 100 mL in the older adult (Weber & Kelley, 2014).

Complications

The retention of urine can lead to chronic infections that if unresolved predispose the patient to renal calculi (urolithiasis or nephrolithiasis), pyelonephritis, sepsis, or hydronephrosis. In addition, urine leakage can lead to perineal skin breakdown, especially if regular hygiene measures are neglected.

Nursing Management

Strategies are instituted to prevent overdistention of the bladder and to treat infection or correct obstruction. However, many complications can be prevented with careful assessment and appropriate nursing interventions. The nurse explains to the patient why normal voiding is not occurring and monitors urine output closely. The nurse also provides reassurance about the temporary nature of retention and successful management strategies.

Promoting Urinary Elimination

Nursing measures to encourage normal voiding patterns include providing privacy, ensuring an environment and body position conducive to voiding, and assisting the patient with the use of the bathroom or bedside commode, rather than a bedpan, to provide a more natural setting for voiding. If his condition allows, the male patient may stand beside the bed to use the urinal; most men find this position more comfortable and natural.

Additional measures include applying warmth to relax the sphincters (i.e., sitz baths, warm compresses to the perineum, showers), giving the patient hot caffeine free beverage and offering encouragement and reassurance. Simple trigger techniques, such as turning on the water faucet while the patient is trying to void, may also be used. Other examples of trigger techniques are stroking the abdomen or inner thighs, tapping above the pubic area, and dipping the patient's hands in warm water. After surgery or childbirth, prescribed analgesic agents should be given because pain in the perineal area can make voiding difficult. A combination of techniques may be necessary to initiate voiding.

When the patient cannot void, bladder scanning is used to assess for distension, then straight catheterization (as prescribed) is used to prevent overdistention of the bladder (see later discussion of neurogenic bladder and catheterization). In the case of prostatic obstruction, attempts at catheterization (by the urologist) may not be successful, requiring insertion of a **suprapubic catheter** (catheter inserted through a small abdominal incision into the bladder). After urinary drainage is restored, bladder retraining is initiated for the patient who cannot void spontaneously.

Promoting Home, Community-Based, and Transitional Care

In addition to the strategies listed for promoting urinary continence found in Chart 55-9, modifications to the home environment can provide simple and effective ways to assist in treating urinary incontinence and retention. For example, the patient may need to remove obstacles, such as throw rugs or other objects, to provide easy, safe access to the bathroom. Other modifications that the nurse may recommend include installing support bars in the bathroom; placing a bedside commode, bedpan, or urinal within easy reach; leaving lights on in the bedroom and bathroom; and wearing clothing that is easy to remove quickly.

Neurogenic Bladder

Neurogenic bladder is a dysfunction that results from a disorder or dysfunction of the nervous system and leads to urinary incontinence. It may be caused by spinal cord injury, spinal tumor, herniated vertebral disc, multiple sclerosis, congenital disorders (spina bifida or myelomeningocele), infection, or complications of diabetes (Bader, Littlejohns, & Olson, 2016) (see Chapters 51, 68, and 69).

Pathophysiology

The two types of neurogenic bladder are spastic (or reflex) bladder and flaccid bladder. Spastic bladder is the more common type and is caused by any spinal cord lesion above the voiding reflex arc (upper motor neuron lesion) (Bader et al., 2016). The result is a loss of conscious sensation and cerebral motor control. A spastic bladder empties on reflex, with minimal or no controlling influence to regulate its activity.

Flaccid bladder is caused by a lower motor neuron lesion, commonly resulting from trauma. This form of neurogenic bladder is also increasingly being recognized in patients with diabetes. The bladder continues to fill and becomes greatly distended, and overflow incontinence occurs. The bladder muscle does not contract forcefully at any time. Because sensory loss may accompany a flaccid bladder, the patient feels no discomfort.

Assessment and Diagnostic Findings

Evaluation for neurogenic bladder involves measurement of fluid intake, urine output, and residual urine volume; urinalysis; and assessment of sensory awareness of bladder fullness and degree of motor control. Comprehensive urodynamic studies are also performed.

Complications

The most common complication of neurogenic bladder is infection resulting from urinary stasis and catheterization. Other complications include renal calculi, impaired skin integrity, and urinary incontinence or retention (Bader et al., 2016).

Medical Management

The problems resulting from neurogenic bladder disorders vary considerably from patient to patient and are a major challenge to the health care team. Several long-term objectives appropriate for all types of neurogenic bladders include preventing overdistention of the bladder, emptying the bladder regularly and completely, maintaining urine sterility with no stone formation, and maintaining adequate bladder capacity with no reflux.

Specific interventions include continuous, intermittent, or self-catheterization (discussed later in this chapter); the use of an external condom-type catheter; a diet low in calcium (to prevent calculi); and encouragement of mobility and ambulation. A liberal fluid intake is encouraged to reduce the urinary bacterial count, reduce stasis, decrease the concentration of calcium in the urine, and minimize the precipitation of urinary crystals and subsequent stone formation.

A bladder retraining program may be effective in treating a spastic bladder or urine retention. The use of a timed, or habit, voiding schedule may be established. To further enhance emptying of a flaccid bladder, the patient may be taught to "double void." After each voiding, the patient is instructed to remain on the toilet, relax for 1 to 2 minutes, and then attempt to void again in an effort to further empty the bladder.

Pharmacologic Therapy

Parasympathomimetic medications, such as bethanechol (Urecholine), may help to increase the contraction of the detrusor muscle.

Surgical Management

Surgery may be carried out to correct bladder neck contractures or vesicoureteral reflux, or to perform a urinary diversion procedure.

Catheterization

In patients with a urologic disorder or with marginal kidney function, care must be taken to ensure that urinary drainage is adequate and that kidney function is preserved. When urine cannot be eliminated naturally and must be drained artificially, catheters may be inserted directly into the bladder, the ureter, or the renal pelvis. Catheters vary in size, shape, length, material, and configuration (Carter et al., 2014). The type of catheter used depends on its purpose.

Catheterization is performed to achieve the following:
- Relieve urinary tract obstruction
- Assist with postoperative drainage in urologic and other surgeries
- Provide a means to monitor accurate urine output in patients who are critically ill
- Promote urinary drainage in patients with neurogenic bladder dysfunction or urine retention
- Prevent urinary leakage in patients with stage III to IV pressure ulcers (see Chapter 10)

A patient should be catheterized only if necessary, because catheterization commonly leads to UTI. Catheters impede most of the natural defenses of the lower urinary tract by obstructing the periurethral ducts, irritating the bladder mucosa, and providing an artificial route for organisms to enter the bladder (Hagerty et al., 2015). Organisms may be introduced from the urethra into the bladder during catheterization, or they may migrate along the epithelial surface of the urethra or external surface of the catheter. In addition, urinary catheters have been associated with other complications, such as bladder spasms, urethral strictures, and pressure necrosis (Bader et al., 2016).

Indwelling Catheters

When an indwelling catheter cannot be avoided, a closed drainage system is essential. This drainage system is designed to prevent any disconnections, thereby reducing the risk of contamination. Triple-lumen catheters are commonly used after transurethral prostate surgery (see Chapter 59). This system has a triple-lumen indwelling urethral catheter attached to a closed sterile drainage system. With the triple-lumen catheter, urinary drainage occurs through one channel. The retention balloon of the catheter is inflated with water or air through the second channel, and the bladder is continuously irrigated with sterile irrigating solution through the third channel.

The spout (or drainage port) of any urinary drainage bag can become contaminated when opened to drain the bag. Bacteria enter the urinary drainage bag, multiply rapidly, and then migrate to the drainage tubing, catheter, and bladder. By keeping the drainage bag lower than the patient's bladder and not allowing urine to flow back into the bladder, this risk is reduced.

Suprapubic Catheters

Suprapubic catheterization allows bladder drainage by inserting a catheter or tube into the bladder through a suprapubic (above the pubis) incision or puncture (see Fig. 55-3). The

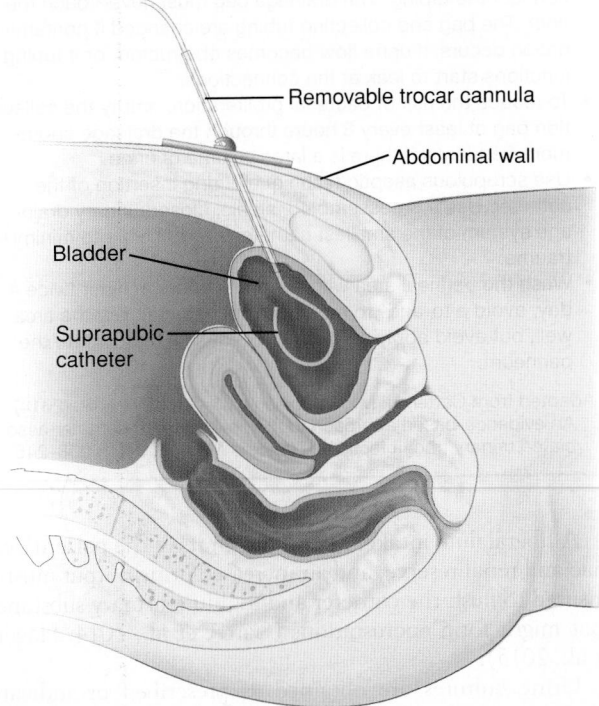

Removable trocar cannula

Abdominal wall

Bladder

Suprapubic catheter

Figure 55-3 • Suprapubic bladder drainage. A trocar cannula is used to puncture the abdominal and bladder walls. The catheter is threaded through the trocar cannula, which is then removed, leaving the catheter in place. The catheter is secured by tape or sutures to prevent unintentional removal.

catheter or suprapubic drainage tube is then threaded into the bladder and secured with sutures or tape, and the area around the catheter is covered with a sterile dressing. The catheter is connected to a sterile closed drainage system, and the tubing is secured to prevent tension on the catheter. This may be a temporary measure to divert the flow of urine from the urethra when the urethral route is impassable (because of injuries, strictures, prostatic obstruction), after gynecologic or other abdominal surgery when bladder dysfunction is likely to occur, and occasionally after pelvic fractures.

Suprapubic bladder drainage may be maintained continuously for several weeks. When the patient's ability to void is to be tested, the catheter is clamped for 4 hours, during which time the patient attempts to void. After the patient voids, the catheter is unclamped, and the residual urine is measured. If the amount of residual urine is less than 100 mL on two separate occasions (morning and evening), the catheter is usually removed. However, if the patient complains of pain or discomfort, the suprapubic catheter is usually left in place until the patient can void successfully.

Suprapubic drainage offers certain advantages. Patients can usually void sooner after surgery than those with urethral catheters, and they may be more comfortable. The catheter allows greater mobility, permits measurement of residual urine without urethral instrumentation, and presents less risk of bladder infection. The suprapubic catheter is removed when it is no longer required, and a sterile dressing is placed over the site.

The patient requires liberal amounts of fluid to prevent encrustation around the catheter. Other potential problems include the formation of bladder stones, acute and chronic infections, and problems collecting urine. A wound-ostomy-continence (WOC) nurse may be consulted to assist the patient and family in selecting the most suitable urine collection system and to educate them about its use and care.

Nursing Management

Assessing the Patient and the System

For patients with indwelling catheters, the nurse assesses the drainage system to ensure that it provides adequate urinary drainage. The color, odor, and volume of urine are also monitored. An accurate record of fluid intake and urine output provides essential information about the adequacy of kidney function and urinary drainage.

Patients at high risk for UTI from catheterization need to be identified and monitored carefully. These include women; older adults; and patients who are debilitated, malnourished, chronically ill, immunosuppressed, or have diabetes (Carter et al., 2014; Hagerty et al., 2015). They are observed for signs and symptoms of UTI: cloudy malodorous urine, hematuria, fever, chills, anorexia, and malaise. Any drainage and excoriation in the area around the urethral orifice is noted. Urine cultures provide the most accurate means of assessing a patient for infection.

Gerontologic Considerations

The older patient with an indwelling catheter may not exhibit the typical signs and symptoms of infection (Eliopoulos, 2018). Therefore, any subtle change in physical condition or mental status must be considered a possible indication of

Physiology/Pathophysiology

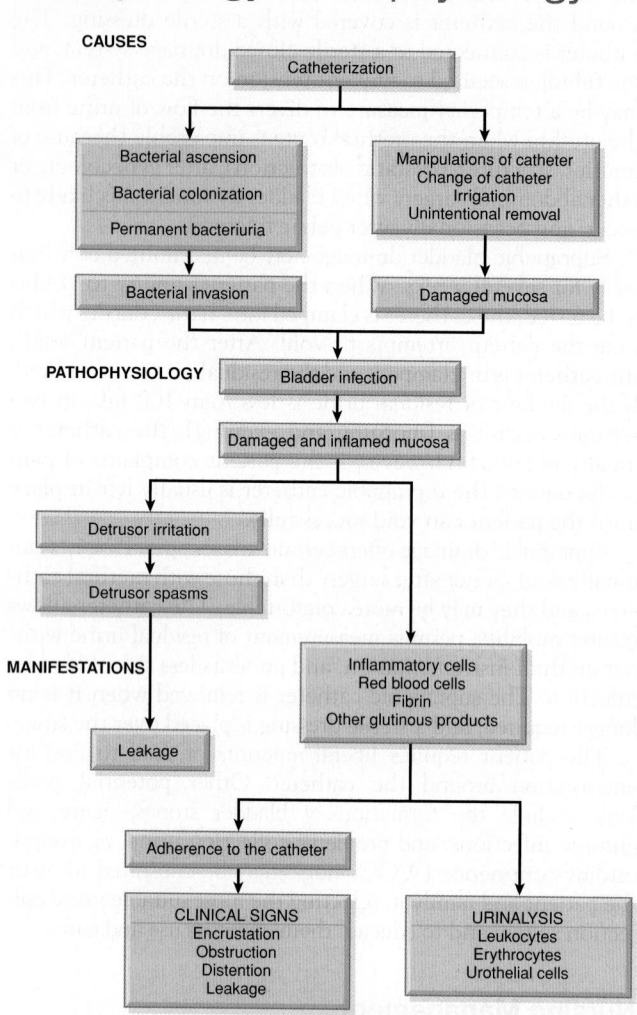

Figure 55-4 • Pathophysiology and manifestations of bladder infection with long-term catheterization in older patients.

infection and promptly investigated because sepsis may occur before the infection is diagnosed. Figure 55-4 summarizes the sequence of events leading to infection and leakage of urine that often follow long-term use of an indwelling catheter in an older patient (Miller, 2015).

Preventing Infection

Certain principles of care are essential to prevent infection in patients with a closed urinary drainage system (see Chart 55-10). The catheter is an object foreign to the body and produces a reaction in the urethral mucosa with some urethral discharge. Vigorous cleansing of the meatus while the catheter is in place is discouraged because the cleansing action can move the catheter back and forth, increasing the risk of infection. To clean the external catheter surface, gentle washing with soap and water or wipes during the daily bath is used by some (Strouse, 2015). Others report that using 2% chlorhexidine gluconate no-rinse wipes during the daily bath helps decrease CAUTI rates (Carter et al., 2014). The catheter is anchored as securely as possible to prevent it from moving in the urethra (Carter et al., 2014; Mori, 2014).

Chart 55-10 Preventing Infection in the Patient With an Indwelling Urinary Catheter

- Avoid contamination of the drainage spout. A receptacle in which to empty the bag is provided for each patient.
- Avoid routine catheter changes. The catheter is changed only to correct problems such as leakage, blockage, or encrustations.
- Avoid unnecessary handling or manipulation of the catheter by the patient or staff.
- Carry out hand hygiene before and after handling the catheter, tubing, or drainage bag.
- Ensure a free flow of urine to prevent infection. Improper drainage occurs when the tubing is kinked or twisted, allowing pools of urine to collect in the tubing loops.
- Evaluate the benefit of placing an indwelling urinary catheter versus the risk the patient developing a catheter-associated urinary tract infection.
- If the collection bag *must* be raised above the level of the patient's bladder, clamp the drainage tube. This prevents backflow of contaminated urine into the patient's bladder from the bag.
- Monitor the patient's voiding when the catheter is removed. The patient must void within 8 hours; if unable to void, the patient may require catheterization with a straight catheter.
- Never disconnect the tubing to obtain urine samples, to irrigate the catheter, or to ambulate or transport the patient.
- Never irrigate the catheter routinely. If the patient is prone to obstruction from clots or large amounts of sediment, use a three-way system with continuous irrigation.
- Never leave the catheter in place longer than is necessary to decrease the risk of CAUTI.
- Obtain a urine specimen for culture at the first sign of infection.
- To prevent contamination of the closed system, *never* disconnect the tubing. The drainage bag must *never* touch the floor. The bag and collecting tubing are changed if contamination occurs, if urine flow becomes obstructed, or if tubing junctions start to leak at the connections.
- To reduce the risk of bacterial proliferation, empty the collection bag at least every 8 hours through the drainage spout—more frequently if there is a large volume of urine.
- Use scrupulous aseptic technique during insertion of the catheter. Use a preassembled, sterile, closed urinary drainage system of the smallest catheter size possible to minimize trauma.
- Wash the perineal area with soap and water at least twice a day; avoid a to-and-fro motion of the catheter. Dry the area well, but avoid applying powder because it may irritate the perineum.

Adapted from Carter, N. M., Reitmeier, L., & Goodloe, L. R. (2014). An evidence-based approach to the prevention of catheter-associated urinary tract infections. *Urologic Nursing, 34*(5), 238–245.

A liberal fluid intake, within the limits of the patient's cardiac and renal reserve, and an increased urine output must be ensured to flush the catheter and to dilute urinary substances that might form encrustations (Carter et al., 2014; Hagerty et al., 2015).

Urine cultures are obtained as prescribed or indicated when monitoring the patient for infection; many catheters have an aspiration (puncture) port from which a specimen can be obtained.

Bacteriuria is considered inevitable in patients with indwelling catheters; therefore, controversy remains about the usefulness of taking cultures and treating asymptomatic bacteriuria, because overtreatment may lead to resistant strains of bacteria. Continual observation for fever, chills, and other signs and symptoms of systemic infection is necessary. Infections are treated aggressively.

Minimizing Trauma

Trauma to the urethra can be minimized by:
- Using an appropriately sized catheter
- Lubricating the catheter adequately with a water-soluble lubricant during insertion
- Inserting the catheter far enough into the bladder to prevent trauma to the urethral tissues when the retention balloon of the catheter is inflated

Manipulation of the catheter is the most common cause of trauma to the bladder mucosa in the catheterized patient. Infection can occur when urine invades the damaged mucosa.

The catheter is secured properly to prevent it from moving, causing traction on the urethra, or being unintentionally removed, and care is taken to ensure that the catheter position permits leg movement. In male patients, the drainage tube (not the catheter) is taped laterally to the thigh to prevent pressure on the urethra at the penoscrotal junction, which can eventually lead to formation of a urethrocutaneous fistula. In female patients, the drainage tubing attached to the catheter is taped to the thigh to prevent tension and traction on the bladder.

Special care should be taken to ensure that any patient who is confused does not remove the catheter with the retention balloon still inflated, because this could cause bleeding and considerable injury to the urethra.

Retraining the Bladder

When an indwelling urinary catheter is in place, the detrusor muscle does not actively contract the bladder wall to stimulate emptying because urine is continuously draining from the bladder. As a result, the detrusor may not immediately respond to bladder filling when the catheter is removed, resulting in either urine retention or urinary incontinence. This condition, known as postcatheterization detrusor instability, can be managed with bladder retraining (see Chart 55-11).

Immediately after the indwelling catheter is removed, the patient is placed on a timed voiding schedule, usually every 2 to 3 hours. At the given time interval, the patient is instructed to void. The bladder is then scanned using a portable ultrasonic bladder scanner, and if the bladder has not emptied completely, straight catheterization may be performed (Carter et al., 2014; Mori, 2014). After a few days, as the nerve endings in the bladder wall become resensitized to the bladder filling and emptying, bladder function usually returns to normal. If the patient has had an indwelling catheter in place for an extended period (e.g., greater than 1 month), bladder retraining will take longer; in some cases, function may never return to normal, and long-term intermittent catheterization may become necessary.

Assisting With Intermittent Self-Catheterization

Intermittent self-catheterization provides periodic drainage of urine from the bladder. By promoting drainage and eliminating excessive residual urine, intermittent catheterization protects the kidneys, reduces the incidence of UTIs, and

---

Chart 55-11

Bladder Retraining After Indwelling Catheterization

- Instruct the patient to drink a measured amount of fluid from 8 am to 10 pm to avoid bladder overdistention. Offer no fluids (except sips) after 10 pm.
- At specific times, ask the patient to void by applying pressure over the bladder, tapping the abdomen, or running water to trigger the bladder.
- Immediately after the voiding attempt, perform a bladder scan to determine the amount of residual urine.
- Measure the volumes of urine voided.
- Palpate the bladder at repeated intervals to assess for distention.
- Instruct the patient who has no voiding sensation to be alert to any signs that indicate a full bladder, such as perspiration, cold hands or feet, or feelings of anxiety.
- Perform straight catheterization, as prescribed, usually for residual urine of >300 mL.
- Lengthen the intervals between catheterizations as the volume of residual urine decreases. Catheterization is usually discontinued when the volume of residual urine is <100 mL.

Adapted from Carter, N. M., Reitmeier, L., & Goodloe, L. R. (2014). An evidence-based approach to the prevention of catheter-associated urinary tract infections. *Urologic Nursing, 34*(5), 238–245.

---

improves continence. It is the treatment of choice in some patients with spinal cord injury and other neurologic disorders, such as multiple sclerosis, when the ability to empty the bladder is impaired. Self-catheterization promotes independence, results in few complications, and enhances self-esteem and quality of life.

When educating the patient about how to perform self-catheterization, the nurse must use aseptic technique to minimize the risk of cross-contamination. However, the patient may use a "clean" (nonsterile) technique at home, where the risk of cross-contamination is reduced. Either antibacterial liquid soap or povidone-iodine (Betadine) solution is recommended for cleaning urinary catheters at home. The catheter is thoroughly rinsed with warm tap water after soaking in the cleaning solution. It must dry before reuse. It should be kept in its own container, such as a plastic food storage bag.

In educating the patient, the nurse emphasizes the importance of frequent catheterization and emptying the bladder at the prescribed time. The average daytime clean intermittent catheterization schedule is every 4 to 6 hours and just before bedtime. If the patient is awakened at night with an urge to void, catheterization may be performed after an attempt is made to void normally.

The female patient assumes a Fowler position and uses a mirror to help locate the urinary meatus. She lubricates the catheter and inserts it 7.5 cm (3 inches) into the urethra, in a downward and backward direction. The male patient assumes a Fowler or sitting position, lubricates the catheter, and retracts the foreskin of the penis with one hand while grasping the penis and holding it at a right angle to the body. (This maneuver straightens the urethra and makes it easier to insert the catheter.) He inserts the catheter 15 to 25 cm (6 to 10 inches) until urine begins to flow. After removal, the catheter is cleaned, rinsed, dried, and placed in a plastic bag or case. Patients who follow an intermittent catheterization routine should consult a primary provider at regular intervals to assess urinary function and to detect complications. If the patient cannot perform intermittent self-catheterization, a family member or caregiver may be taught to carry out the procedure at regular intervals during the day.

An alternative to self-catheterization is creation of the Mitrofanoff umbilical appendicovesicostomy, which provides easy access to the bladder but requires an extensive surgical procedure (Wille, Zagaja, Shalhav, et al., 2011). In this procedure, the bladder neck is closed and the appendix is used to create access to the bladder from the skin surface through a submucosal tunnel created with the appendix. One end of the appendix is brought to the skin surface and used as a stoma, and the other end is tunneled into the bladder. The appendix serves as an artificial urinary sphincter when an alternative is necessary to empty the bladder. A surgically prepared continent urine reservoir with a sphincter mechanism is required in cases of bladder cancer and severe interstitial cystitis. Various types of urinary diversions may be used when a radical **cystectomy** (surgical removal of the bladder) is necessary (see discussion later in chapter).

UROLITHIASIS AND NEPHROLITHIASIS

Urolithiasis and nephrolithiasis refer to stones (calculi) in the urinary tract and kidney, respectively. Urinary stones predominantly occur in the third to fifth decades of life and affect men twice as often as women (Cunningham, Noble, Al-Modhefer, et al., 2016). Stones may develop in one or both kidneys and yearly episodes are increasing (Cunningham et al., 2016).

Pathophysiology

Stones are formed in the urinary tract when urinary concentrations of substances such as calcium oxalate, calcium phosphate, and uric acid increase. Referred to as supersaturation, this depends on the amount of the substance, ionic strength, and pH of the urine. Stones may be found anywhere from the kidney to the bladder and may vary in size from minute granular deposits, called *sand* or *gravel*, to bladder stones as large as an orange. The different sites of calculi formation in the urinary tract are shown in Figure 55-5.

Certain factors favor the formation of stones, including infection, urinary stasis, and periods of immobility, all of which slow kidney drainage and alter calcium metabolism (Grossman & Porth, 2014). In addition, increased calcium concentrations in the blood and urine promote precipitation of calcium and formation of stones (about 80% of all kidney stones are calcium based) (Cunningham et al., 2016). Causes of hypercalcemia (high serum calcium) and hypercalciuria (high urine calcium) may include the following:

- Hyperparathyroidism
- Renal tubular acidosis
- Cancers (e.g., leukemia, multiple myeloma)
- Dehydration
- Granulomatous diseases (e.g., sarcoidosis, tuberculosis), which may cause increased vitamin D production by the granulomatous tissue
- Excessive intake of vitamin D

Figure 55-5 • Examples of potential sites of calculi formation (urolithiasis) in the urinary tract.

- Excessive intake of milk and alkali
- Myeloproliferative diseases such as polycythemia vera, which produce an unusual proliferation of blood cells from the bone marrow

For patients with stones containing uric acid, struvite, or cystine, a thorough physical examination and metabolic workup are indicated because of associated disturbances contributing to the stone formation. Uric acid stones (5% to 10% of all stones) may be seen in patients with gout or myeloproliferative disorders. Struvite stones account for 15% of urinary calculi and form in persistently alkaline, ammonia-rich urine caused by the presence of urease-splitting bacteria such as *Proteus*, *Pseudomonas*, *Klebsiella*, *Staphylococcus*, or *Mycoplasma* species. Predisposing factors for struvite stones include neurogenic bladder, foreign bodies, and recurrent UTIs.

Several conditions, as well as certain metabolic risk factors, predispose patients to stone formation. These include anatomic derangements such as polycystic kidney disease, horseshoe kidneys, chronic strictures, and medullary sponge disease. Urinary stone formation can occur in patients with inflammatory bowel disease and in those with an ileostomy or bowel resection because these patients absorb more oxalate. Medications known to cause stones in some patients include antacids, acetazolamide (Diamox), vitamin D, laxatives, and high doses of aspirin (Comerford, 2015). However, in many patients, no cause may be found.

Clinical Manifestations

Signs and symptoms of stones in the urinary system depend on the presence of obstruction, infection, and edema. When stones block the flow of urine, obstruction develops, producing an increase in hydrostatic pressure and distending the renal pelvis and proximal ureter (Cunningham et al., 2016). Infection (pyelonephritis and UTI with chills, fever, and frequency) can be a contributing factor with struvite stones. Some stones cause few, if any, symptoms while slowly destroying the functional units (nephrons) of the kidney; others cause excruciating pain and discomfort.

Stones in the renal pelvis may be associated with an intense, deep ache in the costovertebral region. Hematuria is often present; pyuria may also be noted. Pain originating in the renal area radiates anteriorly and downward toward the bladder in the female and toward the testes in the male. If the pain suddenly becomes acute, with tenderness over the costovertebral area, and nausea and vomiting occur, the patient is having an episode of renal colic. Diarrhea and abdominal discomfort are due to renointestinal reflexes and the anatomic proximity of the kidneys to the stomach, pancreas, and large intestine.

Stones lodged in the ureter (ureteral obstruction) cause acute, excruciating, colicky, wavelike pain that radiates down the thigh and to the genitalia. Often, the patient has a desire to void, but little urine is passed, and it usually contains blood because of the abrasive action of the stone. This group of symptoms is called *ureteral colic*. Colic is mediated by prostaglandin E, a substance that increases ureteral contractility and renal blood flow and that leads to increased intraureteral pressure and pain. In general, the patient is able to pass stones 0.5 to 1 cm in diameter. Stones larger than 1 cm in diameter usually must be removed or fragmented (broken up by lithotripsy) so that they can be removed or passed spontaneously.

Stones lodged in the bladder usually produce symptoms of irritation and may be associated with UTI and hematuria. If the stone obstructs the bladder neck, urinary retention occurs. If infection is associated with a stone, the condition is far more serious, with the potential for urosepsis developing.

Assessment and Diagnostic Findings

The diagnosis is confirmed by a noncontrast CT scan (Cunningham et al., 2016). Blood chemistries and a 24-hour urine test for measurement of calcium, uric acid, creatinine, sodium, pH, and total volume may be part of the diagnostic workup. Dietary and medication histories and family history of kidney stones are obtained to identify factors predisposing the patient to the formation of stones.

When stones are recovered (whether freely passed by the patient or removed through special procedures), chemical analysis is carried out to determine their composition. Stone analysis can provide a clear indication of the underlying disorder. For example, calcium oxalate or calcium phosphate stones usually indicate disorders of oxalate or calcium metabolism, whereas urate stones suggest a disturbance in uric acid metabolism (Cunningham et al., 2016).

Medical Management

The goals of management are to eradicate the stone, determine the stone type, prevent nephron destruction, control infection, and relieve any obstruction that may be present. The immediate objective of treatment of renal or ureteral colic is to relieve the pain until its cause can be eliminated. Opioid analgesic agents are given to prevent shock and syncope that may result from the excruciating pain. Nonsteroidal anti-inflammatory drugs (NSAIDs) are effective in treating kidney stone pain because they provide specific pain relief (Cunningham et al., 2016). They also inhibit the synthesis of prostaglandin E, reducing swelling and facilitating passage

of the stone. Generally, once the stone has passed, the pain is relieved. Hot baths or moist heat to the flank area may also be helpful. Unless the patient is vomiting or has heart failure or any other condition requiring fluid restriction, fluids are encouraged. This increases the hydrostatic pressure behind the stone, assisting it in its downward passage. A high, around-the-clock fluid intake reduces the concentration of urinary crystalloids, dilutes the urine, and ensures a high urine output.

Nutritional Therapy

Nutritional therapy plays an important role in preventing kidney stones (Cunningham et al., 2016) (see Chart 55-12). Fluid intake is the mainstay of most medical therapy for kidney stones. Unless fluids are contraindicated, patients with kidney stones should drink eight to ten 8-oz glasses of water daily or have IV fluids prescribed to keep the urine dilute. A urine output exceeding 2 L/day is advisable.

Calcium Stones

Historically, patients with calcium-based kidney stones were recommended to restrict calcium in their diet. However, evidence has questioned this practice, except for patients with type II absorptive hypercalciuria (half of all patients with calcium stones), in whom stones are clearly the result of excess dietary calcium. Liberal fluid intake is encouraged. Medications such as ammonium chloride may be used, and if increased parathormone production (resulting in increased serum calcium levels in blood and urine) is a factor in the formation of stones, therapy with thiazide diuretics may be beneficial in reducing the calcium loss in the urine and lowering the elevated parathormone levels (Cunningham et al., 2016).

Uric Acid Stones

For uric acid stones, the patient is placed on a low-purine diet to reduce the excretion of uric acid in the urine. Foods high in

---

Chart 55-12

PATIENT EDUCATION

Preventing Kidney Stones

The nurse instructs the patient to:

- Avoid protein intake to decrease urinary excretion of calcium and uric acid.
- Limit sodium intake to 3–4 g/day. Table salt and high-sodium foods should be reduced, because sodium competes with calcium for reabsorption in the kidneys.
- Be aware that low-calcium diets are not generally recommended, except for true absorptive hypercalciuria. Evidence shows that limiting calcium, especially in women, can lead to osteoporosis and does not prevent stones.
- Avoid intake of oxalate-containing foods (e.g., spinach, strawberries, rhubarb, tea, peanuts, wheat bran).
- Drink fluids (ideally water and one glass of cranberry juice per day) every 1–2 hours during the day.
- Drink two glasses of water at bedtime and an additional glass at each nighttime awakening to prevent urine from becoming too concentrated during the night.
- Avoid activities leading to sudden increases in environmental temperatures that may cause excessive sweating and dehydration.
- Contact the primary provider at the first sign of a urinary tract infection.

purine (shellfish, anchovies, asparagus, mushrooms, and organ meats) are avoided, and other proteins may be limited. Allopurinol (Zyloprim) may be prescribed to reduce serum uric acid levels and urinary uric acid excretion (Comerford, 2015).

Cystine Stones

A low-protein diet is prescribed, the urine is alkalinized, and fluid intake is increased.

Oxalate Stones

A dilute urine is maintained, and the intake of oxalate is limited. Many foods contain oxalate; however, only certain foods increase the urinary excretion of oxalate. These include spinach, strawberries, rhubarb, chocolate, tea, peanuts, and wheat bran.

Interventional Procedures

If the stone does not pass spontaneously or if complications occur, common interventions include endoscopic or other procedures. For example, ureteroscopy, extracorporeal shock wave lithotripsy (ESWL), or endourologic (percutaneous) stone removal may be necessary.

Ureteroscopy (see Fig. 55-6A) involves first visualizing the stone and then destroying it. Access to the stone is accomplished by inserting a ureteroscope into the ureter and then inserting a laser, electrohydraulic lithotriptor, or ultrasound device through the ureteroscope to fragment and remove the stones. A stent may be inserted and left in place for 48 hours or more after the procedure to keep the ureter patent. Length of hospital stay is generally brief, and some patients can be treated as outpatients.

ESWL is a noninvasive procedure used to break up stones in the calyx of the kidney (see Fig. 55-6B). After the stones are fragmented to the size of grains of sand, the remnants of the stones are spontaneously voided. In ESWL, a high-energy amplitude of pressure, or shock wave, is generated by the abrupt release of energy and transmitted through water and soft tissues. When the shock wave encounters a substance of different intensity (a kidney stone), a compression wave causes the surface of the stone to fragment. Repeated shock waves focused on the stone eventually reduce it to many small pieces that are excreted in the urine.

Discomfort from the multiple shocks may occur, although the shock waves usually do not cause damage to other tissue. The patient is observed for obstruction and infection resulting from blockage of the urinary tract by stone fragments. All urine is strained after the procedure; voided gravel or sand is sent to the laboratory for chemical analysis. Several treatments may be necessary to ensure disintegration of stones (Cunningham et al., 2016).

Endourologic methods of stone removal (see Fig. 55-6C) may be used to extract kidney calculi that cannot be removed by other procedures. A percutaneous nephrostomy or a percutaneous nephrolithotomy (which are similar procedures) may be performed. A nephroscope is introduced through a percutaneous route into the renal parenchyma. Depending on its size, the stone may be extracted with forceps or by a stone retrieval basket. If the stone is too large to initially be removed, an ultrasound probe inserted through a nephrostomy tube is used to pulverize the stone. Small stone fragments and stone dust are then removed.

Electrohydraulic lithotripsy is a similar method in which an electrical discharge is used to create a hydraulic shock wave to break up the stone. A probe is passed through the cystoscope, and the tip of the lithotriptor is placed near the stone. The strength of the discharge and pulse frequency can be varied. This procedure is performed under topical anesthesia. After the stone is extracted, the percutaneous nephrostomy tube is left in place for a time to ensure that the ureter is not obstructed by edema or blood clots. The most common complications are hemorrhage, infection, and urinary extravasation. After the tube is removed, the nephrostomy tract usually closes spontaneously.

Chemolysis, stone dissolution using infusions of chemical solutions (e.g., alkylating agents, acidifying agents) for the purpose of dissolving the stone, is an alternative treatment sometimes used in patients who are at risk for complications with other types of therapy, who refuse to undergo other methods, or who have stones (struvite) that dissolve easily. A percutaneous nephrostomy is performed, and the warm chemical solution is allowed to flow continuously onto the stone. The solution exits the renal collecting system by means of the ureter or the nephrostomy tube. The pressure inside the renal pelvis is monitored during the procedure.

Several of these treatment modalities may be used in combination to ensure removal of the stones.

Surgical Management

Surgical removal was the major mode of therapy before the advent of lithotripsy. However, today, surgery is performed in only 1% to 2% of patients (Cunningham et al., 2016). Surgical intervention is indicated if the stone does not respond to other forms of treatment. It may also be performed to correct anatomic abnormalities within the kidney to improve urinary drainage. If the stone is in the kidney, the surgery performed may be a nephrolithotomy (incision into the kidney with removal of the stone) or a nephrectomy, if the kidney is nonfunctional secondary to infection or hydronephrosis. Stones in the kidney pelvis are removed by a pyelolithotomy, those in the ureter by ureterolithotomy, and those in the bladder by cystotomy. If the stone is in the bladder, an instrument may be inserted through the urethra into the bladder, and the stone crushed. Such a procedure is called a *cystolitholapaxy*. Nursing management following kidney surgery is discussed in Chapter 54.

NURSING PROCESS

The Patient With Kidney Stones

Assessment

The patient with suspected kidney stones is assessed for pain and discomfort as well as associated symptoms, such as nausea, vomiting, diarrhea, and abdominal distention. The severity and location of pain are determined, along with any radiation of the pain. Nursing assessment also includes observing for signs and symptoms of UTI (chills, fever, frequency, and hesitancy) and obstruction (frequent urination of small amounts, oliguria, or anuria). The urine is inspected for blood and is strained for stones or gravel.

Figure 55-6 • Methods of treating kidney stones. **A.** During ureteroscopy, which is used for removing small stones located in the ureter close to the bladder, a ureteroscope is inserted into the ureter to visualize the stone. The stone is then fragmented or captured and removed. **B.** Extracorporeal shock water lithotripsy is used for most symptomatic, nonpassable upper urinary stones. Electromagnetically generated shock waves are focused over the area of the kidney stone. The high-energy dry shock waves pass through the skin and fragment the stone. **C.** Percutaneous nephrolithotomy is used to treat larger stones. A percutaneous tract is formed, and a nephroscope is inserted through it. Then, the stone is extracted or pulverized.

The history focuses on factors that predispose the patient to urinary tract stones or that may have precipitated the current episode of renal or ureteral colic. The patient's knowledge about kidney stones and measures to prevent their occurrence or recurrence is also assessed.

Diagnosis

NURSING DIAGNOSES

Based on the assessment data, nursing diagnoses may include the following:

- Acute pain related to inflammation, obstruction, and abrasion of the urinary tract
- Deficient knowledge regarding prevention of recurrence of kidney stones

COLLABORATIVE PROBLEMS/POTENTIAL COMPLICATIONS

Potential complications may include the following:

- Infection and urosepsis (from UTI and pyelonephritis)
- Obstruction of the urinary tract by a stone or edema with subsequent acute kidney injury

Planning and Goals

The major goals for the patient may include relief of pain and discomfort, prevention of recurrence of kidney stones, and absence of complications.

Nursing Interventions

RELIEVING PAIN

Severe acute pain is often the presenting symptom of a patient with kidney and urinary calculi and requires immediate attention. Opioid analgesic agents (IV or intramuscular) may be prescribed and given to provide rapid relief along with an IV NSAID. The patient is encouraged and assisted to assume a position of comfort. If activity brings pain relief, the patient is assisted to ambulate. The pain level is monitored closely, and an increase in severity is reported promptly to the primary provider so that relief can be provided and additional treatment initiated.

MONITORING AND MANAGING POTENTIAL COMPLICATIONS

Increased fluid intake is encouraged to prevent dehydration and increase hydrostatic pressure within the urinary tract to promote passage of the stone. If the patient cannot take adequate fluids orally, IV fluids are prescribed. The total urine output and patterns of voiding are monitored. Ambulation is encouraged as a means of moving the stone through the urinary tract.

All urine is strained because uric acid stones may crumble. Any blood clots passed in the urine should be crushed and the sides of the urinal and bedpan inspected for clinging stones. Because kidney stones increase the risk of infection, sepsis, and obstruction of the urinary tract, the patient is instructed to report decreased urine volume, bloody or cloudy urine, fever, and pain.

Patients with calculi require frequent nursing observation to detect the spontaneous passage of a stone. The patient is instructed to immediately report any sudden increases in pain intensity because of the possibility of a stone fragment obstructing a ureter. Vital signs, including temperature, are monitored closely to detect early signs of infection. UTIs may be associated with kidney stones due to an obstruction from the stone or from the stone itself. All infections should be treated with the appropriate antibiotic agent before efforts are made to dissolve the stone.

PROMOTING HOME, COMMUNITY-BASED, AND TRANSITIONAL CARE

Educating Patients About Self-Care. Because the risk of recurring kidney stones is high, the nurse provides education about the causes of kidney stones and recommendations to prevent their recurrence (see Chart 55-12). The patient is encouraged to follow a regimen to avoid further stone formation, including maintaining a high fluid intake because stones form more readily in concentrated urine. A patient who has shown a tendency to form stones should drink enough fluid to excrete greater than 2000 mL (preferably 3000 to 4000 mL) of urine every 24 hours (Cunningham et al., 2016).

Urine cultures may be performed every 1 to 2 months in the first year and periodically thereafter. Recurrent UTI is treated vigorously. Because prolonged immobilization slows renal drainage and alters calcium metabolism, increased mobility is encouraged whenever possible. In addition, excessive ingestion of vitamins (especially vitamin D) and minerals is discouraged.

If lithotripsy, percutaneous stone removal, ureteroscopy, or other surgical procedures for stone removal have been performed, the nurse instructs the patient about the signs and symptoms of complications (e.g., urinary retention, infection) that need to be reported to the primary provider. The importance of follow-up to assess kidney function and to ensure the eradication or removal of all kidney stones is emphasized to the patient and family.

If ESWL has been performed, the nurse must provide instructions for home care and necessary follow-up. The patient is encouraged to increase fluid intake to assist in the passage of stone fragments, which may occur for 6 weeks to several months after the procedure. The patient and family are instructed about signs and symptoms of complications. It is also important to inform the patient to expect hematuria (it is anticipated in all patients), but it should disappear within 4 to 5 days. If the patient has a stent in the ureter, hematuria may be expected until the stent is removed. The patient is instructed to check their temperature daily and notify the primary provider if the temperature is greater than 38°C (about 101°F) or the pain is unrelieved by the prescribed medication. The patient is also informed that a bruise may be observed on the treated side of the back.

Continuing and Transitional Care. Close monitoring of the patient in follow-up care is essential to ensure that treatment has been effective and that no complications develop. The nurse has the opportunity to assess the patient's understanding of ESWL and possible complications. In addition, the nurse has the opportunity to assess the patient's understanding of factors that increase the risk of recurrence of renal calculi and strategies to reduce those risks.

The nurse must assess the patient's ability to monitor urinary pH and interpret the results during follow-up visits. Because of the high risk of recurrence, the patient with kidney stones needs to understand the signs and symptoms of stone formation, obstruction, and infection and the importance of reporting these signs promptly. If medications are prescribed for the prevention of stone formation, the nurse explains their actions, importance, and side effects to the patient.

Evaluation

Expected patient outcomes may include:

1. Reports relief of pain
2. States increased knowledge of health-seeking behaviors to prevent recurrence
   a. Consumes increased fluid intake (at least eight 8-oz glasses of fluid per day)
   b. Participates in appropriate activity
   c. Consumes diet prescribed to reduce dietary factors predisposing to stone formation
   d. Recognizes symptoms (fever, chills, flank pain, hematuria) to be reported to primary provider
   e. Monitors urinary pH as directed
   f. Takes prescribed medication as directed to reduce stone formation
3. Experiences no complications
   a. Reports no signs or symptoms of infection or urosepsis
   b. Voids 200 to 400 mL per voiding of clear urine without evidence of bleeding
   c. Experiences absence of urgency, frequency, and hesitancy
   d. Maintains normal body temperature

GENITOURINARY TRAUMA

Various types of injuries to the flank, back, or upper abdomen may result in trauma to the ureters, bladder, or urethra. Abdominal trauma is responsible for approximately 90% of all genitourinary trauma (Hallis, Amasyali, Yucak, et al., 2015). Kidney trauma is discussed in Chapter 54.

Specific Injuries

Ureteral Trauma

The main causes are motor vehicle crashes, sports injuries, falls, and assaults (Hallis et al., 2015). Injuries range from contusions to complete transection. Unintentional injury to the ureter may occur during gynecologic or urologic surgery. There are no specific signs or symptoms of ureteral injury; many traumatic injuries are discovered during exploratory surgery. Surgical repair with placement of stents (to divert urine away from an anastomosis) is usually necessary. If the ureteral trauma is not detected and urine leakage continues, fistulas can develop.

Bladder Trauma

Injury to the bladder may occur with pelvic fractures, multiple trauma, or from a blow to the lower abdomen when the bladder is full. Blunt trauma may result in contusion evident as an ecchymosis—a large bruise resulting from escape of blood into the tissues and involving a segment of the bladder wall—or in rupture of the bladder extraperitoneally, intraperitoneally, or both. Complications from these injuries include hemorrhage, shock, sepsis, and extravasation of blood into the tissues, which must be treated promptly.

Urethral Trauma

Urethral injuries usually occur with blunt trauma to the lower abdomen or pelvic region. Many patients also have associated pelvic fractures. The classic triad of symptoms comprises blood at the urinary meatus, inability to void, and a distended bladder.

Medical Management

The goals of management in patients with genitourinary trauma are to control hemorrhage, pain, and infection and to maintain urinary drainage. Genitourinary trauma is frequently associated with kidney trauma (see Chapter 54). Hematocrit and hemoglobin levels are monitored closely; decreasing values can indicate hemorrhage within the genitourinary system. The patient is also monitored for oliguria, signs of hemorrhagic shock, and signs and symptoms of acute peritonitis.

Surgical Management

In urethral trauma, a patient whose condition is unstable and who needs monitoring of urine output may need a suprapubic catheter inserted. The patient is catheterized after urethrography has been performed to minimize the risk of urethral disruption and extensive, long-term complications, such as stricture, incontinence, and impotence. Surgical repair may be performed using either open or laparoscopic approaches (Hallis et al., 2015). After surgery, an indwelling urinary catheter may remain in place for up to 1 month.

Nursing Management

The patient with genitourinary trauma should be assessed frequently during the first few days after injury to detect flank and abdominal pain, muscle spasm, and swelling over the flank.

During this time, patients are instructed about care of the incision and the importance of an adequate fluid intake. In addition, instructions about changes that should be reported to the primary provider, such as fever, hematuria, flank pain, or any signs and symptoms of decreasing kidney function, are provided (Hallis et al., 2015). The patient with a ruptured bladder may have gross bleeding for several days after repair. Guidelines for increasing activity gradually, lifting, and driving are also provided.

Follow-up nursing care includes monitoring the blood pressure to detect hypertension and advising the patient to restrict activities for about 1 month after trauma to minimize the incidence of delayed or secondary bleeding.

URINARY TRACT CANCERS

Urinary tract cancers include those of the urinary bladder; kidney and renal pelvis; ureters; and other urinary structures, such as the prostate. Kidney cancer is discussed in Chapter 54, and prostate cancer is discussed in Chapter 59.

Cancer of the Bladder

Cancer of the urinary bladder is more common in people older than 55 years. It is the third most common cancer in men and the eleventh most common in women (National Cancer Institute [NCI], 2016). Bladder cancer is a leading cause of death, accounting for more than 15,000 deaths in the United States annually (NCI, 2016). Cancers arising from the prostate, colon, and rectum in males and from the lower gynecologic tract in females may metastasize to the bladder.

Tobacco use continues to be a leading risk factor for all urinary tract cancers. People who smoke develop bladder cancer twice as often as those who do not smoke (NCI, 2016) (see Chart 55-13).

Clinical Manifestations

Bladder tumors usually arise at the base of the bladder and involve the ureteral orifices and bladder neck. Visible, painless hematuria is the most common symptom of bladder cancer. Infection of the urinary tract is a common complication, producing frequency and urgency. However, any alteration in voiding or change in the urine may indicate cancer of the bladder. Pelvic or back pain may occur with metastasis.

Assessment and Diagnostic Findings

The diagnostic evaluation includes ureteroscopy (the mainstay of diagnosis), excretory urography, CT and MRI scans, ultrasonography, and bimanual examination with the patient anesthetized. Biopsies of the tumor and adjacent mucosa are the definitive diagnostic procedures (NCI, 2016). Transitional cell carcinomas and carcinomas in situ shed recognizable cancer cells. Cytologic examination of fresh urine and saline bladder washings provide information about the prognosis and staging, especially for patients at high risk for recurrence of primary bladder tumors. See Chapter 15 for more information on cancer grading and staging.

Medical Management

Treatment of bladder cancer depends on the grade of the tumor (the degree of cellular differentiation), the stage of tumor growth (the degree of local invasion and the presence or absence of metastasis) (NCI, 2016). The patient's age and physical, mental, and emotional status are considered when determining treatment modalities.

Surgical Management

Transurethral resection or fulguration (cauterization) may be performed for simple papillomas (benign epithelial tumors).

These procedures (described in more detail in Chapter 59) eradicate the tumors through surgical incision or electrical current with the use of instruments inserted through the urethra. After this bladder-sparing surgery, intravesical administration of bacille Calmette–Guérin (BCG) is the treatment of choice. BCG Live (TheraCys) is an attenuated live strain of *Mycobacterium bovis*, the causative agent in tuberculosis; treatment is recommended for a minimum of 1 year (NCI, 2016). The exact action of BCG is unknown, but it is thought to produce a local inflammatory and a systemic immunologic response.

Management of superficial bladder cancers presents a challenge because there are usually widespread abnormalities in the bladder mucosa. The entire lining of the urinary tract, or urothelium, is at risk because carcinomatous changes can occur in the mucosa of the bladder, kidney pelvis, ureter, and urethra.

A simple cystectomy or a radical cystectomy is performed for invasive or multifocal bladder cancer. Radical cystectomy in men involves removal of the bladder, prostate, and seminal vesicles and immediate adjacent perivesical tissues. In women, radical cystectomy involves removal of the bladder, lower ureter, uterus, fallopian tubes, ovaries, anterior vagina, and urethra. It may include removal of pelvic lymph nodes. Removal of the bladder requires a urinary diversion procedure, which is described later in this chapter.

Although radical cystectomy remains the standard of care for invasive bladder cancer in the United States, clinical trials are exploring trimodality therapy—transurethral resection of the bladder tumor, radiation, and chemotherapy—in an effort to spare patients the need for cystectomy (NCI, 2016). This approach to transitional cell bladder cancer mandates lifelong surveillance with periodic cystoscopy. Although most patients respond completely and their bladders remain free from invasive relapse, one fourth develop a relapse of noninvasive disease. This may be managed with transurethral resection of the bladder tumor and intravesical therapies but carries an additional risk that a late cystectomy may be required.

Pharmacologic Therapy

Chemotherapy with a combination of methotrexate, 5-fluorouracil, vinblastine (Velban), doxorubicin (Adriamycin), and cisplatin (Platinol) has been effective in producing partial remission of transitional cell carcinoma of the bladder in some patients. IV chemotherapy may be accompanied by radiation therapy (NCI, 2016). Topical chemotherapy (intravesical chemotherapy or instillation of antineoplastic agents into the bladder, resulting in contact of the agent with the bladder wall) is considered when there is a high risk of recurrence, when cancer in situ is present, or when tumor resection has been incomplete. Topical chemotherapy delivers a high concentration of medication (thiotepa [Thioplex], doxorubicin, mitomycin [Mutamycin], and BCG Live) to the tumor to promote tumor destruction. Bladder cancer may also be treated by direct infusion of the cytotoxic agent through the bladder's arterial blood supply to achieve a higher concentration of the chemotherapeutic agent with fewer systemic toxic effects (NCI, 2016).

BCG Live is now considered the most predominant and conservative intravesical agent for recurrent bladder cancer, especially superficial transitional cell carcinoma, because it is an immunotherapeutic agent that enhances the body's immune response to cancer. BCG Live has a 43% advantage in preventing tumor recurrence, a significantly better rate than the 16% to 21% advantage of intravesical chemotherapy. In addition, BCG Live is particularly effective in the treatment of carcinoma in situ, eradicating it in more than 80% of cases. In contrast to intravesical chemotherapy, BCG Live has also been shown to decrease the risk of tumor progression. Although BCG Live treatment is the current standard of care, this treatment fails or is not tolerated in a significant proportion of patients (Askeland, Newton, O'Donnell, et al., 2012).

The optimal course of BCG Live appears to be a 6-week course of weekly instillations, followed by a 3-week course at 3 months for tumors that do not respond. In high-risk cancers, maintenance BCG Live given in a 3-week course at 6, 12, 18, and 24 months may limit recurrence and prevent progression. However, the adverse effects associated with this prolonged therapy may limit its widespread applicability.

The patient is allowed to eat and drink before the instillation procedure. Once the bladder is full, the patient must retain the intravesical solution for 2 hours before voiding. At the end of the procedure, the patient is encouraged to void and to drink liberal amounts of fluid to flush the medication from the bladder.

Radiation Therapy

Radiation of the tumor may be performed preoperatively to reduce microextension of the neoplasm and viability of tumor cells, thus decreasing the chances that the cancer may recur in the immediate area or spread through the circulatory or lymphatic systems. Radiation therapy is also used in combination with surgery or to control the disease in patients with inoperable tumors.

For more advanced bladder cancer or for patients with intractable hematuria (especially after radiation therapy), a large, water-filled balloon placed in the bladder produces tumor necrosis by reducing the blood supply of the bladder wall (hydrostatic therapy). The instillation of formalin, phenol, or silver nitrate relieves hematuria and strangury (slow and painful discharge of urine) in some patients.

URINARY DIVERSIONS

Urinary diversion procedures are performed to divert urine from the bladder to a new exit site, usually through a surgically created opening (stoma) in the skin. These procedures are primarily performed when a bladder tumor necessitates cystectomy (NCI, 2016). Urinary diversion has also been used in managing pelvic malignancy, birth defects, strictures, trauma to the ureters and urethra, neurogenic bladder, chronic infection causing severe ureteral and kidney damage, and intractable interstitial cystitis. It may also be used as a last resort in managing incontinence.

Controversy exists about the best method of establishing permanent diversion of the urinary tract. New techniques are frequently introduced in an effort to improve patient outcomes and quality of life. The age of the patient, condition of the bladder, body build, degree of obesity, degree of ureteral dilation, status of kidney function, and the patient's learning ability and willingness to participate in postoperative care are all taken into consideration when determining the appropriate surgical procedure.

The outcome for a patient with a urinary diversion depends to a large degree on the location or position of the stoma, whether the drainage device (pouch or bag) establishes a watertight seal to the skin, and the patient's ability to manage the pouch and drainage apparatus (Rubenwolf, Hampel, Roos, et al., 2016).

There are two types of urinary diversion. In a cutaneous urinary diversion, urine drains through an opening created in the abdominal wall and skin (see Fig. 55-7). In a **continent urinary diversion**, a portion of the intestine is used to create a new reservoir for urine (see Fig. 55-8A).

Cutaneous Urinary Diversions

Ileal Conduit

The **ileal conduit** (ileal loop) is the oldest and most common of the urinary diversion procedures in use because of the low number of complications and surgeons' familiarity with the procedure. In an ileal conduit, the urine is diverted by implanting the ureter into a 12-cm loop of ileum that is led out through the abdominal wall. This loop of ileum is a simple conduit (passageway) for urine from the ureters to the surface. A loop of the sigmoid colon may also be used (Rubenwolf et al., 2016). An ileostomy bag is used to collect the urine. The resected (cut) ends of the remaining intestine are anastomosed (connected) to provide an intact bowel.

Stents, usually made of thin, pliable tubing, are placed in the ureters to prevent occlusion secondary to postsurgical edema. The bilateral ureteral stents allow urine to drain from the kidney to the stoma and provide a method for accurate measurement of urine output. They may be left in place 10 to 21 days postoperatively. Jackson–Pratt drains or other types of drains are inserted to prevent the accumulation of fluid in the space created by removal of the bladder.

After surgery, a skin barrier and a transparent, disposable urinary drainage bag are applied around the conduit and connected to drainage. A custom-cut appliance is used until the edema subsides and the stoma shrinks to normal size. The clear bag allows the stoma to be inspected and the patency of the stent and the urine output to be monitored. The ileal bag drains urine (not feces) continuously. The appliance (bag) usually remains in place as long as it is watertight; it is changed when necessary to prevent leakage of urine.

Complications

Complications that may follow placement of an ileal conduit include wound infection or wound dehiscence, urinary leakage, ureteral obstruction, hyperchloremic acidosis, small bowel obstruction, ileus, and gangrene of the stoma. Delayed complications include ureteral obstruction, contraction or narrowing of the stoma (stenosis), kidney deterioration due to chronic reflux, pyelonephritis, renal calculi, and cancer recurrence (Rubenwolf et al., 2016; Smolar, Salemi, Horst, et al., 2016).

Nursing Management

In the immediate postoperative period, urine volumes are monitored hourly. Throughout the patient's hospitalization,

A Conventional ileal conduit.
The surgeon transplants the ureters to an isolated section of the terminal ileum (ileal conduit), bringing one end to the abdominal wall. The ureter may also be transplanted into the transverse sigmoid colon (colon conduit) or proximal jejunum (jejunal conduit).

— Ileal segment

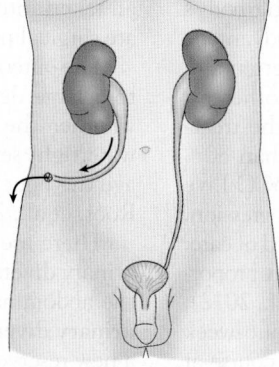

B Cutaneous ureterostomy.
The surgeon brings the detached ureter through the abdominal wall and attaches it to an opening in the skin.

C Vesicostomy.
The surgeon sutures the bladder to the abdominal wall and creates an opening (stoma) through the abdominal and bladder walls for urinary drainage.

D Nephrostomy.
The surgeon inserts a catheter into the renal pelvis via an incision in the flank or by percutaneous catheter placement into the kidney.

Figure 55-7 • Types of cutaneous diversions include the conventional ileal conduit (**A**), cutaneous ureterostomy (**B**), vesicostomy (**C**), and nephrostomy (**D**).

the nurse monitors closely for complications, reports signs and symptoms of them promptly, and intervenes quickly to prevent their progression.

A urine output below 0.5 mL/kg/hr may indicate dehydration or an obstruction in the ileal conduit, with possible backflow or leakage from the ureteroileal anastomosis. A catheter may be inserted through the urinary conduit to monitor the patient for possible stasis or residual urine from a constricted stoma. Urine may drain through the bilateral ureteral stents as well as around the stents. If the ureteral stents are not draining, the nurse may be instructed to carefully irrigate with 5 to 10 mL sterile normal saline solution, being careful not to exert tension that could dislodge the stent. Hematuria may be noted in the first 48 hours after surgery but usually resolves spontaneously.

Providing Stoma and Skin Care

Because the patient requires specialized care, a consultation is initiated with a WOC nurse. The stoma is inspected frequently for color and viability. A healthy stoma is pink or red. A change from this normal color to purple, brown, or black suggests that the vascular supply may be compromised.

If cyanosis and a compromised blood supply persist, surgical intervention may be necessary. The stoma is not sensitive to touch, but the skin around the stoma becomes sensitive if urine or the appliance causes irritation. The skin is inspected for (1) signs of irritation and bleeding of the stoma mucosa, (2) encrustation and skin irritation around the stoma (from alkaline urine coming in contact with exposed skin), and (3) wound infections (Dukes, Lowther, Martin, et al., 2013).

Testing Urine and Caring for the Ostomy

Moisture in bed linens or clothing or the odor of urine around the patient should alert the nurse to the possibility of leakage from the appliance, potential infection, or a problem in hygienic management. Because severe alkaline encrustation can accumulate rapidly around the stoma, the urine pH is kept below 6.5 by administration of ascorbic acid by mouth. Urine pH is determined by testing the urine draining from the stoma, not from the collecting appliance. A properly fitted appliance is essential to prevent exposure of the skin around the stoma to urine. If the urine is foul smelling, the stoma is catheterized, if prescribed, to obtain a urine specimen for culture and sensitivity testing.

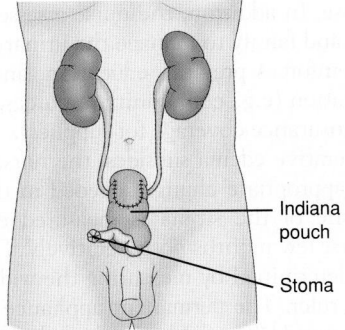

A Indiana pouch.
The surgeon introduces the ureters into
a segment of ileum and cecum. Urine
is drained periodically by inserting a
catheter into the stoma.

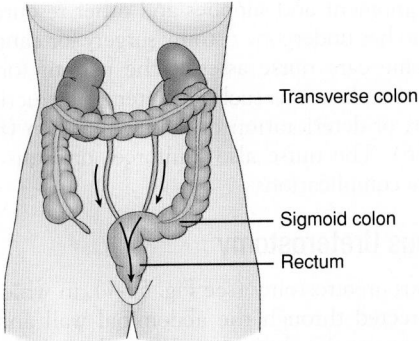

B Ureterosigmoidostomy.
The surgeon introduces the ureters into the
sigmoid colon, thereby allowing urine to flow
through the colon and out of the rectum.

Figure 55-8 • Types of continent urinary diversions include the
Indiana pouch (**A**) and ureterosigmoidostomy (**B**).

Encouraging Fluids and Relieving Anxiety

Because mucous membrane is used in forming the conduit,
the patient may excrete a large amount of mucus mixed with
urine. This causes anxiety in many patients. To help relieve
this anxiety, the nurse reassures the patient that this is a normal occurrence after an ileal conduit procedure. The nurse
encourages adequate fluid intake to flush the ileal conduit and
decrease the accumulation of mucus.

Selecting the Ostomy Appliance

Various urine collection appliances are available, and the
nurse is instrumental (often with consultation with a WOC
nurse) in selecting an appropriate one. The urinary appliance may consist of one or two pieces and may be disposable
(usually used once and discarded) or reusable. The choice of
appliance is determined by the location of the stoma and by
the patient's normal activity, manual dexterity, visual function, body build, economic resources, and preference.

Promoting Home, Community-Based, and Transitional Care

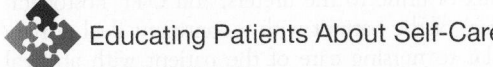 Educating Patients About Self-Care

Patient education begins in the hospital but continues in the
home setting because patients are usually discharged within

days of surgery. The nurse instructs the patient how to assess
and manage the urinary diversion as well as how to deal with
changes in body image. A WOC nurse is invaluable in consulting with the nurse on various aspects of care and patient
education.

Changing the Appliance

The patient and family are educated about how to apply and
change the appliance so that they are comfortable carrying out
the procedure and can do so proficiently. Ideally, the appliance system is changed before the system leaks and at a time
that is convenient for the patient. Many patients find that
early morning is most convenient because the urine output is
reduced. A variety of appliances are available; an average collecting appliance lasts 3 to 7 days before leakage occurs.

Regardless of the type of appliance used, a skin barrier is
essential to protect the skin from irritation and excoriation. To
maintain skin integrity, a skin barrier or leaking pouch is never
patched with tape to prevent accumulation of urine under the
skin barrier or faceplate. The patient is instructed to avoid moisturizing soaps and body washes when cleaning the area because
they interfere with the adhesion of the pouch. The degree to
which the stoma protrudes is not the same in all patients; thus,
there are various accessories and custom-made appliances to
solve individual problems. Patient guidelines for applying reusable and disposable systems are presented in Chart 55-14.

Controlling Odor

The patient is instructed to avoid foods that give the urine
a strong odor (e.g., asparagus, cheese, eggs). Most appliances
contain odor barriers, but, if needed, a few drops of liquid
deodorizer or diluted white vinegar may be introduced through
the drain spout into the bottom of the pouch with a syringe
or eyedropper to reduce odors. Ascorbic acid by mouth helps
acidify the urine and suppress urine odor. Patients should be
cautioned not to put aspirin tablets in the pouch to control
odor, because they may ulcerate the stoma. In addition, the
patient is reminded that odor will develop if the pouch is
worn longer than recommended and not cared for properly.

Managing the Ostomy Appliance

The patient is instructed to empty the pouch by means of a
drain valve when it is one third full because the weight of more
urine will cause the pouch to separate from the skin. Some
patients prefer wearing a leg bag attached with an adapter to
the drainage apparatus. To promote uninterrupted sleep, a
collecting bottle and tubing (one unit) are snapped onto an
adapter that connects to the ileal appliance. A small amount
of urine is left in the bag when the adapter is attached to prevent the bag from collapsing against itself. The tubing may be
threaded down the pajama or pants leg to prevent kinking. The
collecting bottle and tubing are rinsed daily with cool water
and once a week with a 3:1 solution of water and white vinegar.

Cleaning and Deodorizing the Appliance

Usually, the reusable appliance is rinsed in warm water and
soaked in a 3:1 solution of water and white vinegar or a
commercial deodorizing solution for 30 minutes. It is rinsed
with tepid water and air-dried away from direct sunlight.
(Hot water and exposure to direct sunlight dry the pouch and
increase the incidence of cracking.) After drying, the appliance
may be powdered with cornstarch and stored. Two appliances
are necessary—one to be worn while the other is air-drying.

PATIENT EDUCATION
Using Urinary Diversion Collection Appliances

Applying a Reusable Pouch System

The nurse instructs the patient to:

1. Gather all necessary supplies.
2. Prepare new appliance according to the manufacturer's directions:
   - Apply double-faced adhesive disc that has been properly sized to fit the reusable pouch faceplate.
   - Remove paper backing and set pouch aside, or apply thin layer of contact cement to one side of the reusable pouch faceplate.
   - Set pouch aside.
3. Remove soiled pouch gently. Lay aside to clean later.
4. Clean peristomal skin (skin around stoma) with small amount of soap and water. Rinse thoroughly and dry. If a film of soap remains on the skin and the site does not dry, the appliance will not adhere adequately.
5. Use a wick (rolled gauze pad or tampon) over the stoma to absorb urine and keep the skin dry throughout the appliance change.
6. Inspect peristomal skin for irritation.
7. Note that a skin protector wipe or barrier ring may be applied before centering the faceplate opening directly over the stoma.
8. Position appliance over stoma, and press gently into place.
9. If desired, use a pouch cover or apply cornstarch under the pouch to prevent perspiration and skin irritation.
10. Clean soiled pouch, and prepare for reuse.

Applying a Disposable Pouch System

The nurse instructs the patient to:

1. Gather all necessary supplies.
2. Measure stoma, and prepare an opening in the skin barrier about 1/8-inch larger than the stoma and the same shape as the stoma.
3. Remove paper backing from skin barrier, and set aside.
4. Gently remove old appliance, and set aside.
5. Clean peristomal skin with warm water, and dry thoroughly.
6. Inspect peristomal skin (skin around stoma) for irritation.
7. Use a wick (rolled gauze pad or tampon) over the stoma to absorb urine, and keep the skin dry during the appliance change.
8. Center opening of skin barrier over stoma, and apply with firm, gentle pressure to attain a watertight seal.
9. If using a two-piece system, snap pouch onto the flanged wafer that adheres to skin.
10. Close drainage tap or spout at bottom of pouch.
11. Note that a pouch cover can be used or cornstarch applied under pouch to prevent perspiration and skin irritation.
12. Apply hypoallergenic tape around the skin barrier in a picture-frame manner.
13. Dispose of soiled appliance.

Adapted from Dukes, S., Lowther, C., Martin, T., et al. (2013). Guidelines for standardising the treatment of stoma granulomas at the mucocutaneous junction. *World Council of Enterostomal Therapists Journal, 33*(1), 12–15.

Continuing and Transitional Care

Follow-up care is essential to determine how the patient has adapted to the altered body image and lifestyle changes. Referral for home care is indicated to determine how well the patient and family are coping with the urinary drainage diversion. The nurse assesses the patient's physical status and emotional response. In addition, the nurse assesses the ability of the patient and family to manage the urinary diversion and appliance, reinforces previous education, and provides additional information (e.g., community resources, sources of ostomy supplies, insurance coverage for supplies).

As the postoperative edema subsides, the nurse assists in determining the appropriate changes needed in the ostomy appliance. The size of the stoma is measured every 3 to 6 weeks for the first few months postoperatively. The correct appliance size is determined by measuring the widest part of the stoma with a ruler. The permanent appliance should be no more than 1.6 mm (1/8 inch) larger than the diameter of the stoma and the same shape as the stoma to prevent contact of the skin with drainage.

The nurse educates the patient and family about resources (see the Resources section at the end of this chapter). Local chapters of the American Cancer Society (ACS) can provide medical equipment and supplies and other resources for the patient who has undergone ostomy surgery for cancer.

The home care nurse assesses the patient for potential long-term complications such as ureteral obstruction, stenosis, hernias, or deterioration of kidney function (Rubenwolf et al., 2016). The nurse also reinforces previous education about these complications.

Cutaneous Ureterostomy

A cutaneous ureterostomy (see Fig. 55-7), in which the ureters are directed through the abdominal wall and attached to an opening in the skin, is used for selected patients with ureteral obstruction (i.e., advanced pelvic cancer) because it requires less extensive surgery than other urinary diversion procedures. It is also an appropriate procedure for patients who have had previous abdominal irradiation.

A urinary appliance is fitted immediately after surgery. The management of the patient with a cutaneous ureterostomy is similar to the care of the patient with an ileal conduit, although the stomas are usually flush with the skin or retracted.

Continent Urinary Diversions

Continent Ileal Urinary Reservoir (Indiana Pouch)

The most common continent urinary diversion is the Indiana pouch, created for the patient whose bladder is removed or no longer functions. The Indiana pouch uses a segment of the ileum and cecum to form the reservoir for urine (see Fig. 55-8A). The ureters are tunneled through the muscular bands of the intestinal pouch and anastomosed. The reservoir is made continent by narrowing the efferent portion of the ileum and sewing the terminal ileum to the subcutaneous tissue, forming a continent stoma flush with the skin. The pouch is sewn to the anterior abdominal wall around a cecostomy tube. Urine collects in the pouch until a catheter is inserted and the urine is drained.

The pouch must be drained at regular intervals by a catheter to prevent absorption of metabolic waste products from the urine, reflux of urine to the ureters, and UTI. Postoperative nursing care of the patient with a continent ileal urinary pouch is similar to nursing care of the patient with an ileal conduit. However, these patients usually have additional drainage tubes (cecostomy catheter from the pouch, stoma catheter exiting from the stoma, ureteral stents, and Penrose drain, as well as a urethral catheter). All drainage tubes must be carefully monitored for patency and amount and type of drainage. In the immediate postoperative period, the cecostomy tube is irrigated two or three times daily to remove mucus and prevent blockage.

Other variations of continent urinary reservoirs are used occasionally (Crawshaw, Williams, & Woodhouse, 2014). With these methods, the pouch must be drained at regular intervals by inserting a catheter.

 For the procedural guidelines for draining a continent ileostomy (Kock pouch), go to **thepoint.lww.com/Brunner14e.**

Ureterosigmoidostomy

Ureterosigmoidostomy, another form of continent urinary diversion, is a transplantation of the ureters into the sigmoid colon, allowing urine to flow through the colon and out the rectum (see Fig. 55-8B). It is usually performed in patients who have had extensive pelvic irradiation, previous small bowel resection, or coexisting small bowel disease.

After surgery, voiding occurs from the rectum (for life), and an adjustment in lifestyle will be necessary because of urinary frequency. Drainage has a consistency equivalent to watery diarrhea, and the patient has some degree of nocturia. Patients usually need to plan activities around the frequent need to urinate, which in turn may affect the patient's social life. However, patients have the advantage of urinary control without having to wear an external appliance.

Nursing Management

In addition to the usual preoperative regimen, the patient may be placed on a liquid diet for several days preoperatively to reduce residue in the colon. Antibiotic agents (neomycin, kanamycin) are given to disinfect the bowel. Ureterosigmoidostomy requires a competent anal sphincter, adequate kidney function, and active renal peristalsis. The degree of anal sphincter control may be determined by assessing the patient's ability to retain enemas.

The postoperative regimen initially includes placing a catheter in the rectum to drain the urine and prevent reflux of urine into the ureters and kidneys. The tube is taped to the buttocks, and special skin care is given around the anus to prevent excoriation. Irrigations of the rectal tube may be prescribed, but force is never used because of the danger of introducing bacteria into the newly implanted ureters.

Monitoring Fluid and Electrolytes

In ureterosigmoidostomy, larger areas of the bowel mucosa are exposed to urine and electrolyte reabsorption. As a result, electrolyte imbalance and acidosis may occur. Potassium and magnesium in the urine may cause diarrhea. Fluid and electrolyte balance is maintained in the immediate postoperative period by closely monitoring the serum electrolyte levels and administering appropriate IV fluids. Acidosis may be prevented by placing the patient on a low-chloride diet supplemented with sodium potassium citrate.

The patient should be instructed never to wait longer than 2 to 3 hours before emptying urine from the intestine. This keeps rectal pressure low and minimizes the absorption of urinary constituents from the colon. It is essential to educate the patient about the symptoms of UTI: fever, flank pain, urgency, and frequency.

Retraining the Anal Sphincter

After the rectal catheter is removed, the patient learns to control the anal sphincter through special sphincter exercises. At first, urination is frequent. With reassurance and encouragement and the passage of time, the patient gains greater control and learns to differentiate between the need to void and the need to defecate.

Promoting Dietary Measures

Specific dietary instructions include avoidance of gas-forming foods (flatus can cause stress incontinence and offensive odors). Other ways to avoid gas are to avoid chewing gum, smoking, and any other activity that involves swallowing air. Salt intake may be restricted to prevent hyperchloremic acidosis. Potassium intake is increased through foods and medication because potassium may be lost in acidosis.

Monitoring and Managing Potential Complications

Pyelonephritis (upper UTI) due to reflux of bacteria from the colon is fairly common. Long-term antibiotic therapy may be prescribed to prevent infection. A late complication is adenocarcinoma of the sigmoid colon, possibly from cellular changes due to exposure of the colonic mucosa to urine. Urinary carcinogens promote late malignant transformation of the colon after a ureterosigmoidostomy, warranting lifelong medical follow-up.

Other Urinary Diversion Procedures

Variations in urinary diversion surgical procedures are devised frequently in an effort to identify and perfect procedures that will improve patient outcomes and reduce the incidence of postoperative problems (Rubenwolf et al., 2016). These include cecal, patched cecal, and Mainz reservoirs. These techniques involve isolating a part of the large intestine to form a reservoir for urine and creating an abdominal stoma. Another surgical procedure, the Camey procedure, uses a portion of the ileum as a bladder substitute. In this procedure, the isolated ileum serves as the reservoir for urine; it is anastomosed directly to the portion of the remaining urethra after cystectomy. This procedure permits emptying of the bladder through the urethra. However, the Camey procedure applies only to men because the entire urethra is removed when a cystectomy is performed in women.

NURSING PROCESS

The Patient Undergoing Urinary Diversion Surgery

Preoperative Assessment

The following are key preoperative nursing assessment concerns:
- Cardiopulmonary function assessments are performed because patients undergoing cystectomy are often older adults who may be at greater risk for cardiac and respiratory complications.
- A nutritional status assessment is important because of possible poor nutritional intake related to underlying health problems.

- Learning needs are assessed in consultation with a WOC nurse to evaluate the patient's and the family's understanding of the procedure as well as the changes in physical structure and function that result from the surgery. The patient's self-concept and self-esteem are assessed in addition to methods for coping with stress and loss. The patient's mental status, manual dexterity and coordination, vision, and preferred method of learning are noted because they affect postoperative self-care.

Preoperative Diagnosis

NURSING DIAGNOSES

Based on the assessment data, preoperative nursing diagnoses may include the following:

- Anxiety related to anticipated losses associated with the surgical procedure
- Imbalanced nutrition: less than body requirements related to inadequate nutritional intake
- Deficient knowledge about the surgical procedure and postoperative care

Preoperative Planning and Goals

The major goals for the patient may include relief of anxiety; improved preoperative nutritional status; and increased knowledge about the surgical procedure, expected outcomes, and postoperative care.

Preoperative Nursing Interventions

RELIEVING ANXIETY

The threat of cancer and removal of the bladder create anxiety related to changes in body image. Patients may face problems adapting to an external appliance, a stoma, a surgical incision, and altered toileting habits. Men must also adapt to sexual impotency; a penile implant is considered if the patient is a candidate for the procedure. Women also have anxiety related to altered appearance, body image, and self-esteem. A supportive approach, both physical and psychosocial, is needed and includes assessing the patient's self-concept and manner of coping with stress and loss; helping the patient to identify ways to maintain their lifestyle and independence with as few changes as possible; and encouraging the patient to express fears and anxieties about the ramifications of the upcoming surgery. A visitor from the Ostomy Visitation Program of the ACS can provide emotional support and make adaptation easier both before and after surgery.

ENSURING ADEQUATE NUTRITION

A low-residue diet is prescribed to cleanse the bowel to minimize fecal stasis, decompress the bowel, and minimize postoperative ileus. In addition, antibiotic medications are given to reduce pathogenic flora in the bowel and to reduce the risk of infection. Because the patient undergoing a urinary diversion procedure for cancer may be severely malnourished due to the tumor, previous treatments, and anorexia, enteral or parenteral nutrition may be prescribed to promote healing. Adequate preoperative hydration is imperative to ensure urine flow during surgery and to prevent hypovolemia during the prolonged surgical procedure.

EXPLAINING SURGERY AND ITS EFFECTS

Participation of a WOC nurse in patient education and care, is invaluable for informed preoperative education and postoperative planning. Explanations of the surgical procedure, the appearance of the stoma, the rationale for preoperative bowel preparation, the reasons for wearing a collection device, and the anticipated effects of the surgery on sexual functioning are part of patient education. The placement of the stoma site is planned preoperatively with the patient standing, sitting, and lying down to locate the stoma away from bony prominences, skin creases, and folds. The stoma should also be placed away from old scars, the umbilicus, and the belt line.

For ease of self-care, the patient must be able to see and reach the site comfortably. The site is marked with indelible ink so that it can be located easily during surgery. The patient is assessed for allergies or sensitivity to tape or adhesives. Patch testing of certain appliances may be necessary before the ostomy equipment is selected. This is particularly important if the patient is or may be allergic to latex (see Chapter 17; Figure 17-1).

Preoperative Evaluation

To measure the effectiveness of care, the nurse evaluates the patient's preoperative anxiety level and nutritional status as well as pre-existing knowledge and expectations of surgery.

Expected patient outcomes may include:

1. Exhibits reduced anxiety about surgery and expected losses
   a. Verbalizes fears with health care team and family
   b. Expresses positive attitude about outcome of surgery
2. Exhibits adequate nutritional status
   a. Maintains adequate intake before surgery
   b. Maintains body weight
   c. States rationale for enteral or parenteral nutrition if needed
   d. Exhibits normal skin turgor, moist mucous membranes, adequate urine output, and absence of excessive thirst
3. Demonstrates knowledge about the surgical procedure and postoperative course
   a. Identifies limitations expected after surgery
   b. Discusses expected immediate postoperative environment (tubes, equipment, nursing surveillance)
   c. Practices deep-breathing, coughing, and foot exercises

Postoperative Assessment

The role of the nurse in the immediate postoperative period is to prevent complications and to assess the patient carefully for any signs and symptoms of complications. The catheters and any drainage devices are monitored closely. Urine volume, patency of the drainage system, and color of the drainage are assessed. A sudden decrease in urine volume or increase in drainage is reported promptly to the primary provider, because these may indicate obstruction of the urinary tract, inadequate blood volume, or bleeding. In addition, the patient's need for pain control is assessed regularly, as with all postoperative patients.

Postoperative Diagnosis

NURSING DIAGNOSES

Based on the assessment data, major postoperative nursing diagnoses may include the following:

- Risk for impaired skin integrity related to problems in managing the urine collection appliance

- Acute pain related to surgical incision
- Disturbed body image related to urinary diversion
- Ineffective sexuality pattern related to structural and physiologic alterations
- Deficient knowledge about management of urinary function

COLLABORATIVE PROBLEMS/POTENTIAL COMPLICATIONS

Potential complications may include the following:

- Peritonitis due to disruption of anastomosis
- Stoma ischemia and necrosis due to compromised blood supply to stoma
- Stoma retraction and separation of mucocutaneous border due to tension or trauma

Postoperative Planning and Goals

The major goals for the patient may include maintaining skin integrity, relieving pain, increasing self-esteem, developing appropriate coping mechanisms to accept and deal with altered urinary function and sexuality, increasing knowledge about management of urinary function, and preventing potential complications.

Postoperative Nursing Interventions

Postoperative management focuses on monitoring urinary function, preventing postoperative complications (infection and sepsis, respiratory complications, fluid and electrolyte imbalances, fistula formation, and urine leakage), and promoting patient comfort. Catheters or drainage systems are monitored, and urine output is monitored carefully. A nasogastric tube is inserted during surgery to decompress the GI tract and to relieve pressure on the intestinal anastomosis. It is usually kept in place for several days after surgery. As soon as bowel function resumes—as indicated by bowel sounds, the passage of flatus, and a soft abdomen—oral fluids are permitted. Until that time, IV fluids and electrolytes are given. The patient is assisted to ambulate as soon as possible to prevent complications of immobility.

MAINTAINING SKIN INTEGRITY

Strategies to promote skin integrity begin with reducing and controlling those factors that increase the patient's risk of poor nutrition and poor healing. Meticulous skin care and management of the drainage system are provided by the nurse until the patient can manage them and is comfortable doing so. Care is taken to keep the system intact to protect the skin from exposure to drainage. Supplies must be readily available to manage the drainage in the immediate postoperative period. Consistency in implementing the skin care program throughout the postoperative period results in maintenance of skin integrity and patient comfort. In addition, maintenance of skin integrity around the stoma enables the patient and family to adjust more easily to the alterations in urinary function and helps them learn skin care techniques.

RELIEVING PAIN

Analgesic medications are given liberally postoperatively to relieve pain and promote comfort, thereby allowing the patient to turn, cough, and perform deep-breathing exercises. Patient-controlled analgesia and regular administration of analgesic agents around the clock are two options that may be used to ensure adequate pain relief. A pain intensity scale is used to evaluate the adequacy of the medication and the approach to pain management. See Chapter 12 for further discussion of pain management.

IMPROVING BODY IMAGE

The patient's ability to cope with the changes associated with the surgery depends to some degree on their body image and self-esteem before the surgery and the support and reaction of others. Allowing the patient to express concerns and anxious feelings can help, especially in adjusting to the changes in toileting habits. The nurse can also help improve the patient's self-concept by educating about skills needed to be independent in managing the urinary drainage devices. Education about ostomy care is conducted in a private setting to encourage the patient to ask questions without fear of embarrassment. Explaining why the nurse must wear gloves when performing ostomy care can prevent the patient from misinterpreting the use of gloves as a sign of aversion to the stoma.

EXPLORING SEXUALITY ISSUES

Patients who experience altered sexual function as a result of the surgical procedure may mourn this loss. One study of 82 patients reported that sexual function in all domains was negatively affected in both genders (Rubenwolf et al., 2016). Encouraging the patient and partner to share their feelings about this loss with each other and acknowledging the importance of sexual function and expression may encourage the patient and partner to seek sexual counseling and to explore alternative ways of expressing sexuality. A visit from another patient with an ostomy who is functioning fully in society and family life may also assist the patient and family in recognizing that full recovery is possible.

MONITORING AND MANAGING POTENTIAL COMPLICATIONS

Complications are not unusual because of the complexity of the surgery, the underlying reason (cancer, trauma) for the urinary diversion procedure, and the patient's frequently less-than-optimal nutritional status. Complications may include respiratory disorders (e.g., atelectasis, pneumonia), fluid and electrolyte imbalances, breakdown of any anastomosis, sepsis, fistula formation, fecal or urine leakage, and skin irritation. If these occur, the patient will remain hospitalized for an extended length of time and will probably require parenteral nutrition, GI decompression by means of nasogastric suction, and further surgery. The goals of management are to establish drainage, provide adequate nutrition for healing to occur, and prevent sepsis.

Peritonitis. Peritonitis can occur postoperatively if urine leaks at the anastomosis. Signs and symptoms include abdominal pain and distention, muscle rigidity with guarding, nausea and vomiting, paralytic ileus (absence of bowel sounds), fever, and leukocytosis.

Urine output must be monitored closely, because a sudden decrease in output with a corresponding increase in drainage from the incision or drains may indicate urine leakage. In addition, the urine drainage device is observed for leakage. The pouch is changed if a leak is observed. Small leaks in the anastomosis may seal themselves, but surgery may be needed for larger leaks.

Vital signs (blood pressure, pulse and respiratory rates, temperature) are monitored. Changes in vital signs, as well as increasing pain, nausea and vomiting, and abdominal distention, are reported and may indicate peritonitis.

Stoma Ischemia and Necrosis. The stoma is monitored because ischemia and necrosis of the stoma can result from tension on the mesentery blood vessels, twisting of the bowel segment (conduit) during surgery, or arterial insufficiency. The new stoma must be inspected at least every 4 hours to assess the adequacy of its blood supply. The stoma should be red or pink. If the blood supply to the stoma is compromised, the color changes to purple, brown, or black. These changes are reported immediately. The surgeon or WOC nurse may insert a small, lubricated tube into the stoma and shine a flashlight into the lumen of the tube to assess for superficial ischemia or necrosis. A necrotic stoma requires surgical intervention. If the ischemia is superficial, the dusky stoma is observed and may slough its outer layer in several days.

Stoma Retraction and Separation. Stoma retraction and separation of the mucocutaneous border can occur as a result of trauma or tension on the internal bowel segment used for creation of the stoma. In addition, mucocutaneous separation can occur if the stoma does not heal as a result of accumulation of urine on the stoma and mucocutaneous border. Using a collection drainage pouch with an antireflux valve is helpful because the valve prevents urine from pooling on the stoma and mucocutaneous border. Meticulous skin care to keep the area around the stoma clean and dry promotes healing. If a separation of the mucocutaneous border occurs, surgery is not usually needed. The separated area is protected by applying karaya powder, stoma adhesive paste, and a properly fitted skin barrier and pouch. By protecting the separation, healing is promoted. If the stoma retracts into the peritoneum, surgical intervention is mandatory.

If surgery is needed to manage these complications, the nurse provides explanations to the patient and family. The need for additional surgery is usually perceived as a setback by the patient and family. Emotional support of the patient and family is provided along with physical preparation of the patient for surgery.

PROMOTING HOME, COMMUNITY-BASED, AND TRANSITIONAL CARE

Educating Patients About Self-Care. A major postoperative objective is to assist the patient to achieve the highest level of independence and self-care possible. The nurse and WOC nurse work closely with the patient and family to instruct and assist them in all phases of managing the ostomy. Adequate supplies and complete instruction are necessary to enable the patient and a family member to develop competence and confidence in their skills. Written and verbal instructions are provided, and the patient is encouraged to contact the nurse or primary provider with follow-up questions. Follow-up telephone calls from the nurse to the patient and family after discharge may provide added support and provide another opportunity to answer their questions. Follow-up visits and reinforcement of correct skin care and appliance management techniques also promote skin integrity. Specific techniques for managing the appliance are described in Chart 55-14.

The patient is encouraged to participate in decisions regarding the type of collecting appliance and the time of day to change the appliance. The patient is assisted and encouraged to look at and touch the stoma early to overcome any fears. The patient and family need to know the characteristics of a normal stoma:

- Pink or red and moist, like the inside of the mouth

- Insensitive to pain because it has no nerve endings
- Vascular, which means it may bleed when cleaned

In addition, if a segment of the GI tract was used to create the urinary diversion, mucus may be visible in the urine. By learning what is normal, the patient and family become familiar with what signs and symptoms they should report and what problems they can handle themselves.

Information provided to the patient and the extent of involvement in self-care are determined by the patient's physical recovery and ability to accept and acquire the knowledge and skill needed for independence. Verbal and written instructions are provided, and the patient is given the opportunity to practice and demonstrate the knowledge and skills needed to manage urinary drainage.

Continuing and Transitional Care. Follow-up care is essential to determine how the patient has adapted to the changes in body image and lifestyle adjustments. Visits from a nurse are important to assess the patient's adaptation to the home setting and management of the ostomy. Education and reinforcement may assist the patient and family to cope with altered urinary function. It is important to assess for long-term complications that may occur, such as pouch leakage or rupture, stone formation, stenosis of the stoma, deterioration in kidney function, or incontinence.

Long-term monitoring for anemia is performed to identify vitamin B_{12} deficiency, which may occur when a significant portion of the terminal ileum is removed. This may take several years to develop and can be treated with vitamin B_{12} injections. The patient and family are informed about the United Ostomy Associations of America (UOAA) and any local ostomy support groups to provide ongoing support, assistance, and education.

Postoperative Evaluation

Expected patient outcomes may include:

1. Maintains skin integrity
   a. Maintains intact skin and demonstrates skill in managing drainage system and appliance
   b. States actions to take if skin excoriation occurs
2. Reports relief of pain
3. Exhibits improved body image as evidenced by the following:
   a. Voices acceptance of urinary diversion, stoma, and appliance
   b. Demonstrates increasingly independent self-care, including hygiene and grooming
   c. States acceptance of support and assistance from family members, health care providers, and another patient with an ostomy
4. Copes with sexuality issues
   a. Verbalizes concern about possible alterations in sexuality and sexual function
   b. Reports discussion of sexual concerns with partner and appropriate counselor
5. Demonstrates knowledge needed for self-care
   a. Performs self-care and proficient management of urinary diversion and appliance
   b. Asks questions relevant to self-management and prevention of complications
   c. Identifies signs and symptoms needing care from primary provider, nurse, or other health care providers

6. Absence of complications as evidenced by the following:
   a. Reports absence of pain or tenderness in abdomen
   b. Has temperature within normal range
   c. Reports no urine leakage from incision or drains
   d. Has urine output within desired volume limits
   e. Maintains stoma that is red or pink, moist, and appropriate in size without edema
   f. Has intact and healed border of the stoma

CRITICAL THINKING EXERCISES

1 You are caring for a patient in the intensive care unit who has had an indwelling urinary catheter inserted. What strategies should be used to avoid a CAUTI in the patient? Identify the factors that would put this patient at risk for CAUTI.

2 **ebp** You are a nurse in a busy urology practice who often cares for patients with incontinence. Describe the major types of incontinence, and compare and contrast each. What are the evidence-based management techniques used in treating the different types of incontinence? How do practices differ for men and women? Identify the criteria used to evaluate the strength of the evidence for these practices.

3 **pq** A 55-year-old woman is admitted to a medical-surgical nursing unit with bladder cancer. She is scheduled for a radical cystectomy and urinary diversion. Identify the priorities, approach, and techniques you would use to provide care for this patient in the pre-operative phase of care. How will your priorities, approach, and techniques differ in the post-operative phase of care?

REFERENCES

*Asterisk indicates nursing research.

Books

Bader, M. K., Littlejohns, L. R., & Olson, D. M. (2016). *AANN core curriculum for neuroscience nursing* (6th ed.). Chicago, IL: American Association of Neuroscience Nurses.
Booker, K. (2015). *Critical care nursing: Monitoring and treatment for advanced nursing practice.* Oxford: Wiley Blackwell.
Comerford, K. C. (2015). *Nursing 2015 drug handbook.* Philadelphia, PA: Wolters Kluwer.
Eliopoulos, C. (2018). *Gerontological Nursing* (9th ed.). Philadelphia, PA: Lippincott Williams & Wilkins.
Fischbach, F., & Dunning, M. B. (2015). *A manual of laboratory and diagnostic tests* (9th ed.). Philadelphia, PA: Lippincott Williams & Wilkins.
Grossman, S. C., & Porth, C. M. (2014). *Porth's pathophysiology: Concepts of altered health states* (9th ed.). Philadelphia, PA: Lippincott Williams & Wilkins.
Miller, C. A. (2015). *Nursing for wellness in older adults* (7th ed.). Philadelphia, PA: Lippincott Williams & Wilkins.
Weber, J., & Kelley, J. (2014). *Health assessment in nursing* (5th ed.). Philadelphia, PA: Lippincott Williams & Wilkins.

Journals and Electronic Documents

*Anderson, R., & Zinkgraf, K. (2013). Use and effectiveness of complementary therapies among women with interstitial cystitis. *Urologic Nursing, 33*(6), 306–309.

Askeland, E. J., Newton, M. R., O'Donnell, M. A., et al. (2012). Bladder cancer immunotherapy: BCG and beyond. *Advances in Urology, 2012,* 181987. Retrieved 12/13/2016 at: www.ncbi.nlm.nih.gov/pmc/articles/PMC3388311/?tool = pubmed
*Bass-Ware, A., Weed, D., Johnson, T., et al. (2014). Evaluation of the effect of cranberry juice on symptoms associated with a urinary tract infection. *Urologic Nursing, 34*(3), 121–127.
Carter, N. M., Reitmeier, L., & Goodloe, L. R. (2014). An evidence-based approach to the prevention of catheter-associated urinary tract infections. *Urologic Nursing, 34*(5), 238–245.
Chisholm, A. H. (2015). Probiotics in preventing recurrent urinary tract infections in women: A literature review. *Urologic Nursing, 35*(1), 18–21, 29.
Crawshaw, A., Williams, J., & Woodhouse, F. (2014). The Kock pouch reconsidered: An alternative surgical technique. *British Journal of Nursing, 23*(17), S26–S29.
Cunningham, P., Noble, H., Al-Modhefer, A., et al. (2016). Kidney stones: Pathophysiology, diagnosis and management. *British Journal of Nursing, 25*(20), 1112–1116.
*Day, M. R., Leahy-Warren, P., Loughran, S., et al. (2014). Community-dwelling women's knowledge of urinary incontinence. *British Journal of Community Nursing, 19*(11), 534–538.
Dukes, S., Lowther, C., Martin, T., et al. (2013). Guidelines for standardising the treatment of stoma granulomas at the mucocutaneous junction. *World Council of Enterostomal Therapists Journal, 33*(1), 12–15.
*Hagerty, T., Kertesz, L., Schmidt, J. M., et al. (2015). Risk factors for catheter associated urinary tract infections in critically ill patients with subarachnoid hemorrhage. *Journal of Neuroscience Nursing, 47*(1), 51–54.
Hallis, F., Amasyali, A.S., Yucak, A., et al. (2015). Intrathoracic kidney after blunt abdominal trauma: A case report and review of the literature. *Case Reports in Urology, 2015,* 1–3.
Hopkins, L., McCroskey, D., Reeves, G., et al. (2014). Implementing a urinary tract infection clinical practice guideline in an ambulatory urgent care practice. *The Nurse Practitioner, 39*(4), 50–54.
Matsuoka, P. K., Locali, R. F., Pacetta, A. M., et al. (2016). The efficacy and safety of urethral injection therapy for urinary incontinence in women: A systematic review. *Clinics, 71*(2), 94–100.
*McCooty, S., & Latthe, P. (2014). Electronic pelvic floor assessment questionnaire: A systematic review. *British Journal of Nursing, 23*(18), S32–S37.
Mori, C. (2014). A-Voiding catastrophe: Implementing a nurse-driven protocol. *MEDSURG Nursing, 23*(1), 15–21, 28.
National Cancer Institute (NCI). (2016). Bladder cancer treatment (PDQ®)–Health professional version. Retrieved 12/13/2016 at: www.cancer.gov/types/bladder/hp/bladder-treatment-pdq#section/all
Robinson, J. P., Bradway, C. W., Bunting-Perry, L., et al. (2013). Lower urinary tract symptoms in men with Parkinson's disease. *Journal of Neuroscience Nursing, 45*(6), 382–392.
Rubenwolf, P. C., Hampel, C., Roos, F., et al. (2016). Continent anal urinary diversion in Classic bladder exstrophy: 45-year experience. *Urology, 100*:249–254.
Smolar, J., Salemi, S., Horst, H., et al. (2016). Stem cells in functional bladder engineering. *Transfusion Medicine and Hemotherapy 43,* 328–335.
Strouse, A. (2015). Appraising the literature on bathing practices and catheter-associated urinary tract infection prevention. *Urologic Nursing, 35*(1), 11–17.
Wille, M. A., Zagaja, G. P., Shalhav, A. L., & Gundeti, M. S. (2011). Continence outcomes in patients undergoing robotic assisted laparoscopic Mitrofanoff appendicovesicostomy. *Journal of Urology, 185*(4), 1438–1443.

Resources

American Cancer Society (ACS), www.cancer.org
American Urological Association, www.auanet.org
National Association for Continence (NAFC), www.nafc.org
National Cancer Institute (NCI), www.cancer.gov
National Institute of Diabetes and Digestive and Kidney Diseases (NIDDK), National Institutes of Health, www.niddk.nih.gov
National Kidney and Urologic Diseases Information Clearinghouse (NKUDIC), kidney.niddk.nih.gov/
National Kidney Foundation, www.kidney.org
Wound Ostomy and Continence Nurses Society, www.wocn.org

UNIT
13

Reproductive Function

INCORPORATING TECHNOLOGY IN MANAGING A PATIENT WITH NEWLY DIAGNOSED PROSTATE CANCER

The nurse working in an infusion clinic is assigned to care for a 68-year-old patient who is retired and newly diagnosed with prostate cancer. He is accompanied by his wife and prescribed a course of chemotherapy that necessitates close monitoring of several key laboratory values. The patient and his wife live in a rural area with harsh, snowy winters. Their home is 50 miles from the infusion center. Through a state-funded grant, the patient and his wife are invited to enroll in a telehealth program. The program will provide education webinars about prostate cancer; it also will have access to chat rooms with other patients who have a diagnosis of prostate cancer and offer chat rooms for spouses. In addition, the patient will be able to provide periodic data to his primary provider on his laboratory values.

QSEN Competency Focus: Informatics

The complexities inherent in today's health care system challenges nurses to demonstrate integration of specific inter-disciplinary core competencies. These competencies are aimed at ensuring the delivery of safe, quality patient care (Institute of Medicine, 2003). The Quality and Safety Education for Nurses project (QSEN, 2017; Cronenwett, Sherwood, Barnsteiner, et al., 2007) provides a framework for the knowledge, skills, and attitudes (KSA) required for nurses to demonstrate competency in these key areas, which include *patient-centered care, interdisciplinary teamwork and collaboration, evidence-based practice, quality improvement, safety,* and *informatics.*

Informatics Definition: Use information and technology to communicate, manage knowledge, mitigate error, and support decision making.

SELECTED PRE-LICENSURE KSAs	APPLICATION AND REFLECTION
Knowledge	
Explain why information and technology skills are essential for safe patient care.	Describe the differences in this patient's ability to self-manage his therapeutic regimen with and without the telehealth system. How can telehealth improve the quality of care that he receives?
Skills	
Apply technology and information management tools to support safe processes of care.	Identify the skillset required by both the patient and his health care providers if the telehealth system is to be effective in improving his health
Attitudes	
Appreciate the necessity for all health professionals to seek lifelong, continuous learning of information technology skills.	Reflect on your attitudes towards use of technology by older adult patients. Do you feel threatened by monitoring patients from a distance, rather than having face-to-face encounters? If so, how might this attitude create barriers to effective patient care?

Cronenwett, L., Sherwood, G., Barnsteiner, J., et al. (2007). Quality and safety education for nurses. *Nursing Outlook, 55*(3), 122–131.
Institute of Medicine. (2003). *Health professions education: A bridge to quality.* Washington, DC: National Academies Press.
QSEN Institute. (2017). *QSEN Competencies: definitions and pre-picensure KSAs.* Retrieved on 3/1/2017 at: www.qsen.org/competencies/pre-licensure-ksas

56

Assessment and Management of Patients With Female Physiologic Processes

LEARNING OBJECTIVES

On completion of this chapter, the learner will be able to:

1 Describe the structures and functions of the female reproductive system.
2 Explain approaches to effective assessment of female physiologic processes.
3 Identify the diagnostic examinations and tests used to determine alterations in female reproductive function, and describe the nurse's role before, during, and after these examinations and procedures.

4 Recognize common female physiologic processes and related nursing implications.
5 Compare and contrast the different methods of contraception and implications for care and education.
6 Discuss the causes and management of infertility.
7 Use the nursing process to plan for care of the patient with an ectopic pregnancy.
8 Develop an education plan for women who are approaching or have completed menopause.

GLOSSARY

adnexa: the fallopian tubes and ovaries
amenorrhea: absence of menstrual flow
cervix: bottom (inferior) part of the uterus that is located in the vagina
corpus luteum: site within a follicle that changes after ovulation to produce progesterone
cystocele: displacement of the bladder downward into the vagina
dysmenorrhea: painful menstruation
dyspareunia: difficult or painful sexual intercourse
endometrial ablation: procedure performed through a hysteroscope in which the lining of the uterus is burned away or ablated to treat abnormal uterine bleeding
endometrium: mucous membrane lining of the uterus
estrogens: several hormones produced in the ovaries that develop and maintain the female reproductive system
follicle-stimulating hormone (FSH): hormone released by the pituitary gland to stimulate estrogen production and ovulation
fornix: upper part of the vagina
fundus: the rounded upper portion of the uterus
graafian follicle: cystic structure that develops on the ovary as ovulation begins
hymen: tissue that covers the vaginal opening partially or completely before vaginal penetration
hysteroscopy: an endoscopic procedure performed using a long telescope like instrument inserted through the cervix to diagnose uterine problems

introitus: perineal opening to the vagina
luteal phase: stage in the menstrual cycle in which the endometrium becomes thicker and more vascular
luteinizing hormone (LH): hormone released by the pituitary gland that stimulates progesterone production
menarche: beginning of menstrual function
menopause: permanent cessation of menstruation resulting from the loss of ovarian follicular activity
menstruation: sloughing and discharge of the lining of the uterus if conception does not take place
ovaries: almond-shaped reproductive organs that produce eggs at ovulation and play a major role in hormone production
ovulation: discharge of a mature ovum from the ovary
perimenopause: the period around menopause
progesterone: hormone produced by the corpus luteum that prepares the uterus for receiving the fertilized ovum
proliferative phase: stage in the menstrual cycle before ovulation when the endometrium increases
rectocele: bulging of the rectum into the vagina
secretory phase: stage of the menstrual cycle in which the endometrium becomes thickened, becomes more vascular, and ovulation occurs
uterine prolapse: the cervix and uterus descend into the lower vagina

Nurses who work with women need an understanding of the physical, developmental, psychological, and sociocultural influences on women's health, as well as health practices. It is necessary to consider how medications and diseases specifically affect women. In addition, women's sexuality is complex and often affected by many factors, and related issues need careful evaluation and treatment.

ROLE OF NURSES IN WOMEN'S HEALTH

As their presence in the labor market continues to increase, women face challenges in their roles, lifestyles, and family patterns. Furthermore, they encounter environmental hazards and stress, prompting greater attention on health and health-promoting practices. As a result, many women are taking a greater interest in and responsibility for their own health and health care. Because nurses in all settings encounter women with health care needs, they need a solid understanding of the unique issues related to women's health to provide optimal care. The Affordable Care Act (ACA) had made major changes to the health insurance market and millions of women have gained coverage in the first two full years of implementation (Kaiser Family Foundation, 2015).

The ACA expands coverage to the uninsured through a combination of Medicaid expansions, private insurance reforms and tax credits (Ranji & Salganicoff, 2015). The affordability of health coverage and care is a problem that affects both sexes; however, women consistently are more likely than men to report cost-related barriers to care (Salganicoff, Ranji, Beamesderfer, et al., 2014). The vast majority of women enrolled in market place plans are income eligible for some level of financial assistance such as tax credits to offset their premium costs (94%) or caps on their out-of-pocket costs for deductibles, coinsurance, and copayments (75%). Among the 97 million American women ages 19 to 64, most had some form of insurance coverage in 2014. However, gaps in private sector and publicly funded programs still leave almost one in eight women uninsured. Women with low incomes, women of color, and immigrants are still at greater risk of being uninsured. Single mothers are much more likely to be uninsured (18%) than women in two-parent households (10%) (Kaiser Family Foundation, 2015).

The ACA set new standards for the scope of benefits offered in private plans. In addition to the broad categories of essential health benefits (EHBs) offered by the state-based marketplace plans, the law also requires that new private plans cover preventive services without co-payments or other cost sharing. This includes Pap tests, mammograms, bone density tests, as well as the human papilloma virus (HPV) vaccine. New plans are required to cover additional preventive services for women, including prescribed contraceptives, breast feeding supplies, and resources such as breast pumps, screening for domestic violence, well woman visits, and several counseling and screening services (Kaiser Family Foundation, 2015).

ASSESSMENT OF THE FEMALE REPRODUCTIVE SYSTEM

Anatomic and Physiologic Overview

The female reproductive system is complex because it involves many external and internal structures that are under hormonal control.

Anatomy of the Female Reproductive System

The female reproductive system consists of external and internal pelvic structures. Other anatomic structures that affect the female reproductive system include the hypothalamus and pituitary gland of the endocrine system. The female breast is included in discussions of reproductive health and is covered in Chapter 57.

External Genitalia

The female external genitalia are composed of a variety of tissue types starting with the mons pubis, which is a thick pad

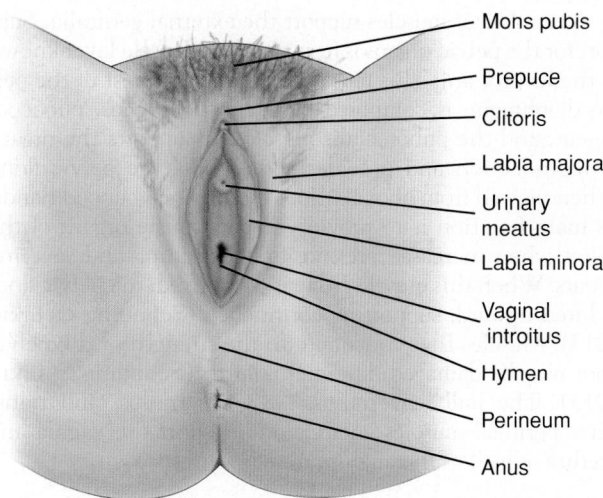

Figure 56-1 • External female genitalia.

of adipose tissue that covers the symphysis pubis and cushions it during intercourse (see Fig. 56-1). Moving downward are two thick folds of connective tissue covered with pubic hair known as the labia majora, which extend from the mons pubis to the perineum. The labia majora cover the oval-shaped area known as the vestibule, where the labia minora originate. The labia minora are two narrow folds of hairless skin, beginning at the clitoris and extending to the fourchette. This area is highly vascular and rich in nerve supply and glands that lubricate the vulva, the collective name for the external genitalia. The labia minora join at the top to form the prepuce, a hood-like structure that partially covers the clitoris. The clitoris, an erectile organ located beneath the pubic arch, consists of a shaft and glans. It secretes smegma, a pheromone (olfactory erotic stimulant), and is sensitive to touch and temperature. Below the clitoris is the urinary meatus, the external opening of the female urethra that has a slit appearance. Below the meatus is the **introitus** (vaginal opening). On each side of the introitus are Bartholin glands, which secrete mucus through tiny ducts that lie within the labia minora and are external to the **hymen** (membrane that encircles the introitus). The vestibule is bounded by the clitoris, fourchette, and labia minora and contains the urethral meatus. Skene gland, located within the urethral meatus, produce mucus for lubrication (Ball, Dains, Flynn, et al., 2015).

 Concept Mastery Alert

The Bartholin glands on either side of the entrance to the vagina can become blocked (cyst formation) or infected (abscess formation). Treatment is different for each, but pain is common with both. Pain can interfere with sitting and walking.

The hymen opening varies widely among women, and the size of the opening is an unreliable indicator of sexual experience (Ball et al., 2015). The fourchette is located in the midline below the vaginal opening where the labia majora and labia minor merge. The perineum is the area between the vagina and the rectum or anus; it is a skin-covered muscular tissue (Ball et al., 2015).

A number of muscles support the external genitalia. Support for the pelvic organs is from the deep muscle layer known as the levator ani. This muscle, which forms most of the pelvic diaphragm, is composed of the iliococcygeus, pubococcygeus, and the puborectalis muscles. It supports the organs of reproduction and provides elasticity of the pelvic floor. When viewed from above, it looks like joined cupped hands. Its main function is to provide support to the organs of the pelvis when increased pressure from coughing and sneezing occurs. When this muscle group is contracted, the pelvic floor is lifted upward, supporting continence (Schuiling & Likis, 2013). Muscles that contribute to the strength of the pelvic floor may be damaged during childbirth (Schuiling & Likis, 2013). The bulbocavernosus, ischiocavernosus, and transverse perineal muscles encircle and support the vagina and urethra as well as the anal sphincter.

Internal Reproductive Structures

The internal structures consist of the vagina, uterus, ovaries, and fallopian or uterine tubes (see Fig. 56-2).

Vagina

The vagina, a tubular-shaped canal lined with glandular mucous membrane, is 7.5 to 10 cm (3 to 4 inches) long and extends upward and backward from the vulva to the cervix. It is thin walled and can be distended during birth. It is highly vascular and has little sensation. Anterior to it are the bladder and the urethra, and posterior to it lies the rectum. The anterior and posterior walls of the vagina normally touch each other. The **fornix** (the upper part of the vagina) surrounds the **cervix** (the inferior part of the uterus) (Ball et al., 2015).

Uterus

The uterus, a pear-shaped, muscular organ, is about 7.5 cm (3 inches) long and 5 cm (2 inches) wide at its upper part. Its walls are about 1.25 cm (0.5 inch) thick. The size of the uterus varies, depending on parity (number of pregnancies), size of the infants, and uterine abnormalities (e.g., fibroids, which are a type of tumor that may distort the uterus). A woman who is nulliparous (one who has not completed a pregnancy to the stage of fetal viability) usually has a smaller uterus than a woman who is multiparous (one who has completed two or more pregnancies to the stage of fetal viability). The uterus lies posterior to the bladder and is held in position by several ligaments. The round ligaments extend anteriorly and laterally to the internal inguinal ring and down the inguinal canal, where they blend with the tissues of the labia majora. The broad ligaments are folds of peritoneum extending from the lateral pelvic walls and enveloping the fallopian tubes. The uterosacral ligaments extend posterior to the sacrum (Schuiling & Likis, 2013).

The uterus has four parts: the cervix, **fundus**, corpus, and isthmus. The cervix is the opening to the uterus and projects into the vagina. A larger upper part, the fundus, is the rounded portion above the insertion of the fallopian tubes. The corpus or body is the main portion of the uterus located between the fundus and the isthmus. The isthmus is referred to as the lower uterine segment during pregnancy and joins the corpus to the cervix.

The cervix is divided into two portions. The portion above the site of attachment of the cervix to the vaginal vault is known as the supravaginal portion; the portion below the attachment site that protrudes into the vagina is known as the vaginal portion. The cervix is composed of fibrous connective tissue. The diameter varies from 2 to 5 cm depending on the childbearing history. The length is usually 2.5 to 3 cm in the woman who is not pregnant. The vaginal portion is smooth, firm, and doughnut shaped with a visible central opening referred to as the external os. The external os is round before the first birth and is often slitlike in shape after childbirth. The internal os is the opening in the cervix to the uterine cavity. In response to cyclic hormones, the cervix produces mucus, which is an important factor in fertility awareness. The vaginal surface of the cervix is covered with squamous epithelium, a rapid cellular growth site of cervical cancer and precancerous changes.

The uterine wall has three layers. The **endometrium**, the innermost layer, is highly vascular and responds to hormone stimulation to prepare to receive the developing ovum. It sloughs if pregnancy does not occur, resulting in menstruation; if pregnancy occurs, it sloughs after delivery. The myometrium, the middle layer, is made up of several smooth muscle layers. The outer layer of the myometrium is composed of longitudinal fibers, chiefly in the fundus, which provide the power to expel the fetus. The middle layer of the myometrium is composed of fibers interlaced with blood vessels in a figure-eight pattern called a *living ligature* because it contracts after childbirth to help control blood loss (Schuiling & Likis, 2013). The inner layer of the myometrium is composed of circular fibers that are concentrated around the internal cervical os to help keep the cervix closed during pregnancy. The other layer of the uterus is composed of parietal peritoneum, which covers most of the uterus. From here, the oviducts or fallopian (or uterine) tubes extend outward, and their lumina are internally continuous with the uterine cavity (Grossman & Porth, 2014). The fallopian tubes or oviducts are the passageway for eggs from the ovary to the uterus. They curve around each ovary and are attached to the uterine fundus. Fallopian tubes are about 10 cm in length and are comprised of four parts. The infundibulum, the most distal portion, is covered in fimbriae, whose wavelike motion helps to pull the egg into the tube. The ampulla is usually the site of fertilization of the egg or ovum. The fallopian tube then narrows from its 0.6 cm diameter in the isthmus, ending in the narrowest part of the interstitial portion, which opens into the uterine cavity. The fallopian tube also secretes nutrients for growth and

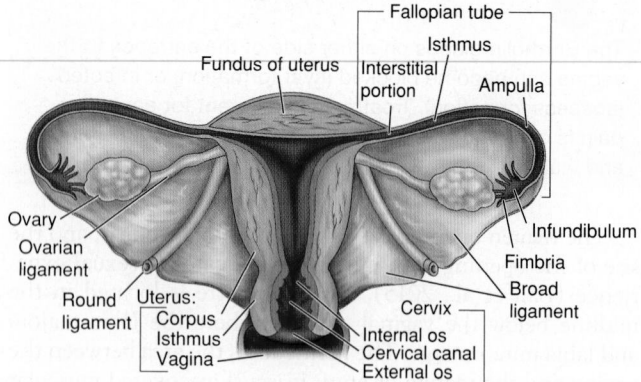

Figure 56-2 • Internal female reproductive structures.

development of the ovum after fertilization while it passes down the tube to the uterus.

Ovaries

The **ovaries** lie behind the broad ligaments and behind and below the fallopian tubes. They are almond-shaped bodies about 3 cm (1.2 inches) long. At birth, they contain thousands of tiny egg cells, or ova. The ovaries and the fallopian tubes together are referred to as the **adnexa.**

Function of the Female Reproductive System

Ovulation

At puberty (usually between 11 and 13 years of age), the ova begin to mature and menstrual cycles begin. In the follicular phase, an ovum enlarges into a cystic structure called a **graafian follicle** until it reaches the surface of the ovary, where transport occurs. The ovum (or oocyte) is discharged into the peritoneal cavity. This periodic discharge of matured ovum is referred to as **ovulation.** The ovum usually finds its way into the fallopian tube, where it is carried to the uterus. If it is penetrated by a spermatozoon, the male reproductive cell, a union occurs and conception takes place. After the discharge of the ovum, the cells of the graafian follicle undergo a rapid change. Gradually, they become yellow and produce **progesterone**, a hormone that prepares the uterus for receiving the fertilized ovum. Ovulation usually occurs 2 weeks prior to the next menstrual period (Grossman & Porth, 2014).

Menstrual Cycle

The menstrual cycle is a complex process involving the reproductive and endocrine systems. The ovaries produce steroid hormones, predominantly **estrogens** and progesterone. Several different estrogens are produced by the ovarian follicle, which consists of the developing ovum and its surrounding cells. The most potent of the ovarian estrogens is estradiol. Estrogens are responsible for developing and maintaining the female reproductive organs and the secondary sex characteristics associated with the adult female. Estrogens play an important role in breast development and in monthly cyclic changes in the uterus (Schuiling & Likis, 2013).

Progesterone is also important in regulating the changes that occur in the uterus during the menstrual cycle. It is secreted by the **corpus luteum** (site within a follicle) or the ovarian follicle after the ovum has been released. Progesterone is the most important hormone for conditioning the endometrium (the mucous membrane lining of the uterus) in preparation for implantation of a fertilized ovum. If pregnancy occurs, the progesterone secretion becomes largely a function of the placenta and is essential for maintaining a normal pregnancy. In addition, progesterone, working with estrogen, prepares the breast for producing and secreting milk. Androgens are hormones produced by the ovaries and adrenal glands in small amounts. These hormones affect many aspects of female health, including follicle development, libido, oiliness of hair and skin, and hair growth (Schuiling & Likis, 2013).

Two gonadotropic hormones are released by the pituitary gland: **follicle-stimulating hormone (FSH)** and **luteinizing hormone (LH).** FSH is primarily responsible for stimulating the ovaries to secrete estrogen. LH is primarily responsible for stimulating progesterone production. Feedback mechanisms,

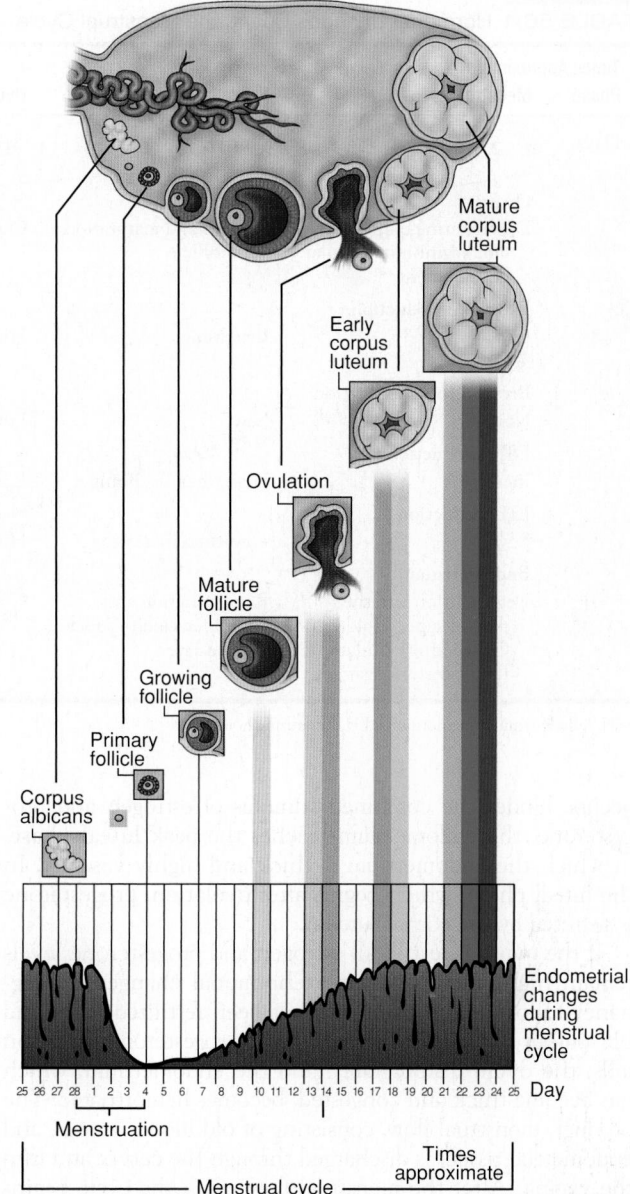

Figure 56-3 • The menstrual cycle and corresponding changes in the endometrium.

in part, regulate FSH and LH secretion. For example, elevated estrogen levels in the blood inhibit FSH secretion but promote LH secretion, whereas elevated progesterone levels inhibit LH secretion. In addition, gonadotropin-releasing hormone (GnRH) from the hypothalamus affects the rate of FSH and LH release (Schuiling & Likis, 2013).

The secretion of ovarian hormones follows a cyclic pattern that results in changes in the uterine endometrium and in menstruation (see Fig. 56-3 and Table 56-1). This cycle is typically 28 days in length, but there are many normal variations (from 21 to 42 days). In the **proliferative phase** at the beginning of the cycle (just after menstruation), FSH output increases, and estrogen secretion is stimulated. This causes the endometrium to thicken and become more vascular. In the **secretory phase** near the middle portion of the cycle (day 14 in a 28-day cycle), LH output increases, and ovulation

TABLE 56-1 Hormonal Changes During the Menstrual Cycle

Phase	Menstrual	Follicular	Ovulation	Luteal	Premenstrual
Times Approximate					
Days	1 2 3 4 5 6 7 8	9 10 11 12 13	14 15 16 17 18	19 20 21 22 23 24	25 26 27 28 1 2
Ovary	Degenerating corpus luteum; beginning follicular development	Growth and maturation of follicle	Ovulation	Active corpus luteum	Degenerating corpus luteum
Estrogen production	Low	Increasing	High	Declining, then a secondary rise	Decreasing
Progesterone production	None	Low	Low	Increasing	Decreasing
FSH production	Increasing	High, then declining	Low	Low	Increasing
LH production	Low	Low, then increasing	High	High	Decreasing
Endometrium	Degeneration and shedding of superficial layer. Coiled arteries dilate, then constrict again.	Reorganization and proliferation of superficial layer	Continued growth	Active secretion and glandular dilation; highly vascular; edematous	Vasoconstriction of coiled arteries; beginning degeneration

FSH, follicle-stimulating hormone; LH, luteinizing hormone.

occurs. Under the combined stimulus of estrogen and progesterone, the endometrium reaches the peak **luteal phase**, in which the endometrium is thick and highly vascular. In the luteal phase, which begins after ovulation, progesterone is secreted by the corpus luteum.

If the ovum is fertilized, estrogen and progesterone levels remain high, and the complex hormonal changes of pregnancy follow. If the ovum has not been fertilized, FSH and LH output diminishes; estrogen and progesterone secretion falls; the ovum disintegrates; and the endometrium, which has become thick and congested, becomes hemorrhagic. The product, menstrual flow, consisting of old blood, mucus, and endometrial tissue, is discharged through the cervix and into the vagina. After the menstrual flow stops, the cycle begins again; the endometrium proliferates and thickens from estrogenic stimulation, and ovulation recurs (Schuiling & Likis, 2013).

Menopausal Period

The menopausal period marks the end of a woman's reproductive capacity. It usually occurs between 45 and 55 years of age (Grossman & Porth, 2014). Perimenopause precedes this and can begin as early as 35 years of age. Physical, emotional, and menstrual changes may occur, and this transition offers another opportunity for health promotion and disease prevention education and counseling. Menopause is a normal part of aging and maturation. Menstruation ceases, and because the ovaries are no longer active, the reproductive organs become smaller. No more ova mature; therefore, no ovarian hormones are produced. (An earlier menopause may occur if the ovaries are surgically removed or are destroyed by radiation or chemotherapy or because of an unknown etiology.) Multifaceted changes also occur throughout the woman's body. These changes are neuroendocrine, biochemical,

and metabolic and are related to normal maturation or aging (see Table 56-2).

Assessment

A nurse who is obtaining information from a woman for the health history and performing physical assessment is in an ideal position to discuss the woman's general health issues, health promotion, and health-related concerns. Relevant topics include fitness, nutrition, cardiovascular risks, health screening, sexuality, menopause, abuse, health risk behaviors, emotional well-being, and immunizations. Selected health screening and counseling issues are summarized in Chart 56-1.

Health History

In addition to the general health history, the nurse asks about past illnesses and experiences specific to a woman's health. Data should be collected about the following:

- Menstrual history (including **menarche**, length of cycles, duration and amount of flow, presence of cramps or pain, bleeding between periods or after intercourse, bleeding after menopause)
- Pregnancies (number of pregnancies, outcomes of pregnancies)
- Exposure to medications (diethylstilbestrol [DES], immunosuppressive agents, others)
- **Dysmenorrhea** (pain with menses), **dyspareunia** (pain with intercourse), pelvic pain
- Symptoms of vaginitis (i.e., odor or itching)
- Problems with urinary function, including frequency, urgency, and incontinence
- Bowel problems
- Sexual history

TABLE 56-2 Age-Related Changes in the Female Reproductive System

The age-related changes described below pertain to women ages 45 years and older.

Changes	Physiologic Effects	Signs and Symptoms
Cessation of ovarian function and decreased estrogen production	Decreased ovulation	Decreased/loss of ability to conceive; increased infertility
	Onset of menopause	Irregular menses with eventual cessation of menses
	Vasomotor instability and hormonal fluctuations	Hot flashes or flushing; night sweats, sleep disturbances; mood swings; fatigue
	Decreased bone formation	Bone loss and increased risk for osteoporosis and osteoporotic fractures; loss of height
	Decreased vaginal lubrication	Dyspareunia, resulting in lack of interest in sex
	Thinning of urinary and genital tracts	Increased risk for urinary tract infection
	Increased pH of vagina Thinning of pubic hair and shrinking of labia	Increased incidence of inflammation (atrophic vaginitis) with discharge, itching, and vulvar burning
Relaxation of pelvic musculature	Prolapse of uterus, cystocele, rectocele	Dyspareunia, incontinence, feelings of perineal pressure

Chart 56-1 Selected Health Screening and Counseling Issues for Women

Ages 19–39 Years

Sexuality and Reproductive Issues

Annual pelvic examination to begin at 21 years of age
Annual clinical breast examination
Contraceptive options
High-risk sexual behaviors

Health and Risk Behaviors

Hygiene
Injury prevention
Nutrition
Exercise patterns
Risk for abuse, maltreatment, and neglect
Use of tobacco, drugs, and alcohol
Life stresses
Immunizations

Diagnostic Testing*

Cervical cytology (Pap smear) alone every 3 years from ages 21 to 29. From ages 30 to 64: Cervical cytology alone every 3 years; or cytology and HPV testing every 5 years.
Sexually transmitted infection screening as indicated

Ages 40–64 Years

Sexuality and Reproductive Issues

Annual pelvic examination
Annual clinical breast examination
Contraceptive options
High-risk sexual behaviors
Menopausal concerns

Health and Risk Behaviors

Hygiene
Bone loss and injury prevention
Nutrition
Exercise patterns
Risk for abuse, maltreatment, and neglect
Use of tobacco, drugs, and alcohol
Life stresses
Immunizations

Diagnostic Testing*

Cervical cytology (Pap smear) every 3 years; or cytology and HPV testing every 5 years.
Annual mammography for women age 45–54 years.
• Women 55 and older should switch to mammograms every 2 years, or can continue yearly screening.
• Screening should continue as long as a woman is in good health and is expected to live 10 more years or longer

Cholesterol and lipid profile
Colorectal cancer screening beginning at age 50 years
Bone mineral density testing
Thyroid-stimulating hormone testing
Hearing and eye examinations

Age 65 Years and Older

Sexuality and Reproductive Issues

Annual pelvic examination
Annual clinical breast examination
High-risk sexual behaviors

Health and Risk Behaviors

Hygiene
Injury prevention, falls
Nutrition
Exercise patterns
Risk for abuse, maltreatment, and neglect
Use of tobacco, drugs, and alcohol
Life stresses
Immunizations

Diagnostic Testing*

No cervical cytology (Pap smear) following adequate negative prior screenings
Mammography
Cholesterol and lipid profile
Colorectal cancer screening
Bone mineral density testing
Thyroid-stimulating hormone testing
Hearing and eye examinations

HPV, human papilloma virus.
*Each individual's risks (family history, personal history) influence the need for specific assessments and their frequency.
Adapted from Smith, R. A., Cokkinides, V., & Brawley, O. W. (2012). Cancer screening in the United States, 2012. *CA: A Cancer Journal for Clinicians,* 62(2), 129–142; Eliopoulos, C. (2018). *Gerontological nursing* (9th ed.). Philadelphia, PA: Lippincott Williams & Wilkins.

Chart 56-2

GENETICS IN NURSING PRACTICE
Female Reproductive Processes

Various female reproductive disorders are influenced by genetic factors. Some examples include:

- Hereditary breast or ovarian cancer syndromes
- Hereditary nonpolyposis colon cancer syndrome (risk for uterine cancer)
- Kallmann syndrome
- Müllerian aplasia
- 21-Hydroxylase deficiency (female masculinization)
- Turner syndrome (45,XO)

Nursing Assessments

Refer to Chapter 5, Chart 5-2: Genetics in Nursing Practice: Genetic Aspects of Health Assessment

Family History Assessment Specific to Female Reproductive Processes

- Assess family history for other family members with similar reproductive problems/abnormalities. If the female is a carrier of fragile X, she may be at risk for premature ovarian failure.
- Ask about age at the start and completion of puberty. Failure to complete puberty can lead to infertility.
- The absence of the sense of smell is noted with Kallmann syndrome which, if untreated, can lead to infertility.
- Inquire about ethnic background (e.g., Ashkenazi Jewish populations and hereditary breast/ovarian cancer mutations).

- Inquire about relatives with other cancers, including early-onset ovarian, uterine, renal, prostate cancers.
- Obtain family history that includes a thorough review of reproductive history which addresses spontaneous abortions (miscarriages), infant deaths, or difficulties during pregnancy.
- If possible, obtain ages of the parents during pregnancy.

Patient Assessment Specific to Female Reproductive Processes

- In females with delayed puberty or primary amenorrhea, assess for clinical features of Turner syndrome (short stature, webbing of the neck, widely spaced nipples).
- Assess for other congenital anomalies in females with Müllerian defect, including renal and vertebral anomalies.
- Assess for exposure to toxic chemicals, radiation, or medications during pregnancy.
- Obtain prior reproductive history.
- Inquire about use and frequency of alcohol or tobacco during pregnancy.

Genetics Resources

American Cancer Society, www.cancer.org
Association for X and Y Chromosome Variations, www.genetic.org
March of Dimes Birth Defects Foundation, www.marchofdimes.org
Turner Syndrome Society, www.turnersyndrome.org
See Chapter 8, Chart 8-7 for components of genetic counseling.

- STIs and methods of treatment
- Current or previous sexual abuse or physical abuse
- Past surgery or other procedures on reproductive tract structures (including female genital mutilation [FGM] or female circumcision)
- Chronic illness or disability that may affect health status, reproductive health, need for health screening, or access to health care
- Presence or family history of a genetic disorder. Chart 56-2 presents information about genetic reproductive disorders.

In collecting data related to reproductive health, the nurse can educate the patient about normal physiologic processes, such as menstruation and menopause, and assess possible abnormalities. Many problems experienced by young or middle-aged women can be corrected easily. However, if they are not treated, they may result in anxiety and health problems. Issues related to sexuality and sexual function are typically more often brought to the attention of the gynecologic or women's health care provider than other health care providers; however, nurses caring for all women should consider these issues part of routine health assessment.

Sexual History

A sexual assessment includes both subjective and objective data and should be included in care of individuals from adolescence through advanced age. Health and sexual histories, physical examination findings, and laboratory results are all part of the database. The purpose of a sexual history is to obtain information that provides a picture of a woman's sexuality and sexual practices and to promote sexual health. It may lead to discussion about sexually transmitted illnesses, unintended pregnancies, and ways of reducing

high-risk sexual behaviors (Sargant, Smallwood, Finley, et al., 2014). The sexual history may enable a patient to discuss sexual matters openly and to discuss sexual concerns with an informed health professional. This information can be obtained after the gynecologic–obstetric or genitourinary history is completed. By incorporating the sexual history into the general health history, the nurse can move from areas of lesser sensitivity to areas of greater sensitivity after establishing initial rapport.

Taking the sexual history becomes a dynamic process reflecting an exchange of information between the patient and the nurse and provides the opportunity to clarify myths and explore areas of concern that the patient may not have felt comfortable discussing in the past. In obtaining a sexual history, the nurse must not assume the patient's sexual preference until clarified. When asking about sexual health, the nurse also cannot assume that the patient is married or unmarried. Asking a patient to label herself as single, married, widowed, or divorced may be considered by some women as inappropriate. Asking about a partner or about current meaningful relationships may be a less offensive way to initiate a sexual history.

The PLISSIT (permission, limited information, specific suggestions, intensive therapy) model of sexual assessment and intervention may be used to provide a framework for nursing interventions (Annon, 1976). The assessment begins by introducing the topic and asking the woman for permission to discuss issues related to sexuality with her.

The nurse can begin by explaining the purpose of obtaining a sexual history (e.g., "I ask all my patients about their sexual health. May I ask you some questions about this?"). History taking continues by inquiring about present sexual activity and sexual orientation (e.g., "Are you currently having sex? With a man, a woman, or both?"). Inquiries about possible sexual dysfunction may include, "Are you having any problems related to your current sexual performance?" Such problems may be related to medication, life changes, disability, or the onset of physical or emotional illness. A patient can be asked about her thoughts on what is causing the current problem (Weber & Kelley, 2014).

Information about sexual function can be introduced during the health history (see Chapter 5). By initiating an assessment about sexual concerns, the nurse communicates to the patient that issues about changes or problems in sexual functioning are valid health issues, which provides a safe environment for discussing these sensitive topics. Young women may be apprehensive about having irregular periods, may be concerned about STIs, or may need contraception. They may want information about using tampons, emergency contraception, or issues related to pregnancy. Women who are perimenopausal may have concerns about irregular menses. Women who are menopausal may be concerned about vaginal dryness and discomfort with intercourse. Women of any age may have concerns about relationships, sexual satisfaction, orgasm, or masturbation.

Risk of STIs can be assessed by asking about the number of sexual partners in the past year or in the patient's lifetime. An open-ended question related to the patient's need for further information should be included (e.g., "Do you have any questions or concerns about your sexual health?"). Women can be advised that intercourse should never be painful; pain should be investigated by a care provider. They should also be encouraged to talk openly about their sexual feelings with their partner; in an intimate relationship, feelings are facts.

Female Genital Mutilation or Cutting

FGM comprises all procedures that involve partial or total removal of the external female genitalia, or other injury to the female genital organs for nonmedical reasons. FGM is recognized internationally as a violation of the human rights of girls and women. It reflects deep-rooted inequality between the sexes, and constitutes an extreme form of discrimination against women. It is nearly always carried out on minors and is a violation of the rights of children. The practice also violates a person's rights to health, security and physical integrity, the right to be free from torture and cruel, inhuman or degrading treatment, and the right to life when the procedure results in death (World Health Organization [WHO], 2016).

Complications for patients who have undergone FGM can include infertility, childbirth complications, impaired bladder function, and urinary complications. The practice is most common in the western, eastern, and north-eastern regions of Africa, in some countries in Asia and the Middle East, and among migrants from these areas (WHO, 2016).

Nurses caring for patients who have undergone FGM need to be sensitive, empathetic, knowledgeable, culturally competent, and nonjudgmental. Respect for others' health beliefs, practices, and behaviors, as well as recognition of the complexity of issues involved, is crucial. The nurse should use terminology with which the woman is familiar; *cutting* is usually a more acceptable term than *mutilation*. Speculums are not used in some developing countries; the function of this instrument should be explained and an appropriately sized speculum used to examine women who have experienced FGM.

Intimate Partner Violence

Intimate partner violence (IPV) is a public health problem that affects millions of Americans each year. In the United States, 24 people per minute are victims of IPV (Centers for Disease Control and Prevention [CDC], 2014). IPV involves four main types of violence: Physical violence, sexual violence, stalking, and psychological aggression (CDC, 2014).

Approximately 27% of women in the United States have experienced one or more of the four forms of IPV, costing more than $8.3 billion (CDC, 2014). Violence is rarely a one-time occurrence in a relationship; it usually continues and escalates in severity. This is an important point to emphasize when a woman states that her partner has hurt her but has promised to change. Perpetrators can change their behavior, although not without extensive counseling and motivation. If a woman states that she is being hurt, sensitive care is required (see Chart 56-3).

By knowing about this major public health problem, being alert to abuse-related problems, and learning how to elicit information from women about abuse, maltreatment, and neglect in their lives, nurses can intervene to assist the patient in addressing a problem that might otherwise go undetected and thus save lives by making women safer through education and support. As part of a comprehensive assessment, the nurse should ensure a safe environment (i.e., a private room with the door closed) and ask each woman about violence in her life. More information on family violence, abuse, and neglect, including sexual assault and rape, can be found in Chapter 72; see Chart 72-8 for information on questions to ask when assessing for abuse, maltreatment, and neglect.

No specific signs or symptoms are diagnostic of abuse; however, nurses may see an injury that does not fit the account of how it happened (e.g., a bruise on the side of the upper arm after "I walked into a door"). Manifestations of abuse, maltreatment, and neglect may involve suicide attempts, drug and alcohol abuse, frequent emergency department visits, vague pelvic pain, somatic complaints, and depression. However, there may be no obvious signs or symptoms. Women in abusive situations have higher levels of depression and often report that they "do not feel well," possibly due to the stress or fear and anticipation of impending abuse.

Incest and Childhood Sexual Abuse

Nurses may encounter women who have been sexually traumatized. Female survivors of sexual abuse are reported to have more mental and physical health problems than women who were not victims of abuse (Pyra, Weber, Wilson, et al., 2014). Victims of childhood sexual abuse are reported to experience more depression (Pyra et al., 2014), posttraumatic stress disorder, morbid obesity, marital instability, gastrointestinal problems, and headaches, as well as use health care services more frequently than people who were not victims. In women, chronic pelvic pain is often associated with physical violence, emotional neglect, and sexual abuse in childhood (Schuiling & Likis, 2013). Women who have experienced rape or sexual abuse may be very anxious about pelvic examinations, labor, pelvic or breast irradiation, or any treatment or examination that involves hands-on treatment or requires

Chart 56-3 Strategies for Providing Sensitive Care Following Abuse, Maltreatment, and Neglect	
Strategy	**Rationale**
Reassure the woman that she is not alone	Women often believe that they are alone in experiencing abuse, maltreatment, and neglect at the hands of their partners.
Express your belief that no one should be hurt, that abuse is the fault of the batterer and is against the law.	Doing so lets the woman know that no one deserves to be abused and that she has not caused the abuse.
Assure the woman that her information is confidential, although it does become part of her medical record. *If children are suspected of being abused or are being abused, the law requires that this be reported to the authorities.* Some states require reporting of spousal or partner abuse. Domestic violence agencies and medical and nursing groups disagree with this policy and are trying to have it changed. Serious opposition is based on the fact that reporting does not and cannot currently guarantee a woman's safety and may place her in more danger. It may also interfere with a patient's willingness to discuss her personal life and concerns with health care providers. This places a serious barrier in the way of comprehensive nursing care. If nurses are in doubt about laws on reporting abuse, they need to check with their local or state domestic violence agency.	Women are often afraid that their information will be reported to the police or protective services and their children may be taken away.
Document the woman's statement of abuse and take photographs of any visible injuries if written formal consent has been obtained. (Emergency departments usually have a camera available if one is not on the nursing unit.)	Doing so provides documentation of injuries that may be needed for later legal or criminal proceedings.
Provide education that includes the following: • Inform the woman that shelters are available to ensure safety for her and her children. (Lengths of stay in shelters vary by state but are often up to 2 months. Staff often assists with housing, jobs, and the emotional distress that accompanies the breakup of the family.) Provide list of shelters. • Inform the woman that violence gets worse, not better. • If the woman chooses to go to a shelter, let her make the call. • If the woman chooses to return to the abuser, remain nonjudgmental and provide information that will make her safer than she was before disclosing her situation. • Make sure that the woman has a 24-hour hotline telephone number that provides information and support (Spanish translation and a device for the deaf are also available), police number, and 911. • Assist her to set up a safety plan in case she decides to return home. (A safety plan is an organized plan for departure with packed bags and important papers hidden in a safe spot.)	Options may be lifesaving for the woman and her children.

Adapted from Centers for Disease Control and Prevention (CDC). (2014). *Understanding intimate partner violence fact sheet.* Retrieved on 11/18/16 at: www.cdc.gov/violenceprevention/pdf/ipv-factsheet.pdf

removal of clothing. Nurses should be prepared to offer support and referral to psychologists, community resources, and self-help groups.

Health Issues in Women With Disabilities

Approximately 20% of women have disabilities and encounter physical, architectural, and attitudinal barriers that may limit their full participation in society (Courtney-Long, Carroll, Znang, et al., 2013). Women with disabilities may experience stereotyping and increased risk of abuse, maltreatment, and neglect. They have reported that others, including health care providers, often equate them with their disability. Studies have reported that women with disabilities receive less primary health care and preventive health screening than other women, often because of access problems and health care providers who focus on the causes of disability rather than on health issues that are of concern to all women (Courtney-Long et al., 2013; Smeltzer, Mitra, Iezzoni, et al., 2016). To address these issues, the health history must include questions about barriers to health care encountered by women with disabilities and the effect of their disability on their health status and health care.

In 2013, the CDC and the Association of Maternal Child Health Programs partnered to develop a central resource tool made of existing resources for nurses, physicians, physician assistants, and nurse practitioners who work with women with disabilities. The Toolbox launched in May 2013 and provides links to existing tools to help facilitate preventive services (such as routine physical examinations, teeth cleanings, hepatitis B vaccinations, cervical cancer and breast cancer screenings, and family planning services) to women

Chart 56-4 — ASSESSMENT
Assessing a Woman With a Disability

Health History

Address questions directly to the woman herself rather than to people accompanying her. Ask about:

- Self-care limitations resulting from her disability (ability to feed and dress self, the use of assistive devices, transportation requirements, other assistance needed)
- Sensory limitations (lack of sensation, low vision, deaf or hard of hearing)
- Accessibility issues (ability to get to health care provider, transfer to examination table, accessibility of office/clinic of health care provider, previous experiences with health care providers, health screening practices; her understanding of physical examination)
- Cognitive or developmental changes that affect understanding
- Limitations secondary to disability that affect general health issues and reproductive health and health care
- Sexual function and concerns (those of all women and those that may be affected by the presence of a disabling condition)
- Menstrual history and menstrual hygiene practices
- Physical, sexual, or psychological abuse (including abuse by care providers; abuse by neglect, withholding or withdrawing assistive devices or personal or health care) (see Chart 56-3)
- Presence of secondary disabilities (i.e., those resulting from the patient's primary disability: pressure ulcers, spasticity, osteoporosis, etc.)
- Health concerns related to aging with a disability

Physical Assessment

Provide instructions directly to the woman herself rather than to people accompanying her; provide written or audiotaped instructions.

Ask the woman what assistance she needs for the physical examination and provide assistance if needed:

- Undressing and dressing
- Providing a urine specimen
- Standing on scale to be weighed (provide alternative means of obtaining weight if she is unable to stand on scale)
- Moving on and off the examination table
- Assuming, changing, and maintaining positions

Consider the fatigue experienced by the woman during a lengthy examination and allow rest.

Provide assistive devices and other aids/methods needed to allow adequate communication with the patient (interpreters, signers, large-print written materials).

Complete examination that would be indicated for any other woman; having a disability is *never* justification for omitting parts of the physical examination, including the pelvic examination.

Adapted from Smeltzer, S. C., Mitra, M., Iezzoni, L. I., et al. (2016). Perinatal experiences of women with physical disabilities and their recommendations for Clinicians. *Journal of Obstetric, Gynecologic & Neonatal Nursing, 45*(6), 781–789.

Chart 56-5 — Health Care for Those Who Identify as LGBT

Nurses working with those who identify as LGBT should consider that these individuals:

- Are found in every ethnic group and socioeconomic class
- Are seen in all age groups, including teens and seniors.
- Can be single, celibate, or divorced.
- Have often encountered insensitivity in health care encounters.
- Are typically offered contraception when asked if they are sexually active and respond affirmatively, as health care providers may assume incorrectly that they practice heterosexual intercourse.
- Have lower health screening rates than other women.
- Often feel invisible and underuse health care, similar to many other marginalized groups of women.

Nurses need to:

- Use gender-neutral questions and terms that are nonjudgmental and accepting.
- Recognize that lesbian teens are at risk for suicide and screen for those at risk.
- Recognize that many lesbians do participate in heterosexual activity but consider themselves at low risk for STIs. Because human papilloma virus, herpes infections, and other organisms implicated in STIs are transmitted by secretions and contact, lesbians may need information on STIs and contraception. If sex toys are used and not cleaned, pelvic infections can occur.

Women who identify as LGBT are at high risk for cancer, heart disease, depression, and alcohol abuse. They may have a higher body mass index, may bear fewer or no children, and often have fewer health preventive screenings than women who are heterosexual. These factors may increase the risk of colon, endometrial, ovarian, and breast cancer, as well as cardiovascular disease and diabetes. Adolescents are at risk for smoking and suicide/depression.

Adapted from Johnson, M. J. & Amella, E. J. (2014). Isolation of lesbian, gay, bisexual and transgender youth: A dimensional concept analysis. *Journal of Advanced Nursing, 70*(3), 523–532. Rager Zuzelo, P. (2014). Improving nursing care for lesbian, bisexual and transgender women. *Journal of Obstetric, Gynecologic and Neonatal Nursing, 43*, 520–530.

with disabilities (Sinclair, Taft, Sloan, et al., 2015). Other issues to be addressed regarding the care of women with disabilities are identified in Chart 56-4.

Lesbians, Gay, Bisexual, and Transgender (LGBT)

Many health care providers are insufficiently prepared to meet the health needs of patients who identify as lesbian, gay, bisexual, or transgender (LGBT) and those who are questioning their gender (Rager Zuzelo, 2014). Many health assessments presume a heterosexual orientation. Nursing organizations have called for recognition of LGBT health disparities (Rager Zuzelo, 2014).

Those who identify themselves as LGBT may have concerns about disclosure and confidentiality, discriminatory attitudes, and treatment (Bosse, Nesteby, & Randall, 2015; Johnson & Amella, 2014; Rager Zuzelo, 2014) (see Chart 56-5). Youth who identify as LGBT are at higher risk of human immune deficiency virus (HIV) and sexually transmitted infections (STIs) (Bosse et al., 2015). Some research has reported that lesbians abuse alcohol and drugs to a greater degree than women who are heterosexual because their social venues may contribute to alcohol and drug use. In addition, youth who self-identify as lesbian, gay, or bisexual or who lack support from parents and families may experience increased physical and mental health issues (e.g., depression and substance abuse) as well as isolation

Chart 56-6 · NURSING RESEARCH PROFILE
Isolation in LGBT Youth

Johnson, M. J., & Amella, E. J. (2014). Isolation of lesbian, gay, bisexual and transgender youth: A dimensional concept analysis. *Journal of Advanced Nursing, 70*(3), 523–532.

Purpose

Few nursing studies have looked at isolation in youth who identify as lesbian, gay, bisexual or transgender (LGBT) despite the fact that nurses have many interactions with them in hospitals, community and school settings. Some research suggests isolation in youth who identify as LGBT is related to increased risk for mental and physical health disparities. The aim of this dimensional concept analysis was to understand isolation in the context, and from the perspective of youth identifying as LGBT.

Design

Procedures for the concept analysis included describing the social construction of the concept, describing the logic of a concept from multiple perspectives and as part of multiple contexts, differentiating the relationship between perspectives and use or definition of the concept and identifying and examining assumptions. To accomplish the analysis, the two authors read each

paper in its entirety and then identified the findings of each article using a table. Additional tables allowed for the identification of patterns or relationships across dimensions, discipline perspectives and publication dates.

Results

The analysis revealed five socially constructed dimensions and four sub-dimensions. These findings indicate that there is substantial variability in the concept of isolation in LGBT youth. These differences and variations are most notably observed in the 20 articles (57%) that had more than one dimension. Although some articles were explicit about the different meanings and use of the concept, most of the papers had wide variability in the use and meaning of the concept.

Nursing Implications

It is imperative that nurses and other professionals understand the significance of isolation in youth who identify as LGBT. Nurses who understand the concept have the potential, in their interactions with these youth in hospitals, community, and school settings, to intervene and suggest strategies to mitigate the isolation.

(Johnson & Amella, 2013) (see Chart 56-6). Nurses need to understand the unique needs of this population and provide appropriate and sensitive care.

 Gerontologic Considerations

Older women function at various levels across the health spectrum; some function at a high level in their jobs or families, whereas others may be very ill. Nurses need to be prepared to care for older women who may be bright, energetic, and ambitious or who are coping with multiple family crises, including their own health issues, as well as for those who are experiencing a life-altering or life-threatening health problem. Older women are at risk for several conditions, including diabetes, dyslipidemia, hypertension, and thyroid disease, all of which have symptoms that may be dismissed as typical aging. Nurses can help prevent morbidity and mortality from these conditions by encouraging women to obtain regular health screenings (Eliopoulos, 2018). Knowledge about heart disease prevention, pharmacology, diet, signs of dementia or cognitive decline, fall prevention, osteoporosis prevention, gynecologic and breast cancers, and sexuality are important for providing high-level nursing care. Health disparities, cultural competency, and end-of-life issues also need to be considered.

Physical Assessment

Periodic examinations and routine cancer screening are important for all women. Annual breast and pelvic examinations are important for all women 21 years or older and for those who are sexually active, regardless of age (US Preventive Services Task Force [USPSTF], 2016). Patients deserve understanding and support because of the emotional and physical considerations associated with gynecologic examinations. Women may be embarrassed by the usual questions asked by a gynecologist or women's health care provider.

Because gynecologic conditions are of a personal and private nature to most women, such information is shared only with those directly involved in patient care.

The approach to the gynecologic examination needs to be systematic and thorough (Weber & Kelley, 2014). The nurse can alleviate feelings of anxiety with explanations and education (see Chart 56-7). It may be helpful to emphasize that a pelvic examination should not usually be uncomfortable. Before the examination begins, the patient is asked to empty her bladder and to provide a urine specimen if urine tests are

Chart 56-7 · PATIENT EDUCATION
The Pelvic Examination

A pelvic examination includes assessment of the appearance of the vulva, vagina, and cervix and the size and shape of the uterus and ovaries to ensure reproductive health and absence of illness. Providing education for the patient should make the examination proceed more smoothly.

The nurse instructs the patient to:

- Expect to have a feeling of fullness or pressure during the examination, but you should not feel pain. It is important to relax, because if you are very tense, you may feel discomfort.
- Recognize that it is normal to feel uncomfortable and apprehensive.
- Be aware that a narrow, warmed speculum will be inserted to visualize the cervix and a Papanicolaou (Pap) smear will be obtained, if indicated, and should not be uncomfortable.
- Note that you may watch the examination with a mirror if you choose; the examination usually takes no longer than 5 minutes.
- Understand that draping will be used to minimize exposure and reduce embarrassment.

Adapted from Weber, J., & Kelley, J. (2014). *Health assessment in nursing* (5th ed.). Philadelphia, PA: Lippincott Williams & Wilkins.

part of the total assessment. Voiding ensures patient comfort and eases the examination because a full bladder can make palpation of pelvic organs uncomfortable for the patient and difficult for the examiner.

Positioning

The supine lithotomy position is used most commonly (Weber & Kelley, 2014). If the patient chooses, alternative positions are sometimes used (Ball et al., 2015). The lithotomy position offers several advantages:

- It is more comfortable for some women.
- It allows better eye contact between patient and examiner.
- It may provide an easier means for the examiner to carry out the bimanual examination.
- It enables the woman to use a mirror to see her anatomy (if she chooses) to visualize any conditions that require treatment or to learn about using certain contraceptive methods.

Inspection

After the patient is prepared, the examiner inspects the external genitalia by looking at the labia majora and minora, noting the epidermal tissue of the labia majora; the skin fades to the pink mucous membrane of the vaginal introitus. Lesions of any type (e.g., genital warts, pigmented lesions [melanoma]) are evaluated. In the woman who is nulliparous, the labia minora come together at the opening of the vagina. In a woman who has delivered children vaginally, the labia minora may gape and vaginal tissue may protrude.

Trauma to the anterior vaginal wall during childbirth may have resulted in incompetency of the musculature, and **cystocele** (a bulge caused by the bladder protruding into the submucosa of the anterior vaginal wall) may be seen. Childbirth trauma may also have affected the posterior vaginal wall, producing a **rectocele** (a bulge caused by rectal cavity protrusion). **Uterine prolapse**, in which the cervix and uterus descend under pressure through the vaginal canal and may be seen at the introitus, may also occur. To identify such protrusions, the examiner asks the patient to "bear down."

The introitus should be free of superficial mucosal lesions. The labia minora may be separated by the fingers of the gloved hand and the lower part of the vagina palpated. In women who have not had vaginal intercourse, a hymen of variable thickness may be felt circumferentially within the vaginal opening. The hymeneal ring usually permits the insertion of one finger. Rarely, the hymen totally occludes the vaginal entrance (imperforate hymen).

Examination

Examination techniques include the speculum examination and several palpation methods.

Speculum Examination

The bivalve speculum, either metal or plastic, is available in many sizes (Ball et al., 2015). Metal specula are cleaned and sterilized between patients; plastic specula are for one-time use. Water-soluble lubricant or warm water is used to lubricate the speculum (Ball et al., 2015).

The speculum is gently inserted into the posterior portion of the introitus and slowly advanced to the top of the vagina;

this should not be painful or uncomfortable for the woman. The speculum is then slowly opened. In the metal types, a set-screw of the thumb rest is tightened; in the plastic types, a clip is locked to hold the blades in place (Ball et al., 2015).

Inspecting the Cervix

The cervix is inspected for color, position, size, surface characteristics, discharge, and size and shape of the cervical os (Ball et al., 2015). In women who are nulliparous, the cervix usually is 2 to 3 cm wide and smooth. In women who have borne children, the cervix may have a laceration, usually transverse, giving the cervical os a "fishmouth" appearance. Epithelium from the endocervical canal may have grown onto the surface of the cervix, appearing as beefy-red surface epithelium circumferentially around the os. Occasionally, the cervix of a woman whose mother took DES during pregnancy has a hooded appearance (a peaked aspect superiorly or a ridge of tissue surrounding it); this is evaluated by colposcopy when identified.

Malignant changes may not be obviously differentiated from the rest of the cervical mucosa. Small, benign cysts may appear on the cervical surface. Called *nabothian (retention) cysts,* these are usually bluish or white and are a normal finding after childbirth (Ball et al., 2015). A polyp of endocervical mucosa may protrude through the os and usually is dark red. Polyps can cause irregular bleeding; they are rarely malignant and usually are removed easily in an office or clinic setting. A carcinoma may appear as a cauliflowerlike growth (Ball et al., 2015). Bluish coloration of the cervix is a sign of early pregnancy (Chadwick sign).

Obtaining Pap Smears and Other Samples

A Pap smear is a screening test for abnormal cells of the cervix. Usually, a Pap test is obtained using liquid-based cytology. A broomlike collection device is rotated in the cervical os. The nurse or provider should be sure to follow the manufacturer's instructions to collect and preserve the specimen appropriately. The liquid sample is also used to test for the presence of HPV (Ball et al., 2015). Immediately after the Pap smear, DNA testing for organisms or a wet mount and potassium hydroxide procedures can be completed before the speculum is removed (Ball et al., 2015).

 For the procedural guidelines for obtaining an optimal Pap smear, go to **thepoint.lww.com/Brunner14e.**

A specimen of any purulent material appearing at the cervical os is obtained for culture. A sterile applicator is used to obtain the specimen, which is immediately placed in an appropriate medium for transfer to a laboratory. In a patient who has a high risk for infection, routine cultures for gonococcal and chlamydial organisms are recommended because of the high incidence of both diseases and the complications of pelvic infection, fallopian tube damage, and subsequent infertility.

Vaginal discharge, which may be normal or may result from vaginitis, may be present. Table 56-3 summarizes the characteristics of vaginal discharge found in different conditions.

TABLE 56-3 Characteristics of Vaginal Discharge

Cause of Discharge	Symptoms	Odor	Consistency/Color
Physiologic	None	None	Mucus/white
Candida species infection	Itching, irritation	Yeast odor or none	Thin to thick, curdlike/white
Bacterial vaginosis	Odor	Fishy, often noticed after intercourse	Thin/grayish or yellow
Trichomonas species infection	Irritation, odor	Malodorous	Copious, often frothy/yellow-green
Atrophic	Vulvar or vaginal dryness	Occasional mild malodor	Usually scant and mucoid/may be blood tinged

Inspecting the Vagina

The vagina is inspected as the examiner withdraws the speculum. It is smooth in young girls and thickens after puberty, with many rugae (folds) and redundancy in the epithelium. In women who are menopausal, the vagina thins and has fewer rugae because of decreased estrogen.

Bimanual Palpation

To complete the pelvic examination, the examiner performs a bimanual examination. The examiner should inform the woman that she will be examined internally with the examiners' fingers. The gloved fingers are then advanced vertically along the vaginal canal, and the vaginal wall is palpated. Any firm part of the vaginal wall may represent old scar tissue from childbirth trauma but may also require further evaluation (Ball et al., 2015).

Cervical Palpation

The cervix is palpated and assessed for its consistency, mobility, size, and position. The normal cervix is uniformly firm but not hard. Softening of the cervix is a finding in early pregnancy. Hardness and immobility of the cervix may reflect invasion by a neoplasm. Pain on gentle movement of the cervix is called a *positive chandelier sign* (positive cervical motion tenderness; recorded as + CMT) and usually indicates a pelvic infection.

Uterine Palpation

To palpate the uterus, the examiner places the opposite hand on the abdominal wall halfway between the umbilicus and the pubis and presses firmly toward the vagina. Movement of the abdominal wall causes the body of the uterus to descend, and the organ becomes freely movable between the hand used to examine the abdomen and the fingers of the hand used to examine the pelvis. Uterine size, mobility, and contour can be estimated through palpation. Fixation of the uterus in the pelvis may be a sign of endometriosis or malignancy.

The body of the uterus is normally twice the diameter and twice the length of the cervix, curving anteriorly toward the abdominal wall. Some women have a retroverted or retroflexed uterus, which tips posteriorly toward the sacrum, whereas others have a uterus that is neither anterior nor posterior and is described as midline.

Adnexal Palpation

The right and left adnexal areas are palpated to evaluate the fallopian tubes and ovaries. The fingers of the hand examining the pelvis are moved first to one side, then to the other, while the hand palpating the abdominal area is moved correspondingly to either side of the abdomen and downward. The adnexa (ovaries and fallopian tubes) are trapped between the two hands and palpated for an obvious mass, tenderness, and mobility. Commonly, the ovaries are slightly tender, and the patient is informed that slight discomfort on palpation is normal.

Vaginal and Rectal Palpation

Bimanual palpation of the vagina and cul-de-sac is accomplished by placing the index finger in the vagina and the middle finger in the rectum. To prevent cross-contamination between the vaginal and rectal orifices, the examiner puts on new gloves. A gentle movement of these fingers toward each other compresses the posterior vaginal wall and the anterior rectal wall and assists the examiner in identifying the integrity of these structures. During this procedure, the patient may sense an urge to defecate. The nurse assures the patient that this is unlikely to occur. Ongoing explanations are provided to reassure and educate the patient about the procedure.

 ### Gerontologic Considerations

Yearly examinations aid early identification of reproductive system disorders in aging women (Eliopoulos, 2018). Nurses play an important role in encouraging all women to have an annual gynecologic examination. Women older than 65 years may stop cervical cancer screening if they have had a hysterectomy or have had three normal cytology tests and no abnormal test in the past 10 years (USPSTF, 2016) (see Chapter 15, Table 15-3).

Perineal pruritus is abnormal in older women and should be evaluated because it may indicate a disease process (diabetes or malignancy). Vulvar dystrophy (a thickened or whitish discoloration of tissue) may be visible, and biopsy is needed to rule out abnormal cells. Topical cortisone and hormone creams may be prescribed for symptomatic relief.

With relaxing pelvic musculature, uterine prolapse and relaxation of the vaginal walls can occur (Eliopoulos, 2018). Appropriate evaluation and surgical repair can provide relief if the patient is a candidate for surgery. After surgery, the patient should know that tissue repair and healing may require more time with aging. Pessaries (latex devices that provide support) are often used if surgery is contraindicated or before surgery to see if surgery can be avoided. They are fitted by a health care provider and may reduce discomfort and pressure. The use of a pessary requires the patient to have routine gynecologic examinations to monitor for irritation or infection. The patient must be assessed for allergy prior to insertion of a latex pessary. See Chapter 57 for details about pessaries.

Diagnostic Evaluation

A wide range of diagnostic studies may be performed in the management of female physiologic processes. The nurse should educate the patient about the purpose, what to expect, and any possible side effects related to these examinations prior to testing. The nurse should be aware of contraindications, potential complications, and trends in results. Trends provide information about disease progression as well as the patient's response to therapy.

Cytologic Test for Cancer (Pap Smear)

The Papanicolaou (Pap) smear is used to detect cervical cancer. Cervical secretions are gently removed from the cervical os and may be transferred to a glass slide and fixed immediately by spraying with a fixative or immersed in solution. If the Pap smear reveals atypical cells, the liquid method allows for HPV testing. See Chapter 57 for further discussion of HPV.

Terminology used to describe findings includes the following categories:

- No abnormal or atypical cells
- Atypical squamous cells of undetermined significance
- Inflammatory reactions and microbes identified
- Positive deoxyribonucleic acid (DNA) test for HPV
- Precancerous and cancerous lesions of the cervix identified

The patient may incorrectly assume that an abnormal Pap smear signifies cancer. If the Pap smear (liquid immersion method) shows atypical cells and no high-risk HPV types, the next Pap smear is performed in 1 year. If a specific infection is causing inflammation, it is treated appropriately, and the Pap smear is repeated. If the repeat Pap smear reveals atypical squamous cells with high-risk HPV types, colposcopy may be indicated. Pap smears that indicate precancerous lesions should be repeated in 4 to 6 months and colposcopy performed if the lesion has not resolved. Patients with Pap smears that indicate cancerous lesions require prompt colposcopy (Fischbach & Dunning, 2015).

If the Pap smear results are abnormal, prompt notification, evaluation, and treatment are crucial. Notification of patients is often the responsibility of nurses in a women's health care practice or clinic. Pap smear follow-up is essential because it can prevent cervical cancer. Interventions are tailored to meet the needs and health beliefs of the particular patient. Intensive telephone counseling, tracking systems, brochures, videos, and financial incentives have all been used to encourage follow-up. The nurse provides clear explanations and emotional support along with a carefully designed setting-specific follow-up protocol designed to meet the needs of the patient.

Colposcopy and Cervical Biopsy

If the cervical cytology screening result requires evaluation, a colposcopy is performed. The colposcope is an instrument with a magnifying lens that allows the examiner to visualize the cervix and obtain a sample of abnormal tissue for analysis (Fischbach & Dunning, 2015). Nurse practitioners and gynecologists require special training in this diagnostic technique.

After inserting a speculum and visualizing the cervix and vaginal walls, the examiner applies acetic acid to the cervix. Subsequent abnormal findings that indicate the need for biopsy include leukoplakia (white plaque visible before applying acetic acid), acetowhite tissue (white epithelium after applying acetic acid), punctation (dilated capillaries occurring in a dotted or stippled pattern), mosaicism (a tile-like pattern), and atypical vascular patterns. If biopsy specimens show precancerous cells, the patient usually requires cryotherapy, laser therapy, or a cone biopsy (excision of an inverted tissue cone from the cervix).

Cryotherapy and Laser Therapy

Cryotherapy (freezing cervical tissue with nitrous oxide) and laser treatment are used in the outpatient setting. Cryotherapy may result in cramping and occasional feelings of faintness (vasovagal response). A watery discharge is normal for a few weeks after the procedure as the cervix heals; however, excessive bleeding, pain, or fever should be reported to the primary provider (Fischbach & Dunning, 2015).

Cone Biopsy and Loop Electrosurgical Excision Procedure

If endocervical curettage findings indicate abnormal changes or if the lesion extends into the canal, the patient may undergo a cone biopsy. This can be performed surgically or with a procedure called *loop electrosurgical excision procedure* (LEEP), which uses a laser beam (Fischbach & Dunning, 2015).

Usually performed in the outpatient setting, LEEP is associated with a high success rate in removal of abnormal cervical tissue. The gynecologist excises a small amount of cervical tissue, and the pathologist examines the borders of the specimen to determine if disease is present. A patient who has received anesthesia for a surgical cone biopsy is advised to rest for 24 hours after the procedure and to leave any vaginal packing in place until it is removed (usually the next day). The patient is instructed to report any excessive bleeding.

The nurse or primary provider provides guidelines regarding postoperative sexual activity, bathing, and other activities. Because open tissue may be potentially exposed to HIV and other pathogens, the patient is cautioned to avoid intercourse until healing is complete and verified at follow-up.

Endometrial (Aspiration) Biopsy

Endometrial biopsy, a method of obtaining endometrial tissue, is performed as an outpatient procedure. This procedure is usually indicated in cases of midlife irregular bleeding, postmenopausal bleeding, and irregular bleeding while taking hormone therapy (HT) or tamoxifen. A tissue sample obtained through biopsy permits diagnosis of cellular changes in the endometrium. The only absolute contraindication to an endometrial biopsy is the presence of a viable and desired pregnancy (Del Priore, 2015).

Women who undergo endometrial biopsy may experience slight discomfort. The examiner may apply a tenaculum (a clamplike instrument that stabilizes the uterus) after the pelvic examination and then inserts a thin, hollow, flexible suction tube (Pipelle or sampler) through the cervix into the uterus.

Findings on aspiration may include normal endometrial tissue, hyperplasia, or endometrial cancer. Simple hyperplasia is an overgrowth of the uterine lining and is usually treated with progesterone. Complex hyperplasia, which refers to overgrowth of cells with abnormal features, is a risk factor for uterine cancer and is treated with progesterone and careful follow-up. Women who are overweight, who are older than 45 years, who have a history of nulliparity and infertility, or who have a family history of colon cancer seem to be at higher risk for hyperplasia. See Chapter 57 for discussion of endometrial cancer.

Dilation and Curettage

Dilation and curettage (D&C) may be diagnostic (identifies the cause of irregular bleeding) or therapeutic (often temporarily stops irregular bleeding). The cervical canal is widened with a dilator, and the uterine endometrium is scraped with a curette. The purpose of the procedure is to secure endometrial or endocervical tissue for cytologic examination, to control abnormal uterine bleeding, and as a therapeutic measure for incomplete abortion.

Because D&C is usually carried out under anesthesia and requires surgical asepsis, it is usually performed in the operating room. However, it may take place in the outpatient setting with the patient receiving a local anesthetic supplemented with diazepam (Valium) or midazolam (Versed).

The nurse explains the procedure, preparation, and expectations regarding postoperative discomfort and bleeding. The patient is instructed to void before the procedure. The patient is placed in the lithotomy position, the cervix is dilated with a dilating instrument, and endometrial scrapings are obtained by a curette. A perineal pad is placed over the perineum after the procedure, and excessive bleeding is reported. No restrictions are placed on dietary intake. If pelvic discomfort or low back pain occurs, mild analgesic medications usually provide relief. The primary provider indicates when sexual intercourse may be safely resumed. To reduce the risk of infection and bleeding, most gynecologists advise no vaginal penetration or use of tampons for 2 weeks.

Endoscopic Examinations

Laparoscopy (Pelvic Peritoneoscopy)

A laparoscopy involves inserting a laparoscope (a tube about 10 mm wide and similar to a small periscope) into the peritoneal cavity through a 2-cm (0.75-inch) incision below the umbilicus to allow visualization of the pelvic structures (see Fig. 56-4). Laparoscopy may be used for diagnostic purposes (e.g., in cases of pelvic pain when no cause can be found) or treatment. Laparoscopy facilitates many surgical procedures, such as tubal ligation, ovarian biopsy, myomectomy, hysterectomy, and lysis of adhesions (scar tissue that can cause pelvic discomfort) (Sharp, 2016). A surgical instrument (intrauterine sound or cannula) may be positioned inside the uterus to permit manipulation or movement during laparoscopy, affording better visualization. The pelvic organs can be visualized after the injection of carbon dioxide intraperitoneally into the cavity. Called *insufflation*, this technique separates the intestines from the pelvic organs (Sharp, 2016). If a patient is undergoing sterilization, the fallopian or uterine tubes may be electrocoagulated, sutured, or ligated and a segment removed for histologic verification (clips are an alternative device for occluding the tubes).

After the laparoscopy is completed, the laparoscope is withdrawn, carbon dioxide is allowed to escape through the outer cannula, the small skin incision is closed with sutures or a clip, and the incision is covered with an adhesive bandage.

Figure 56-4 • Laparoscopy. The laparoscope (*right*) is inserted through a small incision in the abdomen. A forceps is inserted through the scope to grasp the fallopian tube. To improve the view, a uterine cannula (*left*) is inserted into the vagina to push the uterus upward. Insufflation of gas creates an air pocket (pneumoperitoneum), and the pelvis is elevated (note the angle), which forces the intestines higher in the abdomen.

The patient is carefully monitored for several hours to detect any untoward signs indicating bleeding (most commonly from vascular injury to the hypogastric vessels), bowel or bladder injury, or burns from the coagulator. These complications are rare, making laparoscopy a cost-effective and safe short-stay procedure. The patient may experience abdominal or shoulder pain related to the use of carbon dioxide gas.

Hysteroscopy

Hysteroscopy (transcervical intrauterine endoscopy) allows direct visualization of all parts of the uterine cavity by means of a lighted optical instrument. The procedure is best performed about 5 days after menstruation ceases, in the estrogenic phase of the menstrual cycle. The vagina and vulva are cleansed, and a paracervical anesthetic block is performed or lidocaine spray is used. The instrument used for the procedure, a hysteroscope, is passed into the cervical canal and advanced 1 or 2 cm under direct vision. Uterine-distending fluid (normal saline solution or dextrose 5% in water) is infused through the instrument to dilate the uterine cavity and enhance visibility. Hysteroscopy, which has few complications, is useful for evaluating endometrial pathology or for evaluating and treating retained products of conception (Bradley, 2016).

Hysteroscopy may be indicated as an adjunct to a D&C and laparoscopy in cases of infertility, unexplained bleeding, retained intrauterine device (IUD), and recurrent early pregnancy loss (Bradley, 2016). Treatment for some conditions (e.g., fibroid tumors) can be accomplished during this procedure, and sterilization may also be performed. Hysteroscopy is contraindicated in patients with cervical or endometrial carcinoma or acute pelvic inflammation.

An **endometrial ablation** (destruction of the uterine lining) procedure is performed with a hysteroscope and resector (cutting loop), roller ball (a barrel-shaped electrode), or laser beam in cases of severe bleeding not responsive to other therapies. Completed in an outpatient setting under general, regional, or local anesthesia, this rapid procedure is an alternative to hysterectomy for some patients. Following uterine distension with fluid infusion, the lining of the uterus is destroyed. Hemorrhage, perforation, and burns can occur.

Other Diagnostic Procedures

Additional diagnostic procedures may be helpful in evaluating pelvic conditions; these include x-rays, barium enemas, gastrointestinal x-ray series, intravenous (IV) urography, and cystography studies. In addition, because the uterus, ovaries, and fallopian tubes are near the structures of the urinary tract, urologic diagnostic studies, such as x-ray study of the kidney, ureters, and bladder (KUB) and pyelography are used, as are angiography and radioisotope scanning, if needed. Other diagnostic procedures include hysterosalpingography (HSG) and computed tomography (CT) scanning.

Hysterosalpingography or Uterotubography

HSG is an x-ray study of the uterus and the fallopian tubes after injection of a contrast agent. The diagnostic procedure is performed to evaluate infertility or tubal patency and to detect any abnormal condition in the uterine cavity. Sometimes, the procedure is therapeutic because the flowing contrast agent flushes debris or loosens adhesions.

Prior to HSG, laxatives and an enema may be given to evacuate the intestinal tract so that gas shadows do not distort the x-ray findings. A mild sedative or an analgesic agent, such as ibuprofen (Advil, Motrin) may be prescribed. The patient is placed in the lithotomy position and the cervix is exposed with a bivalve speculum. A cannula is inserted into the cervix, and the contrast agent is injected into the uterine cavity and the fallopian tubes. X-rays are taken to show the path and the distribution of the contrast agent.

Some patients experience nausea, vomiting, cramps, and faintness. After the test, the patient is advised to wear a perineal pad for several hours, because the radiopaque contrast agent may stain clothing.

Computed Tomography

CT scans have several advantages over ultrasonography, but they involve radiation exposure and are more costly. They are more effective than ultrasonography for patients with obesity or for patients with a distended bowel. CT scans can also demonstrate a tumor and any extension into the retroperitoneal lymph nodes and skeletal tissue, although they have limited value in diagnosing other gynecologic abnormalities (Fischbach & Dunning, 2015).

Ultrasonography

Ultrasonography (or ultrasound) is a useful adjunct to the physical examination, particularly in patients receiving obstetric care or in patients with abnormal pelvic examination findings. It is a simple procedure based on sound wave transmission that uses pulsed ultrasonic waves at frequencies exceeding 20,000 Hz (formerly cycles per second) by way of a transducer placed in contact with the abdomen (abdominal scan) or a vaginal probe (vaginal ultrasound). Mechanical energy is converted into electrical impulses, which in turn are amplified and recorded on an oscilloscope screen while a photograph or video recording of the patterns is taken. The entire procedure takes 15 to 30 minutes and involves no ionizing radiation and no discomfort other than a full bladder, which is necessary for good visualization during an abdominal scan. A vaginal ultrasound or sonogram does not require a full bladder; however, the vaginal probe may cause mild discomfort in some women (Fischbach & Dunning, 2015).

Magnetic Resonance Imaging

Magnetic resonance imaging (MRI) produces patterns that are finer and more definitive than other imaging procedures, and it does not expose patients to radiation. However, MRI is more costly.

 Quality and Safety Nursing Alert

All metal devices, including medication skin patches with foil backing, must be removed before MRI is performed to avoid burns.

MANAGEMENT OF FEMALE PHYSIOLOGIC PROCESSES

Many health concerns of women are related to normal changes or abnormalities of the menstrual cycle and may result from women's lack of understanding of the menstrual cycle, developmental changes, and factors that may affect the pattern of the menstrual cycle. Educating women about the menstrual cycle and changes over time is an important aspect of the nurse's role in providing quality care to women. Education should begin early so that menstruation and the lifelong changes in the menstrual cycle can be anticipated and accepted as a normal part of life.

Menstruation

Menstruation, the sloughing and discharge of the lining of the uterus that takes place if conception does not occur, happens about every 28 days during the reproductive years, although normal cycles can vary from 25 to 35 days (Schuiling & Likis, 2013) (see Fig. 56-3). The flow usually lasts 4 to 5 days, during which time 50 to 60 mL of blood is lost.

A perineal pad or tampon is generally used to absorb menstrual discharge. Tampons are used extensively. There is no significant evidence of untoward effects from their use, provided that there is no difficulty in inserting them. However, a tampon should not be used for more than 4 to 6 hours, and the lowest absorbency should be used to prevent toxic shock syndrome (Mayo Clinic, 2014). If a tampon is difficult to remove or shreds when removed, less absorbent tampons should be used. If the string breaks or retracts, the woman should squat in a comfortable position, insert one finger into the vagina, try to locate the tampon, and remove it. If she feels uncomfortable attempting this maneuver or cannot remove the tampon, she should consult a gynecologic health care provider promptly.

Psychosocial Considerations

Girls who are approaching menarche (the onset of menstruation) should be educated about the normal process of the menstrual cycle before it occurs. Psychologically, it is much healthier and appropriate to refer to this event as a "period" rather than as "being sick." With adequate nutrition, rest, and exercise, most women feel little discomfort, although some report breast tenderness and a feeling of fullness 1 or 2 days before menstruation begins. Others report fatigue and some discomfort in the lower back, legs, and pelvis on the first day and temperament or mood changes. Slight deviations from a usual pattern of daily living are considered normal, but excessive deviation may require evaluation. Regular exercise and a healthy diet have been found to decrease discomfort for some women. Heating pads or nonsteroidal anti-inflammatory drugs (NSAIDs) may be very effective for cramps. For women with excessive cramping or dysmenorrhea, referral to a women's health care provider is appropriate; following evaluation, providers may prescribe oral contraceptive agents.

Cultural Considerations

Culture refers to knowledge, beliefs, customs, and values acquired as members of a racial, ethnic, religious, or social group. The United States is becoming more culturally diverse. Various aspects of culture affect many health care encounters, and these encounters can be positive if nurses understand the various cultures of their patients.

Cultural views and beliefs about menstruation differ. Some women believe that it is detrimental to change a pad or tampon too frequently; they think that allowing the discharge to accumulate increases the flow, which is considered desirable. Some women believe they are vulnerable to illness during menstruation. Others believe it is harmful to swim, shower, have their hair "permed," have their teeth filled, or eat certain foods during menstruation. They may also avoid using contraception during menstruation.

In such situations, nurses are in a position to provide women with facts in an accepting and culturally sensitive manner. The objective is to be mindful of these unexpressed, deep-rooted beliefs and to provide the facts with care. Aspects of gynecologic problems cannot always be expressed easily. The nurse needs to convey confidence and openness and to offer facts to facilitate communication. Suggestions to improve care include overcoming language barriers, providing appropriate materials in the patient's language, asking about traditional beliefs and dietary practices, and asking about fears regarding care. Patience, sensitivity, and a desire to learn about other cultures and groups will enhance the nursing care of all women.

Menstrual Disorders

Menstrual disorders may include premenstrual syndrome (PMS); dysmenorrhea; **amenorrhea** (absence of menstrual flow); and excessive bleeding, irregular bleeding, or bleeding between cycles or unrelated to cycles. These disorders need to be discussed with a health care provider and managed individually.

Premenstrual Syndrome

PMS is a cluster of physical, emotional, and behavioral symptoms that are usually related to the luteal phase of the menstrual cycle. PMS is very common, affecting many women at some time in their lives (Tharpe, Farley, & Jordan, 2013) (see Chart 56-8).

Clinical Manifestations

Major symptoms of PMS include physical symptoms such as headache, fatigue, low back pain, painful breasts, and a feeling of abdominal fullness. Behavioral and emotional symptoms may include general irritability, mood swings, fear of losing control, binge eating, and crying spells. Symptoms vary widely from one woman to another and from one cycle to the next in the same woman. Great variability is found in the degree of symptoms. Many women are affected to some degree, but some are severely affected. Premenstrual dysphoric disorder (PMDD) is a severe form of PMS with significant severity of symptoms (Hawkins et al., 2012).

Medical Management

Because there is no single treatment or known cure for PMS, it is helpful for women to keep a record of their symptoms so they can anticipate and therefore cope with them. Regular exercise may be helpful. Although women have been advised to avoid caffeine, high-fat foods, and refined sugars, little research demonstrates the efficacy of dietary changes.

Chart 56-8 Causes, Manifestations, and Treatment of Premenstrual Syndrome

Cause

- Unknown; may be related to hormonal changes combined with other factors (diet, stress, and lack of exercise)
- Many women have some symptoms related to menses, but premenstrual syndrome affects 75–95% of women at some point and is a complex of symptoms that result in dysfunction.

Physical Symptoms

- Fluid retention (e.g., bloating, breast tenderness)
- Headache
- Low back pain

Affective Symptoms

- Depression
- Anger
- Irritability
- Anxiety
- Confusion
- Withdrawal
- Symptoms begin in the 5 days preceding menses, and relief occurs within 4 days of onset of menses. Dysfunction usually occurs in relationships, parenting, work, or school.

Treatment

- The use of social support and family resources
- Nutritious diet consisting of whole grains, fruits, and vegetables; increased water intake may help.
- Selective serotonin reuptake inhibitors
- Alprazolam (Xanax) has been effective, but risk of physical and psychological dependence is high.
- Spironolactone, a diuretic agent, may be effective in treating fluid retention
- Initiation/maintenance of exercise program
- Stress reduction techniques

Adapted from Hawkins, J. W., Roberto-Nichols, D. M., & Stanley-Haney, J. L. (2012). *Guidelines for nurse practitioners in gynecologic settings* (10th ed.). New York: Springer; Tharpe, N., Farley, C., & Jordan, R. (2013). *Clinical practice guidelines for midwifery & women's health*. Boston, MA: Jones & Bartlett.

Alternative therapies that have been used include vitamins B_6 (pyridoxine) and E, calcium, magnesium, and oil of primrose capsules (Hawkins et al., 2012).

Pharmacologic treatments include selective serotonin reuptake inhibitors (e.g., fluoxetine [Prozac, Sarafem]), prostaglandin inhibitors (e.g., ibuprofen and naproxen [Anaprox, Aleve]), diuretic agents, antianxiety agents, and calcium supplements. Oral contraceptives containing drospirenone (a synthetic progestin) and extended regimens also may be effective (Tharpe et al., 2013).

Nursing Management

The nurse obtains a health history, noting the time when symptoms began and their nature and intensity. The nurse then determines whether symptoms occur before or shortly after the menstrual flow begins. In addition, the nurse can show the patient how to record the timing and intensity of symptoms. A nutritional history is also elicited to determine if the diet is high in salt, caffeine, or alcohol or low in essential nutrients.

The patient's goals may include reduction of anxiety, mood swings, crying, binge eating, fear of losing control, improved coping with day-to-day stressors, improved relationships with family and coworkers, and increased knowledge about PMS. Positive coping measures are promoted. This may involve encouraging the woman's partner to offer support and assistance with child care. The patient can try to plan her working time to accommodate the days she is less productive because of PMS. The nurse encourages the patient to use exercise, meditation, imagery, and creative activities to reduce stress. The nurse also encourages the patient to take medications as prescribed and provides instructions about the desired effects of the medications. Enrolling in a PMS support group may help the patient learn to recognize and cope with this condition.

If the patient has severe symptoms of PMS or PMDD, the nurse assesses her for suicidal, uncontrollable, and violent behavior. An immediate psychiatric evaluation is necessary for women with any suggestions of suicidal tendencies. In rare cases, uncontrollable behavior may lead to violence toward family members. If abuse, maltreatment, and neglect of any member of a patient's family are suspected, it is important to implement and follow reporting protocols.

Dysmenorrhea

Primary dysmenorrhea is painful menstruation, with no identifiable pelvic pathology. It occurs at the time of menarche or shortly thereafter. It is characterized by crampy pain that begins before or shortly after the onset of menstrual flow and continues for 48 to 72 hours. Pelvic examination findings are normal. Dysmenorrhea is thought to result from excessive production of prostaglandins, which causes painful contraction of the uterus. In secondary dysmenorrhea, pelvic pathology such as endometriosis, tumors such as leiomyomata or malignancies, polyps, or pelvic inflammatory disease (PID) contributes to symptoms. Patients frequently have pain that occurs several days before menses, with ovulation, and occasionally with intercourse. It may be accompanied by nausea, diarrhea, dizziness, and backache (Hawkins et al., 2012).

Assessment and Diagnostic Findings

A pelvic examination is performed to rule out possible disorders, such as endometriosis, PID, adenomyosis, and uterine fibroids. A laparoscopy may be performed to identify organic causes (see Fig. 56-4).

Management

In primary dysmenorrhea, the reason for the discomfort is explained, and the patient is assured that menstruation is a normal function of the reproductive system. If the patient is young and accompanied by her mother, the mother may also need reassurance. Many young women expect to have painful periods if their mothers did. The discomfort of cramps can be treated once anxiety and concern about its cause are dispelled by adequate explanation. Symptoms usually subside with appropriate medication. Useful medications include prostaglandin antagonists such as NSAIDs (e.g., ibuprofen [Motrin], naproxen [Anaprox], and mefenamic acid [Ponstel] or aspirin). If one medication does not provide relief, another may be recommended. Usually, these medications are well tolerated, but some women experience gastrointestinal side effects. Contraindications include allergy, peptic ulcer history, sensitivity to aspirin-containing medications, asthma, and pregnancy. Low-dose oral contraceptives provide relief in more than 90% of patients and may be prescribed for women with dysmenorrhea who are sexually active but do not desire pregnancy (Hawkins et al., 2012).

Continuous low-level local heat may also be effective in relieving primary dysmenorrhea. Heat therapy and medication have been found to work well in combination. The patient is encouraged to continue her usual activities and to increase physical exercise if possible because this relieves discomfort for some women. Taking analgesic agents before cramps start, in anticipation of discomfort, is advised.

Management of secondary dysmenorrhea is directed at diagnosis of and treatment for the underlying cause (e.g., endometriosis or PID) (see Chapter 57.)

Amenorrhea

Amenorrhea, or the absence of menstrual flow, is a symptom of a variety of disorders and dysfunctions. Primary amenorrhea (delayed menarche) refers to the situation in which a young woman who by age 15 years has not begun developing secondary sex characteristics or who by age 16 years or older has developed secondary sex characteristics but has not started menstruation (Welt & Barbieri, 2016). There are many reasons for primary amenorrhea, including genetic and anatomical disorders, Turner syndrome, anorexia, and polycystic ovarian syndrome (Welt & Barbieri, 2016).

The nurse encourages the patient to express her concerns and anxiety about this problem because the patient may feel that she is different from her peers. A complete physical examination, careful health history, and simple laboratory tests help rule out possible causes, such as metabolic or endocrine disorders and systemic diseases. Treatment is directed toward correcting any abnormalities.

Secondary amenorrhea (an absence of menses for three cycles or 6 months after a normal menarche) may be caused by functional hypothalamic amenorrhea, pituitary disease, primary ovarian failure, pregnancy, breast-feeding, menopause, too little body fat (about 22% required for menses), eating disorder, thyroid disease, or polycystic ovary syndrome (Welt & Barbieri, 2016). In adolescents, secondary amenorrhea can be caused by minor emotional upset related to being away from home, attending college, tension due to schoolwork, or interpersonal problems.

Secondary nutritional disturbances may also be factors. Obesity can result in anovulation and subsequent amenorrhea. Eating disorders, such as anorexia and bulimia, often result in lack of menses because the decrease in body fat and caloric intake affects hormonal function. Intense exercise can induce menstrual disturbances. Females who are competitive athletes often experience amenorrhea. Infrequent periods (oligomenorrhea) may be related to thyroid disorders, polycystic ovarian syndrome, or premature ovarian failure. Women who are HIV positive are apt to miss menstrual periods and need to be evaluated for pregnancy, thyroid disorders, hyperprolactinemia, and menopause.

Abnormal Uterine Bleeding

Dysfunctional uterine bleeding is defined as irregular, painless bleeding of endometrial origin that may be excessive, prolonged, or without pattern. Dysfunctional uterine bleeding can occur at any age but is most common at opposite ends of the reproductive lifespan. It is usually secondary to anovulation (lack of ovulation) and is common in adolescents and women approaching menopause.

Adolescents account for many cases of abnormal uterine bleeding; they often do not ovulate regularly as the pituitary–ovarian axis matures. Women who are perimenopausal also experience this condition because of irregular ovulation secondary to decreasing ovarian hormone production. Other causes may include fibroids, obesity, and hypothalamic dysfunction.

Abnormal or unusual vaginal bleeding that is atypical in time or amount must be evaluated because it could possibly be a manifestation of a major disorder. A physical examination is performed, and the patient is evaluated for conditions such as pregnancy, neoplasm, infection, anatomic abnormalities, endocrine disorders, trauma, blood dyscrasias, platelet dysfunction, and hypothalamic disorders.

Menorrhagia

Menorrhagia is prolonged or excessive bleeding at the time of the regular menstrual flow. In young women, the cause is usually related to endocrine disturbance; in later life, it usually results from inflammatory disturbances, tumors of the uterus, or hormonal imbalance.

Women with menorrhagia are urged to see a primary provider and to describe the amount of bleeding by pad count and saturation (i.e., absorbency of perineal pad or tampon and number saturated hourly). Persistent heavy bleeding can result in anemia. It can also be a sign of a bleeding disorder or a result of anticoagulant therapy. Treatment may involve endometrial ablation or hysterectomy.

Metrorrhagia

Metrorrhagia (vaginal bleeding between regular menstrual periods) is probably the most significant form of menstrual dysfunction because it may signal cancer, benign tumors of the uterus, or other gynecologic problems. This condition warrants prompt evaluation and treatment. Although bleeding between menstrual periods by women taking oral contraceptive agents is usually not serious, irregular bleeding by women taking HT should be evaluated.

Menometrorrhagia is heavy vaginal bleeding between and during periods. It, too, requires evaluation.

Dyspareunia

Dyspareunia (difficult or painful intercourse) can be superficial, deep, primary, or secondary and may occur at the beginning of, during, or after intercourse. Dyspareunia may be related to many factors, including injury during childbirth; lack of vaginal lubrication; a history of incest, sexual abuse, or assault; endometriosis; pelvic or vaginal infection; vaginal dryness due to breast-feeding or menopause; gastrointestinal disorders; fibroids; urinary tract infection; STIs; or vulvodynia (vulvar pain that affects women of all ages without any discernible physical cause). Depending on the cause of dyspareunia, counseling, extra lubrication, or antidepressant medications may be prescribed (Schuiling & Likis, 2013). Women's health issues related to sexuality may be affected by many factors. Thus, these issues need to be taken seriously, carefully assessed, and treated.

Contraception

Approximately 61 million women in the United States are in their childbearing years (i.e., between the ages of 15 and 44 years). Those who are sexually active and do not want to become pregnant, but could become pregnant if they and their partners fail to use a contraceptive method, are at risk of unintended pregnancy. Thus, approximately 43 million women of childbearing age are at risk for unintended pregnancy (Alan Guttmacher Institute, 2016). Approximately 51% of the 6 million pregnancies each year are unintended and can result in negative health consequences and are an enormous financial burden to the health care system (American College of Obstetricians and Gynecologists [ACOG], 2016a). Family planning benefits mothers, newborns, families, and communities.

Initiatives have been put into place by ACOG to reduce the number of unintended pregnancies over the next 10 years. One of the initiatives involves reproductive life planning. A reproductive life plan (RLP) is a set of personal goals regarding whether, when, and how to have children based on individual priorities, resources, and values (ACOG, 2016a). A campaign called "Every Woman, Every Time" was launched to encourage health care providers to address reproductive health choices every time a woman has contact with the health care system. Nurses can initiate the RLP conversation by asking all women between the ages of 18 and 50 a key question, "Would you like to become pregnant in the next year?" Nursing education is then based upon the answer to that question. It is recommended that the following three questions be asked of women of childbearing age: "Do you have any children now?" "Do you want to have more children?" And, "How many (more) children would you like to have and when?" (ACOG, 2016a). Nurses who are involved in helping patients make contraceptive choices need to listen, take time to answer questions, and educate and assist patients in choosing the contraceptive method they prefer (see Chart 56-9). It is important for women to receive unbiased and nonjudgmental information, understand the benefits and risks of each contraceptive method, learn about alternatives and how to use them, and receive positive reinforcement and acceptance of their choice. Nurses also have the opportunity to dispel myths and misinformation surrounding contraception. Figure 56-5 provides an overview of the effectiveness of family planning methods.

Contraindications

Coexisting medical disorders may make contraception a complex issue. Contraception needs to be addressed individually in women with pre-existing conditions. With the aid of a thorough history, nurses are well positioned to aid patients in choosing the safest, most effective method of contraception to meet their individual needs. A valuable resource when

---

Chart 56-9

PATIENT EDUCATION

Using Contraceptives

The nurse provides education to enhance the chosen method of contraception.

The nurse instructs patients who have chosen male or female sterilization to:

- Use another contraceptive method for the first 3 months.
- Use condoms to protect against sexually transmitted infections.

The nurse instructs women who have chosen an injectable method to:

- Use condoms to protect against sexually transmitted infections.
- Obtain repeat injections on time.

The nurse instructs women who have chosen pills to:

- Use condoms to protect against sexually transmitted infections.
- Take the pill at exactly the same time every day.

The nurse instructs women who have chosen the patch to:

- Use condoms to protect against sexually transmitted infections.
- Change the patch once a week.

The nurse instructs women who have chosen a ring to:

- Use condoms to protect against sexually transmitted infections.
- Remove the vaginal ring after 3 weeks.

The nurse instructs women who have chosen a diaphragm to:

- Use correctly each time you have sex.

The nurse instructs women who have chosen condoms, a sponge, withdrawal, or spermicides to:

- Use correctly each time you have sex.

Adapted from Centers for Disease Control and Prevention (CDC). (2016). U.S. selected practice recommendations for contraceptive use, 2016. *Morbidity and Mortality Weekly Report, 65*(4), 1–72.

---

counseling patients about contraceptive method choice is the U.S. Medical Eligibility Criteria (USMEC) for Contraceptive Use (CDC, 2016). Specifically, the USMEC provides guidance on the safety of a contraceptive method for women with a wide variety of pre-existing conditions (CDC, 2016).

Abstinence

Abstinence, or celibacy, is the only completely effective means of preventing pregnancy. Abstinence may not be a desired or available option for many women because of cultural expectations and their own and their partner's values and sexual needs.

Long-Acting Reversible Contraceptive (LARC) Methods

Long-acting reversible contraception (LARC) methods are the most effective reversible methods for pregnancy prevention. Encouraging the use of LARC methods for appropriate candidates may help lower unintended pregnancy rates in the United States. Over time, LARC methods are 20 times more effective than birth control pills, the patch or the ring (see later discussion in this chapter) (ACOG, 2016a).

Figure 56-5 • Overview of the effectiveness of family planning methods. Adapted from Centers for Disease Control and Prevention (CDC). (2016). U.S. selected practice recommendations for contraceptive use, 2016. *Morbidity and Mortality Weekly Report, 65*(4), 1–72.

LARC methods include the IUD and the single-rod implant (ACOG, 2016b).

Intrauterine Device

An IUD is a small device, usually T-shaped that is inserted into the uterine cavity to prevent pregnancy. A string attached to the IUD is visible and palpable at the cervical os. Two types of IUDs are the hormonal and nonhormonal. The hormonal IUD releases progestin; a 3-year type and a 5-year are approved for use (ACOG, 2016b). The nonhormonal IUD is effective for up to 10 years (ACOG, 2016b).

Advantages include effectiveness over a long period of time, few if any systemic effects, and reduction of patient error. Almost all women are able to use an IUD. This reversible method of birth control is as effective as sterilization and more effective than barrier methods (ACOG, 2016b).

Disadvantages include possible excessive bleeding, cramps, and backaches; a slight risk of tubal pregnancy; slight risk of pelvic infection on insertion; displacement of the device; and, rarely, perforation of the cervix and uterus. If a pregnancy

occurs with an IUD in place, the device is removed immediately to avoid infection. Spontaneous abortion (miscarriage) may occur on removal (ACOG, 2016b).

Implants

One type of single-rod subdermal implant, effective for 3 years, is approved for use in the United States and is usually placed inside the upper arm using a small incision (CDC, 2016). It has been reported that 22% of etonogestrel implant users experienced amenorrhea and 34% experienced infrequent spotting, whereas 7% reported frequent bleeding (CDC, 2016). Women should be warned about possible discomforts that can be treated with NSAIDs. Heavy or prolonged bleeding should be evaluated for an underlying gynecologic problem, such as interactions with other medications, an STI pregnancy, or new pathologic uterine conditions (e.g., polyps or fibroids) (CDC, 2016).

Almost all women are able to use the implant, even those who are lactating. The implant is very convenient as once it is in place the patient does not have to do anything else to prevent pregnancy.

TABLE 56-4 Comparison of Sterilization Methods

Sterilization Method	Advantages	Disadvantages
Vasectomy	• Highly effective • Relieves female of contraceptive burden • Inexpensive in long run • Permanent • Highly acceptable procedure to most patients • Very safe • Quickly performed	• Expensive in short term • Serious long-term effects suggested (although currently unproved) • Permanent (Although reversal is possible, it is expensive and requires highly technical and major surgery, and results cannot be guaranteed.) • Regret in 5–10% of patients • No protection against STIs, including HIV • Not effective until sperm remaining in reproductive system are ejaculated
Hysteroscopic and laparoscopic tubal sterilization	• Low incidence of complications • Short recovery • Leaves small or no scar • Quickly performed	• Permanent • Reversal difficult and expensive • Sterilization procedures technically difficult • Requires surgeon, operating room (aseptic conditions), trained assistants, medications, surgical equipment. (Essure [insertion of coil or spring in fallopian tubes] requires hysteroscopy rather than surgery.) • Expensive at the time performed • If failure, high probability of ectopic pregnancy • No protection against STIs, including HIV

STIs, sexually transmitted infections; HIV, human immune deficiency virus.

Sterilization

Among women who practice contraception, approximately 25% rely on female and 8% on male sterilization (Alan Guttmacher Institute, 2016). Women and men who choose sterilization should be certain that they no longer wish to have children, no matter how the circumstances in their life may change. Vasectomy (male sterilization) and tubal ligation (female sterilization) are compared in Table 56-4. See Chapter 59 for discussion of vasectomy.

Hormonal Contraception

Oral contraceptives block ovarian stimulation by preventing the release of FSH from the anterior pituitary gland. In the absence of FSH, a follicle does not ripen, and ovulation does not occur. Progestins (synthetic forms of progesterone) suppress the LH surge, prevent ovulation, and also render the cervical mucus impenetrable to sperm. Hormonal contraceptive agents may be intrauterine, implantable, injectable, oral, transdermal, or intravaginal. (See previous discussion of LARC methods.) These methods contain either a combination of estrogen and progestin or progestin-only. The combined methods include combination oral contraceptives, the transdermal patch, and the intravaginal ring. The progestin-only methods include the intrauterine system, the implant, the injectable, and the "mini" pill. Hormonal contraception methods work by inhibiting ovulation (with the exception of the mini-pill and the intrauterine system). The progestin-only methods also thicken the cervical mucus (Schuiling & Likis, 2013).

Chart 56-10 describes the benefits and risks of hormonal contraceptive use.

Hormonal Contraception

A wide variety of hormonal methods of birth control are available. Combination methods include the combination of oral contraceptive pills, vaginal ring (NuvaRing), and transdermal patch (Ortho Evra). Progestin-only methods include the progestin-only pills or "minipills," once-every-3-month injection (Depo-Provera), levonorgestrel-releasing intra-uterine system (Mirena and Skyla), and single-rod subdermal implant (Nexplanon) (CDC, 2016).

> ### Quality and Safety Nursing Alert
>
> Patients need to be aware that hormonal contraceptives protect them from pregnancy but not from STIs or HIV infection. In addition, sex with multiple partners or sex without a condom may also result in chlamydial and other infections, including HIV infection.

Chart 56-10 PHARMACOLOGY
Benefits and Risks of Hormonal Contraceptives

Benefits
• Prevents unintended pregnancy
• Decreased cramps and bleeding
• Regular bleeding cycle
• Decreased incidence of anemia
• Decrease in acne with some formulations
• Protection from uterine and ovarian cancer
• Decreased incidence of ectopic pregnancy
• Protection from benign breast disease
• Decreased incidence of pelvic infection

Risks
• Rare in women who are healthy
• Bothersome side effects (e.g., breakthrough bleeding, breast tenderness)
• Nausea, weight gain, mood changes
• Small increased risk of developing blood clots, stroke, or heart attack, related more to smoking than to oral contraceptive use alone
• Possible increased incidence of benign liver tumors and gallbladder disorders
• No protection from sexually transmitted infections (possible increased risk with unsafe sex)

Oral Contraceptives

Many women use oral contraceptive preparations of synthetic estrogens and progestins. A variety of formulations are available. Extended regimens of oral hormonal contraceptive agents are an option for women who have heavy or uncomfortable menstrual bleeding or who wish to have fewer periods. With the use of these regimens, women may have an increased occurrence of breakthrough bleeding; the blood may be dark brown rather than red. It may be more difficult to tell if a pregnancy occurs with this method, although pregnancy is unlikely if pills are taken as prescribed (CDC, 2016).

Transdermal Contraceptives

Ortho Evra is a thin, beige, matchbook-size skin patch that releases an estrogen and a progestin continuously. It is changed every week for 3 weeks, and no patch is used during the fourth week, resulting in withdrawal bleeding. The effectiveness of Ortho Evra is comparable to that of oral contraceptives. Its risks are similar to those of oral contraceptives and include an increased risk of venous thromboemboli formation. The patch may be applied to the torso, chest, arms, or thighs; it should not be applied to the breasts. The patch is convenient and more easily remembered than a daily pill but is not as effective for women who weigh more than 90 kg (198 lb). One additional side effect with the patch includes possible skin reaction such as irritation, redness, pigment changes, or rash at the site of the patch (CDC, 2016).

Vaginal Contraceptives

NuvaRing (etonogestrel/ethinyl estradiol vaginal ring) is a combination hormonal contraceptive that releases estrogen and progestin. It is as effective as oral contraceptive agents and results in lower hormone blood levels than oral contraceptives. NuvaRing is flexible, does not require sizing or fitting, and is effective when placed anywhere in the vagina. Patients are occasionally reluctant to consider vaginal methods of contraception unless discussed openly and as a convenient alternative to other routes of administration. Some women are uncomfortable with this method and may fear that the ring may migrate or be uncomfortable or be noticed by a partner. NuvaRing is usually more expensive than oral contraceptives.

Injectable Contraceptives

An intramuscular injection of Depo-Provera (a long-acting progestin) every 3 months inhibits ovulation and provides a reliable, private, and convenient contraceptive method (CDC, 2016). A subcutaneous formulation is also available. It can be used by lactating women and those with hypertension, liver disease, migraine headaches, heart disease, and hemoglobinopathies. With continued use, women must be prepared for irregular bleeding episodes and spotting decrease, or amenorrhea.

Advantages of Depo-Provera include reduction of menorrhagia, dysmenorrhea, and anemia due to heavy menstrual bleeding. It may reduce the risk of pelvic infection, has been associated with improvement in hematologic status in women with sickle cell disease, and does not interfere with the efficacy of seizure agents. It decreases the risk of endometrial cancer, PID, endometriosis, and uterine fibroids (CDC, 2016).

Possible side effects of Depo-Provera include irregular menstrual bleeding, bloating, headaches, hair loss, decreased sex drive, bone loss, and weight loss or weight gain. The contraceptive does not protect against STIs. Bone loss may occur while using the injection. When the injections are stopped, sometimes all of the bone loss is regained. Use of Depo-Provera should be limited to 2 years of use because of loss of bone mineral density (Comerford, 2015).

Depo-Provera is contraindicated in women who are pregnant and those who have abnormal vaginal bleeding of unknown cause, breast or pelvic cancer, or sensitivity to synthetic progestin.

Mechanical Barriers

Diaphragm

The diaphragm is an effective contraceptive device that consists of a round, flexible spring (50 to 90 mm wide) covered with a domelike latex rubber cup. A spermicidal (contraceptive) jelly or cream is used to coat the concave side of the diaphragm before it is inserted deep into the vagina, covering the cervix completely. The spermicide inhibits spermatozoa from entering the cervical canal. The diaphragm is not felt by the user or her partner when properly fitted and inserted. Because women vary in size, the diaphragm must be sized and fitted by an experienced clinician. The woman is instructed in using and caring for the device. A return demonstration ensures that the woman can insert the diaphragm correctly and that it covers the cervix.

Each time the woman uses the diaphragm, she should examine it carefully. By holding it up to a bright light, she should ensure that it has no pinpoint holes, cracks, or tears; if any are present, the diaphragm should not be used. She then applies spermicidal jelly or cream and inserts the diaphragm. The diaphragm should remain in place at least 6 hours after coitus (no more than 12 hours). Additional spermicide is necessary if more than 6 hours have passed before intercourse occurs and before each act of repeated intercourse. On removal, the diaphragm should be cleansed thoroughly with mild soap and water, rinsed, and dried before being stored in its original container.

Disadvantages include allergic reactions in those who are sensitive to latex and an increased incidence of urinary tract infections. Toxic shock syndrome has been reported in some diaphragm users but is rare.

 Quality and Safety Nursing Alert

The nurse must assess the woman for possible latex allergy because the use of latex barrier methods (e.g., diaphragm, cervical cap, male condoms) may cause severe allergic reactions, including anaphylaxis, in patients with latex allergy.

Cervical Cap

The cervical cap is much smaller (22 to 35 mm) than the diaphragm and covers only the cervix. If a woman can feel her cervix, she can usually learn to use a cervical cap. The chief advantage is that the cap may be left in place for 2 days after coitus. Although convenient to use, the cervical cap may

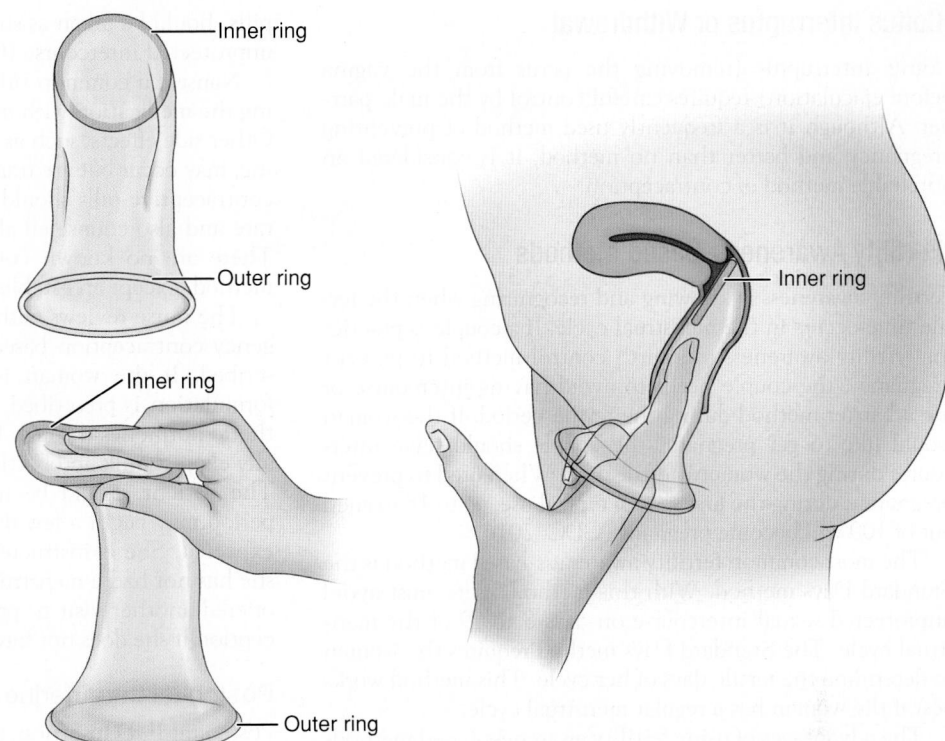

Figure 56-6 • Female condom. To insert the female condom, hold the inner ring between the thumb and middle finger. Put the index finger on the pouch between the thumb and other fingers, and squeeze the ring. Slide the condom into the vagina as far as it will go. The inner ring keeps the condom in place.

cause cervical irritation; therefore, before fitting a cap, most primary providers obtain a Pap smear and repeat the smear after 3 months. The cap is used with a spermicide and does not require additional spermicide for repeated intercourse.

Female Condom

The female condom was developed to give control of barrier protection to women—to provide them with protection from STIs and HIV as well as pregnancy. The female condom (Reality and FC2) consists of a cylinder of polyurethane enclosed at one end by a closed ring that covers the cervix and at the other end by an open ring that covers the perineum (see Fig. 56-6). Advantages include some degree of protection from STIs (i.e., HPV, herpes simplex virus, and HIV) (CDC, 2016). Disadvantages are that female condoms are more costly than male condoms and the inability to use the female condom with some positions (i.e., standing).

Spermicides

Spermicides are made from nonoxynol-9 or octoxynol and are available over the counter as foams, gels, films, and suppositories and also on condoms. Spermicides do not protect women from HIV or other STIs (Alan Guttmacher Institute, 2016; CDC, 2016). Advantages of spermicides include they are nonhormonal, are user controlled, do not cause systemic side effects, and are immediately effective (Alan Guttmacher Institute, 2016).

Male Condom

The male condom is an impermeable, snug-fitting cover applied to the erect penis before it enters the vaginal canal. The tip of the condom is pinched while being applied to leave space for ejaculate. If no space is left, ejaculation may cause a tear or hole in the condom and reduce its effectiveness. The penis, with the condom held in place, is removed from the vagina while still erect to prevent the ejaculate from leaking. Condoms are available in large and small sizes.

The latex condom also creates a barrier against transmission of STIs (gonorrhea, chlamydial infection, and HIV) by body fluids and may reduce the risk of herpes virus transmission. However, natural condoms (those made from animal tissue) do not protect against HIV infection. Nurses need to reassure women that they have a right to insist that their male partners use condoms and a right to refuse sex without condoms, although women in abusive relationships may increase their risk of abuse, maltreatment, and neglect by doing so. Some women carry condoms with them to be certain that one is available. Nurses should be familiar and comfortable with instructions about using condoms because many women need to know about this way of protecting themselves from HIV and other STIs. Condoms do not provide complete protection from STIs, however, because HPV may be transmitted by skin-to-skin contact. Other STIs may be transmitted if any abraded skin is exposed to body fluids. This information should be included in patient education.

The nurse needs to consider the possibility of latex allergy. Swelling and itching can also occur. Possible warning signs of latex allergy include oral itching after blowing up a balloon or eating kiwis, bananas, pineapples, passion fruit, avocados, or chestnuts. Because many contraceptives are made of latex, patients who experience burning or itching while using latex contraceptives are instructed to see their primary provider. Alternatives to latex condoms include the female condom (Reality) and the male condom (Avanti), made of polyurethane.

Coitus Interruptus or Withdrawal

Coitus interruptus (removing the penis from the vagina before ejaculation) requires careful control by the male partner. Although it is a frequently used method of preventing pregnancy and better than no method, it is considered an unreliable method of contraception.

Fertility Awareness-Based Methods

Fertility awareness is knowing and recognizing when the fertile time occurs in the menstrual cycle. If a couple is practicing fertility awareness as a birth control method to prevent pregnancy, the couple needs to avoid having intercourse or use a barrier method during the fertile period. If the woman would like to get pregnant, the couple should have intercourse during the women's fertile days. When used to prevent pregnancy, during the first year of typical use, up to 18 women out of 100 will become pregnant (CDC, 2016).

The most common fertility awareness-based method is the Standard Days method. With this method, users must avoid unprotected sexual intercourse on days 8 to 19 of the menstrual cycle. The Standard Days method requires the woman to determine the fertile days of her cycle. This method works best if the woman has a regular menstrual cycle.

The advantages of using fertility awareness-based methods to prevent pregnancy include: (1) they are not hazardous to health, (2) they are inexpensive, and (3) they are approved by some religions that do not approve of other methods of contraception. The disadvantage is that they require discipline by the couple, who must monitor the menstrual cycle and abstain from sex during the fertile phase.

Ovulation detection methods (e.g., Clearblue Fertility Monitor) are available in most pharmacies. The presence of the enzyme guaiacol peroxidase in cervical mucus signals ovulation 6 days beforehand and also affects mucosal viscosity. Over-the-counter test kits are easy to use and reliable but can be expensive. Ovulation prediction kits are more effective for planning conception than for avoiding it.

Emergency Contraception

Emergency contraception are methods that can be used by women after unprotected sexual intercourse to prevent pregnancy (CDC, 2016). Nurses need to be aware of emergency contraception as an option for women and the indications for its use. It is clearly not suitable for long-term avoidance of pregnancy because it is not as effective as oral contraceptives or other reliable methods used regularly. However, it is valuable following intercourse when a pregnancy is not intended and in emergency situations such as rape, a defective or torn condom or diaphragm, or other situations that may result in unintended conception.

Methods of Emergency Contraception

Emergency Contraceptive Pills

Three kinds of emergency contraceptive pills are available in the United States. A properly timed, adequate dose of medication after intercourse without effective contraception, or when a method has failed, can prevent pregnancy by inhibiting or delaying ovulation. Emergency contraceptive pills should be taken as soon as possible and within 5 days of unprotected intercourse (CDC, 2016).

Nausea, a common side effect, can be minimized by taking the medication with meals and with an antiemetic agent. Other side effects, such as breast soreness and irregular bleeding, may occur but are transient. Patients who use emergency contraceptive pills should be advised of the potential failure rate and also counseled about other contraceptive methods. There are no known contraindications to the use of this method, except an established pregnancy (CDC, 2016).

The nurse reviews with the patient instructions for emergency contraception based on the medication regimen prescribed. If the woman is breast-feeding, a progestin-only formulation is prescribed. To avoid exposing infants to synthetic hormones through breast milk, the patient can manually express milk and bottle-feed for 24 hours after treatment. The patient should be informed that her next menstrual period may begin a few days earlier or a few days later than expected. She is instructed to return for a pregnancy test if she has not had a menstrual period in 3 weeks and should be offered another visit to provide a regular method of contraception if she does not have one currently.

Postcoital Intrauterine Device Insertion

Postcoital IUD insertion, another form of emergency contraception, involves insertion of a copper-bearing IUD within 5 days of coitus (CDC, 2016). The copper-bearing IUD prevents fertilization by causing a chemical change in sperm and egg before they can meet. This method is the most effective form of emergency contraception available (CDC, 2016). The patient may experience discomfort on insertion and may have heavier menstrual periods and increased cramping. Contraindications include a confirmed or suspected pregnancy or any contraindication to regular IUD use. The patient must be informed that there is a risk that insertion of an IUD may disrupt a pregnancy that is already present.

Nursing Management

Patients who use emergency contraception may be anxious, embarrassed, and lacking information about birth control. The nurse must be supportive and nonjudgmental and provide facts and appropriate patient education. If the patient repeatedly uses this method of birth control, she should be informed that the failure rate with this method is higher than with a regularly used method. Nurses can educate and inform women about emergency contraception options to reduce unintended pregnancies and abortions. See the Resources section at the end of this chapter for more information.

Abortion

Interruption of pregnancy or expulsion of the product of conception before the fetus is viable is called *abortion*. The fetus is generally considered to be viable any time after the fifth to sixth month of gestation.

Spontaneous Abortion

It is estimated that 1 of every 5 to 10 conceptions ends in spontaneous abortion. Most of these occur because an abnormality in the fetus makes survival impossible. Other causes may include systemic diseases, hormonal imbalance, or anatomic abnormalities. If a woman who is pregnant experiences bleeding and cramping, a threatened abortion is diagnosed because an actual abortion is usually imminent. Spontaneous abortion occurs most commonly in the second or third month of gestation.

There are various types of spontaneous abortion, depending on the nature of the process (threatened, inevitable, incomplete, or complete). In a threatened abortion, the cervix does not dilate. With bed rest and conservative treatment, the abortion may be prevented. If not, an abortion is imminent. If only some of the tissue is passed, the abortion is referred to as incomplete. An emptying or evacuation procedure (D&C, or dilation and evacuation [D&E]) or administration of oral misoprostol (Cytotec) is usually required to remove the remaining tissue. If the fetus and all related tissue are spontaneously evacuated, the abortion is termed *complete*, and no further treatment is required.

Habitual Abortion

Habitual or recurrent abortion is defined as successive, repeated, spontaneous abortions of unknown cause. As many as 60% of abortions may result from chromosomal anomalies. After two consecutive abortions, the patient is referred for genetic counseling and testing, and other possible causes are explored.

If bleeding occurs in a woman who is pregnant with a past history of habitual abortion, conservative measures, such as bed rest and administration of progesterone to support the endometrium, are attempted to save the pregnancy. Supportive counseling is crucial in this stressful condition. Bed rest, sexual abstinence, a light diet, and no straining on defecation may be recommended in an effort to prevent spontaneous abortion. If infection is suspected, antibiotic agents may be prescribed.

In the condition known as incompetent or dysfunctional cervix, the cervix dilates painlessly in the second trimester of pregnancy, often resulting in a spontaneous abortion. In such cases, a surgical procedure called *cervical cerclage* may be used to prevent the cervix from dilating prematurely. It involves placing a purse-string suture around the cervix at the level of the internal os. Bed rest is usually advised to keep the weight of the uterus off the cervix. About 2 to 3 weeks before term or at the onset of labor, the suture is cut. Delivery is usually by cesarean section.

Medical Management

After a spontaneous abortion, all tissue passed vaginally is saved for examination, if possible. The patient and all personnel who care for her are alerted to save any discharged material. In the rare case of heavy bleeding, the patient may require blood component transfusions and fluid replacement. An estimate of the bleeding volume can be determined by recording the number of perineal pads and the degree of saturation over 24 hours. When an incomplete abortion occurs, oxytocin may be prescribed to cause uterine contractions before D&E or uterine suctioning.

Nursing Management

Because patients experience loss and anxiety, emotional support and understanding are important aspects of nursing care. Women may be grieving or relieved, depending on their feelings about the pregnancy. Providing opportunities for the patient to talk and express her emotions is helpful and also provides clues for the nurse in planning more specific care.

Induced Abortion

A voluntary induced termination of pregnancy is performed by skilled health care providers. Decisions about abortion reside with a woman and her physician in the first trimester. During the second trimester, the state may regulate practice in the interest of a woman's health and during the final weeks of pregnancy may choose to protect the life of the fetus, except when necessary to preserve the life or health of the woman.

In the United States, nearly half of all pregnancies are unintended and about 4 in 10 of these were terminated by abortion (Allan Guttmacher Institute, 2016). These numbers indicate the need for effective contraceptive education, information about emergency contraception, and counseling.

Medical Management

Before the abortion procedure is performed (see Chart 56-11), a nurse or counselor trained in pregnancy counseling should talk with the patient and explore her fears, feelings, and options. The nurse then identifies the patient's choice (i.e., continuing pregnancy and parenthood, continuing pregnancy followed by adoption, or terminating pregnancy by abortion). If abortion is chosen, the patient has a pelvic examination to determine uterine size. A pelvic ultrasound may also be performed. Laboratory studies before an abortion must include a pregnancy test to confirm the pregnancy, hematocrit to rule out anemia, and Rh determination. Patients with anemia will require an iron supplement, and patients who are Rh negative may require Rho(D) immune globulin (RhoGAM) to prevent isoimmunization. Before the procedure, all patients should be screened for STIs to prevent introducing pathogens upward through the cervix during the procedure.

> ### ⚑ *Quality and Safety Nursing Alert*
>
> *Women who have resorted to unskilled attempts to end a pregnancy may become critically ill because of infection, hemorrhage, or uterine rupture. If a woman has undergone such efforts to end a pregnancy, prompt medical attention, broad-spectrum antibiotics, and replacement of fluids and blood components may be required before careful attempts are made to evacuate the uterus.*

Surgical terminations include D & C or vacuum aspiration of uterine contents. Medications can also be used. Mifepristone (Mifeprex), formerly known as RU-486, is used only in early pregnancy (up to 49 days from the last menstrual period). It works by blocking progesterone. Cramping and bleeding similar to a heavy menstrual period occur. After counseling and consent and often a sonogram to confirm the pregnancy, mifepristone is given. This is followed by a dose of misoprostol orally or vaginally. If the pregnancy persists, a suction aspiration is performed. Contraindications include ectopic pregnancy, adrenal failure, allergy to the medications, bleeding disorder, irritable bowel syndrome, or uncontrolled

---

Chart 56-11

Types of Induced Abortions

Vacuum Aspiration

- The cervix is dilated manually with instrumentation or by laminaria (small suppositories made of seaweed that swells as it absorbs water).
- A uterine aspirator is introduced.
- Suction is applied, and tissue is removed from the uterus.

This is the most common type of termination procedure and is used early in pregnancy, up to 14 weeks. Laminaria may be used to soften and dilate the cervix prior to the procedure.

Dilation and Evacuation

Cervical dilation with laminaria followed by vacuum aspiration

Labor Induction

These procedures account for fewer than 1% of all terminations and generally take place in an inpatient setting.

1. Installation of normal saline or urea results in uterine contractions.
   - Although rare, serious complications can occur, including cardiovascular collapse, cerebral edema, pulmonary edema, kidney disease, and disseminated intravascular coagulopathy.
2. Prostaglandins
   - Prostaglandins are introduced into the amniotic fluid or by vaginal suppository or intramuscular injection in later pregnancy.
   - Strong uterine contractions begin within 4 hours and usually result in abortion.
   - Gastrointestinal side effects (e.g., nausea, vomiting, diarrhea, and abdominal cramping) and fever can occur.
3. IV oxytocin
   - Used for later abortions for genetic indications. Requires patient to go through labor.

Medical Abortion

Mifepristone

- Mifepristone (formerly known as RU-486) is a progesterone antagonist that prevents implantation of the ovum.
- Given orally within 10 days of an expected menstrual period, mifepristone produces a medical abortion in most patients.
- Combined with a prostaglandin suppository, mifepristone causes abortion in up to 95% of patients.
- Prolonged bleeding may occur. Other side effects may include abdominal pain, nausea, vomiting, and diarrhea. This method may not be used in women with adrenal failure, asthma, long-term corticosteroid therapy, an intrauterine device in place, porphyria, or a history of allergy to mifepristone or other prostaglandins. It is less effective when used in pregnancies more than 49 days from the beginning of the last menstrual period.

Methotrexate

- Methotrexate has also been used to terminate pregnancy because it is lethal to the fetus. It has been found to have minimal risk and few side effects in the woman. Its low cost may provide an alternative for some women.

Misoprostol

- Misoprostol is a synthetic prostaglandin analog that produces cervical effacement and uterine contractions.
- Inserted vaginally, misoprostol is effective in terminating a pregnancy in about 75% of cases.
- When combined with methotrexate or mifepristone, misoprostol's effectiveness rate is high.

---

seizure disorders. Several deaths from sepsis have occurred following medical abortion; researchers and the FDA are closely monitoring the morbidity and mortality associated with medical abortion. Medical and surgical abortions used in the first trimester are both highly effective with low complication rates (Ireland, Geffen, & Chen, 2015).

Nursing Management

Patient education is an important aspect of care for women who elect to terminate a pregnancy. A patient undergoing induced abortion is informed about what the procedure entails and the expected course after the procedure. The patient is scheduled for a follow-up appointment 2 weeks after the procedure and is instructed about signs and symptoms (i.e., fever, heavy bleeding, or pain) that should be reported.

Available contraceptive methods are reviewed with the patient at this time. Effectiveness depends on the method used and the extent to which the woman and her partner follow the instructions for use. A woman who has used any method of birth control should be assessed for her understanding of the method and its potential side effects as well as her satisfaction with the method. If the woman has not been using contraception, the nurse explains all methods and their benefits and risks and helps the patient make a contraceptive choice for use after abortion. Related education issues, such as

the need to use barrier contraceptive devices (i.e., condoms) for protection against transmission of STIs and HIV infection and the availability of emergency contraception, are becoming increasingly important.

Psychological support is another important aspect of nursing care. The nurse needs to be aware that women terminate pregnancies for many reasons. Some women terminate pregnancies because of severe genetic defects. Women who have been raped or impregnated in incestuous relationships or by an abusive partner may elect to terminate their pregnancies. The care of a woman undergoing termination of pregnancy is stressful, and assistance needs to be provided in a safe and nonjudgmental way. Nurses have the right to refuse to participate in a procedure that is against their religious beliefs but are professionally obligated not to impose their beliefs or judgments on their patients.

Infertility

Infertility is defined as a couple's inability to achieve pregnancy after 1 year of unprotected intercourse (Tarin, Garci-Perez, Hamatani, et al., 2015). Approximately 12% of women ages 15 to 44 have reported ever having received any infertility services (Kessler, Craig, Plosker, et al., 2013). Primary infertility refers to a couple who has never had a child. Secondary infertility means that at least one conception has occurred, but currently the couple cannot achieve a pregnancy. It is often a complex physical problem and causes are related to endometriosis, uterine factors, anovulation, tubal obstruction, and male factors.

Diagnostic Findings

Ovarian and Ovulation Factors

Diagnostic studies performed to determine if ovulation is regular and whether the progestational endometrium is adequate for implantation may include a serum progesterone level and an ovulation index. The ovulation index involves a urine dipstick test to determine whether the surge in LH that precedes follicular rupture has occurred.

Tubal and Uterine Factors

HSG is used to rule out uterine or tubal abnormalities. A contrast agent injected into the uterus through the cervix produces an outline of the shape of the uterine cavity and the patency of the tubes. This process sometimes removes mucus or tissue that is lodged in the tubes. Laparoscopy permits direct visualization of the tubes and other pelvic structures and can assist in identifying conditions that may interfere with fertility (e.g., endometriosis).

Fibroids, polyps, and congenital malformations are possible causative factors affecting the uterus. Their presence may be determined by pelvic examination, hysteroscopy, saline sonogram (a variation of a sonogram), and HSG. Endometriosis, even if mild, is associated with reduced fertility (Schuiling & Likis, 2013).

Male Factors

An analysis of semen provides information about the number of sperm (density), percentage of moving forms, quality of forward movement (forward progression), and morphology (shape and form). From 2 to 6 mL of watery alkaline semen is normal. A normal count has 60 to 100 million sperm/mL. However, the incidence of impregnation is lessened only when the count decreases to fewer than 20 million sperm/mL.

Men may also be affected by varicoceles (varicose veins around the testicle), which decrease semen quality by increasing testicular temperature. Retrograde ejaculation or ejaculation into the bladder is assessed by urinalysis after ejaculation. Blood tests for male partners may include measuring testosterone, FSH and LH (both of which are involved in maintaining testicular function), and prolactin levels.

Medical Management

The treatment of infertility is complex and often requires advanced technology. The specific type of treatment depends on the cause of the problem, if it can be identified. Many infertile couples have normal test results for ovulation, sperm production, and fallopian tube patency.

Ovulatory dysfunction is complex, but many women with ovulation disorders have polycystic ovary syndrome (see Chapter 57) and may be treated with 5 days of clomiphene (Clomid) to induce ovulation (Comerford, 2015). Insulin sensitizing agents are sometimes used, and once insulin levels are normalized, ovulation often occurs. Some women have high prolactin levels, which inhibit ovulation, and they are treated with dopaminergic drugs after a pituitary adenoma is

ruled out by MRI. If a woman has premature ovarian failure, oocyte donation may be considered.

Pharmacologic Therapy

Pharmacologically induced ovulation is undertaken when women do not ovulate on their own or ovulate irregularly. These couples are often treated with clomiphene to stimulate ovulation. Gonadotropin treatment may also be used if conception does not occur. Various other medications are used, depending on the main cause of infertility (see Chart 56-12).

Blood tests and ultrasounds are used to monitor ovulation. Multiple pregnancies (i.e., twins, triplets, or more) may occur with the use of these medications. Ovarian hyperstimulation syndrome (OHSS) may also occur. This condition is characterized by enlarged multicystic ovaries and is complicated by a shift of fluid from the intravascular space into the abdominal cavity. The fluid shift can result in ascites,

---

Chart 56-12

PHARMACOLOGY

Medications That Induce Ovulation

- Clomiphene citrate (Clomid, Serophene) is an estrogen antagonist that increases gonadotropin release, resulting in follicular rupture or ovulation. Clomiphene is used when the hypothalamus is not stimulating the pituitary gland to release follicle-stimulating hormone (FSH) and luteinizing hormone (LH). This medication stimulates follicles in the ovary. It is usually taken for 5 days beginning on the 5th day of the menstrual cycle. Ovulation should occur 4–8 days after the last dose. Patients receive instructions about timing intercourse to facilitate fertilization.
- Menotropins (Repronex, Pergonal), a combination of FSH and LH, may be used to stimulate the ovaries to produce eggs. These agents are used for women with deficiencies in FSH and LH. When followed by administration of human chorionic gonadotropin, menotropins stimulates the ovaries, so monitoring by ultrasound and hormone levels is essential because overstimulation may occur.
- Follitropin alfa (Gonal-F), follitropin beta (Follistim), and urofollitropin (Bravelle) may be used to treat ovulation disorders or to stimulate a follicle and egg production for intrauterine insemination or in vitro fertilization or other assisted reproductive technologies.
- Gonadotropin-releasing hormone agonists (leuprolide [Lupron], nafarelin acetate [Synarel]) suppress FSH, prevent premature egg release, and shrink fibroids.
- Bromocriptine (Parlodel) may be used in treatment for infertility due to elevated prolactin levels.
- Progesterone (Prometrium Crinone, progesterone in oil) vaginal suppositories help improve the uterine lining after ovulation.
- Urofollitropin (Metrodin, Bravelle), which contains FSH with a small amount of LH, is used in some disorders (e.g., polycystic ovarian syndrome) to stimulate follicle growth. Clomiphene is then used to stimulate ovulation.
- Chorionic gonadotropin (Ovidrel, Novarel, Pregnyl), which mimics LH, releases an egg after hyperstimulation and supports the corpus luteum.
- Metformin (Glucophage, Fortamet) may be used in polycystic ovarian syndrome to induce regular ovulation.
- Aspirin and heparin may be used to prevent recurrent pregnancy loss in patients with elevated antiphospholipid antibodies.

Adapted from Comerford, K. C. (2015). *Nursing 2015 drug handbook*. Philadelphia, PA: Wolters Kluwer.

pleural effusion, and edema; hypovolemia may also occur. Risk factors include younger age, history of polycystic ovarian syndrome, high serum estradiol levels, a larger number of follicles, and pregnancy.

Artificial Insemination

Artificial insemination is the deposit of semen into the female genital tract by artificial means. If the sperm cannot penetrate the cervical canal normally, artificial insemination using a partner's or husband's semen or that of a donor may be considered. When the sperm of the woman's partner is defective or absent (azoospermia) or when there is a risk of transmitting a genetic disease, donor sperm may be used. Safeguards are put in place to address legal, ethical, emotional, and religious issues. Written consent is obtained to protect all parties involved, including the woman, the donor, and the resulting child. The donor's semen is frozen, and the donor is evaluated to ensure that he is free of genetic disorders and STIs, including HIV infection (Ginsburg & Srouji, 2016).

Conditions must be optimal for conception before semen is transferred to the vagina or uterus. The woman must have no abnormalities of the genital system, the fallopian tubes must be patent, and ova must be available. In the male, sperm need to be normal in shape, amount, motility, and endurance. The time of ovulation should be determined as accurately as possible so that the 2 or 3 days during which fertilization is possible each month can be targeted for the treatment.

Ultrasonography and blood studies of varying hormone levels are used to pinpoint the best time for insemination and to monitor for OHSS. Fertilization seldom occurs from a single insemination. Usually, insemination is attempted between days 10 and 17 of the cycle; three different attempts may be made during one cycle. The woman may have received clomiphene or other medications to stimulate ovulation before insemination. The recipient is placed in the lithotomy position on the examination table, a speculum is inserted, and the vagina and cervix are swabbed with a cotton-tipped applicator to remove any excess secretions. The sperm are washed before insertion to remove biochemicals and to select the most active sperm. Semen is drawn into a sterile syringe, and a cannula is attached. The semen is then directed to the external os. In intrauterine insemination, semen is placed into the uterine cavity.

Assisted Reproductive Technologies

Assisted reproductive technologies include in vitro fertilization (IVF) and its modifications. Currently, between 1% and 3% of all live births each year in the United States are achieved through assisted technology (Paulson, 2016).

IVF refers to a set of procedures that, if successful, results in a pregnancy. These procedures involve ovarian stimulation, egg retrieval, fertilization, and embryo transfer. The ovaries are stimulated to produce multiple eggs or ova, usually with medications, because success rates are greater with more than one embryo. Many different protocols exist for inducing ovulation with one or more agents (Paulson, 2016). Patients are carefully selected and evaluated, and cycles are carefully monitored using ultrasound and monitoring hormone levels. At the appropriate time, the ova are recovered by transvaginal ultrasound retrieval. Sperm and eggs are coincubated for up to 36 hours, and the embryos are transferred about 48 hours after retrieval. Implantation should occur in 3 to 5 days.

Gamete intrafallopian transfer (GIFT), a variation of IVF, is the treatment of choice for patients with ovarian failure. GIFT is considered in unexplained infertility and when there is religion-based discomfort with IVF. The most common indications for IVF and GIFT are irreparable tubal damage, endometriosis (see Chapter 57), unexplained infertility, inadequate sperm, and exposure to DES. Success rates for GIFT are similar to those for IVF (Paulson, 2016).

Additional Assisted Reproductive Technologies

In intracytoplasmic sperm injection (ICSI), an ovum is retrieved, and a single sperm is injected through the zona pellucida, through the egg membrane, into the cytoplasm of the oocyte. The fertilized egg is then transferred back to the donor. ICSI is the treatment of choice in severe male factor infertility.

Women who cannot produce their own eggs (i.e., premature ovarian failure) have the option of using the eggs of a donor after stimulation of the donor's ovaries. The recipient also receives hormones in preparation for these procedures. Couples may also choose this modality if the female partner has a genetic disorder that may be passed on to children.

Tubal embryo transfer (TET) involves the placement of fertilized eggs or embryos into the fallopian tube. A laparoscopic procedure is needed to place the embryos in the fallopian tubes. Some women choose TET after IVF failure (Paulson, 2016).

Nursing Management

Nursing interventions when working with couples during infertility evaluations include assisting in reducing stress in the relationship, encouraging cooperation, protecting privacy, fostering understanding, and referring the couple to appropriate resources when necessary. Because infertility evaluations and treatments are expensive, time-consuming, invasive, stressful, and not always successful, couples need support in working together to deal with this process.

Smoking cessation is encouraged because smoking has an adverse effect on the success of assisted reproduction. Diet, exercise, stress reduction techniques, folic acid supplementation, health maintenance, and disease prevention are emphasized in many infertility programs. Couples may also consider adoption, child-free living, and gestational carriers (the use of a surrogate to carry the fetus for the infertile couple). Nurses can be helpful listeners and information resources in these deliberations.

Infertility and undergoing assisted reproduction procedures causes significant stress for couples, and women in particular (Frederiksen, Farver-Vestergaard, Skovgård, et al., 2015). Nurses have an opportunity to promote psychosocial interventions for women and couples who are experiencing infertility. A meta-analysis suggested that cognitive-behavioral therapy and mind–body intervention reduce stress and improves pregnancy outcomes of assisted reproductive technologies (Ferderiksen et al., 2015).

Preconception/Periconception Health Care

Nurses can be instrumental in encouraging all women of childbearing age, including those with chronic illness or

Preconception Wellness Strategies

Nurses can help advance pre- and periconception care of women by establishing the following:

- Pregnancy intention
- Access to care
- Preconception multivitamin with folic acid
- Tobacco avoidance
- Absence of uncontrolled depression
- Healthy weight
- Absence of sexually transmitted infections
- Optimal glycemic control in women with pregestational diabetes
- Teratogenic medication avoidance

Adapted from Frayne, D., Verbiest, S., Chelmow, D., et al. (2016). Health care system measures to advance preconception wellness: Consensus recommendations of the clinical workgroup of the national preconception health and health care initiative. *Obstetrics & Gynecology, 127*(5), 863–872.

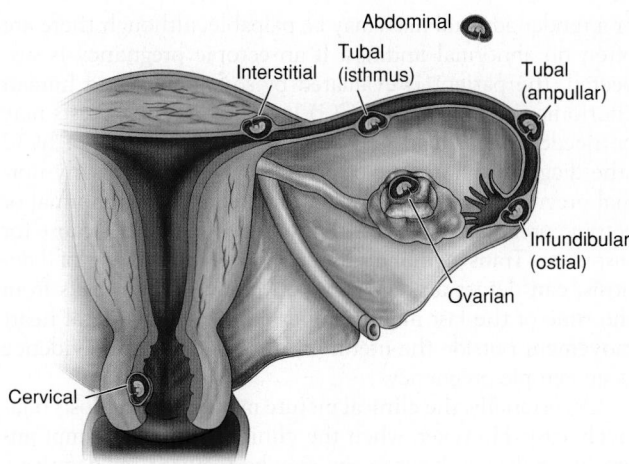

Figure 56-7 • Sites of ectopic pregnancy.

disabilities, to consider issues that may affect health during pregnancy (Smeltzer et al., 2016). Preconception health care is a concept that expands on the definition of prenatal care to include the time before conception (Waggoner, 2013). Women who plan their pregnancies and are healthy and well informed tend to have better outcomes. There are currently nine consensus recommendations for advancing preconception health (see Chart 56-13).

Nurses can make a difference in preconception health through education and counseling. Women who use tobacco products should be encouraged to stop their use; it may help to offer cessation classes. Women should take folic acid supplements to prevent neural tube defects. Women with diabetes should have good glycemic control prior to conception. It is necessary to assess rubella immunity and other immunizations as well as a family history of genetic defects; genetic counseling may be appropriate. Women taking teratogenic medications and women concerned about genetic disorders should be encouraged to discuss effective contraception and childbearing plans with their primary provider (see Chart 56-2).

Ectopic Pregnancy

The incidence of ectopic pregnancy and the risk of death due to ectopic pregnancy are decreasing. However, ectopic pregnancy remains the leading cause of pregnancy-related death in the first trimester (Grossman & Porth, 2014). Ectopic pregnancy occurs when a fertilized ovum (a blastocyst) becomes implanted on any tissue other than the uterine lining, most commonly along the fallopian tube (Grossman & Porth, 2014) (see Fig. 56-7).

Possible causes of ectopic pregnancy include salpingitis, peritubal adhesions (after pelvic infection, endometriosis, appendicitis), structural abnormalities of the fallopian tube, previous ectopic pregnancy, previous tubal surgery, multiple previous induced abortions, and tumors that distort the tube (Grossman & Porth, 2014). Additional risk factors include smoking, IUD use, history of PID, and use of fertility drugs to induce ovulation (Grossman & Porth, 2014).

Risk factors are important, but all women need to be educated about early treatment and have a high index of suspicion in the case of a period that does not seem normal, the presence of pain, or pain with a suspected pregnancy. Women may have fatal hemorrhage with ruptured ectopic pregnancies if they delay seeking attention or if their primary providers are not alert to the possibility of this diagnosis.

Clinical Manifestations

Signs and symptoms vary depending on whether tubal rupture has occurred. Delay in menstruation from 1 to 2 weeks followed by slight bleeding (spotting) or a report of a slightly abnormal period suggests the possibility of an ectopic pregnancy. Symptoms may begin late, with vague soreness on the affected side (probably due to uterine contractions and distention of the tube), and may proceed to sharp, colicky pain. Most patients experience some pelvic or abdominal pain and some spotting or bleeding. Gastrointestinal symptoms, dizziness, or lightheadedness may occur. Patients may think the abnormal bleeding is a menstrual period, especially if a recent period occurred and was normal.

If implantation occurs in the fallopian tube, the tube becomes more and more distended and can rupture if the ectopic pregnancy remains undetected for 4 to 6 weeks or longer after conception. When the tube ruptures, the ovum is discharged into the abdominal cavity, and the woman experiences agonizing pain, dizziness, faintness, and nausea and vomiting due to the peritoneal reaction to blood escaping from the tube. Air hunger and symptoms of shock may occur, and the signs of hemorrhage—rapid and thready pulse, decreased blood pressure, subnormal temperature, restlessness, pallor, and sweating—are evident. Later, the pain becomes generalized in the abdomen and radiates to the shoulder and neck because of accumulating intraperitoneal blood that irritates the diaphragm.

Assessment and Diagnostic Findings

Ectopic pregnancies must be diagnosed promptly to prevent life-threatening hemorrhage, which is the major complication of rupture. During vaginal examination, a large mass of clotted blood that has collected in the pelvis behind the uterus or a tender adnexal mass may be palpable, although there are often no abnormal findings. If an ectopic pregnancy is suspected, the patient is evaluated by sonography and human chorionic gonadotropin (hCG) levels. Serial hCG tests may be needed (Grossman & Porth, 2014). The levels of hCG (the diagnostic hormone of pregnancy) double in early normal pregnancies every 3 days but are reduced in abnormal or ectopic pregnancies. A less-than-normal increase is cause for suspicion. Transvaginal ultrasound, the usual method of diagnosis, can detect a pregnancy between 5 and 6 weeks from the time of the last menstrual period. Detectable fetal heart movement outside the uterus on ultrasound is firm evidence of an ectopic pregnancy.

Occasionally, the clinical picture makes the diagnosis relatively easy. However, when the clinical signs and symptoms are inconclusive, laparoscopy may be required for definitive diagnosis (Grossman & Porth, 2014).

Medical Management

Surgical Management

When surgery is performed early, almost all patients recover rapidly; if tubal rupture occurs, mortality increases. The type of surgery is determined by the size and extent of local tubal damage. Resection of the involved fallopian tube with end-to-end anastomosis may be effective. Some surgeons attempt to salvage the tube with a salpingotomy, which involves opening and evacuating the tube and controlling bleeding. More extensive surgery includes removing the tube alone (salpingectomy) or with the ovary (salpingo-oophorectomy).

Pharmacologic Therapy

Another option is the use of methotrexate without surgery (Grossman & Porth, 2014). Because methotrexate stops the pregnancy from progressing by interfering with DNA synthesis and the multiplication of cells, it interrupts early, small, unruptured ectopic pregnancies. The patient must be hemodynamically stable; have no active renal or hepatic disease; have no evidence of thrombocytopenia or leukopenia; and have a very small, unruptured ectopic pregnancy on ultrasound. Other indications may include no fetal cardiac activity and no active abdominal bleeding. Methotrexate is occasionally used to eliminate residual ectopic pregnancy tissue following a laparoscopy (Grossman & Porth, 2014).

NURSING PROCESS

The Patient With an Ectopic Pregnancy

Assessment

The health history includes the menstrual pattern and any (even slight) bleeding since the last menstrual period. The nurse elicits the patient's description of pain and its location. The nurse asks the patient whether any sharp, colicky pains have occurred and whether pain radiates to the shoulder and neck (possibly caused by rupture and pressure on the diaphragm).

In addition, the nurse monitors vital signs, level of consciousness, and the nature and amount of vaginal bleeding. If possible, the nurse assesses how the patient is coping with the abnormal pregnancy and likely loss.

Diagnosis

NURSING DIAGNOSES

Based on the assessment data, major nursing diagnoses may include the following:

- Acute pain related to the progression of the tubal pregnancy
- Grieving related to the loss of pregnancy and anticipatory effect on future pregnancies
- Deficient knowledge related to the treatment and effect on future pregnancies

COLLABORATIVE PROBLEMS/POTENTIAL COMPLICATIONS

Potential complications may include:

- Hemorrhage
- Hemorrhagic shock

Planning and Goals

The major goals may include relief of pain; acceptance and resolution of grief and pregnancy loss; increased knowledge about ectopic pregnancy, its treatment, and its outcome; and absence of complications.

Nursing Interventions

RELIEVING PAIN

The abdominal pain associated with ectopic pregnancy may be described as cramping or severe continuous pain. If the patient is to have surgery, preanesthetic medications may provide pain relief. Postoperatively, analgesic agents are given liberally; this promotes early ambulation and enables the patient to cough and take deep breaths.

SUPPORTING THE GRIEVING PROCESS

Patients experience varying levels of distress. If the pregnancy was desired, loss may or may not be expressed verbally by the patient and her partner. The impact may not be fully realized until much later. The nurse should be available to listen and provide support. The patient's partner, if appropriate, should participate in this process. Even if the pregnancy was unintended, a loss has been experienced, and a grief reaction may occur.

MONITORING AND MANAGING POTENTIAL COMPLICATIONS

Potential complications of ectopic pregnancy are hemorrhage and shock. Careful assessment is essential to detect the development of these complications. Continuous monitoring of vital signs, level of consciousness, amount of bleeding, and intake and output provide information about the possibility of hemorrhage and the need to prepare for IV therapy. Bed rest is indicated. Hematocrit, hemoglobin, and blood gases are monitored to assess hematologic status and adequacy of tissue perfusion. Significant deviations in these laboratory values are reported immediately, and the patient is prepared for possible surgery. Blood component therapy may be required if blood loss has been rapid and extensive. If hypovolemic shock occurs, the treatment is directed toward reestablishing tissue perfusion and adequate blood volume. See Chapter 14 for a discussion of the IV fluids and medications used in treating shock.

The nurse has an important role in prevention by being alert to patients with abnormal bleeding who may be at risk for an ectopic pregnancy and referring them immediately for care. It is necessary to keep a high index of suspicion in daily practice when a woman of childbearing age, particularly one who is not using an effective method of contraception consistently, reports abdominal discomfort or abnormal bleeding.

PROMOTING HOME, COMMUNITY-BASED, AND TRANSITIONAL CARE

Educating Patients About Self-Care. If the patient has experienced life-threatening hemorrhage and shock, these complications are addressed and treated before education can begin. At this time, the patient's and the nurse's attention is focused on the crisis, not on learning. Once hemodynamically stable, the patient begins to ask questions about what happened and why certain procedures were performed. Procedures are explained in terms that are understandable to a patient who is distressed and apprehensive. The patient's partner is included in education when possible. After the patient recovers from postoperative discomfort, it may be more appropriate to address any questions and concerns that she and her partner have, including the effect of this pregnancy or its treatment on future pregnancies. The patient should be advised that ectopic pregnancies may recur. The patient is educated about possible complications and instructed to report early signs and symptoms. It is important to review signs and symptoms with the patient and instruct her to report an abnormal menstrual period promptly.

Continuing and Transitional Care. Because of the risk of subsequent ectopic pregnancies, the patient is advised to seek preconception counseling before considering future pregnancies and to seek early prenatal care. Follow-up contact allows the nurse to answer questions and clarify information for the patient and her partner.

Evaluation

Expected patient outcomes may include:

1. Experiences relief of pain
   a. Reports a decrease in pain and discomfort
   b. Ambulates as prescribed; performs coughing and deep breathing
2. Begins to accept loss of pregnancy and expresses grief by verbalizing feelings and reactions to loss
3. Verbalizes an understanding of the causes of ectopic pregnancy
4. Experiences no complications
   a. Exhibits no signs of bleeding, hemorrhage, or shock
   b. Has decreased amounts of discharge (on perineal pad)
   c. Has normal skin color and turgor
   d. Exhibits stable vital signs and adequate urine output
   e. Levels of beta-hCG return to normal

Perimenopause

Perimenopause is the period around menopause, lasting between 3 and 6 years before the last menstrual period (Eliopoulos, 2018). Women often have varied beliefs about aging, and these must be considered when caring for or educating patients who are perimenopausal.

Nursing Management

Women who are perimenopausal often benefit from information about the subtle physiologic changes they are experiencing.

Perimenopause has been described as an opportune time for educating women about health promotion and disease prevention strategies. When discussing health-related concerns with women who are in midlife, nurses should consider the following issues:

- Sexuality, fertility, contraception, and STIs
- Unintended pregnancy (if contraception is not used correctly and consistently)
- Oral contraceptive use. Oral contraceptives provide women with protection against uterine cancer, ovarian cancer, anemia, pregnancy, and fibrocystic breast changes as well as relief from perimenopausal symptoms (Eliopoulos, 2018). This option should be discussed with women who are perimenopausal. Women who smoke and are 35 years or older should not take oral contraceptive agents because of an increased risk of CVD. Contraception is discussed in detail earlier in this chapter.
- Breast health. About 16% of cases of breast cancer occur in women who are perimenopausal, so breast self-examination, routine physical examinations, and mammograms are essential.

Menopause

Menopause is the permanent physiologic cessation of menses associated with declining ovarian function (Ball et al., 2015). Most women stop menstruating between 48 and 55 years of age. Postmenopause is the period beginning from about 1 year after menses cease. Due to a decrease in estrogen levels, menopause may be associated with some atrophy of breast tissue and genital organs, loss in bone density, and vascular changes.

Menopause starts gradually and is usually signaled by changes in menstruation. The monthly flow may increase or decrease, become irregular, and finally cease. Often, the interval between periods is longer; a lapse of several months between periods is not uncommon. Ovulation occurs less frequently, estrogen levels fluctuate, and FSH levels increase in an attempt to stimulate estrogen production (Ball et al., 2015).

Postmenopausal Bleeding

Bleeding 1 year after menses cease at menopause must be investigated, and a malignant condition must be considered until proven otherwise. A transvaginal ultrasound can be used to measure the thickness of the endometrial lining (Fischbach & Dunning, 2015). The uterine lining in women who are postmenopausal should be thin because of low estrogen levels. A thicker lining warrants further evaluation by endometrial biopsy or a D&C.

Clinical Manifestations

Menopause has systemic effects that include an increase in body fat and intra-abdominal deposition of body fat. Also, levels of total and LDL cholesterol increase. Hot flashes occur in many women going through menopause due to alterations in thermoregulation. Because of these hormonal changes, some women notice irregular menses, breast tenderness, and mood changes long before menopause occurs (Eliopoulos, 2018). The hot or warm flashes and night sweats reported by some women are thought to be caused by hormonal changes and denote vasomotor instability. They may vary in intensity from a barely perceptible warm feeling to a sensation of extreme warmth accompanied by profuse sweating, causing discomfort, sleep disturbances, and subsequent fatigue. Other physical changes may include increased bone loss (see Chapter 41).

The entire genitourinary system is affected by the reduced estrogen level. Changes in the vulvovaginal area may include a gradual thinning of pubic hair and a gradual shrinkage of the labia. Vaginal secretions decrease, and women may report dyspareunia (discomfort during intercourse). The vaginal pH increases during menopause, predisposing women to bacterial infections and atrophic vaginitis. Discharge, itching, and vulvar burning may result.

Some women report fatigue, forgetfulness, weight gain, irritability, trouble sleeping, feeling "blue," and feelings of panic. Menopausal complaints need to be evaluated carefully because they may indicate other disorders. Most women have few problems and are relieved to be free from menstrual periods. Nurses should provide women with education and health promotion strategies appropriate for those approaching menopause (see Chart 56-14).

Psychological Considerations

Women's reactions and feelings related to loss of reproductive capacity may vary. Some women may experience role confusion, whereas others experience a sense of sexual and personal freedom. Women may be relieved that the childbearing phase of their lives is over. Each woman's personal views about menopause and circumstances affect her response and must be considered on an individual basis. Nurses need to be sensitive to all possibilities and take their cues from the patient.

Medical Management

Women approaching menopause often have many concerns about their health. Some have concerns based on a family history of heart disease, osteoporosis, or cancer. Each woman needs to be as knowledgeable as possible about her health options and should be encouraged to discuss her concerns with her primary provider so that she can make an informed decision about managing menopausal symptoms and maintaining her health.

Hormone Therapy

HT or menopausal hormonal therapy (previously referred to as hormone replacement therapy [HRT]) is medication that contains estrogen or estrogen and progestin together, to replace the ones the body is no longer making. HT is controversial but it is prescribed to treat moderate to severe menopause-related vasomotor symptoms (hot flashes and night sweats) in women without contraindications to estrogen and progesterone whose quality of life is being affected (Eliopoulos, 2018; Fantasia & Sutherland, 2014). The current recommendation for treatment of hot flashes with HT is to use the lowest dose possible for the shortest time possible (Eliopoulos, 2018).

Methods of Administration

Both estrogen and progestin are prescribed for women who have not had a hysterectomy; progestin prevents proliferation of the uterine lining and hyperplasia. Women who no longer have a uterus because of hysterectomy can take estrogen without progestin (i.e., unopposed estrogen) because there is no longer a risk of estrogen-induced hyperplasia of the uterine lining. Although there is a slight increase of risk of stroke in

---

Chart 56-14

HEALTH PROMOTION

Strategies for Women Approaching Menopause

- An annual physical examination can help screen for problems and promote general health.
- Changes in lifestyle (e.g., diet, activity) to promote health and wellness.
  - A nutritious diet (decrease fat and calories, increase fiber and whole grains) and weight control will enhance physical and emotional well-being.
  - Exercise for at least 30 minutes 3 or 4 times a week to maintain good health.
  - Involvement in outside activities is beneficial in reducing anxiety and tension.
- Recognize the following about sexual activity:
  - Sexual functioning may be enhanced at midlife.
  - Frequent sexual activity helps to maintain the elasticity of the vagina.
  - Contraception is advised until 1 year passes without menses.
  - Safer sex is important at any age.
- Strategies and methods to prevent or manage potential problems:
  - *Hot flashes:* See primary provider to discuss hormone replacement therapy (HRT) indications (lowest dose for shortest period of time) and alternative therapy (e.g., vitamin therapy, black cohosh, and other herbal preparations). Fatigue and stress may worsen hot flashes.
  - *Itching or burning of vulvar areas:* See primary provider to rule out dermatologic abnormalities and, if appropriate, to obtain a prescription for a lubricating or hormonal cream.

- *Dyspareunia (painful intercourse) due to vaginal dryness:* Use a water-soluble lubricant (e.g., K-Y Jelly, Astroglide, Replens), hormone cream, or contraceptive foam.
- *Decreased perineal muscle tone and bladder control:* Practice Kegel exercises daily (contract the perineal muscles as though stopping urination; hold for 5–10 seconds and release; repeat frequently during the day).
- *Dry skin:* Use mild emollient skin cream and lotions to prevent dry skin.
- *Weight control:* Join a weight reduction support group such as Weight Watchers or a similar group if appropriate, or consult a registered dietitian for guidance about the tendency to gain weight, particularly around the hips, thighs, and abdomen.
- *Osteoporosis:* Observe recommended calcium and vitamin D intake, including calcium supplements, if indicated, to slow the process of osteoporosis; avoid smoking, alcohol, and excessive caffeine, all of which increase bone loss. Perform weight-bearing exercises. Undergo bone density testing when appropriate.
- *Risk for urinary tract infection (UTI):* Drink 6–8 glasses of water daily as a possible way to reduce the incidence of UTI related to atrophic changes of the urethra.
- *Vaginal bleeding:* Report any bleeding after 1 year of no menses to the primary provider *immediately, no matter how minimal.*

women taking estrogen alone following hysterectomy, the risk of breast cancer is unchanged (Fantasia & Sutherland, 2014).

Some women take both estrogen and progestin daily; others take estrogen for 25 consecutive days each month, with progestin taken in cycles (e.g., 10 to 14 days of the month). Women who take HT for 25 days often experience bleeding after completing the progestin. Other women take estrogen and progestin every day and usually experience no bleeding. They occasionally have irregular spotting, which should be evaluated by their primary provider. Progestin administration may be oral, transdermal, vaginal, or intrauterine.

Estrogen patches, which are replaced once or twice weekly, are another option but require a progestin along with them if the woman still has a uterus. Another type of patch provides estrogen and progestin treatment (Comerford, 2015). Skin should be dry at the area of application, and cleansing the site with alcohol may improve adhesiveness. Vaginal treatment with an estrogen cream, suppository, or a vaginal ring may be used for vasomotor symptoms, vaginal dryness, or atrophy (Comerford, 2015).

Risks and Benefits

HT is contraindicated in women with a history of breast cancer, vascular thrombosis, impaired liver function, uterine cancer, and undiagnosed abnormal vaginal bleeding. The risk of venous thromboembolism is increased with HT (Santen, Loprinzi, & Casper, 2016). Women who elect to take HT should be educated about the signs and symptoms of deep vein thrombosis (DVT) and pulmonary embolism (PE) and instructed to report these signs and symptoms (i.e., leg redness, tenderness, chest pain, shortness of breath) immediately. See Chapter 30 for discussion of DVT and Chapter 23 for discussion of PE. Women who take HT need to be informed about the importance of regular follow-up care, including a yearly physical examination and mammogram. An endometrial biopsy is indicated for any irregular bleeding. Because the risk of complications increases the longer HT is used, HT should be used for the shortest time possible (Eliopoulos, 2018). Estrogen alone or in combination with a progestin does not reduce the risk of dementia or cognitive impairment.

Alternative Therapy for Hot Flashes

Because women often seek information about alternatives to the use of HT, nurses must be knowledgeable about other approaches that women can use to promote their health in the peri- and postmenopausal periods. Problematic hot flashes have been treated with low-dose venlafaxine (Effexor), psychoeducational approaches, and diet and lifestyle changes (Santen, Loprinzi, & Casper, 2016). Similarly, vitamin B_6 and vitamin E may be effective. Some women have expressed interest in other alternative treatments (e.g., natural estrogens and progestins, black cohosh, ginseng, dongquai, soy products, and several other herbal preparations); however, scant data exist about their safety or effectiveness. A few studies have shown some improvement in vasomotor symptoms (hot flashes and night sweats) with the use of complementary therapies. These include reflexology, aromatherapy, yoga, hypnotherapy, breathing exercises, and meditation (Eliopoulos, 2018; Santen, Loprinzi, & Casper, 2016). When taking a medical history of a patient who is perimenopausal or

menopausal, the nurse should always address their use of complementary and alternative therapies and supplements.

Maintaining Bone Health

Acceleration of bone loss resulting in osteoporosis and microarchitectural deterioration of bone tissue occurs at menopause and leads to increased bone fragility and risk of fracture (see Chapter 41).

Maintaining Cardiovascular Health

A variety of strategies can help to lower the risk of heart disease in women, including lifestyle changes and behavioral strategies (see Chapter 25).

Behavioral Strategies

As stated previously, regular physical exercise is beneficial. It may also reduce stress, enhance well-being, and improve self-image. In addition, weight-bearing exercise may prevent loss of muscle tissue and bone tissue.

Women are also encouraged to participate in other health-promoting activities. These include regular health screening recommended for women at the time of menopause: gynecologic examinations, mammograms, colonoscopy, fecal occult blood testing, and bone mineral density testing if at risk for osteoporosis.

Nutritional Therapy

Women are encouraged to decrease their fat and caloric intake and increase their intake of whole grains, fiber, fruit, and vegetables.

Nursing Management

Nurses can encourage women to view menopause as a natural change resulting in freedom from symptoms related to menses. No relationship exists between menopause and mental health problems; however, social circumstances (e.g., adolescent children, ill partners, and dependent or ill parents) that may coincide with menopause can be stressful.

Measures should be taken to promote general health (Eliopoulos, 2018). The nurse explains to the patient that cessation of menses is a normal occurrence that is rarely accompanied by nervous symptoms or illness. The current expected lifespan after menopause for the average woman is 30 to 35 years, which may encompass as many years as the childbearing phase of her life. Normal sexual urges continue, and women retain their usual response to sex long after menopause. Many women enjoy better health after menopause than before, especially those who have experienced dysmenorrhea. The individual woman's evaluation of herself and her worth, now and in the future, is likely to affect her emotional reaction to menopause. Patient education and counseling regarding healthy lifestyles, health promotion, and health screening are of paramount importance (Santen, Loprinzi, & Casper, 2016).

CRITICAL THINKING EXERCISES

1 **ebp** A 20-year-old female college student comes to the student health clinic for a gynecologic examination and contraception. She asks you for advice about the most reliable method of contraception. She would like a method that is convenient. What is the evidence base for contraceptive methods for this college student? Specify the criteria used to evaluate the strength of the evidence for the practices that you identify.

2 You receive report that a 32-year-old patient will be arriving on your unit post-surgery for an ectopic pregnancy. Describe the nursing plan of care. What specific interventions and nursing management strategies are indicated? Develop a plan of patient education, and identify outcomes measures to assess the effectiveness of the education.

3 **pq** During her annual physical examination, a 55-year-old woman complains of night sweats and hot flashes. What are the immediate nursing priorities in providing care to this patient? What assessment data are needed to determine if this patient is in perimenopause or menopause?

REFERENCES

*Asterisk indicates nursing research.
**Double asterisk indicates classic reference.

Books

**Annon, J. S. (1976). The behavioral treatment of sexual problems. Honolulu, HI: Enabling Systems.

Ball, J., Dains, J., Flynn, J., et al. (2015). Seidel's guide to physical examination. (8th ed.). St. Louis, MO: Elsevier Mosby.

Comerford, K. C. (2015). Nursing 2015 drug handbook. Philadelphia, PA: Wolters Kluwer.

Eliopoulos, C. (2018). Gerontological nursing (9th ed.). Philadelphia, PA: Lippincott Williams & Wilkins.

Fischbach, F. T., & Dunning, M. B. (2015). A manual of laboratory and diagnostic tests (9th ed.). Philadelphia, PA: Lippincott Williams & Wilkins.

Grossman & Porth. (2014). Pathophysiology: Concepts of altered health states (9th ed.). Philadelphia, PA: Lippincott Williams & Wilkins.

Hawkins, J. W., Roberto-Nichols, D. M., & Stanley-Haney, J. L. (2012). Guidelines for nurse practitioners in gynecologic settings (10th ed.). New York: Springer.

Schuiling, K., & Likis, F. (2013). Women's gynecologic health. Boston, MA: Jones & Bartlett.

Tharpe, N., Farley, C., & Jordan, R. (2013). Clinical practice guidelines for midwifery & women's health. Boston, MA: Jones & Bartlett.

Weber, J., & Kelley, J. (2014). Health assessment in nursing (5th ed.). Philadelphia, PA: Lippincott Williams & Wilkins.

Journals and Electronic Documents

Alan Guttmacher Institute. (2016). Contraceptive use in the United States. Retrieved on 8/16/2016 at: www.guttmacher.org/fact-sheet/contraceptive-use-united-states

American College of Obstetricians and Gynecologists (ACOG). (2016a). Committee Opinion Number 654. Reproductive life planning to reduce unintended pregnancy. Retrieved on 10/21/16 at: www.acog.org/About-ACOG/News-Room/News-Releases/2016/Ob-Gyns-Encourage-Reproductive-Life-Planning.

American College of Obstetricians and Gynecologists (ACOG). (2016b). Long-acting reversible contraception: implants and intrauterine devices. Retrieved on 11/16/16 at: https://www.acog.org/-/media/For-Patients/faq184.pdf?dmc=1&ts=20161116T1056519865 .

Bosse, J. D., Nesteby, A., & Randall, C. E. (2015). Integrating sexual minority health issues into a health assessment class. Journal of Professional Nursing, 31(6) 498–507.

Bradley, L. D. (2016). Overview of hysteroscopy. Retrieved on 11/10/16 at: www.uptodate.com/contents/overview-of-hysteroscopy?source=search_result&search=Overview+of+GynecOverview+of+Hysteroscopy%2C+ologic+Laparoscopic+Surgery+and+Non-umbilical+Entry+Sites&selectedTitle=1%7E150

Centers for Disease Control and Prevention (CDC). (2014). Understanding intimate partner violence fact sheet. Retrieved on 11/18/16 at: https://www.cdc.gov/violenceprevention/pdf/ipv-factsheet.pdf

Centers for Disease Control and Prevention (CDC). (2016). U.S. selected practice recommendations for contraceptive use, 2016. Morbidity and Mortality Weekly Report, 65(4), 1–72.

Courtney-Long, E., Carroll, D., Znang, O., et al. (2013.) Prevalence of disability and disability types among adults. Morbidity and Mortality Weekly Report, 64(29), 777–783.

Del Priore, G. (2015). Endometrial sampling procedure. Retrieved on 11/01/16 at: www.uptodate.com/contents/endometrial-sampling-procedures

Fantasia, H. C., & Sutherland, M. A. (2014). Hormone therapy for the management of menopause symptoms. Journal of Obstetric, Gynecologic and Neonatal Nursing, 43(2), 226–235

Frayne, D., Verbiest, S., Chelmow, D., et al. (2016). Health care system measures to advance preconception wellness: Consensus recommendations of the clinical workgroup of the national preconception health and health care initiative. Obstetrics & Gynecology, 127(5), 863–872.

Frederiksen, Y., Farver-Vestergaard, I., Skovgård, N., et al. (2015). Efficacy of psychosocial interventions for psychological and pregnancy outcomes in infertile women and men: a systematic review and meta-analysis. BMJ Open, 5(1), e006592.

Ginsburg, E. S., & Srouji, S. S. (2016). Donor insemination. Retrieved on 11/23/16 at: www.uptodate.com/contents/donor-insemination

Ireland, L. D., Geffen, D., & Chen, A. Y. (2015). Medical compared with surgical abortion for effective pregnancy termination in the first trimester. Obstetrics and Gynecology, 126(1), 22–28.

*Johnson, M. J., & Amella, E. J. (2013). Isolation of lesbian, gay, bisexual and transgender youth: A dimensional concept analysis. Journal of Advanced Nursing, 70(3), 523–532.

Kaiser Family Foundation. (2015). Women's health insurance coverage: Fact sheet. Retrieved on 8/16/2016 at: www.kff.org/womens-health-policy.

Kessler, L., Craig, B., Plosker, S., et al. (2013). Infertility evaluation and treatment among women in the United States. Fertility and Sterility, 100(4), 1025–1032.

Mayo Clinic. (2014). Toxic shock syndrome: Prevention. Retrieved on 8/16/2016 at: www.mayoclinic.com/health/toxic-shock-syndrome/DS00221/DSECTION=prevention

Paulson, R. (2016). In Vitro fertilization. Retrieved on 11/23/16 at: www.uptodate.com/contents/in-vitro-fertilization?source=search_result&search=In+Vitro+Fertilitzation&selectedTitle=1%7E150

*Pyra, M., Weber, K. M., Wilson, T. E., et al. (2014). Sexual minority women and depressive symptoms throughout adulthood. American Journal of Public Health, 104(12), E83-E90.

Rager Zuzelo, P. (2014). Improving nursing care for lesbian, bisexual and transgender women. Journal of Obstetric Gynecologic and Neonatal Nursing, 43, 520–530.

Ranji, U., & Salganicoff, A. (2015). Medicaid and women's health coverage two years into the Affordable Care Act. Women's Health Issues, 25, 604–607.

Salganicoff, A, Ranji, U., Beamesderfer, A., et al. (2014. Women and health care in the early years of the ACA: key findings from the 2013 Kaiser Women's Survey. Retrieved on 8/11/2016 at: kff.org/womens-health-policy/report/women-and-health-care-in-the-early-years-of-the-aca-key-findings-from-the-2013-kaiser-womens-health-survey/

Santen, R. J., Loprinzi, C. L., & Casper, R. F. (2016). Menopausal hot flashes. Retrieved on 11/28/16 at: www.uptodate.com/contents/menopausal-hot-flashes?source=search_result&search=Managing+menopausal+symptoms&selectedTitle=1%7E150

Sargant, N., Smallwood, N., Finley, F., et al. (2014). Sexual history taking: A dying skill? Journal of Palliative Medicine. 17(7), 829–831.

Sharp, H. T. (2016). Overview of gynecologic laparoscopic surgery and non-umbilical entry sites. UpToDate. Retrieved on 11/10/16 at: www.uptodate.com/contents/overview-of-gynecologic-laparoscopic-surgery-and-non-umbilical-entry-sites?source=search_result&search=Overview+of+Gynecologic+Laparoscopic+Surgery+and+Non-umbilical+Entry+Sites&selectedTitle=1%7E150

Sinclair, L. B., Taft, K. E., Sloan, M. L., et al. (2015). Tools for improving clinical preventive services receipt among women with disabilities of child-bearing age and beyond. *Maternal Child Health Journal, 19*, 1189–1201.

*Smeltzer, S. C., Mitra, M., Iezzoni, L. I., et al. (2016). Perinatal experiences of women with physical disabilities and their recommendations for clinicians. *Journal of Obstetric, Gynecologic & Neonatal Nursing, 45*(6), 781–789.

Smith, R. A., Cokkinides, V., & Brawley, O. W. (2012). Cancer screening in the United States, 2012. *CA: A Cancer Journal for Clinicians, 62*(2), 129–142.

Tarin, J., Garcia-Perez, M., Hamatani, T., et al. (2015). Infertility etiologies are genetically and clinically linked with other diseases in single meta-diseases.*Reproductive Biology and Endocrinology, 13*(1), 31–42.

U.S. Preventive Services Task Force (USPSTF). (2016). The Guide to Clinical Preventive Service. 2016. Recommendations of the U.S. Preventive Services Task Force. Retrieved on 10/29/16 at: www.uspreventiveservicestaskforce.org/Page/Name/uspstf-a-and-b-recommendations/

Waggoner, M. (2013). Mother preconceived: The emergence of the preconception health and health care initiative. *Journal of Health Politics, Policy and Law.* 38(2), 345–371.

Welt, C. K., & Barbieri, R. L. (2016). Evaluation and management of primary amenorrhea. Retrieved on 11/15/16 at: www.uptodate.com/contents/evaluation-and-management-of-primary-amenorrhea

World Health Organization (WHO). (2016). *Female genital mutilation. Fact sheet number 241.* Retrieved on 8/13/2016 at: www.who.int/mediacentre/factsheets/fs241/en/

Resources

American Congress of Obstetricians and Gynecologists (ACOG), www.acog.org

American Society for Reproductive Medicine (ASRM), www.asrm.org

Amnesty International (resource for activists to end FGM), www.amnesty.org

Association of Reproductive Health Professionals (ARHP), www.arhp.org

Association of Women's Health, Obstetric and Neonatal Nurses (AWHONN), www.awhonn.org

DES Action USA, www.desaction.org

Emergency Contraception, ec.princeton.edu

Female Genital Cutting Education and Networking Project (provides fact sheets, state policies, periodicals), www.fgmnetwork.org

Futures Without Violence (formerly Family Violence Prevention Fund), www.endabuse.org

Guttmacher Institute, www.guttmacher.org

Health Promotion for Women With Disabilities, Villanova University College of Nursing, www.nurseweb.villanova.edu/womenwithdisabilities

National Coalition Against Domestic Violence (NCADV), www.ncadv.org

North American Menopause Society (NAMS), www.menopause.org

Nurse Practitioners in Women's Health (NPWH), www.npwh.org

Planned Parenthood Federation of America, www.plannedparenthood.org

57

Management of Patients With Female Reproductive Disorders

LEARNING OBJECTIVES

On completion of this chapter, the learner will be able to:

1 Compare the various types of vaginal infections and the signs, symptoms, and treatments of each.
2 Use the nursing process as a framework for care of the patient with a vulvovaginal infection.
3 Apply the nursing process as a framework for care of the patient with genital herpes.
4 Discuss the signs and symptoms, management, and nursing care of patients with inflammatory processes and structural disorders of the female reproductive tract.

5 Explain the signs and symptoms, management, and nursing care implications of benign and malignant conditions of the female reproductive tract.
6 Use the nursing process as a framework for care of the patient undergoing a hysterectomy.
7 Describe the nursing management of the patient undergoing radiation therapy for cancer of the female reproductive tract.

GLOSSARY

abscess: a collection of purulent material

Bartholin cyst: a cyst in a paired Bartholin or vestibular gland in the vulva

brachytherapy: delivery of radiation therapy through internal implants to a localized area of tissue

candidiasis: infection caused by *Candida* species or yeast; also referred to as monilial vaginitis or yeast infection

condylomata: warty growths indicative of the human papillomavirus

cryotherapy: destruction of tissue by freezing (e.g., with liquid nitrogen)

cystocele: displacement of the bladder downward into the vagina

douche: rinsing the vaginal canal with fluid

dysplasia: term related to abnormal cell changes; may be found on Pap smear and cervical biopsy reports

endocervicitis: inflammation of the mucosa and the glands of the cervix

endometriosis: endometrial tissue in abnormal locations; causes pain with menstruation, scarring, and possible infertility

enterocele: a protrusion of the intestinal wall into the vagina

fibroid tumor: usually benign tumor arising from the muscle tissue of the uterus

fistula: abnormal opening between two organs or sites (e.g., vesicovaginal, between bladder and vagina; rectovaginal, between rectum and vagina)

hyphae: long, branching filamentous structures characteristic of fungi such as *Candida* seen under microscopic examination

hysterectomy: surgical removal of the uterus

loop electrocautery excision procedure (LEEP): procedure in which a laser is used to remove a thin layer of cervical tissue after abnormal biopsy findings

myomectomy: surgical removal of uterine fibroids

oophorectomy: surgical removal of an ovary

pelvic exenteration: major surgical procedure in which the pelvic organs are removed

pelvic inflammatory disease (PID): inflammatory condition of the pelvic cavity, usually from a sexually transmitted infection

polycystic ovary syndrome (PCOS): complex endocrine condition resulting in chronic anovulation, androgen excess, and multiple ovarian cysts

rectocele: bulging of the rectum into the vagina

salpingitis: inflammation of the fallopian tube

salpingo-oophorectomy: removal of the ovary and its fallopian tube (removal of the fallopian tube alone is a salpingectomy)

vaginitis: inflammation of the vagina, usually secondary to infection

vulvar dystrophy: thickening or lesions of the vulva; usually causes itching and may require biopsy to exclude malignancy

vulvectomy: removal of the tissue of the vulva

vulvitis: inflammation of the vulva, usually secondary to infection or irritation

vulvodynia: painful condition that affects the vulva

Disorders of the female reproductive system can be minor or serious but are often anxiety producing and distressing. Some disorders are self-limited and cause only minor inconvenience; others are life threatening and require immediate attention and long-term therapy. Many disorders are managed by the patient at home, whereas others require hospitalization and surgical intervention. Nurses not only need to be knowledgeable about these disorders but need to be sensitive to patient concerns and possible discomfort in discussing and dealing with these disorders.

VULVOVAGINAL INFECTIONS

Vulvovaginal infections are common, and nurses have an important role in providing information that may prevent their occurrence. To help prevent these infections, women need to understand their anatomy and normal vulvovaginal health.

The vagina is protected against infection by its normally low pH (3.5 to 4.5), which is maintained in part by the actions of *Lactobacillus acidophilus*, the dominant bacteria in a healthy vaginal ecosystem. These bacteria suppress the growth of anaerobes and produce lactic acid, which maintains normal pH. They also produce hydrogen peroxide, which is toxic to anaerobes (Powell & Nyirjesy, 2015). The risk of infection increases if a woman's resistance is reduced by stress or illness, if the pH is altered, or if a pathogen is introduced (see Chart 57-1). Continued research into causes and treatments is needed, along with better ways to encourage growth of lactobacilli.

The epithelium of the vagina is highly responsive to estrogen, which induces glycogen formation. The subsequent breakdown of glycogen into lactic acid assists in producing a low vaginal pH. When estrogen decreases during lactation and menopause, glycogen also decreases. With reduced glycogen formation, infections may occur. In addition, as estrogen production ceases during the peri- and postmenopausal

---

Chart 57-1 ⚠️ **RISK FACTORS:**
Vulvovaginal Infections

- Allergies
- Diabetes
- Frequent douching
- HIV infection
- Intercourse with infected partner
- Long-term or repeated use of broad-spectrum antibiotics
- Low estrogen levels
- Oral–genital contact (yeast can inhabit the mouth and intestinal tract)
- Perimenopause/Menopause
- Poor personal hygiene
- Pregnancy
- Premenarche
- Synthetic clothing
- Tight undergarments
- Use of oral contraceptives

HIV, human immune deficiency virus
Adapted from Beckmann, C. R., Ling, F. W., & Herbert, W. N., et al. (Eds). (2014). *Obstetrics and gynecology* (7th ed.). Philadelphia, PA: Wolters Kluwer.

---

periods, the vagina and labia may atrophy (thin), making the vaginal area more susceptible to infection. When patients are treated with antibiotic agents, the normal vaginal flora are reduced. This results in altered pH and growth of fungal organisms. Other factors that may initiate or predispose to infections include contact with an infected partner and wearing tight, nonabsorbent, and heat- and moisture-retaining clothing.

Vaginitis (inflammation of the vagina) is a group of conditions that cause vulvovaginal symptoms such as itching, irritation, burning, and abnormal discharge. Bacterial vaginitis is the most common cause, followed by trichomoniasis and vulvovaginal candidiasis (Centers for Disease Control and Prevention [CDC], 2015a) (see Table 57-1). Other types include desquamative vaginitis, atrophic vaginitis, various vulvar dermatologic conditions, and vulvodynia. Normal vaginal discharge, which may occur in slight amounts during ovulation or just before the onset of menstruation, is clear to white, odorless, and viscous. It becomes more profuse when vaginitis occurs. Urethritis may accompany vaginitis because of the proximity of the urethra to the vagina. Discharge that occurs with vaginitis may produce itching, odor, redness, burning, or edema, which may be aggravated by voiding and defecation. After the causative organism has been identified, appropriate treatment (discussed later) is prescribed. This may include an oral medication or a local medication that is inserted into the vagina using an applicator.

Candidiasis

Vulvovaginal **candidiasis** is a fungal or yeast infection caused by strains of *Candida* (see Table 57-1). An estimated 75% of women will experience at least one yeast infection, and 40% to 45% will experience two or more in their lifetime (CDC, 2014a; CDC, 2015a). *Candida albicans* accounts for approximately 90% of the cases, but other strains, such as *Candida glabrata*, may also be implicated (Beckmann, Ling, Herbert, et al., 2014). Many women with a healthy vaginal ecosystem harbor *Candida* but are asymptomatic. Certain conditions favor the change from an asymptomatic state to colonization with symptoms. For example, the use of antibiotic agents decreases bacteria, thereby altering the natural protective organisms usually present in the vagina. Although infections can occur at any time, they occur more commonly in pregnancy or with a systemic condition such as diabetes or human immune deficiency virus (HIV) infection, or when patients are taking medications such as corticosteroids or oral contraceptive agents (Beckmann et al., 2014).

Clinical Manifestations

Clinical manifestations include a vaginal discharge that causes pruritus (itching) and subsequent irritation. The discharge may be watery or thick but usually has a white, cottage cheese–like appearance. Symptoms are usually more severe just before menstruation and may be less responsive to treatment during pregnancy. Diagnosis is made by microscopic identification of spores and **hyphae** (long, branching filamentous structures) on a glass slide prepared from a discharge specimen mixed with potassium hydroxide. With candidiasis, the pH is 4.5 or less (Beckmann et al., 2014). Manifestations

TABLE 57-1 Vaginal Infections and Vaginitis

Infection	Cause	Clinical Manifestations	Management Strategies
Candidiasis	*Candida albicans, glabrata,* or *tropicalis*	Inflammation of vaginal epithelium, producing itching, reddish irritation White, cheeselike discharge clinging to epithelium	Eradicate the fungus by administering an antifungal agent. Some more frequently used vaginal creams and suppositories are miconazole (Monistat) and clotrimazole (Gyne-Lotrimin). Review other causative factors (e.g., antibiotic therapy, nylon underwear, tight clothing, pregnancy, oral contraceptive agents). Assess for diabetes and HIV infection in patients with recurrent monilia.
Gardnerella-associated bacterial vaginosis	*Gardnerella vaginalis* and vaginal anaerobes	Usually no edema or erythema of vulva or vagina Gray-white to yellow-white discharge clinging to external vulva and vaginal walls	Administer metronidazole (Flagyl), with instructions about avoiding alcohol while taking this medication. If infection is recurrent, may treat partner.
Trichomonas vaginalis vaginitis	*Trichomonas vaginalis*	Inflammation of vaginal epithelium, producing burning and itching Frothy yellow-white or yellow-green vaginal discharge	Relieve inflammation, restore acidity, and reestablish normal bacterial flora; provide oral metronidazole for patient and partner.
Bartholinitis (infection of greater vestibular gland)	*Escherichia coli* *T. vaginalis* Staphylococcus Streptococcus Gonococcus	Erythema around vestibular gland Swelling and edema Abscessed vestibular gland	Drain the abscess; provide antibiotic therapy; excise gland of patients with chronic bartholinitis.
Cervicitis—acute and chronic	Chlamydia Gonococcus Streptococcus Many pathogenic bacteria	Profuse purulent discharge Backache Urinary frequency and urgency	Determine the cause—perform cytologic examination of cervical smear and appropriate cultures. Eradicate the gonococcal organism, if present: penicillin (as directed) or spectinomycin or tetracycline, if patient is allergic to penicillin. Tetracycline, doxycycline (Vibramycin) to eradicate chlamydia. Eradicate other causes.
Atrophic vaginitis	Lack of estrogen; glycogen deficiency	Discharge and irritation from alkaline pH of vaginal secretions	Provide topical vaginal estrogen therapy; improve nutrition if necessary; relieve dryness through the use of moisturizing medications.

HIV, human immune deficiency virus.
Adapted from Karch, A. M. (2015). *Lippincott nursing drug guide.* Philadelphia, PA: Wolters Kluwer.

may be fairly uncomplicated, occurring sporadically in women who are healthy, or recurrent and complicated in women who have diabetes, are pregnant, have a compromised immune system, or have obesity.

Medical Management

The goal of management is to eliminate symptoms. Treatments include antifungal agents such as miconazole (Monistat), nystatin (Mycostatin), clotrimazole (Gyne-Lotrimin), and terconazole (Terazol) cream. These agents are inserted into the vagina with an applicator at bedtime. There are 1-night, 3-night, and 7-night treatment courses available (Karch, 2015). Oral medication (fluconazole [Diflucan]) is also available in a one-pill dose. Relief should be noted within 3 days.

Some vaginal creams are available without a prescription; however, patients are cautioned to use these creams only if they are certain that they have a yeast or monilial infection. Patients often use these remedies for problems other than yeast infections. If a woman is uncertain about the cause of her symptoms or if relief has not been obtained after using these creams, she should be instructed to seek health care promptly. Yeast infections can become recurrent or complicated. Women may have more than four infections in a year and severe symptoms due to pre-existing conditions such as diabetes or immunosuppression. Cell-mediated immunity may be a factor. Women with recurrent yeast infections benefit from a comprehensive gynecologic assessment.

Bacterial Vaginosis

Bacterial vaginosis is caused by an overgrowth of anaerobic bacteria and *Gardnerella vaginalis* normally found in the vagina and an absence of lactobacilli (see Table 57-1). Risk factors include douching after menses, smoking, multiple sex partners, and other sexually transmitted infections (STIs) (also referred to as sexually transmitted diseases [STDs]). Bacterial vaginosis is not considered an STI but is associated with sexual activity, and incidence is increased in female same-sex partners (Schuiling & Likis, 2013).

Clinical Manifestations

Bacterial vaginosis can occur throughout the menstrual cycle and does not produce local discomfort or pain. More than half of patients with bacterial vaginosis do not notice any symptoms. Discharge, if noticed, is heavier than normal and gray to yellowish white in color. It is characterized by a fishlike odor that is particularly noticeable after sexual intercourse or during menstruation as a result of an increase in vaginal pH. The pH of the discharge is usually greater than 4.7 because of the amines that result from enzymes from anaerobes. The fishlike odor can be detected readily by adding a drop of potassium hydroxide to a glass slide with a sample of vaginal discharge, which releases amines; this is referred to as a positive "whiff" test. Under the microscope, vaginal cells are coated with bacteria and are described as "clue cells." Lactobacilli, which serve as a natural host defense, are usually absent. Bacterial vaginosis is not usually considered a serious condition, although it can be associated with premature labor, premature rupture of membranes, endometritis, and pelvic infection (Schuiling & Likis, 2013).

Medical Management

Metronidazole (Flagyl), given orally twice a day for 1 week, is effective; a vaginal gel is also available. Clindamycin (Cleocin) vaginal cream or ovules (oval suppositories) are also effective. Treatment of patients' partners does not seem to be effective, but the use of condoms may be helpful. Bacterial vaginosis is highly persistent and tends to recur after treatment; therefore, women are encouraged to seek follow-up care if symptoms recur (CDC, 2015a).

Trichomoniasis

Trichomonas vaginalis is a flagellated protozoan that causes a common STI often called *trich*. About 3.7 million cases occur each year in the United States (CDC, 2015b). Trichomoniasis may be transmitted by an asymptomatic carrier who harbors the organism in the urogenital tract (see Table 57-1). It may increase the risk of contracting HIV from an infected partner and may play a role in development of cervical neoplasia, postoperative infections, adverse pregnancy outcomes, pelvic inflammatory disease (PID), and infertility. Incidence is 10 times higher in African-American women, and approximately 70% to 85% of those affected are asymptomatic (CDC, 2015b).

Clinical Manifestations

Clinical manifestations include a vaginal discharge that is thin (sometimes frothy), yellow to yellow-green, malodorous, and very irritating. An accompanying vulvitis may result, with vulvovaginal burning and itching. Diagnosis is made most often by microscopic detection of the motile

causative organisms or less frequently by culture. Inspection with a speculum often reveals vaginal and cervical erythema (redness) with multiple small petechiae ("strawberry spots") (Beckman et al., 2014). Testing of a trichomonal discharge demonstrates a pH greater than 4.5.

Medical Management

The most effective treatment for trichomoniasis is metronidazole or tinidazole (Tindamax). Both partners receive a one-time loading dose or a smaller dose twice a day for 7 days (CDC, 2015a). The one-time dose is more convenient; consequently, adherence tends to be greater. The week-long treatment has occasionally been noted to be more effective. Some patients complain of an unpleasant but transient metallic taste when taking metronidazole. Nausea and vomiting, as well as a hot, flushed feeling can occur when this medication is taken with an alcoholic beverage. Patients are strongly advised to abstain from alcohol during treatment and for 24 hours after taking metronidazole or 72 hours after completion of a course of tinidazole (CDC, 2015a).

 Gerontologic Considerations

After menopause, the vaginal mucosa becomes thinner and may atrophy. While vulvovaginal atrophy can occur at any time in a woman's life, it is most common in women who are postmenopausal, with an incidence of nearly 50% (Lev-Sagie, 2015; Nyirjesy, 2014). This condition can be complicated by infection from phylogenic bacteria, resulting in atrophic vaginitis (see Table 57-1). Leukorrhea (vaginal discharge) may cause itching and burning. Management is similar to bacterial vaginosis. Estrogenic hormones, either taken orally or inserted into the vagina in a cream form, can also be effective in restoring the epithelium.

Desquamative inflammatory vaginitis is an uncommon but severe purulent form of vaginal infection that occurs mostly in Caucasian women who are perimenopausal. It results in vaginal inflammation, burning, discharge, and dyspareunia. Topical anti-inflammatory and antibiotic treatment is usually effective (Nyirjesy, 2014; Reichman & Sobel, 2014).

NURSING PROCESS

The Patient With a Vulvovaginal Infection

Assessment

The woman with vulvovaginal symptoms should be examined as soon as possible after the onset of symptoms. She should be instructed not to **douche** (rinse the vaginal canal), because doing so removes the discharge needed to make the diagnosis. The area is observed for erythema, edema, excoriation, and discharge. Each of the infection-producing organisms produces its own characteristic discharge and effect (see Table 57-1). The patient is asked to describe any discharge and other symptoms, such as odor, itching, or burning. Dysuria often occurs as a result of local irritation of the urinary meatus. A urinary tract infection may need to be ruled out by obtaining a urine specimen for culture and sensitivity testing.

The patient is asked about the occurrence of factors that may contribute to vulvovaginal infection:

- Physical and chemical factors, such as constant moisture from tight or synthetic clothing, perfumes and powders, soaps, bubble bath, poor hygiene, and the use of feminine hygiene products
- Psychogenic factors (e.g., stress, fear of STIs, abuse)
- Medical conditions or endocrine factors, such as a predisposition to *Monilia* in a patient who has diabetes
- The use of medications such as antibiotics, which may alter the vaginal flora and allow an overgrowth of monilial organisms
- New sex partner, multiple sex partners, previous vaginal infection

The patient is also asked about factors that could contribute to infection, including hygiene practices (douching) and the use or nonuse of condoms.

The nurse may prepare a vaginal smear (wet mount) to assist in diagnosing the infection. A common method for preparing the smear is to collect vaginal secretions with an applicator and place the secretions on two separate glass slides. A drop of saline solution is added to one slide and a drop of 10% potassium hydroxide is added to another slide for examination under a microscope. If bacterial vaginosis is present, the slide with normal saline solution added shows epithelial cells dotted with bacteria (clue cells). If *Trichomonas* species is present, small motile cells are seen. In the presence of yeast, the potassium hydroxide slide reveals branching hyphae (Beckman at al., 2014). Discharge associated with bacterial vaginosis produces a strong odor when mixed with potassium hydroxide. Testing the pH of the discharge with Nitrazine paper assists in proper diagnosis (Beckman et al., 2014).

Diagnosis

Nursing Diagnoses

Based upon the assessment data, major nursing diagnoses may include the following:

- Impaired comfort related to burning, odor, or itching from the infectious process
- Anxiety related to stressful symptoms
- Risk for infection or spread of infection
- Deficient knowledge about proper hygiene and preventive measures

Planning and Goals

Major goals may include increased comfort, reduction of anxiety related to symptoms, prevention of reinfection or infection of sexual partner, and acquisition of knowledge about methods for preventing vulvovaginal infections and managing self-care.

Nursing Interventions

Relieving Impaired Comfort

Treatment with the appropriate medication usually relieves discomfort. Sitz baths may be occasionally recommended and may provide temporary relief of symptoms.

Reducing Anxiety

Vulvovaginal infections are upsetting and require treatment. The patient who experiences such an infection may be very anxious about the significance of the symptoms and possible causes. Explaining the cause of symptoms may reduce anxiety related to fear of a more serious illness. Discussing ways to help prevent vulvovaginal infections may help patients adopt specific strategies to decrease infection and the related symptoms.

Preventing Reinfection or Spread of Infection

Patient education should include the fact that vulvovaginal candidiasis is not an STI and incidence can be decreased by completing treatment, avoiding unnecessary antibiotic agents, wearing cotton underwear, and not douching. Prevention strategies for vaginal infections include promotion of adequate rest, reduction of life stress, and a healthy diet low in refined sugars (Schuiling & Likis, 2013).

The patient needs to be informed about the importance of adequate treatment for herself and her partner, if indicated. Other strategies to prevent persistence or spread of infection include abstaining from sexual intercourse when infected, treatment for sexual partners, and minimizing irritation of the affected area. When medications such as antibiotic agents are prescribed for any infection, the nurse instructs the patient about the usual precautions related to using these agents. If vaginal itching occurs several days after use, the patient can be reassured that this is usually not an allergic reaction but may be a yeast or monilial infection resulting from altered vaginal bacteria. Treatment for monilial infection is prescribed if indicated.

Another goal of treatment is to reduce tissue irritation caused by scratching or wearing tight clothing. The area needs to be kept clean by daily bathing and adequate hygiene after voiding and defecation. The use of a hair dryer on a cool setting will dry the area, and application of topical corticosteroids may decrease irritation.

When educating the patient about medications such as suppositories and devices such as applicators to dispense cream or ointment, the nurse may demonstrate the procedure by using a plastic model of the pelvis and vagina. The nurse should also stress the importance of hand hygiene before and after each administration of medication. To prevent the medication from escaping from the vagina, the patient should recline for 30 minutes after it is inserted, if possible. The patient is informed that seepage of medication may occur, and the use of a perineal pad may be helpful.

Promoting Home, Community-Based, and Transitional Care

Educating Patients About Self-Care. Vulvovaginal conditions are treated on an outpatient basis unless a patient has other medical problems. Patient education, tact, and reassurance are important aspects of nursing care. Women may express embarrassment, guilt, or anger and may be concerned that the infection could be serious or that it may have been acquired from a sex partner. In some instances, treatment plans include the partner.

The nurse assesses the patient's learning needs about the immediate problem. The patient needs to know the characteristics of normal as opposed to abnormal discharge. Questions often arise about douching. Normally, douching and the use of feminine hygiene sprays are unnecessary because daily baths or showers and proper hygiene after voiding and defecating keep the perineal area clean. Douching tends to eliminate normal flora, reducing the body's ability to ward off infection. In addition, repeated douching may result in vaginal epithelial breakdown and chemical irritation and has been associated with other pelvic disorders. In the case of recurrent yeast infections, the perineum should be kept as dry as possible. Loose-fitting cotton instead of tight-fitting synthetic, nonabsorbent, heat-retaining underwear is recommended.

Vulvar self-examination is a good health practice for all women. Becoming familiar with one's own anatomy and reporting anything that seems new or different may result in early detection and treatment of any new disorders. Nurses can also play a role in educating women about the risks of unprotected intercourse, particularly with partners who have had sex with others.

Evaluation

Expected patient outcomes may include:

1. Experiences increased comfort
   a. Cleans the perineum as instructed
   b. Reports that itching is relieved
   c. Maintains urine output within normal limits and without dysuria
2. Experiences relief of anxiety
3. Remains free from infection
   a. Has no signs of inflammation, pruritus, odor, or dysuria
   b. Notes that vaginal discharge appears normal (thin, clear, not frothy)
4. Participates in self-care
   a. Takes medication as prescribed
   b. Wears absorbent underwear
   c. Avoids unprotected sexual intercourse
   d. Douches only as prescribed
   e. Performs vulvar self-examination regularly and reports any new findings to primary provider

Human Papillomavirus

Human papillomavirus (HPV) is the most common STI in the United States, affecting 79 million Americans and about 14 million newly acquired infections each year. Most adults who are sexually active will be infected with at least one type of HPV during their lifetime (CDC, 2014b). Most infections are self-limiting and without symptoms, and others can cause cervical and anogenital cancers. Infections can be latent (asymptomatic and detected only by deoxyribonucleic acid [DNA] hybridization tests for HPV), subclinical (visualized only after application of acetic acid followed by inspection under magnification), or clinical (visible condylomata acuminata).

Pathophysiology

HPV can be found in lesions of the skin, cervix, vagina, anus, penis, and oral cavity. Of the more than 100 genotypes of HPV that exist, about 30 genotypes affect the anogenital tract (Beckman et al., 2014). Some are low risk in that they are unlikely to cause cancerous changes. These include types 6, 11, 42, 43, 44, 54, 61, 70, and 72. The most common strains of HPV, 6 and 11, usually cause **condylomata** (warty growths) that can appear on the vulva, vagina, cervix, and anus. These are often visible or may be palpable by patients. Condylomata are rarely premalignant but are an outward manifestation of the virus (Beckman et al., 2014). High-risk oncogenic types, including 16, 18, 31, 33, 45, and 52 affect the cervix, causing abnormal cell changes or **dysplasia** (found on a Papanicolaou [Pap] smear). HPV types 16 and 18 account for 66% of cervical cancer cases, while types 31, 33, 45, and 52 account for another 15% (American College of Obstetricians and Gynecologists [ACOG], 2015a). The incidence of HPV in young women who are sexually active is high. The infection often disappears as the result of an effective immune system response. It is thought that two proteins produced by high-risk types of HPV interfere with tumor suppression by normal cells. Risk factors include being young, being sexually active, having multiple sex partners, and having sex with a partner who has or has had multiple partners. It can be transmitted by other means, however, as it has been found in young girls who have not been sexually active.

Medical Management

Options for the treatment of external genital warts by a primary provider include topical application of trichloroacetic acid, podophyllin (Podofin, Podocon), cryotherapy, as well as surgical removal. Topical agents that can be applied by patients to external lesions include podofilox (Condylox) and imiquimod (Aldara). Because the safety of podophyllin, imiquimod, and podofilox during pregnancy has not been determined, these agents should not be used during pregnancy. Electrocautery and laser therapy are alternative therapies that may be indicated for patients with a large number or area of genital warts.

Treatment usually eradicates perineal warts or condylomata. However, they may resolve spontaneously without treatment and may also recur even with treatment. Genital warts are more resistant to treatment in patients with diabetes, those who are pregnant, who smoke, or are immunocompromised (Beckmann et al., 2014).

If the treatment includes application of a topical agent by the patient, she needs to be carefully instructed in the use of the agent prescribed and must be able to identify the warts and be able to apply the medication to them. The patient is instructed to anticipate mild pain or local irritation with the use of these agents.

Women with HPV should have annual Pap smears because of the potential of HPV to cause dysplasia. Much remains unknown about subclinical and latent HPV disease. Women are often exposed to HPV by partners who are unknowing carriers. The use of condoms can reduce the likelihood of transmission, but transmission can also occur during skin-to-skin contact in areas not covered by condoms.

In many cases, patients are angry about having warts or HPV and do not know who infected them because the incubation period can be long and partners may have no symptoms. Acknowledging the emotional distress that occurs when an STI is diagnosed and providing support and facts are important nursing actions.

Prevention

The best strategy is prevention of HPV. The Advisory Committee on Immunization Practices (ACIP) of the CDC recommends routine vaccination of boys and girls 11 to 12 years of age, before they become sexually active. Vaccination is also recommended for females aged 13 through 26 years and males aged 13 through 21 years (Petrosky, Bocchini, Heriri, et al., 2015). The ACIP recommends the newly approved 9-valent human papillomavirus (9vHPV) vaccine as one of the three used for routine vaccinations. In addition to the four noninfectious virus–like particles (VLP) HPV 6, 11, 16, and 18 found in 4vHPV, 9vHPV also contains HPV 31, 33, 45, 52, and 58 VLPs (Petrosky et al., 2015). The vaccination is given in 3 intramuscular doses, with the initial dose followed by a second dose in 2 months and a third dose 6 months after the first dose. Completion of all 3 doses of the vaccine is important for immunity to develop. The vaccination is contraindicated for use in women who are pregnant (Petrosky et al., 2015).

Although this vaccine is considered an important medical breakthrough with the potential to decrease the impact of HPV-related disease in men and women, it does not replace other strategies important in prevention of HPV. Women still need cervical cancer screening (CDC, 2014b).

Herpes Virus Type 2 Infection (Herpes Genitalis, Herpes Simplex Virus)

Herpes simplex virus 2 (HSV2) is a recurrent, lifelong viral infection that causes herpetic lesions (blisters) on the external genitalia and occasionally the vagina and cervix. It is an STI but possibly may also be transmitted asexually from wet surfaces or by self-transmission (i.e., touching a cold sore and then touching the genital area). The initial infection is usually very painful and blisters may take 2 to 4 weeks to heal, but it can also be asymptomatic. Over 87% of infected individuals are unaware of their infection; most HSV transmission occurs from asymptomatic viral shedding (Bechtel & Trout, 2015; CDC, 2015c). Recurrences are less painful, self-limited and usually produce less severe symptoms. Some patients have few or no recurrences, whereas others have frequent bouts (CDC, 2015c). Recurrences can be associated with stress, sunburn, dental work, or inadequate rest or poor nutrition, or any situations that tax the immune system.

At least 50 million people in the United States have genital herpes infection, and most have not been diagnosed (CDC, 2015c). The prevalence of other STIs has decreased slightly, possibly because of increased condom use, but herpes can be transmitted by contact with skin that is not covered by a condom. Transmission is possible even when a carrier does not have symptoms (subclinical shedding). Lesions increase vulnerability to HIV infection and other STIs. Vaccines for herpes genitalis are in clinical trials; however, at this time, there is no commercially available vaccine (CDC, 2015c).

Pathophysiology

There are nine types of herpes viruses belonging to three different groups that cause infections in humans (Beckmann et al., 2014). These include herpes simplex type 1 (HSV-1), usually associated with cold sores of the lips; herpes simplex type 2 (HSV-2), usually associated with genital herpes; varicella zoster or shingles; Epstein–Barr virus; cytomegalovirus; human B-lymphotropic virus; and others.

Close human contact by the mouth, oropharynx, mucosal surface, vagina, or cervix appears necessary to acquire the infection. Other susceptible sites are skin lacerations and conjunctivae. Usually, the virus is killed at room temperature by drying. When viral replication diminishes, the virus ascends the peripheral sensory nerves and remains inactive in the nerve ganglia. Another outbreak may occur when the host is subjected to stress. In women who are pregnant and have active herpes, infants delivered vaginally may become infected with the virus. There is a risk of fetal morbidity and mortality if this occurs; therefore, a cesarean delivery may be performed if the virus recurs near the time of delivery.

Clinical Manifestations

Itching and pain occur as the infected area becomes red and edematous. Infection may begin with macules and papules and progress to vesicles and ulcers. The vesicular state often appears as a blister, which later coalesces, ulcerates, and encrusts. In women, the labia are the usual primary site, although the cervix, vagina, and perianal skin may be affected. In men, the glans penis, foreskin, or penile shaft is typically affected. Influenza like symptoms may occur 3 or 4 days after the lesions appear. Inguinal lymphadenopathy (enlarged lymph nodes in the groin), minor temperature elevation, malaise, headache, myalgia (aching muscles), and dysuria (pain on urination) are often noted. Pain is evident during the first week and then decreases. The lesions last 2 to 12 days before crusting over (Bechtel & Trout, 2015).

Rarely, complications may arise from extragenital spread, such as to the buttocks, upper thighs, or even the eyes, as a result of touching lesions and then touching other areas. Patients should be advised to wash their hands after contact with lesions. Other potential problems are aseptic meningitis, neonatal transmission, and severe emotional stress related to the diagnosis.

Medical Management

Currently, there is no cure for genital herpes infection, but treatment is aimed at relieving the symptoms. Management goals include preventing the spread of infection, making patients comfortable, decreasing potential health risks, and initiating a counseling and education program. Three oral antiviral agents—acyclovir (Zovirax), valacyclovir (Valtrex), and famciclovir (Famvir)—can suppress symptoms and shorten the course of the infection (Bechtel & Trout, 2015). These agents are effective at reducing the duration of lesions and preventing recurrences. Analgesics and a saline compress can provide additional relief of symptoms. Resistance and long-term side effects do not appear to be major problems. Recurrent episodes are often milder than the initial episode. Prophylactic vaccine and topical gel development for genital herpes continues to be investigated in clinical trials (Bechtel & Trout, 2015; National Institute of Allergy & Infectious Disease [NIAID], 2015).

NURSING PROCESS

The Patient With a Genital Herpes Infection

Assessment

The health history and a physical and pelvic examination are important in establishing the nature of the infectious condition. In addition, patients are assessed for risk of STIs. The perineum is inspected for painful lesions. Inguinal nodes are assessed and are often enlarged and tender during an occurrence of genital herpes.

Diagnosis

NURSING DIAGNOSES

Based on the assessment data, major nursing diagnoses may include the following:

- Acute pain related to the genital lesions
- Risk for infection or spread of infection
- Anxiety related to the diagnosis
- Deficient knowledge about the disease and its management

Planning and Goals

Major goals may include relief of pain and discomfort, control of infection and its spread, relief of anxiety, knowledge of and adherence to the treatment regimen and self-care, and knowledge about implications for the future.

Nursing Interventions

RELIEVING PAIN

The lesions should be kept clean, and proper hygiene practices are advocated. Sitz baths may ease discomfort. Additional strategies for relieving pain during a herpes outbreak can be found in Chart 57-2.

The patient is encouraged to increase fluid intake, to be alert for possible bladder distention, and to contact her primary provider immediately if she cannot void because of discomfort. Painful voiding may occur if urine comes in contact with the herpes lesions. Discomfort with urination can be reduced by pouring warm water over the vulva during voiding. When oral antiviral agents are prescribed, the patient is instructed about when to take the medication and what side effects to note, such as rash and headache.

PREVENTING INFECTION AND ITS SPREAD

The risk of reinfection and spread of infection to others or to other structures of the body can be reduced by proper hand hygiene, the use of barrier methods with sexual contact, and adherence to prescribed medication regimens. Avoidance of contact when obvious lesions are present does not eliminate the risk because the virus can be shed in the absence of symptoms, and lesions may not be visible.

RELIEVING ANXIETY

Concern about the presence of herpes infection, future occurrences of lesions, and the impact of the infection on future relationships and childbearing may cause considerable patient anxiety. Nurses serve as important sources of support by listening to patients' concerns and providing information and instruction. The patient may be angry with her partner if the partner is the probable source of the infection. The patient may need assistance in discussing the infection and its implications with her current sexual partners and in future sexual relationships. The nurse can refer the patient to a support group to assist in coping with the diagnosis (see the Resources section).

INCREASING KNOWLEDGE ABOUT THE DISEASE AND ITS TREATMENT

Patient education is an essential part of nursing care of the patient with a genital herpes infection. This includes an adequate explanation about the infection and how it is transmitted, management and treatment strategies, strategies to minimize spread of infection, the importance of adherence to the treatment regimen, and self-care strategies. Because of the increased risk of HIV and other STIs in the presence of

---

Chart 57-2	**HEALTH PROMOTION**

Strategies for The Patient With Genital Herpes

Herpes is transmitted mainly by direct contact. Intercourse during a herpes outbreak not only increases the risk of transmission but also increases the likelihood of contracting HIV and other STIs. Women therefore take the following measures:

- Abstains from sexual intercourse during treatment for active disease (other options such as hand holding and kissing are acceptable).
- Avoids exposure to the sun, which can cause recurrences (and skin cancer).
- Avoids self-infection by not touching lesions during an outbreak.
- Uses barrier methods when engaging in intercourse to provide protection against viral transmission.
- Informs sexual partners of herpes diagnosis as transmission is possible even in the absence of active lesions.
- Informs obstetric care provider about the history of genital herpes. In cases of recurrence at time of delivery, cesarean section may be considered.

- Joins a support group to share solutions and experiences and hear about newer treatments (see Resources section).
- Keeps follow-up appointments with health care provider, and reports repeated recurrences (may not be as severe as the initial episode).
- Takes medication prescribed for outbreaks and avoids occlusive ointments, strong perfumed soaps, or bubble bath.
- Takes aspirin and other analgesic agents to control pain during outbreaks.
- Uses the appropriate hygiene practices including hand hygiene, perineal cleanliness, gentle washing of lesions with mild soap and running water and lightly drying lesions (i.e., lesions can become infected from germs on the hand, and the virus from the lesion can be transmitted from the hand to another area of the body or another person).
- Wears loose, comfortable clothing; eats a balanced diet; ingests adequate fluids gets adequate rest during outbreaks.

HIV, human immune deficiency virus; STIs, sexually transmitted infections.

skin lesions, an important part of education involves informing the patient of strategies to protect herself from exposure to HIV and other STIs.

PROMOTING HOME, COMMUNITY-BASED,
AND TRANSITIONAL CARE

Educating Patients About Self-Care. Health promotion strategies and self-care measures for the patient with genital herpes are described in Chart 57-2.

Evaluation

Expected patient outcomes may include:

1. Experiences a reduction in pain and discomfort
2. Keeps infection under control
   a. Demonstrates proper hygiene techniques
   b. Takes medication as prescribed
   c. Consumes adequate fluids
   d. Assesses own current lifestyle (diet, adequate fluid intake, safer sex practices, stress management)
3. Uses strategies to reduce anxiety
   a. Verbalizes issues and concerns related to genital herpes infection
   b. Discusses strategies to deal with issues and concerns with current and future sexual partners
   c. Initiates contact with support group if indicated
4. Demonstrates knowledge about genital herpes and strategies to control and minimize recurrences
   a. Identifies methods of transmission of herpes infection and strategies to prevent transmission to others
   b. Discusses strategies to reduce recurrence of lesions
   c. Takes medications as prescribed
   d. Reports no recurrence of lesions

Endocervicitis and Cervicitis

Endocervicitis is an inflammation of the mucosa and the glands of the cervix that may occur when organisms gain access to the cervical glands after intercourse and, less often, after procedures such as abortion, intrauterine manipulation, or vaginal delivery. If untreated, the infection may extend into the uterus, fallopian tubes, and pelvic cavity. Inflammation can irritate the cervical tissue, resulting in spotting or bleeding and mucopurulent cervicitis (inflammation of the cervix with exudate).

Chlamydia and Gonorrhea

Chlamydia and gonorrhea are the most common causes of endocervicitis, although *Mycoplasma* may also be involved. Chlamydia causes about 2.86 million infections every year in the United States; it is most commonly found in young people who are sexually active with more than one partner and is transmitted through sexual contact (CDC, 2015d). Untreated chlamydia infections can spread to the fallopian tubes and uterus leading to serious complications including PID, an increased risk of ectopic pregnancy, and infertility (CDC, 2015d). Chlamydial infections of the cervix often produce no symptoms, but cervical discharge, dyspareunia, dysuria, and bleeding may occur. Other complications include conjunctivitis and perihepatitis (Fitz–Hugh–Curtis

syndrome) (CDC, 2015d). Gonorrhea is the second most commonly reported STI, with an estimated 820,000 new infections each year (CDC, 2015e). The inflamed cervix that results from infection may leave a woman more vulnerable to HIV transmission from an infected partner. Gonorrhea is often asymptomatic and a major cause of PID, tubal infertility, ectopic pregnancy, and chronic pelvic pain (CDC, 2015e). Diagnosis can be confirmed by urine culture or other methods such as using a swab to obtain a sample of cervical or penile discharge from the patient's partner (CDC, 2015e).

Medical Management

The CDC recommends treating chlamydia with doxycycline (Vibramycin) for 1 week or with a single dose of azithromycin (Zithromax) (CDC, 2015a). Antimicrobial resistance to fluoroquinolones in the treatment of gonorrhea has left cephalosporins as the remaining recommended treatment (ACOG, 2015b; CDC, 2015e). Dual therapy with azithromycin and ceftriaxone given simultaneously on the same day is the recommended first-line treatment for gonorrhea infection (ACOG, 2015b; CDC, 2015e). Partners must also be treated. Women who are pregnant are cautioned not to take tetracycline because of potential adverse effects on the fetus. In these cases, erythromycin may be prescribed. Results are usually good if treatment begins early. Possible complications from delayed or no treatment are tubal disease, ectopic pregnancy, PID, and infertility.

Cultures for chlamydia and other STIs should be obtained from all patients who have been sexually assaulted when they first seek medical attention; patients are treated prophylactically. Cultures should then be repeated in 2 weeks. Annual screening for chlamydia is recommended for all young women who are sexually active and older women with new sex partners or multiple partners (CDC, 2015d).

Nursing Management

All women who are sexually active may be at risk for chlamydia, gonorrhea, and other STIs, including HIV. Nurses can assist patients in assessing their own risk. Recognition of risk is a first step before changes in behavior occur. Patients should be discouraged from assuming that a partner is "safe" without open, honest discussion. Nonjudgmental attitudes, educational counseling, and role-playing may be helpful.

Because chlamydia, gonorrhea, and other STIs may have a serious effect on future health and fertility, and because many of these disorders can be prevented by the use of condoms and spermicides and careful choice of partners, nurses can play a major role in counseling patients about safer sex practices. Exploring options with patients, addressing knowledge deficits, and correcting misinformation may reduce morbidity and mortality.

Patients should be advised to refer partners for evaluation and treatment. All women aged 25 and younger who are sexually active should be screened annually. Those older than 25 years should be screened if risk factors are present. Repeat testing should occur 3 months after treatment (CDC, 2015d).

Promoting Home, Community-Based, and Transitional Care

Educating Patients About Self-Care

Nurses can educate women and help them improve communication skills and initiate discussions about sex with their partners. Communicating with partners about sex, risk, postponing intercourse, and using safer sex behaviors, including the use of condoms, may be lifesaving. Some young women report having sex but not being comfortable enough to discuss sexual risk issues. Nurses can help women to advocate for their own health by discussing safety with partners prior to sexual activity.

Reinforcing the need for annual screening for chlamydia and other STIs is an important part of patient education. Instructions also include the need for the patient to abstain from sexual intercourse until all of her sex partners are treated (CDC, 2015d).

Pelvic Inflammatory Disease

Pelvic inflammatory disease (PID) is an inflammatory condition of the pelvic cavity that may begin with cervicitis and involve the uterus (endometritis), fallopian tubes (salpingitis), ovaries (oophoritis), pelvic peritoneum, or pelvic vascular system. Infection, which may be acute, subacute, recurrent, or chronic and localized or widespread, is usually caused by bacteria but may be attributed to a virus, fungus, or parasite. Gonorrheal and chlamydial organisms are common causes, but most cases of PID are polymicrobial. While incidence has been declining over the past decades, there are an estimated 750,000 cases of PID each year (Brunham, Gottlieb, & Paavonen, 2015; CDC, 2015f).

Short- and long-term consequences can occur. The fallopian tubes become narrow and scarred, which increases the risk of ectopic pregnancy (fertilized eggs trapped in the tube), infertility, recurrent pelvic pain, tubo-ovarian **abscess** (a collection of purulent material), and recurrent disease.

Pathophysiology

The exact pathogenesis of PID has not been determined, but it is presumed that organisms usually enter the body through the vagina, pass through the cervical canal, colonize the endocervix, and move upward into the uterus. Under various conditions, the organisms may proceed to one or both fallopian tubes and ovaries and into the pelvis. In bacterial infections that occur after childbirth or abortion, pathogens are disseminated directly through the tissues that support the uterus by way of the lymphatics and blood vessels (see Fig. 57-1A). In pregnancy, the increased blood supply required by the placenta provides a wider pathway for infection. These postpartum and postabortion infections tend to be unilateral. Infections can cause perihepatic inflammation when the organism invades the peritoneum.

In gonorrheal infections, the gonococci pass through the cervical canal and into the uterus, where the environment, especially during menstruation, allows them to multiply rapidly and spread to the fallopian tubes and into the pelvis (see Fig. 57-1B). The infection is usually bilateral.

In rare instances, organisms (e.g., tuberculosis) gain access to the reproductive organs by way of the bloodstream from the lungs (see Fig. 57-1C). One of the most common causes of **salpingitis** (inflammation of the fallopian tube) is chlamydia, possibly accompanied by gonorrhea.

Pelvic infection is most often sexually transmitted but can also occur with invasive procedures such as endometrial biopsy, abortion, hysteroscopy, or insertion of an intrauterine device. Bacterial vaginosis (a vaginal infection) may predispose women to pelvic infection. Risk factors include early age at first intercourse, multiple sexual partners, frequent intercourse, intercourse without condoms, sex with a partner with an STI, and a history of STIs or previous pelvic infection.

Clinical Manifestations

Symptoms of pelvic infection usually begin with vaginal discharge, dyspareunia, dysuria, pelvic or lower abdominal pain, tenderness that occurs after menses and postcoital bleeding. Other symptoms include fever, general malaise, anorexia, nausea, headache, and possibly vomiting. On pelvic examination, intense tenderness may be noted on palpation of the uterus or movement of the cervix (cervical motion tenderness). Symptoms may be acute and severe or low grade and subtle (Brunham et al., 2015; CDC, 2015f).

Complications

Pelvic or generalized peritonitis, abscesses, strictures, and fallopian tube obstruction may develop. Obstruction may

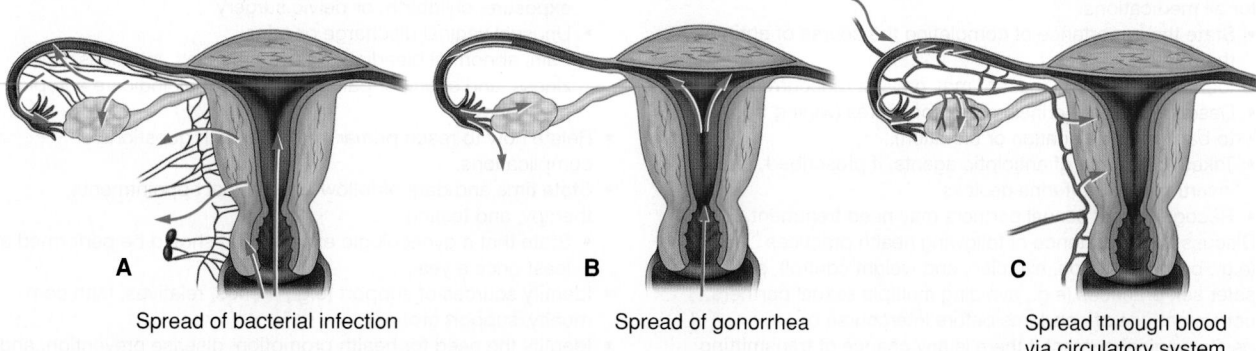

A Spread of bacterial infection   **B** Spread of gonorrhea   **C** Spread through blood via circulatory system

Figure 57-1 • Pathway by which microorganisms spread in pelvic infections. **A.** Bacterial infection spreads up the vagina into the uterus and through the lymphatics. **B.** Gonorrhea spreads up the vagina into the uterus and then to the tubes and ovaries. **C.** Bacterial infection can reach the reproductive organs through the bloodstream (hematogenous spread).

cause an ectopic pregnancy in the future if a fertilized egg cannot pass a tubal stricture, or scar tissue may occlude the tubes, resulting in sterility. Adhesions are common and often result in chronic pelvic pain; they eventually may require removal of the uterus, fallopian tubes, and ovaries.

Medical Management

Broad-spectrum antibiotic therapy is prescribed, usually a combination of ceftriaxone (Rocephin), doxycycline, and metronidazole (Flagyl). Women are most often treated as outpatients and monitored carefully. Indications for hospitalization include surgical emergencies, pregnancy, no clinical response to oral antimicrobial therapy, inability to follow or tolerate an outpatient oral regimen, severe illness (i.e., nausea, vomiting, or high fever), and tubo-ovarian abscess (Brunham et al., 2015). Treatment of sexual partners is necessary to prevent reinfection.

Nursing Management

The nurse assesses for both the physical and emotional effects of PID. The patient may feel well one day and experience vague symptoms and discomfort the next. She may also suffer from constipation and menstrual difficulties.

If the patient is hospitalized, the nurse prepares the patient for further diagnostic evaluation and surgical intervention as prescribed. Accurate recording of vital signs, intake and output, and the characteristics and amount of vaginal discharge is necessary as a guide to therapy.

The nurse administers analgesic agents as prescribed for pain relief. Adequate rest and a healthy diet are encouraged. In addition, the nurse minimizes the transmission of infection by adhering to appropriate infection control practices and performing meticulous hand hygiene.

Promoting Home, Community-Based, and Transitional Care

Educating Patients About Self-Care

The patient must be informed of the need for precautions and must be encouraged to take part in procedures to prevent infecting others and protect herself from reinfection. The use of condoms is essential to prevent infection and sequelae. If reinfection occurs or if the infection spreads, symptoms may include abdominal pain, nausea and vomiting, fever, malaise, malodorous purulent vaginal discharge, and leukocytosis. Patient education consists of explaining how pelvic infections occur, how they can be controlled and avoided, and the associated signs and symptoms. Guidelines and instructions provided to the patient are summarized in Chart 57-3.

All patients who have had PID need to be informed of the signs and symptoms of ectopic pregnancy (pain, abnormal bleeding, delayed menses, faintness, dizziness, and shoulder pain), because they are prone to this complication. See Chapter 56 for a discussion of ectopic pregnancy.

Human Immune Deficiency Virus Infection and Acquired Immune Deficiency Syndrome

Any discussion of vulvovaginal infections and STIs must include the topic of HIV and acquired immune deficiency syndrome (AIDS). The CDC (2015g) estimates approximately one in four people living with HIV are women and 84% of new HIV infections in women are from heterosexual contact. Because HIV infection may be detected during prenatal testing and screening for STIs, nurses and other women's health care clinicians may be the first professionals to provide care for a woman with HIV infection. Thus, clinicians need to be

---

Chart 57-3

HOME CARE CHECKLIST

The Patient With Pelvic Inflammatory Disease

At the completion of education, the patient and/or caregiver will be able to:

- State the impact of pelvic inflammatory disease on physiologic functioning, ADLs, IADLs, roles, relationships, and spirituality.
- Identify the name, dose, side effects, frequency, and schedule for all medications.
  - State the importance of completing the course of antibiotic therapy.
- Understand interventions that may prevent reoccurrence:
  - Describe proper perineal care procedures (wiping from front to back after defecation or urination).
  - Takes full course of antibiotic agents, if prescribed, after insertion of intrauterine devices.
  - Recognize that sexual partners may need treatment.
- Discuss the importance of following health practices (e.g., proper nutrition, exercise, and weight control), and safer sex practices (e.g., avoiding multiple sexual partners, consistent use of condoms before intercourse or any penile–vaginal contact if there is any chance of transmitting infection).

- State symptoms which require evaluation by a health care provider:
  - Pelvic pain or abnormal discharge, particularly after sexual exposure, childbirth, or pelvic surgery.
  - Unusual vaginal discharge or odor.
  - Pain, abnormal bleeding, delayed menses, faintness, dizziness, and shoulder pain (symptoms may indicate ectopic pregnancy).
- Relate how to reach primary provider with questions or complications.
- State time and date of follow-up medical appointments, therapy, and testing.
  - State that a gynecologic examination should be performed at least once a year.
- Identify sources of support (e.g., friends, relatives, faith community, support groups).
- Identify the need for health promotion, disease prevention, and screening activities.

ADL, activities of daily living; IADL, independent activities of daily living.

knowledgeable about this disorder and sensitive to women's issues and concerns.

After informed consent is obtained, women who are at risk for HIV are offered testing by a nurse or counselor. Because patients may be reluctant to discuss risk-taking behavior, routine screening should be offered to all women between the ages of 13 and 64 years in all health care settings (Shuiling & Likis, 2013). Early detection permits early treatment to delay progression of the disease. The nurse needs to remember that many women do not see themselves as at risk for acquiring HIV infection. See Chapter 36 for further discussion of HIV infection and AIDS.

Research suggests that African-American women living with HIV infection experience the effects of the infection in all aspects of their lives (Peltzer, Domain, & Teel, 2015) (see Chart 57-4). Women with HIV and women with partners who have HIV must be counseled about safer sex and informed about the dangers of unprotected sex. Inconsistent use of condoms results in a higher seroconversion rate. Because there is a risk of perinatal transmission, decisions to conceive or to use contraception must be based on education, accurate information, and care. Women who are pregnant are advised to have an HIV test. The use of antiretroviral agents by women who are pregnant significantly decreases perinatal transmission of HIV infection. Therefore, the use of these agents during pregnancy is critical and must also be discussed. For women who choose to avoid conception, the use of condoms alone and with oral contraceptives are possible choices.

STRUCTURAL DISORDERS

Fistulas of the Vagina

A **fistula** is an abnormal opening between two internal hollow organs or between an internal hollow organ and the exterior of the body. The name of the fistula indicates the two areas that are connected abnormally—for example, a vesicovaginal fistula is an opening between the bladder and the vagina,

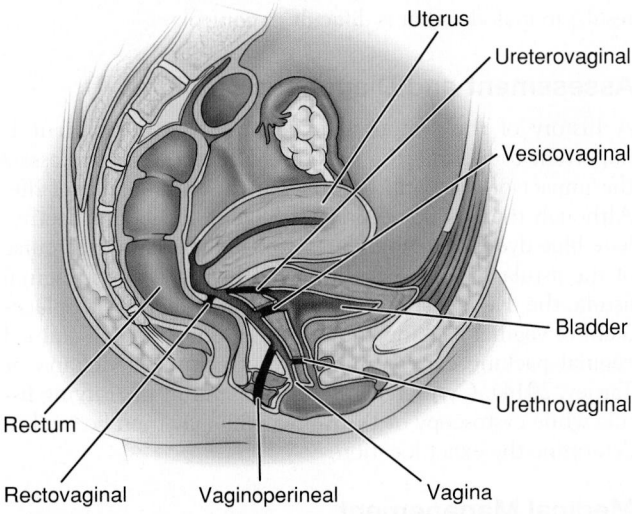

Figure 57-2 • Common sites for vaginal fistulas. *Vesicovaginal*—bladder and vagina. *Urethrovaginal*—urethra and vagina. *Vaginoperineal*—vagina and perineal area. *Ureterovaginal*—ureter and vagina. *Rectovaginal*—rectum and vagina.

and a rectovaginal fistula is an opening between the rectum and the vagina (see Fig. 57-2). Fistulas may be congenital in origin but are most common in developing countries due to obstructed labor complications. In developed countries, they occur most often as a result of injury during pelvic surgery, vaginal delivery, radiation therapy, complications from surgical insertion of vaginal mesh, or disease processes such as carcinoma (Mellano & Tarney, 2014).

Clinical Manifestations

Symptoms depend on the specific defect. For example, in a patient with a vesicovaginal fistula, urine escapes continuously into the vagina. With a rectovaginal fistula, there is fecal incontinence, and flatus is discharged through the

---

NURSING RESEARCH PROFILE

Chart 57-4

Life With HIV Infection

Peltzer, J., Domain, E., & Teel, C. (2015). Living in the everydayness of HIV infection: Experiences of young African-American women. *Medsurg Nursing, 24*(2), 111–118.

Purpose

The purpose of this study was to understand the lived experience of being a young African-American woman infected with HIV, and how she defines and practices both spirituality and self-care. Of US females who are HIV positive, 64% are African Americans; yet, little research has been done examining the self-care behaviors among African-American women who are infected with HIV.

Design

This study used a qualitative phenomenologic methodology. In-depth interviews were conducted with 11 African-American women, 18–35 years of age, who were HIV positive. The women were recruited through links provided from case managers at a safety net clinic and through an infectious disease clinic in a Midwestern, metropolitan city.

Findings

The study characterized the lived experiences of the women with HIV infection as infected lives. This predominant pattern portrays how living with HIV has impacted every aspect of their lives. The women were for the most part physically able to continue their daily routines. However, mentally and emotionally, the women were experiencing significant distress leading to chronic depression, isolation, and strained family and community relations.

Nursing Implications

Nurses should receive comprehensive HIV education that includes an overview of common, everyday experiences of women with HIV infection. Themes throughout this study clearly indicate that African-American women with HIV infection are affected in every aspect of their lives. Nurses should use the results from this study to add depression screening and assessments regarding self-care and spiritual beliefs and practices to their care of these women.

vagina. The combination of fecal discharge with leukorrhea results in malodor that is difficult to control.

Assessment and Diagnostic Findings

A history of the symptoms experienced by the patient is important to identify the structural alterations and to assess the impact of the symptoms on the patient's quality of life. Although there is no reported specificity for its use, methylene blue dye is commonly used to help delineate the course of the fistula (Mellano & Tarney, 2014). In a vesicovaginal fistula, the dye is instilled into the bladder along with placement of vaginal packing known as the "tampon test"; stained vaginal packing can be indicative of a fistula (Mellano & Tarney, 2014). Cystourethroscopy is useful in identifying fistula while cystoscopy or IV pyelography may then be used to determine the exact location.

Medical Management

The goal is to eliminate the fistula and to treat infection and excoriation. A fistula may heal without surgical intervention, but surgery is often required. If the primary provider determines that a fistula will heal without surgical intervention, care is planned to relieve discomfort, prevent infection, and improve the patient's self-concept and self-care abilities. Measures to promote healing include proper nutrition, cleansing douches and enemas, rest, and administration of prescribed intestinal antibiotic agents. A rectovaginal fistula heals faster when the patient eats a low-residue diet and when the affected tissue drains properly. Warm perineal irrigations promote healing.

Sometimes, a fistula does not heal and cannot be surgically repaired. In this situation, care must be planned and implemented on an individual basis. Cleanliness, frequent sitz baths, and deodorizing douches are required, as are perineal pads and protective undergarments. Meticulous skin care is necessary to prevent excoriation. Applying bland creams or lightly dusting with cornstarch may be soothing. In addition, attending to the patient's social and psychological needs is an essential aspect of care.

If the patient is to have a fistula repaired surgically, preoperative treatment of any existing vaginitis is important to ensure success. Usually, the vaginal approach is used to repair vesicovaginal and urethrovaginal fistulas; the abdominal approach is used to repair fistulas that are large or complex. Fistulas that are difficult to repair or very large may require surgical repair with a urinary or fecal diversion. Tissue transfer techniques (skin or tissue grafting) may be used (Mellano & Tarney, 2014).

Because fistulas usually are related to obstetric, surgical, or radiation trauma, occurrence in a patient without previous vaginal delivery or a history of surgery must be evaluated carefully. Crohn's disease and lymphogranuloma venereum are other possible causes.

Despite the best surgical intervention, fistulas may recur. After surgery, medical follow-up continues for at least 2 years to monitor for a possible recurrence.

Pelvic Organ Prolapse: Cystocele, Rectocele, Enterocele

Age and parity can put strain on the ligaments and structures that make up the female pelvis and pelvic floor. Childbirth can result in tears of the levator sling musculature, resulting in structural weakness. Hormone deficiency also may play a role. Some degree of prolapse (weakening of the vaginal walls allowing the pelvic organs to descend and protrude into the vaginal canal) may be found in older women. Risk factors include age, parity (particularly vaginal delivery), menopause, previous pelvic surgery, and possibly a genetic predisposition (Beckmann et al., 2014).

Cystocele is a downward displacement of the bladder toward the vaginal orifice (see Fig. 57-3) from damage to the anterior vaginal support structures. It usually results from injury and strain during childbirth. The condition usually appears years later when genital atrophy associated with aging occurs, but younger women who are multiparous and premenopausal may also be affected.

Rectocele is an upward pouching of the rectum that pushes the posterior wall of the vagina forward. Both rectoceles and perineal lacerations, which occur because of muscle tears below the vagina, may affect the muscles and tissues of the pelvic floor and may occur during childbirth. Sometimes, the lacerations may completely sever the fibers of the anal sphincter (complete tear). An **enterocele** is a protrusion of

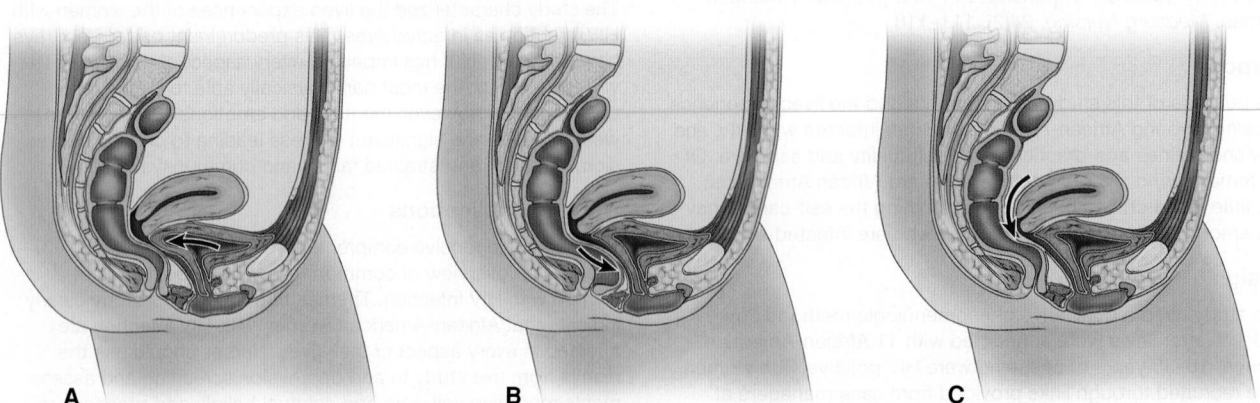

Figure 57-3 • Diagrammatic representation of the three most common types of pelvic floor relaxation. **A.** Cystocele. **B.** Rectocele. **C.** Enterocele. *Arrows* depict sites of maximum protrusion.

Performing Kegel (Pelvic Muscle) Exercises

Purposes: To strengthen and maintain the tone of the pubo-coccygeal muscle, which supports the pelvic organs; reduce or prevent stress incontinence and uterine prolapse; enhance sensation during sexual intercourse; and hasten postpartum healing.

The nurse instructs the patient to:

1. Become aware of pelvic muscle function by "drawing in" the perivaginal muscles and anal sphincter as if to control urine or defecation, but not contracting the abdominal, buttock, or inner thigh muscles.
2. Sustain contraction of the muscles for up to 10 seconds, followed by at least 10 seconds of relaxation.
3. Perform these exercises 30–80 times a day.

the intestinal wall into the vagina. Prolapse results from a weakening of the support structures of the uterus itself; the cervix drops and may protrude from the vagina. If complete prolapse occurs (cervix descending beyond vulva), it may also be referred to as procidentia.

Clinical Manifestations

Because a cystocele causes the anterior vaginal wall to bulge downward, the patient may report a sense of pelvic pressure and urinary problems such as incontinence, frequency, and urgency. Back pain and pelvic pain may occur as well. The symptoms of rectocele resemble those of cystocele, with one exception: Instead of urinary symptoms, patients may experience rectal pressure. Constipation, uncontrollable gas, and fecal incontinence may occur in patients with complete tears. Prolapse can result in feelings of pressure and ulcerations and bleeding. Dyspareunia may occur with these disorders.

Medical Management

Kegel exercises, which involve contracting or tightening the vaginal muscles, are prescribed to help strengthen these weakened muscles (Beckmann et al., 2014). The exercises are more effective in the early stages of a cystocele. Kegel exercises are easy to perform and are recommended for all women, including those with strong pelvic floor muscles (see Chart 57-5).

A pessary can be used alone or in conjunction with other treatments to avoid surgery (McIntosh, Andersen, & Reekie, 2015). This device is inserted into the vagina and positioned to keep an organ, such as the bladder, uterus, or intestine, properly aligned when a cystocele, rectocele, or prolapse has occurred. Pessaries are usually ring- or doughnut shaped and are made of various materials, such as rubber or plastic (see Fig. 57-4). Rubber pessaries must be avoided in women with latex allergy. The size and type of pessary are selected and fitted by a gynecologic health care provider. The patient should have the pessary removed, examined, and cleaned by her health care provider at prescribed intervals. At these checkups, vaginal walls should be examined for pressure points or signs of irritation. Normally, the patient experiences no pain, discomfort, or discharge with a pessary, but if chronic irritation, excessive discharge, or bleeding occurs, alternative measures may be needed (McIntosh et al., 2015).

A Colpexin Sphere is another nonsurgical device used to treat pelvic organ prolapse. This intravaginal device is similar to a pessary, but it supports the pelvic floor muscles and facilitates exercise of these muscles. It is removed daily for cleaning.

Surgical Management

In many cases, surgery helps correct structural abnormalities. The procedure to repair the anterior vaginal wall is called anterior colporrhaphy, repair of a rectocele is referred to as a posterior colporrhaphy, and repair of perineal lacerations is called a perineorrhaphy. These repairs are frequently

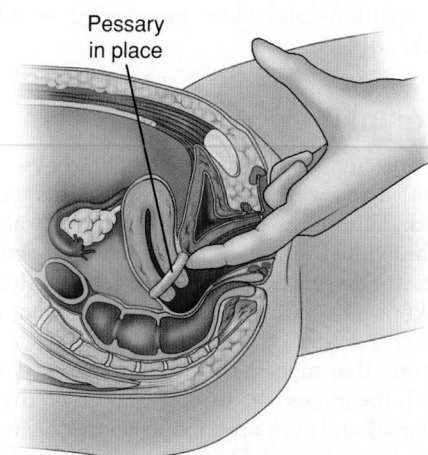

Pessary in place

A **B**

Figure 57-4 • Examples of pessaries. **A.** Various shapes and sizes of pessaries available. **B.** Insertion of one type of pessary.

Figure 57-5 • Positions of the uterus. **A.** The most common position of the uterus detected on palpation. **B.** In *retroversion,* the uterus turns posteriorly as a whole unit. **C.** In *retroflexion,* the fundus bends posteriorly. **D.** In *anteversion,* the uterus tilts forward as a whole unit. **E.** In *anteflexion,* the uterus bends anteriorly.

performed laparoscopically, resulting in short hospital lengths of stay and good outcomes. A laparoscope is inserted through a small abdominal incision, the pelvis is visualized, and surgical repairs are performed. Transvaginal surgical mesh as a treatment option has been associated with the complications of vaginal erosion, pain and infection leading to recommendations from the U.S. Food and Drug Administration (FDA) for regulatory solutions and close monitoring of adverse outcomes (FDA, 2014).

Uterine Prolapse

Usually, the uterus and the cervix lie at right angles to the long axis of the vagina with the body of the uterus inclined slightly forward. The uterus is normally freely movable on examination. Individual variations may result in an anterior, middle, or posterior uterine position. A backward positioning of the uterus, known as retroversion and retroflexion, is not uncommon (see Fig. 57-5).

If the structures that support the uterus weaken (typically from childbirth), the uterus may work its way down the vaginal canal (prolapse) and even appear outside the vaginal orifice (procidentia) (see Fig. 57-6). As the uterus descends, it may pull the vaginal walls and even the bladder and rectum

Figure 57-6 • Complete prolapse of the uterus through the introitus.

with it. Symptoms include pressure and urinary problems (incontinence or retention) from displacement of the bladder. The symptoms are aggravated when a woman coughs, lifts a heavy object, or stands for a long time. Normal activities, even walking up stairs, may aggravate the symptoms.

Medical Management

There are surgical and nonsurgical options for treatment. With surgery, the uterus is sutured back into place and repaired to strengthen and tighten the muscle bands. In women who are postmenopausal, the uterus may be removed (hysterectomy) or repaired by colpopexy. Colpocleisis, or vaginal closure, may be an option for women who do not wish to have sexual intercourse or to bear children. Conservative treatments and mechanical options, including lifestyle changes, pessaries, and pelvic floor muscle training, can usually result in symptomatic improvement. These options may be the treatment of choice for women with a mild prolapse, who desire additional children, or who are unable to tolerate surgery (Jepson & Sung, 2014).

Nursing Management

Implementing Preventive Measures

Some disorders related to "relaxed" pelvic muscles (cystocele, rectocele, and uterine prolapse) may be prevented. During pregnancy, early visits to the primary provider permit early detection of problems. During the postpartum period, the woman can be educated to perform pelvic muscle exercises, commonly known as Kegel exercises, to increase muscle mass and strengthen the muscles that support the uterus and then to continue them as a preventive action (Beckmann et al., 2014).

Delays in obtaining evaluation and treatment may result in complications such as infection, cervical ulceration, cystitis, and hemorrhoids. The nurse encourages the patient to obtain prompt treatment for these structural disorders.

Implementing Preoperative Nursing Care

Before surgery, the patient needs to know the extent of the proposed surgery, the expectations for the postoperative period, and the effect of surgery on future sexual function. In addition, the patient having a rectocele repair needs to know that before surgery, a laxative and a cleansing enema may be prescribed. She may be asked to administer these at home the day before surgery. The patient is usually placed in a lithotomy position for surgery, with special attention given to moving both legs in and out of the stirrups simultaneously to prevent muscle strain and excess pressure on the legs and thighs. Other preoperative interventions are similar to those described in Chapter 17.

Initiating Postoperative Nursing Care

Immediate postoperative goals include preventing infection and pressure on any existing suture line. This may require perineal care and may preclude using dressings. The patient is encouraged to void within a few hours after surgery for cystocele and complete tear. If the patient does not void within this period and reports discomfort or pain in the bladder region after 6 hours, she needs to be catheterized. An indwelling catheter may be indicated for 2 to 4 days, so some women may return home with a catheter in place. Various other bladder care methods are described in Chapter 55. After each voiding or bowel movement, the perineum may be cleaned with warm, sterile saline solution and dried with sterile absorbent material if a perineal incision has been made.

After an external perineal repair, the perineum is kept as clean as possible. Commercially available sprays containing combined antiseptic and anesthetic solutions are soothing and effective, and an ice pack applied locally may relieve discomfort. However, the weight of the ice bag must rest on the bed, not on the patient.

Routine postoperative care is similar to that given after abdominal surgery. The patient is positioned in bed with her head and knees elevated slightly. The patient may go home the day of or the day after surgery; the length of hospital stay depends on the surgical approach used.

After surgery for a complete perineal laceration (through the rectal sphincter), special care and attention are required. The bladder is drained through the catheter to prevent strain on the sutures. Throughout recovery, stool-softening agents are given nightly after the patient begins a soft diet.

Promoting Home, Community-Based, and Transitional Care

 Educating Patients About Self-Care

Prior to discharge, education is provided about cleanliness, prevention of constipation, recommended exercises, and avoiding lifting heavy objects or standing for prolonged periods. The patient is instructed to report any pelvic pain, unusual discharge, inability to carry out personal hygiene, and vaginal bleeding.

Continuing and Transitional Care

The patient is advised to continue with perineal exercises, which are recommended to improve muscle strength and tone. She is reminded to return to the gynecologist for a follow-up visit and to consult with the primary provider about when it is safe to resume sexual activity.

BENIGN DISORDERS

Vulvitis and Vulvodynia

Vulvitis (an inflammation of the vulva) may occur with other disorders, such as diabetes, dermatologic problems, or poor hygiene, or it may be secondary to irritation from a vaginal discharge related to a specific vaginitis.

Vulvodynia is a chronic vulvar pain syndrome. Symptoms may include burning, stinging, irritation, or stabbing pain. The syndrome has been described as primary, with onset at first tampon insertion or sexual experience, or secondary, beginning months or years after first tampon insertion or sexual experience. Women affected by this are usually between 18 and 25 years of age. Vulvodynia may be classified as organic if it has a known cause (infection, trauma, or irritants) or idiopathic if no cause is known. It can be chronic or unremitting, intermittent or episodic, or may occur only in response to contact (Hoffstetter & Shah, 2015). The pathophysiology is unknown. Vestibulodynia is the most frequent type of vulvodynia, producing sharp pain on pressure on the vestibule or posterior aspect of the vaginal opening.

Medical Management

Treatment methods for vulvodynia vary and depend on cause. Topical treatments, self-management care (strict vulvar care/hygiene), surgery, as well as biofeedback and dietary changes, have been used. Some cases seem to be similar to peripheral neuralgia and may respond to treatment with tricyclic antidepressant agents. Patients with dyspareunia or painful intercourse may benefit from referral to a behavioral or mental health professional. Research continues on the use of hypnotherapy for symptom management (Hoffstetter & Shah, 2015).

Vulvar Cysts

Bartholin cyst results from the obstruction of a duct in one of the paired Bartholin or vestibular mucus-secreting glands located in the posterior third of the vulva, near the vestibule. This cyst is the most common vulvar disorder. A simple cyst may be asymptomatic, but an infected cyst or abscess may cause discomfort. Infection may be due to a gonococcal organism, *Escherichia coli*, or *Staphylococcus aureus* and can cause an abscess with or without involving the inguinal lymph nodes. Skene duct cysts may result in pressure, dyspareunia, altered urinary stream, and pain, especially if infection is present. Vestibular cysts, located inferior to the hymen, may also occur. Cysts can be treated by resection or with laser, ablation with silver nitrate, and puncture. Asymptomatic cysts do not require treatment. Malignancy can occur, usually in women older than 40 years, so drainage and biopsy may be considered (Maldonado, 2014).

Medical Management

The usual treatment for a symptomatic Bartholin cyst or abscess is drainage. If a cyst is asymptomatic, treatment is unnecessary. Moist heat or sitz baths may promote drainage and resolution.

If drainage is necessary, several techniques are available. The simplest technique is incision and drainage. Using a Word catheter provides another method. This catheter, which is a short latex stem with an inflatable bulb at the distal end, creates a tract that preserves the gland and allows for drainage. A nonopioid analgesic agent may be given before this outpatient procedure. A local anesthetic agent is injected, and the cyst is incised or lanced and irrigated with normal saline; the catheter is inserted and inflated with 2 to 3 mL of water. The catheter stem is then tucked into the vagina to allow freedom of movement. The catheter is left in place for 4 to 6 weeks (Maldonado, 2014). The patient is informed that discharge should be expected because the catheter allows drainage of the cyst. She is instructed to contact her primary provider if pain occurs, in which case the bulb may be too large for the cavity and fluid may need to be removed. Routine hygiene is encouraged. Marsupialization (creation of small pouch) and gland removal are additional treatment options (Maldonado, 2014).

Vulvar Dystrophy

Vulvar dystrophy is a condition found in older women that causes dry, thickened skin on the vulva or slightly raised, whitish papules, fissures, or macules. Symptoms usually consist of varying degrees of itching, but some patients have no symptoms. A few patients with vulvar cancer have associated dystrophy (vulvar cancer is discussed later in this chapter). Biopsy with careful follow-up is the standard intervention. Benign dystrophies include lichen planus, lichen simplex chronicus, lichen sclerosus (benign disorder of the vulva), squamous cell hyperplasia, vulvar **vestibulitis** (inflammation of the vulvar vestibule), and other dermatoses (Beckmann et al., 2014).

Medical Management

Topical corticosteroids (i.e., hydrocortisone creams) are the usual treatment. Petrolatum jelly may relieve pruritus. Use is decreased as symptoms resolve. Topical corticosteroids are effective in treating squamous cell hyperplasia. Treatment is often complete in 2 to 3 weeks, but ongoing assessment for vulvar atrophy should occur at least annually (Beckmann et al., 2014).

If malignant cells are detected on biopsy, local excision, laser therapy, local chemotherapy, and immunologic treatment are used. Vulvectomy is avoided, if possible, to spare the patient from the stress of disfigurement and possible sexual dysfunction.

Nursing Management

Key nursing responsibilities for patients with vulvar dystrophies focus on education. Important topics include hygiene and self-monitoring for signs and symptoms of complications.

Promoting Home, Community-Based, and Transitional Care

 Educating Patients About Self-Care

Instructions for patients with benign vulvar dystrophies include the importance of maintaining good personal hygiene and keeping the vulva dry. Lanolin or hydrogenated vegetable oil is recommended for relief of dryness. Sitz baths may help but should not be overused because dryness may result or increase. The patient is instructed to notify her primary provider about any change or ulceration because biopsy may be necessary to rule out squamous cell carcinoma.

By encouraging all patients to perform genital self-examinations regularly and have any itching, lesions, or unusual symptoms assessed by a primary provider, nurses can help prevent complications and progression of vulvar lesions. Ongoing assessment should occur at least annually.

Ovarian Cysts

The ovary is a common site for cysts, which may be simple enlargements of normal ovarian constituents, the graafian follicle, or the corpus luteum, or they may arise from abnormal growth of the ovarian epithelium. Ovarian cysts are often detected on routine pelvic examination. Although these cysts are typically benign, they nevertheless should be evaluated to exclude ovarian cancer, particularly in women who are postmenopausal (ACOG, 2007, reaffirmed 2015).

The patient may or may not report acute or chronic abdominal pain. Symptoms of a ruptured cyst mimic various acute abdominal emergencies, such as appendicitis or ectopic pregnancy. Larger cysts may produce abdominal swelling and exert pressure on adjacent abdominal organs.

Postoperative nursing care after surgery to remove an ovarian cyst is similar to that after abdominal surgery, with one exception. The marked decrease in intra-abdominal pressure resulting from removal of a very large cyst usually leads to considerable abdominal distention. This may be prevented to some extent by applying a snug-fitting abdominal binder.

Some surgeons discuss the option of a hysterectomy when a woman is undergoing bilateral ovary removal because of a suspicious mass; it may increase life expectancy and avoid a later second surgery. Patient preference is a priority in determining its appropriateness.

Polycystic ovary syndrome (PCOS) is a type of hormonal imbalance or cystic disorder that affects the ovaries. This complex endocrine condition involves a disorder in the hypothalamic–pituitary and ovarian network or axis, resulting in chronic anovulation and hyperandrogenism, often along with multiple small ovarian cysts. It is common and occurs in approximately 6% to 15% of women of childbearing age (Trikudanathan, 2015). Features can include obesity, insulin resistance, glucose intolerance, dyslipidemia, sleep apnea, and infertility. Symptoms are related to androgen excess. Irregular menstrual periods, resulting from lack of regular ovulation, infertility, obesity, and hirsutism, may be a presenting complaint. Cysts form in the ovaries because the hormonal milieu cannot cause ovulation on a regular basis.

Diagnosis is based on clinical criteria, including hyperandrogenism, chronic anovulation, and polycystic ovaries on ultrasound examination. Two out of three of these criteria must be present to make the diagnosis (Trikudanathan, 2105). Women with PCOS are at increased risk for diabetes, increased blood lipids, cardiovascular disease, nonalcoholic fatty liver disease as well as anxiety and depression (Trikudanathan, 2015).

Medical Management

The treatment of large ovarian cysts is usually surgical removal. However, oral contraceptives may be used in young, healthy patients to suppress ovarian activity and resolve small cysts that appear to be fluid filled or physiologic.

Oral contraceptive agents are also usually prescribed to treat PCOS (Trikudanathan, 2015). When pregnancy is desired, medications to stimulate ovulation (clomiphene citrate [Clomid]) are often effective. Lifestyle modification is critical, and weight management is part of the treatment plan.

Weight loss as little as 5% to 10% of total body weight can help with hormone imbalance and infertility. Metformin (Glucophage) often regulates periods and can help with weight loss. (Trikudanathan, 2015). Women with this diagnosis are at increased risk for endometrial cancer due to anovulation.

Benign Tumors of the Uterus: Fibroids (Leiomyomas, Myomas)

Most women will develop myomatous or **fibroid tumors** of the uterus at some point in their life. It is estimated that by the age of 50, up to 70% of Caucasian women and 80% of African-American women will experience uterine fibroids (National Institute of Health [NIH], 2013). It is thought that women are genetically predisposed to develop this condition, which is almost always benign. Fibroids arise from the muscle tissue of the uterus and can be solitary or multiple, in the lining (intracavitary), muscle wall (intramural), and outside surface (serosal) of the uterus. They usually develop slowly in women between 25 and 40 years of age and may become quite large. A growth spurt with enlargement of the fibroid tumor may occur in the decade before menopause, possibly related to anovulatory cycles and high levels of unopposed estrogen. Fibroids are a common reason for hysterectomy because they often result in menorrhagia, which can be difficult to control.

Clinical Manifestations

Fibroids may cause no symptoms, or they may produce abnormal vaginal bleeding. Other symptoms result from pressure on the surrounding organs and include pain, backache, pressure, bloating, constipation, and urinary problems. Menorrhagia (excessive bleeding) and metrorrhagia (irregular bleeding) may occur because fibroids may distort the uterine lining (see Fig. 57-7). Fibroids may interfere with fertility.

Medical Management

Treatment of uterine fibroids may include medical or surgical intervention and depends to a large extent on the size, symptoms, and location, as well as the woman's age and her reproductive plans. Fibroids usually shrink and disappear during menopause, when estrogen is no longer produced. Simple observation and follow-up may be all the management that is necessary. The patient with minor symptoms is closely monitored. If she plans to have children, treatment is as conservative as possible. As a rule, **myomectomy** (surgical removal of uterine fibroids) is performed for large tumors that produce pressure symptoms. A hysterectomy may be

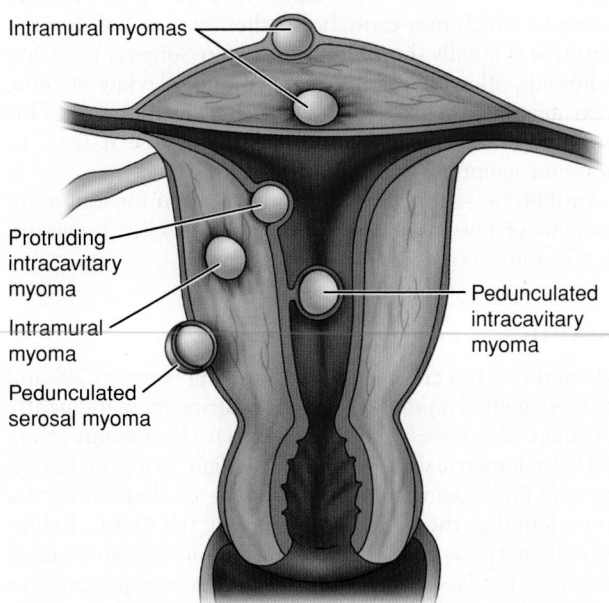

Figure 57-7 • Myomas (fibroids). Those that impinge on the uterine cavity are called *intracavitary myomas*.

performed if symptoms are severe and childbearing is completed (see later discussion of nursing care for a patient having a hysterectomy).

Several alternatives to hysterectomy have been developed for the treatment of excessive bleeding due to fibroids (Schuiling & Likis, 2013). These include the following:

- *Hysteroscopic resection of myomas:* A laser is used through a hysteroscope passed through the cervix; no incision or overnight stay is needed.
- *Laparoscopic myomectomy:* Removal of a fibroid through a laparoscope inserted through a small abdominal incision.
- *Laparoscopic myolysis:* The use of a laser or electrical needles to cauterize and shrink the fibroid.
- *Laparoscopic cryomyolysis:* Electric current is used to coagulate the fibroid.
- *Uterine artery embolization (UAE):* Polyvinyl alcohol or gelatin particles are injected into the blood vessels that supply the fibroid via the femoral artery, resulting in infarction and resultant shrinkage. This percutaneous image-guided therapy offers an alternative to hormone therapy or surgery. UAE may result in infrequent but serious complications such as pain, infection, amenorrhea, necrosis, and bleeding. Although rare, deaths and ovarian failure may occur. Women need to weigh the risks and benefits carefully, especially if they have not completed childbearing.
- *Magnetic resonance–guided focused ultrasound surgery (MRgFUS):* Ultrasonic energy is passed through the abdominal wall to target and destroy the fibroid. This noninvasive procedure is approved by the FDA for women who are premenopausal with bothersome symptoms due to fibroids and who do not want more children. It is an outpatient treatment.

Medications (e.g., leuprolide [Lupron]) or other gonadotropin-releasing hormone (GnRH) analogs, which induce a temporary menopauselike environment, may be prescribed to shrink the fibroids. This treatment consists of monthly injections, which may cause hot flashes and vaginal dryness. Treatment is usually short term (i.e., before surgery) to shrink the fibroids, allowing easier surgery, and to alleviate anemia, which may occur as a result of heavy menstrual flow. This treatment is used on a temporary basis because it leads to vasomotor symptoms and loss of bone density.

Antifibrotic agents are under investigation for long-term treatment of fibroids. Mifepristone (Mifeprex), a progesterone antagonist is also utilized.

Endometriosis

Endometriosis is a chronic disease affecting between 7% and 10% of women of reproductive age, occurring more frequently in women who have never had children (Beckmann et al., 2014). **Endometriosis** consists of a benign lesion or lesions that contain endometrial tissue (similar to that lining the uterus) found in the pelvic cavity outside the uterus. Extensive endometriosis may cause few symptoms, or an isolated lesion may produce severe symptoms. It is a major cause of chronic pelvic pain and infertility.

Endometriosis has been diagnosed more frequently as a result of the increased use of laparoscopy. There is a high incidence among patients who bear children late and among those who have fewer children. In countries where tradition favors early marriage and early childbearing, endometriosis is rare. There also appears to be a familial predisposition to endometriosis; it is more common in women whose close female relatives are affected. Other factors that may suggest increased risk include a shorter menstrual cycle (less than every 27 days), flow longer than 7 days, outflow obstruction, and younger age at menarche.

Pathophysiology

Misplaced endometrial tissue responds to and depends on ovarian hormonal stimulation. During menstruation, this ectopic tissue bleeds, mostly into areas having no outlet, which causes pain and adhesions. The lesions are typically small and puckered, with a blue/brown/gray powder-burn appearance and brown or blue-black appearance, indicating concealed bleeding.

Endometrial tissue contained within an ovarian cyst has no outlet for the bleeding; this formation is referred to as a pseudocyst or chocolate cyst. Adhesions, cysts, and scar tissue may result, causing pain and infertility (Beckmann et al., 2014). Endometriosis may increase the risk of ovarian cancer.

Currently, the best-accepted theory regarding the origin of endometrial lesions is the transplantation theory, which suggests that a backflow of menses (retrograde menstruation) transports endometrial tissue to ectopic sites through the fallopian tubes. Why some women with retrograde menstruation develop endometriosis and others do not is unknown. Endometrial tissue can also be spread by lymphatic or venous channels.

Clinical Manifestations

Symptoms vary but include dysmenorrhea, dyspareunia, and pelvic discomfort or pain. Dyschezia (pain with bowel movements) and radiation of pain to the back or leg may occur. Depression, loss of work due to pain, and relationship difficulties may result. Infertility may occur because of fibrosis and adhesions or because of a variety of substances (prostaglandins, cytokines, other factors) produced by the implants of endometriosis and scar tissue on anatomical sites.

Assessment and Diagnostic Findings

A health history, including an account of the menstrual pattern, is necessary to elicit specific symptoms. On bimanual pelvic examination, fixed tender nodules are sometimes palpated, and uterine mobility may be limited, indicating adhesions. Laparoscopic examination confirms the diagnosis and helps stage the disease. In stage 1, patients have superficial or minimal lesions; stage 2, mild involvement; stage 3, moderate involvement; and stage 4, extensive involvement and dense adhesions, with obliteration of the cul-de-sac. Ultrasonography, magnetic resonance imaging (MRI), and CT scans may also be useful to visualize endometriosis (Beckmann et al., 2014).

Medical Management

Treatment depends on the symptoms, the patient's desire for pregnancy, and the extent of the disease. If the woman does not have symptoms, routine examination may be all that is required. Other therapy for varying degrees of symptoms may be NSAIDs, oral contraceptive agents, GnRH agonists, or surgery. Pregnancy often alleviates symptoms, because neither ovulation nor menstruation occurs.

Pharmacologic Therapy

Palliative measures include the use of medications, such as analgesic agents and prostaglandin inhibitors, for pain. Hormonal therapy is effective in suppressing endometriosis and relieving dysmenorrhea (menstrual pain). Oral contraceptive agents provide effective pain relief and may prevent disease progression (Beckmann et al., 2014). Infrequently, side effects may occur with oral contraceptives, such as fluid retention, weight gain, and nausea. These can usually be managed by changing brands or formulations.

Several types of hormonal therapy are also available in addition to oral contraceptive agents. A synthetic androgen, danazol (Danocrine), causes atrophy of the endometrium and subsequent amenorrhea. The medication inhibits the release of gonadotropin with minimal overt sex hormone stimulation. The drawbacks of this medication are that it is expensive and may cause troublesome side effects such as fatigue, depression, weight gain, oily skin, decreased breast size, mild acne, hot flashes, and vaginal atrophy (Beckmann et al., 2014). GnRH agonists decrease estrogen production and cause subsequent amenorrhea. Side effects are related to low estrogen levels (e.g., hot flashes and vaginal dryness). Loss of bone density is often offset by concurrent use of estrogen. If side effects from GnRH develop, treatment is needed long-term or repeated treatments are necessary, additional therapy should be considered. Norethindrone acetate (Aygestin) (low-dose hormone) given along with GnRH agonist will mitigate the bone density side effects as well as not affect the drug's control of pelvic pain. Aromatase inhibitor therapy is emerging as an alternative therapy (Beckmann et al., 2014). Most women continue treatment despite side effects, and symptoms diminish for 80% to 90% of women with mild to moderate endometriosis. Hormonal medications are not used in patients with a history of abnormal vaginal bleeding or liver, heart, or kidney disease. Bone density is followed carefully because of the risk of bone loss; hormone therapy is usually short term.

Surgical Management

If conservative measures are not helpful, surgery may be necessary to relieve pain and improve the possibility of pregnancy. Surgery may be combined with the use of medical therapy. The procedure selected depends on the patient. Laparoscopy may be used to fulgurate (cut with high-frequency current) endometrial implants and to release adhesions. Laser surgery is another option made possible by laparoscopy. Laser therapy vaporizes or coagulates the endometrial implants, thereby destroying this tissue. Other surgical options include endocoagulation and electrocoagulation, laparotomy, abdominal hysterectomy, **oophorectomy** (removal of the ovary), bilateral **salpingo-oophorectomy** (removal of the ovary and its fallopian tube), and appendectomy. Many women need further intervention following conservative surgeries; therefore, total hysterectomy is the definitive procedure (Beckmann et al., 2014).

Nursing Management

The health history and physical examination focus on specific symptoms (e.g., pelvic pain), the effect of prescribed medications, and the woman's reproductive plans. This information helps in determining the treatment plan. Explaining the various diagnostic procedures may help to alleviate the patient's anxiety. Patient goals include relief of pain, dysmenorrhea, dyspareunia, and avoidance of infertility.

As the treatment progresses, the woman with endometriosis and her partner may find that pregnancy is not easily possible, and the psychosocial impact of this realization must be recognized and addressed. Alternatives, such as assisted reproductive technologies or adoption, may be discussed at an appropriate time and referrals offered.

The nurse's role in patient education is to dispel myths and encourage the patient to seek care if dysmenorrhea or dyspareunia occurs. The Endometriosis Association (see the Resources section) is a helpful resource for patients seeking further information and support for this condition, which can cause disabling pain and severe emotional distress.

Chronic Pelvic Pain

Chronic pelvic pain is a common disorder of women that may be related to several of the previously discussed gynecologic disorders. Chronic pelvic pain is defined as noncyclic pain concentrated in the pelvis, anterior abdominal wall, and buttock or lumbosacral region for a period greater than 6 months (Steege & Siedhoff, 2014). Causes may be of reproductive, genitourinary, or gastrointestinal origin. A history of sexual and physical abuse, PID, endometriosis, interstitial cystitis, musculoskeletal disorders, irritable bowel syndrome, and previous surgery resulting in abdominal adhesions may be associated with chronic pelvic pain. Dysmenorrhea, dyspareunia, and lower abdominal pain may also be associated with sexual and physical abuse.

Chronic pelvic pain is often difficult to treat. Treatment depends on physical and diagnostic test results and may include antidepressant, analgesic, anxiolytics, and oral contraceptive agents; GnRH agonists; exercise; diet modification; and various surgical procedures (Steege & Siedhoff, 2014).

Adenomyosis

In adenomyosis, the tissue that lines the endometrium invades the uterine wall. Symptoms include hypermenorrhea (excessive and prolonged bleeding), dysmenorrhea, polymenorrhea (abnormally frequent bleeding), and pelvic pain. Physical examination findings on palpation include a symmetrically enlarged, tender, and boggy uterus (Beckmann et al., 2014). Treatment depends on the severity of bleeding and pain. Hysterectomy may be the best option in providing relief of symptoms.

Endometrial Hyperplasia

Endometrial hyperplasia (a buildup of endometrial tissue) is the most common precursor to endometrial cancer and often results from unopposed estrogen from any source. Estrogen therapy alone without progesterone in a woman with a uterus can cause this condition. Women with anovulatory cycles, PCOS, or obesity may have high circulating levels of estrogen. Tamoxifen (Nolvadex) may also be a causative factor. Diagnosis is by biopsy or ultrasound findings of thickness of the endometrium. Hyperplasia with atypia on a pathology or biopsy report indicates risk of progression. Progestin treatment may be effective, but hysterectomy may be advised if pathology from an endometrial biopsy shows atypia. Abnormal bleeding is the most common symptom.

MALIGNANT CONDITIONS

Gynecologic cancer is any cancer that starts in a woman's reproductive organs (CDC, 2014c). According to the American Cancer Society (ACS, 2015a), the projected incidence for female reproductive cancers in the United States includes about 54,870 new cases of uterine cancer; 21,290 new cases of ovarian cancer; 12,900 new cases of cervical cancer; 5150 new cases of vulvar cancer; and 4070 new cases of vaginal cancer per year. Ovarian cancer is responsible for 5% of all cancer deaths in women and is the leading cause of death in female reproductive cancers.

Although some cancers are difficult to detect or prevent, annual pelvic examination with a Pap smear is a painless and relatively inexpensive method of early detection (CDC, 2014c). Primary providers can encourage women to follow this health practice by providing examinations that are educational and supportive and offer women an opportunity to ask questions and clarify misinformation.

Women diagnosed with gynecologic malignancies experience anxiety related to their prognosis. The occurrence of physical symptoms may cause more psychological distress. Intervention directed toward physical and psychological symptoms requires a multidisciplinary approach.

Nurses should be aware of ongoing clinical trials to identify options for many conditions. They are often in a position to answer questions about clinical trials and to encourage patients to consider participation if appropriate. Women's participation in cancer research may not occur in part because women are unaware of ongoing relevant research (see ClinicalTrials.gov in the Resources section).

Cancer of the Cervix

Death from cervical cancer is less common due to early detection of cell changes by Pap smear (CDC, 2014c). However, it is still the third most common female reproductive cancer and is estimated to affect nearly 13,000 women in the United States every year (CDC, 2014c). Risk factors are presented in Chart 57-6.

Preventive measures include regular pelvic examinations and Pap tests for all women, especially older women past childbearing age. Preventive counseling should encourage delaying first intercourse, avoiding HPV infection, engaging only in safer sex, ceasing smoking, and receiving HPV immunization.

There are several different types of cervical cancer. Most of these cancers are squamous cell carcinomas, and the rest are adenocarcinomas or mixed adenosquamous carcinomas. Adenocarcinomas begin in mucus-producing glands and are often

Chart 57-6 ⚠ RISK FACTORS — Cervical Cancer

- Chronic cervical infection
- Early childbearing
- Exposure to diethylstilbestrol in utero
- Exposure to human papillomavirus, types 16 and 18
- Family history of cervical cancer
- HIV infection and other causes of immune deficiency
- Low socioeconomic status (may be related to early marriage and early childbearing)
- Nutritional deficiencies (folate, beta-carotene, and vitamin C levels are lower in women with cervical cancer than in women without it)
- Overweight status
- Prolonged use of oral contraceptives
- Sexual activity:
  - Multiple sex partners
  - Early age (<20 years) at first coitus (exposes the vulnerable young cervix to potential viruses from a partner)
- Sexual contact with men whose partners have had cervical cancer
- Sex with uncircumcised men
- Smoking and exposure to secondhand smoke

HIV, human immune deficiency virus.
Adapted from American Cancer Society. (2015b). *Cervical Cancer.* Retrieved on 11/27/2015 at www.cancer.org/acs/groups/cid/documents/webcontent/003094-pdf.pdf; Barakat, R. R., Berchuk, A., & Markman, M., et al. (Eds). (2013). *Principles and practice of gynecologic oncology* (6th ed). Philadelphia, PA: Lippincott Williams & Wilkins

due to HPV infection. Most cervical cancers, if not detected and treated, spread to regional pelvic lymph nodes, and local recurrence is not uncommon.

Clinical Manifestations

Early cervical cancer rarely produces symptoms. If symptoms are present, they may go unnoticed as a thin, watery vaginal discharge often noticed after intercourse or douching. When symptoms such as discharge, irregular bleeding, or pain or bleeding after sexual intercourse occur, the disease may be advanced. Advanced disease should not occur if all women have access to gynecologic care and avail themselves to it. The nurse's role in access to care and its utilization is crucial.

In advanced cervical cancer, the vaginal discharge gradually increases and becomes watery and, finally, dark and foul smelling from necrosis and infection. The bleeding, which occurs at irregular intervals between periods (metrorrhagia) or after menopause, may be slight (just enough to spot the undergarments) and occurs usually after mild trauma or pressure (e.g., intercourse, douching, or bearing down during defecation). As the disease continues, the bleeding may persist and increase. Leg pain, dysuria, rectal bleeding, and edema of the extremities signal advanced disease.

As the cancer advances, it may invade the tissues outside the cervix, including the lymph glands anterior to the sacrum. In one third of patients with invasive cervical cancer, the disease involves the fundus. The nerves in this region may be affected, producing excruciating pain in the back and the legs that is relieved only by large doses of opioid analgesic agents. If the disease progresses, it often produces extreme emaciation and anemia that usually is accompanied by fever (due to secondary infection and abscesses in the ulcerating mass) and by fistula formation. Because the survival rate for in situ cancer is 100% and the rate for women with more advanced stages of cervical cancer decreases dramatically, early detection is essential.

Assessment and Diagnostic Findings

Diagnosis may be made on the basis of abnormal Pap smear results, followed by biopsy results identifying severe dysplasia (cervical intraepithelial neoplasia type III [CIN III], high-grade squamous intraepithelial lesions [HGSILs, also referred to as HSILs], or carcinoma in situ). HPV infections are usually implicated in these conditions. Carcinoma in situ is technically classified as severe dysplasia and is defined as cancer that has extended through the full thickness of the epithelium of the cervix, but not beyond. This is often referred to as preinvasive cancer.

In its very early stages, cervical cancer is found microscopically by Pap smear. In later stages, pelvic examination may reveal a large, reddish growth or a deep, ulcerating lesion. The patient may report spotting or bloody discharge.

When the patient has been diagnosed with invasive cervical cancer, clinical staging estimates the extent of the disease so that treatment can be planned more specifically and prognosis reasonably predicted. Staging is based on the International Federation of Gynecology and Obstetrics (FIGO) Staging Classification (Beckmann et al., 2014):

- Stage I, the carcinoma is strictly confined to the cervix.
- Stage II, the carcinoma invades beyond the uterus but not the pelvic wall or vagina.
- Stage III, the tumor spreads to the pelvic wall and/or the vagina, and/or causes hydronephrosis of the kidneys.
- Stage IV, the tumor has extended beyond the pelvis and involves the bladder or rectum.

Signs and symptoms are evaluated, and x-rays, laboratory tests, and special examinations, such as biopsy and colposcopy, are performed (Beckmann et al., 2014). Depending on the stage of the cancer, other tests and procedures may be performed to determine the extent of disease and appropriate treatment. These tests may include dilation and curettage (D&C), CT scan, MRI scan, IV urography, cystography, positron emission tomography (PET) scan, and barium x-ray studies. Treatment depends on the stage of the disease.

Medical Management

Precursor or Preinvasive Lesions

When precursor lesions, such as low-grade squamous intraepithelial lesions (LGSILs, also referred to as LSILs; CIN I and II or mild to moderate dysplasia), are found by colposcopy and biopsy, careful monitoring by frequent Pap smears or conservative treatment is possible. Conservative treatment may consist of monitoring, **cryotherapy** (freezing with liquid nitrogen), or laser therapy. A **loop electrocautery excision procedure (LEEP)** may also be used to remove abnormal cells. In this procedure, a thin wire loop with laser is used to cut away a thin layer of cervical tissue. LEEP is an outpatient procedure that usually is performed in a gynecologist's office; it takes only a few minutes. Analgesia is given

before the procedure, and a local anesthetic agent is injected into the area. This procedure allows the pathologist to examine the removed tissue sample to determine if the borders of the tissue are disease free. Another procedure referred to as a cone biopsy or conization (removing a cone-shaped portion of the cervix) is performed when biopsy findings demonstrate CIN III or HGSIL (equivalent to severe dysplasia) and carcinoma in situ.

If preinvasive cervical cancer (carcinoma in situ) occurs when a woman has completed childbearing, a simple hysterectomy (removal of the uterus only) is usually recommended (Beckmann et al., 2014). If a woman is pregnant or wishes to have children and invasion is less than 1 mm, conization may be sufficient. Frequent follow-up examinations are necessary to monitor for recurrence (Beckmann et al., 2014).

Patients who have precursor or premalignant lesions need reassurance that they do not have invasive cancer. However, the importance of close follow-up is emphasized because the condition, if untreated for a long time, may progress to cancer. Patients with cervical cancer in situ also need to know that this is usually a slow-growing and nonaggressive type of cancer that is not expected to recur after appropriate treatment.

Invasive Cancer

Treatment of invasive cervical cancer depends on the stage of the lesion, the patient's age and general health, and the judgment and experience of the provider. Surgery and radiation treatment (intracavitary and external) are most often used. Surgical procedures that may be used to treat cervical cancer are summarized in Chart 57-7. Robot-assisted technology for the treatment of cervical cancer is a rapidly growing alternative to more invasive surgical options with decreased length of stay, recovery time, decreased blood loss, and increase in total number of retrievable lymph nodes (ACOG, 2015c).

Chart 57-7 **Surgical Procedures for Cervical Cancer**

- Total hysterectomy—removal of the uterus, cervix, and ovaries
- Radical hysterectomy—removal of the uterus, ovaries, fallopian tubes, proximal vagina, and bilateral lymph nodes through an abdominal incision (*Note:* "Radical" indicates that an extensive area of the paravaginal, paracervical, parametrial, and uterosacral tissues is removed with the uterus.)
- Radical vaginal hysterectomy—vaginal removal of the uterus, ovaries, fallopian tubes, and proximal vagina
- Bilateral pelvic lymphadenectomy—removal of the common iliac, external iliac, hypogastric, and obturator lymphatic vessels and nodes
- Pelvic exenteration—removal of the pelvic organs, including the bladder or rectum and pelvic lymph nodes, and construction of diversional conduit, colostomy, and vagina
- Radical trachelectomy—removal of the cervix and selected nodes to preserve childbearing capacity in a woman of reproductive age with cervical cancer

Adapted from American Cancer Society. (2015b). *Cervical Cancer.* Retrieved on 11/27/2015 at www.cancer.org/acs/groups/cid/documents/webcontent/003094-pdf.pdf; Barakat, R. R., Berchuk, A., & Markman, M., et al. (Eds). (2013). *Principles and practice of gynecologic oncology* (6th ed.) Philadelphia, PA: Lippincott Williams & Wilkins

Chart 57-8	**ETHICAL DILEMMA**
	What If the Patient Refuses to Autonomously Make Decisions?

Case Scenario

You work on a gynecology-oncology unit in a small rural community hospital. The patient, a 60-year-old woman, has been admitted with a diagnosis of cancer of the vulva. She has been married to her husband since she was 16 years old. Both the patient and her husband are Mexican migrant workers. It has been determined that her disease is advanced and that she will need surgical removal of the vulva and radical node dissection. In addition, it is likely she will need chemotherapy and may be a candidate for enrollment in a clinical trial. After the treatment is explained using a medical translator, she asks her physician, "What would you do if it was your mother?" The physician reiterates the information about the surgery, and the patient states, "It is up to my husband to decide; he always makes our important decisions."

Discussion

Some cultures adhere to paternalistic tenets; the male "head of household" makes all major decisions, including health care decisions. The patient may be adhering to her cultural norms when she tells you that she will acquiesce to whatever decision her husband makes for her. Arguably, however, she may feel coerced or obligated to acquiesce to his decisions.

Analysis

- Describe the ethical principles that are in conflict in this case (see Chapter 3, Chart 3-3). Which principle should have preeminence as you proceed with your assessment of this patient?
- Describe any concerns you may have regarding beneficence and autonomy.
- Discuss any concerns that you may have about the patient's refusal to make a health care decision that will have a significant impact on her life. Assume that you have spoken in private with the patient and have verified that she understands that failure to have this surgery may put her life in jeopardy but she still refuses to make the decision. How can you professionally reconcile her decision to put her life at greater risk so that she may adhere to her cultural norms (i.e., decision-making done solely by the spouse)? Does this type of decision truly preserve her autonomy?
- What resources are available to help you, your professional colleagues, the patient, and her husband reach consensus on the best treatment or care in this situation?

Resources

See Chapter 3, Chart 3-6 for ethics resources.

Ethical issues often arise in the treatment of invasive cancers. These issues are summarized in Chart 57-8.

Frequent follow-up after surgery is imperative because the risk of recurrence is high and usually occurs within the first 2 years. Recurrences are often in the upper quarter of the vagina, and ureteral obstruction may be a sign. Weight loss, leg edema, and pelvic pain may be signs of lymphatic obstruction and metastasis.

Radiation, which is often part of treatment to reduce recurrent disease, may be delivered by an external beam or by **brachytherapy** (method by which the radiation source is placed near the tumor in a sealed source) or both. The field to be irradiated as well as the dose and method of radiation are determined by stage, volume of tumor, and lymph node involvement (Beckmann et al., 2014).

A variety of chemotherapeutic approaches are used to treat advanced cervical cancer. They are often used in combination with surgery and radiation. Vaginal stenosis is a frequent side effect of radiation. Preventive therapy (i.e., vaginal dilator) can be used to avoid severe permanent vaginal stenosis.

Some patients with recurrences of cervical cancer are considered for **pelvic exenteration**, in which several pelvic organs are removed. This is a complex, extensive surgical procedure that is reserved for women with a high likelihood of cure. Unilateral leg edema, sciatica, and ureteral obstruction indicate likely disease progression. Patients with these symptoms have advanced disease and are not considered candidates for this major surgical procedure. Surgery is complex because it is performed close to the bowel, bladder, ureters, and great vessels. Possible complications include pulmonary embolism (PE), pulmonary edema, myocardial infarction, cerebrovascular disease, hemorrhage, sepsis, small bowel obstruction, fistula formation, obstruction of the ileal conduit, bladder dysfunction, and pyelonephritis, most often in the first 18 months postoperatively. Vein constriction must be avoided postoperatively. Patients with varicose veins or a history of thromboembolic disease may be treated prophylactically with heparin. Antiembolism stockings are prescribed to reduce the risk of deep vein thrombosis (DVT). Nursing care of these patients is complex and requires coordination and care by experienced health care professionals. Pelvic exenteration is discussed in further detail later in this chapter.

Cancer of the Uterus (Endometrium)

Over the last decade there has been an increase in both the incidence and death rates of cancer of the uterine endometrium (fundus or corpus), possibly because of increased lifespan and coexisting comorbidities. This cancer is the most frequently occurring gynecologic cancer in the United States. After breast, colorectal, and lung cancer, endometrial cancer is the fourth most common cancer in women. More than 54,870 new cases of uterine cancer occur each year, with more than 10,170 deaths (ACS, 2015a). More than 80% of women are diagnosed after menopause, with the average age of diagnosis being 63 years of age (ACOG, 2015d). Many women with endometrial cancer have obesity, which increases the risk of morbidity and mortality from this disease. Cumulative exposure to estrogen is considered the major risk factor (see Chart 57-9). This exposure occurs with the use of estrogen therapy without the use of progestin, early menarche, late menopause, nulliparity, and anovulation. Other risk factors include infertility, diabetes, and the use of tamoxifen. Tamoxifen, which is taken for treatment or prevention of breast cancer, may cause proliferation of the uterine lining (ACOG, 2015d). Women who take tamoxifen should be monitored by their oncologists and/or gynecologic health care providers.

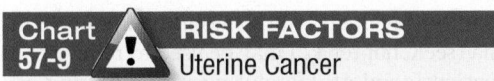

Pathophysiology

Most uterine cancers are endometrioid (i.e., originating in the lining of the uterus). There are two types. Type 1, which accounts for about 90% of cases, is estrogen dependent. It is usually low grade with a favorable prognosis. Type 2, which occurs in about 10% of cases, is high grade and usually serous cell or clear cell. Type 2 is considered to be estrogen independent. Older and African-American women are at higher risk for type 2 (ACOG, 2015d; Beckmann et al., 2014).

Assessment and Diagnostic Findings

All women should be encouraged to have annual checkups, including a gynecologic examination. Any woman who is experiencing irregular bleeding should be evaluated promptly. If a menopausal woman experiences bleeding, an endometrial aspiration or biopsy is performed to rule out hyperplasia, which is a possible precursor of endometrial cancer. The procedure is quick and usually not painful. Transvaginal ultrasound can also be used to measure the thickness of the endometrium (ACOG, 2015d). (Women who are postmenopausal should have a very thin endometrium due to low levels of estrogen; a thicker lining warrants further investigation.) A biopsy or aspiration for tissue pathology is diagnostic.

Medical Management

Treatment for endometrial cancer consists of surgical staging, total or radical hysterectomy (discussed later in this chapter), and bilateral salpingo-oophorectomy and lymph node sampling. Laparoscopy or a robot-assisted laparoscopic surgery is less invasive than abdominal surgery (ACOG, 2015d). Lymph node sampling and visualization of the peritoneum can be accomplished in many women in this manner. Cancer antigen 125 (CA-125) levels must be monitored, because elevated levels are a significant predictor of extrauterine disease or metastasis. Depending on the stage, the therapeutic approach is individualized and is based on stage, type, differentiation, degree of invasion, and node involvement. Radiation may be used in the form of external-beam radiation or vaginal brachytherapy (ACOG, 2015d). Whole pelvis radiotherapy may be used if there is any spread beyond the uterus. Recurrent cancer usually occurs inside the vaginal vault or in the upper vagina, and metastasis usually occurs in lymph nodes or the ovary. Recurrent lesions in the vagina are treated with surgery and radiation. Recurrent lesions beyond the vagina are treated with hormonal therapy or chemotherapy. Progestin therapy is used frequently. Patients should be prepared for such side effects as nausea, depression, rash, or mild fluid retention with progestin therapy.

Cancer of the Vulva

Primary cancer of the vulva is rare, representing 5% of all gynecologic malignancies and 1% of cancer in women (Zweizig, Korets, & Cain, 2014). More than 5150 new cases of vulvar carcinoma occur each year, with more than 1080 deaths (ACS, 2015a). It is most common in women who are postmenopausal, although its incidence in younger women is increasing. Possible risk factors include smoking, HPV infection, HIV infection, and immunosuppression. Squamous cell carcinoma accounts for most primary vulvar tumors. Less common are Bartholin gland cancer, vulvar sarcoma, and malignant melanoma. Little is known about what causes this disease; however, increased risk may be related to chronic vulvar irritation. In younger women, HPV infection may be implicated, especially types 16, 18, and 31. Prevention includes delaying onset of sexual activity to avoid early exposure to HPV, administration of the HPV vaccine, and avoidance of smoking. Regular pelvic examinations, Pap smears, and vulvar self-examination are helpful in early detection. Women with persistent irritation or itching should be encouraged to seek evaluation.

Clinical Manifestations

Vulvar cancers are rarely asymptomatic (Zweizig et al., 2014). Long-standing pruritus and soreness are the most common symptoms of vulvar cancer. Itching occurs in half of all patients with vulvar malignancy. Bleeding, dysuria, foul-smelling discharge, and pain may also be present and are usually signs of advanced disease. Cancerous lesions of the vulva are visible and accessible and grow relatively slowly. Early lesions appear as a chronic dermatitis; later, patients may note a lump that continues to grow and becomes a hard, ulcerated, cauliflower like growth. Biopsy should be performed on any vulvar lesion that persists, ulcerates, or fails to heal quickly with proper therapy. Vulvar malignancies may appear as a lump or mass, redness, or a lesion that fails to heal.

Medical Management

Vulvar intraepithelial lesions are preinvasive and are also called *vulvar carcinoma in situ*. They may be treated by local excision, laser ablation, application of chemotherapeutic creams, or cryosurgery.

When invasive vulvar carcinoma exists, treatment may include wide excision of the vulva and **vulvectomy** (removal of the vulva). An effort is made to individualize treatment, depending on the extent of the disease. A wide excision is performed only if lymph nodes are normal. More pervasive lesions require vulvectomy with deep pelvic node dissection. Vulvectomy is very effective at prolonging life but is frequently followed by complications (i.e., scarring, wound breakdown, leg swelling, vaginal stenosis, or rectocele). To reduce complications, only necessary tissue is removed. External-beam radiation may be used, resulting in sunburnlike irritation that usually resolves in 6 to 12 months. Laser therapy and chemotherapy are other possible treatment options.

If a widespread area is involved or the disease is advanced, a radical vulvectomy with bilateral groin dissection may be performed. Antibiotic and heparin prophylaxis may be prescribed preoperatively and continued postoperatively to prevent infection, DVT, and PE. Sequential compression devices (SCDs) are applied to reduce the risk of venous thromboembolism (VTE).

Although the role of systemic chemotherapy in the treatment of vulvar cancer remains to be determined, chemotherapy may be helpful when used in combination with radiation therapy in treatment for advanced disease. The combination of radiation and chemotherapy may reduce the size of the cancer, resulting in less extensive subsequent surgery (Zweizig et al., 2014).

Clinical trials to determine the most effective treatment are difficult to conduct because there are few patients with this condition. Morbidity with recurrence of the disease is high, and patterns of recurrence vary. Reconstruction after vulvectomy is performed by plastic surgeons when appropriate and desired.

Nursing Management

Obtaining the Health History

The health history is a valuable tool for establishing rapport with the patient. The reason the patient is seeking health care is apparent. What the nurse can tactfully elicit is the reason a delay, if any, occurred in seeking health care—for example, because of modesty, economics, denial, neglect, or fear (partners who are abusive sometimes prevent women from seeking health care). Factors involved in any delay in seeking health care and treatment may also affect recovery. The patient's health habits and lifestyle are assessed, and her receptivity to education is evaluated. Psychosocial factors are also assessed. Preoperative preparation and psychological support begin at this time.

Providing Preoperative Care

Relieving Anxiety

Prior to surgery, the patient must be allowed time to talk and ask questions. Fear often decreases when a woman who is to undergo wide excision of the vulva or vulvectomy learns that the possibility for subsequent sexual relations is good. The nurse reinforces the information the surgeon has given to the patient and addresses the patient's questions and concerns.

Preparing Skin for Surgery

Skin preparation may include cleansing the lower abdomen, inguinal areas, upper thighs, and vulva with chlorhexidine for several days before the surgical procedure. The patient may be instructed to do this at home.

Providing Postoperative Care

Relieving Pain

Because of the wide excision, the patient may experience severe pain and discomfort even with minimal movement. Therefore, analgesic agents are given preventively (i.e., around the clock at designated times) to relieve pain, increase the patient's comfort level, and allow mobility. Patient-controlled analgesia (see Chapter 12) may be used to relieve pain and promote patient comfort. Careful positioning using pillows usually increases comfort, as do soothing back rubs. A low Fowler position or, occasionally, a pillow placed under the knees reduces pain by relieving tension on the incision; however, efforts must be made to avoid pressure behind the knees, which increases the risk of DVT. Positioning the patient on her side, with pillows between her legs and against the lumbar region, provides comfort and reduces tension on the surgical wound.

Improving Skin Integrity

A pressure-reducing mattress may be used to prevent pressure ulcers. Moving from one position to another requires time and effort; the use of an overbed trapeze bar may help the patient move herself more easily. The extent of the surgical incision and the type of dressing are considered when choosing strategies to promote skin integrity. Intact skin needs to be protected from drainage and moisture. Dressings are changed as needed to ensure patient comfort, to perform wound care and irrigation (if prescribed), and to permit observation of the surgical site.

The wound is usually cleansed daily with warm, normal saline irrigations or other antiseptic solutions as prescribed, or a transparent dressing may be in place over the wound to minimize exposure to the air and subsequent pain. The appearance of the surgical site and the characteristics of drainage are assessed and documented. After the dressings are removed, a bed cradle may be used to keep the bed linens away from the surgical site.

Supporting Positive Sexuality and Sexual Function

The patient who undergoes vulvar surgery usually experiences concerns about body image, sexual attractiveness, and functioning. Establishing a trusting nurse–patient relationship is important for the patient to feel comfortable with expressing her concerns and fears. The patient is encouraged to discuss her concerns with her sexual partner as well.

Because alterations in sexual sensation and functioning depend on the extent of surgery, the nurse needs to know about any structural and functional changes resulting from the surgery. Referral of the patient and her partner to a sex counselor may help them address these changes and resume satisfying sexual activity.

Monitoring and Managing Potential Complications

Location, extent, and exposure of the surgical site and incision put the patient at risk for contamination of the site, infection and sepsis. The patient is monitored closely for local and systemic signs and symptoms of infection: purulent drainage, redness, increased pain, fever, and increased white blood cell count. The nurse assists in obtaining specimens for culture if infection is suspected and administers antibiotic agents as prescribed. Hand hygiene—always a crucial infection-preventing measure—is of particular importance along with wearing masks whenever there is an extensive area of exposed tissue. Catheters, drains, and dressings are handled carefully with gloves on to avoid cross-contamination. A low-residue diet prevents straining on defecation and wound contamination.

The patient is at risk for complications of VTE, which include DVT and PE, because of the positioning required during surgery, postoperative edema, and the immobility needed to promote healing. SCDs are applied, and other prophylactic measures may be prescribed for patients at high risk. The patient is encouraged and reminded to perform ankle exercises to minimize venous pooling, which leads to VTE. The patient is encouraged and assisted in changing positions by using the overbed trapeze bar. Pressure behind the knees is avoided when positioning the patient, because this may increase venous pooling. The patient is assessed for signs and symptoms of DVT (leg pain, redness, warmth, edema) and PE (chest pain, tachycardia, dyspnea). Fluid intake is encouraged to prevent dehydration, which also increases the risk of DVT.

The extent of the surgical incision and possibly wide excision of tissue increase the risk of postoperative bleeding and hemorrhage. Pressure dressings are applied after surgery to minimize this risk.

◥ Quality and Safety Nursing Alert

The patient must be monitored closely for signs of hemorrhage and resulting hypovolemic shock. These signs may include decreased blood pressure; increased pulse rate; decreased urine output; decreased mental status; and cold, clammy skin.

If hemorrhage and shock occur, interventions include fluid replacement, blood component therapy, and vasopressor medications. Laboratory results (e.g., hematocrit and hemoglobin levels) and hemodynamic monitoring are used to assess the patient's response to treatment. Depending on the specific cause of hemorrhage, the patient may be returned to the operating room. See Chapter 14 for a detailed discussion of shock.

Promoting Home, Community-Based, and Transitional Care

 ### Educating Patients About Self-Care

Preparing the patient for hospital discharge begins before hospital admission. The patient and family are informed about what to expect during the immediate postoperative and recovery periods. Depending on the changes resulting from the surgery, the patient and her family may need instruction about wound care, urinary catheterization, and possible complications. The patient is encouraged to share her concerns and to assume increasing responsibility for her own care. She is encouraged and assisted in learning to care for the surgical site. A referral for transitional, home, or community-based care is made as indicated.

Nurses are in an ideal position to educate women about performing regular vulvar self-examinations. Using a mirror, patients can see what constitutes normal female anatomy and learn about changes that should be reported (e.g., lesions, ulcers, masses, and persistent itching). Nurses must urge women to seek health care if they notice anything abnormal, because vulvar cancer is one of the most curable of all malignant conditions.

Continuing and Transitional Care

Patients may be discharged early in their postoperative recovery to home or a subacute facility. During this phase, the patient's physical status and psychological responses to the surgery are assessed. In addition, the patient is assessed for complications and healing of the surgical site. During home visits, the nurse assesses the home to determine if modifications are needed to facilitate care. The home visit is used to reinforce previous education and to assess the patient's and the family's understanding of and adherence to the prescribed treatment strategies. Follow-up phone calls by the nurse to the patient between home visits are usually reassuring to the patient and family, who may be responsible for performing complex care procedures. Attention to the patient's psychological responses is important because the patient may become discouraged and depressed because of alterations in body image and a slow recovery. Communication between the nurse involved in the patient's immediate postoperative care and the home care nurse is essential to ensure continuity of care.

Cancer of the Vagina

Cancer of the vagina is uncommon, representing 1% to 3% of gynecologic cancers; it is usually squamous in origin (Beckmann et al., 2014). Malignant melanoma and sarcomas can occur. Most vaginal cancers are secondary and invasive at the time of diagnosis. Risk factors include previous cervical cancer, in utero exposure to diethylstilbestrol (DES), previous vaginal or vulvar cancer, previous radiation therapy, history of HPV, or pessary use. Any patient with previous cervical cancer should be examined regularly for vaginal lesions.

Vaginal pessaries, which are used to support prolapsed tissues, can be a source of chronic irritation. As such, they have been associated with vaginal cancer, but only when the devices were not cared for properly (i.e., the device was not cleaned regularly or the patient did not return to the primary provider regularly for vaginal examinations).

Patients often do not have symptoms but may report slight bleeding after intercourse, spontaneous bleeding, vaginal discharge, pain, and urinary or rectal symptoms (or both). Diagnosis is often by Pap smear. Encouraging close follow-up is the focus of nursing interventions with women who were exposed to DES in utero. Emotional support for mothers who received DES before its risks were discovered and their daughters who were exposed to DES in utero is essential.

Medical Management

Treatment of early lesions may include local excision, topical chemotherapy, or laser. Laser therapy is a common treatment option in early vaginal and vulvar cancer. Surgery for more advanced lesions depends on the size and the stage of the cancer. If radical vaginectomy is required, a vagina can be reconstructed with tissue from the intestine, muscle, or skin grafts. After vaginal reconstructive surgery and radiation, regular intercourse may be helpful in preventing vaginal stenosis. Water-soluble lubricants are helpful in reducing pain with intercourse (dyspareunia).

Following surgery, radiation therapy may be given by a variety of methods, including external-beam radiation, which is usually an outpatient procedure, or brachytherapy, which is internal radiation therapy. Internal radiation may be given with intracavitary radioactive material contained in a seed, wire, needle, or tube, which is placed into a cavity such as the uterus or vagina. Interstitial radiation is another type of internal radiation treatment in which the radioactive material is placed in or near the cancer but not into a body cavity and is used in cervical and ovarian malignancies. These treatments may be high dose for a short period or low dose, which may take longer. Treatment during hospitalization or during outpatient therapy depends on several factors, including the status of the patient and the mode of delivery.

Cancer of the Fallopian Tubes

Malignancies of the fallopian tube are the least common type of genital cancer (ACS, 2015a). Although this type of cancer can occur at any age, it is most common in women who are postmenopausal. Symptoms are often minimal, causing diagnosis to be made at an advanced stage (Beckmann et al., 2014). Symptoms include abdominal pain, abnormal bleeding, and vaginal discharge. An enlarged fallopian tube may be found on sonogram if dilated and fluid filled, or it may appear or be palpated as a mass. Surgery followed by radiation therapy is the usual treatment.

Cancer of the Ovary

Ovarian cancer is the leading cause of gynecologic cancer deaths in the United States, and the fifth deadliest cancer for women following lung, breast, colorectal, and pancreatic (Beckmann et al., 2014; McAlpine, Hanley, Woo, et al., 2014). Despite careful physical examination, ovarian tumors are often difficult to detect because they are usually deep in the pelvis. No early screening mechanism exists at present. Tumor-associated antigens are helpful in determining follow-up care after diagnosis and treatment and to evaluate for recurrent disease but are not useful in early general screening (Beckmann et al., 2014).

Epidemiology

One in 70 women will develop ovarian cancer in her lifetime. The incidence of this type of cancer increases with age until 70 years, with most cases diagnosed by age 60 (Beckmann et al., 2014). The frequency of ovarian cancer is highest in industrialized countries and affects women of all races and ethnic backgrounds.

Family history is the most significant risk factor. Most cases are random, but 5% to 10% of ovarian cancers are familial (Beckmann et al., 2014). In most cases, the mutations are in the *BRCA1* gene and sometimes in the *BRCA2* gene. A family history in a first-degree relative (mother, daughter, or sister), older age, early menarche, late menopause, and obesity may increase the risk of ovarian cancer. However, most women who develop ovarian cancer have no known risk factors, and no definitive causative factors have been determined.

Patients with concerns about their family history should be referred to a cancer genetics center to obtain information and testing, if indicated (see Chapter 8). Women with inherited types of ovarian cancer tend to be younger when the diagnosis is made than the average age at the time of diagnosis. Hereditary nonpolyposis colorectal cancer (HNPCC, also known as Lynch syndrome) increases the risk of ovarian cancer 13-fold

(Beckmann et al., 2014). Lifetime risk of developing ovarian cancer has been shown to be decreased by one half with long-term suppression (greater than 5 years) of ovulation through use of oral contraceptives (Beckmann et al., 2014).

Pathophysiology

Types of tumors include germ cell tumors, which arise from the cells that produce eggs and are the most common cause of ovarian cancer in women younger than 20 years (Beckmann et al., 2014); stromal cell tumors, which arise in connective tissue cells that produce hormones; and epithelial tumors, which originate from the outer surface of the ovary. Most ovarian cancers are epithelial in origin. Of the many different cell types in ovarian cancer, epithelial tumors constitute 90%. Germ cell and stromal tumors make up the other 10% (Beckmann et al., 2014).

Primary peritoneal carcinoma is closely related to ovarian cancer. Extraovarian primary peritoneal carcinoma (EOPPC) resembles ovarian cancer histologically and can occur in women with and without ovaries. Symptoms and treatment are similar. Because of the possibility of EOPPC, oophorectomy lessens the chance, but does not guarantee, that the patient will not develop carcinoma.

Clinical Manifestations

Symptoms of ovarian cancer are nonspecific and may include increased abdominal girth, pelvic pressure, bloating, back pain, constipation, abdominal pain, urinary urgency, indigestion, flatulence, increased waist size, leg pain, and pelvic pain. Symptoms are often vague, so many women tend to ignore them. Ovarian cancer is often silent, but enlargement of the abdomen from an accumulation of fluid is a common sign. All women with gastrointestinal symptoms without a known cause must be evaluated for potential ovarian cancer. Vague, undiagnosed, persistent gastrointestinal symptoms should alert the nurse to the possibility of an early ovarian malignancy. A palpable ovary in a woman who has gone through menopause is investigated immediately, because ovaries normally become smaller and less palpable after menopause.

Assessment and Diagnostic Findings

Any enlarged ovary must be investigated. Pelvic examination often does not detect early ovarian cancer, and pelvic imaging techniques are not always definitive. Ovarian tumors are classified as benign if there is no proliferation or invasion, borderline if there is proliferation but no invasion, and malignant if there is invasion. Of all new cases of ovarian tumors, 20% are classified as borderline and have low malignancy potential. However, by the time of diagnosis, most ovarian cancers are advanced (ACS, 2015a; Beckmann et al., 2014).

Diagnostic test may include an MRI scan, transvaginal and pelvic ultrasound, chest x-rays, and a blood test for CA-125. An abdominal CT scan with and without contrast may be used to rule out metastasis (Beckmann et al., 2014).

Medical Management

Surgical Management

Surgical staging, exploration, and reduction of tumor mass are the basics of treatment. Surgical removal is the treatment

Main Stages of Ovarian Cancer

I. Cancer is contained within the ovary (or ovaries).

II. Cancer is in one or both ovaries and has involved other organs (i.e., uterus, fallopian tubes, bladder, the sigmoid colon, or the rectum) within the pelvis.

III. Cancer involves one or both ovaries, and one or both of the following are present: (1) cancer has spread beyond the pelvis to the lining of the abdomen; (2) cancer has spread to lymph nodes.

IV. The most advanced stage of ovarian cancer. Cancer is in one or both ovaries. There is distant metastasis to the liver, lungs, or other organs outside the peritoneal cavity; ovarian cancer cells in the pleural cavity are evidence of stage IV disease.

Adapted from Beckmann, C. R., Ling, F. W., Herbert, W. N., et al. (Eds.). (2014). *Obstetrics and gynecology* (7th ed.). Philadelphia, PA: Wolters Kluwer.

of choice. Staging the tumor by the FIGO staging system is performed to guide treatment (see Chart 57-10). Likely treatment involves a total abdominal hysterectomy with removal of the fallopian tubes and ovaries and possibly the omentum (bilateral salpingo-oophorectomy and omentectomy), tumor debulking, para-aortic and pelvic lymph node sampling, diaphragmatic biopsies, random peritoneal biopsies, and cytologic washings. Postoperative management may include taxanes or platinum-based chemotherapy (discussed in the next section).

Borderline tumors resemble ovarian cancer but have much more favorable outcomes. Women diagnosed with this type of cancer tend to be younger (early 40s). A conservative surgical approach is used. The affected ovary is removed, but the uterus and the contralateral ovary may remain in place. Adjuvant therapy may not be warranted.

Pharmacologic Therapy

Chemotherapy is usually administered IV on an outpatient basis using a combination of platinum and taxane agents. Paclitaxel (Taxol) plus carboplatin (Paraplatin) are most often used because of their excellent clinical benefits and manageable toxicity. Leukopenia, neurotoxicity, and fever may occur.

Because paclitaxel often causes leukopenia, patients may need to take granulocyte colony-stimulating factor as well. Paclitaxel is contraindicated in patients with hypersensitivity to medications formulated in polyoxyethylated castor oil and in patients with baseline neutropenia. Because of possible adverse cardiac effects, paclitaxel is not used in patients with cardiac disorders. Hypotension, dyspnea, angioedema, and urticaria indicate severe reactions that usually occur soon after the first and second doses are given. Nurses who administer chemotherapy are prepared to assist in treating anaphylaxis. Patients should be prepared for inevitable hair loss.

Carboplatin may be used in the initial treatment and in patients with recurrence. It is used with caution in patients with renal impairment. Usually, six cycles are given. A positive clinical response is normalization of the tumor marker CA-125, negative CT results, and a normal physical and gynecologic examination.

Liposomal therapy, delivery of chemotherapy in a liposome, allows the highest possible dose of chemotherapy to the tumor target with a reduction in adverse effects. Liposomes are used as drug carriers because they are nontoxic, biodegradable, easily available, and relatively inexpensive. This encapsulated chemotherapy allows increased duration of action and better targeting. The encapsulation of doxorubicin (Doxil) lessens the incidence of nausea, vomiting, and alopecia. Patients must be monitored for bone marrow suppression and gastrointestinal and cardiac effects.

Combination IV and intraperitoneal chemotherapy is an option for some patients. However, this treatment is more toxic and side effects are more severe than regular chemotherapy (ACS, 2015c). Intraperitoneal chemotherapy is reserved for women with good kidney function (ACS, 2015c).

Genetic engineering and identification of cancer genes may make gene therapy a future possibility; gene therapy is under investigation. Emerging proteomic technologies (tissue-based protein analysis) look promising; they may allow earlier diagnosis and treatment decision making. New biomarkers need further validation, but protein signature patterns are now being tested. These technologies may result in individualized treatment strategies for epithelial ovarian cancer (ACS, 2105c).

Recurrence of ovarian cancer is common, and many patients may require treatment with multiple agents. Treatment is directed toward control of the cancer, maintenance of quality of life, and palliation. Liposomal preparations, intraperitoneal drug administration, anticancer vaccines, monoclonal antibodies directed against cancer antigens, gene therapy, and antiangiogenic treatments (to prevent formation of new blood vessels in an effort to halt growth of ovarian cancer) may be used in the treatment for recurrence.

Nursing Management

Nursing measures involve those related to the patient's treatment plan, which may include surgery, chemotherapy, palliative care, or a combination of these. Nursing interventions after pelvic surgery to remove the tumor are similar to those after other abdominal surgeries. If ovarian cancer occurs in a young woman and the tumor is unilateral, it is removed. Childbearing, if desired, is encouraged in the near future. After childbirth, surgical reexploration may be performed, and the remaining ovary may be removed. If both ovaries are involved, bilateral oophorectomy is performed and chemotherapy follows.

Patients with advanced ovarian cancer may develop ascites and pleural effusion. Nursing care may include administering IV fluids prescribed to alleviate fluid and electrolyte imbalances, administering parenteral nutrition to provide adequate nutrition, providing postoperative care after intestinal bypass to alleviate any obstruction, controlling pain, and managing drainage tubes. Comfort measures for women with ascites may include providing small frequent meals, decreasing fluid intake, administering diuretic agents, and providing rest. Patients with pleural effusion may experience shortness of breath, hypoxia, pleuritic chest pain, and cough. Thoracentesis is usually performed to relieve these symptoms. The patient with ovarian cancer often has complex needs and benefits from the assistance and support of an oncology clinical nurse specialist.

Hysterectomy

Hysterectomy is the surgical removal of the uterus to treat cancer, dysfunctional uterine bleeding, endometriosis, nonmalignant growths, persistent pain, pelvic relaxation and prolapse, and previous injury to the uterus. Hysterectomies have been steadily declining over the last decade as the number of other therapeutic options (i.e., laser therapy, endometrial ablation, UAE, and medications to shrink fibroid tumors) has increased (Wright, Herzog, Tsui, et al., 2013). Despite the decline in hysterectomies, it is still the most common gynecologic procedure affecting one in nine women in their lifetime; 90% of all hysterectomies are for benign causes (Clark-Pearson & Geller, 2013).

A total hysterectomy involves removal of the uterus and the cervix. Hysterectomy can be supracervical or subtotal, in which the uterus is removed but the cervix is spared. Radical hysterectomy involves removal of the uterus as well as the surrounding tissue, including the upper third of the vagina and pelvic lymph nodes. The procedure can be performed through the vagina, through an abdominal incision, or laparoscopically (in which the uterus is removed in sections through small incisions using a laparoscope). Malignant conditions usually require a total abdominal hysterectomy and bilateral salpingo-oophorectomy.

A laparoscopically assisted approach can also be used for vaginal hysterectomy. This procedure is performed as a short-stay procedure or ambulatory surgery in patients who are carefully selected. Robot-assisted hysterectomies are performed in more than 20% of cases, with similar outcomes compared to laparoscopic and vaginal methods at a higher cost (Ridgeway & Falcone, 2014).

Preoperative Management

Patients are advised to discontinue anticoagulant medications, NSAIDs such as aspirin, and vitamin E prior to surgery to reduce the risk of bleeding. Pregnancy is ruled out on the day of surgery. Prophylactic antibiotic agents may be given prior to surgery and discontinued the next day. Prevention of thromboembolic events is critical, and methods depend on the risk profile of the patient.

Postoperative Management

The principles of general postoperative care for abdominal surgery apply. Major risks are infection and hemorrhage. In addition, because the surgical site is close to the bladder, voiding problems may occur, particularly after a vaginal hysterectomy. Edema or nerve trauma may cause temporary loss of bladder tone (bladder atony), and an indwelling catheter may be inserted.

NURSING PROCESS

The Patient Undergoing a Hysterectomy

Assessment

The health history and the physical and pelvic examination are completed, and laboratory tests are performed. Additional assessment data include the patient's psychosocial responses, because the need for a hysterectomy may elicit strong emotional reactions. If the hysterectomy is performed to remove a malignant tumor, anxiety related to fear of cancer and its consequences adds to the stress of the patient and her family. Women who have had a hysterectomy may be at risk for psychological and physical symptoms. Alternatively, women may note improved physical and mental health after hysterectomy as troublesome symptoms may be alleviated.

Diagnosis

NURSING DIAGNOSES

Based on the assessment data, major nursing diagnoses may include the following:

- Anxiety related to the diagnosis of cancer, fear of pain, possible perception of loss of femininity or childbearing potential
- Disturbed body image related to altered fertility and fears about sexuality and relationships with partner and family
- Acute pain related to surgery and other adjuvant therapy
- Deficient knowledge of the perioperative aspects of hysterectomy and postoperative self-care

COLLABORATIVE PROBLEMS/POTENTIAL COMPLICATIONS

Potential complications may include the following:

- Hemorrhage
- VTE
- Bladder dysfunction
- Infection

Planning and Goals

The major goals may include relief of anxiety, acceptance of loss of the uterus, absence of pain or discomfort, increased knowledge of self-care requirements, and absence of complications.

Nursing Interventions

RELIEVING ANXIETY

Anxiety stems from several factors: unfamiliar environment; the effects of surgery on body image and reproductive ability; fear of pain and other discomfort; and, possibly, feelings of embarrassment about exposure in the perioperative period. The nurse determines what the experience means to the patient and encourages her to verbalize her concerns. Throughout the preoperative, postoperative, and recovery periods, explanations are given about physical preparations and procedures that are performed.

Patient education addresses the outcomes of surgery, possible feelings of loss, and options for management of any symptoms that occur. Women vary in their preferences for information and participation in decision making, including choice of treatment options, accurate and useful information at the appropriate time, support from their health care providers, and access to professional and lay support systems.

IMPROVING BODY IMAGE

The patient may have strong emotional reactions to having a hysterectomy and personal feelings related to the diagnosis, views of significant others who may be involved (family, partner), religious beliefs, and fears about prognosis. Concerns such as the inability to have children and the effect on femininity may surface, as may questions about the effects of surgery on sexual relationships, function, and satisfaction. The patient needs reassurance that she will still have a vagina and that she can experience sexual activity after temporary postoperative abstinence while tissues heal. Information that sexual satisfaction and orgasm arise from clitoral stimulation rather than from the uterus reassures many women. Most women note some change in sexual feelings after hysterectomy, but they vary in intensity. In some cases, the vagina is shortened by surgery, and this may affect sensitivity or comfort.

When hormonal balance is upset, as often occurs with reproductive system disorders, the patient may experience depressed mood and heightened emotional sensitivity to people and situations. The nurse needs to approach and evaluate each patient individually in light of these factors. A nurse who exhibits interest, concern, and willingness to listen to the patient's fears will help the patient progress through the surgical experience.

RELIEVING PAIN

Postoperative pain and discomfort are common. Therefore, the nurse assesses the intensity of the patient's pain and assists the patient with analgesia as prescribed. If the patient has abdominal distention or flatus, a rectal tube and application of heat to the abdomen may be prescribed. When abdominal auscultation reveals return of bowel sounds and peristalsis, additional fluids and a soft diet are permitted. Early ambulation facilitates the return of normal peristalsis.

MONITORING AND MANAGING POTENTIAL COMPLICATIONS

Hemorrhage. Vaginal bleeding and hemorrhage may occur after hysterectomy. To detect these complications early, the nurse counts the perineal pads used or checks the incision site, assesses the extent of saturation with blood, and monitors vital signs. Abdominal dressings are monitored for drainage if an abdominal surgical approach has been used. In preparation for hospital discharge, the nurse gives prescribed guidelines for activity restrictions to promote healing and to prevent postoperative bleeding. Because many women may go home the day of surgery or within a day or two, they are instructed to contact the nurse or surgeon if bleeding is beyond what is expected, which should be minimal.

Venous Thromboembolism. Because of positioning during surgery, postoperative edema, and decreased activity postoperatively, the patient is at risk for DVT and PE. To minimize the risk, antiembolism stockings are applied. In addition, the patient is encouraged and assisted to change positions frequently, although pressure under the knees is avoided, and to exercise her legs and feet while in bed. The nurse helps the patient ambulate early in the postoperative period. The nurse also assesses for DVT (leg pain, redness, warmth, edema) and PE (chest pain, tachycardia, dyspnea). If the patient is being discharged home soon after surgery, she is instructed to avoid prolonged sitting in a chair with pressure at the knees, sitting with crossed legs, and inactivity. Furthermore, she is instructed to contact her primary provider if symptoms of DVT or PE occur.

Bladder Dysfunction. Because of possible difficulty in voiding postoperatively, occasionally an indwelling catheter may be inserted before or during surgery and is left in place in the immediate postoperative period. If a catheter is in place, it is usually removed shortly after the patient begins to ambulate. After the catheter is removed, urinary output is monitored; additionally, the abdomen is assessed for distention. If the patient does not void within a prescribed time, measures are initiated to encourage voiding (e.g., assisting the patient to the bathroom, pouring warm water over the perineum). If the patient cannot void, catheterization may be necessary. On rare occasions, the patient may be discharged home with the catheter in place and is instructed in its management.

PROMOTING HOME, COMMUNITY-BASED, AND TRANSITIONAL CARE

Educating Patients About Self-Care. The information provided to the patient is tailored to her needs. She must know what limitations or restrictions, if any, to expect. She is instructed to check the surgical incision daily and to contact her primary provider if redness or purulent drainage or discharge occurs. She is informed that her periods are now over but that she may have a slightly bloody discharge for a few days; if bleeding recurs after this time, it should be reported immediately. The patient is instructed about the importance of an adequate oral intake and of maintaining bowel and urinary tract function. The patient is informed that she is likely to recover quickly but that postoperative fatigue is not unusual.

The patient should resume activities gradually. This does not mean sitting for long periods, because doing so may cause blood to pool in the pelvis, increasing the risk of VTE. The nurse explains that showers are preferable to tub baths to reduce the possibility of infection and to avoid the dangers of injury that may occur when getting in and out of the bathtub. The patient is instructed to avoid straining, lifting, having sexual intercourse, or driving until permitted. Vaginal discharge, foul odor, excessive bleeding, any leg redness or pain, or an elevated temperature should be reported, and the nurse reinforces education regarding activities and restrictions.

Continuing and Transitional Care. Follow-up telephone contact provides the nurse with the opportunity to determine whether the patient is recovering without problems and to answer any questions that may have arisen. The patient is reminded about postoperative follow-up appointments. If the patient's ovaries were removed and she finds vasomotor symptoms troublesome, hormone therapy may be considered at a low dose for a short amount of time. The patient is reminded to discuss risks and benefits of hormone therapy and alternative therapies with her primary provider and gynecologic care provider. Decisions about use of hormone therapy need to be made individually in consultation with these providers.

Evaluation

Expected patient outcomes may include:
1. Experiences decreased anxiety
2. Has improved body image
   a. Discusses changes resulting from surgery with her partner
   b. Verbalizes understanding of her disorder and the treatment plan
   c. Displays minimal depression or anxiety
3. Experiences minimal pain and discomfort
   a. Reports relief of abdominal pain and discomfort
   b. Ambulates without pain

4. Verbalizes knowledge and understanding of self-care
   a. Practices deep-breathing, turning, and leg exercises as instructed
   b. Increases activity and ambulation daily
   c. Reports adequate fluid intake and adequate urinary output
   d. Identifies reportable symptoms
   e. Schedules and keeps follow-up appointments
5. Absence of complications
   a. Has minimal vaginal bleeding and exhibits normal vital signs
   b. Ambulates early
   c. Notes no chest or calf pain and no redness, tenderness, or swelling in the extremities
   d. Reports no urinary problems or abdominal distention

Unfolding Patient Stories: Doris Bowman • Part 2

 Recall from Chapter 15 **Doris Bowman,** who is undergoing a total abdominal hysterectomy with bilateral salpingo-oophorectomy. What are potential postoperative complications that the nurse should consider? What assessments and interventions are done by the nurse to monitor for early detection or to prevent these complications? Describe the discharge education provided by the nurse on self-care monitoring required of the patient at home and what should be reported to the health care provider.

Care for Doris and other patients in a realistic virtual environment: **vSim** *for Nursing* **(thepoint.lww. com/vSimMedicalSurgical).** Practice documenting these patients' care in DocuCare **(thepoint.lww.com/ DocuCareEHR).**

Radiation Therapy

Radiation may be used in the treatment of cervical, uterine, and less frequently in ovarian cancers either alone or in combination with surgery and chemotherapy. Several approaches are used to deliver radiation to the female reproductive system: external radiation, intraoperative radiation therapy (IORT), and internal (intracavitary) irradiation or brachytherapy (Halperin, Wazer, Perez, et al. 2013). The cervix and uterus can serve as a receptacle for radioactive sources for internal radiation therapy.

Methods of Radiation Therapy

External Radiation Therapy

This method of delivering radiation destroys cancerous cells at the skin surface or deeper in the body. Other methods of delivering radiation therapy are more commonly used to treat cancer of the female reproductive system than this method.

Intraoperative Radiation Therapy

IORT allows radiation to be applied directly to the affected area during surgery. An electron beam is directed at the disease site. This direct-view irradiation may be used when para-aortic nodes are involved or for unresectable (inoperable) or partially resectable neoplasms. Benefits include accurate beam direction (which precisely limits the radiation to the tumor) and the ability during treatment to block sensitive organs from radiation. IORT is usually combined with external-beam irradiation pre- or postoperatively.

Internal (Intracavitary) Irradiation

After the patient receives an anesthetic agent and an examination, specially prepared applicators are inserted into the endometrial cavity and vagina. These devices are not loaded with radioactive material until the patient returns to her room. X-rays are obtained to verify the precise relationship of the applicator to the normal pelvic anatomy and to the tumor. When this step is completed, the radiation oncologist loads the applicators with predetermined amounts of radioactive material. This procedure, called *afterloading,* allows for precise control of the radiation exposure received by the patient, with minimal exposure of physicians, nurses, and other health care personnel. A patient undergoing internal radiation treatment remains isolated in a private room until the application is completed. Adjacent rooms may need to be evacuated and a lead shield placed at the doorway to the patient's room.

Of the various applicators developed for intracavitary treatment, some are inserted into the endometrial cavity and endocervical canal as multiple small irradiators (e.g., Heyman capsules). Others consist of a central tube (a tandem or intrauterine "stem") placed through the dilated endocervical canal into the uterine cavity, which remains in a fixed relationship with the irradiators placed in the upper vagina on each side of the cervix (vaginal ovoids) (see Fig. 57-8).

When the applicator is inserted, an indwelling urinary catheter is also inserted. Vaginal packing is inserted to keep the applicator in place and to keep other organs, such as the bladder and rectum, as far from the radioactive source as possible. The objective of the internal treatment is to maintain the distribution of internal radiation at a fixed dosage throughout

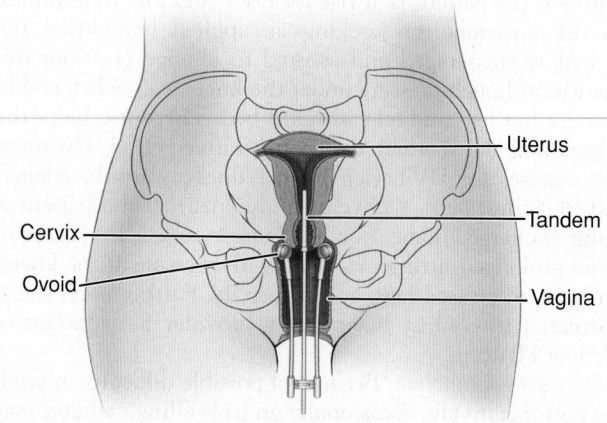

Figure 57-8 • Placement of tandem and ovoids for internal radiation therapy.

the application, which may last 24 to 72 hours, depending on dose calculations made by the radiation physicist.

Automated high-dose rate intracavitary brachytherapy systems have been developed that allow outpatient radiation therapy. Treatment time is shorter, thereby decreasing patient discomfort. Staff exposure to radiation is also avoided. Isotopes of radium and cesium are used for intracavitary irradiation.

Nursing Considerations for Radiation Safety

Special precautions for the safety of the patient and the nurse are important considerations when the patient is receiving radiation therapy. The radiation safety department will identify specific safety precautions to those people who will be in contact with the patient, including health care providers and family. Nursing concerns include providing the patient with emotional support and physical comfort. Further details about nursing management are provided in Chapter 15.

CRITICAL THINKING EXERCISES

1 **ebp** A 60-year-old woman has been diagnosed with ovarian cancer. She reports a strong family history of cancer; her mother and a sister both died from breast cancer. She is concerned of the health status of her two daughters, both of whom are in their 30s. She has asked you to discuss the risks of cancer with them. Explain what counseling and education you will provide to the patient and her daughters. Identify the evidence base for the counseling and education and the strength of that evidence.

2 **pq** Identify the priorities, approach, and techniques you would use to provide care for a 25-year-old woman who is being seen in an outpatient clinic for a new diagnosis of genital herpes. How will your priorities, approach, and techniques differ if the patient says she is not in a monogamous relationship? If the patient is from a culture with very different values from your own? Describe your priorities, approach, and techniques to prevent reinfection or spread of the infection.

3 A 46-year-old woman has been admitted to your unit for repair of a prolapsed uterus. Describe the preoperative education for her and the postoperative care that can be anticipated. What modifications in care, postoperative education, and discharge planning may be necessary if repair of a rectocele is also done?

REFERENCES

*Asterisk indicates nursing research.

Books

American Cancer Society. (2015a). *Cancer facts and figures 2015*. Atlanta, GA: Author.

Barakat, R. R., Berchuk, A., Markman, M., et al. (Eds). (2013). *Principles and practice of gynecologic oncology* (6th ed.). Philadelphia, PA: Lippincott Williams & Wilkins.

Beckmann, C. R., Ling, F. W., Herbert, W. N., et al. (Eds). (2014). *Obstetrics and gynecology* (7th ed.). Philadelphia, PA: Wolters Kluwer.

Halperin, E. C., Wazer, D. E., Perez, C. A., et al. (Eds.). (2013). *Perez and Brady's principles and practice of radiation oncology* (6th ed.). Philadelphia, PA: Lippincott Williams and Wilkins.

Karch, A. M. (2015). *Lippincott nursing drug guide*. Philadelphia, PA: Wolters Kluwer.

Schuiling, K. D., & Likis, F. E. (2013). *Women's gynecologic health* (2nd ed.). Burlington, MA: Jones & Bartlett.

Journals and Electronic Documents

American Cancer Society (ACS). (2015b). *Cervical Cancer*. Retrieved on 11/27/2015 at: www.cancer.org/acs/groups/cid/documents/webcontent/003094-pdf.pdf

American Cancer Society (ACS). (2015c). *Ovarian Cancer*. Retrieved on 12/06/2015 at www.cancer.org/cancer/ovariancancer/detailedguide/ovarian-cancer-new-research

American College of Obstetricians and Gynecologists (ACOG). (2007, reaffirmed 2015). Practice Bulletin No. 83: Management of adnexal masses. *Obstetrics and Gynecology, 110*(1), 201–214.

American College of Obstetricians and Gynecologists (ACOG). (2015a). Human papillomavirus vaccination. *Committee Opinion No. 641*. Retrieved on 11/1/2015 at: www.acog.org/Resources-And-Publications/Committee-Opinions/Committee-on-Adolescent-Health-Care/Human-Papillomavirus-Vaccination

American College of Obstetricians and Gynecologists (ACOG). (2015b). Dual therapy for gonococcal infections. *Committee Opinion No. 645*. Retrieved on 11/1/2015 at: www.acog.org/Resources-And-Publications/Committee-Opinions/Committee-on-Gynecologic-Practice/Dual-Therapy-for-Gonococcal-Infections

American College of Obstetricians and Gynecologists (ACOG). (2015c). Robotic surgery in gynecology. Committee Opinion No. 628. Retrieved on 11/27/2015 at: www.acog.org/Resources-And-Publications/Committee-Opinions/Committee-on-Gynecologic-Practice/Robotic-Surgery-in-Gynecology

American College of Obstetricians and Gynecologists (ACOG). (2015d). Practice Bulletin No. 149: Endometrial cancer. *Obstetrics and Gynecology, 125*(4), 1006–10026.

Bechtel, M. A., & Trout, W. (2015). Sexually transmitted diseases. *Clinical Obstetrics and Gynecology, 58*(1), 172–184.

Brunham, R. C., Gottlieb, S. L., & Paavonen, J. (2015). Pelvic inflammatory disease. *The New England Journal of Medicine, 372*(21), 2039–2043.

Centers for Disease Control and Prevention (CDC). (2014a). *Genital/vulvavaginal candidiasis*. Retrieved on 10/29/2015 at: www.cdc.gov/fungal/diseases/Candidiasis/genital/

Centers for Disease Control and Prevention (CDC). (2014b). *Genital HPV infection—CDC fact sheet*. Retrieved on 11/1/2015 at: www.cdc.gov/std/hpv/default.htm

Centers for Disease Control and Prevention (CDC). (2014c). Basic information about gynecologic cancers. Retrieved on 11/27/2015 at: www.cdc.gov/cancer/gynecologic/basic_info/what-is-gynecologic-cancer.htm

Centers for Disease Control and Prevention (CDC). (2015a). *2015 Sexually transmitted disease treatment guidelines*. Retrieved on 10/29/2015 at: www.cdc.gov/std/tg2015/

Centers for Disease Control and Prevention (CDC). (2015b). *Trichomoniasis—CDC fact sheet*. Retrieved on 10/29/2015 at: www.cdc.gov/std/trichomonas/STDFact-Trichomoniasis.htm

Centers for Disease Control and Prevention (CDC). (2015c). *Genital herpes—CDC fact sheet*. Retrieved on 11/1/2015 at: www.cdc.gov/std/herpes/stdfact-herpes-detailed.htm

Centers for Disease Control and Prevention (CDC). (2015d). *Chlamydia—CDC fact sheet*. Retrieved on 11/7/2015 at: www.cdc.gov/std/chlamydia/stdfact-chlamydia-detailed.htm

Centers for Disease Control and Prevention (CDC). (2015e). *Gonorrhea—CDC fact sheet*. Retrieved on 11/7/2015 at: www.cdc.gov/std/gonorrhea/stdfact-gonorrhea-detailed.htm

Centers for Disease Control and Prevention (CDC). (2015f). *Pelvic Inflammatory Disease (PID)—CDC fact sheet*. Retrieved on 11/7/2015 at: www.cdc.gov/std/pid/stdfact-pid-detailed.htm

Centers for Disease Control and Prevention (CDC). (2015g). *HIV among women*. Retrieved on 11/19/2015 at: www.cdc.gov/hiv/pdf/risk_women.pdf

Clark-Pearson, D. L., & Geller, E. J. (2013). Complications of hysterectomy. *Obstetrics & Gynecology, 121*(3), 654–673.

Hoffstetter, S., & Shah, M. (2015). Vulvodynia. *Clinical Obstetrics and Gynecology, 58*(3), 536–545.

Jepson, P. C., & Sung, V. W. (2014). Hysterectomy for pelvic organ prolapse: Indications and treatments. *Clinical Obstetrics and Gynecology, 57*(1), 72–82.

Lev-Saige, A. (2015). Vulvar and vaginal atrophy: Physiology, clinical presentation, and treatment considerations. *Clinical Obstetrics and Gynecology, 58*(3), 476–491.

Maldonado, V. A. (2014). Benign vulvar tumors. *Best Practices & Research: Clinical Obstetrics & Gynecology, 28*(7), 1088–1097.

*McAlpine, J. N., Hanley, G. E., Woo, M. M., et al. (2014). Opportunistic salpingectomy: Uptake, risks, and complications of a regional initiative for ovarian cancer prevention. *American Journal of Obstetrics & Gynecology, 210*(5), 471.e1–471.e11.

*McIntosh, L., Andersen, E., & Reekie, M. (2015). Conservative treatment of stress urinary incontinence in women: A 10-year (2004-2013) scoping review of the literature. *Urologic Nursing, 35*(4), 179–186, 203.

Mellano, E. M., & Tarney, C. M. (2014). Management of genitourinary fistula. *Current Opinions in Obstetrics & Gynecology, 26*(5), 415–423.

National Institute of Allergy & Infectious Disease (NIAID). (2015). NIAID research on genital herpes. Retrieved on 11/7/2015 at: www.niaid.nih.gov/topics/genitalHerpes/research/Pages/research.aspx

National Institute of Health (NIH). (2013). *Uterine Fibroids- NIH Fact Sheet.* Retrieved on 11/25/2015 at: report.nih.gov/nihfactsheets/ViewFactSheet.aspx?csid = 50

Nyirjesy, P. (2014). Management of persistent vaginitis. *Obstetrics and Gynecology, 124*(6), 1135–1146.

*Peltzer, J., Domain, E., & Teel, C. (2015). Living in the everydayness of HIV infection: Experiences of young African-American women. *Medsurg Nursing, 24*(2), 111–118.

Petrosky, E., Bocchini, J. A., Hariri, S., et al. (2015). Use of 9-Valent human papillomavirus (HPV) vaccine: Updated HPV vaccination recommendations of the advisory committee on immunization practices. *CDC: Morbidity and Mortality Weekly Report, 64*(11), 300–304.

Powell, A. M., & Nyirjesy, P. (2015). New perspectives on the normal vagina and noninfectious causes of discharge. *Clinical Obstetrics and Gynecology, 58*(3), 453–463.

Reichman, O., & Sobel, J. (2014). Desquamative inflammatory vaginitis. *Best Practice & Research: Clinical Obstetrics and Gynecology, 28*(7), 1042–1050.

Ridgeway, B., & Falcone, T. (2014). Innovations in minimally invasive hysterectomies. *Clinical Obstetrics & Gynecology, 57*(1), 83–94.

Steege, J. F., & Siedhoff, M. T. (2014). Chronic pelvic pain. *Obstetrics and Gynecology, 124*(3), 616–629.

Trikudanathan, S. (2015). Polycystic ovarian syndrome. *Medical Clinics of North America, 99*(1), 221–235.

U.S. Food and Drug Administration (FDA). (2014). Medical devices: Update on serious complications associated with transvaginal placement of surgical mesh for pelvic organ prolapse: FDA safety communication. Retrieved on 11/23/15 at: www.fda.gov/MedicalDevices/Safety/AlertsandNotices/ucm262435.htm

Wright, J. D., Herzog, T. J., Tsui, J., et al. (2013). Nationwide trends in the performance of inpatient hysterectomies in the United States. *Obstetrics & Gynecology, 122*(2), 233–241.

Zweizig, S., Korets, S., & Cain, J. (2014). Key concepts in management of vulvar cancer. *Best Practices & Research: Clinical Obstetrics & Gynecology, 28*(7), 959–966.

Resources

American Cancer Society, www.cancer.org

American Congress of Obstetricians and Gynecologists (ACOG), www.acog.org

American Sexual Health Association (ASHA; formerly the American Social Health Organization), www.ashasexualhealth.org

Association of Reproductive Health Professionals (ARHP), www.arhp.org

Association of Women's Health, Obstetric and Neonatal Nurses (AWHONN), www.awhonn.org

California STD/HIV Prevention Training Center, www.stdhivtraining.org

Centers for Disease Control and Prevention (CDC), Office of Women's Health, www.cdc.gov/women/

ClinicalTrials.gov, National Institutes of Health, www.clinicaltrials.gov

Effective Interventions, www.effectiveinterventions.org

Endo-Online, Endometriosis Association, www.endometriosisassn.org

Foundation for Women's Cancer (formerly the Gynecologic Cancer Foundation), Foundationforwomenscancer.org

Gay and Lesbian Medical Association (GLMA), www.glma.org

Herpes Hotline, 1-919-361-8488

National Ovarian Cancer Coalition (NOCC), www.ovarian.org

National STD Hotline, 1-800-232-4636

Oncology Nursing Society (ONS), www.ons.org

Ovarian Cancer National Alliance, www.ovariancancer.org

Planned Parenthood Federation of America, Plannedparenthood.org

RESOLVE: The National Infertility Association, www.resolve.org

58

Assessment and Management of Patients With Breast Disorders

LEARNING OBJECTIVES

On completion of this chapter, the learner will be able to:

1 Describe the anatomy and physiology of the breast.
2 Identify the assessment and diagnostic studies used to diagnose breast disorders.
3 Compare and contrast the pathophysiology of benign and malignant breast disorders.
4 Summarize evidence-based guidelines for the early detection of breast cancer.

5 Develop a plan for educating patients and consumer groups about breast self-awareness.
6 Explain the different modalities used to treat breast cancer.
7 Use the nursing process as a framework for care of the patient undergoing surgery for the treatment of breast cancer.
8 Recognize the physical, psychosocial, and rehabilitative needs of the patient who has had breast surgery for the treatment of breast cancer.

GLOSSARY

adjuvant chemotherapy: the use of anticancer medications in addition to other treatments to delay or prevent a recurrence of the disease

adjuvant hormonal therapy: the use of synthetic hormones or other medications given after primary treatment to increase the chances of a cure by stopping or slowing the growth of certain cancers that are affected by hormone stimulation (sometimes called *endocrine* or *antiestrogen therapy*)

aromatase inhibitors: medications that block the production of estrogens by the adrenal glands

atypical hyperplasia: abnormal increase in the number of cells in a specific area within the ductal or lobular areas of the breast; this abnormal proliferation increases the risk for cancer

benign proliferative breast disease: various types of atypical, yet noncancerous, breast tissue that increase the risk of breast cancer

brachytherapy: delivery of radiation therapy through internal implants to a localized area of tissue

BRCA1 and *BRCA2*: genes on chromosome 17 that, when damaged or mutated, increase a woman's risk for breast and/or ovarian cancer compared with women without the mutation

breast conservation treatment: surgery to remove a breast tumor and a margin of tissue around the tumor without removing any other part of the breast; may or may not include lymph node removal and radiation therapy

dose-dense chemotherapy: administration of chemotherapeutic agents at standard doses with shorter time intervals between each cycle of treatment

ductal carcinoma in situ (DCIS): cancer cells starting in the ductal system of the breast but not penetrating surrounding tissue

fibrocystic breast changes: term used to describe certain benign changes in the breast, typically palpable nodularity, lumpiness, swelling, or pain

fine-needle aspiration (FNA): removal of fluid for diagnostic analysis from a cyst or cells from a mass using a needle and syringe

gynecomastia: firm, overdeveloped breast tissue typically seen in adolescent boys

HER-2/neu: a protein, when found in larger amounts, indicates an aggressive tumor

lobular carcinoma in situ (LCIS): atypical change and proliferation of the lobular cells of the breast

lymphedema: chronic swelling of an extremity due to interrupted lymphatic circulation, typically from an axillary lymph node dissection

mammoplasty: surgery to reconstruct or change the size or shape of the breast; can be performed for reduction or augmentation

mastalgia: breast pain, usually related to hormonal fluctuations or irritation of a nerve

mastectomy: removal of the breast tissue and nipple–areola complex

mastitis: inflammation or infection of the breast

modified radical mastectomy: removal of the breast tissue, nipple–areola complex, and a portion of the axillary lymph nodes

Paget disease: form of breast cancer that begins in the ductal system and involves scaly changes in the nipple, areola, and surrounding skin

sentinel lymph node: first lymph node(s) in the lymphatic basin that receives drainage from the primary tumor in the breast; identified by a radioisotope and/or blue dye

stereotactic core biopsy: computer-guided method of core needle biopsy that is useful when masses or calcifications in the breast cannot be felt but can be visualized using mammography

surgical biopsy: surgical removal of all or a portion of a mass for microscopic examination by a pathologist

transverse rectus abdominal myocutaneous (TRAM) flap: method of breast reconstruction in which a flap of skin, fat, and muscle from the lower abdomen, with its attached blood supply, is rotated to the mastectomy site

Nurses care for patients with breast disorders in many settings. To care for these patients effectively, nurses require an understanding of the assessment, diagnostic testing, nursing management, and rehabilitation needs of patients with multiple processes that affect the breasts. A breast disorder, whether benign or malignant, can cause great anxiety and fear of potential disfigurement, loss of sexual attractiveness, and even death. Nurses, therefore, must have expertise in the assessment and management of not only the physical symptoms but also the psychosocial symptoms associated with various breast disorders.

BREAST ASSESSMENT

Anatomic and Physiologic Overview

Male and female breasts mature comparably until puberty, when estrogen and other hormones initiate breast development in females. This development usually occurs from 10 to 16 years of age, although the range can vary from 9 to 18 years. Stages of breast development are described as Tanner stages 1 through 5:

- Stage 1 describes a prepubertal breast.
- Stage 2 is breast budding, the first sign of puberty in a female.
- Stage 3 involves further enlargement of breast tissue and the areola (a darker tissue ring around the nipple).
- Stage 4 occurs when the nipple and areola form a secondary mound on top of the breast tissue.
- Stage 5 is the continued development of a larger breast with a single contour.

The breasts are located between the second and sixth ribs over the pectoralis muscle from the sternum to the midaxillary line. An area of breast tissue, called the *tail of Spence*, extends into the axilla (Osborne & Boolbol, 2014). Fascial bands, called *Cooper ligaments*, support the breast on the chest wall. The inframammary fold (or crease) is a ridge of fat at the bottom of the breast.

Each breast contains 12 to 20 cone-shaped lobes, which are made up of glandular elements (lobules and ducts) and separated by fat and fibrous tissue that binds the lobes together. Milk is produced in the lobules and then carried through the ducts to the nipple. Figure 58-1 shows the anatomy of the fully developed breast.

Assessment

Health History

When a patient presents with a breast problem, the nurse conducts a general health assessment, including history of medical disorders and previous surgery; family history of diseases, particularly cancer; gynecologic and obstetric history; present medications (including prescriptions, vitamins, and herbals); past and present use of hormonal contraceptives, hormone therapy (HT) (formerly referred to as hormone replacement therapy [HRT]), or fertility treatments; and social habits (e.g., smoking, drinking alcohol, illicit drug use). Psychosocial information, such as the patient's marital status, occupation, and availability of resources and support people, is obtained. Any recent x-rays or other diagnostic tests are noted. Focused questions pertaining to the breast disorder are asked concerning the onset of the disorder and the length of time it has been present. In addition, the patient is asked if any masses are palpable and if there is any associated pain, swelling, redness, nipple discharge, or change in the skin. Knowledge and comfort related to breast self-awareness, which can include breast self-examination (BSE), should also be ascertained from the patient.

Physical Assessment: Female Breast

A female breast examination can be conducted during any general physical or gynecologic examination or whenever the patient reports an abnormality. The American Cancer Society (ACS) screening guidelines for early detection of cancer (ACS, 2012) state that an annual clinical breast examination for women 40 years and older is preferable. A clinical breast

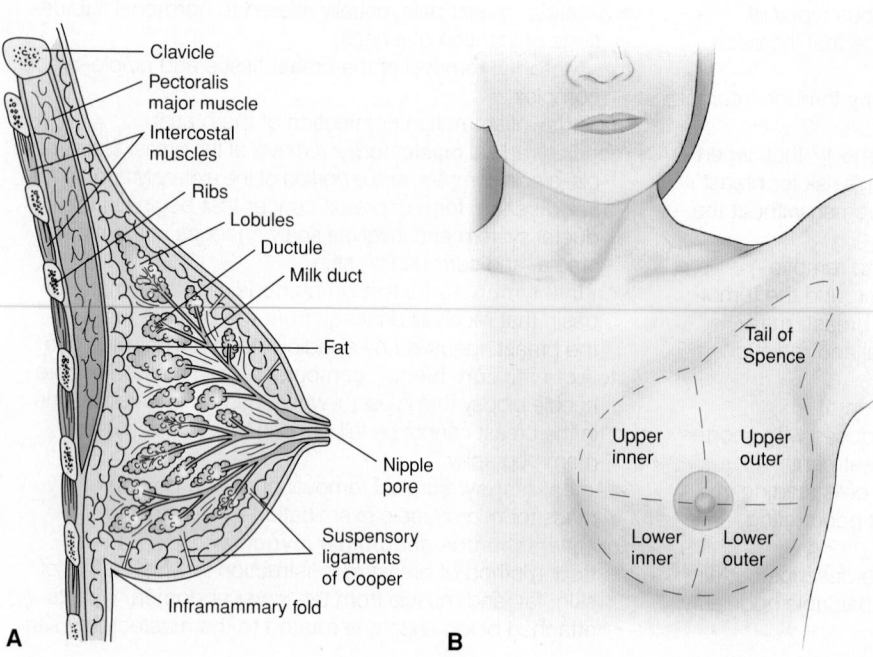

A

B

Figure 58-1 • **A.** Anatomy of the breast. **B.** Areas of breast, including the tail of Spence.

examination every 1 to 3 years for women between the ages of 20 and 39 years is preferable as part of a periodic health examination (ACS, 2012). A thorough breast examination, including instruction in breast awareness and BSE, takes at least 10 minutes.

Inspection

Examination begins with inspection. The patient is asked to disrobe to the waist and sit in a comfortable position facing the examiner. The breasts are inspected for size and symmetry. A slight variation in the size of each breast is common and generally normal. The skin is inspected for color, venous pattern, thickening, or edema. Erythema (redness) may indicate benign local inflammation or superficial lymphatic invasion by a neoplasm. A prominent venous pattern can signal increased blood supply required by a tumor. Edema and pitting of the skin may result from a neoplasm blocking lymphatic drainage, giving the skin an orange peel appearance (peau d'orange)—a classic sign of advanced breast cancer. Nipple inversion of one or both breasts is not uncommon and is significant only when of recent origin. Ulceration, rashes, or spontaneous nipple discharge requires evaluation. Examples of abnormal breast findings on inspection can be found in Chart 58-1.

To elicit skin dimpling or retraction that may otherwise go undetected, the examiner instructs the patient to raise both arms overhead. This maneuver normally elevates both breasts equally. The patient is then instructed to place her hands on her waist and push in. These movements, which cause contraction of the pectoral muscles, do not normally alter the breast contour or nipple direction. Any dimpling or retraction during these position changes suggests an underlying mass. The clavicular and axillary regions are inspected for swelling, discoloration, lesions, or enlarged lymph nodes (Morrow, 2014).

Palpation

The breasts are palpated with the patient sitting up (upright) and lying down (supine). In the supine position, the patient's shoulder is first elevated with a small pillow to help balance the breast on the chest wall. Failure to do this allows the breast tissue to slip laterally, and a breast mass may be missed. The entire surface of the breast and the axillary tail is systematically palpated using the flat part (pads) of the second, third, and fourth fingertips, held together, making dime-size circles. The examiner may choose to proceed in a clockwise direction, following imaginary concentric circles from the outer limits of the breast toward the nipple. Other acceptable methods are to palpate from each number on the face of the clock toward the nipple in a clockwise fashion or along imaginary vertical lines on the breast (see Fig. 58-2).

Palpation of the axillary and clavicular areas is easily performed with the patient seated (see Fig. 58-3). To examine the axillary lymph nodes, the examiner gently abducts the patient's arm from the thorax. With the left hand, the patient's right forearm is grasped and supported. The right hand is then free to palpate the axilla. Any lymph nodes that may be lying against the thoracic wall are noted. Normally, these lymph nodes are not palpable, but if they are enlarged, their location, size, mobility, and consistency are noted. During palpation, the examiner notes any patient-reported tenderness or masses. If a mass is detected, it is described by its location (e.g., right breast, 2 cm from the nipple at 2 o'clock position). Size, shape, consistency, border delineation, and mobility are included in the description (Morrow, 2014). The examiner then modifies these steps to use the right hand to grasp the patient's left forearm, and then uses the left hand to palpate the axilla of the left breast.

The breast tissue of the adolescent is usually firm and lobular, whereas that of the postmenopausal woman is more likely to feel thinner and fattier. During pregnancy and lactation, the breasts are firmer and larger with lobules that are more distinct. Hormonal changes cause the areola to darken.

Obesity may have a proinflammatory effect on the breast that can contribute to increased rates of atypia. Atypia in breast ductal lavage and C-reactive protein levels in the nipple are significantly correlated with body mass index (BMI). Excessive body weight, as reflected by a BMI of 25 kg/m^2 or higher, is associated with postmenopausal breast cancer and increases the risk of dying of this disease (Gucalp, Morris, Hudis, et al., 2014).

Cysts are commonly found in women who are menstruating and are usually well defined and freely movable. In the premenstrual period, cysts may be larger and more tender. Malignant tumors, on the other hand, tend to be hard, poorly defined, and nontender. A clinician should further evaluate any abnormalities detected during inspection and palpation.

Physical Assessment: Male Breast

Breast cancer can occur in men. Assessment of the male breast and axilla is brief but important and should be included in a physical examination. The nipple and areola are inspected for swelling, nodules, ulcerations, and nipple discharge. The flat disc of undeveloped breast tissue under the nipple is palpated. The same procedure for palpating the female axilla is used when assessing the male axilla (Weber & Kelley, 2014).

Gynecomastia is the firm enlargement of glandular tissue beneath and immediately surrounding the areola of the male (see later discussion). This is different from the enlargement of soft, fatty tissue, which is caused by obesity.

Diagnostic Evaluation

A wide range of diagnostic studies may be performed in patients with breast conditions. The nurse should educate the patient about the purpose, what to expect, and any possible side effects related to these examinations prior to testing. The nurse should note trends in the patient's test results, because they often provide information about disease progression as well as the patient's response to therapy.

Breast Self-Examination

The nurse plays a critical role in breast awareness education—a modality used for the early detection of breast cancer. BSE can be taught in a variety of settings, either on a one-to-one basis or in a group. It can also be initiated by a health care provider during a patient's routine physical examination. Regular self-examinations may result in early identification of problems and may also result in more diagnostic work-ups for benign or malignant problems.

Variations in breast tissue occur during the menstrual cycle, pregnancy, and the onset of menopause. Women on

Chart 58-1 ASSESSMENT
Abnormal Assessment Findings During Inspection of the Breasts

Retraction Signs

- Signs include skin dimpling, creasing, or changes in the contour of the breast or nipple
- They may be secondary to contraction of fibrotic tissue that can occur with underlying malignancy
- They may be secondary to scar tissue formation after breast surgery
- Retraction signs may appear only with position changes

Dimpling

Flattening of nipple

Retraction signs   Retraction with compression

Increased Venous Prominence

- Unilateral localized increase in venous pattern associated with malignant tumors
- Normal with bilateral and symmetrical breast enlargement associated with pregnancy and lactation

Increased venous prominence

Peau d'Orange (Edema)

- Associated with inflammatory breast cancer
- Caused by interference with lymphatic drainage
- Breast skin has orange peel appearance
- Skin pores enlarge
- May be noted on the areola
- Skin becomes thick, hard, and immobile

Peau d'orange

Nipple Inversion

- Considered normal if long-standing
- Associated with fibrosis and malignancy if recent development

Nipple inversion

Acute Mastitis (Inflammation of the Breasts)

- Associated with lactation but may occur at any age
- Nipple cracks or abrasions noted
- Breast skin reddened and warm to touch
- Tenderness
- Systemic signs include fever and increased pulse

Paget Disease (Malignancy of Mammary Ducts)

- Early signs—erythema of nipple and areola
- Late signs—thickening, scaling, and erosion of the nipple and areola

Paget's disease

Figure 58-2 • Breast examination with the woman in a supine position. The entire surface of the breast is palpated from the outer edge of the breast to the nipple; palpation patterns are circular or clockwise (**A**), wedge (**B**), and vertical strip (**C**).

HT can also experience fluctuations. Normal changes must be distinguished from those that may signal disease. Most women notice increased tenderness and lumpiness before their menstrual periods; therefore, BSE is best performed after menses (day 5 to day 7, counting the first day of menses as day 1). In addition, many women have grainy-textured breast tissue, but such areas are usually less nodular after menses. Younger women may find BSE particularly difficult because of the density of their breast tissue. As women age, their breasts become fattier and may be easier to examine.

Current practice is shifting from educating about BSE to promoting breast self-awareness, which is a woman's attentiveness to the normal appearance and feel of her breasts. However, self-examination still may be appropriate for some women who are at high risk and for those who prefer it. Breast self-awareness can include self-examination. For every woman, knowing how her breasts normally feel helps detect any changes or signs of a problem. BSE may play an important role in screening, especially for women who develop cancer in the interval after a negative result on mammography or clinical breast examination or who have a false-negative imaging or clinical examination result. It can also promote detection in women who have not been screened. The goal, with or without BSE, is to report any breast changes to a primary provider.

Family history can increase the risk of breast cancer in men, particularly if other men in the family have had breast cancer. The risk is also higher if there is a breast cancer gene abnormality in the family. An abnormal *BRCA2* gene accounts for up to 40% of male breast cancers (Jain & Gradishar, 2014). Instructions about BSE should be provided to men if they have a family history of breast cancer.

Patients who elect to perform BSE should receive proper instruction on technique (see Chart 58-2). They should be informed that routine, monthly BSE will help them become familiar with their "normal abnormalities." If a change is detected, they should seek medical attention.

Patients should be instructed about optimal timing for BSE (5 to 7 days after menses begin for women who are premenopausal and once monthly for women who are postmenopausal). When demonstrating examination techniques, the feel of normal breast tissue should be reviewed and ways to identify breast changes discussed. Patients should then perform a BSE demonstration on themselves or on a breast model. Patients who have had breast cancer surgery should be instructed to examine their breast or chest wall for any new changes or nodules that may indicate a recurrence of the disease.

Mammography

Mammography is a breast imaging technique used to visualize the breast to detect small abnormalities that could suggest

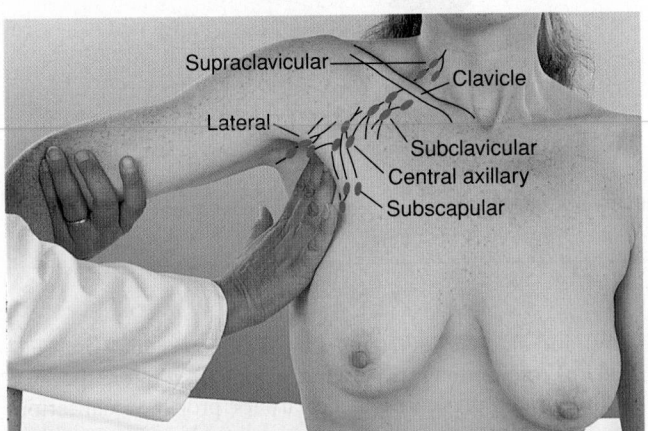

Figure 58-3 • Palpating axillary nodes in breast examination.

Chart 58-2 **PATIENT EDUCATION**
Breast Self-Examination

The nurse instructs the patient to perform the following steps:

Step 1

1. Stand in front of a mirror.
2. Check both breasts for anything unusual.
3. Look for discharge from the nipple, puckering, dimpling, or scaling of the skin.

Step 2

Steps 2 and 3 are done to check for any changes in the contour of your breasts. As you do them, you should be able to feel your muscles tighten.

1. Watch closely in the mirror as you clasp your hands behind your head and press your hands forward.
2. Note any change in the contour of your breasts.

Step 3

1. Next, press your hands firmly on your hips and bow slightly toward the mirror as you pull your shoulders and elbows forward.
2. Note any change in the contour of your breasts.

Step 4

Some women do step 4 of the examination in the shower. Your fingers will glide easily over soapy skin, so you can concentrate on feeling for changes inside the breast.

1. Raise your left arm.
2. Use three or four fingers of your right hand to feel your left breast firmly, carefully, and thoroughly.
3. Beginning at the outer edge, press the flat part of your fingers in small circles, moving the circles slowly around the breast.
4. Gradually work toward the nipple.
5. Be sure to cover the whole breast.
6. Pay special attention to the area between the breast and the underarm, including the underarm itself.
7. Feel for any unusual lumps or masses under the skin.
8. If you have any spontaneous discharge during the month—whether or not it is during your breast self-examination—see your primary provider.
9. Repeat the examination on your right breast.

Step 5

1. Step 5 should be repeated lying down.
2. Lie flat on your back with your left arm over your head and a pillow or folded towel under your left shoulder. (This position flattens your breast and makes it easier to check.)
3. Use the same circular motion described earlier.
4. Repeat on your right breast.

Adapted from U.S. Department of Health and Human Services, Public Health Service. (2012). *What you need to know about breast cancer.* Bethesda, MD: National Institutes of Health.

malignant or benign disease (Fischbach & Dunning, 2015). The procedure takes about 15 minutes and can be performed in a hospital radiology department or independent imaging center. Two views are taken of each breast. The breast is mechanically compressed from top to bottom (craniocaudal view) and side to side (mediolateral oblique view) (see Fig. 58-4). Women may experience some discomfort because maximum compression is necessary for proper visualization. The new mammogram is compared with previous mammograms, and any changes may indicate a need for further

Figure 58-4 • The mammography procedure (**A**) relies on x-ray imaging to produce the mammogram (**B**), which in this case reveals a breast lump.

investigation. Mammography may detect a breast tumor before it is clinically palpable (i.e., smaller than 1 cm); however, it has limitations (Fischbach & Dunning, 2015). The false-negative rate ranges between 5% and 10% (Helvie & Patterson, 2014). Younger women, or those taking HTs, may have dense breast tissue, making it more difficult to detect lesions with mammography.

Patients scheduled for a mammogram may voice concern about exposure to radiation. The radiation exposure is equivalent to about 1 hour of exposure to sunlight, so patients would have to have many mammograms in a year to increase their cancer risk. To ensure that a mammogram is reliable, it is important that a woman find a reputable facility. Mammographic facilities are certified by the U.S. Food and Drug Administration (FDA), and the machines are accredited by the American College of Radiology (Fischbach & Dunning, 2015).

In 2015, the ACS changed the mammography recommendations to state that healthy women should have mammography every year beginning at age 45 years (ACS, 2015). Women 55 and older may continue yearly screening or transition to every 2 years. This change was based on calculations that starting annual screening mammography later and getting it less often would cause less harm and be as safe as starting it earlier and getting it more often. Screening every other year may, however, result in a missed diagnosis and a small increase in the probability of being diagnosed with later-stage cancer (Kerlikowske, 2015).

The ACS, however, continues to recommend that women 45 years and older have a mammogram every year and that they continue to do so for as long as they do not have serious, chronic health problems such as congestive heart failure, end-stage kidney disease, chronic obstructive pulmonary disease, and moderate to severe dementia. Age alone should not be the reason to stop having regular mammograms (ACS, 2012).

Newer techniques for breast screening include digital mammography and 3D mammography. Digital mammography records x-ray images on a computer instead of on film, thus allowing radiologists to adjust the contrast and focus on an image without having to take additional x-rays. Although the accuracy of both film and digital screening mammography is similar for most women, digital mammography has been shown to be better at detecting estrogen receptor–negative tumors and cancer in extremely dense breasts. Both of these subgroups are more common in younger women, who may therefore choose digital mammography if they wish to have screening mammography. The 3D mammography obtains multiple projections of the compressed breast and results in fewer call backs for additional imaging (Jochelson, 2014). Computer-aided detection (CAD) is an option for radiologists and can be helpful in finding abnormal areas that should be checked more closely for early cancers. Refinements and improvements have been made to CAD software with a focus on increasing sensitivity for masses and reducing false-positive rates.

Contrast Mammography

A contrast mammography (i.e., ductogram, galactogram) is a diagnostic procedure that involves injection of less than 1 mL of radiopaque material through a cannula inserted into a ductal opening on the areola, which is followed by a mammogram (Fischbach & Dunning, 2015). It is performed to evaluate an abnormality within the duct when the patient has bloody nipple discharge on expression, spontaneous nipple discharge, or a solitary dilated duct noted on mammography.

Ultrasonography

Ultrasonography (ultrasound) is used as a diagnostic adjunct to mammography to help distinguish fluid-filled cysts from other lesions. A thin coating of lubricating jelly is spread over the area to be imaged. A transducer is then placed on the breast. The transducer transmits high-frequency sound waves through the skin toward the area of concern. The sound waves that are reflected back form a two-dimensional image, which is then displayed on a computer screen. No radiation is emitted during the procedure. Ultrasound is also used as an adjunct to mammography in women with dense breast tissue.

Ultrasonography has advantages and disadvantages. Although it can diagnose cysts with great accuracy, it cannot definitively rule out malignant lesions. Microcalcifications, which are detectable on mammography, cannot be identified on ultrasonography. Finally, examination techniques and interpretation criteria are not standardized.

Magnetic Resonance Imaging

Magnetic resonance imaging (MRI) of the breast is a highly sensitive test that has become a useful diagnostic adjunct to mammography. A magnet is linked to a computer that creates detailed images of the breast without exposure to radiation. An intravenous (IV) injection of gadolinium, a contrast dye, is given to improve visibility. The patient lies face down, and the breast is placed through a depression in the table. A coil is placed around the breast, and the patient is placed inside the MRI machine. The entire procedure takes about 30 to 40 minutes.

Breast MRI is useful for evaluation of contralateral disease, invasive lobular carcinoma, and assessment of chemotherapeutic response. The ACS recommends an annual MRI scan in addition to mammography in women at high risk for breast cancer (i.e., those with greater than 20% lifetime risk). Candidates include women who have a *BRCA1* or *BRCA2* mutation, a first-degree relative with either of these mutations, certain rare genetic syndromes, or radiation to the chest between 10 and 30 years of age (ACS, 2012). MRI should be used in addition to mammography, not instead of it.

Some disadvantages of MRI include high cost, variations in technique and interpretation, and the potential for patient claustrophobia. The procedure cannot always accurately distinguish between malignant and benign breast conditions, so false positive results may occur. MRI is contraindicated in patients with implantable metal devices (e.g., aneurysm clips, pacemakers, ports of tissue expanders) because of the metallic force. Foil-backed medication patches (e.g., nicotine, nitroglycerin, fentanyl) must be removed prior to MRI to avoid burns to the skin.

Procedures for Tissue Analysis

Percutaneous Biopsy

Percutaneous biopsy is performed on an outpatient basis to sample palpable and nonpalpable lesions. Less invasive than a surgical biopsy, percutaneous biopsy is a needle or core biopsy that obtains tissue by making a small puncture in the skin. Table 58-1 outlines the different types of biopsies that can be performed to obtain a tissue diagnosis.

 Concept Mastery Alert

It is important to understand the differences between common procedures used for patients with breast disorders. Mammography is used to detect breast abnormalities, whereas biopsy is performed to confirm a diagnosis of breast cancer.

Fine-Needle Aspiration

Fine-needle aspiration (FNA) is a biopsy technique that is generally well tolerated by most women. A local anesthetic

may or may not be used. A small-gauge needle (25 or 22 gauge) attached to a syringe is inserted into the mass or area of nodularity. Suction is applied to the syringe, and multiple passes are made through the mass. A simple cyst often disappears on aspiration, and the fluid is usually discarded. If no fluid is obtained, any cellular material obtained in the hub of the needle is spread on a glass slide or placed in a preservative and sent to the laboratory for analysis (CancerQuest, 2015). For nonpalpable masses, the same procedure can be performed by a radiologist using ultrasound guidance (ultrasound-guided FNA).

FNA is less expensive than other diagnostic methods, and results are usually available quickly. However, false-negative or false-positive results are possible, and appropriate follow-up depends on the clinical judgment of the treating physician.

Core Needle Biopsy

Core needle biopsy is similar to FNA, except a larger-gauge needle is used (usually 14 gauge). A local anesthetic is applied, and tissue cores are removed via a spring-loaded device. This procedure allows for a more definitive diagnosis than FNA, because actual tissue, not just cells, is removed. It is often performed for relatively large tumors that are close to the skin surface, but is also utilized for smaller, deeper lesions that are visible on ultrasound.

Stereotactic Core Biopsy

Stereotactic core biopsy is performed on nonpalpable lesions detected by mammography. The patient lies prone on the stereotactic table. The breast is suspended through an opening in the table and compressed between two x-ray plates. Images are then obtained using digital mammography. The exact coordinates of the lesion to be sampled are located with the aid of a computer. Next, a local anesthetic is injected into the entry site on the breast. A small nick is made in the skin, a core needle is inserted, and samples of the tissue are taken for pathologic examination. Often, several passes are taken to ensure that the lesion is well sampled. Post-biopsy images are then taken to check that sampling has been adequate. A small titanium clip is almost always placed at the biopsy site so that the site can easily be located if further treatment is indicated.

TABLE 58-1 Types of Breast Biopsies

Procedure	Palpable Mass	Health Professional Who Performs Procedure	Nature of Breast Tissue Removed
Fine-needle aspiration	Yes	Surgeon	Cellular material
Core needle biopsy	Yes	Surgeon	Tissue core
Stereotactic core biopsy	No	Radiologist	Tissue core
Ultrasound-guided core biopsy	No	Radiologist	Tissue core
Magnetic resonance imaging (MRI)-guided core biopsy	No	Radiologist	Tissue core
Excisional biopsy	Yes	Surgeon	Entire mass
Incisional biopsy	Yes	Surgeon	Tissue core
Wire needle localization biopsy; may be guided by mammogram, ultrasound, or MRI	No	Radiologist inserts wire; surgeon performs biopsy	Entire mass

Stereotactic biopsy is quite accurate and often allows the patient to avoid a surgical biopsy. However, there is a small false-negative rate. Appropriate follow-up depends on the final pathologic diagnosis and the clinical judgment of the primary provider. The use of a titanium clip does not preclude subsequent MRIs.

Ultrasound-Guided Core Biopsy

The principles for ultrasound-guided core biopsy are similar to those of stereotactic core biopsy, but by using ultrasound guidance, computer coordination and mammographic compression are not necessary. An ultrasound-guided core biopsy does not use radiation and is also usually faster and less expensive than stereotactic core biopsy.

Magnetic Resonance Imaging–Guided Core Biopsy

MRI-guided core biopsy can be performed by a radiologist and technologist when the abnormal area in the breast is too small to be felt but is visible on MRI.

Surgical Biopsy

Surgical biopsy is usually performed using local anesthesia and intravenous (IV) sedation. After an incision is made, the lesion is excised and sent to a laboratory for pathologic examination. Surgical biopsy is usually preceded by a core biopsy or stereotactic biopsy for pathologic determination.

Types of Surgical Breast Biopsy

Excisional Biopsy

Excisional biopsy is the standard procedure for complete pathologic assessment of a palpable breast mass. The entire mass, plus a margin of surrounding tissue, is removed. This type of biopsy may also be referred to as a lumpectomy. Depending on the clinical situation, a frozen-section analysis of the specimen may be performed at the time of the biopsy by the pathologist, who does an immediate reading intraoperatively and provides a provisional diagnosis. This can help confirm a diagnosis in a patient who has had no previous tissue analysis performed.

Incisional Biopsy

Incisional biopsy surgically removes a portion of a mass. This is performed to confirm a diagnosis and to conduct special studies (e.g., ER/PR, HER-2/neu [also referred to as ERBB2]; see later discussion for explanation of these terms) that will aid in determining treatment, which is discussed later in this chapter. Complete excision of the area may not be possible or immediately beneficial to the patient, depending on the clinical situation. This procedure is often performed on women with locally advanced breast cancer or on women with suspected cancer recurrence, whose treatment may depend on the results of these special studies. However, pathologic information may be easily obtained from core needle biopsy, and incisional biopsy is becoming less common.

Wire Needle Localization

Wire needle localization is a technique used to locate nonpalpable masses or suspicious calcium deposits detected on a mammogram, ultrasound, or MRI that require an excisional biopsy. The radiologist inserts a long, thin wire through a needle, which is then inserted into the area of abnormality using x-ray or ultrasound guidance (whichever imaging technique originally identified the abnormality). The wire remains in place after the needle is withdrawn to ensure the precise location. The patient is then taken to the operating room, where the surgeon follows the wire to the tip and excises the area.

Nursing Management

During the preoperative or preprocedure visit, the nurse assesses the patient for any specific educational, physical, or psychosocial needs. This can be accomplished by reviewing the medical and psychosocial history and encouraging the patient to verbalize fears, concerns, and questions. Patients are often worried not only about the procedure but also about the potential implications of the pathology results. Providing a thorough explanation about what to expect in a supportive manner can help alleviate anxiety. Patients often have difficulty absorbing all the information given to them; therefore, written materials to take home are often provided to reinforce and clarify education.

The nurse instructs the patient to discontinue any agents that can increase the risk of bleeding, including products containing aspirin, nonsteroidal anti-inflammatory drugs, vitamin E supplements, herbal substances (such as ginkgo biloba and garlic supplements). Patients on prescription anticoagulants may need to check with the prescriber prior to temporary cessation for the procedure, as biopsies done without cessation of these drugs can result in prolonged bleeding and hematomas. The patient may be instructed not to eat or drink for several hours prior to the procedure or after midnight the night before the procedure, depending on the type of biopsy and anesthesia planned. Most breast biopsy procedures are performed with the use of moderate sedation and local anesthesia.

Immediate assessment after the procedure includes monitoring the effects of the anesthesia and inspecting the surgical dressing for any signs of bleeding. Once the sedation has worn off, the nurse reviews the care of the biopsy site, pain management, and activity restrictions with the patient. Prior to discharge from the ambulatory surgical center or the office, the patient must be able to tolerate fluids, ambulate, and void. The patient must be accompanied home. The dressing covering the incision is usually removed after 48 hours, but the Steri-Strips, which are applied directly over the incision, should remain in place for approximately 7 to 10 days or until they fall off. The use of a supportive bra following surgery is encouraged to limit movement of the breast and reduce discomfort. A follow-up telephone call from the nurse 24 to 48 hours after the procedure can provide the patient with the opportunity to ask any questions and can be a source of great comfort and reassurance.

Most women return to their usual activities the day after the procedure but are encouraged to avoid jarring or high-impact activities for 1 week to promote healing of the biopsy site. Discomfort is usually minimal, and most women find acetaminophen (Tylenol) sufficient for pain relief, although a mild opioid analgesic agent may be prescribed if needed.

Follow-up after the biopsy includes a return visit to the surgeon for discussion of the final pathology report and assessment of the healing of the biopsy site. Depending on the results of the biopsy, the nurse's role varies. If the pathology report is benign, the nurse reviews incision care and explains what the patient should expect as the biopsy site heals (i.e., changes in sensation may occur weeks or months after the biopsy due to nerve injury within the breast tissue). If a diagnosis of cancer is made, the nurse's role changes dramatically. This is discussed in depth later in this chapter.

CONDITIONS AFFECTING THE NIPPLE

Nipple Discharge

Nipple discharge in a woman who is not lactating may be related to many causes, such as carcinoma, papilloma, pituitary adenoma, cystic breasts, and various medications. Oral contraceptives, pregnancy, HT, chlorpromazine (Thorazine)-type medications, and frequent breast stimulation may be contributing factors. In some women, nipple discharge may occur during running or aerobic exercises. Nipple discharge should be evaluated by a health care provider, but it is not often a cause for alarm. One in three women has clear discharge on expression, which is usually normal. A green discharge could indicate an infection. Any discharge that is spontaneous, persistent, or unilateral is of concern. Although bloody discharge can indicate a malignancy, it is often caused by a benign wartlike growth on the lining of the duct called an *intraductal papilloma*.

Nipple discharge should be evaluated for the presence of occult (hidden) blood by performing a guaiac test. A negative test can be reassuring as it indicates there is no blood, but it does not prove there is no malignancy. A galactogram can also be performed to detect abnormalities within the duct that may be causing the discharge. If there is a high level of suspicion, an excisional biopsy may be indicated. (See procedures for tissue analysis earlier in this chapter.)

Fissure

A fissure is a longitudinal ulcer that may develop in women who are breast-feeding. If the nipple becomes irritated, a painful, raw area may form and become a site of infection. Daily washing with water, massage with breast milk or lanolin, and exposure to air are helpful. Breast-feeding can continue with the use of a nipple shield. However, if the fissure is severe or extremely painful, the woman may be advised to stop breast-feeding. A breast pump can be used until breast-feeding can be resumed. Persistent ulceration requires further diagnosis and therapy. Guidance from a nurse or lactation consultant may be helpful, because nipple irritation can result from improper positioning or poor latching on (i.e., the infant has not grasped the areola fully) during breast-feeding.

BREAST INFECTIONS

Mastitis

Mastitis, an inflammation or infection of breast tissue, occurs most commonly in women who are breast-feeding, although it may also occur in women who are nonlactating. The infection may result from a transfer of microorganisms to the breast by the patient's hands or from a breast-fed infant with an oral, eye, or skin infection. Mastitis may also be caused by bloodborne organisms. As inflammation progresses, the breast texture becomes tough or doughy, and the patient complains of dull to severe pain in the infected region. A nipple that is discharging purulent material, serum, or blood should be investigated promptly.

Treatment consists of antibiotics and local application of cold compresses to relieve discomfort. A broad-spectrum antibiotic agent may be prescribed for 7 to 10 days. The patient should wear a snug bra and perform personal hygiene carefully. Adequate rest and hydration are important aspects of management.

Lactational Abscess

A breast abscess may develop as a consequence of acute mastitis. The area affected becomes tender and red. Purulent matter can usually be aspirated with a needle, but incision and drainage may be required. Specimens of the aspirated material are obtained for culture so that an organism-specific antibiotic agent can be prescribed.

BENIGN CONDITIONS OF THE BREAST

Breast Pain

Mastalgia (breast pain) may be cyclical or noncyclical. Cyclical pain is usually related to hormonal fluctuations, usually during the menstrual cycle, and accounts for the majority of complaints. Noncyclical pain is far less common and does not vary with the menstrual cycle. Women who experience injury or trauma to the breast or those who have had a breast biopsy may experience noncyclical pain. Patients should be reassured that breast pain is rarely indicative of cancer. However, if the pain persists after menses begin, the patient should see her primary provider.

Nursing Management

The nurse may recommend that the patient wear a supportive bra both day and night for a week, decrease her salt and caffeine intake, and take ibuprofen (Advil) as needed for its anti-inflammatory actions. Vitamin E supplements may also be helpful.

Cysts

Cysts are fluid-filled sacs that develop as breast ducts dilate. Cysts occur most commonly in women 30 to 55 years of age and may be exacerbated during perimenopause. Although their cause is unknown, cysts usually disappear after menopause, suggesting that estrogen is a factor. Cystic areas often fluctuate in size and are usually larger premenstrually. They may be painless or may become very tender premenstrually. Occasionally, a patient may report an intermittent shooting sensation or a dull ache. Various breast masses are compared in Table 58-2. Cysts that are confirmed on an ultrasound and are not bothersome can often be left alone. To confirm a diagnosis or to relieve pain, FNA can be performed. Cysts do not increase the risk of breast cancer (ACS, 2015).

Fibrocystic breast changes, often incorrectly called *fibrocystic breast disease*, is a nonspecific term used to describe an array of benign findings including palpable nodularity, lumpiness, swelling, or pain. The changes do not necessarily indicate a cystic or disease process.

Fibroadenomas

Fibroadenomas are firm, round, movable, benign tumors. They can occur from puberty to menopause with a peak

TABLE 58-2 Comparison of Various Breast Masses

The most common breast masses are due to cysts, fibroadenomas, or malignancy. Biopsy is usually needed for confirmation, but the following characteristics are diagnostic clues:

Characteristics	Cysts	Fibroadenomas	Malignancy
Age	30–55 years, regress after menopause except with use of estrogen therapy	Puberty to menopause	30–90 years; most common, 40–80 years
Number	Single or multiple	Usually single	Usually single
Shape	Round	Round, disc, or lobular	Irregular or stellate
Consistency	Soft to firm, usually elastic	Usually firm	Firm or hard
Mobility	Mobile	Mobile	May be fixed to skin or underlying tissues
Tenderness	Usually tender	Usually nontender	Usually nontender
Retraction signs	Absent	Absent	May be present

Adapted from Weber, J., & Kelley, J. (2014). *Health assessment in nursing* (5th ed.). Philadelphia, PA: Lippincott Williams & Wilkins.

incidence at 30 years of age. These masses are nontender and are sometimes biopsied or removed for definitive diagnosis.

Benign Proliferative Breast Disease

The two most common types of **benign proliferative breast disease** (atypical, yet noncancerous, breast tissue) found on biopsy are atypical hyperplasia and lobular carcinoma in situ (LCIS). These diagnoses increase a woman's risk of breast cancer.

Atypical Hyperplasia

Atypical hyperplasia can be ductal or lobular and is a premalignant lesion of the breast. It is recognized as a precursor lesion to both noninvasive and invasive breast cancer. Imbalance in the normal regulation of cell proliferation is a defining feature. Women with atypical hyperplasia have a fourfold increased risk of breast cancer compared to women in the general population, with a cumulative incidence approaching 30% at 25 years of age (Collins & Schnitt, 2014).

Lobular Carcinoma in Situ

Lobular carcinoma in situ (LCIS) is an incidental microscopic finding of abnormal tissue growth in the lobules of the breast. LCIS is a risk indicator and some studies describe half of affected women will develop breast cancer within 15 to 30 years (King & Reis-Filho, 2014). Affected women should undergo rigorous breast cancer surveillance that consists of annual mammography and clinical breast examination every 6 months (National Comprehensive Cancer Network [NCCN], 2015). Patients should be offered information about chemoprevention with selective estrogen receptor modulators (SERMs), such as tamoxifen (Soltamox, Nolvadex). See the discussion of chemoprevention later in this chapter.

Other Benign Conditions

Cystosarcoma phyllodes is a rare fibroepithelial tumor that tends to grow rapidly. It is rarely malignant and is treated with surgical excision. If it is malignant, mastectomy may follow. Lymph node removal is usually not performed, because metastasis is rare.

Fat necrosis is a condition of the breast that is often associated with a history of trauma. Surgical procedures such as a breast biopsy, lumpectomy or mastectomy can cause fat necrosis. It may be indistinguishable from carcinoma, and the entire mass may be excised or biopsied. If excision is not indicated, it is followed with regular breast imaging.

Intraductal papilloma is a wartlike growth that often involves the large milk ducts near the nipple, causing bloody nipple discharge. Surgery usually involves removal of the papilloma and a segment of the duct where the papilloma is found.

Superficial thrombophlebitis of the breast (Mondor disease) is an uncommon condition that is usually associated with pregnancy, trauma, or breast surgery. Pain and redness occur as a result of a superficial thrombophlebitis in the vein that drains the outer part of the breast. The mass is usually linear, tender, and erythematous. Treatment consists of analgesic agents and heat.

MALIGNANT CONDITIONS OF THE BREAST

Breast cancer is a major health problem in the United States. Current statistics indicate that over a lifetime (birth to death), a woman's risk of developing breast cancer is about 12%, or one in eight. Currently, about 231,840 new cases of invasive breast cancer are diagnosed in women each year. Risk of developing breast cancer increases with increasing age. About two of three invasive breast cancers are found in women 55 years or older. About 5% to 10% of breast cancer cases are thought to be hereditary, resulting directly from gene defects (cell mutations) inherited from a biologic parent (ACS, 2015).

Female breast cancer incidence rates vary substantially by race and ethnicity. Higher death rates in African Americans have been attributed to later stage at diagnosis and poorer stage-specific survival. Research suggests that racial disparities in cancer mortality are driven in large part by differences in socioeconomic status (ACS, 2013).

Types of Breast Cancer

Ductal Carcinoma in Situ

Ductal carcinoma in situ (DCIS) is characterized by the proliferation of malignant cells inside the milk ducts without invasion into the surrounding tissue. Unlike invasive breast cancer, DCIS does not metastasize and a woman generally does not die of DCIS unless it develops into invasive breast cancer. DCIS can develop into invasive breast cancer if left untreated. The best estimates are that 14% to 53% of untreated DCIS progresses to invasive breast cancer over a period of 10 years or more. However, the natural history of DCIS is not well understood, and it is currently not possible to accurately predict which women with DCIS will go on to develop invasive breast cancer (ACS, 2015). DCIS is frequently manifested on a mammogram with the appearance of calcifications and is considered breast cancer stage 0.

Medical Management

Current management takes into account (1) assurance of an accurate diagnosis, (2) assessment of DCIS size and grade, and (3) careful margin evaluation. The pathologist analyzes the piece of breast tissue removed to determine the type and grade of the DCIS or how abnormal the cells look when compared with normal breast cells and how fast they are growing. Grade III (high-grade DCIS) cells tend to grow more quickly than grade I (low-grade) and grade II (moderate-grade) cells

and look much different from normal breast cells. Accurate grading of DCIS is critical, because high nuclear grade and the presence of necrosis (the premature death of cells in living tissue) are highly predictive of the inability to achieve adequate margins or borders of healthy tissue around the cancer, of local recurrence, and of the probability of missed areas of invasion. The pros and cons of irradiating patients with DCIS who are treated conservatively should be carefully weighed on a case-by-case basis, considering recent trials have shown that radiation has a beneficial effect on distant recurrence, breast cancer–specific mortality, and overall survival. Breast conservation (treatment of a breast cancer without the loss of the breast) can be curative for well-defined subsets of women with DCIS (ACS, 2015).

Invasive Cancer

The NCCN (2015), a nonprofit group of the world's 21 leading cancer centers, disseminates estimates for various types of cancer.

Infiltrating Ductal Carcinoma

Infiltrating ductal carcinoma—the most common histologic type of breast cancer—accounts for 80% of all cases. The tumors arise from the duct system and invade the surrounding tissues. They often form a solid irregular mass in the breast.

Infiltrating Lobular Carcinoma

Infiltrating lobular carcinoma accounts for 10% to 15% of breast cancers. The tumors arise from the lobular epithelium and typically occur as an area of ill-defined thickening in the breast. They are often multicentric and can be bilateral.

Medullary Carcinoma

Medullary carcinoma accounts for about 5% of breast cancers, and it tends to be diagnosed more often in women younger than 50 years. The tumors grow in a capsule inside a duct. They can become large and may be mistaken for a fibroadenoma. The prognosis is often favorable.

Mucinous Carcinoma

Mucinous carcinoma accounts for about 3% of breast cancers and often presents in women who are postmenopausal and are 75 years and older. A mucin producer, the tumor is also slow growing; thus, the prognosis is more favorable than in many other types.

Tubular Ductal Carcinoma

Tubular ductal carcinoma accounts for about 2% of breast cancers. Because axillary metastases are uncommon with this histology, prognosis is usually excellent. Micropapillary invasive ductal carcinoma is a rare type of aggressive ductal cancer characterized by a high rate of axillary node metastasis and skin involvement.

Inflammatory Carcinoma

Inflammatory carcinoma is a rare (1% to 3%) and aggressive type of breast cancer that has unique symptoms. The cancer is characterized by diffuse edema and erythema of the skin, often referred to as peau d'orange (resembling an orange peel). This is caused by malignant cells blocking the lymph channels in the skin. An associated mass may or may not be present; if there is a mass, it is often a large area of indiscrete thickening. Inflammatory carcinoma can be confused with an infection because of its presentation. The disease can spread to other parts of the body rapidly. Chemotherapy often plays an initial role in controlling disease progression, but radiation and surgery may also follow.

Paget Disease

Paget disease of the breast accounts for 1% of diagnosed cases of breast cancer (Grossman & Porth, 2014). Symptoms typically include a scaly, erythematous, pruritic lesion of the nipple. Paget disease often represents DCIS of the nipple but may have an invasive component. If no lump can be felt in the breast tissue and the biopsy shows DCIS without invasion, the prognosis is very favorable.

Risk Factors

There is no single, specific cause of breast cancer. A combination of genetic, hormonal, and possibly environmental factors may increase the risk of its development (see Table 58-3). More than 80% of all cases of breast cancer are sporadic,

meaning that patients have no known family history of the disease. The remaining cases are either familial (there is a family history of breast cancer, but it is not passed on genetically) or genetically acquired. There is no evidence that smoking, silicone breast implants, the use of antiperspirants, underwire bras, or abortion (induced or spontaneous) increases the risk of the disease. There is some evidence that long-term smoking, starting before first pregnancy, and night shift work may increase the risk for breast cancer (ACS, 2015).

As stated previously, breast cancer can be genetically inherited, resulting in significant risk. Approximately 5% to 10% of breast cancer cases have been linked to specific genetic mutations. Factors that may indicate a genetic link include multiple first-degree relatives with early-onset breast cancer, breast and ovarian cancer in the same family, male breast cancer, and Ashkenazi Jewish background. **BRCA1 and BRCA2** are tumor suppressor genes that normally function to identify damaged deoxyribonucleic acid (DNA) and thereby restrain abnormal cell growth (Yarbo, Wujcik, & Gobel, 2013). Mutations in these genes on chromosome 17 are responsible for the majority of hereditary breast cancer

TABLE 58-3 Risk Factors for Breast Cancer

Risk Factor	Comments
Female gender	99% of cases occur in women.
Increasing age	Increasing age is associated with an increased risk.
Personal history of breast cancer	Once treated for breast cancer, the risk of developing breast cancer in same or opposite breast is significantly increased.
Family history of breast cancer	Having first-degree relative with breast cancer (mother, sister, daughter) increases the risk twofold; having two first-degree relatives increases the risk fivefold. The risk is higher if the relative was premenopausal at the time of diagnosis. The risk is increased if a father or brother had breast cancer (exact risk is unknown).
Genetic mutation	*BRCA1* and *BRCA2* mutations account for majority of inherited cases of breast cancer (see additional information in text).
Hormonal Factors • Early menarche • Late menopause • Nulliparity • Late age at first full-term pregnancy • Hormone therapy (formerly referred to as hormone replacement therapy)	 Before 12 years of age After 55 years of age No full-term pregnancies After 30 years of age Current or recent use of combined postmenopausal hormone therapy (estrogen and progesterone) Long-term use (several years or more)
Exposure to ionizing radiation during adolescence and early adulthood	The risk is highest if breast tissue was exposed while still developing (during adolescence), such as women who received mantle radiation (to the chest area) for treatment of Hodgkin lymphoma in their younger years.
History of benign proliferative breast disease	Having had atypical ductal or lobular hyperplasia or lobular carcinoma in situ increases the risk.
Obesity	Obesity and weight gain during adulthood increases the risk of postmenopausal breast cancer. During menopause, estrogen is primarily produced in fat tissue. More fat tissue can increase estrogen levels, thereby increasing breast cancer risk.
High-fat diet	More research is needed.
Alcohol intake (beer, wine, or liquor)	Two to five drinks daily increases the risk about one and a half times.

Adapted from National Comprehensive Cancer Network (NCCN). (2015). Clinical practice guidelines: Breast. Retrieved on 3/7/2016 at: www.nccn.org/professionals/physician_gls/PDF/infections.pdf

in the United States. *BRCA* mutations in women have been associated with an overall risk of breast cancer up to 65% (ACS, 2015). Currently, women who are *BRCA* positive are counseled to start screening, typically using mammography, once a year and then MRI 6 months after the yearly mammography by 25 years of age, or 5 to 10 years earlier than their youngest affected family member. Mutations in the PALB2 gene confer similar risk. Males who carry the *BRCA2* mutation may have a lifetime risk of 6% to 7% of developing breast cancer (Jain & Gradishar, 2014).

Protective Factors

Certain factors may be protective against the development of breast cancer. Breast feeding for at least 1 year, regular or moderate physical activity and maintaining a healthy body weight are cited as protective (ACS, 2015). Some research suggests that the use of extra virgin olive oil regularly in one's diet may be preventive (Toledo, Salas-Salvad, Donat-Vargas, et al., 2015).

Breast Cancer Prevention Strategies in the Patient Who Is at High Risk

Patients often over- or underestimate their risk of developing breast cancer. A consultation with a breast specialist is of paramount importance prior to embarking on any of the prevention strategies that follow. Once patients have an accurate assessment of their risk, along with the knowledge of the pros and cons of each prevention strategy, they can make a decision that is most appropriate for their situation.

Long-Term Surveillance

Long-term surveillance focuses on early detection. As recommended by the ACS (2012), women at high risk for breast cancer benefit from additional screening using MRI along with a yearly mammogram. Clinical breast examinations may be performed twice a year starting as early as 25 years of age. Mammograms may also be performed as early as 25 years of age. Data concerning the effectiveness of BSE are limited. In addition to yearly mammography and MRI, other screening tests, including ultrasonography, may be useful.

Chemoprevention

Chemoprevention is the main modality that aims to prevent the disease. Several national, randomized clinical trials in the past two decades have led to FDA approval of tamoxifen and raloxifene (Evista) as effective chemopreventive agents for use in women who are at high risk (Cummings, Eckert, Krueger, et al., 1999; Fisher, Constantino, Wickerham, et al., 1998; Vogel, Costantino, Wickerham, et al., 2006). In addition, anastrozole (Arimidex) and exemestane (Aromasin) are now used for chemoprevention (Comerford, 2015). Nurses can help women who are considering chemoprevention by providing them with information about the benefits, risks, and possible side effects of these medications.

Prophylactic Mastectomy

Prophylactic mastectomy is another primary prevention modality that can reduce the risk of breast cancer by 90% (National Cancer Institute [NCI], 2013) and is sometimes referred to as a "risk-reducing" mastectomy. The procedure consists of a total **mastectomy** (removal of breast tissue) and is usually accompanied by immediate breast reconstruction. Possible candidates include women with a strong family history of breast cancer, a diagnosis of LCIS or atypical hyperplasia, a mutation in a *BRCA* gene, and previous cancer in one breast. Because of physical and psychological ramifications including anxiety, depression, and altered body image, this procedure should be undertaken only after extensive counseling related to its risks and benefits. The procedure does not confer 100% protection against the development of breast cancer (NCI, 2013).

A multidisciplinary approach should be used to help the patient arrive at a decision that is best for her. Consultation with a genetic counselor, plastic surgeon, medical oncologist, and psychiatrist can be invaluable. The patient needs to understand that this surgery is elective and not emergent. The nurse can play a valuable role in providing the patient with information, clarification, and support during the decision-making process.

Clinical Manifestations

Breast cancers can occur anywhere in the breast but are usually found in the upper outer quadrant, where the most breast tissue is located. In general, the lesions are nontender, fixed rather than mobile, and hard with irregular borders. Complaints of diffuse breast pain and tenderness with menstruation are usually associated with benign breast disease.

With the increased use of mammography, more women are seeking treatment at earlier stages of the disease. These women often have no signs or symptoms other than a mammographic abnormality. Some women with advanced disease seek initial treatment after ignoring symptoms. Advanced signs may include skin dimpling, nipple retraction, or skin ulceration.

Assessment and Diagnostic Findings

Techniques to determine the diagnosis of breast cancer include various types of biopsy, which have been described previously. Tumor staging and analysis of additional prognostic factors are used to determine the prognosis and optimal treatment regimen (see below).

Staging

Staging involves classifying the cancer by the extent of the disease in the body. It is based on whether the cancer is invasive or noninvasive, the size of the tumor, how many lymph nodes are involved, and if it has spread to other parts of the body. The stage of a cancer is one of the most important factors in determining prognosis and treatment options. The most common system used to describe the stages of breast cancer is the American Joint Committee on Cancer (AJCC) TNM (tumor, nodes, metastasis) system (see Chapter 15, Chart 15-3). Other factors considered in staging include hormone receptors and genetic mutations.

Other diagnostic tests may be performed before or after surgery to help in the staging of the disease. The extent of testing often depends on the clinical presentation of the disease and may include chest x-rays, computed tomography (CT) scan, MRI scan, positron emission tomography (PET) scan, bone scans, and blood work (complete blood count, comprehensive metabolic panel, and tumor markers [i.e., carcinoembryonic antigen, cancer antigen 15-3]).

Prognosis

Several different factors must be taken into consideration when determining the prognosis of a patient with breast cancer. Two of the most important factors are tumor size and whether the tumor has spread to the lymph nodes under the arm (axilla).

In general, the smaller the tumor appears, the better the prognosis. A tumor starts with a genetic alteration in a single cell and takes time to divide and double in size. A carcinoma may double in size 30 times to become 1 cm or larger, at which point it becomes clinically apparent. Doubling time varies, but breast tumors are often present for several years before they become palpable. Nurses can reassure patients that once breast cancer is diagnosed, they have a safe period of several weeks to make decisions regarding treatment; however, a lengthy delay is not advisable.

Prognosis also depends on the extent of spread of the breast cancer. The 5-year survival rate is approximately 88% for a stage I breast cancer and 15% for a stage IV breast cancer (ACS, 2015). The most common route of regional spread is to the axillary lymph nodes. Other sites of lymphatic spread include the internal mammary and supraclavicular nodes (see Fig. 58-5). Distant metastasis can affect any organ, but the most common sites are bone, lung, liver, pleura, adrenals, skin, and brain (ACS, 2015).

In addition to the type of breast cancer and the stage, other factors may help determine prognosis (see Chart 58-3). Excessive number of copies of certain genes (amplification) or excessive amounts of their protein product (overexpression) may represent a poorer prognosis. The HER-2/neu (also known as ERBB2) oncogene is the classic example; approximately 25% of invasive breast cancers, which typically involve the more aggressive tumors, have amplification or overexpression of this gene (Press & Ma, 2015). The proliferative rate or rapidity in growth rate (S-phase fraction) and DNA content (ploidy) of a tumor are factors that are also associated with overall survival rate.

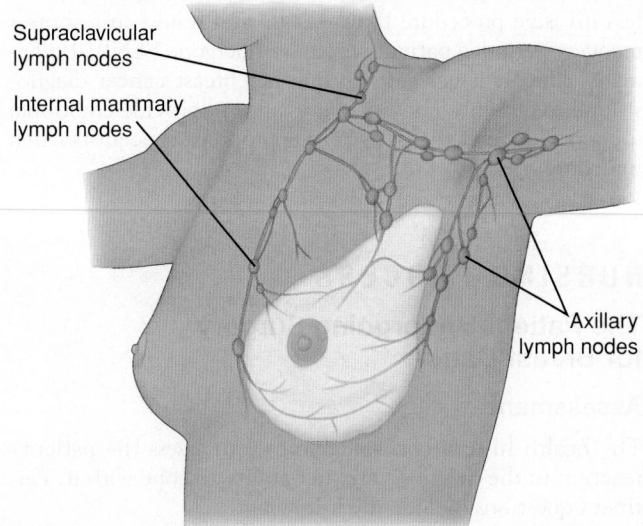

Figure 58-5 • Lymphatic drainage of the breast.

Supraclavicular lymph nodes

Internal mammary lymph nodes

Axillary lymph nodes

> ### Chart 58-3 Pathologic Factors Associated With Favorable Prognosis for Breast Cancer
>
> - Noninvasive tumors or invasive tumors <1 cm
> - Negative axillary lymph nodes
> - Estrogen receptor (ER) and progesterone receptor (PR) proteins
> - Well-differentiated tumors
> - Low expression of HER-2/neu oncogene (also known as ERBB2)
> - No vascular or lymphatic invasion
> - Diploid tumors with low S-phase fraction
>
> Adapted from U.S. Department of Health and Human Services, Public Health Service. (2012). *What you need to know about breast cancer.* Bethesda, MD: National Institutes of Health.

Surgical Management

The main goal of surgery is to gain local control of the disease. With breast cancer being diagnosed today at earlier stages, options for less invasive, breast conserving surgical procedures are available. Surgical treatment options for noninvasive and invasive breast cancer are summarized in Table 58-4.

Modified Radical Mastectomy

Modified radical mastectomy is performed to treat invasive breast cancer. The procedure involves removal of breast tissue, including the nipple–areola complex. In addition, a portion of the axillary lymph nodes are also removed in axillary lymph node dissection (ALND). If immediate breast reconstruction is desired, the patient is referred to a plastic surgeon prior to the mastectomy so that she has the opportunity to explore all available options. In modified radical mastectomy, the pectoralis major and pectoralis minor muscles are left intact, unlike in radical mastectomy, in which the muscles are removed.

Total Mastectomy

Like modified radical mastectomy, total mastectomy (i.e., simple mastectomy) also involves removal of the breast and nipple–areola complex but does not include ALND. Total mastectomy may be performed in patients with noninvasive breast cancer (e.g., DCIS), which does not have a tendency to spread to the lymph nodes. It may also be performed

TABLE 58-4 Surgical Treatment Options for Noninvasive and Invasive Breast Cancer

Noninvasive Breast Cancer	Invasive Breast Cancer
Breast conservation[a] alone	Breast conservation[a] with one of the following: Sentinel lymph node biopsy Axillary lymph node dissection
Total mastectomy alone	Total mastectomy with sentinel lymph node biopsy or Modified radical mastectomy

[a]Breast conservation treatment includes lumpectomy, wide excision, partial or segmental mastectomy, and quadrantectomy. These are relatively synonymous terms that describe removal of varying amounts of breast tissue.

TABLE 58-5 Comparison of Sentinel Lymph Node Biopsy and Axillary Lymph Node Dissection

Sentinel Lymph Node Biopsy	Axillary Lymph Node Dissection
Shorter operating room time (~15–30 minutes)	Longer operating room time (~60–90 minutes)
No surgical drain	Surgical drain
Local anesthesia with IV moderate sedation as outpatient surgery (unless being performed in conjunction with total mastectomy)	General anesthesia; usually overnight admission (sometimes done as outpatient surgery)
Lymphedema incidence approximately 0–7%	Lymphedema incidence approximately 0–20%
Presence of neuropathic sensations postoperatively (prevalence lower than after axillary lymph node dissection)	Presence of neuropathic sensations postoperatively
Decreased range of motion in affected arm unlikely postoperatively but may occur	Decreased range of motion likely postoperatively
Seroma (collection of serous fluid in the axilla) may occur postoperatively.	Seroma may occur postoperatively

prophylactically in patients who are at high risk for breast cancer (e.g., LCIS, *BRCA* mutation). A total mastectomy may also be performed in conjunction with sentinel lymph node biopsy (SLNB) for patients with invasive breast cancer.

Breast Conservation Treatment

The goal of **breast conservation treatment** (i.e., lumpectomy, wide excision, partial or segmental mastectomy, quadrantectomy) is to excise the tumor in the breast completely and obtain clear margins while achieving an acceptable cosmetic result. If the procedure is being performed to treat a noninvasive breast cancer, lymph node removal is not necessary. For an invasive breast cancer, lymph node removal (SLNB or ALND) is indicated. The lymph nodes are removed through a separate semicircular incision in the axilla.

Sentinel Lymph Node Biopsy

The status of the lymph nodes is the most important prognostic factor in breast cancer. The SLNB is a less invasive alternative to ALND and is considered a standard of care for the treatment of early-stage breast cancer. ALND is associated with potential morbidity, including lymphedema, cellulitis, decreased arm mobility, and sensory changes. Studies suggest that SLNB is highly accurate and is associated with a local recurrence rate similar to that of ALND (Chung & Giuliano, 2014). Table 58-5 compares SLNB and ALND.

The **sentinel lymph node**, which is the first node (or nodes) in the lymphatic basin that receives drainage from the primary tumor in the breast, is identified by injecting a radioisotope and/or blue dye into the breast; the radioisotope or dye then travels via the lymphatic pathways to the node. In SLNB, the surgeon uses a handheld probe to locate the sentinel lymph node, excises it, and sends it for pathologic analysis, which is often performed immediately during the surgery using frozen-section analysis. If the sentinel lymph node is positive, the surgeon can proceed with an immediate ALND, thus sparing the patient a return trip to the operating room and additional anesthesia. (The patient could also return for additional surgery at a later time.) If the sentinel lymph node is negative, a standard ALND is not needed, thus sparing the patient the possible complications of the procedure. After the procedure is complete, all specimens are sent to pathology for more thorough analysis.

Nursing Management

Patients who undergo SLNB in conjunction with breast conservation treatments are generally discharged the same day. Patients who undergo SLNB with total mastectomy usually stay in the hospital overnight, possibly longer if breast reconstruction is being performed. The patient must be informed that although frozen-section analysis is highly accurate, false-negative results can occur. A negative sentinel lymph node on frozen-section analysis may show metastatic disease on subsequent analysis, indicating that ALND is still necessary. The patient should also be reassured that the radioisotope and blue dye are generally safe. The nurse informs patients that they may notice a blue-green discoloration in the urine or stool for the first 24 hours as the blue dye is excreted. The incidence of lymphedema, decreased arm mobility, and seroma formation (collection of serous fluid) in the axilla is generally low, but the patient should be prepared for these possibilities. Women who have SLNB alone have neuropathic sensations similar to those who undergo ALND, although the prevalence and severity of these sensations and the resulting distress are lower with SLNB (Chung & Giuliano, 2014).

The nurse must not overlook the psychosocial needs of the patient who has undergone SLNB. Although SLNB is a less invasive procedure than ALND and results in a shorter recovery period, a patient who has undergone SLNB also has many difficult issues surrounding her breast cancer diagnosis and treatment. The nurse must listen, provide emotional support, and refer the patient to appropriate specialists when indicated.

NURSING PROCESS

The Patient Undergoing Surgery for Breast Cancer

Assessment

The health history is a valuable tool to assess the patient's reaction to the diagnosis and her ability to cope with it. Pertinent questions include the following:

- How is the patient responding to the diagnosis?
- What coping mechanisms does she find most helpful?

- What psychological or emotional supports does she have and use?
- Is there a partner, family member, or friend available to assist her in making treatment choices?
- What are her educational needs?
- Is she experiencing any discomfort?

Diagnosis

PREOPERATIVE NURSING DIAGNOSES

Based on the assessment data, major preoperative nursing diagnoses may include the following:

- Deficient knowledge about the planned surgical treatments
- Anxiety related to the diagnosis of cancer
- Fear related to specific treatments and body image changes
- Risk for defensive or ineffective coping related to the diagnosis of breast cancer and related treatment options
- Decisional conflict related to treatment options

POSTOPERATIVE NURSING DIAGNOSES

Based on the assessment data, major postoperative nursing diagnoses may include the following:

- Acute pain and discomfort related to surgical procedure
- Peripheral neurovascular dysfunction related to nerve irritation in affected arm, breast, or chest wall
- Disturbed body image related to loss or alteration of the breast
- Risk for ineffective coping related to the diagnosis of cancer and surgical treatment
- Self-care deficit related to partial immobility of upper extremity on operative side
- Risk for sexual dysfunction related to loss of body part, change in self-image, and fear of partner's responses
- Deficient knowledge: drain management after breast surgery, arm exercises to regain mobility of affected extremity, hand and arm care after ALND

COLLABORATIVE PROBLEMS/POTENTIAL COMPLICATIONS

Potential complications may include the following:

- Lymphedema
- Hematoma/seroma formation
- Infection

Planning and Goals

The major goals may include increased knowledge about the disease and its treatment; reduction of preoperative and postoperative fear, anxiety, and emotional stress; improvement of decision-making ability; pain management; neurovascular function management; maintenance of a positive body image; improvement in coping abilities; increased self-care abilities; improvement in sexual function; and the absence of complications.

Preoperative Nursing Interventions

PROVIDING EDUCATION AND PREPARATION ABOUT SURGICAL TREATMENTS

Patients with newly diagnosed breast cancer are expected to absorb an abundance of new information during a very emotionally difficult time, and this may lead to difficulty in making treatment decisions. The nurse plays a key role in reviewing treatment options by reinforcing information provided to the patient and answering any questions. The nurse fully prepares the patient for what to expect before, during, and after surgery. Patients undergoing breast conservation with ALND, or a total or modified radical mastectomy, generally remain in the hospital overnight (or longer if they have immediate reconstruction). Surgical drains will be inserted in the mastectomy incision and in the axilla if the patient undergoes ALND. A surgical drain is generally not needed after SLNB. The patient should be informed that she will go home with the drain(s) and that complete instructions about drain care will be provided prior to discharge. In addition, the patient should be informed that she will often have decreased arm and shoulder mobility after ALND and that she will be shown range-of-motion exercises prior to discharge. The patient should also be reassured that appropriate analgesia and comfort measures will be provided to alleviate any postoperative discomfort.

REDUCING FEAR AND ANXIETY AND IMPROVING COPING ABILITY

The nurse helps the patient cope with the physical and emotional effects of surgery. Many fears may emerge during the preoperative phase. These can include fear of pain, mutilation (after mastectomy), and loss of sexual attractiveness; concern about inability to care for oneself and one's family; concern about taking time off from work; and coping with an uncertain future. Providing the patient with realistic expectations about the healing process and expected recovery can help alleviate fears. Maintaining open communication and assuring the patient that she can contact the nurse at any time with questions or concerns can be a source of comfort. The patient should also be made aware of available resources at the treatment facility as well as in the breast cancer community such as social workers, psychiatrists, and support groups. Some women find it helpful and reassuring to talk to a survivor of breast cancer who has undergone similar treatments.

PROMOTING DECISION-MAKING ABILITY

The patient may be eligible for more than one therapeutic approach; she may be presented with treatment options and then asked to make a choice. This can be very frightening for some patients, and they may prefer to have someone else make the decision for them (e.g., surgeon, family member). The nurse can be instrumental in ensuring that the patient and family members truly understand their options. The nurse can then help the patient weigh the risks and benefits of each option. The patient may be presented with the option of having breast conservation treatment followed by radiation or a mastectomy. The nurse can explore the issues with the patient by asking questions such as the following:

- How do you think you might feel about losing your breast?
- Are you considering breast reconstruction?
- If you choose to retain your breast, would you consider undergoing radiation treatments 5 days a week for 5 to 6 weeks?

Questions such as these can help the patient focus. Once the patient's decision is made, it is very important to support it.

Postoperative Nursing Interventions

RELIEVING PAIN AND DISCOMFORT

Many patients tolerate breast surgery well and have minimal pain during the postoperative period. This is particularly true of less invasive procedures such as breast conservation treatment with SLNB. However, all patients must be carefully assessed, because individual patients can have varying degrees of pain. Patients who have had more invasive procedures, such as a modified radical mastectomy with immediate reconstruction, may have considerably more pain. All patients are discharged home with analgesic medication (e.g., oxycodone and acetaminophen [Percocet]) and are encouraged to take it if needed. An over-the-counter analgesic agent such as acetaminophen may provide sufficient relief. Patients sometimes complain of a slight increase in pain after the first few days of surgery; this may occur as patients regain sensation around the surgical site and become more active. However, patients who report more than moderate pain must be evaluated to rule out any potential complications such as infection or hematoma. Postoperative pain may be more common in patients who have had axillary dissection and correlates with the number of nodes removed (Cherny & Truong, 2014). Alternative methods of pain management, such as taking warm showers (if permitted by the surgeon) and using distraction methods (e.g., guided imagery), may also be helpful. See Chapter 12 for further discussion of methods that relieve pain.

Managing Postoperative Sensations

Because nerves in the skin and axilla are often ligated or injured during breast surgery, patients experience a variety of sensations. Common sensations include tenderness, soreness, numbness, tightness, pulling, and twinges. These sensations may occur along the chest wall, in the axilla, and along the inside aspect of the upper arm. After mastectomy, some patients experience phantom sensations and report a feeling that the breast or nipple is still present. Overall, patients do not find these sensations severe or distressing. Sensations usually persist for several months and then begin to diminish, although some may persist for as long as 5 years and possibly longer. Patients should be reassured that this is a normal part of healing and that these sensations are not indicative of a problem.

Promoting Positive Body Image

Patients who have undergone mastectomy may find it difficult to view the surgical site for the first time. No matter how prepared the patient may think she is, the appearance of an absent breast can be very emotionally distressing. Ideally, the patient sees the incision for the first time when she is with the nurse or another health care provider who is available for support.

The nurse first assesses the patient's readiness and provides gentle encouragement. It is important to maintain the patient's privacy while assisting her as she views the incision; this allows her to express feelings safely to the nurse. Asking the patient what she perceives, acknowledging her feelings, and allowing her to express her emotions are important nursing actions. Reassuring the patient that her feelings are a normal response to breast cancer surgery may be comforting. If the patient has not had immediate reconstruction, providing her with a temporary breast form or soft padding to place in her bra on discharge can help alleviate feelings of embarrassment or self-consciousness.

Promoting Positive Adjustment and Coping

Providing ongoing assessment of how the patient is coping with her diagnosis of breast cancer and her surgical treatment is important in determining her overall adjustment. Assisting the patient in identifying and mobilizing her support systems can be beneficial to her well-being. The patient's spouse or partner may also need guidance, support, and education. The patient and partner may benefit from a wide network of available community resources, including the Reach to Recovery program of the ACS, advocacy groups, social worker, or a spiritual advisor. Encouraging the patient to discuss issues and concerns with other patients who have had breast cancer may help her to understand that her feelings are normal and that other women who have had breast cancer can provide invaluable support and understanding.

The patient may also have considerable anxiety about the treatments that will follow surgery (i.e., chemotherapy and radiation) and their implications. Providing her with information about the plan of care and referring her to the appropriate members of the health care team also promote coping during recovery. Some women require additional support to adjust to their diagnosis and the changes that it brings. If a woman displays ineffective coping, consultation with a mental health provider may be indicated. Research suggests that nurse navigators can help those undergoing breast biopsy to cope (Harding, 2015) (see Chart 58-4).

Improving Sexual Function

Once discharged from the hospital and feeling well, most patients are physically allowed to engage in sexual activity, if interested. However, any change in the patient's body image, self-esteem, or the response of her partner may increase her anxiety level and affect sexual function. Some partners may have difficulty looking at the incision, whereas others may be completely unaffected. Encouraging the patient to openly discuss how she feels about herself and about possible reasons for a decrease in libido (e.g., fatigue, anxiety, self-consciousness) may help clarify issues for her. Helpful suggestions for the patient may include varying the time of day for sexual activity (when the patient is less tired), assuming positions that are more comfortable, and expressing affection using alternative measures (e.g., hugging, kissing, manual stimulation).

Most patients and their partners adjust with minimal difficulty if they openly discuss their concerns. However, if issues cannot be resolved, a referral for counseling (e.g., psychologist, psychiatrist, psychiatric clinical nurse specialist, social worker, sex therapist) may be helpful. The ambulatory care nurse in the outpatient clinic or hospital should inquire whether the patient who was sexually active prior to surgery has resumed activities, because many patients are reluctant or embarrassed to bring this topic up themselves.

Monitoring and Managing Potential Complications

Lymphedema. **Lymphedema** is a complication characterized by a chronic swelling of an extremity due to interrupted lymphatic circulation. The swelling is due to the accumulation of protein-rich fluid in the interstitial space and is a somewhat common postoperative complication after ALND. It often affects both the breast and ipsilateral limb. It is associated with a painful swelling of the arm as well as weakness, shoulder pain, and tingling sensations in the arm and shoulder. Research results suggest that within 5 years of ALND, there is a 20% risk of lymphedema. Because sentinel lymph node dissection (SLND) involves more focused surgery and less disruption of the axilla, the risk is only up to 7% within

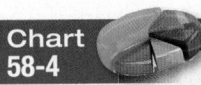

Chart 58-4 NURSING RESEARCH PROFILE
Nurse Navigators and Breast Biopsy

Harding, M. (2015). Effect of nurse navigation on patient care satisfaction and distress associated with breast biopsy. *Clinical Journal Oncology Nursing, 19*(1), E15–E20.

Purpose

This study was conducted to evaluate the impact of nurse navigation on satisfaction with care and level of stress in patients having a breast biopsy.

Design

This study used a descriptive cross sectional survey design. Two outpatient radiology sites were utilized including a community center and a breast center in Appalachia, following institutional review board (IRB) approval. The breast center used a multidisciplinary approach coordinated by a nurse navigator; the community center had no nurse navigator. Patients were invited to participate in the study prior to their biopsy. Study instruments included the Hospital Anxiety and Depression Scale (HADS), the State Trait Anxiety Inventory Scale (STAI-S), and the Patient Satisfaction Questionnaire (PSQ-18). Descriptive statistics were used to analyze demographic characteristics, t tests, chi square tests and Pearson correlations were used to examine variables.

Findings

One hundred and thirty seven women completed the study instruments at home following a core needle biopsy. The majority (68%) of the women were older than 50 years of age. Women who received navigation services (N = 85) had lower scores on all three distress measures (HAD-A [anxiety subscale], HAD-D [depression subscale], & STAI-S), with significantly lower anxiety levels on the HADS-A. There were no significant differences in patient satisfaction between the two groups. Sixty-six women (48%) sought outside information regarding an aspect of the diagnostic experience. Women not receiving navigation services were significantly more likely to seek outside information (X^2 = 7.949; $p < 0.01$), with a majority (67%) using the internet as an information source.

Nursing Implications

This study suggests that nurse navigators providing information and support can improve decision making and help prepare women for explanatory educational sessions with radiologists and surgeons. Nurses working with women having a breast biopsy should also keep in mind that this study reported women seeking additional information commonly used internet sources.

---

5 years. Risk factors for lymphedema in mixed-age groups include ALND, concomitant radiation therapy, increased age, presence of a concomitant infection, pre-existing cardiovascular conditions, and obesity (McLaughlin, 2014).

Lymphedema results if functioning lymphatic channels are inadequate to ensure a return flow of lymph fluid to the general circulation. After axillary lymph nodes are removed, collateral circulation must assume this function. Transient edema in the postoperative period occurs until collateral circulation has completely taken over this function, which generally occurs within a month. Performing prescribed exercises, elevating the arm above the heart several times a day, and gentle muscle pumping (making a fist and releasing) can help reduce the transient edema. The patient needs reassurance that this transient swelling is not lymphedema.

Once lymphedema develops, it tends to be chronic, so preventive strategies are vital. After ALND, the patient is taught hand and arm care to prevent injury or trauma to the affected extremity, thus decreasing the likelihood for development of lymphedema (see Chart 58-5). The patient is instructed to follow these guidelines for the rest of her life. She is also instructed to contact her primary provider immediately if she suspects that she has lymphedema, because early intervention provides the best chance for control. If allowed to progress without treatment, the swelling can become more difficult to manage. Treatment may consist of a course of antibiotic agents if an infection is present. A referral to a rehabilitation specialist (e.g., occupational or physical therapist) may be necessary for a compression sleeve or glove, exercises, manual lymph drainage, and a discussion of ways to modify daily activities to avoid worsening lymphedema. Ongoing research is seeking to identify which lymph nodes drain the arm before surgery so that they can be preserved when possible, helping to prevent the development of lymphedema.

Hematoma or Seroma Formation. Hematoma formation (collection of blood inside a cavity) may occur after either mastectomy or breast conservation and usually develops within the first 12 hours after surgery. The nurse assesses for signs and symptoms of hematoma at the surgical site, which may include swelling, tightness, pain, and bruising of the skin. The surgeon should be notified immediately if there is gross swelling or increased bloody output from the drain. Depending on the surgeon's assessment, a compression wrap may be applied to the incision for approximately 12 hours, or the patient may be returned to the operating room so that the incision may be reopened to identify the source of bleeding. Some hematomas are small, and the body absorbs the blood naturally. The patient may take warm showers (if permitted

Chart 58-5 PATIENT EDUCATION
Hand and Arm Care After Axillary Lymph Node Dissection

The nurse instructs the patient to:

- Avoid blood pressures, injections, and blood draws in affected extremity.
- Use sunscreen (higher than 15 SPF) for extended exposure to sun.
- Apply insect repellent to avoid insect bites.
- Wear gloves for gardening.
- Use cooking mitt for removing objects from oven.
- Avoid cutting cuticles; push them back during manicures.
- Use electric razor for shaving armpit.
- Avoid lifting objects heavier than 5–10 pounds.
- If a trauma or break in the skin occurs, wash the area with soap and water, and apply an over-the-counter antibacterial ointment (Bacitracin or Neosporin). Observe the area and extremity for 24 hours; if redness, swelling, or a fever occurs, call the surgeon or nurse.

by the surgeon) or apply warm compresses to help increase the absorption. A hematoma usually resolves in 4 to 5 weeks.

A seroma, a collection of serous fluid, may accumulate under the breast incision after mastectomy or breast conservation or in the axilla. Signs and symptoms may include swelling, heaviness, discomfort, and a sloshing of fluid. Seromas may develop temporarily after the drain is removed or if the drain is in place and becomes obstructed. Seromas rarely pose a threat and may be treated by unclogging the drain or manually aspirating the fluid with a needle and syringe. Large, long-standing seromas that have not been aspirated may lead to infection. Small seromas that are not bothersome to the patient usually resolve on their own.

Infection. Although infection is rare, it is a risk after any surgical procedure. This risk may be higher in patients with conditions such as diabetes, immune disorders, and advanced age, as well as in those with poor hygiene. Patients are taught to monitor for signs and symptoms of infection (redness, warmth around incision, tenderness, foul-smelling drainage, temperature greater than 40°C [100.4°F], chills) and to contact the surgeon or nurse for evaluation. Treatment consists of oral or IV antibiotics (for more severe infections) for 1 or 2 weeks. Cultures are taken of any foul-smelling discharge.

PROMOTING HOME, COMMUNITY-BASED, AND TRANSITIONAL CARE

 Educating Patients About Self-Care. Patients who undergo breast cancer surgery receive a tremendous amount of information both pre- and postoperatively. It is often difficult for the patient to absorb all of the information, partly because of the emotional distress that often accompanies the diagnosis and treatment. Prior to discharge, the nurse must assess the patient's readiness to assume self-care responsibilities and identify any gaps in knowledge. A review of education provided in written and oral forms, with reinforcement, may be required to ensure that the patient and family are prepared to manage the necessary care at home. The nurse reiterates symptoms that the patient should report, such as infection, seroma, hematoma, or arm swelling. All instruction should be reinforced during office visits and by telephone.

Most patients are discharged 1 or 2 days after ALND or mastectomy (possibly later if they have had immediate reconstruction) with surgical drains in place. Initially, the drainage fluid appears bloody, but it gradually changes to a serosanguineous and then a serous fluid over the next several days. The patient is given instructions about drainage management at home (see Chart 58-6). If the patient lives alone and drainage management is difficult, a referral for a home care nurse should be made. The drains are usually removed when the output is less than 30 mL in a 24-hour period (approximately 7 to 10 days). The home care nurse also reviews pain management and incision care.

In general, the patient may shower on the second postoperative day and wash the incision and drain site with soap and water to prevent infection. Some surgeons do not permit showers until 48 hours after drains are removed. If immediate reconstruction has been performed, showering may be contraindicated until the drain is removed. A dry dressing may be applied to the incision each day for 7 days. The patient should realize that sensation may be decreased in the operative area because the nerves were disrupted during surgery, and she should be informed that gentle care is needed to avoid injury. After the incision has completely healed (usually after 4 to 6 weeks), lotions or creams may be applied to the area to increase skin elasticity. The patient can begin to use deodorant on the affected side, although many women note that they no longer perspire as much as before the surgery.

Chart 58-6

HOME CARE CHECKLIST

Patient With a Drainage Device Following Breast Surgery

At the completion of education, the patient and/or caregiver will be able to:

- Name the procedure that was performed and identify changes in anatomic structure or function as well as changes in ADLs, IADLs, roles, relationships, and spirituality.
- Identify interventions and strategies (e.g., prosthesis) used in adapting to any permanent changes in structure or function.
- Describe ongoing postoperative therapeutic regimen, including diet and activities to perform (e.g., when to shower, arm exercises) and to limit or avoid (e.g., lifting weights, driving a car, contact sports).
- State the name, dose, side effects, frequency, and schedule for all medications.
- Describe approaches to controlling pain (e.g., take analgesics as prescribed; use nonpharmacologic interventions).
- State how to obtain medical supplies and carry out dressing changes, wound care, and other prescribed regimens.
  - Care for the drain site and incision as per surgeon's recommendation.

- Demonstrate how to empty and measure fluid from the drainage device.
- Demonstrate how to milk clots through the tubing of the drainage device.
- Identify when the drain is ready for removal (usually when draining <30 mL for a 24-hour period).
- Describe signs and symptoms of complications.
  - State observations that require contacting the physician or nurse (e.g., sudden change in color of drainage, sudden cessation of drainage, signs or symptoms of an infection).
- Relate how to reach primary provider with questions or complications.
- State time and date of follow-up appointments, therapy, and testing.
- Identify sources of support (e.g., friends, relatives, faith community, cancer support groups, caregiver support).
- Identify the need for health promotion, disease prevention, and screening activities (e.g.. gynecologic examination, mammogram).

ADL, activities of daily living; IADL, independent activities of daily living.

After ALND, patients are taught arm exercises on the affected side to restore range of motion (see Chart 58-7). After SLNB, patients may also benefit from these exercises, although they are less likely to have decreased range of motion than those who have undergone ALND. Range-of-motion exercises are initiated on the second postoperative day; however, instruction often occurs on the first postoperative day. The goals of the exercise regimen are to increase circulation and muscle strength, prevent joint stiffness and contractures, and restore full range of motion. The patient is instructed to perform range-of-motion exercises at home three times a day for 20 minutes at a time until full range of motion is restored (generally 4 to 6 weeks). Most patients find that after the drain is removed, range of motion returns quickly if they have adhered to their exercise program.

If the patient is having any discomfort, taking an analgesic agent 30 minutes before beginning the exercises can be helpful. Taking a warm shower before exercising can also

---

Chart 58-7 — PATIENT EDUCATION

Exercise After Breast Surgery

The nurse instructs the patient to perform the following exercises:

1. *Wall handclimbing.* Stand facing the wall with feet apart and toes as close to the wall as possible. With elbows slightly bent, place the palms of the hand on the wall at shoulder level. By flexing the fingers, work the hands up the wall until arms are fully extended. Then reverse the process, working the hands down to the starting point.

2. *Rope turning.* Tie a light rope to a doorknob. Stand facing the door. Take the free end of the rope in the hand on the side of surgery. Place the other hand on the hip. With the rope-holding arm extended and held away from the body (nearly parallel with the floor), turn the rope, making as wide swings as possible. Begin slowly at first; speed up later.

3. *Rod or broomstick lifting.* Grasp a rod with both hands, held about 2 feet apart. Keeping the arms straight, raise the rod over the head. Bend elbows to lower the rod behind the head. Reverse maneuver, raising the rod above the head, then return to the starting position.

4. *Pulley tugging.* Toss a light rope over a shower curtain rod or doorway curtain rod. Stand as close to the rope as possible. Grasp an end in each hand. Extend the arms straight and away from the body. Pull the left arm up by tugging down with the right arm, then the right arm up and the left down in a see-sawing motion.

loosen stiff muscles and provide comfort. When exercising, the patient is encouraged to use the muscles in both arms and to maintain proper posture. Specific exercises may need to be prescribed and introduced gradually if the patient has had skin grafts; has a tense, tight surgical incision; or has had immediate reconstruction. Self-care activities, such as brushing the teeth, washing the face, and brushing the hair, are physically and emotionally therapeutic because they aid in restoring arm function and provide a sense of normalcy for the patient.

The patient is instructed about postoperative activity limitation. In general, heavy lifting (more than 5 to 10 pounds) is avoided for about 4 to 6 weeks, although normal household and work-related activities are promoted to maintain muscle tone. Brisk walking, the use of stationary bikes and stepping machines, and stretching exercises may begin as soon as the patient feels comfortable. Once the drain is removed, the patient may begin to drive if she has full arm range of motion and is no longer taking opioid analgesic agents. General guidelines for activity focus on the gradual introduction of previous activities (e.g., bowling, weight training) once fully healed.

Continuing and Transitional Care. Patients who have difficulty managing their postoperative care at home may benefit from a referral for home health, transitional, or community-based care. The nurse making a home visit assesses the patient's incision and surgical drain(s), adequacy of pain management, adherence to the exercise plan, and overall physical and psychological functioning. In addition, the home care nurse reinforces previous education and communicates important physiologic findings and psychosocial issues to the patient's primary provider, nurse, or surgeon.

The frequency of follow-up visits after surgery may vary but generally should occur every 3 to 6 months for the first several years. The patient may alternate visits with the surgeon, medical oncologist, or radiation oncologist, depending on the treatment regimen. The ambulatory care nurse can also be a great source of education for the patient and family and should encourage them to telephone if they have any questions or concerns. It is common for people to ignore routine health care when a major health issue arises, so women who have been treated for breast cancer should be reminded of the importance of participating in routine health screening.

Evaluation

Expected preoperative patient outcomes may include:
1. Exhibits knowledge about diagnosis and surgical treatment options
   a. Asks relevant questions about diagnosis and available surgical treatments
   b. States rationale for surgery
   c. Describes advantages and disadvantages of treatment options
2. Verbalizes willingness to deal with anxiety and fears related to the diagnosis and the effects of surgery on self-image and sexual functioning
3. Demonstrates ability to cope with diagnosis and treatment
   a. Verbalizes feelings appropriately and recognizes normalcy of mood lability

   b. Proceeds with treatment in timely fashion
   c. Discusses impact of diagnosis and treatment on family and work
4. Makes decisions regarding treatment options in timely fashion

Expected postoperative patient outcomes may include:
1. Reports that pain has decreased and states pain and discomfort management strategies are effective
2. Identifies postoperative sensations and recognizes that they are a normal part of healing
3. Exhibits clean, dry, and intact surgical incisions without signs of inflammation or infection
4. Lists the signs and symptoms of infection to be reported to the nurse or surgeon
5. Verbalizes feelings regarding change in body image
6. Discusses meaning of the diagnosis, surgical treatment, and fears appropriately
7. Participates actively in self-care measures
   a. Performs exercises as prescribed
   b. Participates in self-care measures as prescribed
8. Discusses issues of sexuality and resumption of sexual relations
9. Demonstrates knowledge of post discharge recommendations and restrictions
   a. Describes follow-up care and activities
   b. Demonstrates appropriate care of incisions and drainage system
   c. Demonstrates arm exercises, and describes exercise regimen and activity limitations during postoperative period
   d. Describes care of affected arm and hand, and lists indications to contact the surgeon or nurse
10. Experiences no complications
    a. Identifies signs and symptoms of reportable complications (e.g., fever, redness, heat, pain, edema)
    b. Explains how to contact appropriate providers in case of complications

Radiation Therapy

Radiation therapy is used to decrease the chance of a local recurrence in the breast by eradicating residual microscopic cancer cells. Breast conservation treatment followed by radiation therapy for stages I and II breast cancer results in a survival rate equal to that of a modified radical mastectomy (NCCN, 2015). If radiation therapy, which is part of breast conservation treatment (see Chart 58-8), is contraindicated, a mastectomy would then be indicated.

External-beam radiation (the most common type) typically begins about 6 weeks after breast conservation to allow the surgical site to heal. If systemic chemotherapy is indicated, radiation therapy usually begins after its completion. Before radiation begins, the patient undergoes a planning session called a *simulation,* in which the anatomic areas to be treated are mapped out and then identified with small permanent ink markings. External-beam radiation, which delivers high-energy photons from a linear accelerator, is given to the entire breast region (whole breast radiation). Each treatment lasts only a few minutes and is generally given 5 days a week

Contraindications to Breast Conservation Treatment

Note: Breast-conservation treatment includes both surgery and radiation.

Absolute Contraindications

- First or second trimester of pregnancy
- Presence of multicentric disease in the breast
- Prior radiation to the breast or chest region

Relative Contraindications

- History of collagen vascular disease
- Large tumor-to-breast ratio
- Tumor beneath nipple

Adapted from Harris, J., & Morrow, M. (2014). Breast-conserving therapy. In J. Harris, M. Lippman, M. Morrow, et al. (Eds.). *Diseases of the breast* (5th ed.). Philadelphia, PA: Wolters Kluwer.

for 5 to 6 weeks. After completion of radiation to the entire breast, many patients receive a "boost"—a dose of radiation to the lumpectomy site where the cancer cells were located. The boost consists of the same dose of radiation but is less penetrating and directed to a smaller area. The treatments are not painful.

Because most breast cancer recurrences appear at or near the lumpectomy site, the need for whole breast radiation has been questioned. Partial breast radiation (radiation to the lumpectomy site alone) continues be evaluated at some institutions in patients who have been carefully selected. One approach is **brachytherapy**, in which radiation is delivered by an internal device that is placed close to the tumor within the breast. This technique can lead to an improved quality of life because the treatments are given over 4 to 5 days instead of 5 to 6 weeks. After mastectomy, postoperative radiation may be indicated for women at high risk for cancer recurrence (i.e., chest wall involvement, four or more positive lymph nodes, tumors larger than 5 cm, positive surgical margins).

Side Effects

In general, radiation therapy is well tolerated. Acute side effects consist of mild to moderate erythema, breast edema, and fatigue. Occasionally, skin breakdown may occur in the inframammary fold or near the axilla toward the end of treatment. Fatigue can be depressing, as can the frequent trips to the radiation oncology unit for treatment. The patient needs to be reassured that the fatigue is normal and not a sign of recurrence. Side effects usually resolve within a few weeks to a few months after treatment is completed. Rare long-term effects of radiation therapy include pneumonitis, rib fracture, heart disease, breast fibrosis or necrosis (Harris & Morrow, 2014).

Nursing Management

Nurses play a significant role in supporting patients throughout their treatment with radiation therapy. See Chapter 15 for discussion of radiation therapy.

Self-care instructions for patients receiving radiation are provided to assist in the maintenance of skin integrity during the treatments and for several weeks after completion. They pertain only to the area being treated and not to the rest of the body. Instructions include:

- Use mild soap with minimal rubbing.
- Avoid perfumed soaps or deodorants.
- Use hydrophilic lotions (Lubriderm, Eucerin, Aquaphor) for dryness.
- Use a nondrying, antipruritic soap (Aveeno) if pruritus occurs.
- Avoid tight clothes, underwire bras, excessive temperatures, and ultraviolet light.

Follow-up care includes educating the patient to minimize sun exposure to the treated area (i.e., using sunblock with sun protection factor [SPF] of 15 or higher) and reassuring the patient that short-term minor twinges and pain in the breast are normal after radiation treatment.

Systemic Treatments

Chemotherapy

Adjuvant chemotherapy involves the use of anticancer agents in addition to other treatments (i.e., surgery, radiation) to delay or prevent a recurrence of breast cancer. It is recommended for patients who have positive lymph nodes or who have invasive tumors greater than 1 cm in size, regardless of nodal status. It is considered in patients with tumors that are 0.6 to 1 cm, are moderately to poorly differentiated, or have unfavorable features (NCCN, 2015). Table 58-6 outlines general indications for adjuvant chemotherapy. A survival benefit has been shown in both women who are pre- and postmenopausal and who have received chemotherapy,

TABLE 58-6 General Indications for Adjuvant Chemotherapy for Breast Cancer

Nodal Status, Tumor Size	Adjuvant Chemotherapy
Node negative, ≤0.5 cm	None
Node negative 0.6–1 cm (well differentiated)	None
Node negative, 0.6–1 cm (moderately or poorly differentiated and/or unfavorable features)	Consider chemotherapy
Node negative, >1 cm	Chemotherapy
Node positive, any tumor size	Chemotherapy

- In addition to chemotherapy, patients with HER-2/neu-positive tumors will receive trastuzumab if they have node-positive disease; or node-negative disease with a tumor >1 cm. Trastuzumab is a monoclonal antibody that targets and inactivates the HER-2/neu protein. HER-2/neu is overproduced in 25–30% of tumors and is associated with rapid growth and poor prognosis.
- Following chemotherapy, patients with hormone receptor positive (ER+/PR+) tumors will receive hormonal therapy (tamoxifen or aromatase inhibitor) if they have either node-positive disease; node-negative disease with a tumor >1 cm; or node-negative disease with a tumor 0.6–1 cm and moderately or poorly differentiated and/or unfavorable features.

Note: These are only general guidelines. Recommendations may vary depending on factors such as prognostic variables, patient age, and comorbid conditions.
Adapted from National Comprehensive Cancer Network (NCCN). (2015). Clinical practice guidelines: Breast. Retrieved on 3/7/2016 at: www.nccn.org/professionals/physician_gls/PDF/infections.pdf

although data are limited in women older than 70 years. Chemotherapy is most commonly initiated after breast surgery and before radiation. Patients who delay initiation of chemotherapy beyond 90 days postsurgery have an increased risk of adverse outcomes (Chavez-McGregor, Clarke, Lichtensztajn, et al., 2016). Nurses encourage and assist in facilitating timely treatment to optimize outcomes.

Chemotherapy regimens for breast cancer combine several agents (polychemotherapy), generally given over a period of 3 to 6 months. Decisions regarding the optimal regimen are based on a variety of factors, including tumor characteristics (i.e., tumor size, lymph node status, hormone receptor status, HER-2/neu status) and the patient's age, physical status, and existing comorbid conditions. A regimen that includes cyclophosphamide (Cytoxan), methotrexate (Trexall), and fluorouracil (Fluoroplex) (collectively referred to as CMF) has been the most widely used adjuvant therapy. It is usually well tolerated and may be considered for patients with a low risk of recurrence. CMF also may be considered for use in patients who have a high risk of cardiac toxicity or who have other limiting comorbidities. Anthracycline-based regimens (e.g., doxorubicin [Adriamycin], epirubicin [Ellence]) have shown longer survival in patients. However, the benefit relative to CMF is modest and is accompanied by increased toxicity (Meneses & Walker, 2014). Selection of patients most likely to benefit from anthracycline therapy would allow better use of current cytotoxic agents and reduce the risk of patients receiving toxicity with little or no effect. Identifying biomarkers that can accurately predict benefit from anthracyclines will also highlight key resistance/susceptibility pathways that can then be exploited clinically to further increase efficacy (Meneses & Walker, 2014). Cyclophosphamide, doxorubicin, and fluorouracil (CAF) and doxorubicin and cyclophosphamide (AC) are examples of combination regimens often given to patients who are at high risk.

The taxanes (paclitaxel [Taxol], docetaxel [Taxotere]) are generally incorporated into treatment regimens for patients with larger, node-negative cancers and for those with positive axillary lymph nodes. The addition of four cycles of paclitaxel after a standard course of AC (regimen known as ACT) has been found to increase the disease-free period and improve overall survival in patients with operable breast cancer and positive lymph nodes (Meneses & Walker, 2014).

Much attention has been focused on **dose-dense chemotherapy**, which is the administration of chemotherapeutic agents at standard doses with shorter time intervals between each cycle of treatment. A systematic review and meta-analysis of existing data from randomized controlled trials that compared dose-dense chemotherapy with a standard chemotherapy schedule in women with nonmetastatic breast cancer demonstrated that dose-dense chemotherapy results in better overall and disease-free survival, particularly in women with hormone receptor–negative breast cancer (Bonilla, Ben-Aharon, Vidal, et al., 2010). However, additional data from randomized controlled trials are needed before dose-dense chemotherapy can be considered the standard of care (Bardia & Baselga, 2014).

Side Effects

Many of the side effects of adjuvant chemotherapy can be managed well, allowing patients to maintain their daily routines and work schedules. In large part, this is the a result of the meticulous educational and psychological preparation provided to patients and their families by oncology nurses, oncologists, social workers, and other members of the health care team. In addition, strides have been made in the effectiveness of antiemetic agents used to alleviate nausea and vomiting and the use of hematopoietic growth factors to treat neutropenia and anemia.

Common physical side effects of chemotherapy for breast cancer may include nausea, vomiting, bone marrow suppression, taste changes, alopecia (hair loss), mucositis, neuropathy, skin changes, and fatigue. A weight gain of more than 10 pounds occurs in about half of all patients; the cause is unknown. Women who are premenopausal may also experience temporary or permanent amenorrhea.

Specific side effects vary with the type of chemotherapeutic agent used. In general, CMF and the taxanes are better tolerated than the anthracyclines. However, the taxanes can cause peripheral neuropathy, arthralgias, and myalgias, particularly at high doses. During taxane administration, hypersensitivity reactions may occur; therefore, the patient must be premedicated. Alopecia is also common. The side effects of the anthracyclines may be severe and include cardiotoxicity in addition to nausea and vomiting, bone marrow suppression, and alopecia. Their vesicant properties can lead to tissue necrosis if infiltration of the medication infusion occurs.

Nursing Management

Nurses play an important role in helping patients manage the physical and psychosocial sequelae of chemotherapy. (Chapter 15 provides an in-depth discussion of side effect management.) Instructing the patient about the use of antiemetic agents and reviewing the optimal dosage schedule can help minimize nausea and vomiting. The different classes of antiemetic agents include serotonin (5-HT-3) receptor antagonists (palonosetron [Aloxi], granisetron [Kytril], ondansetron [Zofran]); neurokinin-1 receptor antagonists (aprepitant [Emend]); dopamine receptor antagonists (prochlorperazine [Compazine], metoclopramide [Reglan]); benzodiazepines (lorazepam [Ativan]); and corticosteroids (dexamethasone [Decadron]). Measures to ease the symptoms of mucositis may include rinsing with normal saline or sodium bicarbonate solution, avoiding hot and spicy foods, and using a soft toothbrush.

Some patients may require hematopoietic growth factors to minimize the effects of chemotherapy-induced neutropenia and anemia. Granulocyte colony-stimulating factors boost the white blood cell count, helping to reduce the incidence of neutropenic fever and infection. The short-acting form, filgrastim (Neupogen), is injected subcutaneously or IV for 7 to 10 days after chemotherapy administration. The long-acting form, pegfilgrastim (Neulasta), is injected once, no earlier than 24 hours after chemotherapy (Comerford, 2015). Erythropoietin growth factor increases the production of red blood cells, thus decreasing the symptoms of anemia. The short-acting form, epoetin alfa (Epogen) is usually given weekly. The long-acting form, darbepoetin alfa (Aranesp), can be given every 2 to 3 weeks. The nurse instructs the patient and family on proper injection technique of hematopoietic growth factors and about symptoms that require follow-up with a primary provider (see Chart 58-9).

Chart 58-9

HOME CARE CHECKLIST

Self-Administration of Hematopoietic Growth Factors

At the completion of education, the patient and/or caregiver will be able to:

- State the impact of treatment on physiologic functioning, ADLs, IADLs, roles, relationships, and spirituality.
- Identify the benefits and expected outcome of hematopoietic growth factors.
- Locate list of names and telephone numbers of resource personnel involved in care (e.g., health care professionals, home care nurse, hematopoietic growth factor and supply vendor).
- Identify the equipment necessary for self-injection and how to obtain hematopoietic growth factor and supplies.
- Demonstrate how to give an injection properly, including:
  - How to draw up the solution in a syringe if indicated. (*Note:* Darbepoetin and pegfilgrastim come in prefilled syringes).
  - Identify appropriate body sites for self-injection.
  - Demonstrate correct disposal of sharps.
  - Describe proper storage of supplies.
- State what types of lifestyle and environmental changes are needed (if any) to maintain a clean home environment and prevent infection.

- State the name, dose, side effects, frequency, and schedule for all medications.
- List complications of medications/therapeutic regimen necessitating a call to the nurse or primary provider. (e.g., excessive pain, fever).
- List complications of medications/therapeutic regimen necessitating a visit to the emergency department.
- Explain treatment plan and importance of follow-up care to all health care providers.
- State time and date of follow-up appointments, therapy, and testing.
- Identify community resources for peer and caregiver/family support:
  - Identify sources of support (e.g., friends, relatives, faith community).
  - Identify phone numbers of support groups for people with cancer and their caregivers/families.
  - State meeting locations and times.
- Identify the need for health promotion, disease prevention, and screening activities.

ADL, activities of daily living; IADL, independent activities of daily living.

To prevent some of the emotional trauma associated with alopecia, it often helps to have a patient obtain a wig before hair loss begins to occur. The nurse may provide a list of wig suppliers in the patient's geographic region. Familiarity with creative ways to use scarves and turbans may also help minimize the patient's distress. The patient needs reassurance that new hair will grow back when treatment is completed, although the color and texture may be different. The ACS offers the Look Good Feel Better program, which provides useful tips for applying cosmetics during the period a patient is receiving chemotherapy (see Resources section).

Chemotherapy may negatively affect the patient's self-esteem, sexuality, and sense of well-being. This, combined with the stress of a potentially life-threatening disease, can be acute. Providing support and promoting open communication are important aspects of nursing care. Referring the patient to the dietitian, social worker, psychiatrist, or spiritual advisor can provide additional support. Numerous community support and advocacy groups are available for patients and their families. Complementary therapies, such as guided imagery, meditation, and relaxation exercises, can also be used in conjunction with conventional treatments.

Hormonal Therapy

The use of **adjuvant hormonal therapy**, with or without the addition of chemotherapy, is considered in women who have hormone receptor–positive tumors. Its use can be determined by the results of an estrogen and progesterone receptor assay (a test to determine whether the breast tumor is nourished by hormones). About two thirds of breast cancers depend on estrogen for growth and express a nuclear receptor that binds to the estrogen; thus, they are estrogen receptor positive (ER+). Similarly, tumors that express the progesterone receptor are progesterone receptor positive (PR+). Hormonal

therapy involves the use of synthetic hormones or other medications that compete with estrogen by binding to the receptor sites (SERMs), or the use of **aromatase inhibitors**, which block estrogen production by the adrenal glands. In general, tumors that are ER+/PR+ have the greatest likelihood of responding to hormonal therapy and have a more favorable prognosis than those that are ER–/PR–. Women who are pre- and perimenopausal are more likely to have non–hormone-dependent lesions, whereas women who are postmenopausal are more likely to have hormone-dependent lesions.

Traditionally, the SERM tamoxifen has been the main hormonal agent used in treatment of pre- and postmenopausal breast cancer and remains the mainstay in women who are premenopausal. As an SERM, tamoxifen has estrogen antagonistic (estrogen-blocking) and agonistic (estrogen-like) effects on certain tissues. Its antagonistic effects in the breast prevent estrogen from binding to the receptor sites, thus preventing tumor growth. Tamoxifen has positive agonistic effects on blood lipid profiles and bone mineral density in women who are postmenopausal. It also has agonistic effects on endometrial tissue and blood coagulation processes, leading to an increased incidence of endometrial cancer and thromboembolic events (e.g., deep vein thrombosis, superficial phlebitis, pulmonary embolism). Nevertheless, the benefits in most women with breast cancer outweigh the risks.

The aromatase inhibitors anastrozole (Arimidex), letrozole (Femara), and exemestane (Aromasin) are important components in the hormonal management of women who are postmenopausal. Most of the circulating estrogens in women who are postmenopausal are derived from the conversion of the adrenal androgen androstenedione to estrone and the conversion of testosterone to estradiol. Aromatase inhibitors work by blocking the enzyme aromatase from performing the conversion, thereby decreasing the level of circulating

Chart 58-10 **PATIENT EDUCATION**

Managing Side Effects of Adjuvant Hormonal Therapy in Breast Cancer

The nurse instructs the patient in strategies to manage the following side effects:

Hot Flashes

- Wear breathable, layered clothing.
- Avoid caffeine and spicy foods.
- Perform breathing exercises (paced respirations).
- Consider medications (vitamin E, antidepressants) or acupuncture.

Vaginal Dryness

- Use vaginal moisturizers for everyday dryness (e.g., Replens, vitamin E suppository).
- Apply vaginal lubrication during intercourse (e.g., Astroglide, K-Y Jelly).

Nausea and Vomiting

- Consume a bland diet.
- Try to take medication in the evening.

Musculoskeletal Symptoms

- Take nonsteroidal analgesic agents as recommended.
- Take warm baths.

Risk of Endometrial Cancer

- Report any irregular bleeding to a gynecologist for evaluation.

Risk for Thromboembolic Events

- Report any redness, swelling, or tenderness in the lower extremities, or any unexplained shortness of breath.

Risk for Osteoporosis or Fractures

- Undergo a baseline bone density scan.
- Perform regular weight-bearing exercises.
- Take calcium supplements with vitamin D.
- Take bisphosphonates (e.g., alendronate) or calcitonin as prescribed.

---

estrogen in peripheral tissues. Clinical trials have demonstrated that the aromatase inhibitors are superior to tamoxifen in terms of overall response rate and clinical benefit and that inhibitors appear to be effective and feasible compared with tamoxifen as first-line hormonal therapy in women who are postmenopausal with advanced breast cancer (Rimawi & Osborne, 2014). These data ensure that aromatase inhibitors will play an increasingly central role in the long-term management of breast cancer. Trials are ongoing to determine the optimal treatment regimen and the timing of the treatment. Table 58-7 outlines the adverse effects of adjuvant hormonal therapy. Chart 58-10 outlines appropriate patient education to manage the adverse effects.

Targeted Therapy

An exciting area of research in the systemic treatment of breast cancer involves the use of targeted therapies. Trastuzumab (Herceptin) is a monoclonal antibody that binds specifically to the **HER-2/neu** protein. This protein, which regulates cell growth, is present in small amounts on the surface of normal breast cells and in most breast cancers. Approximately 25% to 30% of tumors overexpress (overproduce) the HER-2/neu protein and are associated with rapid growth and poor

prognosis. Trastuzumab targets and inactivates the HER-2/neu protein, thus slowing tumor growth.

Unlike chemotherapy, trastuzumab spares the normal cells and has limited adverse reactions, which may include fever, chills, nausea, vomiting, diarrhea, and headache. However, when trastuzumab is given to patients who have previously been treated with an anthracycline, the risk of cardiac toxicity is increased. The medication has been shown to improve survival rates in women with HER-2/neu–positive metastatic breast cancer and is now regarded as standard therapy. It may be given as a single agent or in combination with chemotherapy. More recently, trastuzumab has been shown to be effective in treating early-stage breast cancer that is HER-2/neu positive. Assessing the benefits and risks of trastuzumab is complex, and medical oncologists often use a variety of aids in their decision making (Kimmick, Hughes, & Muss, 2014).

Treatment of Recurrent and Metastatic Breast Cancer

Despite the advances made in the treatment of breast cancer, it may recur locally (on the chest wall or in the conserved

---

TABLE 58-7 Adverse Reactions Associated With Adjuvant Hormonal Therapy Used to Treat Breast Cancer

Therapeutic Agent	Adverse Reactions/Side Effects
Selective Estrogen Receptor Modulator	
tamoxifen (Soltamox)	Hot flashes, vaginal dryness/discharge/bleeding, irregular menses, nausea, mood disturbances, rashes; increased risk for endometrial cancer; increased risk for thromboembolic events (deep vein thrombosis, pulmonary embolism, superficial phlebitis)
Aromatase Inhibitors	
anastrozole (Arimidex) letrozole (Femara) exemestane (Aromasin)	Musculoskeletal symptoms (arthritis, arthralgia, myalgia), increased risk of osteoporosis/fractures, nausea/vomiting, hot flashes, fatigue, mood disturbances, rashes

Adapted from Comerford, K. C. (2015). *Nursing 2015 drug handbook*. Philadelphia, PA: Wolters Kluwer.

breast), regionally (in the remaining lymph nodes), or systemically (in distant organs). In metastatic disease, the bone, usually the hips, spine, ribs, skull, or pelvis, is the most common site of spread. Other sites of metastasis include the lungs, liver, pleura, and brain.

The overall prognosis and optimal treatment are determined by a variety of factors such as the site and extent of recurrence, the time to recurrence from the original diagnosis, history of prior treatments, the patient's performance status, and any existing comorbid conditions. Patients with bone metastases generally have a longer overall survival compared with metastases in visceral organs.

Local recurrence in the absence of systemic disease is treated aggressively with surgery, radiation, and hormonal therapy. Chemotherapy may also be used for tumors that are not hormonally sensitive. Local recurrence may be an indicator that systemic disease will develop in the future, particularly if it occurs within 2 years of the original diagnosis (NCCN, 2015).

Metastatic breast cancer involves control of the disease rather than cure (NCCN, 2015). Treatment includes hormonal therapy, chemotherapy, and targeted therapy. Surgery or radiation may be indicated in select situations. Women who are premenopausal and who have hormonally dependent tumors may eliminate the production of estrogen by the ovaries through oophorectomy (removal of the ovaries) or suppression of estrogen production by medications such as leuprolide (Lupron) or goserelin (Zoladex).

Patients with advanced breast cancer are monitored closely for signs of disease progression. Baseline studies are obtained at the time of recurrence. These may include complete blood count; comprehensive metabolic panel; tumor markers (i.e., carcinoembryonic antigen, cancer antigen 15-3); bone scan; CT of the chest, abdomen, and pelvis; and MRI of symptomatic areas. Additional x-rays may be performed to evaluate areas of pain or abnormal areas seen on bone scan (e.g., long bones, pelvis). These studies are repeated at regular intervals to assess for effectiveness of treatment and to monitor progression of disease.

Nursing Management

Nurses play an important role in not only educating patients and managing their symptoms but also in providing emotional support. Many patients find that recurrence of the disease is more distressing than the initial cancer diagnosis. They not only have to contend with another round of treatments but are also faced with a greater uncertainty about their future and long-term survival. The nurse can help the patient identify coping strategies and set priorities to optimize quality of life. Family members and significant others should be included in the treatment plan and follow-up care. Referrals to support groups, as well as psychiatry or psychiatric clinical nurse specialist, social work, and complementary medicine programs (e.g., guided imagery, meditation, yoga), should be made as indicated.

Nurses can also be instrumental in providing palliative care, if indicated. The highest priorities include alleviating pain and providing comfort measures. A frank discussion with the patient and family regarding their preferences for end-of-life care should occur before the need arises to ensure a smooth transition without disruption of care. Referrals to

hospice and home health care should be initiated as necessary (see Chapters 15 and 16).

Reconstructive Procedures After Mastectomy

Breast reconstruction can provide a significant psychological benefit for women who are already struggling with the emotional distress of losing a breast. A consultation with a plastic surgeon can help the patient understand procedures for which she is a candidate and the pros and cons of each. Factors to consider include body size and shape, comorbid conditions (e.g., hypertension, diabetes, obesity), personal habits such as smoking, and patient preference. The patient must be informed that although breast reconstruction can provide a good cosmetic result, it will never precisely duplicate the natural breast. Realistic preparation can help the patient avoid unrealistic expectations. Once reconstruction is complete, the opposite breast may require augmentation, reduction, or mastopexy to achieve symmetry on both sides. The patient must also be informed that breast reconstruction neither will interfere with breast cancer treatments nor affect the risk of cancer recurrence. Reconstruction is considered an integral component in the surgical treatment of breast cancer and is usually covered by insurance companies.

Many women elect immediate reconstruction at the time of the mastectomy operation. This can be beneficial in that it saves the woman from undergoing general anesthesia a second time and saves the cost and stress of future hospitalizations. However, it does increase the length of the surgical procedure. Delayed reconstruction is preferable in women who are having a difficult time deciding on the type of reconstruction that they desire. It may also be preferable in patients with advanced disease such as inflammatory breast cancer, where the breast cancer treatments should begin without delay. Any delays in healing after immediate reconstruction may interfere with the initiation of treatment.

Tissue Expander Followed by Permanent Implant

Breast reconstruction using a tissue expander followed by a permanent implant is the simplest and most common method used today (see Fig. 58-6). To accommodate an implant, the skin remaining after a mastectomy and the underlying muscle must gradually be stretched by a process called *tissue expansion*. The surgeon places a tissue expander (a balloon-like device) through the mastectomy incision underneath the pectoralis muscle. A small amount of saline is injected through a metal port intraoperatively to partially inflate the expander. Then, for about 6 to 8 weeks, at weekly intervals, the patient receives additional saline injections through the port until the expander is fully inflated. It remains fully expanded for about 6 weeks to allow the skin to loosen. The expander is then exchanged for a permanent implant. This is usually performed as an outpatient surgical procedure.

Advantages of the expansion procedure are a shorter operating time and a shorter recuperation period than for autologous reconstruction (see the Tissue Transfer Procedures section). A disadvantage is a tendency for the implant to feel firm and round, with little natural ptosis (sag). Women with a small to medium opposite breast with little ptosis are good candidates for this procedure. Women who have had radiation or who have connective tissue disease are not good candidates because of the decreased elasticity of the skin.

A **B** **C**

Figure 58-6 • Breast reconstruction with tissue expander. **A.** Mastectomy incision line prior to tissue expansion. **B.** The expander is placed under the pectoralis muscle and is gradually filled with saline solution through a port to stretch the skin enough to accept a permanent implant. **C.** The breast mound is restored. Although permanent, scars will fade with time. The nipple and areola are reconstructed later. Adapted from American Society of Plastic Surgeons.

> ### Quality and Safety Nursing Alert
>
> *The patient must be cautioned not to have an MRI while the tissue expander is in place because the port contains metal. This is not an issue once the permanent implant is in place because it does not contain any metal.*

The patient should be informed that for the rest of her life she should not engage in any exercises that will develop the pectoralis muscle, because this can result in distortion of the reconstructed breast.

Tissue Transfer Procedures

Autologous reconstruction is the use of the patient's own tissue to create a breast mound. A flap of skin, fat, and muscle with its attached blood supply is rotated to the mastectomy site to create a mound that simulates the breast. Donor sites may include the **transverse rectus abdominal myocutaneous (TRAM) flap** (abdominal muscle) (see Fig. 58-7), gluteal flap (buttock muscle), or the latissimus dorsi flap (back muscle) (see Fig. 58-8). The results more closely resemble a

real breast because the skin and fat from the donor sites are similar in consistency to a natural breast. These procedures avoid the use of synthetic material. However, they involve longer recuperation than a tissue expander procedure. The risk of potential complications (e.g., infection, bleeding, flap necrosis) is also greater. Therefore, patients must be in relatively good health, and those with medical conditions (e.g., atherosclerosis, pulmonary disease, heart failure) that affect circulation or compromise oxygen delivery are not good candidates. Other candidates who are poor risks include those with poorly controlled diabetes or morbid obesity and those who smoke.

The TRAM flap is the most commonly performed tissue transfer procedure. A free TRAM procedure may also be performed; in this case, the skin, fat, muscle, and blood supply are completely detached from the body and then transplanted to the mastectomy site using microvascular surgery (the use of a microscope to reconnect the vessels). Postoperatively, patients who have undergone TRAM procedures often face a lengthy recovery (often 6 to 8 weeks) and have incisions both at the mastectomy site and at the donor site

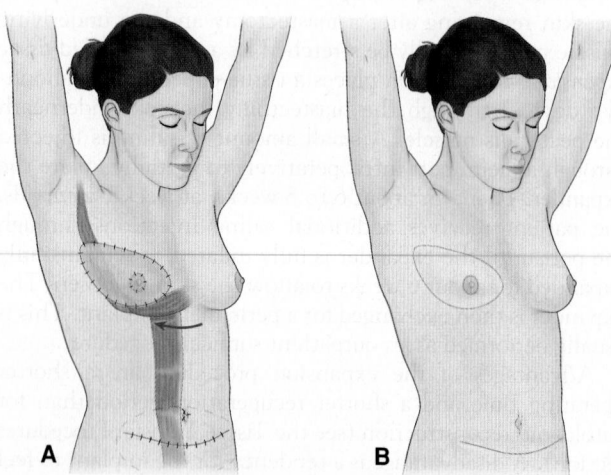

A **B**

Figure 58-7 • Breast reconstruction: transverse rectus abdominal myocutaneous flap. **A.** A breast mound is created by tunneling abdominal skin, fat, and muscle to the mastectomy site. **B.** Final location of scars. Adapted from American Society of Plastic Surgeons.

A **B**

Figure 58-8 • Breast reconstruction: latissimus dorsi flap. **A.** The latissimus muscle with an ellipse of skin is rotated from the back to the mastectomy site. **B.** Because the flap is usually not bulky enough to provide an adequate breast mound, an implant is often also required. Adapted from American Society of Plastic Surgeons.

in the abdomen. Other free flap procedures include deep inferior epigastric perforator flap (DIEP) and superficial inferior epigastric artery flap (SIEA) depending on whether the superior gluteal artery perforator or the inferior one is utilized. Free flaps involve microsurgery for blood vessel transfer.

Deep breathing and leg exercises are essential because the patient is more limited in her activity and is at greater risk for respiratory complications and deep vein thrombosis. Measures to help the patient reduce tension on the abdominal incision during the first postoperative week include elevating the head of the bed 45 degrees and flexing the patient's knees.

Once the patient is able to ambulate, she can protect the surgical incision by splinting it and will gradually achieve a more upright position. The patient is instructed to avoid high-impact activities and lifting (more than 5 to 10 pounds for 6 to 8 weeks after surgery) to prevent stress on the incision.

Nipple–Areola Reconstruction

After the breast mound has been created and the site has healed, some women choose to have nipple–areola reconstruction. This is a minor surgical procedure carried out either in the physician's office or at an outpatient surgical facility. The most common method of creating a nipple is with the use of local flaps (skin and fat from the center of the new breast mound), which are wrapped around each other to create a projecting nipple. The areola is created using a skin graft. The most common donor site is the upper inner thigh, because this skin has darker pigmentation than the skin on the reconstructed breast. After the nipple graft has healed, micropigmentation (tattooing) can be performed to achieve a more natural color. The surgeon can usually match the reconstructed nipple–areola complex with that of the contralateral breast for an acceptable cosmetic result.

Prosthetics

Not all patients desire or are candidates for reconstructive surgery. A breast prosthesis—an external form that simulates the breast—is another option. Prostheses are available in different shapes, sizes, colors, and materials, although they are most often made of silicone. They can be placed inside a pocket in a bra or can adhere directly to the chest wall. The nurse can provide the patient with the names of shops where she can be fitted for a prosthesis, or the patient can call the Reach to Recovery program of the ACS for appropriate referrals. The patient should be encouraged to find a shop with a comfortable, supportive atmosphere that employs a certified prosthetics consultant. In general, medical supply shops are not recommended because often they do not have the appropriate resources to ensure the proper fitting of a prosthesis.

Prior to discharge from the hospital, the nurse usually provides the patient with a temporary, lightweight, cotton-filled form that can be worn until the surgical incision is well healed (4 to 6 weeks). After that, the patient can be fitted for a prosthesis. Insurance companies generally cover the cost of the prosthesis and the special bras that hold it in place. A breast prosthesis can provide a psychological benefit and assist the woman in resuming proper posture because it helps balance the weight of the remaining breast.

Special Issues in Breast Cancer Management

Implications of Genetic Testing

The rapid advancement in genetics not only has brought new knowledge about inherited breast cancer, but it has also raised potential ethical and psychosocial issues. Although the actual testing for the *BRCA1* and *BRCA2* and several other genes that increase risk involves a simple blood or saliva test, ethical and psychosocial issues must first be addressed. Before undergoing genetic testing, a person should meet either with a clinician who has expertise in this area or with a certified genetic counselor to discuss risk factors as well as the benefits, sequelae, and limitations of testing.

How people react when they receive their actual test results is not always easy to predict. A negative test in a person who comes from a family with a known mutation may lead to enormous relief. However, a negative test in a family with no known mutation may be a source of undue reassurance; the possibility of existing genes that cannot yet be detected remains. A negative test may also lead to feelings of guilt in a person whose family members did not receive favorable test results; this is known as survivor's guilt. A positive test could act as a motivator in a person to pursue appropriate screening or treatment, or it could cause tremendous anxiety, depression, and worry.

In addition, test results may be ambiguous, leading to feelings of confusion and uncertainty. People must be informed that not all gene carriers develop breast cancer (incomplete penetrance) and that not all noncarriers are protected or immune.

People must be well informed of all issues and potential implications prior to undergoing genetic testing (see Chapter 8). Nurses play a role in educating and counseling patients and their family members about the implications of genetic testing. Nurses provide support and clarification and make referrals to appropriate specialists when indicated.

Pregnancy and Breast Cancer

Breast cancer during pregnancy is defined as breast cancer diagnosed during gestation or within 1 year of childbirth and occurs in 1 in 3000 women (NCCN, 2015). Because of increased levels of hormones produced during pregnancy and subsequent lactation, the breast tissue becomes tender and swollen, making it more difficult to detect a mass. If a mass is found during pregnancy, ultrasound is the preferred diagnostic method because it involves no exposure to radiation. If indicated, mammography with appropriate shielding, FNA, and biopsy can be performed. Modified radical mastectomy remains the most common form of surgical treatment. SLNB is typically not performed because of the unknown effects of the radioisotope and the blue dye on the fetus. Breast conservation treatment may be considered if the breast cancer is diagnosed during the third trimester. Radiation can then be delayed until after delivery because it is contraindicated during pregnancy. If a woman is close to term, a cesarean section may be performed as soon as maturation of the fetus allows and then treatment is initiated. If aggressive disease is detected early in pregnancy and chemotherapy is advised, termination of the pregnancy may be considered. If a mass is found while a woman is breast-feeding, she is urged to stop to allow the breast to involute (return to its baseline state) before any type of surgery is performed (NCCN, 2015).

Fertility issues and the future desire for children are major concerns of young women who are survivors of breast cancer. Most cancer therapies have a substantial morbidity on reproductive function, not only because they increase the risk of early menopause but also because they are associated with a decreased ovarian reserve and a loss of fertility. It is estimated that physiologic age of the ovaries in a survivor of cancer may be 10 years older than the actual chronologic age.

Chemotherapy causes a progressive dose-related depletion of ovarian follicles and granulosa cells that translates into oligomenorrhea and subsequent premature ovarian failure, ultimately leading to what is known as chemotherapy-induced amenorrhea (CIA). Regardless of the beneficial effects that hormonal changes can have as part of the adjuvant endocrine strategy, CIA is an adverse event to consider when selecting the best adjuvant treatment. Patients with cancer need to be informed about their reproductive future and options to preserve fertility before treatment (Ruddy & Ginsburg, 2014). Fertile Hope, a national nonprofit organization, can also provide updated information on reproduction (see the Resources section).

Quality of Life and Survivorship

With increased early detection and improved treatment modalities, women with breast cancer have become the largest group of cancer survivors. However, the treatment or simply the diagnosis of breast cancer may have long-term effects that negatively affect the patient and her family. The patient should be prepared early on for the potential long-term effects of the disease so that she has realistic expectations and can make informed decisions.

Survivors of breast cancer may experience a variety of issues as a result of their diagnosis and treatment. Estrogen withdrawal from chemotherapy-induced menopause and hormonal treatments can lead to a variety of symptoms, including hot flashes, vaginal dryness, urinary tract infections, weight gain, decreased sex drive, and increased risk of osteoporosis. HT to alleviate symptoms is contraindicated in women with breast cancer. Certain chemotherapeutic agents can cause long-term cardiac effects and neuropathy. In addition, patients may experience impaired cognitive functioning, such as difficulty concentrating (often referred to as "chemo brain"). Rare long-term effects of radiation can include pneumonitis, rib fractures, heart disease, and breast fibrosis or necrosis (Harris & Morrow, 2014). Long-term sequelae after breast surgery may include lymphedema (mainly after ALND), pain, and sensory disturbances. Once lymphedema develops, it tends to be a chronic problem, so prevention strategies (discussed earlier) are vital. Weight gain and infections are risk factors for lymphedema (Ahn & Port, 2016). Nurses need to encourage patients to maintain an active lifestyle and avoid weight gain.

Long-term psychosocial sequelae may include fears of recurrence, mood changes (e.g., worry, sadness, anger, frustration), an increased sense of vulnerability, uncertainty, feelings of loss (e.g., fertility), concerns about body image, self-concept, and sexuality; emotional distress related to role adjustments and family response; and concerns about finances and employment. Depression and anxiety have been documented in 20% to 30% of women with breast cancer. Interventions should be targeted to meet informational needs, manage uncertainty, control symptoms, address cultural differences, and enhance social and emotional support (Heinz, & Williams, 2015; Ligabel & Denlinger, 2013).

 Gerontologic Considerations

Breast cancer reconstruction in older women with breast cancer is a feasible option that should be offered to patients. Most women tolerate the procedure well and have good cosmetic outcomes. Patients can be offered both implant-based reconstruction and autologous tissue transfer with minimal complications as long as appropriate preoperative selection criteria are used. The safety of reconstruction, together with increase in life expectancy and healthier lifestyles, makes breast reconstruction after mastectomy desirable at any age (NCCN, 2015).

A thorough assessment must be performed before any treatment is initiated, and careful monitoring must occur throughout the course of treatment to avoid complications. The physical and psychosocial assessment of the older woman should include general health, currently existing comorbidities, performance status, cognitive status, current medications, available resources, and support systems.

Breast Health of Women With Disabilities

Disparities in obtaining a mammogram at recommended screening intervals persist for many women, including those with disabilities. Prevalence of self-reported use of mammography is lower for women with a disability. Twenty seven million women in the United States are disabled (Courtney-Long, Carroll, Znang, et al., 2013). Efforts to reduce disparities in breast cancer screening might be more effective if all segments of the population are targeted. Possible barriers to the use of mammography in women with disabilities include physical inaccessibility of office space and medical equipment; limited transportation and parking options; and time and assistance constraints associated with undressing, transferring, and positioning for medical examinations. Lesbian, gay, bisexual, transgender and those questioning their gender may also be uncomfortable with the health care system and avoid screening (Bosse, Nesteby, & Randall, 2015). To promote health and wellness, health agencies, providers, and health care plans must promote cancer prevention and educational programs that are inclusive and responsive to the special needs of women with disabilities (Swaine, Parish, Luken, et al., 2014).

An essential role of the nurse is to assist all women, including those with disabilities, to identify accessible health screening and to advocate for greater accessibility of imaging centers and other health care facilities. Reminding women of the need for recommended clinical breast examinations and mammograms is an important part of nursing care.

RECONSTRUCTIVE BREAST SURGERY

Breast reconstruction surgery, called **mammoplasty**, is an elective procedure that can enhance a woman's self-image and sense of well-being. Women desire reconstruction for a variety of physical and psychological reasons. Therefore, it is important for the health care team to conduct a thorough assessment prior to reconstructive surgery to evaluate the woman's underlying desire, motivation, and expectations. Preparing a woman realistically could help her to avoid potential disappointment. A variety of reconstructive options are available today for women who desire a correction in the size or the shape of the breast, including reduction mammoplasty (breast reduction), augmentation mammoplasty (breast enlargement), and mastopexy (breast lift). Several options are also available to reconstruct the breast after a mastectomy.

Reduction Mammoplasty

Reduction mammoplasty is usually performed on women who have breast hypertrophy (excessively large breasts). The weight of the enlarged breasts can cause discomfort, fatigue, embarrassment, and poor posture.

Reduction mammoplasty is an outpatient procedure that is performed under general anesthesia. Most commonly, an anchor-shaped incision that circles the areola is made, extending downward and following the natural curve of the crease beneath the breast (inframammary fold). Depending on the size of the breast, the nipple may be moved up to a higher position while still attached to the breast tissue, or it may be separated and transplanted to a new location. Drains are placed in the incision and remain for 2 to 5 days.

During the preoperative consultation, the patient should be informed that there is a possibility that sensory changes of the nipple (such as numbness) may occur. These sensations are normal and usually resolve after several months but can sometimes persist. The procedure may also make breastfeeding impossible, although some women have breast-fed successfully. The patient must also be aware that if she gains weight (usually more than 10 pounds), her breasts may also enlarge.

After reduction mammoplasty, many women verbalize feelings of extreme satisfaction, possibly because of the relief they experience. The patient is instructed to wear a supportive bra 24 hours a day for 2 weeks to prevent tension on the swollen breast and incision line. Vigorous exercise (e.g., jumping, jogging) should be avoided for about 6 weeks after surgery.

Augmentation Mammoplasty

Augmentation mammoplasty is requested by women who desire larger or fuller breasts. The procedure is performed by placing a breast implant either under the pectoralis muscle (subpectoral) or under the breast tissue (subglandular). The subpectoral approach is preferred because it interferes less with clinical breast examinations and mammograms. The incision line can be placed in the inframammary fold, in the axilla, or around the areola. The procedure is performed as an outpatient procedure under general anesthesia. A drain is not necessary. Postoperative instructions are the same as for reduction mammoplasty.

Saline implants are typically used for augmentation mammoplasty. The FDA has approved the use of silicone gel–filled implants manufactured by three companies. FDA approval for use of these implants applies to women of all ages for breast reconstruction, and women 22 years and older for breast augmentation (FDA, 2013). Women with breast implants should be aware that mammograms may be more difficult to read, so they should seek experienced breast radiologists.

Mastopexy

Mastopexy is performed when the patient is happy with the size of her breasts but wishes to have the shape improved and a lift performed. This is also an outpatient surgical procedure, and postoperative instructions are the same as for reduction mammoplasty.

DISEASES OF THE MALE BREAST

Gynecomastia

Gynecomastia is the most common breast condition in the male. Adolescent boys can be affected because of hormones secreted by the testes. This type of gynecomastia is virtually always benign and resolves spontaneously in 1 to 2 years. Gynecomastia can also occur in older men and usually presents as a firm, tender mass underneath the areola. In these patients, gynecomastia may be diffuse and related to the use of certain medications (e.g., digitalis, ranitidine [Zantac]). It may also be associated with certain conditions, including feminizing testicular tumors, infection in the testes, and liver disease resulting from factors such as alcohol abuse or a parasitic infection.

Patients in their late teens to late 40s presenting with idiopathic (unknown cause) gynecomastia should have a testicular examination and possibly a testicular ultrasound. Treatment of the enlarged breast tissue is based on patient preference and is usually reserved for those men who cannot tolerate the cosmetic appearance of the breast or who have severe pain associated with the condition. Mammography and ultrasound are utilized if there is a concern about malignancy. Observation is acceptable in most cases because gynecomastia may resolve on its own. Surgical removal of the tissue through a small incision around the areola is the best treatment option. Liposuction performed by a plastic surgeon is another possibility, although this does not allow for pathologic examination of the tissue.

Male Breast Cancer

The lifetime risk of breast cancer in men is about 1 in 1000. The number of breast cancer cases in men relative to the population has been fairly stable over the past 30 years. Nearly 2350 new cases of invasive breast cancer were expected to be diagnosed in men in 2015 (ACS, 2015). Although breast carcinoma in both genders shares certain characteristics, notable differences have emerged. Familial cases in men usually have BRCA2 rather than BRCA1 mutations. Klinefelter syndrome, a chromosomal condition reflecting decreased testosterone levels, is the strongest risk factor for developing male breast carcinoma. Presentation is usually a painless lump, but is often late, with more than 40% of individuals having stage III or IV disease. When survival is adjusted for age at diagnosis and stage of disease, outcomes for male and female patients with breast cancer is similar (Jain & Gradishar, 2014).

Early detection is uncommon in male breast cancer because of the rare nature of the disease. Often, neither patient nor provider suspects male breast cancer early in its development. Treatment generally consists of a total mastectomy with either SLNB or ALND. As in women with breast cancer, prognosis depends on the stage of disease at presentation. Involvement of the axillary lymph nodes is the most important prognostic indicator. Male breast cancers are very likely to be ER+, and tamoxifen, although it has several side effects, is a mainstay of treatment.

Because breast cancer is primarily a disease of women, men may feel that a certain stigma is attached to their diagnosis. Health care professionals must be sensitive to their needs and provide information and support.

CRITICAL THINKING EXERCISES

1 `ebp` A 27-year-old woman has no significant medical history but has a positive family history for breast cancer. What evidence-based recommendations are indicated for the regularity of assessments and screening for this woman? Identify the criteria to evaluate the strength of the evidence for these recommendations.

2 `pq` A 64-year-old woman with a new diagnosis of breast cancer is admitted for a mastectomy. What are the priorities for care of this patient in the preoperative phase? How will your priorities change in the postoperative phase? What are the priorities for discharge instructions and education for this patient? How will your priorities change if the patient is being discharged with a drain?

3 A 54-year-old woman with breast cancer has been prescribed adjuvant hormonal therapy. What would be most important to include in patient education? Describe at least three topics that need to be addressed.

REFERENCES

*Asterisk indicates nursing research.
**Double asterisk indicates classic reference.

Books

American Cancer Society. (2012). *Cancer prevention & early detection facts and figures 2012.* Atlanta, GA: Author.

Bardia, A., & Baselga, J. (2014). Preoperative chemotherapy for operable breast cancer. In J. Harris, M. Lippman, M. Morrow, et al. (Eds.). *Diseases of the breast* (5th ed.). Philadelphia, PA: Wolters Kluwer.

Cherny, N., & Truong, P. (2014). Brachial plexopathy in patients with breast cancer. In J. Harris, M. Lippman, M. Morrow, et al. (Eds.). *Diseases of the breast* (5th ed.). Philadelphia, PA: Wolters Kluwer.

Chung, A., & Giuliano, A. (2014). Sentinel lymph node biopsy. In J. Harris, M. Lippman, M. Morrow, et al. (Eds.). *Diseases of the breast* (5th ed.). Philadelphia, PA: Wolters Kluwer.

Collins, L., & Schnitt, S. (2014). Pathology of benign breast disorders. In J. Harris, M. Lippman, M. Morrow, et al. (Eds.). *Diseases of the breast* (5th ed.). Philadelphia, PA: Wolters Kluwer.

Comerford, K. C. (2015). *Nursing 2015 drug handbook.* Philadelphia, PA: Wolters Kluwer.

Fischbach, F., & Dunning, M. B. (2015). *A manual of laboratory and diagnostic tests* (9th ed.). Philadelphia, PA: Wolters Kluwer.

Grossman, S., & Porth, C. M. (2014). *Porth's pathophysiology: Concepts of altered health states* (9th ed.). Philadelphia, PA: Lippincott Williams & Wilkins.

Gucalp, A., Morris, P., Hudis, C., et al. (2014). Implications of obesity in breast cancer. In J. Harris, M. Lippman, M. Morrow, et al. (Eds.). *Diseases of the breast* (5th ed.). Philadelphia, PA: Wolters Kluwer.

Harris, J., & Morrow, M. (2014). Breast-conserving therapy. In J. Harris, M. Lippman, M. Morrow, et al. (Eds.). *Diseases of the breast* (5th ed.). Philadelphia, PA: Wolters Kluwer.

Helvie, M., & Patterson, S. (2014). Imaging analysis: Mammography. In J. Harris, M. Lippman, M. Morrow, et al. (Eds.). *Diseases of the breast* (5th ed.). Philadelphia, PA: Wolters Kluwer.

Jain, S., & Gradishar, W. (2014). Male breast cancer. In J. Harris, M. Lippman, M. Morrow, et al. (Eds.). *Diseases of the breast* (5th ed.). Philadelphia, PA: Wolters Kluwer.

Jochelson, M. (2014). New breast imaging techniques. In J. Harris, M. Lippman, M. Morrow, et al. (Eds.). *Diseases of the breast* (5th ed.). Philadelphia, PA: Wolters Kluwer.

Kimmick, G., Hughes, K., & Muss, H. (2014). Breast cancer in older women. In J. Harris, M. Lippman, M. Morrow, et al. (Eds.). *Diseases of the breast* (5th ed.). Philadelphia, PA: Wolters Kluwer.

King, T., & Reis-Filho, J. (2014). Lobular carcinoma in situ: Biology and management. In J. Harris, M. Lippman, M. Morrow, et al. (Eds.). *Diseases of the breast* (5th ed.). Philadelphia, PA: Wolters Kluwer.

McLaughlin, S. (2014). Lymphedema. In J. Harris, M. Lippman, M. Morrow, et al. (Eds.). *Diseases of the breast* (5th ed.). Philadelphia, PA: Wolters Kluwer.

Meneses, K., & Walker, D. (2014). Nursing care in patient management and quality of life. In J. Harris, M. Lippman, M. Morrow, et al. (Eds.). *Diseases of the breast* (5th ed.). Philadelphia, PA: Wolters Kluwer.

Morrow, M. (2014). Physical examination of the breast. In J. Harris, M. Lippman, M. Morrow, et al. (Eds.). *Diseases of the breast* (5th ed.). Philadelphia, PA: Wolters Kluwer.

Osborne, M., & Boolbol, S. (2014). Breast anatomy and development. In J. Harris, M. Lippman, M. Morrow, et al. (Eds.). *Diseases of the breast* (5th ed.). Philadelphia, PA: Wolters Kluwer.

Press, M., & Ma, Y. (2014). HER2/ERBB2 testing: Assessment of status for targeted therapies. In J. Harris, M. Lippman, M. Morrow, et al. (Eds.). *Diseases of the breast* (5th ed.). Philadelphia, PA: Wolters Kluwer.

Rimawi, M., & Osborne, C. (2014). Adjuvant systemic therapy: Endocrine therapy. In J. Harris, M. Lippman, M. Morrow, et al. (Eds.). *Diseases of the breast* (5th ed.). Philadelphia, PA: Wolters Kluwer.

Ruddy, K., & Ginsburg, E. (2014). Reproductive issues in breast cancer survivors. In J. Harris, M. Lippman, M. Morrow, et al. (Eds.). *Diseases of the breast* (5th ed.). Philadelphia, PA: Wolters Kluwer.

U.S. Department of Health and Human Services, Public Health Service. (2012). *What you need to know about breast cancer.* Bethesda, MD: National Institutes of Health.

Weber, J., & Kelley, J. (2014). *Health assessment in nursing* (5th ed.). Philadelphia, PA: Lippincott Williams & Wilkins.

Yarbo, C. H., Wujcik, D., & Gobel, B. H. (Eds.). (2013). *Breast Cancer.* Sudbury, MA: Jones & Bartlett.

Journals and Electronic Documents

Ahn, S., & Port, E. (2016) Lymphedema precautions: Time to abandon old practices? *Journal of Clinical Oncology, 34*(12), 655–658.

American Cancer Society. (2013). Cancer Facts & Figures for African Americans 2013–2014. Retrieved on 2/22/2016 at: www.cancer.org/acs/groups/content/@epidemiologysurveilance/documents/document/ac spc-036921.pdf

American Cancer Society. (2015). Cancer facts and figures 2015. Retrieved on 2/22/2016 at: www.cancer.org/acs/groups/content/@editorial/documents/document/acspc-044552.pdf

Bonilla, L., Ben-Aharon, I., Vidal, L., et al. (2010). Dose-dense chemotherapy in nonmetastatic breast cancer: A systematic review and meta-analysis of randomized controlled trials. *Journal of the National Cancer Institute, 102*(24), 1845–1854.

Bosse, J. D., Nesteby, A., & Randall, C. E. (2015). Integrating sexual minority health issues into a health assessment class. *Journal of Professional Nursing, 31*(6), 498–507.

CancerQuest. (2015). Introduction to patient information, detection and diagnosis, fine needle aspiration. Retrieved on 5/22/2016 at: www.cancerquest.org

Chavez-McGregor, M., Clarke, C. A., Lichtensztajn, D. Y., et al. (2016). Delayed initiation of adjuvant chemotherapy among patients with breast cancer. *JAMA Oncology, 2*(3), 322–329.

Courtney-Long, E., Carroll, D., Znang, O., et al. (2013). Prevalence of disability and disability types among adults. *Morbidity and Mortality Weekly Report, 64*(29), 777–783.

**Cummings, S. R., Eckert, S., Krueger, K. A., et al. (1999). The effect of raloxifene on risk of breast cancer in postmenopausal women: Results from the MORE randomized trial. *JAMA, 281*(23), 2189–2197.

**Fisher, B., Costantino, J. P., Wickerham, D. L., et al. (1998). Tamoxifen for prevention of breast cancer. Report of the National Surgical Adjuvant Breast and Bowel Project P-1 study. *Journal of the National Cancer Institute, 90*(18), 1371–1388.

*Harding, M. (2015). Effect of nurse navigation on patient care satisfaction and distress associated with breast biopsy. *Clinical Journal Oncology Nursing, 19*(1), E15–E20.

*Heinz, S., & Williams, P. (2015). Symptom alleviation and self-care among breast cancer survivors after treatment completion. *Clinical Journal of Oncology Nursing, 19*(3), 343–349.

Kerlikowske, K. (2015). Progress toward consensus on breast cancer screening guidelines and reducing harms. *JAMA Internal Medicine, 173*(12), 1970–1971.

Ligabel, J., & Denlinger, C. (2013). New NCCN guidelines for survivorship care. *Journal of the National Comprehensive Care Network, 11*(5 Suppl), 640–644.

National Cancer Institute (NCI). (2013). Surgery to reduce the risk of breast cancer. Retrieved on 2/26/16 at: www.cancer.gov/types/breast/risk-reducing-surgery-fact-sheet

National Comprehensive Cancer Network (NCCN). (2015). Clinical practice guidelines: Breast. Retrieved on 3/7/2016 at: www.nccn.org/professionals/physician_gls/PDF/infections.pdf

Swaine, J., Parish, S., Luken, K., et al. (2014). Test of an intervention to improve knowledge of women with intellectual disability about cervical and breast cancer screening. *Journal of Intellectual Disability Research, 58*(7), 651–663.

Toledo, E., Salas-Salvad, J., Donat-Vargas, C., et al. (2015). Mediterranean diet and invasive breast cancer risk among women at high cardiovascular risk in the PREDIMED trial: A randomized clinical trial. *JAMA Internal Medicine, 175*(11), 1752–1760.

U.S. Food and Drug Administration. (2013). FDA approves new silicone gel-filled breast implant. Retrieved on 8/18/2016 at: www.fda.gov/NewsEvents/Newsroom/PressAnnouncements/ucm340447.htm

**Vogel, V. G., Costantino, J. P., Wickerham, D. L., et al. (2006). Effects of tamoxifen vs. raloxifene on the risk of developing invasive breast cancer and other disease outcomes. The NSABP Study of Tamoxifen and Raloxifene (STAR) P-2 trial. *JAMA, 295*(23), 2727–2741.

Resources

ABCD: After Breast Cancer Diagnosis, abcdbreastcancersupport.org
American Cancer Society, www.cancer.org
American Society of Plastic Surgeons (ASPS), www.plasticsurgery.org
Cancer Care, Inc., www.cancercare.org
Fertile Hope, www.fertilehope.org
National Breast Cancer Coalition, www.breastcancerdeadline2020.org/homepage.html
National Cancer Institute (NCI), www.cancer.gov/cancertopics/types/breast
NCCN National Comprehensive Cancer Network. www.nccn.org
National Lymphedema Network (NLN), www.lymphnet.org
Oncology Nursing Society (ONS), www.ons.org
Reach to Recovery Program—I Can Cope Program, www.cancer.org/cancer/breastcancer/more-information/breastreconstructionaftermastectomy/breast-reconstruction-after-mastectomy-reach-to-recovery
Susan G. Komen for the Cure, www.komen.org
Young Survival Coalition (YSC), www.youngsurvival.org

59

Assessment and Management of Patients With Male Reproductive Disorders

LEARNING OBJECTIVES

On completion of this chapter, the learner will be able to:

1 Describe structures and function of the male reproductive system.
2 Discuss nursing assessment of the male reproductive system; identify diagnostic tests used and their related nursing implications.
3 Explain the causes and management of male sexual dysfunction.
4 Compare the types of prostatectomy with regard to advantages and disadvantages.

5 Use the nursing process as a framework for care of the patient with prostate cancer or undergoing prostatectomy.
6 Identify the nursing management of patients with testicular cancer.
7 Compare and contrast the various disorders of the penis, including pathophysiology, clinical manifestations, and management.

GLOSSARY

androgen deprivation therapy (ADT): surgical (orchiectomy) or medical castration (e.g., with luteinizing hormone–releasing hormone agonists)

benign prostatic hyperplasia (BPH): noncancerous enlargement or hypertrophy of the prostate; the most common pathologic condition in older men

brachytherapy: delivery of internal radiation therapy to a localized area of tissue

circumcision: excision of the foreskin, or prepuce, of the glans penis

cystostomy: surgical creation of an opening into the urinary bladder

epididymitis: infection of the epididymis that usually descends from an infected prostate or urinary tract; also may develop as a complication of gonorrhea, chlamydia, or *Escherichia coli*

erectile dysfunction: the inability to either achieve or maintain an erection sufficient to accomplish sexual intercourse; also called *impotence*

hydrocele: a collection of fluid, generally in the tunica vaginalis of the testis, although it also may collect within the spermatic cord

orchiectomy: surgical removal of one or both of the testes

orchitis: acute inflammation of the testes (testicular congestion) caused by pyogenic, viral, spirochetal, parasitic, traumatic, chemical, or unknown factors

phimosis: condition in which the foreskin is constricted so that it cannot be retracted over the glans; can occur congenitally or from inflammation and edema

priapism: an uncontrolled, persistent erection of the penis from either neural or vascular causes, including

medications, sickle cell thrombosis, leukemic cell infiltration, spinal cord tumors, and tumor invasion of the penis or its vessels

prostatectomy: surgical removal of the entire prostate, the prostate urethra, and the attached seminal vesicles plus the ampulla of the vas deferens

prostate-specific antigen (PSA): substance that is produced by the prostate gland; is used in combination with digital rectal examination to screen for prostate cancer

prostatitis: inflammation of the prostate gland caused by infectious agents (bacteria, fungi, mycoplasma) or various other problems (e.g., urethral stricture, prostatic hyperplasia)

retrograde ejaculation: during ejaculation, semen travels to the urinary bladder instead of exiting through the penis

spermatogenesis: production of sperm in the testes

testosterone: male sex hormone secreted by the testes; induces and preserves the male sex characteristics

transurethral resection of the prostate (TURP): resection of the prostate through endoscopy; the surgical and optical instrument is introduced directly through the urethra to the prostate, and the gland is then removed in small chips with an electrical cutting loop

varicocele: an abnormal dilation of the veins of the pampiniform venous plexus in the scrotum (the network of veins from the testis and the epididymis, which constitute part of the spermatic cord)

vasectomy: ligation and transection of part of the vas deferens, with or without removal of a segment of the vas, to prevent the passage of the sperm from the testes; also called *male sterilization*

Disorders of the male reproductive system include a wide variety of conditions that usually affect both urinary and reproductive systems. Because these disorders involve the genitalia and often affect sexuality, the patient may experience anxiety and embarrassment. The nurse must be aware of the patient's need for privacy as well as his need for education and support. This requires an openness to discuss critical and sensitive issues with the patient, including his partner when appropriate, as well as effective assessment, management, and communication. Nurses must be comfortable when examining male genitalia and must recognize their own attitudes and perceptions about male reproductive disorders. Education of the patient and partner about treatment and self-care strategies is essential (Tabloski, 2014).

ASSESSMENT OF THE MALE REPRODUCTIVE SYSTEM

Anatomic and Physiologic Overview

In the male, several organs serve as parts of both the urinary tract and the reproductive system. Disorders in the male reproductive organs may interfere with the functions of one or both of these systems. As a result, diseases of the male reproductive system are usually treated by a urologist. The structures in the male reproductive system include the (1) external male genitalia, consisting of the testes, epididymis, scrotum, and penis, and the (2) internal male genitalia, consisting of the vas deferens (ductus deferens), ejaculatory duct, and prostatic and membranous sections of the urethra, seminal vesicles, and certain accessory glands, such as the prostate gland and Cowper glands (bulbourethral glands) (see Fig. 59-1).

The testes have a dual function: **spermatogenesis** (production of sperm) and secretion of the male sex hormone **testosterone**, which induces and preserves the male sex characteristics. The testes are formed in the embryo, within the abdominal cavity near the kidney. During the last month of

fetal life, they descend posterior to the peritoneum and pierce the abdominal wall in the groin. Later, they progress along the inguinal canal into the scrotal sac. In this descent, they are accompanied by blood vessels, lymphatics, nerves, and ducts, which support the tissue and make up the spermatic cord. This cord extends from the internal inguinal ring through the abdominal wall and the inguinal canal to the scrotum. As the testes descend into the scrotum in the final 2 to 3 months of gestation, a tubular extension of peritoneum accompanies them (Hall, 2015). Normally, this tissue is obliterated during fetal development; only the tunica vaginalis, which covers the testes, remains. If the peritoneal process remains open into the abdominal cavity, a potential sac remains into which abdominal contents may enter to form an indirect inguinal hernia.

The testes, or ovoid sex glands, are encased in the scrotum, which keeps them at a slightly lower temperature than the rest of the body to facilitate spermatogenesis (Hall, 2015). The testes consist of numerous seminiferous tubules in which the spermatozoa form. Collecting tubules transmit the spermatozoa into the epididymis, a hoodlike structure lying on the testes and containing winding ducts that lead into the vas deferens. This firm, tubular structure passes upward through the inguinal canal to enter the abdominal cavity behind the peritoneum. It then extends downward toward the base of the bladder. An out-pouching from this structure is the seminal vesicle, which acts as a reservoir for testicular secretions. The tract is continued as the ejaculatory duct, which passes through the prostate gland to enter the urethra. Testicular secretions take this pathway when they exit the penis during ejaculation.

The penis is the organ for both copulation and urination. It consists of the glans penis, the body, and the root. The glans penis is the soft, rounded portion at the distal end of the penis. The urethra (the tube that carries urine) opens at the tip of the glans. The glans is naturally covered by elongated penile skin—the foreskin—which may be retracted to expose the glans. However, many men as newborns have undergone **circumcision**, which is a procedure to remove the

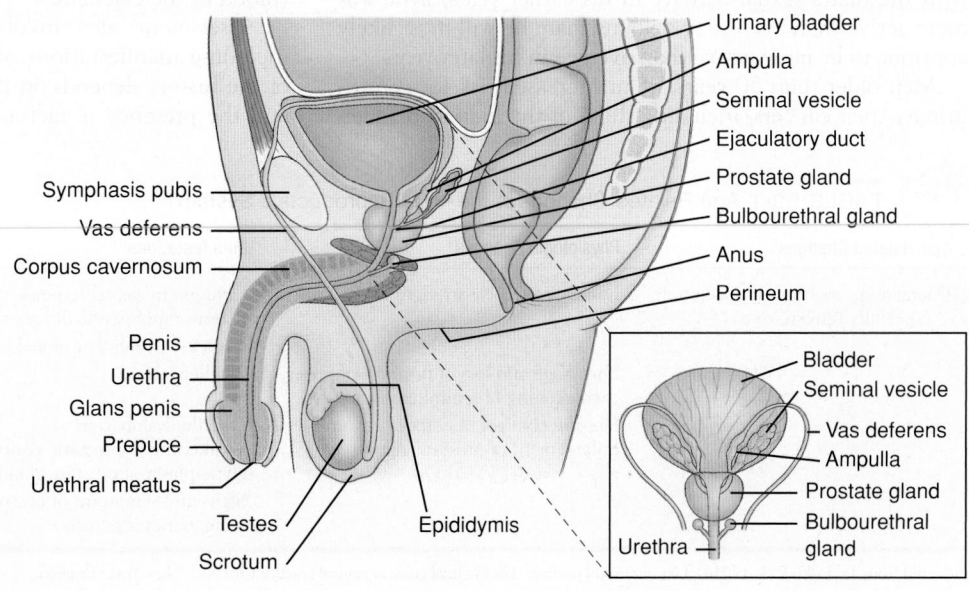

Figure 59-1 • Structures of the male reproductive system.

Labels (left side): Symphasis pubis, Vas deferens, Corpus cavernosum, Penis, Urethra, Glans penis, Prepuce, Urethral meatus, Testes, Scrotum, Epididymis

Labels (right side): Urinary bladder, Ampulla, Seminal vesicle, Ejaculatory duct, Prostate gland, Bulbourethral gland, Anus, Perineum

Inset labels: Bladder, Seminal vesicle, Vas deferens, Ampulla, Prostate gland, Bulbourethral gland, Urethra foreskin. The body of the penis is composed of erectile tissues containing numerous blood vessels that become dilated, leading to an erection during sexual excitement. The urethra, which passes through the penis, extends from the bladder through the prostate to the distal end of the penis.

The prostate gland, lying just below the neck of the bladder, is composed of four zones and four lobes. It surrounds the urethra and is traversed by the ejaculatory duct, a continuation of the vas deferens. This gland produces a secretion that is chemically and physiologically suitable to the needs of the spermatozoa in their passage from the testes. Cowper glands lie below the prostate, within the posterior aspect of the urethra. This gland empties its secretions into the urethra during ejaculation, providing lubrication.

Gerontologic Considerations

As men age, the prostate gland enlarges; prostate secretion decreases; the scrotum hangs lower; the testes decrease in weight, atrophy, and become softer; and pubic hair becomes sparser and stiffer. Changes in gonadal function include a decline in plasma testosterone levels and reduced production of progesterone (see Table 59-1). Libido and potency often decrease in as many as two thirds of men older than 70 years (Tabloski, 2014). Vascular problems cause about half of the cases of impotence in men older than 50 years.

However, male reproductive capability is maintained with advancing age. Although degenerative changes occur in the seminiferous tubules and sperm production decreases, spermatogenesis continues, allowing men to produce viable sperm throughout their lives (McCance, Huether, Braskers, et al., 2013).

Male hypogonadism (decreased function of the testes) starts gradually at approximately 50 years of age, resulting in decreased testosterone production. The older man notices that the sexual response slows, erection takes longer, full erections may not be attained, and ejaculation takes longer to occur and control or resolution may occur without orgasm. Sexual function can be affected by psychological problems, illnesses, and medications (Mulhall & Hsiao, 2014). In general, the entire sexual act takes longer. Sexual activity is closely correlated with the man's sexual activity in his earlier years; if he was more active than average as a young man, he will most likely continue to be more active than average in his later years.

Men older than 50 years are at increased risk for genitourinary tract cancers, including those of the kidney, bladder, prostate, and penis. The digital rectal examination (DRE), prostate-specific antigen (PSA) test, and urinalysis, which screens for hematuria, may uncover a higher percentage of malignancies at earlier stages and lead to lower treatment-associated morbidity as well as a lower mortality.

Urinary incontinence occurs in one fifth of community-dwelling older men and rises to nearly 50% in men in long-term care settings (Tabloski, 2014). Older adults admitted to acute care settings should be screened for this problem. Urinary incontinence may have many causes, including medications, neurologic disease, or benign prostatic hyperplasia (BPH). Incontinence may also be linked to erectile dysfunction when there is damage to the neural pathways that initiate an erection (Lim, 2013). Diagnostic tests are performed to exclude reversible causes. New-onset urinary incontinence is a nursing priority that requires evaluation.

Assessment

Health History

Male sexuality is a complex phenomenon that is strongly influenced by personal, cultural, religious, and social factors. Sexuality and male reproductive function become concerns in the presence of illness and disability (Norton & Tremayne, 2015). Throughout the assessment process, the nurse must recognize the importance of sexuality to the patient. Assessment of male reproductive function begins with an evaluation of urinary function and symptoms. The patient is asked about his usual state of health and any recent change in general physical and sexual activity. Any symptoms or changes in function are explored fully and described in detail. Symptoms related to bladder function and urination, collectively referred to as prostatism, are explored further. They may occur with an obstruction caused by an enlarged prostate gland: increased urinary frequency, decreased force of urine stream, and "double" or "triple" voiding (the patient needs to urinate two or three times over a period of several minutes to completely empty his bladder). The patient is also assessed for dysuria (painful urination), hematuria (blood in the urine), nocturia (urination during the night), and hematospermia (blood in the ejaculate).

Assessment also involves addressing sexual function, including manifestations of sexual dysfunction. The extent of the history depends on the patient's presenting symptoms and the presence of factors that may affect sexual function

TABLE 59-1 Age-Related Changes in the Male Reproductive System

Age-Related Changes	Physiologic Changes	Manifestations
Decrease in sex hormone secretion, especially testosterone	Decreased muscle strength and sexual energy	Changes in sexual response—prolonged time to reach full erection, rapid penile detumescence, and prolonged refractory period
		Decrease in number of viable sperm
	Shrinkage and loss of firmness of testes; thickening of seminiferous tubules	Smaller testes
	Fibrotic changes of corpora cavernosa	Erectile dysfunction
	Enlargement of prostate gland	Weakening of prostatic contractions
		Hyperplasia of prostate gland
		Signs and symptoms of obstruction of lower urinary tract (urgency, frequency, nocturia)

Adapted from Tabloski, P. A. (2014). *Gerontological nursing: The essential guide to clinical practice* (3rd ed.). New York: Pearson.

such as chronic illnesses or disability (e.g., diabetes, multiple sclerosis, stroke, cardiac disease), the use of medications that affect sexual function (e.g., antihypertensive and anticholesterolemic medications, psychotropic agents), stress, the use of alcohol, and the patient's willingness to discuss sexual issues.

By initiating an assessment about sexual concerns, the nurse conveys the message that changes in sexual functioning are valid topics and provides a safe environment for discussing these sensitive topics. A number of models are available to assist in assessing patient's problems and concerns. The PLISSIT (*p*ermission, *l*imited *i*nformation, *s*pecific *s*uggestions, *i*ntensive *t*herapy) model of sexual assessment and intervention may be used to provide a framework for nursing interventions (Norton & Tremayne, 2015). It provides a graded counseling approach that allows health care professionals to deal with sexual issues with a level of comfort and expertise. The model begins by asking the patient's permission (P) to discuss sexual functioning. Limited information (LI) about sexual function may then be provided to the patient. As the discussion progresses, the nurse may offer specific suggestions (SS) for interventions. A professional who specializes in sex therapy may provide more intensive therapy (IT) as needed. The BETTER (*b*ringing up the topic, *e*xplaining, *t*elling, *t*iming, *e*ducate about treatment-related sexual side effects, *r*ecording) model was developed more recently to assist health care professionals to include sexuality in the assessment of patients with cancer (Tannenbaum, 2015).

Patients may find it difficult to express their feelings and concerns regarding their sexuality, especially after a body image change (e.g., after major surgery such as amputation). Discussing sexuality with patients who have an illness or disability can be uncomfortable for nurses and other health care providers; this, in turn, makes discussion of these issues more difficult and uncomfortable for patients. Health care professionals may unconsciously have stereotypes about the sexuality of people who are ill or have a disability (e.g., the belief that people with disabilities are asexual or should be sexually inactive). In addition, patients are often embarrassed to initiate a discussion about sexual issues with their health care providers (Gledhill & Schweitzer, 2013; Mitchell, Mercer, Ploubidis, et al., 2013).

Physical Assessment

In addition to the usual aspects of the physical examination, two essential components address disorders of the male genital or reproductive system: the DRE and the testicular examination.

Digital Rectal Examination

The DRE is used to screen for prostate cancer and is recommended annually for every man older than 50 years (45 years for men at high risk [African American men and men with a family history of prostate cancer in first-degree relatives]) (American Cancer Society [ACS], 2015). The DRE enables the skilled examiner, using a lubricated, gloved finger placed in the rectum, to assess the size, symmetry, shape, and consistency of the posterior surface of the prostate gland (see Fig. 59-2). The clinician assesses for tenderness of the prostate gland on palpation and for the presence and

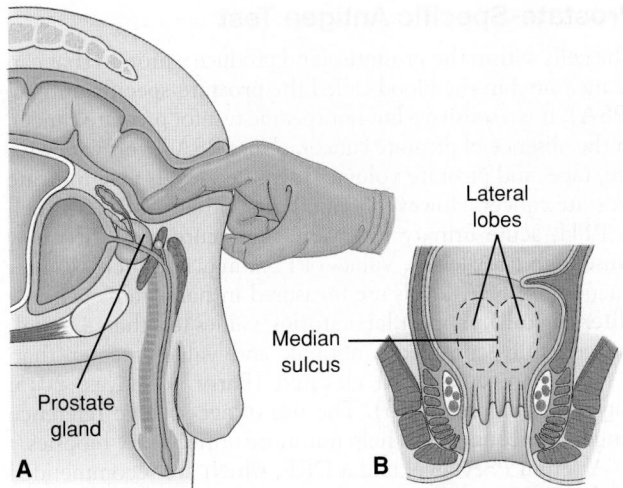

Figure 59-2 • A. Palpation of the prostate gland during digital rectal examination enables the examiner to assess the size, shape, and texture of the gland. **B.** The prostate is round, with a palpable median sulcus or groove separating the lateral lobes. It should feel rubbery and free of nodules and masses.

consistency of any nodules. The DRE may be performed with the patient leaning over an examination table or positioning the man in a side-lying position with legs flexed toward the abdomen or supine with legs resting in stirrups. To minimize discomfort and relax the anal sphincter during the rectal examination, the patient is instructed to take a deep breath and exhale slowly as the practitioner inserts a finger. If possible, he should turn his feet inward so his toes are touching. Although this examination may be uncomfortable and embarrassing for the patient, it is an important screening tool.

Testicular Examination

The male genitalia are inspected for abnormalities and palpated for masses. The scrotum is palpated carefully for nodules, masses, or inflammation. Examination of the scrotum can reveal such disorders as hydrocele, inguinal hernia, testicular torsion, orchitis, epididymitis, or a tumor of the testis. The penis is inspected and palpated for ulcerations, nodules, inflammation, discharge, and curvature. If the patient is uncircumcised, the foreskin should be retracted for visualization of the glans penis. The testicular examination provides an excellent opportunity to instruct the patient on how to perform a testicular self-examination (TSE) and its importance in early detection of testicular cancer. TSE should begin during adolescence. For more details on TSE, see later discussion in the chapter and Chart 59-6.

Diagnostic Evaluation

A wide range of diagnostic studies may be performed in men with reproductive disorders. The nurse should educate the patient about the purpose, what to expect, and any possible side effects related to these tests and examinations prior to testing. The nurse should note trends in results because they provide information about disease progression as well as the patient's response to therapy.

Prostate-Specific Antigen Test

The cells within the prostate gland produce a protein that can be measured in the blood called the **prostate-specific antigen (PSA)**. It is a sensitive but not specific test for prostate cancer. In the absence of prostate cancer, serum PSA levels vary with age, race, and prostate volume. Increased levels may indicate prostate cancer. However, a number of other conditions such as BPH, acute urinary retention, and acute prostatitis may cause high PSA levels. Values of PSA may also increase after ejaculation. PSA levels are measured in nanograms per milliliter (ng/mL). In most laboratories, values less than 4 ng/mL are generally considered normal, and values greater than 4 ng/mL are considered elevated (Barry & Hayes, 2015; Pagana & Pagana, 2013). The use of age-specific reference ranges is encouraged to help minimize unnecessary biopsies.

A serum PSA level and a DRE, which are recommended by the ACS (2015), are used to screen for prostate cancer for men with at least a 10-year life expectancy and for men at high risk, including those with a strong family history of prostate cancer and of African American ethnicity. The perceptions of some African American men and women reflect the belief that PSA screening saves lives and needs to be done despite recommendations against screening due to a number of false positives resulting in unnecessary treatment (Hunter, Vines, & Carlisle, 2015). The PSA test is also used to monitor patients for recurrence after treatment for cancer of the prostate, based on evidence-based guidelines (National Comprehensive Cancer Network [NCCN], 2016b). Neither the DRE nor PSA is 100% accurate, but when used together, their accuracy increases.

Ultrasonography

Transrectal ultrasound (TRUS) may be performed in patients with abnormalities detected by DRE and in those with elevated PSA levels. After DRE has been completed, a lubricated, condom-covered, rectal probe transducer is inserted into the rectum (Itano, Brant, Conde, et al., 2016). Water may be introduced into the condom to help transmit sound waves to the prostate. TRUS may be used in detecting nonpalpable prostate cancers and in staging localized prostate cancer. Needle biopsies of the prostate are commonly guided by TRUS.

Prostate Fluid or Tissue Analysis

Specimens of prostate fluid or tissue may be obtained for culture if disease or inflammation of the prostate gland is suspected. A biopsy of the prostate gland may be necessary to obtain tissue for histologic examination. This may be performed at the time of prostatectomy or by means of a perineal or transrectal needle biopsy. Six to 12 biopsies from all four prostate zones may be obtained during a TRUS-guided biopsy.

Tests of Male Sexual Function

If the patient cannot engage in sexual intercourse to his satisfaction, a detailed history is obtained. Nocturnal erections occur in healthy males of all ages. Nocturnal penile tumescence tests may be conducted in a sleep laboratory to monitor changes in penile circumference during sleep using various methods to determine number, duration, rigidity, and circumference of penile erections; the results help identify whether the erectile dysfunction is caused by physiologic or psychological factors. Additional tests, including psychological evaluations, are also part of the diagnostic workup and are usually conducted by a specialized team of health care providers.

DISORDERS OF MALE SEXUAL FUNCTION

Erectile Dysfunction

Erectile dysfunction, also called *impotence,* is the inability to achieve or maintain an erect penis (Grossman & Porth, 2014). The man may report decreased frequency of erections, inability to achieve a firm erection, or rapid detumescence (subsiding of erection). In the United States, 30 million men experience erectile dysfunction; more than half of men 40 to 70 years of age are unable to attain or maintain an erection sufficient for satisfactory sexual performance (Keane & Graham, 2016). The physiology of erection and ejaculation is complex and involves parasympathetic and sympathetic components. Erection involves the release of nitric oxide into the corpus cavernosum during sexual stimulation. Its release activates cyclic guanosine monophosphate (cGMP), causing smooth muscle relaxation. This allows flow of blood into the corpus cavernosum, resulting in erection (Grossman & Porth, 2014; McDougal, Wein, Kavoussi, et al., 2016).

Erectile dysfunction has both psychogenic and organic causes. Psychogenic causes include anxiety, fatigue, depression, pressure to perform sexually, negative body image, absence of desire, and privacy, as well as trust and relationship issues. Organic causes include cardiovascular disease, endocrine disease (diabetes, pituitary tumors, testosterone deficiency, hyperthyroidism, and hypothyroidism), cirrhosis, chronic kidney injury, genitourinary conditions (radical pelvic surgery), hematologic conditions (Hodgkin lymphoma, leukemia), neurologic disorders (neuropathies, parkinsonism, spinal cord injury [SCI], multiple sclerosis), trauma to the pelvic or genital area, alcohol, smoking, medications (see Chart 59-1), and drug abuse.

Assessment and Diagnostic Findings

The diagnosis of erectile dysfunction requires a sexual and medical history; an analysis of presenting symptoms; a physical examination, including a neurologic examination; a detailed assessment of all medications, alcohol, and drugs used; and various laboratory studies. Nocturnal penile tumescence tests are conducted to monitor changes in penile circumference. This test can help to determine if erectile impotence has an organic or a psychological cause. In healthy men, nocturnal penile erections closely parallel rapid eye movement (REM) sleep in occurrence and duration. Organically impotent men show inadequate sleep-related erections that correspond to their waking performance. Arterial blood flow to the penis is measured using a Doppler probe. In addition, nerve conduction tests and extensive psychological evaluations may be carried out. Figure 59-3 describes the evaluation and treatment of erectile dysfunction.

Medical Management

Treatment can be medical, surgical, or both, depending on the cause. Treatment of erectile dysfunction includes therapy for

Chart 59-1 · PHARMACOLOGY

Medications Associated With Erectile Dysfunction

- *Antiadrenergics and antihypertensives:* guanethidine (Ismelin), clonidine (Catapres), hydralazine (Apresoline)
- *Anticholinergics and phenothiazines:* prochlorperazine (Compazine), trihexyphenidyl (Artane)
- *Antidepressants:* tricyclic antidepressants: amitriptyline (Elavil), desipramine (Norpramin); selective serotonin reuptake inhibitors: fluoxetine (Prozac), sertraline (Zoloft)
- *Antifungals:* ketoconazole (Nizoral)
- *Antihistamines:* diphenhydramine (Benadryl), dimenhydrinate (Dramamine)
- *Antihormone (prostate cancer treatment):* flutamide (Eulexin), leuprolide (Lupron)
- *Antipsychotics:* haloperidol (Haldol), chlorpromazine (Thorazine)
- *Anticonvulsant agents:* carbamazepine (Tegretol)
- *Antispasmodics:* oxybutynin (Ditropan)
- *Anxiolytics, sedative–hypnotics, tranquilizers:* lorazepam (Ativan), triazolam (Halcion)
- *Beta-blockers:* nadolol (Corgard), metoprolol (Lopressor)
- *Calcium channel blockers:* nifedipine (Adalat, Procardia)
- *Carbonic anhydrase inhibitors:* acetazolamide (Diamox)
- *Chemotherapeutic agents:* busulfan (Myleran), cyclophosphamide (Cytoxan)
- *Diuretics:* hydrochlorothiazide (HydroDIURIL), furosemide (Lasix), spironolactone (Aldactone), verapamil (Calan)
- *Histamine-2 antagonists:* nizatidine (Axid), ranitidine (Zantac)
- *Nonsteroidal anti-inflammatory drugs:* naproxen (Naprosyn), indomethacin (Indocin)
- *Other substances:* alcohol, amphetamines, barbiturates, cocaine, marijuana, methadone, nicotine, opioids
- *Parkinson disease medications:* carbidopa/levodopa (Sinemet), benztropine (Cogentin)

Adapted from Karch, A. M. (2016). *2016 Lippincott pocket drug guide for nurses.* (4th ed.). Philadelphia, PA: Wolters Kluwer.

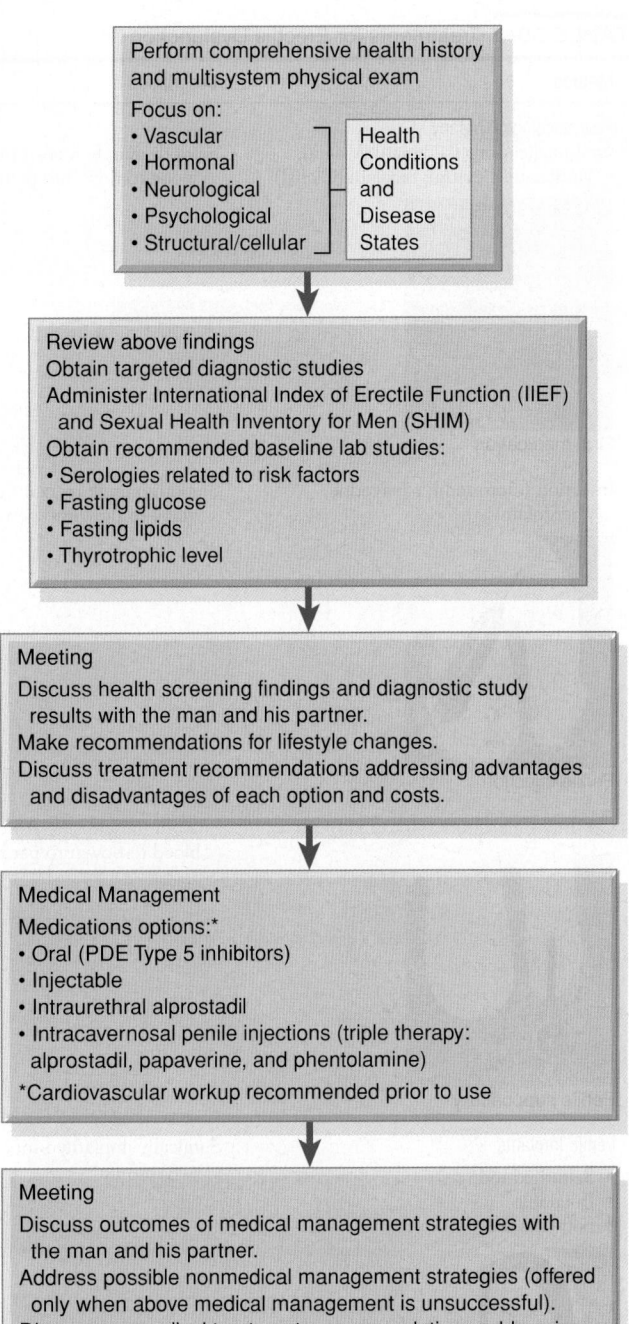

Figure 59-3 • Evaluation and treatment of erectile dysfunction.

associated disorders (e.g., alcoholism, diabetes) or adjustment of medications (Mola, 2015). Endocrine therapy instituted to treat erectile dysfunction secondary to hypothalamic–pituitary–gonadal dysfunction may reverse the condition. Insufficient penile blood flow may be treated with vascular surgery. Patients with erectile dysfunction from psychogenic causes are referred to a health care provider or therapist who specializes in sexual dysfunction. Patients with erectile dysfunction secondary to organic causes may be candidates for penile implants.

Currently available therapies for the treatment of erectile dysfunction include pharmacologic therapy (including urethral suppositories), penile implants, and vacuum constriction devices (see Table 59-2). These options should be considered in a stepwise fashion, with increasing invasiveness and risk balanced against the likelihood of efficacy. The patient and, if possible, his partner, should be informed of the relevant treatment options and their associated risks and benefits. The choice of treatment is made jointly by the primary provider, patient, and partner, taking into consideration patient preferences and expectations.

Pharmacologic Therapy

Phosphodiesterase type 5 (PDE-5) inhibitors (oral medications that are used to treat erectile dysfunction) are first-line therapy (Hsu, Tang, & Lu, 2014). Currently available PDE-5 inhibitors include sildenafil (Viagra), vardenafil (Levitra),

and tadalafil (Cialis). Each of these agents has a similar mechanism of action but a different pharmacologic action and clinical use. Erection involves the release of nitric oxide in the vasculature of the corpus cavernosum as a result of sexual stimulation. This subsequently leads to smooth muscle

TABLE 59-2 Treatments for Erectile Dysfunction

Method	Description	Advantages and Disadvantages	Duration
Pharmacologic Therapy Oral medications (sildenafil [Viagra]; vardenafil [Levitra]; tadalafil [Cialis])	Smooth muscle relaxant causing blood to flow into penis	Can cause headache flushing, dyspepsia, diarrhea, nasal congestion, and lightheadedness See contraindications in Table 59-3	Taken orally before intercourse Stimulation is required to achieve erection. Erection can last 1 hour.
Oral medication			
Injection (alprostadil, papaverine, phentolamine)	Smooth muscle relaxant causing blood to flow into penis	Firm erections are achievable in >50% of cases. Pain at injection site; plaque formation, risk of priapism	Injection 20 minutes before intercourse Erection can last up to 1 hour.
Penile injection			
Urethral suppository (alprostadil)	Smooth muscle relaxant causing blood to flow into penis	May be used twice a day Urethral and genital pain; risk of hypertension and syncope Not recommended with pregnant partners	Inserted 10 minutes before intercourse Erection can last up to 1 hour.
Penile suppository			
Penile Implants • Semirigid rod • Inflatable • Soft silicone	Surgically implanted into corpus cavernosum	Reliable Requires surgery Healing takes up to 3 weeks. Subsequent cystoscopic surgery is difficult. Semirigid rod results in permanent semierection.	Indefinite Inflatable prosthesis— saline returns from penile receptacle to reservoir.
Penile implant			
Negative-Pressure (Vacuum) Devices	Induction of erection with vacuum; maintained with constriction band around base of penis	Few side effects Cumbersome to use before intercourse Vasocongestion of penis can cause pain or numbness.	To prevent penile injury, constriction band must not be left in place >1 hour.
Penile vacuum pump			

relaxation in blood vessels supplying the corpus cavernosum, resulting in increased blood flow and an erection. During sexual stimulation, PDE-5 inhibitors increase blood flow to the penis (Grossman & Porth, 2014).

When PDE-5 inhibitors are taken about 1 hour before sexual activity, they are effective in producing an erection with sexual stimulation; the erection can last about 1 to 2 hours. The most common side effects of these medications include headache, flushing, dyspepsia, diarrhea, nasal congestion, and lightheadedness. These agents are contraindicated in men who take organic nitrates (e.g., isosorbide [Isordil], nitroglycerin), because taken together, these medications can cause side effects such as severe hypotension (Grossman & Porth, 2014; McDougal et al., 2016). In addition, PDE-5 inhibitors must be used with caution in patients with retinopathy, especially in those with diabetic retinopathy. Patient education about the use of these medications and their side effects is summarized in Table 59-3.

For patients in whom PDE-5 inhibitors are contraindicated or ineffective, other pharmacologic measures to induce erections include injecting vasoactive agents, such as alprostadil, papaverine, and phentolamine, directly into the penis. Complications include **priapism** (a persistent abnormal erection) and development of fibrotic plaques at the injection sites. Alprostadil is also formulated in a gel pellet that can be inserted into the tip of the urethra with an applicator to create an erection.

Penile Implants

Two general types of penile implants are available: the malleable, noninflatable, nonhydraulic prosthesis (also called the *semirigid rod*) and the inflatable, hydraulic prostheses (Keane & Graham, 2016). The semirigid rod (e.g., the Small-Carrion prosthesis) results in a permanent semierection but can be bent into an unnoticeable position when appropriate. The inflatable prosthesis simulates natural erections and natural flaccidity. Complications after implantation include infection, erosion of the prosthesis through the skin (more common with the semirigid rod than with the inflatable prosthesis), and persistent pain, which may require removal of the

TABLE 59-3 Pharmacologic Treatment of Erectile Dysfunction

	Sildenafil (Viagra)	Vardenafil (Levitra)	Tadalafil (Cialis)
When to take	Take the medication 30 minutes to 4 hours before intercourse. *There must be sexual stimulation to produce an erection.*	Follow the same directions as with sildenafil; take the medication 1 hour before intercourse. The peak action occurs in 30–120 minutes. *There must be sexual stimulation to produce an erection.*	Take the medication before sexual activity. Effect peaks at 30 minutes to 6 hours; effect may last up to 36 hours. *There must be sexual stimulation to produce an erection.*
Frequency of use	If you take this medication more than once a day, it will not have an increased effect. You may take it 7 days per week if you wish, but only once in 24 hours. It does not build up in your bloodstream. Remember to take it only when you want to have intercourse.	The recommended frequency for this medication is 10 mg in 24 hours.	The effects of this medication may last up to 36 hours. This allows for increased spontaneity in the sexual experience.
Side effects	Side effects include headache, flushing, indigestion, nasal congestion, abnormal vision, diarrhea, dizziness, and rash. You may also have low blood sugar and abnormal liver function tests; your primary provider can determine this.	Side effects include headache, flushing, runny nose, indigestion, sinusitis, flulike syndrome, dizziness, nausea, back pain, and joint pain. Tell your primary provider if you experience any of these effects. You may also have abnormally elevated liver enzymes; your primary provider can determine this.	Side effects are similar to those of sildenafil and vardenafil. Tadalafil may also cause back pain and muscle aches. Tell your primary provider if you experience any of these side effects.
Contraindications	Do not take if you are taking nitrate medications such as nitroglycerin (e.g., Nitro-Bid) or isosorbide mononitrate (e.g., Imdur). Do not take if you have high uncontrolled blood pressure, coronary artery disease, or have had a heart attack within the past 6 months. Do not take if you have been diagnosed with a cardiac dysrhythmia or kidney or liver dysfunction.		
Drug interactions	This medication can react with other medications that you may be taking. Provide your primary provider and pharmacist with a complete list of all prescribed and over-the-counter medications that you are using.		
Use of PDE-5 inhibitors with penile injections or urethral suppositories	The use of PDE-5 inhibitors with other forms of therapy for erectile dysfunction has not been tested and should be avoided.		

PDE-5, phosphodiesterase type 5.
Adapted from Hsu, J. C., Tang, D. H., & Lu, C. Y. (2014). Risk-benefit assessment of oral phosphodiesterase type 5 inhibitors for treatment of erectile dysfunction: A multiple criteria decision analysis. *International Journal of Clinical Practice, 69*(4), 436–443.

implant. Subsequent cystoscopic surgery is more difficult with a semirigid rod than with the inflatable prosthesis.

Factors to consider in choosing a penile prosthesis are the patient's activities of daily living, social activities, and the expectations of the patient and his partner. Ongoing counseling for the patient and his partner is usually necessary to help them adapt to the prosthesis.

Penis Transplants

The first successful penis transplant was performed in 2014 in Cape Town, South Africa. In the United States, a few medical centers have protocols for penis transplants. Candidates for transplantation include military veterans and other men who have suffered traumatic penile injuries. It is believed that men undergoing this surgery will have their ability to urinate and their sexual functioning restored (Kuehn, 2016; Kumnig & Jowsey-Gregoire, 2016). For more details on organ transplantation, see discussion in Chapter 54.

Negative-Pressure Devices

Negative-pressure (vacuum) devices may also be used to induce an erection. A plastic cylinder is placed over the flaccid penis, and negative pressure is applied. When an erection is attained, a constriction band is placed around the base of the penis to maintain the erection. To avoid penile injury, the patient is instructed not to leave the constricting band in place for longer than 1 hour. Only devices with a vacuum limiter are recommended for use (Mulhall & Hsiao, 2014). Although many men find this method satisfactory, others experience premature loss of penile rigidity or pain when applying suction or during intercourse.

Nursing Management

Personal satisfaction and the ability to sexually satisfy a partner are common concerns of patients. Men with illnesses and disabilities may need the assistance of a sex therapist to identify, implement, and integrate their sexual beliefs and behaviors into a healthy and satisfying lifestyle. The nurse can inform patients about support groups for men with erectile dysfunction and their partners.

Disorders of Ejaculation

Premature ejaculation (PE) is defined as the occurrence of ejaculation sooner than desired, either before or shortly after penetration, causing distress to either one or both partners. It is one of the most common complaints of men or couples, affecting 20% to 30% of men (Keane & Graham, 2016; McDougal et al., 2016). The spectrum of responses ranges from occasional ejaculation with intercourse or self-stimulation to complete inability to ejaculate under any circumstances. Various forms of PE have been identified: (1) lifelong PE caused by neurobiologic or genetic conditions, (2) acquired PE (medical or psychological), (3) natural variable PE (normal variation), and (4) prematurelike ejaculatory dysfunction (psychological). In young men ages 18 to 25 years, factors associated with PE and erectile dysfunction include smoking, use of illegal drugs or medications without prescriptions, poor physical and mental health, lack of physical activity and lack of sexual experience (Akre, Berchtold, Gmel, et al., 2014). Other ejaculatory problems may include inhibited (delayed or retarded) ejaculation, which is the involuntary inhibition of the ejaculatory reflex (see Chart 59-2). **Retrograde ejaculation** occurs when semen travels toward the bladder instead of exiting through the penis, resulting in infertility. This form of PE may occur after prior prostate or urethral surgery, with diabetes, or with the use of medications such as antihypertensive agents.

Evaluation of PE involves a thorough sexual history focusing on the duration of symptoms, time to ejaculation, degree of voluntary control over ejaculation, frequency of occurrence, and course of the problem since the first sexual encounter (Keane & Graham, 2016; McDougal et al., 2016).

Chart 59-2	**GENETICS IN NURSING PRACTICE**
	Male Reproductive Disorders

Various male reproductive disorders are influenced by genetic factors. Some examples are:

- 21-Hydroxylase deficiency
- Congenital absence of the vas deferens, prostate gland or seminal vesicles
- Kallmann syndrome
- Klinefelter syndrome (47, XXY)
- Prostate cancer
- Y chromosome deletions

Nursing Assessments

Refer to Chapter 5, Chart 5-2: Genetics in Nursing Practice: Genetic Aspects of Health Assessment

Family History Assessment Specific to Male Reproductive Disorders

- Collect a three-generation family history on both maternal and paternal sides of the family.
- Assess family history for other family members with similar reproductive problems/abnormalities.

Patient Assessment Specific to Male Reproductive Disorders

- In males with delayed puberty or infertility, assess for clinical features of Klinefelter syndrome (tall stature, gynecomastia, learning disabilities).
- Assess males with delayed or absent puberty for clinical features of Kallmann syndrome (cleft lip with or without cleft palate, abnormal eye movements, hearing loss, and abnormalities of tooth development).
- Assess males for history of early growth spurt, which is a symptom of 21-hydroxylase deficiency.
- Inquire about history of prostate inflammation, genital infections, medication use (steroids), or prior history of mumps.
- Assess for physical abnormalities of the genitalia

Genetics Resources

Association for X and Y Chromosome Variations, www.genetic.org
Klinefelter Syndrome Support Group, www.klinefeltersyndrome.org
See Chapter 8, Chart 8-7 for components of genetic counseling.

Treatment, which depends on the nature and severity of PE and perceived distress that it causes, includes behavioral and psychological approaches, as well as pharmacologic therapy that attempts to alter the sensory input or retard the ejaculatory response. Behavioral therapy (e.g., counseling, sex therapy, psychoeducation, and couples therapy) often involves both the man and his sexual partner. The couple is encouraged to identify their sexual needs and to communicate those needs to each other. Pharmacologic management involves selective serotonin reuptake inhibitors dapoxetine (Priligy), alpha$_1$ adrenoceptor antagonists, the tricyclic antidepressant clomipramine (Anafranil), and topical anesthetic agents. In some cases, a combination of pharmacologic and behavioral therapy may be effective.

Inhibited ejaculation is most often caused by psychological factors, neurologic disorders (e.g., SCI, multiple sclerosis, neuropathy secondary to diabetes), surgery (prostatectomy), and medications. Chemical, vibratory, and electrical methods of stimulation have been used with some success. Treatment usually addresses the physical and psychological factors involved in inhibited ejaculation (Wincze & Weisberg, 2015). Although outpatient therapy may involve numerous sessions (12 to 18), it often results in a success rate of 70% to 80%. The outcome depends on a previous satisfying sexual experience history, a short duration of the ejaculatory problem, feelings of sexual desire, feelings of attraction to one's sexual partner, motivation for treatment, and absence of serious psychological problems.

For men with retrograde ejaculation, the urine may be collected shortly after ejaculation, revealing a large amount of sperm in the urine. This urine may also be collected to obtain adequate viable sperm for use in artificial insemination. In men with SCI, techniques that may be used to obtain sperm for artificial insemination include self-stimulation, vibratory stimulation, or electroejaculation. Electroejaculation involves the use of a specially designed probe that is inserted into the rectum next to the prostate. The probe delivers a current that stimulates the nerves and produces contraction of the pelvic muscles and ejaculation. However, spontaneous or stimulated ejaculation may cause autonomic dysreflexia (overstimulation of the autonomic nervous system) in patients with SCI at T6 or higher, creating a life-threatening situation (see Chapter 68). If this disorder is not treated promptly, it may lead to seizures, stroke, and even death.

INFECTIONS OF THE MALE GENITOURINARY TRACT

Acute uncomplicated cystitis in adult men is uncommon but occasionally occurs. Asymptomatic bacteriuria may also result from genitourinary manipulation, catheterization, or instrumentation. Urinary tract infections (UTIs) are discussed in Chapter 55.

According to the Centers for Disease Control and Prevention (CDC, 2015), more than 19 million people develop sexually transmitted infections (STIs) annually in the United States; almost half of all STIs occur in people 18 to 24 years of age. The incidence of STIs has declined over the past several years, except in specific populations, including men who have sex with men. Routine human papillomavirus (HPV)

vaccination for all males has become the standard of preventative care since 2011, as recommended by the Advisory Committee on Immunization Practices (ACIP) (Gerend, Madkins, Phillips, et al., 2016).

STIs affect people from all walks of life—from all social, educational, economic, and racial backgrounds. The single greatest risk factor for contracting an STI is the number of sexual partners. As the number of partners increases, so does the risk of exposure to a person infected with an STI. For men who have sex with men, the CDC recommends annual testing for human immune deficiency virus (HIV), syphilis, *Chlamydia*, gonorrhea, hepatitis B viral infection, and herpes simplex virus type 2, along with counseling (CDC, 2015; Owusu-Edusei, Gift, Patton, et al., 2015).

There are many causes of urethritis (gonococcal and nongonococcal), genital ulcers (genital herpes infections, primary syphilis, chancroid, granuloma inguinale, and lymphogranuloma venereum), genital warts (HPV), scabies, pediculosis pubis, molluscum contagiosum, hepatitis and enteric infections, proctitis, and acquired immune deficiency syndrome (AIDS). Trichomoniasis and STIs characterized by genital ulcers are thought to increase susceptibility to HIV infection. Trichomoniasis is associated with nonchlamydial, nongonococcal urethritis.

Current treatment guidelines for STIs are available from the CDC (2015; Lanier & Sutton, 2013). Treatment must target the patient as well as his sexual partners and sometimes an unborn child. A thorough history, including a sexual history, is crucial to identify patients at risk and to direct care and education. It is essential for patient education to focus on partner safety as people can misjudge partner safety with known acquaintances, thus causing individuals to be at greater risk of STI/HIV transmission (Sparling & Cramer, 2015).

Partners of men with STIs must also be examined, treated, and counseled to prevent reinfection and complications in both partners and to limit the spread of the disease. Sexual abstinence during treatment and recovery is advised to prevent the transmission of STIs. The use of synthetic condoms for at least 6 months after completion of treatment is recommended to decrease transmission of HPV infection as well as other STIs. It is important to assess and test for other STIs because patients who have one STI may also have another. The use of spermicides with nonoxynol-9 (known as N-9) is discouraged; these agents do not protect against HIV infection and may increase the risk of transmission of the virus. See Chapters 36 and 71 for more detailed discussions of HIV infection, AIDS, and other STIs.

PROSTATIC DISORDERS

Prostatitis

Prostatitis is an inflammation of the prostate gland that is often associated with lower urinary tract symptoms and symptoms of sexual discomfort and dysfunction. The condition affects 5% to 10% of men. It is the most common urologic diagnosis in men younger than 50 years and the third most common such diagnosis in men older than 50 years (McDougal et al., 2016). Prostatitis may be caused by infectious agents (bacteria, fungi, mycoplasma) or other conditions (e.g., urethral stricture, BPH). *Escherichia coli* is the most commonly isolated organism, although *Klebsiella* and *Proteus* species are also found (Chen, Hu, Peng, et al., 2015). The microorganisms colonize the urinary tract and ascend to the prostate, ultimately causing infection. The causal pathogen is usually the same in recurrent infections.

There are four types of prostatitis: acute bacterial prostatitis (type I), chronic bacterial prostatitis (type II), chronic prostatitis/chronic pelvic pain syndrome (CP/CPPS) (type III), and asymptomatic inflammatory prostatitis (type IV). Type III, which occurs in more than 90% of cases, is further classified as type IIIA or type IIIB, depending on the presence (type IIIA) or absence (type IIIB) of white blood cells in semen after prostate massage (Chen et al., 2015).

Clinical Manifestations

Acute prostatitis is characterized by the sudden onset of fever, dysuria, perineal prostatic pain, and severe lower urinary tract symptoms: dysuria, frequency, urgency, hesitancy, and nocturia. Approximately 5% of cases of type I prostatitis (acute bacterial prostatitis) progress to type II prostatitis (chronic bacterial prostatitis) (McDougal et al., 2016). Patients with type II disease are typically asymptomatic between episodes. Patients with type III prostatitis often have no bacteria in the urine in the presence of genitourinary pain. Patients with type IV prostatitis are usually diagnosed incidentally during a workup for infertility, an elevated PSA test, or other disorders.

Medical Management

The goal of treatment is to eradicate the causal organisms. Hospital admission may be necessary for patients with unstable vital signs, sepsis, or intractable pelvic pain; those who are frail or immunosuppressed; or those who have diabetes or renal insufficiency. Specific treatment is based on the type of prostatitis and on the results of culture and sensitivity testing of the urine (Wagenlehner, Weidner, Pilatz, et al., 2014). If bacteria are cultured from the urine, antibiotic agents, including trimethoprim-sulfamethoxazole (Bactrim) or a fluoroquinolone (e.g., ciprofloxacin [Cipro]), may be prescribed, and continuous therapy with low-dose antibiotic agents may be used. If the patient is afebrile and has a normal urinalysis, anti-inflammatory agents may be used. Alpha-adrenergic blocker therapy (e.g., tamsulosin [Flomax]), may be prescribed to promote bladder and prostate relaxation.

Factors contributing to prostatitis, including stress, neuromuscular factors, and myofascial pain, are also addressed. Supportive, nonpharmacologic therapies may be prescribed. These include biofeedback, pelvic floor training, physical therapy, reduction of prostatic fluid retention by ejaculation through sexual intercourse or masturbation, sitz baths, stool softeners, and evaluation of sexual partners to reduce the possibility of cross-infection.

Nursing Management

If the patient experiences symptoms of acute prostatitis (fever, severe pain and discomfort, inability to urinate, malaise), he may be hospitalized for intravenous (IV) antibiotic therapy. Nursing management includes administration of prescribed antibiotic agents and provision of comfort measures, including prescribed analgesic agents and sitz baths.

The patient with chronic prostatitis is usually treated on an outpatient basis and needs to be educated about the importance of continuing antibiotic therapy and recognizing recurrent signs and symptoms of prostatitis.

Promoting Home, Community-Based, and Transitional Care

 Educating Patients About Self-Care

The nurse educates the patient about the importance of completing the prescribed course of antibiotic therapy. If IV antibiotic agents are to be given at home, the nurse educates the patient and family about correct and safe administration. Arrangements for a home care nurse to oversee administration may be needed. Warm sitz baths (10 to 20 minutes) may be taken several times daily. Fluids are encouraged to satisfy thirst but are not "forced," because an effective medication level must be maintained in the urine. Foods and liquids with diuretic action or that increase prostatic secretions, such as alcohol, coffee, tea, chocolate, cola, and spices, should be avoided. A suprapubic catheter may be necessary for severe urinary retention. During periods of acute inflammation, sexual arousal and intercourse should be avoided. To minimize discomfort, the patient should avoid sitting for long periods. Medical follow-up is necessary for at least 6 months to 1 year, because prostatitis caused by the same or different organisms can recur. The patient is advised that the UTI may recur and is educated to recognize its symptoms.

Benign Prostatic Hyperplasia (Enlarged Prostate)

Benign prostatic hyperplasia (BPH), a noncancerous enlargement or hypertrophy of the prostate, is one of the most common diseases in aging men. It can cause bothersome lower urinary tract symptoms that affect quality of life by interfering with normal daily activities and sleep patterns (McDougal et al., 2016). BPH typically occurs in men older than 40 years. By the time they reach 60 years, 50% of men have BPH. It affects as many as 90% of men by 85 years of age. BPH is the second most common cause of surgical intervention in men older than 60 years.

Pathophysiology

The cause of BPH is not well understood, but testicular androgens have been implicated. Dihydrotestosterone (DHT), a metabolite of testosterone, is a critical mediator of prostatic growth. Estrogens may also play a role in the cause of BPH; BPH generally occurs when men have elevated estrogen levels and when prostate tissue becomes more sensitive to estrogens and less responsive to DHT. Smoking, heavy alcohol consumption, obesity, reduced activity level, hypertension, heart disease, diabetes, and a Western diet (high in animal fat and protein and refined carbohydrates, low in fiber) are risk factors for BPH (McDougal et al., 2016; Tantamango-Bartley, Knutsen, Knutsen, et al., 2016).

BPH develops over a prolonged period; changes in the urinary tract are slow and insidious. BPH is a result of complex interactions involving resistance in the prostatic urethra to mechanical and spastic effects, bladder pressure during voiding, detrusor muscle strength, neurologic functioning, and general physical health (McCance et al., 2013). The hypertrophied lobes of the prostate may obstruct the bladder neck or urethra, causing incomplete emptying of the bladder and urinary retention. As a result, a gradual dilation of the ureters (hydroureter) and kidneys (hydronephrosis) can occur. Urinary retention may result in UTIs because urine that remains in the urinary tract serves as a medium for infective organisms.

Clinical Manifestations

BPH may or may not lead to lower urinary tract symptoms; if symptoms occur, they may range from mild to severe. Severity of symptoms increases with age, and half of men with BPH report having moderate to severe symptoms. Obstructive and irritative symptoms may include urinary frequency, urgency, nocturia, hesitancy in starting urination, decreased and intermittent force of stream and the sensation of incomplete bladder emptying, abdominal straining with urination, a decrease in the volume and force of the urinary stream, dribbling (urine dribbles out after urination), and complications of acute urinary retention and recurrent UTIs. Normally, residual urine amounts to no more than 50 mL in the middle-aged adult and less than 50 to 100 mL in the older adult (Weber & Kelley, 2014). Ultimately, chronic urinary retention and large residual volumes can lead to azotemia (accumulation of nitrogenous waste products) and kidney failure.

Generalized symptoms may also be noted, including fatigue, anorexia, nausea, vomiting, and pelvic discomfort. Other disorders that produce similar symptoms include urethral stricture, prostate cancer, neurogenic bladder, and urinary bladder stones.

Assessment and Diagnostic Findings

The health history focuses on the urinary tract, previous surgical procedures, general health issues, family history of prostate disease, and fitness for possible surgery (Pearson, 2014). A patient voiding diary is used to record voiding frequency and urine volume. A DRE often reveals a large, rubbery, and nontender prostate gland. A urinalysis to screen for hematuria and UTI is recommended. A PSA level is obtained if the patient is without a terminal disease and for whom knowledge of the presence of prostate cancer would change management. The American Urological Association (AUA) Symptom Index or International Prostate Symptom Score (IPSS) can be used to assess the severity of symptoms (Keane & Graham, 2016).

Other diagnostic tests may include recording urinary flow rate and the measurement of postvoid residual urine. If invasive therapy is considered, urodynamic studies, urethrocystoscopy, and ultrasound may be performed. Complete blood studies are performed. Cardiac status and respiratory function are assessed because a high percentage of patients with BPH have cardiac or respiratory disorders due to their age.

Medical Management

The goals of medical management of BPH are to improve quality of life, improve urine flow, relieve obstruction, prevent disease progression, and minimize complications. Treatment depends on the severity of symptoms, the cause of disease, the severity of the obstruction, and the patient's condition.

If a patient is admitted on an emergency basis because he is unable to void, he is immediately catheterized. The ordinary catheter may be too soft and pliable to advance through the urethra into the bladder. In such cases, a thin wire (stylet) is introduced (by a urologist) into the catheter to prevent the catheter from collapsing when it encounters resistance. A metal catheter with a pronounced prostatic curve may be used if obstruction is severe. A **cystostomy** (incision into the bladder) may be needed to provide urinary drainage.

Discussion of all treatment options by the primary provider enables the patient to make an informed decision based on symptom severity, the effect of BPH on his quality of life, and preference. Patients with mild symptoms and patients with moderate or severe symptoms who are not bothered by them and have not developed complications may be managed with "watchful waiting." With this approach, the patient is monitored and reexamined annually but receives no active intervention (Pearson, 2014). Other therapeutic choices include pharmacologic treatment, minimally invasive procedures, and surgery.

Pharmacologic Therapy

Pharmacologic treatment for BPH includes the use of alpha-adrenergic blockers and 5-alpha-reductase inhibitors (McDougal et al., 2016). Alpha-adrenergic blockers, which include alfuzosin (Uroxatral), terazosin (Hytrin), doxazosin (Cardura), and tamsulosin, relax the smooth muscle of the bladder neck and prostate. This improves urine flow and relieves symptoms of BPH. Side effects include dizziness, headache, asthenia/fatigue, postural hypotension, rhinitis, and sexual dysfunction (Keane & Graham, 2016; McDougal et al., 2016).

Another method of treatment involves hormonal manipulation with antiandrogen agents. The 5-alpha-reductase inhibitors finasteride (Proscar) and dutasteride (Avodart) are used to prevent the conversion of testosterone to DHT and decrease prostate size. Side effects include decreased libido, ejaculatory dysfunction, erectile dysfunction, gynecomastia (breast enlargement), and flushing. Combination therapy (doxazosin and finasteride) has decreased symptoms and reduced clinical progression of BPH (Keane & Graham, 2016; McDougal et al., 2016).

The use of alternative and complementary phytotherapeutic agents and other dietary supplements (*Serenoa repens* [saw palmetto berry] and *Pygeum africanum* [African plum]) are not recommended by the medical community, although they are commonly used (Allkanjari & Vitalone, 2015). They may function by interfering with the conversion of testosterone to DHT. In addition, *S. repens* may directly block the ability of DHT to stimulate prostate cell growth. These agents should not be used with finasteride, dutasteride, or estrogen-containing medications (Allkanjari & Vitalone, 2015).

Surgical Management

Other treatment options include minimally invasive procedures and resection of the prostate gland.

Minimally Invasive Therapy

Several forms of minimally invasive therapy may be used to treat BPH. Transurethral microwave thermotherapy (TUMT) involves the application of heat to prostatic tissue.

High-energy TUMT devices (CoreTherm, Prostatron, Targis) and low-energy devices (TherMatrx) are available (McDougal et al., 2016). A transurethral probe is inserted into the urethra, and microwaves are directed to the prostate tissue. The targeted tissue becomes necrotic and sloughs. To minimize damage to the urethra and decrease the discomfort from the procedure, some systems have a water-cooling apparatus.

Other minimally invasive treatment options include (transurethral needle ablation [TUNA]) by radiofrequency energy and the UroLume stent. TUNA uses low-level radiofrequencies delivered by thin needles placed in the prostate gland to produce localized heat that destroys prostate tissue while sparing other tissues. The body then reabsorbs the dead tissue. Prostatic stents are associated with significant complications (e.g., encrustation, infection, chronic pain); therefore, they are used only for patients with urinary retention and in patients who are poor surgical risks (McDougal et al., 2016).

Surgical Resection

Surgical resection of the prostate gland is another option for patients with moderate to severe lower urinary tract symptoms of BPH and for those with acute urinary retention or other complications. The specific surgical approach (open or endoscopic) and the energy source (electrocautery vs. laser) are based on the surgeon's experience, the size of the prostate gland, the presence of other medical disorders, and the patient's preference. If surgery is to be performed, all clotting defects must be corrected and medications for anticoagulation withheld because bleeding is a potential complication of prostate surgery.

Transurethral resection of the prostate (TURP) remains the benchmark for surgical treatment for BPH. It involves the surgical removal of the inner portion of the prostate through an endoscope inserted through the urethra; no external skin incision is made. It can be performed with ultrasound guidance. The treated tissue either vaporizes or becomes necrotic and sloughs. The procedure is performed in the outpatient setting and usually results in less postoperative bleeding than a traditional surgical prostatectomy.

Other surgical options for BPH include transurethral incision of the prostate (TUIP), transurethral electrovaporization, laser therapy, and open prostatectomy (Keane & Graham, 2016; McDougal et al., 2016). TUIP is an outpatient procedure used to treat smaller prostates. One or two cuts are made in the prostate and prostate capsule to reduce constriction of the urethra and decrease resistance to flow of urine out of the bladder; no tissue is removed. Open **prostatectomy** involves the surgical removal of the inner portion of the prostate via a suprapubic, retropubic, or perineal (rare) approach for large prostate glands. Prostatectomy may also be performed laparoscopically or by robotic-assisted laparoscopy.

Nursing management of patients undergoing these procedures is described later in this chapter.

Cancer of the Prostate

Prostate cancer is the most common cancer in men other than nonmelanoma skin cancer. It is the second most common cause of cancer death in American men, exceeded only by lung cancer, and is responsible for 10% of cancer-related deaths in men. Among men diagnosed with prostate cancer, 98% survive at least 5 years, 84% survive at least 10 years, and 56% survive 15 years (ACS, 2015).

Prostate cancer is common in the United States and northwestern Europe but is rare in Africa, Central America, South America, China, and other parts of Asia. African American men have a high risk of prostate cancer; furthermore, they are more than twice as likely to die of prostate cancer as men of other racial or ethnic groups. Health care providers need to provide education about prostate cancer and appropriate screening in African American men, who are at higher risk compared to all other ethnic communities (Cremin, 2015). Health care providers should also ensure the delivery of culturally sensitive education programs and counseling about prostate cancer screening to not only the African American patient at risk for prostate cancer, but also to his friends and family (Mulheim, Fulbright, & Duncan, 2015).

Other risk factors for prostate cancer include increasing age; the incidence of prostate cancer increases rapidly after the age of 50 years. More than 70% of cases occur in men older than 65 years. A familial predisposition may occur in men who have a father or brother previously diagnosed with prostate cancer, especially if their relatives were diagnosed at a young age. Genes that may be associated with increased risk of prostate cancer include hereditary prostate cancer 1 (*HPC1*) and *BRCA1* and *BRCA2* mutations (McDougal et al., 2016). The risk of prostate cancer is also greater in men whose diet contains excessive amounts of red meat or dairy products that are high in fat (ACS, 2015). Endogenous hormones, such as androgens and estrogens, also may be associated with the development of prostate cancer.

Clinical Manifestations

Cancer of the prostate in its early stages rarely produces symptoms. Usually, symptoms that develop from urinary obstruction occur in advanced disease. Prostate cancer tends to vary in its course. If the cancer is large enough to encroach on the bladder neck, signs and symptoms of urinary obstruction occur (difficulty and frequency of urination, urinary retention, and decreased size and force of the urinary stream). Other symptoms may include blood in the urine or semen and painful ejaculation. Hematuria may occur if the cancer invades the urethra or bladder. Sexual dysfunction is common before the diagnosis is made.

Prostate cancer can spread to lymph nodes and bone. Symptoms of metastases include backache, hip pain, perineal and rectal discomfort, anemia, weight loss, weakness, nausea, oliguria (decreased urine output), and spontaneous pathologic fractures. These symptoms may be the first indications of prostate cancer.

Assessment and Diagnostic Findings

If prostate cancer is detected early, the likelihood of cure is high (Itano et al., 2016). It can be diagnosed through an abnormal finding with the DRE, serum PSA, and ultrasound-guided TRUS with biopsy. Detection is more likely with the use of combined diagnostic procedures. Routine repeated DRE (preferably by the same examiner) is important because early cancer may be detected as a nodule within the gland or as an extensive hardening in the posterior lobe. The more advanced lesion is "stony hard" and fixed. DRE also provides useful clinical information about the rectum, anal sphincter, and quality of stool.

The diagnosis of prostate cancer is confirmed by a histologic examination of tissue removed surgically by TURP, open prostatectomy, or ultrasound-guided transrectal needle biopsy. Fine-needle aspiration is a quick, painless method of obtaining prostate cells for cytologic examination and determining the stage of disease.

Most prostate cancers are detected when a man seeks medical attention for symptoms of urinary obstruction or are found by routine DRE and PSA testing. Cancer detected incidentally when TURP is performed for clinically benign disease and lower urinary tract symptoms occurs in about 1 of 10 cases.

 Concept Mastery Alert

DRE and PSA testing are important screening procedures, because abnormal DRE and elevated levels of PSA may raise suspicion of prostate cancer. However, a diagnosis of cancer requires confirmation with a prostate biopsy.

TRUS helps detect nonpalpable prostate cancers and assists with staging of localized prostate cancer. Needle biopsies of the prostate are commonly guided by TRUS. The biopsies are examined by a pathologist to both determine if cancer is present and to grade the tumor. The most commonly used tumor grading system is the Gleason score. This system assigns a grade of 1 to 5 for the most predominant architectural pattern of the glands of the prostate and a secondary grade of 1 to 5 to the second most predominant pattern. The Gleason score is then reported as, for example, 2 + 4; the combined value can range from 2 to 10. With each increase in Gleason score, there is an increase in tumor aggressiveness. Lower Gleason scores indicate well-differentiated and less aggressive tumor cells; higher Gleason scores indicate undifferentiated cells and more aggressive cancer. A total score of 8 to 10 indicates a high-grade cancer (Keane & Graham, 2016).

Categorization of low-, intermediate-, and high-risk prostate cancer is determined by the extent of cancer in the prostate gland, whether or not the cancer is localized to the prostate, the aggressiveness of the cells, and the spread to the lymph nodes and beyond. Level of risk, in turn, is used to determine treatment options.

Bone scans, skeletal x-rays, and magnetic resonance imaging (MRI) may be used to identify metastatic bone disease. Pelvic computed tomography (CT) scans may be performed to determine if the cancer has spread to the lymph nodes. The radiolabeled monoclonal antibody capromab pendetide with indium 111 (ProstaScint) is an antibody that can be used to detect either recurrent prostate cancer at low PSA levels or metastatic disease (NCCN, 2016b).

Medical Management

Treatment is based on the patient's life expectancy, symptoms, risk of recurrence after definitive treatment, size of the tumor, Gleason score, PSA level, likelihood of complications, and patient preference. Therapy is often guided by the use of a nomogram or risk stratification scheme suggested by the NCCN (2016b) clinical practice guidelines. A multidisciplinary team approach is essential for the development of appropriate treatment. Management may be nonsurgical and involve watchful waiting or be surgical and entail prostatectomy. Nursing care of the patient with cancer of the prostate is summarized in Chart 59-3.

For patients with prostate cancer who choose nonsurgical watchful waiting, this approach involves actively monitoring the course of disease and intervening only if the cancer progresses or if symptoms warrant other intervention. It is an option for patients with life expectancy of less than 5 years and low-risk cancers. Advantages include absence of side effects of more aggressive treatment, improved quality of life, avoidance of unnecessary treatment, and decreased initial costs. Disadvantages include missed chance at cure, risk of metastasis, subsequent need for more aggressive treatment, anxiety about living with untreated cancer, and need for frequent monitoring (NCCN, 2016b; Thakur, 2016).

Therapeutic vaccines kill existing cancer cells and provide long-lasting immunity against further cancer development. In 2010, the U.S. Food and Drug Administration (FDA) approved the first therapeutic cancer vaccine, sipuleucel-T (Provenge), for use in men with metastatic prostate cancer that is no longer responding to hormone therapy. In addition, two other medications, abiraterone acetate (Zytiga) and cabazitaxel (Jevtana injection) are treatments options for patients requiring care for the management of metastatic castration-resistant prostate cancer, which does not respond to sipuleucel-T or the usual treatment options (Simondsen & Kolesar, 2013).

Surgical Management

Radical prostatectomy is considered first-line treatment for prostate cancer and is used with patients whose tumor is confined to the prostate (McDougal et al., 2016). It is the complete surgical removal of the prostate, seminal vesicles, tips of the vas deferens, and often the surrounding fat, nerves, and blood vessels. Laparoscopic radical prostatectomy and robotic-assisted laparoscopic radical prostatectomy have become the standard surgical approaches for localized cancer of the prostate. Although sexual impotence is a common side effect, these laparoscopic radical prostatectomy approaches result in low morbidity and more favorable postoperative outcomes, including improved quality of life and less sexual dysfunction if the nerves are spared. Surgical approaches are discussed in detail later in this chapter.

Radiation Therapy

Two major forms of radiation therapy are used to treat cancer of the prostate: teletherapy (external) and **brachytherapy** (internal). Teletherapy (external-beam radiation therapy [EBRT]) is prescribed by the radiation oncologist for a total dose over a certain time frame—for example, 28 treatments over 5½ weeks (Itano et al., 2016). It is a treatment option for patients with low-risk prostate cancer; progression-free survival is similar to that of low-risk patients treated with radical prostatectomy. Patients with intermediate- and high-risk cancers receive higher doses of EBRT. They may also be candidates both pelvic lymph node irradiation and **androgen deprivation therapy (ADT)** that entails surgical (orchiectomy) or medical castration (e.g., with luteinizing

(*text continued on page 1769*)

PLAN OF NURSING CARE

Chart 59-3

The Patient With Prostate Cancer

NURSING DIAGNOSIS: Anxiety related to concern and lack of knowledge about the diagnosis, treatment plan, and prognosis
GOAL: Reduced stress and improved ability to cope

Nursing Interventions	Rationale	Expected Outcomes

1. Obtain health history to determine the following:
  a. Patient's concerns
  b. His level of understanding of his health problem
  c. His past experience with cancer
  d. Whether he knows his diagnosis of malignancy and its prognosis
  e. His support systems and coping methods
	1. Nurse clarifies information and facilitates patient's understanding and coping.	• Appears relaxed
		• States that anxiety has been reduced or relieved
		• Demonstrates understanding of illness, diagnostic tests, and treatment when questioned
		• Verbalizes adequate coping ability
		• Engages in open communication with others

2. Provide education about diagnosis and treatment plan.
  a. Explain in simple terms what diagnostic tests to expect, how long they will take, and what will be experienced during each test.
  b. Review treatment plan, and encourage patient to ask questions.
	2. Helping the patient to understand the diagnostic tests and treatment plan will help decrease his anxiety and promote cooperation.	

3. Assess his psychological reaction to his diagnosis/prognosis and how he has coped with past stresses.	3. This information provides clues in determining appropriate measures to facilitate coping.	
4. Provide information about institutional and community resources for coping with prostate cancer: social services, support groups, community agencies.	4. Institutional and community resources can help the patient and family cope with the illness and treatment on an ongoing basis.	

NURSING DIAGNOSIS: Urinary retention related to urethral obstruction secondary to prostatic enlargement or tumor and loss of bladder tone due to prolonged distention/retention
GOAL: Improved pattern of urinary elimination

Nursing Interventions	Rationale	Expected Outcomes
1. Determine patient's usual pattern of urinary function.	1. Provides a baseline for comparison and goal to work toward.	• Voids at normal intervals • Reports absence of frequency, urgency, or bladder fullness • Displays no palpable suprapubic distention after voiding • Maintains balanced intake and output
2. Assess for signs and symptoms of urinary retention: amount and frequency of urination, suprapubic distention, complaints of urgency and discomfort.	2. Voiding 20–30 mL frequently and output less than intake suggest retention.	
3. Catheterize patient to determine amount of residual urine.	3. Determines amount of urine remaining in bladder after voiding.	

4. Initiate measures to treat retention.
  a. Encourage assuming normal position for voiding.
  b. Recommend using Valsalva maneuver preoperatively, if not contraindicated.
  c. Administer prescribed cholinergic agent.
  d. Monitor effects of medication.
	4. Promotes voiding:
	  a. Usual position provides relaxed conditions conducive to voiding.
	  b. Valsalva maneuver exerts pressure to force urine out of bladder.
	  c. Stimulates bladder contraction.
	  d. If unsuccessful, another measure may be required.	

5. Consult with primary provider regarding intermittent or indwelling catheterization; assist with procedure as required.	5. Catheterization will relieve urinary retention until the specific cause is determined; it may be an obstruction that can be corrected only surgically.	
6. Monitor catheter function; maintain sterility of closed system; irrigate as required.	6. Adequate functioning of catheter is to be ensured to empty bladder and to prevent infection.	
7. Prepare patient for surgery if indicated.	7. Surgical removal of obstruction may be necessary.	

Chart 59-3

PLAN OF NURSING CARE (Continued)

The Patient With Prostate Cancer

NURSING DIAGNOSIS: Deficient knowledge related to the diagnosis of: cancer, urinary difficulties, and treatment modalities
GOAL: Understanding of the diagnosis and ability to care for self

Nursing Interventions	Rationale	Expected Outcomes
1. Encourage communication with the patient.	1. This is designed to establish rapport and trust.	• Discusses his concerns and problems freely
2. Review the anatomy of the involved area.	2. Orientation to one's anatomy is basic to understanding its function.	• Asks questions and shows interest in his disorder
3. Be specific in selecting information that is relevant to the patient's particular treatment plan.	3. This is based on the treatment plan; because it varies with each patient, individualization is desirable.	• Describes activities that help or hinder recovery
4. Identify ways to reduce pressure on the operative area after prostatectomy.	4. This is to prevent bleeding; such precautions are in order for 6–8 weeks postoperatively.	• Identifies ways of attaining/maintaining bladder control
a. Avoid prolonged sitting (in a chair, long automobile rides), standing, walking.		• Demonstrates satisfactory technique and understanding of catheter care
b. Avoid straining, such as during exercises, bowel movement, lifting, and sexual intercourse.		• Lists signs and symptoms that must be reported should they occur (e.g., abnormal bleeding, infection)
5. Familiarize patient with ways of attaining/maintaining bladder control.	5. These measures will help control frequency and dribbling and aid in preventing retention.	
a. Encourage urination every 2–3 hours; discourage voiding when supine.	a. By sitting or standing, patient is more likely to empty his bladder.	
b. Avoid drinking cola and caffeine beverages; urge a cutoff time in the evening for drinking fluids to minimize frequent voiding during the night.	b. Spacing the kind and amount of liquid intake will help to prevent frequency.	
c. Describe perineal exercises to be performed every hour.	c. Exercises will assist him in starting and stopping the urinary stream.	
d. Develop a schedule with patient that will fit into his routine.	d. A schedule will assist in developing a workable pattern of normal activities.	
6. Demonstrate catheter care; encourage his questions; stress the importance of position of urinary receptacle.	6. By requiring a return demonstration of care, collection, and emptying of the device, he will become more independent and also can prevent backflow of urine, which can lead to infection.	

NURSING DIAGNOSIS: Imbalanced nutrition: less than body requirements related to decreased oral intake because of anorexia, nausea, and vomiting caused by cancer or its treatment
GOAL: Maintain optimal nutritional status

Nursing Interventions	Rationale	Expected Outcomes
1. Assess the amount of food eaten.	1. This assessment will help determine nutrient intake.	• Responds positively to his favorite foods
2. Routinely weigh patient.	2. Weighing the patient on the same scale under similar conditions can help monitor changes in weight.	• Assumes responsibility for his oral hygiene
		• Reports absence of nausea and vomiting
		• Notes increase in weight after improved appetite
3. Elicit patient's explanation of why he is unable to eat more.	3. His explanation may present easily corrected practices.	
4. Cater to his individual food preferences (e.g., avoiding foods that are too spicy or too cold).	4. He will be more likely to consume larger servings if food is palatable and appealing.	
5. Recognize effect of medication or radiation therapy on appetite.	5. Many chemotherapeutic agents and radiation therapy promote anorexia.	
6. Inform patient that alterations in taste can occur.	6. Aging and the disease process can reduce taste sensitivity. In addition, smell and taste can be altered as a result of the body's absorption of by-products of cellular destruction (brought on by malignancy and its treatment).	

(continued on page 1768)

Chart 59-3

PLAN OF NURSING CARE (Continued)

The Patient With Prostate Cancer

Nursing Interventions	Rationale	Expected Outcomes
7. Educate patient about appropriate oral hygiene interventions	7. Food will be more palatable and appealing following good oral hygiene.	
8. Use measures to control nausea and vomiting. a. Administer prescribed antiemetic agents, around the clock if necessary. b. Provide oral hygiene after vomiting episodes. c. Provide rest periods after meals.	8. Prevention of nausea and vomiting can stimulate appetite.	
9. Provide frequent small meals and a comfortable and pleasant environment.	9. Smaller portions of food are less acute to the patient.	
10. Assess patient's ability to obtain and prepare foods.	10. Disability or lack of social support can hinder the patient's ability to obtain and prepare foods.	

NURSING DIAGNOSIS: Sexual dysfunction related to effects of therapy: chemotherapy, hormonal therapy, radiation therapy, surgery
GOAL: Ability to resume/enjoy modified sexual functioning

Nursing Interventions	Rationale	Expected Outcomes
1. Determine from nursing history what effect patient's medical condition is having on his sexual functioning.	1. Usually, decreased libido and, later, impotence may be experienced.	• Describes the reasons for changes in sexual functioning • Discusses with appropriate health care personnel alternative approaches and methods of sexual expression • Includes partner in discussions related to changes in sexual function
2. Inform patient of the effects of prostate surgery, orchiectomy (when applicable), chemotherapy, irradiation, and hormonal therapy on sexual function.	2. Treatment modalities may alter sexual function, but each is evaluated separately with regard to its effect on a particular patient.	
3. Include his partner in developing understanding and in discovering alternative, satisfying close relations with each other.	3. The bond between a couple may be strengthened with new appreciation and support that had not been evident before the current illness.	

NURSING DIAGNOSIS: Acute pain related to progression of disease and treatment modalities
GOAL: Relief of pain

Nursing Interventions	Rationale	Expected Outcomes
1. Evaluate nature of patient's pain, its location, and intensity using pain rating scale.	1. Determining nature and causes of pain and its intensity help to select proper pain relief modality and provide baseline for later comparison.	• Reports relief of pain • Expects exacerbations, reports their quality and intensity, and obtains relief • Uses pain relief strategies appropriately and effectively • Identifies strategies to avoid complications of analgesic use (e.g., constipation)
2. Avoid activities that aggravate or worsen pain.	2. Bumping the bed is an example of an action that can intensify the patient's pain.	
3. Because pain is usually related to bone metastasis, ensure that patient's bed has a bed board on a firm mattress. In addition, protect the patient from falls/injuries.	3. This will provide added support and is more comfortable. Protecting the patient from injury protects him from additional pain.	
4. Provide support for affected extremities.	4. More support, coupled with reduced movement of the part, helps in pain control.	
5. Prepare patient for radiation therapy if prescribed.	5. Radiation therapy may be effective in controlling pain.	
6. Administer analgesic or opioid agents at regularly scheduled intervals as prescribed.	6. Analgesic agents alter perception of pain and provide comfort. Regularly scheduled analgesics around the clock rather than PRN (as needed) provide more consistent pain relief.	
7. Initiate bowel program to prevent constipation.	7. Opioid analgesic agents and inactivity contribute to constipation.	

Chart 59-3	**PLAN OF NURSING CARE** (Continued)
	The Patient With Prostate Cancer

NURSING DIAGNOSIS: Impaired physical mobility related to tissue hypoxia, malnutrition, and exhaustion and to spinal cord or nerve compression from metastases

GOAL: Improved physical mobility

Nursing Interventions	Rationale	Expected Outcomes
1. Assess for factors causing limited mobility (e.g., pain, hypercalcemia, limited exercise tolerance).	1. This information offers clues to the cause; if possible, cause is treated.	• Achieves improved physical mobility • Relates that short-term goals are encouraging him because they are attainable
2. Provide pain relief by administering prescribed medications.	2. Analgesic/opioid agents allow the patient to increase his activity more comfortably.	
3. Encourage the use of assistive devices: cane, walker.	3. Support may offer the security needed to become mobile.	
4. Involve significant others in helping patient with range-of-motion exercises, positioning, and walking.	4. Assistance from partner or others encourages patient to repeat activities and achieve goals.	
5. Provide positive reinforcement for achievement of small gains.	5. Encouragement stimulates improvement of performance.	
6. Assess nutritional status.	6. See Nursing Diagnosis: Imbalanced nutrition: less than body requirements.	

COLLABORATIVE PROBLEMS: Hemorrhage, infection, bladder neck obstruction

GOAL: Absence of complications

Nursing Interventions	Rationale	Expected Outcomes
1. Alert the patient to changes that may occur (after discharge) and that need to be reported:	1. Certain changes signal beginning complications, which call for nursing and medical interventions.	• Experiences no bleeding or passage of blood clots • Reports no infection or pain around the catheter • Experiences normal frequency or urination • Reports normal urinary output • Maintains bladder control
a. Continued bloody urine; passing blood clots	a. Hematuria with or without blood clot formation may occur postoperatively.	
b. Pain; burning around the catheter	b. Indwelling urinary catheters may be a source of pain or infection.	
c. Frequency of urination	c. Urinary frequency may be caused by urinary tract infections or by bladder neck obstruction, resulting in incomplete voiding.	
d. Diminished urinary output	d. Bladder neck obstruction decreases the amount of urine that is voided.	
e. Increasing loss of bladder control	e. Urinary incontinence may be a result of urinary retention.	

hormone–releasing hormone agonists) (NCCN, 2016b). Intensity-modulated radiation therapy (IMRT) is one method of delivery of EBRT. IMRT sets a dose for the target volume and restricts the dose to surrounding tissue. Another approach to delivery of radiation uses a computer-controlled robotic arm to deliver a course of radiotherapy (i.e., stereotactic radiosurgery) to localized prostate cancer. This method, referred to as the CyberKnife®, is now considered a safe and reliable method of delivering radiation to treat prostate cancer (Detti, Bonomo, Masi, et al., 2016).

Brachytherapy involves the implantation of interstitial radioactive seeds under anesthesia. It has become a commonly used monotherapy treatment option for early, clinically organ-confined prostate cancer. The surgeon uses ultrasound guidance to place 80 to 100 seeds (depending on the prostate volume), and the patient returns home after the procedure. Exposure of others to radiation is minimal, but the patient should avoid close contact with pregnant women and infants

for up to 2 months. Radiation safety guidelines include straining urine for seeds and using a condom during sexual intercourse for 2 weeks after implantation to catch any seeds that pass through the urethra. This approach can be completed in 1 day, with little lost time from normal activities. Brachytherapy may be combined with EBRT with or without neoadjuvant ADT for patients considered at intermediate risk. High-risk patients are considered poor candidates for permanent brachytherapy (Itano et al., 2016).

Although cure rates with radiation are comparable to those of radical prostatectomy, radiation therapy possesses its own unique set of side effects, which differ depending on the method of radiation administration. Patients receiving EBRT or brachytherapy may experience inflammation of the rectum, bowel, and bladder (proctitis, enteritis, and cystitis) because of the proximity of these structures to the prostate and the radiation doses. Inflammation and mucosal loss at the bladder neck, prostate, and urethra can cause acute urinary dysfunction. Both irritative and obstructive urinary symptoms can cause pain with urination and ejaculation until the irritation subsides. Rectal urgency, diarrhea, and tenesmus may occur as a result of radiation of the anterior rectal wall. Late side effects include rectal proctitis, bleeding, and rectal fistula; painless hematuria; chronic interstitial cystitis; urethral stricture erectile dysfunction; and, rarely, secondary cancers of the rectum and bladder (Thakur, 2016).

Hormonal Strategies

The number of survivors of prostate cancer in the United States is estimated at 2 million; approximately one third of these men currently receive ADT (Simpson, 2015). ADT is commonly used to suppress androgenic stimuli to the prostate by decreasing the level of circulating plasma testosterone or interrupting the conversion to or binding of DHT. As a result, the prostatic epithelium atrophies (decreases in size). This effect is accomplished either by surgical castration (bilateral **orchiectomy**, removal of one or both of the testes), which has traditionally been the mainstay of hormonal treatment, or by medical castration with the administration of medications, such as luteinizing hormone–releasing hormone (LHRH) agonists. Bilateral orchiectomy decreases plasma testosterone levels significantly because approximately 93% of circulating testosterone is of testicular origin (7% is from the adrenal glands). Thus, the testicular stimulus required for continued prostatic growth is removed, resulting in prostatic atrophy.

However, orchiectomy often results in significant morbidity. Although the procedure does not cause the side effects associated with other hormonal therapies (described later), it is associated with considerable emotional impact. Because patients who have prostate cancer are living longer with the disease, health care providers are focusing on effective therapeutic modalities that promote an acceptable quality of life. Patients may be given the option for testicular prostheses to be placed during surgery.

LHRH agonists include leuprolide (Lupron) and goserelin (Zoladex). Additional hormonal manipulation with antiandrogens may be prescribed for patients who do not show adequate serum testosterone suppression (less than 50 ng/mL) with medical or surgical castration. Antiandrogen receptor antagonists include flutamide (Eulexin), bicalutamide (Casodex), and nilutamide (Nilandron). LHRH agonists suppress testicular androgen, whereas antiandrogen receptor antagonists cause adrenal androgen suppression. When LHRH agonists are initiated, a testosterone flare may occur, causing pain in bony metastatic disease. Antiandrogens given for the first 7 days may reduce this uncomfortable symptom. The most common uses of LHRH agonists are as follows: (1) in the adjuvant and neoadjuvant setting in combination with radiation therapy, (2) after radical prostatectomy, and (3) in the treatment of recurrence indicated by an elevation in the PSA but without clinical or x-ray evidence. Medical and surgical castration causes hot flushing because these treatment modalities increase hypothalamic activity, which stimulates the thermoregulatory centers of the body (Baker, 2014; Jones, 2016; Scher, 2016).

The management of hormone-refractory prostate cancer remains somewhat controversial. Another category of medication used as a second-line hormonal intervention is the adrenal ablating drugs. Ketoconazole (Nizoral) is used to inhibit cytochrome P450 enzymes, which are required for the synthesis of androgens and other steroids. High-dose ketoconazole lowers testosterone by decreasing both testicular and endocrine production of androgen. Administration of this medication requires steroid supplementation to prevent adrenal insufficiency.

Hypogonadism is responsible for the adverse effects of ADT, which include vasomotor flushing, loss of libido, decreased bone density (resulting in osteoporosis and fractures), anemia, fatigue, increased fat mass, lipid alterations, decreased muscle mass, gynecomastia (increased breast tissue), and mastodynia (breast/nipple tenderness). Hypogonadism is associated with an increased risk of diabetes, resulting from insulin resistance, metabolic syndrome, and cardiovascular disease (McDougal et al., 2016).

Chemotherapy

Recent studies have shown clear benefits in terms of survival with chemotherapy treatment that includes a docetaxel-based regimen for non–androgen-dependent prostate cancer (NCCN, 2016b). Other studies are under way to determine the importance of the vascular endothelial growth factor system. Tumor angiogenesis is essential for tumor growth, including growth of prostate carcinomas and other high-grade cancers. Therefore, antiangiogenic treatment in combination with conventional therapies may play a future role in treatment. Gene-based therapy in prostate cancer is an emerging and promising adjuvant to conventional treatment strategies.

Possible complications related to chemotherapy are specific to the type of chemotherapy given (see Chapter 15, Chart 15-3).

Other Therapies

Cryosurgery of the prostate is used to ablate prostate cancer in patients who cannot tolerate surgery and in those with recurrent prostate cancer. Transperineal probes are inserted into the prostate under ultrasound guidance to freeze the tissue directly.

Keeping the urethral passage patent may require repeated TURPs. If this is impractical, catheter drainage is instituted by way of the suprapubic or transurethral route. For men with advanced prostate cancer, palliative measures are indicated. Although cure is unlikely with advanced prostate cancer, many men survive for long periods, free of debilitating symptoms.

Bone lesions that result from metastasis of prostate cancer can be very painful and result in pathologic fractures. Opioid and nonopioid medications are used to control bone pain. EBRT can be delivered to skeletal lesions to relieve pain. Radiopharmaceuticals, such as strontium or samarium, can be injected IV to treat multiple sites of bone metastasis. Antiandrogen therapies are used in an effort to reduce the circulating androgens. If antiandrogen therapies are not effective, medications such as prednisone have been effective in reducing pain and improving quality of life (Lycken, Garmo, Adolfsson, et al., 2013; Rathkopf & Scher, 2013). Bisphosphonate therapy with pamidronate (Aredia) can be given to reduce the risk of pathologic fracture. In advanced prostate cancer, blood transfusions are given to maintain adequate hemoglobin levels when bone marrow is replaced by tumor.

More than one third of men with a diagnosis of prostate cancer elect to use some form of complementary and integrative health. Acupuncture has been used to treat both PE and erectile dysfunction with some limited, anecdotal success (Tsai, Liu, Chang, et al., 2014). Because research on many forms of complementary, alternative, and integrative health is lacking, patients often rely on anecdotal information to make decisions about its use. Nurses and other health care professionals play a vital role in assisting patients to locate and evaluate available information about these practices to ensure that harmful forms are avoided (Braun, Gupta, Birdsall, et al., 2013). The National Center for Complementary and Integrative Health (NCCIH) website can assist nurses in providing patients with evidence-based information (see the Resources section at the end of the chapter).

The Patient Undergoing Prostate Surgery

Prostate surgery may be indicated for the patient with BPH or prostate cancer. The objectives before prostate surgery are to assess the patient's general health status and to establish optimal kidney function. Prostate surgery should be performed before acute urinary retention develops and damages the upper urinary tract and collecting system or, in the case of prostate cancer, before cancer progresses.

Surgical Procedures

Several approaches can be used to remove the hypertrophied portion of the prostate gland: TURP, suprapubic prostatectomy, perineal prostatectomy, retropubic prostatectomy, TUIP, and laparoscopic radical prostatectomy and robotic-assisted laparoscopic radical prostatectomy (see Table 59-4). With these approaches, all cancerous or hyperplastic tissue is removed, leaving behind only the capsule of the prostate.

Transurethral Resection of the Prostate

TURP, which is the most common procedure used, can be carried out through endoscopy. The prostate gland is removed in small chips with an electrical cutting loop (see Fig. 59-4A). This procedure eliminates the risk of transurethral resection syndrome (hyponatremia, hypovolemia). Transurethral resection syndrome is a potential but rare complication of TURP that occurs in approximately 2% of men who undergo the procedure (Lycken, et al., 2013; Rathkopf & Scher, 2013) (see Chart 59-4).

TURP usually requires an overnight hospital stay. Urethral strictures are more frequent than with nontransurethral procedures, and repeated procedures may be necessary because the residual prostatic tissue grows back. TURP rarely causes erectile dysfunction but may trigger retrograde ejaculation, because removal of prostatic tissue at the bladder neck can cause the seminal fluid to flow backward into the bladder rather than forward through the urethra during ejaculation.

Suprapubic Prostatectomy

A suprapubic prostatectomy is an open surgical procedure (see Fig. 59-4B). Disadvantages include blood loss, the need for an abdominal incision, and the risks associated with any major abdominal surgical procedure (see Fig. 59-4B).

Perineal Prostatectomy

A perineal prostatectomy (see Fig. 59-4C) is practical when other approaches are not possible and is useful for an open biopsy. However, incontinence, sexual dysfunction, and rectal injury are more likely to occur with this approach.

Retropubic Prostatectomy

Retropubic prostatectomy is used more commonly than the suprapubic approach (see Fig. 59-4D). This procedure is suitable for large glands located high in the pelvis. Although blood loss can be better controlled and the surgical site is easier to visualize, infections can readily start in the retropubic space.

Transurethral Incision of the Prostate

TUIP is indicated when the prostate gland is small (30 g or less), and it is an effective treatment for many cases of BPH (see Fig. 59-4E). TUIP can be performed on an outpatient basis and has a lower complication rate than other more invasive prostate procedures.

Laparoscopic Radical Prostatectomy

A laparoscopic radical prostatectomy has fewer risks compared with open radical prostatectomy (Simpson, 2015).

Robotic-Assisted Laparoscopic Radical Prostatectomy

Robotic-assisted laparoscopic radical prostatectomy is a minimally invasive approach that uses a computer console and a robot to move instruments, replicating the movements of the surgeon's hands (Simpson, 2015; Sohn, Lee, & Ahlering, 2013).

Pelvic Lymph Node Dissection

Pelvic lymph node dissection (PLND) is not always performed. It may be used in some patients to provide information for staging the tumor and to remove an area of microscopic metastasis. The planned treatment may influence the surgeon's decision to perform PLND and the extent (limited vs. extended) of the dissection. Dissection of nodes anterior and lateral to the external iliac vessels is associated with an increased risk of lymphedema (NCCN, 2016a).

Complications

Postoperative complications depend on the type of prostatectomy performed and may include hemorrhage, clot formation, catheter obstruction, and sexual dysfunction. All prostatectomies carry a risk of impotence because of potential damage to the pudendal nerves. In most instances, sexual activity may be resumed in 6 to 8 weeks, which is the time required for the prostatic fossa to heal. The anatomic changes in the posterior urethra can lead to retrograde ejaculation. During ejaculation, the seminal fluid goes into the bladder and is excreted with the urine. A vasectomy may be performed during surgery to prevent infection from spreading from the prostatic urethra through the vas and into the epididymis.

After total prostatectomy (usually for cancer), the risk of impotence is high. If this is unacceptable to the patient, options are available to produce erections sufficient for sexual intercourse: prosthetic penile implants, negative-pressure (vacuum) devices, and pharmacologic interventions (see earlier discussion and Table 59-2).

TABLE 59-4 Surgical Approaches for Treatment of Prostate Disorders

The surgical approach of choice depends on (1) the size of the gland, (2) the severity of the obstruction, (3) the age of the patient, (4) the condition of the patient, and (5) the presence of associated diseases.

Surgical Approach	Advantages	Disadvantages	Nursing Implications
Transurethral Resection (TURP) Removal of prostatic tissue by optical instrument introduced through urethra; used for glands of varying size. Ideal for patients who are poor surgical risks.	Avoids abdominal incision Safer for surgical-risk patient Shorter length of hospital stay and recovery periods Lower morbidity rate Causes less pain Can be used as a palliative approach with history of radiation therapy	Requires highly skilled surgeon. Recurrent obstruction, urethral trauma, and stricture may develop. Delayed bleeding may occur.	Monitor for hemorrhage. Observe for symptoms of urethral stricture (dysuria, straining, weak urinary stream).
Open Surgical Removal			
Suprapubic approach Removal of prostatic tissue through abdominal incision; can be used for gland of any size	Technically simple Offers wide area of exploration Permits exploration for cancerous lymph nodes Allows more complete removal of obstructing gland Permits treatment of associated bladder lesions	Requires surgical approach through the bladder Control of hemorrhage is difficult Urine may leak around the suprapubic tube Recovery may be prolonged and uncomfortable	Monitor for indications of hemorrhage and shock. Provide meticulous aseptic care to the area around suprapubic tube.
Perineal approach Removal of gland through an incision in the perineum; preferred approach for patients who are obese	Offers direct anatomic approach Permits gravity drainage Particularly effective for radical cancer therapy Allows hemostasis under direct vision Low mortality rate Low incidence of shock Ideal for patients with large prostate who are very old, frail, and poor surgical risks	Higher postoperative incidence of impotence and urinary incontinence Possible damage to rectum and external sphincter Restricted operative field Greater potential for contamination and infection of incision	Avoid using rectal tubes or thermometers and enemas after perineal surgery. Use drainage pads to absorb excess urinary drainage. Provide foam rubber ring for patient comfort in sitting. Anticipate urinary leakage around the wound for several days after the catheter is removed.
Retropubic approach Low abdominal incision; bladder is not entered.	Avoids incision into the bladder Permits surgeon to see and control bleeding Shorter recovery period Less bladder sphincter damage Suitable for removal of large glands	Cannot treat associated bladder disease Increased incidence of hemorrhage from prostatic venous plexus; osteitis pubis	Monitor for hemorrhage. Anticipate posturinary leakage for several days after removing the catheter.
Transurethral Incision (TUIP) Urethral approach; 1–2 cuts are made in the prostate and prostate capsule to reduce pressure on the urethra and to reduce urethral constriction.	Results comparable to TURP Low incidence of erectile dysfunction and retrograde ejaculation No bladder neck contracture	Recurrent obstruction and urethral trauma Delayed bleeding	Monitor for hemorrhage.
Laparoscopic Radical Prostatectomy In this approach, 4–6 small (1 cm [0.5 inch]) incisions are made in the abdomen; laparoscopic instruments inserted through the incisions are used to dissect the prostate.	Minimally invasive technique Improved patient satisfaction and quality of life Shorter length of hospital stay Short convalescence More rapid return to normal activity Short indwelling catheter duration Decreased blood loss to 400 mL Reduced infection risk Less scarring Better visualization of surgical field than other approaches	Lack of tactile sensation available with open prostatectomy Inability to palpably assess for induration and palpable nodules Inability to delineate the proximity of involvement of the neurovascular bundles due to lack of palpation Long surgical time (4–5 hours)	Observe for symptoms of urethral stricture (dysuria), straining, weak urinary stream. Monitor for hemorrhage and shock. Provide meticulous aseptic care to area around suprapubic tube. Monitor for changes in bowel function. Avoid using rectal tubes or thermometers and enemas after perineal surgery. Use drainage pads to absorb excess urinary drainage. Provide foam rubber ring for patient comfort in sitting. Anticipate urinary leakage around the wound for several days after the catheter is removed.

Surgical Approach	Advantages	Disadvantages	Nursing Implications
Robotic-Assisted Laparoscopic Radical Prostatectomy Involves using computer console and da Vinci. In this approach, 6 small (1 cm [0.5 inch]) incisions are made in the abdomen; laparoscopic instruments inserted through the incisions are used to dissect the prostate.	Minimally invasive technique Improved patient satisfaction and quality of life Shorter length of hospital stay Short convalescence More rapid return to normal activity Short indwelling catheter duration Decreased blood loss to 150 mL Improved magnification of operative field, using a 3-dimensional view (includes, magnification, high resolution, and depth perception) Less postoperative pain Reduced risk of infection Less scarring Laparoscopic instruments have 6 degrees of movement with joints, allowing extensive range of motion and precision. Nerve sparing with less incontinence and sexual dysfunction	Lack of tactile sensation available with open prostatectomy Inability to palpably assess for induration and palpable nodules Inability to delineate the proximity of involvement of the neurovascular bundles due to lack of palpation	Observe for symptoms of urethral stricture (dysuria), straining, weak urinary stream. Monitor for hemorrhage and shock. Provide meticulous aseptic care to the area around suprapubic tube. Monitor for changes in bowel function. Avoid using rectal tubes or thermometers and enemas after perineal surgery. Use drainage pads to absorb excess urinary drainage. Provide foam rubber ring for patient comfort in sitting. Anticipate urinary leakage around the wound for several days after the catheter is removed.

Adapted from Keane, T. E., & Graham, S. D. (Eds.) (2016). *Glenn's urologic surgery.* Philadelphia, PA: Wolters Kluwer; McDougal, W. J., Wein, A. J., Kavoussi, L. R., et al. (Eds.). (2016). *Campbell-Walsh urology* (11th ed.). Philadelphia, PA: Elsevier.

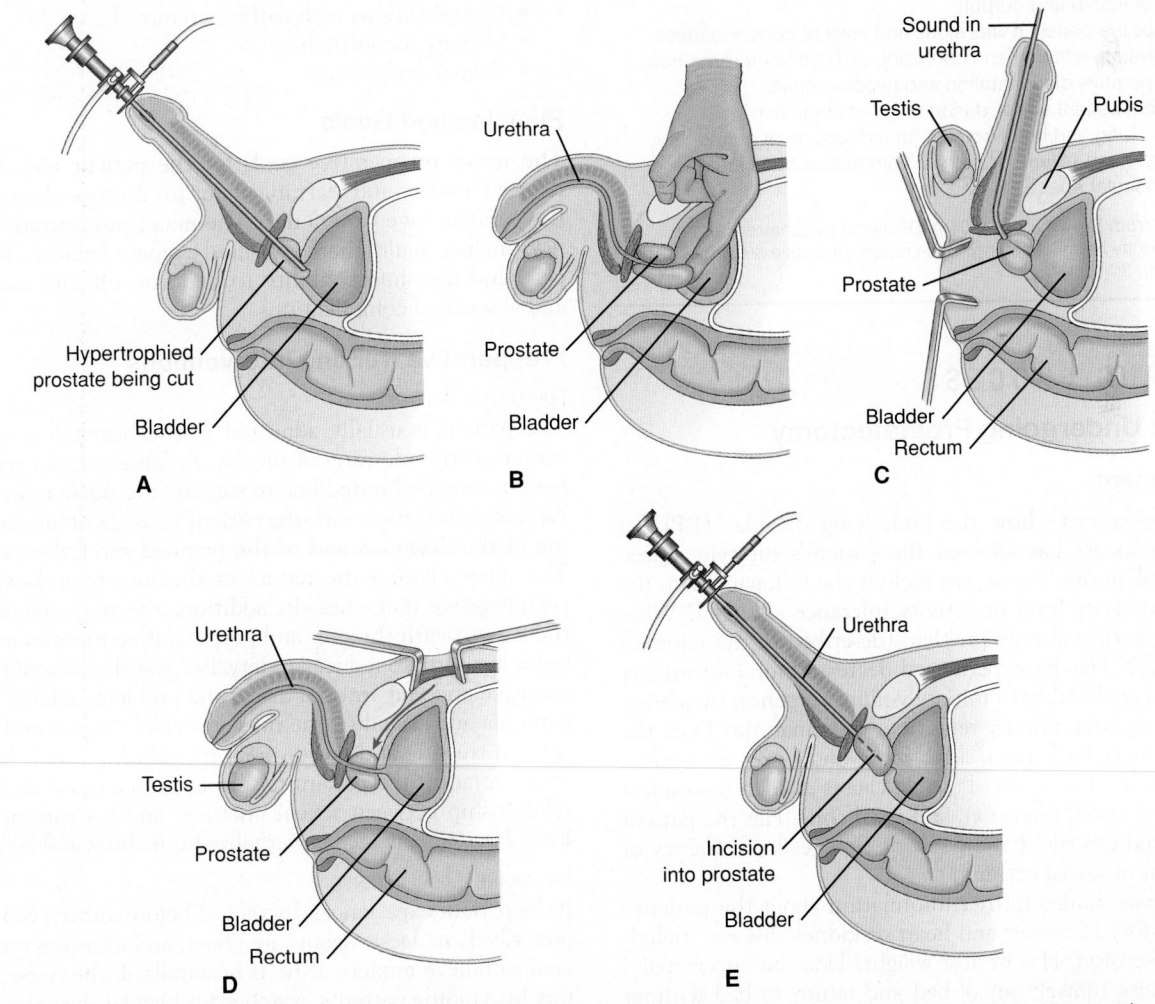

Figure 59-4 • Prostate surgery procedures. **A.** Transurethral resection of the prostate. A loop of wire connected with a cutting current is rotated in the cystoscope to remove shavings of prostate at the bladder orifice. **B.** Suprapubic prostatectomy. With an abdominal approach, the prostate is shelled out of its bed. **C.** Perineal prostatectomy. Two retractors on the left spread the perineal incision to provide a view of the prostate. **D.** Retropubic prostatectomy is performed through a low abdominal incision. Note two abdominal retractors and *arrow* pointing to the prostate gland. **E.** Transurethral incision of the prostate involves one or two incisions into the prostate to reduce pressure on the urethra.

Chart 59-4	Transurethral Resection Syndrome

Transurethral resection syndrome is a rare but potentially serious complication of transurethral prostatectomy (TURP). Signs and symptoms are caused by neurologic, cardiovascular, and electrolyte imbalances associated with absorption of the solution used to irrigate the surgical site during the surgical procedure. Hyponatremia, hypovolemia, and occasionally hyperammonemia may occur.

Signs and Symptoms

- Collapse
- Headache
- Hypotension
- Lethargy and confusion
- Muscle spasms
- Nausea and vomiting
- Seizures
- Tachycardia

Interventions

- Discontinue irrigation.
- Administer diuretic agents as prescribed.
- Replace bladder irrigation with normal saline.
- Monitor intake and output.
- Monitor the patient's vital signs and level of consciousness.
- Differentiate lethargy and confusion of TURP syndrome from postoperative disorientation and hyponatremia.
- Maintain patient safety during times of confusion.
- Assess lung and heart sounds for indications of pulmonary edema, heart failure, or both as fluid moves back into the intravascular space.

Adapted from Brown, C. S. (2014). Dilutional hyponatremia in a community hospital setting: Case report. *Intensive & Critical Care Nursing, 30*(1), 1–5.

NURSING PROCESS

Patient Undergoing Prostatectomy

Assessment

The nurse assesses how the underlying disorder (BPH or prostate cancer) has affected the patient's lifestyle. Questions to ask during assessment include the following: Has the patient's activity level or activity tolerance changed? What is his presenting urinary problem (described in the patient's own words)? Has he experienced decreased force of urinary flow, decreased ability to initiate voiding, urgency, frequency, nocturia, dysuria, urinary retention, or hematuria? Does the patient report back pain, flank pain, and lower abdominal or suprapubic discomfort? Possible causes of such discomfort include infection, retention, and renal colic. Has the patient experienced erectile dysfunction or changes in frequency or enjoyment of sexual activity?

The nurse obtains further information about the patient's family history of cancer and heart or kidney disease, including hypertension. Has he lost weight? Does he appear pale? Can he raise himself out of bed and return to bed without assistance? Can he perform usual activities of daily living? A comprehensive functional assessment helps determine how soon the patient will be able to return to normal activities after prostatectomy.

Diagnosis

PREOPERATIVE NURSING DIAGNOSES

Based on the assessment data, major preoperative nursing diagnoses may include the following:

- Anxiety about surgery and its outcome
- Acute pain related to bladder distention
- Deficient knowledge about factors related to the disorder and the treatment protocol

POSTOPERATIVE NURSING DIAGNOSES

Based on the assessment data, major postoperative nursing diagnoses may include the following:

- Risk for imbalanced fluid volume
- Acute pain related to the surgical incision, catheter placement, and bladder spasms
- Deficient knowledge about postoperative care

COLLABORATIVE PROBLEMS/POTENTIAL COMPLICATIONS

Potential complications may include the following:

- Hemorrhage and shock
- Infection
- Venous thromboembolism (VTE)
- Catheter obstruction
- Complications with catheter removal
- Urinary incontinence
- Sexual dysfunction

Planning and Goals

The major preoperative goals for the patient may include reduced anxiety and learning about his prostate disorder and the perioperative experience. The major postoperative goals may include maintenance of fluid volume balance, relief of pain and discomfort, ability to perform self-care activities, and absence of complications.

Preoperative Nursing Interventions

REDUCING ANXIETY

The patient is usually admitted to the hospital or surgical center on the morning of surgery. Because contact with the patient may be limited before surgery, the nurse must establish communication with the patient to assess his understanding of the diagnosis and of the planned surgical procedure. The nurse clarifies the nature of the surgery and expected postoperative outcomes. In addition, the nurse familiarizes the patient with the pre- and postoperative routines and initiates measures to reduce anxiety. Because the patient may be sensitive and embarrassed discussing problems related to the genitalia and sexuality, the nurse provides privacy and establishes a trusting and professional relationship. Guilt feelings often surface if the patient falsely assumes a cause-and-effect relationship between sexual practices and his current problems. He is encouraged to verbalize his feelings and concerns.

RELIEVING DISCOMFORT

If the patient experiences discomfort before surgery, bed rest is prescribed, analgesic agents are given, and measures are initiated to relieve anxiety. If he is hospitalized, the nurse monitors his voiding patterns, watches for bladder distention, and assists with catheterization if indicated. An indwelling catheter is inserted if the patient has continuing urinary retention or if close monitoring is needed because of laboratory test results that indicate azotemia (accumulation of nitrogenous waste products in the blood). The catheter can help decompress the bladder gradually over several days, especially if the patient is an older adult and hypertensive and has diminished kidney function or urinary retention that has existed for many weeks. For a few days after the bladder begins draining, the blood pressure may fluctuate and kidney function may decline. If the patient cannot tolerate a urinary catheter, he is prepared for a cystostomy (and insertion of a suprapubic catheter).

PROVIDING EDUCATION

Before surgery, the nurse reviews with the patient the anatomy of the affected structures and their function in relation to the urinary and reproductive systems, using diagrams and other educational aids as indicated. Web-based prostate cancer education both before and after surgery, along with phone and internet communication, promotes self-care management and support for patients and their partners and families (Song, Rini, Deal, et al., 2015). This education can occur during the preadmission testing visit, with the nurse in prescribed settings, or in the urologist's office. The nurse explains what will take place while the patient is prepared for diagnostic tests and then for surgery (depending on the type of prostatectomy planned). The nurse also reinforces information given by the surgeon about the type of incision, which varies with the surgical approach (see Table 59-4), and describes the likely type of urinary drainage system (urethral or suprapubic) and the recovery room procedure. The amount of information given is based on the patient's needs and questions. The nurse explains procedures expected to occur during the immediate perioperative period; answers questions the patient, family, or significant other may have; and provides emotional support. In addition, the nurse provides the patient with information about postoperative care and pain management.

PREPARING THE PATIENT

If the patient is scheduled for a prostatectomy, the preoperative preparation described in Chapter 17 is provided. Antiembolism stockings are applied before surgery and are particularly important to prevent VTE if the patient is placed in a lithotomy position during surgery. An enema is usually given at home on the evening before surgery or on the morning of surgery to prevent postoperative straining, which can induce bleeding.

Postoperative Nursing Interventions

MAINTAINING FLUID BALANCE

During the postoperative period, the patient is at risk for imbalanced fluid volume because of the irrigation of the surgical site during and after surgery. With irrigation of the urinary catheter to prevent its obstruction by blood clots, fluid may be absorbed through the open surgical site and retained, increasing the risk of excessive fluid retention, fluid imbalance, and water intoxication. The urine output and the amount of fluid used for irrigation must be closely monitored to determine whether irrigation fluid is being retained and to ensure an adequate urine output. An intake and output record, including the amount of fluid used for irrigation, must be maintained. The patient is also monitored for electrolyte imbalances (e.g., hyponatremia), increasing blood pressure, confusion, and respiratory distress. These signs and symptoms are documented and reported to the surgeon. The risk of fluid and electrolyte imbalance is greater in older patients with pre-existing cardiovascular or respiratory disease.

RELIEVING PAIN

After a prostatectomy, the patient is assisted to sit and dangle his legs over the side of the bed on the day of surgery. The next morning, he is assisted to ambulate. If pain is present, the cause and location are determined, and the severity of pain and discomfort is assessed (Carter, Miller, Murphy, et al., 2014). The pain may be related to the incision or may be the result of excoriation of the skin at the catheter site. It may be in the flank area, indicating a kidney problem, or it may be caused by bladder spasms. Bladder irritability can initiate bleeding and result in clot formation, leading to urinary retention.

Patients experiencing bladder spasms may report urgency to void, a feeling of pressure or fullness in the bladder, and bleeding from the urethra around the catheter. Medications that relax the smooth muscles can help ease the spasms, which can be intermittent and severe; these medications include flavoxate (Urispas) and oxybutynin (Ditropan). Warm compresses to the pubis or sitz baths may also relieve the spasms.

The nurse monitors the drainage tubing and irrigates the system as prescribed to relieve any obstruction that may cause discomfort. Usually, the catheter is irrigated with 50 mL of irrigating fluid at a time. It is important to make sure that the same amount is recovered in the drainage receptacle. Securing the catheter drainage tubing to the leg or abdomen can help decrease tension on the catheter and prevent bladder irritation. Discomfort may be caused by dressings that are too snug, saturated with drainage, or improperly placed. Analgesic agents are given as prescribed. The nurse notifies the primary provider if the analgesic medications do not relieve the patient's pain and obtains a prescription for new doses or different medications.

After the patient is ambulatory, he is encouraged to walk but not to sit for prolonged periods, because this increases intra-abdominal pressure and the possibility of discomfort and bleeding. Prune juice and stool softeners are provided to ease bowel movements and to prevent excessive straining. An enema, if prescribed, is given with caution to avoid rectal perforation.

MONITORING AND MANAGING POTENTIAL COMPLICATIONS

After prostatectomy, the patient is monitored for major complications such as hemorrhage, infection, VTE, catheter problems, and sexual dysfunction.

Hemorrhage. Although patients are advised to discontinue all aspirin, nonsteroidal anti-inflammatory drugs, and platelet inhibitors 10 to 14 days before the surgery to prevent excessive bleeding, bleeding and hemorrhagic shock remain risks. The risk is increased with BPH because a hyperplastic prostate gland is very vascular. Bleeding may occur from the prostatic bed. Bleeding may also result in the formation of clots, which then obstruct urine flow. The drainage normally begins as reddish-pink and then clears to a light pink within 24 hours after surgery. Bright red bleeding with increased viscosity and numerous clots usually indicates arterial bleeding. Venous blood appears darker and less viscous. Arterial hemorrhage usually requires surgical intervention (e.g., suturing or transurethral coagulation of bleeding vessels), whereas venous bleeding may be controlled by applying prescribed traction to the catheter so that the balloon holding the catheter in place applies pressure to the prostatic fossa. The surgeon applies traction by securely taping the catheter to the patient's thigh if hemorrhage occurs. Less blood loss (150 mL) is expected with robotic-assisted laparoscopic radical prostatectomy, compared to the 500 to 900 mL loss that may occur with open prostatectomy.

Nursing management includes assistance in implementing strategies to stop the bleeding and to prevent or reverse hemorrhagic shock. If blood loss is extensive, fluids and blood component therapy may be given. If hemorrhagic shock occurs, treatments described in Chapter 14 are initiated.

Nursing interventions include closely monitoring vital signs; administering medications, IV fluids, and blood component therapy as prescribed; maintaining an accurate record of intake and output; and carefully monitoring drainage to ensure adequate urine flow and patency of the drainage system. The patient who experiences hemorrhage and his family are often anxious and benefit from explanations and reassurance about the event and the procedures that are performed.

Infection. After perineal prostatectomy, the surgeon usually changes the dressing on the first postoperative day. Further dressing changes may become the responsibility of the nurse in the inpatient setting or the home care nurse upon discharge. Careful aseptic technique is used because the potential for infection is great. Dressings can be held in place by a double-tailed, T-binder bandage or a padded athletic supporter. The tails cross over the incision to give double thickness and then each tail is drawn up on either side of the scrotum to the waistline and fastened.

Rectal thermometers, rectal tubes, and enemas are avoided because of the risk of injury and bleeding in the prostatic fossa. After the perineal sutures are removed, the perineum is cleansed as indicated. A heat lamp may be directed to the perineal area to promote healing. The scrotum is protected with a towel while the heat lamp is in use. Sitz baths are also used to promote healing.

UTIs and epididymitis are possible complications after prostatectomy. The patient is assessed for their occurrence; if they occur, the nurse administers antibiotic agents as prescribed. Because the risk of infection continues after discharge from the hospital, the patient and family need to be educated to monitor for signs and symptoms of infection (fever, chills, sweating, myalgia, dysuria, urinary frequency, and urgency). The patient and family are instructed to contact the urologist if these symptoms occur.

Venous Thromboembolism. Patients undergoing prostatectomy are at risk for VTE, including deep vein thrombosis and pulmonary embolism; therefore, the nurse assesses the patient frequently after surgery for manifestations of VTE. Early postoperative ambulation is essential to reduce the risk of VTE. Medical and nursing management of VTE are described in Chapters 23 and 30, respectively. In addition, if the patient is at high risk for clot formation, additional antithrombotic interventions may be prescribed (Goodman, 2013).

Potential Catheter Problems. After TURP, the catheter must drain well; an obstructed catheter produces distention of the prostatic capsule and resultant hemorrhage. Furosemide (Lasix) may be prescribed to promote urination and initiate postoperative diuresis, thereby helping to keep the catheter patent.

The nurse observes the lower abdomen to ensure that the catheter has not become blocked. A distinct, rounded swelling above the pubis is a manifestation of an overdistended bladder. If the nurse ascertains that the client's bladder is distended, a portable bladder scanner may be used to determine if urine retention is a problem (see Chapter 53).

The drainage bag is monitored for bloody urine, and the dressings and surgical incision are examined for bleeding. The

Figure 59-5 • A three-way system for bladder irrigation.

color of the urine is carefully noted and documented; a change in color from pink to amber indicates reduced bleeding. Blood pressure, pulse, and respirations are monitored and compared with baseline preoperative vital signs to detect hypotension. The nurse also observes the patient for restlessness, diaphoresis, pallor, any drop in blood pressure, and an increasing pulse rate.

Drainage of the bladder may be accomplished by gravity through a closed sterile drainage system. A three-way drainage system is useful in irrigating the bladder and preventing clot formation (see Fig. 59-5). Continuous irrigation may be used with TURP. Some urologists leave an indwelling catheter attached to a dependent drainage system. Gentle irrigation of the catheter may be prescribed to remove any obstructing clots.

If the patient complains of pain, the tubing is examined. The drainage system is irrigated with irrigating fluid (usually 50 mL), if indicated and prescribed, to clear any obstruction.

▶ **Quality and Safety Nursing Alert**

The amount of fluid recovered in the drainage bag must equal the amount of fluid instilled. Overdistention of the bladder should be avoided because it can induce secondary hemorrhage by stretching the coagulated blood vessels in the prostatic capsule.

To prevent traction on the bladder, the drainage tube (not the catheter) is secured to the inner thigh. If a cystostomy catheter is in place, it is secured to the abdomen. The nurse explains the purpose of the catheter to the patient and assures him that the urge to void results from the presence of the catheter and from bladder spasms. Reassurance is given to the patient that medication (anticholinergics) will be given to control his bladder spasms. He is cautioned not to pull on the catheter, because this causes bleeding and subsequent catheter blockage, which leads to urinary retention.

After the catheter is removed (usually when the urine appears clear), urine may leak around the wound for several days in the patient who has undergone perineal, suprapubic, or retropubic surgery. The cystostomy tube may be removed before or after the urethral catheter is removed. Some urinary incontinence may occur after catheter removal, and the patient is informed that this is likely to subside over time.

Urinary Incontinence. Postoperative urinary incontinence is a complication that can be reduced through the use of a surgical technique called puboprostatic ligament-sparing, or through the use of a male sling (Sandhu, 2015). Even without these techniques, current surgical procedures have decreased the incidence of urinary incontinence following surgery. Factors associated with postoperative continence are younger age, preservation of both neurovascular bundles, absence of an anastomotic stricture, eversion of the bladder neck, and a smaller prostate volume. The nurse can encourage the patient who experiences incontinence to take steps to prevent incontinence, improve continence, anticipate leakage, and cope with lack of complete control (Dorey, 2013). Preventing incontinence involves increasing voiding frequency, avoiding positions that encourage the urge to void, and decreasing fluid intake prior to activities. Promoting continence involves pelvic floor exercises (see the Educating Patients About Self-Care section that follows), biofeedback, and electrical stimulation. Anticipating leakage may entail lifestyle modifications such as using absorbent pads and carrying extra clothes to prevent urinary accidents; this can improve confidence when bathroom access is limited. It also helps to know the location of public bathrooms. Coping long term with complete lack of control may involve collagen injections, artificial sphincter implants, medications, and leg bags (Dorey, 2013; McDougal et al., 2016).

Sexual Dysfunction. Depending on the type of surgery, the patient may experience sexual dysfunction related to erectile dysfunction, decreased libido, and fatigue. These issues may become a concern to the patient soon after surgery or in the weeks to months of rehabilitation. With nerve-sparing radical prostatectomy, the likelihood of recovering the ability to have erections is better for men who are younger and men in whom both neurovascular bundles are spared. A decrease in libido is usually related to the impact of the surgery on the body. Reassurance that the usual level of libido will return after recuperation from surgery is often helpful to the patient and his partner. The patient should be aware that he may experience fatigue during rehabilitation from surgery. This fatigue may also decrease his libido and alter his enjoyment of usual activities.

Several options to restore erectile function are discussed with the patient by the surgeon or urologist. These options may include medications, surgically placed implants, or negative-pressure devices. PDE-5 inhibitors (see Table 59-3) may be effective for treatment of erectile dysfunction in men after radical prostatectomy, especially if the neurovascular bundles have been preserved. They may also improve erectile function in men with partial or moderate erectile dysfunction after radiation therapy for localized prostate cancer.

Nursing interventions include assessing for sexual dysfunction after surgery. Providing a private and confidential environment to discuss issues of sexuality is important. The emotional challenges of prostate surgery and its consequences need to be carefully explored with the patient and his partner. Providing the opportunity to discuss these issues can be very beneficial to the patient. For patients who have significant difficulty adjusting to sexual dysfunction, a referral to a sex therapist may be indicated.

PROMOTING HOME, COMMUNITY-BASED, AND TRANSITIONAL CARE

Educating Patients About Self-Care. The length of the hospital stay for the patient undergoing prostatectomy depends on the surgical approach used and ranges from 1 to 2 days for robotic-assisted laparoscopic prostatectomy to 3 to 5 days for open prostatectomy. The patient and family require education about how to manage the drainage system, how to assess for complications, and how to promote recovery. The nurse provides verbal and written education about the need to maintain the drainage system and to monitor urinary output; about wound care; and about strategies to prevent complications, such as infection, bleeding, and thrombosis. In addition, the patient and family need to know about signs and symptoms that should be reported to the primary provider (e.g., blood in urine, decreased urine output, fever, change in wound drainage, calf tenderness).

As the patient recovers and drainage tubes are removed, he may become discouraged and depressed because he cannot regain bladder control immediately. Furthermore, urinary frequency and burning may occur after the catheter is removed. Educating the patient about the following exercises may help him regain urinary control:

- Tense the perineal muscles by pressing the buttocks together, hold this position, and then relax. This exercise can be performed 10 to 20 times each hour while sitting or standing (Itano et al., 2016).
- Try to interrupt the urinary stream after starting to void; wait a few seconds and then continue to void.

Perineal exercises should continue until the patient gains full urinary control. The patient is educated to urinate as soon as he feels the first urge to do so. It is important to let the patient know that regaining urinary control is a gradual process; he may continue to "dribble" after being discharged from the hospital, but this should gradually diminish (usually within 1 year). The urine may be cloudy for several weeks after surgery but should clear as the prostate area heals.

While the prostatic fossa heals (6 to 8 weeks), the patient should avoid activities that produce Valsalva effects (straining, heavy lifting) because they may increase venous pressure and produce hematuria. He should avoid long motor trips and strenuous exercise, which increase the tendency to bleed. He should also know that spicy foods, alcohol, and coffee may cause bladder discomfort. The patient should be cautioned to drink enough fluids to avoid dehydration, which increases the tendency for a blood clot to form and obstruct the flow of urine. Signs of complications, such as bleeding, passage of blood clots, a decrease in the urinary stream, urinary retention, or symptoms of UTIs, should be reported to the primary provider (see Chart 59-5). Patients who have undergone robotic-assisted prostatectomy are often able to return to their usual activities in approximately 7 to 10 days (Sohn et al., 2013).

Continuing and Transitional Care. Referral for home, community-based or transitional care may be indicated if the patient is an older adult or has other health problems, if the patient and family cannot provide care in the home, or if the patient lives alone without available supports. The nurse making a home visit assesses the patient's physical status (cardiovascular and respiratory status, fluid and nutritional status,

Chart 59-5 — HOME CARE CHECKLIST

Postprostatectomy Care

At the completion of home care education, the patient and/or caregiver will be able to:

- Name the procedure that was performed and identify any permanent changes in anatomic structure or function as well as changes in ADLs, IADLs, roles, relationships, and spirituality.
- Locate list of names and telephone numbers of resource personnel involved in care (e.g., health care professionals, home care nurse, urinary catheter/dressing supply vendor).
- Identify the equipment necessary and how to obtain medical supplies to carry out dressing changes, wound care, and other prescribed regimens.
- Describe ongoing postoperative therapeutic regimen, including diet and activities to perform (e.g., increased activity and ambulation, perineal exercises) and to limit or avoid (e.g., lifting weights, driving a car, contact sports).
  - Describe measures to relieve postoperative pain and discomfort (e.g., take analgesics as prescribed; use nonpharmacologic interventions).
  - Demonstrate appropriate care of urinary catheter and collection receptacle.
  - Demonstrate appropriate dressing change/wound care.
  - When appropriate, demonstrate performance of perineal muscle exercises to facilitate bladder control.

- State the name, dose, side effects, frequency, and schedule for all medications.
- Identify signs and symptoms of complications that should be reported to surgeon (e.g., decreased output, blood or clots in urine or urine drainage system, change in wound drainage, fever or symptoms of urinary tract infections, calf tenderness).
- Explain treatment plan and importance of follow-up care to all health care providers.
- State time and date of follow-up appointments, therapy, and testing.
- Identify community resources for peer and caregiver/family support:
  - Identify sources of support (e.g. friends, relatives, faith community).
  - Identify phone numbers of support groups for people with cancer and their caregivers/families.
  - State meeting locations and times for support groups.
- Identify the need for health promotion, disease prevention, and screening activities.

ADL, activities of daily living; IADL, independent activities of daily living.

---

patency of the urinary drainage system, wound and nutritional status) and provides catheter and wound care, if indicated. The nurse reinforces previous education, assesses the ability of the patient and family to manage required care, and encourages the patient to ambulate and to carry out perineal exercises as prescribed. The patient may need to be reminded that return of bladder control may take time.

The patient is reminded about the importance of routine health screening and other health promotion activities. If the prostatectomy was performed to treat prostate cancer, the patient and family are also instructed about the importance of follow-up and monitoring with the primary provider.

Evaluation

Expected preoperative patient outcomes may include:
1. Demonstrates reduced anxiety
2. States that pain and discomfort are decreased
3. Relates understanding of the surgical procedure and postoperative course and practices perineal muscle exercises and other techniques useful in facilitating bladder control

Expected postoperative patient outcomes may include the following:
1. Reports relief of discomfort
2. Exhibits fluid and electrolyte balance
   a. Irrigation fluid and urinary output are within parameters determined by surgeon
   b. Experiences no signs or symptoms of fluid retention
3. Participates in self-care measures
   a. Increases activity and ambulation daily
   b. Produces urine output within normal ranges and consistent with intake
   c. Performs perineal exercises and interrupts urinary stream to promote bladder control
   d. Avoids straining and lifting heavy objects

4. Is free of complications
   a. Maintains vital signs within normal limits
   b. Exhibits wound healing, without signs of inflammation or hemorrhage
   c. Maintains acceptable level of urinary elimination
   d. Maintains optimal drainage of catheter and other drainage tubes
   e. Reports understanding of changes in sexual function

DISORDERS AFFECTING THE TESTES AND ADJACENT STRUCTURES

Orchitis

Orchitis is a rare, acute inflammatory response of one or both testes as a complication of systemic infection or as an extension of an associated epididymitis caused by bacterial, viral, spirochetal, or parasitic organisms. Micro-organisms may reach the testes through the blood, lymphatic system, or, more commonly, by traveling through the urethra, vas deferens, and epididymis; bacteria usually spread from an associated epididymitis in sexually active men. Causative organisms include *Neisseria gonorrhoeae*, *Chlamydia trachomatis*, *E. coli*, *Klebsiella*, *Pseudomonas aeruginosa*, *Staphylococcus* species, and *Streptococcus* species.

Signs and symptoms of orchitis include fever; pain, which may range from mild to severe; tenderness in one or both testicles; bilateral or unilateral testicular swelling; penile discharge; blood in the semen; and leukocytosis.

Treatment of orchitis is based on whether the causative organism is bacterial or viral. Bacterial orchitis is treated with antibiotic agents and supportive comfort measures. If the cause of the orchitis is an STI, the partner should be treated as well. Viral orchitis is treated using supportive treatments of rest, elevation of the scrotum, ice packs to reduce scrotal edema, analgesic agents, and anti-inflammatory medications. Bilateral orchitis can cause sterility in some men. Mumps vaccination is recommended for postpubertal men who have not had mumps or received inadequate immunization in childhood. Orchitis develops in approximately 30% of postpubertal men with mumps 4 to 6 days after parotitis starts, and one third of men have some testicular atrophy.

Epididymitis

Epididymitis is an infection of the epididymis, which usually spreads from an infected urethra, bladder, or prostate. The incidence is less than 1 in 1000 males per year. Prevalence is greatest in men 19 to 35 years of age. Acute epididymitis occurs bilaterally in 5% to 10% of affected patients (McDougal et al., 2016). Risk factors for epididymitis include recent surgery or a procedure involving the urinary tract, participation in high-risk sexual practices, personal history of an STI, past prostate infections or UTIs, lack of circumcision, history of an enlarged prostate, and the presence of a chronic indwelling urinary catheter.

Pathophysiology

A causative organism can be identified in 80% of patients. In prepubertal males, older men, and men who are homosexual, the predominate causal organism is *E. coli*, although in older men, the condition may also be a result of urinary obstruction. In sexually active men 35 years and younger, the pathogens usually are related to bacteria associated with STIs (e.g., *C. trachomatis*, *N. gonorrhoeae*). The infection moves in an upward direction, through the urethra and the ejaculatory duct, and then along the vas deferens to the epididymis (Taylor, 2015).

Clinical Manifestations

Epididymitis often slowly develops over 1 to 2 days, beginning with a low-grade fever, chills, and heaviness in the affected testicle. The testicle becomes increasingly tender to pressure and traction. The patient may report unilateral pain, soreness in the inguinal canal along the course of the vas deferens, and pain and swelling in the scrotum and the groin. The epididymis becomes increasingly swollen, with extreme pain in the lower abdomen and pelvis. Occasionally, there may be discharge from the urethra, blood in the semen, pus (pyuria) and bacteria (bacteriuria) in the urine, and pain during intercourse and ejaculation. The patient may report urinary frequency, urgency, or dysuria, and testicular pain aggravated by bowel movement.

Assessment and Diagnostic Findings

Laboratory assessment includes urinalysis, complete blood cell count, Gram stain of urethral drainage, urethral culture or deoxyribonucleic acid (DNA) probe, and referral for syphilis and HIV testing in sexually active patients. Acute testicular pain should never be ignored, and it should be distinguished from testicular torsion, which is a surgical emergency.

Medical Management

The selection of an antibiotic depends on the causative organism; if epididymitis is associated with an STI, the patient's partner should also receive antimicrobial therapy. The spermatic cord may be infiltrated with a local anesthetic agent to relieve pain if the patient is seen within the first 24 hours after onset of pain. Supportive interventions also include reduction in physical activity, scrotal support and elevation, ice packs, anti-inflammatory agents, analgesics (including nerve blocks), and sitz baths. Urethral instrumentation (e.g., catheter insertion) is avoided. The patient is observed for scrotal abscess formation as well.

In chronic epididymitis, a 4- to 6-week course of antibiotic therapy for bacterial pathogens is prescribed. An epididymectomy (excision of the epididymis from the testis) may be performed for patients who have recurrent, refractory, incapacitating episodes of this infection. With long-term epididymitis, the passage of sperm may be obstructed. If the obstruction is bilateral, infertility may result.

Nursing Management

Bed rest is prescribed, and the scrotum is elevated with a scrotal bridge or folded towel to prevent traction on the spermatic cord, to promote venous drainage, and to relieve pain. Antimicrobial agents are given as prescribed until the acute inflammation subsides. Intermittent cold compresses to the scrotum may help ease the pain. Later, local heat or sitz baths may help resolve the inflammation. Analgesic medications are given for pain relief as prescribed.

The nurse instructs the patient to avoid straining, lifting, and sexual stimulation until the infection is under control. He should continue taking analgesic agents and antibiotics as prescribed and using ice packs if necessary to relieve discomfort. He needs to know that it may take 4 weeks or longer for the inflammation to resolve.

Testicular Torsion

Testicular torsion is a surgical emergency requiring immediate diagnosis to avoid loss of the testicle. Torsion of the testis is rotation of the testis, which twists the blood vessels in the spermatic cord and therefore impedes the arterial and venous supply to the testicle and surrounding structures in the scrotum. The patient presents with sudden pain in the testicle, developing over 1 to 2 hours, with or without a predisposing event. Nausea, lightheadedness, and swelling of the scrotum may develop. On physical examination, testicular tenderness, an elevated testis, a thickened spermatic cord, and a swollen, painful scrotum may be present. If the torsion cannot be reduced manually, surgery to untwist the spermatic cord and anchor both testes in their correct position to prevent recurrence should occur within 6 hours of the onset of symptoms in order to save the testis. After 6 hours of impaired blood supply, the risk of loss of the testicle increases.

Testicular Cancer

Although only accounting for about 1% of all cancers in men, testicular cancer is the most common cancer diagnosed in men between 15 and 35 years of age; approximately 8400 new cases and 380 deaths occur in the United States annually (ACS, 2015). It is the second most common malignancy in those 35 to 39 years of age. For unknown reasons, worldwide incidence of testicular tumors has more than doubled in the past 40 years.

Because of advances in cancer therapy, testicular cancer is a highly treatable and usually curable form of cancer. The 5-year relative survival rate for all testicular cancers is more than 95% and approaches 99% if the cancer has not spread outside of the testes (ACS, 2015). After treatment, most patients with testicular cancer have a near-normal life expectancy.

Classification of Testicular Tumors

The testicles contain several types of cells, each of which may develop into one or more types of cancer. The type of cancer cell determines the appropriate treatment and affects the prognosis. Testicular cancer is classified as germinal or nongerminal (stromal). Secondary testicular cancers may also occur.

Germinal Tumors

Germinal tumors make up approximately 90% of all cancers of the testis; germinal tumors are further classified as seminomas or nonseminomas. These cancers grow from the germ cells that produce sperm, thus the name *germinal tumors*. Seminomas are slow-growing forms of testicular cancer that are usually found in men in their 30s and 40s (ACS, 2015; NCCN, 2016c). Although seminomas can spread to the lymph nodes, the cancer is usually localized in the testes. Nonseminomas are more common and tend to grow more quickly than seminomas. Nonseminomas are often made up of different cell types and are identified according to the cells in which they start to grow. Nonseminoma testicular cancers include choriocarcinomas (rare), embryonal carcinomas, teratomas, and yolk sac tumors. It is crucial to distinguish between seminomas and nonseminomas because the differences affect prognosis and treatment.

Nongerminal Tumors

Nongerminal tumors account for less than 10% of testicular cancers. These cancers may develop in the supportive and hormone-producing tissues, or stroma, of the testicles. The two main types of stromal tumors are Leydig cell tumors and Sertoli cell tumors. Although these tumors infrequently spread beyond the testicle, a small number metastasize and tend to be resistant to chemotherapy and radiation therapy.

Secondary Testicular Tumors

Secondary testicular tumors are those that have metastasized to the testicle from other organs. Lymphoma is the most common cause of secondary testicular cancer. Cancers may also spread to the testicles from the prostate gland, lung, skin (melanoma), kidney, and other organs. The prognosis with these cancers is usually poor because they typically also spread to other organs. Treatment depends on the specific type of cancer (ACS, 2015).

Risk Factors

Risk factors for testicular cancer include cryptorchidism (undescended testicles), family history of testicular cancer, and personal history of testicular cancer (ACS, 2015; Fuller, 2014). Other risk factors include race and ethnicity: Caucasian American men have a five times greater risk than African American men and more than two to three times greater risk than Asian, Native American, and Hispanic American men. The risk of developing testicular cancer is higher in HIV-positive men (ACS, 2015). Occupational hazards, including exposure to chemicals encountered in mining, oil and gas production, and leather processing, have been suggested as possible risk factors. No evidence has linked testicular cancer to prenatal exposure to diethylstilbestrol or to vasectomy (ACS, 2015).

Clinical Manifestations

The symptoms appear gradually, with a mass or lump on the testicle and usually painless enlargement of the testis. The patient may report heaviness in the scrotum, inguinal area, or lower abdomen. Backache (from retroperitoneal node extension), abdominal pain, weight loss, and general weakness may result from metastasis. Enlargement of the testis without pain is a significant diagnostic finding. Some testicular tumors tend to metastasize early, spreading from the testis to the lymph nodes in the retroperitoneum and to the lungs.

Assessment and Diagnostic Findings

Educating young men about testicular cancer and the need for urgent evaluation of any mass or enlargement or unexplained testicular pain is key to early detection (Fuller, 2014). Education about TSE, starting in adolescence, alerts men to the importance of seeking medical attention if a testicle becomes indurated, enlarged, atrophied, nodular, or painful (see Chart 59-6). TSE should be performed monthly. Testicular cancers generally grow rapidly and are easily detected against a typically smooth and homogeneous texture. Annual testicular examination by a clinician can reveal signs and lead to early diagnosis and treatment of testicular cancer. Promoting awareness of this disease is an important health promotion intervention; men should seek medical evaluation for signs or symptoms of testicular cancer without delay (Akar & Bebis, 2014). Any suspicious testicular mass warrants prompt evaluation with a thorough history and physical examination, focusing on palpation of the affected testicle.

The tumor markers alpha-fetoprotein (AFP) and beta-human chorionic gonadotropin (beta-hCG) may be elevated in patients with testicular cancer. Tumor marker levels in the blood are used for diagnosis, staging, and monitoring the response to treatment. Blood chemistry, including lactate dehydrogenase, is also necessary.

A chest x-ray to assess for metastasis in the lungs and a transscrotal testicular ultrasound will be performed. Microscopic analysis of tissue is the only definitive way to determine if cancer is present, but it is usually performed at the time of surgery rather than as a part of the diagnostic workup to reduce the risk of promoting spread of the cancer (ACS, 2015). Inguinal orchiectomy is the standard way to establish the diagnosis of testicular cancer. Other staging tests to determine the extent of the disease in the retroperitoneum, pelvis, and chest include an abdominal/pelvic CT scan and chest CT scan (if the abdominal CT or chest x-ray is abnormal). A brain MRI and bone scan may be obtained if indicated (NCCN, 2016c). Discussion of the option to bank sperm should take place prior to orchiectomy and treatment.

Medical Management

Testicular cancer—one of the most curable solid tumors—is highly responsive to treatment. Early-stage disease is curable more than 95% of the time; thus, prompt diagnosis and treatment are essential. The NCCN practice consensus guidelines for testicular cancer are used to guide diagnostic workup,

Chart 59-6 ◆ PATIENT EDUCATION
Testicular Self-Examination

Testicular self-examination is to be performed once a month. The test is neither difficult nor time-consuming. A convenient time is usually after a warm bath or shower when the scrotum is more relaxed.

The nurse instructs the patient to:

1. Use both hands to palpate the testis. The normal testicle is smooth and uniform in consistency.
2. Place the index and middle fingers under the testis and the thumb on top; roll the testis gently in a horizontal plane between the thumb and fingers (**A**).
3. Feel for any evidence of a small lump or abnormality.
4. Follow the same procedure and palpate upward along the testis (**B**).
5. Locate and palpate the epididymis (**C**), a cordlike structure on the top and back of the testicle that stores and transports sperm. In addition, locate and palpate the spermatic cord.
6. Repeat the examination for the other testis, epididymis, and spermatic cord. It is normal to find that one testis is larger than the other.
7. If you find any evidence of a small, pealike lump or if the testis is swollen (possibly from an infection or tumor), consult your primary provider.

Adapted from Weber, J. R., & Kelley, J. H. (2014). *Health assessment in nursing* (5th ed.). Philadelphia, PA: Lippincott Williams & Wilkins.

---

primary treatment, follow-up, and salvage therapy (treatment given when the cancer does not respond to standard treatment) for both seminomas and nonseminomas (NCCN, 2016c). The goals of management are to eradicate the disease and achieve a cure. Therapy is based on the cell type, the stage of the disease, and risk classification tables (determined as good, intermediate, and poor risk). Primary treatment includes removal of the affected testis by orchiectomy through an inguinal incision with a high ligation of the spermatic cord. The patient is offered the option of implantation of a testicular prosthesis during the orchiectomy. Although most patients experience no impairment of endocrine function after unilateral orchiectomy for testicular cancer, some patients have decreased hormonal levels, suggesting that the unaffected testis is not functioning normally. Retroperitoneal lymph node dissection (RPLND) may be performed after orchiectomy to diagnose and prevent lymphatic spread of the cancer. Alternatives to the more invasive open RPLND for early-stage germ cell testicular cancer include nerve-sparing and laparoscopic RPLND, which improve sexual function and promote rapid recovery (Hanna & Einhorn, 2014). Although libido and orgasm are usually unimpaired after RPLND, ejaculatory dysfunction with resultant infertility may develop. Two thirds of men who are newly diagnosed with testicular cancer may be considering future fatherhood, and sperm quality is reduced in men with testicular cancer; therefore, sperm banking before treatment may be considered (Martin, Turner, Bourne, et al., 2013). Half of patients will not recover fertility as a result of radiation therapy, cytotoxic therapy, unilateral excision of a testis, and RPLND. Counseling about fertility issues may help the patient make the appropriate choices (Brand, Williams, & Braybrooke, 2015).

Radiation therapy is more effective with seminomas than with nonseminomas. Postoperatively, radiation may be used in early-stage seminomas. It is delivered only to the affected side; the other testis is shielded from radiation to preserve fertility. Radiation is also used in patients whose disease does not respond to chemotherapy and in those for whom lymph node surgery is not recommended.

Chemotherapy may be used for seminomas, nonseminomas, and advanced metastatic disease. Cisplatin (Platinol-AQ) can be used in combination with other chemotherapeutic agents, such as etoposide (Toposar), bleomycin (Blenoxane), paclitaxel (Taxol), ifosfamide (Ifex), and vinblastine (Velban), and results in a high percentage of complete remissions. With nonseminomas, aggressive surgical resection of all residual masses following chemotherapy is standard therapy. Good results may also be obtained by combining different types of treatment, including surgery, radiation therapy, and chemotherapy. Even with metastatic testicular cancer, the prognosis is favorable because of advances in treatment. However, for patients who do not respond to high-dose salvage chemotherapy, the cancer is nearly always incurable.

A patient with a history of one testicular tumor has a greater chance of developing subsequent tumors. Late relapse of testicular cancer is currently defined as tumor recurrence more than 2 years after complete remission following primary treatment that included chemotherapy. The most common site of recurrence is the retroperitoneum. Follow-up studies include chest x-rays, excretory urography, radioimmunoassay of beta-hCG and AFP levels, and examination of lymph nodes.

Long-term side effects associated with treatment for testicular cancer include renal insufficiency from kidney damage, hearing problems, gonadal damage, peripheral neuropathy, and, rarely, secondary cancers. Management of a patient with testicular carcinoma is therapy aimed at cure followed by

Saab, M., Noureddine, S., Hujer, H. A., et al. (2014). Surviving testicular cancer: The Lebanese lived experience. *Nursing Research, 63*(3), 203–209.

Purpose

There is limited research and other literature available about what it means to live with testicular cancer. Although there are a few studies on survivors of testicular cancer in the United States and in several other European countries, there are no studies on men residing in the Arab region, particularly men in the country of Lebanon. The purpose of this study was to describe the experience of Lebanese survivors of testicular cancer and to obtain an understanding of the psychosexual dimensions of their experience.

Design

A hermeneutic, phenomenologic, qualitative research design was used to interview eight men recruited from the clinics of a urologist and an oncologist. The inclusion criteria specified that the participant: (1) was a resident of Lebanon who was of Lebanese nationality, as it was believed that the participant's cultural background played a major role in shaping their experiences, (2) was between 18 and 50 years of age, (3) was amenable to sharing personal information about the experience, (4) was willing to consent to digitally recording the interview, and (5) was willing to provide informed consent. A purposive sampling method was used. Prior to initiating the interview, the researcher asked several icebreaker questions about the participant's state of health and engagement in various types of daily activities. The main interview question was: Tell me about your life since you were diagnosed with testicular cancer. Specifically, the researchers asked participants about their lives since being diagnosed and receiving treatment, about their personal relationships, how their sex life, fertility, and sexual performance was affected, and if any problems were occurring. To ensure privacy for the interview,

the researcher met with the men in a place of the participant's choice. Interviews were conducted in the participants' homes, workplaces, researcher's office, and one was held by participant request in the researcher's car. After each interview field notes were written by the researcher.

Findings

The study participants were 32–50 years of age, with a mean age of 41 years. The participants were interviewed approximately 6 years after they had completed treatment. Five men reported undergoing a unilateral orchiectomy with chemotherapy, two reported only a bilateral orchiectomy, and one had a bilateral orchiectomy with radiation therapy. The participants were primarily businessmen, managers, skilled workers, an engineer and a bank employee. Six participants were married and two were identified as single. Six themes emerged from the interview data: (1) cancer perception in the Lebanese culture, (2) "do not show, do not tell," (3) the cancer experience is a turning point, (4) fertility, manhood and relationships, (5) coping with cancer, (6) preserved aspects of life.

Nursing Implications

It is important for nurses and other health care providers to address the patients' need for education and the cultural aspects of care related to testicular cancer and its treatment. The topics of fertility and sexuality must be included in all educational programs since these two topics were major areas of concern to the participants. Since fertility was a key determinant to the man's sexual identity, the need to discuss the option of sperm banking was viewed as an important care recommendation. The need for support groups with possible contact between newly diagnosed men and testicular cancer survivors, sexual counseling, and instruction on testicular self-examination during adolescence and young adulthood were important components to integrate into health care practice.

---

close monitoring to detect and promptly treat any recurrences (NCCN, 2016c). Investigations of new medications, combinations of chemotherapeutic agents, and stem cell transplantation are ongoing.

Nursing Management

Nursing management includes assessment of the patient's physical and psychological status and monitoring of the patient for response to and possible effects of surgery, chemotherapy, and radiation therapy (see Chapter 15). Pre- and postoperative care is described in Chapters 17 and 19, respectively. In addition, because the patient may have difficulty coping with his condition, issues related to body image and sexuality should be addressed.

Patients may be required to endure a long course of therapy and will need encouragement to maintain a positive attitude. After completing treatment, patients enter a follow-up surveillance period. Nurses educate these cancer survivors about the importance of adhering to follow-up appointments for early detection of cancer recurrence (most often occurring within 2 years posttreatment) and evaluation of late effects of treatment (including secondary cancers). Additional concerns include infertility, cardiotoxicity, neurotoxicity, nephrotoxicity, pulmonary toxicity, and metabolic syndrome; and altera-

tions in quality of life (Russell, 2014; Schover, van der Kaaij, van Dorst, et al., 2014). The nurse carefully assesses cultural aspects of care related to testicular cancer and its treatment (see Chart 59-7). The nurse reminds the patient about the importance of performing TSE in the treated or remaining testis. The patient is encouraged to participate in healthy behaviors, including smoking cessation, healthy diet, minimization of alcohol intake, and cancer screening activities. Most experts agree that couples should use birth control for 18 to 24 months after the last cycle of chemotherapy as this is the usual period of time after treatment for sperm to return to normal (Brand et al., 2015).

Hydrocele

A **hydrocele** is a collection of fluid most commonly located between the visceral and parietal layers of the tunica vaginalis of the testis, although it may also collect within the spermatic cord. This condition is the most common cause of scrotal swelling. At birth, 1 in 10 infants has a hydrocele, which usually resolves without treatment within the first year of life. Acute hydroceles primarily develop in adults older than 40 years; they may occur in association with inflammation (e.g., radiation therapy), infection, epididymitis, local injury, or systemic infectious disease (e.g., mumps). Chronic hydroceles may occur related to the imbalance between fluid secretion and reabsorption in the tunica vaginalis. On physical examination, an easily transilluminated, painless, extratesticular mass is found. Hydrocele can be differentiated from a hernia by transillumination; a hydrocele transmits light, whereas a hernia does not. Ultrasonography is recommended for large hydroceles to differentiate them from testicular tumors (Crawford, 2014).

Treatment is usually not required unless the hydrocele is large, bulky, tense, or uncomfortable; compromises testicular circulation; or causes an undesirable appearance. Treatment may involve surgical excision or needle aspiration. Surgical excision (hydrocelectomy) may be performed in an outpatient setting under general or spinal anesthesia with the goal of prevention of recurrence by excising the tunica vaginalis or sclerosing the visceral and parietal layers. Surgical excision involves resection or suturing together the two layers. A drainage tube may be required, and the patient is advised to wear a bulky dressing over the incisional site for a few days after the procedure. To reduce swelling, ice packs are applied to the scrotal area during the first 24 hours. A scrotal athletic supporter may be worn for a period of time postoperatively for comfort and support. Surgical risks include hematoma in the loose scrotal tissues, infection, or injury to the scrotum.

Needle aspiration is another option used to remove the fluid in the scrotum. Because it is common for fluid to reaccumulate, this treatment may be followed by the injection of a sclerosing agent to prevent this recurrence. This option may be used for men who are poor surgical risks. Potential risks include infection and scrotal pain.

Varicocele

A **varicocele** is an abnormal dilation of the pampiniform venous plexus and the internal spermatic vein in the scrotum (the network of veins from the testis and the epididymis, which constitute part of the spermatic cord). Varicoceles occur in approximately 15% to 20% of healthy adult men and 40% of infertile men; the large majority (95%) are in the left testicle because incompetent valves are more common in the left internal spermatic veins (Grossman & Porth, 2014). Although men may report scrotal pain, tenderness, heaviness in the inguinal area, and infertility, varicoceles are often asymptomatic.

If the varicocele is mild and fertility is not an issue, no treatment is required, and a scrotal support is usually sufficient to relieve symptoms of heaviness. If the condition results in ongoing distressing symptoms or fertility is an issue, the varicocele can be corrected surgically. Postprocedural education and care include an ice pack applied to the scrotum for the first few hours after surgery to relieve edema, dressing removal after 48 hours, nonstrenuous exercise for the first 2 days, scrotal support, pain control, and reporting complications such as infection and hematoma.

Vasectomy

Vasectomy, or male sterilization, involves the surgical interruption of both vas deferens—the tubes that carry the sperm from the testicles and epididymis to the seminal vesicles—to prevent fertilization of an egg after ejaculation. During the outpatient procedure, the surgeon exposes the vas deferens through a small surgical opening or puncture in the scrotum using a sharp, curved hemostat (see Fig. 59-6). The vas is

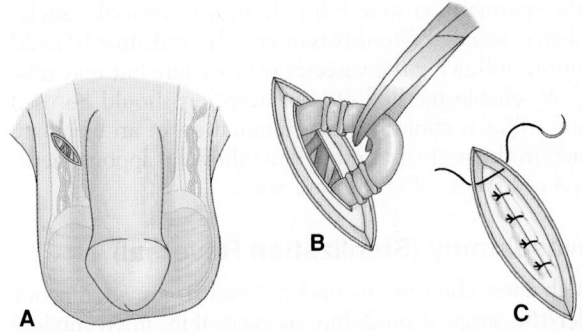

Figure 59-6 • A vasectomy is a resection of the vas deferens to prevent passage of sperm from the testes to the urethra during ejaculation. **A.** An incision or small puncture is made to expose the vas deferens. **B.** The vas deferens is isolated and severed. **C.** The severed ends are occluded with ligatures or clips, or the lumen of each vas is sealed by electrocautery and the incision is sutured closed. (Suturing may not be required if a puncture approach has been used.)

then ligated (cut) or cauterized (burned), with the severed ends occluded by ties or clips to seal the lumens and then placed back into the scrotum. A section of the vas deferens may or may not be removed. The spermatozoa, which are manufactured in the testes, cannot travel up the vas deferens after this surgery (McDougal et al., 2016).

Because seminal fluid is manufactured predominantly in the seminal vesicles and prostate gland, which are unaffected by vasectomy, no noticeable decrease in the amount of ejaculate occurs (volume decreases approximately 3%), even though it contains no spermatozoa. Because the sperm cells have no exit, they are resorbed into the body. A vasectomy usually has no effect on sexual potency, erection, ejaculation, or production of male hormones and provides no protection against STIs.

Couples who were once worried about pregnancy resulting from contraceptive failure often report a decrease in concern and an increase in spontaneous sexual arousal after vasectomy. Concise and factual preoperative explanations may minimize or relieve the patient's concerns related to pain and reduced masculinity. The patient is advised that he will be sterile but that potency will not be altered after a bilateral vasectomy. On rare occasions, a spontaneous reanastomosis of the vas deferens occurs, making it possible to impregnate a partner.

Complications of vasectomy include scrotal ecchymoses and swelling, superficial wound infection, vasitis (inflammation of the vas deferens), epididymitis or epididymo-orchitis, hematomas, chronic pain, and spermatic granuloma. A spermatic granuloma is an inflammatory response to the collection of sperm leaking from the severed end of the proximal vas deferens into the scrotal tissue. A painless small lump is formed, which usually does not require surgical intervention.

Nursing Management

Nursing education focuses on self-management of swelling and discomfort post vasectomy. Applying ice bags intermittently to the scrotum for several hours after surgery can reduce swelling and relieve discomfort. The nurse advises the patient to wear snug cotton underwear or a scrotal support for added comfort and support. Explanation of expected discoloration of the scrotal skin and superficial swelling may alleviate anxiety and concerns. These conditions may be relieved by sitz baths.

Sexual intercourse may be resumed as desired, usually after 1 week. Fertility remains for a varying time after vasectomy until the spermatozoa stored distally in the seminal vesicles have been evacuated. Sterility is often achieved after 10 to 20 ejaculations following the vasectomy procedure but may take longer. A reliable method of contraception should be used until infertility is confirmed by examination of an ejaculate specimen in the urologist's office at a follow-up appointment, usually 4 to 8 weeks after the vasectomy.

Vasovasostomy (Sterilization Reversal)

Although men choosing to undergo vasectomy should not consider the surgical procedure as reversible, microsurgical techniques can be used to reverse a vasectomy (vasovasostomy) and restore patency to the vas deferens. Many men have sperm in their ejaculate after a reversal, and 50% to 70% can impregnate a partner. The success of the procedure depends on the vasectomy method performed and the amount of time since the vasectomy. The procedure can be very costly, is not covered by insurance, is not permanent with occlusion of the vas recurring 2 or more years after vasovasostomy, and results in sperm counts at lower than prevasectomy levels (Lindsey, Herrela, Goodman, et al., 2015).

Semen Cryopreservation (Sperm Banking)

Storing fertile semen in a sperm bank before a vasectomy is an option for men who experience a major life change and may want to father a child at a later time. In addition, if a man has just sustained an injury to the spinal cord or is about to undergo a procedure or treatment (e.g., radiation therapy to the pelvis, chemotherapy, orchiectomy) that may affect his fertility, sperm banking may be considered (Kelvin, 2015). This procedure usually requires several visits to the facility where the sperm is stored under hypothermic conditions. The semen is obtained by masturbation and collected in a sterile container for storage. Insurance carriers rarely cover the cost of semen collection and banking. The costs of semen cryopreservation vary according to facility, method of sperm retrieval, number of specimens, and length of time in storage, making the process cost-prohibitive for some men.

DISORDERS AFFECTING THE PENIS

Phimosis

Phimosis is a condition in which the foreskin (prepuce) cannot be retracted over the glans in uncircumcised males. With the decrease in routine circumcision of newborns, early instruction should be given to parents about cleansing the foreskin and the need for retraction to cleanse the glans. If the glans is not cleaned, secretions accumulate, causing inflammation of the glans penis (balanitis), which can later lead to adhesions and fibrosis. Phimosis often develops in adults as a result of inflammation, edema, and constriction because of poor hygiene or underlying medical conditions such as diabetes. The thickened secretions (smegma) can become encrusted with urinary salts and calcify, forming calculi in the prepuce and increasing the risk of penile carcinoma. Treatment for phimosis secondary to inflammation is the application of steroidal cream to the foreskin to soften and correct the narrowness, resulting in decreased constriction. Although phimosis is the most common indication for

adult circumcision, it is rarely necessary to surgically correct the condition by loosening or removing the foreskin.

Paraphimosis is a condition in which the foreskin, once retracted over the glans, cannot be returned to its usual position. Chronic inflammation under the foreskin leads to formation of a tight ring of skin when the foreskin is retracted behind the glans, causing venous congestion, edema, and enlargement of the glans, which makes the condition worse. As the condition progresses, arterial occlusion and necrosis of the glans may occur. Paraphimosis usually can be treated by firmly compressing the glans for 5 minutes to reduce the tissue edema and size and then pushing the glans back while simultaneously moving the foreskin forward (manual reduction). The constricting skin ring may require incision under local anesthesia. Circumcision is usually indicated after the inflammation and edema subside (Keane & Graham, 2016).

Cancer of the Penis

Penile cancer is rare, occurring in less than 1% of cancers among men in the United States. It accounts for an estimated 1290 new cancer cases and 300 expected deaths each year (ACS, 2015). The 5-year survival rates for cancer localized to the penis approaches 80%, but this statistic drops to 52% if the lymph nodes are involved and to 18% if the cancer has spread beyond the inguinal lymph nodes (Keane & Graham, 2016). Penile cancer is much more common in some parts of Africa and South America, where it accounts for up to 10% of cancers in men. Because the penis contains different cell types, penile cancer can arise in each type of cell, which determines the prognosis. Types of penile cancer include squamous cell carcinoma (most common; 95% of cases), epidermoid penile cancer, verrucous carcinoma, adenocarcinoma, in situ carcinomas (erythroplasia of Queyrat and Bowen disease), basal cell penile cancer, melanoma, and sarcomas (McDougal et al., 2016). Several risk factors for penile cancer have been identified, including lack of circumcision, poor genital hygiene, phimosis, HPV, smoking, ultraviolet light treatment of psoriasis on the penis, increasing age (two thirds of cases occur in men older than 65 years), penile metastasis secondary to bladder cancer, lichen sclerosus, and balanitis xerotica obliterans (Kumar, Bhattacharyya, Mandal, et al., 2014; Turner, Drudge-Coates, & Henderson, 2013). However, the exact cause remains unclear. Because penile cancer is rare, there has been little improvement in diagnostic and staging tests, understanding of risk factors, and development of treatment modalities.

Clinical Manifestations

The penile lesion usually alerts the patient to the presence of penile cancer; however, men may delay seeking treatment for more than a year because of embarrassment, fear, or lack of understanding. Common clinical presentations are a painless lump, ulcer, or wartlike growth on the skin of the penis; a change in skin color such as a red rash, bluish growths, or whitish patches; and malodorous and persistent discharge in late stages.

Assessment and Diagnostic Findings

Penile cancer involves the glans most frequently (48%), followed by lesions of the foreskin (21%), the coronal sulcus (6%), the penile shaft (less than 2%), the urethra, and regional or distant lymph nodes (McDougal et al., 2016). A thorough physical examination is necessary, including assessment and palpation of the penis and the inguinal lymph nodes. The size, location, borders, consistency, fixation, and character and time of onset of the penile lesions should be noted. Incisional or excisional biopsy is performed to determine the cell types of the penile cancer. Further staging tests using ultrasonography, MRI, or CT scan may be obtained to determine the extent of local lesions, if metastatic disease is present, and treatment options.

Prevention

The best way to reduce the risk of penile cancer is to avoid known risk factors whenever possible (ACS, 2015). Avoidance of sexual practices that are likely to result in HPV infection may reduce the risk of penile cancer. Gardasil, a vaccine that protects against infection with HPV, the cause of 90% of genital warts, is recommended for males 9 through 26 years old (CDC, 2015). Although uncircumcised men have a greater incidence of penile cancer than circumcised men, the more important factor in preventing penile cancer is good genital hygiene. Circumcision is not recommended as a prevention strategy (ACS, 2015).

Medical Management

Treatment varies depending on the type and stage of penile cancer, location of the lesion, overall physical health, and personal preferences about treatments and side effects. Treatment emphasis is on minimizing the cancer's invasiveness and preserving organ function (Khoo, 2013). The goal of treatment in invasive penile cancer is complete excision with adequate margins. Surgery is the most common treatment method used in all forms of the disease. Depending on the stage and invasiveness of the cancer, therapeutic options may include simple excision, electrodesiccation and curettage, cryosurgery, Mohs surgery (microscopically controlled surgery), yttrium aluminum garnet (YAG) laser surgery, wide local excision, circumcision, and surgical removal of part of the penis or the entire penis (penectomy). Organ-sparing surgical approaches are preferable. Partial penectomy is preferred to total penectomy because patients can then participate in sexual intercourse, stand for urination, and maintain cosmesis. Modern reconstructive surgical techniques are providing more options for patients. The shaft of the penis can still respond to sexual arousal with an erection and has the sensory capacity for orgasm and ejaculation. Total penectomy is indicated if the tumor is not amenable to conservative treatment. After a total penectomy, the patient may still experience orgasm with stimulation of the perineum and scrotal area.

Topical chemotherapy with 5-fluorouracil cream or biologic therapy may also be effective. Radiation therapy is used to treat small squamous cell carcinomas of the penis and for palliation in advanced tumors or cases of lymph node metastasis.

Penile cancer spreads primarily to the inguinal lymph nodes; thus, appropriate lymph node management plays a significant role in survival. Because enlarged inguinal lymph nodes are caused by inflammation in 50% of cases, patients who present with enlarged lymph nodes should undergo treatment of the primary lesion followed by a 4- to 6-week course of oral broad-spectrum antibiotic agents. Persistent enlarged lymph nodes after antibiotic therapy should be considered to be metastatic disease and treated with either a sentinel lymph node biopsy (to determine presence of cancer) or with pelvic and bilateral inguinal lymph node dissection. If extensive pelvic lymph node involvement is present, the patient should receive adjuvant or neoadjuvant chemotherapy and postoperative radiation therapy (Khoo, 2013).

Priapism

Priapism, a relatively uncommon disorder, is defined as a persistent penile erection that may or may not be related to sexual stimulation. The penis becomes large, hard, and painful. Priapism results from either neural or vascular causes, including sickle cell disease, leukemic cell infiltration, polycythemia, spinal cord tumors or injury, and tumor invasion of the penis or its vessels. It may also occur with use of vasoactive agents that affect the central nervous system, antihypertensive agents, antipsychotic and antidepressant medications, substances injected into the penis to treat erectile dysfunction, alcohol, and cocaine. There are three forms of priapism: ischemic (veno-occlusive; low flow), nonischemic (high flow), and stuttering (intermittent).

The ischemic form, which is described as nonsexual, persistent erection with little or no cavernous blood flow, must be treated promptly to prevent permanent damage to the penis. The goal of therapy is to improve venous drainage of the corpora cavernosa to prevent ischemia, fibrosis, and impotence. The initial treatment is directed at relieving the erection, preventing penile damage and simultaneously treating the underlying disease. Recommended treatment is aspiration of the corpora cavernosa (with or without irrigation) or intracavernous injection of sympathomimetic agents (e.g., phenylephrine). Repeated injections may be needed to resolve priapism. Surgical shunts are used to reestablish penile circulation if repeated injections of the sympathomimetic are ineffective (McDougal et al., 2016).

Nonischemic priapism and stuttering are generally not considered emergencies and often resolve without treatment. Conservative treatment (e.g., application of ice and site-specific compression to the injury) may be used. If repeated episodes occur, surgical shunting is considered. Patients with the intermittent form of priapism may be instructed in intracavernosal self-injection of phenylephrine.

Peyronie's Disease

Peyronie's disease is an acquired, benign condition that involves the buildup of fibrous plaques in the sheath of the corpus cavernosum. These plaques are not visible when the penis is relaxed. However, when the penis is erect, curvature occurs that can be painful and can make sexual intercourse difficult or impossible. Peyronie's disease typically begins between 45 and 65 years of age. Medical management in the first year of active disease includes systemic, topical, intralesional, or extracorporeal techniques, with 50% of men experiencing spontaneous resolution. Surgical removal of mature plaques is used to treat severe disease. Patients should be fully informed of available treatment options and their likely outcomes (McDougal et al., 2016).

Urethral Stricture

Urethral stricture is a condition in which a section of the urethra is narrowed. It can occur congenitally or from a scar along the urethra. Traumatic injury to the urethra (e.g., from instrumentation or infections) can result in strictures that restrict urine flow and decrease the urinary stream, leading to spraying or double stream, postvoiding dribbling, and dilation of the proximal urethra and prostatic ducts. Prostatitis is a common complication. Treatment involves dilation of the urethra or, in severe cases, urethrotomy (surgical removal of the stricture). Antimicrobial agents are necessary for resolution of UTIs, followed by long-term prophylactic therapy until the stricture is corrected. Treatment should not be considered successful until at least 1 year has passed, because strictures may recur anytime during that period (Keane & Graham, 2016).

Circumcision

Circumcision is the surgical excision of the foreskin (prepuce) of the glans penis. According to the CDC, approximately 80% of men are circumcised in the United States, and circumcision is one of the oldest surgical procedures performed worldwide (CDC, 2015). There is controversy about the guidelines to determine the validity of male circumcision as a prevention of disease transmission (Earp, 2015). In adults, circumcision may be indicated as part of treatment for phimosis, paraphimosis, and recurrent infections of the glans and foreskin. It also may be performed at the patient's request.

The primary method of circumcision in adults is surgical excision. Postoperatively, a petrolatum (Vaseline) gauze dressing is applied and changed as indicated. The patient is observed for bleeding. Because considerable pain may occur after circumcision, analgesic agents are given as needed.

CRITICAL THINKING EXERCISES

1 **pq** Identify the priorities, approach, and techniques you would use to perform a health assessment on a 24-year-old male graduate student from Africa who speaks English as a second language and who has been diagnosed with squamous cell carcinoma of the penis. How will your priorities, approach, and techniques integrate cultural considerations into the nursing care?

2 **ebp** A 65-year-old male patient who has a history of thyroid disease, hypertension and type II diabetes is diagnosed with prostate cancer with a Gleason score of 4 post biopsy. What evidence-based information would you provide to the patient and his spouse to assist in preventing postoperative complications during the recovery period? Identify the evidence for and the criteria used to evaluate the strength of the evidence for the nursing care identified.

3 **ebp** You are caring for a 30-year-old man who has been recently advised by his urologist to undergo a circumcision due to repeated episodes of epididymitis. What is the evidence base for his treatment options? Identify the criteria used to evaluate the strength of the evidence. How would you explain the various treatment options to the patient and his significant other?

REFERENCES

*Asterisk indicates nursing research.

Books

American Cancer Society. (2015). *Cancer facts and figures 2015*. Atlanta, GA: Author.

Centers for Disease Control and Prevention. [CDC]. (2015). *National Center for HIV/AIDS, viral hepatitis, STD, and TB prevention: Strategic plan through 2020*. Atlanta, GA: Author.

Grossman, S., & Porth, C. M. (2014). *Pathophysiology: Concepts of altered health states* (9th ed.). Philadelphia, PA: Lippincott, Williams & Wilkins.

Hall, J. E. (2015). *Guyton & Hall textbook of medical physiology* (13th ed.). Philadelphia, PA: Saunders Elsevier.

Itano, J. K., Brant, J. M., Conde, F. A., et al. (2016). *Core curriculum for oncology nursing* (5th ed.). St. Louis, MO: Mosby Elsevier.

Karch, A. M. (2016). *2016 Lippincott pocket drug guide for nurses*. (4th ed.). Philadelphia, PA: Wolters Kluwer.

Keane, T. E., & Graham, S. D. (Eds.) (2016). *Glenn's urologic surgery*. Philadelphia, PA: Wolters Kluwer.

McCance, K. L., Huether, S. E., Braskers, V. L., et al. (Eds.). (2013). *Pathophysiology: The biologic basis for disease in adults and children* (7th ed.). St. Louis, MO: Mosby Elsevier.

McDougal, W. J., Wein, A. J., Kavoussi, L. R., et al. (Eds.). (2016). *Campbell-Walsh urology* (11th ed.). Philadelphia, PA: Elsevier.

Mulhall, J. P., & Hsiao, W. (Eds.) (2014). *Men's sexual health and fertility: A clinician's guide*. New York: Springer.

Pagana, K. D., & Pagana, T. J. (2013). *Mosby's diagnostic and laboratory test reference* (11th ed.). St. Louis, MO: Mosby Elsevier.

Sandhu, J. S. (2015). *Urinary dysfunction in prostate cancer*. New York: Springer.

Tabloski, P. A. (2014). *Gerontological nursing: The essential guide to clinical practice* (3rd ed.). New York: Pearson.

Weber, J. R., & Kelley, J. H. (2014). *Health assessment in nursing* (5th ed.). Philadelphia, PA: Lippincott Williams & Wilkins.

Wincze, J. P., & Weisberg, R. B. (2015). *Sexual dysfunction: A guide for assessment and treatment*. New York: Guildford Press.

Journals and Electronic Documents

Allkanjari, O., & Vitalone, A. (2015). What do we know about phytotherapy of benign prostatic hyperplasia? *Life Sciences, 126*(1), 42–56.

Akar, S. Z., & Bebis, H. (2014). Evaluation of the effectiveness of testicular cancer and testicular self-examination training for patient care personnel: Intervention study. *Health Education Research, 29*(6), 966–976.

Akre, C., Berchtold, A., Gmel, G., et al. (2014). The evolution of sexual dysfunction in young men aged 18–25 years. *Journal of Adolescent Health, 55*(14), 736–743.

Baker, H. (2014). Choosing a prostate cancer drug. *British Journal of Nursing, 23*(16), S14–S16.

Barry, M. J., & Hayes, J. H. (2015). Evaluating an elevated screening PSA test. *JAMA 314*(19), 2073–2074.

*Brand, S., Williams, H., & Braybrooke, J. (2015). How has early testicular cancer affected your life? A study of sexual function in men attending active surveillance for stage one testicular cancer. *European Journal of Oncology Nursing, 19*(15), 278–281.

Braun, D. P., Gupta, D., Birdsall, T. C., et al. (2013). Effect of naturopathic and nutritional supplement treatment on tumor response, control, and recurrence in patients with prostate cancer treated with radiation therapy. *Journal of Alternative & Complementary Medicine, 19*(3), 198–203.

Brown, C. S. (2014). Dilutional hyponatremia in a community hospital setting: Case report. *Intensive & Critical Care Nursing, 30*(1), 1–5.

*Carter, N., Miller, P. A., Murphy, B. R., et al. (2014). Healthcare providers' perspectives of the supportive care needs of men with advanced prostate cancer. *Oncology Nursing Forum, 41*(4), 421–430.

*Cremin, M. (2015). Meeting the unmet support needs of BME men with prostate cancer. *British Journal of Nursing, 24*(20), 1010–1014.

Chen, X., Hu, Y., Peng, J., et al. (2015). Association of diet and lifestyle with chronic prostatitis/chronic pelvic pain syndrome and pain severity: A case–control study. *Prostate Cancer and Prostatic Disease, 19*, 92–99.

Crawford, P. (2014). Evaluation of scrotal masses. *American Family Physician, 89*(9), 723–727.

Detti, B., Bonomo, P., Masi, L. (2016). CyberKnife stereotactic radio-therapy for isolated recurrence in the prostatic bed. *World Journal of Urology, 34*(3), 311–317.

Dorey, G. (2013). Pelvic floor exercises after radical prostatectomy. *British Journal of Nursing, 22*(9), 4–9.

Earp, B. D. (2015). Do the benefits of male circumcision outweigh the risks? A critique of the proposed CDC Guidelines. *Frontier Pediatrics, 3*(18), 1–3.

Fuller, K. (2014). Diagnosis of testicular cancer. *The Journal of Nurse Practitioners, 10*(6), 437–438.

Gerend, M. A., Madkins, K., Phillips, G., et al. (2016). Predictors of human papillomavirus vaccination among men who have sex with men. *Sexually Transmitted Disease, 43*(3), 185–191.

*Gledhill, S. & Schweitzer, R. D. (2013). Sexual desire, erectile dysfunction and the biomedicalization of sex in older heterosexual men. *Journal of Advanced Nursing, 70*(4), 894–903.

Goodman, A., (2013). Anticoagulant use predicts survival in metastatic prostate cancer. *Formulary, 48*(5), 1–2.

Hanna, N. H., & Einhorn, L. (2014). Testicular cancer–Discoveries and updates. *The New England Journal of Medicine, 371*(21), 2005–2016.

Hsu, J. C., Tang, D. H., & Lu, C. Y. (2014). Risk-benefit assessment of oral phosphodiesterase type 5 inhibitors for treatment of erectile dysfunction: A multiple criteria decision analysis. *International Journal of Clinical Practice, 69*(4), 436–443.

Hunter, J. C., Vines, A. I., & Carlisle, V. (2015). African Americans' perceptions of prostate-specific antigen prostate cancer screening. *Health Education and Behavior, 42*(4), 539–544.

Jones, S. (2016). Nurse-led clinic for men receiving targeted therapies for metastatic hormone-relapsed prostate cancer. *Cancer Nursing Practice, 15*(5), 32–36.

Kelvin, J. F. (2015). Sperm banking: Fertility preservation for male patients with cancer. *Clinical Journal of Oncology Nursing, 19*(1), 108–110.

Khoo, V. (2013). Modern management of penile cancer. *European Journal of Cancer, Supplement, 11*(2), 303–306.

Kuehn, B. M. (2016). US hospitals prepare for penis transplants. *Medical News and Perspectives of the American Medical Association, 315*(13), 1322–1324.

Kumar, N., Bhattacharyya, T., Mandal, A. K., et al. (2014). Penile metastasis secondary to bladder cancer: A report of two cases. *Indian Journal of Palliative Care, 20*(1), 57–60.

Kumnig, M., & Jowsey-Gregoire, S. G. (2016). Key psychosocial challenges in vascularized composite allotransplanatation. *World Journal of Transplantation, 6*(1), 91–102.

Lanier, Y., & Sutton, M. Y. (2013). Reframing the context of preventive health care services and prevention of HIV and other sexually transmitted infections for young men: New opportunities to reduce racial/ethnic sexual health disparities. *American Journal of Public Health, 103*(2), 262–269.

Lim, P. H. (2013). How incontinence affects sexual health. *Australian and New Zealand Continence Journal, 19*(4), 117–121.

Lindsey, A. Herrela, M., Goodman, M., et al. (2015). Outcomes of microsurgical vasovasostomy for vasectomy reversal: A meta-analysis and systematic review. *Urology, 85*(4), 819–825.

Lycken, M., Garmo, H., Adolfsson, J., et al. (2013). Patterns of androgen deprivation therapies among men diagnosed with localized prostatic cancer: A population based study. *European Journal of Cancer, 49*(9), 1789–1798.

*Martin, F., Turner, A., Bourne, C., et al., (2013). Development and qualitative evaluation of a self-management workshop for testicular cancer survivor-initiated follow-up. *Oncology Nursing Forum, 40*(1), 14–23.

Mitchell, K. R., Mercer, C. H., Ploubidis, G. B., et al. (2013). Sexual function in Britain: Findings from the Third National Survey of Sexual Attitudes and Lifestyles (Natsal-3). *The Lancet, 382*, 1817–1829.

Mola, J. R. (2015). Erectile dysfunction in the older adult male. *Urologic Nursing, 35*(2), 87–93.

Mulheim, E., Fulbright, N., & Duncan, N. (2015). Prostate cancer screening. *American Family Physician, 92*(8), 683–688.

National Comprehensive Cancer Network. [NCCN]. (2016a). Cancer guidelines. Retrieved on 3/6/2017 at: www.nccn.org/patients/guidelines/cancers.aspx

National Comprehensive Cancer Network [NCCN]. (2016b). Clinical practice guidelines in oncology: Prostate cancer. Retrieved on 3/6/2017 at: www.nccn.org/professionals/default.aspx

National Comprehensive Cancer Network. [NCCN]. (2016c). Clinical practice guidelines in oncology: Testicular cancer. Retrieved on 3/6/2017 at: www.nccn.org/professionals/default.aspx

Norton, W., & Tremayne, P. (2015). Sex and the older man. *British Journal of Nursing, 24*(4), 218–221.

Owusu-Edusei, K., Gift, T. L., Patton, M. E., et al. (2015). Estimating the total annual cost of providing sexually transmitted infection and HIV testing and counseling for men who have sex with men in the United States. *Sexually Transmitted Diseases, 42*(10), 586–589.

Pearson, R. (2014). Common questions about the diagnosis and management of benign prostatic hyperplasia. *American Family Physician, 90*(11), 769–774.

Rathkopf, D., & Scher, H. I. (2013). Androgen receptor antagonists in castration-resistant cancer. *The Cancer Journal, 19*(1), 43–49.

Russell, S. S. (2014). Testicular cancer: Overview and implications for health care providers. *Urologic Nursing, 34*(4), 172–192.

*Saab, M., Noureddine, S., Hujer, H. A., et al. (2014). Surviving testicular cancer: The Lebanese lived experience. *Nursing Research, 63*(3), 203–209.

Scher, H. I. (2016). Defining new standards of care for men with prostate cancer. *The Lancet, 387*, 1135–1137.

Schover, L. R., van der Kaaij, M., van Dorst, E., et al. (2014). Sexual dysfunction and infertility as late effects of cancer treatment. *European Journal of Cancer Supplement, 12*(1), 41–53.

Simondsen, K., & Kolesar, J. (2013). New treatment options for castration-resistant prostate cancer. *American Journal of Health-System Pharmacy, 70*(10), 856–865.

Simpson, P. (2015). Prostatectomy: Information provision and education for patients. *British Journal of Nursing, 24*(9), 24–28.

Sohn, W., Lee, H. J., & Ahlering, T. E. (2013). Robotic surgery: Review of prostate and bladder cancer. *Cancer Journal, 19*(2), 133–139.

*Song, L., Rini, C., Deal, A. M., et al. (2015). Improving couples' quality of life through a web-based prostate cancer education intervention. *Oncology Nursing Forum, 42*(2), 183–192.

Sparling, S. & Cramer, K. (2015). Choosing the danger we think we know: Men's and women's faulty perceptions of sexually transmitted infection risk with familiar and unfamiliar new partners. *The Canadian Journal of Human Sexuality, 24*(3), 237–242.

Tannenbaum, C. (2015), Associations between urinary symptoms and sexual health in older adults. *Clinics in Geriatric Medicine, 31*(4), 581–590.

Tantamango-Bartley, Y., Knutsen, S. F., Knutsen, R., et al. (2016). Are strict vegetarians protected against cancer? *American Journal of Clinical Nutrition, 103*, 153–160.

Taylor, S. N. (2015). *Epididymitis. Clinical Infectious Diseases, 61*(8), 770–773.

Thakur, M. K., (2016). Multifaceted and personalized therapy of advanced prostate cancer. *Current Opinion in Oncology, 28*(3), 222–231.

Tsai, M., Liu, C., Chang, C., et al. (2014). Overview of the relevant literature on the possible role of acupuncture in treating male sexual dysfunction. *Acupuncture Medicine, 32*, 406–410.

Turner, B., Drudge-Coates, L., & Henderson, S. (2013). Penile cancer: Diagnosis, clinical features and management. *Nursing Standard, 27*(29), 50–57.

Wagenlehner, F. M. E; Weidner, W., Pilatz, A., et al. (2014). Urinary tract infections and bacterial prostatitis in men. *Current Opinion in Infectious Diseases, 27*(1), 97–101.

Resources

American Cancer Society, www.cancer.org/cancer/prostatecancer/
American Urological Association, www.auanet.org
CancerCare, www.cancercare.org
Centers for Disease Control and Prevention (CDC), www.cdc.gov/cancer
Hartford Institute for Geriatric Nursing, Consult Geri website, www.consultgerirn.org/topics/urinary_incontinence/want_to_know_more
National Institutes of Health, National Center for Complementary and Integrative Health (NCCIH), nccih.nih.gov
National Cancer Institute (NCI), www.cancer.gov
National Comprehensive Cancer Network (NCCN), www.nccn.org
Prostate Cancer Foundation, www.pcf.org
Testicular Cancer Society (TCS), www.testicularcancersociety.org
Urology Care Foundation, www.urologyhealth.org
Us TOO International Prostate Cancer Education and Support Network, www.ustoo.org

UNIT 14

Integumentary Function

The nurse is caring for an 85-year-old female who was living with her husband at home. The patient was admitted to a medical unit for smoke inhalation after a house fire. While doing a morning assessment, the nurse notes and documents that the patient has a stage II pressure ulcer on her sacral area. No pressure ulcer was documented during the patient's admission assessment. Upon further investigation, the nurse notes that three other patients on this unit in the last two quarters had stage II and III pressure ulcers that were not documented as present upon hospital admission.

QSEN Competency Focus: Evidence-Based Practice (EBP)

The complexities inherent in today's health care system challenges nurses to demonstrate integration of specific interdisciplinary core competencies. These competencies are aimed at ensuring the delivery of safe, quality patient care (Institute of Medicine, 2003). The Quality and Safety Education for Nurses project (QSEN, 2017; Cronenwett, Sherwood, Barnsteiner, et al., 2007) provides a framework for the knowledge, skills, and attitudes (KSA) required for nurses to demonstrate competency in these key areas, which include *patient-centered care, interdisciplinary teamwork and collaboration, evidence-based practice, quality improvement, safety,* and *informatics.*

Evidence-Based Practice Definition: Integrate best current evidence with clinical expertise and patient/family preferences and values for delivery of optimal health care.

SELECTED PRE-LICENSURE KSAs	APPLICATION AND REFLECTION
Knowledge	
Describe reliable sources for locating evidence reports and clinical practice guidelines.	Identify the sources you would use to find evidence-based reports and clinical guidelines for managing stage II pressure ulcers in this patient as well as others admitted to the medical unit.
Skills	
Read original research and evidence reports related to area of practice. Locate evidence reports related to clinical practice topics and guidelines.	Access the source or sources you have identified, and find research and evidence reports that describe how to best manage this patient's skin breakdown. What is the strength of the evidence for these management strategies? What criteria will you use to judge the strength of the evidence you have identified?
Attitudes	
Appreciate the importance of regularly reading relevant professional journals.	Reflect upon what you learned by engaging in this exercise. Think about how the best evidence you found may change in time. If you were treating a patient with a stage II pressure ulcer in ten years' time, do you think you would likely be using these same evidence-based guidelines or reports to guide your practice? Why is the nature of clinical practice ever changing?

Cronenwett, L., Sherwood, G., Barnsteiner, J., et al. (2007). Quality and safety education for nurses. *Nursing Outlook, 55*(3), 122–131.
Institute of Medicine. (2003). *Health professions education: A bridge to quality.* Washington, DC: National Academies Press.
QSEN Institute, (2017). *QSEN Competencies: Definitions and pre-licensure KSAs.* Retrieved on 3/1/2017 at: www.qsen.org/competencies/pre-licensure-ksas

60 Assessment of Integumentary Function

LEARNING OBJECTIVES

On completion of this chapter, the learner will be able to:

1 Identify the structures and functions of the skin, hair, and nails.
2 Describe the normal aging process of the skin and skin changes common in older adult patients.
3 Use appropriate parameters for assessment of the skin, hair, and nails.

4 Compare and contrast primary and secondary skin lesions and their pattern and distribution.
5 Recognize common skin eruptions and manifestations associated with systemic disease.
6 Discuss common diagnostic tests and procedures used in diagnosing skin and related disorders.

GLOSSARY

alopecia: loss of hair from any cause
erythema: redness of the skin caused by dilation of the capillaries due to injury, irritation, inflammation, or various skin conditions
hirsutism: the condition of having excessive hair growth
hyperpigmentation: increase in the melanin of the skin, resulting in an increase in pigmentation
hypopigmentation: decrease in the melanin of the skin, resulting in a loss of pigmentation
keratin: an insoluble, fibrous protein that forms the outer skin layer
keratinocytes: arising from the innermost layer of the epidermis, synthesize the insoluble protein, keratin
Langerhans cells: dendritic clear cells in the epidermis that carry surface receptors for immunoglobulin and complement and that are active participants in delayed hypersensitivity of the skin
melanin: the substance responsible for coloration of the skin

melanocytes: cells of the skin that produce melanin
Merkel cells: cells of the epidermis that play a role in transmission of sensory messages
petechiae: pinpoint red spots that appear on the skin as a result of blood leakage into the skin
rete ridges: undulations and furrows that appear at the lower edge of the epidermis at the dermal junction where these two skin layers are cemented together
sebaceous glands: glands that exist within the epidermis and secrete sebum to keep the skin soft and pliable
sebum: fatty secretion of the sebaceous glands
telangiectasias: venous stars; red marks on the skin caused by distention of the superficial blood vessels
vitiligo: a localized or widespread condition characterized by destruction of the melanocytes in circumscribed areas of the skin, resulting in white patches
Wood light: ultraviolet light used for diagnosing skin conditions

In the United States, as many as one in three persons will have a skin disorder or disease at any given time. Skin disorders are encountered frequently in nursing practice in inpatient and outpatient settings. The assessment of the skin can provide important information about the general health of the patient or clues to systemic conditions that manifest in the skin.

Any patient may suddenly develop itching and a rash from a treatment regimen. The psychological stress of illness or various personal and family problems may be exhibited outwardly as dermatologic disorders. In certain systemic conditions, such as hepatitis and some cancers, dermatologic manifestations may be the first sign of the disorder and the main reason a patient seeks health care.

Anatomic and Physiologic Overview

The skin is the largest organ system of the body and is essential for human life. It participates in many vital body functions; it forms a barrier between the internal and external environment protecting the body from pathogens, helps regulate temperature and water loss, and provides sensory input.

Anatomy of the Skin, Hair, Nails, and Glands of the Skin

Skin

The skin is composed of three layers: epidermis, dermis, and subcutaneous tissue (see Fig. 60-1). The epidermis is an outermost layer of stratified epithelial cells, composed predominantly of keratinocytes. It ranges in thickness from about 0.05 mm on the eyelids to about 1.5 mm on the palms of the hands and soles of the feet. Four distinct layers compose the epidermis; from innermost to outermost, they are the stratum germinativum, stratum granulosum, stratum lucidum, and stratum corneum. Each layer becomes more differentiated

Figure 60-1 • Anatomic structures of the skin.

Labels: Hair, **Epidermis**, Sebaceous gland, **Dermis**, Hair follicle, Bulb, Papilla, **Subcutaneous tissue**, Sweat pore, Arrector pili muscle, Eccrine sweat gland, Nerve, Arteriole, Venule

(i.e., mature and with more specific functions) as it rises from the basal stratum germinativum layer to the outermost stratum corneum layer.

Epidermis

The epidermis, which is contiguous with the mucous membranes and the lining of the ear canals, consists of live, continuously dividing cells called **keratinocytes**, which differentiate and randomly migrate upward. These cells synthesize keratin; eventually they become metabolically inactive and form a thick and protective outer layer. This external layer, called the stratum corneum, is almost completely replaced every 3 to 4 weeks. The dead cells contain large amounts of **keratin**, an insoluble, fibrous protein that forms the outer barrier of the skin and has the capacity to repel pathogens and prevent excessive fluid loss from the body. Keratin is the principal hardening ingredient of the hair and nails.

Melanocytes are the special cells of the epidermis that are primarily involved in producing the pigment **melanin**, which colors the skin and hair. An individual's normal skin color is determined by the amount of melanin produced. Most of the skin of people who are dark skinned and the darker areas of the skin on people who are light skinned (e.g., the nipple) contain larger amounts of melanin and are not related to numbers of melanocytes. Normal skin color depends on race and varies from pale, almost ivory, to deep brown, almost pure black. Systemic disease affects skin color as well. For example, the skin in those who are light skinned appears bluish when there is insufficient oxygenation of the blood, yellow-green in people with jaundice, or red or flushed when there is inflammation or fever.

Production of melanin is influenced by a number of factors including a hormone secreted from the hypothalamus of the brain called *melanocyte-stimulating hormone*. It is believed that melanin production responds in a protective manner with ultraviolet light in sunlight.

Two other types of cells are common to the epidermis: Merkel and Langerhans cells. **Merkel cells** are not fully understood, but may have a role as receptors that transmit stimuli to the axon through a chemical synapse. **Langerhans cells** are believed to play a significant role in cutaneous immune system reactions. These accessory cells of the afferent immune system process invading antigens and transport the antigens to the lymph system to activate the T lymphocytes.

The characteristics of the epidermis vary in different areas of the body. It is thickest over the palms of the hands and soles of the feet and contains increased amounts of keratin. The thickness of the epidermis can increase with friction and pressure, and can result in calluses forming on the hands or corns forming on the feet.

The junction of the epidermis and dermis is an area of undulations and furrows called **rete ridges** on the epidermal side and dermal papillae on the dermal side. This junction is where anchors are found that hold together the epidermis and dermis and permits the free exchange of essential nutrients between the two layers. This interlocking between the dermis and epidermis produces ripples on the surface of the skin. On the fingertips, these ripples are called *fingerprints*. They are a person's most individual physical characteristic, and they rarely change over time (Wilhelmi & Molnar, 2014).

Dermis

The dermis makes up the largest portion of the skin, the connective tissue between the epidermis and subcutaneous tissue. It provides strength and structure in the form of collagen and elastic fibers. It is composed of two layers: papillary and reticular. Collagen fibers are loosely organized in the papillary dermis and are more tightly packed in the reticular dermis. The dermis also contains blood and lymph vessels, nerves, sweat and sebaceous glands, and hair roots.

Subcutaneous Tissue

The subcutaneous tissue, or hypodermis, is the innermost layer of the skin. It is primarily adipose and connective tissue, which provides a cushion between the skin layers and the muscles and bones. This layer also protects the nerve and vascular structures that transect the layers. It promotes skin mobility, molds body contours, and insulates the body. The subcutaneous tissues and the amount of fat deposited are important factors in body temperature regulation.

Hair

An outgrowth of the skin, hair is present over the entire body except for the palms and soles. The hair consists of a root formed in the dermis and a hair shaft that projects beyond the skin. It grows in a cavity called a *hair follicle*. Proliferation of cells in the bulb portion of the follicle causes the hair to form (see Fig. 60-1).

Hair follicles undergo continuous cycles of growth, transition, and rest throughout a person's life. The rate of growth varies; beard growth is the most rapid, followed by hair on the scalp, axillae, thighs, and eyebrows. The growth (anagen) phase may last 2 to 6 years for scalp hair, the involution (catagen) phase lasts 2 to 3 weeks, followed by the telogen or resting phase, which lasts 2 to 3 months. During telogen, hair is shed from the body. The hair follicle recycles into the growing phase spontaneously, or it can be induced by plucking hairs. Growing and resting hairs can be found side by side on all parts of the body. About 90% to 95% of the hair follicles on a normal scalp are in the growing (anagen) phase, around 1% are involuting (catagen), and 5% to 10% are in the shedding (telogen) phase at any one time. It is usual to shed approximately 100 scalp hairs each day (Habif, 2016).

There is a small bulge on the side of the hair follicle that houses the stem cells that migrate down to the follicle root and begin the cycle of reproducing the hair shaft. These bulges also contain the stem cells that migrate upward to reproduce skin. The location of these cells on the side of the hair shaft, rather than at the base, is a factor in hair loss. In conditions in which inflammation causes damage to the root of the hair, regrowth is possible. However, if inflammation causes damage to the side of the hair follicle, stem cells are destroyed and the hair will not grow.

In certain locations on the body, hair growth is controlled by sex hormones. The most obvious example is the growth of hair on the face (i.e., beard and mustache), chest, and back, which is controlled by the male hormones known as androgens. Both men and women produce and need androgens, but in differing amounts. Women with higher levels of the androgen testosterone have hair in the areas generally thought of as masculine, such as the face, chest, and lower abdomen. This is often a normal genetic variation, but if it appears along with irregular menses and weight changes, it may indicate a hormonal imbalance (Habif, 2016).

Hair in different parts of the body serves different functions. The hairs of the eyes (i.e., eyebrows and lashes), nose, and ears filter out dust, bugs, and airborne debris. The hair of the skin provides thermal insulation in mammals with hair or fur. This function is enhanced during cold or fright by

piloerection (i.e., hairs standing on end), caused by contraction of the tiny erector muscles attached to the hair follicle. The piloerector response that occurs in humans is probably vestigial (i.e., rudimentary), no longer serving its original purpose.

Hair color is supplied by various amounts of melanin within the hair shaft. Gray or white hair reflects the loss of pigment. Hair quantity and distribution can be affected by endocrine conditions. For example, Cushing syndrome causes **hirsutism** (i.e., excessive hair growth), especially in women, and hypothyroidism (i.e., underactive thyroid) causes changes in hair texture. **Alopecia** is the general loss of hair caused by various factors. Chemotherapy and radiation therapy cause reversible hair thinning or weakening of the hair shaft. Several autoimmune disorders, including systemic lupus erythematosus and alopecia areata, cause hair loss in smaller defined areas. Folliculitis of the scalp will cause inflammation of the hair roots and may result in scarring alopecia.

Nails

On the dorsal surface of the fingers and toes, a hard, transparent plate of keratin, called the *nail*, overlies the skin. The nail grows from its root, which lies under a thin fold of skin called the *cuticle*. The nail protects the fingers and toes by preserving their highly developed sensory functions, such as for picking up small objects.

Nail growth is continuous throughout life, with an average growth of 0.1 mm daily. Growth is faster in fingernails than toenails and tends to slow with aging. Complete renewal of a fingernail takes about 6 months, whereas toenail renewal takes approximately 18 months (Bolognia, Jorizzo, & Schaffer, 2012).

Glands of the Skin

There are two types of skin glands: **sebaceous glands** and sweat glands (see Fig. 60-1). The sebaceous glands are associated with hair follicles. The ducts of the sebaceous glands empty **sebum** (fatty secretions) onto the space between the hair follicle and the hair shaft, thus lubricating the hair and rendering the skin soft and pliable.

Sweat glands are found in the skin over most of the body surface, but they are most heavily concentrated in the palms of the hands and soles of the feet. Only the glans penis, clitoris, labia minora, the margins of the lips, the external ear, and the nail bed are devoid of sweat glands. Sweat glands are subclassified into two categories: eccrine and apocrine.

The eccrine sweat glands are found in all areas of the skin. Their ducts open directly onto the skin surface. The thin, watery secretion called *sweat* is produced in the basal coiled portion of the eccrine gland and is released into its narrow duct. Sweat is composed predominantly of water and contains about half of the salt content of blood plasma. Sweat is released from eccrine glands in response to elevated ambient temperature and elevated body temperature. The rate of sweat secretion is under the control of the sympathetic nervous system. Excessive sweating of the palms and soles, axillae, forehead, and other areas may occur in response to pain and stress.

The apocrine sweat glands are larger than eccrine sweat glands and are located in the axillae, periumbilical, nipple, anal region, scrotum, and labia majora. Their ducts generally open onto hair follicles. The apocrine glands become active at puberty. In women, they enlarge and recede with each menstrual cycle. Apocrine glands produce an oily sweat that is sometimes broken down by bacteria, such as *Corynebacterium* species, to produce the characteristic underarm odor. Specialized apocrine glands called *ceruminous glands* are found in the external ear, where they produce cerumen (i.e., wax).

Functions of the Skin

Protection

The skin covering most of the body is no more than 1 mm thick, but it provides very effective protection against invasion by bacteria and other foreign matter. The thickened skin of the palms and soles protects against the effects of the constant trauma that occurs in these areas.

The stratum corneum—the outer layer of the epidermis—provides the most effective barrier to epidermal water loss and penetration of environmental factors such as ultraviolet radiation, chemicals, microbes, and insect bites.

Various lipids are synthesized in the stratum corneum and are the basis for the barrier function of this layer. These are long-chain lipids that are suited for water resistant ceramides, cholesterol, and free fatty acids (Bolognia et al., 2012). The presence of these lipids in the stratum corneum creates a relatively impermeable barrier for water loss and for the entry of toxins, microbes, and other substances that come in contact with the surface of the skin.

Some substances do penetrate the skin but meet resistance in trying to move through the channels between the cell layers of the stratum corneum. Microbes and fungi, which are part of the body's normal flora, cannot penetrate unless there is a break in the skin barrier.

The basal layer, at the junction of the epidermis and dermis, is composed of collagen, anchoring fibers, and macromolecules. The basal layer serves four functions. It acts as a support structure for tissue organization and a template for regeneration; it provides selective permeability for migration of cells and proteins; it is a physical barrier between different types of cells; and it binds the epithelium to underlying cell layers (Bolognia et al., 2012).

Sensation

The receptor endings of nerves in the skin allow the body to constantly monitor the conditions of the immediate environment. The main functions of the receptors in the skin are to sense temperature, pain, light touch, and pressure (or heavy touch). Different nerve endings respond to each of the different stimuli. Although the nerve endings are distributed over the entire body, they are more concentrated in the head and distal extremities.

Fluid Balance

The stratum corneum—the outermost layer of the epidermis—has the capacity to absorb water, thereby preventing an excessive loss of water and electrolytes from the internal body and retaining moisture in the subcutaneous tissues. When skin is damaged, as occurs with a severe burn, large quantities of fluids and electrolytes may be lost rapidly, possibly leading to circulatory collapse, shock, and death (see Chapter 62).

The skin is not completely impermeable to water. Small amounts of water continuously evaporate from the skin surface.

This evaporation, called *insensible perspiration*, amounts to approximately 500 mL daily in an average-sized adult (Grossman & Porth, 2014). Insensible water loss varies with temperature, both body and ambient. In a person with a fever, the loss can increase in a predictable fashion, approximately 12% for every 1°C (1.8°F) increase in body temperature (Grossman & Porth, 2014).

Temperature Regulation

The body, in the process of creating energy, continuously produces heat as a result of the metabolism of food. This heat is dissipated primarily through the skin. Three major physical processes are involved in loss of heat from the body to the environment. The first process—radiation—is the transfer of heat to another object of lower temperature situated at a distance. The second process—conduction—is the transfer of heat from the body to a cooler object in contact with it. The third process—convection, which consists of movement of warm air molecules away from the body—is the transfer of heat by conduction to the air surrounding the body.

Evaporation from the skin aids heat loss by conduction. Heat is conducted through the skin into water molecules on its surface, causing the water to evaporate. The water on the skin surface may be from insensible perspiration, sweat, or the environment.

Normally, all of these mechanisms for heat loss are used. However, when the ambient temperature is very high, radiation and convection are ineffective, and evaporation becomes the only means of heat loss.

Under normal conditions, metabolic heat production is balanced by heat loss, and the internal temperature of the body is maintained constant at approximately 37°C (98.6°F). The rate of heat loss depends primarily on the surface temperature of the skin, which is a function of the skin blood flow. Under normal conditions, the total blood circulated through the skin is approximately 450 mL/min, or 10 to 20 times the amount of blood required to provide necessary metabolites and oxygen. Blood flow through these skin vessels is controlled primarily by the sympathetic nervous system. Increased blood flow to the skin results in more heat delivered to the skin and a greater rate of heat loss from the body. In contrast, decreased skin blood flow decreases the skin temperature and helps conserve heat for the body. When the temperature of the body begins to fall, as occurs on a cold day, the blood vessels of the skin constrict, thereby reducing heat loss from the body (Bolognia et al., 2012).

Sweating is another process by which the body can regulate the rate of heat loss. Sweating does not occur until the core body temperature exceeds 37°C (98.6°F), regardless of skin temperature. In extremely hot environments, the rate of sweat production may be as high as 1 L per hour. Under some circumstances (e.g., emotional stress), sweating may occur as a reflex and may be unrelated to the need to lose heat from the body (LeBlond, Brown, Suneja, et al., 2014).

Vitamin Production

Skin exposed to ultraviolet light can convert substances necessary for synthesizing vitamin D (cholecalciferol). Vitamin D is essential for preventing osteoporosis and rickets, a condition that causes bone deformities and results from a deficiency of vitamin D, calcium, and phosphorus. It is estimated that most people need 5 to 30 minutes of sun exposure twice a week in order for this synthesis to occur; however, numerous individual and environmental variables make a uniform recommendation difficult. As yet, no studies have determined if vitamin D synthesis in the skin can occur without increasing skin cancer risk (Office of Dietary Supplements, National Institutes of Health, 2016). Adequate amounts of Vitamin D should be obtained from a healthy diet and supplementation rather than intentional sun exposure (American Academy of Dermatology, 2010).

Immune Response Function

The skin functions not only as a barrier defense against environmental hazards, but also produces immune responses. The skin has the capacity to generate innate and adaptive immune responses (Bolognia et al., 2012). Innate immune functions of the skin include the closely packed layers of the stratum corneum, the nonspecific inflammatory response of pattern recognition receptors, and a chemical environment that inhibits microbial colonization (Grossman & Porth, 2014). The Langerhans cells of the skin are part of adaptive immunity. They function as antigen-presenting cells, with the ability to transport foreign substances to nearby lymph nodes for cell-mediated immune reaction (Grossman & Porth, 2014).

 Gerontologic Considerations

The skin undergoes many physiologic changes associated with normal aging that affect functioning; decreased dermal thickness, degeneration of collagen, decreased sebum production, and increased vascular fragility (Grossman & Porth, 2014). Other factors such as lifetime of excessive sun exposure, systemic diseases, and poor nutrition can increase the range of skin conditions and the rapidity with which they appear. In addition, certain medications (e.g., antihistamine, antibiotic, and diuretic agents) are photosensitizing and increase the damage that results from sun exposure.

The visible changes in the skin of older adults include dryness, wrinkling, uneven pigmentation, and various proliferative lesions. Cellular changes associated with aging include a thinning at the junction of the dermis and epidermis. The result of this thinning is fewer anchoring sites between the two skin layers, which mean that even minor injury or stress to the epidermis can cause it to shear away from the dermis. This phenomenon may account for the increased vulnerability of aged skin to trauma. With increasing age, the epidermis and dermis thin and flatten, causing wrinkles, sags, and overlapping skin folds (see Fig. 60-2).

Loss of the subcutaneous tissue substances of elastin, collagen, and fat diminishes the protection and cushioning of underlying tissues and organs, decreases muscle tone, and results in the loss of the insulating properties of fat.

Cellular replacement slows as a result of aging. As the dermal layers thin, the skin becomes fragile and transparent. The blood supply to the skin also changes with age. Vessels, especially the capillary loops, decrease in number and size. These vascular changes contribute to the delayed wound healing commonly seen in the older adult patient. The dry scaly skin common in aging is likely the consequence of decreased water retention by an impaired stratum corneum and the decreased number and functional ability of sweat and sebaceous glands

Figure 60-2 • Hands with skin atrophy common to aging skin.

(Bolognia et al., 2012). Reduced androgen levels are thought to contribute to declining sebaceous gland function.

Hair growth gradually diminishes, especially over the lower legs and dorsum of the feet. Thinning is common in the scalp, axillae, and pubic areas. Other functions affected by normal aging include the barrier function of skin, sensory perception, and thermoregulation.

Damage from excessive sun exposure (photoaging) has detrimental effects on the normal aging of skin. A lifetime of outdoor work or outdoor activities (e.g., construction work, lifeguarding, sunbathing) without prudent use of covering clothing and sunscreens can lead to profound wrinkling; increased loss of elasticity; mottled, pigmented areas; cutaneous atrophy; and benign or malignant lesions.

Many skin lesions are part of normal aging. Recognizing and differentiating these lesions enables the examiner to assist the patient to feel less anxious about changes in skin. Chart 60-1 summarizes some skin lesions that are expected to appear as the skin ages. These are normal and require no special attention unless the skin becomes infected or irritated.

Assessment

When caring for patients with dermatologic disorders, the nurse obtains important information through the health

---

Chart 60-1 **Benign Changes in the Skin of the Older Adult**

- Cherry angiomas (bright red "moles")
- Diminished hair, especially on scalp and pubic area
- Dyschromias (color variations)
  - Solar lentigo (liver spots)
  - Melasma (dark discoloration of the skin)
  - Lentigines (freckles)
- Neurodermatitis (itchy spots)
- Seborrheic keratoses (crusty brown "stuck-on" patches)
- Spider angiomas (see Fig. 49-3)
- Telangiectasias (red marks on skin caused by stretching of the superficial blood vessels)
- Wrinkles
- Xerosis (dryness)
- Xanthelasma (yellowish waxy deposits on upper and lower eyelids)

ASSESSMENT

Chart 60-2

Assessing for Skin Disorders

Patient history relevant to skin disorders may be obtained by asking the following questions:

- When did you first notice this skin problem? (In addition, investigate duration and intensity.)
- Has it occurred previously?
- Are there any other symptoms?
- What site was first affected?
- What did the rash or lesion look like when it first appeared?
- Where and how fast did it spread?
- Do you have any itching, burning, tingling, or crawling sensations?
- Is there any loss of sensation?
- Is the problem worse at a particular time or season?
- How do you think it started?
- Do you have a history of hay fever, asthma, hives, eczema, or allergies?
- Who in your family has skin problems or rashes?

- Did the eruptions appear after certain foods were eaten? Which foods?
- When the problem occurred, had you recently consumed alcohol?
- What relation do you think there may be between a specific event and the outbreak of the rash or lesion?
- What medications are you taking?
- What topical medication (ointment, cream, salve) have you put on the lesion (including over-the-counter medications)?
- What skin products or cosmetics do you use?
- What is your occupation?
- What in your immediate environment (plants, animals, chemicals, infections) might be precipitating this disorder? Is there anything new, or are there any changes in the environment?
- Does anything touching your skin cause a rash?
- How has this affected you (or your life)?
- Is there anything else you wish to talk about in regard to this disorder?

---

history and direct observations. The nurse's skill in physical assessment and an understanding of the anatomy and function of the skin can ensure that deviations from normal are recognized, reported, and documented.

Health History

During the health history interview, the nurse asks about use of hair and skin products, as well as any family and personal history of skin allergies; allergic reactions to food, medications, and chemicals; previous skin conditions; and skin cancer (Bobonich & Nolen, 2014). The health history addresses the onset, signs and symptoms, location, and duration of any pain, itching, rash, or other discomfort experienced by the patient. The names of cosmetics, soaps, shampoos, and other personal hygiene products are obtained if there have been any recent skin conditions noticed with the use of these products. The patient is questioned about nonprescription or herbal preparations that are being used. Chart 60-2 lists selected questions useful in obtaining appropriate information, and Chart 60-3 provides genetic factors influencing skin conditions.

Unfolding Patient Stories: Vincent Brody • Part 2

Recall from Chapter 4 **Vincent Brody,** with chronic obstructive pulmonary disease (COPD), who spends most of the day in a recliner chair smoking and has a poor nutritional intake due to shortness of breath. He is admitted to the hospital with COPD exacerbation. What are factors related to his diagnosis? What background information can influence skin breakdown? Describe the skin assessment performed by the nurse.

Care for Vincent and other patients in a realistic virtual environment: **vSim for Nursing (thepoint.lww. com/vSimMedicalSurgical).** Practice documenting these patients' care in DocuCare **(thepoint.lww.com/ DocuCareEHR).**

Physical Assessment

Assessment of the skin involves the entire skin area, including the mucous membranes, scalp, hair, and nails. The skin is a reflection of a person's overall health, and alterations commonly correspond to disease in other organ systems. Inspection and palpation are techniques commonly used in examining the skin. The room must be well lighted and warm. A penlight may be used to highlight lesions. The patient completely disrobes and is adequately draped. Gloves are worn during skin examination.

The general appearance of the skin is assessed by observing color, temperature, moisture or dryness, skin texture (rough or smooth), lesions, vascularity, mobility, and the condition of the hair and nails. Skin turgor, possible edema, and elasticity are assessed by palpation.

Assessing Skin Color

The color gradations that occur in people with dark skin are largely determined by genetics; they may be described as light, medium, or dark. In people with dark skin, melanin is produced at a faster rate and in larger quantities than in people with light skin. Healthy dark skin has a reddish base or undertone. The buccal mucosa, tongue, lips, and nails normally are pink. The skin of exposed portions of the body, especially in sunny, warm climates, tends to be more pigmented than the rest of the body. Almost every process that occurs on the skin causes some color change. For example, **hypopigmentation** (i.e., loss of pigmentation) may be caused by a fungal infection, eczema, or **vitiligo** (i.e., white patches); **hyperpigmentation** (i.e., increase in pigmentation) can occur after sun injury or as a result of aging. Dark pigment responds with discoloration after injury or inflammation, and patients with dark skin more often experience postinflammatory hyperpigmentation than those with lighter skin. The hyperpigmentation eventually fades but may require months to do so.

Changes in skin color in people with dark skin are more noticeable and may cause more concern because the discoloration is more readily visible. Because of the increased activity

Chart 60-3 GENETICS IN NURSING PRACTICE
Integumentary Conditions

Integumentary conditions influenced by genetic factors include the following:

Autosomal Dominant:

- Ehlers–Danlos
- Legius syndrome
- Loeys–Dietz syndrome
- Neurofibromatosis type 1
- Tuberous sclerosis

Autosomal Recessive:

- Albinism
- Congenital ichthyosis

X-Linked Dominant:

- Incontinentia pigmenti

X-Linked Recessive:

- Hypohidrotic ectodermal dysplasia
- Pseudoxanthoma elasticum

Inheritance pattern is not distinct; however, there is a genetic predisposition for the disease:

- Ectodermal dysplasias
- Eczema
- Port wine stain
- Psoriasis

Nursing Assessments

Refer to Chapter 5, Chart 5-2: Genetics in Nursing Practice: Genetic Aspects of Health Assessment

Family History Assessment Specific to Skin Disorders

- Assess for family members in the past three generations with integumentary impairment or abnormalities.
- Inquire about the nature and type of skin lesions and age at onset (e.g., skin involvement with incontinentia pigmenti occurs in the first few weeks of life with blistering of the skin, whereas lesions of neurofibromatosis type 1 may appear in early childhood through adulthood).
- Note gender of affected individuals (e.g., mostly females with incontinentia pigmenti, mostly males with hypohidrotic ectodermal dysplasia).
- Inquire about the presence of other clinical features, such as unusual hair, teeth, or nails; thrombocytopenia; recurrent infections.

Patient Assessment

- Assess for related clinical features, such as sparse eyebrows and eyelashes, abnormally shaped teeth, alopecia, nail abnormalities (e.g., hypohidrotic ectodermal dysplasia).
- Assess for related alterations in vision, such as nystagmus or strabismus; albinism; retinal abnormalities (e.g., pseudoxanthoma elasticum); Lisch nodules and/or optic glioma (neurofibromatosis type 1).
- Perform a thorough skin assessment.
- Inquire about sensitivity to the sun.
- Obtain history of wounds and delayed healing time.
- Assess for receding gum line (as seen with Ehlers–Danlos).
- Assess, record location and size of all skin lesions (e.g., café au lait spots, port wine stains, bruises).
- Assess for abdominal pulsations or distention (abdominal aneurysm common in Loeys–Dietz syndrome).
- Inspect skin for presence and location of freckles (axillary freckles are associated with genetic disorders). Inquire if freckles were present upon birth and if the amount or location of freckles has grown.

Genetics Resources

The Ehlers–Danlos Society, ehlers-danlos.com
Neurofibromatosis Network, www.nfnetwork.org
See Chapter 8, Chart 8-7 for components of genetic counseling.

---

of melanocytes in darker skin, pigment changes can become quite obvious and cause great psychological discomfort. Some variation in skin pigment levels is considered normal. Examples include the pigmented crease across the bridge of the nose, some pigmented streaks in the nails, and pigmented spots on the sclera of the eye. Women often develop a dark line along the midline of the lower abdomen during pregnancy (Taylor, Kelly, Lim, et al., 2016).

Table 60-1 provides an overview of color changes in people who are light and dark skinned.

Cyanosis

Cyanosis is the bluish discoloration that results from a lack of oxygen in the blood (see Fig. 60-3). It appears with shock or with respiratory or circulatory compromise. In people with light skin, cyanosis manifests as a bluish hue to the lips, fingertips, and nail beds. Other indications of decreased tissue perfusion include cold, clammy skin; a rapid, thready pulse; and rapid, shallow respirations. The conjunctivae of the eyelids are examined for pallor and **petechiae** (i.e., pinpoint red spots that result from blood leakage into skin).

In a person with dark skin, the skin usually assumes a grayish cast. To detect cyanosis, the areas around the mouth and lips and over the cheekbones and earlobes should be observed.

Erythema

Erythema is redness of the skin caused by the dilation of capillaries. In people who are light skinned, it is easily observable. To determine possible inflammation, the skin is palpated for increased warmth and for smoothness (i.e., edema) or hardness (i.e., intracellular infiltration). Because dark skin tends to assume a purple-gray cast when an inflammatory process is present, it may be difficult to detect erythema.

Jaundice

Jaundice, a yellowing of the skin, is directly related to elevations in serum bilirubin and is often first observed in the sclerae and mucous membranes (see Fig. 60-3).

Assessing Rash

In instances of pruritus (i.e., itching), the patient is asked to indicate which areas of the body are involved. The skin is then stretched gently to decrease the reddish tone and make the rash more visible. Pointing a penlight laterally across the skin may highlight the rash, making it easier to observe. The differences in skin texture are then assessed by running the tips of the fingers lightly over the skin. The borders of the rash may be palpable. The patient's mouth and ears are included in the examination (rubeola, or measles, causes a red cast to appear on the ears, and skin cancers are quite common on the top of the ears). The patient's temperature is assessed, and the lymph

TABLE 60-1 Color Changes in Light and Dark Skin

Etiology	Light Skin	Dark Skin
Pallor		
Anemia—decreased hematocrit		
Shock—decreased perfusion, vasoconstriction	Generalized pallor	Brown skin appears yellow-brown, dull; black skin appears ashen gray, dull. (Observe areas with least pigmentation: conjunctivae, mucous membranes.)
Local arterial insufficiency	Marked localized pallor (lower extremities, especially when elevated)	Ashen gray, dull; cool to palpation
Albinism—total absence of pigment melanin	Whitish pink	Tan, cream, white
Vitiligo—a condition characterized by destruction of the melanocytes in circumscribed areas of the skin (may be localized or widespread)	Patchy, milky white spots, often symmetric bilaterally	Same
Cyanosis		
Increased amount of unoxygenated hemoglobin:	Dusky blue	Dark but dull, lifeless; only severe cyanosis is apparent in skin, and may appear grayish. (Observe conjunctivae, oral mucosa, nail beds.)
Central—chronic heart and lung diseases cause arterial desaturation	Nail beds dusky	
Peripheral—exposure to cold, anxiety		
Erythema		
Hyperemia—increased blood flow through engorged arterial vessels, as in inflammation, fever, alcohol intake, blushing	Red, bright pink	Purplish-gray tinge, but difficult to see. (Palpate for increased warmth with inflammation, taut skin, and hardening of deep tissues.)
Polycythemia—increased red blood cells, capillary stasis	Ruddy blue in face, oral mucosa, conjunctivae, hands and feet	Well concealed by pigment. (Observe for redness in lips.)
Carbon monoxide poisoning	Bright, cherry red in face and upper torso	Cherry red nail beds, lips, and oral mucosa
Venous stasis—decreased blood flow from area, engorged venules	Dusky rubor of dependent extremities (a prelude to necrosis with pressure ulcer)	Easily masked. (Use palpation to identify warmth or edema.)
Jaundice		
Increased serum bilirubin concentration (>2 mg/dL) due to liver dysfunction or hemolysis, as after severe burns or some infections	Yellow first in sclerae, hard palate, and mucous membranes; then over skin	Check sclerae for yellow near limbus; do not mistake normal yellowish fatty deposits in the periphery under eyelids for jaundice. (Jaundice is best noted at junction of hard and soft palate, on palms.)
Carotenemia—increased level of serum carotene from ingestion of large amounts of carotene-rich foods	Yellow-orange tinge in forehead, palms and soles, and nasolabial folds, but no yellowing in sclerae or mucous membranes	Yellow-orange tinge in palms and soles
Uremia—Kidney injury causes retained urochrome pigments in the blood	Orange-green or gray overlying pallor of anemia; may also have ecchymoses and purpura	Easily masked. (Rely on laboratory and clinical findings.)
Brown-Tan		
Addison disease—cortisol deficiency stimulates increased melanin production	Bronzed appearance, an "external tan"; most apparent around nipples, perineum, genitalia, and pressure points (inner thighs, buttocks, elbows, axillae)	Easily masked. (Rely on laboratory and clinical findings.)
Café au lait spots—caused by increased melanin pigment in basal cell layer	Tan to light brown, irregularly shaped, oval patch with well-defined borders	Often not visible in the very dark skinned person

Adapted from Taylor, S. C., Kelly, A. P., Lim, H., et al. (2014). *Dermatology for skin of color* (2nd ed.). New York: McGraw-Hill Medical.

Figure 60-3 • Examples of skin color changes: (**A**) the bluish tint of cyanosis and (**B**) the yellow hue of jaundice. From Weber, J. W., & Kelley, J. (2014). *Health assessment in nursing* (5th ed.). Philadelphia, PA: Lippincott Williams & Wilkins.

nodes are palpated especially in the axillae, inguinal fold, and behind the knees (popliteal area).

Assessing Skin Lesions

Skin lesions are the most prominent characteristics of dermatologic conditions. They vary in size, shape, and cause and are classified according to their appearance and origin. Skin lesions can be described as primary or secondary. Primary lesions are the initial lesions and are characteristic of the disease itself. Secondary lesions result from changes in primary lesions resulting from external causes, such as scratching, trauma, infections, or changes caused by wound healing. Depending on the stage of development, skin lesions are further categorized by type and appearance (see Table 60-2).

TABLE 60-2 **Primary and Secondary Skin Lesions**

Lesion	Description	Examples
Primary Lesions		
MACULE, PATCH Macule / Patch	Flat, nonpalpable skin color change (color may be brown, white, tan, purple, red) • *Macule:* <1 cm; circumscribed border • *Patch:* >1 cm; may have irregular border	Freckles, flat moles, petechia, rubella, vitiligo, port wine stains, ecchymosis
PAPULE, PLAQUE Papule / Plaque	Elevated, palpable, solid mass with a circumscribed border Plaque may be coalesced papules with flat top • *Papule:* <0.5 cm • *Plaque:* >0.5 cm	*Papules:* Elevated nevi, warts, lichen planus *Plaques:* Psoriasis, actinic keratosis
NODULE, TUMOR Tumor	Elevated, palpable, solid mass that extends deeper into the dermis than a papule • *Nodule:* 0.5–2 cm; circumscribed • *Tumor:* >1–2 cm; tumors do not always have sharp borders	*Nodules:* Lipoma, squamous cell carcinoma, poorly absorbed injection, dermatofibroma *Tumors:* Larger lipoma, carcinoma
VESICLE, BULLA Bulla / Vesicle	Circumscribed, elevated, palpable mass containing serous fluid • *Vesicle:* <0.5 cm • *Bulla:* >0.5 cm	*Vesicles:* Herpes simplex/zoster, varicella, poison ivy, second-degree burn (blister) *Bulla:* Pemphigus, contact dermatitis, large burn blisters, poison ivy, bullous impetigo
WHEAL	Elevated mass with transient borders; often irregular; size and color vary Caused by movement of serous fluid into the dermis; does not contain free fluid in a cavity (e.g., as a vesicle does)	Urticaria (hives), insect bites
PUSTULE	Pus-filled vesicle or bulla	Acne, impetigo, furuncles, carbuncles
CYST	Encapsulated fluid-filled or semisolid mass in the subcutaneous tissue or dermis	Sebaceous cyst, epidermoid cysts

Lesion	Description	Examples
Secondary Lesions		
EROSION	Loss of superficial epidermis that does not extend to dermis; depressed, moist area	Ruptured vesicles, scratch marks
ULCER	Skin loss extending past epidermis; necrotic tissue loss; bleeding and scarring possible	Stasis ulcer of venous insufficiency, pressure ulcer
FISSURE	Linear crack in the skin that may extend to dermis	Chapped lips or hands, tinea pedis
SCALES	Flakes secondary to desquamated, dead epithelium that may adhere to skin surface; color varies (silvery, white); texture varies (thick, fine)	Dandruff, psoriasis, dry skin, pityriasis rosea
CRUST	Dried residue of serum, blood, or pus on skin surface Large, adherent crust is a scab	Residue left after vesicle rupture: impetigo, herpes, eczema
SCAR (CICATRIX)	Skin mark left after healing of a wound or lesion; represents replacement by connective tissue of the injured tissue • *Young scars:* Red or purple • *Mature scars:* White or glistening	Healed wound or surgical incision
KELOID	Hypertrophied scar tissue secondary to excessive collagen formation during healing; elevated, irregular, red Greater incidence among African Americans	Keloid of ear piercing or surgical incision
ATROPHY	Thin, dry, transparent appearance of epidermis; loss of surface markings; secondary to loss of collagen and elastin; underlying vessels may be visible	Aged skin, arterial insufficiency
LICHENIFICATION	Thickening and roughening of the skin or accentuated skin markings that may be secondary to repeated rubbing, irritation, scratching	Contact dermatitis

Adapted from Bickley, L. S. (2013). *Bates' guide to physical examination and history taking* (11th ed.). Philadelphia, PA: Lippincott Williams & Wilkins; Weber, J. W., & Kelley, J. (2014). *Health assessment in nursing* (5th ed.). Philadelphia, PA: Lippincott Williams & Wilkins.

A preliminary assessment of the eruption or lesion helps identify the type of dermatosis (i.e., abnormal skin condition) and indicates whether the lesion is primary or secondary. At the same time, the anatomic distribution of the eruption or lesion should be observed because certain diseases more regularly affect certain sites of the body and are distributed in characteristic patterns and shapes (see Figs. 60-4 and 60-5). To determine the extent of the regional distribution, the left and right sides of the body should be compared while the color and shape of the lesions are assessed. The degree of pigmentation of the patient's skin may affect the appearance of a lesion. Lesions may be black, purple, or gray on dark skin and tan or red in patients with light skin. A metric ruler is used to measure the size of the lesions so that any further extension can be compared with this baseline measurement. After observation, the lesions are palpated to determine their texture, shape, and border and to see if they are soft and filled with fluid or hard and fixed to the surrounding tissue.

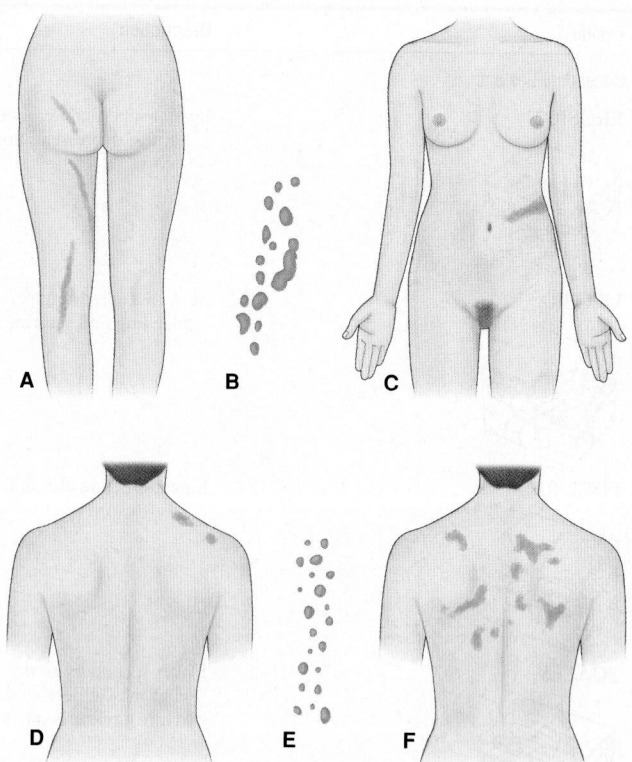

Figure 60-5 • Skin lesion configurations. **A.** Linear (in a line). **B.** Annular and arciform (circular or arcing). **C.** Zosteriform (linear along a nerve route). **D.** Grouped (clustered). **E.** Discrete (separate and distinct). **F.** Confluent (merged).

Skin lesions are described clearly and in detail on the patient's health record, using precise terminology:
- Color of the lesion
- Any redness, heat, pain, or swelling
- Size and location of the involved area
- Pattern of eruption (e.g., macular, papular, scaling, oozing, discrete, confluent)
- Distribution of the lesion (e.g., bilateral, symmetric, linear, circular)

If acute open wounds or lesions are found on inspection of the skin, a comprehensive assessment should be made and documented. This assessment should address the following issues:
- *Wound bed:* Inspect for necrotic and granulation tissue, epithelium, exudate, color, and odor.
- *Wound edges and margins:* Observe for undermining (i.e., extension of the wound under the surface skin), and evaluate for condition of skin (i.e., necrotic).
- *Wound size:* Measure in centimeters, as appropriate, to determine diameter and depth of the wound and surrounding erythema.
- *Surrounding skin:* Assess for color, suppleness and moisture, irritation, and scaling.

Assessing Vascularity and Hydration

After the color of the skin has been evaluated and lesions have been inspected, an assessment of vascular changes in the skin is performed. A description of vascular changes includes location, distribution, color, size, and the presence of pulsations.

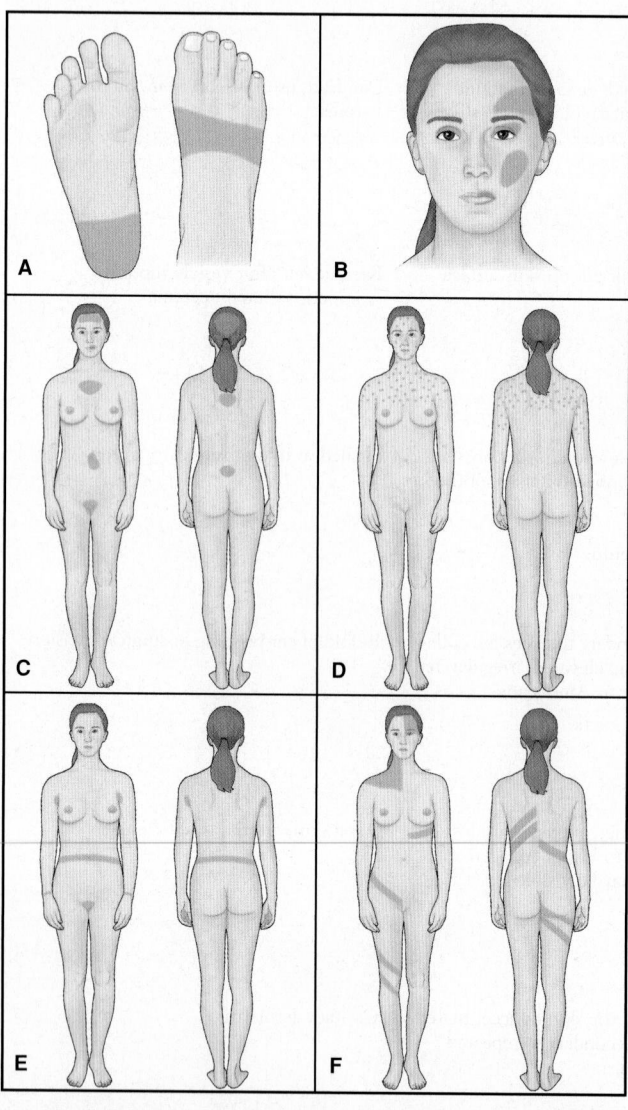

Figure 60-4 • Anatomic distribution of common skin disorders. **A.** Contact dermatitis (shoes). **B.** Contact dermatitis (cosmetics, perfumes, earrings). **C.** Seborrheic dermatitis. **D.** Acne. **E.** Scabies. **F.** Herpes zoster (shingles).

TABLE 60-3 Vascular Lesions

PETECHIA (PL. PETECHIAE)	Round red or purple macule Small (1–2 mm) Secondary to blood extravasation Associated with bleeding tendencies or emboli to skin
ECCHYMOSIS (PL. ECCHYMOSES)	Round or irregular macular lesion Larger than petechia Color varies and changes—black, yellow, and green hues Secondary to blood extravasation Associated with trauma, bleeding tendencies
CHERRY ANGIOMA	Papular and round Red or purple Noted on trunk, extremities May blanch with pressure Normal age-related skin alteration Usually not clinically significant
SPIDER ANGIOMA	Red, arteriole lesion Central body with radiating branches Noted on face, neck, arms, trunk Rare below the waist May blanch with pressure Associated with liver disease, pregnancy, vitamin B deficiency
TELANGIECTASIA (VENOUS STAR)	Shape varies—spider like or linear Color bluish or red Does not blanch when pressure is applied Noted on legs, anterior chest Secondary to superficial dilation of venous vessels and capillaries Associated with increased venous pressure states (varicosities)

Adapted from Bickley, L. S. (2013). *Bates' guide to physical examination and history taking* (11th ed.). Philadelphia, PA: Lippincott Williams & Wilkins; Weber, J. W., & Kelley, J. (2014). *Health assessment in nursing* (5th ed.). Philadelphia, PA: Lippincott Williams & Wilkins.

Common vascular changes include petechiae, ecchymoses, **telangiectasias** (venous stars), and angiomas (see Table 60-3).

Skin moisture, temperature, and texture are assessed primarily by palpation. The turgor (i.e., elasticity) of the skin, which decreases in normal aging, may be a factor in assessing the hydration status of a patient. To assess skin turgor, the skin should be gently pinched between the thumb and forefinger. The skin is observed to see how long it takes to return to baseline. People who are dehydrated or those with dry skin will display decreased skin turgor, where the skin remains tented after being pinched rather than returning to normal almost immediately. Edema is indicated when the skin appears tense and shiny, when a finger gently pressed into the skin leaves an indentation or "pit." Assessing the depth of the pit and length of time to resolution indicates the extent of edema (LeBlond et al., 2014).

Assessing the Nails

A brief inspection of the nails includes observation of configuration, color, and consistency. Many alterations in the nail or nail bed reflect local or systemic abnormalities in progress or resulting from past events (see Fig. 60-6). Beau lines, a transverse depression in the nails, may reflect retarded growth of the nail matrix because of severe illness or, more commonly, local trauma. Ridging, hypertrophy, and other changes may also be visible because of local trauma. Paronychia, an inflammation of the skin around the nail, is usually accompanied by tenderness and erythema. Pitted surface of the nails is a definite indication of psoriasis. Spoon-shaped nails can indicate severe iron-deficiency anemia. The angle between the normal nail and its base is 160 degrees. When palpated, the nail base is usually firm. Clubbing of the nails is manifested by a straightening of the normal angle (180 degrees or greater) and softening of the nail base. The softened area feels sponge like when palpated (Bickley, 2013). Clubbing can be a normal variant, but it is most often associated with pulmonary disease and can be a sign of chronic hypoxia (Habif, 2016).

Assessing the Hair

The hair assessment is carried out by inspection and palpation. Gloves are worn by the examiner, and the examination room should be well lighted. The hair is separated so that the condition of the skin underneath can be easily seen. The examiner notes the color, texture, and distribution of hair shafts. The wooden end of a cotton swab can be used to make small parts in the hair so that the scalp can be inspected. Any abnormal lesions, evidence of itching, inflammation, scaling, or signs of infestation (i.e., lice or mites) are documented.

Color and Texture

Natural hair color ranges from white to black. Hair begins to turn gray or white with age, when loss of melanin in the hair shaft becomes apparent. Loss of melanin in hair can occur at a younger age and may be due to heredity or genetic traits. The person with albinism (i.e., partial or complete absence of pigmentation) has a genetic predisposition to white hair from birth. The natural state of the hair can be altered by using hair dyes, bleaches, and curling or relaxing products. The use of these products has varying impact on hair, depending on its natural characteristics. For example, the use of straightening chemicals on the hair of most people can cause extensive breakage and hair loss (Bobonich & Nolen, 2014).

The texture of scalp hair ranges from fine to coarse, silky to brittle, oily to dry, and shiny to dull, and hair can be straight, curly, or kinky. Dry, brittle hair may result from the overuse of hair dyes, hair dryers, and curling irons or from endocrine disorders, such as thyroid dysfunction. Oily hair is usually caused by increased secretion from the sebaceous glands close to the scalp. If the patient reports a recent change in hair texture, the underlying reason is pursued; the alteration may arise simply from the overuse of commercial hair products or from changing to a new shampoo.

Distribution

Body hair distribution varies with location. Hair over most of the body is fine, except in the axillae and pubic areas, where it is coarse. Pubic hair, which develops at puberty, forms a diamond shape extending up to the umbilicus in boys and

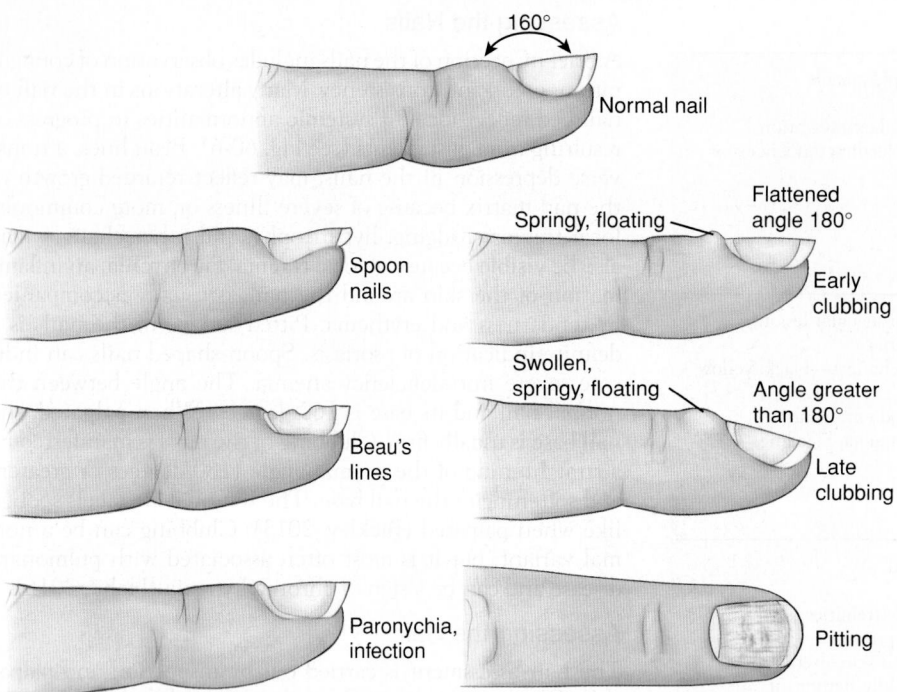

Figure 60-6 • Common nail disorders.

men. Female pubic hair resembles an inverted triangle. If the pattern found is more characteristic of the opposite gender, it may indicate an endocrine disorder and further investigation is in order. Racial differences in hair are expected, such as straight hair in Asians and curly, coarse hair in people of African descent.

Men tend to have more body and facial hair than women. Alopecia can occur over the entire body or be localized to a specific area. Scalp hair loss may be patchy or may range from generalized thinning to total baldness. When assessing scalp hair loss, it is important to investigate the underlying cause with the patient. Patchy hair loss may be from habitual hair pulling or twisting; excessive traction on the hair (e.g., braiding too tightly); excessive use of dyes, straighteners, and oils; chemotherapeutic agents (e.g., doxorubicin [Adriamycin], cyclophosphamide [Cytoxan]); bacterial or fungal infection; or moles or lesions on the scalp. Well-defined patches of hair loss generally indicate the condition called *alopecia areata*. The precise mechanism is unknown, but may be triggered by an interaction between genetic and environmental factors.

Regrowth in most cases is spontaneous and occurs in 1 to 3 months, though in some rarer patterns, the hair loss is recurrent or even permanent (Habif, 2016).

Hair Loss

The most common cause of hair loss is male pattern baldness (i.e., androgenic alopecia), which affects more than half of the male population and is believed to be related to heredity, aging, and androgen (male hormone) levels. Androgen is necessary for male pattern baldness to develop. The pattern of hair loss begins with receding of the hairline in the frontal temporal area and may progress to gradual thinning and complete loss of hair over the top of the scalp and crown. The typical pattern of male hair loss is illustrated in Figure 60-7. Although androgenic alopecia is considered a male disorder, millions of women experience female pattern hair loss, which is typically not seen with other signs of hyperandrogenism. Most women tend to retain hair at the frontal border and do not become completely bald (Bobonich & Nolen, 2014).

Figure 60-7 • The progression of male pattern baldness.

Other Changes

Male pattern hair distribution may be seen in some women at the time of menopause, when the hormone estrogen is no longer produced by the ovaries. In women with hirsutism, excessive hair may grow on the face, chest, shoulders, and pubic area. If menopause is ruled out as the underlying cause, other hormonal changes related to pituitary or adrenal dysfunction must be investigated.

Because patients with skin conditions may be viewed negatively by others, these patients may become distraught and avoid interaction with people. Skin conditions can lead to isolation, job loss, and economic hardship as well as poor self-esteem.

Some conditions may lead to feelings of depression, frustration, self-consciousness, poor self-image, and rejection. Itching and skin irritation (features of many skin diseases) may be constant annoyances. These discomforts may result in loss of sleep, anxiety, and depressive symptoms, all of which reinforce the general distress and fatigue that frequently accompany skin disorders.

For patients experiencing physical and psychological discomforts, the nurse needs to provide understanding, explanations of the problem, appropriate instructions related to treatment, nursing support, and encouragement. It is imperative to overcome any aversion that may be felt when caring for patients with unattractive skin disorders. The nurse should show no sign of hesitancy when approaching patients with skin disorders. Such hesitancy only reinforces the psychological trauma of the disorder.

Skin Consequences of Selected Systemic Diseases

Diabetes

Because diabetes causes changes in circulation and cell nutrition, it can have a great impact on skin status. Some of the more common skin conditions encountered in diabetes are discussed in this section. Further information can be found in Chapter 51.

Diabetic Dermopathy

Diabetic dermopathy (shin spots or pigmented pretibial papules) is a frequent occurrence in people with diabetes. These lesions are found on the lower anterior legs, forearms, and thighs and over other bony prominences. They are thought to be caused by diabetes-associated changes in the small vessels that supply the skin and trauma. Each spot starts as a dull red bump, smaller than a pencil eraser. It slowly spreads to about 1 inch (the size of a quarter), becomes scaly, and eventually leaves a brownish, slightly depressed scar on the skin (Bobonich & Nolen, 2014).

Stasis Dermatitis

Stasis dermatitis is an eczematous eruption that occurs on the lower legs of patients with venous insufficiency. It is very common in patients with diabetes. Large vessels are damaged, compromising circulation to the lower arms and legs. The skin suffers from lack of nutrients, becoming very dry and fragile. Minor injuries heal slowly, and ulcers form easily. It initially presents with variable erythema and scale and pruritus. When chronic, it leads to permanent changes in skin color, hyper or hypopigmentation, and either fragile or thicker skin texture (fibrosis).

Skin Infections

Bacterial infections may appear as small pimples around hair follicles (i.e., folliculitis). The most frequently affected sites include the lower legs, lower abdomen, and buttocks. Sometimes, these lesions enlarge to become furuncles or carbuncles. Furuncles begin in a hair follicle, progressively enlarging and invading deeper into tissue to form an abscess. Carbuncles are formed by multiple contiguous lesions (Habif, 2016). The skin of patients with diabetes is prone to bacterial and fungal infections. If the blood glucose level is not well controlled, these infections may be very slow to heal.

Fungal infections are quite common in areas that remain moist (under breasts, upper thighs, in axillae). *Candida* (i.e., yeast) infections appear beefy red and often have small pustules around the border of the area, with the skin appearing moist and raw.

Dermatophyte infections are dry and only minimally red, with more scale. Common sites are the toenails and feet.

Nurses must be alert to the signs of these common infections. If necessary, they should bring them to the attention of the patient's primary provider and help the patient or family learn basic skin maintenance techniques.

Leg and Foot Ulcers

Because of changes in peripheral nerves, patients with diabetes do not always sense minor injuries to the lower legs and feet. Infections begin and if left untreated may lead to ulcerations. Ulcerations are often not noticed and become quite large before being treated. Ulcerations unresponsive to treatment are a leading cause of diabetic foot and leg amputations.

Human Immune Deficiency Virus Disease

Cutaneous signs may be the first manifestation of human immune deficiency virus (HIV), appearing in more than 90% of people who are HIV infected as immune function deteriorates. These skin signs correlate with low CD4+ counts. Some disorders such as Kaposi sarcoma, oral hairy leukoplakia, facial molluscum contagiosum, and oral candidiasis may suggest that CD4+ counts are less than 200 to 300 cells/mcL. Skin infections, both bacterial and viral, are common and will appear more severe than expected. Acute flare of chronic conditions such as seborrhea or acne may indicate a new infection. Being sensitive to these changes can alert the nurse so that early interventions can be initiated (Schwartz, 2015).

Diagnostic Evaluation

A wide range of diagnostic studies may be performed in patients with altered integumentary function. The nurse educates the patient about the purpose, what to expect, and any possible side effects related to these examinations prior to testing. The nurse also notes trends in results because they provide information about whether lesions are primary or secondary, disease progression, and the patient's response to therapy.

Skin Biopsy

Performed to obtain tissue for microscopic examination, a skin biopsy may be obtained by shave, excision, or by a skin punch instrument that removes a small core of tissue. Biopsies are performed on skin nodules, plaques, blisters, and other lesions to rule out malignancy, to aid in diagnosis, and to perform additional testing such as Gram stain for bacteria or periodic acid–Schiff (PAS) for fungal elements.

Patch Testing

Performed to identify substances to which the patient has developed an allergy, patch testing involves applying the suspected allergens, such as nickel or fragrances, to normal skin under occlusive patches. Patients wear these occluded strips on their backs for 48 hours, and the area is assessed after 72 hours. The development of redness, fine elevations, or itching is considered a weak positive reaction; fine blisters, papules, and severe itching indicate a moderately positive reaction; and blisters, pain, and ulceration indicate a strong positive reaction. The nurse educates the patient with a positive reaction to avoid the allergen, which is often quite difficult, due to the prevalence of many allergens.

Skin Scrapings

Tissue samples are scraped from suspected fungal lesions with a scalpel blade that has been moistened with oil so that the scraped skin adheres to the blade. The scraped material is transferred to a glass slide, covered with a coverslip, and examined microscopically. The spores and hyphae of dermatophyte infections, as well as infestations such as scabies, can be visualized.

Tzanck Smear

The Tzanck smear is a test used to examine cells from blistering skin conditions, such as herpes zoster, varicella, herpes simplex, and all forms of pemphigus. The secretions from a suspected lesion are applied to a glass slide, stained, and examined.

Wood Light Examination

Wood light is a special lamp that produces long-wave ultraviolet rays, which result in a characteristic blue to dark purple fluorescence. The color of the fluorescent light is best seen in a darkened room, where it is possible to differentiate epidermal from dermal lesions and hypo- and hyperpigmented lesions from normal skin. The patient is reassured that the light is not harmful to skin or eyes. Lesions that still contain melanin almost disappear under ultraviolet light, whereas lesions that are devoid of melanin increase in whiteness with ultraviolet light.

Clinical Photographs

Photographs are taken to document the nature and extent of the skin condition and are used to determine progress or improvement resulting from treatment. They are sometimes used to track the status of moles to document if the characteristics of the mole are changing.

Nursing Implications

The nurse may be responsible to ensure that consent forms are completed for surgical procedures and for clinical photography, that all specimens collected are managed according to protocol, that a log is maintained tracking specimens to and from the laboratory, and that results are received in a timely manner. The nurse educates the patient regarding appropriate care of surgical sites and implication of test results.

CRITICAL THINKING EXERCISES

1 **ebp** A neighbor of yours tells you that her 8-year-old twin daughters have joined the swim team that is affiliated with the local pool in your community. She is looking forward to enjoying time at the pool with her daughters, but is worried that she will get sunburned. She tells you that she is thinking about getting a tan at a tanning salon before she begins to take her daughters to the pool. Is this an advisable practice that might diminish her risk of getting sunburned or from getting skin cancer? Describe evidence-based measures she might take that can reduce her risk of getting sunburned and reduce her future risk of skin cancer.

2 **pq** A 79-year-old man admitted to an acute rehabilitation facility is going to be discharged home to the care of his 40-year-old daughter. You suspect that the patient's daughter may not be familiar with the changes in the skin of older adults. What changes are important for her to recognize as she assists her father with his activities of daily living? What changes are normal with age? What skin signs may be important for her to report to her father's primary provider?

3 A 55-year-old woman presents to the family practice clinic where you work as a staff nurse for her periodic health screening. She tells you that she has been healthy since her last health screening, but notes that she is concerned that she is losing hair, much as her mother did at the same age. Hair assessment is an important part of the evaluation of the integument. Discuss the important questions you will ask the patient as you continue to gather data for her health history. Describe the important foci of her physical and psychosocial assessment.

REFERENCES

Books

Bickley, L. S. (2013). *Bates' guide to physical examination and history taking* (11th ed.). Philadelphia, PA: Lippincott Williams & Wilkins.

Bobonich, M. A., & Nolen, M. E. (2014). *Dermatology for advanced practice clinicians*. Philadelphia, PA: Wolters Kluwer. Kindle Edition.

Bolognia, J., Jorizzo, J., & Schaffer, J. (2012). *Dermatology* (3rd ed.). Philadelphia, PA: Elsevier Saunders.

Grossman, S., & Porth, C. M. (2014). *Porth's pathophysiology: Concepts of altered health states* (9th ed.). Philadelphia, PA: Lippincott Williams & Wilkins.

Habif, T. P. (2016). *Clinical dermatology* (6th ed.). St. Louis, MO: Elsevier Health Sciences. Kindle Edition.

LeBlond, R. F., Brown, D. D., Suneja, M., et al. (2014). *DeGowin's diagnostic examination* (10th ed.). New York: McGraw-Hill.

Taylor, S. C., Kelly, A. P., Lim, H., et al. (2016). *Dermatology for skin of color* (2nd ed.). New York: McGraw-Hill Medical.

Weber, J. W., & Kelley, J. (2014). *Health assessment in nursing* (5th ed.). Philadelphia, PA: Lippincott Williams & Wilkins.

Journals and Electronic Documents

American Academy of Dermatology. (2010). Position statement on Vitamin D. Retrieved on 6/10/2016 at: www.aad.org/Forms/Policies/Uploads/PS/PS-Vitamin%20D%20Postition%20Statement.pdf

Office of Dietary Supplements, National Institutes of Health. (2016). *Vitamin D; Fact sheet for health professionals.* Retrieved on 6/10/2016 at: ods.od.nih.gov/factsheets/VitaminD-HealthProfessional/

Schwartz, R. A. (2015). Cutaneous manifestations of HIV. *Medscape.* Retrieved on 6/10/2016 at: emedicine.medscape.com/article/1133746-overview

Wilhelmi, B. J., & Molnar, J. A. (2014). Finger nail and tip injuries. *Medscape.* Retrieved on 6/10/2016 at: emedicine.medscape.com/article/1285680-overview

Resources

American Academy of Dermatology (AAD), www.aad.org

Centers for Disease Control and Prevention, Skin Cancer Facts, www.cdc.gov/cancer/skin/basic_info/index.htm, www.cdc.gov/cancer/skin/

Dermatology Atlas (DermIS), a cooperation between the Department of Clinical Social Medicine (University of Heidelberg) and the Department of Dermatology (University of Erlangen), www.dermis.net

National Institutes of Health, National Institute on Aging, Skin Care and Aging, www.nia.nih.gov/health/publication/skin-care-and-aging

New Zealand Dermatology Society (DermNet NZ), www.dermnetnz.org

Skin Cancer Foundation (lists approved sunscreens and other sun protection products), www.skincancer.org

Management of Patients With Dermatologic Disorders

LEARNING OBJECTIVES

On completion of this chapter, the learner will be able to:

1 Describe the management of the patient with a wound, pruritus, or a dermatologic secretory disorder.
2 Discuss the management and nursing care of the patient with infections of the skin or parasitic skin diseases.
3 Identify the management and nursing care of the patient with noninfectious inflammatory dermatoses, including contact dermatitis or psoriasis.
4 Use the nursing process as a framework for care of patients with blistering disorders, including

toxic epidermal necrolysis and Stevens–Johnson syndrome.
5 Describe the management and nursing care of the patient with skin tumors (benign, malignant, and metastatic).
6 Apply the nursing process as a framework for care of the patient with melanoma.
7 Compare the various types of dermatologic and plastic reconstructive procedures.
8 Identify the management and nursing care of patients undergoing plastic and cosmetic procedures.

GLOSSARY

acantholysis: separation of epidermal cells from each other due to damage or abnormality of the intracellular substance
bullae: large, fluid-filled blisters
carbuncle: localized skin infection involving several hair follicles
cheilitis: inflammation of the lips (when dry, cracking, inflamed skin occurs at the corners of the mouth, it is called *angular cheilitis;* when caused by sun exposure, it is called *solar cheilitis*)
comedones: the primary lesions of acne, caused by sebum blockage in the hair follicle
cytotoxic: destructive of cells
débridement: removal of necrotic or dead tissue by mechanical, surgical, chemical, or autolytic means
dermatitis: any inflammation of the skin
dermatosis: any abnormal skin lesion
epidermopoiesis: development of epidermal cells

furuncle: localized skin infection of a single hair follicle; also known as a boil
hydrophilic: a material that absorbs moisture
hydrophobic: a material that repels moisture
hygroscopic: a material that absorbs moisture from the air
lichenification: thickening of the horny layer of the skin; also known as scaling
liniments: lotions with added oil for increased softening of the skin
pruritus: itching
pyodermas: pus-forming bacterial skin infections
striae: bandlike streaks on the skin, distinguished by color, texture, depression, or elevation from the tissue in which they are found; usually purplish or white
suspensions: liquid preparations in which powder is suspended, requiring shaking before use
tinea: a common superficial fungal infection on the skin or scalp; also called ringworm
xerosis: overly dry skin

Dermatologic disorders are encountered frequently by nurses across many practice settings. Nursing management of patients with dermatologic problems includes administering topical and systemic medications and managing dressings. The nurse can also be instrumental in educating patients how to care for their skin. The objectives of nursing interventions are to prevent additional skin damage, prevent secondary infection, reverse the inflammatory process, and relieve the symptoms.

PATIENTS WITH SKIN DISORDERS

Some skin problems are markedly aggravated by soap and water; therefore, bathing routines are modified according to the

condition. Denuded skin, whether the area of desquamation is large or small, is excessively prone to damage by chemicals, trauma, and even bathing. The friction of a towel, if applied with vigor, is often sufficient to produce a brisk inflammatory response that can cause a lesion to flare (Inamadar & Palit, 2013).

Protecting the Skin

Basic skin care in bathing a patient with skin problems is as follows:

- A mild, lipid-free soap or soap substitute is used (e.g., Dove Sensitive Skin, Cetaphil, Cerave, Vanicream).
- The area is rinsed completely and blotted dry with a soft cloth.

- Deodorant soaps are avoided.
- Laundry detergents and fabric softener free of fragrance are used.

Special care is necessary when changing dressings. The use of pledgets saturated with oil, sterile saline, or another prescribed solution helps loosen crusts, remove exudates, or free an adherent dry dressing (Dabiri, Damstetter, & Phillips, 2014).

Preventing Secondary Infection

Skin lesions should be regarded as potentially infectious, and proper safety precautions should be observed until the diagnosis is established. Most lesions with purulent drainage contain infectious material. The nurse and primary provider must adhere to standard precautions and wear gloves when inspecting the skin or changing a dressing. The use of standard personal protective equipment (PPE) and proper disposal of any contaminated dressing is carried out according to Occupational Safety and Health Administration (OSHA) regulations (OSHA, 2012).

Reversing the Inflammatory Process

The type of skin lesion (e.g., oozing, infected, or dry) usually determines the type of local medication or treatment that is prescribed. As a rule, if the skin is acutely inflamed (i.e., hot, red, and swollen) and oozing, it is best to apply soothing lotions. For chronic conditions in which the skin surface is dry and scaly, water-soluble emulsions, creams, ointments, and pastes are used (Dabiri et al., 2014). The therapy is modified as the responses of the skin indicate. The patient and the nurse note whether the medication, tape, or dressings irritate the skin (Landriscina, Rosen, & Friedman, 2015).

Wound Dressing Care for Skin Disorders

There are three types of wound dressings: passive, interactive, and active. *Passive dressings* have only a protective function and maintain a moist environment for natural healing. They include those that just cover the area (e.g., DuoDERM, Tegaderm) and may remain in place for several days. *Interactive dressings* are capable of absorbing wound exudate while (1) maintaining a moist environment in the area of the wound and (2) allowing the surrounding skin to remain dry. They include hydrocolloids, alginates, and hydrogels. It is thought that interactive dressings are able to modify the physiology of the wound environment by modulating and stimulating cellular activity and by releasing growth factors (Dabiri et al., 2014). *Active dressings* improve the healing process and decrease healing time. They include skin grafts and biologic skin substitutes. Both interactive and active dressings create a moist environment at the interface of the wound with the dressing.

Because so many wound care products are available, it is often difficult to select the most appropriate product for a specific wound. Selection of products should be made carefully because of their expense. Both clinical efficacy and health-related outcomes (e.g., decreased pain, increased mobility) should be used to measure the success of a product for a wound. Even with the availability of a large variety of dressings, an appropriate selection can be made if certain

principles are maintained. These principles are referred to as the five rules of wound care (Dabiri et al., 2014).

1. *Rule 1: Categorization.* The nurse learns about dressings by generic category and compares new products with those that already make up the category. The nurse becomes familiar with indications, contraindications, and side effects. The best dressing may be created by combining products in different categories to achieve several goals at the same time. These categories are discussed in subsequent sections.
2. *Rule 2: Selection.* The nurse selects the safest and most effective, easy-to-use, and cost-effective dressing possible. Nurses follow the primary provider's prescriptions for dressings. They must be prepared to give the primary provider feedback about the dressing's effect on the wound, ease of use for the patient, and other considerations when applicable.
3. *Rule 3: Change.* The nurse changes dressings based on patient, wound, and dressing assessments, not on standardized routines.
4. *Rule 4: Evolution.* As the wound progresses through the phases of wound healing, the dressing protocol is altered to optimize healing. It is rare, especially in cases of chronic wounds, that the same dressing material is appropriate throughout the healing process. The nurse educates the patient or family caregiver about wound care and ensures that the family has access to appropriate dressing choices.
5. *Rule 5: Practice.* Practice with dressing material is required for the nurse to learn the performance parameters of the particular dressing. Refining the skills of applying appropriate dressings correctly and learning about new dressing products are essential nursing responsibilities. Dressing changes should not be delegated to unlicensed personnel; these techniques require the knowledge base and assessment skills of professional nurses.

Autolytic Débridement

Autolytic **débridement** is a process that uses the body's own digestive enzymes to break down necrotic tissue. The wound is kept moist with occlusive dressings. Eschar and necrotic debris are softened, liquefied, and separated from the bed of the wound.

Several commercially available products mirror the enzymes that the body produces naturally and are referred to as enzymatic débriding agents; an example is collagenase (Santyl). Application of these products speeds the rate at which necrotic tissue is removed. This method, although slower than surgical débridement, is more discriminating for tissue removal and does not damage healthy tissue surrounding the wound. When enzymatic débridement is being used under an occlusive dressing, a foul odor and exudate is produced by the breakdown of cellular debris. This odor does not indicate that the wound is infected. The nurse should expect this reaction and help the patient and family understand the reason for the odor (Landriscina et al., 2015; McCallon, Weir, & Lantis, 2015).

Categories of Dressings

Table 61-1 provides a guide to the function and action of wound dressings.

TABLE 61-1 Quick Guide to Function and Action of Wound Dressings

Function	Action	Example
Absorption	Absorbs exudates	Alginates, composite dressings, foams, gauze, hydrocolloids, hydrogels
Cleansing	Removes purulent drainage, foreign debris, and devitalized tissue	Wound cleansers
Débridement	*Autolytic*—covers a wound and allows enzymes to self-digest sloughed skin	Absorption beads, pastes, powders; alginates; composite dressings; foams; hydrate gauze; hydrogels; hydrocolloids; transparent films; wound care systems
	Chemical or enzymatic—applied topically to break down devitalized tissue	Enzymatic débridement agents
	Mechanical—removes devitalized tissue with mechanical force	Wound cleansers, gauze (wet to dry), whirlpool
Diathermy	Produces electrical current to promote warmth and new tissue growth	
Hydration	Adds moisture to a wound	Gauze (saturated with saline solution), hydrogels, wound care systems
Maintain moist environment	Manages moisture levels in a wound and maintains a moist environment	Composites, contact layers, foams, gauze (impregnated or saturated), hydrogels, hydrocolloids, transparent films, wound care systems
Manage high-output wounds	Manages excessive quantities of exudates	Pouching systems
Pack or fill dead space	Prevents premature wound closure or fills shallow areas and provides absorption	Absorbent beads, powders, pastes; alginates; composites, foams; gauze (impregnated and nonimpregnated)
Protect and cover wound	Provides protection from the external environment	Composites, compression bandages/wraps, foams, gauze dressings, hydrogels, hydrocolloids, transparent film dressings
Protect periwound skin	Prevents moisture and mechanical trauma from damaging delicate tissue around wound	Composites, foams, hydrocolloids, pouching systems, skin sealants, transparent film dressings
Provide therapeutic compression	Provides appropriate levels of support to the lower extremities in venous stasis disease	Compression bandages, wraps, graduated compression stockings

Adapted from Krasner, D., Rodeheaver, G., Sibbald, G., et al. (2012). *Chronic wound care: A clinical source book for healthcare professionals* (5th ed.). Malvern, PA: HMP Communications.

Occlusive Dressings

Occlusive dressings may be commercially produced or made inexpensively from sterile or nonsterile gauze squares or wrap. Occlusive dressings cover topical medication that is applied to a skin lesion. The area is kept airtight by using plastic film (e.g., plastic wrap). Plastic film is thin and readily adapts to all sizes, body shapes, and skin surfaces. In general, plastic wrap should be used no more than 12 hours each day. Plastic surgical tape containing a corticosteroid in the adhesive layer can be cut to size and applied to individual lesions.

Moisture-Retentive Dressings

Commercially produced moisture-retentive dressings are efficient at removing exudate because of their higher moisture-vapor transmission rate; some have reservoirs that can hold excessive exudate. A number of moisture-retentive dressings are already impregnated with saline solution, petrolatum, zinc-saline solution, hydrogel, or antimicrobial agents, thereby eliminating the need to coat the skin to avoid maceration. The main advantages of moisture-retentive dressings are improved fibrinolysis, accelerated epidermal resurfacing, reduced pain, fewer infections, less scar tissue, gentle

autolytic débridement, and decreased frequency of dressing changes. Depending on the product used and the type of dermatologic conditions encountered, most moisture-retentive dressings may remain in place from 12 to 24 hours; some can remain in place as long as a week (Landriscina et al., 2015).

Hydrogels

Hydrogels are polymers with 90% to 95% water content. They are available in impregnated sheets or as a gel. Their high moisture content makes them ideal for autolytic débridement of wounds. They are semitransparent, allowing for wound inspection without dressing removal. They are comfortable and soothing for the painful wound. They require a secondary dressing to keep them in place. Hydrogels are appropriate for superficial wounds with high serous output, such as abrasions, skin graft sites, and draining venous ulcers (Landriscina et al., 2015).

Hydrocolloids

Hydrocolloids are composed of a water-impermeable, polyurethane outer covering separated from the wound by a hydrocolloid material. They are adherent and nonpermeable to water vapor and oxygen. As water evaporates over the wound, it is absorbed into the dressing, which softens and discolors with the increased water content. The dressing can be removed without damage to the wound. As the dressing absorbs water, it produces a foul-smelling, yellowish covering over the wound. This is a normal chemical interaction between the dressing and wound exudate and should not be confused with purulent drainage from the wound. Unfortunately, most of the hydrocolloid dressings are opaque, preventing inspection of the wound without removal of the dressing.

Available in sheets and in gels, hydrocolloids are a good choice for both exudative and acute wounds. Easy to use and comfortable, hydrocolloid dressings promote débridement and formation of granulation tissue. Most can be left in place for as long as 7 days and can be submerged in water for bathing or showering. Hydrocolloid dressings are more effective than saline gauze or paraffin gauze dressings in completely healing chronic wounds (Landriscina et al., 2015).

Foam Dressings

Foam dressings consist of microporous polyurethane with an absorptive **hydrophilic** (water-absorbing) surface that covers the wound and a **hydrophobic** (water-resistant) backing to block leakage of exudate. They are nonadherent and require a secondary dressing to keep them in place. Moisture is absorbed into the foam layer, decreasing maceration of surrounding tissue. A moist environment is maintained, and removal of the dressing does not damage the wound. The foams are opaque and must be removed for wound inspection. Foams are a good choice for exudative wounds. They are especially helpful over bony prominences because they provide contoured cushioning (Landriscina et al., 2015).

Calcium Alginates

Calcium alginates are derived from algae or kelp polysaccharides and consist of very absorbent calcium alginate fibers (Dabiri et al., 2014). They are hemostatic and bioabsorbable and can be used as sheets or mats of absorbent material. As the exudate is absorbed, the fibers turn into a viscous hydrogel. They are useful in areas where the tissue is more irritated or macerated. The alginate dressing forms a moist pocket over the wound while the surrounding skin stays dry. The dressing also reacts with wound fluid, which forms a foul-smelling coating. Alginates work well when packed into a deep cavity, wound, or sinus tract with heavy drainage. They are nonadherent and require a secondary dressing. Wound experts

suggest that alginates are superior to other modern dressings for débriding necrotic wounds (Landriscina et al., 2015).

Medical Management

Medical management of skin disorders includes a host of prescribed and over-the-counter therapies.

Pharmacologic Therapy

Topical medications are often used to treat skin conditions. High concentrations of some medications can be applied directly to the affected site with little systemic absorption and therefore with few systemic side effects. However, some medications are readily absorbed through the skin and can produce systemic effects. Because topical preparations may induce allergic contact **dermatitis** (skin inflammation) in patients who are sensitive, any untoward response should be reported immediately and the medication discontinued.

Medicated lotions, creams, ointments, gels, and powders are frequently used to treat skin lesions. In general, moisture-retentive dressings, with or without medication, are used in the acute stage; lotions and creams are reserved for the subacute stage; and ointments are used when inflammation has become chronic and the skin is dry with scaling or **lichenification** (thickening of the horny layer of the skin).

With all types of topical medication, the patient is educated to apply the medication gently but thoroughly and, when necessary, to cover the medication with a dressing to protect clothing. Table 61-2 lists commonly used topical preparations and medications.

Lotions

Lotions are frequently used to replenish lost skin oils or to relieve pruritus. They must be applied every 3 or 4 hours for sustained therapeutic effect. They are usually applied directly to the skin, but a dressing soaked in the lotion can be placed on the affected area. However, if left in place for a longer period, it may crust and cake on the skin.

Lotions are of two types: suspensions and liniments. **Suspensions** consist of either a powder in water that requires shaking before application, or clear solutions, which contain completely dissolved active ingredients. A suspension such as calamine lotion provides a rapid cooling and drying effect as it evaporates, leaving a thin, medicinal layer of powder on the affected skin. **Liniments** are lotions with oil added to prevent

TABLE 61-2 Common Topical Preparations and Medications

Preparation	Product Name
Moisturizer creams	AcidMantle Cream, Curel Cream, Dermasil, Eucerin, Lubriderm, Noxzema Skin Cream
Moisturizer ointments	Aquaphor Ointment, Eutra Swiss Skin Cream, Vaseline Ointment
Topical anesthetic agents	Lidocaine (Xylocaine) of various strengths in the form of spray, ointment, gel; lidocaine 2.5% and prilocaine 2.5% (EMLA cream)
Topical antibiotic agents	Bacitracin, bacitracin and polymyxin B (Polysporin), mupirocin 2% (Bactroban ointment or cream), erythromycin 2% (Emgel, Eryderm solution), clindamycin phosphate 1% (Cleocin cream, gel, solution), gentamicin sulfate 1% (Garamycin cream or ointment), 1% silver sulfadiazine cream (Silvadene)

Adapted from Goldsmith, L., Katz, S. I., Gilchrist B. A., et al. (2012). *Fitzpatrick's dermatology in general medicine* (8th ed.). New York: McGraw-Hill.

crusting. Because lotions are easy to use, therapeutic adherence is generally good.

Powders

Powders usually have a talc, zinc oxide, bentonite, or cornstarch base and are dusted on the skin with a shaker or with cotton sponges. Although their therapeutic action is brief, powders act as **hygroscopic** agents that absorb and retain moisture from the air and reduce friction between skin surfaces and clothing or bedding.

Creams

Creams may be suspensions of oil in water or emulsions of water in oil, with additional ingredients to prevent bacterial and fungal growth. Both may cause an allergic reaction such as contact dermatitis. Oil-in-water creams are easily applied and usually are the most cosmetically acceptable to the patient. Although they can be used on the face, they tend to have a drying effect. Water-in-oil emulsions are greasier and are preferred for drying and flaking dermatoses. Creams usually are rubbed into the skin by hand. They are used for their moisturizing and emollient effects.

Gels

Gels are semisolid emulsions that become liquid when applied to the skin or scalp. They are cosmetically acceptable to the patient because they are not visible after application, and they are greaseless and nonstaining. The newer water-based gels appear to penetrate the skin more effectively and cause less stinging on application. They are especially useful for acute dermatitis in which there is weeping exudate (e.g., poison ivy) and are applied the same way as creams.

Pastes

Pastes are mixtures of powders and ointments and are used in inflammatory blistering conditions. They adhere to the skin and may be difficult to remove without using an oil (e.g., olive oil, mineral oil). Pastes are applied with a wooden tongue depressor or gloved hand.

Ointments

Ointments retard water loss and lubricate and protect the skin. They are the preferred vehicle for delivering medication to chronic or localized dry skin conditions, such as eczema or psoriasis. Ointments are applied with a wooden tongue depressor or gloved hand.

Sprays and Aerosols

Spray and aerosol preparations may be used on any widespread dermatologic condition. They evaporate on contact and are used infrequently.

Topical Corticosteroids

Corticosteroids are widely used in treating dermatologic conditions to provide anti-inflammatory, antipruritic, and vasoconstrictive effects. The patient is educated to apply this medication according to strict guidelines, using it sparingly but rubbing it into the prescribed area thoroughly. Absorption of topical corticosteroids is enhanced when the skin is hydrated or the affected area is covered by an occlusive or moisture-retentive dressing (Karch, 2015). Inappropriate use of topical corticosteroids can result in local and systemic side effects, especially when the medication is absorbed through inflamed and excoriated skin, is used under occlusive dressings, or is used for long periods on sensitive areas. Local side effects may include skin atrophy and thinning, **striae** (band-like streaks), and telangiectasias (dilated blood vessels). Thinning of the skin results from the ability of corticosteroids to inhibit skin collagen synthesis. The thinning process can be reversed by discontinuing the medication, but striae and telangiectasia are permanent. Systemic side effects may include hyperglycemia and symptoms of Cushing syndrome (see Chapter 52). Caution is required when applying corticosteroids around the eyes because long-term use may cause glaucoma or cataracts, and the anti-inflammatory effect of corticosteroids may mask existing viral or fungal infections.

Concentrated (fluorinated) corticosteroids should never be applied on the face or intertriginous areas (i.e., axillae and groin) because these areas have a thinner stratum corneum and therefore absorption is enhanced. Persistent use of concentrated topical corticosteroids in any location may produce acne-like dermatitis, known as steroid-induced acne, and hypertrichosis (excessive hair growth). Because some topical corticosteroid preparations are available without prescription, patients should be cautioned about prolonged and inappropriate use. Table 61-3 lists topical corticosteroid preparations according to potency.

Intralesional Therapy

Intralesional therapy consists of injecting a sterile suspension of medication (usually a corticosteroid) into or just below a lesion. Although this treatment may have an anti-inflammatory effect, local atrophy and discoloration may result if the medication is injected into subcutaneous fat. Skin lesions treated with intralesional therapy include psoriasis, keloids, and cystic acne. Occasionally, immunotherapeutic and antifungal agents are given as intralesional therapy.

Systemic Medications

Systemic medications are also prescribed for skin conditions. These include corticosteroids for short-term therapy for contact dermatitis or for long-term treatment of a chronic **dermatosis** (skin lesion), such as pemphigus vulgaris. Other frequently used systemic medications include antibiotic, antifungal, antihistamine, sedative, analgesic, tranquilizing, **cytotoxic** (destructive of cells), and immunosuppressive agents.

Nursing Management

Management begins with a health history, direct observation, and a complete physical examination (see Chapter 60). Because of its visibility, a skin condition is usually difficult to ignore or conceal from others and may therefore cause the patient emotional distress. The major goals for the patient may include maintenance of skin integrity, relief of discomfort, promotion of restful sleep, self-acceptance, knowledge about skin care, and avoidance of complications.

Nursing management for patients who must perform self-care for skin problems, such as applying medications and dressings, focuses on educating the patient about how to cleanse the affected area and pat it dry, apply medication to the lesion while the skin is moist, cover the area with plastic

TABLE 61-3 Potency: Topical Corticosteroids

Potency	Topical Corticosteroid	Preparations
OTC	0.5–1% hydrocortisone	Cream, lotion, ointment
Lowest	Dexamethasone 0.1% (Decaderm)	Cream, ointment, aerosol, gel
	Alclometasone 0.05% (Aclovate)	Cream, ointment
	Hydrocortisone 2.5% (Hytone)	Cream, lotion, ointment
Low–medium	Desonide 0.05% (DesOwen, Tridesilon)	Cream, lotion, ointment
	Fluocinolone acetonide 0.025% (Synalar)	Cream, solution
	Hydrocortisone valerate 0.2% (Westcort)	Cream, solution
	Betamethasone valerate 0.1% (Valisone)	Cream, ointment
	Fluticasone propionate 0.05% (Cutivate)	Cream, ointment
Medium–high	Triamcinolone acetonide 0.1–0.5% (Aristocort)	Cream, ointment, lotion
	Fluocinonide 0.05% (Lidex)	Cream, ointment, gel
	Desoximetasone 0.05–0.25% (Topicort)	Cream, ointment, gel
	Fluocinolone 0.2% (Synalar)	Cream, ointment
	Diflorasone diacetate 0.05% (Psorcon)	Cream, ointment
Very high	Clobetasol propionate 0.05% (Dermovate)	Cream, ointment, gel
	Betamethasone dipropionate 0.05% (Diprolene)	Cream, ointment, gel
	Halobetasol propionate 0.05% (Ultravate)	Cream, ointment

OTC, over the counter.
Adapted from Karch, A. M. (2015). *2015 Lippincott's nursing drug guide.* Philadelphia, PA: Lippincott Williams & Wilkins.

(e.g., Telfa pads, plastic wrap, vinyl gloves, plastic bag) if recommended, and cover it with an elastic bandage, dressing, or paper tape to seal the edges. Dressings that contain or cover a topical corticosteroid should be removed for 12 of every 24 hours to prevent adverse events.

Other forms of dressings, such as those used to cover topical medications, include soft cotton cloth and stretchable cotton dressings (e.g., Surgitube, Tubegauz) that can be used for fingers, toes, hands, and feet. The hands can be covered with disposable polyethylene or vinyl gloves sealed at the wrists; the feet can be wrapped in plastic bags covered by cotton socks. Gloves and socks that are already impregnated with emollients, making application to the hands and feet more convenient, are also available. When large areas of the body must be covered, cotton cloth topped by an expandable stockinette can be used. Disposable diapers or cloths folded in diaper fashion are useful for dressing the groin and the perineal areas. Axillary dressings can be made of cotton cloth, or a commercially prepared dressing may be used and taped in place or held by dress shields. A turban or plastic shower cap is useful for holding dressings on the scalp. A face mask, made from gauze with holes cut out for the eyes, nose, and mouth, may be held in place with gauze ties looped through holes cut in the four corners of the mask.

PRURITUS

General Pruritus

Pruritus (itching) is the most common symptom of patients with dermatologic disorders (Carr, Veledar, & Chen, 2014; Tarikci, Kocatürk, Güngör, et al., 2015). Itch receptors are unmyelinated, penicillate (brushlike) nerve endings that are found exclusively in the skin, mucous membranes, and cornea. Although pruritus is usually caused by primary skin disease with resultant rash or lesions, it may occur without a rash or lesion. This is referred to as essential pruritus, which generally has a rapid onset, may be severe, and interferes with normal daily activities.

Pruritus may be the first indication of a systemic internal disease such as diabetes, blood disorders, or cancer (occult malignancy of the breast or colon, lymphoma). It may also accompany kidney, hepatic, and thyroid diseases (see Chart 61-1). Some common oral medications such as aspirin,

---

Chart 61-1

Systemic Disorders Associated With Generalized Pruritus

- Chronic kidney disease
- Endocrine disease (thyrotoxicosis, hypothyroidism, diabetes)
- Folliculitis (bacterial, candidiasis, dermatophyte)
- Hematologic disorders (iron deficiency anemia)
- Infestations (scabies, lice, other insects)
- Malignancies (polycythemia vera, Hodgkin lymphoma, lymphoma, leukemia, multiple myeloma, mycosis fungoides, and cancers of the lung, breast, central nervous system, and gastrointestinal tract)
- Neurologic disorders (multiple sclerosis, brain abscess, brain tumor)
- Obstructive biliary disease (primary biliary cirrhosis, extrahepatic biliary obstruction, drug-induced cholestasis)
- Pruritus of pregnancy (pruritic urticarial papules of pregnancy, cholestasis of pregnancy, pemphigoid of pregnancy)
- Psychiatric disorders (emotional stress, anxiety, neurosis, phobias)
- Skin conditions (seborrheic dermatitis, folliculitis, atopic dermatitis)

Adapted from Tarikci, N., Kocaturk, E., Gungor, F., et al. (2015). Pruritus in systemic diseases: A review of etiological factors and new treatment modalities. *The Scientific World Journal.* 2015, 1–8.

antibiotics, hormones (e.g., estrogens, testosterone, or oral contraceptives), and opioids (e.g., morphine) may cause pruritus directly or by increasing sensitivity to ultraviolet light. Certain soaps and chemicals, radiation therapy, prickly heat (miliaria), and contact with woolen garments are associated with pruritus as well. Pruritus may also be caused by psychological factors, such as excessive stress in family or work situations, and is called *psychodermatosis* (Tarikci et al., 2015).

 Gerontologic Considerations

Pruritus occurs frequently in older adults as a result of dry skin. Older adults are also more likely to have a systemic illness that triggers pruritus, are at higher risk for occult malignancy, and are more likely to be taking multiple medications than younger people. All of these factors increase the incidence of pruritus in older adults (Eliopoulos, 2018).

Pathophysiology

Scratching the pruritic area causes the inflamed cells and nerve endings to release histamine, which produces more pruritus, generating a vicious itch–scratch cycle. If the patient responds to an itch by scratching, the integrity of the skin may be altered, and excoriation, redness, raised areas (i.e., wheals), infection, or changes in pigmentation may result. Pruritus usually is more severe at night and is less frequently reported during waking hours, probably because the person is distracted by daily activities. At night, when there are fewer distractions, the slightest pruritus cannot be easily ignored. Severe itching can be debilitating (Bolier, Elferink, & Beuers, 2016).

Medical Management

A thorough history and physical examination usually provide clues to the underlying cause of the pruritus, such as hay fever, allergy, recent administration of a new medication, or a change of cosmetics or soaps. After the cause has been identified, treatment of the condition should relieve the pruritus. Signs of infection and environmental clues, such as warm, dry air or irritating bed linens, should be identified. In general, washing with soap and hot water is avoided. Bath oils containing a surfactant that allows the oil to mix with bathwater (e.g., Lubath, Alpha Keri) may be sufficient for cleaning. However, an older adult patient or a patient with unsteady balance should avoid adding oil because it increases the danger of slipping in the bathtub. A warm bath with a mild soap followed by application of a bland emollient to moist skin can control **xerosis** (overly dry skin). Applying a cold compress, ice cube, or cool agents that contain menthol and camphor (which constrict blood vessels) may also help relieve pruritus (Tarikci et al., 2015).

Pharmacologic Therapy

Topical antipruritic agents (e.g., lidocaine, prilocaine) or capsaicin cream (Capzasin) may be useful in providing relief from localized pruritus. Topical corticosteroids are effective when used to diminish pruritus that occurs secondary to inflammatory conditions because of their anti-inflammatory effects. Oral antihistamines are frequently prescribed and may be effective when the pruritus is nocturnal, particularly agents such as diphenhydramine (Benadryl) or hydroxyzine

(Atarax), which also cause somnolence, resulting in a restful and comfortable sleep. Other nonsedating antihistamines are not beneficial in relieving pruritus. Selective serotonin reuptake inhibitor antidepressants (e.g., fluoxetine [Prozac], sertraline [Zoloft]) may be effective, particularly in patients with pruritus that is secondary to cholestasis or the uremia of chronic kidney disease (Bolier et al., 2016; Chan, Li, Wong, et al., 2013; Hong, Buddenkotte, Berger, et al., 2013).

Nursing Management

The nurse reinforces the reasons for the prescribed therapeutic regimen and educates the patient about specific points of care. The effectiveness of therapy may be gauged by asking the patient to rate the extent of itching pre- and post-therapy with a visual analog scale (VAS; see Chapter 20, Table 20-3 for an example of a VAS) (Bolier et al., 2016). If baths have been prescribed, the patient is reminded to use tepid (not hot) water and to shake off the excess water and blot between intertriginous areas (body folds) with a towel. Rubbing vigorously with the towel is avoided because this overstimulates the skin and causes more itching. It also removes water from the stratum corneum. Immediately after bathing, the skin should be lubricated with an emollient to trap moisture.

The patient is instructed to avoid situations that cause vasodilation. Examples include exposure to an overly warm environment and ingestion of alcohol or hot foods and liquids. All can induce or intensify pruritus. Using a humidifier is helpful if environmental air is dry. Activities that result in perspiration should be limited because perspiration may irritate and promote pruritus. If the patient is troubled at night with itching that interferes with sleep, the nurse can advise wearing cotton clothing next to the skin rather than synthetic materials. The room should be kept cool and humidified. Vigorous scratching should be avoided and nails kept trimmed to prevent skin damage and infection. When the underlying cause of pruritus is unknown and further testing is required, the nurse explains each test and the expected outcome.

Perineal and Perianal Pruritus

Pruritus of the genital and anal regions may be caused by small particles of fecal material lodged in the perianal crevices or attached to anal hairs. Alternatively, it may result from perianal skin damage caused by scratching, moisture, and decreased skin resistance as a result of corticosteroid or antibiotic therapy. Other possible causes of perianal itching include local lesions such as hemorrhoids, fungal or yeast infections, and pinworm infestation. Conditions reviewed in Chart 61-1 may also result in pruritus. Occasionally, no cause can be identified.

Nursing Management

The patient is instructed to follow proper hygiene measures and to discontinue home and over-the-counter remedies. The perineal or anal area should be rinsed with lukewarm water and blotted dry with cotton balls. Premoistened tissues may be used after defecation. Cornstarch can be applied in the skinfold areas to absorb perspiration.

As part of health education, the nurse instructs the patient to avoid bathing in water that is too hot and to avoid using bubble baths, sodium bicarbonate, and detergent soaps, all of which aggravate dryness. To keep the perineal or perianal skin as dry as possible, patients should avoid wearing underwear made of synthetic fabrics. The patient should also avoid vasodilating agents or stimulants (e.g., alcohol, caffeine) and mechanical irritants such as rough or woolen clothing. A diet that includes adequate fiber may help maintain soft stools and prevent minor trauma to the anal mucosa.

SECRETORY DISORDERS

The main secretory function of the skin is performed by the sweat glands, which help regulate body temperature. These glands excrete perspiration that evaporates, thereby cooling the body. The sweat glands are located in various parts of the body and respond to different stimuli. Those on the trunk generally respond to thermal stimulation; those on the palms and soles respond to nervous stimulation; and those in the axillae and on the forehead respond to both kinds of stimulation. Normal perspiration has no odor. Body odor is produced by the increase in bacteria on the skin and the interaction of bacterial waste products with the chemicals of perspiration. As a rule, moist skin is warm, and dry skin is cool, but this is not always true. It is not unusual to observe warm, dry skin in patients who are dehydrated and very hot, dry skin in patients with some febrile states.

Normally, sweat can be controlled with the use of antiperspirants and deodorants. Most antiperspirants are aluminum salts that block the opening to the sweat duct. Pure deodorants inhibit bacterial growth and block the metabolism of sweat; they have no antiperspirant effect. Fragrance-free deodorants are available for those with sensitive skin.

Hidradenitis Suppurativa

Hidradenitis suppurativa (HS) is a chronic suppurative folliculitis of the perianal, axillary, and genital areas or under the breasts. It can produce abscesses or sinuses with scarring. It develops after puberty and diminishes in incidence after 50 years of age. African Americans are at greater risk for HS. In addition, men are at greater risk for anogenital HS, whereas women are at greater risk for axillary HS. The cause is unknown, but it appears to have a genetic basis (Wollina, Koch, Heinig, et al., 2013).

Pathophysiology

It had been assumed for many years that HS was caused by an abnormal blockage and infection of the sweat glands. However, recent evidence suggests that it is a primary disorder of follicular occlusion that causes eventual hypertrophic formation of scar tissue in the area of the sweat glands (Wollina et al., 2013).

Clinical Manifestations

HS occurs more frequently in the axillae but also appears in inguinal folds, on the mons pubis, around the buttocks, areolae of the breasts, submammary fold, nape of the neck, and shoulders. The patient may present with a firm, pea-sized nodule that causes discomfort, or with a history of this type of nodule that then ruptures and discharges purulent drainage. The nodule then propagates, and multiple similar nodules will form adjacent to the initial nodule. These nodules become deep seated and, as they rupture, form scars. The nodules may coalesce or form "bridges," become infected, and result in abscesses. As they coalesce, the patient will present with complaints of persistent pain (Wollina et al., 2013).

Medical Management

The patient is educated to use warm compresses and wear loose-fitting clothes over the nodules or lesions. Oral antibiotic agents such as erythromycin (E-Mycin), tetracycline, minocycline (Minocin), and doxycycline (Vibramycin) are frequently prescribed. Nonsteroidal anti-inflammatory drugs (NSAIDs) may be indicated to relieve the pain. Silver-impregnated alginate dressings may be useful with some lesions. Incision and drainage of large suppurating areas with gauze packs inserted to facilitate drainage are often necessary. Rarely, the entire area is excised, removing the scar tissue and any infection. This surgery is drastic in that it may require the use of skin grafts (see later discussion) and is performed only as a last resort. Carbon dioxide laser surgery (see later discussion) may be more effective than this type of excisional surgery (Wollina et al., 2013).

Seborrheic Dermatoses

Seborrhea is excessive production of sebum (secretion of sebaceous glands) in areas where sebaceous glands are normally found in large numbers, such as the face, scalp, eyebrows, eyelids, sides of the nose and upper lip, malar regions (cheeks), ears, axillae, under the breasts, groin, and gluteal crease of the buttocks. Seborrheic dermatitis is a chronic inflammatory disease of the skin with a predilection for areas that are well supplied with sebaceous glands or lie between skin folds, where the bacterial count is high (Borda & Wikramanayake, 2015).

Clinical Manifestations

Two forms of seborrheic dermatoses can occur: an oily form and a dry form. Either form may start in childhood and continue throughout life. The oily form appears moist or greasy. There may be patches of sallow, greasy skin, with or without scaling, and slight erythema, predominantly on the forehead, nasolabial fold, beard area, scalp, and between adjacent skin surfaces in the regions of the axillae, groin, and breasts. Small pustules or papulopustules resembling acne may appear on the trunk. The dry form, consisting of flaky desquamation of the scalp with a profuse amount of fine, powdery scales, is commonly called *dandruff*. The mild forms of the disease are asymptomatic. When scaling occurs, it is often accompanied by pruritus, which may lead to scratching and secondary infections and excoriation.

Seborrheic dermatitis has a genetic predisposition. Hormones, nutritional status, infection, and emotional stress influence its course. The remissions and exacerbations of this condition should be explained to the patient. If a person has not previously been diagnosed with this condition and suddenly appears with a severe outbreak, a complete history and physical examination should be conducted.

Medical Management

Because there is no known cure for seborrhea, the objectives of therapy are to control the disorder and allow the skin to repair itself. Seborrheic dermatitis of the body and face may respond to a topically applied corticosteroid cream, which allays the secondary inflammatory response. However, this medication should be used with caution near the eyelids because it can lead to glaucoma and cataracts. As an alternative treatment, patients can wash the eyelids using baby shampoo and cotton swabs (Handler, 2017).

Patients with seborrheic dermatitis may develop a secondary candidal (yeast) infection in body creases or folds. To avoid this, patients should be advised to ensure maximum aeration of the skin and to clean carefully areas where there are creases or folds in the skin (Borda & Wikramanayake, 2015). Patients with persistent candidiasis should be evaluated for diabetes.

The mainstay of dandruff treatment is proper, frequent shampooing (at least three times weekly) with medicated shampoos. Two or three different types of shampoo should be used in rotation to prevent the seborrhea from becoming resistant to a particular shampoo. The shampoo is left on at least 5 to 10 minutes. As the condition of the scalp improves, the treatment can be less frequent. Antiseborrheic shampoos include those containing selenium sulfide suspension, zinc pyrithione, salicylic acid, or sulfur compounds, and tar shampoo that contains sulfur or salicylic acid (Borda & Wikramanayake, 2015; Handler, 2017).

Nursing Management

The patient is educated that seborrheic dermatitis is a chronic condition that tends to reappear. The goal is to keep it under control through adherence to the treatment program (Borda & Wikramanayake, 2015). The patient is advised to avoid external irritants, excessive heat, and perspiration; rubbing and scratching prolong the disorder. To avoid secondary infection, the patient should air the skin and keep skin folds clean and dry.

Instructions for using medicated shampoos are reinforced for people with dandruff who require treatment. Frequent shampooing is contrary to some cultural practices; the nurse should be sensitive to these differences when educating the patient.

Acne Vulgaris

Acne vulgaris is a common disorder affecting susceptible hair follicles, most commonly on the face, back, chest, and upper arms (Well, 2013). It is a chronic dermatosis characterized by **comedones** (primary acne lesions), both closed and open, and by papules, pustules, nodules, and cysts (Zaenglein, Pathy, Schlosser, et al., 2016) (see Chapter 60, Table 60-2).

Acne is the most commonly encountered skin condition that affects up to 80% of Americans at some time during their lives. Acne is most prevalent during adolescence among males but is more prevalent in adulthood among females. Acne is traditionally considered a skin disorder of adolescence; however, by age 45 years, up to 5% of adults report having acne (Rao & Chen, 2016; Well, 2013). Acne appears to stem from an interplay of genetic, hormonal, and bacterial factors (Al-Hammadi, Al-Ismaily, Al-Ali, et al., 2016).

Pathophysiology

During puberty, androgens stimulate the sebaceous glands, causing them to enlarge and secrete a natural oil (sebum) that rises to the top of the hair follicle and flows out onto the skin surface. In adolescents who develop acne, androgenic stimulation produces a heightened response in the sebaceous glands so that acne occurs when accumulated sebum plugs the pilosebaceous ducts. Sebaceous plugging then causes a localized inflammatory response (Al-Hammadi et al., 2016).

Clinical Manifestations

The main lesions of acne are comedones. Closed comedones (whiteheads) form from impacted lipids or oils and keratin that plug the dilated follicle. Closed comedones may evolve into open comedones (blackheads), in which the contents of the ducts are in open communication with the external environment. The color of open comedones results from an accumulation of lipid, bacterial, and epithelial debris. Some closed comedones may rupture, resulting in an inflammatory reaction caused by leakage of follicular contents (e.g., sebum, keratin, bacteria) into the dermis. The resultant inflammation is seen clinically as erythematous papules, inflammatory pustules, and inflammatory cysts. Mild papules and cysts drain and heal without treatment. Deeper papules and cysts cause scarring of the skin. Acne is usually graded as mild, moderate, or severe based on the number and type of lesions (Al-Hammadi et al., 2016).

Assessment and Diagnostic Findings

The diagnosis of acne is based on the history and physical examination, evidence of lesions characteristic of acne, and age. Women may report a history of flare-ups a few days before menses. The presence of the typical comedones along with oily skin is characteristic (Rao & Chen, 2016; Well, 2013). Oiliness is more prominent in the midfacial area; other parts of the face may appear dry.

There is at present no consensus on manifestations that constitute mild, moderate, and severe acne (Zaenglein et al., 2016). Generally speaking, mild acne is characterized by the presence of comedones and a few papulopustules; moderate acne is characterized by a greater number of papulopustules and comedones along with the presence of inflammatory pustules; and, severe acne is characterized by the presence of cysts (also called nodules or nodulocysts) that are greater than 5 mm in diameter (Rao & Chen, 2016).

Medical Management

The goals of management are to reduce bacterial colonies, decrease sebaceous gland activity, prevent the follicles from becoming plugged, reduce inflammation, combat secondary infection, minimize scarring, and eliminate factors that predispose the person to acne. The therapeutic regimen depends on the type of lesion (e.g., comedones, papule, pustule, cyst). The duration of treatment depends on the extent and severity of the acne. In severe cases, treatment may extend over years.

Nutrition and Hygiene Therapy

The association between diet and acne is not established. In particular, the association between acne and milk products, chocolate, and fried foods is not well defined. However, there does appear to be a correlation between foods high in refined sugars and acne; therefore, these foods should be avoided (Zaenglein et al., 2016). In general, maintenance of good nutrition equips the immune system for effective action against bacteria and infection.

For mild cases of acne, washing twice each day with a cleansing soap and use of over-the-counter products that contain benzoyl peroxide or salicylic acid (see later discussion) may be all that is required (Well, 2013). Oil-free cosmetics and creams should be chosen. These products are usually designated as useful for acne-prone skin.

Pharmacologic Therapy

Pharmacologic treatments for acne are based upon the severity of the acne (Zaenglein et al., 2016). Table 61-4 summarizes the first-line treatment modalities for acne vulgaris based upon severity.

Topical Therapy

Recommended over-the-counter acne medications contain benzoyl peroxide, which is very effective at removing the sebaceous follicular plugs. Benzoyl peroxide preparations produce

TABLE 61-4 First-Line Medications Indicated for Treatment of Acne Vulgaris

Classification	Recommended Medications
Mild Acne	Benzoyl Peroxide -or- Topical Retinoid -or- Combination[a] Topical Antibiotic and Benzoyl Peroxide -or- Combination[a] Topical Retinoid and Benzoyl Peroxide -or- Combination[a] Topical Retinoid and Benzoyl Peroxide and Topical Antibiotic
Moderate Acne	Combination[a] Topical Antibiotic and Benzoyl Peroxide -or- Combination[a] Topical Retinoid and Benzoyl Peroxide -or- Combination[a] Topical Retinoid and Benzoyl Peroxide and Topical Antibiotic -or- Oral Antibiotic and Combination[a] Topical Retinoid and Benzoyl Peroxide -or- Oral Antibiotic and Combination[a] Topical Retinoid and Benzoyl Peroxide and Topical Antibiotic
Severe Acne	Oral Antibiotic and Combination[a] Topical Retinoid and Benzoyl Peroxide -or- Oral Antibiotic and Combination[a] Topical Antibiotic and Benzoyl Peroxide -or- Oral Antibiotic and Combination[a] Topical Retinoid and Benzoyl Peroxide and Topical Antibiotic -or- Oral Antibiotic and Oral Isotretinoin

[a]May be prescribed as combination products or as singular products
Adapted from Zaenglein, A. L., Pathy, A. L., Schlosser, B. J., et al. (2016). Guidelines of care for the management of acne vulgaris. *Journal of the American Academy of Dermatology, 74*(5), 945–973.

a rapid and sustained reduction of inflammatory lesions. They depress sebum production and promote breakdown of comedo plugs and have an antibacterial effect (Zaenglein et al., 2016). Initially, benzoyl peroxide causes redness and scaling, but the skin usually adjusts quickly to its use. However, the skin of some people can be overly sensitive to these products, which can cause irritation or excessive dryness, especially when used with some prescribed topical medications. The patient should be instructed to discontinue use of the product if severe irritation occurs. Typically, the patient applies a gel of benzoyl peroxide once daily. In many instances, this is the only treatment needed (Karch, 2015).

Over-the-counter salicylic acid preparations are also available for use by patients with mild acne. The effects of these agents are similar to those of benzoyl peroxide products. Although salicylic acid products have long been used by patients with acne, their efficacy has not been demonstrated in clinical trials (Zaenglein et al., 2016). Prescription topical agents used for years that have also not demonstrated efficacy in clinical trials include zinc, sulfur, and resorcinol, and are therefore not recommended for treatment (Zaenglein et al., 2016).

Synthetic vitamin A acids, also called retinoids (e.g., tretinoin [Retin-A], adapalene [Differin], tazarotene [Tazorac]) are applied topically to clear the keratin plugs from the pilosebaceous ducts. The patient should be informed that symptoms may worsen during early weeks of therapy because inflammation, erythema, and peeling may occur. The patient is cautioned against sun exposure while using this topical medication because it may cause sunburn. Package insert directions should be followed carefully. Improvement may take 8 to 12 weeks. Some patients may benefit from being treated with both a retinoid and benzoyl peroxide and may be prescribed a combination topical gel (e.g., adapalene benzoyl peroxide [Epiduo]) (Zaenglein et al., 2016).

Topical antibiotic treatment for acne is common. Topical antibiotic agents suppress bacterial growth; reduce superficial free fatty acid levels; decrease comedones, papules, and pustules; and produce no systemic side effects (Karch, 2015). The most commonly prescribed agents include clindamycin (Cleocin-T) and erythromycin (Erythra-Derm) (Well, 2013). Topical combination gels that include both benzoyl peroxide and an antibiotic (e.g., benzoyl erythromycin [Benzamycin]) are commonly prescribed and can be very effective treatment (Zaenglein et al., 2016).

Other less commonly prescribed topical agents that may be effective in treating acne vulgaris include azelaic acid (Azelex) and dapsone gel (Aczone). Azelaic acid has comedolytic, antibacterial, and anti-inflammatory effects. It may also have a lightening effect on skin that can be hyperpigmented as a consequence of acne (Zaenglein et al., 2016). Dapsone reduces inflammatory lesions and for reasons poorly understood, seems to work better in female adult patients than in adolescent or male patients (Zaenglein et al., 2016).

Systemic Therapy

Oral antibiotic agents given in small doses over a long period are very effective in treating moderate and severe acne, especially when the acne is inflammatory and results in pustules, abscesses, and scarring. Therapy may continue for months to years. Antibiotics most commonly selected are of the tetracycline class (e.g., tetracycline, doxycycline, minocycline) (Zaenglein et al., 2016). The tetracycline family of antibiotics is contraindicated in pregnant women. Side effects of tetracyclines include photosensitivity, nausea, diarrhea, cutaneous infection in either gender, and vaginitis in women (Karch, 2015). Alternative antibiotics that may be selected include erythromycin, azithromycin (Zithromax), and trimethoprim-sulfamethoxazole (Bactrim) (Zaenglein et al., 2016).

Oral retinoids (e.g., isotretinoin [Claravis]) are used with dramatic results in patients with nodular cystic acne unresponsive to conventional therapy. This may prevent scarring that can result from cyst formation. Retinoids reduce sebaceous gland size and inhibit sebum production. They also cause the epidermis to shed (epidermal desquamation), thereby unseating and expelling existing comedones. The most common side effect is **cheilitis** (inflammation of the lips). Dry and chafed skin and mucous membranes are also frequent side effects. These changes are reversible with the withdrawal of the medication. Retinoids are teratogenic, meaning that they may cause fetal defects. Effective contraceptive measures for women of childbearing age are mandatory during treatment and for about 4 to 8 weeks thereafter (Well, 2013). To avoid additive toxic effects, patients are cautioned not to take vitamin A supplements while taking retinoids (Karch, 2015).

Estrogen therapy (including progesterone–estrogen preparations) suppresses sebum production and reduces skin oiliness. It is usually reserved for young women when the acne begins somewhat later than usual and tends to flare up at certain times in the menstrual cycle. Estrogen-dominant oral contraceptive compounds may be given on a prescribed cyclic regimen. Estrogen is not given to male patients because of undesirable side effects such as enlargement of the breasts and decrease in body hair (Al-Hammadi et al., 2016).

Surgical Management

Treatment includes comedo extraction; injections of corticosteroids into the inflamed lesions; and incision and drainage of large, fluctuant (moving in palpable waves), nodular cystic lesions. Patients with deep scars may be treated with deep abrasive therapy (dermabrasion), in which the epidermis and some superficial dermis are removed down to the level of the scars (Al-Hammadi et al., 2016).

Comedones may be removed with a comedo extractor. The site is first cleaned with alcohol. The opening of the extractor is then placed over the lesion, and direct pressure is applied to cause extrusion of the plug through the extractor. Removal of comedones leads to erythema, which may take several weeks to subside. Recurrence of comedones after extraction is common (Rao & Chen, 2016).

Nursing Management

Nursing care of patients with acne includes monitoring and managing potential complications of skin treatments. Major nursing activities include providing patient education, particularly in proper skin care techniques, and managing potential problems related to the skin disorder or therapy. Providing positive reassurance, listening attentively, and being sensitive to the feelings of the patient with acne are essential to the patient's psychological well-being and understanding of the disease and treatment plan. Having acne, particularly if

it persists into adulthood, can lead to adverse psychological well-being. In particular, women with acne frequently report diminished quality of life, more anxiety, and depression (Gorelick, Daniels, Kawata, et al., 2015; Zaenglein et al., 2016) (see Chart 61-2).

Preventing Scarring

Prevention of scarring is the ultimate goal of therapy. The chance of scarring increases with the severity of the grade of acne. Severe acne usually requires longer-term therapy with systemic antibiotic agents and other treatments that may include combination topical agents or isotretinoin (see Table 61-4). Patients should be warned that discontinuing these medications may lead to more flare-ups and increase the chance of deep scarring. Furthermore, manipulation of the comedones, papules, and pustules increases the potential for scarring.

When acne surgery is prescribed to extract deep-seated comedones or inflamed lesions or to incise and drain cystic lesions, the intervention itself may result in further scarring. Dermabrasion, which levels existing scar tissue, can also increase scar formation. Hyper- or hypopigmentation also may affect the tissue involved. The patient should be informed of these potential outcomes before choosing surgical intervention for acne.

Promoting Home, Community-Based, and Transitional Care

 Educating Patients About Self-Care

In addition to providing instructions for taking prescribed medications, the nurse informs patients to wash the face and other affected areas with mild soap and water twice each day to remove surface oils and prevent obstruction of the oil glands. Mild abrasive soaps and drying agents are prescribed to eliminate the oily feeling that troubles many patients. At the same time, patients are cautioned to avoid excessive abrasion, because it makes acne worse.

All forms of friction and trauma are avoided, including propping the hands against the face, rubbing the face, and wearing tight collars and helmets. Patients are instructed to avoid manipulation of pimples or blackheads. Squeezing merely worsens the problem, because a portion of the blackhead is pushed down into the skin, which may cause the follicle to rupture. Because cosmetics, shaving creams, and lotions can aggravate acne, these should be avoided.

INFECTIOUS DERMATOSES

Bacterial Skin Infections

Also called **pyodermas**, pus-forming bacterial infections of the skin may be primary or secondary. Primary skin infections originate in previously normal-appearing skin and are usually caused by a single organism. Secondary skin infections arise from a pre-existing skin disorder or from disruption of the skin integrity from injury or surgery. In either case, several microorganisms may be implicated (e.g., *Staphylococcus aureus*, group A streptococci). Common primary bacterial skin infections are impetigo and folliculitis. Folliculitis may lead to furuncles or carbuncles.

NURSING RESEARCH PROFILE

Quality of Life Among Women With Acne

Gorelick, J., Daniels, S. R., Kawata, A. K., et al. (2015). Acne-related quality of life among female adults of different races/ethnicities. *Journal of the Dermatology Nurses Association, 7*(3), 154–162.

Purpose

Acne vulgaris is a common chronic dermatosis that is traditionally considered a disorder of adolescence. However, it frequently persists into adulthood, with an estimated prevalence of 43% among adults in their third decade of life. Women are more commonly affected than men, and women of color are affected more commonly than Caucasian women. Acne is also associated with depression, distress, and lower quality of life (QOL). However, little is known about the effects of acne on QOL among women of different racial groups. The purpose of this study was to describe the QOL of women with facial acne and find whether or not there existed differences in QOL among participants based upon their racial background.

Design

This was a descriptive cross-sectional web-based study that solicited participants who were part of a preregistered YouGov pool of panelists in the United States. The study was approved by a centralized institutional review board before prospective participants were invited to join the study. Eligibility criteria included women between 25 and 45 years of age with an active email address who could read and understand English and who self-reported having at least 25 visible facial acne lesions. After screening, eligible participants were invited to complete an online survey with items that provided information on demographics, comorbid health conditions, clinical characteristics of the acne, and self-assessed reports of work or school productivity. The Acne-Specific QOL Questionnaire (Acne-QOL) was a component of the survey, as were psychological symptoms measured by items included from the Patient Health Questionnaire-4 (PHQ-4).

Findings

Participants (*N* = 312) reflected a diverse racial mix including Caucasian (34.3%), African American (30.8%), Hispanic (17.6%), and Asian American (17.3%). The mean age of the sample was 35.3 years of age (SD 5.9). Caucasian participants reported more concern with lesions (i.e., "pimples," "bumps") whereas African American, Hispanic, and Asian American participants reported greater concern with postinflammatory hyperpigmentation, in addition to lesions ($p < 0.0001$). More Caucasian participants reported anxiety ($p < 0.0001$), depression ($p < 0.001$), and migraines ($p < 0.05$) than participants from other racial groups. Participants from all racial groups reported that acne hampered their QOL, and more than one third reported moderate to severe symptoms of anxiety and depression. Acne also negatively affected the ability of participants from all racial groups to concentrate on work or school.

Nursing Implications

Results from this study indicate that having acne can adversely affect QOL in women. In particular, women with acne may have different concerns, based upon their racial background/skin type. African American, Hispanic, and Asian American women are more prone to the adverse consequence of hyperpigmentation from acne lesions. Results from this study confirm that this is a top concern among these women who have acne, whereas Caucasian women are primarily concerned about the appearance of lesions. Conversely, Caucasian women express more symptoms consistent with depression and anxiety related to having acne than women from other racial groups. Nurses can use information gleaned from this study to tailor individualized care toward women with acne.

Impetigo

Impetigo is a superficial infection of the skin caused by staphylococci, streptococci, or multiple bacteria. Bullous impetigo, a more deep-seated infection of the skin caused by *S. aureus*, is characterized by the formation of **bullae** (i.e., large, fluid-filled blisters) from original vesicles. The bullae rupture, leaving raw, red areas. Nonbullous impetigo accounts for approximately 70% of cases. This type of impetigo tends to affect skin that has already been disrupted by cuts, abrasions, bites, or other types of trauma. *S. aureus* is also commonly implicated, including methicillin-resistant *Staphylococcus aureus* (MRSA), as well as *Streptococcus pyogenes* (Lewis, 2016).

The exposed areas of the body, face, hands, neck, and extremities are most frequently involved. Impetigo is contagious and may spread to other parts of the patient's skin or to other members of the family who touch the patient or use towels or combs that are soiled with the exudate of the lesions (Lewis, 2016).

Impetigo is seen in people of all races and ages. It is particularly common in children living in poor hygienic conditions. Chronic health problems, poor hygiene, and malnutrition may predispose an adult to impetigo. It is more prevalent in warm, humid climates and is therefore more commonly seen in the southeastern United States than in northern climates (Lewis, 2016).

Clinical Manifestations

The lesions of impetigo are most commonly seen on the face or extremities. They begin as small, red macules, which quickly become discrete, thin-walled vesicles that rupture and become covered with a loosely adherent honey-yellow crust (see Fig. 61-1). These crusts are easily removed to reveal smooth, red, moist surfaces on which new crusts soon develop (Lewis, 2016).

Medical Management

Topical antibacterial therapy (e.g., mupirocin [Bactroban], retapamulin [Altabax]) is typically prescribed when the disease

Figure 61-1 • Impetigo of the nostril.

is limited to a small area. The medication must be applied to the lesions several times daily for 5 to 7 days. Lesions are first soaked or washed with soap solution to remove the central site of bacterial growth, giving the topical antibiotic an opportunity to reach the infected site. After the crusts are removed, the prescribed topical antibiotic cream is applied. Gloves are worn when providing patient care (Lewis, 2016).

Systemic antibiotic agents may be prescribed to treat infections that are widespread or in cases where there are systemic manifestations (e.g., fever is present). These antibiotics are effective in reducing contagious spread, treating deep infections, and preventing acute glomerulonephritis (kidney infection), which may occur as a consequence of streptococcal skin diseases. Amoxicillin–clavulanate (Augmentin), cloxacillin (Cloxapen), or dicloxacillin (Dynapen) may be prescribed. In cases where MRSA is present, antibiotics prescribed may include clindamycin (Cleocin), trimethoprim–sulfamethoxazole (Bactrim), levofloxacin (Levaquin), or ciprofloxacin (Cipro) (Lewis, 2016).

Nursing Management

The nurse educates the patient and family members to bathe at least once daily with bactericidal soap. Cleanliness and good hygiene practices help to prevent the spread of the lesions from one skin area to another and from one person to another. In particular, patients and family members must be educated to practice hand hygiene every time after a lesion is touched. Each person should have a separate towel and washcloth. Because impetigo is a contagious disorder, infected people should avoid contact with other people until the lesions heal (Lewis, 2016).

Folliculitis, Furuncles, and Carbuncles

Folliculitis is an inflammatory condition of the cells within the wall and ostia of the hair follicles that may be caused by a bacterial, viral, fungal, or parasitic infection. Lesions may be superficial or deep. Single or multiple papules or pustules appear close to the hair follicles. Folliculitis commonly affects the beard area of men who shave, as well as women's legs, if they shave. Other areas include the axillae, trunk, and buttocks (Van Bijnen, Paget, den Heijer, et al., 2014).

Pseudofolliculitis barbae (shaving bumps) occur predominately on the faces of African Americans and other curly-haired men as a result of shaving. The sharp ingrowing hairs have a curved root that grows at a more acute angle and pierces the skin, provoking an irritative reaction. The only entirely effective treatment is to avoid shaving. Other treatments include using special lotions or antibiotics or using a hand brush to dislodge the hairs mechanically. If the patient must remove facial hair, a depilatory cream or electric razor may be used.

A **furuncle** (boil) is an acute inflammation arising deep in one or more hair follicles and spreading into the surrounding dermis (see Fig. 61-2). This inflammation is a deep form of folliculitis. Furunculosis refers to multiple or recurrent lesions. Furuncles may occur anywhere on the body but are more prevalent in areas subjected to irritation, pressure, friction, and excessive perspiration, such as the back of the neck, the axillae, and the buttocks.

Figure 61-2 • Painful furuncle on the thigh. From Goodheart H. P. (2003). *Goodheart's photoguide of common skin disorders* (2nd ed.). Philadelphia, PA: Lippincott Williams & Wilkins.

A furuncle may start as a small, red, raised, painful pimple. Frequently, the infection progresses and involves the skin and subcutaneous fatty tissue, causing tenderness, pain, and surrounding cellulitis. The area of redness and induration represents an effort of the body to keep the infection localized. The bacteria (usually staphylococci) produce necrosis of the invaded tissue. The characteristic pointing of a boil follows in a few days. When this occurs, the center becomes yellow or black, and the boil is said to have "come to a head."

A **carbuncle** is an abscess of the skin and subcutaneous tissue that represents an extension of a furuncle that has invaded several follicles and is large and deep seated. It is usually caused by a staphylococcal infection. Carbuncles appear most commonly in areas where the skin is thick and inelastic; the back of the neck and the buttocks are common sites. The extensive inflammation frequently prevents a complete walling off of the infection; purulent material may be absorbed, resulting in high fever, pain, leukocytosis, and sepsis.

Furuncles and carbuncles are more likely to occur in patients with underlying systemic diseases, such as diabetes or hematologic malignancies, and in those receiving immunosuppressive therapy for other diseases. Both are more prevalent in hot climates, especially on skin beneath occlusive clothing.

Medical Management

In treating staphylococcal infections, it is important not to rupture or destroy the protective wall of induration that localizes the infection. The boil or pimple should never be squeezed. Systemic antibiotic therapy, selected by culture and sensitivity study, is generally indicated. Oral dicloxacillin and cephalosporins are first-line medications. If MRSA is suspected, antibiotic agents selected may include clindamycin, trimethoprim–sulfamethoxazole, or minocycline (Peebles, Morris, & Chafe, 2014).

When the pus has localized and is fluctuant, a small incision with a scalpel can speed resolution by relieving the tension and ensuring direct evacuation of the pus and debris. The patient is instructed to keep the draining lesion covered with a dressing.

Nursing Management

Intravenous (IV) fluids, fever reduction, and other supportive treatments are indicated for patients who are acutely ill from infection. Warm, moist compresses hasten resolution of the furuncle or carbuncle. The surrounding skin may be cleaned gently with antibacterial soap, and an antibacterial ointment may be applied. Soiled dressings are handled according to standard precautions. Nursing personnel should carefully follow standard precautions to avoid becoming carriers of staphylococci.

 Quality and Safety Nursing Alert

Nurses must take special precautions in caring for boils on the face because the skin area drains directly into the cranial venous sinuses. Sinus thrombosis can develop after manipulating a boil in this location. The infection can travel through the sinus tract and penetrate the brain cavity, causing a brain abscess.

Promoting Home, Community-Based, and Transitional Care

Educating Patients About Self-Care

To prevent and control staphylococcal skin infections such as boils and carbuncles, the staphylococcal pathogen must be eliminated from the skin and environment. Efforts must be made to provide a hygienic environment. If lesions are actively draining, the mattress and pillow should be covered with plastic material and wiped with disinfectant daily; the bed linens, towels, and clothing should be laundered after each use; and the patient should use an antibacterial soap and shampoo for an indefinite period, often several months.

Viral Skin Infections

Herpes Zoster

Herpes zoster, also called *shingles*, is an infection caused by the varicella-zoster virus (VZV), which are members of a group of deoxyribonucleic acid (DNA) viruses. The disease is characterized by a painful vesicular eruption along the area of distribution of the sensory nerves (i.e., dermatome) from one or more posterior ganglia. After a case of chickenpox, or primary varicella, runs its course, the VZV responsible for the outbreak lies dormant inside nerve cells near the brain and spinal cord. Later, when these latent viruses are reactivated because of declining cellular immunity, they travel by way of the peripheral nerves to the skin, where the viruses multiply and create a red rash of small, fluid-filled blisters.

It is thought that during the aging process, natural immunity to the varicella virus wanes, allowing the virus to reactivate. Herpes zoster develops over the lifetime of about 10% to 20% of all adults who had chickenpox earlier in life, usually after 50 years of age. The rates of occurrence tend to be the same in both men and women but are slightly higher in Caucasians compared to African Americans. There is an increased frequency of herpes zoster infections in patients with weakened immune systems, including those with human immune deficiency virus (HIV) infection and in those with cancer. In these patients, the infection can become widespread and cause significant complications (Janniger, Eastern, Hospenthal, et al., 2016).

Clinical Manifestations

Manifestations typically occur in three phases, including the preeruptive, acute eruptive, and postherpetic neuralgia (PHN) phases. During the preeruptive phase, the previously dormant VZV becomes reactivated within the dorsal root ganglia of the spinal cord. Manifestations that follow, therefore, tend to follow the dermatome that corresponds with the ganglion or ganglia that are affected. The patient will typically complain of pain, or sometimes pruritus or paresthesias, over the sensory region that follows that dermatome. This phase lasts from 1 to 10 days, with 48 hours being typical (Janniger et al., 2016).

The acute eruptive phase is heralded by the appearance of unilateral patchy erythematous areas in the dermatomal area that is affected. Vesicles develop that appear initially clear, then become cloudy, and eventually rupture and crust (see Fig. 61-3). The pain that accompanies this stage is typically described as severe and unrelenting. This phase typically lasts between 10 and 15 days (Janniger et al., 2016).

The last phase—PHN—is variable in terms of both duration and manifestations. The pain is typically localized to the dermatomal area that was affected. Approximately 50% of adults older than 60 years with herpes zoster experience PHN pain for longer than 60 days (Janniger et al., 2016).

Herpes zoster ophthalmicus (HZO) is a rare subtype of herpes zoster that causes severe consequences. Typically in HZO, a branch of the trigeminal nerve is affected that innervates the ocular and periocular structures. This may cause significant pain and morbid ocular complications, including blindness (Janniger et al., 2016).

Medical Management

Herpes zoster infection can be arrested if oral antiviral agents such as acyclovir (Zovirax), valacyclovir (Valtrex), or famciclovir (Famvir) are given within 24 hours of the initial eruption. IV acyclovir may be indicated in patients who are immunocompromised (Janniger et al., 2016).

Figure 61-3 • Herpes zoster (shingles).

The goals of herpes zoster management are to relieve the pain and to reduce or avoid complications, which include infection, scarring, and PHN and eye complications. Pain is controlled with analgesic agents because adequate pain control during the acute phase helps prevent persistent pain patterns. Systemic corticosteroids may be prescribed to reduce the incidence and duration of PHN. Healing usually occurs more quickly in those who have been treated with corticosteroids. Triamcinolone (Aristocort, Kenalog) injected subcutaneously under painful areas is effective as an anti-inflammatory agent. Patients with HZO require emergent treatment by an ophthalmologist (Janniger et al., 2016).

People who have been exposed to varicella by primary infection or by vaccination are not at risk for infection with VZV after exposure to patients with herpes zoster.

Since 1995, the widespread vaccination of children with the VZV vaccine (Varivax) has led to a marked reduction in the incidence of primary varicella, which presumably will result in marked decrease in rates of herpes zoster eventually. The VZV vaccine (Zostavax) was developed to boost VZV cellular immunity in adults older than 50 years. This vaccination is now recommended as part of prevention strategies in adults who are not immunocompromised, including those with a history of herpes zoster, because it may recur (Janniger et al., 2016).

Nursing Management

The patient and family members are instructed about the importance of taking antiviral agents as prescribed and in keeping follow-up appointments with the primary provider. The nurse assesses the patient's discomfort and response to medication and collaborates with the primary provider to make necessary adjustments to the treatment regimen. The patient is educated about how to apply dressings or medication to the lesions and to follow proper hand hygiene techniques to avoid spreading the virus.

Diversionary activities and relaxation techniques are encouraged to ensure restful sleep and to alleviate discomfort. A caregiver may be required to assist with dressings, particularly if the patient is an older adult and unable to apply them. Food preparation for patients who cannot care for themselves or prepare nourishing meals must be arranged.

Herpes Simplex

Herpes simplex is a common skin infection. There are two types of the causative virus, which are identified by viral typing. In general, herpes simplex type 1 occurs on the skin of the lips, mouth, gums, or tongue (or on the skin around the mouth) and type 2 occurs in the genital area, but both viral types can be found in both locations. See Chapters 22 and 57 for discussion of herpes simplex type 1 and type 2, respectively.

Fungal (Mycotic) Skin Infections

Fungi, tiny members of a subdivision of the plant kingdom that thrive on organic matter, cause various common skin infections. In some cases, they affect only the skin and its appendages (hair and nails). In other cases, internal organs are involved, and the diseases may be life threatening. However, superficial infections rarely cause even temporary disability and respond readily to treatment. Secondary infection with bacteria, *Candida,* or both organisms may occur.

The most common fungal skin infection is **tinea**, which is also called *ringworm* because of its characteristic appearance of a ring or rounded tunnel under the skin. Tinea infections affect the head, body, groin, feet, and nails (Sahoo & Mahajan, 2016). Table 61-5 summarizes the tinea infections and treatments.

To obtain a specimen for diagnosis, the lesion is cleaned and a scalpel or glass slide is used to remove scales from the margin of the lesion. The scales are dropped onto a slide to which potassium hydroxide has been added. The diagnosis is made by examination of the infected scales microscopically for spores and hyphae or by isolating the organism in culture. Under Wood's light, a specimen of infected hair appears fluorescent; this may be helpful in diagnosing some cases of tinea capitis (Sahoo & Mahajan, 2016).

Parasitic Skin Infestations

Parasitic skin infestations include those of the skin by lice (pediculosis) and the itch mite (scabies).

Pediculosis: Lice Infestation

Lice infestation affects people of all ages. Three varieties of lice infest humans: *Pediculus humanus capitis* (head louse), *Pediculus humanus corporis* (body louse), and *Pediculosis pubis* (pubic louse or "crab"). Lice are called *ectoparasites* because they live on the outside of the host's body. They depend on the host for their nourishment, feeding on human blood approximately five times each day. They inject their digestive juices and excrement into the skin, which causes severe itching (Dunphy, Winland-Brown, Porter, et al., 2015).

Pediculosis Capitis

Pediculosis capitis is an infestation of the scalp by the head louse. The female louse lays her eggs (nits) close to the scalp. The nits become firmly attached to the hair shafts with a tenacious substance. The young lice hatch in about 10 days and reach maturity in 2 weeks. Head lice may be transmitted directly by physical contact or indirectly by infested combs, brushes, wigs, hats, helmets, and bedding (Dunphy et al., 2015).

Pediculosis Corporis and Pubis

Pediculosis corporis is an infestation of the body by the body louse. This is a disease of those who live in close quarters. Pediculosis pubis is extremely common. The infestation is generally localized in the genital region and is transmitted chiefly by sexual contact (Guenther & Maguiness, 2016).

Clinical Manifestations

Head lice are found most commonly along the back of the head and behind the ears. To the naked eye, the eggs look like silvery, glistening oval bodies. The bite of the insect causes intense pruritus, and the resultant scratching often leads to secondary bacterial infection, such as impetigo or furunculosis. The infestation is more common in children and people with long hair (Bonilla, Durden, Eremeeva, et al., 2013; Dunphy et al., 2015).

TABLE 61-5 Tinea (Ringworm) Infections

Type and Location	Clinical Manifestations	Treatment
Tinea capitis (scalp; contagious fungal infection of the hair shaft)	• Oval, scaling, erythematous patches • Small papules or pustules on the scalp • Brittle hair that breaks easily; patchy alopecia	• Griseofulvin for 4–6 weeks or terbinafine (Lamisil) for 2–4 weeks • Shampoo hair twice weekly with selenium sulfide shampoo for 2 weeks
Tinea corporis (body)	• Begins with red macule, which spreads to a ring of papules or vesicles with central clearing • Lesions found in clusters; many spread to the hair, scalp, or nails • Pruritis is a common complaint	• Local infections—topical antifungal creams once or twice daily (e.g., clotrimazole [Lotrimin], econazole [Spectazole], ketoconazole [Nizoral]) • Extensive infections or concomitant tinea capitis or immunosuppressive conditions (e.g., active neoplasms)—oral antifungal medications (e.g., fluconazole [Diflucan] for 2–4 weeks, itraconazole for 1 week, terbinafine for 2 weeks)
Tinea cruris (groin area; "jock itch")	• Begins with small, red scaling patches, which spread to form circular elevated plaques • Very pruritic • Clusters of pustules may be seen around borders	• Local infections—see treatment for tinea corporis • Extensive infections or concomitant tinea pedis or immunosuppressive conditions (e.g., active neoplasms)—see treatment for tinea corporis • Educate patients to avoid wearing clothing that is tight over the groin; patients should pat dry skin folds thoroughly (avoid rubbing) after bathing and use separate towels for groin and other body parts

Tinea pedis (foot; "athlete's foot")	• Soles of one or both feet have scaling and mild redness with maceration in the toe webs
	• More acute infections may have clusters of clear vesicles on dusky base
		• Local infections—see treatment for tinea corporis.
		• Extensive infections or concomitant tinea pedis or immunosuppressive conditions (e.g., active neoplasms)—see treatment for tinea corporis
		• Educate patients:
		  • to put on socks before underwear to avoid cross-contamination to groin
		  • to either dispose of old shoes or treat them with antifungal powder to prevent reinfection
		  • to wear protective footwear at communal pools and tubs

Tinea unguium (toenails; onychomycosis)	• Nails thicken, crumble easily, and lack luster • Whole nail may be destroyed • If untreated, can result in pain, loss of balance, and candida infection	• Oral antifungal medications for 12 weeks (e.g., itraconazole, terbinafine) with or without concomitant topical ciclopirox olamine nail lacquer (Penlac) • Nail avulsion may be indicated, either surgically or chemically using a 40–50% urea compound

Adapted from Handler, M. Z., Stephany, M. P., & Schwarts, R. A. (2016). Tinea capitis. *Medscape.* Retrieved on 2/11/2017 at: emedicine.medscape.com/article/1091351-overview; Lesher, J. L. (2016). Tinea corporis. *Medscape.* Retrieved on 2/11/2017 at: emedicine.medscape.com/article/1091473-overview; Robbins, C. M., & Elewski, B. E. (2016). Tinea pedis. *Medscape.* Retrieved on 2/11/2017 at: emedicine.medscape.com/article/1091684-overview; Tosti, A. (2016). Onychomycosis. *Medscape.* Retrieved on 2/11/2017 at: emedicine.medscape.com/article/1105828-overview; and Weiderkehr, M., & Schwartz, R. A. (2016). Tinea cruris. *Medscape.* Retrieved on 2/11/2017 at: emedicine.medscape.com/article/1091806-overview

With body lice, the areas of the skin that come in closest contact with the underclothing (i.e., neck, trunk, and thighs) are chiefly involved. The body louse lives primarily in the seams of underwear and clothing, to which it clings as it pierces the skin with its proboscis. Its bites cause characteristic minute hemorrhagic points. Widespread excoriation may appear as a result of intense pruritus and scratching, especially on the trunk and neck. Among the secondary lesions produced are parallel linear scratches and a slight degree of eczema. In long-standing cases, the skin may become thick, dry, and scaly, with dark pigmented areas (Bonilla et al., 2013).

Pruritus, particularly at night, is the most common symptom of pediculosis pubis. Reddish-brown dust (i.e., excretions of the insects) may be found in the patient's underclothing. The pubic area should be examined with a magnifying glass for lice crawling down a hair shaft or nits cemented to the hair or at the junction with the skin. Infestation by pubic lice may coexist with sexually transmitted infections (STI) such as gonorrhea, herpes, or syphilis. There may also be infestation of the hairs of the chest, axillae, beard, and eyelashes. Gray-blue macules may sometimes be seen on the trunk, thighs, and axillae as a result of either the reaction of the insects' saliva with bilirubin (converting it to biliverdin) or an excretion produced by the salivary glands of the louse (Bonilla et al., 2013; Dunphy et al., 2015).

Medical Management

Treatment of head and pubic lice involves washing the hair with a shampoo containing pyrethrin compounds with piperonyl butoxide (RID or R&C Shampoo) or rinsing with permethrin (Nix). Although it had been first-line treatment for many years, lindane (Kwell) is no longer recommended because of its neurotoxic adverse effects (Dunphy et al., 2015). The patient is instructed to shampoo the scalp and hair according to the product directions. After the hair is rinsed thoroughly, it is combed with a fine-toothed comb dipped in vinegar to remove any remaining nits or nit shells freed from the hair shafts. They are extremely difficult to remove and may have to be picked off one by one (Dunphy et al., 2015; Gellatly, Krim, Palenchar, et al., 2016).

The patient with body lice is instructed to bathe with soap and water. Typically, no medications are indicated because the lice live on the patient's clothing. Topical medications used to treat head and pubic lice may be applied to the clothing, however, particularly in the seams of garments (see following discussion about general hygiene measures). If the eyelashes are involved, petrolatum may be thickly applied twice daily for 8 days, followed by mechanical removal of any remaining nits (Bonilla et al., 2013).

All articles of clothing, towels, and bedding that may have lice or nits should be washed in hot water—at least 54°C (130°F)—or dry-cleaned to prevent reinfestation. Upholstered furniture, rugs, and floors should be vacuumed frequently. Combs, brushes, and helmets are disinfected or discarded. All family members and close contacts are treated (Bonilla et al., 2013; Dunphy et al., 2015).

Complications, such as severe pruritus, pyoderma, and dermatitis, are treated with antipruritics, systemic antibiotics, and topical corticosteroids. Body lice can transmit epidemic rickettsial disease (e.g., epidemic typhus, relapsing fever, and trench fever) to humans. The causative organism may be in the gastrointestinal tract of the insect and may be excreted on the skin surface of the infested person (Bonilla et al., 2013).

Nursing Management

The nurse informs the patient that head lice may infest anyone and are not a sign of uncleanliness. Because the condition spreads rapidly, treatment must be started immediately. Epidemics among those living in close quarters (e.g., dormitories, military barracks) may be managed by having everyone shampoo their hair on the same night. Cohabitants and family members should be warned not to share combs, brushes, and hats; they should be inspected for head lice daily for at least 2 weeks.

Treatment is necessary for all family members and sexual contacts of patients with body and/or pubic lice. The nurse educates them about personal hygiene and methods to prevent or control infestation. The patient and partner must also be scheduled for a diagnostic workup for coexisting STIs.

Scabies

Scabies is an infestation of the skin by the itch mite *Sarcoptes scabei*. The disease is most commonly found in people living in substandard hygienic conditions and in people who are sexually active. The mites frequently involve the fingers, and hand contact may produce infection (Mounsey, Murray, Bielefeldt-Ohmann, et al., 2015).

Clinical Manifestations

It takes approximately 4 weeks from the time of contact for the patient's symptoms to appear. The patient complains of severe itching caused by a delayed type of immunologic reaction to the mite or its fecal pellets. During examination, the patient is asked where the pruritus is most severe. A magnifying glass and a penlight are held at an oblique angle to the skin while a search is made for the small, raised burrows created by the mites. The burrows may be multiple, straight

or wavy, brown or black, threadlike lesions, most commonly observed between the fingers and on the wrists. Other sites are the extensor surfaces of the elbows, the knees, the edges of the feet, the points of the elbows, around the nipples, in the axillary folds, under pendulous breasts, and in or near the groin or gluteal fold, penis, or scrotum. Red, pruritic eruptions usually appear between adjacent skin areas. However, the burrow is not always visible (Dunphy et al., 2015; Mounsey et al., 2015).

One classic sign of scabies is the increased itching that occurs during the evening hours, perhaps because the increased warmth of the skin has a stimulating effect on the parasite. Hypersensitivity to the organism and its products of excretion also may contribute to the pruritus. If the infection has spread, other members of the family and close friends also complain of pruritus about 1 month later (Dunphy et al., 2015; Mounsey et al., 2015).

Secondary lesions are quite common and include vesicles, papules, excoriations, and crusts. Bacterial superinfection may result from persistent excoriation of the burrows and papules (Dunphy et al., 2015; Mounsey et al., 2015).

 ## Gerontologic Considerations

Older adult patients living in long-term care facilities are susceptible to outbreaks of scabies because of close living quarters, poor hygiene due to limited physical ability, and the potential for incidental spread of the organisms by staff members. The vivid inflammatory reaction seen in younger people seldom occurs; rather, the older adult may have peripheral sensory deficits and be less prone to scratch or may be physically unable to scratch. Scratching is an effective mechanism that partially eradicates mite infestation; thus, this results in a more severe subtype. The lesions crust over (causing "crusted scabies") and, in time, may become hyperkeratotic (Dunphy et al., 2015).

Health care personnel in extended-care facilities should wear gloves when providing hands-on care to a patient suspected of having scabies until the diagnosis is confirmed and treatment completed. It is advisable to treat all residents, staff, and families of patients at the same time to prevent reinfection. The scales that are present with crusted scabies must be removed so that the antiscabicidal medication may be effective. Crusts may be removed with warm water soaks followed by application of 5% salicylic acid in petrolatum cream (Thomas, Peterson, Walton, et al., 2015).

Assessment and Diagnostic Findings

The diagnosis is confirmed by recovering *S. scabei* or the mites' by-products from the skin. A sample of superficial epidermis is scraped from the top of the burrows or papules with a small scalpel blade. The scrapings are placed on a microscope slide and examined through a microscope at low power to demonstrate evidence of the mite (Dunphy et al., 2015; Thomas et al., 2015).

Medical Management

The patient is instructed to take a warm, soapy bath or shower to remove the scaling debris from the crusts and then to pat the skin dry thoroughly and allow it to cool. A prescription scabicide, 5% permethrin, is considered the medication of choice. It is applied thinly to the entire skin from the neck down, sparing only the face and scalp (which are not affected in scabies). The medication is left on for 12 to 24 hours, after which the patient is instructed to wash thoroughly. One application may be curative, but it is advisable to repeat the treatment in 1 week (Thomas et al., 2015).

Nursing Management

The patient should wear clean clothing and sleep between freshly laundered bed linens. All bedding and clothing should be washed in hot water and dried on the hot dryer cycle. If bed linens or clothing cannot be washed in hot water, dry cleaning is advised.

After treatment is completed, the patient may apply an ointment, such as a topical corticosteroid, to skin lesions because the scabicide may irritate the skin. The patient's hypersensitivity does not cease on destruction of the mites. Pruritus may continue for several weeks as a manifestation of hypersensitivity, particularly in people who are atopic (allergic). This is not a sign that the treatment has failed. The patient is instructed not to apply more scabicide, because it will cause more irritation and increased itching, and not to take frequent hot showers, because they can dry the skin and produce pruritus. Oral antihistamines such as diphenhydramine or hydroxyzine can help control the pruritus. If a secondary infection is present, treatment with oral antibiotic agents may be indicated (Dunphy et al., 2015; Thomas et al., 2015).

All family members and close contacts should be treated simultaneously to eliminate the mites. Some scabicides are approved for use in infants and pregnant women. If scabies is sexually transmitted, the patient may require treatment for coexisting STI. Scabies may also coexist with pediculosis.

NONINFECTIOUS INFLAMMATORY DERMATOSES

Irritant Contact Dermatitis

Contact dermatitis (also called *eczema*) is an inflammatory reaction of the skin to physical, chemical, or biologic agents. The epidermis is damaged by repeated physical and chemical irritations. Contact dermatitis may be of the primary irritant type, in which a nonallergic reaction results from exposure to an irritating substance, or it may be an allergic reaction resulting from exposure of sensitized people to contact allergens (see Chapter 37).

Common causes of irritant dermatitis are soaps, detergents, scouring compounds, and industrial chemicals. Predisposing factors include extremes of heat and cold, frequent contact with soap and water, and a pre-existing skin disease. Persons at risk include those whose occupations require repeated handwashing (e.g., nurses) or repeated exposure to food or other irritants (e.g., cleaners, hairdressers, food preparation workers). Women tend to be affected more commonly than men (Cohen, 2014).

Clinical Manifestations

The eruptions begin when the causative agent contacts the skin. The first reactions include pruritus, burning, and erythema, followed closely by edema, papules, vesicles, and oozing or weeping. In the subacute phase, these vesicular changes are less marked, and they alternate with crusting, drying, fissuring, and peeling. If repeated reactions occur or if the patient continually scratches the skin, lichenification and pigmentation occur. Secondary bacterial invasion may follow (Cohen, 2014).

Medical Management

The objectives of management are to soothe and heal the involved skin and protect it from further damage. The distribution pattern of the reaction is identified to differentiate between allergic and irritant contact dermatitis. A detailed history is obtained. If possible, the offending irritant is removed. Local irritation should be avoided, and soap is not generally used until healing occurs.

Many preparations are advocated for relieving dermatitis. In general, a barrier cream that contains ceramide (e.g., Impruv, CeraVe) or dimethicone (e.g., Cetaphil) is used for small patches of erythema. A thin layer of cream or ointment containing a corticosteroid is commonly used, although the efficacy of corticosteroids has not been demonstrated in research (Cohen, 2014). The patient is educated about how to treat and prevent future bouts of irritant dermatitis (see Chart 61-3).

Psoriasis

Psoriasis is a chronic inflammatory multisystem disorder of the skin that affects approximately 3.2% of Americans (Nicpon, 2017). Although the primary manifestation of this

---

Chart 61-3

PATIENT EDUCATION

Strategies for Avoiding Contact Dermatitis

The precautions listed below may help prevent repeated cases of contact dermatitis and should be followed for at least 4 months after skin appears to be completely healed.

The nurse instructs the patient to:

- Study the pattern and location of your dermatitis and think about which things have touched your skin and which things may have caused the problem; try to avoid contact with these materials.
- Avoid heat, soap, and rubbing, all of which are external irritants.
- Choose bath soaps, laundry detergents, and cosmetics that do not contain fragrance.
- Avoid using a fabric softener dryer sheet (Bounce, Cling Free). Fabric softeners that are added to the washer may be used.
- Avoid topical medications, lotions, or ointments, except those specifically prescribed for your condition.
- Wash your skin thoroughly immediately after exposure to possible irritants.
- Ensure that when wearing gloves (such as for washing dishes or general cleaning), they are cotton lined. Do not wear them more than 15 or 20 minutes at a time.

Adapted from Hogan, D. J. (2016). Irritant contact dermatitis. *Medscape*. Retrieved on 2/11/2017 at: emedicine.medscape.com/article/1049352-overview noncommunicable disease tends to involve the skin, psoriasis may involve the oral cavity, eyes (including the lids, conjunctivae, and corneas), and joints. Psoriasis is typically characterized by the appearance of silvery plaques that most commonly appear on the skin over the elbows, knees, scalp, lower back, and buttocks (Meffert, 2016). Onset may occur at any age, with a median onset at 28 years. It is more prevalent among women and Caucasians. It is thought that most patients with psoriasis have a genetic predisposition to develop the disease. Psoriasis is characterized by periods of remission and exacerbation throughout life (Meffert, 2016).

Pathophysiology

Current evidence supports an autoimmune basis for psoriasis. Periods of emotional stress and anxiety aggravate the condition, and trauma, infections, and seasonal and hormonal changes may also serve as triggers (Meffert, 2016).

In this disease, the epidermis becomes infiltrated by activated T cells and cytokines, resulting in both vascular engorgement and proliferation of keratinocytes. Epidermal hyperplasia results. These epidermal cells tend to improperly retain their nuclei, crippling their ability to release lipids that encourage cellular adhesion. This results in rapid turnover of poorly matured cells that do not adhere well to each other, resulting in the classic presentation of plaquelike lesions that have a silvery, scaly, flaky appearance (Meffert, 2016).

Clinical Manifestations

Psoriasis may range in severity from a cosmetic source of annoyance to a physically disabling and disfiguring disorder. Lesions appear as red, raised patches of skin covered with silvery scales. The scaly patches are formed by the buildup of living and dead skin (see Fig. 61-4). If the scales are scraped away, the dark red base of the lesion is exposed, producing multiple bleeding points. The patches are not moist and may be pruritic. In many cases, the nails are also involved, with pitting, discoloration, crumbling beneath the free edges, and separation of the nail plate (Meffert, 2016). Psoriasis is classified as mild if the plaques involve less than 5% body surface area (BSA), moderate if they involve between 5% and

Figure 61-4 • Psoriasis.

10% of BSA, and severe if more than 10% BSA is affected by plaque formation (Nicpon, 2017).

Complications

Asymmetric rheumatoid factor–negative arthritis of multiple joints occurs in up to 42% of people with psoriasis, most typically after the skin lesions appear (Nicpon, 2017). The most typical joints affected include those in the hands or feet, although sometimes larger joints such as the elbows, knees, or hips may be affected (Meffert, 2016). A rheumatologist should be consulted to assist in the diagnosis and long-term treatment of this disorder. See Chapter 38 for further discussion of spondyloarthropathies, including psoriatic arthritis.

Generalized exfoliative dermatitis, also called *erythroderma*, may also result from psoriasis (see discussion later in this chapter).

Assessment and Diagnostic Findings

The presence of the classic plaque-type lesions generally confirms the diagnosis of psoriasis. If in doubt, the health care provider should assess for signs of nail and scalp involvement and for a positive family history. Biopsy of the skin is of little diagnostic value. The presence and extent of plaque should be assessed carefully, to calculate BSA involvement.

Medical Management

The goals of management are to slow the rapid turnover of epidermis, to promote resolution of the psoriatic lesions, and to control the natural cycles of the disease. There is no known cure.

The therapeutic approach should be one that the patient understands; it should be cosmetically acceptable and minimally disruptive of lifestyle. Treatment involves the commitment of time and effort by the patient and possibly the family. Any precipitating or aggravating factors are addressed. An assessment is made of lifestyle because psoriasis is significantly affected by stress. Management of emotional factors should be addressed as part of the overall treatment of psoriasis. The patient is informed that treatment of severe psoriasis can be time-consuming, expensive, and aesthetically unappealing at times. Many patients report difficulty adhering to treatment plans, either for time reasons or lack of response to the treatment (Mease & Armstrong, 2014).

Gentle removal of scales is an important principle of psoriasis treatment. This can be accomplished by taking baths with added oils (e.g., olive oil, mineral oil), colloidal oatmeal preparations, or coal tar preparations. A soft brush may be used to gently scrub the psoriatic plaques. After bathing, the application of emollient creams containing alpha-hydroxy acids (e.g., Lac-Hydrin, Penederm) or salicylic acid can soften thick scales. The patient and family should be encouraged to establish a regular skin care routine that can be maintained even when the psoriasis is not in an acute stage (Mease & Armstrong, 2014).

Pharmacologic Therapy

Three types of therapy are commonly indicated: topical, phototherapy, and systemic. Topical agents, possibly in tandem with phototherapy, are recommended for mild disease.

Patients with moderate or severe disease should receive topical agents, phototherapy, and systemic treatment (Nicpon, 2017).

Topical Agents

Topically applied agents are used to slow the overactive epidermis. Topical corticosteroids may be applied for their anti-inflammatory effects (see Table 61-3). Choosing the correct strength of corticosteroid for the involved site and choosing the most effective vehicle base are important aspects of topical treatment. In general, high-potency topical corticosteroids should not be used on the face and intertriginous areas, and their use on other areas should be limited to a 4-week course of twice-daily applications. A 4-week break should be taken before repeating treatment with the high-potency corticosteroids. For long-term therapy, moderate-potency corticosteroids are used. On the face and intertriginous areas, only low-potency corticosteroids are appropriate for long-term use (Bronckers, Paller, van Geel, et al., 2015; Mease & Armstrong, 2014).

Occlusive dressings may be applied to increase the effectiveness of the corticosteroid. Large plastic bags may be used—one for the upper body with openings cut for the head and arms and one for the lower body with openings for the legs. Large rolls of tubular plastic can be used to cover the arms and legs. Another option is a vinyl jogging suit. The medication is applied, and the suit is put on over it. The hands can be wrapped in gloves, the feet in plastic bags, and the head in a shower cap. Occlusive dressings should not remain in place longer than 8 hours. The skin should be inspected carefully for the appearance of atrophy, hypopigmentation, striae, and telangiectasias—all of which are side effects of corticosteroids.

When psoriasis involves large areas of the body, topical corticosteroid treatment can be expensive and involve some systemic risk. The more potent corticosteroids, when applied to large areas of the body, have the potential to cause adrenal suppression through percutaneous absorption of the medication. In this event, other treatment modalities (e.g., nonsteroidal topical medications, ultraviolet light) may be used instead or in combination to decrease the need for corticosteroids (Bronckers et al., 2015; Mease & Armstrong, 2014).

Treatment with topical nonsteroidal agents, such as calcipotriene (Dovonex) and tazarotene (Tazorac), can suppress **epidermopoiesis** (i.e., development of epidermal cells) and cause sloughing of the rapidly growing epidermal cells. Calcipotriene 0.05% is a derivative of vitamin D_2. It works by decreasing the mitotic turnover of the psoriatic plaques. Its most common side effect is local irritation. The intertriginous areas and face should be avoided when using this medication. The patient should be monitored for symptoms of hypercalcemia. Calcipotriene is available as a cream for use on the body and a solution for the scalp. It is not recommended for use by older adult patients because of their more fragile skin or by pregnant or lactating women (Meffert, 2016).

Tazarotene, a retinoid, causes sloughing of the scales covering psoriatic plaques. As with other retinoids, it causes increased sensitivity to sunlight by loss of the outermost layer of skin, so the patient should be cautioned to use an effective sunscreen and avoid other photosensitizers (e.g., tetracycline, antihistamines). Tazarotene is listed as a category X drug in pregnancy; reports indicate evidence of fetal risk, and the risk of use in pregnant women clearly outweighs any possible benefits. A negative result on a pregnancy test should be obtained before initiating this medication in women of childbearing age, and an effective contraceptive should be continued during treatment. Side effects include burning, erythema, or irritation at the site of application, and worsening of psoriasis (Meffert, 2016).

Intralesional injections of the corticosteroid triamcinolone (Aristocort) can be given directly into highly visible or isolated patches of psoriasis that are resistant to other forms of therapy. Care must be taken to ensure that the medication is not injected into normal skin (Meffert, 2016).

Phototherapy

For patients who do not respond well to topical treatments, phototherapy using narrow-band ultraviolet-B (UVB) therapy may be effective as a single-therapy modality. However, phototherapy is generally more effective when it is given as ultraviolet-A (UVA) in conjunction with a photosensitizing oral medication (a combination referred to as PUVA). Here, the patient takes a photosensitizing medication (i.e., psoralen) in a standard dose and is subsequently exposed to long-wave ultraviolet light as the medication plasma levels peak. It is thought that when psoralen-treated skin is exposed to UVA light, the psoralen binds with DNA and decreases epidermal cellular proliferation. PUVA has been associated with long-term risks of skin cancer, cataracts, and premature aging of the skin (Bronckers et al., 2015; Meffert, 2016).

The patient is usually treated two or three times each week until the psoriasis clears. An interim period of 48 hours between treatments is necessary to allow any burns resulting from PUVA therapy to become evident. After the psoriasis clears, the patient begins a maintenance program. Once little or no disease is active, less potent therapies are used to keep minor flare-ups under control (Meffert, 2016).

Systemic Agents

Although systemic corticosteroids may cause rapid improvement of psoriasis, the usual risks and the possibility of triggering a severe flare-up on withdrawal limit their use; therefore, they are not indicated for treatment of psoriasis.

Methotrexate, a systemic cytotoxic agent, is the first-line drug for treating moderate to severe psoriasis (Nicpon, 2017). Methotrexate appears to inhibit DNA synthesis in epidermal cells, thereby reducing the turnover time of the psoriatic epidermis. However, the medication can be toxic, especially to the liver, kidneys, and bone marrow. Laboratory studies must be monitored to ensure that the hepatic, hematopoietic, and renal systems are functioning adequately. The patient should avoid drinking alcohol while taking methotrexate because alcohol ingestion increases the possibility of liver damage. The medication is teratogenic and thus should not be given to pregnant women.

Cyclosporine (Neoral), a cyclic peptide immunosuppressive agent, may be considered in treatment of severe, therapy-resistant cases of psoriasis. However, its use is limited by side effects such as hypertension and nephrotoxicity and is only indicated for short-term use, generally no longer than 3 to 6 months (Bronckers et al., 2015; Meffert, 2016).

Another line of treatments for psoriasis includes a group called *biologic agents* because of their derivation from immunomodulators and bioengineered proteins (such as antibodies or recombinant cytokines) and their targeted action directly on the T cells. These agents act by inhibiting activation and migration, eliminating the T cells completely, slowing postsecretory cytokines or inducing immune deviation.

Infliximab (Remicade) is a monoclonal antibody that binds to tumor necrosis factor-alpha (TNF-α) and can only be given by IV infusion. Ustekinumab (Stelara) is also a monoclonal antibody that specifically interferes with the effect of interleukins (ILs), particularly IL-12 and IL-23. Etanercept (Enbrel) is a fusion protein that binds to soluble TNF-α and blocks its interaction with cell surface receptors. Alefacept (Amevive) is a fusion protein that inhibits T-cell proliferation. Adalimumab (Humira) is a recombinant human immunoglobulin G1 (IgG1) monoclonal antibody against TNF-α. These biologic agents have significant side effects, making close monitoring essential (Bronckers et al., 2015; Meffert, 2016).

Nursing Management

Psoriasis may cause despair and frustration for the patient; observers may stare, comment, ask embarrassing questions, or even avoid the person. The disease can eventually exhaust the patient's resources, interfere with their job, and negatively affect many aspects of life.

The nurse assesses the impact of the disease on the patient and the coping strategies used for conducting normal activities and interactions with family and friends (Bronckers et al., 2015). Many patients need reassurance that the condition is not infectious, not a reflection of poor personal hygiene, and not skin cancer. The nurse can create an environment in which the patient feels comfortable discussing important quality-of-life issues related to their psychosocial and physical response to this chronic illness.

The nurse explains with sensitivity that although there is no cure for psoriasis and lifetime management is necessary, the condition can usually be controlled. The pathophysiology of psoriasis is reviewed, as are the factors that provoke it—irritation or injury to the skin (e.g., cut, abrasion, sunburn), current illness (e.g., pharyngeal streptococcal infection), and emotional stress. It is emphasized that repeated trauma to the skin and an unfavorable environment (e.g., cold) may exacerbate psoriasis. The patient is cautioned about taking any nonprescription medications because some may aggravate mild psoriasis. As well, the patient is advised to seek treatment from the same primary provider for any acute illnesses or chronic conditions to minimize chances of receiving prescriptions that may interfere with each other (Meffert, 2016; Nicpon, 2017).

Reviewing and explaining the treatment regimen are essential to ensure adherence to the therapeutic regimen. For example, if the patient has a mild condition confined to localized areas, such as the elbows or knees, application of an emollient to maintain softness and minimize scaling may be all that is required. Most patients need a comprehensive plan of care that ranges from using topical medications and shampoos to more complex and lengthy treatment with systemic medications and photochemotherapy, such as PUVA therapy. Patient education materials that include a description of the

therapy and specific guidelines are helpful but cannot replace face-to-face discussions of the treatment plan.

To avoid injuring the skin, the patient is advised not to pick at or scratch the affected areas. Measures to prevent dry skin are encouraged because dry skin worsens psoriasis. Too-frequent washing produces more soreness and scaling. Water should be warm, not hot, and the skin should be dried by patting with a towel rather than by rubbing. Emollients have a moisturizing effect, providing an occlusive film on the skin surface so that normal water loss through the skin is halted and allowing the trapped water to hydrate the stratum corneum. A bath oil or emollient cleansing agent can comfort sore and scaling skin. Softening the skin can prevent fissures.

A therapeutic relationship between health care professionals and the patient with psoriasis includes education and support. Introducing the patient to successful coping strategies used by others with psoriasis and making suggestions for reducing or coping with stressful situations at home, school, and work can facilitate a more positive outlook and acceptance of the chronicity of the disease (Bronckers et al., 2015).

Promoting Home, Community-Based, and Transitional Care

 Educating Patients About Self-Care

Printed patient education materials may be provided to reinforce face-to-face discussions about treatment guidelines and other considerations. Patients using topical corticosteroid preparations repeatedly on the face and around the eyes should be aware that cataract development is possible. Strict guidelines for applying these medications should be emphasized, because overuse can result in skin atrophy, striae, and medication resistance.

PUVA, which is reserved for moderate to severe psoriasis, produces photosensitization. If exposure to the sun is unavoidable, the skin must be protected with sunscreen and clothing. Gray- or green-tinted wraparound sunglasses should be worn to protect the eyes during and after treatment, and ophthalmologic examinations should be performed on a regular basis (Meffert, 2016; Nicpon, 2017).

If indicated, referral may be made to a mental health professional who can help to ease emotional strain and give support. Belonging to a support group may also help patients recognize that they are not alone in experiencing life adjustments in response to a visible, chronic disease. The National Psoriasis Foundation publishes periodic bulletins and reports about new and relevant developments in this condition (see Resources section at the end of this chapter).

Generalized Exfoliative Dermatitis

Generalized exfoliative dermatitis, also called *erythroderma*, is characterized by a scaling erythematous dermatitis that may involve more than 90% of the skin (César, Cruz, Mota, et al., 2016). Generalized exfoliative dermatitis has a variety of causes. It may occur as a result of a reactive process (e.g., drug allergy) or may be secondary to an underlying skin disease (e.g., psoriasis, contact dermatitis, atopic dermatitis) or a systemic disease (e.g., lymphoma, leukemia). The cause is idiopathic (i.e., unknown) in approximately 16% of cases

(Kellen & Berlin, 2016); idiopathic generalized exfoliative dermatitis is also called *red man syndrome* (Umar & Kelly, 2016). Although generalized exfoliative dermatitis may occur at any age, it more commonly appears in those between the ages of 41 and 61 years. It occurs two to four times more commonly in men than in women (Kellen & Berlin, 2016).

Clinical Manifestations

This condition starts as a patchy or generalized erythematous eruption accompanied by fever, malaise, and chills. The skin color changes from pink to dark red. Afterward, the characteristic exfoliation (i.e., scaling) begins, usually in the form of thin flakes that leave the underlying skin smooth and red, with new scales forming as the older ones come off. It may be associated with chills, fever, prostration, and severe pruritus. There is a profound loss of stratum corneum (i.e., outermost layer of the skin), which causes capillary leakage, hypoalbuminemia, and negative nitrogen balance. Because of widespread dilation of cutaneous vessels, large amounts of body heat can be lost. Hair loss may accompany this disorder. The progression of these clinical manifestations varies, depending on the underlying cause. For instance, the progression from fever and scaling may be acute and progress over hours or a couple of days when generalized exfoliative dermatitis results from a drug reaction, or may be insidious and progress over weeks when it is secondary to a skin disease, such as psoriasis (Umar & Kelly, 2016).

Assessment and Diagnostic Findings

The presence of scaling erythematous dermatitis, particularly when it occurs in tandem with a known skin disease or a new prescription medication, increases the suspicion that generalized exfoliative dermatitis may be diagnosed. The patient frequently also presents with hypoalbuminemia and a negative nitrogen balance, as described previously, as well as an increased erythrocyte sedimentation rate that is consistent with an underlying acute inflammatory process. A skin biopsy is indicated, because it may confirm the underlying cause and diagnosis (Umar & Kelly, 2016).

Medical Management

The objectives of management are to discern and treat any underlying disorder, to maintain fluid and electrolyte balance, and to prevent infection. The treatment is individualized and supportive and should be initiated as soon as the condition is diagnosed.

The patient may be hospitalized. All medications that may be implicated are discontinued. A comfortable room temperature should be maintained because the patient does not have normal thermoregulatory control as a result of temperature fluctuations caused by vasodilation and evaporative water loss. Fluid and electrolyte balance must be maintained because there is considerable water and protein loss from the skin surface. Administration of plasma volume expanders may be indicated. Patients in a negative nitrogen balance may be prescribed enteral or parenteral therapy (Umar & Kelly, 2016) (see Chapter 44).

Nursing Management

Continual nursing assessment is carried out to prevent sepsis. The disrupted, erythematous, moist skin is susceptible to infection and becomes colonized with pathogenic organisms, which produce more inflammation. Antibiotic agents, which are prescribed if infection is present, are selected on the basis of culture and sensitivity.

Hypothermia may occur because increased blood flow in the skin, coupled with increased water loss through the skin, leads to heat loss by radiation, conduction, and evaporation. Changes in vital signs are closely monitored and reported.

Topical therapy is used to provide symptomatic relief. Soothing baths, compresses, and lubrication with emollients are used to treat the extensive dermatitis. Topical corticosteroids are the mainstay of treatment (see Table 61-3). The patient is likely to be extremely irritable because of the severe pruritus; sedating antihistamines to be given before bedtime may be prescribed to relieve the itching and promote sleep (e.g., hydroxyzine [Atarax, Vistaril]) (Umar & Kelly, 2016).

The use of oral or parenteral corticosteroids may be prescribed; however, their use is controversial. They are contraindicated when the cause of the condition is either not known or is suspected to be secondary to an underlying skin disease, such as psoriasis. When generalized exfoliative dermatitis occurs as a complication of psoriasis, systemic corticosteroids can exacerbate the condition (Umar & Kelly, 2016). When a specific cause is known, more specific therapy may be used. The patient is advised to avoid all irritants in the future, particularly medications that are known to cause the condition (Kellen & Berlin, 2016).

BLISTERING DISEASES

Blisters of the skin have many origins, including bacterial, fungal, or viral infections; allergic contact reactions; burns; metabolic disorders; and immunologically mediated (i.e., autoimmune) reactions. Some of these have been discussed previously (e.g., herpes simplex and zoster infections, contact dermatitis).

In the past, blistering diseases that resulted from immunoglobulin G (IgG)-mediated autoimmune reactions were generally classified as *pemphigus*. Today, there are three recognized subsets of these types of IgG-mediated skin disorders, including pemphigus vulgaris, pemphigus foliaceus, and paraneoplastic pemphigus. Pemphigus vulgaris accounts for 70% of these blistering diseases, whereas the others are much less common (Santoro, Stoopler, & Werth, 2013). Bullous pemphigoid, another type of IgG-mediated blistering disorder, has distinct characteristics that make this disease different from the pemphigus disorders. Blistering diseases that result from other autoimmune responses may also occur. For instance, dermatitis herpetiform occurs as a consequence of an immunoglobulin A (IgA)-mediated response from gluten sensitivity. The diagnosis for these types of disorders is made by histologic examination of a biopsy specimen, usually by a dermatopathologist (Santoro et al., 2013).

Pemphigus Vulgaris

Pemphigus vulgaris is characterized by the appearance of bullae (blisters) of various sizes on apparently normal skin and mucous membranes. Pemphigus vulgaris is an autoimmune disease where the IgG antibody is directed against a specific cell surface antigen in epidermal cells. A blister forms from the antigen–antibody reaction. The level of serum antibody is predictive of disease severity. Genetic factors may also have a role in its development, with the highest incidence in people of Jewish or Mediterranean descent. This disorder usually occurs in men and women in middle and late adulthood. The condition may be associated with other concomitant autoimmune diseases, most commonly myasthenia gravis (Santoro et al., 2013).

Assessment and Diagnostic Findings

Most patients present with oral lesions appearing as irregularly shaped erosions that are painful, bleed easily, and heal slowly. The skin bullae enlarge, rupture, and leave large, painful eroded areas that are accompanied by crusting and oozing. A characteristic odor emanates from the bullae and the exuding serum. There is blistering or sloughing of uninvolved skin when minimal pressure is applied (Nikolsky sign). The eroded skin heals slowly, and large areas of the body eventually are involved.

Specimens from the blister and surrounding skin demonstrate **acantholysis** (separation of epidermal cells from each other because of damage to or an abnormality of the intracellular substance), and immunofluorescent studies show intraepidermal presence of IgG (Santoro et al., 2013).

The most common complications arise when the disease process is widespread. Skin bacteria have relatively easy access to the bullae as they ooze, rupture, and leave denuded areas exposed to the environment. Fluid and electrolyte imbalance results from fluid and protein loss as the bullae rupture.

Medical Management

The goals of therapy are to bring the disease under control as rapidly as possible, to prevent loss of serum and the development of secondary infection, and to promote re-epithelization (i.e., renewal of epithelial tissue).

Corticosteroids are given to control the disease and keep the skin free of blisters. The dosage level is maintained until remission is apparent. Immunosuppressive agents (e.g., azathioprine [Imuran], mycophenolate mofetil [CellCept]) are prescribed early in the course of the disease to help control the disease and reduce the corticosteroid dose. The monoclonal antibody rituximab (Rituxan) may be chosen as an alternative agent, as well as intravenous immunoglobulin (IVIG). The immunosuppressant agent cyclophosphamide (Cytoxan) may be tried when other medications fail to induce remission (Santoro et al., 2013; Zeina, Mansoor, & Sakka, 2016).

Bullous Pemphigoid

Bullous pemphigoid is a chronic disease that is characterized by periodic flare-up and remission. If untreated, it may be fatal. It is most commonly seen in the older adult, with a peak incidence at about 65 years of age. There is no gender or racial predilection, and the disease can be found throughout the world (Chan, 2016).

Assessment and Diagnostic Findings

Bullous pemphigoid is characterized most commonly by the general appearance of tense bullae that have a particular tendency to appear on the flexor surfaces of the arms. When the blisters break, the skin has shallow erosions that heal fairly quickly. Pruritus can be intense, even before the appearance of the blisters (Chan, 2016).

Immunofluorescent studies of skin biopsy specimens from patients with bullous pemphigoid reveal depositions of IgG and complement C3 at the junction of the dermis and epidermis (Chan, 2016).

Medical Management

Medical treatment includes topical corticosteroids for localized eruptions and systemic anti-inflammatory or immunosuppressant medications for widespread involvement. Systemic corticosteroids (e.g., prednisone) may be continued for months, in alternate-day doses. The patient needs to understand the implications of long-term corticosteroid therapy (see Chapter 52, Table 52-4). Tetracycline may be prescribed, although not for its antimicrobial effectiveness but because its anti-inflammatory properties are believed to be particularly efficacious in treating this disorder. Alternative medications may include immunosuppressive agents (e.g., azathioprine) or monoclonal antibodies (e.g., rituximab). Most patients will achieve remission, although this may require from 6 to 60 months of treatment (Chan, 2016).

Dermatitis Herpetiformis

Dermatitis herpetiformis is an intensely pruritic, chronic disease that manifests with small, tense blisters that are distributed over the extensor surfaces of the elbows and knees, as well as the buttocks and back. It most commonly occurs between 20 and 40 years of age but can appear at any age. It is more common in people of northern European heritage and is slightly more common in men. Patients with dermatitis herpetiformis have a defect in gluten metabolism; many have a concomitant diagnosis of celiac disease (Antiga & Caproni, 2015).

Assessment and Diagnostic Findings

Patients typically present with erythematous papules with small, clustered (i.e., herpetiform) vesicles that tend to have a symmetrical distribution on affected extensor surfaces of the skin. Erosions and crusts may also be present, which may result from excoriation and scratching as a reaction to the intense pruritus (Antiga & Caproni, 2015).

Immunofluorescent studies of skin biopsy specimens from patients with dermatitis herpetiformis reveal granular patterns of IgA deposits in the papillary dermis (Antiga & Caproni, 2015).

Medical Management

Most patients respond to dapsone (Aczone) and to a gluten-free diet. All patients should be screened for glucose-6-phosphate dehydrogenase deficiency because dapsone can induce severe hemolysis in those with this deficiency. Patients benefit from dietary counseling because the dietary restrictions are lifelong, and a gluten-free diet is often difficult to follow (Antiga & Caproni, 2015). Patients need emotional support as they deal with the process of learning new habits and accepting major changes in their lives.

NURSING PROCESS

Care of the Patient With Blistering Diseases

Assessment

Patients with blistering disorders may experience significant disability. There is constant itching and possible pain in the denuded areas of skin. There may be drainage from the denuded areas, which may be malodorous. Effective assessment and nursing management become a challenge.

Disease activity is monitored clinically by examining the skin for the appearance of new blisters. Particular attention is given to assessing for signs and symptoms of infection. Hyperpigmentation may be seen in areas of resolving blisters.

Diagnosis

NURSING DIAGNOSES

Based on the assessment data, major nursing diagnoses may include the following:

- Acute pain of skin and oral cavity related to blistering and erosions
- Impaired skin integrity related to ruptured bullae and denuded areas of the skin
- Disturbed body image related to the appearance of the skin
- Risk for infection related to loss of protective barrier of skin and mucous membranes
- Deficient fluid volume related to loss of tissue fluids

Planning and Goals

The major goals for the patient may include relief of discomfort from lesions, skin healing, improved body image, absence of infection, and achievement of fluid and electrolyte balance.

Nursing Interventions

RELIEVING ORAL DISCOMFORT

Depending on the skin disorder, the patient's entire oral cavity may be affected with erosions and denuded surfaces. Necrotic tissue may develop over these areas, adding to the patient's discomfort and interfering with eating. Weight loss and hypoproteinemia may result. Meticulous oral hygiene is important to keep the oral mucosa clean and allow the epithelium to regenerate. Frequent rinsing of the mouth with chlorhexidine solution is prescribed to rid the mouth of debris and to soothe ulcerated areas. Commercial mouthwashes are avoided. The lips are kept moist with petrolatum. Cool mist therapy helps humidify environmental air.

ENHANCING SKIN INTEGRITY AND RELIEVING DISCOMFORT

The patient with painful and extensive lesions should be premedicated with analgesic agents before skin care is initiated. Patients with large areas of blistering have a characteristic odor that decreases when secondary infection is controlled. After the patient's skin is bathed, it is dried carefully and dusted liberally with nonirritating powder (e.g., cornstarch), which enables the patient to move about freely in bed. Fairly large amounts are necessary to keep the patient's skin from adhering to the sheets. Tape should never be used because it may produce more blisters. Hypothermia is common, and measures to keep the patient warm and comfortable

are priority nursing activities. The nursing management of patients with bullous skin conditions can be similar to that for patients with extensive burns (see Chapter 62).

PROMOTING A POSITIVE BODY IMAGE

Attention to the psychological needs of the patient requires listening to the patient, being available, providing expert nursing care, and educating the patient and the family. The patient is encouraged to express anxieties, discomfort, and feelings of hopelessness. Arranging for a family member or a close friend to spend more time with the patient can be supportive. When patients receive information about the disease and its treatment, uncertainty and anxiety often decrease, and the patient's capacity to act on their own behalf is enhanced. Psychological counseling may assist the patient in dealing with fears, anxiety, and promote positive self-esteem.

PREVENTING INFECTION

The patient is susceptible to infection because the barrier function of the skin is compromised. Bullae are also susceptible to infection, and sepsis may follow (see Chapter 14). The skin is cleaned to remove debris and dead skin and to prevent infection.

Secondary infection may be accompanied by an unpleasant odor from skin or oral lesions. *Candida albicans* of the mouth (i.e., thrush) commonly affects patients receiving corticosteroid therapy. The oral cavity is inspected daily, and any changes are reported. Oral lesions are slow to heal.

> ▶ **Quality and Safety Nursing Alert**
>
> *Because infection is the leading cause of death in patients with blistering diseases, meticulous assessment for signs and symptoms of local and systemic infection is required. Seemingly trivial complaints or minimal changes are investigated because corticosteroids can mask or alter typical signs and symptoms of infection.*

The patient's vital signs are monitored, and temperature fluctuations are documented. The patient is observed for chills, and all secretions and excretions are monitored for changes suggesting infection. Results of culture and sensitivity tests are monitored. Antimicrobial agents are given as prescribed, and response to treatment is assessed. Health care personnel must perform effective hand hygiene and wear gloves.

In patients who are hospitalized, environmental contamination is reduced as much as possible. Isolation measures, standard precautions, and the use of appropriate PPE are warranted. See Chapter 36, Chart 36-5 for a description of standard precautions.

PROMOTING FLUID BALANCE

Extensive denudation of the skin leads to fluid and electrolyte imbalance because of significant loss of fluids and sodium chloride from the skin. This sodium chloride loss is responsible for many of the systemic symptoms associated with the disease and is treated by IV administration of saline solution.

A large amount of protein and blood is also lost from the denuded skin areas. Blood component therapy may be prescribed to maintain the blood volume, hemoglobin level, and plasma protein concentration. Serum albumin, protein, hemoglobin, and hematocrit values are monitored.

The patient is encouraged to maintain adequate oral fluid intake. Cool, nonirritating fluids are encouraged to maintain hydration. Small, frequent meals or snacks of high-protein, high-calorie foods (e.g., oral nutritional supplements, eggnog, milk shakes) help maintain nutritional status. Parenteral nutrition is considered if the patient cannot eat an adequate diet.

Evaluation

Expected patient outcomes may include:
1. Reports relief from pain of oral lesions
   a. Identifies therapies that reduce pain
   b. Uses mouthwashes and anesthetic or antiseptic aerosol mouth spray
   c. Drinks chilled fluids at 2-hour intervals
2. Achieves skin healing
   a. States purpose of therapeutic regimen
   b. Adheres to soaks and bath regimen
   c. Reminds caregivers to use liberal amounts of nonirritating powder on bed linens
3. Reports body image has improved
   a. Verbalizes concerns about condition, self, and relationships with others
   b. Participates in self-care
4. Remains free of infections and sepsis
   a. Has cultures from bullae, skin, and orifices that are negative for pathogenic organisms
   b. Has no purulent drainage
   c. Shows signs that skin is clearing
   d. Has normal body temperature
5. Maintains fluid and electrolyte balance
   a. Keeps intake record to ensure adequate fluid intake and normal fluid and electrolyte balance
   b. Verbalizes the rationale for IV infusion therapy
   c. Has urine output that is greater than 0.5 mL/kg/hr
   d. Has serum chemistry and hemoglobin and hematocrit values within normal limits

Toxic Epidermal Necrolysis and Stevens–Johnson Syndrome

Toxic epidermal necrolysis (TEN) and Stevens–Johnson syndrome (SJS) are potentially fatal acute skin disorders characterized by widespread erythema and macule formation with blistering, resulting in epidermal detachment or sloughing and erosion formation. These diseases are believed to be one and the same but manifest along a spectrum of reactions, with TEN being the most severe. The mortality rate from TEN is estimated to be 25% to 35% and from SJS is 1% to 5% (Kellen & Berlin, 2016). Up to 75% of cases of TEN and SJS are triggered by a reaction to medications, with antibiotics (especially sulfonamides), anticonvulsants, NSAIDs, allopurinol (Zyloprim), and oxicam NSAIDs (e.g., meloxicam [Mobic]) frequently implicated (Kellen & Berlin, 2016).

TEN and SJS occur in all ages and both genders, with a slight predilection for women. The mean age for patients with TEN and SJS is reported to be between 46 and 63 years. However, older adults who take multiple medications may be at greater risk. There appears to be a genetic component to developing TEN and SJS. The mechanism leading to TEN and SJS seems to be a cell-mediated cytotoxic reaction (Cohen, Jellinek, & Schwartz, 2016).

Clinical Manifestations

TEN and SJS are characterized initially by conjunctival burning or itching, cutaneous tenderness, fever, cough, sore throat, headache, extreme malaise, and myalgias (i.e., aches and pains). These signs are followed by a rapid onset of erythema involving much of the skin surface and mucous membranes, including the oral mucosa, conjunctiva, and genitalia. In severe cases of mucosal involvement, there may be danger of damage to the larynx, bronchi, and esophagus from ulcerations. Large, flaccid bullae develop in some areas; in other areas, large sheets of epidermis are shed, exposing the underlying dermis. Fingernails, toenails, eyebrows, and eyelashes may be shed along with the surrounding epidermis. The skin is excruciatingly tender, and the loss of skin leaves a weeping surface similar to that of a total-body, partial-thickness burn (Cohen et al., 2016; Kellen & Berlin, 2016).

Complications

Keratoconjunctivitis, sepsis, and multiple organ dysfunction syndrome (MODS) are potential complications of TEN and SJS. Keratoconjunctivitis can impair vision and result in conjunctival retraction, scarring, and corneal lesions. Sepsis and MODS can be life threatening (Cohen et al., 2016; Kellen & Berlin, 2016) (see Chapter 14).

Assessment and Diagnostic Findings

Histologic studies of frozen skin cells from a fresh lesion and cytodiagnosis of collections of cellular material from a freshly denuded area are conducted. A history of the use of medications known to precipitate TEN or SJS may confirm medication reaction as the underlying cause, especially if the medications were prescribed within 4 weeks prior to the onset of illness (Cohen et al., 2016).

Results from a complete blood count (CBC) may show leukopenia and a normochromic normocytic anemia. Skin biopsy results confirm the diagnosis, showing necrotic keratinocytes with full-thickness epithelial necrosis and detachment (Cohen et al., 2016).

Medical Management

The goals of treatment include control of fluid and electrolyte balance, prevention of sepsis, and prevention of ophthalmic complications. Supportive care is the mainstay of treatment.

Any medications that may be implicated as precipitating TEN or SJS are discontinued immediately. The patient is treated in a regional burn center because aggressive treatment similar to that for severe burns is required. Tissue samples from the nasopharynx, eyes, ears, blood, urine, skin, and unruptured blisters are obtained for culture to identify pathogenic organisms. IV crystalloid fluids are prescribed to maintain fluid and electrolyte balance, using parameters similar to those used to guide care of patients with burns. Similarly, thermoregulation, wound care, and pain management guidelines used to treat patients with burns are also implemented (Cohen et al., 2016) (see Chapter 62). Patients frequently require nutritional and metabolic support with total parenteral nutrition (see Chapter 44).

Initial treatment with systemic corticosteroids (e.g., methylprednisolone [Solu-Medrol]), although frequently tried, remains controversial. In many cases, the risk of infection, fluid and electrolyte imbalance, delayed healing, and difficulty in initiating oral corticosteroids early in the course of the disease outweigh its benefits. Administration of IVIG may provide rapid improvement and skin healing at dosages of 1 g/kg/day for 4 days. Other medications that may be effective include the immunosuppressive agents cyclosporine or cyclophosphamide (Cohen et al., 2016; Kellen & Berlin, 2016).

Protecting the skin with topical agents is crucial. Various topical antibacterial and anesthetic agents are used to prevent wound sepsis and to assist with pain management. Temporary biologic dressings (e.g., pigskin, amniotic membrane) or plastic semipermeable dressings (e.g., Vigilon) may be used to reduce pain, decrease evaporation, and prevent secondary infection until the epithelium regenerates. Meticulous oropharyngeal and eye care is essential when there is involvement of the mucous membranes and the eyes.

NURSING PROCESS

Care of the Patient With Toxic Epidermal Necrolysis or Stevens–Johnson Syndrome

Assessment

A careful inspection of the skin is made, including its appearance and the extent of involvement. The normal skin is closely observed to determine if new areas of blisters are developing. Drainage from blisters is monitored for amount, color, and odor. The oral cavity is inspected daily for blistering and erosive lesions; the patient is assessed daily for itching, burning, and dryness of the eyes. The patient's ability to swallow and drink fluids, as well as speak normally, is determined.

The patient's vital signs are monitored, and special attention is given to the presence and character of fever and the respiratory rate, depth, rhythm, and cough. The characteristics and amount of respiratory secretions are observed. Assessment for high fever, tachycardia, and extreme weakness and fatigue is essential because these factors indicate the process of epidermal necrosis, increased metabolic needs, and possible gastrointestinal and respiratory mucosal sloughing. Urine volume, specific gravity, and color are monitored. The insertion sites of IV lines are inspected for signs of local infection. Body weight is recorded daily.

The patient is asked to describe fatigue and pain levels. An attempt is made to evaluate the patient's level of anxiety. The patient's basic coping mechanisms are assessed, and effective coping strategies are identified.

Diagnosis

NURSING DIAGNOSES

Based on the assessment data, major nursing diagnoses may include the following:

- Impaired tissue integrity (i.e., oral, eye, and skin) related to epidermal shedding
- Deficient fluid volume and electrolyte losses related to loss of fluids from denuded skin

- Risk for imbalanced body temperature (i.e., hypothermia) related to heat loss secondary to skin loss
- Acute pain related to denuded skin and oral lesions
- Anxiety related to the physical appearance of the skin and prognosis

COLLABORATIVE PROBLEMS/POTENTIAL COMPLICATIONS

Potential complications may include the following:

- Sepsis
- Conjunctival retraction, scars, and corneal lesions

PLANNING AND GOALS

The major goals for the patient may include skin and oral tissue healing, fluid balance, prevention of heat loss, relief of pain, reduced anxiety, and absence of complications.

Nursing Interventions

MAINTAINING SKIN AND MUCOUS MEMBRANE INTEGRITY

The local care of the skin is an important area of nursing management. The skin denudes easily, especially when the patient is lifted and turned. The nursing staff must take special care to avoid friction involving the skin when moving the patient in bed. The skin should be checked after each position change to ensure that no new denuded areas have appeared. The nurse applies the prescribed topical agents to reduce the bacterial population of the wound surface. Warm compresses, if prescribed, should be applied gently to denuded areas. The topical antibacterial agent may be used in conjunction with hydrotherapy in a tank, bathtub, or shower. The nurse monitors the patient's condition during the treatment and encourages the patient to exercise the extremities during hydrotherapy.

The painful oral lesions make oral hygiene difficult. Careful oral hygiene is performed to keep the oral mucosa clean. Prescribed chlorhexidine mouthwashes, anesthetics, or coating agents are used frequently to rid the mouth of debris, soothe ulcerative areas, and control foul mouth odor. The oral cavity is inspected several times each day, and any changes are documented and reported. Petrolatum or a prescribed ointment is applied to the lips.

ATTAINING FLUID BALANCE

The patient's vital signs, urine output, and mental status are assessed for indications of hypovolemia. Mental changes from fluid and electrolyte imbalance, sensory overload, or sensory deprivation may occur. Laboratory test results are evaluated, and abnormal results are reported. The patient is weighed daily.

Oral lesions may result in dysphagia, making tube feeding or parenteral nutrition necessary until oral ingestion can be tolerated. A daily calorie count and accurate recording of all intake and output are essential.

PREVENTING HYPOTHERMIA

The patient with TEN is prone to chilling. Dehydration may be made worse by exposing the denuded skin to a continuous current of warm air. The patient is usually sensitive to changes in room temperature. Measures similar to those implemented for a patient with burns, such as cotton blankets, ceiling-mounted heat lamps, and heat shields, are useful in maintaining body temperature. To minimize shivering and heat loss, the nurse should work rapidly and efficiently when large wounds are exposed for wound care. The patient's temperature is monitored frequently.

RELIEVING PAIN

The nurse assesses the patient's pain, its characteristics, factors that influence the pain, and the patient's behavioral responses. Prescribed analgesic agents are given on a regular schedule, and the nurse documents pain relief and any side effects. Analgesics are given before painful treatments are performed. Providing thorough explanations and speaking calmly to the patient during treatments can allay the anxiety that may intensify pain. Offering emotional support and reassurance and implementing measures that promote rest and sleep are basic in achieving pain control. As the pain diminishes and the patient has more physical and emotional energy, the nurse may educate the patient in self-management techniques for pain relief, such as progressive muscle relaxation and imagery (see Chapter 12).

REDUCING ANXIETY

Because the lifestyle of the patient with TEN or SJS has been abruptly changed to one of complete dependence, an assessment of their emotional state may reveal anxiety, depression, and fear of dying. The patient can be reassured that these reactions are normal. The patient also needs nursing support, honest communication, and hope that the situation can improve. The patient is encouraged to express their feelings. Listening to the patient's concerns and being readily available with skillful and compassionate care are important anxiety-relieving interventions. Emotional support by a psychiatric nurse, spiritual advisor, psychologist, or psychiatrist may be helpful to promote coping during the long recovery period.

MONITORING AND MANAGING POTENTIAL COMPLICATIONS

Sepsis. The major cause of death from TEN is from sepsis. Monitoring vital signs closely and noticing changes in respiratory, kidney, and gastrointestinal function may quickly detect the beginning of an infection. Strict asepsis is always maintained during routine skin care measures. Hand hygiene and wearing sterile gloves when carrying out procedures are essential. Visitors should wear protective garments and wash their hands before and after coming into contact with the patient. People with any infections or infectious disease should not visit the patient until they are no longer a danger to the patient. The nurse is critical in identifying early signs and symptoms of infection and notifying the primary provider. Antibiotic agents are not generally begun until there is indication for their use (Cohen et al., 2016).

Conjunctival Retraction, Scars, and Corneal Lesions. The eyes are inspected daily for signs of pruritus, burning, and dryness, which may indicate progression to keratoconjunctivitis—the principal eye complication. Applying a cool, damp cloth over the eyes may relieve burning sensations. The eyes are kept clean and observed for signs of discharge or discomfort, and the progression of symptoms is documented and reported. Administering an eye lubricant, when prescribed, may alleviate dryness and prevent corneal abrasion. Using eye patches or reminding the patient to blink periodically may also counteract dryness. The patient is instructed to avoid rubbing the eyes or putting any medication into the eyes that has not been prescribed or recommended by the primary provider.

PROMOTING HOME, COMMUNITY-BASED, AND TRANSITIONAL CARE

Educating Patients About Self-Care. Patients with TEN or SJS with involvement of large areas of the skin require care that is similar to that of patients with thermal burns. As the patient completes the acute inpatient stage of illness, the focus is directed toward rehabilitation and outpatient care or care in a rehabilitation center. Throughout this care, the patient and family members are involved in the care and are instructed in the procedures, such as wound care and dressing changes that will need to be continued at home. The patient and family members are assisted in acquiring dressing supplies that will be needed at home.

The patient and family members are also provided with education about pain management; nutrition; measures to increase mobility; and prevention of complications, including prevention of infection. They are educated about the signs and symptoms of complications and instructed when to notify the health care provider. Instructions are provided in writing to the patient and family so that they can refer to these instructions when necessary at later times.

Continuing and Transitional Care. Interdisciplinary follow-up care is imperative to ensure that the patient's progress continues. Some patients will require care in a rehabilitation center before returning home. Others will require outpatient physical and occupational therapy for an extended period. When the patient returns home, the home care nurse coordinates the care provided by the various members of the health care team (e.g., physician, physical therapist, occupational therapist, dietician). The nurse also monitors the patient's progress, provides ongoing assessment to identify complications, and monitors the patient's adherence to the plan of care. The patient's adaptation to the home care environment and the patient's and family's needs for support and assistance are also assessed. Referrals to community agencies are made as appropriate.

Evaluation

Expected patient outcomes may include:

1. Achieves increasing skin and oral tissue healing
   a. Demonstrates areas of healing skin
   b. Swallows fluids and speaks clearly
2. Attains fluid balance
   a. Demonstrates laboratory values within normal ranges
   b. Maintains urine volume and specific gravity within acceptable range
   c. Shows stable vital signs
   d. Increases intake of oral fluids without discomfort
   e. Maintains weight or gains weight, if appropriate
3. Attains thermoregulation
   a. Registers body temperature within normal range
   b. Reports no chills
4. Achieves pain relief
   a. Uses analgesic agents as prescribed
   b. Applies self-management techniques for relief of pain
5. Reports less anxiety
   a. Discusses concerns freely
   b. Sleeps for progressively longer periods
6. Absence of complications, such as sepsis and impaired vision
   a. Has body temperature within normal range
   b. Demonstrates laboratory values within normal ranges
   c. Has no abnormal discharges or signs of infection
   d. Continues to see objects at baseline acuity level
   e. Shows no signs of keratoconjunctivitis

SKIN TUMORS

Tumors of the skin are common and occur along a spectrum from those that are benign to those that are highly malignant.

Benign Skin Tumors

Cysts

Cysts of the skin are epithelium-lined cavities that contain fluid or solid material. Epidermal cysts (epidermoid cysts) occur frequently and may be described as slow-growing, firm, elevated tumors found most frequently on the face, neck, upper chest, and back. Removal of the cysts provides a cure (Song, Burm, Yang, et al., 2014).

Pilar cysts (trichilemmal cysts), formerly called *sebaceous cysts*, are most frequently found on the scalp. They originate from the middle portion of the hair follicle and from the cells of the outer hair root sheath. Treatment is surgical removal (Song et al., 2014).

Seborrheic and Actinic Keratoses

Seborrheic keratoses are benign, wartlike lesions of various sizes and colors, ranging from light tan to black. They are usually located on the face, shoulders, chest, and back and are the most common skin tumors seen in middle-aged and older adults. Although these lesions are benign, they should be assessed periodically for changes in appearance that may suggest malignant transformation (see later discussion) (Grossman & Porth, 2014). They may be cosmetically unacceptable to the patient. Treatment is removal of the tumor tissue by excision, electrodesiccation (destruction of the skin lesions by monopolar high-frequency electric current) and curettage, or application of carbon dioxide or liquid nitrogen.

Actinic keratoses are premalignant skin lesions that develop in chronically sun-exposed areas of the body. They appear as rough, scaly patches with underlying erythema. These lesions may gradually transform into squamous cell carcinoma (SCC) (see later discussion); they are usually removed by cryotherapy, electrodesiccation, or lasers, or they may be treated with topical chemotherapeutic creams (e.g., 5-fluorouracil cream) (Rosso, Kircik, Goldenberg, et al., 2014).

Verrucae: Warts

Warts are common, benign skin tumors caused by infection with the human papillomavirus, which belongs to the DNA virus group. People of all ages may be affected, but the warts occur most frequently between the ages of 12 and 16 years. There are many types of warts.

As a rule, warts are asymptomatic, except when they occur on weight-bearing areas, such as the soles of the feet. They may be treated with locally applied laser therapy, liquid nitrogen, salicylic acid plasters, or electrodesiccation (Akram & Zaman, 2015).

Warts occurring on the genitalia and perianal areas are known as condylomata acuminata. They may be transmitted sexually and are treated with liquid nitrogen, cryosurgery, electrosurgery, topically applied trichloroacetic acid, and curettage. Condylomata that affect the uterine cervix predispose the patient to cervical cancer (see Chapter 57).

Angiomas

Angiomas are benign vascular tumors that involve the skin and the subcutaneous tissues. They are present at birth and may occur as flat, violet-red patches (port-wine angiomas) or as raised, bright red, nodular lesions (i.e., hemangiomas of infancy, formerly known as strawberry angiomas). The latter tend to involute spontaneously within the first few years of life, but port-wine angiomas usually persist indefinitely. Most patients use masking cosmetics to camouflage the lesions. Cherry angiomas are small, smooth deep red papules found on the trunk of most adults older than 30 years of age that are benign and generally not considered cosmetically problematic (Grossman & Porth, 2014).

Pigmented Nevi: Moles

Moles are common skin tumors of various sizes and shades, ranging from yellowish brown to black. They may be flat, macular lesions or elevated papules or nodules that occasionally contain hair. Most pigmented nevi are harmless lesions. However, in rare cases, malignant changes occur, and a melanoma develops at the site of the nevus. Nevi that show a change in color or size, become symptomatic (e.g., itch), or develop irregular borders should be removed to determine if malignant changes have occurred. Moles that occur in unusual places should be examined carefully for any irregularity and for notching of the border and variation in color. Early melanomas may display some redness and irritation and areas of bluish pigmentation where the pigment-containing cells have spread deeper into the skin. Late melanomas have areas of paler color, where pigment cells have stopped producing melanin. Nevi larger than 5 mm should be examined carefully. Excised nevi should be examined histologically (Sardana, Chakravarty, & Goel, 2014).

Keloids

Keloids are benign overgrowths of fibrous tissue at the site of a scar or trauma. They appear to be more common among people with dark skin. Keloids are asymptomatic but may cause disfigurement and cosmetic concern (Hochman, Isoldi, Furtado, et al., 2015). The treatment may consist of surgical excision, intralesional corticosteroid therapy, and radiation.

Dermatofibroma

A dermatofibroma is a common, benign tumor of connective tissue that occurs predominantly on the extremities. It is a firm, dome-shaped nodule that may be skin colored or pinkish brown (Alves, Matos, Barreiros, et al., 2014). Excisional biopsy is the recommended method of treatment.

Neurofibromatosis: Von Recklinghausen Disease

Neurofibromatosis is a hereditary condition manifested by pigmented patches (*café-au-lait* macules), axillary freckling, and cutaneous neurofibromas that vary in size. Developmental changes may occur in the nervous system, muscles, and bone. Malignant degeneration of the neurofibromas occurs in some patients (Friedman, 2014).

Malignant Skin Tumors

Skin cancer is the most common cancer in the United States. Nearly 5 million people are treated for skin cancer each year, which incurs an annual cost of approximately $8.1 billion dollars (U.S. Department of Health and Human Services [HHS], 2014). Because the skin is easily inspected, skin cancer is readily seen and detected and is therefore believed to be amenable to early intervention. However, the U.S. Preventive Services Task Force notes that there remains a gap in the evidence-based literature to support the assertion that early detection reduces skin cancer rates; clearly, more studies are indicated (Wernli, Henrikson, Morrison, et al., 2016).

Exposure to ultraviolet (UV) radiation, including the sun and artificial UV rays (e.g., tanning booths) is the leading preventable cause of skin cancer; incidence is related to the total amount of exposure to the sun. Sun damage is cumulative, and harmful effects may be severe by 20 years of age (HHS, 2014). Most skin cancers manifest after a 20- to 50-year latency period post-UV radiation exposure (Bader, Kennedy, Santacroce, et al., 2016) (see Chart 61-4). Over 99% of all skin cancers include melanoma and the two most common types of nonmelanoma skin cancers (NMSCs), basal cell carcinoma (BCC), and SCC (HHS, 2014).

Basal Cell Carcinoma and Squamous Cell Carcinoma

BCC is the most prevalent skin cancer in the United States. It is rarely associated with any morbidity and rarely causes death. It is estimated that up to 80% of NMSCs among men and up to 90% of NMSCs among women are BCCs. Although less common than BCC, SCC is the second most prevalent skin cancer in the United States. Although less aggressive than melanoma, SCC is believed to be responsible for at least 4000 deaths annually (HHS, 2014).

Clinical Manifestations

BCC generally appears on sun-exposed areas of the body, such as the face, neck, hands, and scalp. BCC usually begins as a small, waxy nodule with rolled, translucent, pearly borders; telangiectatic vessels may be present. As it grows, it undergoes central ulceration and sometimes crusting (see Fig. 61-5A). The tumors appear most frequently on the face. BCC is characterized by invasion and erosion of contiguous (adjoining) tissues. It rarely metastasizes, but recurrence is common. However, a neglected lesion can result in the loss of a nose, an ear, or a lip. Other variants of BCC may appear as shiny, flat, gray, or yellowish plaques (Bader et al., 2016).

SCC is a malignant proliferation arising from the epidermis. Its precursor is typically actinic keratosis (see previous discussion). Although it usually appears on sun-damaged skin, it may arise from normal skin or from pre-existing skin lesions. It is of greater concern than BCC because it is an invasive carcinoma, metastasizing in 4% to 8% of cases by the blood or lymphatic system (Najjar, 2016).

SCC appears as a rough, thickened, scaly tumor that may be asymptomatic or may involve bleeding (see Fig. 61-5B). The border of an SCC lesion may be wider, more infiltrated, and more inflammatory than that of a BCC lesion. Secondary infection can occur. Exposed areas, especially of the upper extremities and of the face, lower lip, ears, nose, and forehead, are common sites (Najjar, 2016). The prognosis for SCC depends on the incidence of metastases, which is related

Figure 61-5 • Basal cell carcinoma (**A**) and squamous cell carcinoma (**B**). From Goodheart, H. P. (2011). *Goodheart's same-site differential diagnosis: A rapid method of diagnosing and treating common skin disorders*. Philadelphia, PA: Lippincott Williams & Wilkins.

to the histologic type and the level or depth of invasion. Regional lymph nodes should be evaluated for metastases (Najjar, 2016).

Medical Management

The goal of treatment is to eradicate the tumor. The treatment method depends on the tumor location; the cell type, location, and depth; the cosmetic desires of the patient; the history of previous treatment; whether the tumor is invasive; and whether metastatic nodes are present. The management of BCC and SCC includes surgical excision, which may include Mohs micrographic surgery, electrosurgery, or cryosurgery. In those patients who are not surgical candidates, alternatives such as radiation therapy, photodynamic therapy (PDT), or topical chemotherapeutic creams may be viable options (Bader et al., 2016).

Surgical Management

The main goal is to remove the tumor entirely. The best way to maintain cosmetic appearance is to place the incision properly along natural skin tension lines and natural anatomic body lines. In this way, scars are less noticeable. The size of the incision depends on the tumor size and location but usually involves a length-to-width ratio of 3:1.

The adequacy of the surgical excision is verified by microscopic evaluation of sections of the specimen. When the tumor is large, reconstructive surgery with the use of a skin flap or skin grafting may be required. The incision is closed in layers to enhance cosmetic effect. A pressure dressing applied over the wound provides support. Infection after a simple excision is uncommon if proper surgical asepsis is maintained.

Mohs Micrographic Surgery

This technique is the most accurate surgical technique and best conserves normal tissue. The procedure removes the tumor layer by layer. The first layer excised includes all evident tumor and a small margin of normal-appearing tissue. The specimen is frozen and analyzed by section to determine if all of the tumor has been removed. If not, additional layers of tissue are shaved and examined until all tissue margins are tumor free. In this manner, only the tumor and a safe, normal tissue margin are removed. Mohs surgery is the recommended tissue-sparing procedure, with extremely high cure rates for BCC and SCC. It is the treatment of choice and the most effective for tumors around the eyes, nose, upper lip, and auricular and periauricular areas (Najjar, 2016).

Electrosurgery

Electrosurgery is the destruction or removal of tissue by electrical energy. The current is converted to heat, which then passes to the tissue from a cold electrode. Electrosurgery may be preceded by curettage (excising the skin tumor by scraping its surface with a curette). Electrodesiccation is then implemented to achieve hemostasis and to destroy any viable malignant cells at the base of the wound or along its edges. Electrodesiccation and curettage is useful for lesions smaller than 1 to 2 cm (0.4 to 0.8 inch) in diameter.

This method takes advantage of the fact that the tumor is softer than surrounding skin and therefore can be outlined by a curette, which "feels" the extent of the tumor. The tumor is removed and the base cauterized. The process is repeated twice. Usually, healing occurs within 1 month (Bader et al., 2016).

Cryosurgery

Cryosurgery destroys the tumor by deep-freezing the tissue. A thermocouple needle apparatus is inserted into the skin, and liquid nitrogen is directed to the center of the tumor until the tumor base is −40° to −60°C (−40° to −76°F). Liquid nitrogen has the lowest boiling point of all cryogens, is inexpensive, and is easy to obtain. The tumor tissue is frozen, allowed to thaw, and then refrozen. The site thaws naturally and then becomes gelatinous and heals spontaneously. Swelling and edema follow the freezing. The appearance of the lesion varies. Normal healing, which may take 4 to 6 weeks, occurs faster in areas with a good blood supply (Bader et al., 2016).

Nonsurgical Alternative Therapies

Some older adult patients may defer surgical treatment options. Furthermore, in some cases, lesions may be extensive or are located on sites where wide surgical excision is not practical to achieve (e.g., cancer of the eyelid, tip of the nose). In these cases, local radiation therapy (see Chapter 15) or PDT may prove reasonable alternatives. PDT involves application of 5-aminolevulinic acid (ALA-PDT) to the lesion, which is then followed by photoactivation with directed blue light for approximately 1 hour. This has the effect of locally destroying the neoplastic cells, with good cosmetic results. Topical application of 5-fluorouracil cream (a chemotherapeutic agent) may be tried as another alternative to managing superficial BCC (Bader et al., 2016).

The patient should be informed that the skin may become red and blistered after any of these therapies. A bland skin ointment prescribed by the primary provider may be applied to relieve discomfort. The patient should also be cautioned to avoid exposure to the sun.

Nursing Management

Because many skin cancers are removed by excision, patients are usually treated in outpatient surgical units. The role of the nurse is to educate the patient about prevention of skin cancer (see Chart 61-5) and self-care after treatment.

Promoting Home, Community-Based, and Transitional Care

Educating Patients About Self-Care

The wound is usually covered with a dressing to protect the site from physical trauma, external irritants, and contaminants. The patient is advised when to report for a dressing change or is given written and verbal information on how to change dressings, including the type of dressing to purchase, how to remove dressings and apply fresh ones, and the importance of hand hygiene before and after the procedure.

The patient is advised to watch for excessive bleeding and tight dressings that compromise circulation. If the lesion is in the perioral area, the patient is instructed to drink liquids through a straw and limit talking and facial movement. Dental work should be avoided until the area is completely healed.

Chart 61-5 HEALTH PROMOTION
Preventing Skin Cancer

Minimize sun exposure:

- To the extent possible, avoid sun between the hours of 10 am and 4 pm.
- Wear protective clothing (e.g., long-sleeved clothing, broad-brimmed hats).
- Seek shady areas when outdoors.
- Use caution around snow and water because of reflective sun rays.

Use sunscreen:

- Use a sunscreen with a sun protection factor (SPF) of 15 or higher that protects against both ultraviolet-A (UVA) and ultraviolet-B (UVB) rays.
- Apply generously 20 minutes prior to sun exposure (e.g., going outdoors).
- Reapply every 2 hours, or immediately after swimming.
- Use lip balm with SPF of 15 or higher.

Do not use artificial ultraviolet sources (e.g., tanning beds and booths).

Check your skin regularly:

- Perform self-examination monthly.
- Schedule an examination by primary provider yearly, if over the age of 50 years.

Adapted from the Centers for Disease Control and Prevention (CDC). (2016b). What can I do to reduce my risk of skin cancer? Retrieved on 11/13/2017 at: www.cdc.gov/cancer/skin/basic_info/prevention.htm

Figure 61-6 • Two forms of melanoma: superficial spreading (*left*) and nodular (*right*).

After the sutures are removed, an emollient cream may be used to help reduce dryness. Applying a sunscreen over the wound is advised to prevent postoperative hyperpigmentation if the patient spends time outdoors.

Follow-up examinations should be at regular intervals, usually every 3 months for a year, and should include palpation of the adjacent lymph nodes. The patient should also be instructed to seek treatment for any moles that are subject to repeated friction and irritation and to watch for indications of potential malignancy in moles as described previously. The importance of lifelong follow-up evaluations is emphasized.

Melanoma

A melanoma is a cancerous neoplasm characterized by neoplastic melanocytes present in the epidermis and the dermis (and sometimes the subcutaneous cells). Although it only accounts for 2% of all skin cancers, it is the most lethal, and is responsible for nearly 10,000 deaths annually (Tan, Talavera, Schulman, et al., 2016). It may strike adults of any age; however, the average age at diagnosis is 57 years. It is more prevalent among women than men younger than 50 years of age; by 65 years of age, it is twice as common among men than women (Tan et al., 2016). Risk factors for melanoma are noted in Chart 61-4.

Clinical Manifestations

Melanoma may manifest as a change in a nevus or a new growth on the skin, arising from cutaneous epidermal melanocytes. A malignant melanoma is dark, red, or blue colored, or a mix of any of these, and irregular in shape. It may be associated with itching, rapid growth, ulceration, or bleeding. This type of malignancy may be found more frequently in the lower extremities in women, and in the trunk, neck, or head in men (National Cancer Institute [NCI], 2016).

Melanoma can occur in one of several forms: superficial spreading melanoma (SSM), lentigo maligna melanoma (LMM), nodular melanoma (NM), acral lentiginous melanoma (ALM), and mucosal lentiginous melanoma (MLM) (see Fig. 61-6). These types have specific histologic features; however, they do not dictate treatment options and are not associated with differential prognoses (NCI, 2016). In some rare instances, melanomas may develop in the uveal tract of the eye or from the mucosal lining of the gastrointestinal or genitourinary tract (Tan et al., 2016).

Melanomas spread in two growth phases: radial and vertical. During the first growth phase—the radial phase—cutaneous melanomas tend to spread radially within the layer of the epidermis. It is during this earlier phase of radial growth that the tumor is most amenable to treatment. The second growth phase—the vertical phase—is characterized by vertical tumor growth into the dermal layer and eventual metastasis. Those melanomas that progress more rapidly from the radial to the vertical growth phase are considered more aggressive types and have a poorer prognosis (Tan et al., 2016).

Assessment and Diagnostic Findings

Biopsy results confirm the diagnosis of melanoma. An excisional biopsy specimen provides information on the type, level of invasion, and thickness of the lesion. An excisional biopsy specimen that includes a 1- to 2-cm margin of normal tissue and a portion of underlying subcutaneous fatty tissue is sufficient for staging a melanoma in situ or an early, noninvasive melanoma. Incisional biopsy should be performed when the suspicious lesion is too large to be removed safely without extensive scarring. Biopsy specimens obtained by shaving, curettage, or needle aspiration are not considered reliable histologic proof of disease (Tan et al., 2016).

A thorough history and physical examination should include a meticulous skin examination and palpation of regional lymph nodes that drain the lesional area. Because melanoma occurs in families, a positive family history of melanoma is investigated so that first-degree relatives, who may be at high risk for melanoma, can be evaluated for atypical lesions. After the diagnosis of melanoma has been confirmed, a chest x-ray, CBC, complete chemistry panel with creatinine, liver function tests, and lactate dehydrogenase (LDH) are usually performed. The LDH may be elevated in the presence of metastatic disease. Depending on the results of these tests, magnetic resonance imaging of the brain, computed tomography scans of the chest, abdomen, or pelvis, and positron emission tomography scans of the lymphatics may be indicated to further stage the extent of disease (Tan et al., 2016).

Staging of the tumors follows the TNM (tumor, nodes, metastasis) classification system (see Chapter 15) and is used to determine appropriate treatment and prognosis. Patients with stage I disease (i.e., tumor less than 2 mm thick and without lymph node involvement or metastases) have a better than 92% survival 5 years post diagnosis, whereas those with stage II disease (i.e., tumor less than 4 mm thick and without lymph node involvement or metastases) and stage III disease (i.e., tumor of any thickness with lymph node involvement but no metastasis) have a likelihood of surviving 5 years post diagnosis between 53% and 81% and between 40% and 78%, respectively. The prognosis is grim for patients who present with stage IV disease (i.e., tumors with associated distant metastases), with less than 20% survival after 5 years (American Cancer Society [ACS], 2016b).

Medical Management

Treatment depends on the stage of the tumor and the tumor type. Surgical excision is the treatment of choice for small, superficial lesions. Deeper lesions require wide local excision, after which skin grafting may be necessary. Sentinel lymph node biopsy is commonly performed to examine the nodes nearest the tumor and to spare the patient the long-term sequelae of extensive removal of lymph nodes if the sample nodes are negative. If these are positive, lymph node dissection may be indicated (Tan et al., 2016).

Recently, greater understanding of the stem cells of melanoma indicates that effective therapies should be individualized for each patient. The observation that 60% of all patients with melanoma have a *BRAF* genetic mutation is useful in guiding targeted therapy. Clinical observations suggest that very few single-agent therapies provide significant clinical benefits because of the complex molecular nature of melanoma and the need to further define individual cell variations (Nguyen, Couts, Luo, et al., 2015).

Patients with a Stage II or Stage III tumor considered at risk for relapse are typically prescribed high-dose interferon alpha-2 intravenously for 4 weeks, followed by subcutaneous dosing for an additional 48 weeks. This adjuvant immunotherapeutic agent is associated with decreased rates of relapse and overall improved survival (NCI, 2016). Some patients with Stage III tumor may also benefit from receiving the monoclonal antibody, ipilimumab (Yervoy). This agent primes the patient's T cells so that they are more adept at identifying and killing tumor cells.

Monoclonal antibodies that could be indicated for later stage tumors (i.e., late Stage III and Stage IV) include pembrolizumab (Keytruda) and nivolumab (Opdivo); these agents are associated with tumor regression (Tan et al., 2016). Other treatments may include traditional chemotherapeutic agents, such as dacarbazine (DTIC-Dome), or therapies that are demonstrating promise in some patients with advanced disease including, IL-2, and granulocyte-macrophage colony-stimulating factor (Tan et al., 2016).

NURSING PROCESS

Care of the Patient With Melanoma

Assessment

Assessment of the patient with melanoma is based on the patient's history and symptoms. The patient is asked specifically about pruritus, tenderness, and pain, which are not features of a benign nevus. The patient is also questioned about changes in pre-existing moles or the development of new, pigmented lesions. People at risk are assessed carefully.

A magnifying lens and good lighting are needed for inspecting the skin for irregularity and changes in the mole. Signs that suggest malignant changes are referred to as the ABCDEs of moles (see Chart 61-6).

Chart 61-6

ASSESSMENT

Assessing the ABCDEs of Moles

Melanomas may be distinguished from benign nevi, using the following characteristics:

A for Asymmetry

- The lesion does not appear balanced on both sides. If an imaginary line was drawn down the middle, the two halves would not look alike.
- The lesion has an irregular surface with uneven elevations (irregular topography) either palpable or visible. A change in the surface may be noted from smooth to scaly.

B for Irregular Border

- Angular indentations or multiple notches appear in the border.
- The border is fuzzy or indistinct, as if rubbed with an eraser.

C for Variegated Color

- Benign moles are usually a uniform light to medium brown. Darker coloration indicates that the melanocytes have penetrated to a deeper layer of the dermis.
- Colors that may indicate malignancy if found together within a single lesion are shades of red, white, and blue; shades of blue are ominous.
- White areas within a pigmented lesion are suspicious.
- Some melanomas, however, are not variegated but are uniformly colored (bluish-black, bluish-gray, bluish-red).

D for Diameter

- A diameter >6 mm (about the size of a pencil eraser) is considered more suspicious, although this finding without other signs is not significant. Many benign skin growths are larger than 6 mm, whereas some early melanomas may be smaller.

E for Evolving

- Benign moles appear the same over time; when a mole starts to change in appearance, in size, shape, color, or elevation, it may suggest malignancy.

Adapted from Skin Cancer Foundation. (2016). Warning signs: The ABCDEs of melanoma. Retrieved on 2/13/2017 at: www.skincancer.org/skin-cancer-information/melanoma

Common sites of melanomas are the skin of the back; the legs (especially in women); between the toes; and on the feet, face, scalp, fingernails, and backs of hands. In people with dark skin, melanomas are most likely to occur in less pigmented sites: palms, soles, subungual areas, and mucous membranes. Satellite lesions (i.e., those situated near the mole) are inspected.

Diagnosis

NURSING DIAGNOSES

Based on the assessment data, major nursing diagnoses may include the following:

- Acute pain related to surgical excision and grafting
- Anxiety related to possible life-threatening consequences of melanoma and disfigurement
- Deficient knowledge about early signs of melanoma

Collaborative Problems/Potential Complications. Potential complications may include the following:

- Metastasis

PLANNING AND GOALS

The major goals for the patient may include relief of pain and discomfort, reduced anxiety, increased knowledge of early signs of melanoma, and absence of complications.

NURSING INTERVENTIONS

Relieving Pain and Discomfort. Surgical removal of melanoma in different locations presents different challenges, taking into consideration the removal of the primary melanoma, the intervening lymphatic vessels, and the lymph nodes to which metastases may spread. Nursing management of the patient having surgery in these regions is discussed in the appropriate chapters.

Nursing interventions after surgery for a melanoma center on promoting comfort, because wide excision surgery may be necessary. A split- or full-thickness skin graft may be necessary when large defects are created by surgical removal of a melanoma. Anticipating the need for and administration of appropriate analgesic medications is important.

Reducing Anxiety. Psychological support is essential when disfiguring surgery is performed. Support includes encouraging the patient to express anxieties and feelings about the seriousness of the neoplasm and conveying understanding of these feelings. During the diagnostic workup and staging of the depth, type, and extent of the tumor, the nurse answers questions, provides information, and helps clarify misconceptions. Learning that he or she has a melanoma can cause the patient considerable fear and anguish. Pointing out the patient's resources, past effective coping mechanisms, and social support systems helps the patient cope with the diagnosis and need for treatment and continuing follow-up. Family members should be included in all discussions to enable them to clarify information, ask questions that the patient might be reluctant to ask, and provide emotional support to the patient.

Monitoring and Managing Potential Complications. Metastasis of melanoma is closely related to prognosis: the deeper and thicker (more than 4 mm) the melanoma, the greater the likelihood of metastasis. The role of the nurse in caring for the patient with metastatic disease is to provide holistic care. The nurse must be knowledgeable about the most effective current therapies and must deliver supportive care, provide and clarify information about the

therapy and the rationale for its use, identify potential side effects of therapy and ways to manage them, and instruct the patient and family about the expected outcomes of treatment. The nurse monitors and documents symptoms that may indicate metastasis: lung (e.g., difficulty breathing, shortness of breath, increasing cough), bone (e.g., pain, decreased mobility and function, pathologic fractures), and liver (e.g., change in liver enzyme levels, pain, jaundice). Nursing care is based on the patient's symptoms and emotional needs.

Although the chance of a cure for melanoma that has metastasized is poor, the nurse encourages hope while maintaining a realistic perspective about the disease and ultimate outcome. Furthermore, the nurse provides time for the patient to express fears and concerns regarding future activities and relationships, offers information about support groups and contact people, and arranges palliative and hospice care if appropriate (see Chapter 16).

PROMOTING HOME, COMMUNITY-BASED, AND TRANSITIONAL CARE

Educating Patients About Self-Care. The best hope of decreasing the incidence of skin cancer lies in educating patients about the early signs. Patients at risk are educated to examine their skin and scalp monthly in a systematic manner and to seek prompt medical attention if changes are detected. The American Academy of Dermatology (AAD) provides multimedia resources on performing skin self-examination (see the Resources section at the end of this chapter). The nurse also points out that a key factor in the development of melanoma is exposure to sunlight. Because melanoma is thought to be genetically linked, the family and the patient should be educated about sun-avoiding measures and the importance of annual assessment by a primary provider.

Evaluation

Expected patient outcomes may include:

1. Experiences relief of pain and discomfort
   a. States pain is diminishing
   b. Exhibits healing of surgical scar without heat, redness, or swelling
2. Is less anxious
   a. Expresses fears and perceptions
   b. Asks questions about medical condition
   c. Requests facts about melanoma
   d. Identifies support and comfort provided by family member or significant other
3. Demonstrates understanding of the means for detecting and preventing melanoma
   a. Demonstrates how to conduct self-examination of skin on a monthly basis
   b. Verbalizes the following danger signals of melanoma: change in size, color, shape, or outline of mole, mole surface, or skin around mole
   c. Identifies measures to protect self from exposure to sunlight
4. Experiences absence of complications
   a. Recognizes abnormal signs and symptoms that should be reported to the primary provider
   b. Adheres to recommended follow-up procedures and prevention strategies

Metastatic Skin Tumors

The skin is an important yet uncommon site of metastatic cancer. All types of cancer may metastasize to the skin. Cancers with a predilection to metastasize to the skin include melanomas and cancers of the breast, nasal sinuses, larynx, and oral cavity. Of these, skin metastases from carcinoma of the breast are most frequently seen, accounting for 30% of all cases. The clinical appearance of metastatic skin lesions is not distinctive, except perhaps in some cases of breast cancer in which diffuse, brawny hardening of the skin of the involved breast is seen. In most instances, metastatic lesions occur as multiple cutaneous or subcutaneous nodules of various sizes that may be skin colored or different shades of red (Cho, Park, Lee, et al., 2014).

Kaposi Sarcoma

Kaposi sarcoma (KS) is a malignancy of endothelial cells that line the small blood vessels. KS is manifested clinically by lesions of the skin, oral cavity, gastrointestinal tract, and lungs. The skin lesions consist of reddish-purple to dark blue macules, plaques, or nodules. KS is subdivided into four categories (Radu & Pantanowitz, 2013):

- *Classic KS* occurs predominantly in older adult men of Mediterranean or Jewish ancestry. Most patients have nodules or plaques on the lower extremities that rarely metastasize beyond this area. Classic KS is chronic, relatively benign, and rarely fatal.
- *Endemic (African) KS* affects people predominantly in the eastern half of Africa near the equator. Men are affected more often than women, and children can be affected as well. The disease may resemble classic KS, or it may infiltrate and progress to lymphadenopathic forms.
- *Iatrogenic/organ transplant–associated KS* occurs in transplant recipients and in patients receiving long-term immunosuppressants, such as azathioprine, cyclosporine, or corticosteroids (e.g., prednisone).
- *AIDS-related or epidemic KS* occurs in people with AIDS. This form of KS is characterized by local skin lesions and disseminated visceral and mucocutaneous diseases. This is a more aggressive tumor type than other forms of KS (Radu & Pantanowitz, 2013). More information on AIDS-related KS can be found in Chapter 36.

PLASTIC, RECONSTRUCTIVE, AND COSMETIC PROCEDURES

The word *plastic* comes from a Greek word meaning "to form." Plastic or reconstructive procedures are performed to reconstruct or alter congenital or acquired defects to restore or improve the body's form and function. Often the terms *plastic* and *reconstructive* are used interchangeably. This type of surgery includes closure of wounds, removal of skin tumors, repair of soft tissue injuries or burns, correction of deformities, and repair of cosmetic defects. Plastic surgery can be used to repair many parts of the body and numerous structures, such as bone, cartilage, fat, fascia, mucous membrane, muscle, nerve, and cutaneous structures. Bone inlays and transplants for deformities and nonunion can be performed, muscle can be transferred, nerves can be reconstructed and spliced, and cartilage can be replaced. As important as any of these measures is the reconstruction of the cutaneous tissues around the neck and the face; this is usually referred to as aesthetic or cosmetic surgery.

Cosmetic procedures are generally considered to be ones that correct defects that are not life threatening or caused by disease. An example would be removal of a benign mole or sebaceous cyst from the face. Most health insurance plans do not cover procedures deemed to be cosmetic, and these procedures can be expensive. Procedures that are performed to correct a surgical defect, such as removal of a skin cancer or correction of a significant congenital defect such as a cleft lip, are generally covered by insurance.

Wound Coverage: Grafts and Flaps

Various surgical techniques, including skin grafts and flaps, are used to cover skin wounds.

Skin Grafts

Skin grafting is a technique in which a section of skin is detached from its own blood supply and transferred as free tissue to a distant (recipient) site. Skin grafting can be used to repair almost any type of wound and is the most common form of reconstructive surgery.

Skin grafts are commonly used to repair surgical defects such as those that result from excision of skin tumors, to cover areas denuded of skin (e.g., burns), and to cover wounds in which insufficient skin is available to permit wound closure. They are also used when primary closure of the wound increases the risk of complications or when primary wound closure would interfere with function.

Skin grafts may be classified as autografts, homografts, or xenografts. An autograft is tissue obtained from the patient's own skin. A homograft is tissue obtained from a donor of the same species. These grafts are also referred to as allogeneic or allografts. A xenograft or heterograft is tissue obtained from another species. A common xenograft for human skin is the pig.

Grafts are also referred to by their thickness. A skin graft may be a split-thickness (i.e., thin, intermediate, or thick) or a full-thickness graft, depending on the amount of dermis included in the specimen. A split-thickness graft can be cut at various thicknesses and is commonly used to cover large wounds or defects for which a full-thickness graft or flap is impractical (see Fig. 61-7). A full-thickness graft consists of epidermis and the entire dermis without the underlying fat. It is used to cover wounds that are too large to be closed directly (Urden, Stacy, & Lough, 2014).

Site Selection

The site where the intact skin is harvested is called the *donor site*. Selection of the donor site is made to match the color and texture of skin at the surgical site and to leave as little scarring as possible.

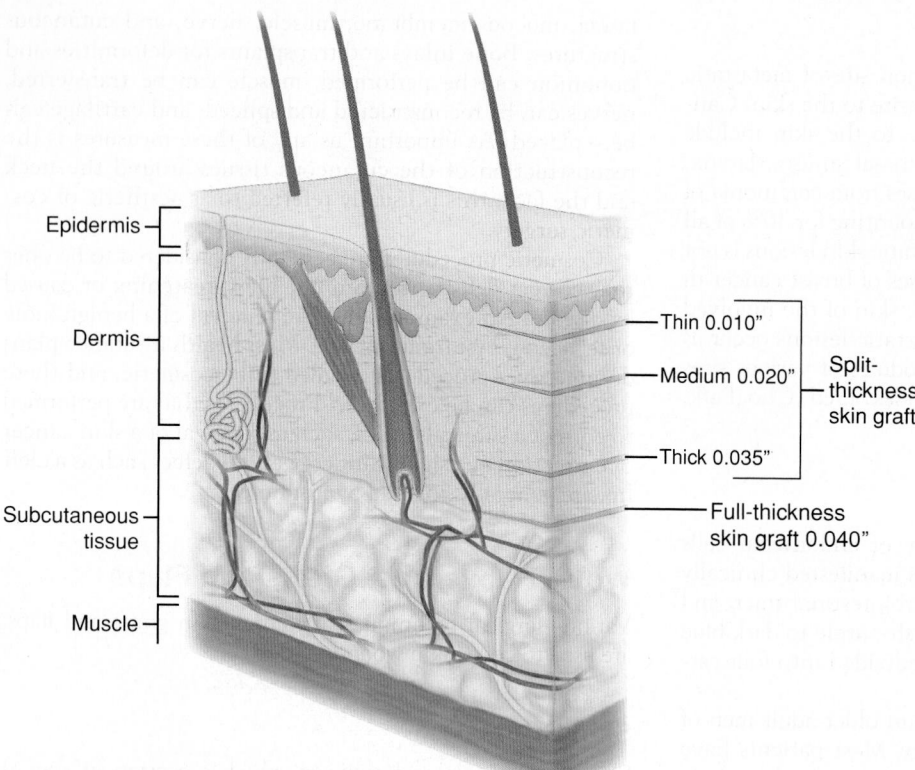

- Epidermis
- Dermis
- Subcutaneous tissue
- Muscle
- Thin 0.010"
- Medium 0.020"
- Thick 0.035"
- Split-thickness skin graft
- Full-thickness skin graft 0.040"

Figure 61-7 • Layers of skin appropriate for split- and full-thickness graft.

Graft Application

The skin graft is taken from the donor or host site and applied to the desired site, called the *recipient site bed* or *recipient graft bed*.

For a graft to survive and be effective, certain conditions must be met:

- The recipient site must have an adequate blood supply so that normal physiologic function can resume.
- The graft must be in close contact with its bed to avoid accumulation of blood or fluid between the graft and the recipient site.
- The graft must be fixed firmly (immobilized) so that it remains in place on the recipient site.
- The area must be free of infection.

The graft, when applied to the recipient site, may be sutured in place; alternatively, it may be slit and spread apart to cover a greater area. The process of revascularization (establishing the blood supply) and reattachment of a skin graft to a recipient site bed is referred to as a "take." After a skin graft is put in place, it may be left exposed (in areas that are impossible to immobilize) or covered with a light dressing or a pressure dressing, depending on the area of the body (Urden et al., 2014).

Nursing Management

The nurse must ensure that both the surgical and the donor sites receive proper postoperative care. The surgical site is covered by the harvested skin, and the donor site heals by re-epithelization of the raw, exposed dermis. Both sites are protected by dressings as they heal. Prevention of infection is essential, as it is with all surgical sites. Both sites can be kept soft and pliable with cream (e.g., lanolin).

> ⚑ **Quality and Safety Nursing Alert**
>
> *Both the donor site and the grafted area must be protected from exposure to extremes in temperature, external trauma, and sunlight because these areas are sensitive, especially to thermal injuries.*

Flaps

Another form of wound coverage is provided by flaps. A flap is a segment of tissue that remains attached at one end (i.e., a base or pedicle) while the other end is moved to a recipient area. Its survival depends on functioning arterial and venous blood supplies and lymphatic drainage in its pedicle or base (Clark, Wang, & Terris, 2015). A flap differs from a graft in that a portion of the tissue is attached to its original site and retains its blood supply. An exception is the free flap, which is described later.

Flaps may consist of skin, mucosa, muscle, adipose tissue, omentum, and bone. They are used for wound coverage and provide bulk, especially when bone, tendon, blood vessels, or nerve tissue is exposed. Flaps are used to repair defects caused by congenital deformity, trauma, or tumor ablation (removal, usually by excision) in an adjacent part of the body (Clark et al., 2015).

Flaps offer an aesthetic solution because a flap retains the color and texture of the donor area; is more likely to survive than a graft; and can be used to cover nerves, tendons, and blood vessels. However, several surgical procedures are usually required to advance a flap. The major complication is necrosis of the pedicle or base as a result of failure of the blood supply.

A striking advance in reconstructive surgery is the use of free flaps or free tissue transfer achieved by microvascular techniques. A free flap is completely severed from the body and transferred to another site. A free flap receives early vascular supply from microvascular anastomosis with vessels at the recipient site. The procedure usually is completed in one step, eliminating the need for a series of surgical procedures to move the flap. Microvascular surgery allows surgeons to use a variety of donor sites for tissue reconstruction (Clark et al., 2015).

Cosmetic Procedures

Chemical Face Peeling

Chemical face peeling involves application of a chemical mixture to the face for superficial destruction of the epidermis and the upper layers of the dermis to treat fine wrinkles, keratoses, and pigment problems. It is especially useful for wrinkles at the upper and lower lip, forehead, and periorbital areas. The type of chemical used depends on the planned depth of the peel. The patient who is conscious feels a burning sensation that continues for 12 to 24 hours. Frequent small doses of analgesic and tranquilizing agents are prescribed to keep the patient comfortable. The most common complications include discoloration of the skin, infection of the burned area, persistent sensory changes or itching, and occasionally permanent scarring of the skin (Arif, 2015).

Dermabrasion

Dermabrasion is a form of skin abrasion used to treat acne scarring, aging, and sun-damaged skin. A special instrument (e.g., motor-driven wire brush, diamond-impregnated disc) is used. The epidermis and some superficial dermis are removed by a sanding-type action, and enough of the dermis is preserved to allow re-epithelization of the treated areas. Results are best in the face because it is rich in intradermal epithelial elements (Hession & Graber, 2015).

Patients with a history of herpes simplex viral infection are typically prescribed prophylactic antiviral medications (e.g., valacyclovir [Valtrex]) preprocedurally so that the physiologic stress of the procedure is less likely to cause a cutaneous herpes eruption. Tretinoin cream (Renova) may be prescribed with instructions to apply it 2 to 3 weeks preoperatively; this is associated with accelerating re-epithelialization post dermabrasion. Patients must be educated preprocedurally about the postprocedural dressing regimen and when to return to the primary provider to have dressing changes performed (Wong, Arnold, & Boeckman, 2016).

Facial Reconstructive Surgery

Reconstructive procedures on the face are individualized to the patient's needs and desired outcomes. They are performed to repair deformities or restore normal function. They may vary from closure of small defects to complicated procedures involving implantation of prosthetic devices to conceal a large defect or reconstruct a lost part of the face (e.g., nose, ear, jaw). Each surgical procedure is customized and involves a variety of incisions, flaps, and grafts. Multiple surgical procedures may be required.

The process of facial reconstruction is often slow and tedious. Because a person's facial appearance affects self-esteem so greatly, this type of reconstruction is often a very emotional experience for the patient.

Face-Lift

Rhytidectomy (face-lift) is a surgical procedure that removes soft tissue folds and minimizes cutaneous wrinkles on the face. It is performed to create a more youthful appearance. Psychological preparation requires that the patient recognize the limitations of surgery and the fact that miraculous rejuvenation will not occur. The patient is informed that the face may appear bruised and swollen after the dressings are removed and that several weeks may pass before the edema subsides. Corticosteroids (e.g., methylprednisolone) and vitamin C are prescribed postoperatively to minimize edema. Prophylactic antibiotic agents such as cephalexin (Keflex) may also be prescribed postoperatively (Warren & Neligan, 2013).

Laser Treatment of Cutaneous Lesions

Lasers are devices that amplify or generate highly specialized light energy. They can mobilize immense heat and power when focused at close range and are valuable tools in providing dermatologic abrasion therapy. The laser modalities used for this purpose today include scanned carbon dioxide laser, pulsed carbon dioxide laser, pulsed erbium/yttrium-aluminum-garnet (Er:YAG) laser, fractional Er:YAG laser resurfacing, combination carbon dioxide and Er:YAG lasers, and fractionated photothermolysis (Husain & Alster, 2016).

Each of these lasers is a precise surgical instrument that vaporizes and excises water-containing tissues with minimal damage. Because the beams used can seal blood and lymphatic vessels, they create a dry surgical field that makes many procedures easier and quicker. Therefore, these lasers are generally safe to use on patients with bleeding disorders or those receiving anticoagulant therapy. They are primarily used to improve the appearance of facial wrinkles, although they are also useful in removing epidermal nevi, tattoos, certain warts, skin cancer, ingrown toenails, and keloids. Incisions made with the laser beam heal and scar much like those made by a scalpel. Patients with a history of herpes simplex viral infection typically receive preprocedural antiviral prophylaxis (Husain & Alster, 2016).

Nursing Management

The majority of dermatologic and reconstructive procedures are performed in the physician's office or in an outpatient surgical department; therefore, most care takes place in the home. Most procedures, except very extensive reconstruction, are performed under local anesthesia or moderate sedation, therefore requiring a very short recovery time. Unless there are complications, the patient does not need hospitalization. The nurse must prepare both the patient and family for what to expect during the postoperative recovery time. Table 61-6 lists a few of the nursing considerations that must be reviewed in educating the patient and family.

TABLE 61-6 Nursing Considerations in Cosmetic Procedures

Nursing Consideration	Interventions and Patient Education
Maintaining airway and pulmonary function	Cosmetic surgeries involving the face and neck can cause considerable swelling; bandages can restrict breathing or eating. Check dressings frequently, and ensure that no constriction occurs as swelling develops.
Relieving pain and achieving comfort	Procedures that involve a large surface area will cause considerable pain. Cool compresses or ice packs will relieve the burning of dermabrasion or chemical peels. Oral analgesic agents should be given regularly to control pain.
Maintaining adequate nutrition	When the face is involved, the patient may be unable to fully open the mouth, and chewing may be painful. Provide soft or liquid diet that is high in protein to assist with healing.
Enhancing communication	Depending on the type of cosmetic procedure, a nonverbal method of communication might be necessary until pain and swelling have subsided.
Improving self-concept	Recovery time from cosmetic procedures is slow. Expected results will take weeks to become apparent. Persons of color will experience increased pigmentation long after the initial wounds have healed. Helping patients to understand postoperative expectations will allow them to feel more comfortable with the healing process.
Promoting family coping	Most cosmetic procedures are performed in an outpatient facility; therefore, family members are integral to postoperative care. They should understand what to expect as the patient emerges from the procedure room: the type of dressings that will be in place, the skin care plan that is prescribed, and how to cope with the patient's pain.
Monitoring and managing potential complications	Infection is the most common complication, but excessive pain, nerve damage, and emotional distress about appearance are also common. If opioid analgesic agents are used, there may be gastrointestinal upset, mental status changes, or allergic reaction to the medication. Alert the caregiver to signs of these complications and how and when to report changes in status.

CRITICAL THINKING EXERCISES

1 You are caring for an 18-year-old female college student with chronic, cystic acne. She has been prescribed oral isotretinoin. What side effects should you review with this patient? What type of screening should be done before she is started on the isotretinoin? What are some self-care strategies you could recommend?

2 ebp You work in a dermatology clinic. A 46-year-old woman presents to the clinic with a new onset of silvery plaques and is diagnosed with moderate psoriasis. The dermatologist has prescribed methotrexate therapy. The patient says to you "My daughter takes that drug for her Crohn's disease. How can this also work for treating what I have?" How you would answer the patient? What is the strength of the evidence that methotrexate is effective in treating moderate to severe psoriasis? Describe components of your plan to educate this woman on how to best self-manage her disease.

3 pq A 44-year-old construction worker presenting to the family practice clinic where you work states that his father had melanoma and that now he is concerned about several pigmented lesions on his arms and neck. He also has red, scaly, nonhealing lesions on his scalp and face. Describe your focused priority assessments and interventions. What are the priorities for education that you should provide to this patient about preventing melanoma and performing self-examination of the skin?

REFERENCES

*Asterisk indicates nursing research.

Books

Dunphy, L., Winland-Brown, J., Porter, B., et al. (2015). *Primary care: Art and science of advanced practice nursing* (4th ed.). Philadelphia, PA: FA Davis.

Eliopoulos, C. (2018). *Gerontological nursing* (9th ed.). Philadelphia, PA: Lippincott Williams & Wilkins.

Goldsmith, L., Katz, S. I., Gilchrist B. A., et al. (2012). *Fitzpatrick's dermatology in general medicine* (8th ed.). New York: McGraw-Hill.

Goodheart, H. P. (2003). *Goodheart's photoguide of common skin disorders* (2nd ed.). Philadelphia, PA: Lippincott Williams & Wilkins.

Goodheart, H. P. (2011). *Goodheart's same-site differential diagnosis: A rapid method of diagnosing and treating common skin disorders*. Philadelphia, PA: Lippincott Williams & Wilkins.

Grossman, S. C., & Porth, C. M. (2014). *Pathophysiology: Concepts of altered health states* (9th ed.). Philadelphia, PA: Lippincott Williams & Wilkins.

Karch, A. M. (2015). *2015 Lippincott's nursing drug guide*. Philadelphia, PA: Lippincott Williams & Wilkins.

Krasner, D., Rodeheaver, G., Sibbald, G., et al. (2012). *Chronic wound care: A clinical source book for healthcare professionals* (5th ed.). Malvern, PA: HMP Communications.

Urden, L. D., Stacy, K. M., & Lough, M. E. (2014). *Critical care nursing: Diagnosis and management* (7th ed.). St. Louis, MO: Elsevier Mosby.

U.S. Department of Health and Human Services (USHHS). (2014). *The Surgeon General's call to action to prevent skin cancer*. Washington, DC: HHS, Office of the Surgeon General.

Warren, R. J., & Neligan, P. C. (2013). *Plastic surgery* (3rd ed.). St. Louis, MO: Elsevier Mosby.

Wong, B., Arnold, M., & Boeckmann, J. (2016). *Facial plastic and reconstructive surgery*. New York: Springer.

Journals and Electronic Documents

Akram, S., & Zaman, H. (2015). Warts and verrucas: Assessment and treatment. *The Pharmaceutical Journal, 294*(7867). doi:10.1211/PJ.2015.20068680

Al-Hammadi, A., Al-Ismaily, A., Al-Ali, S., et al. (2016). Topical, biological and clinical challenges in the management of patients with acne vulgaris. *Sultan Qaboos University Medical Journal, 16*(2), e152–e160.

Alves, J. V., Matos, D. M., Barreiros, H. F., et al. (2014). Variants of dermatofibroma - A histopathological study. *Anais Brasileiros de Dermatologia, 89*(3), 472–477.

American Cancer Society (ACS). (2016a). Risk factors for melanoma skin cancer. Retrieved on 11/29/2016 at: www.cancer.org/cancer/melanoma-skin-cancer/causes-risks-prevention/risk-factors.html

American Cancer Society (ACS). (2016b). Survival rates for melanoma skin cancer, by stage. Retrieved on 2/13/2017 at: www.cancer.org/cancer/melanoma-skin-cancer/detection-diagnosis-staging/survival-rates-for-melanoma-skin-cancer-by-stage.html

Antiga, E., & Caproni, M. (2015). The diagnosis and treatment of dermatitis herpetiformis. *Journal of Clinical, Cosmetic and Investigational Dermatology, 8*, 257–265.

Arif, T. (2015). Salicylic acid as a peeling agent: A comprehensive review. *Clinical, Cosmetic and Investigational Dermatology, 8*, 455–461.

Bader, R. S., Kennedy, A. S., Santacroce, L., et al. (2016). Basal cell carcinoma. Medscape. Retrieved on 11/4/2016 at: emedicine.medscape.com/article/276624-overview

Bolier, R., Elferink, R. P., & Beuers, U. (2016). Advances in pathogenesis and treatment of pruritus. *Clinics in Liver Disease, 17*(2), 319–329.

Bonilla, D. L., Durden, L. A., Eremeeva, M. E., et al. (2013). The biology and taxonomy of head and body lice—Implications for louse-borne disease prevention. *PLoS Pathogens, 9*(11), e1003724.

Borda, L. J., & Wikramanayake, T. C. (2015). Seborrheic dermatitis and dandruff: A comprehensive review. *Journal of Clinical and Investigative Dermatology, 3*(2).

Bronckers, I. M., Paller, A. S., van Geel, M. J., et al. (2015). Psoriasis in children and adolescents: Diagnosis, management and comorbidities. *Paediatric Drugs, 17*, 373–384.

Carr, C., Veledar, E., & Chen, S. (2014). Factors mediating the impact of chronic pruritus on quality of life. *JAMA Dermatology, 150*(6), 613–620.

Centers for Disease Control and Prevention (CDC). (2016a). What are the risk factors for skin cancer? Retrieved on 11/29/106 at: www.cdc.gov/cancer/skin/basic_info/risk_factors.htm

Centers for Disease Control and Prevention (CDC). (2016b). What can I do to reduce my risk of skin cancer? Retrieved on 11/13/2017 at: www.cdc.gov/cancer/skin/basic_info/prevention.htm

César, A., Cruz, M., Mota, A., et al. (2016). Erythroderma. A clinical and etiological study of 103 patients. *Journal of Dermatological Case Reports, 10*(1), 1–9.

Chan, L. S. (2016). Bullous pemphigoid. Medscape. Retrieved on 11/4/2016 at: emedicine.medscape.com/article/1062391-overview

Chan, K. Y., Li, C. W., Wong, H., et al. (2013). Use of sertraline for antihistamine-refractory uremic pruritus in renal palliative care patients. *Journal of Palliative Medicine, 16*(8), 966–970.

Cho, J., Park, Y., Lee, J. -C., et al. (2014). Case series of different onset of skin metastasis according to the breast cancer subtypes. *Cancer Research and Treatment: Official Journal of Korean Cancer Association, 46*(2), 194–199.

Clark, J. M., Wang, T. D., & Terris, D. J. (2015). Skin flap design. Medscape. Retrieved on 2/3/2017 at: emedicine.medscape.com/article/875968-overview

Cohen, P. R. (2014). Follicular contact dermatitis revisited: A review emphasizing neomycin-associated follicular contact dermatitis. *World Journal of Clinical Cases: WJCC, 2*(12), 815–821.

Cohen, V., Jellinek, S. P., & Schwartz, R. A. (2016). Toxic epidermal necrolysis. Medscape. Retrieved on 2/12/2017 at: emedicine.medscape.com/article/229698-overview

Dabiri, G., Damstetter, E., & Phillips, T. (2014). Choosing a wound dressing based on common wound characteristics. *WHS Wound Healing Society, 5*(1), 32–40.

Friedman, J. M. (2014). Neurofibromatosis. GeneReviews. Retrieved on 10/14/2016 at: www.ncbi.nlm.nih.gov/books/NBK1109/

Gellatly, K. J., Krim, S., Palenchar, D. J., et al. (2016). Expansion of the knockdown resistance frequency map for human head lice (Phthiraptera: Pediculidae) in the United States using quantitative sequencing. *Journal of Medical Entomology, 53*(3), 653–659.

*Gorelick, J., Daniels, S. R., Kawata, A. K., et al. (2015). Acne-related quality of life among female adults of different races/ethnicities. *Journal of the Dermatology Nurses Association, 7*(3), 154–162.

Guenther, L., & Maguiness, S. (2016). Pediculosis (lice). Medscape. Retrieved on 11/4/2016 at: emedicine.medscape.com/article/225013-overview

Handler, M. Z. (2017). Seborrheic dermatitis treatment and management. MedScape. Retrieved on 2/4/2017 at: emedicine.medscape.com/article/1108312-treatment

Handler, M. Z., Stephany, M. P., & Schwarts, R. A. (2016). Tinea capitis. Medscape. Retrieved on 2/11/2017 at: emedicine.medscape.com/article/1091351-overview

Hession, M. T., & Graber, E. M. (2015). Atrophic acne scarring: A review of treatment options. *The Journal of Clinical and Aesthetic Dermatology, 8*(1), 50.

Hochman, B., Isoldi, F. C., Furtado, F., et al. (2015). New approach to the understanding of keloid: Psychoneuroimmune–endocrine aspects. *Clinical, Cosmetic and Investigational Dermatology, 8*, 67–73.

Hogan, D. J. (2016). Irritant contact dermatitis. Medscape. Retrieved on 2/11/2017 at: emedicine.medscape.com/article/1049352-overview

Hong, J., Buddenkotte, J., Berger, T. G., et al. (2013). Management of itch in atopic dermatitis. *Seminars in Cutaneous Medicine and Surgery, 30*(2), 71–86.

Husain, Z., & Alster, T. S. (2016). The role of lasers and intense pulsed light technology in dermatology. *Clinical, Cosmetic and Investigational Dermatology, 9*, 29–40.

Inamadar, A. C., & Palit, A. (2013). Sensitive skin: An overview. *Indian Journal of Dermatology, Venereology, and Leprology, 79*(1), 9–16.

Janniger, C. K., Eastern, J. S., Hospenthal, D. R., et al. (2016). Herpes zoster. Medscape. Retrieved on 11/4/2016 at: emedicine.medscape.com/article/1132465-overview

Kellen, R., & Berlin, J. M. (2016). Dermatology emergencies. *Journal of the Dermatology Nurses Association, 8*(3), 193–202.

Landriscina, A., Rosen, J., & Friedman, A. (2015). Systemic approach to wound dressings. *Journal of Drugs in Dermatology, 14*(7), 740–744.

Lesher, J. L. (2016). Tinea corporis. Medscape. Retrieved on 2/11/2017 at: emedicine.medscape.com/article/1091473-overview

Lewis, L. S. (2016). Impetigo. Medscape. Retrieved on 2/11/2017 at: emedicine.medscape.com/article/965254-overview

McCallon, S., Weir, D., & Lantis, J. (2015). Optimizing wound bed preparation with collagenase enzymatic debridement. *Journal of the American College of Clinical Wound Specialists, 6*(1–2), 14–23.

Mease, P. J., & Armstrong, A. W. (2014). Managing patients with psoriatic disease: The diagnosis and pharmacologic treatment of psoriatic arthritis in patients with psoriasis. *Drugs, 74*(4), 423–441.

Meffert, J. (2016). Psoriasis. Medscape. Retrieved on 11/4/2016 at: emedicine.medscape.com/article/1943419-overview

Mounsey, K. E., Murray, H. C., Bielefeldt-Ohmann, H., et al. (2015). Prospective study in a porcine model of Sarcoptes scabiei indicates the association of Th2 and Th17 pathways with the clinical severity of scabies. *PLoS Neglected Tropical Diseases, 9*(3), e0003498.

Najjar, T. (2016). Cutaneous squamous cell carcinoma. Medscape. Retrieved on 2/13/2017 at: emedicine.medscape.com/article/1965430-overview

National Cancer Institute (NCI). (2016). Melanoma treatment – Health professional version. Retrieved on 2/13/2017 at: www.cancer.gov/types/skin/hp/melanoma-treatment-pdq

Nguyen, N., Couts, K. L., Luo, Y., et al. (2015). Understanding melanoma stem cells. *Melanoma Management, 2*(2), 179–188.

Nicpon, J. (2017). Psoriasis management: Quality, cost, and coordination. *Journal of the Dermatology Nurses Association, 9*(1), 21–25.

Occupational Safety and Health Administration (OSHA). (2012). Toxic and hazardous substances: Bloodborne pathogens. Retrieved on 10/11/2016 at: www.osha.gov/pls/oshaweb/owadisp.show_document?p_table = STANDARDS&p_id = 10051

Peebles, E., Morris, R., & Chafe, R. (2014). Community-associated methicillin-resistant Staphylococcus aureus in a pediatric emergency department in Newfoundland and Labrador. *The Canadian Journal of Infectious Diseases & Medical Microbiology, 25*(1), 13–16.

Radu, O., & Pantanowitz, L. (2013). Kaposi sarcoma. *Archives of Pathology & Laboratory Medicine, 137*(2), 289–294.

Rao, J., & Chen, J. (2016). Acne vulgaris. Medscape. Retrieved on 11/4/2016 at: emedicine.medscape.com/articles/1069804-overview/showall

Robbins, C. M., & Elewski, B. E. (2016). Tinea pedis. Medscape. Retrieved on 2/11/2017 at: emedicine.medscape.com/article/1091684-overview

Rosso, J., Kircik, L., Goldenberg, G., et al. (2014). Comprehensive management of actinic keratoses. *The Journal of Clinical and Aesthetic Dermatology, 7*(9 Suppl), S2–S12.

Sahoo, A. K., & Mahajan, R. (2016). Management of tinea corporis, tinea cruris, and tinea pedis: A comprehensive review. *Indian Dermatology Online Journal, 7*(2), 77–86.

Santoro, F., Stoopler, E., & Werth, V. (2013). Pemphigus. *Dental Clinics of North America, 57*(4), 597–610.

Sardana, K., Chakravarty, P., & Goel, K. (2014). Optimal management of common acquired melanocytic nevi (moles): Current perspectives. *Clinical, Cosmetic and Investigational Dermatology, 7*, 89–103.

Skin Cancer Foundation (2016). Warning signs: The ABCDEs of melanoma. Retrieved on 2/13/2017 at: www.skincancer.org/skin-cancer-information/melanoma

Song, S. W., Burm, J. S., Yang, W. Y., et al. (2014). Minimally invasive excision of epidermal cysts through a small hole made by a CO2 laser. *Archives of Plastic Surgery, 41*(1), 85–88.

Tan, W. W., Talavera, F., & Schulman, P., et al. (2016). Malignant melanoma. Medscape. Retrieved on 2/13/2017 at: emedicine.medscape.com/article/280245-overview

Tarikci, N., Kocaturk, E., Gungor, F., et al. (2015). Pruritus in systemic diseases: A review of etiological factors and new treatment modalities. *The Scientific World Journal, 2015*, 1–8.

Thomas, J., Peterson, G. M., Walton, S. F., et al. (2015). Scabies: An ancient global disease with a need for new therapies. *BMC Infectious Diseases, 15*, 250.

Tosti, A. (2016). Onychomycosis. Medscape. Retrieved on 2/11/2017 at: emedicine.medscape.com/article/1105828-overview

Umar, S. H., & Kelly, A. P. (2016). Erythroderma (generalized exfoliative dermatitis). Medscape. Retrieved on 11/4/2016 at: emedicine.medscape.com/article/1106906-overview

Van Bijnen, E. M., Paget, W. J., & den Heijer, C. D., et al. (2014). Primary care treatment guidelines for skin infections in Europe: Congruence with antimicrobial resistance found in commensal Staphylococcus aureus in the community. *BMC Family Practice, 15*(175).

Weiderkehr, M., & Schwartz, R. A. (2016). Tinea cruris. Medscape. Retrieved on 2/11/2017 at: emedicine.medscape.com/article/1091806-overview

Well, D. (2013). Acne vulgaris: A review of causes and treatment options. *The Nurse Practitioner, 38*(10), 22–31.

Wernli, K. J., Henrikson, N. B., Morrison, C. C., et al. (2016). Screening for skin cancer in adults: Updated evidence report and systematic review for the US preventive services task force. *JAMA, 316*(4), 436–447.

Wollina, U., Koch, A., Heinig, B., et al. (2013). Acne inversa (Hidradenitis suppurativa): A review with a focus on pathogenesis and treatment. *Indian Dermatology Online Journal, 4*(1), 2–11.

Zaenglein, A. L., Pathy, A. L., Schlosser, B. J., et al. (2016). Guidelines of care for the management of acne vulgaris. *Journal of the American Academy of Dermatology, 74*(5), 945–973.

Zeina, B., Mansoor, S., & Sakka, N. (2016). Pemphigus vulgaris. Medscape. Retrieved on 2/12/2017 at: emedicine.medscape.com/article/1064187-overview

Resources

American Academy of Dermatology (AAD), www.aad.org

American Melanoma Foundation (AMF), www.melanomafoundation.org

Dermatology Atlas (DermIS), a cooperation between the Department of Clinical Social Medicine (University of Heidelberg) and the Department of Dermatology (University of Erlangen), www.dermis.net

Foundation for Ichthyosis and Related Skin Types (FIRST), www.firstskinfoundation.org

National Eczema Association, nationaleczema.org

National Psoriasis Foundation, www.psoriasis.org

New Zealand Dermatology Society (DermNET NZ), www.dermnetnz.org

Skin Cancer Foundation, www.skincancer.org

62

Management of Patients With Burn Injury

LEARNING OBJECTIVES

On completion of this chapter, the learner will be able to:

1 Identify the incidence of burn injury in the United States.
2 Explain the factors that affect the severity of burn injury.
3 Describe the local and systemic effects of a major burn injury.
4 Compare priorities of care and potential complications for each phase of burn recovery.

5 Plan fluid replacement requirements during the emergent/resuscitative phase of a burn injury.
6 Discuss the nurse's role in burn wound management during the acute/intermediate phase of burn care.
7 Use the nursing process as a framework of care for the patient with burns.
8 Recognize the psychosocial challenges associated with burn injuries and identify strategies for intervention.

GLOSSARY

autograft: a graft derived from one part of a patient's body and used on another part of that same patient's body
carboxyhemoglobin: a compound of carbon monoxide and hemoglobin, formed in the blood with exposure to carbon monoxide
collagen: a protein present in skin, tendon, bone, cartilage, and connective tissue
contracture: shrinkage of burn scar through collagen maturation
débridement: removal of foreign material and devitalized tissue until surrounding healthy tissue is exposed
donor site: the area from which skin is taken to provide a skin graft for another part of the body

eschar: devitalized tissue resulting from a burn or wound
escharotomy: a linear excision made through eschar to release constriction of underlying tissue
excision: surgical removal of tissue
fasciotomy: an incision made through the fascia to release constriction of underlying muscle
homograft: a graft transferred from one human (living or cadaveric) to another human; also called *allograft*
xenograft: a graft obtained from an animal of a species other than that of the recipient (e.g., pigskin); also called *heterograft*

Burn injuries are painful, costly, disfiguring, require intensive and extensive rehabilitation therapy, and are often associated with long-term disability. Advances in burn care that include optimal fluid resuscitation, infection control, early excision and grafting, an enhanced team approach, and the emergence of specialized burn centers have contributed to significant improvements in morbidity and mortality of patients with burns (Meyerson, Coffey, Jones, et al. 2015; Sen, Palmieri, & Greenhalgh, 2015). The role of the nurse in the interdisciplinary treatment team includes provision of holistic evidence-based care during all phases of burn injury recovery to optimize patient outcomes.

Overview of Burn Injury

Incidence

A burn injury can affect people of all ages and socioeconomic groups. An estimated 486,000 people are treated for burns and approximately 40,000 are hospitalized annually (American Burn Association [ABA], 2015). The largest proportion, 43%, were reported as flame related, 34% were scalds, 9% were from

direct source contact, 4% were electrical, 3% were chemical contact, 2% were inhalation only, and the remaining 5% were from unspecified or miscellaneous categories. Of those admitted to burn centers, men have more than twice the incidence of burn injury than women; for both men and women, the most frequent age group for burns is between 20 and 30 years. Burn centers in the United States reported the race and ethnicity of patients treated is as follows: 59% Caucasian, 20% African American, 14% Hispanic, 3% Asian American, 1% Native American, and 3% identified as "other"; 73% had injuries that occurred at home, 8% had industry-related injuries, 5% had recreationally related injuries, and the remaining 14% had injuries from other sources (American Burn Association National Burn Repository [ABA NBR], 2015).

Patients with burns have particularly prolonged hospital lengths of stay (LOS). Many patients require multiple surgical interventions, extensive pain control, immobilization and rehabilitation, and prolonged intravenous (IV) medication regimens, particularly with antibiotics and opioids. Veeravagu, Yoon, Jiang, et al. (2015) reviewed over 500,000 admissions from national databases of burn injuries from 1988 to 2008 that indicated a 2.5% increase in LOS for each one percent of total body surface area (TBSA) burned, a 0.9% increase of TBSA per each year of patient age, and a 33% increase for those with inhalation injury. Adults with greater than 40% TBSA burned are at high risk for morbidity and mortality based on a recent review of 307 patients across 6 burn centers (Jeschke, Pinto, Kraft, et al., 2015).

Gerontologic Considerations

Age-related changes such as diminished mobility, postural stability, strength, coordination, sensation, visual acuity, and declining memory predispose older adults to burn injury. Registry data from 203,422 hospitalized burn patients over a 10-year period suggest that 13% of burn injuries requiring hospitalization occurred in patients 60 years and older. Mortality associated with burns is greater in older adult patients than in younger adult patients when comparing injuries with similar severity. The overall mortality from burns in the adult aged 60 and over is approximately 12%, compared to a 3.2% overall mortality rate for all ages. Fire/flame is the most common etiology of burns in the older adult, accounting for 56% of reported injuries. Among patients who are 60 years and older with burns, 61% are male. Complications associated with burn injuries are also highest in patients 60 years and older. Of all reported complications, pneumonia was the most common, followed closely by urinary tract infections. Other reported complications include respiratory failure, septicemia, cellulitis, wound infection, Kidney injury, dysrhythmias, septicemia, and other infections (ABA NBR, 2015).

The skin of the older adult is thinner and less elastic, which affects the depth of injury and its ability to heal. Delayed wound healing, another consequence of aging, is associated with higher morbidity and mortality (Nitzschke, Aden, Serio-Melvin, et al., 2014). Pulmonary function becomes impaired with age; therefore, airway exchange, lung elasticity, and ventilation may be altered and can be exacerbated by a history of smoking. Decreased cardiac output, coronary artery disease, and decreased cardiovascular compensatory response may increase the risk of complications in older adult patients with burn injuries. There may be a fine line between adequate fluid resuscitation and fluid overload in this population. Decreased kidney and hepatic function can impact medication dosing due to altered medication clearance. Malnutrition may impact morbidity and mortality in older adults, especially those who are institutionalized. Additionally, older patients may have varying degrees of mental capacity on admission or through the course of care, making assessment of pain, anxiety, and delirium a challenge for the burn team.

A recent retrospective review of 1461 patients with burns admitted to a burn center between 2006 and 2015 revealed the Lethal Dose 50 (LD50) (i.e., lethal burn dose) for patients over 65 years of age is 35% of the TBSA, unchanged in the last 30 years, despite advances in burn care. Although there was no significant difference in incidence of pneumonia, bacteremia, sepsis, wound infection, kidney injury, abdominal compartment syndrome (ACS), acute respiratory distress syndrome (ARDS), or deep vein thrombosis (DVT), there was a statistical increase in LOS, gastrointestinal (GI) bleeding, and mortality when compared to patients less than 65 years of age. Furthermore older adult patients displayed impaired capacity for wound healing, impaired immune response, increased risk for multiple organ failure, an inability to respond to stressors, and profound alterations in metabolism (Jeschke, Patsouris, Stanojcic, et al., 2015).

Comorbidities and the resultant treatment polypharmacy (i.e., multiple medication prescriptions) contribute to in-hospital complications as well as increase the need for discharge to a facility other than the patient's home after acute recovery (Justiniano, Coffey, Evans, et al., 2015). Nurses need to assess an older adult patient's ability to safely perform activities of daily living (ADLs), assist older adult patients and families to modify their environment to ensure safety, and make referrals as needed.

Prevention

Burns are preventable. An important goal of nurses in community and home settings is to provide education about the prevention of burn injury (see Chart 62-1). Nurses should capitalize on the teachable moment, an opportunity using a recent injury event, as a prime time people "are likely to be more receptive to accept guidance on how to change their behavior to avoid future injury" (Klas, Smith, Matherly, et al., 2015, p. 434). High-risk behaviors such as alcohol consumption and alcohol abuse often precipitate many burn injuries (Sen et al., 2015). Smoking materials, particularly cigarettes, are a leading cause of fire death in the United States (ABA, 2011). The World Health Organization (WHO) recommends heightened awareness of the burden of burn injury and risk factors as imperatives to develop an effective burn prevention program (WHO, 2014).

Chart 62-1 **HEALTH PROMOTION**
Burn Prevention

- Advise that matches and lighters be kept out of the reach of children.
- Emphasize the importance of never leaving children unattended around fire or in bathroom/bathtub.
- Educate about the installation and maintenance of smoke and carbon monoxide detectors on every level of the home and changing batteries annually on birthday.
- Recommend the development and practice of a home exit fire drill with all members of the household.
- Advocate setting the water heater temperature no higher than 48.9°C (120°F).
- Educate about the perils of smoking in bed, smoking while using home oxygen, or falling asleep while smoking.
- Caution against using flammable liquids to start fires and/or throwing flammable liquids onto an already burning fire.
- Warn of the danger of removing the radiator cap from a hot car engine.
- Recommend avoidance of overhead electrical wires and underground wires when working outside.
- Advise that hot irons and curling irons be kept out of the reach of children.
- Discourage running electric cords under carpets or rugs.
- Recommend storage of flammable liquids well away from a fire source, such as a pilot light.
- Educate about the importance of being aware of loose clothing when cooking over a stovetop or flame.
- Recommend having a working fire extinguisher in the home and knowing how to use it.

Outlook for Survival and Recovery

WHO (2014) estimated 265,000 annual deaths worldwide are caused by burns, the majority occurring in middle- to low-income populations, while nonfatal burns are a leading cause of morbidity including disfigurement, disability, and social stigma. The overall mortality rate for all TBSA burns in the United States is 3.2% (ABA NBR, 2015). The strongest predictors for mortality in burn injuries included increased percent of TBSA burned, presence of inhalation injury, and increased age. Provision of evidenced-based, multidisciplinary, holistic care is crucial to improving both survival and recovery, culminating in re-integration of the survivor into society.

Great strides in research on treatment have helped to increase the survival rate of patients with burn injuries. Long-term outcomes can now be evaluated because patients with very large burns are surviving their injuries. Improvements in fluid resuscitation, infection control, nutrition delivery, early burn **excision** (i.e., surgical removal of tissue), wound closure, modulation of the metabolic response, and development of burn centers have contributed to the survivability and recovery from burn injuries (Rousseau, Massion, Laungani, et al., 2014; Snell, Loh, Mahambrey, et al., 2013). Continued research and advances in the areas of critical care, rehabilitation, and psychosocial and scar management are essential for continued progress in burn care.

Severity

The severity of each burn injury is determined by multiple factors. These factors include age of the patient; depth of the burn; amount of surface area of the body that is burned; the presence of inhalation injury; presence of other injuries; location of the injury in areas such as the face, the perineum, hands, or feet; and the presence of comorbid conditions. Even in specialized burn centers, adults with more than 40% TBSA burned are at high risk for mortality and morbidity (Jeschke et al., 2015). Careful assessment enables the burn team to estimate the likelihood of survival and develop an individualized plan of care for each patient.

Age

Young children and older adults continue to have increased morbidity and mortality when compared to other age groups with similar injuries and present a challenge for the burn team. Thinner skin at both ends of the age spectrum leads to deeper burns with more complications. This is an important factor when determining the severity of injury and possible outcome for the patient.

Burn Depth

Burns are classified according to the depth of tissue destruction as depicted in Table 62-1. First-degree burns are superficial injuries that involve only the outermost layer of skin.

TABLE 62-1 Characteristics of Burns According to Depth

Causes	Skin Involvement	Clinical Manifestations	Wound Appearance	Recuperative Course and Treatment
First Degree (Superficial)				
Sunburn Low-intensity flash Superficial scald	Epidermis	Tingling Hyperesthesia (hypersensitivity) Pain that is soothed by cooling Peeling Itching	Reddened; blanches with pressure; dry Minimal or no edema Possible blisters	Complete recovery within a few days Oral pain medications, cool compresses, skin lubricants (e.g., ointments, emollients); topical antimicrobial agents not indicated
Second Degree (Partial Thickness)				
Scalds Flash flame Contact	Epidermis, portion of dermis	Pain Hyperesthesia Sensitive to air currents	Blistered, mottled red base; disrupted epidermis; weeping surface Edema	Recovery in 2–3 weeks Some scarring and depigmentation possible; may require grafting
Third Degree (Full Thickness)				
Flame Prolonged exposure to hot liquids Electric current Chemical Contact	Epidermis, dermis, and sometimes subcutaneous tissue; may involve connective tissue, and muscle	Insensate Shock Myoglobinuria (red pigment in urine) and possible hemolysis (blood cell destruction) Possible contact points (entrance or exit wounds in electrical burns)	Dry; pale white, red brown, leathery, or charred Coagulated vessels may be visible. Edema	Eschar may slough Grafting necessary Scarring and loss of contour and function
Fourth Degree (Full Thickness That Includes Fat, Fascia, Muscle, and/or Bone)				
Prolonged exposure or high voltage electrical injury	Deep tissue, muscle and bone	Shock Myoglobinuria (red pigment in urine) and possible hemolysis (blood cell destruction)	Charred	Amputations likely Grafting of no benefit, given depth and severity of wound(s)

Adapted from American Burn Association. (2011). *Advanced burn life support (ABLS) course provider manual 2011*. Chicago, IL: Author; Kearns, R. D., Cairns, C. B., Holmes, J. H., et al. (2013). Thermal burns: A review of best practice. *EMS World, 42*(1), 43–51.

These burns are erythematous, but the epidermis is intact; if rubbed, the burned tissue does not separate from the underlying dermis. This is known as a negative Nikolsky's sign. A typical first-degree burn is a sunburn or superficial scald.

Second-degree burns involve the entire epidermis and varying portions of the dermis. They are painful and are typically associated with blister formation. Healing time depends on the depth of dermal injury and typically ranges from 2 to 3 weeks. Hair follicles and skin appendages remain intact.

Third-degree (full-thickness) burns involve total destruction of the epidermis, dermis, and, in some cases, damage of underlying tissue. Wound color ranges widely from pale white to red, brown, or charred. The burned area lacks sensation because nerve fibers are damaged. The wound appears leathery and dry due to the destruction of the microcirculation; hair follicles and sweat glands are destroyed. The severity of this burn is often deceiving to patients because they have no pain in the injury area (see Fig. 62-1).

Fourth-degree burns (deep burn necrosis) are those injuries that extend into deep tissue, muscle, or bone (see Fig. 62-2) (Kearns, Cairns, Holmes, et al., 2013).

Burn depth determines whether spontaneous re-epithelialization will occur. Determining burn depth can be difficult even for the experienced burn care provider. The following factors are considered in determining the depth of a burn: how the injury occurred, causative agent (such as flame or scalding liquid), temperature and duration of contact with the causative agent, and thickness of the skin at the injury site.

Extent of Body Surface Area Injured

Various methods are used to estimate the TBSA affected by burns; among them are the rule of nines, the Lund and Browder method, and the palmer method. These tools assist the treatment team in making decisions about the plan of care, which may include transfer of the patient to a burn center. Burn centers are hospital based and are specially equipped with the resources and personnel to treat patients with burns from the time of injury through their rehabilitation. Burn center designation is jointly conferred by the ABA and the

Figure 62-2 • Fourth-degree burn to second digit. Used with permission from University of Texas Medical Branch, Galveston, TX.

American College of Surgeons (ABA, 2014). Chart 62-2 provides the ABA criteria for referral to a burn center.

Rule of Nines

The most common method used to estimate the extent of burns in adults is the rule of nines (see Fig. 62-3). This system is based on anatomic regions, each representing approximately 9% of the TBSA, allowing clinicians to quickly obtain an estimate of burn size. If a portion of an anatomic area is burned, the TBSA is calculated accordingly—for example, if approximately half of one arm were burned, the TBSA burned would be 4.5% (Kearns et al., 2013).

Lund and Browder Method

A more precise method of estimating the extent of a burn is the Lund and Browder method (Kearns et al., 2013), which recognizes the percentage of surface area of various anatomic parts, especially the head and legs, as it relates to the age of the patient. By dividing the body into very small areas and

Figure 62-1 • Third-degree (full-thickness) burn to arm and upper back with surrounding second-degree (partial-thickness) burn. Used with permission from University of Texas Medical Branch, Galveston, TX.

Chart 62-2 **American Burn Association Criteria for Referral to a Burn Center**

- Partial-thickness burns covering 10% of total body surface area or greater
- Burns involving the face, hands, feet, genitalia, perineum, or major joints
- Third-degree burns
- Electrical burns, including lightning injury
- Chemical burns
- Inhalation injury
- Burn injury in patients with preexisting medical disorders
- Any patients with burns and concomitant trauma
- Children with burn injuries in facilities that do not specialize in pediatric care
- Patients who will require special social, emotional, or long-term rehabilitation

Adapted from American Burn Association. (2011). *Advanced burn life support (ABLS) course provider manual 2011.* Chicago, IL: Author.

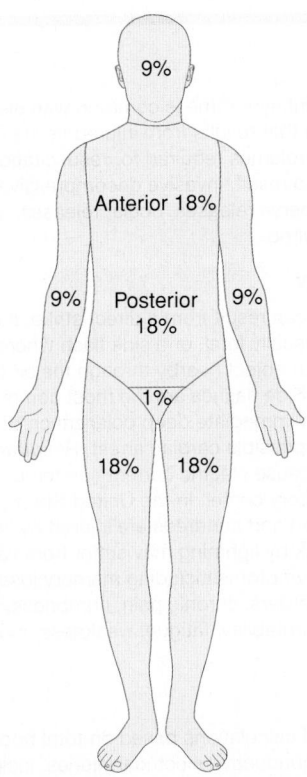

Figure 62-3 • The rule of nines. Estimated percentage of total body surface area (TBSA) in the adult is calculated by sectioning the body surface into areas with a numerical value related to nine. (*Note:* The anterior and posterior head total 9% of TBSA.)

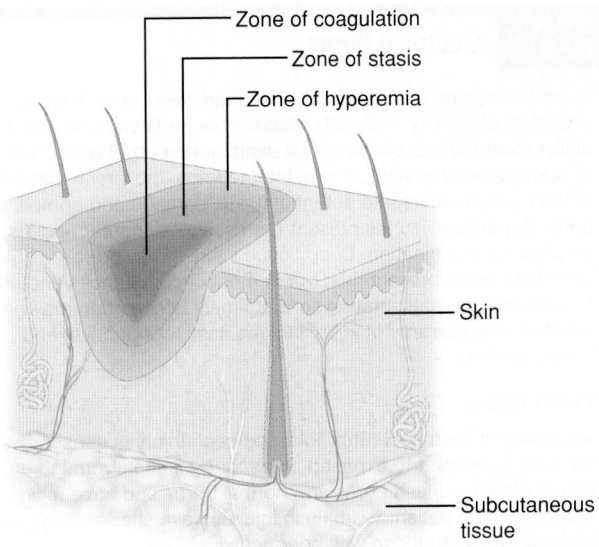

Figure 62-4 • Zones of burn injury. Each burned area has three zones of injury. The zone of coagulation (the innermost area, where cellular death occurs) sustains the most damage. The zone of stasis (the middle area) has a compromised blood supply, inflammation, and tissue injury. The zone of hyperemia (the outermost area) sustains the least damage.

providing an estimate of the proportion of TBSA accounted for by each body part, clinicians can obtain a reliable estimate of TBSA burned. The initial evaluation is made on arrival of the patient to the hospital and should be revised within the first 72 hours, because demarcation of the wound and its depth present themselves more clearly by this time. The Lund and Browder chart is readily available in both printed and electronic formats.

Palmer Method

In patients with scattered burns, the Palmer method may be used to estimate the extent of the burns. The size of the patient's hand, including the fingers, is approximately 1% of that patient's TBSA (ABA, 2011).

Pathophysiology

Burn injuries are very traumatic injuries as the initial injury can evolve and worsen over time. Burn injury is the result of a chemical injury or heat transfer from one site to another, causing tissue destruction through coagulation, protein denaturation, or ionization of cellular contents. The burn wound is not homogenous; rather, tissue necrosis occurs at the center of the injury with regions of tissue viability toward the periphery. The central area of the wound is termed the *zone of coagulation* due to the characteristic coagulation necrosis of cells that occurs (see Fig. 62-4). The surrounding zone, the *zone of stasis*, describes an area of injured cells that may remain viable but, with persistent ischemia, will undergo necrosis within 24 to 48 hours. The outermost zone, the *zone of hyperemia*, sustains minimal injury and may fully recover spontaneously over time.

The skin and the mucosa of the upper airways are the most common sites of tissue destruction, although deep tissues, including the viscera, can be damaged by electrical burns (see Chart 62-3) or by prolonged contact with a heat or chemical source. The release of local mediators and changes in blood flow, tissue edema, and infection can cause progression of the burn injury.

Another potential mechanism of burn injury is radiation exposure. This has received increased attention because of threats of terrorism and recent world events. Radiation injuries produce two detrimental effects. The first is a thermal effect, which results in cutaneous burn injuries. The second effect is damage to the cellular deoxyribonucleic acid (DNA), which may be localized or affect the whole body. Morbidity and mortality are dose dependent (see Chapter 73). Treatment for the cutaneous injury is the same as other burns discussed in this chapter.

The depth of a burn injury depends on the temperature of the burning agent and the duration of contact with the agent. In adults, exposure to temperatures of 54°C (130°F) for 30 seconds will result in burn injury. At 60°C (140°F), tissue destruction occurs in 5 seconds (this is a common setting for home water heaters; see Chart 62-1 for discussion of appropriate water heater setting). At 71°C (160°F) or higher, a full-thickness burn occurs instantaneously (ABA, 2011).

Major burn injuries, those that affect more than 30% TBSA, produce both local and systemic effects characterized by burn wound edema, generalized edema formation in noninjured tissue, increased metabolic rate (hypermetabolism), hyperdynamic circulation, increased oxygen and glucose consumption, catabolism of muscle and bone, immune dysfunction, insulin resistance, and impaired organ perfusion (Flores, Stockton, Roberts, et al., 2015; Snell et al., 2013). Severe injuries ultimately encompass changes

Chart 62-3 Electrical Burns

Electrical injuries are devastating and complex burns. Heat generated by electricity is directly responsible for tissue damage, but unlike most thermal burns, visual examination is not predictive of burn size and severity. It is helpful to know the circumstances of the injury to anticipate potential tissue damage and complications. Superficial injuries present themselves as contact points on physical examination. Deep tissue injuries may not be visible on initial clinical presentation but in most circumstances should be assumed on presentation so that timely intervention may be initiated. Mechanisms of injury include flash, conductive, and lightning injury.

Flash Injury

An electrical flash generates light and heat. Injury is caused by the heat generated to exposed areas, or by flames from ignition of clothing. Flash burns are thermal burns and have fewer complications; patients with flash injuries have shorter lengths of hospital stay than those with conductive injuries.

Conductive Injury

Conductive electrical injuries occur when the current overcomes the skin's resistance and travels through the body. The amount and severity of tissue damage is directly proportional to the strength of the current (voltage), duration of contact with the source, which organs lay along the pathway of current, and whether the current is direct or alternating. Conduction of electricity through the nerves and vessels and along the outside of bones generates heat, causing damage to adjacent tissues and direct injury to the peripheral nerves. Deep muscle injury may be present without injury to superficial muscles, masking the true extent of the injury. In addition, electrical current immediately contracts muscles as it travels through the body causing possible skeletal and joint injuries in high-voltage contact. Although the majority of reported electrical injuries are high voltage (>1000 volts) injuries, significant physical and psychological morbidity also occur with low voltage (<1000 volts) injuries as well.

Entrance and exit wounds or contact points can help identify the probable current path and therefore anticipated tissue and organ involvement. Direct current (DC) travels in one direction, is associated with an explosion and likely concomitant trauma from the blast. Alternating current (AC) passes back and forth from the point of contact, through the body and back to the source many times per second and can hold the victim to it, increasing contact time. Compartment syndrome is common with electrical injuries due to the edema that results from injured tissue compounded by the large fluid volumes required for resuscitation to prevent kidney failure. As a result, invasive decompressive therapies such as fasciotomies, nerve releases, ocular releases, and laparotomies may be required.

Lightning Injury

Lightning injuries can result from a direct strike, a high-voltage DC injury that is usually fatal, or a side flash wherein the current discharges from an object nearby through the air to an adjacent object or person. Side flashes are the most common cause of injury and result in immediate deep polarization of the entire myocardium with possible cardiac arrest. Respiratory arrest is also expected because electric current can temporarily inactivate the brain's respiratory center. In the United States, an average of 49 people are killed and hundreds are injured by lightning each year. People struck by lightning may suffer from various debilitating long-term symptoms including memory loss, attention deficits, sleep disorders, chronic pain, numbness, dizziness, stiffness in joints, irritability, fatigue, weakness, muscle spasms, and depression.

Management

Resuscitation fluid calculations based on total body surface area are inaccurate in conductive electrical injuries, including some lightning injuries. It is difficult to quantify the extent of tissue injury without surgical exploration because the damage may not be visible on physical examination. Serum creatinine kinase levels are useful in determining the degree of muscle injury in the early phases of care. Myoglobinuria, common with muscle damage, may cause kidney failure if not treated. IV fluid administration titrated to a higher target of urine output per hour than usual may be indicated until the urine is no longer red. It is common practice to add 50 mEq of sodium bicarbonate per liter of IV fluid in an effort to assist in alkalinizing the urine. Serum myoglobin and urine myoglobin levels may be monitored as indicators of the need for continued resuscitation.

Finally, the surgical treatment of an electrical injury is as complex as the injury itself. Vasculature is commonly affected; thus, progressive tissue necrosis occurs over time. Sequential surgical débridement may be necessary, using caution to preserve viable tissue.

Adapted from Cahill, K. C., Tiong, W. H. C. & Conroy, F. J. (2013). Trineural injury to the right hand after domestic electrocution. *Journal of Burn Care and Research*, 35(5), e353–e356; Kwon, K. H., Kim, S. H., & Minn Y. K. (2014). Electrodiagnostic study of peripheral nerves in high-voltage electrical injury. *Journal of Burn Care and Research*, 35, e230–233; National Oceanic and Atmospheric Administration. (2015). *Lightning safety*. Retrieved on 6/10/2016 at: www.lightningsafety.noaa.gov/index.shtml; Russell, K. W., Cochran, A. L., Mehta, S. T., et al. (2013). Lightning burns. *Journal of Burn Care and Research*, 35(6), e436–e438; Stergiou-Kita, M., Mansfield, E., Bayley, M., et al. (2014). Returning to work after electrical injuries: Workers' perspectives and advice to others. *Journal of Burn Care and Research*, 35(6), 498–507.

in pathophysiology of all body systems as presented in Table 62-2. Initially, these responses are compensatory adaptive responses to the burn injury, but quickly become counterproductive events negatively impacting recovery (Abdullahi & Jeschke, 2014). These pathologic responses are also seen in trauma, but the magnitude, duration, and severity are significantly higher with burn injuries.

Cardiovascular Alterations

When a burn injury occurs, there is an immediate decrease in cardiac output that precedes the loss of plasma volume, although the exact mechanism why this occurs is unknown. Due to vasoconstrictive compensatory responses secondary to plasma volume loss, the workload of the heart and oxygen demand increase.

Hypovolemia is the immediate consequence of ensuing plasma volume loss and results in decreased perfusion and oxygen delivery. As fluid loss continues due to capillary leakage, and vascular volume decreases, cardiac output continues to decrease and the blood pressure drops. This is the onset of burn shock. Burn shock is initially a type of hypovolemic shock. The systemic inflammation causes the release of free oxygen radicals that increase capillary permeability, causing increased plasma loss and subsequent peripheral edema. As a compensatory response to intravascular fluid loss, the sympathetic nervous system releases catecholamines, resulting in

TABLE 62-2 Pathophysiologic Changes With Severe Burns

Body System	Physiologic Changes
Cardiovascular	Cardiac depression, edema, hypovolemia
Pulmonary	Vasoconstriction, edema
Gastrointestinal	Impaired motility and absorption, vasoconstriction, loss of mucosal barrier function with bacterial translocation, increased pH
Kidney	Vasoconstriction
Other	Altered thermoregulation, immunodepression, hypermetabolism

Adapted from Abdullahi, A., & Jeschke, M. G. (2014). Nutrition and anabolic pharmacotherapies in the care of burn patients. *Nutrition in Clinical Practice, 29*(5), 621–630; Snell, J. A., Loh N. W., Mahambrey, T, et al. (2013). Clinical review: The critical care management of the burn patient. *Critical Care, 17*(5), 241.

Figure 62-5 • Escharotomy of forearm. Used with permission from University of Texas Medical Branch, Galveston, TX.

an increase in peripheral resistance (vasoconstriction) and an increase in pulse rate that further decreases tissue perfusion.

Prompt, appropriate fluid resuscitation maintains the blood pressure in the low to normal range and improves cardiac output (see later discussion). But, despite adequate fluid resuscitation, cardiac filling pressures (central venous pressure, pulmonary artery pressure, and pulmonary artery wedge pressure) remain low during the initial burn shock period. Unlike traumatic injuries, which are often characterized by blood loss, only plasma is lost in the burn injury. If adequate IV fluids are not given to maintain vascular volume, distributive shock occurs (see Chapter 14).

Generally, the greatest volume of fluid leak occurs in the first 24 to 36 hours after the burn, peaking by 6 to 8 hours. As the capillaries begin to regain their integrity, burn shock resolves and fluid returns to the vascular compartment. Intrinsic diuresis will begin and continue for several days to 2 weeks in the previously healthy adult.

Fluid and Electrolyte Alterations

Edema forms rapidly after a burn injury. A superficial burn will cause edema to form within 4 hours, whereas a deeper burn will continue to form edema up to 18 hours post-injury. This is caused by increased perfusion to the injured area in the presence of increased capillary permeability and reflects the amount of microvascular and lymphatic damage to the tissue. In burns greater than 30% TBSA, inflammatory mediators stimulate local and systemic reactions resulting in extensive shift of intravascular fluid, electrolytes, and proteins into the surrounding interstitium (Snell et al., 2013).

Treatments for edema may include elevation of the extremity or, in severe cases, removal of **eschar** (i.e., devitalized tissue) via **escharotomy** (i.e., surgical incision through eschar), or decompression of edema formation via **fasciotomy** (i.e., surgical incision through fascia to relieve constricted muscle) to restore tissue perfusion (see Figs. 62-5 and 62-6).

Reabsorption of edema begins at about 4 hours post-injury and is complete by 4 days post-burn injury. However, the rate of reabsorption depends on the depth of injury to the tissue. Although adequate fluid resuscitation is paramount to maintaining tissue perfusion, excessive fluid administration increases edema formation in both burned and nonburned tissue causing ischemia and necrosis.

Immediately after burn injury, hyperkalemia (excessive potassium) may result from massive cell destruction. Hypokalemia (potassium depletion) may occur later with fluid shifts and inadequate potassium replacement. Serum sodium levels vary in response to fluid resuscitation. Hyponatremia (serum sodium depletion) may be present as a result of plasma loss or may also occur during the first week of the acute phase, as water shifts from the interstitial space and returns to the vascular space.

 Concept Mastery Alert

For patients in the emergent/resuscitative phase, nurses should do a primary survey and monitor circulation. As the taut, burned tissue becomes unyielding to the edema underneath its surface, it begins to act like a tourniquet, especially if the burn is circumferential. As edema increases, pressure on small blood vessels in the distal extremities causes an obstruction of blood flow and consequent tissue ischemia and compartment syndrome. See Chapter 42 for discussion of compartment syndrome. Patients in the acute/intermediate phase must be monitored for the development of venous thromboembolism (VTE).

Figure 62-6 • Fasciotomy of upper arm. Used with permission from University of Texas Medical Branch, Galveston, TX.

At the time of burn injury, some red blood cells may be destroyed and others damaged, resulting in anemia. Despite this, the hematocrit may be elevated due to plasma loss. Abnormalities in coagulation, including a decrease in platelets (thrombocytopenia) and prolonged clotting and prothrombin times, also occur.

Pulmonary Alterations

Inhalation injury is caused by inhalation of thermal and/or chemical irritants. Inhalation injuries are categorized as upper airway injury (above the glottis) or lower airway injury (below the glottis). Injuries above the vocal cords can be thermal or chemical, whereas injuries below the vocal cords are usually chemical (ABA, 2011). Approximately 6% to 30% of patients admitted to burn centers have an inhalation injury (ABA, 2011). The presence of inhalation injury is important to recognize. History of the injury, such as a flame injury occurring in an enclosed space, and clinical signs such as singed facial hair or carbonaceous sputum should be considered indicators for the presence of a smoke inhalation injury. Bronchoscopy is considered the standard test for definitive diagnosis as initial chest x-rays appear normal. The extent of damage is directly related to the temperature and the concentration of toxic gases.

Upper Airway Injury

Upper airway injury is obstructive and is caused by severe upper airway edema from direct thermal injury or secondary edema from face or neck burns in the early post-burn period. Because of the cooling effect of rapid vaporization in the oropharynx, direct heat injury does not normally occur below the level of the glottis. However, with steam exposure, thermal injury to the lower airways is possible because the upper airway cannot effectively protect the lower airway from steam.

Lower Airway Injury

Inhalation injury below the glottis results from inhaling the products of incomplete combustion or noxious gases and is often the source of death at the scene of a fire. Smoke inhalation injuries cause loss of ciliary action, trigger an inflammatory response causing hypersecretion, and produce severe mucosal edema and possibly bronchospasm. Alveolar surfactant production is reduced, resulting in atelectasis (collapse of alveoli). Expectoration of carbon particles in the sputum is the cardinal sign of this injury.

Noxious gases, such as carbon monoxide and hydrogen cyanide, contribute to lower airway injuries. Carbon monoxide poisoning is a factor in most fatalities at the scene of a fire as it combines with hemoglobin and displaces oxygen to form **carboxyhemoglobin**. The affinity of hemoglobin for carbon monoxide is 200 times greater than that for oxygen, and if significant quantities of carbon monoxide are present, then tissue hypoxia will occur (ABA, 2011). Treatment is administration of 100% oxygen to displace the carbon monoxide molecules bound to hemoglobin. Hydrogen cyanide is a systemic toxin also associated with mortality. Signs and symptoms of hypoxia in light of normal arterial oxygen tension (PaO_2) is an indicator of cyanide poisoning (Snell et al., 2013).

Bronchoconstriction (caused by release of histamine, serotonin, and thromboxane [a powerful vasoconstrictor]) and chest constriction secondary to circumferential torso burns can contribute to deterioration. Even without pulmonary injury, hypoxia may be present. Early in the post-burn period, catecholamine release in response to the stress of the burn injury alters peripheral blood flow, thereby reducing oxygen delivery to the periphery. Later, hypermetabolism and continued catecholamine release lead to increased tissue oxygen consumption, which can also lead to hypoxia. To ensure that adequate oxygen is available to the tissues, supplemental oxygen may be needed. Restrictive pulmonary excursion may occur with full-thickness burns encircling the thorax resulting in decreased tidal volume. In such situations, an escharotomy may be necessary to restore adequate chest excursion.

Kidney Alterations

Kidney function may be altered as a result of decreased blood volume post-burn injury due to the compensatory response to intravascular volume loss. Adequate fluid volume replacement can restore renal blood flow, increasing the glomerular filtration rate and urine volume. Additionally, destruction of red blood cells at the injury site results in free hemoglobin in the urine. If muscle damage occurs (e.g., from electrical burns), myoglobin is released from the muscle cells and excreted by the kidneys causing the urine to be red. If there is inadequate blood flow through the kidneys caused by the hemoglobin and myoglobin occluding the renal tubules, acute tubular necrosis and acute kidney injury will occur (see Chapter 54). Increased abdominal pressure from the injury can also cause kidney ischemia.

Immunologic Alterations

The immunologic defenses of the body are greatly altered by a burn injury. The skin is the largest barrier to infection, and when it is compromised, the patient is continually exposed to the environment. The burn injury itself produces systemic release of cytokines and other substances that cause leukocyte and endothelial cell dysfunction. Burn centers provide an infection-controlled environment to protect the patient and minimize exposure to potentially harmful organisms.

Thermoregulatory Alterations

Integumentary loss also results in an inability to regulate body temperature. Patients with burn injuries may, therefore, exhibit low body temperatures in the early hours after injury. Hostler, Weaver, Ziembicki, et al. (2013) found that hypothermia (i.e., core temperature less than 36.5°C [97.7°F]), on admission of patients to the hospital was an independent predictor of mortality. Intraoperative hypothermia, exacerbated by exposure during prolonged surgeries, combined with general anesthesia's blunting of metabolic and neurologic hypothermic responses, also poses challenges to successfully treating patients with major burns (Davis, Rodriquez, Quintana, et al., 2013). Burn centers have heat panels at the bedside as additional heating sources to help maintain the patient's body temperature through environmental warming. After the initial few hours, persistent increases in baseline core temperature ensues as part of the physiologic and metabolic response to a burn injury (Snell et al., 2013).

Gastrointestinal Alterations

Patients who are critically ill, including those with burns, are predisposed to altered GI motility. Impaired enteric nerve and smooth muscle function, inflammation, surgery, medications such as vasopressors, and inadequate tissue perfusion are some causes of GI dysfunction. Indicators of GI organ ischemia include increased bladder pressure, increasing serum lactate, and feeding intolerance (Trexler, Lundy, Chung, et al., 2014). Three of the most common GI alterations in patients with burns are paralytic ileus (absence of intestinal peristalsis), Curling's ulcer, and translocation of bacteria. Decreased peristalsis and bowel sounds are manifestations of paralytic ileus. Gastric distention and nausea may lead to vomiting; therefore, gastric decompression is advised. Gastric bleeding secondary to massive physiologic stress may be signaled by occult blood in the stool, regurgitation of "coffee ground" material from the stomach, or bloody vomitus. These signs suggest gastric or duodenal erosion (Curling's ulcer).

Patients with large TBSA burns are also at risk for life-threatening ACS due to large volumes of fluid required for resuscitation, fluid shifts to the interstitium causing edema formation, and decreased abdominal wall compliance due to eschar formation. Increased pressure in the abdominal cavity contributes to GI tract and abdominal organ ischemia (see Chapter 14).

Management of Burn Injury

Burn care is typically categorized into three phases of care: emergent/resuscitative, acute/intermediate, and rehabilitation. Although priorities exist for each of the phases, assessment and management of problems and complications will overlap. Table 62-3 summarizes the priorities of care for each phase.

 Emergent/Resuscitative Phase

On-the-Scene Care

The first step in management is to remove the patient from the source of injury and stop the burning process while preventing injury to the rescuer. Rescue workers' priorities include establishing an airway, supplying oxygen (100% oxygen if carbon monoxide poisoning is suspected), inserting at least one large-bore IV line, and covering the wound with a clean, dry cloth or gauze. Continuous irrigation of chemical injury must begin immediately. Chart 62-4 describes the procedures and care required at the burn scene. The outward physical appearance of the person who has been burned is often distracting, but it is the internal systemic effects that pose greater threats to life.

An immediate primary survey of the patient is carried out to assess the ABCDEs: airway (A) with consideration given to protecting the cervical spine, gas exchange or breathing (B), circulatory and cardiac status (C), disability (D) including neurologic deficit, and expose and examine (E) while maintaining a warm environment (ABA, 2011).

> ### Quality and Safety Nursing Alert
>
> Airway patency and breathing must be assessed during the initial minutes of emergency care. Immediate therapy is directed toward establishing a patent airway and giving humidified 100% oxygen. If qualified personnel and equipment are available and the victim has severe respiratory distress and/or airway edema, the rescuers must insert an endotracheal tube and initiate mechanical ventilation.

> ### Quality and Safety Nursing Alert
>
> No food or fluid is given by mouth, and the patient is placed in a position that will prevent aspiration of vomitus, because nausea and vomiting may occur and protection of the airway is always a priority.

The secondary survey focuses on obtaining a history, the completion of the total body system assessment, initial fluid resuscitation, and provision of psychosocial support of the conscious patient (see Chapter 72) (ABA, 2011).

Medical Management

Long-term outcomes are impacted by the quality of care received in the first few hours after injury (Kearns et al., 2013). Initially, the patient is transported to the nearest emergency department (ED) so that lifesaving measures can be initiated, and early referral to a burn center is made if indicated.

Initial priorities in the ED remain airway, breathing, and circulation. For mild pulmonary injury, 100% humidified oxygen is given, and the patient is encouraged to cough so that secretions can be expectorated or removed by suctioning. For more severe situations, it may be necessary to remove

---

TABLE 62-3 Phases of Burn Care

Phase	Duration	Priorities
Emergent/resuscitative	From onset of injury to completion of fluid resuscitation	• Primary survey: A, B, C, D, E • Prevention of shock • Prevention of respiratory distress • Detection and treatment of concomitant injuries • Wound assessment and initial care
Acute/intermediate	From beginning of diuresis to near completion of wound closure	• Wound care and closure • Prevention or treatment of complications, including infection • Nutritional support
Rehabilitation	From major wound closure to return to individual's optimal level of physical and psychosocial adjustment	• Prevention and treatment of scars and contractures • Physical, occupational, and vocational rehabilitation • Functional and cosmetic reconstruction • Psychosocial counseling

Adapted from American Burn Association. (2011). *Advanced burn life support (ABLS) course provider manual 2011.* Chicago, IL: Author; Serghiou, M. A., Ott, S., Whitehead, C., et al. (2012). Comprehensive rehabilitation of the burn patient. In D. Herndon (Ed.). *Total burn care* (4th ed.). Edinburgh: Saunders Elsevier.

Chart 62-4 Emergency Procedures at the Burn Scene

- **Extinguish the flames or remove from source.** When clothing catches fire, the flames can be extinguished if the person drops to the floor or ground and rolls ("stop, drop, and roll"); anything available to smother the flames, such as a blanket, rug, or coat, may be used. The older adult, or others with impaired mobility, could be instructed to "stop, sit, and pat" to prevent concomitant musculoskeletal injuries. Standing still forces the person to breathe flames and smoke, and running fans the flames. If the burn source is electrical, the electrical source must be disconnected safely before moving the patient.
- **Cool the burn.** After the flames are extinguished, the burned area and adherent clothing are soaked with *cool* water, *briefly*, to cool the wound and halt the burning process. However, *never* apply ice directly to the burn, *never* wrap the person in ice, and *never* use cold soaks or dressings for longer than several minutes; such procedures may worsen tissue damage and lead to hypothermia in people with large burns.
- **Remove restrictive objects.** If possible, remove clothing immediately. Adherent clothing may be left in place once cooled. Other clothing and all jewelry, including all piercings, should be removed to allow for assessment and to prevent constriction secondary to rapidly developing edema.
- **Cover the wound.** The burn should be covered as quickly as possible to minimize bacterial contamination, maintain body temperature, and decrease pain by preventing air currents from coming in contact with the injured surface. Any clean, dry cloth can be used as an emergency dressing. Ointments and salves should *not* be used. Other than the dressing, no medication or material should be applied to the burn wound at the scene.
- **Irrigate chemical burns.** Chemical burns resulting from contact with a corrosive material are irrigated immediately. Most chemical laboratories have a high-pressure shower for such emergencies. If such an injury occurs at home, brush off the chemical agent, remove clothes immediately, and rinse all areas of the body that have come in contact with the chemical. Rinsing can occur in the shower or any other source of continuous running water. If a chemical gets in or near the eyes, the eyes should be flushed with cool, clean water immediately. Outcomes for the patient with chemical burns are significantly improved by rapid, sustained flushing of the injury at the scene.

Adapted from American Burn Association. (2011). *Advanced burn life support (ABLS) course provider manual* 2011. Chicago, IL: Author.

secretions by bronchial suctioning and to give bronchodilators and mucolytic agents. It is essential to continuously monitor airway patency, because a previously stable airway may rapidly deteriorate as edema increases and toxic effects of smoke inhalation become apparent.

Once urgent respiratory needs are appropriately addressed, fluid resuscitation is initiated in burns greater than 20% TBSA to maintain adequate organ perfusion. Baseline weight and laboratory test results are obtained, and these parameters must be monitored closely in the immediate post-burn (resuscitation) period. Both under-resuscitation and over-resuscitation with IV fluids are associated with poor outcomes. Shock, ischemic complications, and multiple organ dysfunction syndrome (MODS) occur with under-resuscitation (see Chapter 14), and heart failure and pulmonary edema occur with over-resuscitation (see Chapter 29).

In order to facilitate fluid administration, peripheral IV access may be initially obtained; however, in larger burns, central venous access is recommended due to the large volume required. TBSA is calculated and fluid resuscitation with lactated Ringers (LR) should be initiated using ABA fluid resuscitation formulas. LR is the crystalloid of choice because its pH and osmolality most closely resemble human plasma.

The ABA (2011) fluid resuscitation formula for adults within 24 hours post thermal or chemical burn is as follows:

2 mL LR × patient's weight in kilograms × %TBSA second-, third-, and fourth-degree burns

For adults with electrical burns:

4 mL LR × patient's weight in kilograms ×% TBSA second-, third-, and fourth-degree burns

Timing is one of the most important considerations in calculating fluid needs in the first 24 hours post burn. The starting point is the time of injury—not the time of arrival to the treating facility (ABA, 2011). The infusion is regulated so that one half of the total calculated volume is given in the first 8 hours post-burn injury. The second half of the calculated volume is given over the next 16 hours.

These formulas are only a guideline. It is imperative that the rate of infusion be titrated hourly as indicated by physiologic monitoring of the patient's response. For adults, a urine output of 0.5 to 1 mL/kg/h is used as an indication of appropriate resuscitation in thermal and chemical injuries, whereas in electrical injuries a urine output of 75 to 100 mL/h is the goal (ABA, 2011). Other indicators such as blood pressure and heart rate are not useful in assessing adequate intravascular volume in patients with major burns.

After adequate respiratory function and circulatory status have been established, the patient is assessed for cervical spine and/or head injuries if involved in a traumatic or electrical injury. All clothing and jewelry are removed because they may contain chemicals, retain heat, or become constrictive as edema rapidly develops. For chemical burns, flushing of the exposed areas with copious amounts of clean water is continued. The patient is checked for contact lenses. These are removed immediately if chemicals have come in contact with the eyes or if facial burns have occurred. In addition, the eyes are examined promptly for injury to the corneas. An ophthalmologist may be consulted for complete assessment via fluorescent staining to assess for corneal damage.

The patient's temperature must be monitored because hypothermia may develop rapidly and manipulation of the environment may be necessary. A temperature less than 35°C (95°F) causes vasoconstriction, which may increase tissue ischemia and necrosis.

It is important to validate an account of the burn scenario provided by the patient, witnesses at the scene, and first responders. Information should include the time and the source of the burn injury, the scene of injury (particularly if the patient was in an enclosed space), length of exposure, prior treatment, and any history of concomitant traumatic injury. A history of preexisting medical conditions, allergies, medications, and the use of drugs, alcohol, and tobacco is obtained to assist with the treatment plan.

An indwelling urinary catheter is inserted to permit accurate monitoring of urine output and as a measure of kidney function and fluid needs for patients with moderate to severe burns. If the burn exceeds 20% to 25% TBSA, a nasogastric tube is inserted and connected to low intermittent suction. All patients who are intubated should have a nasogastric tube inserted to decompress the stomach, and to prevent vomiting and aspiration. Often, patients with large burns become nauseated as a result of the GI effects of the burn injury, such as paralytic ileus, and the effects of medications such as opioids.

Clean sheets are placed under and over the patient to protect the burn wound from contamination, maintain body temperature, and reduce pain caused by air currents passing over exposed nerve endings. Baseline height, weight, arterial blood gases, hematocrit, serum electrolytes, blood alcohol level, drug panel, urinalysis, and chest x-rays may be obtained. Because poor tissue perfusion accompanies burn injuries, only IV analgesia is given in small repeated doses, which is crucial for pain reduction in the emergent phase. If the patient has an electrical burn, a baseline electrocardiogram is also obtained and continuous cardiac monitoring is initiated. Because burns are contaminated wounds, tetanus prophylaxis is given if the patient's immunization status is not current or is unknown.

> ### ▶ Quality and Safety Nursing Alert
>
> *If necessary, a blood pressure cuff can be placed around a patient's burned extremity. The cuff must be of the correct size with accommodations made for edema.*

Although the major focus of care during the emergent phase is physical stabilization, the nurse must also attend to the patient's and the family's psychological needs. Anxiety accompanies burn injuries and must be addressed on an ongoing basis. Burn injury is a crisis—one that causes varying emotional responses that may result in conflicts that may cause ethical dilemmas (see Chart 62-5). The patient's and

---

Chart 62-5 ETHICAL DILEMMA
How Much Is Enough and What Is Comfort Care?

Case Scenario

A 66-year-old man was transported to the nearest burn center, where you work as a staff nurse. He was drinking beer and cooking steaks on top of a propane grill. He inexplicably threw lighter fluid on the grill and it engulfed his upper torso and face in flames. He sustained a full-thickness burn to 42% of his body (face, neck, both arms, and chest). He was awake at the scene of injury when paramedics arrived and indicated a past medical history of hypertension, hypercholesterolemia, and gout. He was in little pain at the time due to the depth of the burn injury; however, he was asking the team questions related to the survivability of his injury, "Am I going to die?"

Given the extensiveness of his facial burns, he was intubated upon admission to the burn center. Family arrived, and the burn surgeon explained the extent of injury. A decision was made to proceed with care and assess his progress post resuscitation. They were prepared for a future decision regarding withdrawal of care if survival becomes futile.

Initial resuscitation has occurred, and approximately 4 days post burn, the patient begins to show signs of acute kidney injury. He has had one surgical procedure for débridement and grafting to his chest, and although grafts are intact, they do not look healthy. He is showing increased signs of discomfort and pain due to the operative procedure and the addition of another wound (the new donor site). In a team meeting, the family decides that they do not want to initiate hemodialysis and therefore place the patient on comfort measures. Approximately 3 days later, he remains on comfort care and has increased signs of restlessness and pain. You are caring for the patient and request that the physician prescribe an increase in pain medication from 5 mg morphine to 8 mg IV. Within 2 hours after administration, the patient expired without discomfort. Six months later, the facility is contacted by an attorney and informed that the family is taking legal action against you and the physician for performing euthanasia on the patient.

Discussion

Clinicians on burn teams commonly face these types of ethical dilemmas. Whenever possible, the team should attempt to elicit the patient's wishes as early as possible, including any advance directives. It is important to collaborate and communicate with the family regarding end of life care. Although the family agreed to "comfort care," there may have been ambiguity regarding what this entails. The problem in this case is that due to absence of pain, it is often difficult for a patient to understand the severity of their burn injury. The patient begins to experience increased pain as care progresses, and increased medication is expected. As the medication is increased to relieve pain and suffering but death ensued, the *Doctrine of Double Effect* comes into play. The medication given relieved the pain and suffering but the "bad" effect or death occurred. In such cases, the outcome may be predicted but it is not the intention of the intervention.

Analysis

- Describe the ethical principles that are in conflict in this case (see Chapter 3, Chart 3-3). Which principle should have preeminence as you proceeded to work with this family?
- Would you describe your role in this case as complicit with assisted suicide, active euthanasia, or providing palliation? What distinction, if any, might there be among these three acts? Do you believe that this was a survivable injury?
- Describe how the ethical principles of autonomy, beneficence, and nonmaleficence may intersect or be at odds with each other in this case (see Chapter 3, Chart 3-3). As a member of the burn team when the patient arrived at your facility, what could you have done differently to ensure that the patient's autonomy was preserved before he was intubated?
- What were the "intentions" in this case? How might intentionality be instrumental in making this act of titrating medications that provided palliation morally defensible? Is this nursing intervention morally defensible according to the principle of double effect (see Chapter 3, Chart 3-3)?
- Note that the American Nurses Association (2015) *Code of Ethics* clearly states that nurses should not *intentionally* cause a patient's death.

References

American Nurses Association. (2015). *Code of ethics for nurses with interpretive statements.* Washington, DC: American Nurses Publishing, American Nurses Foundation/American Nurses Association.

Beauchamp, T. L., & Childress, J. F. (2012). *Principles of biomedical ethics* (7th ed.). New York: Oxford University Press.

Resources

See Chapter 3, Chart 3-6, for ethics resources.

family's coping abilities and available supports are assessed. The nurse must consider special circumstances surrounding the burn injury when providing care. Examples include cases of abuse, neglect, suicide attempts, and injury/death of other family members or friends from the same event.

Nursing Management

Nursing assessment in the emergent phase of burn injury focuses on the major priorities for any trauma patient; the burn wound is a secondary consideration to stabilization of airway, breathing, and circulation. Respiratory status is monitored closely, and pulses are evaluated, particularly in areas of circumferential burn injury to an extremity. Cardiac monitoring is indicated initially if the patient has a history of cardiac disease, electrical injury, or respiratory conditions. Vital signs and hemodynamic status are monitored closely with awareness of expected abnormalities consistent with burn injury such as tachycardia and tachypnea.

If all extremities are burned, determining blood pressure may be difficult. A clean dressing applied under the blood pressure cuff protects the wound from contamination. Because increasing edema makes blood pressure difficult to auscultate, a Doppler (ultrasound) device or a noninvasive electronic blood pressure device may be helpful. In patients with severe burns, an arterial catheter is used for blood pressure measurement and for collecting blood specimens. Peripheral pulses of burned extremities are checked frequently, either by palpation or the use of a Doppler if necessary. Elevation of burned extremities above the level of the heart is necessary to decrease edema. Large-bore IV catheters (e.g., 14 to 18 gauge) and an indwelling urinary catheter are inserted, if not already in place, and the nurse's assessment must include hourly assessment of intake and urine output.

Red-colored urine suggests the presence of hemochromogens from damage to red blood cells and myoglobin resulting from muscle damage. These are associated with deep burns caused by electrical injury or prolonged contact with heat or flame. Glycosuria, a common finding in the early post-burn hours, results from the release of liver glycogen stores in response to stress.

The nurse assists with calculating the patient's expected fluid requirements and monitoring the patient's response to fluid resuscitation. Nurse-driven resuscitation protocols can improve patient outcomes in the emergent/resuscitative phase (Fahlstrom, Boyle, & Makic, 2013). Nursing responsibilities include administration of fluids, strict monitoring of fluid intake and output, monitoring patient response, and notifying the treatment team of significant assessment findings and any abnormal laboratory values.

To help guide treatment, the following are essential: documentation of body temperature, body weight, and pre-burn weight; history of allergies, tetanus immunization, past medical and surgical history, and current illnesses; and a list of current medications. A head-to-toe assessment is performed, focusing on signs and symptoms of concomitant illness, associated injury, or developing complications. Assessing the extent of the burn wound using the rule of nines or facilitated with anatomic diagrams (described previously) is performed. In addition, the nurse works with the primary provider to clinically assess the initial areas of full- and partial-thickness injury. Psychosocial consid-

erations of the patient and family and communication with the treatment team are imperative early in the course of care.

Nursing care of the patient during the emergent/resuscitative phase of burn injury is detailed in Chart 62-6.

 ## Acute/Intermediate Phase

The acute/intermediate phase of burn care follows the emergent/resuscitative phase and begins 48 to 72 hours after the burn injury. During this phase, attention is directed toward continued assessment and maintenance of respiratory and circulatory status, fluid and electrolyte balance, and GI and kidney function. Infection prevention, burn wound care (e.g., wound cleaning and débridement, topical antibacterial therapy, application of dressings, and wound grafting), pain management, modulation of the hypermetabolic response, and early positioning/mobility are priorities at this stage and are discussed in detail in the following sections.

Medical Management

Pulmonary complications are common in burn injury. Airway obstruction caused by upper airway edema can take as long as 48 hours to develop. Changes detected by x-ray and arterial blood gas analysis may occur as the effects of resuscitative fluid and the chemical reactions of smoke ingredients with lung tissues become apparent. Diagnosis is largely based on history and clinical presentation, monitoring of arterial blood gases with carboxyhemoglobin levels, and direct observation of the airway by fiberoptic bronchoscopy (Dries & Endorf, 2013). To lessen the effects of upper airway edema, elevation of the patient's head of the bed may be helpful. Stridor and dyspnea are ominous because they are late signs of impending airway obstruction. Early protective intubation to maintain airway patency should be considered as obstruction may occur very rapidly. However, intubation and mechanical ventilation are significant contributors to pulmonary infections. Ideally, the best practice is to remove the endotracheal tube as soon as possible so that a route for pathogens is not accessible to the lungs.

Late pulmonary complications secondary to inhalation injuries include mucosal sloughing of the airway and casts formed from cellular debris, which can lead to obstruction, increased secretions, inflammation, atelectasis, airway ulceration, pulmonary edema, and tissue hypoxia (Snell et al., 2013). Pneumonia, acute lung injury (ALI), and ARDS may also occur.

Ventilator-associated pneumonia (VAP) is one complication of any patient who is hospitalized and mechanically ventilated, and is particularly exacerbated in the patient with an inhalation injury. It affects as many as 10% to 20% of patients on mechanical ventilation longer than 48 hours. See Chapter 21, Chart 21-11, for discussion of "bundled" strategies to prevent VAP and Chapter 23 for discussion of respiratory failure and ARDS.

As capillaries regain integrity, 48 or more hours after the burn, fluid moves from the interstitial to the intravascular compartment and intrinsic diuresis begins. If cardiac or kidney function is inadequate, fluid overload may occur and symptoms of heart failure may result (see Chapter 29). Administration of fluids and electrolytes continues cautiously during this phase of burn care due to fluid shifts, evaporative fluid loss from large burn wounds, and the patient's physi-

Chart 62-6

PLAN OF NURSING CARE
Care of the Patient During the Emergent/Resuscitative Phase of Burn Injury

NURSING DIAGNOSIS: Impaired gas exchange related to carbon monoxide poisoning, smoke inhalation, and upper airway obstruction
GOAL: Maintenance of adequate tissue oxygenation

Nursing Interventions	Rationale	Expected Outcomes
1. Provide 100% humidified oxygen.	1. Humidification provides moisture to injured tissues; supplemental oxygen increases alveolar oxygenation.	• Absence of dyspnea • Arterial oxygen saturation >95% by pulse oximetry • Arterial blood gas levels within normal limits • Respiratory rate, pattern, and breath sounds normal
2. Assess breath sounds, and respiratory rate, rhythm, depth, and symmetry of chest excursion. Monitor patient for signs of hypoxia. Report abnormalities to primary provider	2. These factors provide baseline data of assessment and evidence of increasing respiratory compromise.	

3. Observe for the following:
  a. Erythema or blistering of lips or buccal mucosa
  b. Singed nasal hairs
  c. Burns of face, neck, or chest
  d. Increasing hoarseness
  e. Soot in sputum or tracheal tissue in respiratory secretions
	3. These signs indicate possible inhalation injury and risk of respiratory dysfunction.	

4. Monitor arterial blood gas values, pulse oximetry readings, and carboxyhemoglobin levels.	4. Increasing $PaCO_2$ and decreasing PaO_2 and O_2 saturation may indicate need for mechanical ventilation.	
5. Prepare to assist with intubation and escharotomies of chest.	5. Intubation allows airway protection and mechanical ventilation. Escharotomy enables adequate chest excursion in circumferential chest burns.	

NURSING DIAGNOSIS: Ineffective airway clearance related to edema and effects of smoke inhalation
GOAL: Maintain patent airway and adequate airway clearance

Nursing Interventions	Rationale	Expected Outcomes
1. Maintain patent airway through proper patient positioning, removal of secretions, and artificial airway if needed.	1. A patent airway is crucial to respiration.	• Patent airway • Respiratory secretions are minimal, colorless, and thin
2. Provide humidified oxygen as prescribed.	2. Humidification liquefies secretions and facilitates expectoration.	
3. Encourage patient to turn, cough, and deep breathe. Encourage patient to use incentive spirometry. Suction as needed.	3. These activities promote mobilization and removal of secretions.	

NURSING DIAGNOSIS: Deficient fluid volume related to increased capillary permeability and evaporative losses from the burn wound
GOAL: Restoration of optimal fluid and electrolyte balance and perfusion of vital organs

Nursing Interventions	Rationale	Expected Outcomes
1. Monitor vital signs, hemodynamics, and urine output, as well as strict intake and output and daily weight.	1. Hypovolemia is a major risk immediately after the burn injury. Overresuscitation might cause fluid overload.	• Urine output between 0.5 and 1.0 mL/kg/h (30–50 mL/h; 75–100 mL/h if electrical burn injury) • Mean arterial pressure ≥60 mm Hg • Voids clear yellow urine with specific gravity within normal limits • Serum electrolytes within normal limits
2. Maintain IV lines and regulate fluids at appropriate rates, as prescribed.	2. Adequate fluids are necessary for perfusion of vital organs and maintenance of fluid and electrolyte balance.	
3. Observe for symptoms of deficiency or excess of serum sodium, potassium, calcium, phosphorus, and bicarbonate.	3. Rapid shifts in fluid and electrolyte status are possible in the post-burn period.	
4. Elevate head of patient's bed, and elevate burned extremities.	4. Elevation promotes venous return.	
5. Notify physician immediately of decreased urine output and hemodynamic changes.	5. Rapid fluid shifts must be detected early to prevent complications.	

(continued on page 1858)

Chart 62-6

PLAN OF NURSING CARE (Continued)
Care of the Patient During the Emergent/Resuscitative Phase of Burn Injury

NURSING DIAGNOSIS: Hypothermia related to loss of skin microcirculation and open wounds
GOAL: Maintenance of adequate body temperature

Nursing Interventions	Rationale	Expected Outcomes
1. Assess core body temperature frequently.	1. Frequent temperature assessments help detect hypothermia.	• Body temperature remains >37°C (98.6°F)
2. Provide a warm environment by increasing room temperature or adjunct therapies as needed (overbed warmers, blankets, heat lamps, etc.)	2. Minimizes energy expenditure.	• Absence of chills or shivering
3. Work quickly when wounds must be exposed.	3. Limiting exposure minimizes evaporative heat loss from wound.	

NURSING DIAGNOSIS: Acute pain related to tissue and nerve injury
GOAL: Control of pain

Nursing Interventions	Rationale	Expected Outcomes
1. Use pain intensity scale to assess pain level. Differentiate restlessness due to pain from restlessness due to hypoxia.	1. Pain level provides baseline for evaluating effectiveness of pain relief measures. Hypoxia can cause similar signs and must be ruled out before analgesic medication is given.	• States pain level is decreased and is acceptable to patient's pain goal
2. Administer IV analgesics as prescribed and assess for effectiveness.	2. IV administration is necessary because of altered tissue perfusion from burn injury.	• Absence of nonverbal cues of pain
3. Provide emotional support and reassurance.	3. Fear and anxiety increase the perception of pain.	

NURSING DIAGNOSIS: Anxiety related to fear and the emotional impact of burn injury
GOAL: Minimization of patient's and family's anxiety

Nursing Interventions	Rationale	Expected Outcomes
1. Assess patient's and family's understanding of burn injury, coping skills, and family dynamics.	1. Previous successful coping strategies can be fostered for use in the present crisis. Assessment allows planning of individualized interventions.	• Patient and family verbalize understanding of emergent burn care
2. Explain all procedures to the patient and the family in clear, simple terms.	2. Increased understanding alleviates fear of the unknown. High levels of anxiety may interfere with understanding of complex explanations.	• Patient and family's anxiety levels will be minimized
3. Consider administering prescribed antianxiety medications if the patient remains extremely anxious despite nonpharmacologic interventions.	3. Anxiety levels during the emergent phase may exceed the patient's coping abilities.	

COLLABORATIVE PROBLEMS: Acute respiratory failure, distributive shock, acute kidney injury, compartment syndrome, paralytic ileus, Curling's ulcer
GOAL: Absence of complications

Nursing Interventions	Rationale	Expected Outcomes

Acute Respiratory Failure

Nursing Interventions	Rationale	Expected Outcomes
1. Assess for increasing dyspnea, stridor, changes in respiratory patterns.	1. Such signs reflect deteriorating respiratory status.	• Breathes spontaneously with adequate tidal volume
2. Monitor pulse oximetry, arterial blood gas values.	2. Abnormal findings may indicate respiratory failure.	• Arterial blood gas values within acceptable limits
3. Monitor chest x-ray results.	3. X-ray may disclose pulmonary injury.	• Chest x-ray findings normal
4. Assess for restlessness, confusion, difficulty attending to questions, or decreasing level of consciousness.	4. Such manifestations may indicate cerebral hypoxia.	• Absence of cerebral signs of hypoxia
5. Report deteriorating respiratory status immediately to primary provider.	5. Acute respiratory failure is life threatening, and immediate intervention is required.	
6. Prepare to assist with intubation or escharotomies as indicated.	6. Intubation allows mechanical ventilation. Escharotomies allow adequate chest excursion with respirations.	

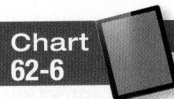

PLAN OF NURSING CARE (Continued)

Chart 62-6

Care of the Patient During the Emergent/Resuscitative Phase of Burn Injury

Nursing Interventions	Rationale	Expected Outcomes
Distributive Shock 1. Assess for decreasing urine output and alterations in vital signs and hemodynamics. 2. Assess for progressive edema as fluid shifts occur. 3. Adjust fluid resuscitation in collaboration with the primary provider in response to physiologic findings.	1. Such signs and symptoms may indicate distributive shock and inadequate intravascular volume. 2. As fluid shifts into the interstitial spaces in burn shock, edema occurs and may compromise tissue perfusion. 3. Optimal fluid resuscitation prevents distributive shock and improves patient outcomes.	• Urine output between 0.5 and 1.0 mL/kg/h (30–50 mL/h; 75–100 mL/h if electrical burn injury) • Blood pressure within patient's normal range • Hemodynamics remain within normal limits • No signs or symptoms of impaired perfusion
Acute Kidney Injury 1. Monitor urine output, blood urea nitrogen (BUN), and serum creatinine levels. 2. Report decreased urine output or increased BUN and creatinine values to primary provider. 3. Assess urine for hemoglobin or myoglobin. Administer increased fluids as prescribed.	1. These values reflect renal function. 2. These laboratory values indicate possible kidney failure. 3. Hemoglobin or myoglobin in the urine predisposes patient to increased risk of kidney failure. Fluids help to flush hemoglobin and myoglobin from renal tubules.	• Adequate urine output • BUN and serum creatinine values remain normal
Compartment Syndrome 1. Assess peripheral pulses frequently with Doppler ultrasound device if needed. 2. Assess warmth, capillary refill, sensation, and movement of extremity frequently. Compare affected with unaffected extremity. 3. Remove blood pressure cuff after each reading. 4. Elevate burned extremities. 5. Report loss of pulse or sensation or presence of pain to primary provider immediately. 6. Prepare to assist with escharotomies.	1. Pulse assessments are crucial to assess for adequate perfusion. 2. These assessments may signal worsening peripheral perfusion. 3. Cuff may act as a tourniquet as extremities swell. 4. Elevation reduces edema formation. 5. These signs and symptoms may indicate impaired tissue perfusion. 6. Escharotomies relieve the constriction caused by edema.	• Peripheral pulses detectable • Signs of adequate peripheral perfusion
Paralytic Ileus 1. Auscultate for bowel sounds, abdominal distention. 2. Maintain nasogastric tube on low intermittent suction until bowel sounds resume.	1. Presence of bowel sounds indicates normal peristalsis. Abdominal distention reflects inadequate decompression. 2. This measure relieves gastric and abdominal distention.	• Normal bowel sounds • Absence of abdominal distention
Curling's Ulcer 1. Assess gastric aspirate and stools for blood. 2. Administer histamine-2 blockers and/or antacids as prescribed.	1. Blood indicates possible gastric or duodenal ulcer bleeding. 2. Such medications reduce gastric acidity and risk of ulceration.	• Gastric aspirate and stools do not contain blood

ologic responses to the burn injury. Blood components are given as needed to treat surgical blood loss and anemia.

Hyperthermia is common in patients after burn shock resolves. A resetting of the core body temperature in patients who are severely burned results in a body temperature a few degrees higher than normal for several weeks after the burn.

This can be compounded by body temperature increases from sepsis.

Central venous, peripheral arterial, or specialty catheters may be required for monitoring hemodynamics. It is not uncommon for patients with major burns to have multiple invasive line sites due to the amount and frequency of fluid and medication that need to be given. Whenever possible, burned areas of the body are avoided as insertion sites for invasive lines.

One of the most important medical interventions for patients with burns that has positively impacted mortality is early excision. Through surgical excision, the necrotic tissue is removed and underlying viable tissue is preserved. Early excision of dead tissue with wound closure and/or application of biologic or synthetic wound covering reduces the effects of inflammatory mediators that cause pathophysiologic abnormalities (Rousseau et al., 2014).

Infection Prevention

There are multifactorial reasons why patients with burns incur some of the highest risks for health care–associated infections (HAIs). These reasons may include loss of the barrier function of the skin for protection against invasive microorganisms; necrotic tissue in burn eschar combines with serum proteins to produce an environment conducive to bacterial growth; and the effects of thermal injury compromise both cell-mediated and systemic intrinsic immunity, thus promoting an environment conducive to pathogen proliferation (Abdullahi & Jeschke, 2014). Pathogens can be transmitted directly by health care staff through contact or droplets, or indirectly through the environment or equipment (Meyerson et al., 2015). It is, therefore, critical that the nurse prioritizes infection prevention in the plan of care.

Causative agents of burn infections may include bacteria, fungi, or viruses. Common sources of potential contamination in a burn unit that require hypervigilance include hydrotherapy equipment, direct or indirect contamination from health care workers' hands, environmental surfaces, and translocation of microorganisms from other body systems—most notably, the GI tract. Whether the burn wound is healing through spontaneous re-epithelialization or is being prepared for skin grafting, it must be protected from pathogens. Infection impedes burn wound healing by promoting excessive inflammation and damaging tissue. Clinical signs of infection include progressive erythema, warmth, tenderness, and malodorous exudate.

A multiple-strategy approach is crucial in prevention and control of burn wound infections. Such strategies include (Mayhall, 2012):

- The use of barrier techniques (e.g., gowns, gloves, eye protection, and masks if needed)
- Environmental cleaning with periodic cultures of patient care equipment (with special attention to hydrotherapy equipment)
- Application of appropriate topical antimicrobial agents
- Appropriate use of systemic antibiotic and antifungal agents (careful use and close monitoring of culture sensitivities are needed due to increasing challenges of antibiotic resistance in health care environments)
- Early excision and closure of the burn wound
- Control of hyperglycemia (with insulin as indicated, even in a patient without a prior diagnosis of diabetes)
- Management of the hypermetabolic response (see Chapter 14)

There are varying practices in the burn community regarding environmental and patient cultures for surveillance. In some burn centers, patients may be cultured on admission to screen for the presence of methicillin-resistant

Staphylococcus aureus and vancomycin-resistant enterococci. Wounds are generally cultured on admission, with each surgical case, and for clinical suspicion of infection. Antimicrobial therapy is tailored to culture results.

Wound Cleaning

Proper management of burn wounds is required to prevent wound deterioration. The goal of wound care is to remove nonviable tissue and wound exudate, and eliminate previously applied topical agents. Gentle cleaning with mild soap, water, and a washcloth can prevent infection by decreasing bacteria and debris on the wound surface. Hair in and around the burn area, except the eyebrows, should be clipped short or shaved.

Various processes are used to clean the burn wound. Patients who are hemodynamically unstable may have their wounds washed at the bedside, whereas patients who are ambulatory may shower. The wounds of patients who are nonambulatory can be cleaned using shower carts—mobile stretchers made with removable sides, drainage holes, and positioning capabilities. Retractable shower hoses suspended from walls and ceilings provide the nurse with easy access to a clean water source for washing the wounds. Whatever method is used, the goal is to protect the wound from acute proliferation of pathogenic organisms on the surface and invasion of deeper tissues until either spontaneous healing or skin grafting can be achieved. Strategies for the prevention of cross-contamination include the use of plastic liners, water filters, and thorough decontamination of equipment.

Patient comfort and ability to participate in the prescribed treatment are important considerations. During bathing, patient participation is encouraged to promote exercise of the extremities. At the time of wound cleaning, all skin is inspected for any signs of redness, breakdown, or local infection. This also provides the nurse an opportunity for patient education. Encouraging family presence during wound care can improve patient and family satisfaction, nursing communication, and optimize patient outcomes (see Chart 62-7) (Bishop, Walker, & Spivak, 2013).

During treatment, the patient is continuously assessed for signs of hypothermia. The temperature of the water is maintained at 37.8°C (100°F), and the temperature of the room should be maintained between 26.6° and 29.4°C (80° and 85°F) to prevent hypothermia. Other assessment considerations include patient fatigue, changes in hemodynamic status, and pain unrelieved by analgesic medications or relaxation techniques.

Topical Antibacterial Therapy

Variations in topical wound care for nonsurgical burn wounds exist among burn centers across the country, and choices are made based on the individualized needs of each patient. The goal of topical therapy is to provide a dressing with the following characteristics:

- Is effective against gram-positive and gram-negative organisms and fungi
- Penetrates the eschar but is not systemically toxic
- Is cost-effective, available, and acceptable to the patient
- Is easy to apply and remove, and decreases the frequency of dressing changes, decreases pain, and minimizes nursing time

NURSING RESEARCH PROFILE

Chart 62-7

Family Presence During Dressing Changes in the Burn Unit

Bishop, S. M., Walker, M. D., & Spivak, I. M. (2013). Family presence in the adult burn intensive care unit during dressing changes. *Critical Care Nurse, 33*(1), 14–23.

Purpose

Severe burn injuries are often devastating events that can disrupt family dynamics. Staff working in burn units have traditionally forbidden visitation during dressing changes, even though the American Association of Critical Care Nurses and the American College of Critical Care Medicine both recommend family presence during procedures. However, there is no evidence that family presence during dressing changes in burn units has any effect on patient satisfaction with care. This quality improvement project sought to find out if family presence during dressing changes would have any association with patient satisfaction and rates of infections.

Design

The setting for this quality improvement project was a five-bed burn intensive care unit located within a 404-bed urban level 1 trauma center, which admits, on average, 130 patients with burns each year. This academic medical center utilizes a patient- and family-centered care (PFCC) model. The central tenet of the PFCC model is that the patient is a reflection of the family unit and that the family is central to the patient's well-being. Core concepts inherent in this model include dignity and respect, collaboration, participation, and information sharing. Although there was no research-based evidence that demonstrated that family presence during dressing changes would improve patient satisfaction, tenets of the PFCC model supported that this would be the case. Patients and their family members were invited to observe

dressing changes, and, if they consented, were instructed in appropriate infection control protocols. Patient satisfaction scores on key Press Ganey Likert scale metrics were used pre- and postimplementation to find if patient satisfaction improved postintervention. Likewise, rates of hospital care–associated infections (HAIs) pre- and postintervention were compared.

Findings

Thirty seven Press Ganey patient satisfaction survey results obtained postintervention (March 2009 through December 2011) were compared to thirty five survey results obtained preintervention (January 2007 through February 2009). Each of the six metrics that were selected as indicative of satisfaction were higher postintervention, including "staff attitudes toward visitors," "nurses kept you informed," "overall rating of nursing care," "included in decisions regarding treatment," "instructions for care at home," and "extent felt ready for discharge." The rate of HAIs dropped from 13.5 per 1000 patient days in 2008 to 6.25 per 1000 patient days in 2011.

Nursing Implications

The results from this quality improvement project support the continued study of family presence during dressing changes in burn units. Family presence during dressing changes could potentially diminish anxiety in the patient, which could mitigate the pain experienced by the patient. Furthermore, most patients with burns rely upon family members to aid with dressing changes once they are discharged to the home setting. Involving family members in the dressing change process earlier may facilitate their comfort in taking on this vitally important caretaking responsibility.

No single topical medication is universally effective, and the use of different agents at different times in the post-burn period may be necessary.

▶ *Quality and Safety Nursing Alert*

Prudent use and alternation of antimicrobial agents can result in reduction of resistant strains of bacteria, greater effectiveness of the agents, and a decreased risk of sepsis. Table 62-4 describes selected topical antimicrobial agents.

Wound Dressing

After the prescribed topical agents are applied, the wound is covered with several layers of dry dressings with lighter dressing over joints to allow for mobility. Dressings may also need to be modified to accommodate splints or other positioning devices. Circumferential dressings should always be applied distally to proximally in order to promote return of excess fluid to the central circulation. If the hand or foot is burned, the fingers and toes should be wrapped individually to promote mobility and function while healing.

Burns to the face may be left open to air once they have been cleaned and the topical agent has been applied. Careful attention is required to ensure that the topical agent does not come in contact with the eyes or mouth. A light dressing can be applied to the face to absorb excess exudates if needed.

Occlusive dressings, gauze, and a topical antimicrobial agent may be used over areas with new skin grafts to protect

the new graft and promote an optimal condition for its adherence to the recipient site. Ideally, these surgical dressings remain in place for 3 to 5 days, at which time they are removed for examination of the graft. When occlusive dressings are applied, precautions are taken to prevent two body surfaces from touching, such as fingers or toes, ear and scalp, the areas under the breasts, any point of flexion, or between the genital folds. Functional body alignment positions are maintained by using splints or by regular repositioning of the patient.

▶ *Quality and Safety Nursing Alert*

Dressings can impede circulation if they are wrapped too tightly. The peripheral pulses must be checked frequently and burned extremities elevated. If the patient's pulse is diminished, this is a critical situation and must be addressed immediately.

Dressings that adhere to the wound bed may be removed more comfortably and with less damage to healing tissue by moistening the dressing with water. The patient may participate in removing the dressings, providing some degree of control over this painful procedure. The wounds are then cleaned and débrided to remove any remaining topical agent, exudate, and nonviable tissue. Sterile scissors and forceps may be used to trim loose eschar and encourage separation of devitalized tissue. During this procedure, the wound and surrounding skin are carefully inspected. Documentation should include color, odor,

TABLE 62-4 Overview of Select Topical Antimicrobial Agents Used for Burn Wounds

Agent	Indication/Comment	Application	Nursing Implications
General			
Antimicrobial ointment	Antibacterial coverage and promotion of a moist wound environment	Apply 1/16-inch layer of ointment with a clean glove daily.	Ensure removal of old ointment at the time of wound cleaning prior to applying a new layer. Monitor closely for signs and symptoms of local infection.
Specific Agents			
Silver sulfadiazine 1% (Silvadene) water-soluble cream	Bactericidal agent for many gram-positive and gram-negative organisms, as well as yeast and *Candida albicans* Minimal penetration of eschar	Apply 1/16-inch layer of cream with a clean glove 1–3 times daily.	Anticipate formation of pseudo-eschar (proteinaceous gel), which can be removed.
Mafenide acetate 5%–10% (Sulfamylon) hydrophilic-based solution or cream	Antimicrobial agent for gram-positive and gram-negative organisms Diffuses through eschar and avascular tissue (e.g., cartilage)	Apply twice a day with a clean glove as prescribed.	Is a strong carbonic anhydrase inhibitor and may cause metabolic acidosis. Application may cause considerable pain initially.
Silver nitrate 0.5% aqueous solution	Effective against most strains of *Staphylococcus* and *Pseudomonas* and many gram-negative organisms. Does not penetrate eschar	Apply solution to gauze dressing and place over wound. Keep the dressing wet but covered with dry gauze and dry blankets to decrease vaporization.	Monitor serum sodium (Na$^+$) and potassium (K$^+$) levels, and replace as prescribed. Silver nitrate solution is hypotonic and acts as a wick for sodium and potassium. Protect bed linens and clothing from contact with silver nitrate, which stains everything it touches.
Silver-impregnated dressings (sheets or mesh)	Broad antimicrobial effects (product specific) Delivers a uniform, antimicrobial concentration of silver ions to the burn wound.	Apply directly to wound. Cover with absorbent secondary dressing if needed.	May produce a pseudo-eschar from silver after application. Can be left in place for several days (product specific).

Adapted from Micromedex 2.0. (2015). *Formulary Advisor*, University of Texas–Medical Branch Galveston. Retrieved on 7/10/2015 (pass-protected) at: www.micromedicsolutions.com/micromedex2/librarian

size, exudate, signs of re-epithelialization, any changes from the previous dressing change, and other key characteristics.

Wound Débridement

The goals of **débridement** (the removal of *devitalized* tissue) are:

- Removal of devitalized tissue or burn eschar in preparation for grafting and wound healing
- Removal of tissue contaminated by bacteria and foreign bodies, thereby protecting the patient from invasion of bacteria

There are four types of débridement—natural, mechanical, chemical, and surgical.

Natural Débridement

With natural débridement, the devitalized tissue separates from the underlying viable tissue spontaneously. Bacteria present at the interface of the burned tissue and the viable tissue gradually liquefy the fibrils of **collagen** that hold the eschar in place. Collagen is a protein present in skin, tendon, bone, cartilage, and connective tissue. Proteolytic and other natural enzymes cause this phenomenon. The process may take weeks to months to occur.

Mechanical Débridement

Mechanical débridement involves the use of surgical tools to separate and remove the eschar. This technique can be performed by physicians, specially trained nurses, or physical therapists and is usually done with daily dressing changes. If bleeding occurs, hemostatic agents or pressure can be applied to achieve hemostasis. Dressing changes and wound cleaning aid the removal of wound debris. Wet-to-dry dressings are not advocated in burn care because of the possibility of removing viable cells along with necrotic tissue.

Chemical Débridement

Topical enzymatic agents are available to promote débridement of burn wounds. Because such agents usually do not have antimicrobial properties, they may be used together with topical antibacterial therapy to protect the patient from bacterial invasion. Heavy metals such as silver can deactivate débriding agents; therefore, caution is necessary to ensure that the topical antimicrobial agent does not interfere with the chemical débridement. Alternating topical medications with dressing changes may also be considered.

Surgical Débridement

Early surgical excision to remove devitalized tissue along with early burn wound closure is now recognized as one of the most important factors contributing to survival in a patient with a major burn injury. Surgical débridement is carried out before the natural separation of eschar occurs. This may be performed as soon as possible after the burn, once the patient is hemodynamically stable and edema has decreased. Ideally, the wound is then covered immediately with a skin graft (if necessary) and a dressing. If the wound bed is not ready for a skin graft at the time of excision, a temporary biologic or synthetic dressing may be used until a skin graft can be applied during a subsequent surgery.

The use of surgical excision carries with it risks and complications, especially with large burns. The procedure creates a high risk of extensive blood loss and lengthy operating and anesthesia times. Furthermore, blood losses sustained during surgical procedures, wound care, and ongoing hemolysis exacerbate anemia. Blood transfusions may be required periodically to maintain adequate hemoglobin levels for oxygen delivery to the myocardium. See Chapter 32 for discussion of blood component therapy.

When conducted in a timely and efficient manner, surgical excision results in shorter lengths of hospital stay and possibly a decreased risk of complications from invasive burn wound sepsis. Once débrided, granulation tissue fills the space created by the wound, creates a barrier to bacteria, and serves as a bed for epithelial cell growth. A wound covering is then applied to keep the wound bed moist and promote the granulation process.

Wound Grafting

The patient with deep partial- or full-thickness burns may be a candidate for skin grafting to decrease the risk of infection; prevent further loss of protein, fluid, and electrolytes through the wound; and minimize evaporative heat loss. Special attention is warranted when grafting the face (for cosmetic, functional, and psychological reasons); functional areas, such as the hands and feet; and areas that involve joints. Grafting permits earlier functional ability and reduces scar **contractures** (shrinkage of burn scar through collagen maturation). When burns are very extensive, the order in which areas are grafted is chosen based on the ability to achieve wound closure as soon as possible; therefore, the chest and abdomen or back may be grafted first to reduce the total body burn surface area.

Autografts

Autografting remains the preferred autologous method for definitive burn wound closure after excision. **Autografts** are the ideal means of covering burn wounds because the grafts are the patient's own skin and therefore are not rejected by the patient's immune system. They can be split-thickness, full-thickness, or epithelial grafts. Because the **donor site** (the area from which skin is taken to provide the autograft) for a full-thickness graft includes both the epidermis and dermis, its use must be cautiously considered because the donor site cannot heal spontaneously.

Split-thickness autografts are most commonly used and can be applied in sheets (see Fig. 62-7), or they can be expanded by meshing so that they cover more than a given donor site area (see Fig. 62-8). Skin meshers enable the surgeon to cut tiny slits into a sheet of donor skin, making it possible to expand to cover larger areas with smaller amounts of donor skin. These expanded grafts adhere to the recipient site more easily than sheet grafts and prevent the accumulation of blood, serum, air, or purulent material under the graft that would prevent revascularization and adherence. However, any kind of graft other than a sheet graft contributes to scar formation as it heals. The use of expanded grafts may be

Figure 62-7 • Split-thickness sheet graft. Used with permission from University of Texas Medical Branch, Galveston, TX.

necessary in large wounds but should be viewed as a compromise in terms of cosmesis.

If blood, serum, air, fat, or necrotic tissue is present between the recipient site and the graft, there may be partial or total loss of the graft. Infection, mishandling of the graft, sheer injury with mobilization or trauma during dressing changes account for most other instances of graft loss. The use of split-thickness grafts allows the remaining donor site to retain sweat glands and hair follicles, minimizing healing time.

Cultured epithelial autograft (CEA) has emerged as an important procedure in the management of massive burns. In burns that cover more than 90% TBSA, CEA may be the only option because the availability of nonburned skin as donor sites will not be sufficient for grafting. CEA involves obtaining full-thickness biopsies of the patient's unburned skin that are cultured to promote growth of keratinocytes. The final product is available approximately 3 weeks later for grafting (see Fig. 62-9). Meticulous attention is required to CEA applied to body surfaces because it is very fragile and prone to graft loss. Optimal application of CEA requires

Figure 62-8 • Split-thickness meshed graft. Used with permission from University of Texas Medical Branch, Galveston, TX.

Figure 62-9 • Application of cultured epithelial autologous grafts. Used with permission from University of Texas Medical Branch, Galveston, TX.

aggressive, early application of allograft to prepare and protect the wound bed (Kym, Yim, Yoon, et al., 2015). CEA can be cost prohibitive and requires extended LOS.

Care of the Graft Site

Protection is key in caring for skin grafts postoperatively. Occlusive dressings are commonly used initially after grafting to immobilize the graft and support a humid environment. Occupational therapists may construct splints to immobilize newly grafted areas. Homograft, xenograft, or synthetic dressings (discussed later) may also be used to protect fragile grafts.

The first dressing change is usually performed 2 to 5 days after surgery, or earlier in the case of clinical signs of infection or bleeding. Infection, bleeding beneath the graft, and shearing forces are the most common reasons for graft loss in the early postoperative period. The patient is positioned and turned carefully to avoid disturbing the graft or putting pressure on the graft site. If an extremity has been grafted, it is elevated to minimize edema. The patient may begin exercising the grafted area 5 to 7 days after surgery. This may vary with individual burn center's protocols.

Care of the Donor Site

The donor site is a clean wound created in a surgical environment. After the donor skin is excised, a hemostatic agent such as thrombin or epinephrine may be applied directly to the site to promote hemostasis. A myriad of dressings are available to cover donor sites. Donor sites must remain clean, dry, and free from pressure. Because a donor site is usually a partial-thickness wound, it is very painful and an additional potential site of infection. With proper care, the donor site should heal spontaneously within 7 to 14 days in a previously healthy, nonsmoking adult.

Homografts and Xenografts

Homografts (or allografts) and **xenografts** (or heterografts) are also referred to as biologic dressings and are intended as temporary wound coverage. Homografts are skin obtained from recently deceased or living humans other than the patient. Xenografts consist of skin taken from animals (usually pigs). Therefore, the body's immune response will eventually reject them as a foreign substance.

Biologic dressings protect the wound from physical trauma and loss of fluid, protein and heat; provide pain relief; and hasten re-epithelialization and, therefore, healing (Hermans,

2014). In extensive burns, they provide temporary wound coverage and protection of granulation tissue until autografting is possible. They may also be used as a test graft in preparation for autografting to determine if the bed will accept the graft. Once the biologic dressing appears to be "taking," or adhering to the granulating surface with minimal underlying exudation, the patient is ready for an autologous skin graft. As a temporary dressing, they also decrease the wound's evaporative water and protein loss, provide an effective barrier for entry of bacteria, and decrease pain by protecting nerve endings. Biologic dressings can be left open or covered. They stay in place for varying lengths of time but are removed in instances of infection or rejection. Another advantage of biologic dressings is that fewer dressing changes may be required.

Homografts tend to be the most expensive biologic dressings. They are available from skin banks in fresh and cryopreserved (frozen) forms. Homografts are thought to provide the best infection control of all biologic or biosynthetic dressings available. Revascularization occurs within 48 hours, and the graft may be left in place for several weeks.

Pigskin, an effective xenograft, is available from commercial suppliers. It is available fresh, frozen, or lyophilized (freeze-dried) for longer shelf life. Pigskin is used for temporary covering of clean wounds such as superficial partial-thickness wounds and donor sites. Although pigskin does not vascularize, it adheres to clean superficial wounds, providing pain control and reducing evaporative fluid loss while the underlying wound re-epithelializes (Lee, Dibildox, Jimenez, et al., 2012).

When grafting is not possible, skin substitutes have been created that surgically replace the epidermis and the dermis either temporarily or permanently. Each provides advantages and disadvantages that are important to consider in product selection.

Biosynthetic and Synthetic Dressings

Problems with availability, sterility, and cost have prompted the search for biosynthetic and synthetic dressings, which may eventually replace biologic dressings as temporary wound coverings. One widely used synthetic dressing is Biobrane® a dual-layer dressing of nylon and silicone (Jeschke, Finnerty, Shahrokhi, et al., 2013). The material is porous, semi-transparent, and sterile. It has an indefinite shelf life and is less costly than homograft or xenograft. Like biologic dressings, Biobrane® protects the wound from fluid loss and bacterial invasion and decreases pain at the site. It can remain in place until spontaneous re-epithelialization and wound healing occur, alleviating pain associated with frequent dressing changes. It can also be laid on top of a wide-meshed autograft to protect the wound until the autograft epithelium grows to close the interstices. As the Biobrane® gradually separates, it is trimmed away, leaving a healed wound (see Fig. 62-10).

Pain Management

A burn injury is considered one of the most painful types of trauma that a patient can experience. The nature of the injury may expose nerve endings; and the patient may require multiple débridements, surgeries, and treatments. Moving, changing position, and receiving occupational and physical therapy cause additional discomfort. Adequate pain management must address background, procedural, and breakthrough pain.

Figure 62-10 • Biobrane® applied to hand and forearm. Used with permission from University of Texas Medical Branch, Galveston, TX.

Background pain is a continuous level of discomfort even when the patient is inactive or not undergoing any procedures. The goal of treatment is to provide a long-acting analgesic agent that will provide even coverage for this long-term discomfort. It is helpful to use escalating doses when initiating the medication to reach the level of pain control that is acceptable to the patient and facilitates participation in their recovery. The use of patient-controlled analgesia gives control to the patient and achieves this goal. Breakthrough pain is described as acute, intense, and episodic. It is generally related to an activity or movement of the affected area. Short-acting agents are used for breakthrough pain to achieve pain control if needed. Procedural pain is discomfort that occurs with procedures such as daily wound treatments, invasive line insertions, and physical and occupational therapy. The goal is to plan proper analgesia that will place the patient in a state of comfort throughout the procedure.

Most severe burns are a combination of partial- and full-thickness burns that influence the amount of pain the patient experiences. Superficial and partial-thickness burns are very painful because the nerve endings are not covered, resulting in excruciating pain with exposure to temperature, pressure, air currents, and movement. In a full-thickness burn, the nerve endings are destroyed, and upon admission there is numbness and decreased sensation to that area. Thus, the patient often underestimates severe injuries. Memories of the pain patients experience may persist for a long time. Educating patients and their families about burn pain and its relationship to the depth of injury as well as the pain management plan is an important priority for the nurse.

Pharmacologic treatment for the management of burn pain includes the use of opioids, nonsteroidal anti-inflammatory drugs, anxiolytics, and anesthetic agents. These and other pain management strategies are discussed in Chapter 12. Treatment of anxiety with benzodiazepines may be used along with opioids. The use of anesthetics in a nonoperative setting (i.e., moderate sedation) requires administration and monitoring by qualified personnel. Recent advances include the use of agents with rapid onset and short duration, which have been very effective in pain control during a planned

procedure. In the provision of holistic patient care, the use of nonpharmacologic pain and anxiety interventions must not be overlooked. Nonpharmacologic therapies include relaxation techniques, distraction, guided imagery, hypnosis, therapeutic touch, humor, music therapy, and more recently virtual reality techniques.

Modulation of Hypermetabolism

Burn injuries produce profound metabolic abnormalities fueled by the exaggerated stress response to the injury. The body's response has been classified as hyperdynamic, hypermetabolic, and hypercatabolic. Hypermetabolism can affect morbidity and mortality by increasing the risk of infection and slowing the healing rate. Early nutritional support is essential to recovery for the patient with burns in order to attenuate the hypercatabolism and hypermetabolism that occurs (Abdullahi & Jeschke, 2014). Improvements in cellular defense, mucosal barrier function of the GI tract, and decreased inflammation have been seen with immune-modulating nutritional support (Sen et al., 2015).

Nutrition should be provided upon arrival to the burn center and may require placement of a feeding tube to deliver adequate calories. Patients who are critically ill may even have their feedings continued intraoperatively if the airway is protected. Several formulas exist for estimating the daily metabolic expenditure and caloric requirements of patients with burn injuries. Carbohydrates are the most important energy source and should account for 55% to 60% of nutrition delivery to decrease protein catabolism (Abdullahi & Jeschke, 2014). Fat, although a required nutrient, should be provided in more limited quantities. When the oral route is used, high-protein, high-calorie meals and supplements are given. Dietary consultations are useful in helping patients meet their nutritional needs. Daily calorie counts aid in assessing the adequacy of nutritional intake.

Early excision and grafting of the burn wound is one of the most important factors in ameliorating hypermetabolism by removing eschar, thereby lessening the effects of inflammatory mediators. Appropriate manipulation of environmental temperatures may decrease energy expenditure by the patient. Insulin therapy in patients with burns is needed to treat the hyperglycemia that occurs from accelerated gluconeogenesis and is beneficial in muscle protein synthesis. Oxandrolone (Oxandrin), an anabolic steroid, is commonly given to patients with burns because it improves protein synthesis and metabolism. Administration of propranolol (Inderal) (a beta-blocker) decreases heart rate and blocks harmful catecholamine effects. Lastly, exercise is described as an essential adjunct in the plan of care for patients with burns, because it attenuates the hypermetabolic response and increases lean muscle mass (Abdullahi & Jeschke, 2014).

Nursing Management

Nursing management of the patient in the acute/intermediate phase is focused on the following priorities: restoring fluid balance, preventing infection, modulating hypermetabolism, promoting skin integrity, relieving pain and discomfort, promoting mobility, strengthening coping strategies, supporting patient and family processes, and monitoring and managing complications.

Restoring Normal Fluid Balance

To reduce the risk of fluid overload and consequent heart failure and pulmonary edema, daily weights and careful calculation of intake and output measurement are utilized to guide therapy. Changes in physical assessment and hemodynamic indicators are also useful in evaluating the patient's response to treatment.

Preventing Infection

The patient with burns is at risk for infection from multiple sources, which may include open wounds, lung injury, GI ischemia, and indwelling catheters. Therapeutic interventions are complex due to the patient's altered physiology. Signs of infection including increased temperature, tachycardia, tachypnea, and leukocytosis may be present in the patient with burns without underlying infection, making infections more difficult to recognize.

A major part of the nurse's role during the acute phase of burn care is detection and prevention of infection. The nurse is responsible for providing a clean environment, including the promotion of protective isolation interventions. The nurse protects the patient from sources of contamination, including other patients, staff members, visitors, and equipment. Patients can inadvertently promote migration of microorganisms from one burned area to another by touching their wounds or dressings. Bed linens can also spread infection through either colonization with wound microorganisms or fecal contamination. Regular bathing of unburned areas and changing of linens can help prevent infection. Fresh flowers, plants, and fresh fruit baskets are not permitted in the patient's room because of the risk of microorganism growth. Invasive lines and tubing must be routinely changed according to CDC recommendations, and prompt removal of all indwelling catheters when no longer indicated can prevent HAIs.

Modulating Hypermetabolism

The nurse collaborates with the dietitian or nutrition support team to develop a plan that meets the needs of the patient. Family members may be encouraged to bring nutritious and favorite foods to the hospital. High-calorie nutritional supplements may be necessary. Nutritional intake must be accurately documented. Vitamin and mineral supplements may be prescribed.

If caloric goals cannot be met by oral feeding, a feeding tube is inserted and used for continuous or bolus feedings of specific formulas. The volume of residual gastric secretions should be checked to ensure absorption. The patient should be weighed each day and the results tracked to properly assess appropriate weight parameters and to attenuate catabolism of lean muscle mass.

Promoting Skin Integrity

Wound care is usually the single most time-consuming element of burn care after the emergent phase. The primary provider prescribes the desired topical antibacterial agents and specific biologic, biosynthetic, or synthetic wound coverings and plans for surgical excision and grafting. The nurse needs to make astute assessments of wound status, use creative approaches to wound dressings, and support the patient during the emotionally distressing and significantly painful experience of wound care.

Assessment of the burn wound requires an experienced eye, hand, and sense of smell. Important wound assessment features include size, color, odor, presence of eschar and exudate, epithelial buds (small pearl-like clusters of cells on the wound surface), bleeding, granulation tissue, the status of graft take, healing of the donor site, and the condition of the surrounding skin. Any significant changes in the wound are reported to the primary provider because they may indicate burn wound infection and require immediate intervention.

The nurse also assists the patient and family by providing instruction, support, and encouragement to take an active part in dressing changes and wound care when appropriate. Discharge planning needs for wound care must be anticipated early in the course of burn management, and the strengths of the patient and family are assessed and used in preparing for the patient's eventual discharge and home care needs. Family presence during dressing changes promotes feelings of readiness for discharge (see Chart 62-7) (Bishop et al., 2013).

Relieving Pain and Discomfort

Pain management continues to be a priority during the acute phase of burn recovery. Frequent assessment of pain is required, and analgesic and anxiolytic medications are given as prescribed. To increase its effectiveness, analgesic medication is provided before the pain becomes severe. Nonpharmacologic interventions can be used to alter the patient's perceptions of and responses to pain. Frequent reassessment of responses to interventions, whether pharmacologic or nonpharmacologic, is essential.

Post-burn pruritus (itching) affects almost all patients with burns and is one of the most distressing symptoms in the post-burn period. Oral antipruritic agents, environmental conditions, frequent lubrication of the skin with water or silica-based lotion, and diversion activities all help to promote comfort in this phase. The instructions "pat, don't scratch" must be reinforced with patients in order to prevent further discomfort and infectious complications. Although gabapentin (Neurontin) had been prescribed to treat both pain and pruritus in patients' post burns, results from a recent double-blinded, randomized controlled trial does not support its effectiveness (Wibbenmeyer, Eid, Liao, et al., 2014).

Lack of sleep and rest interfere with healing, comfort, and restoration of energy. If necessary, sleep aids are prescribed on a regular basis in addition to analgesic and anxiolytic agents.

Promoting Physical Mobility

An early priority is to prevent complications of immobility. Deep breathing, turning, and proper positioning are essential nursing practices that prevent atelectasis and pneumonia, control edema, and prevent pressure ulcers and contractures. Specialty beds may be useful, and early mobility is strongly encouraged. If the lower extremities are burned, elastic pressure bandages should be applied before the patient is placed in an upright position to promote venous return and minimize edema formation. A review of over 36,000 patients with burns showed a DVT rate of 0.8%. Risk factors that were identified included a TBSA greater than 20%, previous history of DVT, African American race, and use of blood transfusions and mechanical ventilation (Satahoo, Parikh, Naranjo, et al., 2015).

The burn wound is in a dynamic state for at least 1 year after wound closure. During this time, aggressive efforts must be made to prevent contracture and hypertrophic scarring. Both passive and active range-of-motion exercises are initiated from the day of admission and are continued after grafting within prescribed limitations. Splints or functional devices may be applied to the extremities for contracture control. The nurse monitors the splinted areas for signs of vascular insufficiency, nerve compression, and skin breakdown. Occupational and physical therapists are consulted to develop a patient-specific plan of care throughout hospitalization and recovery.

Strengthening Coping Strategies

Much of the patient's energy goes into maintaining vital physical functions and wound healing in the early post-burn weeks, leaving little emotional energy for coping. In the acute phase of burn care, the patient is facing the reality of the burn injury. Grief, depression, anger, regression, and manipulative behavior are common responses of patients who have burn injuries. Withdrawal from participation in required treatments and regression must be viewed with an understanding that such behavior may help the patient cope with an enormously stressful event.

The patient may experience feelings of anger. At times, the anger may be directed inward because of a sense of guilt, perhaps for causing the fire or even for surviving when others perished. The anger may also be directed outward toward those who escaped unharmed or those who are now providing care. One way to help the patient handle these emotions is to enlist someone to whom the patient can express feelings without fear of retaliation. A nurse, social worker, psychiatric liaison nurse, peer supporter, spiritual advisor, or counselor who is not involved in direct care activities may fill this role successfully.

Patients with burn injuries are very dependent on health care team members during the long period of treatment and recovery. However, even when physically unable to contribute much to self-care, they should be included in decisions regarding care and encouraged to assert their individuality in terms of preferences and recognition of their unique identities. As the patient improves in mobility and strength, the nurse works with the patient to set realistic expectations for self-care and planning for the future. Many patients respond positively to the use of contractual agreements and other strategies that recognize their independence, set expectations for behavior, and encourage positive communication.

Supporting Patient and Family Processes

The burn injury has tremendous psychological, economic, and life-altering impact on the patient and family. The nurse is instrumental in providing support to the patient and family as they adapt to the burn injury. Referrals for social services or psychological counseling should be made as appropriate. This support continues into the rehabilitation phase. Some burn centers offer a structured peer support program in which a patient who has survived a burn injury visits the patient while hospitalized to provide psychosocial support. Many patients appreciate the opportunity to be able to share their experience with another person who has had a burn injury.

Patients who experience major burns are commonly sent to burn centers far from home. Because burn injuries are sudden and unexpected, family roles are disrupted. If the primary caregiver or wage earner in the family is injured, roles may change, which adds more stress to the family. Therefore, both the patient and the family need thorough information regarding the patient's burn care and expected course of treatment. Barriers to learning and preferred learning styles are assessed and considered. This information is used to tailor education activities. Patient and family education is a priority and is best provided with a multimedia approach.

Monitoring and Managing Potential Complications

Acute Respiratory Failure and Acute Respiratory Distress Syndrome

The patient's respiratory status is monitored closely for increased difficulty in breathing, change in respiratory pattern, or onset of adventitious (abnormal) breath sounds. Typically, at this stage, signs and symptoms of injury to the respiratory tract become apparent. As described previously, signs of hypoxia, diminished breath sounds, wheezing, tachypnea, stridor, and sputum tinged with soot (or in some cases containing sloughed tracheal tissue) are among the many possible findings. Medical management of the patient with acute respiratory failure requires intubation and mechanical ventilation (if not already in use). If ARDS has developed, higher oxygen levels, positive end-expiratory pressure, and pressure support are used with mechanical ventilation to promote gas exchange across the alveolar–capillary membrane (see Chapters 21 and 23).

Heart Failure and Pulmonary Edema

If the cardiac and renal systems cannot compensate for the excess vascular volume as fluid shifts back to the intravascular space, heart failure and pulmonary edema may result. The patient is assessed for signs of heart failure, including decreased cardiac output, oliguria, jugular vein distention, persistent edema, and the onset of an S_3 or S_4 heart sound. If invasive hemodynamic monitoring is used, increasing central venous, pulmonary artery, and pulmonary artery wedge pressures indicate increased fluid volume.

Crackles in the lungs and increased difficulty with breathing may indicate pulmonary edema, which should be reported promptly to the primary provider. In the meantime, the patient is positioned comfortably, with the head of the bed raised (if not contraindicated by other treatments or injuries) to promote lung expansion and gas exchange. Management of this complication includes providing supplemental oxygen, administering IV diuretic agents, carefully assessing the patient's response, and providing vasoactive medications, if indicated (see Chapter 29).

Sepsis

Sepsis is a leading cause of morbidity and mortality in patients with burn injuries. The signs of early sepsis are subtle and require a high index of suspicion and very close monitoring of changes in the patient's status. One of the challenges in the recognition of sepsis is the lack of definition of sepsis in the population of patients with burns. Because patients with burns are hypermetabolic, this results in tachycardia, tachypnea, and elevated body temperature. These physiologic norms in patients with burns make the diagnosis of sepsis more challenging. A recent retrospective study of burn admissions over a 5-year period found that temperature less than 36°C (96.8°F), heart rate greater than130 bpm, base deficit less than −6 mEq/L, a mean arterial pressure less than 60 mm Hg, serum glucose greater than 150 mg/dL, and utilization of vasopressors were predictive of sepsis in patients with burns (Mann-Salinas, Baun, Meininger, et al., 2013). See Chapter 14 for treatment recommendations for sepsis.

Rehabilitation Phase

Rehabilitation begins immediately after the burn has occurred and often extends for years after the initial injury. For nurses who care for patients with burns, this can be one of the more physically demanding and challenging phases. One important focus of the burn team is to evaluate the patient carefully for late complications related to burn injuries as described in Table 62-5.

Burn rehabilitation is comprehensive, complex, and requires a multidisciplinary approach to optimize the patient's physical and psychosocial recovery related to the injury. As patients begin to recover, they become more aware of the injuries and the challenges they face. Individualized plans of care that are specific to the severity and location of injury are developed and reevaluated frequently. The increased survival of patients with significant burn injuries has translated into the need for additional and comprehensive burn rehabilitation programs worldwide. The ultimate goal is to return patients to the highest level of function possible within the context of their injuries. Occupational and physical therapists are essential to optimize patient goals and outcomes.

Psychological Support

A patient's outlook, motivation, and support system are important to their overall well-being and ability to progress through the rehabilitation phase. Psychiatric disorders may have contributed to the cause of the burn injury itself. Examples include self-inflicted burns, suicide attempts, or intentional infliction on one individual by another in cases of abuse. These are a few examples that illustrate the critical need for psychosocial resources in burn recovery. Although psychiatric disorders are not contributory to all burn injuries, the life-altering nature of burn injuries almost always causes temporary or permanent impairment of psychosocial adaptation.

In the acute phase of the injury, acute shock, terror, disbelief, confusion, and anxiety are common. Patients may be at risk for delirium and may experience temporary psychoses. Patients may be confused from medications they are taking, but they have an underlying sense of fear, anxiety, and pain. Early consultation with mental health professionals will assist to best meet individual needs, which may include pharmaceutical interventions with concurrent counseling.

The rehabilitation phase may present a new set of challenges. While the patient is physically recovering, the reality and impact of the injury begin to set in as patients recognize that survival is expected. Patients may experience devastating grief and loss. The sense of loss may originate from physical injury, loss of control from the forced dependency on others for care, or loss of family members/friends who may have perished in the injury. In residential fires, survivors may have lost their homes and all of their possessions.

Posttraumatic stress disorder (PTSD) is the most common psychiatric disorder in patients with burns, with a prevalence of 8% to 30% (Hobbs, 2014). Other psychological disorders that may be experienced by patients with burns include anxiety, depression, and sleep disturbances. The symptoms and psychological responses to stress are discussed further in Chapter 6.

As recovery progresses, discharge planning must include strategies to assist the patient in reintegrating into their home, community, workplace, and school. For many patients, issues regarding quality of life may become very real at this point in

---

TABLE 62-5 Complications in Rehabilitation Phase of Burn Care

Complications	Contributing Factors	Interventions
Neuropathies and nerve entrapment	Electrical injury, large deep burns, improper positioning, edema, scar tissue	Assess peripheral pulses and sensation (neurovascular checks). Prevent edema and pressure by elevation, positioning, and prevention of constricting dressings. Assess splints for proper fit and application. Consult OT and PT departments for positioning.
Wound breakdown and/or pressure ulcer formation	Shearing, pressure, inadequate nutrition	Protect wound from pressure and shearing forces. Educate patient about importance of good nutrition.
Hypertrophic scarring	Partial- and full-thickness burns	Keep skin pliable and soft by using emollients. Apply pressure garments as prescribed. Massage.
Contractures	Partial- and full-thickness burns	Maintain position of joints in alignment. Perform gentle range-of-motion exercises. Consult OT and PT departments for exercises and positioning recommendations.
Joint instability	Burn wound, burn scar, and contractures	Maintain appropriate joint positioning through appropriate application of splints. Monitor joint pinning if indicated.
Complex pain	Trauma and burns	Provide adequate pain management. Consult OT and PT departments for exercises and desensitization. Promote gentle motion of affected extremities.

OT, occupational therapy; PT, physical therapy.

recovery. This is an emotional time as the patient and family begin to live with new physical limitations and challenges in relationships. In addition to preparing the patient's support system, the patient and family must also prepare for the reactions from strangers.

Organizations such as the Phoenix Society for Burn Survivors, an international support group for patients with burns, offer a myriad of resources, education, opportunities for peer support, and strategies for reintegration. The Phoenix Society was founded in 1977 by Alan Breslau, a survivor of burn injuries, who recognized the importance of peer support in psychosocial recovery (see the Resources section). Peer support provides opportunities for reflection and personal growth, and gives new meaning for the patient with burns through sharing experiences with others with similar burn injuries (Tolley & Foroushani, 2014). Each year, the Phoenix Society hosts the World Burn Congress, which is a conference for survivors, their families, caregivers, burn care professionals, and firefighters. This forum offers education as well as an opportunity for patients with burns and their families to connect with others who have experienced similar life-changing events. Such interaction allows the patient and family to see that adaptation to a burn injury is possible.

Organizations that provide support for reintegration are able to offer education and training geared specifically to patients with burn injuries. Workshops on application of makeup to reduce the appearance of scars can benefit those with obvious facial scarring is just one example of strategies available to assist patients with burns who have body image disturbances. Cultural influences play a strong factor in this process, because some cultures are particularly sensitive to physical appearance, which is reinforced by current media. The role of the nurse is to encourage patients to voice their concerns, provide empathy, and provide them with assistive resources.

Abnormal Wound Healing

Partial-thickness wounds involving the epidermis and superficial dermis tend to heal without scarring. Deeper wounds will likely develop scarring of variable degrees. As with other disorders, risk factors may be stratified as modifiable or nonmodifiable. For example, a nonmodifiable risk factor for scarring is heredity, because some patients are simply more prone to hypertrophic scar formation. The focus of patient education for nurses must be on how to best change or adapt risk factors that are modifiable. Patients should be strongly encouraged to follow occupational therapist recommendations for scar prevention and management.

Normal scarring occurs in a superficial tissue injury and begins forming within 7 to 10 days post-injury and progresses over the next 6 to 12 months. Abnormal scarring occurs after a longer period of wound healing and may form either hypertrophic or keloid scars.

Hypertrophic and Keloid Scars

Hypertrophic scars form within the boundaries of the initial wound and push outward on the perimeter of the wound. They are common in areas over joints and in the younger population. The scar becomes red (because of its hypervascular nature), raised, and hard.

Keloid scars are irregularly formed and extend beyond the margins of the original wound. They are large, nodular, and ropelike, often causing itching and tenderness. They are more common in dark-pigmented skin, uncommon in children and older adults, and have familial tendencies.

Prevention and Treatment of Scars

Preventive treatment modalities are used to prevent scar contractures and excess hypertrophic tissue. Compression is introduced early in burn wound treatment. Elastic bandage wraps are used initially to help promote adequate circulation, but they can also be used as the first form of compression for scar management, followed by elasticized tubular bandages until the patient can be measured for a customized garment. Application of elastic pressure garments loosens collagen bundles and encourages parallel orientation of the collagen to the skin surface. As pressure continues over time, collagen restructures and vascularity decreases. Although this therapy is somewhat controversial, pressure has shown to be beneficial in controlling scar formation over time. Garments are worn continuously (i.e., 23 hours per day).

Many areas of the body are difficult to compress due to the contours or location of the injury. Inserts, such as silicone sheets, are helpful for these small troublesome areas and are placed beneath the garment or compression dressing to enhance scar compression. Gentle superficial scar massage can be performed with a moisturizer several times a day.

Burn reconstruction is a treatment option after scars have matured and is discussed within the first few years after injury. This decision requires individualized planning, realistic expectations, and patience. The treatment team and the patient will ultimately decide on the best approach for long-term functionality and cosmesis.

NURSING PROCESS

Care of the Patient During the Rehabilitation Phase

Assessment

The nurse obtains information about the patient's education level, occupation, leisure activities, cultural background, religion, and family interactions. The patient's self-concept, mental status, emotional response to the injury and subsequent hospitalization, level of intellectual functioning, previous hospitalizations, response to pain and pain relief measures, and sleep pattern are also essential components of a comprehensive assessment. Information about the patient's general self-concept, self-esteem, and coping strategies in the past are valuable in assessing emotional needs.

Ongoing physical assessments related to rehabilitation goals include range of motion of affected joints, functional abilities in ADLs, early signs of skin breakdown, evidence of neuropathies (nerve damage), activity tolerance, and quality or condition of healing skin. The patient's participation in care and ability to demonstrate self-care in such areas as ambulation, eating, wound cleaning, toileting, and applying pressure wraps are documented on a regular basis.

Diagnosis

NURSING DIAGNOSES

Based on the assessment data, nursing diagnoses may include the following:

- Activity intolerance related to pain with exercise, limited joint mobility, muscle wasting, and limited endurance
- Disturbed body image related to altered physical appearance and self-concept
- Impaired physical mobility due to contractures or hypertrophic scarring
- Deficient knowledge about postdischarge home care and recovery needs

COLLABORATIVE PROBLEMS/POTENTIAL COMPLICATIONS

Potential complications may include the following:

- Inadequate psychological adaptation to burn injury

Planning and Goals

The major goals for the patient include increased mobility and participation in ADLs; adaptation and adjustment to alterations in body image, self-concept, and lifestyle; increased understanding and knowledge of the injury, treatment, and planned follow-up care; and absence of complications.

Nursing Interventions

PROMOTING ACTIVITY TOLERANCE

The extensive physical rehabilitation can be painful and acute for the patient. Strategies to maintain motivation and participation may be beneficial during this critical phase. The nurse incorporates physical and occupational therapy exercises in the patient's care to prevent muscle atrophy and to maintain the mobility required for daily activities. The patient's activity tolerance, strength, and endurance gradually increase if activity occurs over increasingly longer periods. Fatigue and pain tolerance are monitored and used to determine the amount of activity to be encouraged on a daily basis. Activities such as family visits and recreational therapy (e.g., video games, radio, television) can provide diversion, improve the patient's outlook, and increase tolerance for physical activity. In older adult patients and those with chronic illnesses and disabilities, rehabilitation must take into account preexisting functional abilities and limitations.

The nurse must schedule care in such a way that the patient has periods of rest and uninterrupted sleep. A good time for planned patient rest is after the stress of dressing changes and exercise, while pain interventions and sedatives are still effective. This plan must be communicated to family members and other care providers. The patient may have insomnia related to frequent nightmares about the burn injury or other fears and anxieties about the outcome of the injury. The nurse reassures the patient and administers agents, as prescribed, to promote sleep. Reducing metabolic stress by relieving pain, preventing chilling or fever, and promoting the physical integrity of all body systems help the patient conserve energy for therapeutic activities and wound healing.

IMPROVING BODY IMAGE AND SELF-CONCEPT

Patients who have survived burn injuries may lack the benefit of anticipatory grief often seen in a patient who is approaching surgery or dealing with the terminal illness of a loved one.

As care progresses, the patient who is recovering from burns becomes aware of daily improvement and begins to exhibit basic concerns: Will I be disfigured or be disabled? How long will I be in the hospital? What about my job and family? Will I ever be independent again? How will this injury affect my sexual relationships? How can I pay for my care? Was my burn the result of my carelessness? Where will I live now?

When caring for a patient with a burn injury, the nurse needs to be aware that there are prejudices and misunderstandings in society about those who are viewed as different. Opportunities and accommodations available to others are often denied to those who are disfigured by scarring associated with burn injury. These include social participation, employment, prestige, various roles, and status. The health care team must actively promote a healthy body image and self-concept in patients with burn injuries so that they can accept or challenge others' perceptions of those who are disfigured or disabled. Survivors themselves must show others who they are, how they function, and how they want to be treated.

PROMOTING PHYSICAL MOBILITY THROUGH PREVENTING CONTRACTURES OR HYPERTROPHIC SCAR FORMATION

With early and aggressive physical and occupational therapy, contractures or hypertrophic scars are rarely a long-term complication. However, surgical intervention is indicated if full range of motion in the patient with burns is not achieved. See Chapter 10 for a discussion of prevention of contractures and deformities.

MONITORING AND MANAGING POTENTIAL COMPLICATIONS

Impaired Psychological Adaptation to the Burn Injury. Some patients, particularly those with limited coping skills or psychological function, or a history of psychiatric problems before the burn injury, may not achieve adequate psychological adaptation to the burn injury. Psychological counseling or psychiatric referral may be made to assess the patient's emotional status, to help the patient develop coping skills, and to intervene if major psychological issues or ineffective coping is identified.

PROMOTING HOME, COMMUNITY-BASED, AND TRANSITIONAL CARE

Educating the Patient About Self-Care. The focus of rehabilitative interventions is directed toward outpatient care, home care, or care in a rehabilitation center. This includes wound care, dressing changes, pain management, nutrition, prevention of complications, and other care needs. Information and written instructions are provided about specific exercises and the use of pressure garments and splints. The patient and family are provided education to assist them in their continued care needs after discharge (see Chart 62-8).

Continuing and Transitional Care. After discharge, care by a multidisciplinary treatment team is necessary. Some patients may require the services of an inpatient rehabilitation center before returning home. Patients should receive follow-up from a burn center when possible for periodic evaluation by the burn team, modification of outpatient treatment plan, and evaluation for reconstructive surgery. Many patients require outpatient physical or occupational therapy several times a week. The nurse coordinates all aspects of care and ensures that the patient's needs are met. Such coordination is an important aspect of assisting the patient to achieve independence.

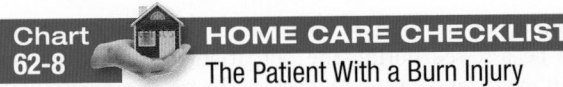

Chart
62-8

HOME CARE CHECKLIST
The Patient With a Burn Injury

At the completion of education, the patient and/or caregiver will be able to:

- State the impact of the burn injury and treatment on physiologic functioning, ADLs, IADLs, roles, relationships, and spirituality.
- State how to contact all members of the treatment team (e.g., interdisciplinary burn team, healthcare providers, home care professionals, and durable medical equipment and supply vendor).
- State the name, dose, side effects, frequency, and schedule for all medications.
- Demonstrate psychosocial adaptation and social integration through verbalizing understanding of the following:
  - Changes in lifestyle and emotional adjustment to injury take time. It is not uncommon for patients to report nightmares or "flashbacks" of the injury. If this becomes disruptive, it should be discussed with the treatment team.
  - Resume previous interests and activities gradually.
  - Consider community and other resources such as burn support groups. Many books, videos, and Web sites are also available and may be invaluable in assisting with burn recovery.
  - Programs are available to assist with school reintegration and return to work. The treatment team should be consulted as needed.
  - Burn care (dressings, medications, therapy) can be very expensive. A social worker or care manager may find funding assistance programs if needed.
- Demonstrate adaptation of the home environment, assisted as needed by team members (e.g., social worker, care manager).
- State burn skin precautions:
  - Wear sunblock with the highest sun protection factor (SPF) possible to protect exposed burned skin from the sun. Light-colored clothing, long pants, and long-sleeved shirts may also be necessary to protect from the sun.
  - Wear wide-brimmed hats if face or ears have been burned to protect the area from the sun.
  - Avoid further trauma to burned skin; leave blisters that may form intact.
  - Lubricate healed burned skin with mild lotion (as prescribed); avoid scratching.
  - Use only mild soap and lotion (i.e., products without perfume) on burned areas. Keeping skin clean overall is important to support good hygiene and prevent infection.
  - Avoid tight clothing over burned areas so as not to restrict movement or irritate newly healed areas.
  - Select white cotton, loose-fitting clothing so that dyes in colored clothes do not irritate healing skin.
  - Wear clothing and gloves to protect healing skin from unnecessary bruises, bumps, and scratches.
  - Be aware that tolerance to extremes in temperatures may be affected.
  - Itching is a normal, uncomfortable part of healing and burn recovery; do not scratch, pat areas; apply mild moisturizers

to decrease itching from dryness. Medications for itching can be discussed with the treatment team.
- Demonstrate wound care technique:
  - Take prescribed pain medications if needed 30 min prior to wound care to achieve maximum effectiveness.
  - Use mild soap, water, and a clean washcloth to clean wounds.
  - Apply prescribed topical medications and dressings as instructed.
  - Inspect wounds carefully with each dressing change for signs of infection, including increased redness, swelling, drainage, or foul odor.
- State aspects of ADLs and exercise:
  - Perform as much of own care as possible.
  - Adhere to the exercise regimen given by the therapists.
  - Although physical rehabilitation is tiring, daily participation is essential.
  - Plan for adequate rest and sleep.
  - When at rest, swollen limbs should be elevated.
- Describe approaches to controlling pain (e.g., take analgesics as prescribed; use nonpharmacologic interventions).
- States changes in diet necessary to promote health (e.g., nutrient rich foods, rather than empty calories).
- States changes in fluid intake needed to prevent constipation associated with the use of analgesic medications.
- Discusses management of burn scar:
  - Massage with mild lotion or cream to stretch skin to maintain/increase its elasticity.
  - Wear compression garments 23 hours a day if instructed.
  - Discoloration of the skin for many months is an expected normal part of healing.
- Discusses resumption of sexual relations:
  - Resumption of sexual relationships is the rule rather than the exception and should occur when comfortable for all.
  - Expect sensitivity of and around the genital area for several months if these areas were burned.
- States correct use of medical devices:
  - Follow occupational therapist's instructions for splint use and cleaning.
  - Use crutches, walkers, or other assistive devices as instructed.
  - If devices such as shower chairs or grab bars are needed in the home, this should be arranged prior to discharge.
- State time and date of follow-up appointments, therapy, and testing:
  - Keep a list of questions to ask team members.
  - Bring medications, or a list of current medications, to each visit for the team to review.
- Identify sources of support (e.g. friends, relatives, faith community, burn support groups, Phoenix Society, caregiver support).
- Identify the need for health promotion, disease prevention, and screening activities.

ADL, activities of daily living; IADL, independent activities of daily living.

Some patients may require referral for transitional care after discharge. The nurse assesses the patient's physical and psychological status as well as the adequacy of the home setting for safe and adequate care. The nurse monitors the patient's progress; assesses adherence to the plan of care; and assists the patient and family with wound care, exercises, and other physical needs. Patients experiencing difficulties with psychosocial adjustments are identified and appropriate referrals are made.

Evaluation

Expected patient outcomes may include:
1. Demonstrates adequate activity tolerance
   a. Has energy available to perform daily activities
   b. Shows gradual increased tolerance and endurance in physical activities
   c. Obtains adequate sleep and rest daily

2. Adapts to altered body image
   a. Verbalizes accurate description of alterations in body image and accepts physical appearance
   b. Demonstrates interest in resources that may improve function and perception of body appearance (e.g., cosmetics, wigs, and prostheses as appropriate)
   c. Socializes with significant others, peers, and usual social group
   d. Seeks and achieves return to role in family, school, and community as a contributing member
3. Demonstrates physical mobility adequate to perform ADLs
   a. Demonstrates range of motion appropriate for injury
   b. Absence of complications from wound healing
4. Demonstrates knowledge of required self-care and follow-up care
   a. Verbalizes detailed plan for follow-up care
   b. Demonstrates ability to perform or direct wound care and prescribed exercises
   c. Returns for follow-up appointments as scheduled
   d. Identifies resource people and agencies to contact for specific problems
5. Exhibits no complications
   a. Exhibits psychosocial adaptation to burn injury
   b. Verbalizes understanding of diagnosis and treatment plan

Outpatient Burn Care

The increased availability of outpatient surgery and access to expert burn care in outpatient settings make this option possible for the treatment of minor burns as well as follow-up for the patient with more severe burns who is discharged. The goals for treatment in an outpatient setting may include burn wound management, pain management, scar and reconstructive care, psychosocial care, and rehabilitation. However, a number of factors must be considered when determining if outpatient care is appropriate for the patient: age, past medical history, extent and depth of the burn, location of the burn wounds, availability of family support systems and community resources, the patient's ability and willingness to adhere to a therapeutic regimen, distance from home, and availability of transportation from home to the outpatient setting.

The frequency of follow-up visits is individualized. The initial outpatient visit for a discharged patient with burn injuries is usually scheduled within 2 to 3 days after hospital discharge. Follow-up appointments will vary and over time decrease in frequency, based on the patient's needs. Patient and family education is paramount and should include verbal and written instructions as well as return demonstration of the wound or scar care required. The importance of notifying the outpatient setting about early complications and of keeping follow-up appointments is emphasized to the patient and family. Physical therapy and occupational therapy are often provided in the outpatient burn setting. The rehabilitation goals are to increase range of motion, strengthen muscles, and build the patient's activity tolerance. This is accomplished by a specific plan of care and includes routine visits for up to 2 years or more following the injury.

Adaptation to lifestyle changes and emotional status should be assessed during the outpatient visits and proper referrals made for counseling services. These assessments may be difficult to recognize due to the infrequent nature of the visits; therefore, it is helpful to incorporate family response and interactions into the assessment. The health care team must also be alert to issues of substance abuse, safety concerns, suicidal thoughts, depression, and PTSD.

CRITICAL THINKING EXERCISES

1 **pq** A 45-year-old man sustains a steam burn while working on an offshore oil platform in the Gulf of Mexico. He sustains third-degree burns over 65% of his body. Inclement weather has delayed transportation to the nearest burn center. What should be the priorities of the first responders on the scene? On arrival to the treating facility, the patient's temperature is 35.2°C (95.3°F), and his weight is 62 kg (137 lb). How should the treatment team at the burn treating facility prioritize this patient's care?

2 **ebp** A 34-year-old woman is roasting a turkey for Thanksgiving. In the process of removing the turkey from the oven, grease spills from the roasting pan onto her right hand and forearm, and both lower legs and feet. She is transported by EMS to the hospital for care. Using the rule of nines, what is her estimated TBSA? Based on the best evidence, what type of fluid should be used for resuscitation and why? What other information would you need to calculate her fluid requirements in the emergent/resuscitative phase?

3 **ebp** A 69-year-old man was found down in the hallway of his apartment by firefighters, who extracted him from the smoke-filled building after being called to the scene by neighbors. He does not sustain obvious cutaneous burns. Upon interview and examination, he is tachypneic and exhibits hoarseness when speaking. You note singed nasal hair and lips. What is your immediate concern? What treatment should you expect the physician to prescribe first? Based on the current best evidence, what tests or procedures would most likely be prescribed to assist in the diagnosis and management of this patient?

REFERENCES

*Asterisk indicates nursing research.

Books

American Burn Association (ABA). (2011). *Advanced burn life support (ABLS) course provider manual 2011*. Chicago, IL: Author.

American Nurses Association. (2015). *Code of ethics for nurses with interpretive statements*. Washington, DC: American Nurses Publishing, American Nurses Foundation/American Nurses Association

Beauchamp, T. L., & Childress, J. F. (2012). *Principles of biomedical ethics* (7th ed.). New York: Oxford University Press.

Lee, J. O., Dibildox, M., Jimenez, C. J., et al. (2012). Operative wound management. In D. Herndon (Ed.): *Total burn care* (4th ed.). Edinburgh: Saunders Elsevier.

Mayhall, C. G. (2012). Healthcare-associated burn wound infections. In C. G. Mayhall (Ed.): *Hospital epidemiology and infection control* (4th ed.). Philadelphia, PA: Lippincott Williams & Wilkins.

Serghiou, M. A., Ott, S., Whitehead, C., et al. (2012). Comprehensive rehabilitation of the burn patient. In D. Herndon (Ed.): *Total burn care* (4th ed.). Edinburgh: Saunders Elsevier.

Journals and Electronic Documents

Abdullahi, A., & Jeschke, M. G. (2014). Nutrition and anabolic pharmacotherapies in the care of burn patients. *Nutrition in Clinical Practice, 29*(5), 621–630.

American Burn Association (ABA). (2014). *Burn center verification.* Retrieved on 6/12/2016 at: www.ameriburn.org/verification_verified-centers.php

American Burn Association (ABA). (2015). *Burn incidence and treatment in the United States: 2015 fact sheet.* Retrieved on 6/12/2016 at: www.ameriburn.org/resources_factsheet.php

American Burn Association National Burn Repository (ABA NBR). (2015). *Report of data from 2051–2014.* Retrieved on 6/12/2016 at: www.ameriburn.org/2015NBRAnnualReport.pdf

*Bishop, S. M., Walker, M. D., & Spivak, I. M. (2013). Family presence in the adult burn intensive care unit during dressing changes. *Critical Care Nurse, 33*(1), 14–23.

Cahill, K. C., Tiong, W. H. C. & Conroy, F. J. (2013). Trineural injury to the right hand after domestic electrocution. *Journal of Burn Care and Research, 35*(5), e353-e356.

Davis, J. S., Rodriquez, L. I., Quintana, O. D., et al. (2013). Use of a warming catheter to achieve normothermia in large burns. *Journal of Burn Care and Research, 34*(1), 191–195.

Dries, D. J., & Endorf, F. W. (2013). Inhalation injury: Epidemiology, pathology, treatment strategies. *Scandinavian Journal of Trauma, Resuscitation & Emergency Medicine, 21,* 31. doi: 10.1186/1757-7241-21-31

*Fahlstrom, K., Boyle, C., & Makic, M. B. F. (2013). Implementation of a nurse-driven burn resuscitation protocol: A quality improvement project. *Critical Care Nurse, 33*(1), 25–35.

Flores, O., Stockton, K., Roberts, J. A., et al. (2015). The efficacy and safety of adrenergic blockade after burn injury: A systematic review and meta-analysis. *Journal of Trauma and Acute Care Surgery, 80*(1), 146–155.

Hermans, M. E. (2014). Porcine xenografts vs. (cryopreserved) allografts in the management of partial thickness burns: Is there a clinical difference? *Burns, 40*(3), 408–415.

*Hobbs, K. (2014). Which factors influence the development of post-traumatic stress disorder in patients with burn injuries? A systematic review of the literature. *Burns, 41*(3), 421–430.

Hostler, D., Weaver, M. D., Ziembicki, J. A., et al. (2013). Admission temperature and survival in patients admitted to burn centers. *Journal of Burn Care and Research, 34*(5), 498–506.

Jeschke, M. G., Finnerty, C. C., Shahrokhi, S., et al. (2013). Wound coverage technologies in burn care: Novel techniques. *Journal of Burn Care and Research, 34*(6), 612–620.

Jeschke, M. G., Patsouris, D., Stanojcic, M., et al. (2015, August 6). Pathophysiologic response to burns in the elderly. *EBioMedicine, 2*(10), 1536–1548. Retrieved on 8/31/2015 at: www.ebiomedicine.com/action/doSearch?searchType=quick&searchText=pathophysiologic+response+to+burns+in+the+elderly&occurrences=all&journalCode=ebiom&searchScope = fullSite

Jeschke, M. G., Pinto, R., Kraft, R., et al. (2015). Morbidity and survival probability in burn patients in modern burn care. *Critical Care Medicine, 43*(4), 808–815.

Justiniano, C. F., Coffey, R. A., Evans, D. C., et al. (2015). Comorbidity-polypharmacy score predicts in-hospital complications and the need for discharge to extended care facility in older burn patients. *Journal of Burn Care and Research, 36*(1), 193–196.

Kearns, R. D., Cairns, C. B., Holmes, J. H., et al. (2013). Thermal burns: A review of best practice. *EMS World, 42*(1), 43–51.

*Klas, K. S., Smith, S. J., Matherly, A. F., et al. (2015). Multicenter assessment of burn team injury prevention knowledge. *Journal of Burn Care and Research, 36*(3), 434–439.

Kwon, K. H., Kim, S. H., & Minn Y. K. (2014). Electrodiagnostic study of peripheral nerves in high-voltage electrical injury. *Journal of Burn Care and Research, 35*(4), e230–233

Kym, D., Yim, H., Yoon, J., et al. (2015). The application of cultured epithelial autografts improves survival in burns. *Wound Repair and Regeneration, 23,* 340–344.

Mann-Salinas, E. A., Baun, M. M., Meininger, J. C., et al. (2013) Novel predictors of sepsis outperform the American Burn Association sepsis criteria in the burn intensive care unit patient. *Journal of Burn Care and Research, 34*(1), 31–43.

Micromedex 2.0. (2015). *Formulary advisor,* University of Texas–Medical Branch Galveston. Retrieved on 7/10/2015 (pass-protected) at: www.micromedicsolutions.com/micromedex2/librarian

Meyerson, J. M., Coffey, R, Jones, L. M., et al. (2015). Burn center barrier protocols during dressing change: A national survey. *Journal of Burn Care and Research, 36*(4), 238–234.

National Oceanic and Atmospheric Administration. (2015). *Lightning safety.* Retrieved on 6/10/2016 at: www.lightningsafety.noaa.gov/index.shtml

Nitzschke, S. L., Adem, J., K., Serio-Melvin, M. L., et al. (2014). Wound healing trajectories in burn patients and their impact on mortality. *Journal of Burn Care and Research, 35*(6), 474–479.

Rousseau, A., Massion, P. B., Laungani, A., et al. (2014). Toward targeted early burn care: Lessons from a European survey. *Journal of Burn Care and Research, 35*(4), e234–e239.

Russell, K. W., Cochran, A. L., Mehta, S. T., et al. (2013). Lightning burns. *Journal of Burn Care and Research, 35*(6), e436–e438.

Satahoo, S. S., Parikh, P. P., Naranjo, D., et al. (2015). Are burn patients really at risk for thrombotic events? *Journal of Burn Care and Research, 36*(1), 100–104.

Sen, S., Palmieri, T., & Greenhalgh, D. (2015). Review of burn research for year 2014. *Journal of Burn Care and Research, 36*(6), 587–594.

Snell, J. A., Loh N. W., Mahambrey, T, et al. (2013). Clinical review: The critical care management of the burn patient. *Critical Care, 17*(5), 241.

Stergiou-Kita, M., Mansfield, E., Bayley, M., et al. (2014). Returning to work after electrical injuries: Workers' perspectives and advice to others. *Journal of Burn Care and Research, 35*(6), 498–507.

Tolley, J. S., & Foroushani, P. S. (2014) What do we know about one-to-one peer support for adults with burn injury? A scoping review. *Journal of Burn Care and Research, 35*(4), 233–242.

Trexler, S. T., Lundy, J. B., Chung, K. K., et al. (2014). Prevalence and impact of late defecation in the critically ill, thermally injured adult patient. *Journal of Burn Care and Research, 35*(4), e224–e229.

Veeravagu, A., Yoon, B. C., Jiang, B., et al. (2015). National trends in burn and inhalation injury in burn patients: Results of analysis of the nationwide inpatient sample database. *Journal of Burn Care and Research, 36*(2), 258–265.

Wibbenmeyer, L., Eid, A., Liao, J. et al. (2014). Gabapentin is ineffective as an analgesic agent in the immediate postburn period. *Journal of Burn Care and Research, 35*(2), 136–142.

World Health Organization (WHO). (2014). *Fact sheet No. 365. Burns.* Retrieved on 6/12/2016 at: www.who.int/mediacentre/factsheets/fs365/en/

Resources

Alisa Ann Ruch Burn Foundation, www.aarbf.org
American Burn Association (ABA), www.ameriburn.org
American Red Cross, www.redcross.org
Burn Foundation, www.burnfoundation.org
Burn Institute, www.burninstitute.org
Burn Prevention Network, www.burnprevention.org
Firefighters Burn Institute, www.ffburn.org
International Association of Fire Fighters, www.iaff.org
International Society for Burn Injuries (ISBI), www.worldburn.org
Lund-Browder Classification, medical-dictionary.thefreedictionary.com/Lund-Browder+classification
National Fire Protection Association (NFPA), www.nfpa.org
Phoenix Society for Burn Survivors, www.phoenix-society.org
U.S. Fire Administration, www.usfa.fema.gov

UNIT 15

Sensory Function

Case Study SUPPORTING A PATIENT WHO VALUES INDEPENDENCE

A 33-year-old patient was admitted to a surgical unit after being hit by a car crossing the street. The patient has been deaf since birth and did not hear the on-coming traffic. He lives alone with his hearing service dog and is used to being very independent. He is awaiting surgery to repair his shoulder fracture. He either does not understand or did not hear the instructions to call for help to get out of bed and got himself up to the bathroom to urinate despite the fact that he was instructed to use a bedside urinal. The nurse is concerned that he may fall while getting up alone and tried to communicate to him the importance of calling for assistance to get out of bed.

QSEN Competency Focus: Patient-Centered Care

The complexities inherent in today's health care system challenges nurses to demonstrate integration of specific inter-disciplinary core competencies. These competencies are aimed at ensuring the delivery of safe, quality patient care (Institute of Medicine, 2003). The Quality and Safety Education for Nurses project (QSEN, 2017; Cronenwett, Sherwood, Barnsteiner, et al., 2007) provides a framework for the knowledge, skills, and attitudes (KSA) required for nurses to demonstrate competency in these key areas, which include **patient-centered care, interdisciplinary teamwork and collaboration, evidence-based practice, quality improvement, safety,** and **informatics.**

Patient-Centered Care Definition: Recognize the patient or designee as the source of control and full partner in providing compassionate and coordinated care based on respect for patient's preferences, values, and needs.

SELECTED PRE-LICENSURE KSAs	APPLICATION AND REFLECTION
Knowledge	
Integrate understanding of multiple dimensions of patient-centered care: • Patient/family/community preferences, values • Coordination and integration of care • Information, communication, and education • Physical comfort and emotional support • Involvement of family and friends	Describe the factors that are impacting the patient's decision to get out of bed on his own. Identify the factors that should be incorporated into his care to best support him so that he is empowered to make the decision that is best for him.
Skills	
Communicate patient values, preferences and expressed needs to other members of the health care team.	Discuss how you would advocate for this patient so that he receives the care that is best for him. How would you coordinate his care with other members of the health care team so that it reflects his wishes and desires?
Attitudes	
Value seeing health care situations "through patient's eyes." Respect and encourage individual expression of patient values, preferences, and expressed needs.	Reflect on a time you felt a loss of control. How did that fear affect your decision making? Think about how individual preferences and values affect how health care decisions are made. Can you respect decisions that others make that are different from decisions you would make in a similar situation? Why is it important for nurses to demonstrate respect for patients' autonomous decision-making?

Cronenwett, L., Sherwood, G., Barnsteiner, J., et al. (2007) Quality and safety education for nurses. *Nursing Outlook, 55*(3), 122–131.

Institute of Medicine. (2003). *Health professions education: A bridge to quality.* Washington, DC: National Academies Press.

QSEN Institute. (2017). *QSEN Competencies: Definitions and pre-licensure KSAs.* Retrieved on 3/1/2017 at: www.qsen.org/competencies/pre-licensure-ksas

63 Assessment and Management of Patients With Eye and Vision Disorders

LEARNING OBJECTIVES

On completion of this chapter, the learner will be able to:

1 Identify the major structures and function of the eye.
2 Specify assessment and diagnostic findings used in the evaluation of ocular disorders.
3 Describe assessment and management strategies for patients with low vision and blindness.
4 List the pharmacologic actions and nursing management of common ophthalmic medications.

5 Recognize the clinical features, assessment and diagnostic findings, and medical or surgical management of glaucoma, cataracts, and other ocular disorders.
6 Explain the nursing management of patients with glaucoma, cataracts, and ocular trauma.
7 Discuss general discharge education for patients after ocular surgery.

GLOSSARY

anterior chamber: aqueous-containing space in the eye between the posterior (endothelial) cornea and the anterior iris and pupil
aqueous humor: transparent nutrient-containing fluid that fills the anterior and posterior chambers of the eye
astigmatism: refractive error due to an irregularity in the curvature of the cornea
binocular vision: normal ability of both eyes to focus on one object and fuse the two images into one
blindness: inability to see, defined as corrected visual acuity of 20/400 or less, or a visual field of no more than 20 degrees in the better eye
cataract: progressive opacity of the lens of the eye
chemosis: edema of the conjunctiva
diplopia: seeing one object as two; double vision
ectropion: turning out of the lower eyelid
emmetropia: normal refractive condition resulting in clear focus on retina; no optical defects
endophthalmitis: intraocular infection
entropion: turning in of the lower eyelid
enucleation: removal of the eyeball and part of the optic nerve
evisceration: removal of the intraocular contents through a corneal or scleral incision; the optic nerve, sclera, extraocular muscles, and sometimes the cornea are left intact
exenteration: surgical removal of the entire contents of the orbit, surrounding soft tissue, and most or all of the eyelids
glaucoma: group of conditions characterized by increased intraocular pressure

hyperemia: red eyes resulting from dilation of the vasculature of the conjunctiva
hyperopia: farsightedness; light rays focus behind the retina
hyphema: blood in the anterior chamber
hypopyon: collection of inflammatory cells in the anterior chamber of the eye
injection: congestion of blood vessels
keratoconus: cone-shaped deformity of the cornea
myopia: nearsightedness; light rays focus in front of the retina
neovascularization: growth of abnormal new blood vessels
nystagmus: involuntary oscillation of the eyeball
papilledema: swelling of the optic disc usually due to increased intracranial pressure
photophobia: ocular pain on exposure to light
presbyopia: the loss of accommodative power in the lens due to age
proptosis or exophthalmos: abnormal protrusion of the eyeball
ptosis: drooping eyelid
refraction: determination of the refractive errors of the eye for the purpose of vision correction
scotomas: blind or partially blind areas in the visual field
sympathetic ophthalmia: an inflammatory condition created in the fellow eye by the affected eye
trachoma: an infectious disease caused by the bacterium *Chlamydia trachomatis*—the leading cause of preventable blindness in the world
trichiasis: turning in of the eyelashes
vitreous humor: transparent, colorless gelatinous material that fills the vitreous chamber behind the lens

Note: Common abbreviations related to vision and eye health are OD (oculus dexter, right eye), OS (oculus sinister, left eye), and OU (oculus uterque, both eyes).

The eye is a sensitive, highly specialized sense organ subject to various disorders, many of which can lead to impaired vision. Impaired vision may affect individuals in many ways, including their independence in self-care, sense of self-esteem,

safety, and overall quality of life. Many of the leading causes of visual impairment are associated with aging (e.g., cataracts, glaucoma, and macular degeneration). Younger people are also at risk for eye disorders, particularly traumatic injuries.

Although most people with eye disorders are treated in an ambulatory care setting, various eye disorders are seen in many settings. In addition to understanding the prevention, treatment, and consequences of eye disorders, nurses in all settings assess visual acuity in patients at risk (e.g., older adults, those with hypertension, diabetes or acquired immune deficiency syndrome [AIDS]), refer patients to eye care specialists as appropriate, implement measures to prevent further visual loss, and help patients adapt to impaired vision.

ASSESSMENT OF THE EYE

Anatomic and Physiologic Overview

Unlike most organs of the body, the eye is available for external examination, and its anatomy is more easily assessed than other body parts (see Fig. 63-1). The eyeball, or globe, sits in the bony protective orbit (Hogan, 2014). Lined with muscle and connective and adipose tissues, the orbit is shaped like a four-sided pyramid, surrounded on three sides by the sinuses: ethmoid (medially), frontal (superiorly), and maxillary (inferiorly). The optic nerve and the ophthalmic artery enter the orbit at its apex through the optic foramen. The eyeball is moved through all fields of gaze by the extraocular muscles. The four rectus muscles and two oblique muscles (see Fig. 63-2) are innervated by cranial nerves (CNs) III, IV, and VI. Normally, the movements of the two eyes are coordinated and the brain perceives a single image.

The eyelids are composed of thin, elastic skin that covers striated and smooth muscles and protect the anterior portion of the eye. The eyelids contain multiple glands (sebaceous, sweat, and lacrimal). The upper lid normally covers the uppermost portion of the iris and is innervated by the oculomotor nerve (CN III). The lid margins contain meibomian

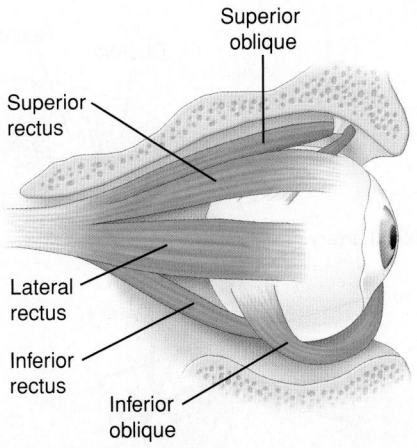

Figure 63-2 • The extraocular muscles responsible for eye movement. The medial rectus muscle (not shown) is responsible for opposing the movement of the lateral rectus muscle.

glands, the inferior and superior puncta, and the eyelashes. The triangular spaces formed by the junction of the eyelids are known as the inner or medial canthus and the outer or lateral canthus. With every blink, the eyelids wash the cornea and conjunctiva with tears.

Tears are vital to eye health. Formed by the lacrimal gland and the accessory lacrimal glands, tears are secreted in response to reflex or emotional stimuli. A healthy tear is composed of three layers: lipoid, aqueous, and mucoid. These layers nourish the cornea and create a smooth optical surface of the cornea and conjunctival epithelium. If there is a defect in the composition of any of these layers, the integrity of the cornea may be compromised.

The conjunctiva, a thin transparent mucous membrane, provides a barrier to the external environment extending under the eyelids (palpebral conjunctiva) and over the sclera (bulbar conjunctiva). The junction of the two portions is known as the fornix. The conjunctiva meets the cornea at the limbus on the outermost edge of the iris.

The eyeball is composed of the following three layers:
- The outer dense fibrous layer, including the sclera and transparent cornea
- The middle vascular layer, containing the iris, ciliary body, and choroid
- The inner neural layer, including the retina, optic nerve, and visual pathway

The eyeball is divided anatomically into two segments. The anterior segment is between the anterior cornea and posterior iris, including the anterior and posterior chamber. The posterior segment is between the posterior lens and the retina, including the vitreous chamber. The eyeball also has three fluid-containing chambers. The aqueous-filled **anterior chamber** lies between the posterior cornea and the anterior iris and pupil. The posterior chamber is a small aqueous containing space between the posterior iris and pupil and anterior lens. The vitreous chamber, containing clear gelatinous vitreous fluid, is the largest chamber in the ocular fundus between the lens and retina (see Fig. 63-3).

The **aqueous humor** (transparent nutrient-containing fluid that fills the anterior and posterior chambers of the eye) is produced in the posterior chamber by the ciliary

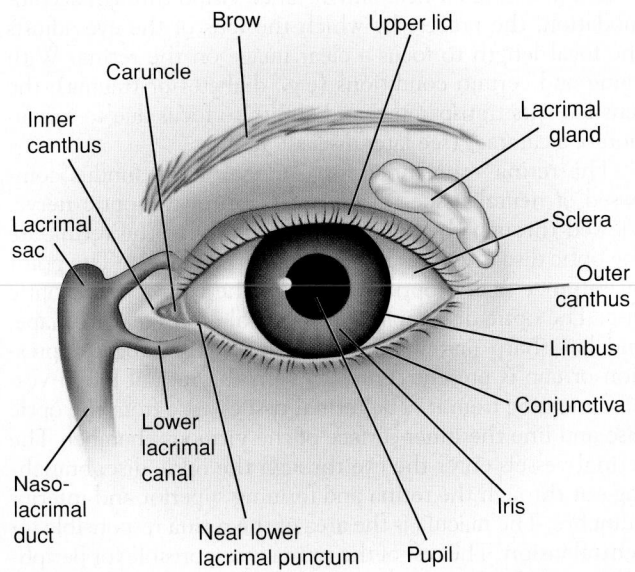

Figure 63-1 • External structures of the eye and position of the lacrimal structures.

Figure 63-3 • Three-dimensional cross-section of the eye.

Labels (clockwise): Sclera, Choroid, Retina, Lateral rectus muscle, Conjunctiva, Zonules, Canal of Schlemm, Posterior chamber, Anterior chamber, Cornea, Pupil, Lens, Iris muscle, Ciliary body, Medial rectus muscle, Vitreous body, Macular area, Central retinal artery and vein, Optic nerve, Retinal vein, Retinal artery

body (Grossman & Porth, 2014). It flows through the pupil into the anterior chamber and drains through the trabecular meshwork into the canal of Schlemm. Production of aqueous humor is related to the intraocular pressure (IOP). Normal IOP is less than 21 mmHg (Eldaly, Bunce, El Sheikha, et al., 2014). **Vitreous humor**, which is composed mostly of water and encapsulated by a hyaloid membrane, helps maintain the shape of the eye. The vitreous is attached to the retina by scattered collagenous filaments. The vitreous shrinks and shifts with age. Through this degenerative process, the gel-like characteristics liquefy, causing stringy debris known as floaters.

The sclera is the white avascular dense fibrous structure that helps maintain the shape of the eyeball and protects the intraocular contents. Scleral thinning and changes of the scleral collagen fibers can cause the underlying uveal pigment to be seen, resulting in a blue or gray sclera. The episclera is a vascularized loose elastic tissue that overlies the sclera supplying nutritional support and reacting to inflammation.

The cornea, a vulnerable transparent avascular domelike structure, forms the most anterior portion of the eyeball and is the main refracting surface of the eye. It is composed of five layers: the epithelium, Bowman membrane, stroma, Descemet membrane, and endothelium. It contains high concentrations of nerve fibers and is extremely sensitive to pain. The epithelium, the outermost protective layer, absorbs oxygen and nutrients from the tear film nourishing the cornea. The epithelial cells readily regenerate, unlike the innermost endothelial cells, which do not regenerate and result in corneal edema when injured.

The uveal tract is the vascular middle layer of the eye consisting of the iris, ciliary body, and the choroid.

The iris surrounding the pupil is a highly vascularized pigmented collection of fibers that give the eye color. The dilator and sphincter muscles of the iris control pupil size. The dilator muscles are controlled by the sympathetic nervous system.

The sphincter muscles are controlled by the parasympathetic nervous system.

The ciliary body consists of ciliary processes, ciliary muscles, and zonular fibers (ligaments) that work together to form aqueous fluid and control focusing through the zonular fibers that suspend the crystalline lens.

The choroid lies between the retina and the sclera, supplying blood and oxygen to the outer retina. Pigmented cells containing melanocytes in the choroid assist to absorb scattered light.

Directly behind the pupil and iris lies the lens, an avascular and almost completely transparent biconvex structure held in position by zonular fibers in the ciliary body. The lens enables focusing for near and distance vision through accommodation, the process by which the lens of the eye adjusts the focal length to focus a clear image on the retina. With aging and certain conditions (e.g., diabetes or trauma), the lens loses its transparency and ability to focus due to formation of a cataract (see later discussion).

The retina—the innermost surface of the fundus composed of neural tissue—is an extension of the optic nerve. Viewed through the pupil, the landmarks of the retina are the optic disc, the retinal vessels, and the macula. The point of entrance of the optic nerve into the retina is the optic disc. The optic disc is pink, either oval or circular in shape, and has sharp margins. In the disc, a physiologic depression or cup is present centrally, with the retinal blood vessels emerging from it. The retinal tissues arise from the optic disc and line the inner surface of the vitreous chamber. The retinal vessels enter the eye through the optic disc, branching out through the retina and forming superior and inferior branches. The macula is the area of the retina responsible for central vision. The rest of the retina is responsible for peripheral vision. In the center of the macula is the most sensitive area—the fovea—which is avascular and surrounded by the superior and inferior vascular arcades. Two important layers of the retina are the retinal pigment epithelium (RPE) and the sensory retina. A single layer of cells constitutes the RPE. These cells have numerous functions, including the absorption of light. The sensory retina contains the photoreceptor cells: rods and cones. The rods are responsible for night or low light vision. The cones are retinal photoreceptor cells essential for visual acuity, color discrimination, and fine detail. Cones are distributed throughout the retina, with their greatest concentration in the fovea. Rods are absent in the fovea.

Visual acuity depends on a healthy functioning eye and an intact visual pathway. This pathway is made up of the retina, optic nerve, optic chiasm, optic tracks, lateral geniculate bodies, optic radiations, and the visual cortex area of the brain. The visual pathway is part of the central nervous system (see Fig. 63-4).

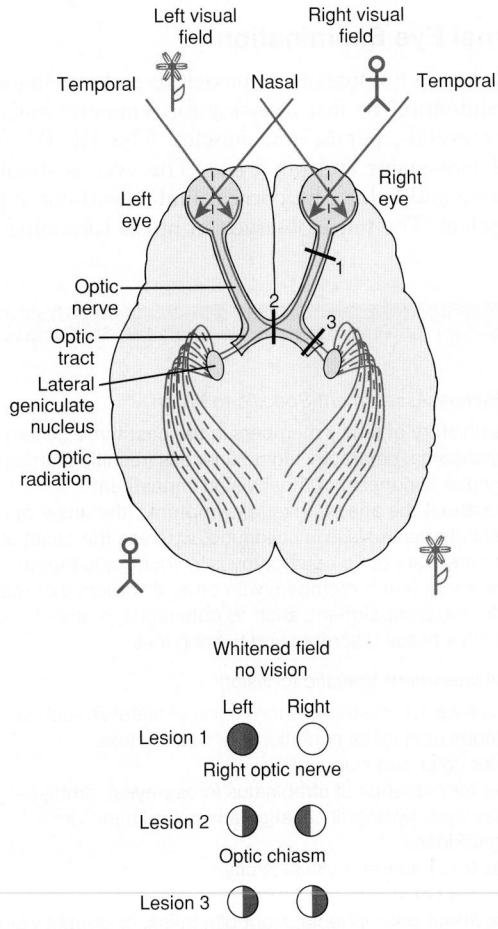

Figure 63-4 • Diagram of optic pathways. The *red* lines indicate the right visual field and the *blue* lines the left visual field. Note the crossing of the fibers from the medial half of each retina at the optic chiasm. Lesion 1 (right optic nerve) produces unilateral blindness. Lesion 2 (optic chiasm) may involve only those fibers that originate in the nasal half of each retina and cross to the opposite side in each field (bitemporal hemianopia). Lesion 3 (right optic tract) interrupts fibers (and vision) originating on the same side of both eyes (homonymous) with loss of vision from half of each field (hemianopia). Reprinted with permission from Grossman, S. C., & Porth, C. M. (2014). *Porth's pathophysiology: Concepts of altered health states* (9th ed.). Philadelphia, PA: Lippincott Williams & Wilkins.

The optic nerve (CN II) transmits impulses from the retina to the occipital lobe of the brain. The optic nerve head, or optic disc, is the physiologic blind spot in each eye. The optic nerve leaves the eye and then meets the optic nerve from the other eye at the optic chiasm. The chiasm is the anatomic point at which the nasal fibers from the nasal retina of each eye cross to the opposite side of the brain. The nerve fibers from the temporal retina of each eye remain uncrossed. Fibers from the right half of each eye, which would be the left visual field, carry impulses to the right occipital lobe. Fibers from the left half of each eye, or the right visual field, carry impulses to the left occipital lobe. Beyond the chiasm, these fibers are known as the optic tract. The optic tract continues on to the lateral geniculate body. The lateral geniculate body is connected by the optic radiations to the cortex of the occipital lobe of the brain.

Assessment

Ocular History

The nurse, through careful questioning, elicits the necessary information that can assist in diagnosis of an ophthalmic condition. Pertinent questions to ask when taking an ocular history are presented in Chart 63-1. Genetics plays a role in many eye and vision disorders (Lee & Garg, 2015) (see Chart 63-2).

Visual Acuity

Following the health history, the patient's visual acuity is assessed. This is an essential part of the eye examination and a measure against which all therapeutic outcomes are based.

Visual acuity is tested for both near (14 inches away) and distance (20 feet away) vision and is performed on each eye separately with a standardized Snellen chart for distance and a Rosenbaum pocket screener for near vision. A tumbling "E," "illiterate E," number, or picture chart is used if the person is illiterate or unable to read the English alphabet (Weber & Kelley, 2014).

The Snellen chart is composed of a series of progressively smaller rows of letters; the person is asked to read the lowest line possible. The fraction 20/20 is considered the standard of normal vision. Most people can see the letters on the line designated as 20/20. The patient should be encouraged to read every letter possible.

Visual acuity is then recorded. The following would be an example of visual acuity documentation: A patient reads all five letters from the 20/20 line on the Snellen chart with the right eye (OD) and three of the five letters on the 20/30 line with the left eye (OS); the visual acuity is documented as OD: 20/20 and OS: 20/30 (Weber & Kelley, 2014).

If the patient cannot see the big "E" at the top of the Snellen chart, the examiner should determine next if the patient can count fingers ("CF" in documentation). Initially, the examiner stands 5 feet from the person, holds up a random number of fingers, and then asks the patient to count the number of fingers seen. If the patient is unable to count fingers at 5 feet, the examiner keeps moving a foot closer until either 1 foot away or the person can correctly count fingers. If the patient correctly counts the number of fingers at 3 feet, for example, the examiner would record vision as CF/3 ft.

ASSESSMENT
Chart 63-1
Taking a History of Patients With Eye and Vision Disorders

- What does the patient perceive to be the problem?
- Is visual acuity diminished?
- Does the patient experience blurred, double, or distorted vision?
- Is there pain? Is it sharp or dull? Is it worse when blinking?
- Is the discomfort an itching sensation or more of a foreign-body sensation?
- Are both eyes affected?
- Is there a history of discharge? If so, inquire about color, consistency, and odor.
- Describe the onset of the problem (sudden, gradual). Is it worsening?

- What is the duration of the problem?
- Is this a recurrence of a previous condition?
- How has the patient self-treated?
- What makes the symptoms improve or worsen?
- Has the condition affected performance of activities of daily living?
- Are there any systemic diseases? What medications are used in their treatment?
- What other eye conditions does the patient have?
- Is there a history of eye surgery?
- Have other family members had the same symptoms or condition?

Adapted from Weber, J., & Kelley, J. (2014). *Health assessment in nursing* (5th ed.). Philadelphia, PA: Lippincott Williams & Wilkins.

If the patient cannot count fingers, the examiner raises one hand up and down or moves it side to side and asks in which direction the hand is moving. This level of vision is known as hand motion. A patient who can perceive only light is described as having light perception. The vision of a patient who cannot perceive light is described as no light perception.

External Eye Examination

The nurse uses a systematic approach to perform an external eye examination by first assessing for symmetry and placement of eyelids, pupils, and muscles. CNs III, IV, and VI control movement and pupil size. The eyelids should rest just above and below the corneal limbus without exposure of the sclera. The nurse observes for **ptosis** (drooping of the

---

GENETICS IN NURSING PRACTICE
Chart 63-2
Eye and Vision Disorders

Several eye and vision disorders are associated with genetic abnormalities. Some examples include:

Autosomal dominant:

- Aniridia
- Vitelliform macular dystrophy

Autosomal recessive:

- Achromatopsia
- Homocystinuria
- Leber congenital amaurosis

X linked:

- Choroideremia
- Color blindness

Mitochondrial inheritance:

- Leber hereditary optic neuropathy

Multiple inheritance patterns identified:

- Glaucoma
- Macular degeneration
- Retinitis pigmentosa

Other genetic illness that will impact vision:

- Albinism
- Isolated familial congenital cataracts
- Marfan syndrome
- Stickler syndrome
- Tay–Sachs disease
- Usher syndrome

Nursing Assessments

Refer to Chapter 5, Chart 5-2: Genetics in Nursing Practice: Genetic Aspects of Health Assessment

Family History Assessment Specific to Vision

- Assess history of family members in the past three generations with glaucoma, cataracts, night blindness (retinitis pigmentosa), color blindness, or other vision impairment.
- Inquire about the age of onset of symptoms (the onset of Leber congenital amaurosis is in childhood, whereas the onset of Leber hereditary optic neuropathy is in young adulthood).
- Inquire about family members with other disorders that may include visual impairment, such as cutaneous, metabolic, or connective tissue disorders and hearing loss.

Patient Assessment Specific to Vision

- Assess for other systemic and/or clinical features such as cutaneous or skeletal conditions, or hearing loss.
- Look for color and clarity of iris.
- Assess for presence of strabismus (cross-eyes), amblyopia (lazy eye), nystagmus, astigmatism, and near- or far-sightedness.
- Assess for changes in visual acuity.
- Assess field of vision.
- Inquire about photophobia, night blindness, or double vision.

Genetics Resources

National Opthalmic Disease Genotyping Network, https://eyegene.nih.gov

See Chapter 8, Chart 8-7 for additional components of genetic counseling.

eyelid), **ectropion** (turning out of the lower eyelid), or **entropion** (turning in of the lower eyelid). Entropion may involve **trichiasis** (turning in of the eyelashes). Eyelids and lashes should be free of drainage or scaling.

The room should be darkened so that the pupils can be examined. The pupillary response is checked with a penlight to determine if the pupils are equally reactive and regular. A normal pupil is black. An irregular pupil may result from trauma, previous surgery, or a disease process.

The patient's eyes are observed in primary or direct gaze, and any head tilt is noted. A head tilt may indicate cranial nerve palsy. The patient is asked to stare at a target; each eye is covered and uncovered quickly while the examiner looks for any shift in gaze. The examiner observes for **nystagmus** (involuntary oscillating movement of the eyeball). The extraocular movements of the eyes are tested by having the patient follow the examiner's finger, pencil, or a hand light through the six cardinal directions of gaze (i.e., up, down, right, left, and both diagonals). This is especially important when screening patients for ocular trauma or for neurologic disorders such as stroke or myasthenia gravis (Hickey, 2014).

Diagnostic Evaluation

A wide range of diagnostic studies may be performed in patients with eye disorders. The nurse should educate the patient about the purpose, what to expect, and any possible side effects related to these examinations prior to testing. The nurse should be aware of contraindications, potential complications, and trends in results. Trends provide information about disease progression as well as the patient's response to therapy.

Direct Ophthalmoscopy

A direct ophthalmoscope is a handheld instrument with various plus and minus lenses (Weber & Kelley, 2014). The lenses can be rotated into place, enabling the examiner to bring the cornea, lens, and retina into focus sequentially. The examiner holds the ophthalmoscope in the right hand and uses the right eye to examine the patient's right eye. The examiner switches to the left hand and left eye when examining the patient's left eye. During this examination, the room should be darkened, and the patient's eye should be on the same level as the examiner's eye. The patient and the examiner should be comfortable, and both should breathe normally. The patient is given a target to gaze at and is encouraged to keep both eyes open and steady.

When the fundus is examined, the vasculature comes into focus first. The veins are larger in diameter than the arteries. The examiner focuses on a large vessel and then follows it toward the midline of the body, which leads to the optic nerve. The central depression in the disc is known as the cup. The normal cup is about one third the size of the diameter of the disc. The size of the physiologic optic cup should be estimated and the disc margins described as sharp or blurred. A silvery or coppery appearance, which indicates arteriolosclerosis, should be noted. The periphery of the retina is examined by having the patient shift their gaze. The last area of the fundus to be examined is the macula, because this area is the most sensitive to light. The retina of a young person often

has a glistening effect, sometimes referred to as a cellophane reflex.

The healthy fundus should be free of any lesions. The examiner looks for intraretinal hemorrhages, which may appear as red smudges, and, if the patient has hypertension, they may be somewhat flame shaped. Lipid with a yellowish appearance may be present in the retina of patients with hypercholesterolemia or diabetes. Soft exudates that have a fuzzy, white appearance (cotton-wool spots) should be noted. The examiner looks for microaneurysms, which look like little red dots, and nevi. Drusen (small, hyaline, globular deposits), commonly found in macular degeneration, appear as yellowish areas with indistinct edges. Small drusen have a more distinct edge. The examiner should sketch the fundus and document any abnormalities.

Indirect Ophthalmoscopy

The indirect ophthalmoscope is an instrument commonly used by the ophthalmologist to see larger areas of the retina, although in an unmagnified state. It produces a bright and intense light. The light source is affixed with a pair of binocular lenses mounted on the examiner's head. The ophthalmoscope is used with a handheld, 20-diopter lens.

Slit-Lamp Examination

The slit lamp is a binocular microscope mounted on a table. This instrument enables the user to examine the eye with magnification of 10 to 40 times the real image. The illumination can be varied from a broad to a narrow beam of light for different parts of the eye. For example, by varying the width and intensity of the light, the anterior chamber can be examined for signs of inflammation. Cataracts may be evaluated by changing the angle of the light. When a handheld contact lens, such as a three-mirror lens, is used with the slit lamp, the angle of the anterior chamber may be examined, as may the ocular fundus.

Tonometry

Tonometry is an essential part of a diagnostic evaluation; it measures IOP to screen for and manage glaucoma. The device used for measuring IOP is an accurately calibrated applanation tonometer, which measures the pressure needed to flatten the cornea. Because the probe or prism touches the highly sensitive cornea, a topical anesthetic is given prior to measurement (Hogan, 2014).

Nursing Interventions

Providing patient education prior to tonometry helps avoid possible errors in IOP measurement. Patients are cautioned to avoid squeezing the eyelids, holding their breath, or performing a Valsalva maneuver, because these may result in abnormally increased IOP.

Color Vision Testing

The ability to differentiate colors has a dramatic effect on the activities of daily living (ADLs). For example, the inability to differentiate between red and green can compromise traffic safety. Some careers (e.g., commercial artist, [color] photographer, airline pilot, and electrician) may be closed to people with significant color deficiencies. The photoreceptor cells responsible for color vision are the cones, and the greatest area of color sensitivity is in the macula—the area of densest cone concentration.

A screening test, such as the polychromatic plates discussed in the next paragraph, can be used to establish whether a person's color vision is within normal range. Color vision deficits can be inherited. For example, red–green color deficiencies are inherited in an X-linked manner, affecting approximately 8% of men and 0.5% of women (Colour Blind Awareness, 2016). Acquired color vision losses may be caused by medications (e.g., digitalis) or pathology (e.g., cataracts). A simple test, such as asking a patient if the red top on a bottle of eye drops appears redder to one eye than the other, can be an effective tool. A difference in the perception of the intensity of the color red between the two eyes can be a symptom of a neurologic problem and may provide information about the location of the lesion.

Because alteration in color vision sometimes indicates conditions of the optic nerve, color vision testing is often performed in a neuro-ophthalmologic workup. The most common color vision test is performed using Ishihara polychromatic plates. These plates are bound together in a booklet. On each plate of this booklet are dots of primary colors that are integrated into a background of secondary colors. The dots are arranged in simple patterns, such as numbers or geometric shapes. Patients with diminished color vision may be unable to identify the hidden shapes. Patients with central vision conditions (e.g., macular degeneration) have more difficulty identifying colors than those with peripheral vision conditions (e.g., glaucoma) because central vision identifies color.

Amsler Grid

The Amsler grid is a test often used for patients with macular problems, such as macular degeneration. It consists of a geometric grid of identical squares with a central fixation point. The grid should be viewed by the patient wearing normal reading glasses. Each eye is tested separately. The patient is instructed to stare at the central fixation spot on the grid and report any distortion in the squares of the grid itself. For patients with macular problems, some of the squares may look faded, or the lines may be wavy. Patients with age-related macular degeneration (AMD) are commonly given these Amsler grids to take home. The patient is encouraged to check the grids frequently, as often as daily, to monitor macular function for early detection of changes requiring immediate attention (Gerstenblith & Rabinowitz, 2017; Weber & Kelley, 2014).

Ultrasonography

Lesions in the globe or the orbit may not be directly visible and are evaluated by ultrasonography. Ultrasonography is a valuable diagnostic technique, especially when the view of the retina is obscured by opaque media such as cataract or hemorrhage. An ultrasonography B-scan identifies pathology such as orbital tumors, retinal detachment, and vitreous hemorrhage. Ultrasonography A-scans are used to measure the axial length for implants prior to cataract surgery (Gerstenblith & Rabinowitz, 2017).

Optical Coherence Tomography

Optical coherence tomography is a technology that involves low-coherence interferometry (Boyd, 2015; Gerstenblith & Rabinowitz, 2017). Light is used to evaluate retinal and macular diseases as well as anterior segment conditions. This method is noninvasive and involves no physical contact with the eye.

Fundus Photography

Fundus photography is used to detect and document retinal lesions. The patient's pupils are usually widely dilated before the procedure. The resulting fundus photographs can be viewed stereoscopically so that elevations such as macular edema can be identified.

Laser Scanning

Various scanning techniques use laser light in the diagnostic evaluation of eye disorders. Confocal laser scanning ophthalmoscopy provides a three-dimensional image of the optic nerve topography and is used alone or in conjunction with fundus photography to provide comparative data for suspected optic nerve disease such as glaucoma and **papilledema** (swelling of the optic disc due to increased intracranial pressure) (Gerstenblith & Rabinowitz, 2017). Laser scanning polarimetry is used to measure nerve fiber layer thickness and is an important indicator of glaucoma progression.

Angiography

Angiography is done using fluorescein or indocyanine green as contrast agents. Fluorescein angiography is used to evaluate clinically significant macular edema, document macular capillary nonperfusion, and identify retinal and choroidal **neovascularization** (growth of abnormal new blood vessels) in AMD. It is an invasive procedure in which fluorescein dye is injected, usually into an antecubital vein. Within 10 to 15 seconds, this dye can be seen coursing through the retinal vessels. Over a 10-minute period, serial black-and-white photographs are taken of the retinal vasculature.

Indocyanine green angiography is used to evaluate abnormalities in the choroidal vasculature, which often are seen in macular degeneration. Indocyanine green dye is injected intravenously (IV), and multiple images are captured using digital video angiography over a period of 30 seconds to 20 minutes.

Nursing Interventions

Prior to the angiography, the patient's blood urea nitrogen and creatinine should be checked to ensure that the kidneys will excrete the contrast agent (Fischbach & Dunning, 2015). The patient should be well hydrated, and clear liquids are usually permitted up to the time of the test. The patient is instructed to remain immobile during the angiogram process and is told to expect a brief feeling of warmth in the face, behind the eyes, or in the jaw, teeth, tongue, and lips, and a metallic taste when the contrast agent is injected.

Nursing care after angiography includes observation of the injection site (usually the antecubital vein) for bleeding or hematoma formation (a localized collection of blood). Fluorescein may impart a gold tone to the skin in some patients, and urine may turn deep yellow or orange. This discoloration usually disappears in 24 hours. Indocyanine green dye is generally well tolerated, but some patients experience nausea and vomiting. Allergic reactions are rare; however, indocyanine green angiography is contraindicated in patients with a history of iodide reactions. Fluids are encouraged following the procedure to facilitate excretion of the contrast agent (Fischbach & Dunning, 2015).

Perimetry Testing

Perimetry testing evaluates the field of vision. Visual field testing (i.e., perimetry) helps identify which parts of the patient's central and peripheral visual fields have useful vision. It is most helpful in detecting central **scotomas** (blind or partially blind areas in the visual field) in macular degeneration and the peripheral field defects in glaucoma and retinitis pigmentosa. Visual field evaluation and optic nerve assessment are major components of monitoring and detecting glaucoma progression.

IMPAIRED VISION

Refractive Errors

In refractive errors, vision is impaired because a shortened or elongated eyeball prevents light rays from focusing sharply on the retina. Blurred vision from refractive error can be corrected with eyeglasses or contact lenses. Ophthalmic **refraction** is the determination of the refractive errors of the eye for the purpose of vision correction and consists of placing various types of lenses in front of the patient's eyes to determine which lens best improves the patient's vision.

The depth of the eyeball is important in determining refractive error (see Fig. 63-5). Patients for whom the visual image focuses precisely on the macula and who do not need eyeglasses or contact lenses are said to have **emmetropia**, a normal refractive condition resulting in clear focus on retina with no optical defects (normal vision). Some people have deeper eyeballs, in which case the distant visual image focuses in front of, or short of, the retina; those with **myopia** are said to be nearsighted and have blurred distance vision. Other people have shallower eyeballs, in which case the visual image focuses beyond the retina; those with **hyperopia** are said to be farsighted and have excellent distance vision but blurry near vision (Weber & Kelley, 2014).

Wavefront technology to measure unique refractive imperfections of the cornea or higher aberrations (i.e., myopia, hyperopia, astigmatism) can be used to customize laser-assisted in situ keratomileusis (LASIK) procedures. These procedures are described later in this chapter.

Vision Impairment and Blindness

Vision impairment is defined as having best corrected visual acuity of 20/40 or worse in the better-seeing eye. *Low vision* describes visual impairment that requires the use of devices and strategies to perform visual tasks.

Blindness is having best corrected visual acuity that can range from 20/400 to no light perception. The clinical definition of absolute blindness is the absence of light perception. Legal blindness is a condition of impaired vision in which a

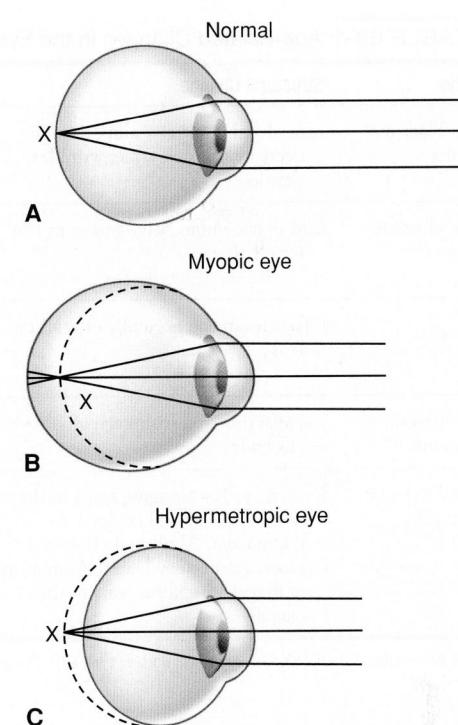

Figure 63-5 • Eyeball shape determines visual acuity in refractive errors. **A.** Normal eye. **B.** Myopic eye. **C.** Hypermetropic eye.

person has best corrected visual acuity that does not exceed 20/200 in the better eye or whose widest visual field diameter is 20 degrees or less (Prevent Blindness America, 2012). This definition neither equates with functional ability nor classifies the degrees of visual impairment. Legal blindness ranges from an inability to perceive light to having some vision remaining. A person who meets the criteria for legal blindness may be eligible for government financial assistance through disability.

Assessment and Diagnostic Testing

Assessment of vision impairment includes a thorough history and examination of distance and near visual acuity, visual field, contrast sensitivity, glare, color perception, and refraction. Specially designed, low vision visual acuity charts are used to evaluate patients.

Patient Interview

During history taking, the cause and duration of the patient's visual impairment are identified. Patients with retinitis pigmentosa, for example, have a genetic abnormality. Patients with diabetic macular edema typically have fluctuating visual acuity. Patients with macular degeneration have central acuity problems that cause difficulty in performing activities that require finer vision, such as reading. People with peripheral field defects have more difficulties with mobility. The patient's customary ADLs, medication regimen, habits (e.g., smoking), acceptance of the physical limitations brought about by the visual impairment, and realistic expectations of low vision aids are identified and included in the plan of care, as well as provision of guidelines for safety and referrals to social services.

TABLE 63-1 Age-Related Changes in the Eye

External Eye	Structural Change	Functional Change	History and Physical Findings
Eyelids and lacrimal structures	Loss of skin elasticity and orbital fat, decreased muscle tone; wrinkles develop	Lid margins turn in, causing entropion; or lid margins turn out, resulting in ectropion.	Reports of burning, foreign-body sensation, epiphora; injection, inflammation, and ulceration may occur.
Refractive changes; presbyopia	Loss of accommodative power in the lens with age	Reading materials must be held at increasing distance in order to focus.	Patient reports, "Arms are too short!"; need for increased light; reading glasses or bifocals needed.
Cataract	Opacities in the normally crystalline lens	Interference with the focus of a sharp image on the retina.	Patients report increased glare, decreased vision, changes in color values (blue and yellow especially affected).
Posterior vitreous detachment	Liquefaction and shrinkage of vitreous body	May lead to retinal tears and detachment.	Reports light flashes, cobwebs, floaters.
Age-related macular degeneration (AMD)	Drusen (yellowish aging spots in the retina) appear and coalesce in the macula. Abnormal choroidal blood vessels may lead to formation of fibrotic disciform scars in the macula	Central vision is affected; onset is more gradual in dry AMD, more rapid in wet AMD; distortion and loss of central vision may occur.	Reading vision is affected; words may be missing letters, faded areas appear on the page, straight lines may appear wavy; drusen, pigmentary changes in retina; abnormal submacular choroidal vessels.

Adapted from Eliopoulos, C. (2018). *Gerontological nursing* (9th ed.). Philadelphia, PA: Lippincott Williams & Wilkins.

Contrast-Sensitivity Testing and Glare Testing

Contrast-sensitivity testing measures visual acuity in different degrees of light and dark contrast to determine visual function. Glare testing is also used to determine visual function. Glare can reduce a person's ability to see, especially in patients with cataracts. Those affected by loss of contrast sensitivity and glare have difficulty functioning in low light, or driving at night or in foggy conditions. People with a loss of contrast sensitivity may benefit from better illumination.

 Gerontologic Considerations

Approximately half of all individuals who are identified as legally blind each year are 65 years of age or older (Eliopoulos, 2018). With aging, structural and functional changes occur in the eye. **Presbyopia**, the loss of accommodative power in the lens, interferes with the ability to adequately focus and is the factor responsible for most older adults requiring some form of corrective lenses (Eliopoulos, 2018). Age-related changes in the eye are summarized in Table 63-1.

Impaired vision is often accompanied by difficulty in performing functional activities. People with visual acuity of 20/80 to 20/100 with a visual field restriction of 60 degrees to greater than 20 degrees can read at a nearly normal level with optical aids. Their visual orientation is near normal but requires increased scanning of the environment (i.e., systematic use of head and eye movements). In a visual acuity range of 20/200 to 20/400 with a 20-degree to greater than 10-degree visual field restriction, the person can read slowly with optical aids.

The most common causes of blindness and visual impairment among adults 40 years and older are diabetic retinopathy, macular degeneration, glaucoma, and cataracts (Prevent Blindness America, 2012). Macular degeneration is more prevalent among Caucasians, whereas glaucoma is more prevalent among African Americans (Eliopoulos, 2018).

Medical Management

Managing vision impairment involves magnification and image enhancement through the use of low vision aids and strategies, as well as referrals to social services and community agencies. The goals are to optimize the patient's remaining vision and assist the patient to perform customary activities. Table 63-2 presents low vision aids. Medications are prescribed for glaucoma. Ongoing research suggests that gene therapy may replace or be an adjunct to pharmacologic or surgical treatment for ocular disorders in the near future (Lee & Garg, 2015).

Referrals to community agencies may be necessary for patients with low vision who live alone and cannot self-administer their medications. Community agencies, such as the Lighthouse Guild, offer a wide variety of vision and health care services to patients with low vision and blindness.

Nursing Management

Nurses need to increase their sensitivity to the challenges faced by patients with visual impairments. Coping with blindness involves emotional, physical, and social adaptation. The emotional adjustment to blindness or severe visual impairment determines the success of the physical and social adjustments of the patient. Successful emotional adjustment means acceptance of blindness or severe visual impairment.

Promoting Coping

Effective coping may not occur until the patient recognizes the permanence of the low vision or blindness. A patient who is newly visually impaired and their family members undergo the various steps of grieving: denial and shock, anger and protest, restitution, loss resolution, and acceptance. The ability to accept the changes that must come with visual loss and willingness to adapt to those changes influence the successful rehabilitation of the patient with vision loss. Additional

TABLE 63-2 Activities Affected by Visual Impairment and Suggestions for Low Vision Aids

Activity	Optical Aids	Nonoptical Aids
Shopping	Hand magnifier	Lighting, color cues
Fixing a snack	Bifocals	Color cues; consistent food storage plan
Eating out	Hand magnifier	Flashlight, portable lamp
Identifying money	Bifocals, hand magnifier	Arrange paper money in wallet compartments
Reading print	High-power spectacle, bifocals, hand magnifier, stand magnifier, closed-circuit television	Lighting, high-contrast print, large print, reading slit
Writing	Hand magnifier	Lighting, bold-tip pen, black ink
Using a telephone	Hand magnifier	Large-print buttons, hand-printed directory Braille phones, picture/photo phones, and talking phones
Crossing streets	Lightweight handheld monoscopes/telescopes	Cane; ask directions
Finding taxis and bus signs	Lightweight handheld monoscopes/telescopes	Ask for assistance
Reading medication labels	Hand magnifier	Color codes, large print
Reading stove dials	Hand magnifier	Color codes, raised dots
Adjusting the thermostat	Hand magnifier	Enlarged-print model
Using a computer	Spectacles	High-contrast color, large-print program. Screen-reader programs convert text on the computer screen to synthesized speech
Reading signs	Spectacles	Move closer
Watching sporting event	Lightweight handheld monoscopes/telescopes	Sit in front rows

Adapted from Pagliuca, L. M., Macedo-Costa, K. N., Reboucas, G. B., et al. (2014). Validation of the general guidelines of communication between the nurse and the blind. *Reviews Bras Enferm,*67(5), 715–725.

aspects to consider are value changes, independence–dependence conflicts, coping with stigma, and learning to function in social settings without visual cues and landmarks.

Promoting Spatial Orientation and Mobility

A person who is blind or severely visually impaired requires strategies for adapting to the environment. ADLs, such as walking to a chair from a bed, require spatial concepts. The person needs to know where he or she is in relation to the rest of the room, to understand the changes that may occur, and to know how to approach the desired location safely. This requires a collaborative effort between the patient and the responsible adult who serves as the sighted guide. The nurse must assess the degree of physical assistance the person with vision loss requires and communicate this to other health care personnel.

The nurse should be aware of the importance of techniques in providing physical assistance, encouraging independence, and ensuring safety. Strategies for interacting with the patient with vision loss are presented in Chart 63-3. Research supports the use of a validated protocol to educate staff to perform therapeutic communication, deliver services, and minimize communication barriers with patients who are blind (Pagliuca, Macedo-Costa, Reboucas, et al., 2014). The readiness of the patient and family to learn

must be assessed before initiating orientation and mobility training.

Promoting Home, Community-Based, and Transitional Care

The nurse, social worker, family, and others collaborate to assess the patient's home condition and support system. A low vision specialist or occupational therapist should be consulted, particularly for patients for whom identifying and administering medications pose challenges. Referral for vision rehabilitation should be provided for appropriate patients (American Academy of Ophthalmology Vision Rehabilitation Committee, 2012).

Other interventions that are appropriate for some people with visual impairment or blindness include Braille and service animals. There has been an ever-increasing reliance on print magnification technology as well as computer-assisted speech output. However, although the use of Braille may be less important for adults who have already learned language and grammar skills, educators and low vision specialists have continued to advocate that children who are legally blind be given the opportunity to learn Braille.

Guide dogs, also known as service dogs, are dogs that are specially bred, raised, and rigorously trained to assist people who are blind. The guide dog is a constant companion to

Chart 63-3 · Strategies for Interacting With People Who Are Blind or Have Low Vision

- Remember that the only difference between you and people who are blind or have low vision is that they are not able to see through their eyes what you are able to see through yours.
- Do not be uncomfortable when in the company of a person who is blind or has low vision. Talk with the person as you would talk with any other individual, honestly and without pity; do not be concerned about using words like "see" and "look." There is no need to raise your voice unless the person asks you to do so.
- Identify yourself as you approach the person and before you make physical contact. Tell the person your name and your role. If another person approaches, introduce him or her. When you leave the room, be sure to tell the person that you are leaving and if anyone else remains in the room.
- Keep in mind that it is often appropriate to touch the person's hand or arm lightly to indicate that you are about to speak.
- When talking, face the person and speak directly to him or her using a normal tone of voice.
- Be specific when communicating direction. Mention a specific distance or use clock cues when possible (e.g., walk left about 2 yards; walk about 20 feet to the right; the telephone is at 2 o'clock). Avoid using phrases such as "over there."
- When you offer to assist someone, allow the person to hold on to your arm just above the elbow and to walk a half-step behind you.

- When offering the person a seat, place the person's hand on the back or the arm of the seat.
- When you are about to go up or down a flight of stairs, tell the person and place their hand on the banister.
- Make sure that the environment is free of obstacles; close doors and cabinets so that they are not in the path.
- Offer to read written information, such as a menu.
- If you serve food to the person, use clock cues to specify where everything is on the plate.
- When the person who is blind or has low vision is a patient in a health care facility:
  - Make sure all objects the person will need are close at hand.
  - Identify the location of objects that the person may need (e.g., "The call light is near your right hand"; "The telephone is on the table on the left side of your bed.")
  - Remove obstacles that may be in the person's pathway and could cause a fall.
  - Place all assistive devices that the person uses close at hand; let the person feel the devices so that he or she knows their location.
- Do not distract a service animal unless the owner has given permission.
- Ask the person, "How can I help you?" At some times, the person needs help; at other times, help may not be needed.

Adapted from Pagliuca, L. M., Macedo-Costa, K. N., Reboucas, G. B., et al. (2014). Validation of the general guidelines of communication between the nurse and the blind. *Reviews Bras Enferm*, 67(5), 715–725.

---

the person who is blind (also referred to as the animal's handler) and is allowed on airplanes and in restaurants, stores, hotels, and other public places. With the assistance of the guide dog, the person who is blind can be extremely mobile and accomplish normal activities both within and outside of the home and workplace. A dog in harness is a working dog, not a pet. The dog should not be distracted from his job by well-intentioned strangers who want to pet, feed, or play with the animal. The dog's handler should always be consulted before approaching the working guide dog. Most health care facilities have a service animal policy that outlines the responsibilities of the handler with regard to the care of the animal.

Unfolding Patient Stories: Vernon Watkins • Part 2

Recall from Chapter 17 **Vernon Watkins,** who came to the emergency department with severe abdominal pain and underwent a hemicolectomy for a bowel perforation. During postoperative care the nurse determines that he has poor vision. What measures can the nurse take to maintain a safe environment for a patient with visual impairment? How will the discovery of impaired vision impact the nursing plan of care, discharge planning, and delivery of patient education? Care for Vernon and other patients in a realistic virtual environment: *vSim for Nursing* **(thepoint.lww. com/vSimMedicalSurgical).** Practice documenting these patients' care in DocuCare **(thepoint.lww.com/ DocuCareEHR).**

OCULAR MEDICATION ADMINISTRATION

Because medications are often prescribed to treat ocular disorders, nurses must understand the actions of the commonly used medications and effective administration. The main objective of ocular medication delivery is to maximize the amount of medication that reaches the ocular site of action in sufficient concentration to produce a beneficial therapeutic effect. This is determined by the dynamics of ocular pharmacokinetics: absorption, distribution, metabolism, and excretion.

Ocular absorption involves the entry of a medication into the aqueous humor through the different routes of ocular medication administration. The rate and extent of aqueous humor absorption are determined by the characteristics of the medication and the anatomy and physiology of the eye. Natural barriers of absorption that diminish the efficacy of ocular medications include the following:

- *Limited size of the conjunctival sac.* The conjunctival sac can hold only 50 mcL, and any excess is wasted. The volume of one eye drop from commercial topical ocular solutions typically ranges from 20 to 35 mcL.
- *Corneal membrane barriers.* The epithelial, stromal, and endothelial layers are barriers to absorption.
- *Blood–ocular barriers.* Blood–ocular barriers prevent high ocular tissue concentration of most ophthalmic medications because they separate the bloodstream from the ocular tissues and keep foreign substances from entering the eye, thereby limiting a medication's efficacy.
- *Tearing, blinking, and drainage.* Increased tear production and drainage due to ocular irritation or an ocular condition may dilute or wash out an instilled eye drop;

blinking expels an instilled eye drop from the conjunctival sac.

Distribution of an ocular medication into the various ocular tissues varies by tissue type—the conjunctiva, cornea, lens, iris, ciliary body, and choroids absorb medications to varying degrees. Medications penetrate the corneal epithelium by diffusion by passing through the cells (intracellular) or by passing between the cells (intercellular). Water-soluble (hydrophilic) medications diffuse through the intracellular route, and fat-soluble (lipophilic) medications diffuse through the intercellular route. Topical administration usually does not reach the retina in significant concentrations. Because the space between the ciliary process and the lens is small, medication diffusion in the vitreous is slow. When high concentrations of medication in the vitreous are required, intraocular injection is often chosen to bypass the natural ocular anatomic and physiologic barriers (American Society of Ophthalmic Registered Nurses [ASORN], 2013).

Aqueous solutions are most commonly used for the eye. They are the least expensive medications and interfere the least with vision. However, corneal contact time is brief because tears dilute the medication. Ophthalmic ointments have extended retention time in the conjunctival sac and provide a higher concentration than eye drops. The major disadvantage of ointments is the blurred vision that results after application. In general, eyelids and eyelid margins are best treated with ointments. The conjunctiva, limbus, cornea, and anterior chamber are treated most effectively with instilled solutions or suspensions. Subconjunctival injection may be necessary for better absorption in the anterior chamber. If high medication concentrations are required in the posterior chamber, intravitreal injections or systemically absorbed medications are considered. Contact lenses and collagen shields soaked in antibiotic agents are alternative delivery methods for treating corneal infections.

Of all these delivery methods, the topical route of administration—instilled eye drops and applied ointments—remains the most common (ASORN, 2013). Topical instillation, which is the least invasive method, permits self-administration of medication and produces fewer side effects.

Preservatives are commonly used in ocular medications. Benzalkonium chloride, for example, prevents the growth of organisms and enhances the corneal permeability of most medications; however, some patients are allergic to this preservative. This may be suspected even if the patient had never before experienced an allergic reaction to systemic use of the medication in question. Eye drops without preservatives can be prepared by pharmacists.

Common Ocular Medications

Common ocular medications include topical anesthetic, mydriatic, and cycloplegic agents that reduce IOP; anti-infective medications; corticosteroids; nonsteroidal anti-inflammatory drugs (NSAIDs); antiallergy medications; eye irrigants; and lubricants.

Topical Anesthetic Agents

One or two drops of proparacaine hydrochloride (Ophthaine 0.5%) and tetracaine hydrochloride (Pontocaine 0.5%) are instilled before diagnostic procedures such as tonometry and minor ocular procedures such as removal of sutures or conjunctival or corneal scrapings. Topical anesthetic agents are also used for severe eye pain to allow the patient to open their eyes for examination or treatment (e.g., eye irrigation for chemical burns). Anesthesia occurs within 20 seconds to 1 minute and lasts 10 to 20 minutes. The nurse must educate the patient not to rub the eyes while anesthetized because this may result in corneal damage.

Mydriatic and Cycloplegic Agents

Mydriasis, or pupil dilation, is the main objective of the administration of mydriatics and cycloplegics (see Table 63-3). These two types of medications function differently and are used in combination to achieve the maximal dilation that is needed during surgery and fundus examinations to give the ophthalmologist a better view of the internal eye structures. Mydriatics potentiate alpha-adrenergic sympathetic effects that result in the relaxation of the ciliary muscle. This causes the pupil to dilate. However, this sympathetic action alone is not enough to sustain mydriasis because of its short duration of action. The strong light used during an eye examination also stimulates miosis (i.e., pupillary contraction). Cycloplegic medications are given to paralyze the iris sphincter.

The patient is educated about the temporary effects of mydriasis on vision, such as glare and the inability to focus properly. The patient may have difficulty reading. The effects of the various mydriatics and cycloplegics can last 3 hours to several days. The patient is advised to wear sunglasses (most eye clinics provide protective sunglasses). The ability to drive depends on the person's age, vision, and comfort level. Some patients can drive safely with the use of sunglasses, whereas others may need to be driven home.

Mydriatic and cycloplegic agents affect the central nervous system. Their effects are most prominent in younger and older adult patients; these patients must be assessed closely for symptoms, such as increased blood pressure, tachycardia, dizziness, ataxia, confusion, disorientation, incoherent speech, and hallucination. These medications are contraindicated in patients with narrow angles or shallow anterior chambers and in patients taking monoamine oxidase inhibitors or tricyclic antidepressants.

Medications Used to Treat Glaucoma

Therapeutic medications for glaucoma are used to lower IOP by decreasing aqueous production or increasing aqueous outflow. Because glaucoma calls for lifetime therapy, the patient must be educated with regard to both the ocular and systemic side effects of the medications. See section on glaucoma later in this chapter.

Anti-Infective Medications

Anti-infective medications include antibiotic, antifungal, and antiviral agents. Most are available as drops, ointments, or subconjunctival or intravitreal injections. Antibiotics include penicillin, cephalosporins, aminoglycosides, and fluoroquinolones. The main antifungal agent is amphotericin B. Side effects of amphotericin are serious and include severe pain, conjunctival necrosis, iritis, and retinal toxicity. Antiviral medications include acyclovir (Zovirax) and ganciclovir (Cytovene). They are used to treat ocular infections associated with herpes virus and cytomegalovirus (CMV). Patients

TABLE 63-3 Mydriatics and Cycloplegics

Medication	Available Preparation/ Concentration	Indication/Dosage	Peak		Recovery Time	
			Mydriasis (Minutes)	Cycloplegia (Minutes)	Mydriasis	Cycloplegia
phenylephrine (Neo-Synephrine)	Solutions (2.5%, 10%)	Given with cycloplegics in pupillary dilation for ophthalmoscopy and surgical procedures every 5–10 minutes × 3 or until the pupils are fully dilated	10–60	—	3–6 hours	—
atropine (Isopto Ophthalmic)	Ointment (0.5–2%) Solutions (0.5–3%)	In uveitis, or after surgery, 2–4 × daily	30–40	60–180	7–10 days	6–12 days
scopolamine (Isopto Hyoscine Ophthalmic)	Solution (0.25%)	Same as atropine	20–30	30–60	3–7 days	3–7 days
homatropine (Homatropine HBr)	Solution (5–2.5%)	Same as atropine and scopolamine	40–60	30–60	1–3 days	1–3 days
cyclopentolate (AK-Pentolate)	Solution (0.5–2%)	Given with mydriatics every 5–10 minutes × 3 or until the pupils are fully dilated for ophthalmoscopy and surgical procedures	30–60	25–75	1 day	6–24 hours
tropicamide (Myrdal)	Solution (0.25–1%)		20–40	20–35	6 hours	<6 hours

Adapted from Comerford, K. C. (2015). *Nursing 2015 drug handbook*. Philadelphia, PA: Wolters Kluwer.

receiving ocular anti-infective agents are subject to the same side effects and adverse reactions as those receiving oral or parenteral medications.

Corticosteroids and Nonsteroidal Anti-Inflammatory Drugs

Topical preparations of corticosteroids are commonly used in inflammatory conditions of the eyelids, conjunctiva, cornea, anterior chamber, lens, and uvea. In posterior segment diseases that involve the posterior sclera, retina, and optic nerve, topical agents are less effective and parenteral and oral routes are preferred. When a suspension is prescribed, the patient is instructed to shake the bottle several times to promote mixture of the medication and maximize its therapeutic effect. The most common ocular side effects of long-term topical corticosteroid administration are glaucoma, cataracts, susceptibility to infection, impaired wound healing, mydriasis, and ptosis. High IOP may develop, which is reversible after corticosteroid use is discontinued. To avoid the side effects of corticosteroids, NSAIDs are used as an alternative in controlling inflammatory eye conditions and postoperatively to reduce inflammation.

Antiallergy Medications

Ocular hypersensitivity reactions, such as allergic conjunctivitis, are extremely common. These conditions result primarily from responses to environmental allergens. Most allergens are airborne or carried to the eye by the hand or by other means, although allergic reactions may also be drug induced. Corticosteroids are commonly used as anti-inflammatory and immunosuppressive agents to control ocular hypersensitivity reactions.

Ocular Irrigants and Lubricants

Most irrigating solutions are used to cleanse the external lids to maintain lid hygiene, to irrigate the external corneal surface to regain normal pH (e.g., in chemical burns), to irrigate the corneal surface to eliminate debris, or to inflate the globe intraoperatively. These solutions have various compositions that include sodium, potassium, magnesium, calcium, bicarbonate, glucose, and glutathione (i.e., substance found in the aqueous humor). Sterile irrigating solutions, such as Dacriose, for lid hygiene are available. Irrigating solutions are safe to use with an intact corneal surface; however, the corneal surface should not be irrigated in cases of threatened corneal perforation. For patients with severe corneal ulcer, specific instructions from the ophthalmologist must be obtained regarding whether it is safe to irrigate the corneal surface or just to cleanse the external lids. Although it is good practice to promote hygiene, prevention of complications must be the primary concern. Normal saline solutions are commonly used to irrigate the corneal surface when chemical burns occur.

Lubricants, such as artificial tears, help alleviate corneal irritation, such as dry eye syndrome. Artificial tears are topical preparations of carboxymethylcellulose or hydroxypropyl methylcellulose that are prepared as eye drop solutions, ointments, or ocular inserts (inserted at the lower conjunctival cul-de-sac once each day). The eye drops can be instilled as often as every hour, depending on the severity of symptoms.

Nursing Management

The objectives in administering ocular medications are to ensure proper administration to maximize the therapeutic effects and to ensure the safety of the patient by monitoring for systemic and local side effects (ASORN, 2013). Absorption of eye drops by the nasolacrimal duct is undesirable because of the potential systemic side effects of ocular medications. To diminish systemic absorption and minimize the side effects, it is important to occlude the puncta (see Chart 63-4). This is especially important for patients who are most vulnerable to medication overdose, including older adults; women who are pregnant or lactating; and patients with cardiac, pulmonary, hepatic, or kidney disease. A 5-minute interval between instillation of different types of ocular drops is recommended.

Before the administration of ocular medications, the nurse warns the patient that blurred vision, stinging, and a burning sensation are symptoms that ordinarily occur after instillation and are temporary. Risk for interactions of the ocular medication with other ocular and systemic medications must be emphasized; therefore, a careful patient interview regarding the medications being taken must be obtained.

🚩 **Quality and Safety Nursing Alert**

To prevent infection, meticulous hand hygiene before and after medication instillation is crucial. In addition, the tip of the eye drop bottle or the ointment tube must never touch any part of the eye, and the medication must be recapped immediately after each use.

Chart 63-4 — PATIENT EDUCATION
Instilling Eye Medications

The nurse instructs the patient to:

- Never use eye solutions that have changed colors.
- Perform hand hygiene before and after the procedure.
- Ensure adequate lighting.
- Read the label of the eye medication to verify that it is the correct medication.
- Remove contact lens as needed.
- Assume a comfortable position.
- Avoid touching the tip of the medication container to any part of the eye or face.
- Hold the lower lid down; do not press on the eyeball. Apply gentle pressure to the cheekbone to anchor the finger holding the lid.

- Instill eye drops before applying ointments.
- Apply a 0.25–0.5-inch ribbon of ointment to the lower conjunctival sac.

- Keep the eyelids closed, and apply gentle pressure on the inner canthus (punctal occlusion) near the bridge of the nose for 1 or 2 minutes immediately after instilling eye drops.
- Use a clean tissue to gently pat skin to absorb excess eye drops that run onto the cheeks.
- Wait 5 minutes before instilling another eye drop and 10 minutes before instilling another ointment.
- Reinsert contact lens if applicable.

Adapted from American Society of Ophthalmic Registered Nurses (ASORN). (2013). *Recommended practice for registered nurses–Use of multi-dose medications*. San Francisco, CA: Author; Comerford, K. C. (2015). *Nursing 2015 drug handbook*. Philadelphia, PA: Wolters Kluwer.

If a patient who instills their own medications cannot feel the eye drops when they are instilled, the eye medication may be refrigerated, because a cold drop is easier to detect. A 5-minute interval between successive administrations allows adequate drug retention and absorption. The patient or the caregiver at home should be asked to demonstrate actual eye drop or ointment instillation and punctal occlusion.

GLAUCOMA

The term **glaucoma** is used to refer to a group of ocular conditions characterized by elevated IOP (Eldaly et al., 2014). If left untreated, the increased IOP damages the optic nerve and nerve fiber layer, but the degree of harm is highly variable (Eliopoulos, 2018). The optic nerve damage is related to the IOP caused by congestion of aqueous humor in the eye. A range of IOPs are considered "normal," but these may also be associated with vision loss in some patients.

Glaucoma is estimated to affect 3 million Americans, approximately 50% of whom are undiagnosed (Grossman & Porth, 2014). Glaucoma is more prevalent in people older than 40 years, and it is the third most common age-related eye disease in the United States. Chart 63-5 presents the risk factors for glaucoma. There is no cure for glaucoma, but the disease can be controlled (Glaucoma Research Foundation, 2016).

Physiology

Aqueous humor flows between the iris and the lens, nourishing the cornea and lens. Most (90%) of the fluid then flows out of the anterior chamber, draining through the spongy trabecular meshwork into the canal of Schlemm and the episcleral veins (see Fig. 63-6). About 10% of the aqueous fluid exits through the ciliary body into the suprachoroidal space and then drains into the venous circulation of the ciliary body, choroid, and sclera (Grossman & Porth, 2014). Unimpeded outflow of aqueous fluid depends on an intact drainage system and an open angle (about 45 degrees) between the iris and the cornea. A narrower angle places the iris closer to the trabecular meshwork, diminishing the angle. The amount of aqueous humor produced tends to decrease with age, in systemic diseases such as diabetes, and in ocular inflammatory conditions.

Chart 63-5 ⚠	**RISK FACTORS** Glaucoma

- African American race
- Cardiovascular disease
- Diabetes
- Family history of glaucoma
- Migraine syndromes
- Nearsightedness (myopia)
- Older age
- Previous eye trauma
- Prolonged use of topical or systemic corticosteroids
- Thin cornea

Adapted from Grossman, S. C., & Porth, C. M. (2014). *Porth's Pathophysiology: Concepts of altered health states* (9th ed.). Philadelphia, PA: Lippincott Williams & Wilkins.

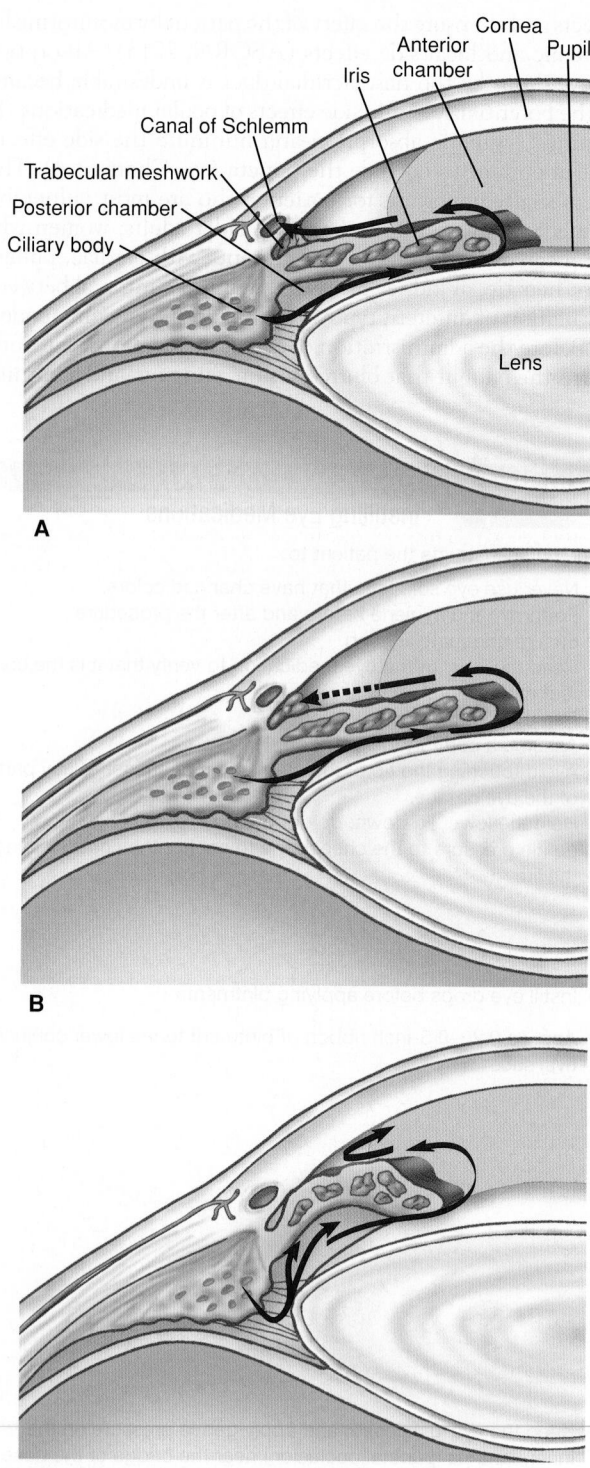

Figure 63-6 • **A.** Normally, aqueous humor, which is secreted in the posterior chamber, gains access to the anterior chamber by flowing through the pupil. In the angle of the anterior chamber, it passes through the canal of Schlemm into the venous system. **B.** In wide-angle glaucoma, the outflow of aqueous humor is obstructed at the trabecular meshwork. **C.** In narrow-angle glaucoma, the aqueous humor encounters resistance to flow through the pupil. Increased pressure in the posterior chamber produces a forward bowing of the peripheral iris so that the iris blocks the trabecular meshwork. Reprinted with permission from Grossman, S. C., & Porth, C. M. (2014). *Porth's pathophysiology: Concepts of altered health states* (9th ed.). Philadelphia, PA: Lippincott Williams & Wilkins.

IOP is determined by the rate of aqueous production, the resistance encountered by the aqueous humor as it flows out of the passages, and the venous pressure of the episcleral veins that drain into the anterior ciliary vein. When aqueous fluid production and drainage are in balance, the IOP is between 10 and 21 mmHg. When aqueous fluid is inhibited from flowing out, pressure builds up within the eye. Fluctuations in IOP occur with time of day, exertion, diet, and medications. IOP tends to increase with blinking, tight lid squeezing, and upward gazing. Systemic conditions such as diabetes and intraocular conditions such as uveitis and retinal detachment have been associated with elevated IOP. Glaucoma may not be recognized in people with thin corneas because measurement of the IOP may be falsely low as a result of this thinness.

Pathophysiology

There are two theories regarding how increased IOP damages the optic nerve in glaucoma. The direct mechanical theory suggests that high IOP damages the retinal layer as it passes through the optic nerve head. The indirect ischemic theory suggests that high IOP compresses the microcirculation in the optic nerve head, resulting in cell injury and death. Some glaucomas appear as exclusively mechanical, and some are exclusively ischemic types. Typically, most cases are a combination of both.

Classification of Glaucoma

There are several types of glaucoma. Forms of glaucoma are identified as wide-angle glaucoma; narrow-angle glaucoma; congenital glaucoma; and glaucoma associated with other conditions, such as developmental anomalies or corticosteroid use. Glaucoma can be primary or secondary, depending on whether associated factors contribute to the rise in IOP. The two common clinical forms of glaucoma in adults are wide- and narrow-angle glaucoma, which are differentiated by the mechanisms that cause impaired aqueous outflow (Grossman & Porth, 2014). Table 63-4 summarizes the characteristics of the different types of adult glaucoma.

Clinical Manifestation

Glaucoma is often called the "silent thief of sight" because most patients are unaware that they have the disease until they have experienced visual changes and vision loss. The patient may not seek health care until he or she experiences blurred vision or "halos" around lights, difficulty focusing, difficulty adjusting eyes in low lighting, loss of peripheral vision, aching or discomfort around the eyes, and headache.

Assessment and Diagnostic Findings

The purpose of a glaucoma workup is to establish the diagnostic category, assess the optic nerve damage, and

TABLE 63-4 Selected Glaucoma Types, Clinical Manifestation, and Treatment

Types of Glaucoma	Clinical Manifestations	Treatment
Wide Angle		
Usually bilateral, but one eye may be more severely affected than the other. In wide-angle glaucoma, the anterior chamber angle is open and appears normal.		
Normal tension glaucoma	IOP ≤21 mmHg. Optic nerve damage, visual field defects.	If medical treatment is unsuccessful, LT can decrease IOP by 20%. Glaucoma filtering surgery if continued optic nerve damage despite medication therapy and LT.
Ocular hypertension	Elevated IOP. Possible ocular pain or headache.	The best management for normal tension glaucoma management is yet to be established. Goal is to lower the IOP by at least 30%.
Narrow Angle		
Obstruction in aqueous humor outflow due to the complete or partial closure of the angle from the forward shift of the peripheral iris to the trabecula. The obstruction results in an increased IOP.		
Acute angle–closure glaucoma	Rapidly progressive visual impairment, periocular pain, conjunctival hyperemia, and congestion. Pain may be associated with nausea, vomiting, bradycardia, and profuse sweating. Reduced central visual acuity, severely elevated IOP, corneal edema. Pupil is vertically oval, fixed in a semidilated position, and unreactive to light and accommodation.	Ocular emergency; administration of hyperosmotics, acetazolamide, and topical ocular hypotensive agents, such as pilocarpine and beta-blockers (betaxolol). Possible laser incision in the iris (iridotomy) to release blocked aqueous and reduce IOP. Other eye is also treated with pilocarpine eye drops and/or surgical management to avoid a similar spontaneous attack.
Subacute angle–closure glaucoma	Transient blurring of vision, halos around lights; temporal headaches and/or ocular pain; pupil may be semidilated.	Prophylactic peripheral laser iridotomy. Can lead to acute or chronic angle–closure glaucoma if untreated.
Chronic angle–closure glaucoma	Progression of glaucomatous cupping and significant visual field loss; IOP may be normal or elevated; ocular pain and headache.	Management includes laser iridotomy and medications.

IOP, intraocular pressure; LT, laser trabeculoplasty.

Adapted from Eldaly, M. A., Bunce, C., El Sheikha, O. Z., et al. (2014). Non-penetrating filtration surgery versus trabeculectomy for open-angle glaucoma. *Cochrane Database of Systematic Reviews*, (2), CD007059. Grossman, S. C., & Porth, C. M. (2014). *Porth's Pathophysiology: Concepts of altered health states* (9th ed.). Philadelphia, PA: Lippincott Williams & Wilkins.

Glaucoma

Figure 63-7 • Visual changes associated with glaucoma. Photo courtesy of the National Eye Institute, National Institutes of Health.

formulate a treatment plan. The patient's ocular and medical history must be detailed to investigate the history of predisposing factors. The types of examinations used in glaucoma include tonometry to measure the IOP, ophthalmoscopy to inspect the optic nerve, and central visual field testing (Glaucoma Research Foundation, 2016; Grossman & Porth, 2014).

The changes in the optic nerve related to glaucoma are pallor and cupping of the optic nerve disc. The pallor of the optic nerve is caused by a lack of blood supply. Cupping is characterized by exaggerated bending of the blood vessels as they cross the optic disc, resulting in an enlarged optic cup that appears more basin like compared with a normal cup. The progression of cupping in glaucoma is caused by the gradual loss of retinal nerve fibers and the loss of blood supply.

As the optic nerve damage increases, visual perception decreases. The localized areas of visual loss (i.e., scotomas) represent loss of retinal sensitivity and nerve fiber damage and are measured and mapped on a graph. In patients with glaucoma, the graph has a distinct pattern that is different from other ocular diseases and is useful in establishing the diagnosis. Figure 63-7 shows the visual changes caused by glaucoma.

Medical Management

The aim of all glaucoma treatment is prevention of optic nerve damage. Lifelong therapy is necessary because glaucoma cannot be cured. Treatment focuses on pharmacologic therapy, laser procedures, surgery, or a combination of these approaches, all of which have potential complications and side effects. The object is to achieve the greatest benefit at the least risk, cost, and inconvenience to the patient. Although treatment cannot reverse optic nerve damage, further damage can be controlled. The goal is to maintain an IOP within a range unlikely to cause further damage (Eldaly et al., 2014).

The initial target for IOP among patients with elevated IOP and those with low-tension glaucoma with progressive visual field loss is typically set at 30% lower than the current pressure. The patient is monitored for changes in the appearance of the optic nerve. If there is evidence of progressive damage, the target IOP is again lowered until the optic nerve shows stability.

Pharmacologic Therapy

Medical management of glaucoma relies on systemic and topical ocular medications that lower IOP. Periodic follow-up examinations are essential to monitor IOP, the appearance of the optic nerve, the visual fields, and side effects of medications. Therapy takes into account the patient's health and stage of glaucoma. Comfort, affordability, convenience, lifestyle, and functional ability are factors to consider in the patient's adherence to the medical regimen (Eliopoulos, 2018).

The patient is usually started on the lowest dose of topical medication and then advanced to increased concentrations until the desired IOP level is reached and maintained. Beta-blockers are the preferred initial topical medications because of their efficacy, minimal dosing (can be used once each day), and low cost. One eye is treated first, with the other eye used as a control in determining the efficacy of the medication; once efficacy has been established, treatment of the other eye is started. If the IOP is elevated in both eyes, both are treated. When results are not satisfactory, a new medication is substituted. The main markers of the efficacy of the medication in glaucoma control are lowering of the IOP to the target pressure, stable appearance of the optic nerve head, and the visual field.

Many ocular medications are used to treat glaucoma (see Table 63-5), including miotics, beta-blockers, alpha$_2$-agonists (i.e., adrenergic agents), carbonic anhydrase inhibitors, and prostaglandins. Cholinergics (i.e., miotics) increase the outflow of the aqueous humor by affecting ciliary muscle contraction and pupil constriction, allowing flow through a larger opening between the iris and the trabecular meshwork. Beta-blockers and carbonic anhydrase inhibitors decrease aqueous production. Prostaglandin analogs reduce IOP by increasing aqueous humor outflow (Comerford, 2015; Grossman & Porth, 2014).

Surgical Management

Surgery is reserved for patients in whom pharmacologic treatment has not controlled the IOP. This minimally invasive procedure is specifically designed to improve fluid drainage from the eye to balance IOP. By restoring the eye's natural fluid balance, trabeculectomy surgery stabilizes the optic nerve and minimizes further visual field damage (Eldaly et al., 2014). The surgery is performed through a small incision and does not require creation of a permanent hole in the eye wall or an external filtering bleb or an implant.

In laser trabeculoplasty for glaucoma, a laser beam is applied to the inner surface of the trabecular meshwork to open the intratrabecular spaces and widen the canal of Schlemm, promoting outflow of aqueous humor and decreasing IOP. The procedure is indicated when IOP is inadequately controlled by medications, and it is contraindicated when the trabecular meshwork cannot be fully visualized because of a narrow angle.

In peripheral iridotomy for pupillary block glaucoma, an opening is made in the iris to eliminate the pupillary blockage. Laser iridotomy is contraindicated in patients with corneal edema, which interferes with laser targeting and strength. Potential complications include burns to the cornea, lens, or retina; transient elevated IOP; closure of the iridotomy; uveitis; and blurring.

Filtering procedures for glaucoma are used to create an opening or fistula in the trabecular meshwork to drain aqueous humor from the anterior chamber to the subconjunctival

TABLE 63-5 Medications Used in the Management of Glaucoma

Medication	Action	Side Effects	Nursing Implications
Cholinergics (miotics) (pilocarpine, carbachol)	Increase aqueous fluid outflow by contracting the ciliary muscle and causing miosis (constriction of the pupil) and opening of trabecular meshwork	Periorbital pain, blurry vision, difficulty seeing in the dark	Caution patients about diminished vision in dimly lit areas. Pilocarpine can be stored at room temperature for up to 8 weeks and then should be discarded.
Beta-blockers (timolol maleate)	Decrease aqueous humor production	Can have systemic effects, including bradycardia, exacerbation of pulmonary disease, and hypotension	Contraindicated in patients with asthma, chronic obstructive pulmonary disease, 2nd- or 3rd-degree heart block, bradycardia, or cardiac failure; educate patients about punctal occlusion to limit systemic effects (see Chart 63-4).
Alpha-adrenergic agonists (apraclonidine, brimonidine)	Decrease aqueous humor production	Eye redness, dry mouth and nasal passages	Educate patients about punctal occlusion to limit systemic effects (see Chart 63-4).
Carbonic anhydrase inhibitors (acetazolamide, dorzolamide)	Decrease aqueous humor production	Oral medications (acetazolamide) are associated with serious side effects, including anaphylactic reactions, electrolyte loss, depression, lethargy, gastrointestinal upset, impotence, and weight loss; side effects of topical form (dorzolamide) include topical allergy	Do not administer to patients with sulfa allergies; monitor electrolyte levels.
Prostaglandin analogs (latanoprost, bimatoprost)	Increase uveoscleral outflow	Darkening of the iris, conjunctival redness, possible rash	Instruct patients to report any side effects.

Adapted from Comerford, K. C. (2015). *Nursing 2015 drug handbook.* Philadelphia, PA: Wolters Kluwer.

space into a bleb (fluid collection on the outside of the eye), thereby bypassing the usual drainage structures. This allows the aqueous humor to flow and exit by different routes (i.e., absorption by the conjunctival vessels or mixing with tears). Trabeculectomy is the standard filtering technique used to remove part of the trabecular meshwork (Eldaly et al., 2014). Complications include hemorrhage, an extremely low (hypotony) or extremely elevated IOP, uveitis, cataracts, bleb failure, bleb leak, and **endophthalmitis** (i.e., intraocular infection).

Drainage implants or *shunts* are tubes implanted in the anterior chamber to shunt aqueous humor to the episcleral plate in the conjunctival space. Implants are used when failure has occurred with one or more trabeculectomies in which antifibrotic agents were used. A fibrous capsule develops around the episcleral plate and filters the aqueous humor, thereby regulating the outflow and controlling IOP.

Nursing Management

Nurses in all settings encounter patients with glaucoma. Even patients with long-standing disease and those with glaucoma as a secondary diagnosis should be assessed for knowledge level and adherence to their prescribed therapeutic regimen.

Promoting Home, Community-Based, and Transitional Care

Educating Patients About Self-Care

The medical and surgical management of glaucoma slows the progression of the disease but does not cure it. The lifelong therapeutic regimen mandates patient education. The nature of the disease and the importance of strict adherence to the medication regimen must be included in an individualized education plan. A structured self-management program may increase adherence to the treatment regime. A thorough discussion of the medication program, particularly the interactions of glaucoma-control medications with other medications, is essential. For example, the diuretic effect of acetazolamide (Diamox) may have an additive effect on the diuretic effects of other antihypertensive medications (Comerford, 2015). The effects of glaucoma-control medications on vision must also be explained. Miotics and sympathomimetics result in altered focus; therefore, patients need to be cautious in navigating their surroundings. Chart 63-4 presents patient education about instilling eye medications and preventing systemic absorption with punctal occlusion. Chart 63-6 contains additional educational information to review with patients with glaucoma.

Continuing and Transitional Care

Patients with severe glaucoma and impaired function may need referral to home, community-based or transitional services that provide assistance in the home. The loss of peripheral vision impairs mobility the most. These patients also benefit from a referral for low vision and rehabilitation services. Patients who meet the criteria for legal blindness should be offered referrals to agencies that can assist them in obtaining federal assistance.

Reassurance and emotional support are important aspects of care. A lifelong disease involving possible loss of sight has psychological, physical, social, and vocational ramifications.

PATIENT EDUCATION
Managing Glaucoma

The nurse instructs the patient to:

- Know your intraocular pressure measurement and the desired range.
- Be informed about the extent of your vision loss and optic nerve damage.
- Keep a record of your eye pressure measurements and visual field test results to monitor your own progress.
- Review all of your medications (including over-the-counter and herbal medications) with your ophthalmologist, and mention any side effects each time you visit.
- Ask about potential side effects and drug interactions of your eye medications.
- Ask whether generic or less costly forms of your eye medications are available.
- Review the dosing schedule with your ophthalmologist, and inform him or her if you have trouble following the schedule.
- Participate in the decision-making process. Let your primary provider know what dosing schedule works for you and other preferences regarding your eye care.
- Have the nurse observe you instilling eye medication to determine whether you are administering it properly (see Chart 63-4).
- Be aware that glaucoma medications can cause adverse effects if used inappropriately. Eye drops are to be given as prescribed, not when eyes feel irritated.
- Ask your ophthalmologist to send a report to your primary provider after each appointment.
- Keep all follow-up appointments.

The family must be integrated into the plan of care, and because the disease has a familial tendency, family members should be encouraged to undergo examinations at least once every 2 years to detect glaucoma early.

CATARACTS

A **cataract** is a lens opacity or cloudiness (see Fig. 63-8). Cataracts are responsible for visual disability in 18 million people worldwide (Grossman & Porth, 2014). By 80 years of age, more than half of all Americans have cataracts. Cataracts are

Figure 63-8 • A cataract is a cloudy or opaque lens. On visual inspection, the lens appears gray or milky. Reprinted with permission from Rubin, R., Strayer, D. S., & Rubin, E. (2012). *Rubin's pathology: Clinicopathologic foundations of medicine* (6th ed.). Philadelphia, PA: Lippincott Williams & Wilkins.

RISK FACTORS
Cataract Formation

Aging

- Accumulation of a yellow-brown pigment due to the breakdown of lens protein
- Clumping or aggregation of lens protein (which leads to light scattering)
- Decreased oxygen uptake
- Decrease in levels of vitamin C, protein, and glutathione (an antioxidant)
- Increase in sodium and calcium
- Loss of lens transparency

Associated Ocular Conditions

- Infection (e.g., herpes zoster, uveitis)
- Myopia
- Retinal detachment and retinal surgery
- Retinitis pigmentosa

Toxic Factors

- Alkaline chemical eye burns, poisoning
- Aspirin use
- Calcium, copper, iron, gold, silver, and mercury, which tend to deposit in the pupillary area of the lens
- Cigarette smoking
- Corticosteroids, especially at high doses and in long-term use
- Ionizing radiation

Nutritional Factors

- Obesity
- Poor nutrition
- Reduced levels of antioxidants

Physical Factors

- Blunt trauma, perforation of the lens with a sharp object or foreign body, electric shock
- Dehydration associated with chronic diarrhea, the use of purgatives in anorexia nervosa, and the use of hyperbaric oxygenation
- Ultraviolet radiation in sunlight and x-ray

Systemic Diseases and Syndromes

- Diabetes
- Disorders related to lipid metabolism
- Down syndrome
- Musculoskeletal disorders
- Renal disorders

Adapted from Grossman, S. C., & Porth, C. M. (2014). *Porth's Pathophysiology: Concepts of altered health states* (9th ed.). Philadelphia, PA: Lippincott Williams & Wilkins.
Kumar, C. M., Seet, E., Eke, T., et al. (2016). Glycaemic control during cataract surgery under loco-regional anesthesia: A growing problem and we are none the wiser. *British Journal of Anesthesia, 117*(6), 687–691.

a leading cause of blindness in the world (Prevent Blindness America, 2012).

Pathophysiology

Cataracts can develop in one or both eyes at any age. The three most common types are traumatic, congenital, or senile cataract (Grossman & Porth, 2014). There are a variety of risk factors, the most common one being age (see Chart 63-7).

Clinical Manifestations

Painless, blurry vision is characteristic of cataracts. The person perceives that surroundings are dimmer, as if their glasses need cleaning. Light scattering is common, and the person experiences reduced contrast sensitivity, sensitivity to glare, and reduced visual acuity. Other effects include myopic shift (return of ability to do close work [e.g., reading fine print] without eyeglasses), **astigmatism** (refractive error due to an irregularity in the curvature of the cornea), monocular **diplopia** (double vision), and color changes as lens becomes more brown in color (Cash & Glass, 2016; Eliopoulos, 2018).

Assessment and Diagnostic Findings

Decreased visual acuity is directly proportionate to cataract density. The Snellen visual acuity test, ophthalmoscopy, and slit-lamp biomicroscopic examination are used to establish the degree of cataract formation. The degree of lens opacity does not always correlate with the patient's functional status. Some patients can perform normal activities despite clinically significant cataracts. Others with less lens opacification have a disproportionate decrease in visual acuity; hence, visual acuity is an imperfect measure of visual impairment.

Medical Management

No nonsurgical treatment (e.g., medications, eye drops, eyeglasses) cures cataracts or prevents age-related cataracts. Optimal medical management is prevention. Patients should be educated by primary providers about risk reduction strategies such as smoking cessation, weight reduction, optimal blood sugar control for patients with diabetes, and should be advised to wear sunglasses outdoors to prevent early cataract formation (Cash & Glass, 2016).

Surgical Management

In general, if reduced vision from cataract does not interfere with normal activities, surgery may not be needed. In deciding when cataract surgery is to be performed, the patient's functional and visual status should be a primary consideration (Eliopoulos, 2018). Cataract removal is common, with more than 1 million such surgeries performed in the United States each year (Prevent Blindness America, 2012). Surgery is performed on an outpatient basis and usually takes less than 1 hour, with the patient being discharged in 30 minutes or less afterward. Although complications from cataract surgery are uncommon, they can have significant effects on vision (see Table 63-6). Restoration of visual function through a safe and minimally invasive procedure is the surgical goal, which is achieved with advances in topical anesthesia, smaller wound incision (i.e., clear cornea incision), and lens design (i.e., foldable and more accurate intraocular lens [IOL] measurements).

Injection-free topical and intraocular anesthesia, such as 1% lidocaine gel applied to the surface of the eye, eliminates the hazards of regional (retrobulbar and peribulbar) anesthesia, such as ocular perforation, retrobulbar hemorrhage, optic injuries, diplopia, and ptosis, and is ideal for patients receiving anticoagulants. Furthermore, patients can communicate and cooperate during surgery.

IV moderate sedation may be used to minimize anxiety and discomfort.

When both eyes have cataracts, one eye is treated first, with at least several weeks, preferably months, separating the two procedures. Because cataract surgery is performed to improve visual functioning, the delay for the other eye gives time for the patient and the surgeon to evaluate whether the results from the first surgery are adequate to preclude the need for a second operation. The delay also provides time for the first eye to recover; if there are any complications, the surgeon may decide to perform the second procedure differently.

Phacoemulsification

In this method of extracapsular cataract surgery, a portion of the anterior capsule is removed, allowing extraction of the lens nucleus and cortex while the posterior capsule and zonular support are left intact. An ultrasonic device is used to liquefy the nucleus and cortex, which are then suctioned out through a tube. An intact zonular–capsular diaphragm provides the needed safe anchor for the posterior chamber IOL. The pupil is dilated to 7 mm or greater (Peng, Fong, Phaik, et al., 2012). The surgeon makes a small incision on the upper edge of the cornea and a viscoelastic substance (clear gel) is injected into the space between the cornea and the lens. This prevents the space from collapsing and facilitates insertion of the IOL. Because the incision is smaller than the manual extracapsular cataract extraction, the wound heals more rapidly, and there is early stabilization of refractive error and less astigmatism.

Lens Replacement

After removal of the crystalline lens, the patient is referred to as aphakic (i.e., without lens). The lens, which focuses light on the retina, must be replaced for the patient to see clearly. There are three lens replacement options: aphakic eyeglasses, contact lenses, and IOL implants.

Aphakic glasses, although effective, are rarely used. Objects are magnified by 25%, making them appear closer than they actually are. This magnification creates distortion. Peripheral vision is also limited, and **binocular vision** (i.e., ability of both eyes to focus on one object and fuse the two images into one) is impossible if the other eye is aphakic (without a natural lens).

Contact lenses provide patients with almost normal vision, but because contact lenses need to be removed occasionally, the patient also needs a pair of aphakic glasses. Contact lenses are not advised for patients who have difficulty inserting, removing, and cleaning them. Frequent handling and improper disinfection increase the risk of infection.

Insertion of IOLs during cataract surgery is the most common approach to lens replacement (Eliopoulos, 2018). After cataract extraction, or phacoemulsification, the surgeon implants an IOL. Cataract extraction and posterior chamber IOLs are associated with a relatively low incidence of complications (e.g., eye infection, loss of vitreous humor, and slipping of the implant) (Eliopoulos, 2018). IOL implantation is contraindicated in patients with recurrent uveitis, proliferative diabetic retinopathy, neovascular glaucoma, or rubeosis iridis.

TABLE 63-6 Potential Complications of Cataract Surgery

Complication	Effects	Management and Outcome
Immediate Preoperative		
Retrobulbar hemorrhage—can result from retrobulbar infiltration of anesthetic agents if the short ciliary artery is located by the injectia	Increased IOP, proptosis, lid tightness, and subconjunctival hemorrhage with or without edema	Emergent lateral canthotomy (slitting of the canthus) is performed to stop central retinal perfusion when the IOP is dangerously elevated. If this procedure fails to reduce IOP, a puncture of the anterior chamber with removal of fluid is considered. The patient must be closely monitored for at least a few hours. Postponement of cataract surgery for 2–4 weeks is advised. Complications such as iris prolapse, vitreous loss, and choroidal hemorrhage could result in a catastrophic visual outcome.
Intraoperative		
Rupture of the posterior capsule	May result in loss of vitreous	Anterior vitrectomy is required if vitreous loss occurs.
Suprachoroidal (expulsive) hemorrhage—profuse bleeding into the suprachoroidal space	Extrusion of intraocular contents from the eye or opposition of retinal surfaces	Closure of the incision and administration of a hyperosmotic agent to reduce IOP or corticosteroids to reduce intraocular inflammation. Vitrectomy is performed 1–2 weeks later. Visual prognosis is poor; some useful vision may be salvaged on rare occasions.
Early Postoperative		
Acute bacterial endophthalmitis—devastating complication that occurs in about 1 in 1000 cases; the most common causative organisms are *Staphylococcus epidermidis*, *Staphylococcus aureus*, *Pseudomonas*, and *Proteus* species	Characterized by marked visual loss, pain, lid edema, hypopyon, corneal haze, and chemosis	Managed by aggressive antibiotic therapy. Broad-spectrum antibiotics are given while awaiting culture and sensitivity results. Once results are obtained, the appropriate antibiotics are given via intravitreal injection. Corticosteroid therapy is also given.
Toxic anterior segment syndrome—noninfectious inflammation that is a complication of anterior chamber surgery; caused by a toxic agent such as an agent used to sterilize surgical instruments	Corneal edema occurs <24 hours after surgery; symptoms include reduced visual acuity and pain	If there is no growth of microorganisms, the treatment is topical steroids alone.
Late Postoperative		
Suture-related problems	Toxic reactions or mechanical injury from broken or loose sutures	Suture removal relieves the symptoms. Topical corticosteroids are used when the incision is not healed and sutures cannot be removed.
Malposition of the IOL	Results in astigmatism, sensitivity to glare, or appearance of halos	Miotics are used for mild cases, whereas IOL removal and replacement is necessary for severe cases.
Chronic endophthalmitis	Persistent, low-grade inflammation, and granuloma	Corticosteroids and antibiotics are given systemically. If the condition persists, removal of the IOL and capsular bag, vitrectomy, and intravitreal injection of antibiotics are required.
Opacification of the posterior capsule—most common late complication of extracapsular cataract extraction	Visual acuity is diminished	Nd:YAG laser is used to create a hole in the posterior capsule. Blurred vision is cleared immediately.

IOP, intraocular pressure; IOL, intraocular lens; Nd:YAG, Neodymium: yttrium aluminum garnet.

Nursing Management

Providing Preoperative Care

The patient with cataracts receives the usual preoperative care for ambulatory surgical patients undergoing eye surgery. The standard battery of preoperative tests (e.g., complete blood count, electrocardiogram, and urinalysis) commonly performed for most surgeries is prescribed only if indicated by the patient's medical history.

Alpha-antagonists (particularly tamsulosin [Flomax], which is used for treatment of enlarged prostate) are known to cause a condition called *intraoperative floppy iris syndrome*.

Alpha-antagonists can interfere with pupil dilation during the surgical procedure, resulting in miosis and iris prolapse and leading to complications. Intraoperative floppy iris syndrome can occur even though a patient has stopped taking the drug. The nurse needs to ask patients about a history of taking alpha-antagonists. Surgical team members are then alerted to the risk of this complication (Comerford, 2015).

Dilating drops are given prior to surgery. Nurses in the ambulatory surgery setting begin patient education about eye medications (antibiotic, corticosteroid, and anti-inflammatory drops) that will need to be self-administered to prevent postoperative infection and inflammation.

At the completion of education, the patient and/or caregiver will be able to:

- Name the procedure that was performed and identify any permanent changes in anatomic structure or function as well as changes in ADLs, IADLs, roles, relationships, and spirituality.
- State the name, dose, side effects, frequency, and schedule for all medications.
- Describe ongoing postoperative therapeutic regimen and activities to limit or avoid (e.g., lifting weights, driving a car, contact sports).
  - Wear glasses or eye shield following surgery as instructed.
  - Always wash hands before touching or cleaning the postoperative eye.
  - Clean postoperative eye with a clean tissue; wipe the closed eye with a single gesture from the inner canthus outward.
  - When bathing or showering, shampoo hair cautiously or seek assistance.
  - Avoid lying on the side of the affected eye the night after surgery.

- Keep activity light (e.g., walking, reading, watching television). Resume the following activities only as directed by the ophthalmologist: driving, sexual activity, unusually strenuous activity.
- Avoid lifting, pushing, or pulling objects heavier than 15 pounds.
- Avoid bending or stooping for an extended period.
- Be careful when climbing or descending stairs.
- Describe signs and symptoms of complications (e.g., vision change, continuous flashing lights appear to the affected eye, redness, swelling or increased pain near the eye, change in amount or type of eye drainage, any eye injury, significant pain not relieved by prescribed analgesia).
- Relate how to reach ophthalmologist with questions or complications.
- State time and date of follow-up appointments.
- Identify sources of assistance (e.g., meals, transportation) and support (e.g., friends, relatives, faith community).
- Identify the need for health promotion, disease prevention, and screening activities

ADL, activities of daily living; IADL, independent activities of daily living.

Providing Postoperative Care

Before discharge, the patient receives verbal and written education regarding eye protection, administration of medications, recognition of complications, activities to avoid, and obtaining emergency care (see Chart 63-8). An eye shield is usually worn at night for the first week to avoid injury. The nurse also explains that there should be minimal discomfort after surgery and educates the patient about taking a mild analgesic agent, such as acetaminophen, as needed. Antibiotic, anti-inflammatory, and corticosteroid eye drops or ointments are prescribed postoperatively. Patients prescribed anti-inflammatory or corticosteroid eye drops are monitored for possible increases in IOP (Kusne, Kang, & Fintelmann, 2016).

Promoting Home, Community-Based, and Transitional Care

 Educating Patients About Self-Care

To prevent accidental rubbing or poking of the eye, the patient wears a protective eye patch for about the first 24 hours after surgery, followed by eyeglasses worn during the day and an eye shield at night. The nurse educates the patient and family about applying and caring for the eye shield, if one is recommended. Sunglasses should be worn while outdoors during the day because the eye is sensitive to light.

Slight morning discharge, some redness, and a scratchy feeling may be expected for a few days. A clean, damp washcloth may be used to remove slight morning eye discharge. Because cataract surgery increases the risk of retinal detachment, the patient must know to notify the surgeon if new floaters (dots) in vision, flashing lights, decrease in vision, pain, or increase in redness occurs.

Continuing and Transitional Care

If an eye patch is worn, it is removed after the first follow-up appointment, which should occur within 48 hours of surgery.

Nurses should educate patients about the importance of keeping their follow-up appointments, because monitoring of visual status and prompt intervention of postoperative complications enhance good visual outcome. Vision is stabilized when the eye is completely healed, usually within 6 to 12 weeks, when final corrective prescription is completed. Visual correction may still be needed for any remaining refractive errors. Patients who choose multifocal IOLs should be aware that there may be increased night glare and contrast sensitivity.

CORNEAL DISORDERS

Corneal Dystrophies

Corneal dystrophies are inherited as autosomal dominant traits and manifest when the person is about 20 years of age. They are characterized by deposits in the corneal layers. Decreased vision is caused by the irregular corneal surface and corneal deposits. Corneal endothelial decomposition leads to corneal edema and blurring of vision. Persistent edema leads to bullous keratopathy or the formation of blisters that cause pain and discomfort on rupturing. The two main types are keratoconus and Fuchs endothelial dystrophy.

Keratoconus

Keratoconus, the most common type of corneal dystrophy, is characterized by a conical protuberance of the cornea with progressive thinning on protrusion and irregular astigmatism. This hereditary condition has a higher incidence among women. Onset occurs at puberty; the condition may progress for more than 20 years and is bilateral. Corneal scarring occurs in severe cases. Blurred vision is a prominent symptom. Rigid, gas-permeable contact lenses correct irregular astigmatism and improve vision. Advances in contact lens design have reduced the need for surgery. Penetrating keratoplasty (PKP) is indicated when contact lens correction is no longer effective.

Fuchs Endothelial Dystrophy

Fuchs (pronounced *Fooks*) dystrophy is manifested by a slow death of cells in the endothelial cornea. It affects women more than men and is usually not noted until 50 years of age. Corneal endothelial cell death leads to corneal edema and blurring of vision. Persistent edema leads to bullous keratopathy. A bandage contact lens is used to flatten the bullae, protect the exposed corneal nerve endings, and relieve discomfort. Symptomatic treatments, such as hypertonic drops or ointment (5% sodium chloride), may reduce epithelial edema. Currently, the only cure is a corneal transplant (Dickman, Peeters, Van Den Biggelaar, et al., 2016).

Corneal Surgeries

Among the surgical procedures used to treat diseased corneal tissue are phototherapeutic keratectomy (PTK), PKP and corneal endothelial transplantation, and Descemet's stripping endothelial keratoplasty (DSEK).

Phototherapeutic Keratectomy

PTK is a laser procedure that is used to treat diseased corneal tissue by removing or reducing corneal opacities and smoothing the anterior corneal surface to improve functional vision. PTK is contraindicated in patients with active herpetic keratitis because the ultraviolet rays may reactivate latent virus. Common side effects are induced hyperopia and stromal haze. Complications are delayed re-epithelialization (particularly in patients with diabetes) and bacterial keratitis. Postoperative management consists of oral analgesic agents for eye pain. Re-epithelialization is promoted with a pressure patch or therapeutic soft contact lens. Antibiotic and corticosteroid ointments and NSAIDs are prescribed postoperatively. Follow-up examinations are required for up to 2 years.

Penetrating Keratoplasty

PKP (corneal transplantation or corneal grafting) involves replacing abnormal host tissue with healthy donor (cadaver) corneal tissue. Common indications are keratoconus, corneal scarring from herpes simplex, keratitis, and chemical burns.

Several factors affect the success of the graft: the condition of the ocular structures (e.g., lids, conjunctiva), quality of the tears, adequacy of blinking, and viability of the donor endothelium. Contraindications for the use of donor tissue are outlined in Chart 63-9.

In PKP, the surgeon determines the graft size before the procedure, and the appropriate size is marked on the surface of the cornea. The surgeon prepares the donor cornea and the recipient bed, removes the diseased cornea, places the donor cornea on the recipient bed, and sutures it in place. Sutures remain in place for 12 to 18 months and are then removed. Potential complications include early graft failure due to poor quality of donor tissue, surgical trauma, acute infection, and persistently increased IOP and late graft failure due to rejection.

Postoperatively, the patient receives mydriatics for 2 weeks and topical corticosteroids for 12 months (daily doses for 6 months and tapered doses thereafter). These mydriatics and

Chart 63-9

Contraindications to the Use of Donor Tissue for Corneal Transplantation: Donor Characteristics

Systemic Disorders

- Death from unknown cause
- History or suspected history of the following:
  - Acquired immune deficiency syndrome or high-risk for human immune deficiency virus infection
  - Creutzfeldt–Jacob disease
  - Eye infection
  - Hepatitis
  - Rabies
  - Systemic infection

Intrinsic Eye Disease

- Disorders of the conjunctiva or corneal surface involving the optical zone of the cornea
- Malignant tumors of anterior segment
- Ocular inflammation
- Retinoblastoma

Other

- Corneal scars
- History of eye trauma
- Previous surgical eye procedures such as corneal graft or LASIK eye surgery

corticosteroid drops should be preservative free to prevent a reactive inflammation. Patients typically describe a sensation of postoperative eye discomfort rather than acute pain.

Additional Keratoplasty Surgeries

For many years, PKP was the standard of care for patients with corneal endothelial failure but with poor refractive results. Subsequently, other techniques have been developed. Anterior lamellar keratoplasty (ALK) involves a partial-thickness graft for disorders such as anterior corneal dystrophies or scarring not involving the endothelial portion of the cornea. Deep anterior lamellar keratoplasty (DALK) involves replacement of only anterior corneal layers and not Descemet's membrane or endothelial layers for disorders such as keratoconus. Posterior lamellar keratoplasty (PLK or EK) and DSEK (which replaces only the endothelial layer of the cornea) are procedures indicated for conditions such as Fuchs endothelial dystrophy or bullous keratopathy (Dickman, et al., 2016). In DSEK, layers of the cornea are dissected and selectively replaced by donor cornea tissue. DSEK offers several advantages, such as less postoperative astigmatism, faster visual recovery, and stronger wound integrity. Theoretically, the risk of rejection is less because less of the patient's tissue is replaced.

Keratoprosthesis

An additional therapeutic option for patients with multiple graft failures or severe corneal disease is keratoprosthesis (artificial cornea; e.g., U.S. Food and Drug Administration [FDA]-approved Boston Keratoprosthesis [KPro] and Alpha-Cor). The design of the keratoprosthesis consists of a central optic core and an outer rim that secures the prosthesis. This procedure has serious potential complications (e.g., glaucoma, endophthalmitis) and requires close follow-up and monitoring (Patel, Moster, Kishfy, et al., 2016).

Nursing Management

For corneal surgeries, the nurse reinforces instructions regarding visual rehabilitation and visual improvement. A technically successful graft may initially produce disappointing results because the procedure has produced a new optical surface. Only after several months do patients start seeing the natural and true colors of their environment. Correction of a resultant refractive error with eyeglasses or contact lenses determines the final visual outcome. The nurse assesses the patient's support system and their ability to comply with long-term follow-up, which includes frequent clinic visits for several months for tapering of topical corticosteroid therapy, selective suture removal, and ongoing evaluation of the graft site and visual acuity. The nurse also initiates appropriate referrals to community services as indicated.

Because graft failure is an ophthalmic emergency that can occur at any time, the primary goal of nursing care is to educate the patient to identify signs and symptoms of graft failure. The early symptoms are blurred vision, discomfort, tearing, or redness of the eye. Decreased vision results after graft destruction. The patient must contact the ophthalmologist as soon as symptoms occur. Treatment of graft rejection usually involves prompt administration of hourly topical corticosteroids and periocular corticosteroid injections. Systemic immunosuppressive agents may be necessary for severe, resistant cases.

Refractive Surgeries

Refractive surgeries are elective procedures performed to correct refractive errors (myopia or hyperopia) and astigmatism by reshaping the cornea (Li, Zhan, Li, et al., 2016). Laser vision correction alters the major optical function of the eye and carries risks. Refractive surgery does not alter the normal aging process of the eye. If the reason for the procedure is to meet vision requirements for the patient's occupation, the results must satisfy both the patient and the employer. Precise visual outcome cannot be guaranteed.

The corneal structure must be normal, and the refractive error must be stable. The patient is required to discontinue using contact lenses for a period before the procedure (2 to 3 weeks for soft lenses and 4 weeks for hard lenses). Patients with conditions that are likely to adversely affect corneal wound healing (e.g., corticosteroid use, immunosuppression, elevated IOP) are not good candidates for the procedure. Any superficial eye disease must be diagnosed and fully treated before a refractive procedure.

Patient satisfaction is the ultimate goal; therefore, patient education and counseling about potential risks, complications, and postoperative follow-up are critical. Minimal postoperative care includes topical corticosteroid or NSAID and antibiotic drops.

Laser Vision Correction Photorefractive Keratectomy

Photorefractive keratectomy (PRK) is used to treat myopia and hyperopia with or without astigmatism (Li et al., 2016).

The excimer laser is applied directly to the cornea according to carefully calculated measurements. For myopia, the relative curvature is decreased; for hyperopia, the relative curvature is increased. A bandage contact lens is placed over the cornea to promote epithelial healing and reduce pain, which is similar to that of a severe corneal abrasion.

Laser-Assisted In Situ Keratomileusis

LASIK involves flattening the anterior curvature of the cornea by removing a stromal lamella or layer. The surgeon creates a corneal flap with a microkeratome, which is an automatic corneal shaper. The surgeon retracts a flap of corneal tissue less than one third the thickness of a human hair to access the corneal stroma and then uses the excimer laser on the stromal bed to reshape the cornea according to calculated measurements (see Fig. 63-9). Data are insufficient to determine whether LASIK or PRK is better at correcting nearsightedness (Li et al., 2016). There are few adverse outcomes of either procedure.

Perioperative Complications
Surgically Induced Abnormalities

Corneal surface irregularities can occur after LASIK treatment. These include central islands (central areas of stiffness or elevation), decentered ablations resulting from misalignment of the laser treatment or from involuntary eye movement during laser treatment, and forms of irregular astigmatism. Symptoms of central islands and decentered ablations include monocular diplopia or ghost images, halos, glare, and decreased visual acuity.

Phakic Intraocular Lenses

Increasingly, phakic IOL implantation has been used for patients with moderate to severe myopia (Barsam & Allan, 2014). Phakic IOLs may be used in either the anterior or posterior chamber. The implantation of such devices is reversible because the natural lens is left in place and the normal architecture of the cornea is preserved. This procedure provides more predictable refractive results than procedures that alter the corneal curvature, is safer, and has higher patient satisfaction scores (Barsam & Allan, 2014). Potential complications

Laser pulse

"Flap"

Figure 63-9 • LASIK combines delicate surgical procedures and laser treatment. A flap is surgically created and lifted to one side. A laser is then applied to the cornea to reshape it. With permission from the Wilmer Laser Vision Center, Lutherville, MD.

include cataract, iritis or uveitis, endothelial cell loss, and increased IOP.

Conductive Keratoplasty

Another innovation in refractive surgery for the correction of low to mild hyperopia uses the principles of thermal keratoplasty by applying radiofrequency current to the peripheral cornea using a thin, handheld probe. It does not involve the removal of cornea tissue.

RETINAL DISORDERS

Although the retina is composed of multiple microscopic layers, the two innermost layers—the sensory retina and the RPE—are most commonly implicated in retinal disorders (Grossman & Porth, 2014).

Retinal Detachment

Retinal detachment refers to the separation of the RPE from the neurosensory layer (Grossman & Porth, 2014). The four types of retinal detachment are rhegmatogenous, traction, a combination of rhegmatogenous and traction, and exudative. *Rhegmatogenous detachment* is the most common form. In this condition, a hole or tear develops in the sensory retina, allowing some of the liquid vitreous to seep through the sensory retina and detach it from the RPE (see Fig. 63-10). People at risk for this type of detachment include those with high myopia or those who have aphakia (absence of the natural lens) after cataract surgery. Trauma may also play a role in rhegmatogenous retinal detachment. Between 5% and 10% of all rhegmatogenous retinal detachments are associated with proliferative retinopathy—a retinopathy associated with diabetic neovascularization (see Chapter 51).

Tension, or a pulling force, is responsible for *traction retinal detachment.* An ophthalmologist must ascertain all of the areas of retinal break and identify and release the scars or bands of fibrous material providing traction on the retina. In general, patients with this condition have

developed fibrous scar tissue from conditions such as diabetic retinopathy, vitreous hemorrhage, or the retinopathy of prematurity. The hemorrhages and fibrous proliferation associated with these conditions exert a pulling force on the delicate retina.

Patients can have both rhegmatogenous and traction retinal detachment. *Exudative retinal detachments* are the result of the production of a serous fluid under the retina from the choroid. Conditions such as uveitis and macular degeneration may cause the production of this serous fluid.

Clinical Manifestations

Patients may report the sensation of a shade or curtain coming across the vision of one eye, cobwebs, bright flashing lights, or the sudden onset of a great number of floaters. Patients do not complain of pain but retinal detachment is an ocular emergency, requiring immediate surgical intervention for optimal outcomes.

Assessment and Diagnostic Findings

After visual acuity is determined, the patient must have a dilated fundus examination using an indirect ophthalmoscope as well as slit-lamp biomicroscopy. Stereo fundus photography and fluorescein angiography are commonly used during the evaluation.

Increasingly, optical coherence tomography and ultrasound are used for the complete retinal assessment, especially if the view is obscured by a dense cataract or vitreal hemorrhage. All retinal breaks, all fibrous bands that may be causing traction on the retina, and all degenerative changes must be identified.

Surgical Management

In rhegmatogenous detachment, an attempt is made to surgically reattach the sensory retina to the RPE. In traction retinal detachment, the source of traction must be removed and the sensory retina reattached. The most commonly used surgical interventions are the scleral buckle and vitrectomy (Boyd, 2016).

Scleral Buckle

The retinal surgeon compresses the sclera (often with a scleral buckle [see Fig. 63-11] or a silicone band) to indent the scleral wall from the outside of the eye and bring the two retinal layers in contact with each other (Boyd, 2016).

Vitrectomy

A vitrectomy is an intraocular procedure that allows the introduction of a light source through an incision; a second incision serves as the portal for the vitrectomy instrument. The surgeon dissects preretinal membranes under direct visualization while the retina is stabilized by an intraoperative vitreous substitute.

Traction on the retina may be relieved through vitrectomy and may be combined with scleral buckling to repair retinal detachments. A gas bubble, silicone oil, or perfluorocarbon and liquids may be injected into the vitreous cavity to help push the sensory retina up against the RPE. Argon laser photocoagulation or cryotherapy is also used to hold the retina in place (Boyd, 2016).

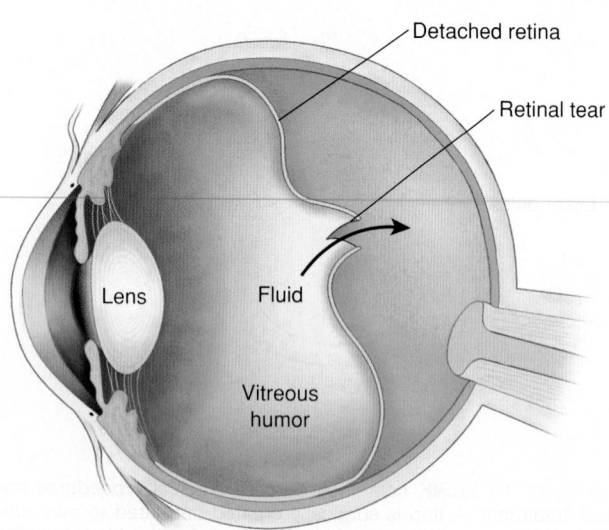

Figure 63-10 • Retinal detachment.

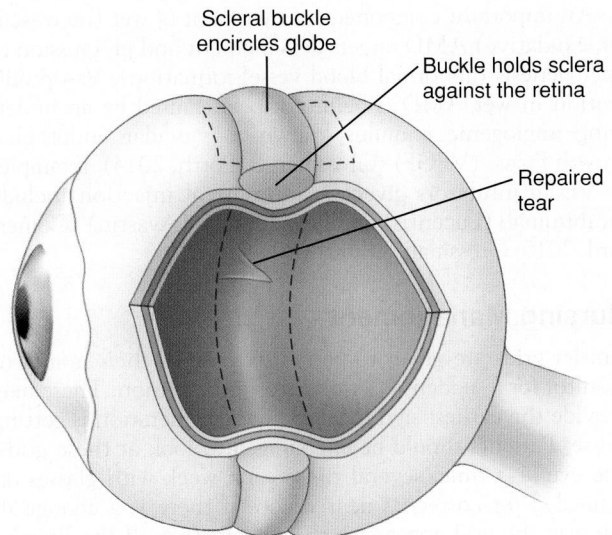

Figure 63-11 • Scleral buckle.

Nursing Management

Nursing management consists of educating the patient and providing supportive care. Postoperative positioning of the patient is critical when a gas bubble is used because the injected bubble must remain in position overlying the area of detachment, providing consistent pressure to reattach the sensory retina. The patient must maintain a prone position that would allow the gas bubble to act as a tamponade for the retinal break (Boyd, 2016). Patients and family members should be made aware of these needs beforehand so that the patient can be made as comfortable as possible.

In most cases, vitreoretinal procedures are performed on an outpatient basis, and the patient is seen the next day for a follow-up examination. Postoperative complications may include increased IOP, endophthalmitis, retinal detachment, and development of cataracts. Patients must be educated about the signs and symptoms of complications, particularly of increasing IOP and postoperative infection. Contact details for the ophthalmic team are provided and the patient is encouraged to call immediately if complications occur.

Retinal Vascular Disorders

Loss of vision can occur from occlusion of a retinal artery or vein. Such occlusions may result from atherosclerosis, valvular heart disease, venous stasis, hypertension, or increased blood viscosity. Associated risk factors include diabetes, glaucoma, and aging.

Central Retinal Vein Occlusion

Blood supply to and from the ocular fundus is provided by the central retinal artery and vein. Central retinal vein occlusions (CRVOs) are found most often in people older than 50 years. Patients who suffer a CRVO report decreased visual acuity ranging from mild blurring to severely limited.

Direct ophthalmoscopy of the retina shows optic disc swelling, venous dilation and tortuousness, retinal hemorrhages, cotton-wool spots, and a bloody appearance of the retina. The better the initial visual acuity, the better the general prognosis.

Fluorescein angiography may show extensive areas of capillary closure. The patient should be monitored carefully over the ensuing several months for signs of neovascularization and neovascular glaucoma. Laser panretinal photocoagulation may be necessary to treat the abnormal neovascularization. Neovascularization of the iris may cause neovascular glaucoma. Macular edema, macular nonperfusion, and vitreous hemorrhage from the neovascularization are among the potential complications of CRVO.

Branch Retinal Vein Occlusion

Some patients with branch retinal vein occlusion (BRVO) are symptom free, whereas others complain of a sudden loss of vision if the macular area is involved. A more gradual loss of vision may occur if macular edema associated with BRVO develops.

On examination, the ocular fundus appears similar to that found in CRVO. The occlusions generally occur at the arteriovenous crossings. The diagnostic evaluation and follow-up assessments and complications are the same as for CRVO. Associated conditions include glaucoma, systemic hypertension, diabetes, and hyperlipidemia.

Central Retinal Artery Occlusion

Patients with central retinal artery occlusion, a relatively rare disorder that accounts for approximately 1 in 10,000 ophthalmologic visits, present with a sudden loss of vision. Visual acuity is reduced to being able to count the examiner's fingers, or the field of vision is tremendously restricted. A relative afferent pupillary defect is present. Examination of the ocular fundus reveals a pale retina with a cherry-red spot at the fovea. The retinal arteries are thin, and emboli are occasionally seen in the central retinal artery or its branches. Central retinal artery occlusion is a true ocular emergency. Various treatments are used: ocular massage, anterior chamber paracentesis, IV administration of hyperosmotic agents such as acetazolamide (Diamox), and high concentrations of oxygen. An aggressive stepwise approach may be beneficial, depending on the underlying cause of the occlusion and the amount of time from onset of occlusion to treatment. Most visual loss associated with central retinal artery occlusion is severe and permanent.

Age-Related Macular Degeneration

AMD accounts for 54% of all blindness in older adults (Centers for Disease Control [CDC], 2016). AMD is characterized by tiny, yellowish spots called *drusen* beneath the retina (see Fig. 63-12). Most people older than 60 years have at least a few small drusen, which are clusters of debris or waste material. When drusen are located in the macular area, they can affect vision. Patients with AMD have a wide range of visual loss, but only a small portion experience total blindness. Central vision is generally the most affected, with most patients retaining peripheral vision (see Fig. 63-13). There are two types of AMD: the dry type and the wet type (CDC, 2016).

Between 85% and 90% of people with AMD have the dry (nonneovascular, nonexudative) type of the condition, in

Figure 63-12 • Retina showing drusen and age-related macular degeneration.

which the outer layers of the retina slowly break down. With this breakdown comes the appearance of drusen. When the drusen occur outside of the macular area, patients generally have no symptoms. When the drusen occur within the macula, however, there is a gradual blurring of vision that patients may notice when they try to read.

The second type of AMD, the wet (neovascular, exudative) type, may have an abrupt onset and is more damaging to the vision (CDC, 2016). Patients report that straight lines appear crooked and distorted or that letters in words appear broken. This effect results from proliferation of abnormal blood vessels growing under the retina, within the choroid layer of the eye, a condition known as choroidal neovascularization. The affected vessels can leak fluid and blood, elevating the retina. Some patients can be treated with laser therapy to stop leakage from these vessels.

Medical Management

There is no known effective therapy for the dry (nonneovascular, nonexudative) type of AMD (Grossman & Porth, 2014).

Age-related Macular Degeneration

Figure 63-13 • Visual changes resulting from age-related macular degeneration. Photo courtesy of the National Eye Institute, National Institutes of Health.

An important component of treatment of wet (neovascular, exudative) AMD targets development and progression of angiogenesis (abnormal blood vessel formation). Vasoproliferation in wet AMD is believed to be caused by an underlying angiogenic stimulus known as vascular endothelial growth factor (VEGF) (Grossman & Porth, 2014). Examples of VEGF inhibitors given by intravitreal injection include ranibizumab (Lucentis) and bevacizumab (Avastin) (Comerford, 2015; Grossman & Porth, 2014).

Nursing Management

Amsler grids are given to patients to use in their homes to monitor for a sudden onset or distortion of vision. These may provide the earliest sign that macular degeneration is getting worse. Patients should be encouraged to look at these grids, one eye at a time, several times each week with glasses on if needed for corrected near vision. If there is a change in the way the grid appears to the patient (e.g., if the lines or squares appear distorted or faded), the patient should notify the ophthalmologist immediately and should arrange to be seen promptly.

Orbital and Ocular Trauma

Whether affecting the eye or the orbit, trauma to the eye and surrounding structures may have devastating consequences for vision. It is preferable to prevent injury rather than treat it. Chart 63-10 details measures to prevent eye injuries.

Orbital Trauma

Injury to the orbit is usually associated with a head injury; hence, the patient's general medical condition must first be stabilized before conducting an ocular examination (Hickey, 2014). Only then is the globe assessed for soft tissue injury. During inspection, the face is meticulously assessed for underlying fractures, which should always be suspected in cases of blunt trauma. To establish the extent of ocular injury, visual acuity is assessed as soon as possible, even if it is only a rough estimate. Soft tissue orbital injuries often result in damage to the optic nerve. Major ocular injuries indicated by a soft globe, prolapsing tissue, ruptured globe, and hemorrhage require immediate surgical attention.

Soft Tissue Injury and Hemorrhage

The signs and symptoms of soft tissue injury from blunt or penetrating trauma include tenderness, ecchymosis, lid swelling, **proptosis or exophthalmos** (abnormal protrusion of the eyeball), and hemorrhage. Closed injuries lead to contusions with subconjunctival hemorrhage, commonly known as a black eye. Blood accumulates in the tissues of the conjunctiva. Hemorrhage may be caused by a soft tissue injury to the eyelid or by an underlying fracture.

Management of soft tissue hemorrhage that does not threaten vision is usually conservative and consists of thorough inspection, cleansing, and repair of wounds. Cold compresses are used in the early phase, followed by warm compresses. Hematomas that appear as swollen, fluctuating areas may be surgically drained or aspirated; if they are causing significant orbital pressure, they may be surgically evacuated.

Chart 63-10

PATIENT EDUCATION

Education for Patients About Preventing Eye Injuries

The nurse instructs the patient in the following measures to prevent eye injuries:

In and Around the House

- Make sure that all spray nozzles are directed away from yourself before pressing down on the handle.
- Read instructions carefully before using cleaning fluids, detergents, ammonia, or harsh chemicals, and wash hands thoroughly after use.
- Use grease shields on frying pans to decrease spattering.
- Use opaque goggles to avoid burns from sunlamps.
- Wear special goggles to shield the eyes from fumes and splashes when using powerful chemicals.

In the Workshop

- Protect the eyes from flying fragments, fumes, dust particles, sparks, and splashed chemicals by wearing safety glasses.
- Read instructions thoroughly before using tools and chemicals, and follow precautions for their use.

Around Children

- Educate children about the correct way to handle potentially dangerous items, such as scissors and pencils.
- Pay attention to age and maturity level of a child when selecting toys and games, and avoid projectile toys, such as darts and pellet guns.
- Supervise children when they are playing with toys or games that can be dangerous.

In the Garden

- Avoid letting anyone stand at the side of or in front of a moving lawn mower.

- Avoid low-hanging branches.
- Direct pesticide spray can nozzles away from the face.
- Pick up rocks and stones before going over them with the lawn mower (stones can be hurled out of the rotary blades and rebound off curbs or walls, causing severe injury to the eye).

Around the Car

- Put out all smoking materials and matches before opening the hood of the car.
- Take standard safety precautions when using jumper cables (wear goggles; make sure the cars are not touching one another; make sure the jumper cable clamps never touch each other; never lean over the battery when attaching cables; and never attach a cable to the negative terminal of a dead battery).
- Use a flashlight, not a match or lighter, to look at the battery at night.
- Wear goggles when grinding metal or striking metal against metal while performing auto body repair.

In Sports

- Wear protective caps, helmets, or face protectors when appropriate, especially for sports such as ice hockey.
- Wear protective safety glasses, especially for sports such as racquetball, squash, tennis, baseball, and basketball.

Around Fireworks

- Avoid explosive fireworks.
- Avoid standing near others when lighting fireworks.
- Douse firework duds in water instead of attempting to relight them.
- Never allow children to ignite fireworks.
- Wear eyeglasses or safety goggles.

Orbital Fractures

Orbital fractures are detected by facial x-rays. Depending on the orbital structures involved, orbital fractures can be classified as blowout, zygomatic or tripod, maxillary, midfacial, orbital apex, and orbital roof fractures. Blowout fractures result from compression of soft tissue and the sudden increase in orbital pressure when the force is transmitted to the orbital floor, which is the area of least resistance (Hickey, 2014).

The inferior rectus and inferior oblique muscles, with their fat and fascial attachments, or the nerve that courses along the inferior oblique muscle may become entrapped, and the globe may be displaced inward (i.e., enophthalmos). Computed tomography (CT) scanning can identify the muscle and its auxiliary structures that are entrapped. These fractures are usually caused by the blunt force from a fist or baseball (Hickey, 2014).

Orbital roof fractures are dangerous because of potential complications to the brain. Surgical management of these fractures requires a neurosurgeon and an ophthalmologist. The most common indications for surgical intervention are displacement of bone fragments disfiguring the normal facial contours, interference with normal binocular vision caused by extraocular muscle entrapment, interference with mastication in zygomatic fracture, and obstruction of the nasolacrimal duct. Surgery is usually nonemergent, and a period of 10 to 14 days gives the ophthalmologist time to assess ocular

function, especially the extraocular muscles and the nasolacrimal duct. Emergency surgical repair is usually not performed unless the globe is displaced into the maxillary sinus. Surgical repair is primarily directed at freeing the entrapped ocular structures and restoring the integrity of the orbital floor.

Foreign Bodies

Foreign bodies that enter the orbit are usually tolerated, except for copper, iron, and vegetable materials such as those from plants or trees, which may cause purulent infection. X-rays and CT scans are used to identify the foreign body. A careful history is important, especially if the foreign body has been in the orbit for a period of time and the incident forgotten. It is important to identify metallic foreign bodies because they prohibit the use of magnetic resonance imaging (MRI) as a diagnostic tool.

After the extent of the orbital damage is assessed, the decision to use conservative treatment or surgical removal is made. In general, orbital foreign bodies are removed if they are superficial and anterior in location; have sharp edges that may affect adjacent orbital structures; or are composed of copper, iron, or vegetable material. Surgical intervention is directed at preventing further ocular injury and maintaining the integrity of the affected areas. Cultures are usually obtained, and the patient is placed on prophylactic IV antibiotic medications that are later changed to an oral route.

Ocular Trauma

Ocular trauma is a leading cause of blindness among children and young adults, especially male trauma victims. Ocular trauma occurs with occupational injuries (e.g., construction industry), contact sports, weapons (e.g., air guns, BB guns), assaults, motor vehicle crashes (e.g., broken windshields), and explosions (e.g., blast fragments).

There are two types of ocular trauma in which the first response is critical: chemical burn and foreign object in the eye. With a chemical burn, the eye should be immediately irrigated with tap water or normal saline. With a foreign body, no attempt should be made to remove the foreign object. The object should be protected from jarring or movement to prevent further ocular damage. No pressure or patch should be applied to the affected eye. All other traumatic eye injuries should be protected using a patch or shield if available or a stiff paper cup until medical treatment can be obtained (see Fig. 63-14).

Assessment and Diagnostic Findings

A thorough history is obtained, particularly assessing the patient's ocular history, such as pre-injury vision in the affected eye or past ocular surgery. Details related to the injury that help in the diagnosis and assessment of the need for further tests include the nature of the ocular injury (i.e., blunt or penetrating trauma); the type of activity that caused the injury to determine the nature of the force striking the eye; and whether onset of vision loss was sudden, slow, or progressive. For chemical eye burns, the chemical agent must be identified and tested for pH if the agent is available. The corneal surface is examined for foreign bodies, wounds, and abrasions, after which the other external structures of the eye are examined. Pupil size, shape, and light reaction of the pupil of the affected eye are compared with the other eye. Ocular motility (ability of the eyes to move synchronously up, down, right, and left) is also assessed.

Medical Management

Splash Injuries

Splash injuries are irrigated with normal saline solution before further evaluation occurs. In cases of a ruptured globe, cycloplegic agents (agents that paralyze the ciliary muscle) or topical antibiotics must be deferred because of potential

Figure 63-14 • Two kinds of eye patches. A. Aluminum shield. **B.** Stiff paper cup shield (innovative substitute when aluminum shield is unavailable).

toxicity to exposed intraocular tissues. Further manipulation of the eye must be avoided until the patient is under general anesthesia. Parenteral, broad-spectrum antibiotics are initiated. Tetanus antitoxin is given, if indicated, as well as analgesic agents. (Tetanus prophylaxis is recommended for full-thickness ocular and skin wounds.) Any topical ophthalmic medication (e.g., anesthetic, dyes) must be sterile.

Foreign Bodies and Corneal Abrasions

After removal of a foreign body from the surface of the eye, an antibiotic ointment is applied and the eye is patched. The eye is examined daily for evidence of infection until the wound is completely healed.

Contact lens wear is a common cause of corneal abrasion. The patient experiences severe pain and **photophobia** (ocular pain on exposure to light). Corneal epithelial defects are treated with antibiotic ointment and, in some instances, a pressure patch to immobilize the eyelids. Topical anesthetic eye drops must not be given to the patient to take home for repeated use after corneal injury because their effects mask further damage, delay healing, and can lead to corneal scarring.

Penetrating Injuries and Contusions of the Eyeball

Sharp penetrating injury or blunt contusion force can rupture the eyeball. When the globe, cornea, and sclera rupture, rapid decompression or herniation of the orbital contents into adjacent sinuses can occur. Blunt traumatic injuries (with an increased incidence of retinal detachment, intraocular tissue avulsion, and herniation) have a worse prognosis than penetrating injuries. Most penetrating injuries result in marked loss of vision with the following signs: hemorrhagic **chemosis** (edema of the conjunctiva), conjunctival laceration, shallow anterior chamber with or without an eccentrically placed pupil, **hyphema** (blood within the anterior chamber), or vitreous hemorrhage.

Hyphema is caused by contusion forces that tear the vessels of the iris and damage the anterior chamber angle. Preventing rebleeding and prolonged increased IOP are the goals of treatment for hyphema. In severe cases, the patient is hospitalized with moderate activity restriction. An eye shield is applied. Topical corticosteroids are prescribed to reduce inflammation. An antifibrinolytic agent (aminocaproic acid [Amicar]) stabilizes clot formation at the site of hemorrhage. Aspirin is contraindicated. A ruptured globe and severe injuries with intraocular hemorrhage require surgical intervention. Vitrectomy is performed for traumatic retinal detachments (Boyd, 2016). Primary **enucleation** (complete removal of the eyeball and part of the optic nerve) is considered only if the globe is irreparable and has no light perception. It is a general rule that enucleation is performed within 2 weeks of the initial injury (in an eye that has no useful vision after sustaining penetrating injury) to prevent the risk of **sympathetic ophthalmia** (an inflammation created in the uninjured eye by the affected eye that can result in blindness of the uninjured eye).

Intraocular Foreign Bodies

A patient who complains of blurred vision and discomfort should be questioned carefully about recent injuries and exposures. Patients may be injured in a number of different situations and experience an intraocular foreign body

(IOFB). Precipitating circumstances can include working in construction, striking metal against metal, being involved in a motor vehicle crash with facial injury, a gunshot wound, grinding-wheel work, and explosions.

IOFB is diagnosed and localized by slit-lamp biomicroscopy and indirect ophthalmoscopy, as well as CT or ultrasonography scanning. MRI is contraindicated because most foreign bodies are metallic and magnetic. It is important to determine the composition, size, and location of the IOFB and affected eye structures. Every effort should be made to identify the type of IOFB and whether it is magnetic. Iron, steel, copper, and vegetable matter may cause intense inflammatory reactions. The incidence of endophthalmitis is high. Surgical excision of the foreign body depends on its location and composition and associated ocular injuries. Specially designed IOFB forceps and magnets are used to grasp and remove the foreign body. Any damaged area of the retina is treated to prevent retinal detachment.

Ocular Burns

Alkali, acid, and other chemically active organic substances, such as Mace and tear gas, cause chemical burns. Alkali burns (e.g., lye, ammonia) result in the most severe injury because they penetrate the ocular tissues rapidly and continue to cause long-term damage. Increased IOP also occurs. Acids (e.g., bleach, car batteries, refrigerant) generally cause less damage because the precipitated necrotic tissue proteins form a barrier to further penetration and damage. Chemical burns may appear as superficial punctate keratopathy (i.e., spotty damage to the cornea), subconjunctival hemorrhage, or complete marbleizing of the cornea.

In treating chemical burns, every minute counts. Immediate irrigation with tap water should be started on site before transport of the patient to an emergency department. A brief history and examination are performed. Critical information, if available, is the name of the substance that went into the eye (the actual container is best). Material safety data sheets (MSDS) should be accessed for reference (see Chapter 73). The corneal surfaces and conjunctival fornices are immediately and copiously irrigated with normal saline or any neutral solution. A local anesthetic is instilled, and a lid speculum is applied to overcome blepharospasm (i.e., spasms of the eyelid muscles that result in closure of the lids). Particulate matter must be removed from the fornices using moistened, cotton-tipped applicators and minimal pressure on the globe. Irrigation continues until the conjunctival pH normalizes (between 7.3 and 7.6). The pH of the corneal surface is checked by placing a pH paper strip in the fornix. Antibiotic agents are instilled, and the eye usually is patched.

The goal of intermediate treatment is to prevent tissue ulceration and promote re-epithelialization of the cornea. Intense lubrication using artificial tears without preservatives (to avoid allergic reactions) is essential. Patching or therapeutic soft lenses may also be used to promote corneal healing, and the patient is closely monitored. Prognosis depends on the type of injury and adequacy of the irrigation immediately after exposure. Long-term treatment consists of two phases: restoration of the ocular surface through grafting procedures and surgical restoration of corneal integrity and optical clarity.

Thermal injury is caused by exposure to a hot object (e.g., curling iron, tobacco, ash), whereas photochemical injury results from ultraviolet irradiation or infrared exposure (e.g., exposure to the reflections from snow, sun gazing, viewing an eclipse of the sun without an adequate filter). These injuries can cause corneal epithelial defect, corneal opacity, conjunctival chemosis and **injection** (congestion of blood vessels), and burns of the eyelids and periocular region. Antibiotic agents and a patch for 24 hours constitute the treatment of mild injuries.

INFECTIOUS AND INFLAMMATORY CONDITIONS

Inflammation and infections of eye structures are common. Table 63-7 summarizes selected common infections and their treatment.

Dry Eyes

Dry eyes can be caused by decreased tear production or increased tear evaporation, which can be episodic or chronic (Grossman & Porth, 2014). Decreased tear production (aqueous deficiency) can be caused by systemic disease (Sjögren's, connective tissue disease), lacrimal gland obstruction, and systemic drugs (e.g., diuretics, antihistamines, psychotropic drugs). Increased tear evaporation (evaporative dry eye) can be caused by meibomian gland deficiency, lid aperture disorder, vitamin A deficiency, reduced lid blinking rate, preservatives from topical drugs, ocular surface disease (allergy), and contact lens wear. Risk factors include increasing age, smoking, recent refractive surgery, and postmenopausal status (in women). An increase in the intake of omega-3 fatty acids may be beneficial in reducing the risk (Grossman & Porth, 2014).

Clinical Manifestations

The most common complaints are photophobia, foreign-body sensation, burning and stinging, redness, and decreased tearing.

Assessment and Diagnostic Findings

Chronic dry eyes may result in chronic conjunctival and corneal irritation that can lead to corneal erosion, scarring, ulceration, thinning, or perforation that can seriously threaten vision. Secondary bacterial infection can occur.

Management

Management of dry eyes requires the cooperation of the patient with a regimen that needs to be followed at home for a long period; otherwise, complete relief of symptoms is unlikely. Instillation of artificial tears during the day and an ointment at night is the usual regimen to hydrate and lubricate the eye and preserve a moist ocular surface. Cyclosporine ophthalmic emulsion (Restasis) is an effective agent that increases tear production and is used once daily. Anti-inflammatory medications are also used, and moisture chambers (e.g., moisture chamber spectacles, swim goggles) may provide additional relief.

Patients may become hypersensitive to chemical preservatives such as benzalkonium chloride and thimerosal. For these patients, preservative-free ophthalmic solutions are

TABLE 63-7 Common Infections and Inflammatory Disorders of Eye Structures

Disorder	Description	Management
Hordeolum (stye)	Acute suppurative infection of the glands of the eyelids caused by *Staphylococcus aureus*. The lid is red and edematous with a small collection of pus in the form of an abscess. There is considerable discomfort.	Warm compresses are applied directly to the affected lid area 3–4 times a day for 10–15 minutes. If the condition is not improved after 48 hours, incision and drainage may be indicated. Application of topical antibiotics may be prescribed thereafter.
Chalazion	Sterile inflammatory process involving chronic granulomatous inflammation of the meibomian glands; can appear as a single granuloma or multiple granulomas in the upper or lower eyelids.	Warm compresses applied 3–4 times a day for 10–15 minutes may resolve the inflammation in the early stages. Most often, however, surgical excision is indicated. Corticosteroid injection to the chalazion lesion may be used for smaller lesions.
Blepharitis	Chronic bilateral inflammation of the eyelid margins. There are 2 types: staphylococcal and seborrheic. Staphylococcal blepharitis is usually ulcerative and is more serious due to the involvement of the base of hair follicles. Permanent scarring can result.	The seborrheic type is chronic and is usually resistant to treatment, but the milder cases may respond to lid hygiene. Staphylococcal blepharitis requires topical antibiotic treatment. Instructions on lid hygiene (to keep the lid margins clean and free of exudates) are given to the patient.
Bacterial keratitis	Infection of the cornea by *S. aureus*, *Streptococcus pneumoniae*, and *Pseudomonas aeruginosa*.	Fortified (high-concentration) antibiotic eye drops are given every 30 minutes around the clock for the first few days, then every 1–2 hours. Systemic antibiotics may be given. Cycloplegics are given to reduce pain caused by ciliary spasm. Corticosteroid therapy and subconjunctival injections of antibiotics are controversial.
Herpes simplex keratitis	Leading cause of corneal blindness in the United States. Symptoms are severe pain, tearing, and photophobia. The dendritic ulcer has a branching, linear pattern with feathery edges and terminal bulbs at its ends. Herpes simplex keratitis can lead to recurrent stromal keratitis and persist to 12 months with residual corneal scarring.	Many lesions heal without treatment and residual effects. The treatment goal is to minimize the damaging effect of the inflammatory response and eliminate viral replication within the cornea. Penetrating keratoplasty is indicated for corneal scarring and must be performed when the herpetic disease has been inactive for many months.

used. Management of dry eyes also includes the concurrent treatment of infections, such as chronic blepharitis and acne rosacea, and treating the underlying systemic disease, such as Sjögren syndrome (an autoimmune disease).

Surgical treatment includes punctal occlusion, grafting procedures, and lateral tarsorrhaphy (uniting the edges of the lids). Punctal plugs are made of silicone material for the temporary or permanent occlusion of the puncta. These help to preserve the volume of natural tears and prolong the effects of artificial tears (Grossman & Porth, 2014).

Conjunctivitis

Conjunctivitis (inflammation of the conjunctiva) is a common ocular disorder worldwide. It is characterized by a pink appearance (hence the common term *pink eye*) because of subconjunctival blood vessel congestion.

Clinical Manifestations

General symptoms include foreign-body sensation, scratching or burning sensation, itching, and photophobia. Conjunctivitis may be unilateral or bilateral, but the infection usually starts in one eye and then spreads to the other eye by hand contact.

Assessment and Diagnostic Findings

The four main clinical features important to evaluate are the type of discharge (watery, mucoid, purulent, or mucopurulent), type of conjunctival reaction (follicular or papillary),

presence of pseudomembranes or true membranes, and presence or absence of lymphadenopathy (enlargement of the preauricular and submandibular lymph nodes where the eyelids drain). Pseudomembranes consist of coagulated exudate that adheres to the surface of the inflamed conjunctiva. True membranes form when the exudate adheres to the superficial layer of the conjunctiva, and removal results in bleeding. Follicles are multiple, slightly elevated lesions encircled by tiny blood vessels; they look like grains of rice. Papillae are hyperplastic conjunctival epithelium in numerous projections that are usually seen as a fine mosaic pattern under slit-lamp examination. Diagnosis is based on the distinctive characteristics of ocular signs, acute or chronic presentation, and identification of any precipitating events. Positive results of swab smear preparations and cultures confirm the diagnosis.

Types of Conjunctivitis

Conjunctivitis is classified according to its cause. The major causes are microbial infection, allergy, and irritating toxic stimuli. A wide spectrum of organisms can cause conjunctivitis, including bacteria (e.g., *Chlamydia*), viruses, fungus, and parasites. Conjunctivitis can also result from an existing ocular infection or can be a manifestation of a systemic disease.

Microbial Conjunctivitis
Bacterial Conjunctivitis

Bacterial conjunctivitis can be acute or chronic. The acute type can develop into a chronic condition. Signs and symptoms can vary from mild to severe. Chronic bacterial conjunctivitis is usually seen in patients with lacrimal duct obstruction, chronic dacryocystitis, and chronic blepharitis. The most common causative microorganisms are *Streptococcus pneumoniae*, *Haemophilus influenzae*, and *Staphylococcus aureus*.

Bacterial conjunctivitis manifests with an acute onset of redness, burning, and discharge. There is papillary formation, conjunctival irritation, and injection in the fornices. The exudates are variable but are usually present on waking in the morning. The eyes may be difficult to open because of adhesions caused by the exudate. Purulent discharge occurs in severe acute bacterial infections, whereas mucopurulent discharge appears in mild cases. In gonococcal conjunctivitis, the symptoms are more acute. The exudate is profuse and purulent, and there is lymphadenopathy. Pseudomembranes may be present.

Trachoma is an infectious disease caused by the bacterium *Chlamydia trachomatis*, an ancient disease and the leading cause of preventable blindness in the world (Grossman & Porth, 2014). It is prevalent in areas with hot, dry, and dusty climates and in areas with poor living conditions. It is spread by direct contact or by carrier (e.g., insects such as flies and gnats). The onset of trachoma in children is usually insidious, but it can be acute or subacute in adults. The initial symptoms include red inflamed eyes, tearing, photophobia, ocular pain, purulent exudates, preauricular lymphadenopathy, and lid edema. Initial ocular signs include follicular and papillary formations. At the middle stage of the disease, there is an acute inflammation with papillary hypertrophy and follicular necrosis, after which trichiasis and entropion begin to develop. The lashes that are turned in rub against the cornea and, after prolonged irritation, cause corneal erosion and ulceration. The late stage of the disease is characterized by scarred conjunctiva, subepithelial keratitis, abnormal vascularization of the cornea (pannus), and residual scars from the follicles that look like depressions in the conjunctiva (Herbert pits). Severe corneal ulceration can lead to perforation and blindness.

Inclusion conjunctivitis affects sexually active people who have genital chlamydial infection. Transmission is by oral–genital sex or hand-to-eye transmission. Indirect transmission can occur in inadequately chlorinated swimming pools. The eye lesions usually appear a week after exposure and may be associated with a nonspecific urethritis or cervicitis. The discharge is mucopurulent, follicles are present, and there is lymphadenopathy.

Viral Conjunctivitis

Viral conjunctivitis can be acute and chronic. The discharge is watery, and follicles are prominent. Severe cases include pseudomembranes. The common causative organisms are adenovirus and herpes simplex virus. Conjunctivitis caused by adenovirus is highly contagious. The condition is usually preceded by symptoms of upper respiratory infection. Corneal involvement causes extreme photophobia. Symptoms include tearing, redness, and foreign-body sensation that can involve one or both eyes. There is lid edema, ptosis, and conjunctival **hyperemia** (red eyes caused by dilation of blood vessels) (see Fig. 63-15). These signs and symptoms vary from mild to severe. Viral conjunctivitis, although self-limited, tends to last longer than bacterial conjunctivitis.

Figure 63-15 • Conjunctival hyperemia in viral conjunctivitis.

Epidemic keratoconjunctivitis (EKC) is a highly contagious viral conjunctivitis that is easily transmitted from one person to another among household members, schoolchildren, and health care workers. The outbreak of epidemics is seasonal, especially during the summer when people use swimming pools. EKC is most often accompanied by preauricular lymphadenopathy and occasionally periorbital pain. There are marked follicular and papillary formations. This type of conjunctivitis can lead to keratopathy.

Allergic Conjunctivitis

Immunologic or allergic conjunctivitis is a hypersensitivity reaction that occurs as part of allergic rhinitis (hay fever), or it can be an independent allergic reaction. The patient usually has a history of an allergy to pollens and other environmental allergens. There is extreme pruritus, epiphora (excessive secretion of tears), injection, and usually severe photophobia. The stringlike mucoid discharge is usually associated with rubbing the eyes because of severe pruritus. Vernal conjunctivitis is also known as seasonal conjunctivitis because it appears mostly during warm weather. There may be large formations of papillae that have a cobblestone appearance. It is more common in children and young adults. Most affected people have a history of asthma or eczema.

Toxic Conjunctivitis

Chemical conjunctivitis can be the result of medications; chlorine from swimming pools; exposure to toxic fumes among industrial workers; or exposure to other irritants such as smoke, hair sprays, acids, and alkalis.

Medical Management

The management of conjunctivitis depends on the type. Most types of mild and viral conjunctivitis are self-limiting, benign conditions that may not require treatment and laboratory procedures. For more severe cases, topical antibiotic agents, eye drops, or ointments are prescribed. Patients with gonococcal conjunctivitis require urgent antibiotic therapy. If left untreated, this ocular disease can lead to corneal perforation and blindness. The systemic complications can include meningitis and sepsis.

Bacterial Conjunctivitis

Acute bacterial conjunctivitis is almost always self-limiting, lasting 2 weeks if left untreated. If treated with antibiotics, it may last a few days, except for gonococcal and staphylococcal conjunctivitis.

For trachoma, usually broad-spectrum antibiotic agents are given topically and systemically. Surgical management includes the correction of trichiasis to prevent conjunctival scarring.

Adult inclusion conjunctivitis requires 1 week of antibiotics. Prevention of reinfection is important, and affected people and their sexual partners must seek treatment for sexually transmitted infection, if indicated.

Viral Conjunctivitis

Viral conjunctivitis is not responsive to any treatment. Cold compresses may alleviate some symptoms. Viral conjunctivitis, especially EKC, is highly contagious. Patients must be made aware of the contagious nature of the disease, and adequate education must be provided (see Chart 63-11).

Proper steps must be taken to avoid health care–associated infections. Frequent hand hygiene and procedures for environmental cleaning and disinfection of equipment used for eye examination must be strictly followed at all times. To prevent spread during outbreaks of conjunctivitis caused by adenovirus, health care facilities must set aside specified areas for treating patients diagnosed with or suspected of having conjunctivitis caused by adenovirus. All forms of tonometry must be avoided unless medically indicated. All multidose ophthalmic medications must be discarded at the end of each day or when contaminated. Employees who are infected and others must not be allowed to work or attend school until symptoms have resolved, which can take 3 to 7 days.

Allergic Conjunctivitis

Patients with allergic conjunctivitis, especially recurrent vernal or seasonal conjunctivitis, are usually given corticosteroids in ophthalmic preparations. Depending on the severity of the disease, they may be given oral preparations. The use of vasoconstrictors, such as topical epinephrine solution, cold compresses, ice packs, and cool ventilation usually provide comfort by decreasing swelling.

Toxic Conjunctivitis

For conjunctivitis caused by chemical irritants, the eye must be irrigated immediately and profusely with saline or sterile water.

Uveitis

Inflammation of the uveal tract (uveitis) can affect the iris, the ciliary body, or the choroid. There are two types of uveitis: nongranulomatous and granulomatous.

The more common form of uveitis is the nongranulomatous type, which manifests as an acute condition with pain, photophobia, and a pattern of conjunctival injection, especially around the cornea. The pupil is small or irregular, and vision is blurred. There may be small, fine precipitates on the posterior corneal surface and cells in the aqueous humor (i.e., cell and flare). If the uveitis is severe, a **hypopyon** (accumulation of inflammatory cells in the anterior chamber of the eye) may develop. The condition may be unilateral or bilateral and may be recurrent. Repeated attacks of nongranulomatous anterior uveitis can cause anterior synechiae (peripheral iris adheres to the cornea and impedes outflow of aqueous humor). Posterior synechiae (adherence of the iris and lens) block aqueous outflow from the posterior chamber. Secondary glaucoma can result from either anterior or posterior synechiae. Cataracts may also occur as a sequela to uveitis.

Granulomatous uveitis can have a more insidious onset and can involve any portion of the uveal tract. It tends to be chronic. Symptoms such as photophobia and pain may be minimal. Vision is markedly and adversely affected. Conjunctival injection is diffuse, and there may be vitreous clouding. In a severe posterior uveitis, such as chorioretinitis, there may be retinal and choroidal hemorrhages.

Medical Management

Because photophobia is a common symptom, patients should wear dark glasses outdoors. Ciliary spasm and synechia are best avoided through mydriasis; cyclopentolate (Cyclogyl) and atropine are commonly used. Local corticosteroid drops, such as Pred Forte 1% and Flarex 0.1%, instilled four to six times a day are also used to decrease inflammation.

If the uveitis is recurrent, a careful history should be initiated to discover any underlying causes. This evaluation should include a complete history, physical examination, and

---

Chart 63-11

PATIENT EDUCATION

Education for Patients With Viral Conjunctivitis

Viral conjunctivitis is a highly contagious eye infection that can easily spread from one person to another. The symptoms can be alarming but are not serious.

The nurse instructs the patient about this eye condition and the following self-care strategies:

- Be aware that your eyes will look red and will have watery discharge, and your lids will be swollen for about a week.
- Expect to experience eye pain, a sandy sensation in your eye, and sensitivity to light.
- Keep in mind that symptoms will resolve after about 1 week.
- Use lightweight cold compresses over your eyes for about 10 minutes 4–5 times a day to soothe the pain.
- Use artificial tears for the sandy sensation in your eye and mild pain medications such as acetaminophen (Tylenol).
- Stay at home and not go outside. You may return to work or school after 7 days, when the redness and discharge have cleared. Obtain a note from your primary provider to return to work or school.
- Do not share towels, linens, makeup, or any items that have come in contact with your eyes.
- Wash your hands thoroughly with soap and water frequently, including before and after you apply artificial tears or cold compresses.
- Use a new tissue every time you wipe the discharge from your eye. Dampen the tissue with clean water to clean the outside of the eye.
- Wash your face and take a shower as you normally do.
- Discard all of your makeup articles and do not apply makeup until the infection has resolved.
- Wear dark glasses if bright lights bother you.
- Note if the discharge from your eye turns yellowish and purulent or if your vision changes and return to the primary provider for an examination.

diagnostic tests, including a complete blood count, erythrocyte sedimentation rate, antinuclear antibodies, and Venereal Disease Research Laboratory (VDRL) and Lyme disease titers. Underlying causes include autoimmune disorders such as ankylosing spondylitis and sarcoidosis as well as toxoplasmosis, herpes zoster virus, ocular candidiasis, histoplasmosis, herpes simplex virus, tuberculosis, and syphilis.

Orbital Cellulitis

Orbital cellulitis is inflammation of the tissues surrounding the eye that may result from bacterial, fungal, or viral inflammatory conditions of contiguous structures, such as the face, oropharynx, dental structures, or intracranial structures. It can also result from foreign bodies and pre-existing ocular infection, such as dacryocystitis and panophthalmitis, or from sepsis. Infection of the sinuses is the most frequent cause. Infection originating in the sinuses can spread easily to the orbit through the thin bony walls and foramina or by means of the interconnecting venous system of the orbit and sinuses. The most common causative organisms are staphylococci and streptococci in adults. The symptoms include pain, eyelid swelling, conjunctival edema, proptosis, and decreased ocular motility. With such edema, optic nerve compression can occur and IOP may increase.

The severe intraorbital tension caused by abscess formation and the impairment of optic nerve function in orbital cellulitis can result in permanent visual loss. Because of the orbit's proximity to the brain, orbital cellulitis can lead to life-threatening complications, such as intracranial abscess and cavernous sinus thrombosis.

Medical Management

Immediate administration of high-dose, broad-spectrum, systemic antibiotics is indicated. Cultures and Gram-stained smears are obtained. Monitoring changes in visual acuity, degree of proptosis, central nervous system function (e.g., nausea, vomiting, fever, cognitive changes), displacement of the globe, extraocular movements, pupillary signs, and the fundus is extremely important. Consultation with an otolaryngologist is necessary, especially when rhinosinusitis is suspected. In the event of abscess formation or progressive loss of vision, surgical drainage of the abscess or sinus is performed. Sinusotomy and antibiotic irrigation are also performed.

ORBITAL AND OCULAR TUMORS

Benign Tumors of the Orbit

Benign tumors can develop from infancy and grow rapidly or slowly and present in later life. Some benign tumors are superficial and are easily identifiable by external presentation, palpation, and x-rays, but some are deep and may require a CT scan to diagnose. There can be significant proptosis, and visual function may be jeopardized. Benign tumors are masses characterized by the lack of infiltration in the surrounding tissues. Examples are cystic dermoid cysts and mucocele, hemangiomas, lymphangiomas, lacrimal tumors, and neurofibromas.

To prevent recurrence, benign masses are excised completely when possible. Excision may be difficult because of the involvement of some portions of the orbital bones, such as deep dermoid cysts, in which dissection of the bone is required. Subtotal resection may be indicated in deep benign tumors that intertwine with other orbital structures, such as optic nerve meningiomas. Complete removal of the tumor may endanger visual function.

Benign Tumors of the Eyelids

There are a wide variety of benign tumors that increase in frequency with age. Nevi may be unpigmented at birth and may enlarge and darken in adolescence or may never acquire any pigment at all. Hemangiomas are vascular capillary tumors that may be bright, superficial, red lesions (formerly known as strawberry angiomas) or bluish and purplish deeper lesions. Milia are small, white, slightly elevated cysts of the eyelid that may occur in multiples. Xanthelasma are yellowish, lipoid deposits on both lids that commonly appear as a result of the aging of the skin or a lipid disorder. Molluscum contagiosum lesions are flat, symmetric growths along the lid margin caused by a virus that can result in conjunctivitis and keratitis if the lesion grows into the conjunctival sac.

Treatment of benign congenital lid lesions is rarely indicated except when visual function is affected. Corticosteroid injection to the hemangioma lesion is usually effective, but surgical excision may be performed. Benign lid lesions usually present aesthetic problems rather than visual function problems. Surgical excision, or electrocautery, is primarily performed for cosmetic reasons, except for cases of molluscum contagiosum, for which surgical intervention is performed to prevent an infectious process that may ensue.

Benign Tumors of the Conjunctiva

Conjunctival nevus, a congenital benign neoplasm, is a flat, slightly elevated, brown spot that becomes pigmented during late childhood or adolescence. This should be differentiated from the pigmented lesion melanosis, which is acquired at middle age and may become melanoma. Keratin- and sebum-containing dermoid cysts are congenital and can be found in the conjunctiva. Dermolipoma is a congenital tumor that manifests as a smooth, rounded growth in the conjunctiva near the lateral canthus. Papillomas are usually soft with irregular surfaces and appear on the lid margins. Treatment consists of surgical excision.

Malignant Tumors of the Orbit

Rhabdomyosarcoma is the most common malignant primary orbital tumor in childhood; it can also develop in older adults. The symptoms of rhabdomyosarcoma include sudden painless proptosis of one eye followed by lid swelling, conjunctival chemosis, and impairment of ocular motility. CT or MRI scans of these tumors establish the size, configuration, location, and stage of the disease; delineates the degree of bone destruction; and is useful in estimating the field for radiation therapy. The most common site of metastasis is the lung.

Management of these primary malignant orbital tumors involves three major therapeutic modalities: surgery, radiation therapy, and adjuvant chemotherapy. The degree of orbital destruction is important in planning the surgical approach. Resection often involves removal of the eyeball. The psychological needs of the patient and family are paramount in planning the management approach.

Malignant Tumors of the Eyelid

Basal cell carcinoma is the most common malignant tumor of the eyelid. Squamous cell carcinoma occurs less frequently but is considered the second most common malignant tumor. Melanoma is rare. Malignant eyelid tumors occur more frequently among people with a fair complexion who have a history of chronic exposure to the sun (Grossman & Porth, 2014).

Basal cell carcinoma appears as a painless nodule that may ulcerate. The lesion is invasive, spreads to the surrounding tissues, and grows slowly but does not metastasize. It usually appears on the lower lid margin near the inner canthus with a pearly white margin. Squamous cell carcinoma of the eyelids may resemble basal cell carcinoma initially because it also grows slowly and painlessly. It tends to ulcerate and invade the surrounding tissues, but it can metastasize to the regional lymph nodes. Melanoma may not be pigmented and can arise from nevi. It spreads to the surrounding tissues and metastasizes to other organs.

Complete excision of these carcinomas is followed by reconstruction with skin grafting if the surgical excision is extensive. The ocular postoperative site and the graft donor site are monitored for bleeding. Donor graft sites may include the buccal mucosa, the thigh, or the abdomen. The patient is referred to an oncologist for evaluation of the need for radiation therapy and monitoring for metastasis. Early diagnosis and surgical management are the basis of a good prognosis. These conditions have life-threatening consequences, and surgical excisions may result in facial disfigurement. Emotional support is an extremely important aspect of nursing management.

Malignant Tumors of the Conjunctiva

Conjunctival carcinoma most often grows in the exposed areas of the conjunctiva. The typical lesions are usually gelatinous and whitish due to keratin formation. They grow gradually, and deep invasion and metastasis are rare. Melanoma is rare but may arise from a pre-existing nevus or acquired melanosis during middle age. Squamous cell carcinoma is also rare but invasive.

The management is surgical incision. Some benign tumors and most malignant tumors recur. To avoid recurrences, patients usually undergo radiation therapy and cryotherapy after the excision of malignant tumors. Cosmetic disfigurement may result from extensive excision when deep invasion by the malignant tumor is involved.

Malignant Tumors of the Globe

Ocular melanoma is a rare malignant choroidal tumor sometimes discovered on a retinal examination. In its early stages, it could be mistaken for a nevus. In addition to a complete physical examination to discover any evidence of metastasis (to the liver, lung, and breast), retinal fundus photography, fluorescein angiography, and ultrasonography are performed. The diagnosis is confirmed at biopsy after enucleation.

Tumors are classified according to boundary lines (apical height and basal diameter) as small, medium, or large. Small tumors are generally monitored, whereas medium and large tumors require treatment. Treatment consists of radiation, enucleation, or both. Radiation therapy may be achieved by external beam performed in repeated episodes over several days or through the implantation of a small plaque that contains radioactive iodine (I-125) pellets over the tumor.

SURGICAL PROCEDURES AND ENUCLEATION

Orbital Surgeries

Orbital surgeries may be performed to repair fractures, remove a foreign body, or remove benign or malignant growths. Surgical procedures involving the orbit and lids affect facial appearance (cosmesis). The goals are to recover and preserve visual function and to maintain the anatomic relationship of the ocular structures to achieve cosmesis. During the repair of orbital fractures, the orbital bones are realigned to follow the anatomic positions of facial structures.

Orbital surgical procedures involve working around delicate structures of the eye, such as the optic nerve, retinal blood vessels, and ocular muscles. Complications of orbital surgical procedures may include blindness as a result of damage to the optic nerve and its blood supply. Sudden pain and loss of vision may indicate intraorbital hemorrhage or compression of the optic nerve. Ptosis and diplopia may result from trauma to the extraocular muscles during the surgical procedure, but these conditions typically resolve after a few weeks.

Prophylaxis with IV antibiotic agents is the usual postoperative regimen after orbital surgery, especially with repair of orbital fractures and intraorbital foreign-body removal. IV corticosteroids may be used if there is concern about optic nerve swelling. Topical ocular antibiotics are typically instilled, and antibiotic ointments are applied externally to the skin suture sites.

For the first 24 to 48 hours postoperatively, ice compresses are applied over the periocular area to decrease periorbital swelling, facial swelling, and hematoma. The head of the patient's bed should be elevated to a comfortable position (30 to 45 degrees).

Discharge education should include information about oral antibiotic agents, instillation of ophthalmic medications, and application of ocular compresses.

Enucleation

Enucleation is removal of the eyeball (globe) from the orbit, leaving the muscles and orbital contents intact. It may be surgically performed for the following conditions:

- Injury resulting in prolapse of uveal tissue or loss of light perception
- A blind, painful, deformed, or disfigured eye, usually caused by glaucoma, retinal detachment, or chronic inflammation
- An eye without useful vision that is producing or has produced sympathetic ophthalmia in the other eye
- Intraocular tumors that are untreatable by other means

The procedure for enucleation involves the separation and cutting of each of the ocular muscles and surrounding soft tissue and cutting of the optic nerve from the eyeball. The insertion of an orbital implant typically follows, and the conjunctiva is closed. A large pressure dressing is applied over the area.

Evisceration involves the removal of the intraocular contents through an incision or opening in the cornea or sclera. Evisceration may be surgically performed to treat severe ocular trauma with ruptured globe, severe ocular inflammation, or severe ocular infection. The optic nerve, sclera, extraocular muscles, and sometimes the cornea are left intact. The main advantage of evisceration over enucleation is that the final cosmetic result and motility after fitting the ocular prosthesis are enhanced.

Exenteration is the surgical removal of the entire contents of the orbit, surrounding soft tissue, and most or all of the eyelids. This surgery is indicated in malignancies of the orbit that are life threatening or when more conservative modalities of treatment have failed or are inappropriate. An example is squamous cell carcinoma of the paranasal sinuses, skin, and conjunctiva with deep orbital involvement. In its most extensive form, exenteration may include the removal of all orbital tissues and resection of the orbital bones.

Ocular Prostheses

Orbital implants and conformers (ocular prostheses usually made of silicone rubber) maintain the shape of the eye after enucleation or evisceration to prevent a contracted, sunken appearance. The temporary conformer is placed over the conjunctival closure after the implantation of an orbital implant. A conformer is placed after the enucleation or evisceration procedure to protect the suture line, maintain the fornices, prevent contracture of the socket in preparation for the ocular prosthesis, and promote the integrity of the eyelids.

All ocular prosthetics have limitations in their motility. There are two designs of eye prostheses. The anophthalmic ocular prostheses are used in the absence of the globe. Scleral shells look just like the anophthalmic prosthesis (see Fig. 63-16) but are thinner and fit over a globe with intact corneal sensation. An eye prosthesis usually lasts about 6 years, depending on the quality of fit, comfort, and cosmetic appearance. When the anophthalmic socket is completely healed, conformers are replaced with prosthetic eyes.

An ocularist is a specially trained and skilled professional who makes prosthetic eyes. After the ophthalmologist is satisfied that the anophthalmic socket is completely healed and is ready for prosthetic fitting, the patient is referred to

an ocularist. The healing period is usually 6 to 8 weeks. It is advisable for the patient to have a consultation with the ocularist before the fitting. Obtaining accurate information and verbalizing concerns can lessen anxiety about wearing an ocular prosthesis.

Medical Management

Removal of an eye has physical, social, and psychological ramifications for any person. The significance of loss of the eye and vision must be addressed in the plan of care. The patient's preparation should include information about the surgical procedure and placement of orbital implants and conformers and the availability of ocular prosthetics to enhance cosmetic appearance. In some cases, patients may choose to see an ocularist before the surgery to discuss ocular prosthetics.

Nursing Management

Providing Education About Postsurgical and Prosthetic Care

Patients who undergo eye removal need to know that they will usually have a large ocular pressure dressing, which is typically removed after a week, and that an ophthalmic topical antibiotic ointment is applied in the socket three times daily.

After the removal of an eye, there is a loss of depth perception. Patients must be advised to take extra caution in their ambulation and movement to avoid miscalculations that may result in injury. It may take some time to adjust to monocular vision.

The patient must be advised that conformers may accidentally fall out of the socket. If this happens, the conformer must be washed, wiped dry, and placed back in the socket.

When surgical eye removal is unexpected, such as in severe ocular trauma, leaving no time for the patient and family to prepare for the loss, the nurse's role in providing emotional support is crucial.

Promoting Home, Community-Based, and Transitional Care

The patient with a new prosthetic eye may need referral to home, community-based or transitional services that provide assistance in the home. These patients also benefit from a referral for rehabilitation services.

 Educating Patients About Self-Care

Patients need to be educated about how to insert, remove, and care for the prosthetic eye. Proper hand hygiene must be observed before inserting and removing an ocular prosthesis. A suction cup may be used if there are problems with manual dexterity. Precautions, such as draping a towel over the sink and closing the sink drain, must be taken to avoid loss of the prosthesis. When instructing patients or family members, a return demonstration is important to assess the level of understanding and ability to perform the procedure.

Before insertion, the inner punctal or outer lateral aspects and the superior and inferior aspects of the prosthesis must be identified by locating the identifying marks, such as a reddish color in the inner punctal area. For people with low vision, other forms of identifying markers, such as dots or notches, are used. The upper lid is raised high enough to

Figure 63-16 • Eye prostheses. (*Left*) Anophthalmic ocular prosthesis. (*Right*) Scleral shell.

create a space and then the patient learns to slide the prosthesis up, underneath, and behind the upper eyelid. Meanwhile, the patient pulls the lower eyelid down to help put the prosthesis in place and to have its inferior edge fall back gradually to the lower eyelid. The lower eyelid is checked for correct positioning.

To remove the prosthesis, the patient cups one hand on the cheek to catch the prosthesis, places the forefinger of the free hand against the midportion of the lower eyelid, and gazes upward. Gazing upward brings the inferior edge of the prosthesis nearer the inferior eyelid margin. With the finger pushing inward, downward, and laterally against the lower eyelid, the prosthesis slides out into the cupped hand.

Continuing and Transitional Care

An eye prosthesis can be worn and left in place for several months. Hygiene and comfort are usually maintained with daily irrigation of the prosthesis in place with normal saline solution, hard contact lens solution, or artificial tears. In the case of dry eye symptoms, the use of ophthalmic ointment lubricants or oil-based drops, such as vitamin E and mineral oil, can be helpful. Removing crusting and mucus discharge that accumulate overnight is performed with the prosthesis in place. Malpositions may occur when wiping or rubbing the prosthesis in the socket. The prosthesis can be repositioned with the use of clean fingers. Proper wiping of the prosthesis should be a gentle temporal-to-nasal motion to avoid malpositions.

The prosthesis needs to be removed and cleaned when it becomes uncomfortable and when there is increased mucus discharge. The socket should also be rendered free of mucus and inspected for any signs of infection. Any unusual discomfort, irritation, or redness of the globe or eyelids may indicate excessive wear, debris under the shell, or lack of proper hygiene. Any infection or irritation that does not resolve needs medical attention.

OCULAR CONSEQUENCES OF SYSTEMIC DISEASE

Diabetic Retinopathy

Advancements in the treatment of diabetes have enabled patients to have a relatively a normal lifespan, but many have complications of long-term diabetes. One of the most serious complications of diabetes is retinopathy. Patients with diabetes are also at higher risk of cataracts and best practices for glycemic control during cataract surgery are not known (Kumar, Seet, Eke, et al., 2016). See Chapter 51 for a detailed discussion of diabetic retinopathy.

Cytomegalovirus Retinitis

Many ophthalmic complications have been associated with AIDS, and CMV is the most common cause of retinal inflammation in patients with AIDS. Early symptoms of CMV retinitis vary from patient to patient. Some patients complain of floaters or a decrease in peripheral vision. Some have a paracentral or central scotoma, whereas others have fluctuations in vision from macular edema. The retina often becomes thin and atrophic and susceptible to retinal tears and breaks.

CMV retinitis generally takes one of three forms: hemorrhagic, brushfire, or granular. In the hemorrhagic type, large areas of white, necrotic retina may be associated with retinal hemorrhage. In the brushfire type, a yellow-white margin begins at the edge of burned-out atrophic retina. This retinitis expands and, if untreated, involves the entire retina. In the granular type, white granular lesions in the periphery of the retina gradually expand. The white, feathery infiltration of the retina destroys sensory retina and leads to necrosis, optic atrophy, and retinal detachment.

Medical Management

Management of CMV retinitis consists of prescribing the appropriate pharmacologic agent.

Pharmacologic Therapy

Pharmacologic agents available for the treatment of CMV retinitis include ganciclovir, foscarnet (Foscavir), and cidofovir (Vistide).

Ganciclovir is administered IV, orally, or intravitreously in the acute stage of CMV retinitis. The intravitreous form is available as a 4-mm intraocular implant or insert containing the medication embedded in a polymer-based system that slowly releases the medication. The insert is surgically placed in the posterior segment of the eye, and the medication diffuses locally to the site of the infection over a period of 5 to 8 months before the insert must be replaced. When given systemically, ganciclovir is a very potent medication; it can cause neutropenia, thrombocytopenia, anemia, and elevated serum creatinine levels. The surgically implanted sustained-release insert enables higher concentrations of ganciclovir to reach the CMV retinitis, but there are risks and complications associated with the inserts, including endophthalmitis, retinal detachment, and hypotony.

Foscarnet inhibits viral deoxyribonucleic acid (DNA) replication. It may be the medication of choice when ganciclovir is ineffective. It may be administered by IV or intravitreal injections. The combination of foscarnet and ganciclovir has been more effective than either medication alone. Nephrotoxicity may occur with systemic foscarnet, and renal function must be monitored carefully.

Cidofovir impedes CMV replication and is administered IV. Cidofovir has been shown to delay the progression of CMV retinitis significantly. Nephrotoxicity, proteinuria, and increased serum creatinine levels are significant side effects.

A nucleoside analog such as zidovudine (Retrovir) given in combination with one or more protease inhibitors such as ritonavir (Norvir) in the management of patients with AIDS has led to a suppression of human immune deficiency virus (HIV) replication for sustained periods. The immune system can then recover to a functional level. Some patients develop immune recovery uveitis, characterized by intraocular inflammation, cystoid macular edema, and the formation of epiretinal membranes. Immune recovery uveitis is managed by corticosteroids or by injection of corticosteroids into the sub-Tenon area of the eye.

Hypertension-Related Eye Changes

Long-standing hypertension is associated with atherosclerosis, and retinal changes are evidenced by the development of retinal arteriolar changes, such as tortuousness, narrowing, and a change in light reflex (Weber & Kelley, 2014). Funduscopic examination reveals a copper or silver coloration of the arterioles and venous compression (arteriovenous nicking) at the arteriolar and venous crossings. Intraretinal hemorrhages from hypertension appear flame shaped because they occur in the nerve fiber layer of the retina.

Hypertension can also occur as an acute consequence of conditions such as pheochromocytoma, acute kidney injury, and pregnancy-induced hypertension. The retinopathy associated with these crisis states is extensive, and the manifestations include cotton-wool spots, retinal hemorrhages, retinal edema, and retinal exudates, often clustered around the macula (Weber & Kelley, 2014).

The choroid is also affected by the profound and abrupt rise in blood pressure and resulting vasoconstriction, and ischemia may result in serious retinal detachments and infarction of the RPE. Ischemic optic neuropathy and papilledema may also result. Blood pressure in these more severe stages should be lowered in a controlled gradual fashion to avoid ischemia of the optic nerve and brain secondary to a too-rapid fall in blood pressure. See Chapter 31 for further information about hypertension.

CRITICAL THINKING EXERCISES

1 **pq** You are making a home visit to a 75-year-old male who has a long history of diabetes and complains that recently he is having trouble with his vision. Describe what priority assessment data you would focus on obtaining during your initial visit. What are your priorities of care of this patient with low vision? How would your priorities change if the man were blind?

2 **pq** A 45-year-old woman presents to the emergency department with family members, complaining she has had progressive loss of vision of her right eye since this morning. What are your priority assessments for this patient? What focused questions would you ask her? How would you focus your physical assessment? What surgical interventions could be appropriate to treat her? How would you prepare the patient and her family members for possible surgery?

3 **ebp** A 56-year-old patient reports to you that he has been diagnosed with glaucoma but it is "no big deal" since his vision is fine. Although prescribed ophthalmic medications to treat glaucoma, he has not been self-administering them. What is the strength of the evidence that prescriptive medications are useful in preventing glaucoma-related complications? Identify the risk he is taking by not adhering to his prescribed medication regimen. Describe how you would educate him to gain his adherence to his prescribed regimen.

REFERENCES
*Asterisk indicates nursing research.

Books

American Society of Ophthalmic Registered Nurses (ASORN). (2013). *Recommended practice for registered nurses –Use of multi-dose medications.* San Francisco, CA: Author.
Cash, J., & Glass, C. (2016). *Adult-gerontology practice guidelines.* New York: Springer Publishing Company.
Comerford, K. C. (2015). *Nursing 2015 drug handbook.* Philadelphia, PA: Wolters Kluwer.
Eliopoulos, C. (2018). *Gerontological nursing* (9th ed.). Philadelphia, PA: Lippincott Williams & Wilkins.
Fischbach, F. T., & Dunning, M. B. (2015). *A manual of laboratory and diagnostic tests* (9th ed.). Philadelphia, PA: Lippincott Williams & Wilkins.
Gerstenblith, A. T., & Rabinowitz, M. P. (2017). *The Wills eye manual: Office and emergency room diagnosis and treatment of eye disease* (7th ed.). Philadelphia, PA: Lippincott Williams & Wilkins.
Grossman, S. C., & Porth, C. M. (2014). *Porth's Pathophysiology: Concepts of altered health states* (9th ed.). Philadelphia, PA: Lippincott Williams & Wilkins.
Hickey, J. V. (2014). *The clinical practice of neurological and neurosurgical nursing* (7th ed.). Philadelphia, PA: Wolters Kluwer Health/Lippincott Williams & Wilkins.
Hogan, M. (2014). *Pearson's review & rationales: Pathophysiology with nursing reviews & rationales* (3rd ed). New Jersey: Prentice Hall, Inc.
Prevent Blindness America. (2012). *Vision problems in the U.S.: Update to the fifth edition.* Schaumberg, IL: Prevent Blindness America/National Eye Institute.
Rubin, R., Strayer, D. S., & Rubin, E. (2012). *Rubin's pathology: Clinicopathologic foundations of medicine* (6th ed.). Philadelphia, PA: Lippincott Williams & Wilkins
Weber, J., & Kelley, J. (2014). *Health assessment in nursing* (5th ed.). Philadelphia, PA: Lippincott Williams & Wilkins.

Journals and Electronic Documents

Barsam, A., & Allan, B. D. (2014). Excimer laser refractive surgery versus phakic intraocular lenses for the correction of moderate to high myopia. *Cochrane Database of Systematic Reviews,* (6):CD007679.
Boyd, K. (2015). What is optical coherence tomography? Retrieved on 10/5/2016 at: www.aao.org/eye-health/treatments/what-is-optical-coherence-tomography
Boyd, K. (2016). Retinal detachment: Torn or detached retina treatment. Retrieved on 1/3/2017 at: www.aao.org/eye-health/diseases/detached-torn-retina-treatment
Centers for Disease Control (CDC). (2016). Learn about age related macular degeneration. Retrieved on 12/27/2016 at: www.cdc.gov/features/healthyvisionmonth/index.html
Colour Blind Awareness. (2016). Inherited colour vision deficiency. Retrieved on 10/5/2016 at: www.colourblindawareness.org/colour-blindness/inherited
Dickman, M. M., Peeters, J. M., Van Den Biggelmaar, F., et al. (2016). Changing practice patterns and long-term outcomes of endothelial versus penetrating keratoplasty: A prospective Dutch registry study. *American Journal of Ophthalmology, 170,* 133–142.
Eldaly, M. A., Bunce, C., El Sheikha, O. Z., et al. (2014). Non-penetrating filtration surgery versus trabeculectomy for open-angle glaucoma. *Cochrane Database of Systematic Reviews,* (2), CD007059.
Glaucoma Research Foundation. (2016). Five common glaucoma tests. Retrieved on 10/11/2016 at: www.glaucoma.org/glaucoma/diagnostic-tests.php
Kumar, C. M., Seet, E., Eke, T., et al. (2016). Glycaemic control during cataract surgery under loco-regional anesthesia: A growing problem and we are none the wiser. *British Journal of Anesthesia, 117*(6), 687–691.
Kusne, Y., Kang, P., & Fintelmann, R. E. (2016). A retrospective analysis of intraocular pressure changes after cataract surgery with the use of prednisolone acetate 1% versus difluprednate 0.05%. *Clinical Ophthalmology, 10,* 2326–2336.

Lee, K., & Garg, S. (2015). Navigating the current landscape of clinical genetic testing for inherited retinal dystrophies. *Genetics in Medicine*, *17*(4), 245–252.

Li, S. M., Zhan, S., Li, S. Y., et al. (2016). Laser-assisted subepithelial keratectomy (LASEK) versus photorefractive keratectomy (PRK) for correction of myopia. *Cochrane Database of Systematic Reviews*, (2), Art. No.: CD009799.

*Pagliuca, L. M., Macedo-Costa, K. N., Reboucas, G. B., et. al. (2014). Validation of the general guidelines of communication between the nurse and the blind. *Reviews Bras Enferm*, *67*(5), 715–725.

Patel, V., Moster, M., Kishfy, L., et al. (2016). Sequential versus concomitant surgery of glaucoma drainage implant and Boston keratoprosthesis type 1. *European Journal of Ophthalmology*, *26*(6), 556–563.

Peng, L. H., Fong, A., Phaik, C. S., et al. (2012). Improving presurgical pupil dilation for cataract surgery patients. *Joint Commission Journal on Quality and Patient Safety*, *38*(9), 420–425.

Resources

American Academy of Ophthalmology, www.aao.org
American Foundation for the Blind (AFB), www.afb.org
American Society of Ophthalmic Registered Nurses (ASORN), www.asorn.org
Foundation Fighting Blindness, www.blindness.org
Glaucoma Research Foundation, www.glaucoma.org
Lighthouse Guild, www.lighthouseguild.org
MAB Community Services, www.mabcommunity.org
Macular Degeneration Foundation,www.eyesight.org
National Diabetes Information Clearinghouse (NDIC), diabetes.niddk.nih.gov/dm/pubs/statistics/
National Eye Institute Information Office, www.nei.nih.gov
Prevent Blindness America, www.preventblindness.org
Research to Prevent Blindness, www.rpbusa.org

64 Assessment and Management of Patients With Hearing and Balance Disorders

LEARNING OBJECTIVES

On completion of this chapter, the learner will be able to:

1 Describe the anatomy and physiology of the ear.
2 Explain methods used to assess hearing and balance disorders.
3 List the manifestations that may be exhibited by a person with hearing and balance disorders.
4 Identify ways to communicate effectively with a person with a hearing disorder.
5 Differentiate problems of the external ear from those of the middle ear and inner ear.

6 Compare the various types of surgical procedures used for managing middle ear disorders and appropriate nursing care.
7 Use the nursing process as a framework of care for patients undergoing mastoid surgery.
8 Apply the nursing process as a framework of care for patients with vertigo.
9 Recognize the different types of inner ear disorders, including the clinical manifestations, diagnosis, and management.

GLOSSARY

acute otitis media: inflammation in the middle ear lasting less than 6 weeks
cholesteatoma: tumor of the middle ear or mastoid, or both, that can destroy structures of the temporal bone
chronic otitis media: repeated episodes of acute otitis media causing irreversible tissue damage
conductive hearing loss: loss of hearing in which efficient sound transmission to the inner ear is interrupted by some obstruction or disease process
deafness: partial or complete loss of the ability to hear
dizziness: altered sensation of orientation in space
endolymphatic hydrops: dilation of the endolymphatic space of the inner ear; the pathologic correlate of Ménière disease
exostoses: small, hard, bony protrusions in the lower posterior bony portion of the ear canal
external otitis (i.e., otitis externa): inflammation of the external auditory canal
labyrinthitis: inflammation of the labyrinth of the inner ear
Ménière disease: condition of the inner ear characterized by a triad of symptoms: episodic vertigo, tinnitus, and fluctuating sensorineural hearing loss

middle ear effusion: fluid in the middle ear without evidence of infection
myringotomy (i.e., tympanotomy): incision in the tympanic membrane
nystagmus: involuntary rhythmic eye movement
ossiculoplasty: surgical reconstruction of the middle ear bones to restore hearing
otalgia: sensation of fullness or pain in the ear
otorrhea: drainage from the ear
otosclerosis: a condition characterized by abnormal spongy bone formation around the stapes
presbycusis: progressive hearing loss associated with aging
rhinorrhea: drainage from the nose
sensorineural hearing loss: loss of hearing related to damage to the end organ for hearing or cranial nerve VIII, or both
tinnitus: subjective perception of sound with internal origin; unwanted noises in the head or ear
tympanoplasty: surgical repair of the tympanic membrane
vertigo: illusion of movement in which the individual or the surroundings are sensed as moving

The ear is a delicate sensory organ with the dual functions of hearing and balance. The sense of hearing is essential for normal development and maintenance of speech as well as the ability to communicate with others. Balance, or equilibrium, is essential for maintaining body movement, position, and coordination.

The early detection and accurate diagnosis of disorders is necessary for preservation of normal hearing and balance. The diagnosis and treatment of these disorders requires skilled health care professionals such as otolaryngologists, internists, audiologists, and nurses. This chapter provides an overview

of the anatomy and physiology of the ear and addresses the general assessment and management of hearing and balance disorders common to adults seen in many health care settings.

ASSESSMENT OF THE EAR

Anatomic and Physiologic Overview

The cranium encloses and protects the brain and surrounding structures, providing attachment for various muscles that

Figure 64-1 • **A.** Anatomy of the ear. **B.** The inner ear.

control head and jaw movements. The ears are located on either side of the cranium at approximately eye level.

Anatomy of the External Ear

The external ear includes the auricle (pinna) and the external auditory canal (see Fig. 64-1). The external ear is separated from the middle ear by a disc-shaped structure called the *tympanic membrane* (eardrum).

Auricle

The auricle, attached to the side of the head by skin, is composed mainly of cartilage, except for the fat and subcutaneous tissue in the earlobe. The auricle collects the sound waves and directs vibrations into the external auditory canal.

External Auditory Canal

The external auditory canal is approximately 2 to 3 cm long (Grossman & Porth, 2014). The lateral third is an elastic cartilaginous and dense fibrous framework to which thin skin is attached. The medial two thirds is bone lined with thin skin. The external auditory canal ends at the tympanic membrane.

The skin of the canal contains hair, sebaceous glands, and ceruminous glands, which secrete a brown, waxlike substance called *cerumen* (ear wax). The ear's self-cleaning mechanism moves old skin cells and cerumen to the outer part of the ear.

Just anterior to the external auditory canal is the temporomandibular joint. The head of the mandible can be felt by placing a fingertip in the external auditory canal while the patient opens and closes the mouth.

Anatomy of the Middle Ear

The middle ear, an air-filled cavity, includes the tympanic membrane laterally and the otic capsule medially. The middle ear cleft lies between the two. The middle ear is connected to the nasopharynx by the eustachian tube and is continuous with air-filled cells in the adjacent mastoid portion of the temporal bone.

The eustachian tube, which is approximately 1 mm wide and 35 mm long, connects the middle ear to the nasopharynx. Normally, the eustachian tube is closed, but it opens by action of the tensor veli palatini muscle when the person performs a Valsalva maneuver, yawns, or swallows. It drains normal and abnormal secretions of the middle ear and equalizes pressure in the middle ear with that of the atmosphere.

Tympanic Membrane

The tympanic membrane (eardrum), about 1 cm in diameter and very thin, is normally pearly gray and translucent (Weber & Kelley, 2014). It consists of three layers of tissue: an outer layer, continuous with the skin of the ear canal; a fibrous middle layer; and an inner mucosal layer, continuous

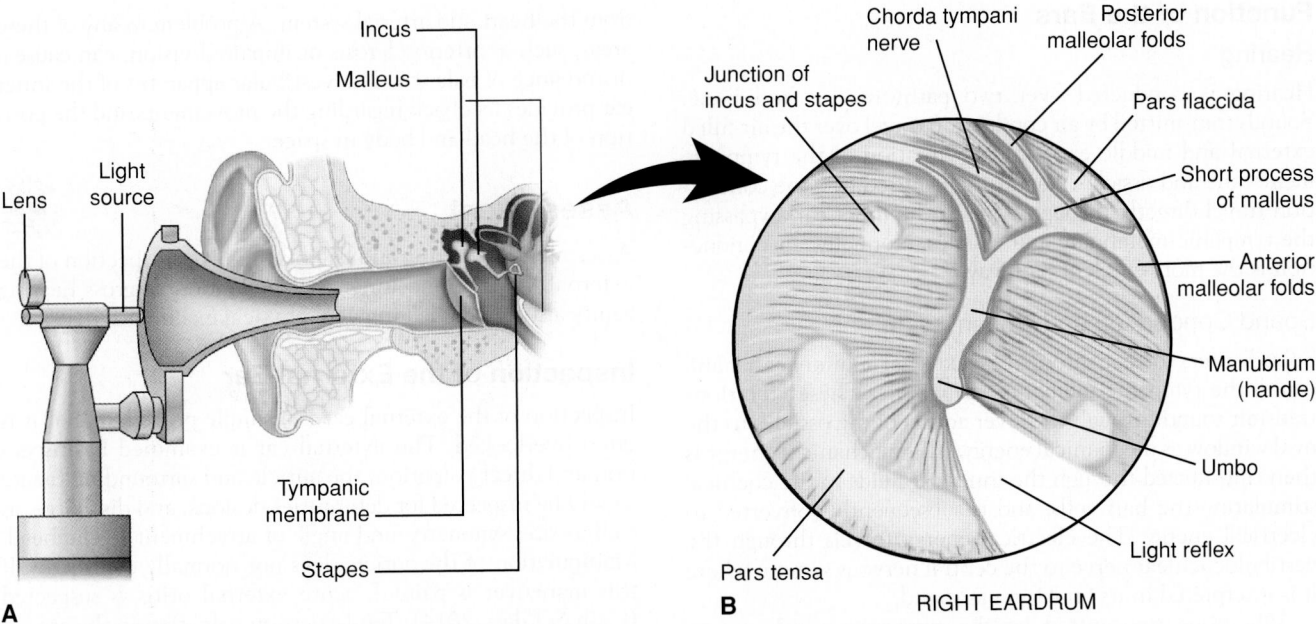

Figure 64-2 • Technique for using the otoscope (**A**) to see the tympanic membrane (**B**).

with the lining of the middle ear cavity. Approximately 80% of the tympanic membrane is composed of all three layers and is called the *pars tensa*. The remaining 20% lacks the middle layer and is called the *pars flaccida*. The absence of this fibrous middle layer makes the pars flaccida more vulnerable to pathologic disorders than the pars tensa. Distinguishing landmarks include the annulus, the fibrous border that attaches the eardrum to the temporal bone; the short process of the malleus; the long process of the malleus; the umbo of the malleus, which attaches to the tympanic membrane in the center; the pars flaccida; and the pars tensa (see Fig. 64-2).

The tympanic membrane protects the middle ear and conducts sound vibrations from the external canal to the ossicles. The sound pressure is magnified 22 times as a result of transmission from a larger area to a smaller one.

Ossicles

The middle ear contains the three smallest bones (the ossicles) of the body: the malleus, the incus, and the stapes (Grossman & Porth, 2014). The ossicles, which are held in place by joints, muscles, and ligaments, assist in the transmission of sound. Two small fenestrae (oval and round windows), located in the medial wall of the middle ear, separate the middle ear from the inner ear. The footplate of the stapes sits in the oval window, secured by a fibrous annulus (ring-shaped structure). The footplate transmits sound to the inner ear. The round window, covered by a thin membrane, provides an exit for sound vibrations (see Fig. 64-1).

Anatomy of the Inner Ear

The inner ear is housed deep within the temporal bone. The organs for hearing (cochlea) and balance (semicircular canals), as well as cranial nerves VII (facial nerve) and VIII (vestibulocochlear nerve), are all part of this complex anatomy (see Fig. 64-1). The cochlea and semicircular canals are housed in the bony labyrinth. The bony labyrinth surrounds

and protects the membranous labyrinth, which is bathed in a fluid called *perilymph*.

Membranous Labyrinth

The membranous labyrinth is composed of the utricle, the saccule, the cochlear duct, the semicircular canals, and the organ of Corti, all of which are surrounded by a fluid called *endolymph*. The three semicircular canals—posterior, superior, and lateral, which lie at 90-degree angles to one another—contain sensory receptor organs that are arranged to detect rotational movement. These receptor end organs are stimulated by changes in the rate or direction of a person's movement. The utricle and saccule are involved with linear movements.

Organ of Corti

The organ of Corti is housed in the cochlea, a snail-shaped, bony tube about 3.5 cm long with two and a half spiral turns. Membranes separate the cochlear duct (scala media) from the scala vestibuli and the scala tympani from the basilar membrane. The organ of Corti is located on the basilar membrane that stretches from the base to the apex of the cochlea. As sound vibrations enter the perilymph at the oval window and travel along the scala vestibuli, they pass through the scala tympani, enter the cochlear duct, and cause movement of the basilar membrane. The organ of Corti, also referred to as the end organ for hearing, transforms mechanical energy into neural activity and separates sounds into different frequencies. This electrochemical impulse travels through the acoustic nerve to the temporal cortex of the brain to be interpreted as meaningful sound. In the internal auditory canal, the cochlear (acoustic) nerve, arising from the cochlea, joins the vestibular nerve, arising from the semicircular canals, utricle, and saccule, to become the vestibulocochlear nerve (cranial nerve VIII). This canal also houses the facial nerve and the blood supply from the ear to the brain.

Function of the Ears

Hearing

Hearing is conducted over two pathways: air and bone. Sounds transmitted by air conduction travel over the air-filled external and middle ear through vibration of the tympanic membrane and ossicles. Sounds transmitted by bone conduction travel directly through bone to the inner ear, bypassing the tympanic membrane and ossicles. Normally, air conduction is the more efficient pathway.

Sound Conduction and Transmission

Sound enters the ear through the external auditory canal and causes the tympanic membrane to vibrate. These vibrations transmit sound through the lever action of the ossicles to the oval window as mechanical energy. This mechanical energy is then transmitted through the inner ear fluids to the cochlea, stimulating the hair cells, and is subsequently converted to electrical energy. The electrical energy travels through the vestibulocochlear nerve to the central nervous system, where it is interpreted in its final form as sound.

Vibrations transmitted by the tympanic membrane to the ossicles of the middle ear are transmitted to the cochlea, located in the labyrinth of the inner ear. The stapes rocks, causing vibrations (waves) in fluids contained in the inner ear. These fluid waves cause movement of the basilar membrane, stimulating the hair cells of the organ of Corti in the cochlea to move in a wavelike manner. The movements of the tympanic membrane set up electrical currents that stimulate the various areas of the cochlea. The hair cells set up neural impulses that are encoded and then transferred to the auditory cortex in the brain, where they are decoded into a sound message.

The footplate of the stapes receives impulses transmitted by the incus and the malleus from the tympanic membrane. The round window, which opens on the opposite side of the cochlear duct, is protected from sound waves by the intact tympanic membrane, permitting motion of the inner ear fluids by sound wave stimulation. For example, in the normally intact tympanic membrane, sound waves stimulate the oval window first, and a lag occurs before the terminal effect of the stimulus reaches the round window. However, this lag phase is changed when a perforation of the tympanic membrane allows sound waves to impinge on the oval and round windows simultaneously. This effect cancels the lag and prevents the maximal effect of inner ear fluid motility and its subsequent effect in stimulating the hair cells in the organ of Corti. The result is a reduction in hearing ability (see Fig. 64-3).

Bone conduction occurs by directly stimulating the bones of the skull that sends sound to the inner ear. An example of how this occurs can be done by striking a tuning fork and placing the tuning fork directly on the skull above the ear. Sound is transmitted to the inner ear.

Balance and Equilibrium

Body balance is maintained by the cooperation of the muscles and joints of the body (proprioceptive system), the eyes (visual system), and the labyrinth (vestibular system). These areas send their information about equilibrium, or balance, to the brain (cerebellar system) for coordination and perception in the cerebral cortex. The brain obtains its blood supply from the heart and arterial system. A problem in any of these areas, such as arteriosclerosis or impaired vision, can cause a disturbance of balance. The vestibular apparatus of the inner ear provides feedback regarding the movements and the position of the head and body in space.

Assessment

Assessment of hearing and balance involves inspection of the external, middle, and inner ear. Evaluation of gross hearing acuity also is included in every physical examination.

Inspection of the External Ear

Inspection of the external ear is a simple procedure, but it is often overlooked. The external ear is examined by inspection and direct palpation; the auricle and surrounding tissues should be inspected for deformities, lesions, and discharge, as well as size, symmetry, and angle of attachment to the head. Manipulation of the auricle does not normally elicit pain. If this maneuver is painful, acute external otitis is suspected (Cash & Glass, 2014). Tenderness on palpation in the area of the mastoid may indicate acute mastoiditis or inflammation of the posterior auricular node. Occasionally, sebaceous cysts and tophi (subcutaneous mineral deposits) are present on the pinna. A flaky scaliness on or behind the auricle usually indicates seborrheic dermatitis and can be present on the scalp and facial structures as well.

Otoscopic Examination

The tympanic membrane is inspected with an otoscope and indirect palpation with a pneumatic otoscope. To examine the external auditory canal and tympanic membrane, the otoscope should be held in the examiner's right hand, in a pencil-hold position, with the examiner's hand braced against the patient's face (see Fig. 64-4). This position prevents the examiner from inserting the otoscope too far into the external canal. Using the opposite hand, the auricle is grasped and gently pulled back to straighten the canal in the adult.

The speculum is slowly inserted into the ear canal, with the examiner's eye held close to the magnifying lens of the otoscope to visualize the canal and tympanic membrane. The largest speculum that the canal can accommodate (usually 5 mm in an adult) is guided gently down into the canal and slightly forward. Because the distal portion of the canal is bony and covered by a sensitive layer of epithelium, only light pressure can be used without causing pain. The external auditory canal is examined for discharge, inflammation, or a foreign body.

The healthy tympanic membrane is pearly gray and is positioned obliquely at the base of the canal. The following landmarks are identified, if visible (see Fig. 64-2): the pars tensa, the umbo, the manubrium of the malleus, and its short process. A slow, circular movement of the speculum allows further visualization of the malleolar folds and periphery. The position and color of the membrane and any unusual markings or deviations from normal are documented. The presence of fluid, air bubbles, blood, or masses in the middle ear also should be noted.

Proper otoscopic examination of the external auditory canal and tympanic membrane requires that the canal be free of large amounts of cerumen. Cerumen is normally present in

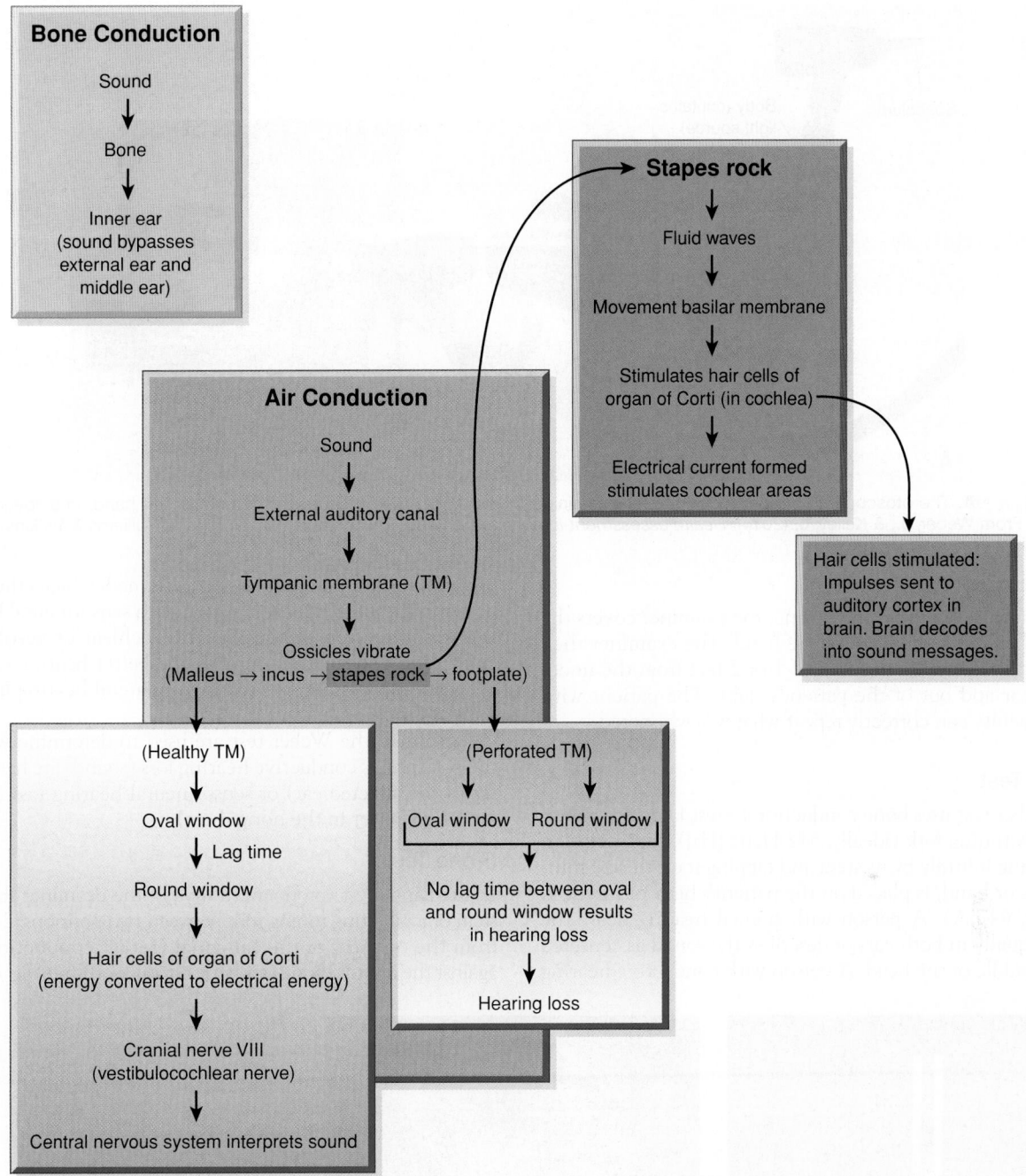

Figure 64-3 • Bone conduction compared to air conduction.

the external canal, and small amounts should not interfere with otoscopic examination. If the tympanic membrane cannot be visualized because of cerumen, the cerumen may be removed by gently irrigating the external canal with warm water (unless contraindicated). If adherent cerumen is present, a small amount of mineral oil or over-the-counter cerumen softener may be instilled into the ear canal and the patient instructed to return for subsequent removal of the cerumen and inspection of the ear. The use of instruments such as a cerumen curette for cerumen removal is reserved for otolaryngologists and nurses with specialized training because of the danger of perforating the tympanic membrane or excoriating the external auditory canal. Cerumen buildup is a

common cause of hearing loss and local irritation (Grossman & Porth, 2014).

Evaluation of Gross Auditory Acuity

A general estimate of hearing can be made by assessing the patient's ability to hear a whispered phrase, testing one ear at a time. The Weber and Rinne tests may be used to distinguish conductive loss from sensorineural loss when hearing is impaired (Weber & Kelley, 2014). These tests are part of the usual screening physical examination and are useful if a more specific assessment is needed, if hearing loss is detected, or if confirmation of audiometric results is desired.

Figure 64-4 • **A.** The otoscope. **B.** Proper technique for examining the ear. Hold the otoscope in the right or left hand, in a "pencil-hold" position. From Weber, J., & Kelley, J. (2014). *Health assessment in nursing* (5th ed.). Philadelphia, PA: Lippincott Williams & Wilkins.

Whisper Test

To exclude one ear from the testing, the examiner covers the untested ear with the palm of the hand. The examiner then whispers softly from a distance of 1 or 2 feet from the unoccluded ear and out of the patient's sight. The patient with normal acuity can correctly repeat what was whispered.

Weber Test

The Weber test uses bone conduction to test lateralization of sound. A tuning fork (ideally, 512 Hertz [Hz]), set in motion by grasping it firmly by its stem and tapping it on the examiner's knee or hand, is placed on the patient's head or forehead (see Fig. 64-5A). A person with normal hearing hears the sound equally in both ears or describes the sound as centered in the middle of the head. A person with conductive hearing

loss, such as from otosclerosis or otitis media, hears the sound better in the affected ear. A person with sensorineural hearing loss, resulting from damage to the cochlear or vestibulocochlear nerve, hears the sound in the better-hearing ear. The Weber test is useful for detecting unilateral hearing loss (see Table 64-1).

Results of the Weber test are used to determine whether the patient has conductive hearing loss (sounds are heard better in the affected ear) or sensorineural hearing loss (sounds are heard better in the normal ear).

Rinne Test

In the Rinne test (pronounced *rin-ay*), the examiner shifts the stem of a vibrating tuning fork between two positions: 2 inches from the opening of the ear canal (for air conduction) and against the mastoid bone (for bone conduction) (see Fig. 64-5B).

Figure 64-5 • **A.** The Weber test assesses bone conduction of sound. **B.** The Rinne test assesses both air and bone conduction of sound.

TABLE 64-1 Comparison of Weber and Rinne Tests

Hearing Status	Weber	Rinne
Normal hearing	Sound is heard equally in both ears.	Air conduction is audible longer than bone conduction in both ears.
Conductive hearing loss	Sound is heard best in affected ear (hearing loss).	Sound is heard as long or longer in affected ear (hearing loss).
Sensorineural hearing loss	Sound is heard best in normal hearing ear.	Air conduction is audible longer than bone conduction in affected ear.

Adapted from Weber, J., & Kelley, J. (2014). *Health assessment in nursing* (5th ed.). Philadelphia, PA: Lippincott Williams & Wilkins.

TABLE 64-2 Severity of Hearing Loss

Loss in Decibels	Interpretation
0–15	Normal hearing
>15–25	Slight hearing loss
>25–40	Mild hearing loss
>40–55	Moderate hearing loss
>55–70	Moderate to severe hearing loss
>70–90	Severe hearing loss
>90	Profound hearing loss

As the position changes, the patient is asked to indicate which tone is louder or when the tone is no longer audible.

The Rinne test is useful for distinguishing between conductive and sensorineural hearing loss. A person with normal hearing reports that air-conducted sound is louder than bone-conducted sound. A person with a conductive hearing loss hears bone-conducted sound as long as or longer than air-conducted sound. A person with a sensorineural hearing loss hears air-conducted sound longer than bone-conducted sound.

Diagnostic Evaluation

Many diagnostic procedures are available to measure the auditory and vestibular systems indirectly. These tests are usually performed by a certified audiologist. The nurse educates the patient about the purpose, what to expect, and any possible side effects related to testing. The nurse notes trends in results because they provide information about disease progression as well as the patient's response to therapy.

Audiometry

In detecting hearing loss, audiometry is the single most important diagnostic instrument. Audiometric testing is of two kinds: pure-tone audiometry, in which the sound stimulus consists of a pure or musical tone (the louder the tone before the patient perceives it, the greater the hearing loss), and speech audiometry, in which the spoken word is used to determine the ability to hear and discriminate sounds and words.

When evaluating hearing, three characteristics are important: frequency, pitch, and intensity. *Frequency* refers to the number of sound waves emanating from a source per second, measured as cycles per second, or Hertz. The normal human ear perceives sounds ranging in frequency from 20 to 20,000 Hz. The frequencies from 500 to 2000 Hz are important in understanding everyday speech and are referred to as the speech range or speech frequencies. *Pitch* is the term used to describe frequency; a tone with 100 Hz is considered of low pitch, and a tone of 10,000 Hz is considered of high pitch.

The unit for measuring loudness (*intensity* of sound) is the decibel (dB), the pressure exerted by sound. Hearing loss is measured in decibels—a logarithmic function of intensity that is not easily converted into a percentage. The critical level of loudness is approximately 30 dB. The shuffling of papers in quiet surroundings is about 15 dB; a low conver-

sation, 40 dB; and a jet plane 100 feet away, about 150 dB. Sound louder than 80 dB is perceived by the human ear to be harsh and can be damaging to the inner ear. Table 64-2 classifies hearing loss based on decibel level. In surgical treatment of patients with hearing loss, the aim is to improve the hearing level to 30 dB or better within the speech frequencies.

With audiometry, the patient wears earphones and signals to the audiologist when a tone is heard. When the tone is applied directly over the external auditory canal, air conduction is measured. When the stimulus is applied to the mastoid bone, bypassing the conductive mechanism (i.e., the ossicles), nerve conduction is tested. For accuracy, testing is performed in a soundproof room. Responses are plotted on a graph known as an audiogram, which differentiates conductive from sensorineural hearing loss.

Tympanogram

A tympanogram, or impedance audiometry, measures middle ear muscle reflex to sound stimulation and compliance of the tympanic membrane by changing the air pressure in a sealed ear canal. Compliance is impaired with middle ear disease.

Auditory Brain Stem Response

The auditory brain stem response is a detectable electrical potential from cranial nerve VIII and the ascending auditory pathways of the brain stem in response to sound stimulation. Electrodes are placed on the patient's scalp and on each earlobe (Fischbach & Dunning, 2015). Acoustic stimuli (e.g., clicks) are made in the ear. The resulting electrophysiologic measurements can determine at which decibel level a patient hears and whether there are any impairments along the nerve pathways (e.g., tumor on cranial nerve VIII). Patients are instructed to wash and rinse their hair prior to this study but to avoid applying any other hair product. Auditory brain stem response assessment should be used in conjunction with audiometry for the most accurate results (Bhattacharyya & Meyers, 2015).

Electronystagmography

Electronystagmography is the measurement and graphic recording of the changes in electrical potentials created by eye movements during spontaneous, positional, or calorically evoked nystagmus. It is also used to assess the oculomotor and vestibular systems and their corresponding interaction. It helps to diagnose causes of unilateral hearing loss of unknown origin, vertigo, or tinnitus. Any vestibular suppressants, such as caffeine and alcohol, are withheld for 48 hours before testing. Medications such as tranquilizers, stimulants, or antivertigo agents are withheld for 5 days before the test (Fischbach & Dunning, 2015).

Platform Posturography

Platform posturography is recommended for patients with dizziness and balance disorders (American Academy of Otolaryngology – Head and Neck Surgery, 2014). It can be used to determine if a patient's vertigo is worsening or to evaluate a patient's response to treatment. The integration of visual, vestibular, and proprioceptive cues (i.e., sensory integration) with motor response output and coordination of the lower limbs is tested. The patient stands on a platform, surrounded by a screen, and different conditions such as a moving platform with a moving screen or a stationary platform with a moving screen are presented. The responses from the patient on six different conditions are measured and indicate which of the anatomic systems may be impaired. Preparation for the testing is the same as for electronystagmography.

Sinusoidal Harmonic Acceleration

Sinusoidal harmonic acceleration, or a rotary chair, is used to assess the vestibulo-ocular system by analyzing compensatory eye movements in response to the clockwise and counterclockwise rotation of the chair. Although such testing cannot identify the side of the lesion in unilateral disease, it helps to identify disease (e.g., Ménière disease and

tumors of the auditory canal) and evaluate the course of recovery. The same patient preparation is required as that for electronystagmography.

Middle Ear Endoscopy

Using endoscopes with very small diameters and acute angles, the ear can be examined by an endoscopist specializing in otolaryngology. Middle ear endoscopy is performed safely and effectively as an office procedure to evaluate suspected perilymphatic fistula and new-onset conductive hearing loss, the anatomy of the round window before transtympanic treatment of Ménière disease, and the tympanic cavity before ear surgery to treat chronic middle ear and mastoid infections.

The tympanic membrane is anesthetized topically for about 10 minutes before the procedure. Then, the external auditory canal is irrigated with sterile normal saline solution. With the aid of a microscope, a tympanotomy is created with a laser beam or a myringotomy knife so that the endoscope can be inserted into the middle ear cavity. Video and photo documentation can be accomplished through the scope.

HEARING LOSS

In the United States, hearing impairment has been reported to occur in 2 to 3 of every 1000 births, and approximately one half of the time it is related to genetic factors (U.S. Department of Health and Human Services [HHS], 2016). Genetic syndromes associated with hearing impairment include Waardenburg syndrome, Usher syndrome, Pendred syndrome, and Jervell and Lange-Nielsen syndrome (Antonio,

---

Chart 64-1 GENETICS IN NURSING PRACTICE
Hearing Disorders

Several hearing disorders are associated with genetic abnormalities and have various patterns of inheritance:

Autosomal dominant:

- Branachiootorenal syndrome
- Neurofibromatosis type 2
- Otosclerosis
- Stickler syndrome
- Waardenburg syndrome

Autosomal recessive:

- Connexin 26 gene hearing loss (the majority of cases are recessive; however, there is an autosomal dominant form that occurs less commonly)
- Jervell and Lange-Nielsen syndrome
- Pendred syndrome
- Refsum disease
- Usher syndrome

X-Linked syndromic hearing loss:

- Alport syndrome

Nursing Assessments

Refer to Chapter 5. Chart 5-2: Genetics in Nursing Practice: Genetic Aspects of Health Assessment

Family History Assessment Specific to Hearing Disorders

- Assess for other family members in several generations with hearing loss (autosomal dominant hearing loss).

- Inquire about genetic relatedness (e.g., individuals who are related, such as first cousins, have a higher chance to share the same recessive genes—autosomal recessive hearing loss).
- Inquire about age at onset of hearing loss.

Patient Assessment Specific to Genetic Hearing Disorders

- Assess for:
  - Dizziness
  - Facial numbness or weakness
  - Headaches
  - Tinnitus
- Assess for related genetic conditions, such as vision impairment (e.g., retinitis pigmentosa in Usher syndrome; thyroid disorder in Pendred syndrome).
- Assess for iris, pigment, and hair alterations (white forelock) seen in Waardenburg syndrome.
- Assess for exposure to loud noises (e.g., industrial).
- Assess for presence of rubella, toxoplasmosis, herpes, or cytomegalovirus during pregnancy.
- Determine if patient had taken medications associated with ototoxicity.

Genetics Resources

Hear-It, www.Hear-it.org/Genetic-hearing-loss
Neurofibromatosis Network, www.nfnetwork.org/
See Chapter 8, Chart 8-7 for components of genetic counseling.

2016). Chart 64-1 contains more information about hearing disorders that have a genetic cause. There are also acquired causes of hearing loss which may be caused by TORCH infections (TOxoplasmosis, Rubella, Cytomegalovirus, Herpes) during pregnancy as well as trauma or chronic exposure to loud noise (Antonio, 2016). Most hospitals or birthing centers offer universal hearing screenings for newborns after birth and prior to discharge.

Hearing loss occurs in men more often than women. Approximately 2% of adults between the ages of 45 and 54 years have disabling hearing loss. This percentage increases to 8.5% in the 55 to 64 age group, to 25% of adults in the 65 to 74 age group and up to 50% for those over 75 years of age (HHS, 2016). Hearing loss is an important health issue, and as people age, hearing screening and treatment are indicated.

Many people are exposed on a daily basis to noise levels that produce high-frequency hearing loss. Occupations such as carpentry, plumbing, and coal mining have the highest risk of noise-induced hearing loss. Wise Ears was developed by the National Institute on Deafness and Other Communication Disorders (NIDCD) and the National Institute for Occupational Safety and Health (NIOSH). It aims to educate the public about noise-induced hearing loss and ways to prevent this hearing loss (NIDCD, 2010).

Conductive hearing loss usually results from an external ear disorder, such as impacted cerumen, or a middle ear disorder, such as otitis media or otosclerosis. In such instances, the efficient transmission of sound by air to the inner ear is interrupted. A **sensorineural hearing loss** involves damage to the cochlea or vestibulocochlear nerve.

Mixed hearing loss and functional hearing loss also may occur. Patients with mixed hearing loss have conductive loss and sensorineural loss, resulting from dysfunction of air and bone conduction. A functional (or psychogenic) hearing loss is nonorganic and unrelated to detectable structural changes in the hearing mechanisms; it is usually a manifestation of an emotional reaction.

Clinical Manifestations

Deafness is the partial or complete loss of the ability to hear. Early manifestations may include tinnitus, increasing inability to hear when in a group, and a need to turn up the volume of the television. Hearing impairment can also trigger changes in attitude, the ability to communicate, the awareness of surroundings, and even the ability to protect oneself, thus affecting a person's quality of life. In a classroom, a student with impaired hearing may be uninterested and inattentive and have failing grades. A person at home may feel isolated because of an inability to hear the clock chime or to hear the telephone. A pedestrian who is hearing impaired may attempt to cross the street and fail to hear an approaching car. People with impaired hearing may miss parts of a conversation. Many people are unaware of their gradual hearing impairment. Often, it is not the person with the hearing loss but the people with whom he or she is communicating who recognizes the impairment first (see Chart 64-2).

For various reasons, some people with hearing loss refuse to seek medical attention or wear a hearing aid. They may feel self-conscious about wearing a hearing aid. Other people, however, may feel comfortable asking those with whom they are

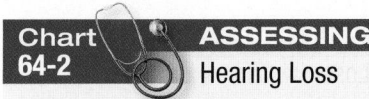

Chart 64-2 **ASSESSING**
Hearing Loss

The nurse should be alert to the following:

Speech deterioration: The person who slurs words, drops word endings, or produces flat-sounding speech may not be hearing correctly. The ears guide the voice, both in loudness and in pronunciation.

Fatigue: If a person tires easily when listening to conversation or to a speech, fatigue may be the result of straining to hear. Under these circumstances, the person may become irritable very easily.

Indifference: It is easy for the person who cannot hear what others say to become depressed and disinterested in life in general.

Social withdrawal: Not being able to hear what is going on causes the person who is hearing impaired to withdraw from situations that might prove embarrassing.

Insecurity: Lack of self-confidence and fear of mistakes create a feeling of insecurity in many people who are hearing impaired. No one likes to say the wrong thing or do anything that might appear foolish.

Indecision and procrastination: Loss of self-confidence makes it increasingly difficult for a person who is hearing impaired to make decisions.

Suspiciousness: The person who is hearing impaired—who often hears only part of what is being said—may suspect that others are talking about him or her, or that portions of the conversation are deliberately spoken softly so that he or she will not hear them.

False pride: The person who is hearing impaired wants to conceal the hearing loss and thus often pretends to be hearing when he or she actually is not.

Loneliness and unhappiness: Although everyone wishes for quiet now and then, *enforced* silence can be boring and even somewhat frightening. People with a hearing loss often feel isolated.

Tendency to dominate the conversation: Many people who are hearing impaired tend to dominate the conversation, knowing that as long as it is centered on them and they can control it, they are not so likely to be embarrassed by some mistake.

trying to communicate to let them know whether difficulties in communication exist. The attitudes and behaviors of patients who need hearing assistance should be taken into account when counseling them. The decision to wear a hearing aid is a personal one that is affected by these attitudes and behaviors.

Prevention

Many environmental factors have an adverse effect on the auditory system and with time result in permanent sensorineural hearing loss. The most common is noise. Noise (unwanted and unavoidable sound) has been identified as one of today's environmental hazards. The volume of noise that surrounds us daily has increased into a potentially dangerous source of physical and psychological damage.

Loud, persistent noise has been found to cause constriction of peripheral blood vessels, increased blood pressure and heart rate (because of increased secretion of adrenalin), and increased gastrointestinal activity. Although research is needed to address the overall effects of noise on the human body, a quiet environment is more conducive to peace of

Chart 64-3 RISK FACTORS
Hearing Loss

- Family history of sensorineural impairment
- Congenital malformations of the cranial structure (ear)
- Low birth weight (<1500 g)
- Use of ototoxic medications (e.g., gentamicin, loop diuretics)
- Recurrent ear infections
- Bacterial meningitis
- Chronic exposure to loud noises
- Perforation of the tympanic membrane

mind. A person who is ill feels more at ease when noise is kept to a minimum.

Numerous factors contribute to hearing loss (see Chart 64-3). *Noise-induced hearing loss* refers to hearing loss that follows a long period of exposure to loud noise (e.g., heavy machinery, engines, artillery, rock-band music). *Acoustic trauma* refers to hearing loss caused by a single exposure to an extremely intense noise, such as an explosion. Usually, noise-induced hearing loss occurs at a high frequency (about 4000 Hz). However, with continued noise exposure, the hearing loss can become more severe and include adjacent frequencies. The minimum noise level known to cause noise-induced hearing loss, regardless of duration, is about 85 to 90 dB.

Noise exposure is inherent in many jobs (e.g., mechanics, printers, pilots, flight attendants, musicians) and in hobbies such as woodworking and hunting. Noise level regulations are based on the amount of noise a person is exposed to, with the maximum legal amount being exposure to noise over an average working day or week of 80 dB, with a peak sound pressure of 135 dB (HHS, 2016). The Occupational Safety and Health Administration (OSHA) requires that workers wear ear protection to prevent noise-induced hearing loss when exposed to noise above the legal limits. Ear protection against noise is the most effective preventive measure available. Hearing loss due to noise is permanent because the hair cells in the organ of Corti are destroyed.

Gerontologic Considerations

With aging, changes occur in the ear that may eventually lead to hearing deficits. Although few changes occur in the external ear, cerumen tends to become harder and drier, posing a greater chance of impaction. In the middle ear, the tympanic membrane may atrophy or become sclerotic. In the inner ear, cells at the base of the cochlea degenerate. A familial predisposition to sensorineural hearing loss is also seen, manifested by inability to hear high-frequency sounds, followed in time by the loss of middle and lower frequencies. The term **presbycusis** is used to describe this progressive hearing loss (Eliopoulos, 2018).

In addition to age-related changes, other factors can affect hearing in the older adult population, such as lifelong exposure to loud noises. Certain medications, such as aminoglycosides, aspirin, loop diuretics, and platinum-based antineoplastic medications have ototoxic effects when kidney changes result in delayed medication excretion and increased levels of the medications in the blood.

Psychogenic factors, other disease processes (e.g., diabetes), and medications may be partially responsible for sensorineural hearing loss. The Individuals with Disabilities Education Act (IDEA) was developed to ensure that children and adults, including older adults, receive the same opportunities in the educational system as those without hearing impairment (U.S. Department of Education, 2012). Chart 64-4 describes ethical issues surrounding older adults with hearing loss (Brock, Park, & Wendler, 2014).

Even with the best health care, people with hearing loss must learn to adjust to it. Care of older patients includes

Chart 64-4 ETHICAL DILEMMA
When Might Someone's Commitment to an Independent Lifestyle Put Himself or Others at Risk?

Case Scenario

You work as a nurse manager in a family practice clinic in the neighborhood where you also live. A 67-year patient tells you that he continues to work full time in a large automotive factory, where he has been employed for the past 40 years. He expresses that he feels incompetent at times and stressed by the noise level. He states, "My boss wants to reassign me from the floor because I can't always hear the alarms when they go off which could cause an accident." He further states, "I think they are just trying to get rid of me because of my age." After reviewing the patient's electronic health record, you find that the patient has a documented history of significant hearing loss. Although he was screened by an audiologist 3 years ago and fitted with hearing aids, he does not wear them.

Discussion

Most adults who have adult onset hearing loss are 65 years of age or older and have been exposed to excessive noise. Hearing loss may put them at risk for injury because they may miss hearing signals that herald changes in the work environment, which could result in injury. Failure to adhere to safety codes and restrictions could also place other employees in the workplace at jeopardy.

Analysis

- Describe the ethical principles that are in conflict in this case (see Chapter 3, Chart 3-3). Which principle should have preeminence as you proceed to work with this patient?
- Is it possible to preserve this patient's autonomy? If so, what steps you might take to ensure that the patient's rights to "self-rule" are maintained?
- The employer recommends a change of workplace environment, which is perceived by the patient as ageism. Are there any indicators of paternalism or ageism in this scenario?
- How could the American Disability Act be utilized in this situation? Are there other agencies or support services that you may be able to mobilize for him (e.g., if he is a veteran, there are veterans' benefits that he may be able to draw from

Resources

See Chapter 3, Chart 3-6 for ethics resources.

Adapted from Brock, D. W., Park, J. K., & Wendler, D. (2014). Making treatment decisions for oneself: Weighing the value. *The Hastings Center Report*, 46(3), 22–30.

recognizing emotional reactions related to hearing loss, such as suspicion of others because of an inability to hear adequately; frustration and anger, with repeated statements such as "I didn't hear what you said!"; and feelings of insecurity because of the inability to hear the telephone or alarms. The Americans with Disabilities Act (ADA) of 1990 requires that all emergency services are accessible to people who have text message telephones (teletypewriters [TTYs]). In addition, all 911 centers in the United States must be accessible to people with TTYs.

Depression, isolation, and a decrease in cognitive function can have a negative impact on quality of life in the older adult with hearing loss. Feelings of social isolation, confusion, alterations in daily living activities, and increasing risk of falls have all been associated with hearing loss in older adults (Mener, Betz, Genther, et al., 2013). Hearing loss can also interfere with relationships due to a loss of communication. A hearing screening is recommended as one component of the physical examination for the older adult when joining Medicare for the first time. "Welcome to Medicare" examinations and annual screenings are also important.

Medical Management

If a hearing loss is permanent or untreatable or if the patient elects not to be treated, aural rehabilitation (discussed at the end of the chapter) may be beneficial.

Nursing Management

Early detection of hearing loss is one of the objectives of *Healthy People 2020*, and nurses are in a position to assist in meeting this goal (HHS, 2010). Another objective is for people diagnosed with hearing loss or deafness to use rehabilitation services and supplemental devices to improve communication with other people. Resources are available in workplaces and in schools. Questions used to assess for hearing loss may include:

- Have you experienced any hearing loss in the past?
- Are you experiencing any hearing loss now?
- Do your family members think that you are having difficulty hearing and/or experiencing any hearing loss?

These questions should be included in any routine nursing assessment and referrals made for further evaluation as needed.

Nurses who understand the different types of hearing loss are more successful in adopting a communication style to fit the needs and preferences of each patient. Trying to speak in a loud voice to a person who cannot hear high-frequency sounds only makes understanding more difficult. However, strategies such as talking into the less impaired ear and using gestures and facial expressions can help (see Chart 64-5).

A major issue for many people who are deaf or hearing impaired is that they have other health problems that often do not receive attention, in large part because of communication barriers with their health care providers. To meet the health care needs of these patients, providers are legally obligated to make accommodations for a patient's inability to hear. Providing interpreters for those who can communicate through sign language is essential in many situations so that effective communication occurs.

During health care and screening procedures, the provider (e.g., dentist, physician, nurse) must be aware that patients who are deaf or hearing impaired are unable to read lips, see a signer, or read written materials in the dark rooms required during some diagnostic tests. The same situation exists if the provider is wearing a mask or is not in sight (e.g., x-ray studies, magnetic resonance imaging [MRI], colonoscopy).

Nurses and other health care providers must work with patients who are deaf or hearing impaired and their families to identify practical and effective means of communication.

Chart 64-5 **Communicating With People Who Are Hearing Impaired**

For the Person Who is Hearing Impaired Whose Speech is Difficult to Understand

- Determine how the person prefers to communicate with others. Do not assume that writing, gestures, or other means are the best or preferred technique.
- Consider if the person uses sign language. Interpreters are available from American Sign Language Services, Inc. (ASLI). These specialists provide the best means of communication, providing accurate, professional services.
- Devote full attention to what the person is saying. Look and listen—do not try to attend to another task while listening.
- Engage the speaker in conversation when it is possible for you to anticipate the replies. This enables you to become accustomed to any peculiarities in speech patterns.
- Try to determine the essential context of what is being said; you can often fill in the details from context.
- Do not try to appear as if you understand if you do not.
- If you cannot understand at all or have serious doubt about your ability to understand what is being said, have the person write the message rather than risk misunderstanding. Having the person repeat the message in speech, after you know its content, also aids you in becoming accustomed to the person's pattern of speech.

- Written communication is an excellent resource. Material should be written at a third-grade level so that the majority of people can understand it.

For the Person Who is Hearing Impaired Who Speech Reads

- When speaking, always face the person as directly as possible.
- Make sure that your face is as clearly visible as possible. Locate yourself so that your face is well lighted; avoid being silhouetted against strong light. Do not obscure the person's view of your mouth in any way; avoid talking with any object held in your mouth.
- Be sure that the patient knows the topic or subject before going ahead with what you plan to say. This enables the person to use contextual clues in speech reading.
- Speak slowly and distinctly, pausing more frequently than you would normally.
- If you question whether some important direction or instruction has been understood, check to be certain that the patient has the full meaning of your message.
- If for any reason your mouth must be covered (as with a mask) and you must direct or instruct the patient, write the message.

Nurses can serve as catalysts throughout the health care system to ensure that accommodations are made to meet the communication needs of these patients.

CONDITIONS OF THE EXTERNAL EAR

Cerumen Impaction

Cerumen normally accumulates in the external canal in various amounts and colors. Although wax does not usually need to be removed, impaction occasionally occurs, causing **otalgia** (a sensation of fullness or pain in the ear) with or without a hearing loss. Accumulation of cerumen as a cause of hearing loss is especially significant in older adult patients (Eliopoulos, 2018). Attempts to clear the external auditory canal with matches, hairpins, and other implements are dangerous because trauma to the skin, infection, and damage to the tympanic membrane can occur.

Management

Cerumen can be removed by irrigation, suction, or instrumentation. Unless the patient has a perforated eardrum or an inflamed external ear (i.e., otitis externa), gentle irrigation with warm water usually helps remove impacted cerumen, particularly if it is not tightly packed in the external auditory canal. For successful removal, the water stream must flow behind the obstructing cerumen to move it first laterally and then out of the canal. To prevent injury, the lowest effective pressure should be used. However, if the eardrum behind the impaction is perforated, water can enter the middle ear, producing acute vertigo and infection. If irrigation is unsuccessful, direct visual, mechanical removal can be performed by a trained health care provider on a patient who is cooperative.

> ◤ **Quality and Safety Nursing Alert**
>
> Warm water (never cold or hot) and gentle (not forceful) irrigation should be used to remove cerumen. Irrigation that is too forceful can cause perforation of the tympanic membrane, and ice water causes vomiting.

Instilling a few drops of warmed glycerin, mineral oil, or half-strength hydrogen peroxide into the ear canal for 30 minutes prior to irrigation can soften cerumen before its removal. Ceruminolytic agents, such as peroxide in glyceryl (Debrox), are available. The use of any softening solution two or three times a day for several days is generally sufficient. If the cerumen cannot be dislodged by these methods, instruments, such as a cerumen curette, aural suction, and a binocular microscope for magnification, can be used.

Foreign Bodies

Some objects are inserted intentionally into the ear by adults who may have been trying to clean the external canal or relieve itching, or by children who introduce peas, beans, pebbles, toys, and beads. Insects may also enter the ear canal. In either case, the effects may range from no symptoms to profound pain and decreased hearing.

Management

Removing a foreign body from the external auditory canal can be quite challenging. The three standard methods for removing foreign bodies are the same as those for removing cerumen: irrigation, suction, and instrumentation. The contraindications for irrigation are also the same. Foreign vegetable bodies and insects tend to swell; thus, irrigation is contraindicated. Usually, an insect can be dislodged by instilling mineral oil, which will kill the insect and allow it to be removed.

Attempts to remove a foreign body from the external canal may be dangerous in unskilled hands. The object may be pushed completely into the bony portion of the canal, lacerating the skin and perforating the tympanic membrane. In rare circumstances, the foreign body may have to be extracted in the operating room with the patient under general anesthesia.

External Otitis (Otitis Externa)

External otitis (i.e., **otitis externa**), refers to an inflammation of the external auditory canal. Causes include water in the ear canal (swimmer's ear); trauma to the skin of the ear canal, permitting entrance of organisms into the tissues; and systemic conditions, such as vitamin deficiency and endocrine disorders. Bacterial or fungal infections are most frequently encountered. The most common bacterial pathogens associated with external otitis are *Staphylococcus aureus* and *Pseudomonas* species. The most common fungus isolated in both normal and infected ears is *Aspergillus* (Grossman & Porth, 2014). External otitis is often caused by a dermatosis such as psoriasis, eczema, or seborrheic dermatitis. Even allergic reactions to hair spray, hair dye, and permanent wave lotions can cause dermatitis, which clears when the offending agent is removed.

Clinical Manifestations

Patients usually report pain; discharge from the external auditory canal; aural tenderness (usually not present in middle ear infections); and occasionally fever, cellulitis, and lymphadenopathy. Other symptoms may include pruritus and hearing loss or a feeling of fullness in the ear. On otoscopic examination, the ear canal is erythematous and edematous. Discharge may be yellow or green and foul smelling. In fungal infections, hairlike black spores may be visible.

Medical Management

The principles of therapy are aimed at relieving the discomfort, reducing the swelling of the ear canal, and eradicating the infection. Patients may require analgesic medications for the first 48 to 96 hours. Treatment most often includes antimicrobial or antifungal otic medications given by dropper at room temperature. In bacterial infection, a combination antibiotic and corticosteroid agent may be used to soothe the inflamed tissues (Grossman & Porth, 2014).

Nursing Management

Nurses should instruct patients not to clean the external auditory canal with cotton-tipped applicators and to avoid events that traumatize the external canal, such as scratching the canal with the fingernail or other objects. Trauma may

PATIENT EDUCATION

Prevention of Otitis Externa

The nurse instructs the patient to:

- Protect the external canal when swimming, showering, or washing hair. Use ear plugs or place a cotton ball covered in petrolatum jelly in the ear, and wear a swim cap. The external canal may be dried afterward with a hair dryer on low heat.
- Place alcohol drops in the external canal to act as an astringent to help prevent infection after water exposure.
- Prevent trauma to the external canal. Procedures, foreign objects (e.g., bobby pin), scratching, or any other trauma to the canal that breaks the skin integrity may cause infection.
- Be aware that if otitis externa is diagnosed, refrain from any water sport activity for approximately 7–10 days to allow the canal to heal completely. Recurrence is highly likely unless you allow the external canal to heal completely.

lead to infection of the canal. Patients should also avoid getting the canal wet when swimming or shampooing the hair. A cotton ball or lamb's wool can be covered in a water-insoluble gel such as petrolatum jelly and placed in the ear as a barrier to the canal getting wet. Infection can be prevented by using antiseptic otic preparations after swimming (e.g., Swim-Ear, Ear Dry), unless there is a history of tympanic membrane perforation or a current ear infection (see Chart 64-6).

Malignant External Otitis

A more serious, although rare, external ear infection is malignant external otitis (temporal bone osteomyelitis). This is a progressive, debilitating, and occasionally fatal infection of the external auditory canal, the surrounding tissue, and the base of the skull. *Pseudomonas aeruginosa* is usually the infecting organism in patients with low resistance to infection (e.g., patients with acquired immune deficiency virus). Successful treatment includes administration of antibiotics (usually intravenously [IV]), and aggressive local wound care. Standard parenteral antibiotic treatment includes the combination of an antipseudomonal agent and an aminoglycoside, both of which have potentially serious side effects. Because aminoglycosides are nephrotoxic and ototoxic, serum aminoglycoside levels and kidney and auditory function must be monitored during therapy. Local wound care includes limited débridement of the infected tissue, including bone and cartilage, depending on the extent of the infection.

Masses of the External Ear

Exostoses are small, hard, bony protrusions found in the lower posterior bony portion of the ear canal; they usually occur bilaterally. The skin covering the exostosis is normal. It is believed that exostoses are caused by an exposure to cold water, as in scuba diving or surfing. The usual treatment, if any, is surgical excision.

Malignant tumors also may occur in the external ear. Most common are basal cell carcinomas on the pinna and squamous cell carcinomas in the ear canal. If untreated, squamous cell carcinoma may spread through the temporal bone, causing facial nerve paralysis and hearing loss. Carcinomas must be treated surgically.

CONDITIONS OF THE MIDDLE EAR

Tympanic Membrane Perforation

Perforation of the tympanic membrane is usually caused by infection or trauma. Sources of trauma include skull fracture, injury from explosion, or a severe blow to the ear. Less frequently, perforation is caused by foreign objects (e.g., cotton-tipped applicators, hairpins, keys) that have been pushed too far into the external auditory canal. In addition to tympanic membrane perforation, injury to the ossicles and even the inner ear may result from this type of trauma. During infection, the tympanic membrane can rupture if the pressure in the middle ear exceeds the atmospheric pressure in the external auditory canal.

Medical Management

Although most tympanic membrane perforations heal spontaneously within weeks after rupture, some may take several months to heal. Some perforations persist because scar tissue grows over the edges of the perforation, preventing extension of the epithelial cells across the margins and final healing. In the case of a head injury or temporal bone fracture, a patient is observed for evidence of cerebrospinal fluid **otorrhea** or **rhinorrhea**—a clear, watery drainage from the ear or nose, respectively. While healing, the ear must be protected from water getting into the ear canal.

Surgical Management

Perforations that do not heal on their own may require surgery. The decision to perform a tympanoplasty (see later section in this chapter) is usually based on the need to prevent potential infection from water entering the ear or the desire to improve the patient's hearing. Performed on an outpatient basis, tympanoplasty may involve a variety of surgical techniques. In all techniques, tissue (commonly from the temporalis fascia) is placed across the perforation to allow healing. Surgery is usually successful in closing the perforation permanently and improving hearing.

Acute Otitis Media

Ear infections can occur at any age; however, they are most commonly seen in children. **Acute otitis media (AOM)** is an acute infection of the middle ear, lasting less than 6 weeks. Pathogens that cause AOM are usually bacterial or viral and enter the middle ear after eustachian tube dysfunction caused by obstruction related to upper respiratory infections, inflammation of surrounding structures (e.g., rhinosinusitis, adenoid hypertrophy), or allergic reactions (e.g., allergic rhinitis) (Grossman & Porth, 2014). Bacteria can enter the eustachian tube from contaminated secretions in the nasopharynx and the middle ear from a tympanic membrane perforation. A purulent exudate is usually present in the middle ear, resulting in a conductive hearing loss.

Clinical Manifestations

Symptoms of otitis media vary with the severity of the infection. The condition, usually unilateral in adults, may be accompanied by otalgia. The pain is relieved after spontaneous

TABLE 64-3 Clinical Features of Otitis

Feature	Acute Otitis Externa	Acute Otitis Media
Otorrhea	May or may not be present	Present if tympanic membrane perforates; discharge is profuse.
Otalgia	Persistent; may awaken patient at night	Relieved if tympanic membrane ruptures
Aural tenderness	Present on palpation of auricle	Usually absent
Systemic symptoms	Absent	Fever, upper respiratory infection, rhinitis
Edema of external auditory canal	Present	Absent
Tympanic membrane	May appear normal	Erythema, bulging, may be perforated
Hearing loss	Conductive type	Conductive type

perforation or therapeutic incision of the tympanic membrane. Other symptoms may include drainage from the ear, fever, and hearing loss. Table 64-3 differentiates acute otitis externa from AOM. Risk factors for AOM include younger age, chronic upper respiratory infections, medical conditions that predispose the patient to ear infections (e.g., Down syndrome, cystic fibrosis, cleft palate), and chronic exposure to secondhand cigarette smoke.

Medical Management

The outcome of AOM depends on the efficacy of therapy (the prescribed dose of an oral antibiotic and the duration of therapy), the virulence of the bacteria, and the physical status of the patient. With early and appropriate broad-spectrum antibiotic therapy, otitis media may resolve with no serious sequelae. If drainage occurs, an antibiotic otic preparation is usually prescribed. The condition may become subacute (lasting 2 weeks to 3 months), with persistent purulent discharge from the ear. Rarely does permanent hearing loss occur. Secondary complications involving the mastoid and other serious intracranial complications, such as meningitis or brain abscess, although rare, can occur.

Surgical Management

A **myringotomy** (i.e., tympanotomy) is an incision in the tympanic membrane. The tympanic membrane is numbed with a local anesthetic agent such as phenol or by iontophoresis (i.e., in which electrical current flows through a lidocaine and epinephrine solution to numb the ear canal and tympanic membrane). The procedure is painless and takes less than 15 minutes. Under microscopic guidance, an incision is made through the tympanic membrane to relieve pressure and to drain serous or purulent fluid from the middle ear.

Normally, this procedure is unnecessary for treating AOM, but it may be performed if pain persists. Myringotomy also allows the drainage to be analyzed (by culture and sensitivity testing) so that the infecting organism can be identified and

appropriate antibiotic therapy prescribed. The incision heals within 24 to 72 hours.

If AOM recurs and there is no contraindication, a ventilating, or pressure-equalizing, tube may be inserted. The ventilating tube, which temporarily takes the place of the eustachian tube in equalizing pressure, is retained for 6 to 18 months. The ventilating tube is then extruded with normal skin migration of the tympanic membrane, with the hole healing in nearly every case. Ventilating tubes are used to treat recurrent episodes of AOM.

Serous Otitis Media

Middle ear effusion, or serous otitis media, involves the presence of fluid, without evidence of active infection, in the middle ear. In theory, this fluid results from a negative pressure in the middle ear caused by eustachian tube obstruction. When this condition occurs in adults, an underlying cause for the eustachian tube dysfunction must be sought. Middle ear effusion is frequently seen in patients after radiation therapy or barotrauma and in patients with eustachian tube dysfunction from a concurrent upper respiratory infection or allergy. Barotrauma results from sudden pressure changes in the middle ear caused by changes in barometric pressure, as in scuba diving or airplane descent. A carcinoma (e.g., nasopharyngeal cancer) obstructing the eustachian tube should be ruled out in adults with persistent unilateral serous otitis media.

Clinical Manifestations

Patients may complain of hearing loss, fullness in the ear or a sensation of congestion, or popping and crackling noises that occur as the eustachian tube attempts to open. The tympanic membrane appears dull on otoscopy, and air bubbles may be visualized in the middle ear. Usually, the audiogram shows a conductive hearing loss.

Management

Serous otitis media need not be treated medically unless infection (i.e., AOM) occurs. If the hearing loss associated with middle ear effusion is significant, a myringotomy can be performed, and a tube may be placed to keep the middle ear ventilated. Corticosteroids in small doses may decrease the edema of the eustachian tube in cases of barotrauma. Decongestants have not proved to be effective. A Valsalva maneuver, which forcibly opens the eustachian tube by increasing nasopharyngeal pressure, may be cautiously performed; this maneuver may cause worsening pain or perforation of the tympanic membrane.

Chronic Otitis Media

Chronic otitis media is recurrent AOM that causes irreversible tissue pathology. Chronic infections of the middle ear damage the tympanic membrane, destroy the ossicles, and involve the mastoid but are rare in developed countries.

Clinical Manifestations

Symptoms may be minimal, with varying degrees of hearing loss and a persistent or intermittent, foul-smelling otorrhea.

Pain is not usually experienced, except in cases of acute mastoiditis, when the postauricular area is tender and may be erythematous and edematous. Otoscopic examination may show a perforation, and cholesteatoma can be identified as a white mass behind the tympanic membrane or coming through to the external canal from a perforation.

Cholesteatoma is a tumor of the external layer of the eardrum into the middle ear. It is generally caused by a chronic retraction pocket of the tympanic membrane, creating a persistently high negative pressure of the middle ear. The skin forms a sac that fills with degenerated skin and sebaceous materials. The sac can attach to the structures of the middle ear, mastoid, or both.

Chronic otitis media can cause chronic mastoiditis and lead to the formation of cholesteatoma. It can occur in the middle ear, mastoid cavity, or both, often dictating the type of surgery to be performed. If untreated, cholesteatoma will continue to enlarge, possibly causing damage to the facial nerve and horizontal canal and destruction of other surrounding structures.

Cholesteatomas are cystlike lesions of the inner ear (Grossman & Porth, 2014). They usually do not cause pain; however, if treatment or surgery is delayed, they may burst or destroy the mastoid bone. These fast-growing lesions may cause severe sequelae such as hearing loss. Cholesteatomas found in older adult patients generally develop in the external canal.

Cholesteatomas may be asymptomatic, or they may cause hearing loss, facial pain and paralysis, tinnitus, or vertigo. Audiometric tests often show a conductive or mixed hearing loss. Based on presenting symptoms, diagnosis may be made by visual examination or by computed tomography (CT) or MRI scan. Therapy includes treatment of the acute infection and surgical removal of the mass to restore hearing.

Medical Management

Local treatment for chronic otitis media consists of careful suctioning of the ear under otoscopic guidance. Instillation of antibiotic drops or application of antibiotic powder is used to treat purulent discharge. Systemic antibiotic agents are prescribed only in cases of acute infection.

Surgical Management

Surgical procedures, including tympanoplasty, ossiculoplasty, and mastoidectomy, are used if medical treatments are ineffective.

Tympanoplasty

The most common surgical procedure for chronic otitis media is **tympanoplasty**, or surgical reconstruction of the tympanic membrane. Reconstruction of the ossicles may also be required. The purposes of a tympanoplasty are to reestablish middle ear function, close the perforation, prevent recurrent infection, and improve hearing.

There are five types of tympanoplasties. The simplest surgical procedure, type I (myringoplasty), is designed to close a perforation in the tympanic membrane. The other procedures, types II through V, involve more extensive repair of middle ear structures. The structures and the degree of involvement can differ, but all tympanoplasty procedures include restoring the continuity of the sound conduction mechanism.

Tympanoplasty is performed through the external auditory canal with a transcanal approach or through a postauricular incision. The contents of the middle ear are carefully inspected, and the ossicular chain (malleus and incus unit) is evaluated. Ossicular interruption is most frequent in chronic otitis media, but problems of reconstruction can also occur with malformations of the middle ear and ossicular dislocations due to head injuries. Dramatic improvement in hearing can result from closure of a perforation and reestablishment of the ossicles. Surgery is usually performed in an outpatient facility under moderate sedation or general anesthesia.

Ossiculoplasty

Ossiculoplasty is the surgical reconstruction of the middle ear bones to restore hearing. Prostheses made of materials such as Teflon, stainless steel, and hydroxyapatite are used to reconnect the ossicles, thereby reestablishing the sound conduction mechanism. However, the greater the damage, the lower the success rate for restoring normal hearing.

Mastoidectomy

The objectives of mastoid surgery are to remove the cholesteatoma, gain access to diseased structures, and create a dry (noninfected) and healthy ear. If possible, the ossicles are reconstructed during the initial surgical procedure. Occasionally, extensive disease or damage dictates that this be performed as part of a two-stage operation.

A mastoidectomy is usually performed through a postauricular incision. Infection is eliminated by removing the mastoid air cells. A second mastoidectomy may be necessary to check for recurrent or residual cholesteatoma. The hearing mechanism may be reconstructed at this time. The success rate for correcting this conductive hearing loss is approximately 75%. Surgery is usually performed in an outpatient setting. The patient has a mastoid pressure dressing, which can be removed 24 to 48 hours after surgery. Although infrequently injured, the facial nerve, which runs through the middle ear and mastoid, is at some risk for injury during mastoid surgery. As the patient awakens from anesthesia, any evidence of facial paresis should be reported to the primary provider.

NURSING PROCESS

The Patient Undergoing Mastoid Surgery

Although several otologic surgical procedures are performed under moderate sedation, mastoid surgery is performed using general anesthesia.

Assessment

The health history includes a complete description of the ear disorder, including infection, otalgia, otorrhea, hearing loss, and vertigo. Data are collected about the duration and intensity of the disorder, its causes, and previous treatments. Information is obtained about other health problems and all medications that the patient is taking. Medication allergies and family history of ear disease also should be obtained.

Physical assessment addresses erythema, edema, otorrhea, lesions, and characteristics such as odor and color of discharge. The results of the audiogram are reviewed.

Nursing Diagnoses

Based on the assessment data, major nursing diagnoses may include the following:

- Anxiety related to surgical procedure, potential loss of hearing, potential taste disturbance, and potential loss of facial movement
- Acute pain related to mastoid surgery
- Risk for infection related to mastoidectomy; placement of grafts, prostheses, and electrodes; and surgical trauma to surrounding tissues and structures
- Impaired verbal communication related to ear disorder, surgery, or packing
- Risk for injury related to impaired balance or vertigo during the immediate postoperative period, dislodgment of the graft or prosthesis, or injury to facial nerve (cranial nerve VII) and chorda tympani nerve
- Deficient knowledge about mastoid disease, surgical procedure, and postoperative care and expectations

Planning and Goals

The major goals of caring for a patient undergoing mastoidectomy include reduction of anxiety; freedom from pain and discomfort; prevention of infection; stable or improved hearing and communication; absence of vertigo and related injury; and increased knowledge regarding the disease, surgical procedure, and postoperative care.

Nursing Interventions

REDUCING ANXIETY

The nurse reinforces the information discussed by the otologic surgeon with the patient, including anesthesia, the location of the incision (postauricular), and expected surgical results (e.g., hearing, balance, taste, facial movement). The patient also is encouraged to discuss any anxieties and concerns about the surgery.

RELIEVING PAIN

Although most patients complain very little about incisional pain after mastoid surgery, they do have some ear discomfort. Aural fullness or pressure after surgery is caused by residual blood or fluid in the middle ear. The prescribed analgesic medication may be taken for the first 24 hours after surgery and then only as needed.

A wick or external auditory canal packing is used if tympanoplasty was performed at the time of the mastoidectomy. For the next 2 to 3 weeks after surgery, the patient may experience sharp, shooting pains intermittently as the eustachian tube opens and allows air to enter the middle ear. Constant, throbbing pain accompanied by fever may indicate infection and should be reported to the primary provider.

PREVENTING INFECTION

Measures are initiated to prevent infection in the operated ear. The external auditory canal wick, or packing, may be impregnated with an antibiotic solution before instillation. Prophylactic antibiotic agents are given as prescribed, and the patient is instructed to prevent water from entering the external auditory canal for 6 weeks. A cotton ball or lamb's wool covered with a water-insoluble substance (e.g., petrolatum jelly) and placed loosely in the ear canal usually prevents water from entering the ear canal and should be used when the patient showers or washes their hair, or

in any situations in which water may enter the ear canal. The postauricular incision should be kept dry for the first 2 days. Signs of infection such as an elevated temperature and purulent drainage should be reported. Some serosanguineous drainage from the external auditory canal is normal after surgery.

IMPROVING HEARING AND COMMUNICATION

Hearing in the operated ear may be reduced for several weeks because of edema, accumulation of blood and tissue fluid in the middle ear, and dressings or packing. Measures are initiated to improve hearing and communication, such as reducing environmental noise, facing the patient when speaking, speaking clearly and distinctly without shouting, providing good lighting if the patient relies on speech reading, and using nonverbal clues (e.g., facial expression, pointing, gestures) and other forms of communication. Family members or significant others are instructed about effective ways to communicate with the patient. If the patient uses assistive hearing devices, one can be used in the unaffected ear.

PREVENTING INJURY

Vertigo may occur after mastoid surgery if the semicircular canals or other areas of the inner ear are traumatized. Antiemetic or antivertiginous medications (e.g., antihistamines) can be prescribed if a balance disturbance or vertigo occurs. Safety measures such as assisted ambulation are implemented to prevent falls and injury. The patient is instructed to avoid heavy lifting, straining, exertion, and nose blowing for 2 to 3 weeks after surgery to prevent dislodging the tympanic membrane graft or ossicular prosthesis.

Facial nerve injury is a potential, although rare, complication of mastoid surgery. The patient is instructed to report immediately any evidence of facial nerve (cranial nerve VII) weakness, such as drooping of the mouth on the operated side, slurred speech, decreased sensation, and difficulty swallowing. A more frequent occurrence is a temporary disturbance in the chorda tympani nerve, which is a small branch of the facial nerve that runs through the middle ear. Patients experience a taste disturbance and dry mouth on the side of surgery for several months until the nerve regenerates.

PROMOTING HOME, COMMUNITY-BASED, AND TRANSITIONAL CARE

Educating Patients About Self-Care. Patients require education about medication therapy, such as analgesic and antivertiginous agents (e.g., antihistamines) prescribed for balance disturbance. Education includes information about the expected effects and potential side effects of the medication. Patients also need instruction about any activity restrictions. Possible complications such as infection, facial nerve weakness, or taste disturbances, including the signs and symptoms to report immediately, are included (see Chart 64-7).

Continuing and Transitional Care. Some patients, particularly older adult patients, who have had mastoid surgery may require the services of a home, community-based, or transitional care nurse for a few days after returning home. However, most people find that assistance from a family member or a friend is sufficient. The caregiver and patient are cautioned that the patient may experience some vertigo and will therefore require help with ambulation to avoid falling. Any

PATIENT EDUCATION

Self-Care After Middle Ear or Mastoid Surgery

Postoperative instructions for patients who have had middle ear and mastoid surgery may vary among otolaryngologists. The nurse instructs the patient in the following general guidelines:

- Take antibiotics and other medications as prescribed.
- Avoid nose blowing for 2–3 weeks after surgery.
- Sneeze and cough with the mouth open for a few weeks after surgery.
- Avoid heavy lifting (>10 pounds), straining, and bending over for a few weeks after surgery.
- Be aware that popping and crackling sensations in the operative ear are normal for approximately 3–5 weeks after surgery.
- Note that temporary hearing loss is normal in the operative ear due to fluid, blood, or packing in the ear.
- Report excessive or purulent ear drainage to the physician.
- Avoid getting water in the operative ear for 2 weeks after surgery. You may shampoo the hair 2–3 days postoperatively if the ear is protected from water by saturating a cotton ball with petrolatum jelly (or some other water-insoluble substance) and loosely placing it in the ear. If the postauricular suture line becomes wet, pat (not rub) the area and cover it with a thin layer of antibiotic ointment.

6. Verbalizes the reasons for and methods of care and treatment
    a. Discusses the discharge plan formulated with the nurse with regard to rest periods, medication, and activities permitted and restricted
    b. Lists symptoms that should be reported to the primary provider
    c. Keeps follow-up appointments

Otosclerosis

Otosclerosis involves the stapes and is thought to result from the formation of new, abnormal spongy bone, especially around the oval window, with resulting fixation of the stapes (Grossman & Porth, 2014). The efficient transmission of sound is prevented because the stapes cannot vibrate and carry the sound as conducted from the malleus and incus to the inner ear. Otosclerosis is more common in women, is a familial condition, and can progress to complete deafness (Eliopoulos, 2018; Grossman & Porth, 2014).

Clinical Manifestations

Otosclerosis may involve one or both ears and manifests as a progressive conductive or mixed hearing loss. The patient may or may not complain of tinnitus. Otoscopic examination usually reveals a normal tympanic membrane. Bone conduction is better than air conduction on Rinne testing. The audiogram confirms conductive hearing loss or mixed loss, especially in the low frequencies.

Medical Management

The management of otosclerosis can be surgical or medical. Amplification with a hearing aid may help (Grossman & Porth, 2014).

Surgical Management

One of two surgical procedures may be performed: the stapedectomy or the stapedotomy. A stapedectomy involves removing the stapes superstructure and part of the footplate and inserting a tissue graft and a suitable prosthesis (see Fig. 64-6). In a stapedotomy, the surgeon drills a small hole into the stapes, instead of removing it, to hold a prosthesis. In both procedures, the prosthesis bridges the gap between the incus and the inner ear, providing better sound conduction. The majority of patients experience resolution of conductive hearing loss following stapes surgery. The use of sodium fluoride in the postoperative period increases the success rate and hearing ability postoperatively (Grossman & Porth, 2014). Balance disturbance or true vertigo may occur during the postoperative period for several days. Long-term balance disorders are rare.

Middle Ear Masses

Other than cholesteatoma, masses in the middle ear are rare. Glomus tympanicum is a tumor that arises from Jacobson nerve (in the temporal bone of the skull) and remains limited to the middle ear. On otoscopy, a red blemish on or behind the tympanic membrane is seen. Glomus jugulare tumors are rarely malignant; however, because of their location, treatment may be necessary to relieve symptoms. The treatment

symptoms of complications are to be reported promptly to the primary provider. The importance of scheduling and keeping follow-up appointments is also stressed.

Evaluation

Expected patient outcomes may include:

1. Demonstrates reduced anxiety about surgical procedure
    a. Verbalizes and exhibits less stress, tension, and irritability
    b. Verbalizes acceptance of the results of surgery and adjustment to possible hearing impairment
2. Remains free of discomfort or pain
    a. Exhibits no facial grimacing, moaning, or crying, and reports absence of pain
    b. Uses analgesic agents appropriately
3. Demonstrates no signs or symptoms of infection
    a. Has normal vital signs, including temperature
    b. Demonstrates absence of purulent drainage from the external auditory canal
    c. Describes method for preventing water from contaminating packing
4. Exhibits signs that communication and hearing have stabilized or improved
    a. Describes surgical goal for hearing and judges whether the goal has been met
    b. Verbalizes that hearing has improved
5. Remains free of injury and trauma
    a. Reports absence of vertigo or balance disturbance
    b. Experiences no injury or fall
    c. Avoids activities that can cause dislodgement of graft or prosthesis
    d. Reports no taste disturbance, mouth dryness, or facial weakness

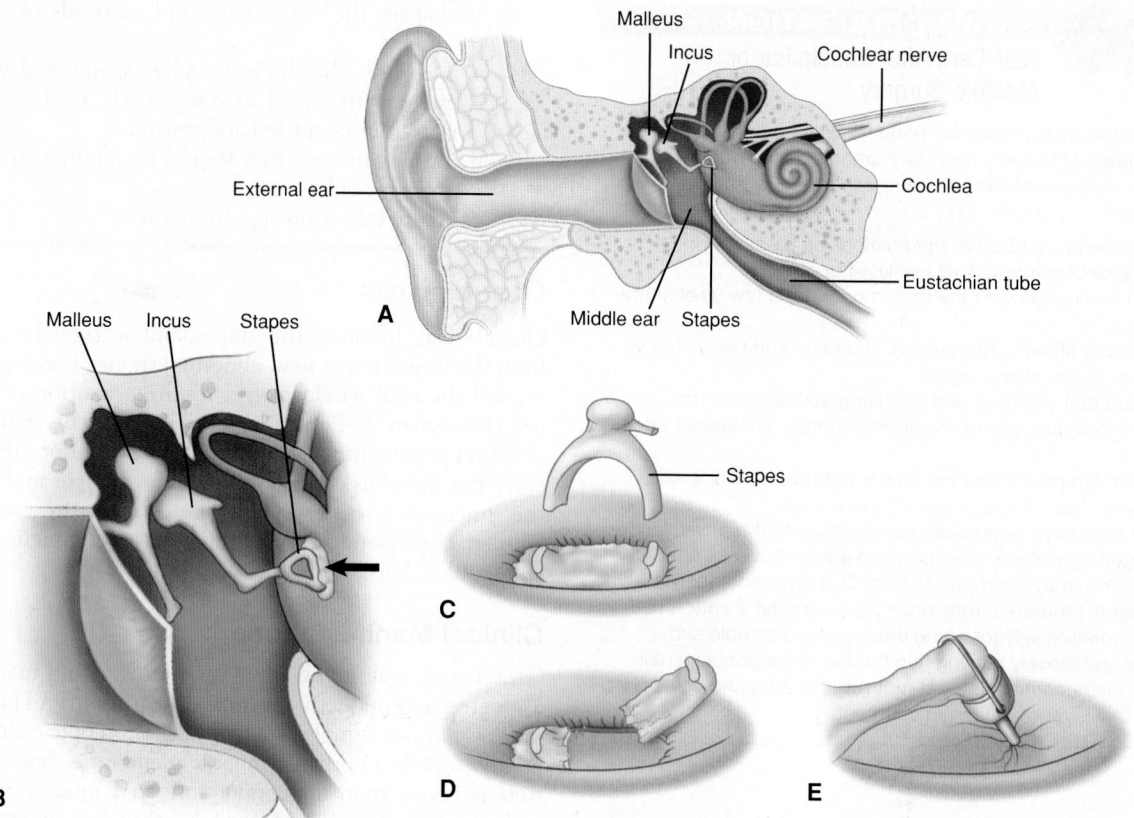

Figure 64-6 • Stapedectomy for otosclerosis. **A.** Normal anatomy. **B.** *Arrow* points to sclerotic process at the foot of the stapes. **C.** Stapes broken away surgically from its diseased base. The hole in the footplate provides an area where an instrument can grasp the plate. **D.** The footplate is removed from its base. Some otosclerotic tissue may remain, and tissue is placed over it. **E.** Robinson stainless steel prosthesis in position.

is surgical excision, except in patients who are poor surgical candidates, in whom radiation therapy is used.

A facial nerve neuroma is a tumor on cranial nerve VII. These types of tumors are usually not visible on otoscopic examination but are suspected when a patient presents with a facial nerve paresis. X-ray evaluation is used to identify the site of the tumor along the facial nerve. The treatment is surgical removal.

CONDITIONS OF THE INNER EAR

Disorders of balance are common (NIDCD, 2015a), and dizziness may increase the risk of falls. The term **dizziness** is used frequently by patients and health care providers to describe any altered sensation of orientation in space and is more commonly referred to as lightheadedness (Weber & Kelley, 2014). **Vertigo** is the misperception or illusion of motion of the person or the surroundings. Most patients with vertigo describe a spinning sensation or say they feel as though objects are moving around them. Ataxia is a failure of muscular coordination and may be present in patients with vestibular disease. Syncope, fainting, and loss of consciousness are not forms of vertigo and usually indicate disease in the cardiovascular system.

Nystagmus is an involuntary rhythmic movement of the eyes. Nystagmus occurs normally when a person watches a rapidly moving object (e.g., through the side window of a moving car or train). However, pathologically, it is an ocular disorder associated with vestibular dysfunction. Nystagmus can be horizontal, vertical, or rotary and can be caused by a disorder in the central or peripheral nervous system.

Motion Sickness

Motion sickness is a disturbance of equilibrium caused by constant motion. For example, it can occur aboard a ship, while riding on a merry-go-round or swing, or in a car (Brainard & Gresham, 2014).

Clinical Manifestations

The syndrome manifests itself in sweating, pallor, nausea, and vomiting caused by vestibular overstimulation. These manifestations may persist for several hours after the stimulation stops.

Management

Over-the-counter antihistamines such as dimenhydrinate (Dramamine) or meclizine (Antivert) may provide some relief of nausea and vomiting by blocking the conduction of the vestibular pathway of the inner ear. Anticholinergic medications, such as scopolamine patches (Transderm Scop), may also be effective because they antagonize the histamine response. These must be applied several hours before exposure to motion and replaced every 3 days (Brainard & Gresham, 2014). Side effects such as dry mouth and drowsiness may occur. Potentially hazardous activities such as driving a car or operating heavy machinery should be avoided if drowsiness occurs.

Ménière Disease

Ménière disease is an abnormality in inner ear fluid balance caused by a malabsorption in the endolymphatic sac or a blockage in the endolymphatic duct (NIDCD, 2015b). **Endolymphatic hydrops** (dilation of the endolymphatic space) develops, and either increased pressure in the system or rupture of the inner ear membrane occurs, producing symptoms of Ménière disease (Hansson & Brattmo, 2013).

Ménière disease affects 10 to 12 of 1000 people in the United States. It is estimated that there are 615,000 cases in the United States, with approximately 45,500 new cases diagnosed annually (NIDCD, 2015b). More common in adults, onset is generally seen when adults reach their 40s, with symptoms usually beginning between the ages of 20 and 60 years. Ménière disease appears to be equally common in men and women, and is usually bilateral (Grossman & Porth, 2014).

Clinical Manifestations

Ménière disease is characterized by a triad of symptoms: episodic vertigo, **tinnitus** (unwanted noises in the head or ear), and fluctuating sensorineural hearing loss. It may also include a feeling of pressure or fullness in the ear and incapacitating vertigo, often accompanied by nausea and vomiting (Hansson & Brattmo, 2013; NIDCD, 2015b). These symptoms range in severity from a minor nuisance to extreme disability, especially if the attacks of vertigo are severe. At the onset of the disease, usually only one or two of the symptoms are manifested.

Some characterize the disease into two subsets: cochlear and vestibular. Cochlear Ménière disease is recognized as a fluctuating, progressive sensorineural hearing loss associated with tinnitus and aural pressure in the absence of vestibular symptoms or findings. Vestibular Ménière disease is characterized as the occurrence of episodic vertigo associated with aural pressure but no cochlear symptoms. Patients may experience either cochlear or vestibular disease symptoms; however, eventually all of these symptoms develop.

Assessment and Diagnostic Findings

Vertigo is usually the most troublesome complaint related to Ménière disease. A careful history is taken to determine the frequency, duration, severity, and character of the vertigo attacks. Vertigo may last minutes to hours, possibly accompanied by nausea or vomiting. Diaphoresis and a persistent feeling of imbalance or disequilibrium may awaken patients at night. Some patients report that these feelings last for days. However, they usually feel well between attacks. Hearing loss may fluctuate, with tinnitus and aural pressure waxing and waning with changes in hearing. These feelings may occur during or before attacks, or they may be constant.

Physical examination findings are usually normal, with the exception of those of cranial nerve VIII. Sounds from a tuning fork (Weber test) may lateralize to the ear opposite the hearing loss, the one affected with Ménière disease. An audiogram typically reveals a sensorineural hearing loss in the affected ear. This can be in the form of a "Pike's Peak"

pattern, which looks like a hill or mountain. A sensorineural loss in the low frequencies occurs as the disease progresses. The electronystagmogram may be normal or may show reduced vestibular response.

Medical Management

Most patients with Ménière disease can be successfully treated with diet and medication. Many patients can control their symptoms by adhering to a low-sodium (1000 to 1500 mg/day or less) diet. Chart 64-8 describes dietary guidelines that may be useful in Ménière disease. The amount of sodium is one of many factors that regulate the balance of fluid within the body. Sodium and fluid retention disrupts the delicate balance between endolymph and perilymph in the inner ear. Psychological evaluation and cognitive therapy may be indicated if a patient is anxious, uncertain, fearful, or depressed (NIDCD, 2015b).

Pharmacologic Therapy

Pharmacologic therapy for Ménière disease consists of antihistamines, such as meclizine, which shortens the attack (NIDCD, 2015b). Tranquilizers such as diazepam (Valium) may be used in acute instances to help control vertigo. Antiemetic agents such as promethazine (Phenergan) suppositories help control the nausea and vomiting and the vertigo because of their antihistamine effect. Diuretic therapy (e.g., hydrochlorothiazide [Dyazide], triamterene, spironolactone) may relieve symptoms by lowering the pressure in the endolymphatic system (Grossman & Porth, 2014). Intratympanic injection of gentamicin (Garamycin) is used to cause ablation of the vestibular hair cells; however, the risk of significant hearing loss is high (NIDCD, 2015b).

Chart 64-8

PATIENT EDUCATION

Dietary Guidelines for Patients with Ménière Disease

The nurse instructs the patient to:

- Limit foods high in salt or sugar. Be aware of foods with hidden salts and sugars.
- Eat meals and snacks at regular intervals to stay hydrated. Missing meals or snacks may alter the fluid level in the inner ear.
- Eat fresh fruits, vegetables, and whole grains. Limit the amount of canned, frozen, or processed foods with high sodium content.
- Drink plenty of fluids daily. Water, milk, and low-sugar fruit juices are recommended. Limit intake of coffee, tea, and soft drinks. Avoid caffeine because of its diuretic effect.
- Limit alcohol intake. Alcohol may change the volume and concentration of the inner ear fluid and may worsen symptoms.
- Avoid monosodium glutamate (MSG), which may increase symptoms.
- Pay attention to the intake of foods containing potassium (e.g., bananas, tomatoes, oranges) if taking a diuretic that causes potassium loss.
- Avoid aspirin and aspirin-containing medications. Aspirin may increase tinnitus and dizziness.

Adapted from National Institute on Deafness and Other Communication Disorders (NIDCD). (2015b). Ménière's disease. Retrieved on 6/12/2012 at: www.nidcd.nih.gov/health/balance/meniere.html

Surgical Management

Although most patients respond well to conservative therapy, some continue to have disabling attacks of vertigo. If these attacks reduce their quality of life, patients may elect to undergo surgery for relief. Surgical procedures include endolymphatic sac procedures and vestibular nerve section (NIDCD, 2015b). However, hearing loss, tinnitus, and aural fullness may continue, because the surgical treatment of Ménière disease is aimed at eliminating the attacks of vertigo.

Endolymphatic Sac Decompression

Endolymphatic sac decompression, or shunting, theoretically equalizes the pressure in the endolymphatic space. A shunt or drain is inserted in the endolymphatic sac through a postauricular incision. This procedure is favored by many otolaryngologists as a first-line surgical approach to treat the vertigo of Ménière disease because it is relatively simple and safe and can be performed on an outpatient basis.

Vestibular Nerve Sectioning

Vestibular nerve sectioning provides the greatest success rate (approximately 98%) in eliminating the attacks of vertigo. It can be performed by a translabyrinthine approach (i.e., through the hearing mechanism) or in a manner that can conserve hearing (i.e., suboccipital or middle cranial fossa), depending on the degree of hearing loss. Most patients with incapacitating Ménière disease have little or no effective hearing. Cutting the nerve prevents the brain from receiving input from the semicircular canals. This procedure may require a brief hospital stay. A plan of nursing care for the patient with vertigo is presented in Chart 64-9.

Benign Paroxysmal Positional Vertigo

Benign paroxysmal positional vertigo is a brief period of incapacitating vertigo that occurs when the position of the patient's head is changed with respect to gravity, typically by placing the head back with the affected ear turned down (Hansson & Brattmo, 2013; NIDCD, 2015b). The onset is sudden and followed by a predisposition for positional vertigo, usually for hours to weeks but occasionally for months or years.

Benign paroxysmal positional vertigo is thought to be due to the disruption of debris within the semicircular canal. This debris is formed from small crystals of calcium carbonate from the inner ear structure (the utricle). This is frequently stimulated by head trauma, infection, or other events. In severe cases, vertigo may easily be induced by any head movement. The vertigo is usually accompanied by nausea and vomiting; however, hearing impairment does not generally occur.

Bed rest is recommended for patients with acute symptoms. Repositioning techniques can be used to treat vertigo. The canalith repositioning procedure, also known as the Epley maneuver, is commonly used (Hansson & Brattmo, 2013). This noninvasive procedure, which involves quick movements of the body, rearranges the debris in the canal. The procedure is performed by placing the patient in a sitting position, turning the head to a 45-degree angle on the affected side, and then quickly moving the patient to the supine position. The procedure is safe, inexpensive, and easy to perform.

Patients with acute vertigo may be treated with meclizine for 1 to 2 weeks. After this time, the meclizine is stopped and the patient is reassessed. Patients who continue to have severe positional vertigo may be premedicated with prochlorperazine (Compazine) 1 hour before the canalith repositioning procedure is performed.

Vestibular rehabilitation can be used in the management of vestibular disorders. This strategy promotes active use of the vestibular system through an interdisciplinary team approach, including medical and nursing care, stress management, biofeedback, vocational rehabilitation, and physical therapy. A physical therapist prescribes balance exercises that help the brain compensate for the impairment to the balance system.

Tinnitus

Tinnitus is a symptom of an underlying disorder of the ear that is associated with hearing loss. This condition affects approximately 25 million people in the United States and is most prevalent in adults (NIDCD, 2015c). The severity of tinnitus may range from mild to severe. Patients describe tinnitus as a roaring, buzzing, or hissing sound in one or both ears. Numerous factors may contribute to the development of tinnitus, including several ototoxic substances (see Chart 64-10). Underlying disorders that contribute to tinnitus may include cardiovascular disease, thyroid disease, hyperlipidemia, vitamin B_{12} deficiency, psychological disorders (e.g., depression, anxiety), fibromyalgia, otologic disorders (Ménière disease, acoustic neuroma), and neurologic disorders (head injury, multiple sclerosis).

A physical examination should be performed to determine the cause of tinnitus. Diagnostic testing determines if hearing loss is present. An audiograph speech discrimination test or a tympanogram may be used to help determine the cause. Some forms of tinnitus are irreversible; therefore, patients may need education and counseling about ways of adjusting to their treatment and dealing with tinnitus in the future.

Labyrinthitis

Labyrinthitis, an inflammation of the labyrinth of the inner ear, can be bacterial or viral in origin. Bacterial labyrinthitis is rare because of antibiotic therapy, but it sometimes occurs as a complication of otitis media. The infection can spread to the inner ear by penetrating the membranes of the oval or round windows. Viral labyrinthitis is a common diagnosis, but little is known about this disorder, which affects hearing and balance. The most common viral causes are mumps, rubella, rubeola, and influenza. Viral illnesses of the upper respiratory tract and herpetiform disorders of the facial and acoustic nerves (i.e., Ramsay Hunt syndrome) also cause labyrinthitis.

Clinical Manifestations

Labyrinthitis is characterized by a sudden onset of incapacitating vertigo, usually with nausea and vomiting, various degrees of hearing loss, and possibly tinnitus. The first episode is usually the worst; subsequent attacks, which usually occur over a period of several weeks to months, are less severe.

Management

Treatment of bacterial labyrinthitis includes IV antibiotic therapy, fluid replacement, and administration of an antihistamine (e.g., meclizine) and antiemetic medications. Treatment of viral labyrinthitis is based on the patient's symptoms.

PLAN OF NURSING CARE

Chart 64-9

Care of the Patient With Vertigo

NURSING DIAGNOSIS: Risk for injury related to altered mobility because of gait disturbance and vertigo
GOAL: Remains free of any injuries associated with imbalance and/or falls

Nursing Interventions	Rationale	Expected Outcomes
1. Assess for vertigo, including history, onset, description of attacks, duration, frequency, and any associated ear symptoms (hearing loss, tinnitus, aural fullness).	1. Health history provides basis for interventions.	• Experiences no falls due to balance disturbance • Fear and anxiety are reduced • Performs exercises as prescribed • Takes prescribed medications appropriately • Assumes safe position when vertigo is present • Keeps head still when vertigo is present • Identifies a characteristic fullness or sense of pressure in the ear as occurring before an attack occurs • Reports measures that help reduce vertigo
2. Assess extent of disability in relation to activities of daily living.	2. Extent of disability indicates risk of falling.	
3. Instruct or reinforce vestibular/balance therapy as prescribed.	3. Exercises hasten labyrinthine compensation, which may decrease vertigo and gait disturbance.	
4. Administer, or educate about administration of, antivertiginous medications and/or vestibular sedation medication; instruct patient about side effects.	4. Alleviates acute symptoms of vertigo.	
5. Encourage patient to sit down and restrict activity when dizzy.	5. Decreases possibility of falling and injury.	
6. Place pillow on each side of head to restrict movement.	6. Movement aggravates vertigo.	
7. Assist patient in identifying aura that suggests an impending attack.	7. Recognition of aura may trigger the need to take medication before an attack occurs, thereby minimizing the severity of effects.	
8. Recommend that the patient keep eyes open and stare straight ahead when lying down and experiencing vertigo.	8. Sensation of vertigo decreases and motion decelerates if eyes are kept in a fixed position.	

NURSING DIAGNOSIS: Risk-prone health behavior related to disability requiring change in lifestyle due to unpredictability of vertigo
GOAL: Modifies lifestyle to decrease disability and exert maximum control and independence within limits posed by chronic vertigo

Nursing Interventions	Rationale	Expected Outcomes
1. Encourage patient to identify personal strengths and roles that can still be fulfilled.	1. Maximizes sense of regaining control and independence.	• Exerts maximum control of environment and independence within limits imposed by vertigo • Is informed about condition • Family and significant others are included in rehabilitation process • Uses strengths and potentials to engage in the most independent and constructive lifestyle
2. Provide information about vertigo and what to expect.	2. Reduces fear and anxiety.	
3. Include family and significant others in rehabilitative process.	3. Perceived beliefs of significant others are important for patient's adherence to medical regimen.	
4. Encourage patient to maintain sense of control by making decisions and assuming more responsibility for care.	4. Reinforces positive psychological and social outcomes.	

NURSING DIAGNOSIS: Risk for deficient fluid volume related to increased fluid output, altered intake, and medications
GOAL: Maintains normal fluid and electrolyte balance

Nursing Interventions	Rationale	Expected Outcomes
1. Assess, or have patient assess, intake and output (including emesis, liquid stools, urine, and diaphoresis). Monitor laboratory values of electrolytes.	1. Accurate records provide basis for fluid replacement.	• Laboratory values within normal limits • Alert and oriented; vital signs within normal limits, skin turgor normal; electrolytes normal • Mucous membranes are moist • Vomiting has stopped; usual oral intake is resumed
2. Assess indicators of dehydration, including blood pressure (orthostasis), pulse, skin turgor, mucous membranes, and level of consciousness.	2. Prompt recognition of dehydration allows early intervention.	
3. Encourage oral fluids as tolerated; discourage beverages containing caffeine (a vestibular stimulant).	3. Oral replacement is begun as soon as possible to replace losses.	

(continued on page 1936)

Chart 64-9

PLAN OF NURSING CARE (Continued)
Care of the Patient with Vertigo

Nursing Interventions	Rationale	Expected Outcomes
4. Administer, or educate about administration of, antiemetic medications as prescribed and needed. Educate patient about side effects.	4. Antiemetic medications reduce nausea and vomiting, reducing fluid losses and improving oral intake.	

NURSING DIAGNOSIS: Anxiety related to threat of, or change in, health status and disability effects of vertigo
GOAL: Experiences less or no anxiety

Nursing Interventions	Rationale	Expected Outcomes
1. Assess level of anxiety. Help patient identify coping skills used successfully in the past.	1. Guides therapeutic interventions and participation in self-care. Past coping skills can relieve anxiety.	• Fear and anxiety about attacks of vertigo reduced or eliminated
2. Provide information about vertigo and its treatment.	2. Increased knowledge helps to decrease anxiety.	• Acquires knowledge and skills to deal with vertigo
3. Encourage patient to discuss anxieties and explore concerns about vertigo attacks.	3. Promotes awareness and understanding of relationship between anxiety level and behavior.	• Feels less tension, apprehension, and uncertainty
4. Educate patient about stress management techniques or make appropriate referral.	4. Improved stress management can reduce the frequency and severity of some vertiginous attacks.	• Uses stress management techniques when needed
5. Provide comfort measures, and avoid stress-producing activities.	5. Stressful situations may exacerbate symptoms of the condition.	• Avoids upsetting encounters
6. Instruct patient in aspects of treatment regimen.	6. Patient knowledge helps to decrease anxiety.	• Repeats instructions given and verbalizes understanding of treatments

NURSING DIAGNOSIS: Risk for trauma related to impaired balance
GOAL: Reduces the risk of trauma by adapting the home environment and by using assistive devices as necessary

Nursing Interventions	Rationale	Expected Outcomes
1. Assess for balance disturbance and/or vertigo by taking history and by examination for nystagmus, positive Romberg, and inability to perform tandem Romberg.	1. Peripheral vestibular disorders cause these signs and symptoms.	• Has adapted home environment or uses rehabilitative devices to reduce risk of falling
2. Assist with ambulation when indicated.	2. Abnormal gait can predispose patient to unsteadiness and falls.	• Ambulates with needed assistance
3. Assess for visual acuity and proprioceptive deficits.	3. Balance depends on visual, vestibular, and proprioceptive systems.	• Visual and proprioceptive risks identified
4. Encourage increased activity level with or without use of assistive devices.	4. Increased activity may help retrain balance system.	• Activity level increased
5. Help identify hazards in home environment.	5. Adaptation of home environment can reduce risk of falls during rehabilitative process.	• Home environment free of hazards

NURSING DIAGNOSIS: Self-care deficit: feeding, bathing/hygiene, dressing/grooming, toileting, related to labyrinth dysfunction and episodes of vertigo
GOAL: Able to care for self

Nursing Interventions	Rationale	Expected Outcomes
1. Administer, or educate about administration of, antiemetic and other prescribed medications to relieve nausea and vomiting associated with vertigo.	1. Antiemetic and sedative-type medications depress stimuli in the cerebellum.	• Carries out necessary functions during symptom-free periods and takes medications to relieve nausea, vomiting, or vertigo
2. Encourage patient to perform self-care when free of vertigo.	2. Spacing activities is important because episodes of vertigo vary in occurrence.	• Carries out daily activities
3. Review diet with patient and caregivers. Offer fluids as necessary.	3. Sodium restriction helps improve an inner ear fluid imbalance in some patients, thereby decreasing vertigo. Fluids help prevent dehydration.	• Accepts dietary plan and reports its effectiveness • Drinks fluids in sufficient amounts

Chart 64-9

PLAN OF NURSING CARE (Continued)

Care of the Patient with Vertigo

NURSING DIAGNOSIS: Powerlessness related to illness regimen and being helpless in certain situations due to vertigo/balance disturbance

GOAL: Experiences increased sense of control over life and activities despite vertigo/balance disturbance

Nursing Interventions	Rationale	Expected Outcomes
1. Assess patient's needs, values, attitudes, and readiness to initiate activities. 2. Provide opportunities for patient to express feelings about self and illness. 3. Help patient identify previous coping behaviors that were successful.	1. Involving patient in planning activities and care enhances potential for mastery. 2. Expressing feelings increases understanding of individual coping styles and defense mechanisms. 3. Awareness increases understanding of stressors that trigger feeling of powerlessness. Awareness of past successes enhances self-confidence.	• Does not restrict activities unnecessarily due to vertigo • Verbalizes positive feelings about own ability to achieve a sense of power and control • Identifies previous successful coping behaviors

Chart 64-10 Selected Ototoxic Substances

- **Aminoglycoside antibiotic agents:** amikacin, gentamicin, kanamycin, netilmicin, neomycin, streptomycin, tobramycin
- **Anti-inflammatory agents:** salicylates (aspirin), indomethacin
- **Antimalarial agents:** quinine, chloroquine
- **Chemicals:** alcohol, arsenic
- **Chemotherapeutic (antineoplastic) agents:** cisplatin, nitrogen mustard, carboplatin
- **Loop diuretic agents:** ethacrynic acid, furosemide, acetazolamide
- **Metals:** gold, mercury, lead
- **Other antibiotic agents:** erythromycin, minocycline, polymyxin B, vancomycin

Adapted from Mudd, P. (2016). Ototoxicity. Medscape. Retrieved on 9/12/2016 at: emedicine.medscape.com/article/857679-overview

Ototoxicity

A variety of medications may have adverse effects on the cochlea, vestibular apparatus, or cranial nerve VIII. All but a few, such as aspirin and quinine, cause irreversible hearing loss. Aspirin toxicity can produce bilateral tinnitus. IV medications, especially the aminoglycosides, are a common cause of ototoxicity, because they destroy the hair cells in the organ of Corti (see Chart 64-10). Antineoplastic agents also cause hair cell death in the cochlea, which can lead to hearing loss (Mudd, 2016). These medications can be found in the body several months later; side effects are dose dependent, with higher doses causing increased ototoxicity. Therefore, hearing loss may occur at any time, even several months after the last dose of the medication was given.

To prevent loss of hearing or balance, patients receiving potentially ototoxic medications should be counseled about their side effects (Lewis, McMillan, Hutter, et al., 2014) (see Chart 64-11). These medications should be used with

Chart 64-11

NURSING RESEARCH PROFILE

Does Interferon Beta-1a Contribute to Hearing Loss in Patients with Multiple Sclerosis (MS)?

Lewis, M. S., McMillan, G. P., Hutter, M., et al. (2014). Does Interferon Beta-1a impact pure-tone hearing sensitivity among individuals with multiple sclerosis? *Journal of Neuroscience Nursing, 46*(6), 352–359.

Purpose

Previous studies reported that interferon medications, commonly used to treat multiple sclerosis (MS), might contribute to hearing loss. The purpose of this study was to assess participants with MS taking intramuscular interferon beta-1a and who have significantly poorer hearing compared to those not currently using any disease-modifying therapies.

Design

The design of this study was a secondary analysis of data that had been collected during two other large studies that evaluated hearing in those with MS. A linear mixed model was fit to the hearing thresholds of participants. The model included interferon use, MS subtype, gender, age, test frequency, MS duration in years and a disability score.

Findings

With all participants included (*N* = 52), there was insufficient evidence to infer that intramuscular interferon-beta 1a was not ototoxic compared to nonuse of a disease-modifying therapy at all frequencies at which participants had their hearing tested. After removing two participants who were outliers, the results indicated that there was support for no ototoxic effect of intramuscular interferon beta-1a at test frequencies from 250 to 6000 Hz. There was insufficient evidence, however, to rule out an ototoxic effect at 8000 Hz.

Nursing Implications

More research is needed to evaluate the ototoxic effects of interferon on hearing in patients with MS. Nurses should be aware of the potential for ototoxicity with interferon use and remind patients with MS to have their hearing evaluated on a regular basis throughout the course of treatment.

caution in patients who are at high risk for complications, such as children, older adults, patients who are pregnant, patients with kidney or liver problems, and patients with current hearing disorders. Blood levels of the medications should be monitored, and patients receiving long-term IV antibiotics should be monitored with an audiogram twice each week during therapy.

Acoustic Neuroma

Acoustic neuromas, also referred to as vestibular schwannomas, are slow-growing, benign tumors of cranial nerve VIII, usually arising from the Schwan cells of the vestibular portion of the nerve. Most acoustic tumors arise within the internal auditory canal and extend into the cerebellopontine angle to press on the brain stem, possibly destroying the vestibular nerve (Bader, Littlejohns, & Olson, 2016). Most acoustic neuromas are unilateral, except in von Recklinghausen disease (neurofibromatosis type 2), in which bilateral tumors occur (Grossman & Porth, 2014).

Acoustic neuromas develop in 1 of every 100,000 people per year. These neuromas account for 6% of all intracranial tumors and seem to occur with equal frequency in men and women at any age, although most occur during middle age (Hio, Kitahara, Uno, et al., 2013).

Assessment and Diagnostic Findings

The most common assessment findings of patients with acoustic neuromas are unilateral tinnitus and hearing loss with or without vertigo or balance disturbance. It is important to identify asymmetry in audiovestibular test results so that further workup can be performed to rule out an acoustic neuroma. Although conflicting data exist, the only known risk factor for acoustic neuroma is cell phone usage (Park, Vernick, & Ramakrishna, 2015). An MRI scan with a contrast agent (i.e., gadolinium or gadopentetate [Magnevist]) is the imaging study of choice. If the patient is claustrophobic or cannot undergo an MRI scan for other reasons, or if the scan is unavailable, a CT scan with contrast dye is performed. However, MRI is more sensitive than CT in delineating a small tumor.

Management

Conservative treatment is recommended for patients with tumors less than 1.5 cm and in those who are older. In addition, routine monitoring is recommended for these patients. For patients who are at low risk, surgical removal of the acoustic tumor is the treatment of choice because these tumors do not respond well to radiation or chemotherapy. Because treatment of acoustic tumors crosses several specialties, the interdisciplinary treatment approach involves a neurologist and a neurosurgeon. The objective of the surgery is to remove the tumor while preserving facial nerve function. Most acoustic tumors have damaged the cochlear portion of cranial nerve VIII, and hearing is impaired. In these patients, the surgery is performed using a translabyrinthine approach, and the hearing mechanism is destroyed. If hearing is still good before surgery, a suboccipital or middle cranial fossa approach to removing the tumor may be used. This procedure exposes the lateral third of the internal auditory canal and preserves hearing (Park et al., 2015).

Potential complications of surgery include facial nerve paralysis, cerebrospinal fluid leakage, meningitis, and cerebral edema. Death from acoustic neuroma surgery is rare (Park et al., 2015).

AURAL REHABILITATION

If hearing loss is permanent or cannot be treated by medical or surgical means or if the patient elects not to undergo surgery, aural rehabilitation may be beneficial. The purpose of aural rehabilitation is to maximize the communication skills of the person with hearing impairment. Aural rehabilitation includes auditory training, speech reading, speech training, and the use of hearing aids and hearing guide dogs.

Auditory training emphasizes listening skills, so the person who is hearing impaired concentrates on the speaker. Speech reading (also known as lip reading) can help fill the gaps left by missed or misheard words. The goals of speech training are to conserve, develop, and prevent deterioration of current communication skills.

It is important to identify the type of hearing impairment a person has so that rehabilitative efforts can be directed at their particular need. Surgical correction may be all that is necessary to treat and improve a conductive hearing loss by eliminating the cause of the hearing loss. With advances in hearing aid technology, amplification for patients with sensorineural hearing loss is more helpful than ever.

Hearing Aids

A hearing aid is a device through which speech and environmental sounds are received by a microphone, converted to electrical signals, amplified, and reconverted to acoustic signals. Many aids available for sensorineural hearing loss depress the low frequencies, or tones, and enhance hearing for the high frequencies. A general guideline for assessing the patient's need for a hearing aid is a hearing loss exceeding 30 dB in the range of 500 to 2000 Hz in the better-hearing ear.

A hearing aid makes sounds louder, but it does not improve a patient's ability to discriminate words or understand speech. People who have low discrimination scores (i.e., 20%) on audiograms may derive little benefit from a hearing aid. Hearing aids amplify all sounds, including background noise, which may be particularly disturbing to the first-time wearer. Chart 64-12 identifies additional problems associated with hearing aid use. Computerized hearing aids are available to compensate for background noise or allow amplification at certain programmed frequencies rather than at all frequencies. Occasionally, depending on the type of hearing loss, binaural aids (i.e., one for each ear) may be indicated. Chart 64-13 provides tips for hearing aid care.

A hearing aid should be fitted according to the patient's needs (e.g., type of hearing loss, manual dexterity, and preferences), rather than the brand name, by a certified audiologist licensed to dispense hearing aids. Many states have consumer protection laws that allow the hearing aid to be returned after a trial use if the patient is not completely satisfied. In addition, to protect the health and safety of people with hearing impairments, the U.S. Food and Drug Administration (FDA) has established certain regulations. A medical evaluation of

Chart 64-12	Hearing Aid Problems

Whistling Noise

- Loose ear mold
- Improperly made
- Improperly worn
- Worn out

Improper Aid Selection

- Too much power required in aid, with inadequate separation between microphone and receiver
- Open mold used inappropriately
- Inadequate amplification
- Dead batteries
- Cerumen in ear
- Cerumen or other material in mold
- Wires or tubing disconnected from aid
- Aid turned off or volume too low
- Improper mold
- Improper aid for degree of loss

Pain From Mold

- Improperly fitted mold
- Ear skin or cartilage infection
- Middle ear infection
- Ear tumor
- Unrelated conditions of the temporomandibular joint, throat, or larynx

Chart 64-13	**PATIENT EDUCATION** Tips for Hearing Aid Care

The nurse instructs the patient how to clean a hearing aid, check for malfunctions, and recognize complications:

Cleaning

- Keep in mind that the ear mold is the only part of the hearing aid that may be washed frequently.
- Wash the ear mold daily with soap and water.
- Allow the ear mold to dry completely before it is snapped into the receiver.
- Clean the cannula with a small pipe cleaner–like device.
- Note that properly caring for the ear device and keeping the ear canal clean and dry can prevent complications.

Checking for Malfunctions

- Be aware that inadequate amplification, a whistling noise, or pain from the mold can occur when a hearing aid is not functioning properly.
- Check for malfunctions:
  - Is the switch on properly?
  - Are the batteries charged and positioned correctly?
  - Is the ear mold clogged with cerumen? Ear wax can be easily removed with pin, pipe cleaner, or wax loop.
- Notify the hearing aid dealer if the hearing aid is still not working properly.
- Keep in mind that if the unit requires extended time for repair, the dealer may lend you a hearing aid until the repair can be accomplished.

Recognizing Complications

- Understand that common medical complications include external otitis media and pressure ulcers in the external auditory canal. Signs and symptoms of these infections include painful ear, especially when the external ear is touched; canal swelling; redness; difficulty hearing; pain radiating to the jaw area; and fever.
- Notify your health care provider for evaluation if any of these symptoms are present. You may need medication to treat infection, pain, or both.

the impairment by a physician must be obtained within 6 months before the purchase of a hearing aid. However, the written statement from a physician may be waived if the patient (a fully informed adult 18 years or older) signs a document to this effect. Health care professionals who dispense hearing aids are required to refer prospective users to a physician if any of the following otologic conditions are evident:

- Visible congenital or traumatic deformity of the ear
- Active drainage from the ear within the previous 90 days
- Sudden or rapidly progressive hearing loss within the previous 90 days
- Complaints of dizziness or tinnitus
- Unilateral hearing loss that has occurred suddenly or within the previous 90 days
- Audiometric air–bone gap of 15 dB or more at 500, 1000, and 2000 Hz
- Significant accumulation of cerumen or a foreign body in the external auditory canal
- Pain or discomfort in the ear

A user instruction brochure is provided with every hearing aid device. In this brochure, the following information is presented:

- Notification that good health practice requires a medical evaluation before purchasing a hearing aid
- Notification that any of the otologic conditions listed previously should be investigated by a physician before purchase of a hearing aid
- Instructions for proper use, maintenance, and care of the hearing aid, as well as instructions for replacing or recharging the batteries
- Repair service information
- Description of avoidable conditions that could damage the hearing aid
- List of any known side effects that may warrant physician consultation (e.g., skin irritation, accelerated cerumen accumulation)

The evolution in technology has led to the availability of many smaller and more effective devices as well as different options and features of hearing aids (FDA, 2014) (see Chart 64-14). The majority of hearing aids sold today are behind-the-ear, in-the-ear, or in-the-canal types (see Table 64-4). One model is the Lyric, which is placed in the ear canal just 4 mm from the tympanic membrane. Its volume is controlled by a magnet, and when its batteries no longer function (1 to 4 months), a physician can remove it with the magnet and reinsert a new device. This device does not have many of the problems (e.g., feedback noise, overamplification of background noise) associated with other hearing aids, and it does not involve the expense and uncertainty of surgical procedures. However, it is not an option for a person whose ear canal is too narrow to accommodate it.

Options and Features of Hearing Aids to Consider

- *T-Coil:* May improve hearing on the telephone by switching the settings from normal to telephone setting. This feature also assists in amplifying voices when the patient is in larger areas, such as theaters, auditoriums, and gymnasiums. Background noise may be toned down to adequately hear close conversation.
- *Directional Microphone:* Useful in environments with a lot of background noise and activity. The microphone may be directed toward the speaker and amplifies conversation while diminishing background noise.
- *Direct Audio Input:* Directly plugs into another device, such as a computer, television, or stereo, that is attached with an extension cord.
- *Feedback Suppression:* Suppresses whistling feedback noise.

Adapted from U.S. Food and Drug Administration. (2014). Medical devices: Types of hearing aids. Retrieved on 8/19/2016 at: www.fda.gov/MedicalDevices/ProductsandMedicalProcedures/HomeHealthandConsumer/ConsumerProducts/HearingAids/ucm181470.htm

Implanted Hearing Devices

There are several types of implanted hearing devices, ranging from implantable to semi-implantable devices (FDA, 2015).

Bone conduction devices, which transmit sound through the skull to the inner ear, are used in patients with a conductive hearing loss if a hearing aid is contraindicated (e.g., those with chronic infection). The device is implanted postauricularly under the skin into the skull, and an external device—worn above the ear, not in the canal—transmits the sound through the skin. There are two types of implantable hearing aids. The bone-anchored hearing aid (BAHA) is implanted behind the ear in the mastoid area. The middle ear implantation (MEI) is implanted in the middle ear cavity. The BAHA is used for conductive or mixed hearing loss, whereas the MEI is used for sensorineural hearing loss (FDA, 2015).

The implantable middle ear hearing device (IMEHD) comes in two styles: piezoelectric and electromagnetic, which are partially or totally implanted. Patients must be 18 years or older, must be diagnosed with mild to severe sensorineural loss, and must have tried other conventional devices but achieved poor results to be considered candidates for this type of device. The implantable device has several advantages—for example, it may eliminate feedback, achieve good cosmetic results, and allow the patient to perform most preferred leisure activities (e.g., dancing, swimming). Disadvantages are that this device is expensive, necessitates surgery, requires periodic recharging of batteries, and has unpredictable power output (FDA, 2015).

The FDA has also approved the semi-implantable Vibrant Soundbridge (electromagnetic) and the total implantable Envoy Esteem (piezoelectric) devices. The Vibrant Soundbridge has an external device attached to the postauricular bone that transmits sound to the magnet in the middle ear that is attached to the long process of the incus. The magnet surrounds the long axis of the stapes, which in turn vibrates and sound is heard. The Envoy Esteem works similarly to the natural ear. The piezoelectric transducer is located at the head of the incus, which sends a signal that is amplified, filtered, and then converted back to a vibration signal. This vibration is delivered by the driver (piezoelectric transducer) and attached to the stapes capitulum; then, via the stapes bone, the inner ear receives the signal and is converted into a nerve impulse and translated into sound by the brain. The incus is removed prior to insertion of this device to prevent feedback from the sensor. It is estimated that sound is amplified up to 110 dB with this device (Shohet & Myers, 2011).

A cochlear implant is an auditory prosthesis used for people with profound sensorineural hearing loss bilaterally who do not benefit from conventional hearing aids. The cochlear implant directly stimulates the auditory nerve and has made it possible for people who are severely hearing impaired or who are deaf to hear sound (NIDCD, 2016). The hearing loss may be congenital or acquired. An implant does not restore normal hearing; rather, it helps the person detect medium to

TABLE 64-4 **Hearing Aids**

Site (Range of Hearing Loss)	Advantages	Disadvantages
Body, usually on the trunk (mild–profound)	Separation of receiver and microphone prevents acoustic feedback, allowing high amplification; generally used in a school setting	Bulky; requires long wire, which may be cosmetically displeasing; some loss of high-frequency response
Behind the ear (mild–profound)	Economical; powerful, with no long wires; easily used by children—adapts easily as the child grows, with only the ear mold needing replacement	Large size
In the ear (mild–moderately severe)	One-piece custom fit to contour of ear; no tubes or cords; miniature microphone located in the ear, which is a more natural placement; more cosmetically appealing due to easy concealment	Smaller size limits output; patients who have arthritis or cannot perform tasks requiring good manual dexterity may have difficulty with the small size of aid and/or battery; can require more repair than the behind-the-ear aid.
In the canal (mild–moderately severe)	Same as in-the-ear aids; less visible, so more cosmetically pleasing	Even smaller than in-the-ear aids; requires good manual dexterity and good vision

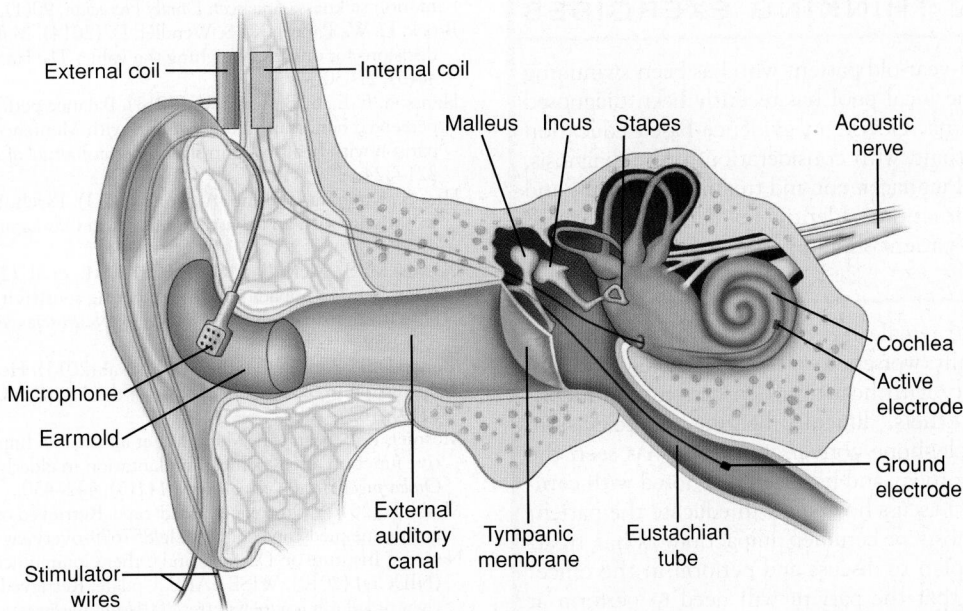

Figure 64-7 • The cochlear implant. The internal coil has a stranded electrode lead. The electrode is inserted through the round window into the scala tympani of the cochlea. The external coil (the transmitter) is held in alignment with the internal coil (the receiver) by a magnet. The microphone receives the sound. The stimulator wire receives the signal after it has been filtered, adjusted, and modified so that the sound is at a comfortable level for the patient. Sound is passed by the external transmitter to the inner coil receiver by magnetic conduction and is then carried by the electrode to the cochlea.

loud environmental sounds and conversation. The implant provides stimulation directly to the auditory nerve, bypassing the nonfunctioning hair cells of the inner ear. The microphone and signal processor, worn outside the body, transmit electrical stimuli to the implanted electrodes. The electrical signals stimulate the auditory nerve fibers and then the brain, where they are interpreted.

Worldwide, more than 324,200 people have received cochlear implants. In the United States, more than 42,600 adults and 28,000 children have received cochlear implants (NIDCD, 2014). Studies report that older adult patients with cochlear implants experience improved understanding of speech and better cognition. Patients with cochlear implants were also noted to have more social interactions with others and improved quality of life. Research has reported that hearing improvement with a cochlear implant delays the occurrence as well as the progression of dementia (Mosnier, Bebear, Marx, et al., 2015). Candidates for a cochlear implant, who are usually at least 1 year of age, are selected after careful screening by otologic history, physical examination, audiologic testing, x-rays, and psychological testing. Criteria for choosing adults who may benefit from a cochlear implant include:

- Profound sensorineural hearing loss in both ears
- Inability to hear and recognize speech well with hearing aids
- No medical contraindication to a cochlear implant or general anesthesia
- Indications that being able to hear would enhance the patient's life

The surgery involves implanting a small receiver in the temporal bone through a postauricular incision and placing electrodes into the inner ear (see Fig. 64-7). The microphone and transmitter are worn on an external unit. The patient undergoes extensive cochlear rehabilitation with the multidisciplinary team, which includes an audiologist and speech pathologist. Several months may be needed to learn to interpret the sounds heard. Children and adults who lost their hearing before they learned to speak take much longer to acquire speech. There are wide variations of success with cochlear implants, and there is also controversy about their use, especially among the deaf community. Patients who have had a cochlear implant are cautioned that an MRI scan will inactivate the implant; MRI should be used only when there is no other diagnostic option.

Hearing Guide Dogs

Specially trained dogs (service dogs) are available to assist the person with a hearing loss. People who live alone are eligible to apply for a dog trained by International Hearing Dog, Inc. The dog reacts to the sound of a telephone, a doorbell, an alarm clock, a baby's cry, a knock at the door, a smoke alarm, or an intruder. The dog alerts its master by physical contact; the dog then runs to the source of the noise. In public, the dog positions itself between the person with hearing impairment and any potential hazard that the person cannot hear, such as an oncoming vehicle or a loud, hostile person. A certified hearing guide dog is legally permitted access to public transportation, public eating places, and stores, including food markets.

CRITICAL THINKING EXERCISES

1 `ebp` A 45-year-old patient who has been swimming frequently in the local pool has recently been diagnosed with otitis externa. Devise an evidence-based education plan for this patient, with consideration to the diagnosis, possible medical management and treatment options, and home care instructions. Identify evidence-based techniques that the patient should perform to prevent future infections.

2 A 91-year-old female has complained of hearing loss that has gradually worsened over the past few months. She has difficulty with hearing when carrying on a conversation with others, difficulty hearing the television, and having a telephone conversation. She has seen the primary provider today and has been diagnosed with cerumen impaction. Discuss how you will educate the patient about the diagnosis of cerumen impaction. What treatments will you plan to discuss and perform in the office? List treatments that the patient will need to perform at home. Should she expect to regain her previous hearing ability? What measures can she use to prevent cerumen impaction in the future?

3 `pq` You are providing home care for a 55-year-old patient with hypertension, diabetes, and a new diagnosis of vertigo. Identify the priorities, approach, and techniques you would use to provide nursing care to this patient. How would your priorities, approach, and techniques change if the patient was 85 years old and lived alone?

REFERENCES

*Asterisk indicates nursing research.

Books

Bader, M., Littlejohns, L. R., & Olson, D. (2016). *AANN core curriculum for neuroscience nursing* (6th ed.). Chicago, IL: American Association of Neuroscience Nurses.
Cash, J. C., & Glass, C. A. (2014). *Family practice guidelines*. New York: New York: Springer Publishing.
Eliopoulos, C. (2018). *Gerontological nursing* (9th ed.). Philadelphia, PA: Lippincott Williams & Wilkins.
Fischbach, F., & Dunning, M. B. (2015). *A manual of laboratory and diagnostic tests* (9th ed.). Philadelphia, PA: Lippincott Williams & Wilkins.
Grossman, S. C., & Porth, C. M. (2014). *Pathophysiology: Concepts of altered health states* (9th ed.). Philadelphia, PA: Lippincott Williams & Wilkins.
Weber, J., & Kelley, J. (2014). *Health assessment in nursing* (5th ed.). Philadelphia, PA: Lippincott Williams & Wilkins.

Journals and Electronic Documents

American Academy of Otolaryngology- Head and Neck Surgery (2014). Position Statement: Posturography. Retrieved on 8/19/2016 at: www.entnet.org/content/position-statement-posturography.
Antonio, S. (2016). Genetic sensorineural hearing loss clinical presentation. Retrieved on 8/19/2016 at: emedicine.medscape.com/article/855875-clinical#b5.
Bhattacharyya, N., & Meyers, A. D. (2015). Auditory brainstem response auditometry. Retrieved on 8/19/2016 at: emedicine.medscape.com/article/836277-overview#a6.

Brainard, A., & Gresham, C. (2014). Prevention and treatment of motion sickness. *American Family Physician, 90*(1), 41–46.
Brock, D. W., Park, J. K., & Wendler, D. (2014). Making treatment decisions for oneself: Weighing the value. *The Hastings Center Report, 46*(3), 22–30.
Hansson, E. E., & Brattmo, M. (2013). Balance performance and self-perceived handicap among patients with Meniere's disease- A comparison with healthy controls. *European Journal of Physiotherapy, 15*(4), 221–224.
Hio, S., Kitahara, T., Uno, A., et al. (2013). Psychological condition in patients with an acoustic tumor. *Acta Oto-Layngologica, 133*(1), 42–46.
*Lewis, M. S., McMillan, G. P., Hutter, M., et al. (2014). Does Interferon Beta-1a impact pure-tone hearing sensitivity among individuals with multiple sclerosis? *Journal of Neuroscience Nursing, 46*(6), 352–359.
Mener, D. J., Betz, J., Genther, D. J., et al.(2013). Hearing loss and depression in older adults. *Journal of the American Geriatrics Society, 61*(9), 1627–1629.
Mosnier, I., Bebear, J. P., Marx, M., et al. (2015). Improvement of cognitive function after cochlear implantation in elderly patients. *JAMA Otolaryngol Head Neck Surgery, 141*(5), 442–450.
Mudd, P. (2016). Ototoxicity. Medscape. Retrieved on 9/12/2016 at: emedicine.medscape.com/article/857679-overview
National Institute on Deafness and Other Communication Disorders (NIDCD) (2010). WISE EARS. Update. Retrieved on 8/23/2016 at: www.nidcd.nih.gov/newsletter/2001/summer/wise-ears-update
National Institute on Deafness and Other Communication Disorders (NIDCD). (2014). Cochlear implants. Retrieved on 6/12/2016 at: www.nidcd.nih.gov/about/strategic-plan/2012-2016/2012-2016-nidcd-strategic-plan
National Institute on Deafness and Other Communication Disorders (NIDCD). (2015a). *NIDCD fact sheet:* Balance disorders. Retrieved on 6/12/2012 at: www.nidcd.nih.gov/staticresources/health/balance-disorders.
National Institute on Deafness and Other Communication Disorders (NIDCD). (2015b). Ménière's disease. Retrieved on 6/12/2012 at: www.nidcd.nih.gov//health/balance/meniere.html
National Institute on Deafness and Other Communication Disorders (NIDCD). (2015c). Tinnitus. Retrieved on 6/12/2012 at: www.nidcd.nih.gov.
National Institute on Deafness and Other Communication Disorders (NIDCD) (2016). Strategic plan: FY 2012–2016. Retrieved on 9/12/2016 at: www.nidcd.nih.gov/staticresources/about/plans/strategic/FY2009–2011NIDCDStrategicPlan.pdf
Park, J. K., Vernick, D. M., & Ramakrishna, N. (2015). Vestibular schwannoma (acoustic neuroma). UpToDate. Retrieved on 8/25/2016 at: www.uptodate.com/contents/search?search = Vestibular+schwannoma+%28acoustic+neuroma% 29.+&x = 16&y = 8
Shohet, J., & Myers, A. (2011). Implantable hearing devices. Medscape. Retrieved on 9/12/2016 at: emedicine.medscape.com/article/860444-overview
U.S. Department of Education. (2012). Department of education issues ADA amendment act dear colleague letter to provide guidance under amended legal standards. Retrieved on 6/12/2016 at: www.ed.gov/news/press-releases/department-education-issues-ada-amendments-act-dear-colleague-letter-provide-gui
U.S. Department of Health and Human Services (HHS). (2010). Healthy People 2020. Retrieved on 9/12/2016 at: www.healthypeople.gov/2020/topics-objectives/topic/hearing-and-other-sensory-or-communication-disorders
U.S. Department of Health & Human Services (HHS). (2016). National Institute on Deafness & Other Communication Disorders: Statistics About Hearing. Retrieved on 8/23/2016 at: www.nidcd.nih.gov/health/statistics/quick-statistics-hearing.
U.S. Food and Drug Administration. (2014). Medical devices: Types of hearing aids. Retrieved on 8/19/2016 at: www.fda.gov/MedicalDevices/ProductsandMedicalProcedures/HomeHealthandConsumer/ConsumerProducts/HearingAids/ucm181470.htm
U.S. Food and Drug Administration. (2015). Medical devices: Other products and devices to improve hearing. Retrieved on 8/19/2016 at: www.fda.gov/MedicalDevices/ProductsandMedicalProcedures/HomeHealthandConsumer/ConsumerProducts/HearingAids/ucm181482.htm

Resources

Acoustic Neuroma Association (ANA), www.anausa.org

Alexander Graham Bell Association for the Deaf and Hard of Hearing, www.agbell.org

American Academy of Audiology, www.audiology.org

American Academy of Facial Plastic and Reconstructive Surgery, www.aafprs.org

American Academy of Otolaryngology–Head and Neck Surgery, www.entnet.org

American Board of Facial Plastic and Reconstructive Surgery, www.abfprs.org

American Speech-Language-Hearing Association, www.asha.org

American Tinnitus Association (ATA), www.ata.org

International Hearing Dog, Inc., www.ihdi.org

National Institute on Deafness and Other Communication Disorders (NIDCD), National Institutes of Health, www.nidcd.nih.gov

Society of Otorhinolaryngology and Head-Neck Nurses, www.sohnnurse.com

Vestibular Disorders Association, www.vestibular.org

UNIT
16

Neurologic Function

Case Study

EVALUATING INCREASED HYPERTENSION IN A NEUROLOGY CLINIC

A nurse who works in a neurology clinic notes that most of the patients who are returning for care after having a stroke also have hypertension, and thus are at increased risk for another stroke. Although these patients received education while in acute care about strategies to control their hypertension, the nurse notes that this education does not seem to have been effective. The nurse wonders if a different type of intervention aimed at decreasing hypertension and the risk for another stroke should be considered.

QSEN Competency Focus: Quality Improvement (QI)

The complexities inherent in today's health care system challenges nurses to demonstrate integration of specific inter-disciplinary core competencies. These competencies are aimed at ensuring the delivery of safe, quality patient care (Institute of Medicine, 2003). The Quality and Safety Education for Nurses project (QSEN, 2017; Cronenwett, Sherwood, Barnsteiner, et al., 2007) provides a framework for the knowledge, skills, and attitudes (KSA) required for nurses to demonstrate competency in these key areas, which include *patient-centered care, interdisciplinary teamwork and collaboration, evidence-based practice, quality improvement, safety,* and *informatics.*

Quality Improvement Definition: Use data to monitor the outcomes of care processes and use improvement methods to design and test changes to continuously improve the quality and safety of health care systems.

SELECTED PRE-LICENSURE KSAs	APPLICATION AND REFLECTION
Knowledge	
Explain the importance of variation and measurement in assessing quality of care.	How can the nurse verify the observations made about increased hypertension rates among patients poststroke? Identify the sources of data that could be accessed to demonstrate the need for a change in the processes of care.
Skills	
Use quality measures to understand performance	Specify the main objective that the nurse in the neurology clinic hopes to achieve with this population of patients who have had strokes. Specify measurable, time-oriented expected outcomes. Might there be an opportunity for the nurse to do a pilot test of change in this clinic? If so, how would the nurse go about designing this type of project? Who else from the neurology clinic team might need to be involved in this type of project?
Attitudes	
Value measurement and its role in good patient care.	Reflect upon the process you might follow if you were the nurse in this clinic. How would you analyze the rates of hypertension and recurrent stroke? How would you approach the patients? Would you mobilize other members of the clinic team to find a root cause for this phenomenon? Think about how mobilizing other team members could result in measurable improvements in quality of life for this population of patients.

Cronenwett, L., Sherwood, G., Barnsteiner, J., et al. (2007). Quality and safety education for nurses. *Nursing Outlook, 55*(3), 122–131.

Institute of Medicine. (2003). *Health professions education: A bridge to quality.* Washington, DC: National Academies Press.

QSEN Institute, (2017). QSEN competencies: Definitions and pre-licensure KSAs. Retrieved on 3/1/2017 at: www.qsen.org/competencies/pre-licensure-ksas

Assessment of Neurologic Function

LEARNING OBJECTIVES

On completion of this chapter, the learner will be able to:

1 Describe the structures and functions of the central and peripheral nervous systems.
2 Differentiate between pathologic changes that affect motor control and those that affect sensory pathways.
3 Compare and contrast the functioning of the sympathetic and parasympathetic nervous systems.
4 Explain the significance of physical assessment to the diagnosis of neurologic dysfunction.
5 Identify changes in neurologic function associated with aging and their impact on neurologic assessment findings.
6 Discuss diagnostic tests used for assessment of suspected neurologic disorders and the related nursing implications.

GLOSSARY

agnosia: loss of ability to recognize objects through a particular sensory system; may be visual, auditory, or tactile
ataxia: inability to coordinate muscle movements, resulting in difficulty in walking, talking, and performing self-care activities
autonomic nervous system: division of the nervous system that regulates the involuntary body functions
axon: portion of the neuron that conducts impulses away from the cell body
Babinski reflex (sign): a reflex action of the toes; in adults is indicative of abnormalities in the motor control pathways leading from the cerebral cortex
clonus: abnormal movement marked by alternating contraction and relaxation of a muscle occurring in rapid succession
delirium: an acute, confused state that begins with disorientation and if not recognized and treated early can progress to changes in level of consciousness, irreversible brain damage, and sometimes death
dendrite: portion of the neuron that conducts impulses toward the cell body

flaccidity: displaying lack of muscle tone; limp, floppy
parasympathetic nervous system: division of the autonomic nervous system active primarily during nonstressful conditions, controlling mostly visceral functions
position (postural) sense: awareness of position of parts of the body without looking at them; also referred to as proprioception
reflex: an automatic response to stimuli
rigidity: increase in muscle tone at rest characterized by increased resistance to passive stretch
Romberg test: test for cerebellar dysfunction that can be done with the patient seated or standing; inability to maintain position for 20 seconds is a positive test
spasticity: sustained increase in tension of a muscle when it is passively lengthened or stretched
sympathetic nervous system: division of the autonomic nervous system with predominantly excitatory responses; the "fight-or-flight" system
vertigo: illusion of movement in which the individual or the surroundings are sensed as moving

Nurses in many practice settings encounter patients with altered neurologic function. Disorders of the nervous system can occur at any time during the lifespan and can vary from mild, self-limiting symptoms to devastating, life-threatening disorders. Nurses must be skilled in the general assessment of neurologic function and be able to focus on specific areas as needed. Assessment requires knowledge of the anatomy and physiology of the nervous system and an understanding of the array of tests and procedures used to diagnose neurologic disorders. Knowledge about the nursing implications and interventions related to assessment and diagnostic testing is also essential.

Anatomic and Physiologic Overview

The nervous system consists of two major parts: the central nervous system (CNS), including the brain and spinal cord, and the peripheral nervous system, which includes the cranial nerves, spinal nerves, and autonomic nervous system. The function of the nervous system is to control motor, sensory, autonomic, cognitive, and behavioral activities. The brain itself contains more than 100 billion cells that link the motor and sensory pathways, monitor the body's processes, respond to the internal and external environment, maintain homeostasis, and direct all psychological, biologic, and physical

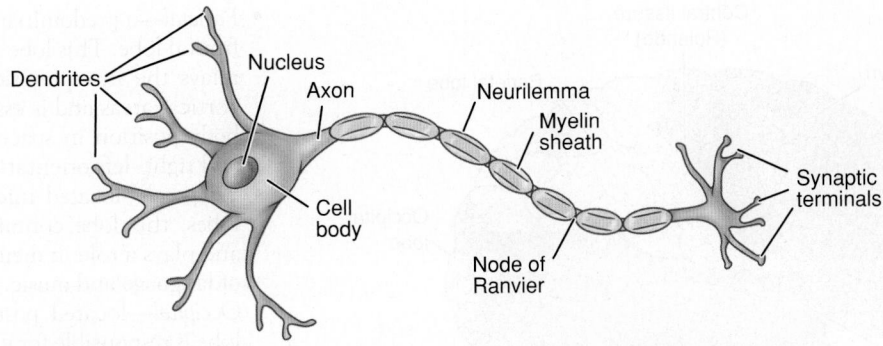

Figure 65-1 • Neuron.

Cells of the Nervous System

The basic functional unit of the brain is the neuron (see Fig. 65-1). It is composed of dendrites, a cell body, and an axon. The **dendrites** are branch-type structures for receiving electrochemical messages. The **axon** is a long projection that carries electrical impulses away from the cell body. Some axons have a myelinated sheath that increases speed of conduction. Nerve cell bodies occurring in clusters are called *ganglia* or *nuclei*. A cluster of cell bodies with the same function is called a *center* (e.g., the respiratory center). Neurons are supported, protected, and nourished by glial cells, which are 50 times greater in number than neurons (Hickey, 2014).

Neurotransmitters

Neurotransmitters communicate messages from one neuron to another or from a neuron to a target cell, such as muscle or endocrine cells. Neurotransmitters are manufactured and stored in synaptic vesicles. As an electrical action potential moves along the axon and reaches the nerve terminal, neurotransmitters are released into the synapse. The neurotransmitter is transported across the synapse, binding to receptors on the postsynaptic cell membrane. A neurotransmitter can either excite or inhibit activity of the target cell. Usually, multiple neurotransmitters are at work in the neural synapse. The source and action of major neurotransmitters are described in Table 65-1. Once released, enzymes either destroy the neurotransmitter or reabsorb it into the neuron for future use.

Many neurologic disorders are due, at least in part, to an imbalance in neurotransmitters. For example, Parkinson disease develops from decreased availability of dopamine, whereas acetylcholine binding to muscle cells is impaired in myasthenia gravis (Porth, 2014). All brain functions are modulated through neurotransmitter receptor site activity, including memory and other cognitive processes (Hickey, 2014).

Ongoing research is evaluating diagnostic tests that can detect abnormal levels of neurotransmitters in the brain. Positron emission tomography (PET), for example, can detect dopamine, serotonin, and acetylcholine. Single-photon emission computed tomography (SPECT), similar to PET, can detect changes in some neurotransmitters, such as dopamine in Parkinson disease (Fischbach & Dunning, 2015). Both PET and SPECT are discussed in more detail later in this chapter.

The Central Nervous System

The Brain

The brain accounts for approximately 2% of the total body weight; in an average young adult, the brain weighs

activity through complex chemical and electrical messages (Klein & Stewart-Amidei, 2012).

TABLE 65-1 Major Neurotransmitters

Neurotransmitter	Source	Action
Acetylcholine (major transmitter of the parasympathetic nervous system)	Many areas of the brain; autonomic nervous system	Usually excitatory; parasympathetic effects sometimes inhibitory (stimulation of heart by vagal nerve)
Serotonin	Brain stem, hypothalamus, dorsal horn of the spinal cord	Inhibitory; helps control mood and sleep, inhibits pain pathways
Dopamine	Substantia nigra and basal ganglia	Usually inhibitory; affects behavior (attention, emotions) and fine movement
Norepinephrine (major transmitter of the sympathetic nervous system)	Brain stem, hypothalamus, postganglionic neurons of the sympathetic nervous system	Usually excitatory; affects mood and overall activity
Gamma-aminobutyric acid	Spinal cord, cerebellum, basal ganglia, some cortical areas	Inhibitory
Enkephalin, endorphin	Nerve terminals in the spine, brain stem, thalamus and hypothalamus, pituitary gland	Excitatory; pleasurable sensation, inhibits pain transmission

Adapted from Porth, C. M. (2014). *Essentials of pathophysiology* (4th ed.). Philadelphia, PA: Lippincott Williams & Wilkins.

Figure 65-2 • View of the external surface of the brain showing lobes, cerebellum, and brain stem.

approximately 1400 g, whereas in an average older adult, the brain weighs approximately 1200 g (Hickey, 2014). The brain is divided into three major areas: the cerebrum, the brain stem, and the cerebellum. The cerebrum is composed of two hemispheres, the thalamus, the hypothalamus, and the basal ganglia. The brain stem includes the midbrain, pons, and medulla. The cerebellum is located under the cerebrum and behind the brain stem (see Fig. 65-2).

Cerebrum

The outside surface of the hemispheres has a wrinkled appearance that is the result of many folded layers or convolutions called *gyri*, which increase the surface area of the brain, accounting for the high level of activity carried out by such a small-appearing organ. Between each gyrus is a sulcus or fissure that serves as an anatomic division. In between the cerebral hemispheres is the great longitudinal fissure that separates the cerebrum into the right and left hemispheres. The two hemispheres are joined at the lower portion of the fissure by the corpus callosum. The external or outer portion of the hemispheres (the cerebral cortex) is made up of gray matter approximately 2 to 5 mm in depth; it contains billions of neuron cell bodies, giving it a gray appearance. White matter makes up the innermost layer and is composed of myelinated nerve fibers and neuroglia cells that form tracts or pathways connecting various parts of the brain with one another. These pathways also connect the cortex with lower portions of the brain and spinal cord. The cerebral hemispheres are divided into pairs of lobes as follows (see Fig. 65-2):

- *Frontal*—the largest lobe, located in the front of the brain. The major functions of this lobe are concentration, abstract thought, information storage or memory, and motor function. It contains Broca area, which is located in the left hemisphere and is critical for motor control of speech. The frontal lobe is also responsible in large part for a person's affect, judgment, personality, and inhibitions (Hickey, 2014).

- *Parietal*—a predominantly sensory lobe posterior to the frontal lobe. This lobe analyzes sensory information and relays the interpretation of this information to other cortical areas and is essential to a person's awareness of body position in space, size and shape discrimination, and right–left orientation (Hickey, 2014).

- *Temporal*—located inferior to the frontal and parietal lobes, this lobe contains the auditory receptive areas and plays a role in memory of sound and understanding of language and music.

- *Occipital*—located posterior to the parietal lobe, this lobe is responsible for visual interpretation and memory.

The corpus callosum (see Fig. 65-3), a thick collection of nerve fibers that connects the two hemispheres of the brain, is responsible for the transmission of information from one side of the brain to the other. Information transferred includes sensation, memory, and learned discrimination. Right-handed people and some left-handed people have cerebral dominance on the left side of the brain for verbal, linguistic, arithmetic, calculation, and analytic functions. The nondominant hemisphere is responsible for geometric, spatial, visual, pattern, and musical functions. Nuclei for cranial nerves I and II are also located in the cerebrum.

The thalami lie on either side of the third ventricle and act primarily as a relay station for all sensation except smell. All memory, sensation, and pain impulses pass through this section of the brain. The hypothalamus (see Fig. 65-3) is located anterior and inferior to the thalamus, and beneath and lateral to the third ventricle. The infundibulum of the hypothalamus connects it to the posterior pituitary gland. The hypothalamus plays an important role in the endocrine system because it regulates the pituitary secretion of hormones that influence metabolism, reproduction, stress response, and urine production. It works with the pituitary to maintain fluid balance through hormonal release and maintains temperature regulation by promoting vasoconstriction or vasodilatation. In addition, the hypothalamus is the site of the hunger center and is involved in appetite control. It contains centers that

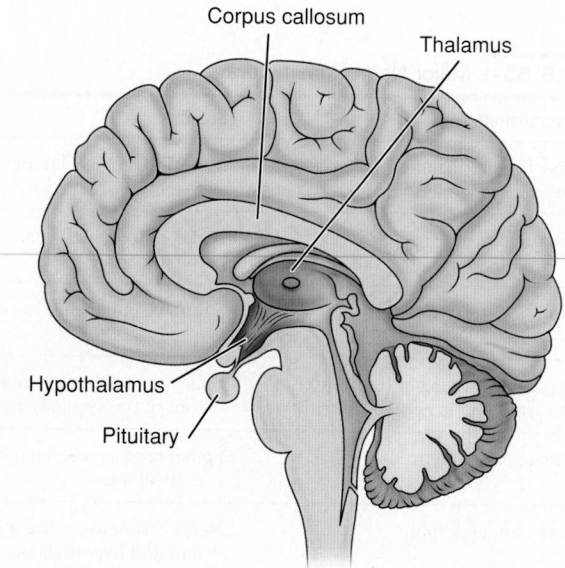

Figure 65-3 • Medial view of the brain.

regulate the sleep–wake cycle, blood pressure, aggressive and sexual behavior, and emotional responses (i.e., blushing, rage, depression, panic, and fear). The hypothalamus also controls and regulates the autonomic nervous system. The optic chiasm (the point at which the two optic tracts cross) and the mammillary bodies (involved in olfactory reflexes and emotional response to odors) are also found in this area.

The basal ganglia are masses of nuclei located deep in the cerebral hemispheres that are responsible for control of fine motor movements, including those of the hands and lower extremities.

Brain Stem

The brain stem consists of the midbrain, pons, and medulla oblongata (see Fig. 65-2). The midbrain connects the pons and the cerebellum with the cerebral hemispheres; it contains sensory and motor pathways and serves as the center for auditory and visual reflexes. Cranial nerves III and IV originate in the midbrain. The pons is situated in front of the cerebellum between the midbrain and the medulla and is a bridge between the two halves of the cerebellum, and between the medulla and the midbrain. Cranial nerves V through VIII originate in the pons. The pons also contains motor and sensory pathways. Portions of the pons help regulate respiration.

Motor fibers from the brain to the spinal cord and sensory fibers from the spinal cord to the brain are located in the medulla. Most of these fibers cross, or decussate, at this level. Cranial nerves IX through XII originate in the medulla. Reflex centers for respiration, blood pressure, heart rate, coughing, vomiting, swallowing, and sneezing are also located in the medulla. The reticular formation, responsible for arousal and the sleep–wake cycle, begins in the medulla and connects with numerous higher structures.

Cerebellum

The cerebellum is posterior to the midbrain and pons, and below the occipital lobe (see Fig. 65-2). The cerebellum integrates sensory information to provide smooth coordinated movement. It controls fine movement, balance, and **position (postural) sense** or proprioception (awareness of position of extremities without looking at them).

Structures Protecting the Brain

The brain is contained in the rigid skull, which protects it from injury. The major bones of the skull are the frontal, temporal, parietal, occipital, and sphenoid bones. These bones join at the suture lines (see Fig. 65-4) and form the base of the skull. Indentations in the skull base are known as fossae. The anterior fossa contains the frontal lobe, the middle fossa contains the temporal lobe, and the posterior fossa contains the cerebellum and brain stem.

The meninges (fibrous connective tissues that cover the brain and spinal cord) provide protection, support, and nourishment. The layers of the meninges are the dura mater, arachnoid, and pia mater (see Fig. 65-5):

- *Dura mater*—the outermost layer; covers the brain and the spinal cord. It is tough, thick, inelastic, fibrous, and gray. There are three major extensions of the dura: the falx cerebri, which folds between the two hemispheres; the tentorium, which folds between the occipital lobe and cerebellum to form a tough, membranous shelf; and

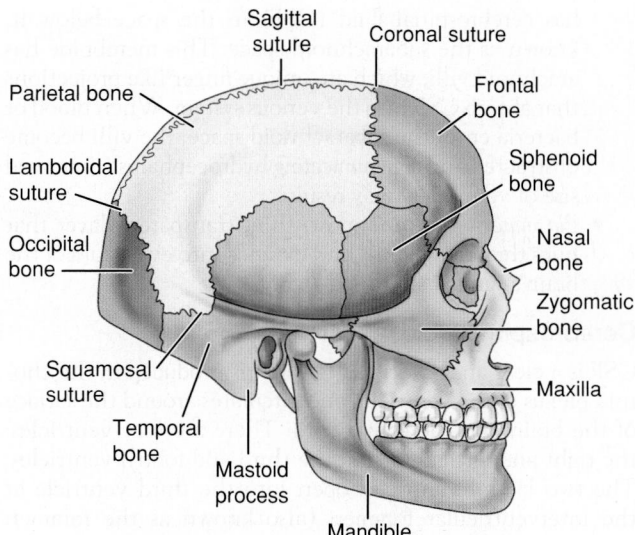

Figure 65-4 • Bones and sutures of the skull.

the falx cerebelli, which is located between the right and left side of the cerebellum. When excess pressure occurs in the cranial cavity, brain tissue may be compressed against these dural folds or displaced around them, a process called *herniation*. A potential space exists between the dura and the skull, and between the periosteum and the dura in the vertebral column, known as the epidural space. Another potential space, the subdural space, also exists below the dura. Blood or an abscess can accumulate in these potential spaces.

- *Arachnoid*—the middle membrane; an extremely thin, delicate membrane that closely resembles a spider web (hence the name *arachnoid*). The arachnoid membrane

Figure 65-5 • Meninges and related structures.

has cerebrospinal fluid (CSF) in the space below it, known as the subarachnoid space. This membrane has arachnoid villi, which are unique finger-like projections that absorb CSF into the venous system. When blood or bacteria enter the subarachnoid space, the villi become obstructed and *communicating* hydrocephalus (increased size of ventricles) may result.

- *Pia mater*—the innermost, thin, transparent layer that hugs the brain closely and extends into every fold of the brain's surface.

Cerebrospinal Fluid

CSF is a clear and colorless fluid that is produced in the choroid plexus of the ventricles and circulates around the surface of the brain and the spinal cord. There are four ventricles: the right and left lateral and the third and fourth ventricles. The two lateral ventricles open into the third ventricle at the interventricular foramen (also known as the foramen of Monro). The third and fourth ventricles connect via the aqueduct of Sylvius. The fourth ventricle drains CSF into the subarachnoid space on the surface of the brain and spinal cord, where it is absorbed by the arachnoid villi. Blockage of the flow of CSF anywhere in the ventricular system produces *obstructive* hydrocephalus.

CSF is important in immune and metabolic functions in the brain. It is produced at a rate of about 500 mL/day; the ventricles and subarachnoid space contain approximately 150 mL of fluid (Hickey, 2014). The composition of CSF is similar to other extracellular fluids (such as blood plasma), but the concentrations of the various constituents differ. A laboratory analysis of CSF indicates color (clear), specific gravity (normal 1.007), protein count, cell count, glucose, and other electrolyte levels (see Table A-5 in Appendix A on thePoint). Normal CSF contains a minimal number of white blood cells and no red blood cells. The CSF may also be tested for immunoglobulins or the presence of bacteria. A CSF sample may be obtained through a lumbar puncture or intraventricular catheter (Hickey, 2014).

Cerebral Circulation

The brain does not store nutrients and requires a constant supply of oxygen. These needs are met through cerebral circulation; the brain receives approximately 15% of the cardiac output, or 750 mL per minute of blood flow. Brain circulation is unique in several aspects. First, arterial and venous vessels are not parallel as in other organs in the body; this is due in part to the role the venous system plays in CSF absorption. Second, the brain has collateral circulation through the circle of Willis (see later discussion), allowing blood flow to be redirected on demand. Third, blood vessels in the brain have two rather than three layers, which may make them more prone to rupture when weakened or under pressure.

Arteries

Arterial blood supply to the anterior brain originates from the common carotid artery, which is the first bifurcation off the aorta. The internal carotid arteries arise at the bifurcation of the common carotid. Branches of the internal carotid arteries (the anterior and middle cerebral arteries) and their connections (the anterior and posterior communicating arteries) form the circle of Willis (see Fig. 65-6).

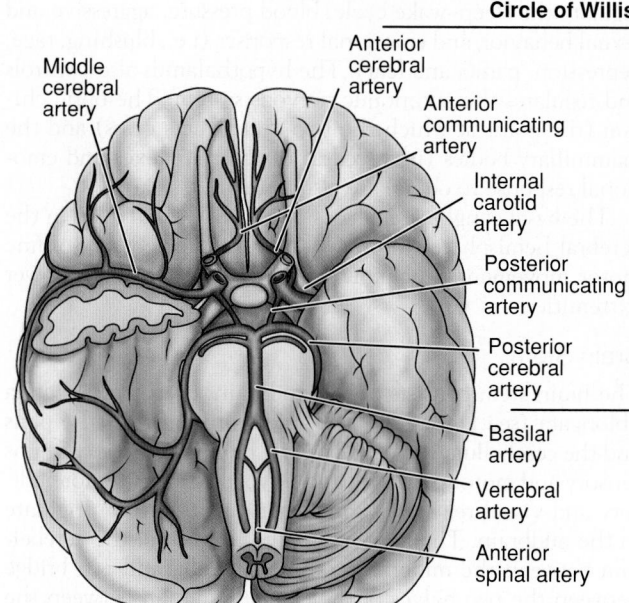

Circle of Willis

Middle cerebral artery

Anterior cerebral artery

Anterior communicating artery

Internal carotid artery

Posterior communicating artery

Posterior cerebral artery

Basilar artery

Vertebral artery

Anterior spinal artery

Figure 65-6 • Arterial blood supply of the brain, including the circle of Willis, as viewed from the ventral surface.

The vertebral arteries branch from the subclavian arteries to supply most of the posterior circulation of the brain. At the level of the brain stem, the vertebral arteries join to form the basilar artery. The basilar artery divides to form the two branches of the posterior cerebral arteries. Functionally, the posterior and anterior portions of the circulation usually remain separate. However, the circle of Willis can provide collateral circulation through communicating arteries if one of the vessels supplying it becomes occluded or is ligated.

The bifurcations along the circle of Willis are frequent sites of aneurysm formation. Aneurysms are outpouchings of the blood vessel due to vessel wall weakness. Aneurysms can rupture and cause a hemorrhagic stroke. See Chapter 67 for a more detailed discussion of aneurysms.

Veins

Venous drainage for the brain does not follow the arterial circulation as in other body structures. The veins reach the brain's surface, join larger veins, and then cross the subarachnoid space and empty into the dural sinuses, which are the vascular channels embedded in the dura (see Fig. 65-5). The network of the sinuses carries venous outflow from the brain and empties into the internal jugular veins, returning the blood to the heart. Cerebral veins are unique, because unlike other veins in the body, they do not have valves to prevent blood from flowing backward and depend on both gravity and blood pressure for flow.

Blood–Brain Barrier

The CNS is inaccessible to many substances that circulate in the blood plasma (e.g., dyes, medications, and antibiotic agents) because of the blood–brain barrier. This barrier is formed by the endothelial cells of the brain's capillaries, which form continuous tight junctions, creating a barrier to macromolecules and many compounds. All substances entering the CSF must filter through the capillary endothelial cells and astrocytes. The blood–brain barrier has a protective function but can be altered by trauma, cerebral edema, and cerebral hypoxemia; this has implications for treatment and selection of medications for CNS disorders (Hickey, 2014).

The Spinal Cord

The spinal cord is continuous with the medulla, extending from the cerebral hemispheres and serving as the connection between the brain and the periphery. Approximately 45 cm (18 inches) long and about the thickness of a finger, it extends from the foramen magnum at the base of the skull to the lower border of the first lumbar vertebra, where it tapers to a fibrous band called the *conus medullaris*. Continuing below the second lumbar space are the nerve roots that extend beyond the conus, which are called the *cauda equina* because they resemble a horse's tail. Meninges surround the spinal cord.

In a cross-sectional view, the spinal cord has an H-shaped central core of nerve cell bodies (gray matter) surrounded by ascending and descending tracts (white matter) (see Fig. 65-7). The lower portion of the H is broader than the upper portion and corresponds to the anterior horns. The anterior horns contain cells with fibers that form the anterior (motor) root and are essential for the voluntary and reflex activity of the muscles they innervate. The thinner posterior (upper horns) portion contains cells with fibers that enter over the posterior (sensory) root and thus serve as a relay station in the sensory/reflex pathway.

The thoracic region of the spinal cord has a projection from each side at the crossbar of the H-shaped structure of gray matter called the *lateral horn*. It contains the cells that give rise to the autonomic fibers of the sympathetic division. The fibers leave the spinal cord through the anterior roots in the thoracic and upper lumbar segments.

The Spinal Tracts

The white matter of the spinal cord is composed of myelinated and unmyelinated nerve fibers. The fast-conducting myelinated fibers form bundles; fiber bundles with a common function are called *tracts*.

There are six ascending tracts (see Fig. 65-7). Two tracts, known as the fasciculus cuneatus and gracilis or the posterior columns, conduct sensations of deep touch, pressure, vibration, position, and passive motion from the same side of the body. Before reaching the cerebral cortex, these fibers cross to the opposite side in the medulla. The anterior and posterior spinocerebellar tracts conduct sensory impulses from muscle spindles, providing necessary input for coordinated muscle contraction. They ascend uncrossed and terminate in the cerebellum. The anterior and lateral spinothalamic tracts are responsible for conduction of pain, temperature, proprioception, fine touch, and vibratory sense from the upper body to the brain. They cross to the opposite side of the cord and then ascend to the brain, terminating in the thalamus (Klein & Stewart-Amidei, 2012).

There are eight descending tracts (see Fig. 65-7). The anterior and lateral corticospinal tracts conduct motor impulses to the anterior horn cells from the opposite side of the brain, cross in the medulla, and control voluntary muscle activity. The three vestibulospinal tracts descend uncrossed and are involved in some autonomic functions (sweating, pupil dilation, and circulation) and involuntary muscle control. The corticobulbar tract conducts impulses responsible for voluntary head and facial muscle movement and crosses at the level of the brain stem. The rubrospinal and reticulospinal tracts conduct impulses involved with involuntary muscle movement.

Vertebral Column

The bones of the vertebral column surround and protect the spinal cord and normally consist of 7 cervical, 12 thoracic, and 5 lumbar vertebrae, as well as the sacrum (a fused mass of 5 vertebrae), and terminate in the coccyx. Nerve roots exit from the vertebral column through the intervertebral foramina (openings). The vertebrae are separated by discs, except for the first and second cervical, the sacral, and the coccygeal vertebrae. Each vertebra has a ventral solid body and a dorsal segment or arch, which is posterior to the body. The arch is composed of two pedicles and two laminae supporting seven processes. The vertebral body, arch, pedicles, and laminae all encase and protect the spinal cord.

The Peripheral Nervous System

The peripheral nervous system includes the cranial nerves, the spinal nerves, and the autonomic nervous system.

Cranial Nerves

Twelve pairs of cranial nerves emerge from the lower surface of the brain and pass through openings in the base of the skull. Three cranial nerves are entirely sensory (I, II, VIII), five are motor (III, IV, VI, XI, and XII), and four are mixed sensory and motor (V, VII, IX, and X). The cranial nerves are numbered in the order in which they arise from the brain (see Fig. 65-8). The cranial nerves innervate the head, neck, and special sense structures. Table 65-2 identifies primary functions of the cranial nerves.

Spinal Nerves

The spinal cord is composed of 31 pairs of spinal nerves: 8 cervical, 12 thoracic, 5 lumbar, 5 sacral, and 1 coccygeal. Each spinal nerve has a ventral root and a dorsal root. The dorsal roots are sensory and transmit sensory impulses from specific areas of the body known as dermatomes (see Fig. 65-9) to the dorsal horn ganglia. The sensory fiber may be somatic, carrying information about pain, temperature, touch, and position sense

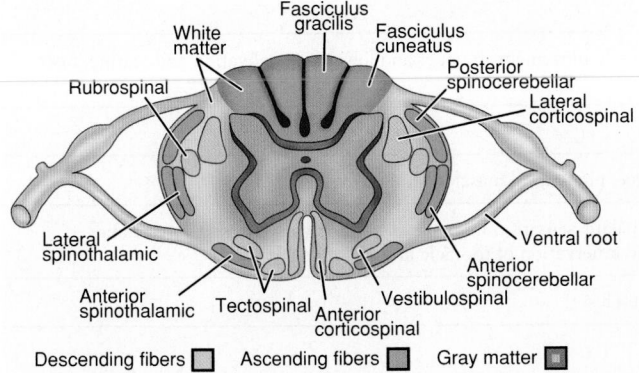

Figure 65-7 • Cross-sectional diagram of the spinal cord showing major spinal tracts.

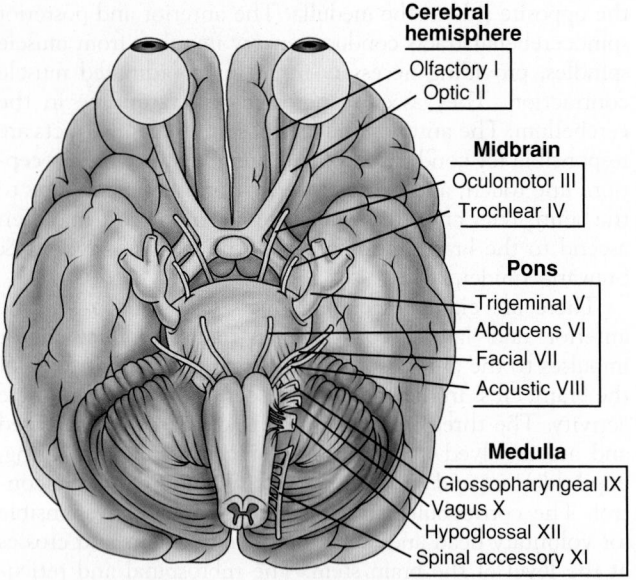

Cerebral hemisphere
- Olfactory I
- Optic II

Midbrain
- Oculomotor III
- Trochlear IV

Pons
- Trigeminal V
- Abducens VI
- Facial VII
- Acoustic VIII

Medulla
- Glossopharyngeal IX
- Vagus X
- Hypoglossal XII
- Spinal accessory XI

Figure 65-8 • Diagram of the base of the brain showing location of the cranial nerves.

(proprioception) from the tendons, joints, and body surfaces; or visceral, carrying information from the internal organs.

The ventral roots are motor and transmit impulses from the spinal cord to the body; these fibers are also either somatic or visceral. The visceral fibers include autonomic fibers that control the cardiac muscles and glandular secretions.

Autonomic Nervous System

The **autonomic nervous system** regulates the activities of internal organs such as the heart, lungs, blood vessels, digestive organs, and glands (see Fig. 65-10). Maintenance and restoration of internal homeostasis is largely the responsibility of the autonomic nervous system. There are two major divisions: the **sympathetic nervous system**, with predominantly excitatory responses (most notably the "fight-or-flight" response), and the parasympathetic nervous system, which controls mostly visceral functions.

The autonomic nervous system innervates most body organs. Although usually considered part of the peripheral nervous system, this system is regulated by centers in the spinal cord, brain stem, and hypothalamus.

The hypothalamus is the major subcortical center for the regulation of autonomic activities, serving an inhibitory–excitatory role. The hypothalamus has connections that link the autonomic system with the thalamus, the cortex, the olfactory apparatus, and the pituitary gland. Located here are the mechanisms for the control of visceral and somatic reactions that were originally important for defense or attack and are associated with emotional states (e.g., fear, anger, and anxiety); for the control of metabolic processes, including fat, carbohydrate, and water metabolism; for the regulation of body temperature, arterial pressure, and all muscular and glandular activities of the gastrointestinal tract; for control of genital functions; and for the sleep cycle.

The autonomic nervous system is separated into the anatomically and functionally distinct sympathetic and parasympathetic divisions. Most of the tissues and the organs under autonomic control are innervated by both systems. For example, the parasympathetic division causes contraction (stimulation) of the urinary bladder muscles and a decrease (inhibition) in heart rate, whereas the sympathetic division produces relaxation (inhibition) of the urinary bladder and an increase (stimulation) in the rate and force of the heartbeat.

TABLE 65-2 Cranial Nerves

Cranial Nerve	Type	Function
I (olfactory)	Sensory	Sense of smell
II (optic)	Sensory	Visual acuity and visual fields
III (oculomotor)	Motor	Muscles that move the eye and lid, pupillary constriction, lens accommodation
IV (trochlear)	Motor	Muscles that move the eye
V (trigeminal)	Mixed	Facial sensation, corneal reflex, mastication
VI (abducens)	Motor	Muscles that move the eye
VII (facial)	Mixed	Symmetry of facial expression and muscle movement in upper and lower face, salivation and tearing, taste, sensation in the ear
VIII (acoustic)	Sensory	Hearing and equilibrium
IX (glossopharyngeal)	Mixed	Taste, sensation in pharynx and tongue, pharyngeal muscles, swallowing
X (vagus)	Mixed	Muscles of pharynx, larynx, and soft palate; sensation in external ear, pharynx, larynx, thoracic and abdominal viscera; parasympathetic innervation of thoracic and abdominal organs
XI (spinal accessory)	Motor	Sternocleidomastoid and trapezius muscles
XII (hypoglossal)	Motor	Movement of the tongue

Adapted from Bader, M., Littlejohns, L. R., & Olson, D. (2016). *AANN core curriculum for neuroscience nursing* (6th ed.). Chicago, IL: American Association of Neuroscience Nurses.

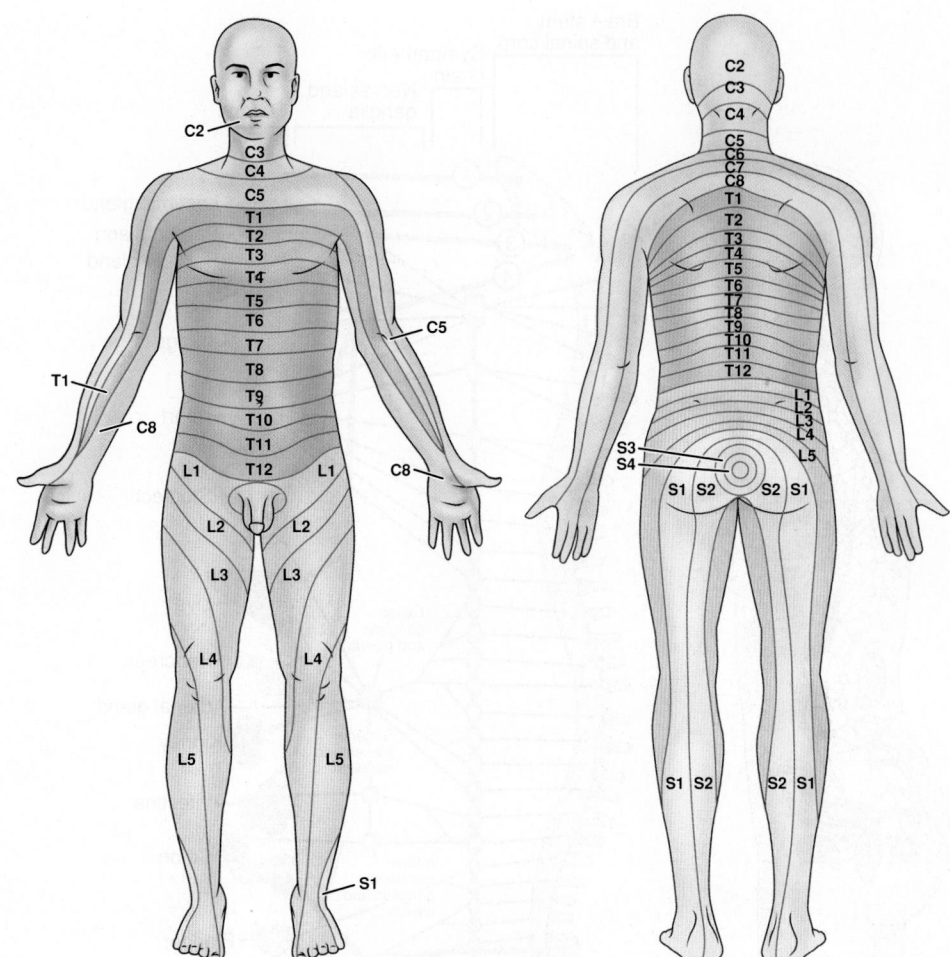

Figure 65-9 • Dermatome distribution.

Table 65-3 compares the sympathetic and the parasympathetic effects on the different systems of the body.

Sympathetic Nervous System

The sympathetic division of the autonomic nervous system is best known for its role in the body's fight-or-flight response. Under stress from either physical or emotional causes, sympathetic impulses increase greatly. As a result, the bronchioles dilate for easier gas exchange; the heart's contractions are stronger and faster; the arteries to the heart and voluntary muscles dilate, carrying more blood to these organs; peripheral blood vessels constrict, making the skin feel cool but shunting blood to essential organs; the pupils dilate; the liver releases glucose for quick energy; peristalsis slows; hair stands on end; and perspiration increases. The main sympathetic neurotransmitter is norepinephrine (noradrenaline). A sympathetic discharge releases epinephrine (adrenalin)—hence, the term *adrenergic* is often used to refer to this division.

Sympathetic neurons are located primarily in the thoracic and lumbar segments of the spinal cord, and their axons, or the preganglionic fibers, emerge by way of anterior nerve roots from the eighth cervical or first thoracic segment to the second or third lumbar segment. A short distance from the cord, these fibers diverge to join a chain, composed of 22 linked ganglia, that extends the entire length of the spinal column, adjacent to the vertebral bodies on both sides. Some form

multiple synapses with nerve cells within the chain. Others traverse the chain without making connections or losing continuity to join large "prevertebral" ganglia in the thorax, the abdomen, or the pelvis or one of the "terminal" ganglia in the vicinity of an organ, such as the bladder or the rectum at the end of the colon (see Fig. 65-10). Postganglionic nerve fibers originating in the sympathetic chain rejoin the spinal nerves that supply the extremities and are distributed to blood vessels, sweat glands, and smooth muscle tissue in the skin. Postganglionic fibers from the prevertebral plexuses (e.g., the cardiac, pulmonary, splanchnic, and pelvic plexuses) supply structures in the head and neck, thorax, abdomen, and pelvis, respectively, having been joined in these plexuses by fibers from the parasympathetic division.

The adrenal glands, kidneys, liver, spleen, stomach, and duodenum are under the control of the giant celiac plexus, commonly known as the solar plexus. This receives its sympathetic nerve components by way of the three splanchnic nerves, composed of preganglionic fibers from nine segments of the spinal cord (T4 to L1), and is joined by the vagus nerve, representing the parasympathetic division. From the celiac plexus, fibers of both divisions travel along the course of blood vessels to their target organs.

Certain syndromes are distinctive to the sympathetic nervous system. For example, sympathetic storm is a syndrome associated with changes in level of consciousness, altered

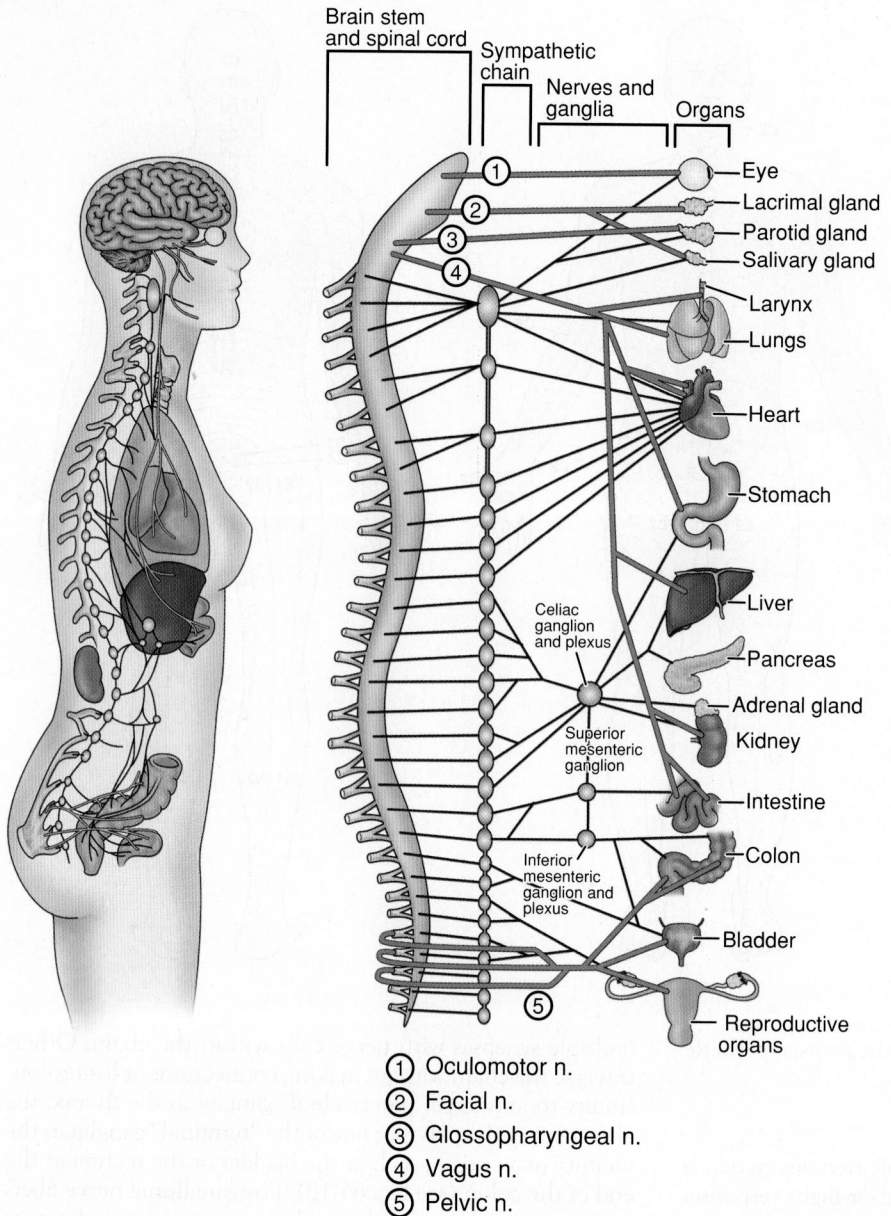

Brain stem
and spinal cord
Sympathetic
chain
Nerves and
ganglia
Organs

- Eye
- Lacrimal gland
- Parotid gland
- Salivary gland
- Larynx
- Lungs
- Heart
- Stomach
- Liver
- Pancreas
- Adrenal gland
- Kidney
- Intestine
- Colon
- Bladder
- Reproductive organs

Celiac
ganglion
and plexus

Superior
mesenteric
ganglion

Inferior
mesenteric
ganglion and
plexus

① Oculomotor n.
② Facial n.
③ Glossopharyngeal n.
④ Vagus n.
⑤ Pelvic n.

Figure 65-10 • Anatomy of the autonomic nervous system.

vital signs, diaphoresis, and agitation that may result from hypothalamic stimulation of the sympathetic nervous system following traumatic brain injury (Fischbach & Dunning, 2015).

Parasympathetic Nervous System

The **parasympathetic nervous system** functions as the dominant controller for most visceral functions; the primary neurotransmitter is acetylcholine. During quiet, nonstressful conditions, impulses from parasympathetic fibers (cholinergic) predominate. The fibers of the parasympathetic system are located in two sections: one in the brain stem and the other from spinal segments below L2. Because of the location of these fibers, the parasympathetic system is referred to as the craniosacral division, as distinct from the thoracolumbar (sympathetic) division of the autonomic nervous system.

The parasympathetic nerves arise from the midbrain and the medulla oblongata. Fibers from cells in the midbrain travel with the third oculomotor nerve to the ciliary ganglia, where postganglionic fibers of this division are joined by those of the sympathetic system, creating controlled opposition, with a delicate balance maintained between the two at all times.

Motor and Sensory Pathways of the Nervous System

Motor Pathways

The corticospinal tract begins in the motor cortex, a vertical band within each frontal lobe, and controls voluntary movements of the body. The exact locations within the brain at which the voluntary movements of the muscles of the face, thumb, hand, arm, trunk, and leg originate are known (see Fig. 65-11). To initiate movement, these particular cells must send the stimulus along their fibers. Stimulation of these cells with an electric current also results in muscle contraction.

TABLE 65-3 Effects of the Autonomic Nervous System

Structure or Activity	Parasympathetic Effects	Sympathetic Effects
Pupil of the Eye	Constricted	Dilated
Circulatory System		
Rate and force of heartbeat	Decreased	Increased
Blood vessels		
In heart muscle	Constricted	Dilated
In skeletal muscle	a	Dilated
In abdominal viscera and the skin	a	Constricted
Blood pressure	Decreased	Increased
Respiratory System		
Bronchioles	Constricted	Dilated
Rate of breathing	Decreased	Increased
Digestive System		
Peristaltic movements of digestive tube	Increased	Decreased
Muscular sphincters of digestive tube	Relaxed	Contracted
Secretion of salivary glands	Thin, watery saliva	Thick, viscid saliva
Secretions of stomach, intestine, and pancreas	Increased	a
Conversion of liver glycogen to glucose	a	Increased
Genitourinary System		
Urinary bladder		
Muscle walls	Contracted	Relaxed
Sphincters	Relaxed	Contracted
Muscles of the uterus	Relaxed; variable	Contracted under some conditions; varies with menstrual cycle and pregnancy
Blood vessels of external genitalia	Dilated	a
Integumentary System		
Secretion of sweat	a	Increased
Pilomotor muscles	a	Contracted (goose flesh)
Adrenal Medulla	a	Secretion of epinephrine and norepinephrine

a No direct effect.

Adapted from Hickey, J. (2014). *Clinical practice of neurological and neurosurgical nursing* (6th ed.). Philadelphia, PA: Lippincott Williams & Wilkins.

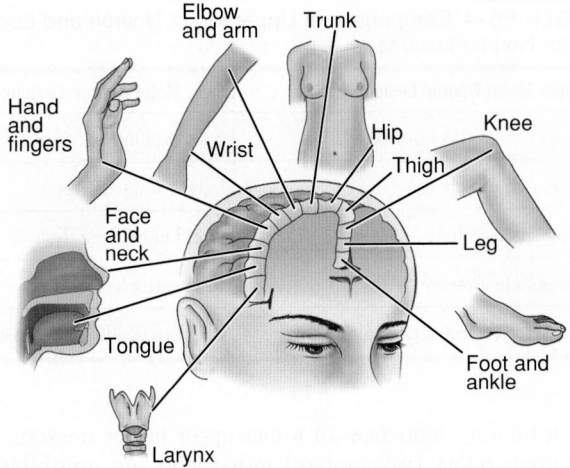

Figure 65-11 • Diagrammatic representation of the cerebrum showing locations for control of motor movement of various parts of the body.

part of the cord and run to the myoneural junction located in the peripheral muscle.

Involuntary motor activity is also possible and is mediated through reflex arcs. Synaptic connections between anterior horn cells and sensory fibers that have entered adjacent or neighboring segments of the spinal cord serve as protective mechanisms. These connections are seen during deep tendon reflex testing.

Upper and Lower Motor Neurons

The voluntary motor system consists of two groups of neurons: upper motor neurons and lower motor neurons. Upper motor neurons originate in the cerebral cortex, the cerebellum, and the brain stem. Their fibers make up the descending motor pathways, are located entirely within the CNS, and modulate the activity of the lower motor neurons. Lower motor neurons are located either in the anterior horn of the spinal cord gray matter or within cranial nerve nuclei in the brain stem. Axons of lower motor neurons in both sites extend through peripheral nerves and terminate in skeletal muscle. Lower motor neurons are located in both the CNS and the peripheral nervous system.

The motor pathways from the brain to the spinal cord, as well as from the cerebrum to the brain stem, are formed by upper motor neurons. They begin in the cortex of one side of the brain, descend through the internal capsule, cross to the opposite side in the brain stem, descend through the corticospinal tract, and synapse with the lower motor neurons in the cord. The lower motor neurons receive the impulse in the posterior part of the cord and run to the myoneural junction located in the peripheral muscle. The clinical features of lesions of upper and lower motor neurons are discussed in the following sections and in Table 65-4.

Upper Motor Neuron Lesions

Upper motor neuron lesions can involve the motor cortex, the internal capsule, the spinal cord gray matter, and other structures of the brain through which the corticospinal tract descends. If the upper motor neurons are damaged or destroyed, as frequently occur with stroke or spinal cord injury, paralysis (loss of voluntary movement) results. However, because

En route to the pons, the motor fibers converge into a tight bundle known as the internal capsule. A comparatively small injury to the internal capsule results in a more severe paralysis than does a larger injury to the cortex itself.

At the medulla, the corticospinal tracts cross to the opposite side, continuing to the anterior horn of the spinal cord, in proximity to a motor nerve cell. Until this point, neurons are known as upper motor neurons. As they connect to motor fibers of the spinal nerves, they become lower motor neurons. The lower motor neurons receive the impulse in the posterior

TABLE 65-4 Comparison of Upper Motor Neuron and Lower Motor Neuron Lesions

Upper Motor Neuron Lesions	Lower Motor Neuron Lesions
Loss of voluntary control	Loss of voluntary control
Increased muscle tone	Decreased muscle tone
Muscle spasticity	Flaccid muscle paralysis
No muscle atrophy	Muscle atrophy
Hyperactive and abnormal reflexes	Absent or decreased reflexes

the inhibitory influences of intact upper motor neurons are impaired, **reflex** (involuntary) movements are uninhibited, and hence hyperactive deep tendon reflexes, diminished or absent superficial reflexes, and pathologic reflexes such as a Babinski response occur. Severe leg spasms can occur as the result of an upper motor neuron lesion; the spasms result from the preserved reflex arc, which lacks inhibition along the spinal cord below the level of injury. There is little or no muscle atrophy, and muscles remain permanently tense, exhibiting spastic paralysis.

Paralysis associated with upper motor neuron lesions can affect a whole extremity, both extremities, or an entire half of the body. *Hemiplegia* (paralysis of an arm and leg on the same side of the body) can be the result of an upper motor neuron lesion. If hemorrhage, an embolus, or a thrombus destroys the fibers from the motor area in the internal capsule, the arm and the leg of the opposite side become stiff, weak, or paralyzed, and the reflexes are hyperactive (see further discussion of hemiplegia in Chapter 67). If both legs are paralyzed, the condition is called *paraplegia*. If all four extremities are paralyzed, the condition is called *tetraplegia* (quadriplegia). See Chapter 68 for additional discussion of these disorders.

Lower Motor Neuron Lesions

A patient is considered to have lower motor neuron damage if a motor nerve is damaged between the spinal cord and muscle. The result of lower motor neuron damage is muscle paralysis. Reflexes are lost, and the muscle becomes flaccid (limp) and atrophied from disuse. If the patient has injured the spinal trunk and it can heal, the use of muscles connected to that section of the spinal cord may be regained. However, if the anterior horn motor cells are destroyed, the nerves cannot regenerate and the muscles are never useful again.

Flaccid paralysis and atrophy of the affected muscles are the principal signs of lower motor neuron disease. Lower motor neuron lesions can be the result of trauma, infection (poliomyelitis), toxins, vascular disorders, congenital malformations, degenerative processes, and neoplasms. Compression of nerve roots by herniated intervertebral discs is a common cause of lower motor neuron dysfunction.

Coordination of Movement

The motor system is complex, and motor function depends not only on the integrity of the corticospinal tracts but also on other pathways from the basal ganglia and cerebellum that control and coordinate voluntary motor function. The smoothness, accuracy, and strength that characterize the muscular movements of a normal person are attributable to the influence of the cerebellum and the basal ganglia.

Through the action of the cerebellum, the contractions of opposing muscle groups are adjusted in relation to each other to maximal mechanical advantage; muscle contractions can be sustained evenly at the desired tension and without significant fluctuation, and reciprocal movements can be reproduced at high and constant speed, in stereotyped fashion and with relatively little effort.

The basal ganglia play an important role in planning and coordinating motor movements and posture. Complex neural connections link the basal ganglia with the cerebral cortex. The major effect of these structures is to inhibit unwanted muscular activity.

Impaired cerebellar function, which may occur as a result of an intracranial injury or some type of an expanding mass (e.g., a hemorrhage, an abscess, or a tumor), results in loss of muscle tone, weakness, and fatigue. Depending on the area of the brain affected, the patient has different motor symptoms or responses. The patient may demonstrate abnormal flexion, abnormal extension, or flaccid posturing. **Flaccidity** (lack of muscle tone) preceded by abnormal posturing in a patient with cerebral injury indicates severe neurologic impairment, which may herald brain death (Klein & Stewart-Amidei, 2012; Posner, Saper, Schiff, et al., 2007). See Figure 66-1 in Chapter 66 for further explanation of posturing.

Destruction or dysfunction of the basal ganglia leads not to paralysis but to muscle rigidity, disturbances of posture, and difficulty initiating or changing movement. The patient tends to have involuntary movements. These may take the form of coarse tremors, most often in the upper extremities, particularly in the distal portions; athetosis, which is movement of a slow, squirming, writhing, twisting type; or chorea, marked by spasmodic, purposeless, irregular, uncoordinated motions of the trunk and the extremities, and facial grimacing. Disorders affecting basal ganglia activity include Parkinson and Huntington diseases (see Chapter 70).

Sensory System Function

Receiving Sensory Impulses

Afferent impulses travel from their points of origin to their destinations in the cerebral cortex via the ascending pathways directly, or they may cross at the level of the spinal cord or in the medulla, depending on the type of sensation carried. Knowledge of these pathways is important for neurologic assessment and for understanding symptoms and their relationship to various lesions.

Sensory impulses convey sensations of heat, cold, and pain; position; and vibration. The axons enter the spinal cord by way of the posterior root, specifically in the posterior gray columns of the spinal cord, where they connect with the cells of secondary neurons. Pain and temperature fibers (located in the spinothalamic tract) cross immediately to the opposite side of the cord and course upward to the thalamus. Fibers carrying sensations of touch, light pressure, and localization do not connect immediately with the second neuron but ascend the cord for a variable distance before entering the gray matter and completing this connection. The axon of the secondary neuron traverses the cord, crosses in the medulla, and proceeds upward to the thalamus.

Position and vibratory sensations are produced by stimuli arising from muscles, joints, and bones. These stimuli are conveyed, uncrossed, all the way to the brain stem by the axon of the primary neuron. In the medulla, synaptic connections are made with cells of the secondary neurons, whose axons cross to the opposite side and then proceed to the thalamus.

Integrating Sensory Impulses

The thalamus integrates all sensory impulses except olfaction. It plays a role in the conscious awareness of pain and the recognition of variation in temperature and touch. The thalamus is responsible for the sense of movement and position as well as the ability to recognize the size, shape, and quality of objects. Sensory information is relayed from the thalamus to the parietal lobe for interpretation.

Sensory Losses

Destruction of a sensory nerve results in total loss of sensation in its area of distribution (see Fig. 65-9). Lesions affecting the posterior spinal nerve roots may impair tactile sensation, causing intermittent severe pain that is referred to their areas of distribution. Destruction of the spinal cord yields complete anesthesia below the level of injury. Selective destruction or degeneration of the posterior columns of the spinal cord is responsible for a loss of position and vibratory sense in segments distal to the lesion, without loss of touch, pain, or temperature perception. A cyst in the center of the spinal cord causes dissociation of sensation—loss of pain at the level of the lesion. This occurs because the fibers carrying pain and temperature cross within the cord immediately on entering; thus, any lesion that divides the cord longitudinally divides these fibers. Other sensory fibers ascend the cord for variable distances, some even to the medulla, before crossing, thereby bypassing the lesion and avoiding destruction. Lesions in the thalamus or parietal lobe result in impaired touch, pain, temperature, and proprioceptive sensations.

Assessment of the Nervous System

Health History

An important aspect of the neurologic assessment is the history of the present illness. The initial interview provides an excellent opportunity to systematically explore the patient's current condition and related events while simultaneously observing overall appearance, mental status, posture, movement, and affect. Depending on the patient's condition, the nurse may need to rely on yes-or-no answers to questions, a review of the medical record, input from witnesses or the family, or a combination of these.

Neurologic disorders may be stable or progressive, characterized by symptom-free periods as well as fluctuations in symptoms. The health history therefore includes details about the onset, character, severity, location, duration, and frequency of symptoms and signs; associated complaints; precipitating, aggravating, and relieving factors; progression, remission, and exacerbation; and the presence or absence of similar symptoms among family members.

Common Symptoms

The symptoms of neurologic disorders are as varied as the disease processes. Symptoms may be subtle or intense, fluctuating

or permanent, inconvenient or devastating. This chapter discusses the most common signs and symptoms associated with neurologic disease; the relationship of specific signs and symptoms to a particular disorder is presented in later chapters in this unit.

Pain

Pain is considered an unpleasant sensory perception and emotional experience associated with actual or potential tissue damage or described in terms of such damage. Pain is therefore considered multidimensional and entirely subjective. Pain can be acute or chronic. In general, acute pain lasts for a relatively short period of time and remits as the pathology resolves. In neurologic disease, acute pain may be associated with brain hemorrhage, spinal disc disease (Jarvis, 2015), or trigeminal neuralgia. In contrast, chronic or persistent pain extends for long periods of time and may represent a broader pathology. This type of pain can occur with many degenerative and chronic neurologic conditions (e.g., multiple sclerosis). See Chapter 12 for a more detailed discussion of pain.

Seizures

Seizures are the result of abnormal electrical discharges in the cerebral cortex, which then manifest as an alteration in sensation, behavior, movement, perception, or consciousness. The alteration may be short, such as in a blank stare that lasts only a second, or of longer duration, such as a tonic–clonic grand mal seizure that can last several minutes. The seizure activity reflects the area of the brain affected. Seizures can occur as isolated events, such as when induced by a high fever, alcohol or drug withdrawal, or hypoglycemia. A seizure may also be the first obvious sign of a brain lesion (Hickey, 2014).

Dizziness and Vertigo

Dizziness is an abnormal sensation of imbalance or movement. It is fairly common in the older adult and a common complaint encountered by health professionals (Jarvis, 2015). Dizziness can have a variety of causes, including viral syndromes, hot weather, roller-coaster rides, and middle ear infections, to name a few. One difficulty confronting health care providers when assessing dizziness is the vague and varied terms that patients use to describe the sensation.

About 50% of all patients with dizziness have **vertigo**, or the illusion of movement in which the individual or the surroundings are sensed as moving, usually as rotation (Jarvis, 2015). Vertigo is usually a manifestation of vestibular dysfunction. It can be so severe as to result in spatial disorientation, lightheadedness, loss of equilibrium (staggering), and nausea and vomiting.

Visual Disturbances

Visual defects that cause people to seek health care can range from the decreased visual acuity associated with aging to sudden blindness caused by glaucoma. Normal vision depends on functioning visual pathways through the retina and optic chiasm and the radiations into the visual cortex in the occipital lobes. Lesions of the eye itself (e.g., cataract), lesions along the pathway (e.g., tumor), or lesions in the visual cortex (e.g., stroke) interfere with normal visual acuity. Abnormalities of eye movement (as in the nystagmus associated with multiple sclerosis) can also compromise vision by causing diplopia or double vision. See Chapter 63 for a more detailed discussion of disorders that affect vision.

Muscle Weakness

Muscle weakness is a common manifestation of neurologic disease. It frequently coexists with other symptoms of disease and can affect a variety of muscles, causing a wide range of disability. Weakness can be sudden and permanent, as in stroke, or progressive, as in neuromuscular diseases such as amyotrophic lateral sclerosis. Any muscle group can be affected.

Abnormal Sensation

Abnormal sensation is a neurologic manifestation of both central and peripheral nervous system disease. Altered sensation can affect small or large areas of the body. It is frequently associated with weakness or pain and is potentially disabling. Lack of sensation places a person at risk for falls and injury.

Past Health, Family, and Social History

The nurse may inquire about any family history of genetic diseases (see Chart 65-1). A review of the medical history, including a system-by-system evaluation, is part of the health history. The nurse should be aware of any history of trauma or falls that may have involved the head or spinal cord. Questions regarding the use of alcohol, medications, and illicit drugs are also relevant. The history-taking portion of the neurologic assessment is critical and, in many cases of neurologic disease, leads to an accurate diagnosis.

Physical Assessment

The neurologic examination is a systematic process that includes a variety of clinical tests, observations, and assessments designed to evaluate the neurologic status of a complex system. Many neurologic rating scales exist (Herndon, 2006), and some of the more common ones are discussed in this chapter.

The brain and spinal cord cannot be examined as directly as other systems of the body. Therefore, much of the neurologic examination is an indirect evaluation that assesses the function of the specific body part or parts controlled by the nervous system. A neurologic assessment is divided into five components: consciousness and cognition, cranial nerves, motor system, sensory system, and reflexes. One or more

---

Chart 65-1 GENETICS IN NURSING PRACTICE
Neurologic Disorders

Several neurologic disorders are associated with genetic abnormalities. Neurologic impairment is noted with many other genetic illnesses. Some examples include:

Autosomal Dominant:

- Cerebral arteriopathy
- Familial Alzheimer disease
- Huntington disease
- Myotonic dystrophies
- Neurofibromatosis
- Von Hippel–Lindau syndrome

Autosomal Recessive:

- Canavan disease
- Familial dysautonomia
- Friedreich ataxia

X Linked:

- Duchenne muscular dystrophy
- Fragile X syndrome

Inheritance pattern is not distinct; however, there is a genetic predisposition for the disease:

- Amyotrophic lateral sclerosis (ALS)
- Epilepsy
- Neural tube defects (e.g., spina bifida, anencephaly)
- Parkinson disease
- Tourette syndrome

Other genetic disorders that also impact the neurologic system:

- Bipolar disease
- Downs syndrome
- Phenylketonuria (PKU)
- Schizophrenia
- Tay–Sachs disease
- Tuberous sclerosis complex

Nursing Assessments

Refer to Chapter 5, Chart 5-2: Genetics in Nursing Practice: Genetic Aspects of Health Assessment

Family History Assessment Specific to Neurologic Disorders

- Assess for other similarly affected relatives with neurologic impairment.
- Inquire about age of onset (e.g., present at birth—spina bifida; developed in childhood—Duchenne muscular dystrophy; developed in adulthood—Huntington disease, Alzheimer disease, ALS).
- Inquire about the presence of related conditions such as intellectual disability and/or learning disabilities (neurofibromatosis type 1).

Patient Assessment

- Assess for the presence of other physical features suggestive of an underlying genetic condition, such as skin lesions seen in neurofibromatosis (*café au lait* spots).
- Assess attention span, and the presence of hyperactivity or withdrawn behavior.
- Assess for other congenital abnormalities (e.g., cardiac, ocular).
- Inspect for presence of freckles in the axillary or inguinal areas.
- Assess for presence of uncoordinated movement of extremities, muscle twitching, or history of seizures.
- Assess for poor or hyperactive muscle tone.
- Assess for episodes of forgetfulness or uncharacteristic changes in behavior or mood.
- Inspect for disproportionate facial features (fragile X or Downs syndrome).
- Observe for presence of "tics" or uncontrolled body movement.
- Ask about history of seizures or head trauma.

Genetics Resources

Epilepsy Foundation, www.epilepsy.com/learn/diagnosis/genetic-testing
Huntington's Disease Society of America, hdsa.org/what-is-hd/#genetic
Muscular Dystrophy Association, www.mda.org
See Chapter 8, Chart 8-7 for components of genetic counseling.

components may become the priority assessment, depending on the patient's condition. For example, motor, sensory, and reflex assessments are the priority in patients with spinal injury, whereas in a patient who is comatose, the cranial nerves and level of consciousness become the priority.

Assessing Consciousness and Cognition

Cerebral abnormalities may cause disturbances in mental status, intellectual functioning, thought content, and emotional status. There may also be alterations in language abilities as well as lifestyle. The examiner must also be aware of the patient's overall level of consciousness and any changes over time (Posner et al., 2007).

The examiner records and reports specific observations regarding mental status, intellectual function, thought content, and emotional status, all of which permit comparison by others over time. Alterations should be described in specific and nonjudgmental terms. The use of terms such as "inappropriate" or "demented" is avoided, because they often mean different things to different people and are therefore not useful when describing behavior. Analysis and the conclusions that may be drawn from these findings usually depend on the examiner's knowledge of neuroanatomy, neurophysiology, and neuropathology.

Mental Status

An assessment of mental status begins by observing the patient's appearance and behavior, noting dress, grooming, and personal hygiene. Posture, gestures, movements, and facial expressions often provide important information about the patient. Does the patient appear to be aware of and interact with the surroundings?

Assessing orientation to time, place, and person assists in evaluating mental status. Does the patient know what day it is, what year it is, and the name of the president of the United States? Is the patient aware of where he or she is? Is the patient aware of who the examiner is and of their purpose for being in the room? Assessment of immediate and remote memory is also important. Is the capacity for immediate memory intact? See Chapter 11.

Intellectual Function

A person with an average intelligence quotient (IQ) can repeat seven digits without faltering and can recite five digits backward. The examiner might ask the patient to count backward from 100 or to subtract 7 from 100, then 7 from that, and so forth (referred to as serial 7s). The capacity to interpret well-known proverbs tests abstract reasoning, which is a higher intellectual function—for example, does the patient know what is meant by "a stitch in time saves nine"? The intellectual function of patients with damage to the frontal cortex appears intact until one or more tests of intellectual capacity are performed. Questions designed to assess this capacity might include the ability to recognize similarities—for example, how are a mouse and dog or pen and pencil alike? Can the patient make judgments about situations—for example, if the patient arrives home without a house key, what alternatives are there?

Thought Content

During the interview, it is important to assess the patient's thought content. Are the patient's thoughts spontaneous, natural, clear, relevant, and coherent? Does the patient have any fixed ideas, illusions, or preoccupations? What are their insights into these thoughts? Preoccupation with death or morbid events, hallucinations, and paranoid ideation are examples of unusual thoughts or perceptions that require further evaluation.

Emotional Status

An assessment of consciousness and cognition also includes the patient's emotional status. Is the patient's affect (external manifestation of mood) natural and even, or irritable and angry, anxious, apathetic or flat, or euphoric? Does their mood fluctuate normally, or does the patient unpredictably swing from joy to sadness during the interview? Is affect appropriate to words and thought content? Are verbal communications consistent with nonverbal cues?

Language Ability

The person with normal neurologic function can understand and communicate in spoken and written language. Does the patient answer questions appropriately? Can he or she read a sentence from a newspaper and explain its meaning? Can the patient write their name or copy a simple figure that the examiner has drawn? A deficiency in language function is called *aphasia*. Different types of aphasia result from injury to different parts of the brain (see Table 65-5). See Chapter 67 for a detailed discussion of aphasia.

Impact on Lifestyle

The nurse assesses the impact of any impairment on the patient's lifestyle. Issues to consider include the limitations imposed on the patient by any cognitive deficit and the patient's role in society, including family and community roles. The plan of care that the nurse develops needs to address and support adaptation to the neurologic deficit and continued function to the extent possible within the patient's support system.

Level of Consciousness

Consciousness is the patient's wakefulness and ability to respond to the environment. Level of consciousness is the most sensitive indicator of neurologic function. To assess level of consciousness, the examiner observes for alertness and ability to follow commands.

If the patient is not alert or able to follow commands, the examiner observes for eye opening; verbal response and motor response to stimuli, if any; and the type of stimuli needed to obtain a response. Noxious stimuli should be used first, then painful stimuli if no response is observed. In the patient with decreased level of consciousness, motor and cranial nerve

TABLE 65-5 Types of Aphasia and Region of Brain Involved

Type of Aphasia	Brain Area Involved
Auditory receptive	Temporal lobe
Visual receptive	Parietal and occipital area
Expressive speaking	Inferior-posterior frontal areas
Expressive writing	Posterior frontal area

functions become the priority assessments, because abnormalities can indicate the area of involvement in the absence of responsiveness. See Chapter 66 for further discussion of changes in level of consciousness.

Examining the Cranial Nerves

Cranial nerves are assessed when level of consciousness is decreased, with brain stem pathology, or in the presence of peripheral nervous system disease (Weber & Kelley, 2014). Right and left cranial nerve functions are compared throughout the examination.

For the procedural guidelines for assessing cranial nerve function, go to **thepoint.lww.com/Brunner14e.**

Examining the Motor System
Motor Ability

A thorough examination of the motor system includes an assessment of muscle size and tone as well as strength, coordination, and balance. The patient is instructed to walk across the room, if possible, while the examiner observes posture and gait. The muscles are inspected, and palpated if necessary, for their size and symmetry. Any evidence of atrophy or involuntary movements (tremors, tics) is noted. Muscle tone (the tension present in a muscle at rest) is evaluated by palpating various muscle groups at rest and during passive movement. Resistance to these movements is assessed and documented. Abnormalities in tone include **spasticity** (increased muscle tone), **rigidity** (resistance to passive stretch), and flaccidity.

Muscle Strength

Assessing the patient's ability to flex or extend the extremities against resistance tests muscle strength. The function of an individual muscle or group of muscles is evaluated by placing the muscle at a disadvantage. The quadriceps, for example, is a powerful muscle responsible for straightening the leg. Once the leg is straightened, it is exceedingly difficult for the examiner to flex the knee. If the knee is flexed and the patient

is asked to straighten the leg against resistance, weakness can be elicited. The evaluation of muscle strength compares the sides of the body to each other. For example, the right upper extremity is compared to the left upper extremity. Subtle differences in strength may be evaluated by testing for drift. For example, both arms are out in front of the patient with palms up; drift is seen as pronation of the palm, indicating a subtle weakness that may not have been detected on the resistance examination.

Clinicians use a five-point scale to rate muscle strength. A 5 indicates full power of contraction against gravity and resistance or normal muscle strength; 4 indicates fair but not full strength against gravity and a moderate amount of resistance or slight weakness; 3 indicates just sufficient strength to overcome the force of gravity or moderate weakness; 2 indicates the ability to move but not to overcome the force of gravity or severe weakness; 1 indicates minimal contractile power (weak muscle contraction can be palpated but no movement is noted) or very severe weakness; and 0 indicates no movement (Jarvis, 2015).

Concept Mastery Alert

When recording muscle strength, a stick figure is used as a precise form to document findings. The five-point scale is used to rate and record distal and proximal strength in both upper and lower extremities. Figure 65-12 provides further details.

Assessment of muscle strength may be as detailed as necessary. One may quickly test the strength of the proximal muscles of the upper and lower extremities, always assessing both sides by comparing one side to the other. The strength of the finer muscles that control the function of the hand (hand grasp) and the foot (dorsiflexion and plantar flexion) can then be assessed.

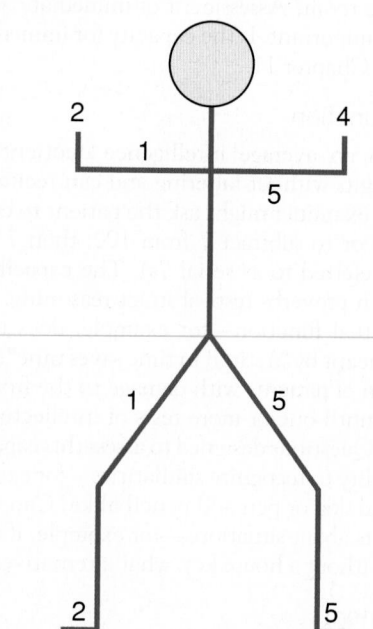

Figure 65-12 • A stick figure may be used to record muscle strength.

Balance and Coordination

Cerebellar and basal ganglia influence on the motor system is reflected in balance control and coordination. Coordination in the hands and upper extremities is tested by having the patient perform rapid, alternating movements and point-to-point testing. First, the patient is instructed to pat their thigh as fast as possible with each hand separately. Then, the patient is instructed to alternately pronate and supinate the hand as rapidly as possible. Last, the patient is asked to touch each of the fingers with the thumb in a consecutive motion. Speed, symmetry, and degree of difficulty are noted. Point-to-point testing is accomplished by having the patient touch the examiner's extended finger and then their own nose. This is repeated several times.

Coordination in the lower extremities is tested by having the patient run the heel down the anterior surface of the tibia of the other leg. Each leg is tested in turn. **Ataxia** is an incoordination of voluntary muscle action, particularly of the muscle groups used in activities such as walking or reaching for objects. Tremors (rhythmic, involuntary movements) noted at rest or during movement suggest a problem in the anatomic areas responsible for balance and coordination.

The **Romberg test** is a screening test for balance that can be done with the patient seated or standing. The patient can be seated or stand with feet together and arms at the side, first with eyes open and then with both eyes closed for 20 seconds (Bader, Littlejohns, & Olson, 2016; Weber & Kelley, 2014). The examiner stands close to support the standing patient if he or she begins to fall. Slight swaying is normal, but a loss of balance is abnormal and is considered a positive Romberg test. Additional cerebellar tests for balance in the patient who is ambulatory include hopping in place, alternating knee bends, and heel-to-toe walking (both forward and backward).

Examining the Sensory System

The sensory system is even more complex than the motor system, because sensory modalities are more widespread throughout the central and peripheral nervous systems. The sensory examination is largely subjective and requires the cooperation of the patient. The examiner should be familiar with dermatomes that represent the distribution of the peripheral nerves that arise from the spinal cord (see Fig. 65-9) (Jarvis, 2015).

Assessment of the sensory system involves tests for tactile sensation, superficial pain, temperature, vibration, and position sense (proprioception). During the sensory assessment, the patient's eyes are closed. Simple directions and reassurance that the examiner will not hurt or startle the patient encourage the cooperation of the patient.

Tactile sensation is assessed by lightly touching a cotton wisp or fingertip to corresponding areas on each side of the body. The sensitivity of proximal parts of the extremities is compared with that of distal parts, and the right and left sides are compared.

Pain and temperature sensations are transmitted together in the lateral part of the spinal cord, so it is unnecessary to test for temperature sense in most circumstances. Determining the patient's sensitivity to a sharp object can assess superficial pain perception. However, pain sensation is usually reserved for patients who do not respond to or cannot discriminate touch stimulation. The patient is asked to differentiate between the sharp and dull ends of a broken wooden cotton swab or tongue blade; using a safety pin is inadvisable because it breaks the integrity of the skin. Both the sharp and dull sides of the object are applied with equal intensity at all times, and the two sides are compared. In the patient with an altered level of consciousness alternate methods of assessing pain may need to be used (see Chart 65-2) (Arbour, Gelinas, Loiselle, et al., 2015; Poulsen, Brix, Andersen, et al., 2016).

Vibration and proprioception are transmitted together in the posterior part of the cord. Vibration may be evaluated through the use of a low-frequency (128 or 256 Hz) tuning fork. The handle of the vibrating fork is placed against a bony prominence, and the patient is asked if he or she feels a

---

Chart 65-2 — NURSING RESEARCH PROFILE

BIS Monitoring for Pain Assessment

Arbour, C., Gelinas, C., Loiselle, C. G., et al. (2015). An exploratory study of the Bilateral Bispectral Index for pain detection in traumatic brain injured patients with altered level of consciousness. *Journal of Neuroscience Nursing, 47*(3), 166–177.

Purpose

The purpose of neurologic assessment is to identify alterations in neurologic function so that interventions may be implemented in a timely manner, but accurate assessment is not always possible in patients with an altered level of consciousness. This study sought to validate the bilateral bispectral index system (BIS) for pain assessment in patients with Traumatic Brain Injury (TBI) with an altered level of consciousness.

Design

The study used a repeated measure within-subject design utilizing a convenience sample of patients with TBI. Pain behaviors and BIS readings were observed during two procedures, one being noninvasive blood pressure monitoring the other during turning. Participants were observed for 1 minute before

for a baseline, then during, and at 15 minutes after the two procedures.

Findings

The sample included 25 participants 18 years of age and older with Glasgow Coma Scores of 3 to 13 who were in ICU between 24 hours and 30 days. Stable BIS readings were found during the use of the noninvasive blood pressure monitoring. There was a significant increase in bilateral BIS from baseline during turning as well as an increase in observed pain behaviors (+3.00). However, only increased BIS readings recorded in the right hemisphere of the brain correlated with the pain behaviors of participants, those with a left-sided TBI.

Nursing Implications

More research is needed but nurses should know that there is potential for the use of bilateral BIS monitoring in the assessment of pain in patients who are nonverbal. This study provides beginning evidence that bilateral BIS has the potential for pain detection in those with a left-sided lesion.

sensation and is instructed to signal the examiner when the sensation ceases. Common locations used to test for vibratory sense include the distal joint of the great toe and the proximal thumb joint. If the patient does not perceive the vibrations at the distal bony prominences, the examiner progresses upward with the tuning fork until the patient perceives the vibrations. As with all measurements of sensation, a side-to-side comparison is made.

Position sense or proprioception may be determined by asking the patient to close both eyes and indicate, as the great toe or index finger is alternately moved up and down, in which direction movement has taken place. Vibration and position sense are often lost together, frequently in circumstances in which all other sensation remains intact.

Integration of sensation in the brain is evaluated by testing two-point discrimination. When the patient is touched with two sharp objects simultaneously, are they perceived as two or as one? If touched simultaneously on opposite sides of the body, the patient should normally report being touched in two places. If only one site is reported, the one not being recognized is said to demonstrate extinction. Another test of higher cortical sensory ability is tactile identification. The patient is instructed to close both eyes and identify an object (e.g., key, coin) that is placed in one hand by the examiner; inability to identify an object by touch is known as tactile agnosia or astereognosis. **Agnosia** is the general loss of ability to recognize objects through a particular sensory system. The patient can also be shown a familiar object and asked to identify it by name; inability to identify a visualized object is known as visual agnosia. Each of these dysfunctions implicates a different part of the brain (see Table 65-6).

Decreased or absent sensations occur with problems anywhere along the sensory pathway. Sensory deficits resulting from peripheral neuropathy or spinal cord injury follow anatomic dermatomes. Destructive lesions of the brain may affect sensation on an entire side of the body. Stroke affecting a portion of the sensory cortex will produce altered sensory discrimination.

Examining the Reflexes

Reflexes are involuntary contractions of muscles or muscle groups in response to a stimulus. Reflexes are classified as deep tendon, superficial, or pathologic. Testing reflexes enables the examiner to assess involuntary reflex arcs that depend on the presence of afferent stretch receptors, spinal or brain stem synapses, efferent motor fibers, and a variety of modifying influences from higher levels.

Deep Tendon Reflexes

A reflex hammer is used to elicit a deep tendon reflex. The handle of the hammer is held loosely between the thumb and index finger, allowing a full swinging motion. The wrist motion is similar to that used during percussion. The extremity is positioned so that the tendon is slightly stretched. This requires a sound knowledge of the location of muscles and their tendon attachments. The tendon is then struck briskly (see Fig. 65-13), and the response is compared with that on the opposite side of the body. A wide variation in reflex response may be considered normal; however, it is more important that the reflexes be symmetrically equivalent. When the comparison is made, both sides should be equivalently relaxed and each tendon struck with equal force.

Valid findings depend on several factors: proper use of the reflex hammer, proper positioning of the extremity, and a patient who is relaxed (Jarvis, 2015). If the reflexes are symmetrically diminished or absent, the examiner may use isometric contraction of other muscle groups to increase reflex activity. For example, if lower extremity reflexes are diminished or absent, the patient is instructed to lock the fingers together and pull in opposite directions. Having the patient clench the jaw or press the heels against the floor or examining table may similarly elicit more reliable biceps, triceps, and brachioradialis reflexes.

The absence of reflexes is significant, although ankle jerks (Achilles reflex) may be normally absent in older adults. Deep tendon reflex responses are often graded on a scale of 0 to 4+, with 2+ considered normal (see Chart 65-3) but scale ratings are highly subjective. Findings can be recorded as a fraction, indicating the scale range (e.g., 2/4). Some examiners prefer to use the terms *present*, *absent*, and *diminished*

TABLE 65-6 Types of Agnosia and Corresponding Sites of Lesions

Type of Agnosia	Affected Cerebral Area
Visual	Occipital lobe
Auditory	Temporal lobe (lateral and superior portions)
Tactile	Parietal lobe
Body parts and relationships	Parietal lobe (posteroinferior regions)

Chart 65-3 Documenting Reflexes

Deep tendon reflexes are graded on a scale of 0–4:

0 No response
1+ Diminished (hypoactive)
2+ Normal
3+ Increased (may be interpreted as normal)
4+ Hyperactive (hyperreflexia)

The deep tendon responses and plantar reflexes are commonly recorded on stick figures. The arrow points downward if the plantar response is normal and upward if the response is abnormal.

Figure 65-13 • Techniques for eliciting major reflexes. **A.** Eliciting the biceps reflex. **B.** Eliciting the triceps reflex. **C.** Eliciting the patellar reflex. **D.** Eliciting the Achilles reflex. Parts **A–D** from Weber, J., & Kelley, J. (2014). *Health assessment in nursing* (5th ed.). Philadelphia, PA: Lippincott Williams & Wilkins.

when describing reflexes. As with muscle strength recording, a stick figure may be used to record numerical findings.

Biceps Reflex
The biceps reflex is elicited by striking the biceps tendon over a slightly flexed elbow (see Fig. 65-13A). The examiner supports the forearm at the elbow with one arm while placing the thumb against the tendon and striking the thumb with the reflex hammer. The normal response is flexion at the elbow and contraction of the biceps.

Triceps Reflex
To elicit a triceps reflex, the patient's arm is flexed at the elbow and hanging freely at the side. The examiner supports the patient's arm and identifies the triceps tendon by palpating 2.5 to 5 cm (1 to 2 inches) above the elbow. A direct blow on the tendon (see Fig. 65-13B) normally produces contraction of the triceps muscle and extension of the elbow.

Brachioradialis Reflex
With the patient's forearm resting on the lap or across the abdomen, the brachioradialis reflex is assessed. A gentle strike of the hammer 2.5 to 5 cm (1 to 2 inches) above the wrist results in flexion and supination of the forearm (Jarvis, 2015).

Patellar Reflex
The patellar reflex is elicited by striking the patellar tendon just below the patella. The patient may be in a sitting or a lying position. If the patient is supine, the examiner supports the legs to facilitate relaxation of the muscles (see Fig. 65-13C). Contractions of the quadriceps and knee extension are normal responses.

Achilles Reflex
To elicit an Achilles reflex, the foot is dorsiflexed at the ankle and the hammer strikes the stretched Achilles tendon (see Fig. 65-13D). This reflex normally produces plantar flexion. If

the examiner cannot elicit the ankle reflex and suspects that the patient cannot relax, the patient is instructed to kneel on a chair or similar elevated, flat surface. This position places the ankles in dorsiflexion and reduces any muscle tension in the gastrocnemius. The Achilles tendons are struck in turn, and plantar flexion is usually demonstrated (Jarvis, 2015).

Clonus

When reflexes are hyperactive, a movement called **clonus** may be elicited. If the foot is abruptly dorsiflexed, it may continue to "beat" two or three times before it settles into a position of rest. Occasionally with CNS system disease, this activity persists, and the foot does not come to rest while the tendon is being stretched but persists in repetitive activity. The unsustained clonus associated with normal but hyperactive reflexes is not considered pathologic. Sustained clonus always indicates the presence of CNS disease and requires further evaluation.

Superficial Reflexes

The major superficial reflexes include corneal, palpebral, gag, upper/lower abdominal, cremasteric (men only), and perianal. These reflexes are graded differently than the motor reflexes and are noted to be present (+) or absent (–). Of these, only the corneal, gag, and plantar reflexes are commonly tested.

The corneal reflex is tested carefully using a clean wisp of cotton and lightly touching the outer corner of each eye on the sclera. The reflex is present if the action elicits a blink. A stroke or brain injury might result in loss of this reflex, either unilaterally or bilaterally. Loss of this reflex indicates the need for eye protection and possible lubrication to prevent corneal damage.

The gag reflex is elicited by gently touching the back of the pharynx with a cotton-tipped applicator, first on one side of the uvula and then the other. Positive response is an equal elevation of the uvula and "gag" with stimulation. Absent response on one or both sides can be seen following a stroke and requires careful evaluation and treatment of the resultant swallowing dysfunction to prevent aspiration of food and fluids.

Pathologic Reflexes

Pathologic reflexes are seen in the presence of neurologic disease; they often represent emergence of earlier reflexes that disappeared with maturity of the nervous system. A pathologic reflex indicative of CNS disease affecting the corticospinal tract is the **Babinski reflex (sign)**. In a person with an intact CNS, if the lateral aspect of the sole of the foot is stroked, the toes contract and draw together. However, in a person who has CNS disease of the motor system, the toes fan out and draw back (see Fig. 65-13E) (Jarvis, 2015). This is normal in newborns but represents a serious abnormality in adults. Other pathologic reflexes include the suck (sucking motions in response to touching the lips), snout (lip pursing in response to touching the lips), palmar (grasp in response to stroking the palm), and palmomental (contraction of the facial muscle in response to stimulation of the thenar eminence near the thumb) reflexes in adults. These reflexes often signify progressive nervous system degeneration (Klein & Stewart-Amidei, 2012).

Gerontologic Considerations

During the normal aging process, the nervous system undergoes many changes and is more vulnerable to illness. Age-related changes in the nervous system vary in degree and must be distinguished from those due to disease. It is important for clinicians not to attribute abnormality or dysfunction to aging without appropriate investigation. For example, although diminished strength and agility are a normal part of aging, localized weakness can only be attributed to disease.

Structural and Physiologic Changes

As the brain ages, neurons are lost, leading to a decrease in the number of synapses and neurotransmitters. This results in slowed nerve conduction and response time. Brain weight is decreased, and the ventricle size increases to maintain cranial volume. Cerebral blood flow and metabolism are reduced, leading to slower mental functions. Temperature regulation becomes less efficient. In the peripheral nervous system, myelin is lost, resulting in a decrease in conduction velocity in some nerves. Visual and auditory nerves degenerate, leading to loss of visual acuity and hearing. Taste buds atrophy, and nerve cell fibers in the olfactory bulb degenerate (Jarvis, 2015). Nerve cells in the vestibular system of the inner ear, cerebellum, and proprioceptive pathways also degenerate, leading to balance difficulties. Deep tendon reflexes can be decreased or in some cases absent. Hypothalamic function is modified such that stage IV sleep is reduced. There is an overall slowing of autonomic nervous system responses. Pupillary responses are reduced or may not appear at all in the presence of cataracts.

Motor Alterations

Reduced nerve input into muscle contributes to an overall reduction in muscle bulk, with atrophy most easily noted in the hands. Changes in motor function often result in decreased strength and agility, with increased reaction time. Gait is often slowed and wide based. These changes can create difficulties in maintaining balance, predisposing the older person to falls.

Sensory Alterations

Tactile sensation is dulled in the older adult due to a decrease in the number of sensory receptors. There may be difficulty in identifying objects by touch, because fewer tactile cues are received from the bottom of the feet and the person may become confused about body position and location (Bates & Wolbers, 2014).

Sensitivity to glare, decreased peripheral vision, and a constricted visual field occur due to degeneration of visual pathways, resulting in disorientation, especially at night when there is little or no light in the room. Because the older adult takes longer to recover visual sensitivity when moving from a light to dark area, nightlights and a safe and familiar arrangement of furniture are essential.

Loss of hearing can contribute to confusion, anxiety, disorientation, misinterpretation of the environment, feelings of inadequacy, and social isolation. A decreased sense of taste and smell may contribute to weight loss and disinterest in food. A decreased sense of smell may present a safety hazard, because older adults living alone may be unable to detect household gas leaks or fires. Smoke and carbon monoxide detectors—important in every residence—are critical for the older adult.

Temperature Regulation and Pain Perception

The older adult patient may feel cold more readily than heat and may require extra covering when in bed; a room temperature somewhat higher than usual may be desirable. Reaction to painful stimuli may be decreased with age. Because pain is an important warning signal, caution must be used when hot or cold packs are used. The older patient may be burned or suffer frostbite before being aware of any discomfort. Complaints of pain such as abdominal discomfort or chest pain may be more serious than the patient's perception might indicate and thus require careful evaluation. In older adults, two common pain syndromes that affect the neurologic system are diabetic and postherpetic neuropathies. These frequently occur due to the high rate of these comorbid conditions in older adults. See Chapter 51 for a discussion of diabetic neuropathy.

Mental Status

Although mental processing time decreases with age, memory, language, and judgment capacities remain intact. Change in mental status should never be assumed to be a normal part of aging. **Delirium** is an acute confused state that begins with disorientation and if not recognized and treated early can progress to changes in level of consciousness, irreversible brain damage, and sometimes death. Older age is a risk, but delirium is also seen in patients who have underlying CNS damage or are experiencing an acute condition such as infection, adverse medication reaction, or dehydration. Drug toxicity and depression may produce impairment of attention and memory and should be evaluated as a possible cause of mental status change. The Confusion Assessment Method (CAM) is a commonly used screening tool (Inouye, van Dyck, Alessi, et al., 1990; Layne, Haas, Davidson, et al., 2015) (see Chapter 11, Chart 11-7). Delirium must be differentiated from dementia, which is a chronic and irreversible deterioration of cognitive status. See Chapter 11, Table 11-3 for further discussion of delirium and dementia.

Nursing Implications

Nursing care for patients with age-related changes to the nervous system and for patients with long-term neurologic disability who are aging should include the modifications described previously. In addition, the consequences of any neurologic deficit and its impact on overall function such as activities of daily living, the use of assistive devices, and individual coping should be assessed and considered in planning patient care. Fall risk must be evaluated and fall prevention measures instituted for the patient who is hospitalized as well as in the home.

The nurse must understand the altered responses and the changing needs of the older adult patient before providing education. Visual and hearing deficits require adaptations in activities such as preoperative education, diet therapy, and education about new medications. When using visual materials for education or menu selection, adequate lighting without glare, contrasting colors, and large print are used to offset visual difficulties caused by rigidity and opacity of the lens in the eye and slower pupillary reaction. Procedures and preparations needed for diagnostic tests are explained, taking into account the possibility of impaired hearing and slowed responses in the older adult. Even with hearing loss, the older adult patient often hears adequately if the speaker uses a low-pitched, clear voice; shouting only makes it harder for the patient to understand the speaker. Providing auditory and visual cues aids understanding; if the patient has a significant hearing or visual loss, assistive devices, a signer, an interpreter, or a translator may be needed.

Providing instruction at an unrushed pace and using reinforcement enhance learning and retention. Material should be short, concise, and concrete. Vocabulary is matched to the patient's ability, and terms are clearly defined. The older adult patient requires adequate time to receive and respond to stimuli, learn, and react. These measures allow comprehension, memory, and formation of association and concepts.

Diagnostic Evaluation

A wide range of diagnostic studies may be performed in patients with altered neurologic function. The nurse should educate the patient about the purpose, what to expect, and any possible side effects related to these examinations prior to testing. Women who are premenopausal are advised to practice effective contraception before and for several days after any diagnostic procedure using contrast, and the woman who is breast-feeding is instructed to stop for the time period recommended by the nuclear medicine department (Pagana & Pagana, 2013). The nurse should note trends in results, because they provide information about disease progression as well as the patient's response to therapy.

Computed Tomography Scanning

Computed tomography (CT) scanning uses a narrow x-ray beam to scan body parts in successive layers. The images provide cross-sectional views of the brain, distinguishing differences in tissue densities of the skull, cortex, subcortical structures, and ventricles. An intravenous (IV) contrast agent may be used to highlight differences further. The brightness of each slice of the brain in the final image is proportional to the degree to which it absorbs x-rays. The image is displayed on an oscilloscope or television monitor and is photographed and stored digitally (Fischbach & Dunning, 2015). CT scanning is usually performed first without contrast material and then with IV contrast, if needed. The patient lies on an adjustable table with the head in a headrest while the scanning system rotates around the head and produces cross-sectional images. The patient must lie with the head held perfectly still without talking or moving the face, because head motion distorts the image. CT scanning is quick and painless and uses a small amount of radiation to produce images; it has a high degree of sensitivity for detecting lesions.

Brain lesions have a different tissue density from the surrounding normal brain tissue. Abnormalities detected on brain CT include tumor or other masses, infarction, hemorrhage, displacement of the ventricles, and cortical atrophy (Fischbach & Dunning, 2015). CT angiography allows visualization of blood vessels; in some situations, this eliminates the need for formal angiography. Whole-body CT scanners allow cross-sections of the spinal cord to be visualized. The injection of a water-soluble iodinated contrast agent into the subarachnoid space through lumbar puncture improves the visualization of the spinal and intracranial contents on these images. The CT scan, along with magnetic resonance imaging (MRI), has largely replaced myelography as a diagnostic procedure for the diagnosis of herniated lumbar discs.

Nursing Interventions

Essential nursing interventions include preparation for the procedure and patient monitoring. Preparation includes educating the patient about the need to lie quietly throughout the procedure. A review of relaxation techniques may be helpful for patients with claustrophobia. Sedation can be used if agitation, restlessness, or confusion interferes with a successful study. Ongoing patient monitoring during sedation is necessary. If a contrast agent is used, the patient must be assessed before the CT scan for an iodine/shellfish allergy, because the contrast agent used may be iodine based. Kidney function must also be evaluated because the contrast material is cleared through the kidneys. A suitable IV line for contrast injection and a period of fasting (usually 4 hours) are required prior to the study. Patients who receive an IV contrast agent are monitored during and after the procedure for allergic reactions and changes in kidney function (Fischbach & Dunning, 2015). Fluid intake is also encouraged after IV contrast to facilitate contrast clearance through the kidney.

Magnetic Resonance Imaging

MRI uses a powerful magnetic field to obtain images of different areas of the body. The magnetic field causes the hydrogen nuclei (protons) within the body to align like small magnets in a magnetic field. In combination with radiofrequency pulses, the protons emit signals, which are converted to images. An MRI scan can be performed with or without a contrast agent and can identify a cerebral abnormality earlier and more clearly than other diagnostic tests (Fischbach & Dunning, 2015). It can provide information about the chemical changes within cells, allowing the clinician to monitor a tumor's response to treatment. It is particularly useful in the diagnosis of brain tumor, stroke, and multiple sclerosis and does not involve ionizing radiation. An MRI scan may take an hour or longer to complete, so its use in emergency situations is limited.

Several MRI applications allow imaging of brain blood flow and metabolism via special imaging techniques added to the MRI. Such techniques include diffusion-weighted imaging (DWI), perfusion-weighted imaging (PWI), magnetic resonance spectroscopy, and fluid attenuation inversion recovery (FLAIR) (Fischbach & Dunning, 2015). Magnetic resonance angiography (MRA) allows separate visualization of the cerebral vasculature without the administration of an arterial contrast agent. Both MRI and CT images are used as tools to plan and direct surgical intervention.

Nursing Interventions

Patient preparation includes providing education and obtaining an adequate history. Ferromagnetic substances in the body may become dislodged by the magnet, so history of working with metal fragments must be reviewed. The patient is questioned about any implants of any metal objects (e.g., aneurysm clips, orthopedic hardware, pacemakers, artificial heart valves, intrauterine devices). These objects could malfunction, be dislodged, or heat up as they absorb energy. Cochlear implants will be inactivated by MRI; therefore, other imaging procedures are considered. A complete list of metal compatibility may be found on MRI manufacturer Web sites.

Before the patient enters the room where the MRI is to be performed, all metal objects and credit cards (the magnetic field can erase them) must be removed. This includes medication patches that have a metal backing and metallic lead wires; these can cause burns if not removed (Fischbach & Dunning, 2015). No metal objects may be brought into the room where the MRI is located; this includes oxygen tanks, IV poles, ventilators, or even stethoscopes. The magnetic field generated by the unit is so strong that any metal-containing items will be strongly attracted and literally can be pulled away with such force that they fly like projectiles toward the magnet. There is a risk of severe injury and death. Further, damage to expensive equipment may occur.

> ⚑ **Quality and Safety Nursing Alert**
>
> For patient safety, the nurse prevents any patient care equipment containing metal or metal parts (e.g., portable oxygen tanks) from entering the room where the MRI is located. The nurse also assesses the patient for the presence of medication patches with foil backing (such as nicotine patches) that may cause a burn while an MRI scan is being performed.

For the MRI, the patient lies with the head in a frame on a flat platform that is moved into a tube housing the magnet (see Fig. 65-14). The tube is narrow; persons with a wide girth may not fit into the scanner. Patients who are unable to lie flat will not be able to tolerate an MRI. The scanning process is painless, but the patient hears loud thumping of the magnetic coils as the magnetic field is being pulsed. Patients may experience claustrophobia while inside the narrow tube; sedation may be prescribed in these circumstances. "Open" MRI machines are less claustrophobic than the other devices

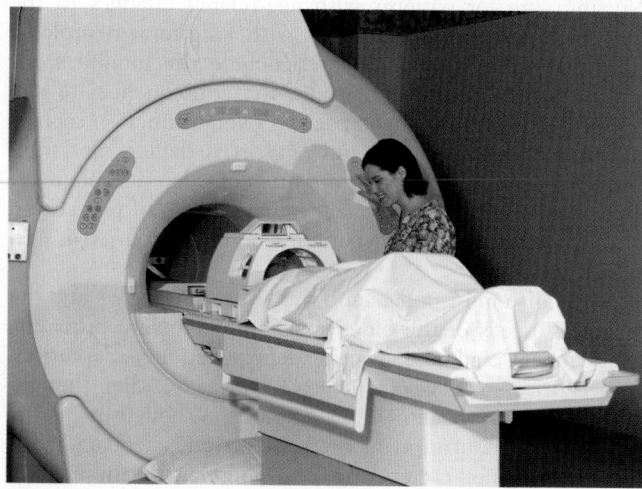

Figure 65-14 • Technician explains what to expect during a magnetic resonance imaging procedure.

and are available in many locations. However, the images produced on these machines are sometimes not so detailed, and traditional devices are preferred for accurate diagnosis. The patient may be educated about the use of relaxation techniques while in the scanner. The patient is informed that he or she will be able to talk to the staff during the scan through a microphone inside the scanner (Fischbach & Dunning, 2015).

Positron Emission Tomography

PET is a computer-based nuclear imaging technique that produces images of actual organ functioning. The patient either inhales a radioactive gas or is injected with a radioactive substance that emits positively charged particles. When these positrons combine with negatively charged electrons (normally found in the body's cells), the resultant gamma rays can be detected by a scanning device that produces a series of two-dimensional views at various levels of the brain. This information is integrated by a computer and gives a composite picture of the brain at work.

PET permits the measurement of blood flow, tissue composition, and brain metabolism and thus indirectly evaluates brain function. The brain is one of the most metabolically active organs, consuming 80% of the glucose the body uses (Bader et al., 2016). PET measures this activity in specific areas of the brain and can detect changes in glucose use.

PET is useful in showing metabolic changes in the brain (Alzheimer disease), locating lesions (brain tumor, epileptogenic lesions), identifying blood flow and oxygen metabolism in patients with strokes, distinguishing tumor from areas of necrosis, and revealing biochemical abnormalities associated with mental illness. The isotopes used have a very short half-life and are expensive to produce, requiring specialized equipment for production. Improvement in the scanning procedure and production of isotopes, as well as the advent of reimbursement by third-party payers, has increased the clinical applications of PET studies.

Nursing Interventions

Key nursing interventions include patient preparation, which involves explaining the test and educating the patient about inhalation techniques and the sensations (e.g., dizziness, lightheadedness, and headache) that may occur. The IV injection of the radioactive substance produces similar side effects. Relaxation exercises may reduce anxiety during the test.

Single-Photon Emission Computed Tomography

SPECT is a three-dimensional imaging technique that uses radionuclides and instruments to detect single photons. It is a perfusion study that captures a moment of cerebral blood flow at the time of injection of a radionuclide. Gamma photons are emitted from a radiopharmaceutical agent given to the patient and are detected by a rotating gamma camera or cameras; the image is sent to a minicomputer. This approach allows areas behind overlying structures or background to be viewed, greatly increasing the contrast between normal and abnormal tissue. It is relatively inexpensive, and the duration is similar to that of a CT scan.

SPECT is useful in detecting the extent and location of abnormally perfused areas of the brain, thus allowing detection, localization, and sizing of stroke (before it is visible by CT scan); localization of seizure foci in epilepsy; detection of tumor progression (Fischbach & Dunning, 2015); and evaluation of perfusion before and after neurosurgical procedures.

Nursing Interventions

The nursing interventions for SPECT primarily include patient preparation and patient monitoring. Providing education about what to expect before the test can allay anxiety and ensure patient cooperation during the test. Pregnancy and breast-feeding are contraindications to SPECT.

The nurse may need to accompany and monitor the patient during transport to the nuclear medicine department for the scan. Patients are monitored during and after the procedure for allergic reactions to the radiopharmaceutical agent.

Cerebral Angiography

Cerebral angiography is an x-ray study of the cerebral circulation with a contrast agent injected into a selected artery. A valuable tool in investigating vascular disease or anomalies, it is used to determine vessel patency, identify presence of collateral circulation, and provide detail on vascular anomalies that can be used in planning interventions. With the advent of additional imaging techniques, formal cerebral angiography is less frequently performed.

Cerebral angiograms are performed by threading a catheter through the femoral artery in the groin and up to the desired vessel. Alternatively, direct puncture of the carotid artery may be performed. X-ray images are obtained as the contrast agent flows through the vessels; the carotid and vertebral arterial systems are visualized, as well as venous drainage. Arterial access may also be used for interventional procedures, such as placing coils in an aneurysm or arteriovenous malformation.

Nursing Interventions

Prior to the angiography, the patient's blood urea nitrogen and creatinine should be checked to ensure the kidneys will be able to excrete the contrast agent. The patient should be well hydrated, and clear liquids are usually permitted up to the time of the test. The patient is instructed to void immediately before the test, and locations of the appropriate peripheral pulses are marked with a felt-tip pen. The patient is instructed to remain immobile during the angiogram process and is told to expect a brief feeling of warmth in the face, behind the eyes, or in the jaw, teeth, tongue, and lips, and a metallic taste when the contrast agent is injected.

After the hair in the groin is clipped and prepared, a local anesthetic agent is given to minimize pain at the insertion site and to reduce arterial spasm. A catheter is introduced into the femoral artery, flushed with heparinized saline, and filled with contrast agent. Fluoroscopy is used to guide the catheter to the appropriate vessels. Neurologic assessment is conducted during and immediately following cerebral angiography to observe for embolism or arterial dissection that may occur during the test. Signs of these complications include new onset of alterations in the level of consciousness, weakness on one side of the body, motor or sensory deficits, and speech disturbances.

Nursing care after cerebral angiography includes observation of the injection site for bleeding or hematoma formation (a localized collection of blood). Because a hematoma at the puncture site or embolization to a distal artery affects peripheral pulses, the peripheral pulses that were marked prior to the test are monitored frequently. The color and temperature of the involved extremity are assessed to detect possible embolism (Fischbach & Dunning, 2015). Fluids are encouraged to facilitate clearance of the contrast through the kidney. The nurse also monitors for an allergic reaction to the contrast agent.

Myelography

A myelogram is an x-ray of the spinal subarachnoid space taken after the injection of a contrast agent into the spinal subarachnoid space through a lumbar puncture. The water-based contrast agent disperses upward through the CSF to outline the spinal subarachnoid space and shows any distortion of the spinal cord or spinal dural sac caused by tumors, cysts, herniated vertebral discs, or other lesions. Myelography is performed infrequently today because of the sensitivity of CT and MRI scanning (Fischbach & Dunning, 2015).

Nursing Interventions

The patient is educated about what to expect during the procedure and made aware that changes in position may be made during the procedure. After myelography, the patient lies in bed with the head of the bed elevated 30 to 45 degrees. The patient is advised to remain in bed in the recommended position for 3 hours or as prescribed. Drinking liberal amounts of fluid for rehydration and replacement of CSF may decrease the incidence of post–lumbar puncture headache. The blood pressure, pulse, respiratory rate, and temperature are monitored, as well as the patient's ability to void. Untoward signs include headache, fever, stiff neck, photophobia (sensitivity to light), seizures, and signs of chemical or bacterial meningitis (Hickey, 2014).

Noninvasive Carotid Flow Studies

Noninvasive carotid flow studies use ultrasound imagery and Doppler measurements of arterial blood flow to evaluate carotid and deep orbital circulation. The graph produced indicates blood velocity. Increased blood velocity can indicate stenosis or partial obstruction. These tests are often obtained before more invasive tests such as arteriography or are used as screening tools. Carotid Doppler, carotid ultrasonography, oculoplethysmography, and ophthalmodynamometry are four common noninvasive vascular techniques that permit evaluation of arterial blood flow and detection of arterial stenosis, occlusion, and plaques. These vascular studies allow noninvasive imaging of extra- and intracranial circulation (Fischbach & Dunning, 2015).

Transcranial Doppler

Transcranial Doppler uses the same noninvasive techniques as carotid flow studies but records the blood flow velocities of the intracranial vessels. Arterial flow velocities can be measured through thin areas of the temporal and occipital bones of the skull. A handheld Doppler probe emits a pulsed beam; the signal is reflected by the moving red blood cells within the blood vessels. Transcranial Doppler is a noninvasive technique that is helpful in assessing vasospasm (a complication following subarachnoid hemorrhage), altered cerebral blood flow found in occlusive vascular disease, other cerebral pathology, and brain death.

Nursing Interventions

When a carotid flow study or transcranial Doppler is scheduled, the procedure is described to the patient. The patient is informed that this is a noninvasive test, that a handheld transducer will be placed over the neck and the orbits of the eyes, and that a water-soluble gel or lubricant is used on the transducer (Fischbach & Dunning, 2015). Either of these two low-risk tests can be performed at the patient's bedside.

Electroencephalography

An electroencephalogram (EEG) represents a record of the electrical activity generated in the brain (Hickey, 2014). It is obtained through electrodes applied on the scalp or through microelectrodes placed within the brain tissue. It provides an assessment of cerebral electrical activity. It is useful for diagnosing and evaluating seizure disorders, coma, or organic brain syndrome. Tumors, brain abscesses, blood clots, and infection may cause abnormal patterns in electrical activity. The EEG is also used in making a determination of brain death.

Electrodes are applied to the scalp to record the electrical activity in various regions of the brain. The amplified activity of the neurons between any two of these electrodes is recorded on continuously moving paper; this record is called the *encephalogram*.

For a baseline recording, the patient lies quietly with both eyes closed. The patient may be asked to hyperventilate for 3 to 4 minutes or to look at a bright, flashing light for photic stimulation. These activation procedures are performed to evoke abnormal electrical discharges, such as seizure potentials. A sleep EEG may be recorded after sedation because some abnormal brain waves are seen only when the patient is asleep. If the epileptogenic area is inaccessible to conventional scalp electrodes, nasopharyngeal electrodes may be used.

Depth recording of EEG is performed by introducing electrodes stereotactically (radiologically placed using instrumentation) into a target area of the brain, as indicated by the patient's seizure pattern and scalp EEG. It is used to identify patients who may benefit from surgical excision of epileptogenic foci. Special transsphenoidal, mandibular, and nasopharyngeal electrodes can be used, and video recording combined with EEG monitoring and telemetry is used in hospital settings to capture epileptiform abnormalities and their sequelae. Some epilepsy centers provide long-term ambulatory EEG monitoring with portable recording devices (Bader et al., 2016).

Nursing Interventions

To increase the chances of recording seizure activity, it is sometimes recommended that the patient be deprived of sleep the night before the EEG. Anticonvulsant agents, tranquilizers, stimulants, and depressants should be withheld 24 to 48 hours before an EEG, because these medications can alter the EEG wave patterns or mask the abnormal wave patterns of seizure disorders (Pagana & Pagana, 2013).

Coffee, tea, chocolate, and cola drinks are omitted from the meal before the test because of their stimulating effect. However, the meal itself is not omitted, because an altered blood glucose level can cause changes in brain wave patterns.

The patient is informed that the standard EEG takes 45 to 60 minutes; a sleep EEG requires 12 hours. The patient is assured that the procedure does not cause an electric shock and that the EEG is a diagnostic test, not a form of treatment. An EEG requires the patient to lie quietly during the test. Sedation is not advisable, because it may lower the seizure threshold in patients with a seizure disorder and it alters brain wave activity in all patients. The nurse needs to check the prescription regarding the administration of anticonvulsant medication prior to testing.

Routine EEGs use a water-soluble lubricant for electrode contact, which can be wiped off and removed by shampooing later. Sleep EEGs involve the use of collodion glue for electrode contact, which requires acetone for removal.

Electromyography

An electromyogram (EMG) is obtained by inserting needle electrodes into the skeletal muscles to measure changes in the electrical potential of the muscles (Pagana & Pagana, 2013). The electrical potentials are shown on an oscilloscope and amplified so that both the sound and appearance of the waves can be analyzed and compared simultaneously.

An EMG is useful in determining the presence of neuromuscular disorders and myopathies. It helps distinguish weakness due to neuropathy (functional or pathologic changes in the peripheral nervous system) from weakness resulting from other causes.

Nursing Interventions

The procedure is explained, and the patient is warned to expect a sensation similar to that of an intramuscular injection as the needle is inserted into the muscle. The muscles examined may ache for a short time after the procedure.

Nerve Conduction Studies

Nerve conduction studies are performed by stimulating a peripheral nerve at several points along its course and recording the muscle action potential or the sensory action potential that results. Surface or needle electrodes are placed on the skin over the nerve to stimulate the nerve fibers. This test is useful in the study of peripheral neuropathies and is often included as part of the EMG.

Evoked Potential Studies

Evoked potential studies involve application of an external stimulus to specific peripheral sensory receptors with subsequent measurement of the electrical potential generated. Electrical changes are detected with the aid of computerized devices that extract the signal, display it on an oscilloscope, and store the data on magnetic tape or disc. In neurologic diagnosis, they reflect nerve conduction times in the peripheral nervous system. In clinical practice, the visual, auditory, and somatosensory systems are most often tested.

In visual evoked responses, the patient looks at a visual stimulus (flashing lights, a checkerboard pattern on a screen).

The average of several hundred stimuli is recorded by EEG leads placed over the occipital lobe. The transit time from the retina to the occipital area is measured using computer-averaging methods.

Brainstem auditory evoked responses (BAERs) are measured by applying an auditory stimulus (repetitive auditory click) and measuring the transit time via the brain stem into the cortex. Specific lesions in the auditory pathway modify or delay the response. BAERs may be used in the diagnosis of brain stem abnormalities and in determination of brain death.

In somatosensory evoked responses (SERs), the peripheral nerves are stimulated (electrical stimulation through skin electrodes) and the transit time along the spinal cord to the cortex is measured and recorded from scalp electrodes. SERs are used to detect deficits in spinal cord or peripheral nerve conduction and to monitor spinal cord function during surgical procedures. It is also useful in the diagnosis of demyelinating diseases, such as multiple sclerosis and polyneuropathies, where nerve conduction is slowed.

Nursing Interventions

The nurse explains the procedure and reassures the patient and encourages him or her to relax. The patient is advised to remain perfectly still throughout the recording to prevent artifacts (signals not generated by the brain) that interfere with the recording and interpretation of the test.

Lumbar Puncture and Examination of Cerebrospinal Fluid

A lumbar puncture (spinal tap) is carried out by inserting a needle into the lumbar subarachnoid space to withdraw CSF. The test may be performed to obtain CSF for examination, to measure and reduce CSF pressure, to determine the presence or absence of blood in the CSF, and to administer medications intrathecally (into the spinal canal).

The needle is usually inserted into the subarachnoid space between the third and fourth or fourth and fifth lumbar vertebrae. Because the spinal cord ends at the first lumbar vertebra, insertion of the needle below the level of the third lumbar vertebra prevents puncture of the spinal cord.

A successful lumbar puncture requires that the patient be relaxed; a patient who is anxious is tense, and this may increase the pressure reading. CSF pressure with the patient in a lateral recumbent position is normally 80 to 100 mm H_2O or 8 to 14 Hg (Hickey, 2014).

A lumbar puncture may be risky in the presence of an intracranial mass lesion because intraspinal pressure is decreased by removal of CSF, and the brain may herniate downward through the foramen magnum. Chart 65-4 provides instructions for assisting with a lumbar puncture.

Cerebrospinal Fluid Analysis

The CSF should be clear and colorless. Pink, blood-tinged, or grossly bloody CSF may indicate a subarachnoid hemorrhage. The CSF may be bloody initially because of local trauma but becomes clearer as more fluid is drained. Specimens are obtained for cell count, culture, glucose, protein, and other tests as indicated. The specimens should be sent to the laboratory immediately because changes will take place and alter the result if the specimens are allowed to stand. See

Chart 65-4 Assisting With a Lumbar Puncture

A needle is inserted into the subarachnoid space through the third and fourth or fourth and fifth lumbar interface to withdraw spinal fluid.

Preprocedure

1. Determine whether written consent for the procedure has been obtained.
2. Explain the procedure to the patient, and describe sensations that are likely during the procedure (i.e., a sensation of cold as the site is cleansed with solution, a needle prick when local anesthetic agent is injected).
3. Determine whether the patient has any questions or misconceptions about the procedure; reassure the patient that the needle will not enter the spinal cord or cause paralysis.
4. Instruct the patient to void before the procedure.

Procedure

1. The patient is positioned on one side at the edge of the bed or examining table with the back toward the physician; the thighs and legs are flexed as much as possible to increase the space between the spinous processes of the vertebrae, for easier entry into the subarachnoid space.

2. A small pillow may be placed under the patient's head to maintain the spine in a horizontal position; a pillow may be placed between the legs to prevent the upper leg from rolling forward.
3. The nurse assists the patient to maintain the position to avoid sudden movement, which can produce a traumatic (bloody) tap.

4. The patient is encouraged to relax and is instructed to breathe normally, because hyperventilation may lower an elevated pressure.
5. The nurse describes the procedure step by step to the patient as it proceeds.
6. The physician cleanses the puncture site with an antiseptic agent solution and drapes the site.
7. The physician injects local anesthetic agent to numb the puncture site and then inserts a spinal needle into the subarachnoid space through the third and fourth or fourth and fifth lumbar interspace. A pressure reading may be obtained.
8. A specimen of cerebrospinal fluid (CSF) is removed and usually collected in three test tubes, labeled in order of collection. The needle is withdrawn.
9. The physician applies a small dressing to the puncture site.
10. The tubes of CSF are sent to the laboratory immediately.

Third lumbar vertebra
Dura mater
Subarachnoid space
Cauda equina

Postprocedure

1. Instruct the patient to lie prone to separate the alignment of the dural and arachnoid needle punctures in the meninges, to reduce leakage of CSF.
2. Monitor the patient for complications of lumbar puncture; notify primary provider if complications occur.
3. Encourage increased fluid intake to reduce the risk of postprocedure headache.

Table A-5 in Appendix A on {thepoint icon} for the normal values of CSF.

Post–Lumbar Puncture Headache

A post–lumbar puncture headache, ranging from mild to severe, may occur a few hours to several days after the procedure. It is a throbbing bifrontal or occipital headache that is dull and deep in character. It is particularly severe on sitting or standing but lessens or disappears when the patient lies down.

The headache is caused by CSF leakage at the puncture site. The fluid continues to escape into the tissues by way of the needle track from the spinal canal. As a result of a leak, the supply of CSF in the cranium is depleted to a point at which it is insufficient to maintain proper mechanical stabi-

lization of the brain. When the patient assumes an upright position, tension and stretching of the venous sinuses and pain-sensitive structures occur.

Post–lumbar puncture headache may be avoided if a small-gauge needle is used and if the patient remains prone after the procedure. The patient is positioned supine for 4 to 8 hours (Hickey, 2014). A postpuncture headache is usually managed by bed rest, analgesic agents, and hydration.

Other Complications of Lumbar Puncture

Herniation of the intracranial contents, spinal epidural abscess, spinal epidural hematoma, and meningitis are rare but serious complications of lumbar puncture. Other complications include temporary voiding problems, slight elevation of temperature, backache or spasms, and stiffness of the neck.

Promoting Home, Community-Based, and Transitional Care

 Educating Patients About Self-Care

Many diagnostic tests that were once performed as part of a hospital stay are now carried out in short-procedure units or outpatient testing settings or units. As a result, family members often provide the postprocedure care. Therefore, the patient and family must receive adequate education about precautions to take after the procedure, complications to watch for, and steps to take if complications occur. Because many patients undergoing neurologic diagnostic studies are older adults or have neurologic deficits, provisions must be made to ensure that transportation, postprocedure care, and appropriate monitoring are available.

Continuing and Transitional Care

Contacting the patient and family after diagnostic testing enables the nurse to determine whether they have any questions about the procedure or whether the patient had any untoward results. Education is reinforced and the patient and family are reminded to make and keep follow-up appointments. Patients, family members, and health care providers are focused on the immediate needs, issues, or deficits that necessitated the diagnostic testing.

CRITICAL THINKING EXERCISES

1 **pq** Identify the priorities, approach, and techniques you would use to perform a neurologic assessment on a 82-year-old patient with confusion. How will your priorities, approach, and techniques differ if the patient has a visual impairment, is hard of hearing, or has lower extremity weakness?

2 **ebp** A 40-year-old patient is scheduled for an electroencephalogram (EEG). What resources would you use to identify the current guidelines for EEG ? What is the evidence base for these practices? Identify the criteria used to evaluate the strength of the evidence for these practices.

3 A 35-year-old female patient is having a lumbar puncture at the bedside. Identify the nursing interventions indicated before, during, and after the procedure. What patient education is indicated? How will your nursing interventions and patient education change if the patient is pregnant or lactating?

REFERENCES

*Asterisk indicates nursing research.
**Double asterisk indicates classic reference

Books

Bader, M., Littlejohns, L. R., & Olson, D. (2016). *AANN core curriculum for neuroscience nursing* (6th ed.). Chicago, IL: American Association of Neuroscience Nurses.

Fischbach, F. T., & Dunning, M. B. (2015). *Nurse's quick reference to common laboratory and diagnostic tests* (6th ed.). Philadelphia, PA: Lippincott Williams & Wilkins.

**Herndon, R. M. (2006). *Handbook of neurologic rating scales* (2nd ed.). New York: Demos Medical Publishing.

Hickey, J. (2014). *Clinical practice of neurological and neurosurgical nursing* (6th ed.). Philadelphia, PA: Lippincott Williams & Wilkins.

Hickey, J. V. (2014). *The clinical practice of neurological and neurosurgical nursing* (7th ed.). Philadelphia, PA: Wolters Kluwer Health/Lippincott Williams & Wilkins.

Jarvis, C. (2015). *Physical examination and health assessment* (7th ed.). Philadelphia, PA: Saunders.

Klein, D. G., & Stewart-Amidei, C. (2012). Nervous system alterations. In M. L. Sole, D. G. Klein, & M. J. Moseley (Eds.). *Introduction to critical care nursing* (6th ed.). St. Louis, MO: Elsevier Saunders.

Pagana, K. D., & Pagana, T. J. (2013). *Manual of diagnostic and laboratory tests* (5th ed.). St. Louis, MO: Mosby Elsevier.

Porth, C. M. (2014). *Essentials of pathophysiology* (4th ed.). Philadelphia, PA: Lippincott Williams & Wilkins.

**Posner, J. B., Saper, C. B., Schiff, N. D., et al. (2007). *Plum and Posner's diagnosis of stupor and coma* (4th ed.). Oxford, UK: Oxford University Press.

Weber, J., & Kelley, J. (2014). *Health assessment in nursing* (5th ed.). Philadelphia, PA: Lippincott Williams & Wilkins.

Journals and Electronic Documents

*Arbour, C., Gelinas, C., Loiselle, C. G., et al. (2015). An exploratory study of the Bilateral Bispectral Index for pain detection in traumatic brain injured patients with altered level of consciousness. *Journal of Neuroscience Nursing, 47*(3), 166–177.

Bates, S. L., & Wolbers, T. (2014). How cognitive aging affects multisensory integration of navigational cues. *Neurobiology of Aging, 35*(12), 2761–2767.

**Inouye, S. K., van Dyck, C. H., Alessi, C. A., et al. (1990). Clarifying confusion: The confusion assessment method. *Annals of Internal Medicine, 113*(12), 941–948.

Layne, T., Haas, S. A., Davidson, J. E., et al. (2015). Postoperative delirium prevention in the older adult: An evidence-based process improvement project. *MedSurg Nursing, 24*(4), 256–263.

Poulsen, I., Brix, P., Andersen, S., et al. (2016). Pain assessment scale for patients with disorders of consciousness: A preliminary validation study. *Journal of Neuroscience Nursing, 48*(3), 124–131.

Resources

American Headache Society, www.americanheadachesociety.org
Brain Injury Association of America, www.biausa.org
Brain Trauma Foundation, www.braintrauma.org
Epilepsy Foundation, www.epilepsy.com
Harvard Health Publications, Harvard Medical School Office of Public Affairs, www.health.harvard.edu/diagnostic-tests/#brain
National Headache Foundation, www.headaches.org

66 Management of Patients With Neurologic Dysfunction

LEARNING OBJECTIVES

On completion of this chapter, the learner will be able to:

1 Describe the causes, clinical manifestations, and medical management of various neurologic dysfunctions.
2 Use the nursing process as a framework for care of the multiple needs of the patient with altered level of consciousness.
3 Identify the early and late clinical manifestations of increased intracranial pressure.
4 Apply the nursing process as a framework for care of the patient with increased intracranial pressure.
5 Compare and contrast the indications for intracranial or transsphenoidal surgery.
6 Use the nursing process as a framework for care of the patient undergoing intracranial or transsphenoidal surgery.
7 Explain the various types and causes of seizures and develop a plan of care for the patient experiencing seizures.
8 Recognize the causes, clinical manifestations, and medical and nursing management of the patient experiencing various types of headaches.

GLOSSARY

akinetic mutism: unresponsiveness to the environment; the patient makes no movement or sound but sometimes opens the eyes

altered level of consciousness (LOC): when a patient is not oriented, does not follow commands, or needs persistent stimuli to achieve a state of alertness

brain death: irreversible loss of all functions of the entire brain, including the brainstem

coma: prolonged state of unconsciousness

craniectomy: a surgical procedure that involves removal of a portion of the skull

craniotomy: a surgical procedure that involves entry into the cranial vault

Cushing's response: the brain's attempt to restore blood flow by increasing arterial pressure to overcome the increased intracranial pressure

decerebration: an abnormal body posture associated with a severe brain injury, characterized by extreme extension of the upper and lower extremities

decortication: an abnormal posture associated with severe brain injury, characterized by abnormal flexion of the upper extremities and extension of the lower extremities

epilepsy: at least two unprovoked seizures occurring more than 24 hours apart

herniation: abnormal protrusion of tissue through a defect or natural opening

intracranial pressure (ICP): pressure exerted by the volume of the intracranial contents within the cranial vault

locked-in syndrome: condition resulting from a lesion in the pons in which the patient lacks all distal motor activity (paralysis) but cognition is intact

migraine: a severe, unrelenting headache often accompanied by symptoms such as nausea, vomiting, and visual disturbances

minimally conscious state: a state in which the patient demonstrates awareness but cannot communicate thoughts or feelings

Monro–Kellie hypothesis: theory that states that due to limited space for expansion within the skull, an increase in any one of the cranial contents—brain tissue, blood, or cerebrospinal fluid (CSF)—causes a change in the volume of the others; also referred to as Monro–Kellie doctrine

persistent vegetative state: condition in which the patient is wakeful but devoid of conscious content, without cognitive or affective mental function

primary headache: a headache for which no specific organic cause can be found

secondary headache: headache identified as a symptom of another organic disorder (e.g., brain tumor, hypertension)

seizures: paroxysmal transient disturbance of the brain resulting from a discharge of abnormal electrical activity

status epilepticus: episode in which the patient experiences multiple seizures with no recovery time in between

transsphenoidal: surgical approach to the pituitary via the sphenoid sinuses

This chapter presents an overview of care of the patient with an altered level of consciousness (LOC); the patient with increased intracranial pressure (ICP); and the patient who is undergoing neurosurgical procedures, experiencing seizures, or experiencing headaches. Some of the disorders in this chapter, such as headaches and seizures, may be symptoms of dysfunction in another body system. Alternatively, headaches and seizures can be symptoms of a disruption of the neurologic system. These disorders can also be diagnosed at times as "idiopathic," or without an identifiable cause.

The commonalities of these disorders are often the behaviors and needs of the patient and the approaches nurses use to support the patient.

The central nervous system (CNS) contains a vast network of neurons that control the body's vital functions. However, this system is vulnerable, and its optimal function depends on several key factors. First, the neurologic system relies on its structural integrity for support and homeostasis, but this integrity may be disrupted. Examples of structural disruption include head injury, brain tumor, intracranial hemorrhage, infection, and stroke. As brain tissue expands in the inflexible cranium, **intracranial pressure (ICP)** (pressure exerted by the volume of the intracranial contents within the cranial vault) rises, and cerebral perfusion is impaired. Further expansion places pressure on vital centers, which can cause permanent neurologic deficits or lead to brain death.

Second, the neurologic system relies on the body's ability to maintain a homeostatic environment. It requires the delivery of the essential elements of oxygen and glucose, as well as filtration of substrates that are toxic to the neurons. The functions of the neurologic system may be decreased or absent because of the effect of toxic substrates or the body's inability to provide essential substrates. Sepsis, hypovolemia, myocardial infarction, cardiopulmonary arrest, hypoglycemia, electrolyte imbalance, drug and/or alcohol overdose, encephalopathy, and ketoacidosis are examples of such circumstances. Some conditions can be treated and reversed; others result in permanent neurologic deficits and disabilities.

Although the specialty of neuroscience nursing requires an understanding of neuroanatomy, neurophysiology, neurodiagnostic testing, critical care nursing, and rehabilitation nursing, nurses in all settings care for patients with neurologic disorders (Hickey, 2014). Ongoing assessment of the patient's neurologic function and health needs, identification of problems, mutual goal setting, development and implementation of care plans (including education, counseling, and coordinating activities), and evaluation of the outcomes of care are nursing actions integral to the recovery of the patient. The nurse also collaborates with other members of the health care team to provide essential care, offer a variety of solutions to problems, help the patient and family gain control of their lives, and explore the educational and supportive resources available in the community. The goals are to achieve as high a level of function as possible and to enhance the quality of life for the patient with neurologic impairment and their family.

ALTERED LEVEL OF CONSCIOUSNESS

An **altered level of consciousness (LOC)** is present when the patient is not oriented, does not follow commands, or needs persistent stimuli to achieve a state of alertness. LOC is gauged on a continuum, with a normal state of alertness and full cognition (consciousness) on one end and coma on the other end. **Coma** is a clinical state of unarousable unresponsiveness in which there are no purposeful responses to internal or external stimuli, although nonpurposeful responses to painful stimuli and brainstem reflexes may be present. The usual duration of coma is variable. **Akinetic mutism** is a state of unresponsiveness to the environment in which the patient makes no voluntary movement. **Persistent vegetative state** is a condition in which the unresponsive patient resumes sleep–wake cycles after coma but is devoid of cognitive or affective mental function. A **minimally conscious state** differs from persistent vegetative state in that the patient has inconsistent but reproducible signs of awareness (Bruno, Laureys, & Demertzi, 2013). **Locked-in syndrome** results from a lesion affecting the pons and results in paralysis and the inability to speak, but vertical eye movements and lid elevation remain intact and are used to indicate responsiveness (Bruno et al., 2013). The level of responsiveness and consciousness is the most important indicator of the patient's condition.

Pathophysiology

Altered LOC is not a disorder itself; rather, it is a result of multiple pathophysiologic phenomena. The cause may be neurologic (head injury, stroke), toxicologic (drug overdose, alcohol intoxication), or metabolic (hepatic or kidney injury, diabetic ketoacidosis).

The underlying cause of neurologic dysfunction is disruption in the cells of the nervous system, neurotransmitters, or brain anatomy (see Chapter 65). Disruptions result from cellular edema or other mechanisms, such as disruption of chemical transmission at receptor sites by antibodies.

Intact anatomic structures of the brain are needed for normal function. The two hemispheres of the cerebrum must communicate, via an intact corpus callosum, and the lobes of the brain (frontal, parietal, temporal, and occipital) must communicate and coordinate their specific functions (see Chapter 65). Other anatomic structures of importance are the cerebellum and the brainstem. The cerebellum has both excitatory and inhibitory actions and is largely responsible for coordination of movement. The brainstem contains areas that control the heart rate, respiration, and blood pressure. Disruptions in the anatomic structures result from trauma, edema, pressure from tumors, or other mechanisms, such as an increase or decrease in the circulation of blood or CSF.

Clinical Manifestations

Alterations in LOC occur along a continuum, and the clinical manifestations depend on where the patient is on this continuum. As the patient's state of alertness and consciousness decreases, changes occur in the pupillary response, eye opening response, verbal response, and motor response. However, initial alterations in LOC may be reflected by subtle behavioral changes, such as restlessness or increased anxiety. The pupils, normally round and quickly reactive to light, become sluggish (response is slower); as the patient becomes comatose, the pupils become fixed (no response to light). The patient in a coma does not open the eyes to voice or command, respond verbally, or move the extremities in response to a request to do so.

Assessment and Diagnostic Findings

The patient with an altered LOC is at risk for alterations in every body system. A complete assessment is performed, with particular attention to the neurologic system. The neurologic examination should be as complete as the LOC allows. It includes an evaluation of mental status, cranial nerve function, cerebellar function (balance and coordination), reflexes, and motor and sensory function. LOC, a sensitive indicator of neurologic function, is assessed based on the criteria in the Glasgow Coma Scale: eye opening, verbal response, and motor response (Hickey, 2014). The patient's responses are rated on a scale from 3 to 15. A score of 3 indicates severe impairment of neurologic function, brain death, or pharmacologic inhibition of the neurologic response. A score of 15 indicates that the patient is fully responsive (see Chapter 68).

If the patient is comatose and has localized signs such as abnormal pupillary and motor responses, it is assumed that neurologic disease is present until proven otherwise. If the patient is comatose but pupillary light reflexes are preserved, a toxic or metabolic disorder is suspected. Common diagnostic procedures used to identify the cause of unconsciousness include computed tomography (CT) scanning, perfusion CT (PCT), magnetic resonance imaging (MRI), magnetic resonance spectroscopy (MRS), and electroencephalography (EEG). Additional procedures include positron emission tomography (PET) and single-photon emission computed tomography (SPECT) (see Chapter 65). Emerging research identifies EEG, MRI, and PET as important technologies in determining brain function through the evaluation of metabolic and electrical activity (Van Der Naalt, 2015). Laboratory tests include analysis of blood glucose, electrolytes, serum ammonia, and liver function tests; blood urea nitrogen (BUN) levels; serum osmolality; calcium level; and partial thromboplastin and prothrombin times. Other studies may be used to evaluate serum ketones, alcohol and drug concentrations, and arterial blood gases.

Medical Management

The first priority of treatment for the patient with altered LOC is to obtain and maintain a patent airway. The patient may be orally or nasally intubated, or a tracheostomy may be performed. Until the ability of the patient to breathe is determined, a mechanical ventilator is used to maintain adequate oxygenation and ventilation. The circulatory status (blood pressure, heart rate) is monitored to ensure adequate perfusion to the body and brain. An intravenous (IV) catheter is inserted to provide access for IV fluids and medications. Neurologic care focuses on the specific neurologic pathology, if known. Nutritional support, via a feeding tube or a gastrostomy tube, is initiated as soon as possible. In addition to measures designed

to determine and treat the underlying causes of altered LOC, other medical interventions are aimed at pharmacologic management and prevention of complications.

NURSING PROCESS

The Patient With an Altered Level of Consciousness

Assessment

Assessment of the patient with an altered LOC often starts with assessing the verbal response through determining the patient's orientation to time, person, and place. Patients are asked to identify the day, date, or season of the year, as well as where they are or the clinicians, family members, or visitors present. Other questions such as "Who is the president?" or "What is the next holiday?" may be helpful in determining the patient's processing of information. Verbal response cannot be evaluated if the patient is intubated or has a tracheostomy, and this should be clearly documented.

Alertness is measured by the patient's ability to open the eyes spontaneously or in response to a vocal or noxious stimulus (pressure or pain). Patients with severe neurologic dysfunction cannot do this. The nurse assesses for periorbital edema (swelling around the eyes) or trauma, which may prevent the patient from opening the eyes, and documents any such condition that interferes with eye opening.

Motor response includes spontaneous, purposeful movement (e.g., the awake patient can move all four extremities with equal strength on command), movement only in response to painful stimuli, or abnormal posturing. If the patient is not responding to commands, the motor response is tested by applying a painful stimulus (firm but gentle pressure) to the nail bed or by squeezing a muscle. If the patient attempts to push away or withdraw, the response is recorded as purposeful or appropriate ("Patient withdraws to painful stimulus"). This response is considered purposeful if the patient can cross the midline from one side of the body to the other in response to a painful stimulus. An inappropriate or nonpurposeful response is random and aimless. Posturing may be decorticate

Figure 66-1 • Abnormal posture response to stimuli. **A.** Decorticate posturing and flexion of the upper extremities, internal rotation of the lower extremities, and plantar flexion of the feet. **B.** Decerebrate posturing, involving extension and outward rotation of upper extremities and plantar flexion of the feet. Adapted from Posner, J. B., Saper, C. B., Schiff, N. D., et al. (2007). *Plum and Posner's diagnosis of stupor and coma* (4th ed.). Oxford, UK: Oxford University Press.

or decerebrate (see Fig. 66-1; see also Chapter 65). The most severe neurologic impairment results in flaccidity. The motor response cannot be elicited or assessed when the patient has been given pharmacologic paralyzing agents (i.e., neuromuscular blocking agents).

In addition to LOC, the nurse monitors parameters such as respiratory status, eye signs, and reflexes on an ongoing basis. Table 66-1 summarizes the assessment and the clinical significance of the findings. Body functions (circulation, respiration, elimination, fluid and electrolyte balance) are examined in a systematic and ongoing manner.

Diagnosis

NURSING DIAGNOSES

Based on the assessment data, major nursing diagnoses may include the following:

- Ineffective airway clearance related to inability to maintain an airway due to altered LOC
- Risk for injury related to lack of adaptive and defensive resources due to decreased LOC
- Deficient fluid volume related to inability to take fluids by mouth
- Risk for imbalanced nutrition: less than body requirements related to inability to ingest nutrients to meet metabolic needs
- Impaired oral mucous membrane related to mouth breathing, absence of pharyngeal reflex, and altered fluid intake
- Risk for impaired skin integrity related to prolonged immobility
- Risk for impaired tissue integrity of cornea related to diminished or absent corneal reflex
- Ineffective thermoregulation related to damage to hypothalamic center
- Impaired urinary elimination (incontinence or retention) related to impairment in neurologic sensing and control
- Bowel incontinence related to impairment in neurologic sensing and control and also related to changes in nutritional delivery methods
- Ineffective health maintenance related to neurologic impairment
- Interrupted family processes related to health crisis

COLLABORATIVE PROBLEMS/POTENTIAL COMPLICATIONS

Potential complications may include the following:

- Respiratory distress or failure
- Pneumonia
- Aspiration
- Pressure ulcer
- Venous thromboembolism (VTE)
- Contractures

Planning and Goals

The patient with altered LOC is subject to all of the complications associated with immobility. Therefore, the goals of care for the patient with altered LOC include maintenance of a clear airway, protection from injury, attainment of fluid volume balance, maintenance of nutritional needs, achievement of intact oral mucous membranes, maintenance of normal skin integrity, absence of corneal irritation, attainment of effective thermoregulation, and effective urinary elimination.

Additional goals include bowel continence, restoration of health maintenance, maintenance of intact family or support system, and absence of complications.

Because the protective reflexes of the patient who is unconscious are impaired, the quality of nursing care provided may mean the difference between life and death. The nurse must assume responsibility for the patient until the basic reflexes (coughing, blinking, and swallowing) return and the patient becomes conscious and oriented. Therefore, the major nursing goal is to compensate for the absence of these protective reflexes.

Nursing Interventions

MAINTAINING THE AIRWAY

The most important consideration in managing the patient with altered LOC is to establish an adequate airway and ensure ventilation. Obstruction of the airway is a risk because the epiglottis and tongue may relax, occluding the oropharynx, or the patient may aspirate vomitus or nasopharyngeal secretions.

The accumulation of secretions in the pharynx presents a serious problem. Because the patient cannot swallow and lacks pharyngeal reflexes, these secretions must be removed to eliminate the danger of aspiration. Elevating the head of the bed to 30 degrees helps prevent aspiration. Positioning the patient in a lateral or semiprone position also helps because it allows the jaw and tongue to fall forward, thus promoting drainage of secretions.

Positioning alone is not always adequate, however. Suctioning and oral hygiene may be required. Suctioning is performed to remove secretions from the posterior pharynx and upper trachea. Before and after suctioning, the patient is adequately ventilated to prevent hypoxia (Hickey, 2014). Chest physiotherapy and postural drainage may be initiated to promote pulmonary hygiene, unless contraindicated by the patient's underlying condition. The chest should be auscultated at least every 8 hours to detect adventitious breath sounds or absence of breath sounds.

Despite these measures, or because of the severity of impairment, the patient with altered LOC often requires intubation and mechanical ventilation. Nursing actions for the patient who is mechanically ventilated include maintaining the patency of the endotracheal tube or tracheostomy, providing frequent oral care, monitoring arterial blood gas measurements, and maintaining ventilator settings (see Chapter 21).

PROTECTING THE PATIENT

For the protection of the patient, side rails are padded. Two rails are kept in the raised position during the day and three at night; however, raising all four side rails is considered a restraint by the Joint Commission if the intent is to limit the patient's mobility. Care should be taken to prevent injury from invasive lines and equipment, and other potential sources of injury should be identified, such as restraints, tight dressings, environmental irritants, damp bedding or dressings, and tubes and drains.

Protection also includes ensuring the patient's dignity during altered LOC. Simple measures such as providing privacy and speaking to the patient during nursing care activities preserve the patient's dignity. Not speaking negatively about the patient's condition or prognosis is also important, because

TABLE 66-1 Nursing Assessment of the Patient Who Is Unconscious

Examination	Clinical Assessment	Clinical Significance
Level of responsiveness or consciousness	Eye opening; verbal and motor responses; pupils (size, equality, reaction to light)	Obeying commands is a favorable response and demonstrates a return to consciousness
Pattern of respiration	Respiratory pattern	Disturbances of respiratory center of brain may result in various respiratory patterns
	Cheyne–Stokes respiration	Suggests lesions deep in both hemispheres; area of basal ganglia and upper brainstem
	Hyperventilation	Suggests onset of metabolic problem or brainstem damage
	Ataxic respiration with irregularity in depth/rate	Ominous sign of damage to medullary center
Eyes		
Pupils (size, equality, reaction to light)	Equal, normally reactive pupils	Suggests that coma is toxic or metabolic in origin
	Equal or unequal diameter	Helps determine location of lesion
	Progressive dilation	Indicates increasing intracranial pressure
	Fixed dilated pupils	Indicates injury at level of midbrain
Eye movements	Normally, eyes should move from side to side	Functional and structural integrity of brainstem is assessed by inspection of extraocular movements; usually absent in deep coma
Corneal reflex	When cornea is touched with a wisp of clean cotton, blink response is normal	Tests cranial nerves V and VII; helps determine location of lesion if unilateral; absent in deep coma
Facial symmetry	Asymmetry (sagging, decrease in wrinkles)	Sign of paralysis
Swallowing reflex	Drooling vs. spontaneous swallowing	Absent in coma Paralysis of cranial nerves X and XII
Neck	Stiff neck Absence of spontaneous neck movement	Subarachnoid hemorrhage, meningitis Fracture or dislocation of cervical spine
Response of extremity to noxious stimuli	Firm pressure on a joint of the upper and lower extremity Observe spontaneous movements	Asymmetric response in paralysis Absent in deep coma
Deep tendon reflexes	Tap patellar and biceps tendons	Brisk response may have localizing value. Asymmetric response in paralysis Absent in deep coma
Pathologic reflexes	Firm pressure with blunt object on sole of foot, moving along lateral margin and crossing to the ball of foot	Flexion of the toes, especially the great toe, is normal except in newborn Dorsiflexion of toes (especially great toe) indicates contralateral pathology of corticospinal tract (Babinski reflex) Helps determine location of lesion in brain
Abnormal posture	Observation for posturing (spontaneous or in response to noxious stimuli) Flaccidity with absence of motor response Decorticate posture (flexion and internal rotation of forearms and hands) Decerebrate posture (extension and external rotation)	Deep extensive brain lesion Seen with cerebral hemisphere pathology and metabolic depression of brain function Decerebrate posturing indicates deeper and more severe dysfunction than does decorticate posturing; implies brain pathology; poor prognostic sign

patients in a coma may be able to hear. The patient who is comatose has an increased need for advocacy, and the nurse is responsible for seeing that these advocacy needs are met.

> ### ▶ Quality and Safety Nursing Alert
>
> *If the patient begins to emerge from unconsciousness, every measure that is available and appropriate for calming and quieting the patient should be used. Any form of restraint is likely to be countered with resistance, leading to self-injury or to a dangerous increase in ICP. Therefore, physical restraints are avoided, if possible; a written prescription must be obtained if their use is essential for the patient's well-being.*

MAINTAINING FLUID BALANCE AND MANAGING NUTRITIONAL NEEDS

Hydration status is assessed by examining tissue turgor and mucous membranes, assessing intake and output trends, and analyzing laboratory data. Fluid needs are met initially by administering the required IV fluids. However, IV solutions (and blood component therapy) for patients with intracranial conditions must be given slowly. If they are given too rapidly, they can increase ICP. The quantity of fluids given may be restricted to minimize the possibility of cerebral edema.

If the patient does not recover quickly and sufficiently enough to take adequate fluids and calories by mouth, a feeding or gastrostomy tube will be inserted for the administration of fluids and enteral feedings. Research suggests that patients fed within 48 hours of injury have improved outcomes over those in whom nutrition is delayed (Wang, Dong, Han, et al., 2013).

PROVIDING MOUTH CARE

The mouth is inspected for dryness, inflammation, and crusting. The patient who is unconscious requires careful oral care, because there is a risk of parotitis if the mouth is not kept scrupulously clean. The mouth is cleansed and rinsed carefully to remove secretions and crusts and to keep the mucous membranes moist. A thin coating of petrolatum on the lips prevents drying, cracking, and encrustations. If the patient has an endotracheal tube, the tube should be moved to the opposite side of the mouth daily to prevent ulceration of the mouth and lips. If the patient is intubated and mechanically ventilated, good oral care is also necessary. Research suggests that comprehensive mouth care with antiseptic such as chlorhexidine and head of bed elevation decreases ventilator-associated pneumonia and improves the oral health in patients who are intubated (Munro & Ruggiero, 2014).

MAINTAINING SKIN AND JOINT INTEGRITY

Preventing skin breakdown requires continuing nursing assessment and intervention. Special attention is given to patients who are unconscious, because they cannot respond to external stimuli. Assessment includes a regular schedule of turning to avoid pressure, which can cause breakdown and necrosis of the skin. Turning also provides kinesthetic (sensation of movement), proprioceptive (awareness of position), and vestibular (equilibrium) stimulation. After turning, the patient is carefully repositioned to prevent ischemic necrosis over pressure areas. Dragging or pulling the patient up in bed must be avoided, because this creates a shearing force and friction on the skin surface (see Chapter 10).

Maintaining correct body position is important; equally important is passive exercise of the extremities to prevent contractures. The use of splints or foam boots aids in the prevention of footdrop and eliminates the pressure of bedding on the toes. The use of trochanter rolls to support the hip joints keeps the legs in proper alignment. The arms are in abduction, the fingers lightly flexed, and the hands in slight supination. The heels of the feet are assessed for pressure areas. Specialty beds, such as fluidized or low-air-loss beds, may be used to decrease pressure on bony prominences (Hickey, 2014).

PRESERVING CORNEAL INTEGRITY

Some patients who are unconscious have their eyes open and have inadequate or absent corneal reflexes. The cornea may become irritated, dry, or scratched, leading to ulceration. The eyes may be cleansed with cotton balls moistened with sterile normal saline to remove debris and discharge. If artificial tears are prescribed, they may be instilled every 2 hours. Periorbital edema often occurs after cranial surgery. If cold compresses are prescribed, care must be exerted to avoid contact with the cornea. Eye patches should be used cautiously because of the potential for corneal abrasion from contact with the patch.

MAINTAINING BODY TEMPERATURE

High fever in the patient who is unconscious may be caused by infection of the respiratory or urinary tract, drug reactions, or damage to the hypothalamic temperature-regulating center. A slight elevation of temperature may be caused by dehydration. The environment can be adjusted, depending on the patient's condition, to promote a normal body temperature. If body temperature is elevated, a minimum amount of bedding is used. The room may be cooled to 18.3°C (65°F). However, if the patient is an older adult and does not have an elevated temperature, a warmer environment is needed.

Because of damage to the temperature-regulating center in the brain or severe intracranial infection, patients who are unconscious often develop very high temperatures. Such temperature elevations must be controlled, because the increased metabolic demands of the brain can exceed cerebral circulation and oxygen delivery, potentially resulting in cerebral deterioration (Hickey, 2014). Studies suggest that hyperthermia may contribute to poor outcome after brain injury but not through a decreased brain oxygen level (Madden & DeVon, 2015). Persistent hyperthermia with no identified clinical source of infection indicates brainstem damage and a poor prognosis.

> ### ▶ Quality and Safety Nursing Alert
>
> *The body temperature of a patient who is unconscious is never taken by mouth. Rectal, tympanic (if not contraindicated), or core temperature measurement is preferred to the less accurate axillary temperature.*

Strategies for reducing fever include:
- Removing all bedding over the patient (with the possible exception of a light sheet, towel, or small drape)
- Administering acetaminophen or ibuprofen as prescribed
- Giving cool sponge baths
- Using a hypothermia blanket
- Monitoring temperature frequently to assess the patient's response to the therapy and to prevent an excessive decrease in temperature and shivering

PREVENTING URINARY RETENTION

The patient with an altered LOC is often incontinent or has urinary retention. The bladder is palpated or scanned at intervals to determine whether urinary retention is present, because a full bladder may be an overlooked cause of overflow incontinence. A portable bladder ultrasound instrument is a useful tool in bladder management and retraining programs.

If the patient is not voiding, a program of intermittent catheterization should be devised in order to reduce the patient's risk of urinary tract infection. A catheter may be inserted during the acute phase of illness to monitor urinary output. Because catheters are a major cause of urinary tract infection, the patient is observed for fever and cloudy urine. The area around the urethral orifice is inspected for drainage and cleansed routinely. The urinary catheter is usually removed if the patient has a stable cardiovascular system and if no diuresis, sepsis, or voiding dysfunction existed before the onset of coma. Although many patients who are unconscious urinate spontaneously after catheter removal, the bladder should be palpated or scanned with a portable ultrasound device periodically for urinary retention (see Chapter 53, Fig. 53-8).

An external catheter (condom catheter) for the male patient and absorbent pads for the female patient can be used for patients who are unconscious and can urinate spontaneously, although involuntarily. As soon as consciousness is regained, a bladder training program is initiated (Hickey, 2014). The patient who is incontinent is monitored frequently for skin irritation and skin breakdown. Appropriate skin care is implemented to prevent these complications.

PROMOTING BOWEL FUNCTION

The abdomen is assessed for distention by listening for bowel sounds and measuring the girth of the abdomen with a tape measure. There is a risk of diarrhea from infection, antibiotic agents, and hyperosmolar fluids. Frequent loose stools may also occur with fecal impaction. Commercial fecal collection bags are available for patients with fecal incontinence (see Chapter 47, Fig. 47-1).

Immobility and lack of dietary fiber can cause constipation. The nurse monitors the number and consistency of bowel movements and performs a rectal examination for signs of fecal impaction. Stool softeners may be prescribed and can be given with tube feedings. To facilitate bowel emptying, a glycerin suppository may be indicated. The patient may require an enema every other day to empty the lower colon.

RESTORING HEALTH MAINTENANCE

Once increased ICP is not a problem, the nurse assists the patient and family to restore the health of the patient who is unconscious. This involves using auditory, visual, olfactory, gustatory, tactile, and kinesthetic activities to stimulate the patient emerging from coma (Megha, Harpreet, & Nayeem, 2013). Efforts are made to restore the sense of daily rhythm by maintaining usual day and night patterns for activity and sleep. The nurse touches and talks to the patient and encourages family members and friends to do so. Communication is extremely important and includes touching the patient and spending enough time with the patient to become sensitive to their needs. It is also important to avoid making any negative comments about the patient's status or prognosis in the patient's presence.

The nurse orients the patient to time and place at least once every 8 hours. Sounds from the patient's usual environment may be introduced using a tape recorder. Family members can read to the patient from a favorite book and may suggest radio and television programs that the patient previously enjoyed as a means of enriching the environment and providing familiar input.

When arousing from coma, many patients experience a period of agitation, indicating that they are becoming more aware of their surroundings but still cannot react or communicate in an appropriate fashion. Although this is disturbing for many family members, it is actually a positive clinical sign. At this time, it is necessary to minimize stimulation by limiting background noises, having only one person speak to the patient at a time, giving the patient a longer period of time to respond, and allowing for frequent rest or quiet times. After the patient has regained consciousness, videotaped family or social events may assist the patient in recognizing family and friends and allow him or her to experience missed events.

Programs of sensory stimulation for patients with brain injury have been developed in an effort to improve outcomes. Although these are controversial programs with inconsistent results, some research supports the concept of providing structured stimulation (Megha et al., 2013).

MEETING THE FAMILY'S NEEDS

The family of the patient with altered LOC may be thrown into a sudden state of crisis and go through the process of severe anxiety, denial, anger, remorse, grief, and reconciliation. Depending on the disorder that caused the altered LOC and the extent of the patient's recovery, the family may be unprepared for the changes in the cognitive and physical status of their loved one. If the patient has significant residual deficits, the family may require considerable time, assistance, and support to come to terms with these changes. To help family members mobilize resources and coping skills, the nurse reinforces and clarifies information about the patient's condition, encourages the family to be involved in care, and listens to and encourages ventilation of feelings and concerns while supporting decision making about management and placement after hospitalization. Families may benefit from participation in support groups offered through the hospital, rehabilitation facility, or community organizations.

The family may need to face the death of their loved one. The patient with a neurologic disorder is often pronounced brain dead before the heart stops beating. The term **brain death** describes irreversible loss of all functions of the entire brain and absence of brainstem reflexes (Wijdicks, 2013). The term may be misleading to the family because, although brain function has ceased, the patient appears to be alive, with the heart rate and blood pressure sustained by vasoactive medications and breathing continued by mechanical ventilation. When discussing a patient who is brain dead with family members, it is important to provide accurate, timely, understandable, and consistent information. See Chapter 16 for discussion of end-of-life care.

MONITORING AND MANAGING POTENTIAL COMPLICATIONS

Pneumonia, aspiration, and respiratory failure are potential complications in any patient who has a depressed LOC and who cannot protect the airway or turn, cough, and take deep breaths. The longer the period of unconsciousness, the greater the risk of pulmonary complications.

Vital signs and respiratory function are monitored closely to detect any signs of respiratory failure or distress. Complete blood count and arterial blood gas measurements are assessed to determine whether there are adequate red blood cells to carry oxygen and whether ventilation is effective. Chest physiotherapy and suctioning are initiated to prevent respiratory complications such as pneumonia. Oral care interventions are performed for patients receiving mechanical ventilation to maintain oral health and decrease the incidence of pneumonia (Kiyoshi-Teo & Blegen, 2015). If pneumonia develops, cultures are obtained to identify the organism so that appropriate antibiotic agents can be given.

The patient with altered LOC is monitored closely for evidence of impaired skin integrity, and strategies to prevent skin breakdown and pressure ulcers are continued through all phases of care, including hospitalization, rehabilitation, and home care. Factors that contribute to impaired skin integrity (e.g., incontinence, inadequate dietary intake, pressure on bony prominences, edema) are addressed. If pressure ulcers develop, strategies to promote healing are undertaken. Care is taken to prevent bacterial contamination of pressure ulcers, which may lead to sepsis and septic shock. See Chapter 10 for assessment and management of pressure ulcers.

The patient should also be monitored for signs and symptoms of VTE, which may manifest as a deep vein thrombosis (DVT) or pulmonary embolism (PE). Prophylaxis with subcutaneous heparin or low–molecular-weight heparin (dalteparin [Fragmin], danaparoid [Orgaran]) as well as antiembolism stockings or pneumatic compression devices are prescribed according to the patient's risk factors for thrombosis and bleeding (Foreman, Schmalz, & Griessenauer, 2014). The nurse observes for signs and symptoms of DVT or PE.

Patients with a prolonged decrease in LOC are at risk for developing contractures. During acute care, the patient is turned every 2 hours and passive range of motion performed at least twice a day. Splints, provided by occupational therapy, are applied to the hands and feet in a rotating manner to maintain functional joint alignment. Hand splints have been reported to be safe and beneficial for patients in decreasing spasticity and improving hand opening (Thibault, Deltombe, Wannez, et al., 2015). See Chapter 10 for further information about management of contractures.

Evaluation

Expected patient outcomes may include:

1. Maintains clear airway and demonstrates appropriate breath sounds
2. Experiences no injuries
3. Attains or maintains adequate fluid balance and nutritional status
   a. Has no clinical signs or symptoms of dehydration
   b. Demonstrates normal range of serum electrolytes
   c. Has no clinical signs or symptoms of overhydration or malnutrition
4. Achieves healthy oral mucous membranes
5. Maintains normal skin integrity
6. Has no corneal irritation
7. Attains or maintains thermoregulation
8. Has no urinary retention
9. Has no diarrhea or fecal impaction
10. Receives appropriate sensory stimulation
11. Has family members who cope with crisis
    a. Verbalize fears and concerns
    b. Participate in patient's care and provide sensory stimulation by talking and touching
12. Is free of complications
    a. Has arterial blood gas values or oxygen saturation levels within normal range
    b. Displays no signs or symptoms of pneumonia
    c. Exhibits intact skin over pressure areas
    d. Does not develop VTE such as DVT or PE

 INCREASED INTRACRANIAL PRESSURE

The rigid cranial vault contains brain tissue (1400 g), blood (75 mL), and CSF (75 mL). The volume and pressure of these three components are usually in a state of equilibrium and produce the ICP. ICP is usually measured in the lateral ventricles, with the normal pressure being 0 to 10 mm Hg, and 15 mm Hg being the upper limit of normal (Hickey, 2014).

The **Monro–Kellie hypothesis**, also known as the Monro–Kellie doctrine, explains the dynamic equilibrium of cranial contents. The hypothesis states that because of the limited space for expansion within the skull, an increase in any one of the components causes a change in the volume of the others. Because brain tissue has limited space to expand, compensation typically is accomplished by displacing or shifting CSF, increasing the absorption or diminishing the production of CSF, or decreasing cerebral blood volume. Without such changes, ICP begins to rise. Under normal circumstances, minor changes in blood volume and CSF volume occur constantly as a result of alterations in intrathoracic pressure (coughing, sneezing, straining), posture, blood pressure, and systemic oxygen and carbon dioxide levels (Hickey, 2014).

Pathophysiology

Increased ICP affects many patients with acute neurologic conditions because pathologic conditions alter the relationship between intracranial volume and ICP. Although elevated ICP is most commonly associated with head injury, it also may be seen as a secondary effect in other conditions, such as brain tumors, subarachnoid hemorrhage, and toxic and viral encephalopathies. Increased ICP from any cause decreases cerebral perfusion, stimulates further swelling (edema), and may shift brain tissue, resulting in herniation—a dire and frequently fatal event.

Decreased Cerebral Blood Flow

Increased ICP may reduce cerebral blood flow, resulting in ischemia and cell death. In the early stages of cerebral ischemia, the vasomotor centers are stimulated and the systemic pressure rises to maintain cerebral blood flow. Usually, this is accompanied by a slow bounding pulse and respiratory irregularities. These changes in blood pressure, pulse, and respiration are important clinically because they suggest increased ICP.

The concentration of carbon dioxide in the blood and in the brain tissue also plays a role in the regulation of cerebral blood flow. An increase in the partial pressure of arterial carbon dioxide ($PaCO_2$) causes cerebral vasodilation, leading to increased cerebral blood flow and increased ICP. A decrease in $PaCO_2$ has a vasoconstrictive effect, limiting blood flow to the brain. Decreased venous outflow may also increase cerebral blood volume, thus raising ICP.

Cerebral Edema

Cerebral edema or swelling is defined as an abnormal accumulation of water or fluid in the intracellular space, extracellular space, or both, associated with an increase in the volume of brain tissue. Edema can occur in the gray, white, or interstitial matter. As brain tissue swells within the rigid skull, several mechanisms attempt to compensate for the increasing ICP. These compensatory mechanisms include autoregulation as well as decreased production and flow of CSF. **Autoregulation** refers to the brain's ability to change the diameter of its blood vessels to maintain a constant cerebral blood flow during alterations in systemic blood pressure. This mechanism can be impaired in patients who are experiencing a pathologic and sustained increase in ICP.

Cerebral Response to Increased Intracranial Pressure

As ICP rises, compensatory mechanisms in the brain work to maintain blood flow and prevent tissue damage. The brain can maintain a steady perfusion pressure if the arterial systolic blood pressure is 50 to 150 mm Hg and the ICP is less than 40 mm Hg. Changes in ICP are closely linked with cerebral perfusion pressure (CPP). The CPP is calculated by subtracting the ICP from the mean arterial pressure (MAP). For example, if the MAP is 100 mm Hg and the ICP is 15 mm Hg, then the CPP is 85 mm Hg. The normal CPP is 70 to 100 mm Hg (Hickey, 2014). As ICP rises and the autoregulatory mechanism of the brain is overwhelmed, the CPP can increase to greater than 100 mm Hg or decrease to less than 50 mm Hg. Patients with a CPP of less than 50 mm Hg experience irreversible neurologic damage. Therefore, the CPP must be maintained at 70 to 80 mm Hg to ensure adequate blood flow to the brain. If ICP is equal to MAP, cerebral circulation ceases.

A clinical phenomenon known as the **Cushing's response** (or Cushing's reflex) is seen when cerebral blood flow decreases significantly. When ischemic, the vasomotor center triggers an increase in arterial pressure in an effort to overcome the increased ICP. A sympathetically mediated response causes an increase in the systolic blood pressure with a widening of the pulse pressure and cardiac slowing. This response is seen clinically as an increase in systolic blood pressure, widening of the pulse pressure, and reflex slowing of the heart rate. It is a late sign requiring immediate intervention; however, perfusion may be recoverable if the Cushing's response is treated rapidly.

At a certain point, the brain's ability to autoregulate becomes ineffective and decompensation (ischemia and infarction) begins. When this occurs, the patient exhibits significant changes in mental status and vital signs. The bradycardia, hypertension, and bradypnea associated with this deterioration are known as Cushing's triad, which is a grave sign. At this point, herniation of the brainstem and occlusion of the cerebral blood flow occur if therapeutic intervention is not initiated. **Herniation** refers to the shifting of brain tissue

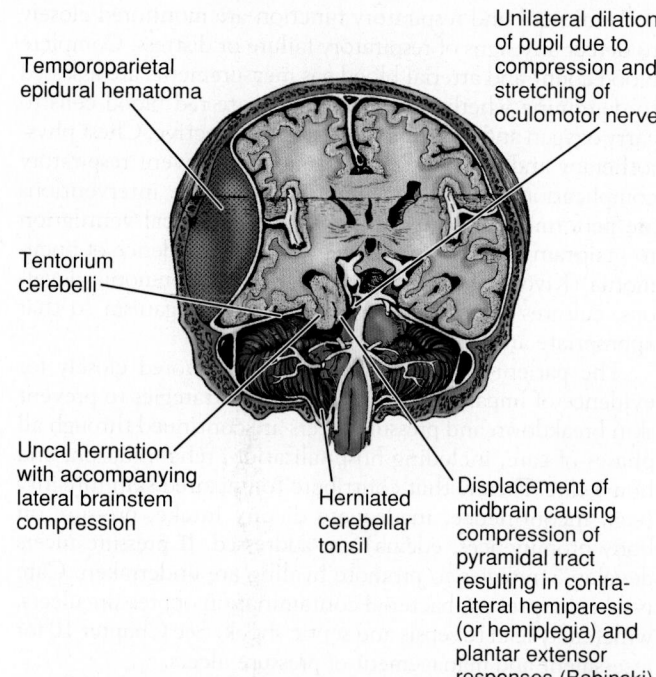

Figure 66-2 • Cross-section of the brain showing herniation of part of the temporal lobe through the tentorium as a result of a temporoparietal epidural hematoma. Reprinted with permission from Hickey, J. V. (2014). *The clinical practice of neurological & neurosurgical nursing* (7th ed.). Philadelphia, PA: Lippincott Williams & Wilkins.

from an area of high pressure to an area of lower pressure (see Fig. 66-2). The herniated tissue exerts pressure on the brain area into which it has shifted, which interferes with the blood supply in that area. Cessation of cerebral blood flow results in cerebral ischemia, infarction, and brain death.

Clinical Manifestations

If ICP increases to the point at which the brain's ability to adjust has reached its limits, neural function is impaired; this may be manifested at first by clinical changes in LOC and later by abnormal respiratory and vasomotor responses.

> **Quality and Safety Nursing Alert**
>
> *The earliest sign of increasing ICP is a change in LOC. Agitation, slowing of speech, and delay in response to verbal suggestions may be early indicators.*

Any sudden change in the patient's condition, such as restlessness (without apparent cause), confusion, or increasing drowsiness, has neurologic significance. These signs may result from compression of the brain due to swelling from hemorrhage or edema, an expanding intracranial lesion (hematoma or tumor), or a combination of both.

As ICP increases, the patient becomes stuporous, reacting only to loud or painful stimuli. At this stage, serious impairment of brain circulation is probably taking place, and immediate intervention is required. As neurologic function deteriorates further, the patient becomes comatose and exhibits abnormal motor responses in the form of **decortication** (abnormal flexion of the upper extremities and extension of the lower extremities), **decerebration** (extreme extension of the upper and lower extremities), or flaccidity (see Fig. 66-1). If the coma is profound and irreversible with no known confounding factors, brainstem reflexes are absent, and respirations are impaired or absent, the patient may be evaluated for brain death (Wijdicks, 2013).

Assessment and Diagnostic Findings

The diagnostic studies used to determine the underlying cause of increased ICP are discussed in detail in Chapter 65. The most common diagnostic tests are CT scanning and MRI. The patient may also undergo cerebral angiography, PET, or SPECT. Transcranial Doppler studies provide information about cerebral blood flow. The patient with increased ICP may also undergo electrophysiologic monitoring to observe cerebral blood flow indirectly. Evoked potential monitoring measures the electrical potentials produced by nerve tissue in response to external stimulation (auditory, visual, or sensory). Lumbar puncture is avoided in patients with increased ICP, because the sudden release of pressure in the lumbar area can cause the brain to herniate (Hickey, 2014). See Chapter 65 for further discussion of lumbar puncture and other diagnostic tests.

Complications

Complications of increased ICP include brainstem herniation, diabetes insipidus, and syndrome of inappropriate antidiuretic hormone (SIADH).

Brainstem herniation results from an excessive increase in ICP in which the pressure builds in the cranial vault and the brain tissue presses down on the brainstem. This increasing pressure on the brainstem results in cessation of blood flow to the brain, leading to irreversible brain anoxia and brain death.

Neurogenic diabetes insipidus is the result of decreased secretion of antidiuretic hormone (ADH). The patient has excessive urine output, decreased urine osmolality, and serum hyperosmolarity (Grossman & Porth, 2014). Therapy consists of administration of fluids, electrolyte replacement, and administration of a synthetic vasopressin (desmopressin [DDAVP]). See Chapters 13 and 52 for a discussion of diabetes insipidus.

SIADH is the result of increased secretion of ADH. The patient becomes volume overloaded, urine output diminishes, and serum sodium concentration becomes dilute. Treatment of SIADH includes fluid restriction (less than 800 mL/day with no free water), which is usually sufficient to correct the hyponatremia. In severe cases, careful administration of a 3% hypertonic saline solution may be therapeutic (Aylwin, Burst, Peri, et al., 2015). The change in serum sodium concentration should not exceed a correction rate of approximately 1.3 mEq/L/hr. See Chapters 13 and 52 for further discussion of SIADH.

Medical Management

Increased ICP is a true emergency and must be treated promptly. Invasive monitoring of ICP is an important component of management. Immediate management to relieve increased ICP requires decreasing cerebral edema, lowering the volume of CSF, or decreasing cerebral blood volume while maintaining cerebral perfusion. These goals are accomplished by administering osmotic diuretics, restricting fluids, draining CSF, controlling fever, maintaining systemic blood pressure and oxygenation, and reducing cellular metabolic demands. See Chapter 68 for a discussion of the management of increased ICP.

Monitoring Intracranial Pressure and Cerebral Oxygenation

The purposes of ICP monitoring are to identify increased pressure early in its course (before cerebral damage occurs), to quantify the degree of elevation, to initiate appropriate treatment, to provide access to CSF for sampling and drainage, and to evaluate the effectiveness of treatment. ICP can be monitored with the use of an intraventricular catheter (ventriculostomy), a subarachnoid bolt, an epidural or subdural catheter, or a fiberoptic transducer-tipped catheter placed in the subdural space or in the ventricle (see Fig. 66-3).

When a ventriculostomy or intraventricular catheter monitoring device is used for monitoring ICP, a fine-bore catheter is inserted into a lateral ventricle, preferably in the nondominant hemisphere of the brain (American Association of Neuroscience Nurses [AANN], 2012). The catheter is connected by a fluid-filled system to a transducer, which records the pressure in the form of an electrical impulse. In addition to obtaining continuous ICP recordings, the ventricular catheter allows CSF to drain, particularly during acute increases in pressure. The ventriculostomy can also be used to drain blood from the ventricle. Continuous drainage of CSF under pressure control is an effective method of treating intracranial hypertension. Another advantage of a ventricular catheter is access for the intraventricular administration of medications and the occasional instillation of air or a contrast agent for ventriculography. Complications associated with its use include infection, meningitis, ventricular collapse, occlusion of the catheter by brain tissue or blood, and problems with the monitoring system.

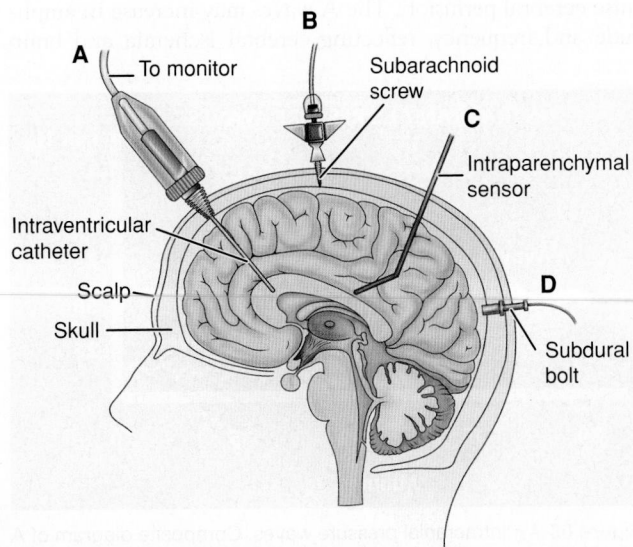

Figure 66-3 • Intracranial pressure monitoring. A device may be placed in the ventricle (**A**), the subarachnoid space (**B**), the intraparenchymal space (**C**), or the subdural space (**D**).

The subarachnoid screw or bolt is a hollow device that is inserted through the skull and dura mater into the cranial subarachnoid space (Hickey, 2014). It has the advantage of not requiring a ventricular puncture. The subarachnoid screw is attached to a pressure transducer, and the output is recorded on an oscilloscope. The hollow screw technique also has the advantage of avoiding complications from brain shift and small ventricle size. Complications include infection and blockage of the screw by clot or brain tissue, which leads to a loss of pressure tracing and a decrease in accuracy at high ICP readings.

An epidural monitor uses a pneumatic flow sensor to detect ICP. The epidural ICP monitoring system has a low incidence of infection and complications and appears to read pressures accurately. Calibration of the system is maintained automatically, and abnormal pressure waves trigger an alarm system. One disadvantage of the epidural catheter is the inability to withdraw CSF for analysis.

A fiberoptic monitor, or transducer-tipped catheter, is an alternative to other intraventricular, subarachnoid, and subdural systems (Sandsmark, Kumar, Park, et al., 2012). The miniature transducer reflects pressure changes, which are converted to electrical signals in an amplifier and displayed on a digital monitor. The catheter can be inserted into the ventricle, subarachnoid space, subdural space, or brain parenchyma or under a bone flap. If inserted into the ventricle, it can also be used in conjunction with a CSF drainage device.

Interpreting Intracranial Pressure Waveforms

Waves of high pressure and troughs of relatively normal pressure indicate changes in ICP. Waveforms are captured and recorded on an oscilloscope. These waves have been classified as A waves (plateau waves), B waves, and C waves (see Fig. 66-4). The plateau waves (A waves) are transient, paroxysmal, recurring elevations of ICP that may last 5 to 20 minutes and range in amplitude from 40 to 100 mm Hg (Dias, Maia, Cerejo, et al., 2014). Plateau waves have clinical significance and indicate changes in vascular volume within the intracranial compartment that are beginning to compromise cerebral perfusion. The A waves may increase in amplitude and frequency, reflecting cerebral ischemia and brain

Figure 66-4 • Intracranial pressure waves. Composite diagram of A (plateau) waves, which indicate cerebral ischemia; B waves, which indicate intracranial hypertension and variations in the respiratory cycle; and C waves, which relate to variations in systemic arterial pressure and respirations.

damage that can occur before overt signs and symptoms of raised ICP are seen clinically. B waves are shorter (30 seconds to 2 minutes) and have smaller amplitude (up to 50 mm Hg). They have less clinical significance, but if seen in a series in a patient with depressed consciousness, they may precede the appearance of A waves. B waves may be seen in patients with intracranial hypertension and decreased intracranial compliance. C waves are small, rhythmic oscillations with frequencies of 4 to 8 per minute and appear to be related to rhythmic variations of the systemic arterial blood pressure and respirations (Hickey, 2014).

Other Neurologic Monitoring Systems

Another trend in neurologic monitoring is microdialysis of the patient with a brain injury (de Lima Oliveira, Kairalla, Fonoff, et al., 2014). Cortical probes are placed near the injured area and are used to measure levels of glutamate, lactate, pyruvate, and glucose, substances that reflect the metabolic function of the brain. Some researchers theorize that direct measurements of glucose and energy by-products in the brain will lead to better management of these patients. Although cerebral microdialysis has reduced the mortality of patients who are brain injured, more study is needed to link it to improved outcomes (de Lima Oliveira et al., 2014).

An additional trend is monitoring of cerebral oxygenation through monitoring of the oxygen saturation in the jugular venous bulb (SjvO$_2$) or via a catheter in the brain. Cerebral oxygenation is thought to be important because changes in cerebral perfusion may reflect an increase in ICP. Readings taken from a catheter residing in the jugular outflow tract allow for a comparison of arterial and venous oxygen saturation, and the balance of cerebral oxygen supply and demand is demonstrated. Venous jugular desaturations can reflect early cerebral ischemia, alerting the clinician before an increase in ICP occurs. Minimizing cerebral desaturations can potentially improve outcomes (Sandsmark et al., 2012). This type of monitoring is now widely available and has been successfully used to identify secondary brain insults. A limiting factor is that this saturation reflects overall perfusion of the brain rather than that of a specific injured area (Oddo, Bosel, & Participants in the International Multidisciplinary Consensus Conference on Multimodality Monitoring, 2014).

Another method of measuring cerebral oxygenation and temperature is by inserting a fiberoptic catheter into the brain matter (Oddo et al., 2014). The most common system is Licox (see Fig. 66-5). The system includes a monitor with a screen for the display of oxygen and temperature values and cables that connect to the monitoring probes in the brain (Hickey, 2014).

Decreasing Cerebral Edema

Osmotic diuretics such as mannitol and hypertonic saline (3%) may be given to dehydrate the brain tissue and reduce cerebral edema (Ong, Keyrouz, & Diringer, 2015). They act by drawing water across intact membranes, thereby reducing the volume of the brain and extracellular fluid. An indwelling urinary catheter is usually inserted to monitor urinary output and to manage the resulting diuresis. If the patient is receiving osmotic diuretics, serum osmolality and electrolytes should be determined to assess hydration status. If a brain tumor is the

Figure 66-5 • Licox catheter system. **A.** The brain tissue oxygen catheter and monitor. **B.** Placement of the catheter in brain white matter. Redrawn with permission of Integra NeuroSciences, Plainsboro, NJ.

cause of the increased ICP, corticosteroids (e.g., dexamethasone) help reduce the edema surrounding the tumor.

Another method for decreasing cerebral edema is fluid restriction (Hickey, 2014). Limiting overall fluid intake leads to dehydration and hemoconcentration, which draws fluid across the osmotic gradient and decreases cerebral edema. Conversely, overhydration of the patient with increased ICP is avoided, because it increases cerebral edema.

Researchers have long hypothesized that lowering body temperature would decrease cerebral edema by reducing the oxygen and metabolic requirements of the brain, thus protecting the brain from continued ischemia. If body metabolism can be reduced by lowering the body temperature, the collateral circulation in the brain may be able to provide an adequate blood supply to the brain. The effect of hypothermia on ICP requires more study; thus far, induced hypothermia has not consistently been shown to be beneficial for patients with brain injury. Inducing and maintaining hypothermia is a major clinical treatment and requires knowledge and skilled nursing observation and management. The type and length of rewarming techniques after hypothermia may also be factors in the outcome of patients with neurologic injuries (Andrews, Sinclair, Rodriguez, et al., 2015; Madden & DeVon, 2015).

Maintaining Cerebral Perfusion

Cardiac output may be manipulated to provide adequate perfusion to the brain. Improvements in cardiac output are made using fluid volume and inotropic agents such as dobutamine (Dobutrex) and norepinephrine (Levophed). The effectiveness of the cardiac output is reflected in the CPP, which is maintained at greater than 70 mm Hg (Oddo et al., 2014). A lower CPP indicates that the cardiac output is insufficient to maintain adequate cerebral perfusion. $SjvO_2$ and Licox, described earlier, assist in monitoring cerebral perfusion.

Decompressive hemicraniectomy may also be considered as a surgical strategy to assist in the management of refractory intracranial hypertension. The removal of a part of the skull allows the brain to expand without the pressure constraints exerted by the cranial vault. Complications of this procedure

include infection and increased potential for injury to the unprotected underlying brain structures. Once the patient is no longer at risk for increased ICP, the bone flap may be surgically replaced (Alali, Naimark, Wilson, et al., 2014).

Reducing Cerebrospinal Fluid and Intracranial Blood Volume

CSF drainage is frequently performed, because the removal of CSF with a ventriculostomy drain can dramatically reduce ICP and restore CPP. Caution should be used in draining CSF, however, because excessive drainage may result in collapse of the ventricles and herniation. The reduction in $PaCO_2$ may result in hypoxia, ischemia, and an increase in cerebral lactate levels. Maintaining the $PaCO_2$ at greater than 30 mm Hg may prove beneficial (Hickey, 2014).

Controlling Fever

Preventing a temperature elevation is critical, because fever increases cerebral metabolism and the rate at which cerebral edema forms. Strategies to reduce body temperature include administration of antipyretic medications, as prescribed, and the use of a hypothermia blanket. Additional strategies for reducing fever were discussed previously in the Nursing Process section on altered LOC. The patient's temperature is monitored closely, and the patient is observed for shivering, which should be avoided because it is associated with increased oxygen consumption, increased levels of circulating catecholamines, and increased vasoconstriction. Shivering is associated with decreased levels of brain oxygenation; however, the association between shivering and neurologic outcome is unknown.

Maintaining Oxygenation and Reducing Metabolic Demands

Arterial blood gases and pulse oximetry are monitored to ensure that systemic oxygenation remains optimal. Metabolic demands may be reduced through the administration of high doses of barbiturates if the patient is unresponsive to conventional treatment. The mechanism by which barbiturates decrease ICP and protect the brain is uncertain, but the resultant comatose state is thought to reduce the metabolic requirements of the brain, thus providing cerebral protection (Alali et al., 2014).

Another method of reducing cellular metabolic demand and improving oxygenation is the administration of medications causing sedation. The patient who receives these agents cannot move; this decreases the metabolic demands and results in a decrease in cerebral oxygen demand. The patient cannot respond to or report pain either. The most common agents used for sedation are pentobarbital (Nembutal), thiopental (Pentothal), propofol (Diprivan), and dexmedetomidine (Precedex) (Majdan, Mauritz, Wilbacher, et al., 2013; Wang, Ji, Fen, et al., 2013).

If sedative agents are used, the ability to perform serial neurologic assessments is lost. Therefore, other monitoring tools are needed to assess the patient's status and response to therapy. Important parameters that must be assessed include ICP, blood pressure, heart rate, respiratory rate, and the patient's response to ventilator therapy (e.g., "fighting or bucking the ventilator"). The level of pharmacologic paralysis is adjusted based on serum levels of the medications given and the assessed parameters. Potential complications of these medications include hypotension caused by decreased sympathetic tone and myocardial depression.

Patients receiving high doses of barbiturates or pharmacologic sedatives require continuous cardiac monitoring, endotracheal intubation, mechanical ventilation, and arterial pressure monitoring, as well as ICP monitoring.

NURSING PROCESS

The Patient With Increased Intracranial Pressure

Assessment

Initial assessment of the patient with increased ICP includes obtaining a history of events leading to the present illness and the pertinent past medical history. It is usually necessary to obtain this information from family or friends. The neurologic examination should be as complete as the patient's condition allows. It includes an evaluation of mental status, LOC, cranial nerve function, cerebellar function (balance and coordination), reflexes, and motor and sensory function. Because the patient is critically ill, ongoing assessment is more focused, including pupil checks, assessment of selected cranial nerves, frequent measurements of vital signs and ICP, and the use of the Glasgow Coma Scale (see Table 66-1).

Diagnosis

NURSING DIAGNOSES
Based on the assessment data, major nursing diagnoses include the following:
- Ineffective airway clearance related to diminished protective reflexes (cough, gag)
- Ineffective breathing patterns related to neurologic dysfunction (brainstem compression, structural displacement)

- Risk for ineffective cerebral tissue perfusion related to the effects of increased ICP
- Deficient fluid volume related to fluid restriction
- Risk for infection related to ICP monitoring system (fiberoptic or intraventricular catheter)

Other relevant nursing diagnoses are included in the earlier section on altered LOC.

COLLABORATIVE PROBLEMS/POTENTIAL COMPLICATIONS
Potential complications may include the following:
- Brainstem herniation
- Diabetes insipidus
- SIADH

Planning and Goals

The goals for the patient include maintenance of a patent airway, normalization of respiration, adequate cerebral tissue perfusion through reduction in ICP, restoration of fluid balance, absence of infection, and absence of complications.

Nursing Interventions

MAINTAINING A PATENT AIRWAY
The patency of the airway is assessed. Secretions that are obstructing the airway must be suctioned with care, because transient elevations of ICP occur with suctioning (Hickey, 2014). Hypoxia caused by poor oxygenation leads to cerebral ischemia and edema. Coughing is discouraged because it increases ICP. The lung fields are auscultated at least every 8 hours to determine the presence of adventitious sounds or any areas of congestion. Elevating the head of the bed may aid in clearing secretions and improve venous drainage of the brain.

ACHIEVING AN ADEQUATE BREATHING PATTERN
The patient must be monitored constantly for respiratory irregularities. Increased pressure on the frontal lobes or deep midline structures may result in Cheyne–Stokes respirations, whereas pressure in the midbrain can cause hyperventilation. If the lower portion of the brainstem (the pons and medulla) is involved, respirations become irregular and eventually cease.

Hyperventilation therapy is a controversial therapy in traumatic brain injury used in some centers to reduce ICP by causing cerebral vasoconstriction and a decrease in cerebral blood volume. The nurse collaborates with the respiratory therapist in monitoring the $PaCO_2$, which is usually maintained at less than 30 mm Hg. Patients undergoing hyperventilation therapy also benefit from multimodality monitoring to determine the overall effect of this therapy on brain perfusion (de Lima Oliveira et al., 2014).

A neurologic observation record (see Fig. 66-6) is maintained, and all observations are made in relation to the patient's baseline condition. Repeated assessments of the patient are made (sometimes minute by minute) so that improvement or deterioration may be noted immediately. If the patient's condition deteriorates, the primary provider is notified emergently and preparations are made for surgical intervention.

OPTIMIZING CEREBRAL TISSUE PERFUSION
In addition to ongoing nursing assessment, strategies are initiated to reduce factors contributing to the elevation of ICP (see Table 66-2).

NURSING NEUROLOGIC CRITICAL CARE FLOWSHEET		ADDRESSOGRAPH											
	Date												
	Time												
	Initials												
Level of orientation (✓)	Person												
	Place												
	Date and time												
	No orientation												
Awakens to (✓)	Voice												
	Touch												
	Noxious stimuli												
	Painful stimuli												
	No response												
Best verbal response (✓)	Clear and appropriate												
	Clear and inappropriate												
	Difficulty speaking*												
	Perseveration												
	Aphasic expressive (non-fluent)												
	Aphasic receptive (fluent)												
	Sounds no speech												
	No verbal response												
	ETT/TRACH												
Best motor response (✓)	Moves all extremities purposefully												
	Withdraws and lifts to painful stimuli												
	Moves to painful stimuli												
	Decorticates (spinal reflex)												
	Decerebrates (spinal reflex)												
	No motor response												
Best motor strength upper extremities (✓)	No drifts (R/L)	R/L	R/L	R/L	R/L	R/L	R/L	R/L	R/L	R/L	R/L	R/L	R/L
	Drift (R/L)	R/L	R/L	R/L	R/L	R/L	R/L	R/L	R/L	R/L	R/L	R/L	R/L
	Can only lift forearm (R/L)	R/L	R/L	R/L	R/L	R/L	R/L	R/L	R/L	R/L	R/L	R/L	R/L
	Trace movement of hand or arm (R/L)	R/L	R/L	R/L	R/L	R/L	R/L	R/L	R/L	R/L	R/L	R/L	R/L
	Trace movement of fingers only (R/L)	R/L	R/L	R/L	R/L	R/L	R/L	R/L	R/L	R/L	R/L	R/L	R/L
	No motor response (R/L)	R/L	R/L	R/L	R/L	R/L	R/L	R/L	R/L	R/L	R/L	R/L	R/L
Best strength lower extremities (✓)	Raises leg off bed (R/L)	R/L	R/L	R/L	R/L	R/L	R/L	R/L	R/L	R/L	R/L	R/L	R/L
	Drags heel on bed and lifts knee (R/L)	R/L	R/L	R/L	R/L	R/L	R/L	R/L	R/L	R/L	R/L	R/L	R/L
	Trace movement of foot or leg (R/L)	R/L	R/L	R/L	R/L	R/L	R/L	R/L	R/L	R/L	R/L	R/L	R/L
	Trace movement of toes only (R/L)	R/L	R/L	R/L	R/L	R/L	R/L	R/L	R/L	R/L	R/L	R/L	R/L
	No response (R/L)	R/L	R/L	R/L	R/L	R/L	R/L	R/L	R/L	R/L	R/L	R/L	R/L
Seizure activity (✓)	No seizure activity												
	With loss of consciousness*												
	Without loss of consciousness*												
Ataxia (✓)	Gross ataxia												
	Fine motor ataxia												
	Does not apply												
ICP monitoring	Ventriculostomy mL												
	ICP mm Hg												
	Not applicable												

***= FURTHER DOCUMENTATION IS REQUIRED TO VALIDATE ASSESSMENT**

Figure 66-6 • A neurologic assessment flowsheet. The nurse fills these out on-line now in most institutions.

PUPIL GAUGE (mm)

•	•	●	●	⬤
2	3	4	5	6

⬤	⬤	⬤
7	8	9

B=Brisk, S=Sluggish, F=Fixed

ADDRESSOGRAPH

Date													
Time													
Initials													

Incision +/−	Dry and intact													
	Drainage													
Pupils: refer to above gauge (✓) (+)=Present (−)=Absent	Size (R/L)	R/L	R/L	R/L	R/L	R/L	R/L	R/L	R/L	R/L	R/L	R/L	R/L
	Regular (R/L)	R/L	R/L	R/L	R/L	R/L	R/L	R/L	R/L	R/L	R/L	R/L	R/L
	Irregular* (R/L)	R/L	R/L	R/L	R/L	R/L	R/L	R/L	R/L	R/L	R/L	R/L	R/L
	Reaction (R/L) (B) - (S) - (F)	R/L	R/L	R/L	R/L	R/L	R/L	R/L	R/L	R/L	R/L	R/L	R/L
	Ptosis (R/L) (+) (−)	R/L	R/L	R/L	R/L	R/L	R/L	R/L	R/L	R/L	R/L	R/L	R/L
	Gaze preference (R/L) (+)* (−)	R/L	R/L	R/L	R/L	R/L	R/L	R/L	R/L	R/L	R/L	R/L	R/L
Meningeal signs (+)=Present (−)=Absent	Headache													
	Nuchal rigidity													
	Photophobia													
Visual fields (+)=Present (−)=Absent* NA=Not applicable	Right upper outer													
	Right lower outer													
	Left upper outer													
	Left lower outer													
Nystagmus (+)=Present (−)=Absent	Lateral (R/L)	R/L	R/L	R/L	R/L	R/L	R/L	R/L	R/L	R/L	R/L	R/L	R/L
	Vertical (R/L)	R/L	R/L	R/L	R/L	R/L	R/L	R/L	R/L	R/L	R/L	R/L	R/L
Cranial nerves (+)=Present (−)=Absent	III, IV, VI, Extraocular movements													
	VII – Peripheral facial droop (R/L)	R/L	R/L	R/L	R/L	R/L	R/L	R/L	R/L	R/L	R/L	R/L	R/L
	XII – Tongue deviation (R/L)	R/L	R/L	R/L	R/L	R/L	R/L	R/L	R/L	R/L	R/L	R/L	R/L
	IX – Gag reflex													
	V, VII – Corneal reflex (R/L)	R/L	R/L	R/L	R/L	R/L	R/L	R/L	R/L	R/L	R/L	R/L	R/L
	X, IX – Cough reflex													
	Doll's eyes if appropriate													
Follows commands	Two step verbal command													
	One step verbal command													
	Unable to follow command													

*= FURTHER DOCUMENTATION IS REQUIRED TO VALIDATE ASSESSMENT

Initials	Signature	Title	Initials	Signature	Title

Figure 66-6 • (*Continued*)

TABLE 66-2 Increased Intracranial Pressure and Interventions

Factor	Physiology	Interventions	Rationale
Cerebral edema	Can be caused by contusion, tumor, or abscess; water intoxication (hypo-osmolality); alteration in the blood–brain barrier (protein leaks into the tissue, causing water to follow)	Administer osmotic diuretics as prescribed (monitor serum osmolality). Maintain head of bed elevation at 30 degrees. Maintain alignment of the head.	Promotes venous return Prevents impairment of venous return through the jugular veins
Hypoxia	A decrease in PaO_2 to <60 mm Hg causes cerebral vasodilation.	Maintain PaO_2 >60 mm Hg. Maintain oxygen therapy. Monitor arterial blood gas values. Suction when needed. Maintain a patent airway.	Prevents hypoxia and vasodilation
Hypercapnia (elevated $PaCO_2$)	Causes vasodilation	Maintain $PaCO_2$ (normally 35–45 mm Hg) by establishing ventilation.	Normalizing $PaCO_2$ minimizes vasodilation and thus reduces the cerebral blood volume.
Impaired venous return	Increases the cerebral blood volume	Maintain head alignment. Elevate head of bed 30 degrees.	Hyperextension, rotation, or hyperflexion of the neck causes decreased venous return.
Increase in intrathoracic or abdominal pressure	An increase in these pressures due to coughing, PEEP, or Valsalva maneuver causes a decrease in venous return.	Monitor arterial blood gas values, and keep PEEP as low as possible. Provide humidified oxygen. Administer stool softeners as prescribed.	To keep secretions loose and easy to suction or expectorate Soft bowel movements will prevent straining or Valsalva maneuver.

PaO_2, partial pressure of arterial oxygen; $PaCO_2$, partial pressure of arterial carbon dioxide; PEEP, positive end-expiratory pressure.

Adapted from American Association of Neuroscience Nurses. (2012). *Care of the patient undergoing intracranial pressure monitoring/external ventricular drainage or lumbar drainage: AANN Clinical Practice Guideline Series.* Glenview, IL: Author; Hickey, J. V. (2014). *The clinical practice of neurological & neurosurgical nursing* (7th ed.). Philadelphia, PA: Lippincott Williams & Wilkins.

Proper positioning helps reduce ICP. The patient's head is kept in a neutral (midline) position, maintained with the use of a cervical collar if necessary, to promote venous drainage. Elevation of the head is maintained at 30 to 45 degrees unless contraindicated. Extreme rotation of the neck and flexion of the neck are avoided, because compression or distortion of the jugular veins increases ICP. Extreme hip flexion is also avoided, because this position causes an increase in intra-abdominal and intrathoracic pressures, which can produce an increase in ICP. Relatively minor changes in position can significantly affect ICP. If monitoring reveals that turning the patient raises ICP, rotating beds, turning sheets, and holding the patient's head during turning may minimize the stimuli that increase ICP. Research suggests that patient response to position change is highly variable and requires close hemodynamic monitoring and individualized care (Mitchell, Kirkness, & Blissitt, 2015).

The Valsalva maneuver, which can be produced by straining at defecation or even moving in bed, raises ICP and is to be avoided. Stool softeners may be prescribed. If the patient is alert and able to eat, a diet high in fiber may be indicated. Abdominal distention, which increases intra-abdominal and intrathoracic pressure and ICP, should be noted. Enemas and cathartics are avoided if possible. When moving or being turned in bed, the patient can be instructed to exhale (which opens the glottis) to avoid the Valsalva maneuver.

Mechanical ventilation presents unique problems for the patient with increased ICP. Before suctioning, the patient should be preoxygenated and briefly hyperventilated using 100% oxygen on the ventilator. Suctioning should not last longer than 15 seconds. High levels of positive end-expiratory pressure (PEEP) must be utilized cautiously, because they may decrease venous return to the heart and decrease venous drainage from the brain through increased intrathoracic pressure (Nemer, Caldeira, Santos, et al., 2015).

Activities that increase ICP, as indicated by changes in waveforms, should be avoided if possible. Spacing of nursing interventions may prevent transient increases in ICP. During nursing interventions, the ICP should not increase above 25 mm Hg, and it should return to baseline levels within 5 minutes. Patients with increased ICP should not demonstrate a significant increase in pressure or change in the ICP waveform. Patients with the potential for a significant increase in ICP may need sedation before initiation of nursing activities (Bader, Littlejohns, & Olson, 2016).

Emotional stress and frequent arousal from sleep are avoided. A calm atmosphere is maintained. Environmental stimuli (e.g., noise, conversation) should be minimal.

MAINTAINING NEGATIVE FLUID BALANCE

The administration of osmotic and loop diuretics is part of the treatment protocol to reduce ICP. Corticosteroids may be used to reduce cerebral edema (except when it results from trauma), and fluids may be restricted. All of these treatment modalities promote dehydration.

Skin turgor, mucous membranes, urine output, and serum and urine osmolality are monitored to assess fluid status. If IV fluids are prescribed, the nurse ensures that they are given at a slow to moderate rate with an IV infusion pump, to prevent too-rapid administration and avoid overhydration. For the patient receiving mannitol, the nurse observes for the possible development of heart failure and pulmonary edema.

The intent of treatment is to promote a shift of fluid from the intracellular to the intravascular compartment and to control cerebral edema. However, this shift of fluid volume to the intravascular compartment may overwhelm the ability of the myocardium to increase workload sufficient to meet these demands, which may cause failure and pulmonary edema.

For patients undergoing dehydrating procedures, vital signs, including blood pressure, must be monitored to assess fluid volume status. An indwelling urinary catheter is inserted to permit assessment of renal function and fluid status. During the acute phase, urine output is monitored hourly. An output greater than 200 mL per hour for 2 consecutive hours may indicate the onset of diabetes insipidus (Hickey, 2014). These patients need careful oral hygiene, because mouth dryness occurs with dehydration. Frequently rinsing the mouth with nondrying solutions, lubricating the lips, and removing encrustations relieve dryness and promote comfort.

PREVENTING INFECTION

The risk of infection is greatest when ICP is monitored with an intraventricular catheter and increases with the duration of the monitoring. Most health care facilities have written protocols for managing these systems and maintaining their sterility; strict adherence to the protocols is essential.

Aseptic technique must be used when managing the system and changing the ventricular drainage bag. The drainage system is also checked for loose connections, because they can cause leakage and contamination of the CSF as well as inaccurate readings of ICP. The nurse observes the character of the CSF drainage and reports increasing cloudiness or blood. The patient is monitored for signs and symptoms of meningitis: fever, chills, nuchal (neck) rigidity, and increasing or persistent headache. See Chapter 69 for a discussion of meningitis.

MONITORING AND MANAGING POTENTIAL COMPLICATIONS

The primary complication of increased ICP is brain herniation resulting in death (see Fig. 66-2). Nursing management focuses on detecting early signs of increasing ICP, because medical interventions are usually ineffective once later signs develop (Bader et al., 2016). Frequent neurologic assessments and documentation and analysis of trends will reveal the subtle changes that may indicate increasing ICP.

Detecting Indications of Increasing Intracranial Pressure. The nurse assesses for and immediately reports any signs or symptoms of increasing ICP (see Chart 66-1). The focus is on detecting early signs of increasing ICP.

Monitoring Intracranial Pressure. Because clinical assessment is not always a reliable guide in recognizing increased ICP, especially in patients who are comatose, monitoring of ICP and cerebral oxygenation is an essential part of management. ICP is monitored closely for continuous elevation or significant increase over baseline. The trend of ICP measurements over time is an important indication of the patient's underlying status. Vital signs are assessed when an increase in ICP is noted (Bader et al., 2016).

Careful attention to aseptic technique is needed when handling any part of the monitoring system. The insertion site is inspected for signs of infection. Temperature, pulse, and respirations are closely monitored for systemic signs of infection. All connections and stopcocks are checked for leaks, because even small leaks can distort pressure readings and lead to infection (AANN, 2012).

Chart 66-1 Detecting Increasing Intracranial Pressure (ICP)

Early Signs and Symptoms of Increasing ICP

- *Disorientation, restlessness, increased respiratory effort, purposeless movements, and mental confusion.* These are early clinical indications of increasing ICP because the brain cells responsible for cognition are extremely sensitive to decreased oxygenation.
- *Pupillary changes and impaired extraocular movements.* These occur as the increasing pressure displaces the brain against the oculomotor and optic nerves (cranial nerves II, III, IV, and VI), which arise from the midbrain and brainstem (see Chapter 65).
- *Weakness in one extremity or on one side of the body.* This occurs as increasing ICP compresses the pyramidal tracts.
- *Headache that is constant, increasing in intensity, and aggravated by movement or straining.* This occurs as increasing ICP causes pressure and stretching of venous and arterial vessels in the base of the brain.

Later Signs and Symptoms of Increasing ICP

- The level of consciousness continues to deteriorate until the patient is comatose (Glasgow Coma Scale score ≤8).
- The pulse rate and respiratory rate decrease or become erratic, and the blood pressure and temperature increase. The pulse pressure (the difference between the systolic and diastolic pressures) widens. The pulse fluctuates rapidly, varying from bradycardia to tachycardia.
- Altered respiratory patterns develop, including Cheyne–Stokes breathing (rhythmic waxing and waning of rate and depth of respirations alternating with brief periods of apnea) and ataxic breathing (irregular breathing with a random sequence of deep and shallow breaths).
- Projectile vomiting may occur with increased pressure on the reflex center in the medulla.
- Hemiplegia or decorticate or decerebrate posturing may develop as pressure on the brainstem increases; bilateral flaccidity occurs before death.
- Loss of brainstem reflexes, including pupillary, corneal, gag, and swallowing reflexes, is an ominous sign of approaching death.

Adapted from Hickey, J. V. (2014). *The clinical practice of neurological & neurosurgical nursing* (7th ed.). Philadelphia, PA: Lippincott Williams & Wilkins.

When ICP is monitored with a fluid system, the transducer is calibrated at a particular reference point, usually 2.5 cm (1 inch) above the ear with the patient in the supine position; this point corresponds to the level of the foramen of Monro (see Fig. 66-7). CSF pressure readings depend on the patient's position. For subsequent pressure readings, the head should be in the same position relative to the transducer. Fiberoptic catheters are calibrated before insertion and do not require further referencing; they do not require the head of the bed to be at a specific position to obtain an accurate reading.

When technology is associated with patient management, the nurse must be certain that the technologic equipment is functioning properly. The most important concern must be the patient to whom equipment is attached. The patient and family must be informed about the technology and the goals of its use. The patient's response is

Figure 66-7 • Location of the foramen of Monro for calibration of the intracranial pressure monitoring system.

monitored, and appropriate comfort measures are implemented to ensure that the patient's stress is minimized.

ICP measurement is only one parameter; repeated neurologic checks and clinical examinations remain important measures. Astute observation, comparison of findings with previous observations, and interventions can assist in preventing life-threatening ICP elevations.

Monitoring for Secondary Complications. The nurse also assesses for complications of increased ICP, including diabetes insipidus and SIADH (see Chapters 13 and 52). Urine output should be monitored closely. Diabetes insipidus requires fluid and electrolyte replacement, along with the administration of vasopressin, to replace and slow the urine output. Serum electrolyte levels are monitored for imbalances. SIADH requires fluid restriction and monitoring of serum electrolyte levels.

Evaluation

Expected patient outcomes may include:
1. Maintains patent airway
2. Attains optimal breathing pattern
   a. Breathes in a regular pattern
   b. Attains or maintains arterial blood gas values within acceptable range
3. Demonstrates optimal cerebral tissue perfusion
   a. Increasingly oriented to time, place, and person
   b. Follows verbal commands; answers questions correctly
4. Attains desired fluid balance
   a. Maintains fluid restriction
   b. Demonstrates serum and urine osmolality values within acceptable range
5. Has no signs or symptoms of infection
   a. Has no fever
   b. Shows no redness, swelling, or drainage at arterial, IV, and urinary catheter sites
   c. Has no redness, swelling, or purulent drainage from invasive intracranial monitoring device
6. Absence of complications
   a. Has ICP values that remain within normal limits
   b. Demonstrates urine output and serum electrolyte levels within acceptable limits

 INTRACRANIAL SURGERY

A **craniotomy** involves opening the skull surgically to gain access to intracranial structures. This procedure is performed to remove a tumor, relieve elevated ICP, evacuate a blood clot, or control hemorrhage. The surgeon cuts the skull to create a bony flap, which can be repositioned after surgery and held in place by periosteal or wire sutures. One of two approaches through the skull is used: (1) above the tentorium (supratentorial craniotomy) into the supratentorial compartment, or (2) below the tentorium into the infratentorial (posterior fossa) compartment. A third approach, the **transsphenoidal** approach (through the mouth and nasal sinuses) is often used to gain access to the pituitary gland (Bader et al., 2016). Table 66-3 compares these three different surgical approaches.

Alternatively, intracranial structures may be approached through burr holes (see Fig. 66-8), which are circular openings made in the skull by either a hand drill or an automatic craniotome (which has a self-controlled system to stop the drill when the bone is penetrated). Burr holes may be used to determine the presence of cerebral swelling and injury and the size and position of the ventricles. They are also a means of evacuating an intracranial hematoma or abscess and for making a bone flap in the skull that allows access to the ventricles for decompression, ventriculography, or shunting procedures. Other cranial procedures include **craniectomy** (excision of a portion of the skull) and cranioplasty (repair of a cranial defect using a plastic or metal plate).

Supratentorial and Infratentorial Approaches

Preoperative Management

Medical Management

Preoperative diagnostic procedures may include a CT scan to demonstrate the lesion and show the degree of surrounding brain edema, the ventricular size, and the displacement. An MRI scan provides information similar to that of a CT scan with improved tissue contrast, resolution, and anatomic definition. Cerebral angiography may be used to study a tumor's blood supply or obtain information about vascular lesions. Transcranial Doppler flow studies are used to evaluate the blood flow within intracranial blood vessels.

Most patients are prescribed an anticonvulsant medication such as phenytoin (Dilantin), levetiracetam (Keppra), or a phenytoin metabolite fosphenytoin sodium (Cerebyx) before surgery to reduce the risk of postoperative **seizures** (paroxysmal transient disturbance of the brain resulting from a discharge of abnormal electrical activity) (Karch, 2015). Before surgery, corticosteroids such as dexamethasone may be given to reduce cerebral edema if the patient has a brain tumor. Fluids may be restricted. A hyperosmotic agent (mannitol) and a diuretic agent such as furosemide (Lasix) may be administered IV immediately before and sometimes during surgery if the patient tends to retain fluid, as do many who have intracranial dysfunction. Antibiotic agents may be given if there is a chance of cerebral contamination; diazepam

TABLE 66-3 Comparison of Cranial Surgical Approaches

Supratentorial	Infratentorial	Transsphenoidal

Pituitary tumor
Tip of forceps

Site of Surgery

Above the tentorium	Below the tentorium, brainstem	Sella turcica and pituitary region

Incision Location

Incision is made above the area to be operated on; usually located behind the hairline.	Incision is made at the nape of the neck, around the occipital lobe.	Incision is made beneath the upper lip to gain access into the nasal cavity.

Selected Nursing Interventions

Maintain head of bed elevated at 30 degrees, with neck in neutral alignment. Position patient on either side or back. (Avoid positioning patient on operative side if a large tumor has been removed.)	Maintain neck in straight alignment. Avoid flexion of the neck to prevent possible tearing of the suture line. Position the patient on either side. (Check surgeon's preference for positioning of patient.)	Maintain nasal packing in place and reinforce as needed. Instruct patient to avoid blowing the nose. Provide oral care according to institutional procedure. Keep head of bed elevated to promote venous drainage and drainage from the surgical site.

Figure 66-8 • Burr holes may be used in neurosurgical procedures to make a bone flap in the skull, to aspirate a brain abscess, or to evacuate a hematoma.

(Valium) or lorazepam (Ativan) may be prescribed before surgery to allay anxiety.

Nursing Management

The preoperative assessment serves as a baseline against which postoperative status and recovery are compared (Bauman & McCourt, 2014). This assessment includes evaluating the LOC and responsiveness to stimuli and identifying any neurologic deficits, such as paralysis, visual dysfunction, alterations in personality or speech, and bladder and bowel disorders. Baseline distal and proximal motor strength in both upper and lower extremities is tested and recorded. See Chapter 65 for a discussion of the testing of motor function.

The patient's and family's understanding of and reactions to the anticipated surgical procedure and its possible sequelae are assessed, as is the availability of support systems for the patient and family. Adequate preparation for surgery, with attention to the patient's physical and emotional status, can reduce the risk of anxiety, fear, and postoperative complications. The patient is assessed for neurologic deficits and their potential impact after surgery. For motor deficits or weakness or paralysis of the arms or legs, trochanter rolls are applied to the extremities, and the feet are positioned against a footboard or the ankles are supported in a neutral position with orthotic boots. A patient who can ambulate is encouraged to do so. If the patient is aphasic, writing materials or picture and word cards showing the bedpan, glass of water, blanket, and other frequently used items may help improve communication.

Preparation of the patient and family includes providing education about what to expect during and after surgery. The patient should plan to shower and wash their hair prior to surgery using the preferred cleansing solution. Hair is removed with the use of clippers and the surgical site prepared immediately before surgery (usually in the operating room), and intravenous antibiotics are given 1 hour prior to the incision to decrease the chance of infection (AANN, 2016b). An indwelling urinary catheter is inserted in the operating room to drain the bladder during the administration of diuretic agents and to permit monitoring of urinary output. The patient may have a central and an arterial line placed for fluid administration and monitoring of pressures after surgery. The large head dressing applied after surgery may impair hearing temporarily. Vision may be limited if the eyes are swollen shut. If a tracheostomy or endotracheal tube is in place, the patient will be unable to speak until the tube is removed, so an alternative method of communication must be established.

An altered cognitive state may make the patient unaware of the impending surgery. Even so, encouragement and attention to the patient's needs are necessary. Whatever the state of awareness of the patient, the family need reassurance and support, because they usually recognize the seriousness of brain surgery.

Postoperative Management

Postoperatively, an arterial line and a central venous pressure line may be in place to monitor and manage blood pressure and central venous pressure. The patient may be intubated and may receive supplemental oxygen therapy. Ongoing postoperative management is aimed at detecting and reducing cerebral edema, relieving pain and preventing seizures, and monitoring ICP and neurologic status.

Reducing Cerebral Edema

Medications to reduce cerebral edema include mannitol, which increases serum osmolality and draws free water from areas of the brain (with an intact blood–brain barrier). The fluid is then excreted by osmotic diuresis. Dexamethasone may be administered IV every 6 hours for 24 to 72 hours; the route is changed to oral as soon as possible, and the dosage is tapered over 5 to 7 days (Karch, 2015).

Relieving Pain and Preventing Seizures

Acetaminophen is usually prescribed for temperatures exceeding 37.5°C (99.6°F) and for mild pain. The patient usually has a headache after a craniotomy as a result of stretching and irritation of nerves in the scalp during surgery. Codeine, administered IV or orally, is often sufficient to relieve headache. Morphine sulfate may also be used in the management of postoperative pain in patients who have undergone a craniotomy with the goal of a patient reporting acceptable pain level (AANN, 2016b).

Anticonvulsant medication (phenytoin, levetiracetam) is often prescribed prophylactically for patients who have undergone supratentorial craniotomy because of the high risk of seizures after these procedures (Hickey, 2014). Serum levels are monitored to check that the medication levels are within the therapeutic range.

Monitoring Intracranial Pressure

A patient undergoing intracranial surgery may have an ICP or cerebral oxygenation monitor inserted during surgery. Strict adherence to written protocols for managing these systems is essential, as discussed earlier, for preventing infection and managing ICP. The system is removed after the ICP or cerebral oxygenation is normal and stable. The neurosurgeon must be notified immediately if the system is not functioning.

NURSING PROCESS

The Patient Who Has Undergone Intracranial Surgery

Assessment

After surgery, the frequency of postoperative monitoring is based on the patient's clinical status. Assessing respiratory function is essential, because even a small degree of hypoxia can increase cerebral ischemia. The respiratory rate and pattern are monitored, and arterial blood gas values are assessed frequently. Fluctuations in vital signs are carefully monitored and documented, because they may indicate increased ICP. The patient's temperature is measured to assess for hyperthermia secondary to infection or damage to the hypothalamus. Neurologic checks are made frequently to detect increased ICP resulting from cerebral edema or bleeding. A change in LOC or response to stimuli may be the first sign of increasing ICP.

The surgical dressing is inspected for evidence of bleeding and CSF drainage. The incision is monitored for redness, tenderness, bulging, separation, or foul odor. Sodium retention may occur in the immediate postoperative period. Serum and urine electrolytes, BUN, blood glucose, weight, and clinical status are monitored. Intake and output are measured in view of losses associated with fever, respiration, and CSF drainage. The nurse must be alert to the development of complications; all assessments are carried out with these problems in mind. Seizures are a potential complication, and any seizure activity is carefully recorded and reported. Restlessness may occur as the patient becomes more responsive, or restlessness may be caused by pain, confusion, hypoxia, or other stimuli.

Diagnosis

NURSING DIAGNOSES

Based on the assessment data, major nursing diagnoses may include the following:

- Risk for ineffective cerebral tissue perfusion related to cerebral edema
- Risk for imbalanced body temperature related to damage to the hypothalamus, dehydration, and infection
- Potential for impaired gas exchange related to hypoventilation, aspiration, and immobility

- Ineffective coping related to sensory perception changes due to periorbital edema, head dressing, endotracheal tube, and effects of ICP
- Disturbed body image related to change in appearance or physical disabilities

Other nursing diagnoses may include impaired communication (aphasia) related to insult to brain tissue and high risk for impaired skin integrity related to immobility, pressure, and incontinence; impaired physical mobility related to a neurologic deficit secondary to the neurosurgical procedure or to the underlying disorder may also occur.

COLLABORATIVE PROBLEMS/POTENTIAL COMPLICATIONS

Potential complications may include the following:

- Increased ICP
- Bleeding and hypovolemic shock
- Fluid and electrolyte disturbances
- Infection
- CSF leak
- Seizures

Planning and Goals

The major goals for the patient include maintaining or restoring neurologic homeostasis to improve cerebral tissue perfusion, adequate thermoregulation, normal ventilation and gas exchange, ability to cope with sensory deprivation, adaptation to changes in body image, and absence of complications.

Nursing Interventions

MAINTAINING CEREBRAL TISSUE PERFUSION

Attention to the patient's respiratory status is essential, because even slight decreases in the oxygen level (hypoxia) or slight increases in the carbon dioxide level (hypercarbia) can affect cerebral perfusion, the clinical course, and the patient's outcome. The endotracheal tube is left in place until the patient shows signs of awakening and has adequate spontaneous ventilation, as evaluated clinically and by arterial blood gas analysis. Secondary brain damage can result from impaired cerebral oxygenation.

Some degree of cerebral edema occurs after brain surgery; it tends to peak 24 to 36 hours after surgery, potentially producing decreased responsiveness on the second postoperative day. The control of cerebral edema was discussed earlier. Nursing strategies used to control factors that may raise ICP were presented in the previous Nursing Process section on increased ICP. Intraventricular drainage is carefully monitored, using strict asepsis when any part of the system is handled.

Vital signs and neurologic status (LOC and responsiveness, pupillary and motor responses) are assessed every 15 to 60 minutes. Extreme head rotation is avoided, because this raises ICP. After supratentorial surgery, the patient is placed on their back or side (on the unoperated side if a large lesion was removed) with one pillow under the head. The head of the bed may be elevated 30 degrees, depending on the level of the ICP and the neurosurgeon's preference. After posterior fossa (infratentorial) surgery, the patient is kept flat on one side (off the back) with the head on a small, firm pillow. The patient may be turned on either side, keeping the neck in a neutral position. When the patient is being turned, the body should be turned as a unit to prevent placing strain on the incision and possibly tearing the sutures. The head of the bed may be elevated slowly as tolerated by the patient.

The patient's position is changed every 2 hours, and skin care is given frequently. During position changes, care is taken to prevent disruption of the ICP monitoring system. A turning sheet or lift sling placed under the patient's head to midthigh makes it easier to move and turn the patient safely.

REGULATING TEMPERATURE

Moderate temperature elevation can be expected after intracranial surgery because of the reaction to blood at the operative site or in the subarachnoid space. Injury to the hypothalamic centers that regulate body temperature can occur during surgery. Fever is treated vigorously to combat the effect of an elevated temperature on brain metabolism and function.

Nursing interventions include monitoring the patient's temperature and using the following measures to reduce body temperature: removing blankets, placing ice packs, and administering prescribed antipyretics to reduce fever (Rockett, Thompson, & Blissitt, 2015).

Conversely, hypothermia may be seen after lengthy neurosurgical procedures. Therefore, frequent measurements of rectal temperatures are necessary. Rewarming should occur slowly to prevent shivering, which increases cellular oxygen demands.

IMPROVING GAS EXCHANGE

The patient undergoing neurosurgery is at risk for impaired gas exchange and pulmonary infections due to immobility, immunosuppression, decreased LOC, and fluid restriction. Immobility compromises the respiratory system by causing pooling and stasis of secretions in dependent areas and the development of atelectasis. The patient whose fluid intake is restricted may be more vulnerable to atelectasis as a result of inability to expectorate thickened secretions. Pneumonia can develop due to aspiration and restricted mobility.

Repositioning the patient every 2 hours helps to mobilize pulmonary secretions and prevent stasis. After the patient regains consciousness, additional measures to expand collapsed alveoli can be instituted, such as yawning, sighing, deep breathing, incentive spirometry, and coughing (unless contraindicated). If necessary, the oropharynx and trachea are suctioned to remove secretions that cannot be raised by coughing; however, coughing and suctioning increase ICP. Therefore, suctioning should be used cautiously. Increasing the humidity in the oxygen delivery system may help to loosen secretions. The nurse and the respiratory therapist work together to monitor the effects of chest physiotherapy.

COPING WITH SENSORY DEPRIVATION

Periorbital edema is a common consequence of intracranial surgery, because fluid drains into the dependent periorbital areas when the patient has been positioned in a prone position during surgery. A hematoma may form under the scalp and spread down to the orbit, producing an area of ecchymosis (black eye).

Before surgery, the patient and family should be informed that one or both eyes may be edematous temporarily after surgery. After surgery, elevating the head of the bed (if not contraindicated) and applying cold compresses over the eyes will help reduce the edema. The surgeon is notified if periorbital edema increases significantly, because this may indicate that a postoperative clot is developing or that there is increasing

ICP and poor venous drainage. Health care personnel should announce their presence when entering the room to avoid startling the patient whose vision is impaired due to periorbital edema or neurologic deficits.

Additional factors that can affect sensation include a bulky head dressing, the presence of an endotracheal tube, and effects of increased ICP. The first postoperative dressing change is usually performed by the neurosurgeon. In the absence of bleeding or a CSF leak, every effort is made to minimize the size of the head dressing. If the patient requires an endotracheal tube for mechanical ventilation, every effort is made to extubate the patient as soon as clinical signs indicate it is possible. The patient is monitored closely for the effects of elevated ICP.

Enhancing Self-Image

The patient is encouraged to verbalize feelings and frustrations about any change in appearance. Nursing support is based on the patient's reactions and feelings. Factual information may need to be provided if the patient has misconceptions about puffiness about the face, periorbital bruising, and hair loss. Attention to grooming, the use of the patient's own clothing, and covering the head with a turban (and later a wig until hair growth occurs) are encouraged. Social interaction with close friends, family, and hospital personnel may increase the patient's sense of self-worth.

The family and social support system can be of assistance while the patient recovers from surgery.

Monitoring and Managing Potential Complications

The nurse must be vigilant for complications that may develop within hours of surgery and require close collaboration with the neurosurgeon. These include increased ICP, bleeding and hypovolemic shock, altered fluid and electrolyte balance (e.g., water intoxication and diabetes insipidus), infection, identification of a CSF leak, and seizures.

Monitoring for Increased Intracranial Pressure and Bleeding. Increased ICP and bleeding are life threatening to the patient who has undergone intracranial surgery. The following points must be kept in mind when caring for any patient who has undergone such surgery:

- An increase in blood pressure and decrease in pulse with respiratory failure may indicate increased ICP.
- An accumulation of blood under the bone flap (extradural, subdural, or intracerebral hematoma) may pose a threat to life. A clot must be suspected in any patient who does not awaken as expected or whose condition deteriorates. An intracranial hematoma is suspected if the patient has any new postoperative neurologic deficits (especially a dilated pupil on the operative side). In these circumstances, the patient is returned to the operating room immediately for evacuation of the clot, if indicated.
- Cerebral edema, infarction, metabolic disturbances, and hydrocephalus are conditions that may mimic the clinical manifestations of a clot.

The patient is monitored closely for indicators of complications, and early signs and trends in clinical status are reported to the surgeon. Treatments are initiated promptly, and the nurse assists in evaluating the patient's response to treatment. The nurse also provides support to the patient and family.

> ### Quality and Safety Nursing Alert
>
> *If signs and symptoms of increased ICP occur, efforts to decrease the ICP are initiated: alignment of the head in a neutral position without flexion to promote venous drainage, elevation of the head of the bed to 30 degrees (when prescribed), administration of mannitol (an osmotic diuretic), and possible administration of pharmacologic paralyzing agents.*

Managing Fluid and Electrolyte Disturbances. Fluid and electrolyte imbalances may occur because of the patient's underlying condition and its management or as complications of surgery. These disturbances can contribute to the development of cerebral edema.

The postoperative fluid regimen depends on the type of neurosurgical procedure and is determined on an individual basis. The volume and composition of fluids are adjusted based on daily serum electrolyte values, along with fluid intake and output. Fluids may have to be restricted in patients with cerebral edema.

Oral fluids are usually resumed after the first 24 hours. The presence of gag and swallowing reflexes must be checked before initiation of oral fluids. Some patients with posterior fossa tumors have impaired swallowing, so fluids may need to be given by alternative routes. The patient should be observed for signs and symptoms of nausea and vomiting as the diet is progressed (AANN, 2016b).

Patients undergoing surgery for brain tumors often receive large doses of corticosteroids and are at risk for hyperglycemia. Serum glucose levels are measured every 4 to 6 hours, and sliding scale insulin is prescribed as needed. These patients are prone to stress ulcers, so histamine-2 receptor antagonists (H_2 blockers) are prescribed to suppress the secretion of gastric acid. Patients also are monitored for bleeding and assessed for gastric pain.

If the surgical site is near to (or causes edema to) the pituitary gland and hypothalamus, the patient may develop symptoms of diabetes insipidus, which is characterized by excessive urinary output, elevated serum osmolality, decreased urine osmolality, hypernatremia, and a low urine-specific gravity. The urine-specific gravity is measured hourly, and fluid intake and output are monitored. Fluid replacement must compensate for urine output, and serum potassium levels must be monitored.

SIADH, which results in water retention with hyponatremia and serum hypo-osmolality, occurs in a wide variety of CNS disorders (e.g., brain tumor, head trauma) causing fluid disturbances. Nursing management includes careful intake and output measurements, specific gravity determinations of urine, and monitoring of serum and urine electrolyte levels while following directives for fluid restriction. SIADH is usually self-limited.

Preventing Infection. The patient undergoing neurosurgery is at risk for infection related to the neurosurgical procedure (brain exposure, bone exposure, wound hematomas) and the presence of IV and arterial lines for fluid administration and monitoring. Risk for infection is increased in patients who undergo lengthy intracranial operations and in those who have external ventricular drains in place.

The dressing is often stained with blood in the immediate postoperative period. Because blood is an excellent culture medium for bacteria, the dressing is reinforced with sterile pads so that contamination and infection are avoided. A heavily stained or displaced dressing should be reported immediately. A drain is sometimes placed in the craniotomy incision to facilitate drainage.

After suboccipital surgical procedures, CSF may leak through the incision. This complication is dangerous because of the possibility of meningitis. After a craniotomy, the patient is instructed to avoid coughing, sneezing, or nose blowing, which can cause CSF leakage by creating pressure on the operative site.

> ### Quality and Safety Nursing Alert
>
> *Any sudden discharge of fluid from a cranial incision is reported at once, because a large leak requires surgical repair. Attention should be paid to the patient who complains of a salty taste or "postnasal drip," because this can be caused by CSF trickling down the throat.*

Aseptic technique is used when handling dressings, drainage systems, and IV and arterial lines. The patient is monitored carefully for signs and symptoms of infection, and cultures are obtained if infection is suspected. Appropriate antibiotic agents are given as prescribed. Other causes of infection in the patient undergoing intracranial surgery, such as pneumonia and urinary tract infections, are similar to those in other patients postoperatively.

Monitoring for Seizure Activity. Seizures may occur as complications after any intracranial neurosurgical procedure. Preventing seizures is essential to avoid further cerebral edema. Administering the prescribed anticonvulsant medication before and after surgery may prevent the development of seizures in subsequent months and years. **Status epilepticus** (prolonged seizures without recovery of consciousness in the intervals between seizures) may occur after craniotomy and also may be related to the development of complications

(hematoma, ischemia). The management of status epilepticus is described later in this chapter.

Monitoring and Managing Other Complications. Other complications may occur during the first 2 weeks or later and may compromise the patient's recovery. The most important of these are VTE (DVT, PE), pulmonary and urinary tract infection, and pressure ulcers. Most of these complications may be avoided with frequent changes of position, adequate suctioning of secretions, thrombosis prophylaxis, early removal of indwelling urinary catheter, early ambulation, and skin care.

PROMOTING HOME, COMMUNITY-BASED, AND TRANSITIONAL CARE

Educating Patients About Self-Care. The recovery at home of a patient who has had neurosurgery depends on the extent of the surgical procedure and its success. The patient's strengths as well as limitations are assessed and explained to the family, along with the family's part in promoting recovery. Because administration of anticonvulsant medication is a priority, the patient and family are educated to use a check-off system, pill boxes, and alarms to ensure that the medication is taken as prescribed.

The patient and family are educated about what to expect after intracranial surgery (see Chart 66-2). Dietary restrictions usually are not required unless another health problem necessitates a special diet. Although showering or tub bathing is permitted, the scalp should be kept dry until all sutures have been removed. A clean scarf or cap may be worn until a wig or hairpiece is purchased. If skull bone has been removed, a protective helmet may be prescribed. The patient may require rehabilitation, depending on the postoperative level of function. The patient may require physical therapy for residual weakness and mobility issues. An occupational therapist is consulted to assist with self-care issues. If the patient has aphasia, speech therapy may be necessary.

Continuing and Transitional Care. The patient is discharged from the hospital as soon as possible. Patients with severe motor deficits require extensive physical therapy and rehabilitation.

Chart 66-2 **HOME CARE CHECKLIST**
Discharge After Intracranial Surgery

At the completion of education, the patient and/or caregiver will be able to:

- Name the procedure that was performed, any complications that occurred, and identify any permanent changes in anatomic structure or function as well as changes in ADLs, IADLs, roles, relationships, and spirituality.
- Identify interventions and strategies (e.g., durable medical equipment, adaptive equipment) used in recovery period.
- Describe ongoing postoperative therapeutic regimen, including diet and activities to perform (e.g., walking and breathing exercises) and to limit or avoid (e.g., lifting weights, driving a car, contact sports).
- State the name, dose, side effects, frequency, and schedule for all medications.
- State how to obtain medical supplies and carry out dressing changes, wound care, and other prescribed regimens.

- Identify durable medical equipment needs, proper usage, and maintenance necessary for safe utilization.
- Describe signs and symptoms of complications.
- State time and date of follow-up appointments.
- Relate how to reach primary provider with questions or complications.
- Identify community resources for peer and caregiver/family support:
  - Identify sources of support (e.g., friends, relatives, faith community).
  - Identify phone numbers, meeting locations/times of community resources for patients and their caregivers/families.
- Identify the need for health promotion (e.g., weight reduction, smoking cessation, stress management), disease prevention and screening activities.

ADL, activities of daily living; IADL, independent activities of daily living.

Those with postoperative cognitive and speech impairments require psychological evaluation, speech therapy, and rehabilitation. The nurse collaborates with the physician and other health care professionals during hospitalization and home or transitional care to achieve as complete a rehabilitation as possible and to assist the patient in living with residual disability.

If tumor, injury, or disease makes the prognosis poor, care is directed toward making the patient as comfortable as possible. With return of the tumor or cerebral compression, the patient becomes less alert and aware. Other possible consequences include paralysis, blindness, and seizures. The home care nurse, hospice nurse, and social worker collaborate with the family to plan for additional services or placement of the patient in an extended care facility (see the Cerebral Metastases section in Chapter 70). The patient and family are encouraged to discuss end-of-life preferences for care; the patient's end-of-life preferences must be respected (see Chapter 16). The nurse involved in home and continuing care of patients after cranial surgery also should remind patients and family members of the need for health promotion activities and recommended health screening.

Evaluation

Expected patient outcomes may include:

1. Achieves optimal cerebral tissue perfusion
   a. Opens eyes on request; uses recognizable words, progressing to normal speech
   b. Obeys commands with appropriate motor responses
2. Maintains normal body temperature
   a. Registers normal body temperature
3. Has normal gas exchange
   a. Has arterial blood gas values within normal ranges
   b. Breathes easily; lung sounds clear without adventitious sounds
   c. Takes deep breaths and changes position as directed
4. Copes with sensory deprivation
5. Demonstrates improving self-concept
   a. Pays attention to grooming
   b. Visits and interacts with others
6. Exhibits absence of complications
   a. Exhibits ICP within normal range
   b. Has minimal bleeding at surgical site; surgical incision healing without evidence of infection
   c. Shows fluid balance and electrolyte levels within desired ranges
   d. Exhibits no evidence of seizures

Transsphenoidal Approach

Tumors within the sella turcica and small adenomas of the pituitary can be removed through a transsphenoidal approach (see Table 66-3). Although an otorhinolaryngologist may make the initial opening, the neurosurgeon completes the opening into the sphenoidal sinus and exposes the floor of the sella. Microsurgical techniques provide improved illumination, magnification, and visualization so that nearby vital structures can be avoided.

The transsphenoidal approach offers direct access to the sella turcica with minimal risk of trauma and hemorrhage

(Bader et al., 2016). It avoids many of the risks of craniotomy, and the postoperative discomfort is similar to that of other transnasal surgical procedures. It may also be used for pituitary ablation (destruction) in patients with metastatic breast or prostatic cancer.

Complications

Manipulation of the posterior pituitary gland during surgery may produce transient diabetes insipidus of several days' duration (Hickey, 2014). It is treated with vasopressin but occasionally persists. Other complications include CSF leakage, visual disturbances, postoperative meningitis, pneumocephalus (air in the intracranial cavity), and SIADH (see Chapter 52).

Preoperative Management

Medical Management

The preoperative evaluation includes a series of endocrine tests, rhinologic evaluation (to assess the status of the sinuses and nasal cavity), and neuroradiologic studies. Funduscopic examination and visual field determinations are performed, because the most serious effect of pituitary tumor is localized pressure on the optic nerve or chiasm. In addition, the nasopharyngeal secretions are cultured, because a sinus infection is a contraindication to an intracranial procedure using this approach. Corticosteroids may be given before and after surgery, because the surgery involves removal of the pituitary, which is the source of adrenocorticotropic hormone (ACTH). Antibiotic agents may or may not be given prophylactically.

Nursing Management

The patient is educated in deep breathing techniques before surgery. In addition, the patient is instructed that after the surgery, they will need to avoid vigorous coughing, blowing the nose, sucking through a straw, or sneezing, because these actions may place increased pressure at the surgical site and cause a CSF leak (Hickey, 2014).

Postoperative Management

Medical Management

Because the procedure disrupts the oral and nasal mucous membranes, management focuses on preventing infection and promoting healing. Medications include antimicrobial agents (which are continued until the nasal packing inserted at the time of surgery is removed), corticosteroids, analgesic agents for discomfort, and agents for the control of diabetes insipidus, if necessary (Hickey, 2014).

Nursing Management

Vital signs are measured to monitor hemodynamic, cardiac, and ventilatory status. Because of the anatomic proximity of the pituitary gland to the optic chiasm, visual acuity and visual fields are assessed at regular intervals. One method is to ask the patient to count the number of fingers held up by the nurse. Evidence of decreasing visual acuity suggests an expanding hematoma.

The head of the bed is raised to decrease pressure on the sella turcica and to promote normal drainage. The patient is cautioned against blowing the nose or engaging in any activity that raises ICP, such as bending over or straining during urination or defecation.

Intake and output are measured as a guide to fluid and electrolyte replacement and to assess for diabetes insipidus. The urine-specific gravity is measured after each voiding. Daily weight is monitored. Fluids are usually given after nausea ceases, and the patient then progresses to a regular diet.

The nasal packing inserted during surgery is checked frequently for blood or CSF drainage. The major discomfort is related to the nasal packing and to mouth dryness and thirst caused by mouth breathing. Oral care is provided every 4 hours or more frequently. Usually, the teeth are not brushed until the incision above the teeth has healed. Warm saline mouth rinses and the use of a cool mist vaporizer are helpful. Petrolatum is soothing when applied to the lips. A room humidifier assists in keeping the mucous membranes moist. The packing is removed in 3 to 4 days, and only then can the area around the nares be cleaned with the prescribed solution to remove crusted blood and moisten the mucous membranes (Hickey, 2014).

Home care considerations include advising the patient to use a room humidifier to keep the mucous membranes moist and to soothe irritation. The head of the bed is elevated at 30 degrees for at least 2 weeks after surgery. The patient is cautioned against blowing the nose or sneezing for at least 1 month (Hickey, 2014).

SEIZURE DISORDERS

Seizures are episodes of abnormal motor, sensory, autonomic, or psychic activity (or a combination of these) that result from sudden excessive discharge from cerebral neurons (Hickey, 2014). A localized area or all of the brain may be involved. The International League Against Epilepsy (ILAE) has defined **epilepsy** as at least two unprovoked seizures occurring more than 24 hours apart (Fisher, Acevedo, Arzimanoglou, et al., 2014). The ILAE differentiates between three main seizure types: focal, generalized, and unknown seizures (see Chart 66-3). Generalized seizures occur in and rapidly engage bilaterally distributed networks. Focal seizures are thought to originate within one hemisphere in the brain. The unknown type includes epileptic spasms. Unclassified seizures are so termed because of incomplete data but are not considered a classification (Fisher et al., 2014) Seizures may also be characterized as "provoked," or related to acute, reversible conditions such as structural, metabolic, immune, infectious or unknown etiologies (Scheffer, French, Hirsch, et al., 2016).

Pathophysiology

The underlying cause is an electrical disturbance (dysrhythmia) in the nerve cells in one section of the brain; these cells emit abnormal, recurring, uncontrolled electrical discharges. The characteristic seizure is a manifestation of this excessive neuronal discharge. Associated loss of consciousness, excess movement or loss of muscle tone or movement, and disturbances of behavior, mood, sensation, and perception may also occur.

The specific causes of seizures are varied and can be categorized as genetic, due to a structural or metabolic

---

Chart 66-3	Classification of Seizures: 2016 Basic Scheme

Focal
- Motor
- Nonmotor
- Awareness
  - Aware
  - Impaired awareness
  - Unknown awareness

Generalized
- Motor
- Absence

Unknown
- Motor
- Non-motor
- Awareness
  - Aware
  - Impaired awareness
  - Unknown awareness
- Unclassified

Adapted from Fisher, R., Cross, H., French, J., et al. (2016). Operational classification of seizure types by the International League Against Epilepsy (ILAE). Retrieved on 9/29/2016 at: www.ilae.org/visitors/centre/documents/ClassificationSeizureILAE-2016.pdf

---

condition, or the cause may be yet unknown etiologies (Scheffer et al., 2016).

Causes of seizures include:
- Cerebrovascular disease
- Hypoxemia of any cause, including vascular insufficiency
- Fever (childhood)
- Head injury
- Hypertension
- CNS infections
- Metabolic and toxic conditions (e.g., kidney injury, hyponatremia, hypocalcemia, hypoglycemia, pesticide exposure)
- Brain tumor
- Drug and alcohol withdrawal
- Allergies

Clinical Manifestations

Depending on the location of the discharging neurons, seizures may range from a simple staring episode (generalized absence seizure) to prolonged convulsive movements with loss of consciousness.

The initial pattern of the seizures indicates the region of the brain in which the seizure originates (see Chart 66-3). Only a finger or hand may shake, or the mouth may jerk uncontrollably. The person may talk unintelligibly; may be dizzy; and may experience unusual or unpleasant sights, sounds, odors, or tastes, but without loss of consciousness (Hickey, 2014).

Generalized seizures often involve both hemispheres of the brain, causing both sides of the body to react. Intense rigidity of the entire body may occur, followed by alternating muscle relaxation and contraction (generalized tonic–clonic contraction). The simultaneous contractions of the diaphragm and chest muscles may produce a characteristic epileptic cry. The tongue is often chewed, and the patient is incontinent of urine and feces. After 1 or 2 minutes, the convulsive movements begin to subside; the patient relaxes and lies in deep coma, breathing noisily. The respirations at this point are chiefly abdominal. In the postictal state (after the seizure), the patient is often confused and hard to arouse and may sleep for hours. Many patients report headache, sore muscles, fatigue, and depression (AANN, 2016a). Other generalized seizures may be absence types of seizures (Fisher, Cross, French et al., 2016).

Focal seizures are subdivided into events characterized by both motor and non-motor symptoms. There may be an impairment of consciousness or awareness or other dyscognitive features, localization, and progression of symptoms (Fisher et al., 2016).

Assessment and Diagnostic Findings

The diagnostic assessment is aimed at determining the type of seizures, their frequency and severity, and the factors that precipitate them. A developmental history is taken, including events of pregnancy and childbirth, to seek evidence of pre-existing injury. The patient is also questioned about illnesses or head injuries that may have affected the brain. In addition to physical and neurologic evaluations, diagnostic examinations include biochemical, hematologic, and serologic studies. MRI is used to detect structural lesions such as focal abnormalities, cerebrovascular abnormalities, and cerebral degenerative changes (AANN, 2016a).

The EEG furnishes diagnostic evidence for a substantial proportion of patients with epilepsy and assists in classifying the type of seizure. Abnormalities in the EEG usually continue between seizures or, if not apparent, may be elicited by hyperventilation or during sleep (AANN, 2016a). Microelectrodes (depth electrodes) can be inserted deep in the brain to probe the action of single brain cells. Some people with clinical seizures have normal EEGs, whereas others who have never had seizures have abnormal EEGs. Telemetry and computerized equipment are used to monitor electrical brain activity while the patient pursues their normal activities and to store the readings on computer tapes for analysis. Video recording of seizures taken simultaneously with EEG telemetry is useful in determining the type of seizure as well as its duration and magnitude (Updyke & Duryea, 2013).

SPECT is an additional tool that is sometimes used in the diagnostic workup. It is useful for identifying the epileptogenic zone so that the area in the brain giving rise to seizures can be removed surgically (AANN, 2016a).

Nursing Management

During a Seizure

A major responsibility of the nurse is to observe and record the sequence of signs. The nature of the seizure usually indicates the type of treatment required (AANN, 2016a). Before and during a seizure, the patient is assessed and the following items are documented:

- Circumstances before the seizure (visual, auditory, or olfactory stimuli; tactile stimuli; emotional or psychological disturbances; sleep; hyperventilation)
- Occurrence of an aura (a premonitory or warning sensation, which can be visual, auditory, or olfactory)

- First thing the patient does in the seizure—where the movements or the stiffness begins, conjugate gaze position, and the position of the head at the beginning of the seizure. This information gives clues to the location of the seizure origin in the brain. (In recording, it is important to state whether the beginning of the seizure was observed.)
- Type of movements in the part of the body involved
- Areas of the body involved (turn back bedding to expose patient)
- Size of both pupils and whether the eyes are open
- Whether the eyes or head are turned to one side
- Presence or absence of automatisms (involuntary motor activity, such as lip smacking or repeated swallowing)
- Incontinence of urine or stool
- Duration of each phase of the seizure
- Unconsciousness, if present, and its duration
- Any obvious paralysis or weakness of arms or legs after the seizure
- Inability to speak after the seizure
- Movements at the end of the seizure
- Whether or not the patient sleeps afterward
- Cognitive status (confused or not confused) after the seizure

In addition to providing data about the seizure, nursing care is directed at preventing injury and supporting the patient, not only physically but also psychologically. Consequences such as anxiety, embarrassment, fatigue, and depression can be devastating to the patient.

After a Seizure

After a patient has a seizure, the nurse's role is to document the events leading to and occurring during and after the seizure and to prevent complications (e.g., aspiration, injury). The patient is at risk for hypoxia, vomiting, and pulmonary aspiration. To prevent complications, the patient is placed in the side-lying position to facilitate drainage of oral secretions, and suctioning is performed, if needed, to maintain a patent airway and prevent aspiration (see Chart 66-4). Seizure precautions are maintained, including having available functioning suction equipment with a suction catheter and oral airway. The bed is placed in a low position with two to three side rails up and padded, if necessary, to prevent injury to the patient. The patient may be drowsy and may wish to sleep after the seizure; they may not remember events leading up to the seizure and for a short time thereafter.

The Epilepsies

Epilepsy is a group of syndromes characterized by unprovoked, recurring seizures (AANN, 2016a). Epileptic syndromes are classified by specific patterns of clinical features, including age at onset, family history, and seizure type. The epilepsies include electroclinical syndromes (a complex of clinical features, signs, and symptoms) and other epilepsies (Institute of Medicine [IOM], 2012). Epilepsy can be primary (idiopathic) or secondary (when the cause is known and the epilepsy is a symptom of another underlying condition, such as a brain tumor).

Epilepsy affects an estimated 3% of people during their lifetime, and most forms of epilepsy occur in children and

Chart 66-4 Care of the Patient During and After a Seizure

Nursing Care During a Seizure

- Provide privacy, and protect the patient from curious onlookers. (The patient who has an aura may have time to seek a safe, private place.)
- Ease the patient to the floor, if possible.
- Protect the head with a pad to prevent injury (from striking a hard surface).
- Loosen constrictive clothing and remove eyeglasses.
- Push aside any furniture that may injure the patient during the seizure.
- If the patient is in bed, remove pillows and raise side rails.
- *Do not attempt to pry open jaws that are clenched in a spasm or attempt to insert anything in the mouth during a seizure.* Broken teeth and injury to the lips and tongue may result from such an action.

- Do not attempt to restrain the patient during the seizure, because muscular contractions are strong and restraint can produce injury.
- If possible, place the patient on one side with head flexed forward, which allows the tongue to fall forward and facilitates drainage of saliva and mucus. If suction is available, use it if necessary to clear secretions.

Nursing Care After the Seizure

- Keep the patient on one side to prevent aspiration. Make sure the airway is patent.
- On awakening, reorient the patient to the environment.
- If the patient is confused or wandering, guide the patient gently to a bed or chair.
- If the patient becomes agitated after a seizure (postictal), stay a distance away, but close enough to prevent injury until the patient is fully aware.

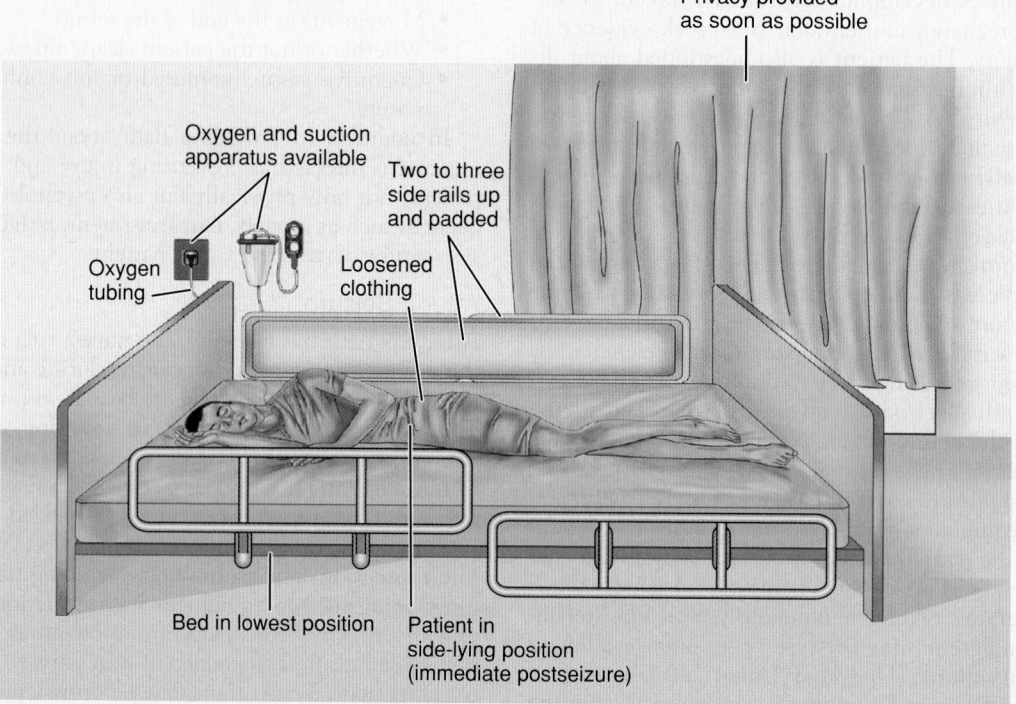

Privacy provided as soon as possible

Oxygen and suction apparatus available

Two to three side rails up and padded

Oxygen tubing

Loosened clothing

Bed in lowest position

Patient in side-lying position (immediate postseizure)

Adapted from American Association of Neuroscience Nurses (AANN). (2016a). *Care of adults and children with seizures and epilepsy: AANN clinical practice guideline series*. Chicago, IL: Author.

older adults (England, Liverman, Schultz, et al., 2012). The improved treatment for cerebrovascular disorders, head injuries, brain tumors, meningitis, and encephalitis has increased the number of patients at risk for seizures after recovery from these conditions. In addition, advances in EEG have aided in the diagnosis of epilepsy. The general public has been educated about epilepsy, which has reduced the stigma associated with it; as a result, more people are willing to acknowledge that they have epilepsy.

Although some evidence suggests that susceptibility to some types of epilepsy may be inherited, the cause of seizures in many people is idiopathic (unknown). Epilepsy can

follow birth trauma, asphyxia neonatorum, head injuries, some infectious diseases (bacterial, viral, parasitic), toxicity (carbon monoxide and lead poisoning), circulatory problems, fever, metabolic and nutritional disorders, or drug or alcohol intoxication. It is also associated with brain tumors, abscesses, and congenital malformations.

Pathophysiology

Messages from the body are carried by the neurons (nerve cells) of the brain by discharges of electrochemical energy that sweep along them. These impulses occur in bursts whenever a nerve cell has a task to perform. Sometimes, these cells or groups of cells continue firing after a task is finished. During the period of unwanted discharges, parts of the body controlled by the errant cells may perform erratically. Resultant dysfunction ranges from mild to incapacitating and often causes loss of consciousness (Hickey, 2014). If these uncontrolled, abnormal discharges occur repeatedly, a person is said to have an epileptic syndrome. Epilepsy is not associated with intellectual level. People who have epilepsy without other brain or nervous system disabilities fall within the same intelligence ranges as the overall population. Epilepsy is not synonymous with intellectual or developmental disabilities, but many people who have these types of disabilities, because of serious neurologic damage, also have epilepsy.

Epilepsy in Women

More than 1 million American women have epilepsy, and they face particular needs associated with the syndrome. Women with epilepsy often note an increase in seizure frequency during menses; this has been linked to the increase in sex hormones that alter the excitability of neurons in the cerebral cortex. The effectiveness of contraceptives is decreased by anticonvulsant medications. Therefore, patients should be encouraged to discuss family planning with their primary provider and to obtain preconception counseling if they are considering childbearing (Lagana, Triolo, D'Amico, et al., 2016).

Women of childbearing age who have epilepsy require special care and guidance before, during, and after pregnancy. Many women note a change in the pattern of seizure activity during pregnancy. The risk of congenital fetal anomaly is two to three times higher in women with epilepsy. Maternal seizures, anticonvulsant medications, and genetic predisposition all contribute to possible malformations. Women who take certain anticonvulsant medications for epilepsy are at risk and need careful monitoring, including blood studies to detect the level of anticonvulsant medications taken throughout pregnancy. Mothers who are at high risk (teenagers, women with histories of difficult deliveries, women who use illicit drugs [e.g., "crack" cocaine, heroin], and women with diabetes or hypertension) should be identified and monitored closely during pregnancy, because damage to the fetus during pregnancy and delivery can increase the risk of epilepsy. All of these issues need further study (Lagana et al., 2016).

Because of bone loss associated with the long-term use of anticonvulsant medications, patients receiving anticonvulsant agents should be assessed for low bone mass and osteoporosis. They should be instructed about strategies to reduce their risks of osteoporosis (AANN, 2016a).

 Gerontologic Considerations

Older adults have a high incidence of new-onset epilepsy (see Chart 66-5) (Hickey, 2014; Miller, Buelow, & Bakas, 2014). Cerebrovascular disease is the leading cause of seizures in the older adult. The increased incidence is also associated with head injury, dementia, infection, alcoholism, and aging. Treatment depends on the underlying cause. Because many older adults have chronic health problems, they may be taking other medications that can interact with medications prescribed for seizure control. In addition, the absorption, distribution, metabolism, and excretion of medications are altered in the older adult as a result of age-related changes in renal and liver function. Therefore, older adult patients must be monitored closely for adverse and toxic effects of

---

Chart 66-5 · NURSING RESEARCH PROFILE

Experiences With a New Diagnosis of Epilepsy in Older Adults

Miller, W., Buelow, J., & Bakas, T. (2014). Older adults and new onset epilepsy: Experiences with diagnosis. *Journal of Neuroscience Nursing, 46*(1), 2–10.

Purpose

Older adults in the United States have a high rate of new-onset epilepsy; however, most research focuses on children and young adults. Older adults may exhibit a different clinical presentation, display age-related cognitive and metabolic changes, and have comorbidities that increase the likelihood of polypharmacy, creating unique challenges. This research was undertaken to identify the experience and characteristics of the older adult with new-onset epilepsy.

Design

A qualitative descriptive approach was undertaken to describe the experiences of 20 community dwelling older adults with new-onset epilepsy living in both urban and rural settings. Eligible participants were diagnosed at or after the age of 60 years, diagnosed within the previous 3 months, took at least one anticonvulsant medication, and spoke and read English. Semi-structured interviews were conducted by one researcher and analyzed and coded using conventional content analysis that identified clusters and themes.

Findings

The mean age of the participants was 70 years; 12 were women and 8 were men. Length of time until diagnosis was the most prominent theme during the interviews and split into two main themes: delayed diagnosis and nondelayed diagnosis. Participants with delayed diagnosis (epilepsy not diagnosed within 3 months of symptoms) attributed the delay to their primary providers not recognizing atypical symptoms or attributing symptoms to another neurologic process, or to their own delay in seeking care. The nondelayed participants reported typical seizure characteristics and rapid referral to a neurologic provider. The seizure events were obvious and interfered with daily life. Participants living in rural areas and women more often experienced delays in diagnosis.

Nursing Implications

Nurses need to be aware that older adults are the group at highest risk for developing new-onset epilepsy, and what might be identified as symptoms of aging may in fact be seizure-related events. Nurses can educate older adults regarding their risk of developing epilepsy and should describe both typical and atypical seizure presentations. Patients should be encouraged to seek specialized care for symptoms such as unexplained changes in mental status, syncopy, and dizziness.

anticonvulsant medications and for osteoporosis. The cost of anticonvulsant medications can lead to poor adherence to the prescribed regimen in older adult patients on fixed incomes.

Prevention

Society-wide efforts are the key to prevention of epilepsy. Head injury is one of the main causes of epilepsy that can be prevented. Through highway safety programs and occupational safety precautions, lives can be saved and epilepsy due to head injury prevented; these programs are discussed in Chapter 68.

Medical Management

The management of epilepsy is individualized to meet the needs of each patient and not just to manage and prevent seizures. Management differs from patient to patient, because some forms of epilepsy arise from brain damage and others result from altered brain chemistry.

Pharmacologic Therapy

Many medications are available to control seizures, although the exact mechanisms of action are unknown. The objective is to achieve seizure control with minimal side effects. Medication therapy controls—rather than cures—seizures. Medications are selected on the basis of the type of seizure being treated and the effectiveness and safety of the medications. If properly prescribed and taken, medications control seizures in 70% to 80% of patients with seizures. However, 20% of patients with generalized seizures and 30% of those with focal seizures do not demonstrate improvement with any prescribed medication or may be unable to tolerate the side effects of medications (AANN, 2016a). Table 66-4 lists select anticonvulsant medications.

Treatment usually starts with a single medication. The starting dose and the rate at which the dosage is increased depend on the occurrence of side effects. The medication levels in the blood are monitored, because the rate of drug absorption varies among patients. Changing to another medication may be necessary if seizure control is not achieved or if

TABLE 66-4 Select Anticonvulsant Medications

Medication	Dose-Related Side Effects	Toxic Effects
carbamazepine (Tegretol)	Dizziness, drowsiness, unsteadiness, nausea and vomiting, diplopia, mild leukopenia	Severe skin rash, blood dyscrasias, hepatitis
clonazepam (Klonopin)	Drowsiness, behavior changes, headache, hirsutism, alopecia, palpitations	Hepatotoxicity, thrombocytopenia, bone marrow failure, ataxia
ethosuximide (Zarontin)	Nausea and vomiting, headache, gastric distress	Skin rash, blood dyscrasias, hepatitis, systemic lupus erythematosus
felbamate (Felbatol)	Cognitive impairments, insomnia, nausea, headache, fatigue	Aplastic anemia, hepatotoxicity
gabapentin (Neurontin)	Dizziness, drowsiness, somnolence, fatigue, ataxia, weight gain, nausea	Leukopenia, hepatotoxicity
lamotrigine (Lamictal)	Drowsiness, tremor, nausea, ataxia, dizziness, headache, weight gain	Severe rash (Stevens–Johnson syndrome)
levetiracetam (Keppra)	Somnolence, dizziness, fatigue	Unknown
oxcarbazepine (Trileptal)	Dizziness, somnolence, double vision, fatigue, nausea, vomiting, loss of coordination, abnormal vision, abdominal pain, tremor, abnormal gait	Hepatotoxicity
phenobarbital (Luminal)	Sedation, irritability, diplopia, ataxia	Skin rash, anemia
phenytoin (Dilantin)	Visual problems, hirsutism, gingival hyperplasia, dysrhythmias, dysarthria, nystagmus	Severe skin reaction, peripheral neuropathy, ataxia, drowsiness, blood dyscrasias
primidone (Mysoline)	Lethargy, irritability, diplopia, ataxia, impotence	Skin rash
tiagabine (Gabitril)	Dizziness, fatigue, nervousness, tremor, difficulty concentrating, dysarthria, weak or buckling knees, abdominal pain	Unknown
topiramate (Topamax)	Fatigue, somnolence, confusion, ataxia, anorexia, depression, weight loss	Nephrolithiasis
valproate (Depakote, Depakene)	Nausea and vomiting, weight gain, hair loss, tremor, menstrual irregularities	Hepatotoxicity, skin rash, blood dyscrasias, nephritis
zonisamide (Zonegran, Excegran)	Somnolence, dizziness, anorexia, headache, nausea, agitation, rash	Leukopenia, hepatotoxicity

Adapted from Karch, A. (2015). *2015 Lippincott's nursing drug guide.* Philadelphia, PA: Lippincott Williams & Wilkins.

toxicity makes it impossible to increase the dosage. The medication may need to be adjusted because of concurrent illness, weight changes, or increases in stress. Side effects of anticonvulsant medications may be divided into three groups: (1) idiosyncratic or allergic disorders, which manifest primarily as skin reactions; (2) acute toxicity, which may occur when the medication is initially prescribed; and (3) chronic toxicity, which occurs late in the course of therapy.

The manifestations of drug toxicity are variable, and any organ system may be involved. For example, gingival hyperplasia (swollen and tender gums) can be associated with long-term use of phenytoin (Karch, 2015). Periodic physical and dental examinations and laboratory tests are performed for patients receiving medications that are known to have hematopoietic, genitourinary, or hepatic effects.

Surgical Management

Surgery is indicated for patients whose epilepsy results from intracranial tumors, abscesses, cysts, or vascular anomalies. Some patients have intractable seizure disorders that do not respond to medication. A focal atrophic process may occur secondary to trauma, inflammation, stroke, or anoxia. If the seizures originate in a reasonably well-circumscribed area of the brain that can be excised without producing significant neurologic deficits, the removal of the area generating the seizures may produce long-term control and improvement (AANN, 2016a).

This type of neurosurgery has been aided by several advances, including microsurgical techniques, EEGs with depth electrodes, improved illumination and hemostasis, and the introduction of neuroleptanalgesic agents (droperidol and fentanyl). These techniques, combined with the use of local anesthetic agents, enable the neurosurgeon to perform surgery on an alert and cooperative patient. Using special testing devices, electrocortical mapping, and the patient's responses to stimulation, the boundaries of the epileptogenic focus (i.e., abnormal area of the brain) are determined. Any abnormal epileptogenic focus is then excised (AANN, 2016a). Resection surgery significantly reduces the incidence of seizures in patients with refractory epilepsy.

When seizures are refractory to medication in adolescents and adults with focal seizures, a vagal nerve stimulator (VNS) may be implanted under the clavicle. The device is connected to the vagus nerve in the cervical area, where it delivers electrical signals to the brain to control and reduce seizure activity. An external programming system is used by the physician to change stimulator settings (Wheless, 2013). Patients can activate the stimulator with a magnet at the time of a seizure or aura. Some patients report that use of the vagal nerve stimulator diminishes the severity or duration of the seizure. Complications such as infection, cardiac dysrhythmias, hoarseness, cough, and laryngeal spasm can occur with the use of this device (AANN, 2016a; Wheless, 2013).

Another surgical option for patients with refractory seizure activity is the responsive neurostimulation system (RNS) (U.S. Food and Drug Administration, 2014). This is a surgically implanted device with electrodes that sense and record brain electrical activity. Electrodes deliver an electrical stimulation to the location of seizure origination within the brain. The RNS works by interrupting brainwave activity before a clinical seizure can occur (AANN, 2016a).

More research is needed to determine the effects of the various surgical approaches on complication rates, quality of life, anxiety, and depression, all of which are issues for patients with epilepsy.

NURSING PROCESS
The Patient With Epilepsy

Assessment

The nurse elicits information about the patient's seizure history. The patient is asked about the factors or events that may precipitate the seizures. Alcohol intake is documented. The nurse determines whether the patient has an aura before an epileptic seizure, which may indicate the origin of the seizure (e.g., seeing a flashing light may indicate that the seizure originated in the occipital lobe). Observation and assessment during and after a seizure assist in identifying the type of seizure and its management.

The effects of epilepsy on the patient's lifestyle are assessed (AANN, 2016a). What limitations are imposed by the seizure disorder? Does the patient participate in any recreational activities? Have any social contacts? Is the patient working, and is it a positive or stressful experience? What coping mechanisms are used?

Diagnosis

Nursing Diagnoses

Based on the assessment data, major nursing diagnoses may include the following:
- Risk for injury related to seizure activity
- Fear related to the possibility of seizures
- Ineffective individual coping related to stresses imposed by epilepsy
- Deficient knowledge related to epilepsy and anticonvulsant medications

Collaborative Problems/Potential Complications

The major potential complications for patients with epilepsy are status epilepticus and medication side effects (toxicity).

Planning and Goals

The major goals for the patient may include prevention of injury, control of seizures, achievement of a satisfactory psychosocial adjustment, acquisition of knowledge and understanding about the condition, and absence of complications.

Nursing Interventions

Preventing Injury

Injury prevention for the patient with seizures is a priority. Patients for whom seizure precautions are instituted should have pads applied to the side rails while in bed. Steps to prevent or minimize injury are presented in Chart 66-4.

Reducing Fear of Seizures

Fear that a seizure may occur unexpectedly can be reduced by the patient's adherence to the prescribed treatment regimen. Cooperation of the patient and family and their trust in the prescribed regimen are essential for control of seizures. The nurse emphasizes that the prescribed anticonvulsant medication must be taken on a continuing basis and that drug dependence or addiction does not occur. Periodic monitoring is necessary to ensure the adequacy of the treatment regimen, to prevent side effects, and to monitor for drug resistance (Hickey, 2014).

In an effort to control seizures, factors that may precipitate them are identified, such as emotional disturbances, new environmental stressors, onset of menstruation in female patients, or fever (AANN, 2016a). The patient is encouraged to follow a regular and moderate routine in lifestyle, diet (avoiding excessive stimulants), exercise, and rest (sleep deprivation may lower the seizure threshold). Moderate activity is therapeutic, but excessive exercise should be avoided. An additional dietary intervention, referred to as the ketogenic diet, may be helpful for control of seizures in some patients. This high-protein, low-carbohydrate, high-fat diet is most effective in children whose seizures have not been controlled with two anticonvulsant medications, but it is sometimes used for adults who have had poor seizure control (Nei, Ngo, Sirven, et al., 2014).

Photic stimulation (e.g., bright flickering lights, television viewing) may precipitate seizures; wearing dark glasses or covering one eye may be preventive. Tension states (anxiety, frustration) induce seizures in some patients. Classes in stress management may be of value. Because seizures are known to occur with alcohol intake, alcoholic beverages should be avoided.

IMPROVING COPING MECHANISMS

The social, psychological, and behavioral problems that frequently accompany epilepsy can be more of a disability than the actual seizures. Epilepsy may be accompanied by feelings of stigmatization, alienation, depression, and uncertainty (IOM, 2012). The patient must cope with the constant fear of a seizure and the psychological consequences (AANN, 2016a). Children with epilepsy may be ostracized and excluded from school and peer activities. These problems are compounded during adolescence and add to the challenges of dating, not being able to drive, and feeling different from other people. Adults face these problems in addition to the burden of finding employment, concerns about relationships and childbearing, insurance problems, and legal barriers. Alcohol abuse may complicate matters. Family reactions may vary from outright rejection of the person with epilepsy to overprotection.

Counseling assists the patient and family to understand the condition and the limitations it imposes. Social and recreational opportunities are necessary for good mental health. Nurses can improve the quality of life for patients with epilepsy by educating them and their families about symptoms and their management (AANN, 2016a).

 PROVIDING PATIENT AND FAMILY EDUCATION

Perhaps the most valuable facets of care contributed by the nurse to the person with epilepsy are education and efforts to modify the attitudes of the patient and family toward the disorder. The person who experiences seizures may consider every seizure a potential source of humiliation and shame. This may result in anxiety, depression, hostility, and secrecy on the part of the patient and family. Ongoing education and encouragement should be given to patients to enable them to overcome these reactions. The patient with epilepsy should carry an emergency medical identification card or wear a medical information bracelet. The patient and family need to be educated about medications as well as care during a seizure.

MONITORING AND MANAGING POTENTIAL COMPLICATIONS

Status epilepticus is the major potential complication and is described later in this chapter. Another complication is the toxicity of medications. The patient and family are instructed about side effects and are given specific guidelines to assess and report signs and symptoms that indicate medication overdose. Anticonvulsant medications require careful monitoring for therapeutic levels. The patient should plan to have serum drug levels assessed at regular intervals. Many known drug interactions occur with anticonvulsant medications. A complete pharmacologic profile should be reviewed with the patient to avoid interactions that either potentiate or inhibit the effectiveness of the medications.

Quality and Safety Nursing Alert

Patients with epilepsy are at risk for status epilepticus from having their medication regimen interrupted.

PROMOTING HOME, COMMUNITY-BASED, AND TRANSITIONAL CARE

 Educating Patients About Self-Care. Thorough oral hygiene after each meal, gum massage, daily flossing, and regular dental care are essential to prevent or control gingival hyperplasia in patients receiving phenytoin. The patient is also educated to inform all health care providers of the medication being taken, because of the possibility of drug interactions. An individualized comprehensive education plan is needed to assist the patient and family to adjust to this chronic disorder. Written patient education materials must be appropriate for the patient's reading level and must be provided in alternative formats if warranted.

Continuing and Transitional Care. Because epilepsy can be lifelong, health promotion is important. See Chart 66-6 for health promotion strategies for the patient with epilepsy.

For many patients with epilepsy, overcoming employment problems is a challenge. State vocational rehabilitation agencies can provide information about job training. The Epilepsy Foundation of America (EFA) has a training and placement service. If seizures are not well controlled, information about sheltered workshops or home employment programs may be obtained. Federal and state agencies and federal legislation may be of assistance to people with epilepsy who experience job discrimination. As a result of the Americans with Disabilities Act, the number of employers who knowingly hire people with epilepsy is increasing, but barriers to employment still exist.

Patients who have uncontrollable seizures accompanied by psychological and social difficulties should be referred as early as possible to a comprehensive epilepsy center where continuous audio-video and EEG monitoring, specialized treatment, and rehabilitation services are available (AANN, 2016a). Patients and their families need to be reminded of the importance of participating in health promotion activities and recommended health screenings to promote a healthy lifestyle. Genetic and preconception counseling is advised.

- Take anticonvulsant medications daily as prescribed to keep the drug level constant to prevent seizures. Never discontinue medications, even if there is no seizure activity.
- Keep a medication and seizure record (in electronic or paper format), noting when medications are taken and any seizure activity.
- Notify the primary provider if unable to take medications due to illness.
- Have anticonvulsant medication serum levels checked regularly. When testing is prescribed, report to the laboratory for blood sampling before taking morning medication.
- Avoid activities that require alertness and coordination (driving, operating machinery) until after the effects of the medication have been evaluated.
- Report signs of toxicity so that dosage can be adjusted. Common signs include drowsiness, lethargy, dizziness, difficulty walking, hyperactivity, confusion, inappropriate sleep, and visual disturbances.

- Avoid over-the-counter medications unless approved by the primary provider.
- Carry a medical alert bracelet or identification card specifying the name of the anticonvulsant medication and primary provider.
- Avoid seizure triggers, such as alcoholic beverages, electrical shocks, stress, caffeine, constipation, fever, hyperventilation, and hypoglycemia.
- Take showers rather than tub baths to avoid drowning if seizure occurs; never swim alone.
- Exercise in moderation in a temperature-controlled environment to avoid excessive heat.
- Develop regular sleep patterns to minimize fatigue and insomnia.
- Be aware of and use the Epilepsy Foundation of America (EFA) special services, including help in obtaining medications, vocational rehabilitation, and coping with epilepsy.

Evaluation

Expected patient outcomes may include:

1. Sustains no injury during seizure activity
   a. Adheres to treatment regimen and identifies the hazards of stopping the medication
   b. Can identify appropriate care during seizure; caregivers can do so as well
2. Indicates a decrease in fear
3. Displays effective individual coping
4. Exhibits knowledge and understanding of epilepsy
   a. Identifies the side effects of medications
   b. Avoids factors or situations that may precipitate seizures (e.g., flickering lights, hyperventilation, alcohol)
   c. Follows a healthy lifestyle by getting adequate sleep and eating meals at regular times to avoid hypoglycemia
5. Absence of complications

Status Epilepticus

Status epilepticus (acute prolonged seizure activity) is a series of generalized seizures that occur without full recovery of consciousness between attacks (Trinka, Cock, Hesdorffer, et al., 2015). The term has been broadened to include continuous clinical or electrical seizures (on EEG) lasting at least 30 minutes, even without impairment of consciousness. It is considered a medical emergency. Status epilepticus produces cumulative effects. Vigorous muscular contractions impose a heavy metabolic demand and can interfere with respirations. Some respiratory arrest at the height of each seizure produces venous congestion and hypoxia of the brain. Repeated episodes of cerebral anoxia and edema may lead to irreversible and fatal brain damage. Factors that precipitate status epilepticus include interruption of anticonvulsant medication, fever, concurrent infection, or other illness.

Medical Management

The goals of treatment are to stop the seizures as quickly as possible, to ensure adequate cerebral oxygenation, and to maintain the patient in a seizure-free state. An airway and adequate oxygenation are established. If the patient remains unconscious and unresponsive, an endotracheal tube is inserted. IV diazepam (Valium), lorazepam (Ativan), or fosphenytoin is given slowly in an attempt to halt seizures immediately. Other medications (phenytoin, phenobarbital) are given later to maintain a seizure-free state.

An IV line is established, and blood samples are obtained to monitor serum electrolytes, glucose, and phenytoin levels. EEG monitoring may be useful in determining the nature of the seizure activity. Vital signs and neurologic signs are monitored on a continuing basis. An IV infusion of dextrose is given if the seizure is caused by hypoglycemia. If initial treatment is unsuccessful, general anesthesia with a short-acting barbiturate may be used. The serum concentration of the anticonvulsant medication is measured, because a low level suggests that the patient was not taking the medication or that the dosage was too low. Cardiac involvement or respiratory depression may be life threatening. The potential for postictal cerebral edema also exists.

Nursing Management

The nurse initiates ongoing assessment and monitoring of respiratory and cardiac function because of the risk for delayed depression of respiration and blood pressure secondary to administration of anticonvulsant medications and sedatives to halt the seizures. Nursing assessment also includes monitoring and documenting the seizure activity and the patient's responsiveness.

The patient is turned to a side-lying position, if possible, to assist in draining pharyngeal secretions. Suction equipment must be available because of the risk of aspiration. The IV line is closely monitored, because it may become dislodged during seizures.

A person who has received long-term anticonvulsant therapy has a significant risk for fractures resulting from bone disease (osteoporosis, osteomalacia, and hyperparathyroidism), which is a side effect of therapy (Karch, 2015). Therefore, during seizures, the patient is protected from injury with the use of seizure precautions and is monitored closely. The patient having seizures can inadvertently injure nearby people, so nurses should protect themselves. Additional nursing interventions for the person having seizures are presented in Chart 66-4.

HEADACHE

Headache, or cephalalgia, is one of the most common of all human physical complaints. Headache is a symptom rather than a disease entity; it may indicate organic disease (neurologic or other disease), a stress response, vasodilation (migraine), skeletal muscle tension (tension headache), or a combination of factors. A **primary headache** is one for which no organic cause can be identified. This type of headache includes migraine, tension-type, and cluster headaches (Hickey, 2014). Cranial arteritis is another common cause of headache. A classification of headaches was issued first by the Headache Classification Committee of the International Headache Society in 1988. The International Headache Society revised the headache classification in 2013; an abbreviated list is shown in Chart 66-7.

Migraine is a complex of symptoms characterized by periodic and recurrent attacks of severe headache lasting from hours to days in adults. The cause of migraine has not been clearly demonstrated, but it is primarily a vascular disturbance that has a strong familial tendency. The typical time of onset is at puberty, and the incidence is higher in women than men (D'Arcy, 2014).

There are many subtypes of migraine headache, including migraine with and without aura. Most patients have migraine without an aura. *Tension-type headaches* tend to be chronic and less severe and are probably the most common type of headache. *Trigeminal autonomic cephalalgias* include cluster headaches and paroxysmal hemicrania. Cluster headaches

---

Chart 66-7	International Headache Society Classification of Headache

- Migraine
- Tension-type headache
- Trigeminal autonomic cephalalgias
- Other primary disorders
- Headache attributed to trauma or injury to the head and/or neck
- Headache attributed to cranial or cervical vascular disorder
- Headache attributed to nonvascular intracranial disorder
- Headache attributed to a substance or its withdrawal
- Headache attributed to infection
- Headache attributed to disorder of homeostasis
- Headache or facial pain attributed to disorder of cranium, neck, eyes, ears, nose, sinuses, teeth, mouth, or other facial or cranial structures
- Headache attributed to psychiatric disorder
- Painful cranial neuropathies and other facial pains
- Other headache disorders

Adapted from Headache Classification Subcommittee of the International Headache Society. (2013). The International Classification of Headache Disorders, 3rd edition (beta version). *Cephalalgia, 33*(9), 629–808.

---

are relatively uncommon and seen more frequently in men than in women (Grossman & Porth, 2014). Types of headaches not subsumed under these categories fall into the *other primary headache* group and include headaches triggered by cough, exertion, and sexual activity.

Cranial arteritis is a cause of headache in the older population, reaching its greatest incidence in those older than 70 years of age. Inflammation of the cranial arteries is characterized by a severe headache localized in the region of the temporal arteries. The inflammation may be generalized (in which case cranial arteritis is part of a vascular disease) or focal (in which case only the cranial arteries are involved).

A **secondary headache** is a symptom associated with other causes, such as a brain tumor, an aneurysm, or lumbar puncture (Destrebecq, Terzoni, & Sala, 2014). Although most headaches do not indicate serious disease, persistent headaches require further investigation. Serious disorders related to headache include brain tumors, subarachnoid hemorrhage, stroke, severe hypertension, meningitis, and head injuries.

Pathophysiology

The cerebral signs and symptoms of migraine result from a hyperexcitable brain that is susceptible to a phenomenon known as cortical spreading depression, a wave of depolarization over the cerebral cortex, cerebellum, and hippocampus. This depolarization activates inflammatory neuropeptides and other neurotransmitters (including serotonin), resulting in the stimulation of meningeal nociceptors. Vascular changes, inflammation, and a continuation of pain signal stimulation occur (Charles, 2015). The initial phase of this process is known as the premonitory phase and may include light, sound, and smell sensitivity. If treatment is initiated at this point, the migraine may be fully terminated. As the attack progresses, central sensitization occurs, and the migraine becomes much harder to treat.

Attacks can be triggered by hormonal changes associated with menstrual cycles, bright lights, stress, depression, sleep deprivation, fatigue, or odors. Certain foods containing tyramine (especially aged cheese), monosodium glutamate, and chocolate may be food triggers (Grossman & Porth, 2014). The use of oral contraceptives may be associated with increased frequency and severity of attacks in some women.

Emotional or physical stress may cause contraction of the muscles in the neck and scalp, resulting in tension headache. The pathophysiology of cluster headache is not fully understood. One theory is that it is caused by dilation of orbital and nearby extracranial arteries. Cranial arteritis is thought to represent an immune vasculitis in which immune complexes are deposited within the walls of affected blood vessels, producing vascular injury and inflammation. A biopsy may be performed on the involved artery to make the diagnosis.

Clinical Manifestations

Migraine

The migraine with aura can be divided into four phases: premonitory, aura, the headache, and recovery (headache termination and postdrome).

Premonitory Phase

The premonitory phase is experienced by more than 80% of adult migraine sufferers, with symptoms that occur hours to days before a migraine headache (Charles, 2013). Symptoms may include depression, irritability, feeling cold, food cravings, anorexia, change in activity level, increased urination, diarrhea, or constipation. Patients may experience the same prodrome with each migraine headache. A current theory regarding premonitory symptoms is that they involve the neurotransmitter dopamine.

Aura Phase

An aura may be a variable feature for patients who experience migraines (Charles & Hansen, 2015). An aura is characterized by focal neurologic symptoms. Visual disturbances (i.e., light flashes and bright spots) are most common and may be hemianopic (affecting only half of the visual field). Other symptoms that may follow include numbness and tingling of the lips, face, or hands; mild confusion; slight weakness of an extremity; drowsiness; and dizziness.

This period of aura was thought to correspond to the phenomenon of cortical spreading depression that is associated with reduced metabolic demand in abnormally functioning neurons. This can be associated with decreased blood flow; however, cerebral blood flow studies performed during migraine headaches demonstrate that although changes in blood vessels occur during phases of migraine, cerebral blood flow is not the main abnormality. In fact, some studies suggest that the aura and headache phases may occur simultaneously (Charles, 2013).

Headache Phase

Migraine headache is severe and incapacitating and is often associated with photophobia (light sensitivity), phonophobia (sound sensitivity), or allodynia (abnormal perception of innocuous stimuli) (Charles, 2013). Research differs in the role of vascular changes (either vasodilatory or vasoconstrictive) with respect to migraine pathophysiology and the experience of migraine headache. Symptoms of migraine can also include nausea and vomiting.

Postdrome Phase

In the postdrome phase, the pain gradually subsides, but patients may experience tiredness, weakness, cognitive difficulties, and mood changes for hours to days. Muscle contraction in the neck and scalp is common, with associated muscle ache and localized tenderness. Physical exertion may exacerbate the headache pain. During this postheadache phase, patients may sleep for extended periods.

Other Headache Types

The tension-type headache is characterized by a steady, constant feeling of pressure that usually begins in the forehead, temple, or back of the neck. It is often bandlike or may be described as "a weight on top of my head."

Cluster headaches are unilateral and come in clusters of one to eight daily, with excruciating pain localized to the eye and orbit and radiating to the facial and temporal regions. The pain is accompanied by watering of the eye and nasal congestion. Each attack lasts 15 minutes to 3 hours and may have a crescendo–decrescendo pattern (Hickey, 2014). The headache is often described as penetrating.

Cranial arteritis often begins with general manifestations, such as fatigue, malaise, weight loss, and fever. Clinical manifestations associated with inflammation (heat, redness, swelling, tenderness, or pain over the involved artery) usually are present. Sometimes a tender, swollen, or nodular temporal artery is visible. Visual problems are caused by ischemia of the involved structures.

Assessment and Diagnostic Findings

The diagnostic evaluation includes a detailed history, a physical assessment of the head and neck, and a complete neurologic examination. Headaches may manifest differently in the same person over the course of a lifetime, and the same type of headache may manifest differently from patient to patient. The health history focuses on assessing the headache itself, with emphasis on the factors that precipitate or provoke it. The patient is asked to describe the headache in their own words.

Because headache is often the presenting symptom of a wider variety of physiologic and psychological disturbances, a general health history is an essential component of the patient database. Therefore, questions addressed in the health history should cover major medical and surgical illness as well as a body systems review.

The medication history can provide insight into the patient's overall health status and indicate medications that may be provoking headaches. Antihypertensive agents, diuretic medications, anti-inflammatory agents, and monoamine oxidase (MAO) inhibitors are a few of the categories of medications that can provoke headaches. Daily use of over-the-counter or prescribed pain medications for 8 to 10 days out of a month can lead to a chronic headache due to medication overuse (Becker, Findlay, Moga, et al., 2015). Emotional factors can play a role in precipitating headaches. Stress is thought to be a major initiating factor in migraine headaches; therefore, sleep patterns, level of stress, recreational interests, appetite, emotional problems, and family stressors are relevant. There is a strong familial tendency for headache disorders, and a positive family history may help in making a diagnosis.

A direct relationship may exist between exposure to toxic substances and headache. Careful questioning may uncover chemicals to which a worker has been exposed. Under the Right-to-Know Law, employees have access to the material safety data sheets (commonly referred to as MSDS) for all substances with which they come in contact in the workplace (see Chapter 72). The occupational history also includes assessment of the workplace as a possible source of stress and for a possible ergonomic basis of muscle strain and headache.

A complete description of the headache itself is crucial. The nurse reviews the age at onset of headaches; this particular headache's frequency, location, and duration; the type of pain; factors that relieve and precipitate the event; and associated symptoms. The data obtained should include the patient's own words about the headache in response to the following questions:

- What is the location? Is it unilateral or bilateral? Does it radiate?
- What is the quality—dull, aching, steady, boring, burning, intermittent, continuous, paroxysmal?
- How many headaches occur during a given period of time?
- What are the precipitating factors, if any—environmental (e.g., sunlight, weather change), foods, exertion, other?

- What makes the headache worse (e.g., coughing, straining)?
- What time (day or night) does it occur?
- How long does a typical headache last?
- Are there any associated symptoms, such as facial pain, lacrimation (excessive tearing), or scotomas (blind spots in the field of vision)?
- What usually relieves the headache (aspirin, nonsteroidal anti-inflammatory drugs, ergot preparation, food, heat, rest, neck massage)?
- Does nausea, vomiting, weakness, or numbness in the extremities accompany the headache?
- Does the headache interfere with daily activities?
- Do you have any allergies?
- Do you have insomnia, poor appetite, loss of energy?
- Is there a family history of headache?
- What is the relationship of the headache to your lifestyle or physical or emotional stress?
- What medications are you taking?

Diagnostic testing often is not helpful in the investigation of headache, because usually there are few objective findings. In patients who demonstrate abnormalities on the neurologic examination, CT scan, cerebral angiography, or MRI scan may be used to detect underlying causes, such as tumor or aneurysm. Electromyography (EMG) may reveal a sustained contraction of the neck, scalp, or facial muscles. Laboratory tests may include complete blood count, erythrocyte sedimentation rate, electrolytes, glucose, creatinine, and thyroid hormone levels.

Prevention

Prevention begins by having the patient avoid specific triggers that are known to initiate the headache syndrome. Preventive medical management of migraine involves the daily use of one or more agents that are thought to block the physiologic events leading to an attack. Treatment regimens vary greatly, as do patient responses; therefore, close monitoring is indicated.

Alcohol, nitrites, vasodilators, and histamines may precipitate cluster headaches. Elimination of these factors helps prevent the headaches.

Medical Management

Therapy for migraine headache is divided into abortive (symptomatic) and preventive approaches. The abortive approach, best used in those patients who have less frequent attacks, is aimed at relieving or limiting a headache at the onset or while it is in progress. The preventive approach is used in patients who experience more frequent attacks at regular or predictable intervals and may have a medical condition that precludes the use of abortive therapies (Becker et al., 2015). Medical management of migraine during pregnancy and lactation includes nonpharmacologic strategies in addition to safe medication practices (Wells, Turner, Lee, et al., 2016). Nonpharmacologic treatments include mainly avoidance of triggers (Grossman & Porth, 2014) (see Chart 66-8).

The triptans, which are serotonin receptor agonists, are the most specific antimigraine agents available. These agents cause vasoconstriction, reduce inflammation, and may reduce pain transmission. The five triptans in routine clinical use include sumatriptan (Imitrex), naratriptan (Amerge), rizatriptan

---

Chart 66-8

PATIENT EDUCATION
Migraine Headaches

The nurse instructs the patient to:

- Be aware of the definition of migraine headaches along with the characteristics and manifestations.
- Recognize triggers of migraine headaches and how to avoid such triggers as:
  - Foods that contain tyramine, such as chocolate, cheese, coffee, dairy products
  - Dietary habits that result in long periods between meals
  - Menstruation and ovulation (caused by hormone fluctuation)
  - Alcohol (causes vasodilation of blood vessels)
  - Fatigue and fluctuations in sleep patterns
- Develop and use a paper or electronic headache diary.
- Implement stress management and lifestyle changes to minimize the frequency of headaches.
- Ensure correct pharmacologic management: acute therapy and prophylaxis to include medication regimen and side effects.
- Use comfort measures during headache attacks, such as resting in a quiet and dark environment, applying cold compresses to the painful area, and elevating the head.
- Seek out resources for education and support, such as the National Headache Foundation.

(Maxalt), zolmitriptan (Zomig), and almotriptan (Axert) (D'Arcy, 2014). Numerous serotonin receptor agonists are under study. Many of the triptan medications are available in a variety of formulations, such as nasal sprays, inhalers, conventional tablet, disintegrating tablet, suppositories, or injections. The nasal sprays are useful for patients experiencing nausea and vomiting (Dahlöf & Van Den Brink, 2012).

The triptans are considered first-line treatment of the management of moderate to severe migraine pain. Best results are achieved with early use of triptans; oral dosing takes effect within 20 to 60 minutes of taking the drug and if needed may be repeated in 2 to 4 hours. Triptans are contraindicated in patients with ischemic heart disease. Careful administration and dosing instructions to patients are important to prevent adverse reactions such as increased blood pressure, drowsiness, muscle pain, sweating, and anxiety. Interactions are possible if the medication is taken in conjunction with St. John wort (Karch, 2015).

Ergotamine preparations (taken orally, sublingually, subcutaneously, intramuscularly, by rectum, or by inhalation) may be effective in aborting the headache if taken early in the migraine process. They are low in cost. Ergotamine tartrate acts on smooth muscle, causing prolonged constriction of the cranial blood vessels. Each patient's dosage is based on individual needs. Side effects include aching muscles, paresthesias (numbness and tingling), nausea, and vomiting. Pretreatment with antiemetic agents may be required. None of the triptan medications should be taken concurrently with medications containing ergotamine because of the potential for a prolonged vasoactive reaction (Karch, 2015).

Many widely used medications for the prevention of migraine are available. An analysis of research in the last decade reported the most effective medications for migraine treatment include anticonvulsant agents (divalproex sodium [Depakote], valproate [Depacon], topiramate [Topamax]), beta-blockers (metoprolol [Lopressor], propranolol [Inderal], timolol [Blocadren]), and triptans (frovatriptan [Frova]). Other medications prescribed for migraine prevention include antidepressant agents (amitriptyline [Elavil], venlafaxine [Effexor]) and additional beta-blockers (atenolol [Tenormin], nadolol [Corgard]) and triptans (naratriptan [Amerge], zolmitriptan [Zomig]) (D'Arcy, 2014).

The medical management of an acute attack of cluster headaches may include 100% oxygen by facemask for 15 minutes, subcutaneous sumatriptan, or intranasal zolmitriptan (Becker et al., 2015).

The medical management of cranial arteritis consists of early administration of a corticosteroid to prevent the possibility of loss of vision due to vascular occlusion or rupture of the involved artery. The patient is instructed not to stop the medication abruptly, because this can lead to relapse. Analgesic agents are prescribed for comfort.

Nursing Management

When migraine or the other types of headaches have been diagnosed, the goal of nursing management is pain relief. It is reasonable to try nonpharmacologic interventions first, but the use of medications should not be delayed. The first priority is to treat the acute event of the headache and the second is to prevent recurrent episodes. Prevention involves patient education regarding precipitating factors, possible lifestyle or habit changes that may be helpful, and pharmacologic measures.

Relieving Pain

Individualized treatment depends on the type of headache and differs for migraine, cluster headaches, cranial arteritis, and tension headache. Nursing care is directed toward treatment of the acute episode. A migraine or a cluster headache in the early phase requires abortive medication therapy instituted as soon as possible. Some headaches can be prevented if the appropriate medications are taken before the onset of pain. Nursing care during an attack includes comfort measures such as a quiet, dark environment; elevation of the head of the bed to 30 degrees; and symptomatic treatment (i.e., administration of antiemetic medication) (Hickey, 2014).

Symptomatic pain relief for tension headache may be obtained by application of local heat or massage. Additional strategies may include administration of analgesic agents, antidepressant medications, and muscle relaxants.

Promoting Home, Community-Based, and Transitional Care

 Educating Patients About Self-Care

Headaches, especially migraines, are more likely to occur when the patient is ill, overly tired, or stressed. Nonpharmacologic therapies are important and include patient education about the type of headache, its mechanism (if known), and appropriate changes in lifestyle to avoid triggers. Regular sleep, meals, exercise, relaxation, and avoidance of dietary triggers may be helpful in avoiding headaches (Becker et al., 2015).

The patient with tension headaches needs education and reassurance that the headache is not the result of a brain tumor or other intracranial disorder. Stress reduction techniques, such as biofeedback, exercise programs, and meditation, are examples of nonpharmacologic therapies that may prove helpful. The patient and family need to be educated about the importance of following the prescribed treatment regimen for headache and keeping follow-up appointments. In addition, the patient is reminded of the importance of participating in health promotion activities and recommended health screenings to promote a healthy lifestyle. Chart 66-8 presents educational topics for the patient with migraine headaches.

Continuing and Transitional Care

The National Headache Foundation (see the Resources section) provides a list of clinics in the United States and the names of physicians who specialize in headache and who are members of the American Headache Society.

CRITICAL THINKING EXERCISES

1 A patient is admitted to your unit for a transsphenoidal cranial procedure. Identify the nursing interventions indicated before, during, and after the procedure. What patient and caregiver education is indicated in preparation for discharge? How will your nursing interventions and patient education change if a supratentorial surgical approach is used?

2 **ebp** As a member of your unit's practice council, you are working on updating interventions to manage increased intracranial pressure. Using your knowledge of evidence-based practice guidelines, list the most important interventions for nurses to implement. Compare and contrast the options supported by the guidelines.

3 **pq** Identify the priorities, approach, and techniques you would use to provide care to a 25-year-old female patient with migraine headaches. How will your priorities, approach, and techniques differ if the patient is male, if the patient has tension-type or cluster headaches?

REFERENCES

*Asterisk indicates nursing research.
**Double asterisk indicates classic reference.

Books

American Association of Neuroscience Nurses (AANN). (2012). *Care of the patient with intracranial pressure monitoring/external ventricular drainage or lumbar drainage: AANN clinical practice guideline series.* Glenview, IL: Author.

American Association of Neuroscience Nurses (AANN). (2016a). *Care of adults and children with seizures and epilepsy: AANN clinical practice guideline series.* Chicago, IL: Author.

American Association of Neuroscience Nurses (AANN). (2016b). *Care of the adult patient with a brain tumor: AANN clinical practice guideline series.* Chicago, IL: Author.

Bader, M., Littlejohns, L. R., & Olson, D. (2016). *AANN core curriculum for neuroscience nursing* (6th ed.). Chicago, IL: American Association of Neuroscience Nurses.

Grossman, S. C., & Porth, C. M. (2014). *Pathophysiology: Concepts of altered health states* (9th ed.). Philadelphia, PA: Lippincott Williams & Wilkins.

Hickey, J. V. (2014). *The clinical practice of neurological & neurosurgical nursing* (7th ed.). Philadelphia, PA: Lippincott Williams & Wilkins.

Karch, A. (2015). *2015 Lippincott's nursing drug guide*. Philadelphia, PA: Lippincott Williams & Wilkins.

**Posner, J. B., Saper, C. B., Schiff, N. D., et al. (2007). *Plum and Posner's diagnosis of stupor and coma* (4th ed.). Oxford, UK: Oxford University Press.

Wheless, J. (2013). Vagus nerve stimulation therapy. In E. Wyllie, G. D. Cascino, B. E. Gidal, & H. P. Goodkin (Eds.). *Wyllie's treatment of epilepsy: Principles and practice* (5th ed.). Philadelphia, PA: Lippincott Williams & Wilkins.

Journals and Electronic Documents

Alali, A., Naimark, D., Wilson, J., et al. (2014). Economic evaluation of decompressive hemicraniectomy versus barbiturate coma for refractory intracranial hypertension following traumatic brain injury. *Critical Care Medicine, 42*(10), 2235–2243.

Andrews, P., Sinclair, L., Rodriguez, A., et al. (2015). Hypothermia for intracranial hypertension after traumatic brain injury. *The New England Journal of Medicine, 373*(25), 2403–2412.

Aylwin, S., Burst, V., Peri, A., et al. (2015). "Do's and dont's" in the management of hyponatremia. *Current Medical Research and Opinion, 31*(9), 1755–1761.

Bauman, M., & McCourt, T. R. (2014). Assessing and managing patients with chronic subdural hematoma, *American Nurse Today, 9*(9), 38–41.

Becker, W., Findlay, T., Moga, C., et al. (2015). Guideline for primary care management of headache in adults. *Canadian Family Physician, 61*(8), 670–679.

Bruno, M., Laureys, S., & Demerttzi, A. (2013). Coma and disorders of consciousness. *Handbook of Clinical Neurology, 118*(2013), 205–213.

Charles, A. (2013). The evolution of migraine attack – a review of recent evidence. *Headache, 53*(2), 413–419.

Charles, A. (2015). Sounding out migraine-related interactions between the brainstem and the cortex. *Cephalalgia, 35*(11), 941–943.

Charles, A., & Hansen, J. (2015). Migraine aura: New ideas about cause, classification, and clinical significance. *Current Opinion in Neurology, 28*(3), 255–260.

Dahlöf, C., & Van Den Brink, A. (2012). Dihydroergotamine, ergotamine, methysergide and sumatriptan – basic science in relation to migraine treatment. *Headache, 52*(4), 707–714.

D'Arcy, Y. (2014). Preventing migraine headaches in adults. *Nursing 2014, 44*(1), 58–61.

de Lima Oliveira, M., Kairalla, A., Fonoff, E., et al. (2014). Cerebral microdialysis in traumatic brain injury and subarachnoid hemorrhage: State of the art. *Neurocritical Care, 21*(1), 152–162.

Destrebecq, A., Terzoni, S., & Sala, E. (2014). Post-lumbar puncture headache: A review of issues for nursing practice. *Journal of Neuroscience Nursing, 46*(3), 180–186.

Dias, C., Maia, I., Cerejo, A., et al. (2014) Pressures, flow, and brain oxygenation during plateau waves of intracranial pressure. *Neurocritical Care, 21*(1), 124–132.

England, M., Liverman, C., Schultz, A., et al. (2012). Epilepsy across the spectrum: Promoting health and understanding. A summary of the Institute of Medicine report. *Epilepsy and Behavior, 25*(2), 266–276.

Fisher, R., Acevedo, C., Arzimanoglou, A., et al. (2014). A practical clinical definition of epilepsy. *Epilepsia, 55*(4), 475–482.

Fisher, R., Cross, H., French, J., et al. (2016). Operational classification of seizure types by the International League Against Epilepsy (ILAE). Retrieved on 9/29/2016 at: www.ilae.org/visitors/centre/documents/ClassificationSeizureILAE-2016.pdf

Foreman, P., Schmalz, P., & Griessenauer, C. (2014). Chemoprophylaxis for venous thromboembolism in traumatic brain injury: A review and evidence based protocol. *Clinical Neurology and Neurosurgery, 123*, 109–116.

Headache Classification Committee of the International Headache Society. (2013). The international classification of headache disorders, 3rd edition (beta version). *Cephalalgia, 33*(9), 629–808.

Institute of Medicine (IOM). (2012). Epilepsy across the spectrum: Promoting health and understanding. Retrieved on 1/5/17 at: www.nationalacademies.org/hmd/Reports/2012/Epilepsy-Across-the-Spectrum.aspx.

Kiyoshi-Teo, H., & Blegen, M. (2015). Influence of institutional guidelines on oral hygiene practices in intensive care units. *American Journal of Critical Care, 24*(4), 309–318.

Lagana, A., Triolo, O., D'Amico, V., et al. (2016). Management of women with epilepsy: From preconception to post-partum. *Archives of Gynecology and Obstetrics, 293*, 493–503.

Madden, L., & DeVon, H. (2015). A systematic review of the effects of body temperature on outcome after adult traumatic brain injury. *Journal of Neuroscience Nursing, 47*(4), 190–203.

Majdan, M., Mauritz, W., Wilbacher, I., et al. (2013). Barbiturates use and its effects in patients with severe traumatic brain injury in five European countries. *Journal of Neurotrauma, 30*(1), 23–29.

Megha, M., Harpreet, S., & Nayeem, Z. (2013). Effect of frequency of multimodal coma stimulation on the consciousness levels of traumatic brain injury comatose patients. *Brain Injury, 27*(5), 570–577.

*Miller, W., Buelow, J., & Bakas, T. (2014). Older adults and new onset epilepsy: Experiences with diagnosis. *Journal of Neuroscience Nursing, 46*(1), 2–10.

*Mitchell, P., Kirkness, C., & Blissitt, P. (2015). Chapter 5 cerebral perfusion pressure and intracranial pressure in traumatic brain injury. *Annual Review of Nursing Research, 33*, 111–117.

Munro, N., & Ruggiero, M. (2014). Ventilator-associated pneumonia bundle. *AACN Advanced Critical Care, 25*(2), 163–175.

Nei, M., Ngo, L., Sirven, J., et al. (2014). Ketogenic diet in adolescents and adults with epilepsy. *Seizure, 23*(6), 439–442.

Nemer, S., Caldeira, J., Santos, R., et al. (2015). Effects of positive end-expiratory pressure on brain tissue oxygen pressure of severe traumatic brain injury patients with acute respiratory distress syndrome – A pilot study. *Journal of Critical Care, 30*(6), 1263–1266.

Oddo, M., Bosel, J., & Participants in the International Multidisciplinary Consensus Conference on Multimodality Monitoring. (2014). Monitoring of brain and systemic oxygenation in neurocritical care patients. *Neurocritical Care, 21*(Supp 2), S103–S120.

Ong, C., Keyrouz, S., & Diringer, M. (2015). The role of osmotic therapy in hemispheric stroke. *Neurocritical Care, 23*(2), 285–291.

Rockett, H., Thompson, H., & Blissitt, P. (2015). Fever management: Practices of neuroscience nurses: What has changed?. *Journal of Neuroscience Nursing, 47*(2), 66–75.

Sandsmark, D., Kumar, M., Park, S., et al. (2012). Multimodal monitoring in subarachnoid hemorrhage. *Stroke, 43*(5), 1440–1445.

Scheffer, I., French, J., Hirsch, E., et al. (2016). Classification of the epilepsies: New concepts for discussion and debate – special report of the ILAE classification task force of the commission for classification and terminology. *Epilepsia Open*, 1–8. doi:10.1002/epi4.5.

Thibault, A., Deltombe, T., Wannez, S., et al. (2015). Impact of soft splints on upper limb spasticity in chronic patients with disorders of consciousness: A randomized, single-blind, controlled trial. *Brain Injury, 29*(7–8), 830–836.

Trinka, E., Cock, H., Hesdorffer, D., et al. (2015). A definition and classification of status epilepticus – Report of the ILAE Task Force on Classification of Status Epilepticus. *Epilepsia, 56*(10), 1515–1523.

Updyke, M., & Duryea, B. (2013). To provoke or not to provoke: Ethical considerations in the epilepsy monitoring unit. *Journal of Neuroscience Nursing, 45*(3), 133–138.

U.S. Food and Drug Administration. (2014). RNS® (Responsive Neurostimulation) System P100026. Retrieved on 9/29/2016 at: www.fda.gov/MedicalDevices/ProductsandMedicalProcedures/DeviceApprovalsandClearances/Recently-ApprovedDevices/ucm376685.htm

Van Der Naalt, J. (2015). Resting functional imaging tools (MRS, SPECT, PET, and PCT). *Handbook of Clinical Neurology, 127*(2015), 295–308.

Wang, X., Dong, Y., Han, X., et al. (2013). Nutritional support for patients sustaining traumatic brain injury: A systematic review and meta-analysis of prospective studies. *PLoS ONE, 8*(3), 1–14.

Wang, X., Ji, J., Fen, L., et al. (2013) Effects of dexmetetomidine on cerebral blood flow in critically ill patients with or without traumatic brain injury: A prospective controlled trial. *Brain Injury, 27*(13–14), 1617–1622.

Wells, R., Turner, D., Lee, M., et al. (2016). Managing migraine during pregnancy and lactation. *Neurology and Neuroscience Reports, 16*(4), 40.

Wijdicks, E. (2013). Brain death. *Handbook of Clinical Neurology, 118*(2013), 191–203.

Resources

American Headache Society, www.americanheadachesociety.org
Brain Injury Association of America, www.biausa.org
Brain Trauma Foundation (BTF), www.braintrauma.org
Epilepsy Foundation of America, www.epilepsy.com
Hydrocephalus Association, www.hydroassoc.org
National Headache Foundation, www.headaches.org

67 Management of Patients With Cerebrovascular Disorders

LEARNING OBJECTIVES

On completion of this chapter, the learner will be able to:

1 Describe the incidence and impact of cerebrovascular disorders.
2 Identify the risk factors for cerebrovascular disorders and related measures for prevention.
3 Compare the various types of cerebrovascular disorders: their causes, clinical manifestations, and medical management.

4 Explain the principles of nursing management as they relate to the care of a patient in the acute stage of an ischemic stroke.
5 Use the nursing process as a framework for care of a patient recovering from an ischemic stroke.
6 Apply the nursing process as a framework for care of a patient with a hemorrhagic stroke.
7 Discuss essential elements for family education and preparation for home care of the patient who has had a stroke.

GLOSSARY

agnosia: loss of ability to recognize objects through a particular sensory system; may be visual, auditory, or tactile
aneurysm: a weakening or bulge in an arterial wall
aphasia: inability to express oneself or to understand language
apraxia: inability to perform previously learned purposeful motor acts on a voluntary basis
dysarthria: defects of articulation due to neurologic causes
dysphagia: difficulty swallowing
expressive aphasia: inability to express oneself; often associated with damage to the left frontal lobe area

hemianopsia: blindness of half of the field of vision in one or both eyes
hemiparesis: weakness of one side of the body, or part of it, due to an injury in the motor area of the brain
hemiplegia: paralysis of one side of the body, or part of it, due to an injury in the motor area of the brain
infarction: tissue necrosis in an area deprived of blood supply
penumbra region: area of low cerebral blood flow
receptive aphasia: inability to understand what someone else is saying; often associated with damage to the temporal lobe area

Cerebrovascular disorders is an umbrella term that refers to a functional abnormality of the central nervous system (CNS) that occurs when the blood supply to the brain is disrupted. Stroke is the primary cerebrovascular disorder in the United States, and while it dropped from the fourth to the fifth leading cause of death, it is still a leading cause of serious, long-term disability. Approximately 795,000 people experience a stroke each year in the United States. Approximately 610,000 of these are new strokes, and 185,000 are recurrent strokes (Mozaffarian, Benjamin, Go, et al., 2016). About 7 million people who have survived a stroke are alive today. The financial impact of stroke is profound, with estimated direct and indirect costs of $33 billion from 2011 to 2012 (Mozaffarian et al., 2016).

Strokes can be divided into two major categories: ischemic (approximately 87%), in which vascular occlusion and significant hypoperfusion occur, and hemorrhagic (approximately 13%), in which there is extravasation of blood into the brain or subarachnoid space (Hickey, 2014). Although there are some similarities between the two types of stroke, differences exist in etiology, pathophysiology, medical management, surgical management, and nursing care. Table 67-1 compares ischemic and hemorrhagic strokes.

Ischemic Stroke

An ischemic stroke, formerly referred to as a cerebrovascular disease (stroke) or "brain attack," is a sudden loss of function resulting from disruption of the blood supply to a part of the brain. The term *brain attack* has been used to suggest to health care practitioners and the public that a stroke is an urgent health care issue similar to a heart attack. With the approval of thrombolytic therapy for the treatment of acute ischemic stroke in 1996 came a revolution in the care of patients after a stroke. Early treatment with thrombolytic therapy for ischemic stroke results in fewer stroke symptoms and less loss of function (National Institute of Neurological Disorders and Stroke [NINDS], 1995). The only U.S. Food and Drug Administration (FDA)-approved thrombolytic therapy has a treatment window of 3 hours after the onset of a stroke, and scientific statements have endorsed its expanded use for up to 4.5 hours (Del Zoppo, Saver, Jauch, et al., 2009; Jauch, Saver, Adams, et al., 2013). Although the time frame for treatment has expanded in some centers, urgency is needed on the part of the public and health care practitioners for rapid transport of the patient to a hospital for assessment and administration of the medication.

TABLE 67-1 Comparison of Major Types of Stroke

Types of Stroke	Causes	Main Presenting Symptoms	Functional Recovery
Ischemic	• Large artery thrombosis • Small penetrating artery thrombosis • Cardiogenic embolic • Cryptogenic (no known cause) • Other	Numbness or weakness of the face, arm, or leg, especially on one side of the body	Usually plateaus at 6 months
Hemorrhagic	• Intracerebral hemorrhage • Subarachnoid hemorrhage • Cerebral aneurysm • Arteriovenous malformation	• "Exploding headache" • Decreased level of consciousness	Slower, usually plateaus at about 18 months

Adapted from Hickey, J. V. (2014). *The clinical practice of neurological & neurosurgical nursing* (7th ed.). Philadelphia, PA: Lippincott Williams & Wilkins.

Ischemic strokes are subdivided into five different types based on the cause: large artery thrombotic strokes (20%), small penetrating artery thrombotic strokes (25%), cardiogenic embolic strokes (20%), cryptogenic strokes (30%), and other (5%) (see Table 67-1). Large artery thrombotic strokes are caused by atherosclerotic plaques in the large blood vessels of the brain. Thrombus formation and occlusion at the site of the atherosclerosis result in ischemia and **infarction** (tissue necrosis in an area deprived of blood supply) (Hickey, 2014).

Small penetrating artery thrombotic strokes affect one or more vessels and are a common type of ischemic stroke. Small artery thrombotic strokes are also called *lacunar strokes* because of the cavity that is created after the death of infarcted brain tissue (Hickey, 2014).

Cardiogenic embolic strokes are associated with cardiac dysrhythmias, usually atrial fibrillation. Embolic strokes can also be associated with valvular heart disease and thrombi in the left ventricle. Emboli originate from the heart and circulate to the cerebral vasculature, most commonly the left middle cerebral artery, resulting in a stroke. Embolic strokes may be prevented by the use of anticoagulation therapy in patients with atrial fibrillation.

The last two classifications of ischemic strokes are cryptogenic strokes, which have no known cause, and strokes from other causes, such as illicit drug use (cocaine), coagulopathies, migraine/vasospasm, and spontaneous dissection of the carotid or vertebral arteries.

Pathophysiology

In an ischemic brain attack, there is disruption of the cerebral blood flow due to obstruction of a blood vessel. This disruption in blood flow initiates a complex series of cellular metabolic events referred to as the ischemic cascade (see Fig. 67-1).

The ischemic cascade begins when cerebral blood flow decreases to less than 25 mL per 100 g of blood per minute. At this point, neurons are no longer able to maintain aerobic respiration. The mitochondria must then switch to anaerobic respiration, which generates large amounts of lactic acid, causing a change in the pH. This switch to the less efficient anaerobic respiration also renders the neuron incapable of producing sufficient quantities of adenosine triphosphate (ATP) to fuel the depolarization processes. The membrane pumps that maintain electrolyte balances begin to fail, and the cells cease to function.

Early in the cascade, an area of low cerebral blood flow, referred to as the **penumbra region**, exists around the area of infarction. The penumbra region is ischemic brain tissue that may be salvaged with timely intervention. The ischemic cascade threatens cells in the penumbra because membrane depolarization of the cell wall leads to an increase in intracellular calcium and the release of glutamate. The influx of calcium and the release of glutamate, if continued, activate a number of damaging pathways that result in the destruction of the cell membrane, the release of more calcium and glutamate, vasoconstriction, and the generation of free radicals. These processes enlarge the area of infarction into the penumbra, extending the stroke. A person experiencing a stroke typically loses 1.9 million neurons each minute that a stroke is not treated, and the ischemic brain ages 3.6 years each hour without treatment (Saver, 2006).

Each step in the ischemic cascade represents an opportunity for intervention to limit the extent of secondary brain damage caused by a stroke. The penumbra area may be revitalized by administration of tissue plasminogen activator (t-PA). Medications that protect the brain from secondary

Figure 67-1 • Some of the processes contributing to ischemic brain cell injury.

injury are called *neuroprotectants*. A number of ongoing clinical trials focus on neuroprotective medications and strategies to improve stroke recovery and survival (Jauch et al., 2013).

Clinical Manifestations

An ischemic stroke can cause a wide variety of neurologic deficits, depending on the location of the lesion (which blood vessels are obstructed), the size of the area of inadequate perfusion, and the amount of collateral (secondary or accessory) blood flow. See Chapter 65 for discussion of anatomy and brain blood supply. The patient may present with any of the following signs or symptoms:

- Numbness or weakness of the face, arm, or leg, especially on one side of the body
- Confusion or change in mental status
- Trouble speaking or understanding speech
- Visual disturbances
- Difficulty walking, dizziness, or loss of balance or coordination
- Sudden severe headache

Motor, sensory, cranial nerve, cognitive, and other functions may be disrupted. Table 67-2 reviews the neurologic deficits frequently seen in patients with strokes. Table 67-3 compares the symptoms and behaviors seen in right hemispheric stroke with those seen in left hemispheric stroke.

Motor Loss

A stroke is an upper motor neuron lesion and results in loss of voluntary control over motor movements. Because the upper motor neurons decussate (cross), a disturbance of voluntary motor control on one side of the body may reflect damage to the upper motor neurons on the opposite side of the brain. The most common motor dysfunction is **hemiplegia** (paralysis of one side of the body, or part of it) caused by a lesion of the opposite side of the brain. **Hemiparesis**, or weakness of one side of the body, or part of it, is another sign. The concept of upper and lower motor neuron lesions is described in more detail in Chapter 65, Table 65-4.

In the early stage of stroke, the initial clinical features may be flaccid paralysis and loss of or decrease in the deep tendon reflexes. When these deep reflexes reappear (usually by 48 hours), increased tone is observed along with spasticity (abnormal increase in muscle tone) of the extremities on the affected side.

Communication Loss

Other brain functions affected by stroke are language and communication. In fact, stroke is the most common cause of **aphasia** (inability to express oneself or to understand language). The following are dysfunctions of language and communication:

- **Dysarthria** (difficulty in speaking) or dysphasia (impaired speech), caused by paralysis of the muscles responsible for producing speech
- Aphasia, which can be **expressive aphasia** (inability to express oneself), **receptive aphasia** (inability to understand language), or global (mixed) aphasia (see Chapter 65, Table 65-5)
- **Apraxia** (inability to perform a previously learned action), as may be seen when a patient makes verbal substitutions for desired syllables or words

Perceptual Disturbances

Perception is the ability to interpret sensation. Stroke can result in visual–perceptual dysfunctions, disturbances in visual–spatial relations, and sensory loss.

Visual–perceptual dysfunctions are caused by disturbances of the primary sensory pathways between the eye and visual cortex. Homonymous **hemianopsia** (blindness in half of the visual field in one or both eyes) may occur from stroke and may be temporary or permanent. The affected side of vision corresponds to the paralyzed side of the body.

Disturbances in visual–spatial relations (perceiving the relationship of two or more objects in spatial areas) are frequently seen in patients with right hemispheric damage.

Sensory Loss

Sensory losses from stroke may be mild, such as a slight impairment of touch, or more severe, with loss of proprioception (ability to perceive the position and motion of body parts) as well as difficulty in interpreting visual, tactile, and auditory stimuli. An **agnosia** is the loss of the ability to recognize objects through a particular sensory system; it may be visual, auditory, or tactile (see Chapter 65, Table 65-6).

Cognitive Impairment and Psychological Effects

If damage has occurred to the frontal lobe, learning capacity, memory, or other higher cortical intellectual functions may be impaired. Such dysfunction may be reflected in a limited attention span, difficulties in comprehension, forgetfulness, and a lack of motivation. These changes can cause the patient to become easily frustrated during rehabilitation. Depression is common and may be exaggerated by the patient's natural response to this catastrophic event. Emotional lability, hostility, frustration, resentment, lack of cooperation, and other psychological problems may occur.

Assessment and Diagnostic Findings

Any patient with neurologic deficits needs a careful history eliciting the last time the patient was seen well (Zanichkowsky, Nascimento, McCune, et al., 2016) and a rapid focused physical and neurologic examination. Initial assessment focuses on airway patency, which may be compromised by loss of gag or cough reflexes and altered respiratory pattern; cardiovascular status (including blood pressure, cardiac rhythm and rate, carotid bruit); and gross neurologic deficits.

Patients may present to the acute care facility with temporary neurologic symptoms. A transient ischemic attack (TIA) is a neurologic deficit typically lasting 1 to 2 hours. A TIA is manifested by a sudden loss of motor, sensory, or visual function. The symptoms result from temporary ischemia (impairment of blood flow) to a specific region of the brain; however, when brain imaging is performed, there is no evidence of ischemia. A TIA may serve as a warning of impending stroke. Approximately 15% of all strokes are preceded by a TIA (Miller & Summers, 2014; Mozaffarian et al., 2016). Lack of evaluation and treatment of a patient who has experienced previous TIAs may result in a stroke and irreversible deficits.

The initial diagnostic test for a stroke is usually a noncontrast computed tomography (CT) scan (Anderson, 2016). This should be performed within 25 minutes or less from the time the patient presents to the emergency department (ED)

TABLE 67-2 Neurologic Deficits of Stroke: Manifestations and Nursing Implications

Neurologic Deficit	Manifestation	Nursing Implications/Patient Education Applications
Visual Field Deficits		
Homonymous hemianopsia (loss of half of the visual field)	• Unaware of persons or objects on side of visual loss • Neglect of one side of the body • Difficulty judging distances	Place objects within intact field of vision. Approach the patient from side of intact field of vision. Instruct/remind the patient to turn head in the direction of visual loss to compensate for loss of visual field. Encourage the use of eyeglasses if available. When educating the patient, do so within patient's intact visual field.
Loss of peripheral vision	• Difficulty seeing at night • Unaware of objects or the borders of objects	Place objects in center of patient's intact visual field. Encourage the use of a cane or other object to identify objects in the periphery of the visual field. Ensure that the patient's driving ability is evaluated.
Diplopia	• Double vision	Explain to the patient the location of an object when placing it near the patient. Consistently place patient care items in the same location.
Motor Deficits		
Hemiparesis	• Weakness of the face, arm, and leg on the same side (due to a lesion in the opposite hemisphere)	Place objects within the patient's reach on the nonaffected side. Instruct the patient to exercise and increase the strength on the unaffected side.
Hemiplegia	• Paralysis of the face, arm, and leg on the same side (due to a lesion in the opposite hemisphere)	Encourage the patient to provide range-of-motion exercises to the affected side. Provide immobilization as needed to the affected side. Maintain body alignment in functional position. Exercise unaffected limb to increase mobility, strength, and use.
Ataxia	• Staggering, unsteady gait • Unable to keep feet together; needs a broad base to stand	Support patient during the initial ambulation phase. Provide supportive device for ambulation (walker, cane). Instruct the patient not to walk without assistance or supportive device.
Dysarthria	• Difficulty in forming words	Provide the patient with alternative methods of communicating. Allow the patient sufficient time to respond to verbal communication. Support patient and family to alleviate frustration related to difficulty in communicating.
Dysphagia	• Difficulty in swallowing	Test the patient's pharyngeal reflexes before offering food or fluids. Assist the patient with meals. Place food on the unaffected side of the mouth. Allow ample time to eat.
Sensory Deficits		
Paresthesia (occurs on the side opposite the lesion)	• Sensation of numbness, tingling, or a "pins and needles" sensation • Difficulty with proprioception	Instruct patient that sensation may be altered. Provide range of motion to affected areas and apply corrective devices as needed.
Verbal Deficits		
Expressive aphasia	• Unable to form words that are understandable; may be able to speak in single-word responses	Encourage patient to repeat sounds of the alphabet. Explore the patient's ability to write as an alternative means of communication.
Receptive aphasia	• Unable to comprehend the spoken word; can speak but may not make sense	Speak clearly and in an unhurried manner to assist the patient in forming the sounds. Explore the patient's ability to read as an alternative means of communication.
Global (mixed) aphasia	• Combination of both receptive and expressive aphasia	Speak clearly and in simple sentences; use gestures or pictures when able. Establish alternative means of communication.
Cognitive Deficits	• Short- and long-term memory loss • Decreased attention span • Impaired ability to concentrate • Poor abstract reasoning • Altered judgment	Reorient patient to time, place, and situation frequently. Use verbal and auditory cues to orient patient. Provide familiar objects (family photographs, favorite objects). Use noncomplicated language. Match visual tasks with a verbal cue; holding a toothbrush, simulate brushing of teeth while saying, "I would like you to brush your teeth now." Minimize distracting noises and views when providing education to the patient. Repeat and reinforce instructions frequently.
Emotional Deficits	• Loss of self-control • Emotional lability • Decreased tolerance to stressful situations • Depression • Withdrawal • Fear, hostility, and anger • Feelings of isolation	Support patient during uncontrollable outbursts. Discuss with the patient and family that the outbursts are due to the disease process. Encourage patient to participate in group activity. Provide stimulation for the patient. Control stressful situations, if possible. Provide a safe environment. Encourage patient to express feelings and frustrations related to disease process.

Adapted from Hickey, J. V. (2014). *The clinical practice of neurological & neurosurgical nursing* (7th ed.). Philadelphia, PA: Lippincott Williams & Wilkins.

TABLE 67-3 Comparison of Left and Right
Hemispheric Strokes

Left Hemispheric Stroke	Right Hemispheric Stroke
Paralysis or weakness on right side of body	Paralysis or weakness on left side of body
Right visual field deficit	Left visual field deficit
Aphasia (expressive, receptive, or global)	Spatial–perceptual deficits
Altered intellectual ability	Increased distractibility
Slow, cautious behavior	Impulsive behavior and poor judgment Lack of awareness of deficits

Adapted from Hickey, J. V. (2014). *The clinical practice of neurological & neurosurgical nursing* (7th ed.). Philadelphia, PA: Lippincott Williams & Wilkins.

to determine if the event is ischemic or hemorrhagic as the type of stroke determines treatment (Anderson, 2016). Further diagnostic workup for ischemic stroke involves attempting to identify the source of the thrombi or emboli. A 12-lead electrocardiogram (ECG) and a carotid ultrasound are standard tests. Other studies may include CT angiography or CT perfusion; magnetic resonance imaging (MRI) and magnetic resonance angiography of the brain and neck vessels; transcranial Doppler flow studies; transthoracic or transesophageal echocardiography; xenon-enhanced CT scan; and single-photon emission CT scan (Summers, Leonard, Wentworth, et al., 2009; Jauch et al., 2013; Miller & Summers, 2014).

Prevention

Primary prevention of ischemic stroke remains the best approach. A healthy lifestyle including not smoking, engaging in physical activity (at least 40 minutes a day, 3 to 4 days a week), maintaining a healthy weight, and following a healthy diet (including modest alcohol consumption), can reduce the risk of having a stroke (Mozaffarian et al., 2016). Specific diets that have decreased risk of stroke include the Dietary Approaches to Stop Hypertension (DASH) diet (high in fruits and vegetables, moderate in low-fat dairy products, and low in animal protein), the Mediterranean diet (supplemented with nuts), and overall diets that are rich in fruits and vegetables. Research findings suggest that low-dose aspirin may lower the risk of a first stroke for those who are at risk (Meschia, Bushnell, Boden-Albala, et al., 2014).

Stroke risk screenings are an ideal opportunity to lower stroke risk by identifying people or groups of people who are at high risk for stroke and by educating patients and the community about recognition and prevention of stroke. Stroke screenings are usually coordinated and run by nurses. Age, gender, and race are well-known nonmodifiable risk factors for stroke. High-risk groups include people older than 55 years, and the incidence of stroke more than doubles in each successive decade. Men have a higher age-adjusted rate of stroke than that of women. However, the magnitude of strokes in women should not be underplayed; 1 in 6 women die of stroke as compared to 1 in 25 who die of breast cancer (Ennen, 2013), and each year 55,000 more women than men

have a stroke (Mozaffarian et al., 2016). Compared to Caucasian Americans, African Americans and some Hispanic/Latino Americans have a higher incidence of stroke and higher mortality (Meschia et al., 2014; Aycock & Clark, 2016). The Nursing Research Profile in Chart 67-1 examines the accuracy of perceived stroke risk in African Americans (Aycock & Clark, 2016).

There are many risk factors for ischemic stroke (see Chart 67-2). For people who are at high risk, interventions that alter modifiable factors, such as treating hypertension and stopping smoking, reduce stroke risk.

Additional treatable conditions that increase risk of stroke include sickle cell diseases, cardiomyopathy (ischemic and nonischemic), and valvular heart disease (e.g., endocarditis, prosthetic heart valves). Lesser known and potentially modifiable risk factors for stroke are migraine (especially migraine with aura), sleep apnea, and inherited and acquired hypercoagulable states. Chronic inflammatory conditions that have been associated with an increased risk of stroke are systemic lupus erythematosus and rheumatoid arthritis (Meschia et al., 2014).

Several methods of preventing recurrent stroke have been identified for patients with TIAs or ischemic stroke. Patients with moderate to severe carotid stenosis are treated with carotid endarterectomy (CEA) or carotid angioplasty and stenting. In patients with atrial fibrillation, which increases the risk of emboli, administration of an anticoagulant that inhibits clot formation may prevent both thrombotic and embolic strokes (Kernan, Ovbiagele, Black, et al., 2014).

Medical Management

Patients who have experienced a TIA or stroke should have medical management for secondary prevention. Those with atrial fibrillation (or cardioembolic strokes) are treated with dose-adjusted warfarin (Coumadin) with a target international normalized ratio (INR) of 2 to 3. Other newer anticoagulants that may be prescribed as alternative drugs include dabigatran (Pradaxa), apixaban (Eliquis), edoxaban (Savaysa), or rivaroxaban (Xarelto), unless they are contraindicated. These newer drugs are also known as new or novel oral anticoagulants (NOACs) (Bentz, 2015). If anticoagulants are contraindicated, aspirin alone is the best option, although the addition of clopidogrel (Plavix) to aspirin is also a reasonable therapy (Kernan et al., 2014).

Platelet-inhibiting medications, including aspirin, extended-release dipyridamole plus aspirin (Aggrenox), and clopidogrel decrease the incidence of cerebral infarction in patients who have experienced TIAs and stroke from suspected embolic or thrombotic causes. The specific medication that is used is based on the patient's health history.

Research suggests that medications known as statins reduce coronary events and ischemic strokes. The most current stroke prevention guideline now includes the recommendation of a statin even if the low-density lipoprotein (LDL) cholesterol is below 100 mg/dL and there is no evidence of atherosclerotic cardiovascular disease (coronary artery disease/myocardial infarction, hypertensive heart disease and peripheral arterial disease) (Kernan et al., 2014). The FDA has included indications for statin medications, such as simvastatin (Zocor), to include secondary stroke prevention.

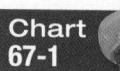

Chart 67-1 · NURSING RESEARCH PROFILE

Awareness of Stroke Risk in Young African Americans

Aycock, D. M., & Clark, P. C. (2016). Incongruence between perceived long-term risk and actual risk of stroke in rural African Americans. *Journal of Neuroscience Nursing*, 48(1), 35–41.

Purpose

African Americans aged 20 to 44 years are twice as likely to have a stroke as Caucasians of the same age. African Americans aged 35 to 64 years also have a higher risk (three to four times) of dying from a stroke than Caucasians. When a stroke occurs in a younger adult, they live longer with disabilities with greater health care costs and loss of productivity. Because up to 80% of strokes can be prevented with recognition and elimination of risk factors, primary prevention is critically important. The purpose of this study was to examine the accuracy of perceived stroke risk of African Americans aged 19 to 54 years.

Design

This study used a descriptive-correlational design. Participants consisted of a nonrandom sample that was recruited from a mobile health clinic (traveling to four rural counties over 4 months). Participants self-identified as African American, were between 19 and 54 years of age, were current residents of a rural county, and could not have a physical impairment that could keep them from exercising. Sixty-six participants were enrolled in the study. Participants were asked to select the risk that represented their risk of having a stroke in the next 10 to 20 years (no risk, little risk, moderate risk, or high risk). This was compared to an individual actual risk assessment that was based on accepted risk factors for stroke. The form that was used included health, social and family histories, and biophysiologic health measures (blood pressure and glucose). A scoring system was used as a guide to obtain a risk factor score. Scores could range between 0 and 8 (zero would be no risk factors). The measures were compared and participants were placed into risk accuracy categories: accurate, underestimate, or overestimate.

Findings

The mean age of participants was 43.3 years. Most of the participants were female (71%). Comparisons of the scores showed that 44% underestimated their risk, 47% were accurate, and 9% overestimated their risk. 67% of participants with a family history of stroke and 69% with a history of hypertension did not identify these as risk factors. Eighty percent of those who smoked cigarettes, 93% of those with diabetes, and 88% of those who were either overweight or who had obesity did not identify these as risk factors. This sample had a high burden of risk factors for stroke. Of the 39 participants who had 3 or more risk factors, only 19 (49%) thought that they were moderate to high risk of stroke.

Nursing Implications

This study suggests that more public education about primary prevention and awareness of modifiable stroke risk factors is needed. Nurses are in an optimal position to provide this education. Nurses in all settings (hospital, community, rehabilitation, outpatient clinics, and industry) should be involved in prevention and wellness activities for the public. This study focused on a young to middle-aged African American sample. Awareness campaigns can be focused and individualized for a younger population, and this study indicates that this type of campaign is needed. More studies are needed to test educational materials and tools that can be of benefit to this young to middle-aged population.

After the acute stroke period, antihypertensive medications are also used, if indicated, for secondary stroke prevention. Preferred drugs include angiotensin-converting enzyme (ACE) inhibitors and diuretics, or a combination of both (Kernan et al., 2014).

Medical management of acute ischemic stroke needs to include consideration for endovascular treatment (Powers, Derdeyn, Biller, et al., 2015). The FDA has approved several devices that open the blocked artery and restore blood flow to the brain. These devices are used by specialists in the endovascular suite.

Thrombolytic Therapy

Thrombolytic agents are used to treat ischemic stroke by dissolving the blood clot that is blocking blood flow to the brain. Recombinant t-PA is a genetically engineered form of t-PA (a thrombolytic substance made naturally by the body) (Karch, 2014). It works by binding to fibrin and converting plasminogen to plasmin, which stimulates fibrinolysis of the clot. Rapid diagnosis of stroke and initiation of thrombolytic therapy (within 3 hours) in patients with ischemic stroke leads to a decrease in the size of the stroke and an overall improvement in functional outcome after 3 months (NINDS, 1995). The goal is for intravenous (IV) t-PA to be given within 60 minutes of the patient arriving to the ED (Jauch et al., 2013).

Intra-arterial delivery of t-PA is an alternative to IV administration. This type of administration can allow for higher concentrations of the drug to be given directly to the clot, and the time window for treatment may be extended up to 6 hours. Those not eligible for IV delivery may be eligible for intra-arterial delivery, and these methods may also be combined. Treatment using intra-arterial delivery must occur in specialized centers with access to emergent cerebral angiogram and interventional operating rooms/suites (Summers

Chart 67-2 ⚠ MODIFIABLE RISK FACTORS

Ischemic Stroke

- Asymptomatic carotid stenosis
- Atrial fibrillation
- Diabetes (associated with accelerated atherogenesis)
- Dyslipidemia
- Excessive alcohol consumption
- Hypercoagulable states
- Hypertension (controlling hypertension, the major risk factor, is the key to preventing stroke)
- Migraine
- Obesity
- Sedentary lifestyle
- Sleep apnea
- Smoking

Adapted from Meschia, J. F., Bushnell, C., Boden-Albala, B., et al. (2014). Guidelines for the primary prevention of stroke: A statement for healthcare professionals from the American Heart Association/American Stroke Association. *Stroke*, 45(12), 3754–3832.

et al., 2009; Jauch et al., 2013). Ongoing clinical trials continue to investigate the efficacy of other thrombolytic agents.

To realize the full potential of early intervention, community education directed at recognizing the symptoms of stroke and obtaining appropriate emergency care is necessary to ensure rapid transport to a hospital and initiation of therapy within the recommended 3-hour period (which may be extended up to 4.5 hours in some cases) (Del Zoppo et al., 2009). Delays make the patient ineligible for therapies, because revascularization of necrotic tissue (which develops after 3 hours) increases the risk of cerebral edema and hemorrhage.

Endovascular Therapy

It is now recommended that patients with acute ischemic stroke receive endovascular therapy and medical management with a stent retriever if they meet specific criteria (Powers et al., 2015). All of the following criteria need to be met:

- Prestroke status of no deficits
- Acute ischemic stroke receiving IV t-PA within 4.5 hours of onset according to guidelines from professional medical societies
- Causative occlusion of the internal carotid artery or proximal middle cerebral artery
- Age ≥18 years
- NIHSS score of ≥6
- ASPECT (a radiologic assessment of the CT scan) score of ≥6, and treatment can be initiated (groin puncture) within 6 hours of symptom onset

Patients eligible for t-PA should receive IV t-PA even if endovascular treatments are being considered (Powers et al., 2015). Thrombolytic therapy should not be delayed.

Enhancing Prompt Diagnosis

After being notified by emergency medical service personnel, the ED contacts the appropriate staff (neurologist, neuroradiologist, radiology department, nursing staff, ECG, and laboratory technicians) and informs them of the patient's imminent arrival at the hospital. Many institutions have acute stroke teams that respond rapidly, ensuring that treatment occurs within the allotted period. This may be called a Code Stroke.

Initial management requires the definitive diagnosis of an ischemic stroke by brain imaging and a careful history to determine whether the patient meets the criteria for t-PA therapy (see Chart 67-3). The goal is that diagnostic results from imaging are completed within 25 minutes of the patient's arrival to the ED (Middleton, Grimley, & Alexandrov, 2015). Some of the contraindications for thrombolytic therapy include symptom onset greater than 3 hours before admission (expanded to 4.5 hours in some cases), a patient who is anticoagulated (with an INR above 1.7), or a patient who has recently had any type of significant intracranial pathology (e.g., previous stroke, head injury, trauma) in the last 3 months.

Before receiving t-PA, the patient is assessed using the National Institutes of Health Stroke Scale (NIHSS), a standardized assessment tool that helps evaluate stroke severity (see Table 67-4). Total NIHSS scores range from 0 (normal) to 42 (severe stroke). Certification in the administration of the scale is recommended and is available for nurses and other health care professionals.

Chart 67-3	Eligibility Criteria for Tissue Plasminogen Activator Administration

- Age ≥18 years
- Clinical diagnosis of ischemic stroke
- Time of onset of stroke known and is less than 3 hours before treatment
- Systolic blood pressure ≤185 mm Hg; diastolic ≤110 mm Hg
- No minor stroke or rapidly resolving stroke
- No seizure at onset of stroke
- Prothrombin time ≤15 seconds or international normalized ratio ≤1.7 (if taking an anticoagulant, the same guidance is used)
- Not received heparin during the past 48 hours with elevated partial thromboplastin time
- Platelet count ≥100,000/mm³
- Glucose >50 mg/dL
- No prior intracranial hemorrhage, neoplasm, arteriovenous malformation, or aneurysm
- No major surgical procedures or serious trauma within 14 days
- No stroke, serious head injury, or intracranial surgery within 3 months
- No gastrointestinal or urinary bleeding within 21 days
- No pregnancy

Some of these are relative contraindications (the provider administering the medication needs to weigh the risks and benefits of the therapy). There are more stringent criteria if t-PA is considered for those patients in the 3.0- to 4.5-hour time window.

Adapted from Jauch, E. C., Saver, J. L., Adams, H. P., et al. (2013). Guidelines for the early management of patients with ischemic stroke: A guideline from the American Heart Association/American Stroke Association. *Stroke, 44*(1), 870–947.

Dosage and Administration

The patient is weighed to determine the dose of t-PA. Typically, two or more IV sites are established prior to administration of t-PA (one for the t-PA and the other for administration of IV fluids). The dosage for t-PA is 0.9 mg/kg, with a maximum dose of 90 mg. Ten percent of the calculated dose is given as an IV bolus over 1 minute. The remaining dose (90%) is given IV over 1 hour via an infusion pump (Jauch et al., 2013).

The patient is admitted to the intensive care unit or an acute stroke unit, where continuous cardiac monitoring and frequent neurologic assessments are conducted. Vital signs are obtained frequently, with particular attention to blood pressure (with the goal of lowering the risk of intracranial hemorrhage). An example of a standard protocol would be to obtain vital signs every 15 minutes for the first 2 hours, every 30 minutes for the next 6 hours, then every hour until 24 hours after treatment. Blood pressure should be maintained with the systolic pressure less than 180 mm Hg and the diastolic pressure less than 105 mm Hg (Jauch et al., 2013; Middleton et al., 2015). Airway management is instituted based on the patient's clinical condition and arterial blood gas values.

Side Effects

Once it is determined that the patient is a candidate for t-PA therapy, no anticoagulant agents are given for the next 24 hours. Bleeding is the most common side effect of t-PA

TABLE 67-4 Summary of National Institutes of Health Stroke Scale

Category	Description	Score
1a. LOC	Alert	0
	Arousable by minor stimulation	1
	Obtunded, strong stimulation to attend	2
	Unresponsive, or reflexive responses only	3
1b. LOC questions (month, age)	Answers both correctly	0
	Answers one correctly	1
	Both incorrect	2
1c. LOC commands (open, close eyes; make fist, let go)	Obeys both correctly	0
	Obeys one correctly	1
	Both incorrect	2
2. Best gaze (eyes open—patient follows examiner's finger or face)	Normal	0
	Partial gaze palsy	1
	Forced deviation	2
3. Visual (introduce visual stimulus/threat to patient's visual field quadrants)	No visual loss	0
	Partial hemianopsia	1
	Complete hemianopsia	2
	Bilateral hemianopsia	3
4. Facial palsy (show teeth, raise eyebrows, and squeeze eyes shut)	Normal	0
	Minor	1
	Partial	2
	Complete	3
5a. Motor; arm—left (elevate extremity to 90 degrees and score drift/movement)	No drift	0
	Drift but maintains in air	1
	Unable to maintain in air	2
	No effort against gravity	3
	No movement	4
	Amputation, joint fusion (explain)	N/A
5b. Motor; arm—right (elevate extremity to 90 degrees and score drift/movement)	No drift	0
	Drift but maintains in air	1
	Unable to maintain in air	2
	No effort against gravity	3
	No movement	4
	Amputation, joint fusion (explain)	N/A
6a. Motor; leg—left (elevate extremity to 30 degrees and score drift/movement)	No drift	0
	Drift but maintains in air	1
	Unable to maintain in air	2
	No effort against gravity	3
	No movement	4
	Amputation, joint fusion (explain)	N/A
6b. Motor; leg—right (elevate extremity to 30 degrees and score drift/movement)	No drift	0
	Drift but maintains in air	1
	Unable to maintain in air	2
	No effort against gravity	3
	No movement	4
	Amputation, joint fusion (explain)	N/A
7. Limb ataxia (finger-to-nose and heel-to-shin testing)	Absent	0
	Present in one limb	1
	Present in two limbs	2
8. Sensory (pinprick to face, arm, trunk, and leg—compare side to side)	Normal	0
	Mild to moderate loss	1
	Severe to total loss	2
9. Best language (name items, describe a picture, and read sentences)	No aphasia	0
	Mild to moderate aphasia	1
	Severe aphasia	2
	Mute	3
10. Dysarthria (evaluate speech clarity by having patient repeat words)	Normal	0
	Mild to moderate dysarthria	1
	Severe dysarthria, mostly unintelligible or worse	2
	Intubated or other physical barrier	N/A
11. Extinction and inattention (use information from prior testing to score)	No abnormality	0
	Visual, tactile, auditory, or other extinction to bilateral simultaneous stimulation	1
	Profound hemiattention or extinction to more than one modality	2
Total score		___

LOC, level of consciousness; N/A, not applicable.

Adapted from the version available at the National Institute of Neurological Disorders and Stroke, National Institutes of Health, Bethesda, MD 20892. Retrieved on 4/23/17 at: www.ninds.nih.gov/sites/default/files/NIH_Stroke_Scale_Booklet.pdf. It is recommended that the full scale with all instructions be used.

administration, and the patient is closely monitored for any bleeding (IV insertion sites, urinary catheter site, endotracheal tube, nasogastric tube, urine, stool, emesis, other secretions). A 24-hour delay in placement of nasogastric tubes, urinary catheters, and intra-arterial pressure catheters is recommended. Intracranial bleeding is a major complication that occurred in approximately 6.4% of patients in the initial t-PA study (NINDS, 1995). A number of factors are associated with the occurrence of symptomatic intracranial bleeding: age greater than 70 years, baseline NIHSS score greater than 20, serum glucose concentration 300 mg/dL or higher, and edema or mass effect observed on the patient's initial CT scan (NINDS, 1995).

Therapy for Patients With Ischemic Stroke Not Receiving Tissue Plasminogen Activator

Not all patients are candidates for t-PA therapy. In some centers, other treatments may include anticoagulant administration (IV heparin or low–molecular-weight heparin). Because of the risks associated with anticoagulation, their general use is no longer recommended for patients with acute ischemic stroke (Jauch et al., 2013).

Careful maintenance of cerebral hemodynamics to maintain cerebral perfusion is extremely important after a stroke. Increased intracranial pressure (ICP) from brain edema and associated complications may occur after a large ischemic stroke. Interventions during this period include measures to reduce ICP, such as administering an osmotic diuretic (e.g., mannitol) to those that are declining clinically (Wijdicks, Sheth, Carter, et al., 2014). Other treatment measures include the following:

- Providing supplemental oxygen if oxygen saturation is below 95%
- Elevation of the head of the bed to 30 degrees to assist the patient in handling oral secretions and decrease ICP
- Possible hemicraniectomy for increased ICP from brain edema in a very large stroke
- Intubation with an endotracheal tube to establish a patent airway, if necessary
- Continuous hemodynamic monitoring (the goals for blood pressure remain controversial for a patient who has not received thrombolytic therapy; antihypertensive treatment may be withheld unless the systolic blood pressure exceeds 220 mm Hg or the diastolic blood pressure exceeds 120 mm Hg.)
- Frequent neurologic assessments to determine if the stroke is evolving and if other acute complications are developing (such complications may include seizures, bleeding from anticoagulation, or medication-induced bradycardia, which can result in hypotension and subsequent decreases in cardiac output and cerebral perfusion pressure).

Managing Potential Complications

Adequate cerebral blood flow is essential for cerebral oxygenation. If cerebral blood flow is inadequate, the amount of oxygen supplied to the brain will decrease, and tissue ischemia will result. Adequate oxygenation begins with pulmonary care, maintenance of a patent airway, and administration of supplemental oxygen as needed. The importance of adequate gas exchange in these patients cannot be

overemphasized, because many patients are at risk for aspiration pneumonia.

Other potential complications after a stroke include urinary tract infections, cardiac dysrhythmias (ventricular ectopy, tachycardia, and heart blocks), and complications of immobility. Hyperglycemia has been associated with poor neurologic outcomes in acute stroke, therefore blood glucose should be in the range of 140 to 180 mg/dL, and hypoglycemia should be avoided (Jauch et al., 2013).

Surgical Prevention of Ischemic Stroke

The main surgical procedure for selected patients with TIAs and mild stroke is CEA, which currently is the most frequently performed noncardiac vascular procedure. A CEA is the removal of an atherosclerotic plaque or thrombus from the carotid artery to prevent stroke in patients with occlusive disease of the extracranial cerebral arteries (see Fig. 67-2). This surgery is indicated for patients with symptoms of TIA or mild stroke (or those without symptoms) that are found to have severe (70% to 99%) carotid artery stenosis or moderate (50% to 69%) stenosis with other significant risk factors.

Carotid artery stenting (CAS), with or without angioplasty, is a less invasive procedure that is used for treatment of carotid stenosis. This procedure has less discomfort for the patient and a shorter recovery time than CEA. Age can be considered when deciding which procedure will be best for the patient. For older patients (older than 70 years), CEA demonstrated improved outcomes in research studies; for those who were younger, outcomes between CAS and CEA were similar when comparing procedure complications (Kernan et al., 2014).

Nursing Management

The main complications of CEA are stroke, cranial nerve injuries, infection or hematoma at the incision, and carotid artery disruption. It is important to maintain adequate blood

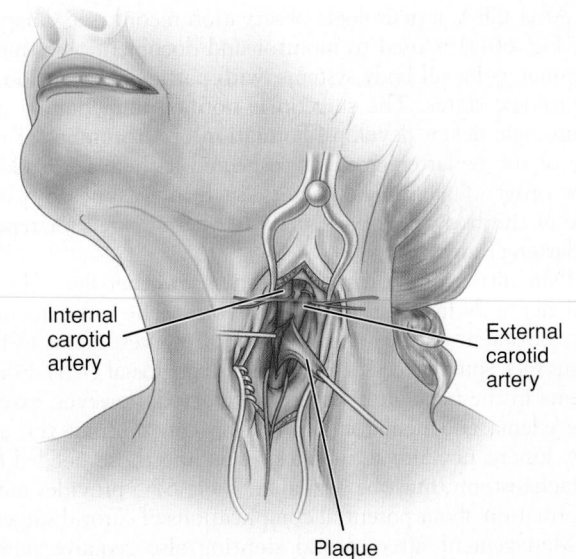

Internal carotid artery

External carotid artery

Plaque

Figure 67-2 • Plaque, a potential source of emboli in transient ischemic attack and stroke, is surgically removed from the carotid artery.

TABLE 67-5 Selected Complications of Carotid Endarterectomy (CEA) and Nursing Interventions

Complication	Characteristics	Nursing Interventions
Incision hematoma	Occurs in 5.5% of patients. Large or rapidly expanding hematomas require emergency treatment. If the airway is obstructed by the hematoma, the incision may be opened at the bedside.	Monitor neck discomfort and wound expansion. Report swelling, subjective feelings of pressure in the neck, difficulty breathing.
Hypertension	Poorly controlled hypertension increases the risk of postoperative complications, including hematoma and hyperperfusion syndrome. There is an increased incidence of neurologic impairment and death due to intracerebral hemorrhage. May be related to surgically induced abnormalities of carotid baroreceptor sensitivity.	Keep in mind that risk is highest in the first 48 hours after surgery. Check blood pressure frequently, and report deviations from baseline. Administer medications, as prescribed, to reduce hypertension. Observe for and report new onset of neurologic deficits.
Postoperative hypotension	Occurs in approximately 5% of patients. Treated with fluids and low-dose phenylephrine infusion. Usually resolves in 24–48 hours. Patients with hypotension should have serial electrocardiograms to rule out myocardial infarction.	Monitor blood pressure, and observe for signs and symptoms of hypotension.
Hyperperfusion syndrome	Occurs when cerebral vessel autoregulation fails. Arteries accustomed to diminished blood flow may be permanently dilated; increased blood flow after endarterectomy coupled with insufficient vasoconstriction leads to capillary bed damage, edema, and hemorrhage.	Observe for severe unilateral headache improved by sitting upright or standing.
Intracerebral hemorrhage	Occurs infrequently but is often fatal (60%) or results in serious neurologic impairment. Can occur secondary to hyperperfusion syndrome. Increased risk with advanced age, hypertension, presence of high-grade stenosis, poor collateral flow, and slow flow in the region of the middle cerebral artery.	Monitor neurologic status, and report any changes in mental status or neurologic functioning immediately.

pressure levels in the immediate postoperative period. Hypotension is avoided to prevent cerebral ischemia and thrombosis. Uncontrolled hypertension may precipitate cerebral hemorrhage, edema, hemorrhage at the surgical incision, or disruption of the arterial reconstruction. Medications are used to reduce the blood pressure to previous levels. Close cardiac monitoring is necessary, because these patients frequently have concomitant coronary artery disease.

After CEA, a neurologic observation record (see Chapter 66, Fig. 66-6) is used to monitor and document assessment parameters for all body systems, with particular attention to neurologic status. The surgeon is notified immediately if a neurologic deficit develops. Formation of a thrombus at the site of the endarterectomy is suspected if there is a sudden new onset of neurologic deficits, such as weakness on one side of the body. The patient should be prepared for repeat endarterectomy.

Difficulty in swallowing, hoarseness, or other signs of cranial nerve dysfunction must be assessed. The nurse focuses on assessment of the following cranial nerves: facial (VII), vagus (X), spinal accessory (XI), and hypoglossal (XII). Some edema in the neck after surgery is expected; however, extensive edema and hematoma formation can obstruct the airway. Emergency airway supplies, including those needed for a tracheostomy, must be available. Table 67-5 provides more information about potential complications of carotid surgery.

Management after carotid stenting also requires monitoring of neurologic status and evaluation for hematoma formation (at the catheterization site). Cardiac monitoring is necessary with assessment for bilateral pulses distal to the catheterization site. Typically, patients are discharged the day after stenting if there are no complications (Treat-Jacobson, Rich, DeVeaux, et al., 2013).

NURSING PROCESS

The Patient Recovering From an Ischemic Stroke

The acute phase of an ischemic stroke may last 1 to 3 days, but ongoing monitoring of all body systems is essential as long as the patient requires care. The patient who has had a stroke is at risk for multiple complications, including deconditioning and other musculoskeletal problems, swallowing difficulties, bowel and bladder dysfunction, inability to perform self-care, and skin breakdown. Nursing management focuses on the prompt initiation of rehabilitation for any deficits.

Assessment

During the acute phase, a neurologic flow sheet is maintained to provide data about the following important measures of the patient's clinical status:

- Change in level of consciousness or responsiveness as evidenced by movement, resistance to changes of position, and response to stimulation; orientation to time, place, and person
- Presence or absence of voluntary or involuntary movements of the extremities, muscle tone and strength, body posture, and position of the head

- Eye opening, comparative size of pupils and pupillary reactions to light, and ocular position
- Color of the face and extremities; temperature and moisture of the skin
- Quality and rates of pulse and respiration; arterial blood gas values as indicated, body temperature, and arterial pressure
- Ability to speak
- Volume of fluids ingested or given; volume of urine excreted each 24 hours
- Presence of bleeding
- Maintenance of blood pressure within the desired parameters
- Monitoring of continuous oxygen saturation

After the acute phase, the nurse assesses mental status (memory, attention span, perception, orientation, affect, speech/language), sensation/perception (the patient may have decreased awareness of pain and temperature), motor control (upper and lower extremity movement), swallowing ability, nutritional and hydration status, skin integrity, activity tolerance, and bowel and bladder function. Ongoing nursing assessment continues to focus on any impairment of function in the patient's daily activities, because the quality of life after stroke is closely related to the patient's functional status.

Diagnosis

NURSING DIAGNOSES

Based on the assessment data, major nursing diagnoses may include the following:

- Impaired physical mobility related to hemiparesis, loss of balance and coordination, spasticity, and brain injury
- Acute pain (painful shoulder) related to hemiplegia and disuse
- Self-care deficits (bathing, hygiene, toileting, dressing, and feeding) related to stroke sequelae
- Impaired comfort related to altered sensory reception, transmission, and/or integration
- Impaired swallowing
- Impaired urinary elimination related to flaccid bladder, detrusor instability, confusion, or difficulty in communicating
- Constipation related to change in mental status or difficulty communicating
- Acute confusion related to brain infarction
- Impaired verbal communication related to brain damage
- Risk for impaired skin integrity related to hemiparesis, hemiplegia, or decreased mobility
- Interrupted family processes related to catastrophic illness and caregiving burdens
- Sexual dysfunction related to neurologic deficits or fear of failure

COLLABORATIVE PROBLEMS/POTENTIAL COMPLICATIONS

Potential complications may include the following:

- Decreased cerebral blood flow due to increased ICP
- Inadequate oxygen delivery to the brain
- Pneumonia

Planning and Goals

Although rehabilitation begins on the day the patient has the stroke, the process is intensified during convalescence and requires a coordinated team effort. It is helpful for the team to know what the patient was like before the stroke: their illnesses, abilities, mental and emotional state, behavioral characteristics, and activities of daily living. It is also helpful for clinicians to be knowledgeable about the relative importance of predictors of stroke outcome (age, NIHSS score, and level of consciousness at the time of admission) in order to provide survivors of stroke and their families with realistic goals (Jauch et al., 2013).

The major goals for the patient (and family) may include improved mobility, avoidance of shoulder pain, achievement of self-care, relief of discomfort, prevention of aspiration, continence of bowel and bladder, decreasing confusion, achieving a form of communication, maintaining skin integrity, restored family functioning, improved sexual function, and absence of complications.

Nursing Interventions

Nursing care has a significant impact on the patient's recovery. Often, many body systems are impaired as a result of the stroke, and conscientious care and timely interventions can prevent debilitating complications. During and after the acute phase, nursing interventions focus on the whole person. In addition to providing physical care, the nurse encourages and fosters recovery by listening to the patient and asking questions to elicit the meaning of the stroke experience.

IMPROVING MOBILITY AND PREVENTING JOINT DEFORMITIES

A patient with hemiplegia has unilateral paralysis (paralysis on one side). When control of the voluntary muscles is lost, the strong flexor muscles exert control over the extensors. The arm tends to adduct (adductor muscles are stronger than abductors) and to rotate internally. The elbow and the wrist tend to flex, the affected leg tends to rotate externally at the hip joint and flex at the knee, and the foot at the ankle joint supinates and tends toward plantar flexion.

Correct positioning is important to prevent contractures; measures are used to relieve pressure, assist in maintaining good body alignment, and prevent compressive neuropathies, especially of the ulnar and peroneal nerves. Because flexor muscles are stronger than extensor muscles, a splint applied at night to the affected extremity may prevent flexion and maintain correct positioning during sleep (see Chapter 10).

Preventing Shoulder Adduction. To prevent adduction of the affected shoulder while the patient is in bed, a pillow is placed in the axilla when there is limited external rotation; this keeps the arm away from the chest. A pillow is placed under the arm, and the arm is placed in a neutral (slightly flexed) position, with distal joints positioned higher than the more proximal joints (i.e., the elbow is positioned higher than the shoulder and the wrist higher than the elbow). This helps to prevent edema and the resultant joint fibrosis that will limit range of motion if the patient regains control of the arm (see Fig. 67-3).

Positioning the Hand and Fingers. The fingers are positioned so that they are barely flexed. The hand is placed in slight supination (palm faces upward), which is its most functional position. If the upper extremity is flaccid, a splint can be used to support the wrist and hand in a functional position. If the upper extremity is spastic, a hand roll is not used, because

Figure 67-3 • Correct positioning to prevent shoulder adduction.

it stimulates the grasp reflex. In this instance, a dorsal wrist splint is useful in allowing the palm to be free of pressure. Every effort is made to prevent hand edema.

Spasticity, particularly in the hand, can be a disabling complication after stroke. Botulinum toxin type A injected intramuscularly into wrist and finger muscles has been shown to be effective in reducing this spasticity (although the effect is temporary, typically lasting 2 to 4 months) (Teasell, Foley, Pereira, et al., 2012). Other treatments for spasticity may include stretching, splinting, and oral medications such as baclofen (Lioresal), diazepam (Valium), dantrolene (Dantrium), and tizanidine (Zanaflex).

Changing Positions. The patient's position should be changed every 2 hours. To place a patient in a lateral (side-lying) position, a pillow is placed between the legs before the patient is turned. To promote venous return and prevent edema, the upper thigh should not be acutely flexed. The patient may be turned from side to side, but if sensation is impaired, the amount of time spent on the affected side should be limited.

If possible, the patient is placed in a prone position for 15 to 30 minutes several times a day. A small pillow or a support is placed under the pelvis, extending from the level of the umbilicus to the upper third of the thigh (see Fig. 67-4). This position helps promote hyperextension of the hip joints, which is essential for normal gait and helps prevent knee and hip flexion contractures. The prone position also helps drain bronchial secretions and prevents contractural deformities of the shoulders and knees. During positioning, it is important to reduce pressure and change position frequently to prevent pressure ulcers.

Establishing an Exercise Program. The affected extremities are exercised passively and put through a full range of motion four or five times a day to maintain joint mobility, regain motor control, prevent contractures in the paralyzed

Figure 67-4 • Prone position with pillow support helps prevent hip flexion.

extremity, prevent further deterioration of the neuromuscular system, and enhance circulation. Exercise is helpful in preventing venous stasis, which may predispose the patient to venous thromboembolism (VTE). VTE includes deep vein thrombosis (DVT) and pulmonary embolus (PE).

Repetition of an activity forms new pathways in the CNS and therefore encourages new patterns of motion. At first, the extremities are usually flaccid. If tightness occurs in any area, the range-of-motion exercises should be performed more frequently (see Chapter 10).

The patient is observed for signs and symptoms that may indicate PE or excessive cardiac workload during exercise; these include shortness of breath, chest pain, cyanosis, and increasing pulse rate with exercise. Frequent short periods of exercise always are preferable to longer periods at infrequent intervals. Regularity in exercise is most important. Improvement in muscle strength and maintenance of range of motion can be achieved only through daily exercise.

The patient is encouraged and reminded to exercise the unaffected side at intervals throughout the day. It is helpful to develop a written schedule to remind the patient of the exercise activities. The nurse supervises and supports the patient during these activities. The patient can be instructed to put the unaffected leg under the affected one to assist in moving it when turning and exercising. Flexibility, strengthening, coordination, endurance, and balancing exercises prepare the patient for ambulation. Quadriceps muscle setting and gluteal setting exercises (see Chapter 40, Chart 40-1) are started early to improve the muscle strength needed for walking; these are performed at least five times daily for 10 minutes at a time.

Preparing for Ambulation. As soon as possible, the patient is assisted out of bed and an active rehabilitation program is started. The patient is first educated to maintain balance while sitting and then to learn to balance while standing. If the patient has difficulty in achieving standing balance, a tilt table, which slowly brings the patient to an upright position, can be used. Tilt tables are especially helpful for patients who have been on bed rest for prolonged periods and have orthostatic blood pressure changes.

If the patient needs a wheelchair, the folding type with hand brakes is the most practical because it allows the patient to manipulate the chair. The chair should be low enough to allow the patient to propel it with the uninvolved foot and narrow enough to permit it to be used at home. When the patient is transferred from the wheelchair, the brakes must be applied and locked on both sides of the chair.

The patient is usually ready to walk as soon as standing balance is achieved. Parallel bars are useful in these first efforts. A chair or wheelchair should be readily available in case the patient suddenly becomes fatigued or feels dizzy.

The training periods for ambulation should be short and frequent. As the patient gains strength and confidence, an adjustable cane can be used for support. In general, a three- or four-pronged cane provides a stable support in the early phases of rehabilitation.

PREVENTING SHOULDER PAIN

The incidence of shoulder pain after stroke can vary widely, but has been measured to be as high as 84% (Zheng & Alexander, 2015). That pain may prevent patients from learning new skills and affect their quality of life. Shoulder function is essential in achieving balance and performing transfers and self-care activities. Problems that can occur include rotator cuff disorders, spasticity of the shoulder muscles, painful shoulder, subluxation of the shoulder, and shoulder–hand syndrome. Development of a condition known as central pain syndrome may also contribute to the development of shoulder pain after a stroke.

A flaccid shoulder joint may be overstretched by the use of excessive force in turning the patient or from overstrenuous arm and shoulder movement. To prevent shoulder pain, the nurse should never lift the patient by the flaccid shoulder or pull on the affected arm or shoulder. Overhead pulleys should also be avoided. If the arm is paralyzed, subluxation (incomplete dislocation) at the shoulder can occur as a result of overstretching of the joint capsule and musculature by the force of gravity when the patient sits or stands in the early stages after a stroke. This results in severe pain. Shoulder–hand syndrome (painful shoulder and generalized swelling of the hand) can cause a frozen shoulder and ultimately atrophy of subcutaneous tissues. When a shoulder becomes stiff, it is usually painful.

Many shoulder problems can be prevented by proper patient movement and positioning. The flaccid arm is positioned on a table or with pillows while the patient is seated. Some clinicians advocate the use of a properly worn sling when the patient first becomes ambulatory, to prevent the paralyzed upper extremity from dangling without support. Range-of-motion exercises are important in preventing painful shoulder. Overstrenuous arm movements are avoided. The patient is instructed to interlace the fingers, place the palms together, and push the clasped hands slowly forward to bring the scapulae forward; he or she then raises both hands above the head. This is repeated throughout the day. The patient is instructed to flex the affected wrist at intervals and move all the joints of the affected fingers. The patient is encouraged to touch, stroke, rub, and look at both hands. Pushing the heel of the hand firmly down on a surface is useful. Elevation of the arm and hand is also important in preventing dependent edema of the hand. Patients with continuing pain after attempted movement and positioning may require the addition of analgesia to their treatment program. Other treatments may include injections to the shoulder joint with corticosteroid medications or botulinum toxin type A, shoulder strapping, acupuncture, electrical stimulation, heat or ice, and soft tissue massage (Zheng & Alexander, 2015).

Medications are often helpful in the management of poststroke pain. The medications that are used include: amitriptyline (Elavil), gabapentin (Neurontin), lamotrigine (Lamictal), and pregabalin (Lyrica) (Flaster, Meresh, Rao, et al., 2013).

ENHANCING SELF-CARE

As soon as the patient can sit up, he or she is encouraged to participate in personal hygiene activities. The patient is helped to set realistic goals; if feasible, a new task is added daily. The first step is to carry out all self-care activities on the unaffected side. Such activities as combing the hair, brushing the teeth, shaving with an electric razor, bathing, and eating can be carried out with one hand and should be encouraged. Although the patient may feel awkward at first, these motor skills can be learned by repetition, and the unaffected

---

Chart 67-4 — Assistive Devices to Enhance Self-Care After Stroke

Bathing and Grooming Devices

- Electric razors with head at 90 degrees to handle
- Grab bars, nonskid mats, handheld shower heads
- Long-handled bath sponge
- Shower and tub seats, stationary or on wheels

Dressing Aids

- Elastic shoelaces
- Long-handled shoehorn
- Velcro closures

Eating Devices

- Nonskid mats to stabilize plates
- Plate guards to prevent food from being pushed off plate
- Wide-grip utensils to accommodate a weak grasp

Mobility Aids

- Canes, walkers, wheelchairs
- Transfer devices such as transfer boards and belts

Toileting Aids

- Grab bars next to toilet
- Raised toilet seat

---

side will become stronger with use. The nurse must be sure that the patient does not neglect the affected side. Assistive devices will help make up for some of the patient's deficits (see Chart 67-4). A small towel is easier to control while drying after bathing, and boxed paper tissues are easier to use than a roll of toilet tissue.

Return of functional ability is important to the patient recovering after a stroke. An early baseline assessment of functional ability with an instrument such as the Functional Independence Measure (FIM™) is important in team planning and goal setting for the patient. The FIM™ is a widely used instrument in stroke rehabilitation and provides valuable information about motor, social, and cognitive function. The patient's morale may improve if ambulatory activities are carried out in street clothes. The family is instructed to bring in clothing that is preferably a size larger than that usually worn. Clothing fitted with front or side fasteners or Velcro closures is the most suitable. The patient has better balance if most of the dressing activities are carried out while seated.

Perceptual problems may make it difficult for the patient to dress without assistance because of an inability to match the clothing to the body parts. To assist the patient, the nurse can take steps to keep the environment organized and uncluttered, because the patient with a perceptual problem is easily distracted. The clothing is placed on the affected side in the order in which the garments are to be put on. The use of a large mirror while dressing promotes the patient's awareness of what he or she is putting on the affected side. The patient has to make many compensatory movements when dressing; these can produce fatigue and painful twisting of the intercostal muscles. Support and encouragement are provided to prevent the patient from becoming overly fatigued and discouraged. Even with intensive training, not all patients can achieve independence in dressing.

ADJUSTING TO PHYSICAL CHANGES

Patients with a decreased field of vision should be approached on the side where visual perception is intact. All visual stimuli (e.g., clock, calendar, television) should be placed on this side. The patient can be educated to turn the head in the direction of the defective visual field to compensate for this loss. The nurse should make eye contact with the patient and draw their attention to the affected side by encouraging the patient to move the head. The nurse may also want to stand at a position that encourages the patient to move or turn to visualize who is in the room. Increasing the natural or artificial lighting in the room and providing eyeglasses are important aids to increasing vision.

The patient with homonymous hemianopsia turns away from the affected side of the body and tends to neglect that side and the space on that side; this is known as amorphosynthesis. In such instances, the patient cannot see food on half of the tray, and only half of the room is visible. It is important for the nurse to constantly remind the patient of the other side of the body; to maintain alignment of the extremities; and, if possible, to place the extremities where the patient can see them.

ASSISTING WITH NUTRITION

Stroke can result in **dysphagia** (difficulty swallowing) due to impaired function of the mouth, tongue, palate, larynx, pharynx, or upper esophagus. Patients must be observed for paroxysms of coughing, food dribbling out of or pooling in one side of the mouth, food retained for long periods in the mouth, or nasal regurgitation when swallowing liquids. Swallowing difficulties place the patient at risk for aspiration, pneumonia, dehydration, and malnutrition.

A swallow assessment should be performed as soon as possible after the patient's arrival to the ED (preferably within 4 to 24 hours). This is done before allowing any oral intake. A speech therapist will evaluate the patient's swallowing ability, but an assessment may also be done by the nurse using a validated and reliable assessment tool (Middleton et al., 2015).

If swallowing function is partially impaired, it may return over time, or the patient may be educated in alternative swallowing techniques, advised to take smaller boluses of food, and educated about types of foods that are easier to swallow. The patient may be started on a thick liquid or pureed diet, because these foods are easier to swallow than thin liquids. Having the patient sit upright, preferably out of bed in a chair, and instructing him or her to tuck the chin toward the chest as he or she swallows will help prevent aspiration. The diet may be advanced as the patient becomes more proficient at swallowing. If the patient cannot resume oral intake, a gastrointestinal feeding tube is placed for ongoing tube feedings and medication administration.

Enteral tubes can be either nasogastric (placed in the stomach) or nasoenteral (placed in the duodenum) to reduce the risk of aspiration. Nursing responsibilities in feeding include elevating the head of the bed at least 30 degrees to prevent aspiration, checking the position of the tube before feeding, ensuring that the cuff of the tracheostomy tube (if in place) is inflated, and giving the tube feeding slowly. The feeding tube is aspirated periodically to ensure that the feedings are passing through the gastrointestinal tract. Retained or residual feedings increase the risk of aspiration. Patients with retained feedings may benefit from the placement of a gastrostomy tube or a percutaneous endoscopic gastrostomy tube. In a patient with a feeding tube, the tube should be placed in the duodenum to reduce the risk of aspiration. For long-term feedings, a gastrostomy tube is preferred (see Chapter 44).

ATTAINING BLADDER AND BOWEL CONTROL

After a stroke, the patient may have transient urinary incontinence due to confusion, inability to communicate needs, and inability to use the urinal or bedpan because of impaired motor and postural control. Occasionally after a stroke, the bladder becomes atonic, with impaired sensation in response to bladder filling. Sometimes, control of the external urinary sphincter is lost or diminished. During this period, intermittent catheterization with sterile technique is carried out. After muscle tone increases and deep tendon reflexes return, bladder tone increases and spasticity of the bladder may develop. Because the patient's sense of awareness is clouded, persistent urinary incontinence or urinary retention may be symptomatic of bilateral brain damage. The voiding pattern is analyzed, and the urinal or bedpan is offered on this pattern or schedule. The upright posture and standing position are helpful for male patients during this aspect of rehabilitation.

Patients may have problems with bowel control, particularly constipation. Unless contraindicated, a high-fiber diet and adequate fluid intake (2 to 3 L/day) should be provided, and a regular time (usually after breakfast) should be established for toileting (see Chapter 10).

IMPROVING THOUGHT PROCESSES

After a stroke, the patient may have problems with cognitive, behavioral, and emotional deficits related to brain damage. However, in many instances, a considerable degree of function can be recovered, because not all areas of the brain are equally damaged; some remain more intact and functional than others.

After assessment that delineates the patient's deficits, the neuropsychologist, in collaboration with the primary provider, psychiatrist, nurse, and other professionals, structures a training program using cognitive-perceptual retraining, visual imagery, reality orientation, and cueing procedures to compensate for losses.

The role of the nurse is supportive. The nurse reviews the results of neuropsychological testing; observes the patient's performance and progress; gives positive feedback; and, most importantly, conveys an attitude of confidence and hope. Interventions capitalize on the patient's strengths and remaining abilities while attempting to improve performance of affected functions. Other interventions are similar to those for improving cognitive functioning after a head injury (see Chapter 68).

IMPROVING COMMUNICATION

Aphasia, which impairs the patient's ability to express him- or herself and to understand what is being said, may become apparent in various ways. The cortical area that is responsible for integrating the myriad pathways required for the comprehension and formulation of language is called *Broca area*. It is located in a convolution adjoining the middle cerebral artery. This area is responsible for control of the combinations of muscular movements needed to speak each word. Broca area is so close to the left motor area that a disturbance in the motor area often affects the speech area. This is why so many patients who are paralyzed on the right side (due to damage or injury to the left side of the brain) cannot speak, whereas those paralyzed on the left side are less likely to have speech disturbances.

The speech therapist assesses the communication needs of the patient who has had a stroke, describes the precise deficit, and suggests the best overall method of communication. Most language intervention strategies can be tailored for the individual patient. The patient is expected to take an active part in establishing goals.

A person with aphasia may become depressed. The inability to talk on the telephone, answer a question, or participate in conversation often causes anger, frustration, fear of the future, and hopelessness. Nursing interventions include strategies to make the atmosphere conducive to communication. This includes being sensitive to the patient's reactions and needs and responding to them in an appropriate manner while always treating the patient as an adult. The nurse provides strong emotional support and understanding to allay anxiety and frustration.

A common pitfall is for the nurse or other health care team member to complete the thoughts or sentences of the patient. This should be avoided, because it causes the patient to become more frustrated at not being allowed to speak and may deter efforts to practice putting thoughts together and completing sentences. A consistent schedule, routines, and repetition help the patient to function despite significant deficits. A written copy of the daily schedule, a folder of personal information (birth date, address, names of relatives), checklists, and an audiotaped list help improve the patient's memory and concentration. The patient may also benefit from a communication board, which has pictures of common needs and phrases. The board may be translated into any language.

When talking with the patient, it is important for the nurse to gain the patient's attention, speak slowly, and keep the language of instruction consistent. One instruction is given at a time, and time is allowed for the patient to process what has been said. The use of gestures may enhance comprehension. Speaking is thinking out loud, and the emphasis is on thinking. Listening and sorting out incoming messages requires mental effort; the patient must struggle against mental inertia and needs time to organize a response.

In working with the patient with aphasia, the nurse must remember to talk to the patient during care activities. This provides social contact for the patient. Chart 67-5 describes points to keep in mind when communicating with the patient with aphasia.

MAINTAINING SKIN INTEGRITY

The patient who has had a stroke may be at risk for skin and tissue breakdown because of altered sensation and inability to respond to pressure and discomfort by turning and moving. Preventing skin and tissue breakdown requires frequent assessment of the skin, with emphasis on bony areas and dependent parts of the body. During the acute phase, a specialty bed (e.g., low air-loss bed) may be used until the patient can move independently or assist in moving.

Chart 67-5

Communicating With the Patient With Aphasia

- Face the patient and establish eye contact.
- Speak in a clear, unhurried manner, and normal tone of voice.
- Use short phrases, and pause between phrases to allow the patient time to understand what is being said.
- Limit conversation to practical and concrete matters.
- Use gestures, pictures, objects, and writing.
- As the patient uses and handles an object, say what the object is. It helps to match the words with the object or action.
- Be consistent in using the same words and gestures each time you give instructions or ask a question.
- Keep extraneous noises and sounds to a minimum. Too much background noise can distract the patient or make it difficult to sort out the message being spoken.

A regular turning schedule (e.g., every 2 hours) is adhered to, even if pressure-relieving devices are used to prevent tissue and skin breakdown. When the patient is positioned or turned, care must be used to minimize shear and friction forces, which cause damage to tissues and predispose the skin to breakdown.

The patient's skin must be kept clean and dry; gentle massage of healthy (nonreddened) skin and adequate nutrition are other factors that help to maintain skin and tissue integrity (see Chapter 10).

IMPROVING FAMILY COPING

Family members play an important role in the patient's recovery. Family members are encouraged to participate in counseling and to use support systems that will help with the emotional and physical stress of caring for the patient. Involving others in the patient's care and providing education about stress management techniques and methods for maintaining personal health also facilitate family coping.

The family may have difficulty accepting the patient's disability and may be unrealistic in their expectations. They are given information about the expected outcomes and are counseled to avoid doing activities for the patient that he or she can do. They are assured that their love and interest are part of the patient's therapy.

The family needs to be informed that the rehabilitation of the patient with hemiplegia requires many months and that progress may be slow. The gains made by the patient in the hospital or rehabilitation unit must be maintained. All caregivers should approach the patient with a supportive and optimistic attitude, focusing on the patient's remaining abilities. The rehabilitation team, the medical and nursing team, the patient, and the family must all be involved in developing attainable goals for the patient at home.

Most relatives of patients with stroke handle the physical changes better than the emotional aspects of care. The family should be prepared to expect occasional episodes of emotional lability. The patient may laugh or cry easily and may be irritable and demanding or depressed and confused. The nurse can explain to the family that the patient's laughter does not necessarily connote happiness, nor does crying reflect sadness, and that emotional lability usually improves with time.

Family-centered care involves seeing patients and family caregivers as a one unit. Nurses can assess caregivers' strengths and ability to provide care. This assessment should be a continual process because needs change throughout the hospitalization period and rehabilitation stay. Providing information about community resources, respite care and adult day care, and mental health issues (for the patient who has had a stroke and for caregivers) will help with the transition to home (Creasy, Lutz, Young, et al., 2015).

HELPING THE PATIENT COPE WITH SEXUAL DYSFUNCTION

Sexual functioning can be profoundly altered by stroke. Although research in this area of stroke management is limited, it appears that patients who have had a stroke consider sexual function important, and many have sexual dysfunction. Sexual dysfunction after stroke is multifactorial. There may be medical reasons for the dysfunction (neurologic and cognitive deficits, previous diseases, medications) as well as various psychosocial factors, including depression. A stroke is such a catastrophic illness that the patient experiences loss of self-esteem and value as a sexual being. These psychosocial factors play an important role in determining sexual drive, activity, and satisfaction after a stroke.

Nurses in the rehabilitation setting play a crucial role in beginning a dialogue between the patient and their partner about sexuality after a stroke. In-depth assessments to determine sexual history before and after the stroke should be followed by appropriate interventions. Interventions for the patient and partner focus on providing relevant information, education, reassurance, adjustment of medications, counseling regarding coping skills, suggestions for alternative sexual positions, and a means of sexual expression and satisfaction.

MONITORING AND MANAGING POTENTIAL COMPLICATIONS

Decreased cerebral blood flow due to increased ICP, leading to inadequate oxygen delivery to the brain, and pneumonia are potential complications in any patient who has had an ischemic stroke. The more severe the stroke (i.e., the higher the NIHSS), the greater the risk of complications.

During the acute phase of care, a neurologic flow sheet (see Chapter 66, Fig. 66-6) is used to monitor and document assessment parameters. Changes in blood pressure, pulse, and respiration are important clinically because they suggest increased ICP and are reported immediately. If signs and symptoms of pneumonia develop, cultures are obtained to identify the organism so that appropriate antibiotic agents can be given.

PROMOTING HOME, COMMUNITY-BASED, AND TRANSITIONAL CARE

Educating Patients About Self-Care. Patient and family education is a fundamental component of stroke recovery. The nurse provides education about stroke, its causes and prevention, and the rehabilitation process. In both acute care and rehabilitation facilities, the focus is on educating the patient to resume as much self-care as possible. This may entail using assistive devices or modifying the home environment to help the patient live with a disability.

An occupational therapist may be helpful in assessing the home environment and recommending modifications to help the patient become more independent. For example, a shower is more convenient than a tub for the patient with hemiplegia because most patients do not gain sufficient strength to get up and down from a tub. Sitting on a stool of medium height with rubber suction tips allows the patient to wash with greater ease. A long-handled bath brush with a soap container is helpful to the patient who has only one functional hand. If a shower is not available, a stool may be placed in the tub and a portable shower hose attached to the faucet. Handrails may be attached alongside the bathtub and the toilet. Other assistive devices include special utensils for eating, grooming, dressing, and writing (see Chart 67-4).

A program of physical therapy can be beneficial, whether it takes place in the home or in an outpatient program. Constraint-induced movement therapy has been used in stroke rehabilitation and involves constraint of the less affected upper limb with a mitt, and intensely training the more affected limb. Robotic-assisted therapy uses sensorimotor training of the upper limb. This method allows patients to train without the presence of a therapist. Recent research has focused on techniques using robotics, virtual reality and video game applications, transcranial magnetic stimulation, and ambulation with body weight support and treadmill training (Brainin & Zorowitz, 2013).

Continuing and Transitional Care. A variety of transitional care models are being used in patients with stroke (Puhr & Thompson, 2015). Some evidence supports positive outcomes using transitional care but more research and standardization of interventions is needed for confirmation (Puhr & Thompson, 2015). Depending on the specific neurologic deficits resulting from the stroke, the patient at home may require the services of a number of health care professionals. The nurse often coordinates the care of the patient at home and considers the many educational needs of caregivers and patients. The family (often the spouse) requires education as well as assistance in planning and providing care.

The family is advised that the patient may tire easily, may become irritable and upset by small events, and may be less interested in events than expected. Emotional problems associated with stroke are often related to speech dysfunction and the frustrations of being unable to communicate. A speech therapist allows the family to be involved and gives the family practical instructions to help the patient between therapy sessions.

Depression is a common and serious problem in the patient who has had a stroke. The incidence of depression in patients who have had a stroke ranges from 25% to 79%. Risk factors include social isolation, gender (more prevalent in women), a history of depression, and cognitive or physical impairment (Miller, Murray, Richards, et al., 2010). Because the length of hospital stays has shortened, depression may not be identified in the acute setting. Nurses in all care settings should identify patients who may be at risk for depression or who show depressive symptoms (Miller et al., 2010). In the home or in the rehabilitation setting, nurses may be involved in coordinating care and referring patients and family to appropriate resources. The family can help by continuing to support the patient and by giving positive reinforcement for the progress that is being made. Antidepressant therapy may be prescribed, and may help with recovery from stroke (Flaster, Sharma, & Rao, 2013).

Community-based stroke support groups may allow the patient and family to learn from others with similar problems and to share their experiences. Support groups take the form of in-person meetings as well as Internet-based support programs. The patient is encouraged to continue hobbies and recreational and leisure interests and to maintain contact with friends to prevent social isolation. All nurses coming in contact with the patient should encourage the patient to keep active, adhere to the exercise program, and remain as self-sufficient as possible.

The nurse should recognize the potential effects of caregiving on the family. Not all families have the adaptive coping skills and adequate psychological functioning necessary for the long-term care of another person. The patient's spouse may be older, with their own health concerns; in some instances, the patient may have been the provider of care to the spouse. A spouse may have to take on new roles and responsibilities in the relationship and around the home. He or she may also feel a sense of loss (of freedom and leisure time as well as of the marital relationship). Caregivers may also experience social isolation and financial burdens. Depression is common in caregivers of patients who have survived a stroke, with rates as high as 30% to 52% (Miller et al., 2010). Nurses should assess caregivers for signs of depression.

Caregivers may require reminders to attend to their own health concerns and well-being. Even healthy caregivers may find it difficult to maintain a schedule that includes being available around the clock. The nurse encourages the family to arrange for respite care services (planned short-term care to relieve the family from having to provide continuous 24-hour care), which may be available from an adult day care center. Some hospitals also offer weekend respite care that can provide caregivers with needed time for themselves. The nurse involved in home and continuing care also needs to remind the patient and family of the need for respite care as well as continuing health promotion and screening practices.

Evaluation

Expected patient outcomes may include:

1. Achieves improved mobility
   a. Avoids deformities (contractures and foot drop)
   b. Participates in prescribed exercise program
   c. Achieves sitting balance
   d. Uses unaffected side to compensate for loss of function of hemiplegic side
2. Reports absence of shoulder pain
   a. Demonstrates shoulder mobility; exercises shoulder
   b. Elevates arm and hand at intervals
3. Achieves self-care; performs hygiene care; uses adaptive equipment
4. Demonstrates techniques to compensate for the discomfort of sensory deficits, such as turning the head to see people or objects
5. Demonstrates safe swallowing
6. Achieves usual pattern of bowel and bladder elimination
7. Participates in cognitive improvement program
8. Demonstrates improved communication
9. Maintains intact skin without breakdown
   a. Demonstrates skin turgor within normal limits
   b. Participates in turning and positioning activities
10. Family members demonstrate a positive attitude and coping mechanisms
    a. Encourage patient in exercise program
    b. Take an active part in rehabilitation process
    c. Contact respite care programs or arrange for other family members to assume some responsibilities for care
11. Develops alternative approaches to sexual expression
12. Absence of complications
    a. Has ICP values that remain within normal limits
    b. Has no signs and symptoms of pneumonia

 Hemorrhagic Stroke

Hemorrhage accounts for approximately 13% of strokes and are primarily caused by intracranial (7%), subarachnoid hemorrhage (8%), and other causes. Hemorrhagic strokes are caused by bleeding into the brain tissue, the ventricles, or the subarachnoid space. Primary intracerebral hemorrhage from a spontaneous rupture of small vessels accounts for approximately 80% of hemorrhagic strokes and is caused chiefly by uncontrolled hypertension. Subarachnoid hemorrhage results from a ruptured intracranial aneurysm (discussed later in this chapter) in about half the cases (Hickey, 2014).

Another common cause of primary intracerebral hemorrhage in the older adult is cerebral amyloid angiopathy (CAA), which involves damage caused by the deposit of beta-amyloid protein in the small- and medium-sized blood vessels of the brain. CAA makes these blood vessels fragile and prone to bleeding. Secondary intracerebral hemorrhage is associated with arteriovenous malformations (AVMs), intracranial aneurysms, intracranial neoplasms, or certain medications (e.g., anticoagulants, amphetamines). The mortality rate has been reported to be as high as 50% after an intracranial hemorrhage (Hickey, 2014). Patients who survive the acute phase of care usually have more severe deficits and a longer recovery phase compared to those with ischemic stroke.

Pathophysiology

The pathophysiology of hemorrhagic stroke depends on the cause and type of cerebrovascular disorder. Symptoms are produced when a primary hemorrhage, aneurysm, or AVM presses on nearby cranial nerves or brain tissue or, more dramatically, when an aneurysm or AVM ruptures, causing subarachnoid hemorrhage (hemorrhage into the cranial subarachnoid space). Normal brain metabolism is disrupted by the brain's exposure to blood; by an increase in ICP resulting from the sudden entry of blood into the subarachnoid space, which compresses and injures brain tissue; or by secondary ischemia of the brain resulting from the reduced perfusion pressure and vasospasm that frequently accompany subarachnoid hemorrhage.

Intracerebral Hemorrhage

An intracerebral hemorrhage, or bleeding into the brain tissue, is most common in patients with hypertension and cerebral atherosclerosis, because degenerative changes from these diseases cause rupture of the blood vessel. An intracerebral hemorrhage may also result from certain types of arterial pathology, brain tumors, and the use of medications (e.g., oral anticoagulants, amphetamines, and illicit drug use).

Bleeding related to hypertension occurs most commonly in the deeper structures of the brain (basal ganglia and thalamus); it occurs less frequently in the brainstem (mostly the pons) and cerebellum (Hickey, 2014). Bleeding in the outer cerebral lobes (lobar hemorrhages) in those 75 or older can be related to CAA. Bleeding from CAA frequently is in the frontal and parietal lobes. Occasionally, the bleeding ruptures the wall of the lateral ventricle and causes intraventricular hemorrhage, which is associated with poor outcomes and death (Hickey, 2014).

Intracranial (Cerebral) Aneurysm

An intracranial (cerebral) **aneurysm** is a dilation of the walls of a cerebral artery that develops as a result of weakness in the arterial wall. The cause of aneurysms is unknown, although research is ongoing. An aneurysm may be due to atherosclerosis, which results in a defect in the vessel wall with subsequent weakness of the wall; a congenital defect of the vessel wall; hypertensive vascular disease; head trauma; or advancing age.

Any artery within the brain can be the site of a cerebral aneurysm, but these lesions usually occur at the bifurcations of the large arteries at the circle of Willis (see Fig. 67-5). The cerebral arteries most commonly affected by an aneurysm are the internal carotid artery, anterior cerebral artery, anterior communicating artery, posterior communicating artery, posterior cerebral artery, and middle cerebral artery. Multiple cerebral aneurysms are not uncommon.

Arteriovenous Malformations

Most AVMs are caused by an abnormality in embryonal development that leads to a tangle of arteries and veins in the brain that lacks a capillary bed (see Fig. 67-5). The absence of a capillary bed leads to dilation of the arteries and veins and

eventual rupture. AVM is a common cause of hemorrhagic stroke in young people (Bader, Littlejohns, & Olson, 2016).

Subarachnoid Hemorrhage

A subarachnoid hemorrhage (hemorrhage into the subarachnoid space) may occur as a result of an AVM, intracranial aneurysm, trauma, or hypertension. The most common causes are a leaking aneurysm in the area of the circle of Willis and a congenital AVM of the brain (Bader et al., 2016).

Clinical Manifestations

The patient with a hemorrhagic stroke can present with a wide variety of neurologic deficits, similar to the patient with ischemic stroke. The conscious patient most commonly reports a severe headache. A comprehensive assessment reveals the extent of the neurologic deficits. Many of the same motor, sensory, cranial nerve, cognitive, and other functions that are disrupted after ischemic stroke are also altered after a hemorrhagic stroke. Table 67-2 reviews the neurologic deficits frequently seen in patients who have had a stroke. Table 67-3 compares the symptoms seen in right hemispheric stroke with those seen in left hemispheric stroke. Other symptoms that may be observed more frequently in patients with acute intracerebral hemorrhage (compared with ischemic stroke) are nausea or vomiting, an early sudden change in level of consciousness, and possibly seizures.

In addition to the neurologic deficits (similar to those of ischemic stroke), the patient with an intracranial aneurysm or AVM may have some unique clinical manifestations. Rupture of an aneurysm or AVM usually produces a sudden, unusually severe headache and often loss of consciousness for a variable period of time. There may be pain and rigidity of the back of the neck (nuchal rigidity) and spine due to meningeal irritation. Visual disturbances (visual loss, diplopia, ptosis) occur if the aneurysm is adjacent to the oculomotor nerve. Tinnitus, dizziness, and hemiparesis may also occur.

At times, an aneurysm or AVM leaks blood, leading to the formation of a clot that seals the site of rupture. In this instance, the patient may show little neurologic deficit. In other cases, severe bleeding occurs, resulting in cerebral damage, followed rapidly by coma and death.

Prognosis depends on the neurologic condition of the patient, the patient's age, associated diseases, and the extent and location of the hemorrhage or intracranial aneurysm. Subarachnoid hemorrhage from an aneurysm is a catastrophic event with significant morbidity and mortality.

Assessment and Diagnostic Findings

Any patient with suspected stroke should undergo a CT scan or MRI scan to determine the type of stroke, the size and location of the hematoma, and the presence or absence of ventricular blood and hydrocephalus. Because hemorrhagic stroke is an emergency, CT scan is usually obtained first because it can be done rapidly. Cerebral angiography using the conventional method or CT (CTA) confirms the diagnosis of an intracranial aneurysm or AVM. These tests show the location and size of the lesion and provide information about the affected arteries, veins, adjoining vessels, and vascular branches. Lumbar puncture may be performed if there is no evidence of increased ICP, the CT scan results

Figure 67-5 • Common sites of intracranial aneurysms and an arteriovenous malformation.

are negative, and subarachnoid hemorrhage must be confirmed. Lumbar puncture in the presence of increased ICP could result in brainstem herniation or rebleeding. When diagnosing a hemorrhagic stroke in a patient younger than 40 years, some clinicians obtain a toxicology screen for illicit drug use.

Prevention

Primary prevention of hemorrhagic stroke is the best approach and includes managing hypertension and ameliorating other significant risk factors. Control of hypertension can reduce the risk of hemorrhagic stroke. Additional risk factors are increased age, male gender, certain ethnicities (Latino, African American, and Japanese) and moderate or excessive alcohol intake (Hickey, 2014). Stroke risk screenings provide an ideal opportunity to lower hemorrhagic stroke risk by identifying individuals or groups at high risk and educating patients and the community about recognition and prevention.

Complications

Potential complications of hemorrhagic stroke include rebleeding or hematoma expansion; cerebral vasospasm resulting in cerebral ischemia; acute hydrocephalus, which results when free blood obstructs the reabsorption of cerebrospinal fluid (CSF) by the arachnoid villi; and seizures.

Cerebral Hypoxia and Decreased Blood Flow

Immediate complications of a hemorrhagic stroke include cerebral hypoxia, decreased cerebral blood flow, and extension of the area of injury. Providing adequate oxygenation of blood to the brain minimizes cerebral hypoxia. Brain function depends on delivery of oxygen to the tissues. Administering supplemental oxygen and maintaining the hemoglobin and hematocrit at acceptable levels will assist in maintaining tissue oxygenation.

Cerebral blood flow depends on the blood pressure, cardiac output, and integrity of cerebral blood vessels. Adequate hydration (IV fluids) must be ensured to reduce blood viscosity and improve cerebral blood flow. Extremes of hypertension or hypotension need to be avoided to prevent changes in cerebral blood flow and the potential for extending the area of injury.

A seizure can also compromise cerebral blood flow, resulting in further injury to the brain. Observing for seizure activity and initiating appropriate treatment are important components of care after a hemorrhagic stroke.

Vasospasm

The development of cerebral vasospasm (narrowing of the lumen of the involved cranial blood vessel) is a serious complication of subarachnoid hemorrhage and is a leading cause of morbidity and mortality in those who survive the initial subarachnoid hemorrhage. Of those with cerebral vasospasm, 15% to 20% die (Wuchner, Bakas, Adams, et al., 2012). The mechanism responsible for vasospasm is not clear, but it is associated with increasing amounts of blood in the subarachnoid cisterns and cerebral fissures, as visualized by CT scan. Monitoring for vasospasm may be performed through the use of bedside transcranial Doppler ultrasonography or follow-up cerebral angiography (Connolly, Rabinstein, Carhuapoma, et al., 2012).

Vasospasm most frequently occurs 7 to 10 days after initial hemorrhage (Connolly et al., 2012), when the clot undergoes lysis (dissolution), and the chance of rebleeding is increased. It leads to increased vascular resistance, which impedes cerebral blood flow and causes brain ischemia (delayed cerebral ischemia) and infarction. The signs and symptoms reflect the areas of the brain involved. Vasospasm is often heralded by a worsening headache, a decrease in level of consciousness (confusion, lethargy, and disorientation), or a new focal neurologic deficit (aphasia, hemiparesis).

Management of vasospasm remains difficult and controversial. It is believed that early surgery to clip the aneurysm prevents rebleeding and that removal of blood from the basal cisterns around the major cerebral arteries may prevent vasospasm.

Medication may be effective in the treatment and prevention of vasospasm. Based on the theory that vasospasm is caused by an increased influx of calcium into the cell, medication therapy may be used either to block or antagonize this action, or to prevent or reverse the action of vasospasm if already present. Nimodipine is the most studied calcium channel blocker for prevention of vasospasm in subarachnoid hemorrhage. An oral solution of nimodipine (Nymalize) was approved by the FDA in 2013; prior to this approval, the medication was only available in a liquid filled gel capsule (Nimotop). Current guidelines recommend that nimodipine be prescribed for all patients with subarachnoid hemorrhage (Connolly et al., 2012). This is currently the only drug approved by the FDA for the prevention and treatment of vasospasm in subarachnoid hemorrhage.

Another therapy for vasospasm and the resulting delayed cerebral ischemia, referred to as triple-H therapy, is aimed at minimizing the deleterious effects of the associated cerebral ischemia and includes (1) fluid volume expanders (hypervolemia), (2) induced arterial hypertension, and (3) hemodilution. However, current research and guidelines now endorse euvolemia to prevent delayed cerebral ischemia and induced arterial hypertension for treatment of delayed cerebral ischemia (Connolly et al., 2012).

Increased Intracranial Pressure

An increase in ICP can occur after either an ischemic or a hemorrhagic stroke but almost always follows a subarachnoid hemorrhage, usually because of disturbed circulation of CSF caused by blood in the basal cisterns. Neurologic assessments are performed frequently, and if there is evidence of deterioration from increased ICP (due to cerebral edema, herniation, hydrocephalus, or vasospasm), CSF drainage may be instituted by ventricular catheter drainage (Hemphill, Greenberg, Anderson, et al., 2015). Mannitol may be given to reduce ICP. When mannitol is used as a long-term measure to control ICP, dehydration and disturbances in electrolyte balance (hyponatremia or hypernatremia; hypokalemia or hyperkalemia) may occur. Mannitol pulls water out of the brain tissue by osmosis and reduces total body water through diuresis. The patient's fluid balance is monitored continuously and is assessed for signs of dehydration and for rebound elevation of ICP. Other interventions may include elevating the head of the bed to 30 degrees, avoidance of hyperglycemia and hypoglycemia, sedation, and use of hypertonic saline in a variety of concentrations (e.g., 3%, 7.5%, or 23%) (Wijdicks et al., 2014).

Hypertension

Hypertension is the most common cause of intracerebral hemorrhage, and its treatment is critical. Specific goals for blood pressure management, which are individualized for each patient, remain controversial. Blood pressure goals may depend on the presence of increased ICP. Recently published guidelines for management of intracerebral hemorrhage recommend early blood pressure lowering (if the systolic blood pressure is between 150 and 220 mm Hg) to a goal systolic of 140 mm Hg, and report that lowering blood pressure can be effective for improving patient outcomes. If systolic blood pressure is above 220 mm Hg, IV continuous infusions of antihypertensives may be prescribed (Hemphill et al., 2015). Nicardipine (Cardene) is one agent that may be used as a continuous IV infusion. Labetalol (Trandate) and hydralazine (Apresoline) are other examples of medications that may be given as an IV bolus. During the administration of antihypertensive agents, hemodynamic monitoring is important to detect and avoid a precipitous drop in blood pressure, which can produce brain ischemia. Stool softeners are used to prevent straining, which can elevate the blood pressure.

Medical Management

The goals of medical treatment for hemorrhagic stroke are to allow the brain to recover from the initial insult (bleeding), to prevent or minimize the risk of rebleeding, and to prevent or treat complications. Management may consist of bed rest with sedation to prevent agitation and stress, management of vasospasm, and surgical or medical treatment to prevent rebleeding. If the bleeding is caused by anticoagulation with warfarin, the INR may be corrected with fresh-frozen plasma and vitamin K. Reversing the anticoagulation effect of the new oral anticoagulants is more complicated. Protocols may include hemodialysis, the use of oral activated charcoal, administration of prothrombin complex concentrates, or administration of recombinant activated factor VII (Kaatz, Kouides, Garcia, et al., 2012). Idarucizumab (Praxbind) is a medication that was recently approved for reversing dabigatran (Pradaxa). If seizures occur, they are treated with anticonvulsant drugs such as phenytoin (Dilantin). Hyperglycemia should also be treated, and hypoglycemia is avoided. Intermittent pneumatic compression devices should be used starting on the first day of the hospital admission to prevent DVT. If the patient is not mobile after 1 to 4 days from the onset of the hemorrhage and there is documentation of the bleeding ceasing, then DVT prevention medications (low–molecular-weight heparin or unfractionated heparin) may be prescribed (Hemphill et al., 2015). Analgesic agents may be prescribed for head and neck pain. Fever should be treated with acetaminophen (Tylenol), iced saline boluses, and devices such as cooling blankets (Bader et al., 2016). After discharge, most patients will require antihypertensive medications to decrease their risk of another intracerebral hemorrhage.

Surgical Management

In many cases, a primary intracerebral hemorrhage is not treated surgically. However, if the patient is showing signs of worsening neurologic examination, increased ICP, or signs of brainstem compression, then surgical evacuation is recommended for the patient with a cerebellar hemorrhage (Hemphill et al., 2015). Surgical evacuation is most frequently accomplished via a craniotomy (see Chapter 66).

The patient with an intracranial aneurysm is prepared for surgical intervention as soon as their condition is considered stable. Surgical treatment of the patient with an unruptured aneurysm is an option. The goal of surgery is to prevent bleeding in an unruptured aneurysm or further bleeding in an already ruptured aneurysm. This objective is accomplished by isolating the aneurysm from its circulation or by strengthening the arterial wall. An aneurysm may be excluded from the cerebral circulation by means of a ligature or a clip across its neck. If this is not anatomically possible, the aneurysm can be reinforced by wrapping it with some substance to provide support and induce scarring.

Advances in technology have led to the introduction of interventional neuroradiology for the treatment of aneurysms. These techniques are now being used more frequently. Endovascular techniques may be used in selected patients to occlude the blood flow from the artery that feeds the aneurysm with coils, liquid embolic agents, or other techniques to occlude the aneurysm itself. If the aneurysm is very large or very wide at its neck, a stent-like device made of a very fine mesh may be used to divert the blood flow away from the aneurysm. The determination of which technique should be used is based on many factors (characteristics of the patient and aneurysm) and is made by experienced endovascular specialists (Connolly et al., 2012; Thompson, Brown, Amin-Hanjani, et al., 2015).

Postoperative complications are rare but can occur. Potential complications include psychological symptoms (disorientation, amnesia, Korsakoff syndrome [disorder characterized by psychosis, disorientation, delirium, insomnia, hallucinations, personality changes]), intraoperative embolization or artery rupture, postoperative artery occlusion, fluid and electrolyte disturbances (from dysfunction of the neurohypophyseal system), and gastrointestinal bleeding.

NURSING PROCESS

The Patient With a Hemorrhagic Stroke

Assessment

A complete neurologic assessment is performed initially and includes evaluation for the following:

- Altered level of consciousness
- Sluggish pupillary reaction
- Motor and sensory dysfunction
- Cranial nerve deficits (extraocular eye movements, facial droop, presence of ptosis)
- Speech difficulties and visual disturbance
- Headache and nuchal rigidity or other neurologic deficits

All patients should be monitored in the intensive care unit after an intracerebral or subarachnoid hemorrhage. Neurologic assessment findings are documented and reported as indicated. The frequency of these assessments varies depending on the patient's condition. Any changes in the patient's condition require reassessment and thorough documentation; changes should be reported immediately.

Concept Mastery Alert

Alteration in level of consciousness often is the earliest sign of deterioration in a patient with a hemorrhagic stroke. Because nurses have the most frequent contact with patients, they are in the best position to detect subtle changes. Drowsiness and slight slurring of speech may be early signs that the level of consciousness is deteriorating.

Diagnosis

NURSING DIAGNOSES
Based on the assessment data, major nursing diagnoses may include the following:

- Risk for ineffective tissue perfusion (cerebral) related to bleeding or vasospasm
- Anxiety related to illness and/or medically imposed restrictions (aneurysm precautions)

COLLABORATIVE PROBLEMS/POTENTIAL COMPLICATIONS
Potential complications may include the following:

- Vasospasm
- Seizures
- Hydrocephalus
- Rebleeding
- Hyponatremia

Planning and Goals

The goals for the patient may include improved cerebral tissue perfusion, relief of anxiety, and the absence of complications.

Nursing Interventions

OPTIMIZING CEREBRAL TISSUE PERFUSION
The patient is closely monitored for neurologic deterioration resulting from recurrent bleeding, increasing ICP, or vasospasm. A neurologic flow record is maintained. The blood pressure, pulse, level of consciousness (an indicator of cerebral perfusion), pupillary responses, and motor function are checked hourly. Respiratory status is monitored, because a reduction in oxygen in areas of the brain with impaired autoregulation increases the chances of a cerebral infarction. Any changes are reported immediately.

Implementing Aneurysm Precautions. Cerebral aneurysm precautions are implemented for the patient with a diagnosis of aneurysm to provide a nonstimulating environment, prevent increases in ICP, and prevent further bleeding. The patient is placed on bed rest in a quiet, nonstressful environment, because activity, pain, and anxiety are thought to elevate the blood pressure, which may increase the risk for bleeding. Visitors may be restricted (American Association of Neuroscience Nurses [AANN], 2009; Hickey, 2014).

The head of the bed is elevated 30 degrees to promote venous drainage and decrease ICP. Any activity that suddenly increases the blood pressure or obstructs venous return is avoided. This includes the Valsalva maneuver, straining, forceful sneezing, pushing oneself up in bed and acute flexion or rotation of the head and neck (which compromises the jugular veins). Stool softeners and mild laxatives are prescribed. Both prevent constipation, which can cause an increase in ICP. Dim lighting is helpful, because photophobia (visual intolerance of light) is common. The purpose of aneurysm precautions should be thoroughly explained to both the patient (if possible) and family. Intermittent pneumatic compression devices are prescribed to decrease the incidence of DVT resulting from immobility. The legs are observed for signs and symptoms of DVT (tenderness, redness, swelling, warmth, and edema), and abnormal findings are reported.

RELIEVING ANXIETY
Sensory stimulation is kept to a minimum for patients on aneurysm precautions. For patients who are awake, alert, and oriented, an explanation of the restrictions helps reduce the patient's sense of isolation. Reality orientation is provided to help maintain orientation.

Keeping the patient well informed of the plan of care provides reassurance and helps minimize anxiety. Appropriate reassurance also helps relieve the patient's fears and anxiety. The family also requires information and support.

MONITORING AND MANAGING POTENTIAL COMPLICATIONS
Vasospasm. The patient is assessed for signs of possible vasospasm: intensified headaches, a decrease in level of responsiveness (confusion, disorientation, lethargy), or evidence of aphasia or partial paralysis. These signs may develop several days after surgery or on the initiation of treatment and must be reported immediately. The calcium channel blocker nimodipine should be given for prevention of vasospasm, and fluid volume expanders in the form of triple-H therapy may be prescribed as well (Connolly et al., 2012).

Seizures. Seizure precautions are maintained for every patient who may be at risk for seizure activity. Should a seizure occur, maintaining the airway and preventing injury are the primary goals. Medication therapy is initiated at this time (see Chapter 68).

Hydrocephalus. Blood in the subarachnoid space or ventricles impedes the circulation of CSF, resulting in hydrocephalus. A CT scan that indicates dilated ventricles confirms the diagnosis. Hydrocephalus can occur within the first 24 hours (acute) after subarachnoid hemorrhage or several days (subacute) to several weeks (delayed) later. Symptoms vary according to the time of onset and may be nonspecific. Acute hydrocephalus is characterized by sudden onset of stupor or coma and is managed with a ventriculostomy drain to decrease ICP. Symptoms of subacute and delayed hydrocephalus include gradual onset of drowsiness, behavioral changes, and ataxic gait. A ventriculoperitoneal shunt is surgically placed to treat chronic hydrocephalus. Changes in patient responsiveness are reported immediately.

Rebleeding. The rate of recurrent hemorrhage is approximately 1% to 5% per patient per year after intracerebral hemorrhage (Hemphill et al., 2015). Hypertension is the most serious and modifiable risk factor, which shows the importance of appropriate antihypertensive treatment.

Aneurysm rebleeding is the highest during the first 2 to 12 hours after the initial hemorrhage (Connolly et al., 2012) and is considered a major complication. Symptoms of rebleeding include sudden severe headache, nausea, vomiting, decreased level of consciousness, and neurologic deficit. Rebleeding is confirmed by CT scan. Blood pressure is carefully maintained with medications. The most effective preventive treatment is to secure the aneurysm if the patient is a candidate for surgery or endovascular treatment.

Hyponatremia. After subarachnoid hemorrhage, hyponatremia is found in 10% to 30% of patients. Hyponatremia has been found to be associated with the onset of vasospasm (Connolly et al., 2012). Laboratory data must be checked frequently, and hyponatremia (defined as a serum sodium concentration less than 135 mEq/L) must be identified as early as possible. The patient's primary provider needs to be notified of a low serum sodium level that has persisted for 24 hours or longer. The patient is then evaluated for syndrome of inappropriate antidiuretic hormone (SIADH) or cerebral salt-wasting syndrome. SIADH is described in Chapter 13. Cerebral salt-wasting syndrome occurs when the kidneys are unable to conserve sodium and volume depletion results. The treatment most often is the use of IV hypertonic 3% saline.

PROMOTING HOME, COMMUNITY-BASED, AND TRANSITIONAL CARE

Educating Patients About Self-Care. The patient and family are provided with education that will enable them to cooperate with the care and restrictions required during the acute phase of hemorrhagic stroke and to prepare them to return home. Patient and family education includes information about the causes of hemorrhagic stroke and its possible consequences. In addition, the patient and family are informed about the medical treatments that are implemented, including surgical intervention if warranted, and the importance of interventions taken to prevent and detect complications (i.e., aneurysm precautions, close monitoring of the patient). Depending on the presence and severity of neurologic impairment and other complications resulting from the stroke, the patient may be transferred to a rehabilitation unit or center for additional patient and family education about strategies to regain self-care ability. Education addresses the use of assistive devices or modification of the home environment to help the patient live with the disability. Modifications of the home may be required to provide a safe environment.

Continuing and Transitional Care. The acute and rehabilitation phase of care focuses on obvious needs, issues, and deficits for the patient with a hemorrhagic stroke. The patient and family are reminded of the importance of following recommendations to prevent further hemorrhagic stroke and keeping follow-up appointments with health care providers for monitoring of risk factors. Referral for home, community-based, or transitional care may be warranted to assess the home environment and the ability of the patient and to ensure that the patient and family are able to manage at home. Home visits provide opportunities to monitor the physical and psychological status of the patient and the ability of the family to cope with any alterations in the patient's status. In addition, the home care nurse reminds the patient and family of the importance of continuing health promotion and screening practices. Chart 67-6 lists education for the patient recovering from a stroke.

Evaluation

Expected patient outcomes may include:
1. Demonstrates stable neurologic status and vital signs and respiratory patterns within normal limits
   a. Is alert and oriented to time, place, and person
   b. Demonstrates understandable speech patterns and stable cognitive processes

---

Chart 67-6 HOME CARE CHECKLIST
The Patient Recovering From a Stroke

At the completion of education, the patient and/or caregiver will be able to:

- State the impact of the stroke on physiologic functioning, ADLs, IADLs, roles, relationships, and spirituality.
- State names, dose, side effects, frequency and schedule for all medications.
- State how to contact all members of the treatment team (e.g., health care providers, home care professionals, rehabilitation team, and durable medical equipment and supply vendor).
- State changes in lifestyle (e.g., diet, ADLs, IADLs, activity) necessary for recovery and health maintenance as applicable.
  - Demonstrate environmental modifications and adaptive techniques for accomplishing activities of daily living.
  - Demonstrate home exercises, the use of splints or orthotics, proper positioning, and frequent repositioning.
  - Identify safety measures to prevent falls.
  - Identify holistic interventions for pain management (e.g., positioning, distraction).
  - Describe procedures for maintaining skin integrity.
  - Demonstrate indwelling catheter care, if applicable. Describe a bowel and bladder elimination program as appropriate.
  - Verbalize dietary adjustments (e.g., thickened liquids, pureed diet, small frequent meals) during recovery.
  - Demonstrate swallowing techniques or care of enteral feeding tube.

- Identify psychosocial consequences of stroke (e.g., depression, emotional lability, frustration, fatigue) and appropriate interventions.
- Discuss measures to prevent subsequent strokes.
- Identify potential complications and discuss measures to prevent them (blood clots, aspiration, pneumonia, urinary tract infection, fecal impaction, skin breakdown, contracture).
- Relate how to reach primary provider with questions or complications.
- State time and date of follow-up medical appointments, therapy, and testing.
- Identify resources and other sources of support (e.g., friends, relatives, faith community, stroke support groups, caregiver support).
- Identify the need for health promotion, disease prevention, and screening activities
- Identify appropriate recreational or diversional activities

Resources
See Chapter 9, Chart 9-9 Home Care Checklist: Managing Chronic Illness and Disability at Home and Chapter 10, Chart 10-8 Home Care Checklist: Managing the Therapeutic Regimen at Home, for additional information.

ADL, activities of daily living; IADL, independent activities of daily living.

   c. Demonstrates usual and equal strength, movement, and sensation of all four extremities
   d. Exhibits deep tendon reflexes and pupillary responses within normal limits
2. Exhibits reduced anxiety level
   a. States rationale for aneurysm precautions
   b. Exhibits clear thought processes
   c. Is less restless
   d. Exhibits absence of physiologic indicators of anxiety (e.g., has vital signs within normal limits; usual respiratory rate; absence of excessive, fast speech)
3. Is free of complications
   a. Exhibits absence of vasospasm
   b. Exhibits vital signs within normal limits and is without seizures
   c. Verbalizes understanding of seizure precautions
   d. Exhibits intact mental, motor, and sensory status
   e. Reports no visual changes

CRITICAL THINKING EXERCISES

1 **pq** A 72-year-old male is in the ED being evaluated for a suspected stroke. Identify the priorities, approach and techniques you would use to provide care for him. What are specific time goals for obtaining a head CT scan? If he is eligible for t-PA, how will your priorities change? If his stroke is a hemorrhagic stroke, how will your approach, techniques, and priorities change?

2 **pq** You are caring for a patient after a large ischemic stroke. The patient has hemiplegia and is beginning to experience shoulder pain on the side affected by the stroke. Identify the priority nursing interventions that can be implemented to prevent shoulder pain. What education can you provide to the patient for interventions that can be done at home once discharged?

3 **ebp** A 69-year-old woman has experienced a brainstem stroke. She has just arrived to the nursing unit from the ED and you are her nurse. She has not had a swallow assessment yet. What is the time goal for obtaining an evaluation of her swallowing function? Evaluate the strength of the evidence to support nurses performing dysphagia screening.

REFERENCES

*Asterisk indicates nursing research.
**Double asterisk indicates classic reference.

Books

American Association of Neuroscience Nurses (AANN). (2009). *Guide to the care of the patient with aneurysmal subarachnoid hemorrhage: AANN clinical practice guideline series.* Glenview, IL: Author.

Bader, M., Littlejohns, L. R., & Olson, D. (2016). *AANN core curriculum for neuroscience nursing* (6th ed.). Chicago, IL: American Association of Neuroscience Nurses.

Hickey, J. V. (2014). *The clinical practice of neurological & neurosurgical nursing* (7th ed.). Philadelphia, PA: Lippincott Williams & Wilkins.

Karch, A. (2014). *2015 Lippincott's nursing drug guide*. Philadelphia, PA: Lippincott Williams & Wilkins.

Journals and Electronic Documents

Anderson, J. (2016). Acute ischemic stroke: The golden hour. *Nursing Critical Care*, 11(3), 28–36.

*Aycock, D. M., & Clark, P. C. (2016). Incongruence between perceived long-term risk and actual risk of stroke in rural African Americans. *Journal of Neuroscience Nursing*, 48(1), 35–41.

Bentz, B. (2015). Nonvitamin K antagonist oral anticoagulants in everyday practice: Stroke prevention in atrial fibrillation and treatment of venous thromboembolism. *Journal of the American Association of Nurse Practitioners*, 27(12), 721–731.

Brainin, M., & Zorowitz, R. (2013). Advances in stroke: Recovery and rehabilitation. *Stroke*, 44(2), 311–313.

Connolly, E., Rabinstein, A., Carhuapoma, J., et al. (2012). Guidelines for the management of aneurysmal subarachnoid hemorrhage: A guideline for healthcare professionals from the American Heart Association/American Stroke Association. *Stroke*, 43(6), 1711–1737.

*Creasy, K. R., Lutz, B. J., Young, M. E., et al. (2015). Clinical implications of family-centered care in stroke rehabilitation. *Rehabilitation Nursing*, 40(6), 349–359.

Del Zoppo, G. J., Saver, J. L., Jauch, E. C., et al; American Heart Association Stroke Council (2009). Expansion of the time window for treatment of acute ischemic stroke with intravenous tissue plasminogen activator: A science advisory from the American Heart Association/American Stroke Association. *Stroke*, 40(8), 2945–2948.

Ennen, K. A. (2013). Taking a second look at stroke in women. *American Nurse Today*, 8(5), 12–15.

Flaster, M., Meresh, E., Rao, M., et al. (2013). Central poststroke pain: Current diagnosis and treatment. *Topics in Stroke Rehabilitation*, 20(2), 116–123.

Flaster, M., Sharma, A., & Rao, M. (2013). Poststroke depression: A review emphasizing the role of prophylactic treatment and synergy with treatment for motor recovery. *Topics In Stroke Rehabilitation*, 20(2), 139–150.

Hemphill, J. C., Greenberg, S. M., Anderson, C. S., et al. (2015). Guidelines for the management of spontaneous intracerebral hemorrhage: A guideline for healthcare professionals from the American Heart Association/American Stroke Association. *Stroke*, 46(7), 2032–2060.

Jauch, E. C., Saver, J. L., Adams, H. P., et al. (2013). Guidelines for the early management of patients with ischemic stroke: A guideline from the American Heart Association/American stroke Association. *Stroke*, 44(1), 870–947.

Kaatz, S., Kouides, P. A., Garcia, D. A., et al. (2012). Guidance on the emergent reversal of oral thrombin and factor Xa inhibitors. *American Journal of Hematology*, 87(Suppl. 1), S141–S145.

Kernan, W. N., Ovbiagele, B., Black, H. R., et al. (2014). Guidelines for the prevention of stroke in patients with stroke and transient ischemic attack: A guideline for healthcare professionals from the American Heart Association/American Stroke Association. *Stroke*, 45(7), 2160–2236.

Meschia, J. F., Bushnell, C., Boden-Albala, B., et al. (2014). Guidelines for the primary prevention of stroke: A statement for healthcare professionals from the American Heart Association/American Stroke Association. *Stroke*, 45(12), 3754–3832.

Middleton, S., Grimley, R., & Alexandrov, A. W. (2015). Triage, treatment, and transfer: Evidence-based clinical practice recommendations and models of nursing care for the first 72 hours of admission to hospital for acute stroke. *Stroke*, 46(2), e18–e25.

Miller, E. L., Murray, L., Richards, L., et al. (2010). Comprehensive overview of nursing and interdisciplinary rehabilitation care of the stroke patient: A scientific statement from the American Heart Association. *Stroke*, 41(10), 2402–2448.

Miller, E. T., & Summers, D. (2014). Update on transient ischemic attack nursing care. *Stroke*, 45(5), e71–e73.

Mozaffarian, D., Benjamin, E. J., Go, A. S., et al. (2016). AHA statistical update: Heart disease and stroke statistics—2016 update: A report from the American Heart Association. *Circulation*, 133(4), e38–e360.

**National Institute of Neurologic Disorders and Stroke. (1995). Tissue plasminogen activator for acute ischemic stroke. The National Institute of Neurological Disorders and Stroke rt-PA Stroke Study Group. *New England Journal of Medicine*, 333(24), 1581–1587.

National Institute of Neurological Disorders and Stroke, National Institutes of Health. National Institutes of Health Stroke Scale. Retrieved on 4/23/17 at: www.ninds.nih.gov/sites/default/files/NIH_Stroke_Scale_Booklet.pdf

Powers, W. J., Derdeyn, C. P., Biller J., et al. (2015). AHA/ASA guideline: 2015 AHA/ASA focused update of the 2013 guidelines for the early management of acute ischemic stroke regarding endovascular treatment. A guideline for healthcare professionals from the American Heart Association/American Stroke Association. *Stroke, 46*(6), 3020–3035.

Puhr, M. I., & Thompson, H. J. (2015). The use of transitional care models in patients with stroke. *Journal of Neuroscience Nursing, 47*(4), 223–234.

**Saver, J. L. (2006). Time is brain quantified. *Stroke, 37*(1), 263–266.

Summers, D., Leonard, A., Wentworth, D., et al. (2009). Comprehensive overview of nursing and interdisciplinary care of the acute ischemic stroke patient: A scientific statement from the American Heart Association. *Stroke, 40*(8), 2911–2944.

Teasell, R., Foley, N., Pereira, S., et al. (2012). Evidence to practice: Botulinum toxin in the treatment of spasticity post stroke. *Topics in Stroke Rehabilitation, 19*(2), 115–121.

Thompson, B. G., Brown, R. J., Amin-Hanjani, S., et al. (2015). Guidelines for the management of patients with unruptured intracranial aneurysms: A guideline for healthcare professionals from the American Heart Association/American Stroke Association. *Stroke, 46*(8), 2368–2400.

Treat-Jacobson, D. J., Rich, K., DeVeaux, T., et al. (2013). Society for vascular nursing clinical practice guideline (CPG) for carotid artery stenting. *Journal of Vascular Nursing, 31*(1), 32–55.

Wijdicks, E. M., Sheth, K. N., Carter, B. S., et al. (2014). Recommendations for the management of cerebral and cerebellar infarction with swelling: A statement for healthcare professionals from the American Heart Association/American Stroke Association. *Stroke, 45*(4), 1222–1238.

*Wuchner, S., Bakas, T., Adams, G., et al. (2012). Nursing interventions and assessments for aneurysmal subarachnoid hemorrhage patients: A mixed methods study involving practicing nurses. *Journal of Neuroscience Nursing, 44*(4), 177–185.

Zanichkowsky, R., Nascimento, J. A., McCune, M., et al. (2016). Where does the time go? The effect of protocols for stroke last known well documentation on intravenous recombinant tissue plasminogen activator delivery in the northeast. *Journal of Neuroscience Nursing, 48*(2), 71–74.

Zheng, L., & Alexander, S. A. (2015). Current evidence in the management of poststroke hemiplegic shoulder pain: A review. *Journal of Neuroscience Nursing, 47*(1), 10–19.

Resources

American Association of Neuroscience Nurses (AANN), www.aann.org

American Stroke Association, a Division of the American Heart Association, www.strokeassociation.org/STROKEORG/

Brain Attack Coalition, www.brainattackcoalition.org

National Institute of Neurological Disorders and Stroke, www.ninds.nih.gov

National Stroke Association, www.stroke.org

68

Management of Patients With Neurologic Trauma

LEARNING OBJECTIVES

On completion of this chapter, the learner will be able to:

1 Describe the mechanisms of injury, clinical signs and symptoms, diagnostic testing, and treatment options for patients with traumatic brain and spinal cord injuries.
2 Use the nursing process as a framework for care of patients with traumatic brain injury.

3 Identify the population at risk for spinal cord injury.
4 Explain the clinical features and management of the patient with neurogenic shock.
5 Discuss the pathophysiology of autonomic dysreflexia and describe the appropriate nursing interventions.
6 Apply the nursing process as a framework for care of patients with spinal cord injury.

GLOSSARY

autonomic dysreflexia: a life-threatening emergency in patients with spinal cord injury that causes a hypertensive emergency; also called *autonomic hyperreflexia*
complete spinal cord lesion: a condition that involves total loss of sensation and voluntary muscle control below the lesion
concussion: a temporary loss of neurologic function with no apparent structural damage to the brain
contusion: bruising of the brain surface
halo vest: external traction device that encircles the head like a halo and stabilizes the cervical spine
incomplete spinal cord lesion: a condition in which there is preservation of the sensory or motor fibers, or both, below the lesion
neurogenic bladder: bladder dysfunction that results from a disorder or dysfunction of the nervous system; may result in either urinary retention or bladder overactivity
paraplegia: paralysis of the lower extremities with dysfunction of the bowel and bladder from a lesion in the thoracic, lumbar, or sacral region of the spinal cord
primary injury: initial damage to the brain that results from the traumatic event

secondary injury: an insult to the brain subsequent to the original traumatic event
spinal cord injury (SCI): an injury to the spinal cord, vertebral column, supporting soft tissue, or intervertebral discs caused by trauma
tetraplegia: varying degrees of paralysis of both arms and legs, with dysfunction of bowel and bladder from a lesion of the cervical segments of the spinal cord; formerly called *quadriplegia*
transection: severing of the spinal cord itself; transection can be complete (all the way through the cord) or incomplete (partially through)
traumatic brain injury: an injury to the skull or brain that is severe enough to interfere with normal functioning
traumatic brain injury, closed (blunt): occurs when the head accelerates and then rapidly decelerates or collides with another object and brain tissue is damaged, but there is no opening through the skull and dura
traumatic brain injury, open (penetrating): occurs when an object penetrates the skull, enters the brain, and damages the soft brain tissue in its path (penetrating injury), or when blunt trauma to the head is so severe that it opens the scalp, skull, and dura to expose the brain

Trauma involving the central nervous system can be life threatening. Even if not life threatening, brain and spinal cord injury (SCI) may result in major physical and psychological dysfunction and can alter the patient's life completely. Neurologic trauma affects the patient, the family, the health care system, and society as a whole because of its major sequelae and the costs of acute and long-term care of patients with trauma to the brain and spinal cord.

Head Injuries

Head injury is a broad classification that encompasses any damage to the head as a result of trauma. A head injury does

not necessarily mean a brain injury is present. **Traumatic brain injury** (TBI) or craniocerebral trauma describes an injury that is the result of an external force and is of sufficient magnitude to interfere with daily life and prompts the seeking of treatment.

The Centers for Disease Control and Prevention (CDC) estimates that there are 2.5 million emergency department (ED) visits in the United States each year, the majority of which are for a mild TBI (CDC, 2016a). As a result of TBI, approximately 52,000 people die (contributing to about 30% of all injury-related deaths), 275,000 are hospitalized, and 80,000 to 90,000 will have long-term disabilities (CDC, 2016a; Hickey, 2014). Approximately 78% of patients are treated in the ED and released (Hemphill & Phan, 2016). The most common causes of TBIs are falls (35.2%), motor vehicle crashes (17.3%), being struck by objects (16.5%), and assaults (10%). Children 0 to 4 years, adolescents 15 to 19 years, and adults 65 years and older are most likely to sustain a TBI. In every age group, TBI rates are higher for males than for females (Hickey, 2014). An estimated 57 million people worldwide are currently living with a TBI-related disability, producing an annual economic impact of approximately $60 to $75 billion due to medical expenses and the cost of lost productivity (CDC, 2016a). The best approach to head injury is prevention (see Chart 68-1).

Pathophysiology

Research suggests that not all brain damage occurs at the moment of impact. Damage to the brain from traumatic injury takes two forms: primary injury and secondary injury. **Primary injury** is defined as the consequence of direct contact to the head/brain during the instant of initial injury, causing extracranial focal injuries (e.g., contusions, lacerations, external hematomas, and skull fractures), as well as possible focal brain injuries from sudden movement of the brain within the cranial vault (e.g., subdural hematomas (SDHs), concussion, diffuse axonal injury [DAI]). The greatest opportunity for decreasing TBI is the implementation of prevention strategies (see Chart 68-1).

Secondary injury evolves over the ensuing hours and days after the initial injury and results from inadequate delivery of nutrients and oxygen to the cells. Identification, prevention, and treatment of secondary injury are the main foci of early management of severe TBI. Contributors to this process include intracranial pathologic processes such as intracranial hemorrhage, cerebral edema, intracranial hypertension, hyperemia, seizures, and vasospasm (Bader, Littlejohns, & Olson, 2016; Hickey, 2014). Systemic effects from hypotension, hyperthermia, hypoxia, hypercarbia, infection, electrolyte imbalances, and anemia can also be factors which add to the complex biochemical, metabolic, and inflammatory changes that further compromise an injured brain (Bader et al., 2016; Hickey, 2014).

Physiology/Pathophysiology

Figure 68-1 • Pathophysiology of traumatic brain injury.

The Monro–Kellie hypothesis, also known as the Monro–Kellie doctrine, explains the dynamic equilibrium of cranial contents. The cranial vault contains three main components: brain, blood, and cerebrospinal fluid (CSF). According to the Monro–Kellie hypothesis, the cranial vault is a closed system, and if one of the three components increases in volume, at least one of the other two must decrease in volume or the pressure will increase. Any bleeding or swelling within the skull increases the volume of contents within the skull and therefore causes increased intracranial pressure (ICP) (see Chapter 66). If the pressure increases enough, it can cause displacement of the brain through or against the rigid structures of the skull. This causes restriction of blood flow to the brain, decreasing oxygen delivery and waste removal. Cells within the brain become anoxic and cannot metabolize properly, producing ischemia, infarction, irreversible brain damage, and eventually brain death (see Fig. 68-1).

Scalp Injury

Isolated scalp trauma is generally classified as a minor injury. Because its many blood vessels constrict poorly, the scalp bleeds profusely when injured. Trauma may result in an abrasion (brush wound), contusion, laceration, or hematoma beneath the layers of tissue of the scalp (subgaleal hematoma) (Hickey, 2014). A large avulsion (tearing away) of the scalp may be potentially life threatening and is a true emergency. Diagnosis of a scalp injury is based on physical examination, inspection, and palpation. Scalp wounds are potential portals of entry for organisms that cause intracranial infections. Therefore, the area is irrigated before the laceration is sutured to remove foreign material and to reduce the risk for infection (Hollander & Camacho, 2014). Subgaleal hematomas (hematomas below the outer covering of the skull) usually reabsorb and do not require any specific treatment.

Skull Fractures

A skull fracture is a break in the continuity of the skull caused by forceful trauma. It may occur with or without damage to the brain. Skull fractures are classified by type and location. Types include linear, comminuted, and depressed skull fractures, whereas location fractures include frontal, temporal, and basal skull fractures. A simple (linear) fracture is a break in the continuity of the bone. A comminuted skull fracture refers to a splintered or multiple fracture line. Depressed skull fractures occur when the bones of the skull are forcefully displaced downward, and can vary from a slight depression to bones of the skull being splintered and embedded within brain tissue. A fracture of the base of the skull is referred to as a basal skull fracture (Hickey, 2014) (see Fig. 68-2). A fracture may be open, indicating a scalp laceration or tear in the dura (e.g., from a bullet or an ice pick), or closed, in which case the dura is intact.

Clinical Manifestations

Symptoms, apart from those of the local injury, depend on the severity and the anatomic location of the underlying brain injury. Persistent, localized pain usually suggests that a fracture is present. Fractures of the cranial vault may or may not produce swelling in the region of the fracture. Fractures of the base of the skull tend to traverse the paranasal sinus of the frontal bone or the middle ear located in the temporal bone (see Fig. 68-2). Therefore, they frequently produce hemorrhage from the nose, pharynx, or ears, and blood may appear under the conjunctiva. An area of ecchymosis (bruising) may

be seen over the mastoid (Battle sign). Basal skull fractures are suspected when CSF escapes from the ears (CSF otorrhea) and the nose (CSF rhinorrhea). Drainage of CSF is a serious problem, because meningeal infection can occur if organisms gain access to the cranial contents via the nose, ear, or sinus through a tear in the dura.

Assessment and Diagnostic Findings

A computed tomography (CT) scan can be used to diagnose a skull fracture. The ease with which a diagnosis of skull fracture is made depends on the site of the fracture. If a fracture is found on CT scan, there is always the question of associated brain injury, and a magnetic resonance imaging (MRI) scan provides better resolution and clearer pictures of the injured area (Hickey, 2014).

Gerontologic Considerations

Older patients with head injuries differ from those who are younger in terms of etiology of injury, higher mortality rates, longer lengths of hospital stay, and poorer functional outcomes. Neurologic assessment can be challenging, as the older adult patient with a TBI can have hearing and/or visual deficits or pre-existing dementia or cognitive issues, making establishment of a neurologic baseline difficult. The most common causes of injury in older adult patients are falls and motor vehicle crashes (Stocchetti & Maas, 2014). Approximately 61% of all TBIs among adults aged 65 years and older result from falls (CDC, 2016a). Physiologic changes related to aging may place the older adult at increased risk for injury, alter the type and severity of injury that occurs, or lead to complications. Two major factors place older adults at increased risk for hematomas. First, brain weight decreases, the dura becomes more adherent to the skull, and reaction times slow with increasing age (Eliopoulos, 2018). Second, many older adults take aspirin and anticoagulant agents as part of routine management of chronic conditions.

Medical Management

Nondepressed skull fractures generally do not require surgical treatment; however, close observation of the patient is essential. Nursing personnel may observe the patient in the hospital, but if no underlying brain injury is present, the patient may be allowed to return home. If the patient is discharged home, specific instructions must be given to the family (see later discussion of concussion).

Depressed skull fractures usually require surgery with elevation of the skull and débridement, usually within 24 hours of injury. Skull fractures can be a combination of open, compound, closed, or simple. Associated injuries include concurrent scalp laceration, dural tears, and brain injury directly below the fracture from compression of the tissue below the bony injury and from lacerations produced by the bony fragments (Hickey, 2014).

Brain Injury

The most important consideration in any head injury is whether the brain is injured. Even seemingly minor injury can cause significant brain damage secondary to obstructed

Figure 68-2 • Basal skull fracture allows cerebrospinal fluid to leak from the nose and ears. Adapted from Hickey, J. V. (2009). *The clinical practice of neurological & neurosurgical nursing* (6th ed.). Philadelphia, PA: Lippincott Williams & Wilkins.

Basilar skull fracture

blood flow and decreased tissue perfusion. The brain cannot store oxygen or glucose to any significant degree. Because the cerebral cells need an uninterrupted blood supply to obtain these nutrients, irreversible brain damage and cell death occur if the blood supply is interrupted for even a few minutes. A **traumatic brain injury, closed (blunt)** occurs when the head accelerates and then rapidly decelerates or collides with another object (e.g., a wall, the dashboard of a car) and brain tissue is damaged but there is no opening through the skull and dura. A **traumatic brain injury, open (penetrating)** occurs when an object penetrates the skull, enters the brain, and damages the soft brain tissue in its path or when blunt trauma to the head is so severe that it opens the scalp, skull, and dura to expose the brain.

Types of Brain Injury

Injuries to the brain can be focal or diffuse. Focal injuries include contusions and several types of hematomas. Concussions and diffuse axonal injuries are the major diffuse injuries (Hickey, 2014).

Contusion

In cerebral **contusion** the brain is bruised and damaged in a specific area because of severe acceleration–deceleration force or blunt trauma. The impact of the brain against the skull leads to a contusion. Clinical manifestations of a contusion are dependent upon size, location, and the extent of surrounding cerebral edema. Although a contusion may occur in any area of the brain, most are usually located in the anterior portions of the frontal and temporal lobes, around the sylvian fissure, and at the orbital areas; less commonly, contusions are located at the parietal and occipital areas.

Contusions can be characterized by loss of consciousness associated with stupor and confusion. The effects of injury, particularly hemorrhage and edema, peak after about 18 to 36 hours. These effects, which can cause secondary effects resulting in increased ICP and possible herniation syndromes, are most pronounced in temporal lobe contusions. Patients are most often managed medically with interventions directed toward prevention of additional insults. Deep contusions are more often associated with hemorrhage and destruction of the reticular activating fibers, altering arousal (Hickey, 2014).

Intracranial Hemorrhage

Hematomas are collections of blood in the brain that may be epidural (above the dura), subdural (below the dura), or intracerebral (within the brain) (see Fig. 68-3). Major symptoms are frequently delayed until the hematoma is large enough to cause distortion of the brain and increased ICP. The signs and symptoms of cerebral ischemia resulting from compression by a hematoma are variable and depend on the speed with which vital areas are affected and the area that is injured. A rapidly developing hematoma, even if small, may be fatal, whereas a larger but slowly developing one may allow compensation for increases in ICP.

Epidural Hematoma

After a head injury, blood may collect in the epidural (extradural) space between the skull and the dura mater. This can

Figure 68-3 • Location of epidural, subdural, and intracerebral hematomas.

result from a skull fracture that causes a rupture or laceration of the middle meningeal artery, the artery that runs between the dura and the skull inferior to a thin portion of temporal bone. Hemorrhage from this artery causes rapid pressure on the brain. Epidural hematomas (EDHs) account for approximately 2.7% to 4% of traumatic head injuries (Hickey, 2014).

Symptoms are caused by the expanding hematoma. EDHs are often characterized by a brief loss of consciousness, followed by a lucid interval in which the patient is awake and conversant. During this lucid interval, compensation for the expanding hematoma takes place by rapid absorption of CSF and decreased intravascular volume, both of which help to maintain the ICP within normal limits. When these mechanisms can no longer compensate, even a small increase in the volume of the blood clot produces a marked elevation in ICP. The patient then becomes increasingly restless, agitated, and confused as the condition progresses to coma. Then, often suddenly, signs of herniation appear (usually deterioration of consciousness and signs of focal neurologic deficits, such as dilation and fixation of a pupil or paralysis of an extremity), and the patient's condition deteriorates rapidly. The most common type of herniation syndrome associated with an EDH is uncal herniation causing pressure on the midbrain (Hickey, 2014).

An EDH is considered an extreme emergency; marked neurologic deficit or even respiratory arrest can occur within minutes. Treatment consists of making openings through the skull (burr holes; see Chapter 66, Fig. 66-8) to decrease ICP emergently, remove the clot, and control the bleeding. A craniotomy may be required to remove the clot and control the bleeding. A drain is usually inserted after creation of burr holes or a craniotomy to prevent reaccumulation of blood.

Subdural Hematoma

An SDH is a collection of blood between the dura and the brain, a space normally occupied by a thin cushion of fluid. The most common cause is trauma, but it can also occur as a result of coagulopathies or rupture of an aneurysm. An SDH is more frequently venous in origin and is caused by the rupture of small vessels that bridge the subdural space (Bauman & McCourt, 2014). SDHs may be acute or chronic depending on the size of the involved vessel and the amount of bleeding on CT scan.

Acute SDH

Approximately 50% of brain injuries and 60% of deaths in patients with brain injuries result from acute SDHs and are associated with major head injury involving contusion or laceration. Clinical symptoms develop rapidly (Bauman & McCourt, 2014). Signs and symptoms include changes in the level of consciousness (LOC), pupillary signs, and hemiparesis. There may be minor or even no symptoms with small collections of blood. Coma, increasing blood pressure, decreasing heart rate, and slowing respiratory rate are all signs of a rapidly expanding mass requiring immediate intervention.

If the patient can be transported rapidly to the hospital, an immediate craniotomy is performed to open the dura, allowing the subdural clot to be evacuated. Successful outcome also depends on the control of ICP and careful monitoring of respiratory function (see Chapter 66). The mortality rate for patients with acute SDH is high because of associated brain damage (Bauman & McCourt, 2014).

Chronic SDH

A chronic SDH can develop from seemingly minor head injuries and is seen most frequently in older adults who are prone to this type of head injury due to brain atrophy, which is a consequence of the aging process (Bauman & McCourt, 2014). Seemingly minor head trauma may produce enough impact to shift the brain contents abnormally. The time between injury and onset of symptoms can be lengthy (e.g., 3 weeks to months), so the actual injury may be forgotten.

A chronic SDH can resemble other conditions—for example, it may be mistaken for a stroke. The bleeding is less profuse, but compression of the intracranial contents still occurs. The blood within the brain changes in character in 2 to 4 days, becoming thicker and darker. In a few weeks, the clot breaks down and has the color and consistency of motor oil. Eventually, calcification or ossification of the clot takes place. The brain adapts to this foreign body invasion, and the clinical signs and symptoms fluctuate. Symptoms include severe headache, which tends to come and go; alternating focal neurologic signs; personality changes; mental deterioration; and focal seizures (Bauman & McCourt, 2014).

The treatment for a chronic SDH consists of surgical evaluation for evacuation of the clot. Consideration must be made for reversal of coagulopathies and iatrogenic anticoagulation (Bauman & McCourt, 2014). The operative procedure may be carried out through multiple burr holes, or a craniotomy may be performed for a sizable subdural mass that cannot be suctioned or drained through burr holes.

Intracerebral Hemorrhage and Hematoma

Intracerebral hemorrhage is bleeding into the parenchyma of the brain. It is commonly seen in head injuries when force is exerted to the head over a small area (e.g., missile injuries, bullet wounds, stab injuries). These hemorrhages within the brain may also result from the following:

- Systemic hypertension, which causes degeneration and rupture of a vessel
- Rupture of an aneurysm
- Vascular anomalies
- Intracranial tumors
- Bleeding disorders such as leukemia, hemophilia, aplastic anemia, and thrombocytopenia
- Complications of anticoagulant therapy

Nontraumatic causes of intracerebral hemorrhage are discussed in Chapter 67.

The onset may be insidious, beginning with the development of neurologic deficits, followed by headache. Management includes supportive care; control of ICP; and careful administration of fluids, electrolytes, and antihypertensive medications. Surgical intervention by craniotomy or craniectomy permits removal of the blood clot and control of hemorrhage, but may not be possible because of the inaccessible location of the bleeding or the lack of a clearly circumscribed area of blood that can be removed.

Concussion

A **concussion** is a temporary loss of neurologic function with no apparent structural damage to the brain. Of the 1.7 million TBIs that occur in the United States each year, it is estimated that approximately 80% of them are concussions, also referred to as "mild TBI" (Hyatt, 2014; CDC, 2016b). The mechanism of injury is usually blunt trauma from an acceleration–deceleration force, a direct blow, or a blast injury. If brain tissue in the frontal lobe is affected, the patient may exhibit bizarre irrational behavior, whereas involvement of the temporal lobe can produce temporary amnesia or disorientation.

The duration of mental status abnormalities is an indicator of the grade of the concussion. The patient is discharged from the hospital or ED once he or she returns to baseline after a concussion. Monitoring includes observing the patient for a decrease in LOC, worsening headache, dizziness, seizures, abnormal pupil response, vomiting, irritability, slurred speech, and numbness or weakness in the arms or legs (West, Bergman, Biggins, et al., 2011). The occurrence of these symptoms is a red flag indicating the need for further intervention. Recovery may appear complete, but long-term sequelae are possible and repeat injuries common.

Repeated concussive incidents can lead to a syndrome known as chronic traumatic encephalopathy. This syndrome has been recognized in those participating in contact sports such as football and boxing. The presentation is similar to Alzheimer disease, characterized by personality changes, memory impairment, and speech and gait disturbances. Imaging findings show gross cerebral, particularly temporal lobe, atrophy (Bailes, Petraglia, Omalu, et al., 2013; Hickey, 2014).

Diffuse Axonal Injury

DAI results from widespread shearing and rotational forces that produce damage throughout the brain—to axons in the cerebral hemispheres, corpus callosum, and brainstem. The injured area may be diffuse with no identifiable focal lesion. DAI is associated with prolonged traumatic coma; it is more serious and is associated with a poorer prognosis than a focal lesion. The patient with DAI in severe head trauma experiences no lucid interval, immediate coma, decorticate and decerebrate posturing (see Chapter 66, Fig. 66-1), and global cerebral edema. Diagnosis is made by clinical signs in conjunction with a CT or MRI scan (Bodanapally, Sours, Zhuo, et al., 2015). Recovery depends on the severity of the axonal injury.

Medical Management

Assessment and diagnosis of the extent of injury are accomplished by the initial physical and neurologic examinations. CT and MRI scans are the main neuroimaging diagnostic tools and are useful in evaluating the brain structure (Bodanapally et al., 2015). Positron emission tomography (PET) is available in some trauma centers for assessing brain function.

Any patient with a head injury is presumed to have a cervical spine injury until proven otherwise. The patient is transported from the scene of the injury on a board with the head and neck maintained in alignment with the axis of the body. A cervical collar should be applied and maintained until cervical spine x-rays have been obtained and the absence of cervical SCI documented.

All therapy is directed toward preserving brain homeostasis and preventing secondary brain injury, which is injury to the brain that occurs after the original traumatic event (Bader et al., 2016). Common causes of secondary injury are cerebral edema, hypotension, and respiratory depression that may lead to hypoxemia and electrolyte imbalance. Treatments to prevent secondary injury include stabilization of cardiovascular and respiratory function to maintain adequate cerebral perfusion, control of hemorrhage and hypovolemia, and maintenance of optimal blood gas values.

 Treatment of Increased Intracranial Pressure

As the damaged brain swells with edema or as blood collects within the brain, an increase in ICP occurs; this requires aggressive treatment (see Chapter 66 for a discussion of the relationship between ICP and cerebral perfusion pressure [CPP]). If the ICP remains elevated, it can decrease the CPP. Initial management is based on preventing secondary injury and maintaining adequate cerebral oxygenation.

Surgery is required for evacuation of blood clots, débridement and elevation of depressed fractures of the skull, and suture of severe scalp lacerations. ICP is monitored closely; if increased, it is managed by maintaining adequate oxygenation, elevating the head of the bed, and maintaining normal blood volume (Stocchetti & Maas, 2014). Devices to monitor ICP or drain CSF can be inserted during surgery or at the bedside using aseptic technique. The patient is cared for in the intensive care unit (ICU), where expert nursing care and medical treatment are readily available.

Supportive Measures

Treatment also includes ventilatory support, seizure prevention, fluid and electrolyte maintenance, nutritional support, and management of pain and anxiety. Patients who are comatose are intubated and mechanically ventilated to ensure adequate oxygenation and protect the airway.

Because seizures can occur after head injury and can cause secondary brain damage from hypoxia, anticonvulsant agents may be given. If the patient is very agitated, benzodiazepines

are the most commonly used sedative agents and do not affect cerebral blood flow or ICP. Lorazepam (Ativan) and midazolam (Versed) are frequently used but have active metabolites that may cause prolonged sedation, making it difficult to conduct a neurologic assessment. Propofol (Diprivan), a sedative–hypnotic agent that is supplied in an intralipid emulsion for intravenous (IV) use, is the sedative of choice. It is an ultrashort acting, rapid onset drug with elimination half-life of less than an hour. It has a major advantage of being titratable to its desired clinical effect but still provides the opportunity for an accurate neurologic assessment (Hickey, 2014). A nasogastric tube may be inserted, because reduced gastric motility and reverse peristalsis are associated with head injury, making regurgitation and aspiration common in the first few hours.

Brain Death

When a patient has sustained a severe head injury incompatible with life, the patient is a potential organ donor. The nurse may assist in the clinical examination for determination of brain death and in the process of organ procurement. The three cardinal signs of brain death on clinical examination are coma, the absence of brainstem reflexes, and apnea. Adjunctive tests, such as cerebral blood flow studies, electroencephalogram (EEG), transcranial Doppler, and brainstem auditory-evoked potential, are often used to confirm brain death (Hickey, 2014). The health care team provides information to the family and assists them with the decision-making process about end-of-life care.

NURSING PROCESS

The Patient With a Traumatic Brain Injury

Assessment

Depending on the patient's neurologic status, the nurse may elicit information from the patient, from the family, or from witnesses or emergency rescue personnel. Although all usual baseline data may not be collected initially, the immediate health history should include the following questions:

- When did the injury occur?
- What caused the injury? A high-velocity missile? An object striking the head? A fall?
- What was the direction and force of the blow?

A history of unconsciousness or amnesia after a head injury indicates a significant degree of brain damage, and changes that occur minutes to hours after the initial injury can reflect recovery or indicate the development of secondary brain damage. The nurse should determine if there was a loss of consciousness, the duration of the unconscious period, and if the patient could be aroused.

In addition to asking questions that establish the nature of the injury and the patient's condition immediately after the injury, the nurse examines the patient thoroughly. This assessment includes determining the patient's LOC using the Glasgow Coma Scale (GCS) and assessing the patient's response to tactile stimuli (if unconscious), pupillary response to light, corneal and gag reflexes, and motor function (Teasdale & Jennett, 1974). The GCS (see Chart 68-2) is based on the three criteria of eye opening, verbal responses, and motor

Chart
68-2

ASSESSMENT
Glasgow Coma Scale

The Glasgow Coma Scale is a tool for assessing a patient's response to stimuli. Scores range from 3 (deep coma) to 15 (normal).

Eye-opening response	Spontaneous	4
	To voice	3
	To pain	2
	None	1
Best verbal response	Oriented	5
	Confused	4
	Inappropriate words	3
	Incomprehensible sounds	2
	None	1
Best motor response	Obeys command	6
	Localizes pain	5
	Withdraws	4
	Flexion	3
	Extension	2
	None	1
Total		3 to 15

Adapted from Teasdale, G., & Jennett, B. (1974). Assessment of coma and impaired consciousness. A practical scale. *Lancet*, 2(7872), 81–84. Used with permission.

responses to verbal commands or painful stimuli. It is particularly useful for monitoring changes during the acute phase, the first few days after a head injury. It does not take the place of an in-depth neurologic assessment.

Detailed assessments are made initially and at frequent intervals throughout the acute phase of care (Hickey, 2014). Monitoring of ICP is crucial to decision making for patients with neurologic injuries, yet research findings indicate that practices for the measurement of ICP vary widely (Olson,

Rogers, & Stutzman, 2015) (see Chart 68-3). Baseline and ongoing assessments are critical in nursing assessment of the patient with brain injury, whose condition can worsen dramatically and irrevocably if subtle signs are overlooked (Arciniegas, Zasler, Vanderploeg, et al., 2013; Booker, 2015). More information on assessment is provided in the following sections and in Figure 68-4 and Table 68-1.

Diagnosis

NURSING DIAGNOSES

Based on the assessment data, major nursing diagnoses may include the following:

- Ineffective airway clearance and impaired gas exchange related to brain injury
- Risk for ineffective cerebral tissue perfusion related to increased ICP, decreased CPP, and possible seizures
- Deficient fluid volume related to decreased LOC and hormonal dysfunction
- Imbalanced nutrition: less than body requirements related to increased metabolic demands, fluid restriction, and inadequate intake
- Risk for injury (self-directed and directed at others) related to seizures, disorientation, restlessness, or brain damage
- Risk for imbalanced body temperature related to damaged temperature-regulating mechanisms in the brain
- Risk for impaired skin integrity related to bed rest, hemiparesis, hemiplegia, immobility, or restlessness
- Ineffective coping related to brain injury
- Disturbed sleep pattern related to brain injury and frequent neurologic checks
- Risk for dysfunctional family processes related to unresponsiveness of patient, unpredictability of outcome, prolonged recovery period, and the patient's residual physical disability and emotional deficit
- Deficient knowledge about brain injury, recovery, and the rehabilitation process

Chart
68-3

NURSING RESEARCH PROFILE
Validating the Electronic Medical Record for Measuring Increased Intracranial Pressure

Olson, D. M., Rogers, M. S., & Stutzman, S. (2015). Electronic medical record validation: Exploring the reliability of intracranial pressure data abstracted from the electronic medical record-pilot. *Journal of Nursing Measurement*, 23(3), 532–540.

Purpose

The most reliable and valid methods of measuring and documenting intracranial pressure (ICP) monitoring for patients with neurologic injuries are not known. The purpose of this pilot study was to compare different methods of ICP monitoring.

Design

This was a nonrandomized, unblinded, observational study that compared three different technologies. The technologies for recording ICP included pen and paper (P&P), electronic medical record (EMR), and video data with continuous data acquisition (CDA).

Findings

Data were obtained from 11 patients who had ICP monitoring and 26 nurses who provided care to these patients. Patients'

mean age was 50.7 years, 6 (54.4%) were female, and 8 (72.7%) were White (two Black, and one not declared). Patient diagnoses included subarachnoid hemorrhage (six), intracranial hemorrhage (two), neoplasm (two), and one patient with cerebral edema following ischemic stroke. Nurses were primarily baccalaureate prepared (n 22, 84.6%) with a mean of 8.3 (SD 9.8) years of nursing experience and 7.5 (SD 1.7) years of experience in critical care. ICP values did not significantly differ between EMR and P&P records, despite an average of 16 minutes' difference in reporting times. ICP values did vary significantly when comparing CDA data to EMR or paper.

Nursing Implications

This pilot study called into question the validity of ICP values as they are currently recorded. Nurses caring for patients with neurologic injuries need to know that significant practice variation exists and there are no best practice standards for recording ICP. With EMRs becoming pervasive, more nursing research is essential in this area.

Figure 68-4 • Assessment parameters for the patient with a head injury include eye opening and responsiveness (**A**), vital signs (**B**), and motor response reflected in hand strength or response to painful stimulus (**C, D**). Photos by B. Proud.

The nursing diagnoses for the patient who is unconscious and the patient with increased ICP also apply (see Chapter 66).

COLLABORATIVE PROBLEMS/POTENTIAL COMPLICATIONS

Potential complications may include the following:

- Decreased cerebral perfusion
- Cerebral edema and herniation
- Impaired oxygenation and ventilation
- Impaired fluid, electrolyte, and nutritional balance
- Risk of posttraumatic seizures

Planning and Goals

The goals for the patient may include maintenance of a patent airway, adequate CPP, fluid and electrolyte balance, adequate nutritional status, prevention of secondary injury, maintenance of body temperature within normal limits, maintenance of skin integrity, improvement of coping, prevention of sleep deprivation, effective family coping, increased knowledge about the rehabilitation process, and absence of complications.

Nursing Interventions

The nursing interventions for the patient with a TBI are extensive and diverse. They include making nursing assessments, setting priorities for nursing interventions, anticipating needs and complications, and initiating rehabilitation.

MAINTAINING THE AIRWAY

One of the most important nursing goals in the management of head injury is to establish and maintain an adequate airway. The brain is extremely sensitive to hypoxia, and a neurologic deficit can worsen if the patient is hypoxic. Therapy is directed toward maintaining optimal oxygenation to preserve cerebral function. An obstructed airway causes carbon dioxide retention and hypoventilation, which can produce cerebral vessel dilation and increased ICP (McNett & Olson, 2013; Mitchell, Kirkness, & Blissitt, 2015).

Interventions to ensure an adequate exchange of air are discussed in Chapter 66 and include the following:

- Maintaining the patient who is unconscious in a position that facilitates drainage of oral secretions, with the head of the bed elevated about 30 degrees to decrease intracranial venous pressure
- Establishing effective suctioning procedures (pulmonary secretions produce coughing and straining, which increase ICP)
- Guarding against aspiration and respiratory insufficiency
- Closely monitoring arterial blood gas values to assess the adequacy of ventilation. The goal is to keep blood gas values within normal limits to ensure adequate cerebral blood flow.
- Monitoring the patient who is receiving mechanical ventilation for pulmonary complications such as acute respiratory distress syndrome and pneumonia (Hickey, 2014)

TABLE 68-1 Multisystem Assessment Measures for the Patient With Traumatic Brain Injury

System-Specific Considerations	Assessment Data
Neurologic System • Severe TBI results in unconsciousness and alters many neurologic functions. • All body functions must be supported. • Increased ICP and herniation syndromes are life threatening. • Measures are instituted to control elevated ICP.	• Assessment of neurologic status • Assessment for signs and symptoms of ICP elevation • Calculation of cerebral perfusion pressure if ICP monitor is in place • Monitoring of anticonvulsant medication blood levels
Integumentary System (Skin and Mucous Membranes) • Immobility secondary to TBI and unconsciousness contributes to the development of pressure areas and skin breakdown. • Intubation causes irritation of the mucous membrane and deterioration of oral health.	• Assessment of skin integrity and character of the skin • Assessment of oral mucous membrane and oral health
Musculoskeletal System • Immobility contributes to musculoskeletal changes. • Decerebrate or decorticate posturing makes proper positioning difficult.	• Assessment of range of motion of joints and development of deformities or spasticity
Gastrointestinal System • Injury to the GI tract can result in paralytic ileus. • Constipation can result from bed rest, NPO status, fluid restriction, and opioids given for pain control. • Bowel incontinence is related to the patient's unconscious state or altered mental state.	• Assessment of abdomen for bowel sounds and distention • Monitoring for decreased hemoglobin
Genitourinary System • Fluid restriction or the use of diuretic agents can alter the amount of urinary output. • Urinary incontinence is related to the patient's unconscious state.	• Intake and output record
Metabolic (Nutritional) System • The patient receives all fluids IV for the first few days until the GI tract is functioning. • A nutritional consultation is initiated within the first 24–48 hours; parenteral or enteral nutrition may be started.	• Assessment of fluid and electrolyte balance • Recording of weight, if possible • Hematocrit • Electrolyte studies

Respiratory System
• Complete or partial airway obstruction will compromise the oxygen supply to the brain.
• An altered respiratory pattern can result in cerebral hypoxia.
• A short period of apnea at the moment of impact can result in spotty atelectasis.
• Systemic disturbances from head injury can cause hypoxemia.
• Brain injury can alter brainstem respiratory function.
• Shunting of blood to the lungs as a result of a sympathetic discharge at the time of injury can cause neurogenic pulmonary edema.
	• Assessment of respiratory function:
	  • Auscultate chest for breath sounds
	  • Note the respiratory pattern, if possible (not possible if a ventilator is being used)
	  • Note the respiratory rate
	  • Note whether the cough reflex is intact
	• Arterial blood gas levels
	• Complete blood count
	• Chest x-ray studies
	• Sputum cultures
	• Oxygen saturation using pulse oximetry

Cardiovascular System
• The patient may develop cardiac dysrhythmias, tachycardia, or bradycardia.
• The patient may develop hypotension or hypertension.
• Because of immobility and unconsciousness, the patient is at high risk for DVT and PE.
• Fluid and electrolyte imbalance can be related to several problems, including alterations in antidiuretic hormone secretion, the stress response, or fluid restriction.
• Specific conditions may occur:
  • Diabetes insipidus
  • Syndrome of inappropriate secretion of antidiuretic hormone
  • Electrolyte imbalance
  • Hyperglycemic hyperosmolar syndrome
	• Assessment of vital signs
	• Monitoring for cardiac dysrhythmias
	• Assessment for venous thromboembolism including PE and DVT
	• Electrocardiogram
	• Electrolyte studies
	• Blood coagulation studies
	• Blood glucose level
	• Blood acetone level
	• Blood osmolality
	• Urine-specific gravity

Psychological/Emotional Response • The patient with TBI is unconscious. • The family needs emotional support to deal with the crisis.	• Alternative methods of assessment for pain are indicated in the patient who is unconscious (see Chapter 65, Chart 65-2) • Collection of information about the family and the role within the family of the person with head injury • Assessment of the family to determine how functional it was before the injury occurred

TBI, traumatic brain injury; ICP, intracranial pressure; GI, gastrointestinal; NPO, nothing by mouth; IV, intravenous; DVT, deep vein thrombosis; PE, pulmonary embolism.
Adapted from Booker, K. (2015). *Critical care nursing: Monitoring and treatment for advanced nursing practice.* Oxford: Wiley Blackwell.

The patient who is intubated is at high risk for ventilator-associated pneumonia, and providing good oral hygiene can help prevent this complication (Larrow & Klich-Heartt, 2016).

MONITORING NEUROLOGIC FUNCTION

Patients with severe TBI are admitted to the ICU for close assessment and monitoring (cardiac monitoring, pulse oximetry, invasive arterial blood pressure monitoring, end-tidal CO_2, and temperature monitoring). Parameters are assessed initially and as frequently as the patient's condition requires. As soon as the initial assessment is made, the use of a neurologic observational flow record is started and maintained.

The importance of ongoing assessment and monitoring of the patient with brain injury cannot be overstated.

Level of Consciousness. The GCS is used to assess LOC at regular intervals, because changes in the LOC precede all other changes in vital and neurologic signs. The patient's best responses to predetermined stimuli are recorded (see Chart 68-2). Each response is scored (the greater the number, the better the functioning), and the sum of these scores gives an indication of the severity of coma and a prediction of possible outcome. The lowest score is 3 (least responsive); the highest is 15 (most responsive). A GCS score between 3 and 8 is generally accepted as indicating a severe head injury (Bader et al., 2016).

Concept Mastery Alert

The GCS is considered the most sensitive indicator of a lapse in neurologic functioning in patients with TBI and is often the earliest sign of acute change in ICP.

Vital Signs. Although a change in LOC is the most sensitive neurologic indication of deterioration of the patient's condition, vital signs also are monitored at frequent intervals to assess the intracranial status. Table 68-1 depicts the general assessment parameters for the patient with a head injury.

Signs of increasing ICP include slowing of the heart rate (bradycardia), increasing systolic blood pressure, and widening pulse pressure (Cushing reflex). As brain compression increases, respirations become rapid, the blood pressure may decrease, and the pulse slows further. This is an ominous development, as is a rapid fluctuation of vital signs (Hickey, 2014). The temperature is maintained at less than 38°C (100.4°F) (Perez-Barcena, Llompart-Pou, & O'Phelan, 2014). Tachycardia and arterial hypotension may indicate that bleeding is occurring elsewhere in the body.

Concept Mastery Alert

In a patient with a head injury, a rapid increase in body temperature is regarded as unfavorable because hyperthermia increases the metabolic demands of the brain and may indicate brainstem damage—a poor prognostic sign.

Motor Function. Motor function is assessed frequently by observing spontaneous movements, asking the patient to raise and lower the extremities, and comparing the strength and equality of the upper and lower extremities at periodic intervals. To assess upper extremity strength, the nurse instructs the patient to squeeze the examiner's fingers tightly. The nurse assesses lower extremity motor strength by placing the hands on the soles of the patient's feet and asking the patient to push down against the examiner's hands. Examination of the motor system is discussed in more detail in Chapter 65. The presence or absence of spontaneous movement of each extremity is also noted, and speech and eye signs are assessed.

If the patient does not demonstrate spontaneous movement, responses to painful stimuli are assessed (Hickey, 2014). Motor response to pain is assessed by applying a central stimulus, such as pinching the pectoralis major muscle, to determine the patient's best response. Peripheral stimulation may provide inaccurate assessment data because it may result in a reflex movement rather than a voluntary motor response. Abnormal responses (lack of motor response; extension responses) are associated with a poorer prognosis.

Other Neurologic Signs. In addition to the patient's spontaneous eye opening, which is evaluated with the GCS, the size and equality of the pupils and their reaction to light are assessed (Booker, 2015). A unilaterally dilated and poorly responding pupil may indicate a developing hematoma, with subsequent pressure on the third cranial nerve due to shifting of the brain. If both pupils become fixed and dilated, this indicates acute injury and intrinsic damage to the upper brainstem and is a poor prognostic sign (Bader et al., 2016).

The patient with a head injury may develop deficits such as anosmia (lack of sense of smell), eye movement abnormalities, aphasia, memory deficits, and posttraumatic seizures or epilepsy. Patients may be left with residual psychological deficits (impulsiveness; emotional lability; or uninhibited, aggressive behaviors) and, as a consequence of the impairment, may lack insight into their emotional responses.

MONITORING FLUID AND ELECTROLYTE BALANCE

Brain damage can produce metabolic and hormonal dysfunctions. The monitoring of serum electrolyte levels is important, especially in patients receiving osmotic diuretics, those with syndrome of inappropriate antidiuretic hormone (SIADH) secretion, and those with posttraumatic diabetes insipidus.

Serial studies of blood and urine electrolytes and osmolality are carried out because head injuries may be accompanied by disorders of sodium regulation. Hyponatremia is common after head injury due to shifts in extracellular fluid, electrolytes, and volume. Hyperglycemia, for example, can cause an increase in extracellular fluid that lowers sodium. Hypernatremia may also occur as a result of sodium retention that may last several days, followed by sodium diuresis. Increasing lethargy, confusion, and seizures may be the result of electrolyte imbalance.

Endocrine function is evaluated by monitoring serum electrolytes, blood glucose values, and intake and output. Urine is tested regularly for acetone. A record of daily weights is maintained, especially if the patient has hypothalamic involvement and is at risk for the development of diabetes insipidus.

PROMOTING ADEQUATE NUTRITION

Head injury results in metabolic changes that increase calorie consumption and nitrogen excretion. Protein demand increases. Early initiation of nutritional therapy has been shown to improve outcomes in patients with head injury. Patients with brain injury are assumed to be catabolic, and nutritional support consultation should be considered as soon as the patient is admitted. Parenteral nutrition via a central line or enteral feedings given via a nasogastric or nasojejunal feeding tube should be considered, though enteral is the preferred route (Hickey, 2014). If CSF rhinorrhea occurs or if there is any suspicion of disruption to the skull base, an oral feeding tube should be inserted instead of a nasal tube.

Laboratory values should be monitored closely in patients receiving parenteral nutrition. Elevating the head of the bed can help prevent distention, regurgitation, and aspiration. A continuous-drip infusion or pump may be used to regulate the feeding. Enteral or parenteral feedings are usually continued until the swallowing reflex returns and the patient can meet caloric requirements orally. See Chapter 45 for the principles and technique of enteral feedings.

PREVENTING INJURY

Often, as the patient emerges from coma, a period of lethargy and stupor is followed by a period of agitation. Each phase is variable and depends on the person, the location of the injury, the depth and duration of coma, and the patient's age. Restlessness may be caused by hypoxia, fever, pain, or a full bladder. It may indicate injury to the brain but may also be a sign that the patient is regaining consciousness. (Some restlessness may be beneficial because the lungs and extremities are exercised.) Agitation may also be the result of discomfort from catheters, IV lines, restraints, and repeated neurologic checks. Alternatives to restraints must be used whenever possible.

Strategies to prevent injury include the following:

- Assessing the patient to ensure that oxygenation is adequate and the bladder is not distended. Dressings and casts are checked for constriction
- Using padded side rails or wrapping the patient's hands in mitts to protect the patient from self-injury and dislodging of tubes. Restraints are used judiciously, because straining against them can increase ICP or cause other injury. Enclosed or floor-level specialty beds may be indicated (see Chart 68-4)
- Avoiding opioids as a means of controlling restlessness, because they depress respiration, constrict the pupils, and alter responsiveness
- Reducing environmental stimuli by keeping the room quiet, limiting visitors, speaking calmly, and providing frequent orientation information (e.g., explaining where the patient is and what is being done)
- Providing adequate lighting to prevent visual hallucinations

- Minimizing disruption of the patient's sleep–wake cycles
- Lubricating the patient's skin with oil or emollient lotion to prevent irritation due to rubbing against the sheet
- Using an external sheath catheter for a male patient if incontinence occurs. Because prolonged use of an indwelling catheter inevitably produces infection, the patient may be placed on an intermittent catheterization schedule.

MAINTAINING BODY TEMPERATURE

Fever in the patient with a TBI can be the result of damage to the hypothalamus, cerebral irritation from hemorrhage, or infection. The nurse monitors the patient's temperature every 2 to 4 hours. If the temperature increases, efforts are made to identify the cause and to control it using acetaminophen and cooling devices to maintain normothermia (Madden & DeVon, 2015; Wilson & DellaPenna, 2015). Cooling devices should be used with caution so as not to induce shivering, which increases ICP. If infection is suspected, potential sites of infection are cultured and antibiotic agents are prescribed and given. Research about intentional hypothermia for patients with TBI suggests there is no clear evidence to guide therapy (Madden & DeVon, 2015; Wilson & DellaPenna, 2015).

MAINTAINING SKIN INTEGRITY

Patients with TBI often require assistance in turning and positioning because of immobility or unconsciousness. Prolonged pressure on the tissues decreases circulation and leads to tissue necrosis. Potential areas of breakdown need to be identified early to avoid the development of pressure ulcers. Specific nursing measures include the following:

- Assessing all body surfaces and documenting skin integrity every 8 hours
- Turning and repositioning the patient every 2 hours (Larrow & Klich-Heartt, 2016)
- Providing skin care every 4 hours
- Assisting the patient to get out of bed to a chair three times a day

IMPROVING COPING

Although many patients with head injury survive because of resuscitative and supportive technology, they frequently have ineffective coping due to cognitive sequelae. Cognitive

---

Chart 68-4 ⚖ ETHICAL DILEMMA
When is it Appropriate to Use Restraints?

Case Scenario

You work as a staff nurse on a rehabilitation unit. A 23-year-old man is admitted to the unit with a brain injury, which occurred as a result of a motorcycle crash. His severe brain injuries caused cerebral hypoxia and ischemia to occur. He has periods of severe agitation, has fallen out of bed twice, and an enclosed bed has been prescribed for his safety.

Discussion

Nurses must weigh carefully the risks of limiting autonomy and increasing the risks of injury by using restraints against the risks of injury if not using restraints, which have been documented as resulting in physical harm and death.

Analysis

- Describe the ethical principles that are in conflict in this case (see Chapter 3, Chart 3-3). Which principle should have pre-eminence when a treatment plan is devised for this patient?
- What are your professional obligations in this case? What steps might you take to ensure that the patient's autonomy is preserved?

Resources

See Chapter 3, Chart 3-6 for ethics resources.

impairment includes memory deficits; decreased ability to focus and sustain attention to a task (distractibility); impulsivity; egocentricity; and slowness in thinking, perceiving, communicating, reading, and writing. Psychiatric, emotional, and relationship problems develop in many patients after head injury. Resulting psychosocial, behavioral, emotional, and cognitive impairments are devastating to the family as well as to the patient (Tam, McKay, Sloan, et al., 2015).

These problems require collaboration among many disciplines. A neuropsychologist (specialist in evaluating and treating cognitive problems) plans a program and initiates therapy or counseling to help the patient reach maximal potential. Cognitive rehabilitation activities help the patient devise new problem-solving strategies. The retraining is carried out over an extended period and may include the use of sensory stimulation and reinforcement, behavior modification, reality orientation, computer training programs, and video games. Assistance from many disciplines is necessary during this phase of recovery. Even if intellectual ability does not improve, social and behavioral abilities may improve.

The patient recovering from a TBI may experience fluctuations in the level of cognitive function, with orientation, attention, and memory frequently affected. Many types of sensory stimulation programs have been tried, and research on these programs is ongoing (Hickey, 2014). When pushed to a level greater than the impaired cortical functioning allows, the patient may show symptoms of fatigue, anger, and stress (headache, dizziness). The Rancho Los Amigos Scale: Levels of Cognitive Functioning is frequently used to assess cognitive function and evaluate ongoing recovery from head injury. Progress through the levels of cognitive function can vary widely for individual patients (Hagen, Malkmus, & Durham, 1972). Nursing management and a description of each level are included in Table 68-2.

PREVENTING SLEEP PATTERN DISTURBANCE

Patients who require frequent monitoring of neurologic status may experience sleep deprivation as they are awakened hourly for assessment of LOC. To allow the patient longer times of uninterrupted sleep and rest, the nurse can group nursing care activities so that the patient is disturbed less frequently. Environmental noise is decreased, and the room lights are dimmed. Measures to increase comfort may promote sleep and rest (Giusti, Tuteri, & Mirella, 2016).

SUPPORTING FAMILY COPING

Having a loved one sustain a TBI produces a great deal of stress in the family. This stress can result from the patient's physical and emotional deficits, the unpredictable outcome, and altered family relationships. Families report difficulties in coping with changes in the patient's temperament, behavior, and personality (Tam et al., 2015). Such changes are associated with disruption in family cohesion, loss of leisure pursuits, and loss of work capacity, as well as social isolation of the caretaker. The family may experience marital disruption, anger, grief, guilt, and denial in recurring cycles.

To promote effective coping, the nurse can ask the family how the patient is different now, what has been lost, and what is most difficult about coping with this situation. Helpful interventions include providing family members with accurate and honest information and encouraging them to continue to set well-defined short-term goals. Family coun-

seling helps address the family members' acute feelings of loss and helplessness and gives them guidance for the management of inappropriate behaviors. Support groups help the family members share problems, develop insight, gain information, network, and gain assistance in maintaining realistic expectations, hope, and a good quality of life (Tam et al., 2015).

The Brain Injury Association of America (see the Resources section) serves as a clearinghouse for information and resources for patients with head injuries and their families, including specific information on coma, rehabilitation, behavioral consequences of head injury, and family issues. This organization can provide names of facilities and professionals who work with patients with head injuries and can assist families in organizing local support groups.

Many patients with severe head injury die of their injuries, and many of those who survive experience long-term disabilities that prevent them from resuming their previous roles and functions. During the most acute phase of injury, family members need factual information and support from the health care team.

Many patients with severe head injuries that result in brain death are young and otherwise healthy and are therefore considered for organ donation. Family members of patients with such injuries need support during this extremely stressful time and assistance in making decisions to end life support and permit donation of organs. They need to know that the patient who is brain dead and whose respiratory and cardiovascular systems are maintained through life support is not going to survive and that the severe head injury, not the removal of the patient's organs or the removal of life support, is the cause of the patient's death. Bereavement counselors and members of the organ procurement team are often very helpful to family members in making decisions about organ donation and in helping them cope with stress.

MONITORING AND MANAGING POTENTIAL COMPLICATIONS

Decreased Cerebral Perfusion Pressure. Maintenance of adequate CPP is important to prevent serious complications of head injury due to decreased cerebral perfusion. Adequate CPP is greater than 50 mm Hg. If CPP falls below a patient's threshold, a vasodilating cascade occurs, causing the volume of blood to increase inside the brain, which causes ICP to increase. Measures to maintain adequate CPP are essential because a decrease in CPP can impair cerebral perfusion and cause brain hypoxia and ischemia, leading to permanent brain damage. Once the threshold CPP is reached, vasoconstriction of the cerebral blood vessels occurs, causing ICP to decrease. Therapy (e.g., elevation of the head of the bed, increased IV fluids, CSF drainage) is directed toward decreasing cerebral edema and increasing venous outflow from the brain. Systemic hypotension, which causes vasoconstriction and a significant decrease in CPP, is treated with increased IV fluids or vasopressors (Griesdale, Ortenwall, Norena, et al., 2015; Perez-Barcena et al., 2014).

Cerebral Edema and Herniation. The patient with a head injury is at risk for additional complications such as increased ICP and brainstem herniation. Cerebral edema is the most common cause of increased ICP in the patient with a head injury, with the swelling peaking approximately 48 to 72 hours after injury. Bleeding also may increase the volume

TABLE 68-2 Rancho Los Amigos Scale: Levels of Cognitive Function

Cognitive Level	Description	Nursing Management
For levels I–III, the key approach is to *provide stimulation*.		
I: No response	Completely unresponsive to all stimuli, including painful stimuli	Multiple modalities of sensory input should be used. Examples are listed here, but management should be individualized and expanded based on available materials and patient preferences (determined by obtaining information from the family).
II: Generalized response	Nonpurposeful response; responds to pain but in a nonpurposeful manner	*Olfactory:* Perfumes, flowers, shaving lotion. *Visual:* Family pictures, card, personal items.
III: Localized response	Responses more focused—withdraws to pain; turns toward sound; follows moving objects that pass within visual field; pulls on sources of discomfort (e.g., tubes, restraints); may follow simple commands but inconsistently and in a delayed manner	*Auditory:* Radio, television, tapes of family voices or favorite recordings, talking to patient (nurse, family members). The nurse should tell patient what is going to be done, discuss the environment, provide encouragement. *Tactile:* Touching of skin, rubbing various textures on skin *Movement:* Range-of-motion exercises, turning, repositioning, the use of water mattress.
For levels IV–VI, the key approach is to *provide structure.*		
IV: Confused, agitated response	Alert, hyperactive state in which patient responds to internal confusion/agitation; behavior nonpurposeful in relation to the environment; aggressive, bizarre behavior common	For level IV, which lasts 2–4 weeks, interventions are directed at decreasing agitation, increasing environmental awareness, and promoting safety. • Approach patient in a calm manner, and use a soft voice. • Screen patient from environmental stimuli (e.g., sounds, sights); provide a quiet, controlled environment. • Remove devices that contribute to agitation (e.g., tubes), if possible. • Functional goals cannot be set because the patient is unable to cooperate.
V: Confused, inappropriate response	When agitation occurs, it is the result of external rather than internal stimuli; focused attention is difficult; memory is severely impaired; responses are fragmented and inappropriate to the situation; there is no carryover of learning from one situation to the other	For levels V and VI, interventions are directed at decreasing confusion, improving cognitive function, and improving independence in performing ADLs. • Provide supervision. • Use repetition and cues to educate about ADLs. Focus the patient's attention, and help to increase their concentration. • Help the patient organize activity. • Clarify misinformation and reorient when confused. • Provide a consistent, predictable schedule (e.g., post daily schedule on large poster board).
VI: Confused, appropriate response	Follows simple directions consistently but is inconsistently oriented to time and place; short-term memory worse than long-term memory; can perform some ADLs	
For levels VII–X, the key approach is *integration into the community*.		
VII: Automatic, appropriate response	Appropriately responsive and oriented within the hospital setting; needs little supervision in ADLs; some carryover of learning; patient has superficial insight into disabilities; has decreased judgment and problem-solving abilities; lacks realistic planning for future	For levels VII–X, interventions are directed at increasing the patient's ability to function with minimal or no supervision in the community. • Reduce environmental structure. • Help the patient plan for adapting ADLs for self into the home environment. • Discuss and adapt home-living skills (e.g., cleaning, cooking) to patient's ability. • Provide standby assistance, as needed, for ADLs and home-living skills.
VIII: Purposeful, appropriate	Alert, oriented, intact memory; has realistic goals for the future. Able to complete familiar tasks for 1 hour in a distracting environment; overestimates or underestimates abilities, argumentative, easily frustrated, self-centered; uncharacteristically dependent/independent	
IX: Purposeful, appropriate	Independently shifts back and forth between tasks and completes them accurately for at least 2 consecutive hours; uses assistive memory devices to recall schedule and activities; aware of and acknowledges impairments and disabilities when they interfere with task completion; depression may continue; may be easily irritable and have a low frustration tolerance	• Provide assistance on request for adapting ADLs and home-living skills.

(continued on page 2046)

TABLE 68-2 Rancho Los Amigos Scale: Levels of Cognitive Function (continued)

Cognitive Level	Description	Nursing Management
X: Purposeful, appropriate	Able to handle multiple tasks simultaneously in all environments but may require periodic breaks; independently initiates and carries out familiar and unfamiliar tasks but may require more than usual amount of time and/or compensatory strategies to complete them; accurately estimates abilities and independently adjusts to task demands; periodic periods of depression may occur; irritability and low frustration tolerance when sick, fatigued, and/or under stress	• Monitor for signs and symptoms of depression. • Help the patient plan, anticipate concerns, and solve problems.

ADLs, activities of daily living.
Adapted from Los Amigos Research and Education Institute, Inc., Downey, CA, 2002. Used with permission.

of contents within the rigid, closed compartment of the skull, causing increased ICP and herniation of the brainstem and resulting in irreversible brain anoxia and brain death (Hickey, 2014; Perez-Barcena et al., 2014). Measures to control ICP are listed in Chart 68-5 and discussed in Chapter 66.

Impaired Oxygenation and Ventilation. Impaired oxygen and ventilation may require mechanical ventilatory support. The patient must be monitored for a patent airway, altered breathing patterns, and hypoxemia and pneumonia. Interventions may include endotracheal intubation, mechanical ventilation, and positive end-expiratory pressure. See Chapters 21 and 66 for a detailed discussion of these topics.

Impaired Fluid, Electrolyte, and Nutritional Balance. Fluid, electrolyte, and nutritional imbalances are common in the patient with a head injury. Common imbalances include hyponatremia, which is often associated with SIADH (see Chapters 13 and 52), hypokalemia, and hyperglycemia. Modifications in fluid intake with tube feedings or IV fluids, including hypertonic saline, may be necessary to treat these imbalances (Hickey, 2014). Insulin administration may be prescribed to treat hyperglycemia; blood glucose levels are maintained between 80 and 160 mg/dL (Perez-Barcena et al., 2014).

Undernutrition is also a common problem in response to the increased metabolic needs associated with severe head injury. Decisions about early feeding should be individualized; options include IV hyperalimentation or placement of a feeding tube (jejunal or gastric). Caloric expenditure can increase up to 120% to 140% with TBI, requiring close monitoring of nutritional status, with a higher concentration of protein if tolerated (Horn, Kinikini, Moore, et al., 2015).

Posttraumatic Seizures. Patients with head injury are at an increased risk for posttraumatic seizures. Posttraumatic seizures are classified as immediate (within 24 hours after injury), early (within 1 to 7 days after injury), or late (more than 7 days after injury) (Hickey, 2014). Seizure prophylaxis is the practice of administering anticonvulsant medications to patients with head injury to prevent seizures. It is important to prevent posttraumatic seizures, especially in the immediate and early phases of recovery, because seizures may increase ICP and decrease oxygenation (Zaman, Dubiel, Driver, et al., 2017). However, many anticonvulsant medications impair cognitive performance and can prolong the duration of rehabilitation. Therefore, the overall benefits of these medications must be weighed against their side effects. Research evidence supports the use of prophylactic anticonvulsant agents to prevent immediate and early seizures after head injury, but not for prevention of late seizures (Hickey, 2014; Zaman et al., 2017). See Chapter 66 for the nursing management of seizures.

PROMOTING HOME, COMMUNITY-BASED, AND TRANSITIONAL CARE

Educating Patients About Self-Care. Education early in the course of head injury often focuses on reinforcing information given to the family about the patient's condition and prognosis. As the patient's status and expected outcome change over time, family education may focus on interpretation and explanation of changes in the patient's physical and psychological responses.

Once the patient's physical status allows discharge to home, a rehabilitation center, or a subacute care facility, the patient and family are educated about limitations that can be expected and complications that may occur. The nurse explains to the patient and family, verbally and in writing, how to monitor for complications that merit contacting the primary provider. Depending on the patient's prognosis and physical and cognitive status, the patient may be included in education about self-care management strategies.

Chart 68-5

Controlling ICP in Patients With Severe Brain Injury

• Elevate the head of the bed as prescribed.
• Maintain the patient's head and neck in neutral alignment (no twisting or flexing the neck).
• Initiate measures to prevent the Valsalva maneuver (e.g., stool softeners).
• Maintain body temperature within normal limits.
• Administer oxygen (O_2) to maintain partial pressure of arterial oxygen (PaO_2) >90 mm Hg.
• Maintain fluid balance with normal saline solution.
• Avoid noxious stimuli (e.g., excessive suctioning, painful procedures).
• Administer sedation to reduce agitation.
• Maintain cerebral perfusion pressure of 50–70 mm Hg.

Adapted from Bader, M. K., Littlejohns, L. R., & Olson, D. (2016). *AANN core curriculum for neuroscience nursing.* (6th ed.). Chicago, IL: American Association of Neuroscience Nurses.

If the patient is at risk for late posttraumatic seizures, anticonvulsant medications may be prescribed at discharge. The patient and family require education about the side effects of these medications and the importance of continuing to take them as prescribed.

Continuing and Transitional Care. The rehabilitation phase of care for the patient with a TBI begins at hospital admission. Admission to the rehabilitation unit is a milestone in a patient's recovery and requires intense work by the patient to complete the daily schedule of therapies. The goals of rehabilitation are to maximize the patient's ability to return to their highest level of functioning and to their home and the community, address concerns before discharge for a smooth transition to home or rehabilitation, and promote independence with adaptation to deficits. The patient is encouraged to continue the rehabilitation program after discharge, because improvement in status may continue 3 or more years after injury. Changes in the patient with a TBI and the effects of long-term rehabilitation on the family and their coping abilities need ongoing assessment. Continued education and support of the patient and family are essential as their needs and the patient's status change. Education to address with the family of the patient who is about to return home is described in Chart 68-6.

Depending on status, the patient is encouraged to return to usual activities gradually. Referral to support groups and to the Brain Injury Association of America may be warranted (see the Resources section).

During the acute and rehabilitation phases of care, the focus of education is on obvious needs, issues, deficits, and complications. Complications after TBI include infections (e.g., pneumonia, urinary tract infection [UTI], sepsis, wound infection, osteomyelitis, meningitis, ventriculitis, brain abscess) and heterotopic ossification (painful bone overgrowth in weight-bearing joints).

The nurse needs to remind the patient and family of the need for continuing health promotion and screening practices after the initial phase of care. Patients who have not been involved in these practices in the past are educated about their importance and are referred to appropriate health care providers.

Evaluation

Expected patient outcomes may include:

1. Attains or maintains effective airway clearance, ventilation, and brain oxygenation
   a. Achieves blood gas values within normal limits and has breath sounds clear on auscultation
   b. Mobilizes and clears secretions
2. Achieves satisfactory fluid and electrolyte balance
   a. Demonstrates serum electrolytes within normal limits
   b. Has no clinical signs of dehydration or overhydration
3. Attains adequate nutritional status
   a. Is free of gastric distention and vomiting
   b. Shows minimal weight loss
4. Avoids injury
   a. Shows lessening agitation and restlessness
   b. Is oriented to person, place, and time
5. Maintains body temperature within normal limits
   a. Absence of fever
   b. Absence of hypothermia
6. Demonstrates intact skin integrity
   a. Exhibits no redness or breaks in skin integrity
   b. Exhibits no pressure ulcers
7. Shows improvement in coping
8. Demonstrates usual sleep–wake cycle
9. Family demonstrates adaptive family processes
   a. Joins support group
   b. Shares feelings with appropriate health care personnel
   c. Makes end-of-life decisions, if needed

Chart 68-6

HOME CARE CHECKLIST

The Patient With a TBI

At the completion of education, the patient and/or caregiver will be able to:

- State the impact of TBI and treatment on physiologic functioning, ADLs, IADLs, roles, relationships, and spirituality.
- State the purpose, dose, route, schedule, side effects, and precautions for prescribed medications.
- State how to contact all members of the treatment team (e.g., health care providers, home care professionals, rehabilitation team, and durable medical equipment and supply vendor).
- State changes in lifestyle (e.g., ADLs, IADLs, activity) necessary for recovery and health maintenance, as applicable.
  - Demonstrate safe techniques to assist patient with self-care, hygiene, and ambulation.
  - Demonstrate safe techniques for eating, feeding patient, or assisting patient with eating.
  - Identify need for close monitoring of behavior due to changes in cognitive functioning.
  - Describe strategies for reinforcing positive behaviors.
  - Describe household modifications needed to ensure safe environment for the patient.
- Explain the need for monitoring for changes in neurologic status and for complications.

- Identify changes in neurologic status and signs and symptoms of complications (e.g., pneumonia, urinary tract infection, meningitis) that should be reported to the neurosurgeon or nurse.
- Relate how to reach primary provider with questions or complications.
- State importance of continuing follow-up by health care team.
- State time and date of follow-up medical appointments, therapy, and testing.
- Identify sources of support (e.g., friends, relatives, faith community, brain injury support groups, caregiver support).
- Identify the need for health-promotion, disease prevention, and screening activities.

Resources

See Chapter 9, Chart 9-9 Home Care Checklist: Managing Chronic Illness and Disability at Home and Chapter 10, Chart 10-8 Home Care Checklist: Managing the Therapeutic Regimen for additional information.

TBI, traumatic brain injury; ADL, activities of daily living; IADL, independent activities of daily living.

10. Demonstrates absence of complications
    a. Demonstrates ICP within normal limits
    b. Exhibits vital signs and body temperature within normal limits and increases orientation to person, place, and time
11. Experiences no posttraumatic seizures
    a. Takes anticonvulsant medications as prescribed
    b. Identifies side effects/adverse effects of anticonvulsant medications
12. Participates in rehabilitation process as indicated for patient and family members
    a. Takes active role in identifying rehabilitation goals and participating in recommended patient care activities
    b. Prepares for discharge

Spinal Cord Injury

Spinal cord injury (SCI), an injury to the spinal cord, vertebral column, supporting soft tissue, or intervertebral discs caused by trauma is a major health disorder. In the United States in 2014, approximately 276,000 persons were living with a disability from SCI. An estimated 17,000 new cases occur annually; common causes are motor vehicle crashes, falls, violence (predominantly gunshot wounds), and sports-related injuries (National Spinal Cord Injury Statistical Center [NSCISC], 2016). Males account for 80% of patients with SCI. The average age of injury has increased from 29 years of age in the 1970s to 42 years in 2010 (NSCISC, 2016). The cost for care of patients with SCI approaches $3 billion every year. Based on 2015 dollars, the cost of lifetime care for a 25-year-old patient with SCI was estimated to approach $4.7 million (NSCISC, 2016). Though tremendous advances have improved the life expectancy of patients with SCI, it still remains lower than that of the general population, particularly during the first year postinjury, as well as for patients who sustain severe SCI (NSCISC, 2016).

The predominant risk factors for SCI include younger age, male gender, and alcohol and drug use (Bader et al., 2016). The frequency with which these risk factors are associated with SCI serves to emphasize the importance of primary prevention. The same interventions suggested earlier in this chapter for head injury prevention help decrease the incidence of SCI (see Chart 68-1). Life expectancy continues to increase for people with SCI because of improved health care but remains slightly lower than for those without SCI. The major causes of death are pneumonia, pulmonary embolism (PE), and sepsis (Hickey, 2014).

Paraplegia (paralysis of the lower body) and **tetraplegia** (paralysis of all four extremities; formerly called *quadriplegia*) can occur, with incomplete tetraplegia being the most frequently occurring injury, followed by complete paraplegia, complete tetraplegia, and incomplete paraplegia.

Pathophysiology

Damage in SCI ranges from transient concussion (from which the patient fully recovers) to contusion, laceration, and compression of the spinal cord tissue (either alone or in combination), to complete **transection** (severing) of the spinal cord

(which renders the patient paralyzed below the level of the injury). The vertebrae most frequently involved are the 5th, 6th, and 7th cervical vertebrae (C5–C7), the 12th thoracic vertebra (T12), and the 1st lumbar vertebra (L1). These vertebrae are most susceptible because there is a greater range of mobility in the vertebral column in these areas (Hickey, 2014).

SCIs can be separated into two categories: primary injuries and secondary injuries. Primary injuries are the result of the initial insult or trauma and are usually permanent. Secondary injuries resulting from SCI include edema and hemorrhage (Bader et al., 2016; Mohit, 2016). The secondary injury is a major concern for critical care nurses. Early treatment is essential to prevent partial damage from becoming total and permanent.

Clinical Manifestations

Manifestations of SCI depend on the type and level of injury (see Chart 68-7). The type of injury refers to the extent of injury to the spinal cord itself. A **complete spinal cord lesion** signifies loss of both sensory and voluntary motor communication from the brain to the periphery, resulting in paraplegia or tetraplegia (Bader et al., 2016). **Incomplete spinal cord lesion** denotes that the ability of the spinal cord to relay messages to and from the brain is not completely absent. Sensory and/or motor fibers are preserved below the lesion. Injuries are classified according to the area of spinal cord damage: central, lateral, anterior, or peripheral (see Chart 68-7).

The American Spinal Injury Association (ASIA) provides classification of SCI according to the degree of sensory and motor function present after injury (see Fig. 68-5; ASIA, 2016). The neurologic level refers to the lowest level at which sensory and motor functions are intact. Below the neurologic level, there may be total or partial, sensory and/or motor paralysis (dependent upon affected tracts), loss of bladder and bowel control (usually with urinary retention and bladder distention), loss of sweating and vasomotor tone, and marked reduction of blood pressure from loss of peripheral vascular resistance.

If conscious, the patient usually complains of acute pain in the back or neck, which may radiate along the involved nerve. However, absence of pain does not rule out spinal injury, and a careful assessment of the spine should be conducted if there has been a significant force and mechanism of injury (i.e., concomitant head injury).

Respiratory dysfunction is related to the level of injury. The muscles contributing to respiration are the diaphragm (C4), intercostals (T1–T6), and abdominals (T6–T12). Injuries at C4 or above (causing paralysis of the diaphragm) often will require ventilator support, since acute respiratory failure is a leading cause of death (Hickey, 2014). Injuries of T12 and above will have impact on respiratory function. Functional abilities by level of injury are described in Table 68-3.

Assessment and Diagnostic Findings

A detailed neurologic examination is performed. Diagnostic x-rays (lateral cervical spine x-rays) and CT scanning are usually performed initially. An MRI scan may be ordered as a further workup if a ligamentous injury is suspected, because significant spinal cord damage may exist even in the absence

Chart 68-7 Effects of Spinal Cord Injuries

Central Cord Syndrome

- *Characteristics:* Motor deficits (in the upper extremities compared to the lower extremities; sensory loss varies but is more pronounced in the upper extremities); bowel/bladder dysfunction is variable, or function may be completely preserved.
- *Cause:* Injury or edema of the central cord, usually of the cervical area. May be caused by hyperextension injuries.

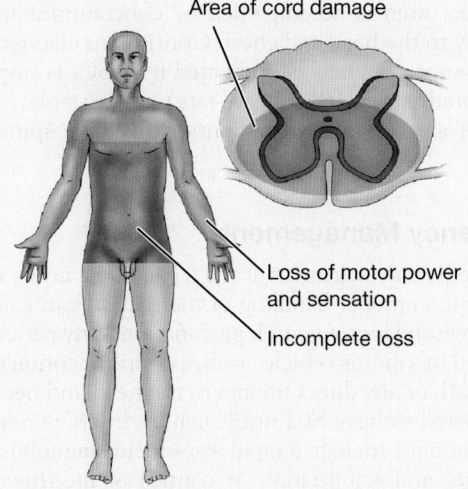

Central cord syndrome

Anterior Cord Syndrome

- *Characteristics:* Loss of pain, temperature, and motor function is noted below the level of the lesion; light touch, position, and vibration sensation remain intact.
- *Cause:* The syndrome may be caused by acute disc herniation or hyperflexion injuries associated with fracture/dislocation of vertebra. It also may occur as a result of injury to the anterior spinal artery, which supplies the anterior two thirds of the spinal cord.

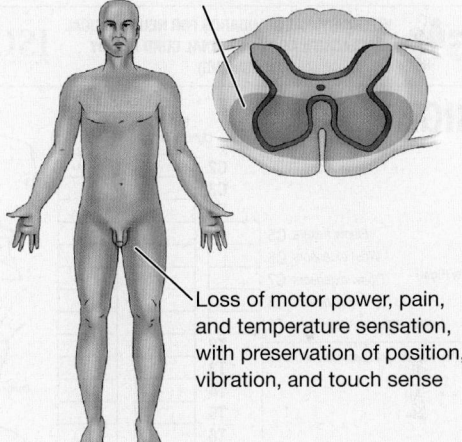

Anterior cord syndrome

Lateral Cord Syndrome (Brown–Séquard Syndrome)

- *Characteristics:* Ipsilateral paralysis or paresis is noted, together with ipsilateral loss of touch, pressure, and vibration and contralateral loss of pain and temperature.
- *Cause:* The lesion is caused by a transverse hemisection of the cord (half of the cord is transected from north to south), usually as a result of a knife or missile injury, fracture/dislocation of a unilateral articular process, or possibly an acute ruptured disc.

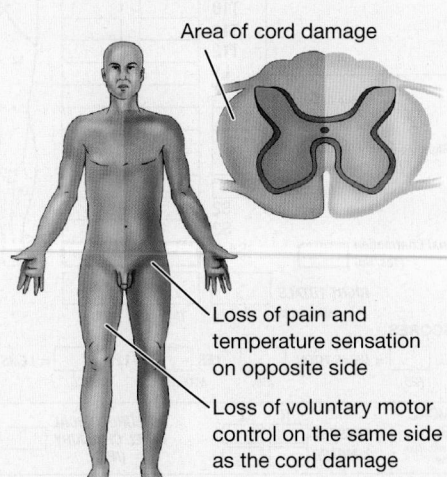

Brown–séquard syndrome

Adapted from Hickey, J. (2014). *The clinical practice of neurological & neurosurgical nursing* (7th ed.). Philadelphia, PA: Lippincott Williams & Wilkins.

of bony injury (Hickey, 2014). If an MRI scan is contraindicated, a myelogram may be used to visualize the spinal axis. An assessment is made for other injuries, because spinal trauma often is accompanied by concomitant injuries, commonly to the head and chest. Continuous electrocardiographic monitoring may be indicated if an SCI is suspected, because bradycardia (slow heart rate) and asystole (cardiac standstill) are common in patients with acute spinal cord injuries.

Emergency Management

The immediate management at the scene of the injury is critical, because improper handling of the patient can cause further damage and loss of neurologic function. Any patient who is involved in a motor vehicle crash, a diving or contact sports injury, a fall, or any direct trauma to the head and neck must be considered to have SCI until such an injury is ruled out. Initial care must include a rapid assessment, immobilization, extrication, and stabilization or control of life-threatening injuries, and transportation to the most appropriate medical facility. Immediate transportation to a trauma center with the capacity to manage major neurologic trauma is then necessary (Hickey, 2014).

At the scene of the injury, the patient must be immobilized on a spinal (back) board, with the head and neck maintained in a neutral position, to prevent an incomplete injury from becoming complete. One member of the team must assume control of the patient's head to prevent flexion, rotation, or extension; this is done by placing the hands on both sides of the patient's head at about ear level to limit movement and maintain alignment while a spinal board and/or cervical immobilizing device is applied. If possible, at least four people should slide the patient carefully onto a board for transfer to the hospital. Head blocks should also be considered, as they will further limit any neck movement. Any twisting movement may irreversibly damage the spinal cord by causing bony fragment or disc movement or exacerbating ligamentous injury, causing further instability (Bader et al., 2016).

The patient is referred to a regional spinal injury or trauma center because of the multidisciplinary personnel and support services required to counteract the destructive

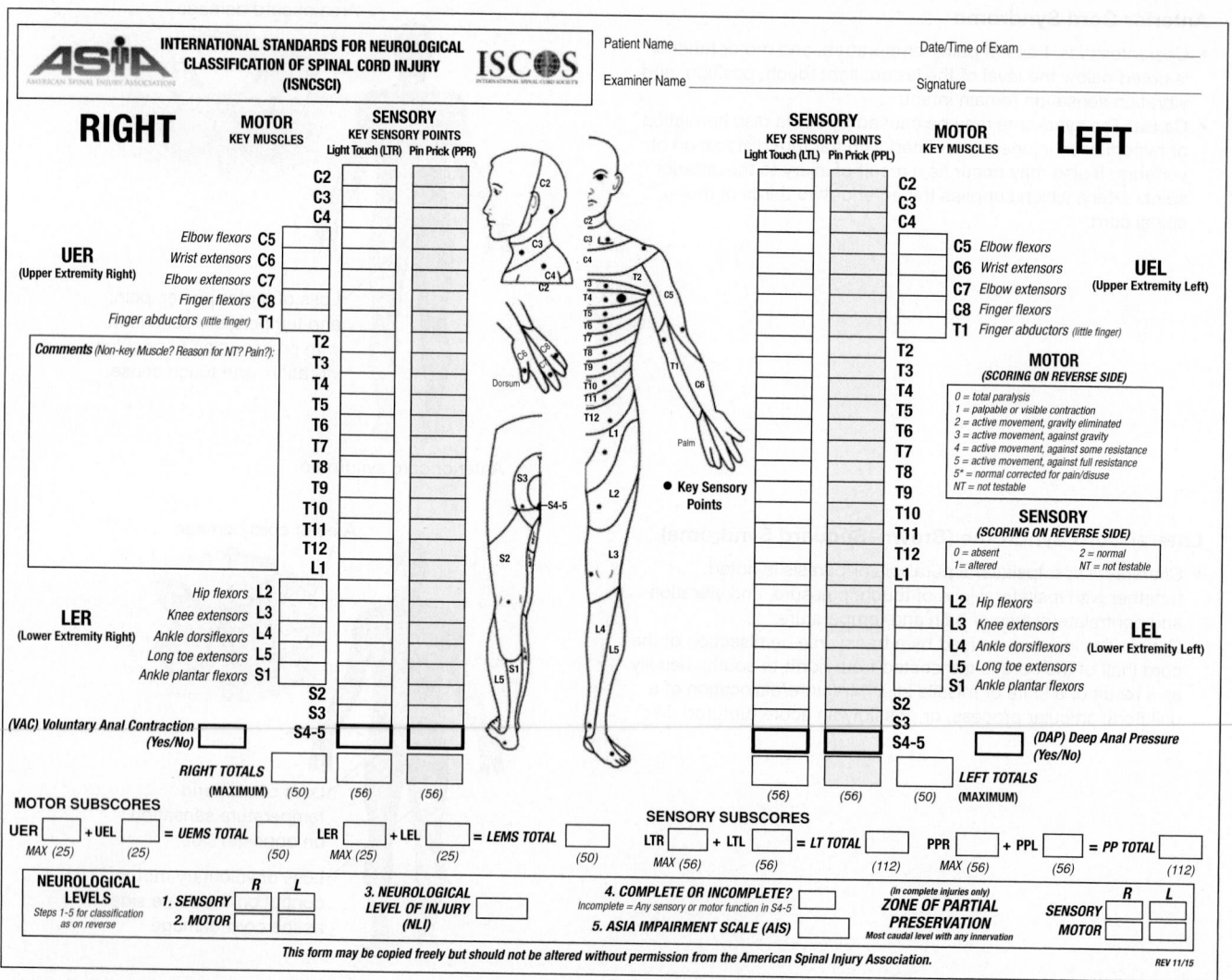

Figure 68-5 • Worksheet for the classification of SCI. Adapted from American Spinal Injury Association (ASIA). (2016). International standards for neurological classification of spinal cord injury. Retrieved on 2/23/17 at: www.asia-spinalinjury.org/wp-content/uploads/2016/02/International_Stds_Diagram_Worksheet.pdf

Muscle Function Grading

0 = total paralysis

1 = palpable or visible contraction

2 = active movement, full range of motion (ROM) with gravity eliminated

3 = active movement, full ROM against gravity

4 = active movement, full ROM against gravity and moderate resistance in a muscle specific position

5 = (normal) active movement, full ROM against gravity and full resistance in a functional muscle position expected from an otherwise unimpaired person

5* = (normal) active movement, full ROM against gravity and sufficient resistance to be considered normal if identified inhibiting factors (i.e. pain, disuse) were not present

NT = not testable (i.e. due to immobilization, severe pain such that the patient cannot be graded, amputation of limb, or contracture of > 50% of the normal ROM)

Sensory Grading

0 = Absent

1 = Altered, either decreased/impaired sensation or hypersensitivity

2 = Normal

NT = Not testable

When to Test Non-Key Muscles:

In a patient with an apparent AIS B classification, non-key muscle functions more than 3 levels below the motor level on each side should be tested to most accurately classify the injury (differentiate between AIS B and C).

Movement	Root level
Shoulder: Flexion, extension, abduction, adduction, internal and external rotation **Elbow:** Supination	C5
Elbow: Pronation **Wrist:** Flexion	C6
Finger: Flexion at proximal joint, extension. **Thumb:** Flexion, extension and abduction in plane of thumb	C7
Finger: Flexion at MCP joint **Thumb:** Opposition, adduction and abduction perpendicular to palm	C8
Finger: Abduction of the index finger	T1
Hip: Adduction	L2
Hip: External rotation	L3
Hip: Extension, abduction, internal rotation **Knee:** Flexion **Ankle:** Inversion and eversion **Toe:** MP and IP extension	L4
Hallux and Toe: DIP and PIP flexion and abduction	L5
Hallux: Adduction	S1

ASIA Impairment Scale (AIS)

A = Complete. No sensory or motor function is preserved in the sacral segments S4-5.

B = Sensory Incomplete. Sensory but not motor function is preserved below the neurological level and includes the sacral segments S4-5 (light touch or pin prick at S4-5 or deep anal pressure) AND no motor function is preserved more than three levels below the motor level on either side of the body.

C = Motor Incomplete. Motor function is preserved at the most caudal sacral segments for voluntary anal contraction (VAC) OR the patient meets the criteria for sensory incomplete status (sensory function preserved at the most caudal sacral segments (S4-S5) by LT, PP or DAP), and has some sparing of motor function more than three levels below the ipsilateral motor level on either side of the body.
(This includes key or non-key muscle functions to determine motor incomplete status.) For AIS C – less than half of key muscle functions below the single NLI have a muscle grade ≥ 3.

D = Motor Incomplete. Motor incomplete status as defined above, with at least half (half or more) of key muscle functions below the single NLI having a muscle grade ≥ 3.

E = Normal. If sensation and motor function as tested with the ISNCSCI are graded as normal in all segments, and the patient had prior deficits, then the AIS grade is E. Someone without an initial SCI does not receive an AIS grade.

Using ND: To document the sensory, motor and NLI levels, the ASIA Impairment Scale grade, and/or the zone of partial preservation (ZPP) when they are unable to be determined based on the examination results.

AMERICAN SPINAL INJURY ASSOCIATION

INTERNATIONAL STANDARDS FOR NEUROLOGICAL CLASSIFICATION OF SPINAL CORD INJURY

ISCOS
INTERNATIONAL SPINAL CORD SOCIETY

Steps in Classification

The following order is recommended for determining the classification of individuals with SCI.

1. Determine sensory levels for right and left sides.
The sensory level is the most caudal, intact dermatome for both pin prick and light touch sensation.

2. Determine motor levels for right and left sides.
Defined by the lowest key muscle function that has a grade of at least 3 (on supine testing), providing the key muscle functions represented by segments above that level are judged to be intact (graded as a 5).
Note: in regions where there is no myotome to test, the motor level is presumed to be the same as the sensory level, if testable motor function above that level is also normal.

3. Determine the neurological level of injury (NLI)
This refers to the most caudal segment of the cord with intact sensation and antigravity (3 or more) muscle function strength, provided that there is normal (intact) sensory and motor function rostrally respectively.
The NLI is the most cephalad of the sensory and motor levels determined in steps 1 and 2.

4. Determine whether the injury is Complete or Incomplete.
(i.e. absence or presence of sacral sparing)
If voluntary anal contraction = **No** AND all S4-5 sensory scores = **0** AND deep anal pressure = **No**, then injury is **Complete.**
Otherwise, injury is **Incomplete.**

5. Determine ASIA Impairment Scale (AIS) Grade:

Is injury Complete? If YES, AIS=A and can record ZPP (lowest dermatome or myotome on each side with some preservation)

NO ↓

Is injury Motor Complete? If YES, AIS=B

NO ↓ (No=voluntary anal contraction OR motor function more than three levels below the motor level on a given side, if the patient has sensory incomplete classification)

Are at least half (half or more) of the key muscles below the neurological level of injury graded 3 or better?

NO ↓   YES ↓

AIS=C   AIS=D

If sensation and motor function is normal in all segments, AIS=E

Note: AIS E is used in follow-up testing when an individual with a documented SCI has recovered normal function. If at initial testing no deficits are found, the individual is neurologically intact; the ASIA Impairment Scale does not apply.

Figure 68-5 • (Continued)

changes that occur in the first 24 hours after injury. During treatment in the emergency and x-ray departments, the patient is kept on the transfer board. The patient must always be maintained in an extended position. No part of the body should be twisted or turned, and the patient is not allowed to sit up. Once the extent of the injury has been determined, the patient may be placed on a rotating specialty bed or in a cervical collar (see Fig. 68-6). Later, if SCI and bone instability have been ruled out, the patient may be moved to a conventional bed or the collar may be removed without harm. If a specialty bed is needed but not available, the patient should be placed in a cervical collar and on a firm mattress.

 ## Medical Management (Acute Phase)

The goals of management are to prevent secondary injury, to observe for symptoms of progressive neurologic deficits, and to prevent complications. The patient is resuscitated as necessary, and oxygenation and cardiovascular stability are maintained. SCI is a devastating event; new treatment methods and medications are continually being investigated for the acute and chronic phases of care (Perez-Barcena et al., 2014; Stocchetti & Maas, 2014).

Pharmacologic Therapy

Administration of high-dose IV corticosteroids (methylprednisolone sodium succinate [Solu-Medrol]) in the first 24 or 48 hours is controversial. The validity of studies has been questioned based on critical analysis of the original and additional data. As a result, there is now a consensus that corticosteroids may offer only a slight benefit. Corticosteroids are no longer considered the standard of care for acute SCI, although some centers continue to use corticosteroid protocols (Hickey, 2014).

Respiratory Therapy

Oxygen is given to maintain a high partial pressure of arterial oxygen (PaO_2), because hypoxemia can create or worsen a neurologic deficit of the spinal cord. If endotracheal intubation is necessary, extreme care is taken to avoid flexing or extending the patient's neck, which can result in extension of a cervical injury.

TABLE 68-3 Functional Abilities by Level of Cord Injury

Injury Level	Segmental Sensorimotor Function	Dressing, Eating	Elimination	Mobility[a]
C1	Little or no sensation or control of head and neck; no diaphragm control; requires continuous ventilation	Dependent	Dependent	Limited. Voice or sip-n-puff controlled electric wheelchair
C2–C3	Head and neck sensation; some neck control; independent of mechanical ventilation for short periods	Dependent	Dependent	Same as for C1
C4	Good head and neck sensation and motor control; some shoulder elevation; diaphragm movement	Dependent; may be able to eat with adaptive sling	Dependent	Limited to voice, mouth, head, chin, or shoulder-controlled electric wheelchair
C5	Full head and neck control; shoulder strength; elbow flexion	Independent with assistance	Maximal assistance	Electric or modified manual wheelchair, needs transfer assistance
C6	Fully innervated shoulder; wrist extension or dorsiflexion	Independent or with minimal assistance	Independent or with minimal assistance	Independent in transfers and wheelchair
C7–C8	Full elbow extension; wrist plantar flexion; some finger control	Independent	Independent	Independent; manual wheelchair
T1–T5	Full hand and finger control; use of intercostal and thoracic muscles	Independent	Independent	Independent; manual wheelchair
T6–T10	Abdominal muscle control, partial to good balance with trunk muscles	Independent	Independent	Independent; manual wheelchair
T11–L5	Hip flexors, hip abductors (L1–L3); knee extension (L2–L4); knee flexion and ankle dorsiflexion (L4–L5)	Independent	Independent	Short distance to full ambulation with assistance
S1–S5	Full leg, foot, and ankle control; innervation of perineal muscles for bowel, bladder, and sexual function (S2–S4)	Independent	Normal to impaired bowel and bladder function	Ambulate independently with or without assistance

[a]*Assistance refers to adaptive equipment, setup, or physical assistance.*
Adapted from Hickey, J. V. (2014). *The clinical practice of neurological & neurosurgical nursing* (7th ed.). Philadelphia, PA: Lippincott Williams & Wilkins.

In high cervical spine injuries, spinal cord innervation to the phrenic nerve, which stimulates the diaphragm, is lost. Diaphragmatic pacing (electrical stimulation of the phrenic nerve) attempts to stimulate the diaphragm to help the patient breathe. Intramuscular diaphragmatic pacing is currently in the clinical trial phase for the patient with a high cervical injury. This is implanted via laparoscopic surgery, usually after the acute phase.

Skeletal Fracture Reduction and Traction

Management of SCI requires immobilization and reduction of dislocations (restoration of preinjury position) and stabilization of the vertebral column. This can be accomplished by surgical and/or nonsurgical interventions; both aim to prevent new or worsening neurologic damage.

Cervical fractures can be reduced, and the cervical spine aligned with some form of skeletal traction, such as with skeletal tongs or with the use of the halo device (Bader et al., 2016). Traction is applied to the skeletal traction device by weights (ensuring the weights are unencumbered); the amount depends on the size of the patient and the degree of fracture displacement (see Fig. 68-7). The traction force is exerted along the longitudinal axis of the vertebral bodies, with the patient's neck in a neutral position. The traction is then gradually increased by adding more weights. As the amount of traction is increased, the spaces between the intervertebral discs widen and the vertebrae are given a chance to slip back into position. Reduction usually occurs after correct alignment has been restored. Once reduction is achieved, as verified by cervical spine x-rays and neurologic examination,

Figure 68-6 • Cervical collar. Used with permission from Aspen Medical Products.

Figure 68-7 • Patient in skeletal traction in a rotating specialty bed. Adapted from Schwartz, E. D., Adam, E., & Flander, S. (2007). *Spinal trauma: Imaging, diagnosis, and management.* Philadelphia, PA: Lippincott Williams & Wilkins.

the weights are gradually removed until the amount of weight needed to maintain the alignment is identified. Traction is sometimes supplemented with manual manipulation of the neck by a surgeon, to help achieve realignment of the vertebral bodies.

A halo device may be used initially with traction or may be applied after removal of the tongs. It consists of a titanium or stainless steel halo ring that is fixed to the skull by four pins, which are inserted into the outer table of the skull. The ring is attached to a removable **halo vest**, a device that suspends the weight of the unit circumferentially around the chest. A frame connects the ring to the chest. Halo devices provide immobilization of the cervical spine while allowing early ambulation (see Fig. 68-8) for patients with adequate function.

Thoracic and lumbar injuries are usually treated with surgical intervention, followed by immobilization with a fitted brace. Traction is often not indicated either before or after surgery, due to the relative stability of the spine in these regions.

> ▶ **Quality and Safety Nursing Alert**
>
> *The patient's vital organ functions and body defenses must be supported and maintained until spinal and neurogenic shock abates and the neurologic system have recovered from the traumatic insult; this can take up to 4 months.*

Surgical Management

Surgery is indicated in any of the following situations:
- Compression of the cord is evident.
- The injury results in a fragmented or unstable vertebral body.
- The injury involves a wound that penetrates the cord.
- Bony fragments are in the spinal canal.
- The patient's neurologic status is deteriorating.

Early surgical stabilization may improve the clinical outcome of patients compared to surgery performed later during

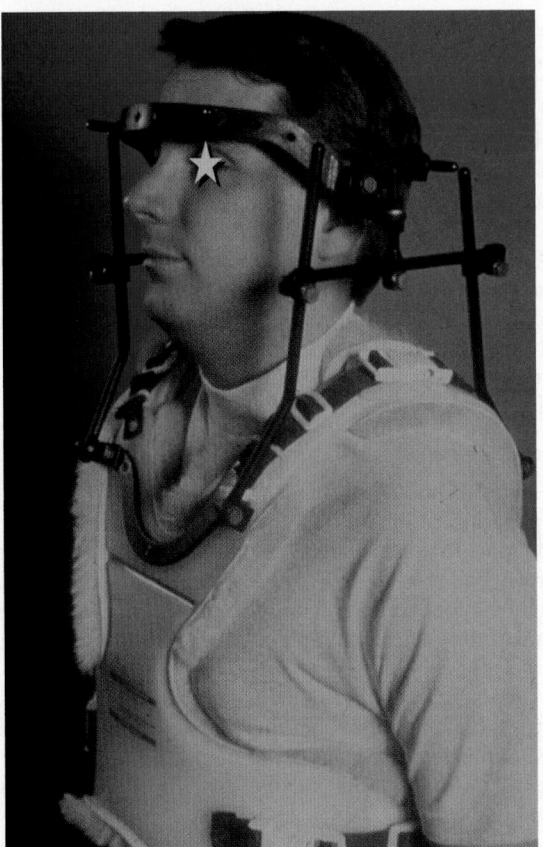

Figure 68-8 • Halo and vest for cervical and thoracic injuries. Adapted from Schwartz, E. D., Adam, E., & Flander, S. (2007). *Spinal trauma: Imaging, diagnosis, and management.* Philadelphia, PA: Lippincott Williams & Wilkins.

the clinical course. The goals of surgical treatment are to preserve neurologic function by removing pressure from the spinal cord and to provide stability.

Management of Acute Complications of Spinal Cord Injury

Spinal and Neurogenic Shock

The spinal shock associated with SCI reflects a sudden depression of reflex activity in the spinal cord (areflexia) below the level of injury. The muscles innervated by the part of the spinal cord segment below the level of the lesion are without sensation, paralyzed, and flaccid, and the reflexes are absent. Blood pressure may be decreased and the patient may be bradycardic. Studies suggest that hypotension and shock can further damage the spinal cord and that the mean arterial pressure (MAP) should be maintained at 85 mm Hg or higher during the hyperacute phase (Jia, Kowalski, Sciubba, et al., 2013). The reflexes that initiate bladder and bowel function are affected. Bowel distention and paralytic ileus can be caused by depression of the reflexes and are treated with intestinal decompression by insertion of a nasogastric tube. A paralytic ileus most often occurs within the first 2 to 3 days after SCI and resolves within 3 to 7 days (Bader et al., 2016).

Neurogenic shock develops as a result of the loss of autonomic nervous system function below the level of the lesion.

The vital organs are affected, causing decreases in blood pressure, heart rate, and cardiac output, as well as venous pooling in the extremities and peripheral vasodilation (Bader et al., 2016). In addition, the patient does not perspire in the paralyzed portions of the body, because sympathetic activity is blocked; therefore, close observation is required for early detection of an abrupt onset of fever. See Chapter 14 for further discussion of neurogenic shock.

With injuries to the cervical and upper thoracic spinal cord, innervation to the major accessory muscles of respiration is lost and respiratory problems develop. These include decreased vital capacity, retention of secretions, increased partial pressure of arterial carbon dioxide ($PaCO_2$) levels and decreased oxygen levels, respiratory failure, and pulmonary edema.

Venous Thromboembolism

The risk of venous thromboembolism (VTE) is a potential complication of immobility and occurs in patients with SCI at the same rate as those having had other types of traumatic injuries (Bader et al., 2016). Patients who develop VTE are at high risk for both deep vein thrombosis (DVT) and PE due to immobility, flaccidity, and decreased vasomotor tone (Jia et al., 2013).

Manifestations of PE include pleuritic chest pain, anxiety, shortness of breath, and abnormal blood gas values (increased $PaCO_2$ and decreased PaO_2). A fatal PE has been reported in up to 2% of patients with SCI within the first 3 months postinjury (Hickey, 2014).

Low-dose anticoagulation therapy usually is initiated to prevent DVT and PE, along with the use of antiembolism stockings or sequential pneumatic compression devices (SCDs). In some cases, permanent indwelling filters (see Chapter 23) may be placed prophylactically in the vena cava to prevent emboli (dislodged clots) from migrating to the lungs and causing PE. Prevention continues into the rehabilitation and chronic phases of SCI care (Abrams & Wakasa, 2014; Jia et al., 2013).

Quality and Safety Nursing Alert

The calves or thighs of a patient who is immobile should never be massaged because of the danger of dislodging an undetected thromboembolus.

Other Complications

In addition to respiratory complications (respiratory failure, pneumonia) and autonomic dysreflexia, other complications that may occur include pressure ulcers and infection (urinary, respiratory, and local infection at the skeletal traction pin sites).

NURSING PROCESS

The Patient With Acute Spinal Cord Injury

Assessment

The patient's breathing pattern and the strength of the cough are assessed and the lungs are auscultated, because paralysis of the diaphragm, in addition to abdominal and respiratory muscles, diminishes coughing and makes clearing of bronchial and pharyngeal secretions difficult. Reduced excursion of the chest also results.

The patient is monitored closely for any changes in motor or sensory function and for symptoms of progressive neurologic damage. In the early stages of SCI, determining whether the cord has been severed may not be possible, because signs and symptoms of cord edema are indistinguishable from those of cord transection. Edema of the spinal cord may occur with any severe cord injury and may further compromise spinal cord function.

Motor and sensory functions are assessed through careful neurologic examination. These findings are recorded on a flow sheet so that changes in the baseline neurologic status can be monitored closely and accurately. The ASIA classification is commonly used to describe the level of function for patients with SCI (see Fig. 68-5). Chart 68-7 also gives examples of the effects of altered spinal cord function. At the minimum:

- Motor ability is tested by asking the patient to spread the fingers, squeeze the examiner's hand, and move the toes or turn the feet.
- Sensation is evaluated by gently pinching the skin or touching it lightly with an object such as a tongue blade, starting at shoulder level and working down both sides of the extremities. The patient should have both eyes closed so that the examination reveals true findings, not what the patient hopes to feel. The patient is asked where the sensation is felt.
- Any decrease in neurologic function is reported immediately.

The patient is also assessed for spinal shock, which is a complete loss of all reflex, motor, sensory, and autonomic activity below the level of the lesion that causes bladder paralysis and distention. The lower abdomen is palpated for signs of urinary retention and overdistention of the bladder. Further assessment is made for gastric dilation and paralytic ileus caused by an atonic bowel, a result of autonomic disruption.

Temperature is monitored because the patient may have periods of hyperthermia as a result of altered temperature control, which is due to the inability to perspire related to autonomic disruption. Body temperature becomes dependent on surroundings (poikilothermia).

Diagnosis

NURSING DIAGNOSES

Based on the assessment data, major nursing diagnoses may include the following:

- Ineffective breathing patterns related to weakness or paralysis of diaphragm, abdominal, and intercostal muscles
- Ineffective airway clearance related to muscle weakness and inability to clear secretions
- Impaired bed and physical mobility related to motor and sensory impairments
- Risk for injury related to motor and sensory impairment
- Risk for impaired skin integrity related to immobility and sensory loss
- Impaired urinary elimination related to inability to void spontaneously
- Constipation related to presence of atonic bowel as a result of autonomic disruption

- Acute pain related to treatment and prolonged immobility
- Autonomic dysreflexia related to uninhibited sympathetic response of the nervous system following SCI

COLLABORATIVE PROBLEMS/POTENTIAL COMPLICATIONS

Potential complications may include the following:

- VTE
- Orthostatic hypotension

Planning and Goals

The goals for the patient may include improved breathing pattern and airway clearance, improved mobility, prevention of injury due to sensory impairment, maintenance of skin integrity, relief of urinary retention, improved bowel function, decreasing pain, early recognition of autonomic dysreflexia, and absence of complications.

Nursing Interventions

PROMOTING ADEQUATE BREATHING AND AIRWAY CLEARANCE

Possible impending respiratory failure is detected by observing the patient, measuring vital capacity, monitoring oxygen saturation through pulse oximetry, and monitoring arterial blood gases. Early and vigorous attention to clearing bronchial and pharyngeal secretions can prevent retention of secretions and atelectasis. Suctioning may be indicated, but it should be used with caution to avoid stimulating the vagus nerve and producing bradycardia and cardiac arrest.

If the patient cannot cough effectively because of decreased inspiratory volume and inability to generate sufficient expiratory pressure, chest physiotherapy and assisted coughing may be indicated. Specific breathing exercises are supervised by the nurse to increase the strength and endurance of the inspiratory muscles, particularly the diaphragm. Assisted coughing promotes clearing of secretions from the upper respiratory tract and is similar to the use of abdominal thrusts to clear an airway. Assisted coughing can be more effective than traditional suctioning because traditional suctioning clears the right mainstem bronchus, whereas sites for atelectasis and pneumonia are most commonly in the left lower lung lobe (Jia et al., 2013). Proper humidification and hydration are important to prevent secretions from becoming thick and difficult to remove even with coughing. The patient is assessed for signs of respiratory infection (e.g., cough, fever, dyspnea). Ascending edema of the spinal cord in the acute phase may cause respiratory difficulty that requires immediate intervention. Therefore, the patient's respiratory status must be monitored closely.

IMPROVING MOBILITY

Proper body alignment is maintained at all times. If not on a specialized rotating bed, the patient should not be turned until the primary provider has indicated that it is safe to do so. Once safe for movement, the patient is repositioned frequently and is assisted out of bed as soon as the spinal column is stabilized. The feet are prone to footdrop; therefore, various types of splints are used to prevent footdrop. When used, the splints are removed and reapplied every 2 hours. Trochanter rolls, applied from the crest of the ilium to the midthigh of both legs, help prevent external rotation of the hip joints. Patients with lesions above the midthoracic level have loss of sympathetic control of peripheral vasoconstrictor activity, leading to hypotension. These patients may tolerate changes

in position poorly and require monitoring of blood pressure when positions are changed.

Contractures can develop rapidly with immobility and muscle paralysis. A joint that is immobilized too long becomes fixed as a result of contractures of the tendon and joint capsule. Atrophy of the extremities results from disuse. Contractures and other complications may be prevented by range-of-motion exercises that help preserve joint motion and stimulate circulation. Passive range-of-motion exercises should be implemented as soon as possible after injury. Toes, metatarsals, ankles, knees, and hips should be put through a full range of motion at least four, or ideally five, times daily.

For most patients who have a cervical fracture without neurologic deficit, reduction in traction followed by rigid immobilization for 6 to 8 weeks restores skeletal integrity. These patients are allowed to move gradually to an erect position. A neck brace or molded collar is applied when the patient is mobilized after traction is removed (see Fig. 68-6).

PREVENTING INJURY DUE TO SENSORY AND PERCEPTUAL ALTERATIONS

The nurse assists the patient to compensate for sensory and perceptual alterations that occur with SCI. The intact senses above the level of the injury are stimulated through touch, aromas, flavorful food and beverages, conversation, and music. Additional strategies include the following:

- Providing glasses to enable the patient to see from the supine position
- Encouraging the use of hearing aids, if indicated, to enable the patient to hear conversations and environmental sounds
- Providing emotional support to the patient and family
- Educating the patient and family about strategies to compensate for, or cope with, sensory deficits

MAINTAINING SKIN INTEGRITY

Pressure ulcers are a significant complication of SCI. The most common sites are over the sacrum (39.0%), heels (13.0%), ischial tuberosity (8.0%), and the occiput (back of head) (6.1%) (Jia et al., 2013). Pressure ulcers may begin within hours of an acute SCI where pressure is continuous and where the peripheral circulation is inadequate as a result of spinal shock and a recumbent position. It is important to move the patient from the backboard as soon as possible and inspect the skin. In addition, patients who wear cervical collars for prolonged periods may develop breakdown from the pressure of the collar under the chin, on the shoulders, and at the occiput. Pressure ulcers can add substantially to the personal and economic costs of living with SCI. The prevalence of this complication ranges from 17% for people 2 months after injury to 33% for those living with SCI.

The most effective approach to addressing this costly complication of SCI is prevention. The patient's position is changed at least every 2 hours (Bader et al., 2016). Turning not only assists in the prevention of pressure ulcers but also prevents pooling of blood and edema in the dependent areas. Careful inspection of the skin is made each time the patient is turned. The skin over the pressure points is assessed for redness or breaks; the perineum is checked for soilage, and the catheter is observed for adequate drainage. The patient's general body alignment and comfort are assessed. Special attention should be given to pressure areas in contact with the transfer board.

In addition, the patient's skin should be kept clean by washing with a mild soap, rinsing well, and blotting dry. Pressure-sensitive areas should be kept well lubricated and soft with oil or emollient lotion. The patient is educated about the danger of pressure ulcers and is encouraged to take control and make decisions about appropriate skin care. See Chapter 10 for other aspects of the prevention of pressure ulcers.

MAINTAINING URINARY ELIMINATION

Immediately after SCI, the urinary bladder becomes atonic and cannot contract by reflex activity. Urinary retention is the immediate result. During the initial acute phase, a Foley catheter is inserted; however, prompt discontinuation is advised due to high risk of catheter-associated UTI. Once discontinued, the patient has no sensation of bladder distention and overstretching of the bladder and detrusor muscle may occur, delaying the return of bladder function.

Intermittent catheterization is carried out to avoid overdistention of the bladder and high risk for UTI due to retention of urine. At an early stage, family members are shown how to carry out intermittent catheterization and are encouraged to participate in this facet of care, because they will be involved in long-term follow-up and must be able to recognize complications so that treatment can be instituted.

The patient is educated to record fluid intake, voiding pattern, amounts of residual urine after voiding, characteristics of urine, and any unusual sensations that may occur. The management of a **neurogenic bladder** (bladder dysfunction that results from a disorder or dysfunction of the nervous system) is discussed in detail in Chapter 10.

IMPROVING BOWEL FUNCTION

Immediately after SCI, a paralytic ileus usually develops as a result of neurogenic paralysis of the bowel; therefore, a nasogastric tube is often required to relieve distention and to prevent vomiting and aspiration (Rodriguez, 2016).

Bowel activity usually returns within the first week. With the intake of nutrition, it is important to establish a bowel program. A bowel program can help to control bowel movements by establishing a pattern of planned evacuation (see Chapter 10). The nurse administers prescribed combinations of stool softeners, stimulant laxatives, bulking laxatives, and rectal laxatives along with rectal stimulation, to counteract the effects of immobility and analgesic agents (Rodriguez, 2016).

PROVIDING COMFORT MEASURES: THE PATIENT IN TRACTION WITH TONGS OR HALO VEST

A patient who has had pins, tongs, or calipers placed for cervical stabilization may have a headache or discomfort for several days after the pins are inserted. Patients initially may be bothered by the rather startling appearance of these devices, but usually they readily adapt to it because the device provides comfort for the unstable neck (see Fig. 68-8). The patient may complain of being caged in and of noise created by any object coming in contact with the frame of a halo device, but they can be reassured that adaptation will occur.

The areas around the four pin sites of a halo device are cleaned at least daily and observed for redness, drainage, and pain. The pins are observed for loosening, which may contribute to infection. If one of the pins becomes detached, the head is stabilized in a neutral position by one person, while another notifies the primary provider. A torque screwdriver should be readily available in case the screws on the frame need tightening.

The skin under the halo vest is inspected for excessive perspiration, redness, and skin blistering, especially on the bony prominences. The vest is opened at the sides to allow the torso to be washed. The liner of the vest should not become wet, because dampness causes skin excoriation. Powder is not used inside the vest, because it may contribute to the development of pressure ulcers. The liner should be changed periodically to promote hygiene and good skin care. If the patient is to be discharged with the vest, detailed instructions must be given to the family, with time allowed for them to demonstrate the necessary skills of halo vest care (see Chart 68-8).

Chart 68-8	**HOME CARE CHECKLIST**
	The Patient With a Halo Vest

At the completion of education, the patient and/or caregiver will be able to:

- Name the procedure that was performed and identify any permanent changes in anatomic structure or function as well as changes in ADLs, IADLs, roles, relationships, and spirituality.
- Describe the rationale for the use of the halo vest.
- State how to contact all members of the treatment team (e.g., health care providers, home care professionals, rehabilitation team, and durable medical equipment and supply vendor).
- State changes in lifestyle (e.g., diet, ADLs, IADLs, activity) necessary for recovery and health maintenance, as applicable.
  - Demonstrate safe techniques to assist the patient with self-care, hygiene, and ambulation.
  - Demonstrate assessment of frame, traction, tongs, and pins.
  - Demonstrate pin care using correct technique.
  - Demonstrate care of skin, including assessment (e.g., reddened or irritated areas, breakdown).
  - Identify signs and symptoms of infection.

- Explain the reasons for and the method for changing the vest liner.
- Identify holistic measures of pain management.
- Identify signs and symptoms of complications (e.g., venous thromboembolism, respiratory impairment, urinary tract infection).
- Describe emergency measures if respiratory or other complications develop while the patient is in the halo vest or if the frame becomes dislodged.
- Relate how to reach primary provider with questions or complications.
- State time and date of follow-up medical appointments, therapy, and testing.
- Identify sources of support (e.g., friends, relatives, faith community, spinal cord injury support groups, caregiver support).
- Identify the need for health-promotion, disease prevention, and screening activities.

ADLs, activities of daily living; IADLs, independent activities of daily living.

RECOGNIZING AUTONOMIC DYSREFLEXIA

Autonomic dysreflexia, also known as autonomic hyperreflexia, is an acute life-threatening emergency that occurs as a result of exaggerated autonomic responses to stimuli that are harmless in people without SCI. It occurs only after spinal shock has resolved. This syndrome is characterized by a severe, pounding headache with paroxysmal hypertension, profuse diaphoresis above the spinal level of the lesion (most often of the forehead), nausea, nasal congestion, and bradycardia. It occurs among patients with cord lesions above T6 (the sympathetic visceral outflow level) after spinal shock has subsided (Bader et al., 2016). The sudden increase in blood pressure may cause retinal hemorrhage, hemorrhagic stroke, myocardial infarction, or seizures (Hickey, 2014). A number of stimuli may trigger this reflex: distended bladder (the most common cause); distention or contraction of the visceral organs, especially the bowel (from constipation, impaction); or stimulation of the skin (tactile, pain, thermal stimuli, pressure ulcer). Because this is an emergency situation, the objectives are to remove the triggering stimulus and to avoid the possibility of serious complications (Wan & Krassioukov, 2014).

The following measures are carried out:

- The patient is placed immediately in a sitting position to lower blood pressure.
- Rapid assessment is performed to identify and alleviate the cause.
- The bladder is emptied immediately via a urinary catheter. If an indwelling catheter is not patent, it is irrigated or replaced with another catheter.
- The rectum is examined for a fecal mass. If one is present, a topical anesthetic agent is inserted 10 to 15 minutes before the mass is removed, because visceral distention or contraction can cause autonomic dysreflexia.
- The skin is examined for any areas of pressure, irritation, or broken skin.
- Any other stimulus that could be the triggering event, such as an object next to the skin or a draft of cold air, must be removed.
- If these measures do not relieve the hypertension and excruciating headache, antihypertensive medications may be prescribed and given slowly by the IV route.
- The medical record is labeled with a clearly visible note about the risk of autonomic dysreflexia.
- The patient is instructed about prevention and management measures.
- Any patient with a lesion above the T6 segment is informed that such an episode is possible and may occur even many years after the initial injury (Bader et al., 2016).

MONITORING AND MANAGING POTENTIAL COMPLICATIONS

Patients are at high risk for VTE after SCI. The patient must be assessed for symptoms of VTE including DVT and PE. Chest pain, shortness of breath, and changes in arterial blood gas values must be reported promptly to the primary provider. The circumferences of the thighs and calves are measured and recorded daily; further diagnostic studies are performed if a significant increase is noted. Patients remain at high risk for thrombophlebitis for several months after the initial injury.

Patients with paraplegia or tetraplegia are at increased risk for the rest of their lives. Immobilization and the associated venous stasis, as well as varying degrees of autonomic disruption, contribute to the high risk and susceptibility for DVT.

Anticoagulation should be initiated within 72 hours of injury and continued for at least 3 months (Jia et al., 2013). The use of low–molecular-weight heparin or low-dose unfractionated heparin may be followed by long-term oral anticoagulation (i.e., warfarin [Coumadin]). Additional measures such as range-of-motion exercises, antiembolism stockings, and adequate hydration are important preventive measures. SCDs may also be used to reduce venous pooling and promote venous return. It is also important to avoid external pressure on the lower extremities that may result from flexion of the knees while the patient is in bed.

Orthostatic Hypotension. For the first 2 weeks after SCI, the blood pressure tends to be unstable and can be quite low. It gradually returns to preinjury levels, but periodic episodes of severe orthostatic hypotension frequently interfere with efforts to mobilize the patient. Interruption in the reflex arcs that normally produce vasoconstriction in the upright position, coupled with vasodilation and pooling in abdominal and lower extremity vessels, can result in hypotension. Orthostatic hypotension is a particularly common problem for patients with lesions above T7. In some patients with tetraplegia, even slight elevations of the head can result in blood pressure dysregulation.

A number of techniques can be used to reduce the frequency of hypotensive episodes. Close monitoring of vital signs before and during position changes is essential. Optimization of fluid status and vasopressor medication can be used to treat the profound vasodilation. Antiembolism stockings should be applied to improve venous return from the lower extremities. Abdominal binders may also be used to encourage venous return and provide diaphragmatic support when the patient is upright (Bader et al., 2016; Mills, Fung, Travios, et al., 2015). Activity should be planned in advance, and adequate time should be allowed for a slow progression of position changes from recumbent to sitting and upright. Tilt tables frequently are helpful in assisting patients to make this transition.

PROMOTING HOME, COMMUNITY-BASED, AND TRANSITIONAL CARE

Educating Patients About Self-Care. In most cases, patients with SCI (i.e., patients with tetraplegia or paraplegia) need long-term rehabilitation. The process begins during hospitalization as acute symptoms begin to subside or come under better control and the overall deficits and long-term effects of the injury become clear. The goals begin to shift from merely surviving the injury to learning strategies necessary to cope with the alterations that the injury imposes on activities of daily living (ADLs). The emphasis shifts from ensuring that the patient is stable and free of complications to specific assessment and planning designed to meet the patient's rehabilitation needs. Patient education may initially focus on the injury and its effects on mobility; dressing; and bowel, bladder, and sexual function. As the patient and family acknowledge the consequences of the injury and the resulting disability, the focus of education broadens to address issues necessary for carrying out the tasks of daily living and taking charge of their lives. Education must begin in the acute phase and continue throughout rehabilitation and the patient's entire life as changes occur, the patient ages, and problems arise (Bader et al., 2016).

Caring for the patient with SCI at home may at first seem a daunting task to the family. They will require dedicated nursing support to gradually assume full care of the patient. Although maintaining function and preventing complications will remain important, goals regarding self-care and preparation for discharge will assist in a smooth transition to rehabilitation and eventually to the community.

Continuing and Transitional Care. The goal of the rehabilitation process is independence. The nurse becomes a support to both the patient and the family, assisting them to assume responsibility for increasing aspects of patient care and management. Care for the patient with SCI involves members of all health care disciplines, which may include nursing, medicine, rehabilitation, respiratory therapy, physical and occupational therapy, case management, and social services. The nurse often serves as coordinator of the management team and as a liaison with rehabilitation centers and home care agencies. The patient and family often require assistance in dealing with the psychological impact of the injury and its consequences; referral to a psychiatric clinical nurse specialist or other mental health care professional often is helpful. Therapeutic horseback riding may help increase balance, muscle strength, and self-esteem (Asselin, Ward, Penning, et al., 2012).

The nurse should reassure female patients with SCI that pregnancy is not contraindicated and fertility is relatively unaffected, but that pregnant women with acute or chronic SCI pose unique management challenges. The normal physiologic changes of pregnancy may predispose women with SCI to many potentially life-threatening complications, including autonomic dysreflexia, pyelonephritis, respiratory insufficiency, thrombophlebitis, PE, and unattended delivery. Preconception assessment and counseling are strongly recommended to ensure that the woman is in optimal health and to increase the likelihood of an uneventful pregnancy and healthy outcomes (Pebdani, Johnson, & Amtmann, 2014).

As more patients survive acute SCI, they face the changes associated with aging with a disability. Three common secondary health problems experienced by persons living with SCI include chronic pain, spasticity, and depression (Abrams & Wakasa, 2014; Saunders, Clarke, Tate, et al., 2015). Education in the home and community focuses on health promotion and addresses the need to minimize risk factors (e.g., smoking, alcohol and drug abuse, obesity). Routine health screening and preventive services are needed for the older adult with SCI for early detection of secondary health problems. Home care nurses and others who have contact with patients with SCI are in a position to educate patients about healthy lifestyles, remind them of the need for health screenings, and make referrals as appropriate. Assisting patients to identify accessible health care providers, clinical facilities, and imaging centers may increase the likelihood that they will participate in health screening.

Evaluation

Expected patient outcomes may include:

1. Demonstrates improvement in gas exchange and clearance of secretions, as evidenced by normal breath sounds on auscultation
   a. Breathes easily without shortness of breath
   b. Performs hourly deep breathing exercises, coughs effectively, and clears pulmonary secretions
   c. Is free of respiratory infection (e.g., has temperature, respiratory rate, and pulse within normal limits; breath sounds clear to auscultation; absence of purulent sputum)
2. Moves within limits of the dysfunction and demonstrates completion of exercises within functional limitations
3. Avoids injury due to sensory, motor, and perceptual alterations
   a. Uses assistive devices (e.g., glasses, hearing aids, computers) as indicated
   b. Describes sensory, motor, and perceptual alterations as a consequence of injury
4. Demonstrates optimal skin integrity
   a. Exhibits normal skin turgor; skin is free of reddened areas or breaks
   b. Participates in skin care and monitoring procedures within functional limitations
5. Regains urinary bladder function
   a. Exhibits no signs of UTI (e.g., has temperature within normal limits; voids clear, dilute urine)
   b. Has adequate fluid intake
   c. Participates in bladder training program within functional limitations
6. Regains bowel function
   a. Reports regular pattern of bowel movement
   b. Consumes adequate dietary fiber and oral fluids
   c. Participates in bowel training program within functional limitations
7. Reports absence of pain and discomfort
8. Recognizes manifestations of autonomic dysreflexia if they occur (e.g., headache, diaphoresis, nasal congestion, bradycardia, or diaphoresis)
9. Is free of complications
   a. Demonstrates no signs of thrombophlebitis, DVT, or PE
   b. Maintains blood pressure within normal limits
   c. Reports no lightheadedness with position changes

Medical Management of Long-Term Complications of Spinal Cord Injury

The patient faces a lifetime of disability, requiring ongoing follow-up and care. The expertise of a number of health professionals, including physicians (specifically a physiatrist), rehabilitation nurses, occupational therapists, physical therapists, psychologists, social workers, rehabilitation engineers, and vocational counselors, is necessary at different times as the need arises.

The patient with an SCI has a shorter life expectancy compared to those who have not had an SCI (Abrams & Wakasa, 2014). As patients with SCI age, they have many of the same medical problems as others. In addition, they face the threat of complications associated with their disability (Hickey, 2014). Usually, patients are encouraged to follow-up at an outpatient spinal cord clinic when complications and other issues arise. Lifetime care includes assessment of the urinary tract at prescribed intervals, because there is the likelihood of continuing alteration in detrusor and sphincter function, and the patient is prone to UTI (Abrams & Wakasa, 2014).

Long-term problems and complications of SCI include disuse syndrome, autonomic dysreflexia (discussed earlier), bladder and kidney infections, spasticity, and depression (Abrams & Wakasa, 2014). Pressure ulcers with potential complications of sepsis, osteomyelitis, and fistulas occur in about 10% of patients. Spasticity may be particularly disabling. Heterotopic ossification (overgrowth of bone) in the hips, knees, shoulders, and elbows occurs in many patients after SCI. Spasticity and heterotopic ossification of these complications are painful and can produce a loss of range of motion (Abrams & Wakasa, 2014). Management includes observing for and addressing any alteration in physiologic status and psychological outlook, as well as the prevention and treatment of long-term complications. The nursing role involves emphasizing the need for vigilance in self-assessment and care.

NURSING PROCESS

The Patient With Tetraplegia or Paraplegia

Assessment

Assessment focuses on the patient's general condition, complications, and how the patient is managing at that particular point in time. A head-to-toe assessment and review of systems should be part of the database, with emphasis on the areas that are prone to problems in this population. A thorough inspection of all areas of the skin for redness or breakdown is critical. The nurse reviews the established bowel and bladder program with the patient, because the program must continue uninterrupted. Patients with tetraplegia or paraplegia have varying degrees of loss of motor power, deep and superficial sensation, vasomotor control, bladder and bowel control, and sexual function. They are faced with potential complications related to immobility, skin breakdown and pressure ulcers, recurring UTIs, and contractures. Knowledge about these particular issues can further guide the assessment in any setting. Nurses in all settings, including home care, must be aware of these potential complications in the lifetime management of these patients.

An understanding of the emotional and psychological responses to tetraplegia or paraplegia is achieved by observing the responses and behaviors of the patient and family and by listening to their concerns (Chuang, Yang, & Kuo, 2015). Documenting these assessments and reviewing the plan with the entire team on a regular basis provide insight into how both the patient and the family are coping with the changes in lifestyle and body functioning. Additional information frequently can be gathered from the social worker or psychiatric/mental health worker.

It takes time for the patient and family to comprehend the magnitude of the disability. They may go through stages of grief, including shock, disbelief, denial, anger, depression, and acceptance. During the acute phase of the injury, denial can be a protective mechanism to shield the patient from the acute reality of what has happened. As the patient realizes the permanent nature of paraplegia or tetraplegia, the grieving process may be prolonged and all-encompassing

because of the recognition that long-held plans and expectations are interrupted or permanently altered. A period of depression often follows as the patient experiences a loss of self-esteem in areas of self-identity, sexual functioning, and social and emotional roles. Exploration and assessment of these issues can assist in developing a meaningful plan of care.

Diagnosis

NURSING DIAGNOSES

Based on the assessment data, major nursing diagnoses may include the following:

- Impaired bed and physical mobility related to loss of motor function
- Risk for disuse syndrome
- Risk for impaired skin integrity related to permanent sensory loss and immobility
- Impaired urinary elimination related to level of injury
- Constipation related to effects of spinal cord disruption
- Sexual dysfunction related to neurologic dysfunction
- Ineffective coping related to impact of disability on daily living
- Deficient knowledge about requirements for long-term management

COLLABORATIVE PROBLEMS/POTENTIAL COMPLICATIONS

Potential complications may include the following:

- Spasticity
- Infection and sepsis

Planning and Goals

The goals for the patient may include attainment of some form of mobility; maintenance of healthy, intact skin; achievement of bladder management without infection; achievement of bowel control; achievement of sexual expression; strengthening of coping mechanisms; knowledge of long-term management; and absence of complications.

Nursing Interventions

The patient requires extensive rehabilitation, which is less difficult if appropriate nursing management has been carried out during the acute phase of the injury or illness. Nursing care is one of the key factors determining the success of the rehabilitation program. The main objective is for the patient to live as independently as possible in the home and community.

INCREASING MOBILITY

Exercise Programs. The unaffected parts of the body are built up to optimal strength to promote maximal self-care. The muscles of the hands, arms, shoulders, chest, spine, abdomen, and neck must be strengthened in the patient with paraplegia, because they must bear full weight on these muscles to ambulate. The triceps and the latissimus dorsi are important muscles used in crutch walking. The muscles of the abdomen and the back also are necessary for balance and for maintaining the upright position.

To strengthen these muscles, the patient can do push-ups when in a prone position and sit-ups when in a sitting position. Extending the arms while holding weights (traction weights can be used) also develops muscle strength. Squeezing rubber balls or crumbling newspaper promotes hand strength.

With encouragement from all members of the rehabilitation team, the patient with paraplegia can develop the increased exercise tolerance needed for gait training and ambulation activities. The importance of maintaining cardiovascular fitness is stressed to the patient. Alternative exercises to increase the heart rate to target levels must be designed within the patient's abilities.

Mobilization. After the spine is stable enough to allow the patient to assume an upright posture, mobilization activities are initiated. A brace or vest may be used, depending on the level of the lesion. The sooner muscles are used, the less chance there is of disuse atrophy. The earlier the patient is brought to a standing position, the less opportunity there is for osteoporotic changes to take place in the long bones. Weight bearing also reduces the possibility of renal calculi and enhances many other metabolic processes.

Braces and crutches enable some patients with paraplegia to ambulate for short distances. Ambulation using crutches requires a high expenditure of energy. Motorized wheelchairs and specially equipped vans can provide greater independence and mobility for patients with high-level SCI or other lesions. Every effort should be made to encourage the patient to be as mobile and active as possible.

Long-term risks include altered body composition, a decrease in lean body mass, decreased bone mineral density, and increased BMI. Patients are at high risk for obesity due to high fat intake combined with decreased physical activity (Lieberman, Goff, Hammond, et al., 2014). This puts patients at higher risk of developing comorbid conditions such as diabetes and cardiovascular disease. Patients benefit from nutrition counseling to prevent these secondary complications. For those who are overweight or who have obesity, weight-loss programs must be designed to accommodate the dietary and physical activity barriers that are unique to this population (Lieberman et al., 2014).

PREVENTING DISUSE SYNDROME

Patients are at high risk for development of contractures as a result of disuse syndrome due to the musculoskeletal system changes (atrophy) brought about by the loss of motor and sensory functions below the level of injury. Range-of-motion exercises must be provided at least four times a day, and care is taken to stretch the Achilles tendon with exercises, to prevent footdrop. The patient is repositioned frequently and is maintained in proper body alignment whether in bed or in a wheelchair.

Contractures can complicate day-to-day care, increasing the difficulty of positioning and decreasing mobility. A number of surgical procedures have been tried, with varying degrees of success. These techniques are used if more conservative approaches fail, but the best treatment is prevention.

PROMOTING SKIN INTEGRITY

Because these patients spend a great portion of their lives in wheelchairs, pressure ulcers are an ever-present threat. Contributing factors are permanent sensory loss over pressure areas; immobility, which makes relief of pressure difficult; trauma from bumps (against the wheelchair, toilet, furniture, and so forth) that cause unnoticed abrasions and wounds; loss of protective function of the skin from excoriation and maceration due to excessive perspiration and possible incontinence; and poor general health (anemia, diabetes), leading to poor tissue perfusion. See Chapter 10 for a detailed discussion of the prevention and management of pressure ulcers.

The person with tetraplegia or paraplegia must take responsibility for monitoring (or directing monitoring) of their skin status. This involves relieving pressure and not remaining in any position for longer than 2 hours, in addition to ensuring that the skin receives meticulous attention and cleansing (Bader et al., 2016). The patient is educated that ulcers develop over bony prominences that are exposed to unrelieved pressure in the sitting and lying positions. The most vulnerable areas are identified. The patient with paraplegia is instructed to use mirrors, if possible, to inspect these areas morning and night, observing for redness, slight edema, or any abrasions. While in bed, the patient should turn at 2-hour intervals and then inspect the skin again for redness that does not fade on pressure. The bottom sheet should be checked for wetness and for creases. The patient with tetraplegia or paraplegia, who cannot perform these activities, is encouraged to direct others to check these areas and prevent ulcers from developing.

The patient is educated to relieve pressure while in the wheelchair by doing push-ups, leaning from side to side to relieve ischial pressure, and tilting forward while leaning on a table. The caregiver for the patient with tetraplegia will need to perform these activities if the patient cannot do so independently. A wheelchair cushion is prescribed to meet individual needs, which may change in time with changes in posture, weight, and skin tolerance. A referral can be made to a rehabilitation engineer, who can measure pressure levels while the patient is sitting and then tailor the cushion and other necessary aids and assistive devices to the patient's needs.

The diet for the patient with tetraplegia or paraplegia should be high in protein, vitamins, and calories to ensure minimal wasting of muscle and the maintenance of healthy skin, and high in fluids to maintain well-functioning kidneys. Excessive weight gain and obesity should be avoided, because they further limit mobility.

IMPROVING BLADDER MANAGEMENT

The effect of the spinal cord lesion on the bladder depends on the level of injury, the degree of cord damage, and the length of time after injury. A patient with tetraplegia or paraplegia usually has either a reflex or a nonreflex bladder (see Chapter 10). Both bladder types increase the risk of UTI.

The nurse emphasizes the importance of maintaining an adequate flow of urine by encouraging a fluid intake of about 2.5 L daily. The patient should empty the bladder frequently so that there is minimal residual urine and should pay attention to personal hygiene, because infection of the bladder and kidneys almost always occurs by the ascending route. The perineum must be kept clean and dry, and attention must be given to the perianal skin after defecation. Underwear should be cotton (which is more absorbent) and should be changed at least once a day.

If an external catheter (condom catheter) is used, the sheath is removed nightly; the penis is cleansed to remove urine and is dried carefully, because warm urine on the periurethral skin promotes the growth of bacteria. Attention also is given to the collection bag. The nurse emphasizes the importance of monitoring for signs of UTI: cloudy, foul-smelling urine or hematuria (blood in the urine); fever; or chills.

The female patient who cannot achieve reflex bladder control or self-catheterization may need to wear pads or waterproof undergarments. Surgical intervention may be indicated in some patients to create a urinary diversion.

Establishing Bowel Control

The objective of a bowel training program is to establish bowel evacuation through reflex conditioning, a technique described in Chapter 10. If the SCI occurs above the sacral segments or nerve roots and there is reflex activity, the anal sphincter may be massaged (digital stimulation) to stimulate defecation. If the cord lesion involves the sacral segment or nerve roots, anal massage is not performed because the anus may be relaxed and lack tone. Massage is also contraindicated if there is spasticity of the anal sphincter. The anal sphincter is massaged by inserting a gloved finger (which has been adequately lubricated) 2.5 to 3.7 cm (1 to 1.5 inches) into the rectum and moving it in a circular motion or from side to side. It soon becomes apparent which area triggers the defecation response. This procedure should be performed at regular time intervals (usually every 48 hours), after a meal, and at a time that will be convenient for the patient at home (Rodriguez, 2016). The patient also is educated about the symptoms of impaction (frequent loose stools; constipation) and is cautioned to watch for hemorrhoids. A diet with sufficient fluids and fiber is essential to developing a successful bowel training program, avoiding constipation, and decreasing the risk of autonomic dysreflexia.

Counseling on Sexual Expression

Many patients with tetraplegia and paraplegia can have some form of meaningful sexual relationship, although modifications are necessary. The patient and partner benefit from counseling about the range of sexual expression possible, special techniques and positions, exploration of body sensations offering sensual feelings, and urinary and bowel hygiene as related to sexual activity. For men with erectile failure, penile prostheses enable them to have and sustain an erection, and impotence drugs may be helpful. Sildenafil (Viagra), vardenafil (Levitra), and tadalafil (Cialis), for example, are oral smooth muscle relaxants that cause blood to flow into the penis, resulting in an erection (see Chapter 59). Patients who are sexually active should undergo counseling in birth control methods, as some methods (e.g., oral contraceptives) may increase risks of complications such as VTE (Hickey, 2014).

Sexual education and counseling services are included in the rehabilitation services at spinal centers. Small group meetings in which patients can share their feelings, receive information, and discuss sexual concerns and practical aspects are helpful in producing effective attitudes and adjustments.

Enhancing Coping Mechanisms

The impact of the disability and loss becomes marked when the patient returns home. Each time something new enters the patient's life (e.g., a new relationship, going to work), the patient is reminded anew of their limitations. Grief reactions and depression are common.

To work through depression, the patient must have some hope for relief in the future. The nurse can encourage the patient to feel confident in their ability to achieve self-care and relative independence. The role of the nurse ranges from caretaker during the acute phase to educator, counselor, and facilitator as the patient gains mobility and independence.

The patient's disability affects not only the patient but also the entire family. In many cases, family therapy is helpful in working through issues as they arise. Adjustment to the disability leads to the development of realistic goals for the future, making the best of the abilities that are left intact, and reinvesting in other activities and relationships. Rejection of the disability causes self-destructive neglect and nonadherence to the therapeutic program, which leads to more frustration and depression. Crises for which interventions may be sought include social, psychological, marital, sexual, and psychiatric problems. The family usually requires counseling, social services, and other support systems to help them cope with the changes in their lifestyle and socioeconomic status.

A major goal of nursing management is to help the patient overcome their sense of futility and to encourage the patient in the emotional adjustment that must be made before they are willing to venture into the outside world. However, an excessively sympathetic attitude on the part of the nurse may cause the patient to develop an overdependence that defeats the purpose of the entire rehabilitation program. The patient is educated and assisted when necessary, but the nurse should avoid performing activities that the patient can do independently with a little effort. This approach to care more than repays itself in the satisfaction of seeing a patient, who is completely demoralized and helpless, become independent and find meaning in a newly emerging lifestyle.

Monitoring and Managing Potential Complications

Spasticity. Muscle spasticity can be a problematic complication of tetraplegia and paraplegia. Flexor or extensor spasms occur below the level of the spinal cord lesion and can interfere with the rehabilitation process, ADLs, and quality of life (Abrams & Wakasa, 2014). Spasticity results from an imbalance between the facilitatory and inhibitory effects on neurons that exist normally. The area of the cord distal to the site of injury or lesion becomes disconnected from the higher inhibitory centers located in the brain, so facilitatory impulses, which originate from muscles, skin, and ligaments, predominate.

Spasticity is defined as a condition of increased muscle tone in a muscle that is weak. Initial resistance to stretching is quickly followed by sudden relaxation. The stimulus that precipitates spasm can be obvious, such as movement or a position change, or subtle, such as a slight jarring of the wheelchair. Most patients with tetraplegia or paraplegia have some degree of spasticity. Because it increases muscle tone, some degree of spasticity can be beneficial in patients who are weak (Abrams & Wakasa, 2014). With SCI, the onset of spasticity usually occurs from a few weeks to 6 months after the injury. The same muscles that are flaccid during the period of spinal shock develop spasticity during recovery. The intensity of spasticity tends to peak approximately 2 years after the injury, after which the spasms tend to regress.

Management of spasticity is based on the severity of symptoms and the degree of incapacitation. Botulinum toxin (Botox) injections, as well as the antispasmodic medication baclofen (Lioresal), available in an oral and an intrathecal form, may be indicated (Comerford et al., 2015).

Oral medications such as diazepam (Valium), dantrolene (Dantrium), and tizanidine (Zanaflex) help control spasms by decreasing sympathetic outflow from the central nervous system. Other forms of adjunctive therapy include oral and transdermal forms of clonidine (Catapres) (Hickey, 2014). All of the antispasmodic medications cause drowsiness, weakness, and vertigo in some patients. Passive range-of-motion exercises and frequent turning and repositioning are helpful, because stiffness tends to increase spasticity. These activities also are essential in the prevention of contractures, pressure ulcers, and bowel and bladder dysfunction.

Infection and Sepsis. Patients with tetraplegia and paraplegia are at increased risk for infection and sepsis from a variety of sources: urinary tract, respiratory tract, and pressure ulcers. Sepsis remains a major cause of complications and death in these patients. Prevention of infection and sepsis is essential through maintenance of skin integrity, complete emptying of the bladder at regular intervals, and prevention of urinary and fecal incontinence. The risk of respiratory infection can be decreased by avoiding contact with people who have symptoms of respiratory infection, performing coughing and deep breathing exercises to prevent pooling of respiratory secretions, receiving yearly influenza vaccines, and giving up smoking. A high-protein diet is important in maintaining an adequate immune system, as is avoiding factors that may reduce immune system function, such as excessive stress, drug abuse, and excessive alcohol intake.

If infection occurs, the patient requires thorough assessment and prompt treatment. Antibiotic therapy and adequate hydration, in addition to local measures (depending on the site of infection), are initiated immediately.

UTIs are minimized or prevented by aseptic technique in catheter management, adequate hydration, a bladder training program, and prevention of overdistention of the bladder and urinary stasis.

Skin breakdown and infection are prevented by maintenance of a turning schedule; frequent back care; regular assessment of all skin areas; regular cleaning and lubrication of the skin; passive range-of-motion exercise to prevent contractures; pressure relief over broken skin areas, bony prominences, and heels; and wrinkle-free bed linen.

Pulmonary infections are managed and prevented by frequent coughing, turning, and deep breathing exercises and chest physiotherapy; aggressive respiratory care and suctioning of the airway if a tracheostomy is present; assisted coughing as needed; and adequate hydration.

Infections of any kind can be life threatening. Aggressive nursing interventions are key to prevention, detection, and early management.

PROMOTING HOME, COMMUNITY-BASED, AND TRANSITIONAL CARE

Educating Patients About Self-Care. Patients with tetraplegia or paraplegia are at risk for complications for the rest of their lives. Therefore, a major aspect of nursing care is educating the patient and family about these complications and about strategies to minimize risks. UTIs, contractures, infected pressure ulcers, and sepsis may necessitate hospitalization. Other late complications that may occur include lower extremity edema, joint contractures, respiratory dysfunction, and pain. To avoid these and other complications, the patient and family members are educated about skin care, catheter care, range-of-motion exercises, breathing exercises, and other care techniques. Education is initiated as soon as possible and extends into the rehabilitation or long-term care facility and home. In all aspects of care, it is important for the nurse and patient to set mutual goals and discuss the tasks the patient is capable of doing independently and which tasks the patient needs assistance to complete. See Chapter 10 for a more detailed discussion of rehabilitation.

Continuing and Transitional Care. Referral for home care is often appropriate for assessment of the home setting, patient education, and evaluation of the patient's physical and emotional status. During visits by the nurse, education about strategies to prevent or minimize potential complications is reinforced. The home environment is assessed for adequacy of care and for safety. Environmental modifications are made, and specialized equipment is obtained, ideally before the patient goes home.

The nurse also assesses the patient's and the family's adherence to recommendations and their use of coping strategies. The use of inappropriate coping strategies (e.g., drug and alcohol use) is assessed, and referrals to counseling are made for the patient and family. Appropriate and effective coping strategies are reinforced. The nurse reviews previous education and determines the need for further physical or psychological assistance. The patient's self-esteem and body image may be very poor at this time. Because people with high levels of social support often report feelings of well-being despite major physical disability, it is beneficial for the nurse to assess and promote further development of the support system and effective coping strategies for each patient. Caregivers and peer mentors play a critical role in helping patients feel less dependent, experience feelings of freedom, and reintegrate into the community (Beauchamp, Scarlett, Ruissen, et al., 2016).

The patient requires continuing, lifelong follow-up by the primary provider, physical therapist, and other rehabilitation team members, because the neurologic deficit is usually permanent and new deficits, complications, and secondary conditions can develop. These require prompt attention before they take their toll in additional physical impairment, time, morale, and financial costs. Research suggests that education and peer mentoring may decrease complications following SCI (Abrams & Wakasa, 2014; Beauchamp et al., 2016). The local counselor for the Office of Vocational Rehabilitation works with the patient with respect to job placement or additional educational or vocational training. The nurse is in a good position to remind patients and family members of the need for continuing health promotion and screening practices. Referral to accessible health care providers and imaging centers is important in health promotion and health screening. See Chapter 9 for more information on chronic illness and disability.

Evaluation

Expected patient outcomes may include:
1. Attains maximum form of mobility
2. Contractures do not develop
3. Maintains healthy, intact skin
4. Achieves bladder control, absence of UTI

5. Achieves bowel control
6. Reports sexual satisfaction
7. Shows improved adaptation to environment and others
8. Exhibits reduction in spasticity
   a. Reports understanding of the precipitating factors
   b. Uses measures to reduce spasticity
9. Describes long-term management required
10. Exhibits absence of complications

CRITICAL THINKING EXERCISES

1 `ebp` An 18-year-old man is brought to the ED by his family, who report that he was "dinged" in a football game 1 week ago. The patient does not recall the event. His family states that he is sleeping more than usual and seems forgetful. What is the evidence base for conducting a comprehensive and focused evaluation for a patient with a sports concussion injury? What evidence-based recommendations may guide return to sports for this patient? Identify the criteria used to evaluate the strength of the evidence for these practices.

2 `pg` A 90-year-old patient on anticoagulant therapy is admitted to your unit with a chronic SDH. Identify the priorities, approach, and techniques you would use to provide care for this patient in the preoperative phase of care. How will your priorities, approach, and techniques differ in the postoperative phase of care?

3 `pg` A 68-year-old woman was involved in a motor vehicle crash 2 days ago and sustained a T6 fracture with SCI. As a result, she has paraplegia and is in a neurologic intensive care unit. Identify the priorities, approach, and techniques you would use to provide care for this patient during the acute phase of care. Identify how your priorities, approach, and techniques will differ once the patient reaches the rehabilitation phase of care.

REFERENCES

*Asterisk indicates nursing research.
**Double asterisk indicate classic reference.

Books

Arciniegas, D. B., Zasler, N. D., Vanderploeg, R. D., et al. (Eds.). (2013). *Management of adults with traumatic brain injury.* Arlington, VA: American Psychiatric Association.
Bader, M. K., Littlejohns, L. R., & Olson, D. (2016). *AANN core curriculum for neuroscience nursing* (6th ed.). Chicago, IL: American Association of Neuroscience Nurses.
Booker, K. (2015). *Critical care nursing: Monitoring and treatment for advanced nursing practice.* Oxford: Wiley Blackwell.
Comerford, K. C. (2015). *Nursing 2015 drug handbook.* Philadelphia, PA: Wolters Kluwer.
Eliopoulos, C. (2018). *Gerontological nursing* (9th ed.). Philadelphia, PA: Wolters Kluwer.
Hickey, J. V. (2014). *The clinical practice of neurological & neurosurgical nursing* (7th ed.). Philadelphia, PA: Lippincott Williams & Wilkins.
West, T. A., Bergman, A., Biggins, M. S., et al. (2011). *Care of the patient with mild traumatic brain injury: AANN and ARN clinical practice guidelines series.* Glenview, IL: American Association of Neuroscience Nurses.

Journals and Electronic Documents

Abrams, G. M., & Wakasa, M. (2014). Chronic complications of spinal cord injury and disease. *UpToDate.* Retrieved on 2/24/17 at: www.uptodate.com/contents/chronic-complications-of-spinal-cord-injury-and-disease
American Spinal Injury Association (ASIA). (2016). International standards for neurological classification of spinal cord injury. Retrieved on 2/23/17 at: www.asia-spinalinjury.org/wp-content/uploads/2016/02/International_Stds_Diagram_Worksheet.pdf
Asselin, G., Ward, C., Penning, J. H., et al. (2012). Therapeutic horse back riding of a spinal cord injured veteran: a case study. *Rehabilitation Nursing, 37*(6), 270–276.
Bailes, J. D., Petraglia, A. L., Omalu, B. I., et al. (2013). Role of subconcussion in repetitive mild traumatic brain injury. *Journal of Neurosurgery, 119*(5), 1235–1245.
Bauman, M., & McCourt T. R. (2014) Assessing and managing patients with chronic subdural hematoma. *American Nurse Today, 9*(9), 38–41.
Beauchamp, M. R., Scarlett, L. J., Ruissen, G. R., et al. (2016). Peer mentoring of adults with spinal cord injury: a transformational leadership perspective. *Disability & Rehabilitation, 38*(19), 1884–1892.
Bodanapally, U. K., Sours, C., Zhuo, J., et al. (2015). Imaging of traumatic brain injury. *Radiologic Clinics of North America, 53*(4), 695–715.
Centers for Disease Control and Prevention (CDC). (2016a). Injury prevention & control: Traumatic brain injury & concussion. Retrieved on 2/9/2017 at: www.cdc.gov/traumaticbraininjury/get_the_facts.html
Centers for Disease Control and Prevention (CDC). (2016b). CDC study finds that adoption of the Brain Trauma Foundation guidelines could result in a substantial reduction in traumatic brain-injury-related deaths. Retrieved on 2/9/2017 at: www.cdc.gov/traumaticbraininjury/brain_trauma_guidelines.html
*Chuang, C., Yang, Y., & Kuo, L. T. (2015). Finding a way to cope: A qualitative study of the experience of persons with spinal cord injury. *Journal of Neuroscience Nursing, 47*(6), 313–319.
*Giusti, G. D., Tuteri, D., & Mirella, G. (2016). Nursing interactions with intensive care unit patients affected by sleep deprivation: an observational study. *Dimensions of Critical Care Nursing, 35*(3), 154–159.
Griesdale, D. E., Örtenwall, V., Norena, M., et al. (2015). Adherence to guidelines for management of cerebral perfusion pressure and outcome in patients who have severe traumatic brain injury. *Journal of Critical Care, 30*(1), 111–115.
**Hagen, C., Malkmus, D., & Durham, P. (1972). *The Rancho levels of cognitive functioning scale.* Downey, CA: Communication Disorders Service, Rancho Los Amigos Hospital. Revised 11/15/74 by: Danese Malkmus and Kathryn Stenderup.
Hemphill, J. C., & Phan, N. (2016). Traumatic brain injury: Epidemiology, classification and pathophysiology. *UpToDate.* Retrieved on 2/18/2017 at: www.uptodate.com/contents/traumatic-brain-injury-epidemiology-classification-and-pathophysiology
Hollander, J. E., & Camacho, M. (2014). Assessment and management of scalp lacerations. *UpToDate.* Retrieved on 2/17/2017 at: www.uptodate.com/contents/assessment-and-management-of-scalp-lacerations
Horn, S. D., Kinikini, M., Moore, L. W., et al. (2015). Enteral nutrition for patients with traumatic brain injury in the rehabilitation setting: Associations with patient preinjury and injury characteristics and outcomes. *Archives of Physical Medicine and Rehabilitation, 96*(8), S245–S255.
Hyatt, K. S. (2014). Mild traumatic brain injury. *American Journal of Nursing, 114*(11), 36–42.
Jia, X., Kowalski, R. G., Sciubba, D. M., et al. (2013). Critical care of the traumatic spinal cord injury. *Journal of Intensive Care Medicine, 28*(1), 12–23.
Larrow, V., & Klich-Heartt, E. I. (2016). Prevention of ventilator-associated pneumonia in the intensive care unit: beyond the basics. *Journal of Neuroscience Nursing, 48*(3), 160–165.
Lieberman, J., Goff, D., Hammond, F., et al. (2014). Dietary intake and adherence to the 2010 guidelines for Americans among individuals with chronic spinal cord injury: a pilot study. *Journal of Spinal Cord Medicine, 37*(6), 751–757.
Madden, L. K., & DeVon, H. (2015). A systematic review of the effects of body temperature on outcome after adult traumatic brain injury. *Journal of Neuroscience Nursing, 47*(4), 190–203.

McNett, M. M., & Olson, D. M. (2013). Evidence to guide nursing interventions for critically ill neurologically impaired patients with ICP monitoring. *Journal of Neuroscience Nursing, 45*(3), 120–123.

Mills, P. B., Fung, C. K., Travios, A., et al. (2015). Nonpharmacologic management of orthostatic hypotension: a systematic review. *Archives of Physical Medicine and Rehabilitation, 96*(2), 366–375.

*Mitchell, P. H., Kirkness, C., & Blissitt, P. A. (2015). Cerebral perfusion pressure and intracranial pressure in traumatic brain injury. *Annual Review of Nursing Research, 33*(1), 111–183.

Mohit, A. A. (2016). Cellular events and pathophysiology of SCI. *Spine (Phila Pa 1976), 41*(Suppl 7), S28.

National Spinal Cord Injury Statistical Center (NSCISC). (2016). Spinal Cord Injury (SCI) facts and figures at a glance. Retrieved on 2/23/2017 at: www.nscisc.uab.edu/Public/Facts%202016.pdf

*Olson, D. M., Rogers, M. S., & Stutzman, S. (2015). Electronic medical record validation: Exploring the reliability of intracranial pressure data abstracted from the electronic medical record-pilot. *Journal of Nursing Measurement, 23*(3), 532–540.

Pebdani, R. N., Johnson, K. L., & Amtmann, D. (2014). Personal experiences of pregnancy and fertility in individuals with spinal cord injury. *Sexuality and Disability, 32*(1), 65–74.

Perez-Barcena, J., Llompart-Pou, J., & O'Phelan, K. H. (2014). Intracranial pressure monitoring and management of intracranial hypertension. *Critical Care Clinics, 30*(4), 735–750.

Rodriguez, G. M. (2016). Bowel function after spinal cord injury. *Archives of Physical Medicine and Rehabilitation, 97*(2), 339–340.

Saunders, L. L., Clarke, A., Tate, D. G., et al. (2015). Lifetime prevalence of chronic health conditions among persons with spinal cord injury. *Archives of Physical Medicine and Rehabilitation, 96*(4), 673–679.

Stocchetti, N., & Maas, A. I. (2014). Traumatic intracranial hypertension. *New England Journal of Medicine, 370*(22), 2121–2130.

Tam, S., McKay, A., Sloan, S., et al. (2015). The experience of challenging behaviours following a severe TBI: a family perspective. *Brain Injury, 29*(7–8), 813–821.

**Teasdale, G., & Jennett, B. (1974). Assessment of coma and impaired consciousness. A practical scale. *Lancet, 2*(7872), 81–84.

Wan, D., & Krassioukov, A. V. (2014). Life-threatening outcomes associated with autonomic dysreflexia: a clinical review. *The Journal of Spinal Cord Medicine, 37*(1), 2–10.

Wilson, M., & DellaPenna, A. (2015). Targeted temperature modulation in the neuroscience patient. *Critical Care Nursing Clinics of North America, 28*(1), 125–136.

Zaman, A., Dubiel, R., Driver, S., et al. (2017). Seizure prophylaxis guidelines following traumatic brain injury: An evaluation of compliance. *Journal of Head Trauma Rehabilitation, 32*(2), E13–E17.

Resources

American Association of Neuroscience Nurses (AANN), www.aann.org
American Academy of Spinal Cord Injury Professionals, Inc., www.academyscipro.org
Association of Rehabilitation Nurses (ARN), www.rehabnurse.org
Brain Injury Association of America, www.biausa.org
Brain Trauma Foundation, www.braintrauma.org
Centers for Disease Control and Prevention (CDC), www.cdc.gov
Information Center for Individuals with Disabilities, www.disability.net
National Spinal Cord Injury Association (NSCIA), www.spinalcord.org
Paralyzed Veterans of America, www.pva.org

69

Management of Patients With Neurologic Infections, Autoimmune Disorders, and Neuropathies

LEARNING OBJECTIVES

On completion of this chapter, the learner will be able to:

1 Differentiate among the infectious disorders of the nervous system according to causes, manifestations, medical care, and nursing management.
2 Describe the pathophysiology, clinical manifestations, and medical and nursing management of multiple sclerosis, myasthenia gravis, and Guillain–Barré syndrome.

3 Use the nursing process as a framework for care of patients with multiple sclerosis and Guillain–Barré syndrome.
4 Explain disorders of the cranial nerves, their manifestations, and indicated nursing interventions.
5 Apply the nursing process as a framework for care of the patient with a cranial nerve disorder.

GLOSSARY

ataxia: impaired coordination of movement during voluntary movement
diplopia: double vision, or the awareness of two images of the same object occurring in one or both eyes
dysphagia: difficulty swallowing
dysphonia: voice impairment or altered voice production
hemiparesis: weakness of one side of the body, or part of it, due to an injury in the motor area of the brain
hemiplegia: paralysis of one side of the body, or part of it, due to an injury in the motor area of the brain

neuropathy: general term indicating a disorder of the nervous system
paresthesia: numbness, tingling, or a "pins and needles" sensation
prion: a pathogen smaller than a virus that is resistant to standard sterilization procedures
ptosis: drooping of the eyelids
spasticity: muscular hypertonicity with increased resistance to stretch often associated with weakness, increased deep tendon reflexes, and diminished superficial reflexes

---

The diverse group of neurologic disorders that make up infectious and autoimmune disorders and cranial and peripheral neuropathies presents unique challenges for nursing care. The nurse who cares for patients with these disorders must have a clear understanding of the pathophysiology, diagnostic testing, medical and nursing care, and rehabilitation processes. Some of the issues nurses must help patients and families confront include adaptation to the effects of the disease, potential changes in family dynamics, and end-of-life issues.

INFECTIOUS NEUROLOGIC DISORDERS

The infectious disorders of the nervous system include meningitis, brain abscesses, various types of encephalitis, Creutzfeldt–Jakob disease (CJD), and variant Creutzfeldt–Jakob disease (vCJD). The clinical manifestations, assessment, and diagnostic findings, as well as the medical and nursing management, are related to the specific infectious process.

Meningitis

Meningitis is inflammation of the meninges, which cover and protect the brain and spinal cord. The three major causes of meningitis are bacterial, viral, and fungal infections (Bader,

Littlejohns, & Olson, 2016). Meningitis can be the main reason a patient is hospitalized, or it can develop during hospitalization; it is classified as septic or aseptic. Septic meningitis is caused by bacteria. The bacteria *Streptococcus pneumoniae* and *Neisseria meningitidis* are responsible for the majority of cases of bacterial meningitis in adults. In aseptic meningitis, the cause is viral or secondary to cancer or having a weakened immune system, such as in human immune deficiency virus (HIV). The most common causative agents are the enteroviruses. Aseptic meningitis occurs more frequently in the summer and early fall.

Outbreaks of *N. meningitidis* infection are most likely to occur in dense community groups, such as college campuses and military installations. Although infections occur year-round, the peak incidence is in the winter and early spring. Factors that increase the risk of bacterial meningitis include tobacco use and viral upper respiratory infection, because they increase the amount of droplet production. Otitis media and mastoiditis increase the risk of bacterial meningitis, because the bacteria can cross the epithelial membrane and enter the subarachnoid space. People with immune system deficiencies are also at greater risk for development of bacterial meningitis (Bader et al., 2016).

Pathophysiology

Meningeal infections generally originate in one of two ways: through the bloodstream as a consequence of other infections or by direct spread, such as might occur after a traumatic injury to the facial bones or secondary to invasive procedures.

The *N. meningitidis* bacteria exists in the throats and nasal passages of approximately 10% of the general population and is transmitted by secretion or aerosol contamination (National Meningitis Association, 2016). Bacterial or meningococcal meningitis also occurs as an opportunistic infection in patients with acquired immune deficiency syndrome (AIDS) and as a complication of Lyme disease (see Chart 69-1). Due to several outbreaks among men who have sex with men, some cities, such as New York City and Chicago, recommend vaccination for all gay, bisexual, and men who have sex with men to help prevent future outbreaks (National Meningitis Association, 2016).

Once the causative organism enters the bloodstream, it crosses the blood–brain barrier and proliferates in the cerebrospinal fluid (CSF). The host immune response stimulates the release of cell wall fragments and lipopolysaccharides, facilitating inflammation of the subarachnoid and pia mater. Because the cranial vault contains little room for expansion, the inflammation may cause increased intracranial pressure (ICP). CSF circulates through the subarachnoid space, where inflammatory cellular materials from the affected meningeal tissue enter and accumulate.

The prognosis for bacterial meningitis depends on the causative organism, the severity of the infection and illness, and the timeliness of treatment. Acute fulminant presentation may include adrenal damage, circulatory collapse, and widespread hemorrhages (Waterhouse–Friderichsen syndrome). This syndrome is the result of endothelial damage and vascular necrosis caused by the bacteria. Complications include visual impairment, deafness, seizures, paralysis, hydrocephalus, and septic shock.

Clinical Manifestations

Headache and fever are frequently the initial symptoms. Fever tends to remain high throughout the course of the illness. The headache is usually either steady or throbbing and very severe as a result of meningeal irritation (Weber & Kelley, 2014). Meningeal irritation results in a number of other well-recognized signs common to all types of meningitis:

- *Neck immobility:* A stiff and painful neck (nuchal rigidity) can be an early sign, and any attempts at flexion of the head are difficult because of spasms in the muscles of the neck. Usually, the neck is supple, and the patient can easily bend the head and neck forward.
- *Positive Kernig sign:* When the patient is lying with the thigh flexed on the abdomen, the leg cannot be completely extended (see Fig. 69-1). When Kernig sign is bilateral, meningeal irritation is suspected (Weber & Kelley, 2014).

Chart 69-1 · Meningitis in Specific Populations

Meningitis can occur as a complication of other diseases and is an opportunistic infection seen with greater frequency in patients who are immunocompromised.

Meningitis in Patients With Acquired Immune Deficiency Syndrome (AIDS)

- Cryptococcal meningitis is the most common fungal infection of the central nervous system in patients with AIDS. Patients may experience headache, nausea, vomiting, seizures, confusion, and lethargy. Treatment consists of IV administration of amphotericin B followed by fluconazole. Maintenance therapy with fluconazole may be necessary to prevent relapse.
- Some patients who are immunosuppressed develop few if any symptoms because of blunted inflammatory responses; others develop atypical features.
- Onset of fever, headache, nausea, and malaise most often occur over a few weeks. Only 25% of patients present with stiff neck and photophobia.

Meningitis in Patients With Lyme Disease

- Lyme disease is a multisystem inflammatory process caused by the tick-transmitted spirochete *Borrelia burgdorferi.*
- Neurologic deficits are seen in later stages (stages 2 or 3). Stage 2 occurs with the start of a characteristic rash or 1–6 months after the rash has disappeared.
- Neurologic comorbidities include aseptic meningitis, chronic lymphocytic meningitis, and encephalitis.
- Cranial nerve inflammation, including Bell palsy and other peripheral neuropathies, is common.
- Stage 3 (the chronic form of the disease) begins years after the initial tick infection and is characterized by arthritis, skin lesions, and neurologic abnormalities.
- Most patients with stage 2 and 3 Lyme disease are treated with IV antibiotics, usually ceftriaxone or penicillin G.
- Meningeal and systemic symptoms begin to improve within days, although other symptoms, such as headache, may persist for weeks.

Adapted from Theroux, N., Phipps, M., Zimmerman, L., & Relf, M. V. (2013). Neurological complications associated with HIV and AIDS: Clinical implications for nursing. *Journal of Neuroscience Nursing*, 45(1), 5–13.

A   Kernig sign

B   Brudzinski sign

Pain

Figure 69-1 • Testing for meningeal irritation. **A.** Kernig sign. Flex the patient's leg at both the hip and knee and then straighten the knee. **B.** Brudzinski sign. As the neck is flexed, watch the hips and knees for a reaction.

- *Positive Brudzinski sign:* When the patient's neck is flexed (after ruling out cervical trauma or injury), flexion of the knees and hips is produced; when the lower extremity of one side is passively flexed, a similar movement is seen in the opposite extremity (see Fig. 69-1). Brudzinski sign is a more sensitive indicator of meningeal irritation than Kernig sign.
- *Photophobia (extreme sensitivity to light):* This finding is common due to irritation of the meninges, especially around the diaphragm sellae (Digre & Brennan, 2012).
- A rash can be a striking feature of *N. meningitidis* infection, occurring in about half of patients with this type of meningitis. Skin lesions develop, ranging from a petechial rash with purpuric lesions to large areas of ecchymosis.

Disorientation and memory impairment are common early in the course of the illness. The changes depend on the severity of the infection as well as the individual response to the physiologic processes. Behavioral manifestations are also common. As the illness progresses, lethargy, unresponsiveness, and coma may develop.

Seizures can occur and are the result of areas of irritability in the brain. ICP increases secondary to diffuse brain swelling or hydrocephalus (Bader et al., 2016). The initial signs of increased ICP include decreased level of consciousness (LOC) and focal motor deficits. If ICP is not controlled, the uncus of the temporal lobe may herniate through the tentorium, causing pressure on the brainstem. Brainstem herniation is a life-threatening event that causes cranial nerve dysfunction and depresses the centers of vital functions, such as the medulla. See Chapter 66 for discussion of the patient with a change in LOC or increased ICP.

An acute fulminant infection occurs in about 10% of patients with meningococcal meningitis, producing signs of sepsis: an abrupt onset of high fever, extensive purpuric lesions (over the face and extremities), shock, and signs of disseminated intravascular coagulation (see Chapter 33). Death may occur within a few hours after onset of the infection.

Assessment and Diagnostic Findings

If the clinical presentation suggests meningitis, diagnostic testing is conducted to identify the causative organism. A computed tomography (CT) scan is used to detect a shift in brain contents (which may lead to herniation) prior to a lumbar puncture in patient with altered LOC, papilledema, neurologic deficits, new onset of seizure, immunocompromised state, or history of central nervous system (CNS) disease. Bacterial culture and Gram staining of CSF and blood are key diagnostic tests (Bader et al., 2016). An overview of CSF values and alterations in bacterial, viral, and fungal meningitis is presented in Table 69-1. Gram staining allows for rapid identification of the causative bacteria and initiation of appropriate antibiotic therapy.

Prevention

The Advisory Committee on Immunization Practices of the Centers for Disease Control and Prevention (CDC, 2016) recommends that the meningococcal conjugated vaccine be given to youth at 11 to 12 years of age, with a booster dose at 16 years of age. First-year college students and members of the military who have not been vaccinated are at higher risk.

People in close contact with patients with meningococcal meningitis should be treated with antimicrobial chemoprophylaxis using rifampin (Rifadin), ciprofloxacin hydrochloride (Cipro), or ceftriaxone sodium (Rocephin). Therapy should be started within 24 hours after exposure because a delay limits the effectiveness of the prophylaxis. Vaccination should also be considered as an adjunct to antibiotic chemoprophylaxis for anyone living with a person who develops meningococcal infection. Vaccination against *Haemophilus influenzae* and *S. pneumoniae* should be encouraged for children and adults who are at-risk (CDC, 2016).

Medical Management

Successful outcomes depend on the early administration of an antibiotic agent that crosses the blood–brain barrier into the subarachnoid space in sufficient concentration to halt the multiplication of bacteria. Penicillin G in combination with one of the cephalosporins (e.g., ceftriaxone sodium, cefotaxime sodium) is most often administered intravenously (IV), optimally within 30 minutes of hospital arrival (Bader et al., 2016).

Dexamethasone has been shown to be beneficial as adjunct therapy in the treatment of acute bacterial meningitis and in pneumococcal meningitis if it is given 15 to 20 minutes

TABLE 69-1 Cerebrospinal Fluid Values Diagnostic for Meningitis

Parameter	Normal CSF	Bacterial Meningitis	Viral Meningitis	Fungal Meningitis
Opening pressure (mm H$_2$O)	100–180	200–500	≤250	>200
Leukocyte count (white blood cell/mm^3)	0–5	Increased 100–5000	Increased 50–1000	Increased >20
Neutrophils (%)	0	≥80	<40	
Protein (mg/dL)	18–45	Elevated 100–500	Elevated <200	Elevated >45
Glucose (mg/dL)	45–80; 0.6 times blood glucose level	<40; <0.4 times blood glucose level	>45	<40

CSF, cerebrospinal fluid.
Adapted from Bader, M., Littlejohns, L. R., & Olson, D. (2016). *AANN core curriculum for neuroscience nursing* (6th ed.). Chicago, IL: American Association of Neuroscience Nurses.

before the first dose of antibiotic and every 6 hours for the next 4 days. Research suggests that dexamethasone improves the outcome in adults and does not increase the risk of gastrointestinal bleeding (Bader et al., 2016).

Dehydration and shock are treated with fluid volume expanders. Seizures, which may occur early in the course of the disease, are treated with anticonvulsant medications. Increased ICP is treated as necessary (see Chapter 66).

 Nursing Management

The patient with meningitis is critically ill; therefore, many of the nursing interventions are collaborative with the physician, respiratory therapist, and other members of the health care team. The patient's safety and well-being depend on sound nursing judgment. Most patients will need the following nursing interventions:

- Instituting infection control precautions until 24 hours after initiation of antibiotic therapy (oral and nasal discharge is considered infectious)
- Assisting with pain management due to overall body aches and neck pain
- Assisting with getting rest in a quiet, darkened room
- Implementing interventions to treat the elevated temperature, such as antipyretic agents and cooling blankets
- Encouraging the patient to stay hydrated either orally or peripherally
- Ensuring close neurologic monitoring (see Chapter 66)

Neurologic status and vital signs are continually assessed. Pulse oximetry and arterial blood gas values are used to quickly identify the need for respiratory support if increasing ICP compromises the brainstem. Insertion of a cuffed endotracheal tube (or tracheotomy) and mechanical ventilation may be necessary to maintain adequate tissue oxygenation.

Blood pressure (usually monitored using an arterial line) is assessed for early manifestations of shock, which precedes cardiac or respiratory failure. Rapid IV fluid replacement may be prescribed, but care is taken to prevent fluid overload. Fever also increases the workload of the heart and cerebral metabolism. ICP will increase in response to increased cerebral metabolic demands. Therefore, measures are taken to reduce body temperature as quickly as possible.

Other important components of nursing care include the following measures:

- Protecting the patient from injury secondary to seizure activity or altered LOC
- Monitoring daily body weight; serum electrolytes; and urine volume, specific gravity, and osmolality, especially if syndrome of inappropriate antidiuretic hormone (SIADH) is suspected
- Preventing complications associated with immobility, such as pressure ulcers and pneumonia

Any sudden, critical illness can be devastating to the family. Because the patient's condition is often critical and the prognosis guarded, the family needs to be informed about the patient's condition. Periodic family visits are essential to facilitate coping of the patient and family. An important aspect of the nurse's role is to support the family and assist them in identifying others who can be supportive to them during the crisis.

Promoting Home, Community-Based, and Transitional Care

After the patient has achieved physiologic homeostasis and has demonstrated achievement of major health care goals, rehabilitation continues either in a rehabilitation facility, skilled nursing facility or at home. Continued support and evaluation by the nurse are essential.

Because patients may have been critically ill and focused on the most obvious needs and issues, the nurse reminds the patient and family about the importance of continuing health-promotion and screening practices, such as regular physical examinations and appropriate diagnostic screening tests.

Brain Abscess

Brain abscesses account for less than 1% of space-occupying brain lesions in the United States (Bader et al., 2016). Brain abscesses are rare in people who are immunocompetent; they are more frequently diagnosed in people who are immunosuppressed as a result of an underlying disease or the use of immunosuppressive medications.

Pathophysiology

A brain abscess is a collection of infectious material within the tissue of the brain. Bacteria are the most common causative organisms. The most common predisposing conditions for abscesses among adults who are immunocompetent are otitis media and rhinosinusitis. It is estimated that 40% of brain abscesses are otogenic in origin (Bader et al., 2016). An abscess can result from intracranial surgery, penetrating head injury, or tongue piercing. Organisms causing brain abscess may reach the brain by hematologic spread from the lungs, gums, tongue, or heart, or from a wound or intra-abdominal infection.

Clinical Manifestations

The clinical manifestations of a brain abscess result from alterations in intracranial dynamics (edema, brain shift), infection, or the location of the abscess. Headache, usually worse in the morning, is the most prevalent symptom. Fever is present 50% of the time (Slazinski, 2013). Vomiting and focal neurologic deficits occur as well. Focal deficits include weakness and decreasing vision reflect the area of brain that is involved. As the abscess expands, symptoms of increased ICP such as decreasing LOC and seizures occur.

Assessment and Diagnostic Findings

The baseline neurologic examination may reveal a variety of signs and symptoms based on the location of the abscess (see Chart 69-2). Neuroimaging with CT scanning with contrast is used most often to identify the size and location of the abscess. Cerebritis is a small infection in the brain that can progress to an abscess if not detected or treated. Aspiration of the abscess, guided by CT or MRI, is often used to culture and identify the infectious organism. MRI is the preferred study, because it is more sensitive to cerebritis and detecting smaller lesions (Slazinski, 2013). Blood cultures are obtained if the abscess is believed to arise from a distant source. Chest x-ray

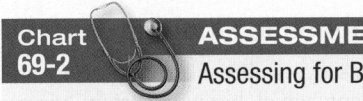

is performed to rule out predisposing lung infections, and electroencephalography (EEG) may help localize the lesion (Hickey, 2014).

Medical Management

Treatment is aimed at controlling increased ICP, draining the abscess, and providing antimicrobial therapy directed at the abscess and the main source of infection. Large IV doses of antibiotic agents are given to penetrate the blood–brain barrier and reach the abscess. The choice of the specific antibiotic medication is based on culture and sensitivity testing and directed at the causative organism. Antibiotics should be started as soon as possible and thus the initial antibiotic started typically is ceftriaxone, which will be adjusted based on the culture and sensitivity results. A stereotactic CT-guided aspiration may be used to drain the abscess and identify the causative organism. Surgical excision is the preferred method, but is not done as often as needle aspiration due to higher risk of neurologic complications (Slazinski, 2013). Corticosteroids may be prescribed to help reduce the inflammatory cerebral edema if the patient shows evidence of an increasing neurologic deficit. Anticonvulsant medications may be prescribed to prevent or treat seizures (see Chapter 66).

Nursing Management

Nursing care focuses on continuing to assess the neurologic status, administering medications, assessing the response to treatment, and providing supportive care.

Ongoing neurologic assessment alerts the nurse to changes in ICP, which may indicate a need for more aggressive intervention. The nurse also assesses and documents the responses to medications. Blood laboratory test results, specifically blood glucose and serum potassium levels, need to be closely monitored when corticosteroids are prescribed (Comerford, 2015). Administration of insulin or electrolyte replacement may be required to return these values to within normal limits.

Patient safety is another key nursing responsibility. Injury may result from decreased LOC or falls related to motor weakness or seizures.

The patient with a brain abscess is very ill, with neurologic deficits, such as **hemiplegia** (paralysis of one side of the body, or part of it), **hemiparesis** (weakness of one side of the body, or part of it), seizures, visual deficits, and cranial nerve palsies that may persist after treatment. The nurse must assess the family's ability to express distress at the patient's condition, cope with the patient's illness and deficits, and obtain support.

Herpes Simplex Encephalitis

Encephalitis is an acute inflammatory process of the brain tissue. The herpes simplex virus (HSV) is the most common cause of acute encephalitis in the United States (Bader et al., 2016).

Pathophysiology

The pathology of encephalitis involves local necrotizing hemorrhage that becomes more generalized, followed by edema. There is also progressive deterioration of nerve cell bodies (Grossman & Porth, 2014).

Clinical Manifestations

The initial symptoms of herpes simplex encephalitis include fever, headache, confusion, and hallucinations. Focal neurologic symptoms reflect the areas of cerebral inflammation and necrosis and include fever, headache, behavioral changes, focal seizures, dysphasia, hemiparesis, and altered LOC (Grossman & Porth, 2014).

Assessment and Diagnostic Findings

Neuroimaging studies, such as EEG, and CSF examination are used to diagnose encephalitis. MRI is used to detect early changes caused by herpes simplex; scans usually show edema in the frontal and temporal lobes. The EEG shows diffuse slowing or focal changes in the temporal lobe in the majority of patients. Lumbar puncture often reveals a high opening pressure, glucose within normal limits, and high protein levels in CSF samples (see Table 69-1). Twenty percent of initial CSF studies have results within normal limits (Bader et al., 2016). Viral cultures are almost always negative. The polymerase chain reaction (PCR) is the standard test for early diagnosis of herpes simplex encephalitis. PCR identifies the deoxyribonucleic acid (DNA) bands of HSV-1 in the CSF. The validity of PCR is very high between the 3rd and 10th days after symptom onset.

Medical Management

Antiviral agents, either acyclovir (Zovirax) or ganciclovir (Cytovene), are the medications of choice in the treatment for HSV (Comerford, 2015). Early administration of antiviral agents (usually well tolerated) improves the prognosis associated with herpes simplex encephalitis. The mode of action is inhibition of viral DNA replication. To prevent relapse, treatment should continue for up to 3 weeks. Slow IV administration over 1 hour prevents crystallization of the medication in the urine. The usual dose of acyclovir is decreased if the patient has a history of renal insufficiency.

Nursing Management

Assessment of neurologic function is key to monitoring the progression of disease. Comfort measures to reduce headache include dimming the lights, limiting noise and visitors, grouping nursing interventions, and administering analgesic agents. Opioid analgesic medications may mask neurologic symptoms; therefore, they are used cautiously. Seizures and altered LOC require care directed at injury prevention and safety. Nursing care addressing patient and family anxieties is ongoing throughout the illness. Monitoring of blood chemistry test results and urinary output alert the nurse to the presence of renal complications related to antiviral therapy.

Arthropod-Borne Virus Encephalitis

Arthropod-borne viruses, or arboviruses, are maintained in nature through biologic transmission between susceptible vertebrate hosts by blood feeding arthropods (mosquitoes, psychodids, ceratopogonids, and ticks). Arthropod vectors transmit several types of viruses that cause encephalitis. The main vector in North America is the mosquito. Arbovirus infection (transmitted by arthropod vectors) occurs in specific geographic areas during the summer and fall. In the United States, there are five main arboviral encephalitides: eastern equine encephalitis, western equine encephalitis, St. Louis encephalitis, La Crosse encephalitis, and West Nile virus encephalitis (Bader et al., 2016).

Pathophysiology

Viral replication occurs at the site of the mosquito bite. The host immune response attempts to control viral replication. If the immune response is inadequate, viremia will ensue. The virus gains access to the CNS via the olfactory tract, resulting in encephalitis. It spreads from neuron to neuron, predominantly affecting the cortical gray matter, the brainstem, and the thalamus. Meningeal exudates compound the clinical presentation by irritating the meninges and increasing ICP.

Clinical Manifestations

St. Louis and West Nile virus encephalitis most commonly affect adults. An arboviral encephalitis occurs along a continuum with some cases having only flulike symptoms (i.e., headache and fever) but others progressing to specific neurologic manifestations that vary depending on the viral type (Bader et al., 2016). A unique clinical feature of St. Louis encephalitis is SIADH with hyponatremia. The incubation period in St. Louis encephalitis is from 4 to 12 days (Bader et al., 2016). Onset of symptoms is abrupt with fever, headache, dizziness, nausea, and malaise. If the disease spreads to the CNS, symptoms include stiff neck, confusion, dizziness, and tremors. Coma can occur in severe cases, and mortality increases with age. Eastern equine encephalitis has the highest mortality rate at 50% to 70% (Bader et al., 2016). Seizures, a poor prognostic indicator, are present in encephalitis and are more common in the St. Louis type.

Assessment and Diagnostic Findings

Preliminary diagnosis is based on clinical presentation and location and dates of recent travel because certain viruses are endemic to certain geographic locales. Neuroimaging and CSF evaluation are useful in the diagnosis of encephalitis. The MRI scan demonstrates inflammation of the basal ganglia in cases of St. Louis encephalitis and inflammation in the periventricular area in cases of West Nile encephalitis. Immunoglobulin M antibodies to West Nile virus are observed in serum and CSF. Serum cultures are not useful, because the viremia is brief. EEG can identify abnormal brain waves, which can help identify some viral infections.

Medical Management

No specific medication for arboviral encephalitis exists; therefore, symptom management is key. Controlling the seizures and the increased ICP are critical components of care in cases with neurologic manifestations. Interferon may be useful in treating St. Louis encephalitis, although no specific drug is indicated. Neuropsychiatric complications, such as emotional outbursts and other behavior changes, occur frequently.

Nursing Management

Many patients, particularly those with only fever and headache, are treated on an outpatient basis. If the patient is very ill, hospitalization may be required. The nurse carefully assesses neurologic status and identifies improvement or deterioration in the patient's condition. Injury prevention is key in light of the potential for falls or seizures. Any encephalitis that progresses may result in death or lifelong residual health issues such as neurologic deficits and seizures. The family will need support and education to cope with these outcomes.

Public education addressing the prevention of arboviral encephalitis is a key nursing role. Clothing that provides coverage and insect repellents containing 20% to 35% diethyltoluamide (DEET) should be used on exposed clothing and skin in high-risk areas to decrease mosquito and tick bites (Bader et al., 2016). Remaining indoors at dawn and dusk when mosquito activity is highest is recommended. Screens should be in good repair in the home, and standing water should be removed. All cases of arboviral encephalitis must be reported to the local health department.

Fungal Encephalitis

Fungal infections of the CNS occur rarely in people who are healthy. The presentation of fungal encephalitis is related to geographic area or to an immune system that is compromised due to disease or immunosuppressive medication. Causes of fungal infections include *Cryptococcus neoformans, Blastomyces dermatitidis, Histoplasma capsulatum, Aspergillus fumigatus, Candida,* and *Coccidioides immitis* (Bader et al., 2016). *C. immitis* is found mainly in California, Arizona, New Mexico, and Texas. *B. dermatitidis* exists in the southeastern United States and in the Ohio, St. Lawrence, and Mississippi River basins. It is a risk for coal miners, construction workers, and farmers. *C. neoformans* is associated with exposure to bird droppings and may be seen in bird handlers.

Pathophysiology

The fungal spores enter the body via inhalation. They initially infect the lungs, causing vague respiratory symptoms or pneumonitis. The fungi may enter the bloodstream, causing a fungemia. If the fungemia overwhelms the person's immune system, the fungus may spread to the CNS. The fungal invasion may cause meningitis, encephalitis, brain abscess, granuloma, or arterial thrombus.

Clinical Manifestations

The common symptoms of fungal encephalitis include fever, malaise, headache, meningeal signs, and change in LOC or cranial nerve dysfunction. Symptoms of increased ICP related to hydrocephalus often occur. *C. neoformans* and *C. immitis* are associated with specific skin lesions. *H. capsulatum* is associated with seizures, and *A. fumigatus* may cause ischemic or hemorrhagic strokes.

Assessment and Diagnostic Findings

A history of immunosuppression associated with AIDS or the use of immunosuppressive medications may indicate fungal disease of the brain (Theroux, Phipps, Zimmerman, et al., 2013). Occupational and travel history may point to a fungal cause of CNS infection. Infections caused by *H. capsulatum* and *C. immitis* will demonstrate fungal antibodies in serologic tests. The CSF usually demonstrates elevated white cell and protein levels; glucose levels are decreased. *C. neoformans* is easily identified in CSF fungal cultures. *Candida* may be cultured from the blood or CSF. To identify *B. dermatitidis*, cisternal or ventricular cultures of CSF may need to be obtained. *A. fumigatus* is difficult to isolate in CSF and is diagnosed by lung biopsy. Neuroimaging is used to identify CNS changes related to fungal infection. MRI is the study of choice; it demonstrates areas of hemorrhage, abscess, or enhanced meninges indicating inflammation.

Medical Management

Medical management is directed at the causative fungus and the neurologic consequences of the infection. Seizures are controlled by standard anticonvulsant medications. Increased ICP is controlled by repeated lumbar punctures or shunting of CSF.

Antifungal agents are given for a specific period to cure the infection in patients with competent immune systems. Patients with compromised immune systems receive antifungal therapy until the infection is controlled, after which they receive a maintenance dose of the medication for an indefinite period. Amphotericin B is used for a progressive fungal infection that does not respond to conventional drug therapy. Dosing depends on the causative organism, and it is usually administered IV. Adverse reactions include fever, nausea and vomiting, anemia, uremia, and electrolyte abnormalities (especially potassium and magnesium). Toxicities may occur, and renal insufficiency is a serious reaction to amphotericin B that can occur (Comerford, 2015).

Fluconazole (Diflucan) or flucytosine (Ancobon) may be given orally in conjunction with amphotericin B as maintenance therapy. Potential side effects of fluconazole include nausea, vomiting, and a transient increase in liver enzymes. The most common adverse reaction to flucytosine is bone marrow depression (Comerford, 2015). Therefore, patients receiving flucytosine should have leukocyte and platelet counts monitored regularly.

Nursing Management

The ICP will increase if hydrocephalus develops and the inflammatory response progresses. Nursing assessment aimed at early identification of increased ICP is necessary to ensure early control and management. See Chapter 66 for management of the patient with increased ICP. Administering nonopioid analgesic agents, limiting environmental stimuli, and positioning may optimize patient comfort. Administering diphenhydramine (Benadryl) and acetaminophen (Tylenol) approximately 30 minutes before giving amphotericin B may prevent flulike side effects. If renal insufficiency develops, the dose may need to be reduced. Increasing levels of serum creatinine and blood urea nitrogen may alert the nurse to the development of renal insufficiency and the need to address the patient's renal status.

Providing support assists the patient and family to cope with the illness. Workup of the patient for immune deficiency diseases such as AIDS may put additional stress on the family. The nurse may need to mobilize community support systems for the patient and family, because the recovery may be long.

Creutzfeldt–Jakob and Variant Creutzfeldt–Jakob Diseases

CJD and vCJD belong to a group of degenerative, infectious neurologic disorders called *transmissible spongiform encephalopathies* (TSE). CJD is very rare and has no identifiable cause. vCJD, the human variation of bovine spongiform encephalopathy (BSE) (commonly known as mad cow disease), results from the ingestion by humans of prions in infected meat. TSEs are caused by **prions**, which are pathogens smaller than a virus that are resistant to standard methods of sterilization (National Institute of Neurological Disorders and Stroke [NINDS], 2016). Although CJD and vCJD have distinct clinical features, one characteristic they share is a lack of CNS inflammation. CJD may lie dormant for decades before causing neurologic degeneration. The incubation period of vCJD seems to be shorter (less than 10 years). In both diseases, the symptoms are progressive, there is no definitive treatment, and the outcome is fatal (Bader et al., 2016).

Almost all cases of vCJD have been reported in the United Kingdom, with a smaller number of cases being identified in 10 other countries worldwide. The risk of vCJD in the United States is thought to be low, because cattle are fed primarily with soy-derived feed as opposed to feed containing animal parts (NINDS, 2016).

Pathophysiology

The prion is a unique pathogen because it lacks nucleic acid, which enables the organism to withstand conventional means of sterilization. It has not been isolated and it is believed to be a protein that takes on a different form (NINDS, 2016). In both CJD and vCJD, the prion crosses the blood–brain barrier and is deposited in brain tissue and causes degeneration of brain tissue. Cell death occurs, and spongiform changes (spongy vacuoles) are produced in the brain. The spongiform vacuoles are surrounded by amyloid plaque.

There are three major forms of CJD. Approximately 85% of cases of CJD appear sporadically; this form is called sporadic CJD. The incidence is one case per 1 million people. Sporadic CJD occurs spontaneously with no risk factors. The second form is familial or hereditary CJD, and this type accounts for 5% to 10% of cases (NINDS, 2016). The final type is acquired CJD. This form is transmitted by contaminated brain, tissue, or neurosurgical instruments and accounts for less than 1% of cases (Vacca, 2016).

The prion exists in lymphoid tissue and blood in both vCJD and CJD. Both prion diseases are believed to be blood-borne. No method is available to screen blood for infectivity. For this reason, the American Red Cross will not accept blood donation from anyone who has stayed more than 3 to 6 months since 1980 in a country where BSE is common (American Red Cross, 2016).

Clinical Manifestations

CJD and vCJD have several clinically distinct features. Psychiatric symptoms occur early in vCJD, whereas they are a late symptom in CJD. The mean age at onset of vCJD is 27 years, whereas the mean age for CJD onset is 65 years. The presenting symptoms of vCJD include affective symptoms (i.e., behavioral changes), sensory disturbance, and limb pain. Muscle spasms and rigidity, dysarthria, incoordination, cognitive impairment, and sleep disturbances follow. Patients with sporadic CJD present with mental deterioration, ataxia, and visual disturbance. Memory loss, involuntary movement, paralysis, and mutism occur as the disease progresses. After clinical presentation, people with vCJD survive an average of 22 months; those with CJD survive for less than 1 year (Bader et al., 2016).

Assessment and Diagnostic Findings

Brain biopsy is not recommended to diagnose CJD. The three diagnostic tests currently used in suspicious clinical presentations to support the diagnosis of CJD are immunologic assessment, EEG, and MRI scanning. Immunologic assessment of CSF detects a protein kinase inhibitor referred to as 14–3–3. The presence of this inhibitor indicates neuronal cell death, which is not specific to CJD but does support the diagnosis. The EEG reveals a characteristic pattern over the duration of the disease. After initial slowing, the EEG shows periodic activity. Later in the course of the disease, the EEG shows burst suppressions characterized by periodic spikes alternating with slow periods. The MRI scan demonstrates symmetric or unilateral hyperintense signals arising from the basal ganglia (Bader et al., 2016).

Medical Management

After the onset of specific neurologic symptoms, progression of disease occurs quickly. There is no effective treatment for CJD or vCJD. The care of the patient is supportive and palliative. Goals of care include prevention of injury related to immobility and dementia, promotion of patient comfort, and provision of support and education for the family.

Nursing Management

The nursing care of patients is primarily supportive and palliative. Psychological and emotional support of the patient and family throughout the course of the illness is needed. Care extends to providing for a dignified death and supporting the family through the processes of grief and loss. Hospice services are appropriate either at home or at an inpatient facility. See Chapter 16 for an in-depth discussion of end-of-life issues.

Prevention of disease transmission is an important part of nursing care. Although patient isolation is not necessary, the use of standard precautions is important. Institutional protocols are followed for handling of brain, spinal cord, pituitary gland, and eye tissue; and for exposure and decontamination of equipment. In the operating room, it is recommended that disposable instruments be used and then incinerated, because conventional methods of sterilization do not destroy the prion (Bader et al., 2016). If disposable instruments cannot be used, stringent sterilization methods such as the use of bleach for cleaning and extended sterilization time for instruments should be used.

AUTOIMMUNE PROCESSES

Autoimmune nervous system disorders include multiple sclerosis (MS), myasthenia gravis, and Guillain–Barré syndrome (GBS).

Multiple Sclerosis

MS is an immune-mediated, progressive demyelinating disease of the CNS. Demyelination refers to the destruction of myelin—the fatty and protein material that surrounds certain nerve fibers in the brain and spinal cord; it results in impaired transmission of nerve impulses (see Fig. 69-2). MS

Figure 69-2 • The process of demyelination. **A, B.** A normal nerve cell and axon with myelin. **C, D.** The slow disintegration of myelin, resulting in a disruption in axon function.

affects nearly 400,000 people in the United States (Bader et al., 2016). MS may occur at any age, but the age of peak onset is between 25 and 35 years; it affects women more frequently than men (Bader et al., 2016).

The cause of MS is an area of ongoing research. Autoimmune activity results in demyelination, but the sensitized antigen has not been identified. Multiple factors play a role in the initiation of the immune process. Geographic prevalence is highest in Europe, New Zealand, southern Australia, the northern United States, and southern Canada. MS is less prevalent in Asians. There is a North–South gradient, with greater frequency in temperate regions and latitudes away from the equator (Bader et al., 2016).

MS is considered to have many risks, including genetic factors. However, it has not been found to be genetically transmitted (Bader et al., 2016). Genetic predisposition is indicated by the presence of a specific cluster (haplotype) of human leukocyte antigens on the cell wall. Its presence may increase susceptibility to factors, such as viruses, that trigger the autoimmune response activated in MS. A specific virus capable of initiating the autoimmune response has not been identified. It is believed that DNA on the virus mimics the amino acid sequence of myelin, resulting in an immune system cross-reaction in the presence of a defective immune system. Environmental risks include smoking, lack of vitamin D exposure, and exposure to the Epstein–Barr virus (Bader et al., 2016).

Pathophysiology

Sensitized T- and B lymphocytes cross the blood–brain barrier; their function is to check the CNS for antigens and then leave. In MS, sensitized T cells remain in the CNS and promote the infiltration of other agents that damage the immune system. The immune system attack leads to inflammation that destroys myelin (which insulates the axon and speeds the conduction of impulses along the axon) and the oligodendroglial cells that produce myelin in the CNS.

Demyelination interrupts the flow of nerve impulses and results in a variety of manifestations, depending on the nerves affected. Plaques appear on demyelinated axons, further interrupting the transmission of impulses. Demyelinated axons are scattered irregularly throughout the CNS. The areas most frequently affected are the optic nerves, chiasm, and tracts; the cerebrum; the brainstem and cerebellum; and the spinal cord. The axons themselves begin to degenerate, resulting in permanent and irreversible damage (Wu & Alvarez, 2016).

Clinical Manifestations

The course of MS may assume many different patterns (Lublin & Reingold, 1996) (see Fig. 69-3). In some patients, the disease follows a benign course, and symptoms are so mild that the patient does not seek health care or treatment. Approximately 85% of patients with MS have a *relapsing-remitting* (RR) course. With each relapse, recovery is usually complete; however, residual deficits may occur and accumulate over time, contributing to functional decline. Over time, most patients with the RR course of MS progress to a *secondary progressive* course, in which disease progression occurs with or without relapses. Approximately 15% of patients have a *primary progressive* course, in which disabling symptoms steadily

Figure 69-3 • Types and courses of multiple sclerosis (MS). **1.** Relapsing-remitting (RR) MS is characterized by clearly acute attacks with full recovery or with sequelae and residual deficit upon recovery. Periods between disease relapses are characterized by lack of disease progression. **2.** Primary progressive MS is characterized by disease showing progression of disability from onset, without plateaus and temporary minor improvements. **3.** Secondary progressive MS begins with an initial RR course, followed by progression of variable rate, which may also include occasional relapses and minor remissions. **4.** Progressive-relapsing MS shows progression from onset but with clear acute relapses with or without recovery. From Lublin, F. D., & Reingold, S. C. (1996). Defining the clinical course of multiple sclerosis: Results of an international survey. *Neurology, 46*(64), 907–911. Used with permission from Lippincott Williams & Wilkins.

increase, with rare plateaus and temporary minor improvement. Primary progressive MS may result in quadriparesis, cognitive dysfunction, visual loss, and brainstem syndromes. The least common presentation (about 5% of cases) is the *progressive-relapsing* course. It is characterized by relapses with continuous disabling progression between exacerbations (Hickey, 2014).

The signs and symptoms of MS are varied and multiple, reflecting the location of the lesion (plaque) or combination of lesions. The main symptoms most commonly reported are fatigue, depression, weakness, numbness, difficulty in coordination, loss of balance, spasticity, and pain (Bader et al., 2016). Visual disturbances due to lesions in the optic nerves or their connections may include blurring of vision, **diplopia** (double vision), scotoma (patchy blindness), and total blindness.

Fatigue affects most people with MS and is often the most disabling symptom (Riley & Vargus, 2015; Morrison & Stuifbergen, 2016). Heat, depression, anemia, deconditioning, and medication may contribute to fatigue. Avoiding hot temperatures, effective treatment of depression and anemia, a change in medication as well as occupational and physical therapies may help manage fatigue.

Pain is another common symptom of MS that can contribute to social isolation. Lesions on the sensory pathways cause pain. Additional sensory manifestations include paresthesias, dysesthesias, and proprioception loss. Many people with

MS need daily analgesic medications. In some cases, pain is managed with opioids, anticonvulsant medications, or antidepressants. Rarely, surgery may be needed to interrupt pain pathways.

Among women who are perimenopausal, those with MS are more likely to have pain related to osteoporosis. In addition to estrogen loss, immobility and corticosteroid therapy play a role in the development of osteoporosis among women with MS. Bone mineral density testing is recommended for this high-risk group. See Chapter 41 for a discussion of the diagnosis of and treatment for osteoporosis.

Spasticity (muscle hypertonicity) occurs in 90% of patients with MS, most often in the lower extremities, and can include loss of the abdominal reflexes. Spasticity results from involvement of the main motor pathways (pyramidal tracts) of the spinal cord. Cognitive and psychosocial problems may reflect frontal or parietal lobe involvement. Some degree of cognitive change (e.g., memory loss, decreased concentration) occurs in about half of patients, but severe cognitive changes with dementia (progressive organic mental disorder) are rare.

Involvement of the cerebellum or basal ganglia can produce **ataxia** (impaired coordination of movements) and tremor. Loss of the control connections between the cortex and the basal ganglia may occur and cause emotional lability and euphoria. Bladder, bowel, and sexual dysfunctions are common.

Researchers reported that patients with MS have higher rates of depression, arthritis, diabetes, coronary artery disease, migraine headaches, and cancer compared to a normative U.S. population (Newland, Jensen, Budhathoki, et al., 2015). Additional complications include urinary tract infections, constipation, pressure ulcers, contracture deformities, dependent pedal edema, pneumonia, and osteoporosis. Emotional, social, marital, economic, and vocational problems may also occur.

Exacerbations and remissions are characteristic of MS. During exacerbations, new symptoms appear and existing ones worsen; during remissions, symptoms decrease or disappear. Relapses may be associated with emotional and physical stress.

Gerontologic Considerations

The life expectancy for patients with MS is 5 to 7 years shorter than patients without MS (Bader et al., 2016). Those diagnosed with secondary progressive disease live an average of 38 years after onset. Older adult patients with MS have specific physical and psychosocial challenges. They may have chronic health problems, for which they may be taking additional medications that could interact with medications prescribed for MS. The absorption, distribution, metabolism, and excretion of medications are altered in the older adult as a result of age-related changes in kidney and liver functions. Therefore, older adult patients must be monitored closely for adverse and toxic effects of MS medications and for osteoporosis (particularly if corticosteroids have been used frequently to treat exacerbations). The cost of medications may lead to poor adherence to the prescribed regimen in older adult patients on fixed incomes.

Older adult patients with MS are particularly concerned about increasing disability, family burden, marital concern, and the possible future need for nursing home care. Immobility resulting in fewer social opportunities contributes to loneliness and depression. Researchers found that 58% of older adults with MS reported frequent depressed feelings and more than 30% contemplated suicide (Buhse, 2015). In addition to functional loss, the physical challenges experienced by older adults with MS include spasticity, pain, bladder dysfunction, impaired sleep, and an increased need for assistance with self-care.

Assessment and Diagnostic Findings

The diagnosis of MS is based on the presence of multiple plaques in the CNS observed with MRI (Hickey, 2014) (see Fig. 69-4). Additional studies augment the diagnosis. Electrophoresis of CSF identifies the presence of oligoclonal banding (several bands of immunoglobulin G bonded together, indicating an immune system abnormality). Evoked potential studies can help define the extent of the disease process and monitor changes. Underlying bladder dysfunction is diagnosed by urodynamic studies. Neuropsychological testing may be indicated to assess cognitive impairment. A sexual history helps identify changes in sexual function.

Medical Management

No cure exists for MS. An individual treatment program is indicated to relieve the patient's symptoms and provide continuing support, particularly for patients with cognitive changes, who may need more structure and support. The goals of treatment are to delay the progression of the disease, manage chronic symptoms, and treat acute exacerbations. Common symptoms requiring intervention include ataxia, bladder dysfunction, depression, fatigue, and spasticity. Management includes pharmacologic and nonpharmacologic strategies.

Figure 69-4 • Multiple sclerosis. Axial T-2 weighted image shows ovoid hyperintense lesions in both hemispheres. From Hickey, J. V. (2014). *The clinical practice of neurological & neurosurgical nursing* (7th ed.). Philadelphia, PA: Lippincott Williams & Wilkins.

Pharmacologic Therapy

Medications prescribed for MS include those for disease modification and those for symptom management. Disease-modifying therapies are available to treat some of the different forms of MS (Hickey, 2014). Many types of medications are used for symptom management in MS.

Disease-Modifying Therapies

The disease-modifying medications reduce the frequency of relapse, the duration of relapse, and the number and size of plaques observed on MRI in the RR form of MS, but are not effective in the primary progressive type of MS (Hickey, 2014).

Interferon beta-1a (Rebif) and interferon beta-1b (Betaseron) may be given subcutaneously every other day. Another preparation of interferon beta-1a (Avonex) may be given intramuscularly once a week. Side effects of all interferon-beta medications include flulike symptoms in approximately half of patients taking these drugs that cause patients to discontinue therapy (Filipi, Beavin, Brillante, et al., 2014). For optimal control of disability, disease-modifying medications should be started early in the course of the disease (Comerford, 2015).

Glatiramer acetate (Copaxone) also reduces the rate of relapse in the RR course of MS. Copaxone is given subcutaneously daily (Hickey, 2014). Copaxone is an option for those with an RR course; however, it may take 6 months for evidence of an immune response to appear. There are oral disease-modifying agents that also reduce disease activity and disease progression. Teriflunomide (Aubagio), fingolimod (Gilenya), and dimethyl fumarate (Tecfidera) are oral alternatives that may be better tolerated by the patient who have difficulty with injection reactions (Hickey, 2014).

IV methylprednisolone, the key agent in treating acute relapse in the RR course, shortens the duration of relapse but has not been found to have long-term benefit (Bader et al., 2016). It exerts anti-inflammatory effects by acting on T cells and cytokines. The medication is given as 1 g IV daily for 3 to 5 days, followed by an oral taper of prednisone. Side effects include mood swings, weight gain, and electrolyte imbalances (Comerford, 2015).

The medication mitoxantrone (Novantrone) is given via IV infusion every 3 months. Mitoxantrone can reduce the frequency of clinical relapses in patients with secondary progressive or worsening RR MS. Patients must be very closely monitored for side effects (i.e., cardiac toxicity), and there is a maximum lifetime dose that can be given (Hickey, 2014).

Symptom Management

Medications are also prescribed for management of specific symptoms. Baclofen (Lioresal), a gamma-aminobutyric acid agonist, is the medication of choice for treating spasticity. It can be given orally or by intrathecal injection for severe spasticity. Benzodiazepines (e.g., diazepam [Valium]), tizanidine (Zanaflex), and dantrolene (Dantrium) may also be used to treat spasticity (Hickey, 2014). Patients with disabling spasms and contractures may require nerve blocks or surgical intervention. Fatigue that interferes with activities of daily living (ADLs) may be treated with amantadine (Symmetrel), pemoline (Cylert), or dalfampridine (Ampyra). Ataxia is a chronic problem most resistant to treatment. Medications used to treat ataxia include beta-adrenergic blockers (e.g., propranolol [Inderal]), the anticonvulsant agent gabapentin (Neurontin), and benzodiazepines (e.g., clonazepam [Klonopin]).

Bladder and bowel problems are often difficult for patients, and a variety of medications (anticholinergic agents, alpha-adrenergic blockers, antispasmodic agents) may be prescribed. Nonpharmacologic strategies also assist in establishing effective bowel and bladder elimination (see later discussion).

Urinary tract infection may be superimposed on the underlying neurologic dysfunction. Ascorbic acid (vitamin C) may be prescribed to acidify the urine, making bacterial growth less likely. Antibiotic agents are prescribed when appropriate.

NURSING PROCESS

The Patient With MS

Assessment

Nursing assessment addresses neurologic deficits, secondary complications, and the impact of the disease on the patient and family. The patient's mobility and balance are observed to determine whether there is risk of falling. Assessment of function is carried out both when the patient is well rested and when fatigued. The patient is assessed for weakness, spasticity, visual impairment, incontinence, and disorders of swallowing and speech. Additional areas of assessment include how MS has affected the patient's lifestyle, how the patient is coping, adherence to the prescribed medication regimen, and what the patient would like to improve.

Diagnosis

Nursing Diagnoses

Based on the assessment data, major nursing diagnoses may include the following:

- Impaired bed and physical mobility related to weakness, muscle paresis, spasticity, increased weight
- Risk for injury related to sensory and visual impairment
- Impaired urinary elimination (urgency, frequency, incontinence), constipation, and bowel incontinence related to nervous system dysfunction
- Impaired verbal communication and risk for aspiration related to cranial nerve involvement
- Chronic confusion related to cerebral dysfunction
- Ineffective coping related to uncertainty of course of MS
- Impaired home maintenance management related to physical, psychological, and social limits imposed by MS
- Ineffective sexuality pattern related to lesions or psychological reaction

Planning and Goals

The major goals for the patient may include promotion of physical mobility, avoidance of injury, achievement of bladder and bowel continence, promotion of speech and swallowing mechanisms, improvement of cognitive function, development of coping strengths, improved home maintenance management, and adaptation to sexual dysfunction.

Nursing Interventions

An individualized program of physical, occupational, and speech-language therapy, rehabilitation, and education is combined with emotional support. An educational plan of care is developed to enable the person with MS to deal with the physiologic, social, and psychological problems that accompany chronic disease. The presence of depression, pain, fatigue, and walking difficulty all decrease physical activity. Assisting patients with management of these symptoms may help increase the level of physical activity and overall sense of well-being.

PROMOTING PHYSICAL MOBILITY

Relaxation and coordination exercises promote muscle efficiency. Progressive resistive exercises are used to strengthen weak muscles, because diminishing muscle strength is often significant in MS.

Exercises. Walking improves the gait, particularly the problem of loss of position sense of the legs and feet. If certain muscle groups are irreversibly affected, other muscles can be trained to compensate. Instruction in the use of assistive devices may be needed to ensure their safe and correct use.

Minimizing Spasticity and Contractures. Muscle spasticity is common and, in its later stages, is characterized by severe adductor spasm of the hips with flexor spasm of the hips and knees. Without relief, fibrous contractures of these joints occur. Warm packs may be beneficial, but hot baths should be avoided because of risk of burn injury secondary to sensory loss and increasing symptoms that may occur with elevation of the body temperature.

Daily exercises for muscle stretching are prescribed to minimize joint contractures. Special attention is given to the hamstrings, gastrocnemius muscles, hip adductors, biceps, and wrist and finger flexors. Muscle spasticity is common and interferes with usual function. Application of prescribed orthotics may help maintain a functional position and reduce contractures. A stretch–hold–relax routine is helpful for relaxing and treating muscle spasticity. Swimming and stationary bicycling are useful, and progressive weight bearing can relieve spasticity in the legs. The patient should not be hurried in any of these activities, because this often increases spasticity.

Activity and Rest. The patient is encouraged to work and exercise to a point just short of fatigue. Very strenuous physical exercise is not advisable, because it raises the body temperature and may aggravate symptoms. The patient is advised to take frequent short rest periods, preferably lying down. Extreme fatigue may contribute to the exacerbation of symptoms. One study reported that functional limitations and depressive symptoms were the strongest predictors of fatigue impact in patients with long-standing MS (see Chart 69-3) (Morrison & Stuifbergen, 2016).

Nutrition. Similar to the population at large, many patients with MS are overweight or have obesity. Contributing factors include the use of corticosteroids for exacerbations of symptoms and mobility impairments as a result of the disease. Interventions to promote healthy eating and weight reduction need to take into account that fatigue and mobility impairments are barriers to engagement in nutritional behaviors for people with MS. Nurses also need to be certain to include family members in interventions and nutrition education, because they are often the gatekeepers for food preparation and selection. Additional strategies include avoidance of alcohol and cigarette smoking (Bader et al., 2016).

Minimizing Effects of Immobility. Because of the decrease in physical activity that often occurs with MS, complications associated with immobility, including pressure ulcers, expiratory muscle weakness, and accumulation of bronchial secretions, need to be considered and steps taken to prevent them. Measures to prevent such complications include assessing and maintaining skin integrity and having the patient perform coughing and deep-breathing exercises.

Chart 69-3

NURSING RESEARCH PROFILE

Predictors of Fatigue in Patients With MS

Morrison, J. D., & Stuifbergen, A. K. (2016). Predictors of fatigue impact in persons with long-standing multiple sclerosis. *Journal of Neuroscience Nursing, 48*(3), 143–150.

Purpose

Fatigue is very common among those with MS and has a negative impact on many aspects of their lives. The underlying mechanisms are poorly understood and treatment is a challenge. The purpose of this study was to explain the physical, cognitive, and psychosocial dimensions of fatigue among those with long-standing MS.

Design

More than 300 people with long-standing MS (for 17 years or more) were surveyed to measure fatigue impact, MS related functional limitations, depressive symptoms, barriers to health promotion, personal resources, and health promoting behaviors. The relationships among fatigue impact, age, MS duration, MS related functional limitations, depressive symptoms, barriers to health promotion, personal resources, and health promoting behaviors were also explored.

Findings

Age and MS duration were not significantly related to fatigue impact. Moderate to strong positive, linear relationships were reported among fatigue impact measures and MS functional limitations (range: r = 0.41–0.58, p < 0.01), depressive symptoms (range: r = 0.58–0.63, p < 0.01), and barriers (range: r = 0.55–0.63, p < 0.01). Moderate inverse linear relationships were reported among fatigue impact measures and personal resources (range: r = –0.40–0.50, p < 0.01) and health-promoting behaviors (range: r = –0.34–0.44, p < 0.01). MS functional limitation was reported as the strongest predictor of physical and psychosocial fatigue impact, while depressive symptoms was the strongest predictor of total and cognitive fatigue impact.

Nursing Implications

Nurses working with patients with MS should know that functional limitations and depressive symptoms were strong predictors of fatigue impact in this study. This illustrates the importance of nurses assessing and monitoring depressive symptoms, functional status, and dimensions of fatigue at each encounter with patients, whether in the in-patient or out-patient setting.

PREVENTING INJURY

If motor dysfunction causes problems of incoordination and clumsiness, or if ataxia is apparent, then the patient is at risk for falling. To overcome this disability, the patient is instructed to walk with feet apart to widen the base of support and to increase walking stability. If loss of position sense occurs, the patient is instructed to watch the feet while walking. Gait training may require assistive devices (walker, cane, braces, crutches, parallel bars) and instruction about their use by a physical therapist. If the gait remains inefficient, a wheelchair or motorized scooter may be the solution. The occupational therapist is a valuable resource person in suggesting and securing aids to promote independence. If incoordination is a problem and tremor of the upper extremities occurs when voluntary movement is attempted (intention tremor), weighted bracelets or wrist cuffs are helpful. The patient is trained in transfer and ADLs.

Because sensory loss may occur in addition to motor loss, pressure ulcers are a continuing threat to skin integrity. The need to use a wheelchair continuously increases the risk. See Chapter 10 for a discussion of the prevention and treatment of pressure ulcers.

ENHANCING BLADDER AND BOWEL CONTROL

In general, bladder symptoms fall into the following categories: (1) inability to store urine (hyperreflexic, uninhibited); (2) inability to empty the bladder (hyporeflexic, hypotonic); and (3) a mixture of both types. The patient with urinary frequency, urgency, or incontinence requires special support. The sensation of the need to void must be heeded immediately, so the bedpan or urinal should be readily available. A voiding time schedule is set up (every 1.5 to 2 hours initially, with gradual lengthening of the interval). The patient is instructed to drink a measured amount of fluid every 2 hours and then attempt to void 30 minutes after drinking. The use of a timer or wristwatch with an alarm may be helpful for the patient who does not have enough sensation to signal the need to empty the bladder. The nurse encourages the patient to take the prescribed medications to treat bladder spasticity, because this allows greater independence. Intermittent self-catheterization (see Chapter 10) has been successful in maintaining bladder control in patients with MS. If a female patient has permanent urinary incontinence, urinary diversion procedures may be considered. The male patient may wear a condom appliance for urine collection.

Bowel problems include constipation, fecal impaction, and incontinence. Adequate fluids, dietary fiber, and a bowel training program are frequently effective in solving these problems. See Chapter 10 for a discussion of promoting bowel continence.

ENHANCING COMMUNICATION AND MANAGING SWALLOWING DIFFICULTIES

If the cranial nerves that control the mechanisms of speech and swallowing are affected, dysarthrias (defects of articulation) marked by slurring, low volume of speech, and difficulties in phonation may occur. **Dysphagia** (difficulty swallowing) may also occur. A speech-language pathologist evaluates speech and swallowing and instructs the patient, family, and health team members about strategies to compensate for speech and swallowing problems. The nurse reinforces this instruction and encourages the patient and family to adhere to the plan.

> ◤ **Quality and Safety Nursing Alert**
>
> *Impaired swallowing increases the patient's risk of aspiration. To reduce that risk, the nurse implements strategies such as having suction apparatus available, ensuring careful feeding, confirming correct food and liquid consistency, and positioning properly for eating.*

IMPROVING COGNITIVE FUNCTION

Measures may be taken if visual defects or changes in cognitive status occur and result in chronic confusion.

Vision. The cranial nerves affecting vision may be affected by MS. An eye patch or a covered eyeglass lens may be used to block the visual impulses of one eye if the patient has diplopia. Prism glasses may be helpful for patients who are confined to bed and have difficulty reading in the supine position. People who are unable to read regular-print materials are eligible for the free "talking book" services of the Library of Congress or may obtain large-print or audio books from local libraries.

Cognition and Emotional Responses. Cognitive impairment and emotional lability occur early in MS in some patients and may impose numerous stresses on the patient and family. Some patients with MS are forgetful and easily distracted and may exhibit emotional lability.

Patients adapt to illness in a variety of ways, including denial, depression, withdrawal, and hostility. Emotional support assists patients and their families to adapt to the changes and uncertainties associated with MS and to cope with the disruption in their lives. The family should be made aware of the nature and degree of cognitive impairment. Patients with MS have identified that the support of family and friends is a major need. The patient is assisted to set meaningful and realistic goals, to remain as active as possible, and to maintain interests and activities. Hobbies may help the patient's morale and provide satisfying interests if the disease progresses to the stage in which formerly enjoyed activities can no longer be pursued. The environment is kept structured, distractions are reduced, and lists and other memory aids are used to help the patient with cognitive changes maintain a daily routine. The occupational therapist can be helpful in formulating a structured daily routine.

STRENGTHENING COPING MECHANISMS

The diagnosis of MS is always distressing to the patient and family. They need to know that no two patients with MS have identical symptoms or courses of illness. Although some patients do experience significant disability early, others have a near-normal lifespan with minimal disability. Some families, however, face acute frustrations and problems. MS affects people who are often in an early stage of life and concerned about career and family responsibilities. Family conflict, disintegration, separation, and divorce are not uncommon. Often, very young family members assume the responsibility of caring for a parent with MS. Nursing interventions in this area include assisting patients and families to manage or reduce stress and making appropriate referrals for counseling and support to minimize the adverse effects of dealing with chronic illness.

The nurse, mindful of these complex problems, initiates home care and coordinates a network of services, including social services, speech therapy, physical therapy, and homemaker services. To strengthen the patient's coping skills, as much information as possible is provided. Patients need an updated list of available assistive devices, services, and resources.

Coping through problem solving involves helping the patient define the problem and develop alternatives for its management. Planning carefully, maintaining flexibility, and preserving a hopeful attitude are useful for psychological and physical adaptation.

IMPROVING HOME MANAGEMENT

MS can affect every facet of daily living. Certain abilities are often impossible to regain after they are lost. Physical function may vary from day to day. Modifications that allow independence in home management should be implemented (e.g., assistive eating devices, raised toilet seat, bathing aids, telephone modifications, long-handled comb, tongs, modified clothing). Exposure to heat increases fatigue and muscle weakness, so air conditioning is recommended in at least one room. Exposure to extreme cold may increase spasticity.

PROMOTING SEXUAL FUNCTIONING

Patients with MS and their partners face problems that interfere with sexual activity, both as a direct consequence of nerve damage and also from psychological reactions to the disease. Easy fatigability, conflicts arising from dependency and depression, emotional lability, and loss of self-esteem compound the problem. Erectile and ejaculatory disorders in men and orgasmic dysfunction and adductor spasms of the thigh muscles in women can make sexual intercourse difficult or impossible. Bladder and bowel incontinence and urinary tract infections add to the difficulties.

Collaboration between the patient, family, and primary provider is essential for supporting intimacy. A sexual counselor can help bring into focus the patient's or partner's sexual resources and suggest relevant information and supportive therapy. Sharing and communicating feelings, planning for sexual activity (to minimize the effects of fatigue), and exploring alternative methods of sexual expression may open up a wide range of sexual enjoyment and experiences.

PROMOTING HOME, COMMUNITY-BASED, AND TRANSITIONAL CARE

Educating Patients About Self-Care. As the disease progresses, the patient and family need to learn new strategies to maintain optimal independence. Educating about self-care techniques may be initiated in the hospital or clinic setting and reinforced in the home. Self-care education may address the use of assistive devices, self-catheterization, and administration of medications that affect the course of the disease or treat complications. An education plan that addresses intramuscular or subcutaneous administration of medications (including side effects) is developed for the patient and their family or caregiver. A panel of experts concluded that flulike symptoms resulting from injectable disease-modifying drugs can be mitigated by dose titration, use of analgesics, evening dosing, drug formulation, solution temperature, adequate hydration, and a nutritious diet (Filipi et al., 2014). The patient and family are educated about exercises that enable the patient to continue some form of activity or that maintain or improve swallowing, speech, or respiratory function (see Chart 69-4).

Continuing and Transitional Care. After discharge, the nurse often provides education and reinforcement of new

---

Chart 69-4 — HOME CARE CHECKLIST

The Patient With MS

At the completion of education, the patient and/or caregiver will be able to:

- State the impact of MS and treatment on physiologic functioning, ADLs, IADLs, roles, relationships, and spirituality.
- State the purpose, dose, route, schedule, side effects, and precautions for prescribed medications.
  - Demonstrate correct techniques of administering injectable medications, if prescribed.
- State how to contact all members of the treatment team (e.g., health care providers, home care professionals, and durable medical equipment and supply vendor).
- State changes in lifestyle (e.g., exercise, activity) necessary to maintain health.
  - Demonstrate environmental modifications and adaptive techniques for accomplishing activities of daily living.
  - Identify strategies to manage symptoms (pain, cognitive responses, dysphagia, tremors, visual disturbances).
  - State how to prevent complications (e.g., pressure ulcers, pneumonia, depression).
  - Identify coping strategies.
  - Identify ways to minimize fatigue.
  - Explain how to prevent injury.

- Identify optimal nutritional intake; consider weight reduction as indicated if patient is overweight or has obesity.
- State ways to promote sexual function.
- Discuss ways to manage bowel and bladder function.
- Name benefits of exercise and physical activity.
- Identify ways to minimize immobility and spasticity.
- Relate how to reach primary provider with questions or complications.
- State time and date of follow-up medical appointments, therapy, and testing.
- Identify sources of support (e.g., friends, relatives, faith community, National MS Society and MS support groups, caregiver support).
- Identify the need for health promotion, disease prevention, and screening activities.

Resources

See Chapter 9, Chart 9-9 Home Care Checklist: Managing Chronic Illness and Disability at Home and Chapter 10 and, Chart 10-8 Home Care Checklist: Managing the Therapeutic Regimen at Home for additional information.

ADL, activities of daily living; IADL, independent activities of daily living; MS, multiple sclerosis.

interventions in the patient's home. Nurses in the home setting assess for changes in the patient's physical and emotional status; provide physical care to the patient if required; coordinate outpatient services and resources; and encourage health promotion, appropriate health screenings, and adaptation. If changes in the disease or its course are noted, the nurse encourages the patient to contact the primary provider, because treatment of an acute exacerbation or new problem may be indicated. Continuing health care and follow-up are recommended.

The patient with MS is encouraged to contact the local chapter of the National MS Society for services, publications, and contact with others who have MS (see the Resources section). Local chapters also provide direct services to patients. Through group participation, the patient has an opportunity to meet others with similar problems, share experiences, and learn self-help methods in a social environment.

Evaluation

Expected patient outcomes may include:

1. Improves physical mobility
   a. Participates in gait training and rehabilitation program
   b. Establishes a balanced program of rest and exercise
   c. Uses assistive devices correctly and safely
2. Is free of injury
   a. Uses visual cues to compensate for decreased sense of touch or position
   b. Asks for assistance when necessary
3. Attains or maintains control of bladder and bowel patterns
   a. Monitors self for urine retention and employs intermittent self-catheterization technique, if indicated
   b. Identifies the signs and symptoms of urinary tract infection
   c. Maintains adequate fluid and fiber intake
   d. Identifies the foods that are constipating versus food that increase gastric motility
4. Participates in strategies to improve speech and swallowing
   a. Practices exercises recommended by speech therapist
   b. Maintains adequate nutritional intake without aspiration
5. Compensates for chronic confusion
   a. Uses lists and other aids to compensate for memory losses
   b. Discusses problems with trusted advisor or friend
   c. Substitutes new activities for those that are no longer possible
6. Demonstrates effective coping strategies
   a. Maintains sense of control
   b. Modifies lifestyle to fit goals and limitations
   c. Verbalizes desire to pursue goals and developmental tasks of adulthood
   d. Demonstrates healthy social interactions
   e. Participates in groups or community activities
7. Adheres to plan for home maintenance management
   a. Uses appropriate techniques to maintain independence
   b. Engages in health-promotion activities and health screenings as appropriate
8. Adapts to changes in sexual function
   a. Is able to discuss problem with partner and appropriate health professional
   b. Identifies alternative means of sexual expression

Myasthenia Gravis

Myasthenia gravis, an autoimmune disorder affecting the myoneural junction, is characterized by varying degrees of weakness of the voluntary muscles. It affects approximately 20 in 1 million people in the United States. More women than men are affected, commonly in the second and third decades of life; however, after age 50, the gender distribution is more equal (American Association of Neuroscience Nurses [AANN], 2013; Bader et al., 2016).

Pathophysiology

Normally, a chemical impulse precipitates the release of acetylcholine from vesicles on the nerve terminal at the myoneural junction. The acetylcholine attaches to receptor sites on the motor endplate and stimulates muscle contraction. Continuous binding of acetylcholine to the receptor site is required for muscular contraction to be sustained.

In myasthenia gravis, antibodies directed at the acetylcholine receptor sites impair transmission of impulses across the myoneural junction. Therefore, fewer receptors are available for stimulation, resulting in voluntary muscle weakness that escalates with continued activity (see Fig. 69-5). These antibodies are found in 80% to 90% of people with myasthenia gravis (Hickey, 2014). Of people with myasthenia gravis, 75% have either thymic hyperplasia or a thymic tumor, and the thymus gland is believed to be the site of antibody production (Bader et al., 2016). In patients who are antibody negative, researchers believe that the offending antibody is directed at a portion of the receptor site rather than the whole complex (AANN, 2013).

Clinical Manifestations

The initial manifestation of myasthenia gravis in 80% of patients involves the ocular muscles. Diplopia and **ptosis** (drooping of the eyelids) are common (Bader et al., 2016). Many patients also experience weakness of the muscles of the face and throat (bulbar symptoms) and generalized weakness. Weakness of the facial muscles results in a bland facial expression. Laryngeal involvement produces **dysphonia** (voice impairment) and dysphagia, which increases the risk of choking and aspiration. Generalized weakness affects all extremities and the intercostal muscles, resulting in decreasing vital capacity and respiratory failure (Mcilvoy, 2014). Myasthenia gravis is purely a motor disorder with no effect on sensation or coordination.

Assessment and Diagnostic Findings

A common test used to diagnose myasthenia gravis is the acetylcholinesterase inhibitor test. It is performed by administering edrophonium chloride (Tensilon) IV; 30 seconds after injection, facial muscle weakness and ptosis should resolve for about 5 minutes (Hickey, 2014). Immediate improvement in

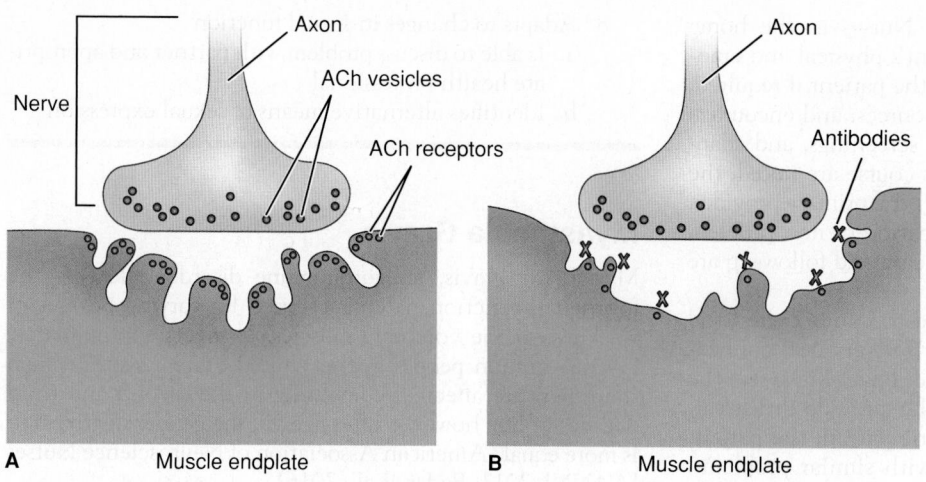

Figure 69-5 • Myasthenia gravis. **A.** Usual acetylcholine (ACh) receptor site. **B.** ACh receptor site in myasthenia gravis.

muscle strength after administration of this agent represents a positive test and usually confirms the diagnosis. Atropine should be available to control potential side effects of this medication, which include bradycardia, asystole, bronchoconstriction, sweating, and cramping.

Another study, the ice test, is indicated in patients who have cardiac conditions or asthma. With this test, an ice pack is held over the patient's eyes for 1 minute; the ptosis should temporarily resolve in a patient with myasthenia gravis (Hickey, 2014).

Several blood tests for acetylcholine antibodies are also used to confirm the diagnosis (AANN, 2013). Repetitive nerve stimulation (RNS) demonstrates a decrease in successive action potentials. A single-fiber electromyography (EMG) detects a delay or failure of neuromuscular transmission and is about 99% sensitive in confirming the diagnosis of myasthenia gravis (Hickey, 2014). This is an uncomfortable test for the patient.

The thymus gland, a site of acetylcholine receptor antibody production, may be enlarged in myasthenia gravis and may be identified by MRI scan.

Medical Management

Management of myasthenia gravis is directed at improving function and reducing and removing circulating antibodies. Therapeutic modalities include administration of anticholinesterase medications and immunosuppressive therapy, intravenous immune globulin (IVIG), therapeutic plasma exchange (TPE), and thymectomy. There is no cure for myasthenia gravis; treatments do not stop the production of the acetylcholine receptor antibodies.

Pharmacologic Therapy

Pyridostigmine bromide (Mestinon), an anticholinesterase medication, is the first line of therapy (Mcilvoy, 2014). It provides symptomatic relief by inhibiting the breakdown of acetylcholine and increasing the relative concentration of available acetylcholine at the neuromuscular junction. The dosage is gradually increased to a daily maximum and is given in divided doses (usually four times a day). Adverse effects of anticholinesterase medications include diarrhea, abdominal cramps, and/or excessive saliva (Comerford, 2015).

Pyridostigmine tends to have fewer side effects than other anticholinesterase medications.

If pyridostigmine bromide does not improve muscle strength and control fatigue, the next agents used are the immunomodulating drugs. The goal of immunosuppressive therapy is to reduce production of the antibody. Corticosteroids suppress the patient's immune response, decreasing the amount of antibody production, and this correlates with clinical improvement. An initial dose of prednisone is given daily and maintained for 1 to 2 months; as symptoms improve, the medication is tapered (Bader et al., 2016). As the corticosteroid medications take effect, the dosage of anticholinesterase medication can usually be lowered. Cytotoxic medications are used to treat myasthenia gravis if there is inadequate response to steroids. Azathioprine (Imuran) inhibits T lymphocytes and B-cell proliferation and reduces acetylcholine receptor antibody levels. Therapeutic effects may not be evident for 3 to 12 months. Leukopenia and hepatotoxicity are serious adverse effects, so monthly evaluation of liver enzymes and white blood cell count is necessary.

Intravenous immune globulin (IVIG) can be used to treat exacerbations; however, in selected patients, it is used on a long-term adjunctive basis. IVIG treatment involves the administration of pooled human gamma-globulin and improvement occurs in a few days (Hickey, 2014). The effects of IVIG typically last only about 28 days after infusion, and complications include headache, migraine exacerbation, aseptic meningitis, and flulike symptoms (Cherin, Marie, Michallet, et al., 2016).

A number of medications are contraindicated for patients with myasthenia gravis because they exacerbate the symptoms. The primary provider and the patient should weigh risks and benefits before any new medications are prescribed. Procaine (Novocaine) should be avoided, and the patient's dentist is informed of the diagnosis of myasthenia gravis.

Therapeutic Plasma Exchange

A technique called TPE, formerly referred to as plasmapheresis, is used to treat exacerbations. The patient's plasma and plasma components are removed through a centrally placed large-bore double-lumen catheter. The blood cells and antibody-containing plasma are separated, after which the cells and a plasma substitute are reinfused. Temporary reduction in the level of circulating antibodies is provided with TPE. A typical course consists of daily or alternate-day treatment, and the number of treatments is determined by the patient's response. Symptoms improve in 75% of patients undergoing TPE; however, improvement lasts only a few weeks after treatment is completed (Hickey, 2014).

 ### Surgical Management

Thymectomy (surgical removal of the thymus gland) can produce antigen-specific immunosuppression and result in clinical improvement. This surgery is frequently performed in patients younger than 65 years who have had myasthenia gravis diagnosed within the past 3 years. It is the only treatment that can result in complete remission, which occurs in approximately 35% of patients (Hickey, 2014). Improvements may take several months to several years after surgery to occur. A course of preoperative TPE decreases the time needed for postoperative mechanical ventilation.

The entire thymus gland must be removed for optimal clinical outcomes. There are three surgical approaches: transsternal, transcervical thymectomy, and video-assisted thoracoscopic surgery (AANN, 2013). After surgery, the patient is monitored in an intensive care unit, with special attention to respiratory function. The patient is weaned from mechanical ventilation after thorough respiratory assessment. After the thymus gland is removed, it may take up to 3 years for the patient to benefit from the procedure because of the long life of circulating T cells. The earlier the surgery in the disease process, the better the prognosis (Bader et al., 2016).

 ## Complications

A myasthenic crisis is an exacerbation of the disease process characterized by severe generalized muscle weakness and respiratory and bulbar weakness that may result in respiratory failure. Crisis may result from disease exacerbation or a specific precipitating event. The most common precipitator is respiratory infection; others include medication change, surgery, pregnancy, and medications that exacerbate myasthenia. A cholinergic crisis caused by overmedication with cholinesterase inhibitors is rare (AANN, 2013).

Neuromuscular respiratory failure is the critical complication in myasthenic and cholinergic crises. Respiratory muscle and bulbar weakness combine to cause respiratory compromise. Weak respiratory muscles do not support inhalation. An inadequate cough and an impaired gag reflex, caused by bulbar weakness, result in poor airway clearance. A downward trend of two respiratory function tests, the negative inspiratory force and vital capacity, is the first clinical sign of respiratory compromise.

Endotracheal intubation and mechanical ventilation may be needed (see Chapter 21). Noninvasive positive-pressure ventilation uses an external device in the form of a vest that provides respiratory support without endotracheal intubation. Cholinesterase inhibitors are stopped when respiratory failure occurs and gradually restarted after the patient demonstrates improvement with a course of TPE or IVIG. Nutritional support may be needed if the patient is intubated for a long period or swallowing ability is affected (see Chapter 44).

Nursing Management

Because myasthenia gravis is a chronic disease and most patients are seen on an outpatient basis, much of the nursing care focuses on patient and family education. Educational topics for outpatient self-care include medication management, energy conservation, strategies to help with ocular manifestations, and prevention and management of complications.

Medication management is a crucial component of ongoing care. Understanding the actions of the medications and taking them on schedule is emphasized, as are the consequences of delaying medication and the signs and symptoms of myasthenic and cholinergic crises. The patient can determine the best times for daily dosing by keeping a diary to determine fluctuation of symptoms and to learn when the medication is wearing off. The medication schedule can then be manipulated to maximize strength throughout the day.

 ### Quality and Safety Nursing Alert

Maintenance of stable blood levels of anticholinesterase medications is imperative to stabilize muscle strength. Therefore, the anticholinesterase medications must be given on time. Any delay in administration of medications may exacerbate muscle weakness and make it impossible for the patient to take medications orally.

Regular administration of IVIG or subcutaneous immunoglobulin (SCIG) may be prescribed. The patient and family are educated about managing immunoglobulin therapy.

 For the procedural guidelines for management of IVIG, go to **thepoint.lww.com/ Brunner14e.**

The patient is also educated about strategies to conserve energy. To do this, the nurse helps the patient identify the optimal times for rest throughout the day. If the patient lives in a two-story home, the nurse can suggest that frequently used items (e.g., hygiene products, cleaning products, snacks) be kept on each floor to minimize travel between floors. The patient is encouraged to apply for a handicapped license plate to minimize walking from parking spaces and to schedule activities to coincide with peak energy and strength levels. Using consistent routines, scheduling periods of rest, monitoring for depression, maintaining good sleep patterns, and incorporating interventions to conserve energy are all strategies to reduce fatigue (Bader et al., 2016).

To minimize the risk of aspiration, mealtimes should coincide with the peak effects of anticholinesterase medication. In addition, rest before meals is encouraged to reduce muscle fatigue. The patient is advised to sit upright during meals, with the neck slightly flexed to facilitate swallowing. Soft foods in gravy or sauces can be swallowed more easily. Eating large meals in the morning and smaller meals in the evening is another good strategy (Bader et al., 2016). Supplemental feedings may be helpful to ensure adequate nutrition.

If choking occurs frequently, the patient should be evaluated by a speech-language pathologist for formal dietary and mechanical techniques to avoid aspiration. Suction should be available at home, with the patient and family instructed in its use.

Impaired vision results from ptosis of one or both eyelids, decreased eye movement, or double vision. To prevent corneal damage when the eyelids do not close completely, the patient is instructed to tape the eyes closed for short intervals and to regularly instill artificial tears. Patients who wear eyeglasses can have "crutches" attached to help lift the eyelids. Patching of one eye can help with double vision.

The patient is reminded of the importance of maintaining health-promotion practices and following health care screening recommendations. Factors that exacerbate symptoms and potentially cause crisis should be noted and avoided: emotional stress, infections (particularly respiratory infections), vigorous physical activity, some medications, and high environmental temperature. The Myasthenia Gravis Foundation of America provides support groups, services, and educational materials for patients, families, and health care providers (see the Resources section).

 Myasthenic Crisis

Respiratory distress and varying degrees of dysphagia, dysarthria (difficulty speaking), eyelid ptosis, diplopia, and prominent muscle weakness are symptoms of myasthenic crisis. The patient is placed in an intensive care unit for constant monitoring because of associated intense and sudden fluctuations in clinical condition.

Providing ventilatory assistance takes precedence in the immediate management of the patient with myasthenic crisis. Ongoing assessment for respiratory failure is essential. The nurse assesses the respiratory rate, depth, and breath sounds and monitors pulmonary function parameters (vital capacity and negative inspiratory force) to detect pulmonary problems before respiratory dysfunction progresses. Blood is drawn for arterial blood gas analysis. Endotracheal intubation and mechanical ventilation may be needed (see Chapter 21).

If the abdominal, intercostal, and pharyngeal muscles are severely weak, the patient cannot cough, take deep breaths, or clear secretions. Chest physiotherapy, including postural drainage to mobilize secretions and suctioning to remove secretions, may have to be performed frequently. (Postural drainage should not be performed for 30 minutes after feeding.)

Assessment strategies and supportive measures include the following:

- Arterial blood gases, serum electrolytes, input and output, and daily weight are monitored.
- If the patient cannot swallow, enteral tube feedings may be prescribed (see Chapter 44).
- Sedative and tranquilizing agents are avoided, because they aggravate hypoxia and hypercapnia and can cause respiratory and cardiac depression.

Guillain–Barré Syndrome (GBS)

GBS, also known as acute idiopathic polyneuritis, is an autoimmune attack on the peripheral nerve myelin. The result is acute, rapid segmental demyelination of peripheral nerves and some cranial nerves, producing ascending weakness with dyskinesia (inability to execute voluntary movements),

hyporeflexia, and **paresthesias** (a sensation of numbness, tingling, or a "pins and needles" sensation). An antecedent event (most often a viral infection) precipitates clinical presentation in approximately 60% to 70% of cases (Bader et al., 2016). *Campylobacter jejuni* (implicated in 24% to 50% of cases), cytomegalovirus, Epstein–Barr virus, *Mycoplasma pneumoniae*, *H. influenzae*, and HIV are the most common infectious agents that are associated with the development of GBS.

There are several types of GBS. With the most well-known type, the patient experiences weakness in the lower extremities, which progresses upward and has the potential for respiratory failure. The second type is purely motor with no altered sensation. A third type, called descending GBS, is much more difficult to diagnose; it mostly affects the head and neck muscles. The rarest type, the Miller–Fisher variant, presents with ataxia, areflexia, and opthalmoplegia (McNair, 2013).

The annual incidence of GBS is 1 to 2 cases per 100,000 people, and it is more frequent in males between 16 and 25 years of age and those older than 55 years (Bader et al., 2016). Death occurs in 5% to 10% of cases, resulting from respiratory failure, autonomic dysfunction, sepsis, or pulmonary embolism (PE) (Hickey, 2014).

Pathophysiology

Myelin is a complex substance that covers nerves, providing insulation and speeding the conduction of impulses from the cell body to the dendrites. The cell that produces myelin in the peripheral nervous system is the Schwann cell. In GBS, the Schwann cell can be spared, allowing for remyelination in the recovery phase of the disease. If damage has occurred to the axons, then regrowth is required and takes months or years and is often incomplete (Hickey, 2014).

GBS is the result of a cell-mediated and humoral immune attack on peripheral nerve myelin proteins that causes inflammatory demyelination. The best-accepted theory of cause is molecular mimicry, in which an infectious organism contains an amino acid that mimics the peripheral nerve myelin protein. The immune system cannot distinguish between the two proteins and attacks and destroys peripheral nerve myelin. The exact location of the immune attack within the peripheral nervous system is the ganglioside GM1b. With the autoimmune attack, there is an influx of macrophages and other immune-mediated agents that attack myelin and cause inflammation and destruction, interruption of nerve conduction, and axonal loss (Hickey, 2014).

Clinical Manifestations

GBS typically begins with muscle weakness and diminished reflexes of the lower extremities. Hyporeflexia and weakness may progress to tetraplegia. Demyelination of the nerves that innervate the diaphragm and intercostal muscles results in neuromuscular respiratory failure. Sensory symptoms include paresthesias of the hands and feet and pain related to the demyelination of sensory fibers.

The antecedent event usually occurs 1 to 3 weeks before symptoms begin. Weakness usually begins in the legs and may progresses upward. Maximum weakness (the plateau) varies in length but usually includes neuromuscular respiratory failure and bulbar weakness. GBS progresses to peak severity typically within 2 weeks and no longer than 4 weeks. If progression is longer, then the patient is classified as having chronic inflammatory demyelinating polyneuropathy (Hickey, 2014). Any residual symptoms are permanent and reflect axonal damage from demyelination.

Cranial nerve demyelination can result in a variety of clinical manifestations. Optic nerve demyelination may result in blindness. Bulbar muscle weakness related to demyelination of the glossopharyngeal and vagus nerves results in the inability to swallow or clear secretions. Vagus nerve demyelination results in autonomic dysfunction, manifested by instability of the cardiovascular system. The presentation is variable and may include tachycardia, bradycardia, hypertension, or orthostatic hypotension. The symptoms of autonomic dysfunction occur and resolve rapidly. GBS does not affect cognitive function or LOC.

Although the classic clinical features include areflexia and ascending weakness, variations in the clinical presentation occurs. There may be a sensory presentation, with progressive sensory symptoms; an atypical axonal destruction; or the Miller–Fisher variant, which includes paralysis of the ocular muscles, ataxia, and areflexia (McNair, 2013).

Assessment and Diagnostic Findings

The patient presents with symmetric weakness, diminished reflexes, and upward progression of motor weakness. A history of a viral illness in the previous few weeks suggests the diagnosis. Changes in vital capacity and negative inspiratory force are assessed to identify impending neuromuscular respiratory failure. Serum laboratory tests are not useful in the diagnosis. However, elevated protein levels are detected in CSF evaluation, without an increase in other cells. Evoked potential studies demonstrate a progressive loss of nerve conduction velocity.

Medical Management

Because of the possibility of rapid progression and neuromuscular respiratory failure, GBS is a medical emergency that may require management in an intensive care unit. After baseline values are identified, assessment of changes in muscle strength and respiratory function alert the clinician to the physical and respiratory needs of the patient. Respiratory therapy or mechanical ventilation may be necessary to support pulmonary function and adequate oxygenation. Some clinicians recommend elective intubation before the onset of extreme respiratory muscle fatigue. Emergent intubation may result in autonomic dysfunction, and mechanical ventilation may be required for an extended period. The patient is weaned from mechanical ventilation after the respiratory muscles can again support spontaneous respiration and maintain adequate tissue oxygenation.

Other interventions are aimed at preventing the complications of immobility. These may include the use of anticoagulant agents and sequential compression boots to prevent venous thromboembolism (VTE), including deep vein thrombosis (DVT) and PE.

TPE and IVIG are used to directly affect the peripheral nerve myelin antibody level. Both therapies decrease circulating antibody levels and reduce the amount of time the patient is immobilized and dependent on mechanical

ventilation. The cardiovascular risks posed by autonomic dysfunction require continuous electrocardiographic (ECG) monitoring. Tachycardia and hypertension are treated with short-acting medications such as alpha-adrenergic blocking agents. The use of short-acting agents is important, because autonomic dysfunction is very labile. Hypotension is managed by increasing the amount of IV fluid administered.

NURSING PROCESS
The Patient With GBS

Assessment

Ongoing assessment for disease progression is critical. The patient is monitored for life-threatening complications (respiratory failure, cardiac dysrhythmias, VTE [including DVT or PE]) so that appropriate interventions can be initiated. Because of the threat to the patient in this sudden, potentially life-threatening disease, the nurse must assess the patient's and family's ability to cope and their use of coping strategies.

Diagnosis

NURSING DIAGNOSES
Based on the assessment data, major nursing diagnoses may include the following:
- Ineffective breathing pattern and impaired gas exchange related to rapidly progressive weakness and impending respiratory failure
- Impaired bed and physical mobility related to paralysis
- Imbalanced nutrition: less than body requirements related to inability to swallow
- Impaired verbal communication related to cranial nerve dysfunction
- Fear and anxiety related to loss of control and paralysis

COLLABORATIVE PROBLEMS/POTENTIAL COMPLICATIONS
Potential complications may include the following:
- Respiratory failure
- Autonomic dysfunction

Planning and Goals

The major goals for the patient may include improved respiratory function, increased mobility, improved nutritional status, effective communication, decreased fear and anxiety, and absence of complications.

Nursing Interventions

MAINTAINING RESPIRATORY FUNCTION
Respiratory function can be maximized with incentive spirometry and chest physiotherapy. Monitoring for changes in vital capacity and negative inspiratory force is key to early intervention for neuromuscular respiratory failure. Mechanical ventilation is required if the vital capacity falls, making spontaneous breathing impossible and tissue oxygenation inadequate.

The potential need for mechanical ventilation should be discussed with the patient and family on admission to provide time for psychological preparation and decision making. Intubation and mechanical ventilation result in less anxiety if they are initiated on a nonemergency basis to a patient who has been well informed. The patient may require mechanical ventilation for a long period. See Chapter 21 for the nursing management of the patient requiring mechanical ventilation.

Bulbar weakness that impairs the ability to swallow and clear secretions is another factor in the development of respiratory failure in the patient with GBS. Suctioning may be needed to maintain a clear airway.

The nurse assesses the blood pressure and heart rate frequently to identify autonomic dysfunction so that interventions can be initiated quickly if needed. Medications are given or a temporary pacemaker placed for clinically significant bradycardia.

ENHANCING PHYSICAL MOBILITY

Nursing interventions to enhance physical mobility and prevent the complications of immobility are key to the function and survival of patients. The paralyzed extremities are supported in functional positions, and passive range-of-motion exercises are performed at least twice daily. DVT and PE are threats to the patient who is paralyzed. Nursing interventions are aimed at preventing VTE. Range-of-motion exercises, position changes, anticoagulation, the use of antiembolism stockings and sequential compression boots, and adequate hydration decrease the risk of VTE.

Padding may be placed over bony prominences, such as the elbows and heels, to reduce the risk of pressure ulcers. The need for frequent position changes cannot be overemphasized. The nurse evaluates laboratory test results that may indicate malnutrition or dehydration, both of which increase the risk of pressure ulcers and decrease mobility. The nurse collaborates with the primary provider and dietitian to develop a plan to meet the patient's nutritional and hydration needs.

PROVIDING ADEQUATE NUTRITION

Paralytic ileus may result from insufficient parasympathetic activity. In this event, the nurse administers IV fluids and parenteral nutrition as a supplement and monitors for the return of bowel sounds. If the patient cannot swallow because of bulbar paralysis (immobility of muscles), a gastrostomy tube may be placed to administer nutrients. The nurse carefully assesses the return of the gag reflex and bowel sounds before resuming oral nutrition.

IMPROVING COMMUNICATION

Because of paralysis, the patient cannot talk, laugh, or cry and therefore has no method for communicating needs or expressing emotion. Although the patient may be unable to speak, cognition is completely intact. Establishing some form of communication with picture cards or an eye blink system provides a means of communication. Collaboration with the speech therapist may be helpful in developing a communication mechanism that is most effective for a specific patient.

DECREASING FEAR AND ANXIETY

The patient and family are faced with a sudden, potentially life-threatening disease; therefore, their levels of anxiety and fear may be high. The impact of disease on the family depends on the patient's role within the family. Referral to a support group may provide information and support to the patient and family.

The family may feel helpless in caring for the patient. Mechanical ventilation and monitoring devices may frighten and intimidate them. Family members often want to participate in physical care; with instruction and support by the nurse, they should be allowed and encouraged to do so.

In addition to fear, the patient may experience isolation, loneliness, and lack of control. Nursing interventions that increase the patient's sense of control include providing information about the condition, emphasizing a positive appraisal of coping resources, and providing instruction about relaxation exercises and distraction techniques. The positive attitude and atmosphere of the multidisciplinary team are important to promote a sense of well-being.

Diversional activities are encouraged to decrease loneliness and isolation. Encouraging visitors, engaging visitors or volunteers to read to the patient, listening to music or books on tape, and watching television are ways to alleviate the patient's sense of isolation.

MONITORING AND MANAGING POTENTIAL COMPLICATIONS

Thorough assessment of respiratory function at regular and frequent intervals is essential, because respiratory insufficiency and subsequent failure due to weakness or paralysis of the intercostal muscles and diaphragm may develop quickly. Respiratory failure is the major cause of mortality. In addition to the respiratory rate and the quality of respirations, vital capacity is monitored frequently and at regular intervals so that respiratory insufficiency can be anticipated. Decreasing vital capacity with associated muscle weakness indicates impending respiratory failure. Signs and symptoms include breathlessness while speaking, shallow and irregular breathing, the use of accessory muscles, tachycardia, weak cough, and changes in respiratory pattern.

Other complications include cardiac dysrhythmias (which necessitate ECG monitoring), transient hypertension, orthostatic hypotension, DVT, PE, urinary retention, and other threats to any patient who is immobilized and paralyzed. These complications require monitoring and attention to prevent them and prompt treatment if indicated.

PROMOTING HOME, COMMUNITY-BASED, AND TRANSITIONAL CARE

Educating Patients About Self-Care. Patients with GBS and their families are usually frightened by the sudden onset of life-threatening symptoms and their severity. Therefore, educating the patient and family about the disorder and its generally favorable prognosis is important (see Chart 69-5).

During the acute phase of the illness, the patient and family are educated about strategies that can be implemented to minimize the effects of immobility and other complications. As function begins to return, family members and other home care providers are educated about care of the patient and their role in the rehabilitation process. Preparation for discharge is an interdisciplinary effort requiring family or caregiver education by all team members, including the nurse, physician, occupational and physical therapists, speech therapist, and respiratory therapist.

Continuing and Transitional Care. Most patients with GBS experience complete recovery. Patients who have experienced total or prolonged paralysis require intensive rehabilitation; the extent depends on the patient's needs. Approaches include a comprehensive inpatient program if deficits are significant, an outpatient program if the patient can travel by car, or a home program of physical and occupational therapy. The recovery phase may be long and requires patience as well as involvement on the part of the patient and family.

Chart 69-5	**HOME CARE CHECKLIST**
	The Patient With GBS

At the completion of education, the patient and/or caregiver will be able to:

- State the impact of GBS and treatment on physiologic functioning, ADLs, IADLs, roles, relationships, and spirituality.
- State the purpose, dose, route, schedule, side effects, and precautions for prescribed medications.
- State how to contact all members of the treatment team (e.g., health care providers, home care professionals, and durable medical equipment and supply vendor).
- State what types of environmental and safety changes or supports are needed for optimum functioning in the home.
  - State changes in lifestyle (e.g., nutrition, skin care, exercise, activity) necessary during recovery period and to maintain health as indicated.
  - Demonstrate environmental modifications and adaptive techniques for accomplishing ADLs (e.g., bathing, hygiene, grooming, dressing) and safely managing self-care.
  - Manage respiratory needs—tracheostomy care, suctioning.
  - Verbalize dietary adjustments and optimum nutrition during recovery.
  - Demonstrate proper body mechanics regarding lifting and transfers.

- Practice gait training and strength endurance.
- Perform range-of-motion exercises.
- Discuss bowel and bladder management.
- Operate and explain function of medical equipment and mobility aids—walkers, wheelchairs, bedside commodes, tub transfer benches, adaptive devices.
- Describe coping mechanisms and diversional activities appropriately.
- Relate how to reach primary provider with questions or complications.
- State time and date of follow-up medical appointments, therapy, and testing.
- Identify sources of support (e.g., friends, relatives, faith community, GBS Foundation International, support groups, caregiver support)
- Identify the need for health promotion, disease prevention, and screening activities

Resources

See Chapter 10, Chart 10-8 Home Care Checklist: Managing the Therapeutic Regimen at Home for additional information.

ADL, activities of daily living; IADL, independent activities of daily living; GBS, Guillain–Barré syndrome.

During acute care, the focus is on immediate issues and deficits. The nurse needs to remind or educate patients and family members of the need for continuing health-promotion and screening practices after this initial phase of care.

Evaluation

Expected patient outcomes may include the following:
1. Maintains effective respirations and airway clearance
   a. Has clear breath sounds on auscultation
   b. Demonstrates gradual improvement in respiratory function
   c. Breathes spontaneously
   d. Has vital capacity within normal range
   e. Exhibits arterial blood gases and pulse oximetry within normal limits
2. Shows increasing mobility
   a. Regains use of extremities
   b. Participates in rehabilitation program
   c. Demonstrates no contractures and minimal muscle atrophy
3. Receives adequate nutrition and hydration
   a. Consumes diet adequate to meet nutritional needs
   b. Swallows without aspiration
4. Demonstrates recovery of speech
   a. Communicates needs through alternative strategies
   b. Practices exercises recommended by the speech therapist
5. Shows lessening fear and anxiety
6. Has absence of complications
   a. Maintains intact skin integrity
   b. Does not develop VTE
   c. Voids without difficulty

CRANIAL NERVE DISORDERS

Because the brainstem and cranial nerves involve vital motor, sensory, and autonomic functions of the body, these nerves may be affected by conditions arising primarily within these structures or in secondary extension from adjacent disease processes. The cranial nerves are examined separately and in sequence (see Chapter 65). Some cranial nerve deficits can be detected by observing the patient's face, eye movements, speech, and swallowing. EMG is used to investigate motor and sensory dysfunction. An MRI scan is used to obtain images of the cranial nerves and brainstem. An overview of disorders that may affect each of the cranial nerves, including clinical manifestations and nursing interventions, is presented in Table 69-2. The following discussion centers on the most common disorders of the cranial nerves: trigeminal neuralgia, a condition affecting the fifth cranial nerve, and Bell palsy, caused by involvement of the seventh cranial nerve.

Trigeminal Neuralgia (Tic Douloureux)

Trigeminal neuralgia is a condition of the fifth cranial nerve that is characterized by paroxysms of sudden pain in the area innervated by any of the three branches of the nerve (Bader et al., 2016) (see Fig. 69-6). The pain ends as abruptly as it starts and is described as a unilateral shooting and stabbing or burning sensation. The unilateral nature of the pain is an important feature. Associated involuntary contraction of the facial muscles can cause sudden closing of the eye or twitching of the mouth, hence the former name *tic douloureux* (painful twitch). Although the cause is not certain, it is thought to

TABLE 69-2 Disorders of Cranial Nerves

Disorder	Clinical Manifestations	Nursing Interventions
Olfactory Nerve—I		
Head trauma Intracranial tumor Intracranial surgery	Unilateral or bilateral anosmia (temporary or persistent) Diminished taste for food	Assess sense of smell. Assess for cerebrospinal fluid rhinorrhea if patient has sustained head trauma.
Optic Nerve—II		
Optic neuritis Increased intracranial pressure Pituitary tumor	Lesions of optic tract producing homonymous hemianopsia	Assess visual acuity. Restructure environment to prevent injuries. Educate patient to accommodate for visual loss.
Oculomotor Nerve—III		Assess extraocular movement and for nonreactive pupil.
Trochlear Nerve—IV		Assess extraocular movement and for nonreactive pupil.
Abducens Nerve—VI		
Vascular Brainstem ischemia Hemorrhage and infarction Neoplasm Trauma Infection	Dilation of pupil with loss of light reflex on one side Impairment of ocular movement Diplopia Gaze palsies Ptosis of eyelid	Assess extraocular movement and for nonreactive pupil.
Trigeminal Nerve—V		
Trigeminal neuralgia Head trauma Cerebellopontine lesion Sinus tract tumor and metastatic disease Compression of trigeminal root by tumor	Pain in face Diminished or loss of corneal reflex Chewing dysfunction	Assess for pain and triggering mechanisms for pain. Assess for difficulty in chewing. Discuss trigger zones and pain precipitants with patient. Protect cornea from abrasion. Ensure good oral hygiene. Educate patient about medication regimen.
Facial Nerve—VII		
Bell palsy Facial nerve tumor Intracranial lesion Herpes zoster	Facial dysfunction; weakness and paralysis Hemifacial spasm Diminished or absent taste Pain	Recognize facial paralysis as emergency; refer for treatment as soon as possible. Discuss protective care for eyes. Select easily chewed foods; patient should eat and drink from unaffected side of mouth. Emphasize importance of oral hygiene. Provide emotional support for changed appearance of face.
Vestibulocochlear Nerve—VIII		
Tumors and acoustic neuroma Vascular compression of nerve Ménière syndrome	Tinnitus Vertigo Hearing difficulties	Assess pattern of vertigo. Provide for safety measures to prevent falls. Ensure that patient can maintain balance before ambulating. Caution patient to change positions slowly. Assist with ambulation. Encourage the use of assistive devices.
Glossopharyngeal Nerve—IX		
Glossopharyngeal neuralgia from neurovascular compression of cranial nerves IX and X Trauma Inflammatory conditions Tumor Vertebral artery aneurysms	Pain at base of tongue Difficulty in swallowing Loss of gag reflex Palatal, pharyngeal, and laryngeal paralysis	Assess for paroxysmal pain in throat, decreased or absent swallowing, and gag and cough reflexes. Monitor for dysphagia, aspiration, and nasal dysarthric speech. Position patient upright for eating or tube feeding.
Vagus Nerve—X		
Spastic palsy of larynx; bulbar paralysis; high vagal paralysis Guillain–Barré syndrome Vagal body tumors Nerve paralysis from malignancy, surgical trauma such as carotid endarterectomy	Voice changes (temporary or permanent hoarseness) Vocal paralysis Dysphagia	Assess for airway obstruction/provide airway management. Prevent aspiration. Support patient having voice reconstruction procedures.

Disorder	Clinical Manifestations	Nursing Interventions
Spinal Accessory Nerve—XI		
Spinal cord disorder Amyotrophic lateral sclerosis Trauma Guillain–Barré syndrome	Drooping of affected shoulder with limited shoulder movement Weakness or paralysis of head rotation, flexion, extension; shoulder elevation	Support patient undergoing diagnostic tests.
Hypoglossal Nerve—XII		
Medullary lesions Amyotrophic lateral sclerosis Polio and motor system disease, which may destroy hypoglossal nuclei Multiple sclerosis Trauma	Abnormal movements of tongue Weakness or paralysis of tongue muscles Difficulty in talking, chewing, and swallowing	Observe swallowing ability. Observe speech pattern. Be aware of swallowing or vocal difficulties. Prepare for alternate feeding methods (tube feeding) to maintain nutrition.

Adapted from Bader, M., Littlejohns, L. R., & Olson, D. (2016). *AANN core curriculum for neuroscience nursing* (6th ed.). Chicago, IL: American Association of Neuroscience Nurses. Hickey, J. V. (2014). *The clinical practice of neurological & neurosurgical nursing* (7th ed.). Philadelphia, PA: Lippincott Williams & Wilkins.

be demyelinaiton of axons in the ganglion, root, and nerve (Grossman & Porth, 2014).

Trigeminal neuralgia occurs most often as people age, most commonly between the fifth and sixth decade of life. It is more common in women and in people with MS compared to the general population (Bader et al., 2016). Patients who develop trigeminal neuralgia before age 50 years should be evaluated for the coexistence of MS, because trigeminal neuralgia occurs in approximately 5% of patients with MS (Bader et al., 2016). Pain-free intervals may be measured in terms of minutes, hours, days, or longer. With advancing years, the painful episodes tend to become more frequent and agonizing. The patient lives in constant fear of attacks.

Paroxysms can occur with any stimulation of the terminals of the affected nerve branches, such as washing the face, shaving, brushing the teeth, eating, and drinking. A draft of cold air or direct pressure against the nerve trunk may also cause pain. Certain areas are called *trigger points* because the slightest touch immediately starts a paroxysm or episode. To avoid stimulating these areas, patients with trigeminal neuralgia try not to touch or wash their faces, shave, chew, or do anything else that might cause an attack. These behaviors are a clue to the diagnosis.

Medical Management

Pharmacologic Therapy

Anticonvulsant agents, such as carbamazepine (Tegretol), relieve pain in most patients with trigeminal neuralgia by reducing the transmission of impulses at certain nerve terminals. Carbamazepine is taken with meals. Serum levels must be monitored to avoid toxicity in patients who require high doses to control the pain. Side effects include nausea, dizziness, drowsiness, and aplastic anemia. Serious drug reactions occur more often in people of Asian ethnicity (Bader et al., 2016). The patient is monitored for bone marrow depression during long-term therapy. Gabapentin and baclofen are also used for pain control. If pain control is still not achieved, phenytoin may be used as adjunctive therapy.

Surgical Management

If pharmacologic management fails to relieve pain, a number of surgical options are available. Although these procedures may relieve facial pain for a few years, recurrence and complication rates are high (Hickey, 2014). The choice of procedure depends on the patient's preference and health status. The procedures are designed to either decompress the nerve and save nerve function or to damage the nerve and destroy nerve function to keep it from malfunctioning (Bader et al., 2016).

Microvascular Decompression of the Trigeminal Nerve

An intracranial approach is used to relieve the contact between the cerebral vessel and the trigeminal nerve root entry. With the aid of an operating microscope, the artery loop is lifted from the nerve to relieve the pressure, and a small prosthetic device is inserted to prevent recurrence of impingement on the nerve. The postoperative management is the same as for other intracranial surgeries (see Chapter 66).

Figure 69-6 • Distribution of trigeminal nerve branches—the fifth cranial nerve.

Radiofrequency Thermal Coagulation

Percutaneous radiofrequency produces a thermal lesion on the trigeminal nerve. Although immediate pain relief is experienced, dysesthesia of the face and loss of the corneal reflex may occur. The use of stereotactic MRI for identification of the trigeminal nerve followed by gamma knife radiosurgery is being used at some medical centers. Gamma knife radiosurgery is a noninvasive method of delivering focused radiation to the trigeminal nerve; it requires 6 to 8 weeks of treatment for maximal effect to occur (Zakrzewska & Akram, 2011).

Percutaneous Balloon Microcompression

Percutaneous balloon microcompression disrupts large myelinated fibers in all three branches of the trigeminal nerve. After its placement, the balloon is filled with a contrast material for fluoroscopic identification. The balloon compresses the nerve root for 1 minute and provides microvascular decompression (Bader et al., 2016).

Nursing Management

Preventing Pain

Preoperative management of a patient with trigeminal neuralgia occurs mostly on an outpatient basis and includes recognizing factors that may aggravate excruciating facial pain, such as food that is too hot or too cold or jarring of the patient's bed or chair. Even washing the face, combing the hair, or brushing the teeth may produce acute pain. The nurse can assist the patient in preventing or reducing this pain by providing instructions about preventive strategies. Providing cotton pads and room temperature water for washing the face, instructing the patient to rinse with mouthwash after eating if toothbrushing causes pain, and performing personal hygiene during pain-free intervals are all effective strategies. The patient is instructed to take food and fluids at room temperature, to chew on the unaffected side, and to ingest soft foods. The nurse recognizes that anxiety, depression, and insomnia often accompany chronic painful conditions and uses appropriate interventions and referrals. See Chapter 12 for management of patients with chronic pain.

Providing Postoperative Care

Postoperative neurologic assessments are conducted to evaluate the patient for facial motor and sensory deficits in each of the three branches of the trigeminal nerve. If the surgery results in sensory deficits to the affected side of the face, the patient is instructed not to rub the eye because the pain of a resulting injury will not be detected. The eye is assessed for irritation or redness. Artificial tears may be prescribed to prevent dryness in the affected eye. The patient is cautioned not to chew on the affected side until numbness has diminished. The patient is observed carefully for any difficulty in eating or swallowing foods of different consistencies.

Bell Palsy

Bell palsy (facial paralysis) is caused by unilateral inflammation of the seventh cranial nerve, which results in weakness or paralysis of the facial muscles on the affected side (see Fig. 69-7). Although the cause is unknown, theories include

Figure 69-7 • Distribution of the facial nerve—the seventh cranial nerve.

vascular ischemia, viral disease (herpes simplex, herpes zoster), autoimmune disease, or a combination of all of these factors. Most adults with Bell palsy are younger than 45 years (Hickey, 2014).

Bell palsy may be a type of pressure paralysis. The inflamed, edematous nerve becomes compressed to the point of damage, or its blood supply is occluded, producing ischemic necrosis of the nerve. The face is distorted from paralysis of the facial muscles; decreased lacrimation (tearing) occurs; and the patient experiences painful sensations in the face, behind the ear, and in the eye. The patient may also experience speech difficulties and may be unable to eat on the affected side because of weakness or paralysis of the facial muscles. The majority of patients recover completely and Bell palsy rarely recurs (Hickey, 2014).

Medical Management

The objectives of treatment are to maintain the muscle tone of the face and to prevent or minimize denervation. The patient should be reassured that no stroke has occurred and that spontaneous recovery occurs within 3 to 5 weeks in most patients.

Corticosteroid therapy (prednisone) may be prescribed to reduce inflammation and edema; this reduces vascular compression and permits restoration of blood circulation to the nerve. Early administration of corticosteroid therapy appears to diminish the severity of the disease, relieve the pain, and prevent or minimize denervation (Gagyor, Madhok, Daly, et al., 2016).

Facial pain is controlled with analgesic agents. Electrical stimulation may be applied to the face to prevent muscle atrophy. Although most patients recover with conservative treatment, surgical exploration of the facial nerve may be indicated if a tumor is suspected, for surgical decompression of the facial nerve, or for surgical treatment of a paralyzed face (Hickey, 2014).

Nursing Management

While the paralysis is present, nursing care involves protection of the eye from injury. Frequently, the eyelid does not close completely and the blink reflex is diminished, so the eye is vulnerable to injury from dust and foreign particles. Corneal irritation and ulceration may occur. Distortion of the lower lid alters the proper drainage of tears. To prevent injury, the eye should be covered with a protective shield at night. The eye patch may abrade the cornea, however, because there is some difficulty in keeping the partially paralyzed eyelids closed. Moisturizing eye drops during the day and eye ointment at bedtime may help prevent injury (Hickey, 2014). The patient can be educated to close the paralyzed eyelid manually before going to sleep. Wraparound sunglasses or goggles may be worn during the day to decrease evaporation from the eye.

After the sensitivity of the nerve to touch decreases and the patient can tolerate touching the face, the nurse can suggest massaging the face several times daily, using a gentle upward motion, to maintain muscle tone. Facial exercises, such as wrinkling the forehead, blowing out the cheeks, and whistling, may be performed with the aid of a mirror to prevent muscle atrophy. Exposure of the face to cold and drafts is avoided.

DISORDERS OF THE PERIPHERAL NERVOUS SYSTEM

Peripheral Neuropathies

A peripheral **neuropathy** (disorder of the nervous system) is a disorder affecting the peripheral motor and sensory nerves. Peripheral nerves connect the spinal cord and brain to all other organs. They transmit motor impulses from the brain and relay sensory impulses to the brain. Peripheral neuropathies are characterized by bilateral and symmetric disturbance of function, usually beginning in the feet and hands. The most common cause of peripheral neuropathy is diabetes with poor glycemic control. The major symptoms of peripheral nerve disorders are loss of sensation, muscle atrophy, weakness, diminished reflexes, pain, and paresthesia of the extremities.

Peripheral nerve disorders are diagnosed by history, physical examination, and electrodiagnostic studies such as EEG. The diagnosis of peripheral neuropathy in the geriatric population is challenging because many symptoms, such as decreased reflexes, can be associated with the normal aging process (Eliopoulos, 2018).

No specific treatment exists for peripheral neuropathy. Elimination or control of the cause may slow progression. Patients with peripheral neuropathy are at risk for falls, thermal injuries, and skin breakdown. The plan of care includes inspection of the lower extremities for skin breakdown. Assistive devices such as a walker or cane may decrease the risk

of falls. Bathwater temperature is checked to avoid thermal injury. Footwear should be accurately sized. Driving may be limited or eliminated, thereby disrupting the patient's sense of independence.

Mononeuropathy

Mononeuropathy is limited to a single peripheral nerve and its branches. It arises when the trunk of the nerve is compressed or entrapped (as in carpal tunnel syndrome), traumatized (as when bruised by a blow), overstretched (as in joint dislocation), punctured by a needle used to inject a drug or damaged by the drugs thus injected, or inflamed because an adjacent infectious process extends to the nerve trunk. Mononeuropathy is frequently seen in patients with diabetes.

Pain is seldom a major symptom of mononeuropathy when the condition is due to trauma, but in patients with complicating inflammatory conditions such as arthritis, pain is prominent. Pain is increased with all body movements that tend to stretch, strain, or cause pressure on the injured nerve and sudden jarring of the body (e.g., from coughing or sneezing). The skin in the areas supplied by nerves that are injured or diseased may become reddened and glossy, the subcutaneous tissue may become edematous, and the nails and hair in this area are altered. Chemical injuries to a nerve trunk, such as those caused by drugs injected into or near it, are often permanent.

The objective of treatment of mononeuropathy is to remove the cause, if possible (e.g., freeing the compressed nerve). Local corticosteroid injections may reduce inflammation and the pressure on the nerve. Aspirin or codeine may be used to relieve pain. Chronic pain can be treated with neuropathic pain medications such as gabapentin (Bader et al., 2016).

Nursing care involves protection of the affected limb or area from injury, as well as appropriate patient education about mononeuropathy and its treatment.

CRITICAL THINKING EXERCISES

1 `pg` A 19-year-old patient is admitted with suspected meningitis. Describe the pathophysiology of meningitis. What are the signs of meningeal irritation the nurse should watch for and how are they tested? What is the priority nursing diagnosis in the patient with meningitis? What history and physical findings are common in the patient with meningitis?

2 `pg` Identify the priorities, approach, and techniques you would use to provide care to the patients in your assignment on an intermediate neuroscience unit. Two of the patients have a diagnosis of myasthenia gravis, one is intubated and on a ventilator, one patient has a diagnosis of GBS and the other has meningitis. What tasks can you delegate and to whom?

3 `ebp` A 35-year-old woman is newly diagnosed with Bell palsy. Identify her treatment options. Describe the evidence base for the options that you have identified and the criteria used to evaluate the strength of the evidence for her various treatment options.

REFERENCES

*Asterisk indicates nursing research.
**Double asterisk indicates classic reference.

Books

American Association of Neuroscience Nurses (AANN). (2013). *Care of the patient with myasthenia gravis: AANN patient guideline series.* Glenview, IL: Author.

Bader, M., Littlejohns, L. R., & Olson, D. (2016). *AANN core curriculum for neuroscience nursing* (6th ed.). Chicago, IL: American Association of Neuroscience Nurses.

Comerford, K. C. (2015). *Nursing 2015 drug handbook.* Philadelphia, PA: Wolters Kluwer.

Eliopoulos, C. (2018). *Gerontological nursing* (9th ed.). Philadelphia, PA: Lippincott Williams & Wilkins.

Grossman, S. C., & Porth, C. M. (2014). *Pathophysiology: Concepts of altered health states* (9th ed.) Philadelphia, PA: Lippincott Williams & Wilkins.

Hickey, J. V. (2014). *The clinical practice of neurological & neurosurgical nursing* (7th ed.). Philadelphia, PA: Lippincott Williams & Wilkins.

Weber, J., & Kelley, J. (2014). *Health assessment in nursing* (5th ed.). Philadelphia, PA: Lippincott Williams & Wilkins.

Journals and Electronic Documents

American Red Cross. (2016). *Eligibility criteria: alphabetically.* Retrieved on 10/16/2016 at: www.redcrossblood.org/donating-blood/eligibility-requirements/eligibility-criteria-alphabetical-listing

Buhse, M. (2015). The elderly person with multiple sclerosis: Clinical implications for the increase life-span. *Journal of Neuroscience Nursing, 47*(6), 333–339.

Centers for Disease Control and Prevention (CDC). (2016). *Recommended adult immunization schedule—United States, 2016.* Retrieved on 8/20/2016 at: www.cdc.gov/vaccines/schedules/hcp/adult.html

Cherin, P., Marie, I., Michallet, M., et al. (2016). Management of adverse events in the treatment of patients with immunoglobulin therapy: A review of evidence. *Autoimmunity Reviews, 15,* 71–81.

Digre, K., & Brennan, K. (2012). Shedding light on photophobia. *Journal of Neuroopthalmology, 32*(1), 68–81.

Filipi, M., Beavin, J., Brillante, R., et al. (2014). Nurses' perspective on approaches to limit flu-like symptoms during interferon therapy for multiple sclerosis. *International Journal of MS Care, 16,* 55–60.

Gagyor, I., Madhok, V., Daly, F., et al. (2016). Corticosteroids for Bell's palsy (idiopathic facial paralysis). *Cochrane Database of Systematic Reviews, 7,* CN-01208827.

**Lublin, F. D., & Reingold, S. C. (1996). Defining the clinical course of multiple sclerosis: Results of an international study. *Neurology, 46*(4), 907–911.

Mcilvoy, L. (2014). Respiratory failure from a myasthenic crisis. *American Nurse Today, 9*(9), 28.

McNair, N. (2013). Treatment of Guillain-Barré syndrome. *The Art and Science of Infusion Nursing, 36*(6), 397–400.

*Morrison, J. D., & Stuifbergen, A. K. (2016). Predictors of fatigue impact in persons with long-standing multiple sclerosis. *Journal of Neuroscience Nursing, 48*(3), 143–150.

National Institute of Neurological Disorders and Stroke (NINDS). (2016). *Creutzfeldt-Jakob Disease Fact Sheet.* Retrieved on 10/03/16 at: www.ninds.nih.gov/disorders/cjd/detail_cjd.htm.

National Meningitis Association. (2016). *Fact sheet: Meningitis.* Retrieved on 12/14/2016 at: www.nmaus.org/disease-prevention-information/is-it-viral-bacterial-or-fungal/

*Newland, P., Jensen, M. P., Budhathoki, C., et al. (2015). Secondary health conditions in individuals with multiple sclerosis: A cross-sectional web-based survey analysis. *Journal of Neuroscience Nursing, 47*(3), 124–130.

Riley, C., & Vargus, W. (2015). Multiple sclerosis in the elderly: Considerations in the geriatric population for diagnosis and management. *Current Geriatrics Reports, 4*(2), 131–141.

Slazinski, T. (2013). Brain abscess. *Critical Care Nursing Clinics of North America, 25,* 381–388.

Theroux, N., Phipps, M., Zimmerman, L., et al. (2013). Neurological complications associated with HIV and AIDS: Clinical implications for nursing. *Journal of Neuroscience Nursing, 45*(1), 5–13.

Vacca, V. (2016). Understanding Creutzfeldt-Jakob disease. *Nursing 2016, 46*(3), 36–42.

Wu, G., & Alvarez, E. (2016). The immune-pathophysiology of MS. Retrieved on 10/03/16 at: www.ncbi.nlm.nih.gov

Zakrzewska, J. M., & Akram, H. (2011). Neurosurgical interventions for the treatment of classical trigeminal neuralgia. *Cochrane Database of Systematic Reviews,* (9), CD007312.

Resources

Creutzfeldt-Jakob Disease Foundation, www.cjdfoundation.org
Guillain–Barré Syndrome Foundation International, www.gbs-cidp.org
Myasthenia Gravis Foundation of America (MGFA), www.myasthenia.org
National Multiple Sclerosis Society, www.nationalmssociety.org
The Foundation for Neuropathy, www.foundationforpn.org

70

Management of Patients With Oncologic or Degenerative Neurologic Disorders

LEARNING OBJECTIVES

On completion of this chapter, the learner will be able to:

1 Describe brain and spinal cord tumors: their classification, pathophysiology, clinical manifestations, diagnosis, and medical and nursing management.
2 Use the nursing process as a framework for care of patients with nervous system metastases or primary brain tumor.

3 Explain the pathophysiologic processes responsible for various neurodegenerative disorders.
4 Apply the nursing process as a framework for care of patients with Parkinson disease.
5 Identify resources for patients and families with oncologic and degenerative neurologic disorders.
6 Use the nursing process as a framework for care of patients following a cervical discectomy.

GLOSSARY

bradykinesia: abnormally slow voluntary movements and speech
chorea: rapid, jerky, involuntary, purposeless movements of the extremities or facial muscles, including facial grimacing
dementia: broad term for a syndrome characterized by a general decline in higher brain functioning, such as reasoning, with a pattern of eventual decline in ability to perform even basic activities of daily living, such as toileting and eating
dyskinesia: impaired ability to execute voluntary movements

dysphonia: voice impairment or altered voice production
neurodegenerative: a disease, process, or condition leading to deterioration of cells or function of the nervous system
papilledema: edema of the optic nerve usually due to increased intracranial pressure (ICP)
paresthesia: numbness, tingling, or a "pins and needles" sensation
sciatica: pain and tenderness that radiates along the sciatic nerve that runs through the thigh and leg
spondylosis: degenerative changes occurring in a disc and adjacent vertebral bodies; can occur in the cervical or lumbar vertebrae

The occurrence of oncologic or degenerative disease processes in the neurologic system produces a unique set of nursing challenges. Thus nurses who care for patients with these disorders must have a clear understanding of the pathophysiology, diagnostic testing, medical and nursing care, and rehabilitation processes. Nurses care for patients with oncologic or degenerative disease processes in many inpatient and outpatient settings. Oncologic disorders include brain and spinal cord tumors. Degenerative neurologic disorders include Parkinson disease (PD), Huntington disease, amyotrophic lateral sclerosis (ALS), muscular dystrophies, and degenerative disc disease. Post-polio syndrome (PPS) is thought to be degenerative in nature and is included in this chapter.

ONCOLOGIC DISORDERS OF THE BRAIN AND SPINAL CORD

There are many types of brain and spinal cord tumors, each with its own biology, prognosis, and treatment options. Because of the unique anatomy and physiology, tumors of the central nervous system (CNS) are challenging to diagnose and treat.

Brain Tumors

A brain tumor occupies space within the skull, growing as a spherical mass or diffusely infiltrating tissue. The effects of brain tumors are caused by inflammation, compression, and infiltration of tissue. A variety of physiologic changes result, causing any or all of the following pathophysiologic events:

- Increased intracranial pressure (ICP) and cerebral edema
- Seizure activity and focal neurologic signs
- Hydrocephalus
- Altered pituitary function

Neoplastic lesions in the brain ultimately cause death by increasing ICP and impairing vital functions, such as respiration.

According to the American Brain Tumor Association (ABTA, 2014), there are over 100 types of brain tumors with an estimated annual occurrence of 78,000 new cases. These include 25,000 malignant and 53,000 nonmalignant brain tumors (ABTA, 2014). Brain tumors are classified as primary or secondary. Primary brain tumors originate from cells within the brain. In adults, most primary brain tumors originate from glial cells (cells that make up the structure and support system of the brain and spinal cord) and are supratentorial (located above the covering of the cerebellum). Primary tumors progress locally and rarely metastasize outside the CNS.

Developed countries have a higher incidence of primary brain tumors, with rates of 5.1 per 100,000 compared to 3.0 per 100,000 in less developed countries. This is most likely due to more frequent diagnosis with improved imaging modalities. Although many risk factors have been investigated, exposure to ionizing radiation is the only known modifiable risk factor (American Association of Neuroscience Nurses [AANN], 2014a). Many genetic factors and genetic syndromes (such as neurofibromatosis) are associated with brain tumor risk in families (AANN, 2014a).

Secondary, or metastatic, brain tumors develop from structures outside the brain and are twice as common as primary brain tumors (AANN, 2014a). Metastatic lesions to the brain can occur from the lung, breast, lower gastrointestinal tract, pancreas, kidney, and skin (melanomas) neoplasms. Single or multiple metastases may occur, and brain metastases may be found at any time during the disease course, even at initial diagnosis of the primary disease. Patient survival rates from primary brains cancers are improving, however, the incidence of brain metastases are increasing (AANN, 2014a; Lovely, Stewart-Amidei, Page, et al., 2013).

The highest incidence of brain tumors in adults occurs in the fifth through seventh decades of life. There is a slight male predominance in the incidence of malignant brain tumors.

Types of Primary Brain Tumors

Brain tumors may be classified into several groups: those arising from the coverings of the brain (e.g., dural meningioma), those developing in or on the cranial nerves (e.g., acoustic neuroma), those originating within brain tissue (e.g., glioma), and metastatic lesions originating elsewhere in the body. Tumors of the pituitary and pineal glands and of cerebral blood vessels are also types of brain tumors. Relevant clinical considerations include the location and the histologic character of the tumor. Tumors may be benign or malignant. A benign tumor, such as a colloid cyst, can occur in a vital area and can grow large enough to have serious effects (Hickey, 2014). See Chart 70-1 for the classification of brain tumors.

Chart 70-1 | **Classification of Brain Tumors in Adults**

I. Intracerebral Tumors
  A. Gliomas—infiltrate any portion of the brain; most common type of brain tumor
   1. Astrocytomas (grades I and II)
   2. Glioblastoma (astrocytoma grades III and IV)
   3. Oligodendroglioma (low and high grades)
   4. Ependymoma (grades I to IV)
   5. Medulloblastoma
II. Tumors Arising From Supporting Structures
  A. Meningiomas
  B. Neuromas (acoustic neuroma, schwannoma)
  C. Pituitary adenomas
III. Developmental Tumors
  A. Angiomas
  B. Dermoid, epidermoid, teratoma, craniopharyngioma
IV. Metastatic Lesions

Gliomas

In adults, gliomas (principally astrocytoma) account for approximately 30% of symptomatic primary brain tumors. Glial tumors, the most common type of intracerebral brain neoplasm, are divided into many categories (Ostrom, Gittleman, Fulop, et al., 2015). Astrocytomas, arising from astrocytic cells, are the most common type of glioma and are graded from I to IV, indicating the degree of malignancy (ABTA, 2014). The grade is based on cellular density, cell mitosis, and degree of differentiation from the original cell type. Grades III and IV tumors are known as glioblastomas and have little resemblance to the original cell type. Astrocytomas infiltrate into the surrounding neural connective tissue and therefore cannot be totally removed without causing considerable damage to vital structures.

Oligodendroglial tumors, arising from oligodendroglial cells (about 4% of primary brain tumors) represent about 10% to15% of the gliomas. Most oligodendrogliomas occur in adults ages 50 to 60, are found in men more often than in women, and are categorized as low or high grade (anaplastic) (ABTA, 2014). The histologic distinction between astrocytomas and oligodendrogliomas is difficult to make but is important, because oligodendrogliomas are more sensitive than astrocytomas to chemotherapy. Tumors originating from ependymal cells, another type of glial cell, are known as ependymomas and are more common in children than adults. Glial tumors may be treated with a combination of surgery, radiation therapy, and chemotherapy, depending on specific cell and patient characteristics.

Meningiomas

Meningiomas, which represent 15% of all primary brain tumors, are common benign encapsulated tumors of arachnoid cells on the meninges (Ostrom et al., 2015). They are slow growing, occur most often in middle-aged adults, and are more common in women. Meningiomas most often occur in areas proximal to the venous sinuses. Manifestations depend on the area involved and are often the result of compression rather than invasion of brain tissue. Preferred treatment for symptomatic lesions is surgery with complete removal or partial dissection, although radiation therapy may be useful for some patients.

Acoustic Neuromas

An acoustic neuroma is a tumor of the eighth cranial nerve—the cranial nerve most responsible for hearing and balance. It usually arises just within the internal auditory meatus, where it frequently expands before filling the cerebellopontine recess. An acoustic neuroma may grow slowly and attain considerable size before it is diagnosed. The patient usually experiences loss of hearing, tinnitus, and episodes of vertigo and staggering gait. As the tumor becomes larger, painful sensations of the face may occur on the same side as a result of the tumor's compression of the fifth cranial nerve (ABTA, 2014). Many acoustic neuromas are benign and can be managed conservatively. Many that continue to grow can be surgically removed and have a good prognosis (see Chapter 64). Some acoustic neuromas may be suitable for stereotactic radiotherapy rather than open craniotomy. Stereotactic radiotherapy is discussed later in this chapter.

Pituitary Adenomas

Pituitary tumors account for about 16% of all primary brain tumors (ABTA, 2014). They can occur at any age, but they are more common in older adults. Women are affected more often than men, particularly during the childbearing years. Pituitary tumors are rarely malignant but cause symptoms as a result of pressure on adjacent structures or hormonal changes (ABTA, 2014).

Pressure Effects of Pituitary Adenomas

Pressure from a pituitary adenoma may be exerted on the optic nerves, optic chiasm, or optic tracts or on the hypothalamus or the third ventricle if the tumor invades the cavernous sinuses or expands into the sphenoid bone. These pressure effects produce headache, visual dysfunction, hypothalamic disorders (disorders of sleep, appetite, temperature, and emotions), increased ICP, and enlargement and erosion of the sella turcica.

Hormonal Effects of Pituitary Adenomas

Functioning pituitary tumors can produce one or more hormones normally produced by the anterior pituitary. Hormonal hypersecretion is caused only by pituitary adenomas. Most adenomas (65% to 70%) secrete an excess amount of hormone including prolactin (prolactinomas), growth hormone (GH) producing acromegaly in adults, adrenocorticotropic hormone (ACTH) resulting in Cushing syndrome, or thyroid-stimulating hormone (TSH) (Melmed, 2016). Adenomas that secrete TSH or follicle-stimulating hormone and luteinizing hormone occur infrequently, whereas adenomas that produce both GH and prolactin are relatively common.

The female patient whose pituitary gland is secreting excessive quantities of prolactin presents with amenorrhea or galactorrhea (excessive or spontaneous flow of milk). Male patients with prolactinomas may present with impotence and hypogonadism. Acromegaly, caused by excess GH, produces enlargement of the hands and feet, distortion of the facial features, and pressure on peripheral nerves (entrapment syndromes). The clinical features of Cushing syndrome, a condition associated with prolonged overproduction of cortisol, occur with excessive production of ACTH. Manifestations include a form of obesity with redistribution of fat to the facial, supraclavicular, and abdominal areas; hypertension; purple striae and ecchymoses; osteoporosis; elevated blood glucose levels; and emotional disorders. See Chapter 52 for a discussion of endocrine disorders resulting from these tumors.

Gerontologic Considerations

The most frequent tumor types in the older adult are anaplastic astrocytoma, glioblastoma, and cerebral metastases from other sites (Perkins & Liu, 2016). The incidence of all brain tumors increases with age. Intracranial tumors can produce personality changes, confusion, speech dysfunction, or disturbances of gait. In older adult patients, early signs and symptoms of intracranial tumors can be easily overlooked or incorrectly attributed to cognitive and neurologic changes associated with normal aging (Eliopoulos, 2018). Neurologic signs and symptoms in the older adult must be carefully evaluated, because brain metastases occur in patients with a history of prior cancer. Regardless of the age of the patient or the decision to proceed or not with treatment, the nurse provides supportive care. Researchers are investigating patterns of care and clinical outcomes of older adult patients with primary brain tumors (Gallego Perez-Larraya & Delattre, 2014).

Clinical Manifestations

Brain tumors can produce both focal or generalized neurologic signs and symptoms. Generalized symptoms reflect increased ICP, and the most common focal or specific signs and symptoms result from tumors that interfere with functions in specific brain regions. Figure 70-1 indicates common brain tumor sites.

Increased Intracranial Pressure

As discussed in Chapter 66, the skull is a rigid compartment containing essential noncompressible contents: brain matter, intravascular blood, and cerebrospinal fluid (CSF). The Monro-Kellie hypothesis or doctrine explains the dynamic equilibrium of the cranial contents. According to this hypothesis, if any one of these skull components increases in volume, ICP increases unless one of the other components decreases in volume. Consequently, any change in volume occupied by the brain (as occurs with disorders such as brain tumor or cerebral edema) produces signs and symptoms of increased ICP (Hickey, 2014).

The enlarging tumor and its associating edema disrupts the equilibrium between the brain, blood, and CSF. As the tumor grows, compensatory adjustments may occur through compression of intracranial veins, reduction of CSF volume (by increased absorption or decreased production), a modest decrease in cerebral blood flow, or reduction of intra- and extracellular brain tissue mass. When these compensatory mechanisms fail, the patient develops signs and symptoms of increased ICP, most often including headache, nausea with or without vomiting, and **papilledema** (swelling of the optic nerve) (Hickey, 2014). Personality changes and a variety of focal deficits, including motor, sensory, and cranial nerve dysfunction, are common.

Headache

Headache, although not always present, is most common in the early morning and is made worse by coughing, straining, or sudden movement. It is thought to be caused by the tumor invading, compressing, or distorting the pain-sensitive structures or by edema that accompanies the tumor. Headaches are usually described as deep, expanding, dull, but unrelenting. Frontal tumors usually produce a bilateral frontal headache; pituitary gland tumors produce pain radiating between the two temples (bitemporal); in cerebellar tumors, the headache may be located in the suboccipital region at the back of the head.

Vomiting

Vomiting, seldom related to food intake, is usually the result of irritation of the vagal centers in the medulla. Forceful vomiting is described as projectile vomiting. Headache may be relieved by vomiting.

Visual Disturbances

The tumor itself or the surrounding edema can compress the third cranial nerve, causing optic disc swelling or papilledema.

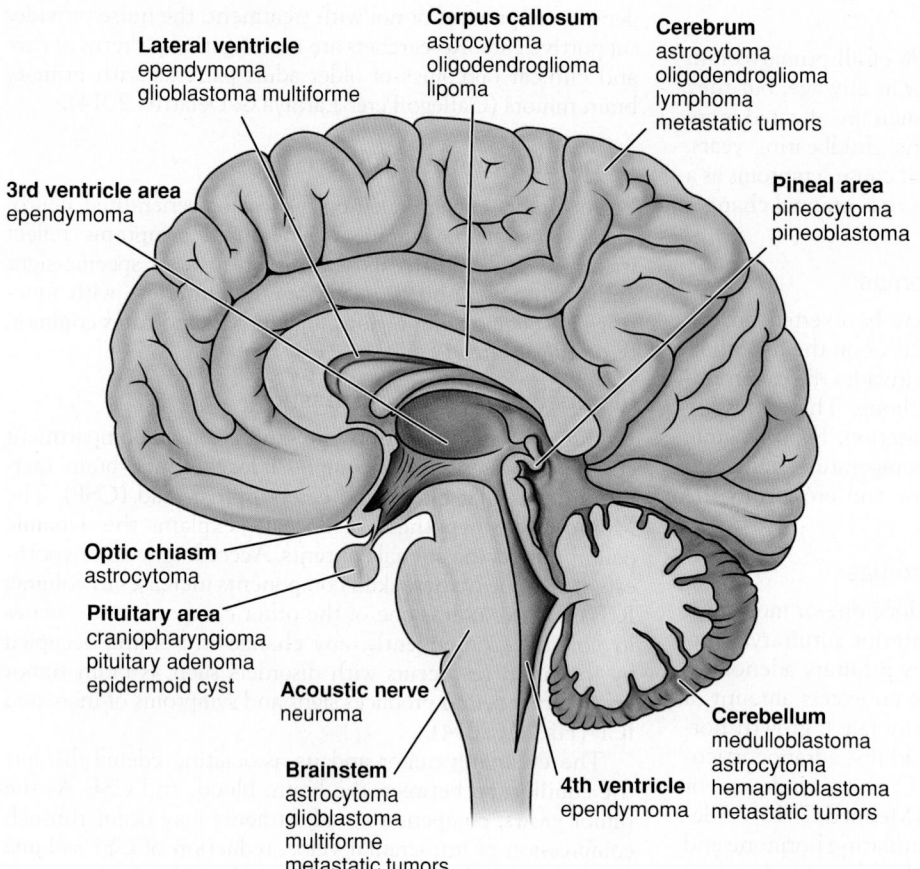

Lateral ventricle
ependymoma
glioblastoma multiforme

Corpus callosum
astrocytoma
oligodendroglioma
lipoma

Cerebrum
astrocytoma
oligodendroglioma
lymphoma
metastatic tumors

3rd ventricle area
ependymoma

Pineal area
pineocytoma
pineoblastoma

Optic chiasm
astrocytoma

Pituitary area
craniopharyngioma
pituitary adenoma
epidermoid cyst

Acoustic nerve
neuroma

Brainstem
astrocytoma
glioblastoma
multiforme
metastatic tumors

4th ventricle
ependymoma

Cerebellum
medulloblastoma
astrocytoma
hemangioblastoma
metastatic tumors

Figure 70-1 • Common brain tumor sites.

This limits the visual acuity along the visual pathway, mildly or profoundly, as diplopia (double vision), hemianopsia (visual field deficits), or varying levels of blindness (Rigi, Almarzbuqi, Morgan, et al., 2015).

Seizures

Seizures are common, occurring in 60% of patients with brain tumors either initially or throughout their disease process (AANN, 2014a). Seizures may be focal or generalized. Tumors of the frontal, parietal, and temporal lobes carry the greatest risk of seizures; seizures are unusual with brainstem or cerebellar tumors. See Chapter 66 for discussion about seizures and related management.

If not the initial presentation, seizures can be a result of metabolic factors (electrolyte imbalances, liver failure or kidney disease, radiation or chemotherapy side effects), structural causes (parenchymal metastases, leptomeningeal disease, dural metastases) or a new hemorrhage, thrombosis, or development of meningitis (Hickey, 2014). If the patient presents with a seizure, then anticonvulsant drugs are prescribed. Medications with the best evidence for controlling seizure activity include levetiracetam (Keppra), carbamazepine (Tegretol), phenytoin (Dilantin), and zonisamide (Zonegran) (Vecht, Kerkhof, & Duran-Pena, 2014).

Localized Symptoms

When specific regions of the brain are affected, local signs and symptoms occur, such as sensory or motor abnormalities, visual alterations, alterations in cognition, or language disturbances (e.g., aphasia). Identifying the signs and symptoms is important, because it can help identify tumor location. Some tumors are not easily localized because they lie in so-called silent areas of the brain (i.e., areas in which functions are not well defined). Many tumors can be localized by correlating the signs and symptoms to specific areas in the brain, as follows:

- A tumor in the motor cortex of the frontal lobe produces hemiparesis and partial seizures on the opposite side of the body or generalized seizures. A frontal lobe tumor may also produce changes in emotional state and behavior, as well as an apathetic mental attitude. The patient often becomes impulsive, inappropriate in speech, gestures, and behavior.
- A parietal lobe tumor may cause decreased sensation on the opposite side of the body or generalized seizures.
- A temporal lobe tumor may cause seizures as well as psychological disorders.
- An occipital lobe tumor produces visual manifestations: contralateral homonymous hemianopsia (visual loss in half of the visual field on the opposite side of the tumor) and visual hallucinations.
- A cerebellar tumor causes dizziness; an ataxic or staggering gait with a tendency to fall toward the side of the lesion; marked muscle incoordination; and nystagmus (involuntary rhythmic eye movements), usually in the horizontal direction.
- A cerebellopontine angle tumor usually originates in the sheath of the acoustic nerve and gives rise to a

Figure 70-2 • Magnetic resonance image of the brain shows an exophytic tectal glioma (*arrow*) in this patient with neurofibromatosis type 1. From Brant, W. E., & Helms, C. A. (2006). *Fundamentals of diagnostic radiology* (3rd ed.). Philadelphia, PA: Lippincott Williams & Wilkins.

characteristic sequence of symptoms. Tinnitus and vertigo appear first, soon followed by progressive nerve deafness (eighth cranial nerve dysfunction). Numbness and tingling of the face and tongue occur (due to involvement of the fifth cranial nerve). Later, weakness or paralysis of the face develops (seventh cranial nerve involvement). Finally, because the enlarging tumor

presses on the cerebellum, abnormalities in motor function may be present.

• Brainstem tumors may be associated with cranial nerve deficits along with complex motor and sensory function impairments (Hickey, 2014).

Assessment and Diagnostic Findings

The history of the illness, the manner, and the time frame in which the symptoms evolved are key components in the diagnosis of brain tumors. A neurologic examination indicates the involved areas of the CNS. To assist in the precise localization of the lesion, a battery of tests is performed. Computed tomography (CT) scans, enhanced by a contrast agent, can give specific information concerning the number, size, and density of the lesions, and the extent of secondary cerebral edema. CT can provide information about the ventricular system. A magnetic resonance imaging (MRI) scan is the most helpful diagnostic tool for detecting brain tumors, particularly smaller lesions, and tumors in the brainstem and pituitary regions, where bone is thick (see Fig. 70-2). MRI is also useful in monitoring response to treatment.

Computer-assisted stereotactic (three-dimensional) biopsy is used to diagnose deep-seated brain tumors and to provide a basis for treatment and prognosis. Stereotactic approaches involve the use of a three-dimensional frame that allows very precise localization of the tumor; a stereotactic frame and multiple imaging studies (x-rays, CT scans, or MRIs) are used to localize the tumor and verify its position (see Fig. 70-3). Brain-mapping technology helps determine the proximity of diseased areas of the brain to structures essential for normal brain function.

Positron emission tomography (PET) is used to supplement MRI scanning in centers where it is available. On PET scans, low-grade tumors are associated with hypometabolism,

Figure 70-3 • **A.** Using stereotactic or "brain-mapping" guided approach, a three-dimensional computer image fuses the computed tomography image and magnetic resonance image to pinpoint the exact location of the brain tumor. This low-grade astrocytoma is localized adjacent to the brainstem, is inoperable, and is treated with radiation. Note the optic chasm and optic nerves. **B.** Computerized image of the prescribed radiation dose.

and high-grade tumors show hypermetabolism. This information can be useful in making treatment decisions (AANN, 2014a). An electroencephalogram can detect abnormal brain waves in regions occupied by or adjacent to tumor; it is used to evaluate temporal lobe seizures and to assist in ruling out other disorders. Cytologic studies of the CSF may be performed to detect malignant cells as CNS tumors can shed cells into the CSF resulting in metastasis.

Medical Management

A variety of medical management approaches, including surgery, chemotherapy, and external-beam radiation therapy, are used alone or in combination (AANN, 2014a).

Secreting tumors may be treated with medications that suppress hormones. Nonfunctioning tumors may have no effect on pituitary function or may suppress hormone production and release. Hormone replacement may be necessary for these patients to restore normal endocrine function.

Surgical Management

The objective of surgical management is to remove as much tumor as possible without increasing the neurologic deficit (paralysis, blindness), or to relieve symptoms by partial removal (decompression). Surgery also provides tissue to establish a definitive diagnosis. A variety of surgical approaches may be used; the specific approach depends on the type of tumor, its location, and its accessibility. Conventional surgical approaches require a craniotomy (incision into the skull). See Chapter 66 for a discussion of care of the patient who has undergone a craniotomy. This approach is used in patients with meningiomas, acoustic neuromas, cystic astrocytomas of the cerebellum, colloid cysts of the third ventricle, congenital tumors such as dermoid cyst, and some of the granulomas. With improved imaging techniques and the availability of the operating microscope and microsurgical instrumentation, even large tumors can be removed through a relatively small craniotomy. For patients with malignant glioma, complete removal of the tumor and cure are not possible, but the rationale for resection includes relief of ICP, removal of any necrotic tissue, and reduction in the bulk of the tumor, which theoretically leaves behind fewer cells to become resistant to radiation or chemotherapy. Most pituitary adenomas are treated by transsphenoidal microsurgical removal (see Chapter 66), and the remainder of tumors that cannot be removed completely are treated by radiation (Hickey, 2014).

Radiation Therapy

Radiation therapy—the cornerstone of treatment for many brain tumors—decreases the incidence of recurrence of incompletely resected tumors (AANN, 2014a). Gamma radiation is delivered via an external beam to the tumor in multiple fractions. Brachytherapy (the surgical implantation of radiation sources to deliver high doses at a short distance) is an option for some types of tumors depending on their location. It is usually used as an adjunct to conventional radiation therapy or as a rescue measure for recurrent disease. Radioisotopes such as iodine 131 (^{131}I) are used to minimize effects on surrounding brain tissue.

Stereotactic procedures may be performed using a linear accelerator or gamma knife to perform radiosurgery (Hickey,

2014). These procedures allow treatment of deep, inaccessible tumors, often in a single session. Precise localization of the tumor is accomplished by the stereotactic approach and by minute measurements and precise positioning of the patient. Multiple narrow beams then deliver a very high dose of radiation. An advantage of this method is that no surgical incision is needed. Disadvantages include the lag time between treatment and the desired result as well as the potential for developing radiation necrosis (AANS, 2014a).

Chemotherapy

Chemotherapy may be used in conjunction with radiation therapy, or as the sole therapy, with the goal of increasing survival time. The greatest challenge in chemotherapy of brain tumors is that the blood–brain barrier prevents drugs from getting to the tumor in effective doses without causing systemic toxicity (AANN, 2014a).

Malignant glioma is usually treated with 6 weeks of oral temozolomide (Temodar) during radiation therapy, followed by 6 to 12 months of oral temozolomide. Low-grade gliomas may be treated with 6 months of oral temozolomide alone. Temozolomide is the first oral chemotherapy that crosses the blood–brain barrier (Hickey, 2014). Several other chemotherapy agents are used alone or in combination depending on the type of tumor (see Chapter 15).

Autologous bone marrow transplantation is used in some patients who will receive chemotherapy or radiation therapy, because it can "rescue" the patient from the bone marrow toxicity associated with high doses of chemotherapy and radiation. A fraction of the patient's bone marrow is aspirated, usually from the iliac crest, and stored. The patient receives large doses of chemotherapy or radiation therapy to destroy large numbers of malignant cells. The marrow is then reinfused intravenously after treatment is completed. See Chapter 34 for discussion of bone marrow transplant.

Pharmacologic Therapy

Corticosteroids are useful in relieving headache and alterations in level of consciousness. Corticosteroids such as dexamethasone (Decadron) are thought to reduce inflammation and edema around tumors (AANN, 2014a). Other medications used include osmotic diuretics (e.g., mannitol [Osmitrol] and hypertonic saline) to decrease the fluid content of the brain, which leads to a decrease in ICP. Anticonvulsant medications are used to treat and control seizures (Vecht et al., 2014). Venous thromboembolic events, such as deep vein thrombosis and pulmonary embolism, occur in about 15% of patients and are associated with significant morbidity. Patients receiving anticoagulant agents must be closely monitored because of the risk of CNS hemorrhage (Farge, 2013).

Nursing Management

Headache characteristics should be assessed. Upright positioning and pain medications may be useful in managing pain; nurses should evaluate effectiveness of pain management interventions. Even if seizure history is absent, the patient and family should be educated about the possibility of seizure and the need to adhere to prophylactic anticonvulsant medications, if prescribed. The patient with a brain tumor may be at increased risk for aspiration as a result of cranial nerve dysfunction. Medications to alleviate nausea and prevent vomiting should be considered. Preoperatively, the gag reflex and ability to swallow are evaluated. In patients with diminished gag response, care includes educating the patient to direct food and fluids toward the unaffected side, having the patient sit upright to eat, offering a semisoft diet, and having suction readily available. The effects of increased ICP caused by the tumor mass are reviewed in Chapter 66. The nurse performs neurologic checks; monitors vital signs; maintains a neurologic observation record (see Fig. 66-6 in Chapter 66); spaces nursing interventions to prevent rapid increase in ICP; and reorients the patient when necessary to person, time, and place. The use of corticosteroids to control headache and neurologic symptoms requires astute nursing assessment and intervention because many adverse effects can occur, including hyperglycemia, electrolyte abnormalities, and muscle weakness (see Table 52-5 in Chapter 52). Patients with changes in cognition caused by their lesion require frequent reorientation and the use of orienting devices (e.g., personal possessions, photographs, lists, a clock), supervision of and assistance with self-care, and ongoing monitoring and intervention for prevention of injury. Patients with seizures are carefully monitored and protected from injury. Motor function is checked at intervals because specific motor deficits may occur, depending on the tumor's location. When muscle weakness is present, a multidisciplinary approach, including the nurse and physical and occupational therapists, can be used to preserve muscle strength, promote range of motion, and facilitate independence in self-care. Sensory disturbances are assessed and any area of numbness should be protected from injury. Speech is evaluated, and patients with speech deficits can be educated to use alternative forms of communication. Eye movement and pupillary size and reaction may be affected by cranial nerve involvement. Fatigue is common during therapy; efforts should be made to conserve energy and promote rest.

The psychosocial effects on family caregivers of a family member who has a primary malignant brain tumor may be significant (Dhandapani, Gupta, Dhandapani, et al., 2015). Caregiving family members should be included in the plan of care.

The nursing process for patients undergoing neurosurgery is discussed in Chapter 66. The patient's functional abilities should be reassessed postoperatively, because changes can occur.

Cerebral Metastases

A significant number of patients with cancer experience neurologic deficits caused by metastasis to the nervous system, which can include the brain, CSF, and meninges. Metastatic lesions to the brain are twice as common as primary brain tumors (Ostrom et al., 2015). This high rate of occurrence is clinically important, as more patients with all forms of cancer live longer because of improved therapies. Neurologic signs and symptoms include headache, gait disturbances, visual impairment, personality changes, altered mentation (memory loss and confusion), focal weakness, paralysis, aphasia, and seizures. These signs and symptoms can be devastating to both patient and family. Metastases to the CSF and meninges, known as leptomeningeal metastases, can produce symptoms of headache and isolated cranial nerve deficits.

Medical Management

The treatment of metastatic nervous system cancer is palliative and involves eliminating or reducing serious symptoms. Even when palliation is the goal, distressing signs and symptoms can be relieved, thereby improving the quality of life for both patient and family. Patients with intracerebral metastases who are not treated have a steady downhill course with a limited survival time. The therapeutic options include whole brain radiation therapy (the foundation of treatment) for multiple metastases or stereotactic radiosurgery for up to three sites of metastases. Surgery may be considered for a single symptomatic metastasis. Systemic chemotherapy directed at the primary cancer may be ineffective in crossing the blood–brain barrier, but chemotherapy that crosses this barrier may be added. Intrathecal chemotherapy, with direct injection of chemotherapy agents into the CSF of the brain or spinal canal, may be useful in persons with leptomeningeal metastases (Lukas, Buerke, & Mrugula, 2016). Some combination of these treatments is usually the optimal method.

Pain can be a significant problem and is managed by means of a stepped progression in the doses and type of analgesic agents needed for relief. If the patient has severe pain, morphine can be infused into the epidural or subarachnoid space through a spinal needle and a catheter placed as near as possible to the spinal segment where the pain is projected. Small doses of morphine are given at prescribed intervals (see Chapter 12).

NURSING PROCESS

The Patient With Nervous System Metastases or Primary Brain Tumor

Assessment

The nursing assessment includes a baseline neurologic examination and focuses on how the patient is functioning, moving, and walking; adapting to weakness or paralysis and to loss of vision and speech; and dealing with seizures. Assessment addresses symptoms that cause distress to the patient and affect the quality of life, including pain, respiratory problems, bowel and bladder disorders, and sleep disturbances, as well as impairment of skin integrity, fluid balance, and temperature regulation (Hickey, 2014). Nutritional status is assessed, because cachexia and cancer-related anorexia-cachexia syndrome are common (see Chapter 15).

The nurse takes a dietary history to assess food intake, intolerance, and preferences. Calculation of body mass index can confirm the loss of subcutaneous fat and lean body mass (see Chapter 5). Biochemical measurements are reviewed to assess the degree of malnutrition, impaired cellular immunity, and electrolyte balance (normal laboratory values are found in Appendix A on {thepoint icon}). A dietitian assists in determining the caloric needs of the patient.

The nurse works with other members of the health care team to assess the impact of the illness on the family in terms of home care, altered relationships, financial problems, time pressures, and family problems. This information is important in helping family members cope with the diagnosis and the changes associated with it.

Diagnosis

NURSING DIAGNOSES

Based on the assessment data, major nursing diagnoses may include the following:

- Self-care deficit (feeding, bathing, and toileting) related to loss or impairment of motor and sensory functions and decreased cognitive abilities
- Imbalanced nutrition: less than body requirements related to cachexia due to treatment and tumor effects, decreased nutritional intake, and malabsorption
- Imbalanced nutrition: more than body requirements related to increased nutritional intake and impaired metabolism
- Anxiety related to fear of dying, uncertainty, change in appearance, or altered lifestyle
- Interrupted family processes related to anticipatory grief and the burdens imposed by the care of the person with a terminal illness

Other nursing diagnoses of the patient with nervous system metastases may include acute pain related to tumor compression; impaired gas exchange related to dyspnea; constipation related to decreased fluid and dietary intake and medications; impaired urinary elimination related to reduced fluid intake, vomiting, and side effects of medications; sleep pattern disturbances related to discomfort and fear of dying; impairment of skin integrity related to cachexia, poor tissue perfusion, and decreased mobility; deficient fluid volume related to fever, vomiting, and low fluid intake; and ineffective thermoregulation related to hypothalamic involvement, fever, and chills. See Chapter 15 for assessment and nursing interventions for the patient with cancer.

Planning and Goals

The goals for the patient include compensating for self-care deficits, improving nutrition, reducing anxiety, enhancing family coping skills, and absence of complications.

Nursing Interventions

COMPENSATING FOR SELF-CARE DEFICITS

The patient may have difficulty participating in goal setting as the tumor metastasizes and affects cognitive function. The nurse should encourage the family to keep the patient as independent as possible for as long as possible (AANN, 2014a). Increasing assistance with self-care activities is to be expected. Because the patient with nervous system metastasis and the family live with uncertainty, they are encouraged to plan for each day and to make the most of each day. The tasks and challenges are to assist the patient to find useful coping mechanisms, adaptations, and compensations for solving problems that arise. This helps patients maintain some sense of control. An individualized exercise program helps maintain strength, endurance, and range of motion. Eventually, referral for home or hospice care may be necessary (see Chapter 16).

IMPROVING NUTRITION

Patients with nausea, vomiting, diarrhea, breathlessness, and pain are rarely interested in eating. These symptoms are managed or controlled through assessment, planning, and care. The nurse educates the family about how to position the patient for comfort and safety during meals. A dietician may help with alternative food choices that are easily tolerated. Meals are planned for times when the patient is rested and in less distress from pain or the effects of treatment.

The patient needs to be clean, comfortable, and free of pain for meals, in an environment that is as attractive as possible. Oral hygiene before meals helps to improve appetite. Offensive sights, sounds, and odors are eliminated. Creative strategies may be required to make food more palatable, provide enough fluids, and increase opportunities for socialization during meals. The family may be asked to keep a log of daily weights and to record the quantity of food eaten to determine the daily calorie count. Dietary supplements, if acceptable to the patient, can be provided to meet increased caloric needs. If the patient is not interested in most usual foods, those foods preferred by the patient should be offered. When the patient shows marked deterioration as a result of tumor growth and effects, some other form of nutritional support (e.g., tube feeding, parenteral nutrition) may be indicated if consistent with the patient's end-of-life preferences (AANN, 2014a). Nursing interventions include assessing the patency of the central and intravenous lines or feeding tube, monitoring the insertion site for infection, checking the infusion rate, monitoring intake and output, and changing the intravenous tubing and dressing. Family members are instructed in these techniques if they will be providing care at home. Parenteral nutrition can be provided at home if indicated. The patient's quality of life may guide the selection, initiation, maintenance, and discontinuation of nutritional support. The nurse and family should not place too much emphasis on eating or on discussions about food, because the patient may not desire aggressive nutritional intervention. The subsequent course of action must be congruent with the wishes and choices of the patient and family.

Increased appetite may occur in patients receiving steroids and may result in weight gain as well as hyperglycemia. Patients and family members should be instructed to monitor weight and blood glucose (if appropriate), as well as maintain a healthy diet with caloric intake appropriate to patient needs.

RELIEVING ANXIETY

Patients may be restless, with changing moods that may include intense depression, euphoria, paranoia, and severe anxiety. The response of patients to terminal illness reflects their pattern of reaction to other crisis situations. Serious illness imposes additional strains that often bring other unresolved problems to light. The patient's own coping strategies can help deal with anxious and depressed feelings. Health care providers need to be sensitive to the patient's concerns and fears.

Patients need the opportunity to exercise some control over their situation. A sense of mastery can be gained as they learn to understand the disease and its treatment and how to deal with their feelings. The presence of family, friends, a spiritual advisor, and health professionals may be supportive. Brain tumor support groups may provide a feeling of support and strength (see the Resources section).

Spending time with patients allows them time to talk and to communicate their fears and concerns. Open communication and acknowledgment of fears are often therapeutic. Touch is also a form of communication. These patients need reassurance that continuing care will be provided and that they will not be abandoned. The situation becomes more endurable when others share in the experience of dying. If a patient's emotional reactions are very intense or prolonged, additional help from a spiritual advisor, social worker, or mental health professional may be indicated.

ENHANCING FAMILY PROCESSES

The family needs to be reassured that their loved one is receiving optimal care and that attention will be paid to the patient's changing symptoms and concerns. When the patient can no longer carry out self-care, the family and additional support systems (social worker, home health aide, home care nurse, hospice nurse) may be needed. Educating family members on how to care for their loved one with additional physical, cognitive, and maybe behavioral impairments is necessary, acute, and challenging. Investigating what supportive and financial resources are available may decrease the burden on the caregivers. These efforts improve quality of life for the patient and family (Dhandapani et al., 2015).

PROMOTING HOME, COMMUNITY-BASED, AND TRANSITIONAL CARE

Educating Patients About Self-Care. The patient and family often have major responsibility for care at home. Caregivers may struggle with a new "normal" while their support systems fluctuate as their relationship with the patient they are caring for is strengthened, maintained, or strained (Ownsworth, Goadby, & Chambers, 2015). In addition to the psychological aspect, education includes pain management strategies, prevention of complications related to treatment strategies, and methods to ensure adequate fluid and food intake (see Chart 70-2). Educational needs of the patient and family regarding care priorities are likely to change as the disease progresses. The nurse should assess the changing needs of the patient and the family and inform them about resources and services early and frequently to assist them in dealing with changes in the patient's condition (see the Resources section).

Continuing and Transitional Care. Home care nursing and hospice services are valuable resources that should be made available to the patient and the family early in the course of a terminal illness. Anticipating needs before they occur can assist in smooth initiation of services. Home care needs and interventions focus on four major areas: palliation of symptoms and pain control, assistance in self-care, control of treatment complications, and administration of specific forms of treatment (e.g., parenteral nutrition). The nurse assesses pain management, respiratory status, complications of the disorder and its treatment, and the patient's cognitive and emotional status. In addition, the nurse assesses the family's ability to perform necessary care and notifies the primary provider about changing needs or complications, if indicated.

The patient and family who elect to care for the patient at home as the disease progresses can benefit from the care and support provided through hospice and palliative care services (Ownsworth et al., 2015). Steps to initiate hospice care, including discussion of hospice care as an option, should not be postponed until death is imminent. Exploration of hospice care as an option should be initiated at a time when hospice services can provide support and care to the patient and family consistent with their end-of-life decisions and can assist in allowing death with dignity. See Chapter 16 for in-depth discussion of end-of-life care.

Evaluation

Expected patient outcomes may include:
1. Engages in self-care activities as long as possible
   a. Uses assistive devices or accepts assistance as needed
   b. Schedules periodic rest periods to permit maximal participation in self-care

---

Chart 70-2 — HOME CARE CHECKLIST
The Patient With Nervous System Metastases

At the completion of education, the patient and/or caregiver will be able to:

- State effects of the tumor according to its type and location in the brain or spinal cord.
- State the impact of the tumor and treatment on physiologic functioning, ADLs, IADLs, roles, relationships, and spirituality.
  - Describe goals and side effects of treatment and suggested management approaches.
- State the name, dose, side effects, frequency, and schedule for all medications.
  - When indicated, use nonpharmacologic pain management techniques in addition to prescribed pharmacologic methods.
- State how to contact all members of the treatment team (e.g., health care providers, home care professionals, and durable medical equipment and supply vendor).
- State changes in lifestyle (e.g., nutritional needs, ADL assistance) necessary to maintain health.
- Identify coping strategies, such as:
  - Taking control, setting daily goals, and staying positive.
  - Rehabilitation to improve self-care.

- Relaxation techniques.
- Family support.
- Support groups.
- American Brain Tumor Association.
- Faith community/religious practices and rituals.
- Identify community resources, including palliative care, home health service, hospice, as appropriate.
- List complications of medications/therapeutic regimen necessitating a call to the nurse or primary provider.
- List complications of medications/therapeutic regimen necessitating a visit to the emergency department.
- Relate how to reach primary provider with questions or complications.
- State time and date of follow-up medical appointments, therapy, and testing.

Resources

See Chapter 15, Chart 15-10 Home Care Checklist: The Client Undergoing Care for an Oncologic Disorder.

ADL, activities of daily living; IADL, independent activities of daily living.

2. Maintains as optimal a nutritional status as possible
   a. Eats and accepts food within limits of condition and preferences
   b. Accepts alternative methods of providing nutrition if indicated
3. Reports being less anxious
   a. Is less restless and is sleeping better
   b. Verbalizes concerns and fears about death
   c. Participates in activities of personal importance as long as feasible
4. Family members seek help as needed
   a. Demonstrate ability to bathe, feed, and care for the patient and participate in pain management and prevention of complications
   b. Express feelings and concerns to appropriate health professionals
   c. Discuss and seek hospice care as an option

Spinal Cord Tumors

Tumors within the spinal canal are classified according to their anatomic relation to the spinal cord (Bader, Littlejohns, Olson, et al., 2016). They include intramedullary lesions (within the spinal cord), extramedullary-intradural lesions (within or under the spinal dura), and extramedullary-extradural lesions (outside the dural membrane). Primary tumors are usually intramedullary, consisting of astrocytoma or ependymoma; meningiomas can occur as extramedullary-intradural lesions. Secondary tumors are far more common and are usually extramedullary-extradural lesions. Tumors that occur within the spinal canal or exert pressure on it cause symptoms ranging from localized or shooting pains, weakness and loss of reflexes below the tumor level to progressive loss of motor function and paralysis. Usually, sharp pain occurs in the area innervated by the spinal roots that arise from the cord in the region of the tumor. In addition, increasing sensory deficits develop below the level of the lesion. Loss of bowel and bladder function is common.

Assessment and Diagnostic Findings

Neurologic examination and diagnostic studies are used to make the diagnosis. Neurologic examination focuses on assessing pain and identifying loss of reflexes, sensation, or motor function. Helpful diagnostic studies include CT scans, MRI scans, and biopsy. The MRI scan is the most commonly used and the most sensitive diagnostic tool (Hickey, 2014) and it is particularly helpful in detecting epidural spinal cord compression and metastases.

Medical Management

Treatment of specific intraspinal tumors depends on the type and location of the tumor and the presenting symptoms and physical status of the patient. Surgical intervention is the primary treatment for most spinal cord tumors followed by chemotherapy and radiation therapy. Research is ongoing with direct, localized drug delivery and nanomedicine treatment (Tobin, Geraghty, Engelhard, et al., 2015).

Extramedullary-extradural spinal cord compression occurs in 5% to 7% of patients who die of cancer and is considered a neurologic emergency. For the patient with spinal cord compression resulting from metastatic cancer (most commonly from breast, prostate, or lung), high-dose dexamethasone (Decadron) combined with radiation therapy is effective in relieving pain (see Chapter 15 for a discussion of care of the patient with spinal cord compression). Palliative care may be an option for the medical management of some patients. Chemotherapy specific to the tumor type may be considered (Perkins & Liu, 2016).

Surgical Management

Tumor removal is desirable but not always possible. The goal is to remove as much tumor as possible while sparing uninvolved portions of the spinal cord. Sudden decrease or loss of motor, sensory, and bowel and bladder function indicates the need for emergent surgery to reestablish function and protect the cord from further damage (Hickey, 2014). Microsurgical techniques have improved the prognosis for patients with intramedullary tumors. Extramedullary-intradural tumors may be completely resected. Prognosis is related to the degree of neurologic impairment at the time of surgery, the speed with which symptoms occurred, and the origin of the tumor. Patients with extensive neurologic deficits before surgery are less likely to regain full functional recovery after successful tumor removal.

Nursing Management
Providing Preoperative Care

The objectives of preoperative care include recognition of neurologic changes through ongoing assessments, pain control, and management of altered activities of daily living (ADLs) resulting from sensory and motor deficits and bowel and bladder dysfunction. The nurse assesses for weakness, muscle wasting, spasticity, sensory changes, bowel and bladder dysfunction, and potential respiratory problems, especially if a cervical tumor is present. The patient is also evaluated for coagulation deficiencies. A history of anticoagulation medication use is obtained and reported, because the use of these may impede hemostasis postoperatively. The patient is educated about breathing exercises, and they are demonstrated preoperatively. Postoperative pain management strategies are discussed with the patient before surgery.

Assessing the Patient After Surgery

The patient is monitored for deterioration in neurologic status. A sudden onset of neurologic deficit is an ominous sign and may be due to spinal cord ischemia or infarction. Frequent neurologic checks are carried out, with emphasis on movement, strength, and sensation of the upper and lower extremities. Assessment of sensory function involves pinching the skin of the arms, legs, and trunk to determine if there is loss of feeling and, if so, at what level. Vital signs are monitored at regular intervals.

Managing Pain

The prescribed pain medication should be given in adequate amounts and at appropriate intervals to relieve pain and prevent its recurrence. Pain is the hallmark of spinal metastasis. Patients with sensory root involvement may suffer excruciating pain, which requires effective pain management.

The bed is usually kept flat initially. The nurse turns the patient as a unit, keeping shoulders and hips aligned and the back straight (also referred to as logrolling) (see Fig. 70-8). The side-lying position is usually the most comfortable, because this position imposes the least pressure on the surgical site. Placement of a pillow between the knees of the patient in a side-lying position helps to prevent extreme knee flexion.

Monitoring and Managing Potential Complications

If the tumor was in the cervical area, respiratory compromise due to postoperative edema may occur (Marchetti, 2014). The nurse monitors the patient for asymmetric chest movement, abdominal breathing, and abnormal breath sounds. For a high cervical lesion, the endotracheal tube remains in place until adequate respiratory function is ensured. The patient is encouraged to perform deep-breathing and coughing exercises.

The area over the bladder is palpated or a bladder scan performed to assess for urinary retention. The nurse also monitors for incontinence, because urinary dysfunction usually implies significant decompensation of spinal cord function. An intake and output record is maintained. In addition, the abdomen is auscultated for bowel sounds.

Staining of the dressing may indicate leakage of CSF from the surgical site, which may lead to serious infection or to an inflammatory reaction in the surrounding tissues that can cause severe pain in the postoperative period. Bulging at the incision may indicate contained CSF leak. The site should be monitored for increasing bulging, known as pseudomeningocele, which may require surgical repair (Hickey, 2014).

Promoting Home, Community-Based, and Transitional Care

 Educating Patients About Self-Care

In preparation for discharge, the patient is assessed for the ability to function independently in the home and for the availability of resources such as family members to assist in caregiving. Patients with residual sensory involvement are cautioned about the dangers of extremes in temperature. They should be educated about the dangers of heating devices (e.g., hot water bottles, heating pads, space heaters) as their sensory integration may be impaired, causing them to lose the ability to detect dangerous stimulations and to react appropriately. The patient is educated to check skin integrity daily. Patients with impaired motor function related to motor weakness or paralysis may require training in ADLs and safe use of assistive devices, such as a cane, walker, or wheelchair (see Chapter 10). The patient and family members are educated about pain management strategies, bowel and bladder management, and assessment for signs and symptoms that should be reported promptly (see Chart 70-2).

Continuing and Transitional Care

Referral for inpatient or outpatient rehabilitation may be warranted to improve self-care abilities. A consultation for home, community-based or transitional care may be indicated and provides the nurse with the opportunity to assess the patient's physical and psychological status and the patient's and family's ability to adhere to recommended management strategies. During the home visit, the nurse determines whether changes in neurologic function have occurred. The patient's respiratory status and nutritional status are assessed. The adequacy of pain management is assessed, and modifications are made to ensure adequate pain relief. The need for hospice services or placement in an extended care facility is discussed with the patient and family if warranted, and the patient is asked about preferences for end-of-life care. In addition, social workers may be consulted to assist the patient and family members in identifying support groups and agencies that can provide help in coping with the disease process (Hickey, 2014).

DEGENERATIVE DISORDERS

Disorders of the central and peripheral nervous system that are **neurodegenerative** (leading to deterioration of normal cells or function of the nervous system) are characterized by the slow onset of signs and symptoms. Patients are managed at home for as long as possible and are admitted to the acute care setting for exacerbations, treatments, and surgical interventions as needed.

Parkinson Disease

PD is a slowly progressing neurologic movement disorder that eventually leads to disability. It affects about 1 million patients who are hospitalized in the United States each year (Moore, Smith, & Cho, 2017). The disease affects men more often than women. Symptoms usually first appear in the fifth decade of life; however, cases have been diagnosed as early as 30 years of age. The degenerative or idiopathic form of PD is the most common; there is also a secondary form with a known or suspected cause. Although the cause of most cases is unknown, research suggests a multifactorial combination of age, environment, and heredity (Moore et al., 2017).

Pathophysiology

PD is associated with decreased levels of dopamine resulting from degeneration of dopamine storage cells in the substantia nigra in the basal ganglia region of the brain (see Fig. 70-4). Fibers or neuronal pathways project from the substantia nigra to the corpus striatum, where neurotransmitters are vital to the control of complex body movements. Through the neurotransmitters acetylcholine (excitatory) and dopamine (inhibitory), striatal neurons relay messages to the higher motor centers that control and refine motor movements. The loss of dopamine stores in this area of the brain results in more excitatory neurotransmitters than inhibitory neurotransmitters, leading to an imbalance that affects voluntary movement (Hickey, 2014).

Clinical symptoms do not appear until 60% of the pigmented neurons are lost and the striatal dopamine level is decreased by 80%. Cellular degeneration impairs the extrapyramidal tracts that control semiautomatic functions and coordinated movements; motor cells of the motor cortex and the pyramidal tracts are not affected. Researchers are working on uncovering the exact mechanism of neurodegeneration. Current theories suggest a combined and complicated

Physiology/Pathophysiology

Figure 70-4 • Pathophysiology of Parkinson disease. The nuclei in the substantia nigra project fibers to the corpus striatum. The nerve fibers carry dopamine to the corpus striatum. The loss of dopamine nerve cells from the brain's substantia nigra is thought to be responsible for the symptoms of parkinsonism.

interweaving of both environmental and genetic factors that affect numerous fundamental cellular processes. Fifteen percent of early PD cases are associated with multiple genetic mutations (Gopalakrishna & Alexander, 2015). Ongoing research includes recognition of biomarkers and development of individualized treatment options (Kalia & Lang, 2015).

Clinical Manifestations

PD has a gradual onset, and symptoms progress slowly over a chronic, prolonged course. The cardinal signs are tremor, rigidity, bradykinesia/akinesia, and postural instability (Hickey, 2014). Two major subtypes of PD are evolving:

tremor dominant (most other symptoms are absent) and nontremor dominant (akinetic-rigid and postural instability) (Kalia & Lang, 2015).

Tremor

Although symptoms are variable, a slow, unilateral resting tremor is present in the majority of patients at the time of diagnosis. Resting tremor characteristically disappears with purposeful movement and during sleep but is evident when the extremities are motionless or at rest. The tremor may manifest as a rhythmic, slow turning motion (pronation–supination) of the forearm and the hand and a motion of the thumb against the fingers as if rolling a pill between the fingers.

Rigidity

Resistance to passive limb movement characterizes muscle rigidity. Passive movement of an extremity may cause the limb to move in jerky increments, referred to as lead-pipe or cogwheel movements. Involuntary stiffness of the passive extremity increases when another extremity is engaged in voluntary active movement. Stiffness of the arms, legs, face, and posture are common. Early in the disease, the patient may complain of shoulder pain due to rigidity (Hickey, 2014).

Bradykinesia

One of the most common features of PD is **bradykinesia**, which refers to the overall slowing of active movement (Gopalakrishna & Alexander, 2015). Patients may also take longer to complete activities and have difficulty initiating movement, such as rising from a sitting position or turning in bed.

Postural Instability

The patient commonly develops postural and gait problems. Due to a loss of postural reflexes, the patient stands with the head bent forward and walks with a propulsive gait. The posture is caused by the forward flexion of the neck, hips, knees, and elbows. The patient may walk faster and faster, trying to move the feet forward under the body's center of gravity (shuffling gait). Difficulty in pivoting causes loss of balance, either forward (propulsion) or backward (retropulsion). Gait impairment and postural instability place the patient at increased risk for falls (Hickey, 2014). Approximately 80% of patients with a 17 years history of symptoms report gait impairment and falls (Kalia & Lang, 2015).

Other Manifestations

The effect of PD on the basal ganglia often produces autonomic symptoms that include excessive and uncontrolled sweating, drooling, paroxysmal flushing, orthostatic hypotension, gastric and urinary retention, constipation, and sexual dysfunction. Dysphagia remains a substantial problem as more than 50% of patients report choking as well as vision and olfactory changes (Hickey, 2014; Kalia & Lang, 2015). Psychiatric changes include depression, anxiety, **dementia** (progressive mental deterioration), delirium, and hallucinations. Depression and anxiety are common; whether these are reactions to the disorder or related to a biochemical abnormality is uncertain (Moore et al., 2017). Stress, medications, and depression contribute to the cognitive changes of diminished executive functions, attention difficulties, decreased thinking, and word-finding challenges. More than 80% of patients with a 20-year disease duration of PD experience dementia (Kalia & Lang, 2015). In addition, auditory and visual hallucinations have been reported in up to 40% of people with PD and may be associated with depression, dementia, lack of sleep, or adverse effects of medications.

Hypokinesia (abnormally diminished movement) is also common and may appear after the tremor. The freezing phenomenon refers to a transient inability to perform active movement and is thought to be an extreme form of bradykinesia. The patient tends to shuffle and exhibits a decreased arm swing as well. As dexterity declines, micrographia (small handwriting) develops. The face becomes increasingly masklike and expressionless, and the frequency of blinking decreases. **Dysphonia** (voice impairment or altered voice production) may occur as a result of weakness and incoordination of the muscles responsible for speech. In many cases, the patient develops dysphagia, begins to drool, and is at risk for choking and aspiration (Hickey, 2014).

Complications associated with PD are common and are typically related to disorders of movement. As the disease progresses, patients are at risk for respiratory and urinary tract infection, skin breakdown, and injury from falls. The adverse effects of medications used to treat the symptoms are associated with numerous complications such as **dyskinesia** (impaired ability to execute voluntary movements) or orthostatic hypotension.

Assessment and Diagnostic Findings

Although laboratory tests and imaging studies are not helpful to the clinician in diagnosing PD ongoing research with PET and single-photon emission computed tomography scanning has been helpful in understanding the disease and advancing treatment. Currently, the disease is diagnosed clinically from the patient's history and the presence of two of the four cardinal manifestations: tremor, rigidity, bradykinesia, and postural changes.

Early diagnosis can be challenging because patients rarely are able to pinpoint when the symptoms started. Often, a family member notices a change such as stooped posture; a stiff arm; a slight limp; tremor; or slow, small handwriting. The medical history, presenting symptoms, neurologic examination, and response to pharmacologic management are carefully evaluated when making the diagnosis. Diagnosis is often confirmed by a positive response to a levodopa (Larodopa) trial (Hickey, 2014).

Medical Management

Treatment is directed toward controlling symptoms and maintaining functional independence, because no medical or surgical approaches in current use prevent disease progression. Care is individualized for each patient based on presenting symptoms and social, occupational, and emotional needs. Pharmacologic management is the mainstay of treatment, although advances in research have led to increased surgical options. Patients are usually cared for at home and are admitted to the hospital only for complications or to initiate new treatments.

Pharmacologic Therapy

Antiparkinsonian medications act by (1) increasing striatal dopaminergic activity; (2) reducing the excessive influence of excitatory cholinergic neurons on the extrapyramidal tract, thereby restoring a balance between dopaminergic and cholinergic activities; or (3) acting on neurotransmitter pathways other than the dopaminergic pathway. PD research efforts are focused on the development of disease-modifying drugs that slow or stop this neurodegenerative process (Kalia & Lang, 2015).

Levodopa is the most effective agent and the mainstay of treatment. Levodopa is converted to dopamine in the basal ganglia, producing symptom relief. Carbidopa is often added to levodopa to avoid metabolism of levodopa before it can reach the brain. The beneficial effects of levodopa therapy are most pronounced in the first year or two of treatment. Benefits begin to wane and adverse effects become more severe over time (Hickey, 2014). Within 5 to 10 years, most patients develop a response to the medication characterized by dyskinesia including facial grimacing, rhythmic jerking movements of the hands, head bobbing, chewing and smacking movements, and involuntary movements of the trunk and extremities. The patient may experience an on–off syndrome in which sudden periods of near immobility ("off effect") are followed by a sudden return of effectiveness of the medication ("on effect"). Changing the drug dosing regimen or switching to other drugs may be helpful in minimizing the on–off syndrome. Other potential adverse effects include nausea, vomiting, appetite loss, decreased BP, dystonia, dyskinesia, and confusion (Moore et al., 2017). To minimize adverse effects of levodopa over time, current practice includes delaying use of levodopa-containing drugs as long as possible, with the use of other drugs for symptom control in the interim.

 Concept Mastery Alert

Nurses caring for patients with PD need a clear understanding of medications that are prescribed. Table 70-1 provides a summary of selected medications used in PD.

Surgical Management

The limitations of levodopa therapy, improvements in surgical techniques, and new approaches in transplantation have renewed interest in the surgical treatment of PD. In patients with disabling tremor, rigidity, or severe levodopa-induced dyskinesia, surgery may be considered. Although surgery provides symptom relief in selected patients, it has not been shown to alter the course of the disease or to produce permanent improvement.

Stereotactic Procedures

Thalamotomy and pallidotomy are ablative procedures that were formerly used to relieve symptoms of PD. However, these procedures permanently destroy brain tissue and are rarely used today. Deep brain stimulation (DBS) has largely replaced ablative procedures in the surgical treatment of PD (Kalia & Lang, 2015). DBS involves surgical implantation of an electrode into the brain in either the globus pallidus or subthalamic nucleus. Stimulation of these areas may increase dopamine release or block anticholinergic release, thereby improving tremor and rigidity. Levodopa medication dose may be able to be reduced, thus improving dyskinesias.

Patients eligible for DBS are those who have responded to levodopa but are impaired by dyskinesias, have had the

TABLE 70-1 Selected Medications Used to Treat Parkinson Disease

Medications	Indications and Therapeutic Effects	Common Side Effects
Anticholinergic Agents		
trihexyphenidyl hydrochloride (Apo-Trihex)	Control of tremor in patients with early-onset disease	Blurred vision, flushing, rash, constipation, urinary retention, and acute confusional states
benztropine mesylate (Cogentin)	Counteract the action of acetylcholine	Contraindicated in patients with narrow-angle glaucoma
Antiviral Agent		
amantadine hydrochloride (Symmetrel)	Reduce rigidity, tremor, bradykinesia, and postural changes in early Parkinson disease (PD)	Psychiatric disturbances (mood changes, confusion, depression, hallucinations), lower extremity edema, nausea, epigastric distress, urinary retention, headache, and visual impairment
Dopamine Agonists		
bromocriptine mesylate (Parlodel)	Early PD as well as secondary drug therapy after carbidopa or levodopa loses effectiveness	Nausea, vomiting, diarrhea, lightheadedness, hypotension, impotence, and psychiatric effects
pergolide (Permax)		
Nonergot Derivatives		
ropinirole hydrochloride (Requip)	Early stages of PD	May cause drowsiness or dizziness
pramipexole (Mirapex)		
Monoamine Oxidase-Inhibitors		
selegiline (Emsam)	Inhibit dopamine breakdown	Agitation, dizziness, nausea, headache, rhinitis, back pain, stomatitis, postural hypotension, insomnia
rasagiline (Azilect)		
Catechol-O-Methyltransferase Inhibitors		
entacapone (Comtan)	Increase the duration of action of carbidopa or levodopa	Abdominal pain, back pain, constipation, nausea, diarrhea, blood in urine
tolcapone (Tasmar)	Reduce motor fluctuations in patients with advanced PD	

Adapted from Moore, D. J., Smith, B. M., & Cho, M. H. (2017). Managing meditations for hospital patients with Parkinson disease. *American Nurse Today*, 12(1), 9–12.

disease for at least 5 years, and are disabled by tremor. Patients with dementia and atypical PD are usually not considered for surgical procedures. PD rating scales and specific neurologic tests are used to identify patients who are eligible. Surgical treatment typically occurs 10 to 13 years after diagnosis. Research is ongoing on the relationship between placing a DBS and patient quality of life (Kalia & Lang, 2015).

A CT or MRI scan is used to localize the appropriate surgical site in the brain. Then, the patient's head is positioned in a stereotactic frame (see Fig. 70-5). After the surgeon makes an incision in the skin and a burr hole, an electrode is passed through to the target area to the subthalamic nuclei or globus pallidus. The desired response of the patient to the electrical stimulation (i.e., a decrease in rigidity) is used to confirm electrode placement. Electrode placement is completed on one side of the brain at a time; bilateral electrodes are usually placed (AANN, 2014b). Electrodes are then connected to a pulse generator that is implanted in a subcutaneous subclavicular or abdominal pouch (see Fig. 70-6). The battery-powered pulse generator sends high-frequency electrical impulses through a wire placed under the skin to a lead anchored to the skull (see Fig. 70-6). These devices are not without

complications that can result from both the surgical procedure needed for implantation (e.g., weakness, paresthesias, confusion, hemorrhage) and the device itself (e.g., infection, lead leakage) (Hickey, 2014).

Figure 70-5 • A stereotactic frame is applied to a patient's head in preparation for deep brain stimulation. The frame provides external points of reference.

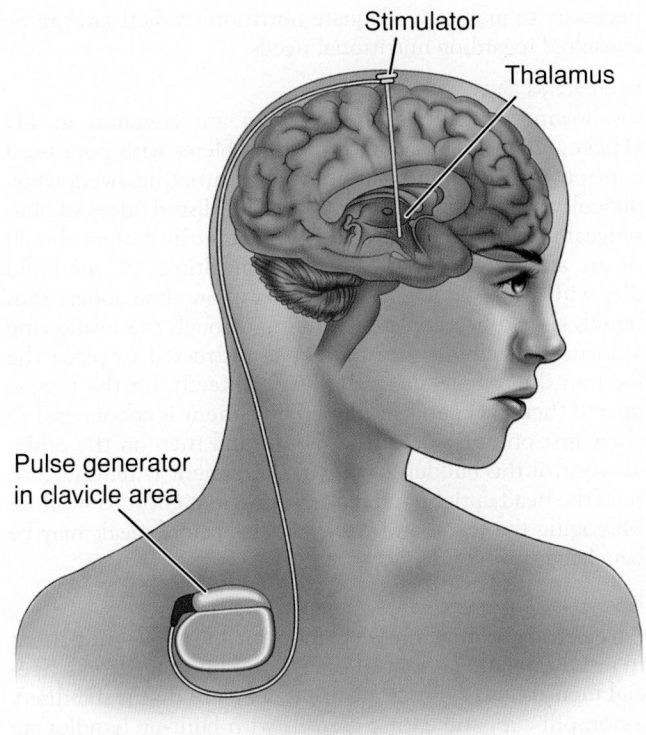

Figure 70-6 • Deep brain stimulation is provided by a pulse generator surgically implanted in a pouch beneath the clavicle. The generator sends high-frequency electrical impulses to the thalamus, thereby blocking the nerve pathways associated with tremors in Parkinson disease.

Neural Transplantation

Ongoing research is exploring transplantation of porcine neuronal cells, human fetal cells, and stem cells to replace degenerated striatal cells (Kim, Lee, & Kim, 2013). Legal, ethical, and political concerns surrounding the use of fetal brain cells and stem cells have limited the exploration of these procedures.

NURSING PROCESS

The Patient With Parkinson Disease

Assessment

Assessment focuses on how the disease has affected the patient's ADLs and functional abilities. The patient is observed for degree of disability and functional changes that occur throughout the day, such as responses to medication. Almost every patient with a movement disorder has some functional alteration and may have some type of behavioral dysfunction. The following questions may be useful to assess alterations:

- Do you have leg or arm stiffness?
- Have you experienced any irregular jerking of your arms or legs?
- Have you ever been "frozen" or rooted to the spot and unable to move?

- Does your mouth water excessively? Have you (or others) noticed yourself grimacing or making faces or chewing movements?
- What specific activities do you have difficulty doing?
- Have you had any recent falls?

During this assessment, the nurse observes the patient for quality of speech, loss of facial expression, swallowing deficits (drooling, poor head control, coughing), tremors, slowness of movement, weakness, forward posture, rigidity, evidence of mental slowness, and confusion. PD symptoms, as well as side effects of medications, put these patients at high risk for falls; therefore, a fall risk assessment should be conducted (Hickey, 2014; Shin & Habermann, 2016a).

Diagnosis

NURSING DIAGNOSES

Based on the assessment data, major nursing diagnoses may include the following:

- Impaired physical mobility related to muscle rigidity and postural impairment
- Self-care deficits (feeding, dressing, bathing, and toileting) related to tremor and muscle rigidity
- Constipation related to medication and reduced activity
- Imbalanced nutrition: less than body requirements related to tremor, slowness in eating, difficulty in chewing and swallowing
- Impaired verbal communication related to decreased speech volume, slowness of speech, inability to move facial muscles
- Ineffective coping related to depression and dysfunction due to disease progression

Other nursing diagnoses may include sleep pattern disturbances, deficient knowledge, risk for injury, risk for activity intolerance, disturbed thought processes, and compromised family coping.

Planning and Goals

The goals for the patient may include improving functional mobility, maintaining independence in ADLs, achieving adequate bowel elimination, attaining and maintaining acceptable nutritional status, achieving effective communication, and developing positive coping mechanisms.

Nursing Interventions

IMPROVING MOBILITY

A progressive program of daily exercise will increase muscle strength, improve coordination and dexterity, reduce muscular rigidity, and prevent contractures that occur when muscles are not used (Hickey, 2014). Walking, riding a stationary bicycle, swimming, and gardening are all exercises that help maintain joint mobility. Stretching (stretch–hold–relax) and range-of-motion exercises promote joint flexibility. Postural exercises are important to counter the tendency of the head and neck to be drawn forward and down. A physical therapist may be helpful in developing an individualized exercise program and can provide instruction to the patient and caregiver on exercising safely. Faithful adherence to an exercise and walking program helps delay the progress of the disease. Warm baths and massage, in addition to passive and active exercises, help relax muscles and relieve painful muscle spasms that accompany rigidity.

Balance may be adversely affected because of the rigidity of the arms (arm swinging is necessary in normal walking). Special walking techniques must be learned to offset the shuffling gait and the tendency to lean forward. The patient is educated to concentrate on walking erect, to watch the horizon, and to use a wide-based gait (i.e., walking with the feet separated). A conscious effort must be made to swing the arms, raise the feet while walking, and use a heel–toe placement of the feet with long strides. The patient is advised to practice walking to marching music or to the sound of a ticking metronome, because this provides sensory reinforcement. Performing breathing exercises while walking provides additional movement of the ribcage and aerates larger parts of the lungs. Frequent rest periods aid in preventing frustration and fatigue.

ENHANCING SELF-CARE ACTIVITIES

Encouraging, educating, and supporting the patient during ADLs promote self-care (Hickey, 2014). See Chapter 10 for rehabilitation techniques.

Environmental modifications are necessary to compensate for functional disabilities. Patients may have severe mobility problems that make normal activities impossible. Adaptive or assistive devices may be useful. A hospital bed at home with bedside rails, an over-bed frame with a trapeze, or a rope tied to the foot of the bed can provide assistance in pulling up without help. An occupational therapist can evaluate the patient's needs in the home, make recommendations regarding adaptive devices, and educate the patient and caregiver how to improvise.

IMPROVING BOWEL ELIMINATION

The patient may have severe problems with constipation. Among the factors causing constipation are weakness of the muscles used in defecation, lack of exercise, inadequate fluid intake, and decreased autonomic nervous system activity. The medications used for the treatment of the disease also inhibit normal intestinal secretions. A regular bowel routine may be established by encouraging the patient to follow a regular time pattern, consciously increase fluid intake, and eat foods with moderate fiber content. Laxatives should be avoided. Psyllium (Metamucil), for example, decreases constipation but carries the risk of bowel obstruction (Moore et al., 2017). A raised toilet seat is useful because the patient has difficulty in moving from a standing to a sitting position.

IMPROVING NUTRITION

Patients may have difficulty maintaining their weight. Eating becomes a very slow process, requiring concentration due to a dry mouth from medications and difficulty chewing and swallowing. These patients are at risk for aspiration because of impaired swallowing and the accumulation of saliva. They may be unaware that they are aspirating; subsequently, bronchopneumonia may develop.

Monitoring weight on a weekly basis indicates whether caloric intake is adequate. Supplemental feedings increase caloric intake. As the disease progresses, a nasogastric or percutaneous endoscopic gastrostomy (PEG) tube may be necessary to maintain adequate nutrition. A dietitian can be consulted regarding nutritional needs.

ENHANCING SWALLOWING

Swallowing difficulties and choking are common in PD (Hickey, 2014). These can lead to problems with poor head control, tongue tremor, hesitancy in initiating swallowing, difficulty shaping food into a bolus, and disturbances in pharyngeal motility. To offset these problems, the patient should sit in an upright position during mealtime. A semisolid diet with thick liquids is easier to swallow than solids; thin liquids should be avoided. Thinking through the swallowing sequence is helpful. The patient is instructed to place the food on the tongue, close the lips and teeth, lift the tongue up and then back, and swallow. The patient is encouraged to chew first on one side of the mouth and then on the other. To control the buildup of saliva, the patient is reminded to hold the head upright and make a conscious effort to swallow. Massaging the facial and neck muscles before meals may be beneficial.

ENCOURAGING THE USE OF ASSISTIVE DEVICES

An electric warming tray keeps food hot and allows the patient to rest during the prolonged time that it may take to eat. Special utensils also assist at mealtime. A plate that is stabilized, a nonspill cup, and eating utensils with built-up handles are useful self-help devices. The occupational therapist can assist in identifying appropriate adaptive devices. Individualized, innovative rehabilitative therapies can increase function in the patient with PD (Abbruzzese, Marchese, Avanzino, et al., 2016).

IMPROVING COMMUNICATION

Speech disorders are present in most patients with PD. The low-pitched, monotonous, soft speech of patients requires that they make a conscious effort to speak slowly, with deliberate attention to what they are saying. The patient is reminded to face the listener, exaggerate the pronunciation of words, speak in short sentences, and take a few deep breaths before speaking. A speech therapist may be helpful in designing speech improvement exercises and assisting the family and health care personnel to develop and use a method of communication that meets the patient's needs. A small electronic amplifier is helpful if the patient has difficulty being heard.

SUPPORTING COPING ABILITIES

Support can be given by encouraging the patient and pointing out that activities will be maintained through active participation. A combination of physiotherapy, psychotherapy, medication therapy, and support group participation may help reduce the depression that often occurs (Hickey, 2014). Patients with PD can become socially and emotionally withdrawn. It is best if patients are active participants in their therapeutic program, including social and recreational events. A planned program of activity throughout the day prevents too much daytime sleeping as well as disinterest and apathy.

Patients often feel embarrassed, apathetic, inadequate, bored, and lonely. In part, these feelings may result from physical slowness and the great effort that even small tasks require. The patient is assisted and encouraged to set achievable goals (e.g., improvement of mobility). Every effort should be made to encourage patients to carry out the tasks involved in meeting their own daily needs and to remain independent. Doing things for the patient merely to save time undermines the basic goal of improving coping abilities and promoting a positive self-concept.

PROMOTING HOME, COMMUNITY-BASED, OR TRANSITIONAL CARE

Educating Patients About Self-Care. Patient and family education is important in the management of PD. The needs depend on the severity of symptoms and the stage of the disease. Care must be taken not to overwhelm the patient and family with too much information early in the disease process. Ongoing assessment, intervention, and evaluation of the patient and family's adaptations and education requirements are necessary with every encounter. The strategies to promote health include a clear explanation of the disease and the goal of assisting the patient to remain functionally independent as long as possible (see Chart 70-3). The patient and family must be educated about the effects and side effects of medications and about the importance of reporting side effects to the primary provider. Nurses in the home help patients and their families enhance self-management and quality of life (Shin & Habermann, 2016b).

Continuing and Transitional Care. Family members and partners often serve as caregivers, with home, community-based or transitional services available to assist in meeting health care needs as the disease progresses. The caregiver may be under considerable stress from living with and caring for a person with a significant disability. Providing information about treatment and care helps anticipate future needs. The caregiver is included in the plan and may be advised to learn stress reduction techniques, to include others in the caregiving process, to obtain periodic relief from responsibilities, and to have a yearly health assessment. Allowing family members and partners to express feelings of frustration,

anger, and guilt is often helpful to them (Martin, 2015) (see Chart 70-4).

The patient should be evaluated in the home for adaptation and safety needs and compliance with the plan of care. In the advanced stages, patients usually enter long-term care facilities. Periodically, admission to an acute care facility may be necessary for changes in medical management or treatment of complications. Nurses provide support, education, and monitoring of patients over the course of the illness (Shin & Habermann, 2016b).

The nurse involved in home and continuing care educates the patient and family members about the importance of addressing health promotion needs such as screening for hypertension and stroke risk assessments in this predominantly older adult population. Patients are referred to appropriate health care providers. Information is available from both the Parkinson Disease Foundation and the American Parkinson's Disease Association (see the Resources section).

Evaluation

Expected patient outcomes may include:

1. Strives toward improved mobility
   a. Participates in exercise program daily
   b. Walks with wide base of support; exaggerates arm swinging when walking
   c. Takes medications as prescribed
2. Progresses toward self-care
   a. Allows time for self-care activities
   b. Uses self-help devices
3. Maintains bowel function
   a. Consumes adequate fluid
   b. Increases dietary intake of fiber
   c. Reports regular pattern of bowel function
4. Attains improved nutritional status
   a. Swallows without aspiration
   b. Takes time while eating

Chart 70-4

NURSING RESEARCH PROFILE
When a Partner Has Parkinson Disease

Martin, S. C. (2015). Psychosocial challenges experienced by partners of people with Parkinson disease. *Journal of Neuroscience Nursing, 47*(4), 211–222.

Purpose

Persons with PD may experience devastating effects that impact those individuals who are close to them as well as the person experiencing the disease. The purpose of this study was to investigate the psychosocial experience of partners of people with PD.

Design

This qualitative descriptive study used in-depth interviews to investigate the psychosocial experience of partners of people with PD. A semistructured interview guide was used with 23 participants (15 women, 8 men) who identified that they were in a committed, romantic relationship with a person with PD.

Findings

Data analysis revealed a multitude of challenges for partners of people with PD. Some challenges included having the person with PD withdraw from communication, being unable to "rescue" the person from their disease (PD), and being the recipient of the person with PD's frustration. Additional challenges included becoming impatient with the person with PD, shouldering increased responsibilities, being confronted with the prospect of losing the person with PD, losing valued activities, being unable to predict the person with PD's daily well-being, and experiencing uncertainty about future caregiving and disease progression.

Nursing Implications

Partners of persons with PD face significant psychosocial challenges related to both caregiving and noncaregiving issues. Nurses should be prepared to provide reassurance to partners of persons with PD that their feelings are normal, as well as offer direction on how to enlist the support of family and friends and access additional support services.

---

5. Achieves a method of communication
   a. Communicates needs
   b. Practices speech exercises
6. Copes with effects of PD
   a. Sets realistic goals
   b. Demonstrates persistence in meaningful activities
   c. Verbalizes feelings to appropriate person

Huntington Disease

Huntington disease is a chronic, progressive, hereditary disease of the nervous system that results in progressive involuntary choreiform movement and dementia. The disease affects approximately 1 in 10,000 men or women of all races at midlife. Every person has the gene that causes Huntington disease; however, only those who inherit the expansion of the gene will develop the disease and pass it onto their children. Because it is transmitted by an autosomal dominant gene, each child of a parent with Huntington disease has a 50% risk of inheriting the disorder (Bader et al., 2016).

A genetic mutation in Huntington disease, the presence of a repeat in the Huntington gene (*HTT*), has been identified. Genetic testing can identify people who will develop this disease but cannot predict timing of disease onset. Although the gene was mapped in 1983, patients may choose not to be tested because of concerns about employment and health care discrimination. People of childbearing age with a family history of Huntington disease often seek information about their risk of disease transmission. Genetic counseling is crucial, and patients and their families may require long-term psychological counseling and emotional, financial, and legal support (see Chapter 8).

Pathophysiology

The basic pathology involves premature death of cells in the striatum (caudate and putamen) of the basal ganglia, the region deep within the brain that is involved in the control of movement. Cells also are lost in the cortex, the region of the brain associated with thinking, memory, perception, judgment, and behavior, and in the cerebellum, the area that coordinates voluntary muscle activity. Why the protein destroys only certain brain cells is unknown, but several theories have been proposed to explain the phenomenon. One possible theory is that glutamine, a building block for protein, abnormally collects in the cell nucleus, causing cell death (Ferrer, 2016).

Clinical Manifestations

This condition is characterized by a triad of symptoms: (1) motor dysfunction (the most prominent is **chorea**, or rapid, jerky, involuntary, purposeless movements); (2) cognitive impairment (problems with attention and emotion recognition); and (3) behavioral features, such as apathy and blunted affect (Bader et al., 2016). As the disease progresses, constant writhing, twisting, and uncontrollable movements may involve the entire body. These motions are devoid of purpose or rhythm, although patients may try to turn them into purposeful movement. All of the body musculature is involved. Facial movements produce tics and grimaces. Speech becomes slurred, hesitant, often explosive, and eventually unintelligible. Chewing and swallowing are difficult, and there is a constant danger of choking and aspiration. Choreiform movements persist during sleep but are diminished (Wilson, Pollock, & Aubeeluck, 2014).

As with speech, the gait becomes disorganized to the point that ambulation eventually is impossible. Although independent ambulation should be encouraged for as long as possible, a wheelchair usually becomes necessary. Eventually, the patient is confined to bed when the chorea interferes with walking, sitting, and all other activities. Bladder and bowel control is lost.

Cognitive impairment, such as problems with attention or emotion recognition, occurs early on while in later stages, marked dementia is present. Initially, the patient is aware that the disease is responsible for the myriad dysfunctions that are occurring.

The behavioral changes may be more devastating to the patient and family than the abnormal movements. Personality changes may result in nervous, irritable, or impatient behaviors. In the early stages, patients are particularly subject to uncontrollable fits of anger, profound and often suicidal depression, apathy, anxiety, psychosis, or euphoria. Judgment and memory are impaired, and dementia eventually ensues (Ross, Aylward, Wild, et al., 2014). Hallucinations, delusions, and paranoid thinking may precede the appearance of disjointed movements. Emotional and cognitive symptoms often become less acute as the disease progresses (Wilson et al., 2014).

Onset usually occurs between 35 and 45 years of age, although about 10% of patients are children. The disease progresses slowly. Despite a ravenous appetite, patients usually become emaciated and exhausted. Patients succumb in 10 to 20 years to heart failure, pneumonia, or infection, or as a result of a fall or choking.

Assessment and Diagnostic Findings

The diagnosis is made based on the clinical presentation of characteristic symptoms, a positive family history, and the known presence of the genetic marker CAG repeats in *HTT* (Bader et al., 2016). CT or MRI scans show symmetrical striatal atrophy before motor symptoms appear (Ross et al., 2014).

Medical Management

No treatment halts or reverses the underlying process; therefore, the focus is on optimizing quality of life with available medication and supportive treatment. Patients experience the most benefit when they have integrated expertise of a Huntington disease multidisciplinary team (Smith, D'Cruz, Gray, et al., 2015). The only medication that is approved by the Food and Drug Administration to treat the symptom of chorea is tetrabenazine (Xenazine) (Kumar, Singh, Kumar, et al., 2015).

Benzodiazepines and neuroleptic drugs have also been reported to control chorea. Motor signs must be assessed and evaluated on an ongoing basis so that optimal therapeutic drug levels can be reached. Akathisia (motor restlessness) in the patient who is overmedicated is dangerous because it may be mistaken for the restless fidgeting of the illness and consequently may be overlooked. In certain types of the disease, hypokinetic motor impairment resembles PD. In patients who present with rigidity, some temporary benefit may be obtained from antiparkinson medications, such as levodopa.

Selective serotonin reuptake inhibitors and tricyclic antidepressants have been recommended for control of psychiatric symptoms. The threat of suicide is present particularly early in the course of the disease. Psychotic symptoms usually respond to antipsychotic medications. Psychotherapy aimed at allaying anxiety and reducing stress may be beneficial. Nurses must look beyond the disease to focus on the patient's needs and capabilities (see Chart 70-5).

Promoting Home, Community-Based, and Transitional Care

 ### Educating Patients About Self-Care

The needs of the patient and family for education depend on the nature and severity of the physical, cognitive, and psychological changes experienced by the patient. The patient and family members are educated about the medications prescribed and about signs indicating a need for change in medication or dosage. The educational plan addresses strategies to manage symptoms such as chorea, swallowing problems, limitations in ambulation, memory loss, irritability, depression, and loss of bowel and bladder function. Consultation with a speech therapist may be indicated to assist in identifying alternative communication strategies if speech is affected. A PEG tube may be considered for nutritional support later in the disease (Wilson et al., 2014).

Continuing and Transitional Care

A program combining medical, nursing, psychological, social, occupational, speech, and physical rehabilitation services and palliative care is needed to help the patient and family cope with this severely disabling illness. Huntington disease exacts enormous emotional, physical, social, and financial tolls on every member of the family. The family needs supportive care as they adjust to the impact of the illness. Regular follow-up visits help allay the fear of abandonment.

Home care assistance, day care centers, respite care, and eventually skilled long-term care can assist the patient and family in coping with the constant strain of the illness. Although the relentless progression of the disease cannot be halted, families can benefit from supportive care. Planning for end-of-life care should occur early in the disease when possible (see Chapter 16).

Voluntary organizations can be major aids to families and have been largely responsible for bringing the illness to national attention. The Huntington's Disease Society of America helps patients and families by providing information, referrals, family and public education, and support for research (see the Resources section).

Amyotrophic Lateral Sclerosis

ALS is a disease of unknown cause in which there is a loss of motor neurons (nerve cells controlling muscles) in the anterior horns of the spinal cord and the motor nuclei of the lower brainstem. It is often referred to as Lou Gehrig disease, after the famous baseball player who suffered from the disease. As motor neuron cells die, the muscle fibers that they supply undergo atrophic changes. Neuronal degeneration may occur in both the upper and lower motor neuron systems (see Chapter 65). The leading theory held by researchers is that overexcitation of nerve cells by the neurotransmitter glutamate results in cell injury and neuronal degeneration. Risk factors that have been identified include smoking, viral infections, autoimmune disease, and environmental exposures to toxins. For example, veterans who deployed during the 1991 Gulf War had an increased number of cases of ALS compared to those who did not serve in that region. However, the

Chart 70-5 Care of the Patient With Huntington Disease

Nursing Diagnosis: Risk for injury from falls and possible skin breakdown (pressure ulcers, abrasions), resulting from constant movement

Nursing Interventions

Pad the sides and head of the bed; ensure that the patient can see over the sides of bed.
Use padded heel and elbow protectors.
Keep the skin meticulously clean.
Apply emollient cleansing agent and skin lotion as needed.
Use soft sheets and bedding.
Have patient wear football padding or other forms of padding.
Encourage ambulation with assistance to maintain muscle tone.
Secure the patient (only if necessary) in bed or chair with padded protective devices, making sure that they are loosened frequently.

Nursing Diagnosis: Imbalanced nutrition: less than body requirements due to inadequate intake and dehydration resulting from swallowing or chewing disorders and danger of choking or aspirating food

Nursing Interventions

Administer phenothiazines (chlorpromazine) as prescribed before meals (calms some patients).
Talk to the patient before mealtime to promote relaxation; use mealtime for social interaction. Provide undivided attention and help the patient enjoy the mealtime experience.
Use a warming tray to keep food warm.
Learn the position that is best for *this* patient. Keep patient as close to upright as possible while feeding. Stabilize patient's head gently with one hand while feeding.
Show the food, explain what the foods are, and temperature (e.g., whether hot or cold).
Encircle the patient with one arm and get as close as possible to provide stability and support while feeding. Use pillows and wedges for additional support.
Do not interpret stiffness, turning away, or sudden turning of the head as rejection; these are uncontrollable choreiform movements.
For feeding, use a long-handled spoon (iced tea spoon). Place spoon on middle of tongue and exert slight pressure.
Place bite-sized food between patient's teeth. Serve stews, casseroles, and thick liquids.
Disregard messiness, and treat the person with dignity.

Wait for the patient to chew and swallow before introducing another spoonful. Make sure that bite-sized food is small.
Give between-meal feedings. Constant movement expends more calories. Patients often have voracious appetites, particularly for sweets.
Use blenderized meals if patient cannot chew; do not repeatedly give the same strained baby foods. Gradually introduce increased textures and consistencies to the diet.
For swallowing difficulties:
   Apply gentle deep pressure around the patient's mouth.
   Rub fingers in circles on the patient's cheeks and then down each side of the patient's throat.
   Develop skill in the abdominal thrust (to be used in the event of choking).

Nursing Diagnosis: Impaired communication from excessive grimacing and unintelligible speech

Nursing Interventions

Read to the patient.
Employ biofeedback and relaxation therapy to reduce stress.
Consult with speech therapist to help maintain and prolong communication abilities.
Try to devise a communication system, perhaps using cards with words or pictures of familiar objects, before verbal communication becomes too difficult. Patients can indicate correct card by hitting it with hand, grunting, or blinking the eyes.
Learn how this particular patient expresses needs and wants—particularly nonverbal messages (widening of eyes, responses).
Patients can understand even if unable to speak. Do not isolate patients by ceasing to communicate with them.

Nursing Diagnosis: Confusion and impaired social interaction

Nursing Interventions

Reorient the patient after awakening.
Have clock, calendar, and wall posters in view to assist in orientation.
Use every opportunity for one-to-one contact.
Use music for relaxation.
Have the patient wear a medical identification bracelet.
Keep the patient in the social mainstream.
Recruit and train volunteers for social interaction. Role-model appropriate and creative interactions.
Do not abandon a patient because the disease is terminal. Patients are *living* until the end.

---

exact cause is still unknown and requires further exploration (Bellomo & Cichminski, 2015).

ALS most commonly occurs between 40 and 60 years of age and affects all social, racial, and ethnic backgrounds, with men being affected at slightly higher rates than women. The majority of cases of ALS arise sporadically, but 5% to 10% of cases are familial ALS resulting from an autosomal dominant trait carried by one parent. Familial ALS occurs 10 years earlier than the ALS average, and those afflicted tend to have a shorter life span (Bellomo & Cichminski, 2015). About 30% of patients with ALS live for 5 years after diagnosis, with 10% to 20% surviving for up to 10 years and 5% surviving greater than 20 years postdiagnosis.

Clinical Manifestations

Clinical manifestations depend on the location of the affected motor neurons, because specific neurons activate specific muscle fibers. The chief symptoms are fatigue, progressive muscle weakness, cramps, fasciculations (twitching), and lack of coordination. Loss of motor neurons in the anterior horns of the spinal cord results in progressive weakness and atrophy of the muscles of the arms, trunk, or legs. Spasticity usually is present, and the deep tendon stretch reflexes become brisk and overactive. Usually, the function of the anal and bladder sphincters remains intact, because the spinal nerves that control muscles of the rectum and urinary bladder are not affected.

In about 25% of patients, weakness starts in the muscles supplied by the cranial nerves, and difficulty in talking, swallowing, and ultimately breathing occurs. When the patient ingests liquids, soft palate and upper esophageal weakness cause the liquid to be regurgitated through the nose. Weakness of the posterior tongue and palate impairs the ability to laugh, cough, or even blow the nose. If bulbar muscles are impaired, speaking and swallowing are progressively difficult, and aspiration becomes a risk. The voice assumes a nasal sound, and articulation becomes so disrupted that speech is unintelligible. Some emotional lability may be present. It was traditionally believed that ALS spared cognitive function, but it is now recognized that some patients experience cognitive impairment.

The prognosis generally is based on the area of CNS involvement and the speed with which the disease progresses. Eventually, respiratory function is compromised. Death usually occurs as a result of infection, respiratory insufficiency, or aspiration.

Assessment and Diagnostic Findings

ALS is diagnosed on the basis of the signs and symptoms, because no clinical or laboratory tests are specific to this disease. Electromyography and muscle biopsy studies of the affected muscles indicate reduction in the number of functioning motor units. An MRI scan may show high signal intensity in the corticospinal tracts; this differentiates ALS from a multifocal motor neuropathy. Neuropsychological testing can assist in assessment and diagnosis (Hickey, 2014).

Management

No cure exists for ALS. The main focus of medical and nursing management is on interventions to maintain or improve function, well-being, and quality of life. Because ALS is a progressive disease, the therapeutic needs are different than those of patients with acute processes. Insurance carriers tend to limit the number of therapy sessions, but with early integration into ALS clinics, alliances are developed for future contact with therapists familiar with the disease process (Majmuder, Wu, & Pagnoni, 2014).

Riluzole (Rilutek), a glutamate antagonist, has been shown to prolong survival for persons with ALS for 3 to 6 months (Hickey, 2014). The action of riluzole is not clear, but its pharmacologic properties suggest that it may have a neuroprotective effect in the early stages of ALS. Symptomatic treatment and rehabilitative measures are used to support the patient and improve the quality of life. Baclofen (Lioresal), dantrolene sodium (Dantrium), or diazepam (Valium) may be useful for patients troubled by spasticity, which causes pain and interferes with self-care. Modafinil (Provigil) may be used for fatigue, and additional medications may be added to manage the pain, depression, drooling, and constipation that often accompany the disease. Research suggests that greater functional impairment is associated with greater depressive symptoms; consequently, managing depression helps to maintain a better quality of life (Rosengren, Gustafusson, & Jarnevi, 2015). Ongoing research for treatment options include neural transplantation (Carletti, Rispoli, DiChirico, et al., 2016).

Most patients with ALS are managed at home and in the community, with hospitalization for acute problems. The most common reasons for hospitalization are dehydration and malnutrition, pneumonia, and respiratory failure; recognizing these problems at an early stage in the illness allows for the development of preventive strategies. End-of-life issues include pain, dyspnea, and delirium (Hickey, 2014).

Mechanical ventilation (using negative-pressure ventilators) is an option if alveolar hypoventilation develops. Noninvasive positive-pressure ventilation is also an option. The use of noninvasive positive-pressure ventilation is particularly helpful at night and postpones the decision about whether to undergo a tracheotomy for long-term mechanical ventilation (Rabinstein, 2016). A patient experiencing aspiration and swallowing difficulties may require enteral feeding. A PEG tube is inserted before the forced vital capacity drops below 50% of the predicted value. The tube can be safely placed in patients who are using noninvasive positive-pressure ventilation for ventilatory support (Hickey, 2014; ProGas Study Group, 2015).

Decisions about life support measures are made by the patient and family and should be based on a thorough understanding of the disease, the prognosis, and the implications of initiating such therapy. Patients are encouraged to complete an advance directive ("living will") to preserve their autonomy in decision making. See Chapter 16 for additional discussion of end-of-life care.

The ALS Association has broad programs of research funding, patient and clinical services, patient information and support, and medical and public information (see the Resources section). The *ALS Association Newsletter* is a source of practical information.

Muscular Dystrophies

The muscular dystrophies are a group of incurable muscle disorders characterized by progressive weakening and wasting of the skeletal or voluntary muscles with 30 different types to date. Most of these diseases are inherited. Duchenne muscular dystrophy, the most common and severe type, occurs in 1 of every 3500 male births (Bader et al., 2016). The pathologic features include degeneration and loss of muscle fibers, variation in muscle fiber size, phagocytosis and regeneration, and replacement of muscle tissue by connective tissue. The common characteristics of these diseases include varying degrees of muscle wasting and weakness and abnormal elevation in serum levels of muscle enzymes. Differences among these diseases center on the genetic pattern of inheritance, the muscles involved, the age at onset, and the rate of disease progression. The symptoms can be diverse and may include muscle stiffness or weakness, dysphagia, mental deficits, vision, or infertility. Prognosis depends on the type of muscular dystrophy. Regardless of age of onset, this disease varies in progression (Dalton & Sampson, 2015). The unique needs of these patients, who in the past did not live to adulthood, must be addressed, considering they live longer because of better supportive care.

Medical Management

Treatment of the muscular dystrophies focuses on supportive care and prevention of complications in the absence of a cure or specific pharmacologic interventions (Kang, Morrison, Iannaccone, et al., 2015). The goal of supportive management is to keep the patient active and functioning as normally as possible and to minimize functional deterioration. An individualized therapeutic exercise program is prescribed to prevent muscle tightness, contractures, and disuse atrophy. Night splints and stretching exercises are used to delay contractures of the joints, especially the ankles, knees, and hips. Braces may compensate for muscle weakness.

Spinal deformity is a severe problem. Weakness of trunk muscles and spinal collapse occur almost routinely in patients with severe neuromuscular disease. To help prevent spinal deformity, the patient is fitted with an orthotic jacket to improve sitting stability and reduce trunk deformity. This measure also supports cardiovascular status. In time, spinal fusion is performed to maintain spinal stability. Other procedures may be carried out to correct deformities.

Compromised pulmonary function may result either from progression of the disease or from deformity of the thorax secondary to severe scoliosis. Upper respiratory infections and fractures from falls must be vigorously treated in a way that minimizes immobilization because joint contractures become worse when the patient's activities are more restricted than usual.

Other difficulties may manifest in relation to the underlying disease. Weakness of the facial muscles makes it difficult to attend to dental hygiene and to speak clearly, and impairs the ability to swallow safely (LaDonna, Koopman, Ray, et al., 2016). Gastrointestinal tract problems may include gastric dilation, rectal prolapse, and fecal impaction. Finally, cardiomyopathy appears to be a common complication in all forms of muscular dystrophy.

Ongoing research is improving the clinical course and survival opportunities. Some research targets specific gene mutations, while other studies deal with the effects of muscle degeneration (Mercuri & Muntoni, 2013). Genetic counseling is advised for parents and siblings of the patient because of the genetic nature of this disease. MDA (the Muscular Dystrophy Association) works to combat neuromuscular disease through research, programs of patient services and clinical care, and professional and public education (see the Resources section).

Nursing Management

The goals of the patient and the nurse are to maintain function at optimal levels and to enhance the quality of life. Therefore, the patient's physical requirements, which are considerable, are addressed without losing sight of emotional and developmental needs. The patient and family are actively involved in decision making, including end-of-life decisions (see Chapter 16).

During hospitalization for treatment of complications, the knowledge and expertise of the patient and family members responsible for caregiving in the home are assessed. Because the patient and family caregivers often have developed caregiving strategies that work effectively for them, these strategies need to be acknowledged and accepted, and provisions must be made to ensure that they are maintained during hospitalization (Piredda, Matarese, & Mastroianni, 2015).

Families of adolescents and young adults with muscular dystrophy need assistance to shift the focus of care from pediatric to adult care and to understand the usual disease course.

Nursing goals include assisting the adolescent to make the transition to adult values and expectations while providing age-appropriate ongoing care. The nurse may need to help build the confidence of an older adolescent or adult patient by encouraging him or her to pursue job training to become economically independent. Other nursing interventions might include guidance in accessing adult health care and finding appropriate programs in sex education.

Promoting Home, Community-Based, and Transitional Care

 Educating Patients About Self-Care

Management goals are addressed in special rehabilitation programs or in the patient's home and community. Therefore, the patient and family require information and instruction about the disorder, its anticipated course, and care and management strategies that will optimize the patient's growth and development and physical and psychological status. Members of a variety of health-related disciplines are involved in patient and family education; recommendations are communicated to all members of the health care team so that they may work toward common goals.

Continuing and Transitional Care

Both the neuromuscular disease and the associated deformities may progress in adolescence and adulthood. Self-help and assistive devices can aid in maintaining maximum independence. These devices, recommended by physical and occupational therapists, often become necessary as more muscle groups are affected.

The family is instructed to monitor the patient for respiratory problems, because respiratory infection and cardiac failure are the most common causes of death. As respiratory difficulties develop, patients and their families need information regarding respiratory support. Options currently exist that can provide ventilatory support (e.g., negative-pressure devices, positive-pressure ventilators) while allowing mobility (Dalton & Sampson, 2015; Rabinstein, 2016). Patients can remain relatively independent in a wheelchair, for example, while being maintained on a ventilator at home for many years.

The patient is encouraged to continue with range-of-motion exercises to prevent contractures, which are particularly disabling. Practical adaptations must be made, however, to cope with the effects of chronic neuromuscular disability. The patient at various stages of the disease may require a manual or an electric wheelchair, gait aids, upper and lower extremity and spinal orthotics, seating systems, bathroom equipment, lifts, ramps, and additional assistive devices, all of which require a team approach. The nurse assesses how the patient and family are managing, makes referrals, and coordinates the activities of the physical therapist, occupational therapist, and social services.

The patient is greatly concerned about issues surrounding the threat of increasing disability and dependence on others, accompanied by a significant deterioration in health-related quality of life. The patient is faced with a progressive loss of function, leading eventually to death. Feelings of helplessness and powerlessness are common. Each functional loss is accompanied by grief and mourning. The patient and family are assessed for depression, anger, or denial. The patient and family are assisted and encouraged to address decisions about end-of-life options before their need arises (see Chapter 16).

A psychiatric nurse clinician or other mental health professional may assist the patient to cope and adapt to the disease. By understanding and addressing clinical concerns that are important for patients and their families, while at the same time assessing caregiver knowledge and burden during every encounter, the nurse provides a hopeful, supportive, and nurturing environment (LaDonna et al., 2016). One study reported that adult patients' illness perceptions are directly connected to their quality of life in muscular dystrophy, and these perceptions influence their overall mood (Graham, Weinman, Sadjadi, et al., 2014).

Degenerative Disc Disease

Low back pain is the second most common neurologic disorder in the United States, with one quarter of all adults reporting recent (within 3 months) back pain (Hickey, 2014). It is frequently associated with depression and anxiety, and it is the most common reason for missed work and decreased productivity while at work. An estimated 500,000 spinal surgeries for herniated discs, stenosis, and degenerative changes were performed in 2010 in the United States. Low back pain results in significant economic costs to patients, their families, and society. Acute pain lasts less than 3 months (see Chart 41-2 in Chapter 41), whereas chronic pain has a duration of 3 months or longer. Most back problems are related to disc disease (Bader et al., 2016).

Pathophysiology

The intervertebral disc is a cartilaginous plate that forms a cushion between the vertebral bodies (see Fig. 70-7A). This tough, fibrous material is incorporated in a capsule. A ball-like cushion in the center of the disc is called the *nucleus pulposus*. In herniation of the intervertebral disc (ruptured disc), the nucleus of the disc protrudes into the annulus (the fibrous ring around the disc), with subsequent nerve compression (Hickey, 2014). Protrusion or rupture of the nucleus pulposus usually is preceded by degenerative changes that occur with aging. Loss of protein polysaccharides in the disc decreases the water content of the nucleus pulposus. The development of radiating cracks in the annulus weakens resistance to nucleus herniation. After trauma (falls and repeated minor stresses such as lifting incorrectly), the cartilage may be injured.

For most patients, the immediate symptoms of trauma are short-lived, and those resulting from injury to the disc do not appear for months or years. Disc degeneration pushes the capsule back into the spinal canal. It could also rupture and allow the nucleus pulposus to be pushed back against the dural sac or against a spinal nerve as it emerges from the spinal column (see Fig. 70-7B). This disease of the spinal root, produces pain and extreme sensitivity to touch due to radiculopathy (pressure in the area of distribution of the involved nerve endings). Continued pressure may produce degenerative changes in the involved nerve, such as changes in sensation and deep tendon reflexes.

Clinical Manifestations

A herniated disc with accompanying pain may occur in any portion of the spine: cervical, thoracic (rare), or lumbar. The clinical manifestations depend on the location, the rate of development (acute or chronic), and the effect on the surrounding structures.

Assessment and Diagnostic Findings

A thorough health history and physical examination are important to rule out potentially serious conditions that may manifest as low back pain, including fracture, tumor, infection, or cauda equina syndrome (Hickey, 2014).

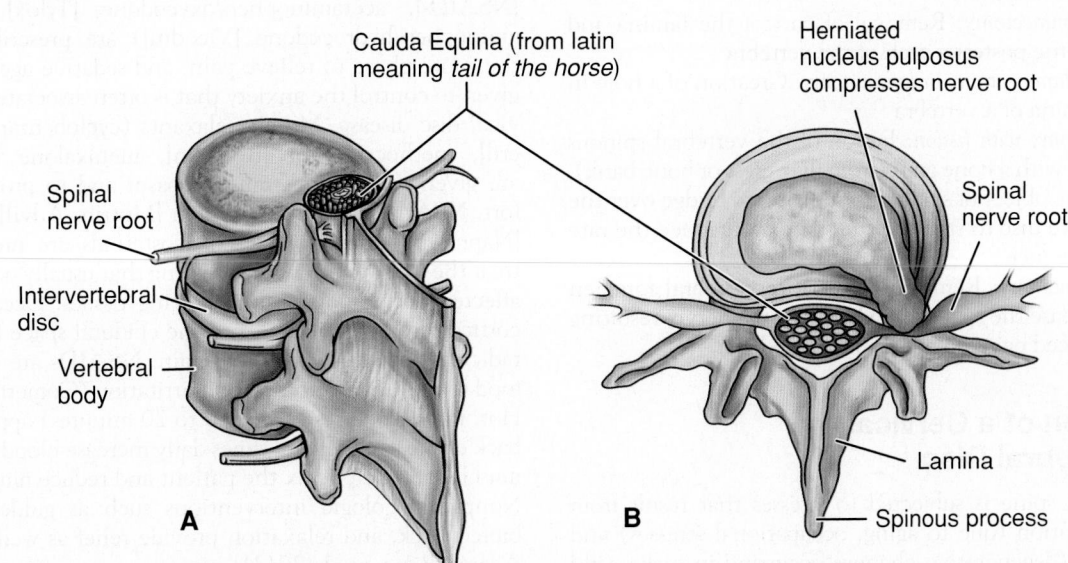

Figure 70-7 • A. Normal lumbar spine vertebrae, invertebral discs, and spinal nerve root. **B.** Ruptured vertebral disc.

The MRI scan has become the diagnostic tool of choice for localizing even small disc protrusions, particularly for lumbar spine disease. If the clinical symptoms are not consistent with the pathology seen on MRI, CT scanning and myelography are performed. A neurologic examination is carried out to determine whether reflex, sensory, or motor impairment from root compression is present and to provide a baseline for future assessment. Electromyography may be used to localize the specific spinal nerve roots involved.

Medical Management

Herniations of the cervical and the lumbar discs occur most commonly and are usually managed conservatively with medication and physical therapy or exercise (Hickey, 2014). Surgery is sometimes necessary.

Surgical Management

Surgical excision of a herniated disc is performed if there is evidence of a progressing neurologic deficit (muscle weakness and atrophy, loss of sensory and motor function, loss of sphincter control) and radicular pain (pain that follows the dermatomal distribution [see Fig. 65-9 in Chapter 65] of the compressed nerve) that are unresponsive to conservative management. The goal of surgical treatment is to reduce the pressure on the nerve root to relieve pain and reverse neurologic deficits. Microsurgical techniques make it possible to remove only the amount of tissue that is necessary, which preserves the integrity of normal tissue better and imposes less trauma on the body. During these procedures, spinal cord function can be monitored electrophysiologically.

Some of the surgical techniques available include:

- *Microdiscectomy:* Removal of herniated or extruded fragments of intervertebral disc material
- *Laminectomy:* Removal of the bone between the spinal process and facet pedicle junction to expose the neural elements in the spinal canal (Hickey, 2014); this allows the surgeon to inspect the spinal canal, identify and remove pathologic tissue, and relieve compression of the cord and roots
- *Hemilaminectomy:* Removal of part of the lamina and part of the posterior arch of the vertebra
- *Partial laminectomy or laminotomy:* Creation of a hole in the lamina of a vertebra
- *Discectomy with fusion:* Fusion of the vertebral spinous process with a bone graft (from iliac crest or bone bank), with the object of spinal fusion being to bridge over the defective disc to stabilize the spine and reduce the rate of recurrence
- *Foraminotomy:* Removal of the intervertebral foramen to increase the space for exit of a spinal nerve, resulting in reduced pain, compression, and edema

Herniation of a Cervical Intervertebral Disc

The cervical spine is subjected to stresses that result from disc degeneration (due to aging, occupational stresses) and **spondylosis** (degenerative changes occurring in a disc and adjacent vertebral bodies). Cervical disc degeneration may lead to lesions that can cause damage to the spinal cord and its roots (Bader et al., 2016).

Clinical Manifestations

A cervical disc herniation usually occurs at the C5–C6 or C6–C7 interspaces and compresses a unilateral nerve root (Bader et al., 2016). Pain and stiffness may occur in the neck, the top of the shoulders, and the region of the scapulae. Patients sometimes interpret these signs as symptoms of heart trouble or bursitis. Pain may also occur in the arm and hand, accompanied by **paresthesia** (numbness, tingling, or a "pins and needles" sensation) of the upper extremity. Cervical MRI usually confirms the diagnosis. Occasionally, the disc herniates centrally onto the spinal cord, causing Lhermitte syndrome, an electriclike shock sensation in the extremities or spine with neck flexion or straining, and bilateral arm and leg weakness (myelopathy).

Medical Management

The goals of treatment are to rest and immobilize the cervical spine to give the soft tissues time to heal and to reduce inflammation in the supporting tissues and the affected nerve roots in the cervical spine (Hickey, 2014). It also reduces inflammation and edema in soft tissues around the disc, relieving pressure on the nerve roots. Proper positioning on a firm mattress may bring dramatic relief from pain.

The cervical spine may be rested and immobilized by a cervical collar, cervical traction, or a brace. A collar allows maximal opening of the intervertebral foramina and holds the head in a neutral or slightly flexed position. The patient may have to wear the collar 24 hours a day during the acute phase. The skin under the collar is inspected for irritation. After the patient is free of pain, cervical isometric exercises are started to strengthen the neck muscles.

Pharmacologic Therapy

Analgesic agents (nonsteroidal anti-inflammatory agents [NSAIDs], acetaminophen/oxycodone [Tylox], or acetaminophen/hydrocodone [Vicodin]) are prescribed during the acute phase to relieve pain, and sedative agents may be given to control the anxiety that is often associated with cervical disc disease. Muscle relaxants (cyclobenzaprine [Flexeril], methocarbamol [Robaxin], metaxalone [Skelaxin]) are given to interrupt muscle spasm and to promote comfort. NSAIDs (aspirin, ibuprofen [Motrin, Advil], naproxen [Naprosyn, Anaprox]) or corticosteroids are prescribed to treat the inflammation and swelling that usually occurs in the affected nerve roots and supporting tissues. Occasionally, a corticosteroid is injected into the epidural space for relief of radicular (spinal nerve root) pain. NSAIDs are given with food to prevent gastrointestinal irritation (Comerford, 2015). Hot, moist compresses (for 10 to 20 minutes) applied to the back of the neck several times daily increase blood flow to the muscles and help relax the patient and reduce muscle spasm. Nonpharmacologic interventions such as guided imagery, biofeedback, and relaxation provide relief as well (Abdulla, Adams, Bone, et al., 2013).

Surgical Management

Surgical excision of the herniated disc may be necessary if there is a significant neurologic deficit, progression of the deficit, evidence of cord compression, or pain that either worsens or fails to improve. A cervical discectomy, with or without fusion, may be performed to alleviate symptoms. An anterior surgical approach may be used through a transverse incision to remove disc material that has herniated into the spinal canal and foramina, or a posterior approach may be used at the appropriate level of the cervical spine. Potential complications with the anterior approach include carotid or vertebral artery injury, recurrent laryngeal nerve dysfunction, esophageal perforation, and airway obstruction (Hickey, 2014). Complications of the posterior approach include damage to the nerve root or the spinal cord due to retraction or contusion of either of these structures, resulting in weakness of muscles supplied by the nerve root or cord.

Microsurgery, such as endoscopic microdiscectomy, may be performed in selected patients through a small incision, using magnification techniques. This usually results in less tissue trauma and pain, and patients consequently have a shorter length of hospital stay compared with those who have conventional surgery (Hickey, 2014).

NURSING PROCESS

The Patient Undergoing a Cervical Discectomy

Assessment

The patient is asked about past injuries to the neck (whiplash), because unresolved trauma can cause persistent discomfort, pain and tenderness, and symptoms of arthritis in the injured joint of the cervical spine. Assessment includes determining the onset, location, and radiation of pain and assessing for paresthesias, limited movement, and diminished function of the neck, shoulders, and upper extremities. It is important to determine whether the symptoms are bilateral; with large herniations, bilateral symptoms may be caused by cord compression. The area around the cervical spine is palpated to assess muscle tone and tenderness. Range of motion in the neck and shoulders is evaluated.

The patient is asked about any health issues that may influence the postoperative course and quality of life. It is also important to assess mood and stress levels. The nurse determines the patient's need for information about the surgical procedure and reinforces what the primary provider has explained. Strategies for pain management are discussed with the patient (Hickey, 2014).

Diagnosis

NURSING DIAGNOSES

Based on the assessment data, major nursing diagnoses may include the following:

- Acute pain related to the surgical procedure

- Impaired physical mobility related to the postoperative surgical regimen
- Deficient knowledge about the postoperative course and home care management

Other nursing diagnoses may include preoperative anxiety, postoperative constipation, urinary retention related to the surgical procedure, self-care deficits related to use of a neck orthosis, and sleep pattern disturbance related to disruption in lifestyle.

Collaborative Problems/Potential Complications

Potential complications may include the following:

- Hematoma at the surgical site, resulting in cord compression and neurologic deficit
- Recurrent or persistent pain after surgery

Planning and Goals

The goals for the patient may include relief of pain, improved mobility, increased knowledge and self-care ability, and prevention of complications.

Nursing Interventions

RELIEVING PAIN

Incisional pain is expected. Radicular pain improves over time as the nerve recovers. If the patient has had a bone fusion with bone removed from the iliac crest, considerable pain may be experienced at the donor site. Interventions consist of monitoring the donor site for hematoma formation, administering the prescribed postoperative analgesic agent, positioning for comfort, and reassuring the patient that the pain can be relieved. If the patient experiences a sudden increase in pain, extrusion of the graft may have occurred, requiring reoperation. A sudden increase in pain should be promptly reported to the surgeon (Hickey, 2014).

The patient may experience a sore throat, hoarseness, and dysphagia due to temporary edema. These symptoms are relieved by throat lozenges, voice rest, and humidification. A pureed diet may be given if the patient has dysphagia.

IMPROVING MOBILITY

Postoperatively, a cervical collar (neck orthosis) may be worn, which contributes to limited neck motion and altered mobility. The patient is instructed to turn the body instead of the neck when looking from side to side. The neck should be kept in a neutral (midline) position. The patient is assisted during position changes to make sure that the head, shoulders, and thorax are kept aligned. When assisting the patient to a sitting position, the nurse supports the patient's neck and shoulders. To increase stability, the patient should wear shoes when ambulating. The patient is encouraged not to lift more than 10 pounds.

MONITORING AND MANAGING POTENTIAL COMPLICATIONS

The patient is evaluated for bleeding and hematoma formation by assessing for swelling, excessive pressure in the neck, or severe pain in the incision area. The dressing is inspected for serosanguineous drainage, which suggests a dural leak. If this occurs, meningitis is a threat. A complaint of headache requires careful evaluation. Neurologic checks are made for swallowing deficits and upper and lower extremity weakness, because cord compression may produce rapid or delayed onset of paralysis (Hickey, 2014). The patient who has had an anterior cervical discectomy is also assessed for a sudden return of radicular (spinal nerve root) pain, which may indicate instability of the spine (AANN, 2014c).

Throughout the postoperative course, the patient is monitored frequently to detect any signs of respiratory difficulty, because retractors used during surgery may injure the recurrent laryngeal nerve, resulting in hoarseness and the inability to cough effectively and clear pulmonary secretions. In addition, the blood pressure and pulse are monitored to evaluate cardiovascular status and optimal circulation to the surgical site.

Bleeding at the surgical site and subsequent hematoma formation may occur. Severe localized pain not relieved by analgesic agents should be reported. A change in neurologic status (motor or sensory function) should be reported promptly, because it suggests hematoma formation that may necessitate surgery to prevent irreversible motor and sensory deficits (Hickey, 2014).

PROMOTING HOME, COMMUNITY-BASED, AND TRANSITIONAL CARE

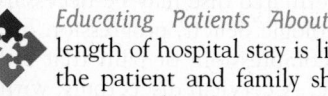

Educating Patients About Self-Care. The patient's length of hospital stay is likely to be short; therefore, the patient and family should understand the care that is important for a smooth recovery. A cervical collar, if prescribed, is usually worn for about 6 weeks. The patient is educated in the use and care of the cervical collar. The patient will need to alternate tasks that involve minimal body movement (e.g., reading) with tasks that require greater body movement.

The patient is educated about strategies to manage the incision and to manage pain, and about signs and symptoms that may indicate complications that should be reported to the primary provider. The nurse assesses the patient's understanding of these management strategies, limitations, and recommendations. In addition, the nurse assists the patient in identifying strategies to cope with ADLs (e.g., self-care, child care) and minimize risks to the surgical site (see Chart 70-6). A discharge

---

Chart 70-6 **HOME CARE CHECKLIST**

The Patient With Cervical Discectomy and Cervical Collar

At the completion of education, the patient and/or caregiver will be able to:

- Name the procedure that was performed and identify any permanent changes in anatomic structure or function as well as changes in ADLs, IADLs, roles, relationships, and spirituality.
- Identify interventions and strategies (e.g., durable medical equipment, adaptive equipment) used in adapting to any permanent changes in structure or function to promote safety and optimum functioning.
  - Use adequate mattress and chair support.
- State the name, dose, side effects, frequency, and schedule for all medications.
  - Describe nonpharmacologic interventions for pain relief used in conjunction to prescribed pain relief preparations.
- State how to obtain medical supplies and carry out dressing changes, wound care, and other prescribed regimens.
- State how to contact all members of the treatment team (e.g., health care providers, home care professionals, and durable medical equipment and supply vendor).
- Describe ongoing postoperative therapeutic regimen, including diet and activities to perform (e.g., exercises) and to limit or avoid (e.g., lifting, stair climbing, driving a car) during rehabilitation.
- Describe care for the surgical incision site.
  - Keep staples or sutures clean and dry and cover with dry dressing.
- Demonstrate proper body mechanics and prescribed exercise techniques.
  - Describe how to modify activity for optimum functioning.
  - Avoid sitting or standing for more than 30 minutes.
  - Avoid twisting, flexing, extending, or rotating the neck.
  - Avoid sleeping in a prone position or the use of pillows to minimize neck flexion in bed; keep head in a neutral position.

- Wear low-heeled shoes.
- Place a wrinkle-free silk scarf under the collar to increase comfort.
- **For men:** Shave without twisting or moving the neck. This may be done with help while lying flat or sitting. Remove only the front part of the collar for shaving.
- Practice stress reduction and relaxation techniques.
- Care of the cervical collar:
  - Wear the collar at all times until directed otherwise by the primary provider.
  - Wash the neck under the collar twice a day with mild soap.
  - Keep the neck still while the collar is open.
  - With the assistance of a helper, wash the neck in steps.
  - Lie flat and supine.
  - Open the Velcro tabs on each side of the collar and remove its front portion.
  - Gently wash and dry the neck.
  - Replace the front part of the collar and refasten the tabs.
  - Turn to one side with a thin pillow under the head.
  - Open one tab.
  - Gently wash and dry the back of the neck. Refasten the tab.
  - Turn to the other side and wash and dry this side. Refasten the tab.
- Notify primary provider if any signs or symptoms of infection occur, such as fever, redness or irritation, drainage, increased pain.
- Relate how to reach primary provider with questions or complications.
- State time and date of follow-up medical appointments, therapy, and testing.
- Identify sources of support (e.g., friends, relatives, faith community, support groups, caregiver support).
- Identify the need for health promotion, disease prevention, and screening activities.

ADL, activities of daily living; IADL, independent activities of daily living.

educational plan is developed collaboratively by members of the health care team to decrease the risk of recurrent disc herniation. Topics include those previously discussed as well as proper body mechanics, maintenance of optimal weight, proper exercise techniques, and modifications in activity.

Continuing and Transitional Care. The patient is instructed to see the primary provider at prescribed intervals so that the provider can document the disappearance of old symptoms and assess the range of motion of the neck. Recurrent or persistent pain may occur despite removal of the offending disc or disc fragments. Patients who undergo discectomy usually have consented to surgery after prolonged pain; they have often undergone repeated courses of ineffective conservative management and previous surgeries to relieve the pain. Therefore, the recurrence or persistence of symptoms postoperatively, including pain and sensory deficits, is often discouraging for the patient and family. The patient who experiences recurrence of symptoms requires emotional support and understanding. In addition, the patient is assisted in modifying activities and in considering options for subsequent treatment. The nurse educates the patient and family members about the need to participate in health-promotion and health-screening practices.

Evaluation

Expected patient outcomes may include:
1. Reports decreasing frequency and severity of pain
2. Demonstrates improved mobility
   a. Demonstrates progressive participation in self-care activities
   b. Identifies prescribed activity limitations and restrictions
   c. Demonstrates proper body mechanics
3. Is knowledgeable about postoperative course, medications, and home care management
   a. Lists the signs and symptoms to be reported postoperatively
   b. Identifies dose, action, and potential side effects of medications
   c. Identifies appropriate home care management activities and any restrictions
4. Has absence of complications
   a. Reports no increase in incision pain or sensory symptoms
   b. Demonstrates normal findings on neurologic assessment

Herniation of a Lumbar Disc

Most lumbar disc herniations occur at the L5–S1 region (AANN, 2014d). A herniated lumbar disc produces low back pain accompanied by varying degrees of sensory and motor impairment.

Clinical Manifestations

The patient complains of low back pain with muscle spasm and **sciatica** (pain and tenderness that radiates along the sciatic nerve that runs through the thigh and leg). Pain is aggravated by actions that increase intraspinal fluid pressure, such as bending, lifting, or straining (as in sneezing or coughing), and usually is relieved by bed rest. There is often some type of postural deformity, because pain causes an alteration of the normal spinal mechanics. If the patient lies on the back and attempts to raise a leg in a straight position, pain radiates into the leg; this maneuver, called the *straight-leg raising test*, stretches the sciatic nerve. Additional signs include muscle weakness, alterations in tendon reflexes, and sensory loss.

Assessment and Diagnostic Findings

The diagnosis of lumbar disc disease is based on the history and physical findings, specifically the location, quality, severity of pain, and the use of imaging techniques such as MRI and CT scans as well as myelography.

Medical Management

The objectives of treatment are to relieve pain, slow disease progression, and increase the patient's functional ability (AANN, 2014d). Bed rest is discouraged because it may weaken muscles, but activities that exacerbate pain should be avoided.

Because muscle spasm is prominent during the acute phase, muscle relaxants are used. NSAIDs and systemic corticosteroids may be given to counter the inflammation and swelling that usually occurs in the supporting tissues and the affected nerve roots. Moist heat and massage help relax muscles. Strategies for increasing the patient's functional ability include weight reduction, physical therapy, and biofeedback. Exercises, prescribed by physical therapists, can help strengthen back muscles and decrease pain (Hickey, 2014). See Chapter 12 for descriptions of nursing interventions for the patient with pain.

Surgical Management

In the lumbar region, surgical treatment includes lumbar disc excision through a posterolateral laminotomy and the techniques of microdiscectomy and percutaneous discectomy. In microdiscectomy, an operating microscope is used to visualize the offending disc and compressed nerve roots; it permits a small incision (2.5 cm [1 inch]) and minimal blood loss and takes about 30 minutes of operating time. In general, the length of hospital stay is short, and the patient makes a rapid recovery. Several minimally invasive techniques in spinal surgery have led to improved patient outcomes and lower hospital costs, and research on these techniques is ongoing. Fusion is considered when vertebral instability is present and contributes to pain. Fusion procedures are longer and cause more postoperative pain. Research suggests that intraoperative wound infiltration with bupivacaine hydrochloride solution decreases pain and the need for opioids postoperatively. Some studies suggest that gel substances for disc replacement may decrease pain and improve spinal function.

A patient undergoing a disc procedure at one level of the vertebral column may have a degenerative process at other levels. A herniation relapse may occur at the same level or elsewhere, so the patient may become a candidate for another disc procedure. Arachnoiditis (inflammation of the arachnoid membrane) may occur after surgery (and after myelography); it involves an insidious onset of diffuse, frequently burning pain in the lower back, radiating into the buttocks. Disc excision can leave adhesions and scarring around the spinal nerves and dura, which then produce inflammatory changes that create chronic neuritis and neurofibrosis. Disc surgery may relieve pressure on the spinal nerves, but it does not reverse the effects of neural injury and scarring and the pain that results. Failed disc syndrome (recurrence of sciatica after lumbar discectomy) remains a cause of disability (Hickey, 2014).

Nursing Management

Providing Preoperative Care

Most patients fear surgery on any part of the spine and therefore need explanations about the surgery and reassurance that it will not weaken the back. When data are being collected for the health history, any reports of pain, paresthesia, or muscle spasm are recorded to provide a baseline for comparison after surgery. Health issues that may influence the postoperative course and quality of life (e.g., fatigue, mood, stress, patient expectations, smoking) are important to assess. Preoperative assessment also includes an evaluation of movement of the extremities as well as bladder and bowel function (Hickey, 2014). To facilitate the postoperative turning procedure, the patient is instructed to turn as a unit (called logrolling) as part of the preoperative preparation (see Fig. 70-8). Before surgery, the patient is also encouraged to take deep breaths, cough, and perform muscle setting exercises to maintain muscle tone.

Assessing the Patient After Surgery

After lumbar disc excision, vital signs are checked frequently and the wound is inspected for hemorrhage, because vascular injury is a complication of disc surgery. Because postoperative neurologic deficits may occur from nerve root injury, the

Figure 70-8 • Before the patient undergoes laminectomy surgery, the logrolling technique that will be used for turning the patient should be demonstrated. The patient's arms will be crossed and the spine aligned. To avoid twisting the spine, the head, shoulders, knees, and hips are turned at the same time so that the patient rolls over like a log. When in a side-lying position, the patient's back, buttocks, and legs are supported with pillows.

sensation and motor strength of the lower extremities are evaluated at specified intervals, along with the color and temperature of the legs and sensation of the toes. It is important to assess for urinary retention, which is another sign of neurologic deterioration (AANN, 2014d). In discectomy with fusion, the patient has an additional surgical incision if bone fragments were taken from the iliac crest or fibula to serve as wedges in the spine. The recovery period is longer than for those patients who underwent discectomy with spinal fusion, because bony union must take place.

Positioning the Patient

To position the patient, a pillow is placed under the head, and the knee rest is elevated slightly to relax the back muscles. When the patient is lying on one side, however, extreme knee flexion must be avoided. The patient is encouraged to move from side to side to relieve pressure and is reassured that no injury will result from moving. When the patient is ready to turn, the bed is placed in a flat position and a pillow is placed between the patient's legs. The patient turns as a unit (logrolls) without twisting the back.

To get out of bed, the patient lies on one side while pushing up to a sitting position. At the same time, the nurse or family member eases the patient's legs over the side of the bed. Coming to a sitting or standing posture is accomplished in one long, smooth motion. Most patients walk to the bathroom on the same day as the surgery. Sitting is discouraged except for defecation.

Promoting Home, Community-Based, and Transitional Care

 Educating Patients About Self-Care

The patient is instructed to increase activity gradually, as tolerated, because it takes up to 6 weeks for the ligaments to heal. Excessive activity may result in spasm of the paraspinal muscles (Hickey, 2014).

Activities that produce flexion strain on the spine (e.g., driving a car) should be avoided until healing has taken place. Heat may be applied to the back to relax muscle spasms. Scheduled rest periods are important, and the patient is advised to avoid heavy work for 2 to 3 months after surgery. Exercises are prescribed to strengthen the abdominal and erector spinal muscles. A back brace or corset may be necessary if back pain persists.

Continuing and Transitional Care

Referral for inpatient or outpatient rehabilitation may be warranted to improve self-care abilities after medical or surgical treatment for herniation of a lumbar disc. A home care referral may be indicated and provides the nurse with the opportunity to assess the patient's physical and psychological status, as well as their ability to adhere to recommended management strategies. During the home visit, the nurse determines whether changes in neurologic function have occurred. The adequacy of pain management is assessed, and modifications are made to ensure adequate pain relief.

Lower back pain can be debilitating and costly. The use of electronic medical records may help physicians identify this earlier so they can develop plans to manage patients differently based on the number of times they seek health care. Maeng, Stewart, Xiaowei, et al. (2015) recognized three trends from reviewing electronic charts: In the first year with low back pain, (1) men were more likely to have a higher cost associated with care than women due to a greater number of visits; (2) workers compensation as the primary payer had more prescriptive opiod use; and (3) patients who were smokers on their first visit tended to have more visits that were more expensive.

Post-Polio Syndrome

Polio has mostly been eradicated globally due to concerted efforts on vaccination. However, people who survived the polio epidemic of the 1950s, many of whom are now older adults, are developing new symptoms of weakness, fatigue, and musculoskeletal pain identified as PPS. This phenomenon, which occurs 30 to 40 years after the polio exposure, affects 25% to 40% of all survivors of polio who were either immediately disabled or who recovered with few or no symptoms (Groce, Banks, & Stein, 2014). Men and women appear to be equally at risk for this condition.

Pathophysiology

The exact cause of PPS is not known, but researchers suspect that with aging or muscle overuse, the neurons not destroyed by the poliovirus continue generating axon sprouts (Woodward, 2014). These new terminal axon sprouts reinnervate the affected muscles after the initial insult but may become more vulnerable as the body ages.

Assessment and Diagnostic Findings

No specific diagnostic test exists for PPS. Clinical diagnosis is made on the basis of the history and physical examination and exclusion of other medical conditions that could be causing the new symptoms. Patients report a history of paralytic poliomyelitis followed by partial or complete recovery of function, with a plateau of function and then the recurrence of symptoms. Signs and symptoms may occur decades after the original onset of poliomyelitis (Woodward, 2014).

Management

No specific medical or surgical treatment is available for this syndrome, and therefore nurses play a pivotal role in the team approach to assisting patients and families in dealing with the symptoms of progressive loss of muscle strength and significant fatigue (McNalley, Yorkston, Jensen, et al., 2015). Pain and weakness may be improved with infusion of intravenous immunoglobulin (Woodward, 2014).

 For the procedural guidelines for managing immunoglobulin therapy, go to **thepoint.lww.com/Brunner14e.**

Other health care professionals who may assist in patient care include physical, occupational, speech, respiratory therapists, social workers, chaplains, and nurses. Nursing interventions are aimed at maintaining the patient's strength as well as physical, psychological, and social well-being.

The patient needs to plan and coordinate activities to conserve energy and reduce fatigue. Rest periods should be planned and assistive devices used to reduce weakness and fatigue. Important activities should be planned for the morning, because fatigue often increases in the afternoon and evening.

Pain in muscles and joints may be a problem. Nonpharmacologic techniques such as the application of heat and cold are most appropriate, because older patients may not tolerate or may have strong reactions to medications.

Maintaining a balance between adequate nutritional intake and avoiding excess calories that can lead to obesity is a challenge in this group of patients who are sedentary. Pulmonary hygiene and adequate fluid intake can help with airway management. Several interventions can improve sleep, including limiting caffeine intake before bedtime and assessing for nocturia. The patient may need to be evaluated for obstructive sleep apnea. Supportive ventilation may be appropriate, with continuous positive airway pressure if sleep apnea is a problem (see Chapter 22).

Bone density testing in patients with PPS has revealed low bone mass and osteoporosis. Therefore, the importance of identifying risks, preventing falls, and treating osteoporosis must be discussed with patients and families. Families also need to be made aware of the possibility of changes in individual and family relationships due to the many symptoms of PPS. The nurse also needs to remind patients and family members of the need for health-promotion activities and health screening (Woodward, 2014).

CRITICAL THINKING EXERCISES

1 A 34-year-old woman, working, married, with three children has been newly diagnosed with a spinal cord tumor. Assess and prioritize the patient's physiologic and psychosocial needs. What nursing interventions and actions would you suggest to assist in managing the treatment of and coping with a spinal cord tumor? How would this be different if the patient lives alone?

2 **ebp** A 65-year-old man is newly diagnosed with ALS. Identify the evidence-based practices for the management of ALS. Describe the evidence base for the practices that you have identified and the criteria used to evaluate the strength of that evidence. Identify the health-promotion activities you would recommend to this patient and the rationale for your recommendations.

3 **pq** A 72-year-old woman is admitted for low back pain that radiates down her leg. What are your priorities for providing care for this patient? Give your rationale. What further diagnostic testing is needed? How will your priorities change if the patient is scheduled for back surgery?

REFERENCES

*Asterisk indicates nursing research.

Books

American Association of Neuroscience Nurses (AANN). (2014a). *Care of the adult patient with a brain tumor: AANN clinical practice guideline series.* Chicago, IL: Author.

American Association of Neuroscience Nurses (AANN). (2014b). *Care of movement disorder patient with deep brain stimulation: AANN clinical practice guideline series.* Chicago, IL: Author.

American Association of Neuroscience Nurses (AANN). (2014c). *Cervical spine surgery: A guide to preoperative and postoperative patient care: AANN clinical practice guideline series.* Chicago, IL: Author.

American Association of Neuroscience Nurses (AANN). (2014d). *Thoracolumbar spine surgery: A guide to preoperative and postoperative care: AANN clinical practice guideline series.* Chicago, IL: Author.

Bader, M., Littlejohns, L. R., & Olson, D. (2016). *AANN core curriculum for neuroscience nursing* (6th ed.). Chicago, IL: American Association of Neuroscience Nurses.

Brant, W. E., & Helms, C. A. (2006). *Fundamentals of diagnostic radiology* (3rd ed.). Philadelphia, PA: Lippincott Williams & Wilkins.

Comerford, K. C. (2015). *Nursing 2015 drug handbook.* Philadelphia, PA: Wolters Kluwer.

Dalton, J., & Sampson, J. B. (2015). Chapter 18. Overview of adult muscular dystrophies. In: *Genetic counseling for adult neurodegenerative disease.* New York: Springer Science and Business.

Eliopoulos, C. (2018). *Gerontological nursing* (9th ed.). Philadelphia, PA: Wolters Kluwer.

Hickey, J. V. (2014). *The clinical practice of neurological & neurosurgical nursing* (7th ed.). Philadelphia, PA: Lippincott Williams & Wilkins.

Journals and Electronic Documents

Abbruzzese, G., Marchese, R., Avanizino, L., et al. (2016). Rehabilitation for Parkinson's disease: Current outlook and future challenges. *Parkisonism and Related Disorders,22*(1), S60–S64.

Abdulla, A., Adams, N., Bone, M., et al. (2013). Guidance on management of pain in older people. *Age and Aging, 42*(1), 1–57.

American Brain Tumor Association (ABTA) (2014). *Brain tumor statistics.* Retrieved on 2/23/17 at: www.abta.org/about-us/news/brain-tumor-statistics/

Bellomo, T., & Cichminski, L. (2015). Amyotrophic lateral sclerosis: What nurses need to know. *Nursing, 45*(10), 47–51.

Carletti, S., Rispoli, R., Di Chirico, A., et al. (2016). Neural stem cells transplantation as a neuroprotective strategy for amyotrophic lateral sclerosis (ALS). *Global Spine Journal, 6*(Suppl 1), 1–20.

Dhandapani, M., Gupta, S., Dhandapani, S., et al. (2015). Study of factors determining caregiver burden among primary caregivers of patients with intracranial tumors. *Surgical Neurology International,6*, 160.

Farge, D. (2013). International clinical practice guidelines for the treatment and prophylaxis of venous thromboembolism in patients with cancer. *Journal of Thrombosis and Haemostasis, 11*(1), 56–70.

Ferrer, I. (2016). Mini-symposium: Huntington's disease. *Brain Pathology, 26*(6), 724–725.

Gallego Perez-Larrraya, J., & Delattre, J. Y. (2014). Management of the elderly patient with gliomas. *Oncologist, 19*(12), 1258–1267.

Gopalakrishna, A., & Alexander, S. A. (2015). Understanding Parkinson disease: A complex and multifaceted illness. *Journal of Neuroscience Nursing, 47*(6), 320–326.

Graham, C. D., Weinman, J., Sadjadi, R., et al. (2014). A multicentre postal survey investigating the contribution of illness perceptions, coping and optimism to quality of life and mood in adults with muscle disease. *Clinical Rehabilitation, 28*(5), 508–519.

Groce, N. E., Banks, L. M., & Stein, M. A. (2014). Surviving polio in a post-polio world. *Social Science and Medicine, 107*, 171–178.

Kalia, L. V., & Lang, A. E. (2015). Parkinson's disease. *Lancet, 386*(9996), 896–912.

Kang, P. B., Morrison, L., Iannaccone, S. T., et al. (2015). Evidence-based guideline summary: Evaluation, diagnosis, and management of congenital muscular dystrophy: Report of the Guideline Development Subcommittee of the American Academy of Neurology and the Practice Issues Review Panel of the American Association of Neuromuscular & Electrodiagnostic Medicine. *Neurology, 84*(13), 1369–1378.

Kim, S. U., Lee, H., & Kim, Y. B. (2013). Neural stem cell-based treatment for neurodegenerative diseases. *Neuropathology, 33*(5), 491–501.

Kumar, A., Singh, S. K., Kumar, V., et al. (2015). Huntington's disease: An update of therapeutic strategies. *Gene, 556*(2), 91–97.

LaDonna, K. A., Koopman, W. J., Ray, S. L., et al. (2016). Hard to swallow: A phenomenological exploration of the experience of caring for individuals with myotonic dystrophy and dysphagia. *Journal of Neuroscience Nursing, 48*(1), 42–51.

Lovely, M. P., Stewart-Amidei, C., Page, M., et al. (2013). A new reality: Long term survivorship with a malignant brain tumor. *Oncology Nursing Forum, 40*(3), 267–274.

Lukas, R. V., Buerki, R., & Mrugula, M. M. (2016). Management of leptomeningeal disease from solid tumors. *Oncology, 30*(8), 724–730.

Maeng, D. D., Stewart, W. F., Xiaowei, Y., et al. (2015). Use of electronic health records for early detection of high-cost low back pain patients. *Pain Research and Management, 20*(5), 234–240.

Majmuder, S., Wu, J., & Paganoni, S. (2014). Rehabilitation in amyotrophic lateral sclerosis: Why it matters. *Muscle Nerve, 50*, 4–13.

Marchetti, B. (2014). Act fast when new neurologic deficits arise. *American Nurse Today, 9*(1), 12.

*Martin, S. C. (2015). Psychosocial challenges experienced by partners of people with Parkinson disease. *Journal of Neuroscience Nursing, 47*(4), 211–222.

McNalley, E., Yorkston, K. M., Jensen, M., et al. (2015). A review of secondary health conditions in post-polio syndrome. *American Journal of Physical Medicine & Rehabilitation, 94*(2), 139–145.

Melmed, S. (2016). Pituitary medicines from discovery to patient focused outcomes. *Journal of Clinical Endocrinology and Metabolism, 101*(3), 769–779.

Mercuri, E., & Muntoni, F. (2013). New challenges and review of the current clinical trials. *Current Opinion in Pediatrics, 25*(6), 701–707.

Moore, D. J., Smith, B. M., & Cho, M. H. (2017). Managing meditations for hospital patients with Parkinson disease. *American Nurse Today, 12*(1), 9–12.

Ostrom, Q. T., Gittleman, H., Fulop, J., et al. (2015). CBTRUS statistical report: Primary brain and central nervous system tumors diagnosed in the United States in 2008–2012. *Journal of Neuro-Oncology, 17* (Suppl 4), 1–63.

Ownsworth, T., Goadby, E., & Chambers, S. K. (2015). Support after brain tumor means different things: Family caregivers' experiences of support and relationship changes. *Frontiers in Oncology, 5*(33), 1–13.

Perkins, A., & Liu, G. (2016). Primary brain tumors in adults: Diagnosis and treatment. *American Family Physician, 93*(3), 211–217.

Piredda, M., Matarese, M., Mastroianni, C., et al. (2015). Adult patients' experiences of nursing care dependence. *Journal of Nursing Scholarship, 47*(5), 397–406.

ProGas Study Group. (2015). Gastrostomy in patients with amyotrophic lateral sclerosis (ProGas): A prospective cohort study. *Lancet Neurology, 14*, 702–709.

Rabinstein, A. A. (2016). Noninvasive ventilation for neuromuscular respiratory failure: When to use and when to avoid. *Current Opinion in Critical Care, 22*(2), 94–99.

Rigi, M., Almarzbuqi, S. J., Morgan, M. L., et al. (2015). Papilledema: Epidemiology, etiology, and clinical management. *Eye and Brain, 2015*(7), 45–57.

Rosengren, K., Gustafusson, I., & Jarnevi, E. (2015). Every second counts: Women's experience of living with ALS in the end-of life situations. *Home Health Care Management & Practice, 27*(2), 76–82.

Ross, C. A., Aylward, E. H., Wild, E. J., et al. (2014). Huntington's disease: National history, biomarkers and prospects for therapeutics. *Nature Reviews Neurology, 10*, 204–216.

*Shin, J. Y., & Habermann, B. (2016a). Medication adherence in people with Parkinson disease. *Journal of Neuroscience Nursing, 48*(4), 185–204.

*Shin, J. Y., & Habermann, B. (2016b). Nursing research in Parkinson's disease from 2006–2015: A systematic review. *Clinical Nursing Research,* (2016), 1–15.

Smith, S., D'Cruz, G., Gray, R., et al. (2015). A concept map of what helps people with HD live with their condition. *Journal of Huntington's Disease,4*(3), 261–270.

Tobin, M. K., Geraghty, J. R., Engelhard, H. H., et al. (2015). Intramedullary spinal cord tumors: A review of current and future treatment strategies. *Neurosurgical Focus, 39*(2), 1–14.

Vecht, C. J., Kerkhof, M., & Duran-Pena, A. (2014). Seizure prognosis in brain tumors: New insights and evidence-based management. *The Oncologist, 19*(7), 751–759.

Wilson, E. Pollock, K., & Aubeeluck, A. (2014). Providing care services to people affected by Huntington's disease an overview of the challenges. *British Journal of Neuroscience Nursing, 10*(3), 139–143.

Woodward, S. (2014). Shining the spotlight on post-polio syndrome. *British Journal of Neuroscience Nursing, 10*(1), 5.

Resources

ALS Association, www.alsa.org
American Brain Tumor Association (ABTA), www.abta.org
American Cancer Society, www.cancer.org
American Association of Neurological Surgeons, www.AANS.org
American Parkinson Disease Association (APDA),
    www.apdaparkinson.org
Cancer Treatment Centers of America (CTCA), www.cancercenter.org
Huntington's Disease Society of America, www.hdsa.org
MDA (Muscular Dystrophy Association), www.mda.org
Michael J. Fox Foundation for Parkinson's Research, www.michaeljfox.org
National Brain Tumor Society, www.braintumor.org
Parkinson's Disease Foundation (PDF), www.pdf.org

Acute Community Based Challenges

ENSURING EQUITABLE PATIENT ASSIGNMENTS IN AN EMERGENCY DEPARTMENT

A new charge nurse has just started a 12-hour night shift in a community emergency department (ED). The first order of business is to make patient assignments for the 32-bed unit. Staffing for this shift includes 3 RNs (1 new and 2 seasoned), 1 LPN and 1 unlicensed assistant. What would be a fair assignment and what can be delegated to each of these staff members? How can the nurse foster open communication, mutual respect, and shared decision-making with the team to achieve quality patient care?

QSEN Competency Focus: Teamwork and Collaboration

The complexities inherent in today's health care system challenges nurses to demonstrate integration of specific interdisciplinary core competencies. These competencies are aimed at ensuring the delivery of safe, quality patient care (Institute of Medicine, 2003). The Quality and Safety Education for Nurses project (QSEN, 2017; Cronenwett, Sherwood, Barnsteiner, et al., 2007) provides a framework for the knowledge, skills, and attitudes (KSA) required for nurses to demonstrate competency in these key areas, which include *patient-centered care, interdisciplinary teamwork and collaboration, evidence-based practice, quality improvement, safety,* and *informatics.*

Teamwork and Collaboration Definition: Function effectively within nursing and interprofessional teams, fostering open communication, mutual respect, and shared decision making to achieve quality patient care.

SELECTED PRE-LICENSURE KSAs	APPLICATION AND REFLECTION
Knowledge	
Describe own strengths, limitations, and values in functioning as a member of the team.	Describe the charge nurse's priorities in making a fair assignment for this night shift. How would these intersect with those of other members of the team? Describe roles of each of the team members and how these roles interplay with each other.
Skills	
Function competently within own scope of practice as a member of the healthcare team.	As a novice charge nurse in the ED setting, whom would you rely on to help you develop your skillset? Identify your professional development growth goals so that you would be an effective member of the emergency health care team.
Attitudes	
Contribute to resolution of conflict and disagreement	Reflect upon your preferred communication style and approach to conflict. How might you react if a seasoned nurse challenges the assignment? What skills might you wish to develop to be most effective in this setting with seasoned nurses and other members of the team?

Cronenwett, L., Sherwood, G., Barnsteiner, J., et al. (2007). Quality and safety education for nurses. *Nursing Outlook, 55*(3), 122–131.
Institute of Medicine. (2003). *Health professions education: A bridge to quality*. Washington, DC: National Academies Press.
QSEN Institute, (2017). *QSEN competencies: Definitions and pre-licensure KSAs*. Retrieved on 3/1/2017 at: www.qsen.org/competencies/pre-licensure-ksas

71

Management of Patients With Infectious Diseases

LEARNING OBJECTIVES

On completion of this chapter, the learner will be able to:

1 Differentiate between the concepts of colonization, infection, and disease.
2 Identify federal and local resources available to the nurse seeking information about infectious diseases.
3 Discuss the benefits of vaccines recommended for health care workers.
4 Compare and contrast standard and transmission-based precautions and discuss the elements of each of these standards.

5 Describe the concept and the nursing management of emerging infectious diseases.
6 Use the nursing process as a framework for care of patients with sexually transmitted infections.
7 Explain measures that reduce the risk of infection in the home.
8 Apply the nursing process as a framework for care of patients with infectious diseases.

GLOSSARY

bacteremia: laboratory-confirmed presence of bacteria in the bloodstream
carrier: person who has an organism without apparent signs and symptoms; one who is able to transmit an infection to others
colonization: microorganisms present in or on a host, without host interference or interaction and without eliciting symptoms in the host
community-associated methicillin-resistant *Staphylococcus aureus* (CA-MRSA): a strain of MRSA infecting persons who have not been treated in a health care setting
emerging infectious diseases: human infectious diseases with an increased incidence within the past two decades, or with a potential to increase in the near future
fungemia: a bloodstream infection caused by a fungal organism
health care–associated infection (HAI): an infection not present or incubating at the time of admission to the health care setting; this term has replaced the term *nosocomial infection*
host: an organism that provides living conditions to support a microorganism
immune: person with protection from a previous infection or vaccination who resists reinfection when re-exposed to the same agent
incubation period: time between contact and onset of signs and symptoms
infection: condition in which the host interacts physiologically and immunologically with a microorganism
infectious disease: the consequences that result from invasion of the body by microorganisms that can produce harm to the body and potentially death

latency: time interval after primary infection when a microorganism lives within the host without producing clinical evidence
methicillin-resistant *Staphylococcus aureus* (MRSA): *Staphylococcus aureus* bacterium that is not susceptible to extended-penicillin antibiotic formulas, such as methicillin, oxacillin, or nafcillin; MRSA may occur in a health care or community setting
normal flora: persistent nonpathogenic organisms colonizing a host
reservoir: any person, plant, animal, substance, or location that provides living conditions for microorganisms and that enables further dispersal of the organism
standard precautions: strategy of assuming all patients may carry infectious agents and using appropriate barrier precautions for all health care worker–patient interactions
susceptible: not possessing immunity to a particular pathogen
transient flora: organisms that have been recently acquired and are likely to be shed in a relatively short period
transmission-based precautions: precautions used in addition to standard precautions when contagious or epidemiologically significant organisms are recognized; the three types of transmission-based precautions are airborne, droplet, and contact precautions
vancomycin-resistant *Enterococcus* (VRE): *Enterococcus* bacterium that is not susceptible to the antibiotic vancomycin
vancomycin-resistant *Staphylococcus aureus* (VRSA): *Staphylococcus aureus* bacterium that is not susceptible to vancomycin
virulence: degree of pathogenicity of an organism

An **infectious disease** is any disease caused by the growth of pathogenic microbes in the body. It may or may not be communicable (i.e., contagious). Modern science has controlled, eradicated, or decreased the incidence of many infectious diseases. However, increases in the incidence of other infections, such as those caused by antibiotic-resistant organisms and emerging infectious diseases, are of growing concern. Examples of these infectious diseases are presented in this chapter. Other infectious diseases are discussed in the appropriate chapters (e.g., see Chapter 23 for information on tuberculosis [TB]). It is important to understand infectious causes and the treatment of contagious, serious, and common infections. Table 71-1 presents selected infectious diseases, their causative organisms, mode of transmission, and usual **incubation periods** (time between contact and development of the first signs and symptoms).

The nurse plays an important role in infection control and prevention. Educating patients may decrease their risk of becoming infected or may decrease the sequelae of infection. Using appropriate barrier precautions, observing prudent hand hygiene, and ensuring aseptic care of intravenous (IV) catheters and other invasive equipment also assists in reducing infections.

The Infectious Process

The Chain of Infection

A complete chain of events is necessary for infection to occur. Six elements are necessary, including a causative organism, a reservoir of available organisms, a portal of exit from the reservoir, a mode of transmission from the reservoir to the **host** (an organism that provides living conditions to support a microorganism) and a mode of entry into a susceptible host.

Nurses must clearly understand the elements of the chain of infection in order to identify points at which they can intervene to interrupt the chain, thus protecting patients, themselves, and others from infectious disease. Figure 71-1 illustrates these concepts.

Causative Organism

The types of microorganisms that cause infections are bacteria, rickettsiae, viruses, protozoa, fungi, and helminths.

Reservoir

Reservoir is the term used for any person, plant, animal, substance, or location that provides nourishment for microorganisms and enables further dispersal of the organism. Infections may be prevented by eliminating the causative organisms from the reservoir.

Mode of Exit

The organism must have a mode of exit from a reservoir. An infected host must shed organisms to another or to the environment for transmission to occur. Organisms exit through the respiratory tract, the gastrointestinal tract, the genitourinary tract, or the blood.

Route of Transmission

A route of transmission is necessary to connect the infectious source with its new host. Organisms may be transmitted through sexual contact, skin-to-skin contact, percutaneous

injection, or infectious particles carried in the air. A person who carries or transmits an organism but does not have apparent signs and symptoms of infection is called a **carrier**.

Specific organisms require specific routes of transmission for infection to occur. For example, *Mycobacterium tuberculosis* is almost always transmitted by the airborne route. Health care providers do not "carry" M. *tuberculosis* bacteria on their hands or clothing. In contrast, bacteria such as *Staphylococcus aureus* are easily transmitted from patient to patient on the hands of health care providers. When appropriate, the nurse should explain routes of disease transmission to patients.

Susceptible Host

For infection to occur, the host must be **susceptible** (not possessing immunity to a particular pathogen). Previous infection or vaccine administration may render the host **immune** (not susceptible) to further infection with an agent. Although exposure to potentially infectious microorganisms occurs essentially on a constant basis, people have elaborate immune systems that generally prevent infection from occurring. A person who is immunosuppressed has much greater susceptibility to infection than a healthy person.

Portal of Entry

A portal of entry is needed for the organism to gain access to the host. Again, specific organisms may require specific portals of entry for infection to occur. For example, airborne M. *tuberculosis* does not cause disease when it settles on the skin of an exposed host; the only entry route for M. *tuberculosis* is through the respiratory tract.

Colonization, Infection, and Infectious Disease

Relatively few anatomic sites (e.g., brain, blood, bone, heart, vascular system) are sterile. Bacteria found throughout the body usually provide beneficial **normal flora** (nonpathogenic organisms colonizing a host) to compete with potential pathogens, to facilitate digestion, or to work in other ways symbiotically with the host.

Colonization

The term **colonization** is used to describe microorganisms present without host interference or interaction. Organisms reported in microbiology test results often reflect colonization rather than infection. The patient's health care team must interpret microbiology test results accurately to ensure appropriate treatment.

Infection

Infection indicates a host interaction with an organism. A patient colonized with S. *aureus* may have staphylococci on the skin without any skin interruption or irritation. However, if the patient has an incision, S. *aureus* could enter the wound, resulting in an immune system reaction of local inflammation and migration of white cells to the site. Clinical evidence of redness, heat, and pain and laboratory evidence of white blood cells on the wound specimen smear suggest infection. In this situation, the host identifies the staphylococci as *foreign*. Infection is recognized by the host reaction (manifested by signs and symptoms) and by laboratory-based

(text continued on page 2128)

TABLE 71-1 Selected Infectious Diseases, Causative Organisms, Modes of Transmission, and Usual Incubation Periods

Disease or Condition	Organism	Usual Mode of Transmission	Usual Incubation Period (Infection to First Symptom)
Acquired immune deficiency syndrome	Human immune deficiency virus	Sexual; percutaneous; perinatal	Median of 10 years
Anthrax	*Bacillus anthracis*	Airborne, contact, or ingestion	1–6 days
Chancroid	*Haemophilus ducreyi*	Sexual	3–5 days
Chickenpox	Varicella zoster	Airborne or contact	~10–21 days
Cytomegalovirus infection	Cytomegalovirus	Transfusion and transplantation; sexual; perinatal	Highly variable: 3–8 weeks after transfusion, 3–12 weeks after delivery of newborn
Diarrheal disease (common causes)	*Campylobacter* species	Ingestion of contaminated food	3–5 days
	Clostridium difficile	Fecal–oral	Variable; in part related to the influence of antibiotic agents
	Salmonella species	Ingestion of contaminated food or drink	12–36 hours
	Shigella species	Ingestion of contaminated food or drink; direct contact with carrier	1–3 days
	Yersinia species	Ingestion of contaminated food or drink; direct contact with carrier	1–3 days
Ebola	Ebola virus	Contact with blood or body fluids	2–21 days
Gonorrhea	*Neisseria gonorrhoeae*	Sexual; perinatal	2–7 days
Hand, foot, and mouth disease	Coxsackievirus	Direct contact with nose and throat secretions and with feces of people who are infected	3–5 days
Hantavirus pulmonary syndrome	Sin Nombre virus	Contact (direct or indirect) with rodents	Unclear
Hepatitis, foodborne	Hepatitis A virus	Ingestion of contaminated food or drink; direct contact with carrier	15–50 days
	Hepatitis E virus	Ingestion of contaminated food or drink; direct contact with carrier	15-65 days
Hepatitis, bloodborne	Hepatitis B virus	Sexual; perinatal; percutaneous	45–160 days
	Hepatitis C virus	Sexual; perinatal; percutaneous	15–160 days
	Hepatitis D	Sexual; perinatal; percutaneous	30–150 days
	Hepatitis G	Percutaneous	14–145 days
Herpes simplex	Human herpes viruses 1 and 2	Contact with mucous membrane secretions	2–12 days
Histoplasmosis	*Histoplasma capsulatum*	Inhalation of airborne spores	5–18 days
Hookworm disease	*Necator americanus; Ancylostoma duodenale*	Contact with soil contaminated with human feces	A few weeks to many months
Impetigo	*Staphylococcus aureus, Streptococcus pyogenes*	Contact with *S. aureus* carrier or with patient's soiled towels or combs	4–10 days
Influenza	Influenza virus A, B, or C	Droplet spread	24–72 hours
Legionnaires disease	*Legionella pneumophila*	Airborne from water source	2–10 days
Lyme disease	*Borrelia burgdorferi*	Tick bite	14–23 days
Lymphogranuloma venereum	*Chlamydia trachomatis*	Sexual	Weeks to years
Malaria	*Plasmodium vivax; Plasmodium malariae; Plasmodium falciparum; Plasmodium ovale*	Bite from *Anopheles* species mosquito	12–30 days

Disease or Condition	Organism	Usual Mode of Transmission	Usual Incubation Period (Infection to First Symptom)
Marburg hemorrhagic fever	Marburg virus	Unknown route of transmission from animals to humans; person-to-person by droplets and direct contact	5–10 days
Meningococcal meningitis or bacteremia	*Neisseria meningitidis*	Contact with pharyngeal secretions; perhaps airborne	2–10 days
Mononucleosis	Epstein–Barr virus	Contact with pharyngeal secretions	4–6 weeks
Mycobacterial diseases (nontuberculosis *Mycobacterium* species)	*Mycobacterium avium; Mycobacterium kansasii; Mycobacterium fortuitum; Mycobacterium gordonae;* other *Mycobacterium* species	Variable; probably contact with soil, water, or other environmental source; none is person-to-person transmissible	Variable
Mycoplasmal pneumonia	*Mycoplasma pneumoniae*	Droplet inhalation	14–21 days
Norovirus	*Norovirus*	Fecal–oral by food or water or by person-to-person spread	24–48 hours
Pediculosis	*Pediculus humanus capitis* (head louse); *Pediculosis pubis* (crab louse)	Direct contact	1–2 weeks
Pertussis (whooping cough)	*Bordetella pertussis*	Contact with respiratory droplets	7–10 days
Pinworm disease	*Enterobius vermicularis*	Direct contact with egg-contaminated articles	4- to 6-week life cycle; often takes months of infection before recognition
Pneumocystis jiroveci pneumonia	*Pneumocystis jiroveci*	Unknown; not transmitted person to person	Infants: 1–2 months; adults: unclear
Pneumococcal pneumonia	*Streptococcus pneumoniae*	Droplet spread	Probably 1–3 days
Rabies	Rabies virus	Bite from rabid animal	2–8 weeks
Respiratory syncytial disease	Respiratory syncytial virus	Self-inoculation by mouth or nose after contact with infectious respiratory secretions	3–7 days
Ringworm	*Microsporum* species; *Trichophyton* species	Direct and indirect contact with lesions	4–10 days
Rocky Mountain spotted fever	*Rickettsia rickettsii*	Bite from infected tick	3–14 days
Roseola infantum	Human herpes virus 6	Saliva	10–15 days
Rotavirus gastroenteritis	*Rotavirus*	Fecal–oral route	~48 hours
Rubella	Rubella virus	Droplet spread; direct contact	14–21 days
Scabies	*Sarcoptes scabei*	Direct skin contact	2–6 weeks
Smallpox	*Variola major and minor*	Airborne and contact	7–14 days
Syphilis	*Treponema pallidum*	Sexual; perinatal	10 days to 10 weeks
Tetanus	*Clostridium tetani*	Puncture wound	4–21 days
Trichinosis	*Trichinella spiralis*	Ingestion of insufficiently cooked foods, especially pork and beef	10–14 days
Tuberculosis	*Mycobacterium tuberculosis*	Airborne	4–12 weeks to the formation of primary lesion
West Nile virus	West Nile virus	Bite of infected mosquitoes; from transfusions and transplants; perinatal	3–14 days
Zika virus	Zika virus	Bite of infected *Aedes* mosquitoes	Unclear

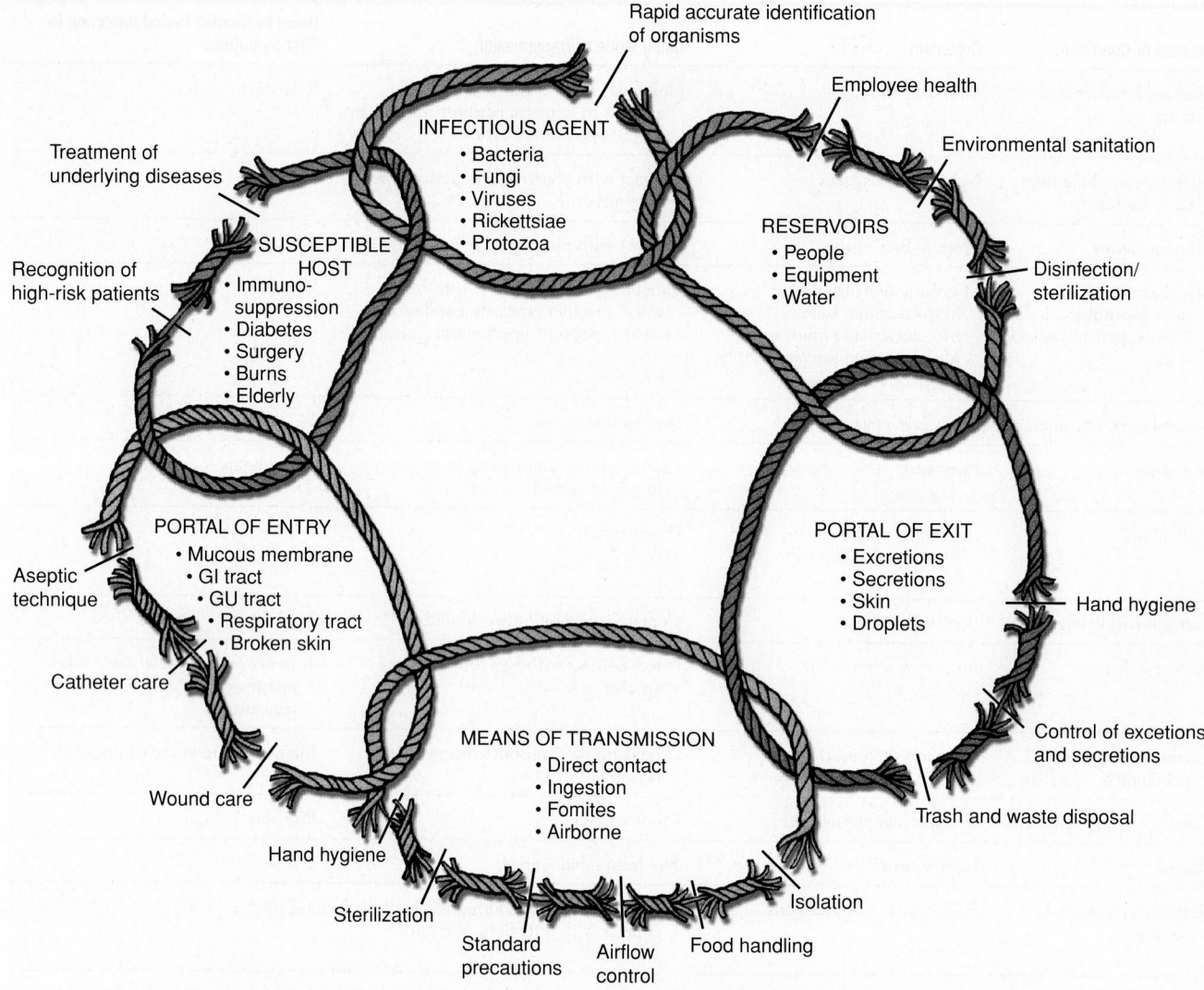

Figure 71-1 • Health care workers' interventions used to break the chain of infection transmission.

evidence of white blood cell reaction and microbiologic organism identification.

Infectious Disease

It is important to recognize the difference between infection and infectious disease. Infectious disease is the state in which the infected host displays a decline in wellness due to the infection. When the host interacts immunologically with an organism but remains symptom free, the definition of infectious disease has not been met. The severity of an infectious disease ranges from mild to life threatening (Grossman & Porth, 2014). Figure 71-2 depicts the range of response to bacterial infection at the cellular and host level.

The primary source of information about most bacterial infections is the microbiology laboratory report, which should be viewed as a tool to be used along with clinical indicators to determine if a patient is colonized, infected, or diseased. Microbiology reports from clinical specimens usually show three components: the smear and stain, the culture and organism identification, and the antimicrobial susceptibility (i.e., sensitivity). As a marker for the likelihood of infection,

the smear and stain generally provide the most helpful information because they describe the mix of cells present at the anatomic site at the time of specimen collection. Culture and sensitivity results specify which organisms are recognized and which antibiotic agents actively affect the bacteria.

Infection Control and Prevention

The World Health Organization (WHO) and the Centers for Disease Control and Prevention (CDC) are the principal agencies involved in setting guidelines about infection prevention. In recent years, the WHO and CDC have focused more attention on **health care–associated infections (HAIs)**, infections acquired in the health care setting. Previously known as nosocomial infections, HAIs have also received increased attention from the Joint Commission, the Institute for Healthcare Improvement (IHI), and Medicare. HAI rates for each hospital are posted on the Medicare Hospital Compare website (see the Resources section).

The impact of infectious diseases changes over time as microorganisms mutate, as human behavior patterns shift,

Cell response	Host response
Death and lysis of cell	Death of host
Dying cell	Septicemic and/or fulminant disease
Severe impairment of cell function	Severe illness requiring hospitalization
Moderate impairment of cell function	Moderate illness requiring medical care
Mild impairment of cell function	Mild, ambulatory illness
Level of cellualr injury	Level of clinical recognition
Attachment, entry, and multiplication without cell injury	Infection without disease (subclinical or inapparent infection)
Attachment with surface multiplication	Colonization without tissue injury
Exposure without attachment to cell	Exposure without multiplication of bacteria

Discernible by studies of growth and metabolism / *Below detectable level of cell injury* — *Apparent illness* / *Inapparent*

Figure 71-2 • Biologic spectrum of response to bacterial infection at the cellular level (*left*) and of the intact host (*right*). Redrawn from Evans, A. S., & Brachman, P. S. (1998). *Bacterial infections in humans* (3rd ed.). New York: Plenum, p. 40.

or as therapeutic options change. The CDC provides timely recommendations about many of the situations that a nurse may face when caring for or educating a patient with an infectious disease. The CDC routinely publishes recommendations, guidelines, and summaries. Through its Internet site and its weekly journal, the *Morbidity and Mortality Weekly Report (MMWR)*, the CDC reports significant cases, outbreaks, environmental hazards, or other public health problems. Examples of important CDC guidelines and summaries are *Sexually Transmitted Diseases Treatment Guidelines* (2015c) and *Immunization Schedule* (CDC, 2016a).

Nurses serve important roles in preventing the transfer of organisms as they have many opportunities for spreading organisms, given their frequent encounters with patients and families. It is essential for the nurse to model appropriate and effective hand hygiene practices in all aspects of patient care. Nurses can also help reduce hand-to-hand spread of organisms by serving as patient advocates. The nurse should observe the hand hygiene activities of other professionals and alert them to lapses in technique that are observed. Nurses need to educate patients and their families to feel comfortable in reminding health care workers to perform hand hygiene before patient contact (Busby, Kennedy, Davis, et al., 2015).

This chapter summarizes several aspects of infectious diseases. However, the field of infection control and prevention changes rapidly. Nurses should seek the most current information when they address patient care concerns or develop infection control policies (see the Resources section).

Preventing Infection in the Hospital

Isolation Precautions

Isolation precautions are guidelines created to prevent transmission of microorganisms in hospitals. The Healthcare Infection Control Practices Advisory Committee (HICPAC) of the CDC recommends two tiers of isolation precautions. The first tier, called **standard precautions**, is designed for the care of *all* patients in the hospital and is the primary strategy for preventing HAIs. The second tier, called **transmission-based**

precautions, is designed for care of patients with known or suspected infectious diseases spread by airborne, droplet, or contact routes. In addition, Occupational Safety and Health Administration (OSHA) regulations are followed to remove toxic and hazardous substances as well as blood-borne pathogens (OSHA, 2012).

Standard Precautions

The premise of standard precautions is that all patients are colonized or infected with microorganisms, whether or not there are signs or symptoms, and that a uniform level of caution should be used in the care of all patients. The health care worker should use additional barriers in the form of personal protective equipment (PPE), including gloves, masks, eye protection, and cover gowns, depending on the expected degree of exposure to patient excretions or secretions. The elements of standard precautions include appropriate hand hygiene, the use of PPE, proper handling of patient care equipment and linen, environmental control, prevention of injury from sharps devices, and patients' room assignments within health care facilities. Hand hygiene, glove use, needlestick prevention, and avoidance of splash or spray of body fluids are discussed in the following sections. See Chapter 36, Chart 36-5 for a description of standard precautions.

Hand Hygiene

The most frequent cause of bacterial transmission in health care institutions is spread of microorganisms by the hands of health care workers. Hands should be washed or decontaminated frequently during patient care. Chart 71-1 describes recommended hand hygiene methods (CDC, 2002).

When hands are visibly dirty or contaminated with biologic material from patient care, the hands should be washed with soap and water. In intensive care units and other locations in which virulent or resistant organisms are likely to be present, antimicrobial agents (e.g., chlorhexidine gluconate, iodophor, chloroxylenol) may be used. Effective handwashing requires at least *15 seconds of vigorous scrubbing*, with special attention to the area around nail beds and between fingers,

Chart 71-1	Hand Hygiene Methods

Hand Decontamination With Alcohol-Based Product

- After contact with body fluids, excretions, mucous membranes, nonintact skin, or wound dressings as long as hands are not visibly soiled
- After contact with a patient's intact skin (e.g., after taking pulse or blood pressure or lifting a patient)
- In patient care, when moving from a contaminated body site to a clean body site
- After contact with inanimate objects in the patient's immediate vicinity
- Before caring for patients with severe neutropenia or other forms of severe immune suppression
- Before donning sterile gloves when inserting central catheters
- Before inserting urinary catheters or other devices that do not require a surgical procedure
- After removing gloves

Handwashing

- When hands are visibly dirty or contaminated with biologic material from patient care
- When health care workers do not tolerate waterless alcohol product

Adapted from Centers for Disease Control and Prevention. (2002). Guideline for hand hygiene in health care settings. *MMWR: Morbidity and Mortality Weekly Report, 51*(RR 16), 1–56.

---

where there is a high bacterial load. Hands should be thoroughly rinsed after washing (CDC, 2002).

If hands are not visibly soiled, health care providers are strongly encouraged to use alcohol-based, waterless antiseptic agents for routine hand decontamination. These solutions are superior to soap or antimicrobial handwashing agents in their speed of action and effectiveness against most microorganisms. Because they are formulated with emollients, they are usually better tolerated than other agents, and because they can be used without sinks and towels, health care workers may be more adherent with their use. Nurses working in home health care or other settings where they are relatively mobile should carry pocket-sized containers of alcohol-based solutions. The spore form of the bacterium *Clostridium difficile* is resistant to alcohol and other hand disinfectants; therefore, the use of gloves and handwashing (soap and water for physical removal) are required when *C. difficile* has been identified (CDC, 2007).

Normal skin flora usually consist of coagulase-negative staphylococci or diphtheroids. In the health care setting, workers may temporarily carry other bacteria such as *S. aureus*, *Pseudomonas aeruginosa*, or other organisms with increased pathogenic potential. These organisms, known as **transient flora**, are typically superficially attached and are shed with hand hygiene and skin regeneration.

Hand hygiene decreases the risk of transfer of bacteria to patients who are vulnerable by reducing bacterial load on health care workers' hands. The Joint Commission includes hand hygiene as one of the National Patient Safety Goals and focuses on this behavior in all surveys of health care facilities (The Joint Commission, 2016). All health care settings should have mechanisms to increase adherence with hand hygiene by all personnel who care for patients (Shabot, Chassin, France, et al., 2016).

When providing patient care, nurses should not wear artificial fingernails or nail extenders because they have been epidemiologically linked to several significant outbreaks of infections. Natural nails should be kept less than 0.6 cm (0.25 inch) long, and nail polish should be removed when chipped because it can support increased bacterial growth (CDC, 2002).

Glove Use

Gloves provide an effective barrier for hands from the microflora associated with patient care. Gloves should be worn when a health care worker has contact with any patient secretions or excretions and must be discarded after each patient care contact. Because microbial organisms colonizing health care workers' hands can proliferate in the warm, moist environment provided by gloves, hands must be washed or disinfected after gloves are removed. As patient advocates, nurses have an important role in promoting hand hygiene and glove use by other hospital workers, such as laboratory personnel, technicians, physicians, and others who have contact with patients.

Compared with vinyl gloves, latex or nitrile gloves are preferred because they resist puncture better and provide greater comfort and fit. Latex gloves have been improved to reduce the incidence of latex hypersensitivity, but some workers continue to experience local skin irritation or more severe reactions, including generalized dermatitis, conjunctivitis, asthma, angioedema, and anaphylaxis (see Chapter 37). The nurse who experiences irritation or an allergic reaction associated with exposure to latex should report symptoms to an occupational health specialist or a primary provider.

Needlestick Prevention

The most important aspect of reducing the risk of bloodborne infection is avoidance of percutaneous injury. Extreme care is essential in all situations in which needles, scalpels, and other sharp objects are handled. Used needles should not be recapped. Instead, they are placed directly into puncture-resistant containers near the place where they are used. If a situation dictates that a needle must be recapped, the nurse must use a mechanical device to hold the cap or use a one-handed approach to decrease the likelihood of skin puncture. OSHA requires use of needleless devices and other instruments designed to prevent injury from sharps when appropriate.

Avoidance of Splash and Spray

When the health care professional is involved in an activity in which body fluids may be sprayed or splashed, appropriate barriers must be used. If a splash to the face may occur, goggles and a facemask are warranted. If the health care worker is involved in a procedure in which clothing may be contaminated with biologic material, a cover gown should be worn (CDC, 2002).

Transmission-Based Precautions

Some microbes are so contagious or epidemiologically significant that in addition to standard precautions, a second tier of precautions—transmission-based precautions—should be used when such organisms have been identified. Isolation categories are airborne, droplet, and contact precautions (CDC, 2007).

Airborne precautions are required for patients with presumed or proven pulmonary TB, varicella, or other airborne pathogens. When hospitalized, patients should be in airborne infection isolation rooms, engineered to provide negative air pressure, rapid turnover of air, and air either highly filtered or exhausted directly to the outside. Health care providers should wear an N95 respirator (i.e., protective mask) at all times while in the patient's room. The nurse should be able to validate negative pressure by reading a pressure manometer placed outside the room and/or by witnessing that a tissue held at the gap between the door and the floor will be pulled toward the room.

Droplet precautions are used for organisms such as influenza or meningococcus that can be transmitted by close contact with respiratory or pharyngeal secretions. When caring for a patient requiring droplet precautions, the nurse should wear a facemask within 3 to 6 feet of the patient; however, because the risk of transmission is limited to close contact, the door may remain open.

Contact precautions are used for organisms that are spread by skin-to-skin contact, such as antibiotic-resistant organisms

or *C. difficile*. Contact precautions are designed to emphasize cautious technique and the use of barriers for organisms that have serious epidemiologic consequences or those easily transmitted by contact between health care worker and patient. When possible, the patient requiring contact isolation is placed in a private room to facilitate hand hygiene and decreased environmental contamination. Masks are not needed, and doors do not need to be closed (see Chart 71-2).

Specific Organisms With HAI Potential

Clostridium difficile

Clostridium difficile is a spore-forming bacterium that has significant HAI potential. An especially virulent strain has affected health care facilities throughout North America in the past several years, and rates of *C. difficile* infection increased significantly in the United States since 2000 (CDC, 2016b). It is considered the most common cause of health care–associated infection in U.S. hospitals (CDC, 2016b). Infection is usually preceded by antibiotic agents that disrupt normal intestinal flora and allow the antibiotic-resistant *C. difficile* spores to proliferate within the intestine. The organism causes pathology

---

Chart 71-2 Summary of Types of Precautions and Patients Requiring the Precautions

Standard Precautions

Use standard precautions for the care of all patients.

Airborne Precautions

In addition to standard precautions, use airborne precautions for patients known or suspected to have serious illnesses transmitted by airborne droplet nuclei. Examples of such illnesses include:
- Measles
- Varicella (including disseminated zoster)[a]
- Tuberculosis

Droplet Precautions

In addition to standard precautions, use droplet precautions for patients known or suspected to have serious illnesses transmitted by large particle droplets. Examples of such illnesses include:
- Invasive *Haemophilus influenzae* type b disease, including meningitis, pneumonia, epiglottitis, and sepsis
- Invasive *Neisseria meningitidis* disease, including meningitis, pneumonia, and sepsis
- Other serious bacterial respiratory infections spread by droplet transmission, including:
  - Diphtheria (pharyngeal)
  - Primary atypical pneumonia (*Mycoplasma pneumoniae*)
  - Pertussis
  - Pneumonic plague
  - Streptococcal (group A) pharyngitis, pneumonia, or scarlet fever in infants and young children
- Serious viral infections spread by droplet transmission, including:
  - Adenovirus[a]
  - Influenza
  - Mumps
  - Parvovirus B19
  - Rubella

Contact Precautions

In addition to standard precautions, use contact precautions for patients known or suspected to have serious illnesses easily transmitted by direct patient contact or by contact with items in the patient's environment. Examples of such illnesses include:
- Gastrointestinal, respiratory, skin, or wound infections or colonization with multidrug-resistant bacteria judged by the infection control program, based on current state, regional, or national recommendations, to be of special clinical and epidemiologic significance
- Enteric infections with a low infectious dose or prolonged environmental survival, including:
  - *Clostridium difficile*
  - For patients who are diapered or incontinent: enterohemorrhagic *Escherichia coli* O157:H7, *Shigella* species, hepatitis A, or rotavirus
- Respiratory syncytial virus, parainfluenza virus, or enteroviral infections in infants and young children
- Skin infections that are highly contagious or that may occur on dry skin, including:
  - Diphtheria (cutaneous)
  - Herpes simplex virus (neonatal or mucocutaneous)
  - Impetigo
  - Major (noncontained) abscesses, cellulitis, or pressure ulcers
  - Pediculosis
  - Scabies
  - Staphylococcal furunculosis in infants and young children
  - Zoster (disseminated or in the immunocompromised host)[a]
- Viral and hemorrhagic conjunctivitis
- Viral hemorrhagic infections (Ebola, Lassa, or Marburg)

[a]Certain infections require more than one type of precaution.
Adapted from Centers for Disease Control and Prevention (CDC). (2007). 2007 *Guideline for isolation precautions: Preventing transmission of infectious agents in healthcare settings.* Retrieved on 5/13/2016 at: www.cdc.gov/hicpac/2007ip/2007ip_part1.html

by releasing toxins into the lumen of the bowel. In pseudomembranous colitis (the most extreme form of *C. difficile* infection), debris from the injured lumen of the bowel and from white blood cells accumulates in the form of pseudomembranes or studded areas of the colon. The destruction of such a large anatomic area can cause sepsis.

Because antibiotic medications are used so extensively in health care settings, many patients are at risk for infection with *C. difficile*. The potential for health care–associated acquisition is increased because the spore is relatively resistant to disinfectants and can be spread on the hands of health care providers after contact with equipment previously contaminated with *C. difficile*. Control is best achieved by using contact precautions for patients who are infected, with use of gowns and gloves for all patient contact. Because the spores are resistant to alcohol, waterless hand products are not as effective as handwashing with soap and water for use in hand hygiene. Bleach-based cleaning products are optimal because bleach can kill spores, whereas other cleaning agents often do not. Frequently touched equipment (such as the overbed table and side rails) should be cleaned daily and whenever visibly soiled. IV poles and other peripheral items should be cleaned when the patient is discharged (CDC, 2016b).

Methicillin-Resistant *Staphylococcus aureus*

Methicillin-resistant *Staphylococcus aureus* (MRSA), a common human pathogen, refers to *S. aureus* that is resistant to methicillin or its comparable pharmaceutical agents, oxacillin and nafcillin. Soon after penicillin was discovered in the 1940s, *S. aureus* became all but universally penicillin resistant. Alternative therapies in the form of cephalosporins and synthetic penicillin solutions such as methicillin were introduced. During the late 1970s, MRSA became increasingly more prevalent, as transmission within hospitals and nursing homes was well documented. However, since 2006, the incidence of serious infections due to MRSA has declined (Dantes, Mu, Belflower, et al., 2013).

Health Care–Associated MRSA

Health care providers transmit MRSA to patients easily because *S. aureus* has an affinity for skin colonization. The patient who is colonized with MRSA has an increased probability of developing health care–associated methicillin-resistant *Staphylococcus aureus* (HA-MRSA) infection, especially when invasive procedures, such as IV therapy, respiratory therapy, or surgery, are performed. The patient who is colonized also serves as a reservoir for MRSA transmission to others. HA-MRSA may persist as normal flora in the patient for an extended time. In recent years, there has been a decreased incidence of invasive HAIs with MRSA (Dantes et al., 2013). Although the exact reasons for the decline are unknown, it is likely that infection control efforts (especially those focused on reduction of bloodstream infections) and declining lengths of hospital stay (therefore decreasing exposure within health care agencies) are important factors.

Community-Associated MRSA

In recent decades, new strains of MRSA caused significant infections and outbreaks of infection in children, members of sports teams, and prison inmates, and in other people who had no apparent health care exposure. These **community-associated methicillin-resistant *Staphylococcus aureus* (CA-MRSA)** infections are typically caused by strains of *S. aureus* that are molecularly distinct from HA-MRSA. The CA-MRSA strains typically produce more toxins than HA-MRSA, and localized skin symptoms can lead to necrotizing fasciitis or bacteremia. Often, skin symptoms are initially mistaken for spider or bug bites. CA-MRSA infections have resulted in serious skin and soft tissue infections; pneumonia; and, in rare cases, death. Once introduced into a health care facility, the virulent CA-MRSA strains can be transmitted to other patients in a manner typically associated with HA-MRSA (Dantes et al., 2013).

Control of MRSA in Health Care Facilities

The CDC recommends contact precautions for patients with MRSA colonization or infection (CDC, 2007). Nurses must be prepared to educate patients and their families about the definitions of colonization and infection and the reason for the vigorous isolation efforts. Vancomycin (Vancocin) and linezolid (Zyvox) are typically the preferred treatment options for serious MRSA infection. However, there is concern that MRSA will eventually become resistant to even these medications because they are used so frequently. A small number of patients have been diagnosed with *S. aureus* infections that are intermediately sensitive to vancomycin (i.e., vancomycin-intermediate *Staphylococcus aureus* [VISA]) or completely resistant to vancomycin (i.e., **vancomycin-resistant *Staphylococcus aureus* [VRSA]**). The threat of VRSA is considered a very serious public health concern because of the incidence and pathogenicity of *S. aureus* infections. With the control of MRSA, the emergence of VRSA strains should decrease.

Vancomycin-Resistant *Enterococcus*

Vancomycin-resistant *Enterococcus* (VRE) is the second most frequently isolated source of HAIs in the United States. This gram-positive bacterium, which is part of the normal flora of the gastrointestinal tract, can produce significant disease when it infects blood, wounds, or the urinary tract (Nealy, McCarty, & Woods, 2016).

Enterococcus has several traits that make it an easily transmittable HAI organism. It is a normal part of the gastrointestinal flora of the host; it is bile resistant and able to withstand harsh anatomic sites, such as the intestine; and it persists well on the hands of health care providers and on environmental objects.

As a relatively resistant organism at baseline, therapy for *Enterococcus* is limited to penicillin formulations (e.g., ampicillin), vancomycin in combination with an aminoglycoside (e.g., gentamicin), or linezolid. Because many strains of VRE are resistant to all other antimicrobial therapies, clinicians are left with few choices for effective therapy. Equally important, VRE colonization and infection may serve as a reservoir of vancomycin-resistant coded genes that may be transferred to the more virulent *S. aureus*. The two most frequently cultured enterococcal strains, *Enterococcus faecalis* and *Enterococcus faecium*, are both increasingly found to be resistant.

Multidrug-Resistant Organisms

The incidence of infections caused by multidrug-resistant organisms (MDROs) has increased since 2000 (Stone, Herzig, Pogorzelska-Maziarz, et al., 2015). Extensive use of antibiotic agents in agriculture and health care has led to a growing prevalence of organisms with fewer effective antibiotics. The bacteria that most commonly develop resistance include *P. aeruginosa* (resistant to fluoroquinolone antibiotics and/or carbapenems), *Acinetobacter* species (resistant to many antibiotics, including carbapenems), and both *Klebsiella pneumoniae* and *Escherichia coli* (resistant to extended-spectrum beta-lactam antibiotics). These pathogens are also associated with outbreaks in health care facilities (Stone et al., 2015).

Concerns about MDROs and the loss of effective antibiotic therapy for serious infections have grown. The Joint Commission National Patient Safety Goals include requirements to have a program to analyze and reduce MDRO infections (The Joint Commission, 2016). In addition, a National Action Plan to Combat Antibiotic Resistant Organisms was established in 2015 (White House, 2015), and in 2016, the United Nations drafted a declaration for a global strategy to reduce the risk of antibiotic resistance (United Nations General Assembly, 2016).

Preventing Health Care–Associated Bloodstream Infections (Bacteremia and Fungemia)

Reducing the risk of health care–associated bloodstream infections requires preventive activities in addition to implementing standard precautions (Fox, Wavra, Drake, et al., 2015) (see Chart 71-3). If a health care–associated bloodstream infection occurs, early diagnosis is important to prevent complications such as endocarditis and brain abscess. Mortality rates associated with infection by some organisms are estimated to average 18%. The estimated average cost per patient attributed to catheter-related bloodstream infections is $16,500 (CDC, 2011).

Bacteremia is defined as laboratory-confirmed presence of bacteria in the bloodstream. **Fungemia** is a bloodstream infection caused by a fungal organism. Any vascular catheter can serve as the source for a bloodstream infection. Vascular catheters are used for most patients who are hospitalized, and increasingly, long-term central catheters are used to provide IV therapy to outpatients in clinic or home settings. In all instances, the nurse must use appropriate care to reduce the risk of bacteremia and to be alert to signs of bacteremia.

Prevention of CLABSI is important in preventing sepsis. A bundle approach is recommended, including (1) hand hygiene; (2) maximal barrier precautions; (3) chlorhexidine skin antisepsis; (4) optimal catheter site selection, with avoidance of the femoral vein for central venous access in adult patients; and (5) daily review of line necessity with prompt removal of unnecessary lines (see Chapter 14, Chart 14-2) (Gilmartin, Sousa, & Battaglia, 2016; Marschall, Mermel, Fakih, et al., 2014).

Preventing Infection in the Community

The CDC as well as state and local public health departments share responsibility for prevention and control of infection in the community. Methods of infection prevention include sanitation techniques (e.g., water purification, disposal of sewage and other potentially infectious materials), regulated health practices (e.g., the handling, storage, packaging, and preparation of food by institutions), and immunization programs. In the United States, immunization programs have markedly decreased the incidence of infectious diseases.

Vaccination Programs

The goal of vaccination programs is to use wide-scale efforts to prevent specific infectious diseases from occurring in a population. Public health decisions about vaccination efforts are complex. Risks and benefits for the person and the community must be evaluated in terms of morbidity, mortality, and financial cost and benefit. Successful vaccine programs have reduced the incidence of many infectious diseases in the United States (see Table 71-2).

More than 50 vaccines are currently licensed in the United States (CDC, 2016a). Vaccines are suspensions of antigen

---

Chart 71-3	**NURSING RESEARCH PROFILE**

Does Washing the Hands of Patients Decrease HAIs?

Fox, C., Wavra, T., Drake, D. A., et al. (2015). Use of a patient hand hygiene protocol to reduce hospital acquired infections and improve nurses' hand washing. *American Journal of Critical Care*, 24(3), 216–224.

Purpose

Patients who are critically ill are at increased risk of health care–associated infections (HAIs) and associated increases in morbidity and mortality. The purpose of this study was to investigate whether a new patient hand hygiene protocol would reduce HAIs in an intensive care unit (ICU).

Design

A posttest with a retrospective comparison group design was used. Data were collected from a single ICU over approximately 2 and a half years. There were three consecutive phases: (1) a comparison 12-month period before protocol implementation, (2) a 10-week protocol training period, and (3) a 12-month period during the protocol implementation. The two HAIs tracked were central line–associated bloodstream infection (CLABSI) and

catheter-associated urinary tract infection (CAUTI). The protocol consisted of the use of 2% chlorhexidine gluconate (CHG) wipes used to wash the hands of patients three times a day.

Findings

There were reductions in 12-month CLABSI and CAUTI rates overall, but the differences were not statistically significant. The rates of nurses washing the hands of the patients with CHG wipes also increased, but the increase was not statistically significant.

Nursing Implications

This study used a unique protocol whereby nurses washed the hands of patient in an ICU with CHG wipes three times each day. While statistically significant results were not found, this protocol deserves further study with a stronger research design. There are no known disadvantages to washing the hands of patients and instructing family members to use CHG wipes on their own hands unless there are breaks in the skin on the hands.

TABLE 71-2 Vaccine Preventable Diseases—Comparison of Cases Reported in Pre-Vaccine Period and 2013

Disease	Comparison Year	Pre-vaccine Average Number of Cases per Year	2013 Number of Cases
Diphtheria	1950	5796	0
Tetanus	1950	486	26
Pertussis	1950	120,718	28,639
Polio (paralytic)	1950	33,300	1
Measles	1950	319,124	187
Rubella	1966	152,209	584
Mumps	1968	46,975	9
Hepatitis A	1972	54,074	1781
Hepatitis B	1972	9402	3050
Varicella	1972	164,114	11,359

Adapted from Centers for Disease Control and Prevention. (2014a). Epidemiology and Prevention of Vaccine Preventable Diseases, *Morbidity and Mortality Weekly Report*, 63(32), 702–715.

preparations that are intended to produce a human immune response to protect the host from future encounters with the organism. Because no vaccine is completely safe for all recipients, contraindications on package inserts of a vaccine and the CDC-produced "Vaccine Information Statements" must be heeded. These documents provide details about studied experiences with allergy and other complications and provide crucial information about refrigeration, storage, dosage, and administration.

The recommended immunization schedules are revised by the CDC (2016a) as epidemiologic evidence warrants. Variations to the recommended immunization schedule should be made on a case-by-case basis, depending on the patient's risk factors as well as likely exposures. An annual influenza vaccine is recommended for all people 6 months or older, unless contraindicated. In addition, adults who are immunosuppressed (including those who have had a splenectomy) should be vaccinated for pneumococcus (*Streptococcus pneumoniae*) and meningococcus (*Neisseria meningitidis*). Health care workers should be immune to measles, mumps, rubella, pertussis, tetanus, hepatitis B, and varicella.

The CDC (2016a) gives information about individual vaccines and vaccine-preventable diseases (see the Resources section). Advice about optimal vaccinations for travelers is available at the CDC and WHO websites as well.

The incidence of vaccine-preventable diseases, such as measles, mumps, rubella, and diphtheria, is affected by immigration from developing countries. Vaccine campaigns in developing countries are often financially and logistically constrained, and immigrants from such areas may be more likely than U.S. residents to be unprotected. Individual risk and epidemic risk are reduced when vaccination campaigns reach all communities, including those with a high proportion of immigrants.

Reporting Problems With Vaccines

Nurses should ask adult vaccine recipients to provide information about any problems encountered after vaccination. As mandated by law, a Vaccine Adverse Event Reporting System (VAERS) form must be completed with the following information: type of vaccine received, timing of vaccination, onset of the adverse event, current illnesses or medication, history of adverse events after vaccination, and demographic information about the recipient. Forms are obtained by telephone or via the Internet (see the Resources section) and can be submitted online.

Contraindications to Vaccines

As a general rule, all vaccines may be given at the same visit, and separating the dosing by time is not indicated. If they must be given on separate visits, it is then wise to separate by at least 4 weeks so that there is no immune reaction interfering with the response to the second vaccine (CDC, 2016a). Patients who have developed anaphylaxis or other moderate or severe sequelae after a previous dose or those who have developed encephalopathy within 7 days of a previous pertussis vaccine dose should not receive further doses. Some live vaccines (e.g., varicella, MMR [against measles, mumps, and rubella], yellow fever) are contraindicated for people who are severely immunosuppressed or pregnant. All decisions about vaccination should be made by the patient's primary provider after careful review of vaccine-specific contraindications.

Common Vaccines

Measles, Mumps, and Rubella Vaccine

Since the time of licensing of the MMR vaccines, endemic rubella has been eliminated in the United States, and mumps and rubella have decreased substantially. To maintain this effective public health strategy, routine MMR vaccination should be given to children at 12 to 15 months of age, with repeat dosing at 4 to 6 years of age (CDC, 2016a). Adults who have not received the MMR vaccine should receive one to two doses (CDC, 2016a).

Patients should be advised that fever, transient lymphadenopathy, or hypersensitivity reaction might occur following an MMR vaccination. The risk of side effects is greater in vaccine recipients who have not previously received the vaccine than in those who have received repeat doses. Antipyretics may be used to decrease the risk of fever.

Varicella (Chickenpox) Vaccine and Zoster (Shingles) Vaccine

Varicella zoster is the virus that causes chickenpox and herpes zoster. In its natural state, the varicella virus often attacks children, causing disseminated disease in the form of chickenpox. Although the incidence of varicella is lower in adults, the severity of chickenpox and possible sequelae, including death, is substantially greater (CDC, 2016d). Transmission occurs by the airborne and contact routes. With rare exception, varicella infects a person only once. The incubation period is about 2 weeks (range, 10 to 21 days). During a prodrome of general malaise (often noticed about 2 days before the rash develops), the newly infected host is capable of transmitting the virus to other susceptible contacts. Typically, the vesicular, pustular rash spreads rapidly from few to many lesions in a matter of hours. New lesions continue to form for 2 to 3 days and appear at different stages throughout this time. By the fourth symptomatic day, the lesions begin to dry, and new lesions usually do not develop. Fever is common during the 4 to 6 days of rash progression. When the lesions have crusted, the patient is no longer contagious.

The vaccine is effective in preventing chickenpox in approximately 90% of people who receive two doses of vaccine (CDC, 2016d). The vaccine should not be given to those who have severely depressed immune function, are pregnant, have moderate or severe concurrent illnesses, or have demonstrated allergy to varicella vaccine.

Herpes zoster, also known as shingles, is a painful, localized rash caused by recurrent varicella. Vesicles are restricted to areas supplied by single associated nerve groups. Varicella may be transmitted from the rash of those with shingles to people who are susceptible to varicella; the new varicella infections are manifested as chickenpox, not shingles. It is estimated that more than 30% of people over age 60 will develop shingles (CDC, 2016e). Zostavax, a vaccine to reduce the risk of shingles, is recommended for people older than 60 years of age because it reduces the risk of shingles by approximately 50% (CDC, 2016e).

Influenza Vaccine

Influenza is an acute viral respiratory disease that predictably and periodically causes worldwide epidemics known as pandemics. Epidemics occur every 2 to 3 years, with a highly variable degree of severity. An estimated 36,000 deaths per year are associated with influenza or its sequelae (i.e., pneumonia, cardiopulmonary collapse). Older adults are more susceptible to influenza, and the incidence of the disease in the United States is increasing as the proportion of older adults increases (CDC, 2016f).

Each year, two influenza vaccine formulations, based on predictions of what strains will likely circulate, are released. The trivalent vaccine is composed of three strains (two type A influenza and one type B influenza); the quadrivalent vaccine is composed of four strains (two of type A and two of type B). The vaccine is given as an injection with inactivated virus or as a nasal spray with live attenuated virus. The nasal spray is recommended for those between 2 and 49 years of age (CDC, 2015d).

The U.S. Food and Drug Administration (FDA) has approved a new manufacturing method for the influenza vaccine called Flublok. The process for Flublok does not use eggs or live influenza virus but rapidly replicates large quantities of a protein component of influenza called *hemagglutinin*—the active ingredient in all inactivated influenza vaccines that is essential for entry of the virus into cells in the body. This improvement in manufacturing will be especially important in years when a new strain of influenza is circulating and a vaccine must be produced quickly. Flublok is approved for the prevention of seasonal influenza in adults 18 to 49 years of age (FDA, 2013).

Although the effectiveness of the vaccine varies from year to year, in general the vaccine reduces the risk of illness from flu by 50% to 60% overall. The vaccine is especially advantageous in preventing hospitalization for children, those with diabetes or pulmonary disease, and those over the age of 50. It also reduces the risk of some cardiac events in those with heart disease and reduces the risk of illness in babies born to mothers who were vaccinated during pregnancy (CDC, 2016f).

Human Papillomavirus Vaccine

Vaccines that reduce the risk of human papillomavirus (HPV), a sexually transmitted infection (STI), have been approved since 2006. HPV is the most prevalent of all sexually transmitted viruses and is the principal cause of cervical cancer (CDC, 2016g) (see Chapter 57).

Vaccination at age 11 or 12 is recommended for both males and females. The vaccines are given in a 3-dose series. They are not recommended for those with a history of hypersensitivity to any vaccine component, those with a history of anaphylactic latex allergy, or for women who are pregnant (Petrosky, Bocchini, Hariri, et al., 2015).

Planning for a Pandemic

A pandemic is a global outbreak of a disease. For example, the H1N1 (named for the characteristics of the viral surface proteins hemagglutinin and neuraminidase) pandemic of 2009 caused between 43 and 89 million infections and between 9,000 and 18,000 influenza-related deaths in the United States (U.S. Department of Health and Human Services [HHS], 2016). Unlike typical years, when more than 90% of deaths occur in those older than 65 years, during the pandemic period, most deaths occurred in those younger than 65 years (HHS, 2016).

Subtypes of influenza viruses have pandemic potential because they constantly change within animals and secondarily within humans. As a result of these changes, essentially new viruses can "emerge" and can expose entire populations who are immunologically unprotected.

Influenza pandemics are likely to be more catastrophic than other anticipated public health problems because they last longer than other emergency events, often occur in "waves," deplete the available health care workforce, and reduce the supply of medical equipment because of their widespread nature. The frequency and severity of pandemics cannot be accurately predicted, but models suggest that a medium-intensity pandemic could quickly overwhelm the existing health care infrastructure. The CDC encourages all health care institutions to have a pandemic plan and to test the components of the plan regularly.

Avian influenza (bird flu) is an infection caused by influenza viruses that chiefly infect birds and poultry. The highly pathogenic Asian avian influenza A (HPAI) H5N1 strain is of particular concern. It has caused a number of outbreaks in poultry since 2003, and the problem is ongoing; flocks of migratory birds have rapidly disseminated the virus throughout much of the world. Although many avian influenza viruses are natural and nonpathogenic in birds, H5N1 is unusual because of its high mortality rate in birds and because it has shown a limited ability to be transmitted from a bird source to mammals, including humans.

Scientists are especially concerned that HPAI may change and become easily transmitted from human to human. If this strain were easily transmissible to humans, it would be likely to cause a severe pandemic because the human population has no immunity to the virus (CDC, 2016h).

The symptoms associated with HPAI in humans have ranged from the symptoms typically seen with seasonal influenza (cough, fever, and muscle aches) to severe pneumonia and multiorgan failure. Influenza antiviral therapy (i.e., oseltamivir [Tamiflu] and zanamivir [Relenza]) and a vaccine for HPAI are stockpiled by the U.S. government to reduce the risk of a pandemic if HPAI were to begin transmitting easily between people. Simple infection control strategies using careful hand hygiene and masks will be especially important in an avian influenza pandemic. Health departments throughout the country are also planning how to implement isolation programs to keep people who are symptomatic away from schools and workplaces (CDC, 2016h).

Home-Based Care of the Patient With an Infectious Disease

The nurse who cares for the patient with an infectious disease in the home should provide information about infection risk prevention to the patient, the family, and the caregiver (see Chart 71-4). Recognizing that a health history may not identify all active or latent infections, the caregiver should carefully follow standard precautions in the home. The nurse should establish a work environment that facilitates hand hygiene and aseptic technique.

Family caregivers should receive an annual influenza vaccine. This is especially true if the caregiver or the patient is older than 50 years, has underlying cardiac or pulmonary disease, or has underlying immunosuppression.

Patients requiring home care are often people with immunosuppression from underlying conditions, such as human immune deficiency virus (HIV) infection or cancer, or those who have treatment-induced immunosuppression, as occurs with many antineoplastic agents. Careful assessment for signs of infection is important.

Reducing Risk to the Patient

Equipment Care

All caregivers must pay careful attention to disinfection and aseptic technique while using medical equipment. Catheter-related sepsis should be suspected in a patient who has unexplained fever, redness, swelling, and drainage around a vascular catheter insertion site. Indwelling urinary catheters should be discontinued whenever possible, because each day of use increases the risk of infection. The nurse should promptly report signs of urinary tract infection or generalized sepsis to the patient's primary provider.

 Patient Education

When assessing the risk of infection in the home environment of the patient who is immunosuppressed, it is important to realize that intrinsic colonizing bacteria and latent viral infections present a greater risk than do extrinsic environmental contaminants. The nurse should reassure the patient and family that their home needs to be clean but not sterile. Family members seldom need to use masks, gowns, or other elements of personal protective equipment. Commonsense approaches to cleanliness and risk reduction are helpful.

Chart 71-4 **HOME CARE CHECKLIST**
Prevention of Infection in the Home Care Setting

At the completion of education, the patient and/or caregiver will be able to:

- State the impact of infectious disease and treatment on physiologic functioning, ADLs, IADLs, roles, relationships, and spirituality.
- State the need for infection risk prevention for the patient (preventing recurrence or new infections) caregivers, and family in the home.
  - Verbalize the route of transmission for agent of infection.
- State the purpose, dose, route, schedule, side effects, and precautions for prescribed medications.
  - Adhere to antibiotic regimen (patient) or completion of vaccination series (patient and caregiver).
- State how to contact all members of the treatment team (e.g., health care providers, home care professionals, and durable medical equipment and supply vendor).
- State changes in lifestyle (e.g., diet, activity) or home environment necessary to decrease risk for infection.
  - Perform satisfactory hand hygiene technique, oral hygiene, total body hygiene, and maintain skin integrity (patient).
  - Ensure thorough hand hygiene (alcohol-based disinfectant or handwashing) after care (family/caregiver)
  - Avoid contact with someone who has a known infectious disease.
  - Cook all foods thoroughly and store meat products separate from other food groups.
  - Use separate eating utensils and towels.

- Demonstrate aseptic technique in the care of technical equipment such as IV catheter and indwelling urinary catheter.
- Identify signs and symptoms of infection to report to the primary provider, such as fever; chills; wet or dry cough; breathing problems; white patches in the mouth; swollen glands; nausea; vomiting; persistent abdominal pain; persistent diarrhea; problems with urination or changes in the character of the urine; red, swollen, or draining wounds; sores or lesions on the body; persistent vaginal discharge with or without itching; and severe fatigue.
- Demonstrate how to monitor for signs of infection.
- Describe to whom, how, and when to report signs of infection.
- Describe appropriate actions to take should infection occur.
- Relate how to reach primary provider with questions or complications.
- State time and date of follow-up medical appointments, therapy, and testing.
- Identify sources of support (e.g., friends, relatives, faith community, support groups, caregiver support).
- Identify the need for health-promotion, disease prevention, and screening activities

Resources

See Chapter 33, Chart 33-7 Home Care Checklist: The Patient at Risk for Infection for additional information.

ADL, activities of daily living; IADL, independent activities of daily living; IV, intravenous.

For patients with neutropenia or T-cell dysfunction (e.g., patients with acquired immune deficiency syndrome [AIDS]), it is wise to restrict visits of people with potentially contagious illnesses. The patient who is immunosuppressed is vulnerable to acquiring bacterial infection with enteric pathogens from food; therefore, family members should be reminded about the need to follow recommendations for hygiene, storage, and safe cooking times and temperatures.

Reducing Risk to Household Members

Establishing reasonable barriers to infection transmission in the household is an important part of home care. The route of transmission of the organism in question must first be determined. The nurse can then educate household members about strategies to reduce their risk of becoming infected. If the patient has active pulmonary TB, the public health department should be contacted to provide screening and treatment for family members. If the patient has shingles (herpes zoster), family members who have had varicella vaccine or who have previously had chickenpox are considered immune and need no precautions. However, if a family member is immunosuppressed or otherwise susceptible to varicella, maintaining physical separation is an important strategy during the time when the patient has draining lesions. When the patient is infected with enteric organisms, the family should be reassured that common household disinfectants are effective in controlling environmental contamination.

Family members who assist in the care of a patient with a blood-borne infection such as HIV or hepatitis C can prevent transmission by carefully handling any sharp objects that are contaminated with blood. Family education may include discussion about the need for caution when shaving the patient; performing dressing changes; or administering any IV, intramuscular, or subcutaneous medication. To collect and dispose of used needles, syringes, and vascular access equipment, the family should use containers designed for sharps disposal. With the exception of TB, the opportunistic infections associated with AIDS do not usually pose a risk to the healthy family member. Family members should be reassured that dishes are safe to use after being washed with hot water and that linens and clothing are safe to use after being washed in a hot water cycle.

Nursing Management

Assessment

Symptoms of infectious diseases vary significantly between and within diseases. For some infections, visible symptoms such as rash, redness, or swelling provide early warnings of infection. In other infections, such as TB and HIV, asymptomatic latency is prolonged, and infection must be determined through diagnostic procedures.

The history is obtained to establish the likelihood and probable source of infection as well as the degree of associated pathology and symptoms. The patient's previous medical record is reviewed when possible. Chart 71-5 outlines questions the nurse should ask when obtaining a health history.

Because infection may occur in any body system, physical examination may reveal signs of infection at any body site. Generalized signs of chronic infection may include significant

Chart 71-5

ASSESSMENT

Assessing for Infectious Disease

The nurse should ask the patient the following questions:
- Do you have a history of previous or recurrent infections?
- Have you had fever? How high has your temperature been? Is your temperature constant, or does it rise and fall? Has fever been associated with chills? Have you taken any medication to relieve fever?
- Do you have a cough? Is the cough chronic or acute? Is it associated with shortness of breath? Does the cough produce sputum? Is the sputum bloody? Have you had a tuberculin skin test recently? If so, what were the results? Have you been given isoniazid (INH) prophylaxis for tuberculosis (TB) infection? Have you been treated for TB in the past?
- Do you have pain? Where is the pain? What is the nature of the pain? Do you have a sore throat, headache, myalgias, or arthralgias? Is there pain on urination or other activity?
- Do you have any swelling? Is there drainage associated with the swelling? Is the swollen area warm to the touch?
- Do you have a draining lesion? Is the drainage associated with trauma or a previous procedure? Is the drainage pus or clear? Does the drainage have an odor?
- Do you have diarrhea, vomiting, or abdominal pain?
- Do you have a rash? What is the nature of the rash—is it flat, raised, red, crusted, weeping or lacelike? Have you taken medications that could have induced the rash? Have you been exposed to another person with an identified infectious disease or rash?
- What is your vaccination history? Are your immunizations up to date?
- Have you had an insect or animal bite? Have you had an animal scratch or other exposure to pets, farm animals, or experimental animals?
- What medications do you use? Have you taken antibiotic agents recently or long term? Are you being treated with corticosteroids, immunosuppressive agents, or chemotherapy?
- Have you been treated for other infectious diseases in the past? Have you been hospitalized for infectious diseases?
- If sexual history is pertinent: Have you had sexual exposure to another person with a known sexually transmitted infection (STI)? Have you been treated for STIs in the past? Are you pregnant, or have you recently been pregnant? Have you been tested for human immune deficiency virus?
- Have you traveled abroad, including developing countries? What was the immunization or antimicrobial prophylaxis used for protection while you were traveling?
- What is your occupation? What are your recreational activities? Hobbies?

weight loss or pallor associated with anemia of chronic diseases. Acute infection may manifest with fever, chills, lymphadenopathy, or rash. Localized signs vary by source of infection. Purulent drainage, pain, edema, and redness are strongly associated with localized infection. Cough and shortness of breath may be caused by influenza, pneumonia, or TB, as well as many noninfectious causes.

Nursing Interventions
Preventing Infection Transmission

Preventing the spread of infection requires an understanding of the usual routes of transmission of the organism. The patient who is hospitalized may pose a contagious risk to others if the disease is easily spread (such as *C. difficile*) or is spread through an airborne route (such as TB). In these situations, strict adherence to isolation measures is important to reduce the opportunity for spread. Preventing transmission of organisms from patient to patient requires participation of all members of the health care team. Transmission of organisms on the hands and gloves of health care workers remains a common source of cross-infection in both inpatient and outpatient settings.

 Quality and Safety Nursing Alert

It is imperative that nurses disinfect their hands before and after contact with patients and after performing a potentially hand-contaminating activity. Hands must be disinfected each time gloves are removed.

 Educating About the Infectious Process

Interruption of transmission requires diagnosis and patient adherence with the treatment regimen. The nurse's role is to educate the patient and, in some situations, to report the case to public health officials for contact tracing and verification of follow-up.

The nurse must stress the importance of immunization to parents of young children and to others for whom vaccines are recommended, such as patients who are older, are immunosuppressed, or have chronic illnesses or disabilities. Nurses should recognize their personal responsibility to receive the hepatitis B vaccine and an annual influenza vaccine to reduce potential transmission to themselves and vulnerable patient groups.

Infectious diseases often seem mysterious and frequently are socially stigmatizing. Patient education requires empathy and sensitivity.

Controlling Fever and Accompanying Discomforts

Fever must always be investigated to determine whether infection is the source. Evidence indicates that fever, mediated by the hypothalamus, may potentiate beneficial functions in the syndrome of reactions known as *acute-phase reaction*. These reactions include changes in liver protein synthesis; alterations in serum metals, such as iron; and increased production of certain classes of white blood cells and other cells of the immune system (Grossman & Porth, 2014). Most fevers are physiologically controlled so that the temperature remains below 41°C (105.8°F). However, severe fever, as often occurs with meningococcal meningitis, may cause complications. Even milder fevers accompanied by fatigue, chills, and diaphoresis are often uncomfortable for the patient. Whether fever is treated or untreated, adequate fluid intake is important during febrile episodes.

 Quality and Safety Nursing Alert

Because fever offers clues about infection severity and the success of antibiotic therapy, outpatients with fever should be instructed to obtain accurate temperature readings. Frequently, family caregivers know that a patient has warm skin but do not take a temperature reading. Body temperature information can be very helpful in adjusting therapy or in reevaluating a preliminary diagnosis.

Monitoring and Managing Potential Complications

The patient with a rapidly progressive infectious disease should have vital signs and level of consciousness closely monitored. X-ray findings and microbiologic, immunologic, hematologic, cytologic, and parasitologic laboratory values must be interpreted in the context of other clinical findings to assess the course of the infectious disease.

Antibiotic therapy is frequently complex, and modifications are necessary because of drug susceptibility test results and disease progression. To rapidly ensure therapeutic blood levels, antibiotic therapy should be initiated as soon as it is prescribed rather than waiting until routine medication scheduling times. Chart 71-6 describes nursing interventions for infection.

Diarrheal Diseases

In the United States, the epidemiology of diarrheal diseases changes constantly. Water disinfection, pasteurization, and appropriate food packaging have decreased the incidence of diseases such as typhoid and cholera. However, importation of foreign foods, environmental and ecologic changes, and changes in diagnostic test modalities have led to recognition of new trends and outbreaks.

Transmission

The portal of entry of all diarrheal pathogens is oral ingestion. Although food is far from sterile, the high acidity of the stomach and the antibody-producing cells of the small bowel generally decrease the potential of pathogens. Infection can occur when the infectious dose is high enough or if the food neutralizes the acidic environment. Decreased gastric acidity with disruption of normal bowel flora (as occurs after surgery), the use of antimicrobial agents, and AIDS all decrease intestinal defenses.

Causes

There are many bacterial, viral, and parasitic causes of diarrheal diseases. Common causes of bacterial infection include *Campylobacter*, *Salmonella*, *Shigella*, and *E. coli*. The most significant viral causes of diarrhea are *Rotavirus* and *Calicivirus* (often called *Norovirus*), a virus associated with outbreaks in long-term care facilities and cruise ships (CDC, 2016j). Parasitic infections of importance include *Giardia* and *Cryptosporidium* species and *Entamoeba histolytica*.

Campylobacter Infections

Campylobacter species are among the most frequent causes of diarrheal disease in the United States (CDC, 2014b). The bacterium, which is abundant in animal foods, is especially common in poultry but can also be found in beef and pork. Direct person-to-person transmission appears to be less common than it is for other enteric pathogens, such as *Shigella*.

Cooking and storing food at appropriate temperatures protect against *Campylobacter*. It is important that kitchen utensils used in meat preparation be kept away from other food to prevent *Campylobacter* transmission (CDC, 2014b).

After a person is infected, the bacterium directly attacks the lumen of the intestine and may cause disease through enterotoxin release. Symptoms can range from mild abdominal

(text continued on page 2144)

NURSING DIAGNOSIS: Risk for infection
GOAL: Prevention of infection

Nursing Interventions	Rationale	Expected Outcomes
1. Prevent patient-to-patient infection spread.	1. Organisms that are spread through an airborne route or are very contagious through direct contact can be transmitted in a health care setting.	• No evidence of patient-to-patient transmission of infection • No evidence of transmission via health care workers • No occupationally acquired infections in nurses and other health care workers • No evidence of transmission due to contaminated equipment • Absence of bacteremia and sepsis • Absence of urinary tract infections • Absence of pneumonia
a. Provide isolation according to CDC guidelines and standard precautions.	a. CDC isolation strategies are developed to reduce the likelihood of transmission from patient to patient.	
b. Ensure that patients with airborne infections remain in private rooms during hospital stay. If they must leave their rooms, arrangements should be made to decrease the likelihood of contact with other patients. Rooms should be ventilated according to CDC criteria. Personal protective equipment in the form of N95 respirators should be worn as indicated.	b. Engineering controls are important in the prevention of airborne diseases. Influenza vaccine safely reduces risk of illness associated with this highly communicable, and frequently virulent, condition. The N95 respirator is the minimal level of personal protection for tuberculosis (TB) control. The "N" indicates the filter resistance to oil aerosols; the "95" indicates that the respirator has 95% effectiveness in filtering test particles.	
c. Ensure that patients with highly transmissible, nonairborne organisms such as *Clostridium difficile* and *Shigella* species are physically separated from other patients if hygiene or institutional policy dictates.	c. Increased prevention strategies are needed when the organism has high epidemic potential.	
2. Prevent health care workers' transfer of organisms from patient to patient.	2. Transfer of organisms on the hands of health care workers is a common route of transmission. Hospital organisms colonizing the hands of health care workers may be virulent.	
a. Perform hand hygiene (by handwashing or by using alcohol-based solution) consistently and thoroughly, disinfecting hands before and after each patient contact, and after procedures that offer contamination risk while caring for an individual patient.	a. Hand hygiene is important in reducing transient flora on outer epidermal layers of skin. Alcohol-based hand disinfectants are effective methods to reduce transient flora.	
b. Use gloves when handling any body fluid from any patient. Change gloves between patient care activities, and disinfect hands after gloves are removed.	b. Gloves provide effective barrier protection. Gloves quickly become contaminated and then become a potential vehicle for the transfer of organisms between patients. Microflora on hands are likely to proliferate while gloves are worn.	
c. Avoid wearing artificial fingernails or extenders when providing patient care. Keep natural nails less than ¼ inch long and remove nail polish when chipped.	c. Artificial fingernails and extenders harbor microorganisms.	
d. Monitor the hand hygiene and glove use behaviors of health care professionals caring for the patient.	d. Poor adherence to hand hygiene among health care workers has been well documented and should be anticipated. It is important for the nurse (as the patient's advocate) to communicate protective behavior.	

(continued on page 2140)

Chart 71-6

PLAN OF NURSING CARE (Continued)

Care of the Patient With an Infectious Disease

Nursing Interventions	Rationale	Expected Outcomes
3. Prevent transmission of infection from patient to health care worker.	**3.** Health care workers may acquire infections occupationally due to close contact with patients.	
a. Avoid risk of infection with TB.	**a.** The most important element in the reduction of TB is early identification. Many of the symptoms of TB are subtle and may be first observed by the nurse who has prolonged contact with the patient.	
(1) Participate in the early identification of patients with active disease. Patients will be asked about risk factors, symptoms, previous exposure, and status of tuberculin skin test or other rapid tests.	(1) Identification of patients at risk can help to prevent exposure.	
(2) Expedite diagnostic workup with chest x-ray, sputum analysis for organisms, and administration of TB testing as appropriate.	(2) Confirmation of diagnosis facilitates development of an appropriate treatment plan, including prevention of spread of infection.	
(3) Maintain engineering controls. Keep the patient in a private room with a closed door.	(3) Confining airflow to the immediate vicinity of the patient and exhausting air to the outside reduces the likelihood of transmission to health care workers in areas outside of the patient room.	
(4) Use protection in isolation room or when participating in procedures that are likely to generate cough, such as suctioning, intubation, or administering nebulized medications.	(4) N95 respirators are designed to reduce health care workers' risk.	
b. Avoid risk of transmission of blood-borne diseases such as hepatitis B, hepatitis C, and the human immune deficiency virus.	**b.** Health care workers can contract blood-borne diseases via percutaneous injury such as needlestick or by contact with blood or body fluids to mucous membranes, such as eyes and mouth.	
(1) Get hepatitis B vaccination.	(1) Hepatitis B vaccine should be given to reduce risk from this contagious blood-borne virus.	
(2) Use standard precautions as defined by the CDC (see Chapter 36, Chart 36-5).	(2) Standard precautions are based on the recognition that most patients are not identified as infected by physical assessment or history taking. Health care workers must assume that all patients may be infected with blood-borne or other infection and must use barrier precautions appropriately for *all* patients.	
(3) Use "needleless" syringes and other injury-preventing devices.	(3) The use of injury-preventing devices decreases risk of transmission of blood-borne diseases.	
c. Avoid risk of airborne diseases. (1) Receive influenza vaccination annually. (2) Get vaccinated or produce proof of immunity to measles, mumps, rubella, and varicella.	**c.** Influenza vaccine is recommended for health care workers to reduce the likelihood of transmission in health care settings where patients who are immunocompromised can be exposed.	

Chart 71-6

PLAN OF NURSING CARE (Continued)

Care of the Patient With an Infectious Disease

Nursing Interventions	Rationale	Expected Outcomes
4. Prevent patient exposure to contaminated medical equipment. a. Ensure that equipment being inserted through intact skin is sterilized between patient uses. b. Ensure that equipment that has contact with mucous membranes is sterilized or receives "high-level disinfection" between patient uses. c. Ensure that equipment used against intact skin is thoroughly cleaned and receives "low-level disinfection" between patient uses. 5. Follow established guidelines for the routine removal and replacement of IV devices. 6. Remove urinary catheters at the earliest time possible. 7. Remove endotracheal and nasogastric tubes as soon as possible.	4. Technologic advances offer increased opportunity for invasive procedures. Equipment may be complex and difficult to clean. a. Sterilization renders equipment free of all microorganisms. b. High-level disinfection renders an object free of all microorganisms with the possible exception of spore-producing organisms. c. The disinfection goal for low-level disinfection is to reduce the load of microorganisms to a level that is not threatening to the host with intact skin. 5. Indwelling IV devices can serve as a conduit for organisms to migrate into the bloodstream. 6. The risk of urinary tract infections is directly proportional to the length of time that a urinary catheter remains in place. 7. The risk for pneumonia is increased as the use of indwelling equipment increases.	

NURSING DIAGNOSIS: Knowledge deficit about disease, cause of infection, and preventive measures
GOAL: Acquisition of knowledge about the infectious process

Nursing Interventions	Rationale	Expected Outcomes
1. Listen carefully to what the patient says about illness and previous treatment. 2. Provide pertinent explanations about: a. Organism and route of transmission b. Treatment goals c. Follow-up schedule d. Prevention of transmission to others 3. Allow opportunities for questions and discussions. 4. Educate the patient and family about: a. Prophylaxis or immunization, if recommended b. Community resources, if necessary c. Means of preventing transmission within the home	1. Listening facilitates detection of misunderstanding and misinformation and provides opportunity for education. 2. Knowledge about specific diagnoses and treatments may promote adherence. 3. The patient's questions indicate issues that need clarification. 4. Understanding of the risks and precautions associated with an infectious disease may reduce the opportunity for further spread.	• Patient actively participates in treatment • Patient adheres to infection control measures

NURSING DIAGNOSIS: Risk for imbalanced body temperature (fever) related to the presence of infection
GOAL: Patient comfort and return of normal temperature

Nursing Interventions	Rationale	Expected Outcomes
1. Monitor temperature, pulse, and respirations at regular intervals. 2. Administer antipyretic agents as prescribed.	1. Graph fever curve to help evaluate when fever occurs, how long it lasts, and whether it responds to therapy. 2. Prompt treatment will improve outcomes.	• Body temperature within normal limits • Maintenance of fluid and electrolyte balance • Patient comfortable

(continued on page 2142)

Chart 71-6

PLAN OF NURSING CARE (Continued)

Care of the Patient With an Infectious Disease

COLLABORATIVE PROBLEMS: Among potential complications are bacteremia or sepsis, septic shock, dehydration, abscess formation, endocarditis, infectious disease–related cancers, and infertility

GOAL: Absence of complications

Nursing Interventions	Rationale	Expected Outcomes
Bacteremia, Sepsis		
1. Monitor patient for evidence of infection at any location.	1. Vigilance for bacterial or fungal infection at any site promotes early recognition and treatment and reduces the likelihood of secondary infections.	• No episode of infection • Effective treatment for identified bacterial and fungal infections without progression to bloodstream infection
2. Assess treatment effectiveness of all identified infections.	2. The natural course of some infections may be rapid unless antibiotic agents are given promptly.	• Early improvement in septic course
3. Administer antibiotic agents as prescribed with first dose given at the earliest time possible.	3. Prompt treatment will improve outcomes.	
Septic Shock		

1. Routinely, and as warranted, monitor vital signs for patients with recognized infections and for patients who are severely immunosuppressed at risk for shock. In particular, be alert to signs of:
a. Fever
b. Tachycardia (>90 bpm)
c. Tachypnea (>20 breaths/min)
d. Evidence of decreased perfusion or dysfunction of vital organs in the form of:
  (1) Change in mental status
  (2) Hypoxemia as measured by arterial blood gases
  (3) Elevated lactate levels
  (4) Urine output (<0.5 mL/kg/hr)
	1. Early recognition of the signs and prompt treatment of impending shock may reduce the associated severity or mortality.	• Absence of symptoms of septic shock
		• Hemodynamic and respiratory status within normal range

2. Administer antibiotic agents, fluid replacement, vasopressors, and oxygen as prescribed.	2. Therapeutic maintenance of hemodynamic and respiratory status is necessary until infection is effectively treated with an antimicrobial regimen.	
Dehydration		
1. Assess for dehydration (thirst, dryness of mucous membranes, loss of skin turgor, reduced peripheral pulses, urine output <0.5 mL/kg/hr).	1. Signs of dehydration provide a basis for fluid replacement and suggest possible further complications of circulatory collapse.	• Attains fluid balance (output approximates intake: body weight unchanged) • Mucous membranes appear moist; normal skin turgor • Serum electrolytes within normal limits
2. Monitor weight.	2. Rapid changes in weight indicate fluid volume changes.	
3. Monitor intake and output and serum electrolyte levels.	3. Dehydration produces a deficit in some electrolytes. Decreased urine production may indicate hypovolemia and decreased renal perfusion.	
4. Replace fluids as needed. If the patient can tolerate oral fluids, offer fluids every 2–4 hours. Administer IV fluids as prescribed.	4. When possible, oral hydration is preferable because the patient can select the beverage, control the rate and interval of replacement, and care for self at home. In addition, the risks associated with vascular devices are avoided. If IV fluid is required, IV solutions are selected to facilitate intestinal reabsorption of fluid and electrolytes.	

Chart 71-6

PLAN OF NURSING CARE (Continued)
Care of the Patient With an Infectious Disease

Nursing Interventions	Rationale	Expected Outcomes
Abscess Formation		
1. Assess vascular access sites, wound sites, pressure ulcers, and other appropriate sites for apparent collections of purulent material.	1. Collections of purulent material often require drainage before antimicrobial therapy is effective.	• Absence of abscess • Takes antibiotic agents as prescribed

2. Assess the patient who has had abdominal surgery or trauma to abdominal area for localized signs of intra-abdominal abscess. These signs include:
  a. Low-grade fever
  b. Elevated peripheral white blood cell count
  c. Localized pain
  d. Abdominal tenderness
  e. Visible or palpable mass
  f. Postoperative diarrhea
  g. GI bleeding
	2. Intra-abdominal abscess formation is most common following traumatic or surgical disruption of the GI tract. Signs are often initially subtle.	

3. Assess patient who has had percutaneous abscess drainage to determine whether drainage has been successful. Be alert to all of the previously mentioned signs and symptoms.	3. After percutaneous drainage, recurrent or persistent signs of abscess may indicate the need for surgical treatment.	
4. Administer antibiotic agents as prescribed.	4. Antibiotic agents, along with drainage, are the most important elements of intra-abdominal abscess management.	
Endocarditis		
Prevention		

1. Educate patients with the following conditions about the importance of antibiotic prophylaxis for events and procedures that may introduce the risk of endocarditis:
  a. Valvular disease
  b. Congenital heart disease
  c. Intracardiac prosthesis
  d. Previous endocarditis
	1. Patients with underlying valvular disease and other cardiac abnormalities are at increased risk for "seeding" of the cardiac valves during procedures that can cause bacteremia.	• Informs health care professionals of cardiac conditions that require antibiotic prophylaxis before invasive procedures
		• Takes prophylactic antibiotics as prescribed

Management		
1. Obtain blood cultures as prescribed; carefully record results. Note persistent bloodstream infections with a particular organism.	1. A definitive diagnosis of endocarditis requires blood culture confirmation.	• Endocarditis is diagnosed, treated, and cured
2. Obtain a detailed history about the duration of fever in the absence of well-recognized cause.	2. Endocarditis should be suspected in patients who report an unexplained fever of more than 1 week's duration.	
3. Administer IV antibiotic therapy at prescribed time schedule.	3. IV therapy is usually required for cure. The goal of therapy is complete eradication of all organisms. Careful adherence to following the scheduled administration is therefore essential.	

Infectious Disease–Related Cancers and Infertility

These potential complications of infectious diseases are prevented by primary avoidance of infection. Management of them is directed toward treating each of them as a noninfectious entity. For example, the management of cancer secondary to hepatitis B is handled as an oncology issue, not as an infectious disease issue.

CDC, Centers for Disease Control and Prevention; GI, gastrointestinal; IV, intravenous; TB, tuberculosis.

cramping and minimal diarrhea to severe disease with profuse watery bloody diarrhea and debilitating abdominal cramping. Antimicrobial therapy is recommended only for patients who are seriously ill (CDC, 2016c).

Salmonella Infection

Salmonella is a gram-negative bacillus with many species, including the very pathogenic *Salmonella typhi* (i.e., typhoid fever). Of the nontyphi species, most organisms are prevalent in animal food sources. Annually in the United States, *Salmonella* species contaminate approximately 2.2 million eggs (1 in 20,000 eggs) and one in eight chickens raised as meat (CDC, 2014b). *Salmonella* outbreaks have also been associated with contaminated sprouts, fruits, and vegetables.

Variable symptoms are associated with *Salmonella* species infection, including an asymptomatic carrier state, gastroenteritis, and systemic infection. Diarrhea with gastroenteritis is common. Disseminated disease and bacteremia, sometimes accompanied by diarrhea, occur less often.

The person with *Salmonella*-caused diarrhea can on rare occasions be a source of transmission to others. The importance of good hygiene should be emphasized, and health care workers should use special care when handling bedpans, stool specimens, or other objects that may be contaminated with feces. Hand hygiene is imperative after any contact with a person with *Salmonella* diarrhea. Although patients with systemic salmonellosis require antimicrobial therapy, those with gastroenteritis only are not usually treated, because antibiotic use may increase the period of time that the patient carries the bacteria while not improving the clinical outcome.

Shigella Infection

The *Shigella* species is a gram-negative organism that invades the lumen of the intestine and causes disease and severe watery (possibly bloody) diarrhea. *Shigella* species are spread through the fecal–oral route, with easy transmission from one person to another. *Shigella* exhibits high levels of **virulence** (degree of pathogenicity of an organism); infection with a very small number of organisms can cause disease. Because transmission occurs easily with improper hygiene, it is not surprising that *Shigella* organisms disproportionately affect pediatric populations. Disease in the very young may infrequently be complicated by pulmonary or neurologic symptoms.

Antimicrobial therapy should be instituted early. Frequently, initial therapy choices must be altered when final microbiologic testing reveals the organism's sensitivity.

Escherichia coli

E. coli is the most common aerobic organism colonizing the large bowel. When *E. coli* bacteria are cultured from fecal specimens, the results usually reflect normal flora. However, certain strains of *E. coli* with increased virulence have been responsible for significant outbreaks of diarrheal disease in recent years. These stronger pathologic strains are subgrouped as Shiga toxin–producing *Escherichia coli* (STEC) because of their production of enterotoxins. STEC strains often cause choleralike disease, with rapid, severe dehydration and an increased risk of death.

Several outbreaks of an *E. coli* STEC species, 0157:H7, have been linked to the ingestion of undercooked beef and to vegetables that have been contaminated by animal wastewater (CDC, 2015a). This bacterium lives in the intestines of cattle and can be introduced into meat at the time of slaughter. Prevention of disease from STEC strains is aimed at educating the public to cook ground beef thoroughly (i.e., until the juices run clear) (CDC, 2016i).

Calicivirus (Norwalklike Virus; Norovirus)

Calicivirus, which is often referred to as the Norwalklike virus or the *Norovirus*, is the most common cause of food-borne illness and gastroenteritis in the United States. Onset of illness is usually acute, with vomiting and watery diarrhea that generally last for approximately 2 days. Most outbreaks occur between November and April. Dehydration is the most common complication. This agent has been associated with important diarrheal outbreaks in schools, day care centers, cruise ships, long-term care facilities, and hospitals.

Calicivirus is transmitted easily from person to person by direct contact and by ingesting contaminated food. Waterborne outbreaks have been associated with sewage-contaminated wells and contaminated swimming pools. Although people with *Calicivirus* infection typically recover within 2 to 3 days, they may continue to transmit the virus to others for approximately 2 more weeks.

Caliciviruses can withstand environmental extremes of heat or cold and are resistant to chemical disinfection, which are significant reasons for their epidemic potential. Control of *Calicivirus* in health care facilities requires a coordinated program with decisions about isolation, environmental disinfection, diagnosis, and coordination with public health officials. Contact precautions should be used when caring for patients with incontinence and during outbreaks of the virus. Workers should wear masks if they are cleaning heavily soiled areas or caring for a patient who is actively vomiting. A number of disinfectants have U.S. Environmental Protection Agency (EPA) approval based on specific effectiveness for *Calicivirus*. However, the CDC recommends that surface disinfection be accomplished with a freshly prepared solution of 1 part bleach to 50 parts water or with the peroxygen compound Virkon-S, which has been approved for feline *Calicivirus* and may be similarly effective for human viruses (CDC, 2016j).

Giardia lamblia

Transmission of the protozoan *Giardia lamblia* occurs when food or drink is contaminated with viable cysts of the organism. People often become infected while traveling to endemic areas or by drinking contaminated water from mountain streams within the United States. The organism can be transmitted by close contact, such as occurs in day care settings. Transmission by sexual contact has also been documented.

Frequently, the infection goes unnoticed. Infection is often recognized more easily in children than in adults. In extreme cases, the patient may experience abdominal pain and chronic diarrhea, usually described as containing mucus and fat but not blood. Microscopic examination of stool specimens reveals the trophozoite or cyst stages of the parasitic life cycle.

Metronidazole (Flagyl) is recommended by the CDC to treat *Giardia* (Comerford, 2015). Patients with *Giardia* infections should be instructed that the organism can be easily transmitted in family or group settings. Personal hygiene measures should be reinforced, and those who travel or camp where water is not treated and filtered should be advised to avoid local water supplies unless water is purified before drinking or using it in cooking.

Vibrio Cholerae

Cholera is rare in the United States. The causative organism is transmitted by contaminated food or water. Cases in the United States have been from contaminated shellfish found in the Gulf of Mexico or from contaminated shellfish brought into the United States by visitors. Cholera causes disease with a very rapid onset of copious diarrhea in which up to 1 L of fluid per hour can be lost. Dehydration, with subsequent cardiopulmonary collapse, may cause rapid progression from onset of signs and symptoms to death. Rehydration efforts should be vigorous and sustained. If oral rehydration cannot be accomplished, the patient needs IV therapy.

Cholera should be suspected in patients who have watery diarrhea after eating shellfish harvested from the Gulf of Mexico. Confirmation of the causative organism can be made by stool culture. It is imperative that all cases are reported to local and state public health authorities.

NURSING PROCESS

The Patient With Infectious Diarrhea

Assessment

The most important element of assessment in the patient with diarrhea is to determine hydration status. The goal of rehydration is to correct the dehydration. Assessment includes evaluation for thirst, dryness of oral mucous membranes, sunken eyes, a weakened pulse, and loss of skin turgor. Careful observation for these signs is especially important in cases of rapidly dehydrating diseases (most notably cholera) and in younger children.

Intake and output measurements are crucial in determining fluid balance. Liquid stool should be measured and recorded, along with the frequency of stools. It is important to note the consistency and appearance of stool as key indicators of the type and severity of the diarrheal disease. The presence of mucus or blood should also be documented.

When conducting a health history, the nurse asks if the patient has recently traveled, if the patient is being treated with antibiotic medications, if the patient has been in contact with anyone who has recently had diarrheal disease, and what the patient has recently eaten. Frequently, patients attribute the most recent meal eaten as the cause of symptoms. However, the incubation period for most diarrheal conditions is longer than the time interval between meals, and the nurse needs to get detailed information about the meal preceding the illness and about all food intake in the previous 3 to 4 days. When eliciting this kind of history, it is helpful to ask the patient to list every food tasted. The nurse also asks the patient if he or she is employed in a food preparation service, because the local public health departments should be notified about any person with infectious diarrhea who works in the food industry.

Diagnosis

NURSING DIAGNOSES

Based on the assessment data, major nursing diagnoses may include the following:
- Deficient fluid volume related to fluid lost through diarrhea
- Deficient knowledge about the infection and the risk of transmission to others

COLLABORATIVE PROBLEMS/POTENTIAL COMPLICATIONS

Potential complications may include the following:
- Bacteremia
- Hypovolemic shock

Planning and Goals

The most important goals are maintenance of fluid and electrolyte balance, increased knowledge about the disease and risk of transmission, and absence of complications.

Nursing Interventions

CORRECTING DEHYDRATION ASSOCIATED WITH DIARRHEA

The patient is assessed to determine the degree of dehydration and the amount and route of rehydration needed. Oral rehydration therapy is a strategy used to reduce the severe complications of diarrheal disease regardless of causative agent. It is inexpensive and effective for most patients, but it is often underused due to some cultural beliefs worldwide discouraging oral intake during episodes of diarrhea. The WHO and the United Nations Children's Fund (UNICEF) recommend zinc replacement and oral rehydration salts (ORS) solution for the treatment of children and adults with dehydration and electrolyte imbalance associated with cholera and other forms of diarrheal disease. The ORS formula contains (in grams per liter) sodium chloride, 2.6; glucose (anhydrous), 13.5; potassium chloride, 1.5; and trisodium citrate (dihydrate), 2.9 (WHO, 2006). Sports drinks do not replace fluid losses correctly and should not be used.

Mild Dehydration. The patient exhibits dry oral mucous membranes of the mouth and increased thirst. The rehydration goal at this level of dehydration is to deliver about 50 mL of ORS per 1 kg of weight over a 4-hour interval (WHO, 2006).

Moderate Dehydration. Common findings are sunken eyes, loss of skin turgor, increased thirst, and dry oral mucous membranes. The rehydration goal at this level of dehydration is to deliver about 100 mL/kg of ORS over 4 hours.

Severe Dehydration. The patient with severe dehydration shows signs of shock (i.e., rapid thready pulse, cyanosis, cold extremities, rapid breathing, lethargy, or coma) and should receive IV replacement until hemodynamic and mental status return to normal. When improvement is evident, the patient can be treated with ORS.

ADMINISTERING REHYDRATION THERAPY

Because diarrheal episodes are often accompanied by vomiting, rehydration and refeeding can be difficult. Oral rehydration therapy should be delivered frequently in small amounts. When patients are persistently vomiting, they often require frequent administration of fluids by spoonfuls. IV therapy is necessary for the patient who is severely dehydrated or in shock.

It is important for children and adults with acute diarrheal symptoms to maintain caloric intake. As soon as dehydration has been corrected, an age-appropriate, unrestricted diet is allowed. Recommended foods include starches, cereals, yogurt, fruits, and vegetables. Foods that are high in simple sugars, such as undiluted apple juice or gelatin, should be avoided.

INCREASING KNOWLEDGE AND PREVENTING SPREAD OF INFECTION

Public health nurses, school nurses, and others who are involved in patient education should emphasize principles of safe food preparation, with special attention to meat preparation and cooking. Ground beef should be thoroughly cooked and all meat should be maintained at temperatures below 40°F or above 140°F (CDC, 2016i). In planning events for groups of people, adequate provision for storage and reheating to temperature thresholds is important. When preparing food, it is important to use different surfaces, knives, and other equipment for meat and nonmeat items.

Diarrheal diseases discussed in this section must be reported to local or state health departments. The goal of reporting is to provide information for determining incidence trends and promptly identifying any restaurants or other food preparation establishments that have served contaminated food.

In both homes and health care delivery settings, good hygiene and principles of standard precautions should be emphasized.

MONITORING AND MANAGING POTENTIAL COMPLICATIONS

Bacteremia. E. coli, *Salmonella,* and *Shigella* are organisms that can enter the bloodstream and disseminate to other organs. Blood cultures are necessary in the patient who is acutely febrile with diarrhea. If initial smear results reveal gram-negative organisms, antibiotic therapy is instituted.

Hypovolemic Shock. Shock associated with diarrheal diseases demands accurate intake and output assessment and vigorous fluid replacement. In rare instances, patients with severe fluid imbalance require intensive care nursing support with aggressive hemodynamic monitoring (see Chapter 14).

Evaluation

Expected patient outcomes may include:
1. Attains fluid balance
   a. Output approximates intake.
   b. Mucous membranes appear moist.
   c. Skin turgor is normal.
   d. Adequate amounts of fluids and calories ingested.
   e. Absence of vomiting.
   f. Stools are of normal color and consistency.
2. Acquires knowledge and understanding about infectious diarrhea and transmission potential
   a. Takes proper precautions to prevent spread of infection to others.
   b. Describes principles and techniques of safe food storage, preparation, and cooking.
3. Absence of complications
   a. Temperature is within normal range.
   b. Blood culture reports are negative.
   c. Fluid balance is achieved.

TABLE 71-3 Sexually Transmitted Infections and Their Routes of Transmission

Sexually Transmitted Infection (STI)	Route(s) of Transmission
Chancroid, *Lymphogranuloma venereum,* and *Granuloma inguinale*	Sexual
Chlamydia	Sexual
Cytomegalovirus	Sexual, less intimate contact
Gonorrhea	Sexual, perinatal
Hepatitis B	Sexual, percutaneous, perinatal
Hepatitis C	Percutaneous, probably sexual, probably perinatal
Herpes simplex	Sexual
HIV infection/AIDS	Sexual, percutaneous, perinatal
Human papillomavirus	Sexual
Syphilis	Sexual, perinatal

HIV, human immune deficiency virus; AIDS, acquired immune deficiency virus.
Adapted from Centers for Disease Control and Prevention (CDC). (2015b). CDC fact sheet: Reported STDs in the United States. Retrieved on 10/24/16 at www.cdc.gov/std/stats14/std-trends-508.pdf

Sexually Transmitted Infections

An STI is a disease acquired through sexual contact with a person who is infected. Table 71-3 identifies STIs and their routes of transmission. Infections caused by organisms not generally considered STIs can also be transmitted during sexual contact—for example, G. *lamblia,* usually associated with contaminated water, can be transmitted through sexual exposure.

STIs are the most common infectious diseases in the United States and are epidemic in most parts of the world. Portals of entry of STI-causing microorganisms and sites of infection include the skin and mucosal linings of the urethra, cervix, vagina, rectum, and oropharynx.

Approximately 20 million Americans become infected with STIs annually. STIs have severe health consequences. In addition, they represent a financial burden estimated to be as high as $16 billion per year (CDC, 2015b).

Education about prevention of STIs includes information about risk factors and behaviors that can lead to infection. Using straightforward language and personal testimonials for targeted audiences (e.g., people who want information about protecting themselves) and conducting presentations in trusted establishments (e.g., churches, health care facilities) are recommended educational strategies. Included in this education is information about the relative value of condoms in reducing the risk of infection. The use of condoms to provide a protective barrier from transmission of STI-related organisms has been broadly promoted, especially since the recognition of HIV/AIDS. At first referred to as a method to ensure *safe sex,* the use of condoms has been shown to reduce but not eliminate the risk of transmission of HIV and other STIs. Thus, the term *safer sex* more appropriately connotes the public health message to be used when promoting the use of condoms. See Chapter 36 for most information about AIDS and HIV.

STIs provide a unique set of challenges for nurses, physicians, and public health officials. Because of perceived stigma and possible threat to emotional relationships, people with symptoms of STIs are often reluctant to seek health care in a timely fashion. STIs may progress without symptoms, and a delay in diagnosis and treatment is potentially harmful because the risk of complications for the person who is infected and the risk of transmission to others increase over time.

Infection with one STI suggests the possibility of infection with other diseases as well. After one STI is identified, diagnostic evaluation for others should be conducted. The possibility of HIV infection should be pursued when any STI is diagnosed.

Syphilis

Syphilis is an acute and chronic infectious disease caused by the spirochete *Treponema pallidum*. It is acquired through sexual contact or may be congenital in origin. The rates of primary and secondary syphilis have been on the rise in men, with a 15% increase between 2013 and 2014 (CDC, 2015b).

Stages of Syphilis

In the person who is untreated, the course of syphilis can be divided into three stages: primary, secondary, and tertiary. These stages reflect the time from infection and the clinical manifestations observed in that period and are the basis for treatment decisions.

Primary syphilis occurs 2 to 3 weeks after initial inoculation with the organism. A painless lesion at the site of infection is called a *chancre*. These lesions usually resolve spontaneously within 3 to 12 weeks, with or without treatment (Grossman & Porth, 2014).

Secondary syphilis occurs when the hematogenous spread of organisms from the original chancre leads to generalized infection. The rash of secondary syphilis occurs from 1 week to 6 months after the chancre and involves the trunk and the extremities, including the palms of the hands and the soles of the feet (Grossman & Porth, 2014). Transmission of the organism can occur through contact with these lesions. Generalized signs of infection may include lymphadenopathy, arthritis, meningitis, hair loss, fever, malaise, and weight loss.

After the secondary stage, there is a period of **latency**, when the person who is infected has no signs or symptoms of syphilis. Latency can be interrupted by a recurrence of secondary syphilis symptoms.

Tertiary syphilis is the final stage in the natural history of the disease. It is estimated that between 20% and 40% of those infected do not exhibit signs and symptoms in this final stage. Tertiary syphilis presents as a slowly progressive inflammatory disease with the potential to affect multiple organs. The most common manifestations at this level are aortitis and neurosyphilis, as evidenced by dementia, psychosis, paresis, stroke, or meningitis.

Assessment and Diagnostic Findings

Because syphilis shares symptoms with many diseases, clinical history and laboratory evaluation are important. The conclusive diagnosis of syphilis can be made by direct identification of the spirochete obtained from the chancre lesions of primary syphilis. Serologic tests used in the diagnosis of secondary and tertiary syphilis require clinical correlation in interpretation. The serologic tests are summarized as follows:

- *Nontreponemal* or *reagin tests*, such as the Venereal Disease Research Laboratory (VDRL) or the rapid plasma reagin circle test (RPR-CT), are generally used for screening and diagnosis. After adequate therapy, the test result is expected to decrease quantitatively until it is read as negative, usually about 2 years after therapy is completed.
- *Treponemal tests*, such as the fluorescent treponemal antibody absorption test (FTA-ABS) and the microhemagglutination test for *Treponema pallidum* (MHA-TP), are used to verify that the screening test did not represent a false-positive result. Positive results usually are positive for life and therefore are not appropriate to determine therapeutic effectiveness.

Medical Management

Treatment of all stages of syphilis is administration of antibiotic medications. Penicillin G benzathine is the medication of choice for early syphilis or early latent syphilis of less than 1 year's duration. It is given by intramuscular injection at a single session. Patients with late latent or latent syphilis of unknown duration should receive three injections at 1-week intervals. Patients who are allergic to penicillin are usually treated with doxycycline (Adoxa). The patient treated with penicillin is monitored for 30 minutes after the injection to observe for a possible allergic reaction.

Treatment guidelines established by the CDC are updated on a regular basis. Recommendations provide special guidelines for treatment in the setting of pregnancy, allergy, HIV infection, pediatric infection, congenital infection, and neurosyphilis (CDC, 2015c).

Nursing Management

Syphilis is a reportable communicable disease. In any health care facility, a mechanism must be in place to ensure that all patients who are diagnosed are reported to the state or local public health department to ensure community follow-up. The public health department is responsible for identification of sexual contacts, contact notification, and contact screening.

Lesions of primary and secondary syphilis may be highly infective. Gloves are worn when direct contact with lesions is likely, and hand hygiene is performed after gloves are removed. Isolation in a private room is not required (see Chart 71-7).

Chlamydia trachomatis and *Neisseria gonorrhoeae* Infections

Chlamydia trachomatis and *Neisseria gonorrhoeae* are the most commonly reported infectious diseases in the United States. Coinfection with *C. trachomatis* often occurs in patients infected with *N. gonorrhoeae*. The greatest risk of *C. trachomatis* infection occurs in young women between 15 and 24 years of age (CDC, 2015b).

The nurse instructs the patient to:
- Complete the full course of therapy if multiple penicillin injections are required.
- Refrain from sexual contact with previous or current partners until the partners have been treated.
- Be aware that if you have primary or secondary syphilis, skin lesions and other sequelae of infection will improve with proper treatment, and serology eventually will reflect cure.
- Recognize that condoms significantly reduce the risk of transmission of syphilis and other sexually transmitted infections.
- Be aware that having multiple sexual partners increases the risk of acquiring syphilis and other sexually transmitted infections.

Clinical Manifestations

Women

Both C. trachomatis and N. gonorrhoeae infections frequently do not cause symptoms in women. When symptoms are present, mucopurulent cervicitis with exudates in the endocervical canal is the most frequent finding. Women with gonorrhea can also present with symptoms of urinary tract infection or vaginitis. See Chapter 57 for more in-depth coverage of STIs in women.

Men

Although men are more likely than women to have symptoms when infected, infection with N. gonorrhoeae or C. trachomatis can be asymptomatic. When symptoms are present, they may include burning during urination and penile discharge. Patients with N. gonorrhoeae infection may also report painful, swollen testicles.

Complications

In women, pelvic inflammatory disease (PID), ectopic pregnancy, endometritis, and infertility are possible complications of either N. gonorrhoeae or C. trachomatis infection. In men, epididymitis, a painful disease that may lead to infertility, may result from infection with either bacterium. In both men and women, arthritis or bloodstream infection may be caused by N. gonorrhoeae.

Assessment and Diagnostic Findings

The patient is assessed for fever, discharge (urethral, vaginal, or rectal), and signs of arthritis. Diagnostic methods used in N. gonorrhoeae infection include Gram stain (appropriate only for male urethral samples), culture, and nucleic acid amplification tests (NAATs). Gram stain and the direct fluorescent antibody test can be used in chlamydia. NAATs are also available for C. trachomatis but demand strict attention to laboratory procedures to ensure test reliability. In the female patient, samples are obtained from the endocervix, anal canal, and pharynx. In the male patient, specimens are obtained from the urethra, anal canal, and pharynx. Because N. gonorrhoeae organisms are susceptible to environmental changes, specimens for culture must be delivered to the laboratory immediately after they are obtained.

Because as many as 70% of chlamydial infections are asymptomatic, the CDC recommends annual Chlamydia testing for all women who are pregnant, women younger than 25 years who are sexually active, and women over 25 years with a new sexual partner or multiple partners (CDC, 2015c).

Medical Management

Because patients are often coinfected with both gonorrhea and chlamydia, the CDC recommends dual therapy even if only gonorrhea has been laboratory proven. CDC guidelines should be used to determine alternative therapy for the patient who is pregnant or allergic or who has a complicated chlamydial infection. The CDC updates STI therapy recommendations regularly because of growing problems with bacterial antibiotic resistance patterns and drug shortages.

Although the number of resistant strains of gonorrhea has increased, that is not the reason for the use of combination antibiotic therapy. Such therapy is prescribed in order to treat both gonorrhea and chlamydia, because many patients with gonorrhea have a coexisting chlamydial infection.

Patients with uncomplicated gonorrhea who are treated with CDC-recommended therapy do not routinely need to return for a proof-of-cure visit. If the patient reports a new episode of symptoms or tests are positive for gonorrhea again, the most likely explanation is reinfection rather than treatment failure. Serologic testing for syphilis and HIV should be offered to patients with gonorrhea or chlamydia, because any STI increases the risk of other STIs.

Nursing Management

Gonorrhea and chlamydia are reportable communicable diseases. In any health care facility, a mechanism should be in place to ensure that all patients who are diagnosed are reported to the local public health department to ensure follow-up of the patient. The public health department also is responsible for interviewing the patient to identify sexual contacts so that contact notification and screening can be initiated.

The target group for preventive patient education about gonorrhea and chlamydia is the adolescent and young adult population. Along with reinforcing the importance of abstinence, when appropriate, education should address postponing the age of initial sexual exposure, limiting the number of sexual partners, and using condoms for barrier protection. Young women and those who are pregnant should also be instructed about the importance of routine screening for chlamydia.

NURSING PROCESS

The Patient With a Sexually Transmitted Infection

Assessment

The patient should be asked to describe the onset and progression of symptoms and to characterize any lesions by location and by describing drainage, if present. Brief explanations of why the information is needed are often helpful. Clarification of terms may be necessary if either the patient or nurse uses words that are unfamiliar to the other.

Protecting confidentiality is important when discussing sexual issues. When a detailed sexual history is necessary, it is important to respect the patient's right to privacy. When obtaining a sexual history, the CDC recommends the following systematic interview of key areas, the "five Ps": partners, prevention of pregnancy, protection from STIs, practices, past history of STIs.

Asking specific information about sexual contacts usually should be done only when the nurse is part of a team that will conduct partner notification. The nurse should describe to the patient the public health notification process and resources that are available to assist sexual partners or infants and children.

During the physical examination, the examiner looks for rashes, lesions, drainage, discharge, or swelling. Inguinal nodes are palpated to elicit tenderness and to assess swelling. Women are examined for abdominal or uterine tenderness. The mouth and throat are examined for signs of inflammation or exudate. The nurse wears gloves while examining the mucous membranes, and gloves are changed and replaced after vaginal or rectal examination.

Diagnosis

NURSING DIAGNOSES

Based on assessment data, major nursing diagnoses may include the following:

- Knowledge deficit about the disease and risk for spread of infection and reinfection
- Anxiety related to anticipated stigmatization and to prognosis and complications
- Noncompliance with treatment

COLLABORATIVE PROBLEMS/POTENTIAL COMPLICATIONS

Potential complications may include the following:

- Ectopic pregnancy
- Infertility
- Transmission of infection to fetus, resulting in congenital abnormalities and other outcomes
- Neurosyphilis
- Gonococcal meningitis
- Gonococcal arthritis
- Syphilitic aortitis
- HIV-related complications

Planning and Goals

Major goals are increased patient understanding of the natural history and treatment of the infection, reduction in anxiety, increased adherence with therapeutic and preventive goals, and absence of complications.

Nursing Interventions

INCREASING KNOWLEDGE AND PREVENTING SPREAD OF DISEASE

Education about STIs and prevention of the spread to others are often accomplished simultaneously. The patient who is infected should be told what the causative organism is and should receive an explanation of the usual course of the infection (including the interval of potential communicability to others) and possible complications. The nurse should stress the importance of following therapy as prescribed and the need to report any side effects or symptom progression.

Discussion should emphasize that the same behaviors that led to infection with one STI increase the risk of any other STI, including HIV. Methods used to contact sexual partners should be discussed. The patient should understand that until the partner has been treated, continued sexual exposure to the same person may lead to reinfection. The relative value of condoms in reducing the risk for infection with STIs should be addressed. When appropriate, the patient should be encouraged to discuss any reasons for resistance to condom use to promote thoughtful decision making about this preventive method.

REDUCING ANXIETY

When appropriate, the patient is encouraged to discuss anxieties and fear associated with the diagnosis, treatment, or prognosis. By individualizing education, factual information applied to specific needs may offer reassurance. Patients may need help in planning discussion with partners. If the patient is especially apprehensive about this aspect, referral to a social worker or other specialist may be appropriate. For example, such support is especially important when the patient has newly diagnosed HIV infection. Patients with HIV may benefit from programs that combine support, education, counseling, and therapeutic goals. Such programs are designed to offer coordinated care throughout the course of disease progression.

INCREASING ADHERENCE

In group settings (e.g., an outpatient obstetric setting) or in a one-to-one setting, open discussion about STI information facilitates patient education. Discomfort can be reduced by factual explanation of causes, consequences, treatments, prevention, and responsibilities. Because most communities have expanded STI prevention resources, referrals to appropriate agencies can complement individual educational efforts and ensure that later questions or uncertainties can be addressed by experts.

MONITORING AND MANAGING POTENTIAL COMPLICATIONS

Infertility and Increased Risk of Ectopic Pregnancy. STIs may lead to PID and, with it, increased risk of ectopic pregnancy and infertility. See Chapters 56 and 57 for additional information.

Congenital Infections. All STIs can be transmitted to infants in utero or at the time of birth. Complications of congenital infection can range from localized infection (e.g., throat infection with *N. gonorrhoeae*), to congenital abnormalities (e.g., stunting of growth or deafness from congenital syphilis), to life-threatening disease (e.g., congenital herpes simplex virus).

Neurosyphilis, Gonococcal Meningitis, Gonococcal Arthritis, and Syphilitic Aortitis. STIs can cause disseminated infection. The central nervous system may be infected, as seen in cases of neurosyphilis or gonococcal meningitis. Gonorrhea that infects the skeletal system may result in gonococcal arthritis. Syphilis can infect the cardiovascular system by forming vegetative lesions on the mitral or aortic valves.

Human Immune Deficiency Virus–Related Complications. HIV infection, if untreated, leads to the profound immunosuppression that is characteristic of AIDS. Complications of HIV infection include many opportunistic infections, including those due to *Pneumocystis jiroveci*, *Cryptococcus neoformans*, cytomegalovirus, and *Mycobacterium avium* (see Chapter 36).

Evaluation

Expected patient outcomes may include:

1. Exhibits knowledge about STIs and their transmission
2. Demonstrates a less anxious demeanor
   a. Discusses anxieties and goals for treatment
   b. Inspects self for lesions, rashes, and discharge
   c. Accepts support, education, and counseling when indicated
   d. Assists with sharing information about infection with sexual partners
   e. Discusses risk reduction behaviors and safer sex practices
3. Adheres to treatment
4. Achieves effective treatment
5. Reports for follow-up examinations if necessary
6. Absence of complications

Emerging Infectious Diseases

As defined by the CDC, **emerging infectious diseases** are human diseases of infectious origin that have increased within the past two decades or that are likely to increase in the near future. Examples of emerging infectious diseases presented here include Zika virus, West Nile virus, Ebola virus disease, Legionnaires disease, and pertussis.

Many factors contribute to newly emerging or re-emerging infectious diseases. These include travel, globalization of food supply and central processing of food, population growth, increased urban crowding, population movements (e.g., those that result from war, famine, or man-made or natural disasters), ecologic changes, human behavior (e.g., risky sexual behavior, IV/injection drug use), antimicrobial resistance, and breakdown in public health measures.

These diseases are important from an epidemiologic standpoint because their incidence has not yet stabilized. When the pattern of disease in a community is not well understood in the medical-scientific community, patients, families, and others in the community often become alarmed about these diseases. During times of increased concern about bioterrorism, whether triggered by actual events or by hoaxes, nurses have responsibility to rationally separate facts from fears. In discussions with patients and other caregivers, it is important to keep the focus on what is known and to clarify the plan for diagnosis, treatment, and containment.

Zika Virus

The Zika virus was first discovered as a pathogen in monkeys in the Zika Forest of Uganda in the 1940s; it was found to cause human disease in the 1950s. The epidemiologic pattern changed as the first large outbreak in humans did not occur until 2007 in Micronesia. The disease was not seen in the Western Hemisphere until July 2015, when a large outbreak began in Brazil. Within the next year, infections were noted in countries throughout the Americas and Pacific Islands (WHO, 2016a).

The incubation period for Zika virus disease appears to be just a few days. There is a wide variation in clinical presentations in those infected. Among patients who are symptomatic, most have self-limiting illness of 2 to 7 days duration with mild fever, rash, headache, conjunctivitis, or joint and muscle pain. The most troubling effect is that Zika has been associated with microcephaly and other congenital abnormalities in infants of some women infected with Zika during pregnancy. The virus can also cause Guillain–Barré syndrome, a condition with nerve and muscle weakness that often quickly progresses to a paralysis (WHO, 2016a).

Zika is primarily transmitted through bites of infected mosquitos from the *Aedes* genus. Sustained outbreaks have been more common in tropical areas where these mosquitos thrive. The *Aedes* mosquito is also the carrier of other mosquito-borne viruses such as dengue, chikungunya, and yellow fever. Unlike these other mosquito-borne diseases, Zika can also be transmitted through sexual transmission. This combination of transmission routes makes prevention efforts especially challenging. People can travel to epidemic areas, and later, as asymptomatic infected carriers, transmit the virus to their sexual partners. Because of the concern about congenital infection, women who are pregnant are advised to avoid travel to endemic areas and to use abstinence or safer sex methods if their sexual partners have traveled to such regions. Similarly, couples with exposure to areas where there is ongoing transmission are counseled in contraceptive options (CDC, 2016k; Morgan, 2017).

West Nile Virus

The West Nile virus was first recognized in the 1930s in Africa and was first seen in humans in the United States in 1999. Although most human infections are mild or asymptomatic, a range of presentations is possible. Approximately 20% of people who are infected have a mild disease called *West Nile fever*. These patients usually experience headache, fever, and a persistent fatigue that may continue for several months. In these patients, fewer than 1 in 150 infections develop into more serious disease, which is characterized by severe neuroinvasive illness, meningitis, encephalitis, and paralysis or poliomyelitis. The mortality rate for people with the milder West Nile fever and meningitis is less than 1%, but this rate increases to approximately 20% for those with encephalitis. Although age-related factors do not appear to affect a person's chances of acquiring West Nile virus, the risk of neuroinvasive disease is greater in those older than 50 years (CDC, 2016l).

The incubation period (i.e., from mosquito bite to onset of symptoms) is between 3 and 14 days. Currently, there is no treatment for West Nile virus infection. Medical and nursing management consists of fluid replacement, airway management, and supportive nursing care when meningitis or symptoms are present.

Birds are the natural reservoir for the virus, and since 1999, the population of infected birds in the United States has increased steadily. Mosquitoes become infected when feeding on birds and can transmit the virus to animals and humans. Although human-to-human transmission of West Nile virus is very rare, transmission has occurred as the result of occupational exposure in laboratory workers, infant exposure transplacentally and from breast-feeding, and blood transfusion or organ transplant from donors who are infected (CDC, 2016l).

Ebola Virus Disease

The first human outbreak of Ebola virus disease occurred in 1976. For decades the virus maintained a pattern of sporadic outbreaks in remote African villages, followed by intervening periods without any recognized cases worldwide. In 2014, the virus broke through this usual pattern and rampaged through the West African countries Liberia, Guinea, and Sierra Leone, with secondary cases in other countries in Africa, Europe, and the United States (Chertow, Kleine, Edwards, et al., 2014).

Pathophysiology

Ebola is spread through direct contact with blood or body fluids (urine, vomit, feces, saliva, sweat, semen, and breast milk) from the person who is ill from the virus and possibly from contact with semen of a man who has recovered from Ebola. It is not spread through an air, water, or insect bite. In Africa, it may occasionally be spread by handling infected bats or infected wild animals that are sometimes hunted for food. Ebola virus is only detected in blood after the patient becomes symptomatic and viral levels rise significantly as the disease progresses (Chertow et al., 2014).

The incubation period from exposure to first symptoms ranges from 2 to 21 days. If there are no symptoms by 21 days after exposure, there is essentially no risk of developing Ebola. Patients are not contagious to others before symptoms occur. Thorough identification of Ebola contacts and careful symptom monitoring can prevent subsequent waves of transmission.

Clinical Manifestations

The initial clinical manifestations include high fever, muscle aches, and fatigue. Between the third and fifth symptomatic day, the patient often develops severe diarrhea, abdominal pain, and vomiting. Patients are at great risk of severe dehydration at this point as many produce over 5 L of liquid stool per day. This stage can persist for a week or more, and many patients develop hemodynamic shock (see Chapter 14). Patients may also show increasing neurologic symptoms during that period, such as confusion, agitation, delirium, or encephalitis. Approximately 5% will develop bleeding or hemorrhage, a very poor prognostic indicator. Patients who do not die during the first 2 weeks of the disease are likely to survive (Chertow et al., 2014).

Medical Management

Treatment is largely supportive maintenance of the circulatory system and respiratory systems. It is likely that the patient who is infected will need ventilator and dialysis support during the acute phase of illness.

Nursing Management

Nursing management mirrors that of medical management and is largely supportive. Supportive care for a patient with such a devastating disease requires psychological support for the patient and family.

Health care workers are at increased risk for acquiring Ebola because they may have contact with body fluids or equipment contaminated from exposure to body fluids. Because so much virus is present, especially in vomit and diarrhea, the patient should be isolated in a private room, away from other patients. Patients must be promptly isolated and health care workers should wear complete PPE. Systems must be set up so that an observer guides each worker to meticulously don PPE before direct contact with a patient who is infected to ensure that all equipment is worn correctly. After a worker has direct contact with a patient who is infected, an observer should direct careful doffing (removal) of PPE to ensure that no exposure occurs in the process. Equipment used for the patient with Ebola virus should be used solely for that patient and should be disposed after use. If equipment must be reused, it should be sterilized or scrupulously cleaned with a bleach-based solution before reuse. Care for the patient with Ebola requires hospitals and transport systems to develop plans to coordinate staffing, supply maintenance, handling of waste, and communication with the public (WHO, 2016b).

Legionnaires Disease

Legionnaires disease is a multisystem illness that usually includes pneumonia and is caused by the gram-negative bacterium *Legionella pneumophila*. Named after an outbreak among people attending a convention of the American Legion in 1976, its potential to cause outbreaks has been demonstrated repeatedly in hospitals and other settings. It continues to be considered an emerging infectious disease because there are new patterns in recent years. There are approximately 5000 new cases each year (CDC, 2016m).

Legionella organisms are found in many man-made and naturally occurring water sources. Although the organisms may initially be introduced to the plumbing system in low numbers, growth is enhanced by water storage, sediment, temperatures ranging from 25°C to 42°C (77°F to 107°F), and certain amoebae frequently present in water that can support intracellular growth of legionellae. Because incidence appears to increase in the summer and autumn months, vacation-related exposure to hotel or cruise ship plumbing and air-conditioning systems, whirlpool spas, and decorative fountains may be the causative risk.

Pathophysiology

L. pneumophila is transmitted by the aerosolized route from an environmental source to a person's respiratory tract. In hospitals, patients may be exposed to aerosols created by cooling towers, water exposure from in-room plumbing, and respiratory therapy equipment. Person-to-person transmission, if it occurs at all, is extremely rare. Because underlying medical conditions can increase host susceptibility and subsequent severity of disease and because hospital plumbing systems are often very complex, outbreaks occur in hospitals more frequently than at other centers within the community. The mortality rate for Legionnaires disease may be as high as 10% in some populations (Cooley, 2016).

Risk Factors

Risk factors for *Legionella* infection include diseases that lead to severe immunosuppression, such as AIDS, hematologic malignancy, end-stage kidney disease, or the use of immunosuppressive agents. Other factors associated with increased risk include diabetes, smoking, exposure to whirlpool spas, and recent travel.

Clinical Manifestations

The lungs are the principal organs of infection; however, other organs may also be involved. The incubation period ranges from 2 to 10 days. Early symptoms may include malaise, myalgias, headache, and dry cough. The patient develops increasing pulmonary symptoms, including productive cough, dyspnea, and chest pain. Patients are usually febrile, and body temperatures may reach or exceed 39.4°C (103°F). Diarrhea and other gastrointestinal symptoms are common. In severe cases, multiorgan involvement and failure may follow.

Assessment and Diagnostic Findings

The diagnostic approach generally involves using information obtained from the history, physical examination, x-rays, laboratory findings, and assessment of therapeutic effectiveness. Chest x-ray abnormalities may vary in severity and in location within the lungs. Laboratory tests available for the diagnosis of *Legionella* include culture or tests that detect either antigen or antibody. The most frequently used test is the urinary antigen. The greatest limitation of the test is that it detects only one subgroup of one of the several species of *Legionella*. The CDC recommends using multiple tests when Legionnaires disease is suspected because none of the tests is completely accurate (CDC, 2016m).

Medical Management

The antibiotic agents of choice are azithromycin (Zithromax) or a fluoroquinolone such as moxifloxacin (Avelox) (CDC, 2016m). The antibiotic doxycycline may also be used.

Nursing Management

The nursing management described for the patient with any pneumonia (see Chapter 23) should form the basis of care for the patient with *Legionella* pneumonia. Isolation is not required because *Legionella* is not usually transmitted between humans. When the patient has acquired the infection in a health care facility, water cultures should be performed to determine if the water supply is contaminated.

Pertussis

Pertussis, also known as whooping cough, a common childhood disease in the pre-vaccine era, is an example of a disease that has re-emerged. Incidence rates declined until the 1980s, when rates for all age groups began to increase steadily for the next three decades. In the short period from 2010 to 2014, the annual incidence of cases in adolescents and adults more than doubled compared with the period from 2000 to 2009 (CDC, 2016n).

Pertussis is caused by the bacterium *Bordetella pertussis*. It is highly contagious, and patients usually present to health care professionals with a sudden (paroxysmal) cough that is accompanied by a characteristic whoop—a high-pitched noise heard when inhaling.

Pathophysiology

B. pertussis is transmitted by droplets. The bacteria easily attach to pharyngeal epithelial cells, where they release a number of antigens, toxins, and other substances that trigger the immune system. Because most of the disease manifestations are caused by this immune reaction, patients are usually contagious only early in the disease (when the bacteria are still present) and not during the protracted period of cough (when the immune reaction is causing the pathology).

Clinical Manifestations

Pertussis causes a range of respiratory symptoms, with cough being the most frequent. It is generally most severe for infants who have not yet been vaccinated. Pneumonia is the most common consequence of infection, but the disease can also lead to seizures, encephalopathy, and, rarely, death. People who have been vaccinated seldom have severe disease.

Assessment and Diagnostic Findings

Most diagnoses of pertussis are made, at least initially, without laboratory confirmation. The clinical case definition, unless there is a pre-existing condition to explain the symptoms, is a new cough lasting at least 2 weeks with inspiratory whoop or vomiting after cough. Laboratory confirmation can be made by clinical culture or by polymerase chain reaction assay for *B. pertussis*. Serologic testing, although less reliable, can also strengthen the diagnostic suspicion. The best source for a culture is a nasopharyngeal specimen obtained by swab or aspirate (CDC, 2016n).

Medical Management

Early treatment for pertussis is important to prevent complications. The antibiotic agents of choice are azithromycin, erythromycin (Erythrocin), or clarithromycin (Biaxin). The antibiotic trimethoprim sulfamethaxasole (TMP-SMZ) (Bactrim) may also be used (CDC, 2016n). Close contacts of a patient with proven or suspected pertussis should receive prophylaxis with one of these agents to reduce the risk of disease.

Nursing Management

Patients who are hospitalized with pertussis should be isolated in droplet precautions until they have received 5 days of appropriate therapy. Household members should receive antimicrobial prophylaxis and should be advised to report any symptoms of an upper respiratory infection.

Because pertussis is most severe for infants, it is important to ensure that all women who are pregnant are vaccinated with Tdap (tetanus, diphtheria, acellular pertussis vaccine). The best time for Tdap for women who have not been vaccinated before becoming pregnant is late in the second trimester or in the third trimester. If a woman has not been vaccinated prior to delivery of the infant, Tdap should be given immediately postpartum. Fathers, siblings, grandparents, and others who are around infants under 12 months should also be vaccinated to reduce the risk of transmitting pertussis.

For the protection of both worker and patient, all health care workers should receive a single dose of Tdap vaccine. Workers who are unsure if they have ever had Tdap should receive the vaccine regardless of the possible interval since the previous vaccination. No redosing for pertussis will be necessary through life, but boosters for tetanus and diphtheria (Td vaccine) should be given every 10 years (CDC, 2016n).

Travel and Immigration

Travel, trade, migration, and wars have led to many epidemics throughout history. The potential for epidemics is greatest when travelers and immigrants introduce microorganisms to which the host population has little or no immunity. Examples of important epidemics in the Western Hemisphere have included yellow fever, malaria, hookworm, leprosy, smallpox, measles, mumps, and syphilis. The HIV epidemic demonstrates the way that travel and immigration allow a disease to spread undetected worldwide. The 2014 Ebola outbreak demonstrates how global travel contributes to a rapidly occurring epidemic involving an unrecognized pathogen.

In the United States, an infrastructure with enforced vaccination, clean water, and insect and rodent control decreases the risk that epidemics will progress even when travel may introduce exotic microorganisms. However, the recent experience with Zika virus has reinforced knowledge that insect transmission can lead to significant human outbreaks. Thus, the concern grows that vector-borne diseases such as dengue and malaria may increase in the United States as mosquitoes can transmit disease locally when a reservoir of infected humans is established. The CDC maintains an active surveillance system to monitor and halt the incidence of many diseases prospectively.

Immigration and Acquired Immune Deficiency Syndrome

The fact that AIDS reached pandemic proportions less than a decade after its recognition attests to the efficiency of world travel in spreading disease. Such rapid transmission rates are especially dramatic because HIV essentially requires intimate contact between two people through sexual activity or sharing blood through needles (see Chapter 36).

Immigration and Tuberculosis

Immigration has always been an important influence in the dynamic epidemiology of TB in the United States. In 2014, the incidence of TB in the United States was 13 times greater in people who were foreign-born than those who were native-born (CDC, 2016o).

The association between immigration and transmission risk is greatest in urban areas, because these locations are frequently heavily populated and frequently visited by people who were foreign-born. These locales are also often the epicenter of the HIV epidemic. Because HIV infection depletes T cells, which are necessary for TB protection, the geographic closeness of these two microorganisms potentiates increased rates of both infections.

A positive TST establishes that TB infection has occurred at some time in a person's life but does not provide information about current infectivity. The reliability of TST interpretation is decreased among people who were foreign-born because the bacille Calmette–Guérin (BCG) vaccine is used in many countries. After receiving BCG, people often have some degree of TST reactivity for a prolonged time.

The QuantiFERON-TB Gold (QFT-G) test is an enzyme-linked immunosorbent assay (ELISA) that detects the release of interferon-gamma by white blood cells when the blood of a patient with TB is incubated with peptides similar to those in *M. tuberculosis*. The results of the QFT-G test are available in less than 24 hours and are not affected by prior vaccination with BCG. Additional rapid tests for TB include the QuantiFERON-TB Gold In-Tube test (QFT-GIT); T-SPOT TB test (T-Spot); and Xpert MTB/RIF, which was endorsed by WHO in 2011 (CDC, 2010). See Chapter 23 for more detailed discussion.

Immigration and Vector-Borne Diseases

Malaria and dengue are diseases that cause significant morbidity and mortality throughout the developing world. These diseases may be "imported" to the United States via travel, immigration, or commerce. They are caused by microorganisms that can be spread to humans by mosquitoes in the United States that thrive in tropical zones and breed in stagnant water sources. Although malaria was eradicated in the United States in the 1950s, limited local outbreaks have occurred regularly when mosquitoes acquire the bacteria from a person recently traveling from an area in which malaria is endemic and transmit it to a small number of people. Similarly, an increase of dengue virus in the Caribbean has caused concern that outbreaks may occur in the United States.

CRITICAL THINKING EXERCISES

1 `ebp` Your unit has had an increase in HAIs in the past 6 months. Identify how HAIs occur. What nursing interventions should be used to reduce the risk of new HAIs? What evidence-based strategies are used to decrease the incidence of HAIs? Identify the criteria used to evaluate the strength of the evidence for the practices you identify.

2 You are a home care nurse caring for a 75-year-old patient with multiple medical conditions. What information should be provided about infection risk prevention to the patient, the family, and the caregiver?

3 `pq` Identify the priorities, approach, and techniques you would use for a 21-year-old woman who presents to student health with symptoms of Zika after traveling to Brazil for spring break. How would your priorities, approach, and techniques differ if the patient is a 21-year-old man? If the female patient is pregnant?

REFERENCES

*Asterisk indicates nursing research.
**Double asterisk indicates classic reference.

Books

Comerford, K. C. (2015). *Nursing 2015 drug handbook*. Philadelphia, PA: Wolters Kluwer.

Evans, A. S., & Brachman, P. S. (1998). *Bacterial infections in humans* (3rd ed.). New York: Plenum, p. 40.

Grossman, S. C., & Porth, C. M. (2014). *Pathophysiology: Concepts of altered health states* (9th ed.). Philadelphia, PA: Lippincott Williams & Wilkins.

Journals and Electronic Documents

*Busby, S. R., Kennedy, B., Davis, S. C., et al. (2015). Assessing patient awareness of proper hand hygiene. *Nursing, 45*(5), 27–30.

**Centers for Disease Control and Prevention (CDC). (2002). Guideline for hand hygiene in health care settings. *MMWR: Morbidity and Mortality Weekly Report, 51*(RR 16), 1–56.

**Centers for Disease Control and Prevention (CDC). (2007). 2007 *Guideline for isolation precautions: Preventing transmission of infectious agents in healthcare settings*. Retrieved on 5/13/2016 at: www.cdc.gov/hicpac/2007ip/2007ip_part1.html

Centers for Disease Control and Prevention (CDC). (2010). Updated guidelines for using interferon gamma release assays to detect *Mycobacterium tuberculosis* infection—United States, 2010. *MMWR: Morbidity Mortality Weekly Report, 59*(RR 5), 1–13.

Centers for Disease Control and Prevention (CDC). (2011). *2011 Guidelines for the prevention of intravascular catheter-related infections*. Retrieved on 10/17/16 at: www.cdc.gov/hicpac/bsi/bsi-guidelines-2011.html

Centers for Disease Control and Prevention (CDC). (2014a). Epidemiology and prevention of vaccine preventable diseases. *Morbidity and Mortality Weekly Report, 63*(32), 702–715.

Centers for Disease Control and Prevention (CDC). (2014b). *Food safety; Campylobacter*. Retrieved on 10/22/16 at cdc.gov/foodsafety/diseases/campylobacter.

Centers for Disease Control and Prevention (CDC). (2015a). *E.coli (Escherichia coli)*. Retrieved on 3/22/17 at: cdc.gov/ecoli/general

Centers for Disease Control and Prevention (CDC). (2015b). *CDC fact sheet: Reported STDs in the United States*. Retrieved on 10/24/16 at: www.cdc.gov/std/stats14/std-trends-508.pdf

Centers for Disease Control and Prevention (CDC). (2015c). *2015 STD treatment guidelines*. Retrieved on 10/4/2016 at: www.cdc.gov/std/tg2015/tg-2015-print.pdf

Centers for Disease Control and Prevention (CDC). (2015d). *Influenza (flu) vaccine (live, intranasal): What you need to know*. Retrieved on 3/22/17 at: www.cdc.gov/vaccines/hcp/vis/vis-statements/flulive.pdf

Centers for Disease Control and Prevention (CDC). (2016a). *Immunization schedules*. Retrieved on 3/16/2017 at: www.cdc.gov/vaccines/schedules

Centers for Disease Control and Prevention (CDC). (2016b). *Frequently asked questions about Clostridium difficile*. Retrieved on 3/16/2017 at: www.cdc.gov/HAI/pdfs/cdiff/Cdiff_tagged.pdf

Centers for Disease Control and Prevention (CDC). (2016c). *Healthcare associated infections: CDC's antibiotic resistance patient safety atlas*. Retrieved on 10/17/16 at: www.cdc.gov/hai/surveillance/ar-patient-safety-atlas.html

Centers for Disease Control and Prevention (CDC). (2016d). *Chickenpox (varicella)*. Retrieved on 10/17/16 at: www.cdc.gov/chickenpox/hcp/clinical-overview

Centers for Disease Control and Prevention (CDC). (2016e). *Shingles (herpes zoster)*. Retrieved on 10/17/16 at: www.cdc.gov/shingles/hcp/clinical-overview

Centers for Disease Control and Prevention (CDC). (2016f). *Influenza (Flu)*. Retrieved on 10/17/16 at: www.cdc.gov/flu

Centers for Disease Control and Prevention (CDC). (2016g). *Human Papillomavirus (HPV)*. Retrieved on 10/22/16 at: www.cdc.gov/hpv/stdfact-hpv

Centers for Disease Control and Prevention (CDC). (2016h). *Highly pathogenic Asian avian influenza A (H5N1)*. Retrieved on 10/22/16 at: www.cdc.gov/flu/avianflu/h5n1-virus

Centers for Disease Control and Prevention (CDC). (2016i). *2015 Food safety report: Measuring progress toward Healthy People 2020 Goals*. Retrieved on 10/22/16 at: www.cdc.gov/foodnet/pdfs/foodnet.mmwr-progress-508-final

Centers for Disease Control and Prevention (CDC). (2016j). *Preventing Norovirus infection*. Retrieved on 10/24/16 at: www.cdc.gov/norovirus/preventing-infection

Centers for Disease Control and Prevention (CDC). (2016k). *Zika virus*. Retrieved on 10/24/16 at: www.cdc.gov/zika

Centers for Disease Control and Prevention (CDC). (2016l). *West Nile virus*. Retrieved on 10/24/16 at: www.cdc.gov/westnile

Centers for Disease Control and Prevention (CDC). (2016m). *Legionnaire's disease*. Retrieved on 10/24/16 at: www.cdc.gov/legionella/about/history.html

Centers for Disease Control and Prevention (CDC). (2016n). *Pertussis (whooping cough)*. Retrieved on 10/24/16 at: www.cdc.gov/pertussis

Centers for Disease Control and Prevention (CDC). (2016o). *Tuberculosis (TB): Fact sheet—trends in tuberculosis, 2014*. Retrieved on 10/24/16 at: www.cdc.gov/tb/publications/factsheets/statistics/TBTrends.htm

Chertow, D. S., Kleine, C., Edwards, J. K., et al. (2014). Ebola virus disease in West Africa – Clinical manifestations and management. *New England Journal of Medicine, 371*(22), 2054–2057.

Cooley L. (2016). Legionnaires disease on rise in US – 2016 Update. *Medscape*. Retrieved on 10/24/16 at: www.medscape.com/viewarticle/864189

Dantes, R., Mu, Y., Belflower, R., et al. (2013). National burden of invasive Methicillin-Resistant Staphylococcus aureus infections, United States, 2011. *JAMA, 173*(21), 1970–1978.

*Fox, C., Wavra, T., Drake, D. A., et al. (2015). Use of a patient hand hygiene protocol to reduce hosptital acquired infections and improve nurses' hand washing. *American Journal of Critical Care, 24*(3), 216–224.

*Gilmartin, H., Sousa, K.H., & Battaglia, C. (2016). Capturing the central line bundle infection prevention interventions. *Nursing Research, 65*(5), 397–407.

Marschall, J., Mermel, L. A., Fakih, M., et al. (2014). Strategies to prevent central-line associated blood stream infections in acute care hospitals: 2014 update. *Infection Control and Hospital Epidemiology, 35*(7), 753–771.

Morgan, S. A. (2017). Spring break? Think Zika. *American Nurse Today, 12*(3), 15.

Nealy, K. L., McCarty, D. J., & Woods, J. A. (2016). Managing drug-resistant organisms in acute care. *The Nurse Practitioner, 41*(2), 38–44.

Occupational Safety and Health Administration (OSHA). (2012). *Toxic and hazardous substances: Bloodborne pathogens*. Retrieved on 10/11/2016 at: www.osha.gov/pls/oshaweb/owadisp.show_document?p_table=STANDARDS&p_id=10051

Petrosky, E., Bocchini, J. A., Hariri S., et al. (2015). Use of 9-Valent Human Papillomavirus (HPV) Vaccine: Updated HPV vaccination recommendations of the Advisory Committee on Immunization Practices. *Morbidity and Mortality Weekly Report, 64*(11), 300–304.

Shabot, M. M., Chassin, M. R., France, A., et al. (2016). Using the Targeted Solutions Tool® to improve hand hygiene compliance is associated with decreased health care–associated infections. *The Joint Commission Journal on Quality and Patient Safety, 42*(1), 6–17.

*Stone, P. W., Herzig, C. T., Pogorzelska-Maziarz, M., et al. (2015). Understanding infection prevention and control in nursing homes: A qualitative study. *Geriatric Nursing, 36*(4), 267–272.

The Joint Commission. (2016). *National Patient Safety Goals; Effective January 1, 2016*. Retrieved 10/17/16 at: www.jointcommission.org/assets/1/6/2016_NPSG_HAP.pdf

U.S. Department of Health and Human Services (HHS) (2016). *Pandemic Flu History*. Retrieved on 10/24/2016 at: www.flu.gov/pandemic/history

United Nations General Assembly. (2016). *Draft Political Declaration of the High-level Meeting of the General Assembly on Antimicrobial Resistance*. Retrieved 10/17/16 at: www.un.org/pga/71/wp-content/uploads/sites/40/2016/09/Draft-AMR-Declaration.pdf

U.S. Food and Drug Administration (FDA). (2013). *FDA news release, January 16, 2013: FDA approves new seasonal influenza vaccine made using novel technology*. Retrieved on 10/17/16 at: www.fda.gov/NewsEvents/Newsroom/PressAnnouncements/ucm335891.htm

White House. (2015). *National action plan to combat antibiotic-resistant bacteria*. Retrieved on 10/24/16 at: www.whitehouse.gov/sites/default/

files/docs/national_action_plan_for_combating_antibotic-resistant_bacteria.pdf

**World Health Organization (WHO). (2006). *Oral rehydration salts. Production of the new ORS*. Retrieved on 3/16/2017 at: www.who.int/maternal_child_adolescent/documents/fch_cah_06_1/en/index.html

World Health Organization (WHO). (2016a). *Zika virus*. Retrieved on 10/24/16 at www.who.int/topics/zika/en/

World Health Organization (WHO). (2016b). *Ebola virus disease*. Retrieved on 10/24/16 at: www.who.int/mediacentre/factsheets/fs103/

Resources

American Lung Association, www.lung.org
American Public Health Association (APHA), www.apha.org

Association for Professionals in Infection Control and Epidemiology (APIC), www.apic.org
Centers for Disease Control and Prevention (CDC), www.cdc.gov
Infectious Diseases Society of America (IDSA), www.idsociety.org
Medicare Hospital Compare, www.medicare.gov/hospitalcompare
National Foundation for Infectious Diseases (NFID), www.nfid.org
National Institute of Allergy and Infectious Diseases (NIAID), www.niaid.nih.gov
Occupational Safety and Health Administration (OSHA), www.osha.gov
Society for Healthcare Epidemiology of America (SHEA), www.shea-online.org
Vaccine Adverse Event Reporting System (VAERS), www.vaers.hhs.gov
World Health Organization (WHO), www.who.int/en/

72 Emergency Nursing

The term *emergency management* traditionally refers to care given to patients with urgent and critical needs. However, because many people lack access to health care, the emergency department (ED) is increasingly used for nonurgent problems. Therefore, the philosophy of emergency management has broadened to include the concept that an emergency is whatever the patient or the family considers it to be.

The emergency nurse has had specialized education, training, experience, and expertise in assessing and identifying patients' health care problems in crisis situations. In addition, the emergency nurse establishes priorities, monitors, and continuously assesses patients who are acutely ill and injured, supports and attends to families, supervises allied health personnel, and educates patients and families within a time-limited, high-pressured care environment. Nursing interventions are accomplished interdependently, in consultation with or under the direction of a physician or advanced practitioner such as a nurse practitioner or physician assistant. The roles of nursing and medicine are complementary in an emergency situation. Appropriate nursing and medical interventions are anticipated based on assessment data. Members of the emergency health care staff work as a team in performing the highly technical, hands-on skills required to care for patients in emergency situations (Emergency Nurses Association [ENA], 2013).

Large numbers of people seek emergency care for serious life-threatening conditions, such as cardiac dysrhythmias, acute coronary syndrome, acute heart failure, pulmonary edema, and

Chart 72-1 Facts About Emergency Department Visits—2013

In 2013, there were 130.4 million visits to emergency departments (EDs), a 4% decrease from 2009. There was a concomitant decrease in injury cases, from 45.4 to 37.2 million patients. Additional relevant statistics included the following:

- The most common reasons for ED visits were abdominal pain, chest pain, cough, and fever.
- Most patients had health insurance, with only 15.1% of patients without insurance
- Approximately 14.5% of patients arrived at the ED by ambulance.
- 12.2 million visits resulted in admission (9.3%); of these, 1.5 million required admission to an intensive care unit (ICU).
- Injuries and poisonings accounted for 21.4% of all ED visits.
- The leading causes of injuries were unintentional, totaling 71.4% of injury admissions, with falls and motor vehicle collisions making up 34.8% of these.
- Nearly 30% of patients were seen by a provider in less than 15 minutes after arrival to the ED.

Adapted from Rui, P., Kang, K., & Albert, M. (2013). National Hospital Ambulatory Medical Care Survey: 2013 emergency department summary tables. Retrieved on 2/22/2017 at: www.cdc.gov/nchs/data/ahcd/nhamcs_emergency/2013_ed_web_tables.pdf

stroke. Priorities for managing these cardiac and other conditions are discussed in Chapters 26, 27, 29, and 67. Emergency management of trauma and conditions not found elsewhere in this book are discussed in this chapter. Facts about ED visits in the United States are presented in Chart 72-1.

ISSUES IN EMERGENCY NURSING CARE

Emergency nursing is demanding because of the diversity of conditions and situations that present unique challenges. These challenges include legal issues, occupational health and safety risks for ED staff, and the challenge of providing holistic care in the context of a fast-paced, technology-driven environment in which serious illness and death are encountered on a daily basis. Another dimension of emergency nursing is nursing in disasters. With the increasing use of weapons of terror and mass destruction, both internationally and at home, the emergency nurse must recognize and treat patients exposed to biologic and other weapons, anticipating nursing care in the event of a mass casualty incident from natural causes or a terrorist event (see Chapter 73).

Documentation of Consent and Privacy

Consent to examine and treat the patient is part of the ED record. The patient needs to give consent for invasive procedures (e.g., angiography, lumbar puncture) unless he or she is unconscious or in a critical condition and unable to make decisions. If the patient is unconscious and brought to the ED without family or friends, this fact must be documented. Monitoring of the patient's condition, as well as all instituted treatments and the times at which they were performed, must be documented. After treatment, a notation is made on the record about the patient's condition, response to the treatment, and condition at discharge or transfer and about instructions given to the patient and family for follow-up care.

The patient is also provided with a statement of the privacy policy of the health care agency, according to federal law. Patients involved in violent events can be provided with an alias, and access to the electronic health record is limited to protect the privacy of the patient. A patient may also request extra privacy by limiting access to their room and by choosing not to receive phone calls, mail, flowers, other gifts, or certain visitors. These practices relate to the federally mandated privacy policy stipulated in the Health Insurance Portability and Accountability Act (HIPAA).

According to the Emergency Medical Treatment and Active Labor Act (EMTALA), every ED with a Medicare provider agreement must perform a medical screening examination on all patients arriving with an emergency medical complaint if their acute signs and symptoms could result in serious injury or death if left untreated. EDs are also required to provide treatment aimed at stabilizing each patient's condition. If the patient must be transferred to another facility, the patient's consent for transfer should be obtained, if possible. In addition, acceptance by the receiving facility and physician must be obtained, and an appropriate method of transfer for the patient should be secured. Documentation of assessment and treatment must be sent with the patient upon transfer (ENA, 2013).

Limiting Exposure to Health Risks

Because of the increasing numbers of people infected with hepatitis, human immune deficiency virus (HIV), tuberculosis, and other infectious diseases, health care providers are at an increased risk for exposure to communicable diseases through blood, respiratory droplets, or other body fluids. This risk is further compounded in the ED because of the common use of invasive treatments in patients who may have a wide range of conditions and are unable to provide a comprehensive medical history. All emergency health care providers must adhere strictly to standard precautions for minimizing exposure.

The re-emergence of tuberculosis as a major health problem is complicated by multidrug-resistant tuberculosis and by tuberculosis concomitant with HIV infection. Nurses in the ED are usually fitted with personal high-efficiency particulate air (HEPA) filter masks to use when treating patients with airborne diseases.

 Quality and Safety Nursing Alert

To limit the risk of exposure to airborne diseases, early identification and strict adherence to transmission-based precautions for patients who are potentially infectious is crucial.

The potential for exposure to highly contagious organisms, hazardous chemicals or gases, and radiation related to acts of terrorism or natural or man-made disasters presents additional risks to ED staff. See Chapter 73 for information about decontamination procedures.

Violence in the Emergency Department

Not only do ED staff members encounter patients who may be violent because of the effects of substance abuse, injury, or other emergencies, they may also encounter other violent situations. Patients and families waiting for assistance may be emotionally volatile. Often, waiting rooms are the sites where feelings of dissatisfaction, fear, and anger are channeled violently. Some EDs assign security officers or off duty police to the area and have installed silent alarm systems or metal detectors to identify weapons in order to protect patients, families, and staff. Safety is the first priority.

Patients and family members under the influence of illicit drugs or alcohol, or who may have psychiatric disorders, including delirium or dementia, or who may be influenced by social situations such as gang membership, are at risk for committing a violent act, whether intentional or not (Avander, Heikki, Bjersa, et al., 2016). The environment of the ED, including being subjected to long wait times and crowded conditions, may also increase their risk of committing violent events. Physical threats are most often accompanied by verbal abuse, which is the most common type of violence (American College of Emergency Physicians [ACEP], 2011). Although not a typical occurrence, a patient or family member may come to the ED armed. To avoid angry confrontations, members of gangs and families who are feuding need to be separated in the ED, in the waiting room, and later in the inpatient nursing unit. Nurses and other personnel must be prepared to deal with these circumstances. The ED should be locked against entry if security is questionable.

Patients who are violent or potentially violent must be vigilantly monitored by the ED staff. Care must be taken to avoid injury. Patients from prison and those who are under guard need to be handcuffed to the bed and appropriately assessed to ensure the safety of hospital staff and other patients. The emergency nurse must understand how to employ safe use of restraints. The Joint Commission has strict standards regarding documentation of the reason, monitoring for safety, and ensuring the dignity of the patient who is restrained (Solheim, 2016). Precautions to be taken to avoid injury include the following situations (ENA 2013; Speroni, Fitch, Dawson, et al., 2014):

- For prisoners, the hand or ankle restraint (handcuff) is never released, and a guard is always present in the room.
- A mask can be placed on the patient to prevent spitting or biting.
- Nonrestraint techniques should be tried when possible—e.g., talking with the patient, minimizing environmental stimulation.
- Physical restraints are used on any patient who is violent only as needed and, if used, should be humanely and professionally given (ACEP, 2014); nonetheless, the staff should be cognizant that the patient could head-butt, even if restrained.
- Distance should be maintained from the patient to avoid grabbing; staff should not wear items that can be grabbed by the patient, such as dangling jewelry and stethoscopes. Furthermore, distance should be maintained between the patient and the door so that an escape route for the staff member is preserved.
- Objects should not be left within patient reach; even an intravenous (IV) line spike can become a tool of violence if the patient is determined.

- Courses on safety (de-escalation and physical restraint techniques) assist the staff with preparing for various violent situations.

In the case of gunfire in the ED, self-protection is a priority. There is no advantage to protecting others if health care providers are injured. Security officers and police must gain control of the situation first, and then care is provided to the injured.

Providing Holistic Care

Patients and families experiencing sudden injury or illness are often overwhelmed by anxiety because they have not had time to adapt to the crisis. They experience real and terrifying fear of death, mutilation, immobilization, and other assaults on their personal identity and body integrity. When confronted with trauma, severe disfigurement, severe illness, or sudden death, the family experiences several stages of crisis. The stages begin with anxiety and progress through denial, remorse and guilt, anger, grief, and reconciliation. The initial goal for the patient and family is anxiety reduction, a prerequisite to effective and appropriate coping. During this stressful time, safety is of prime importance. Close observation and preplanning are essential and security personnel are stationed nearby in the event that a patient or family member responds to stress with physical violence.

Assessment of the patient and family's psychological function includes evaluating emotional expression, degree of anxiety, and cognitive functioning. Possible nursing diagnoses include:

- Anxiety or death anxiety related to uncertain potential outcomes of the illness or trauma
- Ineffective coping related to acute situational crisis

Possible nursing diagnoses for the family include:

- Grieving
- Interrupted family processes
- Compromised or disabled family coping related to acute situational crises

Patient-Focused Interventions

Clinicians caring for the patient should act confidently and competently to relieve anxiety and promote a sense of security. Explanations should be given that the patient can understand. Human contact and reassuring words reduce the panic of the person who is severely injured or ill and aid in dispelling fear of the unknown.

The patient who is unconscious should be treated as if conscious—that is, the patient should be touched, called by name, and given an explanation of every procedure that is performed. As the patient regains consciousness, the nurse should orient the patient by stating their name, the date, and the location. This basic information should be provided repeatedly, as needed, in a reassuring way.

Ensuring patient safety is a major focus in clinical practice settings. Some of the most common **sentinel events** (unanticipated events that result in patient harm) in the ED include delays to care and medication errors. Common root causes for these sentinel events revolve around nurse staffing patterns, patient volume, and specialty availability. Solutions to patient safety issues in the ED include ensuring optimal nurse staffing, pharmacy presence, and rapid diagnostics turnaround times to minimize wait time to diagnosis and fostering teamwork and support by leadership. All errors should be reported and investigated even if a patient was not harmed. In this way, future injury or death may be avoided (ENA, 2013).

Family-Focused Interventions

The family is kept informed about where the patient is, how he or she is doing, and the care that is being given. Encouraging family members to stay with the patient, when possible, also helps allay their anxieties. In many facilities, family presence during resuscitation is permitted to assist the family to cope through this difficult time. Many family members respond very well to this approach. One study found that families view emergency professionals favorably when a family member was resuscitated. They view their role as supportive and protective of the patient. Allowing family presence in the critical care areas of the hospital enhances the family role and builds trust in the caregivers (Leske, McAndrew, & Brasel, 2013). Posttraumatic stress disorder (PTSD) is less likely to occur if the family member is present during resuscitation (Jabre, Belpomme, Azoulay, et al., 2013). The presence of a family facilitator, who is trained to provide support to family members, is vital to the success of a family presence program. Additional interventions are based on the assessment of the stage of crisis that the family is experiencing. Measures to help family members cope with sudden death are presented in Chart 72-2.

Chart 72-2 Helping Family Members Cope With Sudden Death

The nurse takes the following actions:

- Take the family to a private place.
- Talk to the family together so that they can grieve together and hear the information given together.
- Reassure the family that everything possible was done; inform them of the treatment rendered.
- Avoid using euphemisms such as "passed on." Show the family that you care by touching, offering coffee, water, and the services of a chaplain.
- Encourage family members to support each other and to express emotions freely (grief, loss, anger, helplessness, tears, disbelief).
- Avoid giving sedation to family members; this may mask or delay the grieving process, which is necessary to achieve emotional equilibrium and to prevent prolonged depression.
- Encourage the family to view the body if they wish; this action helps to integrate the loss. Cover disfigured and injured areas before the family sees the body. Go with the family and do not leave them alone. Show acceptance by touching the body to give the family "permission" to touch.
- Spend time with the family, listening to them and identifying any needs that they may have for which the nursing staff can be helpful.
- Allow family members to talk about the deceased and what he or she meant to them; this permits ventilation of feelings of loss. Encourage the family to talk about events preceding admission to the emergency department. Do not challenge initial feelings of anger or denial.
- Avoid volunteering unnecessary information (e.g., the patient was drinking).

Anxiety and Denial

During these crises, family members are encouraged to recognize and talk about their feelings of anxiety. Asking questions is encouraged. Honest answers given at the level of the family's understanding must be provided. Although denial is an ego-defense mechanism that protects one from recognizing painful and disturbing aspects of reality, prolonged denial is not encouraged or supported. The family must be prepared for the reality of what has happened and what may come.

Remorse and Guilt

Expressions of remorse and guilt are common, with family members accusing themselves (or each other) of negligence or minor omissions. Family members are urged to verbalize their feelings to help them cope appropriately.

Anger

Expressions of anger, common in crisis situations, are a way of handling anxiety and fear. Anger is frequently directed by the family at the patient, but it is also often expressed toward the physician, the nurse, or admitting personnel. The therapeutic approach is to allow the anger to be expressed and to assist the family members to identify their feelings of frustration.

Grief

Grief is a complex emotional response to anticipated or actual loss. The key nursing intervention is to help family members work through their grief and to support their coping mechanisms, letting them know that it is normal and acceptable for them to cry, feel pain, and express loss. The hospital chaplain and social services staff serve as invaluable members of the team when assisting families to work through their grief (see Chapter 16).

Caring for Emergency Personnel

Concerted efforts have been made to focus on the needs of the ED staff, especially after serious and stressful events (ENA, 2013). Events can range from a local trauma case involving children; to treating someone known to the emergency worker, such as a colleague or family member; to a more complex natural disaster or multicasualty situation. It is important to remember that all staff members may not necessarily respond in the same way; an event that is stressful to one person may not be as stressful to another. Compassion fatigue may result from the continuous exposure to suffering and injury, and energy is expended on a daily basis. Fatigue occurs when the affected staff members cannot replenish the energy stores (Solheim, 2016). In addition, because stress is a daily occurrence in the ED, the staff may not recognize the personal effect of any one event or the cumulative effect of day-to-day crisis interventions. ED leadership should be aware of staff coping patterns and support systems, patterns of interactions between staff members, staff members' health problems, including addiction, and appropriately assist with identifying behaviors caused by workplace stress. The availability of nonjudgmental counseling is essential to promoting a healthy staff.

After serious events, critical incident stress management (CISM) is necessary to critique individual and group performance and to facilitate healthy coping. Optimally, this may consist of three steps: defusing, debriefing, and follow-up.

Defusing occurs immediately after the critical incident. During this session, affected staff are encouraged to discuss their feelings about the incident and are given contact information so that they may talk to someone if they have disturbing symptoms (e.g., sleeplessness, excessive worry). Debriefing typically occurs 1 to 10 days after the critical incident. Debriefing sessions follow a format similar to the initial defusing session; however, during these sessions, participating staff are encouraged to discuss their feelings about the incident and are reassured that their negative reactions and feelings are normal and that their negative feelings will diminish over time. At the end of these sessions, participants should have a feeling of closure and be able to resume their professional roles at an emotional level commensurate to that prior to the critical incident. Some staff may require further professional follow-up, however. Follow-up may occur after the debriefing session is completed for those participants who have persistent negative symptoms and may consist of continued individual or group counseling and therapy (Solheim, 2016).

EMERGENCY NURSING AND THE CONTINUUM OF CARE

A key principle underlying emergency care is that the patient is rapidly assessed, treated, and referred to the appropriate setting for ongoing care. This makes the ED a temporary point on the continuum of care. Only 11.9% of patients who receive emergency care are admitted to the hospital, which means emergency nurses must plan and facilitate the patient's safe discharge and follow-up care in the home, community, and the transitional care environment (Cadogan, Phillips, & Ziminski, 2016).

Discharge Planning

Before discharge, verbal and written instructions for continuing care are given to the patient and the family or significant others. Many EDs have preprinted standard instruction sheets for the more common conditions (i.e., concussion), which can then be individualized. Discharge instructions should be available in a variety of languages. A language interpreter should be used as necessary to provide both written and verbal instructions.

Instructions should include information about prescribed medications, treatments, diet, activity, and when to contact a health care provider or schedule follow-up appointments. Discharge planning is the "teachable moment" for the patient, providing the opportunity to present injury prevention or smoking cessation strategies, alcohol counseling opportunities, and more. It is imperative that instructions are written legibly, use simple language, and are clear in their important points. When providing discharge instructions, the nurse also considers any special needs the patient may have related to hearing or visual impairments. Alternate formats of instruction (e.g., large print, Braille, audiotape) should be available to meet the needs of patients with hearing or visual impairments.

Community and Transitional Services

Before discharge, some patients require the services of a social worker to help them meet continuing health care needs. Home care resources may be contacted before discharge to arrange services. This is particularly important for patients who are older adults or who have disabilities and who need assistance. Identifying continuing health care needs and making arrangements for meeting these needs can prevent return visits to the ED or readmission to the hospital.

For patients who are returning to long-term care facilities and for those who already rely on community agencies for continuing health care, communication about the patient's condition and any changes in health care needs that have occurred must be provided to the appropriate facilities or agencies. This communication is essential to promote continuity of care and to ensure ongoing care that meets the patient's changing health care needs.

Many patients who utilize EDs have health problems that are nonurgent. Moreover, some patients return repeatedly to the ED with nonurgent problems (ENA, 2015a). It is posited that patients who present to the ED with nonurgent problems do so because there is a dearth of outpatient health care resources to fill their needs. In order to fill these gaps, some areas of the United States, particularly rural areas, are offering mobile integrated health-community paramedicine programs. Emergency medical system (EMS) personnel provide in-home visits, without emergency call, to identify needs, and provide education and in-home care. If necessary, they can also transport patients to the ED. These programs have decreased unnecessary EMS calls without transport or unnecessary transports (ENA, 2015a).

 Gerontologic Considerations

The ED is a common point of entry into the health care system for patients 65 years and older. The Centers for Disease Control and Prevention (CDC, 2013) reports that 36.5% of ED visits by patients older than 65 years resulted in hospital admission. As age increases, the percentage of admissions increases. Of these admissions, 29% were related to trauma, primarily falls (CDC, 2013). Older adult patients typically arrive with one or more presenting conditions. Nonspecific symptoms, such as weakness and fatigue, episodes of falling, incontinence, and change in mental status, may be manifestations of acute, potentially life-threatening illness in the older person. Emergencies in this age group may be more difficult to manage because older adult patients may have an atypical presentation, an altered response to treatment, a greater risk of developing complications, or a combination of these factors.

The older adult patient may perceive the emergency as a crisis signaling the end of an independent lifestyle or even resulting in death. The nurse should give attention to the patient's feelings of anxiety and fear.

The older patient may have limited sources of social and financial support during these times of crises. The nurse should assess the psychosocial resources of the patient (and of the caregiver, if necessary) and anticipate discharge needs. Referrals for support services (e.g., to the social service department or a gerontologic nurse specialist) may be necessary.

 Obesity Considerations

The growing rate of obesity in the United States has implications for treating patients with obesity within the ED, in terms of stocking appropriately sized equipment, gowns, and stretchers; ensuring that equipment (e.g., computed tomography [CT] scanners) is able to handle a greater weight capacity; and recognizing specific disorders and complications that may occur in these patients. For instance, research suggests that increased mortality is associated with the degree of obesity (ENA, 2013). Other considerations in ED management of patients with obesity include an understanding that it is generally more challenging to insert IV lines and airways. Ventilation also can be a challenge from the increased weight of the chest wall and the increased incidence of hypoventilation and sleep apnea among patients with obesity. Special consideration must be taken with lipophilic medications, as they take longer to clear from the larger volume of adipose tissue. Weight-based medications must be calculated carefully using ideal body mass. X-rays may be difficult to visualize because of poor penetration.

Complications that patients with obesity are more prone to experience during hospitalization include respiratory failure, acute kidney injury, pneumonia, deep vein thrombosis, and pressure ulcers. Patients with severe obesity who have femur fractures have a significantly higher risk of death, as well as a higher risk of acute respiratory distress syndrome (ARDS) and sepsis than patients of normal weight (Weinlein, Deadrick, & Murphy, 2015). Although many of these complications do not occur until later in the hospital stay, some preventive measures (e.g., encouraging turning, coughing, and deep-breathing exercises to prevent atelectasis) may be initiated in the ED. Functional recovery time is extended in patients with obesity, resulting in longer lengths of stay and increased hospital costs. Initiating prevention measures in the ED, such as early backboard removal and providing early preventive respiratory care, are targeted to improve recovery time (Childs, Nahm, Dolenc, et al., 2015; Dhungel, Liao, Raut, et al., 2015). Arranging transfers of patients with obesity must also take into consideration the availability of appropriately sized equipment.

PRINCIPLES OF EMERGENCY CARE

By definition, emergency care is care that must be rendered without delay. In an ED, several patients with diverse health problems—some life threatening, some not—may present to the ED simultaneously. One of the first principles of emergency care is triage.

Triage

The word **triage** comes from the French word *trier*, meaning "to sort." In the daily routine of the ED, triage is used to sort patients into groups based on the severity of their health problems and the immediacy with which these problems must be treated.

A basic and widely used triage system that had been in use for many years utilized three categories: emergent, urgent, and nonurgent. In this system, emergent patients had the highest priority, urgent patients had serious health problems but not immediately life-threatening ones, and nonurgent patients had episodic illnesses.

A comprehensive, valid, and reliable five-level triage severity rating system that recognizes that EDs are used for both emergency and routine health care is also used. The increased number of triage levels assists the triage nurse to more precisely determine the needs of the patient and the urgency for treatment. Systems that meet these criteria for validity and reliability that are commonly used in the United States are the Emergency Severity Index (ESI) and the Canadian Triage and Acuity Scale (CTAS). The ESI assigns patients into five levels, from level 1 (most urgent) to level 5 (least urgent). With the ESI, patients are assigned to triage levels based on both their acuity and their anticipated resource needs (Gilboy, Tanabe, Travers, et al., 2012). The CTAS system's five levels include time parameters that guide how frequently patients must be reassessed by either a nurse or provider. Patients assigned to the *resuscitation* category must receive continuous nursing surveillance, those in the *emergent* category must be reassessed at least every 15 minutes, patients in the *urgent* category must be reassessed at least every 30 minutes, patients in the *less urgent* category must be reassessed at least every 60 minutes, and those in the *nonurgent* category must be reassessed at least every 120 minutes. The goal of all triage is rapid assessment and decision-making, preferably under 5 minutes (ENA 2013).

Although the ESI and the CTAS are valid and reliable triage severity rating systems, many EDs in the United States have high patient volumes and slow flow. Patients arriving at the ED may experience bottlenecks at triage. To further refine the system, triage bypass moves an incoming patient directly to a bed if open beds are available in the department. This eliminates the patient waiting and the receiving nurse performs the initial assessment and vital signs. In team triage (or provider in triage [PIT]), the triage nurse works with the physician or advanced practitioner within the triage area itself. Team triage can move patients to diagnostics and possibly discharge without full admission to the ED. Both of these additional concepts added to triage decrease wait time for treatment and maintain flow in the department (ENA, 2013). Many patient flow problems are driven by availability of in-house beds. The ED needs to be as efficient as possible to decrease wait times, maintain flow for EMS agencies, and be available for true emergencies.

Triage is an advanced skill. Emergency nurses spend many hours learning to classify different illnesses and injuries to ensure that patients most in need of care do not needlessly wait. Protocols may be followed to initiate laboratory or x-ray studies while the patient is in the triage area. Collaborative protocols are developed and used by the triage nurse based on their level of experience. Nurses in the triage area collect additional crucial baseline data: full vital signs including pain assessment, history of the current event and past medical history, neurologic assessment findings, weight, allergies (especially to latex and medications), domestic violence screening, and necessary diagnostic data. Some facilities collect these data in a computerized system, which help guide the nurse through assessment and documentation. Asking questions is key to appropriate triage decisions. The following questions reflect the minimum information that should be obtained from the patient or from the person who accompanied the patient to the ED (so long as that person is not suspected of abuse or neglect; see later discussion) and then are documented:
- What were the circumstances, precipitating events, location, and time of the injury or illness?
- When did the symptoms appear?
- Was the patient unconscious after the injury or onset of illness?

- How did the patient get to the ED?
- What was the health status of the patient before the injury or illness?
- Is there a history of medical illness or previous surgeries? A history of admissions to the hospital?
- Is the patient currently taking any medications, especially hormones, insulin, digitalis, or anticoagulants? Is the patient using any complementary or alternative therapies such as herbology, naturopathy, Reiki, massage, or acupuncture?
- Does the patient have any allergies, especially to latex, medications, eggs, or nuts?
- Does the patient use tobacco products or recreational drugs? How frequently? What type? When was the last time they were used?
- Does the patient have any fears? Does the patient feel that he or she is in danger or in an unsafe situation?
- When was the last meal eaten? (This is important if general anesthesia is to be given or if the patient is unconscious.)
- When was the last menstrual period?
- Is the patient under a physician's care? What are the name and contact information for the physician?
- What was the date of the patient's most recent tetanus immunization?

In addition to the collection of initial vital signs and medical history, triage consists of providing basic first aid, which may include application of ice, bleeding control, and basic wound care, as well as initiating protocol-based prescriptions (e.g., x-rays, administering antipyretic or mild analgesic agents, obtaining an electrocardiogram [ECG] or urinalysis, removing sutures). The triage nurse also is responsible for and monitors the waiting area, maintains a safe environment, reassesses patients who are waiting, and is the initial liaison to the families of patients.

Routine ED triage protocols differ significantly from the triage protocols used in disasters and mass casualty incidents (field triage). Routine triage directs all available resources to the patients who are most critically ill, regardless of potential outcome. In field triage (or hospital triage during a disaster), scarce resources must be used to benefit the most people possible. This distinction affects triage decisions (see Chapter 73).

Assess and Intervene

For the patient assigned to an urgent or higher triage category, stabilization, provision of critical treatments, and prompt transfer to the appropriate setting (intensive care unit, operating room, general care unit) are the priorities of emergency care. Although treatment is initiated in the ED, ongoing definitive treatment of the underlying problem is provided in other settings, and the sooner the patient is stabilized and moved to that area, the better the outcome.

A systematic approach to effectively establishing and treating health priorities is the primary survey/secondary survey approach. The **primary survey** focuses on stabilizing life-threatening conditions. The ED staff work collaboratively and follow the ABCDE (*a*irway, *b*reathing, *c*irculation, *d*isability, *e*xposure) method:

- Establish a patent airway.
- Provide adequate ventilation, employing resuscitation measures when necessary. Patients who have

experienced trauma must have the cervical spine protected and chest injuries assessed first, immediately after the airway is established.

- Evaluate and restore cardiac output by controlling hemorrhage, preventing and treating shock, and maintaining or restoring effective circulation. This includes the prevention and management of hypothermia. In addition, peripheral pulses are examined, and any immediate closed reductions of fractures or dislocations are performed if an extremity is pulseless.
- Determine neurologic disability by assessing neurologic function using the Glasgow Coma Scale (GCS) (See Chapter 68, Chart 68-2) and a motor and sensory evaluation of the spine (see Chapter 65, Fig. 65-9). A quick neurologic assessment may be performed using the AVPU mnemonic:
  - A—alert. Is the patient alert and responsive?
  - V—verbal. Does the patient respond to verbal stimuli?
  - P—pain. Does the patient respond only to painful stimuli?
  - U—unresponsive. Is the patient unresponsive to all stimuli, including pain?
- Undress the patient quickly but gently so that any wounds or areas of injury are identified; this may entail cutting away articles of clothing (American College of Surgeons [ACS], 2013).

After these priorities have been addressed, the ED team proceeds with the **secondary survey**. This includes the following:

- Complete health history, including the history of the current event
- Head-to-toe assessment (includes a reassessment of airway and breathing parameters and vital signs)
- Diagnostic and laboratory testing
- Insertion or application of monitoring devices such as ECG electrodes, arterial lines, or urinary catheters
- Splinting of suspected fractures
- Cleansing, closure, and dressing of wounds
- Performance of other necessary interventions based on the patient's condition

Once the patient has been assessed, stabilized, and tested, appropriate medical and nursing diagnoses are formulated, initial important treatment is started, and plans for the proper disposition of the patient are made. Many emergent and urgent conditions and priority emergency interventions are discussed in detail in the remaining sections of this chapter.

In addition to the management of the illness or injury, the ED nurse must also focus on providing comfort and emotional support to the patient and family. Included in this is pain management. Effective pain management must be instituted early and should include rapid-acting agents that result in minimal sedation so that the patient can continue to interact with the staff for ongoing assessment. Moderate sedation can help facilitate short procedures in the ED; the patient will not remember the procedure later. The patient is closely monitored during the procedure and then rapidly awakens when it is complete (see Chapter 18).

It is essential that family crisis intervention services are available for families of patients in the ED. Even if a patient's condition is not emergent, the situation may be perceived as such by the family. Every family needs attention and support.

The chaplain and social worker may be available to assist with interventions.

AIRWAY OBSTRUCTION

Acute upper airway obstruction is a life-threatening medical emergency.

Pathophysiology

The airway may be partially or completely occluded. Partial obstruction of the airway can lead to progressive hypoxia, hypercarbia, and respiratory and cardiac arrest. If the airway is completely obstructed, permanent brain injury or death will occur within 3 to 5 minutes secondary to hypoxia. Air movement is absent in the presence of complete airway obstruction. Oxygen saturation of the blood decreases rapidly because obstruction of the airway prevents entry of air into the lungs. Oxygen deficit occurs in the brain, resulting in unconsciousness, with death following rapidly.

Upper airway obstruction has a number of causes, including aspiration of foreign bodies, anaphylaxis, viral or bacterial infection, trauma, and inhalation or chemical burns. For older adult patients, especially those in extended care facilities, sedative and hypnotic medications, diseases affecting motor coordination (e.g., Parkinson disease), and mental dysfunction (e.g., dementia, intellectual disability) are risk factors for asphyxiation by food. As patients age, atrophy of the posterior pharynx occurs, resulting in aspiration or difficulty swallowing. In adults, aspiration of a bolus of meat is the most common cause of airway obstruction. Peritonsillar abscesses, epiglottitis, and other acute infectious processes of the posterior pharynx can also result in airway obstruction. The most common causes of airway obstruction are from an allergic reaction (i.e., causing laryngospasm), infection, or angioedema (ENA, 2013).

Clinical Manifestations

Typically, a person with a foreign-body airway obstruction cannot speak, breathe, or cough. The patient may clutch the neck between the thumb and fingers (i.e., universal distress signal). Other common signs and symptoms include choking, apprehensive appearance, refusing to lie flat, inspiratory and expiratory stridor, labored breathing, the use of accessory muscles (suprasternal and intercostal retraction), flaring nostrils, increasing anxiety, restlessness, and confusion. Cyanosis and loss of consciousness, which develop as hypoxia worsens, are late signs. Action must be taken before these manifestations develop, if possible, or immediately if the patient has already exhibited these signs.

Assessment and Diagnostic Findings

Assessment of the patient who has a foreign object occluding the airway may involve simply asking the person whether he or she is choking and requires help. If the person is unconscious, inspection of the oropharynx may reveal the offending object. X-rays, laryngoscopy, or bronchoscopy also may be performed. Oxygen supplementation should be considered immediately.

Management

If the patient can breathe and cough spontaneously, a partial obstruction should be suspected. The victim is encouraged to cough forcefully and to persist with spontaneous coughing and breathing efforts as long as good air exchange exists. There may be some wheezing between coughs. If the patient demonstrates a weak, ineffective cough, high-pitched noise while inhaling, increased respiratory difficulty, or cyanosis, the patient should be managed as if there were complete airway obstruction.

After the obstruction is removed, rescue breathing is initiated. If the patient has no pulse, cardiac compressions are instituted. These measures provide oxygen to the brain, heart, and other vital organs until definitive medical treatment can restore and support normal heart and ventilatory activity (ENA, 2013). See Chapter 29 for review of current CPR guidelines.

Establishing an Airway

Establishing an airway may be as simple as repositioning the patient's head to prevent the tongue from obstructing the pharynx. Alternatively, other maneuvers, such as the head-tilt/chin-lift maneuver, the jaw-thrust maneuver, or insertion of specialized equipment, may be needed to open the airway, remove a foreign body, or maintain the airway. In all maneuvers, the cervical spine must be protected from injury. After these maneuvers are performed, the patient is assessed for breathing by watching for chest movement and listening and feeling for air movement. In such a case, nursing diagnoses would include ineffective airway clearance related to obstruction of the airway by the tongue, an object, or fluids (blood, saliva) and ineffective breathing pattern related to airway obstruction or injury. See Chapter 21, Chart 21-6 for information regarding how to clear an upper airway obstruction.

Oropharyngeal/Nasopharyngeal Airway Insertion

An oropharyngeal airway is a semicircular tube or tubelike plastic device that is inserted over the back of the tongue into the lower posterior pharynx in a patient who is breathing spontaneously but who is unconscious (see Chart 72-3). This type of airway prevents the tongue from falling back against the posterior pharynx and obstructing the airway. It also allows health care providers to suction secretions. The nasopharyngeal airway provides the same airway access but is inserted through the nares. With an airway in place the patient may breathe spontaneously. If breathing is ineffective or absent, bag-valve-mask ventilation is necessary.

 Quality and Safety Nursing Alert

In the case of potential facial trauma or basal skull fracture, the nasopharyngeal airway should not be used because it could enter the brain cavity instead of the pharynx.

Endotracheal Intubation

The purpose of endotracheal intubation is to establish and maintain the airway in patients with respiratory insufficiency or hypoxia. Endotracheal intubation is indicated to establish an airway for a patient who cannot be adequately ventilated with an oropharyngeal or nasopharyngeal airway, bypass an

Inserting an Oropharyngeal Airway

1. Measure the oral airway alongside the head. The airway should reach from lip to ear.
2. Extend the patient's head by placing one hand under the bony chin (*only if the cervical spine is uninjured*). With the other hand, tilt the head backward by applying pressure to the forehead while simultaneously lifting the chin forward.
3. Open the patient's mouth.
4. **A.** Insert the oropharyngeal airway with the tip facing up toward the roof of the mouth until it passes the uvula.
   B. Rotate the tip 180 degrees so that the tip is pointed

down toward the pharynx. This displaces the tongue anteriorly, and the patient then breathes through and around the airway. An alternate method is to use a tongue blade to hold the tongue and insert the oropharyngeal airway directly without rotation.
5. The distal end of the oropharyngeal airway is in the hypopharynx, and the flange is approximately at the patient's lips. Make sure that the tongue has not been pushed into the airway.

A   **B**

Adapted from Walsh, K & Woten, M. (2016). Oropharyngeal airway: Inserting in adults. In D. Pravikoff (Ed.). *Nursing practice and skill.* Glendale, CA: CINAHL Information Systems.

---

upper airway obstruction, prevent aspiration, permit connection of the patient to a resuscitation bag or mechanical ventilator, or facilitate the removal of tracheobronchial secretions (see Fig. 72-1). Because of the level of skill required, endotracheal intubation is performed only by those who have had extensive training. These may include physicians, nurse anesthetists, respiratory therapists, flight nurses, and nurse practitioners. However, the emergency nurse commonly assists with intubation.

Laryngoscope

Tongue

Tongue
Epiglottis

Vocal
cords

Trachea

Arytenoid
muscle

A   **B**

Figure 72-1 • Endotracheal intubation in a patient without a cervical spine injury. **A.** The primary glottic landmarks for tracheal intubation as visualized with proper placement of the laryngoscope. **B.** Positioning the endotracheal tube.

Rapid sequence intubation may be indicated, which provides management of the patient in a situation similar to that in the operating room. Medications used to facilitate rapid sequence intubation include a sedative, an analgesic, and a neuromuscular blockade agent; these are usually given by the practitioner performing the intubation.

Intubation With a King Tube or Laryngeal Mask Airway

If the patient is not hospitalized and cannot be intubated in the field, emergency medical personnel may insert a King Tube, which rapidly provides pharyngeal ventilation. When the tube is inserted into the trachea, it functions like an endotracheal tube (see Fig. 72-2).

The two balloons that surround the tube are inflated after the tube is inserted. One balloon is large and occludes the oropharynx. This permits ventilation by forcing air through the larynx. The smaller balloon is inflated with air and occludes the esophagus at a site distal to the glottis. Breath sounds are auscultated after balloon inflation to make sure that the oropharyngeal balloon (or cuff) does not obstruct the glottis. One variant type of King Tube is designed so that a gastric tube may also be passed for suction. If it is difficult to establish an airway, a laryngeal mask airway (LMA) may be inserted as an interim airway device. The design of the LMA provides a "mask" in the subglottic airway with a cuff inflated within the esophagus. It allows easy insertion for rapid airway control until a more definitive airway can be placed. Some LMAs also permit removal of secretions from the esophagus (see Chapter 18, Fig. 18-3A).

Gas flow

■ Primary ventilatory outlets
□ Additional side eyelets

Single inflation valve
Hyoid bone
Epiglottis
Vocal cords
Trachea
Esophagus

Hard palate
Soft palate

KingLT(S)-D

Distal cuff
Inflates in the esophagus. Isolates the laryngopharynx from the esophagus.

Proximal cuff
Inflates the base of the tongue. Isolates the laryngopharynx from the oropharynx and nasopharynx.

Figure 72-2 • King Tube (**A**) correctly placed in esophageal position (**B**). Reprinted with permission from King Systems Corporation, Noblesville, Indiana.

Cricothyroidotomy (Cricothyroid Membrane Puncture)

Cricothyroidotomy is the opening of the cricothyroid membrane to establish an airway. This procedure is used in emergency situations in which endotracheal intubation is either not possible or contraindicated, as in airway obstruction from extensive maxillofacial trauma, cervical spine injuries, laryngospasm, laryngeal edema (after an allergic reaction or extubation), hemorrhage into neck tissue, or obstruction of the larynx. A cricothyroidotomy is replaced with a formal tracheostomy when the patient is able to tolerate this procedure.

Maintaining Ventilation

After the airway is determined to be unobstructed, the nurse must ensure that ventilation is adequate by checking for equal bilateral breath sounds. Satisfactory management of ventilations may prevent hypoxia and hypercapnia. The nurse must quickly assess for absent or diminished breath sounds, open chest wounds, and difficulty delivering artificial breaths for the patient. The nurse should monitor pulse oximetry, capnography, and arterial blood gases if the patient requires airway or ventilatory assistance. A tension pneumothorax can mimic hypovolemia, so ventilatory assessment precedes assessment for hemorrhage. A pneumothorax (both simple and tension) or sucking (open) chest wound is managed with a chest tube and occlusion of the sucking wound; immediate relief of increasing positive intrathoracic pressure and maintenance of adequate ventilation should occur.

HEMORRHAGE

Stopping bleeding is essential to the care and survival of patients in an emergency or disaster situation. Hemorrhage that results in the reduction of circulating blood volume is a main cause of shock. Minor bleeding, which is usually venous, generally stops spontaneously unless the patient has a bleeding disorder or has been taking anticoagulant agents. Internal hemorrhage can hide in many anatomic spaces and compartments, resulting in shock without external evidence of hemorrhage. The internal spaces and compartments that are capable of housing large amounts of blood include the retroperitoneum, pelvis, chest, and thighs (ACS, 2013).

The patient is assessed for signs and symptoms of shock: cool, moist skin (resulting from poor peripheral perfusion), decreasing blood pressure, increasing heart rate, delayed capillary refill, and decreasing urine volume (see Chapter 14). The goals of emergency management are to control the bleeding, maintain adequate circulating blood volume for tissue oxygenation, and prevent shock. Patients who hemorrhage are at risk for cardiac arrest caused by hypovolemia with secondary anoxia. Nursing interventions are carried out collaboratively with other members of the emergency health care team.

Management

Fluid Replacement

Whenever a patient is hemorrhaging—whether externally or internally—a loss of circulating blood results in a fluid volume deficit and decreased cardiac output. Therefore, fluid replacement is imperative to maintain circulation. Typically, two large-gauge IV catheters are inserted, preferably in an uninjured extremity, to provide a means for fluid and blood replacement. Blood samples are obtained for analysis, typing, and cross-matching. Replacement fluids are given as prescribed, depending on clinical estimates of the type and volume of fluid lost. Replacement fluids may include isotonic electrolyte solutions (e.g., lactated Ringer's, normal saline), colloids, and blood component therapy.

Packed red blood cells are infused when there is massive blood loss, which may also necessitate transfusion of other blood components, including platelets and clotting factors. See Chapter 32 for full discussion of blood component therapy indications and treatment.

⚑ *Quality and Safety Nursing Alert*

The infusion rate is determined by the severity of the blood loss and the clinical evidence of hypovolemia. Any blood replacement therapy should be given via warmer when possible, because administration of large amounts of blood that has been refrigerated has a core cooling effect that may lead to cardiac arrest and coagulopathy.

Control of External Hemorrhage

If a patient is hemorrhaging externally (e.g., from a wound), a rapid physical assessment is performed as the patient's clothing is cut away in an attempt to identify the area of hemorrhage. Direct, firm pressure is applied over the bleeding area or the involved artery at a site that is proximal to the wound (see Fig. 72-3). Most bleeding can be stopped or at least controlled by application of direct pressure. Otherwise, unchecked arterial bleeding results in death. A firm pressure dressing is applied, and the injured part is elevated to stop venous and capillary bleeding, if possible. If the injured area is an extremity, the extremity is immobilized to control blood loss.

A tourniquet is applied to an extremity when the external hemorrhage cannot be controlled in any other way and until surgery can be performed. The tourniquet is applied just proximal to the wound and tied tightly enough to control arterial blood flow. The patient is tagged with a skin-marking pencil or on adhesive tape on the forehead with a "T," stating the location of the tourniquet and the time applied. If the patient has suffered a traumatic amputation with uncontrollable hemorrhage, the tourniquet remains in place until the patient is in the operating room. Time of tourniquet application and removal should be documented. Tourniquet placement among military personnel with battle-associated trauma has demonstrated clear mortality reduction, although it occasionally has led to amputation or fasciotomy (Inaba, Siboni, Resnick, et al., 2015).

Control of Internal Bleeding

If the patient shows no external signs of bleeding but exhibits tachycardia, falling blood pressure, thirst, apprehension, cool and moist skin, or delayed capillary refill, internal hemorrhage is suspected. Typically, packed red blood cells, plasma, and platelets are given at a rapid rate, and the patient is prepared for more definitive treatment (e.g., surgery, pharmacologic therapy). In addition, arterial blood gas specimens are obtained to evaluate pulmonary function and tissue perfusion and to establish baseline hemodynamic parameters, which are then used as an index for determining the amount of fluid replacement the patient can tolerate and the response to therapy. The patient is maintained in the supine position and monitored closely until hemodynamic or circulatory parameters improve, or until he or she is transported to the operating room or intensive care unit.

Figure 72-3 • Pressure points for control of hemorrhage.

A Temporal

B Facial

C Carotid

D Subclavian

E Brachial

F Radial and ulnar

G Femoral

HYPOVOLEMIC SHOCK

Shock is a condition in which there is loss of effective circulating blood volume. Inadequate organ and tissue perfusion follows, ultimately resulting in cellular metabolic derangements. In any emergency situation, the onset of shock should be anticipated by immediately assessing all people who are injured. The underlying cause of shock (hypovolemic, cardiogenic, neurogenic, anaphylactic, or septic) must be determined. Of these, hypovolemia is the most common cause. See Chapter 14 for further discussion of management of hypovolemic shock.

WOUNDS

Wounds involving injury to soft tissues can vary from minor tears to severe crushing injuries. The types of wounds that may occur are defined in Chart 72-4. The main goal of treatment is to restore the physical integrity and function of the injured tissue while minimizing scarring and preventing infection. Proper documentation of the characteristics of the wound, using precise descriptions and correct terminology, is essential. Such information may be needed in the future for forensic evidence. Photographs are helpful because they provide an accurate, visible depiction of the wound. Photographs also become important for exigent wounds (i.e., wounds that will eventually heal). Patients involved in domestic violence or trauma may need the photographs later to visually describe the extent of injury.

Determining *when* and *how* the wound occurred is important because a treatment delay increases infection risk. Using aseptic technique, the clinician inspects the wound to determine the extent of damage to underlying structures or the presence of a foreign body. Sensory, motor, and vascular function is evaluated for changes that might indicate complications.

Management
Wound Cleansing

Hair around the wound may be clipped (only as directed) if it is anticipated that the hair will interfere with wound closure. Typically, the area around the wound is cleansed with normal saline solution or a polymer agent (e.g., Shur-Clens). The antibacterial agent povidone-iodine (Betadine) should not be allowed to get deep into the wound without thorough

---

Chart 72-4	**Definition of Terms: Wounds**

Laceration: skin tear with irregular edges and vein bridging
Avulsion: tearing away of tissue from supporting structures
Abrasion: denuded skin
Ecchymosis/contusion: blood trapped under the surface of the skin
Hematoma: tumorlike mass of blood trapped under the skin
Stab: incision of the skin with well-defined edges, usually caused by a sharp instrument; a stab wound is typically deeper than long
Cut: incision of the skin with well-defined edges, usually longer than deep
Patterned: wound representing the outline of the object (e.g., steering wheel) causing the wound

---

rinsing. Povidone-iodine is used only for the initial cleansing because it injures exposed and healthy tissue, resulting in further tissue damage (ENA, 2013).

If indicated, the area is infiltrated with a local intradermal anesthetic through the wound margins or by regional block. Patients with soft tissue injuries usually have localized pain at the site of injury. The nurse then assists with cleaning and débriding the wound. The wound is irrigated gently and copiously with sterile isotonic saline solution to remove surface dirt. Devitalized tissue and foreign matter are removed because they impede healing and may promote infection. Any small bleeding vessels are clamped, tied, or cauterized. After wound treatment, a nonadherent dressing is applied to protect the wound and to serve as a splint and as a reminder to the patient that the area is injured.

Primary Closure

The decision to suture a wound depends on the nature of the wound, the time since the injury was sustained, the degree of contamination, and the vascularity of tissues. If primary closure is indicated, the wound is sutured or stapled, usually by the physician, with the patient receiving either local anesthesia or moderate sedation (see Chapter 18). Wound closure begins when subcutaneous fat is brought together loosely with a few sutures to close off the dead space. The subcuticular layer is then closed, and finally the epidermis is closed. Sutures are placed near the wound edge, with the skin edges leveled carefully to promote optimal healing. Instead of sutures, sterile strips of reinforced microporous tape or a bonding agent (skin glue) may be used to close clean, superficial wounds.

Delayed Primary Closure

Delayed primary closure may be indicated if tissue has been lost or there is a high potential for infection. A thin layer of gauze (to ensure drainage and prevent pooling of exudate), covered by an occlusive dressing, may be used. The wound is splinted in a functional position to prevent motion and decrease the possibility of contracture.

If there are no signs of suppuration (formation of purulent drainage), the wound may be sutured (with the patient receiving a local anesthetic). The use of antibiotic agents to prevent infection depends on factors such as how the injury occurred, the age of the wound, and the risk of contamination. The site is immobilized and elevated to limit accumulation of fluid in the interstitial spaces of the wound.

Tetanus prophylaxis is given as prescribed, based on the condition of the wound and the patient's immunization status. If the patient's last tetanus booster was given more than 5 years ago, or if the patient's immunization status is unknown, a tetanus booster must be given (ACS, 2013). The patient is instructed about signs and symptoms of infection and is instructed to contact the primary provider or clinic if there is sudden or persistent pain, fever or chills, bleeding, rapid swelling, foul odor, drainage, or redness surrounding the wound.

TRAUMA

Trauma (an unintentional or intentional wound or injury inflicted on the body from a mechanism against which the body cannot protect itself) is the fourth leading cause of death in the United States. Trauma is the leading cause of death in children and in adults younger than 44 years. The incidence is increasing in adults older than 44 years. Alcohol and drug abuse are often implicated as factors in both blunt and penetrating trauma (ACS, 2013).

Collection of Forensic Evidence

In assessing and managing any patient with an emergency condition, but especially the patient experiencing trauma, meticulous documentation is essential. Included in documentation are descriptions of all wounds, mechanism of injury, time of events, and collection of evidence. In trauma care, the nurse must be exceedingly careful with all potential evidence, handling and documenting it properly.

The basics of care management for patients with traumatic injury include an understanding that trauma in any patient (living or dead) has potential legal or forensic science implications if criminal activity is suspected. Hence, proper management from both a medical and forensic evidence perspective is essential.

When clothing is removed from the patient who has experienced trauma, the nurse must be careful not to cut through or disrupt any tears, holes, blood stains, or dirt present on the clothing if criminal activity is suspected. Each piece of clothing should be placed in an individual paper bag. Plastic bags are not used because they retain moisture; moisture may promote mold and mildew formation, which can destroy evidence. If the clothing is wet, it should be hung to dry. Clothing should not be given to families. Valuables should be inventoried and either placed in the hospital safe or clearly documented to which family member they were given. If a police officer is present to collect clothing or any other items from the patient, each item is labeled and the transfer of custody to the officer, the officer's name, the date, and the time are documented. Evidence cannot be left unattended in the room; a formal chain of custody must be maintained for the evidence to be valid and useful for legal purposes (Foresman-Capuzzi 2014; Nayduch, 2009).

All deaths of patients who experienced trauma are reported to the medical examiner. If suicide or homicide is suspected in a patient who experienced trauma, the medical examiner examines the body on site or has the body moved to the coroner's office for autopsy. All tubes and lines must remain in place. The patient's hands must be covered with paper bags to protect evidence on the hands or under the fingernails. In the patient who has survived trauma, tissue specimens may be swabbed from the hands and nails as potential evidence. Photographs of wounds or clothing are essential and should include a reference ruler in one photo and another without the ruler.

Documentation should also include any statements made by the patient in the patient's own words and surrounded by quotation marks. A chain of evidence is essential. If the patient's case is reviewed in a court of law in the future, clear documentation assists the judicial process and helps to identify the activities that occurred in the ED.

Injury Prevention

Any discussion of trauma management must address injury prevention. A component of the emergency nurse's daily role is to provide injury prevention information to every patient with whom there is contact, including patients admitted for reasons other than injury (Edwards, Stephens-Stidham, Contreras, et al., 2016). The only way to reduce the incidence of trauma is through prevention.

There are three components of injury prevention. The first is education. Providing information and materials to help prevent violence and to maintain safety at home and in vehicles is important. Involvement in local injury prevention organizations, nursing organizations, and health fairs promotes wellness and safety. In practice, nursing and other health care professionals should avoid using the word *accident*, because trauma events are *preventable* and should be viewed as such rather than as "fate" or "happenstance." Responsibility and accountability must be assigned to traumatic incidents, particularly because of the high rate of trauma recidivism (repeated trauma). People who are at risk for trauma and trauma recidivism should be identified and provided with education and counseling directed toward altering risky behaviors and preventing further trauma (ENA, 2013).

The second component of injury prevention is legislation. Nurses should be actively involved in safety legislation at the local, state, and federal levels. Such legislation is meant to provide universal safety measures, not to infringe on rights.

The third component is automatic protection. Airbags and automotive design are included in this category. These mechanisms provide for safety without requiring personal intervention.

Emergency nurses may develop injury prevention programs using a focus similar to the ABCDE approach used in the primary survey in trauma care. In this case, however (ACS, 2013):

- *A*—describes *a*ssessment of the community for common injury mechanisms
- *B*—is used to describe *b*uilding a coalition of key community members
- *C*—refers to *c*ommunicating awareness of the trauma mechanisms and risks prevalent in the local community
- *D*—stands for *d*eveloping and implementing interventions, which may be educational or legislative
- *E*—refers to *e*valuating the injury prevention program soon after it is launched, which may result in either continuation or revision of the program.

 Multiple Trauma

Multiple trauma is caused by a single catastrophic event that causes life-threatening injuries to at least two distinct organs or organ systems. Patients with single-system trauma still receive full assessment, because even single-system injuries can be life threatening or more severe than they initially appear. Mortality in patients with multiple trauma is related to the severity of the injuries, the number of systems and organs involved, and the severity of each injury alone and in combination. Immediately after injury, the body is hypermetabolic, hypercoagulable, and severely stressed.

Care of the patient with multiple injuries requires a team approach, with one person responsible for coordinating the treatment. The nursing staff assumes responsibility for assessing and monitoring the patient, ensuring/maintaining airway and IV access, administering prescribed medications, collecting laboratory specimens, and documenting activities and the patient's subsequent responses.

Assessment and Diagnostic Findings

External evidence of trauma may be sparse or absent. Patients with multiple trauma should be assumed to have a spinal cord injury until it is proven otherwise. The injury regarded as the least significant in appearance may be the most lethal. For example, the pelvic fracture not identified until an x-ray is obtained may cause rapid and massive hemorrhage into the pelvic cavity, but an obvious amputation of the arm may have already stopped bleeding from the body's normal response of vasoconstriction.

Management

The goals of treatment are to determine the extent of injuries and to establish priorities of treatment. Any injury interfering with a vital physiologic function (e.g., airway, breathing, circulation) is an immediate threat to life and has the highest priority for immediate treatment. Essential lifesaving procedures are performed simultaneously by the emergency team. As soon as the patient is resuscitated, clothes are removed or cut off and a rapid physical assessment is performed. Transfer from field management to the ED must be orderly and controlled, with attention and silence given to listen to the verbal report from EMS personnel. Treatment in a trauma center is appropriate for patients experiencing major trauma. Treatment priorities are presented in Chart 72-5.

Intra-Abdominal Injuries

Intra-abdominal injuries are categorized as penetrating or blunt trauma. *Penetrating* abdominal injuries (i.e., gunshot wounds, stab wounds) are serious and usually require surgery. Penetrating abdominal trauma results in a high incidence of injury to hollow organs, particularly the small bowel. The liver is the most frequently injured solid organ due to its size and anterior placement in the right upper quadrant of the abdomen. In gunshot wounds, the most important prognostic factor is the velocity at which the missile enters the body. High-velocity missiles (bullets) produce extensive tissue damage. All abdominal gunshot wounds that cross the peritoneum or are associated with peritoneal signs require surgical exploration. On the other hand, some stab wounds may be managed nonoperatively due to low velocity and less penetration of the implement (i.e., weapon) (ACS, 2013).

Blunt trauma to the abdomen may result from motor vehicle crashes, falls, blows, or explosions. Blunt trauma is commonly associated with extra-abdominal injuries to the chest, head, or extremities. Patients with blunt trauma are a challenge because injuries may be difficult to detect. The incidence of delayed and trauma-related complications is greater than for penetrating injuries. This is especially true of blunt injuries involving the liver, kidneys, spleen, or blood vessels, which can lead to massive blood loss into the peritoneal cavity (ACS, 2013).

Assessment and Diagnostic Findings

As the history of the traumatic event is obtained, the abdomen is inspected as a part of the secondary survey for obvious signs of injury, including penetrating injuries, bruises,

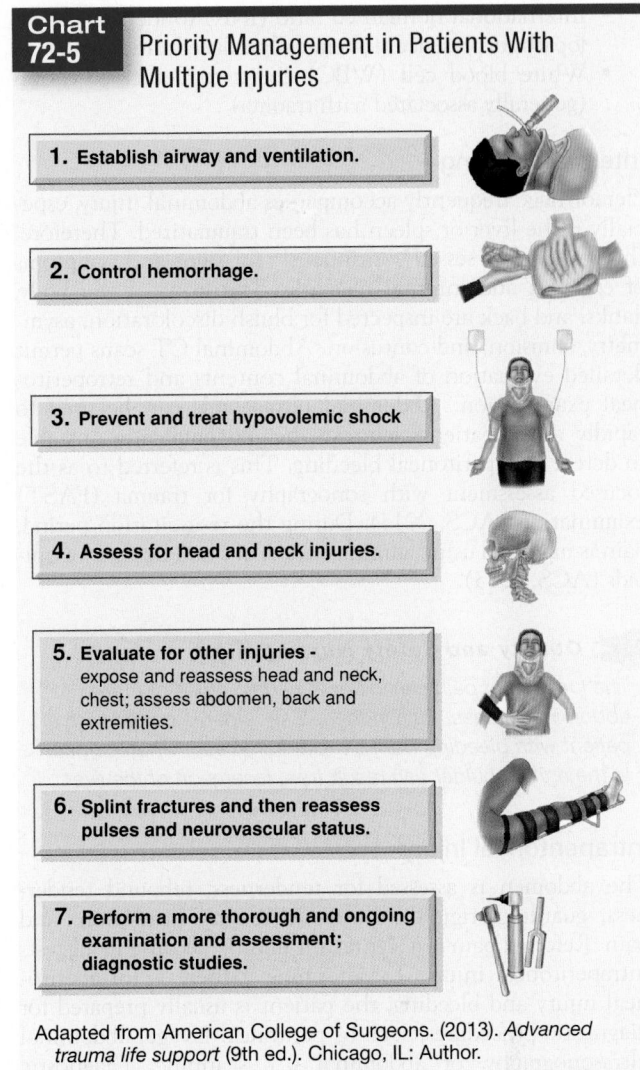

Chart 72-5 Priority Management in Patients With Multiple Injuries

1. **Establish airway and ventilation.**

2. **Control hemorrhage.**

3. **Prevent and treat hypovolemic shock**

4. **Assess for head and neck injuries.**

5. **Evaluate for other injuries -** expose and reassess head and neck, chest; assess abdomen, back and extremities.

6. **Splint fractures and then reassess pulses and neurovascular status.**

7. **Perform a more thorough and ongoing examination and assessment; diagnostic studies.**

Adapted from American College of Surgeons. (2013). *Advanced trauma life support* (9th ed.). Chicago, IL: Author.

and abrasions. Abdominal assessment continues with auscultation of bowel sounds to provide baseline data from which changes can be noted. Absence of bowel sounds may be an early sign of intraperitoneal involvement, although stress can also decrease or halt peristalsis and thus bowel sounds. Further abdominal assessment may reveal progressive abdominal distention, involuntary guarding, tenderness, pain, muscular rigidity, or rebound tenderness along with changes in bowel sounds, all of which are signs of peritoneal irritation. Hypotension and signs and symptoms of shock may also be noted. In addition, the chest and other body systems are assessed for injuries that frequently accompany intra-abdominal injuries (ACS, 2013).

Laboratory studies that aid in assessment include the following:

- Serial hemoglobin and hematocrit levels to evaluate trends reflecting the presence or absence of bleeding
- Lactate to determine acidosis and need for continued resuscitation
- Arterial blood gas (ABG) for pH (acidosis), base deficit for resuscitation evaluation, and ventilation parameters ($PaCO_2$, PaO_2)

- International normalized ratio (INR) to identify coagulopathy or presence of chemically induced anticoagulation
- White blood cell (WBC) count to detect elevation (generally associated with trauma)

Internal Bleeding

Hemorrhage frequently accompanies abdominal injury, especially if the liver or spleen has been traumatized. Therefore, the patient is assessed continuously for signs and symptoms of external and internal bleeding. The front of the body, flanks, and back are inspected for bluish discoloration, asymmetry, abrasion, and contusion. Abdominal CT scans permit detailed evaluation of abdominal contents and retroperitoneal examination. Abdominal ultrasounds can be used to rapidly assess patients who are hemodynamically unstable to detect intraperitoneal bleeding. This is referred to as the focused assessment with sonography for trauma (FAST) examination (ACS, 2013). During the resuscitation period, pain is managed using administration of small dosages of opioids (ACS, 2013).

> **Quality and Safety Nursing Alert**
>
> *The location of pain can indicate certain types of intra-abdominal injuries. Pain in the left shoulder is common in a patient with bleeding from a ruptured spleen, whereas pain in the right shoulder can result from laceration of the liver.*

Intraperitoneal Injury

The abdomen is assessed for tenderness, rebound tenderness, guarding, rigidity, spasm, increasing distention, and pain. Referred pain is a significant finding because it suggests intraperitoneal injury. To determine if there is intraperitoneal injury and bleeding, the patient is usually prepared for diagnostic procedures, such as peritoneal lavage, abdominal ultrasonography, or abdominal CT scanning. Diagnostic peritoneal lavage (DPL), although no longer the standard diagnostic study used to evaluate a traumatized abdomen, remains a backup procedure that is easily performed and is very useful during mass casualty situations when CT scanners may not be readily available. DPL involves the instillation of 1 L of warmed lactated Ringer's or normal saline solution into the abdominal cavity. After a minimum of 400 mL has been returned, a fluid specimen is sent to the laboratory for analysis. Positive laboratory findings include a red blood cell count greater than 100,000/mm^3; a WBC count greater than 500/mm^3; or the presence of bile, feces, or food (ACS, 2013).

In patients with stab wounds, sinography may be performed to detect peritoneal penetration; a purse-string suture is placed around the wound and a small catheter is introduced through the wound. A contrast agent is then introduced through the catheter, and x-rays are taken to identify any peritoneal penetration.

Genitourinary Injury

A focused genitourinary examination, which typically includes a rectal and/or vaginal examination, is performed to determine any injury to the pelvis, bladder, urethra, vagina, or intestinal wall. In the male patient, a high-riding prostate gland (abnormal position) discovered during a rectal examination indicates

a potential urethral injury. A digital vaginal examination is performed on female patients to determine if there is an open pelvic fracture that has torn the vagina.

> **Quality and Safety Nursing Alert**
>
> *To decompress the bladder and monitor urine output in a patient with a genitourinary injury, an indwelling catheter is inserted after a rectal examination has been completed, not before the examination. In addition, urethral catheter insertion when a possible urethral injury is present is contraindicated; a urology consultation and further evaluation of the urethra are required.*

Management

As indicated by the patient's condition, resuscitation procedures (restoration of airway, breathing, and circulation) are initiated as described previously.

With blunt trauma, the patient is kept on a stretcher to immobilize the spine. If the patient has been placed on a backboard, it should be removed as early as possible to prevent skin breakdown. Cervical spine immobilization is maintained until cervical x-rays have been obtained and cervical spine injury has been ruled out. Likewise, once the backboard is removed, logrolling can be used to protect the spine until x-rays are obtained and confirm that there is no evidence of injuries.

Knowing the mechanism of injury (e.g., penetrating force from a gunshot or knife, blunt force from a blow) is essential to determining the type of management needed. All wounds are located, counted, and documented. If abdominal viscera protrude, the area is covered with sterile, moist saline dressings to keep the viscera from drying.

Typically, oral fluids are withheld in anticipation of surgery, and the stomach contents are aspirated with an orogastric tube to reduce the risk of aspiration and to decompress the stomach in preparation for diagnostic procedures.

Trauma predisposes the patient to infection by disruption of mechanical barriers, exposure to exogenous bacteria from the environment at the time of injury, aspiration of vomitus, and diagnostic and therapeutic procedures (hospital-acquired infection). Tetanus prophylaxis and broad-spectrum antibiotics are given as prescribed.

Throughout the stay in the ED, the patient's condition is continuously monitored for changes. If there is continuing evidence of shock, blood loss, free air under the diaphragm, evisceration, hematuria, severe head injury, musculoskeletal injury, or suspected or known abdominal injury, the patient is rapidly transported to surgery. In most cases, blunt liver and spleen injuries are managed nonsurgically. The goal for the management of all patients who have experienced trauma is to minimize the length of stay in the ED. The patient should be moved to the definitive destination quickly so that care and rehabilitation can continue.

Crush Injuries

Crush injuries occur when a person is caught between opposing forces (e.g., run over by a moving vehicle, crushed between two cars, crushed under a collapsed building).

Assessment and Diagnostic Findings

The patient is observed for the following:

- Hypovolemic shock resulting from extravasation of blood and plasma into injured tissues after compression has been released (see Chapter 14)
- Spinal cord injury (see Chapter 68)
- Erythema and blistering of skin
- Fractures (usually an extremity) (see Chapter 42)
- Acute kidney injury (acute tubular necrosis [ATN]) (see Chapter 54)

Management

In conjunction with maintaining the airway, breathing, and circulation, the patient is observed for acute kidney injury (AKI). Injury to the back can cause renal trauma (see Chapter 54). Severe muscular damage may cause **rhabdomyolysis**, a toxic syndrome caused by a release of myoglobin from ischemic skeletal muscle, resulting in ATN. See Chapter 54 for the treatment of AKI and ATN. Rhabdomyolyis may also result from major burns (see Chapter 62), heat stroke, and abuse of illicit drugs, in addition to crush injuries (see later discussions). The classic triad of clinical manifestations suggestive of rhabdomyolysis includes myalgias (muscle cramps), generalized muscle weakness, and darkened urine. The serum creatine kinase (CK) is monitored as the most sensitive indicator of rhabdomyolyis; levels in excess of 6000 IU/L are considered diagnostic (Muscal & DeGuzman, 2016). In addition to treatment aimed at preventing or treating ATN, major soft tissue injuries are splinted promptly to control bleeding and pain. The serum lactic acid level is monitored; a decrease to less than 2.5 mmol/L is an indication of successful resuscitation (Blow, Magliore, Claridge, et al., 1999).

If an extremity is injured, it is elevated to relieve swelling and pressure. If compartment syndrome develops, the physician may perform a **fasciotomy** (i.e., surgical incision to the level of the fascia) to restore neurovascular function (see Chapter 42). Medications for pain and anxiety are then given as prescribed, and the patient is quickly transported to the operating suite for wound débridement and fracture repair. A hyperbaric oxygen chamber (if available) may be used to hyperoxygenate crushed tissue, if indicated.

Fractures

Immediate appropriate management of a fracture may determine the patient's eventual outcome and may mean the difference between recovery and disability. When the patient is being examined for fracture, the body part is handled gently and as little as possible. Clothing is cut off to visualize the affected body part. Assessment is conducted for pain over or near a bone, swelling (from blood, lymph, and exudate infiltrating the tissue), and circulatory disturbance. The patient is assessed for ecchymosis, tenderness, and crepitation (see Chapter 42). The nurse must remember that the patient may have multiple fractures accompanied by head, chest, spine, or abdominal injuries.

Management

Immediate attention is given to the patient's general condition. Assessment of airway, breathing, and circulation (which includes pulses in the extremities) is conducted. The patient is also evaluated for neurologic or abdominal injuries before the extremity is treated, unless a pulseless extremity is detected.

If a pulseless extremity is identified, repositioning of the extremity to proper alignment is required. If the pulseless extremity involves a fractured femur, Hare traction (a portable in-line traction device) may be applied to assist with alignment. If repositioning is ineffective in restoring the pulse, a rapid total-body assessment must be completed, followed by transfer of the patient to the operating room for arteriography and possible arterial repair versus amputation.

After the initial evaluation has been completed, all injuries identified are evaluated and treated. The fractured body part is inspected. Using a systematic head-to-toe approach, the nurse inspects the entire body, observing for lacerations, swelling, and deformities, including angulation (bending), shortening, rotation, and asymmetry. All peripheral pulses, especially those distal to the fractured extremity, are palpated. The extremity is also assessed for coolness, blanching, and decreased sensation and motor function, which are indicative of injury to the extremity's neurovascular supply.

A splint is applied before the patient is moved. Splinting immobilizes the joint at a site distal and proximal to the fracture, relieves pain, restores or improves circulation, prevents further tissue injury, and prevents a closed fracture from becoming an open one. To splint an extremity, one hand is placed distal to the fracture and some traction is applied while the other hand is placed beneath the fracture for support. The splints should extend beyond the joints adjacent to the fracture. Upper extremities must be splinted in a functional position. If the fracture is open, a moist, sterile dressing is applied.

After splinting, the vascular status of the extremity is checked by assessing color, temperature, pulse, and blanching of the nail bed. In addition, the patient is assessed for neurovascular compromise if pain or pressure is reported. See Chapter 42 for a complete description of fracture management.

ENVIRONMENTAL EMERGENCIES

Heat-Induced Illnesses

Heat-induced illnesses may range in severity from mild and self-limiting to life-threatening emergencies. The most serious of these—heat stroke—is an acute medical emergency caused by failure of the heat-regulating mechanisms of the body. It is the inability to maintain cardiac output in the face of moderately high body temperatures and is associated with dehydration. The most common cause of heat stroke is nonexertional, prolonged exposure to an environmental temperature of greater than 39.2°C (102.5°F), although a heat index of greater than 35°C (95°F) is associated with increased mortality (Auerbach, 2017). It usually occurs during extended heat waves, especially when they are accompanied by high humidity. Exertional heat stroke is caused by strenuous physical activity that occurs in a hot environment (Auerbach, 2017; ENA, 2013).

People at risk for nonexertional heat stroke are those not acclimatized to heat, those who are older or very young, those unable to care for themselves, those with chronic and debilitating diseases, and those taking certain medications (e.g.,

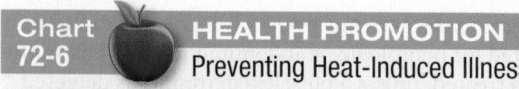

Chart 72-6 · HEALTH PROMOTION
Preventing Heat-Induced Illnesses

The nurse provides the following advice for the patient treated for heat-induced illness:

- Avoid immediate re-exposure to high temperatures; hypersensitivity to high temperatures may remain for a considerable time.
- Maintain adequate fluid intake, wear loose clothing, and reduce activity in hot weather.
- Monitor fluid losses and weight loss during workout activities or exercise and replace fluids and electrolytes.
- Use a gradual approach to physical conditioning, allowing sufficient time for return to baseline temperature.
- Plan outdoor activities to avoid the hottest part of the day (between 10 AM and 2 PM).

For older patients living in urban settings with high environmental temperatures:

- The nurse directs these patients to places where air conditioning is available (e.g., shopping mall, library, church) and advises them that fans alone are not adequate to prevent heat-induced illness.

---

major tranquilizers, anticholinergics, diuretics, beta blockers) (Tintinalli, Stapczynski, Ma, et al., 2016; ENA, 2013). In a study of heat-induced injury from 2006 to 2010, mortality was greater among older adults, men, and patients with pre-existing chronic illnesses. Heat-related events occurred most often in rural areas (Hess, Saha, & Luber, 2014). Exertional heat stroke occurs in healthy individuals during sports or work activities (e.g., exercising in extreme heat and humidity). Hyperthermia results because of inadequate heat loss. Strategies used to prevent heat stroke are reviewed in Chart 72-6.

Less severe forms of heat-induced illnesses include heat exhaustion and heat cramps or heat illness. The causes of heat exhaustion are the same as for heat stroke. Heat illness is caused by a loss of electrolytes, typically during strenuous physical activity in a hot environment (ENA, 2013).

Gerontologic Considerations

Most heat-related deaths occur in older adults because their circulatory systems are unable to compensate for stress imposed by heat. Older adults have a decreased ability to perspire as well as a decreased ability to vasodilate and vasoconstrict. They have less subcutaneous tissue, a decreased thirst mechanism, and a diminished ability to concentrate urine to compensate for heat. Many older adults do not drink adequate amounts of fluid, partly because of fear of incontinence, and thus have a greater risk of heat stroke. In addition, many older adults fear being victims of crime, so even if their residence lacks air conditioning, they tend to keep windows closed despite high temperatures and humidity levels (ENA, 2013).

Assessment and Diagnostic Findings

Heat stroke, whether the cause is exertional or nonexertional, causes thermal injury at the cellular level, resulting in coagulopathies and widespread damage to the heart, liver, and kidneys. Recent patient history reveals exposure to elevated ambient temperature or excessive exercise during extreme heat. When assessing the patient, the nurse notes the following symptoms: profound central nervous system (CNS) dysfunction (manifested by confusion, delirium, bizarre behavior, coma, seizures); elevated body temperature (40.6°C [105°F] or higher); hot, dry skin; and usually anhidrosis (absence of sweating), tachypnea, hypotension, and tachycardia. The patient with heat exhaustion, on the other hand, may exhibit similarly high body temperatures accompanied by headaches, anxiety, syncope, profuse diaphoresis, gooseflesh, and orthostasis. The cardinal manifestations of heat cramps include muscle cramps, particularly in the shoulders, abdomen, and lower extremities; profound diaphoresis; and profound thirst (ENA, 2013).

Management

The main goal is to reduce the high body temperature as quickly as possible, because mortality in heat stroke or morbid progression to heat stroke with less serious forms of heat-induced illnesses is directly related to the duration of hyperthermia. For the patient with heat stroke, simultaneous treatment focuses on stabilizing oxygenation using the CABs (circulation, airway, and breathing) (formerly referred to as the ABCs) of basic life support. This includes establishing IV access for fluid administration.

After the patient's clothing is removed, the core (internal) temperature is reduced to 39°C (102°F) as rapidly as possible, preferably within 1 hour (Auerbach, 2017). One or more of the following methods may be used as prescribed (Auerbach, 2017):

- Cool sheets and towels or continuous sponging with cool water
- Ice applied to the neck, groin, chest, and axillae while spraying with tepid water
- Cooling blankets
- Immersion of the patient in a cold water bath is the optimal method for cooling (if available)

During cooling procedures, an electric fan is positioned so that it blows on the patient to augment heat dissipation by convection and evaporation. The patient's temperature is constantly monitored with a thermistor placed in the rectum, bladder, or esophagus to evaluate core temperature. Caution is used to avoid hypothermia and to prevent hyperthermia, which may recur spontaneously within 3 to 4 hours. The cooling process should stop at 38°C (100.4°F) in order to avoid iatrogenic hypothermia (ENA, 2013).

Throughout treatment, the patient's status is monitored carefully, including vital signs, ECG findings (for possible myocardial ischemia, myocardial infarction, and dysrhythmias), central venous pressure (CVP), and level of responsiveness, all of which may change with rapid alterations in body temperature. A seizure may be followed by recurrence of hyperthermia. To meet tissue needs exaggerated by the hypermetabolic condition, 100% oxygen is given. Endotracheal intubation and mechanical ventilation to support failing cardiopulmonary systems may be required.

IV infusion therapy of normal saline or lactated Ringer solution is initiated as directed to replace fluid losses and maintain adequate circulation. Fluids are given carefully because of the dangers of myocardial injury from high body temperature and poor kidney function. Cooling redistributes fluid volume from the periphery to the core.

Urine output is also measured frequently, because ATN may occur as a complication of heat stroke from rhabdomyolysis (see previous discussion). Blood specimens are obtained for serial testing to detect bleeding disorders, such as disseminated intravascular coagulation, and for serial enzyme studies to estimate thermal hypoxic injury to the liver, heart, and muscle tissue. Permanent liver, cardiac, and CNS damage may occur.

Additional supportive care may include dialysis for AKI, anticonvulsant medications to control seizures, potassium for hypokalemia, and sodium bicarbonate to correct metabolic acidosis. Benzodiazepines such as diazepam (Valium) may be prescribed to suppress seizure activity, while a phenothiazine such as chlorpromazine (Thorazine) may be prescribed to suppress shivering (Auerbach 2017; Tintinalli et al., 2016).

Patients with heat exhaustion or heat cramps may be managed less aggressively. These patients should lie supine in a cool environment. Patients with heat exhaustion may require IV fluids but may also take oral fluids, if they are tolerated. Patients with heat cramps are given oral sodium supplements and oral electrolyte solutions (ENA, 2013). Patients who have experienced a heat-induced illness should receive education to prevent another heat-related illness (see Chart 72-6).

Frostbite

Frostbite is trauma from exposure to freezing temperatures and freezing of the intracellular fluid and fluids in the intercellular spaces. It results in cellular and vascular damage. Frostbite can result in venous stasis and thrombosis. Body parts most frequently affected by frostbite include the feet, hands, nose, and ears. Frostbite ranges from first degree (redness and erythema) to fourth degree (full-depth tissue destruction).

Assessment and Diagnostic Findings

A frozen extremity may be hard, cold, and insensitive to touch and may appear white or mottled blue-white. The extent of injury from exposure to cold is not always initially known. The patient history should include environmental temperature, duration of exposure, clothing worn, humidity, and the presence of wet conditions. Protective clothing may partially prevent exposure to cold environments; however, wearing wet socks and exercise/movement may diminish the protective effects of insulation by 45% (Auerbach 2017; Zafren, 2013).

Management

The goal of management is to restore normal body temperature. Constrictive clothing and jewelry that could impair circulation are removed. Wet clothing is removed as rapidly as possible. If the lower extremities are involved, the patient should not be allowed to ambulate.

Controlled yet rapid rewarming is instituted. Frozen extremities are usually placed in a 37°C to 40°C (98.6°F to 104°F) circulating bath for 30- to 40-minute spans. This treatment is repeated until circulation is effectively restored. Early rewarming appears to decrease the amount of ultimate tissue loss. During rewarming, an analgesic for pain is given as prescribed, because the rewarming process may be very painful. To avoid further mechanical injury, the body part is not handled. Massage is contraindicated.

Once rewarmed, the part is protected from further injury and is elevated to help control swelling. Sterile gauze or cotton is placed between affected fingers or toes to prevent maceration, and a bulky dressing is placed on the extremity. A foot cradle may be used to prevent contact with bedclothes if the feet are involved. Hemorrhagic blebs, which may develop 1 hour to a few days after rewarming, are left intact and not ruptured. Nonhemorrhagic blisters are débrided to decrease the inflammatory mediators found in the blister fluid.

A physical assessment is conducted with rewarming to observe for concomitant injury, such as soft tissue injury, dehydration, alcohol intoxication, or fat embolism. Problems such as hyperkalemia (e.g., from release of potassium in the damaged cells) and hypovolemia, which occur frequently in people with frostbite, are corrected. Risk of infection is also great; therefore, aseptic technique is used during dressing changes, and tetanus prophylaxis is given as indicated. Nonsteroidal anti-inflammatory drugs (NSAIDs) are prescribed for their anti-inflammatory effects and to control pain.

Additional measures that may be carried out when appropriate after emergency stabilization measures have been instituted include the following:

- Whirlpool bath for the affected body parts to aid circulation and débridement of necrotic tissue to help prevent infection
- Escharotomy (incision through the eschar) to prevent further tissue damage, to allow for normal circulation, and to permit joint motion
- Fasciotomy to treat compartment syndrome

After rewarming, hourly active motion of any affected digits is encouraged to promote maximal restoration of function and to prevent contractures. Discharge instructions also include encouraging the patient to avoid tobacco, alcohol, and caffeine because of their vasoconstrictive effects, which further reduce the already deficient blood supply to injured tissues.

Hypothermia

Hypothermia is a condition in which the core (internal) temperature is 35°C (95°F) or less as a result of exposure to cold or an inability to maintain body temperature in the absence of low ambient temperatures. Urban hypothermia (extreme exposure to cold in an urban setting) is associated with a high mortality rate; older adults, infants, people with concurrent illnesses, and those who are homeless are particularly susceptible. Alcohol ingestion increases susceptibility because it causes systemic vasodilation. Some medications (e.g., phenothiazines) or medical conditions (e.g., hypothyroidism, spinal cord injury) decrease the ability to shiver, hampering the body's innate ability to generate body heat. Fatigue and sleep deprivation are also associated with the development of hypothermia. Heat loss of 2% is normal but increases with exposure. Wet clothing accelerates heat loss, and immersion in cold water increases heat loss by 25% (ENA, 2013). Victims of trauma are also at risk for hypothermia resulting from treatment with cold fluids, unwarmed oxygen, and exposure during examination. The patient may also have frostbite, but hypothermia takes precedence in treatment.

Assessment and Diagnostic Findings

Hypothermia leads to physiologic changes in all organ systems. There is progressive deterioration, with apathy, poor judgment, ataxia, dysarthria, drowsiness, pulmonary edema, acid–base abnormalities, coagulopathy, and eventual coma. Shivering may be suppressed at a temperature of less than 32.2°C (90°F), because the body's self-warming mechanisms become ineffective. The heartbeat and blood pressure may be so weak that peripheral pulses become undetectable. Cardiac dysrhythmias may also occur. Other physiologic abnormalities include hypoxemia and acidosis.

Management

Management consists of removal of wet clothing, continuous monitoring, rewarming, and supportive care.

Monitoring

The CABs of basic life support are a priority. The patient's vital signs, CVP, urine output, arterial blood gas levels, blood chemistry determinations (blood urea nitrogen, creatinine, glucose, electrolytes), and chest x-rays are evaluated frequently. Core body temperature is monitored with an esophageal, bladder, or rectal thermistor. Continuous ECG monitoring is performed, because cold-induced myocardial irritability leads to conduction disturbances, especially ventricular fibrillation. An arterial line is inserted and maintained to record blood pressure and to facilitate blood sampling.

Rewarming

Rewarming methods include active internal (core) rewarming and passive (spontaneous) or active external rewarming.

Active internal (core) rewarming methods are used for moderate to severe hypothermia (less than 28°C to 32.2°C [82.5°F to 90°F]) and include cardiopulmonary bypass, warm fluid administration, warmed humidified oxygen by ventilator, and warmed peritoneal lavage. Monitoring for ventricular fibrillation as the patient's temperature increases from 31°C to 32°C (88°F to 90°F) is essential.

Passive or active external rewarming is used for mild hypothermia (32.2°C to 35°C [90°F to 95°F]). Passive external rewarming uses over-the-bed heaters to the extremities and increases blood flow to the acidotic, anaerobic extremities. The cold blood from peripheral tissues has high lactic acid levels. As this blood returns to the core, it causes a significant drop in the core temperature (i.e., core temperature afterdrop) and can potentially cause cardiac dysrhythmias and electrolyte disturbances. Active external rewarming uses forced-air warming blankets. Care must be taken to prevent extremity burn from these devices, because the patient may not have effective sensation to feel the burn.

Supportive Care

Supportive care during rewarming includes the following as directed:

- External cardiac compression (typically performed only as directed in patients with temperatures higher than 31°C [88°F])
- Defibrillation of ventricular fibrillation. A patient whose temperature is less than 32°C [90°F] experiences spontaneous ventricular fibrillation if moved or touched. Defibrillation is ineffective in patients with temperatures lower than 31°C (88°F); therefore, the patient must be rewarmed first.
- Mechanical ventilation with positive end-expiratory pressure (PEEP) and heated humidified oxygen to maintain tissue oxygenation
- Administration of warmed IV fluids to correct hypotension and to maintain urine output and core rewarming, as described previously
- Administration of sodium bicarbonate to correct metabolic acidosis if necessary
- Administration of antiarrhythmic medications
- Insertion of an indwelling urinary catheter to monitor urinary output and kidney function

Nonfatal Drowning

Nonfatal drowning is defined as survival for at least 24 hours after submersion that caused a respiratory arrest. The most common consequence is hypoxemia. Children under 5 years of age and those over the age of 85 have the highest risk of drowning (CDC 2014). An estimated 372,000 drownings occur throughout the world annually, accounting for 7% of global mortality from unintentional injury (World Health Organization [WHO], 2016). Drowning and nonfatal drowning can be prevented by avoiding rip currents offshore; approximately 85% of shore drownings involve a rip current. Pool drownings can be prevented by surrounding the pool with fencing, a self-latching/closing gate, and providing swimming lessons. Supervision near water is still the best prevention measure. When boating, a personal flotation device (PFD), even for swimmers, prevents drowning events. Approximately 50% of nonfatal drownings require hospital admission for management (WHO, 2016).

Factors associated with drowning and nonfatal drowning include alcohol ingestion, inability to swim, diving injuries, hypothermia, and exhaustion. The majority of drowning events occur in pools, lakes, and bathtubs. Suicide by drowning rarely occurs in pools and rarely involves alcohol (Auerbach, 2017).

Efforts to save the patient should not be abandoned prematurely. Successful resuscitation with full neurologic recovery has occurred in patients who have experienced nonfatal drowning after prolonged submersion in cold water. This is possible because of a decrease in metabolic demands and/or the diving reflex. The nonfatal drowning process involves the onset of hypoxia, hypercapnia, bradycardia, and dysrhythmias. If there is a violent struggle associated with the nonfatal drowning episode, exercise-induced acidosis and tachypnea can result in aspiration. Hypoxia and acidosis cause eventual apnea and loss of consciousness. When the victim loses consciousness and makes a final effort to breathe, the terminal gasp occurs. Water then moves passively into the airways prior to death.

After resuscitation, hypoxia and acidosis are the major complications experienced by a person who has experienced nonfatal drowning; immediate intervention in the ED is essential. Resultant pathophysiologic changes and pulmonary injury depend on the type of fluid (fresh or salt water) and the volume aspirated. Freshwater aspiration results in a loss of surfactant and, therefore, an inability to expand the lungs. Salt-water aspiration leads to pulmonary edema from the osmotic effects of the salt within the lungs. If a person survives submersion, acute respiratory distress syndrome (ARDS), resulting in hypoxia, hypercarbia, and respiratory or metabolic acidosis, can occur.

Management

Therapeutic goals include maintaining cerebral perfusion and adequate oxygenation to prevent further damage to vital organs. Cardiopulmonary resuscitation is the factor with the greatest influence on survival. The most important priority in resuscitation is to manage the hypoxia, acidosis, and hypothermia. Prevention and management of hypoxia are accomplished by ensuring an adequate airway and respiration, thus improving ventilation (which helps correct respiratory acidosis) and oxygenation. Arterial blood gases are monitored to evaluate oxygen, carbon dioxide, bicarbonate levels, and pH. These parameters determine the type of ventilatory support needed. The use of endotracheal intubation with PEEP improves oxygenation, prevents aspiration, and corrects intrapulmonary shunting and ventilation–perfusion abnormalities (caused by aspiration of water). If the patient is breathing spontaneously, supplemental oxygen may be given by mask. However, an endotracheal tube is necessary if the patient does not breathe spontaneously.

Because of submersion, the patient is usually hypothermic. A rectal probe or other core measurement device is used to determine the degree of hypothermia. Prescribed rewarming procedures (e.g., extracorporeal warming, warmed peritoneal dialysis, inhalation of warm aerosolized oxygen, torso warming) are started during resuscitation. The choice of warming method is determined by the severity and duration of hypothermia and available resources. Intravascular volume expansion and inotropic agents are used to treat hypotension and impaired tissue perfusion. ECG monitoring is initiated, because dysrhythmias frequently occur. An indwelling urinary catheter is inserted to measure urine output. Hypothermia and accompanying metabolic acidosis may compromise kidney function. Nasogastric intubation is used to decompress the stomach and to prevent the patient from aspirating gastric contents.

Even if the patient appears healthy, close monitoring continues with serial vital signs, serial arterial blood gas values, ECG monitoring, intracranial pressure assessments, serum electrolyte levels, intake and output, and serial chest x-rays. After a nonfatal drowning, the patient is at risk for complications such as hypoxic or ischemic cerebral injury, ARDS, and life-threatening cardiac arrest. The patient is also at heightened risk for aspiration; vomiting frequently occurs in patients requiring rescue breathing and in up to 86% of patients requiring CPR (Auerbach, 2017).

Decompression Sickness

Decompression sickness, also known as "the bends," occurs in patients who have engaged in diving (lake/ocean diving), high-altitude flying, or flying in commercial aircraft within 24 hours after diving. It occurs relatively infrequently in the United States, but its effects can be hazardous. Being aware of decompression sickness and assessing the patient properly ensures appropriate management and results in decreased morbidity.

Decompression sickness results from formation of nitrogen bubbles that occur with rapid changes in atmospheric pressure. They may occur in joint or muscle spaces, resulting in musculoskeletal pain, numbness, or hypesthesia. More significantly, nitrogen bubbles can become air emboli in the bloodstream and thereby produce stroke, paralysis, or death. Taking a rapid history about the events preceding the symptoms is essential.

Assessment and Diagnostic Findings

To identify decompression sickness, a detailed history is obtained from the patient or diving partner. Evidence of rapid ascent, loss of air in the tank, buddy breathing, recent alcohol intake or lack of sleep, or a flight within 24 hours after diving suggests possible decompression sickness. Some patients describe a perfect dive yet still have the signs and symptoms of decompression sickness, in which case they must receive treatment for the condition.

Signs and symptoms include joint or extremity pain, numbness, hypesthesia, and loss of range of motion. Neurologic symptoms mimicking those of a stroke or spinal cord injury can indicate an air embolus. Cardiopulmonary arrest can also occur in severe cases and is usually fatal. Any neurologic symptoms should be rapidly assessed. All patients with decompression sickness need rapid transfer to a hyperbaric chamber.

Management

A patent airway and adequate ventilation are established, as described previously, and 100% oxygen is given throughout treatment and transport. A chest x-ray is obtained to identify aspiration, and at least one IV line is started with lactated Ringer's or normal saline solution. Research findings suggest that among patients requiring air transport (e.g., helicopter), oxygen saturations and symptoms improve when both oxygen and IV fluids are given and the transport flight remains at low altitude (i.e., below 300 m [approximately 1000 feet]) (Oode, Yanagawa, Omori, et al., 2015).

The cardiopulmonary and neurologic systems are supported as needed. If an air embolus is suspected, the head of the bed should be lowered. If the patient's wet clothing is still present, it is removed. The patient is kept warm. Transfer to the closest hyperbaric chamber for treatment is initiated. If air transport is necessary, low-altitude flight (below 300 m) is required (Oode et al., 2015). However, the patient who is awake and alert without central neurologic deficits may be able to travel by ground ambulance or by automobile, depending on the severity of symptoms. Throughout treatment, the patient is continually assessed, and changes are documented. If aspiration is suspected, antibiotic agents and other treatment may be prescribed.

Animal and Human Bites

Bites are a common reason for visits to the ED. Dog bites constitute 80% to 90% of these bites and are responsible for the majority of deaths from bites by a nonvenomous animal (Tintinalli et al., 2016). Cat bites have a high risk of infection because of the presence of *Pasteurella* in their saliva. All animal bites must be reported to public health authorities, which must provide follow-up screening of the offending animal for rabies. If the animal cannot be located and rabies vaccination verified, rabies prophylaxis for the person who has been bitten must be instituted (ENA, 2013).

Human bites are frequently associated with rapes, sexual assaults, or other forms of battery. The human mouth contains more bacteria than that of most other animals, so a high risk of bite-related infection exists. Depending on the circumstances surrounding the event, the victim may delay seeking treatment. The ED nurse should inspect any bitten tissue for pus, erythema, or necrosis. A health care provider should take photographs, which can be used as evidence in criminal and legal proceedings. Guidelines for collecting forensic evidence for photographing with and without a measuring device should be followed. Cleansing with soap and water is then necessary, followed by the administration of antibiotics and tetanus toxoid as prescribed (Tintinalli et al., 2016).

Snakebites

Venomous (poisonous) snakes caused more than 2000 of the 6000 snakebites in the United States annually (Tintinalli et al., 2016). Across the globe, more than 400,000 snakebites occur each year with a 5% mortality rate (Smith, Sammons, Carr, et al. 2014). Children between 1 and 9 years of age are the most likely victims. The greatest number of bites occurs during the daylight hours and early evening of the summer months. The most frequent poisonous snakebite in the United States occurs from Crotalidae, otherwise called pit vipers, such as water moccasins, copperheads, and rattlesnakes. The most common site is the upper extremity (ENA, 2013). Of pit viper bites, 75% to 80% result in **envenomation** (injection of a poisonous material by sting, spine, bite, or other means); the rest result in what are called *dry bites* (Tintinalli et al., 2016). Venomous snakebites are medical emergencies.

Nineteen different species of venomous snakes are found in various regions within the United States. Nurses should be familiar with the types of snakes common to the geographic region in which they practice. However, the exotic pet industry sells atypical snakes as "pets." Because of this, venomous snakes such as cobras and asps may be found outside of their native region.

Clinical Manifestations

Snake venom consists primarily of proteins and has a broad range of physiologic effects. It may affect multiple organ systems, especially the neurologic, cardiovascular, and respiratory systems.

Classic clinical signs of envenomation are edema, ecchymosis, and hemorrhagic bullae, leading to necrosis at the site of envenomation. Symptoms include lymph node tenderness, nausea, vomiting, numbness, and a metallic taste in the mouth. Without decisive treatment, these clinical manifestations may progress to include fasciculations, hypotension, paresthesias, seizures, and coma (Smith et al., 2014).

Management

Initial first aid at the site of the snakebite includes having the person lie down, removing constrictive items such as rings,

providing warmth, cleansing the wound, covering the wound with a light sterile dressing, and immobilizing the injured body part below the level of the heart. Airway, breathing, and circulation are the priorities of care. Ice, incision and suction, or a tourniquet is *not* applied. Tetanus and analgesia should be given as necessary. Initial evaluation in the ED is performed quickly and includes information about the following:

- Whether the snake was venomous or nonvenomous; discourage bringing the snake for identification—even a dead snake's venom is poisonous. Do *not* handle any snake brought to the ED. If the snake is transported to the ED, caution should be taken because the snake is frequently in a stunned, not dead, state. The bite reflex can remain intact for up to 90 minutes after the death of the snake (Auerbach, 2017).
- Where and when the bite occurred and the circumstances of the bite.
- Sequence of events, signs, and symptoms (fang punctures, pain, edema, and erythema of the bite and nearby tissues).
- Severity of poisonous effects. Call the local poison control phone number to gain access to information about an exotic snakebite presentation and management, as necessary. The poison control center may also be able to assist with retrieving antivenin for these particular species (Smith et al., 2014).
- Vital signs.
- Circumference of the bitten extremity or area at several points. The circumference of the extremity that was bitten is compared with the circumference of the opposite extremity.
- Laboratory data (complete blood count, urinalysis, and coagulation studies).

The course and prognosis of snakebite injuries depend on the kind and amount of venom injected; where on the body the bite occurred; and the general health, age, and size of the patient. There is no one specific protocol for treatment of snakebites. In general, ice, tourniquets, heparin, and corticosteroids are not used during the acute stage. Corticosteroids are contraindicated in the first 6 to 8 hours after the bite because they may depress antibody production and hinder the action of **antivenin** (antitoxin manufactured from the snake venom and used to treat snakebites).

Parenteral fluids may be used to treat hypotension. If vasopressors are used to treat hypotension, their use should be short term. Surgical exploration of the bite is rarely indicated. Typically, the patient is observed closely for at least 6 hours. The patient is *never* left unattended.

Administration of Antivenin (Antitoxin)

Although envenomation does not always occur, it should always be suspected with snakebites. An assessment of progressive signs and symptoms is essential before considering administration of antivenin, which is most effective if given within 4 hours and no greater than 12 hours after the snakebite. The decision to administer antivenin depends on worsening tissue injury and evidence of systemic and coagulopathic symptoms. Rattlesnakes are more likely to cause coagulation abnormalities as well as more systemic effects. Coagulation abnormalities are not restricted to severe envenomation (Auerbach, 2017).

The most readily available antivenin in the United States is Crotalidae polyvalent immune Fab antivenom (FabAV or CroFab) (Auerbach, 2017). The dose depends on the type of snake and the estimated severity of the bite. Indications for antivenin depend on the progression of symptoms, including coagulopathy and systemic reaction.

Crotalidae polyvalent immune Fab antivenom does not require pretesting (i.e., skin sensitivity screening for an allergic reaction; see Chapter 37), albeit monitoring for a hypersensitivity reaction is still necessary. Outside of the United States, however, other antivenin formulas that may be commercially available may still result in severe serum sickness. If the dose exceeds 10 vials, serum sickness will most likely occur. Serum sickness is a type of hypersensitivity response that results in fever, arthralgias, pruritus, lymphadenopathy, and proteinuria and can progress to neuropathies (Auerbach, 2017). However, FabAV must be given cautiously to patients receiving anticoagulation therapy. Administration of FabAV may result in a recurring coagulopathy. The dosage and administration of FabAV are different from previously manufactured types of antivenin and should be reviewed carefully before the medication is given.

Before administering antivenin and every 15 minutes thereafter, the circumference of the affected part is measured. Premedication with diphenhydramine (Benadryl) or cimetidine (Tagamet) may be indicated, because these antihistamines may decrease the allergic response to antivenin. Antivenin is given as an IV infusion whenever possible, although intramuscular administration can be used.

Depending on the severity of the snakebite, the antivenin is diluted in 500 to 1000 mL of normal saline solution. The infusion is started slowly, and the rate is increased after 10 minutes if there is no reaction. The total dose should be infused during the first 4 to 6 hours after the bite. The initial dose is repeated until symptoms decrease, after which time the circumference of the affected part should be measured every 30 to 60 minutes for the next 48 hours to detect symptoms of compartment syndrome (swelling, loss of pulse, increased pain, and paresthesias).

There is no limit to the number of antivenin vials that can be given. The decision to continue to administer vials is based upon patient symptoms. Consultation with a snakebite expert is essential at this point; this consultant may be identified and found through contacting the Poison Control Center (see Resources section) or a local zoo reptile center. The most common cause of allergic reaction to the antivenin is too-rapid infusion. Reactions may consist of a feeling of fullness in the face, urticaria, pruritus, malaise, and apprehension. These symptoms may be followed by tachycardia, shortness of breath, hypotension, and shock. In this situation, the infusion should be stopped immediately and IV diphenhydramine given. Vasopressors are used for patients in shock, and resuscitation equipment must be on standby while antivenin is infusing. It is important to note that serum sickness (hypersensitivity) can occur within the first few weeks after discharge. The patient and the patient's family members should be educated about the clinical manifestations of serum sickness (i.e., fever; rash starting on the chest and spreading to the back; arthralgia; GI disturbances [e.g., nausea, vomiting, diarrhea, abdominal pain], and headache) and return to the ED if they occur (Auerbach, 2017; Tintinalli et al., 2016).

Spider Bites

There are two venomous spiders found in the United States that may interact with humans: the brown recluse and the black widow. Both are usually found in dark places such as closets, woodpiles, and attics, as well as in shoes (ENA, 2013).

Brown recluse spider bites are painless. Systemic effects such as fever and chills, nausea and vomiting, malaise, and joint pain develop within 24 to 72 hours. The site of the bite may appear reddish to purple in color within 2 to 8 hours after the bite. Necrosis occurs in the next 2 to 4 days in approximately 10% of cases. The center of the bite may become necrotic, and surgical débridement may be necessary. Wound care consists of cleansing with soap and water, and hyperbaric oxygen treatments may be helpful. Most wounds heal within 2 to 3 months (ENA, 2013; Tintinalli et al., 2016).

Black widow spider bites feel like pinpricks. Systemic effects usually occur within 30 minutes—much more rapidly than with brown recluse spider bites. Signs and symptoms include abdominal rigidity, nausea and vomiting, hypertension, tachycardia, and paresthesias. Severe pain also develops within 60 minutes and increases over 1 to 2 days. Treatment involves application of ice to the site to decrease swelling and discomfort, along with elevation and assessment of tetanus immunization status. Analgesic agents and benzodiazepines may relieve muscle spasms. Cardiopulmonary monitoring is essential. Antivenin is effective for severe black widow spider bites. This antivenin is horse serum based; therefore, testing for sensitivity must be performed prior to administration (Auerbach, 2017; ENA 2013).

Tick Bites

Tick bites are common in many areas of the United States, and they usually occur in grassy or wooded areas. It is important to learn the place where the bite occurred as well as the location of the bite on the body. The tick bite itself is not usually the problem; rather, it is the pathogen transmitted by the tick that can cause serious disease. Ticks can carry diseases such as Rocky Mountain spotted fever, tularemia, west Nile virus, and Lyme disease.

Ticks transmit pathogens through their saliva; therefore, the earlier the tick is removed, the better the prognosis. The tick should be removed with tweezers using a straight upward pull (see Fig. 72-4), and the patient should be informed of the signs and symptoms of diseases carried by ticks, especially if the patient lives in or has visited an area endemic for tick-related diseases (e.g., Lyme disease) (Auerbach 2017; ENA, 2013).

Figure 72-4 • Removal of tick with tweezers using a straight upward pull.

Lyme disease has three stages. Stage I may present with a classic "bull's-eye" rash (i.e., erythema migrans) that typically can be found in the axilla, groin, or thigh area and that appears within 4 weeks after the tick bite, with a peak manifestation time of 7 days after the bite. Classically, this rash is at least 5 cm in diameter with bright red borders. It is accompanied by flulike signs and symptoms that may include chills, fever, myalgia, fatigue, and headache. Without treatment, the rash subsides within 3 to 4 weeks. However, the rash and flulike manifestations can be significantly reduced within days if prompt treatment with antibiotic agents (e.g., doxycycline [Vibramycin]) is initiated. If antibiotics are not given, stage II Lyme disease may present within 4 to 10 weeks following the tick bite and may manifest with joint pain, memory loss, poor motor coordination, adenopathy, and cardiac abnormalities. Facial nerve palsy is the most common manifestation of stage II Lyme disease (Tintinalli et al., 2016). Stage III can begin anywhere from weeks to more than a year after the bite and has serious long-term chronic sequelae, including arthritis, neuropathy, myalgia, and myocarditis. Even after appropriate treatment with antibiotics, 10% to 20% of patients may experience long-term effects including fatigue and arthralgias; some experience neurologic symptoms that may persist for over 10 years (Tintinalli et al., 2016).

POISONING

A poison is any substance that, when ingested, inhaled, absorbed, applied to the skin, or produced within the body in relatively small amounts, injures the body by its chemical action. Poisoning from inhalation and ingestion of toxic materials, both intentional and unintentional, constitutes a major health hazard and an emergency situation. Emergency treatment is initiated with the following goals:

- Removal or inactivation of the poison before it is absorbed
- Provision of supportive care in maintaining vital organ function
- Administration of a specific antidote to neutralize a specific poison
- Implementation of treatment that hastens the elimination of the absorbed poison

Ingested (Swallowed) Poisons

Swallowed poisons may be corrosive. **Corrosive poisons** include alkaline and acid agents that can cause tissue destruction after coming in contact with mucous membranes. Alkaline products include lye, drain cleaners, toilet bowl cleaners, bleach, nonphosphate detergents, oven cleaners, and button batteries (batteries used to power watches, calculators, hearing aids, or cameras). Acid products include toilet bowl cleaners, pool cleaners, metal cleaners, rust removers, and battery acid.

Control of the airway, ventilation, and oxygenation are essential. In the absence of cerebral or renal damage, the patient's prognosis depends largely on successful management of respiration and circulation. Measures are instituted to stabilize cardiovascular and other body functions. ECG, vital signs, and neurologic status are monitored closely for

changes. Shock may result from the cardiodepressant action of the substance ingested, from venous pooling in the lower extremities, or from reduced circulating blood volume resulting from increased capillary permeability (see Chapter 14). An indwelling urinary catheter is inserted to monitor kidney function. Blood specimens are obtained to determine the concentration of drug or poison.

Efforts are made to determine what substance was ingested; the amount; the time since ingestion; signs and symptoms, such as pain or burning sensations, any evidence of redness or burn in the mouth or throat, pain on swallowing or an inability to swallow, vomiting, or drooling; age and weight of the patient; and pertinent health history.

> ### ▶ Quality and Safety Nursing Alert
>
> *The local poison control center should be called if an unknown toxic agent has been taken or if it is necessary to identify an antidote for a known toxic agent.*

Measures are instituted to remove the toxin or decrease its absorption. If there is a specific chemical or physiologic antagonist (antidote), it is given as early as possible to reverse or diminish the effects of the toxin. If this measure is ineffective, procedures may be initiated to remove or dilute the ingested substance. These procedures include administration of multiple doses of activated charcoal, dialysis, or hemoperfusion. Hemoperfusion involves detoxification of the blood by processing it through an extracorporeal circuit and an adsorbent cartridge containing charcoal or resin, after which the cleansed blood is returned to the patient.

The patient who has ingested a corrosive poison, which can be a strong acid or alkaline substance, is given water or milk to drink for dilution. However, dilution is not attempted if the patient has acute airway edema or obstruction; potential for vomiting; or if there is clinical evidence of esophageal, gastric, or intestinal burn or perforation. The following gastric emptying procedures may be used as prescribed:

- Gastric lavage for the patient who is obtunded is only useful within 1 hour of ingestion, for sustained-release substances, or massive life-threatening amounts of a substance; however, complications of aspiration and stomach or esophageal perforation outweigh its usefulness. If performed, gastric aspirate is saved and sent to the laboratory for testing (toxicology screens).
- Activated charcoal administration if the poison is one that is absorbed by charcoal; given orally or by nasogastric tube, it is effective in small intermittent doses to decrease vomiting. It should be diluted as a slurry so that it is easier to drink or pass through the nasogastric tube. Activated charcoal absorbs most commonly ingested poisons except corrosives, heavy metals and hydrocarbons, iron, and lithium.

Cathartics, which had traditionally accompanied the use of activated charcoal, are now rarely indicated because they can result in severe electrolyte imbalances, diarrhea, and hypovolemia (ENA, 2013). Furthermore, syrup of ipecac to induce vomiting in the patient who is alert is not recommended due to the risk of aspiration and should *never* be used with corrosive poisons or with petroleum distillates (e.g., lubricating oil, fuel oil) or further corrosive damage to the upper airway and pharyngeal structures may occur.

Quality and Safety Nursing Alert

Vomiting is never induced after ingestion of caustic substances (acid or alkaline) or petroleum distillates.

Throughout detoxification, the patient's vital signs, CVP, and fluid and electrolyte balance are monitored closely. Hypotension and cardiac dysrhythmias are possible. Seizures are also possible because of CNS stimulation from the poison or from oxygen deprivation. If the patient complains of pain, analgesic agents are given cautiously. Severe pain causes vasomotor collapse and reflex inhibition of normal physiologic functions.

After the patient's condition has stabilized and discharge is imminent, written material should be given to the patient indicating the signs and symptoms of potential problems related to the poison ingested and signs or symptoms requiring evaluation by a health care provider. If poisoning was determined to be a suicide or self-harm attempt, a psychiatric consultation should be requested before the patient is discharged. In cases of inadvertent poison ingestion, poison prevention and home poison-proofing instructions should be provided to the patient and family.

Carbon Monoxide Poisoning

Carbon monoxide poisoning may occur as a result of industrial or household incidents or attempted suicide. It is the most common cause of fatality from poisoning and is frequently under-reported to poison control centers or misdiagnosed (Tintinalli et al., 2016). Carbon monoxide exerts its toxic effect by binding to circulating hemoglobin and thereby reducing the oxygen-carrying capacity of the blood. Hemoglobin absorbs carbon monoxide 200 times more readily than it absorbs oxygen. Carbon monoxide–bound hemoglobin, called **carboxyhemoglobin**, does not transport oxygen.

Clinical Manifestations

Because the CNS has a critical need for oxygen, CNS symptoms predominate with carbon monoxide toxicity. A person with carbon monoxide poisoning may appear intoxicated (from cerebral hypoxia). Other signs and symptoms include headache, muscular weakness, palpitation, dizziness, and confusion, which can progress rapidly to coma. Skin color, which can range from pink or cherry-red to cyanotic and pale, is not a reliable sign. Pulse oximetry may reveal a high hemoglobin saturation, which may be deceiving, since the hemoglobin molecule is saturated with carbon monoxide rather than oxygen (ENA, 2013).

Management

Exposure to carbon monoxide requires immediate treatment. Goals of management are to reverse cerebral and myocardial hypoxia and to hasten elimination of carbon monoxide. Whenever a patient inhales a poison, the following general measures apply:

- Carry the patient to fresh air immediately; open all doors and windows.

- Loosen all tight clothing.
- Initiate traditional cardiopulmonary resuscitation.
- Prevent chilling; wrap the patient in blankets.
- Keep the patient as quiet as possible.
- Do not give alcohol in any form or permit the patient to smoke.

In addition, for the patient with carbon monoxide poisoning, carboxyhemoglobin levels are analyzed on arrival at the ED and before treatment with oxygen if possible. To reverse hypoxia and accelerate the elimination of carbon monoxide, 100% oxygen is given at atmospheric or preferably hyperbaric pressures. Oxygen is given until the carboxyhemoglobin level is less than 5%. The patient is monitored continuously. Psychoses, spastic paralysis, ataxia, visual disturbances, and deterioration of mental status and behavior may persist after resuscitation and may be symptoms of permanent brain damage (Tintinalli et al., 2016).

When unintentional carbon monoxide poisoning occurs, the health department should be contacted so that the dwelling or building in question can be inspected. A psychiatric consultation is warranted if it has been determined that the poisoning was a suicide attempt.

Skin Contamination Poisoning (Chemical Burns)

Skin contamination injuries from exposure to chemicals are challenging because of the large number of possible offending agents with diverse actions and metabolic effects. The severity of a chemical burn is determined by the mechanism of action, the penetrating strength and concentration, and the amount and duration of exposure of the skin to the chemical.

The skin should be drenched immediately with running water from a shower, hose, or faucet, except in the case of lye and white phosphorus, which should be brushed off the skin dry (Moore, 2015).

Quality and Safety Nursing Alert

Water should not be applied to burns from lye or white phosphorus because of the potential for an explosion or for deepening of the burn. All evidence of these chemicals should be brushed off the patient before any flushing occurs.

The skin should be flushed with a constant stream of water as the patient's clothing is removed. The skin of health care personnel assisting the patient should be appropriately protected if the burn is extensive or if the agent is significantly toxic or still present. Prolonged lavage with generous amounts of tepid water is important. The decontamination shower (deluge) in the ED is the optimal place for total body flushing. The staff attending the patient should wear proper personal protective equipment (PPE) to prevent cross-contamination (Moore, 2015).

Attempts to determine the identity and characteristics of the chemical agent are necessary in order to specify future treatment. The standard burn treatment appropriate for the size and location of the wound (antimicrobial treatment, débridement, tetanus prophylaxis, antidote administration as prescribed) is instituted (Moore, 2015) (see Chapter 62). The patient may require plastic surgery for further wound management. The patient is instructed to have the affected area reexamined at 24 and 72 hours and in 7 days because of the risk of underestimating the extent and depth of these types of injuries.

Food Poisoning

Food poisoning is a sudden illness that occurs after ingestion of contaminated food or drink. Botulism is a serious form of food poisoning that requires continual surveillance (see Chapter 73, Table 73-5). Assessment questions for patients with food poisoning are discussed in Chart 72-7.

The key to treatment is determining the source and type of food poisoning. If possible, the suspected food should be brought to the medical facility and a history obtained from the patient or family.

Food, gastric contents, vomitus, serum, and feces are collected for examination. The patient's respirations, blood pressure, level of consciousness (LOC), CVP (if indicated), and muscular activity are monitored closely. Measures are instituted to support the respiratory system. Death from respiratory paralysis can occur with botulism, fish poisoning, and some other food poisonings.

Because large volumes of electrolytes and water are lost by vomiting and diarrhea, fluid and electrolyte status should be assessed. Severe vomiting produces alkalosis, and severe diarrhea produces acidosis. Hypovolemic shock may also occur from severe fluid and electrolyte losses. The patient is assessed for signs and symptoms of fluid and electrolyte imbalances, including lethargy, rapid pulse rate, fever, oliguria, anuria, hypotension, and delirium. Baseline weight and serum electrolyte levels are obtained for future comparisons.

Measures to control nausea are also important to prevent vomiting, which could exacerbate fluid and electrolyte imbalances. An antiemetic medication is given parenterally as prescribed if the patient cannot tolerate fluids or medications by mouth (Tintinalli et al., 2016). For mild nausea, the patient is encouraged to take sips of weak tea, carbonated drinks, or tap water. After nausea and vomiting subside, clear liquids are usually prescribed for 12 to 24 hours, and the diet is gradually progressed to a low-residue, bland diet.

SUBSTANCE ABUSE

Substance abuse is the misuse of specific substances, such as drugs or alcohol, to alter mood or behavior. Drug abuse is the use of drugs for other than legitimate medical purposes. People who abuse drugs often take a variety of drugs simultaneously (such as alcohol, barbiturates, opioids, and tranquilizers), and the combination may have additive and addictive effects.

"Rave parties" are large-scale parties attended by hundreds of people involved in illicit drug use. At these events, one of the most commonly used drugs is 3,4-methylenedioxymethamphetamine (MDMA), or Ecstasy, a methamphetamine-based drug that users believe produces a "harmless high." ED nurses should be aware of rave parties in their geographic area so that they can prepare for a potential influx of patients who abuse this drug. Others may combine Ecstasy with sildenafil (Viagra); this drug combination is nicknamed "sextasy."

Spice is a synthetic cannabinoid sold commercially as a smoking mixture under the names "spice," "incense," or "K2." Its chemical structure and effects are similar to marijuana, targeting the same receptor sites in the brain. Spice is sold with variable concentrations and unregulated potency (National Institute on Drug Abuse, 2015b).

Bath salts are synthetic stimulants similar to Ecstasy known as "mephedrone," "drone," or "MCAT." Their effects are similar to amphetamines, MDMA, and cocaine. Although bath salts are most commonly swallowed or snorted, they may also be smoked or injected; the method of intake affects the severity and duration of effects (Table 72-1). The structural formula 3,4-methylenedioxypyrovalerone (MDPV) is the most common type of bath salt abused (Baumann, Partilla, Lehner, et al., 2013).

Abuse of various inhalants (see Table 72-1) has also increased in popularity; these products generally result more often in cravings than withdrawal when their use is stopped. The method of inhalation varies with the product chosen and requires several deep inhalations to reach euphoria. Methods include sniffing or snorting by directly inhaling the fumes. "Bagging" (from a bag) or "huffing" (from a rag or cloth) provide the greatest concentration; "dusting" is another method that delivers the inhalant by directly spraying it into the nostrils. Long-term use results in cortical atrophy and brainstem dysfunction, in addition to cardiomyopathy and emphysema-like abnormalities of the lung. Significant others or parents may report that the patient has had poor school or work performance or attendance, weight loss, poor hygiene, fatigue, nosebleeds, and decreased appetite (ENA 2013).

Clinical manifestations vary with the substance used, but the underlying principles of management are essentially the same. Table 72-1 identifies commonly abused drugs, listing their clinical manifestations and therapeutic management. Treatment goals for a patient with a drug overdose are to support the respiratory and cardiovascular functions, to enhance clearance of the agent, and to provide for safety of the patient and staff. People who abuse IV/injection drugs are at increased risk for HIV infection, acquired immune deficiency syndrome, hepatitis B and C, and tetanus.

Chart 72-7 **ASSESSMENT**
Food Poisoning

Use the following questions to elicit information about the circumstances surrounding the possibility of food poisoning:
- How soon after eating did the symptoms occur? (Immediate onset suggests chemical, plant, or animal poisoning.)
- What was eaten in the previous meal? Did the food have an unusual odor or taste? (Most foods causing bacterial poisoning *do not* have unusual odor or taste.)
- Did anyone else become ill from eating the same food?
- Did vomiting occur? What was the appearance of the vomitus?
- Did diarrhea occur? (Diarrhea is usually absent with botulism and with shellfish or other fish poisoning.)
- Are any neurologic symptoms present? (These occur in botulism and in chemical, plant, and animal poisoning.)
- Does the patient have a fever? (Fever is characteristic in salmonella, ingestion of fava beans, and some fish poisoning.)

(text continued on page 2185)

TABLE 72-1 Emergency Management of Patients With Drug Overdose

Drug	Clinical Manifestations	Therapeutic Management
Cocaine *Routes may include:* • Intranasally ("snorting")—inhaled into nostrils through straws • By smoking ("freebasing")—cocaine hydrochloride dissolved in ether to yield a pure cocaine alkaloid base ("crack," "rocks"); smoking in a small pipe delivers large quantities of cocaine to lungs. • IV • Polysubstance (cocaine and heroin)	Cocaine is a CNS stimulant that can cause: • Increased heart rate and blood pressure • Hyperpyrexia • Seizures • Sluggish, dilated pupillary response • Muscle rigidity • Increased energy, agitation, aggression • Ventricular dysrhythmias • Intense euphoria, then anxiety, sadness, insomnia, and sexual indifference • Cocaine hallucinations with delusions • Psychosis with extreme paranoia and ideas of persecution • Hypervigilance Chronic psychotic symptoms may persist. Overall psychotic symptoms are short-lived compared to methamphetamines	1. Maintain airway and provide respiratory support. 2. Control seizures. 3. Monitor cardiovascular effects; have antiarrhythmic drugs and defibrillator available. 4. Treat for hyperthermia. 5. If cocaine was ingested, evacuate stomach contents and use activated charcoal to treat. Whole bowel irrigation may be necessary to treat body packers ("mules"). 6. Refer for psychiatric evaluation and treatment in an inpatient unit that eliminates access to the drug. Include drug rehabilitation counseling.
Opioids Heroin Opium or paregoric Morphine, codeine, semisynthetic derivatives: oxycodone (OxyContin), methadone, meperidine (Demerol), tramadol (Ultram), fentanyl (Sublimaze)	Acute intoxication (overdose) can result in: • Pinpoint pupils (may be dilated with severe hypoxia) • Decreased blood pressure • Marked respiratory depression/arrest • Pulmonary edema • Stupor → coma • Seizures Fresh needle marks along course of any superficial vein Skin abscesses (from "popping")	1. Support respiratory and cardiovascular functions. 2. Establish IV lines; obtain blood for chemical and toxicologic analysis. Patient may be given bolus of glucose to eliminate possibility of hypoglycemia. 3. Administer narcotic antagonist (naloxone hydrochloride IV, IM [Narcan]) as prescribed to reverse severe respiratory depression and coma. 4. Continue to monitor level of responsiveness and respirations, pulse, and blood pressure. Duration of action of naloxone hydrochloride is shorter than that of heroin; repeated dosages may be necessary. 5. Send urine for analysis; opioids can be detected in urine. 6. Obtain an ECG. 7. Do not leave patient unattended; he or she may lapse back into coma rapidly. Clinical status may change from minute to minute. Hemodialysis may be indicated for severe drug intoxication. Activated charcoal may be considered if opioids were taken orally and if the patient is alert. 8. Monitor for pulmonary edema, which is frequently seen in patients who abuse/overdose on narcotics. 9. Refer patient for psychiatric and drug rehabilitation evaluation before discharge.

Barbiturates
 	
Pentobarbital (Nembutal), secobarbital (Seconal), amobarbital (Amytal), gamma-hydroxybutyrate (GHB, "liquid Ecstasy")
	Acute intoxication *(may mimic alcohol intoxication)*:
	• Respiratory depression
	• Flushed face
	• Decreased pulse rate; decreased blood pressure
	• Increasing nystagmus (to vertical and horizontal gaze)
	• Sluggish pupils
	• Lack of convergence of eyes
	• Depressed deep tendon reflexes
	• Decreasing mental alertness
	• Difficulty in speaking
	• Poor motor coordination and flaccid muscles
	• Coma, death
	GHB:
	• Sexual disinhibition
	• Amnesia, myoclonus, agitation
	• Overdoses when mixed with alcohol
		1. Maintain airway and provide respiratory support.
		2. Endotracheal intubation or tracheostomy is considered if there is any doubt about the adequacy of airway exchange.
		  a. Check airway frequently.
		  b. Perform suctioning as necessary.
		3. Support cardiovascular and respiratory functions; most deaths result from respiratory depression or shock.
		4. Start infusion through large-gauge needle or IV catheter to support blood pressure; coma and dehydration result in hypotension and respond to infusion of IV fluids with elevation of blood pressure.
		5. Evacuate stomach contents or lavage if within 1 hour of ingestion to prevent absorption; repeated doses of activated charcoal may be given.
		6. Assist with hemodialysis for patient with severe overdose.
		7. Maintain neurologic and vital sign flow sheet.
		8. Patient awakening from overdose may demonstrate combative behavior.
		9. Refer for psychiatric and drug rehabilitation consultation to evaluate suicide potential and drug abuse.

(continued on page 2182)

TABLE 72-1 Emergency Management of Patients With Drug Overdose (continued)

Drug	Clinical Manifestations	Therapeutic Management
Inhalants Amyl nitrate Freon Propane Trichloroethylene Gasoline Perchloroethylene Toluene (metallic paint spray) Helium Canned air Hand sanitizer *Routes may include:* • Sniffing/snorting—direct inhalation of fumes • "Bagging"—sniff from a bag • "Huffing"—sniff from a rag/cloth • "Dusting"—direct spray into the nostrils	Effects mimic those of alcohol, with dizziness and imbalance: • Euphoria, headache, disinhibition, altered level of consciousness to coma • Renal, hepatic, and cardiac toxicity • Aplastic anemia • Fetal growth retardation • Respiratory depression, arrest from CNS depression • Vasodilation • Nosebleeding • Vertical and horizontal nystagmus • Lack of convergence of eyes • Sluggish pupils • Temperature fluctuations • Circumoral red spots/rash • Air embolus	1. Provide airway support, ventilation, and oxygen. 2. Treat cardiac dysrhythmias and hypotension. 3. Provide advanced cardiac life support as needed. 4. Monitor for profound hypotension when amyl nitrate is combined with MDMA and sildenafil or with anesthetic agents. 5. Monitor for hypertension when volatile solvents used.
Amphetamine-Type Drugs (pep pills, "uppers," "speed," "crystal meth") amphetamine (Benzedrine) dextroamphetamine (Dexedrine) methamphetamine (Desoxyn, "speed") 3,4-methylenedioxymethamphetamine (MDMA) ("Ecstasy," "Adam")[a] 3,4-methylenedioxy-*N*-ethylamphetamine (MDEA) ("Eve") 3,4-methylenedioxyamphetamine (MDA); methylphenidate (Ritalin) "ice," "rocks," "crystal meth" 3,4-methylenedioxypyrovalerone (MDPV) or 4-methylmethcathinone (mephedrone); "Bath salts" (synthetic stimulant)	• Nausea, vomiting, anorexia • Palpitations, tachycardia • Increased blood pressure • Tachypnea, anxiety • Nervousness • Diaphoresis, mydriasis • Repetitive or stereotyped behavior • Irritability, insomnia, agitation • Visual misperceptions, auditory hallucinations • Fearfulness, anxiety, depression, hostility, paranoia • Hyperactivity, rapid speech, euphoria, hyperalertness • Decreased inhibition • Seizures, coma, hyperthermia • Cardiovascular collapse • Rhabdomyolysis • MDMA is both a hallucinogenic and stimulant. • MDPV and mephedrone effects last >24 hours.	1. Provide airway support, ventilation, cardiac monitoring; insert IV line. 2. Use GI evacuation in cases of oral overdose; activated charcoal, gastric lavage if within 1 hour of ingestion. 3. Keep in calm, cool, quiet environment; elevated temperature potentiates amphetamine toxicity. Maintain normothermia, cooling the patient as necessary. 4. Administer small doses of diazepam (Valium) (IV) or haloperidol (Haldol) as prescribed for CNS and muscular hyperactivity. 5. Administer appropriate pharmacologic therapy as prescribed for severe hypertension and ventricular dysrhythmias. 6. Treat seizures with benzodiazepines (e.g., diazepam) as prescribed. 7. Treat sympathetic stimulation with beta-blocker agents as prescribed. 8. Try to communicate with patient if delusions or hallucinations are present. 9. Place in a protective environment (preferably psychiatric security room with video monitoring) to observe for suicide attempt. 10. Refer for psychiatric and drug rehabilitation evaluation.

Hallucinogens or Psychedelic-Type Drugs
 	
Lysergic acid diethylamide (LSD)
Phencyclidine HCl (PCP, "angel dust")
Mescaline, psilocybin
Cannabinoids (marijuana)
Ketamine ("special K")
Synthetic cannabinoids ("spice," "incense," "K2")
Butane honey oil (BHo)—"dabs," "shatter"
	• Nystagmus
	• Pupil dilation
	• *Psychedelics*
	  a. Sluggish pupillary response
	  b. Increased pulse and temperature
	  c. Muscle rigidity
	• Mild hypertension
	• Marked confusion bordering on panic
	• Incoherence, hyperactivity
	• Withdrawn
	• Combative behavior; delirium, mania, self-injury (lasts 6–12 hours)
	• Hallucinations, body image distortion
	• Hypertension, hyperthermia, acute kidney injury
	• Flashback—recurrence of LSD-like state without having taken the drug; may occur weeks or months after drug was taken
	• Ketamine—"out-of-body" experience; increased aggressiveness
	• Synthetic cannabinoids—euphoria, increased sensory experience, relaxation
	• Manufacturing can result in burns
		1. Evaluate and maintain patient's circulation, airway, and breathing.
		2. Determine by urine or serum drug screen whether the patient has ingested hallucinogenic drug or has a toxic psychosis.
		3. Try to communicate with and reassure the patient.
		  a. "Talking down" involves understanding the process through which the patient is proceeding and helping the patient overcome fears while establishing contact with reality.
		  b. Remind the patient that fear is common with this problem.
		  c. Reassure the patient that he is not losing his mind but is experiencing the effect of drugs and that this will wear off.
		  d. Instruct the patient to keep the eyes open; this reduces the intensity of reaction.
		  e. Reduce sensory stimuli by minimizing noise, lights, movement, tactile stimulation.
		4. Sedate the patient as prescribed if hyperactivity cannot be controlled; diazepam or a barbiturate may be prescribed.

Drug	Clinical Manifestations	Therapeutic Management

		5. Search for evidence of trauma; patients who use hallucinogens have a tendency to "act out" their hallucinations.
		6. Manage seizures with benzodiazepines (e.g., diazepam) as necessary.
		7. Observe patient closely; patient's behavior may become hazardous. Have safety officers stationed near the patient's room.
		8. Monitor for hypertensive crisis if patient has prolonged psychosis due to drug ingestion.
		9. Place patient in a protected environment under proper medical supervision to prevent self-inflicted bodily harm.
		
		Management for Phencyclidine Abuse
		1. Place patient in a calm, supportive environment to minimize stimuli; protect from self-injury.
		2. Avoid talking down.
		3. Do not leave patient unobserved. Treat symptoms as they occur.
		  a. Drug effects are unpredictable and prolonged.
		  b. Symptoms are likely to exacerbate; patient becomes out of control.
		4. Refer all patients in this category for psychiatric and drug evaluation/rehabilitation.

Drugs Producing Sedation, Intoxication, or Psychological and Physical Dependence (nonbarbiturate sedatives)

Drug	Clinical Manifestations	Therapeutic Management

diazepam (Valium)
chlordiazepoxide (Librium)
oxazepam (Serax)
lorazepam (Ativan)
midazolam (Versed)
flunitrazepam (Rohypnol, "roofies," "date rape drug")[a]
	Seizures, coma, circulatory collapse, death
	Acute intoxication:
	• Respiratory depression
	• Decreasing mental alertness
	• Confusion
	• Slurred speech, decreased blood pressure
	• Ataxia
	• Pulmonary edema
	• Coma, death
	
	Flunitrazepam:
	• Disinhibition with antegrade amnesia
	• Weakness and unsteadiness with impaired judgment
	• Powerlessness
		1. Endotracheal tube is inserted as a precaution; use assisted ventilation to stabilize and correct respiratory depression. Observe for sudden apnea and laryngeal spasm.
		2. Assess for hypotension.
		  a. Insert indwelling urinary catheter for patient who is comatose; decreased urinary volume is an index of reduced renal flow associated with reduced intravascular volume or vascular collapse.
		  b. Start volume expansion with saline or dextrose as prescribed.
		3. Evacuate stomach contents; lavage (if within 1 hour of ingestion); activated charcoal.
		4. Start ECG monitoring. Observe for dysrhythmias.
		5. Administer flumazenil (Romazicon), a benzodiazepine antagonist (reversal agent).
		6. Refer patient for psychiatric evaluation (potential suicide intent).

Salicylate Poisoning

Drug	Clinical Manifestations	Therapeutic Management
Aspirin (present in compound analgesic tablets) • Toxic levels (150–200 mg/kg body weight) • Chronic toxicity (occurs in older adults due to decreased kidney function) • Long-term intoxication (>100 mg/kg/ day for more than 2 days)	• Restlessness • Tinnitus, deafness • Blurring of vision • Hyperpnea • Hyperpyrexia • Sweating • Epigastric pain, vomiting • Dehydration • Respiratory alkalosis and metabolic acidosis • Disorientation, coma • Cardiovascular collapse • Coagulopathy	1. Treat respiratory depression. 2. Induce gastric emptying by lavage (if within 1 hour after ingestion). 3. Give activated charcoal to adsorb aspirin. 4. Support patient with IV infusions as prescribed to establish hydration and correct electrolyte imbalances, including administration of sodium bicarbonate. 5. Enhance elimination of salicylates as directed by forced diuresis, alkalinization of urine, peritoneal dialysis, or hemodialysis, according to severity of intoxication. 6. Monitor serum salicylate level for efficacy of treatment. 7. Administer specific prescribed pharmacologic agent for bleeding and other problems. 8. Recognize that concretions formed in the gut may result in prolonged exposure as they are digested. 9. Refer patient for psychiatric evaluation (potential suicide intent). 10. Monitor thromboelastography for platelet function.

(continued on page 2184)

TABLE 72-1 **Emergency Management of Patients With Drug Overdose** (continued)

Drug	Clinical Manifestations	Therapeutic Management
Acetaminophen (present in prescription and nonprescription analgesics, antipyretics, and cold remedies)	Lethargy to encephalopathy and death GI upset, diaphoresis Right upper quadrant pain Abnormal liver function tests, prolonged prothrombin time, increased bilirubin, disseminated intravascular coagulation Hepatomegaly leading to liver failure Metabolic acidosis Hypoglycemia Stage I—within 24 hours; GI irritation, possible metabolic acidosis and coma if severe ingestion Stage II—24–48 hours; monitor liver and coagulation studies. Stage III—after 48 hours; hepatic encephalopathy/jaundice, vomiting, right upper quadrant pain, coagulopathy, hypoglycemia, acute kidney injury	1. Maintain airway. 2. Obtain acetaminophen level. Levels ≥140 mg/kg are toxic. 3. Laboratory studies—liver function tests, prothrombin time/partial thromboplastin time, complete blood count, blood urea nitrogen, creatinine. 4. Lavage (if within 1 hour after ingestion); activated charcoal. 5. Prepare for possible hemodialysis, which clears acetaminophen but does not halt liver damage. 6. Administer N-acetylcysteine (Mucomyst) as soon as possible. N-acetylcysteine replenishes essential liver enzymes and requires a total of 18 doses every 4 hours. Charcoal absorbs N-acetylcysteine; do not administer together. Repeat N-acetylcysteine dose if patient vomits. 7. Refer patient for psychiatric evaluation (potential suicide intent).
Tricyclic Antidepressants amitriptyline (Elavil) doxepin (Sinequan) nortriptyline (Aventyl) imipramine (Tofranil)	Dysrhythmia: ventricular fibrillation/tachycardia, sinus tachycardia Hypotension Pulmonary edema, hypoxemia, acidosis Confusion, agitation, coma Visual hallucinations Clonus, tremors, hyperactive reflexes, nystagmus, myoclonic jerking Seizures Blurred vision, flushing, hyperthermia	1. Provide airway support, ventilation, cardiac monitoring; insert IV line with normal saline solution. 2. If within 1–2 hours after overdose, insert a nasogastric tube and instill activated charcoal every 4 hours × 3. 3. Administer a sodium bicarbonate drip to decrease dysrhythmias; the alkaline environment increases the protein binding of the metabolite. Synchronized cardioversion may be indicated with some dysrhythmias refractory to sodium bicarbonate. Torsades de pointes should be treated with IV magnesium sulfate. 4. Administer vasopressors. 5. Manage seizure activity with benzodiazepines (e.g., diazepam) as necessary. 6. Refer patient for psychiatric evaluation for potential suicide intent and evaluation of medication regimen for effectiveness.
Selective Serotonin Reuptake Inhibitors and Other Antidepressants trazodone (Desyrel) fluoxetine (Prozac) paroxetine (Paxil) sertraline (Zoloft) venlafaxine (Effexor) escitalopram (Lexapro) bupropion (Wellbutrin)	Decreased level of consciousness, confusion Respiratory depression Increased heart rate Serotonin syndrome may occur if the SSRI was taken in conjunction with dextromethorphan or meperidine Agitation, seizures Hyperthermia, diaphoresis Hypertension, headache, shivering, "goose flesh," cardiac dysrhythmias, loss of consciousness	1. Administer activated charcoal with possibly whole bowel irrigation if a sustained-release medication was taken. 2. Use seizure precautions and administer benzodiazepines (e.g., diazepam) as prescribed.
Anabolic Steroids "roids," "juice," methandrostenolone, stanozolol, nandrolone Synthetic testosterone	Increase in LDL, decrease in HDL Alter carbohydrate metabolism Hyponatremia, hypokalemia Hypocalcemia/osteoporosis Mood swings/violent behaviors Invincibility, depression, potential for suicide attempts Memory loss, cognitive disabilities Immunosuppression Used to bulk up muscles, so skeletal muscle hypertrophy is a common manifestation.	1. Provide supportive therapy appropriate to patient's emotional manifestations. 2. Protect the patient from self-harm/harming others. 3. Encourage the patient to stop use; refer patient for psychiatric evaluation.

CNS, central nervous system; →, precedes; IV, intravenous; IM, intramuscular; ECG, electrocardiogram; GI, gastrointestinal; NAC, N-acetylcysteine; SSRI, selective serotonin reuptake inhibitor; LDL, low-density lipoprotein; HDL, high-density lipoprotein.

[a]Polydrug use at "rave clubs" frequently involves MDMA, alcohol, amphetamines, LSD, and sometimes dextromethorphan. Terms such as "Ecstasy" may refer to flunitrazepam (Rohypnol), GHB, ephedrine, and/or caffeine, in addition to MDMA.

Adapted from Emergency Nurses Association. (2013). *Sheehy's manual of emergency care* (7th ed.). St. Louis, MO: Mosby; National Institute on Drug Abuse (2015a). Drug facts. Retrieved on 2/20/2017 at: www.drugabuse.gov/publications/drugfacts/;; Tintinalli, J. E., Stapczyski, J. S., Ma, O. J, et al., (2016). *Tintinalli's emergency medicine manual* (8th ed.). New York: McGraw-Hill Medical.

Cannabis remains popular, available, and in some states, is now legal. A newer method of cannabis abuse is butane honey oil (BHO) or "dabs." BHO is created at home by heating cannabis with butane to strip the chemical from the plant, which is then heated further to remove the butane. It may be further distilled to "shatter" by being placed in a vacuum to remove any residual butane. The product results in a "dab" which can then be inhaled. Butane in the presence of an ignition source can result in explosion and fire resulting in chemical and thermal burns (Molina, 2017).

Acute Alcohol Intoxication

Alcohol is a psychotropic drug that affects mood, judgment, behavior, concentration, and consciousness. Many people who drink heavily are young adults or those older than 60 years. There is a high prevalence of alcoholism among patients presenting to the ED for management; up to 31% have histories of alcohol abuse. Among patients who present to the ED with various injuries, up to 50% may have histories of alcohol abuse (ENA 2013). Because patients who abuse alcohol return frequently to the ED, they present a challenge to the health professionals who care for them. The CDC advocates routine screening for alcohol abuse in all outpatient settings, including EDs. Therefore, screenings, brief interventions, and referral to treatment (SBIRT) for patients presenting with suspected alcohol abuse are recommended. All level I and II verified trauma centers are required to provide this service. SBIRT is considered cost-effective in saving quality of life-years lost and preventing the morbid consequences of continued alcohol abuse (Kane, Mitchell, Aiello, et al., 2016; Slain, Rickard-Aasen, Pringle, et al., 2014).

Alcohol, or ethanol, is a multisystem toxin and CNS depressant that causes drowsiness, impaired coordination, slurring of speech, sudden mood changes, aggression, belligerence, grandiosity, and uninhibited behavior. In excess, it can also cause stupor and eventually coma and death (i.e., alcohol poisoning). Increasingly, underage minors and college students arrive at the ED with alcohol poisoning from binge drinking.

In the ED, the patient who is intoxicated with alcohol or who presents with alcohol poisoning is assessed for head injury, hypoglycemia (which mimics intoxication), and other health problems. Possible nursing diagnoses include ineffective breathing pattern related to CNS depression and ineffective impulse control related to severe intoxication from alcohol.

Treatment involves detoxification of the acute poisoning, recovery, and rehabilitation. Commonly, the patient uses mechanisms of denial and defensiveness. The nurse should approach the patient in a nonjudgmental manner, using a firm, consistent, accepting, and reasonable attitude. Speaking in a calm and slow manner is helpful because alcohol interferes with thought processes. If the patient appears intoxicated, hypoxia, hypovolemia, and neurologic impairment must be ruled out before it is assumed that the patient is intoxicated. Typically, a blood specimen is obtained for analysis of the blood alcohol level.

If drowsy, the patient should be allowed to sleep off the state of alcoholic intoxication. During this time, maintenance of a patent airway and observation for symptoms of CNS depression are essential. The patient should be undressed and kept warm with blankets. On the other hand, if the patient is noisy or belligerent, sedation may be necessary. If sedation is used, the patient should be monitored carefully for hypotension and decreased LOC.

In addition, the patient is examined for alcohol withdrawal delirium and for injuries and organic disease (such as head injury, seizures, pulmonary infections, hypoglycemia, and nutritional deficiencies) that may be masked by alcoholic intoxication. People with alcoholism suffer more injuries than the general population. Acute alcohol intoxication is the cause of trauma for many patients without alcoholism as well. Pulmonary infections are also more common in patients with alcoholism, resulting from respiratory depression, an impaired defense system, and a tendency toward aspiration of gastric contents. The patient may show little increase in temperature or WBC count. The patient may be hospitalized or admitted to a detoxification center in an effort to examine problems underlying the substance abuse (ENA, 2013).

Alcohol Withdrawal Syndrome/ Delirium Tremens

Alcohol withdrawal syndrome is an acute toxic state that occurs as a result of sudden cessation of alcohol intake after a bout of heavy drinking or, more typically, after prolonged intake of alcohol. Severity of symptoms depends on how much alcohol was ingested and for how long. Delirium tremens may be precipitated by acute injury or infection (pneumonia, pancreatitis, hepatitis) and is the most severe form of alcohol withdrawal syndrome (ENA, 2013). Delirium tremens is a life-threatening condition and carries a high mortality rate if untreated (ENA, 2013).

Patients with alcohol withdrawal syndrome show signs of anxiety, uncontrollable fear, tremor, irritability, agitation, insomnia, and incontinence. They are talkative and preoccupied and experience visual, tactile, olfactory, and auditory hallucinations that often are terrifying. Autonomic overactivity occurs and is evidenced by tachycardia, dilated pupils, and profuse perspiration. Usually, all vital signs are elevated in the alcoholic toxic state.

The goals of management are to give adequate sedation and support to allow the patient to rest and recover without danger of injury or peripheral vascular collapse. A physical examination is performed to identify pre-existing or contributing illnesses or injuries (e.g., head injury, pneumonia). A drug history is obtained to elicit information that may facilitate adjustment of any sedative requirements. Baseline blood pressure is determined, because the patient's subsequent treatment may depend on blood pressure changes.

Usually, the patient is sedated as directed with a sufficient dosage of benzodiazepines to establish and maintain sedation, which reduces agitation, prevents exhaustion, prevents seizures, and promotes sleep. The patient should be calm, able to respond, and able to maintain an airway safely on their own. A variety of medications and combinations of medications are used (e.g., chlordiazepoxide [Librium], lorazepam [Ativan], and clonidine [Catapres]). Haloperidol (Haldol), esmolol (Brevibloc), or midazolam (Versed) may be given for severe acute alcohol withdrawal syndrome. Dosages are adjusted according to the patient's symptoms (agitation, anxiety) and blood pressure response (ENA, 2013).

The patient is placed in a calm, nonstressful environment (usually a private room) and observed closely. The room remains lighted to minimize the potential for illusions (visual misrepresentations) and hallucinations. Homicidal or suicidal responses may result from hallucinations. Closet and bathroom doors are closed to eliminate shadows. Someone is designated to stay with the patient as much as possible. The presence of another person has a reassuring and calming effect, which helps the patient maintain contact with reality. To orient the patient to reality, any illusions are explained.

> ⚑ **Quality and Safety Nursing Alert**
>
> *Restraints are used as prescribed, if necessary, if the patient is aggressive or violent, but only when other alternatives have been unsuccessful. The least restrictive device that will prevent the patient from injuring him- or herself or others is used. Caution is taken to ensure that restraints are applied properly and that they are not impairing circulation to any part of the body or interfering with respirations. Restraints should be used in tandem with verbal intervention to calm the patient and promote adherence. Restraints must be released according to protocol. Physical observation (e.g., skin integrity, circulatory status, respiratory status) is ongoing, and the patient's response is documented.*

Fluid losses may result from gastrointestinal losses (vomiting), profuse perspiration, and hyperventilation. In addition, the patient may be dehydrated as a result of alcohol's effect of decreasing antidiuretic hormone. The oral or IV route is used to restore fluid and electrolyte balance.

Temperature, pulse, respiration, and blood pressure are recorded frequently (every 30 minutes in severe forms of delirium) to monitor for peripheral circulatory collapse or hyperthermia (the two most serious complications).

Frequently seen complications include infections (e.g., pneumonia), trauma, hepatic failure, hypoglycemia, and cardiovascular problems. Hypoglycemia may accompany alcohol withdrawal, because alcohol depletes liver glycogen stores and impairs gluconeogenesis; many patients with alcoholism also are malnourished. Parenteral dextrose may be prescribed if the liver glycogen level is depleted. Orange juice, sports drinks, or other sources of carbohydrates are given to stabilize the blood glucose level and counteract tremulousness. Supplemental vitamin therapy and a high-protein diet are provided as prescribed to counteract nutritional deficits. The patient should be referred to an alcoholic treatment center for follow-up care and rehabilitation.

VIOLENCE, ABUSE, AND NEGLECT

Family Violence, Abuse, and Neglect

EDs are often the first place where victims of family violence, abuse, or neglect go to seek help. In the United States, 18% of women and 1.4% of men have been raped at some time in their lives; however, the percentages are equal by gender if rape was perpetrated by an intimate partner. Most female victims experience rape before the age of 25 years, with 42% of those before the age of 18 years; yet for men, 28% experience rape much younger, before 10 years of age. Intimate partner violence (IPV) many times involves violations beyond rape, including physical assault and stalking. Approximately 35% of women and 28% of men have experienced some component of IPV (Black, Basile, Breiding, et al., 2011). IPV accounts for 38% of murders among women. For those women, 44% had been to the ED in the previous 2 years (Solheim, 2016).

IPV involves fear of one partner by another and control by threats, intimidation, and physical abuse. Most IPV is committed by men against women and can be emotional, physical, sexual, or economic in nature (Black et al., 2011). ED nurses must be vigilant in their assessments of both women and men who present with injuries that may be consistent with IPV. In addition, ED nurses must be aware that men and women with disabilities are at higher risk of domestic violence and abuse than people without disabilities and should include questions that screen for IPV in their evaluations (see Chapter 56, Chart 56-3).

It is estimated that 10% of adults older than 65 years have been abused or neglected, a type of IPV called *elder abuse*, with 90% of elder abuse perpetrated by family (Lachs & Pillemer, 2015; National Center on Elder Abuse, 2016). Elder abuse takes many forms, including physical, sexual, emotional, and verbal abuse; neglect; violation of personal rights; abandonment; and financial abuse (Solheim, 2016) (see Chapter 5).

Clinical Manifestations

When people who have been abused seek treatment, they may present with physical injuries or health problems such as anxiety, insomnia, or gastrointestinal symptoms related to stress. The possibility of abuse should be investigated whenever a person presents with multiple injuries that are in various stages of healing, when injuries are unexplained, and when the explanation does not fit the physical picture (see Chart 72-8). The possibility of neglect should be investigated whenever a person who is dependent shows evidence of inattention to hygiene, to nutrition, or to know medical needs (e.g., unfilled medication prescriptions, missed appointments with health care providers). In the ED, the most common physical injuries seen are unexplained bruises, lacerations, abrasions, head injuries, or fractures. The most common clinical manifestations of neglect are malnutrition and dehydration.

Assessment and Diagnostic Findings

Nurses in EDs are in an ideal position to provide early detection and interventions for victims of IPV. This requires an acute awareness of the signs of possible abuse, maltreatment, and neglect. Nurses must be skilled in interviewing techniques that are likely to elicit accurate information. A careful history is crucial in the screening process. Asking questions in private—away from others—may be helpful in eliciting information about abuse, maltreatment, and neglect (see Chart 72-9). Nurses need to be aware that women may withhold directly answering questions regarding IPV in fear of retaliation, loss of children, and retribution against the children (Amerson, Whittington, & Duggan, 2014).

Whenever evidence leads the nurse to suspect abuse or neglect, an evaluation with careful documentation of

Chart 72-8 ASSESSMENT
Assessing for Abuse, Maltreatment, and Neglect

The following questions may be helpful when assessing a patient for abuse, maltreatment, and neglect:

- I noticed that you have a number of bruises. Can you tell me how they happened? Has anyone hurt you?
- You seem frightened. Has anyone ever hurt you?
- Patients sometimes tell me that they have been hurt by someone at home or at work. Could this be happening to you?
- Are you afraid of anyone at home or work, or of anyone with whom you come in contact?
- Has anyone failed to help you to take care of yourself when you needed help?
- Has anyone prevented you from seeing friends or other people whom you wish to see?
- Have you signed any papers that you did not understand or did not wish to sign?
- Has anyone forced you to sign papers against your will?
- Has anyone forced you to engage in sexual activities within the past year?
- Has anyone prevented you from using an assistive device (e.g., wheelchair, walker) within the past year?
- Has anyone you depend on refused to help you take your medicine, bathe, groom, or eat within the past year?

descriptions of events and drawings or photographs of injuries is important, because the medical record may be used as part of a legal proceeding. Assessment of the patient's general appearance and interactions with significant others, an examination of the entire surface area of the body, and a mental status examination are crucial.

Management

The aims of IPV screening include earlier identification of patients who have been abused and prevention of continued abusive events, including homicide (Day, Fox, Majercik, et al., 2015). Whenever abuse, maltreatment, or neglect is suspected, the health care provider's main concern should be the safety and welfare of the patient. Treatment focuses on the consequences of the abuse, violence, or neglect and on prevention of further injury. Protocols of most EDs require that a multidisciplinary approach be used. Nurses, physicians, social workers, and community agencies work collaboratively to develop and implement a plan for meeting the patient's needs.

If the patient is in immediate danger, he or she should be separated from the person who is abusive or neglectful whenever possible. Referral to a shelter may be the most appropriate action, but many shelters are inaccessible to people with mobility limitations.

When abuse or neglect is the result of stress experienced by a caregiver who is no longer able to cope with the burden of caring for an older adult or a person with chronic disease or a disability, respite services may be necessary. Support groups may be helpful to these caregivers. When mental illness of the person who is abusive or neglectful is responsible for the situation, alternative living arrangements may be required.

Nurses must be mindful that competent adults are free to accept or refuse the help that is offered to them. Some patients insist on remaining in the home environment where the abuse or neglect is occurring. The wishes of patients who are competent and not cognitively impaired should be respected. However, all possible alternatives, available resources, and safety plans should be explored with the patient.

Chart 72-9 NURSING RESEARCH PROFILE
Barriers to Nurses Screening for Intimate Partner Violence

DeBoer, M. I., Kothari, R., Kothari, M. A., et al. (2013). What are barriers to nurses screening for intimate partner violence? *Journal of Trauma Nursing, 20*(3), 155–160.

Purpose

Intimate partner violence (IPV) is a common comorbidity among women who present to emergency departments (EDs) for treatment. It is estimated that between 15% and 30% of all women who present to EDs have experienced IPV within the past year, though few seek care for treatment of IPV-related injuries. Nurses are in a prime position to screen patients for IPV. The purpose of this study was to identify barriers to nurses screening patients for IPV.

Design

This was a descriptive cross-sectional study. Registered nurses (RNs) who worked in a 450-bed level 1 trauma center and who were employed in positions that provided direct patient care were invited to anonymously complete a survey. The survey consisted of 7 demographic and 22 attitude- and knowledge-based Likert scale items. A total of 156 RNs completed the survey, after Institutional Review Board approval was obtained.

Findings

The mean age of participants (*N* = 156) was 43.2 years, with 16.8 mean years of nursing experience. The majority of participants (82.6%) reported taking care of 2 or fewer patients who had been subject to IPV within the past year. The majority (81%) affirmed their feeling that they had sufficient time to screen patients for IPV. However, nearly half (44%) disagreed that they were adequately trained to recognize signs and symptoms of IPV. The majority (95%) affirmed their belief that it is the RN's responsibility to recognize IPV. Results of knowledge-based survey items that confirmed the participants' ability to recognize IPV risks were mixed.

Nursing Implications

Most RNs who participated in this study expressed the belief that recognizing and screening patients for IPV was a key nursing role and felt that they had sufficient time to do so. However, the majority perceived that they cared for few patients with IPV within the past year, although IPV is a prevalent problem. Moreover, many felt that they lacked adequate training to screen for IPV. Many also did not correctly identify knowledge of IPV risks. Providing RNs with education that can enhance their ability to screen patients for IPV may result in earlier detection of patients who have been subjected to IPV.

Mandatory reporting laws in most states require health care workers to report *suspected* child abuse or abuse of older adults to an official agency, usually Adult (or Child) Protective Services. All that is required for reporting is the suspicion of abuse; the health care worker is not required to prove abuse or neglect. Likewise, health care workers who report suspected abuse are immune from civil or criminal liability if the report is made in good faith. Subsequent home visits resulting from the report of suspected abuse are a part of gathering information about the patient in the home environment. In addition, many states have resource hotlines for use by health care workers and by patients who seek answers to questions about abuse and neglect.

Sexual Assault

The definition of *rape* is forced sexual acts, especially if these acts involve vaginal or anal penetration. Attempted rape may include verbal threats of rape (ENA, 2013). Perpetrators and victims may be either male or female. Rape crisis centers offer support and education and help people who have been sexually assaulted through the subsequent police investigation and courtroom experience.

The manner in which the patient is received and treated in the ED is important to their future psychological well-being. Crisis intervention should begin when the patient enters the health care facility. The patient should be seen immediately. Most hospitals have a written protocol that addresses the patient's physical and emotional needs as well as collection of forensic evidence.

In many states, the emergency nurse has the opportunity to become trained as a sexual assault nurse examiner (SANE). Preparing for this role requires specific training in forensic evidence collection, history taking, documentation, and ways to approach the patient and family. Specialized training also includes learning proper photographic methods and the use of colposcopy. Colposcopy facilitates assessment by magnifying tissues and looking for evidence of microtrauma. Evidence is collected through photography, videography, and analysis of specimens. Another tool useful to the SANE is the light-staining microscope, which enables the examiner to identify motile and nonmotile sperm and infectious organisms. This tool saves time and also enhances assessment. The SANE complements the ED staff and can spend more time with both the patient and police officers investigating the incident (ENA, 2013).

Assessment and Diagnostic Findings

The patient's reaction to rape has been termed *rape trauma syndrome* and is seen as an acute stress reaction to a life-threatening situation. The nurse performing the assessment is aware that the patient may go through several phases of psychological reactions, which have been described as follows:

- An acute disorganization phase, which may manifest as an expressed state in which shock, disbelief, fear, guilt, humiliation, anger, and other such emotions are encountered or as a controlled state in which feelings are masked or hidden and the victim appears composed
- A phase of denial and unwillingness to talk about the incident, followed by a phase of heightened anxiety, fear, flashbacks, sleep disturbances, hyperalertness, and psychosomatic reactions that is consistent with PTSD (see later discussion)
- A phase of reorganization, in which the incident is put into perspective. Some victims never fully recover and go on to develop chronic stress disorders and phobias.

Management

The goals of management are to provide support, to reduce the patient's emotional trauma, and to gather available evidence for possible legal proceedings. All of the interventions are aimed at encouraging the patient to gain a sense of control over their life.

Throughout the patient's stay in the ED, the patient's privacy and sensitivity must be respected. The patient may exhibit a wide range of emotional reactions, such as hysteria, stoicism, or feelings of being overwhelmed. Support and caring are crucial. The patient should be reassured that anxiety is natural and asked whether a person who can provide support may be called. Appropriate support is available from professional and community resources. The National Sexual Assault Hotline (see the Resources section) will automatically route the patient to the nearest assault or crisis intervention center for services, as needed. The patient should never be left alone.

Physical Examination

A written, witnessed informed consent must be obtained from the patient (or parent or guardian if the patient is a minor) for examination, for taking of photographs, and for release of findings to police. A history is obtained only if the patient has not already talked to a police officer, social worker, or crisis intervention worker. The patient should not be asked to repeat the history. Any history of the event that is obtained should be recorded in the patient's own words. The patient is asked whether he or she has bathed, douched, brushed his or her teeth, changed clothes, urinated, or defecated since the attack, because these actions may alter interpretation of subsequent findings. The time of admission, time of examination, date and time of the alleged rape, and the patient's emotional state and general appearance (including any evidence of trauma, such as discoloration, bruises, lacerations, secretions, or torn and bloody clothing) are documented. If the patient has no recollection of the event, drugs that induce retrograde amnesia may have been involved, such as alcohol, ketamine, gamma-hydroxybutyrate, benzodiazepines, or flunitrazepam (Rohypnol). Urine drug test must be completed within 96 hours of the event to capture the presence of these drugs. Emesis can also be collected for testing (ENA, 2013).

For the physical examination, the patient is helped to undress and is draped properly. Each item of clothing is placed in a separate paper bag. As noted earlier, plastic bags are not used in order to avoid possible destruction of evidence from mold or mildew formation. The bags are labeled and given to appropriate law enforcement authorities.

The patient is examined (from head to toe) for injuries, especially injuries to the head, neck, breasts, thighs, back, and buttocks. Body diagrams and photographs aid in documenting the evidence of trauma. The physical examination focuses on the following:

- External evidence of trauma (bruises, contusions, lacerations, stab wounds)
- Dried semen stains (appearing as crusted, flaking areas) on the patient's body or clothes
- Broken fingernails and body tissue and foreign materials under nails (if found, samples are taken)
- Oral examination, including a specimen of saliva and cultures of gum and tooth areas

Pelvic and rectal examinations are also performed. The perineum and other areas are examined with a Wood lamp or other filtered ultraviolet light. Areas that appear fluorescent may indicate semen stains. The color and consistency of any discharge present is noted. A water-moistened, rather than lubricated, vaginal speculum is used for the examination. Lubricant contains chemicals that may interfere with later forensic testing of specimens and acid phosphatase determinations. The rectum is examined for signs of trauma, blood, and semen. During the examination, the patient should be advised of the nature and necessity of each procedure and given the rationale for each (ENA, 2013).

Specimen Collection

During the physical examination, numerous laboratory specimens may be collected, including the following:

- Vaginal aspirate, examined for presence or absence of motile and nonmotile sperm.
- Secretions (obtained with a sterile swab) from the vaginal pool for acid phosphatase, blood group antigen of semen, and precipitin test against human sperm and blood.
- Separate smears from the oral, vaginal, and anal areas.
- Culture of body orifices for gonorrhea.
- Blood serum for syphilis and HIV testing and deoxyribonucleic acid (DNA) analysis. A sample of serum for syphilis may be frozen and saved for future testing.
- Pregnancy test if there is a possibility that the female patient may be pregnant.
- Any foreign material (leaves, grass, dirt), which is placed in a clean envelope.
- Pubic hair samples obtained by combing or trimming. Several pubic hairs with follicles are placed in separate containers and identified as the patient's hair.

To preserve the chain of evidence, each specimen is labeled with the name of the patient, the date and time of collection, the body area from which the specimen was obtained, and the names of personnel collecting specimens. The specimens are then given to a designated person (e.g., crime laboratory technician), and an itemized receipt is obtained (ENA, 2013).

Treating Potential Consequences of Rape

After the initial physical examination is completed and specimens have been obtained, any associated injuries are treated as indicated. The patient is given the option of prophylaxis against sexually transmitted infections (STIs) (also referred to as sexually transmitted disease [STDs]). Ceftriaxone (Rocephin), given intramuscularly with 1% lidocaine (Xylocaine), may be prescribed as prophylaxis for gonorrhea. In addition, a single oral dose of metronidazole (Flagyl) and either a single oral dose of azithromycin (Zithromax) or a 7-day oral regimen of doxycycline may be prescribed as prophylaxis for syphilis and chlamydia (ENA, 2013; Solheim, 2016).

Antipregnancy measures may be considered if the patient is a female of childbearing age. A postcoital contraceptive medication, such as an oral contraceptive medication that contains levonorgestrel and ethinyl estradiol (Alesse, Seasonique), may be prescribed after a pregnancy test. To promote effectiveness, the contraceptive medication should be given within 12 to 24 hours and no later than 72 hours after intercourse. The 21-day package is prescribed so that the patient does not mistakenly take the inert tablets included in the 28-day package. An antiemetic agent may be given as prescribed to decrease discomfort from side effects. A cleansing douche, mouthwash, and fresh clothing are usually offered.

Follow-Up Care

The patient is informed of counseling services to prevent long-term psychological effects. Counseling services should be made available to both the patient and the family. A referral is made to the National Sexual Assault Hotline (see the Resources section) or directly to a local crisis intervention center. Appointments for follow-up surveillance for pregnancy and for STI and HIV testing also are made (Solheim, 2016).

The patient is encouraged to return to their previous level of functioning as soon as possible. When leaving the ED, the patient should be accompanied by a family member or friend.

Human Trafficking

The most rapidly growing area of criminal activity in the world is human trafficking, or modern day slavery (ENA, 2015b). Human trafficking is defined as the use of force, fraud, or coercion for the purpose of subjection to involuntary servitude (Solheim, 2016). Human trafficking may involve forced sex or labor or both. Data show approximately 20 million people are trafficked in this form of slavery, with at least 17,000 of these in the United States. These people have limited access to health care and the ED may be the only access point to identify their situation (ENA, 2015b).

A victim of trafficking may present to the ED with injury, accompanied by a significantly older boyfriend or travel partner. The victim may have a history of being a chronic runaway, or of homelessness, and of self-mutilation. Common behaviors exhibited by these patients may include cowering or deferring to the person accompanying them, who may appear controlling, and appearing frightened or agitated. The patient may have a special mark/tattoo present, poor dentition, and multiple injuries in various stages of healing. Common physical complaints include injuries, poor healing or poorly healed old injuries, abdominal pain, dizziness, headaches, rashes or sores. Patients may demonstrate addiction, panic attacks, impulse control, hostility, and suicidal ideation.

The ED nurse may be well positioned to offer an opportunity for the patient to speak, alone without an accompanying companion, who could be a perpetrator of abuse. Targeted, appropriate questions may include asking patients if they are in control of their own money; whether or not they are able to come and go as they please; and who is the person or persons accompanying them (Solheim, 2016). Patients may decline assistance. The National Human Trafficking Hotline may be tapped into as a resource (see Resource section).

PSYCHIATRIC EMERGENCIES

A psychiatric emergency is an urgent, serious disturbance of behavior, affect, or thought that makes the patient unable to cope with life situations and interpersonal relationships. A patient presenting with a psychiatric emergency may display overactive or violent, underactive or depressed, or suicidal behaviors.

The most important concern of the ED personnel is determining whether the patient is at risk for injuring self or others. The aim is to try to maintain the patient's self-esteem (and life, if necessary) while providing care. Determining whether the patient is under psychiatric care is important so that contact can be made with the therapist or physician who works with the patient.

Patients Who Are Overactive

Patients who display disturbed, uncooperative, and paranoid behavior and those who feel anxious and panicky may be prone to assaultive and destructive impulses and abnormal social behavior. Intense nervousness, depression, and crying are evident in some patients. Disturbed and noisy behavior may be exacerbated or compounded by alcohol or drug intoxication.

A reliable source for obtaining an accurate history is needed to identify events leading to the crisis. Past mental illness, hospitalizations, injuries, serious illnesses, the use of alcohol or drugs, crises in interpersonal relationships, or intrapsychic conflicts are explored. Because abnormal thoughts and behavior may be manifestations of an underlying physical disorder, such as hypoglycemia, drug or alcohol toxicity, a stroke, a seizure disorder, or head injury, a physical assessment is also performed.

The immediate goal is to gain control of the situation. If the patient is potentially violent, security or police should be nearby. Restraints are used as a *last* resort and only as prescribed. Approaching the patient with a composed, confident, and firm manner is therapeutic and has a calming effect. Helpful interventions include the following:

- Introduce yourself by name.
- Tell the patient, "I am here to help you."
- Repeat the patient's name from time to time.
- Speak in one-thought sentences, and be consistent.
- Give the patient space and time to slow down.
- Show interest in, listen to, and encourage the patient to talk about personal thoughts and feelings.
- Offer appropriate and honest explanations.

A psychotropic agent (e.g., one that exerts an effect on the mind) may be prescribed for emergency management of functional psychosis. However, a patient with a personality disorder should not be treated with psychotropic medications, and psychotropic medications should not be used if the patient's behavior results from the use of hallucinogens (e.g., lysergic acid diethylamide [LSD]).

Agents such as chlorpromazine and haloperidol act specifically against psychotic symptoms of thought fragmentation and perceptual and behavioral aberrations. The initial dose depends on the patient's body weight and the severity of the symptoms. After administration of the initial dose, the patient is observed closely to determine the degree of change in psychotic behavior. Subsequent doses depend on the patient's response. Typically, after stabilization, the patient is transferred to an inpatient psychiatric unit, or psychiatric outpatient treatment is arranged.

Posttraumatic Stress Disorder

PTSD is the development of characteristic symptoms after a psychologically stressful event that is considered outside the range of normal human experience (e.g., rape, combat, motor vehicle crash, natural catastrophe, terrorist attack). Symptoms of this disorder include intrusive thoughts and dreams, phobic avoidance reaction (avoidance of activities that arouse recollection of the traumatic event), heightened vigilance, exaggerated startle reaction, generalized anxiety, and societal withdrawal. PTSD may be acute, chronic, or delayed. PTSD often presents as multiple readmissions to the ED for minor or recurring complaints without evidence of injury.

Patients Who Are Underactive or Depressed

In the ED, depression may be seen as the main condition bringing the patient to the health care facility, or it may be masked by anxiety and somatic complaints. The person who is depressed has a mood disturbance.

Any patient who is depressed may be at risk for suicide. Attempts are made to find out whether the patient has thought about or attempted suicide. Questions such as "Have you ever thought about taking your own life?" may be helpful. In general, the patient is relieved to have an opportunity to discuss personal feelings. If the patient is seriously depressed, relatives should be notified. The patient should never be left alone, because suicide is usually committed in solitude.

Patients Who Are Suicidal

Attempted suicide is an act that stems from depression (e.g., loss of a loved one, loss of body integrity or status, poor self-image) and can be viewed as a cry for help and intervention. Males are at greater risk of successfully committing suicide than females, who attempt suicide more often (ENA, 2013). Others at risk are older adults; young adults; people who are enduring unusual loss or stress; those who are unemployed, divorced, widowed, or living alone; those showing signs of significant depression (e.g., weight loss, sleep disturbances, somatic complaints, suicidal preoccupation); and those with a history of a previous suicide attempt, suicide in the family, or psychiatric illness.

Being aware of people at risk and assessing for specific factors that predispose a person to suicide are key management strategies. Specific signs and symptoms of potential suicide include the following:

- Communication of *suicidal intent*, such as preoccupation with death or speaking of someone else's suicide (e.g., "I'm tired of living. I've put my affairs in order. I'm better off dead. I'm a burden to my family.")
- History of a previous suicide attempt, with risk being much greater in these cases
- Family history of suicide
- Loss of a parent at an early age

- Specific plan for suicide
- A means to carry out the plan

Emergency management focuses on treating the consequences of the suicide attempt (e.g., gunshot wound, drug overdose) and preventing further self-injury. A patient who has made a suicidal attempt may do so again. Crisis intervention is used to determine suicidal potential, to discover areas of depression and conflict, to find out about the patient's support system, and to determine whether hospitalization or psychiatric referral is necessary. Depending on the patient's potential for suicide, the patient may be admitted to the intensive care unit, referred for follow-up care, or admitted to the psychiatric unit.

Unfolding Patient Stories: Carl Shapiro • Part 2

 Recall from Chapter 27 Carl Shapiro, who was diagnosed with hypertension and hyperlipidemia during a routine visit to his primary provider. He arrives in the ED with a blood pressure of 210/110. The nurse discovers that he stopped his antihypertensive medication due to erectile dysfunction. How does the nurse maintain patient privacy in the ED during discussion of personal issues? What topics should be included in an individualized discharge plan to address his concerns, educational needs, and continuity of care when the nurse receives orders for an ACE inhibitor, captopril (Capoten), and discharge home?

Care for Carl and other patients in a realistic virtual environment: **vSim** for Nursing (thepoint.lww.com/vSimMedicalSurgical). Practice documenting these patients' care in DocuCare (thepoint.lww.com/DocuCareEHR).

CRITICAL THINKING EXERCISES

1 After falling down the stairs, a 25-year-old woman arrives at the ED by car accompanied by an older male. Various parts of her body have bruises, some of which appear to be in various stages of healing. When asked to step to the waiting room, the male refuses; security is required to remove him from the room so that the patient examination can occur privately. The patient is particularly quiet and does not actively participate in her history or questions regarding her injuries. As the nurse interviewing and assessing this patient, what do you suspect? You also note that the patient jumps at a knock on the door and pulls away from touch. She states her occupation is a waitress. How do you evaluate the patient situation? What is expected of the nurse in terms of reporting the patient situation? What strategies should be used to provide sensitive care for this patient?

2 pq A 28-year-old male with a gunshot wound arrives to the hospital lobby after being dropped off by an unknown driver who has abandoned him. He is actively bleeding from multiple wounds in his chest and abdomen and is having difficulty breathing and speaking. The security guard in the lobby calls the ED and a "trauma alert lobby" is announced. The patient is brought rapidly to the ED for assessment and disposition. What are the first measures of the primary survey that you will use to assess and stabilize the patient? Will you expect to administer blood products? What do you anticipate in terms of the ED disposition for this patient? What security measures need to be in place to maintain patient, staff, and visitor safety?

3 ebp Two males in their thirties are transported by EMS to the ED after a house-fire. The EMS agency states suspicious evidence was found in the kitchen, which seemed to be the source of the fire. The patients are hesitant to discuss the events prior to the fire. Both suffered multiple full-thickness burns to their upper extremities, face, neck, and chest. EMS personnel expressed concern about contaminants at the scene, which may be on the patients' clothing. What decision must be made regarding decontamination versus immediate burn care? What is the possible source of the contaminants? As with all patients who have experienced trauma, what is the strength of the evidence that dictates first priorities? In addition to the contaminants, to what other chemical were the patients exposed that may result in inadequate ventilation?

4 It is midsummer and you work in an urban ED. The community includes a large low income and older adult population, and many local residents are concerned about the degree of crime in the area. An 80-year-old woman is brought to the ED unresponsive, skin very dry, pale, with low blood pressure, and with slight tachycardia. Her history includes that she takes a beta blocker and a diuretic for hypertension. Her family states that she lives alone without air conditioning. She rarely opens windows or uses a fan in a window due to fear of a break-in. What do you suspect is the primary problem for this patient? What would you expect her core temperature to be? What will be the immediate treatment for this disorder from which she is suffering? What do you expect her ED disposition to be?

REFERENCES

*Asterisk indicates nursing research.
**Double asterisk indicates classic reference.

Books

American College of Surgeons. (2013). *Advanced trauma life support* (9th ed.). Chicago, IL: Author.

Auerbach, P. S. (2017). *Wilderness medicine* (7th ed.). St. Louis, MO: Elsevier Mosby.

Black, M. C., Basile, K. C., Breiding, M. J., et al. (2011). *The National Intimate Partner and Sexual Violence Survey (NISVS): 2010 Summary Report*. Atlanta, GA: National Center for Injury Prevention and Control, Centers for Disease Control and Prevention.

Emergency Nurses Association. (2013). *Sheehy's manual of emergency care* (7th ed.). St. Louis, MO: Mosby.

Gilboy, N., Tanabe, P., Travers, D., et al. (2012). *Emergency severity index (ESI): A triage tool for emergency department care, version 4. Implementation handbook*. Publication No. 12–0014. Rockville, MD: Agency for Healthcare Research and Quality, Publication.

Nayduch, D. (2009). *Nurse to nurse trauma care.* New York: McGraw-Hill.

Solheim, J. (2016). *Emergency nursing: The profession/the pathway/the practice.* Indianapolis: Sigma Theta Tau International Honor Society of Nursing.

Tintinalli, J. E., Stapczyski, J. S., Ma, O. J., et al., (2016). *Tintinalli's emergency medicine manual* (8th ed.). New York: McGraw-Hill Medical.

Walsh, K., & Woten, M. (2016). Oropharyngeal airway: Inserting in adults. In D. Pravikoff (Ed.): *Nursing practice and skill.* Glendale, CA: CINAHL Information Systems.

Journals and Electronic Documents

American College of Emergency Physicians (ACEP). (2011). Protection from physical violence in the emergency department environment. *ACEP Policy Statement.* Retrieved on 1/8/2017 at: www.acep.org/policystatements/

American College of Emergency Physicians (ACEP). (2014). Use of patient restraints. *ACEP Policy Statement.* Retrieved on 1/8/2017 at: www.acep.org/policystatements/

Amerson, R., Whittington, R., & Duggan, L. (2014). Intimate partner violence affecting Latina women and their children. *Journal of Emergency Nursing, 40*(6), 531–536.

*Avander, K., Heikki, A., Bjersa, K., et al. (2016). Trauma nurses' experience of workplace violence and threats: Short- and long-term consequences in a Swedish setting. *Journal of Trauma Nursing, 23*(2), 51–57.

Baumann, M. H., Patilla, J. S., Lehner, K. R., et al. (2013). Powerful cocaine-like actions of 3,4-methylenedioxypyrovalerone (MDPV), a principal constituent of psychoactive 'bath salts' products. *Neuropsychopharmacology, 38*(4), 552–562.

**Blow, O., Magliore, L., Claridge, J. A., et al. (1999). The golden hour and the silver day: Detection and correction of occult hypoperfusion within 24 hours improves outcome from major trauma. *Journal of Trauma, 47*(5), 964–969.

*Cadogan, M. P., Phillips, L. R., & Ziminski, C. E. (2016). A perfect storm: Care transitions for vulnerable older adults discharged home from the emergency department without a hospital admission. *The Gerontologist, 56*(2), 326–334.

Centers for Disease Control and Prevention (CDC). (2013). Emergency department visits by persons aged 65 and over: United States, 2009-2010. *NCHS Data Brief 130.* Retrieved on 2/16/2017 at: www.cdc.gov/nchs/data/databriefs/db130.htm

Centers for Disease Control and Prevention (CDC). (2014). Unintentional drowning deaths in the United States, 2009-2010. *NCHS Data Brief 149.* Retrieved on 2/16/2017 at: www.cdc.gov/nchs/data/databriefs/db149.pdf

Childs, B. R., Nahm, N. J., Dolenc, A. J., et al. (2015). Obesity is associated with more complications and longer hospital stays after orthopaedic trauma. *Journal of Orthopaedic Trauma, 29*(11), 504–509.

*Day, S., Fox, J., Majercik, S., et al. (2015). Implementing a domestic violence screening program. *Journal of Trauma Nursing, 22*(3), 176–181.

*DeBoer, M. I., Kothari, R., Kothari, M. A., et al. (2013). What are barriers to nurses screening for intimate partner violence? *Journal of Trauma Nursing, 20*(3), 155–160.

Dhungel, V., Liao, J., Raut, H., et al. (2015). Obesity delays functional recovery in trauma patients. *Journal of Surgical Residency, 193*(1), 415–420.

Edwards, C., Stephens-Stidham, S., Contreras, M. A., et al. (2016). Building the conversation for hospital-based injury prevention program capacity. *Journal of Emergency Nursing, 42*(2), 174–176.

Emergency Nurses Association (ENA). (2015a). Emergency nursing interface with mobile integrated health (MIH) and community paramedicine (CP) programs position statement. Retrieved on 1/14/2017 at: www.ena.org/SiteCollectionDocuments/Position%20Statements/MIHAndCP.pdf

Emergency Nurses Association (ENA). (2015b). Human trafficking patient awareness in the emergency setting: Position statement. Retrieved on 1/15/2017 at: www.ena.org/SiteCollectionDocuments/Position%20Statements/HumanTrafficking.pdf

Foresman-Capuzzi, J. (2014). CSI & U: Collection and preservation of evidence in the emergency department. *Journal of Emergency Nursing, 40*(3), 229–236.

Hess, J. J., Saha, S., & Luber, G. (2014). Summertime acute heat illness in U.S. emergency departments from 2006 through 2010: Analysis of a nationally representative sample. *Environmental Health Perspectives, 122*(11), 1209–1215.

Inaba, K., Siboni, S., Resnick, S., et al. (2015). Tourniquet use for civilian extremity trauma. *Journal of Trauma, 79*(2), 232–237.

Jabre, P., Belpomme, V., Azoulay, E., et al. (2013). Family presence during cardiopulmonary resuscitation. *The New England Journal of Medicine, 368*(11), 1008–1018.

Kane, I., Mitchell, A. M., Aiello, J., et al. (2016). Screening, brief intervention, and referral to treatment education for emergency nurses in 5 hospitals: Implementation steps and hurdles. *Journal of Emergency Nursing, 42*(1), 53–60.

Lachs, M., & Pillemer, K. (2015). Elder abuse. *New England Journal of Medicine, 373*(20), 1947–1956.

*Leske, J. S., McAndrew, N. S., & Brasel, K. J. (2013). Experiences of families when present during resuscitation in the emergency department after trauma. *Journal of Trauma Nursing, 20*(1), 77–85.

Molina, G. (2017). Butane hash. *Los Angeles Times.* Retrieved on 2/20/2017 at: www.latimes.com/local/la-me-butane-hash-pictures-20140201-photogallery.html

Moore, K. (2015). Hot topics: Chemical burns in the emergency department. *Journal of Emergency Nursing, 41*(4), 364-365.

Musccal, E., & DeGuzman, M. M. (2016). Rhabdomyolysis. *Medscape.* Retrieved on 5/5/2017 at: www.emedicine.medscape.com/article/1007814-overview

National Center on Elder Abuse. (2016). What we do: Research – Statistics/data. Retrieved on 2/20/2017 at: ncea.acl.gov/whatwedo/research/statistics.html

National Institute on Drug Abuse. (2015a). Drug facts. Retrieved on 2/20/2017 at: www.drugabuse.gov/publications/drugfacts

National Institute on Drug Abuse. (2015b). Drug facts: What are synthetic cannabinoids? Retrieved on 2/20/2017 at: www.drugabuse.gov/publications/drugfacts/synthetic-cannabinoids

Oode, Y., Yanagawa, Y., Omori, K., et al. (2015). Analysis of patients with decompression illness transported via physician-staffed emergency helicopters. *Journal of Emergency Trauma Shock, 8*(1), 26–29.

Rui, P., Kang, K., & Albert, M. (2013). National Hospital Ambulatory Medical Care Survey: 2013 emergency department summary tables. Retrieved on 2/22/2017 at: www.cdc.gov/nchs/data/ahcd/nhamcs_emergency/2013_ed_web_tables.pdf

*Slain, T., Rickard-Aasen, S., Pringle, J. L., et al. (2014). Incorporating screening, brief intervention, and referral to treatment into emergency nursing workflow using an existing computerized physician order entry/clinical decision support system. *Journal of Emergency Nursing, 40*(6), 568–574.

Smith, S., Sammons, S. S., Carr, J., et al. (2014). Bedside management considerations in the treatment of pit viper envenomation. *Journal of Emergency Nursing, 40*(6), 537–545.

*Speroni, K. G., Fitch, T., Dawson, E., et al. (2014). Incidence and cost of nurse workplace violence perpetrated by hospital patients or patient visitors. *Journal of Emergency Nursing, 40*(3), 218–228.

Weinlein, J. C., Deaderick, S., & Murphy, R. F. (2015). Morbid obesity increases the risk for systemic complications in patients with femoral shaft fractures. *Journal of Orthopaedic Trauma, 29*(3), e91–e95.

World Health Organization (WHO). (2016). Drowning: Fact sheet. Retrieved on 2/16/2017 at: www.who.int/mediacentre/factsheets/fs347/en/

Zafren, K. (2013). Frostbite: Prevention and initial management. *High Altitude Medical Biology, 14*(1), 9–12.

Resources

American Association of Poison Control Centers (AAPCC), www.aapcc.org

American College of Emergency Physicians (ACEP), www.acep.org

American College of Surgeons (ACS), Injury Prevention and Control, www.facs.org/quality-programs/trauma/ipc

American Heart Association, www.heart.org

American Trauma Society (ATS), www.amtrauma.org

American Red Cross, Prepare for Emergencies, www.redcross.org/get-help/prepare-for-emergencies/types-of-emergencies

Divers Alert Network (DAN), www.diversalertnetwork.org

Emergency Nurses Association (ENA), www.ena.org

National Center on Elder Abuse (NCEA), www.ncea.acl.gov

National Center for Health Statistics (NCHS), www.cdc.gov/nchs

National Human Trafficking Hotline, www.humantraffickinghotline.org

National Institute on Drug Abuse, www.drugabuse.gov/drugs-abuse/club-drugs

National Safety Council, www.nsc.org

National Capital Poison, Poison Control Center, www.poison.org

Rape, Abuse, and Incest National Network (RAINN), National Sexual Assault Hotline, www.rainn.org

Society of Trauma Nurses (STN), www.traumanurses.org

73 Terrorism, Mass Casualty, and Disaster Nursing

LEARNING OBJECTIVES

On completion of this chapter, the learner will be able to:

1 Identify the necessary components of an emergency operations plan.
2 Discuss how triage in a disaster differs from triage in an emergency department.
3 Evaluate the different levels of personal protection and decontamination procedures that may be necessary during an event involving mass casualties or weapons of mass destruction.
4 Describe the physical injuries that may occur after blast events

5 Explain how to implement isolation precautions necessary for bioterrorism agents.
6 Compare and contrast the differences among various chemical agents used in terrorist events, their effects, and the decontamination and treatment procedures that are necessary.
7 Determine the injuries associated with varying levels of radiation or chemical exposure and the associated decontamination processes.

GLOSSARY

biologic weapon: a biologic agent that is used to spread disease among the general population or the military
chemical weapon: a chemical agent that is used to cause disability and mortality in the general population or the military
decontamination: process of removing, or rendering harmless, contaminants that have accumulated on personnel, patients, and equipment
mass casualty incident (MCI): situation in which the number of casualties exceeds the number of available resources
material safety data sheet (MSDS): provides information to employees and health care providers regarding specific chemical agents; includes chemical name, physical data, chemical ingredients, fire and explosive hazard

data, health and reactive data, spill or leak procedures, special protection information, and special precautions; also known as the Worker's Right to Know
personal protective equipment (PPE): equipment beyond standard precautions; may include different levels of equipment to provide complete protection, depending on the nature of the suspected biologic, chemical or radiologic agent
radiologic weapon: by-products of radiation contamination that are used to cause morbidity and mortality in the general population or the military
terrorism: unlawful, systematic use of violence or threats of violence against people in order to coerce or intimidate
weapons of mass destruction (WMD): weapons used to cause widespread death and destruction

The possibility and reality of mass casualties associated with disasters, terrorism, and biologic warfare are not new to human history, nor is the concept of using **weapons of mass destruction (WMD)** (i.e., weapons used to cause widespread death and destruction). However, geopolitical forces and interests and the availability of destructive technology have brought the possibility of more terrorist events to our doorstep. **Terrorism** involves the systematic use of violence to create feelings of fear. Examples include the destruction of the World Trade Center towers and the damage to the Pentagon on September 11, 2001; the Boston Marathon bombing on April 15, 2013; and, the coordinated series of terrorist attacks in Paris on November 13, 2015 and in Brussels on March 22, 2016. Over 32,000 deaths occurred in 2014 from terrorism-related violence, a nine-fold increase since 2000 (Costa-Roberts, 2015). Since 2000, the number of deaths throughout the globe from terrorism equals the number of deaths from

the bombing of Hiroshima in 1945 (Costa-Roberts, 2015). Terrorists have become increasingly sophisticated, organized, and therefore effective. It is no longer a question of *whether* a terrorist event will again lead to mass casualties, but *when* such an event will occur.

The U.S. Department of Homeland Security was created after the attacks of September 11, 2001, to coordinate federal and state efforts to combat terrorist activity. A plan that adheres to guidelines devised by the National Incident Management System (NIMS), which is directed by the Federal Emergency Management Agency (FEMA), is essential for every community and facility. The preparation based on the NIMS guidelines is effective for terrorist events, as well as any disaster situation, including natural disasters. Natural disasters are caused by environmental forces, including storms, floods, fires, earthquakes, and similar forces of nature (Veenema, 2013).

Chart 73-1

ETHICAL DILEMMA

Who Receives Care First During a Mass Casualty?

Case Scenario

You work as a staff nurse in the emergency department (ED) of a 75-bed community hospital. The unit is notified that an armed man entered the local social security office building and began shooting people in the lobby. There were numerous casualties, including the perpetrator, who was shot by a police officer. Within minutes of the notification, several patients are transported into the trauma bay area with gunshot wounds and other traumatic injuries. A young man appears to be hallucinating and attempts to assault a staff nurse. The perpetrator of the violent assault is transported into the trauma bay on a gurney, with an apparent gunshot wound to the head. An older woman grabs your arm and yells, "You have to take care of my husband first! He has a bad heart and may not be able to survive!" Another patient points at the perpetrator and yells, "He is the one who is responsible for this! How can you treat him?! He doesn't deserve to live!"

Discussion

One of the most difficult and morally distressing situations that nurses working in the ED may face is how to triage and treat patients when medical resources are scarce. Participating in disaster drills may prepare nurses working in the ED in how to respond if an emergency operations plan needs to be executed

for a true mass casualty situation. These drills are intended to assist nurses in the ED to triage and prioritize care in a way that is unbiased. The key principle of triage in these situations is to do the greatest good for the greatest number of people. Medical resources must be distributed to patients in a fair and equitable manner.

Analysis

- Describe the ethical principles that are in conflict in this case (see Chapter 3, Chart 3-3). Which principle should have preeminence as you respond to the patient who feels the perpetrator does not have a right to receive medical care?
- Reflect upon your own desire to do good (i.e., practice beneficence) and how this desire to help an older couple may affect your triage decision. How would you respond to the wife? Should the age of her husband and his past medical history influence the triage process?
- How would you most appropriately triage the patient who has no visible physical injuries but is apparently experiencing a mental health crisis?

Resources

See Chapter 3, Chart 3–6 for ethics resources.

Abbasi, J. (2016). Expanding the health care response to mass violence. *JAMA, 316*(10), 1031–1033.

Warfare, terrorism, and natural disasters are just some of the reasons nurses must plan for mass casualties. Airplane crashes, train crashes, toxic substance spills, and infectious disease outbreaks are other disasters that can result in mass casualties and tax the resources of health care facilities and their communities. Acute care facilities must be prepared for any and all of these disasters. This chapter focuses on disaster preparedness, including information about possible terrorist-related injuries and illnesses that can occur after biologic, chemical, and nuclear or radiation attacks. Information about the process that nurses should follow in order to respond to these emergencies is applicable to other types of mass disasters as well.

Federal, State, and Local Responses to Emergencies

Many resources are available at the federal, state, and local levels to assist in the management of **mass casualty incidents (MCIs)**, disasters, and emergencies. An MCI is defined as any incident that causes a large numbers of casualties to the extent that necessary resources become too scarce (American College of Surgeons [ACS], 2010). When resources to care for casualties become scarce, the greatest good for the greatest number of patients becomes the mode of operation (see Chart 73-1). Local communities must be prepared to act in isolation (i.e., called *sustainability planning*) and provide competent care for up to 5 days before federal or other state resources may become available (ACS, 2010).

Disasters are categorized by type based upon anticipated use of resources and incident duration (see Chart 73-2). A list of local resources with specific instructions about how and when to contact these agencies or organizations should

be readily available to local disaster planning committees and frequently reviewed by those committees for necessary updates.

A disaster response strategy cannot succeed without appropriate physical assets and a staff trained and prepared to carry out the plan. Assets such as increased security; stockpiles of equipment and medications; and planning, drills, and training are essential (Veenema, 2013). Hazard vulnerability assessments should be performed to identify potential and actual threats that involve a particular facility and community. Mutual aid agreements among various communities must take these vulnerabilities into account. Successful execution of a response plan is based on knowledge, confidence, and readiness.

Federal Agencies

In 2009, the National Health Security Strategy was designed to protect the health of all citizens of the United States in

---

Chart 73-2 Disaster Types

Disaster types correspond to anticipated incident duration and number of resources required:

Type 1 & 2: National and State Level
Type 3: State or Metropolitan Area Level
Type 4: City, County, or Fire District Level
Type 5: Local Village and Township Level

Adapted from Federal Emergency Management Agency (2013). *ICS 200 Curriculum*. Retrieved on 6/20/217 at: training.fema.gov/is/courseoverview.aspx?code=IS-200.b the event of any large-scale incident (Veenema, 2013). This is a national strategy targeted at prioritizing the use of limited resources and ensuring a rapid coordinated response by the entire affected community so that the maximum number of lives are saved, property is preserved and protected, and basic health care needs are met in the aftermath of any incident that results in mass casualties (Emergency Nurses Association [ENA], 2014). State authorities must request federal assistance with resources through appropriate government channels. A request for federal resources generally is made when local resources have become or are expected to become depleted.

Federal agencies that may provide resources in response to an MCI or a disaster include the Department of Health and Human Service (HHS), the Department of Justice, the Department of Defense, and the Department of Homeland Security. Each of these federal departments oversees hundreds of agencies that may respond to MCIs. For example, personnel from the Federal Bureau of Investigation (FBI) (structured under the Department of Justice) may be used for scene control and collection of forensic evidence. FEMA, which is overseen by the Department of Homeland Security, can activate teams such as the Urban Search and Rescue Teams (USRTs). HHS administers the Centers for Disease Control and Prevention (CDC) and the National Disaster Medical System. The National Disaster Medical System has many medical support teams, such as Disaster Medical Assistance Teams (DMATs), Disaster Mortuary Operational Response Teams (DMORTs), Veterinary Medical Assistance Teams (VMATs), and National Medical Response Teams for Weapons of Mass Destruction (NMRTs).

The DMAT organizes voluntary medical personnel who can set up and staff a field hospital; DMATs are located across the country. There are four NMRTs: the mobile California, North Carolina, and Colorado teams, and the Washington, DC, team, which is stationary. These specialty teams were developed to respond to situations involving WMD. They consist of specially trained medical and technical personnel. The National Guard Civil Support Teams are specially trained units that may respond to MCIs or disasters.

The Department of Homeland Security, through the National Terrorism Advisory System (NTAS), designates a level of security threat that is intended to alert the country to credible threats of terrorism. Formerly, the NTAS issued levels of threats to the American public using a color-coded system. That system has been replaced with a more simple system, with the belief that its simplicity will result in quicker dissemination of important information to the public. The NTAS notes two levels of terrorism threats, which include *bulletins* and *alerts*. An NTAS bulletin describes trends and developments in threats of terrorism; whereas, an NTAS alert more fully warns of a credible threat of terrorism to the United States. The NTAS alerts may be more specifically designated as an *elevated alert*, meaning that there is indeed a credible alert posted, or an *imminent alert*, meaning that there is a specific pending threat of terrorism to the United States (U.S. Department of Homeland Security NTAS, 2015).

Teams from the CDC may be activated. The CDC is the main federal agency for disease prevention, and it controls activities and provides backup support to state and local health departments. Additional support is available from the American Red Cross, which provides support systems and shelters as needed.

State and Local Agencies

Some state and local agencies may be branches of the same agencies already listed (e.g., local CDC and FBI). Other state and local resources may include the American Red Cross, poison control centers, and other local volunteer organizations. The Metropolitan Medical Response Teams Systems are local teams of health care providers who are located in cities considered possible terrorist targets and are funded for specialty response to WMD. Many state and federal task forces have been developed to assist in the development and improvement of civilian medical response to chemical and biologic terrorism.

Most cities and all states have an Office of Emergency Management (OEM) or Office of Emergency Services (OES). The OEM/OES coordinates the disaster relief efforts at the state and local levels. The OEM/OES is responsible for providing interagency coordination during an emergency. It maintains a corps of emergency management personnel, including a leader, responders, planners, and administrative and support staff.

The Incident Command System

The Incident Command System (ICS) is a federally mandated command structure that coordinates personnel, facilities, equipment, and communication in any emergency situation. The ICS is the center of operations for organization, planning, and transport of patients in the event of a specific local MCI. Successful incident management requires equipment compatibility, effective communication, adequate distribution of resources, and clear differentiation of members' roles. The ICS ensures that any hazardous substances used during an MCI are identified promptly and that appropriate personal protection equipment is distributed. In addition to all of these responsibilities, the ICS is also responsible for determining when an MCI has ended.

The Hospital Incident Command System (HICS) is a modification of the ICS that is used by both hospitals and law enforcement agencies. The HICS incident commander is the hospital emergency preparedness coordinator who oversees and coordinates all efforts surrounding the event. The HICS team includes a safety officer, public information officer, liaison officer, operations chief, logistics chief, planning chief, and finance chief. Each team member has a specific responsibility and communicates directly back to the incident commander (ACS, 2010, 2013).

Hospital Emergency Preparedness Plans

Health care facilities are required by the Joint Commission to create a plan for emergency preparedness and to practice this plan at least twice a year (ACS Committee on Trauma [ACS-COT], 2014). In general, these plans are developed by the facility's safety/disaster management committee and are overseen by an administrative liaison.

Before the basic emergency operations plan (EOP) can be developed, the planning committee of the health care facility first evaluates characteristics of the community to identify the likely types of natural and man-made disasters that might occur. This hazard vulnerability analysis process is the responsibility of the local health care facility and its safety committee, safety officer, or emergency department (ED) manager. This information can be gathered by questioning local law enforcement, fire departments, and emergency medical systems and assessing the patterns of local train traffic, automobile traffic, and flood, earthquake, tornado, or hurricane activity. Consideration is also given to possible mass casualties that could arise because of the community's proximity to chemical plants, nuclear facilities, or military bases. Federal, judicial, or financial buildings, schools, and any places where large groups of people gather can be considered high-risk areas.

The emergency preparedness planning committee must have a realistic understanding of its resources. It must determine, for example, whether the facility has or needs a pharmaceutical stockpile (e.g., vaccinations, antibiotics) available to treat specific chemical or biologic agents (ACS, 2010). Another scenario that might be anticipated may include the dispersal of a pulmonary intoxicant or choking agent, which would require that emergency operations planners determine how many ventilators are available within the facility and throughout the greater community. The committee might also outline how staff would triage and assign priority to patients when the number of ventilators is limited. Multiple factors influence a facility's ability to respond effectively to a sudden influx of injured patients, and the committee must anticipate various scenarios to improve its preparedness.

Components of the Emergency Operations Plan

The principles of emergency management must be a part of the EOP design and include a comprehensive plan for tackling all potential and actual hazards. The main goal is protection of the community. The EOP should be integrated with local, state, and federal government plans and coordinated with the private sector and volunteers. It must be coordinated in advance to achieve a single common purpose, yet the plan must be flexible enough to adapt to any likely situation at hand. Predetermined organization is essential to minimize confusion, ensure that all key operations are directed, identify and correct flaws in the plan, and promote a well-coordinated response. Essential components of the EOP include the following (ACS, 2010):

- *Activation response:* The EOP activation response of a health care facility defines where, how, and when the response is initiated.
- *Internal/external communication plan:* Communication is critical for all parties involved, including communication to and from the prehospital arena.
- *Plan for coordinated patient care:* A response is planned for organized patient care into and out of the facility, including transfers from within the hospital to other facilities. The site of the disaster can determine where the greater number of patients may self-refer.
- *Security plans:* A coordinated security plan involving facility and community agencies is key to the control of an otherwise chaotic situation.

- *Identification of external resources:* Resources outside of the facility are identified, including local, state, and federal resources and information about how to activate these resources.
- *Plan for people management and traffic flow:* "People management" includes strategies to manage the patients, the public, the media, and personnel. Specific areas are assigned and a designated person is delegated to manage each of these groups
- *Data management strategy:* A data management plan for every aspect of the disaster will save time at every step. A backup system for documenting, tracking, and staffing is developed if the facility utilizes an electronic health record.
- *Demobilization response:* Deactivation of the response is as important as activation; resources should not be unnecessarily exhausted. The person who decides when the facility resumes daily activities is clearly identified. Any possible residual effects of a disaster must be considered before this decision is made.
- *After-action report or corrective plan:* Facilities often see increased volumes of patients 3 months or more after an incident. Postincident response must include a critique and a debriefing for all parties involved, immediately and again at a later date.
- *Plan for practice drills:* Practice drills that include community participation allow for troubleshooting any issues before a real-life incident occurs.
- *Anticipated resources:* Food and water must be available for staff, families, and others who may be at the facility for an extended period.
- *MCI planning:* MCI planning includes such issues as planning for mass fatalities and morgue readiness.
- *Education plan for all of the above:* A strong education plan for all personnel regarding each step of the plan allows for improved readiness and additional input for fine-tuning of the EOP.

As noted previously, hospitals are required to periodically hold disaster drills. Results from these drills can identify flaws within the EOP as well as unanticipated needs prior to any real disaster situation. Full-scale regional exercises that coordinate responses from both hospitals and emergency medical services (EMS) have been demonstrated as the most effective drills because they clearly identify breakdowns in communication (Nadworny, Davis, Miers, et al., 2014).

Initiating the Emergency Operations Plan

Notification of a disaster situation to a health care facility varies with each situation. In general, the notification to the facility comes from outside sources unless the initial incident occurred at the facility. The disaster activation plan should clearly state how the EOP is to be initiated. If communication is functioning, field incident command will give notice of the approximate number of patients who are arriving, although the number of patients who are self-referring will not be known.

Identifying Patients and Documenting Patient Information

Patient tracking is a critical component of casualty management. Disaster tags, which are numbered and include triage priority, name, address, age, location and description of injuries, and treatments or medications given, are used to communicate patient information. The tag should be securely placed on the patient and remain with the patient at all times. The tag number and the patient's name, if known, are recorded in a disaster log. The log is used by the command center to track patients, assign beds, and provide families with information.

Triage

Triage is the sorting of patients to determine the priority of their health care needs and the proper site for treatment. In nondisaster situations, health care workers assign a high priority and allocate the most resources to those who are the most critically ill (see Chapter 72). For example, under ordinary circumstances, a young adult who has a chest injury and is in cardiac arrest would receive advanced cardiopulmonary resuscitation, including medications, chest tubes, intravenous (IV) fluids, blood, and possibly emergency surgery in an effort to restore life. However, in a disaster, when health care providers are faced with a large number of casualties, the fundamental principle guiding resource allocation is to do the greatest good for the greatest number of people. Decisions are based on the likelihood of survival and consumption of available resources. Therefore, this same patient, and others with conditions associated with a high mortality rate, will be assigned a low triage priority in a disaster situation, even if the person is conscious. Although this may sound uncaring, from an ethical standpoint the expenditure of limited resources on people with a low chance of survival, and denial of those resources to others with serious but treatable conditions, cannot be justified.

The triage officer rapidly assesses those injured at the disaster scene. Patients are immediately tagged and transported or given lifesaving interventions. One person performs the initial triage while other EMS personnel perform immediate lifesaving measures (e.g., intubation) and transport patients. Although EMS personnel carry out initial field triage, secondary and continuous triage at all subsequent levels of care is essential.

Staff should control all entrances to the acute care facility so that patients who are incoming are directed to the triage area first. Traffic control within the facility is one of the most important components of managing the disaster and resources (ACS, 2010). The triage area may be outside the entry or just at the door of the ED. This facilitates the triage of all patients—those arriving by medical transport and those who walk into the ED. Some patients who have already been seen in the field may be reclassified in the triage area based on their current presentation.

Triage categories separate patients according to severity of injury. A special color-coded tagging system is used during an MCI so that the triage category is immediately obvious. There are several triage systems in use across the country, and every nurse should be aware of the system used by their facility and community. The North Atlantic Treaty Organization (NATO) triage system is one that is widely used. It consists of four colors: red, yellow, green, and black. Each color signifies a different level of priority. Table 73-1 describes each category and gives examples of how different injuries would be classified (see Chapter 72).

Managing Internal Problems

The Red Cross has developed a basic survival/shelter resource kit; however, each facility must determine its supply lists based on its own needs assessment. The EOP committee should determine the top 10 critical medications used during normal day-to-day operations and then anticipate which other medications may be required in a disaster or an MCI.

TABLE 73-1 Triage Categories During a Mass Casualty Incident

Triage Category	Priority	Color	Typical Conditions
Immediate: Injuries are life threatening but survivable with minimal intervention. Individuals in this group can progress rapidly to expectant if treatment is delayed.	1	Red	Sucking chest wound, airway obstruction secondary to mechanical cause, shock, hemothorax, tension pneumothorax, asphyxia, unstable chest and abdominal wounds, incomplete amputations, open fractures of long bones, and 2nd/3rd-degree burns of 15–40% total body surface area
Delayed: Injuries are significant and require medical care but can wait hours without threat to life or limb. Individuals in this group receive treatment only after immediate casualties are treated.	2	Yellow	Stable abdominal wounds without evidence of significant hemorrhage; soft tissue injuries; maxillofacial wounds without airway compromise; vascular injuries with adequate collateral circulation; genitourinary tract disruption; fractures requiring open reduction, débridement, and external fixation; most eye and central nervous system injuries
Minimal: Injuries are minor, and treatment can be delayed hours to days. Individuals in this group should be moved away from the main triage area.	3	Green	Upper extremity fractures, minor burns, sprains, small lacerations without significant bleeding, behavioral disorders or psychological disturbances
Expectant: Injuries are extensive, and chances of survival are unlikely even with definitive care. Persons in this group should be separated from other casualties, but not abandoned. Comfort measures should be provided when possible.	4	Black	Patients who are unresponsive with penetrating head wounds, high spinal cord injuries, wounds involving multiple anatomic sites and organs, 2nd/3rd-degree burns in excess of 60% of body surface area, seizures or vomiting within 24 hours after radiation exposure, profound shock with multiple injuries, agonal respirations; no pulse, no blood pressure, pupils fixed and dilated

Adapted from American College of Surgeons. (2010). *Disaster management and emergency preparedness course.* Chicago: Author.

For example, the health care facility might plan to have available a stockpile of antidotes (e.g., cyanide kits) or antibiotics used in treating biologic agents. Information should be available about stocking or restocking any of the basic and special supplies, how those supplies are requested, and the time required to receive those supplies.

Communicating With the Media and Family

Communication is a key component of disaster management. Communication within the vast team of disaster responders is paramount; however, effective, informative communication with the media and worried family members is also crucial.

Managing Media Requests for Information

Although the media have an obligation to report the news and can play a significant positive role in communication, the number of reporters and newscasters and their support teams can be acute, possibly compromising operations and patient confidentiality. The disaster plan should include a clearly defined process for managing media requests, including a designated spokesperson, the public information officer, a site for the dissemination of information (away from patient care areas), and a regular schedule for providing updates.

The EOP helps prevent the release of contradictory or inaccurate information. Initial statements should focus on current efforts and what is being done to better understand the scope and impact of the situation. Information about casualties should not be released. Security staff should not allow media personnel access to patient care areas. However, media resources may be mobilized to notify the general population when disease containment is needed in case of an epidemic or the potential for one, including the location of shelters, necessity of quarantines, and point of dispensing units in the case of bioterrorism (ACS, 2010).

Caring for Families

Friends and family members converging on the scene must be cared for by the facility. The public information officer's role is to provide direction for the families and provide them with information as it becomes available. They may be feeling intense anxiety, shock, or grief and should be provided with information and updates about their loved ones as soon as possible and regularly thereafter. They should not be in the triage or treatment areas but in a designated area staffed by available social workers, counselors, therapists, or clergy. Access to this area should be controlled to prevent families from being disturbed. Information regarding loved ones can also be obtained at this time, which assists in identification of both the injured and deceased. Chart 73-3 discusses cultural variables to consider when coping with disaster-related injuries and death.

The Nurse's Role in Disaster Response Plans

Nurses make up the largest component of the health care workforce across the globe (Veenema, 2013). The role of the nurse during a disaster varies. Nurses may be asked to perform duties outside their areas of expertise and may take on responsibilities normally held by physicians or advanced practice nurses. For example, a critical care nurse may intubate a patient or even insert a chest tube. A nurse may perform

---

Chart 73-3 | **Cultural Considerations**

Any disaster or mass casualty incident can be expected to involve members of diverse religious, ethnic, and cultural groups or may be targeted at and predominately affect a specific religious or ethnic group. Health care providers likewise include members of all religious, ethnic, and cultural backgrounds and should bear in mind that victims may have needs relating to the following:
- Language difficulties that increase fears and frustrations
- Specific religious practices related to medical treatment, hygiene, or diet
- Specific places/times for prayer
- Rituals about handling the dead
- Timing of funeral services
- Family roles and extended family importance
- Privacy

Some religious communities have plans for emergencies and disasters, and local hospitals should integrate these plans to the extent possible into their emergency operations plans.

---

wound débridement or suturing. A nurse may serve as the triage officer. In these situations, it is imperative that nurses strive to maximize patient safety and be aware of state regulations related to nursing practice (American Nurses Association, 2010).

Although the exact role of a nurse in disaster management depends on the specific needs of the facility at the time, it should be clear which nurse or physician is in charge of a given patient care area and which procedures each individual nurse may or may not perform. Assistance can be obtained through the HICS, and nonmedical personnel can provide services where possible. For example, family members can provide nonskilled interventions for their loved ones. Nurses should remember that nursing care in a disaster focuses on essential care from a perspective of what is best for all patients. In addition, acquiring knowledge of the hospital disaster plan, participating in drills, and honing competencies relating to disaster management are essential (ENA, 2014). Nurse leaders/administrators should be cognizant of potential security issues and assess and plan for surge capacity capability and in-house resources such as water, supplies, pharmaceuticals, and generator power. They also should predetermine means to evacuate the hospital if necessary, including an ultimate destination or destinations. The hospital must take into account in its plans shortages of all kinds—staff, medications, water/food, and equipment (ACS-COT, 2014; ENA, 2014).

New settings and atypical roles for nurses arise during a disaster—for example, the nurse may provide shelter care in a temporary housing area or bereavement support and assistance with identification of deceased loved ones. People may require crisis intervention, or the nurse may participate in counseling other staff members and in Critical Incident Stress Management (CISM). Special care may be warranted for at-risk populations during a disaster (see Chart 73-4).

Considering Ethical Conflicts

Disasters can present a disparity between the resources of the health care agency and the needs of the victims. This

<table>
<tr><td>**Chart 73-4**</td><td>Caring for People With Disabilities During a Disaster</td></tr>
</table>

When a disaster occurs, the multiple agencies involved attempt to provide food, water, and shelter to all those affected. People with disabilities have specific needs that require attention. It is recommended that people with disabilities have a personal support network to check on them after a disaster and to provide needed assistance. They should also have a backup system and an evacuation plan. Agencies need to be aware that service animals are also affected during a disaster and may be brought to shelters with their companions.

Evacuation assistance is imperative for people with disabilities. Directions to personal equipment (e.g., communication aids, medications, oxygen) should be available to rescue personnel. In a rapid evacuation, mobility devices, oxygen, suction, and medications will be needed at the shelters. Special efforts to keep those with vision or hearing impairment informed should be implemented. People skilled in sign language are also valuable resources during a disaster. On their websites, the American Red Cross and the National Organization on Disability provide information for disaster preparedness for people with disabilities (see the Resources section).

Adapted from U.S. Department of Homeland Security Federal Emergency Management Agency (FEMA) & the American Red Cross. (2004). *Preparing for disaster for people with disabilities and other special needs*. Retrieved on 11/26/2016 at: www.redcross.org/images/MEDIA_CustomProductCatalog/m4240199_A4497.pdf; World Health Organization. (2005). *Disasters, disability and rehabilitation*. Retrieved on 11/26/2016 at: www.who.int/violence_injury_prevention/other_injury/disaster_disability2.pdf

generates ethical dilemmas for nurses and other health care providers. Issues include conflicts related to the following:

- Assisted suicide
- Confidentiality
- Consent
- Duty
- Futile therapy
- Rationing care
- Resuscitation

Nurses may find it difficult to not provide care to the dying or to withhold information to avoid spreading fear and panic. Clinical scenarios that are unimaginable in normal circumstances confront the nurse in extreme instances. Other ethical dilemmas may arise out of health care providers' instincts for self-protection and protection of their families. For example, what should a nurse who is pregnant do when incoming disaster victims have been exposed to radiation yet too few nurses are available?

Nurses can plan for the ethical dilemmas they will face during disasters by establishing a framework for evaluating ethical questions before they arise and by identifying and exploring possible responses to difficult clinical situations. They can consider how the fundamental ethical principles of nonmaleficence, beneficence, and distributive justice will influence their decisions and care in disaster response (see Chapter 3).

Managing Behavioral Issues

Although most people pull together and function well during a disaster, both people and communities suffer immediate and sometimes long-term psychological trauma that most often relates to fear and anxiety (ENA, 2014). Common responses to disaster include:

- Anxiety
- Depression
- Impaired performance
- Interpersonal conflicts
- Posttraumatic stress disorder
- Somatization (fatigue, general malaise, headaches, gastrointestinal disturbances, skin rashes)
- Substance abuse

Factors that influence a person's response to disaster include the degree and nature of the exposure to the disaster; loss of friends, family members, and pets; existing coping strategies; available resources and support; and the personal meaning attached to the event. Other factors, such as loss of home and valued possessions, extended exposure to danger, and exposure to toxic contamination, also influence response and increase the risk of adjustment problems. Those exposed to the dead and injured, those endangered by the event, older adults, children, emergency first responders, and health care personnel caring for victims are considered to be at higher risk for emotional sequelae. A person's normal response to stress and bereavement will also affect the response after a disaster. A bioterrorism attack can have psychological effects, resulting in psychogenic illnesses such as panic, fear, and/or anger (ENA, 2013).

Nurses can assist victims of disaster through active listening and providing emotional support, giving information, and referring patients to therapists or social workers. Health care workers must refer people to mental health care services because experience has shown that few victims of disaster seek these services, and early intervention minimizes psychological consequences. Nurses can also discourage victims from subjecting themselves to repeated exposure to the event through media replays and news articles, as well as encourage them to return to normal activities and social roles when appropriate (ENA, 2013).

Critical Incident Stress Management

CISM is an approach to preventing and treating the emotional trauma that can affect emergency responders as a consequence of their jobs and that can also occur to anyone involved in a disaster or MCI. CISM is handled by teams, which are available to the OEM. There are 350 such teams in the United States. All branches of emergency services have CISM teams, as do the military and other industries (e.g., airline industry).

Components of a management plan include education (preparedness) before an incident occurs about critical incident stress and coping strategies; field support (ensuring that staff get adequate rest, food, and fluids, and rotating workloads) during an incident; and defusings, debriefings, demobilization, supportive services to the family, and follow-up care after the incident (Veenema, 2013).

Defusing is a process by which the person receives education about recognition of stress reactions and management strategies for handling stress. Debriefing is a more complicated intervention; it involves a 2- to 3-hour process during which participants are asked about their emotional reactions to the incident, what symptoms they may be experiencing (e.g., flashbacks, difficulty sleeping, intrusive thoughts), and other psychological ramifications. In follow-up, members of the CISM team contact the participants of a debriefing and schedule a follow-up meeting if necessary. People with ongoing stress reactions are referred to mental health specialists.

Preparedness and Response

Recognition and Awareness

Preparedness for natural disasters and acts of terrorism includes devising specific community contingency plans that prepare residents, particularly those who are vulnerable (e.g., older adults, people with disabilities) for access to necessary life-sustaining resources and for evacuation, as necessary (see Chart 73-5). Preparedness also includes an awareness of the potential for covert use of WMD, self-protection, and early detection, containment, or decontamination of substances and agents that may affect others by secondary exposure. The strength of many toxins, mobility of many members of society, and long incubation periods for some organisms and diseases can result in an epidemic that can quickly and silently spread across the entire country. For example, a formerly healthy person with a rapid onset of flulike symptoms can have an ominous illness, such as anthrax (see later discussion).

Nurses should have a heightened awareness of trends that may suggest deliberate dispersal of toxic or infectious agents or pandemic onset that may include the following:

- An unusual increase in the number of people seeking care for fever, respiratory, or gastrointestinal symptoms
- Clusters of patients who present with the same unusual illness from a single location. For example, clusters can be from a specific geographic location, such as a city, or from a single sporting or entertainment event.
- A large number of fatalities, especially when death occurs within 72 hours after hospital admission
- Any increase in disease incidence in a normally healthy population. These cases should be reported to the state health department and to the CDC.

If any of these trends are noted, an extensive patient history is taken in an attempt to identify the possible agent involved. This history includes an occupational, work, and environmental assessment, in addition to the regular admission history. An exposure history contains, at a minimum, information about current and past exposures to possible hazards and an assessment of the patient's typical day and any deviations in routines. The work history includes, at a minimum, a description of all previous jobs, including short-term, seasonal, and part-time employment and any military service. The environmental history includes assessment of present and previous home locations, water supply, and any hobbies, to name a few factors. The admission history should include such information as recent travel and contact with others who have been ill or have recently died of a fatal illness. This is just a brief review of the extensive history that may need to be obtained to identify an exposure agent (Agency for Toxic Substances and Disease Registry, 2016).

Suspicions or findings are reported to the appropriate resources in the facility and to proper authorities in the

---

Chart 73-5 — NURSING RESEARCH PROFILE

Preparedness for Loss of Electricity after a Natural Disaster

Zidek, C., West, E., Holmes, J., et al. (2014). A survey comparison of rural versus urban residents and household preparedness. *Home Healthcare Nurse*, 32(7), 420–429.

Purpose

In 2012, the U.S. Department of Homeland Security began a national campaign to prepare citizens for emergencies, including natural disasters. In response to this, the Pennsylvania State Office of Homeland Security launched the *ReadyPA* campaign, which targeted Pennsylvanians deemed most vulnerable to adverse effects from a natural disaster, including older adults and citizens with disabilities. The aims of this study were to determine the effectiveness of *ReadyPA* in preparing rural and urban residents reliant on electronic medical equipment (ME) and rural and urban ME supply companies for natural disasters that cause loss of electrical power.

Design

This was a descriptive study that used a stratified random sample of adults who resided in one rural and one urban county and who had landline phone numbers listed in the phone book. Those ME supply companies that were listed in the white pages of those same rural and urban county phone books were all sampled. A telephone survey was designed that asked prospective participants whether they used electronic ME and to describe plans made to use ME in the event of power failure. Nursing students were trained to call prospective rural, urban, and ME supply company participants and began to gather data once Institutional Review Board approval was obtained.

Findings

Of the rural county participants ($n = 958$), 128 used electronic ME in their homes; whereas, of the urban county participants ($n = 1000$), 179 used electronic ME in their homes. Commonly used electronic ME included intravenous pumps, oxygen, blood glucose monitors, pressure-relieving mattresses, to name a few. There were eight rural ME and 24 urban ME supply companies that comprised the sample. Results included that 23% of rural participants and 45% of urban participants who used electronic ME had no home preparedness contingency plan made for loss of electrical power. Only 62.5% of both rural and urban ME supply companies indicated they were prepared to supply alternative ME to their users during periods of power failure. Furthermore, only half (50%) of rural ME supply companies and 12.5% of urban ME supply companies kept a nonelectronic list of their most vulnerable customers for retrieval during times of power failure.

Nursing Implications

Findings from this study suggest that one state's efforts to prepare its most vulnerable citizens to be prepared for loss of electrical power from a natural disaster has not resulted in widespread adoption of adequate preparatory practices. Despite the goals of the *ReadyPA* campaign, many Pennsylvanians who use electronic ME and their respective ME supply companies are not adequately prepared to respond to loss of power. Nurses must take the leadership initiative to launch advocacy efforts in their home communities to educate citizens who use electronic ME and the ME supply companies so that they make contingency plans for loss of electric power.

community. Resources can include the infection control department, the state health department, the CDC, the local poison control center, various internet sites, and **material safety data sheets (MSDS)** or the Chemtrac database (see the Resource section). The MSDS provides information to employees and health care providers regarding specific chemical agents; it includes the chemical name, physical data, chemical ingredients, fire and explosive hazard data, health and reactive data, spill or leak procedures, special protection information, and special precautions. Reporting furnishes data elements to those agencies responsible for epidemiology and response. Reporting also allows for sharing of information among facilities and jurisdictions and can help determine the source of infections or exposure and prevent further exposures and even deaths.

Personal Protective Equipment

Another component of preparedness and response involves the protection of the health care provider by additional **personal protective equipment (PPE)**. Chemical or biologic agents and radiation are silent killers and are generally colorless and odorless. The purpose of PPE is to shield health care workers from the chemical, physical, biologic, and radiologic hazards that may exist when caring for patients who have been contaminated. The U.S. Environmental Protection Agency (EPA) has divided protective clothing and respiratory protection into the following four categories, levels A through D:

- *Level A* protection is worn when the highest level of respiratory, skin, eye, and mucous membrane protection is required. This includes a self-contained breathing apparatus (SCBA) and a fully encapsulating, vapor-tight, chemical-resistant suit with chemical-resistant gloves and boots.
- *Level B* protection requires the highest level of respiratory protection but a lesser level of skin and eye protection than with level A situations. This level of protection includes the SCBA and a chemical-resistant suit, but the suit is not vapor tight.
- *Level C* protection requires the air-purified respirator, which uses filters or sorbent materials to remove harmful substances from the air. A chemical-resistant coverall with splash hood, chemical-resistant gloves, and boots are included in level C protection.
- *Level D* protection is the typical work uniform.

Levels C and D PPE are the levels most often used in hospital facilities. Protective equipment must be donned before contact with a patient who has been contaminated. The acute care facility's standard precaution PPE (level D) generally is not adequate for protection from a patient who has been chemically, biologically, or radiologically contaminated. Level C PPE is adequate for the average patient exposure. The health care provider must use equipment that is capable of providing protection against the agent involved. This may mean using a splash suit along with a full-face positive- or negative-pressure respirator (a filter-type gas mask) or even an SCBA for medical personnel in the field.

No single PPE is capable of protecting against all hazards. Under no circumstances should responders wear any PPE without proper training, practice, and fit testing of respirator masks as necessary (Valdez, 2015).

Decontamination

Decontamination, the process of removing accumulated contaminants or rendering them harmless, is critical to the health and safety of health care providers by preventing secondary contamination. The decontamination plan should establish procedures and educate employees about decontamination procedures, identify the equipment needed and methods to be used, and establish methods for disposal of contaminated materials (Veenema, 2013).

Although many principles and theories surround decontamination of a patient, authorities agree that to be effective, decontamination must include a minimum of two steps. The first step is removal of the patient's clothing and jewelry and then rinsing the patient with water. Depending on the type of exposure, this step alone can remove a large amount of the contamination and decrease secondary contamination. The second step consists of a thorough soap-and-water wash and rinse. The hospital must be prepared to perform additional decontamination prior to entry into the facility. The hospital personnel may also treat "walking wounded" who did not receive any decontamination at the scene.

> **Quality and Safety Nursing Alert**
>
> *When patients arrive at the facility after being assessed and treated by a prehospital provider, it should not be assumed that they have been thoroughly decontaminated.*

Natural Disasters

Natural disasters may result in mass casualties. Natural disasters can occur anywhere at any time and include events such as tornadoes, hurricanes, floods, avalanches, tidal waves (e.g., tsunamis), earthquakes, and volcanic eruptions (see Table 73-2). In the event of a natural disaster, loss of communications, potable water, and electricity is usually the greatest obstacle to a well-coordinated emergency response, and preparatory planning is essential. Wireless technology (e.g., cellular phones, computers, other communication devices) may not be functional.

The majority of the immediate casualties are trauma related. These mass casualties tax the trauma system to provide triage, transport of patients (in poor weather and road conditions), and management within the trauma centers. Most patients usually begin arriving within an hour of the event. However, the "walking wounded" may not seek care for 5 days to 2 weeks after the event or may seek care for injuries received during cleanup activities. Casualties arrive at hospitals in three waves. The first wave consists of people who are minimally (generally) injured who arrive of their own accord. The second wave consists of patients who are severely injured. The third wave consists of patients who are injured and who arrive after they are discovered by rescuers. For example, in the event of earthquakes, buildings collapse and cause the majority of fatalities from injuries primarily involving the head and chest (Veenema, 2013).

Excessive exposure to the natural elements and the need for food and water (by both patients and emergency responders) are critical issues. Without cover (e.g., buildings may be unsafe or destroyed) or potable water (e.g., water may be either contaminated or unavailable), injuries from exposure

TABLE 73-2 Natural Disasters

Event	Issues and Injuries
Hurricanes	Causes flooding and tornadoes (see later discussion) Failure to evacuate Food and water safety *Injuries:* From recovery activities (e.g., chainsaws), stress-related disorders, and GI and other vector-borne disease; physical injury; bites from traumatized pets
Earthquakes	Associated with multiple aftershocks, tsunami Buildings require tethering in earthquake-prone areas *Injuries:* Physical injury; dehydration; pulmonary problems
Flooding	Can accompany other natural disasters Results in home and community destruction *Injuries:* Nonfatal drowning/drowning (e.g., people swept away in currents); waterborne and vector-borne disease (e.g., shigellosis, *Escherichia coli* infection, hepatitis A, giardiasis, leptospirosis, malaria, plague, dengue fever); physical injury from debris
Tsunami	As with flooding (above) but with much more rapid onset resulting in immediate large volume of water on land *Injuries:* Physical injury from debris; vector-borne disease (see the Flooding section); cholera
Tornadoes	Minimal warning, fast moving (approximately 30 mph and travel approximately 20 km) Massive destruction, shelter loss *Injuries:* Physical injury; blastlike effects from pressure (see discussion of blast injuries in text)
Volcanic eruptions	Hazards from lava, openings in ground, gases, ash up to a 20 mile radius *Injuries:* Acid rain; toxic gases result in inhalation injury; physical injury
Exposure—heat/cold	*Cold:* Frostbite, hypothermia, (see Chapter 72) *Heat:* Burns, heat exhaustion/stroke (see Chapter 72)
Epidemic/Pandemic	Foodborne poisonings Acute outbreak, unexpected; local or distant transmission due to travel *Risk:* Determined by population density, travel, method of transmission *Illness:* Depends on organism involved (see Chapter 71)

Adapted from American College of Surgeons. (2010). *Disaster management and emergency preparedness course.* Chicago: Author; Veenema, T. G. (2013). *Disaster nursing and emergency preparedness* (3rd ed.). New York: Springer.

to heat, cold, or contaminated food or water can occur. Safety equipment that protects rescue workers from injury, exposure, and potentially dangerous animals (e.g., snakes, alligators, spiders) must be readily available. Rescue workers may also injure themselves in the process of extrication or cleanup (e.g., chain saws, building collapse). Hypothermia can occur rapidly in workers who are exposed to water at temperatures of 23.9°C (75°F) or less. As is true during all disasters, mental health workers and shelters are needed throughout the community. Veterinary assistance is also essential because pets are frequently abandoned and injured. In addition, emergency response workers must be prepared to treat the most common ailments experienced after exposure to a specific natural disaster. For instance, pulmonary problems peak with earthquakes and volcanic eruptions because of the increased particulate matter in the air. Most volcano-related deaths are from suffocation and exposure to noxious gases. After floods or water disasters, waterborne transmission of agents such as *Escherichia coli*, salmonella, shigella, typhoid, leptospirosis, malaria, and tularemia are common and cause widespread disease.

In some instances, early warning systems have assisted in decreasing the number of deaths from tornadoes and hurricanes. Even with the advent of early warning systems, some people are unable or unwilling to leave prior to the occurrence of the natural disaster.

When buildings collapse, rapid response to identify and remove trapped victims is the only means of improving survivability. There is a direct relationship between time trapped and survival; fewer than 50% of people survive if they are trapped more than 2 to 6 hours (ACS, 2010). Water-damaged buildings are not safe and require extensive examination before experts can ensure safe occupancy. Larger-scale issues that can cause significant later morbidity and mortality include the absence of water purification, waste removal, removal of human and animal remains, and vector control. Removal or disposal of biologic, chemical, and nuclear agents must also be considered.

Weapons of Terror

Although biologic, chemical, and radiologic events are not everyday events, they can occur at any facility, and every nurse needs to know the basics of caring for patients who have been affected. An explosion may spread dangerous material. Therefore, treatment of blast injuries must be anticipated and planned.

Blast Injury

A blast may result from terrorism but can also occur anywhere at any time if the right (or wrong) circumstances come together (e.g., welding inside of a tank that formerly contained tar but was not properly cleaned can result in an explosion as well as severe tar burns to the worker).

Types of Explosive Devices

The bomb most commonly utilized by terrorists is the pipe bomb, which contains low-velocity explosives and may also contain nails or other implements that cause more damage when the explosive ignites. Another type of commonly used explosive device is the Molotov cocktail, which uses a common flammable liquid such as gasoline in a glass bottle and a source of ignition, such as a rag. This forms a simple yet effective incendiary device. Other types of explosive devices include fertilizer bombs and dirty bombs, which include a radioactive source that spreads radiation after the initial blast.

Hazards following a bombing include secondary devices (set to explode at a predetermined time, typically after the arrival of rescue personnel); building collapse; contamination from biologic, chemical, or radiologic weapons; and the presence of terrorists among the patients and bystanders. The entire scene of the bombing is a crime scene and is treated as such. Triage of patients involved in a bombing is the same as for all disasters, with a heightened awareness that serious internal injuries from the blast wave may not be immediately evident.

Physical Injuries

Distance from the blast, whether the blast space was enclosed, composition of the explosive, whether a building collapsed, and the efficiency of medical resources available after the blast all affect patient outcomes after a blast injury. The actual blast that occurs during the initial seconds of the bombing or explosion causes a pressure wave or primary blast wave. Injuries can result from the impact of the explosion, the primary blast wave, or shrapnel (i.e., debris from the bomb). The majority of injuries are caused by the primary blast wave (ACS, 2010). A blast wave has four effects. These include spalling, which refers to the pressure wave itself; implosion, which refers to rupture of organs from entrapped gases; shearing, which refers to the blast response of different body tissues, dependent on their density; and irreversible work, which refers to the presence of forces that exceed the tensile strength of an organ or tissue. If the blast occurs in an enclosed space, the wave has the opportunity to be reflected and thus amplified (Veenema, 2013). The various phases of blasts and related injuries are detailed in Table 73-3.

Although approximately 50% to 70% of deaths result from head injuries, most head injuries are not life threatening (ACS, 2010).

Blast Lung

Blast lung results from the blast wave as it passes through air-filled lungs. The result is hemorrhage and tearing of the lung,

TABLE 73-3 Phases of Blasts and Associated Common Injuries

Phase of Blast Injury	Common Injuries
Primary: Results from pressure wave	Pulmonary barotraumas, including pulmonary contusions Head injuries, including concussion, other severe brain injuries Tympanic membrane rupture, middle ear injury Abdominal hollow organ perforation, hemorrhage
Secondary: Results from debris from the scene or shrapnel from the bomb	Penetrating trunk, skin, and soft tissue injuries Fractures, traumatic amputations
Tertiary: Results from pressure wave that causes the victim to be thrown	Head injuries Fractures, including skull
Quaternary: Results from pre-existing conditions exacerbated by the force of the blast or by postblast injury complications	Severe injuries with complex injury patterns—burns, crush injuries, head injuries Common pre-existing conditions that become exacerbated—COPD, asthma, cardiac conditions, diabetes, and hypertension

COPD, chronic obstructive pulmonary disease.

Adapted from Pennardt, A., & Lavonas, E. J. (2016). Blast injuries. *Medscape.* Retrieved on 4/2/2017 at: emedicine.medscape.com/article/822587-overview

ventilation–perfusion mismatch, and possible air emboli. Typical signs and symptoms include dyspnea, hypoxia, tachypnea or apnea (depending on severity), cough, chest pain, and hemodynamic instability. Management involves providing respiratory support that includes administration of supplemental oxygen with nonrebreathing mask but may also require endotracheal intubation and mechanical ventilation. If a hemothorax or pneumothorax is present, a chest tube must be inserted to re-expand the lung. In the event of an air embolus, the patient should be immediately placed in the prone left lateral position to prevent migration of the embolus and will require emergent treatment in a hyperbaric chamber (CDC, 2012). Complications following blast lung can include respiratory failure as well as acute respiratory distress syndrome (see Chapters 21 and 23).

Tympanic Membrane Rupture

TM rupture is the most frequent injury after subjection to a pressure wave because the TM is the body's most sensitive organ to pressure. There is an increased incidence of TM rupture when a blast occurs in close proximity to the patient and when it occurs in an enclosed space. Signs and symptoms include hearing loss, tinnitus, pain, dizziness, and otorrhea (CDC, 2012). The majority of TM ruptures heal spontaneously. Approximately 5% of patients with TM rupture from a blast will require hearing aids, whereas the majority will suffer only mild high-frequency hearing loss (Dodd-Murphy, 2014; ENA, 2014). Other ear injuries may include ossicular disruption and impaction of foreign bodies.

Abdominal and Head Injuries

Blast abdomen may be evidenced by abdominal hemorrhage and internal organ injury. The typical signs and symptoms of internal abdominal injury can include pain, guarding, rebound tenderness, rectal bleeding, nausea, and vomiting (CDC, 2012) (see Chapter 72).

Head injuries are typically minor, but those that are severe result in the majority of postblast deaths. These injuries can occur without a direct blow to the head and may result from the blast itself, building collapse, or flying debris. Concussions commonly occur postblast, and the usual follow-up evaluation and treatment for postconcussive syndrome is indicated (see Chapter 68). Approximately 30% of head injuries involve vascular structures (e.g., arteriovenous fistula, pseudoaneurysm, or dissection) (Veenema, 2013).

Special Populations

Special populations may have different blast-associated risks. For instance, older adults are particularly susceptible to bone fractures because they tend to have decreased bone density. They also tend to have more pre-existing morbid conditions that may be exacerbated by the explosion. Patients who are pregnant are particularly susceptible to placental shear forces that may result in abruptio placentae. People with mobility disabilities may have difficulty extricating themselves from the site of the blast (CDC, 2012).

Biologic Weapons

Biologic weapons are weapons that spread disease among the general population or the military. They can be used for sabotage, such as food or water contamination with a small target

TABLE 73-4 Categories of Biologic Weapons

Category	Mortality and Morbidity	Examples of Biologic Agents That May Be Weaponized
Category A	High mortality	*Bacillus anthracis* (anthrax) *Clostridium botulinum* (botulism) *Francisella tularensis* (tularemia) Viral hemorrhagic fevers (e.g., dengue, Ebola) Variola (i.e., smallpox) *Yersinia pestis* (plague)
Category B	Low mortality, moderate morbidity	*Brucella* species (brucellosis) *Coxiella burnetii* (Q fever) *Staphylococcus aureus*, *Vibrio* species (food poisoning) *Rickettsia typhi* (typhus) Arboviruses (viral encephalitis) *Cryptosporidium parvum* (Cryptosporidiosis)
Category C	Low mortality, low morbidity	Hantavirus

Adapted from Veenema, T. G. (2013). *Disaster nursing and emergency preparedness* (3rd ed.). New York: Springer.

area, or may be used by global terrorists with intentions to enable global objectives.

Effects of Biologic Weapons

Biologic weapons are easily obtained and easily disseminated and can result in significant mortality and morbidity (see Table 73-4). The potential use of biologic weapons calls for continuous increased surveillance by health departments and an increased index of suspicion by clinicians. Many biologic weapons result in signs and symptoms similar to those of common disease processes. Appropriate management of a biologic threat includes rapid recognition of the potential weapon; the use of proper PPE; decontamination, isolation, or quarantine of patients who are infected when appropriate; and the administration of appropriate vaccinations, antidotes, or medications to people at risk.

Biologic weapons are delivered in either a liquid or dry state, applied to foods or water, or vaporized for inhalation or direct contact. Vaporization may be accomplished through spray or explosives loaded with the weapon. Because of increases in business and pleasure travel by people in industrialized nations, a biologic weapon could be released in one city and affect people in other cities thousands of miles away. The vector can be an insect, animal, or person, or there may be direct contact with the weapon itself.

Two of the biologic agents most likely to be used or weaponized are discussed in the next section. Table 73-5 describes other easily weaponized biologic agents.

Types of Biologic Weapons

Anthrax

Anthrax is recognized as the most likely weaponized biologic agent available and has been recognized as a highly debilitating agent for centuries. *Bacillus anthracis* is a naturally occurring gram-positive, encapsulated rod that lives in the soil in the spore state throughout the world. The bacterium sporulates (i.e., is liberated) when exposed to air and is infective only in the spore form. Contact with infected animal products (raw meat) or inhalation of the spores results in infection. Cattle and other herbivores are vaccinated against anthrax to prevent transmission through contaminated meat. As an aerosol, anthrax is odorless and invisible and can travel a great distance before disseminating; hence, the site of release and the site of infection can be miles apart.

Clinical Manifestations

Anthrax is caused by replicating bacteria that release toxin, resulting in hemorrhage, edema, and necrosis. The incubation period is 1 to 6 days. There are three main methods of infection: skin contact, gastrointestinal ingestion, and inhalation. Skin lesions (the most common infection) cause edema with pruritus and macule or papule formation, resulting in ulceration with 1- to 3-mm vesicles. A painless eschar develops, which falls off in 1 to 2 weeks (Auerbach, 2017).

Ingestion of anthrax results in fever, nausea and vomiting, abdominal pain, bloody diarrhea, and occasionally ascites. If severe diarrhea develops, decreased intravascular volume becomes the major treatment concern. The bacterium targets the terminal ileum and cecum. Sepsis can occur.

Inhaling anthrax results in severe clinical manifestations. Its symptoms mimic those of the flu, and usually treatment is sought only when the second stage of severe respiratory distress occurs. Antibiotic therapy does not halt the progress of the disease. Inhaled anthrax can incubate for up to 60 days, making it difficult to identify its source. Initial signs and symptoms include cough, headache, fever, vomiting, chills, weakness, mild chest discomfort, dyspnea, and syncope, without rhinorrhea or nasal congestion. Most patients have a brief recovery period followed by the second stage within 1 to 3 days, characterized by fever, severe respiratory distress, stridor, hypoxia, cyanosis, diaphoresis, hypotension, and shock. These patients require optimization of oxygenation, correction of electrolyte imbalances, and ventilatory and hemodynamic support. More than 50% of these patients have hemorrhagic mediastinitis on a chest x-ray (a hallmark sign). The disease can also progress to include meningitis with subarachnoid hemorrhage. Death results approximately 24 to 36 hours after the onset of severe respiratory distress. The mortality rate approaches 100% (Auerbach, 2017).

Treatment

At present, anthrax is penicillin sensitive; however, strains of penicillin-resistant anthrax are thought to exist. Recommended treatment includes penicillin (Penicillin V), erythromycin (Erythrocin), gentamicin (Garamycin), or doxycycline (Vibramycin). If antibiotic treatment begins within 24 hours after exposure, death can be prevented. In a mass casualty situation, treatment with ciprofloxacin (Cipro) or doxycycline is recommended, because these easily given oral antibiotic agents are stockpiled and there should be sufficient dosages to fully treat many patients who have been anthrax-exposed. Treatment is continued for 60 days. For patients who have been directly exposed to anthrax but have no signs and symptoms of disease, ciprofloxacin or doxycycline is used for prophylaxis for 60 days (Auerbach, 2017).

Standard precautions are the only ones indicated to protect the caregiver exposed to a patient infected with anthrax. The patient is not contagious, and the disease cannot spread from person to person. Equipment should be cleaned using

TABLE 73-5 Selected Examples of Biologic Agents That Can Be Used As Weapons

Agent/Organism	Contagion	Decontamination and Protective Equipment	Signs and Symptoms	Treatment (Mortality Rate)
Tularemia—*Francisella tularensis*: Gramnegative coccobacillus, one of the most infectious bacteria known.	Direct contact with infected animals or aerosolized as a bioterror weapon; bites Not contagious through human-to-human contact Found in Oklahoma, Missouri, Arkansas	Standard barrier precautions. Clothing and linens should be laundered under the usual hospital protocol.	*Initial:* Abrupt onset of fever, fatigue, chills, headache, lower backache, malaise, rigor, coryza, dry cough, and sore throat without adenopathy. Nausea and vomiting or diarrhea possible. *As disease progresses:* Sweating, fever, progressive weakness, anorexia, and weight loss demonstrate continued illness. *Mortality secondary to:* Pneumonitis (if inhalation is the source) with copious watery or purulent sputum, hemoptysis, respiratory insufficiency, sepsis, and shock.	Streptomycin or gentamicin/aminoglycoside for 10–14 days. Inhalation tularemia must be treated within 48 hours of onset. In mass casualty situations, doxycycline or ciprofloxacin is recommended. For persons exposed to tularemia, tetracycline or doxycycline is recommended for 14 days. (Mortality rate = 2%)
Botulism—*Clostridium botulinum*: Botulinum blocks acetylcholine-containing vesicles from fusing with the terminal membranes of the motor neuron end-plate, resulting in a flaccid paralysis.	Direct contact Not contagious through human-to-human contact	Any skin exposure to the botulism toxin can be treated with soap and water or a 0.1% hypochlorite solution. Standard precautions are used when treating patients with botulism.	*Gastrointestinal botulism:* Abdominal cramps, nausea, vomiting, and diarrhea *Inhalation botulism:* Fever; symmetric descending flaccid paralysis with multiple cranial nerve palsies. *Classic signs and symptoms include* diplopia, dysphagia, dry mouth, lack of fever, and alert mental status. *Other possible symptoms include* ptosis of the eyelids, blurred vision, enlarged sluggish pupils, dysarthria, and dysphonia. *Mortality secondary to:* Airway obstruction and inadequate tidal volume	Supportive ventilatory therapy is necessary if respiratory infection occurs. Aminoglycosides and clindamycin are contraindicated because they exacerbate neuromuscular blockage. Equine antitoxin is used to minimize subsequent nerve damage. There is a 2% rate of anaphylaxis to the antitoxin; therefore, diphenhydramine (Benadryl) and epinephrine must be immediately available for use. Supportive care—mechanical ventilation, nutrition, fluids, prevention of complications (Mortality rate = 5%).
Plague—*Yersinia pestis*: nonsporulating gram-negative coccobacillus. The bacterium causes destruction and necrosis of the lymph nodes.	Contagious *Bubonic plague:* Transmitted through flea bites with no person-to-person transmission *Pneumonic plague:* Transmitted through respiratory droplet contact	Isolation barrier precautions with full face respirators; the patient should wear a mask. Rooms should receive a terminal cleaning. Clothing and linens with body fluids on them should be cleaned with the usual disinfectant. Routine precautions should be used in the case of death.	*Bubonic plague:* Sudden fever and chills, weakness, a swollen and tender lymph node (bubo) in the groin, axilla, or cervical area. The resultant bacteremia progresses to septicemia from the endotoxin and, finally, shock and death. *Primary septicemic plague:* Disseminated intravascular coagulation, necrosis of small vessels, purpura, and gangrene of the digits and nose (black death). *Pneumonic plague:* Severe bronchospasm, chest pain, dyspnea, cough, and hemoptysis. There is a 100% mortality associated with pneumonic plague if not treated within the first 24 hours.	Streptomycin or gentamicin for 10–14 days. Start within 12–24 hours. Tetracycline or doxycycline is an acceptable alternative if an aminoglycoside cannot be given. People with close contact exposure (<2 m) require prophylaxis with doxycycline for 7 days. (Mortality rate = 50%)

Adapted from Dire, D. J. (2016). CBRNE—Biological warfare agents. *Medscape.* Retrieved on 11/26/2016 at: emedicine.medscape.com/article/829613-overview; Emergency Nurses Association. (2013). *Sheehy's manual of emergency care* (7th ed.). St. Louis, MO: Elsevier Mosby; Emergency Nurses Association. (2014). *Trauma nursing core course* (7th ed.). Chicago: Author; and Veenema, T. G. (2013). *Disaster nursing and emergency preparedness* (3rd ed.). New York: Springer.

standard hospital disinfectant. After death, cremation is recommended because the spores can survive for decades and represent a threat to morticians and forensic medicine personnel. There is a vaccine for anthrax that has been used in the military; however, it is not yet widely used because it requires multiple time-interval–sensitive boosters.

Smallpox

Smallpox (variola) is classified as a deoxyribonucleic acid (DNA) virus. It has an incubation period of approximately 12 days. It is extremely contagious and is spread by direct contact, by contact with clothing or linens, or by droplets from person to person only after the fever has decreased and the rash phase has begun. Aerosolization of the virus would result in widespread dissemination.

The World Health Organization (WHO) declared smallpox eradicated in 1977 and stopped worldwide vaccination in 1980. In the United States, the last child was vaccinated in 1972. Therefore, a large portion of the current population has no immunity to the virus. A smallpox vaccination plan introduced in 2003 proposed that a designated number of ED staff receive the first vaccinations to ensure that ED staff would be immunized in the event of a smallpox outbreak. The government estimated that 0.1% of those people receiving the vaccine would have serious side effects. Of these, approximately 4% would have life-threatening complications, and 0.1% would die. Currently, only people with a high likelihood of exposure to smallpox are encouraged to receive the vaccination (CDC, 2016).

Clinical Manifestations

Signs and symptoms of smallpox infection include high fever, malaise, headache, backache, and prostration. After 1 to 2 days, a maculopapular rash appears, evolving at the same rate, beginning on the face, mouth, pharynx, and forearms. Only then does the rash progress to the trunk and also become vesicular to pustular (Veenema, 2013). There is a large amount of the virus in the saliva and pustules. Smallpox is contagious only after the appearance of the rash. There are two forms of smallpox: variola major and variola minor. Variola major is more common, results in a higher fever and more extensive rash, and has a 30% case fatality rate (i.e., the

likelihood of fatality per case diagnosed). Hemorrhagic smallpox, a subtype of variola major, includes all of the above signs and symptoms plus a dusky erythema and petechiae leading to frank hemorrhage of the skin and mucous membranes, and it results in death by day 5 or 6 (Veenema, 2013).

Treatment

Treatment includes supportive care with antibiotic agents for any additional infection. The patient must be isolated with the use of transmission precautions. Laundry and biologic wastes should be autoclaved before being washed with hot water and bleach. Standard decontamination of the room is effective. All people who have household or face-to-face contact with the patient after the fever begins should be vaccinated within 4 days to prevent infection and death. A patient with a temperature of 38°C (101°F) or higher within 17 days after exposure must be placed in isolation. Cremation is preferred for all deaths, because the virus can survive in scabs for up to 13 years (Veenema, 2013).

Chemical Weapons

Chemical weapons may be used as agents in warfare or for terrorist purposes; they are overt agents in that the effects are more apparent and occur more quickly than those caused by biologic weapons (see Table 73-6). Poisonous exposure to everyday chemicals also may occur; the same management principles discussed later apply when patients are exposed to these chemical agents even when not used as weapons. Typical

TABLE 73-6 Common Chemical Agents

Agent	Action	Signs and Symptoms	Decontamination and Treatment
Nerve Agents			
Sarin Soman	Inhibition of cholinesterase	Increased secretions (salivation, lacrimation, emesis, urination), gastrointestinal motility, diarrhea, bronchospasm	Soap and water Supportive care Benzodiazepines Pralidoxime Atropine
Blood Agent			
Cyanide	Inhibition of aerobic metabolism	Inhalation—tachypnea, tachycardia, coma, seizures; bright red skin; can progress to respiratory arrest, respiratory failure, cardiac arrest, death	Soap and water Sodium nitrite Sodium thiocyanate Amyl nitrate Hydroxocobalamin
Vesicant Agents			
Lewisite Sulfur mustard Nitrogen mustard Phosgene	Blistering agents	Superficial to partial-thickness burn with vesicles that coalesce; conjunctivitis, nasal irritation	Soap and water Blot; do not rub dry
Pulmonary Agents			
Phosgene Chlorine	Separation of alveoli from capillary bed	Pulmonary edema, bronchospasm, chest tightness, burning sensation, blurry vision; Phosgene can result in pain then blisters followed by partial to full-thickness burn	Copious flushing Move to fresh air—away from gases Airway management Ventilatory support Bronchoscopy

Adapted from Ciottone, G. R., & Arnold, J. L. (2015). CBRNE – Chemical warfare agents. *Medscape.* Retrieved on 11/26/2015 at emedicine.medscape.com/article/829454-overview; Emergency Nurses Association. (2013). *Sheehy's manual of emergency care* (7th ed.). St Louis, MO: Elsevier Mosby; Emergency Nurses Association. (2014). *Trauma nursing core course* (7th ed.). Chicago: Author; and Veenema, T. G. (2013). *Disaster nursing and emergency preparedness* (3rd ed.). New York: Springer.

exposures in these instances include industrial chemicals, gasoline, turpentine, kerosene, and insecticides (ENA, 2014).

Characteristics of Chemicals

Volatility

Volatility is the tendency for a chemical to become a vapor. The most common volatile agents are phosgene and cyanide. Most chemicals are heavier than air, except for hydrogen cyanide. Therefore, in the presence of most chemicals, people should stand up to avoid heavy exposure (because the chemical will sink toward the floor or ground).

Persistence

Persistence means that the chemical is less likely to vaporize and disperse. More volatile chemicals do not evaporate very quickly. Most industrial chemicals (e.g., cyanide) are not very persistent. Weaponized agents (chemicals developed as weapons by the military or terrorists [e.g., mustard gas]) are more likely than industrial chemicals to penetrate skin and mucous membranes and also cause secondary exposure.

Toxicity

Toxicity is the potential of an agent to cause injury to the body. The median lethal dose (LD_{50}) is the amount of the chemical that will cause death in 50% of those who are exposed. For example, cyanogen chloride has the highest LD_{50}, twice that of hydrogen cyanide and eight times higher than sulfur mustard (ACS, 2010). The median effective dose (ED_{50}) is the amount of the chemical that will cause signs and symptoms in 50% of those who are exposed. The concentration time (CT) is the concentration released multiplied by the time exposed (in milligrams per minute). For example, if 1000 mg of a chemical is released and the time a person is exposed to this amount of chemical is 10 minutes, then the CT would be 10,000 mg/min.

Latency

Latency is the time from absorption to the appearance of signs and symptoms. Sulfur mustards and pulmonary agents have the longest latency, whereas other vesicants, nerve agents, and cyanide produce signs and symptoms within seconds.

Limiting Exposure

Evacuation is essential, as is removal of the person's clothing and decontamination as close to the scene as possible and before transport of the person who has been exposed. Soap and water are effective means of decontamination in most cases. Staff involved in decontamination efforts must wear PPE and contain and dispose of the runoff after decontamination procedures (ENA, 2013).

Types of Chemicals

Vesicants

Vesicants are chemicals that cause blistering and result in burning, conjunctivitis, bronchitis, pneumonia, hematopoietic suppression, and death. Examples of vesicants include lewisite, phosgene, nitrogen mustard, and sulfur mustard. In World War I and in the Iran–Iraq conflict of 1980 to 1988, vesicants were used to disable opponents. Vesicants were the main incapacitating agents, resulting in minimal (less than 5%) death but large numbers of injuries (Veenema, 2013).

Liquid sulfur mustard was the most frequently used vesicant in these conflicts.

Clinical Manifestations

The initial presentation after exposure to a vesicant is similar to that of a large superficial to partial-thickness burn in the warm and moist areas of the body (i.e., perineum, axillae, antecubital spaces). There is stinging and erythema for approximately 24 hours, followed by pruritus, painful burning, and small vesicle formation after 2 to 18 hours. These vesicles can coalesce into large, fluid-filled bullae. Lewisite and phosgene result in immediate pain after exposure. Tissue damage occurs within minutes.

If the eye is exposed, there is pain, photophobia, lacrimation, and decreased vision. This progresses to conjunctivitis, blepharospasm, corneal ulcer, and corneal edema.

Respiratory effects are more serious and often are the cause of mortality with vesicant exposure. Purulent fibrinous pseudomembrane discharge may cause obstruction of the airways. Bacterial pneumonia may be the cause of death within approximately a week of pulmonary exposure (ACS, 2010). Gastrointestinal exposure may cause nausea and vomiting, leukopenia, and upper gastrointestinal bleeding.

Treatment

Appropriate decontamination includes soap and water. Scrubbing and the use of hypochlorite solutions should be avoided because they increase penetration. Once the substance has penetrated, it cannot be removed. Eye exposure requires copious irrigation. For respiratory exposure, intubation and bronchoscopy to remove necrotic tissue are essential. With lewisite exposure, dimercaprol (BAL In Oil) is administered IV for systemic toxicity and topically for skin lesions. All persons with sulfur mustard exposures should be monitored for 24 hours for delayed (latent) effects (ENA, 2013).

Nerve Agents

The most toxic agents in existence are the nerve agents such as sarin, soman, tabun, and VX. They are inexpensive, effective in small quantities, and easily dispersed. In the liquid form, nerve agents evaporate into a colorless, odorless vapor. Organophosphates (pesticides) are similar in nature to the nerve agents used in warfare and are readily available in the farming industry.

Nerve agents can be inhaled or absorbed percutaneously or subcutaneously. These agents bond with acetylcholinesterase so that acetylcholine is not inactivated; the adverse result is continuous stimulation (hyperstimulation) of the nerve endings. Carbamates, which are insecticides originally extracted from the Calabar bean, are derivatives of carbamic acid; they are nerve agents that specifically inhibit acetylcholinesterase for several hours and then spontaneously become unbound from the acetylcholinesterase. However, organophosphates require the formation of new enzyme (acetylcholinesterase) before nervous system function can be restored.

A very small drop of a nerve agent is enough to result in sweating and twitching at the site of exposure. A larger amount results in more systemic symptoms. Effects can begin anywhere from 30 minutes up to 18 hours after exposure. The more common organophosphates and carbamates (e.g., Sevin and malathion) that are used in agriculture result in less severe symptoms than do those used in warfare or in terrorist attacks. In an ordinary situation (e.g., nonwarfare, nonterrorist attack situation), a patient could arrive at the ED having been unintentionally exposed to organophosphates or intentionally exposed to these agents in a suicidal attempt (ENA, 2013).

Clinical Manifestations

Signs and symptoms of nerve gas exposure are those of cholinergic crisis and include bilateral miosis, visual disturbances, increased gastrointestinal motility, nausea and vomiting, diarrhea, substernal spasm, indigestion, bradycardia and atrioventricular block, bronchoconstriction, laryngeal spasm, weakness, fasciculations, and incontinence. The patient must be examined in a dark area to truly identify miosis. Neurologic responses include insomnia, forgetfulness, impaired judgment, depression, and irritability. A lethal dose results in loss of consciousness, seizures, copious secretions, fasciculations, flaccid muscles, and apnea (ENA, 2014).

Treatment

Decontamination with copious amounts of soap and water or saline solution for 8 to 20 minutes is essential. The water is blotted off, not wiped off, the skin. Wiping may have the unintended effect of rubbing more of the agent into the skin. Fresh 0.5% hypochlorite solution (bleach) can also be used. The airway is maintained, and suctioning is frequently required. Plastic airway equipment should not be used, because plastic will absorb sarin gas and may result in continued exposure to the agent.

Atropine 2 to 4 mg is administered by IV, followed by 2 mg every 3 to 8 minutes for up to 24 hours of treatment. Alternatively, IV atropine 1 to 2 mg per hour may be given until clear signs of anticholinergic activity have returned (decreased secretions, tachycardia, and decreased gastrointestinal motility). Another medication that may serve as an antidote is pralidoxime (Protopam), which allows cholinesterase to become active against acetylcholine. Pralidoxime 1 to 2 g in 100 to 150 mL of normal saline solution is given over 15 to 30 minutes. Pralidoxime has no effect on secretions and may have any of the following side effects: hypertension, tachycardia, weakness, dizziness, blurred vision, and diplopia. Diazepam (Valium) or other benzodiazepines are used to control seizures, to decrease fasciculations, and to alleviate apprehension and agitation (ENA, 2013).

Blood Agents

Blood agents such as hydrogen cyanide and cyanogen chloride have a direct effect on cellular metabolism, resulting in asphyxiation through alterations in hemoglobin. Cyanide is an agent that has profound systemic effects. It is commonly used in the mining of gold and silver and in the plastics and dye industries.

A cyanide release is often associated with the odor of bitter almonds. In house fires, cyanide is released during the combustion of plastics, rugs, silk, furniture, and other construction materials. There is a significant correlation between blood cyanide and carbon monoxide levels in patients who survive fires, and in some cases, the cause of death is cyanide poisoning.

Clinical Manifestations

Cyanide can be ingested, inhaled, or absorbed through the skin and mucous membranes. Cyanide is protein bound and inhibits aerobic metabolism, leading to respiratory muscle failure, respiratory arrest, cardiac arrest, and death. Its inhalation results in flushing, tachypnea, tachycardia, nonspecific neurologic symptoms, stupor, coma, and seizure preceding respiratory arrest (ENA, 2014).

Treatment

Rapid administration of amyl nitrate, sodium nitrite, and sodium thiosulfate is essential to the successful management of cyanide exposure. First, the patient is intubated and placed on a ventilator. Next, amyl nitrate pearls are crushed and placed in the ventilator reservoir to induce methemoglobinemia. Cyanide has a 20% to 25% higher affinity for methemoglobin than it does for hemoglobin; it binds methemoglobin to form either cyanomethemoglobin or sulfmethemoglobin. The cyanomethemoglobin is then detoxified in the liver by the enzyme rhodanese. Next, IV sodium nitrite is given to induce the rapid formation of methemoglobin. IV sodium thiosulfate is then given; it has a higher affinity for cyanide than methemoglobin and stimulates the conversion of cyanide to sodium thiocyanate, which can be excreted by the kidneys (ENA, 2014; Tintinalli, Stapczyski, Ma, et al., 2016). Although they may be lifesaving, these emergency medications do have side effects—sodium nitrite can result in severe hypotension, and thiocyanate can cause vomiting, psychosis, arthralgia, and myalgia.

The production of methemoglobin is contraindicated in patients with smoke inhalation, because they already have decreased oxygen-carrying capacity secondary to the carboxyhemoglobin produced by smoke inhalation. In facilities where a hyperbaric chamber is available, it may be used to provide oxygenation while the previously discussed therapies are initiated. An alternative suggested treatment for cyanide poisoning is hydroxocobalamin (vitamin B_{12a}). Hydroxocobalamin binds cyanide to form cyanocobalamin (vitamin B_{12}). It must be administered IV in large doses (Tintinalli et al., 2016). Administration of vitamin B_{12} can result in a transient pink discoloration of mucous membranes, skin, and urine. In high doses, tachycardia and hypertension can occur, but they usually resolve within 48 hours.

Pulmonary Agents

Pulmonary agents such as phosgene and chlorine destroy the pulmonary membrane that separates the alveolus from the capillary bed, disrupting alveolar–capillary oxygen transport mechanisms. Capillary leakage results in fluid-filled alveoli. Phosgene and chlorine both vaporize, rapidly causing this pulmonary injury. Phosgene has the odor of freshly mown hay.

Signs and symptoms include pulmonary edema with shortness of breath, especially during exertion. An initial hacking cough is followed by frothy sputum production. A particulate air filter mask is the only protection required to protect health care personnel. Phosgene does not injure the eyes. In a review of a chlorine spill in South Carolina that exposed 155 patients, the most useful tool for identifying worsening symptoms was the pulse oximeter. Ordinary triage systems did not predict the severity of exposure (Culley, Svendsen, Craig, et al., 2014).

Nuclear Radiation Exposure

The threat of nuclear warfare or exposure to a radiologic weapon is very real with the availability of nuclear material and easily concealed simple devices, such as the so-called dirty bomb, for dispersal. A dirty bomb is a conventional explosive (e.g., dynamite) that is packaged with radioactive material that scatters when the bomb is detonated. It disperses radioactive material and may be called a **radiologic weapon**, but it is not a *nuclear* weapon, which uses a complex nuclear fission reaction that is thousands of times more devastating than the dirty bomb.

Sources of radioactive material include not only nuclear weapons but also reactors and simple radioactive samples, such as weapons-grade plutonium or uranium, freshly spent nuclear fuel, or medical supplies (e.g., radium, certain cesium isotopes) used in cancer treatments and radiology. Exposure to a large number of people can be accomplished by placing a radioactive sample in a public place. Thousands may be exposed this way; some may be immediately affected, and others may require health monitoring for many years to assess long-term effects.

Any terrorist act or unintentional radiation release can be sizable and may require the entire hospital and prehospital staff to be prepared, recognize signs and symptoms of exposure, and rapidly treat victims without contamination of personnel, visitors, patients, or the facility itself.

Types of Radiation

Atoms consist of protons, neutrons, and electrons. The protons and neutrons are in balance in the nucleus. The protons repel each other because they are all positively charged. The number of protons is specific for each element in the periodic table. There is a specific ratio of protons and neutrons for each different atom, and the result is element stability. When an element is radioactive, there is an imbalance in the nucleus, resulting from an excess of neutrons.

To achieve stability, a radioactive nuclide can eject particles until the most stable number (an even number) of protons and neutrons exists. A proton can become a neutron by ejecting a positron; conversely, a neutron can become a proton by ejecting a negative electron. An alpha particle is released when two protons and two electrons are ejected (beta particles are electrons).

Alpha particles cannot penetrate the skin. A thin layer of paper or clothing is all that is necessary to protect the skin from alpha radiation. However, this low-level radiation can enter the body through inhalation, ingestion, or injection (open wound). Only localized damage occurs.

Beta particles have the ability to moderately penetrate the skin to the layer in which skin cells are being produced. This high-energy radiation can cause skin damage if the skin is exposed for a prolonged period and can cause injury if beta particles penetrate the skin.

Gamma radiation is a short-wavelength electromagnetic energy that is emitted when there is excess core nucleus energy. Gamma particles are penetrating. Therefore, it is difficult to shield against gamma radiation. X-rays are an example of gamma radiation. Gamma radiation often accompanies both alpha particle and beta particle emission.

Measurement and Detection

Radiation is measured in several different units. The *rad* is the basic unit of measurement. A rad is equivalent to 0.01 J of energy per kilogram of tissue. To determine the damaging effect of the rad, a conversion to the *rem* (roentgen equivalents man) is necessary. The rem reflects the type of radiation absorbed and the potential for damage. For example, 200,000 mrem results in mild radiation sickness (1 rem = 1000 mrem) (ACS, 2010). Typical natural yearly exposure for a person is 360 mrem. Another important concept is *half-life*. The half-life of a radioactive product is the time it takes to lose half of its radioactivity.

The only way to detect radiation is through a device that determines the exposure per minute. There are various devices for this purpose. The Geiger counter (or Geiger-Mueller survey meter) can measure background radiation quickly through detection of gamma radiation and some beta radiation. With high-level radiation, the Geiger counter may underestimate exposure. Other devices include the ionization chamber survey meter, alpha monitors, and dose rate meters. Personal dosimeters are simple tools that identify radiation exposure and are worn by radiology personnel every day.

Exposure

Exposure is affected by time, distance, and shielding. The longer a person is within the radiation area, the higher the exposure. In addition, the larger the amount of radioactive material in the area, the greater the exposure. The farther away the person is from the radiation source, the lower the exposure. Shielding from the radiation source also decreases exposure.

Three types of radiation-induced injury can occur: external irradiation, contamination with radioactive materials, and incorporation of radioactive material into body cells, tissues, or organs:

- *External irradiation* exposure occurs when all or part of the body is exposed to radiation that penetrates or passes completely through the body. In this type of exposure, the person is not radioactive and does not require special isolation or decontamination measures. Irradiation does not necessarily constitute a medical emergency.
- *Contamination* occurs when the body is exposed to radioactive gases, liquids, or solids either externally or internally. If internal, the contaminant can be deposited within the body. Contamination requires immediate medical management to prevent incorporation.
- *Incorporation* is the actual uptake of radioactive material into the cells, tissues, and susceptible organs. The organs involved are usually the kidneys, bones, liver, and thyroid.

Sequelae of contamination and incorporation can occur days to years later. The thyroid gland can be largely protected from radiation exposure by administration of stable iodine (potassium iodide, or KI) before or promptly after the intake of radioactive iodine. Priorities in the treatment of any type of radiation exposure are always treatment for life-threatening injuries and illnesses first, followed by measures to limit exposure, contamination control, and finally decontamination.

Decontamination

Hospital and community disaster plans should be in effect when managing a radiation disaster. Access restriction is essential to prevent contamination of other areas of the hospital. Triage outside the hospital is the most effective means of preventing contamination of the facility itself. Floors are covered to prevent tracking of contaminants throughout the treatment areas. Strict isolation precautions should be in effect. All air ducts and vents must be sealed to prevent spread. Waste is controlled through double-bagging and the use of plastic-lined containers outside of the facility. All radiation-contaminated waste must be disposed in appropriate color-coded yellow and magenta canisters.

Staff are required to wear protective clothing, such as water-resistant gowns, two pairs of gloves, masks, caps, goggles, and booties. Dosimetry devices should be worn by all staff members participating in patient care. The radiation safety officer in the hospital should be notified immediately to assist with surveys (using a radiation survey meter) of the incoming patients and to provide dosimeters to all staff personnel involved in direct care of patients who have been exposed. There is minimal risk to staff if the patients are properly surveyed and decontaminated.

Each patient arriving at the hospital should first be surveyed with the radiation survey meter for external contamination and then directed toward the decontamination area as needed. The majority of patients can be safely decontaminated with soap and water. Decontamination occurs outside of the ED with a shower, collection pool, tarp, and collection containers for patient belongings, as well as soap, towels, and disposable paper gowns for patients. Water runoff needs to be contained. Patients who are uninjured can perform self-decontamination with handheld showers. After the patient has showered, a resurvey is conducted to determine whether the radioactive contaminants have been removed. Additional washings should occur until the patient is free of contamination. It is important to ensure that during showers, previously clean areas are not contaminated with runoff from the washed contaminated areas (e.g., hair should be washed in a position that protects the body from contamination). Wounds are irrigated and then covered with a water-resistant dressing prior to total body decontamination.

Internal contamination or incorporation requires decontamination through catharsis, gastric lavage with chelating agents (agents that bind with radioactive substances and are then excreted), or both. Samples of urine, feces, and vomitus are surveyed to determine internal contamination levels. Biologic samples are taken through nasal and throat swabs, and a complete blood count with differential is obtained.

Acute Radiation Syndrome

Acute radiation syndrome (ARS) can occur after exposure to radiation. It is the dose, rather than the source, that determines whether ARS develops. Factors that determine whether the patient's response to exposure will result in ARS include a high dose (minimum 100 rad) and rate of radiation with total body exposure and penetrating-type radiation. Age, medical history, and genetics also affect the outcome after exposure. The course is predictable. Table 73-7 identifies the phases of ARS.

Each body system is affected differently in ARS. Systems with cells that rapidly reproduce are most commonly affected. The hematopoietic system is the first system affected and serves as an indicator of the severity of radiation exposure (Veenema, 2013). A predictor of outcome is the absolute lymphocyte count at 48 hours after exposure. A significant exposure would be indicated by blood lymphocyte counts of 300 to 1200/mm^3. Barrier precautions should be implemented to protect the patient from infection. Neutrophils decrease within 1 week, platelets decrease within 2 weeks, and red blood cells decrease within 3 weeks. Hemorrhagic complications including fever and sepsis are common.

The gastrointestinal system, with its rapidly reproducing cells, is also readily affected by radiation. Doses of radiation required to produce symptoms are approximately 600 rad or higher. The gastrointestinal symptoms usually occur at the same time as the changes in the hematopoietic system. Nausea and vomiting occur within 2 hours after exposure. Sepsis, fluid and electrolyte imbalance, and opportunistic infections can occur as complications. An ominous sign is the presence of high fever and bloody diarrhea; these typically appear on day 10 after exposure (ENA, 2014).

The central nervous system is affected when the dose exceeds 1000 rad (ENA, 2014). The symptoms occur when damage to the blood vessels of the brain results in fluid

---

TABLE 73-7 Phases of Effects of Radiation Exposure

Phase	Time of Occurrence	Signs and Symptoms
Prodromal phase (presenting symptoms)	48–72 hours after exposure	Nausea, vomiting, loss of appetite, diarrhea, fatigue High-dose radiation—fever, respiratory distress, and increased excitability
Latent phase (a symptom-free period)	After resolution of prodromal phase; can last up to 3 weeks With high-dose radiation, latent period is shorter	Decreasing lymphocytes, leukocytes, thrombocytes, red blood cells
Manifest Illness phase	After latent period phase	Infection, fluid and electrolyte imbalance, bleeding, diarrhea, shock, and altered level of consciousness
Recovery phase OR	After manifest illness phase	Can take weeks to months for full recovery
Death	After manifest illness phase	Increased intracranial pressure is a sign of impending death

Adapted from Centers for Disease Control and Prevention (CDC). (2015). *Acute radiation syndrome: A fact sheet for clinicians*. Retrieved on 11/26/2016 at: www.emergency.cdc.gov/radiation/arsphysicianfactsheet.asp

leakage. Signs and symptoms include cerebral edema; nausea; vomiting; headache; and increased intracranial pressure, which heralds a poor outcome and imminent death. Central nervous system injury with this amount of exposure is irreversible and occurs before hematopoietic or gastrointestinal system symptoms appear. Cardiovascular collapse is usually seen in conjunction with these injuries.

Skin effects can also indicate the dose of radiation exposure. With exposure of 600 to 1000 rad, erythema occurs; it can disappear within hours and then reappear. The patient who has been exposed must be evaluated hourly for the presence of erythema. With exposures greater than 1000 rad, desquamation (radiation dermatitis) of the skin occurs. Necrosis becomes evident within a few days to months at doses greater than 5000 rad.

Secondary injury can occur when the radiation exposure occurs during a traumatic event such as a blast or burn. Trauma in addition to radiation exposure increases patient mortality. Attention must first be directed toward the primary assessment for trauma. Airway, breathing, circulation, and fracture reduction require immediate attention. All definitive treatments must occur within the first 48 hours. Thereafter, all surgical procedures should be delayed for 2 to 3 months because of the potential for delayed wound healing and the possible development of opportunistic infections several weeks after exposure.

Survival

There are three categories of predicted survival after radiation exposure: probable, possible, and improbable. Triage of victims at the scene, after decontamination, is conducted using the routine system for disaster triage. Presenting signs and symptoms determine the potential for survival and therefore the category of predicted survival during triage.

Probable survivors have either no initial symptoms or only minimal symptoms (e.g., nausea and vomiting), or these symptoms resolve within a few hours. These patients should have a complete blood count drawn and may be discharged with instructions to return if any symptoms recur.

Possible survivors present with nausea and vomiting that persist for 24 to 48 hours. They experience a latent period, during which leukopenia, thrombocytopenia, and lymphocytopenia occur. Barrier precautions and protective isolation are implemented if the patient's lymphocyte count is less than 1200/mm^3. Supportive treatment includes administration of blood products, prevention of infection, and provision of enhanced nutrition.

Improbable survivors have received more than 800 rad of total-body penetrating irradiation. People in this group demonstrate an acute onset of vomiting, bloody diarrhea, and shock. Any neurologic symptoms suggest a lethal dose of radiation (ENA, 2014). These patients still require decontamination to prevent further contamination of the area and of others. Personal protection is essential, because it is virtually impossible to fully decontaminate these patients; all of their internal organs have been irradiated. The survival time is variable; however, death usually occurs swiftly due to shock. If there are no neurologic symptoms, patients may be alert and oriented, similar to a patient with extensive burns. In a mass casualty situation, these patients would be triaged into the black category, where they will receive comfort measures

and emotional support. If it is not a mass casualty situation, aggressive fluid and electrolyte therapies are essential.

CRITICAL THINKING EXERCISES

1 **ebp** You work in an occupational health clinic that provides support to a chemical plant that manufactures chlorine. A patient walks to the clinic after being told to report for an examination by his supervisor since he temporarily removed his PPE while at work. Although he walked to the clinic, he tells you that now his eyes are burning and he is experiencing blurry vision. What evidence-based assessments and interventions would you now implement and why?

2 You are a home health nurse. Several patients who comprise your caseload are dependent upon electronic medical equipment, including one patient who requires home mechanical ventilation and three who require home intravenous therapy. You live in a coastal area and a category 4 hurricane is threatening to hit your community within the next 48 hours. Describe the precautions you would take to ensure that these patients are not deprived of the use of their electronic medical equipment in case of a loss of power.

3 **pq** You are working in the emergency department (ED) of a community hospital. One evening, a radio call from EMS sends an alert that there is a possible multiple shooting at a restaurant a block away from the hospital. What are your priorities and first actions? What might be done to ensure safety of the ED staff and patients? How would you prepare for the arrival of patients who may have been injured from this event?

REFERENCES

*Asterisk indicates nursing research.
**Double asterisk indicates classic reference.

Books

American College of Surgeons (ACS). (2010). *Disaster management and emergency preparedness course*. Chicago: Author.
American College of Surgeons (ACS). (2013). *Advanced trauma life support* (9th ed.). Chicago: Author.
American College of Surgeons Committee on Trauma (ACS-COT). (2014). *Resources for optimal care of the injured patient*. Chicago: Author.
Auerbach, P. S. (2017). *Wilderness medicine* (6th ed.). Philadelphia, PA: Mosby Elsevier.
Emergency Nurses Association (ENA). (2013). *Sheehy's manual of emergency care* (7th ed.). St. Louis, MO: Elsevier Mosby.
Emergency Nurses Association (ENA). (2014). *Trauma nursing core course* (7th ed). Chicago: Emergency Nurses Association.
Tintinalli, J. E., Stapczyski, J. S., Ma, O. J., et al. (2016). *Tintinalli's emergency medicine manual* (8th ed.). New York: McGraw-Hill Medical.
Veenema, T. G. (2013). *Disaster nursing and emergency preparedness* (3rd ed.). New York: Springer.

Journals and Electronic Documents

Abbasi, J. (2016). Expanding the health care response to mass violence. *JAMA, 316*(10), 1031–1033.

Agency for Toxic Substances and Disease Registry. (2016). *HazMat emergency preparedness training and tools for responders*. Retrieved on 11/26/2016 at: www.atsdr.cdc.gov/hazmat-emergency-preparedness.html

American Nurses Association. (2010). Who will be there? Ethics, the law, and a nurse's duty to respond in a disaster. *ANA Issue Brief*. Retrieved on 3/27/2017 at: www.nursingworld.org/MainMenuCategories/Workplac-eSafety/Healthy-Work-Environment/DPR/Disaster-Preparedness.pdf

Centers for Disease Control and Prevention (CDC). (2012). *Blast injuries: Fact sheets for professionals*. Retrieved on 3/25/2017 at: stacks.cdc.gov/view/cdc/21571/Print

Centers for Disease Control and Prevention (CDC). (2015). *Acute radiation syndrome: A fact sheet for clinicians*. Retrieved on 11/26/2016 at: www.emergency.cdc.gov/radiation/arsphysicianfactsheet.asp

Centers for Disease Control and Prevention (CDC). (2016). *Smallpox: Who should get vaccination*. Retrieved on 3/23/2017 at: www.cdc.gov/smallpox/vaccine-basics/who-gets-vaccination.html

Ciottone, G. R., & Arnold, J. L. (2015). CBRNE—Chemical warfare agents. *Medscape*. Retrieved on 11/26/2015 at: emedicine.medscape.com/article/829454-overview

Costa-Roberts, D. (2015). 4 surprising facts from the 2015 Global Terrorism Index. *PBS Newshour*. Retrieved on 3/25/2017 at: www.pbs.org/newshour/rundown/4-surprising-facts-from-the-2015-global-terrorism-index/

Culley, J. M., Svendsen, E., Craig, J., et al. (2014). A validation study of 5 triage systems using data from the 2005 Graniteville South Carolina chlorine spill. *Journal of Emergency Nursing, 40*(5), 453–460.

Dire, D. J. (2016). CBRNE—Biological warfare agents. *Medscape*. Retrieved on 11/26/2016 at: emedicine.medscape.com/article/829613-overview

Dodd-Murphy, J. (2014). Auditory effects of blast exposure: Community outreach following an industrial explosion. *American Speech Language Hearing Association*. Retrieved on 3/25/2017 at: www.asha.org/Articles/Auditory-Effects-of-Blast-Exposure/

Federal Emergency Management Agency (2013). *ICS 200 Curriculum*. Retrieved on 6/20/217 at: training.fema.gov/is/courseoverview.aspx?code=IS-200.b

Nadworny, D., Davis, K., Miers, C., et al. (2014). Boston strong—one hospital's response to the 2013 Boston marathon bombings. *Journal of Emergency Nursing, 40*(5), 418–427.

Pennardt, A., & Lavonas, E. J. (2016). Blast injuries. *Medscape*. Retrieved on 4/2/2017 at: emedicine.medscape.com/article/822587-overview

**U.S. Department of Homeland Security Federal Emergency Management Agency (FEMA) & the American Red Cross. (2004). *Preparing for disaster for people with disabilities and other special needs*. Retrieved on 11/26/2016 at: www.redcross.org/images/MEDIA_CustomProduct Catalog/m4240199_A4497.pdf

U.S. Department of Homeland Security National Terrorism Advisory System (NTAS). (2015). *NTAS frequently asked questions*. Retrieved on 4/2/2017 at: www.dhs.gov/ntas-frequently-asked-questions

Valdez, A. M. (2015). Are you covered? Safe practices for the use of personal protective equipment. *Journal of Emergency Nursing, 41*(2), 154–157.

**World Health Organization. (2005). *Disasters, disability and rehabilitation*. Retrieved on 11/26/2016 at: www.who.int/violence_injury_prevention/other_injury/disaster_disability2.pdf

*Zidek, C., West, E., Holmes, J., et al. (2014). A survey comparison of rural versus urban residents and household preparedness. *Home Healthcare Nurse, 32*(7), 420–429.

Resources

Agency for Toxic Substances and Disease Registry, www.atsdr.cdc.gov

American Red Cross, Beat Disaster with Preparedness, www.redcross.org/news/article/Beat-Disaster-with-Preparedness

Centers for Disease Control and Prevention (CDC), Emergency Preparedness and Response, www.emergency.cdc.gov

Chemtrac, www.chemtracglobal.com

Federal Emergency Management Agency (FEMA), www.fema.gov

Global terrorism database, www.start.umd.edu/gtd

National Organization on Disability, www.nod.org

U.S. Department of Homeland Security, www.dhs.gov

Index

Note: Page numbers followed by c indicate charts; those followed by f indicate figures; those followed by t indicate tables.

A

Abacavir (ABC), 1034t
Abatacept (Orencia), 1089t
ABCDE (primary survey), 1853
Abciximab (ReoPro), 683
Abdomen
  acute, 1322
  auscultation, 1232
  blast injuries, 2203
  cardiovascular disorder and, 693
  inspection, 1231
  intra-abdominal injuries, 2169–2190
  pain in (*See* Abdominal pain)
  penetrating injuries, 2169
  percussion and palpation, 1232
  protuberant, 693
  quadrants, 1231, 1231f
  ultrasonography, 1233–1234
  x-ray, 1432
Abdominal aortic aneurysm, 862, 863–864
  assessment and diagnostic findings, 863
  atherosclerosis and, 863
  clinical manifestations, 863
  endovascular and surgical management, 864, 864f
  nursing management, 864
  in older patients, 863
  pathophysiology, 863
  pharmacologic therapy, 864
  risk factors, 863
  rupturing, 863
Abdominal compartment syndrome (ACS), 305, 1853
Abdominal distension, 693
Abdominal pain, 1322
  appendicitis and, 1323–1324
  gallstone and, 1431–1432
  irritable bowel syndrome and, 1318
  pancreatitis and, 1441
Abduction, 171c, 1131, 1147
A-beta (β) fibers, 227
ABI. *See* Ankle-brachial index
Abiraterone acetate (Zytiga), 1765
Ablation, 712
  radiofrequency, 705
ABO incompatibility, 919–920
Abortion
  complete, 1675
  definition of, 1674
  habitual, 1675
  induced, 1675–1676, 1676c
  spontaneous, 1674–1675
ABO system, 916
Above-knee amputation (AKA), 1214
Abrasion, 2060
Abscess, 1311, 1323, 1686
  anorectal, 1351
  brain, 2068–2069, 2069c
  breast, 1728
  lactational, 1728

liver, 1425
  periapical, 1264, 1268–1269
  tubo-ovarian, 1695
Abscessed tooth. *See* periapical abscess
Absolute neutrophil count (ANC), 376, 945, 973
Absorption, 1224, 1225
Abstinence, 1669
Abuse, 7, 25, 57, 68c, 71, 153c, 215, 423, 1421c
  alcohol, 69, 277, 424, 934, 944, 947, 1445
  elder, 193, 217–218
  IV drug, 810
  sexual, 1657–1658
  substance, 62, 69, 208, 2180–2185
  verbal, 2158
Acalculous cholecystitis, 1430
Acantholysis, 1806, 1828
Acarbose (Precose), 1474t
Acceptance, stages of grief, 410t
Accessory muscles, 495
Accidents, 1185
Acculturation, 104
ACE. *See* Angiotensin-converting enzyme
Acebutolol (Sectral), for hypertension, 891t
ACE inhibitors
  for diabetes, 1492
  for heart failure, 824–825, 824t
  for hypertension, 892t
Acetabular fractures, 1202
Acetaminophen, 226
  administration of, 235
  adverse effects of, 235–236
  in fungal encephalitis, 2071
  indications for, 235
  IV (Ofirmev), 235
  in osteoarthritis, 1105
Acetazolamide (Diamox), 1387
Acetylcholinesterase inhibitor test, 2079
Achalasia, 1264, 1279, 1280f
  assessment and diagnostic findings, 1279
  clinical manifestations, 1279
  management, 1279, 1280f
Achilles reflex, 1963–1964
Achilles tendon, rupture of, 1189
Achlorhydria, 1292, 1298
Acid-base balance
  as balance scale, 283f
  blood gas analysis, 287–288
  disorders, 288t
  imbalance, 283–288
  mixed disorders, 287–288
  regulation of, 1552–1553
Acidosis, 271
  metabolic, 284–285
  respiratory, 286–287
Acinetobacter sp., 2133
Acini, 1503
Acne vulgaris, 1814–1816

Acoustic neuromas, 1938, 2092
Acquired cold urticaria (ACU), 1076–1077
Acquired immunity, 1007
  active, 1007
  passive, 1007
Acquired immunodeficiency syndrome (AIDS), 922c, 1025, 1696–1697. *See also* Human immune deficiency virus (HIV) infection
  meningitis and, 2066c
  travel and, 2153
Acquired mutation, 118, 119f
Acral lentiginous melanoma (ALM), 1836
Acrocyanosis, 867
Acromegaly, 1502, 1508
ACS. *See* Acute coronary syndrome; American Cancer Society
ACTH. *See* Adrenocorticotropic hormone
Actinic cheilitis, 1266t
Actinic keratoses, 1833
Activated charcoal administration, 2178
Activated partial thromboplastin time (aPTT), 694t, 703, 910
Activated protein C (APC) resistance, 962
Activated prothrombin complex concentrates (IaPCC, FEIBA), 953
Active body movement, postoperative, 429
Active dressings, skin, 1807
Active internal rewarming method, 2174. *See also* Hypothermia
Active transport, 253
Activities of daily living (ADLs), 1135, 1161, 2075, 2100
  adaptive equipment, 189c
  aging and, 200–201
  definition of, 167, 193
  home care education, 189c–190c
  patient education goals, 169c
  self-care deficits in, 168–170
Activity tolerance, burn injuries and, 1870
Acute alcohol intoxication, 2185
Acute chest syndrome, 936
Acute confusional state. *See* Delirium
Acute coronary syndrome (ACS), 762–771
  assessment of, 763–764, 763c, 767
  cardiac rehabilitation, 766–767
  clinical manifestations, 763
  definition of, 750, 762
  diagnosis of, 763–764, 767
  evaluation, 770–771
  health promotion, 770c
  medical management, 765–766
  nursing interventions, 767–770
  nursing process, 767–771
  pathophysiology, 762–763
  patient goals, 767
  thrombolytic (fibrinolytic) therapy, 766, 766c
Acute decompensated heart failure, 818, 819. *See also* Heart failure (HF)

Acute kidney injury (AKI), 1567, 1576–1581, 2171
  assessment and diagnostic findings, 1578
  causes, 1577c
  clinical manifestations, 1578, 1578t
  intrarenal, 1577
  medical management, 1579–1580
    fluid balance, maintenance of, 1579–1580
    nutritional therapy, 1580
    pharmacologic therapy, 1580
    renal replacement therapy, 1580
  nursing management, 1580–1581
    fluid and electrolyte imbalances, 1581
    infection prevention, 1581
    metabolic rate, 1581
    psychosocial support, 1581
    pulmonary function, 1581
    skin care, 1581
  in older adults, 1579
  pathophysiology, 1576
  phases of
    diuresis period, 1577–1578
    initiation period, 1577
    oliguria period, 1577
    recovery period, 1578
  postrenal, 1577
  prerenal, 1577
  prevention of, 1579, 1579c
  RIFLE classification system, 1576–1577, 1577t
Acute lung injury (ALI), 301–302, 583
Acute lymphocytic leukemia (ALL), 975–976
  clinical manifestations, 975–976
  medical management, 976
  nursing management, 976
Acute myeloid leukemia (AML), 971–974
  assessment and diagnostic findings, 972
  clinical manifestations, 972, 972f
  complications of, 973–974
  medical management, 972–973
  nursing management, 974
Acute nephritic syndrome, 1567, 1570–1572
  assessment and diagnostic findings, 1571
  clinical manifestations, 1570–1571
  complications, 1571
  medical management, 1571
  nursing management, 1571–1572
  pathophysiology, 1570, 1571f
Acute otitis media (AOM), 1927–1928
  clinical features of, 1928t
  medical management of, 1928
Acute radiation syndrome (ARS), 2210–2211, 2210t
Acute respiratory distress syndrome (ARDS), 583, 609–612, 610f, 2161, 2175
  burn injuries and, 1867
Acute respiratory failure, 609–610, 1867
Acute tracheobronchitis, 586–587
  clinical manifestations, 586
  medical management, 586–587
  nursing management, 587
  pathophysiology, 586
Acute tubular necrosis (ATN), 1567, 1577
Acyclovir (Zovirax), 2069
  for genital herpes, 1692
  in herpes zoster infection, 1819
Adalimumab (Humira), 1089t, 1107
  for psoriasis, 1826
Adaptability, anticipatory mourning and, 411c
Adaptation, 84

cellular, 92
  Selye theory of, 87
  stress and, 85
Adaptive devices, 165, 169–170, 169f
Addison disease, 1502, 1534–1536
  assessment and diagnostic findings, 1535
  clinical manifestations, 1534–1535
  continuing and transitional care, 1536
  corticosteroids use and, 1534
  fluid balance in, 1535
  health history and examination, 1535
  home care checklist, 1536c
  medical management, 1535
  nursing management, 1535
  patient education, 1535–1536, 1536c
Addisonian crisis, 1502, 1535, 1539
Adduction, 171c, 1131, 1147
A-delta (d) fibers, 226–227
Adenoiditis, 562–564
Adenoids, 481
Adenomyosis, 1705
Adenosine (Adenocard), 699
Adenosine diphosphate receptor antagonists (P2Y$_{12}$), for angina, 760
Adenosine triphosphate (ATP), 279, 280, 297, 1118
ADH. See Antidiuretic hormone
Adherence, 48, 49
Adiposopathy, 1358, 1360
Adjuvant analgesic agents, 235, 243–244
Adjuvant chemotherapy, 1719
Adjuvant hormonal therapy, 1719
Adnexa, 1650, 1653
Adnexal palpation, 1662
Adrenalectomy, 1502, 1533, 1537
Adrenal enzyme inhibitors, 1538
Adrenal glands, 1531–1543, 1531f
  adrenal cortex, 1531
    androgens, 1532
    glucocorticoids, 1531
    mineralocorticoids, 1531–1532
  adrenal medulla, 1531
  adrenocortical insufficiency, 1534–1536
  Cushing syndrome, 1536–1540
  functions, 256
  pheochromocytoma, 1532–1534
  primary aldosteronism, 1540–1541
Adrenaline, 1531
Adrenergic agents, for allergic rhinitis, 1068
Adrenocorticotropic hormone (ACTH), 85, 87, 89, 1502, 1507, 1531
Adrenogenital syndrome, 1502, 1532
ADT. See Androgen deprivation therapy
Adult-onset conditions, 124–127, 125t
  genomic conditions, 127
  nursing role, 127
  population screening, 127
  single gene conditions, 124–127
Adults
  genetics referrals in, 133c
  older (See Older adults)
Advance directives, 34
Advanced practice registered nurses (APRNs), 12
Adventitious sounds, 498
Adverse drug effects, polypharmacy and, 205
Advisory Committee on Immunization Practices (ACIP), 1692

Aerobacter aerogenes, 474
Aerosol delivery devices, 641t
Aerosol masks, 515
Affordable Care Act (ACA), 25, 1651
Aflatoxin, 1417
Afrezza, 1473
African Americans, hypertension in, 885, 895c
After-death care, 409–410
After-death rituals, 411
Afterload, 678
Age/aging. See also Older adults
  adherence to regimens and, 49–50, 50f
  cardiovascular system and, 195–198
  cellular, 195
  changes related to, 195–207, 197t
  cognitive aspects of, 204–205
  demographics, 193–194
  description of, 193
  with disability, 219
  gastrointestinal system and, 197t, 199
  genitourinary system and, 197t, 199
  health care costs of, 218
  home health care, 218
  hospice services and, 218–219
  and immunologic function, 1014–1015, 1015t
  integumentary system and, 198
  intrinsic, 195
  musculoskeletal system and, 197t, 200–201
  nervous system and, 197t, 201
  overview of, 193–195
  pharmacologic aspects of, 205–207
  physical aspects of, 195–202
  psychosocial aspects of, 201–204
  reproductive system and, 198–199
  respiratory system and, 198
  sensory system and, 197t, 201–202
  theories of, 195
Ageism, 193, 202
Agency for Healthcare Research and Quality (AHRQ), 9
Age-related macular degeneration, 1901–1902, 1902f
Agglutination, 1010
Agitation, reduction of, 213–214
Agnogenic myeloid metaplasia. See Primary myelofibrosis
Agnosia, 1946, 1962t, 2011
Agranulocytes, 907
AIDS-related anorexia, 1042
AIDS-related lymphomas, 1039, 1042
Airborne bacteria, 441
Airborne precautions, 2131, 2131c
Air embolism, 291
Air pressure variances, 484
Air trapping, 645
Airway clearance, 666
  COPD patients, 645, 649t
  cystic fibrosis and, 666
Airway edema, 655
Airway management, 521–537, 522f
  endotracheal intubation, 521–523
  mechanical ventilation, 525–537
  tracheotomy, 523–525
  upper airway obstruction, 521
Airway obstruction, 2115
  assessment and diagnostic findings, 2163

clinical manifestations, 2163
management, 2163–2165
  establishing an airway, 2163–2165
  maintaining ventilation, 2165
pathophysiology, 2163
signs and symptoms of, 2163
Airway pressure release ventilation (APRV), 510, 528
Airway resistance, 484, 484c
Akathisia, 2109
AKI. See Acute kidney injury
Akinetic mutism, 1972, 1973
Alanine aminotransferase (ALT), 1382
Alarm fatigue, 698
Alaryngeal communication, 552, 575
Albumin, 908, 1511
  in ascites, 1387
  leakage in urine, 1492
  nutritional status and, 180
  serum, 305
Albuterol (Proventil, Ventolin), 272, 319, 640, 656, 658t, 661t
Alcoholic cirrhosis, 1406. See also Cirrhosis
Alcoholics Anonymous, 1276
Alcohol use, 695
  and chronic pancreatitis, 1445
  by diabetic patient, 1464–1465
  and liver dysfunction, 1380–1381
  preoperative assessments, 424–425
Alcohol withdrawal syndrome, 2185–2186
Aldosterone, 256, 1532, 1548, 1552
  deficiency of, hyponatremia and, 265
Aldosterone receptor blockers, for hypertension, 890t
Aldrete score form, 462f
Alefacept (Amevive), for psoriasis, 1826
Alemtuzumab (Campath), 978
Alfentanil (Alfenta), 446t
Alfuzosin (Uroxatral), for BPH, 1763
Alginates, 1807, 1808t
  calcium, 1809
Algorithm, use of, 9
Aliskiren (Tekturna), for hypertension, 893t
Alkaline phosphatase (ALP), 1171
Alkalosis, 269
  metabolic, 285–286
  respiratory, 287
Alkylating agents, 343t
ALL. See Acute lymphocytic leukemia
Alleles, 117, 121f
Allen test, 1271
Allergen desensitization, 1070
Allergens, 553c, 1058
Allergic disorder, 1057
  allergic rhinitis, 1066–1074
  anaphylaxis, 1064–1066
  angioneurotic edema, 1076
  assessment form, 1061, 1062c–1063c
  atopic dermatitis, 1074–1075
  atopic diseases, 1064
  cold urticaria, 1076–1077
  contact dermatitis, 1074
  dermatitis medicamentosa, 1075
  diagnostic evaluation, 1061
    complete blood count with differential, 1061
    eosinophil count, 1061
    provocative testing, 1064
    serum-specific IgE test, 1064

skin testing, 1061, 1063–1064, 1063f, 1064f
  total serum IgE levels, 1061
food allergy, 1077–1078
hereditary angioedema, 1076
latex allergy, 1078–1080
nonatopic disorders, 1064
urticaria, 1075–1076
Allergic rhinitis, 1066–1074
  assessment and diagnostic findings, 1067
  clinical manifestations, 1067
  home care checklist, 1073c
  medical management, 1067–1071
    avoidance therapy, 1068
    immunotherapy, 1070–1071, 1071c
    pharmacologic therapy, 1068–1070, 1069t, 1070t
  nursing process
    assessment, 1071–1072
    diagnosis, 1072
    evaluation, 1073–1074
    nursing interventions, 1072–1073
    planning and goals, 1072
  pathophysiology, 1067
Allergy, 654, 1058
  to local anesthetics, 243–244
Allergy vaccine therapy. See Immunotherapy
Alloantibodies, 943
Allodynia, 230
Allogeneic HSCT (AlloHSCT), 349–350
Allogeneic vaccines, 354
Allograft, 1185, 1196
Allopurinol (Zyloprim), 345, 973, 985, 1108, 1109t, 1634
All-trans retinoic acid (ATRA), 973
ALM. See Acral lentiginous melanoma
ALND. See Axillary lymph node dissection
Alogliptin (Nesina), 1475t
Alopecia, 1790, 1792, 1802
  definition of, 324, 340
  nursing interventions, 363c
  nursing management, 370
Alosetron (Lotronex), 1318
Alpha-adrenergic blockers
  for BPH, 1763
  for pheochromocytoma, 1533
Alpha$_1$-antitrypsin deficiency, 126t, 635, 637, 638
Alpha cells, 1457
Alpha-fetoprotein (AFP), 1780
  in primary liver cancer, 1417
Alpha-glucosidase inhibitors, 1474t
Alpha-interferon, in hepatitis B, 1402
Alphanate, 914, 955
Alprostadil, 1759
Alteplase (Activase, t-PA), 866
  for venous thromboembolism, 870t
Altered level of consciousness (LOC)
  assessment of, 1974–1975
  definition of, 1973
  description, 1974
  management, 1975
  manifestation, 1974
  nursing process, 1974–1979, 1976t
  pathophysiolog, 1974
Altretamine (Hexalen), 343t
Aluminum carbonate, 1530
Aluminum hydroxide, 1530
  for GERD, 1284t
Alveoli, 482f, 483, 635, 636, 646, 648

Alzheimer's Association, 215
Alzheimer's disease (AD)
  balanced activity and rest, promotion of, 214–215
  characteristics, 210t
  clinical manifestations of, 211–212
  communication in, improvement of, 214
  community care, 215
  diagnosis of, 212–213
  health history, 212
  home care, 215
  medical management, 213
  nursing management, 213–215
  nutrition, promotion of, 214, 214f
  older adults and, 209–215
  pathophysiology of, 211
  personality changes in, 212
  physical safety in, promotion of, 213
  risk factor for, 209
  self-care activities in, promotion of, 213
  socialization and intimacy needs, 214
  transitional care, 215
  types of, 209–211
Amantadine (Symmetrel), 2075
Ambulation
  with assistive device, 174–175
  benefits of, 473
  postsurgical, 467–468
  preparation for, 173–174
Ambulatory electrocardiography, 696–697
Ambulatory health care, 24
Ambulatory surgery, 418, 419, 422
  attending to family needs, 434
  preoperative education, 431
Amebic liver abscesses, 1425
Amenorrhea, 1650, 1666, 1668
  primary, 1668
  secondary, 1668
America, death and dying in, 388
American Academy of Family Physicians (AFP), 1512
American Academy of Hospice and Palliative Medicine (AAHPM), 390
American Academy of Orthopaedic Surgeons (AAOS), 1131, 1186
American Association of Clinical Endocrinologists (AACE), 1512
American Association of Diabetes Educators (AADE), 1476
American Association of Nurse Anesthetists, 439
American Board of Internal Medicine (ABIM), 1161
American Cancer Society (ACS), 325, 331, 331c, 333t, 388
American College of Cardiology and the American Heart Association (ACC/AHA), 753
American College of Emergency Physicians (ACEP), 2158
American College of Foot and Ankle Surgeons (ACFAS), 1166
American College of Obstetricians and Gynecologists (ACOG), 130
American College of Rheumatology, 1094, 1099, 1109
American College of Surgeons (ACS), 2162, 2194
American Diabetes Association (ADA), 755
American Joint Replacement Registry (AJRR), 1145

American Nurses Association (ANA), 1214
  Center for Ethics and Human Rights, position
      statements from, 32c
  on characteristic of nursing practice, 11
  Code of Ethics for Nurses, 32, 32c
  nursing, definition of, 5, 32
  Nursing's Social Policy Statement, 32
  Scope and Standards of Practice, 35
American Pain Society (APS), 225
American Red Cross, 2195
American Society for Parenteral and Enteral
      Nutrition (ASPEN), 1250
American Society of Anesthesiologists (ASA),
      439
American Society of Clinical Oncology
      (ASCO), 342
American Society of Hematology, 950
American Society of Hypertension (ASH), 884
American Society of PeriAnesthesia Nurses
      (ASPAN), 419, 438
Americans With Disabilities Act, 25
American Thyroid Association (ATA), 1512
American Urological Association (AUA)
      Symptom Index, 1763
Amiloride (Midamor), for hypertension, 890t
Amine hormones, 1504
Aminocaproic acid (Amicar), 947, 950, 953,
      956
Aminosalicylates, for inflammatory bowel
      disease, 1332
Amiodarone
  for atrial fibrillation, 724
  in cardiopulmonary resuscitation, 839t
  for heart failure, 826
  for ventricular fibrillation, 731
Amitriptyline (Elavil), 1087, 1096, 1109, 1197
  in low back pain treatment, 1161
AML. See Acute myeloid leukemia
Amlodipine (Norvasc)
  for angina, 758t, 759
  for hypertension, 893t
Ammonia conversion, role of liver in, 1379
Ammonia, in hepatic encephalopathy, 1394
Ammonium chloride, 1387
Amoxicillin (Amoxil)
  for gastritis, 1295t
  for urinary tract infections, 1619t
Amoxicillin–clavulanate (Augmentin), 1818
Amphiarthrosis joints, 1117
Ampicillin (Principen, Omnipen), for urinary
      tract infections, 1619t
Amputation, 1185, 1214–1220, 1214c, 1215f
  complications, 1215
  defined, 1214
  levels of, 1214–1215
  medical management, 1215
  nursing process, 1216–1220
  patient with, 1219c
  rehabilitation, 1215–1216
Amsler grid testing, 1882
Amylase, 1224, 1226, 1428, 1429
Amyl nitrate pearls, 2208
Amyloid precursor protein, 211
Amyotrophic lateral sclerosis (ALS), 2091
Anagliflozin (Invokana), 1475t
Anagrelide (Agrylin), 985, 987
Anakinra (Kineret), 1089t, 1108
Analgesia
  agents for, 235–244
  groups of, 234

  multimodal, 233–245
  patient-controlled, 234–235
  PRN dosing, 234
  in snakebites, 2176
Anaphylactic shock, 296, 318–319
  medical management, 319
  nursing management, 319
  risk factors, 314c
Anaphylaxis, 1061, 1064–1066
  anesthesia related, 450
  clinical manifestations, 1065
  common causes of, 1065, 1065c
  medical management, 1066
  nursing management, 1066, 1067c
  pathophysiology, 1064–1065
  prevention, 1065–1066
Anaplasia, 324
Anasarca, 264
Anastomosis, 841, 859
Anastrozole (Arimidex), 1732, 1743, 1744t
ANC. See Absolute neutrophil count
Androgen deprivation therapy (ADT), 1752,
      1765, 1770
Androgens, 1502, 1531, 1532, 1653
Anemia, 906, 925–944
  acute kidney injury and, 1578
  aplastic, 932–933
  assessment and diagnostic findings, 927
  of chronic disease, 1557
  cirrhosis and, 1407
  classification of, 925–926, 926t
  clinical manifestations, 926–927
  complications, 927
  definition of, 925
  end-stage kidney disease and, 1582, 1583
  hemolytic, 926, 934–944
  hypoproliferative, 926, 930–934
  immune hemolytic, 943–944
  of inflammation, 932
  iron deficiency, 930–931
  management, 927
  megaloblastic, 933–934
  nursing process, 928–930
    assessment, 928
    diagnosis, 928
    evaluation, 929–930
    nursing interventions, 929
    planning and goals, 929
    potential complications, 928
  in older adults, 927, 932
  pallor in, 928, 928f
  in renal disease, 931–932
  sickle cell, 935–941
  thalassemias, 941–942
Anesthesia
  adverse effects of, 437c
  agents, 448t
    administration of, 444–445
    anaphylaxis, 450
    description of, 436
    doses for older adults, 437
    gas, 444
    inhalation, 444, 444t
    intravenous, 446t–447t
  awareness, 449
  definition of, 436, 443
  delivery methods, 445f
  general, 443–445
  informed consent, 422–423
  intrapleural, 466

  intravenous, 444–445
  local, 243–244, 449
  monitored care, 436, 449
  paravertebral, 448
  perioperative nursing and, 419
  regional, 445–448
  types of, 443–449
Anesthesiologist, 436, 439–440
Aneuploidy, 122
Aneurysm, 841, 849, 862–865, 862f, 2009, 2017,
      2026, 2026f
  abdominal aortic, 863–864
  etiologic classification, 862c
  fusiform, 862
  mycotic, 862
  popliteal artery, 865
  saccular, 862
  thoracic aortic, 862–863
Aneurysmal (widening) bone cysts, 1180
Anger
  emergency care and, 2159
  stages of grief, 410t
Angina pectoris, 757–762
  assessment of, 758, 760, 760c
  chest pain, assessing, 681t
  clinical manifestations, 758
  definition of, 750, 751, 757
  diagnosis, 758, 761
  evaluation, 762
  home care checklist, 762c
  medical management of
    oxygen therapy, 760
    pharmacologic therapy, 758–760, 758t
  nursing interventions, 761
  nursing process, 760–762
  pathophysiology, 757–758
  patient goals, 761
  types of, 757c
Angiogenesis, 987
  cancer invasion and, 326
  definition of, 324
Angiography, 849
  cerebral, 1967–1968
  coronary CT, 701
  eye, 1882
  magnetic resonance, 701–702
Angiomas, 1833
Angioneurotic edema, 1076
Angioplasty, 841, 852
Angiotensin-converting enzyme (ACE), 256,
      820, 844
  for atrial fibrillation, 724
Angiotensin I, 844
Angiotensin II, 820, 844, 1531–1532, 1552,
      1553
Angiotensin receptor blockers (ARBs)
  for atrial fibrillation, 724
  for heart failure, 824t, 825
  for hypertension, 892t
Angiotensin system inhibitors, in cirrhosis, 1408
Animal and human bites, 2175–2176
Ankle-brachial index (ABI), 841, 847–848, 848c
Ankylosing spondylitis (AS), 1106
Ankylosis, 1107
Annexin V, 962
Annuloplasty, 798, 798f
Anorectal disorders, 1350
  anal fissure, 1351, 1351f
  anal fistula, 1351, 1351f
  anorectal abscess, 1351

hemorrhoids, 1351–1352
    nursing management, 1352–1353
        continuing and transitional care, 1353
        patient education, 1352–1353
    pilonidal sinus or cyst, 1352, 1352f
    proctitis, 1350
Anorectal manometry, 1240, 1313
Anorexia, 1143
    management of, 405t
    mouth blindness and, 371
    nursing management, 371
    pharmacologic agents for, 405–406
    serious illness and, 405–406
Anoscopy, 1239–1240
ANP. See Atrial natriuretic peptide
ANS. See Autonomic nervous system
Antacids
    drug interactions, 205
    magnesium-based, 278
    phosphorus binding by, 279
Anterior chamber, 1876, 1877
Anterior cord syndrome, 2081c
Anterior cruciate ligament (ACL), 1188
Anthracyclines, 345–346
Anthrax, 2204
    clinical manifestations of, 2204
    treatment of, 2204–2205
Antibiotics
    and C. difficile. infection, 2132
    drug interactions, 428t
    for pelvic inflammatory disease, 1696
    for peritonitis, 1323
    for total knee arthroplasty, 1154
Antibodies, 1009–1010, 1010t, 1057, 1058
Antibody differentiation tests, 1032
Antibody response, 1007
Anticholinergics, 640, 641t, 656, 661t
Anticoagulant therapy
    for angina, 758t
    drug interactions, 428t
    low-dose, 2054
    thrombosis and, 963–965
Anticonvulsants, 244, 428t, 2000t
Anti-D (WinRho), 950
Antidepressants
    analgesia and, 244
    in irritable bowel syndrome, 1318
Antidiabetic agents, oral, 1473, 1474t–1475t
Antidiuretic hormone (ADH), 85, 87, 89,
        257f, 1508, 1548, 1551–1552. See also
        Vasopressin
    function of, 256
    pituitary gland and, 256
    sodium imbalances and, 265
    and thirst mechanism, 256–257
Antiemetics, 460t
Antifungal agents, 2071
Antigenic determinant, 1010
Antigen-presenting cells (APCs), 330
Antigens, 1007, 1058
    complete protein, 1058
    function of, 1058
    low–molecular-weight substances, 1058
    recognition, 1008–1009
Antihistamines, 701, 1059
    for allergic rhinitis, 1068, 1069t
    for asthma, 640
    long-acting control medications, 656, 658t
    oral, 1812
    systemic, 664

Antileukotrienes, 660
Antimetabolites, 343t
Antineoplastic agents, 343t
    oral, 356t–357t
        promoting adherence to, 356t–357t
        risk for infection, 358c
Antiparkinsonian medications, 2103
Antiphospholipid syndrome, 962
Antiplatelet medications, for angina, 758t, 760
Antiretroviral therapy (ART), 1025, 1033
    adverse effects with, 1033, 1034t–1035t,
        1037, 1037f
    antiretroviral agents, 1033, 1034t–1035t
    drug resistance, 1037
    promoting adherence to, 1036c
Antiseizure medication, drug interactions, 428t
Antithrombin (AT) deficiency, 959, 961
Antithymocyte globulin (ATG), 932, 933
Antithyroid antibody titers, 1513
Antithyroid medications (thionamides), 1521,
        1521t
Anti-TNF therapy, for psoriatic arthritis, 1107
Antitumor antibiotics, 343t
Antivenin, 2156, 2176–2177
    administration of, 2176–2177
    in black widow spider bites, 2177
Antiviral therapy, 2136
Antrectomy, 1292, 1299
Anuria, 818, 829, 1548, 1556t, 1567, 1576
Anus, 1224, 1225, 1225f
Anxiety, 685, 2102
    and ACS, 769–770
    dyspnea and, 404
    dysrhythmia and, 735
    emergency care and, 2159
    expressions of fear, 427
    in postanesthesia units, 459–460
    preoperative, 427
    reduction of, 213–214, 301, 431, 452
AOM. See Acute otitis media
Aorta, 842
Aortic area, 689
Aortic regurgitation, 794–795
Aortic stenosis, 795–796
Aortobifemoral graft, 861
Aortoiliac disease, 861
Aortoiliac endarterectomy, 859, 859f
Aortoiliac graft, 861
Apathy, 1041
Aphasia, 1959t, 2009, 2017, 2023c
Apheresis, 913–914, 913t
Aphonia, 552
Aphthous stomatitis, 1266t
Apixaban (Eliquis), 683, 965
    for venous thromboembolism, 870t, 871
Aplasia, bone marrow, 932
Aplastic anemia, 932–933
    assessment and diagnostic findings, 932
    clinical manifestations, 932
    medical management, 932–933
    nursing management, 933
    pathophysiology, 932
Apligraf, 876
Apnea, 495, 552, 567–569
    definition of, 480
    patterns, 496t
Apocrine sweat glands, 1792–1793
Apoptosis, 821, 1007
    definition of, 324
    initiation of, 326

Appendectomy, 1324
Appendicitis, 1323–1325
    assessment and diagnostic findings, 1324
    clinical manifestations, 1323–1324, 1324f
    complications of, 1324
    medical management, 1324
    nursing management, 1324–1325
    in older adults, 1324
    pathophysiology, 1323
Appendix, perforated, 1324, 1325
Appetite, stimulation of, 405–406
Applied ethics, 31
Apraxia, 2009, 2011
Apremilast (Otezla), 1107
Aqueous humor, 1876, 1877, 1890, 1890f
ARDS. See Acute respiratory distress syndrome
Argatroban, 963
    for venous thromboembolism, 870t
Arginine vasopressin (AVP), 264
Arginine, wound healing and, 425t
Argon laser photocoagulation, for diabetic
        retinopathy, 1491
ARN. See Association of Rehabilitation Nurses
ARN Competency Model for Professional
        Rehabilitation Nurses, 164–165
Aromatase inhibitors, 1705, 1719, 1743–1744,
        1744t
Arrhythmogenic right ventricular
        cardiomyopathy/dysplasia, 803
Arsenic trioxide (Trisenox), 343t
ART. See Antiretroviral therapy
Arterial blood gas (ABG), 502, 2169
Arterial disorders, 850
    aneurysms, 862–865
    aortoiliac disease, 861
    arterial embolism and arterial thrombosis,
        865–867
    arteriosclerosis and atherosclerosis, 850–857
    dissecting aorta, 865
    peripheral arterial occlusive disease, 857–860
    Raynaud phenomenon, 867–868
    upper extremity arterial occlusive disease,
        860–861
Arterial dissections, 865
Arterial embolism and arterial thrombosis,
        865–867
    assessment and diagnostic findings, 866
    clinical manifestations, 865–866
    endovascular management, 866, 866f
    nursing management, 867
    pathophysiology, 865
    pharmacologic therapy, 866–867
Arteries, 842
    walls of, 842
Arterioles, 842
Arteriosclerosis, 841, 850–857. See also
        Atherosclerosis
Arteriovenous fistula (AVF), 1567, 1590–1591,
        1591f
Arteriovenous graft, 1591
Arteriovenous malformation (AVM), 2026,
        2026F
Arthritis, 1082, 1114–1115
Arthrocentesis, 1095, 1128
Arthrodesis, 1095
Arthrography, 1127
Arthroplasty, 1106
Arthroscope, 1185, 1188
Arthroscopic synovectomy, 1164
Artifact, 712

Artificial insemination, 1678
Artificial larynx, 575
Artificial urinary sphincter, 1626
Arytenoid cartilages, 482
Asbestosis, 583
Ascites, 264, 818, 1377, 1382, 1385–1388
    assessment and diagnostic findings, 1386
        abdominal fluid wave, assessment for, 1386,
            1386f
        ballottement technique, 1386, 1386f
    cirrhosis and, 1406–1407
    clinical manifestations, 1386
    home care checklist, 1388c
    medical management, 1386
        bed rest, 1387
        nutritional therapy, 1386
        paracentesis, 1387
        peritoneovenous shunt, 1388
        pharmacologic therapy, 1386–1387
        transjugular intrahepatic portosystemic
            shunt, 1387, 1387f
    nursing management, 1388
    pathophysiology, 1385, 1385f
    patient education, 1388
ASCO. See American Society of Clinical
        Oncology
Asepsis, surgical, 441–442
Asparaginase (Elspar), 343t, 976
Aspartate aminotransferase (AST), 1382
Aspergillus fumigatus, 2070
Aspiration, 583, 599–600, 1243, 1244
    pathophysiology, 599
    pneumonia, 589
    prevention, 599–600, 599c
    risk factors, 599c
Aspiration pneumonia, 1246–1247
Aspirin, 680, 683, 938, 965, 986, 1677c
    for angina, 758t, 760
    function of, 426
    in rheumatic diseases, 1088t
    in total hip arthroplasty treatment, 1152
    for vascular disease, 859
Assessment
    altered elimination patterns, 186
    biochemical, 77
    body mass index, 76–77
    end-of-life care, 400f
    focused, 73–74
    of functional ability, 167–188
    of hospitalized postoperative patient, 463–464
    mobility limitations, 168c
    in nursing process, 35, 36c, 37
        data recording, 38
        health history, 37
        other information, 38
        physical assessment, 37–38
    nutritional, 76–79, 80t
    of older adults, 194, 195
    pain, 230–233
    of respiratory function, 480–508, 500–502
    self-care deficits, 168, 168c
    spiritual, 402
    terminal illness, 403c
Assisted living facilities, 204
Assisted reproductive technologies, 1678
Assisted suicide, 387, 390
Assistive devices, 165, 169f
    ambulation using, 174–175
    in cardiogenic shock, 312
    definition of, 164

nursing actions in use of, 177t
    purpose of, 165
    recommending, 169–170
Association for Professionals in Infection
        Control and Epidemiology (APIC), 441
Association of Operating Room Nurses, 419
Association of PeriOperative Registered Nurses
        (AORN), 419, 438, 440, 441, 442
Association of Rehabilitation Nurses (ARN),
        164
Asterixis, 1377, 1380
    in hepatic encephalopathy, 1395, 1395f
Asthma, 500t, 634, 654–664
    assessment, 655–656
    clinical manifestations, 655
    comorbidities, 658t
    complications, 656
    continuing/transitional care, 664
    deaths from, 654
    diagnostic findings, 655–656
    exacerbations, management of, 660–661
    immunoglobulin E (IgE), 655
    long-term medications for treatment,
        658t–660t
    medical management, 656
        long-acting control medications, 656–660
        pharmacologic treatment, 656
        quick-relief medications, 656
    nursing management, 663
    pathophysiology, 654f, 655
    peak flow monitoring, 661–663, 663c
    prevention, 656
    promoting home/community-based/
        transitional care, 663
    quick-relief medications for treatment, 661,
        661t
    stepwise approach for managing, 657f
Astigmatism, 1876
Astrocytomas, 2092, 2092c
Ataxia, 1946, 1961, 2074
Atazanavir (ATV), 1034t
Atelectasis, 465, 500t, 539c, 583, 584–586, 654,
        656, 1143
    assessment, 584
    clinical manifestations, 584
    collaborative problem, 652t
    diagnostic findings, 584
    management, 585–586
    pathophysiology, 584
    prevention, 584–585, 585c
Atenolol (Tenormin)
    for angina, 758t
    for hypertension, 891t
Atherectomy, 841, 852
Atheroma, 750, 751, 850
Atherosclerosis, 751, 841, 850–857
    clinical manifestations, 852
    collateral circulation, development of, 851
    coronary arteries, 699
    definition of, 750
    development and progression, 695
    development of, 751f
    diabetes-related, 1489
    fatty streaks, 850
    fibrous plaques, 850
    gender considerations, 678
    lipoproteins and development of, 754f
    nursing management, 852–857
    in older adults, 857
    pathophysiology, 850

prevention, 852
    progression of, 850f
    radiologic interventions, 852
    risk factors, 851–852, 851c
    self-care program, 857
    surgical management, 852
ATN. See Acute tubular necrosis
Atonic muscle, 1119
Atopic dermatitis, 1074–1075
Atopic dermatitis/eczema syndrome (AEDS), 1075
Atopy, 1058, 1064
Atorvastatin (Lipitor), 756t
Atracurium besylate (Tracrium), 446t
Atrial depolarization, 696
Atrial dysrhythmias, 720–727
    atrial fibrillation, 720–726
    atrial flutter, 726–727
    premature atrial complex, 720, 722f
Atrial fibrillation, 699, 720–726, 723f
    assessment of, 723
    cardiac rhythm therapies, 725–726
        catheter ablation therapy, 725
        convergent procedure, 725–726
        maze and mini-maze procedures, 725
    characteristics of, 722
    classification system, 723c
    diagnostic findings, 723
    electrical cardioversion for, 725
    left atrial appendage and, 722, 726
    medical management of, 723–725
    pulmonary veins, 701
    pulse deficits, 688, 722
    risk factors in, 722, 723c
    stroke risk assessment in, 724c
    uncertainty among couples with, 736c
    Wolff–Parkinson–White syndrome and, 726
Atrial flutter, 688, 726–727
Atrial natriuretic peptide (ANP), 258, 258f, 821
Atrioventricular (AV), 675
    node, 675, 694t
    opening snaps, 691
    valves, 675
Atrioventricular nodal reentry tachycardia
        (AVNRT), 728–729, 728f
Atrophic gastritis, 1240
Atrophy, 1799t
Atropine, 1237
    in cardiopulmonary resuscitation, 839t
    secretion management and, 409t
Attire, operating room, 440–441, 442
Atypical hyperplasia, 1719, 1729
Audiometry, 1922
Auditory brain stem response, 1922
Auditory canal, external, 1916
Augmentation mammoplasty, 1749
Aural rehabilitation, 1938–1941
Auricle, 1916
Auriculotemporal syndrome. See Frey syndrome
Auscultation, 74f, 521
    abnormal heart sounds, 690–691
    breath sounds, 667
    definition of, 62, 74
    interpretation, 692
    normal heart sounds, 690
    procedure, 692
    thoracic, 498–500
Australasian Society of Clinical Immunology
        and Allergy (ASCIA), 423, 450
Autografts, 800, 1185, 1196
    description, 1845, 1863–1864, 1864f

graft sites, 1864
   wound grafting, 1863–1864, 1864f
Autoimmune disorders, 1017
Autoimmune lymphoproliferative syndrome
   (ALPS), 1024t
Autoimmune polyglandular syndrome type 1
   (APS-1), 1024t
Autoimmune thyroiditis, 1514
Autoimmunity, 1083
Auto-injector system, 1065
Autologous bone marrow transplantation, 2096
Autologous HSCT (AuHSCT), 349, 350
Autologous transfusions, 915–916
Autologous vaccines, 354
Autolytic débridement, 1807
Automated external defibrillators (AEDs), 737,
   838
Automaticity, 712
Autonomic dysreflexia, 2055, 2057
Autonomic nervous system (ANS)
   anatomy of, 952–954, 1954f
   effects of, 1955t
Autonomic neuropathy, 1493–1494
   clinical manifestations, 1493
   hypoglycemic unawareness and, 1493
   management, 1494
   sexual dysfunction and, 1494
   sudomotor neuropathy, 1494
   and urinary retention, 1493
Autonomy, 31c
   acknowledgement of, 389
   definition of, 387
Autosomal dominant inheritance, 114, 119–120
Autosomal recessive inheritance, 114, 120
Autosomes, 117
Auvi-Q, 1065
Avascular necrosis (AVN), 1131, 1144, 1185, 1186
   of bone, 1197
Avian influenza (bird flu), 2135
AVM. *See* Arteriovenous malformation
AVNRT. *See* Atrioventricular nodal reentry
   tachycardia
Avoidance therapy, for allergic rhinitis, 1068
Avonex, 2075
Avulsions, 2134
Awakening and Breathing Coordination, Delirium
   monitoring and management, Early
   mobility bundle (ABCDE), 533, 533c
Awareness contexts, 389
Axillary lymph node dissection (ALND), 1733
   hand and arm care after, 1737c
   and lymphedema, 1737
   sentinel lymph node biopsy and, 1734t
Azacitidine (Vidaza), 973, 983
5-Azacytidine (Vidaza), 343t
Azathioprine (Imuran), 943, 1095, 1610t, 2080
   for bullous pemphigoid, 1828
   for pemphigus vulgaris, 1828
   for rheumatic diseases, 1088t, 1095
   in rheumatic diseases, 1088t
   in SLE nephritis, 1100
Azelaic acid (Azelex), for acne vulgaris, 1815
Azilsartan (Edarbi), for hypertension, 892t
Azithromycin (Zithromax), 2152
   for gonorrhea, 1694
   for rape consequences, 2189
Azoospermia, 1678
Azotemia, 1567, 1570–1571
   with hypervolemia, 263
Aztreonam (AZLI), 666

B
Babinski reflex, 1915, 1954
Bacille Calmette–Guérin (BCG), 352, 1638
Bacillus anthracis, 2204
Baclofen (Lioresal), 2061, 2111
Bacteremia, 2133
   catheter-related, 2133
   definition of, 2133
Bacteria
   carcinogenesis and, 327–328
   gram-negative, 376
   gram-positive, 376
Bacterial infection, biologic spectrum, 2129
Bacterial peritonitis, cirrhosis and, 1407
Bacterial vaginosis, 1688–1689, 1688t, 1695
   clinical manifestations, 1689
   medical management, 1689
   risk factors, 1689
Bacteriuria, 1548, 1556t, 1561, 1615, 1617,
   1630–1631
Bad breath. *See* Halitosis
BAERs. *See* Brainstem auditory evoked responses
BAHA. *See* Bone-anchored hearing aid
BAL (bioartificial liver), 1405
Balanced suspension traction, 1140, 1140f
Ball-and-socket joints, 1117
Balloon sign test, 1124, 1125f
Balloon tamponade, for variceal bleeding,
   1390–1391
Balloon valvuloplasty, 797–798, 797f
Ballottement technique, 1386, 1386f
Bandages. *See also* Dressings
   drainage-soaked, 465
   sterile gauze, 465
Band cells, 906
Bargaining, stages of grief, 410t
Bariatric surgery, 418, 421, 1358, 1368–1369
   and bile reflux, 1373
   bowel/gastric outlet obstruction after, 1373
   and dietary guidelines, 1372c
   dumping syndrome and, 1373
   and dysphagia, 1373
   hemorrhage after, 1372
   nursing process, 1369, 1371–1374
      anastomotic leaks and, 1371–1372
      anxiety reduction, 1371
      assessment, 1369, 1371
      body image changes, 1372
      bowel habits maintenance, 1372
      complications management, 1372–1373
      continuing and transitional care,
         1373–1374
      diagnosis, 1371
      dietary restrictions, 1371
      evaluation, 1374
      fluid volume balance, 1371
      infection prevention, 1371
      nursing interventions, 1371–1374
      nutritional status, 1372
      pain relief, 1371
      patient education, 1373
      planning and goals, 1371
   selection criteria for, 1369, 1369c
   type of procedures, 1369, 1370f
   and venous thromboembolism, 1373
Baroreceptors, 677
Barrel chest, 495, 637
Barrett esophagus (BE), 1283–1284
   assessment and diagnostic findings, 1283
   clinical manifestations, 1283

   GERD and, 1283
   management, 1284
Barthel Index, 167
Bartholin cyst, 1686, 1702
Bartholin glands, 1651
Basal cell carcinoma (BCC), 1834–1836, 1834f
Basal ganglia, 2102
Basal insulin, 1468
Basal metabolic rate, 1502, 1509
Baseline body temperature, for older adults, 217
Basophils, 906, 907
Battery-powered pulse generator, 2104
B cells. *See* B lymphocytes
BCG Live (TheraCys), 1638–1639
BE. *See* Barrett esophagus
Beau lines, 1801
Beclomethasone, 1541t
Beclomethasone propionate (QVAR), 642t,
   658t
Bed rest
   in ascites, 1387
   hepatitis A and, 1399
Behavioral therapy, for urinary incontinence,
   1624–1626, 1625c
Belatacept (Nulojix), 1610t
Beliefs
   cultural
      on death and dying, 396t–397t
      preoperative assessments, 427–428
      respect for, 431
   end-of-life care, 400c
   religious
      on death and dying, 396t–397t
      end-of-life care and, 388
      respect for, 431
   spiritual
      preoperative assessments, 427–428
      respect for, 431
Belimumab (Benlysta), for systemic lupus
   erythematosus, 1100
Bell palsy, 2085, 2088–2089
Below-knee amputation (BKA), 1214
Benazepril (Lotensin), for hypertension, 892t
Beneficence, 31c
Benign bone tumors, 1179–1180
Benign, definition of, 324, 326
Benign paroxysmal positional vertigo, 1934
Benign proliferative breast disease, 1719, 1729
   atypical hyperplasia, 1729
   lobular carcinoma in situ, 1729
Benign prostatic hyperplasia (BPH), 1554, 1752,
   1754, 1762–1764. *See also* Prostate surgery
   assessment and diagnostic findings, 1763
   clinical manifestations, 1763
   medical management, 1763–1764
   minimally invasive therapy, 1763–1764
   pathophysiology, 1762–1763
   pharmacologic treatment, 1763
   surgical resection of prostate gland, 1764
Benign skin tumors
   actinic keratoses, 1833
   angiomas, 1833
   cysts, 1833
   dermatofibroma, 1833
   keloids, 1833
   moles, 1833
   seborrheic keratoses, 1833
   Von Recklinghausen disease, 1833
   warts, 1833
Benson relaxation response, 98, 98c

Benzodiazepines, 407, 2075, 2109, 2173, 2188
  for alcohol withdrawal syndrome, 2185
Benzphetamine (Didrex), for obesity, 1365t
Bereavement
  definition of, 387, 410
  loss and, 410
Beta-adrenergic blockers, 2075
  for angina, 758t, 759
Beta₂-agonists, 272, 640
  long-acting, 640
  short-acting, 640
Beta-blockers
  for heart failure, 824t, 825
  for hypertension, 891t
  for hyperthyroidism, 1521t, 1522
  for pheochromocytoma, 1533
  for variceal bleeding, 1390
Beta cells, 1457
Beta-human chorionic gonadotropin (beta-
      hCG), 1780
Betamethasone, 1541t
Beta-2 microglobulin, 976–977
Betaxolol (Kerlone), for hypertension, 891t
Bethanechol (Urecholine)
  for GERD, 1284t
  for neurogenic bladder, 1628
Bezoars, 1327
Bicarbonate deficit, 1568t
Bicarbonate excess, 1568t
Biceps reflex, 1963
Bilateral pelvic lymphadenectomy, for cervical
      cancer, 1707c
Bile, 1378, 1429
  formation, 1379
Bile acid sequestrants, 756t
Bile reflux
  bariatric surgery and, 1373
  gastric surgery and, 1305
Bilevel positive airway pressure (BiPAP), 510
Biliary cirrhosis, 1406. See also Cirrhosis
Biliary colic, gallstone and, 1431–1432
Biliary disorders, 1428–1454
Biliopancreatic diversion with duodenal switch,
      1369
Bilirubin, 1379, 1429
  excretion of, 1379
Billroth II procedure, 1301t, 1304
Billroth I procedure, 1300t, 1304
Bimanual palpation, 1662
Binocular vision, 1876, 1895, 1903
Bioavailability, 1379–1380
Biobrane®, 1864, 1865f
Biochemical assessment, 77
Biochemical mediators, 296, 297
Biofeedback, 187, 1313, 1317
Biologic response modifier (BRM), 352–354. See
      also Immunomodulators
  monoclonal antibodies, 352–353
  nonspecific, 352
Biologic therapies
  for inflammatory bowel disease, 1332
  for psoriasis, 1826
Biologic weapon, 2193, 2203–2206, 2205t
  categories of, 2204t
  effects of, 2204
  types of, 2204–2206
Biomarkers, cardiac, 693
Bioprostheses, 800
Biopsy
  bone, 1129

liver, 1382
lung, 507–508
skin, 1803–1804
types of
  core needle aspiration, 335–336
  excisional, 335
  fine-needle aspiration, 335
  incisional, 335
  needle, 335
  sentinel lymph node, 335
Biot's respiration patterns, 495, 496t
Bird flu, 2135
Birds, reservoir for virus, 2150
Bisacodyl (Dulcolax), 1314t
Bismuth subsalicylate (Pepto-Bismol), for
      gastritis, 1295t
Bisoprolol (Zebeta)
  for heart failure, 824t
  for hypertension, 891t
Bisphosphonates, in Paget disease, 1175
Bites
  animal, 2127t
  mosquito, 2150
Black widow spider bites, 2177
Bladder cancer, 1637–1639
  assessment and diagnostic findings, 1638
  clinical manifestations, 1638
  pharmacologic therapy, 1638–1639
  radiation therapy, 1639
  risk factors, 1638c
  surgical management, 1638
Bladder compliance, 1553
Bladder distention, 472, 693
Bladder emptying, 1554
Bladder retraining, 1625c
Bladder training, 187
Bladder trauma, 1637
Bladder ultrasonography, 1558, 1562, 1563f
Blast cells, 907, 972
Blast injury
  explosive devices, types of, 2202–2203
  physical injuries, 2203, 2203t
  special populations, 2203
Blast lung, 2203
Blastomyces dermatitidis, 2070
Bleeding, after liver transplantation, 1422–1423
Bleeding disorders, 947
  clinical manifestations, 947, 947f
  medical management, 947
  nursing management, 947–948
  risk factors, 947c
Bleomycin (Blenoxane), 343t, 346
  for corn treatment, 1167
Blindness, 1846–1850
  definition, 1876
  interaction with people, 1886c
Blistering diseases, 1827–1832
  bullous pemphigoid, 1828
  care of patient with, 1829–1830
  dermatitis herpetiformis, 1828
  pemphigus vulgaris, 1827–1828
  Stevens-Johnson syndrome, 1830–1832
  toxic epidermal necrolysis, 1830–1832
Blood, 903
  cells, 903, 905–907
    erythrocytes (red blood cells), 905–906,
      905f
    leukocytes (white blood cells), 906–907
    platelets (thrombocytes), 907
  exposure to, 442–443

function of, 903
  plasma and plasma proteins, 908
Blood agents, 2208
  clinical manifestation, 2208
  treatment, 2208
Blood-brain barrier (BBR), 1950–1951, 2066,
      2067, 2069, 2071, 2096
Blood donation, 914
  autologous donation, 915–916
  blood processing after, 916–917
  complications of, 916
  directed donations, 915
  hemodilution, 916
  intraoperative blood salvage, 916
  standard donation, 915
Blood flow, 843
Blood gas
  analysis, 287–288
  assessment of, 289c
  measurements, 638, 709
Blood glucose monitoring, 1466–1467
Blood pressure, 885, 2068
  autoregulation of, 1553
  intra-arterial monitoring, 705, 709
  measurement of, 894, 894c
  measurements, 709
  postural changes, 685
  systemic arterial, 687
Blood transfusion. See Transfusion
Blood urea nitrogen (BUN)
  hypovolemia and, 259
  laboratory testing, 255
  reference range, 694t
  reference ranges, 694t
Blunt trauma, 626–628, 2136–2137, 2169
  assessment, 626
  diagnostic findings, 626
  medical management, 626–627
  pathophysiology, 626
B lymphocytes, 903, 907, 1005, 1006f
  role of, 1058
BMI. See Body mass index
BNP. See Brain natriuretic peptide
Body fluids
  amount of, 252–253
  composition of, 252–253, 253t
  exposure to, 432, 442–443
  gains and losses, routes of, 254, 254t
  regulation of, 253, 257f
  status of, evaluation of, 255–256
Body mass index (BMI), 682, 1358, 1361, 1361f,
      1361t, 2097
  calculation of, 76c
  definition of, 62
  nutritional assessment and, 76–80
Body temperature
  cardiac surgery and, 787
  maintenance of, 469
Boerhaave syndrome, 1264, 1282
Bolus feedings, 1243, 1246, 1249, 1249f
Bone-anchored hearing aid (BAHA), 1940
Bone densitometry, 1127
Bone integrity, assessment of, 1124
Bone marrow, 903–905, 1005, 1116
  aspiration and biopsy, 910, 912–913, 912f
  failure, 982
Bone mineral density (BMD), 127, 1169
Bones, 1115
  blood supply, 1116
  cells, 1115

flat, 1115
formation, 1116
healing, 1117
irregular, 1115
long, 1115, 1115f
maintenance, 1116–1117
periosteum, 1115–1116
resorption, 1116
short, 1115
Bone scan, 1127–1128
and blood studies, 1161c
Bone tumors, 1179–1183, 1182c
assessment and diagnostic findings, 1180–1181
benign, 1179–1180
clinical manifestations, 1180
malignant, 1180
medical management, 1181
metastatic, 1180
nursing management, 1181–1183
pathophysiology, 1180
Borderline tumors, 1713
Bortezomib (Velcade), 996
Bosentan (Tracleer), 1102
Boston Marathon bombing, 2193
Botulinum toxin (Botox) injections
in achalasia, 1279
in anal fissures, 1351
Bougienage procedure, 1282
Boundaries, anticipatory mourning and, 411c
Bowel function, promotion of, 472
Bowel habits, change in, 1230
Bowel preparation, preoperative, 432
Bowel training programs, 1317, 2061
Bowman capsule, 1550
Boxer's fracture, 1200
BPH. *See* Benign prostatic hyperplasia
Braces, 1131, 1133–1136
home care checklist, 1136c
immobilized lower extremity, 1136–1137
immobilized upper extremity, 1136
nursing management of patient, 1133–1136
Brachial plexus block, 448
Brachioradialis reflex, 1963
Brachytherapy, 1686, 1719, 1752
for breast cancer, 1741
for cervical cancer, 1708
definition of, 324
delivery of, 340
high-dose radiation, 340
interstitial implants, 340
low-dose radiation, 340
for prostate cancer, 1765, 1769–1770
for vaginal cancers, 1711–1712
Bracketing, 29
Bradykinesia, 2102
Bradykinin, 655, 1059
Bradypnea patterns, 496t
Brain
abscesses, 2068, 2069
anatomy of, 1947–1949, 1948f
arterial blood supply, 1950f
circulation, 1950
protection of, 1949–1950, 1949f
Brain death
definition of, 1973
description, 1978
Brain Injury Association of America, 2044
Brain natriuretic peptide (BNP), 258, 695
Brain stem, 1949

Brainstem auditory evoked responses (BAERs), 1969
Brain tumors, 2092
classification of, 2092c
sites, 2094f
Branch retinal vein occlusion (BRVO), 1901
Bravo pH monitoring system, 1241
BRCA1 and *BRCA2*, 1719, 1731
Breakthrough pain (BTP), 226
Breast, 1720
anatomy of, 1720, 1720f
assessment, 1720–1721
health history, 1720
physical assessment, 1720–1721
diagnostic evaluation, 1721
breast self-examination, 1721, 1723
contrast mammography, 1725
magnetic resonance imaging, 1725–1726
mammography, 1723–1725, 1725f
ultrasonography, 1725
female breast examination, 1720–1721
abnormal breast findings on inspection, 1722c
inspection, 1721
palpation, 1721, 1723f
lymphatic drainage of, 1733f
male breast examination, 1721
obesity on, effect of, 1721
percutaneous biopsy, 1726–1727, 1726t
core needle biopsy, 1726
fine-needle aspiration, 1726
MRI-guided core biopsy, 1727
stereotactic core biopsy, 1726–1727
ultrasound-guided core biopsy, 1727
prosthesis, 1747
reconstruction, 1745–1747
latissimus dorsi flap, 1746f
nipple–areola reconstruction, 1747
with tissue expander, 1745–1746, 1746f
TRAM flap, 1746, 1746f
surgical biopsy, 1727
excisional biopsy, 1727
incisional biopsy, 1727
nursing management, 1727–1728
wire needle localization, 1727
tail of Spence, 1720, 1720f
Tanner stages of development, 1720
Breast cancer, 126t, 1730
adjuvant chemotherapy for, 1741–1743
chemotherapy regimens, 1742
dose-dense chemotherapy, 1742
hematopoietic growth factors, self-administration of, 1743c
indications for, 1741t
nursing management, 1742–1743, 1743c
side effects of, 1742
assessment and diagnostic findings, 1732
clinical manifestations, 1732
ductal carcinoma in situ, 1730
genetic testing, implications of, 1747
hormonal therapy for, 1743–1744, 1744c, 1744t
incidence of, 1730
invasive cancer, 1730
infiltrating ductal carcinoma, 1730
infiltrating lobular carcinoma, 1730
inflammatory carcinoma, 1730–1731
medullary carcinoma, 1730
mucinous carcinoma, 1730

Paget disease, 1731
tubular ductal carcinoma, 1730
in men, 1749–1750
nursing process, 1734–1740
assessment, 1734–1735
body image, positive, 1736
diagnosis, 1735
evaluation, 1740
hematoma formation and, 1737–1738
infection and, 1738
lymphedema and, 1736–1737
pain management, 1735–1736
patient preparation, 1735
planning and goals, 1735
positive adjustment and coping, 1736
postoperative nursing interventions, 1735–1740
postoperative sensations and, 1736
preoperative nursing interventions, 1735
sexual function, improving, 1736
in older women, 1748
patient education
drainage management at home, 1738c
exercise after breast surgery, 1739f
home care checklist, 1738c
pregnancy and, 1747–1748
prevention strategies, 1732
chemoprevention, 1732
long-term surveillance, 1732
prophylactic mastectomy, 1732
prognosis, 1733, 1733c
protective factors, 1732
quality of life and survivorship, 1748
radiation therapy for, 1740–1741
breast-conservation treatment and, 1741c
nursing management, 1741
side effects of, 1741
reconstructive surgery after mastectomy, 1745–1747
recurrent and metastatic, treatment of, 1744–1745
risk factors for, 1731–1732, 1731t
staging, 1732–1733
surgical management, 1733, 1733t
breast conservation treatment, 1734
modified radical mastectomy, 1733
sentinel lymph node biopsy, 1734
total mastectomy, 1733–1734
targeted therapies for, 1744
women with disabilities and, 1748
Breast conservation treatment, 1719
Breast disorders, 1720
benign proliferative breast disease, 1729
atypical hyperplasia, 1729
lobular carcinoma in situ, 1729
breast masses, 1728, 1729t
breast pain, 1728
cancer of breast, 1730–1748 (*See also* Breast cancer)
cystosarcoma phyllodes, 1729
cysts, 1728
fat necrosis, 1729
fibroadenomas, 1728–1729
fissure, 1728
intraductal papilloma, 1730
lactational abscess, 1728
mastitis, 1728
nipple discharge, 1728
superficial thrombophlebitis of breast, 1730
Breast reconstruction surgery. *See* Mammoplasty

Breast self-examination (BSE), 1721, 1723, 1724c
Breathing
   airway patency and, 1853
   assessment of, 493–500
   ataxic, 496
   deep, 429
   diaphragmatic, 430c
   exercises, 644
   patterns, 495, 645–646
   retraining, 521
Breath sounds, 498, 499t
Breath tests, 1233
Brentuximab vedotin (Adcetris), 990
Bristol Stool Form Scale (BSFS), 1318, 1319f
Bromocriptine (Parlodel), 1677c
   for pituitary tumors, 1509
Bronchi, anatomy, 483
Bronchiectasis, 648
   assessment/diagnostic findings, 648
   clinical manifestations, 648
   cystic fibrosis (CF), 634
   medical management, 648
   nursing management, 654
   pathophysiology, 648
Bronchioles, anatomy, 483
Bronchitis, 500t
Bronchoconstriction, 1852
Bronchodilators, 640
Bronchophony, 480, 500
Bronchoplastic resection, 538c
Bronchopulmonary infections, 646
Bronchoscopic lung volume reduction therapies, 643
Bronchoscopy
   complications of, 506
   definition of, 480
   endoscopic, 505–506, 506f
   nursing interventions, 506
   procedure, 505–506
Bronchospasm, airway clearance, 645
Brown recluse spider bites, 2177
Brudzinski sign, 2067
Bruit, 841
Brush biopsy, 1565
Brushing, teeth, 1268
Brussels, terrorist attacks in, 2193
BRVO. See Branch retinal vein occlusion
BSE. See Breast self-examination
BSFS. See Bristol Stool Form Scale
B-type natriuretic peptide (BNP), 821
Buck's extension traction, 1140–1141, 1140f, 1203
Budd–Chiari syndrome, 1393
Buddhism, 396t, 438
Budesonide (Pulmicort Flexhaler), 642t, 658t, 659t
Bulbar paralysis, 2084, 2086t
Bullae, 1798t, 1806, 1817
Bullectomy, 643
Bullous impetigo, 1817
Bullous pemphigoid, 1828
Bumetanide (Bumex), for hypertension, 890t
BUN. See Blood urea nitrogen
Bundle of His, 676, 679t
Bundles, of care, 9
Bupivacaine (Marcaine), 234, 448t
Bupropion (Wellbutrin), 207, 639
Buried bumper syndrome, 1255
Burn care, 1853t

Burn centers, 1848c
Burns
   acute/intermediate phase, 1853t, 1856–1868
   age, 1847
   age-related issues, 1846
   comfort care issues, 1855c
   complications, 1868t
   depth of, 1847–1848, 1847t, 1848f
   electrical, 1850c
   emergent care, 1857c–1859c
   extent of, 1848–1849
   first-degree, 1847–1848, 1847t
   fourth-degree, 1847t, 1848, 1848f
   home care checklist, 1871c–1872c
   incidence, 1845–1846
   infection prevention, 1860
   management of, 1853–1868
   memories of pain after, 1865
   ocular, 1905
   outpatient care, 1872
   overview, 1845–1853
   pain management, 1864, 1866
   pathophysiology, 1849–1853, 1851t
   prevention of, 1846, 1846c
   rehabilitation, 166, 1868–1872
   second-degree, 1847t, 1848
   severity, 1847–1849
   shock and, 1859
   supporting patient and family processes, 1867
   survival and recovery, outlook for, 1847
   third-degree, 1847t, 1848, 1848f
   topical antibacterial therapy for, 1860–1861, 1862t
   wound cleaning, 1860
   wound dressing, 1861–1862
Bursa, 1118
Bursitis, 1160, 1164
Busulfan (Busulfex, Myleran), 343t, 346
Butane honey oil (BHO), 2185

C
CAA. See Cerebral amyloid angiopathy
Cabazitaxel (Jevtana injection), 1765
Cachexia, 406
CACS. See Cancer-related anorexia-cachexia syndrome
CAD. See Coronary artery disease
Caffeine (Anacin), 700
Calcipotriene (Dovonex), for psoriasis, 1825
Calcitonin, 276, 1116, 1170, 1502, 1510
Calcitriol, 1116
Calcium acetate, 1583
Calcium alginate, 1809
   dressings, 876
Calcium and phosphorus binders, 1583
Calcium carbonate, 1583
   for GERD, 1284t
Calcium channel blockers
   for angina, 758t, 759
   for esophageal spasm, 1280
   for hypertension, 892t–893t
   for pheochromocytoma, 1533
Calcium deficit, 1568t
Calcium excess, 1568t
Calcium gluconate, 1530
Calcium imbalance, 272–276, 273t
   hypercalcemia, 275–276
   hypocalcemia, 273–275
Calcium stones, 1633. See also Nephrolithiasis
Calculous cholecystitis, 1430

Calf pain, 846
Calicivirus, 2144
Callus, 1166–1167
CAM. See Confusion Assessment Method
Camey procedure, 1643
Campylobacter species, 2082, 2138
Campylobacter transmission, 2138
Canadian Triage and Acuity Scale (CTAS), 2161
Canaliculi, 1379
Cancellous bone, 1115
Cancer
   advanced, 380–383
   age-related changes and, 380t
   biopsy types, 335–336
   body image, improvement of, 375
   care trajectory, 325f
   of cervix, 1706–1708
   classification of, 328t
   community-based care, 378–379
   complications in, 376–378
      infection, 376–377
      neutropenic fever, 376–377, 377t
      septic shock, 377
      thrombocytopenia, 377–378
   description of, 324, 325
   detection of, 330–333
   diagnosis of, 333–334, 334t
   emergencies, management of, 380–383, 381t–383t
   epidemiology of, 325
   of esophagus, 1286–1289
   of fallopian tube, 1712
   fatigue
      management of, 373–375
      sources of, 373c
   genetics of, 327c
   grading, 333–334
   grief, assistance during, 375
   hematopoietic stem cell transplantation, 348–351
   home care checklist, 378c
   home/transitional care, 379
   and immunotherapy, 1013–1014
   of liver, 1417–1420
   management of, 334–348
      chemotherapy, 341–348
      radiation therapy, 338–341
      surgical, 335–338, 336t
   nutrition, promotion of, 371–372
   of oral cavity and pharynx, 1270–1272
   of ovary, 1712–1713
   pain
      algorithm, 374f
      management of, 372–373, 373f
      sources of, 372, 372t
   of pancreas, 1450–1451
   pathophysiology of, 326–330
   of penis, 1784–1785
   plans of care, 358c–370c
   prevention of, 330–333, 331c
      primary, 331
      secondary, 331
      tertiary, 331–333
   proliferative patterns, 327–330
   of prostate, 1764–1771
   psychosocial distress management, 375
   screening guidelines, 333t–334t
   self-esteem, improvement of, 375
   sexuality-based issues, 375

skin, 1834, 1834c
staging, 333, 335c
survivorship care, 379–383, 380t
testicular, 1779–1782
TNM classification system, 335c
of uterus, 1708–1709, 1709c
vaccines, 354
of vagina, 1711–1712
of vulva, 1709–1711
Cancer antigen (CA), 1232
Cancer antigen 125 (CA-125), 1709
Cancer-related anorexia-cachexia syndrome
(CACS), 371
Candesartan (Atacand), for hypertension, 892t
Candida albicans, 376, 1687
Candida vulvovaginitis, HIV infection and, 1039
Candidiasis, 1266t, 1686, 1687–1688, 1688t
clinical manifestations, 1687–1688
HIV infection and, 1039
management, 1688
Canes
ambulation using, 174–175
types of, 175f
use of, 177t
Canker sore, 1266t
CANS. *See* Cardiac autonomic nervous systems
CAPC. *See* Center to Advance Palliative Care
CAPD. *See* Continuous ambulatory peritoneal
dialysis
Capecitabine (Xeloda), 343t, 1346
Capillariasis, 1321t
Capillaries, 842
Capillary leak syndrome, 346
Capillary refill times, 687
Capsaicin (Zostrix), 1089t
Capsaicin cream (Capzasin), in general pruritus,
1812
Captopril (Capoten), for hypertension, 892t
Carbamates, 2207
Carbamazepine (Tegretol), 2087
drug interactions, 428t
Carbidopa, 2103
Carbohydrate
budget, 1464
counting, 1464
in diabetic diet, 1462–1463
metabolism, endocrine control of, 1430
in TLC diet, 755t
wound healing and, 425t
Carbon dioxide (CO2)
partial pressure of, 487f
transport, 488
Carbon monoxide poisoning, 2179
clinical manifestations, 2179
management, 2179
Carboplatin (Paraplatin), 343t, 344
for ovarian cancer, 1713
Carboxyhemoglobin, 1845, 1852, 2156, 2179
Carboxymethylcellulose (MCM), 1317
Carbuncles, 1803, 1806, 1818
Carcinoembryonic antigen (CEA), 1232–1233,
1344
Carcinogenesis
chemical factors, 329
definition of, 324
etiology, 327
genetics/familial factors and, 329
hormonal agents, 329–330
life style factors and, 329
molecular process, 326–327

physical factors associated with, 328–329
radiation therapy and, 328–329
Carcinogens, definition of, 324, 326
Carcinomas, classification of, 328t
CARD9 deficiency, 1024t
Cardiac arrest, 837–839
Cardiac autonomic nervous systems (CANS),
720
Cardiac biomarker analysis, 693
Cardiac catheterization, 703
self-management, 705c
Cardiac conduction system, 675, 676f
Cardiac event recorders, 697
Cardiac illness, 684, 685, 697
Cardiac implantable electronic devices, 697
Cardiac muscle cells, 803
Cardiac output, 677, 885–886
during cardiac surgery
decrease in, 784
maintaining, 785
hypertension and, 886
promotion of, 466–467
Cardiac rehabilitation, 166
in MI, 766–767
phase I, 766–767
phase II, 767
phase III, 767
physical conditioning, 766
Cardiac resynchronization therapy (CRT), 712,
739, 742, 818, 827, 827f
Cardiac sphincter, 1279
Cardiac stress testing, 699–700
Cardiac surgery. *See* Coronary artery bypass graft
Cardiac tamponade, 631, 836–837, 837f
Cardiogenic shock, 296, 310–313, 835
antiarrhythmic medications in, 312
causes of, 310–311
clinical manifestations of, 310
fluid administration in, 311
hemodynamic monitoring in, 311, 312
intra-aortic balloon counterpulsation in,
maintaining, 312
mechanical assistive devices in, 312
medical management, 310–312
nursing management, 312–313
oxygenation in, 311
pain control in, 311
pathophysiology of, 310, 310f
safety and comfort in, 312–313
vasoactive medication therapy, 311–312
Cardiomyopathy, 801, 802f
arrhythmogenic right ventricular
cardiomyopathy/dysplasia, 803
assessment of, 803
clinical manifestation of, 803
diagnosis of, 803
dilated, 801, 802
and heart failure, 819
hypertrophic, 802–803
medical management of, 803–804
nursing process, 807–809
pathophysiology of, 801–803
primary, 801
restrictive, 802
secondary, 801
surgical management of, 804–807
unclassified, 803
Cardiopulmonary bypass system, 774–775, 774f
Cardiopulmonary resuscitation (CPR), 837–839
advanced support interventions in, 838

airway and breathing in, 838
chest compressions in, 837–838, 838f
defibrillation in, 838
follow-up monitoring and care, 838–839
medications used in, 839t
steps in, 837
CardioPulmonary system, chemotherapy-related
effects, 345–346
Cardiorenal syndrome, 820
Cardiovascular alterations, burn injuries and,
1850–1851
Cardiovascular disease (CVD), 126t, 673, 686t,
694t
assessment, 686t
gerontologic considerations, 678
health history, 679
nursing practice, 683c
physical assessment, 685
postural hypotension, 687
signs and symptoms, 679–680
Cardiovascular system
age-related changes, 195–198, 197t, 679t
assessment, 678
postsurgical complications, 473t
preoperative assessments, 426
Cardioversion
definition of, 712
for ventricular tachycardia, 730
Care maps, use of, 9
Care transitions, breakdowns in, 12
CARF. *See* Commission for the Accreditation of
Rehabilitation Facilities
Carfilzomib, 996
Carmustine (BCNU), 343t, 346
Carotid arteries, 2017f
Carotid artery stenting (CAS), 2017
Carotid endarterectomy (CEA), 2013, 2018t
Carpal tunnel syndrome, 1164–1165
causes of, 1164
Carpopedal spasm, 1529
Carrier, 2125
Carriers
definition of, 114
of gene mutation, 120
Carvedilol (Coreg)
for heart failure, 824t
for hypertension, 891t
CAS. *See* Carotid artery stenting
Case management, 12
Case managers, 12
Cast, 1131–1133
body, 1132
fiberglass, 1132
hip spica, 1132
home care checklist, 1136c
immobilized lower extremity, 1136–1137
immobilized upper extremity, 1136
long-arm, 1132, 1132f
long-leg, 1132, 1132f
nursing management of patient,
1133–1136
monitoring and managing, 1134–1135
promoting home, community-based, and
transitional care, 1135–1136
plaster, 1132–1133
short-arm, 1132
short-leg, 1132
shoulder spica, 1132
syndrome, 1131, 1137
walking, 1132

Cataracts, 1894f
  definition of, 1876
  formation of, 1894c
  management, 1895–1896
  pathophysiology, 1894
  surgical complications, 1896t
Catecholamines, 1531
  definition of, 84
  fight-or-flight reaction and, 87
Cathartics, 2178
Catheter-associated urinary tract infections
      (CAUTI), 434, 434c, 1620
  risk factors for, 1621c
Catheterization, 1628–1632
  indwelling, 1629
  nursing management, 1629–1632
    bladder retraining, 1631, 1631c
    infection prevention, 1630, 1630c
    intermittent self-catheterization,
        1631–1632
    patient and drainage system assessment,
        1629
    urethra, minimization of trauma to, 1631
  in older patients, 1629–1630, 1630f
  postcatheterization detrusor instability, 1631
  suprapubic, 1629, 1629f
  and UTI, 1628–1629
Catheters
  external, 187
  indwelling, 187
  nasal endotracheal, 445f
  peripherally inserted central, 372f
  right atrial, 344f
  suprapubic, 187
  transtracheal oxygen, 514
CCPD. See Continuous cycling peritoneal
      dialysis
CCR5 antagonist, 1035t
CCRCs. See Continuing care retirement
      communities
CDC. See Disease Control and Prevention
CEA. See Carotid endarterectomy
Cecostomy, 1329
Cefadroxil (Duricef, Ultracef), for urinary tract
      infections, 1619t
Ceftriaxone (Rocephin)
  for pelvic inflammatory disease, 1696
  for rape consequences, 2189
Celecoxib (Celebrex)
  in rheumatic diseases, 1088t
Celiac disease, 1319–1322, 1321t
  assessment and diagnostic findings, 1321
  clinical manifestations, 1320–1321
  medical management, 1321
  nursing management, 1322
  pathophysiology, 1320
Celibacy. See Abstinence
Cell cycle, phases of, 338f
Cell division, 117
Cellular immune response, 1007, 1010–1012
Cellular immunity, 907
Cellular (cell-mediated) immunity tests, 1020c
Cellulitis, 881
Center for Medicare and Medicaid Services
      (CMS), 7, 33, 218, 393, 419, 1367
Centers for Disease Control and Prevention
      (CDC), 640, 2033, 2067, 2160
Center to Advance Palliative Care (CAPC),
      392
Central cyanosis, 583

Central line-associated bloodstream infections
      (CLABSI), 305, 306c, 434, 434c
Centrally generated pain, 227t
Central nervous system (CNS), 2091
  anatomy of, 1947–1949, 1948f
  parts of, 1947–1951
Central parenteral nutrition (CPN), 1257. See
      also Parenteral nutrition (PN)
Central retinal artery occlusions, 1901
Central retinal vein occlusions (CRVOs), 1901
Central sensitization, 230
Central veins, 1378
Central venous access device (CVAD), 1243
Central venous pressure (CVP), 305, 688, 706,
      2172
Centrilobular (centroacinar), 636
Cephalalgia. See Headache
Cephalexin (Keflex), 1841
Cephalosporin, for urinary tract infections,
      1619t
Cerebellum, anatomy, 1949
Cerebral amyloid angiopathy (CAA), 2025
Cerebral blood flow, 1980
Cerebral circulation, 1950, 1950f
  and cardiac surgery, 785
Cerebral edema, 1980
  decrease in, 1982–1983
Cerebral hypoxia, 2027
Cerebral oxygenation, monitoring of, 1981–
      1982
Cerebral perfusion pressure (CPP), 2038
Cerebrospinal fluid (CSF), 1950, 2034, 2066,
      2093
  analysis, 1970
  reduction in, 1983
Cerebrovascular disease, diabetes and, 1489
Cerebrum
  lobes of, 1948
  motor control and, 1955f
Certified nurse-midwives (CNMs), 12
Certified nurse operating room, 434c
Certified nurse practitioners (CNPs), 12
Certified postanesthesia nurse, 434c
Certified registered nurse anesthetist (CRNA),
      12, 436, 439–440
Certolizumabpegol (Cimzia), 1089t, 1107
Cerumen impaction, 1926
Ceruminous glands, 1793
Cervical biopsy, 1663
Cervical cancer, 1706–1708
  advanced, 1706
  assessment and diagnostic findings, 1707
  clinical manifestations, 1706–1707
  clinical staging, 1707
  HIV infection and, 1041
  low-grade squamous intraepithelial lesions
      (LGSILs), 1707
  medical management
    invasive cancer, 1707–1708
    precursor/preinvasive lesions, 1707
    surgical procedures, 1707c
  preventive measures, 1706
  risk factors, 1706c
  types of, 1706
Cervical cap, 1672–1673
Cervical cerclage, 1675
Cervical collar, 2052f
  home care checklist, 2116c
Cervical fractures, 2052
Cervical injuries, halo and vest for, 2053f

Cervical spine immobilization, 2170
Cervicitis, 1694–1695
Cervix, 1650, 1652
  inspection of, 1661
  palpation of, 1662
Cetirizine (Zyrtec), 1069t
Cetuximab, 344
Cevimeline (Evoxac), 1101
C fibers, 226–227
CFTR gene, 665
Chamber pressures, 674f
Chancre, 1266t
Charcot joints, 1493
Charcot–Marie–Tooth disease, 1168
Cheilitis, 1806, 1816
Chelation therapy, 984
Chemical agents, burns, 1853, 1854
Chemical burns, of esophagus, 1283
Chemical face peeling, 1841
Chemical mediators, of hypersensitivity, 1058,
      1058f, 1059t
  function of, 1058–1060
  primary, 1058–1059
  secondary, 1059–1060
Chemical weapon, 2193, 2206–2208,
      2206t
  characteristics of, 2207
    latency, 2207
    persistence, 2207
    toxicity, 2207
    volatility, 2207
  chemicals, types of, 2207–2208
  limiting exposure, 2207
Chemolysis, 1634
Chemosis, 1876, 1904, 1905
Chemotherapy, 2096
  administration of, 342, 347–348
  agents
    adjunct, 342
    administration of, 342–347
    antineoplastic, 343t
    cell-cycle-nonspecific, 342
    cell-cycle-specific, 342
    classification of, 342
    dosages, 342
    extravasation, 342–344
    hypersensitivity reactions, 344
    protecting caregivers, 348
    toxicity of, 344–347
  for bladder cancer, 1638
  for breast cancer, 1741–1743
  care of patients, 355–379
  definition of, 324, 341
  for gastric cancer, 1305
  goals of, 341
  home care checklist, 378c
  home care settings, 349
  for liver cancer, 1418
  long-term complications, 347c
  nursing management, 347–348
  for ovarian cancer, 1713
  for penile cancer, 1785
  for prostate cancer, 1770
  protecting caregivers, 348
  for testicular cancer, 1781
Chemotherapy-induced amenorrhea (CIA),
      1748
Chemotherapy-induced nausea and vomiting
      (CINV), 345
Chemtrac database, 2201

Chenodeoxycholic acid (chenodiol or CDCA), 1434
Cherry angioma, 1801t
Chest
　configuration, 495
　pain, 490
　percussion, 510, 519–520
　trauma, 625–631
　　blunt trauma, 626–628
　　cardiac tamponade, 631
　　penetrating trauma, 629
　　pneumothorax, 629–631
　　subcutaneous emphysema, 631
　tumors, 620–625
　　lung cancer, 620–624
　　mediastinal tumors, 624–625
　vibration, 511, 519–520
Chest discomfort. *See* Chest pain
Chest drainage system, 510, 540–542, 541f, 543f
　comparison of, 540t
　dry suction water seal systems, 542
　types of, 541
　water seal system, 542
Chest pain, 680
　assessment, 681t–682t
Chest physiotherapy (CPT), 510, 517–521, 645
Chest wall, characteristics, 637f
Chest X-ray, 504
Chewing, 1226
Cheyne-Stokes respirations, 495, 496t
Child–Pugh score, 1421
Child Turcotte–Pugh (CTP) score, 1421
Chin halter strap, 1140
Chlamydia, and endocervicitis, 1694
Chlamydia pneumoniae, 936
Chlamydia trachomatis, 2147
Chlorambucil (Leukeran), 343t, 977–978
Chlordiazepoxide (Librium), for alcohol withdrawal syndrome, 2185
Chlorhexidine, in skeletal traction, 1143
Chloride imbalance, 281–283, 281t
　hyperchloremia, 282–283
　hypochloremia, 281–282
Chloroquine (Aralen), in rheumatic diseases, 1088t
Chlorothiazide (Diuril), for hypertension, 890t
Chlorpheniramine (Chlor-Trimeton), 1069t
Chlorpromazine (Thorazine)
　for patients who are overactive, 2190
　suppress shivering, 2173
Chlorpromazine hydrochloride, drug interactions, 428t
Chlorpropamide (Diabinese), in diabetes insipidus, 1510
Chlorthalidone (Hygroton), for hypertension, 890t
Chocolate cyst, 1704
Cholecystectomy, 1428, 1434
Cholecystitis, 1428, 1430
　acalculous, 1430
　calculous, 1430
Cholecystojejunostomy, 1428, 1452
Cholecystokinin (CCK), 1360, 1428
Cholecystostomy, 1428, 1437
Choledocholithiasis, 1428, 1430
Choledochostomy, 1428, 1437
Cholelithiasis, 1428, 1430–1438
　assessment and diagnostic findings, 1432–1434, 1432t
　　abdominal x-ray, 1432

endoscopic retrograde cholangiopancreatography, 1433, 1433f
　　oral cholecystography, 1433
　　percutaneous transhepatic cholangiography, 1433–1434
　　radionuclide imaging/cholescintigraphy, 1432–1433
　　ultrasonography, 1432
　clinical manifestations, 1431–1432
　　jaundice, 1432
　　pain and biliary colic, 1431–1432
　　urine and stool color, changes in, 1432
　　vitamin deficiency, 1432
　medical management, 1434–1435
　　dissolving gallstones, 1434
　　extracorporeal shock wave therapy, 1435
　　intracorporeal lithotripsy, 1435
　　nutritional and supportive therapy, 1434
　　pharmacologic therapy, 1434
　　stone removal by instrumentation, 1435, 1435f
　pathophysiology, 1430–1431
　　cholesterol stones, 1430–1431
　　pigment stones, 1430
　risk factors, 1431, 1431c
　surgical management, 1436–1437
　　cholecystectomy, 1437
　　choledochostomy, 1437
　　laparoscopic cholecystectomy, 1436–1437, 1436f
　　nursing process, 1438–1440
　　in older adult, 1437–1438
　　percutaneous cholecystostomy, 1437
　　preoperative measures, 1436
　　small-incision cholecystectomy, 1437
Cholera, 2145
Cholescintigraphy, 1432–1433
Cholesteatoma, 1915, 1929
Cholesterol abnormalities, 753–755
Cholesterol absorption inhibitor, 756t
Cholesterol, levels, 695
Cholestyramine (Questran), 756t
Cholinesterase inhibitors, 2081
Choline trilisalicylate (Arthropan, Trilisate) in rheumatic diseases, 1088t
Chondrosarcomas, 1180
Chordae tendineae, 791
　anatomy of, 792f
Chordoplasty, 798–799
Chorea, 2108
Choromosomes
　definition of, 114
　genes and, 116–117
　human, 110f
Christianity, traditional, 397t
Christmas disease, 951
Chromosomal differences, 122
Chronic bronchitis, pathophysiology of, 635f
Chronic diseases. *See also* Chronic illness
　causes of, 142–143
　characteristics of, 143–145
　definition of, 139, 141–142
　gerontologic considerations, 146–147
　health disparities, and, 140–141
　interventions, 143c
　managing, implications of, 145
　misconceptions about, 142t
　nursing care of, 147–149
　phases, 145–146

　prevalence of, 142–143
　prevention of, 143–147, 149f
　reality about, 142t
Chronic glomerulonephritis, 1572–1573
Chronic granulomatous disease (CGD), 1024t
Chronic illness, 139–161. *See also* Chronic diseases
　definition of, 139
　educating about self-care, 148
　nursing process application, 147–148
　special populations with, 149
　trajectory model, 146t
　transitional care, 148–149
　in United States, 140c
Chronic kidney disease (CKD), 1567, 1569–1570
　and anemia, 931–932
　assessment and diagnostic findings, 1569
　causes of, 1569
　clinical manifestations, 1569
　diabetes and, 1569
　medical management, 1569–1570
　in older patients, 1570
　pathophysiology, 1569
　stages of, 1569, 1569c
Chronic liver disease, 1383
　detection of, 1384c
Chronic lymphocytic leukemia (CLL), 976–978
　clinical manifestations, 977
　lymphadenopathy in, 977, 977f
　medical management, 977–978
　pathophysiology, 976–977
Chronic myeloid leukemia (CML), 974–975
　clinical manifestations, 974
　medical management, 974
　nursing management, 974–975
　reduced adherence to oral therapy for, 975, 975t
Chronic obstructive pulmonary disease (COPD), 634–635, 638f
　activity pacing, 644
　assessment, 639c
　bronchodilator medications, 640, 642t
　care of patient, 649c–653c
　cigarette smoking, 637
　coping measures, 645
　deaths from, 635
　defined, 634
　grades, 639t
　nutritional therapy, 645
　palliative care, 645
　pathophysiology, 635
　pharmacologic therapy, 640
　physical conditioning, 644–645
　pulmonary rehabilitation, 644
　risk factors for, 636, 636c
　risk reduction, 638
　self-care activities, 644
　sleep and quality of life, 647c
Chronic otitis media, 1928–1929
Chronic pelvic pain, 1705
Chronotropy, 712, 713
Chvostek sign, 274, 274f, 1502, 1530
Chyle fistula, 1278
Chylomicrons, 753
Chyme, 1224, 1227
Cilia, definition of, 480
Cilostazol (Pletal)
　for claudication, 859

Cimetidine (Tagamet), 1059, 1442
 for gastritis, 1295t
 for GERD, 1284t
 in snakebites, 2177
CINV. See Chemotherapy-induced nausea and
 vomiting
Ciprofloxacin (Cipro), 2067
 for anthrax treatment, 2204
 for impetigo, 1818
 for urinary tract infections, 1619t
CircAid, 873
Circulating nurses (circulators), 436, 438
Circumcision, 1752, 1753, 1786
Cirrhosis, 1377, 1380, 1383, 1406–1417
 assessment and diagnostic findings,
 1407–1408
 bleeding and hemorrhage and, 1416
 Child–Pugh classification, 1406, 1406t
 clinical manifestations, 1406
 edema, 1407
 gastrointestinal varices, 1407
 infection and peritonitis, 1407
 liver enlargement, 1406
 mental deterioration, 1407
 portal obstruction and ascites, 1406–1407
 vitamin deficiency and anemia, 1407
 compensated, 1406, 1407c
 decompensated, 1406, 1407c
 and fluid volume excess, 1416
 and hepatic encephalopathy, 1416
 medical management, 1408
 nursing care plan, 1409c–1416c
 nursing management, 1408
 complications monitoring and
 management, 1416
 continuing and transitional care, 1417
 nutritional status, 1408
 patient education, 1416–1417
 reducing risk of injury, 1408
 rest promotion, 1408
 skin care, 1408
 pathophysiology, 1406
 types of, 1406
Cisatracurium besylate (Nimbex), 446t
Cisplatin (Platinol), 343t, 345
Citric acid, 450
CKD. See Chronic kidney disease
CK isoenzymes (CK-MB), 693
CLABSI. See Central line–associated
 bloodstream infection
Cladribine (Leustatin), 343t
Clarithromycin (Biaxin), for gastritis, 1295t
Clavicle, 1198, 1198f
Clawfoot. See Pes cavus
Clearblue Fertility Monitor, 1674
Clevidipine (Cleviprex), for hypertension, 893t
Client. See Patient
Clindamycin
 for acne, 1815
 for impetigo, 1818
Clindamycin (Cleocin) vaginal cream, 1689
Clinical guidelines, use of, 9
Clinical nurse leader (CNL), 12–13
Clinical nurse specialists (CNSs), 12
Clinic managers, 24
Clitoris, 1651
CLL. See Chronic lymphocytic leukemia
Clog Zapper, 1246
Clomiphene citrate (Clomid, Serophene), 1677,
 1677c

Clomipramine (Anafranil), 1761
Clonal stem cell disorders, 971
Clone, 971
Clonidine (Catapres), 639, 1533
 for alcohol withdrawal syndrome, 2185
 for hypertension, 890t
Clonidine patch (Catapres-TTS)
 for hypertension, 890t
Clonidine suppression test, 1533
Clonus, 1124, 1915, 1964
Clopidogrel (Plavix), 683
 for angina, 758t, 760
 laboratory test reference range, 694t
Closed awareness, 389
Closed fractures, 1189
Clostridium difficile, 2130–2131
Clotrimazole (Gyne-Lotrimin), for candidiasis,
 1688
Cloxacillin (Cloxapen), in impetigo, 1818
Clubbing of fingers or toes, 492, 492f, 686t
Clue cells, 1689
Cluster headache, 2005
CML. See Chronic myeloid leukemia
CNL. See Clinical nurse leader
CNP. See C-type natriuretic peptide
CNPs. See Certified nurse practitioners
CNS. See Central nervous system
CNSs. See Clinical nurse specialists
Coccidioides immitis, 2070
Coccidiosis, 1321t
Codeine, 241
Cognitive behavioral therapy, 1109
Cognitive disabilities
 chemotherapy-related, 346
 pressure ulcers and, 180
Cognitive function
 aging and, 204–205
 elimination problems and, 186
 health promotion, 205c
 Los Amigos Scale, 2044, 2045t
 support for, 213
Cognitive impairment, 2077, 2108
Coitus interruptus, 1674
Colchicine (Colcrys), 1108, 1109t
 in cirrhosis, 1408
Colds, 556c
Cold sores, 556c
Cold therapy, 1137
Cold urticaria, 1076–1077
Colestipol (Colestid), 756t
Collaborative problems, 38–39
Collagen (VasoSeal), 704
Collagenase (Santyl), 1807
Collagens, description, 1845, 1862
Collateral circulation, 851, 861
Colloids, 261t, 296
Colonic function, 1228
Colonic J-pouch, 1346
Colonic transit studies, 1313
Colonization, 2125, 2132
Colonoscopy, 1344
Colony-stimulating factors, 1013
Colorectal cancer, 1343–1349
 assessment and diagnostic findings, 1344
 clinical manifestations, 1344
 complications, 1344
 medical management, 1345–1347
 abdominoperineal resection, 1346, 1347f
 adjuvant therapy, 1346–1347
 surgery, 1346, 1346f

 nursing process
 assessment, 1347–1348
 complications management, 1349, 1350t
 continuing and transitional care, 1349
 diagnosis, 1348
 emotional support, 1348
 evaluation, 1349
 fluid volume balance, 1348
 infection prevention, 1348
 nursing interventions, 1348–1349
 optimal nutrition, 1348
 patient education, 1348, 1349
 planning and goals, 1348
 postoperative care, 1348–1349
 preoperative care, 1348
 wound care, 1349
 in older adults, 1344–1345
 pathophysiology, 1344
 prevention strategies, 1345
 risk factors for, 1343, 1343c
 staging of, 1345c
Color vision testing, 1881
Colostomy, 1311, 1336
Colpexin Sphere, 1699
Colpocleisis, 1701
Colporrhaphy, 1699
Colposcopy, 1663, 2188
CoLyte, 1314t
Coma, 1972, 1974
Comedones, 1806, 1814
Comfort care issues, ethical dilemmas, 1855c
Comfort-function goals, 232, 233
Comminuted fractures, 1189
Commission for the Accreditation of
 Rehabilitation Facilities (CARF), 166
Commissurotomy, 797–798
Common variable immunodeficiency (CVID),
 1024t
Communication
 anticipatory mourning and, 411c
 in palliative care, 398c
 with seriously ill, 395–398
 therapeutic, 37, 37t
 translations and, 438
Community. See also Community-based nursing
 definition of, 18, 48
 nurses in, 18
Community-acquired pneumonia, 587–588
Community-associated methicillin-resistant
 Staphylococcus aureus (CA-MRSA),
 2132
Community-based care
 after surgery, 461–463
 needs in AD, 215
 promotion of, 188–190
 targeted therapies, 355
Community-based nursing, 18, 19. See also
 Home health care
 ambulatory centers, 24
 community nurse-managed centers, 25
 components of, 19–20
 home health care, 20–24
 for homeless population, 25–26
 hospice care, 24, 24c
 occupational health programs, 24–25
 school health programs, 25
Community hubs, 25
Community nurse-managed centers, 25
Community-oriented nursing, 18
Community resources, 19–20

Community services, 2160
Comorbidity, definition of, 193, 205
Compartment syndrome, 1134, 1135f, 1194–1196, 1195f
  diagnosis of, 1134
Compensated cirrhosis, 1383
Compensation, 287, 288t
Complement, 1012
  cascading effect, 1012
Complementary and alternative medicine (CAM), cancer-related, 355
Complete blood cell count (CBC), 703
Complex genetic conditions, 121
Complex pain, 1868t
Complex regional pain syndrome (CRPS), 1197
  clinical manifestation, 1197
Compliance
  lung, 480, 484
  older adults and, 206–207
Compression stockings, 173, 872
Computed tomography (CT), 2035
  chest, 504
  for low back pain, 1161c
  for musculoskeletal disorders, 1127
  nervous system, 1965–1966
  for vascular abnormalities, 849
Computer-aided detection (CAD), 1725
Computer-assisted stereotactic, 2095
Concussion, diffuse axonal injury (DAI), 2034
Condom
  female, 1673
  male, 1673
Conduction, 712, 1793
Conduction abnormalities, 732–734
  first-degree AV block, 732
  medical management of, 734
  second-degree AV block
    type I, 732–733, 733f
    type II, 733–734, 733f
  third-degree AV block, 734
Conductive hearing loss, 1923
Conductive injuries, 1850c
Conductive keratoplasty, 1900
Condylomata, 1686, 1691
Condylomata acuminata, 1833
Cone biopsy, for cervical cancer, 1707
Confidentiality, 33
Confusion
  approaching death and, 408c
  postoperative, 461
  terminal illness and, 407
Confusion Assessment Method for the ICU (CAM-ICU), 303, 786, 1965
Congenital infections, 2149
Congenital neutropenia syndromes, 1024t
Congestive heart failure (CHF), 818. *See also* Heart failure (HF)
Conjunctiva
  benign tumors of, 1909
  malignant tumors of, 1910
Conjunctival hyperemia, 1907f
Conjunctivitis, 1906, 1908
  allergic, 1908
  bacterial, 1906–1907, 1908
  toxic, 1908
  viral, 1907, 1907f, 1908c
Conoamine oxidase (MAO) inhibitors, 2005
Consequentialism, 30
Consolidation, 500t, 583
Constipation, 1143

after surgery, 472
age-related issues, 199
appendicitis and, 1324
assessment and diagnostic findings, 1313
causes of, 1312
clinical manifestations, 1312
complications, 1313
defecatory disorders, 1312
definition of, 1311, 1312
diabetic, 1493, 1494
functional, 1312
medical management, 1313, 1314t
nursing management, 1313–1314
in older adults, 1313
pathophysiology of, 1312
patient education, 1315c
prevention of, 188
Rome criteria for, 1312c
slow-transit, 1312
tube feedings and, 1251
Constructional apraxia, 1377, 1395, 1395f
Contact dermatitis, 1074, 1074t, 1266t, 1823, 1823c
Contact precautions, 2131
Continent ileal urinary reservoir (Indiana pouch), 1642–1643
Continent urinary diversion, 1639, 1642–1643
Continuing care retirement communities (CCRCs), 204
Continuous ambulatory peritoneal dialysis (CAPD), 1322, 1567, 1596, 1597f, 1598–1599, 1599c
Continuous central venous oximetry (ScvO$_2$), 300
Continuous cycling peritoneal dialysis (CCPD), 1567, 1596, 1599
Continuous femoral nerve block infusions (CFNBI), 1155
Continuous glucose monitoring system (CGMS), 1467, 1467f
continuous mandatory ventilation (CMV), 510, 527
Continuous passive motion (CPM), 1154
continuous positive airway pressure (CPAP), 510
Continuous renal replacement therapy (CRRT), 1567, 1580, 1594, 1595f
Continuous venovenous hemodialysis (CVVHD), 1595
Continuous venovenous hemofiltration (CVVH), 1594
Continuous wave (CW) Doppler ultrasound, 847–848, 847f
Contraception, 1669
  abstinence, 1669
  coitus interruptus, 1674
  contraindications, 1669
  emergency, 1674
  family planning methods, effectiveness of, 1670f
  fertility awareness-based methods, 1674
  hormonal, 1671–1672, 1671c
  LARC methods, 1669–1670
    intrauterine device, 1670
    single-rod implant, 1670
  mechanical barriers
    cervical cap, 1672–1673
    diaphragm, 1672
    female condom, 1673
    male condom, 1673
    spermicides, 1673
  sterilization, 1671, 1671t

Contractility, 678, 750
Contractures, 1124, 1160, 1165
  burn injuries and, 1868t
  description of, 1845, 1863
  prevention of, 171, 175
Contrast-induced nephropathy (CIN), 703
Contrast mammography, 1725
Contrast phlebography, 849
Contrast-sensitivity testing, 1884
Contusion, 1185–1186
Convection, 1793
Coombs test, 943
Cooper ligaments, 1720
Coping, 685, 2061
  after burn injuries, 1867
  cognitive strategies, 431
  with death and dying, 412
  in grief and mourning, 412c
  stressful event and, 87
Copper, wound healing and, 425t
Cordectomy, 573
Core measures, 9
Core needle biopsy, 335–336
  of breast, 1726, 1726t
Corn, 1167
Corneas
  abrasions, 1903
  anatomy, 1878
  contraindications, 1898c
  dystrophies, 1897
  surgeries, 1898
Coronary angiography, 704
Coronary artery bypass graft (CABG), 773–788, 774f
  alternative, 775
  complications of, 775, 776t–777t
    intraoperative management, 778
    monitoring for, 784–785
    postoperative management, 779–788, 779f
    preoperative management, 775–778
  definition of, 750
  fear and anxiety, management of, 778
  home care checklist, 788c
  indications for, 773
  nursing care, 780c–783c
  patient assessment, 775–778, 784
  patient education, 778
  recommendation for, 773
  saphenous veins in, 773, 774f
  stabilizer device for off-pump, 775f
  traditional, 773–775
Coronary artery disease (CAD), 673, 675, 678, 679, 681, 699, 750–751
  clinical manifestations, 751–752
  definition of, 750
  diabetes and, 1489
  gender and, 757
  gender considerations, 678
  metabolic syndrome and, 753
  prevention of, 753–757
    cessation of tobacco use, promotion of, 755–756
    cholesterol abnormalities, controlling, 753–755
    diabetes, controlling, 757
    hypertension, management of, 756–757
  risk factors, 752–753, 752c
  sudden cardiac death and, 752
Coronary artery stent, 771–772

Coronary atherosclerosis, 751–757
  pathophysiology of, 751
  vulnerable plaque, 751
Coronary sinus, 673, 675
Cor pulmonale, 583, 636, 638, 643
Corpus callosum, 1948, 1948f
Corpus luteum, 1650, 1653
Corrosive poison, 2156, 2178
Cortical bone, 1115
Corticosteroids, 656, 664, 701, 1502, 1503, 1531
  for adrenal insufficiency, 1541
  for allergic rhinitis, 1069–1070
  for bullous pemphigoid, 1828
  commonly used preparations, 1541t
  continuing and transitional care, 1543
  dosage, 1542–1543
  immunosuppression and, 426
  for inflammatory bowel disease, 1332
  injections
      in bursitis and tendonitis treatment, 1164
      in hallux valgus treatment, 1167
      in morton neuroma treatment, 1168
  for myasthenia gravis, 2080
  nursing management, 1543
  nursing practice, implications for, 1542t
  patient and family education, 1543
  for pemphigus vulgaris, 1828
  for rheumatic diseases, 1089t
  risk for adrenal insufficiency, 426
  side effects, 1541
  for SJS, 1831
  for snakebites, 2176
  for systemic lupus erythematosus, 1100
  tapering, 1543
  for TEN, 1831
  therapeutic uses of, 1541–1542
      acute flare-ups and crises, 1541
      dermatologic disorders, 1541–1542
      ophthalmologic treatment, 1541
  wound care, 1810, 1811t
Corticosteroid triamcinolone (Aristocort), for
      psoriasis, 1825
Corticotropin-releasing hormone (CRH),
      1531
Cortisol, 256, 1116
Cortisone, 1541t
Cortrak Enteral Access System, 1246
Corynebacterium parvum, 352
Costochondritis, 682t
Costovertebral angle, 1557, 1558f
Co-trimoxazole (Bactrim, Septra), for urinary
      tract infections, 1619t
Cough, 692
  assessment, 489–490
  causes of, 489–490
  postoperative, 429, 430c
  postsurgical patients, 466
Cowden Syndrome, 126t
Cowper glands, 1754
COX-2 enzyme blockers, 1105
COX-1 inhibitors, 226
COX-2 inhibitors, 226, 1095
CPOT (Critical Care Pain Observation Tool),
      133
CPR. See Cardiopulmonary resuscitation
Crackles, 480, 498, 499t, 693
Cranberry juice, 1619
Cranial arteritis, 2004, 2005
Cranial nerves, 1951, 1952, 2077, 2086t–2087t
  demyelination, 2083

disorders, 2085–2089
  function, 1952t
  location of, 1952f
Craniectomy, 1972, 1973, 1989
Craniotomy, 1972, 1989
C-reactive protein (CRP), 695, 851
Creams, wound care, 1810
Creatine kinase (CK), 693, 764, 2171
Creatinine, 1548, 1551
  reference range, 694t
Crepitus, 1124, 1185, 1189
CREST syndrome, 1102
Creutzfeldt-Jakob disease (CJD), 922c, 2065,
      2071–2072
Cricoid cartilage, 482
Cricothyroidotomy, 2156, 2165
Critical Care Pain Observation Tool. See
      CPOT
Critical incident stress management (CISM),
      2159, 2199–2200
Critical thinking
  in action, 30c
  and clinical reasoning, 29
  components of, 29
  definition of, 27–28
  metacognition in, 28, 29
  in nursing practice, 28
  rationality and insight in, 28–29
  skills involved in, development of, 28, 28c
Crohn's and Colitis Foundation of America
      (CCFA), 1335
Crohn's disease, 1330–1331
  assessment and diagnostic findings, 1331
  clinical manifestations, 1331
  cobblestone appearance, 1330
  complications of, 1331
  medical treatment, 1332–1334
  pathophysiology, 1330
  skip lesions, 1330
  string sign, 1331
  and ulcerative colitis, 1330t
Cromolyn sodium (Crolom, NasalCrom),
      656
Cross-cultural communication, 105–106
Crossing the Quality Chasm: A New Health
      System for the 21st Century (IOM
      report), 8, 9
Cross-reactivity, 1010
Crotalidae polyvalent immune Fab antivenom,
      2177
CRRT. See Continuous renal replacement
      therapy
CRT. See Cardiac resynchronization therapy
Cruciate ligament injury, 1188
Crush injuries, 2170
  assessment and diagnostic findings, 2171
  management, 2171
Crust, 1799t
Crutches, 175f
  ambulation using, 174–175
  gaits, 176c
  use of, 177t
CRVOs. See Central retinal vein occlusions
Cryoprecipitate, 958
Cryosurgery, 1770, 1835
Cryotherapy, 1185, 1188, 1663, 1686
  for cervical cancer, 1707
Cryptococcal meningitis, 1040, 1041–1042
Cryptococcus neoformans, 1040, 2070, 2149
Crystalloids, 296

administration of, 305
  shock management and, 305–306
CSF. See Cerebrospinal fluid
CT. See Computed tomography
CTLA4 deficiency, 1024t
C-type natriuretic peptide (CNP), 258
Cultural awareness
  care of dying and, 389
  definition of, 102
Cultural beliefs
  on death and dying, 396t–397t
  preoperative assessments, 427–428
  respect for, 431
Cultural blindness, 104
Cultural diversity, nursing care and, 438
Cultural humility, definition of, 102
Cultural imposition, 104
Culturally competent nursing care, 102,
      104–105
Culturally mediated characteristics,
      106–109
Cultural nursing assessment, 102, 111, 111c
Cultural sensitivity. See Cultural awareness
Cultural taboos, 104
Culture
  definition of, 102
  health care delivery, influence on, 6, 19
  microbiological, 503
Culture care accommodation, 104
Culture care restructuring, 104
Cultured epithelial autologous grafts (CEA),
      1864f
Curling ulcer, 1297–1298, 1853
Cushing reflex, 2042, 2093
Cushing's response, 1973, 1980
Cushing's triad, 1980
Cushing syndrome, 1502, 1508, 1536–1540
  assessment and diagnostic findings, 1537
      overnight dexamethasone suppression test,
      1537
      serum cortisol test, 1537
      urinary cortisol test, 1537
  causes of, 1536
  clinical manifestations, 1536–1537, 1537c
  corticosteroids and, 1538
  home care checklist, 1539c
  medical management, 1537–1538
  nursing process, 1538–1540
      assessment, 1538
      complications management, 1539
      diagnosis, 1538
      evaluation, 1539–1540
      nursing interventions, 1538–1539
      patient and family education, 1539
      planning and goals, 1538
Cushing ulcer, 1298
Cutaneous ureterostomy, 1642
Cyanide, 2208
Cyanoacrylate embolization, for varicose veins,
      879
Cyanosis, 1796, 2163
  assessment of, 492
  skin, 492
CyberKnife®, 1769
Cyclic 3',5'-adenosine monophosphate (cAMP),
      655
Cyclic feeding, 1243, 1249
Cyclobenzaprine, 1109
  in acute low back pain, 1161
Cyclo-oxygenase, 1095

Cyclophosphamide (Cytoxan), 343t, 345, 943, 1095, 1102
  for pemphigus vulgaris, 1828
  in rheumatic diseases, 1088t
Cyclophosphamide, methotrexate, and fluorouracil (CMF), 1742
Cycloplegics, 1885t, 1887
Cyclosporine (Gengraf, Neoral, Sandimmune), 350, 1095, 1423, 1610t
  for psoriasis, 1825
Cyclosporine (Neoral), 1088t
Cyst, 1798t
Cystectomy, 1615, 1632
Cystic fibrosis (CF), 665–667
  assessment, 666
  bronchiectasis, 634
  clinical manifestations, 666
  diagnostic findings, 666
  medical management, 666–667
  nursing management, 667
  pathophysiology, 665–666
  pulmonary manifestations, 666
Cystic fibrosis transmembrane conductance regulator (CFTR), 665
Cystine stones, 1634
Cystitis, 1615
Cystocele, 1558, 1650, 1661, 1686, 1698, 1698f
Cystography, 1564
Cystolitholapaxy, 1634
Cystosarcoma phyllodes, 1729
Cystostomy, 1752, 1763
Cystourethroscopy, 1698
Cysts, of skin, 1833
Cytarabine (DepoCyt, Tarabine), 343t, 346
Cytochrome P450 (CYP), 128, 128f, 129t
Cytogenetics, 122
Cytokines, 655, 907, 1011, 1011t, 1503
  definition of, 324
  therapy using, 353–354
Cytomegalovirus (CMV), 922c
  retinitis, 1042, 1912
Cytotoxic, definition of, 1806, 1810
Cytotoxic T cells, 1011–1012

D

Dabigatran (Pradaxa), 965
  for venous thromboembolism, 870t
Dacarbazine (DTIC-Dome), 343t, 1837
Dactinomycin (Cosmegen), 343t
Dalfampridine (Ampyra), 2075
Dalteparin (Fragmin), 683
  for angina, 758t
  in total hip arthroplasty treatment, 1152
  for venous thromboembolism, 870t
Danazol (Danocrine), 943, 1705
Dandruff, 1813
Dantrolene (Dantrium), 2075, 2111
Dapagliflozin (Forxiga), 1475t
Dapoxetine (Priligy), 1761
Dapsone (Aczone)
  for acne vulgaris, 1815
  for dermatitis herpetiformis, 1828
Daratumumab (Darzalex), 996
Darbepoetin alfa (Aranesp), 1742
Darunavir (DRV), 1034t
Dasatinib (Sprycel), 974
Daughter cells, 117
Daunorubicin, 343t, 972
Dawn phenomenon, 1471, 1471t
Deafness, 1915, 1923

Death
  in America, 388
  clinicians' attitudes toward, 389
  coping with, 412
  religious/cultural beliefs and, 396t–397t
  signs of approaching, 408c
Death vigils, 409
Débridement, 876, 1185, 1192, 1807, 1808t
  autolytic, 1807
  burn injuries, 1862–1863
  definition of, 1806, 1807
  description of, 1845, 1862–1863
Debulking, 336
Decerebration, 1972, 1981
Decitabine (Dacogen), 983
Decompression, 1243, 1244, 2087
Decompression sickness
  assessment and diagnostic findings, 2175
  management, 2175
  signs and symptoms of, 2175
Decongestants, 1068
Decontamination, 2193, 2201
Decortications, 1972, 1980
Deep brain stimulation (DBS), 2103–2105, 2105f
  stereotactic frame, 2104
Deep breathing, 429
Deep inferior epigastric perforator flap (DIEP), 1747
Deep tissue injury, 184
Deep vein thrombosis (DVT), 835, 1141, 1979, 2083. See also Venous thromboembolism (VTE)
  physical signs of, 1152
  prevention of, 1145–1146, 1866
  venous thromboembolism and, 1156
Defecography, 1240, 1313
Defibrillation
  definition of, 712
  for dysrhythmias, 737, 738, 738c
Defibrillator, 737
Degenerative disorders, 2101–2105
Degenerative joint disease, 1269. See also Osteoarthritis (OA)
Degradation, 1083–1084
Dehiscence
  definition of, 456
  wound, 474, 475f
Dehydration, 703, 2068
  diarrhea and, 2145
  rehydration, 2145
Delayed complications, 1196–1197
Delayed union, 1185, 1196
Delirium, 1965
  characteristics, 210t
  clinical assessment, 209
  definition of, 193
  description of, 406
  end-of-life care and, 406–407
  family care, 209f
  nursing interventions, 407
  older adults and, 208–209
  postoperative, 461
    causes of, 475c
    in older patients, 475
  prevention, 209
  vs. dementia, 210t
Delirium tremens, 2185–2186
Demand oxygen delivery system (DODS), 515

Dementia
  Alzheimer's disease, 209–215, 210t
  assessment, 211c
  characteristics, 210t
  definition of, 193
  description of, 2102
  older adults and, 209–215
  Parkinson disease, 2104
  types of, 209
  vascular, 210t, 215
  vs. delirium, 210t
Demyelination, 2072f, 2073
Dengue fever, 2153
Denial
  emergency care and, 2159
  stages of grief, 410t
Denosumab (Prolia), 1117
Dental plaque and caries, 1265, 1268
  contributing factors, 1265
  extent of damage to teeth, 1265
  prevention of, 1265
    diet, 1268
    fluoridation, 1268
    mouth care, 1265, 1268
    pit and fissure sealants, 1268
  treatment for, 1265
Dentition, preoperative assessments, 424
Denture care, 1230c
Deontologic/formalist theory, 30
Deoxyribonucleic acid (DNA), 117
  definition of, 114
  structure of, 117f
Department of Health and Human Service (HHS), 2195
Department of Homeland Security, 2195
Depolarization, 676, 712, 713
Depo-Provera, 1672
Depressed skull fractures, 2035
Depression, 685, 2102
  antidepressant medications in, 207
  definition of, 193
  end-of-life care, 407
  older adults and, 207–208
  stages of grief, 410t
Dermabrasion, 1841
Dermagraft, 876
Dermatitis, definition of, 1806, 1809
Dermatitis herpetiformis, 1321, 1828
Dermatitis medicamentosa, 1075
Dermatofibroma, 1833
Dermatologic problems, 1806–1842
Dermatomyositis, 1103
Dermatophyte infections, 1803
Dermatosis, 1806, 1810
Dermis, skin, 1791–1792
Desaturate, 643
Desflurane (Suprane), 444t
Desipramine (Norpramin), 244
Desloratadine (Clarinex), 1069t
Desmopressin (DDAVP), 951, 953, 955
  in diabetes insipidus, 1510
Desquamation, 1273
Desquamative inflammatory vaginitis, 1689
Destination therapy, 828
Detrusor hyperactivity, 216
Developmental disabilities, 150
Dexamethasone (Decadron), 976, 1541t, 2067, 2096, 2100
  anorexia management, 405–406
  drug interactions, 428t

Dexlansoprazole (Dexilant), for GERD, 1284t
Dexrazoxane (Zinecard), 346
Diabetes, 680, 682, 695, 1457. *See also*
    Glycosylated hemoglobin
  assessment and diagnostic findings, 1460–
    1461, 1461c
  blood glucose monitoring, 1466–1467
  CF-related, 666
  classification, 1457, 1458t
  clinical manifestations, 1460
  community diabetes education, impact of,
    1478c
  complications of, 1481
    diabetic ketoacidosis, 1483–1485
    diabetic neuropathy, 1493–1494
    diabetic retinopathy, 1489–1491
    foot and leg problems, 1494–1495
    hyperglycemic hyperosmolar syndrome,
      1485–1488
    hypoglycemia, 1482–1483
    long-term, 1488–1495
    macrovascular complications, 1488–1489
    microvascular, 1489–
    nephropathy, 1491–1493
  consequences, 1457
  criteria for diagnosis of, 1460c
  description of, 1456
  economic cost of, 1457
  epidemiology, 1457
  exercise, 1465–1466
    older adults and, 1466
    precautions, 1465–1466
    recommendations, 1465, 1465c
  gestational, 1459–1460
  and heart failure, 819
  hospitalized patients, management of, 1496
    diet, alterations in, 1498
    hygiene, 1499
    hyperglycemia, 1497
    hypoglycemia, 1497–1498
    nursing management, 1499–1500
    older patients, 1499
    self-care issues, 1496–1497
    stress management, 1499
  ketones, testing for, 1467–1468
  latent autoimmune diabetes of adults, 1460
  medical management, 1461–1473
  nursing management, 1473
    home, community-based, and transitional
      care, 1479–1481
    hyperglycemia, management of, 1473,
      1475
    patient education, 1475–1479
  nutritional therapy, 1461–1465
    caloric distribution, 1462–1463
    caloric requirements, 1462
    dietary concerns, 1464–1465
    food classification systems, 1463–1464
    food exchange system, 1462
    goals of, 1461–1462
    meal planning and education, 1462–1464
  in older adults, 1460–1461
  pathophysiology, 1457–1460, 1459f
  and peripheral arterial disease, 851
  pharmacologic management, 1468–1473
    adjunct therapies, 1473
    insulin therapy, 1468–1473
    oral antidiabetic agents, 1473,
      1474t–1475t
  prevention, 1460

  risk factors for, 1457c
  type 1, 1458–1459
  type 2, 1459
  visual complications, 1489, 1490t
Diabetes Control and Complications Trial
    Research Group (DCCT), 1461
Diabetes insipidus (DI), 1502, 1508, 1509
  ADH deficiency and, 1509
  assessment and diagnostic findings, 1509
  causes of, 1509
  clinical manifestations, 1509
  hypernatremia and, 267, 268
  medical management, 1509–1510
  nursing management, 1510
  polydipsia in, 1509
Diabetes mellitus (DM). *See also* Diabetes
  diabetes type 2, 126t
  ketoacidosis, 278
Diabetes patient education programs, 1475
Diabetes Prevention Program Outcomes Study,
    1460
Diabetic dermopathy, 1803
Diabetic diarrhea, 1494
Diabetic ketoacidosis (DKA), 1456, 1459,
    1483–1485
  assessment and diagnostic findings, 1484
  clinical features of, 1483
  and hyperglycemic hyperosmolar syndrome,
    1486t
  and hypokalemia, 1488
  management of, 1485
    electrolyte balance, 1485
    rehydration, 1485
    reversing acidosis, 1485
  nursing process, 1487–1488
    assessment, 1487
    diagnosis, 1487
    nursing interventions, 1487–1488
    planning and goals, 1487
  pathophysiology, 1483–1484, 1483f
  prevention of, 1484
  sick day rules, 1484c
Diabetic neuropathy, 1493
  autonomic neuropathy, 1493–1494
  peripheral neuropathy, 1493
Diabetic osteomyelitis, 1176
Diabetic retinopathy, 1489–1491, 1490f, 1490t,
    1912
  assessment and diagnostic findings, 1490
  clinical manifestations, 1490
  home, community-based, and transitional
    care, 1491
  and macular edema, 1489
  medical management, 1490–1491
  nonproliferative, 1489
  nursing management, 1491
  preproliferative, 1489
  proliferative, 1490
Diagnosis, in nursing process, 35–36, 38
  choosing nursing diagnosis, 38
  collaborative problems, 38–39, 39f
  nursing diagnoses, 38, 39f
Diagnostic peritoneal lavage (DPL), 2170
Dialysate, 1567
  magnesium-free, 279
Dialysis, 1595
  acute kidney injury and, 1580
  continuous renal replacement therapies,
    1594, 1595f
  hemodialysis, 1589–1594

  hospitalization, considerations during, 1601
    blood pressure monitoring, 1602
    cardiac and respiratory complications, 1601
    catheter site, caring for, 1602
    discomfort and pain, 1601
    electrolyte levels and diet, 1601
    infection prevention, 1602
    intravenous therapy, 1601
    medications administration, 1602
    psychological support, 1602
    uremia symptoms, 1601
    vascular access, 1601
  in hypervolemia, 263
  peritoneal dialysis, 1595–1601
  quality of life in patients on, 1593c
Dialyzer, 1567, 1589–1590
Diaphragm, 1672
Diaphragmatic breathing, 430c
Diaphragmatic excursion, 497–498
Diaphysis, 1115
Diarrhea, 1311, 1314–1316, 2146
  acute, 1314
  antibiotic-associated, 1315
  assessment and diagnostic findings, 1315
  chronic, 1314, 1315
  clinical manifestations, 1315
  complications, 1315
  exudative, 1315
  infectious, 1315
  malabsorptive, 1315
  medical management, 1316
  nursing management, 1316
  older patients and, 1315–1316
  osmotic, 1315
  pathophysiology, 1315
  persistent, 1314
  secretory, 1315
Diarthrosis joints, 1117–1118, 1118f
Diastole, 713
Diastolic blood pressure (DBP), 884
Diastolic heart failure, 818, 819. *See also* Heart
    failure (HF)
Diazepam (Valium), 447t, 2111
  drug interactions, 428t
  seizure activity, 2173
DIC. *See* Disseminated intravascular coagulation
Diclofenac, 235
Diclofenac sodium gel (Voltaren gel), 1105
Dicloxacillin (Dynapen), 666
  in impetigo, 1818
Dicyclomine (Bentyl), 1318
Didanosine (ddl), 1034t
Diet
  and bone health, 1116
  cancer risk and, 329
  cultural differences, 108, 108c
  neutropenic, 351c
Dietary Approaches to Stop Hypertension
    (DASH) diet, 888, 889t, 1364
Diethylpropion (Tenuate), for obesity, 1365t
Diethyltoluamide (DEET), 2070
Differentiation, stem cells, 903, 904f
Diffuse connective tissue disease, 1090, 1093
  giant cell arteritis, 1103–1104
  polymyalgia rheumatica, 1103–1104
  polymyositis, 1102–1103
  rheumatoid arthritis, 1093–1098
  scleroderma, 1101–1102
  Sjögren's syndrome, 1101
  systemic lupus erythematosus, 1098–1101

Diffuse esophageal spasm (DES), 1279–1280
Diffusion, 253, 1567
Digestion, 1224, 1226
    waste products of, 1228
Digestive enzymes and secretions, 1226t
Digitalis, for heart failure, 824t, 825–826
Digital mammography, for breast screening, 1725
Digital rectal examination (DRE), 1558, 1755
Digoxin (Lanoxin), for heart failure, 824t
Dihydrotestosterone (DHT), 1762
Dilated cardiomyopathy (DCM), 801, 802, 819
Dilation and curettage (D&C), 1664
Diltiazem extended release (Cardizem CD, Dilacor XR, Tiazac)
    for hypertension, 892t
Diltiazem (Cardizem, Tiazac), for angina, 758t, 759
Diltiazem long acting (Cardizem LA), for hypertension, 892t
Dimenhydrinate (Dramamine), 460t
Dipeptidyl peptidase-4 (DPP-4) inhibitors, 1475t
Diphenhydramine (Benadryl), 242, 319, 1059, 1069t, 1601
    in general pruritus, 1812
    in snakebites, 2177
Diplopia, 1876, 1899, 1910
Dipyridamole (Persantine), 699
Direct-acting oral anticoagulants, for atrial fibrillation, 724
Dirty bomb, 2202
Disability, 139–161
    accepting limitations, 161
    categories of, 150–151
    characteristics of, 150–152
    communicating with people have, 155c
    definitions of, 149–150
    disabling disorders versus, 151–152
    facts, 150c
    federal legislation, 152–154
    medical–surgical nursing practice, 159–160
    models of, 151, 152c
    nursing care of patients, 158–161
    people with
        perioperative period, 421–422
    prevalence of, 150
    substance abuse rates, 167
    types of, 150–151
Disability Rating Scale (DRS), 167
Disarticulation, 1185, 1214
Disaster, caring for people with disabilities, 2199c
Disaster levels, 2194c
Disaster Medical Assistance Teams (DMAT), 2195
Disaster Mortuary Operational Response Teams (DMORT), 2195
Discharge
    after surgery, 461–463, 463c
    planning, 19
        emergency nursing and, 2160
    from postanesthesia care units, 461–463
    preparation for, 461–462
    readiness for, 461
Disease Activity Score-28 (DAS28), 1094
Disease Control and Prevention (CDC), 329
Disease, definition of, 84
Disease-modifying antirheumatic drugs (DMARDs), 1084, 1088t, 1095

Disease transmission, prevention of, 2072
Disk degeneration and back pain, 1160
Dislocation, 1185, 1186
Dissection, 841, 852
Disseminated intravascular coagulation (DIC), 302, 956–959, 1195
    assessment and diagnostic findings, 956, 958, 958t
    care of patient with, 960c–961c
    clinical manifestations, 956, 957c
    medical management, 958–959
    nursing management, 959
    pathophysiology, 956, 957f
    scoring system for, 958, 958t
Dissolution therapy, for gallstones, 1428, 1433, 1434
Distal interphalangeal (DIP) joint, 1105
Distributive justice, 31c
Distributive shock, 296, 313–319
Disuse syndrome, 1135, 1135c
Diuresis, 1548, 1551
Diuretics
    for ascites, 1386–1387, 1408
    drug interactions, 428t
    for heart failure, 824t, 825
    for hypertension, 890t
    loop, 263
    for lymphedema, 881
    for pulmonary edema, 834
    thiazide, 275
Diverticular disease, 1325–1327
    assessment and diagnostic findings, 1326
    clinical manifestations, 1325–1326
    Hinchey classification, 1326t
    medical management, 1326–1327
    nursing management, 1327
    in older adults, 1326
    pathophysiology, 1325
    surgical management, 1326–1327, 1326f
Diverticulitis, 1311
Diverticulosis, 1311, 1325
Diverticulum, 1281–1282, 1281f, 1311, 1325
Dizziness
    definition of, 1915
    ear and, 1932
    in older adults, 216
DKA. See Diabetic ketoacidosis
DMARDs. See Disease-modifying antirheumatic drugs
DNP. See D-type natriuretic peptide
Dobutamine (Dobutrex), 700
    in cardiogenic shock, 311
    for heart failure, 826
Docetaxel (Taxotere), 343t
DOCK8 deficiency, 1024t
Doctor of nursing practice (DNP) programs, 12
Docusate (Colace), 1314t
Dofetilide (Tikosyn), for atrial fibrillation, 724
Dolutegravir (DTG), 1035t
Dominant genetic disorders, 119f
Donor site
    autografts, 1863
    description of, 1845, 1863
Dopamine
    in cardiogenic shock, 311
    in cardiopulmonary resuscitation, 839t
Doppler techniques, 702
Dornase alfa (Pulmozyme), 666

Dorsal recumbent position, 452
Dorsiflexion, 171c
Dose-dense chemotherapy, 1719, 1742
Double-cuffed tube, 524f
Double effect, 31c
Douche, 1686, 1689
Doxazosin (Cardura)
    for BPH, 1763
    for hypertension, 891t
Doxorubicin (Adriamycin), 343t
Doxycycline (Vibramycin)
    for anthrax treatment, 2204
    for gonorrhea, 1694
    for hidradenitis suppurativa, 1813
    for pelvic inflammatory disease, 1696
Dressings
    active, 1807
    biosynthetic, 1864
    burn injuries, 1861–1862
    categories of, 1807–1809, 1808t
    changing of, 469
    foam, 1809
    function and action of, 1808t
    interactive, 1807
    moisture-retentive, 1808–1809
    occlusive, 1808
    passive, 1807
    synthetic, 1864
Dromotropy, 712, 713
Dronabinol (Marinol), 406, 1042
Drone, 2180
Droplet precautions, 2131
Drug abuse, 2180
Drug-induced hepatitis, 1405
Drug interactions, surgical issues, 428t
Drug metabolism, in liver, 1379–1380
Drug overdose, emergency management in, 2181t–2184t
Drug use, preoperative assessments, 424–425
Dry bites, 2176
Dry eye, 1905–1906
Dryness of mouth. See Xerostomia
Dry powder inhaler, 641t
Dry purpura, 949
Dry suction water seal systems, 542
d-Tubocurarin, 447t
D-type natriuretic peptide (DNP), 258
Dual-energy x-ray absorptiometry (DEXA), 1127, 1171, 1205
Dubin—Johnson syndrome, 1385
Duchenne muscular dystrophy, 2111
Ductal carcinoma in situ (DCIS), 1719, 1730
Dulaglutide (Trulicity), 1475t
Duloxetine (Cymbalta), 244
    for diabetic peripheral neuropathy, 1493
    for low back pain, 1161
Dumping syndrome, 1243, 1248, 1292, 1305, 1358, 1373
    prevention of, 1252c
    tube feedings and, 1251
Duodenal ulcers, 1241
Duodenum, 1243, 1244, 1292, 1294
Duplex ultrasonography, 841, 848
Dupuytren disease, 1165, 1165f
Durable power of attorney, for health care
    definition of, 193, 219
Dutasteride (Avodart), for BPH, 1763
DVT. See Deep vein thrombosis
Dwarfism, 1502, 1508

Dying
  in America, 388
  conspiracy of silence about, 389
  coping with, 412
  physiologic changes, 407–409
  religious/cultural beliefs and, 396t–397t
Dying in America: Improving Quality and Honoring Individual Preferences Near the End of Life, 388
Dysarthria, 2009, 2011
Dyschezia, 1704
Dysfunctional uterine bleeding, 1668
Dyskinesias, 2103
  Guillain-Barré syndrome and, 2082
  Parkinson disease, 2103
Dyslipidemia, 885
Dysmenorrhea, 1650, 1654, 1667–1668
  assessment and diagnostic findings, 1667
  management, 1667–1668
  primary, 1667
  secondary, 1667
Dyspareunia, 1650, 1654, 1668–1669, 1711
Dyspepsia, 1224, 1229–1230, 1292, 1293
Dysphagia, 552, 1264, 1269, 1279, 1358, 1373, 2009, 2022, 2077, 2078, 2079
  aging and, 199
Dysphonia, 2079, 2103
  definition of, 2079, 2103
  Parkinson disease, 2103
Dysplasia, 1264, 1283, 1686, 1691
  cellular adaptation, 92
  definition of, 84
Dyspnea
  anxiety and, 404
  description of, 480, 488–489
  end-of-life care, 403–404
  measuring tools for, 489t
  palliative care for, 404c
  pharmacologic management of, 403
Dyspnea on exertion (DOE), 822
Dysrhythmias, 713–748
  adjunctive modalities and management, 736–748
    defibrillation, 737, 738, 738c
    electrical cardioversion, 737–738, 738c
    electrophysiology studies, 738–739
    implantable cardioverter defibrillator, 744–748
    pacemaker therapy, 739–744
  assessment, 734–735
  atrial, 720–727
    atrial fibrillation, 720–726
    atrial flutter, 726–727
    premature atrial complex, 720
  conduction abnormalities and, 732–734
  definition of, 712
  diagnosis, 735
  electrical conduction and, 713
  electrocardiogram and, 713–717
    components of, 715–716, 716f
    interpretation of, 717c
    obtaining, 713–715
    rhythm strip, 716–717
  evaluation, 736
  goals for patient, 735
  influences on heart rate and contractility, 713
  junctional, 727–729, 727f
    atrioventricular nodal reentry tachycardia, 728–729
    junctional rhythm, 727–728

nonparoxysmal junctional tachycardia, 728
    premature junctional complex, 727
  nursing interventions, 735–736
  in postanesthesia units, 459
  sinus node, 718–720
    sinus arrhythmia, 720
    sinus bradycardia, 718–719
    sinus tachycardia, 719–720
  sinus rhythm, 718
    with first-degree AV block, 732, 732f
    with second-degree AV block, 732–734, 733f
    with third-degree AV block, 734, 734f
  types of, 718–734
  ventricular, 729–732
    idioventricular rhythm, 731, 731f
    premature ventricular complex, 729, 729f
    ventricular asystole, 731–732, 732f
    ventricular fibrillation, 730–731, 731f
    ventricular tachycardia, 730
Dysrhythmias atrial, electrophysiologic (EPS) testing, 705
Dysuria, 1548, 1555, 1556t

E
Ear
  anatomy, 1915–1920, 1916f
  function of
    balance and equilibrium, 1918
    hearing, 1918
    sound conduction, 1918, 1919f
Early-onset familial Alzheimer disease (EOFAD), 125t
Eastern equine, 2070
  encephalitis, 2070
  fungal, 2070
  herpes simplex virus, 2069
  La Crosse, 2070
  St. Louis, 2070
  West Nile virus, 2070
Ebola virus, 2126t, 2151
EBPs. *See* Evidence-based practices
EBRT. *See* External-beam radiation therapy
Ecchymoses, 1801, 1801t, 2093
Eccrine sweat glands, 1792
Echocardiography, 699, 700, 702
  nursing interventions, 702–703
  procedure, 702
  stress testing, 699
  transesophageal, 702
  transthoracic, 702
Ecstasy. *See* 3,4-methylenedioxymethamphetamine (MDMA)
Ectoparasites, 1820
Ectopic pregnancy, 1679–1681
  assessment and diagnostic findings, 1679–1680
  causes of, 1679
  clinical manifestations, 1679
  incidence of, 1679
  nursing process, 1680–1681
    assessment, 1680
    complications management, 1680–1681
    diagnosis, 1680
    evaluation, 1681
    grieving process, supporting, 1680
    nursing interventions, 1680–1681
    pain relief, 1680
    patient education, 1681
    planning and goals, 1680

pharmacologic therapy, 1680
  risk factors for, 1679
  sites of, 1679f
  surgical management, 1680
Ectropion, 1876, 1881
Eczema. *See* Contact dermatitis
Edatrexate fludarabine (Fludara), 343t
Edema, 683
  airway, 655
  cirrhosis and, 1407
  and ecchymosis, localized, 1189
  interstitial pulmonary, 693
  liver dysfunction and, 1397
  patient education, 264
  peripheral, 686
  right-sided heart failure, 643
  and total knee arthroplasty, 1155
Edoxaban (Savaysa), 965
  for venous thromboembolism, 870t
Edrophonium chloride (Tensilon), 2079
Education. *See also* Patient education
  adherence to regimens and, 44
  people with disabilities, 53t
Edwards Lifesciences Vigileo monitoring system, 709
EEG. *See* Electroencephalogram
Efavirenz (EFV), 1034t
Effector T cells, 1010–1012
Effluent, 1567
Effort thrombosis, 869
Effusion, 1124, 1125f
EGFR. *See* Epidermal growth factor receptor
Egophony, 480, 500
EHR. *See* Electronic health record
Ejaculation, disorders of, 1760–1761
Ejaculatory duct, 1753
Ejection fraction (EF), 678, 683, 702, 818, 819
ELAD (extracorporeal liver assist devices), 1405
Elbow, 1199–1200
Elder abuse, 193, 217–218, 2186
  definition of, 193
  neglect, 217–218
Elective replacement indicator (ERI), 712
Electrical burns, 1849, 1850c
Electrical cardioversion, for dysrhythmias, 737–738, 738c
Electrocardiogram (ECG)
  ambulatory, 696–697
  cardiac event recorders, 697
  cardiac implantable electronic devices, 697–699
  continuous monitoring, 696, 697
  continuous real-time monitors, 697
  and dysrhythmias, 713–717
    components of, 715–716, 716f
    definition of, 712
    electrode placement., 715, 715f
    electrophysiology study, 714–715
    hardwire monitoring, 714
    heart rate, determination of, 71t
    Holter monitor, 714
    interpretation of, 717c
    obtaining, 713–715
    PP interval, 716
    PR interval, 716
    P wave, 715
    QRS complex, 715–716
    QT interval, 716
    rhythm strip, 716–717
    RR interval, 716

standard 12-lead, 715
ST segment, 716
telemetry, 714
TP interval, 716
T wave, 716
U wave, 716
lead systems, 696
myocardial infarction, 763–764, 764f
Electrocardiographic monitoring
continuous, 696
electrode placement, 697
monitoring system, 696c
real-time monitors, 697
Electrocautery, for genital warts, 1691
Electroconvulsive therapy, 207
Electrode placement, 698
Electroencephalography, 2038, 2069
nervous system, 1968–1969
Electrohydraulic lithotripsy, 1634
Electrolyte balance, 786. See also Body fluids
burn injuries, 1851–1852
in cardiac surgery, 786
glucose and, 93
homeostasis and, 251
kidney functions, 256
Electrolyte imbalance, 251, 264–283
calcium imbalance, 272–276
chloride imbalance, 281–283
magnesium imbalance, 276–279
medications and, 205
medications and, 205
phosphorus imbalance, 279–281
potassium imbalance, 268–272
side effects of diuretics and, 263
sodium imbalance, 264–268
Electrolytes, 252–253
body fluid, 252, 253t
concentration, 252
excretion, regulation of, 1552
hypovolemia and, 259
IV solutions, 288–290
monitoring, 347
selected water and, 261
transport of, 253
Electrolyte solutions, 261t
isotonic, 260
Electromyogram (EMG)
for low back pain, 1161c
for musculoskeletal disorders, 1128–1129
nervous system, 1969
Electron beam CT (EBCT), 701
Electronic health record (EHR), 33, 38, 62
Electronic Health Record (EHR) Incentive
Program, 7
Electronic nicotine delivery systems (ENDS),
492
Electrophysiology study (EPS), 705
Electrosurgery, 1835
Elephantiasis, 880
Elimination, 1224, 1226
altered patterns of, 186–188
Eltrombopag (Promacta), 950, 982
Eluxadoline (Viberzi, Allergan), 1318
Elvitegravir (EVG), 1035t
Embryonic stem cells, 1013
Emergency care
burn injuries, 1853–1856
at burn scene, 1853, 1854c
principles of
triage, 2161–2163

Emergency contraception, 1674
emergency contraceptive pills, 1674
nursing management, 1674
postcoital intrauterine device insertion, 1674
Emergency department (ED), 2156
facts about, 2157c
Emergency management, 2050–2051, 2156
Emergency medical services (EMS), 34, 2160,
2196
Emergency Medical Treatment and Active
Labor Act (EMTALA), 2157
Emergency Nurses Association (ENA), 1198,
2156, 2195
Emergency nursing and the continuum of care
community and transitional services, 2160
discharge planning, 2160
gerontologic considerations, 2160
obesity considerations, 2160–2161
Emergency nursing care, issues in
consent and privacy, 2157
emergency department, violence in,
2157–2158
health risks, exposure to, 2157
holistic care, 2158–2160
family-focused interventions, 2159–2160,
2159c
patient-focused interventions, 2158–2159
Emergency operations plan (EOP),
2195–2196
components of, 2196
initiating, 2196–2200
communicating with media and family,
2198, 2198c
critical incident stress management,
2199–2200
identifying patients and documenting
patient information, 2196–2197
managing internal problems, 2197–2198
nurse's role in disaster response plans,
2198–2199
triage, 2197, 2197t
Emergency personnel, caring for, 2159–2160
Emergency Severity Index (ESI), 2161
Emergency surgery, 422
Emerging infectious diseases, 2150–2153
Emesis, 2188
EMG. See Electromyogram
EMLA (eutectic mixture or emulsion of local
anesthetics), 234
Emmetropia, 1876, 1883
Empagliflozin (Jardiance), 1475t
Empathetic listening, 979
Emphysema, 500t, 636, 636f
Empyema, 583, 608–609
of gallbladder, 1430
Emtricitabine (FTC), 1034t
Enalapril (Vasotec)
for heart failure, 824t
for hypertension, 892t
Encephalitis, arthropod-borne virus, 2070
Enchondroma, 1180
Endocarditis
infective, 810–812
rheumatic, 809–810, 810c
Endocardium, 673, 679t
Endocervicitis, 1686, 1694–1695
Endocrine, definition of, 1428, 1429, 1502,
1503
Endocrine function, preoperative assessments,
426

Endocrine system, 1503
adrenal glands, 1531–1543
anatomy and physiology of, 1503–1504
assessment, 1504–1505
health history, 1504
physical examination, 1504–1505
diagnostic studies, 1505
blood tests, 1505–1506
genetic screening, 1506
imaging studies, 1506
stimulation tests, 1506
suppression tests, 1506
urine tests, 1506
glands of, 1503, 1504f
hormones produced by, 1503–1504, 1505t
parathyroid glands, 1527–1530
pituitary gland, 1506–1510
thyroid gland, 1510–1527
End-of-life care, 634, 645, 667
comfort measures, 403
culturally sensitive, 399–400
death and dying in America, 388
decision making, 401f
ethical dilemmas, 388, 391c
humane approach to, 388
hydration, 404–406
interventions during, 399c
issues, 34
nutrition and, 404–406
preferences, 397c, 400c
settings for, 391–395
sociocultural context, 388–390
technology and, 388
End of Life Options Act, 390
Endolymph, 1917
Endolymphatic hydrops, 1915, 1933
Endolymphatic sac decompression, 1934
Endometrial ablation, 1650, 1665
Endometrial biopsy, 1663–1664
Endometrial hyperplasia, 1705–1706
Endometriosis, 1686, 1704–1705
assessment and diagnostic findings, 1704
clinical manifestations, 1704
medical management, 1704–1705
pharmacologic therapy, 1705
surgical management, 1705
nursing management, 1705
pathophysiology, 1704
risk factors, 1704
transplantation theory, 1704
Endometriosis Association, 1705
Endometrium, 1650, 1652
Endophthalmitis, 1876, 1893, 1905, 1912
Endoscopic bronchoscopy, 505–506, 506f
Endoscopic myotomy, 1279
Endoscopic retrograde
cholangiopancreatography (ERCP),
1237, 1428, 1433, 1433f
in chronic pancreatitis, 1445
in pancreatic carcinoma, 1450
Endoscopic sclerotherapy, for variceal bleeding,
1391, 1391f
Endoscopic thoracoscopy, 506–507, 507f
Endoscopic ultrasonography (EUS), 1233
Endoscopic variceal ligation (EVL), 1377,
1391–1392, 1391f
Endoscopy
for esophageal varices, 1389
middle ear, 1922
Endosteum, 1116

Endotracheal intubation, 510, 521–523, 522f, 523c, 2068, 2101, 2163–2164, 2164f
    preventing complications, 524c
    during surgery, 440
Endourologic methods of stone removal, 1634
Endourology, 1564–1565, 1565f
Endovascular grafting, of abdominal aortic aneurysms, 864, 864f
Endovascular therapy, 2015
End-stage kidney disease (ESKD), 1457, 1567, 1569, 1581–1589
    assessment and diagnostic findings
        acidosis, 1582
        anemia, 1582
        calcium and phosphorus imbalance, 1582–1583
        glomerular filtration rate, 1581–1582
        sodium and water retention, 1582
    cardiovascular disease and, 1581
    clinical manifestations, 1581, 1582c
    complications of, 1583
    medical management, 1583–1584
        dialysis, 1584
        nutritional therapy, 1584
        pharmacologic therapy, 1583–1584
    nursing care plan, 1585c–1588c
    nursing management, 1584
        continuing and transitional care, 1584
        patient education, 1584
    in older patients, 1584, 1589
    pathophysiology, 1581
End-stage liver disease (ESLD)
    with cirrhosis, 1408
    and liver transplantation, 1420
ENFit connections, 1246, 1247f
Enflurane (Ethrane), 444t
Enfuvirtide (T-20), 1035t
Enoxaparin (Lovenox), 683
    for angina, 758t
    in total hip arthroplasty treatment, 1152
    for venous thromboembolism, 870t
Entamoeba histolytica, 1425
Entecavir (ETV), in hepatitis B, 1402
Enteral feedings, in acute pancreatitis, 1442
Enteral nutrition, 1243, 1246. See also Gastrointestinal intubation
    complications of, 1251t
    indications for, 1248t
    during repositioning and incidence of aspiration, 1248c
Enteric, 1243, 1245
Enterocele, 1558, 1686, 1698–1699, 1698f
Enteroclysis, 1309
Enterocutaneous fistula, 1331
Enterohepatic circulation, 1379, 1429
Enteroviruses, 2065
Entropion, 1876, 1899, 1907
Enucleation, 1876, 1904, 1910–1911
Enuresis, 1556t
Envenomation, 2156, 2176
    signs of, 2176
Environment
    interpersonal, 67
    physical, 67
    safe postsurgical, 472–473
    spiritual, 67
    surgical, 440–443
        controls, 441
        health hazards, 442–443

Environmental emergencies
    animal and human bites, 2175–2176
    decompression sickness
        assessment and diagnostic findings, 2175
        management, 2175
    frostbite
        assessment and diagnostic findings, 2173
        management, 2173
    heat-induced illnesses, 2171–2172
        assessment and diagnostic findings, 2172
        gerontologic considerations, 2172
        management, 2172–2173
    hypothermia, 2173
        assessment and diagnostic findings, 2174
        management, 2174
    nonfatal drowning, 2174–2175
        management, 2175
    snakebites, 2176
        clinical manifestations, 2176
        management, 2176–2177
    spider bites, 2177
    tick bites, 2177–2178
Environmental Protection Agency (EPA), 2201
Envoy esteem, 1940. See also Implanted hearing devices
Enzymatic débridement, 876
Enzyme immunoassay (EIA), 1025
Enzyme-linked immunosorbent assay (ELISA), 1025
Eosinophil chemotactic factor of anaphylaxis, 1059, 1059t
Eosinophils, 906, 907, 1059
Epicardium, 673
Epicondylitis, 1187
Epicutaneous immunotherapy (EPIT), 1071
Epicutaneous tests, 1063
Epidermal growth factor receptor (EGFR), 326
Epidermis, skin, 1791
Epidermopoiesis, 1806, 1825
Epididymectomy, 1779
Epididymitis, 1752, 1779
Epidural anesthesia, 445
    advantages of, 445
    injection sites for, 448f
Epidural hematomas (EDHs) symptoms, 2036
Epidural infusions, 466
Epidural monitor, 1982
Epigastric area, 689
Epigastric distress, 1431
Epigenetics, 115
Epiglottis, 481
Epilepsy, 1961–1964
    age related changes, 1999–2000, 1999c
    medical management, 2000–2001, 2000t
    nursing process, 2001–2004
    pathophysiology, 1998–1999
    surgical management, 2001
Epinephrine, 844, 1531
    in cardiopulmonary resuscitation, 839t
    dysrhythmia, 738
    self-administration of, 1067c
    for ventricular fibrillation, 731
EpiPen, 1065
Epiphyseal plate, 1115
Epiphyses, 1115
Epirubicin, 343t
Epistaxis, 552, 569–570, 569c, 570f
Epitopes, 1005
Eplerenone (Inspra), 1540
    for hypertension, 890t

Epoetin alfa (Epogen), 1145, 1583, 1742
Epogen, 1145
Epoprostenol (Flolan), 1102
Eprosartan (Teveten), for hypertension, 892t
Epstein-Barr virus (EBV), cancer and, 328
Eptifibatide (Integrilin), 683
Epzicom (3TC/ABC), 1034t
Equianalgesia, 238
Equilibrium radionuclide angiocardiography (ERNA), 701
ERCP. See Endoscopic retrograde cholangiopancreatography
Erectile dysfunction, 1752, 1756–1760
    assessment and diagnostic findings, 1756
    diabetes and, 1494
    evaluation and treatment of, 1757f
    medications associated with, 1757c
    nursing management, 1760
    organic causes, 1756
    psychogenic causes, 1756
    treatment of, 1756–1760, 1758t
        negative-pressure devices, 1760
        penile implants, 1759–1760
        penis transplant, 1760
        pharmacologic therapy, 1757–1759, 1758t, 1759t
Ergonomic injuries. See Occupation-related musculoskeletal disorder
Erlotinib (Tarceva), in pancreatic carcinoma, 1451
Erosion, 1799t
Erythema, 1063, 1790, 1796
Erythrocytapheresis, 913t
Erythrocytes, 925. See also Red blood cells (RBCs)
Erythrocyte sedimentation rate (ESR), 989, 1172
Erythroderma. See Generalized exfoliative dermatitis
Erythroid cells, 932
Erythroid-stimulating agents, 988
Erythromelalgia, 984
Erythromycin (E-Mycin, Erythra-Derm)
    for acne, 1815
    for anthrax treatment, 2204
    for hidradenitis suppurativa, 1813
Erythroplakia, 1267t
Erythropoiesis, 905–906
Erythropoietin (EPO), 345, 906, 923c, 926, 1503, 1582
    in ESKD, 1583–1584
Eschar, 1845, 1851
Escharotomy, 1845, 1851, 2173
    of forearm, 1851f
Escherichia coli, 1617, 2103
    wound infections, 474
ESKD. See End-stage kidney disease
Esmolol (Brevibloc), 1534
    for alcohol withdrawal syndrome, 2185
Esomeprazole (Nexium), 1169
    for gastritis, 1295t
    for GERD, 1284t
Esophageal adenocarcinoma (EAC), 1283
Esophageal banding therapy. See Endoscopic variceal ligation (EVL)
Esophageal cancer, 1286–1289
    adenocarcinoma, 1286
    assessment and diagnostic findings, 1287
    clinical manifestations, 1287
    medical management, 1287–1288, 1287f

palliative treatment, 1288
reconstruction with free jejunal transfer, 1287, 1287f
surgical resection of esophagus, 1287
transhiatal esophagectomy, 1287, 1288f
nursing management, 1288–1289
risk factors for, 1286–1287
squamous cell carcinoma, 1286
stages of, 1287
Esophageal candidiasis, HIV infection and, 1039
Esophageal Doppler probes, 709
Esophageal manometry, 1240, 1280
Esophageal spasm, 1279–1280
Esophageal speech, 575
Esophageal sphincter
lower, 1279
upper, 1279
Esophageal varices, 1388–1393
assessment and diagnostic findings, 1389
endoscopy, 1389
laboratory tests, 1390
portal hypertension measurements, 1389–1390
bleeding, 1389
cirrhosis and, 1388
clinical manifestations, 1389
medical management, 1390
balloon tamponade, 1390–1391
coated expandable stents, 1392
endoscopic sclerotherapy, 1391, 1391f
endoscopic variceal ligation, 1391–1392, 1391f
pharmacologic therapy, 1390
tissue adhesives and fibrin glue, 1392
transjugular intrahepatic portosystemic shunt, 1392
mortality rate, 1389
nursing management, 1393, 1393t
pathophysiology, 1389, 1389f
surgical management, 1393
devascularization and transection, 1393
surgical bypass procedures, 1392–1393, 1392f
Esophagogastroduodenoscopy (EGD), 1237, 1280–1281
Esophagojejunostomy, 1304
Esophagomyotomy, 1279
Esophagus, 1224, 1225
Esophagus, disorders of, 1279
achalasia, 1279, 1280f
Barrett esophagus, 1283–1284
benign tumors, 1284–1286
chemical burns, 1283
diverticulum, 1281–1282, 1281f
esophageal cancer, 1286–1289
esophageal spasm, 1279–1280
foreign bodies, 1282
gastroesophageal reflux disease, 1283, 1284t
hiatal hernia, 1280–1281, 1281f
home care checklist, 1286c
perforation, 1282
Essential hypertension. See Primary hypertension
Essential thrombocythemia (ET), 985–987
assessment and diagnostic findings, 986
clinical manifestations, 986
complications, 986
medical management, 986–987
nursing management, 987
Estradiol, 1653
Estrogen, 1650, 1653

effects on bone remodeling, 1116–1117
patches, 1683
ESWL. See Extracorporeal shock wave lithotripsy
Etanercept (Enbrel), 1089t, 1107
for psoriasis, 1826
Ethacrynic acid (Edecrin), for hypertension, 890t
Ethical dilemmas
comfort care issues, 1855c
end-of-life care and, 388, 391c
informed consent, 422–423
Ethical problems, in nursing, 32–33
confidentiality, 33
end-of-life issues, 34
refusal to care, 34
restraints, 33
trust issues, 33
Ethics committees, 34
Ethics, in healthcare, 29–35
approaches to
applied ethics, 31
meta-ethics, 31
ethical principles, 31c
ethics vs. morality, 30
moral dilemmas, 31–32
theories related to, 3031
Ethnicity, definition of, 68
Ethnocentrism, 102, 111
Ethylenediaminetetraacetic acid (EDTA), 949
Etomidate (Amidate), 447t
Etoposide (Etopophos, VePesid), 343t, 972
Etravirine (ETR), 1034t
Eupnea, 495, 496t
European League Against Rheumatism guidelines, 1107
Euthanasia
definition of, 387
palliative sedation and, 407
Euthanasia, Assisted Suicide and Aid in Dying, 390
Euthyroid, 1502, 1511
Evaluation phase, of nursing process, 41–42
Everolimus (Afinitor, Zortess), 1610t
Eversion, 171c
"Every Woman, Every Time" campaign, 1669
Evidence-based practices (EBPs), 8–9
bundles, 9
Evisceration, 1876, 1911
definition of, 456
wound, 474, 475f
EVL. See Endoscopic variceal ligation
Exacerbations, 1082, 1098, 2074
Exchange lists, for meal planning, 1463, 1463t
Excision, 1845, 1847
Excisional biopsy, 335
of breast, 1727
Exemestane (Aromasin), 1732, 1743, 1744t
Exenatide (Byetta, Bydureon), for diabetes, 1473
Exenteration, 1876, 1911
Exercises
after breast surgery, 1739c
bed, 467–468
in diabetes management, 1465–1466
of extremities, 429
leg, 430c
range-of-motion, 171–172, 171c
therapeutic, 172, 172t
types of, 172, 172t
Exercise stress test, 699, 1465
Exercise training, 644, 646

Exertional dysnatremia, 267
Exocrine, definition of, 1428, 1429, 1502, 1503
Exophthalmos, 1502, 1504, 1876, 1902
Exostoses, 1915, 1927
Explosive devices, types of, 2202–2203. See also Blast injury
Expressive aphasia, 2011
Extension, 171c
External-beam radiation therapy (EBRT), 339, 341
for prostate cancer, 1765, 1769
External catheters, 187
External ear
anatomy of, 1916
conditions of, 1926
Inspection of, 1918
masses of, 1927
External fixator, 1131, 1137–1139, 1138f
home care checklist, 1139c
patient with, 1137–1138
nursing management, 1138–1139
External otitis
malignant, 1927
manifestations, 1926
medical management, 1926
nursing management, 1926–1927, 1927c
prevention of, 1927c
External rotation deformity, 171
Extracapsular fracture, 1202
Extracellular fluids (ECFs)
body fluid and, 252
buffer systems in, 284
compartment, 252
composition of, 253t
electrolyte concentrations, 252
potassium level, 271
Extracorporeal shock wave lithotripsy (ESWL), 1435, 1634, 1636
Extramedullary-extradural spinal cord, 2100
Extramedullary hematopoiesis, 903
Extraovarian primary peritoneal carcinoma (EOPPC), 1712
Extravasation
chemotherapeutic agents, 342–344
definition of, 324
IV therapy and, 291–292
Eyeballs
chambers of, 1877–1878
contusions, 1904
penetrating injuries, 1904
shape of, 1883
Eye contact, 107
Eyelids
benign tumors of, 1909
exenteration, 1911
malignant tumors of, 1910
Eye patches, 1904f
Eyes
age-related changes, 1884t
anatomy, 1877–1879, 1878f
assessment of, 1877–1883, 1880c
external examination, 1880–1881
foreign bodies, 1903
injury prevention, 1903c
medication administration, 1886–1890, 1888c
prostheses, 1911
splash injuries, 1904
Ezetimibe (Zetia), 756t

F

Face-lift, 1841
Face, paralysis of, 2095
Face peeling, 1841
Faces Pain Scale–Revised (FPS-R), 231
Facial expression, Leg movement, Activity,
    Crying, and Consolability (FLACC), 233
Facial lipoatrophy, 1033, 1037f
Facial nerve (CN VII), 2086t
Facial pain, 2088
Facial reconstructive surgery, 1841
Factor IX concentrate, 914
Factor VIII concentrate, 914
Factor V Leiden mutation, 962
Factor V Leiden thrombophilia, 125t
Factor Xa inhibitors, 965
    for atrial fibrillation, 724
Faith
    definition of, 62
    spirituality and, 67
Fallopian tubes, 1652–1653
Falls, older adults, 216
Famciclovir (Famvir)
    for genital herpes, 1692
    in herpes zoster infection, 1819
Familial adenomatous polyposis (FAP), 1343
Familial amyotrophic lateral sclerosis, 125t
Familial atypical cold urticaria (FACU),
    1076–1077
Family, 84
    anticipatory mourning, 411c
    bad news for, 398
    boundaries, 411c
    cohesion, 411c
    constellation, 411c
    cultural diversity in, 438
    education of, 408c
    living arrangements, 203–204
    older people and, 202–204
    rehabilitation and, 166
    roles of, 204
    source of psychosocial and physical support,
        203f
Family history
    assessment of, 132–133
    respiratory issues, 491–492
Family violence, abuse, and neglect
    assessment and diagnostic findings, 2186–
        2187, 2187c
    clinical manifestations, 2186
    management, 2187–2188
Famotidine (Pepcid)
    for gastritis, 1295t
    for GERD, 1284t
Fascia, 1118
Fasciculation, 1125
Fasciotomy, 2156, 2171, 2173
    description of, 1845, 1851
    of upper arm, 1851f
Fasting plasma glucose (FPG), 1456, 1460
Fat embolism syndrome (FES), 1155, 1193–1194
Fatigue
    acute, 373
    affects, 2073
    anemia and, 929
    cancer-related, 347, 373
    management of, 373–375
    plans of care, 366c–367c
    sickle cell disease and, 940
    sources of, 373c

Fat necrosis, breast, 1729
Fat redistribution syndrome, 1033
Fats
    in diabetic diet, 1463
    metabolism, role of liver in, 1379
    wound healing and, 425t
Fatty liver disease, 1383
Fear
    expressions of, 427
    preoperative, 431
Febrile nonhemolytic reaction, 919
Febuxostat (Uloric), 1108, 1109t
Fecal diversions, 1336. See also Ileostomy
Fecal immunologic tests (FIT), 1233
Fecal impaction, 1313
Fecal incontinence, 1311, 1316–1317
    assessment and diagnostic findings, 1316
    clinical manifestations, 1316
    medical management, 1316–1317
    nursing management, 1317
    pathophysiology, 1316
Fecal incontinence collectors, 1317
Fecal occult blood testing (FOBT), 1233
Federal Bureau of Investigation (FBI), 2195
Federal Emergency Management Agency
    (FEMA), 2193
Federal, state, and local responses to
    emergencies, 2194
    federal agencies, 2194–2195
    incident command system, 2195
    state and local agencies, 2195
Feedback
    definition of, 48
    learning readiness and, 51
Feelings, grief and mourning, 412c
Felodipine (Plendil), for hypertension, 893t
Female condom, 1673
Female genital mutilation (FGM), 1657
Female physiologic processes. See also Women's
        health
    diagnostic studies for, 1663
        colposcopy and cervical biopsy, 1663
        computed tomography, 1665
        cryotherapy, 1663
        dilation and curettage, 1664
        endometrial biopsy, 1663–1664
        endoscopic examinations, 1664–1665
        hysterosalpingography, 1665
        hysteroscopy, 1665
        laparoscopy, 1664–1665
        laser therapy, 1663
        loop electrosurgical excision procedure,
            1663
        magnetic resonance imaging, 1665
        Pap smear, 1663
        ultrasonography, 1665
    genetic factors and, 1656c
    management of, 1665–1666
        abortion, 1674–1676
        contraception, 1669–1674
        dyspareunia, 1668–1669
        ectopic pregnancy, 1679–1681
        infertility, 1676–1678
        menopause, 1681–1683
        menstrual disorders, 1666–1668
        menstruation, 1666
        perimenopause, 1681
        preconception/periconception health care,
            1678–1679
Female reproductive system, 1651

    age-related changes in, 1655t
    anatomy of, 1651
        external genitalia, 1651–1652, 1651f
        ovaries, 1653
        uterus, 1652–1653
        vagina, 1652
    disorders of, 1686–1717 (See also specific
        disorders)
    function of
        menopausal period, 1654
        menstrual cycle, 1653–1654, 1653f, 1654t
        ovulation, 1653
Femoral shaft, 1210–1211
Fenestrated tube, 524f
Fenofibrate (TriCor), 756t
Fentanyl, 239
    characteristics of, 240t, 446t
    equianalgesic dose chart for, 238
Ferric gluconate (Ferrlecit), 1583
Fertility awareness-based methods, 1674
Fertilizer bombs, 2202
Fetor hepaticus, 1377, 1395
Fexofenadine (Allegra), 1069t
Fiberglass, 1131
    casts, 1132
Fiberoptic bronchoscope, 506
Fiberoptic colonoscopy, 1238–1239, 1238f
Fiberoptic monitor, 1982
Fibers, in diabetic diet, 1463
Fibric acids (Fibrates), 756t
Fibrin, 908
Fibrin degradation products, 908–909
Fibrinogen, 903
Fibrinolysis, 903
Fibrin sealants, 450
Fibroadenomas, 1728–1729
Fibrocystic breast changes, 1719, 1728
Fibroid tumors, 1686, 1703–1704, 1703f
Fibromyalgia, 1109
Fibula, 1211
Fight-or-flight response, 84, 1531
Figure-eight bandage, 1198, 1198f
Filgrastim (Neupogen), 973, 1742
Filtration, hydrostatic pressure and, 253
Finasteride (Proscar), for BPH, 1763
Fine-needle aspiration (FNA), 335, 583, 1719
    of breast, 1726, 1726t
    for thyroid masses, 1513
Fingerprints, 1791
Fingers, clubbing of, 492, 492f
Fingolimod (Gilenya), 2075
Fire risks, 440, 442
First-degree burns, 1847–1848, 1847t
First-intention healing
    definition of, 456
    mechanisms of, 468c
    postsurgical, 468
Fish oil capsules, 756t
Fissure, 1311, 1313, 1799t
    anal, 1351, 1351f
Fistula, 1311, 1325, 1686, 1697
    anal, 1351, 1351f
    vagina, 1697–1698
Fitz–Hugh–Curtis syndrome, 1694
FLACC. See Facial expression, Leg movement,
        Activity, Crying, and Consolability
Flaccidity, 1956
Flaccid muscle, 1119
Flail chest, 627–628, 627f
Flaps, plastic surgery, 1840–1841

Flash injuries, 1850c
Flash pulmonary edema, 833
Flatfoot. *See* Pes planus
Flecainide (Tambocor), for atrial fibrillation, 724
Flexibility, anticipatory mourning and, 411c
Flexion, 171c
Flexi-Seal Fecal Management System, 1317, 1317f
FloTrac transducer, 709
Fluconazole (Diflucan), 2071
   for candidiasis, 1688
Flucytosine (Ancobon), 2071
Fludarabine, 977–978
Fluid administration, preoperative, 432
Fluid and electrolyte disturbances, in kidney
      disorders, 1568–1569, 1568t
   clinical manifestations, 1568–1569, 1568t
   older adults and, 1569
Fluid balance
   burn injuries, 1851–1852, 1866
   prevention of infections, 1866
Fluid deprivation test, 1509
Fluid resuscitation formula, 1854
Fluid volume deficit, 1568t
Fluid volume disturbances, 259–264, 259t
Fluid volume excess (FVE), 1568t. *See also*
      Hypervolemia
Flumazenil (Romazicon), in hepatic
      encephalopathy, 1396
Flunitrazepam (Rohypnol), 2188
Fluorescein angiography, 1490
Fluorescent in situ hybridization (FISH), 122
Fluoridation, 1268
Fluoroquinolone, for urinary tract infections,
      1619t
Fluoroscopy, 504–505, 695
5-Fluorouracil (5-FU), 343t
Fluoxetine (Prozac), 241
   in general pruritus, 1812
Flutter valve, 510
FNA. *See* Fine-needle aspiration
Foam dressings, 876, 1809
Focused assessment, 73–74
Focused assessment with sonography for trauma
      (FAST), 2170
Folate
   deficiency, 906
   metabolism, 906
Folfirinox, 1451
Folic acid deficiency, 933
Folk healers, 110
Folk remedies, 110c
Follicle-stimulating hormone (FSH), 1507,
      1650, 1653
Follicular Lymphoma International Prognostic
      Index (FLIPI), 992
Folliculitis, 1806, 1818
Follitropin alfa (Gonal-F), 1677c
Follitropin beta (Follistim), 1677c
Fondaparinux (Arixtra)
   in total hip arthroplasty treatment, 1152
   for venous thromboembolism, 870t, 871
Food allergy, 1077–1078
   assessment and diagnostic findings, 1077
   clinical manifestations, 1077
   medical management, 1077
   nursing management, 1077–1078, 1077c
Food labels, misleading, 1465
Food poisoning, 2180
   assessment, 2180c

Foot and leg care, in peripheral vascular disease,
      857, 857c
Foot and leg problems
   diabetes and, 1494
   foot care tips, 1495c
   management, 1495
   neuropathic ulcers, 1494, 1494f
   neuropathy and, 1494
   peripheral vascular disease and, 1494
Footdrop, prevention of, 171
Foot problems, 1166–1168
   callus, 1166–1167
   causes of, 1166
   corn, 1167
   hallux valgus, 1167, 1167f
   hammer toe, 1167, 1167f
   ingrown toenail, 1167
   morton neuroma, 1168
   nursing management, 1168
   obesity and, 1166
   pes cavus, 1168
   pes planus, 1168
   plantar fasciitis, 1168
Foot ulcers, 1803
Foramen of Monro, 1989f
Forced end expiratory flow, 502t
Forced expiratory flow, 502t
Forced expiratory volume, 502t
Forced midexpiratory flow, 502t
Forced vital capacity (FVC), 501, 502t, 638
Foreign bodies
   ear and, 1926
   in esophagus, 1282
   ocular, 1904–1905
Fornix, 1650, 1652
Fosamprenavir (FPV), 1035t
Fosinopril (Monopril), for hypertension, 892t
Fourth-degree burns, 1847t, 1848, 1848f
Fraction of inspired oxygen (FiO$_2$), 510
Fracture, 1131, 1185, 1189–1197
   clinical manifestation, 1189
   closed, 1189
   comminuted, 1189
   emergency management, 1191
   greenstick, 1189
   healing, 1117
   healing and complications, 1193, 1193c
   intra-articular, 1189
   management, 2171
   medical management, 1191–1192
   nursing management, 1192–1193, 1192c
   open, 1189
   reduction, 1185, 1191
   types of, 1189, 1190f
Fracture Risk Assessment Tool (FRAX), 1122,
      1171
Frank–Starling law, 678
Fremitus
   definition of, 480
   tactile, 495–496
Frequency, voiding, 1548, 1556, 1556t
Frey syndrome, 1264, 1270
Friction
   pressure ulcers and, 179t, 180, 181f
   reduction of, 184
Friction rubs, 499t, 691
Frontal lobes, tumors of, 2094
Frontotemporal dementia with Parkinsonism-17,
      125t
Frostbite

assessment and diagnostic findings, 2173
   management, 2173
FSH. *See* Follicle-stimulating hormone
Fuchs endothelial dystrophy, 1898
Fulminant hepatic failure, 1377, 1398,
      1405–1406
   treatment, 1405–1406
   viral hepatitis and, 1405
Functional Consequences Theory, 194
Functional incontinence, 186, 1624. *See also*
      Urinary incontinence
Functional Independence Measure (FIM"), 167
Fundus, 1650, 1652
Fundus photography, 1882
Fungal encephalitis, 2070–2071
Fungal infections, 1803
Fungemia, 2133
Funnel chest, 495
Furosemide (Lasix), 263, 1510
   in ascites, 1386
   for heart failure, 824t
   for hypertension, 890t
Furuncles, 1803, 1806, 1818
Fusion inhibitor, 1035t
The Future of Nursing: Leading Change,
      Advancing Health (IOM report), 13, 24

G
Gabapentin (Neurontin), 234, 244, 1197, 1866,
      2075, 2087, 2089
   in low back pain treatment, 1161
Gait
   age-related changes
   assessment of, 1123–1124
   crutch, 176c
Gallbladder, 1378, 1378f
   anatomy of, 1428, 1429f
   disorders, 1430
      cholecystitis, 1430
      cholelithiasis, 1430–1438
   function of, 1428–1429
   surgery
      nursing process, 1438–1440
      patient education, 1440c
Gallium scans, lung, 505
Gallop sounds, heart, 690, 691
Gallstones, 1430, 1431f. *See also* Cholelithiasis
Gamete intrafallopian transfer (GIFT), 1678
Gamma-aminobutyric acid (GHB), 2075
Gamma-glutamyl transferase (GGT), 1382
Gamma-hydroxybutyrate, 2188
Gamma knife radiosurgery, 339, 2088
Gamma rays, 339
Ganciclovir (Cytovene), 1912, 2069
Ganglion, 1165
Gardnerella-associated bacterial vaginosis,
      1688–1689, 1688t
GAS. *See* General adaptation syndrome
Gas exchange
   during cardiac surgery
      adequate, promotion of, 785–786
      impaired, 784–785
   nursing diagnosis, 649c
   partial pressure abbreviations, 486c
   partial pressure of gases, 485–486
   respiratory function and, 478, 543
Gastrectomy, for gastric cancer, 1304–1305,
      1307c
Gastric acid stimulation test, 1240–1241
Gastric analysis, 1240–1241

Gastric banding, 1369
Gastric cancer, 1241, 1303–1308
    assessment and diagnostic findings, 1304
    chemotherapy for, 1305
    clinical manifestations, 1304
    incidence of, 1303
    nursing process, 1306–1308
        anxiety reduction, 1306
        assessment, 1306
        continuing and transitional care,
            1307–1308
        evaluation, 1308
        home care checklist, 1308c
        nursing diagnosis, 1306
        nursing interventions, 1306–1308
        nutritional status, 1306
        pain relief, 1306
        patient and family education, 1307
        planning and goals, 1306
        psychosocial support, 1307
    in older adults, 1306
    pathophysiology, 1304
    prognosis for, 1304
    radiation therapy for, 1305–1306
    risk factors for, 1304
    surgical management, 1304–1305
        complications of, 1305
    targeted therapies for, 1305
Gastric function, 1226–1227
Gastric, meaning of, 1292
Gastric outlet obstruction, 1292, 1294, 1303
    bariatric surgery and, 1373
    gastric surgery and, 1305
    peptic ulcer disease and, 1303
Gastric resection, with gastrojejunostomy, 1321t
Gastric residual volumes (GRVs), 1249–1250
Gastric ulcer, 1241
Gastrinomas, 1297
Gastritis, 1292–1296
    acute, 1292–1293
    assessment and diagnostic findings, 1294
    chronic, 1293
    clinical manifestations, 1293–1294, 1294t
    erosive, 1293, 1293f
    medical management, 1294
    nursing management
        anxiety reduction, 1294
        continuing and transitional care, 1296
        fluid balance, 1294
        home care checklist, 1296c
        nutrition, 1294
        pain relief, 1296
        patient education, 1296
    pathophysiology, 1293, 1293f
    stress-related, 1293
Gastrocolic reflex, 1311, 1313
Gastroduodenal, 1240
Gastroesophageal reflux disease (GERD), 1230,
        1264, 1283
    assessment and diagnostic findings, 1283
    clinical manifestations, 1283
    management, 1283, 1284t
Gastroesophageal sphincter, 1279
Gastrointestinal function, 1224
    anatomic and physiologic examination
        digestive system, function of, 1226–1228
        gastrointestinal system, anatomy of,
            1224–1226
        gerontologic considerations, 1228–1229
    diagnostic evaluation

    abdominal ultrasonography, 1233–1234
    breath tests, 1233
    endoscopic procedures, 1237–1240, 1237f
    gastric analysis, gastric acid stimulation
        test, and pH monitoring, 1240–1241
    genetic testing, 1234, 1234c
    imaging studies, 1234–1237
    laparoscopy (peritoneoscopy), 1241
    manometry and electrophysiologic studies,
        1240
    serum laboratory studies, 1232–1233
    stool tests, 1233
Gastrointestinal intubation, 1244–1252
    complications management, 1246–1247
    enteral tubes, 1244t, 1245–1252
    gastric tubes, 1244–1245, 1244t
    oral and nasal hygiene, 1246
    patient monitoring and tube function,
        1246
    tube feedings, 1247–1249
        administration methods, 1249, 1249f
        assessment findings for patients receiving,
            1250c
        bowel elimination pattern, maintaining of,
            1250–1251
        continuing and transitional care, 1252
        delivery systems, 1250
        feeding equipment and nutritional balance,
            1249–1250
        formulas, 1248–1249
        home care checklist, 1256c
        hydration, maintaining of, 1252
        osmolality, 1248
        patient education, 1252
    tube obstruction, clearing, 1246
Gastrointestinal motility studies, 1236–1237
Gastrointestinal regulatory substances, 1227t
Gastrointestinal system, 687
    age-related changes in, 197t, 199, 1228t
    assessment of
        health history, 1229–1231, 1229c
        physical assessment, 1231–1232, 1231f
    burn injuries and, 1852–1853
    chemotherapy-related effects, 344–345
    postsurgical complications, 473t
    postsurgical management, 469–472
Gastrointestinal varices, 1407
Gastroparesis, 1243, 1245
Gastrostomy, 1243, 1252–1253
GATA2 deficiency, 1024t
Gatorade, 1342
G-CSF. See Granulocyte colony-stimulating
        factor
Gelatin sponge (Quick-Seal), 704
Gels, wound care, 1810
Gemcitabine (Gemzar), 343t
    in pancreatic carcinoma, 1451
Gemfibrozil (Lopid), 756t
Gene-based therapy, in prostate cancer,
        1770
Gene mutations, 118, 118f
    acquired, 119f
    hereditary, 118f
General adaptation syndrome (GAS), 86
General anesthesia, 443–445
    stages of, 443
Generalized exfoliative dermatitis, 1826–1827
General older adult population (GOLD) deaths,
        642
General pruritus, 1811–1812

    gerontologic considerations, 1812
    medical management, 1812
    nursing management, 1812
    pathophysiology, 1812
    pharmacologic therapy, 1812
    systemic disorders associated with, 1811c
Genes
    choromosomes and, 116–117
    mutations, 118
    role, 116–118
Gene therapy, 354, 1713
Genetic conditions, and chromosomal
        differences, 122
Genetic counseling, 134c, 135c
Genetic engineering, 1013
Genetic Information Nondiscrimination Act
        (GINA), 130
Genetic makeup, 115
Genetic profile. See Genetic makeup
Genetics
    counseling, 134c, 135c
    cultural concerns, 130–131
    definition of, 115
    ethical concerns, 129–130
    in health assessment, 131–133
    legal aspects, 130
    in nursing practice, 131–135
    referral, 133c
    services, 134
    social concerns, 130–131
    spiritual concerns, 130–131
Genetic screening, 123–124
    applications, 124t
    in endocrine disorders, 1506, 1506c
Genetics-related nursing care, 29
Genetic testing, 122–123, 123c
    nursing research profile, 131c
Genetic variation, 118–119
Genital herpes, 1692–1694
    clinical manifestations, 1692
    medical management, 1692
    nursing process
        anxiety reduction, 1693
        assessment, 1693
        diagnosis, 1693
        evaluation, 1694
        infection prevention, 1693
        nursing interventions, 1693–1694
        patient education, 1693–1694
        planning and goals, 1693
        strategies for relieving pain, 1693c
    pathophysiology, 1692
Genitourinary injury, 2170
Genitourinary pain, 1555–1556, 1556t
Genitourinary system, 2041t. See also Urinary
        tract infections
    age-related changes, 197t, 199
Genitourinary trauma, 1637
Genome, 115, 1358, 1360
Genomic conditions, 127
Genomics
    definition of, 115
    future of, 136
    in health assessment, 131–133
    in nursing, 114–136
Genotype, 116
Gentamicin (Garamycin), for anthrax
        treatment, 2204
GERD. See Gastroesophageal reflux disease
Geriatric Depression Scales (GDS), 207, 208c

Geriatrics, 193, 194
Geriatric syndromes, 193, 215–217
  aging with disability, 219
  altered emotional impact, 217
  altered systemic response, 217
  atypical responses, 217
  dizziness, 216
  ethical and legal issues, 219
  falls and falling, 216
  health care costs of aging, 218
  home health care, 218
  hospice services, 218–219
  impaired mobility, 216
  neglect and abuse, 217–218
  social services, 218
  susceptibility to infection, 217
  urinary incontinence, 216–217
Geriatric triad, 216
Germ cell tumors, ovarian cancer, 1712
Germinal tumors, 1780
Gerontologic/geriatric nursing, 193, 195
Gerontology, 193, 194
Gestational diabetes, 1456, 1459–1460
GH. *See* Growth hormone
Ghrelin, 1360
Giant cell arteritis (GCA), 1103–1104
Giant cell tumors, 1180
Giardia lamblia, 2144
Giardiasis, 1321t
Gilbert syndrome, 1385
Gingivitis, 1264, 1267t
Glare testing, 1884
Glargine (Lantus), 1473
Glasgow Coma Score (GCS), 317, 2038, 2039, 2042, 2162
  level of consciousness, 2042
  neurologic signs, 2042
Glatiramer acetate (Copaxone), 2075
Glaucoma, 1890–1894
  angle-closure, 1890f
  classification of, 1891
  management of, 1892–1893, 1894c
  medications, 1887, 1893t
  risk factors, 1890c
  types of, 1891t
Gleason score, 1765
Glimepiride (Amaryl), 1474t
Glioblastomas, 2092
Gliomas, 2092, 2096
Glipizide (Glucotrol, Glucotrol XL), 1474t
Glitazones, 1475t
Globulins, 908
Glomerular filtration rate (GFR), 1548, 1553, 1567, 1569
Glomerulonephritis, 1567, 1570
  assessment and diagnostic findings, 1572
  chronic, 1572–1573
  clinical manifestations, 1572
  medical management, 1572–1573
  nursing management, 1573
  pathophysiology, 1572
Glomerulus, 1548, 1549
Glossectomy, 1271
Glottis, 481
Gloves, 2130
Glucagon, 1282, 1429, 1457, 1482
Glucagon-like peptide-1 agonist (GLP-1), 1475t
Glucocorticoids, 84, 89, 1502, 1531
  for hypothyroidism, 1515
Gluconeogenesis, 84, 89, 1379, 1457

Glucose
  in hepatic encephalopathy, 1395
  shock and, 297–298
Glucose challenge test (GCT), 1460
Glucose control, during perioperative period, 1496, 1497c
Glucose metabolism
  abnormalities of, 1397
  role of liver in, 1379
Glucose-6-phosphate dehydrogenase deficiency, 942
Glucose tolerance test, 1445
Gluten, 1319, 1322c. *See also* Celiac disease
Gluten-sensitive enteropathy. *See* Celiac disease
Glyburide (Micronase, Glynase, DiaBeta), 1474t
Glycated hemoglobin, 1456
  testing for, 1467
Glycemic index, 1456, 1463, 1464
Glycerin suppository, 1314t
Glycogenolysis, 1379, 1457
Glycoprotein IIb/IIIa agents, for angina, 760
Glycopyrrolate (Robinul)
  secretion management and, 409t
Glycosaminoglycan (GAG), 1616
Glycosuria, 1459
Glycosylated hemoglobin, 682
Glycosylation disorders with immune deficiency, 1024t
GM-CSF. *See* Granulocyte-macrophage colony-stimulating factor
Goals
  for hospitalized postoperative patient, 465
  of palliative care, 400–401, 401c
Goiter, 1502, 1511, 1524–1525
  endemic (iodine-deficient), 1525
  nodular, 1525
Golfer's elbow, 1187
Golimumab (Simponi), 1089t, 1107
GoLYTELY, 1314t
Gonadotropin-releasing hormone (GnRH), 1653
Gonadotropin-releasing hormone agonists, 1677c
Goniometer, 1124
Gonorrhea, 1694, 2148
  and endocervicitis, 1694
Goodpasture syndrome, 1061, 1572
Gore-Tex, 1132
Goserelin (Zoladex), 1745, 1770
Gout, 1107–1108
  pathophysiology, 1107–1108
Gowns, 442
Graafian follicle, 1650, 1653
Grading, definition of, 324
Graft-*versus*-host disease (GVHD), 922c
  definition of, 324
  HSCT and, 350, 351
Graft-*versus*-tumor effects, 324
Gram-positive bacteria, 376
Granulocyte colony-stimulating factor (G-CSF), 345, 923c, 973
Granulocyte-macrophage colony-stimulating factor (GM-CSF), 345, 923c, 973
Granulocytes, 906–907, 971
Graves disease, 1502, 1512, 1519
Greenstick fractures, 1189
Grief
  after death, 411–412

  anticipatory, 410–411
  complicated, 412
  definition of, 387, 410
  emergency care and, 2159
  Kübler-Ross's five stages of, 410t
  nursing interventions, 368c, 412c
  process of, 375
Gross auditory acuity, 1919, 1920f
Growth factor dressings, 876
Growth factors, 923c
Growth hormone (GH), 1508, 2093
  effects on bone remodeling, 1116
  insufficient secretion of, 1508
  oversecretion of, 1508
Guanfacine (Tenex), for hypertension, 890t
Guided imagery, 84, 98
Guillain-Barré syndrome (GBS), 2072, 2082–2085, 2150
  home care checklist, 2085c
Guilt, emergency care and, 2159
Gum Arabic (GA), 1317
Gums, 1231
GVHD. *See* Graft-*versus*-host disease
Gynecomastia, 1719, 1721, 1749

H
Habit retraining, 1625c
Habit training, 187
Habitual abortion, 1675
Hair
  assessment of, 1801–1803
    color and texture, 1801
    distribution, 1801–1802
    hair loss, 1802, 1802f
  color, 1792
  follicles, 1792
  function, 1792
  growth, 1792
  male pattern baldness, 1802, 1802f
Halitosis, 1264, 1281
Hallux valgus, 1167, 1167f
Haloperidol (Haldol)
  for alcohol withdrawal syndrome, 2185
  delirium management, 407
  for patients who are overactive, 2190
Halothane (Fluorothane), 444t
Hammer toe, 1167, 1167f
Hand, 1200–1201
Hand hygiene methods, 2130c
Haptens, 1058
Hardwire cardiac monitoring, 696
Hartmann procedure, for diverticulitis, 1326–1327, 1326f
Hashimoto thyroiditis, 1512
Haversian system, 1115
Havrix, 1399
Hay fever. *See* Allergic rhinitis
Headache, 2093, 2096
  assessment, 2005–2006
  classification of, 2004c
  manifestations, 2004–2005
  nursing management, 2007
  pathophysiology, 2004
Head injury, 2033
  assessment parameters, 2040f
  brain injury, types of, 2036
  in metabolic changes, 2042
  prevention, 2034c
Head-tilt/chin-lift maneuver, 838
Health and Human Services (HHS), 329

Health assessment, 131–133
  family history assessment, 132–133
  genetics of, 67c
  physical assessment, 133
  psychosocial assessment, 133
Health belief model, 56
Health care
  barriers to, 154–157
  federal assistance programs, 157–158
  right of access to, 154–158
Health care–associated infections (HAIs), 2128
  nursing research profile, 2133
Health care–associated methicillin-resistant
    Staphylococcus aureus (HA-MRSA)
    infection, 2132
Health care–associated pneumonia, 588
Health care delivery system
  influences on, 6
    cultural diversity, 6
    gerontologic considerations, 6
    health problems, changes in, 7
    population demographics, 6
    technology and genetics, advances in, 7
  nursing practice in, 11–13
Healthcare Information Management Systems
    Society (HIMSS), 7
Health care workers, 2128f, 2151
Health, definition of, 5
Health disparities, 104
Health education, 48
  definition of, 48
  health promotion and, 55–59
  informed decision-making and, 49
  purposes of, 48–50
Health histories, 63–71
  components of, 64–71
    chief complaints, 65
    family history, 65–66
    past history, 65
    patient profiles, 66, 68c
    present health concern, 65
    review of systems, 66
  definition of, 62, 63
  informants, 64
  people with disabilities, 70c
Health information technology (HIT), 7
Health Insurance Portability and Accountability
    Act (HIPAA), 33, 63, 2157
Health literacy, 48
Health Professions Education: A Bridge to Quality
    (IOM report), 15
Health promotion, 6, 158–159
  in cancer, 331c
  cognitive function, 205c
  components of, 57
  definition of, 48, 55
  health education and, 48—55
  healthy lifestyle, 89, 96–97
  models of, 55–57, 57t
  nursing implications, 60
  patient profile record of, 66–67
  screening for adults, 58t
  strategies, 58–59, 58t
  technology in, use of, 6
Health Resources and Service Administration
    (HRSA), 1029
Health therapies, 108–109
Healthy food choices, 1464
Healthy People initiatives, 7, 55, 2020
  goals of, 55c

Hearing
  age-related changes, 197t, 202
  aids, 1938–1941
  assessment of, 1918–1921
  diagnostic evaluation, 1922
  implanted devices, 1940–1941
Hearing aids, 1938–1941
  care of, 1939c
  options and features of, 1939c
  problems with, 1939c
  types of, 1940t
Hearing disorders, genetics of, 1922c
Hearing guide dogs, 1941
Hearing loss
  age-related changes, 1924–1925
  assessment of, 1923c
  clinical manifestations, 1923
  communicating with people have, 155c
  ethical dilemma, 1924c
  management, 1925, 1925c
  prevention, 1923
  risk factors, 1925c
  severity of, 1921t
Heart
  and blood vessel functions, 256
  coronary arteries, 675
  hemodynamics, 677
  left catheterization, 703–704
  myocardium, 699, 700
  refractory periods, 676–677
  right catheterization, 703
  structure of, 674f
Heart auscultation, 690
Heartburn. *See* Pyrosis
Heart disease, 690, 695, 702
Heart failure (HF), 636, 689, 818–833
  ACC/AHA classification of, 820t
  acute decompensated, 819
  assessment and diagnostic findings, 823
  burn injuries and, 1867
  clinical manifestations, 821–823, 822c
  continuing and transitional care, 832–833
  diastolic, 819
  ejection fraction, assessment of, 819
  end-of-life considerations, 833
  etiology, 819–820
  home care checklist, 832c
  incidence of, 819
  left-sided, 822
  management of, 823
    cardiac resynchronization therapy, 827
    cardiac transplantation, 828
    goals of, 823
    ICD placement, 827
    nutritional therapy, 826–827
    oxygen therapy, 827
    pharmacologic therapy, 824–826, 824t
    ultrafiltration, 827
  New York Heart Association (NYHA)
    classification of, 819t
  nursing process, 828–833
    activity tolerance, promoting, 829, 829c
    assessment, 828–829
    complications management, 831
    diagnosis, 829
    evaluation, 833
    fluid status, 830
    health history, 828
    nursing interventions, 829–833
    patient education, 831–832

    physical comfort and psychological
      support, 830
    physical examination, 828–829
    planning and goals, 829
    powerlessness, minimizing, 831
  older adults and, 828
  pathophysiology, 820–821, 821f
  with preserved EF, 819
  right-sided, 822–823
  systolic, 819
  vicious cycle of, 821
Heart inspection, 689
Heart murmurs, 678, 692c, 702
Heart rate
  dysrhythmias influences on, 713
  electrocardiogram for, 717
  medications control, 724
Heart sounds
  abnormal, 690
    S_3, 691
    S_4, 691
  interpretation of, 692
  normal, 690
    S_1, 690
    S_2, 690
Heat-induced illnesses, 2171–2172
  assessment and diagnostic findings, 2172
  causes of, 2171
  gerontologic considerations, 2172
  management, 2172–2173
  prevention of, 2172c
Helicobacter pylori (*H. pylori*), 328, 949, 1292,
    1293
Helper T cells, 1011
Hemagglutinin, 2135
Hemarthrosis, 1188
Hematemesis, 1292, 1296
Hematochezia, 1292, 1293
Hematocrit, 909
  reference range, 694t
Hematologic disorders, 903
  assessment
    health history, 909, 911t
    physical assessment, 909, 911t
  diagnostic evaluation, 909
    bone marrow aspiration and biopsy, 910,
      912–913, 912f
    hematologic studies, 909–910
  genetic, 910c
  infection and bleeding in, risk of, 946c
  therapeutic approaches to
    apheresis, 913–914, 913t
    blood component therapy, 914, 915t
    hematopoietic stem cell transplantation,
      914
    phlebotomy, 914
    special preparations, 914
    splenectomy, 913
Hematologic system, 903
  blood, 903
    cells, 905–907
    plasma and plasma proteins, 908
  bone marrow, 903–905
  reticuloendothelial system, 908
Hematomas, 293, 686, 1737–1738, 2036, 2036f,
    2135
  location of, 2036f
  postsurgical, 473
  and total knee arthroplasty, 1155
Hematopoiesis, 903, 970, 1116, 1181

Hematopoietic stem cells (HSCs), 348
Hematopoietic stem cell transplantation
        (HSCT), 914, 973
    allogeneic, 349–350
    autologous, 349, 350
    cancer risk and, 342
    donors, care for, 352
    Hodgkin lymphoma, 990
    infections and, 349
    myeloablative, 349
    nonmyeloablative, 349
    nursing management, 350–351
    patient care, 350–351
    primary immune deficiency diseases, 1023
    psychological impact of, 352
    recipients, care for, 352
    sickle cell disease and, 937
    and sleep disturbances, 980c
    types of, 349–350
Hematopoietic system, chemotherapy-related
        effects, 345
Hematuria, 345, 1548, 1555, 1556t, 1561
Hemianopsia, 2009, 2011
Hemilaminectomy, 2114
Hemiparesis, 2009, 2011, 2019, 2069
Hemiplegia, 2009, 2011, 2019, 2069
Hemochromatosis, 944
Hemodialysis, 1580, 1589–1594, 1590f
    complications of, 1591–1592
    in diabetes, 1492
    dialyzers, 1589–1590
    home, 1593–1594
    nursing management, 1592–1594
        continuing and transitional care, 1594
        nutritional and fluid therapy, 1592
        patient education, 1593
        pharmacologic therapy, 1592
        psychosocial needs, 1592–1593
    objectives of, 1589
    principles of, 1589
    vascular access, 1590
        arteriovenous fistula, 1590–1591, 1591f
        arteriovenous graft, 1591
        devices, 1590, 1591f
Hemodilution, 916
Hemodynamic monitoring, 705–709
Hemofilter, 1594
Hemoglobin, 905
    reference range, 694t
Hemolysis, 926
Hemolytic anemias, 926, 927c. See also Anemia
Hemolytic jaundice, 1384
Hemophilia, 951
    classification, 951
    clinical manifestations, 951–953, 953f
    medical management, 953
    nursing management, 953–954
    older adults and, 954
Hemophilic arthropathy, 952, 953f
Hemoptysis, 583, 692
    assessment of, 490–491
    description of, 480
Hemorrhage
    management, 2165–2166
        external hemorrhage, 2166, 2166f
        fluid replacement, 2165
        internal bleeding, 2166
    in postanesthesia units, 459
    types of, 459t
Hemorrhagic blebs, 2173

Hemorrhagic cystitis, 345
Hemorrhagic stroke, 2025–2031
Hemorrhoids, 1311, 1313, 1351–1352, 1351f
    external, 1352
    internal, 1352
    nonsurgical treatment, 1352
    surgical treatment, 1352
Hemosiderin, 874, 944
Hemostasis, 773, 903, 908–909, 909f
Hemothorax, 583
Hemovac drains, 469, 471f
HEPA filter mask. See High-efficiency
        particulate air filter mask
Heparin, 958, 1677c
    for angina, 758t, 760
    for venous thromboembolism, 870t
Heparin-induced thrombocytopenia (HIT),
        870, 963
Hepatic artery port, 1419
Hepatic disorders, 1377–1425
    ascites, 1385–1388
    cirrhosis, 1406–1417
    diagnostic evaluation, 1382
        imaging studies, 1382
        laparoscopy, 1382
        liver biopsy, 1382
        liver function tests, 1382, 1383f
    esophageal varices, 1388–1393
    fulminant hepatic failure, 1405–1406
    hepatic encephalopathy and coma, 1393–
        1397
    jaundice, 1384–1385
    liver cancer, 1417–1420
    nonviral hepatitis, 1404–1405
    portal hypertension, 1385
    viral hepatitis, 1397–1404, 1398t
Hepatic encephalopathy, 1377, 1384, 1393–
        1397
    assessment and diagnostic findings, 1395
    clinical manifestations, 1394–1395, 1395f
    continuing and transitional care, 1396–1397
    medical management, 1395–1396
    nursing management, 1396–1397
    pathophysiology, 1394
    patient education, 1396
    stages of, 1394t
    subclinical/minimal, 1394
Hepatic function, preoperative assessments, 426
Hepatic sinusoidal obstructive syndrome
        (HSOS), 350
Hepatic vein, 1378
Hepatic venous pressure gradient (HVPG), 1390
Hepatitis, 922c
    nonviral, 1404–1405
    viral, 1397–1404, 1398t
Hepatitis A, 1398–1400
    assessment and diagnostic findings, 1399
    clinical manifestations, 1399
    dietary management, 1399, 1400c
    medical management, 1399
    nursing management, 1399–1400
    prevention, 1399, 1400c
    transmission of, 1398
Hepatitis B, 1400–1403
    assessment and diagnostic findings, 1401
    clinical manifestations, 1401
    continuing and transitional care, 1403
    medical management, 1402–1403
    mortality rate, 1401
    nursing management, 1403

    in older adults, 1401
    prevention, 1401–1402
        active immunization, 1401–1402
        passive immunity, 1402
        preventing transmission, 1401
    risk factors, 1400c
    self-care, 1403
    virus transmission, 1400
Hepatitis B immune globulin (HBIG), 1402
Hepatitis B virus (HBV), cancer and, 328
Hepatitis C, 1403–1404, 2137
    medical management, 1403–1404
    risk factors, 1403, 1403c
Hepatitis D virus (HDV), 1404
Hepatitis E virus (HEV), 1404
Hepatitis G virus (HGV)/GB virus-C (GBV-C),
        1404
Hepatocellular carcinoma (HCC), 1401, 1417
Hepatocellular jaundice, 1384
Hepatocytes, 1378
Hepatojugular reflux, 693
Hereditary angioedema, 1076
Hereditary hemochromatosis, 125t
Hereditary hyperbilirubinemia, 1385
Hereditary mutations, 118f
Hereditary nonpolyposis colorectal cancer
        (HNPCC), 1343, 1712
Hering–Breuer reflex, 488
HER-2/neu protein, 1719, 1744
Hernia, 1264
Herniated disc, with accompanying pain, 2113
Herniation, 1980, 1980f
Herniations, 2114
Herpes labialis, 556c
Herpes simplex, 552, 1820
Herpes simplex virus-1, 1266t
Herpes simplex virus 2 (HSV2) infection, 1692
Herpes zoster, 1819–1820, 1819f, 2135
Herpes zoster ophthalmicus (HZO), 1819
Herpetic gingivostomatitis, 1267t
Hesitancy, 1556t
Heterotopic ossification, 1131, 1147, 1197
HF. See Heart failure
HHS. See Health and Human Services;
        Hyperglycemic hyperosmolar
        syndrome
Hiatal hernia, 1280–1281, 1281f
    assessment and diagnostic findings, 1280
    clinical manifestations, 1280
    management for, 1281
    paraesophageal, 1280, 1281f
    sliding, 1280, 1281f
Hidradenitis suppurativa (HS), 1813
Hierarchy of Pain Measures, 232, 232c
High cholesterol, 680
High-density lipoprotein (HDL), 750, 752, 851
    in CAD, 753–754
High-efficiency particulate air (HEPA) filter,
        441, 979, 1068, 2157
Higher health-related quality of life (HRQOL)
        score, 993
High-flux dialysis, 1590
High linear energy transfer (LET), 339
High sensitivity CRP (hs-CRP) test, 695
Hilus, 482
Hinduism, 396t
Hinge joints, 1117
HIPAA. See Health Insurance Portability and
        Accountability Act
Hip, external rotation of, 171

Hip fracture, 1202–1205
  clinical manifestations, 1203
  extracapsular, 1202
  gerontologic considerations, 1203
  intracapsular, 1202
  medical management, 1203
  nursing management, 1203–1204
  older adult patient with, 1206c–1210c
  periprosthetic, 1202
Hip prosthesis, preventing dislocation of, 1147, 1151. *See also* Total hip arthroplasty (THA)
Hip spica casts, 1137
Hiroshima, bombing of, 2193
Hirschsprung disease, 1312
Hirsutism, 1790, 1792
Histamine, 655, 1058–1059, 1059t
Histiocytes, 908
Histoplasma capsulatum, 2070
HIV/AIDS Prevention Research Synthesis Project, 1027
HIV encephalopathy, 1040, 1040c
HIV-1 nucleic acid tests, 1032
HIV wasting syndrome, 1039
HMG-CoA reductase inhibitors, for atrial fibrillation, 724
Hodgkin lymphoma, 988–991
  assessment and diagnostic findings, 989–990
  clinical manifestations, 989, 990f
  medical management, 990–991
  mixed cellularity type, 989
  nodular sclerosis type, 989
  nursing management, 991
  pathophysiology, 989, 989f
  staging, 989
Holidays, observance of, 107–108
Holter monitors, 697, 714
Homan sign, 870
Home care
  after surgery, 462–463
  needs in AD, 215, 218
  patient transfers in, 173
  promotion of, 188–190
  self-care, 160–161
  targeted therapies, 355
  therapeutic regimens, 189c–190c
Home care assistance, 2109
Home care nurses, 19. *See also* Home health care
Home care setting, 2136c
Home health care, 20–24
  home environment, assessment of, 22, 23c
  home visits, 20, 21
    documentation of, 24
    end of, 22–23
    initial, 22
    need and frequency of future visits, 22, 23c
    and personal safety precautions, 22, 22c
    preparation for, 21–22
  infection control in, 21
  nurse-patient relationship and, 21, 22
  patient's assessment in, 21, 21f
  rehospitalization, factor for, 20c
  safety precautions in, 22c
  services provided in, 20–21
  settings and, 21
  telehealth in, use of, 7, 8c, 21
Homeless population, and health care, 25–26
Homeostasis, 84
  aging and, 201

constancy and, 85, 85f
  definition of, 84
  mechanisms, 256–258
Home ventilator care, 534c
Homocysteine, 695, 851–852
Homografts, 800, 1864
  description of, 1845, 1864
Hope
  fostering of, 402
  nursing interventions to support, 402
  terminal illnesses and, 402
Hormonal contraceptives, 1671–1672
  benefits and risks of, 1671c
  combination methods, 1671
  injectable contraceptives, 1672
  oral contraceptives, 1672
  progestin-only methods, 1671
  transdermal contraceptives, 1672
  vaginal contraceptives, 1672
Hormones
  autocrine action, 1504
  classification and action of, 1503–1504
  definition of, 1502, 1503
  by endocrine glands, 1503
  function and regulation of, 1503
  by GI mucosa, 1503
  by kidney, 1503
  paracrine action, 1504
  by white blood cells, 1503
Hormone therapy (HT)
  for menopause-related symptoms, 1682–1683
  methods of administration, 1682–1683
  risks and benefits, 1683
Hospice and Palliative Nurses Association (HPNA), 388
Hospice care, 24, 24c, 393–395
  benefits of, 394–395
  cancer patients, 383
  eligibility criteria for, 393–394, 394c
  federal rules for, 394
  goal of, 393
  home services, 394c
  Medicare-certified, 394
  of older adult, 218–219
  principles of, 393
  in the United States, 393
  use of, 394–395
Hospital-acquired infections, 699
Hospital-acquired pneumonia, 588–589
Hospital Consumer Assessment of Healthcare Providers and Systems (HCAHPS), 9
Hospital Incident Command System (HICS), 2195
Hot flashes, 1681
  alternative treatments for, 1683
  hormone therapy for, 1682–1683
HPNA. *See* Hospice and Palliative Nurses Association
HPV. *See* Human papillomavirus
HPV2 (Cervarix), 354
HPV4 (Gardasil), 354
HPV9 (Gardasil-9), 354
HS. *See* Hidradenitis suppurativa
HSCT. *See* Hematopoietic stem cell transplantation
HSOS. *See* Hepatic sinusoidal obstructive syndrome
Human chorionic gonadotropin (hCG) levels, 1680

Human Genome Project, 114
Human immune deficiency virus (HIV) infection, 1025, 1696–1697, 1697c, 2136, 2149
  antidepressant therapy, 1042
  antidiarrheal therapy, 1042
  assessment and diagnostic findings in, 1031–1033
  blood tests for screening, 1032, 1032t
  chemotherapy, 1042
  clinical manifestations, 1037–1041, 1038c
  complementary, alternative, and integrative therapies, 1042–1043
  depressive manifestations, 1041
  emotional and ethical concerns, 1053, 1054c
  epidemiology, 1025–1026
  follow-up testing, 1032
  gastrointestinal manifestations, 1039
  gynecologic manifestations, 1041
  health care providers, reducing transmission risk in
    post-exposure prophylaxis, 1029
    standard precautions, 1029, 1029c
    vaccination, 1029–1030
  HIV life cycle, 1030–1031, 1030f
  HIV transmission, 1026–1027
  integumentary manifestations, 1041
  neurologic manifestations, 1039–1040, 1040c
  nursing process, 1043
    diagnosis, 1048–1049
    evaluation, 1053
    nursing interventions, 1049–1053
    planning and goals, 1049
    plan of care, 1044c–1048c
  nutrition therapy, 1042
  older adults and, 1027
  oncologic manifestations, 1039
  opportunistic infections, treatment of, 1041–1042
  pathophysiology, 1030–1031
  patient education, 1052, 1052c
  prevention of, 1027–1029, 1028c
    condoms, correct use of, 1027, 1028c
    in LGBT youth, 1029
    preexposure prophylaxis (PrEP), 1027
    preventive education, 1027–1028
    reproductive education, 1028–1029
  respiratory manifestations, 1037–1039
  risks associated with, 1027t
  self-management strategies, 1038c
  stages of infection, 1031
    latent reservoir, 1031
    primary/acute HIV infection, 1031
    stage 2, 1031
    stage 3, 1031
    viral set point, 1031
  supportive care, 1043
  treatment of, 1033–1037
Human immune deficiency virus type 1 (HIV-1), 1026, 1030–1031, 1030f
Human insulins, 1468
Human leukocyte antigen (HLA), 1083
Human papillomavirus (HPV), 1041, 1691–1692
  cancer and, 328
  clinical infection, 1691
  latent infection, 1691
  medical management, 1691
  pathophysiology, 1691

prevention, 1692
  risk factors, 1691
  subclinical infection, 1691
Human trafficking, 2189
Humate-P, 914, 955
Humeral neck, 1198–1199, 1199f
Humeral shaft, 1199, 1199f
Humoral immune response, 1007, 1008–1010
  antibodies, role of, 1009–1010
  antigen–antibody binding, 1010
  antigen recognition, 1008–1009
  and cellular immune response, 1009t
Humoral (antibody-mediated) immunity tests,
    1020c
Huntington disease, 125t, 2091
  care of patient, 2110
Huntington gene (HTT), 2108
Hybridomas, 352–353, 353f
Hydralazine (Apresoline)
  for hypertension, 892t
Hydralazine and isosorbide dinitrate
  for heart failure, 824t, 825
Hydration
  artificial, 406
  end-of-life care, 404–406
  in hyperparathyroidism, 1528
Hydrocele, 1752, 1782–1783
Hydrochloric acid, 1224, 1226
Hydrochlorothiazide (Hydrodiuril), 1530
  for hypertension, 890t
Hydrochlorothiazide (HCTZ), for heart failure,
    824t
Hydrocodone (Vicodin, Lortab), 235, 240
  equianalgesic dose chart for, 238
Hydrocolloids, 1807, 1808–1809
Hydrocortisone, 1089t, 1541t
Hydrogels, 1807, 1808
Hydromorphone (Dilaudid), 234, 240
  characteristics of, 240t
  equianalgesic dose chart for, 238
Hydrophilic, definition of, 1806, 1809
Hydrophilic drug, 239
Hydrophobic, definition of, 1806, 1809
Hydrostatic force, 844
Hydrostatic pressure, 253
Hydrotherapy, 1860
Hydroxychloroquine
  in rheumatic diseases, 1088t
  for systemic lupus erythematosus, 1100
3-Hydroxy-3-methylglutaryl coenzyme A
    (HMG-CoA), 755, 756t
3-hydroxy-3-methylglutaryl coenzyme A
    (HMG-CoA) reductase inhibitors,
    852
Hydroxyurea (Hydrea), 343t, 937, 973, 985,
    986
Hydroxyzine (Atarax), 460t, 1069t
  in general pruritus, 1812
Hygroscopic, definition of, 1806, 1810
Hymen, 1650, 1651
Hyoscyamine (Levsin)
  secretion management and, 409t
Hyperaldosteronism, 269
Hyperbaric oxygenation (HBO), 877
Hypercalcemia, 273t, 275–276
  assessment of, 276
  and bone metastases, 1180
  causes of, 275
  clinical manifestations of, 275
  diagnostic findings, 276

  management of, 382t
  manifestation of, 382t
  medical management, 276
  neuromuscular excitability and, 275
  nursing management, 276
  pathophysiology of, 275
  symptoms of, 1180–1181
  treatment of, 1182
Hypercalcemic crisis, 1529
Hypercapnia, chronic, 643
Hyperchloremia, 281t, 282–283
Hyperemia, 1876
Hyperglycemia, 426, 1456
  during hospitalization, 1497
  postprandial, 1458
  during surgery, 1496
Hyperglycemic hyperosmolar syndrome (HHS),
    1456, 1459, 1485–1488
  assessment and diagnostic findings, 1486
  clinical manifestations, 1486
  DKA and, 1486t
  management, 1486–1487
  nursing process, 1487–1488
    assessment, 1487
    diagnosis, 1487
    nursing interventions, 1487–1488
    planning and goals, 1487
Hyperhomocysteinemia, 851, 959
Hyper-immunoglobulin E syndrome (HIES),
    1024t
Hyper-immunoglobulin M (hyper-IgM)
    syndrome, 1024t
Hyperinsulinism, 1453
Hyperkalemia, 271–272
  acute kidney injury and, 1578, 1580
  assessment of, 271–272
  causes of, 271
  clinical manifestations of, 271
  diagnostic findings of, 271–272
  emergency pharmacologic therapy, 272
  medical management of, 272
  nursing management of, 272
  pathophysiology of, 271
Hyperlipidemia, 126t, 680, 1573
Hypermagnesemia, 277t, 278–279
  assessment of, 278
  clinical manifestations of, 277
  diagnostic findings of, 278
  medical management, 278–279
  nursing management, 279
  pathophysiology of, 278
Hypermetabolism, 1865, 1866
Hypernatremia, 267–268
  assessment of, 268
  causes of, 267
  clinical manifestations of, 267–268
  diagnostic findings, 268
  medical management, 268
  nursing management, 268
  pathophysiology of, 267
Hyperopia, 1876, 1883, 1899, 1900
Hyperparathyroidism, 1527–1529
  assessment and diagnostic findings,
    1528
  clinical manifestations, 1527–1528
  diet and medications, 1528
  home care checklist, 1529c
  hydration therapy, 1528
  mobility, 1528
  nursing management, 1528

  primary, 1527
  secondary, 1527
  surgical management, 1528
Hyperphosphatemia, 279t, 280–281
  assessment of, 280–281
  clinical manifestations of, 280
  diagnostic findings of, 280–281
  medical management, 281
  nursing management, 281
  pathophysiology of, 280
Hyperpigmentation, 1790, 1795
Hyperplasia
  cellular adaptation, 92
  definition of, 84
Hyperpnea, 496t
Hypersensitivity, 1060, 1060f
  anaphylactic (type I), 1061
  cytotoxic (type II), 1061
  delayed-type (type IV), 1061
  immune complex (Type III), 1061
Hypersensitivity reactions (HSRs)
  chemotherapeutic agents, 344
  desensitization procedures, 344
  premedication regimens, 344
Hypersplenism, 1397
Hypertension, 646, 677, 680, 884–898, 2028
  assessment and diagnostic findings, 887
  and atherosclerotic heart disease, 885
  blood pressure classification and, 884–885,
    885t
  and CAD, 756–757
  causes of, 886
  clinical manifestations, 887
  definition of, 884
  genetics and, 886
  JNC 7 on, 884–885, 885t
  management of, 887–894
    lifestyle modifications, 889t
    pharmacologic therapy, 889, 890t–893t
    treatment algorithm, 888f
    treatment goals, 887
  nursing care, 653c
  nursing process, 894–897
    assessment, 894, 894c
    diagnosis, 894–895
    evaluation, 897
    nursing interventions, 895–897
  older adults and, 886–887, 889, 893–894
  pathophysiology of, 885–887, 886f
  and peripheral arterial disease, 852
  in postanesthesia units, 459
  during pregnancy, 885
  prevalence of, 885
  primary, 885
  prolonged, uncontrolled, 885
  risk factors for, 887c
  secondary, 885
  as silent killer, 885
  stage 1, 885, 885t
  stage 2, 885, 885t
Hypertensive crisis, 897–898
Hypertensive emergency, 897
Hypertensive encephalopathy,
    glomerulonephritis and, 1571
Hypertensive peristalsis. See Nutcracker
    esophagus (NE)
Hypertensive urgency, 897–898
Hyperthermia, 352, 2172
  burn shock and, 1859
  malignant, 436, 450–451

Hyperthyroidism, 1511, 1519–1524
  adjunctive therapy, 1521–1522
  antithyroid medications, 1521
  assessment and diagnostic findings, 1519
  causes of, 1519
  clinical manifestations, 1519
  Graves disease and, 1519
  home care checklist, 1524c
  nursing process, 1522–1524
    assessment, 1522
    complications management, 1523
    coping measures, enhancing, 1523
    evaluation, 1524
    normal body temperature, 1523
    nursing diagnoses, 1523
    nursing interventions, 1523–1524
    nutritional status, improving, 1523
    patient education, 1523–1524
    planning and goals, 1523
    self-esteem, improving, 1523
  in older patients, 1522
  pharmacologic therapy, 1519
  radioactive iodine therapy, 1519–1520
  surgical management, 1522
  treatment of, 1519–1522
Hypertonic solutions, 261t, 290
Hypertrichosis, 1810
Hypertrophic cardiomyopathy (HCM), 802–803, 819–820
Hypertrophic scars, 1868t, 1869
Hyperuricemia, 1107
Hyperventilation patterns, 496t
Hypervolemia, 262–264
  assessment and diagnostic findings, 263
  azotemia with, 263
  clinical manifestations of, 263
  detection and control of, 264
  medical management of, 263
  nursing management of, 263–264
  pathophysiology, 262
  prevention of, 264
  sodium-restricted diet in, 263
Hyphae, 1686, 1687
Hyphema, 1876, 1904
Hypoalbuminemia, 1573, 1601
Hypocalcemia, 273–275, 273t
  acute symptomatic, 274
  assessment of, 274
  clinical manifestations of, 273–274
  diagnostic findings of, 274
  medical management, 274–275
  nursing management, 275
  pathophysiology of, 273
  vitamin D therapy, 275
Hypochloremia, 261t, 281–282
Hypochromia, 941
Hypoglycemia, 426, 1456, 1461
  assessment and diagnostic findings, 1482
  clinical manifestations, 1482
  diabetes and, 1482–1483
  during hospitalization, 1497–1498
  management
    carbohydrate, treatment with, 1482
    emergency measures, 1482–1483
    patient education, 1483
  middle-of-the-night, 1482
  mild, 1482
  moderate, 1482
  in older patients, 1482
  in patients undergoing surgery., 1496

postexercise, 1466
severe, 1482
Hypoglycemic unawareness, 1493
Hypogonadism, 1770
Hypokalemia, 268–271, 269t
  assessment of, 269
  burn injuries and, 1851
  clinical manifestations of, 269
  diagnostic findings of, 269
  DKA and, 1488
  medical management, 269–270
  nursing management, 270–271
  pathophysiology of, 269
  risk for, 270
Hypokinesia, 2103
Hypomagnesemia, 277–278, 277t
  alcohol abuse and, 277
  assessment of, 278
  clinical manifestations of, 277
  diagnostic findings of, 278
  medical management, 278
  nursing management, 278
  pathophysiology of, 277
Hyponatremia, 265–267, 2030
  assessment of, 266
  burn injuries and, 1851
  manifestations of, 265
  medical management, 266
  nursing management, 267
  pathophysiology, 265
  sodium replacement, 266
  water restriction, 266
  water retention in, 267
Hypoparathyroidism, 1529–1530
  assessment and diagnostic findings, 1530
  clinical manifestations, 1529
  home care checklist, 1530c
  medical management, 1530
  nursing management, 1530
Hypopharyngeal obstruction, 458, 458f
Hypopharyngeal sphincter, 1279
Hypophosphatemia, 279–280, 279t
  assessment of, 280
  clinical manifestations of, 280
  diagnostic findings of, 280
  medical management, 280
  nursing management, 280
  pathophysiology of, 279–280
Hypophysectomy, 1502, 1508, 1509
Hypophysis. See Pituitary gland
Hypopigmentation, 1790, 1795
Hypopituitarism, 1508
Hypopyon, 1876, 1908
Hypotension, 677, 703, 704
  aging and, 198–200
  orthostatic, 198, 467
  postanesthesia, 458–459
  postprandial, 198
  postural, 467, 693
Hypothalamic–pituitary–thyroid axis, 1511
Hypothermia, 1827, 2043, 2173
  anesthesia-related, 450
  assessment and diagnostic findings, 2174
  burn shock and, 1860
  management, 2174
    monitoring, 2174
    rewarming, 2174
    supportive care, 2174
  urban, 2173

Hypothyroidism, 1511, 1513–1519
  causes of, 1514, 1514c
  central, 1514
  clinical manifestations, 1514–1515
  congenital, 1511
  home care checklist, 1518, 1518c
  home, community-based, and transitional care, 1518
  hypothalamic/tertiary, 1514
  medical management, 1515
    pharmacologic therapy, 1515
    supportive therapy, 1515
  myxedema coma, 1514–1515
  neonatal, 1514
  nursing care plan, 1516c–1517c
  nursing management, 1515, 1518
  in older adults, 1518–1519
  patient and family education, 1518
  pituitary/secondary, 1514
  primary, 1514
  unrecognized, 1514
Hypotonic solutions, 261t, 290
Hypoventilation
  patterns, 496t
  risk factors, 501c
Hypovolemia, 259–262, 259t
  assessment and diagnostic findings, 259–260
  burn injuries, 1850–1851
  clinical manifestations of, 259
  correction of, 262
  medical management, 260
  nursing management, 260–262
  nursing research, 262c
  pathophysiology of, 259
  prevention of, 262
  serum electrolyte changes and, 259
Hypovolemic shock, 296, 308–310, 1193, 2146, 2167, 2180
  blood replacement in, 308–309
  diarrhea and, 2146
  fluid redistribution in, 309
  fluid replacement, 308–309, 309t
  medical management, 308–309
  nursing management, 309–310
  pathophysiology of, 308, 308f
  in postanesthesia units, 459
Hypoxemia, 510
  description of, 480, 488
  episodic, 465
  life-threatening, 655
  postoperative, 465
  pulmonary artery pressures, 636
  subacute, 465
  ventilation–perfusion abnormality, 664
Hypoxia, 510
  anesthesia-related, 450
  causes of, 92–93
  cyanosis and, 492
  definition of, 480
  ventilation–perfusion ratio, 485
Hysterectomy, 1686, 1701, 1714–1716
  definition of, 1714
  laparoscopically assisted approach, 1714
  nursing process, 1714–1716
    anxiety, relief of, 1714
    assessment, 1714
    body image, improving, 1714–1715
    complications management, 1715
    diagnosis, 1714
    evaluation, 1715–1716

nursing interventions, 1714–1715
  pain relief, 1715
  patient education, 1715
  planning and goals, 1714
postoperative management, 1714
preoperative management, 1714
radical, 1714
robot-assisted, 1714
total, 1714
and venous thromboembolism, 1715
Hysterosalpingography (HSG), 1665
Hysteroscopic resection of myomas, 1704
Hysteroscopy, 1650, 1665
HZO. *See* Herpes zoster ophthalmicus

I

Iatrogenic incontinence, 1624. *See also* Urinary
  incontinence
Ibandronate sodium (Boniva), 276
IBD. *See* Inflammatory bowel disease
Ibritumomab tiuxetan (Zevalin), 353
IBS. *See* Irritable bowel syndrome
Ibuprofen (Caldolor), 235
ICOUGH^SM Program, 586c
ICP. *See* Intracranial pressure
Idarubicin (Idamycin), 343t, 972
Idarucizumab (Praxbind), 872
Idiopathic inflammatory myopathies. *See*
  Polymyositis
Idiopathic thrombocytopenic purpura (ITP), 914
Idioventricular rhythm, 731, 731f
Ifosfamide (Ifex), 343t, 345
IGRT. *See* Image-guided radiation therapy
Ileal conduit, 1615, 1639–1642
  complications, 1639
  nursing management, 1639–1642
    fluid intake and relieving anxiety, 1641
    home, community-based, and transitional
     care, 1641–1642
    ostomy appliance, selection of, 1641
    stoma and skin care, 1640
    urine testing and caring for ostomy, 1640
  patient education, 1641, 1642c
Ileal dysfunction, 1321t
Ileal pouch anal anastomosis (IPAA), 1333
Ileostomy, 1311, 1336
  home care checklist, 1343c
  nursing care plan, 1337c–1339c
  in older adults, 1342
  postoperative care, 1340–1342
    changing appliance, 1341
    complications prevention, 1342
    continuing and transitional care, 1342
    dietary and fluid needs, 1341–1342
    drainage from ileostomy, 1340
    emotional support, 1340–1341
    irrigating colostomy, 1341
    NG suction, 1340
    patient education, 1342
    skin and stoma care, 1341
  preoperative care, 1336, 1339
Ilizarov fixation, 1138
Illness, causes of, 109–110
Image-guided radiation therapy (IGRT), 339
Imatinib mesylate (Gleevec), 974, 1102
Imiquimod (Aldara), for HPV infection, 1691
Immobility, pressure ulcers and, 180
Immune function, preoperative assessments, 426
Immune globulin, 914
  for hepatitis A, 1399

Immune hemolytic anemias, 943–944
  assessment and diagnostic findings, 943
  clinical manifestations, 943
  medical management, 943
  nursing management, 943–944
Immune memory, 1005
Immune reconstitution inflammatory syndrome
  (IRIS), 1037
Immune response, 1006
  acquired, 1007
  cellular, 1007, 1010–1012
  chemical barriers and, 1007
  complement-mediated, 1008f
  humoral, 1008–1010
  natural, 1007
  physical surface barriers and, 1007
  regulation of, 1007
  stages of, 1007, 1009f
    effector stage, 1008
    proliferation stage, 1008
    recognition stage, 1008
    response stage, 1008
Immune system, 1005
  anatomy of, 1005–1006, 1005f, 1006f
    bone marrow, 1005
    lymphoid tissues, 1005–1006
  assessment of, 1014, 1014c
    allergies, 1016–1017
    disorders and diseases, 1017–1018
    gender, 1014
    health history, 1014–1018
    immunization, 1016
    infection, 1016
    lifestyle factors, 1018
    medications and blood transfusions, 1018,
     1019t
    nutrition, 1015–1016
    older adults, 1014–1015
    physical assessment, 1018–1019
    psychoneuroimmunologic factors, 1018
  cancer risk and, 330
  diagnostic evaluation, 1019, 1020c
  disorders of, 1005, 1005t
  evasion by cancers, 330
  function of, 1006
    acquired immunity, 1007
    age-related changes in, 1014–1015, 1015t
    cellular response, 1010–1012
    complement System, 1012
    gender and, 1014
    humoral response, 1008–1010
    immunomodulators, 1013
    natural immunity, 1006–1007
    response to invasion, 1007–1008
  nursing management, 1019
Immune thrombocytopenic purpura (ITP),
  949–951
  assessment and diagnostic findings, 949–950
  clinical manifestations, 949
  medical management, 950
  nursing management, 950–951
  pathophysiology, 949
  primary, 949
Immunity, 1005
Immunocompromised hosts, pneumonia in,
  589
Immunoglobulin E (IgE), hypersensitivity
  reactions, 344
Immunoglobulin G (IgG), 1570
Immunoglobulinopathy, 1321t

Immunoglobulins, 907, 993, 1009–1010, 1010t,
  1058
  function of, 1058
  immunoglobulin E
    hypersensitivity reactions, 344
Immunologic alterations, burn injuries and,
  1852
Immunologic disorders, 1017c
Immunomodulators, 660, 1013
  for inflammatory bowel disease, 1332
  for rheumatic diseases, 1088t–1089t
Immunomodulatory drugs (IMiDs), 996, 997
Immunopathology, 1005
Immunoregulation, 1007
Immunosenescence, 1014
Immunosuppressive agents
  for pemphigus vulgaris, 1828
  for systemic lupus erythematosus, 1100
Immunotherapy
  for allergic disorders, 1070–1071, 1071c
  epicutaneous, 1071
  indications and contraindications, 1071c
  subcutaneous, 1071
  sublingual, 1071
Impaired fasting glucose (IFG), 1456, 1457
Impaired glucose tolerance (IGT), 1456, 1457
Impaired skin integrity, 178–186
Impetigo, 1817–1818, 1817f
Impingement syndrome, 1164
  shoulder healing of, 1164c
Implantable cardioverter defibrillators (ICDs),
  684, 745f
  definition of, 712
  for dysrhythmia, 744–748
    complications of implantation, 745–746
    design criteria, 745
    home care checklist, 747c
    nursing management, 746–748
  wearable automatic, 744f
Implanted hearing devices, 1940–1941
  bone-anchored hearing aid, 1940
  cochlear implant, 1940–1941, 1941f
  middle ear implantation, 1940
Implementation phase, of nursing process, 36, 41
Impotence. *See* Erectile dysfunction
IMRT. *See* Intensity-modulated radiation
  therapy
Incentive spirometry, 429, 510, 516
Incident command system (ICS), 2195
Incisional biopsy, 335
  of breast, 1727
Incontinence, 1556t
  age-related changes
  assessment, 186
  bowel, promotion of, 188
  diagnosis of, 186
  functional, 186
  intervention of, 186–188
  reflex, 186
  stress, 186
  urge, 186
  urinary, 186, 193, 199, 216–217
Incontinence pads (briefs), 187–188
Incretins, 1462
Indapamide (Lozol)
  for hypertension, 890t
Independence
  mobility and, 172–173
  promotion of, 213
  self-care issues and, 168

Indigestion, 1229
Indinavir (IDV), 1035t
Indolent neoplasms, 971
Indomethacin (Indocin), 1108
Induced abortion, 1675–1676, 1676c
  dilation and evacuation, 1676c
  labor induction, 1676c
  medical abortion, 1676c
  medical management, 1675–1676
  nursing management, 1676
    patient education, 1676
    psychological support, 1676
  types of, 1676c
  vacuum aspiration, 1676c
Induction therapy, 972
Induration, 583
Indwelling catheters, 187, 1629
Infarction, 2009, 2010
Infection control, operating room, 441
Infections
  after liver transplantation, 1423
  cultures, 503
  local signs of, 474
  surgical site, 473–474, 474t
Infectious disease, 2125, 2126t–2127t, 2137c,
    2138
  nursing care, 2139c–2143c
Infective endocarditis, 810–812
Infertility, 375, 1676–1677
  definition of, 1676
  diagnostic findings, 1677
  male factors in, 1677
  medical management, 1677–1678
    artificial insemination, 1678
    assisted reproductive technologies, 1678
    pharmacologic therapy, 1677–1678, 1677c
  nursing management, 1678
  ovarian and ovulation factors in, 1677
  primary, 1676
  secondary, 1676–1677
  tubal and uterine factors in, 1677
Infiltration
  assessment of, 292c
  and extravasation, 291–292
Inflammation, 1083
  cellular injury in, 94–95
  chemical mediators of, 95
  definition of, 84
  healing, 95
  regeneration, 95
  replacement, 95
  responses to, 94f
  systemic response to, 95
  types of, 95
Inflammatory bowel disease (IBD), 1311,
    1329–1336
  Crohn's disease, 1329 (See also Crohn's
    disease)
  home care checklist, 1336c
  medical management, 1332–1334
    nutritional therapy, 1332
    pharmacologic therapy, 1332
  nursing process, 1334–1336
    anxiety reduction, 1335
    assessment, 1334
    complications management, 1335
    continuing and transitional care,
      1335–1336
    coping measures, 1335
    diagnosis, 1334

elimination patterns, 1334
    evaluation, 1336
    fluid intake, 1334
    nursing interventions, 1334–1336
    nutrition therapy, 1334
    pain relief, 1334
    patient education, 1335
    planning and goals, 1334
    rest promotion, 1335
    skin breakdown prevention, 1335
  prevalence of, 1329
  surgical management, 1332–1334
    continent ileostomy, 1333–1334
    indications for, 1332
    restorative proctocolectomy with IPAA,
      1333, 1333f
    total colectomy with ileostomy, 1333
  ulcerative colitis, 1329 (See also Ulcerative
    colitis)
Inflammatory process, reversing, 1807
Inflammatory response, 1007
Infliximab (Remicade), 1089t, 1107
  for psoriasis, 1826
Influenza, 2135
  in older adults, 217
Information, disclosure of, 106–107
Informed consent
  definition of, 418
  ethics of, 422–423
  valid, 423c
Infratentorial approach, 1990–1995, 1990t
Infusion drip pyelography, 1564
Infusion Nurses Society (INS), 292
Ingested (swallowed) poisons, 2178–2179
Ingestion, 1224, 1226
Ingrown toenail, 1167
Inguinal orchiectomy, 1780
Inhalation injuries, 1852
Inheritance patterns, 119–122
  autosomal dominant inheritance, 119–120
  autosomal recessive inheritance, 120
  complex genetic conditions, 121
  multifactorial inheritance, 121
  nontraditional inheritance, 121–122
  x-linked inheritance, 120–121
Injectable contraceptives, 1672
Injection sclerotherapy. See Endoscopic
  sclerotherapy
Inner ear
  anatomy of, 1916f
  conditions of, 1932–1938
Inoperative (inop) monitoring alarms, 699
Inotropy, 712, 713
Insensible perspiration, 1793
Inspection, 62, 73
Inspiratory force, 501–502
Institute for Healthcare Improvement (IHI), 9,
    2128
Institute for Safe Medication Practices (ISMP),
    1246
Institute of Medicine (IOM), 7, 388
  on quality control in health care system, 7–8
  recommendations for future of nursing, 13
Instrumental activities of daily living (IADLs),
    193, 201
  definition of, 167
Insufflation, 1664
Insulin, 1429, 1456, 1457, 1468
  complications, 1469, 1471
  dawn phenomenon, 1471

delivery, methods of, 1471–1473
  in diabetic ketoacidosis, 1485
  drug interactions, 428t
  functions of, 1457
  hypermetabolism and, 1865
  impaired secretion in type 2 diabetes, 1459
  injection sites, 1479, 1479f
  intermediate-acting, 1468
  lipodystrophy, 1469
  local allergic reaction, 1469
  mixing, 1478–1479
  preparations, 1468–1469, 1468t
  rapid-acting, 1468
  regimens, 1469, 1470t
    conventional, 1469
    intensive, 1469
  resistance, 1469, 1471
  self-injection of, 1477–1479, 1480c, 1481c
  and self-monitoring of blood glucose, 1468
  short-acting, 1468
  skin preparation, 1479
  Somogyi effect, 1471
  storing, 1478
  surgical issues, 428t
  syringes, 1478, 1479
  systemic allergic reactions, 1469
  type 1 diabetes and, 1468
  type 2 diabetes and, 1468
  very long-acting, 1468
  waning, 1471
  withdrawing, 1479
Insulinomas, 1453
Insulin pens, 1471, 1471f
Insulin pumps, 1456, 1461, 1472, 1472f
Insulin resistance, 1459
Integrase inhibitor (INSTIs), 1035t
Integrated Risk Information System (IRIS),
    329
Integrative medicine, 355
Integumentary system, age-related changes,
    197t, 198
Intelligence, age-related changes, 205
Intensity-modulated radiation therapy (IMRT),
    339, 1305
  for prostate cancer, 1769
Interactive dressings, 1807
Interdisciplinary collaboration, 387, 391
Interferon alfa-2b (Intron), 985, 987
Interferon beta-1a (Rebif), 2075
Interferon gamma deficiency, 1024t
Interferons, 1013
  for renal cancer, 1575
  therapy using, 354
Interleukin 2 (IL-2)
  for renal cancer, 1575
Interleukin 12 deficiency, 1024t
Interleukin 23 deficiency, 1024t
Interleukins
  IL-11, 345
  therapy using, 354
Intermittent claudication, 841, 845, 852, 857
Intermittent mandatory ventilation (IMV),
    510, 528
Intermittent pneumatic compression devices,
    873
International Classification of Diseases (ICD)-
    10, 7
International Classification of Diseases for
    Oncology, 327
International Council of Nurses (ICN), 32

International normalized ratio (INR), 910, 963–964, 1155, 2170
International Prognostic Index (IPI), 992
International Prostate Symptom Score (IPSS), 1763
International Society of Hypertension (ISH), 884
Interprofessional collaborative practice, 15–15, 15f
Interprofessional Education Collaborative (IPEC), 5, 15
Interstitial cystitis, 1615
Interstitial nephritis, 1567, 1579
Interstitial pancreatitis, 1440–1441. *See also* Pancreatitis
Intestinal gas, 1230
Intestinal obstruction, 1327
   causes of, 1327, 1327f
   functional/paralytic obstruction, 1327
   large bowel obstruction, 1328
   mechanical causes of, 1328t
   mechanical obstruction, 1327
   small bowel obstruction, 1327–1329
Intestinal peristalsis, 1227
Intestinal transplant, for Crohn's disease, 1333
Intimacy, needs in AD, 214
Intimate partner violence (IPV), 1657, 2186
   barriers to nurses screening for, 2187c
Intra-abdominal injuries, 2169
   assessment and diagnostic findings, 2169–2170
      genitourinary injury, 2170
      internal bleeding, 2170
      intraperitoneal injury, 2170
   management, 2170
Intra-aortic balloon pump (IABP), 835, 835f
Intra-arterial blood pressure monitoring, 709
Intra-articular fractures, 1189
Intracapsular fracture, 1202
Intracavitary irradiation, 1716–1717, 1716f
Intracavitary radioisotopes, 340
Intracellular fluids (ICFs)
   body fluid and, 252
   composition of, 253t
   electrolyte concentrations, 252
Intracerebral hemorrhage, 2025, 2037
Intracompartmental pressure, 1134
Intracorporeal lithotripsy, 1435
Intracranial pressure (ICP), 1936, 2034
   increased, 1976–1989
      assessment, 1981
      complications, 1981
      detection of, 1988c
      interventions, 1987t
      management, 1981–1984
      manifestations, 1980–1981
      monitoring of, 1981–9182, 1981f
      nursing process, 1984–1989
      pathophysiology, 1979–1980
      waveforms, 1982, 1982f
Intracranial surgery
   home care check list, 1994c
   nursing process, 1991–1995
   postoperative management, 1991
   preoperative management, 1989–1991
Intracytoplasmic sperm injection (ICSI), 1678
Intradermal skin testing, 1063, 1063f
Intraductal papilloma, 1728, 1730
Intragastric balloon therapy, 1366
Intralesional therapy, 1810
Intramuscular epinephrine, 319

Intranasal cromolyn sodium (NasalCrom), 1068
Intraocular lens implants, 1897
Intraoperative nursing management, 436–454
Intraoperative phase, 418
   nursing activities in, 420c
   timing of, 419
Intraoperative radiation therapy (IORT), 1716
Intraoperative temperature, monitoring of, 440c
Intraperitoneal chemotherapy, for ovarian cancer, 1713
Intraperitoneal injury, 2170
Intrapleural anesthesia, 466
Intraspinal analgesia, 234
Intrauterine device (IUD), 1670
   hormonal, 1670
   nonhormonal, 1670
Intravascular catheter-related bloodstream infections, 707t
Intravenous fat emulsions (IVFEs), 1243, 1257
Intravenous immunoglobulin (IVIG), 914, 950, 978, 2080
Intravenous pyelography (IVP), 1564
Intravenous (IV) solutions therapy
   air embolism and, 291
   blood clots and, 293
   and bloodstream infections, 291
   complications of, 291–293
   hypertonic solutions, 290
   hypotonic solutions, 290
   isotonic solutions, 288–290
   nursing management of patient, 290–293
   patient education, 293
   self-care, 293
   transitional care, 293
   types of, 288–290
Intrinsic factor, 1224, 1226
Intrinsic factor antibody test, 934
Introitus, 1650, 1651, 1661
Intubation, 1243
   gastrointestinal, 1244–1252
Inversion, 171c
In vitro fertilization (IVF), 1678
Involucrum, 1160, 1176
Iodine, for synthesis of thyroid hormone, 1511
Iodinism, 1522
IOM. *See* Institute of Medicine
Ionizing radiation
   carcinogenesis and, 328–329
   types of, 328
IPEC. *See* Interprofessional Education Collaborative
Ipilimumab (Yervoy), 1837
Ipratropium (Atrovent), 656
Irbesartan (Avapro), for hypertension, 892t
Irinotecan (Camptosar), 343t
IRIS. *See* Integrated Risk Information System
Iron, 905
   absorption, 906
   overload, 921, 983
   stores and metabolism, 906
   supplementation, 930–931, 931c, 1583
Iron deficiency anemia, 906, 930–931
   assessment and diagnostic findings, 930
   causes of, 930
   clinical manifestations, 930
   medical management, 930–931
   nursing management, 931
Iron dextran (INFeD), 1583
Iron formulations, parenteral, 931, 931c
Iron sucrose (Venofer), 1583

Irritable bowel syndrome (IBS), 1311, 1317–1318, 1320c
   abdominal pain and, 1318
   assessment and diagnostic findings, 1318
   clinical manifestations, 1318
   medical management, 1318
   nursing management, 1318
   pathophysiology, 1318
   prevalence of, 1317
Ischemia, 750, 841
   gastrointestinal, 302
Ischemic stroke
   assessment, 2011–2012
   clinical manifestations, 2011
   medical management, 2013–2017
   pathophysiology, 2010–2011, 2010f
   risk factors, 2014c
   self care, 2021c
Islam, 396t, 438
Islet cell transplants, 1473
Isoflurane (Forane), 444t
Isolated scalp trauma, 2034
Isolated systolic hypertension, 693, 887
Isolation precautions, 2129
Isometric contraction, 1118
Isometric exercises, 1135
Isosorbide (Isordil), for variceal bleeding, 1390
Isotonic contraction, 1118
Isotonic solutions, 260, 261t, 288–290
Israelidipine (Dynacirc CR), for hypertension, 893t
Itching. *See* Pruritus
ITP. *See* Immune thrombocytopenic purpura
IUD. *See* Intrauterine device
IV acetaminophen (Ofirmev), 235
IV conivaptan hydrochloride (Vaprisol), 266
IV ibutilide (Corvert), for atrial fibrillation, 724
IV infusion therapy, 2172
Ixabepilone (Ixempra), 343t
Ixazomib (Ninlaro), 996

J

Jackson-Pratt drains, 469, 471f
Janus Kinase (JAK) inhibitors (Xeljanz), in rheumatic diseases, 1088t
Jaundice, 1377, 1380, 1384, 1796
   gallbladder disease and, 1432
   hemolytic, 1384
   hepatocellular, 1384
   obstructive, 1384–1385
Jaw disorders, 1269
   surgical management of, 1269
Jejunostomy, 1243, 1253–1256
Jejunum, 1243, 1244
Jet injectors, 1471
Job syndrome. *See* Hyper-immunoglobulin E syndrome (HIES)
Joint, 1117–1118
   age-related changes, 201
   amphiarthrosis, 1117
   aspiration (*See* Arthrocentesis)
   capsule, 1118
   diarthrosis, 1117
   dislocations, 1186–1187
   effusion, 1124, 1125f
   function, assessment of, 1124
   internal derangement of, 1269
   mobility of, 171–172
   replacement, 1144–1145
   space, 1104
   synarthrosis, 1117

Joint arthroplasty, 1145
Joint Commission, 8, 2128, 2130
    on anesthesia, 443
    core measures by, 9
    National Patient Safety Goals, 8–9
    program for palliative care, 392
Joint Commission National Patient Safety
        Goals, 2133
Joint instability, 1868t
J point, 763
Judaism, 396t, 438
Jugular venous distention (JVD), 823
Junctional dysrhythmias, 727–729, 727f
    atrioventricular nodal reentry tachycardia,
        728–729, 728f
    junctional rhythm, 727–728, 727f
    nonparoxysmal junctional tachycardia, 728
    premature junctional complex, 727
Junctional rhythm, 727–728, 727f
Juxtaglomerular apparatus, 1550

K
Kaposi sarcoma (KS), 1267t, 1839
    AIDS-related, 1039, 1039f, 1042
Kayexalate, 272, 1580
Kegel exercises, 1625c, 1626, 1699, 1699c
Keloids, 1799t, 1833
    burn injuries and, 1869
Keratin, 1790, 1791
Keratinocytes, 1790, 1791
Keratoconus, 1876, 1897–1898
Keratolytic ointment, for callus, 1167
Keratoprosthesis, 1898
Kernig's sign, 2066, 2066f
Kerotoconjunctivitis sicca, 1101
Ketamine (Ketalar), 244, 447t, 2188
Ketoconazole (Nizoral), 1770
Ketone bodies, 1379, 1459
Ketones, 1456
    testing for, 1467–1468
Ketorolac (Toradol), 235
Kidney and urinary systems, 1548, 1568
    diagnostic evaluation, 1559
        biopsy, 1565
        computed tomography, 1562
        cystography, 1564
        intravenous pyelography, 1564
        kidneys, ureters, and bladder (KUB) x-ray,
            1562
        magnetic resonance imaging, 1562–1563,
            1563c
        MAG3 renogram, 1564
        nuclear scans, 1563–1564
        nursing care plan, 1560c
        osmolality, 1561
        renal angiography, 1564
        renal function tests, 1562, 1562t
        retrograde pyelography, 1564
        specific gravity, 1561
        ultrasonography, 1562, 1563f
        urinalysis and urine culture, 1559, 1561,
            1561t
        urologic endoscopic procedures, 1564–1565
        voiding cystourethrography, 1564
    function of
        acid–base balance, regulation of,
            1552–1553
        antidiuretic hormone, 1551–1552
        bladder emptying, 1554
        blood pressure, autoregulation of, 1553

electrolyte excretion, regulation of, 1552
        older adults and, 1554
        osmolarity and osmolality, 1552
        prostaglandin secretion, 1553
        red blood cell production, regulation of, 1553
        renal clearance, 1553
        urine formation, 1551
        urine storage, 1553–1554
        vitamin D synthesis, 1553
        waste products, excretion of, 1553
        water excretion, regulation of, 1552
    health history, 1555–1557
    kidneys, 1548–1549, 1549f
        blood supply to, 1549
        functions of, 1549c
        nephrons, 1549–1550, 1550f
    physical assessment, 1557–1559
        bladder, percussion of, 1558
        costovertebral angle, 1557, 1558f
        kidneys, palpation of, 1557, 1558f
        vulva, urethral meatus, and vagina
            examination, 1558
    ureters, 1550
    urethra, 1551
    urinary bladder, 1550
Kidney biopsy, 1565
Kidney disorders
    acute kidney injury, 1576–1581
    chronic kidney disease, 1569–1570
    end-stage kidney disease, 1581–1589
    fluid and electrolyte disturbances in,
        1568–1569, 1568t
    nephrosclerosis, 1570
    polycystic kidney disease, 1574
    primary glomerular diseases, 1570–1574
    renal cancer, 1574–1576
    and urinary disorders, 1557c
        risk factors for, 1555t
Kidneys
    burn injuries and, 1852
    chemotherapy-related effects, 345
    functions, 256
    urine volume, 254
Kidney surgery, 1602
    nursing care plan, 1603c–1606c
    nursing management, 1603, 1606
        complications management, 1606
        home, community-based, and transitional
            care, 1606–1607
        immediate postoperative care, 1606
    perioperative concerns, 1602
    postoperative management, 1602–1603
    preoperative considerations, 1602
Kidney transplantation, 1607–1612, 1608f
    acute rejection, 1609
    contraindications to, 1607
    hyperacute rejection, 1609
    kidney donation, 1607c
    postoperative management, 1609–1612
        complications management, 1611
        home, community-based, and transitional
            care, 1611–1612
        immunosuppressive agents, 1609–1610,
            1610t
        infection prevention, 1610–1611, 1611c
        psychological concerns, addressing of, 1611
        transplant rejection, assessment for, 1610
        urinary function, monitoring of, 1611
    preoperative management, 1608–1609
        medical management, 1608

nursing management, 1608–1609
        psychosocial evaluation, 1608, 1609c
Killer T cells. *See* Cytotoxic T cells
King Tube, 2164
Kirsten ras (KRAS), 326
Klebsiella pneumoniae, 2133
Knowledge, skills, and attitudes (KSAs), 11, 11t
Kock pouch, 1333–1334, 1340
KRAS. See Kirsten ras
KS. *See* Kaposi sarcoma
KSAs. *See* Knowledge, skills, and attitudes
Kupffer cells, 1378–1379
Kyphoscoliosis, 495
Kyphosis, 1123, 1123f

L
Labetalol (Trandate), for hypertension, 891t
Labia majora, 1651
Labia minora, 1651
Labor induction, 1676c
Labyrinthitis, 1934
Lactational abscess, 1728
Lactobacillus acidophilus, 1687
Lactose intolerance, 1319, 1320c, 1321t
Lactulose (Cephulac), in hepatic
        encephalopathy, 1395
Lamellae, 1115
Laminar airflow units, 441
Lamivudine (3TC), 1034t
Langerhans cells, 1790, 1791, 1794
Language
    nursing care and, 438
    "people-first," 159
Lanreotide (Somatuline Depot)
    for pituitary tumors, 1509
Lansoprazole (Prevacid)
    for gastritis, 1295t
    for GERD, 1284t
Laparoscopes, 436
Laparoscopic cholecystectomy, 1434, 1436–
        1437, 1436f
    self-care after, 1440c
Laparoscopic cryomyolysis, 1704
Laparoscopic myolysis, 1704
Laparoscopic myomectomy, 1704
Laparoscopic radical prostatectomy, 1771, 1772t
Laparoscopy (pelvic peritoneoscopy), 1664–
        1665, 1664f
Laparoscopy (Peritoneoscopy), 1241
Large bowel obstruction, 1328
    assessment and diagnostic findings, 1329
    clinical manifestations, 1329
    medical management, 1329
    nursing management, 1329
    pathophysiology, 1329
Large intestine, 1224, 1225
    anatomy and blood supply of, 1225f
Laryngeal cancer, 572–581, 572c
    symptom severity patterns, 581c
Laryngeal mask airway (LMA), 445f, 2164
    during surgery, 440
Laryngeal obstruction, 571–572
    causes, 571t
Laryngectomy, 552, 573–574
    home care, 580c
Laryngitis, 552, 565–567
Larynx, anatomy, 481–482
Laser ablation, 879
Laser-assisted in situ keratomileusis, 1899, 1899f
Laser hyperthermia, for hepatic metastases, 1418

Lasers, risks of, 442
Laser therapy, 1663
    for cervical cancer, 1707
    for genital warts, 1691
    for vaginal cancers, 1711–1712
L-asparaginase, 344
Latent autoimmune diabetes of adults (LADA),
    1456, 1460
Latent reservoir, 1031
Late-onset familial Alzheimer disease, 125t
Lateral collateral ligament (LCL), 1188
    injury, 1187–1188, 1187f
Lateral epicondylitis, 1187
Late-stage illness, 389
Latex allergy, 423, 1064, 1078–1080
    assessment and diagnostic findings, 1079
    assessment form, 427f
    clinical manifestations, 1079, 1080t
    intraoperative patients, 452
    latex products and alternative products, 1078t
    medical management, 1079
    nursing management, 1079–1080
    surgical environment, 450
Latex condom, 1673
Lavage, 1243, 1244
Laxatives, 1313, 1314t
    drug interactions, 205
Leading Health Care Indicators (LHIs), 7
Leaflet repair, 798, 798f
Learning
    age-related changes
    definition of, 48, 51
    disabilities,
        developmental disability, 53c
        input disability, 53c
        output disability, 53c
    measurement of, 54
    motivation for, 50
    readiness for
        basis of, 51
        definition of, 48
Learning readiness, 48
Lectronystagmography, 1922
Ledipasvir-sofosbuvir (Harvoni), 1404
Leflunomide (Arava), 1088t
Left atrial appendage occlusion (LAAO), 726
Left-sided heart failure, 818, 821, 822, 844. See
    also Heart failure (HF)
Left ventricular failure. See Left-sided heart failure
Legal issues, end-of-life care and, 388
Legg–Calve–Perthes disease, 1147
Legionella pneumophila, 2151
Legionnaires disease, 2151
Legs, postoperative exercises, 430c
Leg ulcers, 874–878, 1803
    arterial ulcers, 875
    assessment and diagnostic findings, 875
    clinical manifestations, 874–875
    compression therapy, 875
    débridement, 876
    hyperbaric oxygenation, 877
    negative pressure wound therapy, 877
    nursing process, 877–878
    pathophysiology, 874
    pharmacologic therapy, 875
    sickle cell disease and, 940
    stimulated healing, 876
    topical therapy, 876
    venous ulcers, 875
    wound dressings, 876

Leininger's Sunrise Model, 105
Leiomyoma, 1284
Lenalidomide (Revlimid), 982
Lente insulin, 1468
Lentigo maligna melanoma (LMM), 1836
Lepirudin (Refludan), for venous
    thromboembolism, 870t
Leptin, 1360
Lesbians, gay, bisexual, and transgender
    (LGBT), 1029, 1659–1660, 1660c
Letrozole (Femara), 1743, 1744t
Leukapheresis, 913t
Leukemia, 927, 971
    acute, 971
        lymphocytic leukemia, 975–976
        myeloid leukemia, 971–974
    chronic, 971
        lymphocytic leukemia, 976–978
        myeloid leukemia, 974–975
    classification of, 328t
    nursing process, 978–981
        assessment, 978
        diagnosis, 978
        evaluation, 981
        nursing interventions, 978–981
        planning and goals, 978
Leukemia cutis, 972, 972f
Leukocyte adhesion deficiency (LAD), 1024t
Leukocytes, 971. See White blood cells (WBCs)
Leukocytosis, 971
Leukopenia, 909, 1272–1273
Leukoplakia, 1266t
Leukopoor, 917
Leukotriene modifiers, 660
    for allergic rhinitis, 1070, 1070t
Leukotrienes, 655, 1059
Leuprolide (Lupron), 1169, 1677c, 1745, 1770
Levalbuterol (Xopenex HFA), 656
Levator ani, 1652
Level of consciousness (LOC), 2037, 2180
Levin tube, 1244
Levocetirizine (Xyzal), 1069t
Levodopa, 2103
Levofloxacin (Levaquin)
    in impetigo, 1818
    for urinary tract infections, 1619t
Levothyroxine (Synthroid), 1169
    drug interactions, 428t
Leydig cell tumors, 1780
LGBT. See Lesbians, gay, bisexual, and
    transgender
Lice infestation, 1820–1822
Lichenification, 1799t
    definition of, 1806, 1809
Lichen planus, 1266t
Licox catheter system, 1982, 1983f
Lidocaine (Xylocaine), 448t, 506, 1534
    for rape consequences, 2189
    for ventricular tachycardia, 730
Lidocaine patches (Lidoderm), 243
Life-change units, 86
Lifestyle factors, and immune system, 1018
Li-Fraumeni syndrome, 126t
Ligaments, 1118
    injuries to, 1187–1189
Ligation and stripping, 879
Lightning injuries, 1850c
Linaglipitin (Tradjenta), 1475t
Liniments, 1806, 1809–1810
Lipase, 1224, 1227, 1428, 1429

Lipid profiles, 695
Lipoatrophy, 1033, 1037f, 1469
Lipohypertrophy, 1033, 1469
Lipoproteins, 695
    atherosclerosis development and, 754f
    high-density, 750, 752
    high-density (HDL), 695
    low-density, 750, 752
    low-density (LDL), 695
    metabolism of, medications affects, 756t
Liposomal therapy, for ovarian cancer, 1713
Liposomes, 1713
Lipotropin, 1507
Lips, 1231
Liraglutide (Victoza), 1475t
Lisinopril (Prinivil)
    for heart failure, 824t
    for hypertension, 892t
Lithotomy position, 452, 453f
Lithotripsy, 1264, 1270, 1428, 1433
Liver, 1377–1378, 1378f
    age-related changes in, 1380, 1380c
    anatomy of, 1378–1379, 1378f
    assessment of
        health history, 1380
        physical assessment, 1380–1382, 1381f
    cancer of, 1417–1420
    changes with age, 437
    dysfunction, 1382–1384 (*See specific diseases*)
    enlargement, 1406
    functions of, 1379–1380
        ammonia conversion, 1379
        bile formation, 1379
        bilirubin excretion, 1379
        drug metabolism, 1379–1380
        fat metabolism, 1379
        glucose metabolism, 1379
        protein metabolism, 1379
        vitamin and iron storage, 1379
    laboratory tests to assess function of, 1382,
        1383f
    palpation of, 1381–1382, 1381f
    tenderness of, 1382
Liver abscesses, 1425
    amebic, 1425
    assessment and diagnostic findings, 1425
    clinical manifestations, 1425
    medical management, 1425
    nursing management, 1425
    pathophysiology, 1425
    pyogenic, 1425
Liver biopsy, 1382
Liver disease, 956
Liver metastases, 1417
    assessment and diagnostic findings, 1417–1418
    clinical manifestations, 1417
    medical management, 1418
        chemotherapy, 1418
        immunotherapy, 1418
        laser hyperthermia, 1418
        percutaneous biliary drainage, 1418
        radiation therapy, 1418
        transcatheter arterial embolization, 1418
    nursing management, 1419–1420
        continuing and transitional care, 1420
        patient education, 1419–1420
    surgical management, 1418–1419
        liver transplantation, 1419
        lobectomy, 1419
        local ablation, 1419

Liver transplantation, 1420–1425
  biliary anastomoses, 1421, 1422f
  complications, 1422
    bleeding, 1422–1423
    infection, 1423
    LDLT procedure, 1423
    rejection, 1423
  end-stage liver disease and, 1420
  ethical issues related to, 1421, 1421c
  immunosuppressive agents after, 1420
  indications for, 1420
  liver cancer and, 1419
  living donor, 1422
  MELD score, 1420–1421
  Milan criteria, 1419
  nursing management, 1423
    continuing and transitional care,
      1424–1425
    patient education, 1424
    postoperative, 1424
    preoperative, 1423–1424
  patient evaluation before, 1420
  split-liver transplant, 1422
  surgical procedure, 1421–1422
  triple therapy, 1420
Living arrangements, 202–204
Living donor liver transplantation (LDLT), 1422
Living ligature, 1652
Living will, 34
LMM. See Lentigo maligna melanoma
L.M.X.4 (lidocaine cream 4%), 234
Lobectomy, 538c
Lobular carcinoma in situ (LCIS), 1719, 1729
Lobules, liver, 1378
Local adaptation syndrome, 87
Local anesthesia, 243–244, 449
Local conduction blocks, 448
Locked-in syndrome, 1972, 1974
Long-acting beta$_2$-agonists (LABA), 656
Long-acting muscarinic antagonists (LAMA),
  640
Long-acting reversible contraception (LARC),
  1669–1670
  intrauterine device, 1670
  single-rod implant, 1670
Long-term care facilities, older adults and, 204
Look Good Feel Better programs, 1276, 1743
Loop diuretics, for hypertension, 890t
Loop electrocautery excision procedure (LEEP),
  1663, 1686
  for cervical cancer, 1707
Loose bodies, 1164
Loperamide (Imodium), 1316, 1317
Lopinavir + ritonavir (LPV/r), 1035t
Loratadine (Alavert, Claritin), 1069t
Lorazepam (Ativan), 2038
  for alcohol withdrawal syndrome, 2185
  delirium management, 407
Lorcaserin (Belviq), for obesity, 1365t
Lordosis, 1123, 1123f
Losartan (Cozaar)
  for heart failure, 824t
  for hypertension, 892t
Lotions, wound treatment, 1809–1810
Low back pain, 1160–1164
  assessment and diagnostic findings, 1161
  causes of, 1160
  clinical manifestations, 1161
  diagnostic procedures for, 1161c
  medical management, 1161

  nursing assessment, 1162
  nursing management, 1162–1164, 1163f
  pathophysiology of, 1160–1161
  preventing acute, 1162c
Low-density lipoprotein (LDL), 750, 752, 851
  in CAD, 753–754
Lower airway injuries, burn-related, 1852
Lower motor neuron, 1955, 1956t
Lower respiratory tract disorders, 583–631
  atelectasis, 584–586
  chest trauma, 625–631
  chest tumors, 620–625
  pleural conditions, 606–619
  pneumoconiosis, 619–620
  respiratory infections, 586–606
Low–molecular-weight heparin (LMWHs), 958,
    963, 1145
  for angina, 758t, 760
  for venous thromboembolism, 870–871, 870t
Low-profile gastrostomy devices (LPGDs), 1253
Low-profile jejunostomy devices (LPJDs), 1253
Lubiprostone (Amitiza), 1314t, 1318
Lugol's solution, 1521
Lumbar disc excision, 2118
Lumbar disc herniations, 2117
Lumbar puncture
  assisting with, 1970c
  cerebrospinal fluid analysis and, 1970
  headache following, 1970
Lumbar spine vertebrae, 2113f
Lumbar support belts, in low back pain, 1161
Lumen, 1243, 1244
Lund and Browder method, 1848–1849
Lung abscess, 605–606
  assessment, 605–606
  clinical manifestations, 605
  diagnostic findings, 605–606
  medical management, 606
  nursing management, 606
  pathophysiology, 605
  prevention, 606
Lung cancer, 620–624
  metastasis, 622f
  radiation therapy, 340
  survival rates, 621t
Lungs, 254
  airway resistance, 484, 484c
  anatomy, 482–483, 482f, 483f
  capacity, 484, 485t
  compliance, 480, 484
  function of, 256, 484
  lobes of, 494c
  mechanoreceptors in, 488
  positioning, 493
  resection, 623c
  volume, 484, 485t
    reduction, 538c
Lung scans, 505
Lung transplantation, 644
Lupus nephritis, 1099
Luteal phase, 1650
Luteinizing hormone (LH), 1507, 1650, 1653
Luteinizing hormone–releasing hormone
    (LHRH) agonists, 1770
Lyme disease, 2177
  stages of, 2178
Lymph, 842, 880
Lymphadenitis, 880
Lymphadenopathy, 972
Lymphangitis, 880

Lymphatic disorders, 880–881
Lymphatic system, 842, 910f
Lymphatic vessels, 843
Lymphedema, 880–881, 1719, 1736–1737
Lymph node biopsy, 508
Lymph nodes, 1006, 1008
Lymphocytes, 903, 907, 971, 1006
Lymphoid, 971
Lymphoid stem cells, 903, 904f, 905
Lymphoid tissues, 1005–1006
Lymphokines, 1011–1012
Lymphoma, classification of, 328t
Lymphomas, 971, 988
  AIDS-related, 1039, 1042
  Hodgkin, 988–991
  non-Hodgkin, 991–993
Lymphopenia, 946–947
Lymphoscintigraphy, 849
Lynch syndrome, 126t, 1343, 1712. See also
    Colorectal cancer
Lyric, 1939
Lysergic acid diethylamide (LSD), 2190
Lysis, 973

M

Macrophages, 907, 908
Macule, 1798t
Magic mouthwash, 1272
Magico-religious view, 109–110
Magnesium
  deficit, 1568t
  excess, 1568t
  wound healing and, 425t
Magnesium-based antacids, 278, 1583
Magnesium-free dialysate, 279
Magnesium hydroxide (Milk of Magnesia),
    1314t
  for GERD, 1284t
Magnesium imbalance, 276–279, 277t
  hypermagnesemia, 278–279
  hypomagnesemia, 277–278
Magnesium sulfate, in cardiopulmonary
    resuscitation, 839t
Magnetic resonance angiography (MRA), 849
Magnetic resonance–guided focused ultrasound
    surgery (MRgFUS), 1704
Magnetic resonance imaging (MRI)
  of brain, 2095f
  of breast, 1725–1726
  of chest, 504
  in gastroenterology, 1236
  for low back pain, 1161c
  for musculoskeletal disorders, 1127
  nervous system, 1966–1967
Magnetic resonance imaging–guided core biopsy,
    of breast, 1727
Malabsorption, 1311, 1315
  disorders of, 1318–1322, 1321t
  nursing management, 371
Malaria, 2153
Male artificial urinary sphincter, 1626, 1626f
Male breast, diseases of, 1749–1750
Male condom, 1673
Male reproductive system, 1753
  age-related changes in, 1754, 1754t
  assessment
    BETTER model, 1755
    digital rectal examination, 1755
    health history, 1754–1755
    physical examination, 1755

PLISSIT model, 1755
  testicular self-examination, 1755
diagnostic evaluation, 1755
  prostate fluid or tissue analysis, 1756
  prostate-specific antigen test, 1756
  tests of male sexual function, 1756
  ultrasonography, 1756
disorders of
  circumcision, 1786
  ejaculation, disorders of, 1760–1761
  epididymitis, 1779
  erectile dysfunction, 1756–1760
  genetic factors in, 1760c
  hydrocele, 1782–1783
  orchitis, 1778–1779
  penile cancer, 1783–1784
  Peyronie's disease, 1785
  phimosis, 1783
  priapism, 1785
  prostatic disorders, 1761–1778
  sexually transmitted infections, 1761
  testicular cancer, 1779–1782
  testicular torsion, 1779
  urethral stricture, 1785–1786
  varicocele, 1783
structures of, 1753–1754, 1753f
Male sterilization. *See* Vasectomy
Malignant bone tumors, 1180
Malignant cells, characteristics of, 326
Malignant, definition of, 324, 327
Malignant hyperthermia, 436, 450–451
Malignant Hyperthermia Association of the
    United States (MHAUS), 451
Malignant skin tumors, 1834, 1834c
  basal cell carcinoma, 1834–1836, 1834f
  melanoma, 1836–1838
  squamous cell carcinoma, 1834–1836, 1834f
Malunion, 1185, 1196, 1196f
Mammography, 1723–1725, 1725f
Mammoplasty, 1719, 1748–1749
  augmentation, 1749
  mastopexy, 1749
  reduction, 1749
Mandibular fractures, 1269
Manual traction, 1140
Maraviroc (MVC), 1035t
Marburg virus, 2127t
Marshall–Bonney maneuver, 1559
Marsupialization, 1702
Masks, 441
Maslow hierarchy of needs, 5, 5f
Mass casualty incident (MCI), 2193, 2194
  triage categories, 2197t
MAST. *See* Michigan Alcohol Screening Test
Mastalgia (breast pain), 1719, 1728
Mast cells, 1058
Mast cell stabilizers, for allergic rhinitis,
    1068–1069
Mastectomy, 1719, 1732
  total, 1733–1734, 1733t
Mastitis, 1719, 1722c, 1728
Mastoidectomy, 1929–1931
Mastopexy, 1749
Material safety data sheet (MSDS), 2005, 2193,
    2201
Maximal voluntary ventilation, 502t
MDS. *See* Myelodysplastic syndromes
Mean arterial pressure (MAP), 298
Measles, mumps and rubella (MMR) vaccine,
    2134

Measures Application Partnership (MAP), 392
Mechanical ventilation, 525–537, 2111
  classification, 525–526
  indications, 525, 525c
  troubleshooting problems, 530t
  ventilator modes, 527–528, 527f
Medial collateral ligament (MCL)
  injury to, 1187–1188, 1187f
Medial epicondylitis, 1187
Mediastinal tumors, 624–625
Mediastinoscopy, 508
Mediastinum, 482
Mediating process, 86
Medicaid
  older adults and, 218
  reimbursement by, 204
Medical abortion, 1675–1676, 1676c
Medical nutrition therapy (MNT), 1456, 1461
Medical-surgical nursing, 11
Medicare, 393
  older adults and, 218
  short-term nursing facilities, 204
Medicare Hospice Benefit, 393–394
  definition of, 387
Medicare Payment Advisory Commission
    (MedPAC), 395
Medications
  analgesic, 466
  to control postoperative nausea and vomiting,
    460t
  drug interactions, 428t
  intravenous, 446–447
  ocular, 1886–1888, 1888t, 1889t
  over-the-counter, 423, 427–428
  preanesthetic, 432
  prescriptions, 424–425
  previous use of, 427–428
Mediterranean Diet, 1364
MedPAC. *See* Medicare Payment Advisory
    Commission
Medroxyprogesterone (Depo-Provera), 1169
Medullary depression, 443
Megacolon, 1313
Megakaryocytes, 907
Megaloblastic anemia, 906, 928, 933–934
  clinical manifestations, 933–934
  folic acid deficiency and, 933
  medical management, 934
  nursing management, 934
  vitamin B_{12} deficiency and, 933
Megaloblastic red cells, 933
Megaloblasts, 906
Megestrol acetate (Megace), 372, 405–406, 1042
MEI. *See* Middle ear implantation
Meiosis, 117
Melanin, 1790, 1791
Melanocytes, 1790, 1791
Melanocyte-stimulating hormone, 1507, 1791
Melanomas, 1836–1838, 1837c
Melena, 1292, 1293
Melphalan (Alkeran), 343t
Membranous labyrinth, 1917
Memory
  age-related changes, 205
  enhancement programs, 205
  older adults and, 205
Memory cells, 1012
Menarche, 1650, 1654
Mendelian inheritance, 119, 120t. *See also*
    inheritance patterns

Ménière disease, 1933–1934
  definition of, 1915
  dietary guidelines, 1933c
Meningeal infections, 2065
Meningeal irritation, 2066f
Meninges, 1949–1950, 1949f, 2065–2068
  arachnoid, 1950
  dura mater, 1949
  pia mater, 1949–1950
Meningiomas, 2092
Meningitis, 2049, 2065–2068
  cerebrospinal fluid values diagnostic, 2067t
  gonococcal, 2149
  specific populations, 2066c
Meningococcus, vaccination, 2131, 2134
Meniscal injuries, 1188
Menisci, 1188
  injuries to, 1187–1189
Menopause, 1650, 1654, 1681
  clinical manifestations, 1681–1682
  definition of, 1681
  health promotion strategies, 1682c
  medical management, 1682
    behavioral strategies, 1683
    bone health, 1683
    cardiovascular health, 1683
    hormone therapy, 1682–1683
    hot flashes and, 1683
    nutritional therapy, 1683
  nursing management, 1683
  postmenopausal bleeding, 1681
  psychological considerations, 1682
Menorrhagia, 1668
Menotropins (Repronex, Pergonal), 1677c
Menstrual cycle, 1653–1654, 1653f
  hormonal changes during, 1654t
Menstruation, 1650, 1666
  cultural considerations, 1666
  psychosocial considerations, 1666
Mental health, 2113
  of older adults, 207–215
Mental health disabilities, communicating with
    people having, 156c
Mental status, 643, 685
Meperidine (Demerol), 241
Mephedrone, 2180
Mercaptans, 1394
6-Mercaptopurine (Purinethol), 343t
Merkel cells, 1790, 1791
Meshed graft, split-thickness, 1863f
Mesna (Mesnex), 345
Metabolic acidosis, end-stage kidney disease
    and, 1582, 1583
Metabolic bone disorders, 1169–1176
  osteomalacia, 1174–1175
  osteoporosis, 1169–1174
  Paget disease, 1175–1176
Metabolic equivalents (METs), 684
Metabolic syndrome, 750, 753, 1459
[131]I-metaiodobenzylguanidine (MIBG)
    scintigraphy, 1533
Metanephrine (MN), 1532
Metaplasia
  cellular adaptation, 92
  definition of, 84
Metaproterenol sulfate (Alupent), 661t
Metastasis, definition of, 324
Metastatic bone disease, 1180
Metastatic skin tumors, 1839
  Kaposi sarcoma, 1839

Metered-dose inhalers (MDIs), 641f
Metformin (Glucophage, Glucophage XL, Fortamet), 1460, 1474t, 1677c, 1703
Metformin with glyburide (Glucovance), 1474t
Methadone, 240–241
  for ventricular tachycardia, 730
Methicillin-resistant *Staphylococcus aureus* (MRSA), 1146, 1176, 1817, 2132
  description of, 2132
Methimazole, 1520, 1521
  for hyperthyroidism, 1521t
Methohexital sodium (Brevital), 447t
Methotrexate, 343t, 345, 350, 1088t, 1095, 1102
  for abortion, 1676c
  in ectopic pregnancy, 1680
  for psoriasis, 1825
Methyclothiazide (Enduron), for hypertension, 890t
Methylcellulose (Citrucel), 1314t
Methyldopa (Aldomet)
  for hypertension, 891t
3,4-methylenedioxymethamphetamine (MDMA), 2180
3,4-methylenedioxypyrovalerone (MDPV), 2180
Methylprednisolone (Medrol), 658t, 661t, 1534, 1541t
Methyl tertiary butyl ether (MTBE), 1434
Methylxanthines, 658t–659t
Metoclopramide (Reglan), 372, 460t, 1288
  for GERD, 1284t
Metocurine (Metubine), 447t
Metolazone (Zaroxolyn)
  for heart failure, 824t
  for hypertension, 890t
Metoprolol (Lopressor)
  for angina, 758t, 759
  for heart failure, 824t
  for hypertension, 891t
Metoprolol extended release (Toprol-XL), for hypertension, 891t
Metronidazole (Flagyl), 2144
  for bacterial vaginosis, 1689
  for gastritis, 1295t
  in hepatic encephalopathy, 1395
  for pelvic inflammatory disease, 1696
  for rape consequences, 2189
  for trichomoniasis, 1689
Metropolitan Medical Response Teams Systems, 2195
Metrorrhagia, 1668, 1706
MEWS. *See* Modified Early Warning System
Michigan Alcohol Screening Test (MAST), 69
Michigan Quality Improvement Consortium (MQIC), 1161
Miconazole (Monistat), for candidiasis, 1688
Microalbuminuria, 1561
Microbicides, 1028
Microbiome, 1358, 1361
Microbiota, 1358, 1360–1361
Micrographia, 2103
Microhemagglutination test for *Treponema pallidum* (MHA-TP), 2147
Micropapillary invasive ductal carcinoma, 1730
Micturition, 1548, 1550, 1554, 1556, 1615
Midazolam (Versed), 407, 447t, 1237, 2038
  for alcohol withdrawal syndrome, 2185
Middle ear
  anatomy of, 1916–1917
  conditions of, 1927–1932

effusion of, 1928
  masses of, 1931–1932
Middle ear implantation (MEI), 1940
Mifepristone (Mifeprex)
  for abortion, 1675, 1676c
  for fibroids, 1704
Miglitol (Glyset), 1474t
Migraine
  manifestations, 2004–2005
  patient education, 2006c
Milk thistle (*Silybum marianum*), 1408
Miller–Fisher variant, 2082
Milrinone (Primacor), for heart failure, 826
Mineralocorticoids, 1502, 1531–1532
Mineral oil, 1314t
Minimally conscious state, 1973
Minimally invasive surgery, 418
Mini-Mental State Examination (MMSE), 204, 205c
Minocycline (Minocin), in hidradenitis suppurativa, 1813
Minorities, 102, 103–104
Minoxidil (Loniten), for hypertension, 892t
Minute ventilation, 501
Mirtazapine (Remeron), 207
Misoprostol (Cytotec), 1675
  for abortion, 1675, 1676c
  for gastritis, 1295t
Mithramycin, 276
Mitomycin, 343t, 345, 346
Mitomycin C, 346
Mitosis, 117
Mitotic spindle inhibitors, 343t
Mitoxantrone (Novantrone), 343t, 972, 2075
Mitral (apical) area, 689, 689f
Mitral valve, 791
  anatomy of, 791, 792f
  heart sound, 690
  regurgitation, 793–794
  stenosis, 794
Mitral valve prolapse, 792–793
  assessment of, 793
  clinical manifestations of, 792–793
  diagnostic findings of, 793
  medical management of, 793
  nursing management of, 793
  pathophysiology of, 792, 792f
Mitrofanoff umbilical appendicovesicostomy, 1632
Mivacurium (Mivacron), 446t
Mixed pain, 227t
Mixed urinary incontinence, 1624. *See also* Urinary incontinence
MLM. *See* Mucosal lentiginous melanoma
Mobility. *See also* Ambulation
  after burn injuries, 1866–1867
  assessments, 168c, 170
  elimination problems and, 186
  goals of, 429
  home care education, 189c
  improvement of, 183
  limitations in, communication and, 155c
  nursing process and, 170–178
  postoperative, 429
  self-care deficits and, 168c
Model for End-Stage Liver Disease (MELD) classification, 1420–1421
Model Spinal Cord Injury Centers, 166
Moderate sedation, 448–449
  description of, 436

patient monitoring in
use of
Modified Early Warning System (MEWS), 317, 318t
Modified radical mastectomy, 1719, 1733
MODS. *See* Multiple organ dysfunction syndrome
Moexipril (Univasc), for hypertension, 892t
Mohs micrographic surgery, 1835
Moisture
  pressure ulcers and, 180–181, 184
  skin breakdown and, 180
Moisture-retentive dressings, 1808–1809
  calcium alginates, 1809
  foam dressings, 1809
  hydrocolloids, 1808–1809
  hydrogels, 1808
Molecular adsorbent recirculating system (MARS), 1405
Moles, 1833
Molluscum contagiosum, 1041
Molotov cocktail, 2202
Mondor disease, 1730
Moniliasis, 1266t
Monitored anesthesia care (MAC), 449
Monoclonal antibodies (MoAbs), 352–353, 1013
  cancer vaccines, 354
  chimeric, 353
  cytokines, 353–354
  human, 353
  hybridomas, 352–353, 353f
  production of, 352
Monoclonal gammopathy of undetermined significance (MGUS), 993–994
Monoclonal protein, 993
Monocytes, 907, 971
Mononuclear leukocytes. *See* Monocytes
Monotherapy, 896
Monro–Kellie hypothesis, 1973, 1979, 2034, 2093
Montana, on assisted suicide, 390
Montelukast (Singulair), 1070, 1070t
Moral dilemmas, 31
Moral distress, 31
Moral integrity, 33
Moral problems, 31
Moral uncertainty, 31
Morbidity and Mortality Weekly Report (MMWR), 2129
Morning hyperglycemia, 1471, 1471t
Morphine, 239–240
  characteristics of, 240t
  equianalgesic dose chart for, 238
  metabolites, 239
Morphine-3-glucuronide (M3G), 239
Morphine-6-glucuronide (M6G), 239
Morphine sulfate (MS), 446t
  drug interactions, 428t
Morton neuroma, 1168
Motion sickness, 1932–1933
Motivation
  adherence to regimens and, 50
  positive reinforcement and, 50
Motor dysfunction, 2077
Motor pathways, 1954–1956
Motor system, examination of, 1960
Mourning
  after death, 411–412
  anticipatory, 410–411, 411c

assessment of, 411c
complicated, 412
definition of, 387, 410
loss and, 411
six processes of, 411–412
Mouth care, 1265, 1268
Mouth, physical assessment, 493
MRI. *See* Magnetic Resonance Imaging
MRSA. *See* Methicillin-resistant *Staphylococcus aureus*
MSDS. *See* Material safety data sheets
Mucosal lentiginous melanoma (MLM), 1836
Mucositis, 979
chemotherapy agents and, 345
definition of, 324
management of, 357
Mucus hypersecretion, 655
Multidetector-computed tomography (MDCT), 848
Multidetector CT (MDCT), 701
Multidisciplinary action plans (MAPs), 9
Multidrug-resistant organisms (MDROs), 2132
Multifactorial inheritance, 121
Multimodal analgesia, 233–245
Multiple chronic conditions (MCC), 140
facts about, 141c
Multiple endocrine neoplasia, 126t
type 1 (MEN 1), 1297
Multiple myeloma, 971, 993–998
assessment and diagnostic findings, 995
clinical manifestations, 994–995, 994f
complications management, 996–997
CRAB features, 993–994
medical management, 995–997
autologous stem cell transplantation, 996
early treatment options, 995
pharmacologic therapy, 996
nursing management, 997–998
older adults and, 997
pathophysiology, 993–994, 993f
and peripheral neuropathy, 998, 998t
staging, 993
Multiple organ dysfunction syndrome (MODS), 296, 319–320, 956
burn injuries and, 1854
clinical manifestations of, 320
medical management, 320
nursing management, 320
pathophysiology of, 319–320
Multiple sclerosis (MS), 2073f, 2074f
home care checklist, 2078c
predictors of fatigue, 2076c
signs and symptoms of, 2073
Multiple-test dipstick, 1561
Multiple trauma, 2156, 2168–2170
assessment and diagnostic findings, 2169
causes of, 2168
management, 2169, 2169c
Mupirocin (Bactroban)
in impetigo, 1817–1818
Murmurs, 691
characteristics of, 692c
Muscle, 1118
actions, 1119
antagonists, 1119
atrophy, 1119
contraction, 1118–1119, 1120f
cramps, 1120
exercise and disuse, 1119
hypertrophy, 1119

skeletal, 1118
strength and size, assessment of, 1124–1125
synergists, 1119
tone, 1119
Muscle relaxants
depolarizing, 446t
nondepolarizing, 446t–447t
Muscle setting exercises, 1135
Muscular dystrophies, 2091, 2111
Musculoskeletal disorders (MSD), 1114–1115
bone tumors, 1179–1183
foot problems, 1166–1168
genetic, 1122c
low back pain, 1160–1164
metabolic bone disorders, 1169–1176
musculoskeletal infections, 1176–1179
musculoskeletal extremity disorders, 1164–1166
Musculoskeletal infections, 1176–1179
osteomyelitis, 1176–1178
septic (infectious) arthritis, 1178–1179
Musculoskeletal sports injuries, 1213t
Musculoskeletal system, 1114
age-related changes, 197t, 200–201
age-related changes of, 1119, 1121t
assessment, 1119–1126
diagnostic evaluation
arthrocentesis, 1128
arthrography, 1127
arthroscopy, 1128
biopsy, 1129
bone densitometry, 1127
bone scan, 1127–1128
computed tomography, 1127
electromyography, 1128–1129
laboratory studies, 1129
magnetic resonance imaging, 1127
x-rays studies, 1126
health history, 1119
altered sensations, 1121
common symptoms, 1119–1121
pain, 1120–1121
past health, social, and family history, 1121
physical assessment, 1122–1123
bone integrity, 1124
gait, 1123–1124
joint function, 1124
muscle strength and size, 1124–1125
neurovascular status, 1126, 1126c
posture, 1123, 1123f
skin, 1126
structure and function of, 1115
articular system, 1117–1118
skeletal muscle system, 1118–1119
skeletal system, 1115–1117, 1115f
Musculoskeletal trauma
amputation, 1214–1220
clavicle, 1198
contusions, strains, and sprains, 1185–1186
elbow, 1199–1200
femoral shaft, 1210–1211
fibula, 1211
fractures, 1189–1197
hand, 1200–1201
hip, 1202–1205
humeral neck, 1198–1199
humeral shaft, 1199
joint dislocations, 1186–1187
ligaments, injury to, 1187–1189
menisci, injury to, 1187–1189
occupation-related, 1212–1214

pelvis, 1201–1202
radial and ulnar shafts, 1200
radial head, 1200
rib, 1211–1212
sports-related, 1212
tendons, injury to, 1187–1189
thoracolumbar spine, 1212
tibia, 1211
wrist, 1200
Mutual pretense awareness, 389
Myasthenia gravis, 1061, 2072, 2079, 2080
Mycobacterium avium complex (MAC) disease
HIV infection and, 1038, 1041
Mycophenolate mofetil (MMF), 350, 1610t
for pemphigus vulgaris, 1828
Mycophenolic acid (Myfortic), 1610t
Mycoplasma pneumoniae, 936
Mycotic aneurysms, 862
Mydriatics, 1885t, 1887
Myelin, 2082
Myelodysplastic syndromes (MDS), 981–984
assessment and diagnostic findings, 982
clinical manifestations, 982
dysplasia of erythrocytes in, 981
medical management, 982–983
nursing management, 983–984
primary, 981–982
secondary, 982
Myelofibrosis, 987–988, 987f
Myelogram, for low back pain, 1161c
Myeloid, 971
Myeloid neoplasms, development of, 971, 971f
Myeloid stem cells, 903, 904f
Myelomas, classification of, 328t
Myelopoiesis, 907
Myeloproliferative neoplasms
essential thrombocythemia, 985–987
polycythemia vera, 984–985
primary myelofibrosis, 987–988
Myelosuppression, 345, 357
definition of, 324
Myocardial infarction (MI), 762–771
assessment of, 763–764, 763c, 767
cardiac rehabilitation, 766–767
clinical manifestations, 763
definition of, 750, 751
diagnosis of, 763–764, 767
electrocardiogram, 763–764, 764f
evaluation, 770–771
health promotion, 770c
medical management, 765–766
nursing care, 768c–769c
nursing interventions, 767–770
nursing process, 767–771
pathophysiology, 762–763
patient goals, 767
serum enzymes and biomarkers, 765f
treatment guidelines for, 765c
Myocardial perfusion, 700
Myocarditis, 812–813
Myofascial pain, 1269
Myoglobin, 764
Myoglobulin, 1119
Myomas (fibroids), 1703–1704, 1703f
Myomectomy, 1686, 1703
Myopia, 1876, 1883
Myotonic muscular dystrophy type 1, 125t
MyPlate Food Guide, 1464
Myringotomy, 1915, 1928
Myxedema, 1502, 1514–1515

N

Nabothian (retention) cysts, 1661
N-acetylcysteine, 1236, 1405
Nadir, definition of, 324
Nadolol (Corgard)
  for hypertension, 891t
  for variceal bleeding, 1390
Nafarelin acetate (Synarel), 1677c
Nails, 1792
  clubbing of, 1801
  cuticle, 1792
  growth, 1792
  inspection, 1801
Nalbuphine (Nubain), 242
Naltrexone/bupropion (Contrave), for obesity, 1365t
NANDA International (NANDA-I), 38
Nanoparticle albumin-bound paclitaxel (nab-paclitaxel), 1451
Nasal cavity, 481f
Nasal corticosteroids, 558t
Nasal endotracheal catheter, 445f
Nasal fractures, 570–571
Nasal obstruction, 570
Nasoduodenal tube, 1243, 1245
Nasoenteric tube, 1243, 1245
Nasogastric (NG) tube, 1243, 1244
Nasojejunal tube, 1243, 1245
NASPE-BPEG code. *See* North American Society of Pacing and Electrophysiology and the British Pacing and Electrophysiology Group code
Nateglinide (Starlix), 1474t
National Association of Orthopaedic Nurses (NAON), 1156, 1186
National Asthma Education and Prevention Program (NAEPP), 1070
National Center for Complementary and Integrative Health (NCCIH), 355, 1771
National Center for Health Statistics (NCHS), 1185
National Cholesterol Education Program (NCEP), 755
National Colorectal Roundtable, 1344
National Comprehensive Cancer Network (NCCN), 331
National Consensus Project for Quality Palliative Care, 388
National Disaster Medical System, 2195
National Guard Civil Support Teams, 2195
National Health and Nutrition Examination Survey (NHANES), 1366
  on hypertension, 885
National Health Security Strategy, 2194
National Heart, Lung, and Blood Institute (NHLBI), 755
National HIV/AIDS Strategy for the United States: Updated to 2020, 1025
National Hospice and Palliative Care Organization (NHPCO), 388, 394
National Hospital Discharge Survey (NHDS), 1202
National Human Trafficking Hotline, 2189
National Incident Management System (NIMS), 2193
National Institute for Occupational Safety and Health (NIOSH), 329, 1923
National Institute of Disability Research and Rehabilitation (NIDRR), 166
National Institute of Health (NIH), 680

National Institute of Neurological Disorders and Stroke (NINDS), 1161, 1197
National Institute on Deafness and Other Communication Disorders (NIDCD), 1923
National Institute on Drug Abuse, 239
National Institutes of Health (NIH), stoke scale, 2016t
National Medical Response Teams for Weapons of Mass Destruction (NMRT), 2195
National Patient Safety Goals (NPSGs), 8, 9, 432c, 438
National Sexual Assault Hotline, 2188, 2189
National Terrorism Advisory System (NTAS), 2195
Natriuretic peptides, 258
Natural disasters, 2201–2202, 2202t
  preparedness and response
    decontamination, 2201
    personal protective equipment, 2201
    recognition and awareness, 2200–2201
  preparedness for loss of electricity after, 2200c
Natural immunity, 1006–1007
Naturalistic medicine, 109
Natural killer (NK) cells, 907, 1006, 1012
Nausea and vomiting
  intraoperative period, 450
  postoperative
    aromatherapy for, 560c
    medications, 460t
NCCIH. *See* National Center for Complementary and Integrative Health
NCCN. *See* National Comprehensive Cancer Network
Nebivolol (Bystolic), for hypertension, 891t
Neck dissection, 1274–1279
  and chyle fistula, 1278
  and hemorrhage, 1277–1278
  lymphatic drainage of head and neck, 1274f
  and nerve injury, 1278
  nursing process
    airway clearance, 1275
    assessment, 1274
    communication methods, 1276
    complications management, 1277–1278
    continuing and transitional care, 1278–1279
    diagnosis, 1274–1275
    evaluation, 1279
    home care checklist, 1278c
    nursing interventions, 1275–1279
    nutritional status, 1275–1276
    pain relief, 1275
    patient education, 1278, 1278c
    physical mobility, 1276–1277
    planning and goals, 1275
    postoperative care, 1275
    preoperative patient education, 1275
    rehabilitation exercises, 1277, 1277f
    supporting patient and caregivers, 1276, 1276c
    wound care, 1275
  radical, 1274
  reconstructive techniques, 1274
  selective, 1274, 1274f
Neck immobility, 2066
Necrotizing gingivitis, 1267t
Necrotizing pancreatitis, 1441. *See also* Pancreatitis
Needle biopsy, 335

Negative feedback, 1502, 1503
  definition of, 84
  mechanisms of, 91–92
Negative-pressure (vacuum) devices, 1760
Negative pressure wound therapy, 877
Neglect, elder, 217–218
Neisseria gonorrhoeae, 2147
Neisseria meningitidis, 2065
Nelfinavir (NFV), 1035t
Neomycin, in hepatic encephalopathy, 1395
Neoplasia, definition of, 324, 327
Neoplastic disease, 1017–1018
Neovascularization, 1876, 1882, 1902
Nephrectomy, 1575
Nephritic syndrome, acute, 1570–1572
Nephritis, 1099
Nephrolithiasis, 1527, 1632–1637
  assessment and diagnostic findings, 1633
  clinical manifestations, 1632–1633
  interventional procedures, 1634, 1635f
  medical management, 1633–1634
    nutritional therapy, 1633–1634
    pain management, 1633
  nursing process, 1634–1637
    assessment, 1634, 1636
    diagnosis, 1636
    evaluation, 1637
    home, community-based, and transitional care, 1636
    nursing interventions, 1636
    planning and goals, 1636
  pathophysiology, 1632
  predisposing factors, 1632
  surgical management, 1634
Nephrons, 1548, 1549–1550, 1550f
Nephropathy, 1456, 1461
  assessment and diagnostic findings, 1492
  clinical manifestations, 1492
  diabetes and, 1491–1493
  management, 1492–1493
Nephrosclerosis, 1567, 1570
  benign, 1570
  malignant, 1570
  treatment of, 1570
Nephrotic syndrome, 1567, 1573–1574
  assessment and diagnostic findings, 1574
  clinical manifestations, 1573–1574
  complications, 1574
  and edema, 1573
  medical management, 1574
  nursing management, 1574
  pathophysiology, 1573
  sequence of events in, 1573f
Nephrotoxic, 1567, 1578
Nerve agents, 2207–2208
  clinical manifestations of, 2208
  treatment of, 2208
Nervous system
  age-related changes, 197t, 201, 1964–1965
  anatomy of, 1947–1957, 1948f
  assessment of, 1957–1958
  cells of, 1947, 1947f
  metastases, 2099c
  physical assessment, 1958–1965
Neuraxial analgesia, 234
Neurodegenerative, 2101
Neuroendocrine tumors (NETs), 1453
Neurofibromatosis, 1833
Neurogenic bladder, 1615, 1617, 1628

flaccid bladder, 1628
spastic bladder, 1628
Neurogenic shock, 296
description of, 318
medical management, 318
nursing management, 318
risk factors, 314c
Neuroimaging, 2068
Neurologic assessment alerts, 2069
Neurologic disorders
critical care flowsheet, 1985f–1986f
genetics of, 1958c
symptoms of, 1957–1958
Neurologic systems
chemotherapy-related effects, 346
postsurgical complications, 473t
Neuromodulation, 1625c
Neuromuscular blockers, 443, 445
Neuromuscular respiratory failure, 2081
Neuropathic pain, 229–230
classification of, 227t
definition of, 224, 226
mechanisms, 230
pathways, 229f
Neuropathy, 1456, 1461
burn injuries and, 1868t
Neuropeptide Y (NPY), 1360
Neuroplasticity, 230
Neurotransmitters, 1947
examples of, 1947t
Neurovascular status, 1131, 1133
Neutropenia, 945–946, 972
causes of, 945c
clinical manifestations, 945
definition of, 324
medical management, 945
nursing management, 945–946
Neutrophils, 903, 906–907, 971, 1006
Nevirapine (NVP), 1034t
NF-kB essential modifier (NEMO) mutations,
1024t
NHL. See Non-Hodgkin lymphomas
NHPCO. See National Hospice and Palliative
Care Organization
NIC. See Nursing Interventions
Classification
Nicardipine (Cardene)
for hypertension, 893t
for pheochromocytoma, 1533
Nicotine stomatitis, 1266t
NIDCD. See National Institute on Deafness
and Other Communication
Disorders
Nifedipine long acting (Procardia XL, Adalat
CC)
for hypertension, 893t
Nightingale, Florence, 5
NIH. See National Institutes of Health
Nikolsky's sign, 1828, 1848
Nilotinib (Tasigna), 974
NIOSH. See National Institute for Occupational
Safety and Health
Nipple discharge, 1728
Nipple inversion, 1722c
Nisoldipine (Sular), for hypertension, 893t
Nissen fundoplication, 1283
Nitrates, for angina, 758t, 759
Nitrofurantoin (Macrodantin, Furadantin), for
urinary tract infections, 1619t
Nitrogen mustard (Mustargen), 343t

Nitroglycerin
for angina, 758t, 759
self-administration of, 759c
for cardiogenic shock, 311
for hypertension, 892t
Nitroprusside (Nitropress), for hypertension, 892t
Nitrosoureas, 343t
Nitrous oxide, 444t
Nivolumab (Opdivo), 1837
Nizatidine (Axid), for gastritis, 1295t
NM. See Nodular melanoma
N-methyl-D-aspartate (NMDA) receptor
antagonist, 227, 244
NOC. See Nursing Outcomes Classification
Nociception
modulation of, 228f
perception of, 228f
transduction of, 228f
transmission of, 228f
Nociceptive pain, 226–229, 227t, 229f
classification of
description of, 225
transduction of, 226
transmission of, 226–227
Nociceptors, 226
Nocturia, 1548, 1554, 1556t, 1615, 1617
Nocturnal penile tumescence tests, 1756
Nodular goiter, 1525
Nodular melanoma (NM), 1836
Nodule, 1798t
Nonalcoholic fatty liver disease (NAFLD),
1380, 1383
Nonalcoholic steatohepatitis (NASH), 1380,
1383–1384
Nonbullous impetigo, 1817
Noncompensatory pause, 720
Noncompliance, older adults and, 206–207
Nondepressed skull fractures, 2035
Nondisjunction, 118
Nonfatal drowning, 2174–2175
management, 2175
Nongerminal tumors, 1780
Non-Hodgkin lymphomas (NHL), 991–993
assessment and diagnostic findings, 991–992
classification system, 991, 992t
clinical manifestations, 991
extranodal location, 991, 991f
medical management, 992
nursing management, 992–993
Noninvasive respiratory therapies, 511–521
chest physiotherapy, 517–521
incentive spirometry, 516
oxygen therapy, 511–516
small-volume nebulizer (mini-nebulizer)
therapy, 517
Nonmaleficence, 31c
Non-nucleoside reverse transcriptase inhibitors,
1034t
Nonnutritive sweeteners, 1465
Nonopioid analgesics, 226, 235–236, 2071
administration of, 235
adverse effects of, 235–236
in skeletal traction, 1142
Nonparoxysmal junctional tachycardia, 728
Nonrebreathing mask, 514f
Nonselective débridement, 876
Nonseminoma testicular cancers, 1780
Nonsteroidal anti-inflammatory drugs
(NSAIDs), 226, 1161, 2173
administration, 235

adverse effects of, 236
benefits of, 235
in bursitis treatment, 1164
in carpal tunnel syndrome treatment,
1164
in hidradenitis suppurativa, 1813
for kidney stone pain, 1633
for pain management, 938
for rheumatic diseases, 1084, 1088t
in rib fractures, 1211
for spondylarthropathies, 1107
in tendonitis treatment, 1164
Non-sulfonylurea insulin secretagogues, 1474t
Nontraditional inheritance, 121–122
Nontreponemal or reagin tests, 2147
Nonunion, 1185, 1196, 1196f
Norepinephrine, 844
in cardiopulmonary resuscitation, 839t
Norethindrone acetate (Aygestin), 1705
Normal flora, 2125
Normal heart sounds, 690
Normal saline (NS), in diabetic ketoacidosis,
1485
Normochromic, normocytic anemia, 932
North American Society of Pacing and
Electrophysiology and the British
Pacing and Electrophysiology Group
code (NASPE-BPEG code), 741c
North Atlantic Treaty Organization (NATO),
2197
Nortriptyline (Aventyl, Pamelor), 244, 639,
1109
Nose
anatomy of, 481, 481f
physical assessment, 492–493
Nosebleed. See Epistaxis
Nothing-by-mouth (NPO), 233
Novarel, 1677c
NPH insulin, 1468
NPSGs. See National Patient Safety Goals
NSAID-induced kidney disease, 1579
NSAIDs. See Nonsteroidal anti-inflammatory
drugs
Nuchal rigidity, 552
Nuclear radiation exposure, 2208–2209
acute radiation syndrome, 2210–2211
decontamination, 2209–2210
exposure, 2209
measurement and detection, 2209
radiation, types of, 2209
survival, 2211
Nucleated RBCs, 906
Nucleic acid amplification tests (NAATs),
2148
Nucleic acid sequence–based amplification
(NAT), 1033
Nucleoside reverse transcriptase inhibitors
(NRTIs), 1034t
Null lymphocytes, 1012
Numeric Rating Scale (NRS), 230–231
Nurse navigators, 12
Nursing, 5, 32
in ambulatory settings, 24
community-based, 18–26
competencies, 112c, 115c
definition of, 5, 32
future of, 13, 13c, 14–15c
hospice care, 24, 24c
interventions, postsurgical, 464c, 465–476
medical-surgical, 11

Nursing care
    educating patients about self-care, 160–161
    gerontologic considerations, 159
    patients with disabilities, 158–161
    transitional care, 161
Nursing diagnoses, 465
    altered elimination patterns, 186
    patients with impaired mobility, 181
    self-care deficits, 168
Nursing Interventions Classification (NIC), 40, 41c
Nursing management
    breathing retraining, 521
    chest percussion, 519–520
    chest physiotherapy, 519
    mechanical ventilation, 529–537
    tracheotomy, 524–525
Nursing Outcomes Classification (NOC), 39, 40c
Nursing practice
    genetics applications, 131–135
    genomics applications, 131–135
Nursing process, 35–46, 36f
    definition of, 35
    documentation of outcomes, 42
    example of plan of nursing care, 42–45c
    hospitalized postoperative patient, 464–476
    steps of, 35–37, 36c
        assessment, 35
        diagnosis, 35–36
        evaluation, 36
        implementation, 36
        planning, 36
    taxonomy of nursing practice, 45–46c
    use of, 37–42
Nutcracker esophagus (NE), 1280
Nutrition
    in acute pancreatitis, 1444
    age-related changes, 199–200
    anemia and, 929
    artificial, 406
    assessment
        components of, 76–79
        dietary data, 77
        mini, 75c
    for cancer prevention, 331c
    definition of, 48
    elimination problems and, 188
    end-of-life care, 404–406
    health promotion and, 57
    HIV infection and, 1042
    imbalanced, 363c–365c
    and immune function, 1015–1016
    improvement of, 184
    needs in AD, 214
    postsurgical, 469–472
    preoperative, 432
    pressure ulcers and, 179t, 180, 184
    status of
        analysis of, 79
        factors influencing, 79, 80t
        physical indicators, 77f
        preoperative assessments, 424
        wound healing and, 425t
Nutritional therapy
    ascites, 1386
    cholelithiasis, 1434
    diabetes, 1461–1465
    heart failure, 826–827
    inflammatory bowel disease, 1332

Nutrition labels, 1463–1464
Nutritive sweeteners, 1465
NuvaRing (etonogestrel/ethinyl estradiol vaginal ring), 1672
Nystagmus, 1932
    definition of, 1876, 1915
    ear and, 1932
Nystatin (Mycostatin), for candidiasis, 1688

O
OA. See Osteoarthritis
Obesity, 680, 695, 1358
    android, 1362, 1362f
    assessment and diagnostic findings, 1361–1362, 1361f, 1361t
        body mass index, 1361, 1361f, 1361t
        waist circumferences, 1361–1362
        waist-to-hip ratio, 1362
    cancer risk and, 329
    definition of, 1358
    diseases/disorders associated with, 1359–1360, 1359f, 1360t
    economic burden of, 1359
    emergency nursing and, 2160–2161
    epidemiology of, 1358–1359
    and foot problems, 1166
    gynoid, 1362, 1362f
    lifestyle modification for, 1362–1364, 1364c
        caloric dietary intake, decreasing, 1363–1364
        healthy eating strategies, 1364c
        healthy sleep habits, 1364
        physical activity, increasing, 1363
    medical management, 1362
    medications associated with, 1363c
    nonsurgical interventions for, 1366
        intragastric balloon therapy, 1366
        vagal blocking, 1366
    nursing management, 1367–1368
    in older adults, 1366–1367
    pathophysiology, 1360–1361
    pharmacologic therapy for, 1364–1366, 1365t
    pressure ulcers and, 1368, 1368c
    prevalence of, 1359, 1359f
    surgical management, 1368–1369 (See also Bariatric surgery)
        and nursing process, 1369–1374
    wound infections and, 421
Obesity hypoventilation syndrome, 1367
Obesogenic, 1358, 1360
Obstructive jaundice, 1384–1385
Obstructive respiration, 496c
Obstructive sleep apnea (OSA), 567–569, 568c, 684, 1367
    description of, 480, 495
Occlusive dressings, 1808
Occupational and Safety Health Administration (OSHA), 348
Occupational health nurses, 24–25
Occupational health programs, 24–25
Occupational Safety and Health Act (OSHA), 24, 2129
Occupation-related musculoskeletal disorder, 1212–1214
Octreotide (Sandostatin), 1042, 1278, 1299
    for pituitary tumors, 1509
    for variceal bleeding, 1390
Odynophagia, 1264, 1279
OEPCR. See Office of End-of-Life and Palliative Care Research

Office of Emergency Management (OEM), 2195
Office of Emergency Services (OES), 2195
Office of End-of-Life and Palliative Care Research (OEPCR), 387
Office of Inspector General (OIG), 393
Off-pump coronary artery bypass (OPCAB) surgery, 775
Ointments, wound care, 1810
Olanzapine (Zyprexa), 407
Older adults
    altered drug responses in, 206
    body tissues of, 437
    care transitions for, 203c
    chronic health conditions of, 194f
    coping with stress and, 202
    doses of anesthetic agents, 437
    ethical issues affecting, 219
    genetic concepts and, 196c
    genitourinary disorders, 199
    health care needs of, 6
    health status of, 194
    intraoperative period, 437
    legal issues affecting, 219
    liver, changes in, 1380, 1380c
    medication regimens, 206–207
    mental health problems in, 207–215
        delirium, 208–209
        dementia, 209–215
        depression, 207–208
        substance abuse, 208
    MyPlate for, 200f
    noncompliance and, 206–207
    nursing care of, 194–195
    oral conditions in, 1265c
    perioperative period, 419–421
    postoperative care for, 461
    preoperative assessment for, 431c
    preoperative education for, 431c
    pseudobulbar affect in, 215
    sexual function in, 198–199
    shock in, 300c
    sleep complaints in, 200
    smoking in, 198
    social services for, 218
    tuberculosis in, 602
    upper respiratory tract disorders, 553c
    urinary incontinence, 199, 216
    vaccinations, 217
Older Americans Act, 218
Oligodendroglial tumors, 2092
Oliguria, 818, 829, 1548, 1556, 1556t, 1567, 1576
Olmesartan (Benicar), for hypertension, 892t
Omalizumab (Xolair), 660, 660t
Ombitasvir-paritaprevir-ritonavir with dasabuvir, 1404
Omega-3-acid ethyl esters, 756t
Omentum, 1292
Omeprazole (Prilosec)
    for gastritis, 1295t
    for GERD, 1284t
Oncology, 324, 325
Oncology Nursing Society (ONS), 342, 348, 390
Oncotic pressure, 253
Ondansetron (Zofran), 460t
On Death and Dying, 389
ONS. See Oncology Nursing Society
Onychocryptosis. See Ingrown toenail

Oophorectomy, 1686, 1705
Open awareness, 389
Open fractures, 1189
Opening snap, heart sounds, 691
Open lung biopsy, 583
Open reduction with internal fixation (ORIF),
    1144, 1198
Operating rooms
    attire, 440–441
    patient in, 436, 437–438
Opioid analgesics, 236–243, 2070
    addiction, 239
    administration of, 236–238
    adverse effects of, 241–243
    characteristics of, 240t
    dual-mechanism of, 241
    effects of, 237
    equianalgesic dose chart for, 238t
    groups of, 236
    mu receptors, 240t
    physical dependence, 238
    selected, 239–241
    in skeletal traction, 1142
    tolerance, 238–239
Opioid dose-sparing effect, 234
Opioid-induced hyperalgesia (OIH), 239
Opioid methadone (Dolophine), 227
Opioid naïve, 234
    vs. opioid tolerant, 240t
Opioids, 2043, 2117
    in acute pancreatitis, 1442, 1443
    analgesic agents, 446t, 466
    anesthetic use of, 443
    to avoid, 241
    binding of, 227
    definition of, 225
    and respiratory depression, 241
    sedation induced by
    surgical issues, 428t
    titration of, 237
    use of, 237c
Opportunistic infections, 1025
    treatment of, 1041–1042, 1051
Opposition, 171c
Opsonization, 1010
Optical coherence tomography, 1882
Oral cancers, 1270–1272
    alcohol and tobacco use and, 1271
    clinical manifestations, 1271
    diagnostic evaluation, 1271
    HPV vaccine and, 1271
    medical management, 1271
    nursing management, 1271–1272
    pathophysiology, 1271
    risk factors for, 1270–1271
Oral cavity, 1264–1265
    abnormalities of, 1266t–1267t
    assessment of, 357
    dental plaque and caries, 1265, 1268
    and nursing management, 1272–1273
        continuing and transitional care, 1273
        food and fluid intake, 1272
        home care checklist, 1273c
        infection prevention, 1272–1273
        mouth care, 1272
        pain and discomfort reduction, 1272
        patient education, 1273, 1273c
        positive self-image, 1272
    periapical abscess, 1268–1269
    structures of, 1265f

Oral cholecystography, 1433
Oral contraceptives, 1671, 1672, 1681
    for endometriosis, 1705
    for polycystic ovary syndrome, 1703
Oral endotracheal intubation, 445f
Oral glucose tolerance test (OGTT), 1460
Oral hairy leukoplakia, 1266t
Oral health, 1264
    and chronic disease, 1268
Oral hygiene, 2098
Oral rehydration salts (ORS), 2145
Orbital cellulitis, 1910
Orbital fractures, 1903
Orbital trauma, 1902
Orbits
    benign tumors of, 1909
    malignant tumors of, 1909–1910
    surgeries, 1910–1911
Orchiectomy, 1752, 1770
Orchitis, 1752, 1778–1779
Oregon Death With Dignity Act, 390
Orexigenic, 1358, 1360
Organ of Corti, 1917
Orientation, definition of, 193, 212
Orlistat (Xenical), for obesity, 1362–1364,
    1364c, 1365t
Orogastric tube, 1243, 1244
Oropharyngeal candidiasis
    HIV infection and, 1039
Oropharyngeal/nasopharyngeal airway insertion,
    2163, 2164c
Ortho Evra, 1672
Orthopedic rehabilitation programs, 166
Orthopedic surgery, patient undergoing, 1144,
    1144c
    joint replacement, 1144–1145
    nursing interventions, 1145–1146
    nursing process, 1155–1157
    total hip arthroplasty, 1147–1154
    total knee arthroplasty, 1154–1155
Orthopnea, 480, 489, 583, 684, 818, 822
Orthoses, 175
Orthostatic hypotension, 172, 173, 467, 687,
    705, 2102, 2103
    older adult and, 198, 693
Orthotopic liver transplantation (OLT), 1377,
    1420
OSHA. See Occupational and Safety Health
    Administration
Osmolality, 253, 255, 255t, 1243, 1248, 1552,
    1561
Osmolarity, 255, 1552
OsmoPrep, 1239
Osmoreceptors, 257–258
Osmosis, 254f, 1567, 1589
Osmotic diuresis, 253, 1459
Osmotic pressure, 253, 844
Ossicles, 1917
Ossiculoplasty, 1915, 1929
Ossification, 1116
Osteitis deformans. See Paget disease
Osteoarthritic nodules, 1124
Osteoarthritis (OA), 1104–1106
    clinical manifestations, 1105
    joint space narrowing and osteophytes, 1104,
        1104f
    medical management, 1105
        exercise, 1105
        goals of management, 1105
        pharmacologic therapy, 1105

    surgical management, 1106
    nursing management, 1106
    pathophysiology, 1104–1105, 1105f
    primary (idiopathic), 1104
    risk factors for, 1105
    secondary, 1104
    x-rays, 1105
Osteoblasts, 1115
Osteochondroma, 1180
Osteoclasts, 1115
Osteocytes, 1115
Osteogenesis, 1116
Osteoid osteoma, 1180
Osteolysis, 1131, 1155
Osteomalacia, 1174–1175
    assessment and diagnostic findings, 1174–
        1175
    gerontologic considerations, 1174
    medical management, 1175
    pathophysiology, 1174
Osteomyelitis, 1131, 1138, 1156, 1176–1178
    acute, 1176
    assessment and diagnostic findings, 1176–
        1177
    causes of, 1176
    chronic, 1176–1177
    clinical manifestations, 1176
    contiguous-focus, 1176
    diabetic, 1176
    hematogenous, 1176
    medical management, 1177
        pharmacologic therapy, 1177
        surgical management, 1177
    nursing process, 1177–1178
    pathophysiology, 1176
    patient with, 1179c
    prevention, 1177
Osteon, 1115
Osteopenia, 1160, 1169
Osteophytes, 1104
Osteoporosis, 1160, 1169–1174
    assessment and diagnostic findings, 1171–
        1172
    associated with intake of calcium, 274
    gerontologic considerations, 1169
    medical management, 1172, 1173t
    nursing process, 1172–1174
    pathophysiology, 1170, 1170f
    prevention, 1169, 1169c
    primary, 1169
    risk factors, 1170–1171, 1171c
    risks in men, 1171c
    secondary, 1169
Osteoporotic vertebral fractures, 1160
Osteoprotegerin (OPG), 1117
Osteosarcoma, 1180
Osteotomy, 1131, 1147
Otalgia, 1915, 1926, 1929
Otitis externa. See External otitis
Otitis media, 2065
Otorrhea, 1915, 1927
Otosclerosis, 1915
    description of, 19315
    stapedectomy, 1931, 1932f
Otoscopic examination, 1917f, 1918–1919,
    1920f
Ototoxicity, 1937–1938
    substances, selected, 1937c
Outcome and Assessment Information Set
    (OASIS), 20

Ovarian cancer, 1712–1713
    and ascites, 1713
    assessment and diagnostic findings, 1712
    clinical manifestations, 1712
    epidemiology, 1712
    family history and, 1712
    nursing management, 1713
    pathophysiology, 1712
    pharmacologic therapy, 1713
    recurrence of, 1713
    risk factors, 1712
    staging of, 1713c
    surgical management, 1712–1713
Ovarian cysts, 1702–1703
Ovarian hyperstimulation syndrome (OHSS),
    1677–1678
Ovaries, 1650, 1653
Overflow incontinence, 1615, 1627
Overflow urinary incontinence, 185
Overweight, 1361, 1361t, 1462
Ovidrel, 1677c
Ovulation, 1650, 1653
Ovulation detection methods, 1674
Ovulation index, 1677
Ovulation, pharmacologically induced,
    1677–1678, 1677c
Oxalate stones, 1634
Oxaliplatin (Eloxatin), 343t, 344
Oxandrolone (Oxandrin), 1865
Oxycodone, 235, 240
    equianalgesic dose chart for, 238
Oxygen (O₂)
    operating room use of, 444t
    partial pressure of, 485–486, 486c
Oxygen administration devices, 513t
Oxygen administration methods, 512–515
Oxygen masks, 514f
Oxygen saturation
    description of, 480
    monitoring of, 503
Oxygen supplementation, in airway obstruction,
    2163
Oxygen therapy, 511–516, 645, 664
    for heart failure, 827
    for pulmonary edema, 834
Oxygen toxicity, 512
Oxygen transport, 483
    effects of pressure on, 486–487
Oxyhemoglobin, 905
Oxyhemoglobin dissociation curve, 487–488,
    487c
Oxymorphone, 240
    equianalgesic dose chart for, 238
Oxytocin, 1508

P
Pacemakers, in dysrhythmia, 739–744
    complications with, 742–744, 743c,
        743t
    design, 739–741
    dual-chamber pacing, 741
    elective replacement indicator, 740
    generator functions, 741–742
    single-chamber atrial pacing, 741
    spike, 741
    surveillance of, 744
    synchronized biventricular pacing, 742
    transcutaneous, 740f
    types of, 739–741
    VVI pacing, 741

Packed red blood cells (PRBCs), 914
Paclitaxel (Taxol), 343t
    for ovarian cancer, 1713
PACU. See Postanesthesia care unit
Paget disease, 1175–1176, 1719, 1722c,
        1731
    assessment and diagnostic findings, 1175
    clinical manifestations, 1175
    gerontologic considerations, 1176
    medical management, 1175–1176
    pathophysiology, 1175
Paget–Schroetter syndrome, 869
Pain, 2073
    acute, 224, 225
    assessment of, 230–233
    breakthrough, 226
    during cardiac surgery, 786
    categories of, 225–230
    chronic, 224, 225
    classification of, 227t
    definition of, 225
    effects of, 225, 226t
    end-of-life care, 403
    and fractures, 1189
    genitourinary, 1555–1556, 1556t
    location of, 230
    management of (See Pain management)
    modulation of, 228f, 229
    musculoskeletal, 1120–1121
    neuropathic, 226, 227t, 229–230
    nociceptive, 226–229, 227t
    patient reports of, 230, 230c
    perception of, 226
    in postanesthesia units, 459–460
    reassessment of, 233
    types of, 225–230
    unrelieved, 226t
PAINAD (Pain Assessment IN Advanced
        Dementia), 233
Pain Assessment IN Advanced Dementia. See
        PAINAD
Pain management
    in acute pancreatitis, 1442, 1443
    case study, 222
    dosing regimens, 234
    nonpharmacologic, 245, 246c
    nonpharmacologic measure, 466
    nursing implications, 247
    pharmacologic, 233–245
    plans of care, 247c
    postsurgical patients, 466, 467f
    preoperative, 429
    rehabilitation programs, 166
    responsibility for, 233
    sickle cell disease and, 940
    subcutaneous system, 467f
Palifermin (Kepavance), 357
Palindromic rheumatism, 1109
Palliation, definition of, 324, 334
Palliative care, 981c
    communication in, framework for, 398c
    definition of, 387, 390–391
    for dyspnea, 404c
    at the end of life, 390–392
    goal setting in, 400–401, 401c
    in hospital setting, 392
    interdisciplinary collaboration in, 391
    outpatient, 393
    in skilled nursing facilities, 392–393
Palliative sedation

    definition of, 387
    at the end of life, 407
Palmar flexion, 171c
Palmar-plantar erythrodysesthesia (PPE),
        1346
Palmer method, 1849
Palpation, 521
    deep, 73f
    definition of, 62
    light, 73f
    for tactile fremitus, 497f
    thoracic, 495–496
Palpitations, 680, 689
    apical impulse, 689f
Pamidronate (Aredia), 276, 997, 1770
Pancreas
    age-related changes, 1430
    anatomy of, 1429, 1429f
    disorders of, 1440–1454
        cancer of pancreas, 1450–1451
        hyperinsulinism, 1453
        pancreatic cysts, 1449–1450
        pancreatic islet tumors, 1453
        pancreatitis, 1440–1449
        tumors of head of pancreas, 1451–1453
        ulcerogenic tumors, 1453–1454
    endocrine, 1429
    exocrine, 1429
    function of, 1429, 1430
Pancreatic cancer, 1450–1451
    assessment and diagnostic findings, 1450
    clinical manifestations, 1450
    and diabetes, 1450
    incidence of, 1450
    medical management, 1450–1451
    nursing management, 1451, 1451c
    risk factors, 1450
    survival rate, 1450
Pancreatic cells, transplantation of, 1473
Pancreatic cysts, 1449–1450
    diagnosis of, 1449
    nursing management, 1449–1450
Pancreatic insufficiency, 1321t
Pancreatic islet tumors, 1453
Pancreatic necrosis, 1444
pancreaticoduodenectomy (Whipple procedure
        or resection), 1452, 1452f
Pancreaticojejunostomy, 1449
Pancreatitis
    acute, 1440–1441
        assessment and diagnostic findings,
            1442
        clinical manifestations, 1441–1442
        complications and management, 1444
        continuing and transitional care, 1445
        medical management, 1442–1443
        nursing care plan, 1446c–1448c
        nursing management, 1443–1444
        in older adults, 1441
        pathophysiology, 1441
        self-care, 1444–1445
    chronic, 1440, 1445
        assessment and diagnostic findings,
            1445
        clinical manifestations, 1445
        medical management, 1445, 1448–1449
        surgical management, 1449
    description of, 1428, 1440
    severity of, prediction of, 1441c
Pancuronium (Pavulon), 447t

Pancytopenia, 987
Panhypopituitarism, 1508
Panobinostat (Farydak), 996
Panretinal photocoagulation, for diabetic
    retinopathy, 1491
Pantoprazole (Protonix), 1442
    for gastritis, 1295t
    for GERD, 1284t
Papanicolaou (Pap) smear, 1661, 1663, 1707
Papaverine, 1759
Papilledema, 1876, 1882
Papule, 1798t
Paracentesis, for ascites, 1387
Paradoxical pulse. See Pulsus paradoxus
Paradoxical tuberculosis-associated immune
    reconstitution inflammatory syndrome
    (TB-IRIS), 1037
Paralysis, 2084
Paranasal sinuses, 481f, 482
Paraphimosis, 1784
Paraplegia, 1956, 2048
Parasympathetic nervous system, 1954
Parathormone (parathyroid hormone),
    1527
Parathyroidectomy, 1528
Parathyroid glands, 1527, 1527f
    functions, 256
    hyperparathyroidism, 1527–1529
    hypoparathyroidism, 1529–1530
    pathophysiology, 1527
Parathyroid hormone (PTH), 1116, 1170
    associated with hyperparathyroidism, 275
    functions, 256
    serum calcium level and, 273
Paravertebral anesthesia, 448
Parenteral fluid therapy, 288–293
    intravenous solutions, 288–293
    purpose of, 288
Parenteral nutrition (PN), 1243, 1256–1262
    administration methods, 1257
        central method, 1257
        implanted vascular access ports, 1259
        percutaneous central catheters, 1257–
            1258, 1258f
        peripherally inserted central catheters,
            1258
        peripheral method, 1257
        surgically placed central catheters, 1258
    complications of, 1259–1260, 1260t
    discontinuation of, 1259
    formulas, 1257
    goals of, 1256
    home care checklist, 1261c
    indications for, 1256, 1257t
    initiation of, 1257
    nursing process, 1259–1261
    older adult patients and, 1261, 1262t
Paresthesia, 1121, 1131, 1134
Paris, terrorist attacks in, 2193
Parkinson disease, 2104t
    nursing research profile, 2108c
    strategies for patient, 2107c
Paronychia, 1801
Parotitis, 1264, 1270
Paroxetine (Paxil), 241, 1096
    for depression, 207
Paroxysmal, 712
Paroxysmal atrial tachycardia (PAT), 728
Paroxysmal nocturnal dyspnea (PND), 684,
    818, 822

Paroxysmal supraventricular tachycardia
    (PSVT), 729
Partial rebreathing mask, 513, 514f
Partial thromboplastin time (PTT)
    reference range, 694t
Pasero Opioid-Induced Sedation Scale (POSS),
    243c
Passive dressings, skin, 1807
Passive external rewarming method, 2174. See
    also Hypothermia
Pastes, wound care, 1810
Patch, 1798t
Patch testing, 1074, 1804
Patellar reflex, 1963
Pathogen-associated molecular patterns
    (PAMPs), 1008
Patient, 5
    basic needs, 5
    as consumer of nursing and health care, 5
    emotional support to, 473
    hospitalized postoperative, 463–476
    in postanesthesia care unit, 456–463
    receiving in clinical unit, 463
    satisfaction with nursing care, 9
    surgical, 437–438
Patient-centered rehabilitation-focused care,
    166
Patient-controlled analgesia (PCA), 234–235,
    429, 466, 1155, 1306
Patient-controlled epidural analgesia (PCEA),
    429
Patient education
    activities of daily living, 169c
    diabetes, 1475–1477
    nursing process for, 52–55, 53c
    pain rating scale use, 231c
    teaching plan, 53–54
    wound care instructions, 471c
Patient Evaluation Conference System (PECS),
    167
Patient positioning
    perioperative injury, 452
    postoperative, 430c
    preventing musculoskeletal complications,
        171
Patient Protection and Affordable Care Act
    (PPACA), 8, 392, 394
Patient Self-Determination Act (PSDA), 34,
    219
Patient transport, to presurgical area, 433
Pay for performance, 8
PCEA. See Patient-controlled epidural
    analgesia
PD. See Peritoneal dialysis
PE. See Pulmonary embolism
Peak flow monitoring, 663c
Peau d'orange, breast, 1722c
Pectus carinatum, 495
Pectus excavatum, 495
Pediatric care, rehabilitation programs, 166
Pediatric, genetics referrals in, 133c
Pediculosis, 1820–1822
Pediculosis capitis, 1820
Pediculosis corporis, 1820
Pediculosis pubis, 1820
Pediculus humanus capitis, 1820
Pediculus humanus corporis, 1820
Pedigree, 119, 120f, 121f
    nursing research profile, 131c
Pegfilgrastim (Neulasta), 1742

Peginterferon alfa-2a (Pegasys), 1402
Peginterferon (Pegasys) and ribavirin, 1404
Pegloticase (Krystexxa), 1108
Pelvic belt, 1140
Pelvic diaphragm, 1652
Pelvic exenteration, 1686
    for cervical cancer, 1707c, 1708
Pelvic floor exercises (Kegel exercises), 187
Pelvic fracture
    signs and symptoms of, 1201
    stable, 1201–1202, 1201f
    unstable, 1202, 1202f
Pelvic inflammatory disease (PID), 1686,
    1695–1696, 2148
    causes of, 1695
    clinical manifestations, 1695
    complications, 1695–1696
    consequences, 1695
    home care checklist, 1696c
    medical management, 1696
    nursing management, 1696
    pathophysiology, 1695, 1695f
    patient education, 1696
Pelvic lymph node dissection (PLND), 1771
Pelvic muscle exercise (PME), 1625c, 1626
Pelvic organ prolapse, 1698–1700, 1698f
    clinical manifestations, 1699
    cystocele, 1698
    enterocele, 1698–1699
    medical management, 1699
        Kegel exercises, 1699, 1699c
        pessaries, 1699, 1699f
    procidentia, 1699
    rectocele, 1698
    risk factors, 1698
    surgical management, 1699–1700
Pelvic pain, chronic, 1705
Pelvic prolapse, 1558
Pelvis, 1201–1202, 1201f
Pembrolizumab (Keytruda), 1837
Pemoline (Cylert), 2075
Pemphigus vulgaris, 1827–1828
Penbutolol (Levatol), for hypertension,
    891t
Penetrating abdominal injuries, 2169
Penetrating keratoplasty, 1898
Penetrating trauma, 628–631
Penicillin
    for anthrax treatment, 2204
    penicillin G, 2067, 2147
    for urinary tract infections, 1619t
Penile cancer, 1784–1785
    assessment and diagnostic findings, 1784–
        1785
    clinical manifestations, 1784
    medical management, 1785
    prevention, 1785
    risk factors for, 1784
    types of, 1784
Penile implants, 1759–1760
Penis, 1753–1754
Penis transplant, 1760
Penrose drains, 469, 471f
Pentagon, damage to, 2193
Pentostatin (Nipent), 343t
Pentoxifylline (Trental), for claudication,
    859
Penumbra region, 2009, 2010
Peppermint oil, 1318
Pepsin, 1224, 1226

Peptic ulcer disease, 1296–1303
    assessment and diagnostic findings, 1298
    clinical manifestations, 1298
    continuing and transitional care, 1303
    follow-up care, 1301
    and gastric outlet obstruction, 1303
    hemorrhage from, 1302
    home care checklist, 1303c
    H. pylori infection and, 1297
    medical management, 1298
        dietary modification, 1299
        pharmacologic therapy, 1298–1299, 1299t
        smoking cessation, 1299
    NSAIDs use and, 1297
    nursing process, 1301–1303
        anxiety reduction, 1301–1302
        assessment, 1301
        complications management, 1302–1303
        diagnosis, 1301
        evaluation, 1303
        nursing interventions, 1301–1303
        nutritional status, 1302
        pain relief, 1301
        planning and goals, 1301
    in older adults, 1297, 1298
    pathophysiology, 1297–1298
    patient education, 1303
    perforation of peptic ulcer, 1302
    predisposing factors, 1297
    silent peptic ulcers, 1298
    silent peptic ulcers, 1298
    surgical management, 1299, 1300t–1301t
    Zollinger–Ellison syndrome and, 1297
Percussion
    definition of, 62
    sounds, 498t
    thorax, 497–498, 498f
Percutaneous balloon microcompression,
        2088
Percutaneous biliary drainage, 1418
Percutaneous cholecystostomy, 1437
Percutaneous coronary interventions (PCIs),
        681t, 686, 771–773
    complications of, 772, 772t
    coronary artery stent, 771–772
    definition of, 750
    postprocedure care, 772–773
    procedures, types of, 771–772
    PTCA, 771
Percutaneous endoscopic gastrostomy (PEG),
        372, 1243, 1252, 2107
Percutaneous needle biopsy, 507–508
Percutaneous transhepatic cholangiography
        (PTC), 1433–1434
    in pancreatic carcinoma, 1450
Percutaneous transluminal angioplasty (PTA), 852
Percutaneous transluminal coronary angioplasty
        (PTCA), 750, 771, 771f
Perforation, esophageal, 1282
Perianal pruritus, 1812–1813
Periapical abscess, 1264, 1268–1269
    acute, 1268
    blind dental abscess, 1268
    chronic, 1268
    clinical manifestations, 1268
    nursing management, 1268–1269
Pericardial effusion, 836–837
    assessment and diagnostic findings, 836
    clinical manifestations, 836
    medical management, 836–837
    pathophysiology, 836

Pericardial space, 673
Pericardiocentesis, 818, 836–837
Pericardiotomy, 818, 837
Pericarditis, 691, 699, 813–816, 1601
    assessments, 681
Pericardium, description, 673
Perilymph, 1915, 1924
Perimenopause, 1650, 1681
Perimetry testing, 1883
Perindopril (Aceon), for hypertension, 892t
Perineal prostatectomy, 1771, 1772t, 1773f
Perineal pruritus, 1662, 1812–1813
Perineorrhaphy, 1699
Perineum, 1651
Perineural anesthesia, 234
Periodontitis, 1264–1265, 1267t
Perioperative nursing, 418–419
    genetics of, 424c
    immediate interventions, 432–434
    interventions, 426–434
    outcomes, 418
    patient education, 426–431
    phases of, 419
    surgical classifications, 419
Perioperative period
    considerations, 419–422
    definition of, 418
    nursing activities, 420c
    timing of, 419
Periosteum, 1115–1116
Peripheral arterial disease (PAD). *See also*
        Arterial disorders; Atherosclerosis
    effects of smoking on walking and quality-of-
        life in, 856c
    foot and leg care in, 857, 857c
    nursing care plan, 854c–855c
    in older adults, 857
Peripheral arterial occlusive disease, 857–860,
        858f
    assessment and diagnostic findings, 858
    clinical manifestations, 857–858
    medical management, 858–860
        endovascular management, 859
        pharmacologic therapy, 859
        surgical management, 859–860
    nursing management, 860
Peripheral dual-energy x-ray absorptiometry
        (pDXA), 1127
Peripheral edema, 686
Peripheral immune response (PIR), 1016, 1016c
Peripherally generated pain, 227t
Peripherally inserted central catheters (PICCs),
        1243, 1258
Peripheral nerve disorders, 2089
Peripheral nerve function, assessing for, 1126,
        1126c
Peripheral nervous system, 1951–1954
Peripheral neuropathies, 998, 998t, 1493, 2089
    HIV infection and, 1040
Peripheral neurovascular dysfunction, 1126, 1126c
Peripheral parenteral nutrition (PPN), 1257. *See
        also* Parenteral nutrition (PN)
Peripheral sensitization, 230
Peripheral smear, manual examination of, 910
Peripheral vascular disease, diabetes and, 1489
Peripheral vascular resistance, 844
Periprosthetic fracture, 1202
Peristalsis, 1243, 1245
Peritoneal dialysis (PD), 1567, 1580, 1595–
        1601, 1595f
    acute intermittent, 1598

    approaches for, 1598–1599
    complications of, 1597
        bleeding, 1597
        hypertriglyceridemia, 1597–1598
        leakage of dialysate, 1597
        peritonitis, 1597
    continuous ambulatory, 1596, 1597f,
        1598–1599, 1599c
    continuous cycling, 1596, 1599
    in diabetes, 1492
    goals of, 1595
    home care checklist, 1600c
    nursing management
        continuing and transitional care,
            1600–1601
        patient education, 1600
        psychosocial needs, 1599
    procedure, 1596
        catheter insertion, 1596
        equipment preparation, 1596
        exchanges, 1596–1597
        patient preparation, 1596
    ultrafiltration in, 1596
Peritoneum, 1292, 1296
Peritonitis, 1311, 1322, 1567, 1596, 1645
    assessment and diagnostic findings, 1323
    bacterial infection and, 1322
    clinical manifestations, 1322–1323
    medical management, 1323
    nursing management, 1323
    pathophysiology, 1322
    primary, 1322
    secondary, 1322
    tertiary, 1322
Peritonsillar abscess, 564–565, 2163
Periurethral bulking, 1626
Pernicious anemia, 933, 1241
Per-oral endoscopic myotomy (POEM), 1279
Persistent vegetative state, 1972, 1973
Personal flotation device (PFD), 2174
Personalized genomic treatments, 128–129
Personalized health care, legal aspects, 130
Personalized medicine, 115t
Personal protective equipment (PPE), 2129,
        2136, 2179, 2193, 2201
Pertussis, 2152
Pes cavus, 1168
Pes planus, 1168
Pessaries, 1662, 1699, 1699f
PET. *See* Positron Emission Tomography
Petechiae, 947, 947f, 972, 1790, 1796, 1801,
        1801t
Peyronie's disease, 1785
Phacoemulsification, 1895
Phagocytic cells, 1006
Phagocytic immune response, 1007
Phagocytosis, 907, 981
Phakic intraocular lenses, 1899
Phantom limb pain, 1185, 1215
Pharmacogenetics, 114, 128
Pharmacogenomics, 128–129
Pharmacokinetics, aging and, 205–206, 206t
Pharmacologic therapy, 1933
    heart failure, 824–826, 824t
    for psoriasis, 1823–1826
Pharyngitis, 552, 560–562, 561f
Pharynx
    anatomy of, 481
    physical assessment, 493
Phase III PACU, 456
Phase II PACU, 456

Phase I PACU, 456

Phenazopyridine (Pyridium), for urinary tract infections, 1619t

Phendimetrazine (Bontril), for obesity, 1365t

Phenothiazines, 428t, 2173

Phenotype, 116

Phenoxybenzamine (Dibenzyline) for pheochromocytoma, 1533

Phentermine (Adipex-P, Fastin) for obesity, 1365t

Phentermine/topiramate-ER (Qsymia) for obesity, 1365t

Phentolamine (OraVerse), 1534, 1759

Phenytoin (Dilantin), 205, 1169, 2094

Pheochromocytoma, 1502, 1506, 1532–1534
    assessment and diagnostic findings, 1532–1533
    clinical manifestations, 1532
    hypertension and, 1532
    nursing management, 1534
    paroxysmal form of, 1532
    pharmacologic therapy, 1533
    surgical management, 1533–1534

Phimosis, 1752, 1784

Phlebitis, 292
    assessment of, 293c

Phlebostatic axis, 706, 706f, 709

Phlebotomy, 914, 915
    in polycythemia vera, 984–985, 984f

Phlegmasia cerulea dolens, 869

pH monitoring, 1240–1241

Phoenix Society for Burn Survivors, 1869

Phosphodiesterase type 5 (PDE-5) inhibitors
    for erectile dysfunction, 1757–1759, 1758t, 1759t

Phosphorus deficit, 1568t

Phosphorus imbalance, 279–281, 279t
    hyperphosphatemia, 280–281
    hypophosphatemia, 279–280

Photoaging, 1794

Photophobia, 1876, 1905, 1907, 2067

Photorefractive keratectomy (PRK), 1899

Phototherapeutic keratectomy (PTK), 1898

Phototherapy, for psoriasis, 1825

Physical abuse, 218

Physical activity
    in CAD, 755
    for cancer prevention, 331c

Physical examinations
    components of, 72–73
    considerations, 65–66
    definition of, 62
    learning readiness and, 52
    people with disabilities, 70c

Physical fitness
    definition of, 48
    health promotion and, 57

Physical Status Classification System, 439

Physician-assisted suicide, 390

Physician Orders for Life-Sustaining Treatment (POLST), 34, 397c

Physiologic dead space, 480, 483

PID. See Pelvic inflammatory disease

PIDDs. See Primary immune deficiency diseases

Pigeon chest, 495

Pigment stones, 1430. See also Cholelithiasis

PI3 kinase disease, 1024t

PillCam ESO, 1237

Pilocarpine, 1272

Pilonidal sinus or cyst, 1352, 1352f

Pindolol (Visken)
    for hypertension, 891t

Pioglitazone (Acto), 1408, 1475t

Pipe bomb, 2202

Pirbuterol (Maxair), 656

Pitting edema, 823, 823f

Pituitary adenomas, 2093

Pituitary gland, 1506–1510, 1507f
    anterior, 1507–1508
    diabetes insipidus, 1509–1510
    pathophysiology, 1508
    posterior, 1508
    SIADH, 1510
    tumors, 1508–1509

Pituitary portal blood system, 1507

Pituitary tumors, 1508–1509
    assessment and diagnostic findings, 1509
    basophilic tumors, 1508
    chromophobic tumors, 1508–1509
    clinical manifestations, 1508–1509
    eosinophilic tumors, 1508
    functional, 1508
    medical management, 1509
    nonfunctional, 1508
    surgical management, 1509

Pivot joints, 1118

PKD. See Polycystic kidney disease

Placebos
    definition of, 244
    use of, 33, 244–245

Planning, in nursing process, 36, 39
    expected outcomes, 39
    goals for nursing actions, 39–40, 40c
    nursing actions, 40, 41c
    setting priorities, 38

Plantar digital neuroma. See Morton neuroma

Plantar fasciitis, 1168

Plantar flexion, 171c, 1141

Plaques, 850, 1798t

Plasma, 903, 908

Plasma albumin, 914

Plasma pH, 283

Plasmapheresis, 913t, 1405, 2080

Plasma proteins, 908

Plasminogen, 908

Plasminogen activator tissue (tPA), 2015c, 2017

Plaster casts, 1132–1133

Plaster of Paris, 1131

Plastic surgery
    cosmetic, 1839–1840, 1841t
    reconstructive, 1839–1840
    skin grafts, 1839–1840, 1839f

Platelet-activating factor, 1059, 1059t

Platelet defects, 951, 952c

Plateletpheresis, 913t

Platelets, 903, 903t, 907

Platelets, reference range, 694t

Platform posturography, 1922

PLCG2-associated antibody deficiency and immune dysregulation (PLAID), 1024t

Pleura, 482

Pleural biopsy, 507

Pleural conditions, 606–619
    acute respiratory failure, 609–612
    empyema, 608–609
    pleural effusion, 607–608
    pleurisy, 606–607
    Pulmonary edema, 609
    Pulmonary embolism, 614–618
    Pulmonary hypertension, 613–614
    sarcoidosis, 618–619

Pleural effusion, 500t, 583, 607–608, 607f

Pleural friction rub, 583

Pleural space, 583

Pleurisy, 606–607

Plicamycin (Mithracin), 343t, 1176

PLISSIT model of sexual assessment, 1656

PLND. See Pelvic lymph node dissection

PMS. See Premenstrual syndrome

Pneumatic dilation, in achalasia, 1279, 1280f

Pneumoconiosis, 619–620, 620t

Pneumocystis pneumonia (PCP), 589
    HIV infection and, 1038, 1041

Pneumonectomy, 538c

Pneumonia, 587–598, 1143, 2054
    assessment, 590–591
    assessments, 681t
    classification, 587–589
    clinical manifestations, 590
    complications, 596
    diagnostic findings, 590–591
    gerontologic considerations, 596
    medical management, 592–596
    nursing process, 596–598
    pathophysiology, 589–590
    prevention, 592
    risk factors, 590

Pneumothorax, 500t, 510, 540, 583, 629–631, 646
    clinical manifestations, 630
    COPD patient, 638, 646
    medical management, 630–631
    nursing care, 652c
    types, 629–630

Podofilox (Condylox), for HPV infection, 1691

Podophyllin (Podofin, Podocon) for HPV infection, 1691

Poikilocytosis, 933

Poison Control Center, 2177

Poisoning
    carbon monoxide, 2179
    emergency treatment of, 2178
    food poisoning, 2180
    ingested (swallowed) poisons, 2178–2179
    skin contamination, 2179–2180

Polio, 2119

Polycystic kidney disease (PKD), 1574
    autosomal dominant, 1574
    autosomal recessive, 1574

Polycystic ovary syndrome (PCOS), 1686, 1703

Polycythemia, 636, 643, 944
    medical management, 945
    primary, 944
    secondary, 945

Polycythemia vera, 984–985
    assessment and diagnostic findings, 984
    clinical manifestations, 984
    complications, 984
    medical management, 984–985, 984f
    nursing management, 985
    phlebotomy in, 984–985, 984f
    symptoms associated with, 985t

Polydipsia, 1460

Polyethylene glycol (PEG), 1314t

Polymerase chain reaction (PCR), 2069

Polymethylmethacrylate (PMMA), 1145, 1172

Polymorphonuclear neutrophils (PMNs), 906

Polymyalgia rheumatica (PMR), 1103–1104

Polymyositis, 1102–1103

Polyphagia, 1460

Polypharmacy, 193
    adverse effects, 205
    definition of, 193
    drug interactions, 205, 216

Polyps of colon and rectum, 1349–1350
Polyurethane resins, 1132
Polyuria, 1460, 1556t, 1567
Pomalidomide (Pomalyst), 988
Popliteal artery aneurysms, 865
Population screening, 127
Portal hypertension, 1377, 1385. *See also* Ascites
    measurement, 1389–1390
Portosystemic encephalopathy. *See* Hepatic
    encephalopathy
Position (postural) sense, 1946, 1949
Positive chandelier sign, 1662
Positive end-expiratory pressure (PEEP), 510,
    2174
Positive feedback, 84, 92
Positron emission tomography (PET), 505, 700,
    1236, 2038
    cardiovascular, 700
    nervous system, 1967
POSS. *See* Pasero Opioid-Induced Sedation
    Scale
Postanesthesia care unit (PACU), 233, 418
    admission to, 457
    airway maintenance, 457–458, 459f
    Aldrete score form, 462f
    cardiovascular stability, maintenance of,
        458–459
    definition of, 456
    discharge from, 461–463
    function of, 419
    nausea and vomiting, control of, 460–461
    nursing management in, 457–461
    pain and anxiety, management of, 459–460
    patient assessments, 457
    phases of care in, 456–457
    record, 462f
    shock in, 459
Postcoital intrauterine device insertion, 1674
Posterior cruciate ligament (PCL), 1188
Post-exposure prophylaxis (PEP), 1029, 1030c
Postinfarction syndrome, 1575
Postmenopausal bleeding, 1681
Postnecrotic cirrhosis, 1406. *See also* Cirrhosis
Postoperative nausea and vomiting (PONV),
    242, 460–461
    aromatherapy for, 460c
    medications for, 460, 460t
    risk of, 461
Postoperative neurologic assessments, 2088
Postoperative nursing, immediate interventions,
    464c
Postoperative phase
    complication prevention, 430c
    complications, 473t
    definition of, 418
    hospitalized patients, 463–476
    nursing activities in, 420c
    timing of, 419
Post-polio syndrome (PPS), 2091
Postthrombotic syndrome, 873–874
Posttraumatic stress disorder (PTSD), 1868,
    2159, 2190
Postural drainage, 517, 518f
    chest physiotherapy, 645, 667
Postural hypotension, 467
    asesment, 687c
    cardiovascular disease, 687
    orthostatic, 687
Postural instability, 2102
Posture, assessment of, 1123, 1123f
Potassium

deficit, 1568t
    effect on electrocardiogram, 270f
    excess, 1568t
    intravenous, 270–271
Potassium chloride, 1596
Potassium imbalance, 268–272, 269t
    hyperkalemia, 271–272
    hypokalemia, 268–271
Potassium iodide (KI), 1521
    for hyperthyroidism, 1521t
Potassium-sparing diuretics for hypertension,
    890t
Powders, wound care, 1810
PPACA. *See* Patient Protection and Affordable
    Care Act
PP interval, 712, 716
Pramlintide (Symlin), for diabetes, 1473
Prasugrel (Effient), for angina, 758t, 760
Prazosin (Minipress), for hypertension, 891t
Preadmission testing (PAT), 418, 419
Prealbumin, serum
    nutritional status and, 180
Preanesthetic medication, 432
Precapillary sphincter, 842
Precision medicine, 7
    definition of, 324
    description of, 325
Precision Medicine Initiative (PMI), 7
Preconception/periconception health care,
    1678–1679, 1679c
Prediabetes, 1456, 1457
Predisposition testing, 127
Prednisolone, 1089t, 1541t
Prednisone (Apo-Prednisone, Deltasone,
    Orasone, Panasol, Winpred), 1089t,
    1541t, 1610t
Preexposure prophylaxis (PrEP), 1027
Pregabalin (Lyrica), 244
    for diabetic peripheral neuropathy, 1493
Pregnancy, genetics referrals in, 133c
Pregnyl, 1677c
Prehypertension, 885, 885t
Preload, 677
Premature atrial complex (PAC), 720, 722f
Premature ejaculation (PE), 1760
Premature junctional complex, 727
Premature ventricular complex (PVC), 729, 729f
Premenstrual dysphoric disorder (PMDD), 1666
Premenstrual syndrome (PMS), 1666
    clinical manifestations, 1666, 1667c
    medical management, 1666–1667
    nursing management, 1667
    pharmacologic treatments, 1667
Prenatal screening, 122
Preoperative assessments, 423–427
    alcohol (ethanol) use, 424–425
    cardiovascular system, 426
    dentition, 424
    drug use, 424–425
    endocrine function, 426
    hepatic function, 426
    immune function, 426
    nutrition status, 424
    psychosocial factors, 427–428
    respiratory function, 425–426
    thyrotoxicosis, 426
Preoperative education, 426–431
    for ambulatory surgery, 431
    for older adults, 431c
Preoperative phase
    checklist, 433f

definition of, 418
    expected outcomes, 434, 434c
    patient activities in, 434c
    records, 433
    timing of, 419
Presbycusis, 1924
    auditory changes, 202
    definition of, 193
Presbyopia, 193, 201
Pressure-reducing mattress, 1710
Pressure-relieving devices, 183
Pressure support ventilation (PSV), 510, 528
Pressure ulcers, 1134–1135, 2059
    areas susceptible to, 180f
    assessment of, 178, 181
    description of, 164, 178
    developmental stages, 182c
    diagnosis of, 181
    healing, promotion of, 184–185
    interventions, 181–185
    nutritional status and, 184
    prevention of recurrence, 185
    risk factors, 178–181, 178c, 179t
    stages of, 184–185
    treatment of, 185
Pressurized metered-dose inhaler (pMDI), 641f,
    647
    aerosol delivery devices, 641t
Presymptomatic testing, 127
Preventive ethics, 34
    ethical decision making, 35
    ethics committees, 34
    patient self-determination, 34
Priapism, 1752, 1759, 1785
    ischemic form, 1785
    nonischemic, 1785
    stuttering, 1785
PRICE, 1185, 1186
Primary aldosteronism, 1540–1541
    assessment and diagnostic findings, 1540
    clinical manifestations, 1540
    medical management, 1540–1541
    nursing management, 1541
Primary headache, 1972, 1973, 2004
Primary hypertension, 885. *See also*
    Hypertension
Primary immune deficiency diseases (PIDDs),
    1022
    assessment and diagnostic findings, 1023
    clinical manifestations, 1023, 1024t
    Ig replacement therapy at home, 1023, 1025c
    medical management, 1023
    nursing management, 1023–1024
    pathophysiology, 1023
    prevention, 1023
Primary injury, 2034
Primary liver tumors, 1417
Primary myelofibrosis, 987–988, 987f, 988t
Primary polycythemia. *See* Polycythemia vera
Primary prevention, 19
Primary survey, 2156, 2162
Primary thrombocythemia. *See* Essential
    thrombocythemia (ET)
PriMatrix, 876
PR interval, 712, 716
Prinzmetal's angina, 757c
Private health information (PHI), 33
PRK. *See* Photorefractive keratectomy
Probenecid (Benemid), 1108, 1109t
Probiotics, 1318
    for hepatic encephalopathy, 1408

Procainamide, for ventricular tachycardia, 730
Procaine (Novocaine), 448t
Procarbazine (Matulane), 343t
Prochlorperazine (Compazine), 460t
Procrit, 1145
Proctitis, 1350
Proctocolectomy with ileostomy, 1333
Proctoscopy, 1239–1240
Progesterone, 1650, 1653
Progesterone in oil, 1677c
Prognosis
    awareness of, 390
    definition of, 387
Programmed cell death. See Apoptosis
Progressive multifocal leukoencephalopathy
        (PML), 1040
Prolactin (PRL), 1507, 1508
Proliferative phase, menstrual cycle, 1650, 1653
Promethazine (Phenergan), 460t
Prometrium Crinone, 1677c
Prompted voiding, 1625c
Pronation, 171c
Propafenone (Rythmol), for atrial fibrillation,
        724
Prophylactic vaccines, 354
Propofol (Diprivan), 447t, 2038
proportional assist ventilation (PAV), 511, 528
Propoxyphene (Darvon), 241
Propranolol (Inderal)
    for hypertension, 891t
    for hyperthyroidism, 1521t, 1522
    for variceal bleeding, 1390
Propranolol long acting (Inderal LA)
    for hypertension, 891t
Proprioceptors, 488
Proprotein convertase subtilisin-kexin type 9
        (PCSK9), 755
Proptosis, 1876, 1902, 1909
Propylthiouracil (PTU), for hyperthyroidism,
        1521, 1521t
Prostaglandin inhibitors, in diabetes insipidus,
        1510
Prostaglandins, 226, 1059, 1059t
Prostanoids, 655
Prostate cancer, 1764–1771. See also Prostate
        surgery
    assessment and diagnostic findings, 1764–
        1765
    clinical manifestations, 1764
    familial predisposition to, 1764
    nursing care plan, 1766c–1769c
    risk factors for, 1764
    treatment for, 1765
        chemotherapy, 1770
        hormonal strategies, 1770
        other therapies, 1770–1771
        radiation therapy, 1765, 1769–1770
        surgical management, 1765
Prostatectomy, 1752, 1764
    and catheter problems, 1776–1777
    and hemorrhage, 1775–1776
    home care checklist, 1778c
    infection after, 1776
    laparoscopic radical, 1771, 1772t
    nursing process, 1774–1778
        anxiety reduction, 1774
        assessment, 1774
        complications management, 1775–1777
        diagnosis, 1774
        discomfort, reducing of, 1774–1775
        evaluation, 1778

    fluid balance, 1775
    pain relief, 1775
    patient education, 1775, 1777
    patient preparation, 1775
    planning and goals, 1774
    postoperative nursing interventions,
        1775–1778
    preoperative nursing interventions,
        1774–1775
    perineal, 1771, 1772t, 1773f
    retropubic, 1771, 1772t, 1773f
    sexual dysfunction after, 1777
    suprapubic, 1771, 1772t, 1773f
    and urinary incontinence, 1777
    and venous thromboembolism, 1776
Prostate gland, 1754
    biopsy of, 1756
Prostate-specific antigen (PSA), 1752, 1756
Prostate surgery, 1771
    complications, 1771
    nursing pocess, 1774–1778
    procedures, 1771, 1772t–1773t
        laparoscopic radical prostatectomy, 1771
        perineal prostatectomy, 1771, 1773f
        retropubic prostatectomy, 1771, 1773f
        suprapubic prostatectomy, 1771, 1773f
        transurethral incision of the prostate,
            1771, 1773f
        transurethral resection of prostate, 1771,
            1773f
Prostatic stents, 1764
Prostatitis, 1615, 1752, 1761–1762
    clinical manifestations, 1762
    medical management, 1762
    nursing management, 1762
    patient education, 1762
    types of, 1762
Prostheses, 175
Protamine sulfate, 963
Protease inhibitors, 1034t–1035t
Proteasome inhibitors, 996
Protein
    deficit, 1568t
    in diabetic diet, 1463
    hormones, 1504
    metabolism, role of liver in, 1379
    wound healing and, 425t
Protein C deficiency, 961–962
Protein S deficiency, 962
Proteinuria, 1548, 1551, 1556t, 1561, 1573
Proteus vulgaris, wound infections, 474
Prothrombin time (PT), 910
    reference range, 694t
Proton-pump inhibitors (PPIs)
    for esophageal spasm, 1280
Proton therapy, 339
Provider in triage (PIT), 2161
Provirus, 1031
Provocative testing, 1064
Proximal interphalangeal (PIP) joint, 1105
Pruritus, 242, 985
    definition of, 1806, 1811
    general, 1811–1812, 1811c
    liver dysfunction and, 1397
    at night, 1821
    perianal, 1812–1813
    perineal, 1812–1813
    post-burn, 1866
6 Ps, 1134
Pseudoaddiction, 239
Pseudobulbar affect, older adults with, 215

Pseudocysts, 1449, 1704. See also Pancreatic
        cysts
Pseudoephedrine sulfate (Sudafed)
    for stress incontinence, 1626
Pseudohyperkalemia, 271
Pseudomonas aeruginosa, 2130
    wound infections, 474
Pseudothrombocytopenia, 949
Psoriasis, 1823–1826, 1824f
    home care checklist, 1826
    management of, 1824–1826
Psoriatic arthritis, 1106–1107
Psychiatric emergencies
    patients who are overactive, 2190
    patients who are suicidal, 2190–2191
    posttraumatic stress disorder, 2190
Psychiatric nurse clinician, 2113
Psychodermatosis, 1812
Psychoneuroimmunology, 89
Psychosocial assessment, 133, 133c
    preoperative, 427–428
Psychosocial interventions, 431–432
Psychotherapy, for depression, 207
Psyllium (Metamucil), 1314t, 1316
PTCA. See Percutaneous transluminal coronary
        angioplasty
PTK. See Phototherapeutic keratectomy
Ptosis, 1876, 1880, 1886
PTSD. See Posttraumatic stress disorder
Pubic hair, 1801–1802
Public health nursing, 18
Pulmonary agents, 2208
Pulmonary angiography, 505
Pulmonary artery (PA) catheter, 706, 707f,
        708f
Pulmonary artery pressure monitoring, 707
Pulmonary contusion, 628
Pulmonary diffusion, 480, 484–485
Pulmonary disorders, assessments, 681t
Pulmonary edema, 500t, 583, 609, 818,
        833–834
    assessment and diagnostic findings, 834
    burn injuries and, 1867
    clinical manifestations, 834
    flash, 833
    medical management, 834
    nursing management, 834
    pathophysiology, 833–834
    prevention, 834
Pulmonary embolism (PE), 583, 614–618,
        835–836, 1979. See also Venous
        thromboembolism (VTE)
    assessment, 681t
Pulmonary function tests (PFTs), 502, 502t
Pulmonary hypertension, 613–614, 613c
    and heart failure, 819
    sickle cell disease and, 936–937
Pulmonary perfusion, 480, 484–485
Pulmonary rehabilitation, 166
Pulmonary tuberculosis, 600–605
    assessment, 601–602
    clinical manifestations, 601
    diagnostic findings, 601–602
    gerontologic considerations, 602
    medical management, 602–604
    medications, 603t
    nursing management, 604–605
    pathophysiology, 600–601
    risk factors, 600, 600c
    transmission, 600
Pulmonary vascular resistance, 678

Pulmonic area, 689
Pulmonic valve, 791
  anatomy of, 792, 792f
Pulse amplitude, 688
Pulse deficits, 688
Pulseless electrical activity (PEA), 818, 837
Pulse oximetry, 503, 503f
Pulse pressure, 687
  analysis, 709
  postural (orthostatic), 687
PULSES profile, 167
Pulsus paradoxus, 818, 836, 1601
Punctum plugs, 1101
Purkinje cells, 676, 676f
Purulent, 583
Pustule, 1798t
PUVA, 1825, 1826
P vera. See Polycythemia vera
P wave, 712, 715
Pyelonephritis, 1615, 1621–1622
  acute, 1622
  chronic, 1622
Pyloric obstruction, 1294
Pyloroplasty, 1292, 1299
Pylorus, 1292, 1294
Pylorus-preserving pancreaticojejunostomy
  (PPPD), 1452
Pyodermas, 1806, 1816
Pyogenic liver abscesses, 1425
Pyridostigmine bromide (Mestinon), 2080
Pyridoxine deficiency, 1397
Pyrosis, 1264, 1279, 1292, 1293
Pyuria, 1548, 1561, 1615, 1618

Q
QRS complex, 712, 715–716, 737
QT interval, 712, 716
Quadriceps muscles
  strengthening of, 172
Quadriplegia, 2048
  ulcer prevention in, 184
Quality and Safety Education for Nurses
  (QSEN), 11
  definition of safety and associated KSAs, 11,
    11t
Quality of life among women, with acne
  vulgaris, 1817c
Quality of life, effect of pain and, 232
QuantiFERON-TB Gold (QFT-G) test, 2153
Quantitative computed tomography (QCT), 1127
Quantitative ultrasound (QUS), 1127
Quetiapine (Seroquel), 407
Quick SOFA (qSOFA) scale, 317
Quinapril (Accupril), for hypertension, 892t

R
RA. See Rheumatoid arthritis
Rabeprazole (AcipHex)
  for gastritis, 1295t
  for GERD, 1284t
Race/ethnicity, 428
  pulmonary health and, 492c
Radial head fractures, 1200
Radial shaft fracture, 1200
Radiation, 1793
  dosage, 329
  external, 339
  internal, 339–340
  ionizing (See Ionizing radiation)
  skin integrity impaired by, 370

Radiation therapy, 1716, 2096
  administration of, 339–340
  for bladder cancer, 1639
  for breast cancer, 1740–1741
  cancer management and, 338–341
  carcinogenesis and, 328–329
  definition of, 324
  dosage, 339
  external, 1716
  for gastric cancer, 1305–1306
  internal, 1716–1717, 1716f
  intraoperative, 1716
  late effects of, 341
  for liver tumors, 1418
  nursing management, 341
  for penile cancer, 1785
  protecting caregivers, 341
  safety considerations, 1717
  side effects of, 340–341
  for testicular cancer, 1781
  for thyroid cancer, 1525
  toxicity associated with, 340–341
  for vaginal cancers, 1711–1712
Radical cystectomy, 1638
Radical hysterectomy, for cervical cancer, 1707c
Radical prostatectomy, for prostate cancer, 1765
Radical trachelectomy, for cervical cancer, 1707c
Radical vaginal hysterectomy, for cervical
  cancer, 1707c
Radiculopathy, 1160, 1161
Radioactive iodine therapy
  for hyperthyroidism, 1519–1520
  for thyroid cancer, 1525
Radioactive iodine uptake test, 1513
Radiocontrast-induced nephropathy (CIN), 1579
Radioimmunoassays, 1506
Radiologic weapon, 2193, 2209
Radiopaque, 1243, 1244
Radiosensitive tumor, 339
Raltegravir (RAL), 1035t
Ramipril (Altace), for hypertension, 892t
Ramucirumab, 1305
Range of motion (ROM), 1186
  active exercises, 171, 172t
  assisted exercises, 171, 172, 172t
  isometric exercises, 172t
  passive exercises, 171, 172, 172t
  performance of exercises, 171–172
  resistive exercises, 172t
  terminology, 171c
Ranitidine (Zantac), 1059, 1442
  for gastritis, 1295t
  for GERD, 1284t
Rape, 2188
  trauma syndrome, 2188
Rapid cycle testing model, 9, 10c
Rasburicase (Elitek), 973
Raynaud phenomenon, 867–868
Raynaud's phenomenon, 1094, 1101, 1102
R-CHOP, 992
Reactive arthritis, 1106
Real-time communication, 7
Rebound hypertension, 896
Recent Life Changes Questionnaire (RLCQ), 86
Receptive aphasia, 2011
Receptor for activated nuclear factor-kappa B
  ligand (RANKL), 1117
Recombinant deoxyribonucleic acid (DNA)
  technology, 1013
Recombinant factor VIIa (Novoseven, Novo
  Nordixk), 953

Recombination, 117
Recombivax HB, 1402
Rectocele, 1558, 1650, 1661, 1686, 1698, 1698f
Recurrent abortion, 1675
Red blood cell production, regulation of, 1553
Red blood cells (RBCs), 903, 903t, 905–906,
    905f, 982
  destruction, 906
Red man syndrome. See Generalized exfoliative
    dermatitis
Reduction mammoplasty, 1749
Reed-Sternberg cells, 989, 989f
Referral, 375
  to cancer patient for home care, 379
Reflexes
  assessment of, 1963f
  documentation of, 1962c
  examination of, 1962–1964
  pathologic, 1964
  superficial, 1964
Reflex hammer, 1962
Reflex (neurogenic) incontinence, 185
Refraction
  definition, 1876
  errors, 1883–1886, 1883f
Refractive surgeries, 1899–1900
Refractometer, 1561
Refusal to care, 34
Regadenoson (Lexiscan), 699, 700
Regional enteritis. See Crohn's disease
Registered nurse, 11
Registered nurse first assistants (RFNAs), 436,
    439
Registered Nurses' Roles and Responsibilities in
    Providing Expert Care and Counseling at
    the End of Life, 390
Regular insulin, 1468, 1485
Regurgitation
  aortic, 794–795
  definition of, 792
  mitral, 793–794
Rehabilitation, 164–191
  burn injury, 1868, 1868t
  cardiac, 166
  continuing care and, 190
  definition of, 164
  home care education, 189c–190c
  impaired mobility, patient with, 170–178
  patient-centered, 166
  patient outcomes, 170
  pressure ulcers, patient with, 178–186
  self-care and, 166
  specialization, 166
  substance abuse issues, 167
  teams, 165–166, 165c
Rehospitalization, 12
Reinforcement, 48
Reiter's syndrome. See Reactive arthritis
Relaxation techniques, 97
  Benson relaxation response, 98, 98c
  guided imagery, 98
Religious beliefs
  on death and dying, 396t–397t
  end-of-life care and, 388
  respect for, 431
Remifentanil (Ultiva), 446t
Remission, 1082
Remodeling, bone, 1116–1117
Remorse, emergency care and, 2159
Renal angiography, 1564
Renal artery embolization, 1575

Renal cancer, 1574–1576
   assessment and diagnostic findings, 1575
   clinical manifestations, 1575
   incidence of, 1574
   nursing management, 1575–1576
   patient education, 1576
   pharmacologic therapy, 1575
   risk factors, 1575c
   surgical management
      nephrectomy, 1575
      renal artery embolization, 1575
Renal clearance, 1548, 1553
Renal function
   age-related changes
      preoperative assessments, 426
Renal function tests, 1562, 1562t
Renal glycosuria, 1548, 1551
Renal osteodystrophy, 1583
Renal replacement therapies, 1589
   continuous renal replacement therapies,
      1594, 1595f
   continuous venovenous hemodialysis, 1595
   continuous venovenous hemofiltration,
      1594
   hemodialysis, 1589–1594
   kidney transplantation, 1595
   peritoneal dialysis, 1595–1601
Renal rickets, 1527
Renal trauma, 1612–1613
   blunt, 1612
   clinical manifestations, 1612
   hematuria and, 1612
   medical management, 1613
   nursing management, 1613
   penetrating, 1612
   surgical management, 1613
Renin, 256, 1550
Renin–angiotensin–aldosterone system, 256
Repaglinide (Prandin), 1474t
Repolarization, 712, 713
Reproductive life plan (RLP), 1669
Reproductive system
   age-related changes, 197t, 198–199
   chemotherapy-related effects, 346
Reservoir, 2125
Residual urine, 1615, 1624, 1627
Resistance (strength) training, 1465
Resorption, bone, 1116
Resource Model of Preventive Health Behavior,
   56
Respiration
   description of, 480
   function of, 483–484
   patterns of, 495, 496t
   rates and depths of, 495, 496t
   resting, 488
Respiratory care, modalities, 510–550
Respiratory depression, 450
   opioid-induced, 242
   opioids and, 241
   sedation and, 242–243
Respiratory disorders
   assessment findings, 500t
   genetics and, 491c
   risk factors, 491c
   symptoms of, 488–491
Respiratory distress, 2082
Respiratory excursion, 495, 497f
Respiratory failure, 2054
Respiratory function, preoperative assessments,
   425–426

Respiratory infections, 586–606
   acute tracheobronchitis, 586–587
   aspiration, 599–600
   lung abscess, 605–606
   pneumonia, 587–598
   Pulmonary tuberculosis, 600–605
Respiratory system
   age-related changes, 197t, 198
   age-related changes in, 488, 489t
   anatomy of, 480–483
      lower respiratory tract, 482–483
      upper respiratory tract, 481–482
   diagnostic evaluation, 502–508
   function of, 483–488
   physical assessment of, 492–500
      lower respiratory structures, 493–500
      patient appearance, 492
      upper respiratory structures, 492–493
   postsurgical complications, 465–466, 473t
   psychosocial factors, 491c
Respiratory weaning, 511, 535–537
Rest pain, 841, 846
Restraints, use of, 33
Restricted zones, 436, 440
Restrictive cardiomyopathy (RCM), 802
Restrictive lung disease, 583, 609
Retapamulin (Altabax), in impetigo, 1817–1818
Reteplase (Retavase), 866
   for venous thromboembolism, 870t
Rete ridges, 1790, 1791
Reticulocytes, 905–906, 935
Reticuloendothelial cells, 1378
Reticuloendothelial system (RES), 903, 908
Retina
   age-related changes, 1902f
   anatomy, 1878–1879
   detachment, 1900–1901
   vascular disorders, 1901
Retinitis, CMV-related, 1912
Retinoids, 1815
Retinopathy, 1456, 1461
Retraction signs, breast, 1722c
Retrograde ejaculation, 1752, 1760
Retrograde pyelography, 1564
Retroperitoneal lymph node dissection
   (RPLND), 1781
Retropubic prostatectomy, 1771, 1772t, 1773f
Retrovirus, 1030
Reverse transcriptase, 1030
Reverse transcriptase–polymerase chain reaction
   (RT-PCR), 1033
Reverse Trendelenburg position, 452, 453f
Rhabdomyolysis, 2156, 2171
Rh antigen, 916
Rheumatic diseases, 1082
   assessment, 1084, 1085c
   exacerbation, 1082
   exercise to promote mobility, 1090t
   laboratory studies, 1084, 1086t
   medical management, 1084
      exercise and activity, 1087
      goals and strategies, 1087t
      nonpharmacologic pain management,
         1084
      pharmacologic therapy, 1084, 1088t–1089t
      sleep, 1087
   nursing care plan, 1091c–1093c
   older adults and, 1087, 1090
   pathophysiology, 1083–1084, 1083f
      autoimmunity, 1083
      clinical manifestations, 1084

      degeneration, 1083–1084
      inflammation, 1083
   remission, 1082
Rheumatic fever, 809–810, 810c
Rheumatoid arthritis (RA), 1093–1098
   assessment and diagnostic findings, 1094–1095
   clinical manifestations, 1094
   home care checklist, 1097c
   medical management, 1095
      advanced, unremitting RA, 1095–1096
      early RA, 1095
      moderate, erosive RA, 1095
      nutrition therapy, 1096
      persistent, erosive RA, 1095
   nodules of, 1124
   nursing management, 1096–1098
   pathophysiology, 1093–1094
   patient education, 1096–1097
   risk factors for, 1093
Rheumatoid cachexia, 1096
Rheumatoid factor, 1094
Rheumatoid nodules, 1094
Rhinitis, 552, 553–555, 554f
   viral, 555–556
Rhinitis medicamentosa, 552, 1073
Rhinorrhea, 552, 1915, 1927
Rhinosinusitis, 552, 554f, 556–560
   causes, 554t
Rho(D) immune globulin (RhoGAM), 1675
Rhonchi, 480, 490
Rhytidectomy, 1841
Ribavirin (Rebetol), 1403
Rib fractures, 1211–1212
Riboflavin deficiency, 1397
Rifaximin (Xifaxan), 1318
   in hepatic encephalopathy, 1395
Right-sided heart failure, 818, 821, 822–823,
      844. See also Heart failure (HF)
Right ventricular failure. See Right-sided heart
      failure
Rigid bronchoscope, 506
Rilpivirine (RPV), 1034t
Riluzole (Rilutek), 2111
Ringworm. See Tinea
Rinne test, 1920–1921, 1920f, 1921t
Risperidone (Risperdal), 407
Ritonavir (RTV), 1035t
Rituximab (Rituxan), 344, 353, 1089t
   for bullous pemphigoid, 1828
   for pemphigus vulgaris, 1828
Rivaroxaban (Xarelto), 683, 965
   for venous thromboembolism, 870t
RLCQ. See Recent Life Changes Questionnaire
Robert Wood Johnson Foundation (RWJF), 11
Robot-assisted technology, 442
   for cervical cancer, 1707
Robotic-assisted laparoscopic radical
      prostatectomy, 1771, 1773t
Rocky Mountain spotted fever, 2177
Rocuronium (Zemuron), 446t
Romberg test, 1961
Romiplostim (Nplate), 950, 982
Ropivacaine (Naropin), 234
Rosiglitazone (Avandia), 1408, 1475t
Rotary chair. See Sinusoidal harmonic acceleration
Rotation, 171c
Rotator cuff tears, 1187
Rotor syndrome, 1385
Round ligaments, 1652
Routes of administration, 233–234
Roux-en-Y gastric bypass (RYGB), 1369

Roux-en-Y hepaticojejunostomy, 1421, 1422f
Rovsing sign, 1324, 1324f
RR interval, 712, 716
Rubber band ligation procedure, 1352
Rubor, 841, 846
Rule of nines, 1848, 1849f
Rules of wounds care, 1807
Ruxolitinib (Jakafi), 988

S
S-1 (oral fluoropyrimidine), 1451
Sacral edema, 823
Sacral nerve stimulation, 1317
Saddle joints, 1117
Safety
    maintenance of, 432
    National Patient Safety Goals, 432c
    during patient transfer, 173
    protection from injury, 452–454
Salem Sump tube, 1244, 1245f
Salicylates, in rheumatic diseases, 1088t
Saline implants, for augmentation
        mammoplasty, 1749
Salivary calculus. *See* Sialolithiasis
Salivary glands, disorders of, 1269–1270
    neoplasms, 1270
    parotitis, 1270
    salivary calculi, 1270
    sialadenitis, 1270
Salmeterol (Serevent Diskus), 642t, 658t, 660,
        667
Salmonella typhi, 2144
    caused diarrhea, 2144
    infection, 2138, 2144
Salpingectomy, 1680
Salpingitis, 1686, 1695
Salpingo-oophorectomy, 1680, 1686, 1705
Salvage surgery, 336
Saquinavir (SQV), 1035t
Sarcoidosis, 618–619, 1109
Sarcomas, classification of, 328t
Sarcoplasmic reticulum, 1118
Sarcoptes scabei, 1822
Sargramostim (Leukine), 973
Sarin, 2207
Satiety, 1358, 1360
Saturated solution of potassium iodide (SSKI)
        for hyperthyroidism, 1521t
Saxagliptin (Onglyza), 1475t
SBP. *See* Spontaneous bacterial peritonitis
SBRT. *See* Stereotactic body radiotherapy
Scabies, 1822–1823
Scales, 1799t
Scaling. *See* Lichenification
Scalp injuries, 2034–2035
Scarring, prevention of, 1816
Scars, 1799t
    burn injuries and, 1869
        prevention of, 1869
        treatment of, 1869
SCC. *See* Squamous cell carcinoma
SCD. *See* Sickle cell disease
Schilling test, 934
School health programs, 25
School nurses, 25
Schwann cells, 2082
Sciatica, 1160, 1161, 2117
Scintigraphy, 1236
SCIP. *See* Surgical Care Improvement Project
Scleral buckle, 1900, 1901

Scleroderma, 1101–1102
    assessment and diagnostic findings, 1102
    clinical manifestations, 1102
    localized, 1101
    nursing management, 1102
    pathophysiology, 1102
    pharmacologic therapy, 1102
    systemic, 1101
Sclerotherapy, 1352, 1377, 1390
Scoliosis, 1123, 1123f
Scope and Standards of Practice (ANA), 48
Scopolamine (Transderm Scop), 460t
    secretion management and, 409t
Scotomas, 1876, 1883
Screenings, brief interventions, and referral to
        treatment (SBIRT), 2185
Scrub role, 436, 438
Seasonal allergic rhinitis. *See* Allergic rhinitis
Sebaceous glands, 1790, 1792
Seborrhea, 1813
Seborrheic dermatoses, 1813–1814
    clinical manifestations of, 1813
    medical management of, 1814
    nursing management of, 1814
Seborrheic keratoses, 1833
Sebum, 1790, 1792, 1813
Secondary headache, 1973, 2004
Secondary health conditions, 151, 151c
Secondary hypertension, 885
Secondary injury, 2034
Secondary prevention, 19
Secondary survey, 2156, 2162
Secondary thrombocytosis, 948
Second-degree burns, 1847t, 1848
Second-intention healing
    definition of, 456
    mechanisms of, 468c
    postsurgical, 468
Secretin, 1428, 1429
Secretory disorders, 1813–1816
    acne vulgaris, 1814–1816
    hidradenitis suppurativa, 1813
    seborrheic dermatoses, 1813–1814
Secretory phase, menstrual cycle, 1650, 1653
Sedation
    assessment of, 242
    informed consent, 422–423
    moderate, 436, 448–449
    opioid-induced, 243c
    and respiratory depression, 242–243
    unwanted, 242
Segmentation contractions, 1227
Segmentectomy, 538c
Segmented bronchial drainage. *See* Postural
        drainage
Segmented neutrophils (segs), 906
Seizure disorders, 1996–1997
Seizures, 274, 274f, 1957
    assessment, 1997
    brain tumors and, 2091
    classification of, 1996c
    definition of, 1946, 1972
    manifestations, 1996–1997
    nursing management, 1997, 1998c
    pathophysiology, 1996
Selective estrogen receptor modulator (SERM),
        1743, 1744t
Selective serotonin reuptake inhibitors (SSRIs),
        241
    in general pruritus, 1812

Self-care
    activities, 644
    clothing adaptations, 168
    deficits, 168–170
    fostering of, 168–169
    rehabilitation and, 166
Self-catheterization, 187, 1631–1632
Self-concept, 62
Self-contained breathing apparatus (SCBA),
        2201
Self-monitoring of blood glucose (SMBG),
        1456, 1466, 1468
    candidates for, 1467
    frequency of, 1467
    insulin therapy and, 1468
    results and dosage adjustments, 1467
Self-reports, 230
Self-responsibility, 48, 57
Semen analysis, 1677
Semen cryopreservation, 1784
Semilunar valves, 675
Seminal vesicle, 1753
Semirestricted zones, 436, 440
Semirigid rod, 1759
Senna (Senokot), 1314t
Sensations, altered, 1121
Sensorimotor polyneuropathy. *See* Peripheral
        neuropathy
Sensorineural hearing loss, 1915, 1923
Sensory perception
    impaired, 180
    improvement of, 183
    pressure ulcer and, 179t
Sensory system
    age-related changes, 197t, 201–202
    examination of, 1961–1962
    function of, 1956–1957
Sentinel event, 2156, 2158
Sentinel lymph node, 1719, 1734
Sentinel lymph node biopsy (SLNB), 335, 1734
    axillary lymph node dissection and, 1734t
    nursing management, 1734
Sepsis, 296, 2062
    burn injuries and, 1867–1868
    postsurgical, 473–474
Sepsis-Related Organ Failure Assessment Score,
        317, 317t
Septic (infectious) arthritis, 1178–1179
    assessment and diagnostic findings, 1178–
        1179
    clinical manifestations, 1178
    medical management, 1179
    nursing management, 1179
Septic meningitis, 2065
Septic shock, 296, 313–318
    fluid replacement in, 316
    medical management, 315–316
    Modified Early Warning System for, 317, 318t
    nursing management, 316–318
    nutritional therapy in, 316
    pathophysiology of, 314–315
    risk factors, 314c
Sequential compression devices (SCDs), 1710
Sequential Organ Failure Assessment (SOFA)
        score, 317, 317t
Sequestrectomy, 1177
Sequestrum, 1160, 1176
Seroma, 1738
Serosa, 1292
Serotonin, 1060

Serotonin and norepinephrine reuptake inhibitors (SNRI), 244
Serous otitis media, 1928
SERs. *See* Somatosensory evoked responses
Sertoli cell tumors, 1780
Sertraline (Zoloft), 1096
   in general pruritus, 1812
Sevelamer hydrochloride (Renagel), 1583
Severe combined immune deficiency (SCID), 1024t
Sevoflurane (Ultane), 444t
Sex hormones, effects on bone remodeling, 1116–1117
Sexual abuse, in childhood, 1657–1658
Sexual assault
   assessment and diagnostic findings, 2188
   management, 2188–2189
      physical examination, 2188–2189
      specimen collection, 2189
      treating potential consequences of rape, 2189
Sexual assault nurse examiner (SANE), 2188
Sexual dysfunction, 684
Sexual education, 2061
Sexual function, aging and, 198–199
Sexual history, 1656–1657
Sexually transmitted disease (STD), 2189
Sexually Transmitted Diseases Treatment Guidelines, 2129
Sexually transmitted infections (STIs), 1016, 1761, 2146t, 2189
   nursing process, 2148c
Shear
   pressure ulcers and, 179t, 180, 181f
   reduction of, 184
Shiga toxin–producing *Escherichia coli* (STEC), 2144
Shingles. *See* Herpes zoster
Shock, 2068
   burn injuries and, 1850
   cardiogenic, 310–313
   clinical findings in, 299t
   clinical manifestations, 299, 301–302
      cardiovascular effects, 302
      hepatic effects, 302
      neurologic effects, 302
      renal effects, 302
      respiratory effects, 301–302
   compensatory mechanisms, 298f
   description of, 296
   distributive, 313–319
   fluid replacement in, 304–305
   general management, 304–307
   hypovolemic, 308–310
   medical management, 299, 302, 304
   multiple organ dysfunction syndrome and, 319–320
   nursing management, 299–301, 302–303, 304
   nutritional support, 307
   in older adults, 300c
   overview of, 296–298
   pathophysiology of, 297–298
      blood pressure regulation, 298
      cellular changes, 297–298, 297f
      vascular responses, 298
   in postanesthesia units, 459
   recognition of, 300c
   self-care, patient education on, 320
   stages of, 298–304
      compensatory stage, 299–301

      irreversible stage, 303–304
      progressive stage, 301–303
   stress response by, 298
   support to family members, 303
   transitional care, 320–321
   vasoactive medication therapy, 306–307, 307t
Short-acting beta2-adrenergic agonists (SABA), 656
Short-acting muscarinic (anticholinergic) antagonists (SAMA), 640
Shoulder spica casts, 1137
Shunt surgery, for variceal bleeding, 1392–1393, 1392f
SIADH. *See* Syndrome of inappropriate antidiuretic hormone; Syndrome of inappropriate secretion of antidiuretic hormone
Sialadenitis, 1264, 1270
Sialolithiasis, 1270
Sickle cell crisis, 935–936
   acute vaso-occlusive crisis, 935
   aplastic crisis, 936
   sequestration crisis, 936
Sickle cell disease (SCD), 935–941
   assessment and diagnostic findings, 937
   clinical manifestations, 935–937
      acute chest syndrome, 936
      pulmonary hypertension, 936–937
      reproductive problems, 937
      sickle cell crisis, 935–936
      stroke, 937
   complications of, 936t
   medical management, 937–939
      hematopoietic stem cell transplant, 937
      pharmacologic therapy, 937–938
      supportive therapy, 938–939
      transfusion therapy, 938
   nursing process, 939–941
      assessment, 939
      diagnosis, 939
      evaluation, 941
      nursing interventions, 940–941
      planning and goals, 940
Sickle cell trait, 935
Sickle hemoglobin (HbS) gene, 935
Sick sinus syndrome, 741
Sigmoidoscopy, 1239–1240, 1350
Sildenafil (Viagra), 1102, 2180
   for erectile dysfunction, 1757–1759, 1758t, 1759t
Silent ischemia, 757c
Simeprevir (Olysio) plus sofosbuvir (Sovaldi), 1403–1404
Simethicone (Maalox), for GERD, 1284t
Sims position, 452, 453f
Simvastatin (Zocor), 756t
Single gene conditions, 124–127
Single photon emission computed tomography (SPECT), 700
Single-Photon Emission Computed Tomography (SPECT)
   nervous system, 1967
Sinoatrial (SA) node, 675
Sinus arrhythmia, 720
Sinus bradycardia, 718–719
Sinuses
   assessment of, 492–493, 493f
   frontal, 493
   maxillary, 493

   palpation technique for, 493f
   paranasal, 481f, 482
Sinus node dysrhythmias, 718–720
   sinus arrhythmia, 720
   sinus bradycardia, 718–719
   sinus tachycardia, 719–720
Sinusoidal harmonic acceleration, 1922
Sinus rhythm
   definition of, 712, 718
   with first-degree AV block, 732, 732f
   with second-degree AV block, 732–734
      type I, 732–733, 733f
      type II, 733–734, 733f
Sinus tachycardia, 719–720
Sipuleucel-T (Provenge), 1765
Sirolimus (Rapamune), 1610t
SIRS. *See* Systemic inflammatory response syndrome
Sitagliptin (Januvia), 1475t
Sitz baths, 1353, 1690
Sjögren's syndrome, 1101
SJS. *See* Stevens-Johnson syndrome
Skeletal system, structure and function of, 1115–1117, 1115f
Skeletal traction, 1141–1142
   nursing interventions, 1142–1143
   in rotating specialty bed, 2053f
Skene duct cysts, 1702
Skene gland, 1651
Skin
   age-related changes in, 1794, 1794c, 1794f
   anatomy of, 1790–1791, 1791f
      dermis, 1791–1792
      epidermis, 1791
      subcutaneous tissue, 1792
   assessment, 1794–1803, 1795c
      health history, 1795, 1795c
      physical assessment, 1795–1803
   bacterial infections, 1816
      carbuncles, 1818–1819
      folliculitis, 1818–1819
      furuncles, 1818–1819, 1818f
      impetigo, 1817–1818, 1817f
   benign skin tumors
      actinic keratoses, 1833
      angiomas, 1833
      cysts, 1833
      dermatofibroma, 1833
      keloids, 1833
      moles, 1833
      seborrheic keratoses, 1833
      Von Recklinghausen disease, 1833
      warts, 1833
   blistering diseases of, 1827–1832
      bullous pemphigoid, 1828
      care of patient with, 1829–1830
      dermatitis herpetiformis, 1828
      pemphigus vulgaris, 1827–1828
      Stevens-Johnson syndrome, 1830–1832
      toxic epidermal necrolysis, 1830–1832
   cancer, 1834, 1834c, 1836c
   color, 1795–1796
      changes in, 1795–1796, 1797f, 1797t
      cyanosis, 1796
      erythema, 1796
      jaundice, 1796
   cyanosis, 492
   diabetes and, 1803
   diagnostic evaluation, 1803
      clinical photographs, 1804

Skin (continued)
    nursing implications, 1804
    patch testing, 1804
    skin biopsy, 1803–1804
    skin scrapings, 1804
    Tzanck smear, 1804
    Wood Light examination, 1804
  examination, 685
  flaps, 1840–1841
  functions of
    fluid balance, 1793
    immune responses, 1794
    protection, 1793
    sensation, 1793
    temperature regulation, 1793
    vitamin production, 1793–1794
  fungal infections, 1820, 1821t
  genetic factors influencing, 1796c
  glands, 1792–1793
  grafts, 1839–1840, 1839f
  hair, 1792
    assessment, 1801–1803
  HIV infection and, 1803
  integrity
    in acute pancreatitis, 1444
    radiation-associated impairment, 362c, 370
    wound care and, 1866
  Kaposi sarcoma, 1839
  laser treatment of, 1841
  layers, 1840f
  lesions, 370–371, 1798–1800, 1798t–1799t,
      1800f
    configurations, 1800f
    primary, 1798
    secondary, 1798
    terminology related to, 1800
  malignant skin tumors, 1834, 1834c
    basal cell carcinoma, 1834–1836, 1834f
    melanoma, 1836–1838
    squamous cell carcinoma, 1834–1836,
      1834f
  metastatic skin tumors, 1839
  nails, 1792
    inspection, 1801
  parasitic infections, 1820
    pediculosis, 1820–1822
    scabies, 1822–1823
  postsurgical complications, 473t
  preparation for surgery, 449
  protection of, 1806–1807
  rash, 1796, 1798
  secondary infections, 1807
  vascularity and hydration, 1800–1801
  viral infections
    herpes simplex, 1820
    herpes zoster, 1819–1820, 1819f
Skin contamination poisoning, 2179–2180
Skin disorders
  medical management of, 1809
    pharmacologic therapy, 1809–1810
  nursing management for, 1810–1811
  wound dressing care for, 1807
Skin infections, 1803
Skin preparation, 698
  preoperative, 432
Skin scrapings, 1804
Skin tests, 1061, 1063–1064, 1063f, 1064f
Skin traction, 1140
  buck's extension traction, 1140–1141, 1140f
  nursing interventions, 1141
Skull fracture, 2035

SLE. See Systemic lupus erythematosus
Sleep, age-related changes, 200
Sleep apnea, aging and, 200
Sleep-disordered breathing (SDB), 684
Sleep hygiene, 204–205
Sleeve gastrectomy, 1369
Sleeve resection, 538c
Sling, 1131, 1136
Slit-lamp examination, 1881
SLNB. See Sentinel lymph node biopsy
Slough
  definition of, 164
  tissue injury and, 184
Small bowel obstruction, 1327–1329
  assessment and diagnostic findings, 1328
  clinical manifestations, 1328
  medical management, 1328
  nursing management, 1328–1329
  pathophysiology, 1327
Small bowel studies, 1240
Small-Carrion prosthesis, 1759
Small-incision cholecystectomy, 1437
Small intestine, 1224, 1225
  function, 1227–1228
  tumors of, 1308–1309
    assessment and diagnostic findings, 1309
    benign tumors, 1308
    clinical manifestations, 1308–1309
    malignant tumors, 1308
    management, 1309
Smallpox, 2205–2206
  clinical manifestations of, 2206
  treatment of, 2206
Small-volume nebulizer (mini-nebulizer)
      therapy, 517
SMBG. See Self-monitoring of blood glucose
Smegma, 1651
Smell, age-related changes, 197t, 202
Smoke evacuators, 442
Smoke inhalation, 1852
Smokeless tobacco products, 329
Smoker's patch. See Nicotine stomatitis
Smoking, 680
  carcinogenesis and, 329
  and chronic pancreatitis, 1445
  respiratory diseases and, 198
Smooth muscle relaxants, for esophageal spasm,
      1280
Smooth muscle, thermal energy, 665
Snakebites, 2176
  clinical manifestations, 2176
  management, 2176–2177
Snellen chart, 1879
Social histories, 491–492
Social services, older adults, 218
Social support, in grief and mourning, 412c
Society of Critical Care Medicine (SCCM), 1250
Socioeconomics, Pulmonary health and, 492c
Sodium bicarbonate
  in cardiopulmonary resuscitation, 839t
  and hypernatremia, 267
  IV administration, 272
Sodium citrate (Bicitra), 450
Sodium deficit, 1568t
Sodium, dietary, 830c
Sodium excess, 1568t
Sodium-glucose co-transporter 2 (SGL-2)
      inhibitors, 1475t
Sodium imbalance, 264–268, 265t
  hypernatremia, 267–268
  hyponatremia, 265–267

Sodium iodide, for hyperthyroidism, 1521t
Sodium nitroprusside (Nitropress), 1534
Sodium–potassium pump, 253
Sodium restriction, in ascites, 1386
Sodium salicylate, in rheumatic diseases, 1088t
Soman, 2207
Somatic pain, 227t
Somatosensory evoked responses (SERs), 1969
Somatostatin, 1360, 1429
Somogyi effect, 1471, 1471t
Sorafenib (Nexavar), 1418
Sotalol, for ventricular tachycardia, 730
Spacers, 640, 641f
Spasticity, 1946, 1960, 2059, 2061, 2074
  definition of, 2061, 2074
  spinal cord injuries and, 2058, 2061
Spastic muscle, 1119
Spatial orientation, 1885
Specific gravity, 1548
Specificity, 1058
Specimen collection, 2128
SPECT. See Single-Photon Emission Computed
      Tomography
Speculum examination, 1661
Speech disorders, 2106
Speech therapy, 574–575
Spermatic granuloma, 1783
Spermatogenesis, 1752, 1753
Sperm banking. See Semen cryopreservation
Spermicides, 1673
Spherocytes, 943
Sphincter of Oddi, 1379, 1428
Spider angioma, 1380, 1381f, 1801t
Spider bites, 2177
Spinal anesthesia, 445–448
  continuous, 448
  injection sites for, 448f
Spinal cord, 1951
Spinal cord compression
  management of, 381t–382t
  manifestation of, 381t–382t
Spinal cord injuries (SCIs), 2033, 2048, 2053
  categories, 2048
  complications of, 2055, 2058
  effects of, 2049, 2055
  emergency management, 2050
  functional abilities by level, 2052t
  long-term complications of, 2058
  oncologic disorders, 2091
  prevention of, 2048
  rehabilitation programs, 166
  traction, 2052
  tumors, 2091–2093
  worksheet for classification, 2050f
Spinal deformity, 2112
Spinal nerves, 1951–1952
Spinal tracts, 1951
Spinocerebellar ataxias, 125t
Spiritual assessment, preoperative, 427–428
Spiritual beliefs
  preoperative assessments, 427–428
  respect for, 431
Spiritual care, end-of-life, 402
Spiritual issues, end-of-life care and, 388
Spirituality, 62
  assessment of, 402
  definition of, 387
  features of, 402
Spirometry, 638
Spironolactone (Aldactone), 1540
  for ascites, 1386, 1408

for heart failure, 824t
for hypertension, 890t
Spleen, 908, 1005–1006
Spleen cells, 352, 353f
Splenectomy, 913, 943, 988
Splenomegaly, 972, 988, 1385
Splints, 1131, 1133–1136
    advantages of, 1133
    home care checklist, 1136c
    immobilized lower extremity, 1136–1137
    immobilized upper extremity, 1136
    nursing management of patient, 1133–1136
Spondyloarthropathies, 1106–1107
    ankylosing spondylitis, 1106
    nursing management, 1107
    pharmacologic management, 1107
    psoriatic arthritis, 1106–1107
    reactive arthritis, 1106
    surgical management, 1107
Spondylosis, 2114
Spongiform, 2071
Spontaneous abortion, 1674–1675
    cervical cerclage, 1675
    habitual abortion, 1675
    medical management, 1675
    nursing management, 1675
Spontaneous bacterial peritonitis (SBP), 1322,
        1407
Spontaneous mutations, 118
Sports-related musculoskeletal trauma, 1212
Sprain, 1185, 1186
Sprays, wound care, 1810
Sputum production, 635, 666
    assessment of, 490
    chronic bronchitis, 635
Sputum studies, 503
Squamous cell carcinoma (SCC), 1834–1836,
        1834f
SSM. See Superficial spreading melanoma
Stages of Change Mode, 56
Staging, definition of, 324
Standard Days method, 1674
Standard precautions, 2129, 2130, 2131c, 2146
Stapedectomy, 1931, 1932f
Staphylococcus aureus, 937, 1816, 1817
    transmission of, 2125
    wound infections, 474
Stapled hemorrhoidopexy, 1352
Stasis dermatitis, 1803
Stasis syndromes, 1321t
Static support devices, 183
Statins
    in cirrhosis, 1408
    for peripheral arterial disease, 852
Status asthmaticus, 656, 664
    assessment, 664
    clinical manifestations, 664
    diagnostic findings, 664
    medical management, 664–665
    nursing management, 665
    pathophysiology, 664
Status epilepticus, 1972, 2003–2004
Stavudine (d4 T), 1034t
Steady state
    control of, 91–92
    definition of, 84
Steatorrhea, 1292, 1297, 1311, 1331, 1428, 1445
Stem cells, 970, 1013
    bone marrow, 903, 1005
    harvest, 913t
Stenosis, 841, 1292, 1293

aortic, 795–796
    definition of, 792
    mitral, 794
Stent
    coronary artery, 771–772
    definition of, 750, 772
    and stent grafts, 852, 853f
Stereotactic body radiotherapy (SBRT), 339
Stereotactic core biopsy, 1719
    of breast, 1726–1727, 1726t
Stereotactic radiation therapy, for pituitary
        tumors, 1509
Sterile drapes, 442, 442f
Sterilization, 1671, 1671t
Sternal fractures, 626–627
Steroid hormones, 1504
Steroid-induced acne, 1810
Stevens–Johnson syndrome (SJS), 1830–1832
Stimulation tests, 1506
St. Louis encephalitis, 2070
Stoma, 1243, 1252, 1339. See also Urinary
        diversions
    inspection of, 1640
    ischemia and necrosis, 1645–1646
    retraction and separation, 1646
Stomach, 1224, 1225
Stomatitis, 1264, 1267t, 1272
    associated with chemotherapy agents, 345
    definition of, 324
    management of, 355–357
    nursing diagnosis, 360c
Stool
    blood in, 683
    characteristics, 1230
    color, 1230t
    tests, 1233
Stool charts, 1317
Straight-leg raising test, 2117
Straight/running traction, 1140
Strain, 1185, 1186
Streptococcus pneumoniae, 2065
    meningitis and, 2065
    vaccination, 2134
Streptococcus pyogenes, 1817
Streptozocin (Zanosar), 343t
Stress
    adaptation to, 85
    appraisal responses, 86–87
    assessing for, 90c
    brain interpretation of, 88–90
    cellular levels of, 91–95, 91f
    coping with, 87
    definition of, 84
    disease and, 86
    enhanced coping strategies, 97, 97c
    health patterns and, 99
    immunological response, 89–90
    indicators of, 90–91
    maladaptive responses to, 90
    nursing management, 95–96, 96c
    overview of, 85
    physiological responses to, 87–90, 88f
    relaxation techniques, 97–98
    sympathetic adrenal-medullary response, 89,
        89t
Stress incontinence, 185, 1623–1624. See also
        Urinary incontinence
Stress management
    definition of, 48
    health promotion and, 57
    patient profile record of, 68c

Stressor
    definition of, 84
    types of, 85–86
Stress-related gastritis, 1293
Stress testing, cardiac, 699–700
    nursing interventions, 700
    pharmacologic stress testing, 699–700
Stress tolerance, 685
Stress ulcers, 1297
Stretch elastic wraps, 872–873
Striae, 1806, 1810
Strictureplasty, laparoscope-guided, 1333
Stridor, 480
Stroke
    home care check list, 2030c
    hypertension and, 887
    left hemisphere, 2013t
    neurologic deficits, 2012t
    right hemisphere, 2013t
    sickle cell disease and, 937
    types of, 2010t
Stroke volume (SV), 677, 709
    cardiac output, effect of, 677–678
Stroma, bone marrow, 905
Stromal cell tumors, 1712
Strongyloidiasis, 1321t
Struvite stones, 1632
ST segment, 712, 716
Study to Understand Prognoses and Preferences
        for Outcomes and Risks of Treatments
        (SUPPORT), 392
Stylet, 1243, 1245
Subarachnoid hemorrhage, 2026
Subchondral bone, 1104
Subclavian steal syndrome, 860
Subculture, 102, 103
Subcutaneous emphysema, 631
Subcutaneous immunoglobulin (SCIG), 2081
Subcutaneous immunotherapy (SIT), 1071
Subcutaneous tissue, skin, 1792
Subdural hematomas (SDHs), 2034
Sublingual immunotherapy (SLIT), 1071
Subluxation, 1185, 1186
Substance abuse, 62, 69, 2180–2185
    acute alcohol intoxication, 2185
    alcohol withdrawal syndrome, 2185–2186
    issue in rehabilitation and, 167
    older adults and, 208
    rehabilitation issues, 167
Substantia nigra, 2101, 2102
Subtotal thyroidectomy, 1522
Succinylcholine, 446t
Sucralfate (Carafate)
    for gastritis, 1295t
    for GERD, 1284t
Sudden cardiac death, definition of, 750, 752
Sudomotor neuropathy, 1494
Sufentanil (Sufenta), 446t
Suicidal depression, 2109
Suicide
    assisted, 390
    in older adults, 207
    physician-assisted, 390
Sulfasalazine (Azulfidine)
    in rheumatic diseases, 1088t
Summation gallop, 690, 691
Superficial inferior epigastric artery flap (SIEA),
        1747
Superficial spreading melanoma (SSM), 1836
Superior mesenteric artery syndrome, 1137
Superior vena cava (SVC), 300

Superior vena cava syndrome (SVCS)
  management of, 381t
  manifestation of, 381t
Supination, 171c
SUPPORT. *See* Study to Understand Prognoses
      and Preferences for Outcomes and Risks
      of Treatments
Suppressor T cells, 1012
Suprapubic catheters, 187, 1615, 1627–1628,
      1629, 1629f
Suprapubic prostatectomy, 1771, 1772t, 1773f
Suprapubic tapping, 187
Supratentorial approach, 1990–1995, 1990t
Supraventricular tachycardia (SVT), 729
Surgeons, roles of, 438–439
Surgery
  adverse effects of, 437c
  ambulatory, 418, 422
  for cancer, 335–338
  categories of, 421t
  complications, 423c
  diagnostic, 335–336
  discharge after, 461–463, 463c
  emergency, 422
  environment for, 440–449
  gerontologic considerations, 437–438
  informed consent, 422–423
  intracranial, 1989–1996, 1990f, 1990t
  intraoperative nursing, 436–454
  laparoscopic, 336
  minimally-invasive, 336
  nursing management after, 463–464
  nursing process, 451–454
  palliative, 337, 337t
  patient recovering from, 463–476
  position for, 452, 453f
  prophylactic, 337
  radical, 336
  reconstructive, 337
  risks involved in, 437, 437c
  safety checklist, 439f
  salvage, 336
  skin preparation for, 449
  thoracic, 537–550
  verification procedures, 438
  video-assisted endoscopic, 336
Surgical abdomen, 1322
Surgical asepsis
  description of, 436
  function of
  guidelines, 441–442
  principles of, 441–442
Surgical biopsy, 1719
Surgical Care Improvement Project (SCIP),
      419, 449
Surgical débridement, 876
Surgical drains
  care of, 469
  types of, 471f
Surgical intensive care units (SICUs), 434c
Surgical site exposure, 442f
Surgical team, 436–437
Surveillance, Epidemiology, and End Results
      registry (SEER), 1343
Susceptible, 2125
Suspected awareness, 389
Suspensions, definition of, 1806, 1809
Sustainability planning, 2194
Sustained maximal inspiration. *See* Incentive
      spirometry
Sutures (Perclose, Techstar), 704

Swallowing, 1226
  aging and, 199
  difficulties, 2106
Sweat, 1792
Sweat glands, 1792
Sweeteners, use of, 1465
Sympathetic nervous system, 1953
  catecholamine release, 1850–1851
  response to stress, 88–89, 88f
Sympathetic ophthalmia, 1876, 1904, 1910
Synarthrosis joints, 1117
Synchronized intermittent mandatory
      ventilation (SIMV), 511, 528
Syncro BlueTube, 1246
Syndrome of inappropriate secretion of
      antidiuretic hormone (SIADH), 1503,
      1510, 1981, 2068
  associated with sodium imbalance, 264, 265,
      266
Synovectomy, 1095
Synovium, 1118
Synthetic levothyroxine (Synthroid or
      Levothroid)
  for hypothyroidism, 1515
Synthetic vitamin A acids, 1815
Syphilis, 2147
  patient education, 2148c
Systemic inflammatory response syndrome
      (SIRS), 296, 315
Systemic lupus erythematosus (SLE), 1098–1101
  assessment and diagnostic findings, 1099–
      1100
  butterfly rash of, 1098f
  clinical manifestations, 1098–1099
  criteria for classification of, 1099c
  medical management, 1100
  nursing management, 1100–1101
  pathophysiology, 1098
  pharmacologic therapy, 1100
Systemic medications, 1810
Systemic vascular resistance, 678
Systole, 713
Systolic blood pressure (SBP), 884
Systolic heart failure, 818, 819. *See also* Heart
      failure (HF)

T

Tabun, 2207
Tachypnea
  description of, 480, 488
  patterns, 496t
  physical assessment, 493
Tacrolimus (Prograf), 350, 1423, 1610t
Tactile fremitus, 495–496, 497f
Tadalafil (Cialis)
  for erectile dysfunction, 1757–1759, 1758t,
      1759t
Tamm–Horsfall protein, 1561
Tamoxifen, 1706
  in breast cancer, 1743, 1744t
  and uterine cancers, 1708
Tampons, 1666
Tampon test, 1698
Tamsulosin, for BPH, 1763
Tapentadol (Nucynta), 241
TARE-transarterial chemoembolization, 1418
Targeted therapies
  biologic response modifiers therapy, 352–354
  definition of, 324
  for gastric cancer, 1305
  gene therapy, 354

  nursing management, 354–355
  therapeutic and adverse effects, 354–355
Taste
  age-related changes, 197t, 202
  impairment of, 371
Tau protein, 211, 212f
Taxanes, 1742
Tazarotene (Tazorac), for psoriasis, 1825
T-cell dysfunction, 2137
T cells. *See* T lymphocytes
Teaching
  definition of, 48, 51
  nursing function of, 52–53
  plan formulation, 53–54
  teaching aids, 52
  techniques, 52
Teaching aids, 52
Teaching-learning process
  assessments, 52
  evaluation, 54–55
  implementation, 54
  planning, 53–54
Team Strategies and Tools to Enhance
      Performance and Patient Safety
      (TeamSTEPPS), 9, 10f
Teamwork, surgical teams, 436–440
Technology
  and end-of-life care, 388
  genetic and genomic, 122–124
  perioperative nursing and, 419
Technology Informatics Guiding Education
      Reform (TIGER) initiative, 7
Telangiectasias, 1790, 1801, 1801t, 1810
Telehealth, use of, 7, 8c
  in home health care, 21
Telemetry, 696
  ECG monitoring, 696
  nursing research, 698c
  transmitters, 699
Teleologic theory, 30
Teletherapy, for prostate cancer, 1765
Telmisartan (Micardis), for hypertension,
      892t
Temozolomide (Temodar), 2096
Temperature, regulation of
  burn injuries and, 1852
Temporal lobes, tumors of, 2094
Temporomandibular disorders, 1264, 1269
  assessment and diagnostic findings, 1269
  causes, 1269
  clinical manifestations, 1269
  medical management, 1269
TEN. *See* Toxic epidermal necrolysis
Tendonitis, 1160, 1164
Tendons, 1118
  injuries to, 1187–1189
Tenecteplase (TNKase), 866
  for venous thromboembolism, 870t
Tenesmus, 1311, 1315
Teniposide (Vumon, VM-26), 343t
Tenofovir (TDF), 1034t
  in hepatitis B, 1402
Tenorrhaphy, 1095
Tensilon test, 2079
Tension pneumothorax, 583, 629–630
Terazosin (Hytrin)
  for BPH, 1763
  for hypertension, 891t
Terconazole (Terazol) cream
  for candidiasis, 1688
Teriflunomide (Aubagio), 2075

Terminal illness
confusion and, 407
definition of, 387
denial of, 389–390
hope and, 402
nursing care during, 395–407
communication, 395–399
psychosocial issues, 395
regulatory issues, 395
patient and family denial, 389–390
physiologic responses to, 402–407
preparation for, 388–389
sociocultural context, 388–390
spiritual care, 402
symptoms associated with, 403c
Termuo TR Band", 704
Terrorism, 2193, 2201–2202
and mortality, 2193
preparedness and response
decontamination, 2201
personal protective equipment, 2201
recognition and awareness, 2200–2201
Tertiary prevention, 19
Testes, 1753
Testicular cancer, 1779–1782
assessment and diagnostic findings, 1780, 1781c
clinical manifestations, 1780
cultural aspects of care related to, 1782c
germinal, 1780
medical management, 1780–1782
nongerminal, 1780
nursing management, 1782
risk factors for, 1780
secondary, 1780
side effects with treatment for, 1781–1782
Testicular self-examination (TSE), 1755, 1780, 1781c
Testicular torsion, 1779
Testosterone, 1752, 1753
effects on bone remodeling, 1117
Tetanus, 2152
prophylaxis, 2167
in snakebites, 2176
Tetany, 1526–1527, 1529
hypocalcemia and, 273
latent, 1529
overt, 1529
Tetrabenazine (Xenatine), 2109
Tetracaine (Pontocaine), 448t
Tetracycline
for gastritis, 1295t
in hidradenitis suppurativa, 1813
Tetraplegia, 1956, 2048
Thalamotomy, 2103
Thalassemia major, 942
Thalassemias, 941–942
alpha-thalassemias, 942
assessment and diagnostic findings, 942
beta-thalassemia, 942
clinical manifestations, 942
medical management, 942
nursing management, 942
Thalidomide (Thalomid), 988, 996
The bends. See Decompression sickness
Theophylline (Slo-Bid, Theo-Dur), 660
asthma treatment, 658t
Therapeutic communication techniques, 37, 37t
Therapeutic Lifestyle Changes (TLC) diet, 754–755, 1364
nutrient content of, 755t

Therapeutic regimen
adherence to, 49–50
definition of, 48
Therapeutic vaccines, 1765
Thermistors, 707f, 708
Thermoregulatory alterations
burn injuries and, 1852
Thiamine deficiency, 1397
Thiazide diuretics, 275
in diabetes insipidus, 1510
for hypertension, 890t
Thiazolidinediones, 1475t
Thin-layer Rapid Use Epicutaneous (T.R.U.E.) test, 1074
6-Thioguanine (Tabloid), 343t
Thiopental sodium (Pentothal), 447t
Thiotepa (Thioplex), 343t
Third-degree burns, 1847t, 1848, 1848f
Third-intention healing
definition of, 456
mechanisms of, 468c
postsurgical, 468
Third-party payers, 24
Thomas splint, 1141
Thoracentesis, 507, 583
Thoracic aortic aneurysm, 862–863
Thoracic injuries, halo/vest for, 2053f
Thoracic surgery, 537–550, 538c, 547f
cardiopulmonary complications after, prevention of, 541c
continuing and transitional care, 550
patient education, 548c
postoperative management, 539–550
preoperative management, 537–539
Thoracolumbar junction, 1212
Thoraco-lumbar-sacral orthosis (TLSO), 1212
Thoracolumbar spine, 1212
Thoracolumbosacral orthotics (TLSO), 1133
Thoracoscopy, 506
endoscopic, 506–507, 507f
nursing interventions, 507
procedure, 506–507
video-assisted, 507
Thoracotomy, 511, 544c
home care, 549c
Thorax
inspection, 493–495
landmarks, 494c
palpation, 495–496
percussion, 497–498, 498f
structures of, 482f
3-dimensional conformal radiation therapy (3D-CRT), 1305
thrifty gene hypothesis, 1360
Thrombelastography, 958
Thrombin inhibitors, 965
Thrombocytes. See Platelets
Thrombocytopenia, 377–378, 948, 982
assessment and diagnostic findings, 949
causes and management, 948t
clinical manifestations, 948–949
description of, 324
medical management, 949
nursing management, 949
Thrombocytosis, 948, 985
Thromboembolism, 835
Thrombolytic therapy, 750, 2014
Thrombophilias, acquired, 962–966
etiology, 962–963
medical management, 963–965
nursing management, 965–966

Thrombophlebitis, 293
Thrombopoietin (TPO), 923c
Thrombotic disorders, 959, 961–966
Thrush, 1266t
Thumbs rest, 1511
Thymectomy, 2081
Thyrocalcitonin. See Calcitonin
Thyroglobulin, 1513
Thyroid-binding globulin, 908
Thyroid-binding hormones, 1511
Thyroid cancer, 1525–1527
assessment and diagnostic findings, 1525
incidence of, 1525
medical management, 1525–1526
nursing management, 1526–1527
complications management, 1526–1527
home, community-based, and transitional care, 1527
postoperative care, 1526
predischarge education, 1527
preoperative care, 1526
Thyroid cartilage, 482
Thyroidectomy, 1503, 1514
Thyroid gland, 1510, 1510f
diagnostic evaluation, 1512
fine-needle aspiration biopsy, 1513
medications affecting test results, 1513, 1514c
radioactive iodine uptake test, 1513
serum free T_4, 1512
serum T_3 and T_4, 1512–1513
serum thyroglobulin, 1513
serum TSH concentration, 1512
thyroid antibodies, 1513
thyroid scan, radioscan, or scintiscan, 1513
T_3 resin uptake test, 1513
hormones of, 1510–1511
function of, 1511
regulation of, 1511
synthesis of, 1511
hyperthyroidism, 1519–1524
hypothyroidism, 1513–1519
pathophysiology, 1511
physical examination, 1511–1512, 1512t
thyroid cancer, 1525–1527
thyroid tumors, 1524–1525
Thyroid hormone, 1116
drug interactions, 428t
Thyroiditis, 1503, 1512
Thyroid-releasing hormone (TRH), 1511, 1511f
Thyroid-stimulating hormone (TSH), 1503, 1507, 1511
Thyroid storm, 1503, 1520, 1520c
Thyroid tumors, 1524–1525
Thyrotoxicosis, 1503, 1519
preoperative assessments, 426
Thyroxine (T_4), 1503, 1510. See also Thyroid gland
Thyroxine-binding globulin (TBG), 1511
TIA. See Transient ischemic attack
Tibia, 1211
Tick bites, 2177–2178, 2177f
Tidal volumes, 480, 501, 511
Time, attitude towards, 107
Timed voiding, 1625c
Timolol (Blocadren), for hypertension, 891t
Tinea, 1806, 1820, 1821t
Tinidazole (Tindamax), for trichomoniasis, 1689
Tinnitus, 1915, 1934
Tipranavir (TPV), 1035t

TIPS. *See* Transjugular intrahepatic portosystemic shunt
Tirofiban (Aggrastat), 683
Tissue integrity, in cancer, 355–371
Tissue perfusion, 180, 184
  monitoring of, 299–300
Tissue perfusion, during cardiac surgery, 787
Tizanidine (Zanaflex), 2075
TLC diet. *See* Therapeutic Lifestyle Changes diet
T lymphocytes, 903, 907, 1005, 1006f. *See also* Cellular immune response
  role of, 1058
  types of, 1010–1012
Tobramycin (TOBI), 666
Tocilizumab (Actemra), 1089t
To Err Is Human: Building a Safer Health System (IOM report), 7–8
Tolerance, 1005
Tolvaptan (Samsca), 266
Tongue, 1231
Tongue turgor, 262
Tonicity, 253
Tonometry, 1881
Tonsilitis, 552, 562–564
Tonsils, anatomy, 481
Tooth decay, 1265, 1268
Tophi, 1108
Topical corticosteroids, wound care, 1810, 1811t
Topoisomerase II inhibitors, 343t
Topoisomerase I inhibitors, 343t
Topotecan (Hycamtin), 343t
Torsades de pointes, 716
Torsemide (Demadex), 263
  for hypertension, 890t
Total hip arthroplasty (THA), 1148c–1150c, 1151f
  avoiding hip dislocation, 1151c
  home care after, 1153c
  nursing interventions
    gerontologic considerations, 1147
    hip prosthesis, 1147, 1151
    home, community-based, and transitional care, 1152–1154, 1153c
    infection prevention, 1152
    monitoring wound drainage, 1152
    promoting ambulation, 1151–1152
    VTE prevention, 1152
Total hysterectomy, for cervical cancer, 1707c
Total joint arthroplasty, 1145
Total joint replacement. *See* Total joint arthroplasty
Total knee arthroplasty (TKA), 1144, 1154
  nursing interventions, 1154–1155
  nursing process, 1155–1157
  post, 1154
Total knee replacement and pain relief, 1146c
Total nutrient admixture (TNA), 1243, 1257
Total pancreatectomy, 1452
Total thyroidectomy, 1525
Total urinary incontinence, 185
Touch, attitude towards, 107
Tourniquet, 1144, 2166
Toxic epidermal necrolysis (TEN), 1830–1832
Toxic hepatitis, 1404
Toxic nodular goiter, 1522
t-pieces, 515f
TP interval, 712, 716
Trabeculae, 1115
Trachea, anatomy, 482
Tracheoesophageal puncture, 575
Tracheostomal stenosis, 579
Tracheostomy collars, 515f

Tracheostomy tube, 511, 523, 524f
Tracheotomy, 511, 523–525
Trachoma
  conjunctivitis, 1907
  definition, 1876, 1877
Traction, 1131, 1139–1144, 1139f
  balanced suspension, 1140, 1140f
  goal of, 1139
  manual, 1140
  patient in
    effective traction, 1139–1140
    nursing management, 1143–1144
    skeletal traction, 1141–1143
    skin traction, 1140–1141
    traction, types of, 1140
  skeletal, 1140
  skin, 1140
  straight/running, 1140
Tramadol (Ultram), 241
Trandolapril (Mavik), for hypertension, 892t
Tranquilizers, 428t
Transarterial chemoembolization (TACE), 1418
Transbronchial brushing, 507
Transbronchial needle aspiration, 507
Transcatheter Arterial Embolization (TAE), 1302
Transcranial doppler, 1968
Transcultural nursing, 102–113
  definition of, 102
  future of, 111–112
  terminology, 104–106
Transcutaneous electrical nerve stimulation (TENS), 1087, 1187
Transdermal contraceptives, 1672
Transducer-tipped catheter, 1982
Transection, 2048
Trans-esophageal echocardiography (TEE), 702
Transfusion, 917
  complications, 919
    acute hemolytic reaction, 919–920
    allergic reaction, 920
    bacterial contamination, 920–921
    delayed hemolytic reactions, 921
    disease acquisition, 921, 922c
    febrile nonhemolytic reaction, 919
    transfusion-associated circulatory overload, 920
    transfusion-related acute lung injury, 921
  informed consent for, 918, 919c
  long-term, 921, 922t
  nursing management for transfusion reactions, 921–922
  of packed red blood cells, 917c
  and patient education, 919
  pharmacologic alternatives to, 922–923, 923c
  of platelets or fresh-frozen plasma, 918c
  pretransfusion assessment
    patient history, 918
    physical assessment, 918
  setting for, 918
  sickle cell disease and, 938
Transfusion-associated circulatory overload (TACO), 920
Transfusion dependence, 982
Transfusion-related acute lung injury (TRALI), 921
Transient flora, 2130
Transient ischemic attack (TIA), 2011
Transitional care
  after surgery, 462–463
  promotion of, 188–190
Transitional care nurse (TCN), 149

Transitional services, 2160
Transjugular intrahepatic portosystemic shunt (TIPS)
  for ascites, 1387, 1387f
  for variceal bleeding, 1392
Translation services, 438
Transmissible spongiform encephalopathies (TSE), 2071
Transmission-based precautions, 2129
Transrectal ultrasound (TRUS), 1756
Transsacral (caudal) block, 448
Transsphenoidal approach, 1990t, 1995–1996
Transtheoretical Model of Change, 56, 57t
Transthyretin, 1511
Transtracheal oxygen catheter, 514
Transurethral incision of prostate (TUIP), 1764, 1771, 1772t, 1773f
Transurethral microwave thermotherapy (TUMT), 1763–1764
Transurethral needle ablation (TUNA), 1764
Transurethral resection of the prostate (TURP), 1752, 1764, 1771, 1772t, 1773f
Transurethral resection syndrome, 1771, 1774c
Transvaginal surgical mesh, 1700
Transvaginal/transrectal electrical stimulation, 1625c
Transvaginal ultrasound, for ectopic pregnancy, 1680
Transverse rectus abdominal myocutaneous (TRAM) flap, 1719, 1746, 1746f
Trapeze, 1131, 1142
Trastuzumab (Herceptin), 353, 1744
Trauma, 2167–2168
  forensic evidence, 2168
  injury prevention, 2168
Traumatic brain injuries (TBI), 2033, 2134
  body temperature maintaining, 2043
  home care checklist, 2047, 2047c
  management of, 2034
  multisystem assessment, 2041t
  nursing process, 2038
  pathophysiology of, 2034, 2034f
  penetrating, 2136
  prevention of, 2034
  rehabilitation programs, 166
  skin integrity, maintaining, 2043
Traumatic pneumothorax, 629
Travel, infectious diseases and, 2153
Tremors, Parkinson disease, 2105
Trench mouth. *See* Necrotizing gingivitis
Trendelenburg position, 452, 453f
Treponemal tests, 2147
Treponema pallidum, 2147
TRH. *See* Thyroid-releasing hormone
Triage, 2156, 2161–2163
  assess and intervene, 2162–2163
  emergent, 2161
  nonurgent, 2161
  protocols, 2162
  urgent, 2161
Triamcinolone, 1541t
Triamcinolone acetonide (Azmacort), 658t
Triamterene (Dyrenium), 1408
  for hypertension, 890t
Triceps reflex, 1963
Trichiasis, 1876, 1881, 1907
Trichloroacetic acid, 1691
Trichomoniasis, 1688t, 1689
Tricuspid area, 689
Tricuspid valve, 791
  anatomy of, 792f

Tricyclic antidepressants (TCAs), 244, 2109
  for depression, 207
  for esophageal spasm, 1280
Trigeminal nerve (CN V), 2086t
Trigeminal neuralgia, 2085, 2087–2088
Triglycerides, 695, 754
Triiodothyronine (T₃), 1503, 1510. See also
      Thyroid gland
Trimethoprim–sulfamethoxazole, 1041
  in impetigo, 1818
  for urinary tract infections, 1619t
Triptans, 2006
Tropical sprue, 1321t
Troponin, 750, 764
Trousseau sign, 274, 274f, 1503, 1530
Truth-telling, 33
Trypsin, 1224, 1227, 1428, 1429
TSE. See Testicular self-examination
TSH. See Thyroid-stimulating hormone
Tubal embryo transfer (TET), 1678
Tubal ligation (female sterilization), 1671,
      1671t
Tuberculin (TB) skin test, 1094
Tuberculosis (TB), 2125. See also Mycobacterium
      sp.
  HIV infection and, 1038–1039
Tuberculous peritonitis, 1322
Tubo-ovarian abscess, 1695
TUIP. See Transurethral incision of prostate
Tularemia, 2177
Tumor, 1798t
  benign vs. malignant, 326t
  grading, 333–334
  radiosensitive, 339
  removal, 2100
  staging, 333–334
  surgical techniques for, 336t
Tumor-associated antigens (TAAs), 330
Tumor lysis syndrome, 351, 973
  management of, 383t
  manifestation of, 383t
Tumor necrosis factor-alpha (TNF-a)
  for psoriasis, 1826
Tumors of head of pancreas, 1451–1453
  assessment and diagnostic findings, 1452
  clinical manifestations, 1452
  continuing and transitional care, 1453
  medical management, 1452
  nursing management, 1452–1453
  self-care, 1453
TURP. See Transurethral resection of the
      prostate
T wave, 712, 716
Twinrix, 1399
Tympanic membrane, 1916–1917, 1917f, 1920f,
      1927
Tympanic membrane (TM) rupture, 2203
Tympanogram, 1922
Tympanoplasty, 1929
Type 1 diabetes, 1456, 1458–1459
Type 2 diabetes, 1456, 1459
Tyrosine kinase inhibitors, 974
Tzanck smear, 1804

U

U-500 insulin, 1471
Ulcer, 1799t
Ulcerative colitis, 1331–1334
  assessment and diagnostic findings, 1331–1332
  clinical manifestations, 1331
  complications of, 1332

Crohn's disease and, 1330t
  medical treatment, 1332–1334
  pathophysiology, 1331
Ulcerogenic tumors, 1453–1454
Ulnar shaft fracture, 1200
Ultrafiltration, 827, 1567, 1589, 1594, 1595
Ultrasonography, 1665, 1882
  of breast, 1725
  for gallstones, 1432
  for kidney disease, 1578
  for low back pain, 1161c
Ultrasound-guided core biopsy, of breast, 1727
Ultraviolet-A (UVA), 1825
Ultraviolet-B (UVB), 1825
Unconsciousness, nursing assessments in, 1976t
Unfractionated heparin, 958, 963
  for venous thromboembolism, 870, 870t
Unicameral (single cavity) bone cysts, 1180
Unintentional injuries, 1185
United Network for Organ Sharing (UNOS)
      computer system, 1423
United Ostomy Associations of America
      (UOAA), 1341, 1646
United States Preventive Services Task Force
      (USPSTF), 1169
Unna boot, 873
Unrestricted zones, 436, 440
Upper airway infections, 552–567
  adenoiditis, 562–564
  laryngitis, 565–567
  peritonsillar abscess, 564–565
  pharyngitis, 560–562
  rhinitis, 553–555
  rhinosinusitis, 556–560
  tonsilitis, 562–564
  viral rhinitis, 555–556
Upper airway injuries, burn-related, 1852
Upper airway obstruction, 521
Upper extremity arterial occlusive disease,
      860–861
  assessment and diagnostic findings, 861
  clinical manifestations, 860
  medical management, 861
  nursing management, 861
Upper extremity disorders, 1164–1166
  bursitis, 1164
  carpal tunnel syndrome, 1164–1165
  Dupuytren disease, 1165, 1165f
  ganglion, 1165
  hand or wrist, surgery of, 1165–1166, 1166c
  impingement syndrome, 1164
  loose bodies, 1164
  tendonitis, 1164
Upper motor neuron, 1955, 1956t
Upper respiratory tract disorders, 552–582
  obstruction and trauma, 567–582
  in older adults, 553c
  upper airway infections, 552–567
Urban Search and Rescue Teams (USRT), 2195
Urea, 1553
Urea nitrogen, 1548, 1562
Uremia, 1567, 1570, 1571
Uremic bone disease, 1583
Ureteral colic, 1633
Ureteral trauma, 1637
Ureteroscopy, 1634
Ureterosigmoidostomy, 1615, 1643
Ureterovesical junction, 1550
Ureterovesical/vesicoureteral reflux, 1615, 1616,
      1617f
Ureters, 1550

Urethra, 1551, 1753
Urethral stricture, 1785–1786
Urethral trauma, 1637
Urethritis, 1615
Urethrocele, 1558
Urethrovesical reflux, 1615, 1616, 1617f
Urge incontinence, 185, 1624. See also Urinary
      incontinence
Urgency, 1556t
Uric acid, 1553
Uric acid stones, 1632, 1633–1634
Uricosuric agents, 1108
Urinary bladder, 1550
Urinary casts, 1567, 1572, 1578
Urinary diversions, 1639–1647
  continent, 1639, 1642–1643
  cutaneous, 1639–1642, 1640f
  nursing process (postoperative)
    body image, improving, 1645
    complications management, 1645–1646
    evaluation, 1646–1647
    nursing assessment, 1644
    nursing diagnoses, 1644–1645
    nursing interventions, 1645–1646
    pain relief, 1645
    patient education, 1646
    planning and goals, 1645
    sexuality issues, 1645
    skin integrity, 1645
  nursing process (preoperative)
    anxiety reduction, 1644
    evaluation, 1644
    explanations of surgical procedure, 1644
    nursing assessment, 1643–1644
    nursing diagnoses, 1644
    nursing interventions, 1644
    nutrition, 1644
    planning and goals, 1644
Urinary frequency, 1615, 1617
Urinary incontinence, 193, 1615, 1623–1627,
      1754
  assessment and diagnostic findings, 1624
  behavioral therapy for, 1624–1626, 1625c
  nursing management, 1626–1627
  in older adults, 1624
  patient education, 1626c
  pharmacologic therapy for, 1626
  postoperative, 1777
  risk factors, 1624c
  surgical management, 1626
  transient, 1624, 1625c
  types of, 1623–1624
Urinary meatus, 1651
Urinary retention, 1627
  assessment and diagnostic findings, 1627
  complications, 1627
  nursing management, 1627
    home, community-based, and transitional
        care, 1628
    urinary elimination, measures for,
        1627–1628
  pathophysiology, 1627
  postsurgical, 472
Urinary stasis and infection, 1143
Urinary tract, disorders of, 1615–1647
  adult voiding dysfunction, 1622–1632
  genitourinary trauma, 1637
  infections of urinary tract, 1615–1622
  urinary diversions, 1639–1647
  urinary tract cancers, 1637–1639
  urolithiasis and nephrolithiasis, 1632–1637

Urinary tract infections (UTIs), 1615–1622, 2075
  classification of, 1615, 1616c
  complicated, 1616, 1617
  hospital-acquired, 1616
  lower, 1615, 1616–1621
    clinical manifestations, 1617
    diagnosis of, 1618
    nursing process, 1619–1621
    in older adults, 1617–1618, 1618c
    pathophysiology, 1616–1617
    pharmacologic therapy, 1618–1619, 1619t
    risk factors for, 1616c
  in older adults, 1617–1618, 1618c
  recurrent, prevention of, 1621c
  upper, 1615, 1621–1622
Urine
  blood in, 683
  culture, 1618, 1630
  examination, 1561, 1561t
  formation of, 1551, 1551f
  ketone testing, 1468
  proteinuria, 1561
  sodium, 256
  specific gravity, 1551, 1561
  storage, 1553–1554
Urine dipstick, 1467
Urine-specific gravity, 255
Urinometer, 1561
Urobilinogen, 1379, 1429
Urofollitropin (Metrodin, Bravelle), 1677c
Urokinase (Abbokinase)
  for venous thromboembolism, 870t
Urolithiasis, 1632–1634
  assessment and diagnostic findings, 1633
  clinical manifestations, 1632–1633
  medical management, 1633–1634
  pathophysiology, 1632
  predisposing factors, 1632
  sites of calculi formation, 1632f
  surgical management, 1634
Urologic endoscopic procedures, 1564–1565, 1565f
Uromodulin, 1561
Uropathogenic bacteria, 1617
Urosepsis, 1615, 1617
Urothelium, 1550
Ursodeoxycholic acid, 1408, 1434
Urticaria (hives), 920, 1075–1076
U.S. Department of Homeland Security, 2193
U.S. Food and Drug Administration (FDA), 2135
U.S. Medical Eligibility Criteria (USMEC) ,for Contraceptive Use, 1669
U.S. Preventive Services Task Force (USPSTF), 1362
  on colorectal cancer screening, 1344
Ustekinumab (Stelara), 1107
  for psoriasis, 1826
Uterine artery embolization (UAE), 1704
Uterine bleeding, abnormal, 1668
Uterine cancers, 1708–1709, 1709c
  assessment and diagnostic findings, 1709
  medical management, 1709
  pathophysiology, 1709
  risk factors, 1708, 1709c
  type 1, 1709
  type 2, 1709
Uterine fibroids, 1703–1704
Uterine prolapse, 1650, 1661, 1700–1701, 1700f
  medical management, 1701
  nursing management, 1701

  patient education, 1701
  positions of uterus, 1700f
    anteflexion, 1700f
    anteversion, 1700f
    retroflexion, 1700f
    retroversion, 1700f
Uterine wall, 1652
Uterotubography, 1665
Uterus, 1652–1653
  palpation of, 1662
Utilitarianism, 30
UVA. *See* Ultraviolet-A
UVB. *See* Ultraviolet-B
Uveitis, 1908–1909
U wave, 712, 716

V

Vaccine Adverse Event Reporting System (VAERS), 2134c
Vaccine Information Statements, 2134
Vaccine preventable diseases, 2134t
Vaccines
  allogeneic, 354
  autologous, 354
  cancer, 354
  hepatitis A, 1399
  hepatitis B, 1402
  human papillomavirus, 1692
  prophylactic, 354
Vacuum aspiration, 1676c
Vacuum-assisted closures (VAC), 185, 1192
Vagal blocking therapy, 1366
Vagina, 1652, 1687
  inspection of, 1662
  palpation of, 1662
Vaginal cancers, 1711–1712
  diagnosis, 1711
  medical management, 1711–1712
  risk factors, 1711
  vaginal pessaries and, 1711
Vaginal cone retention exercises, 1625c
Vaginal contraceptives, 1672
Vaginal discharge, 1661, 1662t, 1687
  vaginitis and, 1687
Vaginal fistulas, 1697–1698
  assessment and diagnostic findings, 1698
  clinical manifestations, 1697–1698
  medical management, 1698
  rectovaginal fistula, 1697
  sites for, 1697f
  vesicovaginal fistula, 1697
Vaginal stenosis, 1708
Vaginitis, 1686, 1687
Vagotomy, 1299, 1300t
Vagotomy syndrome, 1264, 1288
Valacyclovir (Valtrex)
  for genital herpes, 1692
  for herpes zoster infection, 1819
Valsalva maneuver, 1313, 1558–1559
Valsartan (Diovan)
  for heart failure, 824t
Valsartan (Diovan), for hypertension, 892t
Value-based purchasing, 8
Valve replacement, 799–800, 799f
  mechanical valves, 800, 800f
  nursing management, 800–807
  tissue valves, 800, 800f
Valvular disorders, 791–792
  nursing management of, 796
Valvular heart disease, and heart failure, 820
Valvuloplasty

  balloon, 797–798, 797f
  nursing management, 800–807
  procedure, 796–799
Vancomycin-intermediate *Staphylococcus aureus* (VISA), 2132
Vancomycin-resistant *Enterococcus* (VRE), 2132
Vanillylmandelic acid (VMA), 1532
Vaqta, 1399
Vardenafil (Levitra), for erectile dysfunction, 1757–1759, 1758t, 1759t
Varenicline (Chantix), 639
Variable expression, 120
Varicella-zoster virus (VZV), 1819, 2134
  vaccine (Varivax), 1820
  vaccine (Zostavax), 1820
Varicocele, 1752, 1783
Varicose veins, 878–880
  assessment and diagnostic findings, 878
  clinical manifestations, 878
  nursing management, 879–880
  pathophysiology, 878
  prevention and medical management, 878–879
    ligation and stripping, 879
    sclerotherapy, 879
    thermal ablation, 879
Vasa recta, 1553
Vascular access devices, implanted, 344f
Vascular dementia, 215
Vascular lesions, 1801, 1801t
Vascular system, 841–842
  aging, effect of, 845
  anatomy of
    arteries and arterioles, 842
    capillaries, 842
    lymphatic vessels, 843
    veins and venules, 842–843
  diagnostic evaluation, 847
    angiography, 849
    computed tomography, 849
    contrast phlebography, 849
    Doppler ultrasound flow studies, 847–848, 847f
    Duplex ultrasonography, 848
    exercise testing, 848
    lymphoscintigraphy, 849
    magnetic resonance angiography, 849
  disorders of
    arterial disorders, 850–868
    cellulitis, 881
    lymphatic disorders, 880–881
    venous disorders, 868–880
  function of
    blood flow, 843
    blood pressure, 844
    capillary filtration and reabsorption, 844
    circulatory needs of tissues, 843
    hemodynamic resistance, 844
    regulatory mechanism, 844
  health history, 845–846
  lymphatic system, 842
  pathophysiology of, 844
    arterial and venous insufficiency, 845, 845t
    blood and lymphatic vessels, alterations in, 845
    pump failure, 844
  physical assessment, 846
    palpation of pulses, 846–847, 846f
    skin inspection, 846
  systemic and pulmonary circulation, 841, 842f
Vasectomy, 1671, 1671t, 1752, 1783–1784, 1783f

complications of, 1783
nursing management, 1783–1784
procedure, 1783
Vasoactive drugs, for variceal bleeding, 1390
Vasodilators
for hypertension, 892t
for pulmonary edema, 834
Vasopressin (Pitressin), 1503, 1508
in cardiopulmonary resuscitation, 839t
side effects of, 1390
for variceal bleeding, 1390
Vasospasm, 2027
Vasovasostomy, 1784
Vector-borne diseases, 2153
Vecuronium (Norcuron), 446t
Veins, 842–843
deep, 868, 869
perforating, 868
superficial, 868, 869
Velcro straps, 1133
Venlafaxine (Effexor), 244
for hot flashes, 1683
Venography, 849
Venous blood gas (VBG) studies, 502–503
Venous disorders, 868
leg ulcers, 874–878
varicose veins, 878–880
venous insufficiency/postthrombotic
syndrome, 873–874
venous thromboembolism, 868–873
Venous gangrene, 869
Venous insufficiency, 873–874
Venous prominence, breast, 1722c
Venous thromboembolism (VTE), 378, 419,
868–873, 1142–1144, 1188, 1975, 2083
assessment and diagnostic findings, 869–870
and bleeding, 872
clinical manifestations, 869
complications of, 869f
deep vein thrombosis, 868
endovascular management, 871
incidence of, 868
nursing management, 871–873
anticoagulant therapy, monitoring of,
871–872
comfort promotion, 872
complications management, 872
compression therapy, 872–873
patient education, 873, 873c
patient positioning and exercises, 873
and older adults after hip fracture, 1205c
pathophysiology, 868–869
pharmacologic therapy for, 870–871, 870t
factor Xa and direct thrombin inhibitors, 871
low–molecular-weight heparin, 870–871
oral anticoagulants, 871
thrombolytic therapy, 871
unfractionated heparin, 870
prevention of, 473, 870, 1152
pulmonary embolism, 868
risk factors, 868c
Ventilation
description of, 480, 481
minute, 501
neurologic control of, 488
perfusion balance and, 485
suppression, 512
Ventilation-perfusion ratio (V/Q), 485, 583
dead space, 486c
shunts, 486c
silent units, 486c

Ventilator, 510, 525. *See also* Mechanical
ventilation
adjustment, 527
monitoring, 529
settings, 528c
Ventilator-associated pneumonia (VAP), 303,
530c, 589
Ventricular assist device (VAD), 833
Ventricular asystole, 731–732, 732f
Ventricular dysrhythmias, 729–732
idioventricular rhythm, 731, 731f
premature ventricular complex, 729, 729f
ventricular asystole, 731–732, 732f
ventricular fibrillation, 730–731, 731f
ventricular tachycardia, 730
Ventricular escape rhythm, 731
Ventricular fibrillation, 730–731, 731f
Ventricular function tests, 701
Ventricular gallop, 822
Ventricular hypertrophy, 821
Ventricular hypertrophy, hypertension and, 885,
887
Ventricular tachycardia, 730
Ventriculography, 704
Venturi mask, 514f
Venules, 842–843
Verapamil (Covera-HS, Verelan PM), for
hypertension, 892t
Verapamil immediate release (Calan, Isoptin)
for AVNRT, 728
for hypertension, 892t
Verapamil long acting (Calan SR, Isoptin SR),
for hypertension, 892t
Verbal descriptor scale (VDS), 231
Vertebral column, 1951
Vertigo
definition of, 1915
ear and, 1933–1934
plan of care, 1935c–1937c
Vesicants, 2207
administration of, 348
clinical manifestations of, 2207
definition of, 324
description of, 342
treatment of, 2207
Vesicle, 1798t
Vesicoureteral reflux, 1550
Vestibular nerve sectioning, 1934
Vestibular schwannomas. *See* Acoustic neuromas
Vestibulitis, 1702
Vestibulodynia, 1701
Veterinary Medical Assistance Teams (VMAT),
2195
Vibrant sound bridge, 1940. *See also* Implanted
hearing devices
Vibrio cholerae, 2145
Video-assisted surgery, 336, 654
Video-assisted thoracoscopy (VATS), 507, 538c
Vildagliptin (Galvus), 1475t
Villi, 1228
Vinblastine (Velban), 343t
Vincristine (VCR, Oncovin)
characteristics, 343t
neurotoxicity of, 346
vesicant action, 342
Vinorelbine (Navelbine), 343t
Viral hepatitis, 1397–1404, 1398t
hepatitis A virus (HAV), 1398–1400
hepatitis B virus (HBV), 1400–1403
hepatitis C virus (HCV), 1403–1404
hepatitis D virus (HDV), 1404

hepatitis E virus (HEV), 1404
hepatitis G virus (HGV), 1404
Viral load tests, 1032–1033
Viral replication, 2070
Viral rhinitis, 555–556
Viral set point, 1031
Virchow triad, 868
Virkon-S, 2144
Virtual colonoscopy, 1238
Virulence, 2144
Visceral pain, 227t
Viscosupplementation, 1105
Visicol, 1239
Vision
age-related changes, 197t, 201–202, 1884,
1884t
impairment, 1883–1886
low vision aids, 1885t
Visual Analog Scale (VAS), 231, 489t
Vital capacity, 501
Vitamin A
deficiency, 1397
wound healing and, 425t
Vitamin B$_{12}$, 906
assay, 934
deficiency, 933
Vitamin B, wound healing and, 425t
Vitamin C deficiency, 1397
Vitamin D, 1116, 1793–1794
Vitamin K, 1379
deficiency, 956, 1397
wound healing and, 425t
Vitiligo, 1790, 1795
Vitrectomy, 1491
Vitreous humor, 1876, 1878
Vocal cords, 482
Voice sounds, 500
Voiding
changes in, 1556–1557, 1556t
management of, 472
Voiding cystourethrography, 1564
Voiding diary, 1627
Volkmann contracture, 1136, 1199
Vomiting, 1230, 2093
Von Recklinghausen disease, 1833
Von Willebrand disease (vWD), 954–956, 954f
types of, 954
Von Willebrand factor, 914, 954
V/Q lung scan, 505
VTE. *See* Venous thromboembolism
Vulnerable plaque, 751
Vulvar cancer, 1709–1711
clinical manifestations, 1709
HPV infection and, 1709
medical management, 1709–1710
nursing management, 1710–1711
anxiety relief, 1710
complications management, 1710–1711
health history, 1710
pain relief, 1710
patient education, 1711
postoperative care, 1710
preoperative care, 1710
sexual function, 1710
skin integrity, 1710
skin preparation, 1710
risk factors, 1709
vulvar carcinoma in situ, 1709
Vulvar cysts, 1702
Vulvar dystrophy, 1662, 1686, 1702
Vulvar self-examination, 1691

Vulvectomy, 1686, 1709
Vulvitis, 1686, 1701–1702
Vulvodynia, 1686, 1701–1702
Vulvovaginal candidiasis. *See* Candidiasis
Vulvovaginal infections, 1687–1697, 1688t
    bacterial vaginosis, 1688–1689
    candidiasis, 1687–1688
    nursing process, 1689–1691
        anxiety reduction, 1690
        assessment, 1689–1690
        diagnosis, 1690
        evaluation, 1691
        nursing interventions, 1690–1691
        patient education, 1690
        planning and goals, 1690
    risk factors, 1687c
    trichomoniasis, 1689
VZV. *See* Varicella-zoster virus

W
Walkers
    ambulation using, 174–175
    benefits of, 175
    types of, 175f
    use of, 177t
Wall motion tests, 701
Warfarin (Coumadin), 683, 963–965
    agents interaction with, 964t
    antidote for, 965
    for atrial fibrillation, 724
    drug interactions, 428t
    for venous thromboembolism, 870t, 871
Warfarin-induced skin necrosis, 961–962
Warts, 1833
Warts, hypogammaglobulinemia, infections, and
    myelokathexis syndrome (WHIMS),
    1024t
Washington Death With Dignity Act, 390
Waste products, excretion of, 1553
Wasting syndrome, 1039, 1051
WATCHMAN device, 726, 726f
Water excretion, regulation of, 1552
Waterhouse–Friderichsen syndrome, 2066
Water seal system, 542
Water, wound healing and, 425t
Weapons of mass destruction (WMD), 2193
Weapons of terror
    biologic weapons, 2203–2204
        effects of, 2204
        types of, 2204–2206
    blast injury
        explosive devices, 2202–2203
        physical injuries, 2203
        special populations, 2203
    chemical weapons, 2206–2207
        characteristics of, 2207
        chemicals, types of, 2207–2208
        limiting exposure, 2207
    nuclear radiation exposure, 2208–2209
        acute radiation syndrome, 2210–2211
        decontamination, 2209–2210
        exposure, 2209
        measurement and detection, 2209
        radiation, types of, 2209
        survival, 2211
Weber test, 1920, 1920f, 1921f, 1921t
Wedge resection, 538c
Weight-bearing activity, 1116
Weight bearing as tolerated (WBAT), 1188
Weight loss
    and blood glucose levels, 1462

chronic pancreatitis and, 1445
    gastric surgery and, 1306
    medications associated with, 1363c
Weight-resistance exercise, 1116
Wellness
    components of, 6
    definition of, 6
West Nile virus, 2177
Wet purpura, 949
Wheal, 1798t
Wheat dextrin (Benefiber), 1314t
Wheelchairs
    patient transfers, 173, 174f
    pressure ulcer prevention, 181, 183f
Wheezing, 498, 499t
    assessment of, 490
    description of, 480
Whiff test, 1689
Whipple disease, 1321t
Whipple resection (pancreaticoduodenectomy),
    1449
Whispered pectoriloquy, 480, 500
Whisper test, 1920
White blood cells (WBCs), 903, 903t, 906–907,
    1005, 1005f, 2170
    action, 1006
    agranulocytes, 907
        lymphocytes, 907
        monocytes, 907
    function of, 907
    granulocytes, 906–907
    reference range, 694t
Whooping cough, 2152
Window edema, 1135
Wire needle localization, of breast, 1727
Wiskott–Aldrich syndrome (WAS), 1024t
Wolff–Parkinson–White (WPW) syndrome, 726
Women's health
    health history, 1654, 1656
        female genital mutilation, 1657
        incest and childhood sexual abuse,
            1657–1658
        intimate partner violence, 1657
        LGBT and, 1659–1660, 1660c
        older women and, 1660
        sexual history, 1656–1657
        women with disabilities and, 1658–1659,
            1659c
    physical assessment, 1660–1662
        adnexal palpation, 1662
        aging women and, 1662
        bimanual palpation, 1662
        cervical palpation, 1662
        cervix inspection, 1661
        inspection, 1661
        Pap smears and other samples, obtaining
            of, 1661
        pelvic examination, 1660–1661, 1660c
        positioning, 1661
        speculum examination, 1661
        uterine palpation, 1662
        vagina inspection, 1662
        vaginal and rectal palpation, 1662
        vaginal discharge, 1661, 1662t
    role of nurses in, 1650–1651
    screening and counseling issues, 1655c
Wong-Baker FACES Pain Rating Scale, 231
Wood light, 1790, 1804
Word catheter, 1702
World Burn Congress, 1869
World Health Organization (WHO), 2128

Global Oral Health Programme, 1268
    health, definition of, 5
World Trade Center towers, destruction of, 2193
Wound healing
    abnormal, 1869
    factors in, 470t
    mechanisms of, 468c
    nutrition and, 425t
    postsurgical, 468–469
Wound-ostomy-continence (WOC) nurse,
    1368, 1444, 1629
Wounds
    breakdown of, 1868t
    care of, 468–469, 471c, 1807–1811, 1808t
        five rules of, 1807
    classification, 474t
    cleaning, 1860
    coverage, 1839–1841, 1840f
    débridement, 1862–1863
    definition, 2167c
    dehiscence, 474, 475f
    dressings
        active, 1807
        biosynthetic, 1864
        burn injuries, 1861–1862
        categories of, 1807–1809, 1808t
        foam, 1809
        function and action of, 1808t
        moisture-retentive, 1808–1809
        occlusive, 1808
        passive, 1807
        synthetic, 1864
    evisceration, 474, 475f
    grafting, 1863–1864
    management, 2167
        cleansing, 2167
        delayed primary closure, 2167
        primary closure, 2167
Wrist fracture, 1200, 1200c
Wrist splints, for carpal tunnel syndrome, 1164

X
Xanthine oxidase inhibitors, 1108
X choromosomes, 110f
Xenografts, 1377, 1405, 1845, 1864
Xerosis, 1806, 1812
Xerostomia, 552, 574, 1101, 1264, 1272
X-linked inheritance, 121f
    definition of, 114, 119
X-rays
    for musculoskeletal disorders, 1126
    spine, 1161c

Y
Yankauer suction, 1275
Y choromosomes, 110f

Z
Zafirlukast (Accolate), 659t, 660, 1070, 1070t
Zenker diverticulum, 1281–1282, 1281f
Zidovudine (AZT or ZDV), 1034t
Zika virus, 2150
Zileuton (Zyflo), 660, 1070
Zinc
    role of, 1015
    wound healing and, 425t
Zoledronic acid (Zometa), 997
Zollinger–Ellison syndrome (ZES), 1240, 1297,
    1321t, 1428, 1454
Zostavax vaccine, 2135